PEDIATRIC DOSAGE HANDBOOK
with INTERNATIONAL TRADE NAMES INDEX

Including Neonatal Dosing, Drug Administration, and Extemporaneous Preparations

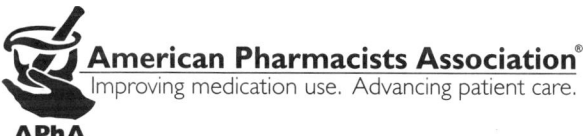

American Pharmacists Association®
Improving medication use. Advancing patient care.

APhA

Lexi-Comp is the official drug reference for the American Pharmacists Association

17th Edition

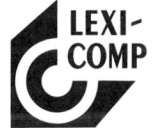
LEXI-COMP

Carol K. Taketomo, PharmD
Jane H. Hodding, PharmD
Donna M. Kraus, PharmD, FAPhA

PEDIATRIC DOSAGE HANDBOOK
with INTERNATIONAL TRADE NAMES INDEX

Including Neonatal Dosing, Drug Administration, & Extemporaneous Preparations

Carol K. Taketomo, PharmD
Director, Pharmacy and Nutritional Services
Children's Hospital Los Angeles
Los Angeles, California

Jane Hurlburt Hodding, PharmD
Executive Director, Pharmacy and Nutritional Services
Long Beach Memorial Medical Center and Miller Children's Hospital
Long Beach, California

Donna M. Kraus, PharmD, FAPhA
Associate Professor of Pharmacy Practice
Departments of Pharmacy Practice and Pediatrics
Pediatric Clinical Pharmacist
University of Illinois at Chicago
Chicago, Illinois

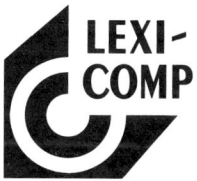

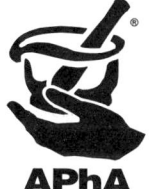

APhA

NOTICE

This data is intended to serve the user as a handy reference and not as a complete drug information resource. It does not include information on every therapeutic agent available. The publication covers over 870 commonly used drugs and is specifically designed to present important aspects of drug data in a more concise format than is typically found in medical literature or product material supplied by manufacturers.

The nature of drug information is that it is constantly evolving because of ongoing research and clinical experience and is often subject to interpretation. While great care has been taken to ensure the accuracy of the information and recommendations presented, the reader is advised that the authors, editors, reviewers, contributors, and publishers cannot be responsible for the continued currency of the information or for any errors, omissions, or the application of this information, or for any consequences arising therefrom. Therefore, the author(s) and/or the publisher shall have no liability to any person or entity with regard to claims, loss, or damage caused, or alleged to be caused, directly or indirectly, by the use of information contained herein. Because of the dynamic nature of drug information, readers are advised that decisions regarding drug therapy must be based on the independent judgment of the clinician, changing information about a drug (eg, as reflected in the literature and manufacturer's most current product information), and changing medical practices. Therefore, this data is designed to be used in conjunction with other necessary information and is not designed to be solely relied upon by any user. The user of this data hereby and forever releases the authors and publishers from this data for any and all liability of any kind that might arise out of the use of this data. The editors are not responsible for any inaccuracy of quotation or for any false or misleading implication that may arise due to the text or formulas as used or due to the quotation of revisions no longer official.

Certain of the authors, editors, and contributors have written this book in their private capacities. No official support or endorsement by any federal or state agency or pharmaceutical company is intended or inferred.

The publishers have made every effort to trace any third party copyright holders, if any, for borrowed material. If they have inadvertently overlooked any, they will be pleased to make the necessary arrangements at the first opportunity.

If you have any suggestions or questions regarding any information presented in this data, please contact our drug information pharmacists at (330) 650-6506. Book revisions are available at our website at http://www.lexi.com/home/revisions/.

This manual was produced using Lexi-Comp's Information Management System™ (LIMS) — A complete publishing service of Lexi-Comp Inc.

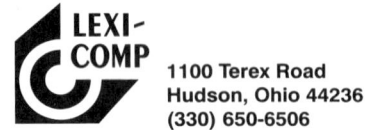

LEXI-COMP

1100 Terex Road
Hudson, Ohio 44236
(330) 650-6506

ISBN 978-1-59195-283-1 (Domestic Edition)

ISBN 978-1-59195-284-8 (International Edition)

TABLE OF CONTENTS

P̦REFACE

This seventeenth edition of the *Pediatric Dosage Handbook* is designed to be a practical and convenient guide to the dosing and usage of medications in children. The pediatric population is a dynamic group, with major changes in pharmacokinetics and pharmacodynamics taking place throughout infancy and childhood. Therefore, the need for the evaluation and establishment of medication dosing regimens in children of different ages is great.

Special considerations must be taken into account when dosing medications in pediatric patients. Unfortunately, due to a lack of appropriate studies, most medications commonly used in children do not have FDA approved labeling for use in pediatric patients. Only 30% of drugs used in children in a 1988 survey carried FDA approval in their labeling. Seventy-five percent of medications listed in the *1990 Physicians Desk Reference* carry some type of precaution or disclaimer statement for use in children.[1]

The FDA Modernization Act of 1997, the Children's Health Act of 2000, the Best Pharmaceuticals for Children Act of 2002, and the Pediatric Research Equity Act of 2003 have all helped to increase pediatric drug studies. The recent FDA Amendment Act of 2007, which was signed into law in September 2007, reauthorizes and amends the Pediatric Research Equity Act and the Best Pharmaceuticals for Children Act (Title IV and Title V, Public Law 110-85, 110th Congress).

The FDA Modernization Act of 1997 (Section 111, Public Law 105-115, 105th Congress) **encouraged** pharmaceutical companies to conduct pediatric drug studies by allowing 6 months of market exclusivity to certain designated drugs. A list of drugs, for which additional pediatric information may produce pediatric healthcare benefits, was required by this law to be developed by the U.S. Department of Health and Human Services (HHS), with input from the American Academy of Pediatrics, the Pediatric Pharmacology Research Unit Network,[2] and the U.S. Pharmacopoeia. To date, the FDA has received 601 proposals from pharmaceutical companies to conduct pediatric drug studies under this Act (and subsequent acts) and has issued 391 written requests for studies. If these pediatric studies are completed as the FDA has specified, then these medications will qualify for the 6 month patent extension or additional market exclusivity. One-hundred seventy-three products have already had their marketing patents extended by this law and to date, 367 pediatric labeling changes have occurred.[3]

The pediatric section of the FDA Modernization Act was renewed by Congress and signed into law January 4, 2002. This new law, called the Best Pharmaceuticals for Children Act, reauthorized the use of the 6-month patent extension to **encourage** pharmaceutical companies to conduct pediatric drug research. This law called for the establishment of an Office of Pediatric Therapeutics within the FDA and established an FDA Pediatric Pharmacology Advisory Committee and a Pediatric Subcommittee of the Oncologic Drugs Advisory Committee. It also created a research fund for pediatric studies of drugs that are off patent, granted a special "priority status" to pediatric labeling changes, required the Department of Health and Human Services (along with the Institute of Medicine) to conduct a study to assess federally funded pediatric research and called for the development of a Final Rule that required drug labeling to include a toll-free number to report adverse events.[4]

The Best Pharmaceuticals for Children Act was reauthorized, amended, and signed into law September 2007, as part of the FDA Amendment Act of 2007.[3] This amended law establishes an internal review committee (the Pediatric Review Committee) within the FDA to review written requests that were issued and the submitted reports from drug manufacturers.[5] It also requires manufacturers who were granted a patent extension to revise pediatric labeling in a timely manner; reduces the patent extension from 6 months to 3 months for drugs with combined gross sales >1 billion dollars; prohibits the extension of market exclusivity for >9 months; requires manufacturers to explain why a pediatric formulation cannot be developed (when requested to perform pediatric studies); requires product labeling to include information about pediatric studies whether or not the studies demonstrate that the drug is safe and effective; requires the government to notify the public of pediatric drug formulations that were developed and studied and found to be safe and effective, but not introduced into the market within 1 year; and requires that a report be submitted to congress that assesses the use of patent extensions in making sure that medications used by pediatric patients are tested and properly labeled.[6]

The 1998 Pediatric Final Rule was an FDA regulation, titled "Regulations Requiring Manufacturers to Assess the Safety and Effectiveness of New Drugs and Biological Products in Pediatric Patients; Final Rule".[7] This important regulation **required** that manufacturers conduct pediatric studies for certain new and marketed drugs and biological products. This requirement was mandatory, and its scope included new drugs (ie, new chemical entities, new dosage forms, new indications, new routes of administration, and new dosing regimens) and certain marketed drugs (ie, where the drug product offered meaningful therapeutic benefit or had substantial use in pediatric patients, AND the absence of pediatric labeling posed a risk). This FDA regulation became effective April 1, 1999, but studies mandated under this rule were not required to be submitted to the FDA before December 2, 2000. The 1998 Pediatric Final Rule and the authority of the FDA to **require** manufacturers to conduct pediatric studies was challenged with a law suit. In March 2002, the FDA requested a 2-month stay on the lawsuit, so it could publish a notice and suspend the 1998 Pediatric Final Rule for 2 years. During the 2 year suspension of the Rule, the FDA planned to study whether the Best Pharmaceuticals for Children Act of 2002 made the 1998 Final Rule unnecessary. After multiple organizations lobbied Congress and the president, the Secretary of Health and Human Services announced in April 2002, that the FDA would continue to defend the Pediatric Final Rule of 1998 in court. However, on October 17, 2002, the U.S. District Court for the District of Columbia barred the FDA from enforcing the Pediatric Final Rule. Fortunately, Congress passed the Pediatric Research Equity Act of 2003 (Public Law S.650, 108th Congress). This law essentially reinstates the Pediatric Final Rule and authorizes the FDA to **require** pharmaceutical manufacturers to conduct pediatric studies of certain drugs and biological products. It also establishes an FDA Pediatric Advisory Committee. The Pediatric Research Equity Act was reauthorized, amended, and signed into law in September 2007, as part of the FDA Amendment Act of 2007.

The Children's Health Act of 2000 was signed into law on October 17, 2000. This important law establishes a Pediatric Research Initiative (headed by the Director of the NIH) and provides funds to increase support for pediatric clinical research. These three important laws, plus other FDA regulations, such as the FDA labeling changes[8] that required expanded information in the Pediatric Use section of the package insert for all prescription drugs, will certainly help to increase and disseminate pediatric drug information.

Currently, however, most commonly used pharmacy references do not include information regarding pediatric dosing, drug administration, or special pediatric concerns. It is, therefore, not surprising that in order to obtain pediatric dosing information, oftentimes the pediatric clinician is faced with extensive literature searches to arrive at a logical dose. This handbook was developed with the intent to serve as a compilation of recommended pediatric doses found in the literature and to provide relevant clinical information regarding the use of drugs in children.

New in This Edition

This new edition incorporates additions and revisions in a format that we hope the user will find beneficial. One new field of information, "Pregnancy Considerations," has been added. "Pregnancy Considerations" is a summary of human and/or animal information pertinent to or associated with the use of the drug as it relates to clinical effects on the fetus, newborn, or pregnant women.

As with each edition, drug monographs have been updated and revised. Twenty-three new monographs have been added. Five monographs have been deleted because the drugs are no longer available in the U.S.: Cephradine, Gonadorelin, Mitomycin, Protirelin, and Triethanolamine Polypeptide Oleate-Condensate. This brings the total number of drug monographs to 873. The 23 new monographs added to this edition include: Abatacept; Adalimumab; Argatroban; Atovaquone and Proguanil; Balsalazide; Basiliximab; Benzyl Alcohol; Besifloxacin; Cholecalciferol; Colesevelam; Diphtheria and Tetanus Toxoids, Acellular Pertussis, Poliovirus and *Haemophilus* b Conjugate Vaccine; Guanfacine; Imatinib; Influenza Virus Vaccine (H1N1, Inactivated); Influenza Virus Vaccine (H1N1, Live/Attenuated); Papillomavirus (Types 16, 18) Vaccine (Human, Recombinant); Peginterferon Alfa-2b; Peramivir; Pneumococcal Conjugate Vaccine (13-Valent); Rabeprazole; Rosuvastatin; Tretinoin (Systemic); and Vigabatrin.

One new appendix piece has been added to this edition: Patient Information for Disposal of Unused Medications. Appendix material has been updated and the following tables were revised: Acid / Base Assessment; Adult and Adolescent HIV; Antihypertensive Agents by Class; Corticosteroids; Cytochrome P450 Enzymes: Substrates, Inhibitors, and Inducers; Emergency Pediatric Drip Calculations; Emetogenic Potential of Antineoplastic Agents; Immunization Guidelines; Laboratory Calculations; Preprocedure Sedatives in Children; Therapeutic Drug Monitoring: Blood Sampling Time Guidelines; and Tumor Lysis Syndrome. The appendix piece Laboratory Calculations is new and replaces Osmolality and Anion Gap in previous editions. Milliequivalent and Millimole Calculations and Conversions is now named Milliequivalent of Selected Ions.

We hope this edition continues to be a valuable and practical source of clinical drug information for the pediatric healthcare professional. We welcome comments to further improve future editions.

Footnotes

1. Food and Drug Letter, Washington Business Information, Inc. November 23, 1990.
2. "NIH Funds Network of Centers for Pediatric Drug Research," *Am J Hosp Pharm*, 1994, 51:2546.
3. http://www.fda.gov/Drugs/DevelopmentApprovalProcess/DevelopmentResources/ucm049867.htm.
4. Birenbaum D, "Pediatric Initiatives: A Regulatory Perspective of the U.S. Experience," June 17, 2002, http://www.fda.gov/cder/pediatric/presentation/Ped_Init_2002_ DB/index.htm.
5. Establishment of the Pediatric Review Committee, http://www.fda.gov/cder/pediatric/Pediatric_Review_Committee_Establishment%20_Memo.pdf.
6. Ref B.S. 1156, "The Best Pharmaceuticals for Children Amendments of 2007," http://www.washingtonwatch.com/bills/show/110 SN 1156.html.
7. Department of Health and Human Services, Food and Drug Administration, 21CFR Parts 201, 312, 314, and 601, Regulations Requiring Manufacturers to Assess the Safety and Effectiveness of New Drugs and Biological Products in Pediatric Patients; Final Rule," *Fed Regist*, 1998, 63(231):66631-72.
8. "Pediatric Use Drug Labeling NDA Supplements Due by December 1996 - FDA Final Rule; Agency Establishing Pediatric Subcommittee to Track Implementation," *F-D-C Reports - The Pink Sheet*, Wallace Werble Jr, Publisher, December 19, 1994.

ACKNOWLEDGMENTS

Special acknowledgement goes to all Lexi-Comp staff for their contributions to this handbook.

The authors wish to thank their families, friends, and colleagues who supported them in their efforts to complete this handbook.

Special thanks goes to Chris Lomax, PharmD, who played a significant role in bringing APhA and Lexi-Comp together.

In addition, Dr Taketomo would like to thank Robert Taketomo, PharmD, MBA, and Chris Lomax, PharmD, for their professional guidance and continued support, and the pharmacy staff at Children's Hospital, Los Angeles, for their assistance.

Dr Kraus would like to especially thank Keith A. Rodvold, PharmD, for his ongoing professional and personal support, and the pediatric clinical pharmacists at the University of Illinois Medical Center for their assistance.

Dr Hodding would like to thank Glenn Hodding, PharmD, Neepa Rai, PharmD, and the pediatric pharmacists at Miller Children's Hospital for their continued professional and personal support.

Some of the material contained in this book was a result of pediatric pharmacy contributors throughout the United States and Canada. Lexi-Comp has assisted many pediatric medical institutions to develop hospital-specific formulary manuals that contain clinical drug information as well as dosing. Working with these pediatric clinical pharmacists, pediatric hospital pharmacy and therapeutics committees, and hospital drug information centers, Lexi-Comp has developed an evolutionary drug database that reflects the practice of pediatric pharmacy in these major pediatric institutions.

Special thanks to Jenny Campbell of Campbell and Co. Cartooning, Chagrin Falls, Ohio, who makes our *Pediatric Dosage Handbook* come alive with her wonderful cover illustrations.

EDITORIAL ADVISORY PANEL

6

Daren Knoell, PharmD
*Associate Professor of Pharmacy Practice
and Internal Medicine*
Davis Heart and Lung Research Institute
The Ohio State University
Columbus, Ohio

Sandra Knowles, RPh, BScPhm
Drug Safety Pharmacist
Sunnybrook and Women's College HSC
Toronto, Ontario

Jill M. Kolesar, PharmD, FCCP, BCPS
Associate Professor
School of Pharmacy
Associate Professor
University of Wisconsin Paul P. Carbone Comprehensive
Cancer Center
University of Wisconsin
Madison, Wisconsin

Donna M. Kraus, PharmD, FAPhA
Associate Professor of Pharmacy Practice
Departments of Pharmacy Practice and Pediatrics
Pediatric Clinical Pharmacist
University of Illinois
Chicago, Illinois

Daniel L. Krinsky RPh, MS
Manager, MTM Services
Giant Eagle Pharmacy
Ravenna, Ohio
Assistant Professor
Department of Pharmacy Practice
College of Pharmacy NEOUCOM
Rootstown, Ohio

Kay Kyllonen, PharmD
Clinical Specialist
The Cleveland Clinic Children's Hospital
Cleveland, Ohio

Charles Lacy, MS, PharmD, FCSHP
Vice President for Executive Affairs
Professor, Pharmacy Practice
Professor, Business Leadership
University of Southern Nevada
Las Vegas, Nevada

Brenda R. Lance, RN, MSN
Program Development Director
Northcoast HealthCare Management Company
Northcoast Infusion Network
Beachwood, Ohio

Leonard L. Lance, RPh, BSPharm
Pharmacist
Lexi-Comp, Inc
Hudson, Ohio

Mandy C. Leonard, PharmD, BCPS
Assistant Professor
Cleveland Clinic Lerner College of Medicine
of Case Western University
Assistant Director, Drug Information Services
Cleveland Clinic
Cleveland, Ohio

John J. Lewin III, PharmD, BCPS
Clinical Specialist, Neurosciences Critical Care
The Johns Hopkins Hospital
Baltimore, Maryland

Jeffrey D. Lewis, PharmD, MACM
*Assistant Dean and
Associate Professor of Pharmacy Practice*
Cedarville University School of Pharmacy
Cedarville, Ohio

Jennifer Lowe, PharmD, BCOP
Pharmacotherapy Specialist, Oncology
Akron General Medical Center
Akron, Ohio

Sherry Luedtke, PharmD
Associate Professor and Associate Dean
Department of Pharmacy Practice
Texas Tech University HSC School of Pharmacy
Amarillo, Texas

Vincent F. Mauro, BS, PharmD, FCCP
Professor of Clinical Pharmacy
College of Pharmacy
Adjunct Professor of Medicine
College of Medicine
The University of Toledo
Toledo, Ohio

Barrie McCombs, MD, FCFP
Medical Information Service Coordinator
The Alberta Rural Physician Action Plan
Calgary, Alberta, Canada

Timothy F. Meiller, DDS, PhD
Professor
Oncology and Diagnostic Sciences
Baltimore College of Dental Surgery
Professor of Oncology
Marlene and Stewart Greenebaum Cancer Center
University of Maryland Medical System
Baltimore, Maryland

Geralyn M. Meny, MD
Medical Director
American Red Cross, Penn-Jersey Region
Philadelphia, Pennsylvania

Julie Miller, PharmD
Pharmacy Clinical Specialist, Cardiology
Columbus Children's Hospital
Columbus, Ohio

Leah Millstein, MD
Assistant Professor
Division of General Internal Medicine
University of Maryland School of Medicine
Baltimore, Maryland

Kevin M. Mulieri, BS, PharmD
Pediatric Hematology/Oncology Clinical Specialist
Penn State Milton S. Hershey Medical Center
Instructor of Pharmacology
Penn State College of Medicine
Hershey, Pennsylvania

Tom Palma, MS, RPh
Medical Science Pharmacist
Lexi-Comp, Inc
Hudson, Ohio

Susie H. Park, PharmD, BCPP
Assistant Professor of Clinical Pharmacy
University of Southern California
Los Angeles, California

8

Nathan Wirick, PharmD
Infectious Disease and Antibiotic Management
Clinical Specialist
Hillcrest Hospital
Cleveland, Ohio

Richard L. Wynn, BSPharm, PhD
Professor of Pharmacology
Baltimore College of Dental Surgery
Dental School
University of Maryland Baltimore
Baltimore, Maryland

Sallie Young, PharmD, BCPS, AQ Cardiology
Clinical Pharmacy Specialist, Cardiology
Penn State Milton S. Hershey Medical Center
Hershey, Pennsylvania

Jennifer Zimmer-Young, PharmD, CCRP
Educator, Clinical Pharmacist
ThedaCare
Appleton, Wisconsin

ABOUT THE AUTHORS

Carol K. Taketomo, PharmD

Dr Taketomo received her doctorate from the University of Southern California School of Pharmacy. Subsequently, she completed a clinical pharmacy residency at the University of California Medical Center in San Diego. With over 30 years of clinical experience at one of the largest pediatric teaching hospitals in the nation, she is an acknowledged expert in the practical aspects of pediatric drug distribution and clinical pharmacy practice. She currently holds the appointment of Adjunct Assistant Professor of Pharmacy Practice at the University of Southern California School of Pharmacy.

In her current capacity as Director of Pharmacy and Nutritional Services at Children's Hospital of Los Angeles, Dr Taketomo plays an active role in the education and training of the medical, pharmacy, and nursing staff. She coordinates the Pharmacy Department's quality assurance and drug use evaluation programs; maintains the hospital's strict formulary program; and is the editor of the house staff manual. Her particular interests are strategies to influence physician prescribing patterns and methods to decrease medication errors in the pediatric setting. She has been the author of numerous publications, and is an active presenter at professional meetings.

Dr Taketomo is a member of the American Pharmacists Association (APhA), American Society of Health-System Pharmacists (ASHP), California Society of Hospital Pharmacists (CSHP), and Southern California Pediatric Pharmacy Group.

Jane Hurlburt Hodding, PharmD

Dr Hodding earned a doctorate and completed her pharmacy residency at the University of California School of Pharmacy in San Francisco. She has held teaching positions as Assistant Clinical Professor of Pharmacy at UCSF as well as Assistant Clinical Professor of Pharmacy Practice at the University of Southern California in Los Angeles. Currently, Dr Hodding is the Executive Director, Pharmacy and Nutritional Services at Long Beach Memorial and Miller Children's Hospital in Long Beach, California.

Throughout her 33 years of pediatric pharmacy practice, Dr Hodding has actively pursued methods to improve the safety of medication use in neonates, children, and adolescents. She has actively practiced as a clinical pharmacy specialist in neonatal intensive care, pediatric intensive care, and pediatric hematology/oncology. Parenteral nutrition is another area of focus. She has published numerous articles covering neonatal medication administration and aminoglycoside and theophylline clearance in premature infants.

Dr Hodding is a member of the American Pharmacists Association (APhA), American Society of Health-System Pharmacists (ASHP), California Society of Hospital Pharmacists (CSHP), Pediatric Pharmacy Advocacy Group (PPAG), Children's Oncology Group, and Southern California Pediatric Pharmacy Group. She is frequently an invited speaker on the topics of Medication Safety in Children, A Multidisciplinary Approach; Monitoring Drug Therapy in the NICU; Fluid and Electrolyte Therapy in Children; Drug Therapy Considerations in Children; and Parenteral Nutrition in the Premature Infant.

Donna M. Kraus, PharmD

Dr Kraus received her Bachelor of Science in Pharmacy from the University of Illinois at Chicago (UIC). She worked for several years as a hospital pediatric/obstetric satellite pharmacist before earning her doctorate degree at the UIC. Dr Kraus then completed a postdoctoral pediatric specialty residency at the University of Texas Health Science Center in San Antonio. She served as a pediatric intensive care clinical pharmacist for 15 years and for the past 12 years has been an ambulatory care pediatric clinical pharmacist, specializing in pediatric HIV pharmacotherapy and patient/parent medication adherence. Dr Kraus has also served as a clinical pharmacist consultant to a pediatric long-term care facility for over 21 years. She currently holds the appointment of Associate Professor of Pharmacy Practice in both the Departments of Pharmacy Practice and Pediatrics at the University of Illinois in Chicago.

In her 33 years of active pharmacy experience, Dr Kraus has dealt with pediatric pharmacy issues and pharmacotherapy problems. She is an active educator and has been a guest lecturer in China, Thailand, and Hong Kong. Dr Kraus has played a leading role in the advanced training of postgraduate pharmacists and has been the Director of the UIC (ASHP accredited) Pediatric Residency and Fellowship Program for 23 years. Dr Kraus' research areas include pediatric drug dosing and developmental pharmacokinetics and pharmacodynamics. She has published a number of articles on various issues of pediatric pharmacy and pharmacotherapy.

Dr Kraus has been an active member of numerous professional associations including the American Pharmacists Association (APhA), American Society of Health-System Pharmacists (ASHP), Illinois Pharmacists Association (IPhA), American College of Clinical Pharmacy (ACCP), and Illinois College of Clinical Pharmacy (ICCP). She has served as Chairperson of the ASHP Commission on Therapeutics; member of the Board of Directors of the Pediatric Pharmacy Advocacy Group (PPAG); Member-at-Large of the Academy of Pharmaceutical Research and Science (APhA); member of the ASHP, Commission on Credentialing, Design/Writing Group, Educational Outcomes, Goals and Objectives for Postgraduate Year Two (PGY2) Pediatric Pharmacy Residency Programs (2007); and a member of the Alliance for Pediatric Quality, Improve First Measures Task Force. Dr. Kraus also served as an Editorial Board member of the *American Journal of Health-System Pharmacy* and the *Journal of Pediatric Pharmacy Practice*. Currently, she serves as an Editorial Board member of *The Journal of Pediatric Pharmacology and Therapeutics*. Dr. Kraus was awarded Fellow status by the American Pharmaceutical Association and is the APhA designated author for this handbook.

DESCRIPTION OF SECTIONS AND FIELDS USED IN THIS HANDBOOK

The *Pediatric Dosage Handbook, 17th Edition* is organized into a drug information section, an appendix, and a therapeutic category & key word index.

Drug information is presented in a consistent format and provides the following:

Generic Name	U.S. adopted name. "Tall Man" lettering appears for look-alike generic drug names as recommended by the FDA. See "FDA Differentiation Project: The Use of "Tall Man" Letters" on page 22. The symbol [DSC] appears after the generic name of drugs that have been recently discontinued.
Pronunciation Guide	Phonetic listing of generic name
Medication Safety Issues	Highlights safety concerns which apply to a particular drug with a focus on name confusion, ie, drug or brand names with the potential to sound or look similar to another drug or brand name
Related Information	Cross-reference to other pertinent drug information found in the Appendix
U.S. Brand Names	Common trade names used in the U.S. The symbol [DSC] appears after trade names that have been recently discontinued.
Canadian Brand Names	Common trade names used in Canada
Therapeutic Category	Unique systematic classification of medications
Generic Available	Indicated by a "Yes" or "No" as to whether a generic form of the drug is available. Specific generic dosage forms (or exceptions) are listed in parentheses.
Use	Information pertaining to appropriate indications or use of the drug. Labeled uses will be indicated in parentheses by "FDA approved in" followed by the specific patient population. "FDA approved in all ages" denotes ages day 0 through adult. This specific FDA approval information is currently being phased in to all monographs. Age-specific FDA approval may not be present in some monographs; product labeling should be consulted for additional detail.
Restrictions	Drug Enforcement Agency (DEA) classification for federally scheduled controlled substances
Medication Guide	Information regarding the FDA-required distribution of patient Medication Guides for select drugs
Pregnancy Risk Factor	Five categories established by the FDA to indicate the potential of a systemically absorbed drug for causing birth defects
Pregnancy Considerations	A summary of human and/or animal information pertinent to or associated with the use of the drug as it relates to clinical effects on the fetus, newborn, or pregnant women.
Lactation	Information regarding the excretion of the drug in breast milk and whether breast-feeding is recommended or not; a notation is made when recommendations differ from the American Academy of Pediatrics
Breast-Feeding Considerations	A summary of available information pertinent to or associated with the human use of the drug as it relates to clinical effects on the nursing infant or postpartum woman.
Contraindications	Information pertaining to inappropriate use of the drug, or disease states and patient populations in which the drug should not be used
Warnings	Hazardous conditions related to use of the drug; the notation **[U.S. Boxed Warning]** immediately follows information which has been adapted from the boxed warnings of the FDA-approved labeling. Consult the product labeling for the exact wording of black box warning through the manufacturer's or the FDA website.
Precautions	Disease states or patient populations in which the drug should be cautiously used
Adverse Reactions	Side effects are grouped by body system and include a listing of the more common and/or serious side effects. Due to space limitations, every reported side effect is not listed.

◀ Drug Interactions

Metabolism/Transport Effects
If a drug has demonstrated involvement with cytochrome P450 enzymes or other metabolism or transport proteins, this field will identify the drug as an inhibitor, inducer, or substrate of the specific enzyme(s) (eg, CYP1A2 or UGT1A1). CYP450 isoenzymes are identified as substrates (minor or major), inhibitors (weak, moderate, or strong), and inducers (weak or strong).

Avoid Concomitant Use
Designates drug combinations which should not be used concomitantly, due to an unacceptable risk:benefit assessment. Frequently, the concurrent use of the agents is explicitly prohibited or contraindicated by the product labeling.

Increased Effect/Toxicity
Drug combinations that result in an increased or toxic therapeutic effect between the drug listed in the monograph and other drugs or drug classes.

Decreased Effect
Drug combinations that result in a decreased therapeutic effect between the drug listed in the monograph and other drugs or drug classes.

Food Interactions
Possible interactions between the drug listed in the monograph and certain foods and/or nutritional substances

Stability
Storage, refrigeration, and compatibility information

Mechanism of Action
How the drug works in the body to elicit a response

Pharmacodynamics
Dose-response relationships including onset of action, time of peak action, and duration of action

Pharmacokinetics
Drug movement through the body over time. Pharmacokinetics deals with absorption, distribution, protein binding, metabolism, bioavailability, half-life, time to peak concentration, elimination, and clearance of drugs. Pharmacokinetic parameters help predict drug concentration and dosage requirements.

Usual Dosage
The amount of the drug to be typically given or taken during therapy

Please note that doses for neonates are often listed by postnatal age (PNA) (eg, PNA ≤7 days) and/or by body weight (eg, 1200-2000 g)

When both milligram doses and weight-based, milligram per kilogram (mg/kg) doses are listed, the milligram per kilogram dosing method is preferred. When weight-based (mg/kg) and maximum doses are provided, use the weight-based (mg/kg) dose to calculate the milligram dose for the patient, but do **not** exceed the maximum dose listed. A *usual* maximum dose may be exceeded only if clinically indicated. If using a milligram dosing guideline according to age, special care and lower doses should be used in children who have a low weight for their age. When ranges of doses are listed, initiate therapy at the lower end of the range and titrate the dose accordingly. References are listed at the end of drug monographs to support doses listed when little dosing information exists.

For select drugs, the dosing adjustment in renal impairment or dosing interval in renal impairment is given according to creatinine clearance (Cl_{cr}). Since most studies that recommend dosing guidelines in renal dysfunction are conducted in adult patients, Cl_{cr} is usually expressed in units of mL/minute. However, in order to extrapolate the adult information to the pediatric population, one must assume that the adults studied were of standard surface area (ie, 1.73 m^2). Therefore, although the value of Cl_{cr} listed for dosing adjustment in renal impairment or dosing interval in renal impairment may be expressed in mL/minute, it is assumed to be equal to the same value in mL/minute/1.73 m^2.

To calculate the dose in a pediatric patient with renal dysfunction, first calculate the normal dose (ie, the dose for a patient without renal dysfunction), then use the guidelines to adjust the dose. For example, the normal piperacillin dose for a 20 kg child is 200-300 mg/kg/day divided every 4-6 hours. If one selected 300 mg/kg/day divided every 6 hours, the dose would be 1.5 g every 6 hours in normal renal function. If Cl_{cr} was 20-40 mL/minute/1.73 m^2, the dose would be 1.5 g every 8 hours and if Cl_{cr} was <20 mL/minute/1.73 m^2, the dose would be 1.5 g every 12 hours.

Administration
Information regarding the recommended final concentrations and rates for administration of parenteral drugs are listed when appropriate, along with pertinent oral, ophthalmic, and topical administration information.

Monitoring Parameters
Laboratory tests and patient physical parameters that should be monitored for safety and efficacy of drug therapy are listed when appropriate.

Reference Range
Therapeutic and toxic serum concentrations are listed when appropriate

Test Interactions
Listing of assay interferences when relevant;
(S) = Serum; (U) = Urine

Patient Information
Advice, warnings, precautions, and other information of which the patient should be informed

Nursing Implications
Comments regarding nursing care of the patient are offered when appropriate

Additional Information
Other data and facts about the drug are offered when appropriate

Product Availability	Provides availability information on products that have been approved by the FDA, but not yet available for use. Estimates for when a product may be available are included when this information is known. This field may also be used to provide any unique or critical drug availability issues (eg, drug shortage of a critical drug).
Dosage Forms	Information with regard to form, strength, and availability of the drug. **Note:** Additional formulation information (eg, excipients, preservatives) is included when available. Please consult product labeling for further information. The symbol [DSC] appears after dosage forms that have been recently discontinued. U.S. brand names appear in this field when more than one brand name exists for a medication. For dosage forms that are available as generic products and multiple brand names, the generic dosage forms are listed first, followed by the U.S. brand names and dosage form descriptions. Important information about ingredients found in specific dosage forms appears in brackets at the end of the dosage form entry. The strength of available products is expressed as base unless otherwise noted (salt form is listed only when strength is expressed as salt form or when more than one salt form exists); available salt forms are listed in Index Terms field.
Extemporaneous Preparations	Directions for preparing liquid formulations from solid drug products. May include stability information and references (listed when appropriate).
References	Bibliographic information referring to specific pediatric literature findings, especially doses

Appendix

The appendix offers a compilation of tables, guidelines, and conversion information which can often be helpful when considering patient care. This section is broken down into various sections for ease of use.

Therapeutic Category & Key Word Index

This index provides a useful listing by an easy-to-use therapeutic classification system. Also listed are controlled substances, preservative free, sugar free, and alcohol free medications.

International Trade Names Index

Alphabetical listing of international trade names covering over 100 countries.

DEFINITION OF AGE GROUP TERMINOLOGY

Information in this handbook is listed according to specific age or by age group. The following are definitions of age groups and age-related terminologies. These definitions should be used unless otherwise specified in the monograph.

Gestational age (GA)	The time from conception until birth. More specifically, gestational age is defined as the number of weeks from the first day of the mother's last menstrual period (LMP) until the birth of the baby. Gestational age at birth is assessed by the date of the LMP and by physical exam (Dubowitz score).
Postnatal age (PNA)	Chronological age since birth
Postconceptional age (PCA)	Age since conception. Postconceptional age is calculated as gestational age plus postnatal age (PCA = GA + PNA).
Neonate	A full-term newborn 0-4 weeks postnatal age. This term may also be applied to a premature neonate whose postconceptional age (PCA) is 42-46 weeks.
Premature neonate	Neonate born at <38 weeks gestational age
Full-term neonate	Neonate born at 38-42 weeks (average ~40 weeks) gestational age
Infant	1 month (>4 weeks) to 1 year of age
Child/Children	1-12 years of age
Adolescent	13-18 years of age
Adult	>18 years of age

FDA PREGNANCY CATEGORIES

Throughout this book there is a field labeled Pregnancy Risk Factor and the letter A, B, C, D, or X immediately following which signifies a category. The FDA has established these five categories to indicate the potential of a systemically absorbed drug for causing birth defects. The key differentiation among the categories rests upon the reliability of documentation and the risk:benefit ratio. Pregnancy Category X is particularly notable in that if any data exists that may implicate a drug as a teratogen and the risk:benefit ratio is clearly negative, the drug is contraindicated during pregnancy.

These categories are summarized as follows:

A   Controlled studies in pregnant women fail to demonstrate a risk to the fetus in the first trimester with no evidence of risk in later trimesters. The possibility of fetal harm appears remote.

B   Either animal-reproduction studies have not demonstrated a fetal risk but there are no controlled studies in pregnant women, or animal-reproduction studies have shown an adverse effect (other than a decrease in fertility) that was not confirmed in controlled studies in women in the first trimester and there is no evidence of a risk in later trimesters.

C   Either studies in animals have revealed adverse effects on the fetus (teratogenic or embryocidal effects or other) and there are no controlled studies in women, or studies in women and animals are not available. Drugs should be given only if the potential benefits justify the potential risk to the fetus.

D   There is positive evidence of human fetal risk, but the benefits from use in pregnant women may be acceptable despite the risk (eg, if the drug is needed in a life-threatening situation or for a serious disease for which safer drugs cannot be used or are ineffective).

X   Studies in animals or human beings have demonstrated fetal abnormalities or there is evidence of fetal risk based on human experience, or both, and the risk of the use of the drug in pregnant women clearly outweighs any possible benefit. The drug is contraindicated in women who are or may become pregnant.

SYMBOLS & ABBREVIATIONS USED IN THIS HANDBOOK*

°C	degrees Celsius (Centigrade)
<	less than
>	greater than
≤	less than or equal to
≥	greater than or equal to
AAP	American Academy of Pediatrics
AAPC	antibiotic associated pseudomembranous colitis
ABG	arterial blood gas
ABMT	autologous bone marrow transplant
ACE	angiotensin-converting enzyme
ACLS	advanced cardiac life support
ADH	antidiuretic hormone
AED	antiepileptic drug
AHCPR	Agency for Health Care Policy and Research
AIDS	acquired immunodeficiency syndrome
ALL	acute lymphoblastic leukemia
ALT	alanine aminotransferase (formerly called SGPT)
AML	acute myeloblastic leukemia
ANA	antinuclear antibodies
ANC	absolute neutrophil count
ANLL	acute nonlymphoblastic leukemia
APTT	activated partial thromboplastin time
ARB	angiotensin receptor blocker
ARDS	adult respiratory distress syndrome
ASA-PS	American Society of Anesthesiologists - Physical Status P1: Normal, healthy patient P2: Patient having mild systemic disease P3: Patient having severe systemic disease P4: Patient having severe systemic disease which is a constant threat to life P5: Moribund patient; not expected to survive without the procedure P6: Patient declared brain-dead; organs being removed for donor purposes
AST	aspartate aminotransferase (formerly called SGOT)
ATP	adenosine triphosphate
AUC	area under the curve (area under the serum concentration-time curve)
A-V	atrial-ventricular
BMT	bone marrow transplant
BPH	benign prostatic hyperplasia
BPD	bronchopulmonary disease
BSA	body surface area
BUN	blood urea nitrogen
CAD	coronary artery disease
CADD	computer ambulatory drug delivery
cAMP	cyclic adenosine monophosphate
CAPD	continuous ambulatory peritoneal dialysis
CBC	complete blood count
CDC	Center for Disease Control and Prevention
CF	cystic fibrosis
CFC	chlorofluorocarbons
CHF	congestive heart failure
CI	cardiac index
Cl_{cr}	creatinine clearance
CLL	chronic lymphocytic leukemia
CML	chronic myelogenous leukemia
CMV	cytomegalovirus
CNS	central nervous system
COPD	chronic obstructive pulmonary disease

CPK	creatine phosphokinase
CPR	cardiopulmonary resuscitation
CRF	chronic renal failure
CRRT	continuous renal replacement therapy
CSF	cerebrospinal fluid
CT	computed tomography
CVA	cerebral vascular accident
CVP	central venous pressure
CYP	cytochrome
CVVH	continuous veno-venous hemofiltration
d	day
D_5/LR	dextrose 5% in lactated Ringer's
D_5/NS	dextrose 5% in sodium chloride 0.9%
D_5W	dextrose 5% in water
$D_5/^1/_4$ NS	dextrose 5% in sodium chloride 0.2%
$D_5/^1/_2$ NS	dextrose 5% in sodium chloride 0.45%
D_{10}W	dextrose 10% in water
DIC	disseminated intravascular coagulation
DL_{co}	pulmonary diffusion capacity for carbon monoxide
DNA	deoxyribonucleic acid
[DSC]	discontinued
DVT	deep vein thrombosis
ECG	electrocardiogram
ECHO	echocardiogram
ECMO	extracorporeal membrane oxygenation
EEG	electroencephalogram
ESR	erythrocyte sedimentation rate
ESRD	end stage renal disease
E.T.	endotracheal
FDA	Food and Drug Administration (United States)
FEV_1	forced expiratory volume exhaled after 1 second
FSH	follicle-stimulating hormone
FVC	forced vital capacity
g	gram
G-6-PD	glucose-6-phosphate dehydrogenase
GA	gestational age
GABA	gamma-aminobutyric acid
GE	gastroesophageal
GERD	gastroesophageal reflux disease
GFR	glomerular filtration rate
GI	gastrointestinal
GVHD	graft versus host disease
GU	genitourinary
h	hour
Hct	hematocrit
HDL-C	high density lipoprotein cholesterol
HF	heart failure
Hgb	hemoglobin
HFA	hydrofluoroalkane
HIV	human immunodeficiency virus
HMG-CoA	hydroxymethyl glutaryl coenzyme A
HPA	hypothalamic-pituitary-adrenal
HPLC	high performance liquid chromatography
HSV	herpes simplex virus
ICP	intracranial pressure
IDDM	insulin-dependent diabetes mellitus
IgG	immune globulin G
I.M.	intramuscular
INR	international normalized ratio

ILCOR	International Liaison Committee on Resuscitation
I.O.	intraosseous
I & O	input and output
IOP	intraocular pressure
IQ	intelligence quotient
I.T.	intrathecal
ITP	idiopathic thrombocytopenic purpura
I.V.	intravenous
IVH	intraventricular hemorrhage
IVP	intravenous push
JRA	juvenile rheumatoid arthritis
kg	kilogram
KOH	potassium hydroxide
L	liter
LDH	lactate dehydrogenase
LDL-C	low density lipoprotein cholesterol
LE	lupus erythematosus
LH	luteinizing hormone
LP	lumbar puncture
LR	lactated Ringer's
LV	left ventricular
M	molar
MAC	*Mycobacterium avium* complex
MAO	monoamine oxidase
MAP	mean arterial pressure
mcg	microgram
mEq	milliequivalent
mg	milligram
MI	myocardial infarction
min	minute
mL	milliliter
mM	millimole
mo	month
MOPP	mustargen (mechlorethamine), Oncovin® (vincristine), procarbazine, and prednisone
mOsm	milliosmoles
MRI	magnetic resonance image
MRSA	methicillin-resistant *Staphylococcus aureus*
NAEPP	National Asthma Education and Prevention Program
NCI	National Cancer Institute
ND	nasoduodenal
ng	nanogram
NG	nasogastric
NIDDM	noninsulin-dependent diabetes mellitus
NIH	National Institutes of Health
NMDA	n-methyl-d-aspartate
nmol	nanomole
NMS	neuroleptic malignant syndrome
NPO	nothing per os (nothing by mouth)
NS	normal saline (0.9% sodium chloride)
1/2NS	0.45% sodium chloride
NSAID	nonsteroidal anti-inflammatory drug
NYHA	New York Heart Association
O.R.	operating room
OTC	over-the-counter (nonprescription)
PABA	para-aminobenzoic acid
PACTG	Pediatric AIDS Clinical Trials Group
PALS	pediatric advanced life support
PCA	postconceptional age
PCP	*Pneumocystis jiroveci* pneumonia (also called *Pneumocystis carinii* pneumonia)

PCWP	pulmonary capillary wedge pressure
PDA	patent ductus arteriosus
PE	pulmonary embolism
PICU	Pediatric Intensive Care Unit
PIP	peak inspiratory pressure
PNA	postnatal age
prn	as needed
PSVT	paroxysmal supraventricular tachycardia
PT	prothrombin time
PTH	parathyroid hormone
PTT	partial thromboplastin time
PUD	peptic ulcer disease
PVC	premature ventricular contraction
PVR	peripheral vascular resistance
qsad	add an amount sufficient to equal
RAP	right arterial pressure
RDA	recommended daily allowance
RIA	radioimmunoassay
RNA	ribonucleic acid
RSV	respiratory syncytial virus
S-A	sino-atrial
S_{cr}	serum creatinine
SIADH	syndrome of inappropriate antidiuretic hormone
S.L.	sublingual
SLE	systemic lupus erythematosus
SNRI	serotonin norepinephrine reuptake inhibitor
SSRI	selective serotonin reuptake inhibitor
STD	sexually-transmitted disease
SubQ	subcutaneous
SVR	systemic vascular resistance
SVT	supraventricular tachycardia
SWI	sterile water for injection
T_3	triiodothyronine
T_4	thyroxine
TCA	tricyclic antidepressant
TIA	transient ischemic attack
TIBC	total iron binding capacity
TNF	tissue necrosis factor
TPN	total parenteral nutrition
TSH	thyroid stimulating hormone
TT	thrombin time
UA	urine analysis
UTI	urinary tract infection
V_d	volume of distribution
V_{dss}	volume of distribution at steady-state
VF	ventricular fibrillation
VMA	vanillylmandelic acid
VT	ventricular tachycardia
VTE	venous thromboembolism
VZV	varicella zoster virus
w/v	weight for volume
w/w	weight for weight
y	year

*Other than drug synonyms

PREVENTING PRESCRIBING ERRORS

Prescribing errors account for the majority of reported medication errors and have prompted healthcare professionals to focus on the development of steps to make the prescribing process safer. Prescription legibility has been attributed to a portion of these errors and legislation has been enacted in several states to address prescription legibility. However, eliminating handwritten prescriptions and ordering medications through the use of technology [eg, computerized prescriber order entry (CPOE)] has been the primary recommendation. Whether a prescription is electronic, typed, or hand-printed, additional safe practices should be considered for implementation to maximize the safety of the prescribing process. Listed below are suggestions for safer prescribing:

- Ensure correct patient by using at least 2 patient identifiers on the prescription (eg, full name, birth date, or address). Review prescription with the patient or patient's caregiver.
- If pediatric patient, document patient's birth date or age and most recent weight. If geriatric patient, document patient's birth date or age.
- Prevent drug name confusion:
    - Use TALLman lettering (eg, buPROPion, busPIRone, predniSONE, prednisoLONE). For more information see: http://www.fda.gov/Drugs/DrugSafety/MedicationErrors/ucm164587.htm.
    - Avoid abbreviated drug names (eg, MSO₄, MgSO₄, MS, HCT, 6MP, MTX), as they may be misinterpreted and cause error.
    - Avoid investigational names for drugs with FDA approval (eg, FK-506, CBDCA).
    - Avoid chemical names such as 6-mercaptopurine or 6-thioguanine, as sixfold overdoses have been given when these were not recognized as chemical names. The proper names of these drugs are mercaptopurine or thioguanine.
    - Use care when prescribing drugs that look or sound similar (eg, look- alike, sound-alike drugs). Common examples include: Celebrex® vs Celexa®, hydroxyzine vs hydralazine, Zyprexa® vs Zyrtec®.
- Avoid dangerous, error-prone abbreviations (eg, regardless of letter-case: U, IU, QD, QOD, µg, cc, @). Do not use apothecary system or symbols. Additionally, text messaging abbreviations (eg, "2Day") should never be used.
    - For more information see: http://www.ismp.org/Tools/errorproneabbreviations.pdf
- Always use a leading zero for numbers less than 1 (0.5 mg is correct and .5 mg is **incorrect**) and never use a trailing zero for whole numbers (2 mg is correct and 2.0 mg is **incorrect**).
- Always use a space between a number and its units as it is easier to read. There should be no periods after the abbreviations mg or mL (10 mg is correct and 10mg is **incorrect**).
- For doses that are greater than 1,000 dosing units, use properly placed commas to prevent 10-fold errors (100,000 units is correct and 100000 units is **incorrect**).
- Do not prescribe drug dosage by the type of container in which the drug is available (eg, do not prescribe "1 amp", "2 vials", etc).
- Do not write vague or ambiguous orders which have the potential for misinterpretation by other healthcare providers. Examples of vague orders to avoid: "resume pre-op medications," "give drug per protocol," or "continue home medications."
- Review each prescription with patient (or patient's caregiver) including the medication name, indication, and directions for use.
- Take extra precautions when prescribing *high alert drugs* (drugs that can cause significant patient harm when prescribed in error). Common examples of these drugs include: Anticoagulants, chemotherapy, insulins, opiates, and sedatives.
    - For more information see: http://www.ismp.org/Tools/highalertmedications.pdf
    To Err is Human: Building a Safer Health System, Kohn LT, Corrigan JM, and Donaldson MS, eds, Washington, D.C.: National Academy Press, 2000.

A Complete Outpatient Prescription[1]

A complete outpatient prescription can prevent the prescriber, the pharmacist, and/or the patient from making a mistake and can eliminate the need for further clarification. The complete outpatient prescription should contain:

- Patient's full name
- Medication indication
- Allergies
- Prescriber name and telephone or pager number
- For pediatric patients: Their birth date or age and current weight
- For geriatric patients: Their birth date or age
- Drug name, dosage form and strength
- For pediatric patients: Intended daily weight-based dose so that calculations can be checked by the pharmacist (ie, mg/kg/day or units/kg/day)
- Number or amount to be dispensed
- Complete instructions for the patient or caregiver, including the purpose of the medication, directions for use (including dose), dosing frequency, route of administration, duration of therapy, and number of refills.
- Dose should be expressed in convenient units of measure.

- When there are recognized contraindications for a prescribed drug, the prescriber should indicate knowledge of this fact to the pharmacist (ie, when prescribing a potassium salt for a patient receiving an ACE inhibitor, the prescriber should write "K serum leveling being monitored").

Upon dispensing of the final product, the pharmacist should ensure that the patient or caregiver can effectively demonstrate the appropriate administration technique. An appropriate measuring device should be provided or recommended. Household teaspoons and tablespoons should not be used to measure liquid medications due to their variability and inaccuracies in measurement; oral medication syringes are recommended.

For additional information see: http://www.ppag.org/attachments/files/111/Guidelines_Peds.pdf
[1]Levine SR, Cohen MR, Blanchard NR, et al, "Guidelines for Preventing Medication Errors in Pediatrics," *J Pediatr Pharmacol Ther*, 2001, 6:426-42.

FDA NAME DIFFERENTIATION PROJECT: THE USE OF "TALL MAN" LETTERS

Confusion between similar drug names is a frequent cause of medication errors. For years, The Institute For Safe Medication Practices (ISMP), has urged generic manufacturers to use a combination of capital and lower case letters (eg, chlorproMAZINE and chlorproPAMIDE) to help distinguish drugs with look-alike names, especially when they share similar strengths. The FDA's Office of Generic Drugs has acted upon this suggestion and initiated the "Name Differentiation Project," to help decrease medication errors that result from look-alike drug names. From March to May 2001, the Office of Generic Drugs issued 142 letters encouraging manufacturers to revise product labeling and labels to visually differentiate the established drug name with the use of "Tall Man" letters.

The ISMP recommends that hospitals follow suit by making similar changes in their pharmacy-prepared labels, preprinted order forms, pharmacy and physician order entry systems, computer-generated medication administration records, drug storage location labels, and other print or electronic use of the drug name.

Lexi-Comp Medical Publishing will use "Tall Man" letters for the drugs suggested by the FDA or recommended by ISMP. The "Tall Man" lettering will appear in the generic name field of the monograph.

The following is a list of generic product names and recommended revisions.

Drug Product	Recommended Revision
acetazolamide	aceta**ZOLAMIDE**
acetohexamide	aceto**HEXAMIDE**
alprazolam	**ALPRAZ**olam
amiloride	a**MIL**oride
amlodipine	am**LODIP**ine
azacitidine	aza**CITID**ine
azathioprine	aza**THIO**prine
bupropion	bu**PROP**ion
buspirone	bus**PIR**one
carbamazepine	car**BAM**azepine
carboplatin	**CARBO**platin
cefazolin	ce**FAZ**olin
ceftriaxone	cef**TRIAX**one
chlordiazepoxide	chlordiaze**POXIDE**
chlorpromazine	chlorpro**MAZINE**
chlorpropamide	chlorpro**PAMIDE**
cisplatin	**CIS**platin
clomiphene	clomi**PHENE**
clomipramine	clomi**PRAMINE**
clonazepam	clonaze**PAM**
clonidine	clo**NID**ine
cycloserine	cyclo**SERINE**
cyclosporine	cyclo**SPORINE**
dactinomycin	**DACTIN**omycin
daptomycin	**DAPTO**mycin
daunorubicin	**DAUNO**rubicin
dimenhydrinate	dimenhy**DRINATE**
diphenhydramine	diphenhydr**AMINE**
dobutamine	**DOBUT**amine
dopamine	**DOP**amine
doxorubicin	**DOXO**rubicin
duloxetine	**DUL**oxetine
ephedrine	e**PHED**rine
epinephrine	**EPINEPH**rine
fentanyl	fenta**NYL**
fluoxetine	**FLU**oxetine
glipizide	glipi**ZIDE**
glyburide	gly**BURIDE**
guaifenesin	guai**FEN**esin
guanfacine	guan**FACINE**

Drug Product	Recommended Revision
hydralazine	hydr**ALAZINE**
hydrocodone	**HYDRO**codone
hydromorphone	**HYDRO**morphone
hydroxyzine	hydr**OXY**zine
idarubicin	**IDA**rubicin
infliximab	in**FLIX**imab
lamivudine	lami**VUD**ine
lamotrigine	lamo**TRI**gine
lorazepam	**LOR**azepam
medroxyprogesterone	medroxy**PROGESTER**one
metformin	met**FORMIN**
methylprednisolone	methyl**PREDNIS**olone
methyltestosterone	methyl**TESTOSTER**one
metronidazole	metro**NIDAZOLE**
nicardipine	ni**CAR**dipine
nifedipine	**NIFE**dipine
nimodipine	ni**MOD**ipine
olanzapine	**OLANZ**apine
oxcarbazepine	**OX**carbazepine
oxycodone	oxy**CODONE**
paroxetine	**PAR**oxetine
pentobarbital	**PENT**obarbital
phenobarbital	**PHEN**obarbital
prednisolone	predniso**LONE**
prednisone	predni**SONE**
quetiapine	**QUE**tiapine
quinidine	qui**NID**ine
quinine	qui**NINE**
rituximab	ri**TUX**imab
sitagliptin	sita**GLIP**tin
sufentanil	**SUF**entanil
sulfadiazine	sulf**ADIAZINE**
sulfisoxazole	sulfi**SOXAZOLE**
sumatriptan	**SUMA**triptan
tiagabine	tia**GAB**ine
tizanidine	ti**ZAN**idine
tolazamide	**TOLAZ**amide
tolbutamide	**TOLBUT**amide
tramadol	tra**MAD**ol
trazodone	tra**ZOD**one
valacyclovir	val**ACY**clovir
valganciclovir	val**GANCI**clovir
vinblastine	vin**BLAS**tine
vincristine	vin**CRIS**tine

Institute for Safe Medication Practices. "New Tall-Man Lettering Will Reduce Mix-Ups Due to Generic Drug Name Confusion," *ISMP Medication Safety Alert*, September 19, 2001. Available at: http://www.ismp.org.

Institute for Safe Medication Practices. "Prescription Mapping, Can Improve Efficiency While Minimizing Errors With Look-Alike Products," *ISMP Medication Safety Alert*, October 6, 1999. Available at: http://www.ismp.org.

Institute for Safe Medication Practices. "Use of Tall Man Letters Is Gaining Wide Acceptance," *ISMP Medication Safety Alert*, July 31, 2008. Available at: http://www.ismp.org.

U.S. Pharmacopeia, "USP Quality Review: Use Caution-Avoid Confusion," March 2001, No. 76. Available at: http://www.usp.org.

ALPHABETICAL LISTING OF DRUGS

◆ **A200® Lice [OTC]** *see* Permethrin *on page 1094*

◆ **A-ase** *see* Asparaginase *on page 139*

Abacavir (uh BACK ah veer)

Related Information
Adult and Adolescent HIV *on page 1620*
Pediatric HIV *on page 1613*
Perinatal HIV *on page 1628*

U.S. Brand Names Ziagen®

Canadian Brand Names Ziagen®

Therapeutic Category Antiretroviral Agent; HIV Agents (Anti-HIV Agents); Nucleoside Reverse Transcriptase Inhibitor (NRTI)

Generic Available No

Use Treatment of HIV-1 infection in combination with other antiretroviral agents. (**Note:** HIV regimens consisting of **three** antiretroviral agents are strongly recommended)

Medication Guide An FDA-approved patient medication guide, which is available with the product information and at http://www.fda.gov/downloads/Drugs/DrugSafety/ucm089831.pdf, must be dispensed with this medication for each new outpatient prescription and refill. A Warning Card (summarizing symptoms of hypersensitivity), which is available with the product information, must also be dispensed with this medication for each new outpatient prescription and refill.

Pregnancy Risk Factor C

Pregnancy Considerations Adverse events have been observed in some animal reproduction studies. It is not known if abacavir crosses the human placenta. No increased risk of overall birth defects has been observed following 1st trimester exposure according to data collected by the antiretroviral pregnancy registry. Cases of lactic acidosis/hepatic steatosis syndrome have been reported in pregnant women receiving nucleoside analogues. It is not known if pregnancy itself potentiates this known side effect; however, pregnant women may be at increased risk of lactic acidosis and liver damage. Hepatic enzymes and electrolytes should be monitored frequently during the 3rd trimester of pregnancy in women receiving nucleoside analogues. Dose adjustment is not needed for pregnancy. The Perinatal HIV Guidelines Working Group considers abacavir to be an alternative NRTI in dual nucleoside combination regimens. Health professionals are encouraged to contact the antiretroviral pregnancy registry to monitor outcomes of pregnant women exposed to antiretroviral medications (1-800-258-4263 or www.-APRegistry.com).

Lactation Excretion in breast milk unknown/contraindicated

Breast-Feeding Considerations In infants born to mothers who are HIV positive, HAART while breast-feeding may decrease postnatal infection. However, maternal or infant antiretroviral therapy does not completely eliminate the risk of postnatal HIV transmission.

In the United States where formula is accessible, affordable, safe, and sustainable, complete avoidance of breast-feeding by HIV-infected women is recommended to decrease potential transmission of HIV.

Contraindications Hypersensitivity to abacavir or any component [**do not rechallenge** patients who have experienced hypersensitivity reactions to abacavir (regardless of *HLA-B*5701* status), potentially fatal hypersensitivity reactions may occur (see Warnings)]; moderate or severe hepatic dysfunction

Warnings Serious and sometimes fatal hypersensitivity reactions may occur [**U.S. Boxed Warning**]. Patients testing positive for the presence of the *HLA-B*5701* allele are at a significantly increased risk for hypersensitivity reactions [**U.S. Boxed Warning**]. Screening for *HLA-B*5701* allele status is recommended prior to initiating therapy or reinitiating therapy in patients of unknown genotype status, including patients who previously tolerated therapy. Abacavir therapy is **not** recommended in patients testing positive for the *HLA-B*5701* allele. If a suspected abacavir hypersensitivity reaction occurs during therapy, regardless of *HLA-B*5701* status, abacavir should be discontinued immediately and permanently. **Note:** Hypersensitivity reactions may also occur in patients who test negative for the *HLA-B*5701* allele, but at a significantly lower rate (see Additional Information).

Abacavir hypersensitivity is a multiorgan clinical syndrome [**U.S. Boxed Warning**]. Discontinue therapy immediately in patients who show signs or symptoms of 2 or more of the following: Fever, skin rash, respiratory symptoms (including cough, dyspnea, or pharyngitis), GI symptoms (including nausea, vomiting, diarrhea, or abdominal pain), and constitutional symptoms (including fatigue, malaise, or achiness). Carefully consider the diagnosis of hypersensitivity reaction in patients who present with acute onset respiratory symptoms, even if other diagnoses, such as bronchitis, flu-like illness, pharyngitis, or pneumonia, are possible. Permanently discontinue abacavir if hypersensitivity reaction cannot be ruled out, even when other diagnoses are possible (regardless of *HLA-B*5701* status) [**U.S. Boxed Warning**]. Skin rash may be maculopapular or urticarial, but can be variable in appearance; erythema multiforme has been reported; hypersensitivity reaction may occur without a rash. Other symptoms may include edema, lethargy, myolysis, paresthesia, shortness of breath, mouth ulcerations, conjunctivitis, lymphadenopathy, and abnormal findings on chest x-ray (ie, infiltrates that can be localized). Anaphylaxis, renal failure, hepatic failure, respiratory failure, ARDS, hypotension, and death may also occur in association with hypersensitivity reactions. Laboratory abnormalities include increases in liver function tests, elevated CPK or serum creatinine, and lymphopenia.

Do not restart abacavir or any other abacavir-containing product after a hypersensitivity reaction occurs [**U.S. Boxed Warning**]; more severe symptoms can recur within hours and may include life-threatening hypotension and death. Fatal hypersensitivity reactions have occurred following the reintroduction of abacavir in patients whose therapy was interrupted for other reasons [**U.S. Boxed Warning**]. These patients had no identified history or had unrecognized symptoms of abacavir hypersensitivity. Reactions occurred within hours. In some cases, signs of a hypersensitivity reaction may have been previously present, but attributed to other medical conditions (acute onset respiratory diseases, gastroenteritis, reactions to other medications). If abacavir or any other abacavir-containing product is to be restarted following an interruption in therapy, the patient must first be evaluated for previously unsuspected symptoms of hypersensitivity. **Do not restart** abacavir or any other abacavir-containing product, if hypersensitivity is suspected or cannot be ruled out (regardless of *HLA-B*5701* status). Hypersensitivity reactions occur in 5% to 8% of adult and pediatric patients (actual incidence varies by race/ethnicity); most hypersensitivity reactions occur within the first 6 weeks of therapy, but can occur at any time; one study reported a higher incidence of severe hypersensitivity reactions with once daily dosing compared with twice daily dosing (see product information); call the Abacavir Hypersensitivity Reaction Registry at 1-800-270-0425 to facilitate reporting and collection of information on patients experiencing abacavir hypersensitivity reactions.

Cases of lactic acidosis, severe hepatomegaly with steatosis and death have been reported with the use of abacavir and other NRTIs **[U.S. Boxed Warning]**; most of these cases have been in women; prolonged nucleoside use, obesity, and prior liver disease may be risk factors; use with extreme caution in patients with other risk factors for liver disease; discontinue abacavir in patients who develop laboratory or clinical evidence of lactic acidosis or pronounced hepatotoxicity

Precautions Use with caution and decrease the dose in patients with mild hepatic dysfunction (see Contraindications). Fat redistribution and accumulation [ie, central obesity, peripheral wasting, facial wasting, breast enlargement, dorsocervical fat enlargement (buffalo hump), and cushingoid appearance] have been observed in patients receiving antiretroviral agents (causal relationship not established). Always use abacavir in combination with other antiretroviral agents; do not add abacavir as a single agent to antiretroviral regimens that are failing; resistance to abacavir develops relatively slowly, but cross resistance between abacavir and other nucleoside reverse transcriptase inhibitors (NRTIs) may occur; limited response may be seen in patients with HIV isolates containing multiple mutations conferring resistance to NRTIs or in patients with a prolonged prior NRTI exposure (see Additional Information)

Immune reconstitution syndrome (an acute inflammatory response to residual or indolent opportunistic infections) may occur in HIV patients during initial treatment with combination antiretroviral agents, including abacavir; this syndrome may require further patient assessment and therapy. Use with caution in patients with risks for coronary heart disease; modifiable risk factors (eg, hypertension, hyperlipidemia, diabetes mellitus, and smoking) should be minimized prior to use. **Note:** Two studies found an increased risk of MI in patients receiving abacavir; however, a subsequent study did not find an increased risk (see Working Group, 2009).

Systemic exposure of abacavir at 6-32 times the normal human exposure, increased the incidence of tumors (malignant and nonmalignant) in mice and rats; myocardial degeneration was seen in mice and rats receiving abacavir for 2 years at 7-24 times the expected human exposure; the clinical relevance of these findings is currently unknown.

Adverse Reactions
Cardiovascular: MI (postmarketing reports; see Precautions)
Central nervous system: Insomnia, fever, headache, malaise, fatigue, anxiety
Dermatologic: Rash (see Warnings); erythema multiforme. **Note:** Suspected toxic epidermal necrolysis and Stevens-Johnson syndrome have been reported but patients also received medications known to be associated with these rashes; due to the similarities between these rashes and abacavir hypersensitivity reactions, abacavir should be discontinued and never restarted in such patients.
Endocrine & metabolic: Mild elevations of blood glucose (may be more frequent in pediatric patients), hypertriglyceridemia, lactic acidosis, fat redistribution and accumulation (see Precautions)
Gastrointestinal: Nausea, vomiting, diarrhea, anorexia; pancreatitis (rare); **Note:** Severe diarrhea may occur at a higher incidence in patients receiving once daily dosing
Hepatic: Hepatomegaly with steatosis; liver enzymes elevated
Neuromuscular & skeletal: Asthenia, musculoskeletal pain
Respiratory: Cough

Miscellaneous: Hypersensitivity reaction (see Warnings); immune reconstitution syndrome

Drug Interactions
Avoid Concomitant Use There are no known interactions where it is recommended to avoid concomitant use.
Increased Effect/Toxicity
The levels/effects of Abacavir may be increased by: Ganciclovir-Valganciclovir; Ribavirin
Decreased Effect
The levels/effects of Abacavir may be decreased by: Protease Inhibitors
Food Interactions Food does not significantly affect AUC.
Stability Store tablets and oral solution at room temperature; oral solution may be refrigerated; do not freeze
Mechanism of Action A carbocyclic analogue that is converted within cells to the active metabolite carbovir triphosphate; carbovir triphosphate serves as an alternative substrate to deoxyguanosine-5'-triphosphate (dGTP), a natural substrate for cellular DNA polymerase and reverse transcriptase; carbovir triphosphate inhibits HIV viral reverse transcriptase by competing with natural dGTP and by becoming incorporated into viral DNA causing chain termination. Abacavir is also a weak inhibitor of cellular DNA polymerases (alpha, beta, and gamma).

Pharmacokinetics (Adult data unless noted)
Absorption: Rapid and extensive
Distribution: Apparent V_d: Adults: 0.86 ± 0.15 L/kg
  CSF to plasma AUC ratio: 27% to 33%
Protein binding: 50%
Metabolism: In the liver by alcohol dehydrogenase and glucuronyl transferase to inactive carboxylate and glucuronide metabolites; not significantly metabolized by cytochrome P450 enzymes
Bioavailability: Tablet: 83%; solution and tablet provide comparable AUCs
Half-life, elimination (serum):
  Infants ≥3 months and Children ≤13 years: 1-1.5 hours
  Adults: 1.54 ± 0.63 hours
  Hepatic impairment: Increases half-life by 58%
Half-life, intracellular: 12-26 hours
Time to peak serum concentration: Infants ≥3 months and Children ≤13 years: Within 1.5 hours
Elimination: ~83% of dose excreted in the urine (1.2% as unchanged drug, 30% as 5'-carboxylic acid metabolite, 36% as the glucuronide, and 15% as other metabolites); 16% eliminated in feces
Clearance (apparent): Single dose 8 mg/kg:
  Infants ≥3 months and Children ≤13 years: 17.84 mL/minute/kg
  Adults: 10.14 mL/minute/kg

Usual Dosage Oral (use in combination with other antiretroviral agents):
Neonates and Infants <3 months: Not approved for use
Infants ≥3 months, Children, and Adolescents ≤16 years: 8 mg/kg twice daily (maximum: 300 mg twice daily); **Note:** Limited data exists for the use of abacavir in adolescents; clinical trials support the use of adult doses of 300 mg twice daily in adolescent patients ≥13 years (see Working Group, 2009); safety and efficacy of once daily dosing have not been established in pediatric patients
Adolescents >16 years and Adults: 300 mg twice daily or 600 mg once daily
Dosing adjustment in hepatic impairment:
  Mild hepatic impairment (Child-Pugh score 5-6): Adults: 200 mg twice daily (using oral solution)
  Moderate to severe hepatic impairment: Drug is contraindicated

Administration Oral: May be administered without regard to food

Monitoring Parameters HLA-B*5701 genotype status prior to initiating therapy or resuming therapy in patients of unknown HLA-B*5701 status (including patients previously tolerating therapy); signs and symptoms of hypersensitivity reaction (in all patients, but especially in those untested for the HLA-B*5701 allele); CBC with differential, serum creatine kinase, CD4 count, HIV RNA plasma levels, serum transaminases, triglycerides, serum amylase

Patient Information Abacavir is not a cure for HIV. Take abacavir everyday as prescribed; do not change dose or discontinue without physician's advice. If abacavir is stopped for any reason, notify physician before restarting therapy. If a dose is missed, take it as soon as possible, then return to normal dosing schedule; if a dose is skipped, do **not** double the next dose

Serious and sometimes fatal allergic reactions may occur. Read the patient Medication Guide that you receive with each prescription and refill of abacavir; carry the Warning Card with you. Stop taking abacavir and notify physician immediately if 2 or more of the following sets of symptoms occur: Fever, rash, GI symptoms (nausea, vomiting, diarrhea or abdominal pain), flu-like symptoms (severe tiredness, achiness, or generally ill feeling), or respiratory symptoms (sore throat, shortness of breath, cough). If you experience an allergic (hypersensitivity) reaction to abacavir (or Ziagen®, Trizivir®, or Epzicom®), **never** take abacavir, Ziagen®, Trizivir®, or Epzicom® again. If you take an abacavir-containing medication after having an allergic reaction, you may get life-threatening symptoms including very low blood pressure or death within hours.

HIV medications may cause changes in body fat, including an increase in fat in the upper back and neck, breasts, and trunk; a loss of fat from the face, arms, and legs may also occur. Some HIV medications (including abacavir) may cause a serious, but rare, condition called lactic acidosis with an increase in liver size (hepatomegaly). Before starting abacavir, inform your physician about your medical conditions, including any liver or heart problems, if you smoke, or have diabetes, high cholesterol, or high blood pressure. Do not take Ziagen® with other abacavir-containing medications (eg, Epzicom® or Trizivir®).

Nursing Implications Inform patients of the possibility of a fatal hypersensitivity reaction and the signs and symptoms (see Warnings)

Additional Information The patient Medication Guide, which includes written manufacturer information, should be dispensed to the patient with each new prescription and refill; the Warning Card describing the hypersensitivity reaction should be given to the patient to carry with them.

The development of the abacavir hypersensitivity reaction has been associated with certain HLA genotypes (eg, HLA-B*5701, HLA-DR7, HLA-DQ3) which may help predict which patients are at risk for developing the abacavir hypersensitivity reaction (see Hetherington, 2002; Lucas, 2007; Mallal, 2002). Patients who test positive for the HLA-B*5701 allele should have an abacavir allergy recorded in their medical record and should **not** receive abacavir. All patients who receive abacavir (and their caregivers) should be educated about the risk of abacavir hypersensitivity reactions (including patients who test negative for the HLA-B*5701 allele, as the risk for the reaction is not completely eliminated). Approximately 4% of patients who test negative for the HLA-B*5701 allele will experience a clinically suspected abacavir hypersensitivity reaction compared to 61% of those who test positive for the HLA-B*5701 allele.

The prevalence of HLA-B*5701 in the United States has been estimated to be 8% in Caucasians, 2.5% in African-Americans, 2% in Hispanics, 1% in Asians; in the sub-Saharan Africa it is <1%. Pretherapy identification of HLA-B*5701-positive patients and subsequent avoidance of abacavir therapy in these patients has been shown to significantly reduce the occurrence of abacavir-associated hypersensitivity reactions. A skin patch test is in development for clinical screening purposes; however, only PCR-mediated genotyping methods are currently in clinical practice use for documentation of this susceptibility marker. A familial predisposition to the abacavir hypersensitivity reaction has also been reported; use abacavir with great caution in children of parents who experience a hypersensitivity reaction to abacavir (see Peyriére, 2001).

Reverse transcriptase mutations of K65R, L74V, Y115F, and M184V have been associated with abacavir resistance; at least 2-3 mutations are needed to decrease HIV susceptibility by 10-fold. The presence of a multiple number of these abacavir resistance-associated mutations, may confer cross-resistance for other nucleoside or nucleotide reverse transcriptase inhibitors (eg, didanosine, emtricitabine, lamivudine, zalcitabine, or tenofovir). A progressive decrease in abacavir susceptibility is associated with an increasing number of thymidine analogue mutations (TAMs; M41L, D67N, K70R, L210W, T215Y/F, K219E/R/H/Q/N).

A recent multicenter study, conducted in previously untreated HIV-infected children (median age: 5.3 years; range: 0.3-16.7 years), demonstrated that abacavir-containing antiretroviral regimens were more effective than regimens containing the NRTI combination of zidovudine and lamivudine; after adjusting for use of nelfinavir and controlling for baseline factors, the NRTI combination of abacavir and lamivudine showed the largest and most durable reduction in viral load, compared to the combination of zidovudine and lamivudine or zidovudine and abacavir; further studies are needed.

A high rate of early virologic failure in therapy-naive adult HIV patients has been observed with the once daily three-drug combination therapy of abacavir, lamivudine, and tenofovir. This combination should not be used as a new treatment regimen for naive or pretreated patients. Any patient currently receiving this regimen should be closely monitored and considered for regimen modification.

A new scored 300 mg abacavir tablet has recently been approved by the FDA; once available, new pediatric dosing recommendations using the scored tablets will be available.

Dosage Forms Excipient information presented when available (limited, particularly for generics); consult specific product labeling.

Solution, oral:
   Ziagen®: 20 mg/mL (240 mL) [strawberry-banana flavor]
Tablet:
   Ziagen®: 300 mg [scored]

References

Briars LA, Hilao JJ, and Kraus DM, "A Review of Pediatric Human Immunodeficiency Virus Infection," *Journal of Pharmacy Practice*, 2004, 17(6):407-31.

Center for Disease Control and Prevention, "Guidelines for Using Antiretroviral Agents Among HIV-Infected Adults and Adolescents. Recommendations of the Panel on Clinical Practices for Treatment of HIV," *MMWR*, 2002, 51(RR-7):1-55.

Collura JM and Kraus DM, "New Pediatric Antiretroviral Agents," *J Pediatr Health Care*, 2000, 14(4):183-90.

Foster RH and Faulds D, "Abacavir," *Drugs*, 1998, 55(5):729-36.

Hetherington S, Hughes AR, Mosteller M, et al, "Genetic Variations in HLA-B Region and Hypersensitivity Reactions to Abacavir," *Lancet*, 2002, 359(9312):1121-2.

Hughes W, McDowell JA, Shenep J, et al, "Safety and Single-Dose Pharmacokinetics of Abacavir (1592U89) in Human Immunodeficiency Virus Type 1-Infected Children," *Antimicrob Agents Chemother*, 1999, 43(3):609-15.

Kline MW, Blanchard S, Fletcher CV, et al, "A Phase I Study of Abacavir (1592U89) Alone and in Combination With Other Antiretroviral Agents in Infants and Children With Human Immunodeficiency Virus Infection," *Pediatrics*, 1999, 103(4):e47; http://www.pediatrics.org/cgi/content/full/103/4/e47.

Lucas A, Nolan D, and Mallal S, "HLA-B*5701 Screening for Susceptibility to Abacavir Hypersensitivity," *J Antimicrob Chemother,* 2007, 59(4):591-3.

Mallal S, Nolan D, Witt C, et al, "Association Between Presence of HLA-B*5701, HLA-DR7, and HLA-DQ3 and Hypersensitivity to HIV-1 Reverse-Transcriptase Inhibitor Abacavir," *Lancet,* 2002, 359 (9308):727-32.

Paediatric European Network for Treatment of AIDS (PENTA), "Comparison of Dual Nucleoside-Analogue Reverse-Transcriptase Inhibitor Regimens With and Without Nelfinavir in Children with HIV-1 Who Have Not Previously Been Treated: The PENTA 5 Randomised Trial," *Lancet,* 2002, 359(9308):733-40.

Panel on Antiretroviral Guidelines for Adults and Adolescents, "Guidelines for the Use of Antiretroviral Agents in HIV-Infected Adults and Adolescents," December 1, 2009, http://www.aidsinfo.nih.gov.

Peyriére H, Nicolas J, Siffert M, et al, "Hypersensitivity Related to Abacavir in Two Members of a Family," *Ann Pharmacother,* 2001, 35 (10):1291-2.

Working Group on Antiretroviral Therapy and Medical Management of HIV-Infected Children, "Guidelines for the Use of Antiretroviral Agents in Pediatric HIV Infection," February 23, 2009. Available at http://www.aidsinfo.nih.gov.

◆ **Abacavir and 3TC** *see* Abacavir and Lamivudine on page 29

Abacavir and Lamivudine
(a BAK a veer & la MI vyoo deen)

Related Information
Adult and Adolescent HIV on page 1620

U.S. Brand Names Epzicom®

Canadian Brand Names Kivexa™

Therapeutic Category Antiretroviral Agent; HIV Agents (Anti-HIV Agents); Nucleoside Analog Reverse Transcriptase Inhibitor (NRTI)

Generic Available No

Use Treatment of HIV-1 infection in combination with other antiretroviral agents (**Note:** HIV regimens consisting of **three** antiretroviral agents are strongly recommended)

Medication Guide An FDA-approved patient medication guide, which is available with the product information and at http://www.fda.gov/downloads/Drugs/DrugSafety/ucm088592.pdf, must be dispensed with this medication for each new outpatient prescription and refill. A Warning Card (summarizing symptoms of hypersensitivity), which is available with the product information, must also be dispensed with this medication for each new outpatient prescription and refill.

Pregnancy Risk Factor C

Pregnancy Considerations See individual agents.

Lactation See individual agents.

Breast-Feeding Considerations HIV-infected mothers are discouraged from breast-feeding to decrease potential transmission of HIV. See individual agents.

Contraindications Hypersensitivity to abacavir, lamivudine, or any component; hepatic impairment. **Do not rechallenge** patients who have experienced hypersensitivity reactions to abacavir (regardless of *HLA-B*5701* status); potentially fatal hypersensitivity reactions may occur (see Warnings).

Warnings Serious and sometimes fatal hypersensitivity reactions to abacavir may occur **[U.S. Boxed Warning]**. Patients testing positive for the presence of the *HLA-B*5701* allele are at a significantly increased risk for hypersensitivity reactions **[U.S. Boxed Warning]**. Screening for *HLA-B*5701* allele status is recommended prior to initiating therapy or reinitiating therapy in patients of unknown genotype status, including patients who previously tolerated therapy. Abacavir therapy is **not** recommended in patients testing positive for the *HLA-B*5701* allele. If a suspected abacavir hypersensitivity reaction occurs during therapy, regardless of *HLA-B*5701* status, abacavir should be discontinued immediately and permanently. **Note:** Hypersensitivity reactions may also occur in patients who test negative for the *HLA-B*5701* allele, but at a significantly lower rate (see Additional Information).

Abacavir hypersensitivity is a multiorgan clinical syndrome **[U.S. Boxed Warning]**. Discontinue therapy immediately in patients who show signs or symptoms of 2 or more of the following: Fever, skin rash, respiratory symptoms (including cough, dyspnea, or pharyngitis), GI symptoms (including nausea, vomiting, diarrhea, or abdominal pain), and constitutional symptoms (including fatigue, malaise, or achiness). Carefully consider the diagnosis of hypersensitivity reaction in patients who present with acute onset respiratory symptoms, even if other diagnoses, such as bronchitis, flu-like illness, pharyngitis, or pneumonia, are possible. Permanently discontinue abacavir-containing medications if hypersensitivity reaction cannot be ruled out, even when other diagnoses are possible (regardless of *HLA-B*5701* status) **[U.S. Boxed Warning]**. Skin rash may be maculopapular or urticarial, but can be variable in appearance; erythema multiforme has been reported; hypersensitivity reaction may occur without a rash. Other symptoms may include edema, lethargy, myolysis, paresthesia, shortness of breath, mouth ulcerations, conjunctivitis, lymphadenopathy, and abnormal findings on chest x-ray (ie, infiltrates that can be localized). Anaphylaxis, renal failure, hepatic failure, respiratory failure, ARDS, hypotension, and death may also occur in association with hypersensitivity reactions. Laboratory abnormalities include increases in liver function tests, elevated CPK or serum creatinine, and lymphopenia.

Do not restart abacavir, Epzicom®, or any other abacavir-containing product after a hypersensitivity reaction occurs **[U.S. Boxed Warning]**; more severe symptoms can recur within hours and may include life-threatening hypotension and death. Fatal hypersensitivity reactions have occurred following the reintroduction of abacavir in patients whose therapy was interrupted for other reasons **[U.S. Boxed Warning]**. These patients had no identified history or had unrecognized symptoms of abacavir hypersensitivity. Reactions occurred within hours. In some cases, signs of a hypersensitivity reaction may have been previously present, but attributed to other medical conditions (acute onset respiratory diseases, gastroenteritis, or reactions to other medications). If abacavir, Epzicom®, or any other abacavir-containing product is to be restarted following an interruption in therapy, the patient must first be evaluated for previously unsuspected symptoms of hypersensitivity. **Do not restart** abacavir, Epzicom®, or any other abacavir-containing product if hypersensitivity is suspected or cannot be ruled out (regardless of *HLA-B*5701* status). Hypersensitivity reactions occur in 5% to 8% of adult and pediatric patients (actual incidence varies by race/ethnicity); most hypersensitivity reactions occur within the first 6 weeks of therapy, but can occur at any time; call the Abacavir Hypersensitivity Reaction Registry at 1-800-270-0425 to facilitate reporting and collection of information on patients experiencing abacavir hypersensitivity reactions.

Cases of lactic acidosis, severe hepatomegaly with steatosis, and death have been reported in patients receiving nucleoside analogues **[U.S. Boxed Warning]**; most of these cases have been in women; prolonged nucleoside use, obesity, and prior liver disease may be risk factors; use with extreme caution in patients with other risk factors for liver disease; discontinue Epzicom® in patients who develop laboratory or clinical evidence of lactic acidosis or pronounced hepatotoxicity.

The major clinical toxicity of lamivudine in pediatric patients is pancreatitis; discontinue therapy if clinical signs, symptoms, or laboratory abnormalities suggestive of pancreatitis occur. HIV-infected patients who are coinfected with hepatitis B may experience severe acute exacerbations and clinical symptoms or laboratory evidence of hepatitis when a lamivudine-containing medication is discontinued [U.S. Boxed Warning]; most cases are self-limited, but fatalities have been reported; monitor patients closely for at least several months after discontinuation of abacavir and lamivudine; initiation of antihepatitis B therapy may be required. Note: HIV-infected patients should be screened for hepatitis B infection prior to starting lamivudine therapy. Concomitant use of combination antiretroviral therapy with interferon alfa (with or without ribavirin) has resulted in hepatic decompensation (with some fatalities) in patients coin-fected with HIV and HCV; monitor patients closely, especially for hepatic decompensation; consider discontin-uation of abacavir and lamivudine if needed; consider dose reduction or discontinuation of interferon alfa, ribavirin, or both if clinical toxicities, including hepatic decompensation, worsen.

Epzicom® contains abacavir and lamivudine as a fixed-dose combination; do not use in patients with renal dysfunction (Cl$_{cr}$ ≤50 mL/minute) who require lamivudine dosage adjustment or in patients with hepatic dysfunction (Note: Abacavir is contraindicated in patients with moderate to severe hepatic dysfunction; patients with mild hepatic impairment require abacavir dosage reduction). Do not administer Epzicom® with abacavir, lamivudine, or emtricitabine-containing products.

Precautions Fat redistribution and accumulation [ie, central obesity, peripheral wasting, facial wasting, breast enlargement, dorsocervical fat enlargement (buffalo hump), and cushingoid appearance] have been observed in patients receiving antiretroviral agents (causal relation-ship not established). Resistance to abacavir develops relatively slowly, but cross resistance between abacavir and other nucleoside reverse transcriptase inhibitors (NRTIs) may occur; limited response may be seen in patients with HIV isolates containing multiple mutations conferring resistance to NRTIs or in patients with a prolonged prior NRTI exposure.

Immune reconstitution syndrome (an acute inflammatory response to residual or indolent opportunistic infections) may occur in HIV patients during initial treatment with combination antiretroviral agents, including abacavir and lamivudine; this syndrome may require further patient assessment and therapy. Use with caution in patients with risks for coronary heart disease; modifiable risk factors (eg, hypertension, hyperlipidemia, diabetes mellitus, smoking) should be minimized prior to use. Note: Two studies found an increased risk of MI in patients receiving abacavir; however, a subsequent study did not find an increased risk (see Working Group, 2009).

Systemic exposure of abacavir at 6-32 times the normal human exposure, increased the incidence of tumors (malignant and nonmalignant) in mice and rats; myocardial degeneration was seen in mice and rats receiving abacavir for 2 years at 7-24 times the expected human exposure; the clinical relevance of these findings is currently unknown

Adverse Reactions See individual agents.

Drug Interactions

Avoid Concomitant Use

Avoid concomitant use of Abacavir and Lamivudine with any of the following: Emtricitabine

Increased Effect/Toxicity

Abacavir and Lamivudine may increase the levels/effects of: Emtricitabine

The levels/effects of Abacavir and Lamivudine may be increased by: Ganciclovir-Valganciclovir; Ribavirin; Trimethoprim

Decreased Effect

The levels/effects of Abacavir and Lamivudine may be decreased by: Protease Inhibitors

Food Interactions Food decreases the rate, but not the extent of absorption; in a single dose study, a high-fat meal did not change bioavailability or peak concentrations.

Stability Store at room temperature 25°C (77°F).

Mechanism of Action See individual agents.

Pharmacokinetics (Adult data unless noted) One Epzicom® tablet is bioequivalent, in the extent (AUC) of absorption and peak concentration, to two abacavir 300 mg tablets and two lamivudine 150 mg tablets; see individual agents

Usual Dosage Oral:

Children and Adolescents <18 years of age: Not intended for pediatric use; product is a fixed-dose combination; safety and efficacy has not been established in pediatric patients

Adolescents ≥18 years of age and Adults: 1 tablet daily

Dosage adjustment in hepatic impairment: Use is contraindicated (use individual antiretroviral agents to reduce dosage)

Dosage adjustment in renal impairment: Cl$_{cr}$ ≤50 mL/minute: Not recommended (use individual antiretroviral agents to reduce dosage)

Administration May be administered without regards to meals.

Monitoring Parameters *HLA-B*5701* genotype status prior to initiating therapy or resuming therapy in patients of unknown *HLA-B*5701* status (including patients previously tolerating therapy); signs and symptoms of abacavir hypersensitivity reaction (in all patients, but especially in those untested for the *HLA-B*5701* allele), lactic acidosis, pronounced hepatotoxicity, and pancreatitis; serum glu-cose, triglycerides, creatine kinase; HIV RNA plasma levels, CD4 counts, CBC with differential, hemoglobin, liver enzymes, serum amylase, bilirubin, renal and hepatic function tests; HIV patients should be screened for hepatitis B before starting lamivudine (see Warnings)

Patient Information Epzicom® is not a cure for HIV. Take Epzicom® every day as prescribed; do not change dose or discontinue without physician's advice. If Epzicom® is stopped for any reason, notify physician before restarting therapy. If a dose is missed, take it as soon as possible, then return to normal dosing schedule; if a dose is skipped, do **not** double the next dose. Avoid alcohol. Notify physician if persistent severe abdominal pain, nausea, or vomiting occurs.

Epzicom® contains abacavir (also called Ziagen®). Abacavir may cause serious and sometimes fatal allergic (hypersensitivity) reactions. Read the Patient Medication Guide that you receive with each prescription and refill of abacavir and lamivudine. Stop taking Epzicom® and notify physician immediately if 2 or more of the following sets of symptoms occur: Fever, rash, GI symptoms (nausea, vomiting, diarrhea, or abdominal pain); flu-like symptoms (severe tiredness, achiness, or generally ill feeling), or respiratory symptoms (sore throat, shortness of breath, cough). If you experience an allergic (hypersensitivity) reaction to Epzicom® (or abacavir, Ziagen®, or Trizivir®), never take Epzicom®, abacavir, Ziagen®, or Trizivir® again.

HIV medications may cause changes in body fat, including an increase in fat in the upper back and neck, breasts, and trunk; a loss of fat from the face, arms, and legs may also occur. Some HIV medications (including abacavir and lamivudine) may cause a serious, but rare, condition called lactic acidosis with an increase in liver size (hepatome-galy). Before starting Epzicom®, inform your physician about your medical conditions, including any kidney, heart, or liver problems (including hepatitis B infection), if you smoke, or have diabetes, high cholesterol, or high blood pressure. Do not take Epzicom® with Combivir®, Emtriva®, Epivir®, Epivir-HBV®, Trizivir®, Truvada®, or Ziagen®.

Nursing Implications Inform patients of the possibility of a fatal abacavir hypersensitivity reaction and the signs and symptoms (see Warnings and Patient Information)

Additional Information The Patient Medication Guide, which includes written manufacturer information, should be dispensed to the patient with each new prescription and refill; a Warning Card describing the hypersensitivity reaction should be given to the patient to carry with them.

The development of the abacavir hypersensitivity reaction has been associated with certain HLA genotypes (eg, *HLA-B*5701, HLA-DR7, HLA-DQ3*) which may help predict which patients are at risk for developing the abacavir hypersensitivity reaction (see Hetherington, 2002; Lucas, 2007; Mallal, 2002). Patients who test positive for the *HLA-B*5701* allele should have an abacavir allergy recorded in their medical record and should **not** receive abacavir. All patients who receive abacavir (and their caregivers) should be educated about the risk of abacavir hypersensitivity reactions (including patients who test negative for the *HLA-B*5701* allele, as the risk for the reaction is not completely eliminated). Approximately 4% of patients who test negative for the *HLA-B*5701* allele will experience a clinically suspected abacavir hypersensitivity reaction compared to 61% of those who test positive for the *HLA-B*5701* allele.

The prevalence of *HLA-B*5701* in the United States has been estimated to be 8% in Caucasians, 2.5% in African-Americans, 2% in Hispanics, <1% in Asians; in the sub-Saharan Africa it is 1%. Pretherapy identification of *HLA-B*5701*-positive patients and subsequent avoidance of abacavir therapy in these patients has been shown to significantly reduce the occurrence of abacavir-associated hypersensitivity reactions. A skin patch test is in development for clinical screening purposes; however, only PCR-mediated genotyping methods are currently in clinical practice use for documentation of this susceptibility marker. A familial predisposition to the abacavir hypersensitivity reaction has been reported; use abacavir with great caution in children of parents who experience a hypersensitivity reaction to abacavir (see Peyriére, 2001).

A high rate of early virologic failure in therapy-naive adult HIV patients has been observed with the once-daily three-drug combination therapy of abacavir, lamivudine, and tenofovir; this antiretroviral regimen is currently **not** recommended; any patient currently receiving this regimen should be closely monitored for virologic failure and considered for treatment modification.

Dosage Forms Excipient information presented when available (limited, particularly for generics); consult specific product labeling.

Tablet:

Epzicom®: Abacavir 600 mg and lamivudine 300 mg

References

Hetherington S, Hughes AR, Mosteller M, et al, "Genetic Variations in HLA-B Region and Hypersensitivity Reactions to Abacavir," *Lancet*, 2002, 359(9312):1121-2.

Lucas A, Nolan D, and Mallal S, "HLA-B*5701 Screening for Susceptibility to Abacavir Hypersensitivity," *J Antimicrob Chemother*, 2007, 59(4):591-3.

Mallal S, Nolan D, Witt C, et al, "Association Between Presence of HLA-B*5701, HLA-DR7, and HLA-DQ3 and Hypersensitivity to HIV-1 Reverse-Transcriptase Inhibitor Abacavir," *Lancet*, 2002, 359 (9308):727-32.

Panel on Antiretroviral Guidelines for Adults and Adolescents, "Guidelines for the Use of Antiretroviral Agents in HIV-Infected Adults and Adolescents," December 1, 2009, http://www.aidsinfo.nih.gov.

Peyriére H, Nicolas J, Siffert M, et al, "Hypersensitivity Related to Abacavir in Two Members of a Family," *Ann Pharmacother*, 2001, 35 (10):1291-2.

Working Group on Antiretroviral Therapy and Medical Management of HIV-Infected Children, "Guidelines for the Use of Antiretroviral Agents in Pediatric HIV Infection," February 23, 2009. Available at http://www.aidsinfo.nih.gov.

Abacavir, Lamivudine, and Zidovudine

(uh BACK ah veer, la MI vyoo deen, & zye DOE vyoo deen)

U.S. Brand Names Trizivir®

Canadian Brand Names Trizivir®

Therapeutic Category Antiretroviral Agent; HIV Agents (Anti-HIV Agents); Nucleoside Analog Reverse Transcriptase Inhibitor (NRTI)

Generic Available No

Use Treatment of HIV-1 infection (either alone or in combination with other antiretroviral agents) (**Note:** HIV regimens consisting of **three** antiretroviral agents are strongly recommended; data on the use of this triple NRTI combination regimen in patients with baseline viral loads >100,000 copies/mL is limited)

Medication Guide An FDA-approved patient medication guide, which is available with the product information and at http://www.fda.gov/downloads/Drugs/DrugSafety/ucm089807.pdf, must be dispensed with this medication for each new outpatient prescription and refill. A Warning Card (summarizing symptoms of hypersensitivity), which is available with the product information, must also be dispensed with this medication for each new outpatient prescription and refill.

Pregnancy Risk Factor C

Pregnancy Considerations See individual agents.

Lactation See individual agents.

Breast-Feeding Considerations See individual agents.

Contraindications Hypersensitivity to abacavir, lamivudine, zidovudine, or any component; hepatic impairment. **Do not rechallenge** patients who have experienced hypersensitivity reactions to abacavir (regardless of *HLA-B*5701* status), potentially fatal hypersensitivity reactions may occur (see Warnings)

Warnings Serious and sometimes fatal hypersensitivity reactions to abacavir may occur **[U.S. Boxed Warning]**. Patients testing positive for the presence of the *HLA-B*5701* allele are at a significantly increased risk for hypersensitivity reactions **[U.S. Boxed Warning]**. Screening for *HLA-B*5701* allele status is recommended prior to initiating therapy or reinitiating therapy in patients of unknown genotype status, including patients who previously tolerated therapy. Abacavir therapy is **not** recommended in patients testing positive for the *HLA-B*5701* allele. If a suspected abacavir hypersensitivity reaction occurs during therapy, regardless of *HLA-B*5701* status, abacavir should be discontinued immediately and permanently. **Note:** Hypersensitivity reactions may also occur in patients who test negative for the *HLA-B*5701* allele, but at a significantly lower rate (see Additional Information).

Abacavir hypersensitivity is a multiorgan clinical syndrome **[U.S. Boxed Warning]**. Discontinue therapy immediately in patients who show signs or symptoms of 2 or more of the following: Fever, skin rash, respiratory symptoms (including cough, dyspnea, or pharyngitis) and GI symptoms (including nausea, vomiting, diarrhea, or abdominal pain), and constitutional symptoms (including fatigue, malaise, or achiness). Carefully consider the diagnosis of hypersensitivity reaction in patients who present with acute onset respiratory symptoms, even if other diagnoses, such as bronchitis, flu-like illness, pharyngitis, or pneumonia, are possible. Permanently discontinue abacavir-containing medications if hypersensitivity reaction cannot be ruled out, even when other diagnoses are possible (regardless of *HLA-B*5701* status) **[U.S. Boxed Warning]**. Skin rash may be maculopapular or urticarial, but can be variable in appearance; erythema multiforme has been reported; hypersensitivity reaction may occur without a rash. Other symptoms may include edema, lethargy, myolysis, paresthesia, shortness of breath, mouth ulcerations, conjunctivitis, lymphadenopathy, and abnormal findings on chest x-ray (ie, infiltrates that can be localized). Anaphylaxis, renal failure, hepatic failure, respiratory failure, ARDS, hypotension, and death may also occur in association with hypersensitivity reactions. Laboratory abnormalities include increases in liver function tests, elevated CPK or serum creatinine, and lymphopenia.

Do not restart abacavir, Trizivir®, or any other abacavir-containing product after a hypersensitivity reaction occurs **[U.S. Boxed Warning]**; more severe symptoms can recur within hours and may include life-threatening hypotension and death. Fatal hypersensitivity reactions have occurred following the reintroduction of abacavir in patients whose therapy was interrupted for other reasons **[U.S. Boxed Warning]**. These patients had no identified history or had unrecognized symptoms of abacavir hypersensitivity. Reactions occurred within hours. In some cases, signs of a hypersensitivity reaction may have been previously present, but attributed to other medical conditions (acute onset respiratory diseases, gastroenteritis, reactions to other medications). If abacavir, Trizivir®, or any other abacavir-containing product is to be restarted following an interruption in therapy, the patient must first be evaluated for previously unsuspected symptoms of hypersensitivity. **Do not restart** abacavir, Trizivir®, or any other abacavir-containing product if hypersensitivity is suspected or cannot be ruled out (regardless of *HLA-B*51701* status). Hypersensitivity reactions occur in 5% to 8% of adult and pediatric patients (actual incidence varies by race/ethnicity); most hypersensitivity reactions occur within the first 6 weeks of therapy, but can occur at any time; call the Abacavir Hypersensitivity Reaction Registry at 1-800-270-0425 to facilitate reporting and collection of information on patients experiencing abacavir hypersensitivity reactions.

Cases of lactic acidosis, severe hepatomegaly with steatosis, and death have been reported in patients receiving nucleoside analogues **[U.S. Boxed Warning]**; most of these cases have been in women; prolonged nucleoside use, obesity, and prior liver disease may be risk factors; use with extreme caution in patients with other risk factors for liver disease; discontinue Trizivir® in patients who develop laboratory or clinical evidence of lactic acidosis or pronounced hepatotoxicity.

The major clinical toxicity of lamivudine in pediatric patients is pancreatitis; discontinue therapy if clinical signs, symptoms, or laboratory abnormalities suggestive of pancreatitis occur. HIV-infected patients who are coinfected with hepatitis B may experience severe acute exacerbations and clinical symptoms or laboratory evidence of hepatitis when a lamivudine-containing medication is discontinued **[U.S. Boxed Warning]**; most cases are self-limited, but fatalities have been reported; monitor patients closely for at least several months after discontinuation of abacavir, lamivudine, and zidovudine; initiation of antihepatitis B therapy may be required. **Note:** HIV-infected patients should be screened for hepatitis B infection prior to starting lamivudine therapy. Concomitant use of combination antiretroviral therapy with interferon alfa (with or without ribavirin) has resulted in hepatic decompensation (with some fatalities) in patients coinfected with HIV and HCV; monitor patients closely, especially for hepatic decompensation, neutropenia, and anemia; consider discontinuation of abacavir, lamivudine, and zidovudine if needed; consider dose reduction or discontinuation of interferon alfa, ribavirin, or both if clinical toxicities, including hepatic decompensation, worsen.

Zidovudine is associated with hematologic toxicity including granulocytopenia and severe anemia requiring transfusions **[U.S. Boxed Warning]**; use with caution in patients with ANC <1000 cells/mm^3 or hemoglobin <9.5 g/dL; discontinue treatment in children with an ANC <500 cells/mm^3 until marrow recovery is observed; use of erythropoietin, or filgrastim may be necessary in some patients; prolonged use of zidovudine may cause myositis and myopathy **[U.S. Boxed Warning]**; zidovudine has been shown to be carcinogenic in rats and mice.

Trizivir® contains abacavir, lamivudine, and zidovudine as a fixed-dose combination; do not use in patients weighing <40 kg, in patients with renal dysfunction (Cl$_{cr}$ ≤50 mL/minute) who require lamivudine and zidovudine dosage adjustment, or in patients with hepatic dysfunction (**Note:** Patients with mild to moderate hepatic dysfunction or liver cirrhosis require zidovudine dosage adjustment; abacavir is contraindicated in patients with moderate to severe hepatic dysfunction; patients with mild hepatic impairment require abacavir dosage reduction). Do not administer Trizivir® with abacavir, lamivudine, emtricitabine, or zidovudine-containing products.

Precautions Fat redistribution and accumulation [ie, central obesity, peripheral wasting, facial wasting, breast enlargement, dorsocervical fat enlargement (buffalo hump), and cushingoid appearance] have been observed in patients receiving antiretroviral agents (causal relationship not established). Resistance to abacavir develops relatively slowly, but cross resistance between abacavir and other nucleoside reverse transcriptase inhibitors (NRTIs) may occur; limited response may be seen in patients with HIV isolates containing multiple mutations conferring resistance to NRTIs or in patients with a prolonged prior NRTI exposure.

Immune reconstitution syndrome (an acute inflammatory response to residual or indolent opportunistic infections) may occur in HIV patients during initial treatment with combination antiretroviral agents, including abacavir, lamivudine, and zidovudine; this syndrome may require further patient assessment and therapy. Use with caution in patients with risks for coronary heart disease; modifiable risk factors (eg, hypertension, hyperlipidemia, diabetes mellitus, smoking) should be minimized prior to use. **Note:** Two studies found an increased risk of MI in patients receiving abacavir; however, a subsequent study did not find an increased risk (see Working Group, 2009).

Systemic exposure of abacavir at 6-32 times the normal human exposure, increased the incidence of tumors (malignant and nonmalignant) in mice and rats; myocardial degeneration was seen in mice and rats receiving abacavir for 2 years at 7-24 times the expected human exposure; the clinical relevance of these findings is currently unknown

Adverse Reactions See individual agents.

Drug Interactions

Avoid Concomitant Use

Avoid concomitant use of Abacavir, Lamivudine, and Zidovudine with any of the following: Emtricitabine; Stavudine

Increased Effect/Toxicity

Abacavir, Lamivudine, and Zidovudine may increase the levels/effects of: Emtricitabine; Ribavirin

The levels/effects of Abacavir, Lamivudine, and Zidovudine may be increased by: Acyclovir-Valacyclovir; Clarithromycin; Divalproex; DOXOrubicin; DOXOrubicin (Liposomal); Fluconazole; Ganciclovir-Valganciclovir; Interferons; Methadone; Probenecid; Ribavirin; Trimethoprim; Valproic Acid

Decreased Effect
Abacavir, Lamivudine, and Zidovudine may decrease the levels/effects of: Stavudine

The levels/effects of Abacavir, Lamivudine, and Zidovudine may be decreased by: Clarithromycin; DOXOrubicin; DOXOrubicin (Liposomal); Protease Inhibitors; Rifamycin Derivatives

Food Interactions Food decreases the rate, but not the extent of absorption (see Yuen, 2001).

Stability Store at room temperature 25°C (77°F)

Mechanism of Action See individual agents.

Pharmacokinetics (Adult data unless noted) One Trizivir® tablet is bioequivalent, in the extent (AUC) and rate of absorption (peak concentration and time to peak concentration), to one abacavir 300 mg tablet, one lamivudine 150 mg tablet, plus one zidovudine 300 mg tablet; see individual agents

Usual Dosage Oral:
Children: Not intended for pediatric use; product is a fixed-dose combination
Adolescents <40 kg: Not recommended; product is a fixed-dose combination
Adolescents ≥40 kg and Adults: 1 tablet twice daily

Dosage adjustment in hepatic impairment: Use is contraindicated (use individual antiretroviral agents to reduce dosage)

Dosage adjustment in renal impairment: Cl_{cr} ≤50 mL/minute: Not recommended (use individual antiretroviral agents to reduce dosage)

Administration May be administered without regard to meals

Monitoring Parameters *HLA-B*5701* genotype status prior to initiating therapy or resuming therapy in patients of unknown *HLA-B*5701* status (including patients previously tolerating therapy); signs and symptoms of abacavir hypersensitivity reaction (in all patients, but especially in those untested for the *HLA-B*5701* allele), lactic acidosis, pronounced hepatotoxicity, anemia, bone marrow suppression, and pancreatitis; serum glucose, triglycerides, creatine kinase; HIV RNA plasma levels, CD4 counts, CBC with differential, platelets, hemoglobin, MCV, reticulocyte count, liver enzymes, serum amylase, bilirubin, renal and hepatic function tests. HIV patients should be screened for hepatitis B infection before starting lamivudine (see Warnings).

Patient Information Trizivir® is not a cure for HIV. Take Trizivir® every day as prescribed; do not change dose or discontinue without physician's advice. If Trizivir® is stopped for any reason, notify physician before restarting therapy. If a dose is missed, take it as soon as possible, then return to normal dosing schedule; if a dose is skipped, do **not** double the next dose. Avoid alcohol. Notify physician if persistent severe abdominal pain, nausea, or vomiting occurs.

Trizivir® contains abacavir (also called Ziagen®). Abacavir may cause serious and sometimes fatal allergic (hypersensitivity) reaction. Read the Patient Medication Guide that you receive with each prescription and refill of abacavir, lamivudine, and zidovudine. Stop taking Trizivir® and notify physician immediately if 2 or more of the following sets of symptoms occur: Fever, rash, GI symptoms (nausea, vomiting, diarrhea, or abdominal pain), flu-like symptoms (severe tiredness, achiness, or generally ill feeling), or respiratory symptoms (sore throat, shortness of breath, cough). If you experience an allergic (hypersensitivity) reaction to Trizivir® (or abacavir, Ziagen®, or Epzicom®), **never** take Trizivir®, abacavir, Ziagen®, or Epzicom® again.

Trizivir® contains zidovudine which may cause a decrease in white blood cells or red blood cells (anemia); routine blood tests can help detect these blood problems.

Zidovudine may also cause muscle weakness with prolonged use, which may be a serious problem; notify physician if muscle weakness occurs.

HIV medications may cause changes in body fat, including an increase in fat in the upper back and neck, breasts, and trunk; a loss of fat from the face, arms, and legs may also occur. Some HIV medications (including abacavir, lamivudine, and zidovudine) may cause a serious, but rare, condition called lactic acidosis with an increase in liver size (hepatomegaly). Before starting Trizivir®, inform your physician about your medical conditions, including any blood, kidney, heart, or liver problems (including hepatitis B infection), if you smoke, or have diabetes, high cholesterol, or high blood pressure. Do not take Trizivir® with Combivir®, Emtriva®, Epivir®, Epivir-HBV®, Epzicom®, Retrovir®, Truvada®, or Ziagen®.

Nursing Implications Inform patients of the possibility of a fatal abacavir hypersensitivity reaction and the signs and symptoms (see Warnings and Patient Information)

Additional Information The Patient Medication Guide, which includes written manufacturer information, should be dispensed to the patient with each new prescription and refill; a Warning Card describing the hypersensitivity reaction should be given to the patient to carry with them.

The development of the abacavir hypersensitivity reaction has been associated with certain HLA genotypes (eg, *HLA-B*5701, HLA-DR7, HLA-DQ3*) which may help predict which patients are at risk for developing the abacavir hypersensitivity reaction (see Hetherington, 2002; Lucas, 2007; Mallal, 2002). Patients who test positive for the *HLA-B*5701* allele should have an abacavir allergy recorded in their medical record and should **not** receive abacavir. All patients who receive abacavir (and their caregivers) should be educated about the risk of abacavir hypersensitivity reactions (including patients who test negative for the *HLA-B*5701* allele, as the risk for the reaction is not completely eliminated). Approximately 4% of patients who test negative for the *HLA-B*5701* allele will experience a clinically suspected abacavir hypersensitivity reaction compared to 61% of those who test positive for the *HLA-B*5701* allele.

The prevalence of *HLA-B*5701* in the United States has been estimated to be 8% in Caucasians, 2.5% in African-Americans, 2% in Hispanics, 1% in Asians; in the sub-Saharan Africa it is <1%. Pretherapy identification of *HLA-B*5701*-positive patients and subsequent avoidance of abacavir therapy in these patients has been shown to significantly reduce the occurrence of abacavir-associated hypersensitivity reactions. A skin patch test is in development for clinical screening purposes; however, only PCR-mediated genotyping methods are currently in clinical practice use for documentation of this susceptibility marker. A familial predisposition to the abacavir hypersensitivity reaction has been reported; use abacavir with great caution in children of parents who experience a hypersensitivity reaction to abacavir (see Peyriére, 2001).

Dosage Forms Excipient information presented when available (limited, particularly for generics); consult specific product labeling.
Tablet:
Trizivir®: Abacavir 300 mg, lamivudine 150 mg, and zidovudine 300 mg

References
Briars LA, Hilao JJ, and Kraus DM, "A Review of Pediatric Human Immunodeficiency Virus Infection," *Journal of Pharmacy Practice*, 2004, 17(6):407-31.
Center for Disease Control and Prevention, "Guidelines for Using Antiretroviral Agents Among HIV-Infected Adults and Adolescents. Recommendations of the Panel on Clinical Practices for Treatment of HIV," *MMWR*, 2002, 51(RR-7):1-55.
Hetherington S, Hughes AR, Mosteller M, et al, "Genetic Variations in HLA-B Region and Hypersensitivity Reactions to Abacavir," *Lancet*, 2002, 359(9312):1121-2.

Lucas A, Nolan D, and Mallal S, "HLA-B*5701 Screening for Susceptibility to Abacavir Hypersensitivity," *J Antimicrob Chemother*, 2007, 59(4):591-3.

Mallal S, Nolan D, Witt C, et al, "Association Between Presence of HLA-B*5701, HLA-DR7, and HLA-DQ3 and Hypersensitivity to HIV-1 Reverse-Transcriptase Inhibitor Abacavir," *Lancet*, 2002, 359 (9308):727-32.

Panel on Antiretroviral Guidelines for Adults and Adolescents, "Guidelines for the Use of Antiretroviral Agents in HIV-Infected Adults and Adolescents," December 1, 2009, http://www.aidsinfo.nih.gov.

Peyriére H, Nicolas J, Siffert M, et al, "Hypersensitivity Related to Abacavir in Two Members of a Family," *Ann Pharmacother*, 2001, 35 (10):1291-2.

Saez-Llorens X, Nelson RP, Emmanuel P, et al, "A Randomized, Double-Blind Study of Triple Nucleoside Therapy of Abacavir, Lamivudine, and Zidovudine Versus Lamivudine and Zidovudine in Previously Treated Human Immunodeficiency Virus Type 1-Infected Children," *Pediatrics*, 2001, 107(1), URL: http://www.pediatrics.org/cgi/content/full/107/1/e4.

Working Group on Antiretroviral Therapy and Medical Management of HIV-Infected Children, "Guidelines for the Use of Antiretroviral Agents in Pediatric HIV Infection," February 23, 2009. Available at http://www.aidsinfo.nih.gov.

Yuen GJ, Lou Y, Thompson NF, et al, "Abacavir/Lamivudine/Zidovudine as a Combined Formulation Tablet: Bioequivalence Compared With Each Component Administered Concurrently and the Effect of Food on Absorption," *J Clin Pharmacol*, 2001, 41(3):277-88.

◆ **Abacavir Sulfate** see Abacavir on page 26

◆ **Abacavir Sulfate and Lamivudine** see Abacavir and Lamivudine on page 29

Abatacept (ab a TA sept)

Medication Safety Issues
Sound-alike/look-alike issues:
Orencia® may be confused with Oracea™

U.S. Brand Names Orencia®

Canadian Brand Names Orencia®

Therapeutic Category Antirheumatic, Disease Modifying

Generic Available No

Use Treatment of moderately- to severely-active rheumatoid arthritis; used as monotherapy or in combination with other DMARDs (FDA approved in adults). Treatment of moderately- to severely-active polyarticular juvenile idiopathic arthritis (used as monotherapy or concomitantly with methotrexate) (FDA approved in ages ≥6-17 years). **Note:** Abatacept should not be used in combination with TNF antagonists or with other biologic rheumatoid arthritis drugs, such as anakinra.

Pregnancy Risk Factor C

Pregnancy Considerations Teratogenic effects were not observed in animal studies. There are no adequate and well-controlled studies in pregnant women. Due to the potential risk for development of autoimmune disease in the fetus, use during pregnancy only if clearly needed. A pregnancy registry has been established to monitor outcomes of women exposed to abatacept during pregnancy (1-877-311-8972).

Lactation Excretion in breast milk unknown/not recommended

Breast-Feeding Considerations Due to the potential for adverse reactions and possible effects on the developing immune system, breast-feeding is not recommended.

Contraindications Hypersensitivity to abatacept or any component

Warnings Use caution when considering the use of abatacept in patients with a history of recurrent infections; with conditions that predispose them to infections; or with chronic, latent, or localized infections. Closely monitor patients who develop a new infection while undergoing treatment. If a patient develops a serious infection, discontinue abatacept. Patients should be evaluated for latent tuberculosis with a tuberculin skin test prior to starting abatacept. Treatment of latent tuberculosis should be initiated before abatacept is used; safety in

tuberculosis-positive patients has not been established. Reactivation of hepatitis B may occur in chronic carriers of the virus; evaluate prior to etanercept initiation and during treatment in patients at risk for hepatitis B infection. Patients receiving abatacept in combination with TNF antagonists had higher rates of infections than patients on TNF antagonists alone (concurrent use with TNF antagonists is not recommended). Due to the effect of T-cell inhibition on host defenses, abatacept may affect immune responses against infections and malignancies.

Precautions Use with caution in patients with chronic obstructive pulmonary disease. May cause hypersensitivity, anaphylaxis, or anaphylactoid reactions; medications for the treatment of hypersensitivity reactions should be readily available for immediate use. Patients should be brought up-to-date with all immunizations before initiating therapy. Live vaccines should not be given concurrently or within 3 months of discontinuation of therapy. Injection formulation contains maltose which may result in falsely-elevated serum glucose readings on the day of infusion.

Adverse Reactions Note: COPD patients experienced a higher frequency of COPD-related adverse reactions (COPD exacerbation, cough, dyspnea, pneumonia, rhonchi)

Cardiovascular: Flushing, hypertension, hypotension

Central nervous system: Dizziness, fever, headache

Dermatologic: Pruritus, rash, urticaria

Gastrointestinal: Abdominal pain, diarrhea, dyspepsia, nausea, ulcerative colitis

Genitourinary: Urinary tract infection

Hematologic: Lymphoma

Neuromuscular & skeletal: Back pain, limb pain

Respiratory: Bronchitis, cough, dyspnea, nasopharyngitis, pneumonia, rhinitis, sinusitis, sore throat, upper respiratory tract infection, wheezing

Miscellaneous: Anaphylactoid reactions, anaphylaxis, infection, influenza, infusion-related reactions (hypertension, hypotension, dizziness, headache), lung cancer, neutralizing antibodies

Drug Interactions

Avoid Concomitant Use
Avoid concomitant use of Abatacept with any of the following: Anti-TNF Agents; BCG; Natalizumab; Pimecrolimus; Tacrolimus (Topical); Vaccines (Live)

Increased Effect/Toxicity
Abatacept may increase the levels/effects of: Leflunomide; Natalizumab; Vaccines (Live)

The levels/effects of Abatacept may be increased by: Anti-TNF Agents; Denosumab; Pimecrolimus; Tacrolimus (Topical); Trastuzumab

Decreased Effect
Abatacept may decrease the levels/effects of: BCG; Sipuleucel-T; Vaccines (Inactivated); Vaccines (Live)

The levels/effects of Abatacept may be decreased by: Echinacea

Food Interactions Avoid echinacea (has immunostimulant properties)

Stability Store intact vial at 2°C to 8°C (36°F to 46°F); protect from light. Reconstitute vial with 10 mL SWI using a silicone-free disposable syringe (translucent particles may develop in solutions prepared with a siliconized syringe). After further dilution in NS, store for up to 24 hours at room temperature or refrigerate. Use within 24 hours of reconstitution.

Mechanism of Action Inhibits T-cell (T-lymphocyte) activation by binding to CD80 and CD86 on antigen presenting cells (APC), thus blocking the required CD28 interaction between APCs and T-cells. Abatacept also blocks the production of inflammatory mediators such as TNF-α, IL-2, and interferon-γ.

Pharmacokinetics (Adult data unless noted)
Distribution: V_{dss}: 0.07 L/kg (range: 0.02-0.13 L/kg)
Half-life elimination: RA: 13.1 days (range: 8-25 days)
Clearance: 0.22-0.23 mL/hour/kg
    Children 6-17 years: 0.4 mL/hour/kg (increases with baseline body weight)

Usual Dosage I.V.:
Children ≥6 years and <75 kg: 10 mg/kg; dose is repeated at 2 weeks and 4 weeks after initial dose and every 4 weeks thereafter
Children >6 years and >75 kg: Use adult dosing (maximum dose: 1000 mg); dose is repeated at 2 weeks and 4 weeks after initial dose and every 4 weeks thereafter
Adults: Dose is based on body weight range; repeat dose at 2 weeks and 4 weeks after initial dose, and every 4 weeks thereafter:
<60 kg: 500 mg
60-100 kg: 750 mg
>100 kg: 1000 mg

Administration I.V.: Prepare abatacept using only the silicone-free disposable syringe provided with each vial [for information on obtaining additional silicone-free disposable syringes contact Bristol-Myers Squibb at (800) 673-6242]. Following reconstitution, remove an equal volume of solution from a 100 mL NS infusion bag before adding the abatacept dose to the bag with the silicone-free syringe. Mix gently; do not shake. Administer through a 0.2-1.2 micron low protein-binding filter. Infuse over 30 minutes at a final concentration not to exceed 10 mg/mL.

Monitoring Parameters Signs and symptoms of infection; signs and symptoms of infusion reaction; hepatitis and TB screening prior to therapy initiation

Test Interactions Contains maltose; may result in falsely-elevated blood glucose levels with glucose dehydrogenase pyrroloquinolinequinone or glucose-dye-oxidoreductase testing methods on the day of infusion.

Patient Information Notify physician if you have symptoms of infection (cough, feeling tired, fever, flu-like symptoms, night sweats, weight loss), hypersensitivity reaction (chest tightness, difficulty breathing, hives, or swollen eyelids, face, lips, throat, tongue), or infusion-related reaction (headache, hypertension or hypotension, lightheadedness). Patient should be informed to discontinue previous anti-TNF-α therapy prior to starting abatacept due to increased risk of serious infection.

Nursing Implications Infusion-related reactions may be alleviated by slowing the infusion rate or temporarily discontinuing the infusion. Administer antihistamines and/or corticosteroids for hypersensitivity reactions.

Dosage Forms Excipient information presented when available (limited, particularly for generics); consult specific product labeling.
Injection, powder for reconstitution [preservative free]:
Orencia®: 250 mg [contains maltose]

References
Bruce SP and Boyce EG, "Update on Abatacept: A Selective Costimulation Modulator for Rheumatoid Arthritis," *Ann Pharmacother,* 2007, 41(7):1153-62.
Ruperto N, Lovell DJ, Quartier P, et al, "Abatacept in Children With Juvenile Idiopathic Arthritis: A Randomised, Double-Blind, Placebo-Controlled Withdrawal Trial," *Lancet,* 2008, 372(9636):383-91.

◆ **Abbott-43818** *see* Leuprolide *on page 805*

◆ **ABC** *see* Abacavir *on page 26*

◆ **ABC and 3TC** *see* Abacavir and Lamivudine *on page 29*

◆ **Abelcet®** *see* Amphotericin B Lipid Complex *on page 102*

◆ **Abenol® (Can)** *see* Acetaminophen *on page 36*

◆ **Abilify®** *see* Aripiprazole *on page 132*

◆ **Abilify Discmelt®** *see* Aripiprazole *on page 132*

◆ **ABLC** *see* Amphotericin B Lipid Complex *on page 102*

◆ **A/B Otic** *see* Antipyrine and Benzocaine *on page 118*

◆ **Abraxane® For Injectable Suspension (Can)** *see* Paclitaxel *on page 1044*

◆ **ABT-378/Ritonavir** *see* Lopinavir and Ritonavir *on page 839*

◆ **Acanya™** *see* Clindamycin and Benzoyl Peroxide *on page 329*

Acarbose (AY car bose)

Medication Safety Issues
Sound-alike/look-alike issues:
Precose® may be confused with PreCare®

International issues:
Precose® may be confused with Precosa® which is a brand name for *Saccharomyces boulardii* in Denmark, Finland, Norway, and Sweden

U.S. Brand Names Precose®
Canadian Brand Names Glucobay™
Therapeutic Category Antidiabetic Agent, Alpha-glucosidase Inhibitor; Antidiabetic Agent, Oral
Generic Available Yes
Use Management of type II diabetes mellitus (noninsulin-dependent, NIDDM) when hyperglycemia cannot be managed by diet alone; may be used concomitantly with metformin, a sulfonylurea, or insulin to improve glycemic control
Pregnancy Risk Factor B
Pregnancy Considerations Adverse events have not been reported in animal reproduction studies; therefore, acarbose is classified as pregnancy category B. Low amounts of acarbose are absorbed systemically which should limit fetal exposure. Maternal hyperglycemia can be associated with adverse effects in the fetus, including macrosomia, neonatal hyperglycemia, and hyperbilirubinemia; the risk of congenital malformations is increased when the Hb A_{1c} is above the normal range. Diabetes can also be associated with adverse effects in the mother. Poorly-treated diabetes may cause end-organ damage that may in turn negatively affect obstetric outcomes. Physiologic glucose levels should be maintained prior to and during pregnancy to decrease the risk of adverse events in the mother and the fetus. Acarbose has been studied for its potential role in treating GDM; however, only limited information is available describing pregnancy outcomes. Until additional safety and efficacy data are obtained, the use of oral agents is generally not recommended as routine management of GDM or type 2 diabetes mellitus during pregnancy. Insulin is the drug of choice for the control of diabetes mellitus during pregnancy.
Lactation Excretion in breast milk unknown/not recommended
Breast-Feeding Considerations It is not known if acarbose is found in breast milk; however, low amounts of acarbose are absorbed systemically in adults, which may limit the amount that could distribute into breast milk. Breast-feeding is not recommended by the manufacturer.
Contraindications Hypersensitivity to acarbose or any component; diabetic ketoacidosis; cirrhosis; patients with inflammatory bowel disease, colonic ulceration, partial intestinal obstruction, or patients predisposed to intestinal obstruction; patients who have chronic intestinal diseases associated with marked disorders of digestion or absorption; patients who have conditions that may deteriorate as a result of increased gas formation in the intestine
Warnings Dose-related elevations in serum transaminases occurred in 15% of acarbose-treated patients in long-term studies; these elevations were asymptomatic, reversible, more common in females, and not associated with other evidence of liver dysfunction; acarbose serum levels are proportionately higher in patients with renal dysfunction ▶

(S$_{cr}$ >2 mg/dL); until long term clinical studies are completed, use in renally-compromised patients is not recommended

Precautions Hypoglycemia may occur when used in combination with sulfonylureas or insulin; oral glucose (absorption is not affected by acarbose) should be used instead of sucrose (table sugar) for the treatment of mild to moderate hypoglycemia

Adverse Reactions
Central nervous system: Headache, vertigo, drowsiness
Dermatologic: Urticaria, erythema
Endocrine & metabolic: Hypoglycemia
Gastrointestinal: Abdominal pain, diarrhea, flatulence
Hepatic: Liver enzymes elevated
Neuromuscular & skeletal: Weakness

Drug Interactions
Avoid Concomitant Use There are no known interactions where it is recommended to avoid concomitant use.
Increased Effect/Toxicity
Acarbose may increase the levels/effects of: Hypoglycemic Agents

The levels/effects of Acarbose may be increased by: Herbs (Hypoglycemic Properties); Pegvisomant
Decreased Effect
Acarbose may decrease the levels/effects of: Digoxin

The levels/effects of Acarbose may be decreased by: Corticosteroids (Orally Inhaled); Corticosteroids (Systemic); Luteinizing Hormone-Releasing Hormone Analogs; Somatropin; Thiazide Diuretics
Mechanism of Action Competitive inhibitor of pancreatic α-glucosidases, resulting in delayed hydrolysis of ingested complex carbohydrates and disaccharides and absorption of glucose; dose-dependent reduction in postprandial serum insulin and glucose peaks; inhibits the metabolism of sucrose to glucose and fructose
Pharmacodynamics Average decrease in fasting blood sugar: 20-30 mg/dL
Pharmacokinetics (Adult data unless noted)
Absorption: <2% absorbed as active drug
Metabolism: Metabolized exclusively within the GI tract, principally by intestinal bacteria and by digestive enzymes; 13 metabolites have been identified
Bioavailability: Low systemic bioavailability of parent compound
Elimination: Fraction absorbed as intact drug is almost completely excreted in urine
Usual Dosage Oral:
Adolescents and Adults: Dosage must be individualized on the basis of effectiveness and tolerance; do not exceed the maximum recommended dose (use slow titration to prevent or minimize GI effects):
Initial: 25 mg 3 times/day; increase in 25 mg/day increments in 2-4 week intervals to maximum dose
Maximum dose:
Patients ≤60 kg: 50 mg 3 times/day
Patients >60 kg: 100 mg 3 times/day
Dosing adjustment in renal impairment: See Warnings
Administration Oral: Administer with first bite of each main meal
Monitoring Parameters Fasting blood glucose; hemoglobin A$_{1c}$; liver enzymes every 3 months for the first year of therapy and periodically thereafter
Reference Range Target range:
Blood glucose: Fasting and preprandial: 80-120 mg/dL; bedtime: 100-140 mg/dL
Glycosylated hemoglobin (hemoglobin A$_{1c}$): <7%
Additional Information Acarbose has been used successfully to treat postprandial hypoglycemia in children with Nissen fundoplications. Six children (4-25 months) initially received 12.5 mg before each bolus feeding of

formula containing complex carbohydrates. The dosage was increased in 12.5 mg increments (dosage range: 12.5-50 mg per dose) until postprandial serum glucose was stable ≥60 mg/dL. Most commonly reported side effects were flatulence, abdominal distension, and diarrhea (Ng, 2001).
Dosage Forms Excipient information presented when available (limited, particularly for generics); consult specific product labeling.
Tablet: 25 mg, 50 mg, 100 mg
Precose®: 25 mg, 50 mg, 100 mg
References
DeFronzo RA, "Pharmacologic Therapy for Type 2 Diabetes Mellitus," *Ann Intern Med*, 1999, 131(4):281-303.
Ng DD, Ferry RJ Jr, Kelly A, et al, "Acarbose Treatment of Postprandial Hypoglycemia in Children After Nissen Fundoplication," *J Pediatr*, 2001, 139(6):877-9.

♦ **Accel-Amlodipine (Can)** *see* AmLODIPine *on page 91*

♦ **Accolate®** *see* Zafirlukast *on page 1439*

♦ **AccuNeb®** *see* Albuterol *on page 57*

♦ **Accutane® [DSC]** *see* Isotretinoin *on page 769*

♦ **Accutane® (Can)** *see* Isotretinoin *on page 769*

♦ **ACE** *see* Captopril *on page 242*

♦ **Acephen™ [OTC]** *see* Acetaminophen *on page 36*

♦ **Acerola [OTC]** *see* Ascorbic Acid *on page 138*

♦ **Acetadote®** *see* Acetylcysteine *on page 43*

Acetaminophen (a seet a MIN oh fen)

Medication Safety Issues
Sound-alike/look-alike issues:
Acephen® may be confused with AcipHex®
FeverALL® may be confused with Fiberall®
Tylenol® may be confused with atenolol, timolol, Tuinal®, Tylenol® PM, Tylox®

International issues:
Paralen® [Czech Republic] may be confused with Aralen® which is a brand name for chloroquine in the U.S.
Duorol® may be confused with Diuril® which is a brand name for chlorothiazide in the U.S.

Duplicate therapy issues: This product contains acetaminophen, which may be a component of combination products. Do not exceed the maximum recommended daily dose of acetaminophen.
Related Information
Acetaminophen Serum Level Nomogram *on page 1708*
U.S. Brand Names Acephen™ [OTC]; APAP 500 [OTC]; Apra [OTC] [DSC]; Aspirin Free Anacin® Extra Strength [OTC]; Cetafen® Extra [OTC]; Cetafen® [OTC]; Excedrin® Tension Headache [OTC]; FeverALL® [OTC]; Genapap™ Extra Strength [OTC] [DSC]; Genapap™ Infant [OTC] [DSC]; Genapap™ [OTC] [DSC]; Genebs Extra Strength [OTC]; Genebs [OTC] [DSC]; Infantaire [OTC]; Little Fevers™ [OTC]; Mapap® Arthritis Pain [OTC]; Mapap® Children's Rapid Tabs [OTC]; Mapap® Children's [OTC]; Mapap® Extra Strength [OTC]; Mapap® Infants [OTC]; Mapap® Junior Rapid Tabs [OTC]; Mapap® [OTC] [DSC]; Nortemp Children's [OTC]; Pain Eze [OTC]; Silapap Children's [OTC]; Silapap Infant's [OTC]; Tycolene Maximum Strength [OTC]; Tycolene [OTC] [DSC]; Tylenol® 8 Hour [OTC]; Tylenol® Arthritis Pain Extended Relief [OTC]; Tylenol® Children's Meltaways [OTC]; Tylenol® Children's [OTC]; Tylenol® Extra Strength [OTC]; Tylenol® Infant's Concentrated [OTC]; Tylenol® Jr. Meltaways [OTC]; Tylenol® [OTC]; Valorin Extra [OTC]; Valorin [OTC]

Canadian Brand Names Abenol®; Apo-Acetaminophen®; Atasol®; Novo-Gesic; Pediatrix; Tempra®; Tylenol®

Therapeutic Category Analgesic, Non-narcotic; Antipyretic

Generic Available Yes: Excludes extended release products

Use Treatment of mild to moderate pain and fever (FDA approved in all ages); **Note:** Acetaminophen does not have antirheumatic or systemic anti-inflammatory effects.

Pregnancy Risk Factor B

Pregnancy Considerations Acetaminophen crosses the placenta. It is generally considered to be safe for use during pregnancy when used at therapeutic doses for short periods of time.

Lactation Enters breast milk/compatible

Breast-Feeding Considerations Acetaminophen is found in breast milk. The AAP considers acetaminophen to be "compatible" with breast-feeding.

Contraindications Hypersensitivity to acetaminophen or any component

Warnings May cause severe hepatic toxicity with overdose. Use with caution in patients with alcoholic liver disease. Chronic daily dosing in adults of 5-8 g of acetaminophen over several weeks or 3-4 g/day· for 1 year have resulted in liver damage. Do not exceed maximum daily doses; consider acetaminophen content of combination products when evaluating the dose of acetaminophen.

Elixir, suspension, and some oral drops and oral liquids contain propylene glycol. Gelcap and geltab contain benzyl alcohol; some elixir preparations contain benzoic acid; liquid preparations (ie, elixir, liquid, suspension, and drops) may contain sodium benzoate (see Dosage Forms); benzoic acid (benzoate) is a metabolite of benzyl alcohol; large amounts of benzyl alcohol (≥99 mg/kg/day) have been associated with a potentially fatal toxicity ("gasping syndrome") in neonates; the "gasping syndrome" consists of metabolic acidosis, respiratory distress, gasping respirations, CNS dysfunction (including convulsions, intracranial hemorrhage), hypotension and cardiovascular collapse; avoid use of acetaminophen products containing sodium benzoate in neonates; *in vitro* and animal studies have shown that benzoate displaces bilirubin from protein binding sites

Precautions Some products (eg, chewable tablets) contain aspartame which is metabolized to phenylalanine and must be avoided (or used with caution) in patients with phenylketonuria.

G-6-PD deficiency: Although several case reports of acetaminophen-associated hemolytic anemia have been reported in patients with G-6-PD deficiency, a direct cause and effect relationship has not been well established (concurrent illnesses such as fever or infection may precipitate hemolytic anemia in patients with G-6-PD deficiency); therefore, acetaminophen is generally thought to be safe when given in therapeutic doses to patients with G-6-PD deficiency.

Adverse Reactions

Dermatologic: Rash

Hematologic: Blood dyscrasias (leukopenia, neutropenia, pancytopenia)

Hepatic: Hepatic necrosis with overdose

Renal: Renal injury with chronic use

Miscellaneous: Hypersensitivity reactions (rare)

Drug Interactions

Metabolism/Transport Effects Substrate (minor) of CYP1A2, 2A6, 2C9, 2D6, 2E1, 3A4; **Inhibits** CYP3A4 (weak)

Avoid Concomitant Use There are no known interactions where it is recommended to avoid concomitant use.

Increased Effect/Toxicity

Acetaminophen may increase the levels/effects of: Vitamin K Antagonists

The levels/effects of Acetaminophen may be increased by: Imatinib; Isoniazid

Decreased Effect

The levels/effects of Acetaminophen may be decreased by: Anticonvulsants (Hydantoin); Barbiturates; CarBAMazepine; Cholestyramine Resin; Peginterferon Alfa-2b

Food Interactions Rate of absorption may be decreased when given with food high in carbohydrates

Mechanism of Action Inhibits the synthesis of prostaglandins in the CNS and peripherally blocks pain impulse generation; produces antipyresis from inhibition of hypothalamic heat-regulating center

Pharmacokinetics (Adult data unless noted)

Protein binding: 20% to 50%

Metabolism: At normal therapeutic dosages the parent compound is metabolized in the liver to sulfate and glucuronide metabolites, while a small amount is metabolized by microsomal mixed function oxidases to a highly reactive intermediate (N-acetyl-imidoquinone) which is conjugated with glutathione and inactivated; at toxic doses (as little as 4 g in a single day) glutathione can become depleted, and conjugation becomes insufficient to meet the metabolic demand causing an increase in N-acetyl-imidoquinone concentration, which is thought to cause hepatic cell necrosis.

Half-life:

Neonates: 2-5 hours

Adults: 1-3 hours

Time to peak serum concentration: 10-60 minutes after normal oral doses, but may be delayed in acute overdoses

Usual Dosage

Neonates: Oral, rectal: 10-15 mg/kg/dose every 6-8 hours as needed

International Evidence-Based Group for Neonatal Pain recommendations (Anand, 2001; Anand, 2002):

Preterm neonates 28-32 weeks:

Oral: 10-12 mg/kg/dose every 6-8 hours; maximum daily dose: 40 mg/kg/day

Rectal: 20 mg/kg/dose every 12 hours; maximum daily dose: 40 mg/kg/day

Preterm neonates 32-36 weeks and term neonates <10 days:

Oral: 10-15 mg/kg/dose every 6 hours; maximum daily dose: 60 mg/kg/day

Rectal: Loading dose: 30 mg/kg; then 15 mg/kg/dose every 8 hours; maximum daily dose: 60 mg/kg/day

Term neonates ≥10 days:

Oral: 10-15 mg/kg/dose every 4-6 hours; maximum daily dose: 90 mg/kg/day

Rectal: Loading dose: 30 mg/kg; then 20 mg/kg/dose every 6-8 hours; maximum daily dose: 90 mg/kg/day

Infants and Children:

Oral: 10-15 mg/kg/dose every 4-6 hours as needed; do **not** exceed 5 doses in 24 hours; alternatively, the following manufacturer recommended doses may be used. See table on next page.

Acetaminophen Dosing (Oral)[1]

Weight (kg)	Weight (lbs)	Age	Dosage (mg)
2.7-5.3	6-11	0-3 mo	40
5.4-8.1	12-17	4-11 mo	80
8.2-10.8	18-23	1-2 y	120
10.9-16.3	24-35	2-3 y	160
16.4-21.7	36-47	4-5 y	240
21.8-27.2	48-59	6-8 y	320
27.3-32.6	60-71	9-10 y	400
32.7-43.2	72-95	11 y	480

[1]Manufacturer's recommendations; use of weight to select dose is preferred; if weight is not available, then use age. Manufacturer's recommendations are based on weight in pounds (OTC labeling); weight in kg listed here is derived from pounds and rounded; kg weight listed also is adjusted to allow for continuous weight ranges in kg. OTC labeling instructs consumer to consult with physician for dosing instructions in children under 2 years of age.

Rectal: 10-20 mg/kg/dose every 4-6 hours as needed. **Note:** Although the perioperative use of high-dose rectal acetaminophen (eg, 25-45 mg/kg/dose) has been investigated in several studies, its routine use remains controversial; optimal doses and dosing frequency to ensure efficacy and safety have not yet been established; further studies are needed (see Buck, 2001).

Children ≥12 years and Adults: Oral, rectal: 325-650 mg every 4-6 hours or 1000 mg 3-4 times/day; do **not** exceed 4 g/day

Administration Oral: Administer with food to decrease GI upset; shake suspension well before use; do not crush or chew extended release products

Reference Range Acute ingestions: Toxic concentration with probable hepatotoxicity: >200 mcg/mL at 4 hours or 50 mcg/mL at 12 hours after ingestion of overdose

Patient Information Avoid alcohol; do not take longer than 10 days without physician's advice. Consult your doctor about dosing instructions in children under 2 years of age.

Additional Information Drops may contain saccharin. Acetaminophen (15 mg/kg/dose given orally every 6 hours for 24 hours) did **not** relieve the intraoperative or the immediate postoperative pain associated with neonatal circumcision; some benefit was seen 6 hours after circumcision (see Howard, 1994).

There is currently no scientific evidence to support alternating acetaminophen with ibuprofen in the treatment of fever (see Mayoral, 2000).

Dosage Forms Excipient information presented when available (limited, particularly for generics); consult specific product labeling. [DSC] = Discontinued product

Caplet, oral: 500 mg
  Cetafen® Extra: 500 mg
  Genapap™ Extra Strength: 500 mg [DSC]
  Genebs Extra Strength: 500 mg
  Mapap® Extra Strength: 500 mg
  Pain Eze: 650 mg
  Tycolene Maximum Strength: 500 mg [DSC]
  Tylenol®: 325 mg
  Tylenol® Extra Strength: 500 mg
Caplet, extended release, oral:
  Tylenol® 8 Hour: 650 mg
  Tylenol® Arthritis Pain Extended Relief: 650 mg
Capsule, oral:
  Mapap® Extra Strength: 500 mg
Captab, oral: 500 mg

Elixir, oral:
  Apra: 160 mg/5 mL (118 mL) [ethanol free; contains benzoic acid, propylene glycol, sodium benzoate, sucrose; grape flavor] [DSC]
  Apra: 160 mg/5 mL (118 mL, 473 mL, 3785 mL) [ethanol free; contains propylene glycol, sodium benzoate, sucrose; cherry flavor] [DSC]
  Mapap® Children's: 160 mg/5 mL (118 mL, 480 mL) [ethanol free; contains benzoic acid, propylene glycol, sodium benzoate; cherry flavor]
Gelcap, oral:
  Tylenol® Extra Strength: 500 mg [contains benzyl alcohol]
Geltab, oral:
  Excedrin® Tension Headache: 500 mg [contains caffeine 65 mg/geltab]
  Mapap® Extra Strength: 500 mg
  Tylenol® Extra Strength: 500 mg [contains benzyl alcohol]
Liquid, oral:
  APAP 500: 500 mg/5 mL (237 mL) [ethanol free, sugar free; cherry flavor]
  Mapap® Children's: 160 mg/5 mL (120 mL) [ethanol free; contains propylene glycol, sodium benzoate; cherry flavor]
  Silapap Children's: 160 mg/5 mL (118 mL, 237 mL, 473 mL) [ethanol free, sugar free; contains propylene glycol, sodium benzoate; cherry flavor]
  Tylenol® Extra Strength: 500 mg/15 mL (240 mL) [ethanol free; contains propylene glycol, sodium benzoate; cherry flavor]
Solution, oral: 160 mg/5 mL (5 mL, 10 mL, 20 mL, 118 mL, 473 mL)
Solution, oral [drops]: 80 mg/0.8 mL (15 mL)
  Genapap™ Infant: 80 mg/0.8 mL (15 mL) [ethanol free; contains propylene glycol; fruit flavor] [DSC]
  Infantaire: 80 mg/0.8mL (15 mL, 30 mL)
  Little Fevers™: 80 mg/1 mL (30 mL) [dye free, ethanol free, gluten free; contains propylene glycol, sodium benzoate; berry flavor]
  Silapap Infant's: 80 mg/0.8 mL (15 mL, 30 mL) [ethanol free; contains propylene glycol, sodium benzoate; cherry flavor]
Suppository, rectal: 120 mg (12s, 50s, 100s); 325 mg (12s); 650 mg (12s, 50s, 100s)
  Acephen™: 120 mg (6s [DSC], 12s, 50s, 100s); 325 mg (6s, 12s, 50s, 100s); 650 mg (12s, 50s, 100s, 500s)
  FeverALL®: 120 mg (6s, 12s, 50s); 325 mg (6s, 12s, 50s); 650 mg (12s, 50s, 500s); 80 mg (6s, 50s)
  Mapap®: 125 mg (12s) [DSC]
Suspension, oral: 160 mg/5 mL (5 mL, 10 mL, 20 mL)
  Mapap® Children's: 160 mg/5 mL (118 mL) [ethanol free; contains propylene glycol, sodium benzoate; cherry flavor]
  Nortemp Children's: 160 mg/5 mL (118 mL) [ethanol free; contains propylene glycol, sodium benzoate; cotton candy flavor]
  Tylenol® Children's Suspension: 160 mg/5 mL (120 mL) [ethanol free; contains propylene glycol, sodium benzoate; bubblegum, strawberry, grape flavors]
  Tylenol® Children's Suspension: 160 mg/5 mL (60 mL, 120 mL, 240 mL [DSC]) [ethanol free; contains propylene glycol, sodium benzoate; cherry flavor]
  Tylenol® Children's Suspension: 160 mg/5 mL (120 mL) [dye free; ethanol free; contains propylene glycol, sodium benzoate; cherry flavor]
Suspension, oral [drops]:
  Mapap® Infant's: 80 mg/0.8 mL (15 mL, 30 mL) [ethanol free; contains propylene glycol, sodium benzoate; cherry flavor]
  Tylenol® Infant's Concentrated: 80 mg/0.8 mL (15 mL, 30 mL) [ethanol free; contains sodium benzoate; cherry, grape flavors]

Tylenol® Infant's Concentrated: 80 mg/0.8 mL (30 mL) [dye free; ethanol free; contains propylene glycol; cherry flavor]
Tablet, oral: 325 mg, 500 mg
Aspirin Free Anacin® Extra Strength: 500 mg
Cetafen®: 325 mg
Genapap™: 325 mg [DSC]
Genapap™ Extra Strength: 500 mg [OTC]
Genebs: 325 mg [DSC]
Genebs Extra Strength: 500 mg
Mapap®: 325 mg, 500 mg
Tycolene: 325 mg [DSC]
Tylenol®: 325 mg
Valorin Extra®: 500 mg [sugar free]
Valorin®: 325 mg [sugar free]
Tablet, chewable, oral: 80 mg
Mapap® Children's: 80 mg [bubblegum flavor] [DSC]
Mapap® Children's: 80 mg [contains phenylalanine 3 mg/tablet; grape flavor] [DSC]
Tablet, extended release, oral:
Mapap® Arthritis Pain: 650 mg
Tablet, orally disintegrating, oral: 80 mg, 160 mg, 325 mg, 500 mg
Mapap® Children's: 80 mg [fruit flavor]
Mapap® Children's Rapid Tabs: 80 mg [grape flavor]
Mapap® Junior Rapid Tabs: 160 mg [bubblegum flavor]
Tylenol® Children's Meltaways: 80 mg [bubblegum, grape flavors]
Tylenol® Jr. Meltaways: 160 mg [bubblegum, grape flavors]

References

American Academy of Pediatrics: Committee on Drugs, "Acetaminophen Toxicity in Children," *Pediatrics*, 2001, 108(4):1020-4.
Anand KJ and International Evidence-Based Group for Neonatal Pain, "Consensus Statement for the Prevention and Management of Pain in the Newborn," *Arch Pediatr Adolesc Med*, 2001, 155(2):173-80.
Anand KJ, Chair, International Evidence-Based Group for Neonatal Pain, personal correspondence, April 2002.
Buck ML, "Perioperative Use of High-Dose Rectal Acetaminophen," *Pediatr Pharm*, 2001, 7(9), http://www.medscape.com/viewarticle/415082.
Howard CR, Howard FM, and Weitzman ML, "Acetaminophen Analgesia in Neonatal Circumcision: The Effect on Pain," *Pediatrics*, 1994, 93(4):641-646.
Mayoral CE, Marino RV, Rosenfeld W, et al, "Alternating Antipyretics: Is This An Alternative?" *Pediatrics*, 2000, 105(5):1009-12.

Acetaminophen and Codeine
(a seet a MIN oh fen & KOE deen)

Medication Safety Issues

Sound-alike/look-alike issues:
Capital® may be confused with Capitrol®
Tylenol® may be confused with atenolol, timolol, Tuinal®, Tylox®

T3 is an error-prone abbreviation (mistaken as liothyronine)

High alert medication: The Institute for Safe Medication Practices (ISMP) includes this medication among its list of drug classes which have a heightened risk of causing significant patient harm when used in error.

Duplicate therapy issues: This product contains acetaminophen, which may be a component of other combination products. Do not exceed the maximum recommended daily dose of acetaminophen.

U.S. Brand Names Capital® and Codeine; Tylenol® with Codeine No. 3; Tylenol® with Codeine No. 4

Canadian Brand Names ratio-Emtec; ratio-Lenoltec; Triatec-30; Triatec-8; Triatec-8 Strong; Tylenol Elixir with Codeine; Tylenol No. 1; Tylenol No. 1 Forte; Tylenol No. 2 with Codeine; Tylenol No. 3 with Codeine; Tylenol No. 4 with Codeine

Therapeutic Category Analgesic, Narcotic

Generic Available Yes

Use Relief of mild to moderate pain (FDA approved in ages ≥3 and adults)

Restrictions C-III; C-V

Pregnancy Risk Factor C

Pregnancy Considerations Refer to Codeine monograph.

Lactation Enters breast milk/use caution

Breast-Feeding Considerations Refer to Codeine monograph.

Contraindications Hypersensitivity to acetaminophen, codeine phosphate, or any component (see Warnings)

Warnings Acetaminophen may cause severe hepatic toxicity with overdose. Use with caution in patients with alcoholic liver disease. Chronic daily dosing in adults of 5-8 g of acetaminophen over several weeks or 3-4 g/day for 1 year have resulted in liver damage. Do not exceed maximum daily doses; consider acetaminophen content of combination products when evaluating the dose of acetaminophen.

Codeine may cause CNS depression which may impair physical or mental abilities; patients must be cautioned about performing tasks which require mental alertness (eg, operating machinery or driving). Respiratory depression may occur even at therapeutic dosages; use with extreme caution in patients with respiratory diseases including asthma, emphysema, COPD, cor pulmonale, hypoxia, hypercapnia, pre-existing respiratory depression, significantly decreased respiratory reserve, other obstructive pulmonary disease, kyphoscoliosis, or other skeletal disorder which may alter respiratory function. Use with extreme caution in patients with head injury, intracranial lesions, or elevated intracranial pressure; exaggerated elevation of ICP may occur. May cause hypotension; use with caution in patients with circulatory shock, hypovolemia, impaired myocardial function, or those receiving drugs which may exaggerate hypotensive effects (including phenothiazines or general anesthetics). Codeine may obscure diagnosis or clinical course of patients with acute abdominal conditions.

Physical and psychological dependence may occur; abrupt discontinuation after prolonged use may result in withdrawal symptoms or seizures. Concurrent use of agonist/antagonist analgesics may precipitate withdrawal symptoms and/or reduce analgesic efficacy in patients following prolonged therapy with mu opioid agonists. Interactions with other CNS drugs may occur (see Drug Interactions). Healthcare provider should be alert to problems of abuse, misuse, and diversion. Infants born to women physically dependent on opioids will also be physically dependent and may experience respiratory difficulties or opioid withdrawal symptoms (neonatal abstinence syndrome). Symptoms of opiate withdrawal may include excessive crying, diarrhea, fever, hyperreflexia, irritability, tremors, or vomiting.

Some tablets contain metabisulfite which may cause allergic reactions in susceptible individuals. Suspension contains propylene glycol. Suspension contains and other liquid products may contain sodium benzoate; benzoic acid (benzoate) is a metabolite of benzyl alcohol; large amounts of benzyl alcohol (≥99 mg/kg/day) have been associated with a potentially fatal toxicity ("gasping syndrome") in neonates; the "gasping syndrome" consists of metabolic acidosis, respiratory distress, gasping respirations, CNS dysfunction (including convulsions, intracranial hemorrhage), hypotension and cardiovascular collapse; avoid use of acetaminophen and codeine products containing sodium benzoate in neonates; *in vitro* and animal studies have shown that benzoate displaces bilirubin from protein binding sites

Precautions Use with caution in patients with hypersensitivity reactions to other phenanthrene derivative opioid agonists (morphine, hydrocodone, hydromorphone, levorphanol, oxycodone, oxymorphone), adrenal insufficiency, biliary tract impairment, CNS depression/coma, morbid obesity, prostatic hyperplasia, urinary stricture, thyroid dysfunction, or severe liver or renal insufficiency. Use with caution in patients with two or more copies of the variant CYP2D6*2 allele (ie, CYP2D6 "ultra-rapid metabolizers"); these patients may have extensive conversion of codeine to morphine with resultant increased opioid-mediated effects.

G-6-PD deficiency: Although several case reports of acetaminophen-associated hemolytic anemia have been reported in patients with G-6-PD deficiency, a direct cause and effect relationship has not been well established (concurrent illnesses such as fever or infection may precipitate hemolytic anemia in patients with G-6-PD deficiency); therefore, acetaminophen is generally thought to be safe when given in therapeutic doses to patients with G-6-PD deficiency.

Use codeine with caution in lactating women. Codeine and its metabolite (morphine) are found in breast milk and can be detected in the serum of nursing infants. Exposure to the nursing infant is generally considered to be low; the relative dose to a nursing infant has been calculated to be ~1% of the weight-adjusted maternal dose. Higher levels of morphine may be found in the breast milk of lactating mothers who are "ultra-rapid metabolizers" of codeine; patients with two or more copies of the variant CYP2D6*2 allele may have extensive conversion to morphine and thus increased opioid-mediated effects. In one case, excessively high serum concentrations of morphine were reported in a breast-fed infant following maternal use of acetaminophen with codeine (see Koren, 2006). The mother was later found to be an "ultra-rapid metabolizer" of codeine; symptoms in the infant included feeding difficulty and lethargy, followed by death. Because exposure to the nursing infant is generally low, the AAP considers codeine to be "usually compatible with breast-feeding." However, caution should be used since most persons are not aware if they have the genotype resulting in "ultra-rapid metabolizer" status. When codeine is used in breast-feeding women, it is recommended to use the lowest dose for the shortest duration of time and observe the infant for increased sleepiness, difficulty in feeding or breathing, or limpness. Medical attention should be sought immediately if the infant develops these symptoms.

Adverse Reactions
Acetaminophen:
Dermatologic: Rash
Hematologic: Blood dyscrasias (leukopenia, neutropenia, pancytopenia)
Hepatic: Hepatic necrosis with overdose
Renal: Renal injury with chronic use
Miscellaneous: Hypersensitivity reactions (rare)
Codeine:
Cardiovascular: Bradycardia, hypotension, palpitations, peripheral vasodilation
Central nervous system: CNS depression, dizziness, drowsiness, intracranial pressure elevated, sedation
Dermatologic: Pruritus
Endocrine & metabolic: Antidiuretic hormone release
Gastrointestinal: Biliary tract spasm, constipation, nausea, vomiting
Genitourinary: Urinary retention
Hepatic: Transaminases elevated
Ocular: Miosis
Respiratory: Respiratory depression
Miscellaneous: Histamine release, physical and psychological dependence with prolonged use

Drug Interactions
Metabolism/Transport Effects Acetaminophen: **Substrate** (minor) of CYP1A2, 2A6, 2C9, 2D6, 2E1, 3A4; **Inhibits** CYP3A4 (weak)
Avoid Concomitant Use There are no known interactions where it is recommended to avoid concomitant use.
Increased Effect/Toxicity
Acetaminophen and Codeine may increase the levels/effects of: Alcohol (Ethyl); Alvimopan; CNS Depressants; Desmopressin; Selective Serotonin Reuptake Inhibitors; Thiazide Diuretics; Vitamin K Antagonists

The levels/effects of Acetaminophen and Codeine may be increased by: Amphetamines; Antipsychotic Agents (Phenothiazines); Imatinib; Isoniazid; Somatostatin Analogs; Succinylcholine
Decreased Effect
Acetaminophen and Codeine may decrease the levels/effects of: Pegvisomant

The levels/effects of Acetaminophen and Codeine may be decreased by: Ammonium Chloride; Anticonvulsants (Hydantoin); Barbiturates; CarBAMazepine; Cholestyramine Resin; CYP2D6 Inhibitors (Moderate); CYP2D6 Inhibitors (Strong); Mixed Agonist / Antagonist Opioids; Peginterferon Alfa-2b
Food Interactions Rate of absorption of acetaminophen may be decreased when given with food high in carbohydrates
Mechanism of Action See individual agents.
Pharmacokinetics (Adult data unless noted) See individual agents.
Usual Dosage Oral (doses should be titrated to appropriate analgesic effect):
Children: Analgesic:
Codeine: 0.5-1 mg codeine/kg/dose every 4-6 hours; maximum dose: 60 mg/dose
Acetaminophen: 10-15 mg/kg/dose every 4-6 hours; do **not** exceed 5 doses in 24 hours; maximum dose: Children ≥12 years: 4 g acetaminophen/24 hours
Alternatively, the following doses may be used:
3-6 years: 5 mL 3-4 times/day as needed
7-12 years: 10 mL 3-4 times/day as needed
>12 years: 15 mL every 4 hours as needed
Adults: Analgesic: 1-2 tablets every 4 hours; maximum dose: 12 tablets/24 hours
Codeine: Usual: 30 mg/dose; range: 15-60 mg every 4-6 hours
Acetaminophen: 325-650 mg every 4-6 hours or 1000 mg 3-4 times/day; do **not** exceed 4 g/day
Administration Oral: Administer with food to decrease GI upset; shake suspension well before use
Patient Information Codeine may be habit-forming; avoid abrupt discontinuation after prolonged use; may cause drowsiness and impair ability to perform activities requiring mental alertness or physical coordination; avoid alcohol
Nursing Implications Observe patient for excessive sedation, respiratory depression
Additional Information Tylenol® With Codeine elixir contains saccharin
Dosage Forms Excipient information presented when available (limited, particularly for generics); consult specific product labeling. [DSC] = Discontinued product; [CAN] = Canadian brand name
Caplet:
ratio-Lenoltec No. 1 [CAN], Tylenol No. 1 [CAN]: Acetaminophen 300 mg, codeine phosphate 8 mg, and caffeine 15 mg [not available in the U.S.]
Tylenol No. 1 Forte [CAN]: Acetaminophen 500 mg, codeine phosphate 8 mg, and caffeine 15 mg [not available in the U.S.]

Solution, oral [C-V]: Acetaminophen 120 mg and codeine phosphate 12 mg per 5 mL (5 mL, 10 mL, 12.5 mL, 15 mL, 120 mL, 480 mL) [contains alcohol 7%]

Tylenol Elixir with Codeine [CAN]: Acetaminophen 160 mg and codeine phosphate 8 mg per 5 mL (500 mL) [contains alcohol 7%, sucrose 31%; cherry flavor; not available in the U.S.]

Suspension, oral [C-V] (Capital® and Codeine): Acetaminophen 120 mg and codeine phosphate 12 mg per 5 mL (480 mL) [alcohol free; contains propylene glycol, sodium benzoate; fruit punch flavor]

Tablet [C-III]: Acetaminophen 300 mg and codeine phosphate 15 mg; acetaminophen 300 mg and codeine phosphate 30 mg; acetaminophen 300 mg and codeine phosphate 60 mg

ratio-Emtec [CAN], Triatec-30 [CAN]: Acetaminophen 300 mg and codeine phosphate 30 mg [not available in the U.S.]

ratio-Lenoltec No. 1 [CAN]: Acetaminophen 300 mg, codeine phosphate 8 mg, and caffeine 15 mg [not available in the U.S.]

ratio-Lenoltec No. 2 [CAN], Tylenol No. 2 with Codeine [CAN]: Acetaminophen 300 mg, codeine phosphate 15 mg, and caffeine 15 mg [not available in the U.S.]

ratio-Lenoltec No. 3 [CAN], Tylenol No. 3 with Codeine [CAN]: Acetaminophen 300 mg, codeine phosphate 30 mg, and caffeine 15 mg [not available in the U.S.]

ratio-Lenoltec No. 4 [CAN], Tylenol No. 4 with Codeine [CAN]: Acetaminophen 300 mg and codeine phosphate 60 mg [not available in the U.S.]

Triatec-8 [CAN]: Acetaminophen 325 mg, codeine phosphate 8 mg, and caffeine 30 mg [not available in the U.S.]

Triatec-8 Strong [CAN]: Acetaminophen 500 mg, codeine phosphate 8 mg, and caffeine 30 mg [not available in the U.S.]

Tylenol® with Codeine No. 3: Acetaminophen 300 mg and codeine phosphate 30 mg [contains sodium metabisulfite]

Tylenol® with Codeine No. 4: Acetaminophen 300 mg and codeine phosphate 60 mg [contains sodium metabisulfite]

References

Khan K and Chang J, "Neonatal Abstinence Syndrome Due to Codeine," *Arch Dis Child Fetal Neonatal Ed*, 1997, 76(1):F59-60.

Koren G, Cairns J, Chitayat D, et al, "Pharmacogenetics of Morphine Poisoning in a Breastfed Neonate of a Codeine-Prescribed Mother," Lancet, 2006, 368(9536):704.

Reynolds EW, Riel-Romero RM, and Bada HS, "Neonatal Abstinence Syndrome and Cerebral Infarction Following Maternal Codeine Use During Pregnancy," *Clin Pediatr (Phila)*, 2007, 46(7):639-45.

Spigset O and Hägg S, "Analgesics and Breast-Feeding: Safety Considerations," *Paediatr Drugs*, 2000, 2(3):223-38.

U.S. Food and Drug Administration Center for Drug Evaluation and Research, "FDA Public Health Advisory: Use of Codeine By Some Breastfeeding Mothers May Lead to Life-Threatening Side Effects in Nursing Babies," available at: http://www.fda.gov/cder/drug/advisory/codeine.htm.

◆ **Acetaminophen and Hydrocodone** see Hydrocodone and Acetaminophen on page 684

◆ **Acetaminophen and Oxycodone** see Oxycodone and Acetaminophen on page 1041

◆ **Acetaminophen and Propoxyphene** see Propoxyphene and Acetaminophen on page 1173

AcetaZOLAMIDE (a set a ZOLE a mide)

Medication Safety Issues
Sound-alike/look-alike issues:
AcetaZOLAMIDE may be confused with aceto-HEXAMIDE

Diamox® Sequels® may be confused with Diabinese®, Dobutrex®, Trimox®

International issues:
Diamox® [Canada and multiple international markets] may be confused with Zimox brand name for amoxicillin [Italy] and carbidopa/levodopa [Greece]

Related Information
Antiepileptic Drugs on page 1693

U.S. Brand Names Diamox® Sequels®

Canadian Brand Names Apo-Acetazolamide®; Diamox®

Therapeutic Category Anticonvulsant, Miscellaneous; Carbonic Anhydrase Inhibitor; Diuretic, Carbonic Anhydrase Inhibitor

Generic Available Yes

Use Reduce elevated intraocular pressure in glaucoma; diuretic; adjunct to the treatment of refractory seizures; prevent acute altitude sickness; treatment of centrencephalic epilepsies; reduce CSF production in hydrocephalus

Pregnancy Risk Factor C

Pregnancy Considerations Teratogenic in animal studies, however, there are no adequate and well-controlled studies in pregnant women.

Lactation Enters breast milk/not recommended (AAP rates "compatible")

Contraindications Hypersensitivity to acetazolamide, any component, or other sulfonamides; patients with hepatic disease or insufficiency; decreased serum sodium and/or potassium; adrenocortical insufficiency; hyperchloremic acidosis; or severe renal disease; long-term administration in patients with chronic noncongestive angle-closure glaucoma

Warnings Fatalities associated with sulfonamides, although rare, have occurred due to severe reactions including Stevens-Johnson syndrome, toxic epidermal necrolysis, hepatic necrosis, agranulocytosis, aplastic anemia, and other blood dyscrasias; discontinue use at first sign of rash or any sign of adverse reaction. Anorexia, tachypnea, lethargy, metabolic acidosis, and death have been reported in patients receiving acetazolamide and high-dose aspirin concomitantly. Tolerance to antiepileptic effects may require dosage adjustment.

Precautions Use with caution in patients with respiratory acidosis, COPD, diabetes mellitus, and gout; reduce dosage in patients with renal impairment; growth retardation has been reported in children receiving chronic therapy (possibly due to chronic acidosis)

Adverse Reactions
Cardiovascular: Cyanosis

Central nervous system: Drowsiness, ataxia, confusion, fatigue, vertigo, fever, seizures, dizziness, depression, malaise, headache, excitement

Dermatologic: Rash, erythema multiforme, photosensitivity, Stevens-Johnson syndrome (see Warnings), urticaria, toxic epidermal necrolysis

Endocrine & metabolic: Hypokalemia, hyperchloremic metabolic acidosis, hyperglycemia, hypoglycemia, growth retardation

Gastrointestinal: GI irritation, anorexia, nausea, vomiting, xerostomia, melena, dysgeusia, metallic taste, black stools

Genitourinary: Dysuria, polyuria

Hematologic: Bone marrow suppression, thrombocytopenia, hemolytic anemia, pancytopenia, agranulocytosis, leukopenia

Hepatic: Hepatic insufficiency, cholestatic jaundice, hepatic necrosis

Local: Pain at injection site

Neuromuscular & skeletal: Paresthesia, muscle weakness

Ocular: Myopia (transient)

Otic: Tinnitus

Renal: Renal calculi, phosphaturia, renal colic, hematuria, renal failure, polyuria

Respiratory: Hyperpnea

◀ **Drug Interactions**
Metabolism/Transport Effects Inhibits CYP3A4 (weak)
Avoid Concomitant Use
Avoid concomitant use of AcetaZOLAMIDE with any of the following: Brinzolamide
Increased Effect/Toxicity
AcetaZOLAMIDE may increase the levels/effects of: Alcohol (Ethyl); Alpha-/Beta-Agonists; Amifostine; Amphetamines; Anticonvulsants (Barbiturate); Anticonvulsants (Hydantoin); Antihypertensives; Brinzolamide; CarBAMazepine; CNS Depressants; Flecainide; Hypotensive Agents; Memantine; Methotrimeprazine; Primidone; QuiNIDine; RiTUXimab

The levels/effects of AcetaZOLAMIDE may be increased by: Diazoxide; Herbs (Hypotensive Properties); MAO Inhibitors; Methotrimeprazine; Pentoxifylline; Phosphodiesterase 5 Inhibitors; Prostacyclin Analogues; Salicylates
Decreased Effect
AcetaZOLAMIDE may decrease the levels/effects of: Lithium; Methenamine; Primidone; Trientine

The levels/effects of AcetaZOLAMIDE may be decreased by: Herbs (Hypertensive Properties); Ketorolac; Ketorolac (Systemic); Mefloquine; Methylphenidate; Yohimbine
Food Interactions Avoid natural licorice (causes sodium and water retention and increases potassium loss)
Stability Store tablets and capsules at room temperature; after reconstitution, acetazolamide injection is stable for 12 hours at room temperature and for 1 week when refrigerated; physically incompatible with parenteral multivitamins
Mechanism of Action Competitive, reversible inhibition of the enzyme carbonic anhydrase resulting in increased renal excretion of sodium, potassium, bicarbonate, and water and decreased formation of aqueous humor; also inhibits carbonic anhydrase in CNS to retard abnormal and excessive discharge from CNS neurons
Pharmacodynamics
Onset of action:
  Capsule, extended release: 2 hours
  Tablet: 1-1.5 hours
  I.V.: 2 minutes
Maximum effect:
  Capsule, extended release: 3-6 hours
  Tablet: 1-4 hours
  I.V.: 15 minutes
Duration:
  Capsule, extended release: 18-24 hours
  Tablet: 8-12 hours
  I.V.: 4-5 hours
Pharmacokinetics (Adult data unless noted)
Absorption: Appears to be dose dependent; erratic with daily doses >10 mg/kg
Distribution: Into erythrocytes, kidneys, and breast milk (breast milk to plasma ratio of 0.25 has been reported); crosses the blood-brain barrier and the placenta
Protein binding: 95%
Half-life: 2.4-5.8 hours
Time to peak serum concentration: Tablet: 2-4 hours
Elimination: 70% to 100% of an I.V. or tablet dose and 47% of an extended release capsule excreted unchanged in urine within 24 hours
Dialysis: 20% to 50% removed by hemodialysis
Usual Dosage
Children:
  Glaucoma:
    Oral: 8-30 mg/kg/day or 300-900 mg/m²/day divided every 8 hours

I.V.: 20-40 mg/kg/day divided every 6 hours, not to exceed 1 g/day
  Edema: Oral, I.V.: 5 mg/kg/dose or 150 mg/m²/dose once daily
  Epilepsy: Oral: 4-16 mg/kg/day in 1-4 divided doses, not to exceed 30 mg/kg/day or 1 g/day; **extended release capsule is not recommended for treatment of epilepsy**
Adults:
  Glaucoma:
    Chronic simple (open-angle): Oral: 250 mg 1-4 times/day or 500 mg once followed by 125-250 mg every 4 hours, or 500 mg sustained release capsule twice daily
    Secondary, acute (closed-angle): I.V.: 250-500 mg, may repeat in 2-4 hours to a maximum of 1 g/day
  Edema: Oral, I.V.: 250-375 mg/day
  Epilepsy: Oral: 4-16 mg/kg/day in 1-4 divided doses, not to exceed 30 mg/kg/day or 1 g/day; **extended release capsule is not recommended for treatment of epilepsy**
  Altitude sickness: Oral: 500-1000 mg daily in divided doses such as 250 mg every 8-12 hours or 500 mg extended release capsules every 12-24 hours; therapy should begin 24-48 hours before and continued during ascent and for at least 48 hours after arrival at the high altitude
  Urine alkalinization: Oral: 5 mg/kg/dose repeated 2-3 times over 24 hours
Dosing interval in renal impairment: Children and Adults:
  Cl_{cr} 10-50 mL/minute: Administer every 12 hours
  Cl_{cr} <10 mL/minute: Avoid use
Administration
Oral: Administer with food to decrease GI upset; tablet may be crushed and suspended in cherry or chocolate syrup to disguise the bitter taste of the drug (see Extemporaneous Preparations)
Parenteral:
  I.V.: Reconstitute with at least 5 mL SWI to provide a solution containing not more than 100 mg/mL; maximum concentration: 100 mg/mL; maximum rate of I.V. infusion: 500 mg/minute
  I.M.: Not generally recommended as the drug's alkaline pH makes it very painful
Monitoring Parameters Serum electrolytes, CBC and platelet counts
Test Interactions May cause false-positive results for urinary protein with Albustix®, Labstix®, Albutest®, Bumintest®; interferes with HPLC method for assaying theophylline
Patient Information Do not crush or chew long-acting capsule; may cause dry mouth. May rarely cause photosensitivity reactions (eg, exposure to sunlight may cause severe sunburn, skin rash, redness, or itching); avoid direct exposure to sunlight; may cause drowsiness and impair ability to perform activities requiring mental alertness or physical coordination
Additional Information Sodium content of 500 mg injection: 2.049 mEq

Extended release capsules are indicated only for use for the adjunctive treatment of open-angle or secondary glaucoma and the prevention of high altitude sickness; avoid using extended release capsules for anticonvulsant or diuretic therapy

Acetazolamide has been used with questionable efficacy to slow the progression of hydrocephalus in neonates and infants who may not be good candidates for surgery. I.V. or oral doses of 5 mg/kg/dose every 6 hours increased by 25 mg/kg/day to a maximum of 100 mg/kg/day, if tolerated, have been used. Furosemide was used in combination with acetazolamide (Libenson, 1999).

Dosage Forms Excipient information presented when available (limited, particularly for generics); consult specific product labeling.

Capsule, extended release: 500 mg
  Diamox® Sequels®: 500 mg
Injection, powder for reconstitution: 500 mg
Tablet: 125 mg, 250 mg

Extemporaneous Preparations

A 25 mg/mL suspension may be made by crushing twelve 250 mg tablets and mixing with 120 mL of a 1:1 mixture of Ora-Sweet® and Ora-Plus® or a 1:1 mixture of Ora-Sweet® SF and Ora-Plus®. The resulting suspension is stable for 60 days refrigerated (Allen, 1996). When diluted in 120 mL solution of cherry syrup concentrate diluted 1:4 with simple syrup, NF, it is stable 60 days refrigerated (preferred) or at room temperature (Nahata, 2004).

A 25 mg/mL suspension may be made by crushing one hundred 250 mg tablets; add 100 mL flavor/purified water; add a mixture of 10 g Veegum (already mixed with 200 mL purified water), 300 mL 1% methylcellulose and 300 mL syrup; qsad to 1000 mL with flavor/purified water and 10 mL paraben concentrate (methylparaben 120 mg, propylparaben 12 mg, propylene glycol qsad to 100 mL); stable 79 days refrigerated (Alexander, 1991).

Allen LV and Erickson MA, "Stability of Acetazolamide, Allopurinol, Azathioprine, Clonazepam, and Flucytosine in Extemporaneously Compounded Oral Liquids," *Am J Health Sys Pharm*, 1996, 53:1944-9.

Alexander KS, Haribhakti RP, and Parker GA, "Stability of Acetazolamide in Suspension Compounded From Tablets," *Am J Hosp Pharm*, 1991, 48(6):1241-4.

Nahata, MC, Pai VB, and Hipple TF, *Pediatric Drug Formulations*, 5th ed, Cincinnati, OH: Harvey Whitney Books Co, 2004.

References

Libenson MH, Kaye EM, Rosman NP, et al, "Acetazolamide and Furosemide for Posthemorrhagic Hydrocephalus of the Newborn," *Pediatr Neurol*, 1999, 20(3):185-91.

Reiss WG and Oles KS, "Acetazolamide in the Treatment of Seizures," *Ann Pharmacother*, 1996, 30(5):514-9.

Shinnar S, Gammon K, Bergman EW Jr, et al, "Management of Hydrocephalus in Infancy: Use of Acetazolamide and Furosemide to Avoid Cerebrospinal Fluid Shunts," *J Pediatr*, 1985, 107(1):31-7.

◆ **Acetoxyl® (Can)** see Benzoyl Peroxide *on page 184*

◆ **Acetoxymethylprogesterone** see MedroxyPROGES-TERone *on page 870*

Acetylcholine (a se teel KOE leen)

Medication Safety Issues
Sound-alike/look-alike issues:
  Acetylcholine may be confused with acetylcysteine
U.S. Brand Names Miochol®-E
Canadian Brand Names Miochol®-E
Therapeutic Category Cholinergic Agent, Ophthalmic; Ophthalmic Agent, Miotic
Generic Available No
Use Produces complete miosis in cataract surgery, keratoplasty, iridectomy and other anterior segment surgery where rapid miosis is required
Pregnancy Risk Factor C
Pregnancy Considerations Acetylcholine is used primarily in the eye and there are no reports of its use in pregnancy. Because it is ionized at physiologic pH, transplacental passage would not be expected.
Contraindications Hypersensitivity to acetylcholine chloride or any component; acute iritis and acute inflammatory disease of the anterior chamber
Warnings Open under aseptic conditions only
Precautions Systemic effects rarely occur, but can cause problems for patients with acute CHF, bronchial asthma, peptic ulcer, hyperthyroidism, GI spasm, and urinary tract obstruction

Adverse Reactions
Cardiovascular: Transient bradycardia and hypotension
Central nervous system: Headache
Ocular: Iris atrophy, temporary lens opacities (attributed to osmotic effect of 5% mannitol present in preparation)
Respiratory: Dyspnea
Miscellaneous: Diaphoresis
Drug Interactions
Avoid Concomitant Use There are no known interactions where it is recommended to avoid concomitant use.
Increased Effect/Toxicity
The levels/effects of Acetylcholine may be increased by:
Acetylcholinesterase Inhibitors
Decreased Effect There are no known significant interactions involving a decrease in effect.
Stability Prepare solution immediately before use; do not use solution which is not clear and colorless
Mechanism of Action Causes contraction of the sphincter muscles of the iris, resulting in miosis and contraction of the ciliary muscle, leading to accommodation
Pharmacodynamics
Onset of action: Miosis occurs promptly
Duration: ~10-20 minutes
Usual Dosage Ophthalmic: Adults: Instill 0.5-2 mL of 1% injection (5-20 mg)
Administration Ophthalmic: Instill into anterior chamber before or after securing one or more sutures; instillation should be gentle and parallel to the iris face and tangential to the pupil border; in cataract surgery, acetylcholine should be used only after delivery of the lens
Dosage Forms Excipient information presented when available (limited, particularly for generics); consult specific product labeling.
Powder for solution, intraocular, as chloride [kit]:
  Miochol®-E: 20 mg [supplied with diluent; reconstitution results in 1:100 solution]

◆ **Acetylcholine Chloride** see Acetylcholine *on page 43*

Acetylcysteine (a se teel SIS teen)

Medication Safety Issues
Sound-alike/look-alike issues:
  Acetylcysteine may be confused with acetylcholine
  Mucomyst® may be confused with Mucinex®
U.S. Brand Names Acetadote®
Canadian Brand Names Acetylcysteine Solution; Mucomyst®; Parvolex®
Therapeutic Category Antidote, Acetaminophen; Mucolytic Agent
Generic Available Yes: Solution for inhalation
Use
Inhalation: Adjunctive therapy in patients with abnormal or viscid mucous secretions in bronchopulmonary diseases, pulmonary complications of surgery, and cystic fibrosis; diagnostic bronchial studies
Injection, Oral: Antidote for acute acetaminophen toxicity; prevention of radiocontrast-induced renal dysfunction
Oral, rectal: Treatment of distal intestinal obstruction syndrome (previously known as "meconium ileus or its equivalent")
Pregnancy Risk Factor B
Pregnancy Considerations Based on limited reports using acetylcysteine to treat acetaminophen poisoning in pregnant women, acetylcysteine has been shown to cross the placenta and may provide protective levels in the fetus.
Lactation Excretion in breast milk unknown/use caution
Contraindications Hypersensitivity to acetylcysteine or any component

Warnings Serious anaphylactoid reactions including death in a patient with asthma have been reported after I.V. use; acute flushing and erythema may occur 30-60 minutes into an I.V. infusion, resolving spontaneously; the infusion may be interrupted until treatment of allergic symptoms is initiated; if acute hypersensitivity reactions occur which do not respond to medical management (eg, antihistamines, H_2 blockers) or temporarily halting infusion, discontinue use and pursue alternative management. Since increased bronchial secretions may develop after inhalation, percussion, postural drainage, and suctioning should follow.

Acetaminophen overdose: The modified Rumack-Matthew nomogram allows for stratification of patients into risk categories based on the relationship between the serum acetaminophen level and time after ingestion. There are several situations where the nomogram is of limited use. Serum acetaminophen levels obtained prior to 4-hour postingestion are not interpretable; patients presenting late may have undetectable serum concentrations, but have received a lethal dose. The nomogram is less predictive in a chronic ingestion or in an overdose with an extended release product. Acetylcysteine should be administered for any signs of hepatotoxicity even if acetaminophen serum level is low or undetectable. The nomogram also does not take into account patients at higher risk of acetaminophen toxicity (eg, alcoholics, malnourished patients) or individuals ingesting higher than recommended acetaminophen doses for extended periods of time (repeated supratherapeutic ingestion).

Precautions Use with caution in patients with asthma or previous history of bronchospasm

Adverse Reactions

Cardiovascular: Tachycardia, hypotension, syncope, chest tightness, vasodilation

Central nervous system: Drowsiness, chills, dysphoria

Dermatologic: Generalized urticaria, rash, pruritus, erythema, angioedema

Gastrointestinal: Stomatitis, nausea, vomiting, dyspepsia, hemoptysis

Hepatic: Mild elevations in liver function tests have occurred after oral therapy

Ocular: Eye pain

Respiratory: Bronchospasm, rhinorrhea, cough

Miscellaneous: Anaphylactoid reactions (I.V. use; 17% in an open label study; 1% reported as severe or moderate in 10% of patients within 15 minutes of the first infusion; severe in 1% or mild to moderate in 6% to 7% of patients after the 60 minute infusion); diaphoresis, unpleasant odor during administration

Drug Interactions

Avoid Concomitant Use There are no known interactions where it is recommended to avoid concomitant use.

Increased Effect/Toxicity There are no known significant interactions involving an increase in effect.

Decreased Effect There are no known significant interactions involving a decrease in effect.

Stability Store at room temperature; I.V. formulation is preservative free and stable 24 hours after dilution at room temperature; opened inhalation solution vials may be stored in the refrigerator; use within 96 hours; contact with rubber, copper, iron, and cork may inactivate the drug; the light purple color of solution does **not** affect its activity. I.V. acetylcysteine is hyperosmolar (2600 mOsm/L) and is compatible with 5% dextrose, 0.45% sodium chloride, and SWI.

Mechanism of Action Exerts mucolytic action through its free sulfhydryl group which opens up the disulfide bonds in the mucoproteins thus lowering the viscosity. The exact mechanism of action in acetaminophen toxicity is unknown. It may act by maintaining or restoring glutathione levels or by acting as an alternative substrate for conjugation with the acetaminophen's toxic metabolite.

Pharmacodynamics

Onset of action: Upon inhalation, mucus liquefaction occurs maximally within 5-10 minutes

Duration of mucus liquefaction: More than 1 hour

Pharmacokinetics (Adult data unless noted)

Distribution: V_d: 0.47 L/kg

Protein binding: 83%

Half-life:

Reduced acetylcysteine: 2 hours

Total acetylcysteine:

Newborns: 11 hours

Adults: 5.6 hours

Time to peak serum concentration: Oral: 1-2 hours

Elimination: Clearance: Adults: 0.11 L/hour/kg

Usual Dosage

Acetaminophen poisoning: Children and Adults: Begin treatment within 8 hours of ingestion to optimize therapy in patients whose serum acetaminophen levels fall above the "possible" toxicity line on the Rumack-Matthew nomogram; (see Acetaminophen Serum Level Nomogram on page 1708 in the appendix). Treatment is also indicated in patients with a history of known or suspected acute acetaminophen ingestion of >150 mg/kg (child) or >7.5 g (adolescent or adult) total dose when plasma levels are not available within 8-10 hours of ingestion or in patients presenting >24 hours after acute ingestion who have a measurable acetaminophen level. See Warnings.

I.V.: 150 mg/kg infused over 60 minutes; followed by a 4-hour infusion of 50 mg/kg; followed by a 16-hour infusion of 100 mg/kg; equivalent to a total dose of 300 mg/kg infused over 21 hours

Oral: 140 mg/kg; followed by 17 doses of 70 mg/kg every 4 hours; repeat dose if emesis occurs within 1 hour of administration; therapy should continue until all doses are administered even though the acetaminophen plasma level has dropped below the toxic range

Nebulized inhalation:

Infants: 1-2 mL of 20% solution or 2-4 mL of 10% solution until nebulized, given 3-4 times/day

Children: 3-5 mL of 20% solution or 6-10 mL of 10% solution until nebulized, given 3-4 times/day

Adolescents: 5-10 mL of 10% to 20% solution until nebulized, given 3-4 times/day

Note: Patients should receive an aerosolized bronchodilator 10-15 minutes prior to acetylcysteine

Intratracheal: Children and Adults: 1-2 mL of 10% to 20% solution every 1-4 hours as needed

Distal intestinal obstruction syndrome (previously known as meconium ileus equivalent): Varying regimens have been reported (polyethylene glycol has become more widely used for this indication):

Oral:

Children <10 years: 30 mL of 10% solution diluted in 30 mL juice or soda 3 times/day for 24 hours

Children 10 years and Adults: 60 mL of 10% solution diluted in 60 mL juice or soda 3 times/day for 24 hours

Note: Prior to treatment, administer a phosphosoda enema. A clear liquid diet should be used during the 24-hour acetylcysteine treatment

Rectal enema: Children: Varying dosages; 100-300 mL of 4% to 6% solution 2-4 times/day; 50 mL of 20% solution 1-4 times/day and 5-30 mL of 10% to 20% solution 3-4 times/day have been used; rectal enemas appear to have less favorable results than oral administration (Mascarenhas, 2003)

Prevention of radiocontrast-induced renal dysfunction: Adults: Oral: 600 mg twice daily for 2 days (beginning the day before the procedure); hydrate patient concurrently

Administration

Parenteral: I.V.: Three infusions (see Usual Dosage) of different lengths: Dilute first dose (150 mg/kg) in 200 mL D$_5$W and infuse over 60 minutes; dilute second dose (50 mg/kg) in 500 mL D$_5$W and infuse over 4 hours; dilute third dose (100 mg/kg) in 1000 mL D$_5$W and infuse over 16 hours; for children <40 kg and patients who are fluid restricted, the manufacturer recommends reducing the diluent to a "proportional" amount. See table for manufacturer's recommended infusion guideline for patients <40 kg. Or as an alternative to proportionally lower the diluent volume, a reasonable approach might be to utilize the concentrations resulting from using the recommended dilution for the dosage in a 50 kg patient. The calculated concentration would range between 5 mg/mL (maintenance infusion) to 37.5 mg/mL (loading dose).

Infusion Guide by Weight for Patients <40 kg

Body Weight (kg)	LOADING Dose 150 mg/kg over 60 min		SECOND Dose 50 mg/kg over 4 h		THIRD Dose 100 mg/kg over 16 h	
	Acetyl-cysteine Dose mg (mL)	5% Dex-trose (mL)	Acetyl-cysteine Dose mg (mL)	5% Dex-trose (mL)	Acetyl-cysteine Dose mg (mL)	5% Dex-trose (mL)
10	1500 (7.5)	30	500 (2.5)	70	1000 (5)	140
15	2250 (11.25)	45	750 (3.75)	105	1500 (7.5)	210
20	3000 (15)	60	1000 (5)	140	2000 (10)	280
25	3750 (18.75)	100	1250 (6.25)	250	2500 (12.5)	500
30	4500 (22.5)	100	1500 (7.5)	250	3000 (15)	500

Oral: For treatment of acetaminophen overdosage, administer as a 5% solution; dilute the 20% solution (inhalation formulation) 1:3 with a cola, orange juice, or other soft drink; use within 1 hour of preparation

Oral inhalation: May be administered by nebulization either undiluted (both 10% and 20%) or diluted in NS

Rectal: Dilute the inhalation solution in NS to the desired final concentration and administer rectally

Monitoring Parameters

When used in acetaminophen overdose, determine acetaminophen level as soon as possible, but no sooner than 4 hours after ingestion of immediate release formulations or 2 hours after ingestion of liquid formulations (to ensure peak levels have been obtained) (see Acetaminophen Serum Level Nomogram on page 1708 in the appendix); coingestion of acetaminophen with other medications which may delay GI peristalsis eg, antihistamines, opioids, may require repeated serum levels to determine the peak serum level; liver function tests

Patient Information

Clear airway by coughing deeply before aerosol treatment

Nursing Implications

Anaphylactoid reactions following I.V. administration have been reported; have emergency treatments such as antihistamines and H$_2$ blockers readily available for potential adverse effects; assess patient for nausea, vomiting, and skin rash following oral administration for treatment of acetaminophen poisoning; intermittent aerosol treatments are commonly given when patient arises, before meals, and just before retiring at bedtime

Dosage Forms

Excipient information presented when available (limited, particularly for generics); consult specific product labeling.

Injection, solution:
Acetadote®: 20% (30 mL) [200 mg/mL; contains disodium edetate]
Solution, inhalation/oral: 10% (4 mL, 10 mL, 30 mL) [100 mg/mL]; 20% (4 mL, 10 mL, 30 mL) [200 mg/mL]

References

Hanly JG and Fitzgerald MX, "Meconium Ileus Equivalent in Older Patients With Cystic Fibrosis," Br Med J (Clin Res Ed), 1983, 286 (6375):1411-3.

Mascarenhas MR, "Treatment of Gastrointestinal Problems in Cystic Fibrosis," Curr Treat Options Gastroenterol, 2003, 6(5):427-441.

Rashid ST, Salman M, Myint F, et al, "Prevention of Contrast-Induced Nephropathy in Vascular Patients Undergoing Angiography: A Randomized Controlled Trial of Intravenous N-Acetylcysteine," J Vasc Surg, 2004, 40(6):1136-41.

Tepel M, van der Giet M, Schwarzfeld C, et al, "Prevention of Radiographic-Contrast-Agent-Induced Reductions in Renal Function by Acetylcysteine," N Engl J Med, 2000, 343(3):180-4.

Walson PD and Groth JF Jr, "Acetaminophen Hepatotoxicity After Prolonged Ingestion," Pediatrics, 1993, 91(5):1021-2.

◆ **Acetylcysteine Sodium** see Acetylcysteine on page 43

◆ **Acetylcysteine Solution (Can)** see Acetylcysteine on page 43

◆ **Acetylsalicylic Acid** see Aspirin on page 141

◆ **Achromycin** see Tetracycline on page 1331

◆ **Aciclovir** see Acyclovir on page 46

◆ **Acid Control (Can)** see Famotidine on page 561

◆ **Acid Reducer (Can)** see Ranitidine on page 1200

◆ **Acid Reducer Maximum Strength Non Prescription (Can)** see Ranitidine on page 1200

◆ **Acidulated Phosphate Fluoride** see Fluoride on page 595

◆ **Acilac (Can)** see Lactulose on page 791

◆ **AcipHex®** see Rabeprazole on page 1197

◆ **Aclovate®** see Alclometasone on page 59

◆ **Acne Clear Maximum Strength [OTC]** see Benzoyl Peroxide on page 184

◆ **ACT** see DACTINomycin on page 383

◆ **ACT® [OTC]** see Fluoride on page 595

◆ **ACT-D** see DACTINomycin on page 383

◆ **ACTH** see Corticotropin on page 359

◆ **ActHIB®** see Haemophilus b Conjugate Vaccine on page 664

◆ **Acticin®** see Permethrin on page 1094

◆ **Actidose-Aqua® [OTC]** see Charcoal, Activated on page 284

◆ **Actidose® with Sorbitol [OTC]** see Charcoal, Activated on page 284

◆ **Actifed® (Can)** see Triprolidine and Pseudoephedrine on page 1388

◆ **Actigall®** see Ursodiol on page 1393

◆ **Actinomycin** see DACTINomycin on page 383

◆ **Actinomycin D** see DACTINomycin on page 383

◆ **Actinomycin CI** see DACTINomycin on page 383

◆ **Actiq®** see FentaNYL on page 567

◆ **Activase®** see Alteplase on page 71

◆ **Activase® rt-PA (Can)** see Alteplase on page 71

◆ **Activated Carbon** see Charcoal, Activated on page 284

◆ **Activated Charcoal** see Charcoal, Activated on page 284

◆ **Activated Dimethicone** see Simethicone on page 1262

◆ **Activated Ergosterol** see Ergocalciferol on page 519

◆ **Activated Methylpolysiloxane** see Simethicone on page 1262

◆ **Activated Protein C, Human, Recombinant** *see* Drotrecogin Alfa (Activated) *on page 484*

◆ **ACT® Plus [OTC]** *see* Fluoride *on page 595*

◆ **ACT® x2™ [OTC]** *see* Fluoride *on page 595*

◆ **Acular®** *see* Ketorolac *on page 781*

◆ **Acular LS®** *see* Ketorolac *on page 781*

◆ **Acular® PF [DSC]** *see* Ketorolac *on page 781*

◆ **Acuvail™** *see* Ketorolac *on page 781*

◆ **ACV** *see* Acyclovir *on page 46*

◆ **Acycloguanosine** *see* Acyclovir *on page 46*

Acyclovir (ay SYE kloe veer)

Medication Safety Issues
Sound-alike/look-alike issues:
Acyclovir may be confused with ganciclovir, Retrovir®, valACYclovir
Zovirax® may be confused with Valtrex®, Zithromax®, Zostrix®, Zyloprim®, Zyvox®

International issues:
Opthavir® [Mexico] may be confused with Optivar® which is a brand name for azelastine in the U.S.

U.S. Brand Names Zovirax®

Canadian Brand Names Apo-Acyclovir®; Mylan-Acyclovir; Novo-Acyclovir; Nu-Acyclovir; ratio-Acyclovir; Zovirax®

Therapeutic Category Antiviral Agent, Oral; Antiviral Agent, Parenteral; Antiviral Agent, Topical

Generic Available Yes: Excludes cream, ointment

Use Treatment of initial and prophylaxis of recurrent mucosal and cutaneous herpes simplex (HSV 1 and HSV 2) infections; herpes simplex encephalitis; herpes zoster infections; varicella-zoster infections in healthy, nonpregnant persons >13 years of age, children >12 months of age who have a chronic skin or lung disorder or are receiving long-term aspirin therapy, and immunocompromised patients

Pregnancy Risk Factor B

Pregnancy Considerations Teratogenic effects were not observed in animal studies. Acyclovir has been shown to cross the human placenta. There are no adequate and well-controlled studies in pregnant women. Results from a pregnancy registry, established in 1984 and closed in 1999, did not find an increase in the number of birth defects with exposure to acyclovir when compared to those expected in the general population. However, due to the small size of the registry and lack of long-term data, the manufacturer recommends using during pregnancy with caution and only when clearly needed. Data from the pregnancy registry may be obtained from GlaxoSmithKline.

Lactation Enters breast milk/use with caution (AAP rates "compatible")

Breast-Feeding Considerations Nursing mothers with herpetic lesions near or on the breast should avoid breast-feeding. Limited data suggest exposure to the nursing infant of ~0.3 mg/kg/day following oral administration of acyclovir to the mother.

Contraindications Hypersensitivity to acyclovir, valacyclovir, or any component

Warnings HSV and VZV with reduced susceptibility to acyclovir have been isolated from immunocompromised patients; thrombocytopenic purpura/hemolytic uremic syndrome [TTP/HUS] has been reported, especially with advanced HIV infection; renal failure, in some cases resulting in death, has occurred with acyclovir

Precautions Use with caution in patients with renal disease, dehydration, and underlying neurologic disease; in patients with hypoxia, hepatic, or electrolyte abnormalities; and in patients receiving other nephrotoxic drugs.

Dosage should be reduced in patients with renal impairment. Maintain adequate hydration during oral or I.V. therapy.

Adverse Reactions
Cardiovascular: DIC, peripheral edema
Central nervous system: Headache, lethargy, delirium, coma, dizziness, seizures, pain, insomnia, fever, hallucinations, aggressive behavior, ataxia, malaise, agitation, consciousness decreased, encephalopathy, fatigue, fever, depression, psychosis, somnolence
Dermatologic: Skin rash, pruritus, alopecia, erythema multiforme, urticaria, photosensitivity, Stevens-Johnson syndrome, angioedema, hives; mild pain, burning, stinging (ointment); alopecia, dry lips, toxic epidermal necrolysis
Gastrointestinal: Nausea, vomiting, diarrhea, abdominal pain, anorexia, GI distress
Hematologic: Bone marrow suppression, neutropenia, thrombotic thrombocytopenic purpura/hemolytic uremic syndrome, anemia, leukocytoclastic vasculitis, leukocytosis, leukopenia, neutrophilia, thrombocytopenia, thrombocytosis
Hepatic: Liver enzymes elevated, hepatitis, jaundice, hyperbilirubinemia
Local: Phlebitis at injection site, tissue necrosis upon extravasation, local pain and stinging with topical use
Neuromuscular & skeletal: Tremulousness, myalgia, paresthesia, dysarthria, tremor
Ocular: Visual disturbance
Renal: Nephrotoxicity, hematuria, BUN and serum creatinine elevated, acute renal failure, renal pain
Respiratory: Sore throat
Miscellaneous: Diaphoresis, anaphylaxis, lymphadenopathy

Drug Interactions
Avoid Concomitant Use
Avoid concomitant use of Acyclovir with any of the following: Zoster Vaccine

Increased Effect/Toxicity
Acyclovir may increase the levels/effects of: Mycophenolate; Tenofovir; Zidovudine

The levels/effects of Acyclovir may be increased by: Mycophenolate

Decreased Effect
Acyclovir may decrease the levels/effects of: Zoster Vaccine

Food Interactions Food does not appear to affect absorption

Stability Incompatible with blood products and protein-containing solutions; reconstitute with SWI 10 mL to a concentration of 50 mg/mL; solution should be used within 12 hours; do not refrigerate reconstituted solutions or solutions for infusion as they may precipitate. Do not use bacteriostatic water-containing benzyl alcohol or parabens to reconstitute. For I.V. infusion, dilute in D_5W, D_5NS, $D_5\frac{1}{4}NS$, $D_5\frac{1}{2}NS$, LR, or NS to a final concentration ≤7 mg/mL; concentrations >10 mg/mL increase the risk of phlebitis

Mechanism of Action Inhibits DNA synthesis and viral replication by competing with deoxyguanosine triphosphate for viral DNA polymerase and by incorporation into viral DNA

Pharmacokinetics (Adult data unless noted)
Absorption: Oral: 15% to 30%
Distribution: Widely distributed throughout the body including brain, kidney, lungs, liver, spleen, muscle, uterus, vagina, and the CSF; CSF acyclovir concentration is 50% of serum concentration; crosses the placenta; excreted into breast milk
V_d:
Neonates to 3 months of age: 28.8 L/1.73 m^2
Children 1-2 years: 31.6 L/1.73 m^2
Children 2-7 years: 42 L/1.73 m^2

Protein binding: <30%

Half-life, terminal phase:

Neonates: 4 hours

Children 1-12 years: 2-3 hours

Adults: 2-3.5 hours (with normal renal function)

Time to peak serum concentration: Oral: Within 1.5-2 hours

Elimination: Primary route is the kidney with 30% to 90% of a dose excreted unchanged in the urine; requires dosage adjustment with renal impairment; hemodialysis removes ~60% of a dose while removal by peritoneal dialysis is to a much lesser extent; supplemental dose recommended after hemodialysis

Usual Dosage

Genital herpes simplex virus (HSV): First infection:

Oral:

Children: 40-80 mg/kg/day in 3-4 divided doses for 5-10 days; maximum dose: 1 g/day

Adolescents and Adults: 200 mg 5 times/day or 400 mg 3 times/day for 5-10 days

I.V.: Children and Adults: 5 mg/kg/dose every 8 hours for 5-7 days

Genital HSV infection: Recurrence: Oral: Adolescents and Adults: 200 mg 5 times/day or 400 mg 3 times/day for 5 days

Recurrent genital and cutaneous (ocular) HSV episodes in a patient with frequent recurrences, chronic suppressive therapy: Oral:

Children: 40-80 mg/kg/day in 3 divided doses for up to 12 months; maximum dose: 1 g/day; re-evaluate after 12 months of treatment

Adolescents and Adults: 400 mg twice daily or 400 mg 3 times/day or 200 mg 3 times/day for as long as 12 continuous months; re-evaluate after 12 months of treatment

HSV in immunocompromised host:

Oral:

Children:1000 mg/day in 3-5 divided doses for 7-14 days; maximum dose: 80 mg/kg/day not to exceed 1 g/day

Adults: 400 mg 5 times/day for 7-14 days

I.V.:

Children <12 years: 10 mg/kg/dose every 8 hours for 7-14 days

Children ≥12 years and Adults: 5 mg/kg/dose every 8 hours for 7-14 days

Prophylaxis of HSV in immunocompromised host:

Oral: Children and Adults: 600-1000 mg/day in 3-5 divided doses during period of risk; maximum dose in children: 80 mg/kg/day not to exceed 1 g/day

HSV encephalitis: I.V.:

Children 3 months to 12 years: 20 mg/kg/dose every 8 hours; some clinicians recommend 500 mg/m^2/dose every 8 hours for 14-21 days

Children >12 years and Adults: 10-15 mg/kg/dose every 8 hours for 14-21 days

Neonatal HSV: I.V.: 20 mg/kg/dose every 8 hours for 14-21 days

Varicella-zoster in immunocompromised host: I.V.:

Note: The AIDS*info* guidelines' recommended duration of therapy is 7-10 days or until no new lesions for 48 hours (for patients with mild varicella and no or moderate immune suppression).

Infants <1 year: 10 mg/kg/dose every 8 hours for 7-10 days or until no new lesions for 48 hours

Children ≥1 year: 500 mg/m^2/dose or 10 mg/kg/dose every 8 hours for 7-10 days or until no new lesions for 48 hours for 7-10 days

Adolescents and Adults: 10-15 mg/kg/dose every 8 hours for 7-10 days

Manufacturer's labeling:

Children <12 years: 20 mg/kg/dose every 8 hours for 7 days

Children ≥12 years and Adults: 10 mg/kg/dose every 8 hours for 7 days

Varicella in immunocompetent host: Oral (initiate treatment within the first 24 hours of rash onset):

Children ≥2 years and ≤40 kg: 20 mg/kg/dose 4 times/day for 5 days; maximum dose: 3200 mg/day

Children >40 kg and Adults: 800 mg 4 times/day for 5 days

Zoster in immunocompetent host: Oral (initiate treatment within 48 hours of rash onset): Children ≥12 years and Adults: 800 mg 5 times/day for 7-10 days

Prophylaxis of HSV in HSCT recipients (seropositive): I.V.:

Children: 250 mg/m^2/dose every 8 hours or 125 mg/m^2/dose every 6 hours

Adults:

Oral 200 mg 3 times/day

I.V.: 250 mg/m^2/dose every 12 hours (per CDC 2000 guidelines)

Children and Adults: Topical: Apply 1/2" ribbon of ointment for a 4" square surface area every 3 hours (6 times/day) for 7 days

Dosing interval in renal impairment:

Neonates: I.V.:

S_{cr} 0.8-1.1 mg/dL: Administer 20 mg/kg/dose every 12 hours

S_{cr} 1.2-1.5 mg/dL: Administer 20 mg/kg/dose every 24 hours

S_{cr} >1.5 mg/dL: Administer 10 mg/kg/dose every 24 hours

Children ≥6 months and Adults:

Oral: See table.

Usual Dose	Creatinine Clearance	Adjusted Dose
200 mg 5 times/day	Cl_{cr} <10 mL/minute	Administer 200 mg q12h
400 mg q12h	Cl_{cr} <10 mL/minute	Administer 200 mg q12h
800 mg 5 times/day	Cl_{cr} 10-25 mL/minute	Administer 800 mg q8h
	Cl_{cr} <10 mL/minute	Administer 800 mg q12h

I.V.:

Cl_{cr} 25-50 mL/minute: Administer normal dose every 12 hours

Cl_{cr} 10-25 mL/minute: Administer normal dose every 24 hours

Cl_{cr} <10 mL/minute: 50% decrease in dose, administer every 24 hours

Hemodialysis: Administer dose after dialysis

CVVHD/CVVH: Adjust dose based upon Cl_{cr} 30 mL/minute

Administration

Oral: May administer with food; shake suspension well before use

Parenteral: Reconstitute vial for injection with paraben-free SWI; administer by slow I.V. infusion over at least 1 hour at a final concentration not to exceed 7 mg/mL since rapid infusions can cause nephrotoxicity and renal tubular damage; in patients who require fluid restriction, a concentration of up to 10 mg/mL has been infused; concentration >10 mg/mL increases the risk of phlebitis. Avoid I.M. or SubQ administration.

Monitoring Parameters Urinalysis, BUN, serum creatinine, I & O; liver enzymes, CBC; neutrophil count at least twice weekly in neonates receiving acyclovir 60 mg/kg/day I.V.

Nursing Implications Maintain adequate hydration and urine output the first 2 hours after I.V. infusion to decrease the risk of nephrotoxicity; check infusion site for phlebitis; avoid extravasation

Additional Information Sodium content of 1 g: 4.2 mEq

Dosage Forms Excipient information presented when available (limited, particularly for generics); consult specific product labeling.
Capsule: 200 mg
  Zovirax®: 200 mg
Cream, topical:
  Zovirax®: 5% (2 g, 5 g)
Injection, powder for reconstitution, as sodium: 500 mg [base strength], 1000 mg [base strength]
Injection, solution, as sodium [preservative free]: 50 mg/mL (10 mL, 20 mL) [base strength]
Ointment, topical:
  Zovirax®: 5% (15 g)
Suspension, oral: 200 mg/5 mL (480 mL)
  Zovirax®: 200 mg/5 mL (480 mL) [banana flavor]
Tablet: 400 mg, 800 mg
  Zovirax®: 400 mg, 800 mg

References

American Academy of Pediatrics Committee on Infectious Diseases, "The Use of Oral Acyclovir in Otherwise Healthy Children With Varicella," *Pediatrics*, 1993, 91(3):674-6.

American Academy of Pediatrics, *Red Book®, 2003 Report of the Committee on Infectious Diseases*, 26th ed, Pickering LK ed, Elk Grove Village, IL: American Academy of Pediatrics, 2003, 729-30.

Desparmet J, Meistelman C, Barre J, et al, "Continuous Epidural Infusion of Bupivacaine for Postoperative Pain Relief in Children," *Anesthesiology*, 1987, 67(1):108-10.

Dunkle LM, Arvin AM, Whitley RJ, et al, "A Controlled Trial of Acyclovir for Chickenpox in Normal Children," *N Engl J Med*, 1991, 325 (22):1539-44.

Englund JA, Fletcher CV, and Balfour HH Jr, "Acyclovir Therapy in Neonates," *J Pediatr*, 1991, 119(1 Pt 1):129-35.

"Guidelines for Prevention and Treatment of Opportunistic Infections Among HIV-Exposed and HIV-Infected Children," June 20, 2008; available at http://aidsinfo.nih.gov.

"Guidelines for Prevention and Treatment of Opportunistic Infections in HIV-Infected Adults and Adolescents," June 18, 2008; available at http://aidsinfo.nih.gov.

Kimberlin DW, Lin CY, Jacobs RF, et al, "Safety and Efficacy of High-Dose Intravenous Acyclovir in the Management of Neonatal Herpes Simplex Virus Infections," *Pediatrics*, 2001, 108(2):230-8.

Meyers JD, Reed EC, Shepp DH, et al, "Acyclovir for Prevention of Cytomegalovirus Infection and Disease After Allogenic Marrow Transplantation," *N Engl J Med*, 1988, 318(2):70-5.

Novelli VM, Marshall WC, Yeo J, et al, "High-Dose Oral Acyclovir for Children at Risk of Disseminated Herpes Virus Infections," *J Infect Dis*, 1985, 151(2):372.

♦ **Aczone®** *see* Dapsone *on page 387*

♦ **Adacel®** *see* Diphtheria, Tetanus Toxoids, and Acellular Pertussis Vaccine *on page 458*

♦ **Adalat® XL® (Can)** *see* NIFEdipine *on page 991*

♦ **Adalat® CC** *see* NIFEdipine *on page 991*

Adalimumab (a da LIM yoo mab)

Medication Safety Issues
Sound-alike/look-alike issues:
Humira® may be confused with Humulin®, Humalog®
Humira® Pen may be confused with HumaPen® Memoir®

U.S. Brand Names Humira®
Canadian Brand Names Humira®
Therapeutic Category Antirheumatic, Disease Modifying; Gastrointestinal Agent, Miscellaneous; Monoclonal Antibody; Tumor Necrosis Factor (TNF) Blocking Agent
Generic Available No
Use Treatment of moderately- to severely-active polyarticular juvenile idiopathic arthritis (JIA) alone or in combination with methotrexate (FDA approved in ages >4 years); moderately- to severely-active rheumatoid arthritis (RA) alone or in combination with methotrexate or other disease-modifying antirheumatic drugs (DMARDs) (FDA approved in adults); active psoriatic arthritis alone or in combination with DMARDs (FDA approved in adults); ankylosing spondylitis (FDA approved in adults); treatment of moderately- to severely-active Crohn's disease in patients with inadequate response to conventional treatment or patients who have lost response to or are intolerant of infliximab (FDA approved in adults); treatment of moderate to severe plaque psoriasis (FDA approved in adults). Has been used in children with idiopathic or JIA-associated uveitis, chronic uveitis, and for treatment of moderately- to severely-active Crohn's disease with inadequate response to conventional treatment.

Medication Guide An FDA-approved patient medication guide, which is available with the product information and at http://www.fda.gov/downloads/Drugs/DrugSafety/ucm088611.pdf, must be dispensed with this medication for each new outpatient prescription and refill.

Pregnancy Risk Factor B

Pregnancy Considerations Teratogenic effects were not observed in animal studies, however, there are no adequate and well-controlled studies in pregnant women. Use during pregnancy only if clearly needed. A pregnancy registry has been established to monitor outcomes of women exposed to adalimumab during pregnancy (877-311-8972).

Lactation Excretion in breast milk unknown/not recommended

Breast-Feeding Considerations It is not known whether adalimumab is secreted in human milk. Because many immunoglobulins are secreted in milk and the potential for serious adverse reactions exists, a decision should be made whether to discontinue nursing or discontinue the drug, taking into account the importance of the drug to the mother.

Contraindications Hypersensitivity to adalimumab or any component

Warnings Serious and potentially fatal infections have been reported with use [**U.S. Boxed Warning**]; reported infections include tuberculosis (TB), bacterial sepsis, invasive fungal infections (such as histoplasmosis), and infections due to other opportunistic pathogens. Adalimumab should be discontinued if a patient develops a serious infection or sepsis during treatment. Caution should be exercised when considering the use in patients with chronic infection, history of recurrent infection, or predisposition to infection. In patients receiving TNF-blocking agents, other commonly reported opportunist pathogens include aspergillosis, candidiasis, coccidioidomycosis, listeriosis, and pneumocystosis. Patients frequently present with disseminated disease rather than localized and concomitant immunosuppressive therapy (eg, methotrexate or corticosteroids) is often present. Do not initiate therapy in patients with active chronic or localized infection.

Tuberculosis (disseminated or extrapulmonary) has been reported in patients receiving etanercept; most cases have been reported within the first 8 months of treatment; higher than recommended doses of adalimumab are associated with increased risk for reactivation; use with caution in patients who have resided in regions where tuberculosis is endemic. Perform test for latent TB before use; if positive, start treatment for TB prior to starting adalimumab, monitor all patients for active TB during treatment, even if initial latent TB is negative [**U.S. Boxed Warning**].

In children and adolescents, lymphomas and other malignancies, some fatal, have been reported with use of TNF blockers [**U.S. Boxed Warning**]. Use may affect defenses against malignancies; impact on the development and course of malignancies is not fully defined. In an analysis of children and adolescents who had received TNF blockers (etanercept and infliximab), the FDA identified 48 cases of malignancy. Of the 48 cases, ~50% were lymphomas (eg, Hodgkin's and non-Hodgkin's lymphoma). Other malignancies such as leukemia, melanoma, and solid organ tumors were reported;

malignancies rarely seen in children (eg, leiomyosarcoma, hepatic malignancies, and renal cell carcinoma) were also observed. Of note, most of these cases (88%) were receiving other immunosuppressive medications (eg, azathioprine and methotrexate). A higher incidence of nonmelanoma skin cancers was noted in adalimumab-treated patients (0.9/100 patient years), when compared to the control group (0.3/100 patient years). As compared to the general population, an increased risk of lymphoma has been noted in clinical trials; however, rheumatoid arthritis has been previously associated with an increased rate of lymphoma. The role of TNF blockers in the development of malignancies in children cannot be excluded. The FDA also reviewed 147 postmarketing reports of leukemia (including acute myeloid leukemia, chronic lymphocytic leukemia, and chronic myeloid leukemia) in patients (children and adults) using TNF blockers. Average onset time to development of leukemia was within the first 1-2 years of TNF blocker initiation. Although most patients were receiving other immunosuppressive agents, the role of TNF blockers in the development of leukemia could not be excluded. The FDA concluded that there is a possible association with the development of leukemia and the use of TNF blockers. Patients should be monitored closely for signs and symptoms suggestive of malignancy, evidence of which should result in prompt discontinuation of the medication and appropriate diagnostic evaluation.

May also cause new-onset psoriasis. Analysis by the FDA identified 69 cases of new-onset psoriasis (including pustular, palmoplantar) occurring in patients using TNF blockers for the treatment of conditions other than psoriasis and psoriatic arthritis. Of the 69 cases, two were reported in children and 12 required hospitalization, the most severe outcome. Improvement was seen when the TNF blocker was discontinued. The FDA concluded that there is a possible association with new-onset psoriasis and the use of TNF blockers. Patients should be monitored closely for signs and symptoms suggestive of new-onset psoriasis, evidence of which should result in prompt discontinuation of the medication and appropriate diagnostic evaluation.

May rarely cause hypersensitivity reactions; anaphylaxis and angioneurotic edema have been reported. Therapy should be immediately discontinued and appropriate therapy initiated if anaphylactic or other serious allergic reaction occurs.

Rare reactivation of hepatitis B virus (HBV) has occurred in chronic HBV carriers; evaluate prior to initiation, during, and for several months after treatment. Determine status of patients at risk for HBV infection prior starting therapy.

Precautions Use of TNF-blocking agents has been associated with rare cases of new onset or exacerbation of demyelinating disease; caution should be used in patients with pre-existing or recent onset CNS demyelinating disorders. Rare cases of pancytopenia (including aplastic anemia) have been reported with TNF-blocking agents. Avoid concomitant use with anakinra (interleukin-1 antagonist); serious infections have been reported with other TNF-blockers (etanercept) when used with anakinra without added clinical benefit versus TNF-blocker used alone. Caution should be exercised in patients with congestive heart failure (CHF) or decreased left ventricular function; worsening or new onset CHF have been reported with TNF blockers. Patients should be brought up to date with all immunizations before initiating therapy; live vaccines should not be given concurrently. There are no data available concerning secondary transmission of infection from live vaccine in patients receiving adalimumab. Positive antinuclear antibody titers have been detected in patients (with negative baselines); rare cases of autoimmune disorder, including lupus-like syndrome,

have been reported; monitor and discontinue if symptoms develop. The needle cover of syringe contains latex; patients with latex allergy should avoid contact.

Adverse Reactions

Cardiovascular: Hypertension

Central nervous system: Headache

Dermatologic: Granuloma annulare, psoriasis (including new onset, palmoplantar, pustular, or exacerbation) (see Warnings), rash

Endocrine & metabolic: Hypercholesterolemia, hyperlipidemia, metrorrhagia

Gastrointestinal: Abdominal pain, appendicitis, nausea

Genitourinary: UTI

Hematologic: Neutropenia

Hepatic: Alkaline phosphatase increased, ALT and AST increased

Local: Injection site reaction (may include erythema, hemorrhage, itching, pain, swelling)

Neuromuscular & skeletal: Back pain, CPK increased, myositis

Renal: Hematuria

Respiratory: Pharyngitis (streptococcal), sinusitis, URI

Miscellaneous: Accidental injury; antibodies to adalimumab; carcinoma (including breast, gastrointestinal, lymphoma, skin, urogenital) (see Warnings); flu-like syndrome; herpes zoster; hypersensitivity reactions; infections (bacterial, viral, fungal and protozoal) (see Warnings); positive ANA; tuberculosis (reactivation of latent infection; miliary, lymphatic, peritoneal,and pulmonary)

<5%, postmarketing, and/or case reports: Adenoma, agranulocytosis, allergic reactions, anaphylactoid reaction, anaphylaxis, angioneurotic edema, aplastic anemia, arrhythmia, arthralgia, arthritis, asthma, atrial fibrillation, bone fracture, bone necrosis, bronchospasm, CAD, cardiac arrest, cataract, cellulitis, chest pain, CHF, cholecystitis, cholelithiasis, confusion, cutaneous vasculitis, cystitis, cytopenia, dehydration, diverticulitis, dyspnea, erysipelas, erythema multiforme, esophagitis, fever, fixed drug eruption, gastroenteritis, gastrointestinal hemorrhage, granulocytopenia, Gullian-Barré syndrome, hepatic necrosis, hypertensive encephalopathy, interstitial lung disease (eg, pulmonary fibrosis), intestinal perforation, joint disorder, ketosis, kidney calculus, leukemias, leukopenia, lung function decreased, lupus erythematosus syndrome, melanoma, menstrual disorder, MI, muscle cramps, multiple sclerosis, myasthenia, pain in extremity, palpitation, pancytopenia, paraproteinemia, parathyroid disorder, paresthesia, pelvic pain, pericardial effusion, pericarditis, peripheral edema, pleural effusion, pneumonia, polycythemia, postsurgical infection, pyelonephritis, pyogenic arthritis, sepsis, septic arthritis, subdural hematoma, syncope, synovitis, tachycardia, tendon disorder, thrombocytopenia, thrombosis (leg), tremor, vascular disorder, vomiting

Drug Interactions

Avoid Concomitant Use

Avoid concomitant use of Adalimumab with any of the following: Abatacept; Anakinra; BCG; Canakinumab; Certolizumab Pegol; Natalizumab; Pimecrolimus; Rilonacept; Tacrolimus (Topical); Vaccines (Live)

Increased Effect/Toxicity Concomitant use with anakinra may increase risk of infections; not recommended.

Decreased Effect Concomitant use with vaccines (live) has not be studied; currently recommended not to administer live vaccines during adalimumab therapy.

Stability Store under refrigeration at 2°C to 8°C (36°F to 46°F); do not freeze. Protect from light.

Mechanism of Action Adalimumab binds to TNF-alpha and blocks its interaction with cell surface TNF receptors rendering TNF biologically inactive; modulates biological responses that are induced or regulated by TNF.

Pharmacokinetics (Adult data unless noted)
Distribution: V_d: 4.7-6 L; synovial fluid concentrations: 31% to 96% of serum
Bioavailability: Absolute: 64%
Half-life: ~2 weeks (range: 10-20 days)
Time to peak serum concentration: SubQ: 131 ± 56 hours
Elimination: Clearance increased in the presence of antiadalimumab antibodies; decreased in patients ≥40 years

Usual Dosage SubQ:
Children:
Juvenile idiopathic arthritis: ≥4 years:
15 kg to <30 kg: 20 mg every other week
≥30 kg: 40 mg every other week
Crohn's disease/ ulcerative colitis: 9-18 years: Limited data available; dose not established; additional clinical trials ongoing (see Noe, 2008; Rosh, 2009; Viola 2009; Wyneski, 2008)
Induction:
<40 kg: 80 mg on day 1 followed by 40 mg on day 14
>40 kg: 160 mg on day 1 followed by 80 mg on day 14
Maintenance dose: Start 2 weeks after induction completed: 20-40 mg every other week. If needed, dose may be increased by decreasing frequency to every week.
Uveitis: >4 years: Limited data available; dose not established (see Biester, 2007; Tynjala, 2008)
<30 kg: 20 mg every other week
>30 kg: 40 mg every other week
Adults:
Rheumatoid arthritis: 40 mg every other week; may be administered with other DMARDs; patients not taking methotrexate may increase dose to 40 mg every week
Ankylosing spondylitis, psoriatic arthritis: 40 mg every other week
Crohn's disease: Initial: 160 mg given as 4 injections on day 1 or over 2 days, then 80 mg 2 weeks later (day 15); maintenance: 40 mg every other week beginning day 29
Plaque psoriasis: Initial: 80 mg as a single dose; maintenance: 40 mg every other week beginning 1 week after initial dose

Administration For SubQ injection; rotate injection sites. Do not use if solution is discolored. Do not administer to skin which is red, tender, bruised, or hard; rotate injection sites. To reduce pain of injection, some centers use 0.2 mL of 1% lidocaine and add adalimumab dose to the lidocaine syringe swirling gently to mix contents prior to administration (see Ayala, 2008).

Monitoring Parameters Place and read PPD before initiation. Monitor improvement of symptoms and physical function assessments; CBC; signs of infection, bleeding, or bruising.

Patient Information May cause headache, nausea, or stomach pain. Notify prescriber of any signs of infection. If self-administered, follow directions for injection and needle/syringe disposal exactly. You may be more susceptible to infection. Do not have any vaccinations while using this medication without consulting prescriber first. Report persistent fever, increased bruising or bleeding, respiratory tract infection, unhealed or infected wounds, urinary tract infection, flu-like symptoms, unexplained weight loss, persistent cough, or unusual bump or sore that does not heal. Stop drug and report immediately persistent nausea, abdominal pain; numbness or tingling; problems with vision; weakness in legs; chest pains; respiratory difficulty; sudden weight gain of >3-5 pounds/ week; swelling of extremities; joint pain; skin rash; redness, swelling, or pain at injection site.

Nursing Implications Perform tuberculin skin test prior to initiating therapy. Monitor for signs of tuberculosis throughout therapy. Do not initiate therapy if active infection (underlying chronic or localized infection) is occurring. Monitor for signs and symptoms of infection. Assess for liver dysfunction. Assess potential for interactions with other prescriptions, OTC medications, and herbal products patient may be taking. Assess results of laboratory tests (PDD), therapeutic effectiveness, and adverse response at regular intervals during treatment. Teach patient proper use if self-injected (appropriate injection technique and syringe/needle disposal), possible side effects/appropriate interventions, and adverse symptoms to report. Latex-sensitive patients: Needle cap of prefilled syringe contains latex.

Additional Information A pregnancy registry has been established to monitor outcomes of women exposed to adalimumab during pregnancy (877-311-8972).

Dosage Forms Excipient information presented when available (limited, particularly for generics); consult specific product labeling.
Injection, solution [pediatric; preservative free]:
Humira®: 20 mg/0.4 mL (0.4 mL) [contains polysorbate 80]
Injection, solution [preservative free]:
Humira®: 40 mg/0.8 mL (0.8 mL) [contains polysorbate 80]

References
Ayala RS, Groh BP, Robbins LM, et al, "The Addition of Injectable Lidocaine to Adalimumab Results in Decreased Injection Site Pain and Increased Acceptance of Therapy," 2008, American College of Rheumatology Annual Scientific Meeting, San Francisco, CA (poster).

Biester S, Deuter C, Michels H, et al, "Adalimumab in the Therapy of Uveitis in Childhood," Br J Ophthalmol, 2007, 91(3):319-24.

Furst DE, Keystone EC, Kirkham B, et al, "Updated Consensus Statement on Biological Agents for the Treatment of Rheumatic Diseases, 2008," Ann Rheum Dis, 2008, 67 Suppl 3:iii2-25.

Lovell DJ, Ruperto N, Goodman S, et al, "Adalimumab With or Without Methotrexate in Juvenile Rheumatoid Arthritis," N Engl J Med, 2008, 359(8):810-20.

Noe JD and Pfefferkorn M, "Short-Term Response to Adalimumab in Childhood Inflammatory Bowel Disease," Inflamm Bowel Dis, 2008, 14(12):1683-7.

Rosh JR, Lerer T, Markowitz J, et al, "Retrospective Evaluation of the Safety and Effect of Adalimumab Therapy (RESEAT) in Pediatric Crohn's Disease," Am J Gastroenterol, 2009, 104(12):3042-9.

Tynjälä P, Kotaniemi K, Lindahl P, et al, "Adalimumab in Juvenile Idiopathic Arthritis-Associated Chronic Anterior Uveitis," Rheumatology (Oxford), 2008, 47(3):339-44.

Viola F, Civitelli F, Di Nardo G, et al, "Efficacy of Adalimumab in Moderate-to-Severe Pediatric Crohn's Disease," Am J Gastroenterol, 2009, 104(10):2566-71.

Wyneski MJ, Green A, Kay M, et al, "Safety and Efficacy of Adalimumab in Pediatric Patients With Crohn Disease," J Pediatr Gastroenterol Nutr, 2008, 47(1):19-25.

♦ **Adamantanamine Hydrochloride** see Amantadine on page 77

Adapalene (a DAP a leen)

U.S. Brand Names Differin®
Canadian Brand Names Differin®; Differin® XP
Therapeutic Category Acne Products
Generic Available Yes: Gel
Use Topical treatment of acne vulgaris
Pregnancy Risk Factor C
Pregnancy Considerations There are no adequate and well-controlled studies in pregnant women. Use only if benefit outweighs the potential risk to fetus.
Lactation Excretion in breast milk unknown/use caution
Contraindications Hypersensitivity to adapalene or any component; sunburn
Warnings Avoid excessive exposure to sunlight and sunlamps; avoid contact with abraded skin, mucous membranes, eyes, mouth, or angles of the nose
Precautions Use with caution in patients with eczema

Adverse Reactions
Dermatologic: Erythema, scaling, dry skin, skin irritation, pruritus, acne flares, photosensitivity, sunburn, skin discoloration

Local: Pruritus or burning immediately after application

Ophthalmic: Eyelid edema, conjunctivitis

Drug Interactions
Avoid Concomitant Use There are no known interactions where it is recommended to avoid concomitant use.

Increased Effect/Toxicity
The levels/effects of Adapalene may be increased by: Vitamin A

Decreased Effect
Adapalene may decrease the levels/effects of: Contraceptives (Progestins)

Stability Store at controlled room temperature

Mechanism of Action Retinoid-like compound which is a modulator of cellular differentiation, keratinization, and inflammatory processes, all of which represent important features in the pathology of acne vulgaris

Pharmacodynamics Onset of action: 8-12 weeks

Pharmacokinetics (Adult data unless noted)
Absorption: Absorption through the skin is very low; only trace amounts have been measured in serum after chronic application

Elimination: Primarily in bile

Usual Dosage Topical: Children >12 years and Adults: Apply topically once daily in the evening

Administration Topical: After cleansing the affected area with mild or soapless cleanser, using gloves, apply a thin film of medication (cream or gel) before retiring in the evening. Avoid contact with eyes, angles of the nose, lips and mucous membranes.

Monitoring Parameters Reduction in lesion size and/or inflammation; reduction in the number of lesions

Patient Information For external use only; apply using gloves; avoid contact with eyes, mouth, mucous membranes, or open wounds. Do not apply occlusive dressing. Moisturizers may be used if necessary; however, products containing alpha hydroxy or glycolic acids should be avoided. Wax epilation should not be performed on treated skin due to the potential for skin erosions. Transient burning or stinging immediately after applying may occur. Mild to moderate redness, dryness, scaling, burning or itching are likely to occur during the first 2-4 weeks and will usually lessen with continued use; report worsening of condition or skin redness, dryness, peeling, or burning that persists between applications to the healthcare provider. May cause photosensitivity reactions (eg, exposure to sunlight may cause severe sunburn, skin rash, redness, or itching); avoid exposure to sunlight and artificial light sources (sunlamps, tanning booth/bed); wear protective clothing, wide-brimmed hats, sunglasses, and lip sunscreen (SPF ≥15); use a sunscreen [broad-spectrum sunscreen or physical sunscreen (preferred) or sunblock with SPF ≥15]; contact physician if reaction occurs.

Dosage Forms Excipient information presented when available (limited, particularly for generics); consult specific product labeling.

Cream, topical:
Differin®: 0.1% (15 g, 45 g)

Gel, topical: 0.1% (45 g)
Differin®: 0.1% (15 g, 45 g) [alcohol free]; 0.3% (45 g) [alcohol free]

◆ **Addaprin [OTC]** *see* Ibuprofen *on page 702*

◆ **Adderall®** *see* Dextroamphetamine and Amphetamine *on page 418*

◆ **Adderall XR®** *see* Dextroamphetamine and Amphetamine *on page 418*

◆ **Adenocard®** *see* Adenosine *on page 51*

◆ **Adenoscan®** *see* Adenosine *on page 51*

Adenosine (a DEN oh seen)

Medication Safety Issues
High alert medication: The Institute for Safe Medication Practices (ISMP) includes this medication among its list of drugs which have a heightened risk of causing significant patient harm when used in error.

Related Information
Adult ACLS Algorithms *on page 1463*
CPR Pediatric Drug Dosages *on page 1455*
Pediatric ALS Algorithms *on page 1460*

U.S. Brand Names Adenocard®; Adenoscan®

Canadian Brand Names Adenocard®; Adenoscan®; Adenosine Injection, USP

Therapeutic Category Antiarrhythmic Agent, Miscellaneous

Generic Available Yes

Use Treatment of paroxysmal supraventricular tachycardia (PSVT); used in adult ACLS algorithms for narrow-complex tachycardias, stable narrow-complex supraventricular tachycardias, and wide-complex tachycardias that are supraventricular in origin; used in PALS algorithms for probable supraventricular tachycardia; investigationally used as a continuous infusion for the treatment of primary pulmonary hypertension in adults and persistent pulmonary hypertension of the newborn (PPHN) (see Additional Information)

Pregnancy Risk Factor C

Pregnancy Considerations Animal reproduction studies have not been conducted. Adenosine is an endogenous substance and adverse fetal effects would not be anticipated. Case reports of administration during pregnancy have indicated no adverse effects on fetus or newborn attributable to adenosine.

Lactation Excretion in breast milk unknown

Contraindications Hypersensitivity to adenosine or any component; second and third degree A-V block or sick sinus syndrome unless pacemaker placed

Warnings Heart block, including transient or prolonged asystole may occur as well as other arrhythmias; episodes of asystole or other arrhythmias may be fatal; if arrhythmia is not due to re-entry pathway through A-V node or sinus node (ie, atrial fibrillation, flutter, or tachycardia or ventricular tachycardia), adenosine will not terminate the arrhythmia but can produce transient ventriculoatrial or A-V block; possible mutagenic effects

Precautions Bronchoconstriction may occur in asthmatics (avoid use in patients with bronchospasm or bronchoconstriction); use with caution in patients with underlying dysfunction of sinus or A-V node, obstructive lung disease, and those taking digoxin or verapamil; initial adenosine dose should be significantly decreased in patients receiving dipyridamole

Adverse Reactions
Cardiovascular: Flushing, arrhythmias, palpitations, chest pain, bradycardia, heart block, minimal hemodynamic disturbances, hypotension (<1%)

Central nervous system: Irritability, headaches, lightheadedness, dizziness

Gastrointestinal: Nausea, metallic taste

Respiratory: Dyspnea, hyperventilation, bronchoconstriction in asthmatics

Drug Interactions
Avoid Concomitant Use There are no known interactions where it is recommended to avoid concomitant use.

Increased Effect/Toxicity
The levels/effects of Adenosine may be increased by: CarBAMazepine; Dipyridamole; Nicotine

Decreased Effect

The levels/effects of Adenosine may be decreased by: Theophylline Derivatives

Stability Do **not** refrigerate, precipitation may occur; contains no preservatives, discard unused portion

Mechanism of Action Slows conduction time through the A-V node, interrupting the re-entry pathways through the A-V node, restoring normal sinus rhythm

Pharmacodynamics

Onset of action: Rapid

Duration: Very brief

Pharmacokinetics (Adult data unless noted)

Metabolism: Removed from systemic circulation primarily by vascular endothelial cells and erythrocytes (by cellular uptake); rapidly metabolized intracellularly; phosphorylated by adenosine kinase to adenosine monophosphate (AMP) which is then incorporated into high-energy pool; intracellular adenosine is also deaminated by adenosine deaminase to inosine; inosine can be metabolized to hypoxanthine, then xanthine and finally to uric acid.

Half-life: <10 seconds

Usual Dosage Note: Adequate controlled studies in pediatric patients have not been conducted.

Manufacturer's recommendations: Rapid I.V.:

Neonates, Infants, Children, and Adolescents weighing <50 kg: Initial dose: 0.05-0.1 mg/kg; if not effective within 1-2 minutes, increase dose by 0.05-0.1 mg/kg increments every 1-2 minutes to a maximum single dose of 0.3 mg/kg or until termination of PSVT

Children and Adolescents weighing ≥50 kg and Adults: 6 mg, if not effective within 1-2 minutes, 12 mg may be given; may repeat 12 mg bolus if needed

Alternative pediatric dosing:

Neonates: Rapid I.V.: Initial dose: 0.05 mg/kg; if not effective within 2 minutes, increase dose by 0.05 mg/kg increments every 2 minutes to a maximum dose of 0.25 mg/kg or until termination of PSVT

Infants and Children: **PALS dose for treatment of SVT**: Rapid I.V.; I.O.: Initial: 0.1 mg/kg (maximum: 6 mg); if not effective, give 0.2 mg/kg (maximum: 12 mg)

Administration Parenteral: For rapid bolus I.V. use, administer over 1-2 seconds at peripheral I.V. site closest to patient's heart (I.V. administration into lower extremities may result in therapeutic failure or requirement of higher doses); follow each bolus with NS flush (infants and children: 5-10 mL; adults: 20 mL); if given peripherally in adults, elevate the extremity for 10-20 seconds after the NS flush. To administer doses <600 mcg (0.2 mL of commercial product), a dilution with NS (final concentration: 300 mcg/mL) may be made. **Note:** Preliminary results in adults suggest adenosine may be administered via a **central line** at lower doses (eg, Adults: Initial dose: 3 mg); FDA approved labeling for pediatric patients weighing <50 kg states that doses listed may be administered either peripherally or centrally (further studies are needed)

Monitoring Parameters Continuous ECG, heart rate, blood pressure, respirations

Nursing Implications Be alert for dyspnea, shortness of breath, and possible exacerbation of asthma

Additional Information Not effective in atrial flutter, atrial fibrillation, or ventricular tachycardia; short duration of action is an advantage as adverse effects are usually rapidly self-limiting; effects may be prolonged in patients with denervated transplanted hearts. Individualize treatment of prolonged adverse effects: Give I.V. fluids for hypotension, aminophylline/theophylline may antagonize effects.

Limited information is available regarding the use of adenosine for the treatment of persistent pulmonary hypertension of the newborn (PPHN); efficacy, optimal dose, and duration of therapy is not established; a randomized, masked, placebo-controlled pilot study of 18 term infants with PPHN used initial doses of 25 mcg/kg/minute (n=9); after 30 minutes, doses were increased to 50 mcg/kg/minute if no improvement in PaO$_2$ was observed; all patients received study drug via central line into the right atrium (inserted via the umbilical vein); significant improvement in oxygenation was observed in 4 of 9 newborns receiving 50 mcg/kg/minute; hypotension or tachycardia were not observed; further studies are needed (Kondur, 1996).

Adenosine is also available as Adenoscan®, which is used in adults as an adjunct to thallium-201 myocardial perfusion scintigraphy; see package insert for further information on this use.

Dosage Forms Excipient information presented when available (limited, particularly for generics); consult specific product labeling.

Injection, solution [preservative free]: 3 mg/mL (2 mL, 4 mL)

Adenocard®: 3 mg/mL (2 mL, 4 mL)

Adenoscan®: 3 mg/mL (20 mL, 30 mL)

References

Eubanks AP and Artman M, "Administration of Adenosine to a Newborn of 26 Weeks' Gestation," *Pediatr Cardiol*, 1994, 15(3):157-8.

"Guidelines 2000 for Cardiopulmonary Resuscitation and Emergency Cardiovascular Care, Part 6: Advanced Cardiovascular Life Support, The American Heart Association in Collaboration With the International Liaison Committee on Resuscitation," *Circulation*, 2000, 102(8 Suppl):I86-171.

"Guidelines 2000 for Cardiopulmonary Resuscitation and Emergency Cardiovascular Care, Part 10: Pediatric Advanced Life Support, The American Heart Association in Collaboration With the International Liaison Committee on Resuscitation," *Circulation*, 2000, 102(8 Suppl): I291-342.

Konduri GG, Garcia DC, Kazzi NJ, et al, "Adenosine Infusion Improves Oxygenation in Term Infants With Respiratory Failure," *Pediatrics*, 1996, 97(3):295-300.

McIntosh-Yellin NL, Drew BJ, and Scheinman MM, "Safety and Efficacy of Central Intravenous Bolus Administration of Adenosine for Termination of Supraventricular Tachycardia," *J Am Coll Cardiol*, 1993, 22(3):741-5.

Paul T and Pfammatter JP, "Adenosine: An Effective and Safe Antiarrhythmic Drug in Pediatrics," *Pediatr Cardiol*, 1997, 18 (2):118-26.

Sherwood MC, Lau KC, and Sholler GF, "Adenosine in the Management of Supraventricular Tachycardia in Children," *J Paediatr Child Health*, 1998, 34(1):53-6.

Till J, Shinebourne EA, Rigby ML, et al, "Efficacy and Safety in the Treatment of Supraventricular Tachycardia in Infants and Children," *Br Heart J*, 1989, 62(3):204-11.

Zeigler V, "Adenosine in the Pediatric Population: Nursing Implications," *Pediatr Nurs*, 1991, 17(6):600-2.

◆ **Adenosine Injection, USP (Can)** see Adenosine on page 51

◆ **ADH** see Vasopressin on page 1410

◆ **Adoxa®** see Doxycycline on page 479

◆ **Adrenaclick™** see EPINEPHrine on page 511

◆ **Adrenalin®** see EPINEPHrine on page 511

◆ **Adrenaline** see EPINEPHrine on page 511

◆ **Adrenocorticotropic Hormone** see Corticotropin on page 359

◆ **ADR (error-prone abbreviation)** see DOXOrubicin on page 477

◆ **Adria** see DOXOrubicin on page 477

◆ **Adriamycin®** see DOXOrubicin on page 477

◆ **Adrucil®** see Fluorouracil on page 598

◆ **Adsorbent Charcoal** see Charcoal, Activated on page 284

◆ **Advagraf™ (Can)** see Tacrolimus on page 1311

◆ **Advair® (Can)** see Fluticasone and Salmeterol on page 611

◆ **Advair Diskus®** *see* Fluticasone and Salmeterol *on page 611*

◆ **Advair® HFA** *see* Fluticasone and Salmeterol *on page 611*

◆ **Advate** *see* Antihemophilic Factor (Recombinant) *on page 112*

◆ **Advil® [OTC]** *see* Ibuprofen *on page 702*

◆ **Advil® (Can)** *see* Ibuprofen *on page 702*

◆ **Advil® Children's [OTC]** *see* Ibuprofen *on page 702*

◆ **Advil® Cold, Children's [OTC] [DSC]** *see* Pseudoephedrine and Ibuprofen *on page 1184*

◆ **Advil® Cold & Sinus [OTC]** *see* Pseudoephedrine and Ibuprofen *on page 1184*

◆ **Advil® Cold & Sinus (Can)** *see* Pseudoephedrine and Ibuprofen *on page 1184*

◆ **Advil® Infants' [OTC]** *see* Ibuprofen *on page 702*

◆ **Advil® Migraine [OTC]** *see* Ibuprofen *on page 702*

◆ **Aerius® (Can)** *see* Desloratadine *on page 403*

◆ **AeroBid®** *see* Flunisolide *on page 592*

◆ **AeroBid®-M** *see* Flunisolide *on page 592*

◆ **Afeditab® CR** *see* NIFEdipine *on page 991*

◆ **Afluria®** *see* Influenza Virus Vaccine (Inactivated) *on page 734*

◆ **Afrin® Extra Moisturizing [OTC]** *see* Oxymetazoline *on page 1043*

◆ **Afrin® Original [OTC]** *see* Oxymetazoline *on page 1043*

◆ **Afrin® Severe Congestion [OTC]** *see* Oxymetazoline *on page 1043*

◆ **Afrin® Sinus [OTC]** *see* Oxymetazoline *on page 1043*

Agalsidase Beta (aye GAL si days BAY ta)

Medication Safety Issues
Sound-alike/look-alike issues:
Agalsidase beta may be confused with agalsidase alfa, alglucerase, alglucosidase alfa

International issues:
Agalsidase beta may be confused with agalsidase alfa, which is available in international markets
U.S. Brand Names Fabrazyme®
Canadian Brand Names Fabrazyme®
Therapeutic Category Enzyme, α-galactosidase A; Fabry's Disease, Treatment Agent
Generic Available No
Use Treatment of Fabry's disease
Pregnancy Risk Factor B
Pregnancy Considerations Animal reproduction studies have not demonstrated adverse effects. There are no adequate and well-controlled studies in pregnant women. Women of childbearing potential are encouraged to enroll in Fabry registry.
Lactation Excretion in breast milk unknown/use caution
Breast-Feeding Considerations Nursing mothers are encouraged to enroll in Fabry registry.
Contraindications Hypersensitivity to agalsidase beta or any component
Warnings Infusion-related reactions (ranging from mild to severe) including fever, rigors, chest tightness, hypertension, hypotension, pruritus, myalgia, dyspnea, urticaria, abdominal pain, and headache have been reported; these reactions may be minimized by pretreatment with acetaminophen and an antihistamine; if an infusion related reaction occurs, regardless of pretreatment, decreasing the infusion rate, temporarily stopping the infusion, and/or additional administration of analgesics, antihistamines, or corticosteroids may ameliorate the reaction.

Precautions Use with caution in patients with compromised cardiac function (seen in advanced Fabry's disease) due to an increased potential for severe infusion related reactions; monitor these patients closely; patients may develop IgG antibodies to agalsidase beta
Adverse Reactions
Cardiovascular: Tachycardia, hypertension, hypotension, chest pain, chest tightness, bradycardia, arrhythmias, cardiac arrest, edema, pallor
Central nervous system: Headache, dizziness, fever, anxiety, depression, chills, rigors, vertigo
Dermatologic: Pruritus, urticaria
Gastrointestinal: Dyspepsia, nausea, abdominal pain, vomiting
Genitourinary: Testicular pain
Neuromuscular & skeletal: Arthrosis, skeletal pain, myalgia
Otic: Hypoacousia
Respiratory: Bronchitis, bronchospasm, laryngitis, pharyngitis, sinusitis, rhinitis, dyspnea
Miscellaneous: Hypersensitivity reactions
Drug Interactions
Avoid Concomitant Use
Avoid concomitant use of Agalsidase Beta with any of the following: Amiodarone; Chloroquine; Gentamicin; Gentamicin (Systemic)
Increased Effect/Toxicity There are no known significant interactions involving an increase in effect.
Decreased Effect
The levels/effects of Agalsidase Beta may be decreased by: Amiodarone; Chloroquine; Gentamicin; Gentamicin (Systemic)
Stability Store in refrigerator 2°C to 8°C (36°F to 46°F); reconstituted solution is stable for 24 hours refrigerated
Mechanism of Action Agalsidase beta is a recombinant human α-galactosidase A enzyme with the same amino acid sequence as the naturally-occurring enzyme. Fabry's disease is an X-linked genetic disorder occurring in 1 in 50,000 male births, which results in a deficiency of α-galactosidase A. Lack of this enzyme leads to a progressive accumulation of glycosphingolipids, predominantly GL-3, in the vascular endothelium, leading to ischemia and infarction, especially in the kidney, heart, and brain. Clinical manifestations of Fabry's disease in childhood include intermittent severe pain in the extremities, characteristic vascular skin lesions (angiokeratomas), corneal and lenticular opacities that do not affect vision, decreased ability to sweat, intolerance to heat, cold, and exercise, mild proteinuria, and GI problems. By adulthood, this progresses to renal failure, cardiomyopathy, and cerebrovascular accidents.
Pharmacokinetics (Adult data unless noted)
Distribution: V_d:
Children: 247-1097 mL/kg
Adults: 80-570 mL/kg
Half-life (dose dependent):
Children: 86-151 minutes
Adults: 45-102 minutes
Clearance:
Children: 1.1-5.8 mL/minute/kg
Adults: 0.8-4.9 mL/minute/kg
Usual Dosage I.V.: Children and Adults: 1 mg/kg/dose every two weeks
Administration I.V.: Reconstitute each 35 mg vial with 7.2 mL SWI and each 5 mg vial with 1.1 mL SWI to result in 5 mg/mL concentrations; swirl to dissolve; do not shake; further dilute dosage in NS (see chart on next page for dilution volumes). Initial infusion not to exceed 15 mg/hour (0.25 mg/minute); after patient tolerance to initial infusion rate is established, the infusion rate may be increased in increments of 3-5 mg/hour (0.05-0.08 mg/minute) with subsequent infusions. Per the manufacturer's recommendation: For patients weighing <30 kg, the maximum

infusion rate should remain at 0.25 mg/minute; for patients weighing >30 kg, the administration duration should not be less than 1.5 hours (based upon individual tolerability). An initial maximum infusion rate of 0.01 mg/minute should be used for rechallenge in patients with IgE antibodies; may increase infusion rate (doubling the infusion rate every 30 minutes) to a maximum rate of 0.25 mg/minute as tolerated. A 0.2 micron low protein-binding filter may be used during administration. Pretreatment with acetaminophen and an antihistamine is recommended to reduce infusion related side effects (see Warnings)

Recommended Minimum Volumes for Dilution

Patient Weight (kg)	Minimum Total Volume (mL)
<35	50
35.1-70	100
70.1-100	250
>100	500

Monitoring Parameters Vital signs during infusion; infusion-related reactions; globotriasylceramide (GL3) plasma levels; improvement in disease symptomatology
Reference Range Normal endogenous activity of alpha-galactosidase A in plasma is approximately 170 nmol/hour/mL; in patients with Fabry's disease this activity is <1.5 nmol/hour/mL

Normal (goal) globotriasylceramide (GL3) <1.2 ng/microliter
Additional Information Agalsidase beta is an orphan drug; a Fabry Patient Support Group (800-745-4447) is available to assist patients in obtaining reimbursement from private insurers, Medicare, and Medicaid, and a Charitable Access Program sponsored by Genzyme provides the drug gratis to those patients in need. Detailed information regarding organizations and websites is also available in the Expert Panel Recommendations (Desnick, 2003)
Dosage Forms Excipient information presented when available (limited, particularly for generics); consult specific product labeling.
Injection, powder for reconstitution:
Fabrazyme®: 5 mg [contains mannitol 33 mg; derived from Chinese hamster cells]; 35 mg [contains mannitol 222 mg; derived from Chinese hamster cells]
References
Desnick RJ, Brady R, Barranger J, et al, "Fabry Disease, an Under-Recognized Multisystemic Disorder: Expert Recommendations for Diagnosis, Management, and Enzyme Replacement Therapy," *Ann Intern Med*, 2003, 138(4):338-46.

◆ **AgNO₃** see Silver Nitrate *on page 1261*
◆ **Agriflu®** see Influenza Virus Vaccine (Inactivated) *on page 734*
◆ **AHF** see Antihemophilic Factor (Human) *on page 109*
◆ **AHF (Human)** see Antihemophilic Factor / von Willebrand Factor Complex (Human) *on page 114*
◆ **AHF (Recombinant)** see Antihemophilic Factor (Recombinant) *on page 112*
◆ **AHG** see Antihemophilic Factor (Human) *on page 109*
◆ **Ahist™** see Chlorpheniramine *on page 296*
◆ **A-hydroCort** see Hydrocortisone *on page 685*
◆ **A-Hydrocort®** see Hydrocortisone *on page 685*
◆ **AICC** see Anti-inhibitor Coagulant Complex *on page 117*
◆ **Airomir (Can)** see Albuterol *on page 57*
◆ **AK-Con™** see Naphazoline *on page 966*
◆ **AK-Dilate®** see Phenylephrine *on page 1102*

◆ **Akne-Mycin®** see Erythromycin *on page 525*
◆ **AK-Pentolate™** see Cyclopentolate *on page 368*
◆ **AK-Poly-Bac™** see Bacitracin and Polymyxin B *on page 170*
◆ **AK Sulf Liq (Can)** see Sulfacetamide *on page 1298*
◆ **Akten™** see Lidocaine *on page 818*
◆ **AK-Tob™** see Tobramycin *on page 1354*
◆ **Akurza [DSC]** see Salicylic Acid *on page 1241*
◆ **Alamag [OTC]** see Aluminum Hydroxide and Magnesium Hydroxide *on page 76*
◆ **Alamast®** see Pemirolast *on page 1075*
◆ **Alavert® Allergy 24 Hour [OTC]** see Loratadine *on page 842*
◆ **Alavert™ Allergy and Sinus [OTC]** see Loratadine and Pseudoephedrine *on page 844*
◆ **Alavert® Children's Allergy [OTC]** see Loratadine *on page 842*
◆ **Alaway™ [OTC]** see Ketotifen *on page 785*

Albendazole (al BEN da zole)

Medication Safety Issues
Sound-alike/look-alike issues:
Albenza® may be confused with Aplenzin™, Relenza®
International issues:
Albenza® may be confused with Avanza® which is a brand name for mirtazapine in Australia
U.S. Brand Names Albenza®
Therapeutic Category Anthelmintic
Generic Available No
Use Treatment of parenchymal neurocysticercosis due to active lesions caused by larval forms of *Taenia solium* and treatment of cystic hydatid disease of the liver, lung, and peritoneum caused by the larval form of *Echinococcus granulosus*. Active against *Ascaris lumbricoides* (roundworm), *Ancylostoma caninum*, *Ancylostoma duodenale*, *Necator americanus* (hookworm), *Enterobius vermicularis* (pinworm), cutaneous larva migrans, *Gnathostoma spinigerum*, *Gongylonema* sp: *Mansonella perstans* (filariasis), *Opisthorchis sinensis* (liver fluke), visceral larva migrans (toxocariasis), *Echinococcus multilocularis*, *Clonorchis sinensis* (Chinese liver fluke), *Giardia lamblia*, *Cysticercus cellulosae*, *Trichuris trichiura* (whipworm), microsporidiosis, and *Capillaria philippinensis*.
Pregnancy Risk Factor C
Pregnancy Considerations Albendazole has been shown to be teratogenic in laboratory animals and should not be used during pregnancy, if at all possible. Women should be advised to avoid pregnancy for at least 1 month following therapy. Discontinue if pregnancy occurs during treatment.
Lactation Excretion in breast milk unknown/not recommended
Contraindications Hypersensitivity to albendazole, any component, or the benzimidazole class of compounds
Warnings Agranulocytosis, aplastic anemia, granulocytopenia, leukopenia, and pancytopenia have occurred leading to fatalities (rare). Patients with liver disease, including hepatic echinococcosis, appear to be at greater risk for bone marrow suppression. Monitor blood counts at the beginning of each 28-day cycle and every 2 weeks while on therapy. Discontinue therapy in all patients who develop clinically significant decreases in blood cell counts. Women of childbearing age should only begin treatment after a negative pregnancy test and should be cautioned against becoming pregnant during and for at least 1 month after treatment cessation with albendazole since it may cause fetal harm.

Precautions Use with caution in patients with abnormal liver function tests or decreased total leukocyte count (increased risk for hepatotoxicity and bone marrow suppression); discontinue albendazole if significant elevation of liver enzymes occur; may restart therapy when liver enzymes decrease to pretreatment values; corticosteroids should be administered 1-2 days before initiating albendazole therapy in patients with neurocysticercosis to minimize inflammatory reactions and should be followed by concurrent steroid and anticonvulsant therapy for the first week of therapy to prevent cerebral hypertension. Albendazole may induce further retinal damage in patients having retinal lesions with neurocysticercosis.

Adverse Reactions

Central nervous system: Headache, dizziness, vertigo, intracranial pressure elevated, meningeal signs, fever, seizures

Dermatologic: Rash, urticaria, alopecia, erythema multiforme, Stevens-Johnson syndrome

Gastrointestinal: Abdominal pain, nausea, vomiting

Hematologic: Leukopenia, pancytopenia, thrombocytopenia, granulocytopenia, neutropenia, agranulocytosis, aplastic anemia

Hepatic: Liver enzymes elevated, hepatotoxicity, acute liver failure

Renal: Acute renal failure

Miscellaneous: Hypersensitivity reactions, migration of *Ascaris* through mouth and nose

Drug Interactions

Metabolism/Transport Effects Substrate (minor) of CYP1A2, 3A4; **Inhibits** CYP1A2 (weak)

Avoid Concomitant Use There are no known interactions where it is recommended to avoid concomitant use.

Increased Effect/Toxicity There are no known significant interactions involving an increase in effect.

Decreased Effect

The levels/effects of Albendazole may be decreased by: Aminoquinolines (Antimalarial)

Food Interactions Bioavailability is increased (up to 5 times) when taken with a fatty meal

Stability Store at room temperature

Mechanism of Action Binds to β-tubulin in parasite cells inhibiting tubulin polymerization which results in the loss of cytoplasmic microtubules and inhibition of glucose uptake

Pharmacokinetics (Adult data unless noted)

Absorption: Poorly absorbed from the GI tract

Distribution: Widely distributed throughout the body including urine, bile, liver, cyst wall, cyst fluid, and CSF

Protein binding: 70%

Metabolism: Extensive first-pass metabolism; hepatic metabolism to albendazole sulfoxide, an active metabolite

Half-life: Albendazole sulfoxide: 8-12 hours

Time to peak serum concentration: 2-5 hours for the metabolite

Elimination: Biliary

Usual Dosage Children and Adults: Oral:

Neurocysticercosis (patients should receive appropriate corticosteroid for the first 2-3 days of albendazole therapy and anticonvulsant therapy as required):

<60 kg: 15 mg/kg/day in 2 divided doses (maximum: 800 mg/day) for 8-30 days

≥60 kg: 400 mg twice daily for 8-30 days

Hydatid disease:

<60 kg: 15 mg/kg/day in 2 divided doses (maximum: 800 mg/day); 28-day cycle followed by a 14-day albendazole-free interval, for a total of 3 cycles

≥60 kg: 400 mg twice daily; 28-day cycle followed by a 14-day albendazole-free interval, for a total of 3 cycles

Ancylostoma caninum, ascariasis (roundworm), hookworm, trichuriasis (whipworm): 400 mg as a single dose

Capillariasis: 400 mg once daily for 10 days

Clonorchis sinensis (Chinese liver fluke): 10 mg/kg/day once daily for 7 days

Cutaneous larva migrans: 400 mg once daily for 3 days

Enterobius vermicularis (pinworm): 400 mg as a single dose; repeat in 2 weeks

Filariasis (*Mansonella perstans*): 400 mg twice daily for 10 days

Gnathostoma spinigerum (Gnathostomiasis): 400 mg twice daily for 21 days

Gongylonema sp (Gongylonemiasis): 10 mg/kg/day once daily for 3 days

Microsporidiosis

Disseminated: 400 mg twice daily

Intestinal: 400 mg twice daily for 21 days

Ocular: 400 mg twice daily in combination with fumagillin

Trichinellosis (*Trichinella spiralis*): 400 mg twice daily for 8-14 days

Visceral larva migrans: 400 mg twice daily for 5 days

Administration Oral: Administer with food. For children who have difficulty swallowing whole tablets, tablet may be crushed or chewed and swallowed with a drink of water.

Monitoring Parameters Monitor liver function tests, CBC at start of each cycle and every 2 weeks during therapy, fecal specimens for ova and parasites; pregnancy test

Patient Information Follow physician's suggestions to prevent reinfection. Notify physician if fever, abdominal pain, vomiting, yellowing of skin or eyes, darkening of urine, or light colored stools occur. Women of childbearing age should be advised to avoid becoming pregnant while on albendazole or within 1 month after discontinuing treatment. May cause dizziness and impair ability to perform activities requiring mental alertness.

Dosage Forms Excipient information presented when available (limited, particularly for generics); consult specific product labeling.

Tablet:

Albenza®: 200 mg

References

Baranwal AK, Singhi PD, Khandelwal N, et al, "Albendazole Therapy in Children With Focal Seizures and Single Small Enhancing Computerized Tomographic Lesions: A Randomized, Placebo-Controlled, Double Blind Trial," *Pediatr Infect Dis J*, 1998, 17(8):696-700.

"Drugs for Parasitic Infections," *Med Lett Drugs Ther*, 1998, 40 (1017):1-12.

Jung H, Sanchez M, Gonzalez-Astiazaran A, et al, "Clinical Pharmacokinetics of Albendazole in Children With Neurocysticercosis," *Am J Ther*, 1997, 4(1):23-6.

Paul I, Gnanamani G, and Nallam NR, "Intestinal Helminth Infections Among School Children in Visakhapatnam," *Indian J Pediatr*, 1999, 66 (5):669-73.

Pengsaa K, Sirivichayakul C, Pojjaroen-anant C, et al, "Albendazole Treatment for *Giardia intestinalis* Infections in School Children," *Southeast Asian J Trop Med Public Health*, 1999, 30(1):78-83.

◆ **Albenza®** *see* Albendazole *on page 54*

◆ **Albert® Pentoxifylline (Can)** *see* Pentoxifylline *on page 1090*

Albumin (al BYOO min)

Medication Safety Issues

Sound-alike/look-alike issues:

Albutein® may be confused with albuterol

Buminate® may be confused with bumetanide

U.S. Brand Names Albuminar®; AlbuRx™; Albutein®; Buminate®; Flexbumin; Human Albumin Grifols®; Plasbumin®

Canadian Brand Names Plasbumin®-25; Plasbumin®-5

Therapeutic Category Blood Product Derivative; Plasma Volume Expander

Generic Available Yes

Use Treatment of hypovolemia; plasma volume expansion and maintenance of cardiac output in the treatment of certain types of shock or impending shock; hypoproteinemia resulting in generalized edema or decreased intravascular volume (eg, hypoproteinemia associated with acute nephrotic syndrome, premature neonates)

Note: PALS and Neonatal Resuscitation 2000 Guidelines recommend isotonic crystalloid solutions (eg, NS or LR) as initial volume expansion; albumin is used less frequently due to limited supply, potential risk of infections, and an association with an increase in mortality (identified by meta-analyses); few studies in these analyses included children, so no firm conclusions in pediatric patients can be made

Pregnancy Risk Factor C

Lactation Excretion in breast milk unknown/compatible

Contraindications Hypersensitivity to albumin or any component; patients with severe anemia or cardiac failure

Warnings Use 25% concentration with extreme caution and infuse slowly in preterm neonates, due to increased risk of IVH (from rapid expansion of intravascular volume). Some products (eg, Albuminar®, Buminate®) contain natural rubber latex (in certain components of the product packaging) which may cause allergic reactions in susceptible individuals; avoid use in patients with allergy to latex

Precautions Rapid infusion of albumin solutions may cause vascular overload. Do not administer albumin to burn patients for the first 24 hours after the burn (capillary exudation of albumin will occur); use with caution in patients with hepatic or renal failure (added protein load) and in patients who require sodium restriction; monitor for signs of hypervolemia

Due to the occasional shortage of 5% human albumin, 5% solutions may at times be prepared by diluting 25% human albumin with NS or with D_5W (if sodium load is a concern); however, **do not use sterile water** to dilute albumin solutions, as this may result in hypotonic-associated hemolysis which can be fatal

Adverse Reactions

Cardiovascular: Precipitation of CHF or pulmonary edema, hypertension, tachycardia, hypervolemia, hypotension due to hypersensitivity reaction

Central nervous system: Fever, chills

Dermatologic: Rash

Gastrointestinal: Nausea, vomiting

Drug Interactions

Avoid Concomitant Use There are no known interactions where it is recommended to avoid concomitant use.

Increased Effect/Toxicity There are no known significant interactions involving an increase in effect.

Decreased Effect There are no known significant interactions involving a decrease in effect.

Stability Use within 4 hours after opening vial, do not use if turbid or contains a deposit; do not use SWI to dilute albumin (see Precautions)

Mechanism of Action Provides increase in intravascular oncotic pressure and causes mobilization of fluids from interstitial into intravascular space

Pharmacodynamics Duration of volume expansion: ~24 hours

Pharmacokinetics (Adult data unless noted) Half-life: 21 days

Usual Dosage Albumin **5%** should be used in hypovolemic or intravascularly depleted patients; albumin **25%** should be used in patients with fluid or sodium restrictions (eg, patients with hypoproteinemia and generalized edema, or nephrotic syndrome) (see Additional Information). Dose depends on condition of patient: I.V.:

Hypoproteinemia: Neonates, Infants, and Children: 0.5-1 g/kg/dose of 25% albumin; may repeat every 1-2 days; up to 1.5 g/kg/day has been added to hyperalimentation solutions; see Administration

Hypovolemia:
Neonates: Usual dose: 0.5 g/kg/dose (10 mL/kg/dose of 5% albumin); range: 0.25-0.5 g/kg/dose (5-10 mL/kg/dose of 5% albumin)

Infants and Children: 0.5-1 g/kg/dose (10-20 mL/kg/dose of 5% albumin); may repeat as needed; maximum dose: 6 g/kg/day (120 mL/kg/day of 5% albumin); see Administration

Nephrotic syndrome: Infants and Children: 0.25-1 g/kg/dose of 25% albumin

Adults: 25 g; no more than 250 g should be administered within 48 hours

Nephrotic syndrome: 12.5-50 g/day in 3-4 divided doses; daily dose has also been added to hyperalimentation solution; see Administration

Administration Parenteral: I.V.: Too rapid infusion may result in vascular overload

Albuminar®: May administer via the administration set provided (in-line 60 micron filter) or via any administration set; use of filter is optional; size of filter may vary according to institutional policy. Method of filter sterilization used by manufacturer includes 0.2 micron filter; however, aggregates may form under storage, shipping, and handling. Administration via very small filter will not damage product, but will slow flow rate.

Albutein®: May administer via the administration set provided (in-line 50 micron filter) or via any administration set; use of filter is optional; size of filter may vary according to institutional policy. Method of production includes passage through 0.22 micron filter. May administer via filter as small as 0.22 microns.

Buminate®: Administer via the administration set provided (in-line 15 micron filter) or via any filtered administration set; use ≥5 micron filter to ensure adequate flow rate

Plasbumin®: May administer with or without an I.V. filter; filter as small as 0.22 microns may be used

Hypoproteinemia: Infuse over 2-4 hours; for neonates, dose may be added to hyperalimentation fluid and infused over 24 hours; **Note:** Hyperalimentation fluid containing >25 g/L of albumin is more likely to occlude 0.22 micron in-line filters; but hyperalimentation solutions containing albumin in concentrations as low as 10.8 g/L have also occluded 0.22 micron filters; use ≥5 micron filter to ensure adequate flow rate; addition of albumin to hyperalimentation solutions may increase potential for growth of bacteria or fungi.

Hypovolemia: Rate of infusion depends on severity of hypovolemia and patient's symptoms; usually infuse dose over 30-60 minutes (faster infusion rates may be clinically necessary)

Maximum rates of I.V. infusion after initial volume replacement:
5%: 2-4 mL/minute
25%: 1 mL/minute

To prepare 5% albumin from 25%, see Precautions.

Monitoring Parameters Observe for signs of hypervolemia, pulmonary edema, cardiac failure, vital signs, I & O, Hgb, Hct, urine specific gravity

Nursing Implications Albumin administration must be completed within 6 hours after entering container, provided that administration is begun within 4 hours of entering the container

Additional Information In certain conditions (eg, hypoproteinemia with generalized edema, nephrotic syndrome), doses of albumin may be followed with I.V. furosemide: 0.5-1 mg/kg/dose.

Both albumin 5% and 25% contain 130-160 mEq/L of sodium; albumin 5% is osmotically equivalent to an equal volume of plasma; albumin 25% is osmotically equivalent to 5 times its volume of plasma.

Dosage Forms Excipient information presented when available (limited, particularly for generics); consult specific product labeling.

Injection, solution [preservative free; human]: 5% (250 mL, 500 mL); 25% (50 mL, 100 mL)

Albuminar®: 5% (50 mL, 250 mL, 500 mL) [50 mg/mL; contains sodium 130-160 mEq/L and potassium ≤1 mEq/L; packaging contains dry natural rubber]; 25% (20 mL, 50 mL, 100 mL) [250 mg/mL; contains sodium 130-160 mEq/L and potassium ≤1 mEq/L; packaging contains dry natural rubber]

AlbuRx™: 5% (250 mL, 500 mL) [50 mg/mL; contains sodium 130-160 mEq/L and potassium ≤2 mEq/L]; 25% (50 mL, 100 mL) [250 mg/mL; contains sodium 130-160 mEq/L and potassium ≤2 mEq/L]

Albutein®: 5% (250 mL, 500 mL) [50 mg/mL; contains sodium 130-160 mEq/L and potassium ≤2 mEq/L]

Buminate®: 5% (250 mL, 500 mL) [50 mg/mL; contains sodium 130-160 mEq/L and potassium ≤2 mEq/L; packaging contains dry natural rubber]; 25% (20 mL, 50 mL, 100 mL) [250 mg/mL; contains sodium 130-160 mEq/L and potassium ≤2 mEq/L; packaging contains dry natural rubber]

Flexbumin: 25% (50 mL, 100 mL) [250 mg/mL; contains sodium 130-160 mEq/L and potassium ≤2 mEq/L]

Human Albumin Grifols®: 25% (50 mL, 100 mL) [250 mg/mL; contains sodium 130-160 mEq/L and potassium ≤2 mEq/L]

Plasbumin®: 5% (50 mL, 250 mL) [50 mg/mL; contains sodium ~145 mEq/L and potassium ≤2 mEq/L]; 25% (20 mL, 50 mL, 100 mL) [250 mg/mL; contains sodium ~145 mEq/L and potassium ≤2 mEq/L]

References

"Guidelines 2000 for Cardiopulmonary Resuscitation and Emergency Cardiovascular Care, Part 10: Pediatric Advanced Life Support, The American Heart Association in Collaboration With the International Liaison Committee on Resuscitation," *Circulation*, 2000, 102(8 Suppl): I306.

"Guidelines 2000 for Cardiopulmonary Resuscitation and Emergency Cardiovascular Care, Part 11: Neonatal Resuscitation, The American Heart Association in Collaboration With the International Liaison Committee on Resuscitation," *Circulation*, 2000, 102(8 Suppl):I352.

"Hemolysis Associated With 25% Human Albumin Diluted With Sterile Water - United States, 1994-1998," *MMWR Morb Mortal Wkly Rep*, 1999, 48(8):157-9.

◆ **Albuminar®** see Albumin on page 55

◆ **Albumin (Human)** see Albumin on page 55

◆ **AlbuRx™** see Albumin on page 55

◆ **Albutein®** see Albumin on page 55

Albuterol (al BYOO ter ole)

Medication Safety Issues

Sound-alike/look-alike issues:

Albuterol may be confused with Albutein®, atenolol

Proventil® may be confused with Bentyl®, Prilosec® Prinivil®

Salbutamol may be confused with salmeterol

Ventolin® may be confused with phentolamine, Benylin®, Vantin

Related Information

Asthma on page 1697

U.S. Brand Names AccuNeb®; ProAir® HFA; Proventil® HFA; Ventolin® HFA; VoSpire ER®

Canadian Brand Names Airomir; Apo-Salvent®; Apo-Salvent® CFC Free; Apo-Salvent® Respirator Solution; Apo-Salvent® Sterules; Mylan-Salbutamol Respirator Solution; Mylan-Salbutamol Sterinebs P.F.; Nu-Salbutamol; PHL-Salbutamol; PMS-Salbutamol; ratio-Ipra-Sal; ratio-Salbutamol; Salbu-2; Salbu-4; Sandoz-Salbutamol; Ventolin®; Ventolin® Diskus; Ventolin® HFA; Ventolin® I.V. Infusion; Ventolin® Nebules P.F.

Therapeutic Category Adrenergic Agonist Agent; Antiasthmatic; Beta$_2$-Adrenergic Agonist Agent; Bronchodilator; Sympathomimetic

Generic Available Yes

Use Prevention and relief of bronchospasm in patients with reversible airway obstruction due to asthma or COPD; prevention of exercise-induced bronchospasm

Pregnancy Risk Factor C

Pregnancy Considerations Albuterol crosses the placenta; tocolytic effects, fetal tachycardia, fetal hypoglycemia secondary to maternal hyperglycemia with oral or intravenous routes reported. Available evidence suggests safe use as an inhalation during pregnancy, and albuterol is the preferred short-acting beta agonist for use in asthma according to the NHLBI 2007 Guidelines for the Diagnosis and Management of Asthma.

Use of the parenteral formulation (not available in the U.S.) as a tocolytic agent has been associated with myocardial ischemia. Patients with a history of cardiac disease should be referred to a cardiologist for evaluation prior to initiating therapy in premature labor. If therapy is initiated, patients should be carefully monitored for ECG changes as well as for changes in fluid balance and cardiopulmonary function. Maternal pulse rate should not exceed 140 beats per minute during I.V. infusion of salbutamol. Consider discontinuing therapy with the development of signs of pulmonary edema or myocardial ischemia. Cautious use of parenteral salbutamol, as with other beta$_2$-agonists, is also warranted when used during labor and delivery for the relief of bronchospasm.

Lactation Excretion in breast milk unknown/use caution

Contraindications Hypersensitivity to albuterol, any component, or adrenergic amine

Warnings Inhaled albuterol can produce paradoxical bronchospasm; discontinue therapy immediately if this occurs. Excessive or prolonged use can lead to tolerance; excessive use has also been associated with deaths, possibly due to cardiac arrest. Increasing use (>2 days/week) for symptom relief (not prevention of exercise-induced asthma) generally indicates inadequate control of asthma and the need for initiating or intensifying anti-inflammatory treatment. Regularly scheduled, daily, chronic use of short-acting beta agonists (eg, albuterol) is not recommended (NAEPP, 2007). Outbreaks of lower respiratory tract colonization and infection have been attributed to contaminated multidose albuterol bottles (see Administration).

Precautions Use with caution in patients with hyperthyroidism, seizure disorders, diabetes mellitus; cardiovascular disorders including coronary insufficiency, hypertension, or arrhythmia

Adverse Reactions

Cardiovascular: Tachycardia, palpitations, hypertension, chest pain, myocardial ischemia

Central nervous system: Nervousness, CNS stimulation, hyperactivity and insomnia occur more frequently in younger children than adults; dizziness, lightheadedness, drowsiness, headache

Dermatologic: Angioedema, urticaria

Endocrine & metabolic: Hypokalemia

Gastrointestinal: GI upset, xerostomia, heartburn, vomiting, nausea, unusual taste, hoarseness (inhalation only)

Genitourinary: Dysuria

Neuromuscular & skeletal: Tremor, weakness, muscle cramping

Respiratory: Irritation of oropharynx, coughing, paradoxical bronchospasm (oral inhalation only)

Miscellaneous: Diaphoresis increased

Drug Interactions

Avoid Concomitant Use

Avoid concomitant use of Albuterol with any of the following: Iobenguane I 123

Increased Effect/Toxicity

Albuterol may increase the levels/effects of: Sympathomimetics

The levels/effects of Albuterol may be increased by: Atomoxetine; Cannabinoids; MAO Inhibitors; Tricyclic Antidepressants

Decreased Effect

Albuterol may decrease the levels/effects of: Iobenguane I 123

The levels/effects of Albuterol may be decreased by: Alpha-/Beta-Blockers; Beta-Blockers (Beta1 Selective); Beta-Blockers (Nonselective); Betahistine

Food Interactions Caffeinated beverages may increase side effects of albuterol

Stability Liquid, tablets, MDIs, and oral inhalation solutions are stable at room temperature; discard Ventolin® HFA MDI canister after 200 actuations or 3 months after removal from moisture protective pouch; discard Accu-Neb™ vial 1 week after removal from foil pouch or if solution is not colorless; oral inhalation solution compatible with cromolyn and ipratropium nebulizer solutions

Mechanism of Action Relaxes bronchial smooth muscle by action on beta$_2$-receptors with little effect on heart rate

Pharmacodynamics

Nebulization/oral inhalation:

Peak bronchodilation: Within 0.5-2 hours nebulization

Duration: 2-5 hours

Oral:

Peak bronchodilatation: 2-3 hours

Duration: 4-6 hours

Extended release tablets: Duration: Up to 12 hours

Pharmacokinetics (Adult data unless noted)

Metabolism: By the liver to an inactive sulfate

Half-life:

Oral: 2.7-5 hours

Inhalation: 3.8 hours

Elimination: 30% appears in urine as unchanged drug

Usual Dosage

Acute asthma exacerbation (NAEPP, 2007):

Nebulization:

Children: 0.15 mg/kg (minimum dose: 2.5 mg) every 20 minutes for 3 doses then 0.15-0.3 mg/kg (not to exceed 10 mg) every 1-4 hours as needed or 0.5 mg/kg/hour by continuous nebulization

Note: Continuous nebulized albuterol at 0.3 mg/kg/hour has also been used safely in the treatment of severe status asthmaticus in children; continuous nebulized doses of 3 mg/kg/hour ± 2.2 mg/kg/hour (Katz, 1993) in children whose mean age was 20.7 months resulted in no cardiotoxicity; the optimal dosage for continuous nebulization remains to be determined

Adults: 2.5-5 mg every 20 minutes for 3 doses then 2.5-10 mg every 1-4 hours as needed or 10-15 mg/hour by continuous nebulization

Inhalation: MDI: 90 mcg/spray:

Children: 4-8 puffs every 20 minutes for 3 doses then every 1-4 hours

Adults: 4-8 puffs every 20 minutes for up to 4 hours then every 1-4 hours as needed

Maintenance therapy (nonacute) (NIH guidelines, 2007):

Inhalation: MDI: 90 mcg/spray: Not recommended for long-term daily maintenance treatment; regular use exceeding 2 days/week for symptom control (not prevention of exercise-induced bronchospasm) indicates the need for additional long-term control therapy

Children 0-4 years: 1-2 inhalations every 4-6 hours as needed

Children ≥5 years and Adults: 2 inhalations every 4-6 hours as needed

Exercise-induced bronchospasm:

Children 0-4 years: 1-2 inhalations 5 minutes before exercising

Children >4 years and Adults: 2 inhalations 5 minutes before exercising

Inhalation: Children and Adults: Nebulization: See dosage table

Albuterol Nebulization Dosage (Maintenance Therapy - Non-Acute)

Age	Dose (mg)	0.5% Solution (mL)	0.083% Solution (mL)	Frequency
Children 0-4 y	0.63-2.5 mg	0.13-0.5 mL	0.76-3 mL	Every 4-6 h
Children ≥5 y and adults	1.25-5 mg	0.25-1 mL	1.5-6 mL	Every 4-8 h

or as an alternative (manufacturer's recommendation):

Children:

10-15 kg: 1.25 mg 3-4 times/day

>15 kg: 2.5 mg 3-4 times/day

AccuNeb™:

Children <12 years: 0.75-1.5 mg 3-4 times/day

Children ≥12 years and Adults: 1.5 mg 3-4 times/day

AccuNeb™ has not been studied in the treatment of acute bronchospasm; a more concentrated form may be necessary for treatment in acute bronchospasm especially in children ≥6 years.

Oral: Not the preferred route for treatment of asthma; per NIH guidelines, inhalation via nebulization or MDI is preferred

Immediate release formulation:

Children 2-6 years: 0.1-0.2 mg/kg/dose 3 times/day; maximum dose not to exceed 4 mg 3 times/day

Children 6-12 years: 2 mg/dose 3-4 times/day

Children >12 years and Adults: 2-4 mg/dose 3-4 times/day

Sustained release formulation:

Children: 0.3-0.6 mg/kg/day in 2 divided doses; not to exceed 8 mg/day

Children >12 years and Adults: 4 mg 2 times/day; may increase to 8 mg 2 times/day

Administration

Inhalation: Nebulization: Using 0.5% solution, dilute dosage in 1-2 mL NS (0.083% solution and AccuNeb™ do not require further dilution; adjust nebulizer flow to deliver dosage over 5-15 minutes; avoid contact of the dropper tip (multidose bottle) with any surface, including the nebulizer reservoir and associated ventilator equipment (see Warnings)

Oral: Administer with food; do not crush or chew extended release tablets (Repetabs® or Volmax®)

Oral inhalation: Prime the inhaler (before first use or if it has not been used for more than 2 weeks) by releasing 4 test sprays into the air away from the face (3 test sprays for ProAir® HFA); shake well before use; use spacer for children <8 years of age

Monitoring Parameters Serum potassium, oxygen saturation, heart rate, pulmonary function tests, respiratory rate, use of accessory muscles during respiration, suprasternal retractions; arterial or capillary blood gases (if patient's condition warrants)

Patient Information Do not exceed recommended dosage; may cause dry mouth; rinse mouth with water following each inhalation to help with dry throat and mouth; if more than one inhalation is necessary, wait at least 1 full minute between inhalations; notify physician if palpitations, tachycardia, chest pain, muscle tremors, dizziness, headache, flushing, or if breathing difficulty persists; limit caffeinated beverages; to prevent medication build-up or blockage in the inhaler, the actuator, with the canister removed, should be washed and air-dried once weekly

Dosage Forms Excipient information presented when available (limited, particularly for generics); consult specific product labeling. [DSC] = Discontinued product; [CAN] = Canadian brand name

Aerosol, for oral inhalation: 90 mcg/metered inhalation (17 g) [200 metered inhalations; contains chlorofluorocarbons] [DSC]

Aerosol, for oral inhalation:
ProAir® HFA: 90 mcg/metered inhalation (8.5 g) [200 metered inhalations; chlorofluorocarbon free]
Proventil® HFA: 90 mcg/metered inhalation (6.7 g) [200 metered inhalations; chlorofluorocarbon free]
Ventolin® HFA: 90 mcg/metered inhalation (8 g) [60 metered inhalation; chlorofluorocarbon free]; (18 g) [200 metered inhalations; chlorofluorocarbon free]

Injection, as sulphate:
Ventolin® I.V. [CAN]: 1 mg/1mL (5 mL) [not available in U.S.]

Solution for nebulization [preservative free]: 0.021% (3 mL); 0.042% (3 mL); 0.083% (3 mL); 0.5% (0.5 mL, 20 mL)
AccuNeb®: 0.021% (3 mL); 0.042% (3 mL)

Syrup, oral: 2 mg/5 mL (480 mL)

Tablet, oral: 2 mg, 4 mg

Tablet, extended release, oral: 4 mg, 8 mg

VoSpire ER®: 4 mg, 8 mg

References

Katz RW, Kelly HW, Crowley MR, et al, "Safety of Continuous Nebulized Albuterol for Bronchospasm in Infants and Children," *Pediatrics*, 1993, 92(5):666-69.

"National Asthma Education and Prevention Program. Expert Panel Report: Guidelines for the Diagnosis and Management of Asthma Update on Selected Topics–2002," *J Allergy Clin Immunol*, 2002, 110 (5 Suppl):S141-219.

National Asthma Education and Prevention Program (NAEPP), "Expert Panel Report 3 (EPR-3): Guidelines for the Diagnosis and Management of Asthma," *Clinical Practice Guidelines*, National Institutes of Health, National Heart, Lung, and Blood Institute, NIH Publication No. 08-4051, prepublication 2007; available at http://www.nhlbi.nih.gov/guidelines/asthma/asthgdln.htm.

O'Callaghan C, Milner AD, and Swarbrick A, "Nebulized Salbutamol Does Have a Protective Effect on Airways in Children Under One Year Old," *Arch Dis Child*, 1988, 63(5):479-83.

Papo MC, Frank J, and Thompson AE, "A Prospective, Randomized Study of Continuous Versus Intermittent Nebulized Albuterol for Severe Status Asthmaticus in Children," *Crit Care Med*, 1993, 21 (10):1479-86.

Rachelefsky GS and Siegel SC, "Asthma in Infants and Children - Treatment of Childhood Asthma: Part II," *J Allergy Clin Immunol*, 1985, 76(3):409-25.

Schuh S, Parkin P, Rajan A, et al, "High- Versus Low-Dose, Frequently Administered, Nebulized Albuterol in Children With Severe, Acute Asthma," *Pediatrics*, 1989, 83(4):513-8.

Schuh S, Reider MJ, Canny G, et al, "Nebulized Albuterol in Acute Childhood Asthma: Comparison of Two Doses," *Pediatrics*, 1990, 86 (4):509-13.

◆ **Albuterol Sulfate** *see* Albuterol *on page 57*

◆ **Alcaine®** *see* Proparacaine *on page 1168*

◆ **Alcalak [OTC]** *see* Calcium Carbonate *on page 232*

◆ **Alcalak [OTC]** *see* Calcium Supplements *on page 239*

Alclometasone (al kloe MET a sone)

Medication Safety Issues
Sound-alike/look-alike issues:
Aclovate® may be confused with Accolate®

International issues:
Cloderm: Brand name for alclometasone [Indonesia], but also brand name for clobetasol [China, India, Malaysia, Singapore, Thailand]; clocortolone [U.S., Canada]; clotrimazole [Germany]

Related Information
Corticosteroids *on page 1487*

U.S. Brand Names Aclovate®

Therapeutic Category Adrenal Corticosteroid; Anti-inflammatory Agent; Corticosteroid, Topical; Glucocorticoid

Generic Available Yes

Use
Treatment of inflammation of corticosteroid-responsive dermatosis (mild to moderate potency topical corticosteroid)

Pregnancy Risk Factor C

Pregnancy Considerations
Teratogenic effects have been observed in animals administered topical corticosteroids.

Contraindications
Hypersensitivity to alclometasone or any component; viral, fungal, or tubercular skin lesions; herpes (including varicella)

Warnings
Infants and small children, due to larger surface area to body weight ratio and particularly if applying to >20% of body surface area, may be more susceptible to adrenal axis suppression from topical corticosteroid therapy; systemic effects may occur when used on large areas of the body, denuded areas, for prolonged periods of time, or with an occlusive dressing. Hypothalamic pituitary adrenal (HPA) axis suppression may occur; acute adrenal insufficiency may occur with abrupt withdrawal after long term use or with stress; withdrawal or discontinuation should be done carefully; patients with HPA axis suppression may require doses of systemic glucocorticosteroids prior to, during, and after unusual stress (eg, surgery).

Precautions
Safety and efficacy have not been established in children <1 year of age; not for use in treatment of diaper dermatitis; generally not for routine use on the face, underarms, or groin areas

Adverse Reactions
Dermatologic: Acne, allergic dermatitis, hypopigmentation, maceration of the skin, skin atrophy, striae, miliaria, telangiectasia

Endocrine & metabolic: HPA suppression, Cushing's syndrome, growth retardation

Local: Burning, erythema, itching, irritation, dryness, folliculitis, hypertrichosis

Systemic: HPA axis suppression, Cushing's syndrome, hyperglycemia; these reactions occur more frequently with occlusive dressings

Miscellaneous: Secondary infection

Drug Interactions

Avoid Concomitant Use
Avoid concomitant use of Alclometasone with any of the following: Aldesleukin

Increased Effect/Toxicity There are no known significant interactions involving an increase in effect.

Decreased Effect
Alclometasone may decrease the levels/effects of: Aldesleukin; Corticorelin

Stability Store between 2°C and 30°C (36°F and 86°F)

Mechanism of Action
Possesses anti-inflammatory, antiproliferative, and immunosuppressive properties

Pharmacodynamics
Initial response:
Eczema: 5.3 days
Psoriasis: 6.7 days
Peak response:
Eczema: 13.9 days
Psoriasis: 14.8 days

Pharmacokinetics (Adult data unless noted)
Absorption: Topical: 3% (when left on intact skin without an occlusive dressing for 8 hours); large variation in absorption depending upon anatomical sites: Forearm 1%; scalp 4%; scrotum 36%

Metabolism: Liver, extensive

Usual Dosage Topical: Children and Adults: Apply to affected area 2-3 times/day. Therapy should be discontinued when control is achieved; if no improvement is seen, reassessment of diagnosis may be necessary. Not recommended for use >3 weeks in children. Occlusive dressings may be used when treating refractory lesions of psoriasis and other deep-seated dermatoses such as localized neurodermatitis (lichen simplex chronicus); see Warnings

Administration Topical: Apply sparingly in a thin film; rub in lightly; for external use only; avoid contact with the eyes. Do not use on open wounds or weeping lesions. Apply sparingly to occlusive dressings.

Monitoring Parameters Clinical signs and symptoms of improvement in condition; assessment of HPA suppression if treatment for prolonged periods

Patient Information Before applying, gently wash area to reduce risk of infection. Apply a thin film to cleansed area and rub in gently and thoroughly until medication vanishes. Do not use for longer than directed; notify physician if condition being treated persists or worsens.

Dosage Forms Excipient information presented when available (limited, particularly for generics); consult specific product labeling.

Cream, as dipropionate: 0.05% (15 g, 45 g, 60 g)
  Aclovate®: 0.05% (15 g, 60 g)
Ointment, as dipropionate: 0.05% (15 g, 45 g, 60 g)
  Aclovate®: 0.05% (15 g, 45 g, 60 g)

◆ **Alclometasone Dipropionate** see Alclometasone on page 59

◆ **Alcohol, Absolute** see Ethyl Alcohol on page 547

◆ **Alcohol, Dehydrated** see Ethyl Alcohol on page 547

◆ **Alcomicin® (Can)** see Gentamicin on page 642

◆ **Aldactazide®** see Hydrochlorothiazide and Spironolactone on page 683

◆ **Aldactazide 25® (Can)** see Hydrochlorothiazide and Spironolactone on page 683

◆ **Aldactazide 50® (Can)** see Hydrochlorothiazide and Spironolactone on page 683

◆ **Aldactone®** see Spironolactone on page 1289

Aldesleukin (al des LOO kin)

Medication Safety Issues
Sound-alike/look-alike issues:
Aldesleukin may be confused with oprelvekin
Proleukin® may be confused with oprelvekin

High alert medication: The Institute for Safe Medication Practices (ISMP) includes this medication among its list of drug classes which have a heightened risk of causing significant patient harm when used in error.

Related Information
Compatibility of Chemotherapy and Related Supportive Care Medications on page 1580
Emetogenic Potential of Antineoplastic Agents on page 1579

U.S. Brand Names Proleukin®
Canadian Brand Names Proleukin®
Therapeutic Category Antineoplastic Agent, Miscellaneous; Biological Response Modulator
Generic Available No
Use Treatment of metastatic renal cell carcinoma and metastatic melanoma (FDA approved in adults); has been used in the treatment of acute myeloid leukemia (AML)
Pregnancy Risk Factor C
Pregnancy Considerations Maternal toxicity and embryocidal effects were noted in animal studies. There are no adequate and well-controlled studies in pregnant women; use during pregnancy only if benefits to the mother outweigh potential risk to the fetus. Contraception is recommended for fertile males or females using this medication.
Lactation Excretion in breast milk unknown/not recommended
Breast-Feeding Considerations Due to the potential for serious adverse reactions in the nursing infant, breast-feeding should be discontinued during treatment.
Contraindications Hypersensitivity to aldesleukin or any component; abnormal thallium stress test or pulmonary function tests; organ allografts (due to increased risk of rejection); **retreatment** in patients who have experienced sustained ventricular tachycardia (≥5 beats), cardiac rhythm disturbances not controlled or unresponsive to management, recurrent chest pain with ECG changes (consistent with angina or MI), intubation required >72 hours, cardiac tamponade; renal dysfunction requiring dialysis >72 hours, coma or toxic psychosis lasting >48 hours, repetitive or difficult to control seizures, bowel ischemia/perforation, and GI bleeding requiring surgery
Warnings Hazardous agent; use appropriate precautions for handling and disposal. High-dose aldesleukin therapy is associated with capillary leak syndrome (CLS), resulting in hypotension and reduced organ perfusion (occurring within 2-12 hours after start of treatment) which may be severe and fatal and is characterized by vascular tone loss and extravasation of plasma proteins and fluid into extravascular space **[U.S. Boxed Warning]**; CLS may be associated with cardiac arrhythmias, angina, MI, respiratory insufficiency requiring intubation, GI bleeding or infarction, renal insufficiency, edema, and mental status changes; therapy should be restricted to patients with normal cardiac and pulmonary functions as defined by thallium stress and formal pulmonary function testing. Monitor fluid status and organ perfusion status carefully; consider fluids and/or pressor agents to maintain organ perfusion. Withhold treatment for signs of organ failure (due to hypoperfusion), altered mental status, reduced urine output, systolic BP <90 mm Hg (in adults), or cardiac arrhythmia. Once blood pressure is normalized, may consider diuretics for excessive weight gain/edema. Recovery from CLS generally begins soon after treatment cessation. Hold aldesleukin administration in patients developing moderate to severe lethargy or somnolence as continued administration may result in coma **[U.S. Boxed Warning]**; may exacerbate disease symptoms in patients with clinically unrecognized or untreated CNS metastases thoroughly evaluate and treat all patients with CNS metastases prior to therapy
Precautions Use with extreme caution in patients with normal thallium stress tests and pulmonary functions tests who have a history of prior cardiac or pulmonary disease **[U.S. Boxed Warning]**; intensive aldesleukin treatment is associated with impaired neutrophil function (reduced

chemotaxis) and with an increased risk of disseminated infection (particularly with *Staphylococcus aureus*) including sepsis and bacterial endocarditis **[U.S. Boxed Warning]**; patients with indwelling central lines are particularly at increased risk of infection; treat pre-existing bacterial infections prior to initiation of aldesleukin therapy; standard supportive care during high-dose aldesleukin treatment includes acetaminophen to relieve fever and chills and an H_2 antagonist to reduce the risk of GI ulceration and/or bleeding; closely monitor for thyroid abnormalities; mental status changes (irritability, confusion, depression) can occur and may indicate bacteremia, sepsis, hypoperfusion, CNS malignancy, or CNS toxicity; use with caution in patients with known seizure disorders; use with caution in patients with autoimmune disease or inflammatory disorders; may exacerbate condition; exacerbation and/or new onset have been reported with aldesleukin and interferon alfa combination therapy; may impair hepatic function; concomitant hepatotoxic agents may increase the risk of hepatotoxicity; adults must have a serum creatinine ≤1.5 mg/dL prior to treatment; may impair renal function; concomitant nephrotoxic agents may increase the risk of renal toxicity; enhancement of cellular immune function may increase the risk of allograft rejection in transplant patients; an acute array of symptoms resembling aldesleukin adverse reactions (fever, chills, nausea, rash, pruritus, diarrhea, hypotension, edema and oliguria) were observed within 1-4 hours after iodinated contrast media administration, usually when given within 4 weeks after aldesleukin treatment, although has been reported several months after aldesleukin treatment

Adverse Reactions Many adverse effects of aldesleukin are dosage and schedule dependent; greater toxicity occurs with high dose, bolus administration and the least toxicity with low dose, subcutaneous administration

Cardiovascular: Angina, arrhythmias, capillary leak syndrome, cardiac arrest, CHF, edema, hypotension (dose-limiting, possibly fatal), MI, peripheral edema, sinus tachycardia, supraventricular tachycardia, vasodilation, ventricular tachycardia

Central nervous system: Anxiety, chills, cognitive changes, coma, confusion, disorientation, dizziness, drowsiness, fatigue, fever, headaches, insomnia, malaise, pain, paranoid delusion, psychosis, seizures, somnolence, stupor, transient memory loss

Dermatologic: Alopecia, dry skin, erythema, exfoliative dermatitis, macular erythematous rash, pruritus, petechiae, purpura, vitiligo

Endocrine & metabolic: Acidosis, hypercalcemia, hyperglycemia, hyperkalemia, hypermagnesemia, hypernatremia, hyperphosphatemia, hypocalcemia, hypoglycemia, hypokalemia, hypomagnesemia, hyponatremia, hypophosphatemia, thyroid dysfunction, weight gain

Gastrointestinal: Abdomen enlarged, abdominal pain, anorexia, diarrhea, GI bleeding, nausea, pancreatitis, stomatitis, vomiting

Hematologic: Anemia, coagulation disorder, eosinophilia, leukopenia, thrombocytopenia

Hepatic: Alkaline phosphatase increased, ascites, bilirubin and liver enzymes increased, clotting factors decreased, jaundice

Neuromuscular & skeletal: Arthralgia, myalgia, rigors, weakness

Renal: Acute renal failure, anuria, creatinine increased, hematuria, oliguria, proteinuria, transient elevation in BUN

Respiratory: Apnea, congestion, cough, dyspnea, pleural effusion, pulmonary edema, rhinitis

Miscellaneous: Allergic reactions, infection, sepsis

<1%, postmarketing, and/or case reports (limited to important or life-threatening): Acute tubular necrosis, allergic interstitial nephritis, anaphylaxis, AV block, blindness (transient or permanent), bowel infarction, bowel necrosis, bowel obstruction, bowel perforation, bradycardia, cardiomyopathy, cellulitis, cerebral edema, cerebral lesions, cerebral vasculitis, cholecystitis, colitis, crescentic IgA glomerulonephritis, delirium, depression (severe; leading to suicide), duodenal ulcer, encephalopathy, endocarditis, extrapyramidal syndrome, hematemesis, hemoptysis, hemorrhage (including cerebral), gastritis, gastrointestinal (retroperitoneal), hepatic failure, hepatitis, hepatosplenomegaly, hypertension, hyperuricemia, hyper-/hypoventilation, hypothermia, hypoxia, injection site necrosis, leukocytosis, malignant hyperthermia, meningitis, myocardial ischemia, myocarditis, myopathy, myositis, neuralgia, neuritis, neuropathy, neutropenia, NPN increased, oculobulbar myasthenia gravis, optic neuritis, organ perfusion decreased, pericardial effusion, pericarditis, peripheral gangrene, phlebitis, pneumonia, pneumothorax, pulmonary embolus, respiratory acidosis, respiratory arrest, respiratory failure, rhabdomyolysis, scleroderma, shock, Stevens-Johnson syndrome, stroke, syncope, thrombosis, tracheoesophageal fistula, transient ischemic attack, urticaria, ventricular extrasystoles

Drug Interactions

Avoid Concomitant Use
Avoid concomitant use of Aldesleukin with any of the following: Corticosteroids

Increased Effect/Toxicity
Aldesleukin may increase the levels/effects of: Hypotensive Agents

The levels/effects of Aldesleukin may be increased by: Contrast Media (Non-ionic); Interferons (Alfa)

Decreased Effect
The levels/effects of Aldesleukin may be decreased by: Corticosteroids

Stability Store in refrigerator; do not freeze; reconstituted solution is stable 48 hours in refrigerator or at room temperature; since aldesleukin contains no preservatives, refrigerated storage of the reconstituted solution is preferred; reconstituted solution packaged in tuberculin syringes for SubQ administration are stable 14 days refrigerated and 6 hours at room temperature; compatible **only** with D_5W; incompatible with sodium chloride solutions; do not mix with other medications; protect from light

Mechanism of Action Aldesleukin, a human recombinant interleukin-2 product, promotes proliferation, differentiation, and recruitment of T and B cells, natural killer cells, and thymocytes; also causes cytolytic activity in some lymphocytes and subsequent interactions between lymphokine-activated killer cells and tumor-infiltrating lymphocytes; causes multiple immunological effects including activation of cellular immunity with lymphocytosis, eosinophilia, and thrombocytopenia; production of cytokines (including tumor necrosis factor, interleukin-1), and inhibition of tumor growth

Pharmacokinetics (Adult data unless noted)
Absorption: Oral: Not absorbed
Distribution: Primarily into plasma, lymphocytes, lungs, liver, kidney, and spleen
V_d: Adults: 4-7 L
Metabolism: Metabolized to amino acids in the cells lining the proximal convoluted tubules of the kidney
Half-life:
Children:
Distribution: 14 ± 6 minutes
Elimination: 51 ± 11 minutes
Adults:
Distribution: 6-27 minutes
Elimination: 85 minutes
Time to peak serum concentration: SubQ: 2-3 hours
Clearance: Adults: 7.2-16.1 L/hour

Usual Dosage A wide variety of dosages have been or are currently under investigation (refer to individual protocols):

AML: Children: (unlabeled use; Lange, 2008): 9 million international units (9×10^6 international units)/m²/day continuous infusion over 24 hours daily for 4 days; repeat 4 days later with 1.6 million international units (1.6×10^6 international units)/m²/day continuous infusion over 24 hours daily for 10 days

Metastatic renal cell carcinoma and metastatic melanoma: Adults: I.V.: Initial: 600,000 international units/kg every 8 hours for a maximum of 14 doses; repeat after 9 days for a total of 28 doses per course; retreat if tumor shrinkage observed (and if no contraindications) at least 7 weeks after previous course

Dosage modification for toxicity (Adults): Hold or interrupt a dose, **do not dose reduce**:

Cardiovascular toxicity:

Withhold dose for atrial fibrillation, supraventricular tachycardia, or bradycardia that is persistent, recurrent, or requires treatment; may resume when asymptomatic with full recovery to normal sinus rhythm

Withhold dose for systolic BP <90 mm Hg (with increasing pressor requirements); may resume treatment when systolic BP ≥90 mm Hg and stable or pressor requirements improve

Withhold dose for any ECG change consistent with MI, ischemia, myocarditis (with or without chest pain), or suspected cardiac ischemia; may resume when asymptomatic, MI/myocarditis have been ruled out, suspicion of angina is low, or there is no evidence of ventricular hypokinesia

CNS toxicity: Withhold dose for mental status change, including moderate confusion or agitation; may resume when resolved completely

Dermatologic toxicity: Withhold dose for bullous dermatitis or marked worsening of pre-existing skin condition; may treat with antihistamines or topical products (do not use topical steroids); may resume with resolution of all signs of bullous dermatitis

Gastrointestinal: Withhold dose for stool guaiac repeatedly >3-4+; may resume with negative stool guaiac

Hepatotoxicity: Withhold dose and discontinue treatment for balance of cycle for signs of hepatic failure, encephalopathy, increasing ascites, liver pain, hypoglycemia; may initiate a new course, if indicated, only after at least 7 weeks past resolution of all signs of hepatic failure (including hospital discharge)

Infection: Withhold dose for sepsis syndrome, clinically unstable; may resume when sepsis syndrome has resolved, patient is clinically stable, and infection is under treatment

Renal toxicity:

Withhold dose for serum creatinine >4.5 mg/dL (or ≥4 mg/dL with severe volume overload, acidosis, or hyperkalemia); may resume when <4 mg/dL and fluid/electrolyte status is stable

Withhold dose for persistent oliguria or urine output <10 mL/hour for 16-24 hours with rising serum creatinine; may resume when urine output >10 mL/hour with serum creatinine decrease of >1.5 mg/dL or normalization

Respiratory toxicity: Withhold dose for oxygen saturation <90%; may resume when >90%

Retreatment with aldesleukin is **contraindicated** with the following toxicities: Sustained ventricular tachycardia (≥5 beats), refractory uncontrolled or unresponsive cardiac arrhythmias, recurrent chest pain with ECG changes consistent with angina or MI, cardiac tamponade, intubation >72 hours, renal failure requiring dialysis for >72 hours, coma or toxic psychosis lasting >48 hours, repetitive or refractory seizures, bowel ischemia/perforation, or GI bleeding requiring surgery

Administration

I.V.: Reconstitute with 1.2 mL preservative-free SWI (swirl, do not shake); resulting concentration is 18 million (18×10^6) international units/mL [1.1 mg/mL]; further dilute dosage in D_5W [plastic (polyvinyl chloride) bags result in more consistent drug delivery and are recommended] to a final concentration between 0.49-1.1 million international units/mL (30-70 mcg/mL) and infuse over 15 minutes; allow solution to reach room temperature prior to administration; for continuous infusions, dilute in D_5W maintaining the same final concentration; final dilutions <0.49 million international units/mL (30 mcg/mL) or >1.1 million international units/mL (70 mcg/mL) have shown increased variability in drug stability and bioactivity and should be avoided; addition of 0.1% albumin has been used to increase stability and decrease the extent of sorption if low final concentrations cannot be avoided; do not use in-line filter when administering; flush line before and after with D_5W

SubQ: Reconstituted solution may be administered subcutaneously without further dilution (**Note**: Subcutaneous administration is a non-FDA approved route)

Monitoring Parameters Baseline chest x-ray, pulmonary function tests and thallium stress study; CBC with differential, platelet counts, electrolytes, BUN, serum creatinine, hepatic enzymes, vital signs, weight, pulse oximetry, arterial blood gases (if pulmonary symptoms), fluid intake and output; cardiac monitoring (in a patient with a decreased blood pressure, especially systolic BP <90 mm Hg); ECG if an abnormal complex or rhythm is seen; monitor for change in mental status, and for signs of infection

Nursing Implications See Warnings and Precautions

Additional Information 18×10^6 int. units = 1.1 mg protein

Dosage Forms Excipient information presented when available (limited, particularly for generics); consult specific product labeling.

Injection, powder for reconstitution:

Proleukin®: 22×10^6 int. units [18 million int. units/mL = 1.1 mg/mL when reconstituted]

References

Bergmann L, Heil G, Kolbe K, et al, "Interleukin-2 Bolus Infusion as Late Consolidation Therapy in Acute Remission of Acute Myeloblastic Leukemia," Leuk Lymphoma, 1995, 16(3-4):271-9.

Lange BJ, Smith FO, Feusner J, et al, "Outcomes in CCG-2961, a Children's Oncology Group Phase 3 Trial for Untreated Pediatric Acute Myeloid Leukemia: A Report From the Children's Oncology Group," Blood, 2008, 111(3):1044-53.

Sievers EL, Lange BJ, Sondel PM, et al, "Feasibility, Toxicity, and Biologic Response of Interleukin-2 After Consolidation Chemotherapy for Acute Myelogenous Leukemia: A Report From the Children's Cancer Group," J Clin Oncol, 1998, 16(3):914-9.

Whittington R and Faulds D, "Interleukin-2: A Review of Its Pharmacological Properties and Therapeutic Use in Patients With Cancer," Drugs, 1993, 46(3):446-514.

◆ **Aldomet** see Methyldopa on page 905
◆ **Aldurazyme®** see Laronidase on page 803
◆ **Aler-Cap [OTC]** see DiphenhydrAMINE on page 448
◆ **Aler-Dryl [OTC]** see DiphenhydrAMINE on page 448
◆ **Aler-Tab [OTC]** see DiphenhydrAMINE on page 448
◆ **Alertec® (Can)** see Modafinil on page 940
◆ **Aleve® [OTC]** see Naproxen on page 967
◆ **Alfenta®** see Alfentanil on page 62

Alfentanil (al FEN ta nil)

Medication Safety Issues

Sound-alike/look-alike issues:

Alfentanil may be confused with Anafranil®, fentanyl, remifentanil, sufentanil

Alfenta® may be confused with Sufenta®

High alert medication: The Institute for Safe Medication Practices (ISMP) includes this medication among its list of drug classes which have a heightened risk of causing significant patient harm when used in error.

Related Information
Opioid Analgesics Comparison *on page 1510*

U.S. Brand Names Alfenta®

Canadian Brand Names Alfentanil Injection, USP; Alfenta®

Therapeutic Category Analgesic, Narcotic; General Anesthetic

Generic Available Yes

Use Analgesia; analgesia adjunct; anesthetic agent

Restrictions C-II

Pregnancy Risk Factor C

Pregnancy Considerations Alfentanil is known to cross the placenta, which may result in respiratory or CNS depression in the newborn. Use during labor and delivery is not recommended.

Contraindications Hypersensitivity to alfentanil hydrochloride or any component; increased intracranial pressure; severe respiratory depression

Warnings Rapid I.V. infusion may result in skeletal muscle and chest wall rigidity → impaired ventilation → respiratory distress/arrest; inject slowly over 3-5 minutes; nondepolarizing skeletal muscle relaxant may be required

Precautions Use with caution in patients with bradycardia

Adverse Reactions
Cardiovascular: Bradycardia, peripheral vasodilation, hypotension
Central nervous system: Drowsiness, dizziness, sedation, CNS depression, intracranial pressure elevated
Dermatologic: Pruritus
Endocrine & metabolic: Antidiuretic hormone release
Gastrointestinal: Nausea, vomiting, constipation, biliary tract spasm
Genitourinary: Urinary tract spasm
Neuromuscular & skeletal: Skeletal muscle and chest wall rigidity especially following rapid I.V. administration
Ocular: Miosis
Respiratory: Respiratory depression, apnea, respiratory arrest
Miscellaneous: Histamine release, physical and psychological dependence with prolonged use

Drug Interactions
Metabolism/Transport Effects Substrate of CYP3A4 (major)

Avoid Concomitant Use
Avoid concomitant use of Alfentanil with any of the following: MAO Inhibitors

Increased Effect/Toxicity
Alfentanil may increase the levels/effects of: Alcohol (Ethyl); Alvimopan; Beta-Blockers; Calcium Channel Blockers (Nondihydropyridine); CNS Depressants; Desmopressin; Fospropofol; MAO Inhibitors; Propofol; Selective Serotonin Reuptake Inhibitors; Thiazide Diuretics

The levels/effects of Alfentanil may be increased by: Amphetamines; Antifungal Agents (Azole Derivatives, Systemic); Antipsychotic Agents (Phenothiazines); Cimetidine; CYP3A4 Inhibitors (Moderate); CYP3A4 Inhibitors (Strong); Dasatinib; Diltiazem; Fluconazole; Macrolide Antibiotics; MAO Inhibitors; Succinylcholine

Decreased Effect
Alfentanil may decrease the levels/effects of: Pegvisomant

The levels/effects of Alfentanil may be decreased by: Ammonium Chloride; Mixed Agonist / Antagonist Opioids; Rifamycin Derivatives

Mechanism of Action Binds with stereospecific receptors at many sites within the CNS, increases pain threshold, alters pain reception, inhibits ascending pain pathways

Pharmacodynamics
Onset of action: Within 5 minutes
Duration: <15-20 minutes

Pharmacokinetics (Adult data unless noted)
Distribution: V_d beta:
Newborns, premature: 1 L/kg
Children: 0.163-0.48 L/kg
Adults: 0.46 L/kg
Protein binding:
Neonates: 67%
Adults: 88% to 92%
Bound to alpha$_1$-acid glycoprotein
Metabolism: Hepatic
Half-life, elimination:
Newborns, premature: 320-525 minutes
Children: 40-60 minutes
Adults: 83-97 minutes

Usual Dosage Doses should be titrated to appropriate effects; wide range of doses is dependent upon desired degree of analgesia/anesthesia

Neonates, Infants, and Children <12 years: Dose not established; A high percent of newborn infants receiving alfentanil (prior to procedures) at doses of 9-15 mcg/kg (mean dose: 11.7 mcg/kg) developed chest wall rigidity; 9 out of 20 newborns (45%) developed mild or moderate rigidity that did not affect ventilation, while 4 out of 20 (20%) had severe rigidity interfering with respiration for ~5-10 minutes; use of a skeletal muscle relaxant to prevent chest wall rigidity is recommended; however, smaller alfentanil doses may be required in newborns. Further studies are needed to determine appropriate doses of alfentanil in pediatric patients.

Adults: Use lean body weight for patients who weigh >20% over ideal body weight; see table.

Alfentanil: Adult Dosing

Indication	Approximate Duration of Anesthesia (min)	Induction Period (Initial Dose) (mcg/kg)	Maintenance Period (Increments/ Infusion)	Total Dose (mcg/kg)	Effects
Incremental injection	≤30	8-20	3-5 mcg/kg or 0.5-1 mcg/kg/min	8-40	Spontaneously breathing or assisted ventilation when required.
	30-60	20-50	5-15 mcg/kg	Up to 75	Assisted or controlled ventilation required. Attenuation of response to laryngoscopy and intubation.
Continuous infusion	>45	50-75	0.5-3 mcg/kg/min; average infusion rate: 1-1.5 mcg/kg/min	Dependent on duration of procedure	Assisted or controlled ventilation required. Some attenuation of response to intubation and incision, with intraoperative stability.
Anesthetic induction	>45	130-245	0.5-1.5 mcg/kg/min or general anesthetic	Dependent on duration of procedure	Assisted or controlled ventilation required. Administer slowly (over 3 minutes). Concentration of inhalation agents reduced by 30% to 50% for initial hour.

Administration Parenteral: I.V.: Inject slowly over 3-5 minutes or by I.V. continuous infusion; maximum concentration: 80 mcg/mL

Monitoring Parameters Respiratory rate, blood pressure, heart rate, neurological status (for degree of analgesia/ anesthesia)

◀ **Nursing Implications** Alfentanil may produce more hypotension compared to fentanyl, therefore, be sure to administer slowly and ensure patient has adequate hydration; may be habit-forming; avoid abrupt discontinuation after prolonged use

Dosage Forms Excipient information presented when available (limited, particularly for generics); consult specific product labeling. [DSC] = Discontinued product

Injection, solution [preservative free]: 500 mcg/mL (2 mL, 5 mL)

Alfenta®: 500 mcg/mL (2 mL, 5 mL; 10 mL [DSC]; 20 mL [DSC])

References

Davis PJ, Killian A, Stiller RL, et al, "Pharmacokinetics of Alfentanil in Newborn Premature Infants and Older Children," *Dev Pharmacol Ther*, 1989, 13(1):21-7.

Marlow N, Weindling AM, Van Peer A, et al, "Alfentanil Pharmacokinetics in Preterm Infants," *Arch Dis Child*, 1990, 65(4 Spec No):349-51.

Meistelman C, Saint-Maurice C, Lepaul M, et al, "A Comparison of Alfentanil Pharmacokinetics in Children and Adults," *Anesthesiology*, 1987, 66(1):13-6.

Pokela ML, Ryhanen PT, Koivisto ME, et al, "Alfentanil-Induced Rigidity in Newborn Infants," *Anesth Analg*, 1992, 75(2):252-7.

◆ **Alfentanil Hydrochloride** *see* Alfentanil *on page 62*

◆ **Alfentanil Injection, USP (Can)** *see* Alfentanil *on page 62*

Alglucerase (al GLOO ser ase)

Medication Safety Issues
Sound-alike/look-alike issues:
Alglucerase may be confused with agalsidase alfa, agalsidase beta, alglucosidase alfa
Ceredase® may be confused with Cerezyme®

U.S. Brand Names Ceredase®

Therapeutic Category Enzyme, Glucocerebrosidase; Gaucher's Disease, Treatment Agent

Generic Available No

Use Long-term enzyme replacement in patients with confirmed Type I Gaucher disease who exhibit one or more of the following conditions: Moderate to severe anemia; thrombocytopenia and bleeding tendencies; bone disease; hepatomegaly or splenomegaly; growth retardation related to Gaucher disease

Pregnancy Risk Factor C

Pregnancy Considerations Animal studies have not been conducted.

Lactation Excretion in breast milk unknown/use caution

Contraindications Hypersensitivity to alglucerase or any component

Precautions Alglucerase is prepared from pooled human placental tissue that may contain the causative agents of some viral diseases; the risk of contamination from slowly active or latent viruses is believed to be remote due to steps taken in the manufacturing process; observe for signs of early virilization in males <10 years of age

Adverse Reactions
Central nervous system: Fever, chills, fatigue
Endocrine & metabolic: Early virilization (males <10 years)
Gastrointestinal: Abdominal discomfort, nausea, vomiting, diarrhea, oral ulcerations
Local: Discomfort, burning, and edema at the site of injection
Neuromuscular: Weakness, backache
Miscellaneous: Hypersensitivity reactions

Drug Interactions
Avoid Concomitant Use There are no known interactions where it is recommended to avoid concomitant use.

Increased Effect/Toxicity There are no known significant interactions involving an increase in effect.

Decreased Effect There are no known significant interactions involving a decrease in effect.

Stability When diluted to 100-200 mL with NS, resultant solution is stable up to 18 hours when stored at 2°C to 8°C

Mechanism of Action Glucocerebrosidase is an enzyme prepared from human placental tissue. Gaucher's disease is an inherited metabolic disorder caused by the defective activity of beta-glucosidase and the resultant accumulation of glucosyl ceramide laden macrophages in the liver, bone, and spleen. Alglucerase acts by replacing the missing enzyme associated with Gaucher's disease.

Pharmacodynamics
Onset of significant improvement in symptoms:
Hepatosplenomegaly and hematologic abnormalities: Occurs within 6 months
Improvement in bone mineralization: Noted at 80-104 weeks of therapy

Pharmacokinetics (Adult data unless noted)
Distribution: V_d: 0.05-0.28 L/kg
Half-life, elimination: ~4-10 minutes

Usual Dosage I.V. Infusion: Children, Adolescents, and Adults: 30-60 units/kg every 2 weeks; range in dosage: 2.5 units/kg 3 times/week to 60 units/kg once weekly to every 4 weeks. Initial dose should be based on disease severity and rate of progression. Children at high risk for complications from Gaucher's disease (one or more of the following: symptomatic disease including manifestations of abdominal or bone pain, fatigue, exertional limitations, weakness, and cachexia; growth failure; evidence of skeletal involvement; platelet count ≤60,000 mm³ and/or documented abnormal bleeding episode(s); Hgb ≥2.0 g/dL below lower limit for age and sex; impaired quality of life) should receive an initial dose of 60 units/kg; failure to respond to treatment within 6 months indicates the need for a higher dosage.
Maintenance: After patient response is well established a reduction in dosage may be attempted; progressive reductions may be made at intervals of 3-6 months; assess dosage frequently to maintain consistent dosage per kg body weight

Administration Parenteral: Dilute to a final volume of 100-200 mL NS and infuse I.V. over 1-2 hours; an in-line filter should be used; do not shake solution as it denatures the enzyme

Monitoring Parameters CBC, platelets, liver function tests, MRI or CT scan (spleen and liver volume), skeletal x-rays

Dosage Forms Excipient information presented when available (limited, particularly for generics); consult specific product labeling.
Injection, solution [preservative free]:
Ceredase®: 80 units/mL (5 mL) [contains human albumin 1%]

References

Barton NW, Brady RO, Dambrosia JM, et al, "Replacement Therapy for Inherited Enzyme Deficiency - Macrophage-Targeted Glucocerebrosidase for Gaucher's Disease," *N Engl J Med*, 1991, 324(21):1464-70.

Charrow J, Andersson HC, Kaplan P, et al, "Enzyme Replacement Therapy and Monitoring for Children With Type 1 Gaucher Disease: Consensus Recommendations," *J Pediatr*, 2004, 144(1):112-20.

◆ **Alglucosidase** *see* Alglucosidase Alfa *on page 64*

Alglucosidase Alfa (al gloo KOSE i dase AL fa)

Medication Safety Issues
Sound-alike/look-alike issues:
Alglucosidase alfa may be confused with agalsidase alfa, agalsidase beta, alglucerase

U.S. Brand Names Lumizyme™; Myozyme®

Canadian Brand Names Myozyme®

Therapeutic Category Enzyme

Generic Available No

Use Replacement therapy of alpha-glucosidase (GAA) for infantile-onset Pompe disease

Pregnancy Risk Factor B

Pregnancy Considerations Animal studies have not demonstrated teratogenicity or fertility impairment. There are no adequate and well-controlled studies in pregnant women. A registry has been established for Pompe patients; women of childbearing potential are encouraged to enroll in the registry (www.pomperegistry.com or 1-800-745-4447).

Lactation Excretion in breast milk unknown/use caution

Breast-Feeding Considerations A registry has been established for Pompe patients; women who are nursing are encouraged to enroll in the registry (www.-pomperegistry.com or 1-800-745-4447)

Contraindications Hypersensitivity to alglucosidase alfa or any component of the formulation

Warnings Life -threatening anaphylactic reactions have been observed in some patients during and within 3 hours after infusions. Therefore, appropriate medical support should be readily available when alglucosidase alfa is administered. **[U.S. Boxed Warning]** Reactions have included anaphylactic shock, cardiac arrest, respiratory distress, hypotension, bradycardia, hypoxia, bronchospasm, throat tightness, dyspnea, angioedema, and urticaria. Experience from clinical trials and expanded access programs has shown approximately 14% of patients treated with alglucosidase alfa develop allergic reaction involving at least 2 of the 3 following body systems: Cardiovascular, respiratory, or cutaneous. If anaphylactic or other severe allergic reaction occurs, immediately discontinue administration and provide appropriate medical treatment. Use extreme caution if readministration is attempted.

Patients with compromised cardiac or respiratory function may be at risk of serious acute exacerbation of their cardiac or respiratory compromise due to infusion reactions and may require additional monitoring. **[U.S. Boxed Warning]**; acute cardiorespiratory failure requiring intubation and inotropic support has been reported up to 72 hours post-infusion in patients with infantile-onset Pompe disease with underlying cardiac hypertrophy which may possibly be secondary to intravenous fluid overload from drug administration.

Infusion-related reactions are common; reactions may occur at any time during administration or for up to 2 hours post-infusion; discontinue immediately for severe hypersensitivity or anaphylactic reaction; mild-to-moderate reactions may be managed by reducing the infusion rate and/or administering antihistamines and/or antipyretics. Appropriate medical support for the management of infusion reactions should be readily available. Use caution with subsequent infusions; infusion reactions have occurred despite premedication with antihistamines, antipyretics, and/or steroids. Patients with acute underlying illness are at greater risk for infusion reactions.

Cardiac arrhythmias (including ventricular fibrillation, ventricular tachycardia, and bradycardia) have been observed in patients with cardiac hypertrophy in patients undergoing general anesthesia during central venous catheter placement; relationship not well established; use caution.

Precautions Systemic immune mediated and severe cutaneous reactions have been reported. Patients should be monitored for the development of systemic immune-complex mediated reactions involving the skin and other organs during therapy.

Adverse Reactions

Cardiovascular: Tachycardia, bradycardia, flushing

Central nervous system: Fever, pain (postprocedural)

Dermatologic: Rash, diaper dermatitis, urticaria

Gastrointestinal: Diarrhea, vomiting, gastroenteritis, oral candidiasis, gastroesophageal reflux, constipation

Hematologic: Anemia

Local: Catheter-related infections

Otic: Otitis media

Respiratory: Cough, pneumonia, upper respiratory tract infection, oxygen saturation decreased, pharyngitis, respiratory distress, respiratory failure, rhinorrhea, RSV bronchiolitis, nasopharyngitis, tachypnea

Miscellaneous: Antibodies to alglucosidase alfa (may affect efficacy), infusion reaction

Drug Interactions

Avoid Concomitant Use There are no known interactions where it is recommended to avoid concomitant use.

Increased Effect/Toxicity There are no known significant interactions involving an increase in effect.

Decreased Effect There are no known significant interactions involving a decrease in effect.

Stability Store vials between 2°C and 8°C (36°F and 46°F); do not freeze. Protect from light. Allow vials to reach room temperature prior to reconstitution. Final solutions for infusion should be used immediately if possible, but may be stored for up to 24 hours between 2°C and 8°C (36°F and 46°F); do not freeze. Protect from light.

Mechanism of Action Alglucosidase alfa is a recombinant form of the enzyme acid alpha-glucosidase (GAA), which is required for glycogen cleavage. Due to an inherited GAA deficiency, glycogen accumulates in the tissues of patients, leading to progressive muscle weakness. In infantile-onset Pompe disease, glycogen accumulates in cardiac and skeletal muscles and hepatic tissue, leading to cardiomyopathy and respiratory failure. Juvenile- and adult-onset Pompe disease are limited to glycogen accumulation in skeletal muscle, leading to respiratory failure. Alglucosidase alfa binds to mannose-6-phosphate receptors on the cell surface and becomes internalized and transported to lysosomes, resulting in increased enzymatic activity and glycogen cleavage.

Pharmacokinetics (Adult data unless noted)

Distribution: V_{ss}: 80-147 mL/kg

Half-life elimination: 2-3 hours

Usual Dosage I.V.: Children 1 month to 3.5 years (at first infusion): 20 mg/kg over ~4 hours every 2 weeks

Administration Visually inspect the powder in the vial for particulate matter prior to reconstitution. After vial reaches room temperature, reconstitute each vial with 10.3 mL SWI. Inject slowly down internal side wall of vial (do not inject into powder; avoid foaming). Roll and tilt gently; do not invert, swirl, or shake. Resulting solution contains 5 mg/mL. Visually inspect the solution following reconstitution for particulate matter. To make final infusion, add the desired dose amount of reconstituted solution to 50-600 mL NS (volume determined by patient's weight; see product labeling for complete details) to make a final concentration of 0.5-4 mg/mL. Do not use filter needle for preparation. Remove airspace from infusion bag prior to admixture to minimize particle formation due to sensitivity of drug to air-liquid interfaces. Do not shake. Final solutions for infusion should be used immediately if possible, but may be stored for up to 24 hours between 2°C and 8°C (36°F and 46°F); do not freeze. Protect from light.

Infuse over ~4 hours; initiate at 1 mg/kg/hour. If tolerated, increase by 2 mg/kg/hour every 30 minutes to a maximum rate of 7 mg/kg/hour. Decrease rate or temporarily hold for infusion reactions. Infuse through a low protein-binding, 0.2 micron in-line filter. Do not administer products with visualized particulate matter.

◀

Monitoring Parameters Liver enzymes (baseline and periodically; elevation may be due to disease process); vital signs during and following infusion; volume overload The manufacturer recommends monitoring for IgG antibody formation every 3 months. No commercial tests are available; however, sampling kits can be obtained by contacting Genzyme Corporation at 1-800-745-4447.

Patient Information This medication can only be administered by intravenous infusion. Report immediately any redness, swelling, pain, or burning at infusion site or any adverse response during infusion (eg, respiratory difficulty, facial edema, pain, restlessness, tremor, wheezing). Report rash, diarrhea, or constipation; nausea or vomiting; change in appetite; mouth sores; respiratory distress, cough, or respiratory tract infection; or other adverse response that occurs between infusions.

Nursing Implications Patient must be monitored closely during and following infusion for hypersensitivity reactions; life-threatening anaphylactic reactions (including anaphylactic shock) have been reported during infusion. Emergency response equipment should be readily available. Premedication with antihistamines and/or antipyretics may be ordered. Prescriber should be notified of any adverse reaction. Decrease rate or temporarily hold for infusion reaction. Teach patient/caregiver possible side effects and adverse symptoms to report. **Note:** A registry has been established for Pompe patients; women who are of childbearing potential or nursing should be encouraged to enroll in the registry.

Additional Information A registry has been established for Pompe patients (www.pomperegistry.com or 1-800-745-4447).

Patients >18 years who may need alglucosidase alfa therapy must enroll in the Myozyme Temporary Access Program (MTAP), as required by prescriber and institution (http://www.myozyme.com/MTAP/mtap_pt.asp).

Patients with sustained positive IgG antibody titers (≥12,800) to alglucosidase alfa may have poorer clinical response. Most patients (89%) develop antibodies within the first 3 months of therapy; concern is with patients with sustained high (≥12,800) antibody titers. Patients developing a decreased motor function should be tested for neutralization of enzyme uptake or activity. Infusion reactions are more common in antibody-positive patients. Patients with moderate-to-severe or recurrent reactions with suspected mast-cell activation may be tested for alglucosidase alfa-specific IgE antibodies.

Product Availability Myozyme®: Information for physicians and patients with Pompe disease in the U.S. regarding product availability, supply, and access is available through the Alglucosidase Alfa Temporary Access Program (ATAP) at http://www.myozyme.com/MTAP/mtap_pt.asp.

Dosage Forms Excipient information presented when available (limited, particularly for generics); consult specific product labeling.

Injection, powder for reconstitution [preservative free]:
  Lumizyme™: 50 mg [contains polysorbate 80; derived from Chinese hamster ovary cells]
  Myozyme®: 50 mg [contains mannitol, polysorbate 80; derived from Chinese hamster ovary cells]

References

Kishnani PS, Corzo D, Nicolino M, et al, "Recombinant Human Acid [Alpha]-Glucosidase: Major Clinical Benefits in Infantile-Onset Pompe Disease," Neurology, 2007, 68(2):99-109.
Kishnani PS, Nicolino M, Voit T, et al, "Chinese Hamster Ovary Cell-Derived Recombinant Human Acid Alpha-Glucosidase in Infantile-Onset Pompe Disease," J Pediatr, 2006, 149(1):89-97.
Schoser B, Hill V, and Raben N, "Therapeutic Approaches in Glycogen Storage Disease Type II/Pompe Disease," Neurotherapeutics, 2008, 5(4):569-78.

◆ **Aliclen™** see Salicylic Acid on page 1241

◆ **Alinia®** see Nitazoxanide on page 993
◆ **Alka-Mints® [OTC]** see Calcium Carbonate on page 232
◆ **Alka-Mints® [OTC]** see Calcium Supplements on page 239
◆ **Alkeran®** see Melphalan on page 875
◆ **All Day Allergy** see Cetirizine on page 283
◆ **Allegra®** see Fexofenadine on page 579
◆ **Allegra® ODT** see Fexofenadine on page 579
◆ **Aller-Chlor® [OTC]** see Chlorpheniramine on page 296
◆ **Allerdryl® (Can)** see DiphenhydrAMINE on page 448
◆ **Allerfrim [OTC]** see Triprolidine and Pseudoephedrine on page 1388
◆ **Allergen®** see Antipyrine and Benzocaine on page 118
◆ **AllerMax® [OTC]** see DiphenhydrAMINE on page 448
◆ **Allernix (Can)** see DiphenhydrAMINE on page 448
◆ **Allfen [OTC]** see GuaiFENesin on page 656
◆ **Allfen DM [OTC]** see Guaifenesin and Dextromethorphan on page 658
◆ **Alloprin® (Can)** see Allopurinol on page 66

Allopurinol (al oh PURE i nole)

Medication Safety Issues
  Sound-alike/look-alike issues:
    Allopurinol may be confused with Apresoline
    Zyloprim® may be confused with Xylo-Pfan®, ZORprin®, Zovirax®

Related Information
  Tumor Lysis Syndrome on page 1599

U.S. Brand Names Aloprim®; Zyloprim®

Canadian Brand Names Alloprin®; Apo-Allopurinol®; Novo-Purol; Zyloprim®

Therapeutic Category Antigout Agent; Uric Acid Lowering Agent

Generic Available Yes

Use Prevention of attacks of gouty arthritis and nephropathy; also used in treatment of secondary hyperuricemia which may occur during treatment of tumors or leukemia; prevention of recurrent calcium oxalate calculi

Pregnancy Risk Factor C

Pregnancy Considerations There are few reports describing the use of allopurinol during pregnancy; no adverse fetal outcomes attributable to allopurinol have been reported in humans; use only if potential benefit outweighs the potential risk to the fetus.

Lactation Enters breast milk/use caution (AAP rates "compatible")

Contraindications Hypersensitivity to allopurinol or any component

Warnings Do not use to treat asymptomatic hyperuricemia; monitor liver function and complete blood counts before initiating therapy and periodically

Precautions Reduce dosage in renal impairment; discontinue drug at the first sign of rash; risk of skin rash may be increased in patients receiving amoxicillin or ampicillin; risk of hypersensitivity may be increased in patients receiving thiazides and possibly ACE inhibitors

Adverse Reactions
  Cardiovascular: (reported with I.V. administration) Hypotension, flushing, hypertension, bradycardia, heart failure
  Central nervous system: Drowsiness, fever, headache, chills, somnolence, agitation
  Dermatologic: Pruritic maculopapular rash, exfoliative dermatitis, erythema multiforme, alopecia
  Gastrointestinal: GI irritation, dyspepsia, nausea, vomiting, diarrhea, abdominal pain, gastritis
  Genitourinary: Hematuria

Hematologic: Leukocytosis, leukopenia, thrombocytopenia, eosinophilia, bone marrow suppression

Hepatic: Hepatitis, liver enzymes elevated, hepatomegaly, hyperbilirubinemia, jaundice

Local: Local injection site reaction

Neuromuscular & skeletal: Peripheral neuropathy, paresthesia, neuritis, arthralgia, myoclonus

Ocular: Cataracts, optic neuritis

Renal: Renal impairment

Respiratory: Epistaxis; (reported with I.V. administration) apnea, hyperpnea, ARDS

Vascular: Necrotizing angiitis, vasculitis

Drug Interactions

Avoid Concomitant Use

Avoid concomitant use of Allopurinol with any of the following: Didanosine

Increased Effect/Toxicity

Allopurinol may increase the levels/effects of: Amoxicillin; Ampicillin; Anticonvulsants (Hydantoin); AzaTHIOprine; CarBAMazepine; ChlorproPAMIDE; Cyclophosphamide; Didanosine; Mercaptopurine; Theophylline Derivatives; Vitamin K Antagonists

The levels/effects of Allopurinol may be increased by: ACE Inhibitors; Loop Diuretics; Thiazide Diuretics

Decreased Effect

The levels/effects of Allopurinol may be decreased by: Antacids

Stability Reconstituted parenteral solution should be stored at room temperature; do not refrigerate; use within 10 hours of preparation; physically **incompatible** when mixed with or infused through the same line with the following: Amikacin, amphotericin B, carmustine, cefotaxime, chlorpromazine, cimetidine, clindamycin, cytarabine, dacarbazine, daunorubicin, diphenhydramine, doxorubicin, doxycycline, droperidol, floxuridine, gentamicin, haloperidol, hydroxyzine, idarubicin, imipenem-cilastatin, mechlorethamine, meperidine, metoclopramide, methylprednisolone sodium succinate, minocycline, nalbuphine, netilmicin, ondansetron, prochlorperazine, promethazine, sodium bicarbonate, streptozocin, tobramycin, vinorelbine

Mechanism of Action Decreases the production of uric acid by inhibiting the action of xanthine oxidase, an enzyme that converts hypoxanthine to xanthine and xanthine to uric acid

Pharmacodynamics Decrease in serum uric acid occurs in 1-2 days with a nadir achieved in 1-3 weeks

Pharmacokinetics (Adult data unless noted)

Absorption: Oral: ~80% from the GI tract

Distribution: Into breast milk; breast milk to plasma ratio: 0.9-1.4

Protein binding: <1%

Metabolism: ~75% of drug metabolized to active metabolites, chiefly oxypurinol

Half-life:

Parent: 1-3 hours

Oxypurinol metabolite: 18-30 hours in patients with normal renal function

Time to peak serum concentration: Within 2-6 hours

Dialysis: Allopurinol and oxypurinol are dialyzable

Usual Dosage

Prevention of acute uric acid nephropathy in myeloproliferative neoplastic disorders (beginning 1-2 days before chemotherapy): Daily doses >300 mg should be administered in divided doses:

Children ≤10 years:

I.V.: 200 mg/m^2/day in 1-3 divided doses; maximum dose: 600 mg/day

Oral: 10 mg/kg/day in 2-3 divided doses or 200-300 mg/m^2/day in 2-4 divided doses; maximum dose: 800 mg/day

Alternative:

<6 years: 150 mg/day in 3 divided doses

6-10 years: 300 mg/day in 2-3 divided doses

Children >10 years and Adults:

I.V.: 200-400 mg/m^2/day in 1-3 divided doses; maximum: 600 mg/day

Oral: 600-800 mg/day in 2-3 divided doses

Gout: Children >10 years and Adults: Oral:

Mild: 200-300 mg/day

Severe: 400-600 mg/day

Recurrent calcium oxalate stones: Children >10 years and Adults: Oral: 200-300 mg daily in divided or single daily dosage

Dosing adjustment in renal impairment:

Cl_{cr} >50 mL/minute: No dosage change

Cl_{cr} 10-50 mL/minute: Reduce dosage to 50% of recommended

Cl_{cr} <10 mL/minute: Reduce dosage to 30% of recommended

Administration

Oral: Administer after meals with plenty of fluid

Parenteral: Reconstitute 500 mg vial with 25 mL SWI; prior to administration, further dilute with D$_5$W or NS to a maximum concentration of 6 mg/mL; rate of infusion is dependent upon the volume of infusate (in research studies, 100-300 mg doses were infused over 30 minutes)

Monitoring Parameters CBC, liver function tests, renal function, serum uric acid; 24-hour urinary urate (when treating calcium oxalate stones)

Reference Range

Uric acid: Male: 3.0-7.0 mg/dL; Female: 2.0-6.0 mg/dL

Urinary urate excretion: Male: <800 mg/day; Female: <750 mg/day

Patient Information Report any skin rash, painful urination, blood in urine, irritation of the eyes, or swelling of lips or mouth; avoid alcohol; drink plenty of fluids; may cause drowsiness and impair ability to perform activities requiring mental alertness or physical coordination

Dosage Forms Excipient information presented when available (limited, particularly for generics); consult specific product labeling

Injection, powder for reconstitution, as sodium: 500 mg (base)

Aloprim®: 500 mg (base)

Tablet: 100 mg, 300 mg

Zyloprim®: 100 mg, 300 mg

Extemporaneous Preparations

A 20 mg/mL suspension may be made by crushing eight 300 mg tablets and mixing with 120 mL of either a 1:1 mixture of Ora-Sweet® and Ora-Plus® or a 1:1 mixture of Ora-Sweet® SF and Ora-Plus® or a 1:4 mixture of cherry syrup concentrate and simple syrup, NF. The resulting suspension is stable for 60 days refrigerated or at room temperature (Allen, 1996; Nahata, 2004).

A 20 mg/mL suspension may be made by crushing one 100 mg tablet; wet crushed tablet with small amount of 1% methylcellulose then add syrup NF to a final volume of 5 mL; stable 56 days refrigerated or at room temperature (Dressman, 1983; Nahata, 2004).

Allen LV and Erickson MA, "Stability of Acetazolamide, Allopurinol, Azathioprine, Clonazepam, and Flucytosine in Extemporaneously Compounded Oral Liquids," *Am J Health Sys Pharm*, 1996, 53:1944-9.

Dressman JB and Poust RI, "Stability of Allopurinol and of Five Antineoplastics in Suspension," *Am J Hosp Pharm*, 1983, 40(4):616-8.

Nahata, MC, Pai VB, and Hipple TF, *Pediatric Drug Formulations*, 5th ed, Cincinnati, OH: Harvey Whitney Books Co, 2004.

References

Bennett WM, Aronoff GR, Golper TA, et al, *Drug Prescribing in Renal Failure*, Philadelphia, PA: American College of Physicians, 1987.

Krakoff IH and Murphy ML, "Hyperuricemia in Neoplastic Disease in Children: Prevention With Allopurinol, A Xanthine Oxidase Inhibitor" *Pediatrics*, 1968, 41(1):52-6.

◆ **Allopurinol Sodium** see Allopurinol on page 66

◆ **All-*trans* Retinoic Acid** see Tretinoin (Systemic) on page 1373

◆ **All-*trans* Vitamin A Acid** see Tretinoin (Systemic) on page 1373

◆ **Almora® [OTC]** see Magnesium Supplements on page 859

◆ **Alocril®** see Nedocromil on page 970

◆ **Alodox™** see Doxycycline on page 479

◆ **Aloe Vesta® Antifungal [OTC]** see Miconazole on page 927

◆ **Alophen® [OTC]** see Bisacodyl on page 194

◆ **Aloprim®** see Allopurinol on page 66

◆ **Alora®** see Estradiol on page 536

◆ **Aloxi®** see Palonosetron on page 1047

◆ **Alpha-Galactosidase-A (Recombinant)** see Agalsidase Beta on page 53

◆ **Alphagan® (Can)** see Brimonidine on page 202

◆ **Alphagan® P** see Brimonidine on page 202

◆ **Alphanate®** see Antihemophilic Factor / von Willebrand Factor Complex (Human) on page 114

◆ **AlphaNine® SD** see Factor IX on page 557

◆ **Alph-E [OTC]** see Vitamin E on page 1427

◆ **Alph-E-Mixed [OTC]** see Vitamin E on page 1427

ALPRAZolam (al PRAY zoe lam)

Medication Safety Issues
Sound-alike/look-alike issues:
ALPRAZolam may be confused with alprostadil, LORazepam, triazolam
Xanax® may be confused with Lanoxin®, Tenex®, Tylox®, Xopenex®, Zantac®, Zyrtec®

Beers Criteria medication: This drug may be inappropriate for use in geriatric patients (high severity risk).
Related Information
Serotonin Syndrome on page 1695
U.S. Brand Names Alprazolam Intensol®; Niravam™; Xanax XR®; Xanax®
Canadian Brand Names Alti-Alprazolam; Apo-Alpraz®; Apo-Alpraz® TS; Mylan-Alprazolam; Novo-Alprazol; Nu-Alpraz; Xanax TS™; Xanax®
Therapeutic Category Antianxiety Agent; Benzodiazepine
Generic Available Yes: Excludes oral solution
Use Treatment of generalized anxiety disorder (GAD); symptoms of anxiety (short-term treatment); anxiety associated with depression; management of panic disorder, with or without agoraphobia
Restrictions C-IV
Pregnancy Risk Factor D
Pregnancy Considerations Benzodiazepines have the potential to cause harm to the fetus, particularly when administered during the first trimester. In addition, withdrawal symptoms may occur in the neonate following *in utero* exposure. Use during pregnancy should be avoided.
Lactation Enters breast milk/not recommended (AAP rates "of concern")
Breast-Feeding Considerations Symptoms of withdrawal, lethargy, and loss of body weight have been reported in infants exposed to alprazolam and/or benzodiazepines while nursing. Breast-feeding is not recommended.
Contraindications Hypersensitivity to alprazolam, any component, or other benzodiazepines; severe uncontrolled pain, narrow-angle glaucoma, severe respiratory depression, pre-existing CNS depression; not to be used in

pregnancy or lactation or in patients taking certain medications (see Drug Interactions)
Warnings Withdrawal symptoms including seizures have occurred 18 hours to 3 days after abrupt discontinuation; when discontinuing therapy, decrease daily dose by no more than 0.5 mg every 3 days; reduce dose in patients with significant hepatic disease. Concentrated oral solution contains propylene glycol.
Precautions Safety and effectiveness have not been established in children <18 years of age
Adverse Reactions
Central nervous system: Drowsiness, dizziness, confusion, sedation, fatigue, headache, ataxia, abnormal coordination, somnolence, dysarthria, memory impairment, depression
Endocrine & metabolic: Weight gain or weight loss
Gastrointestinal: Xerostomia, constipation, diarrhea, nausea, vomiting, appetite increased or decreased
Ocular: Blurred vision
Miscellaneous: Physical and psychological dependence with prolonged use
Drug Interactions
Metabolism/Transport Effects Substrate of CYP3A4 (major)
Avoid Concomitant Use
Avoid concomitant use of ALPRAZolam with any of the following: Indinavir
Increased Effect/Toxicity
ALPRAZolam may increase the levels/effects of: Alcohol (Ethyl); Clozapine; CNS Depressants; Methotrimeprazine

The levels/effects of ALPRAZolam may be increased by: Antifungal Agents (Azole Derivatives, Systemic); Aprepitant; Calcium Channel Blockers (Nondihydropyridine); Cimetidine; Contraceptives (Estrogens); Contraceptives (Progestins); CYP3A4 Inhibitors (Moderate); CYP3A4 Inhibitors (Strong); Dasatinib; Fluconazole; Fosaprepitant; Grapefruit Juice; Indinavir; Isoniazid; Macrolide Antibiotics; Methotrimeprazine; Nefazodone; Protease Inhibitors; Proton Pump Inhibitors; Selective Serotonin Reuptake Inhibitors
Decreased Effect
The levels/effects of ALPRAZolam may be decreased by: CarBAMazepine; CYP3A4 Inducers (Strong); Deferasirox; Rifamycin Derivatives; St Johns Wort; Theophylline Derivatives; Yohimbine
Food Interactions
Extended release tablet: A high-fat meal eaten ≤2 hours before the dose may increase peak concentrations by ~25%. A high-fat meal eaten immediately before the dose may decrease the time to peak concentrations by about 33%. A high-fat meal eaten ≥1 hour after the dose may increase the time to peak concentrations by about 33%. The extent of absorption (AUC) is not affected by food.
Orally-disintegrating tablet: A high-fat meal may decrease peak concentrations by 25% and delay the time to peak concentrations by 2 hours. The AUC is not affected by food.
Stability Orally-disintegrating tablet: Store at room temperature of 20°C to 25°C (68°F to 77°F). Protect from moisture. Discard any cotton packaged inside bottle; reseal bottle tightly.
Mechanism of Action Depresses all levels of the CNS, including the limbic and reticular formation, by binding to the benzodiazepine site on the gamma-aminobutyric acid (GABA) receptor complex and modulating GABA, which is a major inhibitory neurotransmitter in the brain
Pharmacokinetics (Adult data unless noted)
Absorption: Oral:
Immediate release tablet: Rapidly and well absorbed
Extended release tablet: Rate of absorption is increased following night time dosing (versus morning dosing)
Distribution: 0.9-1.2 L/kg; distributes into breast milk

Protein binding: 80%

Metabolism: Extensive in the liver, primarily via cytochrome P450 isoenzyme CYP3A; major metabolites: alpha-hydroxy-alprazolam (about half as active as alprazolam), 4-hydroxyalprazolam (active), and a benzophenone metabolite (inactive). **Note:** Active metabolites are not likely to contribute to pharmacologic effects due to low levels of activity and low concentrations.

Bioavailability: Similar for extended and immediate release tablets (~90%)

Half-life: Adults: 6.3-26.9 hours; mean: 11.2 hours; **Note:** Half-life may be 25% longer in Asians compared to Caucasians.

Time to peak serum concentration:

Immediate release tablet: Within 1-2 hours

Orally-disintegrating tablet: 1.5-2 hours (if given with or without water); **Note:** Time to peak serum concentration occurs ~15 minutes earlier when taken with water (versus without)

Elimination: Excretion of metabolites and parent compound in urine

Usual Dosage Oral: **Note:** Titrate dose to effect; use lowest effective dose

Children <18 years: Immediate release: Dose not established; investigationally in children 7-16 years of age (n=13), initial doses of 0.005 mg/kg or 0.125 mg/dose were given 3 times/day for situational anxiety and increments of 0.125-0.25 mg/dose were used to increase doses to maximum of 0.02 mg/kg/dose or 0.06 mg/kg/day; a range of 0.375-3 mg/day was needed (see Pfefferbaum, 1987). **Note:** A more recent study in 17 children (8-17 years of age) with overanxious disorder or avoidant disorders used initial daily doses of 0.25 mg for children <40 kg and 0.5 mg for those >40 kg. The dose was titrated at 2-day intervals to a maximum of 0.04 mg/kg/day. Required doses ranged from 0.5-3.5 mg/day with a mean of 1.6 mg/day. Based on clinical global ratings, alprazolam appeared to be better than placebo, however, this difference was **not** statistically significant (see Simeon, 1992); further studies are needed.

Adults:

Anxiety: Immediate release: Initial: 0.25-0.5 mg 3 times/day; titrate dose upward as needed every 3-4 days; maximum dose: 4 mg/day given in divided doses

Panic disorder:

Immediate release: Initial: 0.5 mg 3 times/day; titrate dose upward as needed every 3-4 days in increments ≤1 mg/day; mean dose used in controlled trials: 5-6 mg/day; maximum dose: 10 mg/day (rarely required)

Extended release: Initial: 0.5-1 mg once daily; titrate dose upward as needed every 3-4 days in increments ≤1 mg/day; usual dose: 3-6 mg/day; maximum dose: 10 mg/day (rarely required)

Switching from immediate release to extended release: Administer the same total daily dose, but give once daily; if effect is not adequate, titrate dose as above

Administration Oral:

Immediate release tablet: Administer with food to decrease GI upset

Extended release tablet: Administer once daily, preferably in the morning; do not crush, chew, or break; swallow whole

Orally-disintegrating tablet: Do not remove tablets from bottle until right before dose; using dry hands, place tablet on top of tongue; if using one-half of tablet, immediately discard remaining half (half tablet may not remain stable). Administration with water is not necessary (water is not required to aid dissolution or swallowing)

Monitoring Parameters CNS status, respiratory rate

Patient Information May cause drowsiness and impair ability to perform activities requiring mental alertness or physical coordination; may be habit-forming; avoid abrupt discontinuation after prolonged use; avoid alcohol; limit caffeine; may cause dry mouth

Nursing Implications Assist with ambulation during beginning of therapy; allow patient to rise slowly to avoid fainting

Additional Information If used for an extended period of time, long-term usefulness of alprazolam should be periodically re-evaluated for an individual patient.

Dosage Forms Excipient information presented when available (limited, particularly for generics); consult specific product labeling.

Solution, oral [concentrate]:

Alprazolam Intensol®: 1 mg/mL (30 mL) [alcohol free, dye free, sugar free; contains propylene glycol]

Tablet: 0.25 mg, 0.5 mg, 1 mg, 2 mg

Xanax®: 0.25 mg, 0.5 mg, 1 mg, 2 mg

Tablet, extended release: 0.5 mg, 1 mg, 2 mg, 3 mg

Xanax XR®: 0.5 mg, 1 mg, 2 mg, 3 mg

Tablet, orally disintegrating [scored]: 0.25 mg, 0.5 mg, 1 mg, 2 mg

Niravam™: 0.25 mg, 0.5 mg, 1 mg, 2 mg [orange flavor]

References

Bernstein GA, Garfinkel BD, and Borchardt CM, "Comparative Studies of Pharmacotherapy for School Refusal," *J Am Acad Child Adolesc Psychiatry*, 1990, 29(5):773-81.

DeVane CL, Hill M, and Antal EJ, "Therapeutic Drug Monitoring of Alprazolam in Adolescents With Asthma," *Ther Drug Monit*, 1998, 20 (3):257-60.

Pfefferbaum B, Overall JE, Boren HA, et al, "Alprazolam in the Treatment of Anticipatory and Acute Situational Anxiety in Children With Cancer," *J Am Acad Child Adolesc Psychiatry*, 1987, 26 (4):532-5.

Simeon JG and Ferguson HB, "Alprazolam Effects in Children With Anxiety Disorders," *Can J Psychiatry*, 1987, 32(7):570-4.

Simeon JG, Ferguson HB, Knott V, et al, "Clinical, Cognitive, and Neurophysiological Effects of Alprazolam in Children and Adolescents With Overanxious and Avoidant Disorders," *J Am Acad Child Adolesc Psychiatry*, 1992, 31(1):29-33.

◆ **Alprostadil Intensol®** *see* ALPRAZolam *on page 68*

Alprostadil (al PROS ta dill)

Medication Safety Issues

Sound-alike/look-alike issues:

Alprostadil may be confused with alPRAZolam

U.S. Brand Names Caverject Impulse®; Caverject®; Edex®; Muse®; Prostin VR Pediatric®

Canadian Brand Names Caverject®; Muse® Pellet; Prostin® VR

Therapeutic Category Prostaglandin

Generic Available Yes: Solution for injection

Use Temporary maintenance of patency of ductus arteriosus in neonates with ductal-dependent congenital heart disease until surgery can be performed. These defects include cyanotic (eg, pulmonary atresia, pulmonary stenosis, tricuspid atresia, Fallot's tetralogy, transposition of the great vessels) and acyanotic (eg, interruption of aortic arch, coarctation of aorta, hypoplastic left ventricle) heart disease.

Investigationally used for the treatment of pulmonary hypertension in infants and children with congenital heart defects with left-to-right shunts

Adult males: Diagnosis and treatment of erectile dysfunction (see Additional Information)

Pregnancy Risk Factor X/C (Muse®)

Pregnancy Considerations Alprostadil is embryotoxic in animal studies. It is not indicated for use in women. The manufacturer of Muse® recommends a condom barrier when being used during sexual intercourse with a pregnant women.

◄ **Lactation** Not indicated for use in women

Contraindications Hypersensitivity to alprostadil or any component; respiratory distress syndrome or persistent fetal circulation

Warnings Apnea occurs in 10% to 12% of neonates with congenital heart defects (especially in those weighing <2 kg at birth) and usually appears during the first hour of drug infusion **[U.S. Boxed Warnings]**. May cause gastric outlet obstruction in neonates secondary to antral hyperplasia; occurrence is related to duration of therapy and cumulative dose. Infuse alprostadil at lowest effective dose and for shortest period of time; weigh risks of long-term effects versus benefits.

Precautions Use cautiously in neonates with bleeding tendencies. If hypotension or pyrexia occurs, the infusion rate should be reduced until symptoms subside; severe hypotension, apnea, or bradycardia requires drug discontinuation with cautious reinstitution at a lower dose. Tissue necrosis may occur with extravasation of concentrated solutions (due to high osmolality). Cortical proliferation of long bones has been associated with long-term infusions of alprostadil.

Adverse Reactions

Cardiovascular: Systemic hypotension, flushing, bradycardia, rhythm disturbances, tachycardia, edema

Central nervous system: Seizure-like activity, fever

Endocrine & metabolic: Hypocalcemia, hypoglycemia, hypokalemia, hyperkalemia

Gastrointestinal: Diarrhea, gastric-outlet obstruction secondary to antral hyperplasia (occurrence related to duration of therapy and cumulative dose)

Hematologic: Inhibition of platelet aggregation

Neuromuscular & skeletal: Cortical proliferation of long bones (cortical hyperostosis) has been seen with long-term infusions (incidence and severity are related to duration of therapy and cumulative dose); **Note:** Cortical hyperostosis may present with clinical symptoms that mimic cellulitis or osteomyelitis (eg, symptomatic bone tenderness, soft tissue swelling)

Respiratory: Respiratory depression, apnea

Miscellaneous: Pretibial and soft tissue swelling, swelling of upper and lower extremities

Drug Interactions

Avoid Concomitant Use There are no known interactions where it is recommended to avoid concomitant use.

Increased Effect/Toxicity There are no known significant interactions involving an increase in effect.

Decreased Effect There are no known significant interactions involving a decrease in effect.

Stability Compatible in D_5W, $D_{10}W$, and saline solutions; refrigerate ampuls at 2°C to 8°C. Avoid direct contact of undiluted alprostadil with the plastic walls of volumetric infusion chambers because the drug will interact with the plastic and create a hazy solution; discard solution and volumetric chamber if this occurs.

Mechanism of Action Causes vasodilation by means of direct effect on vascular and ductus arteriosus smooth muscle

Pharmacodynamics

Maximum effect:

Acyanotic congenital heart disease: Usual: 1.5-3 hours; range: 15 minutes to 11 hours

Cyanotic congenital heart disease: Usual: ~30 minutes

Duration: Ductus arteriosus will begin to close within 1-2 hours after drug is stopped

Pharmacokinetics (Adult data unless noted)

Metabolism: ~70% to 80% metabolized by oxidation during a single pass through the lungs; metabolite (13,14 dihydro-PGE_1) is active and has been identified in neonates

Half-life: 5-10 minutes; since the half-life is so short, the drug must be administered by continuous infusion

Elimination: Metabolites excreted in urine

Usual Dosage Neonates and Infants: 0.05-0.1 mcg/kg/minute; with therapeutic response, rate is reduced to lowest effective dosage; with unsatisfactory response, rate is increased gradually; maintenance: 0.01-0.4 mcg/kg/minute

PGE_1 is usually given at an infusion rate of 0.1 mcg/kg/minute; but it is often possible to reduce the dosage to 1/2 or even 1/10 without losing the therapeutic effect. The mixing schedule is shown in the table.

Add 1 Ampul (500 mcg) to:	Concentration (mcg/mL)	Infusion Rate to Deliver 0.1 mcg/kg/min		
		mL/kg/min	mL/kg/h	mL/kg/24 h
250 mL	2	0.05	3	72
100 mL	5	0.02	1.2	28.8
50 mL	10	0.01	0.6	14.4
25 mL	20	0.005	0.3	7.2

Administration Parenteral: I.V. continuous infusion into a large vein or alternatively through an umbilical artery catheter placed at the ductal opening; maximum concentration listed (per package insert) for I.V. infusion: 20 mcg/mL; has also been administered via continuous infusion into the right pulmonary artery for investigational treatment of pulmonary hypertension in infants and children with congenital heart defects with left-to-right shunts; rate of infusion (mL/hour) = dose (mcg/kg/minute) x weight (kg) x 60 minutes/hour divided by concentration (mcg/mL)

Monitoring Parameters Arterial pressure, respiratory rate, heart rate, temperature, pO_2; monitor for gastric obstruction in patients receiving PGE_1 for longer than 120 hours; x-rays may be needed to assess cortical hyperostosis in patients receiving prolonged PGE_1 therapy

Nursing Implications Prepare fresh solution every 24 hours; flushing of arm or face may indicate misplacement of intra-arterial catheter and infusion of drug into subclavian or carotid artery; reposition catheter

Additional Information Therapeutic response is indicated by an increase in systemic blood pressure and pH in those with restricted systemic blood flow and acidosis, or by an increase in oxygenation (pO_2) in those with restricted pulmonary blood flow. Most cases of bone changes occurred 4-6 weeks after starting alprostadil, but it has occurred as early as 9 days; cortical hyperostosis usually resolves over 6-12 months after stopping PGE_1 therapy

Other dosage forms of alprostadil [Caverject® injection, Caverject® Impulse™ injection, Edex® injection, and Muse® Pellet (urethral)] are indicated for the diagnosis and treatment of erectile dysfunction in adult males; see package inserts for further information for this use.

Dosage Forms Excipient information presented when available (limited, particularly for generics); consult specific product labeling. [DSC] = Discontinued product

Injection, powder for reconstitution:

Caverject®: 20 mcg, 40 mcg [contains lactose; diluent contains benzyl alcohol]

Caverject Impulse®: 10 mcg, 20 mcg [prefilled injection system; contains lactose; diluent contains benzyl alcohol]

Edex®: 10 mcg, 20 mcg, 40 mcg [contains lactose; packaged in kits containing diluent, syringe, and alcohol swab]

Injection, solution: 500 mcg/mL (1 mL)
Prostin VR Pediatric®: 500 mcg/mL (1 mL) [contains dehydrated alcohol]
Pellet, urethral:
Muse®: 125 mcg (6s) [DSC], 250 mcg (6s), 500 mcg (6s), 1000 mcg (6s)

References

Kaufman MB and El-Chaar GM, "Bone and Tissue Changes Following Prostaglandin Therapy in Neonates," *Ann Pharmacother*, 1996, 30 (3):269-74, 277.

Lewis AB, Freed MD, Heymann MA, et al, "Side Effects of Therapy With Prostaglandin E₁ in Infants With Critical Congenital Heart Disease," *Circulation*, 1981, 64(5):893-8.

Peled N, Dagan O, Babyn P, et al, "Gastric-Outlet Obstruction Induced by Prostaglandin Therapy in Neonates," *N Engl J Med*, 1992, 327 (8):505-10.

Weesner KM, "Hemodynamic Effects of Prostaglandin E₁ in Patients With Congenital Heart Disease and Pulmonary Hypertension," *Cathet Cardiovasc Diagn*, 1991, 24(1):10-5.

Woo K, Emery J, and Peabody J, "Cortical Hyperostosis: A Complication of Prolonged Prostaglandin Infusion in Infants Awaiting Cardiac Transplantation," *Pediatrics*, 1994, 93(3):417-20.

♦ **Altachlore [OTC]** *see* Sodium Chloride *on page 1270*

♦ **Altafrin** *see* Phenylephrine *on page 1102*

♦ **Altamist [OTC]** *see* Sodium Chloride *on page 1270*

♦ **Altaryl [OTC]** *see* DiphenhydrAMINE *on page 448*

Alteplase (AL te plase)

Medication Safety Issues
Sound-alike/look-alike issues:
Activase® may be confused with Cathflo® Activase®, TNKase®
Alteplase may be confused with Altace®
"tPA" abbreviation should not be used when writing orders for this medication; has been misread as TNKase (tenecteplase)

High alert medication: The Institute for Safe Medication Practices (ISMP) includes this medication (I.V.) among its list of drugs which have a heightened risk of causing significant patient harm when used in error.

Related Information
Antithrombotic Therapy in Neonates and Children *on page 1602*

U.S. Brand Names Activase®; Cathflo® Activase®

Canadian Brand Names Activase® rt-PA; Cathflo® Activase®

Therapeutic Category Thrombolytic Agent; Thrombotic Occlusion (Central Venous Catheter), Treatment Agent

Generic Available No

Use
Activase®: Thrombolytic agent used in treatment of acute MI, acute ischemic stroke, and acute massive pulmonary embolism
CathFlo® Activase®: Treatment of occluded central venous catheters

Pregnancy Risk Factor C

Pregnancy Considerations Teratogenic effects were not observed in animal studies. There are no adequate and well-controlled studies in pregnant women. The risk of bleeding may be increased in pregnant women. Use during pregnancy is limited; administer to pregnant women only if the potential benefits justify the risk to the fetus.

Lactation Excretion in breast milk unknown/use caution

Contraindications Hypersensitivity to alteplase or any component (see Additional Information)

Contraindications for use in the treatment of acute MI or pulmonary embolism: Active internal bleeding; known bleeding diathesis; history of CVA; intracranial neoplasm, arteriovenous malformation, or aneurysm; recent intracranial or intraspinal surgery or trauma; severe uncontrolled hypertension

Contraindications for use in the treatment of acute ischemic stroke: Active internal bleeding; known bleeding diathesis (including but not limited to: Current use of oral anticoagulants or an INR >1.7 or PT >15 seconds, use of heparin within 48 hours before the onset of stroke and an elevated aPTT at presentation, platelet count <100,000/mm³); evidence of intracranial hemorrhage on pretreatment evaluation; history of intracranial hemorrhage; suspicion of subarachnoid hemorrhage; recent (within 3 months) intracranial or intraspinal surgery, serious head trauma, or previous stroke; intracranial neoplasm, arteriovenous malformation, or aneurysm; seizure at the onset of stroke; uncontrolled hypertension at time of treatment (eg, adults with blood pressures of >185 mm Hg systolic or >110 mm Hg diastolic)

Warnings Activase®: May cause bleeding (internal, superficial, or surface bleeding); concurrent use of heparin anticoagulation may increase bleeding; monitor all potential bleeding sites. Avoid I.M. injections and nonessential handling of patient; carefully perform venipunctures and only when necessary. If an arterial puncture is required, use vessel in an upper extremity that can be manually compressed. Stop alteplase (and heparin) if serious bleeding occurs (effects of heparin can be reversed by protamine). Do not exceed recommended doses; do not use doses of 150 mg to treat acute MI as this dose has been associated with an increase in intracranial hemorrhage.

Risks from alteplase may be increased in the following conditions (risks versus benefits should be weighed carefully before use): Recent major surgery (eg, organ biopsy, previous puncture of noncompressible vessels, coronary artery bypass graft, obstetrical delivery), recent trauma, recent GI or GU bleeding, current use of oral anticoagulants, cerebrovascular disease, diabetic hemorrhagic retinopathy or other hemorrhagic ophthalmic conditions, hypertension (eg, adults with systolic BP ≥175 mm Hg and/or diastolic BP ≥110 mm Hg), patients with an increased risk of left heart thrombus (eg, mitral stenosis with atrial fibrillation), acute pericarditis, subacute bacterial endocarditis, hemostatic defects including ones caused by severe renal or hepatic dysfunction, significant hepatic dysfunction, pregnancy, septic thrombophlebitis or occluded AV cannula at seriously infected site, advanced age (eg, >75 years old), any other condition in which bleeding would be a significant risk or would be especially difficult to manage due to its location.

Cholesterol embolism may occur (rare). Risk of stroke in acute MI patients who are at low risk for death from cardiac causes and who present with high blood pressure, may be greater than the survival benefit from thrombolytic therapy. Reperfusion arrhythmias may occur following coronary thrombolysis. In patients with pulmonary embolism, alteplase has not been proven to adequately treat underlying DVT; possible re-embolization from DVT may occur.

Acute ischemic stroke: Risks of alteplase therapy may be increased in patients with major early signs of infarct on CT and in those with severe neurological deficit at presentation (risks versus benefits should be weighed carefully); treatment of patients >3 hours after onset of symptoms and those with rapidly improving symptoms or minor neurological deficit is not recommended.

Precautions
Activase®: Use with caution if drug is readministered; discontinue immediately if anaphylactoid reaction occurs. For treatment of acute ischemic stroke, frequent monitoring and control of blood pressure during and after alteplase administration is recommended. For systemic use, pretreatment lab studies should include platelet count, PT/PTT, fibrinogen, fibrin degradation products, plasminogen, antithrombin III, protein S, protein C.

CathFlo® Activase®: Consider other causes of central venous catheter occlusion (eg, mechanical failure, constriction by a suture, catheter malposition, and drug precipitates or lipid deposits within the lumen of the catheter) before use; do not use vigorous suction when determining catheter occlusion (vascular wall damage or collapse of soft-walled catheters may occur); avoid excessive pressure when instilling alteplase into an occluded catheter (catheter may rupture or clot may become dislodged and enter the circulation). The use of CathFlo® Activase® has not been evaluated in patients who are at risk for bleeding; use with caution in patients with active internal bleeding or those who have had any of the following within 48 hours: Surgery, puncture of noncompressible vessels, obstetrical delivery, or percutaneous biopsy of viscera or deep tissues; use with caution in patients with thrombocytopenia, hemostatic defects including ones caused by severe renal or hepatic dysfunction, any condition in which bleeding would be a significant risk or would be especially difficult to manage due to its location, or those who are at a high risk for embolic complications (eg, venous thrombosis in the region of the catheter). Discontinue CathFlo® Activase® and withdraw from catheter if serious bleeding in a critical location occurs. Use with caution in patients with known or suspected catheter infection (use of CathFlo® Activase® in these patients may release a localized infection in the catheter into the systemic circulation). Use of >2 doses of CathFlo® Activase® has not been studied.

Adverse Reactions Note: Adverse reactions listed below have been reported with systemic use. Major adverse events after intracatheter use include: Sepsis, GI bleeding, and venous thrombosis; injection site hemorrhage in a patient with pre-existing thrombocytopenia and rupture of the catheter have also been reported.

Cardiovascular: Hypotension; reperfusion arrhythmias (following coronary thrombolysis)

Central nervous system: Fever, intracranial hemorrhage, cerebral hemorrhage

Dermatologic: Bruising (1%), rash, urticaria (rare)

Gastrointestinal: GI bleeding (5%), nausea, vomiting

Genitourinary: GU bleeding (4%)

Hematologic: Surface bleeding, internal bleeding

Local: Bleeding at catheter puncture site; bruising and inflammation with extravasation

Respiratory: Epistaxis (<1%), laryngeal edema (rare)

Miscellaneous: Anaphylactoid reaction (rare)

Drug Interactions

Avoid Concomitant Use There are no known interactions where it is recommended to avoid concomitant use.

Increased Effect/Toxicity

Alteplase may increase the levels/effects of: Anticoagulants; Drotrecogin Alfa

The levels/effects of Alteplase may be increased by: Antiplatelet Agents; Herbs (Anticoagulant/Antiplatelet Properties); Nonsteroidal Anti-Inflammatory Agents; Salicylates

Decreased Effect

The levels/effects of Alteplase may be decreased by: Aprotinin; Nitroglycerin

Stability

Activase®: Store lyophilized product at room temperature [not to exceed 86°F (30°C)] or under refrigeration; protect from excessive light exposure during extended storage. Reconstituted solution (1 mg/mL) must be used within 8 hours (manufacturer's recommendations).

The 1 mg/mL solution may be diluted further (immediately before use) with an equal volume of NS or D₅W to yield a final concentration of 0.5 mg/mL; swirl gently, do not shake to dilute; diluted solutions are stable for 8 hours at room temperature. Dilutions to concentrations <0.5 mg/mL are not recommended for routine clinical use; dilutions <0.5 mg/mL using D_5W or SWI will result in a precipitate; an immediate formation of a precipitate following dilution of alteplase with D_5W to 0.16 mg/mL has been reported (Frazin, 1990); after reconstitution to 1 mg/mL, alteplase may be further diluted with NS to concentrations as low as 0.2 mg/mL without precipitation (Frazin, 1990); do not dilute <0.2 mg/mL; after reconstitution to 1 mg/mL, further dilution with NS to target concentrations of 0.05 mg/mL, 0.025 mg/mL, and 0.01 mg/mL resulted in <90% recovery of active alteplase (data on file at Genetech).

Solutions of 0.5 mg/mL, 1 mg/mL, and 2 mg/mL in SWI retained ≥94% of fibrinolytic activity at 48 hours when stored at 2°C in plastic syringes; these solutions retained ≥90% of fibrinolytic activity when stored in plastic syringes at -25°C or -70°C for 7 or 14 days, thawed at room temperature and then stored at 2°C for 48 hours (see Davis, 2000). Solutions of 1 mg/mL in SWI were stable for 22 weeks in plastic syringes when stored at -30°C and for ~1 month in glass vials when stored at -20°C; bioactivity remained unchanged for 6 months in propylene containers when stored at -20°C and for 2 weeks in glass vials when stored at -70°C (see review by Generali, 2001).

Do not add other medications to alteplase solutions. Alteplase is incompatible with bacteriostatic water, dobutamine, dopamine, heparin, morphine, and nitroglycerin infusions; physically compatible with lidocaine, metoprolol, and propranolol when administered via Y site.

CathFlo® Activase®: Store lyophilized product at refrigerated temperature [2°C to 8°C (36°F to 46°C)]; protect from excessive light exposure during extended storage. Reconstituted solution (1 mg/mL) must be used within 8 hours when stored at 2°C to 30°C (36°F to 81°F); do not add other medications to CathFlo® Activase® solutions

Mechanism of Action A naturally-occurring serine protease (enzyme) that initiates local fibrinolysis by binding to fibrin in a thrombus (clot) and directly activating entrapped plasminogen to plasmin; plasmin degrades fibrin, fibrinogen, and other procoagulant proteins into soluble fragments

Pharmacokinetics (Adult data unless noted)

Distribution: Initial: Approximates plasma volume; distribution into breast milk is unknown

Metabolism: In the liver

Half-life: Adults:

Initial: <5 minutes

Terminal: 72 minutes

Clearance: Plasma: Adults: 380-570 mL/minute

Usual Dosage

Neonates, Infants, and Children:

Occluded I.V. catheters: Intracatheter:

Chest, 2001 and *Chest*, 2004 dosing recommendations:

Central venous catheter: **Dose listed is per lumen; for multilumen catheters, treat one lumen at a time:** [Note: Some institutions use lower doses (eg, 0.25 mg/0.5 mL) in neonates and infants <3 months]

Patients ≤10 kg: 0.5 mg diluted in NS to a volume equal to the internal volume of the lumen; instill in each lumen over 1-2 minutes; leave in lumen for 1-2 hours, then **aspirate out of catheter, do not infuse into patient**; flush catheter with NS

Patients >10 kg: 1 mg in 1 mL of NS; use a volume equal to the internal volume of the lumen; maximum: 2 mg in 2 mL per lumen; instill in each lumen over 1-2 minutes; leave in lumen for 1-2 hours; then **aspirate out of catheter, do not infuse into patient**; flush catheter with NS

SubQ port:
Patients ≤10 kg: 0.5 mg diluted with NS to 3 mL
Patients >10 kg: 2 mg diluted with NS to 3 mL
Manufacturer's recommendations (CathFlo® Activase®):
Central venous catheter:
Patients <30 kg: Use a 1 mg/mL concentration; instill a volume equal to 110% of the internal lumen volume of the catheter; do not exceed 2 mg in 2 mL; may instill a second dose if catheter remains occluded after 2-hour dwell time (see Administration)
Patients ≥30 kg: 2 mg in 2 mL; may instill second dose if catheter remains occluded ofter 2-hour dwell time (see Administration)
Systemic thromboses: I.V. (**Note:** Dose must be titrated to effect): *Chest*, 2004 recommendations: 0.1-0.6 mg/kg/hour for 6 hours (some patients may require longer or shorter duration of therapy). **Note:** The optimal dose for various thrombotic conditions is not established in pediatric patients; most published papers consist of case reports; few prospective pediatric studies have been conducted; several studies have used the following doses (see Levy, 1991 and Weiner, 1998). **Note:** Bleeding complications were associated with doses in the higher range.
Initial: 0.1 mg/kg/hour for 6 hours; monitor patient closely for bleeding, monitor fibrinogen levels; if no response after 6 hours, increase infusion by 0.1 mg/kg/hour at 6-hour intervals to a maximum of 0.5 mg/kg/hour; maintain fibrinogen >100 mg/dL (**Note:** Some centers maintain fibrinogen >150 mg/dL in newborns); duration of therapy is based on clinical response
Low-dose (local) infusion for occluded catheters:
Note: No pediatric studies have compared local to systemic thrombolytic therapy; therefore, there is no evidence to suggest that local infusions are superior. The pediatric patients' small vessel size may increase the chance of local damage to blood vessels and formation of a new thrombus; however, local infusion may be appropriate for catheter related thromboses if the catheter is already in place (see *Chest*, 2004). Various "low-dose" regimens have been used; the following dosing recommendations are based on Doyle, 1992 and Anderson, 1991:
Initial: 0.01 mg/kg/hour for 6 hours; if no response after 6 hours, increase infusion by 0.01 mg/kg/hour at 6-hour intervals to a maximum of 0.05 mg/kg/hour; monitor patient closely; systemic fibrinolysis (decreased plasma fibrinogen levels) or bleeding has been reported in some neonates and infants receiving 0.05 mg/kg/hour; duration of therapy is based on clinical response
Adults:
Acute MI: I.V. (**Note:** Alteplase should be administered as soon as possible after symptom onset):
Accelerated infusion:
Patients >67 kg: Total dose: 100 mg given in 3 divided doses as follows: Infuse 15 mg I.V. bolus over 1-2 minutes, then infuse 50 mg over the next 30 minutes, then 35 mg over the next 60 minutes. Maximum total dose: 100 mg
Patients ≤67 kg: Infuse 15 mg I.V. bolus over 1-2 minutes, then infuse 0.75 mg/kg (maximum: 50 mg) over the next 30 minutes, then 0.5 mg/kg (maximum: 35 mg) over the next 60 minutes. Maximum total dose: 100 mg
Acute ischemic stroke: I.V. (**Note:** Alteplase therapy should only be started within 3 hours after the onset of symptoms of stroke and after exclusion of intracranial hemorrhage by CT scan or other sensitive diagnostic imaging method): Total dose: 0.9 mg/kg (maximum: 90 mg) given over 1 hour as follows: Infuse 10% of total

dose (0.09 mg/kg) I.V. bolus over 1 minute, then infuse the rest of the total dose (0.81 mg/kg) over 60 minutes
Pulmonary embolism: I.V.: 100 mg infused over 2 hours
Occluded central venous catheter: Intracatheter: Manufacturer's recommendations (CathFlo® Activase®): Patients ≥30 kg: 2 mg in 2 mL; may instill second dose if catheter remains occluded after 2-hour dwell time (see Administration); **Note:** A recent study using escalating doses of 0.5 mg, 1 mg, and 2 mg (60 minute dwell time) found that 86.2% of catheters were cleared with the 0.5 mg dose (see Davis, 2000).

Administration

Parenteral: Activase®: Reconstitute vials with supplied diluent (SWI); do not reconstitute with bacteriostatic water for injection; use large bore needle and syringe to reconstitute 50 mg vial and accompanying transfer device to reconstitute 100 mg vial (100 mg vial does not contain vacuum); swirl gently, do not shake; final concentration after reconstitution: 1 mg/mL

I.V.: May administer at a final concentration of 1 mg/mL or may dilute and administer as 0.5 mg/mL (see Stability). Prepare bolus dose using one of the following methods: 1) Remove bolus dose from reconstituted vial using syringe and needle; for 50 mg vial: do not prime syringe with air, insert needle into vial stopper; for 100 mg vial, insert needle away from puncture mark created by transfer device; 2) Remove bolus dose from a port on the infusion line after priming; 3) Program an infusion pump to deliver the bolus at the beginning of the infusion. Administer the remaining dose as follows: From 50 mg vial: Use polyvinyl chloride I.V. bag or glass vial and infusion set; from 100 mg vial: Use same puncture site made by transfer device to insert spike end of infusion set and infuse from vial.

CathFlo® Activase®: Reconstitute vial with 2.2 mL of SWI; do not reconstitute with bacteriostatic water for injection; allow vial to stand undisturbed so large bubbles may dissipate; swirl gently, do not shake; complete dissolution occurs within 3 minutes; final concentration after reconstitution: 1 mg/mL. Discard any unused solution (solution does not contain preservatives) (see Stability).

Intracatheter: Instill the appropriate dose into the occluded catheter (see Usual Dosage); leave in lumen; evaluate catheter function (by attempting to aspirate blood) after 30 minutes; if catheter is functional, aspirate 4-5 mL of blood out of catheter in patients ≥10 kg or 3 mL in patients <10 kg to remove drug and residual clot, then gently flush catheter with NS; if catheter is still occluded, leave alteplase in lumen and evaluate catheter function after 120 minutes of dwell time; if catheter is functional, aspirate 4-5 mL of blood out of catheter in patients ≥10 kg or 3 mL in patients <10 kg and gently flush with NS; if catheter remains occluded after 120 minutes of dwell time, a second dose may be instilled by repeating the above administration procedure.

Monitoring Parameters

Systemic use: Blood pressure; temperature; CBC, reticulocyte, platelet count; fibrinogen level, plasminogen, fibrin/fibrinogen degradation products, D-dimer, PT, PTT, antithrombin III, protein C; urinalysis, signs of bleeding

Intracatheter use: Catheter function (by attempting to aspirate blood); temperature, signs of sepsis, GI bleeding, bleeding at injection site, and venous thrombosis

Nursing Implications Extravasation may cause bruising or inflammation; monitor infusion site for patency of I.V.; if extravasation occurs, discontinue infusion at site of extravasation and apply local treatment; avoid I.M. injections; assess patient for bleeding

Additional Information Activase® and CathFlo® Activase® also contain L-arginine, polysorbate 80, and phosphoric acid (for pH adjustment).

Advantages of alteplase include: Low immunogenicity, short half-life, direct activation of plasminogen, and a strong and specific affinity for fibrin. Failure of thrombolytic agents in newborns/neonates may occur due to the low plasminogen concentrations (~50% to 70% of adult levels); supplementing plasminogen (via administration of fresh frozen plasma) may possibly help. Osmolality of 1 mg/mL solution is ~215 mOsm/kg.

Appropriate intracatheter use of alteplase for the treatment of occluded central venous catheters is not expected to cause systemic pharmacologic effects; in adults, if a 2 mg dose is administered I.V. (instead of being instilled into the catheter), the serum concentration of alteplase would be expected to return to normal endogenous levels within 30 minutes.

An open-label, single-arm trial of CathFlo® Activase® in pediatric patients, 2 weeks to 17 years of age (n=310), was conducted using the manufacturer's recommended doses (see Usual Dosage); catheter function was restored in 83% of patients (similar to adults); rates of serious adverse events were also similar to adults (see CathFlo® Activase® package insert, 2005).

Dosage Forms Excipient information presented when available (limited, particularly for generics); consult specific product labeling.

Injection, powder for reconstitution, recombinant:

Activase®: 50 mg [29 million int. units; contains polysorbate 80; packaged with diluent]; 100 mg [58 million int. units; contains polysorbate 80; packaged with diluent and transfer device]

CathFlo® Activase®: 2 mg [contains polysorbate 80]

References

Anderson BJ, Keeley SR, and Johnson ND, "Caval Thrombolysis in Neonates Using Low Doses of Recombinant Human Tissue-Type Plasminogen Activator," *Anaesth Intensive Care*, 1991, 19(1):22-7.

Andrew M, Brooker L, Leaker M, et al, "Fibrin Clot Lysis by Thrombolytic Agents is Impaired in Newborns Due to a Low Plasminogen Concentration," *Thromb Haemost*, 1992, 68(3):325-30.

Cada DJ, Levien T, and Baker DE, "Alteplase," *Hospital Pharmacy*, 2002, 37(2): 148-54.

Choi M, Massicotte MP, Marzinotto V, et al, "The Use of Alteplase to Restore Patency of Central Venous Lines in Pediatric Patients: A Cohort Study," *J Pediatr*, 2001, 139(1):152-6.

Davis SN, Vermeulen L, Banton J, et al, "Activity and Dosage of Alteplase Dilution for Clearing Occlusions of Venous-Access Devices," *Am J Health Syst Pharm*, 2000, 57(11):1039-45.

Doyle E, Britto J, Freeman J, et al, "Thrombolysis With Low Dose Tissue Plasminogen Activator," *Arch Dis Child*, 1992, 67(12):1483-4.

Farnoux C, Camard O, Pinquier D, et al, "Recombinant Tissue-Type Plasminogen Activator Therapy of Thrombosis in 16 Neonates," *J Pediatr*, 1998, 133(1):137-40.

Frazin BS, "Maximal Dilution of Activase," *Am J Hosp Pharm*, 1990, 47 (5):1016.

Generali J and Cada DJ, "Alteplase (t-PA) Bolus: Occluded Catheters," *Hospital Pharmacy*, 2001, 36(1):93-103.

Kothari SS, Varma S, and Wasir S, "Thrombolytic Therapy in Infants and Children," *Am Heart J*, 1994, 127(3):651-7.

Levy M, Benson LN, Burrows PE, et al, "Tissue Plasminogen Activator for the Treatment of Thromboembolism in Infants and Children," *J Pediatr*, 1991, 118(3):467-72.

Monagle P, Chan A, Massicotte P, et al, "Antithrombotic Therapy in Children: The Seventh ACCP Conference on Antithrombotic and Thrombolytic Therapy," *Chest*, 2004, 126(3 Suppl):645S-687S.

Monagle P, Michelson AD, Bovill E, et al, "Antithrombotic Therapy in Children," *Chest*, 2001, 119(1 Suppl):344S-370S.

Nowak-Gottl U, Auberger K, Halimeh S, et al, "Thrombolysis in Newborns and Infants," *Thromb Haemost*, 1999, 82 (Suppl 1):112-6.

Ponec D, Irwin D, Haire WD, et al, "Recombinant Tissue Plasminogen Activator (Alteplase) for Restoration of Flow in Occluded Central Venous Access Devices: A Double-Blind Placebo-Controlled Trial - The Cardiovascular Thrombolytic to Open Occluded Lines (COOL) Efficacy Trial," *J Vasc Intern Radiol*, 2001, 12(8):951-5.

Weiner GM, Castle VP, DiPietro MA, et al, "Successful Treatment of Neonatal Arterial Thromboses With Recombinant Tissue Plasminogen Activator," *J Pediatr*, 1998, 133(1):133-6.

♦ **Alteplase, Recombinant** see Alteplase on page 71

♦ **Alteplase, Tissue Plasminogen Activator, Recombinant** see Alteplase on page 71

♦ **ALternaGel® [OTC]** see Aluminum Hydroxide on page 75

♦ **Alti-Alprazolam (Can)** see ALPRAZolam on page 68

♦ **Alti-Captopril (Can)** see Captopril on page 242

♦ **Alti-Clonazepam (Can)** see ClonazePAM on page 337

♦ **Alti-Desipramine (Can)** see Desipramine on page 401

♦ **Alti-Divalproex (Can)** see Valproic Acid and Derivatives on page 1398

♦ **Alti-Flunisolide (Can)** see Flunisolide on page 592

♦ **Alti-Flurbiprofen (Can)** see Flurbiprofen on page 605

♦ **Alti-Fluvoxamine (Can)** see Fluvoxamine on page 615

♦ **Alti-Ipratropium (Can)** see Ipratropium on page 757

♦ **Alti-MPA (Can)** see MedroxyPROGESTERone on page 870

♦ **Alti-Nadolol (Can)** see Nadolol on page 961

♦ **Alti-Nortriptyline (Can)** see Nortriptyline on page 1002

♦ **Alti-Sulfasalazine (Can)** see Sulfasalazine on page 1304

♦ **Alti-Timolol (Can)** see Timolol on page 1351

♦ **Altoprev®** see Lovastatin on page 850

Aluminum Acetate (a LOO mi num AS e tate)

U.S. Brand Names Domeboro®

Therapeutic Category Topical Skin Product

Use Astringent wet dressing for relief of inflammatory conditions of the skin and to reduce weeping that may occur in dermatitis; relieve minor skin irritations due to poison ivy, poison oak, poison sumac, insect bites, athlete's foot, and rashes caused by soaps, detergents, cosmetics, or jewelry

Pregnancy Risk Factor C

Contraindications Use with topical collagenase

Precautions Do not use plastic or other impervious material to prevent evaporation

Adverse Reactions Local: Irritation

Drug Interactions

Avoid Concomitant Use

Avoid concomitant use of Aluminum Acetate with any of the following: BCG

Increased Effect/Toxicity There are no known significant interactions involving an increase in effect.

Decreased Effect

Aluminum Acetate may decrease the levels/effects of: BCG

Usual Dosage Children and Adults: Topical: Soak the affected area in the solution 2-4 times/day for 15-30 minutes or apply wet dressing soaked in the solution 2-4 times/day for 30-minute treatment periods; rewet dressing with solution every few minutes to keep it moist

Administration Topical: Keep away from eyes, external use only; one powder packet dissolved in 16 oz of water makes a modified Burow's solution equivalent to a 1:40 dilution, 2 packets: 1:20 dilution, 3 packets: 1:13 dilution. When used as a compress or wet dressing, soak a clean soft cloth in the solution. Apply cloth loosely to affected area for 15-30 minutes.

Dosage Forms Excipient information presented when available (limited, particularly for generics); consult specific product labeling.

Powder, for topical solution:

Domeboro®: Aluminum sulfate 1191 mg and calcium acetate 839 mg per packet (12s, 100s) [when powder packet is mixed with water, provides active ingredient aluminum acetate]

♦ **Aluminum and Magnesium Hydroxide** see Aluminum Hydroxide and Magnesium Hydroxide on page 76

Aluminum Hydroxide

(a LOO mi num hye DROKS ide)

U.S. Brand Names ALternaGel® [OTC]; Dermagran® [OTC]
Canadian Brand Names Amphojel®; Basaljel®
Therapeutic Category Antacid; Antidote; Gastrointestinal Agent, Gastric or Duodenal Ulcer Treatment; Protectant, Topical
Generic Available Yes: Suspension
Use
Oral: Adjunct for the relief of peptic ulcer pain and to promote healing of peptic ulcers; relief of sour stomach or stomach upset associated with hyperacidity; relief of heartburn; treatment of gastritis, esophagitis, and gastroesophageal reflux disease; reduce phosphate absorption in hyperphosphatemia

Topical: Temporary protection of minor cuts, scrapes, burns, and other skin irritations
Pregnancy Risk Factor C
Pregnancy Considerations No data available on clinical effects on the fetus; available evidence suggests safe use during pregnancy and breast-feeding.
Lactation Excretion in breast milk unknown
Contraindications Hypersensitivity to aluminum salts or any component
Warnings
Oral: Hypophosphatemia may occur with prolonged aluminum hydroxide administration or with large doses; aluminum toxicity and osteomalacia may occur in patients with chronic kidney disease.

Topical: Not for application over deep wounds, puncture wounds, infected areas, or lacerations. When used for self medication (OTC use), consult with healthcare provider if needed for >7 days or for use in children <6 months of age.
Precautions Use oral aluminum hydroxide with caution in patients with decreased bowel motility and dehydration, gastric outlet obstruction, renal failure, CHF, edema, cirrhosis, and in patients who have an upper GI hemorrhage
Adverse Reactions
Central nervous system: Dementia, encephalopathy, malaise, seizures, confusion, coma
Endocrine & metabolic: Hypophosphatemia, hypomagnesemia
Gastrointestinal: Constipation, fecal impaction, anorexia, stomach cramps, nausea, vomiting, bezoar or fecalith formation
Genitourinary: Urinary calculi
Neuromuscular & skeletal: Muscle weakness, osteomalacia, osteoporosis
Drug Interactions
Avoid Concomitant Use
Avoid concomitant use of Aluminum Hydroxide with any of the following: QuiNINE
Increased Effect/Toxicity
Aluminum Hydroxide may increase the levels/effects of: Amphetamines

The levels/effects of Aluminum Hydroxide may be increased by: Ascorbic Acid; Calcium Polystyrene Sulfonate; Citric Acid Derivatives; Sodium Polystyrene Sulfonate
Decreased Effect
Aluminum Hydroxide may decrease the levels/effects of: ACE Inhibitors; Allopurinol; Anticonvulsants (Hydantoin); Antifungal Agents (Azole Derivatives, Systemic); Antipsychotic Agents (Phenothiazines); Atazanavir; Bisacodyl; Bisphosphonate Derivatives; Cefditoren; Cefpodoxime; Cefuroxime; Chloroquine; Corticosteroids (Oral); Dabigatran Etexilate; Dasatinib; Deferasirox; Delavirdine; Eltrombopag; Erlotinib; Ethambutol; Fexofenadine; HMG-CoA Reductase Inhibitors; Iron Salts; Isoniazid; Mesalamine; Methenamine; Mycophenolate; Penicillamine; Phosphate Supplements; Protease Inhibitors; QuiNINE; Quinolone Antibiotics; Tetracycline Derivatives; Trientine; Ursodiol
Food Interactions Forms insoluble salts with dietary phosphorus decreasing phosphorus absorption
Stability Avoid freezing
Mechanism of Action Neutralizes gastric acidity by reacting with hydrochloric acid in the stomach to form aluminum chloride and water. Topical aluminum hydroxide has astringent and demulcent actions.
Pharmacodynamics
Duration: Dependent on gastric emptying time
Fasting state: 20-60 minutes
One hour after meals: Up to 3 hours
Pharmacokinetics (Adult data unless noted) Elimination: Excreted by the kidneys (normal renal function): 17% to 30%; combines with dietary phosphate in the intestine and is excreted in the feces
Usual Dosage
Oral:
Antacid:
Children: 300-900 mg between meals and at bedtime
Adolescents and Adults: 600-1200 mg between meals and at bedtime; or 600 mg 5-6 times/day between meals; maximum daily dose: 3600 mg/day; do not use maximum daily dose for more than 2 weeks without physician consultation
Hyperphosphatemia associated with chronic renal failure:
Children: 30 mg/kg/day in divided doses 3 or 4 times/day; maximum daily dose: 3000 mg/day; titrate to normal serum phosphorus level
Adolescents and Adults: 300-600 mg 3 or 4 times/day; maximum daily dose: 3000 mg/day
Topical: Apply to affected area as needed; reapply at least every 12 hours
Administration
Oral: Shake suspension well before use; dose should be followed with water
Antacid: Administer 1-3 hours after meals
To decrease phosphorus: Administer within 20 minutes of a meal
Topical: For external use only
Monitoring Parameters Monitor for GI complaints, stool frequency; serum phosphate and serum aluminum concentrations in patients with chronic kidney disease
Reference Range Baseline serum aluminum level <20 mcg/L
Patient Information Antacids may impair or increase absorption of many drugs; do not take oral medications within 1-2 hours of an antacid dose unless specifically instructed to do so. Report unresolved nausea, malaise, muscle weakness, blood in stool, or abdominal pain.
Additional Information Sodium content of ALternaGel®: <0.11 mEq per 5 mL

Dosage Forms Excipient information presented when available (limited, particularly for generics); consult specific product labeling.

Ointment:

Dermagran®: 0.275% (120 g)

Suspension, oral: 320 mg/5 mL (473 mL); 600 mg/5 mL (355 mL)

ALternaGel®: 600 mg/5 mL (360 mL)

References

Avner ED, Harmon W, and Niaudet P, "Chronic Renal Disease," *Pediatric Nephrology*, 5th ed, Baltimore, MD: Lippincott Williams & Wilkins, 2003, 1363.

"K/DOQI Clinical Practice Guidelines for Bone Metabolism and Disease in Chronic Kidney Disease. Guideline 11. Aluminum Overload and Toxicity in CKD," 2002, available at www.kidney.org/professionals/kdoqi/guidelines_bone/guide11.htm.

Aluminum Hydroxide and Magnesium Hydroxide

(a LOO mi num hye DROKS ide & mag NEE zhum hye DROK side)

U.S. Brand Names Alamag [OTC]

Canadian Brand Names Diovol®; Diovol® Ex; Gelusil® Extra Strength; Mylanta™

Therapeutic Category Antacid; Gastrointestinal Agent, Gastric or Duodenal Ulcer Treatment

Generic Available Yes

Use Adjunct for the relief of heartburn, peptic ulcer pain, and to promote healing of peptic ulcers; relief of stomach upset associated with hyperacidity

Pregnancy Risk Factor C

Contraindications Hypersensitivity to aluminum hydroxide, magnesium hydroxide, or any component. Aluminum and magnesium-containing antacids should not be used in patients with a creatinine clearance <30 mL/minute.

Precautions Use with caution in patients with decreased bowel motility and dehydration, diarrhea, appendicitis, gastric outlet obstruction, and in patients who have an upper GI hemorrhage. Decreased renal function (Cl$_{cr}$ <30 mL/minute) may result in toxicity of aluminum or magnesium. There are reports of osteomalacia and osteoporosis due to aluminum toxicity associated with use.

Adverse Reactions

Aluminum-containing antacids:

Central nervous system: Dementia, encephalopathy, malaise, seizures, confusion, coma, headache

Endocrine & metabolic: Hypophosphatemia, hyperaluminemia, osteoporosis

Gastrointestinal: Constipation, anorexia, nausea, fecal impaction

Genitourinary: Urinary calculi

Neuromuscular & skeletal: Muscle weakness, osteomalacia

Magnesium-containing antacids:

Endocrine & metabolic: Hypermagnesemia, fluid and electrolyte imbalance, metabolic alkalosis, sodium overload

Gastrointestinal: Laxative effects, diarrhea, flatulence

Drug Interactions

Avoid Concomitant Use

Avoid concomitant use of Aluminum Hydroxide and Magnesium Hydroxide with any of the following: Calcium Polystyrene Sulfonate; QuiNINE; Sodium Polystyrene Sulfonate

Increased Effect/Toxicity

Aluminum Hydroxide and Magnesium Hydroxide may increase the levels/effects of: Alpha-/Beta-Agonists; Amphetamines; Calcium Channel Blockers; Misoprostol; Neuromuscular-Blocking Agents; QuiNIDine

The levels/effects of Aluminum Hydroxide and Magnesium Hydroxide may be increased by: Ascorbic Acid; Calcitriol; Calcium Channel Blockers; Calcium

Polystyrene Sulfonate; Citric Acid Derivatives; Sodium Polystyrene Sulfonate

Decreased Effect

Aluminum Hydroxide and Magnesium Hydroxide may decrease the levels/effects of: ACE Inhibitors; Allopurinol; Anticonvulsants (Hydantoin); Antifungal Agents (Azole Derivatives, Systemic); Antipsychotic Agents (Phenothiazines); Atazanavir; Bisacodyl; Bisphosphonate Derivatives; Cefditoren; Cefpodoxime; Cefuroxime; Chloroquine; Corticosteroids (Oral); Dabigatran Etexilate; Dasatinib; Deferasirox; Delavirdine; Eltrombopag; Erlotinib; Ethambutol; Fexofenadine; HMG-CoA Reductase Inhibitors; Iron Salts; Isoniazid; Mesalamine; Methenamine; Mycophenolate; Penicillamine; Phosphate Supplements; Protease Inhibitors; QuiNINE; Quinolone Antibiotics; Tetracycline Derivatives; Trientine; Ursodiol

The levels/effects of Aluminum Hydroxide and Magnesium Hydroxide may be decreased by: Trientine

Food Interactions Aluminum hydroxide forms insoluble salts with dietary phosphorus decreasing phosphorus absorption.

Stability Store at room temperature; avoid freezing aluminum hydroxide and magnesium hydroxide.

Mechanism of Action Neutralizes gastric acidity increasing gastric pH; inhibits proteolytic activity of pepsin when gastric pH is increased >4; binds bile salts

Pharmacodynamics Duration: Dependent on gastric emptying time

Fasting state: 20-60 minutes

1 hour after meals: May be up to 3 hours

Usual Dosage Oral: Aluminum/magnesium hydroxide combination (for extra strength or concentrated suspension, use half the volume of the stated dose): **Note:** Dosing information for children is limited, very few published clinical trials are available. The following pediatric dose represents suggested dosing from review articles:

Suspension:

Children: 0.5-2 mL/kg/dose after meals and at bedtime (maximum dose: 15 mL)

Adults: 5-10 mL 4-6 times/day, between meals and at bedtime (maximum dose: 20 mL/dose or 90 mL/24 hours); may be used every hour for severe symptoms

Tablet: Children ≥6 years and Adults: 1-2 tablets 4 times/day

Administration Oral:

Suspension: Shake suspensions well before use; administer 1-2 hours after meals when stomach acidity is highest

Tablet: Chew tablet thoroughly before swallowing; follow by a full glass of water.

Monitoring Parameters GI complaints, stool frequency; serum phosphate concentrations in patients on hemodialysis receiving chronic aluminum-containing antacid therapy; serum electrolytes in patients with renal impairment receiving magnesium-containing antacids

Patient Information Antacids may impair or increase absorption of many drugs; do not take oral medications within 1-2 hours of an antacid dose unless specifically instructed to do so. Inform physician if symptoms do not improve within 2 weeks or if they worsen, or if black, tarry stools or coffee ground emesis occurs.

Dosage Forms Excipient information presented when available (limited, particularly for generics); consult specific product labeling.

Suspension: Aluminum hydroxide 225 mg and magnesium hydroxide 200 mg per 5 mL (360 mL)

Alamag: Aluminum hydroxide 225 mg and magnesium hydroxide 200 mg per 5 mL (360 mL)

Tablet, chewable:

Alamag: Aluminum hydroxide 300 mg and magnesium hydroxide 150 mg

References

Nord KS, "Peptic Ulcer Disease in the Pediatric Population," *Pediatr Clin North Am*, 1988, 35(1):117-40.

Orenstein SR and Orenstein DM, "Gastroesophageal Reflux and Respiratory Disease in Children," *J Pediatr*, 1988, 112(6):847-58.

Rudolph CD, Mazur LJ, Liptak GS, et al, "Guidelines for Evaluation and Treatment of Gastroesophageal Reflux in Infants and Children: Recommendations of the North American Society for Pediatric Gastroenterology and Nutrition," *J Pediatr Gastroenterol Nutr*, 2001, 32 (Suppl 2):S1-31.

Sutphen JL, Dillard VL, and Pipan ME, "Antacid and Formula Effects on Gastric Acidity in Infants With Gastroesophageal Reflux," *Pediatrics*, 1986, 78(1):55-7.

Shaffer SE and Levine S, "Gastroesophageal Reflux in Children," *Hosp Pharm*, 2003, 38(3):212-7.

Shapiro GG and Christie DL, "Gastroesophageal Reflux in Steroid-Dependent Asthmatic Youths," *Pediatrics*, 1979, 63(2):207-12.

◆ **Aluminum Hydroxide and Magnesium Hydroxide** *see* Aluminum Hydroxide and Magnesium Hydroxide *on page 76*

◆ **Aluminum Sucrose Sulfate, Basic** *see* Sucralfate *on page 1296*

◆ **Alupent® [DSC]** *see* Metaproterenol *on page 890*

Amantadine (a MAN ta deen)

Medication Safety Issues

Sound-alike/look-alike issues:

Amantadine may be confused with ranitidine, rimantadine

Symmetrel® may be confused with Synthroid®

International issues:

Symmetrel® may be confused with Somatrel® which is a brand name for somatorelin in Denmark

U.S. Brand Names Symmetrel®

Canadian Brand Names Endantadine®; Mylan-Amantadine; PMS-Amantadine; Symmetrel®

Therapeutic Category Anti-Parkinson's Agent; Antiviral Agent, Oral

Generic Available Yes

Use Prophylaxis and treatment of influenza A viral infection (FDA approved in ages ≥1 year and adults); symptomatic and adjunct treatment of parkinsonism (FDA approved in adults)

Pregnancy Risk Factor C

Pregnancy Considerations Teratogenic effects were observed in animal studies; limited data in humans. Impaired fertility has also been reported during animal studies and during human *in vitro* fertilization.

Lactation Enters breast milk/not recommended

Contraindications Hypersensitivity to amantadine hydrochloride or any component

Warnings Deaths due to amantadine overdose have been reported with the lowest lethal dose being 1 gram. Drug overdose has resulted in cardiac (ie, arrhythmia, tachycardia, hypertension), respiratory, renal, or central nervous system toxicity.

Precautions Use with caution in patients with liver disease, epilepsy, history of recurrent eczematoid dermatitis, uncontrolled psychosis, and in patients receiving CNS stimulant drugs; may increase seizure activity or EEG disturbances in patients with pre-existing seizure disorders; neuroleptic malignant syndrome has been reported in patients undergoing dosage reduction or withdrawal of amantadine; modify dosage in patients with renal impairment; may need to modify dose in patients with active seizure disorders, CHF, peripheral edema, and orthostatic hypotension

Adverse Reactions

Cardiovascular: Orthostatic hypotension, edema

Central nervous system: Dizziness, confusion, headache, insomnia, difficulty in concentrating, anxiety, restlessness, irritability, hallucinations, seizures, suicide ideation, neuroleptic malignant syndrome, lightheadedness

Dermatologic: Livedo reticularis

Gastrointestinal: Nausea, vomiting, xerostomia, anorexia, constipation

Genitourinary: Urinary retention

Drug Interactions

Avoid Concomitant Use There are no known interactions where it is recommended to avoid concomitant use.

Increased Effect/Toxicity

Amantadine may increase the levels/effects of: Trimethoprim

The levels/effects of Amantadine may be increased by: Antipsychotics (Typical); MAO Inhibitors; Trimethoprim

Decreased Effect

Amantadine may decrease the levels/effects of: Antipsychotics (Typical); Influenza Virus Vaccine (H1N1, Live/Attenuated); Influenza Virus Vaccine (Live/Attenuated)

The levels/effects of Amantadine may be decreased by: Antipsychotics (Atypical); Metoclopramide

Mechanism of Action As an antiviral, blocks the uncoating of influenza A virus preventing penetration of virus into host and inhibits M_2 protein in the assembly of progeny virions; antiparkinsonian activity may be due to its blocking the reuptake of dopamine into presynaptic neurons and causing direct stimulation of postsynaptic receptors

Pharmacokinetics (Adult data unless noted)

Absorption: Well absorbed from the GI tract

Half-life, patients with normal renal function: 10-28 hours

Time to peak serum concentration: 1-4 hours

Elimination: 80% to 90% excreted unchanged in the urine by glomerular filtration and tubular secretion

Dialysis: 0% to 5% removed by hemodialysis; no supplemental dose needed after hemodialysis or peritoneal dialysis

Usual Dosage Oral:

Children:

Influenza A treatment/prophylaxis: **Note:** Due to issues of resistance, amantadine is no longer recommended for the treatment or prophylaxis of influenza A. Please refer to the current ACIP recommendations. The following is based on the manufacturer's labeling and past ACIP dosing recommendations:

Influenza A treatment:

1-9 years: 5 mg/kg/day in 2 divided doses (manufacturer's range: 4.4-8.8 mg/kg/day); maximum dose: 150 mg/day

≥10 years and <40 kg: 5 mg/kg/day in 2 divided doses; maximum dose: 150 mg/day (CDC, 2003)

≥10 years and ≥40 kg: 100 mg twice daily (CDC, 2003)

Note: Initiate within 24-48 hours after onset of symptoms; continue for 24-48 hours after symptom resolution (duration of therapy is generally 3-5 days)

Influenza A prophylaxis: Refer to "Influenza A treatment" dosing

Note: Continue prophylaxis throughout the peak influenza activity in the community or throughout the entire influenza season in patients who cannot be vaccinated. Development of immunity following vaccination takes ~2 weeks; amantadine therapy should be considered for high-risk patients from the time of vaccination until immunity has developed. For ages <9 years receiving influenza vaccine for the first time, amantadine prophylaxis should continue for 6 weeks (4 weeks after the first dose and 2 weeks after the second dose).

◀ Adults:
Drug-induced extrapyramidal symptoms: 100 mg twice daily; may increase to 300 mg/day in divided doses, if needed

Parkinson's disease: Usual dose: 100 mg twice daily as monotherapy; may increase to 400 mg/day in divided doses, if needed, with close monitoring
Note: Patients with a serious concomitant illness or those receiving high doses of other antiparkinson drugs should be started at 100 mg/day; may increase to 100 mg twice daily, if needed, after one to several weeks

Influenza A treatment/prophylaxis: **Note:** Due to issues of resistance, amantadine is no longer recommended for the treatment or prophylaxis of influenza A. Please refer to the current ACIP recommendations. The following is based on the manufacturer's labeling:
Influenza A treatment: 200 mg once daily **or** 100 mg twice daily (may be preferred to reduce CNS effects)
Note: Initiate within 24-48 hours after onset of symptoms; continue for 24-48 hours after symptom resolution (duration of therapy is generally 3-5 days)
Influenza A prophylaxis: 200 mg once daily **or** 100 mg twice daily (may be preferred to reduce CNS effects)
Note: Continue prophylaxis throughout the peak influenza activity in the community or throughout the entire influenza season in patients who cannot be vaccinated. Development of immunity following vaccination takes ~2 weeks; amantadine therapy should be considered for high-risk patients from the time of vaccination until immunity has developed.

Elderly (≥65 years): Adjust dose based on renal function; some patients tolerate the drug better when it is given in 2 divided daily doses (to avoid adverse neurologic reactions).

Dosing interval in renal impairment:
Cl_cr 30-50 mL/minute: Administer 200 mg on day 1, then 100 mg/day
Cl_cr 15-29 mL/minute: Administer 200 mg on day 1, then 100 mg on alternate days
Cl_cr <15 mL/minute: Administer 200 mg every 7 days
Hemodialysis: Administer 200 mg every 7 days
Peritoneal dialysis: No supplemental dose is needed
Continuous arteriovenous or venous-venous hemofiltration: No supplemental dose is needed

Monitoring Parameters Renal function; monitor for signs of neurotoxicity

Patient Information May cause drowsiness and impair ability to perform activities requiring mental alertness or physical coordination; do not abruptly discontinue therapy, may precipitate a parkinsonian crisis; avoid alcohol; may cause dry mouth

Nursing Implications If insomnia occurs, the last daily dose should be taken several hours before retiring

Dosage Forms Excipient information presented when available (limited, particularly for generics); consult specific product labeling.
Capsule, as hydrochloride: 100 mg
Capsule, softgel, as hydrochloride: 100 mg
Solution, oral, as hydrochloride: 50 mg/5 mL (473 mL)
Syrup, oral, as hydrochloride: 50 mg/5 mL (10 mL, 480 mL)
Tablet, as hydrochloride: 100 mg
Symmetrel®: 100 mg

References
Centers for Disease Control, "Prevention and Control of Influenza. Recommendations of the Advisory Committee on Immunization Practices (ACIP)," *MMWR Recomm Rep*, 2003, 52(RR-8):35.
Centers for Disease Control, "Prevention and Control of Influenza. Recommendations of the Advisory Committee on Immunization Practices (ACIP)," MMWR Recomm Rep, 2008, 56 (early release):1-60. Available at http://www.cdc.gov/mmwr/preview/mmwrhtml/rr57e717a1.htm.

Strong DK, Eisenstat DD, Bryson SM, et al, "Amantadine Neurotoxicity in a Pediatric Patient With Renal Insufficiency," *DICP*, 1991, 25 (11):1175-7.

◆ **Amantadine Hydrochloride** *see* Amantadine *on page 77*
◆ **Ambien®** *see* Zolpidem *on page 1447*
◆ **Ambien CR®** *see* Zolpidem *on page 1447*
◆ **AmBisome®** *see* Amphotericin B Liposome *on page 103*
◆ **AMCA** *see* Tranexamic Acid *on page 1369*
◆ **Americaine® Hemorrhoidal [OTC]** *see* Benzocaine *on page 182*
◆ **A-Methapred** *see* MethylPREDNISolone *on page 912*
◆ **A-Methapred®** *see* MethylPREDNISolone *on page 912*
◆ **Amethocaine Hydrochloride** *see* Tetracaine *on page 1330*
◆ **Amethopterin** *see* Methotrexate *on page 900*
◆ **Ametop™ (Can)** *see* Tetracaine *on page 1330*
◆ **Amicar®** *see* Aminocaproic Acid *on page 82*
◆ **Amidate®** *see* Etomidate *on page 550*

Amifostine (am i FOS teen)

Medication Safety Issues
Sound-alike/look-alike issues:
Ethyol® may be confused with ethanol
Related Information
Compatibility of Chemotherapy and Related Supportive Care Medications *on page 1580*
Emetogenic Potential of Antineoplastic Agents *on page 1579*
U.S. Brand Names Ethyol®
Canadian Brand Names Ethyol®
Therapeutic Category Antidote, Cisplatin; Cytoprotective Agent
Generic Available Yes
Use Cytoprotective agent which scavenges free radicals and binds to reactive drug derivatives due to radiation therapy, cisplatin, carboplatin, cyclophosphamide, ifosfamide, carmustine, melphalan, and mechlorethamine to selectively protect normal tissues against toxicity due to these agents; reduction of moderate to severe xerostomia from radiation treatment of the head and neck where the radiation port includes a substantial portion of the parotid glands
Pregnancy Risk Factor C
Pregnancy Considerations Animal studies have demonstrated embryotoxicity. There are no adequate and well-controlled studies in pregnant women.
Lactation Excretion in breast milk unknown/not recommended
Breast-Feeding Considerations Due to the potential for adverse reactions in the nursing infant, breast-feeding should be discontinued.
Contraindications Hypersensitivity to amifostine, aminothiol compounds, or any component
Warnings Due to limited experience and the possibility of amifostine interference with antineoplastic efficacy, amifostine should not be administered to patients receiving definitive radiation therapy or in settings in which chemotherapy (for malignancies other than ovarian cancer) can produce a significant survival benefit or cure, except in the context of a clinical study. Monitor serum calcium levels in patients at risk of hypocalcemia (eg, those patients receiving multiple doses of amifostine, patients with nephrotic syndrome).

Rare hypersensitivity reactions, including anaphylaxis and allergic reaction, have been reported. Discontinue if allergic reaction occurs; do not rechallenge. Medications for the treatment of hypersensitivity reactions should be available. Serious cutaneous reactions, including erythema multiforme, Stevens-Johnson syndrome, toxic epidermal necrolysis, toxoderma, and exfoliative dermatitis have been reported with amifostine; may be delayed, developing up to weeks after treatment initiation. Cutaneous reactions have been reported more frequently when used as a radioprotectant. Discontinue treatment for severe/serious cutaneous reaction or with fever. Withhold treatment and obtain dermatologic consultation for rash involving lips or mucosa (of unknown etiology outside of radiation port) and for bullous, edematous, or erythematous lesions on hands, feet, or trunk; reinitiate only after careful evaluation.

Precautions Use with caution in patients with pre-existing cardiovascular or cerebrovascular conditions such as ischemic heart disease, arrhythmias, CHF, history of stroke or transient ischemic attacks; may cause hypotension (adequately hydrate prior to treatment and keep in a supine position during the infusion); use special caution in situations where concomitant antihypertensive therapy cannot be interrupted 24 hours prior to starting amifostine or in patients in whom the adverse effects of nausea/vomiting may be more likely to have serious consequences. Infusions >15 minutes are associated with a higher incidence of adverse effects.

Adverse Reactions

Cardiovascular: Transient hypotension (62%; incidence is higher in patients with head and neck cancer, esophageal cancer, nonsmall cell lung cancer, prior neck irradiation, or hypercalcemia), flushing, warm sensation, arrhythmia, atrial fibrillation, atrial flutter, bradycardia, cardiac arrest, chest pain, chest tightness, extrasystoles, hypertension (transient), MI, myocardial ischemia, supraventricular tachycardia, syncope, tachycardia

Central nervous system: Chills, fever, dizziness, somnolence, hiccups, anxiety, malaise, seizure

Dermatologic: Rash, cutaneous eruptions, erythema multiforme, exfoliative dermatitis, pruritus, Stevens-Johnson syndrome, toxic epidermal necrolysis, toxoderma, urticaria

Endocrine & metabolic: Hypocalcemia, hypomagnesemia

Gastrointestinal: Nausea, vomiting, metallic taste in mouth

Genitourinary: Urinary retention (reversible)

Neuromuscular & skeletal: Rigors

Renal: Renal failure

Respiratory: Sneezing, apnea, dyspnea, hypoxia, respiratory arrest

Miscellaneous: Anaphylactoid reactions, anaphylaxis, hypersensitivity reactions (fever, rash, hypoxia, dyspnea, laryngeal edema)

Drug Interactions

Avoid Concomitant Use There are no known interactions where it is recommended to avoid concomitant use.

Increased Effect/Toxicity

The levels/effects of Amifostine may be increased by: Antihypertensives

Decreased Effect There are no known significant interactions involving a decrease in effect.

Stability When 500 mg amifostine is reconstituted with 9.7 mL of NS, the resultant solution is stable for 5 hours at room temperature or up to 24 hours if refrigerated; amifostine solutions diluted to 5-40 mg/mL in NS are chemically stable for 5 hours at room temperature or 24 hours if refrigerated; decreased stability in low pH conditions; incompatible with acyclovir, amphotericin B, chlorpromazine, cisplatin, ganciclovir, hydroxyzine, prochlorperazine

Mechanism of Action Amifostine is a prodrug that is converted by the plasma membrane-bound enzyme alkaline phosphatase to the active free sulfhydryl compound WR-1065, which is further oxidized to a symmetrical disulfide (WR-33278) or to mixed disulfides. The active drug scavenges free radicals, donates hydrogen ions to free radicals, and binds to active derivatives of antineoplastic agents, thus preventing the alkylation of nucleic acid. Selective protection of normal tissue is demonstrated by:
1) decreased alkaline phosphatase activity in tumor cells,
2) decreased vascularity of tumors, and
3) lower pH in tumor tissues due to the predominance of anaerobic metabolism (WR-1065 requires a pH in the range of 6.6-8.2 for uptake into tissues)

Pharmacokinetics (Adult data unless noted)

Distribution: V_d: Adults: 6.4 L; unmetabolized prodrug is largely confined to the intravascular compartment; active metabolite is distributed into normal tissues with high concentrations in bone marrow, GI mucosa, skin, liver, and salivary glands

Protein binding: 4%

Metabolism: Amifostine (phosphorylated prodrug) is hydrolyzed by alkaline phosphatase to an active free sulfhydryl compound (WR-1065)

Half-life:
Children: 9.3 minutes
Adults: 8 minutes

Elimination: Metabolites excreted in urine

Usual Dosage I.V. (refer to individual protocols):

Children: Limited data available on use in pediatric patients; dosing based on a prior clinical phase I trial and single case reports: 740 mg/m^2 once daily administered 30 minutes prior to chemotherapy; doses as high as 600 mg/m^2/dose administered 15 minutes prior to and 2 hours after chemotherapy (total of 1200 mg/m^2/day) have been used in phase I trials in patients treated with ifosfamide, carboplatin, and etoposide chemotherapy; repeat amifostine doses may be required when using a cytotoxic agent with a long half-life or long infusion time

Adults: 910 mg/m^2 once daily administered 30 minutes prior to chemotherapy; reduce dose to 740 mg/m^2 in patients who have a higher incidence of hypotension

Reduction of moderate to severe xerostomia from radiation of the head and neck: 200 mg/m^2 once daily starting 15-30 minutes prior to standard fraction radiation therapy

Administration Parenteral: I.V.: Reconstituted amifostine dose must be further diluted with NS to a final volume of 50 mL (adults) or a final concentration of 5-40 mg/mL (children). Administer amifostine doses >740 mg/m^2 as an I.V. intermittent infusion over 15 minutes since the 15-minute infusion is better tolerated than a more prolonged infusion. Administer 200 mg/m^2 dose as a 3-minute infusion. Amifostine should be interrupted if the blood pressure decreases significantly from baseline or if the patient develops symptoms related to decreased cerebral or cardiovascular perfusion. Patients experiencing decreased blood pressure should receive a rapid infusion of NS and be kept supine or placed in the Trendelenburg position. Amifostine can be restarted if the blood pressure returns to the baseline level.

Monitoring Parameters Baseline blood pressure followed by a blood pressure reading every 3-5 minutes during the 15-minute infusion; monitor electrolytes, urinalysis, serum calcium, serum magnesium; monitor I & O; evaluate for cutaneous reactions prior to each dose

Nursing Implications Pretreat patient with antiemetics; patients should be well hydrated prior to amifostine infusion; patients taking antihypertensive medications should discontinue therapy 24 hours before administration of amifostine; begin chemotherapy or radiation therapy 15 minutes after completion of amifostine

Dosage Forms Excipient information presented when available (limited, particularly for generics); consult specific product labeling.

Injection, powder for reconstitution: 500 mg

Ethyol®: 500 mg

References

Adamson PC, Balis FM, Belasco JE, et al, "A Phase I Trial of Amifostine (WR-2721) and Melphalan in Children With Refractory Cancer," *Cancer Res*, 1995, 55(18): 4069-72.

Fouladi M, Stempak D, Gammon J, et al, "Phase I Trial of a Twice-Daily Regimen of Amifostine With Ifosfamide, Carboplatin, and Etoposide Chemotherapy in Children With Refractory Carcinoma," *Cancer*, 2001, 92(4):914-23.

Schuchter LM, "Guidelines for the Administration of Amifostine," *Semin Oncol*, 1996, 23(4 Suppl 8):40-3.

Shaw LM, Bonner H, and Lieberman R, "Pharmacokinetic Profile of Amifostine," *Semin Oncol*, 1996, 23(4 Suppl 8):18-22.

Amikacin (am i KAY sin)

Medication Safety Issues

Sound-alike/look-alike issues:

Amikacin may be confused with Amicar®, anakinra

Amikin® may be confused with Amicar®, Kineret®

Related Information

Therapeutic Drug Monitoring: Blood Sampling Time Guidelines *on page 1704*

Canadian Brand Names Amikacin Sulfate Injection, USP; Amikin®

Therapeutic Category Antibiotic, Aminoglycoside

Generic Available Yes

Use Treatment of documented gram-negative enteric infection resistant to gentamicin and tobramycin; amikacin is usually effective against *Pseudomonas*, *Klebsiella*, *Enterobacter*, *Serratia*, *Proteus*, and *E. coli*; documented infection of mycobacterial organisms susceptible to amikacin

Pregnancy Risk Factor D

Pregnancy Considerations Adverse events were not observed in the initial animal reproduction studies; however, renal toxicity has been reported in additional studies. Amikacin crosses the placenta, produces detectable serum levels in the fetus, and concentrates in the fetal kidneys. Because of several reports of total irreversible bilateral congenital deafness in children whose mothers received another aminoglycoside (streptomycin) during pregnancy, the manufacturer classifies amikacin as pregnancy risk factor D. Although serious side effects to the fetus have not been reported following maternal use of amikacin, a potential for harm exists.

Due to pregnancy-induced physiologic changes, some pharmacokinetic parameters of amikacin may be altered. Pregnant women have an average-to-larger volume of distribution which may result in lower peak serum levels than for the same dose in nonpregnant women. Serum half-life may also be shorter.

Lactation Enters breast milk/not recommended

Breast-Feeding Considerations Amikacin is excreted into breast milk in trace amounts; however, it is not absorbed when taken orally. This limited oral absorption may minimize exposure to the nursing infant. Nondose-related effects could include modification of bowel flora. Breast-feeding is not recommended by the manufacturer.

Contraindications Hypersensitivity to amikacin sulfate or any component (see Warnings); cross-sensitivity may exist with other aminoglycosides

Warnings Aminoglycosides are associated with significant nephrotoxicity **[U.S. Boxed Warning]**; vestibular and permanent bilateral auditory ototoxicity can occur **[U.S. Boxed Warning]**; tinnitus or vertigo are indications of vestibular injury and impending bilateral irreversible deafness. Risk of nephrotoxicity and ototoxicity is increased in patients with impaired renal function, high dose therapy, or prolonged therapy. Risk of nephrotoxicity increases when used concurrently with other potentially nephrotoxic drugs **[U.S. Boxed Warning]**; renal damage is usually reversible. Risk of ototoxicity increases with use of potent diuretics **[U.S. Boxed Warning]**; may cause neuromuscular blockade and respiratory paralysis **[U.S. Boxed Warning]**; risk increased with concomitant use of anesthesia or muscle relaxants. Aminoglycosides can cause fetal harm when administered to a pregnant woman, and have been associated with several reports of total irreversible bilateral congenital deafness in pediatric patients exposed *in utero*. Some products contain sulfites which may cause allergic reactions in susceptible individuals.

Precautions Use with caution in neonates (due to renal immaturity that results in a prolonged half-life); patients with pre-existing renal impairment, auditory or vestibular impairment, hypocalcemia, myasthenia gravis, and in conditions which depress neuromuscular transmission; dose and/or frequency of administration must be modified in patients with renal impairment. Monitor renal and eighth nerve function in patients with known or suspected renal impairment.

Adverse Reactions

Central nervous system: Fever, headache, dizziness, drowsiness, ataxia, vertigo

Dermatologic: Rash

Gastrointestinal: Nausea, vomiting

Hematologic: Eosinophilia, anemia, leukopenia

Neuromuscular & skeletal: Neuromuscular blockade, tremor, paresthesia, weakness, gait instability

Otic: Ototoxicity

Renal: Nephrotoxicity

Drug Interactions

Avoid Concomitant Use

Avoid concomitant use of Amikacin with any of the following: BCG; Gallium Nitrate

Increased Effect/Toxicity

Amikacin may increase the levels/effects of: AbobotulinumtoxinA; Bisphosphonate Derivatives; CARBOplatin; Colistimethate; CycloSPORINE; CycloSPORINE (Systemic); Gallium Nitrate; Neuromuscular-Blocking Agents; OnabotulinumtoxinA; RimabotulinumtoxinB

The levels/effects of Amikacin may be increased by: Amphotericin B; Capreomycin; CISplatin; Loop Diuretics; Nonsteroidal Anti-Inflammatory Agents; Vancomycin

Decreased Effect

Amikacin may decrease the levels/effects of: BCG; Typhoid Vaccine

The levels/effects of Amikacin may be decreased by: Penicillins

Mechanism of Action Inhibits protein synthesis in susceptible bacteria by binding to ribosomal subunits

Pharmacokinetics (Adult data unless noted)

Distribution: Primarily into extracellular fluid (highly hydrophilic); 12% of serum concentration penetrates into bronchial secretions; poor penetration into the blood-brain barrier even when meninges are inflamed; V_d is increased in neonates and patients with edema, ascites, fluid overload; V_d is decreased in patients with dehydration; crosses the placenta

Half-life:

Infants:

Low birth weight, 1-3 days of age: 7 hours

Full-term >7 days: 4-5 hours

Children: 1.6-2.5 hours

Adolescents: 1.5 ± 1 hour

Adults: 2-3 hours

Anuria: 28-86 hours; half-life and clearance are dependent on renal function

Time to peak serum concentration:
I.M.: Within 45-120 minutes
I.V.: Within 30 minutes following a 30-minute infusion
Elimination: 94% to 98% is excreted unchanged in the urine via glomerular filtration within 24 hours
Dialysis: Dialyzable (50% to 100%); supplemental dose recommended after hemodialysis or peritoneal dialysis
Usual Dosage I.M., I.V. (dosage should be based on an estimate of ideal body weight except in neonates; neonatal dosage should be based on actual weight unless the patient has hydrocephalus or hydrops fetalis):

Neonates:
0-4 weeks, <1200 g: 7.5 mg/kg/dose every 18-24 hours
Postnatal age ≤7 days:
1200-2000 g: 7.5 mg/kg/dose every 12 hours
>2000 g: 7.5-10 mg/kg/dose every 12 hours
Postnatal age >7 days:
1200-2000 g: 7.5-10 mg/kg/dose every 8-12 hours
>2000 g: 10 mg/kg/dose every 8 hours
Infants and Children: 15-22.5 mg/kg/day divided every 8 hours; some consultants recommend initial doses of 30 mg/kg/day divided every 8 hours in patients who may require larger doses; see **Note**
Treatment for nontuberculous mycobacterial infection: 15-30 mg/kg/day divided every 12-24 hours as part of a multiple drug regimen
Adults: 15 mg/kg/day divided every 8-12 hours
Treatment of *M. avium* complex infection: 7.5-15 mg/kg/day divided every 12-24 hours as part of a multiple drug regimen
Dosing interval in renal impairment: Loading dose: 5-7.5 mg/kg; subsequent dosages and frequency of administration are best determined by measurement of serum levels and assessment of renal insufficiency
Note: Some patients may require larger or more frequent doses if serum concentrations document the need (ie, cystic fibrosis or febrile granulocytopenic patients). Manufacturer recommends a maximum daily dose of 15 mg/kg/day (or 1.5 g/day in heavier patients). Higher doses may be warranted based on therapeutic drug monitoring or susceptibility information.
Administration Parenteral: Administer by I.M. or slow intermittent I.V. infusion over 30 minutes at a final concentration not to exceed 10 mg amikacin/mL. Administer other antibiotics such as penicillins and cephalosporins at least 1 hour before or after an amikacin dose.
Monitoring Parameters Urinalysis, urine output, BUN, serum creatinine, peak and trough serum amikacin concentrations; be alert to ototoxicity
Not all infants and children who receive aminoglycosides require monitoring of serum aminoglycoside concentrations. Indications for use of aminoglycoside serum concentration monitoring include:
• treatment course >5 days
• patients with decreased or changing renal function
• patients with poor therapeutic response
• infants <3 months of age
• atypical body constituency (obesity, expanded extracellular fluid volume)
• clinical need for higher doses or shorter intervals (eg, cystic fibrosis, burns, endocarditis, meningitis, critically ill patients, relatively resistant organisms)
• patients on hemodialysis or chronic ambulatory peritoneal dialysis
• signs of nephrotoxicity or ototoxicity
• concomitant use of other nephrotoxic agents
Reference Range
Peak: 20-30 mcg/mL
Trough: <10 mcg/mL
Patient Information Report loss of hearing, ringing or roaring in the ears, or feeling of fullness in head

Nursing Implications Aminoglycoside levels measured from blood taken from Silastic® central catheters can sometimes give falsely elevated readings; peak serum levels should be drawn 30 minutes after the end of a 30-minute infusion; trough levels are drawn within 30 minutes before the next dose; provide optimal patient hydration
Dosage Forms Excipient information presented when available (limited, particularly for generics); consult specific product labeling.
Injection, solution, as sulfate: 50 mg/mL (2 mL); 250 mg/mL (2 mL, 4 mL)
References

Kenyon CF, Knoppert DC, Lee SK, et al, "Amikacin Pharmacokinetics and Suggested Dosage Modifications for the Preterm Infant," *Antimicrob Agents Chemother*, 1990, 34(2):265-8.
Public Health Service Task Force on Prophylaxis and Therapy for *Mycobacterium avium* Complex, "Recommendations on Prophylaxis and Therapy for Disseminated *Mycobacterium avium* Complex Disease in Patients Infected With the Human Immunodeficiency Virus," *N Engl J Med*, 1993, 329(12):898-904.
Starke JR and Correa AG, "Management of Mycobacterial Infection and Disease in Children," *Pediatr Infect Dis J*, 1995, 14(6):455-69.
Vogelstein B, Kowarski A, and Lietman PS, "The Pharmacokinetics of Amikacin in Children," *J Pediatr*, 1977, 91(2):333-9.

◆ **Amikacin Sulfate** *see* Amikacin *on page 80*
◆ **Amikacin Sulfate Injection, USP (Can)** *see* Amikacin *on page 80*
◆ **Amikin® (Can)** *see* Amikacin *on page 80*

AMILoride (a MIL oh ride)

Medication Safety Issues
Sound-alike/look-alike issues:
AMILoride may be confused with amiodarone, amLODIPine, amrinone
Related Information
Antihypertensive Agents by Class *on page 1481*
Canadian Brand Names Apo-Amiloride®; Mylan-Amilazide
Therapeutic Category Antihypertensive Agent; Diuretic, Potassium Sparing
Generic Available Yes
Use Management of edema associated with CHF, hepatic cirrhosis, and hyperaldosteronism; hypertension; primary hyperaldosteronism; hypokalemia induced by kaliuretic diuretics
Pregnancy Risk Factor B
Pregnancy Considerations Teratogenic effects were not observed in animal studies.
Lactation Excretion in breast milk unknown/not recommended
Contraindications Hypersensitivity to amiloride or any component; hyperkalemia; anuria, acute or chronic renal insufficiency, and evidence of diabetic nephropathy; concomitant use of potassium supplements (except in severe and/or refractory hypokalemia) or potassium-sparing diuretics
Warnings Severe hyperkalemia can occur **[U.S. Boxed Warning]**. Incidence is greater in patients with renal impairment, diabetes mellitus, and in elderly patients. Serum potassium levels must be monitored at frequent intervals especially when dosages are changed or with any illness that may cause renal dysfunction. Amiloride should be discontinued in diabetic patients for at least 3 days prior to glucose tolerance testing; discontinue if serum potassium >5.5 mEq/L; risk of hyperkalemia is reduced with concomitant use of thiazide diuretic.
Precautions Use with caution in patients with dehydration, electrolyte imbalance, metabolic or respiratory acidosis, diabetes (particularly those with nephropathy), hyponatremia, impaired renal function, or hepatic dysfunction; patients receiving potassium or other potassium-sparing diuretics; use with caution and modify dosage in patients with decreased renal function

Adverse Reactions

Cardiovascular: Angina, orthostatic hypotension, arrhythmia, palpitations

Central nervous system: Headache, dizziness, encephalopathy, vertigo, nervousness, mental confusion, insomnia, depression, somnolence

Dermatologic: Skin rash, pruritus, alopecia

Endocrine & metabolic: Hyperkalemia, hyperchloremic metabolic acidosis, dehydration, hyponatremia, gynecomastia

Gastrointestinal: Nausea, anorexia, diarrhea, vomiting, abdominal pain, appetite changes, constipation, GI bleeding, xerostomia, heartburn, flatulence, dyspepsia

Genitourinary: Impotence, dysuria, urinary frequency, bladder spasms

Hematologic: Aplastic anemia, neutropenia

Hepatic: Abnormal liver function

Neuromuscular & skeletal: Weakness, muscle cramps, joint and back pain, paresthesia, tremors

Ocular: Visual disturbances, intraocular pressure elevated

Otic: Tinnitus

Renal: Polyuria

Respiratory: Cough, dyspnea, nasal congestion, shortness of breath

Drug Interactions

Avoid Concomitant Use There are no known interactions where it is recommended to avoid concomitant use.

Increased Effect/Toxicity

AMILoride may increase the levels/effects of: ACE Inhibitors; Amifostine; Ammonium Chloride; Antihypertensives; Cardiac Glycosides; Hypotensive Agents; RiTUXimab

The levels/effects of AMILoride may be increased by: Angiotensin II Receptor Blockers; Diazoxide; Drospirenone; Eplerenone; Herbs (Hypotensive Properties); MAO Inhibitors; Nonsteroidal Anti-Inflammatory Agents; Pentoxifylline; Phosphodiesterase 5 Inhibitors; Potassium Salts; Prostacyclin Analogues; Tolvaptan

Decreased Effect

AMILoride may decrease the levels/effects of: Cardiac Glycosides; QuiNIDine

The levels/effects of AMILoride may be decreased by: Herbs (Hypertensive Properties); Methylphenidate; Nonsteroidal Anti-Inflammatory Agents; Yohimbine

Food Interactions Avoid natural licorice (causes sodium and water retention and increases potassium loss) and salt substitutes; food decreases absorption to ~30%

Mechanism of Action Acts directly on the distal renal tubule to inhibit sodium-potassium ion exchange; decreases sodium reabsorption in the distal tubule by inhibiting cellular sodium transport mechanisms such as the conductive sodium influx pathway and possibly the sodium-hydrogen ion exchange system; also inhibits hydrogen ion secretion; its diuretic activity is **independent** of aldosterone.

Pharmacodynamics

Onset of action: 2 hours

Maximum effect: 6-10 hours

Duration: 24 hours

Pharmacokinetics (Adult data unless noted)

Absorption: 50%

Distribution: Adults: V_d: 350-380 L

Metabolism: No active metabolites

Half-life: Adults:

  Normal renal function: 6-9 hours

  End-stage renal disease: 21-144 hours

Elimination: Unchanged drug, equally in urine and feces

Usual Dosage Oral:

Hypertension:

  Children: 0.4-0.625 mg/kg/day; maximum dose: 20 mg/day

  Adults: 5-10 mg/day in 1-2 divided doses (JNC 7)

Edema:

  Children 6-20 kg: 0.625 mg/kg/day in 1-2 divided doses; maximum dose: 10 mg/day

  Children >20 kg and Adults: 5-10 mg/day in 1-2 divided doses; maximum dose: 20 mg/day

Dosing adjustment in renal impairment:

  Cl_{cr} 10-50 mL/minute: Administer at 50% of normal dose

  Cl_{cr} <10 mL/minute: Avoid use

Administration Oral: Administer with food or milk

Monitoring Parameters Serum potassium, sodium, creatinine, BUN, blood pressure, fluid balance

Test Interactions May falsely elevate serum digoxin levels done by radioimmunoassay

Patient Information Report to your physician any muscle cramps, weakness, nausea, or dizziness; may cause drowsiness and impair ability to perform activities requiring mental alertness or physical coordination; may cause dry mouth

Additional Information Studies utilizing aerosolized amiloride (5 mmol/L in 0.3% saline) in adult cystic fibrosis patients (Tomkiewicz, 1993) have suggested that inhaled amiloride is capable of improving the rheologic properties of the abnormally thickened mucus by increasing mucus sodium content

Dosage Forms Excipient information presented when available (limited, particularly for generics); consult specific product labeling.

Tablet, as hydrochloride: 5 mg

Extemporaneous Preparations A 1 mg/mL oral liquid may be prepared from crushed tablets added to a small quantity of sterile water to which glycerin (final concentration of 40% w/v) is added; sterile water is then added in sufficient quantity to make the desired volume; stable 21 days when refrigerated

Fawcett JP, Woods DJ, Ferry DG, et al, "Stability of Amiloride Hydrochloride Oral Liquids Prepared From Tablets and Powder," *Aust J Hosp Pharm*, 1995, 25:10-23.

References

Chobanian AV, Bakris GL, Black HR, et al, "The Seventh Report of the Joint National Committee on Prevention, Detection, Evaluation, and Treatment of High Blood Pressure: The JNC 7 Report," *JAMA*, 2003, 289(19):2560-72.

National High Blood Pressure Education Program Working Group on High Blood Pressure in Children and Adolescents, "The Fourth Report on the Diagnosis, Evaluation, and Treatment of High Blood Pressure in Children and Adolescents," *Pediatrics*, 2004, 114(2 Suppl):555-76.

Tomkiewicz RP, App, EM, Zayas JG, et al, "Amiloride Inhalation Therapy in Cystic Fibrosis. Influence on Ion Content, Hydration, and Rheology of Sputum," *Am Rev Resp Dis*, 1993, 148:1002-7.

van der Vorst MM, Kist JE, van der Heijden AJ, et al, "Diuretics in Pediatrics: Current Knowledge and Future Prospects," *Paediatr Drugs*, 2006, 8(4):245-64.

◆ **Amiloride Hydrochloride** *see* AMILoride *on page 81*

◆ **2-Amino-6-Mercaptopurine** *see* Thioguanine *on page 1339*

◆ **2-Amino-6-Methoxypurine Arabinoside** *see* Nelarabine *on page 974*

◆ **Aminobenzylpenicillin** *see* Ampicillin *on page 104*

Aminocaproic Acid (a mee noe ka PROE ik AS id)

Medication Safety Issues

Sound-alike/look-alike issues:

  Amicar® may be confused with amikacin, Amikin®, Omacor®

U.S. Brand Names Amicar®

Therapeutic Category Hemostatic Agent

Generic Available Yes

Use Treatment of excessive bleeding resulting from systemic hyperfibrinolysis, urinary fibrinolysis, or traumatic ocular hyphema

Pregnancy Risk Factor C

Pregnancy Considerations Animal reproductive studies have not been conducted.

Lactation Excretion in breast milk unknown/use caution

Contraindications Hypersensitivity to aminocaproic acid or any component (see Warnings); disseminated intravascular coagulation; evidence of an intravascular clotting process; use of factor IX concentrate or anti-inhibitor coagulant concentrate

Warnings Aminocaproic acid may accumulate in patients with decreased renal function; intrarenal obstruction may occur secondary to glomerular capillary thrombosis or clots in the renal pelvis and ureters; do not use in hematuria of upper urinary tract origin unless benefits outweigh potential risks; inhibition of fibrinolysis may promote clotting or thrombosis.

Injection contains benzyl alcohol which may cause allergic reactions in susceptible individuals; large amounts of benzyl alcohol (≥99 mg/kg/day) have been associated with a potentially fatal toxicity ("gasping syndrome") in neonates; the "gasping syndrome" consists of metabolic acidosis, respiratory distress, gasping respirations, CNS dysfunction (including convulsions, intracranial hemorrhage), hypotension and cardiovascular collapse; avoid use of injection in neonates; in vitro and animal studies have shown that benzoate, a metabolite of benzyl alcohol, displaces bilirubin from protein-binding sites

Precautions Use with caution in patients with cardiac, renal or hepatic disease; adjust dosage in patients with oliguria or end-stage renal disease; use with caution in patients at risk for veno-occlusive disease of the liver

Adverse Reactions
Cardiovascular: Hypotension, bradycardia and arrhythmias (following rapid I.V. administration), peripheral ischemia, thrombosis, stroke, syncope
Central nervous system: Dizziness, headache, malaise, seizures, confusion, delirium, hallucinations
Dermatologic: Rash, pruritus
Endocrine & metabolic: Hyperkalemia
Gastrointestinal: GI irritation, nausea, cramps, diarrhea, vomiting, abdominal pain
Genitourinary: Dry ejaculation
Hematologic: Platelet function decreased, agranulocytosis, leukopenia
Neuromuscular & skeletal: Myopathy, acute rhabdomyolysis, weakness, myalgia, CPK elevated
Ocular: Glaucoma, watery eyes
Otic: Tinnitus, deafness
Renal: Renal failure, BUN elevated
Respiratory: Nasal congestion, dyspnea, pulmonary embolism

Drug Interactions
Avoid Concomitant Use
Avoid concomitant use of Aminocaproic Acid with any of the following: Anti-inhibitor Coagulant Complex; Factor IX; Factor IX Complex (Human)
Increased Effect/Toxicity
Aminocaproic Acid may increase the levels/effects of: Anti-inhibitor Coagulant Complex; Factor IX; Factor IX Complex (Human); Fibrinogen Concentrate (Human)

The levels/effects of Aminocaproic Acid may be increased by: Fibrinogen Concentrate (Human); Tretinoin (Systemic)
Decreased Effect There are no known significant interactions involving a decrease in effect.

Mechanism of Action Competitively inhibits activation of plasminogen thereby reducing fibrinolysin, without inhibiting lysis of clot

Pharmacodynamics Onset of action: Inhibition of fibrinolysis: Within 1-72 hours (onset shortened substantially if loading dose is used)

Pharmacokinetics (Adult data unless noted)
Distribution: Widely distributes through intravascular and extravascular compartments
Metabolism: Hepatic metabolism is minimal
Bioavailability: Oral: 100%
Half-life: 1-2 hours
Elimination: 40% to 60% excreted as unchanged drug in the urine within 12 hours

Usual Dosage
Children:
Oral, I.V.: Loading dose: 100-200 mg/kg; maintenance: 100 mg/kg/dose every 6 hours; maximum daily dose: 30 g
or as an alternative: I.V. loading dose: 100 mg/kg or 3 g/m^2 followed by a continuous infusion of 33.3 mg/kg/hour or 1 g/m^2/hour; total dosage should not exceed 18 g/m^2/day
Traumatic hyphema: Oral, I.V.: 100 mg/kg/dose every 4 hours (maximum dose: 5 g/dose; maximum daily dose: 30 g/day)
Adults:
Oral: For the treatment of acute bleeding syndromes due to elevated fibrinolytic activity, give 5 g during first hour, followed by 1-1.25 g/hour for about 8 hours or until bleeding stops; daily dose should not exceed 30 g
I.V.: Give 4-5 g during first hour followed by continuous infusion at the rate of 1-1.25 g/hour, continue for 8 hours or until bleeding stops

Dosing adjustment in renal impairment: Oliguria or ESRD: Reduce dose to 25% of normal

Administration
Oral: May administer without regard to food
Parenteral: Maximum concentration for I.V. administration: 20 mg/mL; administer single doses over at least 1 hour

Monitoring Parameters Fibrinogen, fibrin split products, serum creatinine kinase (long-term therapy); serum potassium (may be elevated by aminocaproic acid, especially if the patient has impaired renal function)

Reference Range Therapeutic concentration: >130 mcg/mL (concentration necessary for inhibition of fibrinolysis)

Nursing Implications Rapid I.V. injection (IVP) should be avoided since hypotension, bradycardia, and arrhythmias may result

Dosage Forms Excipient information presented when available (limited, particularly for generics); consult specific product labeling.
Injection, solution: 250 mg/mL (20 mL)
Solution, oral: 1.25 g/5 mL (240 mL, 480 mL)
Syrup:
Amicar®: 1.25 g/5 mL (480 mL) [raspberry flavor]
Tablet [scored]: 500 mg
Amicar®: 500 mg, 1000 mg

References
McGetrick JJ, Jampol LM, Goldberg MP, et al, "Aminocaproic Acid Decreases Secondary Hemorrhage After Traumatic Hyphema," *Arch Ophthalmol*, 1983, 101(7):1031-3.

Aminophylline (am in OFF i lin)

Medication Safety Issues
Sound-alike/look-alike issues:
Aminophylline may be confused with amitriptyline, ampicillin

Related Information
Asthma *on page 1697*
Theophylline *on page 1335*

Canadian Brand Names Phyllocontin®; Phyllocontin®-350

◄ **Therapeutic Category** Antiasthmatic; Bronchodilator; Respiratory Stimulant; Theophylline Derivative

Generic Available Yes

Use Bronchodilator in reversible airway obstruction due to asthma or COPD; increase diaphragmatic contractility; neonatal idiopathic apnea of prematurity

Pregnancy Risk Factor C

Pregnancy Considerations Theophylline crosses the placenta; adverse effects may be seen in the newborn. Theophylline metabolism may change during pregnancy; monitor serum levels.

Lactation Enters breast milk/compatible (AAP rates "compatible")

Breast-Feeding Considerations Irritability may be observed in the nursing infant.

Contraindications Hypersensitivity to aminophylline or any component; uncontrolled arrhythmias

Adverse Reactions See Theophylline on page 1335

Drug Interactions

Metabolism/Transport Effects Substrate of CYP1A2 (major), 2E1 (minor), 3A4 (minor)

Avoid Concomitant Use

Avoid concomitant use of Aminophylline with any of the following: Febuxostat; Iobenguane I 123

Increased Effect/Toxicity

Aminophylline may increase the levels/effects of: Sympathomimetics

The levels/effects of Aminophylline may be increased by: Allopurinol; Atomoxetine; Cannabinoids; Cimetidine; CYP1A2 Inhibitors (Moderate); CYP1A2 Inhibitors (Strong); Disulfiram; Febuxostat; Fluvoxamine; Interferons; Isoniazid; Macrolide Antibiotics; Mexiletine; Pentoxifylline; QuiNINE; Quinolone Antibiotics; Thiabendazole; Ticlopidine

Decreased Effect

Aminophylline may decrease the levels/effects of: Adenosine; Benzodiazepines; Iobenguane I 123; Lithium; Phenytoin; Regadenoson; Zafirlukast

The levels/effects of Aminophylline may be decreased by: Aminoglutethimide; Barbiturates; Beta-Blockers (Beta1 Selective); Beta-Blockers (Nonselective); CarBAMazepine; CYP1A2 Inducers (Strong); Phenytoin; Protease Inhibitors; Thyroid Products

Food Interactions Food does not appreciably affect absorption; avoid extremes of dietary protein and carbohydrate intake; limit charcoal-broiled foods and caffeinated beverages

Mechanism of Action See Theophylline on page 1335

Pharmacokinetics (Adult data unless noted) Aminophylline is the ethylenediamine salt of theophylline, pharmacokinetic parameters are those of **theophylline**; fraction available: 80% (eg, 100 mg aminophylline = 80 mg theophylline); see Theophylline on page 1335

Usual Dosage All dosages based upon **aminophylline**; dose should be based on ideal body weight

Neonates:

Apnea of prematurity: Oral, I.V.:

Loading dose: 5 mg/kg

Maintenance: Initial: 5 mg/kg/day every 12 hours; increased dosages may be indicated as liver metabolism matures (usually >30 days of life); monitor serum levels to determine appropriate dosages

Theophylline levels should be initially drawn after 3 days of therapy; repeat levels are indicated 3 days after each increase in dosage or weekly if on a stabilized dosage

Infants, Children, and Adults: Treatment of acute bronchospasm: I.V.: Loading dose (in patients not currently receiving aminophylline or theophylline): 6 mg/kg (based on aminophylline) given I.V. over 20-30 minutes

Approximate I.V. maintenance dosages are based upon **continuous infusions**; intermittent dosing (often used in children <6 months of age) may be determined by multiplying the hourly infusion rate by 24 hours and dividing by the desired number of doses/day (usually in 3-4 doses/day)

6 weeks to 6 months: 0.5 mg/kg/hour

6 months to 1 year: 0.6-0.7 mg/kg/hour

1-9 years: 1-1.2 mg/kg/hour

9-12 years and young adult smokers: 0.9 mg/kg/hour

12-16 years: 0.7 mg/kg/hour

Adults (healthy, nonsmoking): 0.7 mg/kg/hour

Older patients and patients with cor pulmonale, patients with CHF or liver failure: 0.25 mg/kg/hour

Oral dose: See Theophylline on page 1335 (consider mg theophylline available when using aminophylline products)

Dosage should be adjusted according to serum level measurements during the first 12- to 24-hour period. See table.

Guidelines for Drawing Theophylline Serum Levels

Dosage Form	Time to Draw Level[1]
I.V. bolus	30 min after end of 30-min infusion
I.V. continuous infusion	12-24 h after initiation of infusion
P.O. liquid, fast-release formulation	Peak: 1 h postdose after at least 1 day of therapy Trough: Just before a dose after at least 1 day of therapy

[1]The time to achieve steady-state serum levels is prolonged in patients with longer half-lives (eg, premature neonates, infants, and adults with cardiac or liver failure (see theophylline half-life table). In these patients, serum theophylline levels should be drawn after 48-72 hours of therapy; serum levels may need to be done prior to steady-state to assess the patient's current progress or evaluate potential toxicity.

Administration

Oral: May be administered without regard to meals

Parenteral: Do not administer I.M. (I.M. administration causes intense pain); dilute with I.V. fluid to a concentration of 1 mg/mL and infuse over 20-30 minutes; maximum concentration: 25 mg/mL; maximum rate of infusion: 0.36 mg/kg/minute, and not to exceed 25 mg/minute

Monitoring Parameters Serum theophylline levels, heart rate, respiratory rate, number and severity of apnea spells (when used for apnea of prematurity); arterial or capillary blood gases (if applicable); pulmonary function tests

Reference Range Therapeutic: For asthma 10-20 mcg/mL; for neonatal apnea 6-13 mcg/mL (serum levels are reduced for neonatal apnea due to decreased binding of theophylline to fetal albumin resulting in a greater amount of free "active" theophylline)

Dosage Forms Excipient information presented when available (limited, particularly for generics); consult specific product labeling.

Injection, solution, as dihydrate: 25 mg/mL (10 mL, 20 mL)

Injection, solution, as dihydrate [preservative free]: 25 mg/mL (10 mL, 20 mL)

Tablet, as dihydrate: 100 mg

References

Bhatt-Mehta V and Schumacher RE, "Treatment of Apnea of Prematurity," Paediatr Drugs, 2003, 5(3):195-210.

◆ **5-Aminosalicylic Acid** see Mesalamine on page 887

◆ **Aminoxin [OTC]** see Pyridoxine on page 1190

Amiodarone (a MEE oh da rone)

Medication Safety Issues

Sound-alike/look-alike issues:

Amiodarone may be confused with aMILoride, amrinone

Cordarone® may be confused with Cardura®, Cordran®

High alert medication: The Institute for Safe Medication Practices (ISMP) includes this medication among its list of drugs which have a heightened risk of causing significant patient harm when used in error.

Beers Criteria medication: This drug may be inappropriate for use in geriatric patients (high severity risk).

International issues:
Ambyen [Great Britain] may be confused with Ambien® which is a brand name for zolpidem in the U.S.

Related Information
CPR Pediatric Drug Dosages *on page 1455*
Pediatric ALS Algorithms *on page 1460*

U.S. Brand Names Cordarone®; Pacerone®

Canadian Brand Names Amiodarone Hydrochloride for Injection®; Apo-Amiodarone®; Cordarone®; Dom-Amiodarone; Mylan-Amiodarone; Novo-Amiodarone; PHL-Amiodarone; PMS-Amiodarone; PRO-Amiodarone; ratio-Amiodarone; ratio-Amiodarone I.V.; Riva-Amiodarone; Sandoz-Amiodarone; ZYM-Amiodarone

Therapeutic Category Antiarrhythmic Agent, Class III

Generic Available Yes

Use
Oral: Management of life-threatening recurrent ventricular arrhythmias [eg, recurrent ventricular fibrillation (VF) or recurrent hemodynamically unstable ventricular tachycardia (VT)] unresponsive to other therapy or in patients intolerant to other therapy

I.V.: Initiation of management and prophylaxis of frequently recurrent VF and hemodynamically unstable VT unresponsive to other therapy; VF and VT in patients requiring amiodarone who are not able to take oral therapy

Note: Also has been used to treat supraventricular arrhythmias unresponsive to other therapy. Amiodarone is recommended in the PALS guidelines for SVT (unresponsive to vagal maneuvers and adenosine). It is recommended in both the PALS and ACLS guidelines for cardiac arrest with pulseless VT or VF (unresponsive to defibrillation, CPR, and vasopressor administration) and control of hemodynamically-stable VT or wide-complex tachycardia of uncertain origin. The drug is also recommended in the ACLS guidelines for re-entry SVT (unresponsive to vagal maneuvers and adenosine); control of rapid ventricular rate due to conduction via an accessory pathway in pre-excited atrial arrhythmias; and control of polymorphic VT with a normal QT interval. A benzyl alcohol free and polysorbate free injectable product is currently under development.

Medication Guide An FDA-approved patient medication guide, which is available with the product information and as follows, must be dispensed with this medication for each new outpatient prescription and refill.
Cordarone®: http://www.fda.gov/downloads/Drugs/DrugSafety/UCM152841.pdf
Pacerone®: http://www.fda.gov/downloads/Drugs/DrugSafety/ucm088668.pdf

Pregnancy Risk Factor D

Pregnancy Considerations May cause fetal harm when administered to a pregnant woman, leading to congenital goiter and hypo- or hyperthyroidism.

Lactation Enters breast milk/not recommended (AAP rates "of concern")

Breast-Feeding Considerations Hypothyroidism may occur in nursing infants. Both amiodarone and its active metabolite are excreted in human milk. Breast-feeding may lead to significant infant exposure and potential toxicity.

Contraindications Hypersensitivity to amiodarone, iodine, or any component (see Warnings); severe sinus node dysfunction; marked sinus bradycardia, second or third degree A-V block; cardiogenic shock; bradycardia-induced syncope, except if pacemaker is placed

Warnings Amiodarone has several potentially fatal toxicities **[U.S. Boxed Warning]**; pulmonary and hepatic toxicities may be fatal (see Adverse Reactions). Not considered first-line antiarrhythmic due to high incidence of toxicity **[U.S. Boxed Warning]**; 75% of patients experience adverse effects with large doses; discontinuation is required in 5% to 20% of patients. Reserve for use in life-threatening arrhythmias refractory to other therapy. Amiodarone may worsen or precipitate arrhythmias **[U.S. Boxed Warning]**, including torsade de pointes; when possible, hypokalemia and hypomagnesemia should be corrected prior to I.V. amiodarone use due to increased risk for torsade de pointes. Amiodarone is a potent inhibitor of cytochrome P450 enzymes and p-glycoprotein; serious drug interactions may occur (see Drug Interactions); prolongation of the QT interval, with or without torsade de pointes, has been reported in patients receiving amiodarone concomitantly with macrolide antibiotics, azoles, or fluroquinolones. Hypotension with I.V. product occurs in about 16% of patients, may be associated with infusion rate, and may be fatal. Bradycardia and AV block may occur; temporary pacemaker should be available when I.V. product is used in patients with known predisposition to bradycardia or AV block. Patients should be hospitalized for initiation of therapy and loading dose administration **[U.S. Boxed Warning]**. Chronic administration of antiarrhythmic drugs may affect defibrillation or pacing thresholds in patients with implantable cardiac devices (eg, defibrillators, pacemakers); assess thresholds when initiating amiodarone and during therapy. Optic neuropathy and/or optic neuritis resulting in visual impairment may occur at any time and can progress to permanent blindness; prompt ophthalmic exam is recommended if visual impairment occurs; re-evaluate amiodarone therapy if optic neuropathy or neuritis occurs. Corneal refractive laser surgery is generally contraindicated in patients receiving amiodarone (per manufacturers of the laser surgery devices).

Injectable product contains polysorbate (Tween®) 80 and benzyl alcohol; benzyl alcohol may cause allergic reactions in susceptible individuals; large amounts of benzyl alcohol (≥99 mg/kg/day) have been associated with a potentially fatal toxicity ("gasping syndrome") in neonates; the "gasping syndrome" consists of metabolic acidosis, respiratory distress, gasping respirations, CNS dysfunction (including convulsions, intracranial hemorrhage), hypotension and cardiovascular collapse; use amiodarone products containing benzyl alcohol with caution in neonates (see Precautions); a benzyl alcohol free and polysorbate free injection is currently under development; *in vitro* and animal studies have shown that benzoate, a metabolite of benzyl alcohol, displaces bilirubin from protein binding sites

Precautions Amiodarone HCl contains 37% iodine by weight; avoid use during pregnancy and while breast-feeding (fetal/neonatal goiters, hypothyroidism, and possible cerebral damage may occur); amiodarone may cause hypothyroidism or hyperthyroidism; hyperthyroidism may result in potentially fatal thyrotoxicosis or breakthrough or aggravation of potentially fatal arrhythmias; consider the possibility of hyperthyroidism if any new signs of arrhythmia appear; use with caution and monitor thyroid function closely in patients with thyroid disease (**Note:** Oral amiodarone has caused dose-related thyroid tumors in rats; cases of thyroid nodules/thyroid cancer have been reported in patients treated with amiodarone; hyperthyroidism was also present in some of these patients).

Safety and efficacy of amiodarone have not been established in pediatric patients. I.V. amiodarone has been shown to leach out plasticizers [eg, DEHP or di-(2-ethylhexyl)phthalate] from I.V. tubing, including polyvinyl chloride tubing. Polysorbate (Tween®) 80, an ingredient found in I.V. amiodarone, is also known to leach DEHP from polyvinyl chloride tubing. In immature animals, exposure to DEHP may adversely affect the development of the male reproductive tract. In order to decrease the potential exposure of infants to plasticizers, consider the use of bolus dosing in 1 mg/kg aliquots as described by Perry, 1996; see Usual Dosage. See also http://www.fda.gov/downloads/Safety/MedWatch/SafetyInformation/SafetyAlertsforHumanMedicalProducts/UCM173753.pdf.

Adverse Reactions

Cardiovascular: Proarrhythmia (including torsade de pointes), atropine-resistant bradycardia, heart block, sinus arrest, myocardial depression, CHF, paroxysmal ventricular tachycardia, cardiogenic shock, hypotension [Note: Hypotension may be potentially fatal with I.V. use; in adults, I.V. daily doses >2100 mg are associated with a greater risk of hypotension; in pediatric patients 30 days-15 years of age (n=61), dose-related cardiovascular adverse reactions were common (hypotension 36%, bradycardia 20%, and AV block 15%) and in some cases severe or life-threatening]

Central nervous system (20% to 40% incidence): Lack of coordination, fatigue, malaise, abnormal gait, dizziness, headache, insomnia, nightmares, ataxia, behavioral changes, fever

Dermatologic: Discoloration of skin (slate blue), photosensitivity, rash, angioedema, pruritus; skin cancer (postmarketing reports)

Endocrine & metabolic: Hypothyroidism (or less commonly hyperthyroidism, see Additional Information), hyperglycemia, triglycerides elevated, SIADH

Gastrointestinal: Nausea, vomiting, anorexia, constipation

Genitourinary: Sterile epididymitis

Hematologic: Coagulation abnormalities, thrombocytopenia; neutropenia, pancytopenia, hemolytic anemia, aplastic anemia

Hepatic: Liver enzymes elevated, bilirubin elevated, serum ammonia elevated, severe hepatic toxicity (potentially fatal); **Note:** Hepatocellular necrosis, hepatic coma, acute renal failure, and death have been associated with I.V. loading doses at much higher concentrations and I.V. rates of infusion much faster than recommended

Local: Injection site reactions (25% of pediatric patients); phlebitis (with I.V. formulation; concentration dependent)

Neuromuscular & skeletal: Paresthesia, tremor, peripheral neuropathy (rare), muscle weakness, rhabdomyolysis, parkinsonian symptoms (postmarketing reports); sometimes reversible after discontinuation of treatment)

Ocular: Corneal microdeposits, halos or blurred vision (10% incidence), photophobia, optic neuropathy, optic neuritis, visual impairment, permanent blindness (**Note:** Asymptomatic corneal microdeposits alone do not require dose reduction or discontinuation)

Renal: Renal impairment (postmarketing reports)

Respiratory (potentially fatal): Interstitial pneumonitis, hypersensitivity pneumonitis, pulmonary fibrosis [may present with cough, fever, dyspnea, bronchospasm, wheezing, hemoptysis, hypoxia, malaise, chest x-ray changes (pulmonary infiltrates and/or mass)]; pulmonary alveolar hemorrhage; adult respiratory distress syndrome; **Note:** Use of lower amiodarone doses (loading and maintenance) may be associated with a lower incidence of pulmonary toxicity. Early onset pulmonary toxicity (ie, occurring over days to weeks) has been reported with oral amiodarone (with or without initial I.V. use) and may progress to respiratory failure or death.

Miscellaneous: Anaphylaxis, anaphylactoid reactions (including shock); thyroid nodules/thyroid cancer (postmarketing reports)

Drug Interactions

Metabolism/Transport Effects Substrate of CYP1A2 (minor), CYP12C8 (major at low concentration), CYP12C19 (minor), CYP12D6 (minor), CYP13A4 (major), P-glycoprotein; **Inhibits** CYP1A2 (weak), CYP12A6 (moderate), CYP12B6 (weak), CYP12C9 (moderate), CYP12C19 (weak), CYP12D6 (moderate), CYP13A4 (moderate), P-glycoprotein

Avoid Concomitant Use

Avoid concomitant use of Amiodarone with any of the following: Agalsidase Beta; Artemether; Dronedarone; Grapefruit Juice; Lumefantrine; Nilotinib; Pimozide; Protease Inhibitors; QuiNINE; Silodosin; Tetrabenazine; Thioridazine; Tolvaptan; Topotecan; Ziprasidone

Increased Effect/Toxicity

Amiodarone may increase the levels/effects of: Antiarrhythmic Agents (Class Ia); Beta-Blockers; Cardiac Glycosides; Colchicine; CycloSPORINE; CycloSPORINE (Systemic); CYP2A6 Substrates; CYP2C9 Substrates (High risk); CYP2D6 Substrates; CYP3A4 Substrates; Dabigatran Etexilate; Dronedarone; Eplerenone; Everolimus; FentaNYL; Fesoterodine; Flecainide; HMG-CoA Reductase Inhibitors; Lidocaine; Lidocaine (Systemic); Lidocaine (Topical); Loratadine; P-Glycoprotein Substrates; Phenytoin; Pimecrolimus; Pimozide; QTc-Prolonging Agents; QuiNINE; Rivaroxaban; Salmeterol; Saxagliptin; Silodosin; Tamoxifen; Tetrabenazine; Thioridazine; Tolvaptan; Topotecan; Vitamin K Antagonists; Ziprasidone

The levels/effects of Amiodarone may be increased by: Alfuzosin; Artemether; Azithromycin; Calcium Channel Blockers (Nondihydropyridine); Chloroquine; Cimetidine; Ciprofloxacin; Ciprofloxacin (Systemic); CYP2C8 Inhibitors (Moderate); CYP2C8 Inhibitors (Strong); CYP3A4 Inhibitors (Moderate); CYP3A4 Inhibitors (Strong); Deferasirox; Gadobutrol; Grapefruit Juice; Lumefantrine; Nilotinib; P-Glycoprotein Inhibitors; Protease Inhibitors; QuiNINE

Decreased Effect

Amiodarone may decrease the levels/effects of: Agalsidase Beta; Codeine; Sodium Iodide I131; TraMADol

The levels/effects of Amiodarone may be decreased by: Bile Acid Sequestrants; CYP2C8 Inducers (Highly Effective); CYP3A4 Inducers (Strong); Deferasirox; Grapefruit Juice; Herbs (CYP3A4 Inducers); Orlistat; Peginterferon Alfa-2b; P-Glycoprotein Inducers; Phenytoin; Rifamycin Derivatives

Food Interactions Food increases rate and extent of oral absorption (high fat meal increased AUC by a mean of 2.3 times). Grapefruit juice increases oral amiodarone AUC by 50% and peak serum concentrations by 84%; avoid grapefruit juice during amiodarone therapy.

Stability

Storage:

Tablets: Store at controlled room temperature; protect from light; dispense in a light-resistant, tightly closed container

Injection: Store at controlled room temperature; protect from light during storage; protect from excessive heat; there is no need to protect diluted solutions from light during I.V. administration

Compatibility: Injection is compatible in D$_5$W at concentrations of 1-6 mg/mL for 24 hours in glass or polyolefin bottles and for 2 hours in polyvinyl chloride bags; although amiodarone adsorbs to polyvinyl chloride tubing, all clinical studies used polyvinyl chloride tubing and the recommended doses take adsorption into account, therefore, in adults, polyvinyl chloride tubing is recommended; amiodarone I.V. in D$_5$W is **not** compatible with aminophylline, cefamandole, cefazolin, mezlocillin, heparin, or sodium bicarbonate when administered together at the Y-site (a precipitate will occur)

Mechanism of Action A class III antiarrhythmic agent which inhibits adrenergic stimulation (possesses alpha- and beta-adrenergic-blocking properties); affects sodium, potassium, and calcium channels; prolongs the action potential and refractory period in myocardial tissue; decreases A-V conduction and sinus node function; possesses vasodilatory and negative inotropic effects

Pharmacodynamics

Onset of action: Oral: 2-3 days to 1-3 weeks after starting therapy; I.V.: (electrophysiologic effects) within hours; antiarrhythmic effects: 2-3 days to 1-3 weeks; mean onset of effect may be shorter in children vs adults and in patients receiving I.V. loading doses

Maximum effect: Oral: 1 week to 5 months

Duration of effects after discontinuation of oral therapy: Variable, 2 weeks to months: Children: Less than a few weeks; adults: several months

Pharmacokinetics (Adult data unless noted)

Absorption: Oral: Slow and incomplete

Distribution: Amiodarone and its active metabolite cross the placenta; both distribute to breast milk in concentrations higher than maternal plasma concentrations

I.V.: Rapid redistribution with a decrease to 10% of peak values within 30-45 minutes after completion of infusion

V_{dss}: I.V. single dose in adults: Mean range: 40-84 L/kg

V_d: Oral dose in adults: 66 L/kg: range: 18-148 L/kg

Protein binding: >96%

Metabolism: In the liver and possibly the GI tract via cytochrome P450 enzymes; the major metabolite N-desethylamiodarone is active

Bioavailability: Oral: ~50% (range: 35% to 65%)

Half-life:

Amiodarone:

Single dose in adults: Mean: 58 days (range 15-142 days)

Oral chronic therapy in adults: Mean range: 40-55 days (range: 26-107 days)

I.V. single dose in adults: Mean range: 20-47 days

Half-life is shortened in children vs adults

N-desethylamiodarone (active metabolite):

Single dose in adults: Mean: 36 days (range 14-75 days)

Oral chronic therapy in adults: Mean: 61 days

Elimination: Via biliary excretion; possible enterohepatic recirculation; <1% excreted unchanged in urine

Dialysis: Nondialyzable (parent and metabolite)

Usual Dosage

Infants and Children:

Oral: **Note:** Calculate dose using body surface area for children <1 year of age: Loading dose: 10-15 mg/kg/day or 600-800 mg/1.73 m^2/day in 1-2 divided doses/day for 4-14 days or until adequate control of arrhythmia or prominent adverse effects occur; dosage should then be reduced to 5 mg/kg/day or 200-400 mg/1.73 m^2/day given once daily for several weeks; if arrhythmia does not recur, reduce to lowest effective dosage possible; usual daily minimal dose: 2.5 mg/kg; maintenance doses may be given for 5 of 7 days/week.

Note: A more aggressive dosing regimen was used in neonates and infants (n=50; mean age: 1 ± 1.5 months) <9 months of age, treated for various types of SVT; 90% of patients at discharge and 100% of patients within 3 months of discharge were free of tachycardia; however, patients who received a higher loading dose (20 mg/kg/day in 2 divided doses) were more likely to have a prolongation of the corrected QT interval (see Etheridge, 2001); further studies are needed.

I.V., I.O.: **Note:** Use with caution when administering amiodarone with other drugs that prolong the QT interval (consider consulting expert)

PALS dose for treatment of pulseless VT or VF: 5 mg/kg (maximum: 300 mg/dose) rapid I.V. bolus or I.O.; may repeat up to a maximum daily dose of 15 mg/kg (**Note:** Maximum recommended daily dose in adolescents: 2.2 g)

PALS dose for treatment of perfusing tachycardias: Loading dose: 5 mg/kg (maximum: 300 mg/dose) I.V. given over 20-60 minutes or I.O.; may repeat up to maximum daily dose of 15 mg/kg (**Note:** Maximum recommended daily dose in adolescents: 2.2 g)

I.V.: Limited data is available. Four retrospective studies (Celiker, 1998; Figa, 1994; Raja, 1994; Soult, 1995) used I.V. loading doses of 5 mg/kg. Loading doses were administered over 1 hour in three of these studies to treat various life-threatening tachyarrhythmias including junctional ectopic tachycardia after cardiac surgery (in conjunction with atrial pacing). Soult 1995 used I.V. amiodarone for short-term treatment of paroxysmal supraventricular tachycardia (PSVT) and administered the loading dose via slow I.V. bolus over 5 minutes. For continuous infusion, Figa 1994 and Celiker 1998, used initial maintenance doses of 5 mcg/kg/minute (7.2 mg/kg/day) which was increased incrementally until the desired effect was seen or a maximum dose of 15 mcg/kg/minute (21.6 mg/kg/day) was reached. The mean effective dose in the study by Figa 1994 (n=30) was 9.5 mcg/kg/minute (13.7 mg/kg/day) and in Celiker 1998 (n=12) was 10 ± 4.7 mcg/kg/minute (range: 5-15 mcg/kg/minute).

A multicenter study (Perry, 1996; n=40; mean age 5.4 years with 24 of 40 children <2 years of age) used an I.V. loading dose of 5 mg/kg that was divided into five 1 mg/kg aliquots, with each aliquot given over 5-10 minutes. Additional 1-5 mg/kg doses could be administered 30 minutes later in a similar fashion if needed. The mean loading dose was 6.3 mg/kg. A maintenance dose (continuous infusion of 10-15 mg/kg/day) was administered to 21 of the 40 patients. Further studies are needed.

Adults:

ACLS dose for cardiac arrest due to pulseless VT or VF: I.V., I.O.: Initial: 300 mg diluted in 20-30 mL D$_5$W or NS given rapid I.V. push or given I.O.; one supplemental bolus dose of 150 mg given by rapid I.V. infusion or I.O. may be given for recurring VF or pulseless VT

ACLS doses for perfusing tachycardias: I.V.: See manufacturer's recommendations below for ventricular arrhythmias, for loading dose and continuous infusion; ACLS also recommends: Bolus doses for hemodynamically stable VT or wide QRS tachycardia of uncertain origin (regular rhythm): 150 mg given over 10 minutes; may repeat as needed to a maximum of 2.2 g/24 hours; for pre-excited atrial fibrillation: Consider 150 mg I.V. over 10 minutes

Ventricular arrhythmias (manufacturer's recommendations):

Oral: Loading dose: 800-1600 mg/day divided in 1-2 doses/day for 1-3 weeks, then 600-800 mg/day in 1-2 doses/day for 1 month; maintenance: 400 mg/day; lower doses are recommended for supraventricular arrhythmias.

I.V.: Loading dose: 1050 mg delivered over 24 hours as follows: 150 mg given over 10 minutes (at a rate of 15 mg/minute) followed by 360 mg given over 6 hours (at a rate of 1 mg/minute); follow with maintenance dose: 540 mg given over the next 18 hours (at a rate of 0.5 mg/minute); after the first 24 hours the maintenance dose is continued at 0.5 mg/minute; additional supplemental bolus doses of 150 mg infused over 10 minutes may be given for breakthrough VF or hemodynamically unstable VT; maintenance dose infusion may be increased to control arrhythmia; maximum daily dose: 2.1 g

Atrial fibrillation (see Goldschlager, 2000):
Oral: Loading dose: 600-800 mg/day divided in 2 doses/day for 2-4 weeks, then 400 mg/day; at 3-6 months, dose may be reduced further to 100-300 mg/day based on clinical efficacy and adverse effects; usual maintenance: 200 mg/day; **Note:** Some patients may require higher maintenance doses or increased maintenance doses for short periods of time for breakthrough arrhythmias; some patients can be maintained with 200 mg/day given for 5 of 7 days/week

Transition from I.V. to oral therapy: Optimal initial daily dose depends on I.V. dose administered and oral bioavailability; use the following as a guide for an initial daily dose, assuming patient received 0.5 mg/minute for the listed duration of I.V. infusion:
<1 week infusion: 800-1600 mg/day
1-3 week infusion: 600-800 mg/day
>3 week infusion: 400 mg/day

Dosing adjustment in renal impairment: No adjustment necessary

Administration

Oral: Administer at same time in relation to meals; do not administer with grapefruit juice

I.V.: Adjust administration rate to patient's clinical condition and urgency; give slowly to patients who have a pulse (ie, perfusing arrhythmia); may be given rapidly to patients with ventricular fibrillation or in cardiac arrest. Do not exceed recommended I.V. concentrations or rates of infusion (severe hepatic toxicity may occur; see Adverse Reactions). Slow the infusion rate if hypotension or bradycardia develops. Injection must be diluted before I.V. use. Adults: Usual dilutions: First loading infusion: 150 mg in 100 mL D_5W (1.5 mg/mL) for infusion over 10 minutes; then 900 mg in 500 mL D_5W (1.8 mg/mL) to deliver rest of dose. Administer via central venous catheter, if possible; increased phlebitis may occur with peripheral infusions >3 mg/mL in D_5W, but concentrations ≤2.5 mg/mL may be less irritating; the use of a central venous catheter with concentrations >2 mg/mL for infusions >1 hour is recommended. Maximum concentration for infusion: 6 mg/mL. Use glass or polyolefin bottles for infusions >2 hours; the use of polyvinyl chloride tubing is recommended in adults (see Stability). Must be infused via volumetric infusion device; drop size of I.V. solution may be reduced and underdosage may occur if drop counter infusion sets are used. Use in-line filter during administration. Adults: Do not exceed 30 mg/minute initial infusion rate; infants and children: See Usual Dosage I.V. and Precautions

Monitoring Parameters Heart rate and rhythm, blood pressure, ECG, chest x-ray, pulmonary function tests, thyroid function tests (see Additional Information); serum glucose, electrolytes (especially potassium and magnesium), triglycerides, liver enzymes; ophthalmologic exams including fundoscopy and slit-lamp examinations; physical signs and symptoms of thyroid dysfunction (lethargy, edema of hands and feet, weight gain or loss), and pulmonary toxicity (dyspnea, cough; oxygen saturation, blood gases). Monitor pacing or defibrillation thresholds in patients with implantable cardiac devices (eg, pacemakers, defibrillators) at initiation of therapy and periodically during treatment.

Reference Range Therapeutic: Chronic oral dosing: 1-2.5 mg/L (SI: 2-4 micromoles/L) (parent); desethyl metabolite (active) is present in equal concentration to parent drug; serum levels may not be of great value for predicting toxicity and efficacy; toxicity may occur even at therapeutic concentrations

Patient Information Read the patient Medication Guide that you receive with each prescription and refill of amiodarone. Report the use of other medications, non-prescription medications, and herbal or natural products to your physician and pharmacist. Avoid grapefruit juice and the herbal medicine, St John's wort. Notify physician or get medical help immediately if shortness of breath, wheezing, chest pain, spitting up of blood, yellow eyes, brown or dark-colored urine, heart pounding, lightheadedness, fainting, weakness, heat or cold intolerance, weight gain or loss, sweating, thinning of hair, changes in menses, swelling of neck (goiter), nervousness, irritability, restlessness, decreased concentration, depression, or tremor occurs. Notify physician if persistent dry cough or decreased vision occurs. May discolor skin to a slate blue color. May cause photosensitivity reactions (eg, exposure to sunlight may cause severe sunburn, skin rash, redness, or itching); avoid exposure to sunlight and artificial light sources (sunlamps, tanning booth/bed); wear protective clothing, wide-brimmed hats, sunglasses, and lip sunscreen (SPF ≥15); use a sunscreen [broad-spectrum sunscreen or physical sunscreen (preferred) or sunblock with SPF ≥15]; contact physician if reaction occurs.

Nursing Implications Ambulation of patient may be impaired due to adverse effects; due to possible infusion rate-related hypotension, the I.V. infusion rate should be carefully monitored

Additional Information Intoxication with amiodarone necessitates ECG monitoring; bradycardia may be atropine resistant, I.V. isoproterenol or cardiac pacemaker may be required; hypotension, cardiogenic shock, heart block, QT prolongation and hepatotoxicity may also be seen; patients should be monitored for several days following overdose due to long half-life

I.V. product is used for acute treatment; the duration of I.V. treatment is usually 48-96 hours, however, in adults, infusions may be used cautiously for 2-3 weeks; there is limited experience with administering infusions for >3 weeks

Use of amiodarone 300 mg I.V. in adults with cardiac arrest (out-of-hospital) due to refractory ventricular arrhythmias improved the rate of survival to hospital admission (see Kudenchuk, 1999). In a randomized, double blind, placebo controlled trial in adults with shock-resistant ventricular fibrillation (out-of-hospital), I.V. amiodarone [initial dose: 5 mg/kg; second dose (if needed): 2.5 mg/kg] resulted in higher rates of survival to hospital admission as compared to I.V. lidocaine [initial dose: 1.5 mg/kg; second dose (if needed): 1.5 mg/kg] (see Dorian, 2002).

Thyroid function tests: Amiodarone partially inhibits the peripheral conversion of thyroxine (T_4) to triiodothyronine (T_3); serum T_4 and reverse triiodothyronine (RT_3) concentrations may be increased and serum T_3 may be decreased; most patients remain clinically euthyroid, however, clinical hypothyroidism or hyperthyroidism may occur. **Note:** Amiodarone HCl contains 37% iodine by weight and is a potential source of large amounts of iodine; ~3 mg of inorganic iodine per 100 mg of amiodarone is released into the systemic circulation (RDA for iodine in Adults is 150 mcg).

Dosage Forms Excipient information presented when available (limited, particularly for generics); consult specific product labeling.
Injection, solution, as hydrochloride: 50 mg/mL (3 mL, 9 mL, 18 mL) [contains benzyl alcohol and polysorbate 80]
Tablet, as hydrochloride [scored]: 200 mg, 400 mg
Cordarone®: 200 mg
Pacerone®: 100 mg [not scored], 200 mg, 400 mg

Extemporaneous Preparations
A 5 mg/mL oral suspension can be made from tablets; two stability studies using different vehicles exist; a 5 mg/mL oral suspension made with simple syrup NF containing methylcellulose 1% (50:50, v/v) was stable for 42 days at

room temperature (25°C) and 91 days under refrigeration (4°C) in both glass and plastic prescription bottles (Nahata, 1997); label "shake well" and "protect from light" Five 200 mg tablets were crushed in a mortar; the vehicle (either a 1:1 mixture of Ora-Sweet® and Ora-Plus® or a 1:1 mixture of Ora-Sweet® SF and Ora-Plus®) was adjusted to a pH between 6-7 using a sodium bicarbonate solution (5 g/100 mL of distilled water). A small amount of the vehicle was added to the mortar to make a uniform paste; geometric amounts of the vehicle were added while mixing to **almost** the desired volume; suspension was transferred to a graduate and qsad to 200 mL while mixing. Suspensions prepared in both vehicles were stable for 42 days at room temperature (25°C) and 91 days under refrigeration (4°C) in plastic prescription bottles (Nahata 1999); label "shake well" and "protect from light"

Neither of these 2 studies determined microbial growth; extended storage under refrigeration is recommended

Nahata MC, "Stability of Amiodarone in an Oral Suspension Stored Under Refrigeration and at Room Temperature," *Ann Pharmacother*, 1997, 31(7-8):851-2.

Nahata MC, Morosco RS, and Hipple TF, "Stability of Amiodarone in Extemporaneous Oral Suspensions Prepared From Commercially Available Vehicles," *J Ped Pharmacy Practice*, 1999, 4(4):186-9.

References

American Heart Association Emergency Cardiovascular Care Committee," 2005 American Heart Association (AHA) Guidelines for Cardiopulmonary Resuscitation (CPR) and Emergency Cardiovascular Care (ECC), Part 7.2: Management of Cardiac Arrest, Part 7.3: Management of Symptomatic Bradycardia and Tachycardia, and Part 12: Pediatric Advanced Life Support," *Circulation*, 2005, 112(24 Suppl):IV58-77,167-87.

Celiker A, Ceviz N, and Ozme S, "Effectiveness and Safety of Intravenous Amiodarone in Drug-Resistant Tachyarrhythmias of Children," *Acta Paediatr Jpn*, 1998, 40(6):567-72.

Coumel P and Fidelle J, "Amiodarone in the Treatment of Cardiac Arrhythmias in Children: One Hundred Thirty-Five Cases," *Am Heart J*, 1980, 100(6 Pt 2):1063-9.

Dorian P, Cass D, Schwartz B, et al, "Amiodarone as Compared With Lidocaine for Shock-Resistant Ventricular Fibrillation," *N Engl J Med*, 2002, 346(12):884-90.

Drago F, Mazza A, Guccione P, et al, "Amiodarone Used Alone or in Combination With Propranolol: A Very Effective Therapy for Tachyarrhythmias in Infants and Children," *Pediatr Cardiol*, 1998, 19 (6):445-9.

Etheridge SP, Craig JE, and Compton SJ, "Amiodarone is Safe and Highly Effective Therapy for Supraventricular Tachycardia in Infants," *Am Heart J*, 2001, 141(1):105-10.

Figa FH, Gow RM, Hamilton RM, et al, "Clinical Efficacy and Safety of Intravenous Amiodarone in Infants and Children," *Am J Cardiol*, 1994, 74(6):573-7.

Garson A Jr, Gillette PC, McVey P, et al, "Amiodarone Treatment of Critical Arrhythmias in Children and Young Adults," *J Am Coll Cardiol*, 1984, 4(4):749-55.

Goldschlager N, Epstein AE, Naccarelli G, et al, "Practical Guidelines for Clinicians Who Treat Patients With Amiodarone," *Arch Intern Med*, 2000, 160(12):1741-8.

Kudenchuk PJ, Cobb LA, Copass MK, et al, "Amiodarone for Resuscitation After Out-of-Hospital Cardiac Arrest Due to Ventricular Fibrillation," *N Engl J Med*, 1999, 341(12):871-8.

Paul T and Guccione P, "New Antiarrhythmic Drugs in Pediatric Use: Amiodarone," *Pediatr Cardiol*, 1994, 15(3):132-8.

Pediatric Advanced Life Support, Provider Manual, copyright American Heart Association, 2006

Perry JC, Fenrich AL, Hulse JE, et al, "Pediatric Use of Intravenous Amiodarone: Efficacy and Safety in Critically Ill Patients From a Multicenter Protocol," *J Am Coll Cardiol*, 1996, 27(5):1246-50.

Raja P, Hawker RE, Chaikitpinyo A, et al, "Amiodarone Management of Junctional Ectopic Tachycardia After Cardiac Surgery in Children," *Br Heart J*, 1994, 72(3):261-5.

Shahar E, Barzilay Z, Frand M, et al, "Amiodarone in Control of Sustained Tachyarrhythmias in Children With Wolff-Parkinson-White Syndrome," *Pediatrics*, 1983, 72(6):813-6.

Shuler CO, Case CL, and Gillette PC, "Efficacy and Safety of Amiodarone in Infants," *Am Heart J*, 1993, 125(5 Pt 1):1430-2.

Soult JA, Munoz M, Lopez JD, et al, "Efficacy and Safety of Intravenous Amiodarone for Short-Term Treatment of Paroxysmal Supraventricular Tachycardia in Children," *Pediatr Cardiol*, 1995, 16(1):16-9.

◆ **Amiodarone Hydrochloride** *see* Amiodarone *on page 84*

◆ **Amiodarone Hydrochloride for Injection® (Can)** *see* Amiodarone *on page 84*

◆ **Amitone® [OTC] [DSC]** *see* Calcium Supplements *on page 239*

Amitriptyline (a mee TRIP ti leen)

Medication Safety Issues
Sound-alike/look-alike issues:
Amitriptyline may be confused with aminophylline, imipramine, nortriptyline
Elavil® may be confused with Aldoril®, Eldepryl®, enalapril, Equanil®, Mellaril®, Plavix®

Beers Criteria medication: This drug may be inappropriate for use in geriatric patients (high severity risk).

Related Information
Antidepressant Agents *on page 1484*
Medications for Which A Single Dose May Be Fatal When Ingested By A Toddler *on page 1709*
Serotonin Syndrome *on page 1695*

Canadian Brand Names Apo-Amitriptyline®; Bio-Amitriptyline; Dom-Amitriptyline; Levate®; Novo-Triptyn; PMS-Amitriptyline

Therapeutic Category Antidepressant, Tricyclic (Tertiary Amine); Antimigraine Agent

Generic Available Yes

Use Treatment of various forms of depression, often in conjunction with psychotherapy; analgesic for certain chronic and neuropathic pain; migraine prophylaxis

Medication Guide An FDA-approved patient medication guide, which is available with the product information and at http://www.fda.gov/downloads/Drugs/DrugSafety/ ucm088622.pdf, must be dispensed with this medication for each new outpatient prescription and refill.

Pregnancy Risk Factor C

Pregnancy Considerations Teratogenic effects have been observed in animal studies. Amitriptyline crosses the human placenta; CNS effects, limb deformities and developmental delay have been noted in case reports.

Lactation Enters breast milk/not recommended (AAP rates "of concern")

Breast-Feeding Considerations Generally, it is not recommended to breast-feed if taking antidepressants because of the long half-life, active metabolites, and the potential for side effects in the infant.

Contraindications Hypersensitivity to amitriptyline (cross-sensitivity with other tricyclics may occur) or any component; narrow-angle glaucoma; use of MAO inhibitors within 14 days (potentially fatal reactions may occur, see Drug Interactions); concurrent use of cisapride; use during acute recovery phase after MI

Warnings Amitriptyline is not approved for use in pediatric patients. Clinical worsening of depression or suicidal ideation and behavior may occur in children and adults with major depressive disorder **[U.S. Boxed Warning]**. In clinical trials, antidepressants increased the risk of suicidal thinking and behavior (suicidality) in children, adolescents, and young adults (18-24 years of age) with major depressive disorder and other psychiatric disorders. This risk must be considered before prescribing antidepressants for any clinical use. Short-term studies did **not** show an increased risk of suicidality with antidepressant use in patients >24 years of age and showed a decreased risk in patients ≥65 years.

Patients of all ages who are treated with antidepressants for any indication require appropriate monitoring and close observation for clinical worsening of depression, suicidality, and unusual changes in behavior, especially during the first few months after antidepressant initiation or when the dose is adjusted. Family members and caregivers should be instructed to closely observe the patient (ie, daily) and communicate condition with healthcare provider. Patients should also be monitored for associated behaviors (eg, anxiety, agitation, panic attacks, insomnia, irritability, hostility, aggressiveness, impulsivity, akathisia, hypomania, mania) which may increase the risk for worsening depression or suicidality. Worsening depression or emergence of suicidality (or associated behaviors listed above) that is abrupt in onset, severe, or not part of the presenting symptoms, may require discontinuation or modification of drug therapy.

Do not discontinue abruptly in patients receiving high doses chronically (withdrawal symptoms may occur; see Adverse Reactions). To reduce risk of intentional overdose, write prescriptions for the smallest quantity consistent with good patient care. Screen individuals for bipolar disorder prior to treatment (using antidepressants alone may induce manic episodes in patients with this condition). May worsen psychosis in some patients.

Precautions Use with caution in patients with cardiac conduction disturbances, cardiovascular disease, seizure disorders, diabetes mellitus, narrow-angle glaucoma, increased intraocular pressure, history of urinary retention or bowel obstruction, hepatic or renal dysfunction, hyperthyroidism or those receiving thyroid hormone replacement; degree of sedation, anticholinergic effects, and risk of orthostatic hypotension are very high relative to other antidepressants; manufacturer does not recommend use in children <12 years of age

Adverse Reactions Anticholinergic effects may be pronounced; moderate to marked sedation can occur (tolerance to these effects usually occurs)

Cardiovascular: Postural hypotension, arrhythmias, tachycardia, sudden death, cardiomyopathy (very rare)

Central nervous system: Sedation, fatigue, anxiety, confusion, insomnia, impaired cognitive function, seizures; extrapyramidal symptoms are possible; suicidal thinking and behavior (see Warnings)

Dermatologic: Photosensitivity, urticaria, rash

Endocrine & metabolic: SIADH (rare), weight gain, hyperglycemia, hypoglycemia

Gastrointestinal: Xerostomia, constipation, decrease of lower esophageal sphincter tone, GE reflux, appetite increased

Genitourinary: Urinary retention, discoloration of urine (blue-green)

Hematologic: Rarely agranulocytosis, leukopenia, eosinophilia

Hepatic: Liver enzymes elevated, cholestatic jaundice

Neuromuscular & skeletal: Tremor, weakness

Ocular: Blurred vision, intraocular pressure increased

Miscellaneous: Allergic reactions; withdrawal symptoms following abrupt discontinuation (headache, nausea, malaise)

Drug Interactions

Metabolism/Transport Effects Substrate of CYP1A2 (minor), 2B6 (minor), 2C9 (minor), 2C19 (minor), 2D6 (major), 3A4 (minor); **Inhibits** CYP1A2 (weak), 2C9 (weak), 2C19 (weak), 2D6 (weak), 2E1 (weak)

Avoid Concomitant Use

Avoid concomitant use of Amitriptyline with any of the following: Artemether; Cisapride; Dronedarone; Iobenguane I 123; Lumefantrine; MAO Inhibitors; Metoclopramide; Nilotinib; Pimozide; QuiNINE; Sibutramine; Tetrabenazine; Thioridazine; Ziprasidone

Increased Effect/Toxicity

Amitriptyline may increase the levels/effects of: Alcohol (Ethyl); Alpha-/Beta-Agonists (Direct-Acting); Alpha1-Agonists; Amphetamines; Anticholinergics; Aspirin; Beta2-Agonists; Cisapride; CNS Depressants;

Desmopressin; Dronedarone; NSAID (COX-2 Inhibitor); NSAID (Nonselective); Pimozide; QTc-Prolonging Agents; QuiNIDine; QuiNINE; Serotonin Modulators; Sulfonylureas; Tetrabenazine; Thioridazine; TraMADol; Vitamin K Antagonists; Yohimbine; Ziprasidone

The levels/effects of Amitriptyline may be increased by: Alfuzosin; Altretamine; Artemether; BuPROPion; Chloroquine; Cimetidine; Cinacalcet; Ciprofloxacin; Ciprofloxacin (Systemic); CYP2D6 Inhibitors (Moderate); CYP2D6 Inhibitors (Strong); Dexmethylphenidate; Divalproex; DULoxetine; Gadobutrol; Lithium; Lumefantrine; MAO Inhibitors; Methylphenidate; Metoclopramide; Nilotinib; Pramlintide; Propoxyphene; Protease Inhibitors; QuiNIDine; QuiNINE; Selective Serotonin Reuptake Inhibitors; Sibutramine; Terbinafine; Terbinafine (Systemic); Valproic Acid

Decreased Effect

Amitriptyline may decrease the levels/effects of: Acetylcholinesterase Inhibitors (Central); Alpha2-Agonists; Iobenguane I 123

The levels/effects of Amitriptyline may be decreased by: Acetylcholinesterase Inhibitors (Central); Barbiturates; CarBAMazepine; Peginterferon Alfa-2b; St Johns Wort

Food Interactions Riboflavin dietary requirements may be increased; increased dietary fiber may decrease drug effect

Mechanism of Action Increases the synaptic concentration of serotonin and/or norepinephrine in the CNS by inhibition of their reuptake by the presynaptic neuronal membrane

Pharmacodynamics Onset of action: Therapeutic antidepressant effects begin in 7-21 days; maximum effects may not occur for ≥2 weeks and as long as 4-6 weeks

Pharmacokinetics (Adult data unless noted)

Absorption: Oral: Rapid, well absorbed

Distribution: Crosses placenta; enters breast milk

Protein binding: >90%

Metabolism: In the liver to nortriptyline (active), hydroxy derivatives and conjugated derivatives

Half-life, adults: 9-25 hours (15-hour average)

Time to peak serum concentration: Within 4 hours

Elimination: Renal excretion of 18% as unchanged drug; small amounts eliminated in feces by bile

Dialysis: Nondialyzable

Usual Dosage Oral:

Chronic pain management: Children: Initial: 0.1 mg/kg at bedtime, may advance as tolerated over 2-3 weeks to 0.5-2 mg/kg at bedtime

Depressive disorders: **Note:** Not FDA approved for use in pediatric patients; controlled clinical trials have not shown tricyclic antidepressants to be superior to placebo for the treatment of depression in children and adolescents (see Dopheide, 2006 and Wagner, 2005).

Children: Investigationally initial doses of 1 mg/kg/day given in 3 divided doses with increases to 1.5 mg/kg/day have been reported in a small number of children (n=9) 9-12 years of age; clinically, doses up to 3 mg/kg/day (5 mg/kg/day if monitored closely) have been proposed

Adolescents: Initial: 25-50 mg/day; may give in divided doses; increase gradually to 100 mg/day in divided doses; maximum dose: 200 mg/day

Migraine prophylaxis: Children: Limited studies exist; one small study (n=24; mean age: 8 years; range: 6-12 years) used increasing doses over 5 days to reach a final dose of 1.5 mg/kg/day; effectiveness was seen in 19 of 24 patients, but 5 children dropped out of the trial due to adverse effects (see Sorge, 1982). A recent large open-label trial in 192 children (mean age 12 ± 3 years) with >3 headaches/month (61% with migraine, 8% with migraine with aura, and 10% with tension-type headaches) used an initial dose of 0.25 mg/kg/day given before bedtime;

doses were increased every 2 weeks by 0.25 mg/kg/day to a final dose of 1 mg/kg/day; patients also used appropriate abortive medications and lifestyle adjustments; at initial re-evaluation (mean: 67 days after initiation of therapy), the mean number of headaches per month significantly decreased from 17.1 to 9.2; the mean duration of headaches decreased from 11.5 to 6.3 hours; continued improvement was observed at follow-up visits; minimal adverse effects were reported. **Note:** Mean final dose was 0.99 ± 0.23 mg/kg; range: 0.16-1.7 mg/kg/day; ECGs were obtained on children receiving >1 mg/kg/day or in those describing a cardiac side effect (see Hershey, 2000). Further studies are needed.

Depression: Adults: Initial: 50-100 mg/day single dose at bedtime or in divided doses; dose may be gradually increased up to 300 mg/day; once symptoms are controlled, decrease gradually to lowest effective dose

Administration Oral: May administer with food to decrease GI upset

Monitoring Parameters Heart rate, blood pressure, mental status, weight. Monitor patient periodically for symptom resolution; monitor for worsening depression, suicidality, and associated behaviors (especially at the beginning of therapy or when doses are increased or decreased; see Warnings).

Reference Range Note: Plasma levels do not always correlate with clinical effectiveness

Therapeutic:

Amitriptyline plus nortriptyline (active metabolite): 100-250 ng/mL (SI: 360-900 nmol/L)

Nortriptyline 50-150 ng/mL (SI: 190-570 nmol/L)

Toxic: >500 ng/mL (SI: >1800 nmol/L)

Patient Information Read the patient Medication Guide that you receive with each prescription and refill of amitriptyline. An increased risk of suicidal thinking and behavior has been reported with the use of antidepressants in children, adolescents, and young adults (18-24 years of age). Notify physician if you feel more depressed, have thoughts of suicide, or become more agitated or irritable (see Warnings). Avoid alcohol and the herbal medicine St John's wort; limit caffeine intake; may cause drowsiness and impair ability to perform activities requiring mental alertness or physical coordination; may cause dry mouth; do not discontinue abruptly; may discolor urine to a blue-green color. May cause photosensitivity reactions (eg, exposure to sunlight may cause severe sunburn, skin rash, redness, or itching); avoid exposure to sunlight and artificial light sources (sunlamps, tanning booth/bed); wear protective clothing, wide-brimmed hats, sunglasses, and lip sunscreen (SPF ≥15); use a sunscreen [broad-spectrum sunscreen or physical sunscreen (preferred) or sunblock with SPF ≥15]; contact physician if reaction occurs.

Additional Information Due to promotion of weight gain with amitriptyline, other antidepressants (ie, imipramine or desipramine) may be preferred in heavy or obese children and adolescents

Dosage Forms Excipient information presented when available (limited, particularly for generics); consult specific product labeling.

Tablet, as hydrochloride: 10 mg, 25 mg, 50 mg, 75 mg, 100 mg, 150 mg

References

Dopheide JA, "Recognizing and Treating Depression in Children and Adolescents," *Am J Health Syst Pharm*, 2006, 63(3):233-43.

Elser JM and Woody RC, "Migraine Headache in the Infant and Young Child," *Headache*, 1990, 30(6):366-8.

Hershey AD, Powers SW, Bentti AL, et al, "Effectiveness of Amitriptyline in the Prophylactic Management of Childhood Headaches," *Headache*, 2000, 40(7):539-49.

Kashani JH, Shekim WO, and Reid JC, "Amitriptyline in Children With Major Depressive Disorder: A Double-Blind Crossover Pilot Study," *J Am Acad Child Psychiatry*, 1984, 23(3):348-51.

Levy HB, Harper CR, and Weinberg WA, "A Practical Approach to Children Failing in School," *Pediatr Clin North Am*, 1992, 39 (4):895-928.

Sorge F, Barone P, Steardo L, et al, "Amitriptyline as a Prophylactic for Migraine in Children," *Acta Neurol (Napoli)*, 1982, 4(5):362-7.

Wagner KD, "Pharmacotherapy for Major Depression in Children and Adolescents," *Prog Neuropsychopharmacol Biol Psychiatry*, 2005, 29 (5):819-26.

◆ **Amitriptyline Hydrochloride** *see* Amitriptyline *on page 89*

◆ **AmLactin® [OTC]** *see* Lactic Acid and Ammonium Hydroxide *on page 789*

AmLODIPine (am LOE di peen)

Medication Safety Issues

Sound-alike/look-alike issues:

AmLODIPine may be confused with aMILoride

Norvasc® may be confused with Navane®, Norvir®, Vascor®

Related Information

Antihypertensive Agents by Class *on page 1481*

U.S. Brand Names Norvasc®

Canadian Brand Names Accel-Amlodipine; Apo-Amlodipine®; CO Amlodipine; Dom-Amlodipine; GD-Amlodipine; JAMP-Amlodipine; Mylan-Amlodipine; Norvasc®; Novo-Amlodipine; PHL-Amlodipine; PMS-Amlodipine; RAN™-Amlodipine; ratio-Amlodipine; Riva-Amlodipine; Sandoz Amlodipine

Therapeutic Category Antianginal Agent; Antihypertensive Agent; Calcium Channel Blocker; Calcium Channel Blocker, Nondihydropyridine

Generic Available Yes

Use Treatment of hypertension (FDA approved in ages ≥6 years and adults); chronic stable angina (FDA approved in adults); vasospastic (Prinzmetal's) angina (FDA approved in adults); angiographically documented CAD [to decrease risk of hospitalization (due to angina) and coronary revascularization procedure] (FDA approved in adults)

Pregnancy Risk Factor C

Pregnancy Considerations Embryotoxic effects have been demonstrated in animal studies. No well-controlled studies have been conducted in pregnant women. Use in pregnancy only when clearly needed and when the benefits outweigh the potential hazard to the fetus.

Lactation Excretion in breast milk unknown/not recommended

Contraindications Hypersensitivity to amlodipine or any component

Warnings May increase frequency, duration, and severity of angina or precipitate acute MI during initiation of therapy or dosage increase (particularly in patients with severe obstructive coronary artery disease)

Precautions Use with caution and reduce the dose in patients with hepatic impairment; titrate dose slowly in patients with severe hepatic impairment. Symptomatic hypotension may occur; use with caution in patients with severe aortic stenosis; acute hypotension may rarely occur

Adverse Reactions

Cardiovascular system: Angina, flushing, hypotension, MI, palpitations, peripheral edema, syncope

Central nervous system: Dizziness, fatigue, headache, somnolence

Dermatologic: Pruritus, rash

Endocrine & metabolic: Sexual dysfunction

Gastrointestinal: Abdominal pain, dyspepsia, nausea

Neuromuscular & skeletal: Asthenia, muscle cramps

Respiratory: Dyspnea

Miscellaneous: Hypersensitivity reactions

<1%, postmarketing, and/or case reports: Abnormal dreams, abnormal vision, allergic reactions, angioedema, anorexia, anxiety, arrhythmia, arthralgia, arthrosis, atrial

fibrillation, back pain, bradycardia, chest pain, conjunctivitis, constipation, depersonalization, depression, dysphagia, dyspnea, diarrhea, diaphoresis, diplopia, epistaxis, erythema multiforme, eye pain, flatulence, gingival hyperplasia (may be less than with nifedipine), gynecomastia, hepatitis, hot flushes, hyperglycemia, hypoesthesia, insomnia, jaundice, leukopenia, liver enzymes increased, malaise, micturition disorder, micturition frequency, myalgia, nervousness, nocturia, pain, pancreatitis, paresthesia, peripheral ischemia, peripheral neuropathy, postural dizziness, postural hypotension, purpura, rigors, tachycardia, thirst, thrombocytopenia, tinnitus, tremor, vasculitis, ventricular tachycardia, vertigo, vomiting, weight gain, weight loss, xerostomia

Drug Interactions

Metabolism/Transport Effects Substrate of CYP3A4 (major); **Inhibits** CYP1A2 (moderate), 2A6 (weak), 2B6 (weak), 2C8 (weak), 2C9 (weak), 2D6 (weak), 3A4 (weak)

Avoid Concomitant Use There are no known interactions where it is recommended to avoid concomitant use.

Increased Effect/Toxicity

AmLODIPine may increase the levels/effects of: Amifostine; Antihypertensives; Calcium Channel Blockers (Nondihydropyridine); CYP1A2 Substrates; Hypotensive Agents; Magnesium Salts; Neuromuscular-Blocking Agents (Nondepolarizing); Nitroprusside; Phenytoin; RiTUXimab; Tacrolimus; Tacrolimus (Systemic)

The levels/effects of AmLODIPine may be increased by: Alpha1-Blockers; Antifungal Agents (Azole Derivatives, Systemic); Calcium Channel Blockers (Nondihydropyridine); CycloSPORINE; CycloSPORINE (Systemic); CYP3A4 Inhibitors (Moderate); CYP3A4 Inhibitors (Strong); Dasatinib; Diazoxide; Fluconazole; Grapefruit Juice; Herbs (Hypotensive Properties); Macrolide Antibiotics; Magnesium Salts; MAO Inhibitors; Pentoxifylline; Phosphodiesterase 5 Inhibitors; Prostacyclin Analogues; Protease Inhibitors; Quinupristin

Decreased Effect

AmLODIPine may decrease the levels/effects of: Clopidogrel; QuiNIDine

The levels/effects of AmLODIPine may be decreased by: Barbiturates; Calcium Salts; CarBAMazepine; CYP3A4 Inducers (Strong); Deferasirox; Herbs (CYP3A4 Inducers); Herbs (Hypertensive Properties); Methylphenidate; Nafcillin; Rifamycin Derivatives; Yohimbine

Food Interactions Food does not affect the bioavailability of amlodipine. Grapefruit juice increased amlodipine peak serum concentrations by 15% and AUC by 16% in one single dose study (Josefsson, 1996); however, repeated daily ingestion of grapefruit juice did **not** affect amlodipine pharmacokinetics in another single-dose amlodipine study (Vincent, 2000); multiple dose amlodipine-grapefruit juice interaction studies are needed. Avoid natural licorice (causes sodium and water retention and increases potassium loss)

Stability Store at room temperature of 15°C to 30°C (59°F to 86°F); dispense in tightly-closed, light-resistant container

Mechanism of Action Inhibits calcium ions from entering the "slow channels" or select voltage-sensitive areas of vascular smooth muscle and myocardium during depolarization; produces a relaxation of coronary vascular smooth muscle and coronary vasodilation; increases myocardial oxygen delivery in patients with vasospastic angina

Pharmacodynamics Antihypertensive effects: Duration: ≥24 hours with chronic daily dosing

Pharmacokinetics (Adult data unless noted)

Absorption: Oral: Well absorbed

Distribution: Distribution into breast milk is unknown

Mean V_d:

Children >6 years: Similar to adults on a mg per kg basis; **Note:** Weight-adjusted V_d in younger children (<6 years of age) may be greater than in older children (see Flynn, 2006)

Adults: 21 L/kg

Protein binding: 93%

Metabolism: In the liver with 90% metabolized to inactive metabolites

Bioavailability: Oral: 64% to 90%

Half-life: Terminal: 30-50 hours

Time to peak serum concentrations: 6-12 hours

Elimination: 10% of parent drug and 60% of metabolites are excreted in the urine

Clearance: May be decreased in patients with hepatic insufficiency or moderate to severe heart failure; weight-adjusted clearance in children >6 years of age is similar to adults; **Note:** Weight-adjusted clearance in younger children (<6 years of age) may be greater than in older children (see Flynn, 2006)

Dialysis: Not dialyzable

Usual Dosage Oral:

Children: Hypertension: **Note:** For a summary of other pediatric studies see Additional Information

Children 1-5 years: Limited information exists in the literature. One population pharmacokinetic study found that children <6 years of age had weight-adjusted clearance and V_d of amlodipine that were significantly greater than children ≥6 years of age. This may suggest the need for higher mg/kg/day doses in younger children (<6 years of age); however, the study included only a small number of younger children (n=11) (see Flynn, 2006). One retrospective pediatric study (n=55) that included only eight patients 1-6 years of age used initial doses of 0.05-0.1 mg/kg/day; doses were titrated upwards as needed; mean required dose was significantly higher in patients 1-6 years of age (0.3 ± 0.16 mg/kg/day) compared to older children (6-12 years: 0.16 ± 0.12 mg/kg/day; 12-20 years: 0.14 ± 0.1 mg/kg/day) (see Flynn, 2000a and Additional Information). Further studies are needed.

Children 6-17 years: Manufacturer recommendations: 2.5-5 mg once daily; doses >5 mg daily have not been fully studied.

Note: Limited data exists in the literature. In the only randomized, placebo-controlled trial of amlodipine in children (n=268; mean age: 12.1 years; range: 6-16 years), a significant reduction in systolic blood pressure (compared to placebo) was observed in both the 2.5 mg once daily and the 5 mg once daily amlodipine groups. The authors recommend an initial dose of 0.06 mg/kg/day with a maximum dose of 0.34 mg/kg/day (not to exceed 10 mg/day) (see Flynn, 2004 and Additional Information).

Adults:

Hypertension: Initial: 2.5-5 mg once daily; use initial dose of 2.5 mg once daily in patients who are small or fragile, and when adding amlodipine to other antihypertensive therapy; in general, titrate dose over 7-14 days to fully assess effects; usual dose: 5 mg once daily; maximum dose: 10 mg once daily; usual dosage range (JNC 7): 2.5-10 mg once daily

Angina or CAD: 5-10 mg once daily; use lower dose for patients with hepatic impairment; most patients with CAD require 10 mg once daily

Dosing adjustment in renal impairment: Not needed; patients may receive the usual initial dose

Dosing adjustment in hepatic impairment: Adults: Angina: Initial: 5 mg once daily; Hypertension: Initial: 2.5 mg once daily

Administration Oral: May be administered without regard to food; use caution if administered with grapefruit juice (see Food Interactions)

Monitoring Parameters Blood pressure, liver enzymes

Patient Information Do not discontinue abruptly; report unrelieved headache, vomiting, palpitations, peripheral or facial swelling, weight gain, or respiratory changes; may cause dizziness or drowsiness and impair ability to perform activities requiring mental alertness or physical coordination; may cause dry mouth

Additional Information Summary of additional pediatric studies:

In one prospective study, 21 hypertensive children (mean age: 13.1 years; range: 6-17 years) received the following initial daily doses of amlodipine based on weight groups: Children <50 kg: 0.05 mg/kg/day; children 50-70 kg: 2.5 mg daily; children >70 kg: 5 mg daily; mean initial dose: 0.07 ± 0.04 mg/kg/day; doses were increased by 25% to 50% (rounded to the nearest 2.5 mg) every 5-7 days to a maximum of 0.5 mg/kg/day, as needed to control blood pressure; the mean required dose was almost twice as high for children <13 years of age (0.29 ± 0.13 mg/kg/ day) compared to children ≥13 years of age (0.16 ± 0.11 mg/kg/day) (see Tallian, 1999).

In a small randomized crossover trial, amlodipine was compared to nifedipine or felodipine in 11 hypertensive children (mean age: 16 years; range: 9-17 years); amlodipine was administered once daily as a liquid preparation (tablets dissolved in water immediately prior to administration); an initial daily dose of 0.1 mg/kg/day (maximum: 5 mg daily) was increased by 50% to 100% after 1 week to a maximum of 10 mg/day, as needed for blood pressure control; mean initial dose: 0.09 ± 0.01 mg/ kg/day; mean required dose: 0.12 mg/kg/day (see Rogan, 2000). A third prospective study used fixed mg doses, rather than dosing on a mg/kg basis (see Pfammatter, 1998).

A prospective study in 43 pediatric outpatients with chronic kidney disease (median age: 9 years; range: 1-19 years) used the following initial daily doses of amlodipine based on weight groups: Children 10-30 kg: 2.5 mg once daily; children ≥31 kg: 5 mg once daily. Doses were increased if needed to a maximum of 0.5 mg/kg/day (20 mg/day). Younger patients required significantly higher mg/kg/day doses of amlodipine compared to older children. This relationship was not observed when the dose was expressed as mg/m²/day. The authors recommend a dose of 7-10 mg/m² given once daily (see von Vigier, 2001).

Five retrospective studies used a variety of initial amlodipine doses ranging from 0.05-0.13 mg/kg/day; mean required dose after dosage titration (for all aged pediatric patients) ranged from 0.15-0.23 mg/kg/day (see Andersen, 2006; Flynn, 2000a; Khattak, 1998; Parker 2002; Silverstein, 1999). Two of these studies noted a relationship between dose and age, with younger patients requiring higher mg/kg/day doses. Several retrospective studies used twice daily dosing in younger children, but it is unknown whether this reflects altered pharmacokinetics or physician prescribing habits. One population pharmacokinetic study suggests there is no justification for twice-daily dosing of amlodipine children (see Flynn, 2006). Further pediatric studies are needed.

Dosage Forms Excipient information presented when available (limited, particularly for generics); consult specific product labeling.

Tablet: 2.5 mg, 5 mg, 10 mg

Norvasc®: 2.5 mg, 5 mg, 10 mg

Extemporaneous Preparations A 1 mg/mL oral suspension made from tablets and two different vehicles (a 1:1 mixture of simple syrup and 1% methylcellulose or a 1:1 mixture of OraPlus® and OraSweet®) was stable for 56 days at room temperature (25°C) and 91 days under refrigeration (4°C) when stored in amber plastic prescription bottles; grind fifty 5 mg tablets in a mortar into a fine powder; add a small amount of the vehicle and mix well to form a uniform paste; mix while adding the vehicle in geometric proportions to **almost** 250 mL; transfer to a calibrated bottle and qsad with vehicle to 250 mL. Microbial growth was not determined in this study; extended storage under refrigeration is recommended to minimize microbial contamination. Label "shake well" and "refrigerate"

Nahata MC, Morosco RS, and Hipple TF, "Stability of Amlodipine Besylate in Two Liquid Dosage Forms," *J Am Pharm Assoc*, 1999, 39(3):375-7.

References

Andersen J, Groshong T, and Tobias JD, "Preliminary Experience With Amlodipine in the Pediatric Population," *Am J Ther*, 2006, 13 (3):198-204.

Chobanian AV, Bakris GL, Black HR, et al, "The Seventh Report of the Joint National Committee on Prevention, Detection, Evaluation, and Treatment of High Blood Pressure: The JNC 7 report," *JAMA*, 2003, 289(19):2560-72.

Flynn JT and Pasko DA, "Calcium Channel Blockers: Pharmacology and Place in Therapy of Pediatric Hypertension," *Pediatr Nephrol*, 2000, 15(3-4):302-16.

Flynn JT, Nahata MC, Mahan JD Jr, et al, "Population Pharmacokinetics of Amlodipine in Hypertensive Children and Adolescents," *J Clin Pharmacol*, 2006, 46(8):905-16.

Flynn JT, Newburger JW, Daniels SR, et al, "A Randomized, Placebo-Controlled Trial of Amlodipine in Children With Hypertension," *J Pediatr*, 2004, 145(3):353-9.

Flynn JT, Smoyer WE, and Bunchman TE, "Treatment of Hypertensive Children With Amlodipine," *Am J Hypertens*, 2000a, 13(10):1061-6.

Josefsson M, Zackrisson AL, and Ahlner J, "Effect of Grapefruit Juice on the Pharmacokinetics of Amlodipine in Healthy Volunteers," *Eur J Clin Pharmacol*, 1996, 51(2):189-93.

Khattak S, Rogan JW, Saunders EF, et al, "Efficacy of Amlodipine in Pediatric Bone Marrow Transplant Patients," *Clin Pediatr (Phila)*, 1998, 37(1):31-5.

Meredith PA and Elliott HL, "Clinical Pharmacokinetics of Amlodipine," *Clin Pharmacokinet*, 1992, 22(1):22-31.

National High Blood Pressure Education Program Working Group on High Blood Pressure in Children and Adolescents, "The Fourth Report on the Diagnosis, Evaluation, and Treatment of High Blood Pressure in Children and Adolescents," *Pediatrics*, 2004, 114(2 Suppl 4th Report):555-76.

Parker ML, Robinson RF, and Nahata MC, "Amlodipine Therapy in Pediatric Patients With Hypertension," *J Am Pharm Assoc*, 2002, 42 (1):114-7.

Pfammatter JP, Clericetti-Affolter C, Truttmann AC, et al, "Amlodipine Once-Daily in Systemic Hypertension," *Eur J Pediatr*, 1998, 157 (8):618-21.

Rogan JW, Lyszkiewicz DA, Blowey D, et al, "A Randomized Prospective Crossover Trial of Amlodipine in Pediatric Hypertension," *Pediatr Nephrol*, 2000, 14(12):1083-7.

Silverstein DM, Palmer J, Baluarte HJ, et al, "Use of Calcium-Channel Blockers in Pediatric Renal Transplant Recipients," *Pediatr Transplant*, 1999, 3(4):288-92.

Tallian KB, Nahata MC, Turman MA, et al, "Efficacy of Amlodipine in Pediatric Patients With Hypertension," *Pediatr Nephrol*, 1999, 13 (4):304-10.

Vincent J, Harris SI, Foulds G, et al, "Lack of Effect of Grapefruit Juice on the Pharmacokinetics and Pharmacodynamics of Amlodipine," *Br J Clin Pharmacol*, 2000, 50(5):455-63.

von Vigier RO, Franscini LM, Bianda ND, et al, "Antihypertensive Efficacy of Amlodipine in Children With Chronic Kidney Diseases," *J Hum Hypertens*, 2001, 15(6):387-91.

◆ **Amlodipine Besylate** *see* AmLODIPine *on page 91*

◆ **Ammens® Original Medicated [OTC]** *see* Zinc Oxide *on page 1445*

◆ **Ammens® Shower Fresh [OTC]** *see* Zinc Oxide *on page 1445*

◆ **Ammonapse** *see* Sodium Phenylbutyrate *on page 1275*

Ammonium Chloride (a MOE nee um KLOR ide)

Therapeutic Category Metabolic Alkalosis Agent; Urinary Acidifying Agent

Generic Available Yes

Use Diuretic or systemic and urinary acidifying agent; treatment of hypochloremia

Pregnancy Risk Factor C

Pregnancy Considerations Reproduction studies have not been conducted.

Contraindications Hypersensitivity to ammonium chloride or any component; severe hepatic and renal dysfunction; patients with primary respiratory acidosis

Adverse Reactions

Cardiovascular: Bradycardia

Central nervous system: Mental confusion, coma, headache

Dermatologic: Rash

Endocrine & metabolic: Metabolic acidosis secondary to hyperchloremia

Gastrointestinal: GI irritation

Local: Pain at site of injection

Respiratory: Hyperventilation

Drug Interactions

Avoid Concomitant Use There are no known interactions where it is recommended to avoid concomitant use.

Increased Effect/Toxicity

The levels/effects of Ammonium Chloride may be increased by: Potassium-Sparing Diuretics

Decreased Effect

Ammonium Chloride may decrease the levels/effects of: Amphetamines; Analgesics (Opioid)

Mechanism of Action Its dissociation to ammonium and chloride ions increases acidity by increasing free hydrogen ion concentration which combines with bicarbonate ion to form CO_2 and water; the net result is the replacement of bicarbonate ions by chloride ions

Pharmacokinetics (Adult data unless noted)

Metabolism: In the liver

Elimination: In urine

Usual Dosage

The following equations represent different methods of chloride or alkalosis correction utilizing either the serum HCO_3^-, the serum Cl- or the base excess: Children and Adults: I.V. (**Note:** Ammonium chloride is an alternative treatment and should be used only after sodium and potassium chloride supplementation has been optimized.):

Correction of refractory hypochloremic metabolic alkalosis: mEq NH_4Cl = 0.5 L/kg x wt in kg x [serum HCO_3^- - 24] mEq/L; give $1/2$ to $2/3$ of the calculated dose, then re-evaluate

Correction of hypochloremia: mEq NH_4Cl = 0.2 L/kg x wt in kg x [103 - serum Cl-] mEq/L, give $1/2$ to $2/3$ of calculated dose, then re-evaluate

Correction of alkalosis via base excess method: mEq NH_4Cl = 0.3 L/kg x wt in kg x base excess (mEq/L), give $1/2$ to $2/3$ of calculated dose, then re-evaluate

Children: I.V.: 75 mg/kg/day in 4 divided doses for urinary acidification; maximum daily dose: 6 g

Adults: I.V.: 1.5 g/dose every 6 hours

Administration

Parenteral: Dilute to 0.2 mEq/mL and infuse I.V. over 3 hours; maximum concentration: 0.4 mEq/mL; maximum rate of infusion: 1 mEq/kg/hour

Monitoring Parameters Serum electrolytes, serum ammonia

Nursing Implications Rapid I.V. injection may increase the likelihood of ammonia toxicity

Dosage Forms Excipient information presented when available (limited, particularly for generics); consult specific product labeling.

Injection, solution: Ammonium 5 mEq/mL and chloride 5 mEq/mL (20 mL) [equivalent to ammonium chloride 267.5 mg/mL]

◆ **Ammonium Hydroxide and Lactic Acid** *see* Lactic Acid and Ammonium Hydroxide *on page 789*

◆ **Ammonium Lactate** *see* Lactic Acid and Ammonium Hydroxide *on page 789*

◆ **Ammonium Molybdate** *see* Trace Metals *on page 1366*

◆ **Ammonul®** *see* Sodium Phenylacetate and Sodium Benzoate *on page 1274*

◆ **Amnesteem®** *see* Isotretinoin *on page 769*

Amobarbital (am oh BAR bi tal)

U.S. Brand Names Amytal®

Canadian Brand Names Amytal®

Therapeutic Category Anticonvulsant, Barbiturate; Barbiturate; General Anesthetic; Hypnotic; Sedative

Generic Available No

Use Hypnotic in short-term treatment of insomnia; to reduce anxiety and provide sedation preoperatively. Has been used as an alternative agent for treatment of refractory tonic-clonic seizures. See Additional Information for special uses.

Restrictions C-II

Pregnancy Risk Factor D

Pregnancy Considerations Barbiturates cross the placenta and distribute in fetal tissue. Teratogenic effects have been reported with 1st trimester exposure. Exposure during the 3rd trimester may lead to symptoms of acute withdrawal following delivery; symptoms may be delayed up to 14 days.

Lactation Excretion in breast milk unknown/use caution

Breast-Feeding Considerations Small amounts of barbiturates are excreted in breast milk; information specific for amobarbital is not available.

Contraindications Hypersensitivity to barbiturates or any component; marked hepatic impairment; dyspnea or airway obstruction; porphyria

Warnings Tolerance and/or psychological and physical dependence may occur; abrupt discontinuation after prolonged use may result in withdrawal symptoms or seizures; withdraw gradually if used over extended periods of time; use with caution in patients with depression or suicidal tendencies, or in patients with a history of drug abuse. When used as a hypnotic for the treatment of insomnia, effectiveness is limited to ≤2 weeks. Rapid I.V. administration may cause respiratory depression, apnea, laryngospasm, or hypotension. Solution for injection is highly alkaline and extravasation may cause local tissue damage. May cause CNS depression, which may impair physical or mental abilities; patients must be cautioned about performing tasks which require mental alertness (eg, operating machinery or driving). Effects with other sedative drugs or ethanol may be potentiated.

Precautions Use with caution in patients with acute or chronic pain (paradoxical excitement may occur or important symptoms may be masked), hepatic dysfunction (decreased dosage may be needed; avoid use in patients with premonitory signs of hepatic coma), hypoadrenalism (effects of exogenous or endogenous corticosteroids may be decreased), pregnancy (fetal abnormalities may occur; infants may experience withdrawal symptoms with chronic maternal use), CHF, renal impairment (decreased dosage may be needed), hypovolemic shock, or in children (barbiturates may produce paradoxical excitement). Safety and efficacy have not been established in children <6 years of age.

Adverse Reactions

Cardiovascular: Bradycardia, hypotension, syncope

Central nervous system: Somnolence, agitation, anxiety, ataxia, confusion, CNS depression, dizziness, fever, hallucinations, headache, insomnia, nightmares, nervousness, psychiatric disturbances, abnormal thoughts

Dermatologic: Skin rash, exfoliative dermatitis

Gastrointestinal: Constipation, nausea, vomiting

Hematologic: Megaloblastic anemia (reported following chronic phenobarbital use)

Hepatic: Liver damage

Local: Injection site reaction; local tissue damage and possible necrosis with extravasation; transient pain, possible gangrene with inadvertent intra-arterial injection

Neuromuscular & skeletal: Hyperkinesia

Respiratory: Hypoventilation, apnea, atelectasis (postoperative)

Miscellaneous: Hypersensitivity reactions (eg, angioedema); physical and psychological dependency with chronic use

Drug Interactions

Metabolism/Transport Effects Induces CYP2A6 (strong)

Avoid Concomitant Use

Avoid concomitant use of Amobarbital with any of the following: Voriconazole

Increased Effect/Toxicity

Amobarbital may increase the levels/effects of: Alcohol (Ethyl); CNS Depressants; Meperidine; Thiazide Diuretics

The levels/effects of Amobarbital may be increased by: Chloramphenicol; Divalproex; Felbamate; Primidone; Valproic Acid

Decreased Effect

Amobarbital may decrease the levels/effects of: Acetaminophen; Beta-Blockers; Calcium Channel Blockers; Chloramphenicol; Contraceptives (Estrogens); Contraceptives (Progestins); Corticosteroids (Systemic); CycloSPORINE; CycloSPORINE (Systemic); CYP2A6 Substrates; Disopyramide; Divalproex; Doxycycline; Etoposide; Etoposide Phosphate; Griseofulvin; LamoTRIgine; Methadone; Propafenone; QuiNIDine; Teniposide; Theophylline Derivatives; Tricyclic Antidepressants; Valproic Acid; Vitamin K Antagonists; Voriconazole

The levels/effects of Amobarbital may be decreased by: Pyridoxine; Rifamycin Derivatives

Food Interactions High doses of pyridoxine may decrease drug effect; barbiturates may increase the metabolism of vitamins D and K; dietary requirements of vitamins D, K, C, B_{12}, folate, and calcium may be increased with long-term use

Stability Powder should be stored at 15°C to 30°C (59°F to 86°F). Reconstitute with SWI to make a 10% I.V. solution; a 20% solution can be made for I.M. use. Rotate vial to dissolve, do not shake. Do not use unless a clear solution forms within 5 minutes. Following reconstitution, solution should be used within 30 minutes.

Mechanism of Action Intermediate-acting barbiturate with sedative, hypnotic, and anticonvulsant properties; interferes with transmission of impulses from the thalamus to the cortex of the brain resulting in an imbalance in central inhibitory and facilitatory mechanisms

Pharmacodynamics

Onset of action: Rapid, within minutes

Maximum effect: Hours

Duration: Variable

Pharmacokinetics (Adult data unless noted)

Distribution: Readily crosses placenta; small amounts enter breast milk

Metabolism: Primarily hepatic via microsomal enzymes

Half-life: Adults: 15-40 hours (mean: 25 hours)

Elimination: Metabolites are eliminated in the urine and feces; negligible amounts excreted unchanged in urine

Usual Dosage Note: Dosage should be individualized with consideration of patient's age, weight, and medical condition.

Children:

Sedative: I.M., I.V.: 6-12 years: Manufacturer's dosing range: 65-500 mg

Hypnotic: I.M.: 2-3 mg/kg/dose given before bedtime (maximum: 500 mg)

Adults:

Hypnotic: I.M., I.V.: 65-200 mg at bedtime (mean range: I.M.: 65-500 mg; maximum single dose: 1000 mg)

Sedative: I.M., I.V.: 30-50 mg 2-3 times/day

Dosing adjustment in renal/hepatic impairment: Dosing should be reduced; specific recommendations not available; drug is contraindicated in patients with marked hepatic impairment; avoid use in patients with premonitory signs of hepatic coma

Administration

I.M.: Administer deeply into a large muscle. Do not use more than 5 mL at any single site (may cause tissue damage)

I.V.: Use only when I.M. administration is not feasible. Administer by slow I.V. injection (maximum: 50 mg/minute in adults)

Monitoring Parameters Vital signs should be monitored during injection and for several hours after administration. If using I.V., monitor patency of I.V. access; extravasation may cause local tissue damage (see Adverse Reactions). Monitor hematologic, renal, and hepatic function with prolonged therapy.

Reference Range

Therapeutic: 1-5 mcg/mL (SI: 4-22 µmol/L)

Toxic: >10 mcg/mL (SI: >44 µmol/L)

Lethal: >50 mcg/mL

Patient Information Patient instructions and information are determined by patient condition and therapeutic purpose. Drug may be habit-forming; avoid abrupt discontinuation after prolonged use. While using this medication, avoid alcohol, limit caffeine; do not use other prescription or nonprescription medications (especially pain medications, sedatives, antihistamines, or hypnotics) without consulting prescriber. Medication may cause drowsiness, dizziness, or blurred vision and impair ability to perform activities requiring mental alertness or physical coordination (use caution when driving or engaging in tasks requiring alertness until response to drug is known). May cause nausea, vomiting, or loss of appetite (small, frequent meals, frequent mouth care, chewing gum, or sucking lozenges may help); constipation. Report skin rash or irritation; CNS changes (eg, confusion, depression, increased sedation, excitation, headache, insomnia, or nightmares); respiratory difficulty or shortness of breath; changes in urinary pattern or menstrual pattern; muscle weakness or tremors; or difficulty swallowing or feeling of tightness in throat.

Nursing Implications Parenteral solutions are very alkaline; avoid extravasation (local tissue damage and necrosis may occur); avoid inadvertent intra-arterial injection (various reactions ranging from transient pain to gangrene of the limb may occur); stop injection if patient complains of pain in limb

Additional Information Amobarbital has also been used for therapeutic or diagnostic "amobarbital interviewing" (Kavirajan, 1999) and the "Wada test" (ie, intracarotid amobarbital procedure) to lateralize speech and memory functions prior to brain surgery, in order to prevent or predict the degree of impact of the surgery (Breier, 2001; Grote, 2005; Hamer, 2000; Szabo, 1993).

Dosage Forms Excipient information presented when available (limited, particularly for generics); consult specific product labeling.

Injection, powder for reconstitution, as sodium:
Amytal®: 500 mg

References
Bengner T, Haettig H, Merschhemke M, et al, "Memory Assessment During the Intracarotid Amobarbital Procedure: Influence of Injection Order," Neurology, 2003, 61(11):1582-7.

Breier JI, Simos PG, Wheless JW, et al, "Language Dominance in Children as Determined by Magnetic Source Imaging and the Intracarotid Amobarbital Procedure: A Comparison," J Child Neurol, 2001, 16(2):124-30.

Grote CL and Meador K, "Has Amobarbital Expired? Considering the Future of the Wada," Neurology, 2005, 65(11):1692-3.

Hamer HM, Wyllie E, Stanford L, et al, "Risk Factors for Unsuccessful Testing During the Intracarotid Amobarbital Procedure in Preadolescent Children," Epilepsia, 2000, 41(5):554-63.

Kavirajan H, "The Amobarbital Interview Revisited: A Review of the Literature Since 1966," Harv Rev Psychiatry, 1999, 7(3):153-65.

Kim HS, Wan X, Mathers DA, et al, "Selective GABA-Receptor Actions of Amobarbital on Thalamic Neurons," Br J Pharmacol, 2004, 143 (4):485-94.

Redmond GP, Bell JJ, and Perel JM, "Effect of Human Growth Hormone on Amobarbital Metabolism in Children," Clin Pharmacol Ther, 1978, 24(2):213-8.

Szabó CA and Wyllie E, "Intracarotid Amobarbital Testing for Language and Memory Dominance in Children," Epilepsy Res, 1993, 15 (3):239-46.

◆ **Amobarbital Sodium** see Amobarbital on page 94

◆ **Amoclan** see Amoxicillin and Clavulanic Acid on page 98

Amoxicillin (a moks i SIL in)

Medication Safety Issues

Sound-alike/look-alike issues:
Amoxicillin may be confused with amoxapine, Augmentin®
Amoxil® may be confused with amoxapine

International issues:
Fisamox [Australia] may be confused with Fosamax® which is a brand name for alendronate in the U.S.
Fisamox [Australia] may be confused with Vigamox® which is a brand name for moxifloxacin in the U.S.
Zimox: Brand name for amoxicillin [Italy], but also the brand name for carbidopa/levodopa [Greece]
Zimox [Italy] may be confused with Diamox® which is the brand name for acetazolamide [Canada and multiple international markets]

Related Information
Endocarditis Prophylaxis on page 1610

U.S. Brand Names Amoxil® [DSC]; Moxatag™

Canadian Brand Names Apo-Amoxi®; Gen-Amoxicillin; Lin-Amox; Mylan-Amoxicillin; Novamoxin®; Nu-Amoxi; PHL-Amoxicillin; PMS-Amoxicillin

Therapeutic Category Antibiotic, Penicillin

Generic Available Yes: Excludes drops and extended-release formulation

Use Treatment of otitis media, sinusitis, and infections involving the upper and lower respiratory tract, skin, and urinary tract due to susceptible (beta-lactamase negative) H. influenzae, N. gonorrhoeae, E. coli, P. mirabilis, E. faecalis, streptococci, and nonpenicillinase-producing staphylococci (FDA approved in children and adults); treatment of Lyme disease in children <8 years of age; prophylaxis of bacterial endocarditis; prophylaxis of postexposure inhalational anthrax; H. pylori eradication to reduce the risk of duodenal ulcer recurrence (FDA approved in adults)

Pregnancy Risk Factor B

Pregnancy Considerations Adverse events have not been observed in animal studies; therefore, amoxicillin is classified as pregnancy category B. There is no documented increased risk of adverse pregnancy outcome or teratogenic effects caused by amoxicillin. It is the drug of choice for the treatment of chlamydial infections in pregnancy and for anthrax prophylaxis when penicillin susceptibility is documented.

Due to pregnancy-induced physiologic changes, amoxicillin clearance is increased during pregnancy resulting in lower concentrations and smaller AUCs. Oral ampicillin-class antibiotics are poorly-absorbed during labor.

Lactation Enters breast milk/compatible

Breast-Feeding Considerations Very small amounts of amoxicillin are excreted in breast milk. The manufacturer recommends that caution be exercised when administering amoxicillin to nursing women. The AAP considers amoxicillin to be "usually compatible with breast-feeding." Nondose-related effects could include modification of bowel flora and allergic sensitization of the infant.

Contraindications Hypersensitivity to amoxicillin, penicillin, other beta-lactams, or any component

Warnings Epstein-Barr virus infection, acute lymphocytic leukemia or cytomegalovirus infection increases risk for amoxicillin-induced maculopapular rash; some oral suspensions may contain sodium benzoate; benzoic acid (benzoate) is a metabolite of benzyl alcohol; large amounts of benzyl alcohol (≥99 mg/kg/day) have been associated with a potentially fatal toxicity ("gasping syndrome") in neonates; the "gasping syndrome" consists of metabolic acidosis, respiratory distress, gasping respirations, CNS dysfunction (including convulsions, intracranial hemorrhage), hypotension and cardiovascular collapse; avoid use of amoxicillin products containing sodium benzoate in neonates; in vitro and animal studies have shown that benzoate displaces bilirubin from protein binding sites

Precautions In patients with renal dysfunction, doses and/or frequency of administration should be modified in response to the degree of renal impairment; avoid use of extended release 775 mg tablet and immediate release 875 mg tablet in patients with Cl_{cr} <30 mL/minute or patients requiring hemodialysis; use with caution in patients with history of cephalosporin allergy; chewable tablets contain aspartame which is metabolized to phenylalanine and must be used with caution in patients with phenylketonuria

Adverse Reactions

Central nervous system: Agitation, fever, hyperactivity, seizures

Dermatologic: Acute generalized exanthematous pustulosis, erythema multiforme, exfoliative dermatitis, rash, Stevens-Johnson syndrome, urticaria

Gastrointestinal: Diarrhea, nausea, pseudomembranous colitis, vomiting

Hematologic: Anemia, bleeding time prolonged, eosinophilia, hemolytic anemia, leukopenia, neutropenia, thrombocytopenia

Hepatic: Acute cytolytic hepatitis, AST and ALT increased, cholestatic jaundice

Miscellaneous: Anaphylaxis (rare), hypersensitivity reactions, serum sickness, superinfection, tooth discoloration (brown, yellow, or gray), vasculitis

Drug Interactions

Avoid Concomitant Use

Avoid concomitant use of Amoxicillin with any of the following: BCG

Increased Effect/Toxicity

Amoxicillin may increase the levels/effects of: Methotrexate

The levels/effects of Amoxicillin may be increased by: Allopurinol; Probenecid

Decreased Effect

Amoxicillin may decrease the levels/effects of: BCG; Mycophenolate; Typhoid Vaccine

The levels/effects of Amoxicillin may be decreased by: Fusidic Acid; Tetracycline Derivatives

Food Interactions Food does not interfere with absorption

Stability Suspensions are stable for 14 days at room temperature or if refrigerated; refrigeration is preferred

Mechanism of Action Interferes with bacterial cell wall synthesis during active multiplication by binding to one or more of the penicillin-binding proteins, causing cell wall death and resultant bactericidal activity against susceptible bacteria

Pharmacokinetics (Adult data unless noted)

Absorption: Oral: Rapid and nearly complete (74% to 92% of a single dose is absorbed)

Extended-release tablet: Rate of absorption is slower compared to immediate-release formulation

Distribution: Into liver, lungs, prostate, muscle, middle ear effusions, maxillary sinus secretions, bone, gallbladder, bile, and into ascitic and synovial fluids; excreted into breast milk

Protein binding: 17% to 20%, lower in neonates

Metabolism: Partial

Half-life:

Neonates, full-term: 3.7 hours

Infants and children: 1-2 hours

Adults with normal renal function: 0.7-1.4 hours

Patients with Cl_{cr} <10 mL/minute: 7-21 hours

Time to peak serum concentration:

Capsule: Within 2 hours

Extended release: 3.1 hours

Suspension: Neonates: 3-4.5 hours; children: 1 hour

Elimination: Renal excretion (80% unchanged drug)

Dialysis: Moderately dialyzable (20% to 50%); ~30% removed by 3-hour hemodialysis; supplemental dose is recommended after hemodialysis

Usual Dosage Oral:

Neonates and Infants: ≤3 months: 20-30 mg/kg/day in divided doses every 12 hours

Infants >3 months and Children: 25-50 mg/kg/day in divided doses every 8 hours or 25-50 mg/kg/day in divided doses every 12 hours

Acute otitis media: 80-90 mg/kg/day divided every 12 hours

Community acquired pneumonia: Children 4 months to 4 years: 80-100 mg/kg/day in divided doses every 6-8 hours. **Note:** In children 5-15 years of age, a macrolide antibiotic is a more reasonable first choice since *M. pneumoniae* is the chief cause of pneumonia in this age group.

Primary prevention of rheumatic fever (treatment of streptococcal tonsillopharyngitis):

Children 3-18 years: 50 mg/kg once daily (maximum dose: 1000 mg) for 10 days

Children ≥12 years: Extended release tablets: 775 mg once daily for 10 days

Uncomplicated gonorrhea:

<2 years, probenecid is contraindicated in this age group

≥2 years: 50 mg/kg plus probenecid 25 mg/kg as a single dose

Endocarditis prophylaxis: 50 mg/kg 1 hour before procedure, not to exceed adult dose

Postexposure inhalational anthrax prophylaxis:

<40 kg: 45 mg/kg/day in divided doses every 8 hours

≥40 kg: 500 mg every 8 hours

Adults: 250-500 mg every 8 hours or 500-875 mg tablets twice daily; maximum dose: 2-3 g/day

Uncomplicated gonorrhea: 3 g plus probenecid 1 g as a single dose

Endocarditis prophylaxis: 2 g 1 hour before procedure

H. pylori eradication: 1 g twice daily for 14 days in combination with a proton pump inhibitor and at least one other antibiotic (clarithromycin)

Tonsillitis and/or pharyngitis: Extended release tablets: 775 mg once daily for 10 days

Dosing interval in renal impairment: Note: The immediate-release 875 mg tablet and the extended-release 775 mg tablet should not be used in patients with a Cl_{cr} <30 mL/minute

Cl_{cr} 10-30 mL/minute: Administer every 12 hours

Cl_{cr} <10 mL/minute: Administer every 24 hours

Administration Oral:

Immediate release: May be administered on an empty or full stomach; may be mixed with formula, milk, cold drink, or juice; administer dose immediately after mixing; shake suspension well before use

Extended release: Take within 1 hour of finishing a meal

Monitoring Parameters With prolonged therapy, monitor renal, hepatic, and hematologic function periodically; monitor for diarrhea

Patient Information May cause tooth discoloration (most reports occurred in pediatric patients); tooth brushing or dental cleaning will reduce or eliminate discoloration.

Additional Information Appearance of a rash should be carefully evaluated to differentiate a nonallergic amoxicillin rash from a hypersensitivity reaction. Amoxicillin rash occurs in 5% to 10% of children receiving amoxicillin and is a generalized dull, red, maculopapular rash, generally appearing 3-14 days after the start of therapy. It normally begins on the trunk and spreads over most of the body. It may be most intense at pressure areas, elbows, and knees. Incidence of amoxicillin rash is higher in patients with viral infections, cytomegalovirus infections, infectious mononucleosis, lymphocytic leukemia, or patients with hyperuricemia who are receiving allopurinol.

Dosage Forms Excipient information presented when available (limited, particularly for generics); consult specific product labeling. [DSC] = Discontinued product

Capsule: 250 mg, 500 mg

Amoxil®: 500 mg [DSC]

Powder for suspension, oral: 125 mg/5 mL (80 mL, 100 mL, 150 mL); 200 mg/5 mL (50 mL, 75 mL, 100 mL); 250 mg/5 mL (80 mL, 100 mL, 150 mL); 400 mg/5 mL (50 mL, 75 mL, 100 mL)

Amoxil®: 250 mg/5 mL (100 mL, 150 mL) [contains sodium benzoate; bubble gum flavor] [DSC]; 400 mg/5 mL (100 mL) [contains sodium benzoate; bubble gum flavor] [DSC]

Powder for suspension, oral [drops]:

Amoxil®: 50 mg/mL (30 mL) [contains sodium benzoate; bubble gum flavor] [DSC]

Tablet: 500 mg, 875 mg

Tablet, chewable: 125 mg, 200 mg, 250 mg, 400 mg

Tablet, extended release:

Moxatag™: 775 mg

References

American Academy of Pediatrics Subcommittee on Management of Acute Otitis Media, "Diagnosis and Management of Acute Otitis Media," *Pediatrics*, 2004, 113(5):1451-65.

Boguniewicz M and Leung DY, "Hypersensitivity Reactions to Antibiotics Commonly Used in Children," *Pediatr Infect Dis J*, 1995, 14 (3):221-31.

Canafax DM, Yuan Z, Chonmaitree T, et al, "Amoxicillin Middle Ear Fluid Penetration and Pharmacokinetics in Children with Acute Otitis Media," *Pediatr Infect Dis J*, 1998, 17(2):149-56.

CDC and Johns Hopkins Working Group on Civilian Biodefense, "Commentary on Non-Labeled Dosing of Oral Amoxicillin in Adults and Pediatrics for Post-Exposure Inhalational Anthrax," December 10, 2001, http://www.fda.gov/cder/drugprepare/amox-anthrax.htm.

Dajani AS, Taubert KA, Wilson WW, et al, "Prevention of Bacterial Endocarditis. Recommendations by the American Heart Association," *JAMA*, 1997, 277(22):1794-1801.

Gerber MA, Baltimore RS, Eaton CB, et al, "Prevention of Rheumatic Fever and Diagnosis and Treatment of Acute *Streptococcal pharyngitis*: A Scientific Statement from the American Heart Association Rheumatic Fever, Endocarditis, and Kawasaki Disease Committee of the Council on Cardiovascular Disease in the Young, the Interdisciplinary Council on Functional Genomics and Translational Biology, and the Interdisciplinary Council on Quality of Care and Outcomes Research: Endorsed by the American Academy of Pediatrics," *Circulation*, 2009, 119(11):1541-51.

McIntosh K, "Community-Acquired Pneumonia in Children," *N Engl J Med*, 2002, 346(6):429-37.

Amoxicillin and Clavulanic Acid

(a moks i SIL in & klav yoo LAN ic AS id)

Medication Safety Issues

Sound-alike/look-alike issues:

Augmentin® may be confused with amoxicillin, Azulfidine®

U.S. Brand Names Amoclan; Augmentin ES-600®; Augmentin XR®; Augmentin®

Canadian Brand Names Amoxi-Clav; Apo-Amoxi-Clav®; Augmentin®; Clavulin®; Novo-Clavamoxin; ratio-Aclavulanate

Therapeutic Category Antibiotic, Beta-lactam and Beta-lactamase Combination; Antibiotic, Penicillin

Generic Available Yes

Use Infections caused by susceptible organisms involving the lower respiratory tract, otitis media, sinusitis, skin and skin structure, and urinary tract; spectrum same as amoxicillin in addition to beta-lactamase producing *M. catarrhalis, H. influenzae, N. gonorrhoeae,* and *S. aureus* (not MRSA)

Pregnancy Risk Factor B

Pregnancy Considerations Adverse events have not been observed in animal studies; therefore, amoxicillin/clavulanate is classified as pregnancy category B. Both amoxicillin and clavulanic acid cross the placenta. There is no documented increased risk of teratogenic effects caused by amoxicillin/clavulanate. A potential increased risk of necrotizing enterocolitis in the newborn has been noted after maternal use of amoxicillin/clavulanate for preterm labor or premature prolonged rupture of membranes. When used during pregnancy, pharmacokinetic changes have been observed with amoxicillin alone (refer to the Amoxicillin monograph for details).

Lactation Enters breast milk/use caution

Breast-Feeding Considerations Amoxicillin is found in breast milk. The manufacturer recommends that caution be administered to breast-feeding women. The use of amoxicillin/clavulanate may be safe while breast-feeding; however, the risk of adverse events in the infant may be increased when compared to the use of amoxicillin alone. The risk of adverse events may be related to maternal dose. Nondose-related effects could include modification of bowel flora and allergic sensitization of the infant.

Contraindications Hypersensitivity to amoxicillin, clavulanic acid, penicillins, or any component; history of amoxicillin/clavulanic acid-associated cholestatic jaundice or hepatic dysfunction

Warnings Epstein-Barr virus infection, acute lymphocytic leukemia or cytomegalovirus infection increase the risk for amoxicillin-induced maculopapular rash. Pseudomembranous colitis has been reported; prolonged use may result in superinfection

Precautions Use with caution in patients with history of cephalosporin hypersensitivity; in patients with renal dysfunction, doses and/or frequency of administration should be modified in response to the degree of renal impairment. The "BID" formulation may contain aspartame which is metabolized to phenylalanine and must be avoided or used with caution in patients with phenylketonuria.

Adverse Reactions

Central nervous system: Headache, agitation

Dermatologic: Rash, urticaria, exfoliative dermatitis, Stevens-Johnson syndrome

Gastrointestinal: Nausea, vomiting, abdominal pain, pseudomembranous colitis; incidence of diarrhea (9%) is higher than with amoxicillin alone

Genitourinary: Vaginal candidiasis

Hepatic: AST, ALT, alkaline phosphatase, and bilirubin elevated

Miscellaneous: Superinfection, hypersensitivity reactions, serum sickness, vasculitis, anaphylaxis

Drug Interactions

Avoid Concomitant Use

Avoid concomitant use of Amoxicillin and Clavulanate Potassium with any of the following: BCG

Increased Effect/Toxicity

Amoxicillin and Clavulanate Potassium may increase the levels/effects of: Methotrexate

The levels/effects of Amoxicillin and Clavulanate Potassium may be increased by: Allopurinol; Probenecid

Decreased Effect

Amoxicillin and Clavulanate Potassium may decrease the levels/effects of: BCG; Mycophenolate; Typhoid Vaccine

The levels/effects of Amoxicillin and Clavulanate Potassium may be decreased by: Fusidic Acid; Tetracycline Derivatives

Stability Reconstituted oral suspension should be refrigerated; discard unused suspension after 10 days; store tablets, chewable tablets, and powder for oral suspension at room temperature

Mechanism of Action Clavulanic acid binds and inhibits beta-lactamases that inactivate amoxicillin resulting in amoxicillin having an expanded spectrum of activity; amoxicillin interferes with bacterial cell wall synthesis by binding to one or more of the penicillin-binding proteins and causing cell wall death

Pharmacokinetics (Adult data unless noted)

Absorption: Both amoxicillin and clavulanate are well absorbed

Distribution: Both widely distributed into lungs, pleural, peritoneal, synovial, and ascitic fluid as well as bone, gynecologic tissue, and middle ear fluid; crosses the placenta; excreted in breast milk

Protein binding:

Amoxicillin: 17% to 20%

Clavulanate: 25%

Metabolism: Clavulanic acid: Metabolized in the liver

Half-life of both agents in adults with normal renal function: ~1 hour; amoxicillin pharmacokinetics are not affected by clavulanic acid

Time to peak serum concentration: Within 2 hours

Elimination: Amoxicillin: 60% to 80%; excreted unchanged in the urine

Dialysis: ~30% of amoxicillin removed by 3-hour hemodialysis; supplemental dose recommended after hemodialysis (do **not** use extended release tablets)

Usual Dosage Oral (dosing based on amoxicillin component):

Neonates and Infants <3 months: 30 mg/kg/day divided every 12 hours using the 125 mg/5 mL suspension

Children <40 kg: Less severe infection: 20-40 mg (amoxicillin component)/kg/day in divided doses every 8 hours **or** 25-45 mg (amoxicillin component)/kg/day divided every 12 hours using either 200 mg/5 mL or 400 mg/5 mL suspension, or 200 mg, 400 mg chewable tablet formulation

Community acquired pneumonia: Beta-lactamase positive or nontypable *H. influenza* strains: 80-100 mg/kg/day (amoxicillin component) in divided doses every 8 hours

Acute otitis media or sinusitis: Recurrent or treatment failure after initial antibiotic therapy, severe illness, coverage for B-lactamase positive organisms (*H. influenza*, *M. catarrhalis*) desired: 2 months-12 years: 80-90 mg/kg/day divided every 12 hours (use a 14:1 ratio amoxicillin/clavulanate formulation)

Note: Children <40 kg should not receive the 250 mg film-coated tablets which contain a higher dose of clavulanic acid than the 250 mg chewable tablets.

Children ≥16 years and Adults:

Acute bacterial sinusitis: Extended release tablet: 2000 mg every 12 hours for 10 days

Community-acquired pneumonia: Extended release tablet: 2000 mg every 12 hours for 7-10 days

Adults:

Less severe infection: 250 mg every 8 hours or 500 mg every 12 hours

More severe infections and respiratory tract infections: 500 mg every 8 hours or 875 mg every 12 hours

Dosing interval in renal impairment:

Cl_{cr} <30 mL/minute: Do not use 875 mg tablet or extended release tablet

Cl_{cr} 10-30 mL/minute: Administer 250-500 mg every 12 hours

Cl_{cr} <10 mL/minute: Administer 250-500 mg every 24 hours

Administration Oral: Administer at the start of a meal to decrease the frequency or severity of GI side effects; do not administer with a high fat meal (clavulanate absorption is decreased); may mix with milk, formula, or juice; shake suspension well before use

Monitoring Parameters With prolonged therapy, monitor renal, hepatic, and hematologic function periodically

Test Interactions May interfere with urinary glucose determinations using Clinitest®

Patient Information Adverse GI effects may occur less frequently if taken with food. Report persistent diarrhea to physician.

Additional Information Since both the 250 mg and 500 mg tablets contain the same amount of clavulanic acid, two 250 mg tablets are not equivalent to one 500 mg tablet. Four 250 mg tablets or two 500 mg tablets are **not** equivalent to a single 1000 mg extended release tablet.

Appearance of a rash should be carefully evaluated to differentiate a nonallergic amoxicillin rash from a hypersensitivity reaction. Amoxicillin rash occurs in 5% to 10% of children receiving amoxicillin and is a generalized dull, red, maculopapular rash, generally appearing 3-14 days after the start of therapy. It normally begins on the trunk and spreads over most of the body. It may be most intense at pressure areas, elbows, and knees. Incidence of amoxicillin rash is higher in patients with viral infections, *Salmonella* infections, lymphocytic leukemia, or patients with hyperuricemia who are receiving allopurinol.

Dosage Forms Excipient information presented when available (limited, particularly for generics); consult specific product labeling. [DSC] = Discontinued product

Powder for oral suspension: 200: Amoxicillin 200 mg and clavulanate potassium 28.5 mg per 5 mL (50 mL, 75 mL, 100 mL) [contains phenylalanine]; 400: Amoxicillin 400 mg and clavulanate potassium 57 mg per 5 mL (50 mL, 75 mL, 100 mL) [contains phenylalanine]; 600: Amoxicillin 600 mg and clavulanate potassium 42.9 mg per 5 mL (75 mL, 125 mL, 200 mL)

Amoclan:

200: Amoxicillin 200 mg and clavulanate potassium 28.5 mg per 5 mL (50 mL, 75 mL, 100 mL) [contains phenylalanine 7 mg/5 mL and potassium 0.14 mEq/ 5 mL; fruit flavor]

400: Amoxicillin 400 mg and clavulanate potassium 57 mg per 5 mL (50 mL, 75 mL, 100 mL) [contains phenylalanine 7 mg/5 mL and potassium 0.29 mEq/ 5 mL; fruit flavor]

600: Amoxicillin 600 mg and clavulanate potassium 42.9 mg per 5 mL (75 mL, 125 mL) [contains phenylalanine 7 mg/5 mL, potassium 0.248 mEq/ 5 mL; orange flavor]

Augmentin®:

125: Amoxicillin 125 mg and clavulanate potassium 31.25 mg per 5 mL (75 mL, 100 mL, 150 mL) [contains potassium 0.16 mEq/5 mL; banana flavor]

200: Amoxicillin 200 mg and clavulanate potassium 28.5 mg per 5 mL (50 mL, 75 mL, 100 mL) [contains phenylalanine 7 mg/5 mL and potassium 0.14 mEq/ 5 mL; orange flavor] [DSC]

250: Amoxicillin 250 mg and clavulanate potassium 62.5 mg per 5 mL (75 mL, 100 mL, 150 mL) [contains potassium 0.32 mEq/5 mL; orange flavor]

400: Amoxicillin 400 mg and clavulanate potassium 57 mg per 5 mL (50 mL, 75 mL, 100 mL) [contains phenylalanine 7 mg/5 mL and potassium 0.29 mEq/ 5 mL; orange flavor] [DSC]

Augmentin ES-600®: Amoxicillin 600 mg and clavulanate potassium 42.9 mg per 5 mL (75 mL, 125 mL, 200 mL) [contains phenylalanine 7 mg/5 mL and potassium 0.23 mEq/5 mL; strawberry cream flavor]

Tablet: 250: Amoxicillin 250 mg and clavulanate potassium 125 mg; 500: Amoxicillin 500 mg and clavulanate potassium 125 mg; 875: Amoxicillin 875 mg and clavulanate potassium 125 mg

Augmentin®:

250: Amoxicillin 250 mg and clavulanate potassium 125 mg [contains potassium 0.63 mEq/tablet]

500: Amoxicillin 500 mg and clavulanate potassium 125 mg [contains potassium 0.63 mEq/tablet]

875: Amoxicillin 875 mg and clavulanate potassium 125 mg [contains potassium 0.63 mEq/tablet]

Tablet, chewable; 200: Amoxicillin 200 mg and clavulanate potassium 28.5 mg [contains phenylalanine]; 400: Amoxicillin 400 mg and clavulanate potassium 57 mg [contains phenylalanine]

Tablet, extended release: Amoxicillin 1000 mg and clavulanate potassium 62.5 mg

Augmentin XR®: 1000: Amoxicillin 1000 mg and clavulanate acid 62.5 mg [contains potassium 12.6 mg (0.32 mEq) and sodium 29.3 mg (1.27 mEq) per tablet; packaged in either a 7-day or 10-day package]

References

American Academy of Pediatrics Subcommittee on Management of Acute Otitis Media, "Diagnosis and Management of Acute Otitis Media," *Pediatrics*, 2004, 113(5):1451-65.

Bradley JS, "Management of Community-Acquired Pediatric Pneumonia in an Era of Increasing Antibiotic Resistance and Conjugate Vaccines," *Pediatr Infect Dis J*, 2002, 21(6):592-8.

Gan VN, Kusmiesz H, Shelton S, et al, "Comparative Evaluation of Loracarbef and Amoxicillin-Clavulanate for Acute Otitis Media," *Antimicrob Agents Chemother*, 1991, 35(5):967-71.

Hoberman A, Paradise JL, Burch DJ, et al, "Equivalent Efficiency and Reduced Occurrence of Diarrhea From a New Formulation of Amoxicillin/Clavulanate Potassium (Augmentin®) for Treatment of Acute Otitis Media in Children," *Pediatr Infect Dis J*, 1997, 16 (5):463-70.

Reed MD, "Clinical Pharmacokinetics of Amoxicillin and Clavulanate," *Pediatr Infect Dis J*, 1996, 15(10):949-54.

Thoene DE and Johnson CE, "Pharmacotherapy of Otitis Media," *Pharmacotherapy*, 1991, 11(3):212-21.

Todd PA and Benfield P, "Amoxicillin/Clavulanic Acid. An Update of Its Antibacterial Activity, Pharmacokinetic Properties and Therapeutic Use," *Drugs*, 1990, 39(2):264-307.

◆ **Amoxicillin Trihydrate** *see* Amoxicillin *on page 96*

◆ **Amoxi-Clav (Can)** *see* Amoxicillin and Clavulanic Acid *on page 98*

◆ **Amoxil® [DSC]** *see* Amoxicillin *on page 96*

◆ **Amoxycillin** *see* Amoxicillin *on page 96*

◆ **Amphadase™** *see* Hyaluronidase *on page 679*

◆ **Amphetamine and Dextroamphetamine** *see* Dextroamphetamine and Amphetamine *on page 418*

◆ **Amphojel® (Can)** *see* Aluminum Hydroxide *on page 75*

Amphotericin B (Conventional)
(am foe TER i sin bee con VEN sha nal)

Medication Safety Issues

Safety issues:

Conventional amphotericin formulations (Amphocin®, Fungizone®) may be confused with lipid-based formulations (AmBisome®, Abelcet®, Amphotec®).

Large overdoses have occurred when conventional formulations were dispensed inadvertently for lipid-based products. Single daily doses of conventional amphotericin formulation never exceed 1.5 mg/kg.

High alert medication: The Institute for Safe Medication Practices (ISMP) includes this medication (intrathecal administration) among its list of drugs which have a heightened risk of causing significant patient harm when used in error.

Canadian Brand Names Fungizone®

Therapeutic Category Antifungal Agent, Systemic; Antifungal Agent, Topical

Generic Available Yes

Use Treatment of severe systemic infections and meningitis caused by susceptible fungi such as *Candida* species, *Histoplasma capsulatum*, *Cryptococcus neoformans*, *Aspergillus* species, *Mucor* species, *Blastomyces dermatitidis*, *Torulopsis glabrata*, *Sporothrix schenckii*, *Paracoccidioides brasiliensis*, and *Coccidioides immitis*; fungal peritonitis; irrigant for bladder fungal infections; treatment of amebic meningoencephalitis caused by *Naegleria fowleri*

Pregnancy Risk Factor B

Lactation Excretion in breast milk unknown/ contraindicated

Contraindications Hypersensitivity to amphotericin B or any component

Warnings I.V. amphotericin is used primarily for the treatment of patients with progressive and potentially fatal fungal infections **[U.S. Boxed Warning]**; not to be used for noninvasive forms of fungal disease. Verify the product name and dosage if dose exceeds 1.5 mg/kg **[U.S. Boxed Warning]**; overdosage may result in cardiorespiratory arrest. Anaphylaxis has been reported with amphotericin B-containing drugs; facilities for cardiopulmonary resuscitation should be available during administration due to the possibility of anaphylactic reaction.

Precautions Due to the nephrotoxic potential of amphotericin B, other nephrotoxic drugs should be avoided. Acute pulmonary reactions have been reported in patients simultaneously receiving intravenous amphotericin B and leukocyte transfusions; separate these infusions temporally as much as possible and monitor pulmonary function. Administer by slow I.V. infusion; rapid infusion has been associated with hypotension, hypokalemia, arrhythmias, and shock.

Adverse Reactions

Cardiovascular: Hypotension, hypertension, cardiac arrhythmias, shock, flushing

Central nervous system: Fever, chills, and headache are the most common adverse effects reported with amphotericin B infusion; delirium, seizures, malaise

Dermatologic: Rash, pruritus, urticaria

Endocrine & metabolic: Hypokalemia, hypomagnesemia, weight loss

Gastrointestinal: Anorexia, nausea, vomiting, steatorrhea, diarrhea, abdominal pain

Hematologic: Anemia, leukopenia, thrombocytopenia

Hepatic: Acute hepatic failure, jaundice; AST, ALT, and bilirubin elevated

Local: Phlebitis

Renal: Renal tubular acidosis, renal failure (oliguria, azotemia, serum creatinine elevated)

Respiratory: Wheezing, hypoxemia, bronchospasm, tachypnea

Miscellaneous: Anaphylactoid reaction

Adverse effects due to intrathecal amphotericin B:

Central nervous system: Headache, pain along lumbar nerves, arachnoiditis

Gastrointestinal: Nausea, vomiting

Genitourinary: Urinary retention

Neuromuscular & skeletal: Paresthesia, leg and back pain, foot drop

Ocular: Vision changes

Drug Interactions

Avoid Concomitant Use

Avoid concomitant use of Amphotericin B (Conventional) with any of the following: Gallium Nitrate

Increased Effect/Toxicity

Amphotericin B (Conventional) may increase the levels/ effects of: Aminoglycosides; Colistimethate; CycloSPORINE; CycloSPORINE (Systemic); Flucytosine; Gallium Nitrate

The levels/effects of Amphotericin B (Conventional) may be increased by: Corticosteroids (Orally Inhaled); Corticosteroids (Systemic)

Decreased Effect

Amphotericin B (Conventional) may decrease the levels/ effects of: Saccharomyces boulardii

The levels/effects of Amphotericin B (Conventional) may be decreased by: Antifungal Agents (Azole Derivatives, Systemic)

Stability Store unopened vials in refrigerator at 2°C to 8°C (36°F to 46°F). Protect from light. Reconstitute only with SWI without preservatives, not bacteriostatic water; benzyl alcohol, sodium chloride, or other electrolyte solutions may cause precipitation; can be diluted in D_5W, $D_{10}W$, up to $D_{20}W$; for I.V. infusion, an in-line filter (>1 micron mean pore diameter) may be used; irrigating solutions should be diluted in sterile water; short-term exposure (<24 hours) to light during I.V. infusion does **not** appreciably affect potency

Mechanism of Action Binds to ergosterol altering cell membrane permeability in susceptible fungi and causing leakage of cell components with subsequent cell death

Pharmacokinetics (Adult data unless noted)

Absorption: Poor oral absorption

Distribution: Minimal amounts enter the aqueous humor, bile, amniotic fluid, pericardial fluid, pleural fluid, and synovial fluid; poor CSF penetration

Protein binding: 90%

Half-life: Increased in small neonates and young infants

Initial: 15-48 hours

Terminal phase: 15 days

Elimination: 2% to 4% of dose eliminated in urine unchanged; ~40% eliminated over 7-day period and may be detected in urine for up to 8 weeks after discontinued use

Dialysis: Poorly dialyzed

Usual Dosage Medication errors, including deaths, have resulted from confusion between lipid-based forms of amphotericin (Abelcet®, Amphotec®, AmBisome®) and conventional amphotericin B for injection; conventional amphotericin B for injection doses should not exceed 1.5 mg/kg/day

Neonates, Infants, and Children:

I.V.: Test dose: 0.1 mg/kg/dose to a maximum of 1 mg; infuse over 20-60 minutes; an alternative method to the 0.1 mg/kg test dose is to initiate therapy with 0.25 mg/kg amphotericin administered over 6 hours; frequent observation of the patient and assessment of vital signs during the first several hours of the infusion is recommended

Initial therapeutic dose: If the 0.1 mg/kg test dose is tolerated without the occurrence of serious adverse effects, a therapeutic dose of 0.4 mg/kg can be given the same day as the test dose

The daily dose can then be gradually increased, usually in 0.25 mg/kg increments on each subsequent day until the desired daily dose is reached; in critically ill patients, more rapid dosage acceleration (up to 0.5 mg/kg increments on each subsequent day) may be warranted

Maintenance dose: 0.25-1 mg/kg/day given once daily; infuse over 2-6 hours; rapidly progressing disease may require short-term use of doses to 1.5 mg/kg/day; once therapy has been established, amphotericin B can be administered on an every-other-day basis at 1-1.5 mg/kg/dose

HIV-infected infants and children with invasive candidiasis: May consider addition of oral flucytosine 25-37.5 mg/kg/dose every 6 hours to amphotericin B therapy

Cryptococcal meningitis in HIV-infected infants and children: May consider addition of oral flucytosine 25 mg/kg/dose every 6 hours to amphotericin B therapy

Intrathecal, intraventricular, or intracisternal (preferably into the lateral ventricles through a cisternal Ommaya reservoir): 25-100 mcg every 48-72 hours; increase to 500 mcg as tolerated

Adults:

I.V.: Test dose: 1 mg infused over 20-30 minutes

Initial therapeutic dose (if the test dose is tolerated): 0.25 mg/kg

The daily dose can then be gradually increased, usually in 0.25 mg/kg increments on each subsequent day until the desired daily dose is reached

Maintenance dose: 0.25-1 mg/kg/day once daily, infuse over 2-6 hours; or 1-1.5 mg/kg/dose every other day; do not exceed 1.5 mg/kg/day

HIV-infected adults with invasive candidiasis: May consider addition of oral flucytosine 25-37.5 mg/kg/dose every 6 hours to amphotericin B therapy

Cryptococcosis with CNS involvement in HIV-infected adults: May consider addition of oral flucytosine 25 mg/kg/dose every 6 hours to amphotericin B therapy

Intrathecal, intraventricular, or intracisternal (preferably into the lateral ventricles through a cisternal Ommaya reservoir): 25-100 mcg every 48-72 hours; increase to 500 mcg as tolerated

Children and Adults:

Bladder irrigation: 5-15 mg amphotericin B/100 mL of sterile water irrigation solution at 100-300 mL/day. Fluid is instilled into the bladder; the catheter is clamped for 60-120 minutes and the bladder drained. Perform irrigation 3-4 times/day for 2-5 days.

Dialysate: 1-4 mg/L of peritoneal dialysis fluid either with or without low-dose I.V. amphotericin B therapy

Note: Amphotericin B has been administered intranasally to reduce the frequency of invasive aspergillosis in neutropenic patients; 7 mg amphotericin B in 7 mL sterile water was placed in a De Vilbiss atomizer and the aerosolized solution was instilled intranasally to each nostril 4 times/day delivering an average of 5 mg amphotericin/day

Dosing adjustment in renal impairment: Dosage adjustments are not necessary with pre-existing renal impairment; if decreased renal function is due to amphotericin B, the daily dose can be decreased by 50% or the dose can be given every other day. Therapy may be held until serum creatinine concentrations begin to decline.

Administration Parenteral: Amphotericin B is administered by I.V. infusion over 2-3 hours (range: 1-6 hours); in patients with azotemia or hyperkalemia or in those receiving doses >1 mg/kg, infuse over 3-6 hours; infuse at a final concentration not to exceed 0.1 mg/mL through a peripheral venous catheter; in patients unable to tolerate a large fluid volume, amphotericin B at a final concentration not to exceed 0.5 mg/mL in D_5W or $D_{10}W$ may be administered through a central venous catheter

Monitoring Parameters BUN and serum creatinine levels should be determined every other day while therapy is increased and at least weekly thereafter; serum potassium and magnesium should be monitored closely; monitor electrolytes, liver function, hemoglobin, hematocrit, CBC regularly; monitor I & O; monitor for signs of hypokalemia (muscle weakness, cramping, drowsiness, ECG changes, etc); blood pressure, temperature, pulse, respiration, I.V. site

Nursing Implications Extravasation may cause chemical irritation (monitor infusion site). Hypotension, hypokalemia, arrhythmias, and cardiovascular collapse have been reported after rapid amphotericin B infusion; may premedicate patients who experience mild adverse reactions with acetaminophen and diphenhydramine 30 minutes prior to the amphotericin B infusion. Meperidine and ibuprofen may help to reduce fevers and chills. Hydrocortisone can be added to the infusion solution to reduce febrile and other systemic reactions. Heparin 1 unit per 1 mL of infusion solution can be added to reduce phlebitis. Administration of amphotericin B on alternate days may decrease anorexia and phlebitis.

Additional Information A study by Harbarth, et al, reported that 29% of patients who experienced moderate to severe nephrotoxicity during conventional amphotericin B treatment had 3 or more risk factors which included body weight ≥90 kg, male sex, mean daily amphotericin B dosage ≥35 mg, chronic kidney disease, or concomitant use of amikacin or cyclosporine. Amphotericin B-induced nephrotoxicity may be minimized by sodium loading with 10-15 mL/kg of NS infused prior to each amphotericin B dose or pentoxifylline, and avoiding use of other nephrotoxic agents

Dosage Forms Excipient information presented when available (limited, particularly for generics); consult specific product labeling.

Injection, powder for reconstitution, as desoxycholate: 50 mg

References

Benson JM and Nahata MC, "Pharmacokinetics of Amphotericin B in Children," *Antimicrob Agents Chemother*, 1989, 33(11):1989-93.

Bianco JA, Almgren J, Kern DL, et al, "Evidence That Oral Pentoxifylline Reverses Acute Renal Dysfunction in Bone Marrow Transplant Recipients Receiving Amphotericin B and Cyclosporine," *Transplantation*, 1991, 51(4):925-7.

Branch RA, "Prevention of Amphotericin B-Induced Renal Impairment. A Review on the Use of Sodium Supplementation," *Arch Intern Med*, 1988, 148(11):2389-94.

CDC, NIH, and HIVMA/IDSA, "Guidelines for Prevention and Treatment of Opportunistic Infections Among HIV-Exposed and HIV-Infected Children," 2008; available at http://aidsinfo.nih.gov.

Harbarth S, Pestotnik SL, Lloyd JF, et al, "The Epidemiology of Nephrotoxicity Associated With Conventional Amphotericin B Therapy," *Am J Med*, 2001, 111(7):528-34.

Jeffery GM, Beard ME, Ikram RB, et al, "Intranasal Amphotericin B Reduces the Frequency of Invasive Aspergillosis in Neutropenic Patients," *Am J Med*, 1991, 90(6):685-92.

Kintzel PE and Smith GH, "Practical Guidelines for Preparing and Administering Amphotericin B," *Am J Hosp Pharm*, 1992, 49 (5):1156-64.

Koren G, Lau A, Klein J, et al, "Pharmacokinetics and Adverse Effects of Amphotericin B in Infants and Children," *J Pediatr*, 1988, 113 (3):559-63.

The Ad Hoc Advisory Panel on Peritonitis Management. "Continuous Ambulatory Peritoneal Dialysis (CAPD) Peritonitis Treatment Recommendations: 1989 Update," *Perit Dial Int*, 1989, 9(4):247-56.

◆ **Amphotericin B Desoxycholate** *see* Amphotericin B (Conventional) *on page* 100

Amphotericin B Lipid Complex
(am foe TER i sin bee LIP id KOM pleks)

Medication Safety Issues
Safety issues:
Lipid-based amphotericin formulations (Abelcet®) may be confused with conventional formulations (Amphocin®, Fungizone®)

Large overdoses have occurred when conventional formulations were dispensed inadvertently for lipid-based products. Single daily doses of conventional amphotericin formulation never exceed 1.5 mg/kg.

High alert medication: The Institute for Safe Medication Practices (ISMP) includes this medication among its list of drugs which have a heightened risk of causing significant patient harm when used in error.

U.S. Brand Names Abelcet®

Canadian Brand Names Abelcet®

Therapeutic Category Antifungal Agent, Systemic

Generic Available No

Use Treatment of aspergillosis or invasive fungal infections in patients who are refractory to or intolerant of conventional amphotericin B therapy (refractory to or intolerant is defined as renal dysfunction with a serum creatinine ≥1.5 mg/dL that develops during therapy, or disease progression after a total dose of conventional amphotericin B of at least 10 mg/kg). This indication is primarily based on results of emergency studies for the treatment of aspergillosis; may be useful in the treatment of hepatosplenic candidiasis and cryptococcal meningitis.

Pregnancy Risk Factor B

Lactation Enters breast milk/contraindicated

Breast-Feeding Considerations Due to limited data, consider discontinuing nursing during therapy.

Contraindications Hypersensitivity to amphotericin B, dimyristoylphosphatidylcholine (DMPC) and dimyristoylphosphatidylglycerol (DMPG) which are two phospholipids in the formulation, or any component

Warnings Anaphylaxis has been reported with amphotericin B-containing drugs; facilities for cardiopulmonary resuscitation should be available during administration due to the possibility of anaphylactic reaction

Precautions Due to the nephrotoxic potential of amphotericin B, other nephrotoxic drugs should be avoided. Acute pulmonary reactions have been reported in patients simultaneously receiving intravenous amphotericin B and leukocyte transfusions; separate these infusions temporally as much as possible and monitor pulmonary function.

Adverse Reactions
Cardiovascular: Hypotension, cardiac arrest, arrhythmias, flushing

Central nervous system: Headache; transient chills and fever and during infusion of the drug are the most common effects reported with ABLC

Dermatologic: Rash, pruritus

Endocrine & metabolic: Hypokalemia, bilirubinemia, hypomagnesemia

Gastrointestinal: Diarrhea, abdominal pain

Hematologic: Thrombocytopenia, leukopenia, anemia

Renal: Renal tubular acidosis, serum creatinine elevated (occurs to a lesser degree than with conventional amphotericin B), azotemia, oliguria

Respiratory: Dyspnea, respiratory failure

Miscellaneous: Anaphylactoid and other allergic reactions

Drug Interactions
Avoid Concomitant Use
Avoid concomitant use of Amphotericin B (Lipid Complex) with any of the following: Gallium Nitrate

Increased Effect/Toxicity
Amphotericin B (Lipid Complex) may increase the levels/effects of: Aminoglycosides; Colistimethate; CycloSPORINE; CycloSPORINE (Systemic); Flucytosine; Gallium Nitrate

The levels/effects of Amphotericin B (Lipid Complex) may be increased by: Corticosteroids (Orally Inhaled); Corticosteroids (Systemic)

Decreased Effect
Amphotericin B (Lipid Complex) may decrease the levels/effects of: Saccharomyces boulardii

The levels/effects of Amphotericin B (Lipid Complex) may be decreased by: Antifungal Agents (Azole Derivatives, Systemic)

Stability Prior to admixture, refrigerate vial and protect from light; diluted ABLC infusion solution in D₅W is stable up to 48 hours refrigerated and an additional 6 hours at room temperature. Do not freeze. Do not dilute with saline solutions or mix with other drugs or electrolytes.

Mechanism of Action Binds to ergosterol altering cell membrane permeability in susceptible fungi and causing leakage of cell components with subsequent cell death

Pharmacokinetics (Adult data unless noted) Exhibits nonlinear kinetics; volume of distribution and clearance from blood increases with increasing dose

Distribution: High tissue concentration found in the liver, spleen, and lung

Half-life, terminal: 173 hours

Elimination: 0.9% of dose excreted in urine over 24 hours; effects of hepatic and renal impairment on drug disposition are unknown

Dialysis: ABLC is not hemodialyzable

Usual Dosage Children and Adults: I.V.: 2.5-5 mg/kg given as a once daily infusion

Dosing adjustment in renal failure: Renal toxicity is dose dependent; there are no firm guidelines for dose adjustment based on lab test results (serum creatinine levels).

Administration Parenteral: I.V.: Prior to administration, amphotericin B lipid complex 5 mg/mL concentrated suspension must be diluted in D₅W by gently shaking the vial until solution contains no sediment; the appropriate dose is drawn into one or more sterile 20 mL syringes using an 18 gauge needle. The needle is removed and replaced with a 5 micrometer filter needle which can be used to filter the contents of up to 4 vials of drug. Contents of the syringe are injected via the filter needle into the I.V. container of D₅W diluting amphotericin B lipid complex to a final concentration of 1 mg/mL; a maximum concentration of 2 mg/mL may be used in fluid-restricted patients. Shake the I.V. container of diluted drug to insure that contents are thoroughly mixed then administer at a rate of 2.5 mg/kg/hour (over 2 hours). The manufacturer recommends that an in-line filter should be used NOT be used during administration of amphotericin B lipid complex.

Monitoring Parameters BUN, serum creatinine, liver function tests, serum electrolytes, CBC; vital signs, I & O; monitor for signs of hypokalemia (muscle weakness, cramping, drowsiness, ECG changes, etc)

Nursing Implications If infusion time exceeds 2 hours, mix the contents by gently rotating the infusion bag every 2 hours.

Additional Information Management of side effects is similar to conventional amphotericin B. [See Amphotericin B (Conventional) on page 100 for suggested management guidelines of side effects.]

Dosage Forms Excipient information presented when available (limited, particularly for generics); consult specific product labeling.

Injection, suspension [preservative free]:
    Abelcet®: 5 mg/mL (20 mL)

References

De Marie S, "Clinical Use of Liposomal and Lipid-Complexed Amphotericin B," *J Antimicrob Chemother*, 1994, 33(5):907-16.

Kline S, Larsen TA, Fieber L, et al, "Limited Toxicity of Prolonged Therapy With High Doses of Amphotericin B Lipid Complex," *Clin Infect Dis*, 1995, 21(5):1154-8.

Amphotericin B Liposome

(am foe TER i sin bee LYE po som)

Medication Safety Issues

Safety issues:

Lipid-based amphotericin formulations (AmBisome®) may be confused with conventional formulations (Amphocin®, Fungizone®) or with other lipid-based amphotericin formulations (Abelcet®, Amphotec®)

Large overdoses have occurred when conventional formulations were dispensed inadvertently for lipid-based products. Single daily doses of conventional amphotericin formulation never exceed 1.5 mg/kg.

High alert medication: The Institute for Safe Medication Practices (ISMP) includes this medication among its list of drugs which have a heightened risk of causing significant patient harm when used in error.

U.S. Brand Names AmBisome®

Canadian Brand Names AmBisome®

Therapeutic Category Antifungal Agent, Systemic

Generic Available No

Use Treatment of aspergillosis, candidiasis, or cryptococcosis in patients who are refractory to or intolerant of conventional amphotericin B therapy (refractory to or intolerant is defined as renal dysfunction with a serum creatinine ≥1.5 mg/dL that develops during therapy, or disease progression after a total dose of conventional amphotericin B of at least 10 mg/kg); empiric therapy for presumed fungal infection in febrile, neutropenic bone marrow transplant patients or febrile, neutropenic acute nonlymphocytic leukemia patients after an unsuccessful trial of antibiotics; treatment of cryptococcal meningitis in HIV-infected patients; treatment of visceral leishmaniasis; treatment of suspected or proven fungal infections in patients with renal impairment; has also been used for treatment of systemic *Histoplasmosis* infection, blastomycosis, coccidioidomycosis, and mucormycosis

Pregnancy Risk Factor B

Pregnancy Considerations Animal studies did not demonstrate teratogenicity. There are no adequate and well-controlled studies in pregnant women. Conventional amphotericin B has been used successfully to treat systemic fungal infection in a limited number (case reports) of pregnant women.

Lactation Excretion in breast milk unknown/not recommended

Breast-Feeding Considerations Due to the potential for serious adverse reactions in the nursing infant, breast-feeding is not recommended.

Contraindications Hypersensitivity to amphotericin B desoxycholate or any component

Warnings Anaphylaxis has been reported with amphotericin B-containing drugs; if a severe anaphylactic reaction occurs, discontinue infusion immediately; patient should not receive further infusions of amphotericin B liposome; facilities for cardiopulmonary resuscitation should be available during administration due to the possibility of anaphylactic reaction

Precautions Due to the nephrotoxic potential of amphotericin B, other nephrotoxic drugs should be avoided. Acute infusion reactions (including fever and chills) may occur 1-2 hours after starting infusions; reactions are more common with the first few doses and generally diminish with subsequent doses. Acute pulmonary reactions have been reported in patients simultaneously receiving intravenous amphotericin B and leukocyte transfusions; separate these infusions temporally as much as possible and monitor pulmonary function. Concurrent use with antineoplastic agents may enhance the potential for renal toxicity, bronchospasm, or hypotension.

Adverse Reactions

Cardiovascular: Hypotension, arrhythmias, chest pain, cardiac arrest, vasodilatation, hypertension, tachycardia, edema, peripheral edema, hypervolemia, atrial fibrillation, bradycardia, cardiomegaly, facial swelling, flushing, postural hypotension, valvular heart disease, vascular disorder

Central nervous system: Headache, transient chills or rigors, fever (17%), anxiety, insomnia, dizziness, hallucinations, asthenia, convulsion

Dermatologic: Pruritus, rash, diaphoresis, urticaria

Endocrine & metabolic: Hypokalemia, hypomagnesemia, hyperglycemia, hypocalcemia, hyperphosphatemia, hyponatremia

Gastrointestinal: Diarrhea, nausea, vomiting, abdominal pain, constipation, anorexia, gastrointestinal hemorrhage

Hematologic: Anemia, thrombocytopenia, leukopenia

Hepatic: ALT elevated, AST elevated, alkaline phosphatase elevated, bilirubinemia

Local: Phlebitis, injection site inflammation

Neuromuscular & skeletal: Weakness, back pain, arthralgia, tremor

Renal: Renal tubular acidosis, serum creatinine elevated, BUN elevated (22%; occurs to a lesser degree than with conventional amphotericin B), oliguria, hematuria, nephrotoxicity, renal failure

Respiratory: Dyspnea, respiratory failure, cough, epistaxis, pleural effusion, hypoxia

Miscellaneous: Anaphylactoid and other allergic reactions, infusion reactions

Drug Interactions

Avoid Concomitant Use

Avoid concomitant use of Amphotericin B (Liposomal) with any of the following: Gallium Nitrate

Increased Effect/Toxicity

Amphotericin B (Liposomal) may increase the levels/effects of: Aminoglycosides; Colistimethate; CycloSPORINE; CycloSPORINE (Systemic); Flucytosine; Gallium Nitrate

The levels/effects of Amphotericin B (Liposomal) may be increased by: Corticosteroids (Orally Inhaled); Corticosteroids (Systemic)

Decreased Effect

Amphotericin B (Liposomal) may decrease the levels/effects of: Saccharomyces boulardii

The levels/effects of Amphotericin B (Liposomal) may be decreased by: Antifungal Agents (Azole Derivatives, Systemic)

◄ **Stability** Store unopened vials at temperatures ≤25°C (77°F); reconstituted drug is stable for 24 hours under refrigeration. Do not dilute with saline solutions or mix with other drugs or electrolytes since this may cause precipitation of AmBisome®. AmBisome® is stable when further diluted to a concentration of 0.2-2 mg/mL (0.2-0.5 mg/mL may be used for infants and small children) in D_5W and $D_{10}W$ or 2 mg/mL in $D_{20}W$ and $D_{25}W$ (see table).

AmBisome® Stability

Solution		Temperature	Stability
D_5W	2 mg/mL	2°C to 8°C	14 days
	0.2 mg/mL	2°C to 8°C	11 days
	0.2-2 mg/mL	23°C to 27°C	24 hours
$D_{10}W$	0.2-2 mg/mL	2°C to 8°C	48 hours
$D_{20}W$	2 mg/mL	2°C to 8°C	48 hours
$D_{25}W$	2 mg/mL	2°C to 8°C	48 hours

Mechanism of Action Binds to ergosterol altering cell membrane permeability in susceptible fungi and causing leakage of cell components with subsequent cell death

Pharmacokinetics (Adult data unless noted) Exhibits nonlinear kinetics (greater than proportional increase in serum concentration with an increase in dose)

Distribution: V_d: Adults: 0.1-0.16 L/kg

Half-life (terminal): Adults: 100-153 hours

Usual Dosage Infants ≥1 month, Children, and Adults: I.V.:

Empiric therapy: 3 mg/kg/day given as a once daily infusion

Systemic fungal infections: 3-5 mg/kg/day given as a once daily infusion; doses as high as 10 mg/kg/day have been used in patients with documented *Aspergillus* infection; HIV-infected patients with invasive candidiasis (may consider addition of oral flucytosine 25-37.5 mg/kg/dose every 6 hours)

Cryptococcal meningitis in HIV infected patients: 6 mg/kg/day given as a once daily infusion (may consider addition of oral flucytosine 25 mg/kg/dose every 6 hours).

Visceral leishmaniasis:

Immunocompetent patients:

Days 1-5: 3 mg/kg/day once daily

Days 14 and 21: 3 mg/kg/dose

Note: Repeat course may be given to patients who do not achieve parasitic clearance

Immunocompromised patients:

Days 1-5: 4 mg/kg/day once daily

Days 10, 17, 24, 31, 38: 4 mg/kg/dose

Administration Parenteral: I.V.: Reconstitute with 12 mL SWI to a concentration of 4 mg/mL; shake vigorously for at least 30 seconds, until dispersed into a translucent yellow suspension; a 5-micron filter should be on the syringe used to inject the reconstituted product from the vial into the D_5W diluent. Do not use in-line filter less than 1 micron to administer AmBisome®. Flush line with D_5W prior to infusion; infusion of diluted AmBisome® should start within 6 hours of preparation; infuse over 2 hours; infusion time may be reduced to 1 hour in patients who tolerate the treatment; AmBisome® may be diluted with D_5W, $D_{10}W$, or $D_{20}W$ to a final concentration of 1-2 mg/mL; lower concentrations (0.2-0.5 mg/mL) may be administered to infants and small children to provide sufficient volume for infusion

Monitoring Parameters BUN, serum creatinine, liver function tests, serum electrolytes (particularly magnesium and potassium), CBC, vital signs, I & O; monitor for signs of hypokalemia (muscle weakness, cramping, drowsiness, ECG changes); monitor cardiac function if used concurrently with corticosteroids

Nursing Implications Management of side effects is similar to conventional amphotericin B. [See Amphotericin B (Conventional) on page 100 for suggested management guidelines of side effects.]

Dosage Forms Excipient information presented when available (limited, particularly for generics); consult specific product labeling.

Injection, powder for reconstitution:

AmBisome®: 50 mg [contains soy and sucrose]

References

Burgos A, Zaoutis TE, Dvorak CC, et al, "Pediatric Invasive Aspergillosis: A Multicenter Retrospective Analysis of 139 Contemporary Cases," Pediatrics, 2008, 121(5):e1286-94.

Emminger W, Graninger W, Emminger-Schmidmeir W, et al, "Tolerance of High Doses of Amphotericin B by Infusion of a Liposomal Formulation in Children With Cancer," Ann Hematol, 1994, 68:27-31.

NIH, CDC, and HIVMA/IDSA, "Guidelines for Prevention and Treatment of Opportunistic Infections Among HIV-Exposed and HIV-Infected Children - June 20, 2008." Available at http://aidsinfo.nih.gov.

Ringden O, Andstrom E, Remberger M, et al, "Safety of Liposomal Amphotericin B (AmBisome®) In 187 Transplant Recipients Treated With Cyclosporin," Bone Marrow Transplant, 1994, 14 Suppl 5:S10-4.

Walsh TJ, Goodman JL, Pappas P, et al, "Safety, Tolerance, and Pharmacokinetics of High-Dose Liposomal Amphotericin B (AmBisome®) in Patients Infected With Aspergillus Species and Other Filamentous Fungi: Maximum Tolerated Dose Study," Antimicrob Agents Chemother, 2001, 45(12):3487-96.

Walsh TJ, Finberg RW, Arndt C, et al, "Liposomal Amphotericin B for Empirical Therapy in Patients With Persistent Fever and Neutropenia," N Engl J Med, 1999, 340:764-71.

Ampicillin (am pi SIL in)

Medication Safety Issues

Sound-alike/look-alike issues:

Ampicillin may be confused with aminophylline

Related Information

Endocarditis Prophylaxis on page 1610

Canadian Brand Names Apo-Ampi®; Novo-Ampicillin; Nu-Ampi

Therapeutic Category Antibiotic, Penicillin

Generic Available Yes

Use Treatment of susceptible bacterial infections caused by streptococci, pneumococci, enterococci, nonpenicillinase-producing staphylococci, *Listeria*, meningococci; some strains of *H. influenzae*, *P. mirabilis*, *Salmonella*, *Shigella*, *E. coli*, *Enterobacter*, and *Klebsiella*; initial empiric treatment of neonates with suspected bacterial sepsis or meningitis used in combination with an aminoglycoside or cefotaxime; endocarditis prophylaxis

Pregnancy Risk Factor B

Pregnancy Considerations Adverse events have not been observed in animal studies; therefore, ampicillin is classified as pregnancy category B. Ampicillin crosses the human placenta, providing detectable concentrations in the cord serum and amniotic fluid. Most studies have not identified a teratogenic potential for ampicillin use during pregnancy. Two possible associations (congenital heart disease and cleft palate) have been noted; each of these was observed in a single study, was not substantiated by other studies, and may have been chance associations. Ampicillin is recommended for use in pregnant women for the management of premature rupture of membranes. Ampicillin is considered an acceptable alternative to penicillin for the prevention of early-onset Group B Streptococcal (GBS) disease in newborns.

The volume of distribution of ampicillin is increased during pregnancy and the half-life is decreased. As a result, serum concentrations in pregnant patients are approximately 50% of those in nonpregnant patients receiving the same dose. Higher doses may be needed during pregnancy. Although oral absorption is not altered during pregnancy, oral ampicillin is poorly-absorbed during labor.

Lactation Enters breast milk/use caution

Breast-Feeding Considerations Ampicillin is excreted in breast milk. The manufacturer recommends that caution be exercised when administering ampicillin to nursing women. Due to the low concentrations in human milk, minimal toxicity would be expected in the nursing infant. Nondose-related effects could include modification of bowel flora and allergic sensitization.

Contraindications Hypersensitivity to ampicillin (penicillins) or any component

Warnings Epstein-Barr virus infection, acute lymphocytic leukemia or cytomegalovirus infection increases risk for ampicillin-induced maculopapular rash

Precautions Dosage adjustment may be necessary in patients with renal impairment (Cl_{cr} <10-15 mL/minute); use with caution in patients allergic to cephalosporins

Adverse Reactions

Central nervous system: Seizures, headache, dizziness, drug fever

Dermatologic: Rash, urticaria, exfoliative dermatitis, Stevens-Johnson syndrome

Gastrointestinal: Diarrhea (20%), nausea, vomiting, glossitis, pseudomembranous enterocolitis, oral candidiasis

Hematologic: Eosinophilia, hemolytic anemia, thrombocytopenia, neutropenia, prolongation of bleeding time

Renal: Interstitial nephritis

Miscellaneous: Anaphylaxis, hypersensitivity reactions, serum sickness, vasculitis, superinfection

Drug Interactions

Avoid Concomitant Use

Avoid concomitant use of Ampicillin with any of the following: BCG

Increased Effect/Toxicity

Ampicillin may increase the levels/effects of: Methotrexate

The levels/effects of Ampicillin may be increased by: Allopurinol; Probenecid

Decreased Effect

Ampicillin may decrease the levels/effects of: Atenolol; BCG; Mycophenolate; Typhoid Vaccine

The levels/effects of Ampicillin may be decreased by: Chloroquine; Fusidic Acid; Tetracycline Derivatives

Food Interactions Food decreases rate and extent of absorption

Stability Oral suspension is stable for 14 days under refrigeration; reconstituted solutions for I.M. or direct I.V. should be used within 1 hour; solutions for I.V. infusion will be inactivated by dextrose at room temperature; if dextrose-containing solutions are to be used as a diluent, the resultant solution will only be stable for 2 hours vs 8 hours in solutions containing NS

Mechanism of Action Interferes with bacterial cell wall synthesis by binding to one or more penicillin-binding proteins during active multiplication; inhibits the final transpeptidation step of peptidoglycan synthesis causing cell wall death and resultant bactericidal activity against susceptible bacteria

Pharmacokinetics (Adult data unless noted)

Absorption: Oral: 50%

Distribution: Into bile; penetration into CSF occurs with inflamed meninges only; low excretion into breast milk

Protein binding:

Neonates: 10%

Adults: 15% to 18%

Half-life:

Neonates:

2-7 days: 4 hours

8-14 days: 2.8 hours

15-30 days: 1.7 hours

Children and Adults: 1-1.8 hours

Anuric patients: 8-20 hours

Time to peak serum concentration: Oral: Within 1-2 hours

Elimination: ~90% of drug excreted unchanged in urine within 24 hours; excreted in bile

Dialysis: ~40% is removed by hemodialysis

Usual Dosage

Children: Oral: 50-100 mg/kg/day divided every 6 hours; maximum dose: 2-3 g/day

Adults: Oral: 250-500 mg every 6 hours

Neonates: I.M., I.V.:

Postnatal age ≤7 days:

≤2000 g: 50 mg/kg/day divided every 12 hours; meningitis: 100 mg/kg/day divided every 12 hours

>2000 g: 75 mg/kg/day divided every 8 hours; meningitis: 150 mg/kg/day divided every 8 hours

Group B streptococcal meningitis: 200 mg/kg/day divided every 8 hours

Postnatal age >7 days:

<1200 g: 50 mg/kg/day divided every 12 hours; meningitis: 100 mg/kg/day divided every 12 hours

1200-2000 g: 75 mg/kg/day divided every 8 hours; meningitis: 150 mg/kg/day divided every 8 hours

>2000 g: 100 mg/kg/day divided every 6 hours; meningitis: 200 mg/kg/day divided every 6 hours

Group B streptococcal meningitis: 300 mg/kg/day divided every 6 hours

Infants and Children: I.M., I.V.: 100-200 mg/kg/day divided every 6 hours; meningitis: 200-400 mg/kg/day divided every 6 hours; maximum dose: 12 g/day

Endocarditis prophylaxis:

50 mg/kg within 30 minutes before procedure (dental, oral, respiratory tract, or esophageal procedures); maximum dose: 2 g

50 mg/kg (maximum dose: 2 g) plus gentamicin 1.5 mg/kg (maximum dose: 120 mg) within 30 minutes of starting the procedure; 25 mg/kg 6 hours later (for high-risk patients undergoing genitourinary and GI tract procedures)

Adults: I.M., I.V.: 500 mg to 3 g every 6 hours; maximum dose: 14 g/day

Endocarditis prophylaxis:

2 g within 30 minutes before procedure (dental, oral, respiratory tract, or esophageal procedures)

2 g plus gentamicin 1.5 mg/kg (maximum dose: 120 mg) within 30 minutes of starting the procedure; 1 g 6 hours later (for high-risk patients undergoing genitourinary and GI tract procedures)

Dosing interval in renal impairment: Adults:

Cl_{cr} 10-30 mL/minute: Administer every 6-12 hours

Cl_{cr} <10 mL/minute: Administer every 12 hours

Administration

Oral: Administer with water 1-2 hours prior to food on an empty stomach; shake suspension well before using

Parenteral: Ampicillin may be administered IVP over 3-5 minutes at a rate not to exceed 100 mg/minute or I.V. intermittent infusion over 15-30 minutes; final concentration for I.V. administration should not exceed 100 mg/mL (IVP) or 30 mg/mL (I.V. intermittent infusion)

Monitoring Parameters With prolonged therapy monitor renal, hepatic, and hematologic function periodically; observe for change in bowel frequency

Test Interactions False-positive urinary glucose (Benedict's solution, Clinitest®); + Coombs' [direct]

Nursing Implications Ampicillin and gentamicin should not be mixed in the same I.V. tubing or administered concurrently

Additional Information Appearance of a rash should be carefully evaluated to differentiate a nonallergic ampicillin rash from a hypersensitivity reaction. Ampicillin rash occurs in 5% to 10% of children receiving ampicillin and is a generalized dull red, maculopapular rash, generally appearing 3-14 days after the start of therapy. It normally begins on the trunk and spreads over most of the body. It may be most intense at pressure areas, elbows, and knees. Incidence of ampicillin rash is higher in patients with viral infections, infectious mononucleosis, lymphocytic leukemia, or patients with hyperuricemia who are receiving allopurinol.

Sodium content of suspension (250 mg/5 mL, 5 mL): 10 mg (0.4 mEq)

Sodium content of 1 g: 66.7 mg (3 mEq)

Dosage Forms Excipient information presented when available (limited, particularly for generics); consult specific product labeling.

Capsule: 250 mg, 500 mg

Injection, powder for reconstitution, as sodium [strength expressed as base]: 125 mg, 250 mg, 500 mg, 1 g, 2 g, 10 g

Powder for oral suspension: 125 mg/5 mL (100 mL, 200 mL); 250 mg/5 mL (100 mL, 200 mL)

References

Boguniewicz M and Leung DY, "Hypersensitivity Reactions to Antibiotics Commonly Used in Children," *Pediatr Infect Dis J*, 1995, 14 (3):221-31.

Brown RD, Campoli-Richards DM, "Antimicrobial Therapy in Neonates, Infants, and Children," *Clin Pharmacokinet*, 1989, 17(Suppl 1):105-15.

Ampicillin and Sulbactam
(am pi SIL in & SUL bak tam)

U.S. Brand Names Unasyn®

Canadian Brand Names Unasyn®

Therapeutic Category Antibiotic, Beta-lactam and Beta-lactamase Combination; Antibiotic, Penicillin

Generic Available Yes

Use Treatment of susceptible bacterial infections involved with skin and skin structure, intra-abdominal infections, gynecological infections; spectrum is that of ampicillin plus organisms producing beta-lactamases such as *S. aureus*, *H. influenzae*, *E. coli*, *Klebsiella*, *Acinetobacter*, *Enterobacter*, and anaerobes

Pregnancy Risk Factor B

Pregnancy Considerations Adverse events have not been observed in animal studies; therefore, ampicillin/sulbactam is classified as pregnancy category B. Both ampicillin and sulbactam cross the placenta. When used during pregnancy, pharmacokinetic changes have been observed with ampicillin alone (refer to the Ampicillin monograph for details).

Lactation Enters breast milk/use caution

Breast-Feeding Considerations Ampicillin and sulbactam are both excreted into breast milk in low concentrations. The manufacturer recommends that caution be used if administering to lactating women. Nondose-related effects could include modification of bowel flora and allergic sensitization of the infant. The maternal dose of sulbactam does not need altered in the postpartum period. Also refer to the Ampicillin monograph.

Contraindications Hypersensitivity to ampicillin, sulbactam, any component, or penicillins

Warnings Epstein-Barr virus infection, acute lymphocytic leukemia or cytomegalovirus infection increases risk for ampicillin-induced maculopapular rash; not FDA approved for children <12 years of age

Precautions Modify dosage in patients with renal impairment; use with caution in patients allergic to cephalosporins

Adverse Reactions

Cardiovascular: Chest pain

Central nervous system: Fatigue, malaise, headache, chills, dizziness, seizures

Dermatologic: Rash (2%), itching, urticaria, exfoliative dermatitis, Stevens-Johnson syndrome

Gastrointestinal: Diarrhea (3%), nausea, vomiting, candidiasis, flatulence, pseudomembranous colitis, hairy tongue

Genitourinary: Dysuria, hematuria

Hematologic: WBC decreased, neutrophils, platelets, hemoglobin, and hematocrit

Hepatic: Liver enzymes elevated

Local: Pain at injection site (I.M.: 16%, I.V.: 3%), thrombophlebitis (3%)

Renal: BUN elevated, serum creatinine elevated

Miscellaneous: Hypersensitivity reactions, anaphylaxis, serum sickness, vasculitis, superinfection

Drug Interactions

Avoid Concomitant Use

Avoid concomitant use of Ampicillin and Sulbactam with any of the following: BCG

Increased Effect/Toxicity

Ampicillin and Sulbactam may increase the levels/effects of: Methotrexate

The levels/effects of Ampicillin and Sulbactam may be increased by: Allopurinol; Probenecid

Decreased Effect

Ampicillin and Sulbactam may decrease the levels/effects of: Atenolol; BCG; Mycophenolate; Typhoid Vaccine

The levels/effects of Ampicillin and Sulbactam may be decreased by: Chloroquine; Fusidic Acid; Tetracycline Derivatives

Stability Ampicillin/sulbactam infusion solution is stable for 8 hours in NS at room temperature; incompatible when mixed with aminoglycosides

Mechanism of Action Sulbactam has very little antibacterial activity by itself. The addition of sulbactam, a beta-lactamase inhibitor, to ampicillin extends the spectrum of ampicillin to include beta-lactamase producing organisms; ampicillin acts by inhibiting bacterial cell wall synthesis during the stage of active multiplication

Pharmacokinetics (Adult data unless noted)

Distribution: Into bile, blister and tissue fluids; poor penetration into CSF with uninflamed meninges; higher concentrations attained with inflamed meninges

Protein binding:
Ampicillin: 28%
Sulbactam: 38%

Half-life: Ampicillin and sulbactam are similar: 1-1.8 hours and 1-1.3 hours, respectively in patients with normal renal function

Elimination: ~75% to 85% of both drugs are excreted unchanged in urine within 8 hours following administration

Usual Dosage Unasyn® (ampicillin/sulbactam) is a combination product; each 3 g vial contains 2 g of ampicillin and 1 g of sulbactam. Dosage recommendations are based on the **ampicillin** component.

I.M., I.V.:

Infants ≥1 month: 100-150 mg ampicillin/kg/day divided every 6 hours

Meningitis: 200-300 mg ampicillin/kg/day divided every 6 hours

Children: 100-200 mg ampicillin/kg/day divided every 6 hours

Meningitis: 200-400 mg ampicillin/kg/day divided every 6 hours; maximum dose: 8 g ampicillin/day

Adults: 1-2 g ampicillin every 6-8 hours; maximum dose: 12 g ampicillin/day

Dosing interval in renal impairment:

Cl_cr 15-29 mL/minute: Administer every 12 hours

Cl_cr 5-14 mL/minute: Administer every 24 hours

Administration Parenteral: May be administered by slow I.V. injection over 10-15 minutes at a final concentration for administration not to exceed 45 mg Unasyn® (30 mg ampicillin and 15 mg sulbactam)/mL or by intermittent infusion over 15-30 minutes

Monitoring Parameters With prolonged therapy monitor hematologic, renal, and hepatic function; observe for change in bowel frequency

Test Interactions False-positive urinary glucose levels (Benedict's solution, Clinitest®); positive Coombs' [direct]

Additional Information Sodium content of 1.5 g (1 g ampicillin plus 0.5 g sulbactam): 5 mEq

Dosage Forms Excipient information presented when available (limited, particularly for generics); consult specific product labeling.

Injection, powder for reconstitution: 1.5 g: Ampicillin 1 g and sulbactam 0.5 g [contains sodium 115 mg (5 mEq)/1.5 g)]; 3 g: Ampicillin 2 g and sulbactam 1 g [contains sodium 115 mg (5 mEq)/1.5 g)]; 15 g: Ampicillin 10 g and sulbactam 5 g [bulk package; contains sodium 115 mg (5 mEq)/1.5 g]

Unasyn®:

1.5 g: Ampicillin 1 g and sulbactam 0.5 g [contains sodium 115 mg (5 mEq)/1.5 g)]

3 g: Ampicillin 2 g and sulbactam 1 g [contains sodium 115 mg (5 mEq)/1.5 g)]

15 g: Ampicillin 10 g and sulbactam 5 g [bulk package; contains sodium 115 mg (5 mEq)/1.5 g)]

References

Dajani AS, "Sulbactam/Ampicillin in Pediatric Infections," *Drugs*, 1988, 35(Suppl 7):35-8.

Goldfarb J, Aronoff SC, Jaffé A, et al, "Sultamicillin in the Treatment of Superficial Skin and Soft Tissue Infections in Children," *Antimicrob Agents Chemother*, 1987, 31(4):663-4.

Kulhanjian J, Dunphy MG, Hamstra S, et al, "Randomized Comparative Study of Ampicillin/Sulbactam vs Ceftriaxone for Treatment of Soft Tissue and Skeletal Infections in Children," *Pediatr Infect Dis J*, 1989, 8(9):605-10.

Syriopoulou V, Bitsi M, Theodoridis C, et al, "Clinical Efficacy of Sulbactam/Ampicillin in Pediatric Infections Caused by Ampicillin-Resistant or Penicillin-Resistant Organisms," *Rev Infect Dis*, 1986, 8 (Suppl 5):S630-3.

◆ **Ampicillin Sodium** *see* Ampicillin *on page 104*

◆ **Ampicillin Trihydrate** *see* Ampicillin *on page 104*

◆ **Amrinone Lactate** *see* Inamrinone *on page 722*

◆ **Amrix®** *see* Cyclobenzaprine *on page 367*

◆ **Amylase, Lipase, and Protease** *see* Pancrelipase *on page 1051*

Amyl Nitrite (AM il NYE trite)

Therapeutic Category Antidote, Cyanide; Vasodilator, Coronary

Generic Available Yes

Use Coronary vasodilator in angina pectoris; an adjunct in treatment of cyanide poisoning

Pregnancy Risk Factor C

Lactation Excretion in breast milk unknown/not recommended

Contraindications Hypersensitivity to nitrates or any component; severe anemia; recent head trauma or cerebral hemorrhage; glaucoma; hyperthyroidism; recent MI

Warnings Postural hypotension with episodes of dizziness, weakness, or syncope may occur after inhalation; may cause harm to the fetus if administered to a pregnant woman (may significantly decrease systemic blood pressure and blood flow)

Precautions Use with great caution in patients with increased intracranial pressure or low systolic blood pressure; tolerance to coronary vasodilator effects may occur (to minimize tolerance, use lowest effective initial dose and alternate with another coronary vasodilator); high doses of nitrates may cause methemoglobinemia (especially in patients with methemoglobin reductase deficiency or other metabolic abnormalities)

Adverse Reactions

Cardiovascular: Postural hypotension; cutaneous flushing of head, neck, and clavicular area; tachycardia; palpitations; vasodilation; syncope

Central nervous system: Headache, dizziness, restlessness

Dermatologic: Skin rash (contact dermatitis)

Gastrointestinal: Nausea, vomiting

Hematologic: Hemolytic anemia

Neuromuscular & skeletal: Weakness

Ocular: Intraocular pressure elevated

Miscellaneous: Tolerance to coronary vasodilator effects may occur

Drug Interactions

Avoid Concomitant Use There are no known interactions where it is recommended to avoid concomitant use.

Increased Effect/Toxicity

Amyl Nitrite may increase the levels/effects of: Hypotensive Agents

Decreased Effect There are no known significant interactions involving a decrease in effect.

Stability Store in cool place, protect from light; flammable, avoid exposure to heat or flame

Mechanism of Action Vasodilator (vascular smooth muscle relaxant) which decreases afterload and improves myocardial blood supply via coronary artery vasodilation; antidote for cyanide poisoning: promotes formation of methemoglobin which combines with cyanide molecule to form cyanmethemoglobin (nontoxic)

Pharmacodynamics

Onset of action: Within 30 seconds

Duration: 3-5 minutes

Pharmacokinetics (Adult data unless noted)

Absorption: Inhalation: Readily absorbed through respiratory tract

Metabolism: In the liver to form inorganic nitrates (less potent)

Half-life:

Amyl nitrite: <1 hour

Methemoglobin: 1 hour

Elimination: Renal; ~33%

Usual Dosage Nasal inhalation:

Children and Adults: Cyanide poisoning: Inhale the vapor from a 0.3 mL crushed ampul every minute for 15-30 seconds until I.V. sodium nitrite infusion is available

Adults: Angina: 1-6 inhalations from 1 crushed ampul; may repeat in 3-5 minutes

Administration Give by nasal inhalation with patient in recumbent or seated position; crush ampul in woven covering between finger and hold under patient's nostrils

Monitoring Parameters Blood pressure; with treatment for cyanide poisoning: methemoglobin levels, arterial blood gas

Patient Information Remain seated or lying down during administration because of possible hypotension and dizziness; do not get up suddenly after use; avoid alcohol; if angina pain is not relieved after 2 doses, seek immediate medical attention

Nursing Implications To facilitate recovery from symptoms of postural hypotension, place patient in head-down position; may also use measures such as deep breathing and movement of extremities

Additional Information Amyl nitrite has been used to treat penile erections after urological surgery (eg, circumcisions in adults) and has been used to change the intensity of heart murmurs to aid in their diagnosis

Dosage Forms Excipient information presented when available (limited, particularly for generics); consult specific product labeling.

Liquid, for inhalation: USP: 85% to 103% (0.3 mL) [crushable covered glass capsule]

◆ **Amyl Nitrite, Sodium Nitrite, and Sodium Thiosulfate** *see* Sodium Nitrite, Sodium Thiosulfate, and Amyl Nitrite *on page 1273*

◆ **Amylobarbitone** *see* Amobarbital *on page 94*

◆ **Amytal®** *see* Amobarbital *on page 94*

◆ **Anafranil®** *see* ClomiPRAMINE *on page 334*

Anakinra (an a KIN ra)

Medication Safety Issues
Sound-alike/look-alike issues:
Anakinra may be confused with amikacin, Ampyra™
Kineret® may be confused with Amikin®

U.S. Brand Names Kineret®

Canadian Brand Names Kineret®

Therapeutic Category Antirheumatic, Disease Modifying; Interleukin-1 Receptor Antagonist

Generic Available No

Use Treatment of moderately- to severely-active rheumatoid arthritis in adult patients who have failed one or more disease-modifying antirheumatic drugs (DMARDs); may be used alone or in combination with DMARDs that are not tumor necrosis factor (TNF) blocking agents (eg, etanercept, adalimumab). In children, anakinra has shown efficacy in reducing signs and symptoms of systemic onset juvenile idiopathic arthritic (SOJIA), polyarticular-course juvenile idiopathic arthritis (JIA), and congenital autoinflammatory diseases, such as chronic infantile neurological cutaneous articular syndrome (CINCA) and its less severe forms, which have shown beneficial effects of therapy.

Pregnancy Risk Factor B

Pregnancy Considerations No evidence of impaired fertility or harm to fetus in animal models; however, there are no controlled trials in pregnant women. Women exposed to anakinra during pregnancy may contact the Organization of Teratology Information Services (OTIS), Rheumatoid Arthritis and Pregnancy Study at 1-877-311-8972.

Lactation Excretion in breast milk unknown/use caution

Breast-Feeding Considerations Endogenous interleukin-1 receptor antagonist can be found in breast milk; specific excretion of anakinra is not known.

Contraindications Hypersensitivity to *E. coli*-derived proteins, anakinra, or any component of the formulation

Warnings Use associated with increased risk of developing serious infections; risk is higher if used concurrently with etanercept or if patient has asthma; therapy should be discontinued if serious infection develops. DO not initiate therapy in patients with active infection, including chronic or local infections. Use in immunosuppressed patients has not been evaluated.

Precautions Use may affect defenses against malignancies; impact on the development and course of malignancies is not fully defined. As compared to the general population, an increased risk of lymphoma has been noted in clinical trials; however, rheumatoid arthritis has been previously associated with an increased rate of lymphoma. Use with caution in patients with a history of significant hematologic abnormalities; therapy is associated with uncommon but significant decreases in hematologic parameters (particularly neutrophil counts). Patients should be brought up-to-date with all immunizations before initiating therapy; live vaccines should not be given concurrently. There is no data available concerning the effects of therapy on vaccination or secondary transmission of live vaccines in patients receiving therapy. Patients with latex allergy should not handle the needle cover of the diluent syringe since it contains latex. Use caution in patients with renal impairment; consider increased dosing intervals for severe renal dysfunction (Cl_{cr} <30 mL/minute).

Adverse Reactions
Central nervous system: Headache, fever

Dermatologic: Cellulitis, rash

Gastrointestinal: Nausea, diarrhea, abdominal pain, vomiting

Hematologic: Neutropenia, leukopenia, thrombocytopenia

Local: Injection site reaction (usually mild, typically lasting 14-28 days, characterized by erythema, ecchymosis, inflammation, and pain)

Respiratory: Sinusitis, cough, URI

Miscellaneous: Infection, flu-like syndrome

Drug Interactions

Avoid Concomitant Use
Avoid concomitant use of Anakinra with any of the following: Anti-TNF Agents; BCG; Canakinumab; Natalizumab; Pimecrolimus; Tacrolimus (Topical); Vaccines (Live)

Increased Effect/Toxicity
Anakinra may increase the levels/effects of: Canakinumab; Leflunomide; Natalizumab; Vaccines (Live)

The levels/effects of Anakinra may be increased by: Anti-TNF Agents; Denosumab; Pimecrolimus; Tacrolimus (Topical); Trastuzumab

Decreased Effect
Anakinra may decrease the levels/effects of: BCG; Sipuleucel-T; Vaccines (Inactivated); Vaccines (Live)

The levels/effects of Anakinra may be decreased by: Echinacea

Stability Store in refrigerator at 2°C to 8°C (36°F to 46°F); do not freeze. Do not shake. Protect from light.

Mechanism of Action Antagonist of the interleukin-1 (IL-1) receptor. Endogenous IL-1 is induced by inflammatory stimuli and mediates a variety of immunological responses, including degradation of cartilage (loss of proteoglycans) and stimulation of bone resorption.

Pharmacokinetics (Adult data unless noted)
Bioavailability: SubQ: 95%

Half-life elimination: 4-6 hours

Time to peak: SubQ: 3-7 hours

Usual Dosage SubQ:
Children:

Systemic onset JIA (data based on clinical trials): Initial dose: 1 mg/kg once daily; if no response, may increase to 2 mg/kg (maximum dose: 100 mg). Not studied in children <1 year.

Polyarticular course JIA (data based on clinical trials): 1 mg/kg once daily (maximum dose: 100 mg). Not studied in children <2 years.

CINCA (and similar congenital autoinflammatory diseases): ≥4 years: Initial dose: 1 mg/kg once daily; if no response, may increase up to 2 mg/kg.

Adults: Rheumatoid arthritis: 100 mg once daily; administer at approximately the same time each day

Dosage adjustment in renal impairment: Adults: Cl_{cr} <30 mL/minute and/or end-stage renal disease: 100 mg every other day

Administration SubQ: Rotate injection sites (thigh, abdomen, upper arm); injection should be given at least 1 inch away from previous injection site. Do not shake. Provided in single-use, preservative-free syringes with 27-gauge needles; discard any unused portion.

Monitoring Parameters CBC with differential (baseline, then monthly for 3 months, then every 3 months); serum creatinine

Patient Information If self-injecting, follow instructions for injection and disposal of needles exactly. If redness, swelling, or irritation appears at the injection site, contact prescriber. Do not have any vaccinations while using this medication without consulting prescriber first. Immediately report skin rash, unusual muscle or bone weakness, or signs of respiratory flu or other infection (eg, chills, fever, sore throat, easy bruising or bleeding, mouth sores, unhealed sores).

Additional Information Anakinra is produced by recombinant DNA/*E. coli* technology.

Women exposed to anakinra during pregnancy may contact the Organization of Teratology Information Services (OTIS), Rheumatoid Arthritis and Pregnancy Study at 1-877-311-8972.

Dosage Forms Excipient information presented when available (limited, particularly for generics); consult specific product labeling.

Injection, solution [preservative free]:
Kineret®: 100 mg/0.67 mL (0.67 mL) [prefilled syringe; needle cover contains latex]

References
Callejas JL, Oliver J, Martín J, et al, "Anakinra in Mutation-Negative CINCA Syndrome," *Clin Rheumatol*, 2007, 26(4):576-7.

Gartlehner G, Hansen RA, Jonas BL, et al, "Biologics for the Treatment of Juvenile Idiopathic Arthritis: A Systematic Review and Critical Analysis of the Evidence," *Clin Rheumatol*, 2008, 27(1):67-76.

Gattorno M, Piccini A, Lasigliè D, et al, "The Pattern of Response to Anti-Interleukin-1 Treatment Distinguishes Two Subsets of Patients With Systemic-Onset Juvenile Idiopathic Arthritis," *Arthritis Rheum*, 2008, 58(5):1505-15.

Goldbach-Mansky R, Dailey NJ, Canna SW, et al, "Neonatal-Onset Multisystem Inflammatory Disease Responsive to Interleukin-1Beta Inhibition," *N Engl J Med*, 2006, 355(6):581-92.

Ilowite N, Porras O, Reiff A, et al, "Anakinra in the Treatment of Polyarticular-Course Juvenile Rheumatoid Arthritis: Safety and Preliminary Efficacy Results of a Randomized Multicenter Study," *Clin Rheumatol*, 2009, 28(2):129-37.

Irigoyen P, Olson J, Horn C, et al, "Treatement of Systemic Onset Juvenile Idiopathic Arthritis With Anakinra," *Ped Rheumatol Online J*, 2006, 4(2):123-34

Kashiwagi Y, Kawashima H, Nishimata S, et al, "Extreme Efficiency of Anti-Interleukin 1 Agent (Anakinra) in a Japanese Case of CINCA Syndrome," *Clin Rheumatol*, 2008, 27(2):277-9.

Lequerré T, Quartier P, Rosellini D, et al, "Interleukin-1 Receptor Antagonist (Anakinra) Treatment in Patients With Systemic-Onset Juvenile Idiopathic Arthritis or Adult Onset Still Disease: Preliminary Experience in France," *Ann Rheum Dis*, 2008, 67(3):302-8.

Lovell DJ, Bowyer SL, and Solinger AM, "Interleukin-1 Blockade by Anakinra Improves Clinical Symptoms in Patients With Neonatal-Onset Multisystem Inflammatory Disease," *Arthritis Rheum*, 2005, 52 (4):1283-6.

Matsubayashi T, Sugiura H, Arai T, et al, "Anakinra Therapy for CINCA Syndrome With a Novel Mutation in Exon 4 of the CIAS1 Gene," *Acta Paediatr*, 2006, 95(2):246-9.

Ohlsson V, Baildam E, Foster H, et al, "Anakinra Treatment for Systemic Onset Juvenile Idiopathic Arthritis (SOJIA)," *Rheumatology (Oxford)*, 2008, 47(4):555-6.

Pascual V, Allantaz F, Arce E, et al, "Role of Interleukin-1 (IL-1) in the Pathogenesis of Systemic Onset Juvenile Idiopathic Arthritis and Clinical Response to IL-1 Blockade," *J Exp Med*, 2005, 201 (9):1479-86.

Reiff A, "The Use of Anakinra in Juvenile Arthritis," *Curr Rheumatol Rep*, 2005, 7(6):434-40.

Rigante D, Ansuini V, Caldarelli M, et al, "Hydrocephalus in CINCA Syndrome Treated With Anakinra," *Childs Nerv Syst*, 2006, 22 (4):334-7.

♦ **Anaprox®** see Naproxen on page 967

♦ **Anaprox® DS** see Naproxen on page 967

♦ **Anaspaz®** see Hyoscyamine on page 699

♦ **Anbesol® [OTC]** see Benzocaine on page 182

♦ **Anbesol® Baby [OTC]** see Benzocaine on page 182

♦ **Anbesol® Baby (Can)** see Benzocaine on page 182

♦ **Anbesol® Cold Sore Therapy [OTC]** see Benzocaine on page 182

♦ **Anbesol® Jr. [OTC]** see Benzocaine on page 182

♦ **Anbesol® Maximum Strength [OTC]** see Benzocaine on page 182

♦ **Ancef** see CeFAZolin on page 262

♦ **Anchoic Acid** see Azelaic Acid on page 162

♦ **Ancobon®** see Flucytosine on page 586

♦ **Andehist NR Drops [DSC]** see Carbinoxamine and Pseudoephedrine on page 249

♦ **Andehist NR Syrup [DSC]** see Brompheniramine and Pseudoephedrine on page 205

♦ **Andriol® (Can)** see Testosterone on page 1325

♦ **Androderm®** see Testosterone on page 1325

♦ **AndroGel®** see Testosterone on page 1325

♦ **Andropository (Can)** see Testosterone on page 1325

♦ **Androxy™** see Fluoxymesterone on page 604

♦ **Anectine®** see Succinylcholine on page 1295

♦ **Anestacon® [DSC]** see Lidocaine on page 818

♦ **Anestafoam™ [OTC]** see Lidocaine on page 818

♦ **Aneurine Hydrochloride** see Thiamine on page 1338

♦ **Anexate® (Can)** see Flumazenil on page 590

♦ **Anhydrous Glucose** see Dextrose on page 422

♦ **Ansaid® (Can)** see Flurbiprofen on page 605

♦ **Ansamycin** see Rifabutin on page 1213

♦ **Anti-CD20 Monoclonal Antibody** see RiTUXimab on page 1227

♦ **Antidigoxin Fab Fragments, Ovine** see Digoxin Immune Fab on page 440

♦ **Antidiuretic Hormone** see Vasopressin on page 1410

♦ **Anti-Fungal™ [OTC]** see Clotrimazole on page 344

Antihemophilic Factor (Human)
(an tee hee moe FIL ik FAK tor HYU man)

U.S. Brand Names Hemofil M; Koāte®-DVI; Monarc-M™; Monoclate-P®

Canadian Brand Names Hemofil M

Therapeutic Category Antihemophilic Agent; Blood Product Derivative

Generic Available Yes

Use Prevention and treatment of hemorrhagic episodes in patients with hemophilia A (classical hemophilia); perioperative management of patients with hemophilia A; can provide therapeutic effects in patients with acquired factor VIII inhibitors <10 Bethesda units/mL

Pregnancy Risk Factor C

Pregnancy Considerations Reproduction studies have not been conducted. Safety and efficacy in pregnant women have not been established. Use during pregnancy only if clearly needed. Parvovirus B19 or hepatitis A, which may be present in plasma-derived products, may affect a pregnant woman more seriously than nonpregnant women.

Lactation Excretion in breast milk unknown/use caution

Contraindications

All products: Hypersensitivity to any component (see Warnings and table)

Antihemophilic factor, human (Method M, monoclonal purified); Hemofil M; Monarc-M™; Monoclate-P®: Hypersensitivity to mouse protein

Antihemophilic Factor (Human) [Factor VIII (Human)] Products

Product	Preparation and Purification Methods	Viral Inactivation	Stabilizers and Excipients
Hemofil M	• Method M process • Immunoaffinity chromatography using murine monoclonal antibody • Ion exchange chromatography	• Organic solvent/ detergent treatment	• Albumin (human)[1] • Polyethylene glycol[1] • Histidine[1] • Glycine[1] • Mouse protein • Tri-n-butyl phosphate • Octoxynol 9
Koāte®-DVI	• Purified from cold insoluble fraction of fresh-frozen plasma • Gel permeation chromatography	• Organic solvent/ detergent treatment • Heat treatment (dry; in lyophilized form in final container; 80°C x 72 hours)	• Albumin (human) • Polyethylene glycol • Glycine • Polysorbate 80 • Tri-n-butyl phosphate • Calcium • Aluminum • Histidine
Monarc-M™	• Method M process • Immunoaffinity chromatography using murine monoclonal antibody • Ion exchange chromatography	• Organic solvent/ detergent treatment	• Albumin (human)[1] • Polyethylene glycol[1] • Histidine[1] • Glycine[1] • Mouse protein • Tri-n-butyl phosphate • Octoxynol 9
Monoclate-P®	• Immunoaffinity chromatography using murine monoclonal antibody	• Heat treatment in aqueous solution (pasteurization; 60°C x 10 hours)	• Albumin (human)[1] • Sodium (300-450 millimoles/L) • Calcium chloride • Mannitol • Histidine • Hydrochloric acid and/or sodium hydroxide (pH adjustment) • Mouse protein

Note: Source of all products is pooled human plasma.

[1]Listed as a stabilizer in the product's package insert.

Warnings Hemofil M and Monarc-M™ contain natural rubber latex (in certain components of the product packaging) which may cause allergic reactions in susceptible individuals; avoid use in patients with allergy to latex

Precautions Clinical response to recommended doses may vary; dosage must be individualized based on coagulation studies (performed prior to treatment and at regular intervals during treatment) and clinical response. Human antihemophilic factor is prepared from pooled plasma and even with heat treated or other viral attenuated processes, the risk of viral transmission (ie, viral hepatitis, HIV, parvovirus B19, and theoretically, Creutzfeldt-Jacob disease agent) is not totally eradicated. Hepatitis B vaccination is recommended for all patients receiving human antihemophilic factor and hepatitis A vaccination is recommended for seronegative patients. [Note: The use of recombinant antihemophilic factor products (such as Advate, Helixate® FS, Kogenate® FS, Recombinate™, or ReFacto®) substantially decreases the risk of viral transmission because these products are biosynthetically prepared.] Progressive anemia and hemolysis may occur in individuals with blood groups A, B, and AB who receive large or frequent doses of human antihemophilic factor due to trace amounts of blood group A and B isohemagglutinins (see Monitoring Parameters).

Formation of factor VIII inhibitors (neutralizing antibodies to AHF human) may occur (see Adverse Reactions); monitor patients appropriately (see Monitoring Parameters and Additional Information). Allergic-type hypersensitivity reactions including anaphylaxis may occur; discontinue therapy immediately if urticaria, hives, hypotension, tightness of the chest, wheezing, dyspnea, faintness, or anaphylaxis develop; emergency treatment and resuscitative measures (eg, epinephrine, oxygen) may be needed. Products vary by preparation method (see table); final formulations contain human albumin

Adverse Reactions

Cardiovascular: Flushing, tachycardia, chest tightness

Central nervous system: Headache, fever, chills, lethargy, somnolence, dizziness, nervousness

Dermatologic: Urticaria, rash, pruritus

Gastrointestinal: Nausea, vomiting, GI upset; unusual taste (one patient)

Local: Injection site reactions, stinging; phlebitis

Neuromuscular & skeletal: Paresthesia

Ocular: Blurred vision

Miscellaneous: Hypersensitivity reactions, anaphylaxis (see Precautions); allergic vasomotor reactions, edema, development of inhibitor antibodies (3% to 52%); inhibitor antibodies are IgG immunoglobulins that neutralize the activity of factor VIII; an increase of inhibitor antibody concentration is seen at 2-7 days, with peak concentrations at 1-3 weeks after therapy. Children <5 years of age are at greatest risk; higher doses of AHF may be needed if antibody is present; if antibody concentration is >10 Bethesda units/mL, patients may not respond to larger doses and alternative treatment modalities may be needed (see Additional Information).

Drug Interactions

Avoid Concomitant Use There are no known interactions where it is recommended to avoid concomitant use.

Increased Effect/Toxicity There are no known significant interactions involving an increase in effect.

Decreased Effect There are no known significant interactions involving a decrease in effect.

Stability

Storage: Store unopened vials under refrigeration 2°C to 8°C (36°F to 46°F); avoid freezing (to prevent damage to diluent vial)

Hemofil M: May also be stored at room temperature (≤30°C or 86°F)

Koāte®-DVI: May also be stored at room temperature (≤25°C or 77°F) for up to 6 months

Monarc-M™: May also be stored at room temperature (≤30°C or 86°F) for up to 12 months

Monoclate-P®: May also be stored at room temperature (≤30°C or 86°F) for up to 6 months

Reconstitution: If refrigerated, the dried concentrate and diluent should be warmed to room temperature before reconstitution; see individual product labeling for specific reconstitution guidelines; gently agitate or rotate vial after adding diluent, do not shake vigorously (**Note:** For Koāte®-DVI: Swirl vigorously without creating excessive foaming); use filter needle provided by manufacturer to draw product into syringe; use one filter needle per vial; do **not** refrigerate after reconstitution (precipitation may occur); administer within 3 hours after reconstitution; **Note:** Use plastic syringes, since AHF may stick to the surface of glass syringes

Mechanism of Action Factor VIII is a protein in normal plasma which is necessary for clot formation and maintenance of hemostasis; it activates factor X in conjunction with activated factor IX; activated factor X converts prothrombin to thrombin, which converts fibrinogen to fibrin and with factor XIII forms a stable clot

Pharmacodynamics Maximum effect: 1-2 hours

Pharmacokinetics (Adult data unless noted)

Distribution: Does not readily cross the placenta

Half-life: 4-24 hours; mean = 12 hours (biphasic)

Usual Dosage Children and Adults: I.V.: Individualize dosage based on coagulation studies performed prior to and during treatment at regular intervals:

Hemophilia A: For every 1 international unit per kg body weight of AHF (human) administered, factor VIII level should increase by 2%; calculated dosage should be adjusted to the actual vial size

Formula to calculate dosage required, based on desired increase in factor VIII (% of normal) (**Note:** This formula assumes that the patient's baseline AHF level is <1%):

International units required = Body weight (kg) x 0.5 x desired increase in factor VIII (international units/dL or % of normal)

Hospitalized patients: 20-50 units/kg/dose; may be higher for special circumstances. Dose can be given every 12-24 hours and more frequently in special circumstances.

Hemophilia A with high titer of inhibitor antibody: 50-75 units/kg/hour has been given

General dosing guidelines (consult individual product labeling for specific dosage recommendations):

Minor hemorrhage (required peak postinfusion AHF level: 20% to 40%): 10-20 international units/kg; repeat every 12-24 hours for 1-3 days until bleeding is resolved or healing achieved; mild superficial or early hemorrhages may respond to a single dose

Moderate hemorrhage (required peak postinfusion AHF level: 30% to 60%): 15-30 international units/kg; repeat every 12-24 hours for ≥3 days until pain and disability are resolved

Alternatively (to achieve peak postinfusion AHF level: 50%) Initial: 25 international units/kg; maintenance: 10-15 international units/kg every 8-12 hours

Severe/life-threatening hemorrhage (required peak postinfusion AHF level: 60% to 100%): 30-50 international units/kg; repeat every 8-24 hours until threat is resolved

Alternatively (to achieve peak postinfusion AHF level: 80% to 100%): 40-50 international units/kg; maintenance: 20-25 international units/kg every 8-12 hours

Minor surgery (required peak postinfusion AHF level: Range 30% to 80%): 15-40 international units/kg; dose is highly dependent upon procedure and specific product recommendations; for some procedures, a single dose plus oral antifibrinolytic therapy within 1 hour is sufficient; in other procedures, may repeat dose every 12-24 hours as needed

Major surgery (required peak pre- and postsurgery AHF level: 80% to 100%): 40-50 international units/kg; repeat every 8-24 hours depending on state of healing

Prophylaxis: May also be given on a regular schedule to prevent bleeding

Administration Parenteral: I.V. administration only; see Stability for reconstitution and dosage preparation; administer through a separate line, do not mix with drugs or other I.V. fluids

Maximum rate of administration is product dependent:

Hemofil® M, Monarc-M™: 10 mL/minute

Monoclate-P®: 2 mL/minute

Koate®-DVI: Total dose may be given over 5-10 minutes; adjust administration rate based on patient response

Monitoring Parameters Bleeding; heart rate and blood pressure (before and during I.V. administration); AHF levels prior to and during treatment; monitor for development of inhibitor antibodies by clinical observation (eg, inadequate control of bleeding with adequate doses) and laboratory tests (eg, inhibitor level, Bethesda assay); see Additional Information. In patients with blood groups A, B, or AB who receive large or frequent doses, monitor Hct, direct Coombs' test, and signs of intravascular hemolysis

Reference Range

Plasma antihemophilic factor level:

Normal range: 50% to 150%

Level to prevent spontaneous hemorrhage: 5%

Required peak postinfusion AHF activity in blood (as % of normal or units/dL plasma):

Early hemarthrosis, muscle bleed, or oral bleed: 20% to 40%

More extensive hemarthrosis, muscle bleed, or hematoma: 30% to 60%

Life-threatening bleeds (such as head injury, throat bleed, severe abdominal pain): 80% to 100%

Minor surgery, including tooth extraction: 60% to 80%

Major surgery: 80% to 100% (pre- and postoperative)

Patient Information This medication can only be given intravenously. Stop taking antihemophilic factor human and notify physician immediately if any of the following signs or symptoms of an allergic (hypersensitivity) reaction occur: Itching, hives, low blood pressure, tightness in chest, wheezing, or anaphylaxis. Wear identification indicating that you have a hemophilic condition.

Nursing Implications Reduce rate of administration or temporarily discontinue if patient experiences tachycardia or any other adverse reaction; allergic type hypersensitivity reactions (eg, hives, chest tightness, itching, wheezing, dyspnea, faintness, hypotension, anaphylaxis) may occur (see Precautions)

Additional Information One international unit of AHF is equal to the factor VIII activity present in 1 mL of normal human plasma. If bleeding is not controlled with adequate dose, test for the presence of factor VIII inhibitor; larger doses of AHF may be therapeutic with inhibitor titers <10 Bethesda units/mL; it may not be possible or practical to control bleeding if inhibitor titers >10 Bethesda units/mL (due to the very large AHF doses required); other treatments [eg, antihemophilic factor (porcine), factor IX complex concentrates, recombinant factor VIIa, or anti-inhibitor coagulant complex] may be needed in patients with inhibitor titers >10 Bethesda units/mL.

Dosage Forms Excipient information presented when available (limited, particularly for generics); consult specific product labeling.

Injection, powder for reconstitution:

Hemofil M: Vial labeled with international units [contains albumin; derived from mouse proteins; packaging may contain natural rubber latex]

Koate®-DVI: ~250 int. units, ~500 int. units, ~1000 int. units [contains albumin]

Monarc-M™: Vial labeled with international units [contains albumin; derived from mouse proteins; packaging may contain natural rubber latex]

Monoclate-P®: ~250 int. units, ~500 int. units, ~1000 int. units, ~1500 int. units [contains albumin; derived from mouse proteins]

References

Liesner RJ, "Prophylaxis in Haemophilic Children," *Blood Coagul Fibrinolysis*, 1997, 8(Suppl 1):S7-10.

Scharrer I, Bray GL, and Neutzling O, "Incidence of Inhibitors in Haemophilia A Patients–A Review of Recent Studies of Recombinant and Plasma-Derived Factor VIII Concentrates," *Haemophilia*, 1999, 5 (3):145-54.

Shord SS and Lindley CM, "Coagulation Products and Their Uses," *Am J Health Syst Pharm*, 2000, 57(15):1403-20.

Antihemophilic Factor (Recombinant)

(an tee hee moe FIL ik FAK tor ree KOM be nant)

Medication Safety Issues Confusion may occur due to the omitting of "Factor VIII" from some product labeling. Review product contents carefully prior to dispensing any antihemophilic factor.

U.S. Brand Names Advate; Helixate® FS; Kogenate® FS; Recombinate; ReFacto® [DSC]; Xyntha™

Canadian Brand Names Advate; Helixate® FS; Kogenate®; Kogenate® FS; Recombinate; ReFacto®

Therapeutic Category Antihemophilic Agent

Generic Available No

Use Note: Antihemophilic Factor (Recombinant) is not indicated for the treatment of von Willebrand disease.

Advate: Prevention and control of hemorrhagic episodes in patients with hemophilia A (FDA approved in ages 0-16 years and adults); perioperative management of patients with hemophilia A (FDA approved in ages 0-16 years and adults)

Helixate® FS, Kogenate® FS: Prevention and control of hemorrhagic episodes in patients with hemophilia A (FDA approved in ages 0-16 and adults); perioperative management of patients with hemophilia A (FDA approved in ages 0-16 years and adults); prophylaxis of joint bleeding and reduction of the risk of joint damage in children with hemophilia A with no pre-existing joint damage (FDA approved in ages 0-16 years)

Recombinate™, ReFacto®: Prevention and control of hemorrhagic episodes in patients with hemophilia A (FDA approved in all ages); perioperative management of patients with hemophilia A (FDA approved in all ages)

Xyntha™: Prevention and control of hemorrhagic episodes in patients with hemophilia A (FDA approved in adults); perioperative management of patients with hemophilia A (FDA approved in adults)

Has also been used in patients with acquired factor VIII inhibitors <10 Bethesda units/mL

Pregnancy Risk Factor C

Pregnancy Considerations Animal reproduction studies have not been conducted. Safety and efficacy in pregnant women has not been established. Use during pregnancy only if clearly needed.

Lactation Excretion in breast milk unknown/use caution

Contraindications

All products: Hypersensitivity or intolerance to any component (see Warnings and table)

Advate; Helixate® FS; Kogenate® FS: Hypersensitivity to mouse or hamster protein

Recombinate™; ReFacto®: Hypersensitivity to mouse, hamster, or bovine protein

Warnings Recombinate™ contains natural rubber latex (in certain components of the product packaging) which may cause allergic reactions in susceptible individuals; avoid use in patients with allergy to latex.

Precautions Clinical response to recommended doses may vary; dosage must be individualized based on coagulation studies (performed prior to treatment and at regular intervals during treatment) and clinical response. Formation of factor VIII inhibitors (neutralizing antibodies to AHF recombinant) may occur; antibody formation may occur at any time, but is more common in young children with severe hemophilia during the first years of therapy, or in patients at any age who received little prior therapy with factor VIII; monitor patients appropriately (see Monitoring Parameters and Additional Information). Although remote, formation of antibodies to mouse, hamster, or bovine protein may occur (products may contain trace amounts of these proteins). Allergic type hypersensitivity reactions,

including anaphylaxis may occur; discontinue therapy immediately if urticaria, hives, hypotension, tightness of the chest, wheezing or anaphylaxis develop; emergency treatment and resuscitative measures (eg, epinephrine, oxygen) may be needed. Products vary by preparation method (see table). Recombinate™ formulation is stabilized using human albumin; Helixate® FS, Kogenate® FS, ReFacto®, and Xyntha™ formulations are stabilized using sucrose.

Antihemophilic Factor (Recombinant) [Factor VIII (Recombinant)] Products

Product	Synthesis	Purification Methods	Stabilizers and Excipients
Advate	• Recombinant DNA technology • Chinese hamster ovary (CHO) cell line • Plasma/albumin - free method	• Solvent/detergent virus inactivation • Column chromatography • Monoclonal antibody immunoaffinity chromatography	• Mannitol[1] • Trehalose[1] • Sodium[1] • Histidine[1] • Tris[1] • Calcium[1] • Polysorbate-80[1] • Glutathione[1] • von Willebrand factor (insignificant amounts)[1]
Helixate® FS	• Recombinant DNA technology • Baby hamster kidney (BHK) cells • Human plasma protein solution (HPPS) and recombinant insulin in cell culture medium	• Solvent/detergent virus inactivation • Ion exchange chromatography • Monoclonal antibody immunoaffinity chromatography • Other chromatographic steps	• Sucrose[1] • Glycine[1] • Histidine[1] • Calcium chloride • Sodium • Chloride • Polysorbate-80 • Imidazole • Tri-n-butyl phosphate • Copper
Kogenate® FS	• Recombinant DNA technology • Baby hamster kidney (BHK) cells • Human plasma protein solution (HPPS) and recombinant insulin in cell culture medium	• Solvent/detergent virus inactivation • Ion exchange chromatography • Monoclonal antibody immunoaffinity chromatography • Other chromatographic steps	• Sucrose[1] • Glycine[1] • Histidine[1] • Calcium • Sodium • Chloride • Polysorbate-80 • Imidazole • Tri-n-butyl phosphate • Copper
Recombinate™	• Recombinant DNA technology • Chinese hamster ovary (CHO) cell line	• Column chromatography • Monoclonal antibody immunoaffinity chromatography	• Albumin (human)[1] • Calcium[1] • Polyethylene glycol[1] • Sodium[1] • Histidine[1] • Polysorbate-80[1] • von Willebrand factor[1] (insignificant amounts)
ReFacto®	• Recombinant DNA technology • Chinese hamster ovary (CHO) cell line • Human serum albumin and recombinant insulin in cell culture medium	• Chromatography	• Sodium chloride • Sucrose • L-histadine • Calcium chloride • Polysorbate-80
Xyntha™	• Recombinant DNA technology • Chinese hamster ovary (CHO) cell line	• Chromatography • Solvent/detergent virus inactivation • Virus nanofiltration	• Sodium chloride • Sucrose • L-histadine • Calcium chloride • Polysorbate-80

[1]Listed as a stabilizer in the product's package insert.

Adverse Reactions

Cardiovascular: Angina pectoris, flushing, vasodilation

Central nervous system: Asthenia, chills, dizziness, headache, lethargy

Dermatologic: Pruritus, rash, urticaria

Gastrointestinal: Diarrhea, nausea, sore throat, unusual taste, vomiting

Hepatic: Aminotransferase increased, bilirubin increased

Local: Injection site reactions (burning, erythema, inflammation, pain, pruritus)

Neuromuscular & skeletal: Muscle weakness, paresthesia

Ocular: Abnormal vision

Respiratory: Cough, epistaxis, rhinitis

Miscellaneous: Adenopathy, allergic reactions (including bronchospasm, hypotension), anaphylaxis, cold feet, CPK increased, development of inhibitor antibodies, diaphoresis, permanent venous catheter access complications; **Note:** Inhibitor antibodies are IgG immunoglobulins that neutralize the activity of factor VIII; higher doses of AHF recombinant may be needed if antibody is present; if antibody concentration is >10 Bethesda units/ mL, patients may not respond to larger doses and alternative treatment modalities may be needed (see Additional Information)

<1%, postmarketing, and/or case reports: Abdominal pain, anemia, anorexia, arthralgia, blood pressure decreased, chest discomfort, chest pain, constipation, depersonalization, edema, facial edema, facial flushing, fatigue, fever, GI hemorrhage, hives, hot flashes, hyper-/hypotension (slight), hypersensitivity reaction, infection, joint swelling, otitis media, pallor, restlessness, rigors, shortness of breath, somnolence, tachycardia, urinary tract infection

Drug Interactions

Avoid Concomitant Use There are no known interactions where it is recommended to avoid concomitant use.

Increased Effect/Toxicity There are no known significant interactions involving an increase in effect.

Decreased Effect There are no known significant interactions involving a decrease in effect.

Stability

Storage: Store unopened vials under refrigeration 2°C to 8°C (36°F to 46°F); avoid freezing

Advate: May also be stored at room temperature [22°C to 28°C (72°F to 82°F)] for up to 6 months

Helixate® FS, Kogenate® FS, ReFacto®, Xyntha™: May also be stored at room temperature (≤25°C or 77°F) for up to 3 months. Avoid extreme or prolonged exposure to light during storage (store drug in carton before use). Kogenate® FS: Do not return vials to refrigeration, once removed from refrigeration

Recombinate™: May also be stored at room temperature (≤30°C or 86°F)

Mechanism of Action Antihemophilic factor (recombinant) has the same biological activity as AHF (factor VIII) derived from human plasma; factor VIII is a protein in normal plasma which is necessary for clot formation and maintenance of hemostasis; factor VIII activates factor X in conjunction with activated factor IX; activated factor X converts prothrombin to thrombin, which converts fibrinogen to fibrin, and with factor XIII forms a stable clot

Pharmacokinetics (Adult data unless noted) Half-life:

Children 4-18 years of age (mean age: 12 years): Mean: 10.7 hours (range: 7.8-15.3)

Adults: Mean: 11-16 hours

Usual Dosage Neonates, Infants, Children, and Adults: I.V.: **Individualize dosage based on coagulation studies performed prior to treatment and at regular intervals during treatment;** for every 1 international unit per kg body weight of rAHF administered, factor VIII level should increase by 2%; calculated dosage should be adjusted to the actual vial size

Formula to calculate dosage required, based on desired increase in factor VIII (% of normal) (**Note:** This formula assumes that the patient's baseline AHF level is <1%): International units required = body weight (kg) x 0.5 x desired increase in factor VIII (international units/dL or % of normal)

General dosing guidelines (consult individual product labeling for specific dosage recommendations):

Minor hemorrhage (required peak postinfusion AHF level: 20% to 40%): 10-20 international units/kg; repeat every 12-24 hours for 1-3 days until bleeding is resolved or healing achieved; mild, superficial, or early hemorrhages may respond to a single dose

Moderate hemorrhage (required peak post-infusion AHF level: 30% to 60%): 15-30 international units/kg, repeat every 12-24 hours for 3-4 days until pain and disability are resolved

Severe/life-threatening hemorrhage:

Helixate® FS, Kogenate® FS (required peak post-infusion AHF level: 80% to 100%): Initial: 40-50 international units/kg; maintenance: 20-25 international units/kg every 8-12 hours until bleeding is resolved

Advate, Recombinate™, ReFacto®, Xyntha™ (required peak post-infusion AHF level: 60% to 100%): 30-50 international units/kg; repeat every 8-24 hours until threat is resolved

Minor surgery (required peak postinfusion AHF level: range: 30% to 80%): 15-40 international units/kg; dose is highly dependent upon procedure and specific product recommendations; for some procedures, a single dose plus oral antifibrinolytic therapy within 1 hour is sufficient; in other procedures, may repeat dose every 12-24 hours until bleeding is resolved

Major surgery:

Advate (required peak pre- and postsurgery AHF level: 80% to 120%): 40-60 international units/kg; repeat every 8-24 hours depending on state of healing

Helixate® FS, Kogenate® FS (required peak pre- and postsurgery AHF level: 100%): 50 international units/kg; may repeat every 6-12 hours initially and until healing complete (10-14 days); intensity of regimen is dependent on type of surgery and postoperative care

Recombinate™, ReFacto® (required peak pre- and post-surgery AHF level: 80% to 100%): 40-50 international units/kg; repeat every 8-24 hours depending on state of healing

Xyntha™ (required peak pre- and postsurgery AHF level: 60% to 100%): 30-50 international units/kg; repeat every 8-24 hours depending on state of healing

Prophylaxis: May also be given on a regular schedule to prevent bleeding

Joint bleeding prophylaxis: Children with no pre-existing joint damage: Helixate® FS, Kogenate® FS: 25 international units/kg given every other day

Administration

Reconstitution: If refrigerated, the dried concentrate and diluent should be warmed to room temperature before reconstitution; see individual product labeling for specific reconstitution guidelines; gently agitate or rotate vial after adding diluent, do not shake vigorously. Use filter needle provided by manufacturer to draw product into syringe (all products except Xyntha™); do **not** refrigerate after reconstitution; administer within 3 hours after reconstitution; **Note:** Use plastic syringes, since rAHF may stick to the surface of glass syringes

Parenteral: I.V. administration only; total dose may be administered over 5-10 minutes; Advate may be administered over ≤5 minutes; Helixate® FS and Kogenate® FS may be administered over 1-15 minutes; maximum rate of infusion (all products): 10 mL/minute; adjust administration rate based on patient response (all products); for Advate, Helixate® FS, Kogenate® FS, and ReFacto®, use sterile administration set provided by manufacturer

Monitoring Parameters Bleeding; heart rate and blood pressure (before and during I.V. administration); AHF levels prior to and during treatment; monitor for the development of inhibitor antibodies by clinical observations (eg, inadequate control of bleeding with adequate doses) and laboratory tests (eg, inhibitor level, Bethesda assay); see Additional Information

Reference Range

Plasma antihemophilic factor level:

Normal range: 50% to 150%

Level to prevent spontaneous hemorrhage: 5%

Required peak post-infusion AHF activity in blood (as % of normal or units/dL plasma):

Early hemarthrosis, muscle bleed, or oral bleed: 20% to 40%

More extensive hemarthrosis, muscle bleed, or hematoma: 30% to 60%

Life-threatening bleeds (such as head injury, throat bleed, severe abdominal pain): 80% to 100%

Minor surgery, including tooth extraction: 60% to 80%

Major surgery: 80% to 100% (pre- and postoperative)

Patient Information This medication can only be given intravenously. Stop taking antihemophilic factor recombinant and notify physician immediately if any of the following signs or symptoms of an allergic (hypersensitivity) reaction occur: Itching, hives, low blood pressure, tightness of the chest, wheezing, or anaphylaxis. Wear identification indicating that you have a hemophilic condition.

Nursing Implications Reduce rate of administration, or temporarily discontinue, if patient experiences tachycardia or any other adverse reaction; allergic type hypersensitivity reactions (eg, hives, chest tightness, itching, wheezing, dyspnea, faintness, hypotension, anaphylaxis) may occur (see Precautions)

Additional Information One international unit of rAHF is equal to the factor VIII activity present in 1 mL of fresh pooled human plasma. If bleeding is not controlled with adequate dose, test for the presence of factor VIII inhibitor; larger doses of rAHF may be therapeutic with inhibitor titers <10 Bethesda units/mL; it may not be possible or practical to control bleeding if inhibitor titers >10 Bethesda units/mL (due to the very large rAHF doses required); other treatments [eg, antihemophilic factor (porcine), factor IX complex concentrates, recombinant factor VIIa, or anti-inhibitor coagulant complex] may be needed in patients with inhibitor titers >10 Bethesda units/mL

Dosage Forms Excipient information presented when available (limited, particularly for generics); consult specific product labeling. [DSC] = Discontinued product

Injection, powder for reconstitution, recombinant [preservative free]:

Advate: 250 int. units, 500 int. units, 1000 int. units, 1500 int. units, 2000 int. units, 3000 int. units [plasma/albumin free; contains polysorbate 80, sodium 108 mEq/L, mannitol; derived from hamster or mouse proteins]

Helixate® FS: 250 int. units, 500 int. units, 1000 int. units, 2000 int. unit, 3000 int. units [contains sucrose 28-52 mg/vial, sodium 26-36 mEq/L, polysorbate 80; derived from hamster or mouse protein]

Kogenate® FS: 250 int. units, 500 int. units, 1000 int. units, 2000 int. units, 3000 int. units [contains sucrose 28-56 mg/vial, sodium 27-36 mEq/L, polysorbate 80; derived from hamster or mouse protein]

Recombinate: 250 int. units, 500 int. units, 1000 int. units [contains human albumin, sodium 180 mEq/L, polysorbate 80; derived from bovine, hamster or mouse proteins; packaging contains natural rubber latex]

ReFacto®: 250 int. units, 500 int. units, 1000 int. units, 2000 int. units [contains polysorbate 80, sucrose; derived from hamster or mouse proteins] [DSC]

Xyntha™: 250 int. units, 500 int. units, 1000 int. units, 2000 int. units [albumin free; contains sucrose, polysorbate 80; derived from hamster proteins]

References

Abshire TC, Brackmann HH, Scharrer I, et al, "Sucrose Formulated Recombinant Human Antihemophilic Factor VIII is Safe and Efficacious for Treatment of Hemophilia A in Home Therapy. International Kogenate-FS Study Group," *Thromb Haemost*, 2000, 83(6):811-6.

Bray GL, Gomperts ED, Courter S, et al, "A Multicenter Study of Recombinant Factor VIII (Recombinate): Safety, Efficacy, and Inhibitor Risk in Previously Untreated Patients With Hemophilia A. The Recombinate Study Group," *Blood*, 1994, 83(9):2428-35.

Kelly KM, Butler RB, Farace L, et al, "Superior In Vivo Response of Recombinant Factor VIII Concentrate in Children With Hemophilia A," *J Pediatr*, 1997, 130(4):537-40.

Liesner RJ, "Prophylaxis in Haemophilic Children," *Blood Coagul Fibrinolysis*, 1997, 8(Suppl 1):S7-10.

Scharrer I, Bray GL, and Neutzling O, "Incidence of Inhibitors in Haemophilia A Patients - A Review of Recent Studies of Recombinant and Plasma-Derived Factor VIII Concentrates," *Haemophilia*, 1999, 5 (3):145-54.

Shord SS and Lindley CM, "Coagulation Products and Their Uses," *Am J Health Syst Pharm*, 2000, 57(15):1403-20.

Schwartz RS, Abildgaard CF, Aledort LM, et al, "Human Recombinant DNA-Derived Antihemophilic Factor (Factor VIII) in the Treatment of Hemophilia A. Recombinant Factor VIII Study Group," *N Engl J Med*, 1990, 323(26):1800-5.

Antihemophilic Factor / von Willebrand Factor Complex (Human)

(an tee hee moe FIL ik FAK tor von WILL le brand FAK tor KOM plex HYU man)

U.S. Brand Names Alphanate®; Humate-P®

Canadian Brand Names Humate-P®

Therapeutic Category Antihemophilic Agent; Blood Product Derivative

Generic Available No

Use

Acquired factor VIII deficiency (Alphanate®): Prevention and treatment of hemorrhagic episodes.

Hemophilia A (Alphanate®, Humate-P®): Prevention and treatment of hemorrhagic episodes.

von Willebrand disease (vWD):

Alphanate®: Prophylaxis for surgical and/or invasive procedures in patients with vWD when desmopressin is either ineffective or contraindicated. **Note:** Alphanate® is **not** indicated for patients with severe vWD (type 3) who are undergoing major surgery.

Humate-P®: Treatment of spontaneous and trauma-induced hemorrhagic episodes and prevention of excessive perioperative bleeding in patients with mild-to-moderate and severe vWD where the use of desmopressin is suspected or known to be inadequate.

Pregnancy Risk Factor C

Pregnancy Considerations Reproduction studies have not been conducted. Safety and efficacy in pregnant women have not been established. Use during pregnancy only if clearly needed. Parvovirus B19 or hepatitis A, which may be present in plasma-derived products, may affect a pregnant woman more seriously than nonpregnant women.

Lactation Excretion in breast milk unknown/use caution

Contraindications History of anaphylactic or severe systemic response to antihemophilic factor or von Willebrand factor products; hypersensitivity to any component; see table

Antihemophilic Factor / von Willebrand Factor Complex (Human) Product

Product	Preparation and Purification Methods	Viral Inactivation	Stabilizers and Excipients
Alphanate®	• Purified from pooled human plasma	• Cryoprecipitation • Fractional solubilization • Precipitation with 3.5% polyethylene glycol • Heparin coupled, cross-linked agarose chromatography • Solvent detergent treatment with tri-n-butyl phosphate and polysorbate 80 • Dry heat treatment 80°C x 72 hours	• Albumin (human) • Calcium • Glycine • Heparin • Histidine • Imidazole • Arginine • Polyethylene glycol • Polysorbate 80 • Sodium • Tri-n-butyl phosphate
Humate-P®	• Purified from cold insoluble fraction of fresh-frozen plasma	• Cryoprecipitation • Aluminum hydroxide adsorption, glycine precipitation and sodium chloride precipitation • Heat treatment in aqueous solution (pasteurization; 60°C x 10 hours)	• Glycine • Sodium citrate • Sodium chloride • Albumin (human) • Other proteins • Fibrinogen (<0.2 mg/mL)

Note: Source of all products is pooled human plasma.

Warnings Thromboembolic events in patients with von Willebrand disease receiving antihemophilic factor/von Willebrand factor complex have been reported; risk of these events may be higher in patients with other risk factors for thrombosis and in females; use antihemophilic factor/von Willebrand factor complex with caution in these patients; consider antithrombotic measures

Precautions Human antihemophilic factor/von Willebrand factor complex is prepared from pooled plasma; even with heat treated or other viral attenuated processes, the risk of viral transmission (ie, viral hepatitis, HIV, parvovirus B19, and theoretically, Creutzfeldt-Jacob disease agent) is not totally eradicated. Hepatitis B vaccination is recommended for all patients receiving human antihemophilic factor/von Willebrand factor complex and hepatitis A vaccination is recommended for seronegative patients. Progressive anemia and hemolysis may occur in individuals with blood groups A, B, and AB who receive large or frequent doses of human antihemophilic factor/von Willebrand factor complex due to trace amounts of blood group A and B isohemagglutinins (see Monitoring Parameters).

Formation of factor VIII inhibitors (neutralizing antibodies to AHF human) may occur (see Adverse Reactions); the risk of developing alloantibodies to von Willebrand factor after using this product is not known; monitor patients appropriately (see Monitoring Parameters); optimal dosage should be determined by clinical response. Allergic-type hypersensitivity reactions are possible; discontinue therapy immediately if urticaria, hives, hypotension, tightness of the chest, wheezing, dyspnea, faintness, or anaphylaxis develop.

Adverse Reactions

Cardiovascular: Edema, chest tightness, thromboembolic events, vasodilation, orthostatic hypotension, hypervolemia

Central nervous system: Fever, chills, headache, dizziness, somnolence, lethargy, pain

Dermatologic: Urticaria, rash, pruritus

Gastrointestinal: Nausea, vomiting

Hematologic: Pseudothrombocytopenia (platelet clumping with a false low reading)

Hepatic: SGPT elevated (one possible case reported)

Local: Phlebitis, stinging at infusion site

Neuromuscular & skeletal: Paresthesia, extremity pain, joint pain

Respiratory: Dyspnea, pharyngitis, pulmonary embolus (large doses)

Ocular: Blurred vision

Miscellaneous: Hypersensitivity reactions, anaphylaxis (see Precautions); development of inhibitor antibodies to factor VIII; inhibitor antibodies are IgG immunoglobulins that neutralize the activity of factor VIII; an increase of inhibitor antibody concentration is seen at 2-7 days, with peak concentrations at 1-3 weeks after therapy. Children <5 years of age are at greatest risk; higher doses of AHF may be needed if antibody is present; if antibody concentration is >10 Bethesda units/mL, patients may not respond to larger doses and alternative treatment modalities may be needed (see Additional Information).

Drug Interactions

Avoid Concomitant Use There are no known interactions where it is recommended to avoid concomitant use.

Increased Effect/Toxicity There are no known significant interactions involving an increase in effect.

Decreased Effect There are no known significant interactions involving a decrease in effect.

Stability

Storage: Store unopened vials under refrigeration 2°C to 8°C (36°F to 46°F); avoid freezing (to prevent damage to diluent vial)

Alphanate®: May also be stored at room temperature (≤30°C or 86°F) for up to 2 months

Humate-P®: May also be stored at room temperature (≤30°C or 86°F) for up to 6 months

Reconstitution: If refrigerated, the dried concentrate and diluent should be warmed to room temperature before reconstitution; see product labeling for specific reconstitution guidelines; gently agitate or rotate vial after adding diluent, do not shake vigorously; administer within 3 hours after reconstitution; do **not** refrigerate after reconstitution, precipitation may occur; **Note:** Use plastic syringes, since AHF may stick to the surface of glass syringes. Discard unused contents and administration equipment after use.

Mechanism of Action Factor VIII and von Willebrand factor (vWF), obtained from pooled human plasma, are used to replace endogenous factor VIII and vWF in patients with hemophilia or vWD. Factor VIII is a protein in normal plasma which is necessary for clot formation and maintenance of hemostasis; it activates factor X in conjunction with activated factor IX; activated factor X converts prothrombin to thrombin, which converts fibrinogen to fibrin and with factor XIII forms a stable clot. vWF promotes platelet aggregation and adhesion to damaged vascular endothelium and acts as a stabilizing carrier protein for factor VIII. [Circulating levels of functional vWF are measured as ristocetin cofactor activity (vWF:RCof)]

Pharmacodynamics Maximum effect: 1-2 hours

Pharmacokinetics (Adult data unless noted) Half-life, elimination:

FVIII:C: 8-17 hours (mean: 12 hours) in patients with hemophilia

VWF:RCof: 3-34 hours (median: 10 hours) in patients with vWD

◀ **Usual Dosage** Children and Adults: I.V.: Individualize dosage based on coagulation studies performed prior to and during treatment at regular intervals:

Hemophilia A: For every 1 international unit per kg body weight of factor VIII activity (FVIII) administered, factor VIII level should increase by 2 international units/dL (or 2%); calculated dosage should be adjusted to the actual vial size

Formula to calculate dosage required, based on desired increase in factor VIII (% of normal) (**Note:** This formula assumes that the patient's baseline AHF level is <1%): International units required = Body weight (kg) x 0.5 x desired increase in factor VIII (international units/dL or % of normal)

General dosing guidelines (consult individual product labeling for specific dosage recommendations):

Minor hemorrhage: Loading dose: FVIII:C 15 international units/kg to achieve FVIII:C plasma level ~30% of normal. One infusion may be adequate. If second infusion is needed, half the loading dose may be given once or twice daily for 1-2 days.

Moderate hemorrhage: Loading dose: FVIII:C 25 international units/kg to achieve FVIII:C plasma level ~50% of normal. Maintenance: FVIII:C 15 international units/kg every 8-12 hours for 1-2 days in order to maintain FVIII:C plasma levels at 30% of normal. Repeat the same dose once or twice daily for up to 7 days or until adequate wound healing.

Life-threatening hemorrhage: Loading dose: FVIII:C 40-50 international units/kg. Maintenance: FVIII:C 20-25 international units/kg every 8 hours to maintain FVIII:C plasma levels at 80% to 100% of normal for 7 days. Continue same dose once or twice daily for another 7 days in order to maintain FVIII:C levels at 30% to 50% of normal.

von Willebrand disease (vWD): Treatment (Humate-P®): Children and Adults: I.V.: Individualize dosage based on coagulation studies performed prior to treatment and at regular intervals during treatment. In general, for every 1 international unit per kg body weight of factor VIII administered, von Willebrand factor: Ristocetin cofactor (vWF:RCof) level should increase by approximately 5 international units/dL

Type 1, mild (if desmopressin is not appropriate; baseline vWF:RCof activity usually >30%): Major hemorrhage:

Loading dose: vWF:RCof 40-60 international units/kg

Maintenance dose: vWF:RCof 40-50 international units/kg every 8-12 hours for 3 days, keeping vWF: RCof trough level >50%; follow with vWF:RCof 40-50 international units/kg daily for up to 7 days

Type 1, moderate or severe (baseline vWF:RCof activity usually <30%):

Minor hemorrhage: vWF:RCof 40-50 international units/kg for 1-2 doses

Major hemorrhage:

Loading dose: vWF:RCof 50-75 international units/kg

Maintenance dose: vWF:RCof 40-60 international units/kg every 8-12 hours for 3 days keeping vWF: RCof trough level >50%; follow with vWF:RCof 40-60 international units/kg daily for up to 7 days

Types 2 (all variants) and 3:

Minor hemorrhage: vWF:RCof 40-50 international units/kg for 1-2 doses

Major hemorrhage:

Loading dose: vWF:RCof 60-80 international units/kg

Maintenance dose: vWF:RCof 40-60 international units/kg every 8-12 hours for 3 days, keeping vWF: RCof trough level >50%; follow with vWF:RCof 40-60 international units/kg daily for up to 7 days

von Willebrand disease (vWD): Surgery/procedure prophylaxis (except patients with type 3 undergoing major surgery) (Alphanate®):

Children: I.V.:

Preoperative dose: vWF:RCof 75 international units/kg 1 hour prior to surgery

Maintenance dose: vWF:RCof 50-75 international units/kg every 8-12 hours as clinically needed. May reduce dose after third postoperative day; continue treatment until healing is complete.

Adults: I.V.:

Preoperative dose: vWF:RCof 60 international units/kg 1 hour prior to surgery

Maintenance dose: vWF:RCof 40-60 international units/kg every 8-12 hours as clinically needed. May reduce dose after third postoperative day; continue treatment until healing is complete. For minor procedures, maintain vWF of 40% to 50% during postoperative days 1-3; for major procedures maintain vWF of 40% to 50% for ≥3-7 days postoperative.

von Willebrand disease (vWD): Surgery/procedure prevention of bleeding (Humate-P®): Children and Adults: I.V.:

Emergency surgery: Administer vWF:RCof 50-60 international units/kg; monitor trough coagulation factor levels for subsequent doses

Surgical management (nonemergency): **Note:** Whenever possible, the *in vivo* recovery (IVR) should be measured and baseline plasma vWF:RCof and FVIII:C should be assessed in all patients prior to surgery. The IVR is calculated as follows: Measure baseline plasma vWF: RCof; then infuse vWF:RCof 60 international units/kg I.V. at time zero; measure vWF:RCof at 30 minutes after infusion. IVR = (plasma vWF:RCof at 30 minutes minus plasma vWF:RCof at baseline) divided by 60 international units/kg. If individual IVR is not available, a standardized loading dose can be used based on assumed IVR of 2 international units/dL for every one vWF:RCof international unit/kg administered (see product labeling for further information).

Loading dose calculation is based on baseline target vWF:RCof: (Target peak vWF:RCof - Baseline vWF: RCof) x weight (in kg) / IVR = international units vWF: RCof required. Administer loading dose 1-2 hours prior to surgery.

Target concentrations for vWF:RCof following loading dose:

Major surgery: 100 international units/dL

Minor surgery: 50-60 international units/dL

Maintenance dose: Initial: 1/2 loading dose followed by dosing determined by target trough concentrations, generally every 8-12 hours.

Target maintenance trough vWF:RCof concentrations:

Major surgery: >50 international units/dL for up to 3 days, followed by >30 international units/dL for a minimum total treatment of 72 hours

Minor surgery: ≥30 international units/dL for a minimum duration of 48 hours

Oral surgery: ≥30 international units/dL for a minimum duration of 8-12 hours

Administration Parenteral: I.V. administration only; see Stability for reconstitution and dosage preparation; administer through a separate line, do not mix with drugs or other I.V. fluids. Infuse I.V. slowly. Maximum rate of administration: Alphanate®: 10 mL/minute; Humate-P®: 4 mL/minute

Monitoring Parameters Bleeding; heart rate and blood pressure (before and during I.V. administration). AHF levels prior to and during treatment. Monitor for development of inhibitor antibodies by clinical observation (eg, inadequate control of bleeding with adequate doses) and laboratory tests (eg, inhibitor level, Bethesda assay). In patients with blood groups A, B, or AB who receive large or frequent doses, monitor Hct, direct Coombs' test, and signs of intravascular hemolysis. vWF activity [circulating levels of functional vWF are measured as ristocetin cofactor activity (vWF:RCof)]

Reference Range
Hemophilia: Classification of hemophilia; normal is defined as 1 international unit/mL of factor VII:C:
Severe: Factor level <1% of normal
Moderate: Factor level 1% to 5% of normal
Mild: Factor level >5% to <40% of normal
Plasma antihemophilic factor level:
Normal range: 50% to 150%
Level to prevent spontaneous hemorrhage: 5%
Required peak postinfusion AHF activity in blood (as % of normal or units/dL plasma):
Early hemarthrosis, muscle bleed, or oral bleed: 20% to 40%
More extensive hemarthrosis, muscle bleed, or hematoma: 30% to 60%
Life-threatening bleeds (such as head injury, throat bleed, severe abdominal pain): 80% to 100%
Minor surgery, including tooth extraction: 60% to 80%
Major surgery: 80% to 100% (pre- and postoperative)
Von Willebrand disease: Classification of von Willebrand disease:
Severe forms: vWF:RCof <10 units/dL and factor VIII:C <20 units/dL
Moderate forms: vWF:RCof 10-30 units/dL and factor VIII:C 20-40 units/dL
Mild forms: vWF:RCof 30-50 units/dL and factor VIII:C 40-60 units/dL
Note: Circulating levels of functional VWF are measured as ristocetin cofactor activity (vWF:RCof)]

Patient Information This medication can only be given intravenously. Stop taking this medication and notify physician immediately if any of the following signs or symptoms of an allergic (hypersensitivity) reaction occur: Itching, hives, low blood pressure, tightness in chest, wheezing, or anaphylaxis. Report immediately any sudden-onset headache, chest or back pain, low-grade fever, stomach pain, or nausea/vomiting to prescriber. Wear identification indicating that you have a hemophilic condition.

Nursing Implications Assess potential for interactions with other pharmacological agents patient may be taking that may affect coagulation or platelet function. Hypersensitivity reactions (eg, hives, chest tightness, itching, wheezing, dyspnea, chills, fever, faintness, hypotension, anaphylaxis) may occur (see Precautions). Reduce rate of administration or temporarily discontinue if patient experiences tachycardia or any other adverse reaction. Patient should be monitored closely during and after infusion for any change in vital signs, cardiac and CNS status, or hypersensitivity reactions. Assess response [eg, results of laboratory tests (hematocrit and coagulation studies)], therapeutic effectiveness (bleeding and coagulation status), and adverse reactions (eg, bleeding or anemia).

Additional Information One international unit of AHF is equal to the factor VIII activity present in 1 mL of normal human plasma. If bleeding is not controlled with adequate dose, test for the presence of factor VIII inhibitor; larger doses of AHF may be therapeutic with inhibitor titers <10 Bethesda units/mL; it may not be possible or practical to control bleeding if inhibitor titers >10 Bethesda units/mL (due to the very large AHF doses required); other treatments [eg, antihemophilic factor (porcine), factor IX complex concentrates, recombinant factor VIIa, or anti-inhibitor coagulant complex] may be needed in patients with inhibitor titers >10 Bethesda units/mL.

Dosage Forms Excipient information presented when available (limited, particularly for generics); consult specific product labeling.

Injection, powder for reconstitution [human derived]:
Alphanate®:
250 int. units [Factor VIII and vWF:RCof ratio varies by lot; contains sodium ≥10 mEq/vial, albumin and polysorbate 80; packaged with diluent]
500 int. units [Factor VIII and vWF:RCof ratio varies by lot; contains sodium ≥10 mEq/vial, albumin and polysorbate 80; packaged with diluent]
1000 int. units [Factor VIII and vWF: RCof ratio varies by lot; contains sodium ≥10 mEq/vial, albumin and polysorbate 80; packaged with diluent]
1500 int. units [Factor VIII and vWF:RCof ratio varies by lot; contains sodium ≥10 mEq/vial, albumin and polysorbate 80; packaged with diluent]
Humate-P®:
FVIII 250 int. units and vWF:RCof 600 int. units [contains albumin; packaged with diluent]
FVIII 500 int. units and vWF:RCof 1200 int. units [contains albumin; packaged with diluent]
FVIII 1000 int. units and vWF:RCof 2400 int. units [contains albumin; packaged with diluent]

♦ **Anti-Hist [OTC]** see DiphenhydrAMINE on page 448

Anti-inhibitor Coagulant Complex
(an tee-in HI bi tor coe AG yoo lant KOM pleks)

U.S. Brand Names Feiba VH
Canadian Brand Names Feiba VH Immuno
Therapeutic Category Antihemophilic Agent; Blood Product Derivative
Generic Available No
Use Control of spontaneous bleeding episodes or to cover surgical interventions in hemophilia A and hemophilia B patients with factor VIII inhibitors
Pregnancy Risk Factor C
Pregnancy Considerations Reproduction studies have not been conducted.
Lactation Excretion in breast milk unknown/use caution
Contraindications Patients with a normal coagulation mechanism
Warnings Not for use in patients with bleeding episodes resulting from coagulation factor deficiencies without circulating inhibitors. Product is prepared from pooled human plasma; such plasma may contain the causative agents of viral diseases; risk of transmission is extremely rare. Reserve use for patients with circulating inhibitors to Factor VIII only. aPTT, WBCT, and TEG tests do not correlate with clinical efficacy; dosing to normalize these values may result in DIC. Discontinue immediately if symptoms of DIC occur. Thromboembolic events may occur, particularly following administration of high doses and/or in patients with thrombotic risk factors. Patients receiving single doses >100 units/kg or daily doses >200 units/kg must be monitored for the development of DIC and/or symptoms of acute coronary ischemia. Anamnestic rises in inhibitor (antibody) levels have been observed in 20% of the patients which may result in prolonged refractoriness to subsequent therapy. Transient hypofibrinogenemia has been reported in a few pediatric patients; all patients responded favorably to cryoprecipitate and did not develop DIC; measure fibrinogen levels in pediatric patients prior to initiation of therapy
Precautions Use with extreme caution in patients with thrombotic risk factors; hypotension may be more prevalent if administered more than one hour after reconstitution of anti-inhibitor coagulant complex due to increased prekallikrein activator activity; if infusion-related side effects occur (eg, headache, heart rate changes, hypotension or flushing), temporarily discontinue the infusion until the symptoms disappear and resume at a slower rate

Adverse Reactions
Cardiovascular: Hypotension, flushing, and tachycardia (related to the rate of infusion), chest pain, MI
Dermatologic: Rash, urticaria
Hematologic: DIC, thromboembolic events
Miscellaneous: Anaphylaxis

Drug Interactions

Avoid Concomitant Use
Avoid concomitant use of Anti-inhibitor Coagulant Complex with any of the following: Antifibrinolytic Agents

Increased Effect/Toxicity
The levels/effects of Anti-inhibitor Coagulant Complex may be increased by: Antifibrinolytic Agents

Decreased Effect There are no known significant interactions involving a decrease in effect.

Stability Refrigerate freeze-dried powder at 2°C to 8°C (36°F to 46°F); avoid freezing; do not refrigerate after reconstitution; stable at room temperature for up to 6 months

Mechanism of Action Anti-inhibitor coagulant complex contains varying amounts of factors II (prothrombin), VII (proconvertin or serum prothrombin conversion accelerator), IX (Christmas factor or plasma thromboplastin component), and X (Stuart-Prower factor) prepared from pooled human plasma. Factors VII and X may be activated or partially-activated forms. The exact mechanism of action is not completely known but has been described as "inhibitor bypassing activity".

Usual Dosage Dosage is dependent upon the severity and location of bleeding, type and level of inhibitors, and whether the patient has a history of an anamnestic increase in antihemophilic inhibitor levels following use of preparations containing antihemophilic factor. The two formulations listed below differ from each other in the amounts of their individual components but the clinical significance related to efficacy and/or adverse effects is unknown. In addition, each formulation uses a different method of standardization, so recommended dosages are not considered equivalent. The dosage recommendations below reflect the manufacturer's recommendations with duration of use dependent upon the patient's response.

Children and Adults: I.V.: 50-100 Feiba VH® immuno units/kg; not to exceed 200 Feiba VH® immuno units/kg/day; dosage may vary with the bleeding site and severity; see below:

Joint hemorrhage: 50 Feiba VH® immuno units/kg every 12 hours; may increase to 100 Feiba VH® immuno units/kg

Mucous membrane bleeding: 50 Feiba VH® immuno units/kg every 6 hours; may increase to 100 Feiba VH® immuno units/kg every 6 hours for only two doses; not to exceed 200 Feiba VH immuno units/kg/day

Soft tissue hemorrhage: 100 Feiba VH® immuno units/kg every 12 hours

Other severe hemorrhages: 100 Feiba VH® immuno units/kg every 6-12 hours

Administration I.V.: Reconstitute with provided diluent; swirl gently; do not shake; use within 3 hours of reconstitution; administer without further dilution. Maximum rate of infusion: 2 units/kg/minute

Monitoring Parameters Hemoglobin, hematocrit, bleeding at site, PTT, fibrinogen, platelets, fibrin split products, Factor VIII inhibitor levels

Reference Range Factor VIII inhibitor levels: <2 Bethesda Units (B.U.) antihemophilic factor is the preferred treatment agent; 2-10 B.U. either anti-inhibitor coagulant complex or antihemophilic factor may be used; >10 B.U. anti-inhibitor coagulant complex is the preferred treatment agent

Patient Information Report sudden onset headache, rash, chest or back pain, wheezing or respiratory difficulties, hives, itching, or acute feelings of anxiety. Wear identification indicating that you have a hemophilic condition.

Dosage Forms Excipient information presented when available (limited, particularly for generics); consult specific product labeling.
Injection, powder for reconstitution:
Feiba VH: Each bottle is labeled with Immuno units of factor VIII [heparin free; contains sodium 8 mg/mL; packaging contains natural rubber latex]

Antipyrine and Benzocaine
(an tee PYE reen & BEN zoe kane)

U.S. Brand Names A/B Otic; Allergen®; Aurodex [DSC]
Canadian Brand Names Auralgan®
Therapeutic Category Otic Agent, Analgesic; Otic Agent, Cerumenolytic
Generic Available Yes
Use Temporary relief of pain and reduction of inflammation associated with acute otitis media, swimmer's ear, otitis externa; facilitates ear wax removal
Pregnancy Risk Factor C
Pregnancy Considerations Reproduction studies have not been conducted with this combination.
Lactation Excretion in breast milk unknown/use caution
Contraindications Hypersensitivity to antipyrine, benzocaine, or any component; perforated tympanic membrane
Warnings Use of otic anesthetics may mask symptoms of a fulminating middle ear infection (acute otitis media); not intended for prolonged use
Adverse Reactions
Hematologic: Methemoglobinemia
Local: Burning, stinging, tenderness, edema
Miscellaneous: Hypersensitivity reactions
Drug Interactions
Avoid Concomitant Use There are no known interactions where it is recommended to avoid concomitant use.
Increased Effect/Toxicity There are no known significant interactions involving an increase in effect.
Decreased Effect There are no known significant interactions involving a decrease in effect.
Usual Dosage Infants, Children, and Adults: Otic: Fill ear canal; moisten cotton pledget, place in external ear, repeat every 1-2 hours until pain and congestion is relieved; for ear wax removal instill drops 3-4 times/day for 2-3 days
Dosage Forms Excipient information presented when available (limited, particularly for generics); consult specific product labeling. [DSC] = Discontinued product
Solution, otic [drops]: Antipyrine 5.4% and benzocaine 1.4% (10 mL)
A/B Otic, Allergen®, Aurodex [DSC]: Antipyrine 5.4% and benzocaine 1.4% (15 mL)
References
Rodriguez LF, Smolik LM, and Zbehlik AJ, "Benzocaine-Induced Methemoglobinemia: Report of a Severe Reaction and Review of the Literature," *Ann Pharmacother*, 1994, 28(5):643-9.

◆ **anti-Tac Monoclonal antibody** *see* Daclizumab *on page 382*

Antithymocyte Globulin (Equine)
(LIM foe site i MYUN GLOB yoo lin E kwine)

Medication Safety Issues
Sound-alike/look-alike issues:
Antithymocyte globulin equine (Atgam®) may be confused with antithymocyte globulin rabbit (Thymoglobulin®)
Atgam® may be confused with Ativan®
U.S. Brand Names Atgam®
Canadian Brand Names Atgam®

Therapeutic Category Immunosuppressant Agent; Polyclonal Antibody

Generic Available No

Use Prevention and/or treatment of acute renal allograft rejection [FDA approved in pediatrics (age not specified) and adults]; treatment of moderate to severe aplastic anemia in patients not considered suitable candidates for bone marrow transplantation; [FDA approved in pediatrics (age not specified) and adults]; has also been used in prevention or treatment of graft-vs-host disease following allogenic stem cell transplantation; prevention and treatment of other solid organ (other than renal) allograft rejection; treatment of myelodysplastic syndrome (MDS)

Pregnancy Risk Factor C

Pregnancy Considerations Reproduction studies have not been conducted; use during pregnancy is not recommended. Use in pregnant women is not recommended and should be considered only in exceptional circumstances. Women exposed to Atgam® during pregnancy may be enrolled in the National Transplantation Pregnancy Registry (877-955-6877).

Lactation Excretion in breast milk unknown/use caution

Contraindications Hypersensitivity to ATG (history of severe systemic reaction with prior administration), any component, or other equine gamma globulins

Warnings Should only be used by physicians experienced in immunosuppressive therapy or management of renal transplant patients **[U.S. Boxed Warning]**; adequate laboratory and supportive medical resources must be readily available in the facility for patient management **[U.S. Boxed Warning]**. Anaphylaxis (symptoms can include hypotension, respiratory distress, pain in the chest, rash, and tachycardia) may occur at any time during ATG therapy. Epinephrine and oxygen should be readily available to treat anaphylaxis.

Therapy should be discontinued in patients who experience any symptoms of anaphylaxis (rash, tachycardia, dyspnea, hypotension); severe unremitting hemolysis, or in transplant patients who experience severe, unremitting leukopenia or thrombocytopenia

Precautions Product potency may vary from lot to lot. Product of equine and human plasma; may have a risk of transmitting disease, including a theoretical risk of Creutzfeldt-Jakob disease (CJD). Monitor closely for signs of infection; the incidence of cytomegalovirus (CMV) infection may be increased.

Adverse Reactions

Cardiovascular: Bradycardia, cardiac irregularity, edema, heart failure, hypertension, hypotension, myocarditis, tachycardia

Central nervous system: Agitation, chills, encephalitis (including viral), fever, headache, lethargy, lightheadedness, listlessness, malaise, seizures

Dermatologic: Pruritus, rash, urticaria, wheal and flare

Gastrointestinal: Diarrhea, nausea, stomatitis, vomiting

Hematologic: Hemolysis, hemolytic anemia, leukopenia, thrombocytopenia

Hepatic: Hepatosplenomegaly

Local: Pain, redness, swelling, thrombophlebitis

Neuromuscular & skeletal: Arthralgia, back pain, joint stiffness, myalgia, pain in the chest

Ocular: Periorbital edema

Renal: Abnormal renal function tests, proteinuria

Respiratory: Dyspnea, pleural effusion, respiratory distress

Miscellaneous: Anaphylaxis (may be indicated by hypotension or respiratory distress) (see Warnings), diaphoresis, infection, lymphadenopathy, night sweats, serum sickness, viral infection

<1%, postmarketing, and/or case reports: Abdominal pain, acute renal failure, anemia, apnea, aplasia, confusion, cough, deep vein thrombosis, disorientation, dizziness, epigastric pain, enlarged kidney, eosinophilia, epistaxis, faintness, flank pain, herpes simplex reactivation, GI bleed, GI perforation, granulocytopenia, hiccups, hyperglycemia, ileac vein obstruction, infection, involuntary movement, laryngospasm, neutropenia, pancytopenia, paresthesia, pulmonary edema, renal artery thrombosis, rigidity, sore throat, toxic epidermal necrolysis, tremor, vasculitis, viral hepatitis, weakness, wound dehiscence

Drug Interactions

Avoid Concomitant Use

Avoid concomitant use of Antithymocyte Globulin (Equine) with any of the following: BCG; Natalizumab; Pimecrolimus; Tacrolimus (Topical); Vaccines (Live)

Increased Effect/Toxicity

Antithymocyte Globulin (Equine) may increase the levels/effects of: Leflunomide; Natalizumab; Vaccines (Live)

The levels/effects of Antithymocyte Globulin (Equine) may be increased by: Denosumab; Pimecrolimus; Tacrolimus (Topical); Trastuzumab

Decreased Effect

Antithymocyte Globulin (Equine) may decrease the levels/effects of: BCG; Sipuleucel-T; Vaccines (Inactivated); Vaccines (Live)

The levels/effects of Antithymocyte Globulin (Equine) may be decreased by: Echinacea

Stability Store ampuls at 2°C to 8°C (36°F to 46°F); do not freeze. Dilute in 1/2NS or NS; when diluted to concentrations up to 4 mg/mL, ATG infusion solution is stable for 24 hours if refrigerated; use of dextrose solutions is not recommended; precipitation can occur in solutions with a low salt concentration (ie, D_5W)

Mechanism of Action Immunosuppressant involved in elimination of antigen-reactive T-lymphocytes (killer cells) in peripheral blood or alterations in the functions of T-lymphocytes, which are involved in humoral immunity and partly in cell-mediated immunity; induces complete or partial hematologic response in aplastic anemia

Pharmacokinetics (Adult data unless noted)

Distribution: Poor into lymphoid tissues; binds to circulating lymphocytes, granulocytes, platelets, bone marrow cells

Half-life, plasma: 1.5-12 days

Elimination: ~1% of dose excreted in urine

Usual Dosage Intradermal skin test is recommended prior to administration of the initial dose of ATG; use 0.1 mL of a fresh 1:1000 dilution of ATG in NS; observe the skin test every 15 minutes for 1 hour; a local reaction ≥10 mm diameter with a wheal or erythema or both should be considered a positive skin test; if a positive skin test occurs, the first infusion should be administered in a controlled environment with intensive life support immediately available. A systemic reaction precludes further administration of the drug. The absence of a reaction does **not** preclude the possibility of an immediate sensitivity reaction.

I.V.: Children and Adults:

Aplastic anemia protocol: 10-20 mg/kg/day for 8-14 days; additional every other day therapy can be administered up to a total of 21 doses in 28 days. One study (see Rosenfeld, 1995) used a dose of 40 mg/kg/day once daily over 4 hours for 4 days.

Renal allograft: Dosage range: Children: 5-25 mg/kg/day; Adults: 10-30 mg/kg/day

Induction dose (delaying the onset of allograft rejection): 15 mg/kg/day for 14 days, then every other day for 14 days for a total of 21 doses in 28 days. Initial dose should be administered within 24 hours before or after transplantation.

Treatment of rejection: 10-15 mg/kg/day for 14 days; additional every other day therapy can be administered up to a total of 21 doses

Acute GVHD treatment (unlabeled use): 30 mg/kg/dose every other day for 6 doses (see MacMillan, 2007) or 15 mg/kg/dose twice daily for 10 doses (see MacMillan, 2002)

Dosage adjustment for toxicity:
Anaphylaxis: Stop infusion immediately; administer epinephrine. May require corticosteroids, respiration assistance, and/or other resuscitative measures. Do not resume infusion.

Hemolysis (severe and unremitting): May require discontinuation of treatment

Administration Parenteral: Do not shake diluted or undiluted ATG solution to prevent excessive foaming and denaturation of the product. ATG should be added to an inverted bottle of sterile diluent so that undiluted drug does not contact air inside the bottle. Allow diluted ATG to reach room temperature before infusion. Administer via central line; use of high flow central vein will minimize the occurrence of phlebitis and thrombosis; administer by slow I.V. infusion through a 0.2-1 micron in-line filter over 4-8 hours at a final concentration not to exceed 4 mg ATG/mL

Monitoring Parameters Lymphocyte profile; CBC with differential and platelet count, vital signs during administration, renal function test

Nursing Implications Patient may need to be pretreated with an antipyretic, antihistamine, and/or corticosteroid to prevent chills, fever, itching, and erythema

Dosage Forms Excipient information presented when available (limited, particularly for generics); consult specific product labeling.
Injection, solution:
Atgam®: 50 mg/mL (5 mL)

References
Macmillan ML, Couriel D, Weisdorf DJ, et al, "A Phase 2/3 Multicenter Randomized Clinical Trial of ABX-CBL Versus ATG as Secondary Therapy for Steroid-Resistant Acute Graft-Versus-Host Disease," *Blood*, 2007, 109(6):2657-62.
MacMillan ML, Weisdorf DJ, Davies SM, et al, "Early Antithymocyte Globulin Therapy Improves Survival in Patients With Steroid-Resistant Acute Graft-Versus-Host Disease," *Biol Blood Marrow Transplant*, 2002, 8(1):40-6.
Rosenfeld SJ, Kimball J, Vining D, et al, "Intensive Immunosuppression With Antithymocyte Globulin and Cyclosporine as Treatment for Severe Acquired Aplastic Anemia," *Blood*, 1995, 85(11):3058-65.
Taylor DO, Edwards LB, Aurora P, et al, "Registry of the International Society for Heart and Lung Transplantation: Twenty-Fifth Official Adult Heart Transplant Report–2008," *J Heart Lung Transplant*, 2008, 27 (9):943-56.
Webster A, Chapman JR, Craig JC, et al. "Polyclonal and Monoclonal Antibodies For Preventing Acute Rejection Episodes in Kidney Transplant Recipients," *Cochrane Database of Systematic Reviews*, 2006, Issue 2.
Whitehead B, James I, Helms P, et al, "Intensive Care Management of Children Following Heart and Heart-Lung Transplantation," *Intensive Care Med*, 1990, 16(7):426-30.

◆ **Antithymocyte Globulin (Equine)** *see* Antithymocyte Globulin (Equine) *on page 118*

Antithymocyte Globulin (Rabbit)
(an te THY moe site GLOB yu lin (RAB bit)

Medication Safety Issues
Sound-alike/look-alike issues:
Antithymocyte globulin rabbit (Thymoglobulin®) may be confused with antithymocyte globulin equine (Atgam®)

U.S. Brand Names Thymoglobulin®
Therapeutic Category Immunosuppressant Agent
Generic Available No

Use Treatment of acute rejection of renal transplant; used in conjunction with concomitant immunosuppression (FDA approved in adults); has also been used as induction therapy in renal transplant; treatment of myelodysplastic syndrome (MDS); prevention and/or treatment of acute rejection after bone marrow, heart/lung, liver, intestinal, or multivisceral transplantation in conjunction with other immunosuppressive agents; treatment of aplastic anemia in patients who failed to respond to antithymocyte immunoglobulin (equine)

Pregnancy Risk Factor C
Pregnancy Considerations Reproduction studies have not been conducted.
Lactation Excretion in breast milk unknown/use caution
Contraindications Hypersensitivity to antithymocyte globulin, rabbit proteins, or any component; acute or chronic infection

Warnings Adequate laboratory and supportive medical resources must be readily available in the facility for patient management. Anaphylaxis has been reported with the use of antithymocyte globulin (rabbit). Epinephrine, oxygen, and resuscitative equipment should be readily available to treat anaphylaxis. Release of cytokines by activated monocytes and lymphocytes may cause fatal cytokine release syndrome (CRS) during administration of antithymocyte globulin. Rapid infusion rates have been associated with CRS in case reports. Severe or life-threatening symptoms include hypotension, acute respiratory distress syndrome, pulmonary edema, myocardial infarction, and tachycardia; symptoms range from a mild, self-limiting "flu-like" reaction to severe, life-threatening reactions.

Thrombocytopenia or neutropenia may result from cross-reactive antibodies and is reversible following dose reduction or discontinuation. Risk of post-transplant lymphoproliferative disease or other malignancies may be increased with prolonged use or overdosage of antithymocyte globulin (rabbit) in association with other immunosuppressants.

Precautions Infusion may cause fever and chills. Infuse first dose slowly over a minimum of 6 hours into a high flow vein; 1 hour prior to infusion, premedicate with corticosteroids, acetaminophen, and/or an antihistamine to reduce incidence of side effects during infusion. Reduce dose in patients with WBC between 2000-3000 cells/mm^3 or if the platelet count is between 50,000-75,000 cells/mm^3. Consider discontinuing antithymocyte globulin (rabbit) if WBC <2000 cells/mm^3 or platelets <50,000 cells/mm^3. Patients should not be immunized with attenuated live virus vaccines during or shortly after treatment; safety of immunization following therapy has not been studied.

Adverse Reactions
Cardiovascular: Hypertension, hypotension, peripheral edema, tachycardia

Central nervous system: Asthenia, chills, dizziness, fever, headache, malaise

Endocrine & metabolic: Hyperkalemia

Gastrointestinal: Abdominal pain, diarrhea, nausea, vomiting

Hematologic: Leukopenia, neutropenia (see Warnings), thrombocytopenia (see Warnings)

Respiratory: Dyspnea

Miscellaneous: Anaphylaxis (see Warnings); cytokine release syndrome (see Warnings); diaphoresis; risk of infection increased, lymphoma, post-transplant lymphoproliferative disease (see Warnings)

<1%, postmarketing, and/or case reports: Serum sickness (delayed)

Drug Interactions
Avoid Concomitant Use
Avoid concomitant use of Antithymocyte Globulin (Rabbit) with any of the following: BCG; Natalizumab; Pimecrolimus; Tacrolimus (Topical); Vaccines (Live)

Increased Effect/Toxicity
Antithymocyte Globulin (Rabbit) may increase the levels/ effects of: Leflunomide; Natalizumab; Vaccines (Live)

The levels/effects of Antithymocyte Globulin (Rabbit) may be increased by: Denosumab; Pimecrolimus; Tacrolimus (Topical); Trastuzumab

Decreased Effect

Antithymocyte Globulin (Rabbit) may decrease the levels/effects of: BCG; Sipuleucel-T; Vaccines (Inactivated); Vaccines (Live)

The levels/effects of Antithymocyte Globulin (Rabbit) may be decreased by: Echinacea

Stability Store intact vial in refrigerator; protect from light; do not freeze. Allow diluent and contents of vial to reach room temperature prior to reconstitution; reconstituted product is stable for up to 24 hours at room temperature; however, since it contains no preservatives, it should be used immediately following reconstitution; compatible with D_5W or NS; Y-site injection compatible with hydrocortisone sodium succinate and heparin 100 units/mL in D_5W or NS; incompatible with heparin 2 units/mL in D_5W

Mechanism of Action Possible mechanism may involve elimination of antigen-reactive T-lymphocytes (killer cells) in peripheral blood or alteration of T-cell function

Pharmacodynamics Onset of action (T-cell depletion): Within one day

Pharmacokinetics (Adult data unless noted) Half-life: 2-3 days

Usual Dosage IV: (refer to individual protocols):
Children:
Bone marrow transplantation: 1.5-3 mg/kg/day once daily for 4 consecutive days before transplantation
Treatment of graft-versus-host disease: 1.5 mg/kg/dose once daily or every other day
Renal transplantation:
Induction: 1-2 mg/kg/day once daily for 4-5 days initiated at time of transplant
Acute rejection: 1.5mg/kg/day once daily for 7-14 days
Heart/lung transplantation:
Induction: 1-2 mg/kg/day depending on baseline platelet count once daily for 5 days
Rejection: 2 mg/kg/day once daily for 5 days
Liver, intestinal, or multivisceral transplant:
Preconditioning/induction: Pretransplant: 2 mg/kg; postop day 1: 3 mg/kg
Rejection: 1.5 mg/kg/day once daily for 7-14 days based upon biopsy results; maximum dose: 2 mg/kg/dose
Adults:
Acute renal transplant rejection: 1.5 mg/kg/day once daily for 7-14 days
Aplastic Anemia: 3.5 mg/kg/day once daily for 5 days

Administration Parenteral: Administer by slow I.V. infusion over 6-12 hours for the preconditioning/induction dose or over 6 hours for the initial acute rejection treatment dose; infuse over 4 hours for subsequent doses if first dose tolerated. Administer through an in-line filter with pore size of 0.22 microns via central line or high flow vein at a final concentration of 0.5 to 2 mg/mL in NS or D_5W

Monitoring Parameters Platelet count, CBC with differential, lymphocyte count, vital signs during infusion

Test Interactions Potential interference with rabbit antibody-based immunoassays

Nursing Implications Patient may need to be pretreated with an antipyretic, antihistamine, and corticosteroid 1 hour prior to each dose of antithymocyte globulin (rabbit). Mild itching and erythema can be treated with an antihistamine. Chills and fever can be treated by slowing the infusion rate or administering an additional dose of corticosteroid. If anaphylaxis occurs, terminate infusion immediately.

Additional Information Antiviral therapy should be given prophylactically during antithymocyte globulin (rabbit) use.

Dosage Forms Excipient information presented when available (limited, particularly for generics); consult specific product labeling.

Injection, powder for reconstitution:
Thymoglobulin®: 25 mg

References

Di Filippo S, Boissonnat P, Sassolas F, et al, "Rabbit Antithymocyte Globulin as Induction Immunotherapy in Pediatric Heart Transplantation," *Transplantation*, 2003, 75(3):354-8.

Horan JT, Liesveld JL, Fenton P, et al, "Hematopoietic Stem Cell Transplantation for Multiply Transfused Patients With Sickle Cell Disease and Thalassemia After Low-Dose Total Body Irradiation, Fludarabine, and Rabbit Anti-thymocyte Globulin," *Bone Marrow Transplant*, 2005, 35(2):171-7.

Starzl TE, Murase N, Abu-Elmagd K, et al, "Tolerogenic Immunosuppression for Organ Transplantation," *Lancet*, 2003, 361 (9368):1502-10.

Trissel LA and Saenz CA, "Physical Compatibility of Antithymocyte Globulin (Rabbit) With Heparin Sodium and Hydrocortisone Sodium Succinate," *Am J Health Syst Pharm*, 2003, 60(16):1650-2.

◆ **Antithymocyte Immunoglobulin** *see* Antithymocyte Globulin (Equine) *on page 118*

◆ **Antithymocyte Immunoglobulin** *see* Antithymocyte Globulin (Rabbit) *on page 120*

◆ **Antitumor Necrosis Factor-Alpha** *see* InFLIXimab *on page 728*

◆ **Antitumor Necrosis Factor Apha (Human)** *see* Adalimumab *on page 48*

◆ **Anti-VEGF Monoclonal Antibody** *see* Bevacizumab *on page 192*

◆ **Anti-VEGF rhuMAb** *see* Bevacizumab *on page 192*

Antivenin (*Latrodectus mactans*)
(an tee VEN in lak tro DUK tus MAK tans)

Therapeutic Category Antivenin

Generic Available No

Use Treatment of severe systemic symptoms refractory to supportive measures due to black widow spider bites.

Pregnancy Risk Factor C

Pregnancy Considerations Reproduction studies have not been conducted.

Lactation Excretion in breast milk unknown/use caution

Warnings Anaphylaxis and serum sickness have been reported in patients who received *Latrodectus mactans* antivenin. Patients with atopic sensitivity to horses may have an increased risk of experiencing an immediate sensitivity reaction to the antivenin. Desensitization may need to be performed on patients with positive skin or conjunctival test reaction or history of sensitivity to equine serum; epinephrine and oxygen should be readily available to treat anaphylaxis. *Latrodectus mactans* antivenin contains thimerosal which has been associated with neurologic and renal toxicities.

Adverse Reactions

Cardiovascular: Shock, flushing, hypotension, edema of face, tongue and throat
Dermatologic: Pruritus, urticaria
Gastrointestinal: Vomiting
Respiratory: Cough, dyspnea, bronchospasm
Miscellaneous: Anaphylaxis, serum sickness (occurs 7-14 days after antivenin administration in 75% of patients)

Drug Interactions

Avoid Concomitant Use There are no known interactions where it is recommended to avoid concomitant use.

Increased Effect/Toxicity There are no known significant interactions involving an increase in effect.

Decreased Effect There are no known significant interactions involving a decrease in effect.

Stability Refrigerate; do not freeze

Mechanism of Action Neutralizes the venom of black widow spiders

Pharmacodynamics Onset of action: Within 30 minutes with symptoms subsiding after 1-3 hours

Pharmacokinetics (Adult data unless noted) Data in humans is not available.

Usual Dosage The initial dose of antivenin should be administered as soon as possible for prompt relief of symptoms. Delayed antivenin administration (up to 90 hours after bite) may still be effective in treating patients with prolonged or refractory symptoms resulting from black widow spider bites.

Sensitivity testing: Intradermal skin test or conjunctival test must be performed prior to antivenin administration:

Intradermal skin test: Use 0.02 mL of a 1:10 dilution of normal horse serum in NS. An intradermal control of 0.02 mL NS should also be administered. Read skin test after 10 minutes. Positive reaction consists of an urticarial wheal surrounded by a zone of erythema.

Conjunctival test: Positive reaction consists of reddening of the conjunctiva and itching of the eye 10 minutes following test.

Children: Instill one drop of 1:100 dilution of horse serum into conjunctival sac.

Adults: Instill one drop of 1:10 dilution of horse serum into the conjunctival sac.

Desensitization: (Desensitization is only utilized when antivenin is considered a necessary lifesaving treatment in patients with history of allergy or with mildly positive sensitivity tests): SubQ: Inject 0.1 mL, followed by 0.2 mL and 0.5 mL of a 1:100 antivenin dilution administered in 15- to 30-minute intervals (30 minutes preferably); repeat procedure with a 1:10 dilution of antivenin; then repeat procedure with undiluted antivenin. If a reaction occurs after a desensitization injection, apply tourniquet proximal to the injection site and administer epinephrine proximal to the tourniquet or into another extremity. After 30 minutes, continue desensitization procedure by injecting the last dose that did not evoke a reaction. If no reaction occurs after 0.5 mL of undiluted antivenin is administered, continue to administer 0.5 mL of undiluted antivenin at 15-minute intervals until the entire dose (2.5 mL) has been injected.

If sensitivity test is negative, antivenin may be administered:

Children <12 years: I.V.: Entire contents of a reconstituted vial (2.5 mL); second dose may be needed in some cases

Adults: I.M., I.V.: Entire contents of a reconstituted vial (2.5 mL); administer I.V. to patients in shock or for management of severe cases; second dose may be needed in some cases

Administration Parenteral: Reconstitute vial containing 6000 units of antivenin with 2.5 mL SWI; shake vial (with the needle still in the rubber stopper) to dissolve powder. Visually inspect vial for particulate matter.

I.M.: Administer into the anterolateral thigh. Apply tourniquet if an adverse reaction occurs.

I.V.: Dilute reconstituted antivenin with 10-50 mL of NS; infuse over 15 minutes. If an immediate hypersensitivity reaction occurs, immediately interrupt antivenin infusion and provide appropriate supportive therapy. If administration of antivenin can be resumed after control of the reaction, reinitiate at a slower infusion rate.

Monitoring Parameters Vital signs; signs and symptoms of allergy, anaphylaxis, and serum sickness

Additional Information The venom of the black widow spider is a neurotoxin that causes release of a presynaptic neurotransmitter. Within 1 hour of the bite, clinical effects such as sharp pain, muscle spasm, weakness, tremor, severe abdominal pain with rigidity, hypertension, respiratory distress, diaphoresis, and facial swelling may be seen.

Dosage Forms Excipient information presented when available (limited, particularly for generics); consult specific product labeling.

Injection, powder for reconstitution: 6000 antivenin units [equine origin; contains thimerosal; packaged with diluent and normal horse serum for sensitivity testing]

References

Saucier JR, "Arachnid Envenomation," *Emerg Med Clin North Am*, 2004, 22(2):405-22

◆ **Antivert®** *see* Meclizine *on page 869*

◆ **Antizol®** *see* Fomepizole *on page 620*

◆ **Anucort-HC®** *see* Hydrocortisone *on page 685*

◆ **Anu-Med [OTC]** *see* Phenylephrine *on page 1102*

◆ **Anusol-HC®** *see* Hydrocortisone *on page 685*

◆ **Anusol® HC-1 [OTC]** *see* Hydrocortisone *on page 685*

◆ **Anzemet®** *see* Dolasetron *on page 469*

◆ **APAP** *see* Acetaminophen *on page 36*

◆ **APAP 500 [OTC]** *see* Acetaminophen *on page 36*

◆ **Apidra®** *see* Insulin Glulisine *on page 742*

◆ **Aplenzin™** *see* BuPROPion *on page 217*

◆ **Apo-Acetaminophen® (Can)** *see* Acetaminophen *on page 36*

◆ **Apo-Acetazolamide® (Can)** *see* AcetaZOLAMIDE *on page 41*

◆ **Apo-Acyclovir® (Can)** *see* Acyclovir *on page 46*

◆ **Apo-Allopurinol® (Can)** *see* Allopurinol *on page 66*

◆ **Apo-Alpraz® (Can)** *see* ALPRAZolam *on page 68*

◆ **Apo-Alpraz® TS (Can)** *see* ALPRAZolam *on page 68*

◆ **Apo-Amiloride® (Can)** *see* AMILoride *on page 81*

◆ **Apo-Amiodarone® (Can)** *see* Amiodarone *on page 84*

◆ **Apo-Amitriptyline® (Can)** *see* Amitriptyline *on page 89*

◆ **Apo-Amlodipine® (Can)** *see* AmLODIPine *on page 91*

◆ **Apo-Amoxi® (Can)** *see* Amoxicillin *on page 96*

◆ **Apo-Amoxi-Clav® (Can)** *see* Amoxicillin and Clavulanic Acid *on page 98*

◆ **Apo-Ampi® (Can)** *see* Ampicillin *on page 104*

◆ **Apo-Atenol® (Can)** *see* Atenolol *on page 147*

◆ **Apo-Atorvastatin® (Can)** *see* Atorvastatin *on page 151*

◆ **Apo-Azathioprine® (Can)** *see* AzaTHIOprine *on page 161*

◆ **Apo-Azithromycin® (Can)** *see* Azithromycin *on page 164*

◆ **Apo-Baclofen® (Can)** *see* Baclofen *on page 171*

◆ **Apo-Beclomethasone® (Can)** *see* Beclomethasone *on page 176*

◆ **Apo-Benazepril® (Can)** *see* Benazepril *on page 179*

◆ **Apo-Benztropine® (Can)** *see* Benztropine *on page 185*

◆ **Apo-Bisacodyl® (Can)** *see* Bisacodyl *on page 194*

◆ **Apo-Brimonidine® (Can)** *see* Brimonidine *on page 202*

◆ **Apo-Brimonidine P® (Can)** *see* Brimonidine *on page 202*

◆ **Apo-Bromocriptine® (Can)** *see* Bromocriptine *on page 203*

◆ **Apo-Buspirone® (Can)** *see* BusPIRone *on page 222*

◆ **Apo-Cal® (Can)** *see* Calcium Carbonate *on page 232*

◆ **Apo-Calcitonin® (Can)** *see* Calcitonin *on page 227*

◆ **Apo-Capto® (Can)** *see* Captopril *on page 242*

◆ **Apo-Carbamazepine® (Can)** *see* CarBAMazepine *on page 244*

◆ **Apo-Carvedilol® (Can)** *see* Carvedilol *on page 254*

◆ **Apo-Cefaclor® (Can)** *see* Cefaclor *on page 260*

- **Apo-Cefadroxil®** **(Can)** *see* Cefadroxil *on page 261*
- **Apo-Cefoxitin®** **(Can)** *see* Cefoxitin *on page 269*
- **Apo-Cefprozil®** **(Can)** *see* Cefprozil *on page 271*
- **Apo-Cefuroxime®** **(Can)** *see* Cefuroxime *on page 277*
- **Apo-Cephalex®** **(Can)** *see* Cephalexin *on page 282*
- **Apo-Cetirizine®** **(Can)** *see* Cetirizine *on page 283*
- **Apo-Cimetidine®** **(Can)** *see* Cimetidine *on page 309*
- **Apo-Ciproflox®** **(Can)** *see* Ciprofloxacin *on page 310*
- **Apo-Citalopram®** **(Can)** *see* Citalopram *on page 319*
- **Apo-Clarithromycin®** **(Can)** *see* Clarithromycin *on page 324*
- **Apo-Clindamycin®** **(Can)** *see* Clindamycin *on page 327*
- **Apo-Clomipramine®** **(Can)** *see* ClomiPRAMINE *on page 334*
- **Apo-Clonazepam®** **(Can)** *see* ClonazePAM *on page 337*
- **Apo-Clonidine®** **(Can)** *see* CloNIDine *on page 338*
- **Apo-Clorazepate®** **(Can)** *see* Clorazepate *on page 343*
- **Apo-Clozapine®** **(Can)** *see* Clozapine *on page 345*
- **Apo-Cromolyn®** **(Can)** *see* Cromolyn *on page 363*
- **Apo-Cyclobenzaprine®** **(Can)** *see* Cyclobenzaprine *on page 367*
- **Apo-Cyclosporine®** **(Can)** *see* CycloSPORINE *on page 372*
- **Apo-Desipramine®** **(Can)** *see* Desipramine *on page 401*
- **Apo-Desmopressin®** **(Can)** *see* Desmopressin *on page 404*
- **Apo-Dexamethasone®** **(Can)** *see* Dexamethasone *on page 406*
- **Apo-Diazepam®** **(Can)** *see* Diazepam *on page 424*
- **Apo-Diclo®** **(Can)** *see* Diclofenac *on page 429*
- **Apo-Diclo Rapide®** **(Can)** *see* Diclofenac *on page 429*
- **Apo-Diclo SR®** **(Can)** *see* Diclofenac *on page 429*
- **Apo-Digoxin®** **(Can)** *see* Digoxin *on page 437*
- **Apo-Diltiaz®** **(Can)** *see* Diltiazem *on page 443*
- **Apo-Diltiaz CD®** **(Can)** *see* Diltiazem *on page 443*
- **Apo-Diltiaz® Injectable (Can)** *see* Diltiazem *on page 443*
- **Apo-Diltiaz SR®** **(Can)** *see* Diltiazem *on page 443*
- **Apo-Diltiaz TZ®** **(Can)** *see* Diltiazem *on page 443*
- **Apo-Dimenhydrinate®** **(Can)** *see* DimenhyDRINATE *on page 446*
- **Apo-Dipyridamole FC®** **(Can)** *see* Dipyridamole *on page 461*
- **Apo-Divalproex®** **(Can)** *see* Valproic Acid and Derivatives *on page 1398*
- **Apo-Docusate-Sodium®** **(Can)** *see* Docusate *on page 468*
- **Apo-Doxepin®** **(Can)** *see* Doxepin *on page 475*
- **Apo-Doxy®** **(Can)** *see* Doxycycline *on page 479*
- **Apo-Doxy Tabs®** **(Can)** *see* Doxycycline *on page 479*
- **Apo-Enalapril®** **(Can)** *see* Enalapril/Enalaprilat *on page 499*
- **Apo-Erythro Base®** **(Can)** *see* Erythromycin *on page 525*
- **Apo-Erythro E-C®** **(Can)** *see* Erythromycin *on page 525*
- **Apo-Erythro-ES®** **(Can)** *see* Erythromycin *on page 525*
- **Apo-Erythro-S®** **(Can)** *see* Erythromycin *on page 525*
- **Apo-Famciclovir®** **(Can)** *see* Famciclovir *on page 560*
- **Apo-Famotidine®** **(Can)** *see* Famotidine *on page 561*

- **Apo-Famotidine® Injectable (Can)** *see* Famotidine *on page 561*
- **Apo-Ferrous Gluconate®** **(Can)** *see* Ferrous Gluconate *on page 577*
- **Apo-Ferrous Sulfate®** **(Can)** *see* Ferrous Sulfate *on page 577*
- **Apo-Flecainide®** **(Can)** *see* Flecainide *on page 582*
- **Apo-Fluconazole®** **(Can)** *see* Fluconazole *on page 584*
- **Apo-Flunisolide®** **(Can)** *see* Flunisolide *on page 592*
- **Apo-Fluoxetine®** **(Can)** *see* FLUoxetine *on page 600*
- **Apo-Flurazepam®** **(Can)** *see* Flurazepam *on page 604*
- **Apo-Flurbiprofen®** **(Can)** *see* Flurbiprofen *on page 605*
- **Apo-Fluticasone®** **(Can)** *see* Fluticasone *on page 607*
- **Apo-Fluvoxamine®** **(Can)** *see* Fluvoxamine *on page 615*
- **Apo-Folic®** **(Can)** *see* Folic Acid *on page 619*
- **Apo-Fosinopril®** **(Can)** *see* Fosinopril *on page 627*
- **Apo-Furosemide®** **(Can)** *see* Furosemide *on page 632*
- **Apo-Gabapentin®** **(Can)** *see* Gabapentin *on page 634*
- **Apo-Gain®** **(Can)** *see* Minoxidil *on page 935*
- **Apo-Glyburide®** **(Can)** *see* GlyBURIDE *on page 648*
- **Apo-Granisetron®** **(Can)** *see* Granisetron *on page 653*
- **Apo-Haloperidol®** **(Can)** *see* Haloperidol *on page 666*
- **Apo-Haloperidol LA®** **(Can)** *see* Haloperidol *on page 666*
- **Apo-Hydralazine®** **(Can)** *see* HydrALAZINE *on page 680*
- **Apo-Hydro®** **(Can)** *see* Hydrochlorothiazide *on page 682*
- **Apo-Hydroxyquine®** **(Can)** *see* Hydroxychloroquine *on page 694*
- **Apo-Hydroxyurea®** **(Can)** *see* Hydroxyurea *on page 695*
- **Apo-Hydroxyzine®** **(Can)** *see* HydrOXYzine *on page 697*
- **Apo-Ibuprofen®** **(Can)** *see* Ibuprofen *on page 702*
- **Apo-Imipramine®** **(Can)** *see* Imipramine *on page 716*
- **Apo-Indomethacin®** **(Can)** *see* Indomethacin *on page 726*
- **Apo-Ipravent®** **(Can)** *see* Ipratropium *on page 757*
- **Apo-K®** **(Can)** *see* Potassium Chloride *on page 1136*
- **Apo-Ketoconazole®** **(Can)** *see* Ketoconazole *on page 780*
- **Apo-Ketorolac®** **(Can)** *see* Ketorolac *on page 781*
- **Apo-Ketorolac Injectable®** **(Can)** *see* Ketorolac *on page 781*
- **Apo-Labetalol®** **(Can)** *see* Labetalol *on page 787*
- **Apo-Lactulose®** **(Can)** *see* Lactulose *on page 791*
- **Apo-Lamotrigine®** **(Can)** *see* LamoTRIgine *on page 795*
- **Apo-Lansoprazole®** **(Can)** *see* Lansoprazole *on page 801*
- **Apo-Levetiracetam®** **(Can)** *see* Levetiracetam *on page 808*
- **Apo-Levobunolol®** **(Can)** *see* Levobunolol *on page 811*
- **Apo-Levofloxacin®** **(Can)** *see* Levofloxacin *on page 813*
- **Apo-Lisinopril®** **(Can)** *see* Lisinopril *on page 832*
- **Apo-Lithium® Carbonate (Can)** *see* Lithium *on page 834*

◆ **Apo-Lithium® Carbonate SR (Can)** *see* Lithium *on page 834*

◆ **Apo-Loperamide® (Can)** *see* Loperamide *on page 838*

◆ **Apo-Loratadine® (Can)** *see* Loratadine *on page 842*

◆ **Apo-Lorazepam® (Can)** *see* LORazepam *on page 845*

◆ **Apo-Lovastatin® (Can)** *see* Lovastatin *on page 850*

◆ **Apo-Medroxy® (Can)** *see* MedroxyPROGESTERone *on page 870*

◆ **Apo-Mefloquine® (Can)** *see* Mefloquine *on page 872*

◆ **Apo-Megestrol® (Can)** *see* Megestrol *on page 874*

◆ **Apo-Metformin® (Can)** *see* MetFORMIN *on page 891*

◆ **Apo-Methotrexate® (Can)** *see* Methotrexate *on page 900*

◆ **Apo-Methyldopa® (Can)** *see* Methyldopa *on page 905*

◆ **Apo-Methylphenidate® (Can)** *see* Methylphenidate *on page 908*

◆ **Apo-Methylphenidate® SR (Can)** *see* Methylphenidate *on page 908*

◆ **Apo-Metoclop® (Can)** *see* Metoclopramide *on page 915*

◆ **Apo-Metoprolol® (Can)** *see* Metoprolol *on page 918*

◆ **Apo-Metoprolol SR® (Can)** *see* Metoprolol *on page 918*

◆ **Apo-Metronidazole® (Can)** *see* MetroNIDAZOLE *on page 921*

◆ **Apo-Midazolam® (Can)** *see* Midazolam *on page 928*

◆ **Apo-Minocycline® (Can)** *see* Minocycline *on page 933*

◆ **Apo-Misoprostol® (Can)** *see* Misoprostol *on page 937*

◆ **Apo-Modafinil® (Can)** *see* Modafinil *on page 940*

◆ **Apo-Nadol® (Can)** *see* Nadolol *on page 961*

◆ **Apo-Napro-Na® (Can)** *see* Naproxen *on page 967*

◆ **Apo-Napro-Na DS® (Can)** *see* Naproxen *on page 967*

◆ **Apo-Naproxen® (Can)** *see* Naproxen *on page 967*

◆ **Apo-Naproxen EC® (Can)** *see* Naproxen *on page 967*

◆ **Apo-Naproxen SR® (Can)** *see* Naproxen *on page 967*

◆ **Apo-Nifed® (Can)** *see* NIFEdipine *on page 991*

◆ **Apo-Nifed PA® (Can)** *see* NIFEdipine *on page 991*

◆ **Apo-Nitrofurantoin® (Can)** *see* Nitrofurantoin *on page 995*

◆ **Apo-Nizatidine® (Can)** *see* Nizatidine *on page 999*

◆ **Apo-Nortriptyline® (Can)** *see* Nortriptyline *on page 1002*

◆ **Apo-Oflox® (Can)** *see* Ofloxacin *on page 1011*

◆ **Apo-Ofloxacin® (Can)** *see* Ofloxacin *on page 1011*

◆ **Apo-Omeprazole® (Can)** *see* Omeprazole *on page 1016*

◆ **Apo-Ondansetron® (Can)** *see* Ondansetron *on page 1022*

◆ **Apo-Orciprenaline® (Can)** *see* Metaproterenol *on page 890*

◆ **Apo-Oxaprozin® (Can)** *see* Oxaprozin *on page 1033*

◆ **Apo-Oxcarbazepine® (Can)** *see* OXcarbazepine *on page 1035*

◆ **Apo-Oxybutynin® (Can)** *see* Oxybutynin *on page 1037*

◆ **Apo-Paclitaxel® (Can)** *see* Paclitaxel *on page 1044*

◆ **Apo-Pantoprazole® (Can)** *see* Pantoprazole *on page 1054*

◆ **Apo-Paroxetine® (Can)** *see* PARoxetine *on page 1064*

◆ **Apo-Pentoxifylline SR® (Can)** *see* Pentoxifylline *on page 1090*

◆ **Apo-Pen VK® (Can)** *see* Penicillin V Potassium *on page 1082*

◆ **Apo-Perphenazine® (Can)** *see* Perphenazine *on page 1094*

◆ **Apo-Pimozide® (Can)** *see* Pimozide *on page 1112*

◆ **Apo-Piroxicam® (Can)** *see* Piroxicam *on page 1118*

◆ **Apo-Pravastatin® (Can)** *see* Pravastatin *on page 1145*

◆ **Apo-Prazo® (Can)** *see* Prazosin *on page 1147*

◆ **Apo-Prednisone® (Can)** *see* PredniSONE *on page 1151*

◆ **Apo-Primidone® (Can)** *see* Primidone *on page 1154*

◆ **Apo-Procainamide® (Can)** *see* Procainamide *on page 1156*

◆ **Apo-Prochlorperazine® (Can)** *see* Prochlorperazine *on page 1161*

◆ **Apo-Propranolol® (Can)** *see* Propranolol *on page 1175*

◆ **Apo-Quinidine® (Can)** *see* QuiNIDine *on page 1192*

◆ **Apo-Quinine® (Can)** *see* QuiNINE *on page 1194*

◆ **Apo-Ranitidine® (Can)** *see* Ranitidine *on page 1200*

◆ **Apo-Risperidone® (Can)** *see* Risperidone *on page 1218*

◆ **Apo-Salvent® (Can)** *see* Albuterol *on page 57*

◆ **Apo-Salvent® CFC Free (Can)** *see* Albuterol *on page 57*

◆ **Apo-Salvent® Respirator Solution (Can)** *see* Albuterol *on page 57*

◆ **Apo-Salvent® Sterules (Can)** *see* Albuterol *on page 57*

◆ **Apo-Sertraline® (Can)** *see* Sertraline *on page 1254*

◆ **Apo-Simvastatin® (Can)** *see* Simvastatin *on page 1263*

◆ **Apo-Sotalol® (Can)** *see* Sotalol *on page 1284*

◆ **Apo-Sulfatrim® (Can)** *see* Sulfamethoxazole and Trimethoprim *on page 1302*

◆ **Apo-Sulfatrim® DS (Can)** *see* Sulfamethoxazole and Trimethoprim *on page 1302*

◆ **Apo-Sulfatrim® Pediatric (Can)** *see* Sulfamethoxazole and Trimethoprim *on page 1302*

◆ **Apo-Sulin® (Can)** *see* Sulindac *on page 1307*

◆ **Apo-Sumatriptan® (Can)** *see* SUMAtriptan *on page 1308*

◆ **Apo-Terbinafine® (Can)** *see* Terbinafine *on page 1322*

◆ **Apo-Tetra® (Can)** *see* Tetracycline *on page 1331*

◆ **Apo-Theo LA® (Can)** *see* Theophylline *on page 1335*

◆ **Apo-Timol® (Can)** *see* Timolol *on page 1351*

◆ **Apo-Timop® (Can)** *see* Timolol *on page 1351*

◆ **Apo-Topiramate® (Can)** *see* Topiramate *on page 1360*

◆ **Apo-Trazodone® (Can)** *see* TraZODone *on page 1371*

◆ **Apo-Trazodone D® (Can)** *see* TraZODone *on page 1371*

◆ **Apo-Triazo® (Can)** *see* Triazolam *on page 1381*

◆ **Apo-Trifluoperazine® (Can)** *see* Trifluoperazine *on page 1382*

◆ **Apo-Trimethoprim® (Can)** *see* Trimethoprim *on page 1386*

◆ **Apo-Valacyclovir® (Can)** *see* Valacyclovir *on page 1394*

◆ **Apo-Valproic® (Can)** *see* Valproic Acid and Derivatives *on page 1398*

◆ **Apo-Verap® (Can)** *see* Verapamil *on page 1416*

◆ **Apo-Verap® SR (Can)** *see* Verapamil *on page 1416*

◆ **Apo-Warfarin® (Can)** *see* Warfarin *on page 1432*

◆ **Apo-Zidovudine® (Can)** *see* Zidovudine *on page 1442*

◆ **APPG** *see* Penicillin G Procaine *on page 1081*

◆ **Apra [OTC] [DSC]** *see* Acetaminophen *on page 36*

Aprepitant/Fosaprepitant
(ap RE pi tant, fos a PRE pi tant)

Medication Safety Issues
Sound-alike/look-alike issues:
Aprepitant may be confused with fosaprepitant
Emend® (aprepitant) oral capsule formulation may be confused with Emend® for injection (fosaprepitant).

U.S. Brand Names Emend®

Canadian Brand Names Emend®

Therapeutic Category Antiemetic; Substance P/Neurokinin 1 (NK$_1$) Receptor Antagonist

Generic Available No

Use Prevention of acute and delayed nausea and vomiting associated with initial and repeat courses of moderate and highly emetogenic cancer chemotherapy; prevention of postoperative nausea and vomiting (oral only). FDA approved in ages ≥18 years and adults.

Pregnancy Risk Factor B

Pregnancy Considerations Teratogenic effects were not observed in animal studies. There are no adequate and well-controlled studies in pregnant women; use only if clearly needed. Efficacy of hormonal contraceptive may be reduced; alternative or additional methods of contraception should be used both during treatment with fosaprepitant or aprepitant and for at least 1 month following the last fosaprepitant/aprepitant dose.

Lactation Excretion in breast milk unknown/not recommended

Contraindications Hypersensitivity to aprepitant, fosaprepitant, or any component; concurrent use with pimozide, terfenadine, astemizole, or cisapride

Warnings Has the potential to significantly interact with many medications (see Drug Interactions); potential increased serum levels of pimozide, terfenadine, astemizole, or cisapride could result in serious or life-threatening adverse effects; concomitant use with warfarin may result in clinically significant decrease in INR; patients on warfarin should have INR monitored closely, particularly at 7-10 days following initiation of 3-day aprepitant/fosaprepitant therapy. The efficacy of oral contraceptives may also be reduced during treatment with aprepitant/fosaprepitant; alternative methods of birth control should be used during aprepitant/fosaprepitant therapy. A single 40 mg aprepitant oral dose is not likely to alter plasma concentrations of CYP3A4 substrates.

Precautions A weak to moderate cytochrome P450 isoenzyme CYP3A4 inhibitor; use with caution in patients receiving medications metabolized by CYP3A4 as a reduction in metabolism and consequent elevation of serum levels may occur; the effect of aprepitant/fosaprepitant on the pharmacokinetics of orally administered CYP3A4 substrates may be greater than that seen with I.V. administered CYP3A4 substrates. Use with caution and monitor use closely in patients receiving docetaxel, paclitaxel, etoposide, irinotecan, ifosfamide, imatinib, vinorelbine, vinblastine, and vincristine as they are known to be metabolized by CYP3A4 isoenzymes. Use with caution in patients with severe hepatic insufficiency (Child-Pugh score >9). Not intended for treatment of existing nausea and vomiting or for chronic continuous therapy.

Adverse Reactions
Cardiovascular: Hypertension, hypotension, MI, tachycardia, bradycardia, hot flushing, DVT, edema, palpitation, sinus tachycardia, syncope, tachycardia

Central nervous system: Confusion, depression, anxiety, headache, insomnia, dizziness, fatigue (18% to 22%), fever, disorientation, hypoesthesia, hypothermia, malaise, pain

Dermatologic: Rash, alopecia, urticaria, angioedema, Stevens-Johnson syndrome (rare), acne, pruritus

Endocrine & metabolic: Anorexia, hyperglycemia, hypokalemia, weight loss, hyponatremia, dehydration, albumin decreased, diabetes mellitus, hypovolemia, weight loss

Gastrointestinal: Abdominal pain, constipation (9% to 12%), diarrhea, epigastric discomfort, gastritis, heartburn, nausea (7% to 13%), vomiting, dysgeusia, dyspepsia, dysphagia, flatulence, taste disturbance, vocal disturbance, pharyngitis, salivation increased, hiccups (11%), throat pain, stomatitis, xerostomia, acid reflux, appetite decreased, deglutition disorder, duodenal ulcer (perforating), enterocolitis, eructation, obstipation

Genitourinary: Dysuria, erythrocyturia, glucosuria, leukocyturia, pelvic pain, urinary tract infection

Hematologic: Anemia, thrombocytopenia, neutropenia, leukopenia, hemoglobin decreased, febrile neutropenia, neutropenic sepsis, leukocytes increased

Hepatic: Serum transaminases elevated, alkaline phosphatase increased, bilirubin increased

Local: Infusion site pain and induration (injection)

Neuromuscular & skeletal: Weakness (3% to 18%), myalgia, muscle pain, back pain, arthralgia, sensory disturbance, dysarthria, peripheral neuropathy, rigors, sensory neuropathy, tremor

Ocular: Visual acuity decreased, conjunctivitis, miosis

Otic: Tinnitus

Renal: Renal insufficiency, serum creatinine elevated, BUN increased, proteinuria

Respiratory: Cough, dyspnea, pneumonitis, respiratory insufficiency, hypoxia, wheezing, nasal secretion, pharyngitis, pneumonia, pulmonary embolism, respiratory infection

Miscellaneous: Herpes simplex, anaphylactic reaction, hypersensitivity reaction, candidiasis, diaphoresis, herpes simplex, septic shock

Drug Interactions
Metabolism/Transport Effects Substrate of CYP1A2 (minor), 2C19 (minor), 3A4 (major); **Inhibits** CYP2C9 (weak), 2C19 (weak), 3A4 (moderate); **Induces** CYP2C9 (weak), 3A4 (weak)

Avoid Concomitant Use
Avoid concomitant use of Aprepitant with any of the following: Cisapride; Pimozide; Tolvaptan

Increased Effect/Toxicity
Aprepitant may increase the levels/effects of: Benzodiazepines (metabolized by oxidation); Cisapride; Colchicine; Corticosteroids (Systemic); CYP3A4 Substrates; Diltiazem; Eplerenone; Everolimus; FentaNYL; Halofantrine; Pimecrolimus; Pimozide; Ranolazine; Salmeterol; Saxagliptin; TOLBUTamide; Tolvaptan

The levels/effects of Aprepitant may be increased by: Antifungal Agents (Azole Derivatives, Systemic); CYP3A4 Inhibitors (Moderate); CYP3A4 Inhibitors (Strong); Dasatinib; Diltiazem

Decreased Effect
Aprepitant may decrease the levels/effects of: Contraceptives (Estrogens); Contraceptives (Progestins); CYP2C9 Substrates (High risk); Saxagliptin; Warfarin

The levels/effects of Aprepitant may be decreased by: CYP3A4 Inducers (Strong); Deferasirox; Herbs (CYP3A4 Inducers); Rifamycin Derivatives

Stability Store **aprepitant** capsules at room temperature. Store **fosaprepitant** injection in refrigerator; stable for 24 hours at room temperature after dilution in NS.

Mechanism of Action Aprepitant is a selective high-affinity antagonist of human substance P/neurokinin 1 receptors. Antiemetic activity is via central action with little or no affinity for serotonin, dopamine, and corticosteroid receptors. Fosaprepitant, the prodrug of aprepitant, is rapidly converted to aprepitant after administration.

Pharmacokinetics (Adult data unless noted)
Distribution: V_d: Adults: 70 L
Protein binding: >95%
Metabolism: Extensive hepatic metabolism primarily by CYP3A4 with minor metabolism by CYP1A2 and CYP2C19
Bioavailability:
Oral: **Aprepitant:** 60% to 65%
I.V.: **Fosaprepitant:** Rapidly converted to aprepitant in liver and extrahepatic tissues within 30 minutes following the end of infusion
Half-life: Adults: 9-13 hours
Time to peak serum concentration: Oral: **Aprepitant:** 3-4 hours
Elimination:
Clearance: Adults: 62-90 mL/minute

Usual Dosage Adults:
Prevention of chemotherapy-induced emesis:
Oral: **Aprepitant:** 125 mg 1 hour prior to chemotherapy followed by 80 mg once daily for the next 2 days. Use in combination with a 5-HT$_3$ antagonist and a corticosteroid.
I.V.: **Fosaprepitant:** 115 mg may be substituted for aprepitant (125 mg) 30 minutes prior to chemotherapy on day 1 of chemotherapy only; follow on days 2 and 3 with aprepitant oral therapy as described above.
Note: Aprepitant/fosaprepitant has only been studied in a 3-day regimen combined with a corticosteroid and 5-HT$_3$ antagonist. Efficacy as a single agent or for prolonged treatment of chemotherapy-induced emesis has not been demonstrated. Has not been studied for chronic continuous therapy and its use for chronic therapy is not recommended.
Prevention of postoperative nausea and vomiting: Oral: **Aprepitant:** 40 mg within 3 hours prior to induction of anesthesia
Dosage adjustment in renal impairment: No dosage adjustment needed
Dosage adjustment in hepatic impairment: No dosage adjustment needed in mild to moderate hepatic insufficiency; the pharmacokinetic profile of aprepitant or fosaprepitant in severe hepatic insufficiency (Child-Pugh score >9) has not be studied

Administration
Oral: **Aprepitant:** May be administered without regard to food, 1 hour prior to chemotherapy on day 1 of treatment and in the morning on the subsequent next two days or within 3 hours prior to induction of anesthesia
I.V.: **Fosaprepitant:** Dilute in NS to a final volume of 115 mL resulting in 1 mg/mL concentration; infuse over 15 minutes, 30 minutes prior to chemotherapy

Patient Information Aprepitant may react with many other medications; report all medication use including OTC and herbal products to your physician; due to potential decrease effectiveness of oral contraceptives, alternative contraceptive methods should be used during therapy

Dosage Forms Excipient information presented when available (limited, particularly for generics); consult specific product labeling.
Capsule:
Emend®: Aprepitant: 40 mg, 80 mg, 125 mg
Combination package: Capsule 80 mg (2s), capsule 125 mg (1s)
Injection, powder for reconstitution:
Emend®: Fosaprepitant: 115 mg

References
American Society of Clinical Oncology, Kris MG, Hesketh PJ, et al, "American Society of Clinical Oncology Guideline for Antiemetics in Oncology: Update 2006," *J Clin Oncol,* 2006, 24(18):2932-47.
National Comprehensive Cancer Network (NCCN)®, "Clinical Practice Guidelines in Oncology™: Antiemesis," Version 2, 2009. Available at http://www.nccn.org/professionals/physician_gls/PDF/antiemesis.pdf.

◆ **Apresoline [DSC]** *see* HydrALAZINE *on page 680*

◆ **Apresoline® (Can)** *see* HydrALAZINE *on page 680*

◆ **Apriso™** *see* Mesalamine *on page 887*

◆ **Aprodine [OTC]** *see* Triprolidine and Pseudoephedrine *on page 1388*

Aprotinin (a proe TYE nin)

U.S. Brand Names Trasylol®
Canadian Brand Names Trasylol®
Therapeutic Category Hemostatic Agent
Generic Available No
Use Prophylactic use to reduce perioperative blood loss and the need for blood transfusion in patients undergoing cardiopulmonary bypass in the course of coronary artery bypass graft surgery (CABG); in selected repeat cases of primary CABG surgery where the risk of bleeding is especially high or where transfusion is unavailable or unacceptable
Pregnancy Risk Factor B
Pregnancy Considerations Teratogenic effects were not observed in animal studies. There are no adequate and well-controlled studies in pregnant women.
Lactation Excretion in breast milk unknown/use caution
Contraindications Hypersensitivity to aprotinin or any component
Warnings Aprotinin may cause fatal anaphylactic or anaphylactoid reactions; fatal reactions have occurred with initial (test) doses as well as any time in dosage regimen, including situations where initial dose was tolerated; patients with a previous exposure to aprotinin (particularly when re-exposure is within 12 months) are at an increased risk **[U.S. Boxed Warning]**; test dose should only be done when patient is intubated and in a setting where cardiopulmonary bypass can be rapidly initiated; emergency medications to treat severe hypersensitivity reactions should be readily available; pretreatment with an antihistamine and H2 blocker before administration of the loading dose is recommended in patients with prior exposure; delay the addition of aprotinin into the pump prime solution until the loading dose has safely been administered

The FDA has issued a Public Health Advisory alerting physicians who perform heart bypass surgery and their patients that aprotinin has been linked to an increased risk of death, serious kidney damage, CHF, and stroke in observational studies. The FDA is advising healthcare providers to limit the use of aprotinin to patients where benefit of reducing blood loss is essential to management (outweighs the risks), to carefully monitor patients for the occurrence of toxicity, and to report adverse events associated with its use to the FDA. Safety and efficacy in children have not been established.
Precautions All patients treated with aprotinin should first receive a test dose at least 10 minutes before the loading dose to assess the potential for allergic reactions
Adverse Reactions
Cardiovascular: Atrial fibrillation, MI, CHF, atrial flutter, ventricular tachycardia, ventricular extrasystoles, supraventricular tachycardia, stroke, chest pain, hypotension, pericardial effusion, pulmonary hypertension, pericarditis
Central nervous system: Fever, mental confusion, seizures, agitation, dizziness, anxiety, insomnia
Endocrine & metabolic: Hyperglycemia, hypokalemia, acidosis
Gastrointestinal: Nausea, vomiting, constipation, diarrhea, GI hemorrhage
Hematologic: Hemolysis, anemia, thrombosis, CPK increased
Hepatic: Liver damage, jaundice
Local: Phlebitis
Neuromuscular & skeletal: Arthralgia

Renal: Renal function decreased, renal failure, renal tubular acidosis

Respiratory: Dyspnea, bronchoconstriction, pulmonary edema, apnea, cough increased

Miscellaneous: Anaphylaxis (see Warnings)

Drug Interactions

Avoid Concomitant Use There are no known interactions where it is recommended to avoid concomitant use.

Increased Effect/Toxicity There are no known significant interactions involving an increase in effect.

Decreased Effect

Aprotinin may decrease the levels/effects of: ACE Inhibitors; Thrombolytic Agents

Stability Store between 2°C to 25°C (36°F to 77°F); do not freeze; do not mix with other medications; incompatible with corticosteroids, heparin (see Administration), amino acids, and fat emulsion

Mechanism of Action Aprotinin, a serine protease inhibitor, modulates the systemic inflammatory response associated with cardiopulmonary bypass surgery; inhibits plasmin, kallikrein, and platelet activation producing antifibrinolytic effects; is a weak inhibitor of plasma pseudocholinesterase; inhibits the contact phase activation of coagulation and preserves adhesive platelet glycoproteins making them resistant to damage from increased circulating plasmin or mechanical injury occurring during cardiopulmonary bypass

Pharmacokinetics (Adult data unless noted)

Metabolism: Slowly degraded by lysosomal enzymes

Half-life, elimination: 150 minutes; terminal elimination: 10 hours

Elimination: <10% excreted unchanged in the urine

Usual Dosage I.V.: Test dose: All patients should receive a test dose at least 10 minutes prior to the loading dose to assess the potential for allergic reactions

Infants and Children: No conclusive dosage regimen has been established; variable dosage recommendations in the literature. Test dose: (dosage not well documented in studies) 0.1 mg/kg (maximum: 1.4 mg) has been used. The following dosage ranges have been reported in the literature:

10,000-35,000 Kallikrein inhibitor units/kg (1.4-4.9 mg/kg) loading dose

10,000-35,000 Kallikrein inhibitor units/kg (1.4-4.9 mg/kg) into pump prime volume

10,000-35,000 Kallikrein inhibitor units/kg/hour (1.4-4.2 mg/kg/hour) continuous infusion

Alternative (based upon surface area):

120-240 mg/m^2 (857,142-1,714,284 Kallikrein inhibitor units/m^2) loading dose

120-240 mg/m^2 (857,142-1,714,284 Kallikrein inhibitor units/m^2) into pump prime volume

28-56 mg/m^2/hour (200,000-400,000 Kallikrein inhibitor units/m^2/hour) continuous infusion

Adults: Test dose: 1 mL (1.4 mg)

Regimen A (standard dose):

2 million Kallikrein inhibitor units (280 mg) loading dose

2 million Kallikrein inhibitor units (280 mg) into pump prime volume

500,000 Kallikrein inhibitor units/hour (70 mg/hour) continuous infusion during surgery

Regimen B (low dose):

1 million Kallikrein inhibitor units (140 mg) loading dose

1 million Kallikrein inhibitor units (140 mg) into pump prime volume

250,000 Kallikrein inhibitor units/hour (35 mg/hour) continuous infusion during surgery

Dosage adjustment in renal impairment: No adjustment required

Dosage adjustment in hepatic impairment: No information available

Administration Parenteral: For I.V. use only; all I.V. doses should be administered through a central line; infuse test dose over at least 10 minutes; infuse loading dose over 20-30 minutes with patient in the supine position; add pump priming dose while recirculating the priming fluid of the cardiopulmonary bypass circuit. To avoid physical incompatibility with heparin when adding to pump-prime solution, each agent should be added during recirculation to assure adequate dilution.

Monitoring Parameters Bleeding times, prothrombin time (PT), activated clotting time (ACT), platelet count, CBC, Hct, Hgb, and fibrinogen degradation products; for toxicity also include renal function tests and blood pressure

Because aPPT and ACT are difficult to interpret with aprotinin use, the manufacturer recommends two different ways to administer heparin:

1) Fixed heparin dosing where a standard loading dose of heparin plus the quantity of heparin added to the prime volume of the cardiopulmonary bypass (CPB) circuit should total at least 350 units/kg; additional heparin should be administered based upon the patient's weight and duration of CPB.

2) Heparin dosing based upon a protamine titration method. A heparin dose response, assessed by protamine titration, should be performed prior to administration of aprotinin to determine the heparin loading dose. Additional heparin should be administered on the basis of heparin levels measured by protamine titration. Heparin levels during bypass should not be allowed to drop below 2.7 units/mL (2 mg/kg) or below the level indicated by heparin dose response testing.

Reference Range Antiplasmin effects occur when plasma aprotinin concentrations are 125 kallikrein inhibitor units/mL and antikallikrein effects occur when plasma levels are 250-500 kallikrein inhibitor units/mL; it remains unknown if these plasma concentrations are required for clinical benefits to occur during cardiopulmonary bypass.

While institutional protocols may vary, a minimal celite ACT of 750 seconds or kaolin-ACT of 480 seconds is recommended in the presence of aprotinin. Consult the manufacturer's information on specific ACT test interpretation in the presence of aprotinin.

Test Interactions Aprotinin prolongs whole blood clotting time of heparinized blood as determined by the Hemochrom® method or similar surface activation methods; patients may require additional heparin even in the presence of activated clotting time levels that appear to represent adequate anticoagulation

Additional Information Due to interference with aprotinin and ACT, the amount of protamine administered to reverse heparin activity should be based upon the amount of heparin administered and not the ACT value.

Dosage Forms Excipient information presented when available (limited, particularly for generics); consult specific product labeling.

Injection, solution:

Trasylol®: 1.4 mg/mL [10,000 KIU/mL] (100 mL, 200 mL) [bovine derived]

References

Arnold DM, Fergusson DA, Chan AK, et al, "Avoiding Transfusions in Children Undergoing Cardiac Surgery: A Meta-Analysis of Randomized Trials of Aprotinin," *Anesth Analg*, 2006, 102(3):731-7.

Boldt J, "Endothelial-Related Coagulation in Pediatric Surgery," *Ann Thorac Surg*, 1998, 65(6 Suppl):S56-9.

Carrel TP, Schwanda M, Vogt P, et al, "Aprotinin in Pediatric Cardiac Operations: A Benefit in Complex Malformations and With High-Dose Regimen Only," *Ann Thorac Surg*, 1998, 66(1):153-8.

Miller BE, Tosone SR, Tam VK, et al, "Hematologic and Economic Impact of Aprotinin in Reoperative Pediatric Cardiac Operations," *Ann Thorac Surg*, 1998, 66(2):535-41.

Penkoske P, Entwistle LM, Marchak BE, et al, "Aprotinin in Children Undergoing Repair of Congenital Heart Defects," *Ann Thorac Surg*, 1995, 60(6 Suppl):S529-32.

Spray TL, "Use of Aprotinin in Pediatric Organ Transplantation," *Ann Thorac Surg*, 1998, 65(6 Suppl):S71-3.

◆ **Aquachloral® Supprettes® [DSC]** *see* Chloral Hydrate *on page 286*

◆ **Aquacort® (Can)** *see* Hydrocortisone *on page 685*

◆ **AquaMEPHYTON® (Can)** *see* Phytonadione *on page 1109*

◆ **Aquanil™ HC [OTC]** *see* Hydrocortisone *on page 685*

◆ **Aquasol A®** *see* Vitamin A *on page 1426*

◆ **Aquasol E® [OTC]** *see* Vitamin E *on page 1427*

◆ **Aquavit-E [OTC] [DSC]** *see* Vitamin E *on page 1427*

◆ **Aqueous Procaine Penicillin G** *see* Penicillin G Procaine *on page 1081*

◆ **Ara-C** *see* Cytarabine *on page 377*

◆ **Arabinosylcytosine** *see* Cytarabine *on page 377*

◆ **Aralen®** *see* Chloroquine *on page 293*

◆ **Aranesp®** *see* Darbepoetin Alfa *on page 390*

◆ **ARB** *see* Irbesartan *on page 758*

◆ **ARB** *see* Losartan *on page 847*

◆ **ARB** *see* Valsartan *on page 1402*

◆ **Aredia®** *see* Pamidronate *on page 1048*

◆ **Arepanrix™ H1N1 (Can)** *see* Influenza Virus Vaccine (H1N1, Inactivated) *on page 731*

◆ **Arestin Microspheres (Can)** *see* Minocycline *on page 933*

Argatroban (ar GA troh ban)

Medication Safety Issues
Sound-alike/look-alike issues:
Argatroban may be confused with Aggrastat®, Organan®

High alert medication: The Institute for Safe Medication Practices (ISMP) includes this medication among its list of drugs which have a heightened risk of causing significant patient harm when used in error.

Therapeutic Category Anticoagulant, Thrombin Inhibitor

Generic Available No

Use Prophylaxis or treatment of thrombosis in patients with heparin-induced thrombocytopenia (HIT) (FDA approved in adults); anticoagulant for percutaneous coronary intervention (PCI) in patients who have or are at risk for thrombosis associated HIT (FDA approved in adults). Has also been studied in children with HIT for procedural anticoagulation including cardiac catheterization, extracorporeal membrane oxygenation (ECMO), and hemodialysis/hemofiltration (see Additional Information)

Pregnancy Risk Factor B

Pregnancy Considerations Adverse events were not observed in animal studies. There are no adequate and well-controlled studies in pregnant women. Argatroban should be used in pregnant women only if clearly needed.

Lactation Excretion in breast milk unknown/not recommended

Breast-Feeding Considerations It is not known if argatroban is excreted in human milk. Because of the serious potential of adverse effects to the nursing infant, a decision to discontinue nursing or discontinue argatroban should be considered.

Contraindications Hypersensitivity to argatroban or any component; overt major bleeding

Warnings Prior to initiation of argatroban therapy, all other parenteral anticoagulants should be discontinued and adequate time lapsed. Hemorrhage is the most frequent complication of argatroban; bleeding can occur at any site in the body. Use with extreme caution in patients with increased risk of hemorrhage. Risk factors for hemorrhage include intensity of anticoagulation; bacterial endocarditis; congenital or acquired bleeding disorders; recent puncture of large vessels or organ biopsy; recent CVA, stroke, or intracerebral surgery; severe hypertension; renal impairment; recent major surgery, especially of the brain, spinal cord, or eye; recent major bleeding (intracranial, GI, intraocular, or pulmonary); GI lesions (eg, ulcerations); immediately after lumbar puncture; spinal anesthesia. Monitor for signs and symptoms of bleeding including unexplained decrease in hematocrit or blood pressure. Argatroban is for I.V. use only.

Precautions Use with caution and reduce dose in patients with hepatic impairment; may require >4 hours to achieve full reversal of argatroban anticoagulant effect following treatment in patients with hepatic impairment. Avoid use during PCI in patients with elevations of ALT/AST (≥3 times the upper limit of normal); use in these patients has not been evaluated. Use with caution and reduce the dose in critically ill patients, patients with multiple organ dysfunction, heart failure, severe anascara, or postcardiac surgery; clearance is reduced in these patients. Limited pediatric pharmacokinetic and dosing information is available; the appropriate goals of anticoagulation and duration of treatment in pediatric patients have not been established.

Argatroban prolongs the PT/INR. Concomitant use with warfarin will cause increased prolongation of the PT and INR greater than that of warfarin alone. If warfarin is initiated concurrently with argatroban, initial PT/INR goals while on argatroban may require modification; alternative guidelines for monitoring therapy should be followed (see Usual Dosage). Safety and efficacy for use with thrombolytic agents have not been established.

Adverse Reactions Note: Bleeding from any site is the major adverse effect of argatroban (see Warnings); major bleeding may occur

Cardiovascular: Atrial fibrillation, bradycardia, CABG-related bleeding (minor), cardiac arrest, cerebrovascular disorder, chest pain, hypotension, MI, myocardial ischemia, thrombosis, vasodilation, ventricular tachycardia

Central nervous system: Fever, headache, intracranial bleeding, pain

Dermatologic: Skin reactions (bullous eruption, rash)

Endocrine & metabolic: Hypokalemia (see Young, 2007)

Gastrointestinal: Abdominal pain, constipation (see Young, 2007), diarrhea, GI bleed, nausea, vomiting

Genitourinary: Genitourinary bleed, hematuria, urinary tract infection

Hematologic: Hematocrit decreased, hemoglobin decreased

Local: Bleeding at injection or access site

Neuromuscular & skeletal: Back pain

Renal: Abnormal renal function

Respiratory: Cough, dyspnea, hemoptysis, pneumonia

Miscellaneous: Infection, sepsis

<1%, postmarketing, and/or case reports: Allergic reactions, GERD, limb and below-the-knee amputation stump bleed, multisystem hemorrhage and DIC, pulmonary edema, retroperitoneal bleeding

Drug Interactions

Metabolism/Transport Effects Substrate of CYP3A4 (minor)

Avoid Concomitant Use There are no known interactions where it is recommended to avoid concomitant use.

Increased Effect/Toxicity Drugs which affect platelet function (eg, aspirin, NSAIDs, dipyridamole, ticlopidine, clopidogrel), anticoagulants, or thrombolytics may potentiate the risk of hemorrhage. Sufficient time must pass after heparin therapy is discontinued; allow heparin's effect on the aPTT to decrease

Concomitant use of argatroban with warfarin increases PT and INR greater than that of warfarin alone. Argatroban is commonly continued during the initiation of warfarin therapy to assure anticoagulation and to protect against possible transient hypercoagulability.

Decreased Effect There are no known significant interactions involving a decrease in effect.

Stability Store unused vials at 25°C (77°F) with excursions permitted to 15°C to 30°C (59°F to 86°F) in original carton (to protect from light); do not freeze. Prepared solution is stable for 24 hours at 25°C (77°F) with excursions permitted to 15°C to 30°C (59°F to 86°F) in ambient indoor light. Do not expose to direct sunlight. Prepared solution that is protected from light and kept at controlled room temperature of 20°C to 25°C (68°F to 77°F) or under refrigeration at 2°C to 8°C (36°F to 46°F) is stable for up to 96 hours. Additional light resistant measures (eg, foil protection for I.V. lines) are not needed.

Mechanism of Action Argatroban is highly-selective direct thrombin inhibitor which reversibly binds to the active thrombin site of free and clot-associated thrombin. Anticoagulant effects result from the inhibition of thrombin-catalyzed reactions including fibrin formation; activation of coagulation factors V, VIII, and XIII; activation of protein C; and platelet aggregation.

Pharmacodynamics

Onset of action: Immediate

Pharmacokinetics (Adult data unless noted)

Distribution: Distributes primarily to intracellular fluid

V_d: 174 mL/kg

Protein binding: Total: 54%; Albumin: 20%; α_1-acid glycoprotein: 34%

Metabolism: Hepatic via hydroxylation and aromatization. Metabolism via CYP3A4/5 to four known metabolites plays a minor role. Unchanged argatroban is the major plasma component. Plasma concentration of primary metabolite (M1) is 0% to 20% of the parent drug; M1 is three- to fivefold weaker.

Half-life, terminal: 39-51 minutes; hepatic impairment: 181 minutes

Elimination: Feces via biliary secretion (65%; 14% unchanged); urine (22%; 16% unchanged)

Clearance:

Pediatric patients (seriously ill): 0.16 L/kg/hour; 50% lower than healthy adults

Pediatric patients (seriously ill with elevated bilirubin due to hepatic impairment or cardiac complications; n=4): 0.03 L/kg/hour; 80% lower than pediatric patients with normal bilirubin

Adult: 0.31 L/kg/hour (5.1 mL/kg/minute); hepatic impairment: 1.9 mL/kg/minute

Dialysis: Hemodialysis: 20% dialyzed

Usual Dosage I.V.

Infants and Children ≤16 years: Note: Limited data available; dosing regimens not established. Titration of maintenance dose must consider multiple factors including current argatroban dose, current aPTT, target aPTT, and clinical status of the patient. For specific uses, required maintenance dose is highly variable between patients. Additionally, during the course of treatment, patient's dosing requirements may change as clinical status changes (eg, sicker patients require lower dose); frequent dosage adjustments may be required to maintain desired anticoagulant activity (see Alsoufi, 2004; Boshkov 2006). If argatroban therapy is used concurrently with or following FFP or a thrombolytic, some centers decrease dose by half (see Alsoufi, 2004).

Heparin-induced thrombocytopenia: I.V. continuous infusion: (manufacturer's recommendations):

Initial dose: 0.75 mcg/kg/minute

Maintenance dose: Measure aPTT after 2 hours; adjust dose until the steady-state aPTT is 1.5-3 times the initial baseline value, not exceeding 100 seconds; adjust in increments of 0.1-0.25 mcg/kg/minute for normal hepatic function; reduce dose in hepatic impairment (see Dosing adjustment in hepatic impairment).

Note: A lower initial infusion rate may be needed in other pediatric patients with reduced clearance of argatroban (eg, patients with heart failure, multiple organ system failure, severe anasarca, or postcardiac surgery). This precaution is based on adult studies of patients with these disease states who had reduced argatroban clearance.

Conversion to oral anticoagulant: Because there may be a combined effect on the INR when argatroban is combined with warfarin, loading doses of warfarin should not be used. Warfarin therapy should be started at the expected daily dose. Once combined INR on warfarin and argatroban is >4, stop argatroban. Repeat INR measurement in 4-6 hours; if INR is below therapeutic level, argatroban therapy may be restarted. Repeat procedure daily until desired INR on warfarin alone is obtained. Another option is to use factor X levels to monitor the effect of warfarin anticoagulation. When factor X level is <0.3, warfarin is considered therapeutic and at which time argatroban can be discontinued (see Alsoufi, 2004; Boshkov, 2006).

Adults: Heparin-induced thrombocytopenia: I.V. continuous infusion:

Initial dose: 2 mcg/kg/minute; use actual body weight up to 130 kg (BMI up to 51 kg/m^2) (see Rice, 2007)

Maintenance dose: Patient may not be at steady state but measure aPTT after 2 hours; adjust dose until the steady-state aPTT is 1.5-3.0 times the initial baseline value, not exceeding 100 seconds; dosage should not exceed 10 mcg/kg/minute

Note: Critically-ill patients with normal hepatic function became excessively anticoagulated with FDA approved or lower starting doses of argatroban. Doses between 0.15-1.3 mcg/kg/minute were required to maintain aPTTs in the target range (see Reichert, 2003). In a prospective observational study of critically-ill patients with multiple organ dysfunction (MODS) and suspected or proven HIT, an initial infusion dose of 0.2 mcg/kg/minute was found to be sufficient and safe in this population (see Beiderlinden, 2007). Consider reducing starting dose to 0.2 mcg/kg/minute in critically-ill patients with MODS defined as a minimum number of two organ failures. Another report of a cardiac patient with anasarca secondary to acute renal failure had a reduction in argatroban clearance similar to patients with hepatic dysfunction. Reduced clearance may have been due to reduced liver perfusion (see de Denus, 2003). The American College of Chest Physicians has recommended an initial infusion rate of 0.5-1.2 mcg/kg/minute for patients with heart failure, MODS, severe anasarca, or postcardiac surgery (see Hirsch, 2008).

Conversion to oral anticoagulant: Because there may be a combined effect on the INR when argatroban is combined with warfarin, loading doses of warfarin should not be used. Warfarin therapy should be started at the expected daily dose.

Patients receiving ≤2 mcg/kg/minute of argatroban: Argatroban therapy can be stopped when the combined INR on warfarin and argatroban is >4; repeat INR measurement in 4-6 hours; if INR is below therapeutic level, argatroban therapy may be restarted. Repeat procedure daily until desired INR on warfarin alone is obtained.

Patients receiving >2 mcg/kg/minute of argatroban: In order to predict the INR on warfarin alone, reduce dose of argatroban to 2 mcg/kg/minute; measure INR for argatroban and warfarin 4-6 hours after dose reduction; argatroban therapy can be stopped when the combined INR on warfarin and argatroban is >4. Repeat INR measurement in 4-6 hours; if INR is below therapeutic level, argatroban therapy may be restarted. Repeat procedure daily until desired INR on warfarin alone is obtained.

Note: The American College of Chest Physicians recommends monitoring chromogenic factor X assay when transitioning from argatroban to warfarin (see Hirsh, 2008). Factor X levels <45% have been associated with INR values >2 until the effects of argatroban have been eliminated (see Arpino, 2005).

Dosing adjustment in renal impairment: Dosage adjustment is not required.

Dosing adjustment in hepatic impairment: Decreased clearance is seen with hepatic impairment; dose should be reduced.

Infants and Children ≤16 years: Heparin-induced thrombocytopenia; I.V. continuous infusion:

Initial dose: 0.2 mcg/kg/minute

Maintenance dose: Measure aPTT after 2 hours; adjust dose until the steady-state aPTT is 1.5-3 times the initial baseline value, not exceeding 100 seconds; adjust in increments of ≤0.05 mcg/kg/minute.

Adults: Moderate hepatic impairment: I.V. continuous infusion: Initial dose: 0.5 mcg/kg/minute; monitor aPTT closely; adjust dose as clinically needed. **Note:** During PCI, avoid use in patients with elevations of ALT/AST (>3 times ULN); the use of argatroban in these patients has not been evaluated.

Administration For I.V. use only. Solution must be diluted prior to administration; dilute each 250 mg vial with 250 mL of diluent; final concentration: 1 mg/mL. May be mixed with NS, D₅W, or LR. Mix by repeated inversion for 1 minute. A slight but brief haziness may occur prior to mixing. Do not mix with other medications.

Monitoring Parameters HIT: Obtain baseline aPTT prior to start of therapy. Check aPTT 2 hours after start of therapy and any dosage adjustment. Monitor hemoglobin, hematocrit, platelets, signs and symptoms of bleeding.

Test Interactions Argatroban may elevate PT/INR levels in the absence of warfarin. If warfarin is started, initial PT/INR goals while on argatroban may require modification. The American College of Chest Physicians recommends monitoring chromogenic factor X assay when transitioning from argatroban to warfarin (see Hirsh, 2008). Factor Xa levels <45% have been associated with INR values >2 after the effects of argatroban have been eliminated (see Arpino, 2005).

Nursing Implications
Assess potential for interactions with other pharmacological agents patient may be taking (especially drugs which affect platelet function or coagulation). Assess for therapeutic effectiveness according to purpose for use and adverse reactions (abnormal bleeding, GI pain, epistaxis, hematuria, irritation at infusion site) frequently during therapy. Observe bleeding precautions and teach patient interventions to reduce side effects and adverse reactions to report.

Additional Information Molecular weight: 526.66; argatroban is a synthetic anticoagulant (direct thrombin inhibitor) derived from L-arginine. Increases in aPTT,

ACT, PT, INR, and TT occur in a dose-dependent fashion with increasing doses of argatroban. Adult studies have established the use of aPTT for patients with HIT and ACT for patients with PCI procedures. Therapeutic ranges for PT, INR, and TT have not been identified.

A reversal agent to argatroban is not available. Should life-threatening bleeding occur, discontinue argatroban immediately, obtain an aPTT and other coagulation tests, and provide symptomatic and supportive care.

Infants and Children ≤16 years: Doses reported in the literature for infants and children with HIT for procedural anticoagulation:

Cardiac Catheterization: Dose not established; the following doses have been used in limited reports: Initial I.V. bolus dose: 150-250 mcg/kg, followed by continuous I.V. infusion at an initial rate 5-15 mcg/kg/minute; one case series adjusted the continuous infusion dose to maintain target ACT >300 seconds (n=4). **Note:** Data is limited to an open-labeled study of a mixed population that included six pediatric cardiac catheterization patients and case reports/series (n=4 patients) [see Alsoufi, 2004; GlaxoSmithKline Result Summary, 2007 (manufacturer unpublished data); Young, 2007]. Further studies are required before these doses can be recommended.

ECMO: Dose not established; data is limited to an open-labeled study of a mixed population that included one infant on ECMO, published and submitted abstracts, and case reports/series (n=16 patients) [see Alsoufi, 2004; GlaxoSmithKline Result Summary, 2007 (manufacturer unpublished data); Hursting, 2006; Potter, 2007; Tcheng, 2004]. Further studies are required before these doses can be recommended.

The reported argatroban doses used to prime the ECMO circuit have varied widely; more recent reports utilize an ECMO priming dose between 30-50 mcg based upon patient's clinical status and ACT, followed by a continuous I.V. infusion at an initial rate of 0.5-2 mcg/kg/minute; continuous infusion doses were adjusted to maintain target ACT of at least 200 seconds; reported ACT target ranges varied from 160-300 seconds or aPTT 2 times initial baseline value. Dosing requirements ranging from 0.1-24 mcg/kg/minute have been reported. If patient not previously anticoagulated on heparin prior to starting argatroban, an initial bolus dose may be required.

Hemodialysis/Hemofiltration: Dose not established; clinical data limited to case series/reports (see Alsoufi, 2004; Hursting, 2006; Young, 2007). Further studies are required before these doses can be recommended.

The following doses have been used in limited reports: I.V. continuous infusion: Initial dose: 0.5-2 mcg/kg/minute; infusions were adjusted to maintain target ACT at least >160 seconds or aPTT >50 seconds; when reported, ACT target ranges were 160-200 seconds and aPTT 50-75 seconds. Reported dosing requirements were 0.1-2 mcg/kg/minute. If patient not previously anticoagulated on heparin prior to starting argatroban, an initial bolus dose may be required; initial bolus doses of 65 mcg/kg and 250 mcg/kg have each been reported.

Dosage Forms Excipient information presented when available (limited, particularly for generics); consult specific product labeling.

Injection, solution: 100 mg/mL (2.5 mL) [contains dehydrated alcohol 1000 mg/mL]

References
Alsoufi B, Boshkov LK, Kirby A, et al, "Heparin-Induced Thrombocytopenia (HIT) in Pediatric Cardiac Surgery: An Emerging Cause of Morbidity and Mortality," *Semin Thorac Cardiovasc Surg Pediatr Card Surg Annu*, 2004, 7:155-71.

Arpino PA, Demirjian Z, and Van Cott EM, "Use of the Chromogenic Factor X Assay to Predict the International Normalized Ratio in Patients Transitioning From Argatroban to Warfarin," *Pharmacotherapy*, 2005, 25(2):157-64.

Beiderlinden M, Treschan TA, Gorlinger K, et al, "Argatroban Anticoagulation in Critically Ill Patients," *Ann Pharmacother*, 2007, 41 (5):749-54.

Boshkov LK, Kirby A, Shen I, et al, "Recognition and Management of Heparin-Induced Thrombocytopenia in Pediatric Cardiopulmonary Bypass Patients," *Ann Thorac Surg*, 2006, 81(6):S2355-9.

de Denus S and Spinler SA, "Decreased Argatroban Clearance Unaffected by Hemodialysis in Anasarca," *Ann Pharmacother*, 2003, 37(9):1237-40.

GlaxoSmithKline Result Summary, Study No: SKF105043/013, "An Open-Label Study of Argatroban Injection to Evaluate the Safety and Effectiveness in Pediatric Patients Requiring Anticoagulation Alternatives to Heparin," July 2, 2007. Available at: http://www.gsk-clinicalstudyregister.com/files/pdf/22691.pdf.

Hirsh J, Guyatt G, Albers GW, et al, "Executive Summary: American College of Chest Physicians Evidence-Based Clinical Practice Guidelines (8th Edition)," *Chest*, 2008, 133(6 Suppl):71-109.

Hursting MJ, Dubb J, and Verme-Gibboney CN, "Argatroban Anticoagulation in Pediatric Patients: A Literature Analysis," *J Pediatr Hematol Oncol*, 2006, 28(1):4-10.

Potter KE, Raj A, and Sullivan JE, "Argatroban for Anticoagulation in Pediatric Patients With Heparin-Induced Thrombocytopenia Requiring Extracorporeal Life Support," *J Pediatr Hematol Oncol*, 2007, 29 (4):265-8.

Reichert MG, MacGregor DA, Kincaid EH, et al, "Excessive Argatroban Anticoagulation for Heparin-Induced Thrombocytopenia," *Ann Pharmacother*, 2003, 37(5):652-4.

Rice L, Hursting MJ, Baillie GM, et al, "Argatroban Anticoagulation in Obese Versus Nonobese Patients: Implications for Treating Heparin-Induced Thrombocytopenia," *J Clin Pharmacol*, 2007, 47(8):1028-34.

Scott LK, Grier LR, and Conrad SA, "Heparin-Induced Thrombocytopenia in a Pediatric Patient Receiving Extracorporeal Membrane Oxygenation Managed With Argatroban," *Pediatr Crit Care Med*, 2006, 7(5):473-5.

Tcheng WY and Wong W, "Successful Use of Argatroban in Pediatric Patients Requiring Anticoagulant Alternatives to Heparin," *Blood*, 2004,104:107b-108b.

Young G and Boshkov L, "Prospective Study of Direct Thrombin Inhibition With Argatroban in Pediatric Patients Requiring Non-Heparin Anticoagulation," *Blood*, 2007, 110.

Young G, "New Anticoagulants in Children," *Hematology Am Soc Hematol Educ Program*, 2008, 245-50.

Arginine (AR ji neen)

Medication Safety Issues The Food and Drug Administration (FDA) has identified several cases of fatal arginine overdose in children and has recommended that healthcare professionals always recheck dosing calculations prior to administration of arginine. Doses used in children should not exceed usual adult doses.

U.S. Brand Names R-Gene® 10

Therapeutic Category Diagnostic Agent, Growth Hormone Function; Metabolic Alkalosis Agent; Urea Cycle Disorder (UCD) Treatment Agent

Generic Available No

Use Pituitary function test (stimulant for the release of growth hormone); management of severe, uncompensated, metabolic alkalosis (pH ≥7.55) **after** optimizing therapy with sodium or potassium chloride supplements; treatment agent for urea cycle disorders (FDA approved in children and adults)

Pregnancy Risk Factor B

Pregnancy Considerations Teratogenic effects were not observed in animal studies; however, the manufacturer does not recommend use of arginine during pregnancy.

Lactation Enters breast milk/use caution

Breast-Feeding Considerations Amino acids are excreted in breast milk, the amount following arginine administration is not known.

Contraindications Hypersensitivity to arginine or any component

Warnings Use extreme caution when administering to neonates and children as overdosage has resulted in hyperchloremic metabolic acidosis, cerebral edema, or possibly death. Use with caution in renal or hepatic failure.

Precautions Arginine hydrochloride is metabolized to nitrogen-containing products for excretion; the temporary effect of a high nitrogen load on the kidneys should be evaluated; accumulation of excess arginine may result in an overproduction of nitric oxide, leading to vasodilation and hypotension; each 1 mEq chloride delivers 1 mEq hydrogen; monitor acid base balance closely, particularly in neonates

Adverse Reactions

Cardiovascular: Flushing (after rapid I.V. administration), hypotension

Central nervous system: Cerebral edema, headache (after rapid I.V. administration), lethargy

Dermatologic: Rash

Endocrine & metabolic: Hyperglycemia, hyperkalemia, metabolic acidosis

Gastrointestinal: Abdominal pain, bloating, nausea, perioral tingling, vomiting

Genitourinary: Hematuria

Hematologic: Thrombocytopenia (rare)

Local: Injection site reaction, severe tissue necrosis with extravasation, venous irritation

Miscellaneous: Hypersensitivity reaction, serum gastrin concentration elevated

Drug Interactions

Avoid Concomitant Use There are no known interactions where it is recommended to avoid concomitant use.

Increased Effect/Toxicity There are no known significant interactions involving an increase in effect.

Decreased Effect There are no known significant interactions involving a decrease in effect.

Mechanism of Action Stimulates pituitary release of growth hormone and prolactin and pancreatic release of glucagon and insulin; patients with impaired pituitary function have lower or no increase in plasma concentrations of growth hormone after administration of arginine. Arginine hydrochloride has been used for treatment of hypochloremic metabolic alkalosis due to its high chloride content. Arginine becomes an essential amino acid in ASL deficiency due to a decrease in the conversion of argininosuccinate to arginine; in other urea cycle disorders, exogenous arginine is used to produce increased serum concentrations and to prevent the breakdown of endogenous protein. Arginine is a precursor to nitric oxide and can produce vasodilation and inhibition of platelet aggregation.

Pharmacokinetics (Adult data unless noted)

Absorption: Oral: Well absorbed

Bioavailability: ~68%

Time to peak serum concentration:

Oral: 1.5-2 hours

I.V.: 30 minutes

Half-life: 0.7-1.3 hours

V_d:. 33-100 L/kg

Usual Dosage I.V.:

Growth hormone reserve test:

Children: 0.5 g/kg over 30 minutes

Adults: 30 g (300 mL) over 30 minutes

Treatment of urea cycle disorders: Neonates, Infants, Children, and Adults:

Argininosuccinic acid lyase (ASL) or argininosuccinic acid synthetase (ASS) disorders or pending definitive diagnosis: 600 mg/kg as a loading dose followed by 600 mg/kg/day as a continuous infusion

Carbamyl phosphate synthetase (CPS) or ornithine transcarbamylase (OTC) disorder: 200 mg/kg as a loading dose followed by 200 mg/kg/day as a continuous infusion. A single case using 60 mg/kg/hour for 12 hours has been reported (Kodama, 1996).

Intermittent hyperammonemic crisis in patients with urea cycle disorders: Neonates, Infants, Children, and Adults:
ASL or ASS: 0.6 g/kg or 12 g/m^2 loading dose followed by 0.6 g/kg/day or 12 g/m^2/day continuous infusion
CPS or OTC: 0.2 g/kg or 4 g/m^2 loading dose followed by 0.2 g/kg/day or 4 g/m^2/day continuous infusion

Metabolic alkalosis: Infants, Children, and Adults: Arginine hydrochloride dose (g) = weight (kg) x 0.1 x [HCO$_3^-$ - 24] where HCO$_3^-$ = the patient's serum bicarbonate concentration in mEq/L; give $^1/_2$ to $^2/_3$ of calculated dose and re-evaluate

Note: Arginine hydrochloride is an alternative treatment for uncompensated metabolic alkalosis after sodium chloride and potassium chloride supplementation have been optimized.

To correct hypochloremia: Infants, Children, and Adults: Arginine hydrochloride dose (mEq) = 0.2 x weight (kg) x [103 - Cl$^-$] where Cl$^-$ = the patient's serum chloride concentration in mEq/L; give $^1/_2$ to $^2/_3$ of calculated dose and re-evaluate

Note: Arginine hydrochloride should never be used as initial therapy for chloride supplementation but as an alternative in the patient who is unresponsive to sodium chloride or potassium chloride supplementation.

Administration Parenteral: May be infused without further dilution (however, very irritating to tissues; dilution is recommended; administration through a central line is recommended; maximum rate of I.V. infusion: 1 g/kg/hour (4.75 mEq/kg/hour) (maximum dose: 60 g/hour = 285 mEq over 1 hour); infuse loading doses for urea cycle disorders over 90 minutes

Monitoring Parameters Acid-base status (arterial or capillary blood gases), serum electrolytes, BUN, glucose, plasma growth hormone concentrations (when evaluating growth hormone reserve), plasma ammonia and amino acids (when treating urea cycle disorders)

Reference Range If intact pituitary function, human growth hormone levels should rise after arginine administration to 10-30 ng/mL (control range: 0-6 ng/mL)

Nursing Implications I.V. infiltration of arginine hydrochloride may cause necrosis and phlebitis; prolongation of the infusion may diminish the stimulus to the pituitary gland and nullify the test

Additional Information When treating urea cycle disorders, sodium bicarbonate use may be necessary to neutralize the acidifying effects of arginine HCl.

Dosage Forms Excipient information presented when available (limited, particularly for generics); consult specific product labeling.

Injection, solution, as hydrochloride:
R-Gene® 10: 10% (300 mL) [100 mg/mL = 950 mOsm/L; contains chloride 0.475 mEq/mL]

References

Batshaw ML, MacArthur RB, and Tuchman M, "Alternative Pathway Therapy for Urea Cycle Disorders: Twenty Years Later," *J Pediatr*, 2001, 138(1 Suppl):S46-54.

Bode-Böger SM, Böger RH, Galland A, et al, "L-Arginine-Induced Vasodilation in Healthy Humans: Pharmacokinetic-Pharmacodynamic Relationship," *Br J Clin Pharmacol*, 1998, 46(5):489-97.

Bushinsky DA and Gennari FJ, "Life-Threatening Hyperkalemia Induced by Arginine," *Ann Intern Med*, 1978, 89(5 Pt 1):632-4.

Kodama H, Mori Y, Kubota K, et al, "Intravenous Arginine Dramatically Improved Hyperammonemia in a Patient With Late-Onset Ornithine Transcarbamylase Deficiency," *Tohoku J Exp Med*, 1996, 180 (1):83-6.

Summar M, "Current Strategies for the Management of Neonatal Urea Cycle Disorders," *J Pediatr*, 2001, 138(1 Suppl):S30-9.

◆ **Arginine HCl** *see* Arginine *on page 131*

◆ **Arginine Hydrochloride** *see* Arginine *on page 131*

◆ **8-Arginine Vasopressin** *see* Vasopressin *on page 1410*

Aripiprazole (ay ri PIP ray zole)

Medication Safety Issues
Sound-alike/look-alike issues:
Abilify® may be confused with Ambien®

Aripiprazole may be confused with proton pump inhibitors (dexlansoprazole, esomeprazole, lansoprazole, omeprazole, pantoprazole, rabeprazole)

U.S. Brand Names Abilify Discmelt®; Abilify®

Canadian Brand Names Abilify®

Therapeutic Category Antipsychotic Agent, Atypical

Generic Available No

Use
Oral: Acute and maintenance treatment of schizophrenia (FDA approved in ages ≥13 years and adults); acute and maintenance treatment of bipolar disorder (with acute manic or mixed episodes) (FDA approved in ages ≥10 years and adults); adjunctive therapy (to lithium or valproate) for acute treatment of bipolar disorder (with acute manic or mixed episodes) (FDA approved in ages ≥10 years and adults); treatment of irritability associated with autistic disorder (including symptoms of aggression, deliberate self-injurious behavior, temper tantrums, quickly changing moods) (FDA approved in ages 6-17 years); adjunctive treatment (to antidepressants) of major depressive disorder (FDA approved in adults). Has also been used in children and adolescents for treatment of ADHD, conduct disorders, Tourette's syndrome, and irritability associated with other pervasive developmental disorders.

Injection: Acute treatment of agitation associated with schizophrenia or bipolar disorder (manic or mixed) (FDA approved in adults)

Medication Guide An FDA-approved patient medication guide, which is available with the product information and at http://www.fda.gov/downloads/Drugs/DrugSafety/ucm085804.pdf, must be dispensed with this medication for each new prescription and refill.

Pregnancy Risk Factor C

Pregnancy Considerations Aripiprazole demonstrated developmental toxicity and teratogenic effects in animal models. There are no adequate and well-controlled trials in pregnant women. Should be used in pregnancy only when potential benefit to mother outweighs possible risk to the fetus. Healthcare providers are encouraged to enroll women 18-45 years of age exposed to aripiprazole during pregnancy in the Atypical Antipsychotics Pregnancy Registry (866-961-2388).

Lactation Excretion in breast milk unknown/not recommended

Contraindications Hypersensitivity to aripiprazole or any component

Warnings Aripiprazole is **not** FDA approved for the (adjunctive) treatment of depression in pediatric patients. Clinical worsening of depression or suicidal ideation or behavior may occur in children and adults with major depressive disorder **[U.S. Boxed Warning]**. In clinical trials, antidepressants increased the risk of suicidal thinking and behavior (suicidality) in children, adolescents, and young adults (18-24 years of age) with major depressive disorder and other psychiatric disorders. This risk must be considered before prescribing antidepressants for any clinical use. Short-term studies did **not** show an increased risk of suicidality with antidepressant use in patients >24 years of age and showed a decreased risk in patients ≥65 years.

Patients of all ages who are treated with antidepressants for any indication require appropriate monitoring and close observation for clinical worsening of depression, suicidality, and unusual changes in behavior, especially during the first few months after antidepressant initiation or when the dose is adjusted. Family members and caregivers should be instructed to closely observe the patient (ie, daily) and communicate condition with healthcare provider. Patients should also be monitored for associated behaviors (eg, anxiety, agitation, panic attacks, insomnia, irritability, hostility, aggressiveness, impulsivity, akathisia, hypomania, mania) which may increase the risk for worsening depression or suicidality. Worsening depression or emergence of suicidality (or associated behaviors listed above) that is abrupt in onset, severe, or not part of the presenting symptoms, may require discontinuation or modification of drug therapy. To reduce risk of intentional overdose, write prescriptions for the smallest quantity consistent with good patient care. Screen individuals for bipolar disorder prior to treatment of depression (using antidepressants alone may induce manic episodes in patients with this condition).

May cause neuroleptic malignant syndrome (symptoms include hyperpyrexia, altered mental status, muscle rigidity, autonomic instability, acute renal failure, rhabdomyolysis, and elevated CPK). May cause extrapyramidal reactions, including pseudoparkinsonism, acute dystonic reactions, akathisia, and tardive dyskinesia (risk of these reactions is low relative to other neuroleptics, and is dose-dependent; to decrease risk of tardive dyskinesia: Use smallest dose and shortest duration possible; evaluate continued need periodically; risk of dystonia is increased with the use of high potency and higher doses of conventional antipsychotics and in males and younger patients). May cause hyperglycemia, which may be severe and include potentially fatal ketoacidosis or hyperosmolar coma; use with caution and monitor glucose closely in patients with diabetes mellitus (or with risk factors such as family history or obesity); measure fasting blood glucose at the beginning of therapy and periodically during therapy in these patients; monitor for symptoms of hyperglycemia in all patients treated with aripiprazole; measure fasting blood glucose in patients who develop symptoms. Leukopenia, neutropenia, and agranulocytosis (sometimes fatal) have been reported in clinical trials and postmarketing reports with antipsychotic use; presence of risk factors (eg, pre-existing low WBC or history of drug-induced leuko/neutropenia) should prompt periodic blood count assessment. Discontinue therapy at first signs of blood dyscrasias or if absolute neutrophil count <1000/mm^3.

Pediatric psychiatric disorders are frequently serious mental disorders which present with variable symptoms that do not always match adult diagnostic criteria. Conduct a thorough diagnostic evaluation and carefully consider risks of psychotropic medication before initiation in pediatric patients with schizophrenia, bipolar disorder, or irritability associated with autistic disorder. Medication therapy for pediatric patients with these disorders is indicated as part of a total treatment program that frequently includes educational, psychological, and social interventions.

An increased risk of death has been reported with the use of antipsychotics in elderly patients with dementia-related psychosis **[U.S. Boxed Warning]**; most deaths seemed to be cardiovascular (eg, sudden death, heart failure) or infectious (eg, pneumonia) in nature. An increased incidence of cerebrovascular adverse events (eg, transient ischemic attack, stroke), including fatalities, has been reported with the use of aripiprazole in elderly patients with dementia-related psychosis. Aripiprazole is not approved for the treatment of patients with dementia-related psychosis.

Precautions Use with caution in patients with seizure disorders (seizures have been rarely reported), in suicidal patients, patients with concomitant systemic illnesses, patients with unstable heart disease or a recent history of MI (these patients not adequately studied), and in those at risk of aspiration pneumonia (esophageal dysmotility and aspiration have been associated with antipsychotic agents). May cause orthostatic hypotension; use with caution in patients at risk for this effect or in those who would not tolerate transient hypotensive episodes (eg, cerebrovascular disease, cardiovascular disease, hypovolemia, or concurrent medication use which may predispose to hypotension). May cause somnolence (dose-related). May cause alteration of temperature regulation (use with caution in patients exposed to temperature extremes).

Aripiprazole may cause a higher than normal weight gain in children and adolescents; monitor growth (including weight, height, BMI, and waist circumference) in pediatric patients receiving aripiprazole; compare weight gain to standard growth curves. **Note:** A prospective, nonrandomized cohort study followed 338 antipsychotic naïve pediatric patients (age: 4-19 years) for a median of 10.8 weeks (range: 10.5-11.2 weeks) and reported the following significant mean increases in weight in kg (and % change from baseline): Olanzapine: 8.5 kg (15.2%), quetiapine: 6.1 kg (10.4%), risperidone: 5.3 kg (10.4%), and aripiprazole: 4.4 kg (8.1%) compared to the control cohort: 0.2 kg (0.65%). Increases in metabolic indices (eg, serum cholesterol, triglycerides, glucose) were also reported; however, these changes were not significant in patients receiving aripiprazole. Biannual monitoring of cardiometabolic indices after the first 3 months of therapy is suggested (see Correll, 2009).

Oral solution contains 400 mg fructose and 200 mg sucrose per mL. Orally disintegrating tablets contain aspartame which is metabolized to phenylalanine and must be avoided (or used with caution) in patients with phenylketonuria.

Adverse Reactions Note: Frequency of adverse effects is reported for the oral formulation; incidences given for children are from studies that included children and adolescents.

Cardiovascular: Orthostatic hypotension, tachycardia

Central nervous system: Agitation, akathisia, anxiety, attention disturbances, dizziness, dyskinesia, dystonia, EPS (children: 6% to 20%; adults: 2% to 5%), fatigue (children: 10% to 17%; adults: 6% to 8%), feeling jittery, fever, headache (children: 13%; adults: 27%), insomnia, lethargy, lightheadedness, neuroleptic malignant syndrome (see Warnings), pain, restlessness, sedation, somnolence (children: 10% to 23%; adults: 5% to 6%), suicidal thinking and behavior (see Warnings)

Gastrointestinal: Abdominal discomfort, constipation, diarrhea, drooling, dyspepsia, nausea, salivation increased, stomach discomfort, toothache, vomiting, xerostomia

Dermatologic: Rash

Endocrine & metabolic: Appetite decreased, appetite increased, dysmenorrhea, hyperglycemia (see Warnings), hyperlipidemia, weight gain (see Precautions)

Hematologic: Agranulocytosis, leukopenia, neutropenia (see Warnings)

Neuromuscular & skeletal: Arthralgia, extremity pain, muscle spasm, myalgia, stiffness, tremor, weakness

Ocular: Blurred vision

Respiratory: Cough, nasopharyngitis, pharyngolaryngeal pain, rhinorrhea

Miscellaneous: Hiccups, hypersensitivity reactions

<1%, postmarketing, and/or case reports (limited to important or life-threatening): Aggression, akinesia, alopecia, amenorrhea, anger, angina pectoris, angioedema, anorexia, anorgasmia, aspiration pneumonia, asthenia, atrial fibrillation, atrial flutter, AV- block, bilirubin increased, bradycardia, bradykinesia, breast pain, BUN increased, cardiopulmonary failure, cardiorespiratory arrest, catatonia, cerebrovascular accident, chest pain, choreoathetosis, cogwheel rigidity, coordination abnormal, CPK increased, delirium, diabetes mellitus, diplopia, DKA, dysphagia, dyspnea, edema (eyelid), edema (facial), erectile dysfunction, esophagitis, extrasystoles, falling, GERD, GGT increased, glycosylated hemoglobin increased, gynecomastia, heat stroke, hepatic enzyme increased, hepatitis, hirsutism, homicidal ideation, hyper-/hypotonia, hypoglycemia, hypokalemia, hypokinesia, hyponatremia, hypotension, hypothermia, intentional self injury, irritability, jaundice, LDH increased, libido changes, memory impairment, menstrual irregularities, MI, muscle rigidity, muscle tightness, myocardial ischemia, myoclonus, nasal congestion, nocturia, oropharyngeal spasm, palpitations, pancreatitis, parkinsonism, peripheral edema, photophobia, photopsia, photosensitivity reaction, polydipsia, polyuria, priapism, prolactin increased, pruritus, QT prolongation, rhabdomyolysis, seizure (grand mal), self-mutilation, serum creatinine increased, sleep-talking, somnambulism, speech disorder, suicide, suicide attempt, supraventricular tachycardia, swollen tongue, tardive dyskinesia, thirst, thrombocytopenia, tic, tongue dry, tongue spasm, urinary retention, urticaria, ventricular tachycardia, weight loss

Drug Interactions

Metabolism/Transport Effects Substrate (major) of CYP2D6, 3A4

Avoid Concomitant Use

Avoid concomitant use of Aripiprazole with any of the following: Metoclopramide

Increased Effect/Toxicity

Aripiprazole may increase the levels/effects of: Alcohol (Ethyl); CNS Depressants; Methotrimeprazine

The levels/effects of Aripiprazole may be increased by: Acetylcholinesterase Inhibitors (Central); CYP2D6 Inhibitors (Moderate); CYP2D6 Inhibitors (Strong); CYP3A4 Inhibitors (Moderate); CYP3A4 Inhibitors (Strong); Darunavir; Dasatinib; Lithium formulations; Methotrimeprazine; Metoclopramide; Tetrabenazine

Decreased Effect

Aripiprazole may decrease the levels/effects of: Amphetamines; Anti-Parkinson's Agents (Dopamine Agonist); Quinagolide

The levels/effects of Aripiprazole may be decreased by: CarBAMazepine; CYP3A4 Inducers (Strong); Deferasirox; Herbs (CYP3A4 Inducers); Lithium formulations; Peginterferon Alfa-2b

Food Interactions A high-fat meal delays the time to peak plasma concentrations of aripiprazole by 3 hours and of dehydro-aripiprazole (active metabolite) by 12 hours. However, a high-fat meal does not affect peak concentrations or AUC of either compound.

Stability Store at controlled room temperature of 25°C (77°F); excursions permitted to 15°C to 30°C (59°F to 86°F). Protect injection from light; store in original container; keep in carton until ready to use. Use oral solution within 6 months after opening.

Mechanism of Action Aripiprazole is a quinolinone antipsychotic; its therapeutic effects may be mediated through a combination of partial agonist activity at D_2 and $5-HT_{1A}$ receptors and antagonist activity at $5-HT_{2A}$ receptors; it may cause orthostatic hypotension via its antagonist activity at adrenergic alpha$_1$ receptors. Aripiprazole exhibits high affinity for D_2, D_3, $5-HT_{1A}$, and $5-HT_{2A}$ receptors; moderate affinity for D_4, $5-HT_{2C}$, $5-HT_7$, alpha$_1$ adrenergic, and histamine H_1 receptors. It also possesses moderate affinity for the serotonin reuptake transporter; has no affinity for muscarinic (cholinergic) receptors. Aripiprazole functions as a partial agonist at the D_2 and $5-HT_{1A}$ receptors, and as an antagonist at the $5-HT_{2A}$ receptor.

Pharmacodynamics

Onset: Initial: 1-3 weeks

Pharmacokinetics (Adult data unless noted) Note: In

pediatric patients 10-17 years of age, the pharmacokinetic parameters of aripiprazole and dehydro-aripiprazole have been shown to be similar to adult values when adjusted for weight.

Absorption: Well absorbed

Distribution: V_{dss}: 4.9 L/kg

Protein binding: ≥99%, primarily to albumin

Metabolism: Hepatic, via CYP2D6 and CYP3A4; the dehydro-aripiprazole metabolite has affinity for D_2 receptors similar to the parent drug and represents 40% of the parent drug exposure in plasma

Bioavailability: I.M.: 100%; Oral: Tablet: 87%; **Note:** Orally disintegrating tablets are bioequivalent to tablets; oral solution to tablet ratio of geometric mean for peak concentration is 122% and for AUC is 114%.

Half-life elimination: Aripiprazole: 75 hours; dehydro-aripiprazole: 94 hours

CYP2D6 poor metabolizers: Aripiprazole: 146 hours

Time to peak serum concentration: I.M.: 1-3 hours; tablet: 3-5 hours (see Food Interactions)

Elimination: Feces (55%, ~18% of dose as unchanged drug); urine (25%, <1% unchanged drug)

Usual Dosage Note: Oral solution may be substituted for the oral tablet on a mg-per-mg basis, up to 25 mg. Patients receiving 30 mg tablets should be given 25 mg oral solution. Orally disintegrating tablets (Abilify Discmelt®) are bioequivalent to the immediate release tablets (Abilify®).

Children and Adolescents: Oral:

Bipolar I disorder (acute manic or mixed episodes): Children and Adolescents 10-17 years: Initial: 2 mg daily for 2 days, followed by 5 mg daily for 2 days with a further increase to target dose of 10 mg daily; subsequent dose increases may be made in 5 mg increments, up to a maximum of 30 mg/day

Schizophrenia: Adolescents 13-17 years: Initial: 2 mg daily for 2 days, followed by 5 mg daily for 2 days with a further increase to target dose of 10 mg daily; subsequent dose increases may be made in 5 mg increments up to a maximum of 30 mg/day; **Note:** 30 mg/day was **not** found to be more effective than the 10 mg/day dose

Autism: Treatment of irritability associated with autistic disorder (including aggression, deliberate self-injurious behavior, temper tantrums, and quickly changing moods): Children and Adolescents 6-17 years: Initial dose: 2 mg daily for 7 days, followed by 5 mg daily; subsequent dose increases may be made in 5 mg increments every ≥7 days, up to a maximum of 15 mg/day

Note: See Additional Information for doses used in studies to treat irritability and aggressive behavior in pediatric patients with other pervasive developmental disorders, conduct disorders, and ADHD.

Tourette's syndrome, tic disorders: Children and Adolescents 7-18 years: Limited information exists in literature: Dose is not established; small, open-labeled clinical trials and retrospective observational studies suggest low doses (2.5-5 mg/day) may be efficacious. Studies used the following doses: Initial dose: 1.25-5 mg/day; daily doses were increased by 1.25-2.5 mg weekly or by 5 mg every 2 weeks. Maximum dose: 15-20 mg/day. Reported mean required doses ranged from 3.3-11.7 mg/day (see Budman, 2008; Murphy, 2009; Seo, 2008; Yoo, 2007). See Additional Information for more detailed information. Further studies are needed.

Adults:
Oral:
Bipolar disorder (acute manic or mixed episodes): Initial: 15 mg once daily (as monotherapy or as adjunctive therapy with lithium or valproate); usual: 15 mg once daily; may be increased to a maximum of 30 mg once daily; doses >30 mg/day have not been evaluated.

Depression (adjunctive with antidepressants): Initial: 2-5 mg/day; dosage adjustments of up to 5 mg/day may be made in intervals of ≥1 week; usual dose: 2-15 mg/day.

Schizophrenia: Initial: 10-15 mg once daily; usual: 10-15 mg once daily; may be increased to a maximum of 30 mg once daily. Dosage titration should not be more frequent than every 2 weeks. **Note:** Doses higher than 10-15 mg once daily were **not** found to be more effective.

I.M.: Acute agitation (schizophrenia/bipolar mania): 9.75 mg as a single dose (range: 5.25-15 mg); may repeat (≥2-hour intervals) to a maximum of 30 mg/day); **Note:** A dose of 15 mg was **not** shown to be more effective than 9.75 mg dose.

Dosage adjustment with concurrent CYP450 inducer or inhibitor therapy: Oral:
CYP3A4 inducers (eg, carbamazepine): Aripiprazole dose should be doubled; dose should be subsequently reduced if concurrent inducer agent discontinued.
Strong CYP3A4 inhibitors (eg, ketoconazole, clarithromycin): Aripiprazole dose should be reduced to 1/2 of the usual dose, and proportionally increased upon discontinuation of the inhibitor agent.
CYP2D6 inhibitors (eg, fluoxetine, paroxetine, quinidine): Aripiprazole dose should be reduced to 1/2 of the usual dose, and proportionally increased upon discontinuation of the inhibitor agent. **Note:** When aripiprazole is administered as adjunctive therapy to patients with MDD, the dose should **not** be adjusted, but administered as specified above in the dose for depression field.

Dosage adjustment in renal impairment: No dosage adjustment required.
Dosage adjustment in hepatic impairment: No dosage adjustment required.

Administration
Oral (all dosage forms): May be administered with or without food.
Orally-disintegrating tablet: Do not remove tablet from blister pack until ready to administer; do not push tablet through foil (tablet may become damaged); peel back foil to expose tablet; use dry hands to remove tablet and place immediately on tongue. Tablet dissolves rapidly in saliva and may be swallowed without liquid; if needed, tablet can be taken with liquid. Do not split tablet.
Injection: For I.M. use only; do not administer SubQ or I.V.; inject slowly into deep muscle mass

Monitoring Parameters Vital signs; CBC with differential; fasting lipid profile and fasting blood glucose/Hb A$_{1c}$ (prior to treatment, at 3 months, then annually); weight, growth, BMI, and waist circumference [especially in children (see Precautions)], personal/family history of diabetes, blood pressure, mental status, abnormal involuntary movement scale (AIMS), extrapyramidal symptoms (EPS). Weight should be assessed prior to treatment, at 4 weeks, 8 weeks, 12 weeks, and then at quarterly intervals. Consider titrating to a different antipsychotic agent for a weight gain ≥5% of the initial weight. Monitor patient periodically for symptom resolution; monitor for worsening depression, suicidality, and associated behaviors (especially at the beginning of therapy or when doses are increased or decreased; see Warnings)

Patient Information Read the patient Medication Guide that you receive with each prescription and refill of aripiprazole. An increased risk of suicidal thinking and behavior has been reported with the use of antidepressants in children, adolescents, and young adults (18-24 years of age). Notify physician if you feel more depressed, have thoughts of suicide, or become more agitated or irritable (see Warnings). May cause dizziness or drowsiness and impair ability to perform activities requiring mental alertness or physical coordination; may cause dry mouth; may cause postural hypotension, especially during initial dose titration (use caution when changing position from lying or sitting to standing).

Report the use of other medications, nonprescription medications, and herbal or natural products to your physician and pharmacist; avoid alcohol and the herbal medicine, St John's wort. Report persistent CNS effects (eg, trembling fingers, altered gait or balance, excessive sedation, seizures, unusual muscle or skeletal movements), rapid heartbeat, severe dizziness, vision changes, skin rash, weight gain or loss, or worsening of condition to your physician. If you have diabetes, monitor blood glucose levels closely at beginning of therapy and periodically thereafter (may cause hyperglycemia). Patients may be more vulnerable to overheating and dehydration while taking this medication; maintain adequate hydration unless advised by prescriber to restrict fluids.

Nursing Implications May need to assist patient in rising slowly from lying or sitting to standing position [orthostatic blood pressure changes may occur (see Precautions and Monitoring Parameters)]

Additional Information Long-term usefulness of aripiprazole should be periodically re-evaluated in patients receiving the drug for extended periods of time.

Additional detailed aripiprazole dosing information for Children and Adolescents: Oral:

Note: For each of these indications, limited information exists in the literature; dose is not established; further studies are needed.

Pervasive Developmental Disorder Not Otherwise Specified (PDD-NOS) and Asperger's Disorder: Irritability (aggression, self-injury, tantrums): An open-labeled, pilot study (n=25; mean age: 8.6 years; range: 5-17 years) used initial aripiprazole doses of 1.25 mg/day for 3 days, then 2.5 mg/day until the end of week two; doses were then titrated upward over the next 4 weeks as tolerated or clinically indicated (maximum dose: 15 mg). An 88% response rate was reported (see Stigler, 2009). A retrospective, noncontrolled, open-label study of 34 PDD patients (mean age: 10.2 years; range: 4-15 years) included 10 patients with autistic disorder and 24 patients with PDD-NOS. The following aripiprazole dosing regimen was used: Preschool age: Initial dose: 1.25 mg/day with titration every ≥5 days in 1.25 mg/day increments as tolerated or clinically indicated; prepubertal children: Initial dose: 2.5 mg/day with titration every 5 days in 2.5 mg/day increments as tolerated or clinically indicated; adolescents (>12 years of age): Initial dose: 2.5-5 mg/day with titration every 5 days in 2.5-5 mg/day increments as tolerated or clinically indicated (doses >5 mg/day were divided twice daily; if sleep disorder was reported, the dose was given in morning and/or at lunchtime. Mean final dose: 8.1 ± 4.9 mg/day. An overall response rate of 32.4% (29.2% in patients with PDD-NOS) was reported (see Masi, 2009). In a retrospective chart review of children and adolescents with developmental disability and a wide range of psychiatric disorders (n=32; age: 5-19 years), a mean starting dose of aripiprazole of 7.1 ± 0.32 mg/day and a mean maintenance dose of 10.55 ± 6.9 mg/day was used. A response rate of 56% was reported for the overall population and for children with mental retardation. However, a study population subset analysis in patients with mental retardation (n=18) showed a lower response rate in patients with mental retardation with PDD-NOS (38%) than in patients with mental retardation without PDD-NOS (100%) (see Valicenti-McDermott, 2006).

Aggression, conduct disorder (CD): An open-label, prospective study (n=23; age: 6-17 years) evaluated pharmacokinetics and effectiveness of aripiprazole in patients with a primary diagnosis of CD (with or without comorbid ADHD). Results showed improvement in CD symptom scores with only minor improvements in cognition. Initial dosing was weight-based and after 14 days could be titrated to clinically effectiveness (maximum dose: 15 mg/day). Initial doses were: Patient weight <25 kg: 1 mg/day; 25-50 kg: 2 mg/day; 51-70 kg: 5 mg/day; >70 kg: 10 mg/day (see Findling, 2009). A non-randomized, open-labeled study (n=46; age: 6-17 years) evaluated effectiveness of aripiprazole (n=24) and ziprasidone (n=22) in aggressive behavior in various psychiatric diagnoses; the aripiprazole study arm included 8 patients with CD. Initial doses were 2.5 mg/day in patients <12 years and 5 mg/day in patients ≥12 years; doses were adjusted as needed for clinical effectiveness and/or tolerability (mean final dose: 4.5 ± 2.3 mg). A significant improvement in outcome measures was found with both agents (average improvement 63%) with neither drug showing superiority (see Bastiaens, 2009).

Attention-Deficit/Hyperactivity Disorder (ADHD): An open-label, pilot study (n=23; age: 8-12 years) reported significant improvement in ADHD outcome scores without an impact on cognitive measures (positive or negative). The initial dose was 2.5 mg/day and was increased on a weekly basis by 2.5 mg/day increments (maximum dose: 10 mg/day); doses were adjusted for tolerability; mean final dose: 6.7 ± 2.4 mg/day (see Findling, 2008). Other aripiprazole published reports in pediatric and adolescent patients in which ADHD is a comorbid diagnosis within the study population exist; however, effectiveness in ADHD was not a reported primary outcome measure (see Bastiaens, 2009; Budman, 2008; Findling, 2009; Murphy, 2009; Valicenti-McDermott, 2006).

Tourette's syndrome, tic disorders: One open-label study (n=24, age: 7-18 years) used an initial dose of 5 mg/day; dose was increased by 5 mg/day increments every 2 weeks as tolerated (maximum dose: 20 mg/day); mean final dose: 9.8 ± 4.8 mg/day; range: 2.5-20 mg/day (see Yoo, 2007). In a prospective, open-labeled study (n=16; age: 8-17 years), an initial dose of 1.25 mg/day was used; dose was increased by 1.25-2.5 mg/day increments weekly as tolerated and clinically indicated (maximum dose: 15 mg/day); mean final dose: 3.3 ± 2.1 mg/day; range 1.25-7.5 mg/day (see Murphy, 2009). Another prospective, open-labeled study (n=15; age: 7-19 years) showed significant improvement in tic scores using an initial dose of 2.5-7.5 mg/day (mean 5.33 ± 1.29 mg/day); final mean dose: 8.17 ± 4.06 mg/day (see Seo, 2008). A retrospective, case series (n=37, age 8-18 years) used an initial dose of 1.25-2.5 mg/day in prepubertal children and 2.5-5 mg/day in adolescents; dose was escalated every

5-7 days as tolerated and clinically indicated; mean final dose 11.69 ± 7.15 mg/day (see Budman, 2008).

Dosage Forms Excipient information presented when available (limited, particularly for generics); consult specific product labeling.

Injection, solution:
    Abilify®: 7.5 mg/mL (1.3 mL)
Solution, oral:
    Abilify®: 1 mg/mL (150 mL) [contains propylene glycol, sucrose 400 mg/mL, and fructose 200 mg/mL; orange cream flavor]
Tablet:
    Abilify®: 2 mg, 5 mg, 10 mg, 15 mg, 20 mg, 30 mg
Tablet, orally disintegrating:
    Abilify Discmelt®: 10 mg [contains phenylalanine 1.12 mg; creme de vanilla flavor]; 15 mg [contains phenylalanine 1.68 mg; creme de vanilla flavor]

References

Bastiaens L, "A Non-Randomized, Open Study With Aripiprazole and Ziprasidone for the Treatment of Aggressive Behavior in Youth in a Community Clinic," *Community Ment Health J*, 2009, 45(1):73-7.

Budman C, Coffey BJ, Shechter R, et al, "Aripiprazole in Children and Adolescents With Tourette Disorder With and Without Explosive Outbursts," *J Child Adolesc Psychopharmacol*, 2008, 18(5):509-15.

Correll CU, Manu P, Olshanskiy V, et al, "Cardiometabolic Risk of Second-Generation Antipsychotic Medications During First-Time Use in Children and Adolescents," *JAMA*, 2009, 302(16):1765-73.

Findling RL, Kauffman R, Sallee FR, et al, "An Open-Label Study of Aripiprazole: Pharmacokinetics, Tolerability, and Effectiveness in Children and Adolescents With Conduct Disorder," *J Child Adolesc Psychopharmacol*, 2009, 19(4):431-9.

Findling RL, Short EJ, Leskovec T, et al, "Aripiprazole in Children With Attention-Deficit/Hyperactivity Disorder," *J Child Adolesc Psychopharmacol*, 2008, 18(4):347-54.

Marcus RN, Owen R, Kamen L, et al, "A Placebo-Controlled, Fixed-Dose Study of Aripiprazole in Children and Adolescents With Irritability Associated With Autistic Disorder," *J Am Acad Child Adolesc Psychiatry*, 2009, 48(11):1110-9.

Masi G, Cosenza A, Millepiedi S, et al, "Aripiprazole Monotherapy in Children and Young Adolescents With Pervasive Developmental Disorders: A Retrospective Study," *CNS Drugs*, 2009, 23(6):511-21.

Murphy TK, Mutch PJ, Reid JM, et al, "Open Label Aripiprazole in the Treatment of Youth With Tic Disorders," *J Child Adolesc Psychopharmacol*, 2009, 19(4):441-7.

Owen R, Sikich L, Marcus RN, et al, "Aripiprazole in the Treatment of Irritability in Children and Adolescents With Autistic Disorder," *Pediatrics*, 2009, 124(6):1533-40.

Seo WS, Sung HM, Sea HS, et al, "Aripiprazole Treatment of Children and Adolescents With Tourette Disorder or Chronic Tic Disorder," *J Child Adolesc Psychopharmacol*, 2008, 18(2):197-205.

Stigler KA, Diener JT, Kohn AE, et al, "Aripiprazole in Pervasive Developmental Disorder Not Otherwise Specified and Asperger's Disorder: A 14-Week, Prospective, Open-Label Study," *J Child Adolesc Psychopharmacol*, 2009, 19(3):265-74.

Valicenti-McDermott MR and Demb H, "Clinical Effects and Adverse Reactions of Off-Label Use of Aripiprazole in Children and Adolescents With Developmental Disabilities," *J Child Adolesc Psychopharmacol*, 2006, 16(5):549-60.

Yoo HK, Choi SH, Park S, et al, "An Open-Label Study of the Efficacy and Tolerability of Aripiprazole for Children and Adolescents With Tic Disorders," *J Clin Psychiatry*, 2007, 68(7):1088-93.

◆ **Aristospan®** see Triamcinolone *on page 1376*

◆ **Arranon®** see Nelarabine *on page 974*

◆ **Artemether and Benflumetol** see Artemether and Lumefantrine *on page 136*

Artemether and Lumefantrine

(ar TEM e ther & loo me FAN treen)

U.S. Brand Names Coartem®
Therapeutic Category Antimalarial Agent
Generic Available No
Use Treatment of acute, uncomplicated malaria infections due to *Plasmodium falciparum*, including malaria in geographical regions where chloroquine resistance has been reported [FDA approved in children ≥2 months (and at least 5 kg) and adults to age 65 years]
Pregnancy Risk Factor C

Pregnancy Considerations Safety data from an observational pregnancy study included 500 pregnant women exposed to artemether/lumefantrine and did not show an increased in adverse outcomes or teratogenic effects over background rate. Approximately one-third of these patients were in the third trimester. Efficacy has not been established in pregnant patients. Treatment failures with standard doses have been reported in pregnant women in areas where drug resistant parasites are prevalent. This may be attributed to lower serum concentration of both artemether and lumefantrine in this population (McGready, 2008). Animal studies have demonstrated increased fetal resorption and postimplantation loss during the period of organogenesis. Use during pregnancy only if potential benefit justifies potential risk to the fetus.

Lactation Excretion in breast milk unknown/use caution

Breast-Feeding Considerations The benefits of breast-feeding to mother and infants should be weighed against the potential risk from infant exposure to artemether and lumefantrine.

Contraindications Hypersensitivity to artemether, lumefantrine, or any component

Warnings QT interval prolongation has been reported in patients taking artemether/lumefantrine; avoid use in patients at risk for QT prolongation, including patients with a history of long QT syndrome, family history of congenital QT prolongation or sudden death, symptomatic arrhythmias, clinically-relevant bradycardia, severe heart disease, known hypokalemia, hypomagnesemia, or concurrent administration of antiarrhythmics (eg, Class Ia or III), or other drugs known to prolong the QT interval (eg, antipsychotics, antidepressants, macrolides, fluoroquinolones, triazole antifungals, or cisapride). Concomitant use of agents that prolong the QT interval or promote hypokalemia or hypomagnesemia should be avoided.

Precautions Use with caution in patients receiving CYP3A4 inhibitors, substrates, or inducers as loss of concomitant drug efficacy or QT prolongation may occur. Avoid use in patients receiving medications metabolized by CYP2D6 as plasma concentrations of theses coadministered medications may increase. Do not use within 1 month of halofantrine (not available in the U.S.) due to the potential additive effects on the QT interval. Drugs that prolong the QT interval (including quinidine and quinine) should be used with caution following treatment with artemether/lumefantrine due to lumefantrine's long half-life and potential for additive effects on the QT interval. If mefloquine is administered prior to lumefantrine, decreased lumefantrine exposure may occur due to mefloquine-induced decreased bile production; encourage food consumption and monitor efficacy.

In the event of disease reappearance after treatment with artemether/lumefantrine, patients should be treated with a different antimalarial drug. Use caution in patients with severe hepatic or renal impairment as it has not been studied in these populations.

Adverse Reactions Note: Adverse reactions reported are those reported in pediatric studies.

Cardiovascular: Palpitations

Central nervous system: Chills, dizziness, fatigue, fever, headache

Dermatologic: Angioedema, rash, urticaria

Gastrointestinal: Abdominal pain, anorexia, diarrhea, nausea, splenomegaly, vomiting

Hematologic: Anemia

Hepatic: AST increased, hepatomegaly

Neuromuscular & skeletal: Arthralgia, myalgia, weakness

Otic: Hearing loss

Respiratory: Cough, rhinitis

Drug Interactions

Avoid Concomitant Use

Avoid concomitant use of Artemether and Lumefantrine with any of the following: Antimalarial Agents; Artemether; Dronedarone; Halofantrine; Lumefantrine; Nilotinib; Pimozide; QTc-Prolonging Agents; QuiNINE; Tetrabenazine; Thioridazine; Ziprasidone

Increased Effect/Toxicity

Artemether and Lumefantrine may increase the levels/effects of: Antimalarial Agents; Antipsychotic Agents (Phenothiazines); CYP2D6 Substrates; Dapsone; Dapsone (Systemic); Dapsone (Topical); Dronedarone; Fesoterodine; Halofantrine; Lumefantrine; Nebivolol; Pimozide; QTc-Prolonging Agents; QuiNINE; Tamoxifen; Tetrabenazine; Thioridazine; Ziprasidone

The levels/effects of Artemether and Lumefantrine may be increased by: Alfuzosin; Antimalarial Agents; Artemether; Chloroquine; Ciprofloxacin; Ciprofloxacin (Systemic); CYP3A4 Inhibitors (Strong); Dapsone; Dapsone (Systemic); Gadobutrol; Grapefruit Juice; Lumefantrine; Nilotinib; QuiNINE

Decreased Effect

Artemether and Lumefantrine may decrease the levels/effects of: Codeine; Contraceptives (Estrogens); Contraceptives (Progestins); Saxagliptin; TraMADol

The levels/effects of Artemether and Lumefantrine may be decreased by: Mefloquine

Food Interactions Administration with grapefruit juice may result in increased concentrations of artemether and/or lumefantrine and potentiate QT prolongation (avoid grapefruit juice).

Absorption of artemether/lumefantrine is increased in the presence of food. The bioavailability of artemether increases two- to threefold and lumefantrine increases 16-fold (particularly with a high-fat meal).

Stability Store at controlled room temperature of 25°C (77°F).

Mechanism of Action Artemether and major metabolite dihydroartemisinin (DHA) are rapid schizontocides with activity attributed to the endoperoxide moiety common to each substance. Artemether inhibits an essential calcium adenosine triphosphatase. The exact mechanism of lumefantrine is unknown but may be due to inhibiting the formation of β-hematin by complexing with hemin. Both artemether and lumefantrine inhibit nucleic acid and protein synthesis. Artemether rapidly reduces parasite biomass and lumefantrine eliminates residual parasites.

Pharmacokinetics (Adult data unless noted)

Absorption:

Artemether: Rapid; enhanced with food

Lumefantrine: Initial absorption at 2 hours; enhanced with food

Protein binding:

Artemether: 95%

Dihydroartemisinin (DHA): 47% to 76%

Lumefantrine: 99.7%

Metabolism: Artemether is hepatically metabolized to an active metabolite, dihydroartemisinin (DHA) catalyzed predominantly by CYP3A4/5 and to a lesser extent by CYP2B6, CYP2C9, and CYP2C19. The artemether/DHA AUC ratio is 1.2 after one dose and 0.3 after six doses which may indicate autoinduction. Lemefantrine is hepatically metabolized to desbutyl-lumefantrine by CYP3A4.

Bioavailability: Absorption is increased in the presence of food. The bioavailability of artemether increases two- to threefold and lumefantrine increases 16-fold (particularly a high fat meal)

Half-life:
Artemether: 1-2 hours
DHA: 2 hours
Lumefantrine: 100-120 hours
Time to peak serum concentration:
Artemether: ~2 hours
Lumefantrine: ~6-8 hours
Excretion: No excretion data exist for humans

Usual Dosage Note: 3-day schedule for the treatment of uncomplicated malaria; Oral:

Children 2 months to <16 years:

5 kg to <15 kg: One tablet at hour 0 and at hour 8 on the first day and then one tablet twice daily (in the morning and evening) on days 2 and 3 (total of 6 tablets per treatment course)

15 kg to <25 kg: Two tablets at hour 0 and at hour 8 on the first day and then two tablets twice daily (in the morning and evening) on days 2 and 3 (total of 12 tablets per treatment course)

25 kg to <35 kg: Three tablets at hour 0 and at hour 8 on the first day and then three tablets twice daily (in the morning and evening) on day 2 and 3 (total of 18 tablets per treatment course)

≥35 kg: Four tablets at hour 0 and at hour 8 on the first day and then four tablets twice daily (in the morning and evening) on days 2 and 3 (total of 24 tablets per treatment course)

Adolescents >16 years and Adults (≥35 kg): Four tablets at hour 0 and at hour 8 on the first day and then four tablets twice daily (in the morning and evening) on days 2 and 3 (total of 24 tablets per treatment course). If patient is <35 kg, refer to child dosing.

Administration Administer with a full meal for best absorption. For infants, children, and patients unable to swallow tablets: Crush tablet and mix with 1-2 teaspoons of water in a clean container; administer; rinse container with water and administer remaining contents. The crushed mixture should be followed with food/milk, infant formula, pudding, porridge, or broth if possible. Repeat dose if vomiting occurs within 2 hours of administration; for persistent vomiting, explore alternative therapy.

Monitoring Parameters Monitor for signs and symptoms of efficacy.

Patient Information Food/Drug/Alcohol interactions: Do not take medication with grapefruit juice. Take medication with food. Inform physician if flu-like symptoms, vomiting, fainting, change in heart beat, or loss of appetite occurs.

Dosage Forms Excipient information presented when available (limited, particularly for generics); consult specific product labeling.

Tablet:

Coartem®: Artemether 20 mg and lumefantrine 120 mg

References

Alecrim MG, Lacerda MV, Mourão MP, et al, "Successful Treatment of *Plasmodium falciparum* Malaria With a Six-Dose Regimen of Artemether-Lumefantrine Versus Quinine-Doxycycline in the Western Amazon Region of Brazil," *Am J Trop Med Hyg*, 2006, 74(1):20-5.

Makanga M, Premji Z, Falade C, et al, "Efficacy and Safety of the Six-Dose Regimen of Artemether-Lumefantrine in Pediatrics With Uncomplicated *Plasmodium falciparum* Malaria: a Pooled Analysis of Individual Patient Data," *Am J Trop Med Hyg*, 2006, 74(6):991-8.

McGready R, Tan SO, Ashley EA, et al, "A Randomised Controlled Trial of Artemether-Lumefantrine Versus Artesunate for Uncomplicated *Plasmodium falciparum* Treatment in Pregnancy," *PLoS Med*, 2008, 5 (12):e253.

Omari AA, Gamble C, and Garner P, "Artemether-Lumefantrine (Six-Dose Regimen) for Treating Uncomplicated *Falciparum* Malaria," *Cochrane Database Syst Rev*, 2005, Issue 4, Art. No.: CD005564.

Toovey S and Jamieson A, "Audiometric Changes Associated With the Treatment of Uncomplicated *Falciparum* Malaria With Co-Artemether," *Trans R Soc Trop Med Hyg*, 2004, 98(5):261-7.

"World Health Organization Guidelines for the Treatment of Malaria," Available at http://www.who.int/malaria/docs/TreatmentGuidelines2006.pdf

◆ **ASA** *see* Aspirin *on page* 141

◆ **5-ASA** *see* Mesalamine *on page* 887

◆ **Asacol®** *see* Mesalamine *on page* 887

◆ **Asacol® 800 (Can)** *see* Mesalamine *on page* 887

◆ **Asacol® HD** *see* Mesalamine *on page* 887

◆ **Asaphen (Can)** *see* Aspirin *on page* 141

◆ **Asaphen E.C. (Can)** *see* Aspirin *on page* 141

◆ **Asco-Caps [OTC]** *see* Ascorbic Acid *on page* 138

◆ **Ascocid® [OTC]** *see* Ascorbic Acid *on page* 138

◆ **Ascor L 500®** *see* Ascorbic Acid *on page* 138

◆ **Ascor L NC®** *see* Ascorbic Acid *on page* 138

Ascorbic Acid (a SKOR bik AS id)

Medication Safety Issues

International issues:

Rubex® [Ireland] may be confused with Revex® which is a brand name for nalmefene in the U.S.

Rubex® [Ireland]: Discontinued brand name for doxurbicin in the U.S.

U.S. Brand Names Acerola [OTC]; Asco-Caps [OTC]; Asco-Tabs [OTC]; Ascocid® [OTC]; Ascor L 500®; Ascor L NC®; C-Gel [OTC]; C-Gram [OTC]; C-Time [OTC]; Cecon® [OTC] [DSC]; Cemill [OTC]; Cenolate® [DSC]; Chew-C [OTC]; Dull-C® [OTC]; Mild-C® [OTC]; One Gram C [OTC]; Time-C [OTC]; Time-C-Bio [OTC]; Vicks® Vitamin C [OTC]; Vita-C® [OTC]

Canadian Brand Names Proflavanol C™; Revitalose C-1000®

Therapeutic Category Nutritional Supplement; Urinary Acidifying Agent; Vitamin, Water Soluble

Generic Available Yes

Use Prevention and treatment of scurvy; urinary acidification; dietary supplementation; prevention and reduction in the severity of colds

Pregnancy Risk Factor A/C (dose exceeding RDA recommendation)

Pregnancy Considerations Animal reproduction studies have not been conducted.

Lactation Enters breast milk/compatible

Contraindications Hypersensitivity to ascorbic acid or any component (see Warnings); large doses during pregnancy

Warnings Cenolate® injection contains sulfites which may cause allergic reactions in susceptible individuals

Precautions Some products contain aspartame which is metabolized to phenylalanine and must be avoided (or used with caution) in patients with phenylketonuria.

Adverse Reactions

Cardiovascular: Flushing

Central nervous system: Faintness, dizziness, headache, fatigue

Gastrointestinal: Nausea, vomiting, heartburn, diarrhea

Renal: Hyperoxaluria

Drug Interactions

Avoid Concomitant Use There are no known interactions where it is recommended to avoid concomitant use.

Increased Effect/Toxicity

Ascorbic Acid may increase the levels/effects of: Aluminum Hydroxide; Deferoxamine

Decreased Effect

Ascorbic Acid may decrease the levels/effects of: Amphetamines; Bortezomib

Stability Injectable form should be stored under refrigeration (2°C to 8°C); protect oral dosage forms from light; ascorbic acid solution is rapidly oxidized

Mechanism of Action Necessary for collagen formation and tissue repair in the body; involved in some oxidation-reduction reactions as well as many other metabolic reactions

Pharmacodynamics Reversal of scurvy symptoms: 2 days to 3 weeks

Pharmacokinetics (Adult data unless noted)
Absorption: Oral: Readily absorbed; absorption is an active process and is thought to be dose-dependent
Distribution: Widely distributed
Protein binding: 25%
Metabolism: In the liver by oxidation and sulfation
Elimination: In urine; there is an individual specific renal threshold for ascorbic acid; when blood levels are high, ascorbic acid is excreted in urine, whereas when the levels are subthreshold very little if any ascorbic acid is excreted into urine

Usual Dosage Oral, I.M., I.V., SubQ:
Recommended adequate intake (AI):
0-6 months: 40 mg
6-12 months: 50 mg
Recommended daily allowance (RDA):
1-3 years: 15 mg
4-8 years: 25 mg
9-13 years: 45 mg
14-18 years: Males: 75 mg, females: 65 mg
19 years to Adults: Males: 90 mg, females: 75 mg
Children:
Scurvy: 100-300 mg/day in divided doses
Urinary acidification: 500 mg every 6-8 hours
Dietary supplement (variable): 35-100 mg/day
Adults:
Scurvy: 100-250 mg 1-2 times/day
Urinary acidification: 4-12 g/day in 3-4 divided doses
Dietary supplement (variable): 50-200 mg/day

Administration
Oral: May be administered without regard to meals
Parenteral: Use only in circumstances when the oral route is not possible; I.M. preferred parenteral route due to improved utilization; for I.V. use dilute in equal volume D_5W or NS, and infuse over at least 10 minutes

Reference Range
Normal levels: 10-20 mcg/mL
Scurvy: <1-1.5 mcg/mL

Test Interactions False-positive urinary glucose with cupric sulfate reagent, false-negative urinary glucose with glucose oxidase method, false-negative amine-dependent stool occult blood test

Additional Information Sodium content of 1 g: ~5 mEq

Dosage Forms Excipient information presented when available (limited, particularly for generics); consult specific product labeling. [DSC] = Discontinued product
Caplet: 1000 mg
Caplet, timed release: 500 mg, 1000 mg
Capsule:
Mild-C®: 500 mg
Capsule, softgel:
C-Gel: 1000 mg
Capsule, sustained release:
C-Time: 500 mg
Capsule, timed release: 500 mg
Asco-Caps: 500 mg, 1000 mg [sugar free]
Time-C®: 500 mg
Crystals for solution, oral: 4 g/teaspoonful (170 g, 1000 g)
Mild-C®: 3600 mg/teaspoonful [contains calcium 400 mg/teaspoonful]
Vita-C®: 4 g/teaspoonful (100 g, 454 g)
Injection, solution: 500 mg/mL (50 mL)
Cenolate® [DSC]: 500 mg/mL (1 mL, 2 mL) [contains aluminum, sodium hydrosulfite]

Injection, solution [preservative free]:
Ascor L 500®: 500 mg/mL (50 mL) [contains edetate disodium]
Ascor L NC®: 500 mg/mL (50 mL) [contains edetate disodium]
Liquid, oral: 500 mg/5 mL
Lozenge:
Vicks® Vitamin C: 25 mg [contains sodium 5 mg; orange flavor]
Powder, for solution, oral:
Ascocid®: 4000 mg/5 mL (227 g); 4300 mg/5 mL (227 g, 454 g); 5000 mg/5 mL (227 g, 454 g)
Dull-C®: 4 g/teaspoonful
Solution, oral:
Cecon®: 90 mg/mL [DSC]
Tablet: 100 mg, 250 mg, 500 mg, 1000 mg
Asco-Tabs: 1000 mg [sugar free]
Ascocid®: 500 mg [sugar free]
C-Gram, One Gram C: 1000 mg
Tablet, chewable: 250 mg, 500 mg
Acerola: 500 mg [cherry flavor]
Chew-C: 500 mg [orange flavor]
Mild-C®: 250 mg
Tablet, timed release: 500 mg, 1000 mg
Cemill: 500 mg, 1000 mg
Mild-C®: 1000 mg
Time-C-Bio: 500 mg

References
"Dietary Reference Intakes for Vitamin C, Vitamin E, Selenium, and Carotenoids. A Report of the Panel on Dietary Antioxidants and Related Compounds Food and Nutrition Board, Institute of Medicine," National Academy of Sciences, Washington, DC: National Academy Press, 2000.

◆ **Asco-Tabs [OTC]** *see* Ascorbic Acid *on page 138*

◆ **Ascriptin® [OTC]** *see* Aspirin *on page 141*

◆ **Ascriptin® Maximum Strength [OTC]** *see* Aspirin *on page 141*

◆ **Asmanex® Twisthaler®** *see* Mometasone Furoate *on page 942*

◆ **ASN-ase** *see* Asparaginase *on page 139*

Asparaginase (a SPIR a ji nase)

Medication Safety Issues
Sound-alike/look-alike issues:
Asparaginase may be confused with pegaspargase
Elspar® may be confused with Elaprase™, Oncaspar®

High alert medication: The Institute for Safe Medication Practices (ISMP) includes this medication among its list of classes of drugs which have a heightened risk of causing significant patient harm when used in error.

Related Information
Compatibility of Chemotherapy and Related Supportive Care Medications *on page 1580*
Emetogenic Potential of Antineoplastic Agents *on page 1579*

U.S. Brand Names Elspar®

Canadian Brand Names Kidrolase®

Therapeutic Category Antineoplastic Agent, Miscellaneous

Generic Available No

Use In combination therapy for the treatment of acute lymphoblastic leukemia; treatment of lymphoma, acute myeloid leukemia, chronic lymphocytic leukemia

Pregnancy Risk Factor C

Pregnancy Considerations Decreased weight gain, resorptions, gross abnormalities, and skeletal abnormalities were observed in animal studies. There are no adequate and well-controlled studies in pregnant women. Use during pregnancy only if clearly needed.

Lactation Excretion in breast milk unknown/not recommended

Breast-Feeding Considerations Due to the potential for serious adverse reactions in the nursing infant, breast-feeding is not recommended.

Contraindications Hypersensitivity to *E. coli*, asparaginase, or any component; serious thrombosis with prior asparaginase treatment; pancreatitis with prior asparaginase treatment; serious hemorrhagic events with prior asparaginase treatment. (**Note:** If a reaction to Elspar® occurs, obtain investigational *Erwinia* preparation from Opi SA, Pharmaceuticals for Rare Diseases, Les Jardins d'Eole, France or pegaspargase is another alternative; use with caution)

Warnings Hazardous agent; use appropriate precautions for handling and disposal; asparaginase should be administered under the supervision of a physician experienced in the use of cancer chemotherapy agents; severe allergic reactions may occur; monitor for 1 hour after administration; immediate treatment for anaphylactic reactions should be available during administration. Risk factors for allergic reactions include: I.V. administration, doses >6000-12,000 units/m^2, patients with prior exposure to asparaginase, and intervals of even a few days between doses. Discontinue asparaginase in patients who experience serious allergic reactions. Up to 33% of patients who have an allergic reaction to *E. coli* asparaginase will also react to the *Erwinia* form or pegaspargase. A test dose may be administered prior to the first dose of asparaginase, or prior to restarting therapy after a hiatus of several days. Desensitization may be performed in patients found to be hypersensitive by the intradermal test dose or who have received previous courses of therapy with the drug.

Increased prothrombin time, partial thromboplastin time, and hypofibrinogenemia may occur; cerebrovascular hemorrhage has been reported; monitor coagulation parameters. Fresh frozen plasma may be used to replace coagulation factors in patients with severe coagulopathy. Serious thrombosis, including sagittal sinus thrombosis, may occur; discontinue with serious thrombotic events. May cause hyperglycemia/glucose intolerance (some cases may be irreversible); monitor blood glucose. May cause serious and possibly fatal pancreatitis; evaluate patients with abdominal pain; discontinue if pancreatitis develops. There is a potential for patients to develop asparaginase antibodies which may result in hypersensitivity reactions or lead to faster clearance of asparaginase.

Precautions Use with caution in patients with an underlying coagulopathy, impaired renal function, or in patients with pre-existing liver impairment; discontinue asparaginase at the first sign of renal failure or pancreatitis. Appropriate measures should be taken to prevent hyperuricemia and uric acid nephropathy (consider allopurinol, hydration, and urinary alkalinization).

Adverse Reactions

Cardiovascular: Hypotension, edema, chest pain

Central nervous system: Fever, drowsiness, seizures, chills, malaise, lethargy, coma, fatigue, agitation, headache, stroke, confusion, dizziness, hallucinations, depression, somnolence, cerebrovascular thrombosis, seizures

Dermatologic: Rash, pruritus, urticaria, angioedema

Endocrine & metabolic: Hyperglycemia, transient diabetes mellitus, hyperammonemia, hyperuricemia, hypoalbuminemia; thyroxine and thyroxine-binding globulin concentration decreased

Gastrointestinal: Vomiting, pancreatitis, nausea, anorexia, abdominal cramps, stomatitis

Hematologic: Leukopenia, coagulation abnormalities (prolonged thrombin, PT, and partial prothrombin times), reduced fibrinogen, thrombosis, hemorrhage

Hepatic: Hepatotoxicity (elevated liver enzymes and alkaline phosphatase, hypoalbuminemia, hyperbilirubinemia), hepatic failure

Neuromuscular & skeletal: Arthralgia

Renal: Azotemia, acute renal failure

Respiratory: Coughing, laryngeal edema, bronchospasm

Miscellaneous: Hypersensitivity reactions (incidence in children is 20% with *E. coli* asparaginase and <5% with *Erwinia* asparaginase); anaphylaxis (can occur within 30-60 minutes following the first injection but occurs more frequently between the 5th and 9th dose)

Drug Interactions

Avoid Concomitant Use

Avoid concomitant use of Asparaginase with any of the following: BCG; Natalizumab; Pimecrolimus; Tacrolimus (Topical); Vaccines (Live)

Increased Effect/Toxicity

Asparaginase may increase the levels/effects of: Dexamethasone; Dexamethasone (Systemic); Leflunomide; Natalizumab; Vaccines (Live)

The levels/effects of Asparaginase may be increased by: Denosumab; Pimecrolimus; Tacrolimus (Topical); Trastuzumab

Decreased Effect

Asparaginase may decrease the levels/effects of: BCG; Sipuleucel-T; Vaccines (Inactivated); Vaccines (Live)

The levels/effects of Asparaginase may be decreased by: Echinacea

Stability Store at 2°C to 8°C (36°F to 46°F); no loss in potency was noted after storage for 1 week under refrigeration; however, the manufacturer recommends that reconstituted solutions should be discarded after 8 hours since there is no preservative; discard immediately if solution becomes cloudy; a 5 micron filter may be used to remove fiber-like particles; use of a 0.2 micron filter may result in some loss of potency

Mechanism of Action Inhibits protein synthesis by deaminating asparagine and depriving tumor cells of this essential amino acid

Pharmacokinetics (Adult data unless noted)

Absorption: Not absorbed from GI tract, therefore requires parenteral administration

Distribution: Asparaginase not detected in CSF but CSF asparagine is depleted; asparaginase is detected in lymph

V_d: 4-5 L/kg (~70% to 80% of plasma volume)

Half-life:

E. coli L-asparaginase: 24-36 hours

Patients who have had a hypersensitivity reaction to asparaginase have a decreased half-life

Note: *Erwinia* L-asparaginase: Significantly shorter than for the *E. coli*-derived product; mean half-life *Erwinia* L-asparaginase: 10-15 hours

Time to peak plasma levels: I.M.: 14-24 hours

Elimination: Clearance is unaffected by age, renal function, or hepatic function; only trace amounts appear in the urine

Usual Dosage Children and Adults: Refer to individual protocols

Perform intradermal sensitivity testing with 2 units of asparaginase before the initial dose and when a week or more has elapsed between doses (**Note:** False-negative rates of up to 80% to test doses of 2-5 units have been reported):

I.M. (preferred): 6000-10,000 units/m^2/dose 3 times/week for 3 weeks for combination therapy; high-dose I.M. regimen of 25,000 units/m^2/dose once weekly for 9 doses has also been used

I.V.: 6000 units/m^2/dose 3 times/week for 6-9 doses or 1000 units/kg/day for 10 days for combination therapy or 200 units/kg/day for 28 days if combination therapy is inappropriate

Administration
I.M.: Reconstitute vial with 2 mL NS. Maximum 2 mL volume is recommended for I.M. injections; if the volume to be administered is >2 mL, use multiple injection sites
I.V.: Reconstitute vial with 5 mL SWI or NS. Dilute dose in 50-250 mL of D$_5$W or NS; must be infused over a minimum of 30 minutes

Monitoring Parameters Vital signs during administration, CBC with differential, coagulation parameters, urinalysis, amylase, liver enzymes, bilirubin, prothrombin time, renal function tests, urine glucose, blood glucose, uric acid; monitor for allergic reaction

Patient Information Notify physician if fever, severe headache, leg swelling, chest pain, abdominal pain, excessive thirst, sore throat, painful/burning urination, bruising, bleeding, difficulty breathing, or shortness of breath occurs

Nursing Implications I.M. route is associated with a more delayed, less severe anaphylactoid reaction compared to the I.V. route; patients should be observed for one hour following an I.M. injection for signs of severe hypersensitivity; appropriate agents for maintenance of an adequate airway and treatment of a hypersensitivity reaction (antihistamine, epinephrine, oxygen, I.V. corticosteroids) should be readily available. Asparaginase is irritating to eyes, skin, and the upper respiratory tract; avoid inhalation of aerosols or contact with skin, eyes, or mucous membranes.

Dosage Forms Excipient information presented when available (limited, particularly for generics); consult specific product labeling.
Injection, powder for reconstitution:
Elspar®: 10,000 int. units

References
Amylon MD, Shuster J, Pullen J, et al, "Intensive High-Dose Asparaginase Consolidation Improves Survival for Pediatric Patients With T Cell Acute Lymphoblastic Leukemia and Advanced Stage Lymphoblastic Lymphoma: A Pediatric Oncology Group Study," *Leukemia*, 1999, 13(2):335-42.
Asselin BL, Whitin JC, Coppola DJ, et al, "Comparative Pharmacokinetic Studies of Three Asparaginase Preparations," *J Clin Oncol*, 1993, 11(9):1780-6.
Avramis VI, Sencer S, Periclou AP, et al, "A Randomized Comparison of Native *Escherichia coli* Asparaginase and Polyethylene Glycol Conjugated Asparaginase for Treatment of Children With Newly Diagnosed Standard-Risk Acute Lymphoblastic Leukemia: A Children's Cancer Group Study," *Blood*, 2002, 99(6):1986-94.
Clavell LA, Gelber RD, Cohen HJ, et al, "Four-Agent Induction and Intensive Asparaginase Therapy for Treatment of Childhood Acute Lymphoblastic Leukemia," *N Engl J Med*, 1986, 315(11):657-63.
Nesbit M, Chard R, Evans A, et al, "Evaluation of Intramuscular Versus Intravenous Administration of L-Asparaginase in Childhood Leukemia," *Am J Pediatr Hematol Oncol*, 1979, 1(1):9-13.
Ortega JA, Nesbit ME Jr, and Donaldson MH, "L-Asparaginase, Vincristine, and Prednisone for Induction of First Remission in Acute Lymphocytic Leukemia," *Cancer Res*, 1977, 37(2):535-40.
Stecher AL, de Deus PM, Polikarpov I, et al, "Stability of L-Asparaginase: An Enzyme Used in Leukemia Treatment," *Pharm Acta Helv*, 1999, 74(1):1-9.

◆ **Aspart Insulin** see Insulin Aspart on page 738

◆ **Aspercin [OTC]** see Aspirin on page 141

◆ **Aspergum® [OTC]** see Aspirin on page 141

Aspirin (AS pir in)

Medication Safety Issues
Sound-alike/look-alike issues:
Aspirin may be confused with Afrin®, Asendin®
Ascriptin® may be confused with Aricept®
Ecotrin® may be confused with Akineton®, Edecrin®, Epogen®
Halfprin® may be confused with Halfan®, Haltran®
ZORprin® may be confused with Zyloprim®

International issues:
Cartia® [multiple international markets] may be confused with Cartia XT® which is a brand name for diltiazem in the U.S.

Related Information
Antithrombotic Therapy in Neonates and Children on page 1602

U.S. Brand Names Ascriptin® Maximum Strength [OTC]; Ascriptin® [OTC]; Aspercin [OTC]; Aspergum® [OTC]; Aspirtab [OTC]; Bayer® Aspirin Extra Strength [OTC]; Bayer® Aspirin Regimen Adult Low Dose [OTC]; Bayer® Aspirin Regimen Children's [OTC]; Bayer® Aspirin Regimen Regular Strength [OTC]; Bayer® Genuine Aspirin [OTC]; Bayer® Plus Extra Strength [OTC]; Bayer® with Heart Advantage [OTC] [DSC]; Bayer® Women's Aspirin Plus Calcium [OTC] [DSC]; Bayer® Women's Low Dose Aspirin [OTC]; Buffasal [OTC]; Bufferin® Extra Strength [OTC]; Bufferin® [OTC]; Buffinol [OTC]; Easprin®; Ecotrin® Low Strength [OTC]; Ecotrin® Maximum Strength [OTC]; Ecotrin® [OTC]; Genacote™ [OTC] [DSC]; Halfprin® [OTC]; St. Joseph® Adult Aspirin [OTC]; ZORprin®

Canadian Brand Names Asaphen; Asaphen E.C.; Entrophen®; Novasen; Praxis ASA EC 81 Mg Daily Dose

Therapeutic Category Analgesic, Non-narcotic; Anti-inflammatory Agent; Antiplatelet Agent; Antipyretic; Nonsteroidal Anti-inflammatory Drug (NSAID), Oral; Salicylate

Generic Available Yes: Excludes gum

Use Treatment of mild to moderate pain, inflammation and fever; adjunctive treatment of Kawasaki disease; prevention of vascular mortality during suspected acute MI; prevention of recurrent MI; prevention of MI in patients with angina; prevention of recurrent stroke and mortality following TIA or stroke; management of rheumatoid arthritis, rheumatic fever, osteoarthritis, and gout (high dose); adjunctive therapy in revascularization procedures (coronary artery bypass graft, percutaneous transluminal coronary angioplasty, carotid endarterectomy)

Pregnancy Risk Factor C/D (full-dose aspirin in 3rd trimester - expert analysis)

Pregnancy Considerations Salicylates have been noted to cross the placenta and enter fetal circulation. Adverse effects reported in the fetus include mortality, intrauterine growth retardation, salicylate intoxication, bleeding abnormalities, and neonatal acidosis. Use of aspirin close to delivery may cause premature closure of the ductus arteriosus. Adverse effects reported in the mother include anemia, hemorrhage, prolonged gestation, and prolonged labor. Aspirin has been used for the prevention of preeclampsia; however, the ACOG currently recommends that it not be used in low-risk women. Low-dose aspirin is used to treat complications resulting from antiphospholipid syndrome in pregnancy (either primary or secondary to SLE). In general, low doses during pregnancy needed for the treatment of certain medical conditions have not been shown to cause fetal harm, however, discontinuing therapy prior to delivery is recommended. Use of safer agents for routine management of pain or headache should be considered.

Lactation Enters breast milk/use caution

Breast-Feeding Considerations Low amounts of aspirin can be found in breast milk. Milk/plasma ratios ranging from 0.03-0.3 have been reported. Peak levels in breast milk are reported to be at ~9 hours after a dose. Metabolic acidosis was reported in one infant following an aspirin dose of 3.9 g/day in the mother. The AAP states that aspirin should be used with caution while breast-feeding. The WHO considers occasional doses of aspirin to be compatible with breast-feeding, but to avoid long-term therapy and consider monitoring the infant for adverse effects. Other sources suggest avoiding aspirin while breast-feeding due to the theoretical risk of Reye's syndrome.

Contraindications Hypersensitivity to salicylates or any component; history of asthma, urticaria, or allergic-type reaction to aspirin, or other NSAIDs; patients with the "aspirin triad" [asthma, rhinitis (with or without nasal polyps), and aspirin intolerance] (fatal asthmatic and anaphylactoid reactions may occur in these patients); bleeding disorders; hepatic failure

Warnings Do not use aspirin in children and teenagers who have or who are recovering from chickenpox or flu symptoms (due to the association with Reye's syndrome); when using aspirin, changes in behavior (along with nausea and vomiting) may be an early sign of Reye's syndrome; instruct patients and caregivers to contact their healthcare provider if these symptoms occur. Caplet may contain tartrazine which may cause allergic reactions in susceptible individuals

Precautions Use with caution in patients with impaired renal function, erosive gastritis, peptic ulcer, gout, platelet and bleeding disorders

Adverse Reactions

Dermatologic: Rash, urticaria

Gastrointestinal: Nausea, vomiting, GI distress, GI bleeding, ulcers

Hematologic: Inhibition of platelet aggregation

Hepatic: Hepatotoxicity

Otic: Tinnitus

Renal: Interstitial nephritis, renal papillary necrosis

Respiratory: Bronchospasm

Drug Interactions

Metabolism/Transport Effects Substrate of CYP2C9 (minor)

Avoid Concomitant Use

Avoid concomitant use of Aspirin with any of the following: Ketorolac; Ketorolac (Systemic)

Increased Effect/Toxicity

Aspirin may increase the levels/effects of: Alendronate; Anticoagulants; Carbonic Anhydrase Inhibitors; Collagenase (Systemic); Corticosteroids (Systemic); Divalproex; Drotrecogin Alfa; Heparin; Ibritumomab; Methotrexate; Pralatrexate; Salicylates; Sulfonylureas; Thrombolytic Agents; Tositumomab and Iodine I 131 Tositumomab; Valproic Acid; Varicella Virus-Containing Vaccines; Vitamin K Antagonists

The levels/effects of Aspirin may be increased by: Antidepressants (Tricyclic, Tertiary Amine); Antiplatelet Agents; Calcium Channel Blockers (Nondihydropyridine); Dasatinib; Ginkgo Biloba; Glucosamine; Herbs (Anticoagulant/Antiplatelet Properties); Ketorolac; Ketorolac (Systemic); Loop Diuretics; Nonsteroidal Anti-Inflammatory Agents; NSAID (Nonselective); Omega-3-Acid Ethyl Esters; Pentosan Polysulfate Sodium; Pentoxifylline; Prostacyclin Analogues; Selective Serotonin Reuptake Inhibitors; Serotonin/Norepinephrine Reuptake Inhibitors; Treprostinil

Decreased Effect

Aspirin may decrease the levels/effects of: ACE Inhibitors; Loop Diuretics; NSAID (Nonselective); Probenecid; Tiludronate

The levels/effects of Aspirin may be decreased by: Corticosteroids (Systemic); Nonsteroidal Anti-Inflammatory Agents; NSAID (Nonselective)

Food Interactions Aspirin may increase the renal excretion of vitamin C and may decrease serum folate levels; some suggest increasing the dietary intake of foods that are high in vitamin C and folic acid

Stability Keep suppositories in refrigerator, do not freeze; hydrolysis of aspirin occurs upon exposure to water or moist air, resulting in salicylate and acetate; acetate possesses a vinegar-like odor; do not use if a strong odor is present

Mechanism of Action Inhibits prostaglandin synthesis, acts on the hypothalamus heat-regulating center to reduce fever, blocks prostaglandin synthetase action which prevents formation of the platelet-aggregating substance thromboxane A_2

Pharmacokinetics (Adult data unless noted)

Absorption: From the stomach and small intestine

Distribution: Readily distributes into most body fluids and tissues; hydrolyzed to salicylate (active) by esterases in the GI mucosa, red blood cells, synovial fluid and blood

Metabolism: Primarily by hepatic microsomal enzymes

Half-life: 15-20 minutes; metabolic pathways are saturable such that salicylate half-life is dose-dependent ranging from 3 hours at lower doses (300-600 mg), 5-6 hours (after 1 g) and 10 hours with higher doses

Time to peak serum concentration: Salicylate: ~1-2 hours; may be delayed with controlled or timed-release preparations

Elimination: Renal as salicylate and conjugated metabolites

Dialysis: Dialyzable: 50% to 100%

Usual Dosage

Children:

Analgesic and antipyretic: Oral, rectal: 10-15 mg/kg/dose every 4-6 hours; maximum dose: 4 g/day

Anti-inflammatory: Oral: Initial: 60-90 mg/kg/day in divided doses; usual maintenance: 80-100 mg/kg/day divided every 6-8 hours; monitor serum concentrations

Antiplatelet effects: Adequate pediatric studies have not been performed; pediatric dosage is derived from adult studies and clinical experience and is not well established; suggested doses have ranged from 3-5 mg/kg/day to 5-10 mg/kg/day given as a single daily dose. Doses are rounded to a convenient amount (eg, $^{1}/_{2}$ of 81 mg tablet).

Mechanical prosthetic heart valves: 6-20 mg/kg/day given as a single daily dose (used in combination with an oral anticoagulant in children who have systemic embolism despite adequate oral anticoagulation therapy and used in combination with low-dose anticoagulation when full-dose oral anticoagulation is contraindicated; see Monagle, 2004)

Blalock-Taussig shunts, primary prophylaxis: 5 mg/kg/day given as a single daily dose

Patients following Fontan surgery, primary prophylaxis: 5 mg/kg/day given as a single daily dose

Arterial ischemic stroke: 2-5 mg/kg/day given as single daily dose after anticoagulation therapy has been discontinued

Kawasaki disease: Oral: 80-100 mg/kg/day divided every 6 hours for up to 14 days (until fever resolves for at least 48 hours); then decrease dose to 3-5 mg/kg/day once daily. In patients without coronary artery abnormalities, give lower dose for 6-8 weeks. In patients with coronary artery abnormalities, low-dose aspirin should be continued indefinitely (in addition to therapy with warfarin; see Monagle, 2008)

Adults:

Analgesic and antipyretic: Oral, rectal: 325-1000 mg every 4-6 hours up to 4 g/day

Anti-inflammatory: Oral: Initial: 2.4-3.6 g/day in divided doses; usual maintenance: 3.6-5.4 g/day; monitor serum concentrations

Suspected acute MI: Oral: Initial: 160-162.5 mg as soon as MI is suspected; then 160-162.5 mg once daily for 30 days post MI; then consider further aspirin treatment

MI prophylaxis: Oral: 75-325 mg once daily (continue indefinitely)

Prevention of stroke following ischemic stroke or TIA: Oral: 50-325 mg once daily (continue indefinitely)

Administration Oral: Administer with water, food, or milk to decrease GI upset. Do not crush or chew controlled release, timed release, or enteric coated tablets; these preparations should be swallowed whole

Monitoring Parameters Serum salicylate concentration with chronic use; may not be necessary in Kawasaki disease; **Note:** Decreased aspirin absorption and increased salicylate clearance has been observed in children with acute Kawasaki disease; these patients rarely achieve therapeutic serum salicylate concentrations; thus, monitoring of serum salicylate concentrations is not necessary in most of these children (see Pickering, 2009).

Reference Range

Therapeutic levels:

Anti-inflammatory effect: 150-300 mcg/mL

Analgesic and antipyretic effect: 30-50 mcg/mL

Timing of serum samples: Peak levels usually occur 2 hours after normal doses but may occur 6-24 hours after acute toxic ingestion.

Salicylate serum concentrations correlate with the pharmacological actions and adverse effects observed. See table.

Serum Salicylate: Clinical Correlations

Serum Salicylate Concentration (mcg/mL)	Desired Effects	Adverse Effects / Intoxication
~100	Antiplatelet Antipyresis Analgesia	GI intolerance and bleeding, hypersensitivity, hemostatic defects
150-300	Anti-inflammatory	Mild salicylism
250-400	Treatment of rheumatic fever	Nausea/vomiting, hyperventilation, salicylism, flushing, sweating, thirst, headache, diarrhea, and tachycardia
>400-500		Respiratory alkalosis, hemorrhage, excitement, confusion, asterixis, pulmonary edema, convulsions, tetany, metabolic acidosis, fever, coma, cardiovascular collapse, renal and respiratory failure

Test Interactions False-negative results for glucose oxidase urinary glucose tests (Clinistix®); false-positives using the cupric sulfate method (Clinitest®); interferes with Gerhardt test, VMA determination; 5-HIAA, xylose tolerance test and T_3 and T_4

Patient Information Avoid alcohol; watch for bleeding gums or signs of GI bleeding, (bright red blood in emesis or stool, coffee ground-like emesis, black tarry stools); notify physician if ringing in the ears, persistent GI pain, GI bleeding, or changes in behavior (along with nausea and vomiting) occur (see Warnings)

Dosage Forms Excipient information presented when available (limited, particularly for generics); consult specific product labeling. [DSC] = Discontinued product

Caplet:

Bayer® Aspirin Extra Strength: 500 mg

Bayer® Aspirin Regimen Regular Strength: 325 mg

Bayer® Genuine Aspirin: 325 mg

Bayer® Plus Extra Strength: 500 mg [contains calcium carbonate]

Bayer® with Heart Advantage: 81 mg [contains phytosterols, tartrazine] [DSC]

Bayer® Women's Aspirin Plus Calcium: 81 mg [contains elemental calcium 300 mg] [DSC]

Bayer® Women's Low Dose Aspirin: 81 mg [contains elemental calcium 300 mg]

Caplet, buffered:

Ascriptin® Maximum Strength: 500 mg [contains aluminum hydroxide, calcium carbonate, and magnesium hydroxide]

Gum:

Aspergum®: 227 mg [cherry or orange flavor]

Suppository, rectal: 300 mg, 600 mg

Tablet: 325 mg

Aspercin, Aspirtab: 325 mg

Bayer® Genuine Aspirin: 325 mg

Tablet, buffered: 325 mg

Ascriptin®: 325 mg [contains aluminum hydroxide, calcium carbonate, and magnesium hydroxide]

Buffasal: 325 mg [contains magnesium oxide]

Bufferin®: 325 mg [contains calcium carbonate, magnesium oxide, and magnesium carbonate; contains calcium 65 mg/tablet, magnesium 50 mg/tablet]

Bufferin® Extra Strength: 500 mg [contains calcium carbonate, magnesium oxide, and magnesium carbonate; contains calcium 90 mg/tablet, magnesium 70 mg/tablet]

Buffinol: 325 mg [contains magnesium oxide]

Tablet, chewable: 81 mg

Bayer® Aspirin Regimen Children's: 81 mg [cherry or orange flavor]

St. Joseph® Adult Aspirin: 81 mg [orange flavor]

Tablet, controlled release:

ZORprin®: 800 mg

Tablet, delayed release, enteric coated:

Easprin®: 975 mg

Tablet, enteric coated: 81 mg, 325 mg, 500 mg, 650 mg, 975 mg [DSC]

Bayer® Aspirin Regimen Adult Low Dose, Ecotrin® Low Strength, St. Joseph Adult Aspirin: 81 mg

Ecotrin®, Genacote™ [DSC]: 325 mg

Ecotrin® Maximum Strength: 500 mg

Halfprin®: 81 mg, 162 mg

References

Capone ML, Sciulli MG, Tacconelli S, et al, "Pharmacodynamic Interaction of Naproxen With Low-Dose Aspirin in Healthy Subjects," J Am Coll Cardiol, 2005, 45(8):1295-1301.

Catella-Lawson F, Reilly MP, Kapoor SC, et al, "Cyclooxygenase Inhibitors and the Antiplatelet Effects of Aspirin," N Engl J Med, 2001, 345(25):1809-17.

Cryer B, Verlin RG, Cooper SA, et al, "Double-Blind, Randomized, Parallel, Placebo-Controlled Study Of Ibuprofen Effects On Thromboxane B2 Concentrations In Aspirin-Treated Healthy Adult Volunteers," Clin Ther, 2005, 27 (2):185-191.

Hathaway WE, "Use of Antiplatelet Agents in Pediatric Hypercoagulable States," Am J Dis Child, 1984, 138(3):301-4.

Monagle P, Chalmers E, Chan A, et al, "Antithrombotic Therapy in Neonates and Children: American College of Chest Physicians Evidence-Based Clinical Practice Guidelines (8th Edition)," Chest, 2008, 133(6 Suppl):887S-968S.

Monagle P, Chan A, Massicotte P, et al, "Antithrombotic Therapy in Children: The Seventh ACCP Conference on Antithrombotic and Thrombolytic Therapy," Chest, 2004, 126(3 Suppl):645S-687S.

Pickering LK, ed, 2009 Red Book, Report of the Committee on Infectious Diseases, 28th ed, Elk Grove Village IL: American Academy of Pediatrics, 2000, 360-3417.

◆ **Aspirin and Oxycodone** *see* Oxycodone and Aspirin *on page 1042*

◆ **Aspirin Free Anacin® Extra Strength [OTC]** *see* Acetaminophen *on page 36*

◆ **Aspirtab [OTC]** *see* Aspirin *on page 141*

◆ **Astelin®** *see* Azelastine *on page 163*

◆ **Astepro®** *see* Azelastine *on page 163*

◆ **Astramorph/PF™** *see* Morphine Sulfate *on page 946*

◆ **Atarax® (Can)** *see* HydrOXYzine *on page 697*

◆ **Atasol® (Can)** *see* Acetaminophen *on page 36*

Atazanavir (at a za NA veer)

Related Information
Adult and Adolescent HIV *on page 1620*
Management of Healthcare Worker Exposures to HBV, HCV, and HIV *on page 1661*
Pediatric HIV *on page 1613*
Perinatal HIV *on page 1628*

U.S. Brand Names Reyataz®
Canadian Brand Names Reyataz®
Therapeutic Category Antiretroviral Agent; HIV Agents (Anti-HIV Agents); Protease Inhibitor
Generic Available No
Use Treatment of HIV infection in combination with other antiretroviral agents (FDA approved in ages ≥6 years and adults) [**Note:** HIV regimens consisting of **three** antiretroviral agents are strongly recommended; low-dose ritonavir (booster dose) is recommended in combination with atazanavir in antiretroviral-experienced patients with prior virologic failure; see Usual Dosage]
Pregnancy Risk Factor B
Pregnancy Considerations Teratogenic effects not observed in animal studies. Pregnancy and protease inhibitors are both associated with an increased risk of hyperglycemia. Glucose levels should be closely monitored. Atazanavir crosses the human placenta in low/variable amounts; it is not known if atazanavir will exacerbate hyperbilirubinemia in neonates. Teratogenic effects have not been observed based on information collected by the antiretroviral pregnancy registry. Pharmacokinetic studies suggest that standard dosing during pregnancy may provide decreased plasma concentrations. Atazanavir is a recommended alternative agent for use in pregnancy when combined with low-dose ritonavir boosting; may give as once-daily dosing. In naïve patients unable to tolerate ritonavir, once-daily dosing may be considered; however, efficacy data is insufficient. Must be used with low-dose ritonavir boosting when used in combination with tenofovir. Health professionals are encouraged to contact the antiretroviral pregnancy registry to monitor outcomes of pregnant women exposed to antiretroviral medications (1-800-258-4263 or www.APRegistry.com).
Lactation Excretion in breast milk unknown/contraindicated
Breast-Feeding Considerations In infants born to mothers who are HIV positive, HAART while breast-feeding may decrease postnatal infection. However, maternal or infant antiretroviral therapy does not completely eliminate the risk of postnatal HIV transmission.

In the United States where formula is accessible, affordable, safe, and sustainable, complete avoidance of breast-feeding by HIV-infected women is recommended to decrease potential transmission of HIV.
Contraindications Hypersensitivity (eg, Stevens-Johnson syndrome, erythema multiforme, or toxic skin eruptions) to atazanavir or any component; concurrent therapy with medications that largely rely on cytochrome P450 isoenzyme CYP3A or UGT1A1 for clearance and that

have an association between increased plasma concentrations and serious or life-threatening effects [eg, cisapride, dihydroergotamine, ergotamine, ergonovine, irinotecan, lovastatin, methylergonovine, midazolam (oral), pimozide, simvastatin, triazolam]; concurrent therapy with indinavir, rifampin, or the herbal medicine St John's wort (*Hypericum perforatum*) (see Drug Interactions)

Warnings Atazanavir is an inhibitor of cytochrome P450 isoenzyme CYP3A and uridine diphosphate glucuronosyl transferase (UGT1A1; a glucuronidation enzyme). Administration of atazanavir with drugs that are primarily metabolized by CYP3A or UGT1A1 may result in increased serum concentrations of the other drug and lead to an increase or prolongation of adverse effects. Due to potential serious and/or life-threatening drug interactions, some drugs are contraindicated or not recommended for concurrent use; other drug interactions require dosage or regimen adjustment or monitoring of serum concentrations of drugs coadministered with atazanavir (see Contraindications and Drug Interactions).

Asymptomatic elevations in unconjugated (indirect) bilirubin occur commonly during therapy with atazanavir; this reversible hyperbilirubinemia is related to inhibition of uridine diphosphate glucuronosyl transferase; consider alternative therapy if bilirubin is >5 times upper limits of normal (long-term safety data is not available for such patients) or if jaundice or scleral icterus become a cosmetic concern for the patient; evaluate alternative etiologies if elevated transaminase also occur. Do not use atazanavir in infants <3 months of age due to potential risk of kernicterus. Pharmacokinetic profile of atazanavir in patients 3 months to <6 years of age has not been established.

Skin rash may occur with atazanavir use (median onset: 7.3 weeks); treatment may be continued if rash is mild to moderate (rash may resolve; median duration: 1.4 weeks); discontinue therapy in cases of severe rash. Postmarketing cases of nephrolithiasis have been reported; consider temporary interruption of therapy or discontinuation if signs or symptoms of nephrolithiasis occur.

Precautions Atazanavir may prolong the P-R interval; rare cases of second-degree AV block and other conduction abnormalities have also been reported; use with caution in patients with pre-existing conduction abnormalities or medications which prolong A-V conduction (dosage adjustment is required with some agents; see Drug Interactions). Hyperglycemia, changes in glucose tolerance, exacerbation of diabetes, DKA, and new-onset diabetes mellitus have been reported in patients receiving protease inhibitors (use with caution in patients with diabetes mellitus).

Use atazanavir with caution in patients with mild to moderate hepatic impairment; consider dosage adjustment in patients with moderate hepatic dysfunction; atazanavir is **not** recommended for use in patients with severe hepatic impairment; the use of atazanavir **plus** ritonavir is not recommended in patients with hepatic impairment. Atazanavir may exacerbate pre-existing hepatic dysfunction; use with caution in patients with hepatitis B or C or in patients with marked elevations in hepatic transaminases. Use with caution and adjust dose (and add ritonavir) in antiretroviral-naïve patients with end-stage renal disease managed with hemodialysis; do not use atazanavir in antiretroviral-experienced patients with end-stage renal disease managed with hemodialysis. Use with caution in patients with hemophilia; spontaneous bleeding episodes have been reported in patients with hemophilia type A and B receiving protease inhibitors.

Fat redistribution and accumulation [ie, central obesity, peripheral wasting, facial wasting, breast enlargement, dorsocervical fat enlargement (buffalo hump), and cushingoid appearance] have been observed in patients receiving antiretroviral agents (causal relationship not established). Immune reconstitution syndrome (an acute inflammatory response to residual or indolent opportunistic infections) may occur in HIV patients during initial treatment with combination antiretroviral agents, including atazanavir; this syndrome may require further patient assessment and therapy.

Adverse Reactions Note: Adverse effect profile in children ≥6 years and adolescents <18 years is similar to profile in adults; percent listed indicates incidence in pediatric studies, unless otherwise noted.

Cardiovascular: Prolongation of the P-R interval (concentration and dose dependent), second-degree AV block (2%)

Central nervous system: Depression, dizziness, fever (19%), headache (7%), insomnia

Dermatologic: Rash [pediatric patients: 14% (Grade 2-4); adults: 21% (all grades); usually mild to moderate; maculopapular] (see Warnings); rarely: erythema multiforme, Stevens-Johnson syndrome

Endocrine & metabolic: Exacerbation of diabetes mellitus, fat redistribution and accumulation (less common than with other protease inhibitors; see Precautions), hypercholesterolemia (less common than with other protease inhibitors), hyperglycemia, hypertriglyceridemia, new-onset diabetes

Gastrointestinal: Abdominal pain, diarrhea (8%), nausea, vomiting (8%)

Hematologic: Anemia, neutropenia, thrombocytopenia

Hepatic: Amylase increased, jaundice (pediatric patients: 13%; adults: 5% to 9%), lipase increased, liver enzymes increased, unconjugated hyperbilirubinemia (Grade 3-4 hyperbilirubinemia: pediatric patients: 49%; adults: 35% to 49%)

Neuromuscular & skeletal: Creatine kinase increased, myalgia, peripheral neuropathy

Ocular: Scleral icterus

Renal: Nephrolithiasis (postmarketing case reports)

Respiratory: Cough increased (21%); rhinorrhea (6%)

Miscellaneous: Immune reconstitution syndrome (see Precautions)

<1%, postmarketing, and/or case reports: Alopecia, arthralgia, cholecystitis, cholelithiasis, cholestasis, edema, left bundle branch block, pancreatitis, pruritus, QT_c prolongation, third-degree AV block

Drug Interactions

Metabolism/Transport Effects Substrate of CYP3A4 (major); **Inhibits** CYP1A2 (weak), 2C8 (weak), 2C9 (weak), 3A4 (strong), UGT1A1 (strong)

Avoid Concomitant Use

Avoid concomitant use of Atazanavir with any of the following: Alfuzosin; Amiodarone; Buprenorphine; Cisapride; Dronedarone; Eplerenone; Ergot Derivatives; Etravirine; Everolimus; Halofantrine; Indinavir; Irinotecan; Lovastatin; Midazolam; Nevirapine; Nilotinib; Nisoldipine; Pimozide; QuiNIDine; Ranolazine; Rifampin; Rivaroxaban; Romidepsin; Salmeterol; Silodosin; Simvastatin; St Johns Wort; Tamsulosin; Tolvaptan; Triazolam

Increased Effect/Toxicity

Atazanavir may increase the levels/effects of: Alfuzosin; Almotriptan; Alosetron; ALPRAZolam; Amiodarone; Antifungal Agents (Azole Derivatives, Systemic); Bortezomib; Brinzolamide; Buprenorphine; Calcium Channel Blockers (Dihydropyridine); Calcium Channel Blockers (Nondihydropyridine); CarBAMazepine; Ciclesonide; Cisapride; Clarithromycin; Colchicine; Corticosteroids (Orally Inhaled); CycloSPORINE; CycloSPORINE (Systemic); CYP3A4 Substrates; Dienogest; Digoxin; Dronedarone; Dutasteride; Enfuvirtide; Eplerenone; Ergot Derivatives;

Etravirine; Everolimus; FentaNYL; Fesoterodine; Fusidic Acid; GuanFACINE; Halofantrine; HMG-CoA Reductase Inhibitors; Indinavir; Ixabepilone; Lovastatin; Lumefantrine; Maraviroc; Meperidine; MethylPREDNISolone; Midazolam; Nefazodone; Nevirapine; Nilotinib; Nisoldipine; Paricalcitol; Pazopanib; Pimecrolimus; Pimozide; Pitavastatin; Protease Inhibitors; QuiNIDine; Ranolazine; Rifamycin Derivatives; Rivaroxaban; Romidepsin; Salmeterol; Saxagliptin; Sildenafil; Silodosin; Simvastatin; Sirolimus; Sorafenib; Tacrolimus; Tacrolimus (Systemic); Tacrolimus (Topical); Tadalafil; Tamsulosin; Temsirolimus; Tenofovir; Tolvaptan; TraZODone; Triazolam; Tricyclic Antidepressants; Vardenafil; Warfarin

The levels/effects of Atazanavir may be increased by: Antifungal Agents (Azole Derivatives, Systemic); Clarithromycin; CycloSPORINE; CycloSPORINE (Systemic); CYP3A4 Inhibitors (Moderate); CYP3A4 Inhibitors (Strong); Dasatinib; Delavirdine; Efavirenz; Enfuvirtide; Fusidic Acid; Indinavir

Decreased Effect

Atazanavir may decrease the levels/effects of: Abacavir; Clarithromycin; Contraceptives (Estrogens); Delavirdine; Didanosine; Divalproex; Meperidine; Prasugrel; Theophylline Derivatives; Valproic Acid; Zidovudine

The levels/effects of Atazanavir may be decreased by: Antacids; Buprenorphine; CarBAMazepine; Contraceptives (Estrogens); CYP3A4 Inducers (Strong); Deferasirox; Didanosine; Efavirenz; Etravirine; Garlic; H2-Antagonists; Minocycline; Nevirapine; Proton Pump Inhibitors; Rifampin; Rifamycin Derivatives; St Johns Wort; Tenofovir

Food Interactions Food increases oral bioavailability and decreases interpatient pharmacokinetic variability.

Stability Store at 25°C (77°F); excursions permitted to 15°C to 30°C (59°F to 86°F).

Mechanism of Action An azapeptide protease inhibitor which acts on an enzyme (protease) late in the HIV replication process after the virus has entered into the cell's nucleus. Atazanavir binds to the protease activity site and inhibits the activity of the enzyme, thus preventing cleavage of viral polyprotein precursors (gag-pol protein precursors) into individual functional proteins found in infectious HIV. This results in the formation of immature, noninfectious viral particles.

Pharmacokinetics (Adult data unless noted)

Distribution: CSF: Plasma concentration ratio (range): 0.0021-0.0226

Protein binding: 86%; binds to both alpha$_1$-acid glycoprotein and albumin (similar affinity)

Metabolism: Extensively metabolized in the liver, primarily by cytochrome P450 isoenzyme CYP3A; also undergoes biliary elimination; major biotransformation pathways include mono-oxygenation and deoxygenation; minor pathways for parent drug or metabolites include glucuronidation, N-dealkylation, hydrolysis and oxygenation with dehydrogenation; 3 minor inactive metabolites have been identified

Half-life:

Adults: 6.5 hours

Adults with hepatic impairment: 12 hours

Time to peak serum concentration: 2 hours

Elimination: 13% of the dose is excreted in the urine (7% as unchanged drug); 79% of the dose is excreted in feces (20% as unchanged drug)

Dialysis: Not appreciably removed during hemodialysis. Only 2.1% of the dose was removed during a 4 hour dialysis session; however, mean AUC, peak, and trough serum concentrations were 25% to 43% lower (versus adults with normal renal function) when atazanavir was administered either prior to, or after hemodialysis; mechanism of the decrease is not currently known.

◄ **Usual Dosage** Oral (use in combination with other antiretroviral agents):

Neonates and Infants <3 months: Not recommended due to risk of kernicterus

Infants ≥3 months and Children <6 years: Not approved for use; dose not established (see Additional Information)

Children ≥6 years and Adolescents <18 years: **Note:** Dosage is based on body weight (see Additional Information); do not exceed recommended adult dose; use a combination of the available capsule strengths to achieve the recommended dosage.

Antiretroviral-naïve patients:

Ritonavir unboosted regimen; **Note:** Ritonavir boosted atazanavir dosing regimen is preferred; data from an ongoing Phase II clinical trial indicate that higher atazanavir dosing (ie, higher on a mg/kg or mg/m² basis than predicted by adult dosing guidelines) may be needed when atazanavir is used without ritonavir boosting in children and adolescents (see Additional Information and Working Group, 2009).

Children ≥6 years to <13 years: Dose not established

Children ≥13 years and ≥39 kg who are not able to tolerate ritonavir: Atazanavir 400 mg once daily (without ritonavir)

Ritonavir boosted regimen:

15 kg to <25 kg: Atazanavir 150 mg **plus** ritonavir 80 mg once daily

25 kg to <32 kg: Atazanavir 200 mg **plus** ritonavir 100 mg once daily

32 kg to <39 kg: Atazanavir 250 mg **plus** ritonavir 100 mg once daily

≥39 kg: Atazanavir 300 mg **plus** ritonavir 100 mg once daily

Antiretoviral-experienced patients:

Ritonavir unboosted regimen: Atazanavir **without** ritonavir is **not** recommended in antiretroviral-experienced patients with prior virologic failure

Ritonavir boosted regimen:

<25 kg: Dose not established

25 kg to <32 kg: Atazanavir 200 mg **plus** ritonavir 100 mg once daily

32 kg to <39 kg: Atazanavir 250 mg **plus** ritonavir 100 mg once daily

≥39 kg: Atazanavir 300 mg **plus** ritonavir 100 mg once daily

Adolescents ≥18 years and Adults:

Antiretroviral-naïve patients: Atazanavir 300 mg once daily **plus** ritonavir 100 mg once daily **OR** for patients unable to tolerate ritonavir: Atazanavir 400 mg once daily

Antiretroviral-experienced patients: 300 mg once daily **plus** ritonavir 100 mg once daily (**Note:** Atazanavir **without** ritonavir is **not** recommended in antiretroviral-experienced patients with prior virologic failure)

Coadministration with efavirenz:

Antiretroviral-naïve patients: Atazanavir 400 mg **plus** ritonavir 100 mg once daily (as a single dose, administered with food); give with efavirenz 600 mg (administered on an empty stomach, preferably at bedtime); do **not** use efavirenz and atazanavir without booster doses of ritonavir (see Drug Interactions)

Antiretroviral-experienced patients: Concurrent use not recommended due to decreased atazanavir exposure

Coadministration with tenofovir: Atazanavir 300 mg **plus** ritonavir 100 mg once daily with tenofovir 300 mg (all as a single daily dose); administer with food; do **not** use tenofovir and atazanavir without booster doses of ritonavir (see Drug Interactions); if H₂-receptor antagonist is coadministered, increase atazanavir to 400 mg **plus** ritonavir 100 mg once daily (see Coadministration with H₂-receptor antagonist)

Coadministration with H₂-receptor antagonists:

Antiretroviral-naïve patients: Atazanavir 300 mg **plus** ritonavir 100 mg once daily given simultaneously with, or at least 10 hours after, the H₂-receptor antagonist; dosage of H₂-receptor antagonist must be limited to the equivalent of a 40 mg dose of famotidine twice daily; administer with food (see Drug Interactions)

Patients unable to tolerate ritonavir: Atazanavir 400 mg once daily given at least 2 hours before or at least 10 hours after an H₂ antagonist; dosage of H₂-receptor antagonist must be limited to the equivalent daily dose of ≤40 mg famotidine (single dose: ≤20 mg)

Antiretroviral-experienced patients: Atazanavir 300 mg **plus** ritonavir 100 mg once daily given simultaneously with, or at least 10 hours after, the H₂-receptor antagonist; dosage of H₂-receptor antagonist must be limited to the equivalent of a 20 mg dose of famotidine twice daily; administer with food (see Drug Interactions)

With tenofovir: Increase atazanavir to 400 mg **plus** ritonavir 100 mg once daily given simultaneously with, or at least 10 hours after, the H₂-receptor antagonist; dosage of H₂-receptor antagonist must be limited to the equivalent of a 20 mg dose of famotidine twice daily; administer with food (see Drug Interactions)

Coadministration with proton pump inhibitor:

Antiretroviral-naïve patients: Atazanavir 300 mg **plus** ritonavir 100 mg once daily given 12 hours after the proton pump inhibitor; dosage of proton pump inhibitor must be limited to the equivalent of a 20 mg dose of omeprazole/day; administer with food (see Drug Interactions)

Antiretroviral-experienced patients: Concurrent use **not** recommended

Dosage adjustment in renal impairment: Adults:

Patients with renal impairment, including severe renal impairment who are not managed with hemodialysis: No dosage adjustment required

Patients with end-stage renal disease managed with hemodialysis:

Antiretroviral-naïve patients: Atazanavir 300 mg **plus** ritonavir 100 mg once daily

Antiretroviral-experienced patients: Do not use atazanavir; dosage is not known

Dosage adjustment in hepatic impairment: Adults:

Mild-to-moderate hepatic insufficiency: Use with caution; if moderate hepatic impairment (Child-Pugh class B) and no prior virologic failure, consider dose reduction to 300 mg once daily

Severe hepatic impairment (Child-Pugh Class C): Do not use

Note: Patients with underlying hepatitis B or C or those with marked elevations in transaminases prior to treatment may be at increased risk of hepatic decompensation or further increases in transaminases with atazanavir therapy (monitor patients closely). Combination therapy with ritonavir in patients with hepatic impairment is **not** recommended.

Administration Administer with food to enhance absorption; swallow capsules whole, do not open. Administer atazanavir 2 hours before or 1 hour after didanosine buffered formulations, didanosine enteric-coated capsules, other buffered medications, or antacids. Administer atazanavir (with ritonavir) simultaneously with, or at least 10 hours after, H₂-receptor antagonists; administer atazanavir (without ritonavir) at least 2 hours before or at least 10 hours after H₂-receptor antagonist (see Usual Dosage). Administer atazanavir (with ritonavir) 12 hours after proton pump inhibitor (see Usual Dosage).

Monitoring Parameters CD4 cell count, HIV RNA plasma levels, serum glucose, bilirubin, triglycerides, cholesterol, liver enzyme tests (especially in patients with a history of hepatitis B or C)

Patient Information Before starting atazanavir, tell your doctor if you have liver problems, hepatitis B or C, end stage kidney disease managed with hemodialysis, diabetes, or hemophilia. Atazanavir may cause changes in the ECG (notify physician if dizziness or lightheadedness occur); elevated bilirubin levels and yellowing of the skin or whites of the eye (other medication can be used if these side effects are of concern); kidney stones (notify healthcare provider if you experience pain in your side, blood in the urine, or pain when urinating), gallstones or inflammation of the gallbladder. Atazanavir may cause a skin rash that will usually go away with continued use of the drug (notify healthcare provider if skin rash occurs). In rare cases, the skin rash may be associated with symptoms that can be serious or potentially fatal; stop using atazanavir and notify healthcare provider immediately if a skin rash with any of the following symptoms occurs: Blisters, fever, flu-like symptoms, mouth sores, muscle or joint aches, red or inflamed eyes, shortness of breath, or swelling of face.

Some medicines should not be taken with atazanavir; report the use of other medications, nonprescription medications and herbal or natural products to your physician and pharmacist; avoid the herbal medicine St John's wort. Atazanavir is not a cure for HIV; take atazanavir everyday as prescribed; do not change dose or discontinue without physician's advice; if a dose is missed, take it as soon as possible, then return to normal dosing schedule; if it is within 6 hours of your next dose, do not take the missed dose; if a dose is skipped, do not double the next dose.

HIV medications may cause changes in body fat, including an increase in fat in the upper back and neck, breasts, and trunk; a loss of fat from the face, arms, and legs may also occur.

Additional Information Preliminary studies have shown that appropriate atazanavir serum concentrations are difficult to achieve in pediatric patients even with higher doses (on a mg/kg or m^2 basis). Optimal dosing in children <6 years of age is under investigation; the addition of low-dose ritonavir (booster doses) to increase atazanavir serum concentrations may be required and is currently being evaluated. Results of a pediatric Phase II clinical trial suggest that when used **without** ritonavir boosting, children ≥6 and <13 years of age require atazanavir 520 mg/m^2/day and adolescents ≥13 years of age require atazanavir 620 mg/m^2/day (once daily doses of 600-900 mg/day). When used in combination **with** ritonavir, the study used atazanavir 205 mg/m^2/day (once daily doses of 250-375 mg/day). A powder formulation is also being studied in pediatric patients (Working Group, 2009).

Current FDA labeled dosing for children ≥6 years and Adolescents <18 years is based on the following:

Antiretroviral-naïve patients:

Children 15 kg to <20 kg: Atazanavir 8.5 mg/kg **plus** ritonavir 4 mg/kg once daily

Children ≥20 kg: Atazanavir 7 mg/kg (maximum: 300 mg) **plus** ritonavir 4 mg/kg (maximum: 100 mg) once daily

Antiretroviral-experienced patients: Children ≥25 kg: Atazanavir 7 mg/kg (maximum: 300 mg) **plus** ritonavir 4 mg/kg (maximum: 100 mg) once daily (Product Information, January, 2010)

Dosage Forms Excipient information presented when available (limited, particularly for generics); consult specific product labeling.

Capsule, as sulfate:

Reyataz®: 100 mg, 150 mg, 200 mg, 300 mg

References

Briars LA, Hilao JJ, and Kraus DM, "A Review of Pediatric Human Immunodeficiency Virus Infection," *Journal of Pharmacy Practice*, 2004, 17(6):407-31.

Goldsmith DR and Perry CM, "Atazanavir," *Drugs*, 2003, 63 (16):1679-93.

Morris JL and Kraus DM, "New Antiretroviral Therapies for Pediatric HIV Infection," *J Pediatr Pharmacol Ther*, 2005, 10:215-47.

Musial BL, Chojnacki JK, and Coleman CI, "Atazanavir: A New Protease Inhibitor to Treat HIV Infection," *Am J Health Syst Pharm*, 2004, 61(13):1365-74.

Panel on Antiretroviral Guidelines for Adults and Adolescents, "Guidelines for the Use of Antiretroviral Agents in HIV-Infected Adults and Adolescents," December 1, 2009. Available at: http://www.aidsinfo. nih.gov.

Working Group on Antiretroviral Therapy and Medical Management of HIV-Infected Children, "Guidelines for the Use of Antiretroviral Agents in Pediatric HIV Infection," February 23, 2009. Available at http:// www.aidsinfo.nih.gov.

◆ **Atazanavir Sulfate** *see* Atazanavir *on page 144*

Atenolol (a TEN oh lole)

Medication Safety Issues

Sound-alike/look-alike issues:

Atenolol may be confused with albuterol, Altenol®, timolol, Tylenol®

Tenormin® may be confused with Imuran®, Norpramin®, thiamine, Trovan®

International issues:

Betanol® [Bangladesh] may be confused with Patanol® which is a brand name for olopatadine in the U.S.

Related Information

Antihypertensive Agents by Class *on page 1481*

U.S. Brand Names Tenormin®

Canadian Brand Names Apo-Atenol®; CO Atenolol; Dom-Atenolol; Med-Atenolol; Mylan-Atenolol; Nu-Atenolol; PHL-Atenolol; PMS-Atenolol; RAN™-Atenolol; ratio-Atenolol; Riva-Atenolol; Sandoz-Atenolol; Tenormin®; Teva-Atenolol

Therapeutic Category Antianginal Agent; Antihypertensive Agent; Beta-Adrenergic Blocker

Generic Available Yes

Use Treatment of hypertension, alone or in combination with other agents (FDA approved in adults); management of angina pectoris (FDA approved in adults); post-MI patients (to reduce cardiovascular mortality) (FDA approved in adults); acute alcohol withdrawal; supraventricular and ventricular arrhythmias; migraine headache prophylaxis

Pregnancy Risk Factor D

Pregnancy Considerations Atenolol crosses the placenta; beta-blockers have been associated with persistent bradycardia, hypotension, and IUGR; IUGR is probably related to maternal hypertension. Available evidence suggests beta-blockers are generally safe during pregnancy (JNC 7). Cases of neonatal hypoglycemia have been reported following maternal use of beta-blockers at parturition or during breast-feeding. Monitor breast-fed infant for symptoms of beta-blockade.

Lactation Enters breast milk/use caution

Breast-Feeding Considerations Symptoms of beta-blockade including cyanosis, hypothermia, and bradycardia have been reported in nursing infants.

Contraindications Hypersensitivity to atenolol or any component; pulmonary edema, cardiogenic shock, bradycardia, heart block, or uncompensated CHF

Warnings Exacerbation of angina, arrhythmias, and, in some cases, MI may occur following abrupt discontinuation of beta-blockers **[U.S. Boxed Warning]**; avoid abrupt discontinuation, wean slowly, and monitor for signs and symptoms of ischemia. Atenolol should not be administered to patients with untreated pheochromocytoma. Atenolol may mask clinical signs of hyperthyroidism (exacerbation of symptoms of hyperthyroidism, including thyroid storm, may occur following abrupt discontinuation). Atenolol decreases the ability of the heart to respond to reflex adrenergic stimuli and may increase the risk of general anesthesia and surgical procedures; use caution with anesthetic agents that decrease myocardial function. Beta-blocker use has been associated with induction or exacerbation of psoriasis, but cause and effect have not been firmly established.

Precautions Use with caution and modify dosage in patients with renal impairment; use with caution in patients with CHF, bronchospastic disease, diabetes mellitus, and hyperthyroidism. Use with caution in nursing women; clinically significant bradycardia may occur in breast-fed infants; infants with renal dysfunction and premature infants may be at higher risk for adverse effects; breast-fed infants and neonates born to mothers receiving atenolol may be at increased risk for hypoglycemia. Patients who have a history of anaphylactic hypersensitivity reactions to various substances may be more reactive while receiving beta-blockers; these patients may not be responsive to the normal doses of epinephrine used to treat hypersensitivity reactions.

Adverse Reactions

Cardiovascular: Bradycardia, chest pain, CHF, edema, hypotension, Raynaud's phenomenon, second or third degree A-V block

Central nervous system: Confusion, dizziness, fatigue, headache, insomnia, lethargy, mental impairment, nightmares

Dermatologic: Psoriasiform rash, psoriasis exacerbation

Gastrointestinal: Constipation, diarrhea, nausea

Respiratory: Dyspnea and wheezing have occurred with higher doses (eg, >100 mg/day in adults)

Drug Interactions

Avoid Concomitant Use

Avoid concomitant use of Atenolol with any of the following: Methacholine

Increased Effect/Toxicity

Atenolol may increase the levels/effects of: Alpha-/Beta-Agonists (Direct-Acting); Alpha1-Blockers; Alpha2-Agonists; Amifostine; Antihypertensives; Bupivacaine; Cardiac Glycosides; Hypotensive Agents; Insulin; Lidocaine; Lidocaine (Systemic); Lidocaine (Topical); Mepivacaine; Methacholine; Midodrine; RiTUXimab; Sulfonylureas

The levels/effects of Atenolol may be increased by: Acetylcholinesterase Inhibitors; Amiodarone; Anilidopiperidine Opioids; Calcium Channel Blockers (Nondihydropyridine); Diazoxide; Dipyridamole; Disopyramide; Dronedarone; Herbs (Hypotensive Properties); MAO Inhibitors; Pentoxifylline; Phosphodiesterase 5 Inhibitors; Prostacyclin Analogues; Reserpine

Decreased Effect

Atenolol may decrease the levels/effects of: Beta2-Agonists; Theophylline Derivatives

The levels/effects of Atenolol may be decreased by: Ampicillin; Herbs (Hypertensive Properties); Methylphenidate; Nonsteroidal Anti-Inflammatory Agents; Yohimbine

Mechanism of Action Competitively blocks response to beta-adrenergic stimulation; selectively blocks beta$_1$-receptors with little or no effect on beta$_2$-receptors except at high doses; does not possess membrane stabilizing or intrinsic sympathomimetic (partial agonist) activities

Pharmacodynamics

Beta-blocking effect:

Onset of action: Oral: ≤1 hour

Maximum effect: Oral: 2-4 hours

Duration: Oral: ≥24 hours

Antihypertensive effect:

Duration: Oral: 24 hours

Pharmacokinetics (Adult data unless noted)

Absorption: Incomplete from the GI tract; ~50% absorbed

Distribution: Does not cross the blood-brain barrier; low lipophilicity; distributes into breast milk at a concentration 1.5-6.8 times the maternal plasma concentration (see Precautions)

Protein binding: Low (6% to 16%)

Half-life, beta:

Neonates: Mean: 16 hours, up to 35 hours

Children 5-16 years of age: Mean: 4.6 hours; range: 3.5-7 hours; children >10 years of age may have longer half-life (>5 hours) compared to children 5-10 years of age (<5 hours)

Adults: 6-7 hours

Prolonged half-life with renal dysfunction

Time to peak serum concentration: Oral: Within 2-4 hours

Elimination: 40% as unchanged drug in urine, 50% in feces

Dialysis: Moderately dialyzable (20% to 50%)

Usual Dosage Oral: Hypertension:

Children: Initial: 0.5-1 mg/kg/day given once daily or divided in 2 doses per day; titrate dose to effect; usual range: 0.5-1.5 mg/kg/day; maximum dose: 2 mg/kg/day; do not exceed adult maximum dose of 100 mg/day (National High Blood Pressure Education Program Working Group on High Blood Pressure in Children and Adolescents, 2004)

Adults: Initial: 25-50 mg once daily; titrate dose to effect; usual dose: 50-100 mg once daily; usual dosage range (JNC 7): 25-100 mg once daily; maximum dose: 100 mg once daily

See table for oral dosing interval in renal impairment.

Creatinine Clearance	Maximum Oral Dose	Frequency of Administration
15-35 mL/min	50 mg or 1 mg/kg/dose	Daily
<15 mL/min	50 mg or 1 mg/kg/dose	Every other day

Administration Oral: May be administered without regard to food

Monitoring Parameters Blood pressure, heart rate, ECG, fluid intake and output, daily weight, respiratory rate

Patient Information Abrupt withdrawal of the drug should be avoided

Additional Information In diabetic patients, atenolol may potentiate hypoglycemia and mask signs and symptoms of hypoglycemia; limited data suggests that atenolol may have a shorter half-life and faster clearance in patients with Marfan syndrome. Higher doses (2 mg/kg/day divided every 12 hours) have been used in patients with Marfan syndrome (6-22 years of age) to decrease aortic root growth rate and prevent aortic dissection or rupture; further studies are needed.

Dosage Forms Excipient information presented when available (limited, particularly for generics); consult specific product labeling.

Tablet: 25 mg, 50 mg, 100 mg

Tenormin®: 25 mg, 50 mg, 100 mg

Extemporaneous Preparations

A 2 mg/mL atenolol oral liquid compounded from tablets and a commercially available oral diluent was found to be stable for up to 40 days when stored at 5°C or 25°C (Garner, 1994)

Stability of a 2 mg/mL atenolol oral liquid compounded from tablets and several different vehicles was studied at room temperature in amber prescription bottles. The 2 mg/mL atenolol oral liquid in Ora-Sweet® SF was stable for 90 days; in a vehicle of simple syrup, the preparation was stable for approximately 3 weeks; when formulated in Ora-Sweet® however, the preparation was stable for <1 week (Patel, 1997)

Garner SS, Wiest DB, and Reynolds ER, "Stability of Atenolol in an Extemporaneously Compounded Oral Liquid," *Am J Hosp Pharm*, 1994, 51(4):508-11.

Patel D, Doski DH, and Desai A, "Short-Term Stability of Atenolol in Oral Liquid Formulations," *Int J Pharmaceut Compd*, 1997, 1:437-9.

References

Brauchli YB, Jick SS, Curtin F, et al, "Association Between Beta-Blockers, Other Antihypertensive Drugs and Psoriasis: Population-Based Case-Control Study," *Br J Dermatol*, 2008, 158(6):1299-307.

Buck ML, Wiest D, Gillette PC, et al, "Pharmacokinetics and Pharmacodynamics of Atenolol in Children," *Clin Pharmacol Ther*, 1989, 46(6):629-33.

Case CL, Trippel DL, and Gillette PC, "New Antiarrhythmic Agents in Pediatrics," *Pediatr Clin North Am*, 1989, 36(5):1293-320.

Chobanian AV, Bakris GL, Black HR, et al, "The Seventh Report of the Joint National Committee on Prevention, Detection, Evaluation, and Treatment of High Blood Pressure: The JNC 7 report," *JAMA*, 2003, 289(19):2560-72.

Gold MH, Holy AK, and Roenigk HH Jr, "Beta-Blocking Drugs and Psoriasis. A Review of Cutaneous Side Effects and Retrospective Analysis of Their Effects on Psoriasis," *J Am Acad Dermatol*, 1988, 19 (5 Pt 1):837-41.

National High Blood Pressure Education Program Working Group on High Blood Pressure in Children and Adolescents, "The Fourth Report on the Diagnosis, Evaluation, and Treatment of High Blood Pressure in Children and Adolescents," *Pediatrics*, 2004, 114(2 Suppl 4th Report):555-76.

Schön MP and Boehncke WH, "Psoriasis," *N Engl J Med*, 2005, 352 (18):1899-912.

Trippel DL and Gillette PC, "Atenolol in Children With Supraventricular Tachycardia," *Am J Cardiol*, 1989, 64(3):233-6.

Trippel DL and Gillette PC, "Atenolol in Children With Ventricular Arrhythmias," *Am Heart J*, 1990, 119(6):1312-6.

♦ **ATG** *see* Antithymocyte Globulin (Equine) *on page 118*

♦ **Atgam®** *see* Antithymocyte Globulin (Equine) *on page 118*

♦ **Ativan®** *see* LORazepam *on page 845*

Atomoxetine (AT oh mox e teen)

Medication Safety Issues
Sound-alike/look-alike issues:
Atomoxetine may be confused with atorvastatin

U.S. Brand Names Strattera®

Canadian Brand Names Strattera®

Therapeutic Category Norepinephrine Reuptake Inhibitor, Selective

Generic Available No

Use Treatment of attention deficit/hyperactivity disorder (ADHD); has been used investigationally to treat depression

Medication Guide An FDA-approved patient medication guide, which is available with the product information and at http://www.fda.gov/downloads/Drugs/DrugSafety/ucm089138.pdf, must be dispensed with this medication for each new outpatient prescription and refill.

Pregnancy Risk Factor C

Pregnancy Considerations Decreased pup weight and survival were observed in animal studies. There are no adequate and well-controlled studies in pregnant women. Use only if potential benefit to the mother outweighs possible risk to fetus.

Lactation Excretion in breast milk unknown/use caution

Contraindications Hypersensitivity to atomoxetine or any component; concurrent use or use within 14 days of MAO inhibitors; narrow-angle glaucoma

Warnings Atomoxetine has been associated with an increased risk of suicidal thinking in children and adolescents with ADHD **[U.S. Boxed Warning]**. This risk must be considered before prescribing atomoxetine in pediatric patients. Children and adolescents who start treatment with atomoxetine require close monitoring for suicidal thinking and behavior (ie, suicidality), unusual changes in behavior, or clinical worsening, especially during the first few months after initiation of a course of therapy or when the dosage is changed. Family members and caregivers should be instructed to closely observe the patient and communicate their condition with the health-care provider. Recommended monitoring includes daily observation by family members and caregivers, at least weekly face-to-face visits with patients or their family members or caregivers during the first 4 weeks of treatment, then every other week visits for the next 4 weeks, then at 12 weeks, and then as clinically indicated beyond 12 weeks. In addition, contact by phone may be appropriate between visits. Patients should also be monitored for associated behaviors (eg, agitation, irritability, anxiety, akathisia, aggressiveness, insomnia, hostility, impulsivity, panic attacks, hypomania, mania) which may be precursors to emerging suicidality. Emergence of suicidality or associated behaviors listed above, that is abrupt in onset, severe, or not part of the presenting symptoms, may require discontinuation or modification of drug therapy.

Screen individuals for bipolar disorder prior to treatment (atomoxetine may induce mixed/manic episodes in patients at risk for bipolar disorder). Atomoxetine has been associated with emergent psychotic or manic symptoms in children and adolescents without a prior history of psychotic illness or mania, even at standard doses. Consider discontinuation if such symptoms (eg, delusional thinking, hallucinations, or mania) occur. Although rare, severe liver injury has been reported and may progress to liver failure, death, or the need for liver transplantation; discontinue atomoxetine and do not restart in patients who develop jaundice or laboratory evidence of liver injury; obtain liver enzyme levels if patient develops signs of liver dysfunction (eg, dark urine, jaundice, pruritus, right upper quadrant tenderness, or unexplained flu-like symptoms).

Serious cardiovascular events including sudden death may occur in patients with pre-existing structural cardiac abnormalities or other serious heart problems. Sudden death has been reported in children and adolescents; sudden death, stroke, and MI have been reported in adults. Avoid the use of atomoxetine in patients with known serious structural cardiac abnormalities, cardiomyopathy, serious heart rhythm abnormalities, coronary artery disease, or other serious cardiac problems that could place patients at an increased risk to the noradrenergic effects of atomoxetine. Patients should be carefully evaluated for cardiac disease prior to initiation of therapy. Patients who develop cardiac signs or symptoms while receiving atomoxetine should undergo cardiac evaluation. **Note:** The American Heart Association recommends that all children diagnosed with ADHD who may be candidates for medication, such as atomoxetine, should have a thorough cardiovascular assessment prior to initiation of therapy. This assessment should include a combination of medical history, family history, and physical examination focusing on cardiovascular disease risk factors. An ECG is not mandatory but should be considered.

Allergic reactions (including rash, urticaria, and angioneurotic edema) may occur. Suppression of growth may occur with long-term use in children (monitor carefully; consider interruption of therapy in children who are not growing or gaining weight appropriately). Aggressive behavior or hostility has been observed in patients receiving atomoxetine (causal relationship not established); patients should be monitored for appearance or worsening of such behavior.

Precautions May cause increased heart rate or blood pressure, use with caution in patients with hypertension, tachycardia, or other cardiovascular or cerebrovascular disease. May cause orthostatic hypotension or syncope, use with caution in patients with conditions that predispose to hypotension. May cause new onset or exacerbation of Raynaud's phenomenon. May cause urinary retention or hesitancy, use with caution in patients with a history of urinary retention or bladder outlet obstruction. May rarely cause priapism; prompt medical attention may be required. Use with caution and reduce the dose in patients with hepatic dysfunction. Use with caution in patients who are cytochrome P450 CYP2D6 poor metabolizers; use with caution and modify dose in patients receiving strong CYP2D6 inhibitors (see Drug Interactions and Usual Dosage). Safety and efficacy have not been established in children <6 years of age; safety and efficacy of long-term use have not been established.

Adverse Reactions Note: Adverse reactions reported to be increased in poor metabolizers of CYP2D6 substrates include: Appetite decreased, insomnia, sedation, depression, tremor, early morning awakening, pruritus, and mydriasis

Cardiovascular: Palpitations, tachycardia, hypertension, orthostatic hypotension, syncope, chest pain, Raynaud's phenomenon; QT prolongation (rare). **Note:** Serious cardiovascular events including sudden death may occur in patients with pre-existing structural cardiac abnormalities or other serious heart problems (see Warnings).

Central nervous system: Headache, insomnia, fatigue, lethargy, irritability, somnolence, dizziness, mood swings, abnormal dreams, sleep disorder, pyrexia, rigors, crying, aggression, sedation, depression, early morning awakening; suicidal thinking and behavior (0.4%; see Warnings); emergent psychotic or manic symptoms (see Warnings); seizures (rare)

Dermatologic: Dermatitis, pruritus

Endocrine & metabolic: Weight loss, dysmenorrhea, libido decreased, menstruation disorders, hot flashes

Gastrointestinal: Xerostomia, abdominal pain, vomiting, appetite decreased, dyspepsia, diarrhea, flatulence, constipation, nausea

Genitourinary: Sexual dysfunction, priapism (rare)

Hepatic: Rare: Severe liver injury including liver enzymes elevated, hyperbilirubinemia, jaundice (**Note:** Liver injury may rarely progress to liver failure or death; see Warnings)

Neuromuscular & skeletal: Paresthesia, myalgia, tremor

Ocular: Mydriasis

Renal: Urinary retention, urinary hesitation, difficulty in micturition

Respiratory: Cough, rhinorrhea, sinus headache

Miscellaneous: Diaphoresis increased, sinusitis, ear infection, influenza, hypersensitivity reactions, urticaria, angioedema (rare)

Drug Interactions

Metabolism/Transport Effects Substrate of CYP2C19 (minor), 2D6 (major)

Avoid Concomitant Use

Avoid concomitant use of Atomoxetine with any of the following: Iobenguane I 123; MAO Inhibitors

Increased Effect/Toxicity

Atomoxetine may increase the levels/effects of: Alcohol (Ethyl); Beta2-Agonists; CNS Depressants; Methotrimeprazine; Sympathomimetics

The levels/effects of Atomoxetine may be increased by: CYP2D6 Inhibitors (Moderate); CYP2D6 Inhibitors (Strong); Darunavir; MAO Inhibitors; Methotrimeprazine

Decreased Effect

Atomoxetine may decrease the levels/effects of: Iobenguane I 123

The levels/effects of Atomoxetine may be decreased by: Peginterferon Alfa-2b

Food Interactions A high fat meal decreases the rate, but not the extent of absorption.

Stability Store at room temperature of 25°C (77°F).

Mechanism of Action Enhances norepinephrine activity by selectively inhibiting norepinephrine reuptake; little to no activity at other neuronal reuptake pumps or receptor sites

Pharmacokinetics (Adult data unless noted)

Absorption: Oral: Rapid

Distribution: V_d: Adults: I.V.: 0.85 L/kg

Protein binding: 98%, primarily albumin

Metabolism: Extensive in the liver, primarily by oxidative metabolism via cytochrome P450 CYP2D6 to 4-hydroxyatomoxetine (major metabolite regardless of CYP2D6 status, active, equipotent to atomoxetine) with subsequent glucuronidation; also metabolized via CYP2C19 to N-desmethlyatomoxetine (active, minimal activity); **Note:** CYP2D6 poor metabolizers have atomoxetine AUCs that are ~10-fold higher and peak concentrations that are ~5-fold greater than extensive metabolizers; 4-hyroxyatomoxetine plasma concentrations are very low (extensive metabolizers: 1% of atomoxetine concentrations; poor metabolizers: 0.1% of atomoxetine concentrations)

Bioavailability: Extensive metabolizers: 63%; poor metabolizers: 94%

Half-life: Adults:

Atomoxetine: Extensive metabolizers: 5.2 hours; poor metabolizers: 21.6 hours

4-hydroxyatomoxetine: Extensive metabolizers: 6-8 hours

N-desmethlyatomoxetine: Extensive metabolizers: 6-8 hours; poor metabolizers: 34-40 hours

Time to peak serum concentration: 1-2 hours; delayed 3 hours by high-fat meal

Elimination: Urine: <3% is excreted unchanged; 80% excreted as 4-hydroxyatomoxetine glucuronide; feces: <17%

Usual Dosage Oral:

Children ≥6 years and Adolescents ≤70 kg: Initial: 0.5 mg/kg/day; increase after a minimum of 3 days to approximately 1.2 mg/kg/day; may administer once daily in the morning or divide into two doses and administer in the morning and late afternoon/early evening. Maximum daily dose: 1.4 mg/kg/day or 100 mg/day, whichever is less. **Note:** Doses >1.2 mg/kg/day have not been shown to provide additional benefit.

Note: In patients receiving strong CYP2D6 inhibitors (eg, paroxetine, fluoxetine, quinidine) or patients known to be CYP2D6 poor metabolizers, maintain the above listed initial dose for 4 weeks; increase dose to 1.2 mg/kg/day only if clinically needed and the initial dose is well tolerated; do not exceed 1.2 mg/kg/day

Children ≥6 years and Adolescents >70 kg and Adults: Initial: 40 mg/day; increase after a minimum of 3 days to approximately 80 mg/day; may administer once daily in the morning or divide into two doses and administer in morning and late afternoon/early evening. May increase (if needed) to 100 mg/day in 2-4 additional weeks

Note: In patients receiving strong CYP2D6 inhibitors (eg, paroxetine, fluoxetine, quinidine) or patients known to be CYP2D6 poor metabolizers, maintain the above listed initial dose for 4 weeks; increase dose to 80 mg/day only if clinically needed and the initial dose is well tolerated; do not exceed 80 mg/day

Dosage adjustment in renal impairment: No adjustment needed

Dosage adjustment in hepatic impairment:

Moderate hepatic impairment (Child-Pugh class B): All doses should be reduced to 50% of normal

Severe hepatic impairment (Child-Pugh class C): All doses should be reduced to 25% of normal

Administration Oral: May be administered without regard to food. Do not crush, chew, or open capsule; swallow whole with water or other liquids. **Note:** Atomoxetine is an ocular irritant; see Additional Information.

Monitoring Parameters Evaluate for cardiac disease prior to initiation of therapy with thorough medical history, family history, and physical exam; consider ECG (see Warnings); perform ECG and echocardiogram if findings suggest cardiac disease; promptly conduct cardiac evaluation in patients who develop chest pain, unexplained syncope, or any other symptom of cardiac disease during treatment; monitor weight, height, growth (in children); blood pressure, heart rate, and rhythm; liver enzymes in patients with symptoms of liver dysfunction; sleep, appetite, abnormal movements. Patients should be re-evaluated at appropriate intervals to assess continued need of the medication. Monitor for suicidality and associated behaviors (see Warnings); new psychotic symptoms, appearance or worsening of aggressive behavior, or hostility.

Patient Information An increased risk of suicidal thinking and behavior has been reported with the use of atomoxetine in children and adolescents; notify physician if you feel depressed, have thoughts of suicide, or become more agitated or irritable (see Warnings). Read the patient Medication Guide that you receive with each prescription and refill of atomoxetine. Cases of sudden death and other heart problems have been reported in patients with heart defects or heart problems; inform physician if you have a heart defect, heart problems, high or low blood pressure, or a family history of these problems. Inform physician if you have allergies, narrow-angle glaucoma, or current or past liver problems. Notify physician if you experience problems with rapid or irregular heartbeats, dark urine, yellow skin or eyes, abdominal pain, itching, unexplained flu-like symptoms, new psychotic symptoms (eg, hearing voices), or an increase in aggression or hostility. Some medicines should not be taken with atomoxetine; report the use of other medications, nonprescription medications, and herbal or natural products to your physician and pharmacist. If a dose is missed, take it as soon as possible, but do not take more than the prescribed total daily amount in any 24-hour period. May cause dizziness and impair ability to perform activities requiring mental alertness or physical coordination; may cause weight loss; may cause decreased growth in children; may make it difficult to urinate; may cause dry mouth; may rarely cause prolonged (>4 hours) penile erections (seek prompt medical attention). Do not open capsules or allow capsule or contents to come into contact with eye (see Additional Information).

Additional Information Atomoxetine hydrochloride is the R(-) isomer. Therapy may be discontinued without being tapered. Total daily doses >150 mg/day and single doses >120 mg/dose have not been systematically evaluated. Medications used to treat ADHD should be part of a total treatment program that may include other components such as psychological, educational, and social measures. If used for an extended period of time, long-term usefulness of atomoxetine should be periodically re-evaluated for the individual patient.

Atomoxetine is an ocular irritant; avoid contact with eye; if capsule contents come into contact with eye, flush eye immediately with water and obtain medical advice; wash hands and any potentially contaminated surface as soon as possible

Dosage Forms Excipient information presented when available (limited, particularly for generics); consult specific product labeling.
Capsule:
Strattera®: 10 mg, 18 mg, 25 mg, 40 mg, 60 mg, 80 mg, 100 mg

References

American Academy of Pediatrics/American Heart Association Clarification of Statement on Cardiovascular Evaluation and Monitoring of Children and Adolescents With Heart Disease Receiving Medications for ADHD; available at: http://americanheart.mediaroon.com/index.-php?s=43&item=422.

Biderman J, Heiligenstein JH, Faries DE, at al, "Efficacy of Atomoxetine Versus Placebo in School-Age Girls With Attention-Deficit/Hyperactivity Disorder," Pediatrics, 2002, 110(6), http://www.pediatrics.org/cgi/content/full/110/6/e75.

Dopheide JA and Pliszka SR, "Attention-Deficit-Hyperactivity Disorder: An Update," Pharmacotherapy, 2009, 29(6):656-79.

Kratochvil CJ, Heiligenstein JH, Dittmann R, et al, "Atomoxetine and Methylphenidate Treatment in Children With ADHD: A Prospective, Randomized, Open-Label trial," J Am Acad Child Adolesc Psychiatry, 2002, 41(7):776-84.

Michelson D, Allen AJ, Busner J, et al, "Once-Daily Atomoxetine Treatment for Children and Adolescents With Attention Deficit Hyperactivity Disorder: A Randomized, Placebo-Controlled Study," Am J Psychiatry, 2002, 159(11):1896-901.

Michelson D, Faries D, Wernicke J, et al, "Atomoxetine in the Treatment of Children and Adolescents With Attention-Deficit/Hyperactivity Disorder: A Ramdomized, Placebo-Controlled, Dose-Response Study," Pediatrics, 2001, 108(5), http://www.pediatrics.org/cgi/content/full/108/5/e83.

Newcorn JH, Michelson D, Kratochvil CJ, et al, "Low-Dose Atomoxetine for Maintenance Treatment of Attention-Deficit/Hyperactivity Disorder," Pediatrics, 2006, 118(6):e1701-6.

Spencer T, Heiligenstein JH, Biederman J, et al, "Results From 2 Proof-of-Concept, Placebo-Controlled Studies of Atomoxetine in Children With Attention-Deficit/Hyperactivity Disorder," J Clin Psychiatry, 2002, 63(12):1140-7.

Vetter VL, Elia J, Erickson C, et al, "Cardiovascular Monitoring of Children and Adolescents With Heart Disease Receiving Stimulant Drugs: A Scientific Statement From the American Heart Association Council on Cardiovascular Disease in the Young Congenital Cardiac Defects Committee and the Council on Cardiovascular Nursing," Circulation, 2008, 117(18):2407-23.

Wernicke JF and Kratochvil CJ, "Safety Profile of Atomoxetine in the Treatment of Children and Adolescents With ADHD," J Clin Psychiatry, 2002, 63(Suppl 12):50-5.

◆ **Atomoxetine Hydrochloride** see Atomoxetine on page 149

Atorvastatin (a TORE va sta tin)

Medication Safety Issues
Sound-alike/look-alike issues:
Atorvastatin may be confused with atomoxetine, lovastatin, nystatin, pitavastatin, pravastatin, rosuvastatin, simvastatin
Lipitor® may be confused with labetalol, Levatol®, lisinopril, Loniten®, Lopid®, Mevacor®, Zocor®, Zyrtec®

Related Information
Normal Laboratory Values for Children on page 1672

U.S. Brand Names Lipitor®

Canadian Brand Names Apo-Atorvastatin®; CO Atorvastatin; GD-Atorvastatin; Lipitor®; PMS-Atorvastatin; RAN™-Atorvastatin; Sandoz-Atorvastatin

Therapeutic Category Antilipemic Agent; HMG-CoA Reductase Inhibitor

Generic Available No

Use
Hyperlipidemia: Adjunct to dietary therapy in pediatric patients with heterozygous familial hypercholesterolemia if LDL-C remains ≥190 mg/dL, if ≥160 mg/dL with family history of premature CHD, or if ≥2 cardiovascular risk factors are present (FDA approved in boys and postmenarchal girls 10-17 years) (see Additional Information for recommendations on initiating hypercholesterolemia pharmacologic treatment in children ≥8 years). Adjunct to

dietary therapy to decrease elevated serum total and low density lipoprotein cholesterol (LDL-C), apolipoprotein B (apo-B), and triglyceride levels, and to increase high density lipoprotein cholesterol (HDL-C) in patients with primary hypercholesterolemia (heterozygous, familial and nonfamilial) and mixed dyslipidemia (Fredrickson types IIa and IIb) (FDA approved in adults); treatment of homozygous familial hypercholesterolemia (FDA approved in adults); treatment of isolated hypertriglyceridemia (Fredrickson type IV) and type III hyperlipoproteinemia; treatment of primary dysbetalipoproteinemia (Fredrickson Type III) (FDA approved in adults)

Primary prevention of cardiovascular disease in high risk patients (FDA approved in adults); risk factors include: Age ≥55 years, smoking, hypertension, low HDL-C, or family history of early coronary heart disease; secondary prevention of cardiovascular disease to reduce the risk of MI, stroke, revascularization procedures, and angina in patients with evidence of coronary heart disease and to reduce the risk of hospitalization for heart failure. Has also been used in prevention of graft coronary artery disease in heart transplant patients.

Pregnancy Risk Factor X

Pregnancy Considerations Cholesterol biosynthesis may be important in fetal development. Contraindicated in pregnancy. Administer to women of childbearing potential only when conception is highly unlikely and patients have been informed of potential hazards.

Lactation Excretion in breast milk unknown/contraindicated

Contraindications Hypersensitivity to atorvastatin or any component; active liver disease; unexplained persistent elevations of serum transaminases; pregnancy; breast-feeding

Warnings Rhabdomyolysis with or without acute renal failure secondary to myoglobinuria has occurred rarely. Risk is increased with concurrent use of amiodarone, clarithromycin, danazol, diltiazem, fluvoxamine, amprenavir, delavirdine, indinavir, nefazodone, nelfinavir, ritonavir, verapamil, troleandomycin, cyclosporine, fibric acid derivatives, erythromycin, niacin, or azole antifungals. Assess the risk versus benefit before combining any of these medications with atorvastatin. Temporarily discontinue atorvastatin in any patient experiencing an acute or serious condition predisposing to renal failure secondary to rhabdomyolysis. Patients with a history of hemorrhagic stroke may be at increased risk for another when taking atorvastatin.

Precautions Persistent increases in serum transaminases have occurred (incidence in clinical trials 0.7% overall and highest with the 80 mg dose, 2.3%); liver function tests must be monitored at the initiation of therapy and 12 weeks following initiation of therapy or increase in dosage, and then periodically eg, semiannually, thereafter. Liver enzyme changes generally occur in the first 3 months of treatment. Use with caution in patients who consume substantial quantities of alcohol or have a previous history of liver disease.

Adverse Reactions

Central nervous system: Insomnia

Dermatologic: Acne, alopecia, dry skin, eczema, erythema multiforme, photosensitivity, pruritus, rash, seborrhea, skin ulcer, Stevens-Johnson syndrome, toxic epidermal necrolysis

Endocrine & metabolic: Gout, hyperglycemia, hypoglycemia

Gastrointestinal: Diarrhea, dyspepsia, nausea

Genitourinary: UTI

Hepatic: Cholestatic jaundice, hepatitis, serum transaminases increased

Neuromuscular & skeletal: Arthralgias, CPK elevated, muscle spasms, musculoskeletal pain, myalgias, myopathy, rhabdomyolysis

Respiratory: Nasopharyngitis, pharyngolaryngeal pain

<2% and/or postmarketing: Abdominal pain, anaphylaxis, angioneurotic edema, blurred vision, bullous rash, CPK elevated, depression, dizziness, epistaxis, eructation, erythema multiforme, fatigue, fever, flatulence, hepatic failure, hyperglycemia, joint swelling, malaise, memory impairment, muscle fatigue, neck pain, nightmare, peripheral neuropathy, Stevens-Johnson Syndrome, tendon rupture, tinnitus, toxic epidermal necrolysis, urticaria

Drug Interactions

Metabolism/Transport Effects Substrate of CYP3A4 (major), P-glycoprotein; **Inhibits** CYP3A4 (weak), P-glycoprotein

Avoid Concomitant Use

Avoid concomitant use of Atorvastatin with any of the following: Silodosin; Topotecan

Increased Effect/Toxicity

Atorvastatin may increase the levels/effects of: Aliskiren; DAPTOmycin; Digoxin; Diltiazem; Midazolam; P-Glycoprotein Substrates; Rivaroxaban; Silodosin; Topotecan; Verapamil

The levels/effects of Atorvastatin may be increased by: Amiodarone; Antifungal Agents (Azole Derivatives, Systemic); Colchicine; CycloSPORINE; CycloSPORINE (Systemic); CYP3A4 Inhibitors (Moderate); CYP3A4 Inhibitors (Strong); Danazol; Dasatinib; Diltiazem; Dronedarone; Eltrombopag; Fenofibrate; Fenofibric Acid; Fluconazole; Fusidic Acid; Gemfibrozil; Grapefruit Juice; Macrolide Antibiotics; Nefazodone; Niacin; Niacinamide; P-Glycoprotein Inhibitors; Protease Inhibitors; QuiNINE; Rifamycin Derivatives; Sildenafil; Verapamil

Decreased Effect

Atorvastatin may decrease the levels/effects of: Dabigatran Etexilate

The levels/effects of Atorvastatin may be decreased by: Antacids; Bosentan; CYP3A4 Inducers (Strong); Deferasirox; Etravirine; P-Glycoprotein Inducers; Phenytoin; Rifamycin Derivatives; St Johns Wort

Food Interactions Atorvastatin serum concentration may be increased when taken with large quantities (>1 quart/day) of grapefruit juice; avoid concurrent use

Stability Tablets should be stored in well closed container at controlled room temperature between 20°C to 25°C (68°F to 77°F)

Mechanism of Action Atorvastatin is a selective, competitive inhibitor of 3-hydroxy-3-methylglutaryl-coenzyme A (HMG-CoA) reductase, the enzyme that catalyzes the rate-limiting step in cholesterol biosynthesis

Pharmacodynamics

Onset of action: Within 2 weeks

Maximum effect: After 4 weeks

LDL reduction: 10 mg/day: 39% (for each doubling of this dose, LDL is lowered approximately 6%)

Pharmacokinetics (Adult data unless noted)

Absorption: Oral: Rapidly absorbed; extensive first-pass metabolism in GI mucosa and liver

Distribution: V_d: ~381 L

Protein binding: >98%

Metabolism: Extensive metabolism to ortho- and para-hydroxylated derivatives and various beta-oxidation products with equivalent *in vitro* activity to atorvastatin

Bioavailability: Absolute: 14%

Half-life: 14 hours (half-life of inhibitory activity due to active metabolites is 20-30 hours)

Time to peak serum concentration: 1-2 hours

Elimination: Primarily in bile following hepatic and/or extra-hepatic metabolism; does not appear to undergo enterohepatic recirculation; <2% excreted in urine

Usual Dosage Oral: Dosage should be individualized according to the baseline LDL-C level, the recommended goal of therapy, and patient response; adjustments should be made at intervals of 4 weeks (adults: 2-4 weeks)

Children:

Heterozygous familial and nonfamilial hypercholesterolemia: Children and Adolescents 10-17 years: 10 mg once daily; may increase to a maximum of 20 mg/day

Hyperlipidemia: Children and adolescents 10-17 years: 10 mg once daily; may increase to 20 mg once daily; doses >20 mg have not been studied

Prevention of graft coronary artery disease: 0.2 mg/kg/day rounded to nearest 2.5 mg increment (Chin, 2008)

Adults:

Heterozygous familial and nonfamilial hypercholesterolemia: 10-20 mg once daily; may increase to a maximum of 80 mg/day

Homozygous familial hypercholesterolemia: 10-80 mg/day

Hyperlipidemia:

Initial: 10-20 mg once daily; patients who require a reduction of >45% in LDL-C may be started at 40 mg once daily

Maintenance: Recommended dosage range: 10-80 mg/day

Primary prevention of cardiovascular disease: 10 mg once daily

Dosage adjustment for atorvastatin with concomitant medications:

Cyclosporine: Atorvastatin dose should **not** exceed 10 mg/day

Clarithromycin, itraconazole, ritonavir plus saquinavir, or lopinavir plus ritonavir when atorvastatin dose >20 mg: Ensure that the lowest dose necessary of atorvastatin is used.

Dosing adjustment in renal impairment: Adults: Because atorvastatin does not undergo significant renal excretion, dose modification is not necessary

Dosing adjustment in hepatic impairment: Contraindicated in active liver disease or in patients with unexplained persistent elevations of serum transaminases

Administration Oral: May be taken without regard to meals or time of day

Monitoring Parameters Serum cholesterol (total and fractionated), CPK; liver function tests (see Precautions)

Reference Range See Related Information for age- and gender-specific serum cholesterol, LDL-C, TG, and HDL concentrations.

Patient Information May rarely cause photosensitivity reactions (eg, exposure to sunlight may cause severe sunburn, skin rash, redness, or itching); avoid direct exposure to sunlight. Report severe and unresolved gastric upset, any vision changes, muscle pain and weakness, changes in color of urine or stool, yellowing of skin or eyes, and any unusual bruising. Female patients of childbearing age must be counseled to use 2 effective forms of contraception simultaneously, unless absolute abstinence is the chosen method; this drug may cause severe fetal defects. May cause dry mouth.

Additional Information The current recommendation for pharmacologic treatment of hypercholesterolemia in children is limited to children ≥8 years of age and is based on LDL-C concentrations and the presence of coronary vascular disease (CVD) risk factors (see table and Daniels, 2008). In adults, for each 1% lowering in LDL-C, the relative risk for major cardiovascular events is reduced by ~1%. For more specific risk assessment and treatment recommendations for adults, see NCEP ATPIII, 2001.

Recommendations for Initiating Pharmacologic Treatment in Children ≥8 Years[1]

No risk factors for CVD	LDL ≥190 mg/dL despite 6-month to 1-year diet therapy
Family history of premature CVD or ≥2 CVD risk factors present, including obesity, hypertension, or cigarette smoking	LDL ≥160 mg/dL despite 6-month to 1-year diet therapy
Diabetes mellitus present	LDL ≥130 mg/dL

[1]Adapted from Daniels SR, Greer FR, and Committee on Nutrition, "Lipid Screening and Cardiovascular Health in Childhood," *Pediatrics*, 2008, 122(1):198-208.

Dosage Forms Excipient information presented when available (limited, particularly for generics); consult specific product labeling.

Tablet:

Lipitor®: 10 mg, 20 mg, 40 mg, 80 mg

References

American Academy of Pediatrics Committee on Nutrition, "Cholesterol in Childhood," *Pediatrics*, 1998, 101(1 Pt 1):141-7.

American Academy of Pediatrics, "National Cholesterol Education Program: Report of the Expert Panel on Blood Cholesterol Levels in Children and Adolescents," *Pediatrics*, 1992, 89(3 Pt 2):525-84.

Belay B, Belamarich PF, and Tom-Revzon C, "The Use of Statins in Pediatrics: Knowledge Base, Limitations, and Future Directions," *Pediatrics*, 2007, 119(2):370-80.

Chin C, Gamberg P, Miller J, et al, "Efficacy and Safety of Atorvastatin After Pediatric Heart Transplantation," *J Heart Lung Transplant*, 2002, 21(11):1213-7.

Chin C, Lukito SS, Shek J, et al, "Prevention of Pediatric Graft Coronary Artery Disease: Atorvastatin," *Pediatr Transplant*, 2008, 12(4):442-6.

Daniels SR, Greer FR, and Committee on Nutrition, "Lipid Screening and Cardiovascular Disease in Health in Childhood," *Pediatrics*, 2008, 122(1):198-208.

Duplaga BA, "Treatment of Childhood Hypercholesterolemia With HMG-CoA Reductase Inhibitors," *Ann Pharmacother*, 1999, 33(11):1224-7.

Grundy SM, Cleeman JI, Merz CN, et al, "Implications of Recent Clinical Trials for the National Cholesterol Education Program Adult Treatment Panel III Guidelines," *Circulation*, 2004, 110(2):227-39.

McCrindle BW, Ose L, and Marais AD, "Efficacy and Safety of Atorvastatin in Children and Adolescents With Familial Hypercholesterolemia or Severe Hyperlipidemia: A Multicenter, Randomized, Placebo-Controlled Trial," *J Pediatr*, 2003, 143(1):74-80.

McCrindle BW, Urbina EM, Dennison BA, et al, "Drug Therapy of High-Risk Lipid Abnormalities in Children and Adolescents: A Scientific Statement From the American Heart Association Atherosclerosis, Hypertension, and Obesity in Youth Committee, Council of Cardiovascular Disease in the Young, With the Council on Cardiovascular Nursing," *Circulation*, 2007, 115(14):1948-67.

"Third Report of the National Cholesterol Education Program Expert Panel on Detection, Evaluation, and Treatment of High Blood Cholesterol in Adults (Adult Treatment Panel III)," May 2001, www.nhlbi.nih.gov/guidelines/cholesterol.

◆ **Atorvastatin Calcium** *see* Atorvastatin *on page 151*

Atovaquone (a TOE va kwone)

U.S. Brand Names Mepron®

Canadian Brand Names Mepron®

Therapeutic Category Antiprotozoal

Generic Available No

Use Second-line treatment of mild to moderate *Pneumocystis jiroveci* pneumonia (PCP) in patients intolerant of trimethoprim/sulfamethoxazole (TMP/SMX); mild to moderate PCP is defined as an alveolar-arterial oxygen diffusion gradient ≤45 mm Hg and PaO$_2$ ≥60 mm Hg on room air; patients intolerant of TMP/SMX are defined as having a significant rash (ie, Stevens-Johnson-like syndrome), neutropenia, or hemolysis; prevention of PCP in patients who are intolerant to TMP/SMX; treatment of babesiosis

Pregnancy Risk Factor C

Pregnancy Considerations There are no adequate and well-controlled studies of atovaquone in pregnant women. Use in pregnant women only if the potential benefit outweighs the possible risk to the fetus.

Lactation Excretion in breast milk unknown/use caution

Contraindications Hypersensitivity to atovaquone or any component (see Warnings)

Warnings Clinical experience with atovaquone has been limited to patients with mild to moderate PCP; treatment of more severe episodes of PCP has not been systematically studied

Suspension contains benzyl alcohol which may cause allergic reactions in susceptible individuals; large amounts of benzyl alcohol (≥99 mg/kg/day) have been associated with a potentially fatal toxicity ("gasping syndrome") in neonates; the "gasping syndrome" consists of metabolic acidosis, respiratory distress, gasping respirations, CNS dysfunction (including convulsions, intracranial hemorrhage), hypotension and cardiovascular collapse; avoid use in neonates; in vitro and animal studies have shown that benzoate, a metabolite of benzyl alcohol, displaces bilirubin from protein binding sites

Precautions For patients who have difficulty taking atovaquone with food or who have chronic diarrhea, stomach or intestinal problems which may result in drug malabsorption, parenteral therapy with other agents should be considered since a low serum atovaquone concentration could lead to treatment failure

Adverse Reactions

Central nervous system: Fever, headache, insomnia, dizziness, pain

Dermatologic: Maculopapular rash, erythema multiforme, pruritus

Endocrine & metabolic: Hyponatremia

Gastrointestinal: Nausea, vomiting, diarrhea, abdominal pain, constipation, anorexia, amylase elevated

Hematologic: Rare: Neutropenia, anemia

Hepatic: Hepatic enzymes elevated, cholestasis

Respiratory: Cough, sinusitis

Miscellaneous: Diaphoresis

Drug Interactions

Avoid Concomitant Use There are no known interactions where it is recommended to avoid concomitant use.

Increased Effect/Toxicity

Atovaquone may increase the levels/effects of: Etoposide; Hypoglycemic Agents

The levels/effects of Atovaquone may be increased by: Herbs (Hypoglycemic Properties)

Decreased Effect

Atovaquone may decrease the levels/effects of: Indinavir

The levels/effects of Atovaquone may be decreased by: Rifamycin Derivatives; Ritonavir; Tetracycline

Food Interactions Administration with food increases bioavailability of atovaquone suspension 1.4-fold over that achieved in a fasting state or up to 3-fold with a high fat meal

Stability Store at room temperature; do not freeze

Mechanism of Action The mechanism of action against Pneumocystis jiroveci has not been fully elucidated; in Plasmodium species, atovaquone selectively inhibits the mitochondrial electron-transport system at the cytochrome bc_1 complex resulting in depletion of dihydroorotate dehydrogenase and ultimately resulting in the inhibition of nucleic acid and adenosine triphosphate synthesis

Pharmacokinetics (Adult data unless noted)

Absorption: Oral:

Infants and Children <2 years of age: Decreased absorption

Adults: Oral suspension: Absorption is enhanced 1.4-fold with food; decreased absorption with single doses exceeding 750 mg

Distribution: V_{dss}: 0.6 L/kg; CSF concentration is <1% of the plasma concentration

Protein binding: >99%

Bioavailability: Suspension (administered with food): 47%

Half-life, elimination:

Children (4 months to 12 years): 60 hours (range: 31-163 hours)

Adults: 2.9 days

Adults with AIDS: 2.2 days

Time to peak serum concentration: Dual peak serum concentrations at 1 to 8 hours and at 24 to 96 hours after dose due to enterohepatic cycling

Elimination: ~94% is recovered as unchanged drug in feces; 0.6% excreted in urine

Usual Dosage Oral:

Children:

Treatment: Dose of 40 mg/kg/day divided twice daily (maximum dose: 1500 mg/day) may be necessary to attain comparable plasma concentrations associated with the successful treatment of PCP as seen in adults.

Prophylaxis of Pneumocystis jiroveci pneumonia:

1-3 months of age and >24 months of age: 30 mg/kg/day once daily (maximum dose: 1500 mg/day)

4-24 months of age: 45 mg/kg/day once daily (maximum dose: 1500 mg/day)

Babesiosis: 40 mg/kg/day divided twice daily (maximum dose: 1500 mg/day) with azithromycin 12 mg/kg/day once daily for 7-10 days

Adolescents 13-16 years and Adults:

Treatment: 750 mg/dose twice daily for 21 days

Prophylaxis of Pneumocystis jiroveci pneumonia: 1500 mg once daily

Babesiosis: 750 mg/dose twice daily for 7-10 days with azithromycin 1000 mg once daily for 3 days then 500 mg once daily for 7 days

Administration Oral: Administer with food or a high-fat meal; shake suspension well before using

Monitoring Parameters CBC with differential, liver enzymes, serum chemistries, serum amylase

Additional Information The suspension contains the inactive ingredient poloxamer 188

Dosage Forms Excipient information presented when available (limited, particularly for generics); consult specific product labeling.

Suspension, oral:

Mepron®: 750 mg/5 mL (5 mL, 210 mL) [contains benzyl alcohol; citrus flavor]

References

Centers for Disease Control and Prevention, "2001 USPHS/IDSA Guidelines for the Prevention of Opportunistic Infections in Persons Infected With Human Immunodeficiency Virus," November 28, 2001, http://www.aidsinfo.nih.gov

Haile LG and Flaherty JF, "Atovaquone: A Review," Ann Pharmacother, 1993, 27(12):1488-94.

Hughes W, Dorenbaum A, Yogev R, et al, "Phase I Safety and Pharmacokinetics Study of Micronized Atovaquone Human Immunodeficiency Virus-Infected Infants and Children. Pediatric AIDS Clinical Trials Group," Antimicrob Agents Chemother, 1998, 42(6):1315-8.

Hughes W, Leoung G, Kramer F, et al, "Comparison of Atovaquone (566C80) With Trimethoprim-Sulfamethoxazole to Treat Pneumocystis carinii Pneumonia in Patients With AIDS," N Engl J Med, 1993, 328(21):1521-7.

Atovaquone and Proguanil
(a TOE va kwone & pro GWA nil)

U.S. Brand Names Malarone®

Canadian Brand Names Malarone®; Malarone® Pediatric

Therapeutic Category Antimalarial Agent

Generic Available No

Use Prevention (FDA approved in pediatric patients >11 kg and adults) or treatment (FDA approved in pediatric patients >5 kg and adults) of acute, uncomplicated *P. falciparum* malaria

Pregnancy Risk Factor C

Pregnancy Considerations Teratogenic effects were not observed with the combination of atovaquone/proguanil in animal reproduction studies using concentrations similar to the estimated human exposure. The pharmacokinetics of atovaquone and proguanil are changed during pregnancy. Malaria infection in pregnant women may be more severe than in nonpregnant women. Because *P. falciparum* malaria can cause maternal death and fetal loss, pregnant women traveling to malaria-endemic areas must use personal protection against mosquito bites. Atovaquone/proguanil may be used as an alternative treatment of malaria in pregnant women; consult current CDC guidelines.

Lactation

Atovaquone: Excretion in breast milk unknown/use caution

Proguanil: Enters breast milk/use caution

Breast-Feeding Considerations

Small quantities of proguanil are found in breast milk. This combination is not recommended if nursing infants <5 kg (safety data is limited concerning therapeutic use in infants <5 kg)

Contraindications Hypersensitivity to atovaquone, proguanil, or any component of the formulation; prophylactic use in severe renal impairment (Cl_{Cr} <30 mL/minute)

Warnings Liver function test abnormalities and hepatitis have been reported with use. One case of hepatic failure has been reported. Not indicated for severe or complicated malaria.

Precautions Absorption of atovaquone may be decreased in patients who have diarrhea or vomiting; monitor closely and consider use of an antiemetic. If severe, consider use of an alternative antimalarial. Delayed cases of *P. falciparum* malaria may occur after stopping prophylaxis; travelers returning from endemic areas who develop febrile illnesses should be evaluated for malaria. Recrudescent infections or infections following prophylaxis with this agent should be treated with alternative agent(s). Use with caution in patients with pre-existing renal disease. Parasite relapse is common when used to treat *P. vivax*.

Adverse Reactions The following adverse reactions were reported in patients being treated for malaria. When used for prophylaxis, reactions are similar to those seen with placebo.

Central nervous system: Dizziness, headache

Dermatologic: Pruritus

Gastrointestinal: Abdominal pain, anorexia, diarrhea, nausea, vomiting

Hepatic: Hepatic failure, hepatitis, transaminases increased (typically normalize after ~4 weeks)

Neuromuscular & skeletal: Weakness

Respiratory: Cough

Miscellaneous: Anaphylaxis

<1%, postmarketing, and/or case reports: Anemia, angioedema, cholestasis, erythema multiforme, hallucinations, neutropenia, pancytopenia (with severe renal impairment), photosensitivity, psychotic episodes, rash, seizure, Stevens-Johnson syndrome, stomatitis, urticaria, vasculitis

Drug Interactions

Metabolism/Transport Effects Proguanil: **Substrate** (minor) of 1A2, 2C19, 3A4

Avoid Concomitant Use

Avoid concomitant use of Atovaquone and Proguanil with any of the following: Artemether; Lumefantrine

Increased Effect/Toxicity

Atovaquone and Proguanil may increase the levels/effects of: Antipsychotic Agents (Phenothiazines); Dapsone; Dapsone (Systemic); Dapsone (Topical); Etoposide; Hypoglycemic Agents; Lumefantrine

The levels/effects of Atovaquone and Proguanil may be increased by: Artemether; Dapsone; Dapsone (Systemic); Herbs (Hypoglycemic Properties)

Decreased Effect Metoclopramide decreases bioavailability of atovaquone. Rifabutin decreases atovaquone levels by 34%. Rifampin decreases atovaquone levels by 50%. Tetracycline decreases plasma concentrations of atovaquone by 40%.

Food Interactions Atovaquone taken with dietary fat increases the rate and extent of absorption.

Stability Store tablets at 25°C (77°F)

Mechanism of Action

Atovaquone: Selectively inhibits parasite mitochondrial electron transport.

Proguanil: The metabolite cycloguanil inhibits dihydrofolate reductase, disrupting deoxythymidylate synthesis. Together, atovaquone/cycloguanil affect the erythrocytic and exoerythrocytic stages of development.

Pharmacokinetics (Adult data unless noted)

Atovaquone: See Atovaquone monograph.

Proguanil:

Absorption: Extensive

Distribution: 42 L/kg

Protein binding: 75%

Metabolism: Hepatic to active metabolites, cycloguanil (via CYP2C19) and 4-chlorophenylbiguanide

Half-life elimination: 12-21 hours

Elimination: Urine (40% to 60%)

Usual Dosage Oral:

Children (dosage based on body weight):

Prevention of malaria: Start 1-2 days prior to entering a malaria-endemic area, continue throughout the stay and for 7 days after returning. Take as a single dose, once daily.

11-20 kg: Atovaquone/proguanil 62.5 mg/25 mg

21-30 kg: Atovaquone/proguanil 125 mg/50 mg

31-40 kg: Atovaquone/proguanil 187.5 mg/75 mg

>40 kg: Atovaquone/proguanil 250 mg/100 mg

Treatment of acute malaria: Take as a single dose, once daily for 3 consecutive days.

5-8 kg: Atovaquone/proguanil 125 mg/50 mg

9-10 kg: Atovaquone/proguanil 187.5 mg/75 mg

11-20 kg: Atovaquone/proguanil 250 mg/100 mg

21-30 kg: Atovaquone/proguanil 500 mg/200 mg

31-40 kg: Atovaquone/proguanil 750 mg/300 mg

>40 kg: Atovaquone/proguanil 1 g/400 mg

Adults:

Prevention of malaria: Atovaquone/proguanil 250 mg/100 mg once daily; start 1-2 days prior to entering a malaria-endemic area, continue throughout the stay and for 7 days after returning

Treatment of acute malaria: Atovaquone/proguanil 1 g/400 mg as a single dose, once daily for 3 consecutive days

Dosage adjustment in renal impairment: Should not be used as prophylaxis in severe renal impairment (Cl_{cr} <30 mL/minute). For treatment of malaria, alternative regimens should be used in patients with Cl_{cr} <30 mL/minute unless benefits outweigh the risks. No dosage adjustment required in mild to moderate renal impairment.

Dosage adjustment in hepatic impairment: No dosage adjustment required in mild to moderate hepatic impairment. No data available for use in severe hepatic impairment.

Administration Administer with food or milk at the same time each day. If vomiting occurs within 1 hour of administration, repeat the dose. For children who have difficulty swallowing tablets, tablets may be crushed and mixed with condensed milk just prior to administration.

Patient Information Inform prescriber of all prescriptions, OTC medications, or herbal products you are taking, and any allergies you have. Do not take any new medication during therapy without consulting prescriber. Complete full course of therapy; do not discontinue or alter dosage without consulting prescriber. Take at the same time each day with full glass of milk or food. If vomiting occurs within 1 hour of taking dose, you may repeat the dose. You may experience nausea, vomiting, or loss of appetite (small frequent meals may help); or headache (if persistent, contact prescriber). Follow recommended precautions to avoid malaria exposure (use insect repellent, bednets, protective clothing). Notify prescriber if you develop fever after returning from or while visiting a malaria-endemic area. **Pregnancy/breast-feeding precautions:** Inform prescriber if you are or intend to become pregnant. Consult prescriber if breast-feeding.

Dosage Forms Excipient information presented when available (limited, particularly for generics); consult specific product labeling.

Tablet, oral:
Malarone®: Atovaquone 250 mg and proguanil hydrochloride 100 mg
Tablet, oral [pediatric]:
Malarone®: Atovaquone 62.5 mg and proguanil hydrochloride 25 mg

♦ **Atovaquone and Proguanil Hydrochloride** *see* Atovaquone and Proguanil *on page* 154

♦ **ATRA** *see* Tretinoin (Systemic) *on page* 1373

Atracurium (a tra KYOO ree um)

Medication Safety Issues
High alert medication: The Institute for Safe Medication Practices (ISMP) includes this medication among its list of drugs which have a heightened risk of causing significant patient harm when used in error.

United States Pharmacopeia (USP) 2006: The Interdisciplinary Safe Medication Use Expert Committee of the USP has recommended the following:
- Hospitals, clinics, and other practice sites should institute special safeguards in the storage, labeling, and use of these agents and should include these safeguards in staff orientation and competency training.
- Healthcare professionals should be on high alert (especially vigilant) whenever a neuromuscular-blocking agent (NMBA) is stocked, ordered, prepared, or administered.

Canadian Brand Names Atracurium Besylate Injection
Therapeutic Category Neuromuscular Blocker Agent, Nondepolarizing; Skeletal Muscle Relaxant, Paralytic
Generic Available Yes
Use Eases endotracheal intubation as an adjunct to general anesthesia and relaxes skeletal muscle during surgery or mechanical ventilation
Pregnancy Risk Factor C
Lactation Excretion in breast milk unknown/use caution
Contraindications Hypersensitivity to atracurium besylate or any component
Warnings Reduce initial dosage and inject slowly (over 1-2 minutes) in patients in whom substantial histamine release would be potentially hazardous (eg, patients with clinically important cardiovascular disease); maintenance of an adequate airway and respiratory support is critical; formulation with preservative contains benzyl alcohol which may cause allergic reactions in susceptible individuals; large amounts of benzyl alcohol (≥99 mg/kg/day) have been associated with a potentially fatal toxicity ("gasping syndrome") in neonates; the "gasping syndrome" consists of metabolic acidosis, respiratory distress, gasping respirations, CNS dysfunction (including convulsions, intracranial hemorrhage), hypotension and cardiovascular collapse; avoid use of atracurium products containing benzyl alcohol in neonates; use preservative free product; *in vitro* and animal studies have shown that benzoate, a metabolite of benzyl alcohol, displaces bilirubin from protein binding sites; avoid use of preservative-containing formulation in neonates

Certain clinical conditions may result in potentiation or antagonism of neuromuscular blockade, see table. Increased sensitivity in patients with myasthenia gravis, Eaton-Lambert syndrome; resistance to neuromuscular blockade in burn patients (>30% of body) for period of 5-70 days postinjury; resistance in patients with muscle trauma, denervation, immobilization, infection, chronic treatment with atracurium. When used in conjunction with anesthetics, bradycardia may be more common with atracurium than with other neuromuscular blocking agents; it has no clinically significant effects on heart rate to counteract the bradycardia produced by anesthetics.

Clinical Conditions Affecting Neuromuscular Blockade

Potentiation	Antagonism
Electrolyte abnormalities	Alkalosis
Severe hyponatremia	Hypercalcemia
Severe hypocalcemia	Demyelinating lesions
Severe hypokalemia	Peripheral neuropathies
Hypermagnesemia	Diabetes mellitus
Neuromuscular diseases	
Acidosis	
Acute intermittent porphyria	
Renal failure	
Hepatic failure	

Precautions Due to potential histamine release, use with caution in patients in whom histamine release may be hazardous (eg, cardiovascular disease, asthma); patients with severe electrolyte disorders; patients with myasthenia gravis

Adverse Reactions
Cardiovascular: Effects are minimal and transient
Dermatologic: Erythema, itching, urticaria
Respiratory: Wheezing, bronchial secretions increased

Drug Interactions
Avoid Concomitant Use
Avoid concomitant use of Atracurium with any of the following: QuiNINE
Increased Effect/Toxicity
Atracurium may increase the levels/effects of: Cardiac Glycosides; Corticosteroids (Systemic); OnabotulinumtoxinA; RimabotulinumtoxinB

The levels/effects of Atracurium may be increased by: AbobotulinumtoxinA; Aminoglycosides; Calcium Channel Blockers; Capreomycin; Colistimethate; Inhalational Anesthetics; Ketorolac; Ketorolac (Systemic); Lincosamide Antibiotics; Lithium; Loop Diuretics; Magnesium Salts; Polymyxin B; Procainamide; QuiNIDine; QuiNINE; Spironolactone; Tetracycline Derivatives; Vancomycin
Decreased Effect
The levels/effects of Atracurium may be decreased by: Acetylcholinesterase Inhibitors; Loop Diuretics
Stability Refrigerate; stable at room temperature for 14 days; unstable in alkaline solutions; compatible with D_5W, D_5NS, and NS; do not dilute in LR
Mechanism of Action Blocks neural transmission at the myoneural junction by binding with cholinergic receptor sites

Pharmacodynamics
Onset of action: I.V.: 1-4 minutes
Maximum effect: Within 3-5 minutes
Duration: Recovery begins in 20-35 minutes when anesthesia is balanced

Pharmacokinetics (Adult data unless noted)
Distribution: V_d:
Infants: 0.21 L/kg
Children: 0.13 L/kg
Adults: 0.1 L/kg
Metabolism: Some metabolites are active; undergoes rapid nonenzymatic degradation (Hofmann elimination) in the bloodstream; additional metabolism occurs via ester hydrolysis
Half-life: Elimination:
Infants: 20 minutes
Children: 17 minutes
Adults: 16 minutes
Elimination: Clearance:
Infants: 7.9 mL/kg/minute
Children: 6.8 mL/kg/minute
Adults: 5.3 mL/kg/minute

Usual Dosage I.V.:
Neonates, Infants, and Children ≤2 years:
0.3-0.4 mg/kg initially followed by maintenance doses of 0.3-0.4 mg/kg as needed to maintain neuromuscular blockade
or
Continuous infusion: 0.6-1.2 mg/kg/hour or 10-20 mcg/kg/minute
Children >2 years to Adults:
0.4-0.5 mg/kg then 0.08-0.1 mg/kg 20-45 minutes after initial dose to maintain neuromuscular block
or
Continuous infusion: 0.4-0.8 mg/kg/hour or 6.7-13 mcg/kg/minute (range: 2-15 mcg/kg/minute)
Dosage adjustment in hepatic or renal impairment: Not necessary
Dosage adjustment with enflurane or isoflurane: Reduce dosage by 33%
Dosage adjustment with induced hypothermia (cardiobypass surgery): Reduce dosage by 50%

Administration Parenteral: May be administered without further dilution by rapid I.V. injection; for continuous infusions, dilute to a maximum concentration of 0.5 mg/mL (more concentrated solutions have reduced stability, ie, <24 hours at room temperature); not for I.M. injection due to tissue irritation

Monitoring Parameters Muscle twitch response to peripheral nerve stimulation, heart rate, blood pressure

Additional Information Neuromuscular blockade may be reversed with neostigmine; atropine or glycopyrrolate should be available to treat excessive cholinergic effects from neostigmine

Dosage Forms Excipient information presented when available (limited, particularly for generics); consult specific product labeling.
Injection, as besylate: 10 mg/mL (10 mL) [contains benzyl alcohol]
Injection, as besylate [preservative free]: 10 mg/mL (5 mL)

References
Martin LD, Bratton SL, and O'Rourke PP, "Clinical Uses and Controversies of Neuromuscular Blocking Agents in Infants and Children," *Crit Care Med*, 1999, 27(7):1358-68.

◆ **Atracurium Besylate** *see* Atracurium *on page 156*

◆ **Atracurium Besylate Injection (Can)** *see* Atracurium *on page 156*

◆ **Atralin™** *see* Tretinoin (Topical) *on page 1375*

◆ **Atriance™ (Can)** *see* Nelarabine *on page 974*

◆ **Atripla®** *see* Efavirenz, Emtricitabine, and Tenofovir *on page 493*

◆ **AtroPen®** *see* Atropine *on page 157*

Atropine (A troe peen)

Medication Safety Issues
International issues:
Genatropine® [France] may be confused with Genotropin®

Related Information
Adult ACLS Algorithms *on page 1463*
Asthma *on page 1697*
Compatibility of Medications Mixed in a Syringe *on page 1713*
CPR Pediatric Drug Dosages *on page 1455*

U.S. Brand Names AtroPen®; Atropine-Care®; Isopto® Atropine; Sal-Tropine™

Canadian Brand Names Dioptic's Atropine Solution; Isopto® Atropine

Therapeutic Category Antiasthmatic; Anticholinergic Agent; Anticholinergic Agent, Ophthalmic; Antidote, Organophosphate Poisoning; Antispasmodic Agent, Gastrointestinal; Bronchodilator; Ophthalmic Agent, Mydriatic

Generic Available Yes: Excludes tablet

Use Preoperative medication to inhibit salivation and secretions; treatment of sinus bradycardia; treatment of asystole and pulseless electrical activity (adults); management of peptic ulcer; reversal of the muscarinic effects of cholinergic agents such as neostigmine and pyridostigmine; treatment of exercise-induced bronchospasm; antidote for organophosphate or carbamate pesticide poisoning; used to produce mydriasis and cycloplegia for examination of the retina and optic disk and accurate measurement of refractive errors; treatment of uveitis

Pregnancy Risk Factor C

Pregnancy Considerations Animal reproduction studies have not been conducted. Atropine has been found to cross the human placenta.

Lactation Enters breast milk (trace amounts)/use caution (AAP rates "compatible")

Breast-Feeding Considerations Anticholinergic agents may suppress lactation.

Contraindications Hypersensitivity to atropine sulfate or any component; narrow-angle glaucoma; tachycardia; thyrotoxicosis; obstructive disease of the GI tract; obstructive uropathy

Warnings The AtroPen® formulation is available for use primarily by the Department of Defense as an initial treatment of the muscarinic symptoms of insecticide or nerve agent poisoning; its use should be reserved for individuals who have had adequate training in the recognition and treatment of this type of intoxication.

Precautions Use with caution in children with spastic paralysis or brain damage; children are at increased risk for rapid rise in body temperature due to suppression of sweat gland activity; paradoxical hyperexcitability may occur in children given large doses; infants with Down's syndrome have both increased sensitivity to cardiac effects and mydriasis

Adverse Reactions
Cardiovascular: Tachycardia, palpitations, flushing, arrhythmias
Central nervous system: Fatigue, delirium, headache, restlessness, ataxia, confusion, dizziness, hyperpyrexia
Dermatologic: Dry hot skin, dry mucous membranes, rash
Gastrointestinal: Impaired GI motility, xerostomia, constipation, abdominal distension, nausea, vomiting, loss of libido
Genitourinary: Urinary retention, impotency
Local: Pain at injection site
Neuromuscular & skeletal: Tremor, hypertonia
Ocular: Blurred vision, photophobia, mydriasis, dry eyes

Respiratory: Tachypnea, shallow respirations, stridor, laryngitis, pulmonary edema, respiratory failure

Drug Interactions

Avoid Concomitant Use There are no known interactions where it is recommended to avoid concomitant use.

Increased Effect/Toxicity

Atropine may increase the levels/effects of: AbobotulinumtoxinA; Anticholinergics; Cannabinoids; OnabotulinumtoxinA; Potassium Chloride; RimabotulinumtoxinB

The levels/effects of Atropine may be increased by: Pramlintide

Decreased Effect

Atropine may decrease the levels/effects of: Acetylcholinesterase Inhibitors (Central); Secretin

The levels/effects of Atropine may be decreased by: Acetylcholinesterase Inhibitors (Central)

Stability Store at controlled room temperature; protect AtroPen® from light

Mechanism of Action Blocks the action of acetylcholine at parasympathetic sites in smooth muscle, secretory glands, and the CNS; increases cardiac output, dries secretions, antagonizes histamine and serotonin

Pharmacodynamics

Inhibition of salivation:

Onset of action:

Oral: 30-60 minutes

I.M.: 30 minutes

Maximum effect:

Oral: 2 hours

I.M.: 1-1.6 hours

Duration: Oral, I.M.: Up to 4 hours

Increased heart rate:

Onset of action:

Oral: 30 minutes to 2 hours

I.M.: 5-40 minutes

Maximum effect:

Oral: 1-2 hours

I.M.: 20 minutes to 1 hour

I.V.: 2-4 minutes

Bronchodilation: Oral Inhalation:

Onset of action: 15 minutes

Maximum effect: 15 minutes to 1.5 hours

Pharmacokinetics (Adult data unless noted)

Absorption: Well absorbed from all dosage forms

Distribution: Widely distributes throughout the body; crosses the placenta; trace amounts appear in breast milk; crosses the blood-brain barrier

Protein binding: 14% to 22%

Metabolism: In the liver

Half-life:

Children <2 years: 6.9 ± 3 hours

Children >2 years: 2.5 ± 1.2 hours

Adults: 3 ± 0.9 hours

Elimination: Both metabolites and unchanged drug (13% to 50%) are excreted into urine

Usual Dosage Note: Doses <0.1 mg have been associated with paradoxical bradycardia

Neonates, Infants and Children:

Preanesthetic: Oral, I.M., I.V., SubQ:

<5 kg: 0.02 mg/kg/dose 30-60 minutes preop then every 4-6 hours as needed; use of a minimum dosage of 0.1 mg in neonates <5 kg will result in dosages >0.02 mg/kg; there is no documented minimum dosage in this age group

>5 kg: 0.01-0.02 mg/kg/dose to a maximum 0.4 mg/dose 30-60 minutes preop; minimum dose: 0.1 mg

Bradycardia: I.V., intratracheal, I.O.: 0.02 mg/kg, minimum dose 0.1 mg, maximum single dose: 0.5 mg in children and 1 mg in adolescents; may repeat in 5 minutes; maximum total dose of 1 mg in children or 2 mg in adolescents. (**Note:** For intratracheal administration, must be diluted; see Administration.) When treating bradycardia in neonates, reserve use for those patients unresponsive to improved oxygenation and epinephrine.

Children:

Bronchospasm: Inhalation: 0.03-0.05 mg/kg/dose 3-4 times/day; maximum: 2.5 mg/dose

Refraction: Ophthalmic:

Infants <1 year: Instill 1 drop of 0.25% solution 3 times/day for 3 days before the procedure

Children: 1-5 years: Instill 1 drop of 0.5% solution 3 times/day for 3 days before the procedure

Children >5 years or Children with dark irides: Instill 1 drop of 1% solution 3 times/day for 3 days before the procedure

Organophosphate or carbamate poisoning:

I.V.: 0.02-0.05 mg/kg every 10-20 minutes until atropine effect (dry flushed skin, tachycardia, mydriasis, fever) is observed then every 1-4 hours for at least 24 hours

I.M.: AtroPen®:

Children 6 months to 4 years (15-40 lbs): 0.5 mg (blue pen)

Children 4-10 years (40-90 lbs): 1 mg (dark red pen)

Children >10 years (>90 lbs): 2 mg (green pen)

Mild symptoms: 1 injection as soon as exposure is known or suspected

Severe symptoms: 2 additional injections (3 total) given in rapid succession 10 minutes after receiving the first injection

Uveitis: Ophthalmic: Instill 1 drop of 0.5% solution 1-3 times daily

Adults (doses <0.5 mg have been associated with paradoxical bradycardia):

Asystole and slow pulseless electrical activity: I.V.: 1 mg; may repeat every 3-5 minutes as needed to a total dose of 0.04 mg/kg

Preanesthetic: Oral, I.M., I.V., SubQ: 0.4-0.6 mg 30-60 minutes preop

Bradycardia: I.V.: 0.5-1 mg every 5 minutes, not to exceed a total of 2 mg or 0.04 mg/kg

Bronchospasm: Inhalation: 0.025-0.05 mg/kg/dose every 4-6 hours as needed; maximum: 2.5 mg/dose

Organophosphate or carbamate poisoning: **Note:** The dose of atropine required varies considerably with the severity of poisoning. Total amount of atropine used in carbamate poisoning is usually less. Severely poisoned patients may exhibit significant tolerance to atropine; ≥2 times the suggested doses may be needed. Titrate to pulmonary status (decreased bronchial secretions). Once patient is stable for a period of time, the dose/dosing frequency may be decreased. If atropinization occurs after 1-2 mg of atropine then re-evaluate working diagnosis.

I.V.: Initial: 1-5 mg; doses should be doubled every 5 minutes until signs of muscarinic excess abate (clearing of bronchial secretions, bronchospasm, and adequate oxygenation). Overly aggressive dosing may cause anticholinergic toxicity (eg, delirium, hyperthermia, and muscle twitching).

I.V. Infusion: 0.5-1 mg/hour or 10% to 20% of loading dose/hour

I.M. (AtroPen®): Mild symptoms: Administer 2 mg as soon as exposure is known or suspected. If severe symptoms develop after first dose, 2 additional doses should be repeated in 10 minutes; do not administer more than 3 doses. Severe symptoms: Immediately administer three 2 mg doses.

Refraction: Ophthalmic: Instill 1-2 drops of 1% solution before the procedure

Uveitis: Ophthalmic: Instill 1-2 drops of 1% solution up to 4 times/day

Administration

Intratracheal: Administer and flush with 5 mL NS followed by 5 manual ventilations

Parenteral:

I.V.: Administer undiluted by rapid I.V. injection; slow injection may result in paradoxical bradycardia

I.M.: AtroPen®: Administer to outer thigh. May be given through clothing as long as pockets at the injection site are empty. Hold autoinjector in place for 10 seconds following injection; massage the injection site.

Oral: Administer without regard to food

Ophthalmic: Due to the discontinuance of 0.5% ophthalmic solutions commercially, 0.5% and 0.25% solutions may be prepared under sterile conditions by dilution of 1% atropine ophthalmic solution with artificial tears; 0.5%: An equal part dilution (equal volume of 1% atropine with artificial tears) and 0.25%: Dilute 2.5 mL 1% atropine with 7.5 mL artificial tears; instill solution into conjunctival sac of affected eye(s); avoid contact of bottle tip with eye or skin

Monitoring Parameters Heart rate; organophosphate or carbamate poisoning symptomatology

Patient Information May cause dry mouth

Dosage Forms Excipient information presented when available (limited, particularly for generics); consult specific product labeling.

Injection, solution, as sulfate: 0.05 mg/mL (5 mL); 0.1 mg/mL (5 mL, 10 mL); 0.4 mg/0.5 mL (0.5 mL); 0.4 mg/mL (0.5 mL, 1 mL, 20 mL); 1 mg/mL (1 mL)

AtroPen®: 0.25 mg/0.3 mL (0.3 mL); 0.5 mg/0.7 mL (0.7 mL); 1 mg/0.7 mL (0.7 mL); 2 mg/0.7 mL (0.7 mL) [prefilled autoinjector]

Ointment, ophthalmic, as sulfate: 1% (3.5 g)

Solution, ophthalmic, as sulfate: 1% (2 mL, 5 mL, 15 mL)

Atropine-Care®: 1% (2 mL) [contains benzalkonium chloride]

Isopto® Atropine: 1% (5 mL, 15 mL) [contains benzalkonium chloride]

Tablet, as sulfate:

Sal-Tropine™: 0.4 mg

References

"2005 American Heart Association (AHA) Guidelines for Cardiopulmonary Resuscitation (CPR) and Emergency Cardiovascular Care (ECC) of Pediatric and Neonatal Patients: Pediatric Advanced Life Support," *Pediatrics*, 2006, 117(5):1005-28.

◆ **Atropine and Diphenoxylate** *see* Diphenoxylate and Atropine *on page 450*

◆ **Atropine-Care®** *see* Atropine *on page 157*

◆ **Atropine, Hyoscyamine, Phenobarbital, and Scopolamine** *see* Hyoscyamine, Atropine, Scopolamine, and Phenobarbital *on page 700*

◆ **Atropine Sulfate** *see* Atropine *on page 157*

◆ **Atrovent®** *see* Ipratropium *on page 757*

◆ **Atrovent® HFA** *see* Ipratropium *on page 757*

Attapulgite (at a PULL gite)

Medication Safety Issues

Note: Attapulgite preparations have been discontinued in the U.S.; refer to Bismuth monograph for newly-reformulated Kaopectate® products.

Sound-alike/look-alike issues:

Kaopectate® may be confused with Kayexalate®

Canadian Brand Names Kaopectate® Children's [OTC]; Kaopectate® Extra Strength [OTC]; Kaopectate® [OTC]

Therapeutic Category Antidiarrheal

Use Treatment of uncomplicated diarrhea

Contraindications Hypersensitivity to attapulgite or any component

Warnings Not to be used for self-medication for diarrhea >48 hours or in the presence of high fever in infants and children <3 years of age; do not use for diarrhea associated with pseudomembranous enterocolitis or in diarrhea caused by toxigenic bacteria

Adverse Reactions

Gastrointestinal: Constipation

Respiratory: Pneumoconiosis (from inhalation of the powder chronically as it contains large amounts of silica)

Drug Interactions

Avoid Concomitant Use There are no known interactions where it is recommended to avoid concomitant use.

Increased Effect/Toxicity There are no known significant interactions involving an increase in effect.

Decreased Effect There are no known significant interactions involving a decrease in effect.

Mechanism of Action Controls diarrhea because of its absorbent action

Usual Dosage Adequate controlled clinical studies documenting the efficacy of attapulgite are lacking; its usage and dosage has been primarily empiric; the following are manufacturer's recommended dosages

Oral: Give after each bowel movement

Children:

3-6 years: 300-750 mg/dose; maximum dose: 7 doses/day or 2250 mg/day

6-12 years: 600-1500 mg/dose; maximum dose: 7 doses/day or 4500 mg/day

Children >12 years and Adults: 1200-3000 mg/dose; maximum dose: 8 doses/day or 9000 mg/day

Administration May be administered without regard to meals; shake liquid preparation well before use

Patient Information Do not exceed maximum number of doses per day; drink plenty of fluids; contact your physician if diarrhea persists more than 48 hours or if fever develops in children <3 years of age

Additional Information Kaopectate®, Kaopectate® Advanced Formula, Children's Kaopectate®, and Kaopectate® Maximum Strength have been reformulated. Previously, Kaopectate® contained attapulgite. The new formulation contains only bismuth subsalicylate. Bismuth salicylate has significant contraindications, particularly in children with influenza and chickenpox. Please refer to bismuth monograph for product information. During the transition period, the older formulation may still be available, read product label closely.

Dosage Forms Excipient information presented when available (limited, particularly for generics); consult specific product labeling. [CAN] = Canadian brand name

Suspension, oral:

Kaopectate® [CAN]: 600 mg/15 mL (250 mL, 350 mL) [vanilla flavor] [not available in the U.S.]

Kaopectate® Children's [CAN]: 600 mg/15 mL (180 mL) [cherry flavor] [not available in the U.S.]

Kaopectate® Extra Strength [CAN]: 750 mg/15 mL (250 mL, 350 mL) [peppermint flavor] [not available in the U.S.]

◆ **Attenuvax® [DSC]** *see* Measles Virus Vaccine (Live) *on page 866*

◆ **Augmentin®** *see* Amoxicillin and Clavulanic Acid *on page 98*

◆ **Augmentin ES-600®** *see* Amoxicillin and Clavulanic Acid *on page 98*

◆ **Augmentin XR®** *see* Amoxicillin and Clavulanic Acid *on page 98*

◆ **Auralgan® (Can)** *see* Antipyrine and Benzocaine
on page 118

Auranofin (au RANE oh fin)

Medication Safety Issues
Sound-alike/look-alike issues:
Ridaura® may be confused with Cardura®

U.S. Brand Names Ridaura®

Canadian Brand Names Ridaura®

Therapeutic Category Gold Compound

Generic Available No

Use Management of active stage of classic or definite rheumatoid or psoriatic arthritis in patients who do not respond to or tolerate other agents; adjunctive or alternative therapy for pemphigus

Pregnancy Risk Factor C

Lactation Enters breast milk/contraindicated

Contraindications Any history of gold-induced disorders including anaphylactoid reactions, necrotizing enterocolitis, exfoliative dermatitis, pulmonary fibrosis, bone marrow aplasia, or other severe hematologic disorders

Warnings May be associated with significant toxicity involving dermatologic, gastrointestinal, hematologic, pulmonary, renal, and hepatic systems **[U.S. Boxed Warning]**; patient education is required; signs of gold toxicity include decrease in hemoglobin, leukocytes, granulocytes, and platelets; therapy should be discontinued if platelet count falls to <100,000/mm^3, WBC <4000, granulocytes <1500/mm^3. Dermatitis and lesions of the mucous membranes are common and may be serious; pruritus may precede the early development of a skin reaction; consider alternative therapy in patient with dermatitis. Signs of GI toxicity include persistent diarrhea, stomatitis, and enterocolitis; avoid use in patients with prior inflammatory bowel disease. May be associated with the development of cholestatic jaundice. Consider alternative therapy in patients with hepatic impairment. May be associated with interstitial fibrosis; monitor closely. Renal toxicity ranges from mild proteinuria to nephrotic syndrome.

Precautions Use with caution and modify dose in patients with renal impairment

Adverse Reactions
Central nervous system: Confusion, hallucinations, seizures

Dermatologic: Dermatitis, pruritus, urticaria, alopecia, chrysiasis, rash, angioedema, photosensitivity

Gastrointestinal: Diarrhea, loose stools, stomatitis, abdominal cramping, metallic taste, glossitis, ulcerative enterocolitis, GI hemorrhage, gingivitis, dysphagia

Hematologic: Thrombocytopenia, aplastic anemia, eosinophilia, leukopenia

Hepatic: Liver enzymes elevated, cholestatic jaundice, hepatitis

Neuromuscular & skeletal: Peripheral neuropathy

Ocular: Conjunctivitis, iritis, corneal ulcers

Renal: Proteinuria, hematuria, nephrotic syndrome

Respiratory: Interstitial pneumonitis, fibrosis, gold bronchitis

Drug Interactions
Avoid Concomitant Use There are no known interactions where it is recommended to avoid concomitant use.

Increased Effect/Toxicity There are no known significant interactions involving an increase in effect.

Decreased Effect There are no known significant interactions involving a decrease in effect.

Stability Store in tight, light-resistant containers at 15°C to 30°C.

Mechanism of Action Unknown, acts principally via immunomodulating effects and by decreasing lysosomal enzyme release; may alter cellular mechanisms by inhibiting sulfhydryl systems

Pharmacodynamics Onset of action: Therapeutic response may not be seen for 3-4 months after start of therapy

Pharmacokinetics (Adult data unless noted)
Absorption: Oral: Only about 20% to 25% of gold in a dose is absorbed

Protein binding: 60%

Half-life: 21-31 days (half-life dependent upon single or multiple dosing)

Time to peak serum concentration: Within 2 hours

Elimination: 60% of absorbed gold is eliminated in urine while the remainder is eliminated in feces

Usual Dosage Oral:
Children: Initial: 0.1 mg/kg/day in 1-2 divided doses; usual maintenance: 0.15 mg/kg/day in 1-2 divided doses; maximum dose: 0.2 mg/kg/day in 1-2 divided doses

Adults: 6 mg/day in 1-2 divided doses; after 3 months may be increased to 9 mg/day in 3 divided doses; if still no response after 3 months at 9 mg/day, discontinue drug

Dosing adjustment in renal impairment:
Cl$_{cr}$ 50-80 mL/minute: Reduce dose to 50%
Cl$_{cr}$ <50 mL/minute: Avoid use

Monitoring Parameters Baseline and periodic (at least monthly): CBC with differential, platelet count, urinalysis for protein; baseline renal and liver function tests; skin and oral mucosa examinations; specific questioning for symptoms of pruritus, rash, stomatitis, or metallic taste

Reference Range Gold: Normal: 0-0.1 mcg/mL (SI: 0-0.0064 micromoles/L); Therapeutic: 1-3 mcg/mL (SI: 0.06-0.18 micromoles/L); Urine <0.1 mcg/24 hours

Test Interactions May enhance the response to a tuberculin skin test

Patient Information Notify your physician of pruritus, sore mouth, indigestion, metallic taste; observe careful oral hygiene. May cause photosensitivity reactions (eg, exposure to sunlight may cause severe sunburn, skin rash, redness, or itching); avoid exposure to sunlight and artificial light sources (sunlamps, tanning booth/bed); wear protective clothing, wide-brimmed hats, sunglasses, and lip sunscreen (SPF ≥15); use a sunscreen [broad-spectrum sunscreen or physical sunscreen (preferred) or sunblock with SPF ≥15]; contact physician if reaction occurs.

Additional Information Metallic taste may indicate stomatitis

Dosage Forms Excipient information presented when available (limited, particularly for generics); consult specific product labeling.
Capsule:
Ridaura®: 3 mg [29% gold]

◆ **Auraphene® B [OTC]** *see* Carbamide Peroxide
on page 248

◆ **Auro® [OTC]** *see* Carbamide Peroxide *on page 248*

◆ **Aurodex [DSC]** *see* Antipyrine and Benzocaine
on page 118

◆ **Avagard™ [OTC]** *see* Chlorhexidine Gluconate
on page 291

◆ **Avage™** *see* Tazarotene *on page 1314*

◆ **Avakine** *see* InFLIXimab *on page 728*

◆ **Avamys® (Can)** *see* Fluticasone *on page 607*

◆ **Avandia®** *see* Rosiglitazone *on page 1233*

◆ **Avapro®** *see* Irbesartan *on page 758*

◆ **Avastin®** *see* Bevacizumab *on page 192*

◆ **Avaxim® (Can)** *see* Hepatitis A Vaccine *on page 672*

◆ **Avaxim®-Pediatric (Can)** see Hepatitis A Vaccine on page 672

◆ **Aventyl® (Can)** see Nortriptyline on page 1002

◆ **Avinza®** see Morphine Sulfate on page 946

◆ **Avita®** see Tretinoin (Topical) on page 1375

◆ **AVP** see Vasopressin on page 1410

◆ **Axid®** see Nizatidine on page 999

◆ **Axid® AR [OTC]** see Nizatidine on page 999

◆ **Aygestin®** see Norethindrone on page 1001

◆ **Ayr® Allergy Sinus [OTC]** see Sodium Chloride on page 1270

◆ **Ayr® Baby Saline [OTC]** see Sodium Chloride on page 1270

◆ **Ayr® Saline [OTC]** see Sodium Chloride on page 1270

◆ **Ayr® Saline No-Drip [OTC]** see Sodium Chloride on page 1270

◆ **Azactam®** see Aztreonam on page 167

◆ **Azasan®** see AzaTHIOprine on page 161

◆ **AzaSite®** see Azithromycin on page 164

AzaTHIOprine (ay za THYE oh preen)

Medication Safety Issues
Sound-alike/look-alike issues:
AzaTHIOprine may be confused with azaCITIDine, azatadine, azidothymidine, azithromycin, Azulfidine®
Imuran® may be confused with Elmiron®, Enduron®, Imdur®, Inderal®, Tenormin®

Azathioprine is metabolized to mercaptopurine; concurrent use of these commercially-available products has resulted in profound myelosuppression.

U.S. Brand Names Azasan®; Imuran®

Canadian Brand Names Apo-Azathioprine®; Imuran®; Mylan-Azathioprine; Teva-Azathioprine

Therapeutic Category Immunosuppressant Agent

Generic Available Yes

Use Adjunct with other agents in prevention of solid organ transplant rejection; used as an immunosuppressant in a variety of autoimmune diseases such as SLE, severe rheumatoid arthritis unresponsive to other agents, and nephrotic syndrome; steroid-sparing agent for corticosteroid-dependent Crohn's disease and ulcerative colitis

Pregnancy Risk Factor D

Pregnancy Considerations Azathioprine was found to be teratogenic in animal studies; temporary depression in spermatogenesis and reduction in sperm viability and sperm count were also reported in mice. Azathioprine crosses the placenta in humans; congenital anomalies, immunosuppression, hematologic toxicities (lymphopenia, pancytopenia), and intrauterine growth retardation have been reported. There are no adequate and well-controlled studies in pregnant women. Azathioprine should not be used to treat arthritis during pregnancy. The potential benefit to the mother versus possible risk to the fetus should be considered when treating other disease states.

The National Transplantation Pregnancy Registry (NTPR, Temple University) is a registry for pregnant women taking immunosuppressants following any solid organ transplant. The NTPR encourages reporting of all immunosuppressant exposures during pregnancy in transplant recipients at 877-955-6877.

Lactation Enters breast milk/not recommended

Breast-Feeding Considerations Due to risk of immunosuppression and serious adverse effects in the nursing infant, breast-feeding is not recommended.

Contraindications Hypersensitivity to azathioprine or any component; pregnancy (patients with rheumatoid arthritis); patients with rheumatoid arthritis previously treated with alkylating agents (eg, cyclophosphamide, chlorambucil, melphalan) may have a prohibitive risk of neoplasia with azathioprine treatment

Warnings Chronic immunosuppression increases the risk of neoplasia **[U.S. Boxed Warning]**, particularly lymphoma and skin cancers; mutagenic potential in both men and women; may cause severe leukopenia, thrombocytopenia, anemia, pancytopenia. and bone marrow suppression. hematologic toxicities are dose-related; prompt dosage reduction or temporary discontinuation of azathioprine may be needed if there is a rapid decrease or persistently low leukocyte counts. Patients with genetic deficiency of thiopurine methyltransferase (TPMT) may be sensitive to myelosuppressive effects. Patients with intermediate TPMT activity may be at risk for increased myelosuppression; those with low or absent TPMT activity are at risk for developing severe and life-threatening hematologic toxicity. TPMT genotyping or phenotyping may assist in identifying patients at risk for developing toxicity.

Precautions Use with caution in patients with liver disease, renal impairment, and those with cadaveric kidneys; modify dosage in patients with renal impairment; reduce dosage to 25% to 33% of usual dosage in patients receiving allopurinol and azathioprine concurrently; discontinue azathioprine therapy in patients with hepatic veno-occlusive disease. Hepatotoxicity (transaminase, bilirubin, and alkaline phosphatase elevations) may occur, usually in renal transplant patients and generally within 6 months of transplant; normally reversible with discontinuation; monitor liver function periodically. Should be prescribed by physicians familiar with the risks, including hematologic toxicities and mutagenic potential **[U.S. Boxed Warning]**. Hazardous agent: Use appropriate precautions for handling and disposal.

Adverse Reactions
Central nervous system: Fever, chills, malaise

Dermatologic: Alopecia, erythematous or maculopapular rash

Endocrine & metabolic: Negative nitrogen balance

Gastrointestinal: Nausea, vomiting, anorexia, diarrhea, aphthous stomatitis, pancreatitis, abdominal pain, steatorrhea

Hematologic: Bone marrow depression (leukopenia, thrombocytopenia, anemia), bleeding, pancytopenia

Hepatic: Hepatotoxicity, jaundice, hepatic veno-occlusive disease; serum alkaline phosphatase, bilirubin, and/or serum transaminases elevated

Neuromuscular & skeletal: Arthralgias, myalgias

Ocular: Retinopathy

Respiratory: Interstitial pneumonitis

Miscellaneous: Infection, neoplasia (including lymphoma, hepatosplenic T-cell lymphoma), lymphoproliferative disease, rare hypersensitivity reactions which include myalgias, rigors, dyspnea, hypotension, serum sickness, rash

Drug Interactions
Avoid Concomitant Use
Avoid concomitant use of AzaTHIOprine with any of the following: BCG; Febuxostat; Natalizumab; Pimecrolimus; Tacrolimus (Topical); Vaccines (Live)

Increased Effect/Toxicity
AzaTHIOprine may increase the levels/effects of: Leflunomide; Mercaptopurine; Natalizumab; Vaccines (Live)

The levels/effects of AzaTHIOprine may be increased by: 5-ASA Derivatives; ACE Inhibitors; Allopurinol; Denosumab; Febuxostat; Pimecrolimus; Ribavirin; Sulfamethoxazole; Tacrolimus (Topical); Trastuzumab; Trimethoprim

Decreased Effect

AzaTHIOprine may decrease the levels/effects of: BCG; Sipuleucel-T; Vaccines (Inactivated); Vaccines (Live); Vitamin K Antagonists

The levels/effects of AzaTHIOprine may be decreased by: Echinacea

Stability

Tablet: Store at room temperature of 15°C to 25°C (59°F to 77°F); protect from light.

Powder for injection: Store intact vials at room temperature of 15°C to 25°C (59°F to 77°F); protect from light. Reconstitute each vial with 10 mL SWI; may further dilute for infusion (in D_5W or NS); use within 24 hours of reconstitution. Use appropriate precautions for handling and disposal.

Mechanism of Action Antagonizes purine metabolism and may inhibit synthesis of DNA, RNA, and proteins; may also interfere with cellular metabolism and inhibit mitosis. Cytotoxicity of azathioprine is partially due to incorporation of 6-thioguanine nucleotides into DNA.

Pharmacokinetics (Adult data unless noted)

Absorption: Oral: Well absorbed

Distribution: Crosses the placenta; appears in breast milk

Protein binding: ~30%

Metabolism: Hepatic, to 6-mercaptopurine (6-MP). 6-MP undergoes metabolism via 3 major pathways: Activation via hypoxanthine-guanine phosphoribosyltransferase (HGPRT) to 6-thioguanine nucleotides, oxidation by xanthine oxidase to 6-thiouric acid, and thiol methylation by the enzyme thiopurine 5-methyltransferase (TPMT) which forms 6-methyl mercaptopurine

Half-life:

Parent: 12 minutes

6-mercaptopurine: 0.7-3 hours; with anuria: 50 hours

Elimination: Small amount eliminated as unchanged drug; metabolites eliminated eventually in the urine

Dialysis: Slightly dialyzable (5% to 20%)

Usual Dosage Note: Patients with intermediated TPMT activity may be at risk for increased myelosuppression; those with low or absent TPMT activity are at risk for developing severe myelotoxicity. Dosage reductions are recommended for patients with reduced TPMT activity. **Note:** I.V. dose is equivalent to oral dose (dosing should be transitioned from I.V. to oral as soon as tolerated).

Children and Adults:

Inflammatory bowel disease: Oral: 3 mg/kg/dose once daily has been used in children with Crohn's disease

Transplantation: Oral, I.V.: Initial: 3-5 mg/kg/dose once daily, beginning at the time of transplant; maintenance: 1-3 mg/kg/dose once daily

Lupus nephritis: Oral: 2-3 mg/kg/dose once daily

Rheumatoid arthritis: Oral: 1 mg/kg/dose once daily or divided twice daily for 6-8 weeks; increase by 0.5 mg/kg daily every 4 weeks until response or up to 2.5 mg/kg/day. A minimum of 12 weeks is needed for an adequate therapeutic response trial.

Adults: Reduction of steroid use in Crohn's disease or ulcerative colitis: Oral: Initial: 50 mg daily; may increase by 25 mg/day every 1-2 weeks as tolerated to target dose of 2-3 mg/kg/day

Dosage adjustment for concomitant use with allopurinol: Reduce azathioprine dose to 25% to 33% of the usual dose when used concurrently with allopurinol. Patients with low or absent TPMT activity may require further dose reductions or discontinuation.

Dosage adjustment for toxicity:

Rapid WBC count decrease, persistently low WBC count, or serious infection: Reduce dose or temporarily withhold treatment

Severe toxicity in renal transplantion: May require discontinuation

Hepatic veno-occlusive disease: Permanently discontinue

Dosing interval in renal impairment:

Cl_{cr} 10-50 mL/minute: Administer 75% of dose once daily

Cl_{cr} <10 mL/minute: Administer 50% of dose once daily

Hemodialysis (dialyzable; ~45% removed in 8 hours): Administer 50% of normal dose

CAPD: Administer 50% of normal dose

CRRT: Children: Administer 75% of normal dose

Administration

Oral: Administer with food or in divided doses to decrease GI upset

Parenteral: Administer IVP over 5 minutes at a concentration not to exceed 10 mg/mL; or may be further diluted with NS or D_5W and administered by intermittent infusion over 15-60 minutes

Monitoring Parameters CBC, platelet counts, creatinine, total bilirubin, alkaline phosphatase, liver function tests, TPMT genotyping or phenotyping

Test Interactions TPMT phenotyping results will not be accurate following recent blood transfusions.

Patient Information Response in rheumatoid arthritis may not occur for up to 2-3 months; inform physician of persistent sore throat, signs of infection, unusual bleeding or bruising, or fatigue. Women of childbearing age should avoid becoming pregnant while taking azathioprine.

Nursing Implications Handle and dispose according to guidelines issued for hazardous drugs.

Additional Information

Injection, powder for reconstitution, as sodium: 100 mg

Dosage Forms Excipient information presented when available (limited, particularly for generics); consult specific product labeling.

Injection, powder for reconstitution: 100 mg

Tablet [scored]: 50 mg

Azasan®: 75 mg, 100 mg

Imuran®: 50 mg

Extemporaneous Preparations A 50 mg/mL suspension compounded from one-hundred twenty 50 mg tablets comminuted to a fine powder in a mortar with 40 mL of a 1:1 mixture of Ora-Sweet® and Ora-Plus® added and mixed to a fine paste, and then adding the 1:1 mixture of Ora-Sweet® and Ora-Plus® to a total volume of 120 mL, was stable for 60 days at 5°C and 25°C when protected from light. Label "shake well before using" and "protect from light."

Allen LV Jr and Erickson MA, "Stability of Acetazolamide, Allopurinol, Azathioprine, Clonazepam, and Flucytosine in Extemporaneously Compounded Oral Liquids," *Am J Health Syst Pharm,* 1996, 53 (16):1944-9.

References

American College of Rheumatology Ad Hoc Committee on Clinical Guidelines, "Guidelines for Monitoring Drug Therapy in Rheumatoid Arthritis," *Arthritis Rheum,* 1996, 39(5):723-31.

Aronoff GR, Bennett WM, Berns JS, et al, *Drug Prescribing in Renal Failure: Dosing Guidelines for Adults and Children,* 5th ed. Philadelphia, PA: American College of Physicians, 2007, p. 97, 177.

Baum D, Bernstein D, Starnes VA, et al, "Pediatric Heart Transplantation at Stanford: Results of a 15-Year Experience," *Pediatrics,* 1991, 88(2):203-14.

Fuentes D, Torrente F, Keady S, et al, "High-Dose Azathioprine in Children With Inflammatory Bowel Disease," *Aliment Pharmacol Ther,* 2003, 17(7):913-21.

Johnson CA and Porter WA, "Compatibility of Azathioprine Sodium With Intravenous Fluids," *Am J Hosp Pharm,* 1981, 38(6):871-5.

Leichter HE, Sheth KJ, Gerlach MJ, et al, "Outcome of Renal Transplantation in Children Aged 1-5 and 6-18 Years," *Child Nephrol Urol,* 1992, 12(1):1-5.

◆ **Azathioprine Sodium** *see* AzaTHIOprine *on page 161*

Azelaic Acid (a zeh LAY ik AS id)

U.S. Brand Names Azelex®; Finacea®; Finacea® Plus™

Canadian Brand Names Finacea®

Therapeutic Category Acne Products

Generic Available No

Use Topical treatment of mild to moderate acne vulgaris; treatment of inflammatory papules and pustules of mild to moderate rosacea

Pregnancy Risk Factor B

Lactation Enters breast milk/use caution

Breast-Feeding Considerations Since <4% of a topically applied dose is systemically absorbed, the uptake of azelaic acid into breast milk is not expected to cause a significant change from baseline azelaic acid levels in the milk. However, exercise caution when administering to a nursing mother.

Contraindications Hypersensitivity to azelaic acid, propylene glycol, or any component

Warnings Cream and gel contain benzoic acid; benzoic acid (benzoate) is a metabolite of benzyl alcohol; large amounts of benzyl alcohol (≥99 mg/kg/day) have been associated with a potentially fatal toxicity ("gasping syndrome") in neonates; do not use in neonates; *in vitro* and animal studies have shown that benzoate displaces bilirubin from protein binding sites

Precautions Due to isolated reports of hypopigmentation, use cautiously in patients with dark complexions; for topical use only; avoid contact with eyes, mouth, mucous membranes, or open wounds

Adverse Reactions

Dermatologic: Pruritus, erythema, dry skin, rash, peeling, dermatitis, hypopigmentation (vitiligo depigmentation and small depigmented spots), hypertrichosis

Local: Burning, tingling

Respiratory: Worsening of asthma

Miscellaneous: Exacerbation of recurrent herpes labialis

Drug Interactions

Avoid Concomitant Use There are no known interactions where it is recommended to avoid concomitant use.

Increased Effect/Toxicity There are no known significant interactions involving an increase in effect.

Decreased Effect There are no known significant interactions involving a decrease in effect.

Stability Store at controlled room temperature.

Mechanism of Action Azelaic acid is a dietary constituent of whole grain cereals and animal products; its exact mechanism of action has not been determined; azelaic acid possesses antimicrobial activity against *Propionibacterium acnes* and *Staphylococcus epidermidis*; normalization of keratinization leading to an anticomedonal effect may also contribute to its clinical activity

Pharmacodynamics

Onset of action: Within 4 weeks

Maximum effect: 1-4 months

Pharmacokinetics (Adult data unless noted)

Absorption: ~3% to 5% penetrates stratum corneum; up to 10% found in epidermis and dermis; 4% systemic absorption

Half-life: Adults: 12 hours

Excretion: Primarily unchanged in the urine

Usual Dosage Topical:

Acne vulgaris: Children >12 years and Adults: Apply 20% azelaic acid twice daily in the morning and evening; may reduce to once daily if persistent skin irritation occurs

Rosacea: Adults: Apply 15% azelaic acid gel to affected areas of the face twice daily in the morning and evening

Administration Topical: After skin is thoroughly washed with a mild soap or a soapless cleansing lotion and patted dry, apply a thin film and massage into the affected area. Wash hands following application.

Monitoring Parameters Reduction in lesion size and/or inflammation; reduction in the number of lesions

Patient Information For external use only; avoid contact with eyes, mouth, mucous membranes, or open wounds. Avoid use of alcoholic skin cleansers, tinctures, and astringents, abrasives and peeling agents. Do not apply occlusive dressings; temporary skin irritation may occur when applied to broken or inflamed skin, usually at the start of treatment; report abnormal changes in skin color or persistent skin irritation to the healthcare provider. Gel: Avoid spicy foods, thermally hot foods and drinks, and alcoholic beverages that might cause erythema, flushing, or blushing.

Dosage Forms Excipient information presented when available (limited, particularly for generics); consult specific product labeling.

Cream:

Azelex®: 20% (30 g, 50 g) [contains benzoic acid]

Gel:

Finacea®: 15% (50 g) [contains benzoic acid]

Finacea® Plus™: 15% (50 g) [contains benzoic acid]

Azelastine (a ZEL as teen)

Medication Safety Issues

Sound-alike/look-alike issues:

Astelin® may be confused with Astepro®, Avastin®

Optivar® may be confused with Optiray®, Optive™

International issues:

Optivar® may be confused with Opthavir® which is a brand name for acyclovir in Mexico

U.S. Brand Names Astelin®; Astepro®; Optivar®

Canadian Brand Names Astelin®

Therapeutic Category Antiallergic, Ophthalmic; Antihistamine, Nasal

Generic Available Yes: Ophthalmic solution

Use

Nasal: Treatment of the symptoms of seasonal allergic rhinitis (SAR) and vasomotor rhinitis

Ophthalmic: Treatment of itching of the eye associated with allergic conjunctivitis

Pregnancy Risk Factor C

Pregnancy Considerations Animal reproduction studies have shown toxic effects to the fetus at maternally toxic doses.

Lactation Excretion in breast milk unknown/use caution

Contraindications Hypersensitivity to azelastine or any component

Warnings Ophthalmic solution not for use in contact lens-related irritation; preservative in ophthalmic solution may be absorbed by soft contact lenses; wait at least 10 minutes after instillation before inserting soft contact lenses

Precautions Use with caution in asthmatics; patients with hepatic or renal dysfunction may require lower doses

Adverse Reactions

Cardiovascular: Flushing, hypertension, tachycardia

Central nervous system: Drowsiness, headache, somnolence, fatigue, vertigo, depression, nervousness, hypoesthesia

Dermatologic: Contact dermatitis, eczema, hair and follicle infection, furunculosis

Endocrine & metabolic: Weight gain

Gastrointestinal: Nausea, xerostomia, bitter taste, glossitis, ulcerative stomatitis, aphthous stomatitis, constipation, abdominal pain

Genitourinary: Urinary frequency, hematuria

Neuromuscular & skeletal: Myalgia, hyperkinesia

Ocular: Conjunctivitis, watery eyes, eye pain, transient eye burning/stinging (ophthalmic use)

Respiratory: Nasal burning, paroxysmal sneezing, rhinitis, epistaxis, bronchospasm, coughing, throat burning, laryngitis (nasal use)

◀ **Drug Interactions**

Metabolism/Transport Effects Substrate (minor) of CYP1A2, 2C19, 2D6, 3A4; **Inhibits** CYP2B6 (weak), 2C9 (weak), 2C19 (weak), 2D6 (weak), 3A4 (weak)

Avoid Concomitant Use There are no known interactions where it is recommended to avoid concomitant use.

Increased Effect/Toxicity

Azelastine may increase the levels/effects of: Alcohol (Ethyl); Anticholinergics; CNS Depressants

The levels/effects of Azelastine may be increased by: Pramlintide

Decreased Effect

Azelastine may decrease the levels/effects of: Acetylcholinesterase Inhibitors (Central); Betahistine

The levels/effects of Azelastine may be decreased by: Acetylcholinesterase Inhibitors (Central); Amphetamines; Peginterferon Alfa-2b

Stability Stable 3 months after opening

Mechanism of Action Competes with histamine for H_1-receptor sites on effector cells in the blood vessels and respiratory tract; reduces hyper-reactivity of the airways; increases the motility of bronchial epithelial cilia, improving mucociliary transport

Pharmacodynamics

Onset of action: 30 minutes to 1 hour

Maximum effect: 3 hours

Duration: 12 hours

Pharmacokinetics (Adult data unless noted)

Protein binding: 88%

Metabolism: Metabolized by cytochrome P450 enzyme system; active metabolite desmethylazelastine

Bioavailability: After intranasal administration: 40%

Half-life, elimination: Intranasal: Azelastine: 22 hours; desmethylazelastine: 52 hours

Time to peak serum concentration: 2-3 hours

Elimination: Clearance: 0.5 L/hour/kg

Usual Dosage

Intranasal:

Seasonal allergic rhinitis:

Children 5-11 years: (Astelin®): 1 spray in each nostril twice daily

Children ≥12 years and Adults: (Astelin®, Astepro™): 1-2 sprays in each nostril twice daily

Vasomotor rhinitis: Children ≥12 years and Adults: (Astelin®): 2 sprays in each nostril twice daily

Ophthalmic: Children ≥3 years and Adults: Instill 1 drop into each affected eye twice daily

Administration

Intranasal: Before use, the child-resistant screw cap on the bottle should be replaced with the pump unit and the delivery system should be primed with 4 sprays (Astelin®), 6 sprays (Astepro™) or until a fine mist appears; when 3 or more days have elapsed since the last use, the pump should be reprimed with 2 sprays or until a fine mist appears. Avoid spraying in eyes or mouth.

Ophthalmic: Apply finger pressure to lacrimal sac during and for 1-2 minutes after instillation to decrease risk of systemic effects; avoid contact of bottle tip with skin or eye

Patient Information May cause drowsiness and impair ability to perform activities requiring mental alertness or physical coordination; may cause dry mouth

Dosage Forms Excipient information presented when available (limited, particularly for generics); consult specific product labeling.

Solution, intranasal, as hydrochloride [spray]:

Astelin®: 0.1% [137 mcg/spray] (30 mL) [contains benzalkonium chloride; 200 metered sprays]

Astepro®: 0.1% [137 mcg/spray] (30 mL) [contains benzalkonium chloride; 200 metered sprays]

Astepro®: 0.15% [205.5 mcg/spray] (30 mL) [contains benzalkonium chloride; 200 metered sprays]

Solution, ophthalmic, as hydrochloride: 0.05% (6 mL)

Optivar®: 0.05% (6 mL) [contains benzalkonium chloride]

References

McNeely W and Wiseman LR, "Intranasal Azelastine. A Review of Its Efficacy in the Management of Allergic Rhinitis," *Drugs,* 1988, 56 (1):91-114.

◆ **Azelastine Hydrochloride** *see* Azelastine *on page 163*

◆ **Azelex®** *see* Azelaic Acid *on page 162*

◆ **Azidothymidine** *see* Zidovudine *on page 1442*

◆ **Azidothymidine, Abacavir, and Lamivudine** *see* Abacavir, Lamivudine, and Zidovudine *on page 31*

Azithromycin (az ith roe MYE sin)

Medication Safety Issues

Sound-alike/look-alike issues:

Azithromycin may be confused with azathioprine, erythromycin

Zithromax® may be confused with Fosamax®, Zinacef®, Zovirax®

Related Information

Endocarditis Prophylaxis *on page 1610*

U.S. Brand Names AzaSite®; Zithromax®; Zmax®

Canadian Brand Names Apo-Azithromycin®; CO Azithromycin; Dom-Azithromycin; Mylan-Azithromycin; Novo-Azithromycin; PHL-Azithromycin; PMS-Azithromycin; PRO-Azithromycin; ratio-Azithromycin; Riva-Azithromycin; Sandoz-Azithromycin; Zithromax®

Therapeutic Category Antibiotic, Macrolide; Antibiotic, Ophthalmic

Generic Available Yes: Injection, powder for oral suspension (excludes extended release microspheres), tablet

Use Treatment of mild-to-moderate upper and lower respiratory tract infections, community-acquired pneumonia, bacterial sinusitis, infections of the skin and skin structure, acute otitis media, acute pelvic inflammatory disease, chancroid, and urethritis and cervicitis due to susceptible strains of *C. trachomatis, N. gonorrhoeae, M. catarrhalis, H. influenzae, S. aureus, S. pyogenes, S. pneumoniae, Mycoplasma pneumoniae, M. avium* complex, *C. psittaci,* and *C. pneumoniae;* treatment of babesiosis; pertussis; endocarditis prophylaxis in penicillin allergic patients; treatment of CF lung disease

Used ophthalmically for treatment of bacterial conjunctivitis due to susceptible CDC coryneform group G, *H. influenzae, S. aureus, S. mitis* group, or *S. pneumoniae*

Pregnancy Risk Factor B

Pregnancy Considerations Adverse events were not observed in animal studies; therefore, azithromycin is classified as pregnancy category B. Azithromycin crosses the placenta. Fetal malformations have not been observed following maternal use of azithromycin. The maternal serum half-life of azithromycin is unchanged in early pregnancy and decreased at term; however, high concentrations of azithromycin are sustained in the myometrium and adipose tissue. Azithromycin is recommended for the treatment of several infections, including chlamydia and *Mycobacterium avium* complex (MAC) in pregnant patients.

Lactation Enters breast milk/use caution

Breast-Feeding Considerations Azithromycin is excreted in low amounts into breast milk. The manufacturer recommends that caution be exercised when administering azithromycin to breast-feeding women. Nondose-related effects could include modification of bowel flora.

Contraindications Hypersensitivity to azithromycin or any component, erythromycin, other macrolide or ketolide antibiotics; concurrent use of pimozide due to potential cardiotoxicity (see Drug Interactions)

Warnings Oral azithromycin should not be used to treat pneumonia that is considered inappropriate for outpatient oral therapy; may mask or delay symptoms of incubating gonorrhea or syphilis so appropriate culture and susceptibility tests should be performed prior to initiating azithromycin; pseudomembranous colitis has been reported with use of macrolide antibiotics. Serious allergic reactions including anaphylaxis, angioedema, Stevens-Johnson syndrome, and toxic epidermal necrolysis have been reported; patients who experience allergic reactions to azithromycin may require prolonged periods of observation and symptomatic treatment possibly due to the drug's long tissue half-life

Hepatic impairment with or without jaundice have been reported in older children and adults; it may be accompanied by malaise, nausea, vomiting, abdominal colic, and fever; discontinue use if this occurs

Precautions Use with caution in patients with impaired hepatic function and patients with severe renal impairment (GFR <10 mL/minute). Use with caution in patients at risk of prolonged cardiac repolarization and in patients with myasthenia gravis.

Adverse Reactions
Cardiovascular: Palpitations, chest pain, ventricular arrhythmias, hypotension, QT_c prolongation
Central nervous system: Headache, dizziness, agitation, nervousness, insomnia, fever, fatigue, seizures, malaise, vertigo, anxiety
Dermatologic: Rash, pruritus, angioedema, photosensitivity, Stevens-Johnson syndrome, toxic epidermal necrolysis, urticaria
Gastrointestinal: Diarrhea (6%), nausea (2%), abdominal pain (2.5%), vomiting, constipation, anorexia, pseudomembranous colitis, pancreatitis, oral candidiasis, hypertrophic pyloric stenosis
Genitourinary: Vaginitis
Hematologic: Anemia, leukopenia, thrombocytopenia
Hepatic: Hepatic enzymes elevated, cholestatic jaundice
Local: Pain at injection site, inflammation
Neuromuscular & skeletal: Arthralgia
Ocular: Ophthalmic solution: Eye irritation (stinging, burning), corneal erosion, ocular discharge, ocular dryness, punctate keratitis
Otic: Ototoxicity, tinnitus, hearing loss
Renal: Nephritis, acute renal failure
Miscellaneous: Anaphylaxis

Drug Interactions
Metabolism/Transport Effects Substrate of CYP3A4 (minor); **Inhibits** CYP3A4 (weak)

Avoid Concomitant Use
Avoid concomitant use of Azithromycin with any of the following: Artemether; BCG; Dronedarone; Lumefantrine; Nilotinib; Pimozide; QuiNINE; Tetrabenazine; Thioridazine; Ziprasidone

Increased Effect/Toxicity
Azithromycin may increase the levels/effects of: Amiodarone; Cardiac Glycosides; CycloSPORINE; CycloSPORINE (Systemic); Dronedarone; Pimozide; QTc-Prolonging Agents; QuiNINE; Tacrolimus; Tacrolimus (Systemic); Tacrolimus (Topical); Tetrabenazine; Thioridazine; Vitamin K Antagonists; Ziprasidone

The levels/effects of Azithromycin may be increased by: Alfuzosin; Artemether; Chloroquine; Ciprofloxacin; Ciprofloxacin (Systemic); Gadobutrol; Lumefantrine; Nelfinavir; Nilotinib; QuiNINE

Decreased Effect
Azithromycin may decrease the levels/effects of: BCG; Typhoid Vaccine

Food Interactions Presence of food does not affect bioavailability of the tablet formulation, immediate release oral suspension, or the 1 g suspension regimen. Azithromycin extended release suspension has increased absorption (23%) when given with a high fat meal.

Stability Store intact vials of injection, dry powder for oral suspension, and tablets at room temperature.
Ophthalmic solution: Store unopened bottle in refrigerator at 2°C to 8°C (36°F to 46°F). Once bottle is opened, store in refrigerator for ≤14 days; discard any remaining solution after 14 days.
Oral suspension:
Immediate release: After reconstitution, multiple dose oral suspension may be stored for 10 days at room temperature or in the refrigerator.
Extended release microspheres: After reconstitution, store at room temperature; do not refrigerate or freeze; must be consumed within 12 hours following reconstitution. Any suspension remaining after dosing must be discarded.
Injection: After reconstituting 500 mg vial at a concentration of 100 mg/mL, solution is stable for 24 hours at room temperature. If solution is further diluted with a compatible diluent to a 1-2 mg/mL concentration, this solution is stable for 24 hours at room temperature or 7 days if refrigerated.

Mechanism of Action Inhibits bacterial RNA-dependent protein synthesis by binding to the 50S ribosomal subunit which results in the blockage of transpeptidation

Pharmacokinetics (Adult data unless noted)
Absorption: Oral: Rapid from the GI tract
Distribution: Extensive tissue distribution into skin, lungs, tonsils, bone, prostate, cervix; CSF concentrations are low; crosses the placenta; excreted in breast milk
V_d: Adults: 31.1 L/kg
Protein binding: 7% to 51% (concentration-dependent and dependent on alpha$_1$-acid glycoprotein levels)
Metabolism: In the liver to inactive metabolites
Bioavailability: Tablet, immediate release oral suspension: 34% to 52%; extended release oral suspension: 28% to 43%
Half-life, terminal:
Children 4 months to 15 years: 54.5 hours
Adults: 68 hours
Time to peak serum concentration: Oral:
Immediate release: 2-3 hours
Extended release oral suspension: 3-5 hours
Elimination: 50% of dose is excreted unchanged in bile; 6% of dose is excreted unchanged in urine

Usual Dosage Note: Extended release suspension (Zmax®) is not interchangeable with immediate-release formulations. All doses are expressed as immediate release azithromycin unless otherwise specified.
Oral: Immediate release:
Infants <6 months: Pertussis: 10 mg/kg/dose once daily for 5 days
Children ≥6 months:
Respiratory tract infections: 10 mg/kg on day 1 (maximum dose: 500 mg) followed by 5 mg/kg/day (maximum dose: 250 mg) once daily on days 2-5
Community-acquired pneumonia: 10 mg/kg (maximum dose: 500 mg) once daily for 3 days or 10 mg/kg (maximum dose: 500 mg) as a single dose on the first day followed by 5 mg/kg/day (maximum dose: 250 mg) on days 2 through 5

Alternative regimen for community-acquired pneumonia: Extended release suspension: 60 mg/kg as a single dose (maximum dose: 2 g)

Otitis media:

Single dose regimen: 30 mg/kg as a single dose (maximum dose: 1500 mg)

Three-day regimen: 10 mg/kg (maximum dose: 500 mg/day) once daily for 3 days

Five-day regimen: 10 mg/kg on day 1 (maximum dose: 500 mg), followed by 5 mg/kg (maximum dose: 250 mg/day) once daily on days 2-5

Pertussis: 10 mg/kg on day 1 (maximum dose: 500 mg), followed by 5 mg/kg/day (maximum dose: 250 mg) once daily on days 2-5

Acute bacterial sinusitis: 10 mg/kg (maximum dose: 500 mg/day) once daily for 3 days

Children ≥2 years: Pharyngitis, tonsillitis: 12 mg/kg/day (maximum dose: 500 mg/day) once daily for 5 days

Children:

Chancroid: Single 20 mg/kg dose (maximum dose: 1 g)

Uncomplicated chlamydial urethritis or cervicitis:

Children <8 years and <45 kg: 20 mg/kg as a single dose (maximum dose: 1 g)

Children ≥8 years and ≥45 kg: Single 1 g dose

Primary prevention of disseminated MAC: 5 mg/kg once daily (maximum dose: 250 mg/day) or 20 mg/kg (maximum dose: 1200 mg) once weekly given alone or in combination with rifabutin

Treatment and secondary prevention of disseminated MAC: 5 mg/kg/day (maximum dose: 250 mg/day) once daily in combination with ethambutol, with or without rifabutin

Babesiosis: 12 mg/kg/day (maximum dose: 600 mg) once daily for 7-10 days with oral atovaquone 40 mg/kg/day divided twice daily

Endocarditis prophylaxis: 15 mg/kg/dose (maximum dose: 500 mg) 30-60 minutes before procedure

Children ≥6 years, weight ≥25 kg and Adolescents: CF patients with chronic *Pseudomonas aeruginosa* infection:

≥25 kg to <40 kg: 250 mg on Mondays, Wednesdays, Fridays (MWF). If intolerable side effects occur, decrease dose to twice a week, or if necessary, once weekly.

≥40 kg: 500 mg on Mondays, Wednesdays, Fridays (MWF). If intolerable side effects occur, decrease dose to twice a week, or if necessary, once weekly.

Adolescents ≥16 years and Adults:

Bacterial sinusitis: 500 mg once daily for 3 days

Alternative regimen for bacterial sinusitis: Extended release suspension: Single 2 g dose

Community-acquired pneumonia, pharyngitis/tonsillitis, bacterial exacerbation of COPD, skin and soft tissue infections: 500 mg on day 1 followed by 250 mg/day once daily on days 2-5

Alternative regimen for bacterial exacerbation of COPD: 500 mg once daily for 3 days

Alternative regimen for community-acquired pneumonia: Extended release suspension: Single 2 g dose

Chancroid or nongonococcal urethritis and cervicitis due to *C. trachomatis*: Single 1 g dose

Urethritis and cervicitis due to *N. gonorrhoeae*: Single 2 g dose

Endocarditis prophylaxis: 500 mg dose 30-60 minutes before procedure

Prevention of disseminated MAC: 1200 mg once weekly alone or in combination with rifabutin

Treatment and secondary prevention of disseminated MAC: 500 mg once daily in combination with ethambutol, with or without rifabutin

Pertussis: 500 mg on day 1 followed by 250 mg once daily on days 2-5

I.V.:

Children: Not currently FDA approved; limited published data in children. A pharmacokinetic study of children 6 months to 16 years used 10 mg/kg (maximum dose: 500 mg); however, this was a single-dose pharmacokinetic study meant to guide dosing for larger trials.

Adolescents ≥16 years and Adults: 500 mg once daily for 2 days followed by a switch to **oral** azithromycin therapy (500 mg once daily to complete a 7- to 10-day course of therapy).

Ophthalmic: Children ≥1 year and Adults: Instill 1 drop in the affected eye(s) twice daily (8-12 hours apart) for 2 days, then 1 drop once daily for 5 days.

Administration

Oral: Shake suspension well before use; immediate-release oral suspension, tablet, or the 1 g suspension regimen formulation may be administered with or without food; do not administer with antacids that contain aluminum or magnesium; azithromycin 1 g oral suspension for a single dose regimen should be prepared by mixing contents of 1 packet with approximately 60 mL of water. Have the patient drink the entire contents immediately; add an additional 60 mL of water, mix, and drink.

Extended release oral suspension: Prepare 2 g azithromycin suspension by reconstituting with 60 mL of water (final concentration: 27 mg/mL). Shake suspension well before use; administer on an empty stomach 1 hour before or 2 hours after a meal. May be administered without regard to antacids containing aluminum or magnesium.

Parenteral: **Do not give I.M. or by direct I.V. injection.** Administer I.V. infusion at a final concentration of 1 mg/mL over 3 hours; for a 2 mg/mL concentration, infuse over 1 hour; do not infuse over a period of less than 60 minutes

Ophthalmic: For topical ophthalmic use only. Avoid contacting tip with skin or eye. Invert closed bottle and shake once before each use. Remove cap with bottle still in the inverted position. Tilt head back and gently squeeze inverted bottle to instill drop.

Monitoring Parameters Liver function tests, WBC with differential; number and type of stools/day for diarrhea; monitor patients receiving azithromycin and drugs known to interact with erythromycin (ie, theophylline, digoxin, anticoagulants, triazolam) since there are still very few studies examining drug-drug interactions with azithromycin

Patient Information Report any symptoms of chest pain, heart palpitations, and yellowing of skin or eyes. May cause photosensitivity reactions (eg, exposure to sunlight may cause severe sunburn, skin rash, redness, or itching); avoid exposure to sunlight and artificial light sources (sunlamps, tanning booth/bed); wear protective clothing, wide-brimmed hats, sunglasses, and lip sunscreen (SPF ≥15); use a sunscreen [broad-spectrum sunscreen or physical sunscreen (preferred) or sunblock with SPF ≥15]; contact physician if diarrhea, abnormal heart rhythm, allergic or photosensitivity reaction occurs. Advise patients who are being treated for bacterial conjunctivitis not to wear contact lenses.

Dosage Forms Excipient information presented when available (limited, particularly for generics); consult specific product labeling. [DSC] = Discontinued product

Note: Strength expressed as base

Injection, powder for reconstitution, as dihydrate: 500 mg

Zithromax®: 500 mg [contains sodium 114 mg (4.96 mEq) per vial]

Injection, powder for reconstitution, as hydrogencitrate: 500 mg, 2.5 g

Injection, powder for reconstitution, as monohydrate: 500 mg

Microspheres for oral suspension, extended release, as dihydrate:

Zmax®: 2 g/bottle (60 mL) [contains sodium 148 mg per bottle, sucrose 19 g/bottle; cherry/banana flavor; product contains azithromycin 27 mg/mL after constitution]

Powder for oral suspension, as monohydrate: 100 mg/5 mL (15 mL); 200 mg/5 mL (15 mL, 22.5 mL, 30 mL); 1 g/packet (3s)

Powder for oral suspension, as dihydrate: 100 mg/5 mL (15 mL); 200 mg/5 mL (15 mL, 22.5 mL, 30 mL); 1 g/packet (3s; 10s [DSC])

Zithromax®: 100 mg/5 mL (15 mL) [contains sodium 3.7 mg/ 5 mL; cherry creme de vanilla and banana flavor]; 200 mg/5 mL (15 mL, 22.5 mL, 30 mL) [contains sodium 7.4 mg/5 mL; cherry creme de vanilla and banana flavor]; 1 g/packet (3s, 10s) [single-dose packet; contains sodium 37 mg per packet; cherry creme de vanilla and banana flavor]

Solution, ophthalmic:

AzaSite®: 1% (2.5 mL) [contains benzalkonium chloride]

Tablet, oral, as anhydrous: 250 mg, 500 mg, 600 mg

Tablet, oral, as dihydrate: 250 mg, 500 mg, 600 mg

Zithromax®: 250 mg [contains sodium 0.9 mg per tablet]; 500 mg [contains sodium 1.8 mg per tablet]; 600 mg [contains sodium 2.1 mg per tablet]

Zithromax® TRI-PAK™ [unit-dose pack]: 500 mg (3s) [contains sodium 1.8 mg per tablet]

Zithromax® Z-PAK® [unit-dose pack]: 250 mg (6s) [contains sodium 0.9 mg per tablet]

Tablet, as monohydrate: 250 mg, 500 mg, 600 mg

References

"CDC/NIH/PIDS/AAP/IDSA Guidelines for Prevention and Treatment of Opportunistic Infections Among HIV-Exposed and HIV-Infected Children. USPHS/IDSA Prevention of Opportunistic Working Group," June 20, 2008, http://www.aidsinfo.nih.gov.

Centers for Disease Control and Prevention, Workowski KA, and Berman SM, "Sexually Transmitted Diseases Treatment Guidelines, 2006," *MMWR Recomm Rep*, 2006, 55(RR-11):1-94.

Drew RH and Gallis HA, "Azithromycin-Spectrum of Activity, Pharmacokinetics, and Clinical Applications," *Pharmacotherapy*, 1992, 12(3):161-73.

Foulds G, Shepard RM, and Johnson RB, "The Pharmacokinetics of Azithromycin in Human Serum and Tissues," *J Antimicrob Chemother*, 1990, 25(Suppl A):73-82.

Jacobs RF, Maples HD, Aranda JV, et al, "Pharmacokinetics of Intravenously Administered Azithromycin in Pediatric Patients," *Pediatr Infect Dis J*, 2005, 24(1):34-9.

Nahata MC, Koranyi KI, Gadgil SD, et al, "Pharmacokinetics of Azithromycin After Oral Administration of Multiple Doses of Suspension," *Antimicrob Agents Chemother*, 1993, 37(2):314-16.

Saiman L, Marshall BC, Mayer-Hamblett N, et al, "Azithromycin in Patients With Cystic Fibrosis Chronically Infected With *Pseudomonas aeruginosa*: A Randomized Controlled Trial," *JAMA*, 2003, 290 (13):1749-56.

Starke JR and Correa AG, "Management of Mycobacterial Infection and Disease in Children," *Pediatr Infect Dis J*, 1995, 14(6):455-69.

Tiwari T, Murphy TV, and Moran J, "Recommended Antimicrobial Agents for the Treatment and Postexposure Prophylaxis of Pertussis: 2005 CDC Guidelines," *MMWR*, 2005, 54(RR-14):1-16.

◆ **Azithromycin Dihydrate** *see* Azithromycin *on page 164*

◆ **Azithromycin Hydrogencitrate** *see* Azithromycin *on page 164*

◆ **Azithromycin Monohydrate** *see* Azithromycin *on page 164*

◆ **Azmacort® [DSC]** *see* Triamcinolone *on page 1376*

◆ **AZO-Gesic® [OTC]** *see* Phenazopyridine *on page 1097*

◆ **AZO-Standard® [OTC]** *see* Phenazopyridine *on page 1097*

◆ **AZO-Standard® Maximum Strength [OTC]** *see* Phenazopyridine *on page 1097*

◆ **AZT™ (Can)** *see* Zidovudine *on page 1442*

◆ **AZT, Abacavir, and Lamivudine** *see* Abacavir, Lamivudine, and Zidovudine *on page 31*

◆ **AZT and 3TC** *see* Lamivudine and Zidovudine *on page 794*

◆ **AZT (error-prone abbreviation)** *see* Zidovudine *on page 1442*

◆ **Azthreonam** *see* Aztreonam *on page 167*

Aztreonam (AZ tree oh nam)

Medication Safety Issues

Sound-alike/look-alike issues:

Aztreonam may be confused with azidothymidine

U.S. Brand Names Azactam®; Cayston®

Canadian Brand Names Azactam®

Therapeutic Category Antibiotic, Miscellaneous

Generic Available No

Use

Injection: Treatment of patients with documented multidrug resistant aerobic gram-negative infection in which beta-lactam therapy is contraindicated; used for UTI, lower respiratory tract infections, intra-abdominal infections, and gynecological infections caused by susceptible *Enterobacteriaceae*, *E. coli*, *K. pneumoniae*, *P. mirabilis*, *S. marcescens*, *Citrobacter* species, *H. influenzae*, and *P. aeruginosa* (FDA approved in ages ≥9 months and adults); treatment of susceptible skin and skin-structure infections and septicemia (FDA approved in adults)

Inhalation (nebulized): Improve respiratory symptoms in cystic fibrosis patients with *Pseudomonas aeruginosa* in the lungs (FDA approved in ages ≥7 years and adults)

Pregnancy Risk Factor B

Pregnancy Considerations Adverse events have not been observed in animal reproduction studies; therefore, the manufacturer classifies aztreonam as pregnancy category B. Aztreonam crosses the placenta and enters cord blood during middle and late pregnancy. Distribution to the fetus is minimal in early pregnancy. The amount of aztreonam available systemically following inhalation is significantly less in comparison to doses given by injection.

Lactation Enters breast milk/not recommended (AAP rates "compatible")

Breast-Feeding Considerations Very small amounts of aztreonam are excreted in breast milk. The poor oral absorption of aztreonam (<1%) may limit adverse effects to the infant. Although the manufacturer recommends considering temporary discontinuation of nursing during systemic therapy, the AAP considers aztreonam to be "usually compatible with breast-feeding." Nondose-related effects could include modification of bowel flora. Maternal use of aztreonam inhalation is not likely to pose a risk to breast-feeding infants.

Contraindications Hypersensitivity to aztreonam or any component

Warnings Check for hypersensitivity to other beta-lactams (hypersensitivity reactions to aztreonam have occurred rarely in patients with a history of penicillin or cephalosporin hypersensitivity); prolonged use may result in superinfection. *C. difficile*-associated diarrhea has been reported with the use of aztreonam. Bronchospasm may occur following nebulization; administer a bronchodilator prior to treatment. Safety and efficacy have not been established for nebulized inhalation patients colonized with *Burkholderia cepacia*, for use in children <7 years, or in patients with FEV1 <25% or >75% predicted. To reduce the development of resistant bacteria and maintain efficacy, reserve use of inhalation solution for CF patients with known *Pseudomonas aeruginosa*.

Precautions Use with caution and reduce injectable dose in patients with renal impairment; no dosing adjustment is necessary in patients receiving the inhalation formulation.

Adverse Reactions

Injection:

Central nervous system: Fever

Dermatologic: Rash, toxic epidermal necrolysis

Gastrointestinal: Diarrhea, GI bleeding, nausea, pseudo-membranous colitis, vomiting

Hematologic: Eosinophilia, leukopenia, neutropenia, thrombocytopenia

Hepatic: ALT, AST, and alkaline phosphatase increased

Local: Erythema, induration, pain at injection site, thrombophlebitis

Renal: BUN and serum creatinine increased

Miscellaneous: Allergic reaction, anaphylaxis, hypersensitivity

<1%, postmarketing, and/or case reports: Abdominal cramps, abnormal taste, anemia, angioedema, aphthous ulcer, breast tenderness, bronchospasm, *C. difficile*-associated diarrhea, chest pain, confusion, diaphoresis, diplopia, dizziness, dyspnea, ECG changes (transient), erythema multiforme, exfoliative dermatitis, flushing, halitosis, headache, hepatitis, hypotension, insomnia, jaundice, muscular aches, myalgia, numb tongue, pancytopenia, paresthesia, petechiae, pruritus, purpura, seizure, sneezing, tinnitus, urticaria, vaginitis, vertigo, weakness, wheezing

Inhalation:

Cardiovascular: Chest discomfort

Central nervous system: Fever

Dermatologic: Rash

Gastrointestinal: Abdominal pain, vomiting

Respiratory: Bronchospasm (see Warnings), cough, nasal congestion, pharyngeal pain, wheezing

Drug Interactions

Avoid Concomitant Use

Avoid concomitant use of Aztreonam with any of the following: BCG

Increased Effect/Toxicity There are no known significant interactions involving an increase in effect.

Decreased Effect

Aztreonam may decrease the levels/effects of: BCG; Typhoid Vaccine

Stability

Inhalation: Store intact vials and diluent ampules at 2°C to 8°C (36°F to 46°F). May be stored at 25°C (77°F) for up to 28 days; protect from light. Reconstituted solution must be used immediately.

I.V.: Reconstituted solution is stable 48 hours at room temperature and 7 days when refrigerated; incompatible when mixed with nafcillin or metronidazole. Store aztreonam infusion solution in GALAXY plastic container at or below -20°C (-4°F). The thawed solution is stable for 14 days at 2°C to 8°C (36°F to 46°F) or 48 hours at 25°C (77°F); do not refreeze thawed antibiotics.

Mechanism of Action Binds to penicillin-binding protein 3 which produces filamentation of the bacterium inhibiting bacterial cell wall synthesis and causing cell wall destruction

Pharmacokinetics (Adult data unless noted)

Absorption: I.M.: Well absorbed; Oral inhalation: Poorly absorbed

Distribution: Injection: Widely distributed into body tissues, cerebrospinal fluid, bronchial secretions, peritoneal fluid, bile, bone, and breast milk; crosses the placenta

V_d:

Neonates: 0.26-0.36 L/kg

Children: 0.2-0.29 L/kg

Adults: 0.2 L/kg

Protein binding: 56%

Half-life: Injection:

Neonates:

<7 days, ≤2.5 kg: 5.5-9.9 hours

<7 days, >2.5 kg: 2.6 hours

1 week to 1 month: 2.4 hours

Children 2 months to 12 years: 1.7 hours

Children with cystic fibrosis: 1.3 hours

Adults: 1.3-2.2 hours (half-life prolonged in renal failure)

Time to peak serum concentration: Within 60 minutes after an I.M. dose

Elimination:

Injection: 60% to 70% excreted unchanged in the urine by active tubular secretion and glomerular filtration; 12% excreted in feces

Inhalation: Urine (10% of the total dose)

Dialysis: Moderately dialyzable

Hemodialysis: 27% to 58% in 4 hours

Peritoneal dialysis: 10% with a 6-hour dwell time

Usual Dosage I.M., I.V.:

Neonates:

Postnatal age ≤7 days:

≤2000 g: 60 mg/kg/day divided every 12 hours

>2000 g: 90 mg/kg/day divided every 8 hours

Postnatal age >7 days:

<1200 g: 60 mg/kg/day divided every 12 hours

1200-2000 g: 90 mg/kg/day divided every 8 hours

>2000 g: 120 mg/kg/day divided every 6 hours

Children >1 month: 90-120 mg/kg/day divided every 6-8 hours

Cystic fibrosis: 50 mg/kg/dose every 6-8 hours (ie, up to 200 mg/kg/day); maximum dose: 8 g/day

Adults:

Urinary tract infection: 500 mg to 1 g every 8-12 hours

Moderately severe systemic infections: 1 g I.V. or I.M. or 2 g I.V. every 8-12 hours

Severe systemic or life-threatening infections (especially if caused by *Pseudomonas aeruginosa*): I.V.: 2 g every 6-8 hours; maximum dose: 8 g/day

Oral inhalation: Children ≥7 years and adults: Cystic fibrosis: 75 mg 3 times daily (do not administer doses <4 hours apart); administer in repeated cycles of 28 days on drug, followed by 28 days off drug

Dosing adjustment in renal impairment:

I.V.:

Cl_{cr} 10-30 mL/minute: Reduce dose by 50%; give at the usual interval

Cl_{cr} <10 mL/minute: Reduce dose by 75%; give at the usual interval

Inhalation (nebulized): Dosage adjustment not required for mild, moderate, or severe renal impairment.

Administration Parenteral:

I.V.: Administer by IVP over 3-5 minutes at a maximum concentration of 66 mg/mL or by intermittent infusion over 20-60 minutes at a final concentration not to exceed 20 mg/mL

I.M.: Deep I.M. injection into a large muscle mass such as the upper outer quadrant of the gluteus maximus or lateral part of the thigh

Inhalation: Administer only using an Altera® nebulizer system; dose can be nebulized over 2-3 minutes. Do not mix with other inhaled nebulizer medications. Administer a bronchodilator before administration of aztreonam (short-acting 15 minutes to 4 hours before; long-acting 30 minutes to 12 hours before). Administer doses ≥4 hours apart.

Monitoring Parameters

Injection: Periodic renal and hepatic function tests; monitor for stool frequency

Inhalation: FEV_1

Test Interactions False positive urine glucose (Clinitest®), positive Coombs' test

Patient Information Report persistent diarrhea to physician.

Dosage Forms Excipient information presented when available (limited, particularly for generics); consult specific product labeling. [DSC] = Discontinued product
Infusion premixed iso-osmotic solution:
Azactam®: 1 g (50 mL); 2 g (50 mL)
Injection, powder for reconstitution:
Azactam®: 1 g, 2 g [DSC]
Powder for reconstitution, for oral inhalation [preservative free]:
Cayston®: 75 mg [supplied with diluent]

References

Bosso JA and Black PG, "The Use of Aztreonam in Pediatric Patients: A Review," *Pharmacotherapy*, 1991, 11(1):20-5.
Le J, Ashley ED, Neuhauser MM, et al, "Consensus Summary of Aerosolized Antimicrobial Agents: Application of Guideline Criteria," *Pharmacotherapy*, 2010, 30(6):562-84.
Retsch-Bogart GZ, Quittner AL, Gibson RL, et al, "Efficacy and Safety of Inhaled Aztreonam Lysine for Airway Pseudomonas in Cystic Fibrosis," *Chest*, 2009, 135(5):1223-32.
Stutman HR, Chartrand SA, Tolentino T, et al, "Aztreonam Therapy for Serious Gram-Negative Infections in Children," *Am J Dis Child*, 1986, 140(11):1147-51.

♦ **Azulfidine®** *see* Sulfasalazine *on page 1304*

♦ **Azulfidine® EN-tabs®** *see* Sulfasalazine *on page 1304*

♦ **B6** *see* Pyridoxine *on page 1190*

♦ **Baby Aspirin** *see* Aspirin *on page 141*

♦ **BabyBIG®** *see* Botulism Immune Globulin (Intravenous-Human) *on page 201*

♦ **Bacid® [OTC]** *see* Lactobacillus *on page 790*

♦ **Bacid® (Can)** *see* Lactobacillus *on page 790*

♦ **Baciguent® [OTC]** *see* Bacitracin *on page 169*

♦ **Baciguent® (Can)** *see* Bacitracin *on page 169*

♦ **BaciIM®** *see* Bacitracin *on page 169*

♦ **Baciject® (Can)** *see* Bacitracin *on page 169*

♦ **Baci-Rx** *see* Bacitracin *on page 169*

Bacitracin (bas i TRAY sin)

Medication Safety Issues
Sound-alike/look-alike issues:
Bacitracin may be confused with Bactrim®, Bactroban®
U.S. Brand Names Baci-Rx; Baciguent® [OTC]; BaciIM®
Canadian Brand Names Baciguent®; Baciject®
Therapeutic Category Antibiotic, Miscellaneous; Antibiotic, Topical
Generic Available Yes
Use Treatment of pneumonia and empyema caused by susceptible staphylococci; prevention or treatment of superficial skin infections; due to its toxicity, use of bacitracin systemically or as an irrigant should be limited to situations where less toxic alternatives would not be effective; treatment of antibiotic-associated colitis
Pregnancy Considerations It is unknown if bacitracin crosses the placenta. The minimal absorption after topical use should limit the amount of medication available for transfer to the fetus.
Lactation Excretion in breast milk unknown/use caution
Breast-Feeding Considerations It is unknown if bacitracin is distributed in human milk. The minimal absorption after topical use should limit the amount of medication available for transfer.
Contraindications Hypersensitivity to bacitracin or any component; I.M. use is not recommended in patients with renal impairment
Warnings I.M. use may cause renal failure due to tubular and glomerular necrosis **[U.S. Boxed Warning]**; avoid concurrent use with other nephrotoxic drugs; discontinue use if toxicity occurs; monitor renal function prior to therapy and daily during therapy **[U.S. Boxed Warning]**; ensure adequate fluid intake and urinary output; should only be

used where adequate laboratory facilities are available and when constant supervision is possible; avoid concomitant use with other nephrotoxic drugs if possible; do not administer intravenously because severe thrombophlebitis occurs; bacitracin may be absorbed from denuded areas and irrigation sites
Precautions Prolonged use may result in overgrowth of nonsusceptible organisms
Adverse Reactions
Cardiovascular: Hypotension, tightness of chest
Central nervous system: Pain
Dermatologic: Rash, itching
Gastrointestinal: Anorexia, nausea, vomiting, diarrhea, rectal itching and burning
Hematologic: Blood dyscrasias
Renal: With I.M. use: Renal tubular and glomerular necrosis, azotemia, renal failure
Miscellaneous: Diaphoresis, edema of lips and face
Drug Interactions
Avoid Concomitant Use
Avoid concomitant use of Bacitracin with any of the following: BCG
Increased Effect/Toxicity There are no known significant interactions involving an increase in effect.
Decreased Effect
Bacitracin may decrease the levels/effects of: BCG
Stability Sterile powder should be stored in the refrigerator; once reconstituted, bacitracin is stable for 1 week under refrigeration (2°C to 8°C); incompatible with diluents containing parabens
Mechanism of Action Inhibits bacterial cell wall synthesis by preventing transfer of mucopeptides into the growing cell wall
Pharmacokinetics (Adult data unless noted)
Absorption: Poor from mucous membranes and intact skin; rapid following I.M. administration
Protein binding: Minimally bound to plasma proteins
Time to peak serum concentration: I.M.: Within 1-2 hours
Elimination: Slow elimination into the urine with 10% to 40% of a dose excreted within 24 hours
Usual Dosage
I.M. (not recommended):
Infants:
≤2.5 kg: 900 units/kg/day in 2-3 divided doses
>2.5 kg: 1000 units/kg/day in 2-3 divided doses
Children: 800-1200 units/kg/day divided every 8 hours
Adults: 10,000-25,000 units/dose every 6 hours; not to exceed 100,000 units/day
Children and Adults:
Topical: Apply 1-5 times/day
Irrigation, solution: 50-100 units/mL in NS, LR, or sterile water for irrigation; soak sponges in solution for topical compresses 1-5 times/day or as needed during surgical procedures
Antibiotic-associated colitis: Adults: Oral: 25,000 units every 6 hours for 7-10 days
Administration
Parenteral: For I.M. administration, pH of urine should be kept above 6 by using sodium bicarbonate; bacitracin sterile powder should be dissolved in NS injection containing 2% procaine hydrochloride; administer I.M. injection into the upper outer quadrant of the buttocks; alternate injection sites
Topical: Apply thin layer to the cleansed affected area. May cover with a sterile bandage. For external use only. Do not use topical ointment in the eyes.
Monitoring Parameters I.M.: Urinalysis, renal function tests
Patient Information Topical bacitracin should not be used for longer than 1 week unless directed by a physician

◄ **Dosage Forms** Excipient information presented when available (limited, particularly for generics); consult specific product labeling.

Injection, powder for reconstitution: 50,000 units
 BaciiM®: 50,000 units

Ointment, ophthalmic: 500 units/g (3.5 g)

Ointment, topical, as zinc [strength expressed as base]: 500 units/g (0.9 g, 15 g, 30 g, 120 g, 454 g)
 Baciguent®: 500 units/g (15 g, 30 g)

Powder, for prescription compounding [micronized]:
 Baci-Rx: 5 million units

References

Kelly CP, Pothoulakis C, and LaMont JT, "*Clostridium difficile* Colitis," *N Engl J Med*, 1994, 330(4):257-62.

Bacitracin and Polymyxin B
(bas i TRAY sin & pol i MIKS in bee)

Medication Safety Issues
Sound-alike/look-alike issues:
Betadine® may be confused with Betagan®, betaine

U.S. Brand Names AK-Poly-Bac™; Polysporin® [OTC]

Canadian Brand Names LID-Pack®; Optimyxin®

Therapeutic Category Antibiotic, Ophthalmic; Antibiotic, Topical

Generic Available Yes

Use Treatment of superficial infections involving the conjunctiva and/or cornea caused by susceptible organisms; prevent infection in minor cuts, scrapes and burns

Pregnancy Risk Factor C

Pregnancy Considerations Animal reproduction studies have not been conducted with this combination; therefore, Bacitracin and Polymyxin B is considered pregnancy category C. See individual agents.

Lactation Excretion in breast milk unknown/use caution

Breast-Feeding Considerations It is not known if bacitracin or polymyxin B is found in breast milk. The manufacturer recommends that caution be exercised when administering Bacitracin and Polymyxin B to nursing women. See individual agents.

Contraindications Hypersensitivity to polymyxin, bacitracin, or any component

Precautions Prolonged use may result in overgrowth of nonsusceptible organisms

Adverse Reactions
Local: Rash, itching, burning, edema
Ocular: Conjunctival erythema
Miscellaneous: Anaphylactoid reactions

Drug Interactions
Avoid Concomitant Use
Avoid concomitant use of Bacitracin and Polymyxin B with any of the following: BCG

Increased Effect/Toxicity
Bacitracin and Polymyxin B may increase the levels/effects of: Colistimethate; Neuromuscular-Blocking Agents

The levels/effects of Bacitracin and Polymyxin B may be increased by: Capreomycin

Decreased Effect
Bacitracin and Polymyxin B may decrease the levels/effects of: BCG

Pharmacokinetics (Adult data unless noted) Absorption: Insignificant from intact skin or mucous membrane

Usual Dosage Children and Adults:
Ophthalmic: Instill 1/4" to 1/2" directly into conjunctival sac(s) every 3-4 hours depending on severity of the infection
Topical: Apply a small amount of ointment or dusting of powder to the affected area 1-3 times/day

Administration Ophthalmic: Do not use topical ointment in the eyes; avoid contact of tube tip with skin or eye

Patient Information Do not use longer than 1 week unless directed by physician; ophthalmic ointment may cause blurred vision

Dosage Forms Excipient information presented when available (limited, particularly for generics); consult specific product labeling.

Ointment, ophthalmic: Bacitracin 500 units and polymyxin B 10,000 units per g (3.5 g)
 AK-Poly-Bac™: Bacitracin 500 units and polymyxin B 10,000 units per g (3.5 g)

Ointment, topical: Bacitracin 500 units and polymyxin B 10,000 units per g in white petrolatum (15 g, 30 g)
 Polysporin®: Bacitracin 500 units and polymyxin B 10,000 units per g (0.9 g, 15 g, 30 g)

Powder, topical:
 Polysporin®: Bacitracin 500 units and polymyxin B 10,000 units per g (10 g)

Bacitracin, Neomycin, and Polymyxin B
(bas i TRAY sin, nee oh MYE sin, & pol i MIKS in bee)

U.S. Brand Names Neosporin® Neo To Go® [OTC]; Neosporin® Topical [OTC]

Therapeutic Category Antibiotic, Ophthalmic; Antibiotic, Topical

Generic Available Yes

Use Help prevent infection in minor cuts, scrapes and burns; short-term treatment of superficial external ocular infections caused by susceptible organisms

Pregnancy Risk Factor C

Pregnancy Considerations Reproduction studies have not been conducted with this combination; therefore, Bacitracin, Neomycin, and Polymyxin B is classified as pregnancy category C. See individual agents.

Lactation Excretion in breast milk unknown/use caution

Breast-Feeding Considerations It is not known if bacitracin, neomycin, or polymyxin B is excreted into breast milk. The manufacturer recommends that caution be exercised when administering Bacitracin, Neomycin, and Polymyxin B to nursing women. See individual agents.

Contraindications Hypersensitivity to neomycin, polymyxin B, zinc bacitracin, or any component

Warnings Symptoms of neomycin sensitization include itching, reddening, edema, failure to heal; ophthalmic ointments may retard corneal healing

Precautions Prolonged use may result in overgrowth of nonsusceptible organisms

Adverse Reactions
Local: Rash and hypersensitivity reactions ranging from generalized itching, local edema, and erythema have been reported; contact dermatitis
Ocular: Conjunctival sensitization, blurring of vision (ophthalmic formulation)

Drug Interactions
Avoid Concomitant Use
Avoid concomitant use of Bacitracin, Neomycin, and Polymyxin B with any of the following: BCG; Gallium Nitrate

Increased Effect/Toxicity
Bacitracin, Neomycin, and Polymyxin B may increase the levels/effects of: AbobotulinumtoxinA; Bisphosphonate Derivatives; CARBOplatin; Colistimethate; CycloSPORINE; CycloSPORINE (Systemic); Gallium Nitrate; Neuromuscular-Blocking Agents; OnabotulinumtoxinA; RimabotulinumtoxinB

The levels/effects of Bacitracin, Neomycin, and Polymyxin B may be increased by: Amphotericin B; Capreomycin; CISplatin; Loop Diuretics; Nonsteroidal Anti-Inflammatory Agents; Vancomycin

Decreased Effect

Bacitracin, Neomycin, and Polymyxin B may decrease the levels/effects of: BCG; Cardiac Glycosides

The levels/effects of Bacitracin, Neomycin, and Polymyxin B may be decreased by: Penicillins

Usual Dosage Children and Adults:

Ophthalmic ointment: Instill into the conjunctival sac 1 or more times daily every 3-4 hours for 7-10 days

Topical: Apply 1-3 times/day

Administration

Ophthalmic: Avoid contamination of the tip of the ointment tube

Topical: Apply a thin layer to the cleansed affected area; may cover with a sterile bandage

Patient Information Ophthalmic: May cause sensitivity to bright light; may cause temporary blurring of vision or stinging following administration

Dosage Forms Excipient information presented when available (limited, particularly for generics); consult specific product labeling.

Ointment, ophthalmic: Bacitracin 400 units, neomycin 3.5 mg, and polymyxin B 10,000 units per g (3.5 g)

Ointment, topical: Bacitracin 400 units, neomycin 3.5 mg, and polymyxin B 5000 units per g (0.9 g, 15 g, 30 g, 454 g)

Neosporin®: Bacitracin 400 units, neomycin 3.5 mg, and polymyxin B 5000 units per g (15 g, 30 g)

Neosporin® Neo To Go®: Bacitracin 400 units, neomycin 3.5 mg, and polymyxin B 5000 units per g (0.9 g)

Baclofen (BAK loe fen)

Medication Safety Issues

Sound-alike/look-alike issues:

Baclofen may be confused with Bactroban®

Lioresal® may be confused with lisinopril, Lotensin®

High alert medication: The Institute for Safe Medication Practices (ISMP) includes this medication (intrathecal administration) among its list of drugs which have a heightened risk of causing significant patient harm when used in error.

U.S. Brand Names Lioresal®

Canadian Brand Names Apo-Baclofen®; Dom-Baclofen; Lioresal®; Liotec; Med-Baclofen; Mylan-Baclofen; Novo-Baclofen; Nu-Baclo; PHL-Baclofen; PMS-Baclofen; ratio-Baclofen; Riva-Baclofen

Therapeutic Category Skeletal Muscle Relaxant, Nonparalytic

Generic Available Yes: Tablets only

Use Treatment of cerebral spasticity, reversible spasticity associated with multiple sclerosis or spinal cord lesions; intrathecal use for the management of spasticity in patients who are unresponsive to oral baclofen or experience intolerable CNS side effects; treatment of trigeminal neuralgia; adjunctive treatment of tardive dyskinesia

Pregnancy Risk Factor C

Lactation Enters breast milk (small amounts)/compatible

Contraindications Hypersensitivity to baclofen or any component; injection for intrathecal use is not recommended or intended for I.V., I.M., SubQ, or epidural administration

Warnings Should not be used when spasticity is used to maintain posture or balance; due to the life-threatening complications of intrathecal use, physicians must be adequately trained in its use; abrupt withdrawal of oral baclofen has been reported to precipitate hallucinations and/or seizures. Abrupt discontinuation of intrathecal baclofen regardless of the cause, has resulted in sequelae that include high fever, altered mental status, exaggerated rebound spasticity, and muscle rigidity, that in rare cases, has advanced to rhabdomyolysis, multiple organ system failure, and death **[U.S. Boxed Warning]**. Early symptoms of withdrawal include: Return of baseline spasticity, pruritus, hypotension, and paresthesias. Clinical characteristics of advanced withdrawal may resemble autonomic dysreflexia, sepsis, malignant hyperthermia, neuroleptic-malignant syndrome, and other conditions associated with hypermetabolic state or widespread rhabdomyolysis. Patients at increased risk those include spinal cord injuries at T-6 or above, those with communication difficulties, and those history of withdrawal symptoms from oral baclofen. If restoration of intrathecal baclofen is delayed, oral baclofen or benzodiazepine treatment may be used as a temporary measure.

Precautions Use with caution in patients with seizure disorder, impaired renal function, peptic ulcer disease, stroke, ovarian cysts, psychotic disorders, autonomic dysreflexia (intrathecal therapy); careful attention to programming and monitoring of intrathecal baclofen is recommended to prevent abrupt discontinuation

Adverse Reactions

Cardiovascular: Hypotension, cardiovascular collapse (with intrathecal therapy), chest pain, palpitations

Central nervous system: Drowsiness, fatigue, vertigo, dizziness, psychiatric disturbances, insomnia, slurred speech, headache, hypotonia, ataxia, life-threatening CNS depression (with intrathecal use)

Dermatologic: Rash, pruritus

Gastrointestinal: Nausea, constipation, anorexia, dysgeusia, diarrhea, abdominal pain, xerostomia

Genitourinary: Impotence, urinary frequency, nocturia

Renal: Hematuria

Respiratory: Respiratory failure (with intrathecal administration), dyspnea

Miscellaneous: Diaphoresis

Drug Interactions

Avoid Concomitant Use There are no known interactions where it is recommended to avoid concomitant use.

Increased Effect/Toxicity

Baclofen may increase the levels/effects of: Alcohol (Ethyl); CNS Depressants; Methotrimeprazine

The levels/effects of Baclofen may be increased by: Methotrimeprazine

Decreased Effect There are no known significant interactions involving a decrease in effect.

Mechanism of Action Inhibits the transmission of both monosynaptic and polysynaptic reflexes at the spinal cord level, possibly by hyperpolarization of primary afferent fiber terminals, with resultant relief of muscle spasticity

Pharmacodynamics

Oral: Muscle relaxation effects require 3-4 days and maximal clinical effects are not seen for 5-10 days

Intrathecal:

Bolus:

Onset of action: 30 minutes to 1 hour

Maximum effect: 4 hours

Duration: 4-8 hours

Continuous intrathecal infusion:

Onset of action: 6-8 hours

Maximum activity: 24-48 hours

Pharmacokinetics (Adult data unless noted)

Oral:

Absorption: Rapid; absorption from the GI tract is thought to be dose dependent

Protein binding: 30%

Metabolism: Minimal in the liver (15%)

Half-life: 2.5-4 hours

Time to peak serum concentration: Oral: Within 2-3 hours

Elimination: 85% of dose excreted in urine and feces as unchanged drug

Intrathecal:
Half-life, CSF elimination: 1.5 hours
Clearance, CSF: 30 mL/hour

Usual Dosage

Oral: Dose-related side effects (eg, sedation) may be minimized by slow titration; lower initial doses than described below (2.5-5 mg **daily**) may be used with subsequent titration to 8 hourly doses.

Children: Limited published data in children; the following is a compilation of small prospective studies (Albright, 1996; Milla, 1977; Scheinberg, 2006) and one large retrospective analysis of baclofen use in children (Lubsch, 2006):

<2 years: 10-20 mg **daily** divided every 8 hours; titrate dose every 3 days in increments of 5-15 mg/day to a maximum of 40 mg **daily**

2-7 years: 20-30 mg **daily** divided every 8 hours; titrate dose every 3 days in increments of 5-15 mg/day to a maximum of 60 mg **daily**

≥8 years: 30-40 mg **daily** divided every 8 hours; titrate dosage as above to a maximum of 120 mg **daily**

Note: Lubsch retrospective analysis noted that higher daily dosages of baclofen were needed as the time increased from injury onset, as age increased, and as the number of concomitant antispasticity medications increased. Each of these variables may represent drug tolerance or progressive spasticity. In this review, doses as high as 200 mg **daily** were used.

Adults: 5 mg 3 times/day, may increase 5 mg/dose every 3 days to a maximum of 80 mg/day

Intrathecal: Children and Adults:

Screening dosage: 50 mcg for 1 dose and observe for 4-8 hours; very small children may receive 25 mcg; if ineffective, a repeat dosage increased by 50% (eg, 75 mcg) may be repeated in 24 hours; if still suboptimal, a third dose increased by 33% (eg, 100 mcg) may be repeated in 24 hours; patients who do not respond to 100 mcg intrathecally should not be considered for continuous chronic administration via an implantable pump

Maintenance dose: Continuous infusion: Initial: Depending upon the screening dosage and its duration:

If the screening dose duration >8 hours: Daily dose = effective screening dose

If the screening dose duration <8 hours: Daily dose = **twice** effective screening dose

Continuous infusion dose mcg/hour = daily dose divided by 24 hours

Note: Further adjustments in infusion rate may be done every 24 hours as needed; for spinal cord-related spasticity, increase in 10% to 30% increments/24 hours; for spasticity of cerebral origin, increase in 5% to 10% increments/24 hours

Average daily dose:

Children ≤12 years: 100-300 mcg/day (4.2-12.5 mcg/hour); doses as high as 1000 mcg/day have been used

Children >12 years and Adults: 300-800 mcg/day (12.5-33 mcg/hour); doses as high as 2000 mcg/day have been used

Administration

Oral: Administer with food or milk

Parenteral: Intrathecal: Test dosage: Use dilute concentration (50 mcg/mL) and inject over at least 1 minute; for maintenance infusion via implantable infusion pump, concentrations of 500-2000 mcg/mL may be used; do not abruptly discontinue intrathecal baclofen administration (see Warnings)

Monitoring Parameters Muscle rigidity, spasticity (decrease in number and severity of spasms), modified Ashworth score

Patient Information Avoid alcohol and other CNS depressants; may cause drowsiness and impair ability to perform activities requiring mental alertness or physical coordination; may cause dry mouth; do not abruptly discontinue therapy

Dosage Forms Excipient information presented when available (limited, particularly for generics); consult specific product labeling.

Injection, solution, intrathecal [preservative free]:
Lioresal®: 50 mcg/mL (1 mL); 500 mcg/mL (20 mL); 2000 mcg/mL (5 mL, 20 mL)
Tablet: 10 mg, 20 mg

Extemporaneous Preparations

A 5 mg/mL suspension may be made by crushing thirty 20 mg tablets; levigate with a small amount of glycerin to form a paste. Add simple syrup incrementally to a total volume of 120 mL; shake well; refrigerate; stable 35 days (Johnson, 1993)

A 10 mg/mL oral suspension may be made by crushing one hundred twenty 10 mg tablets; gradually add 60 mL Ora-Sweet® or Ora-Plus® and mix until a uniform paste, then add more vehicle to make a total volume of 120 mL; refrigerate; shake well; stable 60 days (Allen, 1996)

Allen LV Jr and Erickson MA 3rd, "Stability of Baclofen, Captopril, Diltiazem Hydrochloride, Dipyridamole, and Flecainide Acetate in Extemporaneously Compounded Oral Liquids," *Am J Health Syst Pharm*, 1996, 53(18):2179-84.

Johnson CE and Hart SM, "Stability of an Extemporaneously Compounded Baclofen Oral Liquid," *Am J Hosp Pharm*, 1993, 50 (11):2353-5.

References

Albright AL, "Baclofen in the Treatment of Cerebral Palsy," *J Child Neurol*, 1996, 11(2):77-83.

Lubsch L, Habersang R, Haase M, et al, "Oral Baclofen and Clonidine for Treatment of Spasticity in Children," *J Child Neurol*, 2006, 21 (12):1090-2.

Milla PJ and Jackson AD, "A Controlled Trial of Baclofen in Children With Cerebral Palsy," *J Int Med Res*, 1977, 5(6):398-404.

Scheinberg A, Hall K, Lam LT, et al, "Oral Baclofen in Children With Cerebral Palsy: A Double-Blind Cross-Over Pilot Study," *J Paediatr Child Health*, 2006, 42(11):715-20.

◆ **BactoShield® CHG [OTC]** *see* Chlorhexidine Gluconate *on page 291*

◆ **Bactrim™** *see* Sulfamethoxazole and Trimethoprim *on page 1302*

◆ **Bactrim™ DS** *see* Sulfamethoxazole and Trimethoprim *on page 1302*

◆ **Bactroban®** *see* Mupirocin *on page 954*

◆ **Bactroban Cream®** *see* Mupirocin *on page 954*

◆ **Bactroban Nasal®** *see* Mupirocin *on page 954*

◆ **Baking Soda** *see* Sodium Bicarbonate *on page 1269*

◆ **BAL** *see* Dimercaprol *on page 447*

◆ **Balacet 325™** *see* Propoxyphene and Acetaminophen *on page 1173*

◆ **BAL in Oil®** *see* Dimercaprol *on page 447*

◆ **Balmex® [OTC]** *see* Zinc Oxide *on page 1445*

◆ **Balminil Decongestant (Can)** *see* Pseudoephedrine *on page 1183*

◆ **Balminil DM E (Can)** *see* Guaifenesin and Dextromethorphan *on page 658*

◆ **Balminil Expectorant (Can)** *see* GuaiFENesin *on page 656*

◆ **Balnetar® [OTC]** *see* Coal Tar *on page 349*

◆ **Balnetar® (Can)** *see* Coal Tar *on page 349*

Balsalazide (bal SAL a zide)

Medication Safety Issues

Sound-alike/look-alike issues:
Colazal® may be confused with Clozaril®

U.S. Brand Names Colazal®

Therapeutic Category 5-Aminosalicylic Acid Derivative; Anti-inflammatory Agent

Generic Available Yes

Use Short-term treatment of mildly to moderately active ulcerative colitis (FDA approved in ages ≥5 years and adults); Children (5-17 years): 8 weeks of therapy; Adults: 12 weeks of therapy

Pregnancy Risk Factor B

Pregnancy Considerations Teratogenic effects were not observed in animal studies. There are no adequate and well-controlled studies have been done in pregnant women. Balsalazide should be used in pregnant women only if clearly needed.

Lactation Excretion in breast milk unknown/use caution

Contraindications Hypersensitivity to balsalazide or metabolites, salicylates, or any component

Warnings May exacerbate symptoms of ulcerative colitis; reported incidence higher in children than adults (6% vs 1%). Hepatoxicity (some cases fatal) including increased liver function tests, jaundice, cholestatic jaundice, cirrhosis, and hepatocellular damage, including liver necrosis and failure, has been reported with products that contain mesalamine or are metabolized to mesalamine, including balsalazide.

Precautions Use with caution in patients with renal impairment; renal toxicity has been observed with other mesalamine (5-aminosalicylic acid) products. Patients with pyloric stenosis may have prolonged gastric retention of capsules, delaying release of drug in the colon.

Adverse Reactions

Central nervous system: Fatigue, fever, headache (children: 15%; adults: 8%), insomnia

Endocrine & metabolic: Dysmenorrhea

Gastrointestinal: Abdominal pain (children: 12% to 13%; adults: 6%), anorexia, diarrhea, dyspepsia, flatulence, hematochezia, nausea, stomatitis, ulcerative colitis exacerbation (see Warnings), vomiting

Hepatic: Hepatotoxicity (see Warnings)

Neuromuscular & skeletal: Arthralgia

Respiratory: Cough, nasopharyngitis, pharyngitis, pharyngolaryngeal pain, respiratory infection, rhinitis

Miscellaneous: Influenza

≤1%, postmarketing, and/or case reports: Alopecia, alveolitis, constipation, cramps, dry mouth, interstitial nephritis, Kawasaki-like syndrome, myalgia, myocarditis, pancreatitis, pericarditis, pleural effusion, pneumonia (with and without eosinophilia), pruritus, renal failure, urinary tract infection, vasculitis

Drug Interactions

Avoid Concomitant Use There are no known interactions where it is recommended to avoid concomitant use.

Increased Effect/Toxicity

Balsalazide may increase the levels/effects of: Heparin; Heparin (Low Molecular Weight); Thiopurine Analogs; Varicella Virus-Containing Vaccines

Decreased Effect No studies have been conducted. Oral antibiotics may potentially interfere with 5-aminosalicylic acid release in the colon.

Stability Store at 20°C to 25°C (68°F to 77°F); excursions permitted between 15° to 30°C (59° to 86°F)

Mechanism of Action Balsalazide is a prodrug, converted by bacterial azoreduction to mesalamine [5-aminosalicylic acid (5-ASA)]. Mesalamine (5-aminosalicylic acid) is the active component of sulfasalazine; the specific mechanism of action of mesalamine is unknown; however, it is thought that it may modulates local chemical mediators of the inflammatory response, especially leukotrienes; action appears topical rather than systemic

Pharmacodynamics Onset of action: Delayed; may require several days to weeks (2 weeks); similar in adults and children

Pharmacokinetics (Adult data unless noted)

Absorption: Very low and variable; in children, reported systemic absorption of 5-ASA (active) lower than adults (C_{max}: 67% lower, AUC: 64% lower)

Protein binding: ≥99%

Metabolism: Azoreduced in the colon to 5-aminosalicylic acid (active), 4-aminobenzoyl-β-alanine (inert), and N-acetylated metabolites

Half-life: Primary effect is topical (colonic mucosa); systemic half-life not determined

Time to peak serum concentration: 1-2 hours

Elimination: Feces (65% as 5-aminosalicylic acid, 4-aminobenzoyl-β-alanine, and N-acetylated metabolites); urine (11.3% as N-acetylated metabolites); Parent drug: Urine or feces (<1%)

Usual Dosage Oral:

Children (5-17 years): **Note:** Limited blinded clinical trial in children did not demonstrate significant improvement between total daily doses of 6.75 g or 2.25 g (see Quiros, 2009):

2.25 g (three 750 mg capsules) 3 times/day for up to 8 weeks (total daily dose: 6.75 g/day)

or

750 mg (one capsule) 3 times/day for up to 8 weeks (total daily dose: 2.25 g/day)

Adults: 2.25 g (three 750 mg capsules) 3 times/day for 8-12 weeks (total daily dose: 6.75 g/day)

Administration Capsules should be swallowed whole or may be opened and sprinkled on applesauce. Applesauce mixture may be chewed; swallow immediately, do not store mixture for later use. When sprinkled on food, may cause staining of teeth or tongue. Color variation of powder inside capsule (ranging from orange to yellow) is expected.

Patient Information Capsules should be swallowed whole or may be opened and sprinkled on applesauce; may cause staining of teeth or mouth when capsules are opened and sprinkled on food instead of swallowed whole. Report abdominal pain, unresolved diarrhea, or severe headache to prescriber. May cause dry mouth.

Additional Information Balsalazide 750 mg is equivalent to mesalamine 267 mg.

A twice-daily formulation (1.1 g tablet) has been developed; safety and efficacy have been shown with 3.3 g (3 tablets) twice daily (6.6 g/day) dosing for 8 weeks (see Scherl, 2009).

Dosage Forms Excipient information presented when available (limited, particularly for generics); consult specific product labeling.

Capsule, as disodium: 750 mg

Colazal®: 750 mg [contains sodium ~86 mg/capsule]

References

Quiros JA, Heyman MB, Pohl JF, et al, "Safety, Efficacy, and Pharmacokinetics of Balsalazide in Pediatric Patients With Mild-to-Moderate Active Ulcerative Colitis: Results of a Randomized, Double-Blind Study," *J Pediatr Gastroenterol Nutr*, 2009, 49(5):571-9.

Scherl EJ, Pruitt R, Gordon GL, et al, "Safety and Efficacy of a New 3.3 g b.i.d. Tablet Formulation in Patients With Mild-to-Moderately-Active Ulcerative Colitis: A Multicenter, Randomized, Double-Blind, Placebo-Controlled Study," *Am J Gastroenterol*, 2009, 104(6):1452-9.

◆ **Balsalazide Disodium** see Balsalazide *on page 172*

◆ **Band-Aid® Hurt-Free™ Antiseptic Wash [OTC]** *see* Lidocaine *on page 818*

◆ **Banophen™ [OTC]** *see* DiphenhydrAMINE *on page 448*

◆ **Banophen™ Anti-Itch [OTC]** *see* DiphenhydrAMINE *on page 448*

◆ **Baridium® [OTC]** *see* Phenazopyridine *on page 1097*

◆ **Basaljel® (Can)** *see* Aluminum Hydroxide *on page 75*

◆ **Base Ointment** *see* Zinc Oxide *on page 1445*

Basiliximab (ba si LIK si mab)

U.S. Brand Names Simulect®
Canadian Brand Names Simulect®
Therapeutic Category Monoclonal Antibody
Generic Available No
Use In combination with an immunosuppressive regimen (cyclosporine and corticosteroids), induction therapy for the prophylaxis of acute organ rejection in patients receiving renal transplants (FDA approved in pediatric patients [age not specified] and adults); basiliximab has also been used in liver and heart transplant patients

Pregnancy Risk Factor B
Pregnancy Considerations Teratogenic effects were not observed in animal studies. IL-2 receptors play an important role in the development of the immune system. Use in pregnant women only when benefit exceeds potential risk to the fetus. Women of childbearing potential should use effective contraceptive measures before beginning treatment and for 4 months after completion of therapy with this agent. The National Transplantation Pregnancy Registry (NTPR, Temple University) is a registry for pregnant women taking immunosuppressants following any solid organ transplant. The NTPR encourages reporting of all immunosuppressant exposures during pregnancy in transplant recipients at 877-955-6877.

Lactation Excretion in breast milk unknown/not recommended

Breast-Feeding Considerations It is not known whether basiliximab is excreted in human milk. Because many immunoglobulins are secreted in milk and the potential for serious adverse reactions exists, a decision should be made whether to discontinue nursing or discontinue the drug, taking into account the importance of the drug to the mother.

Contraindications Hypersensitivity to basiliximab, murine proteins, or any component of the formulation

Warnings Basiliximab should only be prescribed by physicians experienced in immunosuppression therapy and management of organ transplant patients **[U.S. Boxed Warning]**. Patients receiving basiliximab should be treated at facilities specially equipped and staffed to manage organ transplant patients.

Severe, acute hypersensitivity reactions, including anaphylaxis, have been reported following initial exposure or re-exposure to basiliximab. Patients in whom concomitant immunosuppression was prematurely discontinued (eg, abandoned transplantation or early loss of graft) are at particular risk of developing a severe hypersensitivity reaction upon readministration. If a severe hypersensitivity reaction occurs, basiliximab should be permanently discontinued. Medications for the management of severe allergic reactions should be available for immediate use.

Precautions May result in an increased susceptibility to infection or an increased risk for developing lymphoproliferative disorders. Treatment with basiliximab may result in the development of human antimurine antibodies (HAMA); however, limited evidence suggesting the use of muromonab-CD3 or other murine products is not precluded.

Adverse Reactions Note: Administration of basiliximab did not appear to increase the incidence or severity of adverse effects in clinical trials. Adverse events were reported in 96% of both the placebo and basiliximab groups.
Cardiovascular: Abnormal heart sounds, angina pectoris, arrhythmia, atrial fibrillation, chest pain, facial edema, heart failure, hyper-/hypotension, peripheral edema, tachycardia, thrombosis
Central nervous system: Agitation, anxiety, depression, dizziness, fatigue, fever, headache, hypoesthesia, insomnia, malaise, pain

Dermatologic: Acne, cyst, hypertrichosis, pruritus, rash, skin ulceration, wound complications
Endocrine & metabolic: Acidosis, dehydration, diabetes mellitus, fluid overload, glucocorticoids increased, hyper-/hypocalcemia, hypercholesterolemia, hyper-/hypoglycemia, hyper-/hypokalemia, hyperlipidemia, hypertriglyceridemia, hyperuricemia, hypomagnesemia, hyponatremia, hypophosphatemia, weight gain
Gastrointestinal: Abdomen enlarged, abdominal pain, constipation, diarrhea, dyspepsia, esophagitis, flatulence, gastroenteritis, GI hemorrhage, gingival hyperplasia, melena, moniliasis, nausea, stomatitis (including ulcerative), vomiting
Genitourinary: Bladder disorder, dysuria, genital edema, impotence, ureteral disorder, urinary frequency, urinary retention, urinary tract infection
Hematologic: Anemia, hematoma, hemorrhage, leukopenia, polycythemia, purpura, thrombocytopenia
Neuromuscular & skeletal: Arthralgia, arthropathy, back pain, cramps, fracture, hernia, leg pain, myalgia, neuropathy, paresthesia, rigors, tremor, weakness
Ocular: Cataract, conjunctivitis, vision abnormal
Renal: Albuminuria, hematuria, nonprotein nitrogen increased, oliguria, renal function abnormal, renal tubular necrosis
Respiratory: Bronchitis, bronchospasm, cough, dyspnea, infection (upper respiratory), pharyngitis, pneumonia, pulmonary edema, rhinitis, sinusitis
Miscellaneous: Anaphylaxis, hypersensitivity reactions, lymphoproliferative disease, sepsis, viral infection
<1%, postmarketing, and/or case reports: Capillary leak syndrome, cytokine release syndrome, noncardiogenic pulmonary edema

Drug Interactions
Avoid Concomitant Use
Avoid concomitant use of Basiliximab with any of the following: BCG; Natalizumab; Pimecrolimus; Tacrolimus (Topical); Vaccines (Live)

Increased Effect/Toxicity
Basiliximab may increase the levels/effects of: Hypoglycemic Agents; Leflunomide; Natalizumab; Vaccines (Live)

The levels/effects of Basiliximab may be increased by: Abciximab; Denosumab; Herbs (Hypoglycemic Properties); Pimecrolimus; Tacrolimus (Topical); Trastuzumab

Decreased Effect
Basiliximab may decrease the levels/effects of: BCG; Sipuleucel-T; Vaccines (Inactivated); Vaccines (Live)

The levels/effects of Basiliximab may be decreased by: Echinacea

Stability Store intact vials under refrigeration 2°C to 8°C (36°F to 46°F). Reconstituted solution should be used immediately after reconstitution; however, may be stored at 2°C to 8°C for up to 24 hours or at room temperature for up to 4 hours. Discard the reconstituted solution within 24 hours. Do not shake.

Mechanism of Action Chimeric (murine/human) immunosuppressant monoclonal antibody which blocks the alpha-chain of the interleukin-2 (IL-2) receptor complex; this receptor is expressed on activated T lymphocytes and is a critical pathway for activating cell-mediated allograft rejection

Pharmacodynamics
Duration: 36 days ± 14 days (determined by IL-2R alpha saturation in patients also on cyclosporine and corticosteroids)

Pharmacokinetics (Adult data unless noted) Note:

Values based on data from renal transplant patients

Distribution: V_{dss}:

Children 1-11 years: 4.8 ± 2.1 L

Adolescents 12-16 years: 7.8 ± 5.1 L

Adults: 8.6 ± 4.1 L

Half-life:

Children 1-11 years: 9.5 ± 4.5 days

Adolescents 12-16 years: 9.1 ± 3.9 days

Adults: 7.2 ± 3.2 days

Elimination: Clearance:

Children 1-11 years: 17 ± 6 mL/hour; in pediatric liver transplant patients, significant basiliximab loss through ascites fluid can increase total body clearance and reduce IL-2R (CD25) saturation duration; dosage adjustments may be necessary (see Cintorino, 2006; Kovarik, 2002; Spada, 2006)

Adolescents 12-16 years: 31 ±19 mL/hour

Adults: 41 ± 19 mL/hour

Usual Dosage I.V.: Note: Patients previously administered basiliximab should only be re-exposed to a subsequent course of therapy with extreme caution. I.V. (refer to individual protocols):

Children <35 kg:

Renal transplantation:

Initial dose: 10 mg administered within 2 hours prior to renal transplant surgery

Second dose: 10 mg administered 4 days after transplantation; hold second dose if complications occur (including severe hypersensitivity reactions or graft loss)

Liver transplantation: Limited data available (see Cintorino, 2006; Kovarik, 2002; Spada, 2006); **Note:** Infants included in clinical trials.

Initial dose: 10 mg administered within 6 hours of organ perfusion

Second dose: 10 mg administered 4 days after transplantation; hold second dose if complications occur (including severe hypersensitivity reactions or graft loss)

Third dose: 10 mg has been repeated on postoperative days 8-10 if ascites fluid loss exceeds 70 mL/kg or >5 L.

Heart transplantation: Limited data available (see Ford, 2005; Grundy, 2009); **Note:** Infants included in clinical trials.

Initial dose: 10 mg administered immediately before cardiopulmonary by-pass started or within 6 hours of organ perfusion

Second dose: 10 mg administered 4 days after transplantation; hold second dose if complications occur (including severe hypersensitivity reactions or graft loss)

Children ≥35 kg:

Renal transplantation:

Initial dose: 20 mg administered within 2 hours prior to renal transplant surgery

Second dose: 20 mg administered 4 days after transplantation; hold second dose if complications occur (including severe hypersensitivity reactions or graft loss)

Liver transplantation: Limited data available (see Cintorino, 2006; Kovarik, 2002; Spada, 2006)

Initial dose: 20 mg administered within 6 hours of organ perfusion

Second dose: 20 mg administered 4 days after transplantation; hold second dose if complications occur (including severe hypersensitivity reactions or graft loss)

Third dose: 20 mg has been repeated on postoperative days 8-10 if ascites fluid loss exceeds 70 mL/kg or if total ascites volume ≥5 L

Heart transplantation: Limited data available (see Ford, 2005; Grundy, 2009):

Initial dose: 20 mg administered immediately before cardiopulmonary by-pass started or within 6 hours of organ perfusion

Second dose: 20 mg administered 4 days after transplantation; hold second dose if complications occur (including severe hypersensitivity reactions or graft loss)

Adults: Renal transplantation:

Initial dose: 20 mg administered within 2 hours prior to renal transplant surgery

Second dose: 20 mg administered 4 days after transplantation; hold second dose if complications occur (including severe hypersensitivity reactions or graft loss)

Dosing interval in renal or hepatic impairment: No dosing adjustment recommended

Administration
For intravenous administration only. Reconstitute vials with SWI, USP. Shake the vial gently to dissolve. It is recommended that after reconstitution, the solution should be used immediately. Reconstituted basiliximab solution may be administered without further dilution as a bolus injection over 10 minutes or further dilute in NS or D5W to a final concentration of 0.4 mg/mL and infuse over 20-30 minutes. When mixing the solution, gently invert the bag to avoid foaming. Do not shake the bag. Bolus injection is associated with nausea, vomiting, and local pain at the injection site.

Monitoring Parameters
CBC with differential, vital signs, immunologic monitoring of T cells, renal function, serum glucose, signs or symptoms of hypersensitivity, infection

Reference Range
Serum concentration >0.2 mcg/mL

Patient Information
You will be susceptible to infection (avoid crowds and exposure to infection). Frequent mouth care and small frequent meals may help counteract any GI effects you may experience and will help maintain adequate nutrition and fluid intake. You may experience trouble sleeping or headaches. Report any changes in urination; unusual bruising or bleeding; chest pain or palpitations; acute dizziness; respiratory difficulty; fever or chills; changes in cognition; rash; feelings of pain or numbness in extremities; swelling of extremities; severe GI upset or diarrhea; unusual back or leg pain or muscle tremors; vision changes; or any sign of infection (eg, chills, fever, sore throat, easy bruising or bleeding, mouth sores, unhealed sores, vaginal discharge).

Dosage Forms
Excipient information presented when available (limited, particularly for generics); consult specific product labeling.

Injection, powder for reconstitution [preservative free]:

Simulect®: 10 mg, 20 mg

References

Bamgbola FO, Del Rio M, Kaskel FJ, et al, "Non-Cardiogenic Pulmonary Edema During Basiliximab Induction in Three Adolescent Renal Transplant Patients," *Pediatr Transplant*, 2003, 7(4):315-20.

Cintorino D, Riva S, Spada M, et al, "Corticosteroid-Free Immunosuppression in Pediatric Liver Transplantation: Safety and Efficacy After a Short-Term Follow-Up," *Transplant Proc*, 2006, 38(4):1099-100.

Dolan N, Waldron M, O'Connell M, et al, "Basiliximab Induced Non-Cardiogenic Pulmonary Edema in Two Pediatric Renal Transplant Recipients," *Pediatr Nephrol*, 2009, 24(11):2261-5.

Ford KA, Cale CM, Rees PG, et al, "Initial Data on Basiliximab in Critically Ill Children Undergoing Heart Transplantation," *J Heart Lung Transplant*, 2005, 24(9):1284-8.

Goulet O, Sauvat F, Ruemmele F, et al, "Results of the Paris Program: Ten Years of Pediatric Intestinal Transplantation," *Transplant Proc*, 2005, 37(4):1667-70.

Grundy N, Simmonds J, Dawkins H, et al, "Pre-Implantation Basiliximab Reduces Incidence of Early Acute Rejection in Pediatric Heart Transplantation," *J Heart Lung Transplant*, 2009, 28(12):1279-84.

Ji SQ, Chen HR, Yan HM, et al, "Anti-CD25 Monoclonal Antibody (Basiliximab) for Prevention of Graft-Versus-Host Disease After Haploidentical Bone Marrow Transplantation for Hematological Malignancies," *Bone Marrow Transplant*, 2005, 36(4):349-54.

Kovarik JM, Gridelli BG, Martin S, et al, "Basiliximab in Pediatric Liver Transplantation: A Pharmacokinetic-Derived Dosing Algorithm," *Pediatr Transplant*, 2002, 6(3):224-30.

Spada M, Petz W, Bertani A, et al, "Randomized Trial of Basiliximab Induction Versus Steroid Therapy in Pediatric Liver Allograft Recipients Under Tacrolimus Immunosuppression," *Am J Transplant*, 2006, 6(8):1913-21.

♦ **Bausch & Lomb® Computer Eye Drops [OTC]** *see* Glycerin *on page 650*

♦ **Baycadron™** *see* Dexamethasone *on page 406*

♦ **Bayer® Aspirin Extra Strength [OTC]** *see* Aspirin *on page 141*

♦ **Bayer® Aspirin Regimen Adult Low Dose [OTC]** *see* Aspirin *on page 141*

♦ **Bayer® Aspirin Regimen Children's [OTC]** *see* Aspirin *on page 141*

♦ **Bayer® Aspirin Regimen Regular Strength [OTC]** *see* Aspirin *on page 141*

♦ **Bayer® Genuine Aspirin [OTC]** *see* Aspirin *on page 141*

♦ **Bayer® Plus Extra Strength [OTC]** *see* Aspirin *on page 141*

♦ **Bayer® with Heart Advantage [OTC] [DSC]** *see* Aspirin *on page 141*

♦ **Bayer® Women's Aspirin Plus Calcium [OTC] [DSC]** *see* Aspirin *on page 141*

♦ **Bayer® Women's Low Dose Aspirin [OTC]** *see* Aspirin *on page 141*

♦ **BayGam® (Can)** *see* Immune Globulin (Intramuscular) *on page 718*

♦ **Baza® Antifungal [OTC]** *see* Miconazole *on page 927*

♦ **BCNU** *see* Carmustine *on page 252*

♦ **BCX-1812** *see* Peramivir *on page 1092*

♦ **BD™ Glucose [OTC]** *see* Dextrose *on page 422*

♦ **Bebulin® VH** *see* Factor IX Complex (Human) *on page 558*

Beclomethasone (be kloe METH a sone)

Medication Safety Issues
Sound-alike/look-alike issues:
Vanceril® may be confused with Vancenase®

Related Information
Asthma *on page 1697*

U.S. Brand Names Beconase® AQ; QVAR®

Canadian Brand Names Apo-Beclomethasone®; Gen-Beclo; Mylan-Beclo AQ; Nu-Beclomethasone; Propaderm®; QVAR®; Rivanase AQ; Vanceril® AEM

Therapeutic Category Adrenal Corticosteroid; Anti-inflammatory Agent; Antiasthmatic; Corticosteroid, Inhalant (Oral); Corticosteroid, Intranasal; Glucocorticoid

Generic Available No

Use
Oral inhalation: Long-term (chronic) control of persistent bronchial asthma (FDA approved in ages ≥5 years and adults); **NOT** indicated for the relief of acute bronchospasm. Also used to help reduce or discontinue oral corticosteroid therapy for asthma.

Intranasal: Management of seasonal or perennial rhinitis and nasal polyposis (FDA approved in ages ≥6 years and adults)

Pregnancy Risk Factor C

Pregnancy Considerations Teratogenic effects were observed in animal studies. No human data on beclomethasone crossing the placenta or effects on the fetus. A decrease in fetal growth has not been observed with inhaled corticosteroid use during pregnancy. Inhaled corticosteroids are recommended for the treatment of asthma (most information available using budesonide) and allergic rhinitis during pregnancy.

Lactation Excretion in breast milk unknown/use caution

Breast-Feeding Considerations Other corticosteroids have been found in breast milk; however, information for beclomethasone is not available. Inhaled corticosteroids are recommended for the treatment of asthma (most information available using budesonide) while breast-feeding.

Contraindications Hypersensitivity to beclomethasone or any component; primary treatment of status asthmaticus or other acute episodes of bronchial asthma where intensive treatment is needed

Warnings Fatalities have occurred due to adrenal insufficiency in asthmatic patients during and after switching from systemic corticosteroids to aerosol steroids; several months may be required for full recovery of hypothalamic-pituitary-adrenal (HPA) function; patients receiving higher doses of systemic corticosteroids (eg, adults receiving ≥20 mg of prednisone per day) may be at greater risk; during this period of HPA suppression, aerosol steroids do **not** provide the systemic glucocorticoid or mineralocorticoid activity needed to treat patients requiring stress doses (ie, patients with major stress such as trauma, surgery, or infections, or other conditions associated with severe electrolyte loss). When used at high doses or for a prolonged time, hypercorticism and HPA suppression (including adrenal crisis) may occur; use with inhaled or systemic corticosteroids (even alternate-day dosing) may increase risk of HPA suppression. Acute adrenal insufficiency may occur with abrupt withdrawal after long-term use or with stress; withdrawal and discontinuation of corticosteroids should be done carefully; patients with HPA axis suppression may require doses of systemic glucocorticosteroids prior to, during, and after unusual stress (eg, surgery). Immunosuppression may occur; patients may be more susceptible to infections; avoid exposure to chickenpox and measles. Switching from systemic corticosteroids to inhalation may unmask allergic conditions (such as eczema, conjunctivitis, and rhinitis) that were previously suppressed by systemic steroids. Bronchospasm may occur after use of inhaled asthma medications (see Additional Information).

Precautions Avoid using higher than recommended dosages; suppression of HPA function, suppression of linear growth (ie, reduction of growth velocity), reduced bone mineral density, hypercorticism (Cushing's syndrome), hyperglycemia, or glucosuria may occur. Use with extreme caution in patients with respiratory tuberculosis, untreated systemic infections, or ocular herpes simplex. Use with caution and monitor patients closely with hepatic dysfunction. Rare cases of increased IOP, glaucoma, or cataracts may occur.

Adverse Reactions
Central nervous system: Headache, dizziness, malaise, fatigue, insomnia

Endocrine & metabolic: HPA suppression, Cushing's syndrome, growth suppression, hyperglycemia, dysmenorrhea

Gastrointestinal: Xerostomia, sore throat, pharyngitis, nausea, vomiting, diarrhea, dyspepsia

Local: Growth of *Candida* in the mouth, throat, or nares

Neuromuscular & skeletal: Growth velocity suppression (reported in asthmatic children receiving oral inhalation 2 puffs 4 times/day); muscular soreness, osteoporosis, bone mineral density decreased

Ocular: Cataracts, IOP increased, glaucoma

Respiratory: Cough, sneezing, hoarseness, dysphonia; irritation and burning of the nasal mucosa, nasal ulceration, epistaxis, rhinorrhea, nasal congestion (intranasal use)

Miscellaneous: Immunosuppression, anaphylactoid reactions (rare)

Drug Interactions

Avoid Concomitant Use

Avoid concomitant use of Beclomethasone with any of the following: Aldesleukin; BCG; Natalizumab; Pimecrolimus; Tacrolimus (Topical); Vaccines (Live)

Increased Effect/Toxicity

Beclomethasone may increase the levels/effects of: Amphotericin B; Leflunomide; Loop Diuretics; Natalizumab; Thiazide Diuretics; Vaccines (Live)

The levels/effects of Beclomethasone may be increased by: Denosumab; Pimecrolimus; Tacrolimus (Topical); Trastuzumab

Decreased Effect

Beclomethasone may decrease the levels/effects of: Aldesleukin; Antidiabetic Agents; BCG; Corticorelin; Sipuleucel-T; Vaccines (Inactivated); Vaccines (Live)

The levels/effects of Beclomethasone may be decreased by: Echinacea

Stability Do not store near heat or open flame; store QVAR® so inhaler rests on concave end of canister (with plastic actuator on top); use Vanceril® within 6 months after removal from moisture protective package

Mechanism of Action Controls the rate of protein synthesis, depresses the migration of polymorphonuclear leukocytes and fibroblasts, reverses capillary permeability, and stabilizes lysosomal membranes at the cellular level to prevent or control inflammation

Pharmacodynamics

Onset of action:
Oral inhalation: Within 1-2 days in some patients; usually within 1-2 weeks
Nasal inhalation: Within a few days up to 2 weeks
Maximum effect: Oral inhalation: 3-4 weeks

Pharmacokinetics (Adult data unless noted)

Absorption: Inhalation: Readily absorbed; quickly hydrolyzed by pulmonary esterases to active metabolite, beclomethasone-17-monoproprionate (17-BMP), prior to absorption

Distribution: Secreted into breast milk
V_d: Adults: Beclomethasone dipropionate (BDP): 20 L; 17-BMP: 424 L

Protein binding: BDP 87%; 17-BMP: 94% to 96%

Metabolism: BDP is a prodrug (inactive) which undergoes rapid hydrolysis to 17-BMP (active monoester) during absorption; BDP is also metabolized in the liver via cytochrome P450 isoenzyme CYP3A4 to 17-BMP and two other less active metabolites: Beclomethasone-21-monopropionate (21-BMP) and beclomethasone (BOH)

Bioavailability: Nasal inhalation: 17-BMP: 44% (43% from swallowed portion)

Half-life, elimination: BDP: 0.5 hours; 17-BMP: 2.7 hours

Time to peak serum concentration: Oral inhalation: BDP: 0.5 hours; 17-BMP: 0.7 hours

Elimination: Primary route of excretion is via feces (~60%); <10% to 12% of oral dose excreted in urine as metabolites

Usual Dosage

Aqueous inhalation, nasal:
Beconase® AQ:
Children 6-12 years: Initial: 1 inhalation in each nostril twice daily; may increase if needed to 2 inhalations in each nostril twice daily; once symptoms are adequately controlled, decrease dose to 1 inhalation in each nostril twice daily
Children ≥12 years and Adults: 1-2 inhalations in each nostril twice daily

Oral inhalation (doses should be titrated to the lowest effective dose once asthma is controlled):
QVAR®:
Children 5-11 years: Initial: 40 mcg twice daily; maximum dose: 80 mcg twice daily

Children ≥12 years and Adults:
No previous inhaled corticosteroids: Initial: 40-80 mcg twice daily; maximum dose: 320 mcg twice daily
Previous inhaled corticosteroid use: Initial: 40-160 mcg twice daily; maximum dose: 320 mcg twice daily

Note: Therapeutic ratio between QVAR® and other beclomethasone inhalers has not been established; when switching to QVAR®, monitor patients for efficacy and adverse effects (see Additional Information)

NIH Asthma Guidelines (NAEPP, 2007) [give in divided doses]:
HFA formulation (eg, QVAR®):
Children 5-11 years:
"Low" dose: 80-160 mcg/day (40 mcg/puff: 2-4 puffs/day or 80 mcg/puff: 1-2 puffs/day)
"Medium" dose: >160-320 mcg/day (40 mcg/puff: 4-8 puffs/day or 80 mcg/puff: 2-4 puffs/day)
"High" dose: >320 mcg/day (40 mcg/puff: >8 puffs/day or 80 mcg/puff: >4 puff/day)
Children ≥12 years and Adults:
"Low" dose: 80-240 mcg/day (40 mcg/puff: 2-6 puffs/day or 80 mcg/puff: 1-3 puffs/day)
"Medium" dose: >240-480 mcg/day (40 mcg/puff: 6-12 puffs/day or 80 mcg/puff: 3-6 puffs/day)
"High" dose: >480 mcg/day (40 mcg/puff: >12 puffs/day or 80 mcg/puff: 6 puffs/day)

Administration

Nasal inhalation: Shake container well before use; gently blow nose to clear nasal passages before administration; occlude one nostril with finger while carefully inserting nasal applicator into other nostril to administer dose

Oral inhalation: Prime canister before use. Use a spacer device for children 5-8 years of age; **Note:** Use of Qvar® with a spacer device is not recommended in children <5 years of age due to the decreased amount of medication that is delivered with increasing wait times; patients should be instructed to inhale immediately if using a spacer device. Rinse mouth after use to prevent *Candida* infection. Do not wash or put inhaler in water; mouthpiece may be cleaned with a dry tissue or cloth.

Monitoring Parameters Check mucous membranes for signs of fungal infection. Monitor growth in pediatric patient. Monitor IOP with therapy >6 weeks

Patient Information Notify physician if condition being treated persists or worsens; do not decrease dose or discontinue without physician approval; may cause dry mouth; avoid spraying in eyes; avoid exposure to chicken pox or measles; if exposed, seek medical advice without delay; discard canister when labeled number of metered doses (sprays) have been used. QVAR® may taste differently and have a different feeling during inhalation compared to other inhalers containing chlorofluorocarbons (CFCs).

Oral inhalant: Rinse mouth after inhalation to decrease chance of oral candidiasis; report sore mouth or mouth lesions to physician

Additional Information

Oral inhalation: If bronchospasm with wheezing occurs after use, a fast-acting bronchodilator may be used; discontinue orally inhaled corticosteroid and initiate alternative chronic therapy.

QVAR®: Does not contain chlorofluorocarbons (CFCs), uses hydrofluoroalkane (HFA) as the propellant; is a solution formulation (other beclomethasone inhalers are suspension aerosols); uses smaller-size particles which results in a higher percent of drug delivered to the respiratory tract and lower recommended doses than other products. An open-label, randomized, multicenter, 12-month study in 300 asthmatic children 5-11 years of age indicated that QVAR® provided long-term control of asthma at approximately half the dose compared with a CFC propelled beclomethasone MDI and spacer (see Pederson, 2002). Further studies are needed to define therapeutic ratio between QVAR® and other beclomethasone inhalers.

Aqueous beclomethasone nasal spray (42 mcg/inhalation; 2 sprays in each nostril twice daily for 4 weeks, followed by 1 spray in each nostril twice daily) may be useful in reducing adenoidal hypertrophy and nasal airway obstruction in children 5-11 years of age (Demain, 1995)

Dosage Forms Excipient information presented when available (limited, particularly for generics); consult specific product labeling.

Aerosol for oral inhalation, as dipropionate:
QVAR®: 40 mcg/inhalation [100 metered actuations] (7.3 g); 80 mcg/inhalation [100 metered actuations] (7.3 g)

Suspension, intranasal, as dipropionate [aqueous spray]:
Beconase® AQ: 42 mcg/inhalation [180 metered sprays] (25 g)

References

Demain JG and Goetz DW, "Pediatric Adenoidal Hypertrophy and Nasal Airway Obstruction: Reduction With Aqueous Nasal Beclomethasone," *Pediatrics*, 1995, 95(3):355-64.

Kobayashi RH, Tinkelman DG, Reese ME, et al, "Beclomethasone Dipropionate Aqueous Nasal Spray for Seasonal Allergic Rhinitis in Children," *Ann Allergy*, 1989, 62(3):205-8.

National Asthma Education and Prevention Program (NAEPP), "Expert Panel Report 3 (EPR-3): Guidelines for the Diagnosis and Management of Asthma," *Clinical Practice Guidelines*, National Institutes of Health, National Heart, Lung, and Blood Institute, NIH Publication No. 08-4051, prepublication 2007; available at http://www.nhlbi.nih.gov/guidelines/asthma/asthgdln.htm.

Pedersen S, Warner J, Wahn U, et al, "Growth, Systemic Safety, and Efficacy During 1 Year of Asthma Treatment With Different Beclomethasone Dipropionate Formulations: An Open-Label, Randomized Comparison of Extra Fine and Conventional Aerosols in Children," *Pediatrics*, 2002, 109(6), http://www.pediatrics.org/cgi/content/full/109/6/e92.

Tinkelman DG, Reed CE, Nelson HS, et al, "Aerosol Beclomethasone Dipropionate Compared With Theophylline as Primary Treatment of Chronic, Mild to Moderately Severe Asthma in Children," *Pediatrics*, 1993, 92(1):64-77.

Wyatt R, Waschek J, Weinberger M, et al, "Effects of Inhaled Beclomethasone Dipropionate and Alternate-Day Prednisone on Pituitary-Adrenal Function in Children With Chronic Asthma," *N Engl J Med*, 1978, 299(25):1387-92.

◆ **Beclomethasone Dipropionate** see Beclomethasone on page 176

◆ **Beconase® AQ** see Beclomethasone on page 176

◆ **Belladonna Alkaloids With Phenobarbital** see Hyoscyamine, Atropine, Scopolamine, and Phenobarbital on page 700

Belladonna and Opium (bel a DON a & OH pee um)

Medication Safety Issues
Sound-alike/look-alike issues:
B&O may be confused with beano®

Beers Criteria medication: This drug may be inappropriate for use in geriatric patients (high severity risk).

U.S. Brand Names B&O Supprettes® [DSC]

Therapeutic Category Analgesic, Narcotic; Antispasmodic Agent, Urinary

Generic Available Yes

Use Relief of moderate to severe pain associated with rectal or bladder tenesmus that may occur in postoperative states and neoplastic situations; relief of pain associated with ureteral spasms not responsive to non-narcotic analgesics and to space intervals between injections of opiates

Restrictions C-II

Pregnancy Risk Factor C

Pregnancy Considerations Reproduction studies have not been conducted with this product. Refer to Atropine and Morphine Sulfate monographs for additional information.

Lactation Excretion in breast milk unknown/use caution

Breast-Feeding Considerations It is not known if/how much morphine or atropine may be found in breast milk following rectal administration of this product. Refer to Atropine and Morphine Sulfate monographs for additional information.

Contraindications Hypersensitivity to belladonna, atropine, opium alkaloids, morphine, or any component; glaucoma; severe renal or hepatic disease; obstructive uropathy; obstructive disease of the GI tract; severe respiratory depression; convulsive disorders; acute alcoholism; premature labor

Warnings Opium shares the toxic potential of opiate agonists; usual precautions of opiate agonist therapy should be observed; not recommended for use in children <12 years

Precautions Use with caution in patients with cardiac, respiratory, hepatic, or renal dysfunction, severe prostatic hypertrophy, or history of narcotic abuse; use with caution in patients with increased intracranial pressure

Adverse Reactions
Cardiovascular: Orthostatic hypotension, ventricular fibrillation, tachycardia, palpitations
Central nervous system: Confusion, drowsiness, headache, loss of memory, fatigue, ataxia, CNS depression, physical and psychological dependence
Dermatologic: Dry skin, sensitivity to light increased, rash, pruritus, urticaria
Endocrine & metabolic: Flow of breast milk decreased, antidiuretic hormone release
Gastrointestinal: Constipation, dry throat, xerostomia, dysphagia, bloated feeling, nausea, vomiting, constipation, biliary tract spasm
Genitourinary: Dysuria, urinary retention, urinary tract spasm
Neuromuscular & skeletal: Weakness
Ocular: Intraocular pain, blurred vision, photophobia
Respiratory: Dry nose, respiratory depression
Miscellaneous: Diaphoresis decreased, histamine release

Drug Interactions
Avoid Concomitant Use There are no known interactions where it is recommended to avoid concomitant use.

Increased Effect/Toxicity
Belladonna and Opium may increase the levels/effects of: AbobotulinumtoxinA; Alcohol (Ethyl); Alvimopan; Anticholinergics; Cannabinoids; CNS Depressants; Desmopressin; OnabotulinumtoxinA; Potassium Chloride; RimabotulinumtoxinB; Selective Serotonin Reuptake Inhibitors; Thiazide Diuretics

The levels/effects of Belladonna and Opium may be increased by: Amphetamines; Antipsychotic Agents (Phenothiazines); MAO Inhibitors; Pramlintide; Succinylcholine

Decreased Effect
Belladonna and Opium may decrease the levels/effects of: Acetylcholinesterase Inhibitors (Central); Pegvisomant; Secretin

The levels/effects of Belladonna and Opium may be decreased by: Acetylcholinesterase Inhibitors (Central); Ammonium Chloride; Mixed Agonist / Antagonist Opioids

Food Interactions Avoid ethanol (may increase sedation).

Stability Store at room temperature; avoid freezing

Mechanism of Action Anticholinergic alkaloids act primarily by competitive inhibition of the muscarinic actions of acetylcholine on structures innervated by postganglionic cholinergic neurons and on smooth muscle; resulting effects include antisecretory activity on exocrine glands and intestinal mucosa and smooth muscle relaxation. Contains many narcotic alkaloids including morphine; its mechanism for gastric motility inhibition is primarily due to this morphine content; it results in a decrease in digestive secretions, an increase in GI muscle tone, and therefore a reduction in GI propulsion.

Pharmacodynamics Opium: Onset of action: Within 30 minutes

Pharmacokinetics (Adult data unless noted) Metabolism: Hepatic

Usual Dosage Rectal: Adults: 1 suppository 1-2 times/day, up to 4 doses/day

Administration Rectal: Remove from foil; moisten finger and suppository; insert rectally

Patient Information Drug may cause physical and/or psychological dependence; avoid abrupt discontinuation after prolonged use. Avoid alcohol; may cause drowsiness and impair ability to perform activities requiring mental alertness or physical coordination; may cause dry mouth

Dosage Forms Excipient information presented when available (limited, particularly for generics); consult specific product labeling. [DSC] = Discontinued product

Suppository: Belladonna extract 16.2 mg and opium 30 mg; belladonna extract 16.2 mg and opium 60 mg
B&O Supprettes® #15 A: Belladonna extract 16.2 mg and opium 30 mg [DSC]
B&O Supprettes® #16 A: Belladonna extract 16.2 mg and opium 60 mg [DSC]

◆ **Benadryl® (Can)** see DiphenhydrAMINE on page 448

◆ **Benadryl® Allergy [OTC]** see DiphenhydrAMINE on page 448

◆ **Benadryl® Allergy Quick Dissolve [OTC]** see DiphenhydrAMINE on page 448

◆ **Benadryl® Children's Allergy [OTC]** see DiphenhydrAMINE on page 448

◆ **Benadryl® Children's Allergy Fastmelt® [OTC]** see DiphenhydrAMINE on page 448

◆ **Benadryl® Children's Allergy Perfect Measure™** see DiphenhydrAMINE on page 448

◆ **Benadryl® Children's Dye-Free Allergy [OTC]** see DiphenhydrAMINE on page 448

◆ **Benadryl® Children's Allergy Quick Dissolve [OTC] [DSC]** see DiphenhydrAMINE on page 448

◆ **Benadryl® Dye-Free Allergy [OTC]** see DiphenhydrAMINE on page 448

◆ **Benadryl® Itch Relief Extra Strength [OTC]** see DiphenhydrAMINE on page 448

◆ **Benadryl® Itch Stopping [OTC]** see DiphenhydrAMINE on page 448

◆ **Benadryl® Itch Stopping Extra Strength [OTC]** see DiphenhydrAMINE on page 448

Benazepril (ben AY ze pril)

Medication Safety Issues
Sound-alike/look-alike issues:
Benazepril may be confused with Benadryl®
Lotensin® may be confused with Lioresal®, lovastatin

International issues:
Lotensin® may be confused with Latensin® which is a brand name for bacillus cereus in Germany

Related Information
Antihypertensive Agents by Class on page 1481

U.S. Brand Names Lotensin®

Canadian Brand Names Apo-Benazepril®; Lotensin®

Therapeutic Category Angiotensin-Converting Enzyme (ACE) Inhibitor; Antihypertensive Agent

Generic Available Yes

Use Treatment of hypertension, either alone or in combination with a thiazide diuretic (FDA approved in ages ≥6 years and adults)

Pregnancy Risk Factor D

Pregnancy Considerations Due to adverse events observed in humans, benazepril is considered pregnancy category D. Benazepril crosses the placenta. First trimester exposure to ACE inhibitors may cause major congenital malformations. An increased risk of cardiovascular and/or central nervous system malformations was observed in one study; however, an increased risk of teratogenic events was not observed in other studies. Second and third trimester use of an ACE inhibitor is associated with oligohydramnios. Oligohydramnios due to decreased fetal renal function may lead to fetal limb contractures, craniofacial deformation, and hypoplastic lung development. The use of ACE inhibitors during the second and third trimesters is also associated with anuria, hypotension, renal failure (reversible or irreversible), skull hypoplasia, and death in the fetus/neonate. Chronic maternal hypertension itself is also associated with adverse events in the fetus/infant. ACE inhibitors are not recommended during pregnancy to treat maternal hypertension or heart failure. Those who are planning a pregnancy should be considered for other medication options if an ACE inhibitor is currently prescribed or the ACE inhibitor should be discontinued as soon as possible once pregnancy is detected. The exposed fetus should be monitored for fetal growth, amniotic fluid volume, and organ formation. Infants exposed to an ACE inhibitor in utero, especially during the second and third trimester, should be monitored for hyperkalemia, hypotension, and oliguria.

[U.S. Boxed Warning]: Based on human data, ACE inhibitors can cause injury and death to the developing fetus. ACE inhibitors should be discontinued as soon as possible once pregnancy is detected.

Lactation Enters breast milk

Breast-Feeding Considerations Small amounts of benazepril and benazeprilat are found in breast milk.

Contraindications Hypersensitivity to benazepril, any component, or other ACE inhibitors; patients with a history of angioedema (with or without prior ACE inhibitor therapy)

Warnings Serious adverse effects including angioedema, anaphylactoid reactions, neutropenia, agranulocytosis, hypotension, and hepatic failure may occur (see Adverse Reactions). Angioedema can occur at any time during treatment (especially following first dose). Angioedema may occur in the head, neck, extremities, or intestines; angioedema of the larynx, glottis, or tongue may cause airway obstruction, especially in patients with a history of airway surgery; prolonged monitoring may be required, even in patients with swelling of only the tongue (ie, without respiratory distress) because treatment with corticosteroids and antihistamines may not be sufficient; very rare fatalities have occurred with angioedema of the larynx or tongue; appropriate treatment (eg, establishing patent airway and/or SubQ epinephrine) should be readily available for patients with angioedema of larynx, glottis, or tongue, in whom airway obstruction is likely to occur. Risk of neutropenia may be increased in patients with renal dysfunction and especially in patients with both collagen vascular disease and renal dysfunction. A nonproductive, persistent cough may occur with any ACE inhibitor (presumably due to accumulation of bradykinin).

ACE inhibitors can cause injury and death to the developing fetus when used during pregnancy. ACE inhibitors should be discontinued as soon as possible once pregnancy is detected **[U.S. Boxed Warning]**. Neonatal hypotension, skull hypoplasia, anuria, renal failure, oligohydramnios (associated with fetal limb contractures, craniofacial deformities, hypoplastic lung development), prematurity, intrauterine growth retardation, patent ductus arteriosus, and death have been reported with the use of ACE inhibitors, primarily in the second and third trimesters. The risk of neonatal toxicity has been considered less when ACE inhibitors are used in the first trimester; however, major congenital malformations have been reported. The cardiovascular and/or central nervous systems are most commonly affected.

Precautions Careful blood pressure monitoring is required (hypotension can occur especially in volume-depleted patients). Use with caution in patients with hypovolemia; collagen vascular diseases; valvular stenosis (particularly aortic stenosis); hyperkalemia; or before, during, or immediately after anesthesia (vasodilating anesthesia increases endogenous renin release; use of ACE inhibitors perioperatively will blunt angiotensin II formation and may result in hypotension). Avoid rapid dosage escalation which may lead to renal insufficiency. Rare toxicities associated with ACE inhibitors include cholestatic jaundice (which may progress to hepatic necrosis) and neutropenia/agranulocytosis with myeloid hyperplasia. Hyperkalemia may rarely occur. ACE inhibitors may be associated with deterioration of renal function and/or increases in serum creatinine, particularly in patients dependent on renin-angiotensin-aldosterone system (eg, those with severe CHF). Use with caution and decrease dose in patients with renal impairment. Use with caution in patients with renal artery stenosis or pre-existing renal insufficiency; if patient has renal impairment, then a baseline WBC with differential and serum creatinine should be evaluated and monitored closely during the first 3 months of therapy. Hypersensitivity reactions may be seen during hemodialysis with high-flux dialysis membranes (eg, AN69). ACE inhibitors should not be administered to infants <1 year of age due to possible effects on kidney development; long-term effects of benazepril on growth and development have not be evaluated.

Adverse Reactions Note: The adverse reaction profile for pediatric patients is similar to that observed in adults.

Cardiovascular: Hypotension (see Warnings), postural hypotension

Central nervous system: Dizziness, fatigue, headache, somnolence

Dermatologic: Angioedema (see Warnings). **Note:** The relative risk of angioedema with ACE inhibitors is higher within the first 30 days of use (compared to >1 year of use), for Black Americans (compared to Caucasians), for lisinopril or enalapril (compared to captopril), and for patients hospitalized within 30 days (see Brown, 1996).

Endocrine & metabolic: Hyperkalemia

Gastrointestinal: Nausea

Hematologic: Agranulocytosis, neutropenia (see Warnings)

Hepatic: Cholestatic jaundice, hepatitis, fulminant hepatic necrosis (rare, but potentially fatal) (see Warnings)

Renal: BUN and serum creatinine increased, worsening of renal function (in patients with bilateral renal artery stenosis or hypovolemia)

Respiratory: Cough (see Warnings)

Note: An isolated dry cough lasting >3 weeks was reported in 7 of 42 pediatric patients (17%) receiving ACE inhibitors (see von Vigier, 2000).

Miscellaneous: Anaphylactoid reactions (see Warnings)

<1%, postmarketing, and/or case reports (limited to important or life-threatening): Alopecia, angina, arthralgia, arthritis, asthma, dermatitis, dyspnea, ECG changes, eosinophilia, eosinophilic pneumonitis, flushing, gastritis, hemoglobin decreased, hemolytic anemia, hyperbilirubinemia, hyperglycemia, hypersensitivity, hypertonia, hyponatremia, impotence, insomnia, leukopenia, melena, myalgia, palpitations, pancreatitis, paresthesia, pemphigus, peripheral edema, photosensitivity, postural hypotension, proteinuria, pruritus, rash, shock, Stevens-Johnson syndrome, syncope, thrombocytopenia, transaminases increased, uric acid increased, vomiting

Drug Interactions

Avoid Concomitant Use There are no known interactions where it is recommended to avoid concomitant use.

Increased Effect/Toxicity

Benazepril may increase the levels/effects of: Allopurinol; Amifostine; Antihypertensives; AzaTHIOprine; CycloSPORINE; CycloSPORINE (Systemic); Ferric Gluconate; Gold Sodium Thiomalate; Hypotensive Agents; Iron Dextran Complex; Lithium; RiTUXimab

The levels/effects of Benazepril may be increased by: Angiotensin II Receptor Blockers; Diazoxide; DPP-IV Inhibitors; Eplerenone; Everolimus; Herbs (Hypotensive Properties); Loop Diuretics; MAO Inhibitors; Pentoxifylline; Phosphodiesterase 5 Inhibitors; Potassium Salts; Potassium-Sparing Diuretics; Prostacyclin Analogues; Sirolimus; Temsirolimus; Thiazide Diuretics; Tolvaptan; Trimethoprim

Decreased Effect

The levels/effects of Benazepril may be decreased by: Antacids; Aprotinin; Herbs (Hypertensive Properties); Methylphenidate; Nonsteroidal Anti-Inflammatory Agents; Salicylates; Yohimbine

Food Interactions Food decreases the rate, but does not significantly decrease the extent of absorption. Limit salt substitutes or potassium-rich diet. Avoid natural licorice (causes sodium and water retention and increases potassium loss).

Stability Store at temperatures ≤30°C (86°F); protect from moisture; dispense in tight container

Mechanism of Action Competitive inhibitor of angiotensin-converting enzyme (ACE); prevents conversion of angiotensin I to angiotensin II, a potent vasoconstrictor; results in lower levels of angiotensin II which causes an increase in plasma renin activity and a reduction in aldosterone secretion; a CNS mechanism may also be involved in hypotensive effect as angiotensin II increases adrenergic outflow from CNS; vasoactive kallikreins may be decreased in conversion to active hormones by ACE inhibitors, thus reducing blood pressure

Pharmacodynamics Adults:

Maximum effect:

Reduction in plasma angiotensin-converting enzyme (ACE) activity: 1-2 hours after 2-20 mg dose

Reduction in blood pressure: Single dose: 2-4 hours; Continuous therapy: 2 weeks

Duration: Reduction in plasma angiotensin-converting enzyme (ACE) activity: >90% inhibition for 24 hours after 5-20 mg dose

Pharmacokinetics (Adult data unless noted)

Absorption: Oral: 37%; rapidly absorbed; **Note:** Metabolite (benazeprilat) is unsuitable for oral administration due to poor absorption

Distribution: V_d: ~8.7 L

Protein binding: Benazepril: 97%; benazeprilat: 95%

Metabolism: Rapidly and extensively metabolized (primarily in the liver) to benazeprilat (active metabolite), via cleavage of ester group; extensive first-pass effect. Benazeprilat is about 200 times more potent than benazepril. Parent and active metabolite undergo glucuronide conjugation

Half-life: Benazeprilat: Terminal:

Children 6-16 years: 5 hours

Adults: 22 hours

Time to peak serum concentration: Oral:

Parent drug: 0.5-1 hour

Active metabolite (benazeprilat):

Fasting: 1-2 hours

Nonfasting: 2-4 hours

Elimination: Hepatic clearance is the main elimination route of unchanged benazepril. Only trace amounts of unchanged benazepril appear in the urine; 20% of dose is excreted in urine as benazeprilat, 8% as benazeprilat glucuronide, and 4% as benazepril glucuronide

Clearance: Nonrenal excretion (ie, biliary) appears to contribute to the elimination of benazeprilat (11% to 12% in healthy adults); biliary clearance may be increased in patients with severe renal impairment

Dialysis: ~6% of metabolite removed within 4 hours of dialysis following 10 mg of benazepril administered 2 hours prior to procedure; parent compound not found in dialysate

Usual Dosage Oral: Hypertension: **Note:** Dosage must be titrated according to patient's response; use lowest effective dose

Children <6 years: Dosage not established; manufacturer does not recommend use

Children ≥6 years: Initial: 0.2 mg/kg once daily (up to 10 mg/day) as monotherapy; maintenance: 0.1-0.6 mg/kg once daily (maximum: 40 mg/day)

Adults: Initial: 10 mg once daily in patients not receiving a diuretic; maintenance: 20-40 mg/day as a single dose or 2 divided doses; the need for twice-daily dosing should be assessed by monitoring peak (2-6 hours after dosing) and trough blood pressure responses. Doses >80 mg/ day have not been evaluated.

Note: To decrease the risk of hypotension, patients taking diuretics should have diuretics discontinued 2-3 days prior to starting benazepril; diuretic may be resumed if blood pressure is not controlled with benazepril monotherapy. If diuretics cannot be discontinued prior to starting benazepril, then an initial dose of benazepril of 5 mg once daily should be used.

Dosing adjustment in renal impairment:

Children: Cl_{cr} <30 mL/minute/1.73 m^2: Use is not recommended (insufficient data exists; dose not established)

Adults: Cl_{cr} <30 mL/minute/1.73 m^2: Initial: 5 mg once daily, then increase as required to a maximum of 40 mg/ day

Administration Oral: May be administered without regard to food.

Monitoring Parameters Blood pressure (supervise for at least 2 hours after the initial dose or any dosage increase for significant orthostasis); renal function, WBC, serum potassium; monitor for angioedema and anaphylactoid reactions (see Warnings)

Patient Information Notify physician immediately if swelling of face, lips, tongue, or difficulty in breathing occurs; if these occur, do not take any more doses until a physician can be consulted. Notify physician if vomiting, diarrhea, excessive perspiration, dehydration, or persistent cough occurs. Do not add a salt substitute (potassium-containing) without physician advice. May cause dizziness, fainting, and lightheadedness, especially in first week of therapy. Sit and stand up slowly. May cause changes in taste or rash. Report sore throat, fever, other signs of infection, or other side effects. This medication may cause injury and death to the developing fetus when used during pregnancy; women of childbearing potential should be informed of potential risk; consult prescriber for appropriate contraceptive measures; this medication should be discontinued as soon as possible once pregnancy is detected (see Warnings).

Nursing Implications Discontinue if angioedema occurs; observe closely for hypotension after the first dose or initiation of a new higher dose (keep in mind that maximum effect on blood pressure occurs at 2-4 hours)

Dosage Forms Excipient information presented when available (limited, particularly for generics); consult specific product labeling.

Tablet, as hydrochloride: 5 mg, 10 mg, 20 mg, 40 mg

Lotensin®: 5 mg, 10 mg, 20 mg, 40 mg

Extemporaneous Preparations To prepare a 2 mg/mL suspension, mix fifteen benazepril 20 mg tablets in an amber polyethylene terephthalate bottle with Ora-Plus® 75 mL. Shake for 2 minutes, allow suspension to stand for ≥1 hour, then shake again for at least 1 additional minute. Add Ora-Sweet® 75 mL to suspension and shake to disperse. Will make 150 mL of a 2 mg/mL suspension. Store under refrigeration at 2°C to 8°C (36°F to 46°F) for up to 30 days; label "shake well" prior to each use.

Lotensin® (package insert), Suffern, NY: Novartis Pharmaceuticals Corporation, 2009.

References

ALLHAT Officers and Coordinators for the ALLHAT Collaborative Research Group, "Major Outcomes in High-Risk Hypertensive Patients Randomized to Angiotensin-Converting Enzyme Inhibitor or Calcium Channel Blocker vs Diuretic: The Antihypertensive and Lipid-Lowering Treatment to Prevent Heart Attack Trial (ALLHAT)," *JAMA*, 2002, 288(23):2981-97.

Antman EM, Anbe DT, Armstrong PW, et al, "ACC/AHA Guidelines for the Management of Patients With ST-Elevation Myocardial Infarction - Executive Summary: A Report of the American College of Cardiology/ American Heart Association Task Force on Practice Guidelines (Writing Committee to Revise the 1999 Guidelines for the Management of Patients With Acute Myocardial Infarction)," *Circulation*, 2004, 110:588-636.

Brown NJ, Ray WA, Snowden M, et al, "Black Americans Have an Increased Rate of Angiotensin-Converting Enzyme Inhibitor-Associated Angioedema," *Clin Pharmacol Ther*, 1996, 60(1):8-13.

Chase MP, Fiarman GS, Scholz FJ, et al, "Angioedema of the Small Bowel Due to an Angiotensin-Converting Enzyme Inhibitor," *J Clin Gastroenterol*, 2000, 31(3):254-7.

Chobanian AV, Bakris GL, Black HR, et al, "The Seventh Report of the Joint National Committee on Prevention, Detection, Evaluation, and Treatment of High Blood Pressure: The JNC 7 Report," *JAMA*, 2003, 289(19):2560-72.

Conlin PR, Moore TJ, Swartz SL, et al, "Effect of Indomethacin on Blood Pressure Lowering by Captopril and Losartan in Hypertensive Patients," *Hypertension*, 2000, 36(3):461-5.

"Consensus Recommendations for the Management of Chronic Heart Failure. On Behalf of the Membership of the Advisory Council to Improve Outcomes Nationwide in Heart Failure," *Am J Cardiol*, 1999, 83(2A):1A-38A.

Cooper WO, Hernandez-Diaz S, Arbogast PG, et al, "Major Congenital Malformations After First-Trimester Exposure to ACE Inhibitors," *N Engl J Med*, 2006, 354(23):2443-51.

"Guidelines for the Evaluation and Management of Heart Failure. Report of the American College of Cardiology/American Heart Association Task Force on Practice Guidelines (Committee on Evaluation and Management of Heart Failure)," *Circulation*, 1995, 92(9):2764-84.

Kaiser G, Ackermann R, Brechbühler S, et al, "Pharmacokinetics of the Angiotensin Converting Enzyme Inhibitor Benazepril.HCl (CGS 14 824 A) in Healthy Volunteers After Single and Repeated Administration," *Biopharm Drug Dispos*, 1989, 10(4):365-76.

"K/DOQI Clinical Practice Guidelines for Chronic Kidney Disease: Evaluation, Classification, and Stratification. Kidney Disease Outcome Quality Initiative," *Am J Kidney Dis*, 2002, 39(2 Suppl 2):1-246.

Konstam MA, Dracup K, Baker, DW, et al, "Heart Failure Evaluation and Care of Patients With Left-Ventricular Systolic Dysfunction," *J Card Fail*, 1995, 1(2):183-7.

Mastrobattista JM, "Angiotensin Converting Enzyme Inhibitors in Pregnancy," *Semin Perinatol*, 1997, 21(2):124-34.

National High Blood Pressure Education Program Working Group on High Blood Pressure in Children and Adolescents, "The Fourth Report on the Diagnosis, Evaluation, and Treatment of High Blood Pressure in Children and Adolescents," *Pediatrics*, 2004, 114(2 Suppl):555-76.

Packer M, Poole-Wilson PA, Armstrong PW, et al, "Comparative Effects of Low and High Doses of the Angiotensin-Converting Enzyme Inhibitor, Lisinopril, on Morbidity and Mortality in Chronic Heart Failure," *Circulation*, 1999, 100(23):2312-8.

Quan A, "Fetopathy Associated With Exposure to Angiotensin Converting Enzyme Inhibitors and Angiotensin Receptor Antagonists," *Early Hum Dev*, 2006, 82(1):23-8.

Smoger SH and Sayed MA, "Simultaneous Mucosal and Small Bowel Angioedema Due to Captopril," *South Med J*, 1998, 91(11):1060-3.

von Vigier RO, Mozzettini S, Truttmann AC, et al, "Cough is Common in Children Prescribed Converting Enzyme Inhibitors," *Nephron*, 2000, 84(1):98.

◆ **Benazepril Hydrochloride** *see* Benazepril *on page 179*

◆ **BeneFix®** *see* Factor IX *on page 557*

◆ **Benemid [DSC]** *see* Probenecid *on page 1155*

◆ **Benflumetol and Artemether** *see* Artemether and Lumefantrine *on page 136*

◆ **Benoxyl® (Can)** *see* Benzoyl Peroxide *on page 184*

◆ **Ben-Tann [DSC]** *see* DiphenhydrAMINE *on page 448*

◆ **Bentyl®** *see* Dicyclomine *on page 433*

◆ **Bentylol® (Can)** *see* Dicyclomine *on page 433*

◆ **Benuryl™ (Can)** *see* Probenecid *on page 1155*

◆ **Benylin® D for Infants (Can)** *see* Pseudoephedrine *on page 1183*

◆ **Benylin® DM-E (Can)** *see* Guaifenesin and Dextromethorphan *on page 658*

◆ **Benylin® E Extra Strength (Can)** *see* GuaiFENesin *on page 656*

◆ **Benzac® AC** *see* Benzoyl Peroxide *on page 184*

◆ **Benzac AC® (Can)** *see* Benzoyl Peroxide *on page 184*

◆ **BenzaClin®** *see* Clindamycin and Benzoyl Peroxide *on page 329*

◆ **Benzac W® Gel (Can)** *see* Benzoyl Peroxide *on page 184*

◆ **Benzac W® Wash (Can)** *see* Benzoyl Peroxide *on page 184*

◆ **5 Benzagel®** *see* Benzoyl Peroxide *on page 184*

◆ **10 Benzagel®** *see* Benzoyl Peroxide *on page 184*

◆ **BenzaShave®** *see* Benzoyl Peroxide *on page 184*

◆ **Benzathine Benzylpenicillin** *see* Penicillin G Benzathine *on page 1078*

◆ **Benzathine Penicillin G** *see* Penicillin G Benzathine *on page 1078*

◆ **BenzEFoam™** *see* Benzoyl Peroxide *on page 184*

◆ **Benzene Hexachloride** *see* Lindane *on page 825*

◆ **Benzhexol Hydrochloride** *see* Trihexyphenidyl *on page 1385*

◆ **Benziq™** *see* Benzoyl Peroxide *on page 184*

◆ **Benziq™ LS** *see* Benzoyl Peroxide *on page 184*

◆ **Benzmethyzin** *see* Procarbazine *on page 1159*

Benzocaine (BEN zoe kane)

Medication Safety Issues
Sound-alike/look-alike issues:
Orabase® may be confused with Orinase®

U.S. Brand Names Americaine® Hemorrhoidal [OTC]; Anbesol® Baby [OTC]; Anbesol® Cold Sore Therapy [OTC]; Anbesol® Jr. [OTC]; Anbesol® Maximum Strength [OTC]; Anbesol® [OTC]; Benzodent® [OTC]; Bi-Zets; Boil-Ease® Pain Relieving; Cepacol® Fizzlers™ [OTC]; Cepacol® Sore Throat [OTC]; Chiggerex® Plus; Chiggerex® [OTC]; Chiggertox® [OTC]; Cylex® [OTC] [DSC]; Dent's Extra Strength Toothache [OTC]; Dentapaine [OTC]; Dermoplast® Antibacterial [OTC]; Dermoplast® Pain Relieving [OTC]; Detane® [OTC]; Foille® [OTC]; HDA® Toothache [OTC]; Hurricaine® [OTC]; Ivy-Rid® [OTC]; Kank-A® Soft Brush™ [OTC]; Lanacane® Maximum Strength [OTC]; Lanacane® [OTC]; Little Teethers® [OTC]; Medicone® Hemorrhoidal [OTC]; Mycinettes® [OTC]; Orabase® with Benzocaine [OTC]; Orajel PM® Maximum Strength [OTC]; Orajel® Baby Daytime and Nighttime [OTC]; Orajel® Baby Teething Nighttime [OTC]; Orajel® Baby Teething [OTC]; Orajel® Denture Plus [OTC]; Orajel® Maximum Strength [OTC]; Orajel® Medicated Toothache [OTC]; Orajel® Mouth Sore [OTC]; Orajel® Multi-Action Cold Sore [OTC]; Orajel® Ultra Mouth Sore [OTC]; Outgro® [OTC]; Red Cross™ Canker Sore [OTC]; Rid-A-Pain Dental [OTC]; Sepasoothe®; Skeeter Stik [OTC]; Sting-Kill [OTC]; Tanac® [OTC]; Thorets [OTC]; Trocaine® [OTC]; Zilactin Toothache and Gum Pain® [OTC]; Zilactin®-B [OTC]

Canadian Brand Names Anbesol® Baby; Zilactin Baby®; Zilactin-B®

Therapeutic Category Analgesic, Topical; Local Anesthetic, Oral; Local Anesthetic, Topical

Generic Available Yes: Lozenge

Use Temporary relief of pain associated with pruritic dermatosis, pruritus, minor burns, toothache, minor sore throat pain, canker sores, hemorrhoids, rectal fissures; anesthetic lubricant for passage of catheters and endoscopic tubes

Pregnancy Risk Factor C

Pregnancy Considerations Reproduction studies have not been conducted.

Lactation Excretion in breast milk unknown/use caution

Contraindications Hypersensitivity to benzocaine, other ester-type local anesthetics, or any component (see Warnings); secondary bacterial infection of area; perforated tympanic membrane (otic formulations only)

Warnings Benzocaine sprays used in the mouth, throat, and other mucous membranes, particularly when using higher concentrations (14% to 25%), have been associated with an increased risk for developing methemoglobinemia; patients with asthma, bronchitis, emphysema, mucosal damage or inflammation at the application site, heart disease, malnutrition, and children <4 months of age may be at greater risk for developing methemoglobinemia; use cautiously or select another product for these patients. Patients with a greater tendency for elevated levels of methemoglobin, eg, G6PD deficiency, hemoglobin-M disease, NADH-methemoglobin reductase deficiency, and pyruvate-kinase deficiency may benefit from products with an alternative anesthetic (eg, lidocaine). Monitor for signs and symptoms of methemoglobinemia including pale, gray, or blue colored skin, headache, lightheadedness, shortness of breath, anxiety, fatigue, and tachycardia. The classical clinical finding of methemoglobinemia is chocolate brown-colored arterial blood. However, suspected cases should be confirmed by co-oximetry, which yields a direct and accurate measure of methemoglobin levels (standard pulse oximetry readings or arterial blood gas values are not reliable). Clinically significant methemoglobinemia requires immediate treatment.

Topical use prior to cosmetic procedures can result in high systemic levels and lead to toxic effects (eg arrhythmias, seizures, coma, respiratory depression, and death), particularly when applied in large amounts to cover large areas and/or left on for long periods of time or used with materials, wraps, or dressings to cover the skin after anesthetic application. These practices may increase the degree of systemic absorption and should be avoided. The FDA is recommending consumers consult their healthcare provider for instructions on safe use prior to applying topical anesthetics for medical or cosmetic purposes. Use of products with the lowest amount of anesthetic with the least amount of application possible to relieve pain is also recommended.

Some products contain tartrazine and benzyl alcohol which may cause allergic reactions in susceptible individuals; large amounts of benzyl alcohol (≥99 mg/kg/day) have been associated with a potentially fatal toxicity ("gasping syndrome") in neonates; the "gasping syndrome" consists of metabolic acidosis, respiratory distress, gasping respirations, CNS dysfunction (including convulsions, intracranial hemorrhage), hypotension and cardiovascular collapse; avoid use of injection in neonates. *In vitro* and animal studies have shown that benzoate, a metabolite of benzyl alcohol, displaces bilirubin from protein-binding sites.

Adverse Reactions
Cardiovascular: Edema, arrhythmias (see Warnings)
Central nervous system: Seizures (see Warnings)
Dermatologic: Angioedema, urticaria
Genitourinary: Urethritis
Hematologic: Methemoglobinemia in infants
Local: Contact dermatitis, burning, stinging, tenderness

Drug Interactions
Avoid Concomitant Use There are no known interactions where it is recommended to avoid concomitant use.

Increased Effect/Toxicity There are no known significant interactions involving an increase in effect.

Decreased Effect There are no known significant interactions involving a decrease in effect.

Stability Store at room temperature.

Mechanism of Action Blocks both the initiation and conduction of nerve impulses from sensory nerves by decreasing the neuronal membrane's permeability to sodium ions, which results in inhibition of depolarization with resultant blockade of conduction

Pharmacokinetics (Adult data unless noted)
Absorption: Poor after topical administration to intact skin, but well absorbed from mucous membranes and traumatized skin
Metabolism: Hydrolyzed in plasma and to a lesser extent in the liver by cholinesterase
Elimination: Excretion of the metabolites in urine

Usual Dosage Children and Adults:
Mucous membranes: Dosage varies depending on area to be anesthetized and vascularity of tissues
Oral mouth/throat preparations: Do not administer for >2 days or in children <2 years of age, unless directed by a physician; refer to specific package labeling
Otic: 4-5 drops into ear canal; may repeat every 1-2 hours as needed
Topical: Apply to affected area as needed

Administration
Mucous membranes: Apply to mucous membrane; do not eat for 1 hour after application to oral mucosa
Otic: After instilling into external ear canal, insert cotton pledget into ear canal
Topical: Apply evenly; do not apply to deep or puncture wounds or to serious burns

Monitoring Parameters Monitor patients for signs and symptoms of methemoglobinemia such as pallor, cyanosis, nausea, muscle weakness, dizziness, confusion, agitation, dyspnea, and tachycardia; co-oximetry (see Warnings)

Patient Information Consult healthcare provider for safe application practice prior to application; do not eat for 1 hour after application to oral mucosa; do not chew gum while mouth or throat is anesthetized due to potential biting trauma; do not overuse; do not apply to infected areas or to large areas of broken skin

Dosage Forms Excipient information presented when available (limited, particularly for generics); consult specific product labeling. [DSC] = Discontinued product
Aerosol, oral spray:
  Hurricaine®: 20% (60 mL) [dye free; cherry flavor]
Aerosol, topical spray:
  Dermoplast® Antibacterial: 20% (83 mL) [contains aloe vera, benzethonium chloride, menthol]
  Dermoplast® Pain Relieving: 20% (60 mL, 83 mL) [contains menthol]

Foille®: 5% (92 g) [contains chloroxylenol 0.63% and corn oil]
Ivy-Rid®: 2% (83 mL)
Lanacane® Maximum Strength: 20% (120 mL) [contains ethanol 36%]
Combination package (Orajel® Baby Daytime and Nighttime):
  Gel, oral [Daytime Regular Formula]: 7.5% (5.3 g)
  Gel, oral [Nighttime Formula]: 10% (5.3 g)
Cream, oral:
  Benzodent®: 20% (7.5 g, 30 g)
  Orajel PM® Maximum Strength: 20% (5.3 g, 7 g) [contains menthol]
Cream, topical:
  Lanacane®: 6% (30 g, 60 g)
  Lanacane® Maximum Strength: 20% (30 g)
Gel, oral:
  Anbesol®: 10% (7.5 g) [contains benzyl alcohol; cool mint flavor]
  Anbesol® Baby: 7.5% (7.5 g) [contains benzoic acid; grape flavor]
  Anbesol® Jr.: 10% (7 g) [contains benzyl alcohol; bubble gum flavor]
  Anbesol® Maximum Strength: 20% (7.5 g, 10 g) [contains benzyl alcohol]
  Dentapaine: 20% (11 g) [contains clove oil]
  HDA® Toothache: 6.5% (15 mL) [contains benzyl alcohol]
  Hurricaine®: 20% (5 g) [dye free; wild cherry flavor]; (30 g) [dye free; mint, pina colada, watermelon, and wild cherry flavors]
  Kank-A® Soft Brush™: 20% (2 mL) [packaged in applicator with brush tip]
  Little Teethers®: 7.5% (9.4 g) [cherry flavor]
  Orabase® with Benzocaine®: 20% (7 g) [contains ethanol 48%; mild mint flavor]
  Orajel®: 10% (5.3 g, 7 g, 9.4 g)
  Orajel® Baby Teething: 7.5% (9.4 g, 11.9 g) [cherry flavor]
  Orajel® Baby Teething Nighttime: 10% (5.3 g)
  Orajel® Denture Plus: 15% (9 g) [contains menthol 2%, ethanol 66.7%]
  Orajel® Maximum Strength: 20% (5.3 g, 7 g, 9.4 g, 11.9 g)
  Orajel® Mouth Sore: 20% (5.3 g, 9.4 g, 11.9 g) [contains allantoin, benzalkonium chloride 0.02%, zinc chloride 0.1%]
  Orajel® Multi-Action Cold Sore: 20% (9.4 g) [contains allantoin 0.5%, camphor 3%, dimethicone 2%]
  Orajel® Ultra Mouth Sore: 15% (9.4 g) [contains ethanol 66.7%, menthol 2%]
  Zilactin®-B: 10% (7.5 g)
Gel, topical:
  Detane®: 7.5% (15 g)
Liquid, oral:
  Anbesol®: 10% (9 mL) [contains benzyl alcohol; cool mint flavor]
  Anbesol® Maximum Strength: 20% (9 mL) [contains benzyl alcohol]
  Hurricaine®: 20% (30 mL) [dye free; pina colada and wild cherry flavors]
  Orajel® Baby Teething: 7.5% (13 mL) [very berry flavor]
  Orajel® Maximum Strength: 20% (13 mL) [contains ethanol 44%, tartrazine]
  Tanac®: 10% (13 mL) [contains benzalkonium chloride]
Liquid, oral [drops]:
  Rid-A-Pain Dental: 6.3% (30 mL) [contains ethanol 70%]
Liquid, topical:
  Chiggertox®: 2% (30 mL)
  Outgro®: 20% (9 mL)
  Skeeter Stik: 5% (14 mL) [contains menthol]

Lozenge: 6 mg (18s) [contains menthol]; 15 mg (10s)
Bi-Zets: 15 mg (10s)
Cepacol® Sore Throat: 15 mg (18s) [contains cetylpyridinium, menthol; cherry, citrus, and honey lemon flavors]
Cepacol® Sore Throat: 15 mg (16s) [sugar free; contains cetylpyridinium, menthol; cherry and menthol flavors]
Cylex®: 15 mg (12s) [sugar free; contains cetylpyridinium chloride 5 mg; cherry flavor] [DSC]
Mycinettes®: 15 mg (12s) [sugar free; contains sodium 9 mg; cherry or regular flavor]
Sepasoothe®: 10 mg (6s, 24s, 100s, 250s, 500s) [sugar free; contains cetylpyridium 0.5 mg/lozenge; wild cherry flavor]
Thorets: 18 mg (300s) [sugar free]
Trocaine®: 10 mg (50s, 300s)
Ointment, oral:
Anbesol® Cold Sore Therapy: 20% (7.1 g) [contains benzyl alcohol, allantoin, aloe, camphor, menthol, vitamin E]
Red Cross™ Canker Sore: 20% (7.5 g) [contains coconut oil]
Ointment, rectal:
Americaine® Hemorrhoidal: 20% (30 g)
Medicone® Hemorrhoidal: 20% (28.4 g)
Ointment, topical:
Boil-Ease® Pain Relieving: 20% (30 g)
Chiggerex®: 2% (50 g) [contains aloe vera] [DSC]
Chiggerex® Plus: 6% (50 g) [contains aloe]
Foille®: 5% (3.5 g, 14 g, 28 g) [contains chloroxylenol 0.1%, benzyl alcohol; corn oil base]
Pads, topical:
Sting-Kill: 20% (8s) [contains menthol and tartrazine]
Paste, oral:
Orabase® with Benzocaine: 20% (6 g)
Swabs, oral:
Hurricaine®: 20% (6s, 100s) [dye free; wild cherry flavor]
Orajel® Baby Teething: 7.5% (12s) [berry flavor]
Orajel® Medicated Mouth Sore, Orajel® Medicated Toothache: 20% (8s, 12s) [contains tartrazine]
Zilactin® Toothache and Gum Pain: 20% (8s) [grape flavor]
Swabs, topical:
Boil-Ease® Pain Relieving: 20% (12s) [contains tartrazine]
Sting-Kill: 20% (5s) [contains menthol and tartrazine]
Tablet, orally dissolving:
Cepacol® Fizzlers™: 6 mg (12s) [grape flavor]
Wax, oral:
Dent's Extra Strength Toothache Gum: 20% (1 g)

♦ **Benzocaine and Antipyrine** see Antipyrine and Benzocaine on page 118

♦ **Benzodent® [OTC]** see Benzocaine on page 182

Benzoyl Peroxide (BEN zoe il peer OKS ide)

Medication Safety Issues
Sound-alike/look-alike issues:
Benzoyl peroxide may be confused with benzyl alcohol
Benoxyl® may be confused with Brevoxyl®, Peroxyl®
Benzac® may be confused with Benza®
Brevoxyl® may be confused with Benoxyl®
Fostex® may be confused with pHisoHex®

U.S. Brand Names 10 Benzagel®; 5 Benzagel®; Acne Clear Maximum Strength [OTC]; Benzac® AC; Benza-Shave®; BenzEfoam™; Benziq™; Benziq™ LS; Brevoxyl® Acne Wash Kit [DSC]; Brevoxyl®-4; Brevoxyl®-8; breze™ [DSC]; Clearskin [OTC]; Clinic BPO; Desquam-E™ [DSC]; Desquam-X®; EthexDERM™ BPW-10 [DSC]; EthexDERM™ BPW-5 [DSC]; Inova™; Levoclen™ Acne Wash; Levoclen™-4; Levoclen™-8; NeoBenz® Micro SD [DSC]; NeoBenz® Micro Wash [DSC]; NeoBenz® Micro

[DSC]; Neutrogena® Body Clear® [OTC]; Neutrogena® Clear Pore™ [OTC]; Neutrogena® Oil-Free Acne Wash [OTC]; Neutrogena® On The Spot® Acne Treatment [OTC]; Pacnex™; Palmer's® Skin Success Invisible Acne [OTC]; PanOxyl® Aqua Gel; PanOxyl® Bar [OTC]; Triaz®; Zapzyt® [OTC]; Zoderm®; Zoderm® Hydrating Wash™; Zoderm® Redi-Pads™

Canadian Brand Names Acetoxyl®; Benoxyl®; Benzac AC®; Benzac W® Gel; Benzac W® Wash; Desquam-X®; Oxyderm™; PanOxyl®; Solugel®

Therapeutic Category Acne Products; Topical Skin Product

Generic Available Yes: Excludes cream, foam, pads, and soap

Use Treatment of mild to moderate acne vulgaris (FDA approved in ages ≥12 years and adults)

Pregnancy Risk Factor C

Lactation Excretion in breast milk unknown/use caution

Contraindications Hypersensitivity to benzoyl peroxide, benzoic acid, or any component

Warnings Discontinue if burning, swelling, irritation, or undue dryness occurs.

Precautions For external use only; may bleach hair, carpeting, or colored fabrics; avoid contact with eyes, eyelids, lips, mucous membranes, open wounds, and highly inflamed or denuded skin; use a sunscreen and minimize exposure to sunlight or artificial light sources

Adverse Reactions
Dermatologic: Contact dermatitis
Local: Dryness, erythema, irritation, peeling, stinging

Drug Interactions
Avoid Concomitant Use There are no known interactions where it is recommended to avoid concomitant use.
Increased Effect/Toxicity There are no known significant interactions involving an increase in effect.
Decreased Effect There are no known significant interactions involving a decrease in effect.

Mechanism of Action Releases free-radical oxygen which oxidizes bacterial proteins in the sebaceous follicles decreasing the number of anaerobic bacteria and irritating free fatty acids; exerts a keratolytic activity and a comedolytic effect

Pharmacokinetics (Adult data unless noted)
Absorption: ~5% through the skin
Metabolism: Major metabolite is benzoic acid
Elimination: In the urine as benzoate

Usual Dosage Children ≥12 years, Adolescents, and Adults: Topical:
Topical formulations: Apply sparingly once daily; gradually increase to 2-3 times/day if needed. If excessive dryness or peeling occurs, reduce dose frequency or concentration. If excessive stinging or burning occurs, remove with mild soap and water; resume use the next day
Topical cleansers: Wash once or twice daily; control amount of drying or peeling by modifying dose frequency or concentration

Administration Topical: Shake lotion before using; cleanse skin before applying; for external use only. Avoid contact with eyes, eyelids, lips, and mucous membranes; rinse with water if accidental contact occurs

Patient Information
Notify physician if rash develops or if skin becomes red, itchy, or swollen. Avoid exposure to sunlight and artificial light sources (sunlamps, tanning booth/bed); wear protective clothing or wide-brimmed hat; use sunscreen with SPF >15

Additional Information Granulation may indicate effectiveness; gels are more penetrating than creams and last longer than creams or lotions

Dosage Forms Excipient information presented when available (limited, particularly for generics); consult specific product labeling. [DSC] = Discontinued product

Aerosol, topical [emollient-based, foam]:
  BenzEFoam™: 5.3% (60 g)
Bar, topical [wash]:
  PanOxyl® Bar: 5% (113 g); 10% (113 g)
  Zapzyt®: 10% (113 g)
Cloth, topical [cleanser]:
  Triaz®: 3% (60s); 6% (60s)
Cream, topical:
  BenzaShave®: 5% (120 g); 10% (120 g) [contains sodium coconut sulfate and coconut acid]
  Clearskin: 10% (28 g)
  NeoBenz® Micro: 3.5% (45 g) [DSC]; 5.5% (45 g) [DSC]; 8.5% (45 g) [DSC]
  NeoBenz® Micro SD: 3.5% (0.5 g) [DSC]; 5.5% (0.5 g) [DSC]; 8.5% (0.5 g) [DSC]
  Neutrogena® On The Spot® Acne Treatment: 2.5% (22.5 g) [vanishing and tinted formulas]
  Zoderm®: 4.5% (125 mL) [contains urea 10%]; 6.5% (125 mL) [contains urea 10%]; 8.5% (125 mL) [contains urea 10%]
Cream, topical [cleanser, mask]:
  Neutrogena® Clear Pore™: 3.5% (125 mL)
Gel, topical: 5% (45 g, 60 g); 10% (42.5 g, 45 g, 60 g, 90 g)
  5 Benzagel®: 5% (45 g) [contains ethanol 14%]
  10 Benzagel®: 10% (45 g) [contains ethanol 14%]
  Acne Clear Maximum Strength: 10% (42.5 g)
  Brevoxyl®-4: 4% (42.5 g)
  Brevoxyl®-8: 8% (42.5 g)
  Clinic™ BPO: 7% (45 g)
  Desquam-X®: 5% (42.5 g, 90 g) [DSC]; 10% (42.5 g, 90 g)
  Neutrogena® Oil-Free Acne Wash: 2% (177 mL) [contains tartrazine]
  Zapzyt®: 10% (30 g)
  Zoderm®: 4.5% (125 mL) [contains urea 10%]; 6.5% (125 mL) [contains urea 10%]; 8.5% (125 mL) [contains urea 10%]
Gel, topical [alcohol-based]: 5% (60 g); 10% (60 g)
Gel, topical [cleanser]: 3% (170 g, 340 g); 6% (170 g, 340 g); 9% (170 g, 340 g)
  Triaz®: 3% (170 g, 340 g); 6% (170 g, 340 g); 9% (170 g, 340 g)
Gel, topical [wash]: 5% (150 g, 240 g); 10% (150 g, 240 g)
Gel, topical [water-based]: 2.5% (60 g; 5% (60 g, 90 g); 10% (60 g, 90 g)
  Benzac® AC: 5% (60 g); 10% (60 g)
  Benziq™: 5.25% (50 g) [contains aloe, benzyl alcohol]
  Benziq™ LS: 2.75% (50 g) [contains aloe, benzyl alcohol]
  Desquam-E™: 2.5% (42.5 g) [DSC]; 5% (42.5 g) [DSC] [emollient gel]
  PanOxyl® Aqua Gel: 10% (42.5 g)
Liquid, topical:
  Desquam-X®: 5% (150 mL)
Liquid, topical [body wash]: 5.75% (473 mL)
  Neutrogena® Body Clear®: 2% (250 mL) [contains tartrazine]
Liquid, topical [wash]: 2.5% (240 mL); 5% (120 mL, 150 mL, 240 mL); 10% (150 mL, 240 mL)
  Zoderm® Hydrating Wash™: 5.75% (473 mL) [contains urea 10%]
Liquid, topical [wash/water-based]:
  Benzac® AC: 10% (240 mL)
  Benzac® W: 5% (240 mL); 10% (240 mL)
  Benziq™: 5.25% (175 g) [contains aloe, benzyl alcohol]
  EthexDERM™ BPW-5: 5% (240 mL) [DSC]
  EthexDERM™ BPW-10: 10% (240 mL) [DSC]
Lotion, topical: 5% (30 mL); 10% (30 mL)
  Palmer's® Skin Success Invisible Acne: 10% (30 mL) [contains vitamin E and aloe]
Lotion, topical [wash]: 4% (170 g); 5% (227 g); 8% (170 g); 10% (227 g)
  Brevoxyl® Acne Wash Kit: 4%; 8% [kit includes SFC™ Lotion] [DSC]
  NeoBenz® Micro Wash: 7% (180 g) [DSC]
  Pacnex™: 7% (454 g) [contains aloe]
Pad, topical:
  breze™: 4.75% (30s), 7.75% (30s) [DSC]
  Inova™: 4% (30s); 8% (30s)
  Triaz®: 3% (30s, 60s); 6% (30s, 60s); 9% (30s)
  ZoDerm® Redi-Pads™: 4.5% (30s); 6.5% (30s); 8.5% (30s) [contains urea 10%]
Soap, topical [cleanser/emulsion-based]:
  ZoDerm®: 4.5% (400 mL); 6.5% (400 mL); 8.5% (400 mL) [contains urea 10%]
Wash, topical: 2.5% (227 g); 5% (113 g, 142 g, 227 g); 10% (142 g, 227 g)
  Levoclen™-4: 4% (170 g)
  Levoclen™-8: 8% (170 g)
  Levoclen™ Acne Wash Kit: 4%; 8% [kit includes soap-free cleanser lotion]

References
Winston MH and Shalita AR, "Acne Vulgaris: Pathogenesis and Treatment," *Pediatr Clin North Am*, 1991, 38(4):889-903.

◆ **Benzoyl Peroxide and Clindamycin** *see* Clindamycin and Benzoyl Peroxide *on page 329*

Benztropine (BENZ troe peen)

Medication Safety Issues
  Sound-alike/look-alike issues:
    Benztropine may be confused with bromocriptine
Related Information
  Acute Dystonic Reactions, Management *on page 1687*
U.S. Brand Names Cogentin®
Canadian Brand Names Apo-Benztropine®
Therapeutic Category Anti-Parkinson's Agent; Anticholinergic Agent; Antidote, Drug-induced Dystonic Reactions
Generic Available Yes: Tablet
Use Adjunctive treatment of parkinsonism; also used in treatment of drug-induced extrapyramidal effects (except tardive dyskinesia) and acute dystonic reactions
Pregnancy Risk Factor C
Lactation Excretion in breast milk unknown/use caution
Contraindications Hypersensitivity to benztropine mesylate or any component; children <3 years of age; patients with narrow-angle glaucoma, pyloric or duodenal obstruction, stenosing peptic ulcers; bladder neck obstructions; achalasia; myasthenia gravis
Precautions Use with caution in hot weather or during exercise; may cause anhydrosis and hyperthermia; increased risk of hyperthermia in alcoholics, patients with CNS disease, and with prolonged outdoor exposure
Adverse Reactions
  Cardiovascular: Tachycardia, orthostatic hypotension, ventricular fibrillation, palpitations
  Central nervous system: Drowsiness, nervousness, hallucinations, coma
  Dermatologic: Dry skin
  Endocrine & metabolic: Flow of breast milk decreased
  Gastrointestinal: Nausea, vomiting, xerostomia, constipation, dry throat, dysphagia
  Neuromuscular & skeletal: Weakness
  Ocular: Blurred vision, mydriasis, intraocular pressure elevated, pain
  Respiratory: Dry nose
  Miscellaneous: Diaphoresis decreased
Drug Interactions
  Metabolism/Transport Effects Substrate of CYP2D6 (minor)

◄ **Avoid Concomitant Use** There are no known inter-actions where it is recommended to avoid concomitant use.

Increased Effect/Toxicity
Benztropine may increase the levels/effects of: Abobo-tulinumtoxinA; Anticholinergics; Cannabinoids; Onabotu-linumtoxinA; Potassium Chloride; RimabotulinumtoxinB

The levels/effects of Benztropine may be increased by: Pramlintide

Decreased Effect
Benztropine may decrease the levels/effects of: Acetyl-cholinesterase Inhibitors (Central); Secretin

The levels/effects of Benztropine may be decreased by: Acetylcholinesterase Inhibitors (Central); Peginterferon Alfa-2b

Mechanism of Action Thought to partially block striatal cholinergic receptors to help balance cholinergic and dopaminergic activity

Pharmacodynamics
Onset of action:
Oral: Within 1 hour
Parenteral: Within 15 minutes
Duration: 6-48 hours

Usual Dosage
Drug-induced extrapyramidal reaction: Oral, I.M., I.V.:
Children >3 years: 0.02-0.05 mg/kg/dose 1-2 times/day; use in children <3 years should be reserved for life-threatening emergencies
Adults: 1-4 mg/dose 1-2 times/day
Acute dystonia: Adults: I.M., I.V.: 1-2 mg as a single dose
Parkinsonism: Adults: Oral: 0.5-6 mg/day in 1-2 divided doses; begin with 0.5 mg/day; increase in 0.5 mg increments at 5- to 6-day intervals to achieve the desired effect

Administration
Oral: Administer with food to decrease GI upset
Parenteral: I.V. route should be reserved for situations when oral or I.M. are not appropriate

Patient Information May causes drowsiness and impair ability to perform activities requiring mental alertness or physical coordination; may cause dry mouth.

Dosage Forms Excipient information presented when available (limited, particularly for generics); consult specific product labeling.
Injection, solution, as mesylate (Cogentin®): 1 mg/mL (2 mL)
Tablet, as mesylate: 0.5 mg, 1 mg, 2 mg

♦ **Benztropine Mesylate** *see Benztropine on page 185*

Benzyl Alcohol (BEN zill AL koe hol)

Medication Safety Issues
Sound-alike/look-alike issues:
Benzyl alcohol may be confused with benzoyl peroxide
U.S. Brand Names Ulesfia™; Zilactin®-L [OTC]
Therapeutic Category Analgesic, Topical; Antiparasitic Agent, Topical; Pediculocide; Topical Skin Product
Generic Available No
Use
Lotion: Treatment of head lice infestation (FDA approved in ages ≥6 months and adults)
Liquid (topical): Temporary relief of pain caused by cold sores/fever blisters (FDA approved in ages ≥2 years and adults)
Pregnancy Risk Factor B
Pregnancy Considerations Teratogenic effects were not observed in animal studies. There are no well-controlled human studies with topical benzyl alcohol in pregnancy. Use only if clearly needed.
Lactation Excretion in breast milk unknown/use caution

Breast-Feeding Considerations It is unknown if benzyl alcohol is distributed in human milk. Use with caution.
Contraindications Hypersensitivity to benzyl alcohol or any component
Warnings Large amounts of benzyl alcohol (≥99 mg/kg/day) have been associated with a potentially fatal toxicity ("gasping syndrome") in neonates; the "gasping syndrome" consists of metabolic acidosis, respiratory distress, gasping respirations, CNS dysfunction (including con-vulsions, intracranial hemorrhage), hypotension, and cardiovascular collapse; avoid use in neonates
Precautions For external use only; if contact with eyes occurs, flush immediately with water; allergic or irritant dermatitis may occur
Adverse Reactions Note: Adverse reactions reported are from lotion dosage form.
Dermatologic: Contact dermatitis, erythema, pruritus, pyoderma
Local: Anesthesia, hypoesthesia, irritation, pain
Ocular: Ocular irritation
<1%, postmarketing, and/or case reports: Application site dryness, dandruff, erythema, excoriation, paraesthesia, rash, skin exfoliation, thermal burn

Drug Interactions
Avoid Concomitant Use There are no known inter-actions where it is recommended to avoid concomitant use.
Increased Effect/Toxicity There are no known signifi-cant interactions involving an increase in effect.
Decreased Effect There are no known significant interactions involving a decrease in effect.

Stability
Lotion: Store at 20°C to 25°C (68°F to 77°F); excursions permitted to 15°C to 30°C (59°F to 86°F); do not freeze.
Liquid (topical): Store at 15°C to 20°C (59°F to 86°F). Flammable; keep away from fire or flame.
Mechanism of Action Inhibits respiration of lice by obstructing respiratory spiracles causing lice asphyxiation. No ovicidal activity.
Pharmacokinetics (Adult data unless noted) Absorp-tion: Quantifiable serum plasma concentrations reported following prolonged exposure (30 minutes) in patients 6 months to 11 years of age

Usual Dosage
Lotion (Ulesfia™): Treatment of head lice infestation: Children ≥6 months of age and adults: Apply appropriate volume for hair length to dry hair, saturate the scalp completely, leave on for 10 minutes, rinse thoroughly with water; repeat in 7 days.
Hair length 0-2 inches: 4-6 ounces
Hair length 2-4 inches: 6-8 ounces
Hair length 4-8 inches: 8-12 ounces
Hair length 8-16 inches: 12-24 ounces
Hair length 16-22 inches: 24-32 ounces
Hair length >22 inches: 32-48 ounces
Liquid (topical) [Zilactin®-L (OTC)]: Cold sores/fever blisters: Children ≥2 years of age and adults: Moisten cotton swab with several drops of liquid; apply to affected area up to 4 times/day; do not use for more than 7 days
Administration For topical use only. Do not swallow liquid or lotion.
Lotion (Ulesfia™): Apply under adult supervision to dry hair, until entire scalp and hair are saturated. Leave on for 10 minutes then rinse thoroughly. Avoid contact with eyes. Wash hands after application. A lice comb may be used to remove dead lice after both treatments.
Liquid (topical) [Zilactin®-L (OTC)]: Apply to affected area only with moistened cotton swab. Allow to dry for 15 seconds. Avoid contact with eyes.

Patient Information Lotion should be used in conjunction with overall lice management program. Dry clean or wash all clothing, hats, bedding, and towels in hot water. Wash all personal care items (eg, combs, brushes, hair clips) in hot water. May use a fine-tooth or special nit comb to remove nits and dead lice. May shampoo hair right after treatment. Keep topical liquid away from fire or flame. Inform physician if swelling, rash, or fever develops or if application site irritation occurs.

Dosage Forms Excipient information presented when available (limited, particularly for generics); consult specific product labeling.

Liquid, topical:

Zilactin®-L: 10% (5.9 mL) [contains ethanol 80%]

Lotion, topical:

Ulesfia™: 5% (240 mL)

◆ **Benzylpenicillin Benzathine** *see* Penicillin G Benzathine *on page 1078*

◆ **Benzylpenicillin Potassium** *see* Penicillin G (Parenteral/Aqueous) *on page 1080*

◆ **Benzylpenicillin Sodium** *see* Penicillin G (Parenteral/Aqueous) *on page 1080*

Beractant (ber AKT ant)

Medication Safety Issues
Sound-alike/look-alike issues:
Survanta® may be confused with Sufenta®

U.S. Brand Names Survanta®

Canadian Brand Names Survanta®

Therapeutic Category Lung Surfactant

Generic Available No

Use Prevention and treatment of respiratory distress syndrome (RDS) in premature infants

Prophylactic therapy: Infants with body weight <1250 g who are at risk for developing or with evidence of surfactant deficiency

Rescue therapy: Treatment of infants with RDS confirmed by x-ray and requiring mechanical ventilation

Warnings Rapidly affects oxygenation and lung compliance and should be restricted to a highly supervised use in a clinical setting with immediate availability of clinicians experienced with intubation and ventilatory management of premature infants. If transient episodes of bradycardia and decreased oxygen saturation occur, discontinue the dosing procedure and initiate measures to alleviate the condition; produces rapid improvements in lung oxygenation and compliance that may require immediate reductions in ventilator settings and FiO$_2$.

Precautions Use of beractant in infants <600 g birth weight or >1750 g birth weight has not been evaluated

Adverse Reactions During the dosing procedure:

Cardiovascular: Transient bradycardia, vasoconstriction, hypotension, hypertension, pallor

Respiratory: Oxygen desaturation, endotracheal tube blockage, hypocarbia, hypercarbia, apnea, pulmonary air leaks, pulmonary interstitial emphysema, pulmonary hemorrhage

Miscellaneous: Probability of post-treatment nosocomial sepsis increased

Drug Interactions

Avoid Concomitant Use There are no known interactions where it is recommended to avoid concomitant use.

Increased Effect/Toxicity There are no known significant interactions involving an increase in effect.

Decreased Effect There are no known significant interactions involving a decrease in effect.

Stability Refrigerate; protect from light; prior to administration warm by standing at room temperature for 20 minutes or hold in hand for 8 minutes; artificial warming methods should **not** be used; unused, unopened vials warmed to room temperature may be returned to the refrigerator within 8 hours of warming only once

Mechanism of Action Replaces deficient or ineffective endogenous lung surfactant in neonates with respiratory distress syndrome (RDS) or in neonates at risk of developing RDS. Surfactant prevents the alveoli from collapsing during expiration by lowering surface tension between air and alveolar surfaces.

Usual Dosage Intratracheal: Neonates:

Prophylactic treatment: Give 4 mL/kg as soon as possible; as many as 4 doses may be administered during the first 48 hours of life, no more frequently than 6 hours apart. The need for additional doses is determined by evidence of continuing respiratory distress or if the infant is still intubated and requiring at least 30% inspired oxygen to maintain a PaO$_2$ ≤80 torr.

Rescue treatment: Give 4 mL/kg as soon as the diagnosis of RDS is made; may repeat if needed, no more frequently than every 6 hours to a maximum of 4 doses

Administration Intratracheal: For intratracheal administration only. Do not shake; if settling occurs during storage, gently swirl. Suction infant prior to administration; inspect solution to verify complete mixing of the suspension. Administer intratracheally by instillation through a 5-French end-hole catheter inserted into the infant's endotracheal tube. Administer the dose in four 1 mL/kg aliquots. Each quarter-dose is instilled over 2-3 seconds; each quarter-dose is administered with the infant in a different position; slightly downward inclination with head turned to the right, then repeat with head turned to the left; then slightly upward inclination with head turned to the right, then repeat with head turned to the left.

Monitoring Parameters Continuous heart rate and transcutaneous O$_2$ saturation should be monitored during administration; frequent ABG sampling is necessary to prevent postdosing hyperoxia and hypocarbia.

Dosage Forms Excipient information presented when available (limited, particularly for generics); consult specific product labeling.

Suspension, intratracheal [preservative free; bovine derived]:

Survanta®: 25 mg/mL (4 mL, 8 mL)

Besifloxacin (be si FLOX a sin)

U.S. Brand Names Besivance™

Therapeutic Category Antibiotic, Ophthalmic; Antibiotic, Quinolone; Ophthalmic Agent

Generic Available No

Use Treatment of bacterial conjunctivitis (FDA approved in ages ≥1 year and adults)

Pregnancy Risk Factor C

Pregnancy Considerations Oral besifloxacin has been shown to be fetotoxic in animal studies at doses that were also maternally toxic. Quinolone exposure during human pregnancy has been reported with other agents (refer to Ciprofloxacin and Ofloxacin monographs). The low plasma concentrations of besifloxacin following ophthalmic use (<1.3 ng/mL in nonpregnant patients) should limit fetal exposure.

Lactation Excretion in breast milk unknown/use caution

Breast-Feeding Considerations Other quinolones are known to be excreted in breast milk. The manufacturer recommends using caution if besifloxacin is administered while nursing.

Contraindications Hypersensitivity to besifloxacin or any component

Warnings Do not inject ophthalmic solution subconjunctivally or introduce directly into the anterior chamber of the eye. Prolonged use may result in fungal or bacterial superinfection; discontinue use and initiate alternative therapy if superinfection occurs. Severe hypersensitivity reactions, including anaphylaxis, have occurred with systemic quinolone therapy. Prompt discontinuation of drug should occur if skin rash or other symptoms arise.

Precautions Contact lenses should not be worn during treatment of ophthalmic infections.

Adverse Reactions
Central nervous system: Headache
Ocular: Blurred vision, conjunctival redness, irritation, pain, pruritus

Drug Interactions
Avoid Concomitant Use There are no known interactions where it is recommended to avoid concomitant use.
Increased Effect/Toxicity There are no known significant interactions involving an increase in effect.
Decreased Effect There are no known significant interactions involving a decrease in effect.

Stability Store between 15°C to 25°C (59°F to 77°F); protect from light.

Mechanism of Action Inhibits both DNA gyrase and topoisomerase IV DNA gyrase is an essential bacterial enzyme required for DNA replication, transcription, and repair. Topoisomerase IV is an essential bacterial enzyme required for decatenation during cell division. Inhibition effect is bactericidal.

Pharmacokinetics (Adult data unless noted) Half-life elimination: ~7 hours

Usual Dosage Ophthalmic: Children ≥1 year and Adults: Bacterial conjunctivitis: Instill 1 drop into affected eye(s) 3 times/day (4-12 hours apart) for 7 days

Administration Ophthalmic: Wash hands before and after instillation. Shake bottle once prior to each administration. Avoid contaminating the applicator tip with affected eye(s).

Monitoring Parameters Signs and symptoms of infection or hypersensitivity reaction

Patient Information Avoid contaminating the applicator tip with material from the eye, fingers, or other source. Discontinue use immediately and contact a physician at the first sign of a rash or allergic reaction. Finish the entire course of therapy even if feeling better. Skipping doses can lead to decreased effectiveness of the medication and bacterial resistance. Do not wear contacts when you have an eye infection or when you are using this medication. Wash your hands thoroughly prior to use. Invert closed bottle (upside down) and shake once before each use. Remove cap with bottle still in the inverted position. Tilt head back and, with bottle inverted, gently squeeze bottle to instill one drop into the affected eye(s).

Dosage Forms Excipient information presented when available (limited, particularly for generics); consult specific product labeling.
Suspension, ophthalmic [drops]:
Besivance™: 0.6% (5 mL) [contains benzalkonium chloride]

References
Cambau E, Matrat S, Pan XS, et al, "Target Specificity of the New Fluoroquinolone Besifloxacin in *Streptococcus pneumoniae*, *Staphylococcus aureus* and *Escherichia coli*," *J Antimicrob Chemother*, 2009, 63(3):443-50.
Karpecki P, DePaolis M, Hunter JA, et al, "Besifloxacin Ophthalmic Suspension 0.6% in Patients With Bacterial Conjunctivitis: A Multicenter, Prospective, Randomized, Double-Masked, Vehicle-Controlled, 5-Day Efficacy and Safety Study," *Clin Ther*, 2009, 31 (3):514-26.

♦ **Besifloxacin Hydrochloride** see Besifloxacin on page 187

♦ **Besivance™** see Besifloxacin on page 187

♦ **β,β-Dimethylcysteine** see Penicillamine on page 1076

♦ **9-Beta-D-Ribofuranosyladenine** see Adenosine on page 51

♦ **Betacaine® (Can)** see Lidocaine on page 818

♦ **Betaderm (Can)** see Betamethasone on page 189

♦ **Betagan®** see Levobunolol on page 811

♦ **Beta-HC®** see Hydrocortisone on page 685

Betaine (BAY tayne)

Medication Safety Issues
Sound-alike/look-alike issues:
Betaine may be confused with Betadine®
Cystadane® may be confused with cysteamine, cysteine

U.S. Brand Names Cystadane®
Canadian Brand Names Cystadane®
Therapeutic Category Homocystinuria, Treatment Agent
Generic Available No
Use Treatment agent to reduce elevated homocysteine blood levels in homocystinuria; homocystinuria includes deficiencies or defects in cystathionine beta-synthase (CBS), 5,10-methylenetetrahydrofolate reductase (MTHFR), and cobalamin cofactor metabolism (cbl)
Pregnancy Risk Factor C
Pregnancy Considerations Animal reproduction studies have not been conducted with betaine. It is not known whether betaine can cause fetal harm when administered to a pregnant woman or can affect reproductive capacity. Betaine should be given to a pregnant woman only if needed.
Lactation Excretion in breast milk unknown/use caution
Breast-Feeding Considerations Betaine is found naturally in human breast milk. The influence from betaine therapy is unknown.
Contraindications Hypersensitivity to betaine or any component
Warnings Cerebral edema has been reported in patients with hypermethioninemia, including a few patients treated with betaine. Treatment of CBS with betaine may further increase methionine serum levels (due to remethylation of homocysteine to methionine); monitor methionine serum levels in patients with CBS deficiency; maintain methionine levels <1,000 micromol/L.
Adverse Reactions Gastrointestinal: Nausea, vomiting, diarrhea, GI distress
Drug Interactions
Avoid Concomitant Use There are no known interactions where it is recommended to avoid concomitant use.
Increased Effect/Toxicity There are no known significant interactions involving an increase in effect.
Decreased Effect There are no known significant interactions involving a decrease in effect.
Stability Store at room temperature; protect from moisture
Mechanism of Action Betaine reduces homocysteine blood concentrations by acting as a methyl group donor in the remethylation of homocysteine to methionine
Usual Dosage Oral:
Children <3 years: 100 mg/kg/day divided into 2 doses; increase at weekly intervals in 50 mg/kg/day increments
Children ≥3 years and Adults: 3 g twice daily; doses up to 20 g/day have been needed to control homocysteine plasma concentrations in some patients
Note: Minimal benefit has been shown in patients treated with >150 mg/kg/day or >20 g/day
Administration Oral: Shake bottle lightly before opening; measure prescribed amount with provided measuring scoop and dissolve in 4-6 ounces of water, juice, milk, or formula; administer immediately; do not use if powder does not completely dissolve or gives a colored solution

Monitoring Parameters Plasma homocysteine concentration (should be low or undetectable); plasma methionine (CBS patients)

Additional Information Orphan drug; may only be obtained by contacting Chronimed Inc at 1-800-900-4267; vitamin B$_6$, vitamin B$_{12}$, and folate have been helpful in the management of homocystinuria and are often used in conjunction

Dosage Forms Excipient information presented when available (limited, particularly for generics); consult specific product labeling.

Powder for oral solution, anhydrous:

Cystadane®: 1 g/scoop (180 g) [1 scoop = 1.7 mL]

References

Burns SP, Iles RA, Ryalls M, et al "Methylgenesis From Betaine in Cystathionine-Beta-Synthase Deficiency," *Biochem Soc Trans*, 1993, 21:455S.

Devlin AM, Hajipour L, Gholkar A, "Cerebral Edema Associated With Betaine Treatment in Classical Homocystinuria," *J Pediatr*, 2001,144 (4):545-8.

Kishi T, Kawamura I, Harada Y, et al, "Effect of Betaine on S-Adenosylmethionine Levels in the Cerebrospinal Fluid in a Patient With Methylenetetrahydrofolate Reductase Deficiency and Peripheral Neuropathy," *J Inherit Metab Dis*, 1994, 17(5):560-5.

Lawson-Yuen A and Levy, HL, "The Use of Betaine in the Treatment of Elevated Homocysteine," *Mol Genet Metab*, 2006, 88(3):201-7.

Matthews A, Johnson TN, Rostami-Hodjegan A, et al, "An Indirect Response Model of Homocysteine Suppression by Betaine: Optimising the Dosage Regimen of Betaine in Homocystinuria," *Br J Clin Pharmacol*, 2002, 54(2):140-6.

Smolin LA, Benevenga NJ, and Berlow S, "The Use of Betaine for the Treatment of Homocystinuria," *J Pediatr*, 1981, 99:467-72.

◆ **Betaine Anhydrous** see Betaine on page 188

◆ **Betaject™ (Can)** see Betamethasone on page 189

◆ **Betaloc® (Can)** see Metoprolol on page 918

Betamethasone (bay ta METH a sone)

Medication Safety Issues

Sound-alike/look-alike issues:

Luxiq® may be confused with Lasix®

International issues:

Beta-Val® may be confused with Betanol® which is a brand name for metipranolol in Monaco

Related Information

Corticosteroids on page 1487

U.S. Brand Names Beta-Val®; Celestone®; Celestone® Soluspan®; Diprolene®; Diprolene® AF; Luxiq®

Canadian Brand Names Betaderm; Betaject™; Betnesol®; Betnovate®; Celestone® Soluspan®; Diprolene® Glycol; Diprosone®; Ectosone; Prevex® B; Taro-Sone; Topilene®; Topisone®; Valisone® Scalp Lotion

Therapeutic Category Adrenal Corticosteroid; Anti-inflammatory Agent; Corticosteroid, Systemic; Corticosteroid, Topical; Glucocorticoid

Generic Available Yes: Excludes aerosol, solution

Use Anti-inflammatory; immunosuppressant agent; corticosteroid replacement therapy

Topical: Inflammatory dermatoses such as psoriasis, seborrheic or atopic dermatitis, neurodermatitis, inflammatory phase of xerosis, late phase of allergic dermatitis or irritant dermatitis; Foam: Inflammatory and pruritic symptoms of scalp dermatoses responsive to corticosteroids

Pregnancy Risk Factor C

Pregnancy Considerations Adverse events have been observed with corticosteroids in animal reproduction studies. Betamethasone crosses the placenta; approximately 25% is metabolized by placental enzymes to an inactive metabolite. Due to its positive effect on stimulating fetal lung maturation, the injection is often used in patients with premature labor (24-34 weeks gestation). Topical products are not recommended for extensive use, in large quantities, or for long periods of time in pregnant women. Some studies have shown an association between first trimester systemic corticosteroid use and oral clefts; adverse events in the fetus/neonate have been noted in case reports following large doses of systemic corticosteroids during pregnancy. Women exposed to betamethasone during pregnancy for the treatment of an autoimmune disease may contact the OTIS Autoimmune Diseases Study at 877-311-8972.

Lactation Excretion in breast milk unknown/use caution

Breast-Feeding Considerations Corticosteroids are excreted in human milk. The onset of milk secretion after birth may be delayed and the volume of milk produced may be decreased by antenatal betamethasone therapy; this affect was seen when delivery occurred 3-9 days after the betamethasone dose in women between 28 and 34 weeks gestation. Antenatal betamethasone therapy did not affect milk production when birth occurred <3 days or >10 days of treatment. It is not known if systemic absorption following topical administration results in detectable quantities in human milk. Use with caution while breast-feeding; do not apply to nipples.

Contraindications Hypersensitivity to betamethasone or any component; systemic fungal infections

Warnings Hypothalamic-pituitary-adrenal (HPA) axis suppression may occur; acute adrenal insufficiency (adrenal crisis) may occur with abrupt withdrawal after long-term use or with stress; withdrawal or discontinuation of corticosteroids should be done carefully; patients with HPA axis suppression may require increased doses of systemic glucocorticosteroids prior to, during, and after unusual stress (eg, surgery). Immunosuppression may occur; patients may be more susceptible to infection; avoid exposure to chicken pox and measles. Corticosteroids may mask signs of infection. Corticosteroids may activate latent opportunistic infections or exacerbate systemic fungal infections. May cause osteoporosis (at any age) or inhibition of bone growth in pediatric patients. Acute myopathy may occur with high doses, elevated IOP may occur (especially with prolonged use), CNS effects (ranging from euphoria to psychosis) may occur. Rare cases of anaphylactoid reactions have been reported with corticosteroids.

Topical: Infants and small children may be more susceptible to HPA axis suppression from topical corticosteroid therapy; systemic effects may occur when used on large areas of the body, denuded areas, for prolonged periods of time, or with an occlusive dressing; do not use in diaper area or with occlusive dressings, especially on weeping or exudative lesions; discontinue if skin irritation or contact dermatitis occurs; do not use very high potency topical products for the treatment of rosacea or perioral dermatitis (see Additional Information).

Oral solution contains propylene glycol and sodium benzoate; benzoic acid (benzoate) is a metabolite of benzyl alcohol; large amounts of benzyl alcohol (≥99 mg/kg/day) have been associated with a potentially fatal toxicity ("gasping syndrome") in neonates; the "gasping syndrome" consists of metabolic acidosis, respiratory distress, gasping respirations, CNS dysfunction (including convulsions, intracranial hemorrhage), hypotension and cardiovascular collapse; avoid use of betamethasone products containing sodium benzoate in neonates; in vitro and animal studies have shown that benzoate displaces bilirubin from protein binding sites

Precautions Avoid using higher than recommended doses; suppression of HPA axis, suppression of linear growth (ie, reduction of growth velocity), reduced bone mineral density, hypercorticism (Cushing's syndrome), hyperglycemia, or glucosuria may occur; titrate to lowest effective dose. Reduction in growth velocity may occur when corticosteroids are administered to pediatric patients ▶

by any route (monitor growth). Use with extreme caution in patients with respiratory tuberculosis, untreated systemic infections, or ocular herpes simplex; use with caution in patients with thyroid dysfunction, cirrhosis, nonspecific ulcerative colitis, hypertension, renal impairment, osteoporosis, thromboembolic tendencies, CHF, recent MI, convulsive disorders, myasthenia gravis, thrombophlebitis, peptic ulcer, diabetes, glaucoma, cataracts, or hepatic impairment. Prolonged use may result in cataracts or glaucoma.

Use topical products sparingly in children, systemic effects may be seen; **Note:** Due to the high incidence of developing adrenal suppression, augmented topical products (eg, Diprolene® AF cream, Diprolene® lotion) are not recommended for use in children ≤12 years of age (see Additional Information). Foam is not recommended for children <16 years.

Adverse Reactions

Cardiovascular: Edema, hypertension, CHF

Central nervous system: Convulsions, vertigo, confusion, headache, psychoses, pseudotumor cerebri, euphoria, insomnia, intracranial hypertension, nervousness

Dermatologic: Thin fragile skin, hyperpigmentation or hypopigmentation, acne, impaired wound healing, skin atrophy (bruising, shininess, telangiectasia, thinness, loss of skin markings), erythema, rash, dry skin

Endocrine & metabolic: HPA suppression, Cushingoid state, sodium and water retention, growth suppression, glucose intolerance, hypokalemia

Gastrointestinal: Peptic ulcer, nausea, vomiting

Local: Burning, itching, stinging, sterile abscess, irritation, erythema, folliculitis, vesiculation, acneform eruptions, contact dermatitis

Neuromuscular & skeletal: Muscle weakness, bone mineral density decreased, osteoporosis, fractures

Ocular: Cataracts, IOP elevated, glaucoma

Miscellaneous: Immunosuppression, anaphylactoid reactions (rare)

Drug Interactions

Metabolism/Transport Effects Inhibits CYP3A4 (weak)

Avoid Concomitant Use

Avoid concomitant use of Betamethasone with any of the following: Aldesleukin; BCG; Natalizumab; Pimecrolimus; Tacrolimus (Topical); Vaccines (Live)

Increased Effect/Toxicity

Betamethasone may increase the levels/effects of: Acetylcholinesterase Inhibitors; Amphotericin B; Leflunomide; Loop Diuretics; Natalizumab; NSAID (COX-2 Inhibitor); NSAID (Nonselective); Thiazide Diuretics; Vaccines (Live); Warfarin

The levels/effects of Betamethasone may be increased by: Antifungal Agents (Azole Derivatives, Systemic); Aprepitant; Calcium Channel Blockers (Nondihydropyridine); Denosumab; Estrogen Derivatives; Fluconazole; Fosaprepitant; Macrolide Antibiotics; Neuromuscular-Blocking Agents (Nondepolarizing); Pimecrolimus; Quinolone Antibiotics; Salicylates; Tacrolimus (Topical); Trastuzumab

Decreased Effect

Betamethasone may decrease the levels/effects of: Aldesleukin; Antidiabetic Agents; BCG; Calcitriol; Corticorelin; Isoniazid; Salicylates; Sipuleucel-T; Vaccines (Inactivated); Vaccines (Live)

The levels/effects of Betamethasone may be decreased by: Aminoglutethimide; Antacids; Barbiturates; Bile Acid Sequestrants; Echinacea; Mitotane; Primidone; Rifamycin Derivatives

Food Interactions Systemic use of corticosteroids may require a diet with increased potassium, vitamins A, B₆, C, D, folate, calcium, zinc, and phosphorus and decreased sodium

Stability Store at controlled room temperature; foam canister is flammable; avoid fire, flame, heat; do not store at >120°F (49°C)

Mechanism of Action Controls the rate of protein synthesis, depresses the migration of polymorphonuclear leukocytes and fibroblasts, reverses capillary permeability, and causes lysosomal stabilization at the cellular level to prevent or control inflammation

Pharmacokinetics (Adult data unless noted)

Protein binding: 64%

Metabolism: Hepatic

Elimination: <5% of dose excreted renally as unchanged drug; small amounts eliminated via biliary tract

Usual Dosage Base dosage on severity of disease and patient response

I.M.:

Children: Use lowest dose listed as initial dose for adrenocortical insufficiency (physiologic replacement); 0.0175-0.125 mg base/kg/day divided every 6-12 hours **or** 0.5-7.5 mg base/m²/day divided every 6-12 hours

Adolescents and Adults: 0.6-9 mg/day divided every 12-24 hours

Oral:

Children: Use lowest dose listed as initial dose for adrenocortical insufficiency (physiologic replacement); 0.0175-0.25 mg/kg/day divided every 6-8 hours **or** 0.5-7.5 mg/m²/day divided every 6-8 hours

Adolescents and Adults: 2.4-4.8 mg/day in 2-4 doses; range: 0.6-7.2 mg/day

Topical: Use smallest amount for shortest period of time to avoid HPA suppression; discontinue use once control is achieved; reassess diagnosis if no improvement is seen within 2 weeks

Children and Adults: Apply thin film 1-2 times/day (see Precautions and Additional Information)

Adolescents ≥13 years and Adults:

Diprolene® AF cream: Apply thin film 1-2 times/day; maximum: 45 g of cream/week; do not use >2 weeks

Diprolene® Lotion: Apply a few drops once or twice daily; maximum: 50 mL/week; do not use >2 weeks

Diprolene® Gel: Apply thin film once or twice daily; maximum: 50 g/week; do not use >2 weeks

Adolescents ≥16 years and Adults: Luxiq® foam: Apply twice daily (in morning and at night)

Administration

Oral: Administer with food to decrease GI effects

Parenteral: Do not administer injectable suspension I.V.; shake injectable suspension before use

Topical: Apply sparingly, rub in gently until it disappears; do not apply to face, axillae, or inguinal areas; not for use on broken skin, in areas of infection, or in diaper area. Do not apply to wet skin unless directed; do not cover with occlusive dressing.

Foam: Invert can, dispense small amount of foam onto saucer or other cool surface; foam will melt upon contact with warm skin (do not dispense directly into hands); use fingers to apply small amounts of foam to affected scalp area; rub in gently until it disappears; avoid fire, flame, or smoking during use; contents of can are flammable and under pressure

Test Interactions Skin tests

Patient Information

Systemic use: Avoid alcohol and caffeine; do not decrease dose or discontinue without physician's approval

Topical use: Avoid contact with eyes; do not use occlusive dressings or other corticosteroid-containing products unless directed by physician

Additional Information Long-acting corticosteroid with minimal or no sodium-retaining potential. Topical products: Very high potency: Augmented betamethasone dipropionate ointment and lotion; high potency: Augmented betamethasone dipropionate cream and betamethasone dipropionate cream and ointment; intermediate potency: Betamethasone dipropionate lotion and betamethasone valerate cream. Topical products labeled as augmented use a vehicle that augments (increases) the penetration of the drug into the skin.

Several recent studies conducted in children ≤12 years of age with atopic dermatitis demonstrated a high incidence of adrenal suppression when topical betamethasone products were applied twice daily for 2-3 weeks. Adrenal suppression occurred in 19 of 60 (32%) evaluable patients (3 months to 12 years of age) using Diprolene® AF cream 0.05%. A higher percent incidence of adrenal suppression was noted in younger children and infants (see product package insert). Pediatric patients may be more susceptible to adrenal suppression and other systemic side effects of topical corticosteroids, due to their larger skin surface area to body weight ratio. The smallest effective dose of topical corticosteroids should be used in pediatric patients.

Dosage Forms Excipient information presented when available (limited, particularly for generics); consult specific product labeling.

Note: Potency expressed as betamethasone base.

Aerosol, topical, as valerate [foam]:
Luxiq®: 0.12% (50 g, 100 g, 150 g) [strength expressed as salt; contains ethanol 60.4%]
Cream, topical, as dipropionate: 0.05% (15 g, 45 g)
Cream, topical, as dipropionate augmented: 0.05% (15 g, 50 g)
Diprolene® AF: 0.05% (15 g, 50 g)
Cream, topical, as valerate (Beta-Val®): 0.1% (15 g, 45 g)
Beta-Val®: 0.1% (15 g, 45 g)
Gel, topical, as dipropionate augmented: 0.05% (15 g, 50 g)
Injection, suspension: Betamethasone sodium phosphate 3 mg and betamethasone acetate 3 mg per 1 mL (5 mL)
Celestone® Soluspan®: Betamethasone sodium phosphate 3 mg and betamethasone acetate 3 mg per 1 mL (5 mL) [6 mg/mL]
Lotion, topical, as dipropionate: 0.05% (60 mL)
Lotion, topical, as dipropionate augmented:
Diprolene®: 0.05% (30 mL, 60 mL)
Lotion, topical, as valerate: 0.1% (60 mL)
Beta-Val®: 0.1% (60 mL)
Ointment, topical, as dipropionate: 0.05% (15 g, 45 g)
Ointment, topical, as dipropionate augmented: 0.05% (15 g, 50 g)
Diprolene®: 0.05% (15 g, 50 g)
Ointment, topical, as valerate: 0.1% (15 g, 45 g)
Solution, as base:
Celestone®: 0.6 mg/5 mL (118 mL) [contains alcohol and sodium benzoate; cherry-orange flavor]

◆ **Betamethasone Dipropionate** see Betamethasone on page 189

◆ **Betamethasone Dipropionate, Augmented** see Betamethasone on page 189

◆ **Betamethasone Sodium Phosphate** see Betamethasone on page 189

◆ **Betamethasone Valerate** see Betamethasone on page 189

◆ **Betapace®** see Sotalol on page 1284

◆ **Betapace AF®** see Sotalol on page 1284

◆ **Beta Sal® [OTC]** see Salicylic Acid on page 1241

◆ **Betasept® [OTC]** see Chlorhexidine Gluconate on page 291

◆ **Betatar® Gel [OTC]** see Coal Tar on page 349

◆ **Beta-Val®** see Betamethasone on page 189

◆ **Betaxin® (Can)** see Thiamine on page 1338

Bethanechol (be THAN e kole)

Medication Safety Issues
Sound-alike/look-alike issues:
Bethanechol may be confused with betaxolol

U.S. Brand Names Urecholine®

Canadian Brand Names Duvoid®; PMS-Bethanechol

Therapeutic Category Cholinergic Agent

Generic Available Yes

Use Treatment of nonobstructive urinary retention and retention due to neurogenic bladder; gastroesophageal reflux

Pregnancy Risk Factor C

Pregnancy Considerations Reproduction studies have not been conducted.

Lactation Excretion in breast milk unknown/not recommended

Contraindications Hypersensitivity to bethanechol chloride or any component; do not use in patients with mechanical obstruction of the GI or GU tract; do not use in patients with hyperthyroidism, peptic ulcer, bronchial asthma, or cardiac disease

Adverse Reactions
Cardiovascular: Hypotension, cardiac arrest, flushed skin (vasomotor response)
Central nervous system: Headache, malaise, seizure
Gastrointestinal: Abdominal cramps, belching, borborygmi, colicky pain, diarrhea, nausea, vomiting, salivation
Genitourinary: Urinary frequency
Hepatic: Liver enzymes elevated, bilirubin elevated
Ocular: Miosis, lacrimation
Respiratory: Bronchial constriction
Miscellaneous: Diaphoresis

Drug Interactions
Avoid Concomitant Use There are no known interactions where it is recommended to avoid concomitant use.
Increased Effect/Toxicity
The levels/effects of Bethanechol may be increased by: Acetylcholinesterase Inhibitors
Decreased Effect There are no known significant interactions involving a decrease in effect.

Mechanism of Action Stimulates cholinergic receptors in the smooth muscle of the urinary bladder and GI tract resulting in increased peristalsis, increased GI and pancreatic secretions, bladder muscle contraction, and increased ureteral peristaltic waves

Pharmacodynamics
Onset of action: Oral: 30-90 minutes
Duration: Oral: Up to 6 hours

Pharmacokinetics (Adult data unless noted)
Absorption: Oral: Variable
Metabolic fate and excretion have not been determined

Usual Dosage Oral:
Children:
Abdominal distention or urinary retention: 0.6 mg/kg/day divided 3-4 times/day
Gastroesophageal reflux: 0.1-0.2 mg/kg/dose or 3 mg/m^2/dose given 30 minutes to 1 hour before each meal to a maximum of 4 times/day
Adults: 10-50 mg 2-4 times/day

Administration Oral: Administer on an empty stomach to reduce nausea and vomiting

Patient Information Dizziness, lightheadedness, or fainting may occur especially when getting up from a lying position

◄ **Dosage Forms** Excipient information presented when available (limited, particularly for generics); consult specific product labeling. [CAN] = Canadian brand name
Tablet, as chloride: 5 mg, 10 mg, 25 mg, 50 mg
Duvoid® [CAN]: 10 mg, 25 mg, 50 mg [not available in U.S.]
Urecholine®: 5 mg, 10 mg, 25 mg, 50 mg

Extemporaneous Preparations
A 1 mg/mL solution may be made by crushing twelve 10 mg tablets; add sterile water in increments to a total volume of 120 mL; shake well; refrigerate; stable for 30 days (Schlatter, 1997).
A 5 mg/mL suspension may be made by crushing twelve 50 mg tablets; add to a total volume of 120 mL of a 1:1 mixture of Ora-Plus®:Ora-Sweet® or Ora-Plus®:Ora-Sweet® SF or 1:4 concentrated cherry syrup and simple syrup, NF mixture; stable 60 days refrigerated (preferred) or at room temperature; label "shake well" and protect from light (Allen, 1998; Nahata, 2004).
Allen LV Jr and Erickson MA, "Stability of Bethanechol Chloride, Pyrazinamide, Quinidine Sulfate, Rifampin, and Tetracycline Hydrochloride in Extemporaneously Compounded Oral Liquids," *Am J Health Syst Pharm*, 1998, 55(17):1804-9.
Nahata, MC, Pai VB, and Hipple TF, *Pediatric Drug Formulations*, 5th ed, Cincinnati, OH: Harvey Whitney Books Co, 2004.
Schlatter JL and Saulnier JL, "Bethanechol Chloride Oral Solutions: Stability and Use in Infants," *Ann Pharmacother*, 1997, 31(3):294-6.

◆ **Bethanechol Chloride** *see* Bethanechol *on page 191*

◆ **Betimol®** *see* Timolol *on page 1351*

◆ **Betnesol® (Can)** *see* Betamethasone *on page 189*

◆ **Betnovate® (Can)** *see* Betamethasone *on page 189*

Bevacizumab (be vuh SIZ uh mab)

Medication Safety Issues
Sound-alike/look-alike issues:
Avastin® may be confused with Astelin®
Bevacizumab may be confused with cetuximab, riTUXimab

International issues:
Avastin® [U.S., Canada, and multiple international markets] may be confused with Avaxim®, a brand name for hepatitis A vaccine [Canada and multiple international markets]

High alert medication: This medication is in a class the Institute for Safe Medication Practices (ISMP) includes among its list of drug classes which have a heightened risk of causing significant patient harm when used in error.

Related Information
Emetogenic Potential of Antineoplastic Agents *on page 1579*

U.S. Brand Names Avastin®
Canadian Brand Names Avastin®
Therapeutic Category Antineoplastic Agent, Monoclonal Antibody; Vascular Endothelial Growth Factor (VEGF) Inhibitor
Generic Available No
Use Treatment of metastatic colorectal cancer; treatment of advanced nonsquamous, nonsmall cell lung cancer; treatment of metastatic HER-2 negative breast cancer, glioblastoma with progressive disease following prior therapy as single agent (FDA approved in ages ≥18 years and adults). Has also been studied for use in recurrent ovarian cancer, renal cell cancer, age-related macular degeneration (AMD)
Pregnancy Risk Factor C

Pregnancy Considerations There are no adequate or well-controlled studies in pregnant women; however, bevacizumab is teratogenic in animals. Angiogenesis is of critical importance to fetal development, and bevacizumab inhibits angiogenesis. Adequate contraception during therapy is recommended (and for ≥6 months following last dose of bevacizumab per Canadian labeling). Patients should also be counseled regarding prolonged exposure following discontinuation of therapy due to the long half-life of bevacizumab.

Based on animal studies, bevacizumab may disrupt normal menstrual cycles and impair fertility by several effects, including reduced endometrial proliferation and follicular developmental arrest. Some parameters do not recover completely, or recover very slowly following discontinuation.

Lactation Excretion in breast milk unknown/not recommended
Breast-Feeding Considerations Immunoglobulins are excreted in breast milk, and it is assumed that bevacizumab may appear in breast milk. Due to concerns for effects on the infant, breast-feeding is not recommended. The half-life of bevacizumab is up to 50 days (average 20 days), and this should be considered when decisions are made concerning breast-feeding resumption.

Note: Canadian labeling recommends to discontinue breast-feeding during treatment and to avoid breast-feeding a minimum of 6 months following discontinuation of treatment.

Contraindications Hypersensitivity to bevacizumab, murine proteins, or any component.
Warnings Wound dehiscence/wound healing complications have been reported in patients (not related to treatment duration) **[U.S. Boxed Warning]**; monitor patients for signs/symptoms of improper wound healing. Permanently discontinue in patients who develop these complications. The appropriate intervals between administration of bevacizumab and surgical procedures to avoid impairment in wound healing has not been established. Do not initiate therapy within 28 days of major surgery and only following complete healing of the incision. Bevacizumab should be discontinued at least 28 days prior to elective surgery and the estimated half-life (20 days) should be considered.

May cause CHF and/or potentiate cardiotoxic effects of anthracyclines. CHF is more common with prior anthracycline exposure and/or left chest wall irradiation. Bevacizumab may cause and/or worsen hypertension significantly. Permanent discontinuation is recommended in patients who experience hypertensive crisis or encephalopathy. Temporarily discontinue in patients who develop uncontrolled hypertension. Cases of reversible posterior leukoencephalopathy syndrome (RPLS) have been reported; discontinue therapy if RPLS occurs. Symptoms such as headache, seizure, confusion, lethargy, blindness, or other vision or neurologic disturbances may occur from 16 hours to 1 year after treatment initiation. RPLS may be associated with hypertension; discontinue bevacizumab and begin management of hypertension if present.

Avoid use in patients with recent hemoptysis (>2.5 mL blood) or with CNS metastases **[U.S. Boxed Warning]**; severe or fatal hemorrhage has occurred, including hemoptysis, GI bleed, CNS bleeding, epistaxis, vaginal bleeding, and significant pulmonary bleeding (primarily in patients with nonsmall cell lung cancer with squamous cell histology); discontinuation of treatment is recommended in all patients with serious hemorrhage. Use with caution in patients with CNS metastases; one case of CNS hemorrhage was observed in a study of NSCLC patients with CNS metastases. Use with caution in patients at risk for thrombocytopenia. Bevacizumab may impair fertility and have adverse effects on fetal development; adequate contraception during therapy and following discontinuation is recommended. An increased risk for arterial thromboembolic events (eg, stroke, MI, TIA, angina) is associated with bevacizumab use in combination with chemotherapy. History of arterial thromboembolism or ≥65 years of age may present an even greater risk; permanently discontinue if serious arterial thromboembolic event occurs. Although patients with cancer are at risk for venous thromboembolism, a meta-analysis of 15 controlled trials has demonstrated an increased risk for venous thromboembolism in patients who received bevacizumab.

Interrupt therapy if patient experiences severe infusion reaction which includes hypertension, hypertensive crises associated with neurologic manifestations, wheezing, oxygen desaturation, chest pain, headaches, rigors, and diaphoresis. Proteinuria and/or nephrotic syndrome have been associated with bevacizumab; discontinue in patients with nephrotic syndrome. Microangiopathic hemolytic anemia (MAHA) has been reported when bevacizumab has been used in combination with sunitinib. Gastrointestinal perforation has been reported **[U.S. Boxed Warning]**; may be complicated by fistula formation (including enterocutaneous, esophageal, duodenal, and rectal fistulas), and nongastrointestinal fistulas (including tracheoesophageal, bronchopleural, biliary, vaginal, and bladder fistulas), most commonly within the first 6 months of treatment **[U.S. Boxed Warning]**; discontinue therapy in patients who develop these complications.

Precautions Use with caution in patients with cardiovascular disease, acquired coagulopathy, and patients with pre-existing hypertension (monitor blood pressure).

Adverse Reactions
Cardiovascular: Hypertension (may be dose-dependent), thromboembolism, hypotension, DVT, arterial thrombosis, syncope, intra-abdominal venous thrombosis, cerebrovascular arterial thrombotic event, CHF, chest pain, myocardial infarction, left ventricular dysfunction

Central nervous system: Pain, headache, dizziness, fatigue, confusion, rigors, fever, reversible posterior leukoencephalopathy syndrome

Dermatologic: Alopecia, dry skin, exfoliative dermatitis, erythema, nail disorder, wound dehiscence, skin ulcer

Endocrine & metabolic: Weight loss, hypokalemia, dehydration

Gastrointestinal: Abdominal pain, diarrhea, vomiting, anorexia, constipation, stomatitis, GI hemorrhage, dyspepsia, taste disorder, nausea, flatulence, xerostomia, colitis, ileus, fistulas, GI perforation, intra-abdominal abscess, hemoptysis

Genitourinary: Polyuria/urgency, vaginal hemorrhage

Hematologic: Leukopenia, neutropenia, thrombocytopenia, hemorrhage, anemia

Hepatic: Bilirubinemia

Neuromuscular & skeletal: Weakness, myalgia, paresthesia, abnormal gait, neuropathy (sensory and other)

Renal: Proteinuria, nephrotic syndrome, renal thrombotic microangiopathy

Respiratory: Dyspnea, epistaxis, wheezing

Miscellaneous: Sepsis

Drug Interactions
Avoid Concomitant Use
Avoid concomitant use of Bevacizumab with any of the following: Sunitinib

Increased Effect/Toxicity
Bevacizumab may increase the levels/effects of: Antineoplastic Agents (Anthracycline); Irinotecan; Sorafenib; Sunitinib

The levels/effects of Bevacizumab may be increased by: Sunitinib

Decreased Effect There are no known significant interactions involving a decrease in effect.

Stability Store vials in the refrigerator; protect from light; do not freeze or shake. **Do not mix** with dextrose-containing solutions (concentration-dependent degradation may occur). Diluted solution is stable for up to 8 hours under refrigeration.

Mechanism of Action Bevacizumab is a recombinant, humanized monoclonal antibody which binds and neutralizes vascular endothelial growth factor (VEGF), preventing its association with endothelial receptors. VEGF binding initiates angiogenesis (endothelial proliferation and the formation of new blood vessels). The inhibition of microvascular growth is believed to retard the growth of all tissues, including metastatic tissue.

Pharmacokinetics (Adult data unless noted)
Half-life: Adults: 20 days (range: 11-50 days)

Usual Dosage I.V.: Details concerning dosing in combination regimens should also be consulted:

Children: Solid tumor:
Monotherapy: 15 mg/kg every 2 weeks in 28-day cycles
Combination therapy: 5-10 mg/kg every 2 weeks in combination chemotherapy regimens

Adults:
Colorectal cancer: 5-10 mg/kg every 2 weeks
Non-small cell lung cancer (nonsquamous): 15 mg/kg every 3 weeks
Breast cancer: 10 mg/kg every 2 weeks
Glioblastoma: 10 mg/kg every 2 weeks
Ovarian cancer: 15 mg/kg every 3 weeks
Renal cell cancer: 10 mg/kg every 2 weeks

Administration I.V. infusion: Dilute prescribed dose of bevacizumab in 100 mL NS; infuse the initial dose over 90 minutes; shorten infusion to 60 minutes if the initial infusion is well-tolerated. Third and subsequent infusions may be shortened to 30 minutes if the 60-minute infusion is well-tolerated.

Monitoring Parameters Monitor for signs of an infusion reaction during infusion; blood pressure (continue to monitor blood pressure during and after bevacizumab has been discontinued). Monitor CBC with differential; signs/symptoms of GI perforation or abscess (abdominal pain, constipation, vomiting); signs/symptoms of bleeding including hemoptysis, GI bleeding, CNS bleeding, epistaxis. Urinalysis for proteinuria, nephrotic syndrome

Patient Information Use adequate contraception during therapy and for 6 months following discontinuation of bevacizumab.

Dosage Forms Excipient information presented when available (limited, particularly for generics); consult specific product labeling.

Injection, solution [preservative free]:
Avastin®: 25 mg/mL (4 mL, 16 mL)

References
Glade JL, Adamson PC, Baruchel S, et al, "A Phase I Study of Bevacizumab in Children With Refractory Solid Tumors: A Children's Oncology Group Study," *Journal of Clinical Oncology,* 2006, 24 (18S):9017.

Nalluri SR, Chu D, Keresztes R, et al, "Risk of Venous Thromboembolism With the Angiogenesis Inhibitor Bevacizumab in Cancer Patients: A Meta-Analysis," *JAMA,* 2008, 300(19):2277-85.

◆ **Bio-Carbamazepine (Can)** *see* CarBAMazepine *on page 244*

◆ **Bio-Hydrochlorothiazide (Can)** *see* Hydrochlorothiazide *on page 682*

◆ **Bioniche Promethazine (Can)** *see* Promethazine *on page 1163*

◆ **BioQuin® Durules™ (Can)** *see* QuiNIDine *on page 1192*

Biotin (BYE oh tin)

Therapeutic Category Biotinidase Deficiency, Treatment Agent; Nutritional Supplement; Vitamin, Water Soluble

Use Treatment of primary biotinidase deficiency; nutritional biotin deficiency; component of the vitamin B complex

Contraindications Hypersensitivity to biotin or any component

Food Interactions Large amounts of raw egg whites prevent biotin absorption

Mechanism of Action A member of the B-complex group of vitamins; biotin is required for various metabolic functions such as gluconeogenesis, lipogenesis, fatty acid biosynthesis, propionate metabolism, and the catabolism of branched-chain amino acids; there are 9 known biotin-dependent enzymes; the enzyme biotinidase regenerates biotin in the body and is also required for the release of dietary protein-bound biotin.

Biotinidase deficiency is an autosomal recessively inherited metabolic disorder characterized by deficient activity of the enzyme in serum. Children with the disorder usually exhibit seizures, hypotonia, ataxia, skin rash, alopecia, metabolic ketoacidosis, and organic aciduria.

Usual Dosage Oral:

RDA: Infants, Children, and Adults: There is no official RDA, however 100-200 mcg/day is considered adequate

Biotinidase deficiency: Neonates, Infants, Children, and Adults: 5-10 mg once daily

Biotin deficiency: Children and Adults: 5-20 mg once daily

Administration Oral: May be administered without regard to meals

Reference Range Serum biotinidase activity

Dosage Forms Capsule: 1 mg

References

McVoy JR, Levy HL, Lawler M, et al, "Partial Biotinidase Deficiency: Clinical and Biochemical Features," *J Pediatr*, 1990, 116(1):78-83.

Salbert BA, Pellock JM, and Wolf B, "Characterization of Seizures Associated With Biotinidase Deficiency," *Neurology*, 1993, 43 (7):1351-5.

Wastell HJ, Bartlett K, Dale G, et al, "Biotinidase Deficiency: A Survey of 10 Cases," *Arch Dis Child*, 1988, 63(10):1244-9.

◆ **Biphentin® (Can)** *see* Methylphenidate *on page 908*

◆ **Bisac-Evac™ [OTC]** *see* Bisacodyl *on page 194*

Bisacodyl (bis a KOE dil)

Medication Safety Issues

Sound-alike/look-alike issues:

Doxidan® may be confused with doxepin

Dulcolax® (bisacodyl) may be confused with Dulcolax® (docusate)

Beers Criteria medication: This drug may be inappropriate for use in geriatric patients (high severity risk).

U.S. Brand Names Alophen® [OTC]; Bisac-Evac™ [OTC]; Bisacodyl Uniserts® [OTC] [DSC]; Biscolax™ [OTC]; Correctol® Tablets [OTC]; Dacodyl™ [OTC]; Doxidan® [OTC]; Dulcolax® [OTC]; ex-lax® Ultra [OTC]; Femilax™ [OTC]; Fleet® Bisacodyl [OTC]; Fleet® Stimulant Laxative [OTC]; Veracolate [OTC]

Canadian Brand Names Apo-Bisacodyl®; Carter's Little Pills®; Dulcolax®; Gentlax®

Therapeutic Category Laxative, Stimulant

Generic Available Yes: Excludes enema

Use Treatment of constipation; colonic evacuation prior to procedures or examination

Pregnancy Risk Factor C

Contraindications Hypersensitivity to bisacodyl or any component; do not use in patients with abdominal pain, appendicitis, obstruction, nausea or vomiting; not to be used during pregnancy or lactation

Warnings Stimulant laxatives are habit-forming; long-term use may result in laxative dependence and loss of normal bowel function.

Precautions Bisacodyl tannex powder for preparation as a rectal solution should be used with caution in patients with ulceration of the colon

Adverse Reactions

Endocrine & metabolic: Electrolyte and fluid imbalance (metabolic acidosis or alkalosis, hypocalcemia)

Gastrointestinal: Abdominal cramps, nausea, vomiting, diarrhea, rectal burning, proctitis (rare)

Drug Interactions

Avoid Concomitant Use There are no known interactions where it is recommended to avoid concomitant use.

Increased Effect/Toxicity There are no known significant interactions involving an increase in effect.

Decreased Effect

The levels/effects of Bisacodyl may be decreased by: Antacids

Food Interactions Administration within 1 hour of ingesting antacids, alkaline material, milk, or dairy products will cause premature dissolution of the enteric coating and resultant gastric irritation

Stability Store enteric-coated tablets and rectal suppositories at <30°C.

Mechanism of Action Stimulates peristalsis by directly irritating the smooth muscle of the intestine, possibly the colonic intramural plexus; alters water and electrolyte secretion producing net intestinal fluid accumulation and laxation

Pharmacodynamics Onset of action:

Oral: Within 6-10 hours

Rectal: 15-60 minutes

Pharmacokinetics (Adult data unless noted)

Absorption: Oral, rectal: <5% absorbed systemically

Metabolism: In the liver

Elimination: Conjugated metabolites excreted in breast milk, bile, and urine

Usual Dosage

Bisacodyl (Dulcolax®) tablet: Oral:

Children 3-12 years: 5-10 mg or 0.3 mg/kg/day as a single dose

Children ≥12 years and Adults: 5-15 mg/day as a single dose; maximum dose: 30 mg

Bisacodyl (Dulcolax®) suppository: Rectal:

Children:

<2 years: 5 mg/day as a single dose

2-11 years: 5-10 mg/day as a single dose

Children ≥12 years and Adults: 10 mg/day as a single dose

Administration Oral: Administer on an empty stomach with water; patient should swallow tablet whole; do not break or chew enteric-coated tablet; do not administer within 1 hour of ingesting antacids, alkaline material, milk, or dairy products

Patient Information Should not be used regularly for more than 1 week

Additional Information In a randomized prospective study of 70 patients, bisacodyl tablets were given orally once daily in the morning for 2 days before colonoscopy to 19 patients (dose for children <5 years: 5 mg; 5-12 years: 10 mg; >12 years: 15 mg) with a Fleet® enema given on the morning of the procedure without any dietary restriction. Results showed that bisacodyl without dietary restriction provided unsatisfactory colon cleansing.

Dosage Forms Excipient information presented when available (limited, particularly for generics); consult specific product labeling. [DSC] = Discontinued product

Solution, rectal [enema]:
  Fleet® Bisacodyl: 10 mg/30 mL (37 mL)
Suppository, rectal: 10 mg
  Bisac-Evac™, Bisacodyl Uniserts® [DSC], Biscolax™, Dulcolax®: 10 mg
Tablet [enteric coated]: 5 mg
  Alophen®, Bisac-Evac™, Correctol®, Dacodyl™, Dulco-lax®, ex-lax® Ultra, Femilax™, Veracolate: 5 mg
Tablet, delayed release: 5 mg
  Doxidan®, Fleet® Stimulant Laxative: 5 mg

References

BaKer SS, Liptak GS, Colletti RB, et al, "Constipation in Infants and Children: Evaluation and Treatment," 2000, www.naspgn.org/constipation.

Dahshan A, Lin CH, Peters J, et al, "A Randomized, Prospective Study to Evaluate the Efficacy and Acceptance of Three Bowel Preparations for Colonoscopy in Children," *Am J Gastroenterol*, 1999, 94 (12):3497-501.

◆ **Bisacodyl Uniserts® [OTC] [DSC]** *see* Bisacodyl *on page 194*

◆ **bis-chloronitrosourea** *see* Carmustine *on page 252*

◆ **Biscolax™ [OTC]** *see* Bisacodyl *on page 194*

◆ **Bismatrol** *see* Bismuth *on page 195*

◆ **Bismatrol [OTC]** *see* Bismuth *on page 195*

◆ **Bismatrol Maximum Strength [OTC]** *see* Bismuth *on page 195*

Bismuth (BIZ muth)

Medication Safety Issues

Sound-alike/look-alike issues:
Kaopectate® may be confused with Kayexalate®

Maalox® Total Relief® is a different formulation than other Maalox® liquid antacid products which contain aluminum hydroxide, magnesium hydroxide, and simethicone.

Note: Canadian formulation of Kaopectate® does not contain bismuth; the active ingredient in the Canadian formulation is attapulgite.

U.S. Brand Names Bismatrol Maximum Strength [OTC]; Bismatrol [OTC]; Diotame® [OTC]; Kao-Tin [OTC]; Kaopectate® Extra Strength [OTC]; Kaopectate® [OTC]; Kapectolin [OTC] [DSC]; Maalox® Total Relief® [OTC]; Peptic Relief [OTC]; Pepto Relief [OTC]; Pepto-Bismol® Maximum Strength [OTC]; Pepto-Bismol® [OTC]

Therapeutic Category Antidiarrheal; Gastrointestinal Agent, Gastric or Duodenal Ulcer Treatment

Generic Available Yes

Use

Subsalicylate formulation: Symptomatic treatment of mild, nonspecific diarrhea including traveler's diarrhea; chronic infantile diarrhea; adjunctive treatment of *Helicobacter pylori*-associated antral gastritis

Subgallate formulation: An aid to reduce fecal odors from a colostomy or ileostomy

Pregnancy Risk Factor C/D (3rd trimester)

Lactation Excretion in breast milk unknown (salicylates enter breast milk)/use caution

Contraindications Hypersensitivity to bismuth, salicylates, or any component; history of severe GI bleeding or coagulopathy

Warnings Kaopectate® has been reformulated to contain **only** bismuth subsalicylate; follow dosage recommendations closely. Do not use subsalicylate in patients with a viral infection, such as influenza or chickenpox, because of

the risk of Reye's syndrome; when using bismuth subsalicylate, changes in behavior (along with nausea and vomiting) may be an early sign of Reye's syndrome; instruct patients and caregivers to contact their healthcare provider if these symptoms occur; subsalicylate should be used with caution if patient is taking aspirin, due to additive toxicity; use with caution in children <3 years of age; be aware of salicylate content when prescribing for use in children. May cause bleeding.

Precautions May interfere with radiologic examinations of GI tract as bismuth is radiopaque; should not be used in patients with a history of bleeding disorder, gastrointestinal ulcer disease, or those taking anticoagulants, clopidogrel, NSAIDS, and/or oral antidiabetic agents.

Adverse Reactions

Central nervous system: Anxiety, confusion, headache, mental depression, slurred speech

Gastrointestinal: Darkened tongue, grayish-black stools, impaction (infants and debilitated patients)

Hematologic: Bleeding

Neuromuscular & skeletal: Muscle spasms, weakness

Otic: Loss of hearing, tinnitus

Drug Interactions

Avoid Concomitant Use There are no known interactions where it is recommended to avoid concomitant use.

Increased Effect/Toxicity There are no known significant interactions involving an increase in effect.

Decreased Effect

Bismuth may decrease the levels/effects of: Tetracycline Derivatives

Mechanism of Action Adsorbs extra water in large intestine, as well as toxins; forms a protective coat on the intestinal mucosa; appears to have antisecretory (salicylate moiety) and antimicrobial effects (bismuth moiety) against bacterial and viral pathogens

Pharmacokinetics (Adult data unless noted)

Absorption: Bismuth is minimally absorbed (<1%) across the GI tract while salicylate salt is readily absorbed (80%)

Distribution: Salicylate: V_d: 170 mL/kg

Protein binding, plasma: Bismuth and salicylate: >90%

Metabolism: Bismuth salts undergo chemical dissociation after oral administration; salicylate is extensively metabolized in the liver

Half-life:
  Bismuth: Terminal: 21-72 days
  Salicylate: Terminal: 2-5 hours
Elimination:
  Bismuth: Renal, biliary
  Salicylate: Only 10% excreted unchanged in urine

Usual Dosage Oral: Bismuth subsalicylate: **(bismuth subsalicylate liquid dosages expressed in mL of 262 mg/15 mL concentration):**

Nonspecific diarrhea: Children: 100 mg/kg/day divided into 5 equal doses for 5 days (maximum: 4.19 g/day) **or**

Children: Up to 8 doses/24 hours:
  3-6 years: 1/3 tablet or 5 mL (87 mg) every 30 minutes to 1 hour as needed
  6-9 years: 2/3 tablet or 10 mL (175 mg) every 30 minutes to 1 hour as needed
  9-12 years: 1 tablet or 15 mL (262 mg) every 30 minutes to 1 hour as needed
  Adults: 2 tablets or 30 mL (524 mg) every 30 minutes to 1 hour as needed up to 8 doses/24 hours

Chronic infantile diarrhea:
  2-24 months: 2.5 mL (44 mg) every 4 hours
  24-48 months: 5 mL (87 mg) every 4 hours
  48-70 months: 10 mL (175 mg) every 4 hours

Prevention of traveler's diarrhea: Adults: 2.1 g/day or 2 tablets 4 times/day before meals and at bedtime

◀ *Helicobacter pylori*-associated antral gastritis: Dosage in children is not well established, the following dosages have been used [in conjunction with ampicillin and metronidazole or (in adults) tetracycline and metronidazole]:
Children ≤10 years: 15 mL (262 mg) 4 times/day for 6 weeks
Children >10 years and Adults: 30 mL (524 mg) solution or two 262 mg tablets 4 times/day for 6 weeks
Dosing adjustment in renal impairment: Avoid use in patients with renal failure
Administration Oral: Shake liquid well before using; chew tablets or allow to dissolve in mouth before swallowing
Test Interactions Bismuth absorbs x-rays and may interfere with diagnostic procedures of GI tract
Patient Information May darken stools; if diarrhea persists for more than 2 days, consult a physician; may turn tongue black; notify physician if behavioral changes along with nausea and vomiting occur (see Warnings)
Additional Information Bismuth subsalicylate: 262 mg = 130 mg nonaspirin salicylate; 525 mg = 236 mg non-aspirin salicylate
Dosage Forms Excipient information presented when available (limited, particularly for generics); consult specific product labeling. [DSC] = Discontinued product
Caplet, as subsalicylate:
Kaopectate®: 262 mg
Pepto-Bismol®: 262 mg [sugar free; contains sodium 2 mg/caplet]
Liquid, as subsalicylate: 262 mg/15 mL (240 mL)
Bismatrol: 262 mg/15 mL (240 mL)
Bismatrol Maximum Strength: 525 mg/15 mL (240 mL)
Diotame®: 262 mg/15 mL (30 mL) [sugar free]
Kaopectate®: 262 mg/15 mL (236 mL, 354 mL [DSC]) [contains potassium 5 mg/15 mL, sodium 5 mg/15 mL; peppermint flavor]
Kaopectate®: 262 mg/15 mL (236 mL, 354 mL) [contains potassium 5 mg/15 mL, sodium 5 mg/15 mL; regular flavor]
Kaopectate®: 262 mg/15 mL (177 mL) [contains sodium 4 mg/15 mL; cherry flavor]
Kaopectate®: 262 mg/15 mL (354 mL) [contains sodium 4 mg/15 mL; vanilla flavor]
Kaopectate® Extra Strength: 525 mg/15 mL (236 mL) [contains potassium 5 mg/15 mL, sodium 5 mg/15 mL; peppermint flavor]
Kao-Tin: 262 mg/15 mL (240 mL, 480 mL) [contains sodium benzoate]
Maalox® Total Relief®: 525 mg/15 mL (360 mL) [contains sodium 3.3 mg/15 mL; strawberry and peppermint flavor]
Peptic Relief: 262 mg/15 mL (240 mL) [sugar free; mint flavor]
Pepto-Bismol®: 262 mg/15 mL (120 mL, 240 mL, 360 mL, 480 mL) [sugar free; contains sodium 6 mg/15 mL and benzoic acid; cherry and wintergreen flavors]
Pepto-Bismol® Maximum Strength: 525 mg/15 mL (120 mL, 240 mL, 360 mL) [sugar free; contains sodium 6 mg/15 mL and benzoic acid; wintergreen flavor]
Suspension, as subsalicylate:
Kapectolin: 262 mg/15 mL (480 mL) [mint flavor] [DSC]
Tablet, chewable, as subsalicylate: 262 mg
Bismatrol: 262 mg
Diotame®: 262 mg [sugar free]
Peptic Relief, Pepto Relief: 262 mg
Pepto-Bismol®: 262 mg [sugar free; contains sodium <1 mg; cherry and wintergreen flavors]
References
Drumm B, Sherman P, Karmali M, et al, "Treatment of *Campylobacter pylori*-associated Antral Gastritis in Children With Bismuth Subsalicylate and Ampicillin," *J Pediatr*, 1988, 113(5):908-12.
Soriano-Brucher HE, Avendano P, O'Ryan M, et al, "Use of Bismuth Subsalicylate in Acute Diarrhea in Children," *Rev Infect Dis*, 1990, 12 (Suppl 1):S51-5.

Walsh JH and Peterson WL, "The Treatment of *Helicobacter pylori* Infection in the Management of Peptic Ulcer Disease," *N Engl J Med*, 1995, 333(15):984-91.

◆ **Bismuth Subsalicylate** *see* Bismuth *on page 195*
◆ **Bistropamide** *see* Tropicamide *on page 1390*
◆ **Bivalent Human Papillomavirus Vaccine** *see* Papillomavirus (Types 16, 18) Vaccine (Human, Recombinant) *on page 1058*
◆ **Bi-Zets** *see* Benzocaine *on page 182*
◆ **Black-Draught™ Tablets [OTC]** *see* Senna *on page 1253*
◆ **Black Widow Spider Species Antivenin** *see* Antivenin (*Latrodectus mactans*) *on page 121*
◆ **Blenoxane** *see* Bleomycin *on page 196*
◆ **Blenoxane® (Can)** *see* Bleomycin *on page 196*
◆ **Bleo** *see* Bleomycin *on page 196*

Bleomycin (blee oh MYE sin)

Medication Safety Issues
Sound-alike/look-alike issues:
Bleomycin may be confused with Cleocin®

High alert medication: This medication is in a class the Institute for Safe Medication Practices (ISMP) includes among its list of drugs which have a heightened risk of causing significant patient harm when used in error.
Related Information
Compatibility of Chemotherapy and Related Supportive Care Medications *on page 1580*
Emetogenic Potential of Antineoplastic Agents *on page 1579*
Canadian Brand Names Blenoxane®; Bleomycin Injection, USP
Therapeutic Category Antineoplastic Agent, Antibiotic
Generic Available Yes
Use Palliative treatment of squamous cell carcinoma, testicular carcinoma, and germ cell tumors; Hodgkin's lymphoma, non-Hodgkin's lymphoma, renal carcinoma, and soft tissue sarcoma; sclerosing agent to control malignant effusions
Pregnancy Risk Factor D
Pregnancy Considerations Animal studies have demonstrated teratogenic and abortifacient effects. There are no adequate and well-controlled studies in pregnant women. Women of childbearing potential should avoid becoming pregnant during treatment.
Lactation Excretion in breast milk unknown/not recommended
Breast-Feeding Considerations Due to the potential for serious adverse reactions in the nursing infant, breast-feeding is not recommended.
Contraindications Hypersensitivity to bleomycin sulfate or any component
Warnings Hazardous agent; use appropriate precautions for handling and disposal. Pulmonary toxicity occurs in 10% of patients and can progress to pulmonary fibrosis **[U.S. Boxed Warning]**. Occurrence of pulmonary fibrosis is higher in elderly patients and in those receiving a total cumulative dose >400 units; pulmonary toxicity has occurred at a total dosage <200 units or 250 units/m^2 in younger patients; pulmonary irradiation and use of supplemental oxygen increase the chance for developing toxic pulmonary reactions in patients previously treated with bleomycin; a severe idiosyncratic reaction consisting of hypotension, mental confusion, fever, chills, and wheezing is possible **[U.S. Boxed Warning]**. This reaction may be immediate or delayed, but usually occurs after the first or second dose.

Precautions Use with caution in patients with renal or pulmonary impairment; dosage modification is recommended in patients with renal impairment; dosage modification may be necessary in patients with a 20% decrease from baseline in FEV_1, FVC, or DL_{co}; administer test dose to lymphoma patients prior to starting therapy

Adverse Reactions

Cardiovascular: Cerebrovascular accident, hypotension, Raynaud's phenomenon

Central nervous system: Fever, chills, malaise

Dermatologic: Hyperpigmentation, hyperkeratosis of hands and nails, rash, alopecia, desquamation

Gastrointestinal: Stomatitis, vomiting, anorexia, mild nausea

Hematologic: Thrombocytopenia, leukopenia

Local: Phlebitis

Respiratory: Interstitial pneumonitis (10%), pulmonary fibrosis (cumulative lifetime dose should not exceed 400 units or 250 units/m^2 in younger patients), dyspnea, tachypnea, nonproductive cough, rales

Miscellaneous: Anaphylactoid reactions

Drug Interactions

Avoid Concomitant Use

Avoid concomitant use of Bleomycin with any of the following: BCG; Natalizumab; Pimecrolimus; Tacrolimus (Topical); Vaccines (Live)

Increased Effect/Toxicity

Bleomycin may increase the levels/effects of: Leflunomide; Natalizumab; Vaccines (Live)

The levels/effects of Bleomycin may be increased by: Denosumab; Filgrastim; Gemcitabine; Pimecrolimus; Sargramostim; Tacrolimus (Topical); Trastuzumab

Decreased Effect

Bleomycin may decrease the levels/effects of: BCG; Cardiac Glycosides; Sipuleucel-T; Vaccines (Inactivated); Vaccines (Live)

The levels/effects of Bleomycin may be decreased by: Echinacea

Stability Refrigerate; intact vials are stable 28 days at room temperature; reconstituted solution is stable for 24 hours at room temperature; incompatible with amino acid solutions, ascorbic acid, cefazolin, furosemide, diazepam, hydrocortisone, mitomycin, nafcillin, penicillin G, aminophylline, copper; dilution in dextrose solutions may result in a 10% loss of activity within 24 hours

Mechanism of Action Inhibits synthesis of DNA; binds to DNA leading to single- and double-strand breaks by a Fe^{++}-O_2-catalyzed free radical reaction

Pharmacokinetics (Adult data unless noted)

Distribution: Into skin, lungs, kidneys, peritoneum, and lymphatics

Protein binding: <10%

Half-life: Dependent upon renal function

Children: 2.1-3.5 hours

Adults, with normal renal function: 2-3 hours

Time to peak serum concentration: I.M.: Within 30-60 minutes

Elimination: 60% to 70% of a dose excreted in the urine as active drug

Dialysis: Not removed by hemodialysis

Usual Dosage Refer to individual protocol

Children and Adults:

I.M., I.V., SubQ:

Test dose for lymphoma patients: 1-2 units of bleomycin for the first 2 doses; monitor vital signs every 15 minutes; wait a minimum of 1 hour before administering remainder of dose

Treatment: 10-20 units/m^2 (0.25-0.5 units/kg) 1-2 times/week in combination regimens or once every 2-4 weeks

Germ cell tumors: 15 units/m^2/dose once weekly for 3 weeks per regimen

Hodgkin's disease: 10 units/m^2/dose on days 1 and 15 of cycle

I.V. continuous infusion: 15-20 units/m^2/day over 24 hours for 3-5 days

Adults: Intracavitary injection for pleural effusion: 15-60 units (dose generally does not exceed 1 unit/kg); drug is diluted with 50-100 mL of NS and is instilled into the pleural cavity via a thoracostomy tube

Dosing adjustment in renal impairment:

Cl_{cr} 25-50 mL/minute: Reduce dose by 25%

Cl_{cr} <25 mL/minute: Reduce dose by 50% to 75%

Administration Parenteral:

I.V.: Administer I.V. slowly over at least 10 minutes (no greater than 1 unit/minute) at a concentration not to exceed 3 units/mL; bleomycin for I.V. continuous infusion can be further diluted in NS (preferred) or D_5W; administration by continuous infusion may produce less severe pulmonary toxicity.

I.M., SubQ: 15 units/mL concentration may be used for I.M., SubQ administration

Monitoring Parameters Pulmonary function tests (total lung volume, FEV_1, FVC, DL_{co}), renal function tests, chest x-ray; vital signs and temperature initially; CBC with differential and platelet count

Patient Information Report any coughing, shortness of breath, or wheezing to physician

Nursing Implications Fever and chills can occur 2-6 hours following parenteral administration; pretreatment with acetaminophen, antihistamine, and hydrocortisone may decrease the severity of fever and chills

Dosage Forms Excipient information presented when available (limited, particularly for generics); consult specific product labeling.

Injection, powder for reconstitution, as sulfate: 15 units, 30 units

References

Alberts DS, Chen HS, Liu R, et al, "Bleomycin Pharmacokinetics in Man. I. Intravenous Administration," *Cancer Chemother Pharmacol*, 1978, 1(3):177-81.

Berg SL, Grisell DL, Delaney TF, et al, "Principles of Treatment of Pediatric Solid Tumors," *Pediatr Clin North Am*, 1991, 38(2):249-67.

Bosentan (boe SEN tan)

Medication Safety Issues

Sound-alike/look-alike issues:

Tracleer® may be confused with TriCor®

Related Information
World Health Organization (WHO) Functional Classification of Pulmonary Hypertension *on page 1483*

U.S. Brand Names Tracleer®

Canadian Brand Names Tracleer®

Therapeutic Category Endothelin Receptor Antagonist

Generic Available No

Use Treatment of pulmonary arterial hypertension (PAH) in patients with World Health Organization (WHO) Class II, III, or IV symptoms to improve exercise capacity and decrease the rate of clinical deterioration (FDA approved in ages >12 years and adults).

Restrictions Bosentan (Tracleer®) is available only through a limited distribution program [Tracleer® Access Program (T.A.P.)]. Only prescribers and pharmacies registered with T.A.P. may prescribe and dispense bosentan. Patients who receive the drug must be enrolled in and meet all conditions of T.A.P. Further information may be obtained from the manufacturer, Actelion Pharmaceuticals (1-866-228-3546).

Medication Guide An FDA-approved patient medication guide, which is available with the product information and at http://www.fda.gov/downloads/Drugs/DrugSafety/ucm089801.pdf, must be dispensed with this medication for each new outpatient prescription and refill.

Pregnancy Risk Factor X

Pregnancy Considerations [U.S. Boxed Warning]: Use in pregnancy is contraindicated; may cause birth defects. Exclude pregnancy prior to initiation of therapy, monthly during therapy and one month after stopping bosentan. Two reliable methods of contraception must be used during therapy and for one month after stopping treatment except in patients with tubal ligation or an implanted IUD (Copper T 380A or LNg 20). No other contraceptive measures are required for these patients. Women of childbearing potential should avoid exposure to dust generated from broken or split tablets, especially if repeated exposure is expected (tablet splitting is currently outside of product labeling). Sperm counts may be reduced in men during treatment. No changes in sperm function or hormone levels have been noted.

Lactation Excretion in breast milk unknown/not recommended

Contraindications Hypersensitivity to bosentan or any component; pregnancy (see Warnings); concurrent use of cyclosporine or glyburide

Warnings Serious hepatic injury, including rare reports of cirrhosis and liver failure may occur **[U.S. Boxed Warning]**. Elevations in liver aminotransferases (ALT and AST) of at least 3 times the upper limit of normal may occur in 11% of patients with elevations in bilirubin in some cases. Monitor liver enzymes at baseline and monthly thereafter. Use with caution in patients with mildly impaired liver function; avoid use in moderate-to-severe hepatic impairment. Avoid use in patients with elevated serum transaminases (>3 times upper limit of normal) at baseline; adjust dosage if elevations in liver enzymes occur during therapy. Treatment should be discontinued in patients who develop elevated transaminases (ALT or AST) in combination with symptoms of hepatic injury (unusual fatigue, jaundice, nausea, vomiting, abdominal pain, and/or fever) or elevated serum bilirubin ≥2 times upper limit of normal.

Major birth defects may occur if bosentan is used during pregnancy (use in pregnancy is contraindicated) **[U.S. Boxed Warning]**. Exclude pregnancy prior to initiation of therapy; obtain monthly pregnancy tests in women of childbearing potential during therapy and 1 month after stopping treatment. Two reliable methods of contraception must be used during therapy and for 1 month after stopping treatment except in patients with tubal ligation or an implanted IUD (Copper T 380A or LNg20). One additional method of contraception is still needed if a male partner has had a vasectomy. Efficacy of hormonal contraceptives may be decreased (see Drug Interactions), and should not be the sole contraceptive method in patients receiving bosentan. A missed menses should be reported to healthcare provider and prompt immediate pregnancy testing. Women of childbearing potential should avoid excessive handling of broken tablets and should not be exposed to the drug by crushing the tablets; tablets should be dissolved in water if necessary (see Extemporaneous Preparations).

Patients with WHO Class II symptoms who received bosentan demonstrated a decrease in the rate of clinical deterioration; however, only a trend for improved exercise capacity was observed. The risk of serious hepatic injury should be weighed against these benefits in this group of patients, as serious hepatic injury may preclude future use of bosentan as the disease progresses.

Precautions Use with caution in patients with low hemoglobin levels or ischemic cardiovascular disease. Bosentan may cause dose-related decreases in hemoglobin and hematocrit (monitoring of hemoglobin is recommended). May cause fluid retention, worsening of CHF, weight gain, and leg edema; **Note:** PAH itself may cause fluid retention and edema; if significant fluid retention occurs, further evaluation may be necessary to determine the cause and appropriate treatment or discontinuation of bosentan therapy. If pulmonary edema occurs, consider the possibility of pulmonary veno-occlusive disease and discontinue bosentan. Sperm count may be reduced in men during treatment; no changes in sperm function or hormone levels have been noted; fertility issues may require discussion with patient. Safety and efficacy in pediatric patients ≤12 years have not been established. Limited information exists about the safety and efficacy of bosentan in adolescents 12-18 years of age.

Adverse Reactions Percent incidence is from adult studies:

Cardiovascular: Chest pain, edema, flushing, hypotension, palpitation, syncope

Central nervous system: Fatigue, headache

Endocrine & metabolic: Fluid retention, weight gain

Genitourinary: Sperm count decreased

Hematologic: Anemia, hemoglobin decreased (≥1 g/dL in up to 57% of patients, typically in first 6 weeks of therapy; markedly decreased hemoglobin may occur in up to 6% of patients)

Hepatic: Abnormal hepatic function, bilirubin elevated, hepatic cirrhosis (rare; reported after prolonged use >12 months in patients receiving multiple medications), jaundice, liver enzymes elevated (**Note:** Transaminases are increased >3 times the upper limit of normal in up to 11% of patients; elevations are dose-dependent, may occur at any time, usually progress slowly, typically are asymptomatic, and usually are reversible after drug interruption or discontinuation), liver failure (rare)

Neuromuscular & skeletal: Arthralgia

Respiratory: Respiratory tract infection, sinusitis

<1%, postmarketing, and/or case reports: Angioneurotic edema, dizziness, heart failure (exacerbation), hypersensitivity, leukocytoclastic vasculitis, leukopenia, neutropenia, peripheral edema, rash, thrombocytopenia

Drug Interactions

Metabolism/Transport Effects Substrate of CYP2C9 (major), CYP3A4 (major), SLCO1B1; **Induces** CYP2C9 (strong), 3A4 (strong)

Avoid Concomitant Use

Avoid concomitant use of Bosentan with any of the following: CycloSPORINE; CycloSPORINE (Systemic); Dronedarone; Everolimus; GlyBURIDE; Nilotinib; Nisoldipine; Pazopanib; Ranolazine; Romidepsin; Tolvaptan

Increased Effect/Toxicity

The levels/effects of Bosentan may be increased by: Antifungal Agents (Azole Derivatives, Systemic); CycloSPORINE; CycloSPORINE (Systemic); CYP2C9 Inhibitors (Moderate); CYP2C9 Inhibitors (Strong); CYP3A4 Inhibitors (Moderate); CYP3A4 Inhibitors (Strong); Dasatinib; Eltrombopag; GlyBURIDE; Phosphodiesterase 5 Inhibitors; Ritonavir

Decreased Effect

Bosentan may decrease the levels/effects of: Contraceptives (Estrogens); Contraceptives (Progestins); CycloSPORINE; CycloSPORINE (Systemic); CYP2C9 Substrates (High risk); CYP3A4 Substrates; Dronedarone; Everolimus; GlyBURIDE; GuanFACINE; HMG-CoA Reductase Inhibitors; Maraviroc; NIFEdipine; Nilotinib; Nisoldipine; Pazopanib; Phosphodiesterase 5 Inhibitors; Ranolazine; Romidepsin; Saxagliptin; Sorafenib; Tolvaptan; Vitamin K Antagonists

The levels/effects of Bosentan may be decreased by: CYP2C9 Inducers (Highly Effective); CYP3A4 Inducers (Strong); Deferasirox; GlyBURIDE; Herbs (CYP3A4 Inducers); Peginterferon Alfa-2b

Food Interactions Food does not affect bioavailability.

Stability Store at controlled room temperature of 20°C to 25°C (68°F to 77°F).

Mechanism of Action Bosentan acts as a competitive antagonist and blocks endothelin receptors on vascular endothelium and smooth muscle. Stimulation of endothelin receptors is associated with vasoconstriction and proliferation (**Note:** Patients with PAH have elevated lung tissue and plasma concentrations of endothelin). Although bosentan blocks both ET_A and ET_B receptors, the affinity is slightly higher for the A subtype. In clinical trials, bosentan significantly increased cardiac index and decreased pulmonary artery pressure, pulmonary vascular resistance, and mean right atrial pressure. Improvement in symptoms of PAH and exercise capacity, and a decrease in the rate of clinical deterioration were observed.

Pharmacokinetics (Adult data unless noted)

Distribution: Unknown if distributes into breast milk; does not distribute into RBCs; V_d: Adults: ~18 L

Protein binding: >98% to plasma proteins (primarily albumin)

Metabolism: Extensive in the liver via cytochrome P450 isoenzymes CYP2C9 and CYP3A4 to three metabolites (one has pharmacologic activity and may account for 10% to 20% of drug effect); steady-state plasma concentrations are 50% to 65% of those attained after single dose (most likely due to autoinduction of liver enzymes); steady-state is attained within 3-5 days

Bioavailability: ~50%

Half-life: Healthy subjects: 5 hours; half-life may be prolonged in PAH, as AUC is 2-fold greater in adults with PAH versus healthy subjects

Time to peak serum concentration: Oral: Within 3-5 hours

Elimination: Biliary excretion; <3% of dose is excreted in the urine

Dialysis: Not likely to be removed (due to extensive protein binding and high molecular weight)

Usual Dosage Oral:

Neonates: Very limited information exists; one article describes the short-term use of bosentan in two full-term neonates (8 days and 14 days old) with persistent pulmonary hypertension of the newborn (PPHN) and transposition of the great arteries prior to cardiac surgery; an initial bosentan dose of 1 mg/kg twice daily was used; patients received other therapies; bosentan treatment duration was 8 days and 16 days (see Goissen, 2008)

Infants and Children: Limited information available; several pediatric studies have used the following doses based on body weight in patients as young as 7 months of age (see Barst, 2003; Goissen, 2008; Ivy, 2004; Maiya, 2006; Rosenzweig, 2005):

<10 kg (see Rosenzweig, 2005): Initial: 15.6 mg daily for 4 weeks; increase to maintenance dose of 15.6 mg twice daily; **Note:** Based on an extrapolation of study doses used in Barst, 2003, the following doses are recommended for patients <10 kg: Initial: 1-2 mg/kg twice daily for 4 weeks; increase to maintenance dose of 2-4 mg/kg twice daily (Villanueva, 2006)

10-20 kg: Initial: 31.25 mg daily for 4 weeks; increase to maintenance dose of 31.25 mg twice daily

>20-40 kg: Initial: 31.25 mg twice daily for 4 weeks; increase to maintenance dose of 62.5 mg twice daily

>40 kg: Initial: 62.5 mg twice daily for 4 weeks; increase to maintenance dose of 125 mg twice daily

Note: A smaller pediatric study of 7 patients, 1.5-6.4 years of age (median: 3.8 years) used initial doses of 1.5 mg/kg/day divided into 1-3 doses/day (in capsule form) for 4 weeks; doses were increased to maintenance doses of 3 mg/kg/day (see Gilbert, 2005)

Adolescents >12 years who are <40 kg: Manufacturer's recommendations: Initial and maintenance: 62.5 mg twice daily

Adolescents >12 years who are ≥40 kg: Refer to adult dosing.

Adults: Initial: 62.5 mg twice daily for 4 weeks; increase to maintenance dose of 125 mg twice daily; adults <40 kg should be maintained at 62.5 mg twice daily.

Note: Doses >125 mg twice daily do not provide additional benefit sufficient to offset the increased risk of hepatic injury. When discontinuing treatment, consider a reduction in dosage to 62.5 mg twice daily for 3-7 days (to avoid clinical deterioration).

Dosage adjustment for concurrent use of ritonavir: Adults:

Coadministration of bosentan in patients currently receiving ritonavir: For patients receiving ritonavir for at least 10 days, begin with bosentan 62.5 mg once daily or every other day based on tolerability

Coadministration of ritonavir in patients currently receiving bosentan: Discontinue bosentan at least 36 hours prior to the initiation of ritonavir; after at least 10 days of ritonavir, resume bosentan at a dose of 62.5 mg once daily or every other day based on tolerability

Dosage adjustment in renal impairment: No dosage adjustment required.

Dosage adjustment in hepatic impairment: Use with caution in patients with mild hepatic impairment. Avoid use in patients with moderate-to-severe hepatic insufficiency and in patients with elevated serum transaminases (>3 times upper limit of normal) at baseline

Dosage adjustment in patients who develop elevations of aminotransferases: Adult guidelines: Note: If any elevation, regardless of degree, is accompanied by clinical symptoms of hepatic injury (unusual fatigue, nausea, vomiting, abdominal pain, fever, or jaundice) or a serum bilirubin ≥2 times the upper limit of normal, treatment should be stopped.

AST/ALT >3 times but ≤5 times upper limit of normal: Confirm elevation with additional test; if confirmed, reduce dose or interrupt treatment. Monitor transaminase levels at least every 2 weeks. May continue or reintroduce treatment, as appropriate, following return to pretreatment aminotransferase values. Begin with initial dose (above) and recheck transaminases within 3 days.

AST/ALT >5 times but ≤8 times upper limit of normal: Confirm elevation with additional test; if confirmed, stop treatment. Monitor transaminase levels at least every 2 weeks. May consider reintroduction of treatment, as appropriate, following return to pretreatment amino-transferase values.

AST/ALT >8 times upper limit of normal: Stop treatment.

Administration Oral: May be administered without regard to meals (see Extemporaneous Preparations).

Monitoring Parameters Serum transaminase (AST and ALT) should be determined prior to the initiation of therapy and at monthly intervals thereafter. A woman of child-bearing potential must have a negative pregnancy test prior to the initiation of therapy, monthly thereafter, and 1 month after stopping therapy. Hemoglobin and hematocrit should be measured at baseline, after 1 and 3 months of treatment, and every 3 months thereafter. Monitor for clinical signs and symptoms of liver injury.

Patient Information Read the patient Medication Guide that you receive with each prescription and refill of bosentan. Some medicines should not be taken with bosentan; report the use of other medications, non-prescription medications, and herbal or natural products to your physician and pharmacist; avoid the herbal medicine St John's wort. Bosentan may cause liver damage and low red blood cell levels; blood tests to check for these side effects must be performed frequently. Notify physician if persistent headache or GI problems, swelling of extremities, or unusual weight gain, chest pain or palpitations, unusual fatigue or weakness, yellowing of skin or eyes, change in color of stool or urine, or other persistent reactions occur.

Bosentan may cause major birth defects and must not be taken by women who are pregnant or who may become pregnant. Women who are able to become pregnant must use two effective birth control methods while taking bosentan and for 1 month after stopping treatment [except for patients with tubal ligation or an implanted IUD (copper T 380A or LNg20); no other contraceptive measures are required for these patients]. Bosentan may decrease the effectiveness of hormonal contraceptives, including birth control pills, skin patches, shots, and implants; hormonal contraceptives should not be the only contraceptive method in patients receiving bosentan. Pregnancy tests (either urine or blood tests) must be performed before starting bosentan therapy, every month while taking the medication, and 1 month after stopping therapy in women who are able to become pregnant. Notify physician immediately if you think you might be pregnant. Do not crush tablets; women who are able to become pregnant should avoid exposure to bosentan powder (dust) from cutting tablets; tablets should be dissolved in water if necessary (see Extemporaneous Preparations). Reduced sperm counts may occur in men taking bosentan; talk to your healthcare provider if fertility issues are important.

Nursing Implications Assess results of laboratory tests, therapeutic effectiveness, and adverse reactions on a regular basis during therapy. Assess for fluid retention. Instruct patient on appropriate use, side effects/appro-priate interventions, and adverse symptoms to report.

Bosentan is a teratogen (Pregnancy Risk Factor X); avoid exposure to bosentan powder (dust) when cutting the tablets (use gloves and mask); do not crush the tablets; (see Extemporaneous Preparations).

Additional Information The addition of bosentan to epoprostenol therapy in 8 children (8-18 years of age) with idiopathic PAH allowed for a reduction in the epoprostenol dose (and its associated side effects) in 7 of the 8 children. Epoprostenol was able to be discon-tinued in 3 of the 8 children (see Ivy, 2004). The results from the European postmarketing surveillance program in children 2-11 years of age confirm the need for monthly

measurement of liver aminotransferases in pediatric patients for the duration of bosentan treatment (see Beghetti, 2008).

Clinical studies in adults have shown that bosentan was **not** effective in the treatment of CHF in patients with left ventricular dysfunction; hospitalizations for CHF were more common during the first 1-2 months after initiation of the drug.

Dosage Forms Excipient information presented when available (limited, particularly for generics); consult specific product labeling.

Tablet:

Tracleer®: 62.5 mg, 125 mg

Extemporaneous Preparations Note: Tablets are not scored; a commercial pill cutter should be used to prepare a 31.25 mg dose from the 62.5 mg tablet; the half-cut 62.5 mg tablets are stable for up to 4 weeks, when stored at room temperature in the high-density polyethylene plastic bottle provided by the manufacturer of the drug. Since bosentan is classified as a teratogen (Pregnancy Risk Factor X), individuals should avoid exposure to bosentan powder (dust) by taking appropriate measures (eg, using gloves and mask); women of childbearing potential should avoid all possible exposure to the dust.

Crushing of the tablets is not recommended; bosentan tablets will disintegrate rapidly (within 5 minutes) in 5-25 mL of water, to create a suspension. An appropriate aliquot of the suspension can be used to deliver the prescribed dose. The suspension is stable for up to 24 hours when stored at room temperature in a 10 mL syringe. Bosentan should not be mixed or dissolved in liquids with a low (acidic) pH (eg, fruit juices) due to poor solubility; the drug is most soluble in solutions with a pH >8.5.

Villanueva D. Medical Information Manager, Actelion, personal correspondence, March 2006.

References

Adatia I, "Improving the Outcome of Childhood Pulmonary Arterial Hypertension: The Effect of Bosentan in the Setting of a Dedicated Pulmonary Hypertension Clinic," *J Am Coll Cardiol*, 2005, 46 (4):705-6.

Apostolopoulou SC, Manginas A, Cokkinos DV, et al, "Long-Term Oral Bosentan Treatment in Patients With Pulmonary Arterial Hypertension Related to Congenital Heart Disease: A 2-Year Study," *Heart*, 2007, 93(3):350-4.

Barst RJ, Ivy D, Dingemanse J, et al, "Pharmacokinetics, Safety, and Efficacy of Bosentan in Pediatric Patients With Pulmonary Arterial Hypertension," *Clin Pharmacol Ther*, 2003, 73(4):372-82.

Beghetti M, Hoeper MM, Kiely DG, et al, "Safety Experience With Bosentan in 146 Children 2-11 Years Old With Pulmonary Arterial Hypertension: Results From the European Postmarketing Surveil-lance Program," *Pediatr Res*, 2008, 64(2):200-4.

Gilbert N, Luther YC, Miera O, et al, "Initial Experience With Bosentan (Tracleer®) as Treatment for Pulmonary Arterial Hypertension (PAH) Due to Congenital Heart Disease in Infants and Young Children," *Z Kardiol*, 2005, 94(9):570-4.

Goissen C, Ghyselen L, Tourneux P, et al, "Persistent Pulmonary Hypertension of the Newborn With Transposition of the Great Arteries: Successful Treatment With Bosentan," *Eur J Pediatr*, 2008, 167 (4):437-40.

Ivy DD, Doran A, Claussen L, et al, "Weaning and Discontinuation of Epoprostenol in Children With Idiopathic Pulmonary Arterial Hyper-tension Receiving Concomitant Bosentan," *Am J Cardiol*, 2004, 93 (7):943-6.

Maiya S, Hislop AA, Flynn Y, et al, "Response to Bosentan in Children With Pulmonary Hypertension," *Heart*, 2006, 92(5):664-70.

Rosenzweig EB, Ivy DD, Widlitz A, et al, "Effects of Long-Term Bosentan in Children With Pulmonary Arterial Hypertension," *J Am Coll Cardiol*, 2005, 46(4):697-704.

Villanueva D. Medical Information Manager, Actelion, personal correspondence, March 2006.

◆ **B&O Supprettes® [DSC]** *see* Belladonna and Opium *on page 178*

◆ **Botox®** *see* OnabotulinumtoxinA *on page 1020*

◆ **Botox® Cosmetic** *see* OnabotulinumtoxinA *on page 1020*

- ◆ **Botulinum Toxin Type A** *see* OnabotulinumtoxinA *on page 1020*
- ◆ **Botulinum Toxin Type B** *see* RimabotulinumtoxinB *on page 1216*

Botulism Immune Globulin (Intravenous-Human)

(BOT yoo lism i MYUN GLOB you lin, in tra VEE nus, YU man)

Medication Safety Issues
Sound-alike/look-alike issues:
BabyBIG® may be confused with HBIG

U.S. Brand Names BabyBIG®

Therapeutic Category Immune Globulin

Generic Available No

Use Treatment of infant botulism caused by toxin type A or B in patients <1 year of age.

Restrictions In order to obtain this product, an invoice and purchase agreement must be completed and faxed to the Infant Botulism Treatment and Prevention Program (IBTPP) at 510-231-7609 (normal business hours) or 510-217-4449 (nights, weekends, and holidays).

> After faxing the purchase agreement, the original copy of the purchase agreement must be returned to the IBTPP via overnight courier, and payment must be wired within 5 business days.
>
> Arrange for courier pick-up of BabyBIG® from FFF Enterprises in Temecula, CA.

Pregnancy Considerations Reproduction studies have not been conducted.

Contraindications Hypersensitivity to immune globulin or any component; IgA deficiency (BabyBIG® contains trace amounts of immunoglobulin A)

Warnings Renal dysfunction and/or acute renal failure has been reported with the administration of IVIG; 88% of the cases were associated with the administration of sucrose-containing IVIG products at doses of 400 mg/kg or greater. BabyBIG® contains sucrose as a stabilizer. BabyBIG® is made from human plasma which carries the risk of blood-borne virus transmission, including the disease-causing agent for Creutzfeldt-Jakob disease. Like any other blood product, the risks and benefits of this agent should be discussed between the patient's legal guardian and the attending physician. An aseptic meningitis syndrome has been reported to occur with high total doses of other I.V. immune globulin products (eg, 2 g/kg of IVIG). Symptoms usually present within hours to days of treatment. Signs and symptoms may include severe headache, nuchal rigidity, photophobia, nausea, vomiting, painful eye movement, and fever. Cerebrospinal fluid may be positive with pleocytosis and elevated protein levels.

Precautions Use with caution in patients at increased risk for developing acute renal failure (patients with pre-existing renal insufficiency, diabetes mellitus, volume depletion, sepsis, paraproteinemia, and concomitant nephrotoxic drugs). Assure that patients are not volume depleted prior to the initiation of BabyBIG®.

Adverse Reactions
Dermatologic: Erythematous rash

Renal: Acute renal failure, renal dysfunction, proximal tubular nephropathy, osmotic nephrosis, BUN/serum creatinine elevated

Miscellaneous: Anaphylaxis; infusion rate-related effects: Blood pressure increased, irritability, chills, muscle cramps, back pain, fever, nausea, vomiting, wheezing

Drug Interactions
Avoid Concomitant Use There are no known interactions where it is recommended to avoid concomitant use.

Increased Effect/Toxicity There are no known significant interactions involving an increase in effect.

Decreased Effect
Botulism Immune Globulin (Intravenous-Human) may decrease the levels/effects of: Vaccines (Live)

Stability Store between 2°C to 8°C (35.6°F to 46.4°F). Since BabyBIG® does not contain a preservative, reconstituted vials should be used within 2 hours. Do not mix with other drugs.

Mechanism of Action BabyBIG® contains antibody titers against botulinum toxin type A of at least 15 international units/mL and botulinum toxin type B of at least 4 international units/mL at levels sufficient to neutralize expected levels of circulating neurotoxin.

Pharmacodynamics Duration: ~6 months with a single infusion

Pharmacokinetics (Adult data unless noted) Half-life: ~28 days

Usual Dosage I.V.: Infants <1 year: Total dose is 75 mg/kg as a single I.V. infusion. Start as soon as diagnosis of infant botulism is made.

Administration Do not administer I.M. or SubQ

I.V. infusion: Add 2 mL SWI to 100 mg vial, resulting in 50 mg/mL solution; rotate vial gently to wet all the powder and avoid foaming. Do not shake vial. Allow solution to stand 30 minutes until it clears. Use within 2 hours of reconstitution. Use low volume tubing for administration via a separate line. If this is not possible, piggyback BabyBIG® into a pre-existing line containing either NS or a dextrose solution ($D_{2.5}$W, D_5W, D_{10}W, or D_{20}W) with or without added NaCl. Do not dilute more than 1:2 with any of the above solutions. Drug concentration should be no less than 25 mg/mL. Administer via an in-line 18 micron filter.

> **Initial:** Administer slowly at 25 mg/kg/hour for the first 15 minutes; after 15 minutes, rate may be increased to the maximum infusion rate of 50 mg/kg/hour to the end of the infusion (infusion should conclude within 4 hours of reconstitution). At the recommended infusion rate, infusion of total dose should take 97.5 minutes total elapsed time.

Monitoring Parameters Vital signs and blood pressure monitored continuously during the infusion. BUN and serum creatinine should be monitored prior to initial infusion. Periodic monitoring of renal function tests and urine output in patients at risk for developing renal failure.

Nursing Implications Appropriate agents for treatment of a hypersensitivity reaction (eg, epinephrine) should be readily available; adverse reactions may also be alleviated by decreasing the rate or the concentration of infusion, or temporarily interrupting the infusion

Dosage Forms Excipient information presented when available (limited, particularly for generics); consult specific product labeling.

Injection, powder for reconstitution [preservative free]:
BabyBIG®: ~100 mg [contains albumin and sucrose; packaged with SWFI]

References
Arnon SS, Schechter R, Maslanka SE, et al, "Human Botulism Immune Globulin for the Treatment of Infant Botulism," *N Engl J Med*, 2006, 354(5):462-71.

Infant Botulism Treatment and Prevention Program, Department of Communicable Disease Control, California Department of Health Services, http://infantbotulism.org

- ◆ **Boudreaux's® Butt Paste [OTC]** *see* Zinc Oxide *on page 1445*
- ◆ **Bovine Lung Surfactant** *see* Beractant *on page 187*
- ◆ **Bovine Lung Surfactant** *see* Calfactant *on page 240*
- ◆ **Breathe Free® [OTC]** *see* Sodium Chloride *on page 1270*
- ◆ **Brethaire [DSC]** *see* Terbutaline *on page 1324*
- ◆ **Brethine** *see* Terbutaline *on page 1324*
- ◆ **Brevibloc®** *see* Esmolol *on page 532*

◆ **Brevital® (Can)** *see* Methohexital *on page 899*

◆ **Brevital® Sodium** *see* Methohexital *on page 899*

◆ **Brevoxyl®-4** *see* Benzoyl Peroxide *on page 184*

◆ **Brevoxyl®-8** *see* Benzoyl Peroxide *on page 184*

◆ **Brevoxyl® Acne Wash Kit [DSC]** *see* Benzoyl Peroxide *on page 184*

◆ **breze™ [DSC]** *see* Benzoyl Peroxide *on page 184*

◆ **Bricanyl [DSC]** *see* Terbutaline *on page 1324*

◆ **Bricanyl® (Can)** *see* Terbutaline *on page 1324*

Brimonidine (bri MOE ni deen)

Medication Safety Issues
Sound-alike/look-alike issues:
Brimonidine may be confused with bromocriptine

U.S. Brand Names Alphagan® P

Canadian Brand Names Alphagan®; Apo-Brimonidine P®; Apo-Brimonidine®; PMS-Brimonidine Tartrate; ratio-Brimonidine; Sandoz-Brimonidine

Therapeutic Category Alpha-Adrenergic Agonist, Ophthalmic; Glaucoma, Treatment Agent

Generic Available Yes

Use Lowering of IOP in patients with open-angle glaucoma or ocular hypertension

Pregnancy Risk Factor B

Pregnancy Considerations Teratogenic effects were not observed in animal studies. There are no adequate and well-controlled studies in pregnant women.

Lactation Excretion in breast milk unknown/not recommended

Contraindications Hypersensitivity to brimonidine or any component; use during or within 14 days of MAO inhibitor therapy

Warnings May cause CNS depression, particularly in young children; the most common adverse effect reported in a study of pediatric glaucoma patients was somnolence and decreased alertness (50% to 83% in children 2-6 years of age); these effects resulted in a 16% discontinuation of treatment rate; children >7 years (>20 kg) had a much lower rate of somnolence (25%); apnea, bradycardia, hypotension, hypothermia, hypotonia, and somnolence have been reported in infants receiving brimonidine; brimonidine is not approved for use in children <2 years

Precautions Use with caution in patients with severe cardiovascular disease, hepatic or renal impairment, depression, cerebral or coronary insufficiency, Raynaud's phenomenon, orthostatic hypotension, or thromboangiitis

Adverse Reactions
Cardiovascular: Hypertension, bradycardia, hypotension, tachycardia

Central nervous system: Headache, dizziness, somnolence (see Warnings), alertness decreased, insomnia, hypothermia (in infants only)

Dermatologic: Rash

Gastrointestinal: Xerostomia, taste perversion, dyspepsia, pharyngitis

Local: Stinging, burning sensation

Neuromuscular & skeletal: Hypotonia (in infants only)

Ocular: Allergic conjunctivitis, conjunctival hyperemia, eye pruritus (10% to 20%); conjunctival folliculosis, visual disturbances (5% to 9%); blepharitis, conjunctival edema, conjunctival hemorrhage, conjunctivitis, discharge, dryness, irritation, eye pain, eyelid edema, eyelid erythema, foreign body sensation, photophobia, superficial punctate keratopathy, visual field defect, vitreous floaters, worsened visual acuity, corneal erosion (rare), iritis, miosis

Respiratory: Bronchitis, cough, dyspnea, rhinitis, sinus infection, sinusitis, nasal dryness, apnea

Miscellaneous: Flu-like syndrome, hypersensitivity reactions

Drug Interactions
Avoid Concomitant Use
Avoid concomitant use of Brimonidine with any of the following: MAO Inhibitors

Increased Effect/Toxicity
Brimonidine may increase the levels/effects of: Alcohol (Ethyl); CNS Depressants; Hypotensive Agents; Methotrimeprazine

The levels/effects of Brimonidine may be increased by: MAO Inhibitors; Methotrimeprazine

Decreased Effect There are no known significant interactions involving a decrease in effect.

Stability Store at controlled room temperature (59°F to 77°F)

Mechanism of Action Brimonidine is an alpha-adrenergic receptor agonist that reduces aqueous humor production and increases uveoscleral outflow

Pharmacodynamics Onset of action: Peak effect: 2 hours

Pharmacokinetics (Adult data unless noted)
Metabolism: Extensive in liver
Half-life: 2 hours
Time to peak serum concentration: Ophthalmic: Within 0.5-2.5 hours

Usual Dosage Ophthalmic: Children ≥2 years and Adults: Instill 1 drop into lower conjunctival sac of affected eye(s) 3 times/day (approximately every 8 hours)

Administration Ophthalmic: Instill into conjunctival sac avoiding contact of bottle tip with skin or eye; apply finger pressure to lacrimal sac during and for 1-2 minutes after instillation to decrease risk of absorption and systemic effects. Administer other topical ophthalmic medications at least 5 minutes apart; generic formulation contains benzalkonium chloride which may be absorbed by soft contact lenses; wait at least 15 minutes after administration to insert soft contact lenses.

Monitoring Parameters IOP

Patient Information Brimonidine may cause dizziness, drowsiness, visual disturbances, and impair ability to perform activities requiring mental alertness or physical coordination; may cause dry mouth

Dosage Forms Excipient information presented when available (limited, particularly for generics); consult specific product labeling.
Solution, ophthalmic, as tartrate: 0.2% (5 mL, 10 mL, 15 mL); 0.15% (5 mL, 10 mL, 15 mL)
Alphagan® P: 0.1% (5 mL, 10 mL, 15 mL) [contains Purite® as preservative]; 0.15% (5 mL, 10 mL, 15 mL) [contains Purite® as preservative]

References
Berlin RJ, Lee UT, Samples JR, et al, "Ophthalmic Drops Causing Coma in an Infant," *J Pediatr,* 2001, 138(3):441-3.
Carlsen JO, Zabriskie NA, Kwon YH, et al, "Apparent Central Nervous System Depression in Infants After the Use of Topical Brimonidine," *Am J Ophthalmol,* 1999, 128(2):255-6.
Enyedi LB and Freedman SF, "Safety and Efficacy of Brimonidine in Children With Glaucoma," *J AAPOS,* 2001, 5(5):281-4.

◆ **Brimonidine Tartrate** *see* Brimonidine *on page 202*

◆ **Brioschi® [OTC]** *see* Sodium Bicarbonate *on page 1269*

◆ **British Anti-Lewisite** *see* Dimercaprol *on page 447*

◆ **BRL 43694** *see* Granisetron *on page 653*

◆ **Bromaline® [OTC]** *see* Brompheniramine and Pseudoephedrine *on page 205*

◆ **Bromfenex® [DSC]** *see* Brompheniramine and Pseudoephedrine *on page 205*

◆ **Bromfenex® PD [DSC]** *see* Brompheniramine and Pseudoephedrine *on page 205*

◆ **Bromhist-NR [DSC]** *see* Brompheniramine and Pseudoephedrine *on page 205*

◆ **Bromhist Pediatric [DSC]** *see* Brompheniramine and Pseudoephedrine *on page 205*

Bromocriptine (broe moe KRIP teen)

Medication Safety Issues

Sound-alike/look-alike issues:

Bromocriptine may be confused with benztropine, brimonidine

Cycloset® may be confused with Glyset®

Parlodel® may be confused with pindolol, Provera®

U.S. Brand Names Cycloset®; Parlodel®; Parlodel® SnapTabs®

Canadian Brand Names Apo-Bromocriptine®; Parlodel®; PMS-Bromocriptine

Therapeutic Category Anti-Parkinson's Agent, Dopamine Agonist; Ergot Derivative

Generic Available Yes

Use Treatment of dysfunctions associated with hyperprolactinemia including amenorrhea with or without galactorrhea, infertility, or hypogonadism; treatment of prolactin-secreting adenomas; treatment of acromegaly; treatment of Parkinson's disease; neuroleptic malignant syndrome

Pregnancy Risk Factor B

Pregnancy Considerations No evidence of teratogenicity or fetal toxicity in animal studies. Bromocriptine is used for ovulation induction in women with hyperprolactinemia. In general, therapy should be discontinued if pregnancy is confirmed unless needed for treatment of macroprolactinoma. Data collected from women taking bromocriptine during pregnancy suggest the incidence of birth defects is not increased with use. However, the majority of women discontinued use within 8 weeks of pregnancy. Women not seeking pregnancy should be advised to use appropriate contraception.

Lactation Enters breast milk/not recommended

Breast-Feeding Considerations A previous indication for prevention of postpartum lactation was withdrawn voluntarily by the manufacturer following reports of serious adverse reactions, including stroke, MI, seizures, and severe hypertension. Based on the risk/benefit assessment, other treatments should be considered for lactation suppression.

Contraindications Hypersensitivity to bromocriptine, ergot alkaloids, or any component; hereditary problems of galactose intolerance, severe lactase deficiency, or glucose-galactose malabsorption; ergot alkaloids are contraindicated with potent inhibitors of CYP3A4 (includes protease inhibitors, azole antifungals, and some macrolide antibiotics); concomitant use with serotonin agonists (includes buspirone, SSRIs, TCAs, nefazodone, sumatriptan, and trazodone) and sibutramine (see Drug Interactions); uncontrolled hypertension; severe ischemic heart disease or peripheral vascular disorders; pregnancy (risk to benefit evaluation must be performed in women who become pregnant during treatment for acromegaly, prolactinoma, or Parkinson's disease); hypertensive disorders of pregnancy (including eclampsia, preeclampsia, or pregnancy-induced hypertension) are indications for withdrawing therapy in these patients unless withdrawal is considered to be medically contraindicated

Warnings Complete evaluation of pituitary function should be completed prior to initiation of treatment. Patients not seeking pregnancy or those with large adenomas should be advised to use contraception other than oral contraceptives during treatment with bromocriptine. Pregnancy testing is recommended at least every 4 weeks during the amenorrheic period and, once menses are reinitiated, every time a patient misses a menstrual period.

Symptomatic hypotension may occur in a significant number of patients especially during the first days of treatment. Ergot alkaloids and derivatives have been associated with fibrotic valve thickening (eg, aortic, mitral, tricuspid); usually associated with long-term, chronic use. Hypertension, seizures, MI, and stroke have been rarely associated with therapy. Severe headache or visual changes may precede events. The onset of reactions may be immediate or delayed (often may occur in the second week of therapy). Patients who receive bromocriptine during and immediately following pregnancy as a continuation of previous therapy (eg, acromegaly) should be closely monitored for cardiovascular effects. Prolactin-secreting adenomas may expand and compress the optic or other cranial nerves. Monitoring and careful evaluation of visual changes during the treatment of hyperprolactinemia is recommended to differentiate between tumor shrinkage and traction on the optic chiasm. Rapidly progressing visual field loss requires neurosurgical consultation. In most cases, compression resolves following delivery.

Rare cases of pleural and pericardial effusions as well as pleural and pulmonary fibrosis and constrictive pericarditis have been reported, particularly with long term and high-dose treatment. Retroperitoneal fibrosis has also been reported.

In the treatment of acromegaly, discontinuation is recommended if tumor expansion occurs during therapy. Cold sensitive digital vasospasm may occur in some patients with acromegaly and may be reversed with dosage reduction. Discontinuation of therapy in patients with macroadenomas has been associated with rapid regrowth of tumor and increased prolactin serum levels. Safety and effectiveness have not been established in children <15 years of age for pituitary adenoma. Patients treated with pituitary radiation should have an annual 4-8 week withdrawal from bromocriptine to assess both the clinical effects of radiation on the disease process as well as the effects of bromocriptine. Recurrence of signs and symptoms or increases in growth hormone indicate the need to resume treatment.

Safety has not been established for use >2 years in patients with Parkinson's disease. Concurrent use with levodopa has been associated with an increased risk of hallucinations; consider dosage reduction and/or discontinuation in patients with hallucinations. Hallucinations may require weeks to months before resolution. Bromocriptine has been associated with sudden onset of sleep during daily activities, in some cases without awareness or warning signs. A reduction in dosage or termination of therapy may be necessary.

Precautions Use with caution in patients with cardiovascular disease (myocardial infarction, arrhythmia), peptic ulcer, dementia, hepatic impairment, and psychosis. Should not be used postpartum in women with coronary artery disease or other cardiovascular disease; use to control or prevent lactation or in patients with uncontrolled hypertension is not recommended. Concurrent antihypertensives or drugs which may alter blood pressure should be used with caution.

Adverse Reactions Note: Frequency of adverse effects may vary by dose and/or indication.

Cardiovascular: Hypotension (up to 30%), orthostasis, vasospasm (cold-sensitive), exacerbation of Raynaud's syndrome, syncope, arrhythmias, bradycardia, MI, hypertension, vasovagal reaction, mottled skin, pericardial effusions, constrictive pericarditis (rare)

Central nervous system: Headache (19%), dizziness (17%), fatigue, lightheadedness, drowsiness, hallucinations (visual), seizures, nightmares, paranoia, psychosis, vertigo, insomnia, lassitude, CSF rhinorrhea (rare when treating large prolactinomas), ataxia, psychomotor agitation

Dermatologic: Alopecia, rash

Gastrointestinal: Nausea (49%), constipation, anorexia, vomiting, abdominal cramps, diarrhea, dyspepsia, GI bleeding, xerostomia, retroperitoneal fibrosis (rare), dysphagia

Hepatic: Transaminases increased, CPK increased

Muscular & skeletal: Muscle cramps, paresthesia, tingling, dyskinesia

Ocular: Blepharospasm, visual changes

Renal: BUN increased

Respiratory: Nasal congestion, pulmonary infiltrates, pleural effusion, pulmonary fibrosis, pleural fibrosis

Miscellaneous: Pulmonary infiltrates, pleural effusion

Withdrawal reactions: Abrupt discontinuation has resulted in rare cases of a withdrawal reaction with symptoms similar to neuroleptic malignant syndrome.

Drug Interactions

Metabolism/Transport Effects Substrate of CYP3A4 (major); **Inhibits** CYP1A2 (weak), 3A4 (weak)

Avoid Concomitant Use

Avoid concomitant use of Bromocriptine with any of the following: Efavirenz; Itraconazole; Posaconazole; Protease Inhibitors; Serotonin 5-HT1D Receptor Agonists; Sibutramine; Voriconazole

Increased Effect/Toxicity

Bromocriptine may increase the levels/effects of: Cyclo-SPORINE; CycloSPORINE (Systemic); Serotonin 5-HT1D Receptor Agonists; Serotonin Modulators

The levels/effects of Bromocriptine may be increased by: Alpha-/Beta-Agonists; Antipsychotics (Typical); CYP3A4 Inhibitors (Moderate); CYP3A4 Inhibitors (Strong); Dasatinib; Efavirenz; Itraconazole; Macrolide Antibiotics; MAO Inhibitors; Posaconazole; Protease Inhibitors; Serotonin 5-HT1D Receptor Agonists; Sibutramine; Voriconazole

Decreased Effect

Bromocriptine may decrease the levels/effects of: Antipsychotics (Typical)

The levels/effects of Bromocriptine may be decreased by: Antipsychotics (Atypical); Metoclopramide

Food Interactions The herbal medicine St John's wort (*Hypericum perforatum*) may decrease bromocriptine levels.

Mechanism of Action Semisynthetic ergot alkaloid derivative and a dopamine receptor agonist which activates postsynaptic dopamine receptors in the tuberoinfundibular process which results in inhibition of pituitary prolactin secretion. Stimulation of dopamine receptors in the corpus striatum is beneficial in the treatment of Parkinson's disease, a condition characterized by a progressive deficiency in dopamine synthesis.

Pharmacodynamics Reduction of prolactin levels:

Onset of action: 1-2 hours

Maximum effect: 5-10 hours

Duration: 8-12 hours

Pharmacokinetics (Adult data unless noted)

Bioavailability: 28%

Protein binding: 90% to 96%

Metabolism: Primarily hepatic with extensive first-pass biotransformation

Half-life: Biphasic with terminal half-life: 15 hours; range: 8-20 hours

Time to peak serum concentration: 1-2 hours

Elimination: Feces; urine (2% to 6% as unchanged drug)

Usual Dosage Oral:

Hyperprolactinemia:

Children 11-15 years (based on limited information): Initial: 1.25-2.5 mg daily; dosage may be increased as tolerated to achieve a therapeutic response (range: 2.5-10 mg daily)

Children ≥16 years and Adults: Initial: 1.25-2.5 mg/day; may be increased by 2.5 mg/day as tolerated every 2-7 days until optimal response (range: 2.5-15 mg/day)

Parkinsonism: Adults: 1.25 mg twice daily, increased by 2.5 mg/day in 2- to 4-week intervals (usual dose range is 30-90 mg/day in 3 divided doses), though elderly patients can usually be managed on lower doses

Neuroleptic malignant syndrome: Adults: 2.5-5 mg 3 times/day

Acromegaly: Adults: Initial: 1.25-2.5 mg daily increasing by 1.25-2.5 mg daily as necessary every 3-7 days; usual dose: 20-30 mg/day (maximum: 100 mg/day)

Dosing adjustment in hepatic impairment: No guidelines are available; however, may be necessary

Administration Oral: May be taken with food to decrease GI distress

Monitoring Parameters Monitor blood pressure closely as well as hepatic, hematopoietic, and cardiovascular function; visual field monitoring is recommended (prolactinoma); pregnancy testing (see Warnings); growth hormone and prolactin levels

Patient Information Take exactly as directed (may be prescribed in conjunction with levodopa/carbidopa); do not change dosage or discontinue this medicine without consulting prescriber. Therapeutic effects may take several weeks or months to achieve and you may need frequent monitoring during first weeks of therapy. Take with meals if GI upset occurs, before meals if dry mouth occurs, or after eating if drooling or if nausea occurs. Take at the same time each day. Maintain adequate hydration unless instructed to restrict fluid intake; void before taking medication. Do not use alcohol, prescription or OTC sedatives, or CNS depressants without consulting prescriber. Urine or perspiration may appear darker. You may experience drowsiness, dizziness, confusion, or vision changes (use caution when driving, climbing stairs, or engaging in tasks requiring alertness until response to drug is known); orthostatic hypotension (use caution when rising from sitting or lying position); constipation (increased exercise, fluids, fruit, or fiber may help); nasal congestion (consult prescriber for appropriate relief); or nausea, vomiting, loss of appetite, or stomach discomfort (small frequent meals, frequent mouth care, chewing gum, or sucking lozenges may help). Report unresolved constipation or vomiting; chest pain or irregular heartbeat; acute headache or dizziness; CNS changes (eg, hallucination, loss of memory, seizures, acute headache, nervousness); painful or difficult urination; increased muscle spasticity, rigidity, or involuntary movements; skin rash; or significant worsening of condition.

Additional Information Usually used with levodopa or levodopa/carbidopa to treat Parkinson's disease. When adding bromocriptine, the dose of levodopa/carbidopa can usually be decreased.

Product Availability

Cycloset®: FDA approved May 2009; availability anticipated in the first quarter of 2010

Cycloset® has been approved for the treatment of type 2 diabetes.

Dosage Forms Excipient information presented when available (limited, particularly for generics); consult specific product labeling.

Capsule: 5 mg

Parlodel®: 5 mg

Tablet: 2.5 mg

Parlodel® SnapTabs®: 2.5 mg

References

de Groot AN, van Dongen PW, Vree TB, et al, "Ergot Alkaloids. Current Status and Review of Clinical Pharmacology and Therapeutic Use Compared With Other Oxytocics in Obstetrics and Gynaecology," *Drugs*, 1998, 56(4):523-35.

Gillam MP, Fideleff H, Boquete HR, et al, "Prolactin Excess: Treatment and Toxicity," *Pediatr Endocrinol Rev*, 2004, 2(suppl)1:108-14.

Lejoyeux M, et al, "Serotonin Syndrome: Incidence, Symptoms, and Treatment," *CNS Drugs*, 1994, 2:132-43.

Melmed S and Braunstein GD, "Bromocriptine and Pleuropulmonary Disease," *Arch Intern Med*, 1989, 149(2):258-9.

Molitch ME, "Management of Prolactinomas During Pregnancy," *J Reprod Med*, 1999, 44(12 Suppl):1121-6.

Morgans D, "Re: Parlodel," *Aust N Z J Obstet Gynaecol*, 1995, 35 (2):228-9.

Mueller PS, Vester JW, and Fermaglich J, "Neuroleptic Malignant Syndrome. Successful Treatment With Bromocriptine," *JAMA*, 1983, 249(3):386-8.

Parkes D, "Drug Therapy: Bromocriptine," *N Engl J Med*, 1979, 301 (16):873-8.

◆ **Bromocriptine Mesylate** *see* Bromocriptine *on page 203*

Brompheniramine and Pseudoephedrine

(brome fen IR a meen & soo doe e FED rin)

U.S. Brand Names Andehist NR Syrup [DSC]; Bromaline® [OTC]; Bromfenex® PD [DSC]; Bromfenex® [DSC]; Bromhist Pediatric [DSC]; Bromhist-NR [DSC]; Brotapp; Brovex SR [DSC]; Histex® SR; Lodrane® 12D; Lodrane® 24D; Lodrane® D [DSC]; Lodrane® [DSC]; LoHist 12D; LoHist LQ; LoHist PD [DSC]; Respahist®; Sildec Syrup

Therapeutic Category Antihistamine/Decongestant Combination

Generic Available Yes

Use Temporary relief of nasal congestion, running nose, sneezing, and itchy, watery eyes; also promotes nasal or sinus drainage

Pregnancy Risk Factor C

Lactation Enters breast milk/not recommended

Breast-Feeding Considerations Small amounts of antihistamines and pseudoephedrine are excreted in breast milk. Premature infants and newborns have a higher risk of intolerance to antihistamines. Antihistamines may inhibit lactation.

Contraindications Hypersensitivity to brompheniramine, pseudoephedrine, or any component; MAO inhibitor therapy, severe hypertension, severe coronary artery disease

Warnings Safety and efficacy for the use of cough and cold products in children <2 years of age is limited. Serious adverse effects including death have been reported (in some cases, high blood concentrations of pseudoephedrine were found). The FDA notes that there are no approved OTC uses for these products in children <2 years of age. Healthcare providers are reminded to ask caregivers about the use of OTC cough and cold products in order to avoid exposure to multiple medications containing the same ingredient.

Some products may contain sodium benzoate; benzoic acid (benzoate) is a metabolite of benzyl alcohol; large amounts of benzyl alcohol (≥99 mg/kg/day) have been associated with a potentially fatal toxicity ("gasping syndrome") in neonates; the "gasping syndrome" consists of metabolic acidosis, respiratory distress, gasping respirations, CNS dysfunction (including convulsions, intracranial hemorrhage), hypotension and cardiovascular collapse; avoid use in neonates; *in vitro* and animal studies have shown that benzoate displaces bilirubin from protein binding sites

Precautions Use with caution in patients with mild-moderate hypertension, heart disease, arrhythmias, diabetes mellitus, thyroid disease, asthma, glaucoma, and prostatic hypertrophy

Adverse Reactions See individual monograph for Pseudoephedrine.

Brompheniramine component only:

Cardiovascular: Palpitations

Central nervous system: Paradoxical excitability, drowsiness, dizziness, headache, fever, nervousness, depression

Dermatologic: Rash, photosensitivity, angioedema

Endocrine & metabolic: Weight gain

Gastrointestinal: Nausea, anorexia, xerostomia, appetite increase, diarrhea, abdominal pain

Hepatic: Hepatitis

Neuromuscular & skeletal: Myalgia, paresthesia

Respiratory: Bronchospasm, epistaxis, thickening of bronchial secretions

Drug Interactions

Avoid Concomitant Use

Avoid concomitant use of Brompheniramine and Pseudoephedrine with any of the following: Iobenguane I 123; MAO Inhibitors

Increased Effect/Toxicity

Brompheniramine and Pseudoephedrine may increase the levels/effects of: Bromocriptine; Sympathomimetics

The levels/effects of Brompheniramine and Pseudoephedrine may be increased by: Antacids; Atomoxetine; Cannabinoids; Carbonic Anhydrase Inhibitors; MAO Inhibitors; Serotonin/Norepinephrine Reuptake Inhibitors

Decreased Effect

Brompheniramine and Pseudoephedrine may decrease the levels/effects of: Iobenguane I 123

The levels/effects of Brompheniramine and Pseudoephedrine may be decreased by: Spironolactone

Pharmacodynamics See individual monograph for Pseudoephedrine.

Brompheniramine component only:

Maximum effect: Maximal clinical effects seen within 3-9 hours

Duration: Varies with formulation

Pharmacokinetics (Adult data unless noted) See individual monograph for Pseudoephedrine.

Brompheniramine component only:

Metabolism: Extensive by the liver

Half-life: 12-34 hours

Time to peak serum concentration: Oral: Within 2-5 hours

Elimination: In urine as inactive metabolites

Usual Dosage Oral:

Manufacturer's recommendations:

Lodrane® D suspension:

Children 2-6 years: 1.25 mL (pseudoephedrine 15 mg) every 12 hours

Children 6-12 years: 2.5 mL (pseudoephedrine 30 mg) every 12 hours; not to exceed 2 doses/day

Children >12 years and Adults: 5 mL (pseudoephedrine 60 mg) every 12 hours not to exceed 2 doses/day

Lodrane® 12D:

Children 6-12 years: 1 tablet (pseudoephedrine 45 mg) every 12 hours; not to exceed 2 tablets/day

Children >12 years and Adults: 1-2 tablets (pseudoephedrine 45-90 mg) every 12 hours; not to exceed 4 tablets/day

Lodrane® 24D:

Children 6-12 years: 1 capsule (pseudoephedrine 90 mg) once daily

Children >12 years and Adults: 1-2 capsules (pseudoephedrine 90-180 mg) once daily

Alternative pediatric dosing: May dose according to the pseudoephedrine component:

Infants and Children <2 years: 4 mg/kg/day in divided doses every 6 hours

Children 2-5 years: 15 mg every 6 hours; maximum dose: 60 mg/24 hours

Children 6-12 years: 30 mg every 6 hours or extended release product 60 mg every 12 hours; maximum dose: 120 mg/24 hours

Children >12 years and Adults: 30-60 mg every 6 hours or extended release product 120 mg every 12 hours; maximum dose: 240 mg/24 hours

Administration Oral: Administer with food

Test Interactions False-positive test for amphetamines by EMIT assay

Patient Information May cause drowsiness and impair ability to perform activities requiring mental alertness or physical coordination. May cause photosensitivity reactions (eg, exposure to sunlight may cause severe sunburn, skin rash, redness, or itching); avoid direct exposure to sunlight

Dosage Forms Excipient information presented when available (limited, particularly for generics); consult specific product labeling. [DSC] = Discontinued product

Caplet, extended release:
  Histex® SR: Brompheniramine maleate 10 mg and pseudoephedrine hydrochloride 120 mg

Capsule, extended release:
  Bromfenex®: Brompheniramine maleate 12 mg and pseudoephedrine hydrochloride 120 mg [DSC]
  Bromfenex® PD: Brompheniramine maleate 6 mg and pseudoephedrine hydrochloride 60 mg [DSC]
  Lodrane® 24D: Brompheniramine maleate 12 mg and pseudoephedrine hydrochloride 90 mg

Capsule, sustained release:
  Brovex SR: Brompheniramine maleate 9 mg and pseudoephedrine hydrochloride 90 mg [DSC]
  Respahist®: Brompheniramine maleate 6 mg and pseudoephedrine hydrochloride 60 mg

Liquid: Brompheniramine maleate 4 mg and pseudoephedrine hydrochloride 60 mg per 5 mL (480 mL)

Brotapp: Brompheniramine maleate 1 mg and pseudoephedrine hydrochloride 15 mg per 5 mL (120 mL, 240 mL, 480 mL) [grape flavor]

Lodrane®: Brompheniramine maleate 4 mg and pseudoephedrine hydrochloride 60 mg per 5 mL (480 mL) [alcohol free, dye free, sugar free; cherry flavor] [DSC]

LoHist LQ: Brompheniramine maleate 4 mg and pseudoephedrine hydrochloride 60 mg per 5 mL (480 mL) [cherry flavor]

Liquid, oral [drops]:
  Bromhist NR: Brompheniramine maleate 1 mg and pseudoephedrine hydrochloride 12.5 mg per 1 mL (30 mL) [cherry flavor] [DSC]
  Bromhist Pediatric: Brompheniramine maleate 1 mg and pseudoephedrine hydrochloride 15 mg per 1 mL (30 mL) [cherry flavor] [DSC]
  LoHist PD: Brompheniramine maleate 1 mg and pseudoephedrine hydrochloride 12.5 mg per 1 mL (30 mL) [cherry flavor] [DSC]

Solution:
  Bromaline®: Brompheniramine maleate 1 mg and pseudoephedrine hydrochloride 15 mg per 5 mL (120 mL, 480 mL) [alcohol free; contains sodium benzoate; grape flavor]

Suspension:
  Lodrane® D: Brompheniramine tannate 8 mg and pseudoephedrine tannate 90 mg per 5 mL (480 mL) [alcohol free, sugar free; strawberry flavor] [DSC]

Syrup:
  Andehist NR: Brompheniramine maleate 4 mg and pseudoephedrine sulfate 45 mg per 5 mL (473 mL) [raspberry flavor] [DSC]
  Sildec: Brompheniramine maleate 4 mg and pseudoephedrine hydrochloride 45 mg per 5 mL (480 mL) [raspberry flavor]

Tablet, extended release:
  Lodrane® 12D: Brompheniramine maleate 6 mg and pseudoephedrine hydrochloride 45 mg [dye free]
  LoHist 12D: Brompheniramine maleate 6 mg and pseudoephedrine hydrochloride 45 mg

Tablet, sustained release: Brompheniramine maleate 6 mg and pseudoephedrine hydrochloride 45 mg

♦ **Brompheniramine Maleate and Pseudoephedrine Hydrochloride** see Brompheniramine and Pseudoephedrine on page 205

♦ **Brompheniramine Maleate and Pseudoephedrine Sulfate** see Brompheniramine and Pseudoephedrine on page 205

♦ **Brontex® [DSC]** see Guaifenesin and Codeine on page 657

♦ **Brotapp** see Brompheniramine and Pseudoephedrine on page 205

♦ **Brovex SR [DSC]** see Brompheniramine and Pseudoephedrine on page 205

♦ **BTX-A** see OnabotulinumtoxinA on page 1020

♦ **Budeprion XL®** see BuPROPion on page 217

♦ **Budeprion SR®** see BuPROPion on page 217

Budesonide (byoo DES oh nide)

Related Information
  Asthma on page 1697

U.S. Brand Names Entocort® EC; Pulmicort Flexhaler™; Pulmicort Respules®; Rhinocort® Aqua®

Canadian Brand Names Entocort®; Gen-Budesonide AQ; Mylan-Budesonide AQ; Pulmicort®; Rhinocort® Aqua™; Rhinocort® Turbuhaler®

Therapeutic Category Adrenal Corticosteroid; Anti-inflammatory Agent; Antiasthmatic; Corticosteroid, Inhalant (Oral); Corticosteroid, Intranasal; Corticosteroid, Oral; Glucocorticoid

Generic Available No

Use

Intranasal: Management of seasonal or perennial allergic rhinitis (FDA approved in ages ≥6 years and adults); nonallergic perennial rhinitis

Nebulization: Maintenance therapy and prophylaxis of bronchial asthma (FDA approved in ages 12 months to 8 years); **NOT** indicated for the relief of acute bronchospasm

Oral inhalation: Maintenance therapy and prophylaxis of bronchial asthma (FDA approved in ages ≥6 years and adults); **NOT** indicated for the relief of acute bronchospasm; also indicated in bronchial asthma patients requiring oral corticosteroids (inhalation may decrease or eliminate need for oral steroids over time) (FDA approved in ages ≥6 years and adults)

Oral: Treatment of mild to moderate active Crohn's disease of the ileum and/or ascending colon (FDA approved in adults); maintenance of remission (for up to 3 months) of mild to moderate Crohn's disease of the ileum and/or ascending colon (FDA approved in adults)

Pregnancy Risk Factor C (capsule)/B (inhalation)

Pregnancy Considerations Adverse events have been observed with corticosteroids in animal reproduction studies. Studies of pregnant women using inhaled budesonide have not demonstrated an increased risk of abnormalities. Some studies have shown an association between first trimester systemic corticosteroid use and oral clefts; adverse events in the fetus/neonate have been noted in case reports following large doses of systemic corticosteroids during pregnancy. Budesonide is the preferred inhaled corticosteroid for the treatment of asthma in pregnant women.

Lactation Enters breast milk/use caution

Breast-Feeding Considerations Following use of the powder for oral inhalation, ~0.3% to 1% of the maternal dose was found in breast milk. The maximum concentration appeared within 45 minutes of dosing. Plasma budesonide levels obtained from infants ~90 minutes after breast-feeding (~140 minutes after maternal dose) were below the limit of quantification. Concentrations of budesonide in breast milk are expected to be higher following administration of oral capsules than after an inhaled dose.

Contraindications Hypersensitivity to budesonide or any component (see Warnings); oral inhalation and nebulization: Primary treatment of status asthmaticus or other acute episodes of bronchial asthma where intensive treatment is needed

Warnings

Oral inhalation and nebulization: Fatalities have occurred due to adrenal insufficiency in asthmatic patients during and after switching from systemic corticosteroids to aerosol steroids; several months may be required for full recovery of hypothalamic-pituitary-adrenal (HPA) function; patients receiving higher doses of systemic corticosteroids (eg, adults receiving ≥20 mg of prednisone per day may be at greater risk; during this period of HPA suppression, aerosol steroids do **not** provide the systemic glucocorticoid or mineral corticoid activity needed to treat patients requiring stress doses (ie, patients with major stress such as trauma, surgery, or infections, or other conditions associated with severe electrolyte loss). When used at high doses, HPA suppression may occur; use with inhaled or systemic corticosteroids (even alternate-day dosing) may increase risk of HPA suppression. Acute adrenal insufficiency may occur with abrupt withdrawal after long-term use or with stress; withdrawal and discontinuation of corticosteroids should be done carefully; patients with HPA axis suppression may require doses of systemic gluco-corticosteroids prior to, during, and after unusual stress (eg, surgery). Immunosuppression may occur; patients may be more susceptible to infections; avoid exposure to chickenpox and measles. Bronchospasm may occur after use of inhaled asthma medications (see Additional Information). Powder for oral inhalation (Pulmicort Flexha-lerTM) contains lactose (milk proteins) which may cause allergic reactions in patients with severe milk protein allergy.

Oral: HPA axis suppression may occur; adrenal suppression may occur when switching patients from systemic corticosteroids to oral budesonide (due to lower bioavailability); withdrawal and discontinuation of systemic corticosteroids should be done carefully (monitoring of adrenocorticoid function may be needed); patients with HPA axis suppression may require increased doses of systemic glucocorticosteroids prior to, during, and after unusual stress (eg, surgery). Immunosuppression may occur; patients may be more susceptible to infections; avoid exposure to chickenpox and measles.

Precautions Avoid using higher than recommended dosages; suppression of HPA function, suppression of linear growth (ie, reduction of growth velocity), reduced bone mineral density, or hypercorticism (Cushing's syndrome) may occur; titrate to lowest effective dose. Reduction in growth velocity may occur when corticosteroids are administered to pediatric patients, even at recommended doses via oral, inhaled, nebulized, or intranasal route (monitor growth). Use of oral, inhaled, nebulized, or nasal budesonide in place of systemic corticosteroids may unmask allergies (eg, eczema, rhinitis) that were previously controlled by the systemic corticosteroids. Use oral budesonide with caution in patients with hypertension, tuberculosis, osteoporosis, diabetes mellitus, peptic ulcer disease, glaucoma, cataracts, or a family history of glaucoma or diabetes mellitus; use oral budesonide with caution and consider dosage reduction in patients with hepatic cirrhosis. Use inhaled budesonide with extreme caution in patients with respiratory tuberculosis, untreated systemic infections, or ocular herpes simplex. Rare cases of increased IOP, glaucoma, or cataracts may occur with inhaled corticosteroids.

Adverse Reactions Reaction severity varies by dose and duration; not all adverse reactions have been reported with each dosage form.

Cardiovascular: Chest pain, edema, flushing, hypertension, palpitation, syncope, tachycardia

Central nervous system: Amnesia, dizziness, dysphonia, emotional lability, fatigue, fever, headache, insomnia, malaise, migraine, nervousness, pain, sleep disorder, somnolence, vertigo

Dermatologic: Acne, alopecia, bruising, contact dermatitis, eczema, hirsutism, pruritus, pustular rash, rash, striae

Endocrine & metabolic: Adrenal insufficiency, Cushingoid state, HPA suppression, hypokalemia, menstrual disorder, weight gain

Gastrointestinal: Abdominal pain, anorexia, diarrhea, dyspepsia, flatulence, gastroenteritis (including viral), glossitis, growth suppression, intestinal obstruction, nausea, oral candidiasis, taste perversion, tongue edema, vomiting, weight gain, xerostomia

Genitourinary: Dysuria, hematuria, nocturia, pyuria

Hematologic: Cervical lymphadenopathy, leukocytosis, purpura

Hepatic: Alkaline phosphatase increased

Local: Nasal irritation, burning, or ulceration; nasal septum perforation, pharyngitis; growth of *Candida* in the mouth, throat, or nares

Neuromuscular & skeletal: Arthralgia, back pain, bone mineral density decreased, fracture, hyperkinesis, hypertonia, myalgia, neck pain, paresthesia, tremor, weakness

Ocular: Conjunctivitis, eye infection, visual abnormalities

Otic: Earache, external ear infection, otitis media

Respiratory: Bronchitis, bronchospasm, cough, epistaxis, hoarseness, nasal congestion, respiratory infection, rhinitis, sense of smell decreased, sinusitis, stridor, throat irritation, wheezing

Miscellaneous: Abscess, allergic reaction, C-reactive protein increased, erythrocyte sedimentation rate increased; flu-like syndrome, herpes simplex, immunosuppression, infection, moniliasis, viral infection, voice alteration

<1%, postmarketing, and/or case reports: Aggressive reactions, anaphylactic reactions, angioedema, anxiety, avascular necrosis of the femoral head, benign intracranial hypertension, cataracts, depression, dyspnea, glaucoma, IOP increased, hypersensitivity reactions [immediate and delayed (includes rash, contact dermatitis, angioedema, bronchospasm)], hypocorticism, intermenstrual bleeding, irritability, osteoporosis, psychosis, somnolence, urticaria, wheezing (patients with severe milk allergy)

Drug Interactions

Metabolism/Transport Effects Substrate of CYP3A4 (major)

Avoid Concomitant Use

Avoid concomitant use of Budesonide with any of the following: Aldesleukin; BCG; Natalizumab; Pimecrolimus; Tacrolimus (Topical); Vaccines (Live)

Increased Effect/Toxicity

Budesonide may increase the levels/effects of: Amphotericin B; Leflunomide; Loop Diuretics; Natalizumab; Thiazide Diuretics; Vaccines (Live)

The levels/effects of Budesonide may be increased by: Antifungal Agents (Azole Derivatives, Systemic); CYP3A4 Inhibitors (Moderate); CYP3A4 Inhibitors (Strong); Dasatinib; Denosumab; Pimecrolimus; Protease Inhibitors; Tacrolimus (Topical); Trastuzumab

Decreased Effect

Budesonide may decrease the levels/effects of: Aldesleukin; Antidiabetic Agents; BCG; Corticorelin; Sipuleucel-T; Vaccines (Inactivated); Vaccines (Live)

The levels/effects of Budesonide may be decreased by: Antacids; Bile Acid Sequestrants; Echinacea

Food Interactions Capsules: A high-fat meal delays the time to peak concentration by 2.5 hours, but does not affect the extent of oral absorption. Grapefruit juice significantly increases oral absorption.

Stability

Capsule: Store at room temperature in a tightly closed container

Intranasal inhaler: Store with valve up at 15°C to 30°C (59°F to 86°F). Use within 6 months after opening; avoid storage in high humidity; do not store or use by heat or open flame

Nebulization: Store Respules® upright at room temperature at 20°C to 25°C (68°F to 77°F); protect from light; do not refrigerate or freeze; do not mix with other medications; after foil packet has been opened, Respules® are stable for 2 weeks when protected from light; return unused Respules® to foil packet to protect from light; use opened Respules® promptly

Oral inhaler: Keep clean and dry; store at room temperature at 20°C to 25°C (68°F to 77°F)

Mechanism of Action Controls the rate of protein synthesis, depresses the migration of polymorphonuclear leukocytes and fibroblasts, reverses capillary permeability, and stabilizes lysosomal membranes at the cellular level to prevent or control inflammation

Pharmacodynamics Clinical effects are due to direct local effect, rather than systemic absorption

Onset of action:

Intranasal spray (Rhinocort® Aqua®): Within 10 hours

Nebulization (control of asthma symptoms): Within 2-8 days

Oral inhalation; intranasal inhaler: Within 24 hours

Maximum effect:

Intranasal spray: 2 weeks

Nebulization: 4-6 weeks

Oral inhalation: 1-2 weeks or more

Duration after discontinuation: Intranasal: Several days

Pharmacokinetics (Adult data unless noted)

Absorption:

Intranasal spray: 34% of dose delivered reaches systemic circulation

Oral inhalation: 39% of the metered dose is systemically available

Distribution: Distributes into breast milk (see Breast-Feeding Considerations)

V_d:

Children 4-6 years: 3 L/kg

Adults: ~200 L or 2.2-3.9 L/kg

Protein binding: 85% to 90%

Metabolism: Extensively metabolized by the liver via cytochrome P450 CYP3A isoenzyme to 2 major metabolites: 16α-hydroxyprednisolone and 6β-hydroxy-budesonide; both are <1% as active as parent

Bioavailability:

Nebulization: Children 4-6 years: 6%; **Note:** AUC of single 1 mg dose was comparable to a single 2 mg dose in healthy adults

Oral: ~10% (large first pass effect); **Note:** Oral bioavailability is 2.5-fold higher in patients with hepatic cirrhosis

Oral inhalation: Adults: 39%

Half-life:

Children: 4-6 years: 2.3 hours (after nebulization)

Children 10-14 years: 1.5 hours

Adults: 2-3.6 hours

Time to peak serum concentration: Oral: 30-600 minutes

Nebulization: 10-30 minutes

Oral inhalation (Pulmicort Flexhaler™): Adults: 10 minutes

Elimination: 60% to 66% of dose renally excreted as metabolites; no unchanged drug found in urine

Clearance:

Children 4-6 years: 0.5 L/minute (~50% greater than healthy adults after weight adjustment)

Adults: 0.9-1.8 L/minute

Usual Dosage

Intranasal: Children ≥6 years and Adults:

Rhinocort® Aqua® (32 mcg/spray): Initial: 2 sprays (1 spray/nostril) once daily (64 mcg/day); dose may be increased if needed

Maximum dose:

Children <12 years: 4 sprays (2 sprays/nostril) once daily (128 mcg/day)

Children ≥12 years and Adults: 8 sprays (4 sprays/nostril) once daily (256 mcg/day)

Nebulization: Pulmicort® Respules®: Doses should be titrated to the lowest effective dose once asthma is controlled:

Manufacturer's recommendations: Children 12 months to 8 years:

Previously treated with bronchodilators alone: Initial: 0.25 mg twice daily or 0.5 mg once daily; maximum dose: 0.5 mg/day

Previously treated with inhaled corticosteroids: Initial: 0.25 mg twice daily or 0.5 mg once daily; maximum dose: 1 mg/day

Previously treated with oral corticosteroids: Initial: 0.5 mg twice daily or 1 mg once daily; maximum dose: 1 mg/day

Symptomatic children not responding to nonsteroidal asthma medications: Initial: 0.25 mg once daily may be considered

Oral:

Children ≥6 years: Limited data available; optimal dose and duration of treatment not established; several dosage regimens have been evaluated (see Additional Information):

Active Crohn's disease (treatment): 9 mg/day given once daily for 7-8 weeks (see Escher, 2004; Levine, 2003; Levine, 2009)

Maintenance of remission: 6 mg/day given once daily for 3-4 weeks (see Escher, 2004; Levine, 2009)

Note: One study in children 10-19 years of age showed a trend for higher remission rates using an induction dose of 12 mg/day given once daily for 4 weeks, followed by 9 mg/day for 3 weeks, followed by 6 mg/day for 3 weeks (see Levine, 2009). Further studies are needed to establish optimal dosing regimen.

Adults:

Active Crohn's disease (treatment): 9 mg once daily in the morning for ≤8 weeks; may repeat the 8-week course for recurring episodes of active Crohn's disease; **Note:** When switching patients from oral prednisolone to oral budesonide, do not stop prednisolone abruptly; prednisolone taper should begin at the same time that budesonide is started

Maintenance of remission: Following treatment of active disease and control of symptoms (Crohn's Disease Activity Index <150), use 6 mg once daily for up to 3 months; if symptoms are still controlled at 3 months, taper the dose to complete cessation; continuing remission dose >3 months has not been demonstrated to result in substantial benefit

Oral inhalation: Note: Doses should be titrated to the lowest effective dose once asthma is controlled; Manufacturer's recommendations:

Children ≥6 years:

Pulmicort® Turbuhaler®:

Previously treated with bronchodilators alone or with inhaled corticosteroids: Initial: 200 mcg (1 puff) twice daily; maximum dose: 400 mcg (2 puffs) twice daily

Treated with oral corticosteroids: Initial: 400 mcg (2 puffs) twice daily (maximum dose)

Pulmicort Flexhaler™: Initial: 180 mcg twice daily (some patients may be initiated at 360 mcg twice daily); maximum: 360 mcg twice daily

Adults:

Pulmicort® Turbuhaler®:

Previously treated with bronchodilators alone: Initial: 200-400 mcg (1-2 puffs) twice daily; maximum dose: 400 mcg (2 puffs) twice daily

Treated with inhaled corticosteroids: Initial: 200-400 mcg (1-2 puffs) twice daily; maximum dose: 800 mcg (4 puffs) twice daily

Treated with oral corticosteroids: Initial: 400-800 mcg (2-4 puffs) twice daily; maximum dose: 800 mcg (4 puffs) twice daily

Pulmicort Flexhaler™: Initial: 360 mcg twice daily (selected patients may be initiated at 180 mcg twice daily); maximum: 720 mcg twice daily

NIH Asthma Guidelines (NAEPP, 2007):

Nebulization [give once daily or in divided doses twice daily]:

Children ≤4 years:

"Low" dose: 0.25-0.5 mg/day

"Medium" dose: >0.5-1 mg/day

"High" dose: >1 mg/day

Children 5-11 years:

"Low" dose: 0.5 mg/day

"Medium" dose: 1 mg/day

"High" dose: 2 mg/day

Oral inhalation [give in divided doses twice daily]:

Children 5-11 years:

"Low" dose: 180-400 mcg/day (90 mcg/inhalation: 2-4 inhalations/day or 180 mcg/inhalation: 1-2 inhalations/day)

"Medium" dose: >400-800 mcg/day (90 mcg/inhalation: 4-8 inhalations/day or 180 mcg/inhalation: 2-4 inhalations/day)

"High" dose: >800 mcg/day (90 mcg/inhalation: >8 inhalations/day or 180 mcg/inhalation: >4 inhalations/day)

Children ≥12 years and Adults:

"Low" dose: 180-600 mcg/day (90 mcg/inhalation: 2-6 inhalations/day or 180 mcg/inhalation: 1-3 inhalations/day)

"Medium" dose: >600-1200 mcg/day (90 mcg/inhalation: 6-13 inhalations/day or 180 mcg/inhalation: 3-6 inhalations/day)

"High" dose: >1200 mcg/day (90 mcg/inhalation: >13 inhalations/day or 180 mcg/inhalation: >6 inhalations/day)

Dosage adjustment in moderate to severe liver dysfunction: Oral: Monitor for signs and symptoms of hypercorticism; consider dosage reduction

Administration

Intranasal spray: Clear nasal passage by blowing nose prior to use; shake container gently before use. Prime before first use by actuating 8 times; if spray is not used for ≥2 consecutive days, reprime with one spray or until a fine spray appears; if spray is not used for > 14 days, clean and rinse the applicator according to manufacturer's instructions and reprime with 2 sprays or until a fine spray appears. Do not spray into eyes. Discard after 120 sprays.

Nebulization: Shake gently with a circular motion before use. Administer only with a compressed air driven jet nebulizer; do not use an ultrasonic nebulizer; use adequate flow rates and administer via appropriate size face mask or mouthpiece. Avoid exposure of nebulized medication to eyes. Rinse mouth following treatments to decrease risk of oral candidiasis (wash face if using face mask).

Oral: May be administered without regard to meals; do not chew, crush, break, or open capsule; swallow whole; do not administer with grapefruit juice

Oral inhaler:

Pulmicort Flexhaler™: Hold inhaler in upright position (mouthpiece up) to load dose. Do not shake prior to use. Unit should be primed prior to first use. It will not need primed again, even if not used for a long time. Place mouthpiece between lips and inhale forcefully and deeply. Do not exhale through inhaler; do not use a spacer. Dose indicator does not move with every dose, usually only after 5 doses. Discard when dose indicator reads "0". Rinse mouth with water after use to reduce incidence of candidiasis.

Pulmicort Turbuhaler®: Hold inhaler in upright position (mouthpiece up) to load dose. Do not shake inhaler after dose is loaded. Unit should be primed prior to first use. Place mouthpiece between lips and inhale forcefully and deeply; mouthpiece should face up. Do not exhale through inhaler; do not use a spacer. When a red mark appears in the dose indictor window, 20 doses are left. When the red mark reaches the bottom of the window, the inhaler should be discarded. Rinse mouth with water after use to reduce incidence of candidiasis.

Monitoring Parameters Monitor growth in pediatric patients. Inhalation and intranasal: Check mucous membranes for signs of fungal infection. Asthma: FEV1, peak flow, and/or other pulmonary function tests. Long-term use: Regular eye examinations and IOP

Patient Information Notify physician if condition being treated persists or worsens; do not decrease dose or discontinue without physician approval. Avoid exposure to chicken pox or measles; if exposed, seek medical advice without delay. May cause dry mouth. Report acute nervousness or inability to sleep; severe sneezing or nosebleed; difficulty breathing, sore throat, hoarseness, or bronchitis; respiratory difficulty or bronchospasms; disturbed menstrual pattern; vision changes; loss of taste or smell perception.

Nebulization: This is not a bronchodilator and will not relieve acute asthma attacks; it may take several days for full effects of treatment to occur. Rinse mouth after treatment and wash face after using face mask to decrease chance of oral candidiasis and steroid effects on skin

Oral: Avoid grapefruit juice and grapefruit

Oral inhaler: This is not a bronchodilator and will not relieve acute asthma attacks; it may take several days for full effects of treatment to occur. Rinse mouth after inhalation to decrease chance of oral candidiasis; report sore mouth or mouth lesions to physician.

Additional Information If bronchospasm with wheezing occurs after use of oral inhaler, a fast-acting bronchodilator may be used; discontinue orally inhaled corticosteroid and initiate alternative chronic therapy.

Budesonide nebulization: A 12-week study in infants (n=141; 6-12 months of age) receiving budesonide nebulizations (0.5 mg or 1 mg once daily) versus placebo demonstrated a budesonide dose-dependent suppression of linear growth; in addition, although mean changes from baseline did not indicate budesonide-induced adrenal suppression, 6 infants who received budesonide had subnormal stimulated cortisol levels at week 12. Children and adolescents (n=18; 6-15 years) receiving budesonide nebulizations of 1 and 2 mg twice daily showed a significant reduction in urinary cortisol excretion; this reduction was not seen when patients were dosed at 1 mg/day (maximum recommended dose). Long-term effects of chronic use of budesonide nebulization on immunological or developmental processes of upper airways, mouth, and lung are unknown.

◀ Oral budesonide: A retrospective study of 62 children (mean age: 14.1 ± 2.5 years; range: 9.5-18 years) used oral budesonide in doses of 0.45 mg/kg/day (maximum dose: 9 mg/day) for the treatment of mild to moderate Crohn's disease (see Levine, 2002). In a prospective, randomized, open-labeled comparison of oral budesonide versus prednisone in children 8-18 years of age (weighing >20 kg) with active Chrohn's disease, 19 children (mean age: 13.8 ± 2.4 years) received budesonide 9 mg/day (divided into 3 doses per day) for 8 weeks, followed by 6 mg/day for 1 week and 3 mg/day for 1 week; remission rates were similar for budesonide versus prednisone; adverse effect were less with budesonide (see Levine, 2003). In a randomized, double-blind, double-dummy controlled, comparative study of oral budesonide versus prednisolone in children 6-16 years of age with active Crohn's disease, 22 patients received budesonide 9 mg/day (given once daily in the morning) for 8 weeks, followed by 6 mg/day for 4 weeks; remission rates were similar for budesonide versus prednisolone; a trend existed for prednisolone to be more effective; significantly fewer adverse effects and less adrenal suppression were seen in the budesonide group (see Escher, 2004). In a randomized placebo-controlled trial comparing two oral budesonide dosing regimens in 70 patients 10-19 years of age with mild or moderately active Crohn's disease, 35 patients (mean age: 13.6 years ± 2.8 years) received 9 mg/day for 7 weeks followed by 6 mg/day for 3 weeks; 35 patients (mean age: 14.4 years ± 2.5 years) received 12 mg/day for 4 weeks, then 9 mg/day for 3 weeks, followed by 6 mg/day for 3 weeks; remission rates were not statistically different; however, there was a trend for higher remission rates in the higher dose group; adverse effects were similar between the two groups (see Levine, 2009). Further studies are needed to establish optimal dosing regimen.

Budesonide capsules (Entocort® EC) contain granules in an ethylcellulose matrix; the granules are coated with a methacrylic acid polymer to protect from dissolution in the stomach; the coating dissolves at a pH >5.5 (duodenal pH); the ethylcellulose matrix controls the release of drug in a time-dependent manner (until the drug reaches the ileum and ascending colon)

The manufacturer of Pulmicort® is replacing the Turbuhaler® delivery system with a new device, the Flexhaler™. The new powdered-drug inhalation system is available in two strengths (180 mcg/inhalation and 90 mcg/inhalation) and will include an advanced indicator which will allow users to estimate the doses remaining in the device. Because the Turbuhaler® will continue to be used until current devices are exhausted, this monograph retains currently dosing for both products.

Dosage Forms Excipient information presented when available (limited, particularly for generics); consult specific product labeling. [CAN] = Canadian brand name; [DSC] = Discontinued product

Capsule, enteric coated:

Entocort® EC: 3 mg

Powder for nasal inhalation:

Rhinocort® Turbuhaler® [CAN]: 100 mcg/inhalation [delivers 200 metered actuations] [not available in the U.S.]

Powder for oral inhalation:

Pulmicort Flexhaler™: 90 mcg/inhalation (165 mg) [contains lactose; delivers ~80 mcg/inhalation; 60 actuations]

Pulmicort Flexhaler™: 180 mcg/inhalation (225 mg) [contains lactose; delivers ~160 mcg/inhalation; 120 actuations]

Pulmicort Turbuhaler® [CAN]: 100 mcg/inhalation [delivers 200 metered actuations]; 200 mcg/inhalation [delivers 200 metered actuations]; 400 mcg/inhalation [delivers 200 metered actuations] [not available in the U.S.]

Suspension, intranasal [spray]:

Rhinocort® Aqua®: 32 mcg/inhalation (8.6 g) [120 metered actuations]

Rhinocort® Aqua® [CAN]: 64 mcg/inhalation [120 metered actuations] [not available in the U.S.]

Suspension for nebulization:

Pulmicort Respules®: 0.25 mg/2 mL (2 mL); 0.5 mg/2 mL (2 mL); 1 mg/2 mL (2 mL)

References

Escher JC and the European Collaborative Research Group on Budesonide in Paediatric IBD, "Budesonide Versus Prednisolone for the Treatment of Active Crohn's Disease in Children: A Randomized, Double-Blind, Controlled, Multicentre Trial," *Eur J Gastroenterol Hepatol*, 2004, 16(1):47-54.

Fält A, Bengtsson T, Kennedy BM, et al, "Exposure of Infants to Budesonide Through Breast Milk of Asthmatic Mothers," *J Allergy Clin Immunol*, 2007, 120(4):798-802.

Levine A, Broide E, Stein M, et al, "Evaluation of Oral Budesonide for Treatment of Mild and Moderate Exacerbations of Crohn's Disease in Children," *J Pediatr*, 2002, 140(1):75-80.

Levine A, Kori M, Dinari G, et al, "Comparison of Two Dosing Methods for Induction of Response and Remission With Oral Budesonide in Active Pediatric Crohn's Disease: A Randomized Placebo-Controlled Trial," *Inflamm Bowel Dis*, 2009, 15(7):1055-61.

Levine A, Weizman Z, Broide E, et al, "A Comparison of Budesonide and Prednisone for the Treatment of Active Pediatric Crohn Disease," *J Pediatr Gastroenterol Nutr*, 2003, 36(2):248-52.

National Asthma Education and Prevention Program (NAEPP), "Expert Panel Report 3 (EPR-3): Guidelines for the Diagnosis and Management of Asthma," *Clinical Practice Guidelines*, National Institutes of Health, National Heart, Lung, and Blood Institute, NIH Publication No. 08-4051, prepublication 2007; available at http://www.nhlbi.nih.gov/guidelines/asthma/asthgdln.htm.

Szefler SJ, "A Review of Budesonide Inhalation Suspension in the Treatment of Pediatric Asthma," *Pharmacotherapy*, 2001, 21 (2):195-206.

♦ **Budesonide and Eformoterol** *see* Budesonide and Formoterol *on page 210*

Budesonide and Formoterol
(byoo DES oh nide & for MOH te rol)

Related Information
Asthma *on page 1697*
Budesonide *on page 206*
Formoterol *on page 621*
U.S. Brand Names Symbicort®
Canadian Brand Names Symbicort®
Therapeutic Category Adrenal Corticosteroid; Adrenergic Agonist Agent; Anti-inflammatory Agent; Antiasthmatic; Beta₂-Adrenergic Agonist; Bronchodilator; Corticosteroid; Inhalant (Oral); Glucocorticoid
Generic Available No
Use Maintenance treatment of asthma
Medication Guide An FDA-approved patient medication guide, which is available with the product information and at http://www.fda.gov/downloads/Drugs/DrugSafety/ucm089139.pdf, must be dispensed with this medication for each new outpatient prescription and refill.
Pregnancy Risk Factor C
Pregnancy Considerations Teratogenic and embryocidal effects were observed in animal studies when administered by inhalation at doses less than the maximum equivalent human dose. Also see individual agents.
Lactation
Budesonide: Enters breast milk/use caution
Formoterol: Excretion in breast milk unknown/use caution
Contraindications Hypersensitivity to adrenergic amines, formoterol, budesonide, or any component; acute asthma; status asthmaticus

Warnings Fatalities have occurred due to adrenal insufficiency in asthmatic patients during and after switching from systemic corticosteroids to aerosol steroids; several months may be required for full recovery of the adrenal glands; patients receiving higher doses of systemic corticosteroids (eg, adults receiving ≥20 mg/day of prednisone) may be at greater risk; during this period of adrenal suppression, aerosol steroids do not provide the systemic corticosteroid needed to treat patients requiring stress doses (ie, patients with major stress such as trauma, surgery, or infections); when used at high doses or for a prolonged time, hypercorticism and hypothalamic-pituitary-adrenal (HPA) suppression (including adrenal crisis) may occur; withdrawal and discontinuation of corticosteroid therapy should be done carefully. Immunosuppression may occur. Budesonide/formoterol should not be used for transferring patients from systemic corticosteroid therapy.

Long-acting beta₂ agonists have been associated with an increased risk of serious asthma exacerbations and asthma-related deaths **[U.S. Boxed Warning]**. Long-acting beta₂ agonists should only be prescribed in patients not adequately controlled on other asthma-controller medications or whose disease severity clearly warrants treatment with two maintenance therapies. A medication guide is available to provide information to patients covering the risk of use.

Budesonide/formoterol is not meant to relieve acute asthmatic symptoms, rapidly deteriorating, or potentially life-threatening episodes of asthma. Acute episodes should be treated with short-acting beta₂ agonist. Do not increase the frequency of budesonide/formoterol use. Paroxysmal bronchospasm (which can be fatal) has been reported with this and other inhaled beta₂-agonist agents. If this occurs, discontinue treatment; symptoms of laryngeal spasm, irritation, or swelling, such as stridor and choking, have been reported in patients receiving budesonide/formoterol; if this occurs, discontinue treatment.

Precautions Use with caution in patients with cardiovascular disorders, convulsive disorders, liver dysfunction, thyrotoxicosis, or others who are sensitive to the effects of sympathomimetic amines; avoid using higher than recommended doses; suppression of HPA function, suppression of linear growth, or hypercorticism (Cushing's syndrome) may occur; use with extreme caution in patients with respiratory tuberculosis, untreated systemic infections, or ocular herpes simplex; long-term use of inhaled corticosteroids have been associated with osteoporosis

Adverse Reactions See individual agents.

Drug Interactions

Metabolism/Transport Effects
Budesonide: **Substrate** (minor) of CYP3A4
Formoterol: **Substrate** (minor) of CYP2A6, 2C9, 2C19, 2D6

Avoid Concomitant Use
Avoid concomitant use of Budesonide and Formoterol with any of the following: Aldesleukin; BCG; Iobenguane I 123; Natalizumab; Pimecrolimus; Tacrolimus (Topical); Vaccines (Live)

Increased Effect/Toxicity
Budesonide and Formoterol may increase the levels/effects of: Amphotericin B; Leflunomide; Loop Diuretics; Natalizumab; Sympathomimetics; Thiazide Diuretics; Vaccines (Live)

The levels/effects of Budesonide and Formoterol may be increased by: Antifungal Agents (Azole Derivatives, Systemic); Atomoxetine; Cannabinoids; CYP3A4 Inhibitors (Moderate); CYP3A4 Inhibitors (Strong); Dasatinib; Denosumab; MAO Inhibitors; Pimecrolimus; Protease

Inhibitors; Tacrolimus (Topical); Trastuzumab; Tricyclic Antidepressants

Decreased Effect
Budesonide and Formoterol may decrease the levels/effects of: Aldesleukin; Antidiabetic Agents; BCG; Corticorelin; Iobenguane I 123; Sipuleucel-T; Vaccines (Inactivated); Vaccines (Live)

The levels/effects of Budesonide and Formoterol may be decreased by: Alpha-/Beta-Blockers; Antacids; Beta-Blockers (Beta1 Selective); Beta-Blockers (Nonselective); Betahistine; Bile Acid Sequestrants; Echinacea

Stability Store at controlled room temperature of 20°C to 25°C (68°F to 77°F) with mouthpiece down; do not expose to temperatures >120°F; do not puncture or incinerate.

Mechanism of Action Formoterol is a long-acting selective beta₂-adrenergic receptor agonist. It relaxes bronchial smooth muscle by selective action on beta₂-receptors with little effect on heart rate. Budesonide is a corticosteroid which controls the rate of protein synthesis, depresses the migration of polymorphonuclear leukocytes/fibroblasts, reverses capillary permeability and lysosomal stabilization at the cellular level to prevent or control inflammation.

Pharmacodynamics See individual agents.

Pharmacokinetics (Adult data unless noted) See individual agents.

Usual Dosage Asthma: Maintenance treatment:
Children 5-11 years: Budesonide 80 mcg/formoterol 4.5 mcg (Symbicort® 80/4.5): 2 inhalations twice daily. Do not exceed 4 inhalations/day.
Children ≥12 years not controlled on low-medium dose inhaled corticosteroids: Budesonide 80 mcg/formoterol 4.5 mcg (Symbicort® 80/4.5): 2 inhalations twice daily. Do not exceed 4 inhalations/day.
Children ≥12 years not controlled on medium-high dose inhaled corticosteroids: Budesonide 160 mcg/formoterol 4.5 mcg (Symbicort® 160/4.5): 2 inhalations twice daily. Do not exceed 4 inhalations/day.

Administration Prior to first use, inhaler must be primed by releasing 2 test sprays into the air (away from the face); shake well for 5 seconds before each use. Inhaler must be reprimed if inhaler has not been used for >7 days or has been dropped. Discard after labeled number of inhalations has been used or within 3 months after foil wrap has been removed; do not use immerse in water or use "float test" to determine number of inhalations left.

Monitoring Parameters Pulmonary function tests, check mucous membranes for signs of fungal infection; monitor growth in pediatric patients

Patient Information Do not use to treat acute symptoms; do not exceed the prescribed dose of budesonide/formoterol; report sore mouth or mouth lesions to physician

Dosage Forms Excipient information presented when available (limited, particularly for generics); consult specific product labeling. [CAN] = Canadian product
Aerosol for oral inhalation:
Symbicort® 80/4.5: Budesonide 80 mcg and formoterol fumarate dihydrate 4.5 mcg per actuation (6.9 g) [60 metered inhalations]; budesonide 80 mcg and formoterol fumarate dihydrate 4.5 mcg per actuation (10.2 g) [120 metered inhalations]
Symbicort® 160/4.5: Budesonide 160 mcg and formoterol fumarate dihydrate 4.5 mcg per actuation (6 g) [60 metered inhalations]; budesonide 160 mcg and formoterol fumarate dihydrate 4.5 mcg per actuation (10.2 g) [120 metered inhalations]
Powder for oral inhalation:
Symbicort® 100 Turbuhaler® [CAN]: Budesonide 100 mcg and formoterol dihydrate 6 mcg per inhalation (available in 60 or 120 metered doses) [delivers ~80 mcg budesonide and 4.5 mcg formoterol per inhalation; contains lactose] [not available in the U.S]

Symbicort® 200 Turbuhaler® [CAN]: Budesonide 200 mcg and formoterol dihydrate 6 mcg per inhalation (available in 60 or 120 metered doses) [delivers ~160 mcg budesonide and 4.5 mcg formoterol per inhalation; contains lactose] [not available in the U.S]

References

Expert Panel Report 3, "Guidelines for the Diagnosis and Management of Asthma," Clinical Practice Guidelines, National Institutes of Health, National Heart, Lung, and Blood Institute, NIH Publication No. 08-4051, prepublication 2007. Available at http://www.nhlbi.nih.gov/guidelines/asthma/asthgdln.htm.

Pohunek P, Kuna P, Jorup C, et al, "Budesonide/Formoterol Improves Lung Function Compared With Budesonide Alone in Children With Asthma," Pediatr Allergy Immunol, 2006, 17(6):458-65.

◆ **Buffasal [OTC]** see Aspirin on page 141

◆ **Bufferin® [OTC]** see Aspirin on page 141

◆ **Bufferin® Extra Strength [OTC]** see Aspirin on page 141

◆ **Buffinol [OTC]** see Aspirin on page 141

◆ **Bulk-K [OTC]** see Psyllium on page 1185

Bumetanide (byoo MET a nide)

Medication Safety Issues

Sound-alike/look-alike issues:
Bumetanide may be confused with Buminate®
Bumex® may be confused with Brevibloc®, Buprenex®, Permax®

Related Information

Antihypertensive Agents by Class on page 1481

Canadian Brand Names Burinex®

Therapeutic Category Antihypertensive Agent; Diuretic, Loop

Generic Available Yes

Use Management of edema secondary to CHF or hepatic or renal disease including nephrotic syndrome; may also be used alone or in combination with antihypertensives in the treatment of hypertension

Pregnancy Risk Factor C

Pregnancy Considerations Adverse events have been observed in some animal studies.

Lactation Excretion in breast milk unknown/not recommended

Contraindications Hypersensitivity to bumetanide or any component; anuria or increasing azotemia; hepatic coma; severe electrolyte depletion (until condition is improved or corrected)

Warnings Loop diuretics are potent diuretics; excess amounts can lead to profound diuresis with fluid and electrolyte loss **[U.S. Boxed Warning]**; close medical supervision and dose evaluation is required. Increased risk of ototoxicity with rapid I.V. administration, renal impairment, excessive doses, and concurrent use of other ototoxins.

Precautions Use with caution in patients with cirrhosis; allergy to sulfonamides may result in cross hypersensitivity to bumetanide

Adverse Reactions

Cardiovascular: Hypotension, chest pain
Central nervous system: Dizziness, headache, encephalopathy, vertigo
Dermatologic: Rash, pruritus, urticaria
Endocrine & metabolic: Hyperglycemia, hypokalemia, hypochloremia, hypomagnesemia, hyponatremia, hyperuricemia
Gastrointestinal: Cramps, nausea, vomiting, diarrhea, abdominal pain, xerostomia
Hematologic: Thrombocytopenia (rare)
Hepatic: Liver enzymes elevated
Neuromuscular & skeletal: Weakness, muscle cramps, arthritic pain

Otic: Ototoxicity (with rapid I.V. administration)
Renal: Uric acid excretion decreased, serum creatinine elevated, azotemia

Drug Interactions

Avoid Concomitant Use There are no known interactions where it is recommended to avoid concomitant use.

Increased Effect/Toxicity
Bumetanide may increase the levels/effects of: ACE Inhibitors; Allopurinol; Amifostine; Aminoglycosides; Antihypertensives; CISplatin; Dofetilide; Hypotensive Agents; Lithium; Neuromuscular-Blocking Agents; RiTUXimab; Salicylates

The levels/effects of Bumetanide may be increased by: Corticosteroids (Orally Inhaled); Corticosteroids (Systemic); Diazoxide; Herbs (Hypotensive Properties); MAO Inhibitors; Pentoxifylline; Phosphodiesterase 5 Inhibitors; Probenecid; Prostacyclin Analogues

Decreased Effect
Bumetanide may decrease the levels/effects of: Lithium; Neuromuscular-Blocking Agents

The levels/effects of Bumetanide may be decreased by: Bile Acid Sequestrants; Herbs (Hypertensive Properties); Methylphenidate; Nonsteroidal Anti-Inflammatory Agents; Phenytoin; Probenecid; Salicylates; Yohimbine

Stability Store at room temperature; light sensitive, may discolor when exposed to light

Mechanism of Action Inhibits reabsorption of sodium and chloride in the ascending loop of Henle and proximal renal tubule, interfering with the chloride-binding cotransport system, thus causing increased excretion of water, sodium, chloride, magnesium, calcium, and phosphate

Pharmacodynamics

Onset of action:
Oral, I.M.: Within 30-60 minutes
I.V.: Within a few minutes
Maximum effect:
Oral, I.M.: 1-2 hours
I.V.: 15-30 minutes
Duration:
Oral: 4-6 hours
I.V.: 2-3 hours

Pharmacokinetics (Adult data unless noted)

Distribution: V_d: Neonates and infants: 0.26-0.39 L/kg
Protein binding: 95%
Neonates: 97%
Metabolism: Partial metabolism occurs in the liver
Bioavailability: 59% to 89% (median: 80%)
Half-life:
Premature and full term neonates: 6 hours (range up to 15 hours)
Infants <2 months: 2.5 hours
Infants 2-6 months: 1.5 hours
Adults: 1-1.5 hours
Time to peak serum concentration: 0.5-2 hours
Elimination: Unchanged drug excreted in urine (45%); biliary/fecal (2%)
Clearance:
Preterm and full term neonates: 0.2-1.1 mL/minute/kg
Infants <2 months: 2.17 mL/minute/kg
Infants 2-6 months: 3.8 mL/minute/kg
Adults: 2.9 ± 0.2 mL/minute/kg

Usual Dosage

Oral, I.M., I.V.:
Neonates (see Warnings): 0.01-0.05 mg/kg/dose every 24-48 hours
Infants and Children: 0.015-0.1 mg/kg/dose every 6-24 hours (maximum dose: 10 mg/day)

Adults:

Edema:

Oral: 0.5-2 mg/dose (maximum dose: 10 mg/day) 1-2 times/day

I.M., I.V.: 0.5-1 mg/dose; may repeat in 2-3 hours for up to 2 doses if needed (maximum dose: 10 mg/day)

Continuous I.V. infusion: 0.9-1 mg/hour

Hypertension: Oral: 0.5-2 mg divided twice daily; maximum dose: 5 mg/day

Administration

Oral: Administer with food to decrease GI irritation

Parenteral: Administer without additional dilution by direct I.V. injection over 1-2 minutes; for intermittent I.V. infusion, dilute in D_5W, LR, or NS and infuse over 5 minutes; for continuous infusion, dilute in D_5W to a final concentration of 0.024 mg/mL

Monitoring Parameters Blood pressure, serum electrolytes, renal function, urine output

Patient Information May cause dry mouth

Additional Information Patients with impaired hepatic function must be monitored carefully, often requiring reduced doses; larger doses may be necessary in patients with impaired renal function to obtain the same therapeutic response; 1 mg bumetanide approximately equivalent in potency to 40 mg furosemide

Dosage Forms Excipient information presented when available (limited, particularly for generics); consult specific product labeling. [DSC] = Discontinued product

Injection, solution: 0.25 mg/mL (2 mL, 4 mL, 10 mL)

Tablet: 0.5 mg, 1 mg, 2 mg

References

Brater DC, "Clinical Pharmacology of Loop Diuretics," *Drugs*, 1991, 41 Suppl 3:14-22.

Chobanian AV, Bakris GL, Black HR, et al, "The Seventh Report of the Joint National Committee on Prevention, Detection, Evaluation, and Treatment of High Blood Pressure: The JNC 7 Report," *JAMA*, 2003, 289(19):2560-72.

Cook JA, Smith DE, Cornish LA, et al, "Kinetics, Dynamics, and Bioavailability of Bumetanide in Healthy Subjects and Patients With Congestive Heart Failure," *Clin Pharmacol Ther*, 1988, 44(5):487-500.

Wells TG, "The Pharmacology and Therapeutics of Diuretics in the Pediatric Patient," *Pediatr Clin North Am*, 1990, 37(2):463-504.

♦ **Bumex** *see* Bumetanide *on page 212*

♦ **Buminate®** *see* Albumin *on page 55*

♦ **Buphenyl®** *see* Sodium Phenylbutyrate *on page 1275*

Bupivacaine (byoo PIV a kane)

Medication Safety Issues

Sound-alike/look-alike issues:

Bupivacaine may be confused with mepivacaine, ropivacaine

Marcaine® may be confused with Narcan®

High alert medication: The Institute for Safe Medication Practices (ISMP) includes this medication (epidural administration) among its list of drug classes which have a heightened risk of causing significant patient harm when used in error.

U.S. Brand Names Marcaine®; Marcaine® Spinal; Sensorcaine®; Sensorcaine®-MPF; Sensorcaine®-MPF Spinal

Canadian Brand Names Marcaine®; Sensorcaine®

Therapeutic Category Local Anesthetic, Injectable

Generic Available Yes

Use Local anesthetic (injectable) for peripheral nerve block, infiltration, sympathetic block, caudal or epidural block, retrobulbar block

Pregnancy Risk Factor C

Pregnancy Considerations Decreased pup survival and embryocidal effects were observed in animal studies. Bupivacaine is approved for use at term in obstetrical anesthesia or analgesia. **[U.S. Boxed Warning]: The 0.75% is not recommended for obstetrical anesthesia.** Bupivacaine 0.75% solutions have been associated with cardiac arrest following epidural anesthesia in obstetrical patients and use of this concentration is not recommended for this purpose. Use in obstetrical paracervical block anesthesia is contraindicated.

Lactation Enters breast milk/not recommended

Contraindications Hypersensitivity to bupivacaine hydrochloride, other amide-type anesthetics, or any component (see Warnings); not recommended for I.V. regional anesthesia (Bier block); obstetrical paracervical block anesthesia (use is associated with fetal bradycardia and death); 0.75% concentration in obstetrical anesthesia

Warnings Convulsions due to systemic toxicity leading to cardiac arrest have been reported, presumably following unintentional I.V. injection; some products contain sulfites which may cause allergic reactions in susceptible individuals; **do not use solutions containing preservatives for caudal or epidural block.** Infants may be at greater risk for bupivacaine toxicity because α_1-acidglycoprotein, the major serum protein to which bupivacaine is bound, is lower in infants compared with older children; use epidural infusions with caution in infants and monitor closely; increased toxicity may be minimized by limiting the duration of infusion to ≤48 hours (McCloskey, 1992). Reduce epidural infusion dosage in patients with seizure disorders or at increased risk for seizures (eg, electrolyte imbalance) (Berde, 1992). Chondrolysis has been reported following continuous intra-articular infusion; intra-articular administration of local anesthetics is not an FDA-approved route of administration.

Precautions Use with caution in patients with liver disease and impaired cardiovascular function; when used for epidural anesthesia, a smaller test dose is recommended to evaluate the patient's response

Adverse Reactions

Cardiovascular: Bradycardia, cardiac arrest, hypotension, palpitations

Central nervous system: Anxiety, dizziness, headache, restlessness, seizures

Dermatologic: Angioneurotic edema, pruritus

Gastrointestinal: Nausea, vomiting

Neuromuscular & skeletal: Chondrolysis (continuous intra-articular administration), weakness

Ocular: Blurred vision

Otic: Tinnitus

Respiratory: Apnea, sneezing

Miscellaneous: Hypersensitivity reactions

Drug Interactions

Metabolism/Transport Effects Substrate (minor) of CYP1A2, 2C19, 2D6, 3A4

Avoid Concomitant Use There are no known interactions where it is recommended to avoid concomitant use.

Increased Effect/Toxicity

The levels/effects of Bupivacaine may be increased by: Beta-Blockers

Decreased Effect

The levels/effects of Bupivacaine may be decreased by: Peginterferon Alfa-2b

Stability Store at room temperature; solutions containing epinephrine should be protected from light; bupivacaine 0.4375 mg/mL when mixed with epinephrine 0.6875 mcg/mL and fentanyl 1.25 mcg/mL is stable refrigerated for 20 days and at room temperature for 48 hours; bupivacaine 625 mcg/mL or 1250 mcg/mL mixed with morphine sulfate 100 mcg/mL or 500 mcg/mL in NS is stable for 72 hours at room temperature

Mechanism of Action Blocks both the initiation and conduction of nerve impulses by decreasing the neuronal membrane's permeability to sodium ions, which results in inhibition of depolarization with resultant blockade of conduction

Pharmacodynamics

Onset of anesthetic action: Dependent on total dose, concentration, and route administered, but generally occurs within 4-10 minutes

Duration: 1.5-8.5 hours (depending upon route of administration)

Pharmacokinetics (Adult data unless noted)

Distribution: V_d:

Infants: 3.9 ± 2 L/kg

Children: 2.7 ± 0.2 L/kg

Protein binding: 84% to 95%

Metabolism: In the liver

Half-life (age-dependent):

Neonates: 8.1 hours

Adults: 2.7 hours

Time to peak serum concentration: Caudal, epidural, or peripheral nerve block: 30-45 minutes

Elimination: Small amounts (~6%) excreted in urine unchanged

Clearance:

Infants: 7.1 ± 3.2 mL/kg/minute

Children: 10 ± 0.7 mL/kg/minute

Usual Dosage Dose varies with procedure, depth of anesthesia, vascularity of tissues, duration of anesthesia and condition of patient

Caudal block (with or without epinephrine, **preservative free**):

Children: 1-3.7 mg/kg

Adults: 15-30 mL of 0.25% or 0.5%

Epidural block, **preservative free** (other than caudal block):

Children: 1.25 mg/kg/dose

Adults: 10-20 mL of 0.25%, 0.5%, or 0.75%

Peripheral nerve block: 5 mL dose of 0.25% or 0.5% (12.5-25 mg); maximum dose: 400 mg/day

Sympathetic nerve block: 20-50 mL of 0.25% (no epinephrine) solution

Continuous epidural (caudal or lumbar) infusion (limited information in neonates, infants, and children):

Loading dose: 2-2.5 mg/kg (0.8-1 mL/kg of 0.25% bupivacaine)

Infusion dose: See table

Bupivacaine Infusion Dose

Age	Dose	Dose (using 0.25% solution)	Dose (using 0.125% solution)	Dose (using 0.05% solution)
Neonates and infants ≤4 mo	0.2-0.25 mg/kg/h	0.08-0.1 mL/kg/h	0.16-0.2 mL/kg/h	0.4-0.5 mL/kg/h
Infants >4 mo and children	0.4-0.5 mg/kg/h	0.16-0.2 mL/kg/h	0.32-0.4 mL/kg/h	0.8-1 mL/kg/h
Adults	5-20 mg/h	2-8 mL/h	4-16 mL/h	10-40 mL/h

Administration Solutions containing preservatives should not be used for epidural or caudal blocks; for epidural infusion, may use undiluted or diluted with preservative free NS

Reference Range Toxicity: 2-4 mcg/mL (however, some experts have suggested that the rate of rise of the serum level is more predictive of toxicity than the actual value; Scott, 1975)

Patient Information May experience temporary loss of sensation and motor activity, usually in the lower half of the body following caudal or lumbar epidural anesthesia

Additional Information For epidural infusion, lower dosages of bupivacaine may be effective when used in combination with narcotic analgesics

Dosage Forms Excipient information presented when available (limited, particularly for generics); consult specific product labeling.

Injection, solution, as hydrochloride [preservative free]: 0.25% (10 mL, 20 mL, 30 mL, 50 mL); 0.5% (10 mL, 20 mL, 30 mL); 0.75% (10 mL, 20 mL, 30 mL)

Marcaine®: 0.25% (10 mL, 30 mL, 50 mL); 0.5% (10 mL, 30 mL); 0.75% (10 mL, 30 mL)

Sensorcaine®-MPF: 0.25% (10 mL, 30 mL); 0.5% (10 mL, 30 mL); 0.75% (10 mL, 30 mL)

Injection, solution, premixed in D8.25, as hydrochloride [preservative free]: 0.75% (2 mL)

Marcaine® Spinal: 0.75% (2 mL)

Sensorcaine®-MPF Spinal: 0.75% (2 mL)

Injection, solution, as hydrochloride: 0.25% (50 mL); 0.5% (50 mL)

Marcaine®: 0.5% (50 mL) [contains methylparaben]

Sensorcaine®: 0.25% (50 mL); 0.5% (50 mL) [contains methylparaben]

References

Berde CB, "Convulsions Associated With Pediatric Regional Anesthesia," *Anesth Analg*, 1992, 75(2):164-6.

Desparmet J, Meistelman C, Barre J, et al, "Continuous Epidural Infusion of Bupivacaine for Postoperative Pain Relief in Children," *Anesthesiology*, 1987, 67(1):108-10.

Luz G, Innerhofer P, Bachmann B, et al, "Bupivacaine Plasma Concentrations During Continuous Epidural Anesthesia in Infants and Children," *Anesth Analg*, 1996, 82(2):231-4.

McCloskey JJ, Haun SE, and Deshpande JK, "Bupivacaine Toxicity Secondary to Continuous Caudal Epidural Infusion in Children," *Anesth Analg*, 1992, 75(2):287-90.

Scott DB, "Evaluation of Clinical Tolerance of Local Anaesthetic Agents," *Br J Anaesth*, 1975, 47:328-31.

♦ **Bupivacaine Hydrochloride** *see* Bupivacaine *on page 213*

♦ **Buprenex®** *see* Buprenorphine *on page 214*

Buprenorphine (byoo pre NOR feen)

Medication Safety Issues

Sound-alike/look-alike issues:

Buprenex® may be confused with Brevibloc®, Bumex®

High alert medication: The Institute for Safe Medication Practices (ISMP) includes this medication among its list of drug classes which have a heightened risk of causing significant patient harm when used in error.

U.S. Brand Names Buprenex®; Subutex®

Canadian Brand Names Buprenex®; Subutex®

Therapeutic Category Analgesic, Narcotic; Opioid Partial Agonist

Generic Available Yes

Use

Injection: Management of moderate to severe pain

Sublingual tablet: Treatment of opioid dependence

Restrictions Injection: C-V/C-III; Tablet: C-III

Pregnancy Risk Factor C

Pregnancy Considerations Withdrawal has been reported in infants of women receiving buprenorphine during pregnancy. Onset of symptoms ranged from day 1 to day 8 of life, most occurring on day 1.

Lactation Enters breast milk/not recommended

Contraindications Hypersensitivity to buprenorphine or any component

Warnings Respiratory depression may occur; use with caution and in reduced doses in patients with pre-existing respiratory depression, decreased respiratory reserve, hypoxia, hypercapnia, significant COPD, or cor pulmonale, and in those receiving medications with CNS or respiratory depressant effects; respiratory depression may not be reversible with naloxone; mechanical ventilation may be required.

May cause CNS depression; warn patients of possible impairment of alertness or physical coordination (see Patient Information); interactions with other CNS drugs may occur (see Drug Interactions); physical and psychological dependence may occur; abrupt discontinuation after prolonged use may result in withdrawal symptoms (**Note:** Compared to full opioid agonists, withdrawal from buprenorphine may be milder and may be delayed in onset); narcotic antagonist activity of buprenorphine may precipitate acute narcotic withdrawal in opioid-dependent individuals.

Hepatitis and other hepatic events (see Adverse Reactions) have been reported in patients receiving buprenorphine for the treatment of opioid dependence; infection with viral hepatitis, concomitant use of potentially hepatotoxic drugs, pre-existing liver enzyme abnormalities, ongoing drug use may have contributed to liver abnormalities. Acute and chronic hypersensitivity reactions have also been reported. Orthostatic hypotension may occur in ambulatory patients.

Precautions Use with caution in patients with head injury; increased intracranial pressure; CNS depression; coma; toxic psychosis; seizures; acute abdominal conditions; biliary tract disease, pancreatitis; severe renal, respiratory, or hepatic insufficiency; hypothyroidism; Addison's disease; urethral stricture, prostatic hypertrophy; acute alcoholism; delirium tremens, kyphoscoliosis, and in children or debilitated patients. Safety and efficacy of injection in children <2 years of age and of sublingual tablets in children <16 years of age have not been established.

Adverse Reactions

Cardiovascular: Hypotension, bradycardia, tachycardia, hypertension, Wenckebach block, orthostatic hypotension

Central nervous system: Sedation, dizziness, vertigo, CNS depression, headache, confusion, euphoria, fatigue, nervousness, depression, slurred speech, dreaming, psychosis, anxiety, insomnia

Dermatologic: Pruritus, rash, hives

Gastrointestinal: Nausea, vomiting, constipation, xerostomia, abdominal pain, dyspepsia

Genitourinary: Urinary retention

Hepatic: Sublingual tablets: Liver enzymes elevated, hepatitis with jaundice, cytolytic hepatitis, hepatic failure, hepatic necrosis, hepatorenal syndrome, hepatic encephalopathy

Local: Injection site reaction

Neuromuscular & skeletal: Weakness, paresthesia

Ocular: Miosis, diplopia, visual abnormalities, blurred vision

Otic: Tinnitus

Respiratory: Respiratory depression, hypoventilation, dyspnea, cyanosis

Miscellaneous: Physical and psychological dependence, diaphoresis; hypersensitivity reactions, angioneurotic edema, anaphylactic shock

Drug Interactions

Metabolism/Transport Effects Substrate of CYP3A4 (major); **Inhibits** CYP1A2 (weak), 2A6 (weak), 2C19 (weak), 2D6 (weak)

Avoid Concomitant Use

Avoid concomitant use of Buprenorphine with any of the following: Atazanavir

Increased Effect/Toxicity

Buprenorphine may increase the levels/effects of: Alcohol (Ethyl); Alvimopan; CNS Depressants; Desmopressin; Selective Serotonin Reuptake Inhibitors; Thiazide Diuretics

The levels/effects of Buprenorphine may be increased by: Amphetamines; Antipsychotic Agents (Phenothiazines); Atazanavir; CYP3A4 Inhibitors (Moderate); CYP3A4 Inhibitors (Strong); Dasatinib; Succinylcholine

Decreased Effect

Buprenorphine may decrease the levels/effects of: Analgesics (Opioid); Atazanavir; Pegvisomant

The levels/effects of Buprenorphine may be decreased by: Ammonium Chloride; CYP3A4 Inducers (Strong); Deferasirox; Herbs (CYP3A4 Inducers); Mixed Agonist / Antagonist Opioids

Stability

Injection: Protect from exposure to excessive heat of >40°C (>104°F) or prolonged exposure to light.

Sublingual tablet: Store at room temperature of 25°C (77°F).

Mechanism of Action Binds to opiate receptors in the CNS, causing inhibition of ascending pain pathways, altering perception of and response to pain; produces generalized CNS depression. Can be classified as a partial agonist with both agonist and antagonist activity (ie, partial agonist at the mu opioid receptor and an antagonist at the kappa opioid receptor). When used as recommended, buprenorphine acts as a classic mu receptor agonist (like morphine). In vitro studies demonstrate a very slow rate of dissociation from the mu receptor which may account for buprenorphine's longer duration of action (compared to morphine), unpredictability of reversal by opioid antagonists, and low level of apparent physical dependence.

Pharmacodynamics I.M.:

Onset of action: 15 minutes

Maximum effect: 1 hour

Duration: ≥6 hours

Pharmacokinetics (Adult data unless noted)

Distribution: Distributes into breast milk at concentrations greater than maternal plasma

V_d:

Premature neonates 27-32 weeks GA (n=11) (mean ± SD): 6.2 ± 2.1 L/kg

Children 4-7 years (n=10) (mean ± SD): 3.2 ± 2 L/kg

Protein binding: 96%, primarily to alpha and beta globulin

Metabolism: In the liver, via both N-dealkylation (to an active metabolite, norbuprenorphine) and glucuronidation; norbuprenorphine also undergoes glucuronidation; two other unidentified metabolites have been found; extensive first-pass effect

Half-life:

I.V.:

Premature neonates 27-32 weeks GA (n=11) (mean ± SD): 20 ± 8 hours

Adults: 2.2 hours

Sublingual: Adults: 37 hours

Elimination: 30% of the dose is excreted in the urine (1% as unchanged drug; 9.4% as conjugated drug; 2.7% as norbuprenorphine; and 11% as conjugated norbuprenorphine) and 69% in feces (33% as unchanged drug; 5% as conjugated drug; 21% as norbuprenorphine; and 2% as conjugated norbuprenorphine)

Clearance: Related to hepatic blood flow

Premature neonates 27-32 weeks GA (n=11): 0.23 ± 0.07 L/hour/kg

Children 4-7 years: 3.6 ± 1.1 L/hour/kg

Adults: 0.78-1.32 L/hour/kg

◀ **Usual Dosage** Dose should be titrated to appropriate effect. Use ¹/₂ of the dose listed in patients with pre-existing respiratory depression, decreased respiratory reserve, hypoxia, hypercapnia, significant COPD, or cor pulmonale, and in those receiving medications with CNS or respiratory depressant effects.

Moderate to severe pain:

Children 2-12 years: I.M., slow I.V. injection: 2-6 mcg/kg every 4-6 hours; **Note:** 3 mcg/kg/dose has been most commonly studied (see References); not all children have faster clearance rates than adults; some children may require dosing intervals of every 6-8 hours; observe clinical effects to establish the proper dosing interval

Children ≥13 years and Adults: I.M., slow I.V. injection: Initial: Opiate-naive: 0.3 mg every 6-8 hours as needed; initial dose (up to 0.3 mg) may be repeated once in 30-60 minutes if clinically needed; **Note:** In adults, single doses of up to 0.6 mg administered I.M. may occasionally be required

Opioid dependence: Note: Do not start induction with buprenorphine until objective and clear signs of withdrawal are apparent (otherwise withdrawal may be precipitated). Children ≥16 years and Adults: Sublingual: Induction: Target range: 12-16 mg/day (doses during one induction study used 8 mg on day 1, followed by 16 mg on day 2; other studies accomplished induction over 3-4 days). Treatment should begin at least 4 hours after last use of heroin or short-acting opioid, preferably when first signs of withdrawal appear. Titrating dose to clinical effect should be done as rapidly as possible to prevent undue withdrawal symptoms.

Maintenance: **Note:** Patients should be switched to the buprenorphine/naloxone combination product for maintenance and for unsupervised therapy; initial target dose: 12-16 mg/day; then adjust dose in 2-4 mg increments/decrements to a dose that adequately suppresses opioid withdrawal; usual range: 4-24 mg/day

Administration

Oral: Sublingual: Place tablet under the tongue until dissolved; do not swallow. If 2 or more tablets are needed per dose, all tablets may be placed under the tongue at once, or 2 tablets may be placed under the tongue at a time; to ensure consistent bioavailability, subsequent doses should always be taken the same way.

Parenteral:

I.M.: Administer via deep I.M. injection

I.V.: Administer slowly, over at least 2 minutes

Monitoring Parameters Pain relief, respiratory rate, mental status, blood pressure; liver enzymes (baseline and periodic) with use of sublingual tablets

Patient Information May cause drowsiness and impair ability to perform activities requiring mental alertness or physical coordination; may cause postural hypotension (use caution when changing positions from lying or sitting to standing); avoid alcohol, sedatives, benzodiazepines, tranquilizers, and antidepressants; report the use of other prescription and nonprescription medications to your physician and pharmacist. May be habit-forming; use exactly as directed; do not increase dose or frequency; do not discontinue abruptly, dose should be tapered to prevent withdrawal. May cause dry mouth.

Additional Information Equianalgesic doses (parenteral): Buprenorphine 0.3 mg = morphine 10 mg; buprenorphine has a longer duration of action than morphine

Symptoms of overdose include CNS and respiratory depression, pinpoint pupils, hypotension, and bradycardia; treatment is supportive; naloxone may have limited effects in reversing respiratory depression; doxapram has also been used as a respiratory stimulant.

Neonatal withdrawal symptoms (including tremor, agitation, hypertonia, and myoclonus) have been reported in infants of women receiving buprenorphine sublingual tablets during pregnancy; onset of symptoms ranged from day 1 to day 8 of life, most occurring on day 1 of life; rare cases of convulsions (with one case of apnea and bradycardia) have also been reported

Dosage Forms Excipient information presented when available (limited, particularly for generics); consult specific product labeling.

Injection, solution: 0.3 mg/mL (1 mL) [C-III]

Buprenex®: 0.3 mg/mL (1 mL) [C-V]

Tablet, sublingual: 2 mg, 8 mg

Subutex®: 2 mg, 8 mg

References

Barrett DA, Simpson J, Rutter N, et al, "The Pharmacokinetics and Physiological Effects of Buprenorphine Infusion in Premature Neonates," *Br J Clin Pharmacol*, 1993, 36(3):215-9.

Hamunen K, Olkkola KT, and Maunuksela EL, "Comparison of the Ventilatory Effects of Morphine and Buprenorphine in Children," *Acta Anaesthesiol Scand*, 1993, 37(5):449-53.

Maunuksela EL, Korpela R, and Olkkola KT, "Comparison of Buprenorphine With Morphine in the Treatment of Postoperative Pain in Children," *Anesth Analg*, 1988, 67(3):233-9.

Maunuksela EL, Korpela R, and Olkkola KT, "Double-Blind, Multiple-Dose Comparison of Buprenorphine and Morphine in Postoperative Pain of Children," *Br J Anaesth*, 1988, 60(1):48-55.

Olkkola KT, Leijala MA, and Maunuksela EL, "Paediatric Ventilatory Effects of Morphine and Buprenorphine Revisited," *Paediatr Anaesth*, 1995, 5(5):303-5.

Olkkola KT, Maunuksela EL, and Korpela R, "Pharmacokinetics of Intravenous Buprenorphine in Children," *Br J Clin Pharmacol*, 1989, 28(2):202-4.

Buprenorphine and Naloxone
(byoo pre NOR feen & nal OKS one)

Medication Safety Issues

High alert medication: The Institute for Safe Medication Practices (ISMP) includes this medication among its list of drug classes which have a heightened risk of causing significant patient harm when used in error.

U.S. Brand Names Suboxone®

Therapeutic Category Analgesic, Narcotic; Opioid Partial Agonist

Generic Available No

Use Treatment of opioid dependence

Restrictions C-III

Pregnancy Risk Factor C

Pregnancy Considerations Withdrawal has been reported in infants of women receiving buprenorphine during pregnancy. Onset of symptoms ranged from day 1 to day 8 of life, most occurring on day 1.

Lactation Buprenorphine: Enters breast milk/not recommended

Contraindications Hypersensitivity to buprenorphine, naloxone, or any component

Warnings Respiratory depression may occur; use with caution and in reduced doses in patients with pre-existing respiratory depression, decreased respiratory reserve, hypoxia, hypercapnia, significant COPD, or cor pulmonale, and in those receiving medications with CNS or respiratory depressant effects; respiratory depression may not be reversible with naloxone; mechanical ventilation may be required.

May cause CNS depression; warn patients of possible impairment of alertness or physical coordination (see Patient Information); interactions with other CNS drugs may occur (see Drug Interactions); physical and psychological dependence may occur; abrupt discontinuation after prolonged use may result in withdrawal symptoms (**Note:** Compared to full opioid agonists, withdrawal from buprenorphine may be milder and may be delayed in onset); narcotic antagonist activity of buprenorphine may precipitate acute narcotic withdrawal in opioid-dependent individuals.

Naloxone may precipitate intense withdrawal symptoms in patients addicted to opiates when administered before the opioid effects have subsided, or if misused parenterally in opioid-dependent individuals. Combination product of buprenorphine and naloxone is indicated for maintenance therapy and should not be used for induction. Oral buprenorphine is not approved for management of pain.

Hepatitis and other hepatic events (see Adverse Reactions) have been reported in patients receiving buprenorphine for the treatment of opioid dependence; infection with viral hepatitis, concomitant use of potentially hepatotoxic drugs, pre-existing liver enzyme abnormalities, ongoing drug use may have contributed to liver abnormalities. Acute and chronic hypersensitivity reactions have also been reported. Orthostatic hypotension may occur in ambulatory patients.

Precautions Use with caution in patients with head injury; increased intracranial pressure; CNS depression; coma; toxic psychosis; seizures; acute abdominal conditions; biliary tract disease, pancreatitis; severe renal, respiratory, or hepatic insufficiency; hypothyroidism; Addison's disease; urethral stricture, prostatic hypertrophy; acute alcoholism; delirium tremens, kyphoscoliosis, and in children or debilitated patients. Safety and efficacy in children <16 years of age have not been established.

Adverse Reactions See individual agents.

Drug Interactions

Avoid Concomitant Use

Avoid concomitant use of Buprenorphine and Naloxone with any of the following: Atazanavir

Increased Effect/Toxicity

Buprenorphine and Naloxone may increase the levels/effects of: Alcohol (Ethyl); Alvimopan; CNS Depressants; Desmopressin; Selective Serotonin Reuptake Inhibitors; Thiazide Diuretics

The levels/effects of Buprenorphine and Naloxone may be increased by: Amphetamines; Antipsychotic Agents (Phenothiazines); Atazanavir; CYP3A4 Inhibitors (Moderate); CYP3A4 Inhibitors (Strong); Dasatinib; Succinylcholine

Decreased Effect

Buprenorphine and Naloxone may decrease the levels/effects of: Analgesics (Opioid); Atazanavir; Pegvisomant

The levels/effects of Buprenorphine and Naloxone may be decreased by: Ammonium Chloride; CYP3A4 Inducers (Strong); Deferasirox; Herbs (CYP3A4 Inducers); Mixed Agonist / Antagonist Opioids

Stability Store a room temperature of 25°C (77°F)

Mechanism of Action See individual agents.

Pharmacokinetics (Adult data unless noted) See individual agents.

Absorption: Absorption of the combination product is variable between patients following sublingual use, but variability within each individual patient is low.

Usual Dosage Dose should be titrated to appropriate effect.

Opioid dependence: Children ≥16 years and Adults: Sublingual:

Induction: **Note:** Combination product (buprenorphine and naloxone) is not recommended for use during induction; initial treatment should begin using buprenorphine sublingual tablets (see buprenorphine monograph).

Maintenance: **Note:** Patients should be switched to the buprenorphine and naloxone combination product for maintenance and for unsupervised therapy; initial target dose: 12-16 mg/day (based on buprenorphine content); then adjust dose in 2-4 mg increments/decrements to a dose that adequately suppresses opioid withdrawal; usual range: 4-24 mg/day

Administration Oral: Sublingual: Place tablet under the tongue until dissolved; do not swallow. If 2 or more tablets are needed per dose, all tablets may be placed under the tongue at once, or 2 tablets may be placed under the tongue at a time; to ensure consistent bioavailability, subsequent doses should always be taken the same way.

Monitoring Parameters Symptoms of withdrawal, respiratory rate, mental status, blood pressure; liver enzymes (baseline and periodic)

Patient Information May cause drowsiness and impair ability to perform activities requiring mental alertness or physical coordination; may cause postural hypotension (use caution when changing positions from lying or sitting to standing); avoid alcohol, sedatives, benzodiazepines, tranquilizers, and antidepressants; report the use of other prescription and nonprescription medications to your physician and pharmacist. May be habit-forming; use exactly as directed; do not increase dose or frequency; do not discontinue abruptly, dose should be tapered to prevent withdrawal. May cause dry mouth.

Additional Information Sublingual tablets contain a free base ratio of buprenorphine to naloxone of 4 to 1. Naloxone has been added to the formulation to decrease the abuse potential of crushing and dissolving tablets in water and using as an injection (precipitation of severe withdrawal would occur in opioid dependent patients if the tablets were misused in this manner).

Symptoms of overdose include CNS and respiratory depression, pinpoint pupils, hypotension, and bradycardia; treatment is supportive; parenteral naloxone may have limited effects in reversing respiratory depression; doxapram has also been used as a respiratory stimulant.

Neonatal withdrawal symptoms (including tremor, agitation, hypertonia, and myoclonus) have been reported in infants of women receiving buprenorphine sublingual tablets during pregnancy; onset of symptoms ranged from day 1 to day 8 of life, most occurring on day 1 of life; rare cases of convulsions (with one case of apnea and bradycardia) have also been reported

Dosage Forms Excipient information presented when available (limited, particularly for generics); consult specific product labeling.

Tablet, sublingual: Buprenorphine 2 mg and naloxone 0.5 mg; buprenorphine 8 mg and naloxone 2 mg [lemon-lime flavor]

◆ **Buprenorphine Hydrochloride** *see* Buprenorphine *on page 214*

◆ **Buprenorphine Hydrochloride and Naloxone Hydrochloride Dihydrate** *see* Buprenorphine and Naloxone *on page 216*

◆ **Buproban®** *see* BuPROPion *on page 217*

BuPROPion (byoo PROE pee on)

Medication Safety Issues

Sound-alike/look-alike issues:

Aplenzin™ may be confused with Albenza®, Relenza®

BuPROPion may be confused with busPIRone

Wellbutrin SR® may be confused with Wellbutrin XL®

Wellbutrin XL® may be confused with Wellbutrin SR®

Zyban® may be confused with Zagam®, Diovan®

Related Information

Antidepressant Agents *on page 1484*

U.S. Brand Names Aplenzin™; Budeprion SR®; Budeprion XL®; Buproban®; Wellbutrin SR®; Wellbutrin XL®; Wellbutrin®; Zyban®

Canadian Brand Names Bupropion SR®; Novo-Bupropion SR; PMS-Bupropion SR; ratio-Bupropion SR; Sandoz-Bupropion SR; Wellbutrin® SR; Wellbutrin® XL; Zyban®

Therapeutic Category Antidepressant, Dopamine-Reuptake Inhibitor; Smoking Cessation Aid

Generic Available Yes: Excludes bupropion hydrobromide tablet, sustained release hydrochloride tablet

Use Treatment of major depressive disorder (FDA approved in adults), seasonal affective disorder (SAD) (FDA approved in adults); adjunct in smoking cessation (FDA approved in adults); also used to treat ADHD in children

Medication Guide An FDA-approved patient medication guide, which is available with the product information and as follows, must be dispensed with this medication for each new outpatient prescription and refill.

Aplenzin™: http://www.fda.gov/downloads/Drugs/DrugSafety/ucm085915.pdf

Wellbutrin®: http://www.fda.gov/downloads/Drugs/DrugSafety/ucm089824.pdf

Wellbutrin SR®: http://www.fda.gov/downloads/Drugs/DrugSafety/ucm089826.pdf

Wellbutrin XL®: http://www.fda.gov/downloads/Drugs/DrugSafety/UCM172744.pdf

Zyban®: http://www.fda.gov/downloads/Drugs/DrugSafety/ucm089835.pdf

Pregnancy Risk Factor C

Pregnancy Considerations Due to adverse events observed in some animal studies, bupropion is classified as pregnancy category C. A significant increase in major teratogenic effects has not been observed following exposure to bupropion during pregnancy; however, the risk of spontaneous abortions may be increased (additional studies are needed to confirm). The long-term effects on development and behavior have not been studied.

Pregnancy itself does not provide protection against depression. The ACOG recommends that therapy with antidepressants during pregnancy be individualized and should incorporate the clinical expertise of the mental health clinician, obstetrician, primary care provider, and pediatrician. If treatment is needed, consider gradually stopping antidepressants 10-14 days before the expected date of delivery to prevent potential withdrawal symptoms in the infant. If this is done and the woman is considered to be at risk of relapse from her major depressive disorder, the medication can be restarted following delivery, although the dose should be readjusted to that required before pregnancy. Bupropion has also been evaluated for smoking cessation during pregnancy; current recommendations suggest that pharmacologic treatments be considered only after other therapies have failed. Treatment algorithms have been developed by the ACOG and the APA for the management of depression in women prior to conception and during pregnancy (Yonkers, 2009).

Lactation Enters breast milk/not recommended (AAP rates "of concern")

Breast-Feeding Considerations Bupropion and its metabolites are excreted into breast milk, although neither bupropion nor its metabolites have been detected in the plasma of breast-fed infants. Adverse events have not been reported in older breast-fed infants; however, a seizure was noted in one 6-month old infant (a causal effect could not be confirmed). Breast-feeding is not recommended by the manufacturer. The AAP considers bupropion to be a "drug for which the effect on the nursing infant is unknown, but may be of concern."

Contraindications Hypersensitivity to bupropion or any component (see Warnings); seizure disorder; anorexia/bulimia; use of MAO inhibitors within 14 days; patients undergoing abrupt discontinuation of ethanol or sedatives (including benzodiazepines); patients receiving other dosage forms of bupropion

Warnings Bupropion is not FDA approved for use in children. Use in treating psychiatric disorders: Clinical worsening of depression or suicidal ideation and behavior may occur in children and adults with major depressive disorder **[U.S. Boxed Warning]**. In clinical trials, antidepressants increased the risk of suicidal thinking and behavior (suicidality) in children, adolescents, and young adults (18-24 years of age) with major depressive disorder and other psychiatric disorders. This risk must be considered before prescribing antidepressants for any clinical use. Short-term studies did **not** show an increased risk of suicidality with antidepressant use in patients >24 years of age and showed a decreased risk in patients ≥65 years.

Patients of all ages who are treated with antidepressants for any indication require appropriate monitoring and close observation for clinical worsening of depression, suicidality, and unusual changes in behavior, especially during the first few months after antidepressant initiation or when the dose is adjusted. Family members and caregivers should be instructed to closely observe the patient (ie, daily) and communicate condition with healthcare provider. Patients should also be monitored for associated behaviors (eg, anxiety, agitation, panic attacks, insomnia, irritability, hostility, aggressiveness, impulsivity, akathisia, hypomania, mania) which may increase the risk for worsening depression or suicidality. Worsening depression or emergence of suicidality (or associated behaviors listed above) that is abrupt in onset, severe, or not part of the presenting symptoms, may require discontinuation or modification of drug therapy.

Do not discontinue abruptly in patients receiving high doses chronically (withdrawal symptoms may occur; see Adverse Reactions). To reduce risk of intentional overdose, write prescriptions for the smallest quantity consistent with good patient care. Screen individuals for bipolar disorder prior to treatment (using antidepressants alone may induce manic episodes in patients with this condition). May worsen psychosis in some patients. Bupropion is not FDA approved for the treatment of bipolar depression.

Use in smoking cessation: Serious neuropsychiatric events, including depression, suicidal thoughts, suicide attempt, and suicide, have been reported with use **[U.S. Boxed Warning]**; neuropsychiatric symptoms including psychosis, hallucinations, paranoia, delusions, hostility, agitation, aggression, anxiety, panic, and homicidal ideation have also been reported; some cases may have been complicated by symptoms of nicotine withdrawal following smoking cessation. Smoking cessation (with or without treatment) is associated with nicotine withdrawal symptoms (including depression or agitation), or the exacerbation of underlying psychiatric illness; however, some of the behavioral disturbances reported occurred in treated patients who continued to smoke. These neuropsychiatric symptoms (eg, mood disturbances, psychosis, hostility) have occurred in patients with and without pre-existing psychiatric disease; many cases resolved following therapy discontinuation although in some cases, symptoms persisted. Monitor all patients for behavioral changes and psychiatric symptoms (eg, agitation, depression, suicidal behavior, suicidal ideation); inform patients to discontinue treatment and contact their healthcare provider immediately if they experience any behavioral and/or mood changes.

The American Heart Association recommends that all children diagnosed with ADHD who may be candidates for medication, such as bupropion, should have a thorough cardiovascular assessment prior to initiation of therapy. These recommendations are based upon reports of serious cardiovascular adverse events (including sudden death) in patients (both children and adults) taking usual doses of stimulant medications. Most of these patients were found to have underlying structural heart disease (eg, hypertrophic obstructive cardiomyopathy). This assessment should include a combination of thorough medical history, family history, and physical examination. An ECG is not mandatory but should be considered.

Bupropion may cause seizures; the risk of seizures is dose-dependent; do not exceed maximum recommended doses; increase dose gradually. Risk of seizures is increased in patients with a history of seizures, anorexia/bulimia (see Contraindications), head trauma, CNS tumor, severe hepatic cirrhosis, abrupt discontinuation of sedative-hypnotics or ethanol, and concurrent use of medications which lower seizure threshold (antipsychotics, antidepressants, theophylline, systemic steroids), stimulants, or hypoglycemic agents. Discontinue and do not restart in patients experiencing a seizure. Use with extreme caution in patients at risk for seizures.

Budeprion SR® 100 mg and Budeprion XL® 300 mg tablets contain tartrazine which may cause allergic reactions in susceptible individuals.

Precautions May cause CNS stimulation (restlessness, anxiety, agitation, insomnia) or anorexia. Use in patients with depression may be associated with neuropsychiatric symptoms such as delusions, hallucinations, psychosis, confusion, paranoia, and concentrations disturbance. May increase the risks associated with electroconvulsive therapy. Consider discontinuing, when possible, prior to elective surgery. May cause weight loss; use caution in patients where weight loss is not desirable.

Use with caution in patients with cardiovascular disease, history of hypertension, recent MI, or coronary artery disease; treatment-emergent hypertension (including some severe cases) has been reported, both with bupropion alone and in combination with nicotine transdermal systems. Use with caution and decrease the dose and/or frequency in patients with hepatic or renal dysfunction. May cause motor or cognitive impairment in some patients; use with caution if tasks requiring alertness such as operating machinery or driving are undertaken. May cause allergic reactions; rare cases of erythema multiforme, Stevens-Johnson syndrome, and anaphylactic shock have been reported. Arthralgia, myalgia, and fever with rash and other symptoms suggestive of delayed hypersensitivity resembling serum sickness may occur.

Extended release tablet: Insoluble tablet shell may remain intact and be visible in the stool.

Adverse Reactions

Cardiovascular: Arrhythmias, chest pain, flushing, hypertension, hypotension, palpitation, tachycardia

Central nervous system: Abnormal dreams, agitation, anxiety, CNS stimulation, confusion, depression, dizziness, fever, headache, hostility, insomnia, irritability, memory decreased, migraine, nervousness, pain, psychosis, seizures, sensory disturbance, sleep disturbance, somnolence

Dermatologic: Pruritus, rash, urticaria

Endocrine & metabolic: Hot flashes, libido decreased, menstrual complaints, weight loss

Gastrointestinal: Abdominal pain, anorexia, appetite increased, constipation, diarrhea, dyspepsia, dysphagia, flatulence, nausea, taste perversion, vomiting, xerostomia

Genitourinary: Urinary frequency, urinary urgency, UTI, vaginal hemorrhage

Neuromuscular & skeletal: Akathisia, arthralgia, arthritis, myalgia, neck pain, paresthesia, tics, tremor, twitching, weakness

Ocular: Amblyopia, blurred vision

Otic: Auditory disturbance, tinnitus

Respiratory: Cough increased, pharyngitis, sinusitis, upper respiratory infection

Miscellaneous: Allergic reaction (including anaphylaxis, pruritus, urticaria), diaphoresis increased, infection, serum-sickness

Drug Interactions

Metabolism/Transport Effects Substrate of CYP1A2 (minor), 2A6 (minor), 2B6 (major), 2C9 (minor), 2D6 (minor), 2E1 (minor), 3A4 (minor); **Inhibits** CYP2D6 (strong)

Avoid Concomitant Use

Avoid concomitant use of BuPROPion with any of the following: MAO Inhibitors; Tamoxifen; Thioridazine

Increased Effect/Toxicity

BuPROPion may increase the levels/effects of: Alcohol (Ethyl); Atomoxetine; CNS Depressants; CYP2D6 Substrates; Fesoterodine; Methotrimeprazine; Nebivolol; Tamoxifen; Tetrabenazine; Thioridazine; Tricyclic Antidepressants

The levels/effects of BuPROPion may be increased by: CYP2B6 Inhibitors (Moderate); CYP2B6 Inhibitors (Strong); MAO Inhibitors; Methotrimeprazine; Quazepam

Decreased Effect

BuPROPion may decrease the levels/effects of: Codeine; TraMADol

The levels/effects of BuPROPion may be decreased by: CYP2B6 Inducers (Strong); Lopinavir; Peginterferon Alfa-2b; Ritonavir

Food Interactions

Extended release tablets:

Aplenzin™: Food does not affect peak concentration or time to peak; food increases bioavailability by 19%

Wellbutrin XL®: Food does not affect peak concentration or bioavailability.

Sustained release tablets: Food increases peak concentrations by 11% and AUC by 17% and prolongs the time to peak concentration by 1 hour. These effects are not thought to be clinically significant.

Stability

Aplenzin™, Wellbutrin XL®: Store at 25°C (77°F); excursions permitted to 15°C to 30°C (59°F to 86°F).

Immediate release tablets: Store at 15° to 25°C (59° to 77°F). Protect from light and moisture.

Wellbutrin SR®, Zyban®: Store at controlled room temperature of 20°C to 25°C (68°F to 77°F). Dispense in tight, light-resistant container.

Mechanism of Action Aminoketone antidepressant structurally different from all other marketed antidepressants; like other antidepressants the mechanism of bupropion's activity is not fully understood. Bupropion is a relatively weak inhibitor of the neuronal uptake of norepinephrine and dopamine, and does not inhibit monoamine oxidase or the reuptake of serotonin. Metabolite inhibits the reuptake of norepinephrine. The primary mechanism of action is thought to be dopaminergic and/or noradrenergic.

Pharmacodynamics

Onset of action: 1-2 weeks

Maximum effect: 8-12 weeks

Duration: 1-2 days

Pharmacokinetics (Adult data unless noted)

Absorption: Rapid

Distribution: V_d: Adults: 19-21 L/kg

Protein binding: 82% to 88%

Metabolism: Extensively hepatic via CYP2B6 to hydroxybupropion; non-CYP-mediated metabolism to erythrohydrobupropion and threohydrobupropion; these 3 metabolites are active. Preliminary studies suggest hydroxybupropion is 50% and erythrohydrobupropion and threohydrobupropion are 20% as active as parent drug. Bupropion also undergoes oxidation to form the glycine conjugate of meta-chlorobenzoic acid, the major urinary metabolite.

Half-life:

Distribution: 3-4 hours

Elimination: 21 ± 9 hours; Metabolites: Hydroxybupropion: 20 ± 5 hours; Erythrohydrobupropion: 33 ± 10 hours; Threohydrobupropion: 37 ± 13 hours

Time to peak serum concentration: Bupropion: Sustained release: ~3 hours; extended release: ~5 hours

Metabolites: Hydroxybupropion, erythrohydrobupropion, threohydrobupropion: ~7 hours

Elimination: Urine (87%); feces (10%); only 0.5% of the dose is excreted as unchanged drug

Usual Dosage Oral: **Note:** Safe and effective use in children has not been established; further studies are needed.

Children and Adolescents: ADHD: Hydrochloride salt: Immediate release: Some centers use the following doses: Initial: 3 mg/kg/day in 2 divided doses; titrate dose slowly to response (while monitoring for behavioral activation), up to 6 mg/kg/day in 2 divided doses. Maximum doses studied: Children 20-30 kg: 150 mg/day; 31-40 kg: 200 mg/day; >40 kg: 250 mg/day (Conners, 1996). **Note:** Several studies have used target doses ranging from 1.4-6 mg/kg/day (see Additional Information).

Children and Adolescents <15 years: Depression, ADHD: Hydrochloride salt: Some centers use the following doses: Initial: 37.5 mg twice daily of immediate release or 50 mg twice daily of sustained release; titrate to response with usual daily dose not to exceed 300 mg/day. **Note:** Pharmacokinetic studies demonstrate accelerated hepatic metabolism in children and young adolescents, therefore, divided doses are recommended to provide optimal symptom control.

Adolescents ≥15 years: Depression, ADHD: Hydrochloride salt: Hepatic metabolism is similar to adults; patients may respond well to once daily dosing with sustained release or extended release with maximum daily dose between 300-450 mg/day; see Adult dosing for initial doses and titration.

Adolescents ≥14 years and ≥40.5 kg: Smoking cessation: Hydrochloride salt: **Note:** Limited information exists; one adolescent study demonstrated short-term efficacy of 150 mg twice daily of sustained release for 7 weeks with cessation counseling (Muramoto, 2007).

Initial dose: Sustained release: 150 mg once daily for 3 days; increase to 150 mg twice daily; treatment should start while the patient is still smoking in order to allow drug to reach steady-state levels prior to smoking cessation; generally, patients should stop smoking during the second week of treatment; treatment should continue for 7-12 weeks; maximum dose: 300 mg/day

Adults:

Depression:

Immediate release: Hydrochloride salt: Initial: 100 mg twice daily; increase to recommended dose of 100 mg 3 times/day; maximum dose: 450 mg/day

Sustained release: Hydrochloride salt: Initial: 150 mg/day given once daily in the morning; may increase to 150 mg twice daily by day 4 if tolerated; target dose: 300 mg/day given as 150 mg twice daily; maximum dose: 400 mg/day given as 200 mg twice daily; **Note:** Interval between successive doses should be at least 8 hours

Extended release: Hydrochloride salt: Initial: 150 mg/day given once daily in the morning; may increase to the recommended target dose of 300 mg/day given once daily in the morning; this increase may be made as early as day 4 of dosing; if no improvement is observed after several weeks, may increase to maximum dose of 450 mg/day

Extended release: Hydrobromide salt: Aplenzin™: Target dose: 348 mg/day administered once daily in the morning. Patients not previously on bupropion: Initial: 174 mg/day in the morning; may increase as early as day 4 of dosing to 348 mg/day; maximum dose: 522 mg/day (if no improvement seen after several weeks on 348 mg)

Switching from bupropion hydrochloride (eg, Wellbutrin immediate release, SR®, XL®) to bupropion hydrobromide (Aplenzin™):

Bupropion hydrochloride 150 mg is equivalent to bupropion hydrobromide 174 mg

Bupropion hydrochloride 300 mg is equivalent to bupropion hydrobromide 348 mg

Bupropion hydrochloride 450 mg is equivalent to bupropion hydrobromide 522 mg

Note: Patients being treated twice daily or three times daily with bupropion hydrochloride would be switched to the equivalent once daily dose of bupropion hydrobromide.

SAD (Wellbutrin XL®): Initial: 150 mg/day given once daily in the morning; if tolerated, may increase after 1 week to 300 mg/day

Note: Prophylactic treatment should be reserved for those patients with frequent depressive episodes and/or significant impairment. Initiate treatment in the Autumn prior to symptom onset, and discontinue in early Spring with dose tapering to 150 mg/day for 2 weeks.

Smoking cessation (Zyban®): Initial: 150 mg once daily for 3 days; increase to 150 mg twice daily; treatment should start while the patient is still smoking in order to allow drug to reach steady-state levels prior to smoking cessation; generally, patients should stop smoking during the second week of treatment; treatment should continue for 7-12 weeks; maximum dose: 300 mg/day

Dosage adjustment/comments in renal impairment: Use with caution and consider a reduction in dose and/or dosing frequency; limited pharmacokinetic information suggests elimination of bupropion and/or the active metabolites may be reduced.

Moderate-to-severe renal impairment: Bupropion exposure was ~twofold higher compared to normal subjects following a 150 mg single dose administration of the sustained release product.

End-stage renal failure: Per the manufacturer, the elimination of hydroxybupropion and threohydrobupropion are reduced in patients with end-stage renal failure

Dosage adjustment in hepatic impairment:

Mild-to-moderate hepatic impairment: Use with caution; consider reduced dosage and/or frequency

Severe hepatic cirrhosis: Use with extreme caution; Adults: Maximum dose:

Aplenzin™: 174 mg every other day

Wellbutrin®: 75 mg/day

Wellbutrin SR®: 100 mg/day or 150 mg every other day

Wellbutrin XL®: 150 mg every other day

Zyban®: 150 mg every other day

Administration Oral: May be taken without regard to meals. Sustained-release tablets (Zyban®) and extended-release tablets (Wellbutrin XL®, Aplenzin™) should be swallowed whole; do not crush, chew, or divide. The insoluble shell of the extended-release tablet may remain intact during GI transit and is eliminated in the feces. Data from the manufacturer states that dividing Wellbutrin® SR tablets resulted in an increased rate of release at 15 minutes: "However, the divided tablet retained its sustained-release characteristics with similar increases of released bupropion at each sampling point beyond 15 minutes when compared to the intact Wellbutrin® SR tablet..." Bupropion is hydroscopic and therefore should be stored in a dry place. Splitting of large quantities in advance of administration is not advised since loss of potency may result. If necessary, splitting should be done cleanly without crushing.

Monitoring Parameters Heart rate, blood pressure, mental status, weight. Monitor patient periodically for symptom resolution; monitor for worsening depression, suicidality, and associated behaviors (especially at the beginning of therapy or when doses are increased or decreased; see Warnings), anxiety, social functioning, mania, panic attacks, tics

ADHD: Evaluate patients for cardiac disease prior to initiation of therapy for ADHD with thorough medical history, family history, and physical exam; consider ECG (see Warnings); perform ECG and echocardiogram if findings suggest cardiac disease; promptly conduct cardiac evaluation in patients who develop chest pain, unexplained syncope, or any other symptom of cardiac disease during treatment.

Reference Range Therapeutic levels (trough, 12 hours after last dose): 50-100 ng/mL

Patient Information Read the patient Medication Guide that you receive with each prescription and refill of bupropion. An increased risk of suicidal thinking and behavior has been reported with the use of antidepressants in children, adolescents, and young adults (18-24 years of age). Serious neuropsychiatric events, including depression, suicidal thoughts, suicide attempt, and suicide have been reported with use of bupropion for smoking cessation. Notify physician if you feel more depressed, have thoughts of suicide, or become more agitated or irritable (see Warnings). Be aware that bupropion is marketed under different names and should not be taken together; Zyban® is for smoking cessation and Wellbutrin® is for treatment of depression. **Note:** Excessive use or abrupt discontinuation of alcohol or sedatives may alter seizure threshold.

Depression: Take as directed, in equally divided doses; do not take in larger dose or more often than recommended. Do not discontinue this medicine without consulting prescriber. Do not use alcohol or OTC medications not approved by prescriber. May cause drowsiness, clouded sensorium, headache, restlessness, or agitation (use caution when driving or engaging in tasks requiring alertness or physical coordination until response to drug is known); nausea, vomiting, or dry mouth (small, frequent meals, frequent mouth care, chewing gum, or sucking lozenges may help); weight loss; constipation; or impotence (reversible). Report persistent CNS effects (eg, agitation, confusion, anxiety, restlessness, insomnia, psychosis, hallucinations, seizures); suicidal ideation; muscle weakness or tremor; skin rash, hives, itching or irritation; chest pain or palpitations, abdominal pain or blood in stools; yellowing of skin or eyes; or respiratory difficulty, bronchitis, or unusual cough.

Smoking cessation: Use as directed; do not take extra doses. Do not combine nicotine patches with use of Zyban® unless approved by prescriber. May cause dry mouth and insomnia (these may resolve with continued use). Report any respiratory difficulty, unusual cough, dizziness, or muscle tremors.

Nursing Implications Assess other medications patient may be taking for possible interactions (especially MAO inhibitors, P450 inhibitors, and other CNS active agents). Assess mental status for depression, suicidal ideation, and associated behaviors (see Warnings), especially at the

beginning of therapy or when dose changes occur. If history of cardiac problems, monitor cardiac status closely. Be alert to the potential of new or increased seizure activity. Periodically evaluate need for continued use. Taper dosage slowly when discontinuing (allow 3-4 weeks between discontinuing this medication and starting another antidepressant).

Additional Information ADHD: Children and Adolescents: Bupropion hydrochloride: Doses ranging from 1.4-5.7 mg/kg/day (mean: 3.3 mg/kg/day) were utilized in 15 ADHD subjects 7-17 years of age (Barrickman, 1995); 72 children with ADHD (6-12 years of age) received 3-6 mg/kg/day (Conners, 1996); adolescents with conduct disorder and substance use disorder were titrated to a maximum fixed daily dose of 300 mg (Riggs, 1998). The immediate-release dosage form was studied in clinical trials for indications other than depression in 104 pediatric patients. This limited exposure does not allow for assessment of the safety and efficacy of bupropion in pediatric patients. Further studies are needed.

Dosage Forms Excipient information presented when available (limited, particularly for generics); consult specific product labeling.

Tablet, as hydrochloride: 75 mg [generic for Wellbutrin®], 100 mg [generic for Wellbutrin®]

Wellbutrin®: 75 mg, 100 mg

Tablet, extended release, as hydrobromide:

Aplenzin™: 174 mg, 348 mg, 522 mg

Tablet, extended release, as hydrochloride: 100 mg [generic for Wellbutrin SR®], 150 mg [generic for Wellbutrin SR®], 150 mg [generic for Wellbutrin XL®], 150 mg [generic for Zyban®], 200 mg [generic for Wellbutrin SR®], 300 mg [generic for Wellbutrin XL®]

Budeprion SR®: 100 mg [generic for Wellbutrin SR®; contains tartrazine], 150 mg [generic for Wellbutrin SR®]

Budeprion XL®: 150 mg [generic for Wellbutrin XL®], 300 mg [generic for Wellbutrin XL®; contains tartrazine]

Buproban®: 150 mg [generic for Zyban®]

Wellbutrin XL®: 150 mg, 300 mg

Tablet, sustained release, as hydrochloride:

Wellbutrin SR®: 100 mg, 150 mg, 200 mg

Zyban®: 150 mg

References

American Academy of Pediatrics/American Heart Association Clarification of Statement on Cardiovascular Evaluation and Monitoring of Children and Adolescents With Heart Disease Receiving Medications for ADHD; available at: http://americanheart.mediaroon.com/index.php?s=43&item=422.

Barrickman LL, Petty PJ, Allen AJ, et al, "Bupropion Versus Methylphenidate in the Treatment of Attention-Deficit Hyperactivity Disorder," *J Am Acad Child Adolesc Psychiatry*, 1995, 34(5):649-57.

Conners CK, Casat CD, Gualtieri CT, et al, "Bupropion Hydrochloride in Attention Deficit Disorder With Hyperactivity," *J Am Acad Child Adolesc Psychiatry*, 1996, 35(10):1314-21.

Davidson J, "Seizures and Bupropion: A Review," *J Clin Psychiatry*, 1989, 50(7):256-61.

Daviss WB, Perel JM, Birmaher B, et al, "Steady-State Clinical Pharmacokinetics of Bupropion Extended-Release in Youths," *J Am Acad Child Adolesc Psychiatry*, 2006, 45(12):1503-9.

Dopheide JA, "Recognizing and Treating Depression in Children and Adolescents," *Am J Health Syst Pharm*, 2006, 63(3):233-43.

GlaxoSmithKline [data on file], "Wellbutrin® SR, GAZZ/96/0006/00, Study Report Synopsis," 1996, 1-8.

Hack S, "Pediatric Bupropion-Induced Serum Sickness Like Reaction," *J Child Adolesc Psychopharmacol*, 2004, 14(3):478-80.

Jennison TA, Brown P, Crossett J, et al, "A High-Performance Liquid Chromatographic Method for Quantitating Bupropion in Human Plasma or Serum," *J Anal Toxicol*, 1995, 19(2):69-72.

Kavoussi RJ, Segraves RT, Hughes AR, et al, "Double-Blind Comparison of Bupropion Sustained Release and Sertraline in Depressed Outpatients," *J Clin Psychiatry*, 1997, 58(12):532-7.

Leverich GS, Altshuler LL, Frye MA, et al, "Risk of Switch in Mood Polarity to Hypomania or Mania in Patients with Bipolar Depression During Acute and Continuation Trials of Venlafaxine, Sertraline, and Bupropion as Adjuncts to Mood Stabilizers," *Am J Psychiatry*, 2006, 163(2):232-9.

McIntyre RS, Mancini DA, McCann S, et al, "Topiramate Versus Bupropion SR When Added to Mood Stabilizer Therapy for the Depressive Phase of Bipolar Disorder: A Preliminary Single-Blind Study," *Bipolar Disord*, 2002, 4(3):207-13.

Muramoto ML, Leischow SJ, Sherrill D, et al, "Randomized, Double-Blind, Placebo-Controlled Trial of 2 Dosages of Sustained-Release Bupropion for Adolescent Smoking Cessation," *Arch Pediatr Adolesc Med*, 2007, 161(11):1068-74.

Pass SE and Simpson RW, "Discontinuation and Reinstitution of Medications During the Perioperative Period," *Am J Health Syst Pharm*, 2004, 61(9):899-912.

Pliszka SR, Crismon ML, Hughes CW, et al, "The Texas Children's Medication Algorithm Project: Revision of the Algorithm for Pharmacotherapy of ADHD," *J Am Acad Child Adolesc Psychiatry*, 2006, 45(6):642-57.

Riggs PD, Leon SL, Mikulich SK, et al, "An Open Trial of Bupropion for ADHD in Adolescents With Substance Use Disorders and Conduct Disorder," *J Am Acad Child Adolesc Psychiatry*, 1998, 37(12):1271-8.

Spencer T, Biederman J, Kerman K, et al, "Desipramine Treatment of Children With Attention-Deficit Hyperactivity Disorder and Tic Disorder or Tourette's Syndrome," *J Am Acad Child Adolesc Psychiatry*, 1993, 32(2):354-60.

Turpeinen M, Koivuviita N, Tolonen A, et al, "Effect of Renal Impairment on the Pharmacokinetics of Bupropion and Its Metabolites," *Br J Clin Pharmacol*, 2007, 64(2):165-73.

Van Wyck FJ, Manberg PJ, Miller LL, et al, "Overview of Clinically Significant Adverse Reactions to Bupropion," *J Clin Psychiatry*, 1983, 44(5 Pt 2):191-6.

Vetter VL, Elia J, Erickson C, et al, "Cardiovascular Monitoring of Children and Adolescents With Heart Disease Receiving Stimulant Drugs: A Scientific Statement From the American Heart Association Council on Cardiovascular Disease in the Young Congenital Cardiac Defects Committee and the Council on Cardiovascular Nursing," *Circulation*, 2008, 117(18):2407-23.

Wagner KD, "Pharmacotherapy for Major Depression in Children and Adolescents," *Prog Neuropsychopharmacol Biol Psychiatry*, 2005, 29 (5):819-26.

Wilens TE, Prince JB, Spencer T, et al, "An Open Trial of Bupropion for the Treatment of Adults with Attention-Deficit/Hyperactivity Disorder and Bipolar Disorder," *Biol Psychiatry*, 2003, 54(1):9-16.

◆ **Bupropion Hydrobromide** *see* BuPROPion *on page* 217

◆ **Bupropion Hydrochloride** *see* BuPROPion *on page* 217

◆ **Bupropion SR® (Can)** *see* BuPROPion *on page* 217

◆ **Burinex® (Can)** *see* Bumetanide *on page* 212

◆ **Burn Jel® [OTC]** *see* Lidocaine *on page* 818

◆ **Burn Jel® Plus [OTC]** *see* Lidocaine *on page* 818

◆ **Burn-O-Jel [OTC]** *see* Lidocaine *on page* 818

◆ **Burow's Solution** *see* Aluminum Acetate *on page* 74

◆ **Buscopan® (Can)** *see* Scopolamine *on page* 1248

◆ **BuSpar®** *see* BusPIRone *on page* 222

◆ **Buspirex (Can)** *see* BusPIRone *on page* 222

BusPIRone (byoo SPYE rone)

Medication Safety Issues
Sound-alike/look-alike issues:
BusPIRone may be confused with buPROPion

Related Information
Serotonin Syndrome *on page* 1695

U.S. Brand Names BuSpar®

Canadian Brand Names Apo-Buspirone®; BuSpar®; Buspirex; Bustab®; CO Buspirone; Dom-Buspirone; Gen-Buspirone; Lin-Buspirone; Mylan-Buspirone; Novo-Buspirone; Nu-Buspirone; PMS-Buspirone; ratio-Buspirone; Riva-Buspirone

Therapeutic Category Antianxiety Agent

Generic Available Yes

Use Management of anxiety disorders

Pregnancy Risk Factor B

Pregnancy Considerations No impairment of fertility or fetotoxic effects were noted in animal studies with doses 30 times maximum recommended human dose. There are no adequate and well-controlled studies in pregnant women.

Lactation Excretion in breast milk unknown/not recommended

Contraindications Hypersensitivity to buspirone or any component

Warnings Do not use concurrently with MAO inhibitors or within 10 days of MAO inhibitors as significant increases in blood pressure may occur. Buspirone does not possess antipsychotic activity and should not be used in place of appropriate antipsychotic treatment.

Precautions Use with caution in patients with hepatic or renal dysfunction; use in severe hepatic or renal impairment is not recommended. Buspirone does not prevent or treat withdrawal from benzodiazepines or sedative/hypnotic drugs; if substituting buspirone for these agents, gradually withdraw the other drug(s) prior to initiating buspirone. Buspirone possesses a low potential for cognitive or motor impairment; however, until effects on an individual patient are known, patients should be warned to use caution when performing tasks which require mental alertness (eg, operating machinery or driving). Restlessness syndrome has been reported in a small number of patients; may be attributable to buspirone's antagonism of central dopamine receptors. Monitor for signs of any dopamine-related movement disorders (eg, dystonia, akathisia, pseudo-parkinsonism). Effectiveness of buspirone has not been established in pediatric patients; safety has been established in pediatric patients 6-17 years of age; no long-term safety or efficacy data is available in children.

Adverse Reactions
Cardiovascular: Chest pain, tachycardia

Central nervous system: Dizziness, lightheadedness, headache, fatigue, restlessness, confusion, insomnia, nightmares, sedation (about 1/3 of that with benzodiazepines), disorientation, excitement, fever, drowsiness (more common with ≥20 mg/day), akathisia; possible psychotic deterioration has been reported (two pediatric cases, see Soni, 1992)

Dermatologic: Rash, urticaria

Gastrointestinal: Nausea, vomiting, diarrhea, flatulence, xerostomia

Hematologic: Rare: Leukopenia, eosinophilia, thrombocytopenia

Neuromuscular & skeletal: Muscle weakness, numbness

Ocular: Blurred vision

Otic: Tinnitus

Drug Interactions
Metabolism/Transport Effects Substrate of CYP2D6 (minor), 3A4 (major)

Avoid Concomitant Use
Avoid concomitant use of BusPIRone with any of the following: MAO Inhibitors; Sibutramine

Increased Effect/Toxicity
BusPIRone may increase the levels/effects of: Alcohol (Ethyl); Antidepressants (Serotonin Reuptake Inhibitor/Antagonist); CNS Depressants; MAO Inhibitors; Methotrimeprazine; Selective Serotonin Reuptake Inhibitors; Serotonin Modulators

The levels/effects of BusPIRone may be increased by: Antifungal Agents (Azole Derivatives, Systemic); Calcium Channel Blockers (Nondihydropyridine); CYP3A4 Inhibitors (Moderate); CYP3A4 Inhibitors (Strong); Dasatinib; Grapefruit Juice; Macrolide Antibiotics; Methotrimeprazine; Selective Serotonin Reuptake Inhibitors; Sibutramine

Decreased Effect

The levels/effects of BusPIRone may be decreased by: CYP3A4 Inducers (Strong); Deferasirox; Peginterferon Alfa-2b; Rifamycin Derivatives; Yohimbine

Food Interactions Food may delay oral absorption, decrease the first-pass metabolism effect and increase oral bioavailability; grapefruit juice may greatly increase buspirone concentrations

Stability Store at controlled room temperature of 25°C (77°F). Protect from light.

Mechanism of Action Decreases the spontaneous firing of serotonin-containing neurons in the CNS by selectively binding to and acting as agonist at presynaptic CNS serotonin 5-HT$_1$A receptors; possesses partial agonist activity (mixed agonist/antagonist) at postsynaptic 5-HT$_2$A receptors; does not bind to benzodiazepine-GABA receptors; binds to dopamine$_2$ receptors; may have other effects on other neurotransmitter systems; buspirone is "anxiolytic-select" and does not possess the anticonvulsant, muscle relaxant, or sedative effects of the benzodiazepines; little potential for abuse, tolerance, or withdrawal reactions

Pharmacodynamics

Onset of action: Within 2 weeks

Maximum effect: 3-4 weeks, up to 4-6 weeks

Pharmacokinetics (Adult data unless noted)

Absorption: Rapid and complete, but bioavailability is limited by extensive first-pass effect; only 1.5% to 13% (mean 4%) of the oral dose reaches the systemic circulation unchanged

Protein binding: 86%

Distribution: V_d: Adults: 5.3 L/kg

Metabolism: In the liver by oxidation (by cytochrome P450 isoenzyme CYP3A4) to several metabolites including 1-pyrimidinyl piperazine (about 1/4 as active as buspirone)

Half-life: Adults: Mean: 2-3 hours; increased with renal or liver dysfunction

Time to peak serum concentration: 40-90 minutes

Elimination: 29% to 63% excreted in urine (primarily as metabolites)

Usual Dosage Oral:

Children and Adolescents: Anxiety disorders: Limited information is available; dose is not well established. One pilot study of 15 children, 6-14 years of age (mean 10 years), with mixed anxiety disorders, used initial doses of 5 mg daily; doses were individualized with increases in increments of 5 mg/day every week as needed to a maximum dose of 20 mg/day divided into 2 doses; the mean dose required: 18.6 mg/day (Simeon, 1994). Some authors (Carrey, 1996 and Kutcher, 1992), based on their clinical experience, recommend higher doses (eg, 15-30 mg/day in 2 divided doses). An open-label study in 25 prepubertal inpatients (mean age: 8 ± 1.8 years; range: 5-11 years) with anxiety symptoms and moderately aggressive behavior used initial doses of 5 mg daily; doses were titrated upwards (over 3 weeks) by 5-10 mg every 3 days to a maximum dose of 50 mg/day; doses >5 mg/day were administered in 2 divided doses/day; buspirone was discontinued in 25% of the children due to increased aggression and agitation or euphoric mania; mean optimal dose (n=19): 28 mg/day; range: 10-50 mg/day; median: 30 mg/day (Pfeffer, 1997). Two placebo-controlled 6-week trials in children and adolescents (n=559; age: 6-17 years) with generalized anxiety disorder studied doses of 7.5-30 mg twice daily (15-60 mg/day); no significant differences between buspirone and placebo with respect to generalized anxiety disorder symptoms were observed (see package insert).

Adults: Initial: 7.5 mg twice daily; increase in increments of 5 mg/day every 2-3 days as needed to a maximum of 60 mg/day; usual dose: 20-30 mg/day in 2 or 3 divided doses; **Note:** For patients receiving concomitant therapy with cytochrome P450 CYP3A4 inhibitors, a lower dose of buspirone is recommended (eg, 2.5 mg twice daily for patients receiving erythromycin; 2.5 mg daily for patients receiving itraconazole or nefazodone); with further dosage adjustments based on clinical assessment

Dosing adjustment in renal impairment: Patients with impaired renal function demonstrated increased plasma levels and a prolonged half-life of buspirone. Use in patients with severe renal impairment not recommended.

Dosing adjustment in hepatic impairment: Patients with impaired hepatic function demonstrated increased plasma levels and a prolonged half-life of buspirone. Use in patients with severe hepatic impairment not recommended.

Administration Oral: Administer in a consistent manner in relation to food (ie, either always with food or always without food); may administer with food to decrease GI upset; use caution if administered with grapefruit juice; avoid large amounts of grapefruit juice (see Food Interactions)

Monitoring Parameters Mental status, signs and symptoms of anxiety, liver and renal function; signs of dopamine-related movement disorders (eg, dystonia, akathisia, pseudo-parkinsonism).

Patient Information Avoid alcohol and large amounts of grapefruit juice; may cause drowsiness and impair ability to perform activities requiring mental alertness or physical coordination; may cause dry mouth

Additional Information Not appropriate for "as needed" (prn) use or for brief, situational anxiety; buspirone is equipotent to diazepam on a milligram to milligram basis in the treatment of anxiety; however, unlike diazepam, the onset of buspirone is delayed (see Pharmacodynamics)

Dosage Forms Excipient information presented when available (limited, particularly for generics); consult specific product labeling. [DSC] = Discontinued product

Tablet, as hydrochloride: 5 mg, 7.5 mg, 10 mg, 15 mg, 30 mg

BuSpar®: 5 mg, 10 mg, 15 mg; 30 mg [DSC]

References

Carrey NJ, Wiggins DM, and Milin RP, "Pharmacological Treatment of Psychiatric Disorders in Children and Adolescents," *Drugs*, 1996, 51 (5):750-9.

Gammans RE, Mayol RF, and LaBudde JA, "Metabolism and Disposition of Buspirone," *Am J Med*, 1986, 80(3B):41-51.

Hanna GL, Feibusch EL, and Albright KJ, "Buspirone Treatment of Anxiety, Associated With Pharyngeal Dysphagia in a Four-Year Old," *J Child Adolesc Psychopharmacol*, 1997, 7(2):137-43.

Kutcher SP, Reiter S, Gardner DM, et al, "The Pharmacotherapy of Anxiety Disorders in Children and Adolescents," *Psychiatr Clin North Am*, 1992, 15(1):41-67.

Pfeffer CR, Jiang H, and Domeshek LJ, "Buspirone Treatment of Psychiatrically Hospitalized Prepubertal Children With Symptoms of Anxiety and Moderately Severe Aggression," *J Child Adolesc Psychopharmacol*, 1997, 7(3):145-55.

Simeon JG, Knott VJ, DuBois C, et al, "Buspirone Therapy of Mixed Anxiety Disorders in Childhood and Adolescence: A Pilot Study," *J Child Adolesc Psychopharmacol*, 1994, 4(3):159-70.

Soni P and Weintraub AL, "Buspirone-Associated Mental Status Changes," *J Am Acad Child Adolesc Psychiatry*, 1992, 31(6):1098-9.

◆ **Buspirone Hydrochloride** *see BusPIRone on page 222*

◆ **Bustab® (Can)** *see BusPIRone on page 222*

Busulfan (byoo SUL fan)

Medication Safety Issues

Sound-alike/look-alike issues:

Busulfan may be confused with Butalan®

Myleran® may be confused with Alkeran®, Leukeran®, melphalan, Mylicon®

High alert medication: The Institute for Safe Medication Practices (ISMP) includes this medication among its list of drugs which have a heightened risk of causing significant patient harm when used in error.

Related Information

Compatibility of Chemotherapy and Related Supportive Care Medications *on page 1580*

Emetogenic Potential of Antineoplastic Agents *on page 1579*

U.S. Brand Names Busulfex®; Myleran®

Canadian Brand Names Busulfex®; Myleran®

Therapeutic Category Antineoplastic Agent, Alkylating Agent

Generic Available No

Use Chronic myelogenous leukemia (CML); component of marrow-ablative conditioning regimen prior to bone marrow transplantation (BMT) for refractory leukemias, lymphomas, and pediatric solid tumors

Pregnancy Risk Factor D

Pregnancy Considerations Animal studies have demonstrated teratogenic effects. May cause fetal harm if administered during pregnancy. The solvent in I.V. busulfan, DMA, is associated with teratogenic effects and may impair fertility. There are no adequate and well-controlled studies in pregnant women. Women of child-bearing potential should avoid pregnancy while receiving treatment.

Lactation Excretion in breast milk unknown/not recommended

Breast-Feeding Considerations Due to the tumorigenicity potential and the potential for serious adverse reactions in the nursing infant, breast-feeding is not recommended.

Contraindications Hypersensitivity to busulfan or any component; failure to respond to previous courses; should not be used in pregnancy or lactation

Warnings Hazardous agent; use appropriate precautions for handling and disposal; discontinue busulfan if lung toxicity develops; busulfan is potentially carcinogenic; malignant tumors and acute leukemias have been reported in patients who received busulfan; busulfan is associated with ovarian failure including failure to achieve puberty in females

May cause significant bone marrow suppression even with recommended dosages **[U.S. Boxed Warning]**. Severe granulocytopenia, thrombocytopenia, and anemia are the most frequent serious adverse events. Monitor blood counts frequently. Seizures have been reported in patients receiving high-dose busulfan. Prophylactic anticonvulsant therapy should be initiated prior to high-dose busulfan therapy. High busulfan AUC values (>1500 micromolar/minute) may be associated with an increased risk of developing hepatic veno-occlusive disease (HVOD). Patients who have received prior radiation therapy, ≥3 cycles of chemotherapy, or prior progenitor cell transplant may be at increased risk for developing HVOD. Of the patients who developed HVOD, it was fatal in 40% of the cases.

Precautions May induce severe bone marrow hypoplasia; reduce dosage in patients with bone marrow suppression; use with extreme caution in patients who have recently received other myelosuppressive drugs or radiation therapy; use with caution in patients with a history of seizure disorder, head trauma, or when receiving other epileptogenic drugs

Adverse Reactions

Cardiovascular: Cardiac tamponade (reported in a small number of thalassemia patients who received busulfan and cyclophosphamide as part of a BMT conditioning regimen), edema, tachycardia

Central nervous system: Dizziness, seizures, fever, chills, insomnia, confusion, hallucinations

Dermatologic: Hyperpigmentation, alopecia, rash, urticaria

Endocrine & metabolic: Addisonian-like syndrome (hyperpigmentation, wasting, hypotension), hyperuricemia, gynecomastia, testicular atrophy, amenorrhea, sterility, hyperglycemia, hypomagnesemia, hypokalemia

Gastrointestinal: Nausea, vomiting, mucositis, diarrhea, abdominal pain, constipation, ileus, anorexia, pancreatitis

Genitourinary: Hemorrhagic cystitis

Hematologic: Myelosuppression with nadirs of 14-21 days for leukopenia and thrombocytopenia; anemia, aplastic anemia, thrombosis

Hepatic: Hepatic impairment, hepatic veno-occlusive disease (7.7% to 12% with high-dose busulfan), hyperbilirubinemia, hepatocellular necrosis, ascites

Ocular: Blurred vision, subcapsular cataracts, corneal thinning

Respiratory: Pulmonary fibrosis (may occur 4 months to 10 years after initiation of therapy), dyspnea

Drug Interactions

Metabolism/Transport Effects Substrate of CYP3A4 (major)

Avoid Concomitant Use

Avoid concomitant use of Busulfan with any of the following: BCG; Natalizumab; Pimecrolimus; Tacrolimus (Topical); Vaccines (Live)

Increased Effect/Toxicity

Busulfan may increase the levels/effects of: Leflunomide; Natalizumab; Vaccines (Live); Vitamin K Antagonists

The levels/effects of Busulfan may be increased by: Antifungal Agents (Azole Derivatives, Systemic); CYP3A4 Inhibitors (Moderate); CYP3A4 Inhibitors (Strong); Dasatinib; Denosumab; MetroNIDAZOLE; MetroNIDAZOLE (Systemic); Pimecrolimus; Tacrolimus (Topical); Trastuzumab

Decreased Effect

Busulfan may decrease the levels/effects of: BCG; Sipuleucel-T; Vaccines (Inactivated); Vaccines (Live); Vitamin K Antagonists

The levels/effects of Busulfan may be decreased by: CYP3A4 Inducers (Strong); Deferasirox; Echinacea; Herbs (CYP3A4 Inducers)

Food Interactions No clear or firm data on the effect of food on busulfan bioavailability

Stability Store tablets at room temperature. Store intact ampuls in the refrigerator; diluted busulfan solution is stable for up to 8 hours at room temperature; infusion must be completed within that 8 hour time frame. If diluted in NS, the solution is stable for 12 hours if refrigerated, but the infusion must be completed within that 12-hour time frame.

Mechanism of Action Interferes with the normal function of DNA by alkylation of intracellular nucleophiles and cross-linking the strands of DNA

Pharmacokinetics (Adult data unless noted)

Absorption: Oral: 70% absorbed

Distribution: Crosses into CSF, saliva, placenta, and liver

V_d: Children: 0.64 L/kg

Protein binding: 32% to 55%

Metabolism: Extensive in the liver by conjugation with glutathione

Half-life:
Children: 2.5 hours
Adults: 2.3-2.6 hours

Time to peak serum concentration: Oral: Within 1-2 hours

Elimination: 10% to 50% excreted in urine as metabolites, 1% excreted unchanged in urine within 24 hours; total plasma clearance rate is 2-4 times higher in children than in adults

Clearance:
Children: 3.37 mL/minute/kg
Adults: 2.52 mL/minute/kg (range: 1.49-4.31 mL/minute/kg)

Usual Dosage Refer to individual protocols; dose should be based on ideal body weight:

Children:

Oral:

Remission induction of CML: 0.06-0.12 mg/kg once daily **or** 1.8-4.6 mg/m^2/day once daily; titrate dose to maintain a leukocyte count >40,000/mm^3; discontinue busulfan if counts fall to ≤20,000/mm^3

BMT marrow-ablative conditioning regimen: 1 mg/kg/ dose every 6 hours for 16 doses

Hematopoietic stem cell transplant regimen: Children ≤6 years: 40 mg/m^2/dose every 6 hours for 16 doses

I.V.: High-dose BMT or peripheral blood progenitor cell transplantation conditioning regimen: Dose based on actual body weight:

≤12 kg: 1.1 mg/kg/dose every 6 hours for 16 doses over 4 consecutive days

>12 kg: 0.8 mg/kg/dose every 6 hours for 16 doses over 4 consecutive days

Dosage adjustment based on therapeutic drug monitoring:

Adjusted dose (mg) = Actual dose (mg) x target AUC (micromolar•minute) / actual AUC (micro-molar•minute)

Target AUC = 1125 micromolar•minute

Adults:

Oral:

Remission induction of CML: 4-8 mg/day or 0.06 mg/kg/day

Maintenance dose: Controversial; range is from 1-4 mg/ day to 2 mg/week; reduce dose in proportion to the decrease in leukocyte count or discontinue busulfan when the leukocyte count falls to ≤20,000/mm^3

I.V.: High-dose BMT conditioning regimen: 0.8 mg/kg/ dose every 6 hours for 16 doses over 4 consecutive days

I.V. dose for obese patients: Dose should be based on adjusted ideal body weight (AIBW)

AIBW = Ideal body weight (IBW) + 0.25 x (actual weight - IBW)

Administration

Oral: May be administered without regard to meals. To facilitate ingestion of high doses, insert multiple tablets into clear gelatin capsules for administration.

Parenteral: Filter busulfan using 5 micron syringe filter provided, using one filter per ampul. If using the syringe filter in the forward flow direction, allow for ~0.16 mL of residual busulfan to remain in the filter. Dilute busulfan injection with either NS or D$_5$W to a final concentration of ≥0.5 mg/mL (diluent volume should be 10 times the volume of busulfan injection); infuse over 2 hours through a central venous catheter; flush line before and after each infusion with D$_5$W or NS. Do **not** use polycarbonate syringes or filters.

Monitoring Parameters CBC with differential and platelet count, hemoglobin, liver function tests, bilirubin, alkaline phosphatase; monitor busulfan plasma concentration

Patient Information Report any difficulty in breathing, cough, fever, sore throat, bleeding or bruising to physician. Report any signs of abrupt weakness, fatigue, anorexia, weight loss, nausea, vomiting, and melanoderma. Female patients of childbearing potential should avoid becoming pregnant during and for one month following therapy.

Additional Information One method used to prevent seizures during high-dose busulfan (~4 mg/kg/day for 4 days) is to initiate a standard loading dose of phenytoin (15 mg/kg) 1 day prior to starting busulfan therapy followed by a maintenance dose adjusted to maintain a therapeutic phenytoin concentration until 24 hours after the final busulfan dose

"Juvenile type" chronic myelogenous leukemia which typically occurs in young children and is associated with the absence of Philadelphia chromosome responds poorly to busulfan.

Dosage Forms Excipient information presented when available (limited, particularly for generics); consult specific product labeling.

Injection, solution:

Busulfex®: 6 mg/mL (10 mL) [contains N,N-dimethylace-tamide (DMA)]

Tablet:

Myleran®: 2 mg

Extemporaneous Preparations A 2 mg/mL oral suspension can be prepared in a vertical flow hood using simple syrup; crush one-hundred twenty 2 mg tablets into a fine powder in a mortar; levigate with a small amount of simple syrup and mix to make a uniform paste; mix while adding simple syrup in geometric portions to almost 120 mL; pour contents into a graduated cylinder; rinse mortar and pestle with simple syrup, transfer to the graduated cylinder, and qsad with vehicle to 120 mL. Transfer contents of the graduated cylinder into an amber prescription bottle. Preparation is stable for 30 days when stored under refrigeration; label "shake well" and "caution chemotherapy"

Allen LV, "Busulfan Oral Suspension," *US Pharmacist*, 1990, 15:94-5.

References

Bolinger AM, Zangwill AB, Slattery JT, et al, "An Evaluation of Engraftment, Toxicity and Busulfan Concentration in Children Receiving Bone Marrow Transplantation for Leukemia or Genetic Disease," *Bone Marrow Transplant*, 2000, 25(9):925-30.

Heard BE and Cooke RA, "Busulphan Lung," *Thorax*, 1968, 23 (2):187-93.

Ozkaynak MF, Weinberg K, Kohn D, et al, "Hepatic Veno-Occlusive Disease Post-Bone Marrow Transplantation in Children Conditioned With Busulfan and Cyclophosphamide: Incidence, Risk Factors, and Clinical Outcome," *Bone Marrow Transplant*, 1991, 7(6):467-74.

Regazzi MB, Locatelli F, Buggia I, et al, "Disposition of High Dose Busulfan in Pediatric Patients Undergoing Bone Marrow Transplantation," *Clin Pharmacol Ther*, 1993, 54(1):45-52.

Vassal G, Gouyette A, Hartmann O, et al, "Pharmacokinetics of High-Dose Busulfan in Children," *Cancer Chemother Pharmacol*, 1989, 24 (6):386-90.

◆ **Busulfex®** *see* Busulfan *on page 223*

◆ **1,4-Butanediol Dimethanesulfonate** *see* Busulfan *on page 223*

◆ **BW-430C** *see* LamoTRIgine *on page 795*

◆ **BW524W91** *see* Emtricitabine *on page 496*

◆ **C2B8 Monoclonal Antibody** *see* RiTUXimab *on page 1227*

◆ **CaEDTA** *see* Edetate CALCIUM Disodium *on page 487*

◆ **Cafcit®** *see* Caffeine *on page 225*

◆ **CAFdA** *see* Clofarabine *on page 332*

◆ **Cafergor® (Can)** *see* Ergotamine and Caffeine *on page 522*

◆ **Cafergot®** *see* Ergotamine and Caffeine *on page 522*

Caffeine (KAF een)

U.S. Brand Names Cafcit®; Enerjets [OTC]; No Doz® Maximum Strength [OTC]; Vivarin® [OTC]

Therapeutic Category Central Nervous System Stimulant; Diuretic; Respiratory Stimulant

Generic Available Yes: Tablet, caffeine and sodium benzoate injection, injection, oral solution

Use

Treatment of idiopathic apnea of prematurity **(caffeine citrate)**

Emergency stimulant in acute circulatory failure; diuretic; treatment of spinal puncture headaches **(caffeine sodium benzoate)**

Pregnancy Risk Factor C

◀ **Pregnancy Considerations** Caffeine crosses the placenta; serum levels in the fetus are similar to those in the mother. When large bolus doses are administered to animals, teratogenic effects have been reported. Similar doses are not probable following normal caffeine consumption and moderate consumption is not associated with congenital malformations, spontaneous abortions, preterm birth or low birth weight. According to one source, pregnant women who do not smoke or drink alcohol could consume ≤5 mg/kg of caffeine over the course of a day without reproductive risk. Another source recommends limiting caffeine intake to <150 mg/day. The half-life of caffeine is prolonged during the second and third trimesters of pregnancy.

Lactation Enters breast milk/use caution (AAP rates "compatible")

Breast-Feeding Considerations Irritability and poor sleeping patterns have been reported following maternal consumption of large amounts of caffeine. Moderate intake (2-3 cups/day) is considered to be compatible with breast-feeding.

Contraindications Hypersensitivity to caffeine or any component; sodium benzoate salt form in neonates (see Warnings)

Warnings Do not interchange the caffeine citrate salt formulation with the caffeine sodium benzoate formulation; sodium benzoate has been associated with a potentially fatal toxicity ("gasping syndrome") in neonates; the "gasping syndrome" consists of metabolic acidosis, respiratory distress, gasping respirations, CNS dysfunction (including convulsions, intracranial hemorrhage), hypotension and cardiovascular collapse; *in vitro* and animal studies have shown that benzoate also displaces bilirubin from protein-binding sites; avoid use of products containing sodium benzoate in neonates. During a Cafcit® double-blind, placebo-controlled study, 6 of 85 patients developed necrotizing enterocolitis (NEC); 5 of these 6 patients had received caffeine citrate; although no causal relationship has been established, neonates who receive caffeine citrate should be closely monitored for the development of NEC. Caffeine serum levels should be closely monitored to optimize therapy and prevent serious toxicity.

Precautions Use with caution in patients with a history of peptic ulcer, impaired renal or hepatic function, seizure disorders, or cardiovascular disease; avoid in patients with symptomatic cardiac arrhythmias

Adverse Reactions
Cardiovascular: Cardiac arrhythmias, tachycardia, extrasystoles
Central nervous system: Insomnia, restlessness, agitation, irritability, hyperactivity, jitteriness, headache, nervousness, anxiety
Endocrine & metabolic: Hypoglycemia, hyperglycemia
Gastrointestinal: Nausea, vomiting, gastric irritation, necrotizing enterocolitis, GI hemorrhage
Genitourinary: Urine output increased
Neuromuscular & skeletal: Muscle tremors or twitches

Drug Interactions
Metabolism/Transport Effects Substrate of CYP1A2 (major), 2C9 (minor), 2D6 (minor), 2E1 (minor), 3A4 (minor); **Inhibits** CYP1A2 (weak)

Avoid Concomitant Use
Avoid concomitant use of Caffeine with any of the following: Iobenguane I 123

Increased Effect/Toxicity
Caffeine may increase the levels/effects of: Sympathomimetics

The levels/effects of Caffeine may be increased by: Atomoxetine; Cannabinoids; CYP1A2 Inhibitors (Moderate); CYP1A2 Inhibitors (Strong); Quinolone Antibiotics

Decreased Effect
Caffeine may decrease the levels/effects of: Iobenguane I 123; Regadenoson

The levels/effects of Caffeine may be decreased by: Peginterferon Alfa-2b

Stability Caffeine citrate: Injection and oral solution contain no preservatives; injection is chemically stable for at least 24 hours at room temperature when diluted to 10 mg/mL (as caffeine citrate) with D_5W, $D_{50}W$, Intralipid® 20%, and Aminosyn® 8.5%; also compatible with dopamine (600 mcg/mL), calcium gluconate 10%, heparin (1 unit/mL), and fentanyl (10 mcg/mL) at room temperature for 24 hours

Mechanism of Action Increases levels of 3'5' cyclic AMP by inhibiting phosphodiesterase; CNS stimulant which increases medullary respiratory center sensitivity to carbon dioxide, stimulates central inspiratory drive, and improves skeletal muscle contraction (diaphragmatic contractility); prevention of apnea may occur by competitive inhibition of adenosine

Pharmacokinetics (Adult data unless noted)
Distribution: V_d:
Neonates: 0.8-0.9 L/kg
Children >9 months to Adults: 0.6 L/kg
Protein binding: 17%
Metabolism: Interconversion between caffeine and theophylline has been reported in preterm neonates (caffeine levels are ~25% of measured theophylline after theophylline administration and ~3% to 8% of caffeine would be expected to be converted to theophylline)
Half-life:
Neonates: 72-96 hours (range: 40-230 hours)
Infants >9 months, Children, and Adults: 5 hours
Time to peak serum concentration: Oral: Within 30 minutes to 2 hours
Elimination:
Neonates ≤1 month: 86% excreted unchanged in urine
Infants >1 month and Adults: Extensively liver metabolized to a series of partially demethylated xanthines and methyluric acids
Clearance:
Neonates: 8.9 mL/hour/kg (range: 2.5-17)
Adults: 94 mL/hour/kg

Usual Dosage
Apnea of prematurity: **Caffeine citrate:** Neonates: Oral, I.V.:
Loading dose: 10-20 mg/kg as caffeine citrate (5-10 mg/kg as caffeine base). If theophylline has been administered to the patient within the previous 3 days, a full or modified loading dose (50% to 75% of a loading dose) may be given (caffeine is a significant metabolite of theophylline in the newborn; see Pharmacokinetics).
Maintenance dose: 5 mg/kg/day as caffeine citrate (2.5 mg/kg/day as caffeine base) once daily starting 24 hours after the loading dose. Maintenance dose is adjusted based on patient's response (efficacy and adverse effects), and serum caffeine concentrations.

Stimulant/diuretic: **Caffeine sodium benzoate:** Adults: I.M., I.V.: 500 mg as a single dose
Treatment of spinal puncture headache: **Caffeine sodium benzoate:** Adults: I.V.: 500 mg as a single dose; may repeat in 4 hours if headache unrelieved (see Administration)

Administration
Oral: May be administered without regard to feedings or meals; may administer injectable formulation (caffeine citrate) orally
Parenteral:
Caffeine citrate: Infuse loading dose over at least 30 minutes; maintenance dose may be infused over at least 10 minutes; may administer without dilution or diluted with D_5W to 10 mg caffeine citrate/mL

Caffeine sodium benzoate: I.V. as slow direct injection; for spinal headaches, dilute in 1000 mL NS and infuse over 1 hour; follow with 1000 mL NS, infuse over 1 hour; administer I.M. undiluted

Monitoring Parameters Heart rate, number and severity of apnea spells, serum caffeine levels

Reference Range
Therapeutic: Apnea of prematurity: 8-20 mcg/mL
Potentially toxic: >20 mcg/mL
Toxic: >50 mcg/mL

Dosage Forms Excipient information presented when available (limited, particularly for generics); consult specific product labeling. [DSC] = Discontinued product
Caplet:
NoDoz® Maximum Strength, Vivarin®: 200 mg
Injection, solution, as citrate [preservative free]: 20 mg/mL (3 mL) [equivalent to 10 mg/mL caffeine base]
Cafcit®: 20 mg/mL (3 mL) [equivalent to 10 mg/mL caffeine base]
Injection, solution [with sodium benzoate]: Caffeine 125 mg/mL and sodium benzoate 125 mg/mL (2 mL); caffeine 121 mg/mL and sodium benzoate 129 mg/mL (2 mL) [DSC]
Lozenge:
Enerjets®: 75 mg [classic coffee, hazelnut cream, or mochamint flavor]
Solution, oral, as citrate [preservative free]: 20 mg/mL (3 mL) [equivalent to 10 mg/mL caffeine base]
Cafcit®: 20 mg/mL (3 mL) [equivalent to 10 mg/mL caffeine base]
Tablet: 200 mg
Vivarin®: 200 mg

Extemporaneous Preparations
An oral solution of 20 mg/mL caffeine citrate, prepared from 10 g caffeine (anhydrous) combined with 10 g citric acid USP and 1000 mL SWI is stable for 3 months refrigerated (Nahata, 1987).
An oral solution 20 mg/mL caffeine citrate may be made by dissolving 5 g anhydrous caffeine and 5 g citric acid USP in 250 mL SWI. Stir solution until completely clear; add 2:1 simple syrup:cherry syrup mixture to a final volume of 500 mL; stable refrigerated 90 days (Eisenberg, 1984).
Eisenberg MG and Kang N, "Stability of Citrated Caffeine Solutions for Injectable and Enteral Use," *Am J Hosp Pharm*, 1984, 41(11):2405-6.
Nahata, MC, Pai VB, and Hipple TF, *Pediatric Drug Formulations*, 5th ed, Cincinnati, OH: Harvey Whitney Books Co, 2004.

References
Bhatt-Mehta V and Schumacher RE, "Treatment of Apnea of Prematurity," *Paediatr Drugs*, 2003, 5(3):195-210.
Erenberg A, Leff RD, Haack DG, et al, "Caffeine Citrate for the Treatment of Apnea of Prematurity: A Double-Blind, Placebo-Controlled Study," *Pharmacotherapy*, 2000, 20(6):644-52.
Kriter KE and Blanchard J, "Management of Apnea in Infants," *Clin Pharm*, 1989, 8(8):577-87.

◆ **Caffeine and Ergotamine** *see* Ergotamine and Caffeine *on page 522*

◆ **Caffeine and Sodium Benzoate** *see* Caffeine *on page 225*

◆ **Caffeine Citrate** *see* Caffeine *on page 225*

◆ **Cal-C-Caps [OTC]** *see* Calcium Citrate *on page 234*

Calamine Lotion (KAL a myne loe shun)

Therapeutic Category Topical Skin Product

Use Employed primarily as an astringent, protectant, and soothing agent for conditions such as poison ivy, poison oak, poison sumac, sunburn, insect bites, or minor skin irritations

Pregnancy Risk Factor C

Precautions For external use only

Adverse Reactions
Dermatologic: Rash
Local: Irritation

Usual Dosage Topical: Apply 1-4 times/day as needed; reapply after bathing

Administration Topical: Shake well before using; avoid contact with the eyes; do not use on open wounds or burns

Additional Information Active ingredients: Calamine, zinc oxide

Dosage Forms Lotion:
Topical: Calamine 8%, zinc oxide 8%, glycerin 2% and bentonite magma in calcium hydroxide solution (120 mL, 240 mL, 480 mL)
Topical, phenolated: Calamine 8%, zinc oxide 8%, glycerin 2%, bentonite magma, and phenol 1% in calcium hydroxide solution (120 mL, 240 mL)

◆ **Calan®** *see* Verapamil *on page 1416*

◆ **Calan® SR** *see* Verapamil *on page 1416*

◆ **Calcarb 600 [OTC]** *see* Calcium Carbonate *on page 232*

◆ **Calcarb 600 [OTC]** *see* Calcium Supplements *on page 239*

◆ **Cal-Cee [OTC]** *see* Calcium Citrate *on page 234*

◆ **Calci-Chew® [OTC]** *see* Calcium Carbonate *on page 232*

◆ **Calci-Chew® [OTC]** *see* Calcium Supplements *on page 239*

◆ **Calciferol™ [OTC]** *see* Ergocalciferol *on page 519*

◆ **Calcijex®** *see* Calcitriol *on page 229*

◆ **Calcimar® (Can)** *see* Calcitonin *on page 227*

◆ **Calci-Mix® [OTC]** *see* Calcium Carbonate *on page 232*

◆ **Calci-Mix® [OTC]** *see* Calcium Supplements *on page 239*

◆ **Calcionate [OTC]** *see* Calcium Glubionate *on page 235*

◆ **Calcite-500 (Can)** *see* Calcium Carbonate *on page 232*

Calcitonin (kal si TOE nin)

Medication Safety Issues
Sound-alike/look-alike issues:
Calcitonin may be confused with calcitriol
Miacalcin® may be confused with Micatin®

Calcitonin nasal spray is administered as a single spray into **one** nostril daily, using alternate nostrils each day.

U.S. Brand Names Fortical®; Miacalcin®

Canadian Brand Names Apo-Calcitonin®; Calcimar®; Caltine®; Miacalcin® NS; PRO-Calcitonin; Sandoz-Calcitonin

Therapeutic Category Antidote, Hypercalcemia

Generic Available Yes: Intranasal solution

Use
Parenteral: Treatment of Paget's disease of bone; adjunctive therapy for hypercalcemia; postmenopausal osteoporosis (FDA approved in adults); has also been used for osteogenesis imperfecta
Intranasal: Postmenopausal osteoporosis in women >5 years postmenopause with low bone mass (FDA approved in adults)

Pregnancy Risk Factor C

Pregnancy Considerations Decreased birth weight was observed in animal studies. Calcitonin does not cross the placenta.

Lactation Excretion in breast milk unknown/not recommended

Breast-Feeding Considerations Has been shown to decrease milk production in animals.

Contraindications Hypersensitivity to calcitonin, salmon protein, or any component

◄ **Precautions** Due to potential hypersensitivity reactions, a skin test is recommended prior to initiating parenteral therapy; the skin test is 0.1 mL of 10 unit/mL calcitonin injection in NS (must be prepared) injected intradermally; observe injection site for 15 minutes for wheal or significant erythema; when using intranasal formulation, periodic nasal examinations are recommended. Discontinue for nasal ulcerations >1.5 mm or those that penetrate below the mucosa.

Adverse Reactions

Cardiovascular: Angina, flushing of the face, hypertension, thrombophlebitis

Central nervous system: Agitation, chills, dizziness, fatigue, headache, neuralgia

Dermatologic: Erythematous rash

Gastrointestinal: Abdominal pain, constipation, diarrhea, dyspepsia, metallic taste, nausea, xerostomia

Genitourinary: Cystitis

Local: Injection site reactions (10%)

Neuromuscular & skeletal: Back and joint pain, paresthesia, tingling of palms and soles, weakness

Renal: Diuresis

Respiratory: Epistaxis, nasal sores, nasal ulcerations (nasal spray), rhinitis, sore bridge of nose (nasal spray)

Miscellaneous: Anaphylaxis/anaphylactic shock, hypersensitivity reactions, influenza-like symptoms, lymphadenopathy

<1%, postmarketing, and/or case reports: Allergic rhinitis, alopecia, anaphylactoid reaction, anemia, anorexia, anxiety, appetite increased, arthralgia, arthritis, blurred vision, bronchitis, bundle branch block, cerebrovascular accident, cholelithiasis, cough, diaphoresis, dyspnea, earache, eczema, edema, eye pain, fever, flatulence, gastritis, goiter, hearing loss, hematuria, hepatitis, hyperthyroidism, insomnia, migraine, myocardial infarction, nasal congestion, nasal odor, nocturia, palpitation, parosmia, periorbital edema, pharyngitis, pneumonia, polymyalgia rheumatica, polyuria, pruritus, pyelonephritis, rash, renal calculus, skin ulceration, sneezing, stiffness, tachycardia, taste perversion, thirst, tinnitus, urine sediment abnormality, vertigo, visual disturbances, vitreous floater, vomiting, weight gain

Drug Interactions

Avoid Concomitant Use There are no known interactions where it is recommended to avoid concomitant use.

Increased Effect/Toxicity There are no known significant interactions involving an increase in effect.

Decreased Effect

Calcitonin may decrease the levels/effects of: Lithium

Stability

Injection: Store under refrigeration at 2°C to 8°C (36°F to 46°F); protect from freezing.

Nasal: Store unopened bottle under refrigeration at 2°C to 8°C (36°F to 46°F); do not freeze.

Fortical®: After opening, store for up to 30 days at 20°C to 25°C (68°F to 77°F); excursions permitted to 15°C to 30°C (59°F to 86°F). Store in upright position.

Miacalcin®: After opening, store for up to 35 days at room temperature of 15°C to 30°C (59°F to 86°F). Store in upright position.

Mechanism of Action Calcitonin directly inhibits osteoclastic bone resorption; promotes the renal excretion of calcium, phosphate, sodium, magnesium and potassium by decreasing tubular reabsorption; increases the jejunal secretion of water, sodium, potassium, and chloride

Pharmacodynamics

Onset of action:

Hypercalcemia: I.M., SubQ: ~2 hours

Paget's disease: Within a few months; may take up to 1 year for neurologic symptom improvement

Duration: Hypercalcemia: I.M., SubQ: 6-8 hours

Pharmacokinetics (Adult data unless noted)

Absorption: Intranasal: Rapidly but highly variable and lower than I.M. administration

Metabolism: Rapidly in the kidneys, blood, and peripheral tissues

Bioavailability: I.M. 66%; SubQ: 71%

Half-life, elimination (terminal): I.M.: 58 minutes; SubQ: 59-64 minutes

Time to peak serum concentration: SubQ ~23 minutes

Elimination: As inactive metabolites in urine

Clearance: Salmon calcitonin: 3.1 mL/kg/minute

Usual Dosage

Children >6 months and adults: Osteogenesis imperfecta: I.M., SubQ: 2 international units/kg 3 times/week (see Castells, 1979)

Adults:

Paget's disease: I.M., SubQ: Initial: 100 international units/day; maintenance dose: 50 international units/day or 50-100 international units every 1-2 days

Hypercalcemia: Initial: I.M., SubQ: 4 international units/kg every 12 hours for 1-2 days; may increase up to 8 international units/kg every 12 hours; if the response remains unsatisfactory after 2 additional days, a further increase up to a maximum of 8 international units/kg every 6 hours may be considered

Postmenopausal osteoporosis:

I.M., SubQ: 100 international units every other day

Intranasal: 200 international units (1 spray) into **one** nostril daily

Administration

Intranasal: Spray into **one** nostril daily; alternate nostrils to reduce irritation. Before priming a new pump, allow it to reach room temperature first.

Parenteral: Do not exceed 2 mL volume per injection site; may be administered SubQ or I.M. SubQ is preferred for outpatient self administration; I.M. is preferred for larger injection volumes.

Monitoring Parameters Serum electrolytes and calcium; alkaline phosphatase and 24-hour urine collection for hydroxyproline excretion (Paget's disease); urinalysis (urine sediment); serum calcium; periodic nasal exams (intranasal use only)

Patient Information Nasal spray: Notify physician if you develop significant nasal irritation; alternate nostrils; in treatment of postmenopausal osteoporosis, maintain adequate vitamin D intake and supplemental calcium

Dosage Forms Excipient information presented when available (limited, particularly for generics); consult specific product labeling.

Injection, solution [calcitonin-salmon]:

Miacalcin®: 200 int. units/mL (2 mL)

Solution, intranasal [spray, calcitonin-salmon]: 200 int. units/actuation (3.7 mL, 3.8 mL)

Fortical®: 200 int. units/actuation (3.7 mL) [rDNA origin; contains benzyl alcohol; delivers 30 doses]

Miacalcin®: 200 int. units/actuation (3.7 mL) [contains benzalkonium chloride; delivers 30 doses]

References

Castells S, Colbert C, Chakrabarti C, et al, "Therapy of Osteogenesis Imperfecta With Synthetic Salmon Calcitonin," *J Pediatr*, 1979, 95(5 Pt 1):807-11.

◆ **Calcitonin (Salmon)** *see* Calcitonin *on page 227*

◆ **Cal-Citrate-225** *see* Calcium Citrate *on page 234*

◆ **Cal-Citrate® 250 [OTC]** *see* Calcium Supplements *on page 239*

Calcitriol (kal si TRYE ole)

Medication Safety Issues
Sound-alike/look-alike issues:
Calcitriol may be confused with calcifediol, Calciferol®, calcitonin, calcium carbonate, captopril, colestipol, paricalcitol, ropinirole

Dosage is expressed in mcg (micrograms), **not** mg (milligrams); rare cases of acute overdose have been reported

U.S. Brand Names Calcijex®; Rocaltrol®; Vectical™

Canadian Brand Names Calcijex®; Rocaltrol®

Therapeutic Category Rickets, Treatment Agent; Vitamin D Analog; Vitamin, Fat Soluble

Generic Available Yes: Excludes ointment

Use
Oral/Injection: Management of secondary hyperparathyroidism and resultant metabolic bone disease in patients with moderate-to-severe chronic renal failure not yet on dialysis (FDA approved in ages ≥3 years and adults); management of hypocalcemia and resultant metabolic bone disease in patients on chronic renal dialysis (FDA approved in ages ≥18 years); management of hypocalcemia in patients with hypoparathyroidism (FDA approved in ages ≥1 year and adults) and pseudohypoparathyroidism (FDA approved in ages ≥6 years and adults)

Topical: Management of mild-to-moderate plaque psoriasis (FDA approved in ages ≥18 years)

Pregnancy Risk Factor C

Pregnancy Considerations Teratogenic effects have been observed in animal studies. Mild hypercalcemia has been reported in a newborn following maternal use of calcitriol during pregnancy. If calcitriol is used for the management of hypoparathyroidism in pregnancy, dose adjustments may be needed as pregnancy progresses and again following delivery. Vitamin D and calcium levels should be monitored closely and kept in the lower normal range.

Lactation Enters breast milk/not recommended

Breast-Feeding Considerations Low levels are found in breast milk (~2 pg/mL)

Contraindications Hypersensitivity to calcitriol or any component; hypercalcemia; vitamin D toxicity; abnormal sensitivity to the effects of vitamin D

Warnings Excessive administration may lead to over suppression of PTH, hypercalcemia, hypercalciuria, hyperphosphatemia, and adynamic bone disease. Acute hypercalcemia may increase risk of cardiac arrhythmias and seizures. Chronic hypercalcemia may lead to generalized vascular and other soft-tissue calcification. Phosphate and vitamin D (and its derivatives) should be withheld during therapy to avoid hypercalcemia. Monitor serum calcium levels closely; the calcitriol dosage should be adjusted accordingly; serum calcium times phosphorus product (Ca x P) should not exceed 65 mg^2/dL^2 for infants and children <12 years of age and 55 mg^2/dL^2 for adolescents and adults. Not indicated for use in patients with rapidly worsening kidney function or those who are noncompliant with medications or follow-up (K/DOQI Guidelines, 2003). Topical: May cause hypercalcemia; if alterations in calcium occur, discontinue treatment until levels return to normal.

Precautions Hypercalcemia potentiates digoxin toxicity; use concomitantly with caution

Topical: For external use only; not for ophthalmic, oral, or intravaginal use. Do not apply to facial skin, eyes, or lips. Absorption may be increased with occlusive dressings. Avoid or limit excessive exposure to natural or artificial sunlight or phototherapy. The safety and effectiveness have not been evaluated in patients with erythrodermic, exfoliative, or pustular psoriasis.

Adverse Reactions Effects primarily associated with hypercalcemia

Cardiovascular: Blood pressure elevated, cardiac arrhythmias

Central nervous system: Somnolence, headache, hyperthermia, apathy

Dermatologic: Pruritus

Endocrine & metabolic: Hypercholesterolemia, hypercalcemia, polydipsia, weight loss, hyperphosphatemia

Gastrointestinal: Nausea, vomiting, constipation, anorexia, xerostomia, pancreatitis, metallic taste

Genitourinary: Nocturia

Hepatic: Liver enzymes elevated

Neuromuscular & skeletal: Myalgia, bone pain, weakness

Ocular: Calcific conjunctivitis, photophobia

Renal: Polyuria, uremia, albuminuria, nephrocalcinosis, UTIs, hypercalciuria

Respiratory: Rhinorrhea

Miscellaneous: Hypersensitivity reactions, dehydration

Topical ointment:
Endocrine & metabolic: Hypercalcemia
Dermatologic: Skin discomfort, pruritus

Drug Interactions
Metabolism/Transport Effects Substrate of CYP3A4 (major); **Induces** CYP3A4 (weak)

Avoid Concomitant Use There are no known interactions where it is recommended to avoid concomitant use.

Increased Effect/Toxicity
Calcitriol may increase the levels/effects of: Cardiac Glycosides; Magnesium Salts

The levels/effects of Calcitriol may be increased by: CYP3A4 Inhibitors (Moderate); CYP3A4 Inhibitors (Strong); Dasatinib; Thiazide Diuretics

Decreased Effect
Calcitriol may decrease the levels/effects of: Saxagliptin

The levels/effects of Calcitriol may be decreased by: Bile Acid Sequestrants; Corticosteroids (Systemic); CYP3A4 Inducers (Strong); Deferasirox; Herbs (CYP3A4 Inducers)

Stability Store at room temperature; protect oral and I.V. formulations from light and heat. Do not refrigerate or freeze topical ointment.

Mechanism of Action Calcitriol, the active form of vitamin D (1,25 hydroxyvitamin D_3), binds to and activates the vitamin D receptor in kidney, parathyroid gland, intestine, and bone, stimulating intestinal calcium transport and absorption. It reduces PTH levels and improves calcium and phosphate homeostasis by stimulating bone resorption of calcium and increasing renal tubular reabsorption of calcium. Decreased renal conversion of vitamin D to its primary active metabolite (1,25 hydroxyvitamin D) in chronic renal failure leads to reduced activation of vitamin D receptor, which subsequently removes inhibitory suppression of parathyroid hormone (PTH) release; increased serum PTH (secondary hyperparathyroidism) reduces calcium excretion and enhances bone resorption. The mechanism by which calcitriol is beneficial in the treatment of psoriasis has not been established.

Pharmacodynamics Oral:
Onset of action: 2 hours
Maximum effect: 10 hours
Duration: 3-5 days

Pharmacokinetics (Adult data unless noted)
Distribution: Breast milk: Very low (levels 2.2 ± 0.1 pg/mL)
Protein binding: 99.9%
Metabolism: Primarily to 1,24,25-trihydroxycholecalciferol and 1,24,25-trihydroxy ergocalciferol

Half-life:
Children 1.8-16 years undergoing peritoneal dialysis: 27.4 hours
Adults without renal dysfunction: 5-8 hours
Adults with CRF: 16.2-21.9 hours
Time to peak serum concentration: Oral: 3-6 hours
Elimination: Feces 27% and urine 7% excreted unchanged in 24 hours
Clearance: Children 1.8-16 years undergoing peritoneal dialysis: 15.3 mL/hour/kg

Usual Dosage

Management of hypocalcemia in patients with chronic kidney disease (CKD): Indicated for therapy when serum levels of 25(OH)D are >30 ng/mL (75 nmol/L) and serum levels of intact parathyroid hormone (iPTH) are above the target range for the stage of CKD (see Reference Range); serum levels of corrected total calcium are <9.5-10 mg/dL (2.37 mmol/L) and serum levels of phosphorus in children are less than age-appropriate upper limits of normal or in adults <4.6 mg/dL (1.49 mmol/L) (K/DOQI Guidelines, 2005):

Children and Adolescents: CKD Stages 2-4: Oral:
<10 kg: 0.05 mcg every other day
10-20 kg: 0.1-0.15 mcg daily
>20 kg: 0.25 mcg daily

Dosage adjustment:
If iPTH decrease is <30% after 3 months of therapy and serum levels of calcium and phosphorus are within the target ranges based upon the CKD Stage (see Reference Range), increase dosage by 50%
If iPTH decrease < target range for CKD stage (see Reference Range) hold calcitriol therapy until iPTH increases to above target range; resume therapy at half the previous dosage (if dosage <0.25 mcg capsule or 0.05 mcg liquid, use every other day therapy)
If serum levels of total corrected calcium exceed 10.2 mg/dL (2.37 mmol/L) hold calcitriol therapy until serum calcium decreased to <9.8 mg/dL (2.37 mmol/L); resume therapy at half the previous dosage (if dosage <0.25 mcg capsule or 0.05 mcg liquid, use every other day therapy)
If serum levels of phosphorus increase to > age-appropriate upper limits, hold calcitriol therapy (initiate or increase phosphate binders until the levels of serum phosphorus decrease to age-appropriate limits); resume therapy at half the previous dosage

Children and Adolescents: CKD Stage 5: Oral, I.V.: Serum calcium times phosphorus product (Ca x P) should not exceed 65 mg^2/dL^2 for infants and children <12 years of age and 55 mg^2/dL^2 for adolescents, serum phosphorus should be within target (see Reference Range), serum calcium <10 mg/dL (2.37 mmol/L):

iPTH 300-500 pg/mL: 0.0075 mcg/kg per dialysis session (3 times/week); not to exceed 0.25 mcg daily
iPTH >500-1000 pg/mL: 0.015 mcg/kg per dialysis session (3 times/week); not to exceed 0.5 mcg daily
iPTH >1000 pg/mL: 0.025 mcg/kg per dialysis session (3 times/week); not to exceed 1 mcg daily

Dosage adjustment: If iPTH decrease is <30% after 3 months of therapy and serum levels of calcium and phosphorus are within the target ranges based upon the CKD Stage 5 (see Reference Range), increase dosage by 50%

Adult CKD Stages 3 or 4: Serum calcium <9.5 mg/dL (2.37 mmol/L), serum phosphorus <5.5 mg/dL (1.77 mmol/L), serum calcium times phosphorus product (Ca x P) <55 mg^2/dL^2:

iPTH 300-600 pg/mL: Oral, I.V.: 0.5-1.5 mcg per dialysis session (3 times/week)

iPTH 600-1000 pg/mL: I.V.: 1-3 mcg per dialysis session (3 times/week); Oral: 1-4 mcg per dialysis session (3 times/week)
iPTH >1000 pg/mL: I.V. 3-5 mcg per dialysis session (3 times/week); Oral: 3-7 mcg per dialysis session (3 times/week)

Dosage adjustment:
If iPTH decrease < target range for CKD stage 5 (see Reference Range) hold calcitriol therapy until iPTH increases to above target range; resume therapy at half the previous dosage (if dosage <0.25 mcg capsule or 0.05 mcg liquid, use every other day therapy)
If serum levels of total corrected calcium exceed 9.5 mg/dL (2.37 mmol/L) hold calcitriol therapy until serum calcium decreased to <9.5 mg/dL (2.37 mmol/L); resume therapy at half the previous dosage (if dosage <0.25 mcg capsule or 0.05 mcg liquid, use every other day therapy)
If serum levels of phosphorus increase to >4.6 mg/dL (1.49 mmol/L), hold calcitriol therapy (initiate or increase phosphate binders until the levels of serum phosphorus decrease to 4.6 mg/dL (1.49 mmol/L); resume therapy at prior dosage

Note: Intermittent administration of calcitriol by I.V. or oral routes is more effective than daily oral calcitriol in lowering iPTH levels.

Hypoparathyroidism/pseudohypoparathyroidism: Oral (evaluate dosage at 2- to 4-week intervals):
Children:
<1 year: 0.04-0.08 mcg/kg once daily
1-5 years: 0.25-0.75 mcg once daily
Children >6 years and Adults: 0.5-2 mcg once daily
Vitamin D-dependent rickets: Children and Adults: Oral: 1 mcg once daily
Vitamin D-resistant rickets (familial hypophosphatemia): Children and Adults: Oral: Initial: 0.015-0.02 mcg/kg once daily; maintenance: 0.03-0.06 mcg/kg once daily; maximum dose: 2 mcg once daily
Hypocalcemia in premature infants: Oral: 1 mcg once daily for the first 5 days of life
Hypocalcemic tetany in premature infants: I.V.: 0.05 mcg/kg once daily for 5-12 days
Psoriasis: Adults: Topical: Apply twice daily to affected areas (maximum: 200 g/week)

Administration

Oral: May be administered with or without meals; when administering small doses from the liquid-filled capsules, consider the following concentration for Rocaltrol®:
0.25 mcg capsule = 0.25 mcg per 0.17 mL
0.5 mcg capsule = 0.5 mcg per 0.17 mL
Parenteral: May be administered undiluted as a bolus dose I.V. through the catheter at the end of hemodialysis
Topical: Apply externally; not for ophthalmic, oral, or intravaginal use

Monitoring Parameters Signs and symptoms of vitamin D intoxication

Serum calcium and phosphorus:
I.V.: Twice weekly during initial phase, then at least monthly once dose established
Oral: At least every 2 weeks for 3 months or following dose adjustment, then monthly for 3 months, then every 3 months
Serum or plasma intact parathyroid hormone (iPTH): At least every 2 weeks for 3 months or following dose adjustment, then monthly for 3 months, then as per K/DOQI Guidelines below.
Per Kidney Disease Outcome Quality Initiative Practice Guidelines: Children (K/DOQI, 2005):
Stage 3 CKD: iPTH every 6 months
Stage 4 CKD: iPTH every 3 months
Stage 5 CKD: iPTH every 3 months

Per Kidney Disease Outcome Quality Initiative Practice Guidelines: Adults (K/DOQI, 2003):

Stage 3 CKD: iPTH every 12 months

Stage 4 CKD: iPTH every 3 months

Stage 5 CKD: iPTH every 3 months

Reference Range

Chronic kidney disease (CKD) is defined either as kidney damage or GFR <60 mL/minute/1.73 m^2 for ≥3 months); stages of CKD are described below:

CKD Stage 1: Kidney damage with normal or increased GFR; GFR >90 mL/minute/1.73m^2

CKD Stage 2: Kidney damage with mild decrease in GFR; GFR 60-89 mL/minute/1.73 m^2

CKD Stage 3: Moderate decrease in GFR; GFR 30-59 mL/minute/1.73 m^2

CKD Stage 4: Severe decrease in GFR; GFR 15-29 mL/minute/1.73 m^2

CKD Stage 5: Kidney failure; GFR <15 mL/minute/1.73 m^2 or dialysis

Target range for iPTH:

Stage 2 CKD: Children: 35-70 pg/mL (3.85-7.7 pmol/L)

Stage 3 CKD: Children and Adults: 35-70 pg/mL (3.85-7.7 pmol/L)

Stage 4 CKD: Children and Adults: 70-110 pg/mL (7.7-12.1 pmol/L)

Stage 5 CKD:

Children: 200-300 pg/mL (22-33 pmol/L)

Adults: 150-300 pg/mL (16.5-33 pmol/L)

Serum phosphorous:

Stages 1-4 CKD: Children: At or above the age-appropriate lower limits and no higher than age-appropriate upper limits

Stage 3 and 4 CKD: Adults: ≥2.7 to <4.6 mg/dL (≥0.87 to <1.49 mmol/L)

Stage 5 CKD:

Children 1-12 years: 4-6 mg/dL (1.29-1.94 mmol/L)

Children >12 years and Adults: 3.5-5.5 mg/dL (1.13-1.78 mmol/L)

Patient Information Take as directed; do not increase dosage without consulting healthcare provider. Adhere to diet as recommended (do not take any other phosphate or vitamin D-related compounds while taking calcitriol). You may experience nausea, vomiting, dry mouth (small frequent meals, frequent mouth care, chewing gums, or sucking lozenges may help).

Dosage Forms Excipient information presented when available (limited, particularly for generics); consult specific product labeling.

Capsule, softgel: 0.25 mcg, 0.5 mcg

Rocaltrol®: 0.25 mcg [contains coconut oil]; 0.5 mcg [contains coconut oil]

Injection, solution: 1 mcg/mL (1 mL)

Calcijex®: 1 mcg/mL (1 mL) [contains aluminum]

Ointment, topical:

Vectical™: 3 mcg/g (100 g)

Solution, oral: 1 mcg/mL (15 mL)

Rocaltrol®: 1 mcg/mL (15 mL) [contains palm seed oil]

References

"K/DOQI Clinical Practice Guidelines for Bone Metabolism and Disease in Children With Chronic Kidney Disease," *Am J Kidney Dis*, 2005, 46 (4 Suppl 1):S1-121.

"K/DOQI Clinical Practice Guidelines for Bone Metabolism and Disease in Chronic Kidney Disease. Guideline 1. Evaluation of Calcium and Phosphorus Metabolism," *Am J Kidney Dis*, 2003, 42(4 Suppl 3):52-7.

"K/DOQI Clinical Practice Guidelines for Bone Metabolism and Disease in Chronic Kidney Disease. Guideline 3. Evaluation of Serum Phosphorus Levels," *Am J Kidney Dis*, 2003, 42(4 Suppl 3):62-3.

"K/DOQI Clinical Practice Guidelines for Chronic Kidney Disease: Evaluation, Classification, and Stratification, Part 4. Definition and Classification of Stages of Chronic Kidney Disease," *Am J Kidney Dis*, 2002, 39(2 Suppl 1):46-75.

Sanchez CP, "Secondary Hyperparathyroidism in Children With Chronic Renal Failure: Pathogenesis and Treatment," *Paediatr Drugs*, 2003, 5 (11): 763-76.

Ziolkowska H, "Minimizing Bone Abnormalities in Children With Renal Failure," *Paediatr Drugs*, 2006, 8(4):205-22.

Calcium Acetate (KAL see um AS e tate)

Medication Safety Issues

Sound-alike/look-alike issues:

PhosLo® may be confused with Phos-Flur®, ProSom™

U.S. Brand Names PhosLo®

Canadian Brand Names PhosLo®

Therapeutic Category Calcium Salt; Electrolyte Supplement, Parenteral

Generic Available Yes

Use Treatment and prevention of calcium depletion (injection); treatment of hyperphosphatemia in end-stage renal failure

Pregnancy Risk Factor C

Contraindications See Calcium Supplements on page 239.

Warnings See Calcium Supplements on page 239. Avoid use of calcium acetate in dialysis patients with hypercalcemia or whose plasma PTH concentrations are <150 pg/mL on two consecutive measurements.

Precautions See Calcium Supplements on page 239.

Adverse Reactions See Calcium Supplements on page 239.

Drug Interactions

Avoid Concomitant Use There are no known interactions where it is recommended to avoid concomitant use.

Increased Effect/Toxicity

Calcium Acetate may increase the levels/effects of: CefTRIAXone

The levels/effects of Calcium Acetate may be increased by: Thiazide Diuretics

Decreased Effect

Calcium Acetate may decrease the levels/effects of: Bisphosphonate Derivatives; Calcium Channel Blockers; DOBUTamine; Eltrombopag; Estramustine; Phosphate Supplements; Quinolone Antibiotics; Thyroid Products; Trientine

The levels/effects of Calcium Acetate may be decreased by: Trientine

Food Interactions See Calcium Supplements on page 239.

Stability Store at room temperature; parenteral solutions are incompatible with bicarbonates, phosphates, and sulfate formulations; mixing will result in precipitation. TPN solutions containing phosphate and calcium are compatible depending upon the parenteral amino-acid formulation and its concentration.

Mechanism of Action Calcium moderates nerve and muscle performance via action potential excitation threshold regulation; it is necessary for maintaining the functional integrity of nervous, muscular, and skeletal systems and cell-membrane and capillary permeability. Calcium acetate combines with dietary phosphate to form insoluble calcium phosphate which is excreted in feces and reduces phosphate absorption.

Pharmacokinetics (Adult data unless noted) See Calcium Supplements on page 239.

Usual Dosage

Recommended daily allowance (RDA) and adequate intake: See Calcium Supplements on page 239.

Treatment of hyperphosphatemia in end-stage renal failure: Oral: Adults: Dose expressed in mg of **calcium acetate** (PhosLo®): 1334 mg (two 667 mg capsules) with each meal; may increase up to 2668 mg (four 667 mg capsules) with each meal

Dosage adjustment in renal impairment: Cl_{cr} <25 mL/minute may require dosage adjustment depending upon serum calcium level

Administration

Oral: Administer with plenty of fluids with meals to optimize effectiveness

Parenteral:

I.V.: For direct I.V. injection infuse slow IVP over 3-5 minutes or at a rate not to exceed 0.7-1.8 mEq/minute

I.V. infusion: Infuse 0.6-1.2 mEq/kg over 1 hour

Do not inject calcium salts I.M. or administer SubQ since severe necrosis and sloughing may occur; extravasation of calcium can result in severe necrosis and tissue sloughing. Do not use scalp vein or small hand or foot veins for I.V. administration. Not for endotracheal administration.

Monitoring Parameters See Calcium Supplements on page 239.

Reference Range See Calcium Supplements on page 239.

Additional Information 1 g calcium acetate = 250 mg elemental calcium = 12.7 mEq calcium. Due to a poor correlation between the serum ionized calcium (free) and total serum calcium, particularly in states of low albumin or acid/base imbalances, direct measurement of ionized calcium is recommended. If ionized calcium is unavailable, in low albumin states, the corrected **total** serum calcium may be estimated by this equation (assuming a normal albumin of 4 g/dL); corrected total calcium = total serum calcium + 0.8(4 - measured serum albumin)

Dosage Forms Excipient information presented when available (limited, particularly for generics); consult specific product labeling.

Gelcap: 667 mg

PhosLo®: 667 mg [equivalent to elemental calcium 169 mg (8.45 mEq)]

Calcium Carbonate (KAL see um KAR bun ate)

Medication Safety Issues

Sound-alike/look-alike issues:

Calcium carbonate may be confused with calcitriol

Florical® may be confused with Fiorinal®

Mylanta® may be confused with Mynatal®

Nephro-Calci® may be confused with Nephrocaps®

International issues:

Remegel® [Great Britain, Ireland, Italy] may be confused with Renagel® which is a brand name for sevelamer in the U.S.

U.S. Brand Names Alcalak [OTC]; Alka-Mints® [OTC]; Cal-Gest [OTC]; Cal-Mint [OTC]; Calcarb 600 [OTC]; Calci-Chew® [OTC]; Calci-Mix® [OTC]; Caltrate® 600 [OTC]; Children's Pepto [OTC]; Chooz® [OTC]; Florical® [OTC]; Maalox® Children's [OTC]; Maalox® Regular Chewable [OTC] [DSC]; Mylanta® Children's [OTC] [DSC]; Nephro-Calci® [OTC]; Nutralox® [OTC]; Oysco 500 [OTC]; Oyst-Cal 500 [OTC]; Rolaids® Softchews [OTC]; Titralac™ [OTC]; Tums® E-X [OTC]; Tums® Extra Strength Sugar Free [OTC]; Tums® Smoothies™ [OTC]; Tums® Ultra [OTC]; Tums® [OTC]

Canadian Brand Names Apo-Cal®; Calcite-500; Cal-trate®; Caltrate® Select; Os-Cal®

Therapeutic Category Antacid; Calcium Salt; Electrolyte Supplement, Oral

Generic Available Yes

Use Symptomatic relief of hyperacidity associated with peptic ulcer, gastritis, esophagitis, and hiatal hernia; treatment of hyperphosphatemia in end-stage renal failure; dietary supplement; prevention and treatment of calcium deficiency; topical treatment of hydrofluoric acid burns; adjunctive prevention and treatment of osteoporosis

Pregnancy Considerations Available evidence suggests safe use during pregnancy and breast-feeding.

Contraindications See Calcium Supplements on page 239.

Warnings See Calcium Supplements on page 239. Milk-Alkali syndrome (hypercalcemia, metabolic alkalosis, and rarely, renal insufficiency) has been associated with ingestion of large quantities of milk concomitantly with calcium carbonate; patients with renal impairment or dehydration and electrolyte imbalance are at increased risk for developing this syndrome; monitor calcium serum levels periodically

Precautions See Calcium Supplements on page 239. When used chronically as an antacid, calcium carbonate has been associated with gastric hypersecretion and acid rebound. Some chewable tablets contain phenylalanine which must be avoided in patients with phenylketonuria.

Adverse Reactions See Calcium Supplements on page 239.

Drug Interactions

Avoid Concomitant Use There are no known interactions where it is recommended to avoid concomitant use.

Increased Effect/Toxicity

Calcium Carbonate may increase the levels/effects of: Alpha-/Beta-Agonists; Amphetamines; QuiNIDine

The levels/effects of Calcium Carbonate may be increased by: Calcium Polystyrene Sulfonate; Sodium Polystyrene Sulfonate; Thiazide Diuretics

Decreased Effect

Calcium Carbonate may decrease the levels/effects of: ACE Inhibitors; Allopurinol; Anticonvulsants (Hydantoin); Antifungal Agents (Azole Derivatives, Systemic); Antipsychotic Agents (Phenothiazines); Atazanavir; Bisacodyl; Bisphosphonate Derivatives; Calcium Channel Blockers; Cefditoren; Cefpodoxime; Cefuroxime; Chloroquine; Corticosteroids (Oral); Dabigatran Etexilate; Dasatinib; Delavirdine; DOBUTamine; Eltrombopag; Erlotinib; Estramustine; HMG-CoA Reductase Inhibitors; Iron Salts; Isoniazid; Mesalamine; Methenamine; Mycophenolate; Penicillamine; Phosphate Supplements; Protease Inhibitors; Quinolone Antibiotics; Tetracycline Derivatives; Thyroid Products; Trientine; Ursodiol

The levels/effects of Calcium Carbonate may be decreased by: Trientine

Food Interactions See Calcium Supplements on page 239.

Stability Store at room temperature.

Mechanism of Action Calcium moderates nerve and muscle performance via action potential excitation threshold regulation; it is necessary for maintaining the functional integrity of nervous, muscular, and skeletal systems and cell-membrane and capillary permeability. Calcium carbonate combines with dietary phosphate to form insoluble calcium phosphate which is excreted in feces and reduces phosphate absorption.

Pharmacodynamics Acid neutralizing capacity: Tums® 500 mg: 10 mEq, Tums® E-X 750 mg: 15mEq; Tums® Ultra 1000 mg: 20 mEq

Pharmacokinetics (Adult data unless noted) See Calcium Supplements on page 239.

Usual Dosage Oral:

Recommended daily allowance (RDA) and adequate intake: See Calcium Supplements on page 239.

Antacid:

Children 2-5 years: Children's Pepto, Mylanta® Children's: 1 tablet (400 mg calcium carbonate) as symptoms occur; not to exceed 3 tablets/day

Children >5-11 years: Children's Pepto, Mylanta® Children's: 2 tablets (800 mg calcium carbonate) as symptoms occur; not to exceed 6 tablets/day

Children >11 years and Adults:

Tums®, Tums® E-X: Chew 2-4 tablets as symptoms occur; not to exceed 15 tablets (Tums®) or 10 tablets (Tums® E-X) per day

Tums® Ultra: Chew 2-3 tablets as symptoms occur; not to exceed 7 tablets per day

Hypocalcemia (dose depends on clinical condition and serum calcium level): Dose expressed in mg of **elemental calcium**:

Neonates: 50-150 mg/kg/day in 4-6 divided doses; not to exceed 1 g/day

Children: 45-65 mg/kg/day in 4 divided doses

Adults: 1-2 g or more per day in 3-4 divided doses

Treatment of hyperphosphatemia in end-stage renal failure: Children and Adults: Dose expressed in mg of **calcium carbonate**: 1 g with each meal; increase as needed; range: 4-7 g/day

Adjunctive prevention and treatment of osteoporosis: Adults: 500 mg **elemental calcium** 2-3 times/day; recommended dosage includes dietary intake and should be adjusted depending upon the patient's diet; to improve absorption do not administer more than 500 mg **elemental calcium**/dose

Hydrofluoric acid (HF) burns (HF concentration <20%): Topical: Various topical calcium preparations have been used anecdotally for treatment of dermal exposure to HF solutions; calcium carbonate at concentrations ranging from 2.5% to 33% has been used; a topical calcium carbonate preparation must be compounded (see Extemporaneous Preparations); apply topically as needed

Dosage adjustment in renal impairment: Cl_{cr} <25 mL/minute may require dosage adjustment depending upon serum calcium level

Administration

Oral: Administer with plenty of fluids with or immediately following meals; if using for phosphate-binding, administer with meals

Suspension: Shake well before administration

Chewable tablets: Thoroughly chew tablets before swallowing

Topical: Massage calcium carbonate slurry into exposed area for 15 minutes

Monitoring Parameters See Calcium Supplements on page 239.

Reference Range See Calcium Supplements on page 239.

Additional Information 1 g calcium carbonate = 400 mg elemental calcium = 20 mEq calcium. Due to a poor correlation between the serum ionized calcium (free) and total serum calcium, particularly in states of low albumin or acid/base imbalances, direct measurement of ionized calcium is recommended. If ionized calcium is unavailable, in low albumin states, the corrected **total** serum calcium may be estimated by this equation (assuming a normal albumin of 4 g/dL); corrected total calcium = total serum calcium + 0.8(4 - measured serum albumin)

Dosage Forms Excipient information presented when available (limited, particularly for generics); consult specific product labeling. [DSC] = Discontinued product

Capsule:

Calci-Mix®: 1250 mg [equivalent to elemental calcium 500 mg]

Florical®: 364 mg [equivalent to elemental calcium 145.6 mg; contains sodium fluoride 3.75 mg]

Gum, chewing: 250 mg (30s)

Chooz®: 500 mg (12s) [sugar free; contains phenylalanine 1.4 mg/tablet; mint flavor; equivalent to elemental calcium 200 mg]

Powder: 4000 mg/teaspoonful (480 g) [equivalent to 1600 mg elemental calcium/teaspoonful]

Suspension, oral: 1250 mg/5 mL (5 mL, 500 mL) [equivalent to elemental calcium 500 mg/5 mL; mint flavor]

Tablet: 1250 mg [equivalent to elemental calcium 500 mg]; 1500 mg [equivalent to elemental calcium 600 mg]

Calcarb 600, Caltrate® 600, Nephro-Calci®: 1500 mg [equivalent to elemental calcium 600 mg]

Florical®: 364 mg [equivalent to elemental calcium 145.6 mg; contains sodium fluoride 8.3 mg]

Oysco 500, Oyst-Cal 500: 1250 mg [equivalent to elemental calcium 500 mg]

Tablet, chewable: 500 mg [equivalent to elemental calcium 200 mg]; 650 mg [equivalent to elemental calcium 260 mg]; 750 mg [equivalent to elemental calcium 300 mg]

Alcalak: 420 mg [equivalent to elemental calcium 168 mg; mint flavor]

Alka-Mints®: 850 mg [equivalent to elemental calcium 340 mg; spearmint flavor]

Cal-Gest: 500 mg [equivalent to elemental calcium 200 mg; assorted flavors]

Calci-Chew®: 1250 mg [equivalent to elemental calcium 500 mg; cherry, lemon, and orange flavors]

Cal-Mint: 650 mg [equivalent to elemental calcium 260 mg; mint flavor]

Children's Pepto: 400 mg [equivalent to elemental calcium 161 mg; bubble gum or watermelon flavors]

Maalox® Children's: 400 mg [equivalent to elemental calcium 160 mg; contains phenylalanine 0.3 mg/tablet; wildberry flavor]

Maalox® Regular: 600 mg [equivalent to elemental calcium 222 mg; contains phenylalanine 0.5 mg/tablet; lemon flavor] [DSC]

Mylanta® Children's: 400 mg [equivalent to elemental calcium 160 mg; bubble gum flavor] [DSC]

Nutralox®: 420 mg [equivalent to elemental calcium 168 mg; sugar free; mint flavor]

Titralac™: 420 mg [equivalent to elemental calcium 168 mg; sugar free; contains sodium 1.1 mg/tablet; spearmint flavor]

Tums®: 500 mg [equivalent to elemental calcium 200 mg; contains tartrazine; assorted fruit and peppermint flavors]

Tums® E-X: 750 mg [equivalent to elemental calcium 300 mg; contains tartrazine; assorted fruit, cool relief mint, fresh blend, tropical assorted fruit, wintergreen, and assorted berry flavors]

Tums® Extra Strength Sugar Free: 750 mg [equivalent to elemental calcium 300 mg; sugar free; contains phenylalanine <1 mg/tablet; orange cream flavor]

Tums® Smoothies™: 750 mg [equivalent to elemental calcium 300 mg; contains tartrazine; assorted fruit, assorted tropical fruit, peppermint flavors]

Tums® Ultra®: 1000 mg [equivalent to elemental calcium 400 mg; contains tartrazine; assorted berry, assorted fruit, assorted tropical fruit, peppermint, and spearmint flavors]

Tablet, softchew:

Rolaids®: 1177 mg [equivalent to elemental calcium 471 mg; contains coconut oil and soy lecithin; vanilla creme and wild cherry flavors]

Extemporaneous Preparations Calcium carbonate slurry: 32.5% slurry can be prepared by triturating ten 650 mg tablets into a fine powder and adding 20 mL of water-soluble lubricant gel (eg, K-Y® Jelly)

Calcium Chloride (KAL see um KLOR ide)

Medication Safety Issues

Dosing issues:

Calcium chloride may be confused with calcium gluconate

Confusion with the different intravenous salt forms of calcium has occurred. There is a threefold difference in the primary cation concentration between calcium chloride (in which 1g = 13.6 mEq [270 mg] of elemental Ca++) and calcium gluconate (in which 1g = 4.65 mEq [90 mg] of elemental Ca++).

Prescribers should specify which salt form is desired. Dosages should be expressed either as mEq, mg, or grams of the salt form.

Related Information
CPR Pediatric Drug Dosages *on page 1455*

Therapeutic Category Calcium Salt; Electrolyte Supplement, Parenteral

Generic Available Yes

Use Treatment and prevention of calcium depletion; treatment of hypocalcemic tetany; hypermagnesemia, cardiac disturbances of hyperkalemia, hypocalcemia, or calcium channel blocking agent toxicity

Pregnancy Risk Factor C

Contraindications See Calcium Supplements on page 239.

Warnings See Calcium Supplements on page 239.

Precautions See Calcium Supplements on page 239.

Adverse Reactions See Calcium Supplements on page 239.

Drug Interactions

Avoid Concomitant Use There are no known interactions where it is recommended to avoid concomitant use.

Increased Effect/Toxicity
Calcium Chloride may increase the levels/effects of: CefTRIAXone

The levels/effects of Calcium Chloride may be increased by: Thiazide Diuretics

Decreased Effect
Calcium Chloride may decrease the levels/effects of: Bisphosphonate Derivatives; Calcium Channel Blockers; DOBUTamine; Eltrombopag; Phosphate Supplements; Thyroid Products; Trientine

The levels/effects of Calcium Chloride may be decreased by: Trientine

Food Interactions See Calcium Supplements on page 239.

Stability Store at room temperature; parenteral solutions are incompatible with bicarbonates, phosphates, and sulfate formulations; mixing will result in precipitation. TPN solutions containing phosphate and calcium are compatible depending upon the parenteral amino-acid formulation and its concentration.

Mechanism of Action Calcium moderates nerve and muscle performance via action potential excitation threshold regulation; it is necessary for maintaining the functional integrity of nervous, muscular, and skeletal systems and cell-membrane and capillary permeability.

Pharmacokinetics (Adult data unless noted) See Calcium Supplements on page 239.

Usual Dosage
Hypocalcemia: I.V.: Dosage expressed in mg of **calcium chloride**:
Manufacturer's recommendations: Children: 2.7-5 mg/kg/dose every 4-6 hours
Alternative pediatric dosing: Neonates, Infants, and Children: 10-20 mg/kg/dose, repeat every 4-6 hours if needed
Adults: 500 mg to 1 g/dose every 6 hours

Cardiac arrest in the presence of hyperkalemia or hypocalcemia, magnesium toxicity, or calcium antagonist toxicity: I.V., I.O.: Dosage expressed in mg of **calcium chloride**:
Neonates, Infants, and Children: 20 mg/kg; may repeat in 10 minutes if necessary; if effective, consider I.V. infusion of 20-50 mg/kg/hour
Adults: 500-1000 mg; may repeat as necessary; **Note:** Routine use in cardiac arrest is not recommended due to the lack of improved survival (see ACLS Guidelines, 2005).

Hypocalcemia secondary to citrated blood infusion: I.V.: Give 0.45 mEq **elemental** calcium for each 100 mL citrated blood infused (for conversion factor, see Additional Information)

Tetany: I.V.: Dose expressed in mg of **calcium chloride**:
Neonates, Infants, and Children: 10 mg/kg over 5-10 minutes; may repeat after 6 hours or follow with an infusion with a maximum dose of 200 mg/kg/day
Adults: 1 g over 10-30 minutes; may repeat after 6 hours

Dosage adjustment in renal impairment: Cl_{cr} <25 mL/minute may require dosage adjustment depending upon serum calcium level

Administration Parenteral:
I.V.: For direct I.V. injection infuse slow IVP over 3-5 minutes or at a maximum rate of 50-100 mg calcium chloride/minute; in situations of cardiac arrest, calcium chloride may be administered over 10-20 seconds
I.V. infusion: Dilute to a final concentration of 20 mg/mL; administer 45-90 mg calcium chloride/kg over 1 hour; 0.6-1.2 mEq calcium/kg over 1 hour
Do not inject calcium salts I.M. or administer SubQ since severe necrosis and sloughing may occur; extravasation of calcium can result in severe necrosis and tissue sloughing. Do not use scalp vein or small hand or foot veins for I.V. administration. Not for endotracheal administration.

Monitoring Parameters See Calcium Supplements on page 239.

Reference Range See Calcium Supplements on page 239.

Additional Information 1 g calcium chloride = 270 mg elemental calcium = 13.5 mEq calcium. Due to a poor correlation between the serum ionized calcium (free) and total serum calcium, particularly in states of low albumin or acid/base imbalances, direct measurement of ionized calcium is recommended. If ionized calcium is unavailable, in low albumin states, the corrected **total** serum calcium may be estimated by this equation (assuming a normal albumin of 4 g/dL); corrected total calcium = total serum calcium + 0.8(4 - measured serum albumin)

Dosage Forms Excipient information presented when available (limited, particularly for generics); consult specific product labeling.
Injection, solution [preservative free]: 10% (10 mL) [equivalent to elemental calcium 27.2 mg (1.36 mEq)/mL]
Injection, solution: 10% (10 mL) [equivalent to elemental calcium 27.2 mg (1.36 mEq)/mL]

References
ECC Committee and Subcommittees and Task Forces of the American Heart Association, "2005 American Heart Association Guidelines for Cardiopulmonary Resuscitation and Emergency Cardiovascular Care," *Circulation*, 2005, 112(24 Suppl):IV1-203.

Calcium Citrate (KAL see um SIT rate)

Medication Safety Issues
Sound-alike/look-alike issues:
Citracal® may be confused with Citrucel®

U.S. Brand Names Cal-C-Caps [OTC]; Cal-Cee [OTC]; Cal-Citrate-225; Citracal® Kosher [OTC] [DSC]

Canadian Brand Names Osteocit®

234

Therapeutic Category Calcium Salt; Electrolyte Supplement, Oral

Generic Available Yes

Use Treatment of hyperphosphatemia in end-stage renal failure; dietary supplement; prevention and treatment of calcium deficiency; adjunctive prevention and treatment of osteoporosis

Pregnancy Risk Factor C

Contraindications See Calcium Supplements on page 239.

Warnings See Calcium Supplements on page 239.

Precautions See Calcium Supplements on page 239.

Adverse Reactions See Calcium Supplements on page 239.

Drug Interactions

Avoid Concomitant Use There are no known interactions where it is recommended to avoid concomitant use.

Increased Effect/Toxicity

Calcium Citrate may increase the levels/effects of: Aluminum Hydroxide

The levels/effects of Calcium Citrate may be increased by: Thiazide Diuretics

Decreased Effect

Calcium Citrate may decrease the levels/effects of: Bisphosphonate Derivatives; Calcium Channel Blockers; DOBUTamine; Eltrombopag; Estramustine; Phosphate Supplements; Quinolone Antibiotics; Thyroid Products; Trientine

The levels/effects of Calcium Citrate may be decreased by: Trientine

Food Interactions See Calcium Supplements on page 239.

Stability Store at room temperature.

Mechanism of Action Calcium moderates nerve and muscle performance via action potential excitation threshold regulation; it is necessary for maintaining the functional integrity of nervous, muscular, and skeletal systems and cell-membrane and capillary permeability. Calcium citrate combines with dietary phosphate to form insoluble calcium phosphate which is excreted in feces and reduces phosphate absorption

Pharmacokinetics (Adult data unless noted) See Calcium Supplements on page 239.

Usual Dosage Oral:

Recommended daily allowance (RDA) and adequate intake: See Calcium Supplements on page 239.

Hypocalcemia (dose depends on clinical condition and serum calcium level): Dose expressed in mg of **elemental calcium:**

Neonates: 50-150 mg/kg/day in 4-6 divided doses; not to exceed 1 g/day

Children: 45-65 mg/kg/day in 4 divided doses

Adults: 1-2 g or more per day in 3-4 divided doses

Dietary supplement: Adults: 500 mg to 2 g divided 2-4 times/day

Adjunctive prevention and treatment of osteoporosis: Adults: 500 mg elemental calcium 2-3 times/day; recommended dosage includes dietary intake and should be adjusted depending upon the patient's diet; to improve absorption do not administer more than 500 mg **elemental calcium**/dose

Dosage adjustment in renal impairment: Cl$_{cr}$ <25 mL/minute may require dosage adjustment depending upon serum calcium level

Administration Oral: Administer with plenty of fluids; may administer without regard to food when using to treat/prevent deficiency conditions; administer with food when treating hyperphosphatemia or when administering granule formulation

Monitoring Parameters See Calcium Supplements on page 239.

Reference Range See Calcium Supplements on page 239.

Additional Information 1 g calcium citrate = 211mg elemental calcium = 10.6 mEq calcium. Due to a poor correlation between the serum ionized calcium (free) and total serum calcium, particularly in states of low albumin or acid/base imbalances, direct measurement of ionized calcium is recommended. If ionized calcium is unavailable, in low albumin states, the corrected **total** serum calcium may be estimated by this equation (assuming a normal albumin of 4 g/dL); corrected total calcium = total serum calcium + 0.8(4 - measured serum albumin)

Dosage Forms Excipient information presented when available (limited, particularly for generics); consult specific product labeling. [DSC] = Discontinued product

Capsule:

Cal-C-Caps: Elemental calcium 180 mg

Cal-Citrate-225: Elemental calcium 225 mg

Granules: Elemental calcium 760 mg/teaspoonful (480 g)

Tablet: Elemental calcium 200 mg, 250 mg

Cal-Cee: Elemental calcium 250 mg

Citracal® Kosher: Elemental calcium 200 mg [DSC]

◆ **Calcium Disodium Edetate** *see* Edetate CALCIUM Disodium *on page 487*

◆ **Calcium Disodium Versenate®** *see* Edetate CALCIUM Disodium *on page 487*

Calcium Glubionate (KAL see um gloo BYE oh nate)

Medication Safety Issues

Sound-alike/look-alike issues:

Calcium glubionate may be confused with calcium gluconate

U.S. Brand Names Calcionate [OTC]

Therapeutic Category Calcium Salt; Electrolyte Supplement, Oral

Generic Available Yes

Use Treatment and replacement of calcium deficiency; dietary supplement; adjunctive prevention and treatment of osteoporosis

Contraindications See Calcium Supplements on page 239.

Warnings See Calcium Supplements on page 239.

Precautions See Calcium Supplements on page 239.

Adverse Reactions See Calcium Supplements on page 239.

Drug Interactions

Avoid Concomitant Use There are no known interactions where it is recommended to avoid concomitant use.

Increased Effect/Toxicity

The levels/effects of Calcium Glubionate may be increased by: Thiazide Diuretics

Decreased Effect

Calcium Glubionate may decrease the levels/effects of: Bisphosphonate Derivatives; Calcium Channel Blockers; DOBUTamine; Eltrombopag; Estramustine; Phosphate Supplements; Quinolone Antibiotics; Thyroid Products; Trientine

The levels/effects of Calcium Glubionate may be decreased by: Trientine

Food Interactions See Calcium Supplements on page 239.

Stability Store at room temperature.

Mechanism of Action Calcium moderates nerve and muscle performance via action potential excitation threshold regulation; it is necessary for maintaining the functional integrity of nervous, muscular, and skeletal systems and cell-membrane and capillary permeability.

Pharmacokinetics (Adult data unless noted) See Calcium Supplements on page 239.

Usual Dosage Oral:

Recommended daily allowance (RDA) and adequate intake: See Calcium Supplements on page 239.

Hypocalcemia (dose depends on clinical condition and serum calcium level):

Dose expressed in mg of **elemental calcium**:

Neonates: 50-150 mg/kg/day in 4-6 divided doses; not to exceed 1 g/day

Children: 45-65 mg/kg/day in 4 divided doses

Adults: 1-2 g or more per day in 3-4 divided doses

Dose expressed in mg of **calcium glubionate**:

Neonates: 1200 mg/kg/day in 4-6 divided doses

Infants and Children: 600-2000 mg/kg/day in 4 divided doses up to a maximum of 9 g/day

Adults: 6-18 g/day in divided doses

Adjunctive prevention and treatment of osteoporosis: Adults: 500 mg **elemental calcium** 2-3 times/day; recommended dosage includes dietary intake and should be adjusted depending upon the patient's diet; to improve absorption do not administer more than 500 mg **elemental calcium**/dose

Dosage adjustment in renal impairment: Cl_{cr} <25 mL/ minute may require dosage adjustment depending upon serum calcium level

Administration Oral: Administer with plenty of fluids with or following meals; for phosphate binding, administer on an empty stomach before meals to optimize effectiveness

Monitoring Parameters See Calcium Supplements on page 239.

Reference Range See Calcium Supplements on page 239.

Additional Information 1 g calcium glubionate = 64 mg elemental calcium = 3.2 mEq calcium. Due to a poor correlation between the serum ionized calcium (free) and total serum calcium, particularly in states of low albumin or acid/base imbalances, direct measurement of ionized calcium is recommended. If ionized calcium is unavailable, in low albumin states, the corrected **total** serum calcium may be estimated by this equation (assuming a normal albumin of 4 g/dL); corrected total calcium = total serum calcium + 0.8(4 - measured serum albumin)

Dosage Forms Excipient information presented when available (limited, particularly for generics); consult specific product labeling.

Syrup:

Calcionate: 1.8 g/5 mL (480 mL) [equivalent to elemental calcium 115 mg/5 mL; contains benzoic acid; caramel and orange flavor]

Calcium Gluconate (KAL see um GLOO koe nate)

Medication Safety Issues

Sound-alike/look-alike issues:

Calcium gluconate may be confused with calcium glubionate

U.S. Brand Names Cal-G [OTC]; Cal-GLU™

Therapeutic Category Antidote, Hydrofluoric Acid; Calcium Salt; Electrolyte Supplement, Oral; Electrolyte Supplement, Parenteral

Generic Available Yes

Use Treatment and prevention of calcium depletion; treatment of hypocalcemic tetany; hypermagnesemia, cardiac disturbances of hyperkalemia, hypocalcemia, or calcium channel blocking agent toxicity; adjunctive prevention and treatment of osteoporosis; topical treatment of hydrofluoric acid burns

Pregnancy Risk Factor C

Pregnancy Considerations Reproduction studies have not been completed.

Lactation Enters breast milk

Breast-Feeding Considerations Endogenous calcium is excreted in breast milk.

Contraindications See Calcium Supplements on page 239.

Warnings See Calcium Supplements on page 239.

Precautions See Calcium Supplements on page 239.

Adverse Reactions See Calcium Supplements on page 239.

Drug Interactions

Avoid Concomitant Use There are no known interactions where it is recommended to avoid concomitant use.

Increased Effect/Toxicity

Calcium Gluconate may increase the levels/effects of: CefTRIAXone

The levels/effects of Calcium Gluconate may be increased by: Thiazide Diuretics

Decreased Effect

Calcium Gluconate may decrease the levels/effects of: Bisphosphonate Derivatives; Calcium Channel Blockers; DOBUTamine; Eltrombopag; Estramustine; Phosphate Supplements; Quinolone Antibiotics; Thyroid Products; Trientine

The levels/effects of Calcium Gluconate may be decreased by: Trientine

Food Interactions See Calcium Supplements on page 239.

Stability Store at room temperature; parenteral solutions are incompatible with bicarbonates, phosphates, and sulfate formulations; mixing will result in precipitation. TPN solutions containing phosphate and calcium are compatible depending upon the parenteral amino-acid formulation and its concentration.

Mechanism of Action Calcium moderates nerve and muscle performance via action potential excitation threshold regulation; it is necessary for maintaining the functional integrity of nervous, muscular, and skeletal systems and cell-membrane and capillary permeability.

Pharmacokinetics (Adult data unless noted) See Calcium Supplements on page 239.

Usual Dosage

Recommended daily allowance (RDA) and adequate intake: See Calcium Supplements on page 239.

Hypocalcemia (dose depends on clinical condition and serum calcium level): Oral:

Dose expressed in mg of **elemental calcium**:

Neonates: 50-150 mg/kg/day in 4-6 divided doses; not to exceed 1 g/day

Children: 45-65 mg/kg/day in 4 divided doses

Adults: 1-2 g or more per day in 3-4 divided doses

Dose expressed in mg of **calcium gluconate**:

Neonates: 500-1500 mg/kg/day in 4-6 divided doses

Infants and Children: 500-725 mg/kg/day in 3-4 divided doses

Adults: 500 mg to 2 g 2-4 times/day

Hypocalcemia (dose depends on clinical condition and serum calcium level): I.V.: Dose expressed in mg of **calcium gluconate**:

Neonates: 200-800 mg/kg/day as a continuous infusion or in 4 divided doses

Infants and Children: 200-500 mg/kg/day as a continuous infusion or in 4 divided doses

Adults: 2-15 g/day as a continuous infusion or in divided doses

Cardiac arrest in the presence of hyperkalemia or hypocalcemia, magnesium toxicity, or calcium antagonist toxicity: I.V., I.O.: Dosage expressed in mg of **calcium gluconate**:

Neonates, Infants, and Children: 60-100 mg/kg/dose (maximum: 3 g/dose); may repeat in 10 minutes if necessary; if effective, consider I.V. infusion

Adults: 500-800 mg (maximum: 3 g/dose); may repeat in 10 minutes if necessary

Hypocalcemia secondary to citrated blood infusion: I.V.: Give 0.45 mEq **elemental calcium** for each 100 mL citrated blood infused

Tetany: I.V.: Dose expressed in mg of **calcium gluconate**:

Neonates, Infants, and Children: 100-200 mg/kg/dose; over 5-10 minutes; may repeat after 6 hours or follow with an infusion with a maximum dose of 500 mg/kg/day

Adults: 1-3 g over 10-30 minutes; may repeat after 6 hours

Daily maintenance calcium: I.V.:

Neonates: 3-4 mEq/kg/day

Infants and Children <25kg: 1-2 mEq/kg/day

Children 25-45 kg: 0.5-1.5 mEq/kg/day

Children >45 kg and Adults: 0.2-0.3 mEq/kg/day or 10-20 mEq/day

Adjunctive prevention and treatment of osteoporosis: Oral: Adults: 500 mg **elemental calcium** 2-3 times/day; recommended dosage includes dietary intake and should be adjusted depending upon the patient's diet; to improve absorption, do not administer more than 500 mg **elemental calcium**/dose

Dosage adjustment in renal impairment: Cl_{cr} <25 mL/minute may require dosage adjustment depending upon serum calcium level

Hydrofluoric acid (HF) burns (HF concentration <20%): Topical: Various topical calcium preparations have been used anecdotally for treatment of dermal exposure to HF solutions; calcium gluconate at concentrations ranging from 2.5% to 33% has been used; a topical calcium gluconate preparation must be compounded (see Extemporaneous Preparations); apply topically as needed

Administration

Oral: Administer with plenty of fluids with or following meals; for phosphate-binding, administer on an empty stomach before meals to optimize effectiveness; powder may be added to food

Parenteral:

I.V.: For direct I.V. injection, infuse slow IVP over 3-5 minutes or at a maximum rate of 50-100 mg calcium gluconate/minute; in situations of cardiac arrest, calcium gluconate may be administered over 10-20 seconds

I.V. infusion: Dilute to 50 mg/mL and infuse at 120-240 mg/kg (0.6-1.2mEq calcium/kg) over 1 hour

Do not inject calcium salts I.M. or administer SubQ since severe necrosis and sloughing may occur; extravasation of calcium can result in severe necrosis and tissue sloughing. Do not use scalp vein or small hand or foot veins for I.V. administration. Not for endotracheal administration.

Topical: Massage calcium gluconate gel into exposed area for 15 minutes

Monitoring Parameters See Calcium Supplements on page 239.

Reference Range See Calcium Supplements on page 239.

Additional Information 1 g calcium gluconate = 90 mg elemental calcium = 4.5 mEq calcium. Due to a poor correlation between the serum ionized calcium (free) and total serum calcium, particularly in states of low albumin or acid/base imbalances, direct measurement of ionized calcium is recommended. If ionized calcium is unavailable, in low albumin states, the corrected **total** serum calcium may be estimated by this equation (assuming a normal albumin of 4 g/dL); corrected total calcium = total serum calcium + 0.8(4 - measured serum albumin)

Dosage Forms Excipient information presented when available (limited, particularly for generics); consult specific product labeling.

Capsule, oral:

Cal-G: 700 mg [equivalent to elemental calcium 65 mg; gluten free, wheat free]

Capsule, oral [preservative free]:

Cal-GLU™: 515 mg [equivalent to elemental calcium 50 mg; dye free, sugar free]

Injection, solution [preservative free]: 10% (10 mL, 50 mL, 100 mL, 200 mL) [100 mg/mL; equivalent to elemental calcium 9 mg/mL; calcium 0.46 mEq/mL]

Powder: 347 mg/tablespoonful (480 g)

Tablet: 500 mg [equivalent to elemental calcium 45 mg]; 650 mg [equivalent to elemental calcium 58.5 mg]; 975 mg [equivalent to elemental calcium 87.75 mg]

Extemporaneous Preparations Calcium gluconate gel: Crush 3.5 g calcium gluconate tablets into a fine powder; add to 5 oz tube of water-soluble surgical lubricant (eg, K-Y® Jelly) or add 3.5 g calcium gluconate injection to 5 oz of water-soluble surgical lubricant (calcium carbonate may be substituted; do not use calcium chloride due to potential for irritation)

Calcium Lactate (KAL see um LAK tate)

Therapeutic Category Calcium Salt; Electrolyte Supplement, Oral

Generic Available Yes

Use Prevention and treatment of calcium deficiency; dietary supplement; adjunctive prevention and treatment of osteoporosis

Pregnancy Risk Factor C

Contraindications See Calcium Supplements on page 239.

Warnings See Calcium Supplements on page 239.

Precautions See Calcium Supplements on page 239.

Adverse Reactions See Calcium Supplements on page 239.

Drug Interactions

Avoid Concomitant Use There are no known interactions where it is recommended to avoid concomitant use.

Increased Effect/Toxicity

The levels/effects of Calcium Lactate may be increased by: Thiazide Diuretics

Decreased Effect

Calcium Lactate may decrease the levels/effects of: Bisphosphonate Derivatives; Calcium Channel Blockers; DOBUTamine; Eltrombopag; Estramustine; Phosphate Supplements; Quinolone Antibiotics; Thyroid Products; Trientine

The levels/effects of Calcium Lactate may be decreased by: Trientine

Food Interactions See Calcium Supplements on page 239.

Stability Store at room temperature.

◀ **Mechanism of Action** Calcium moderates nerve and muscle performance via action potential excitation threshold regulation; it is necessary for maintaining the functional integrity of nervous, muscular, and skeletal systems and cell-membrane and capillary permeability.

Pharmacokinetics (Adult data unless noted) See Calcium Supplements on page 239.

Usual Dosage Oral:
Recommended daily allowance (RDA) and Adequate Intake: See Calcium Supplements on page 239.
Hypocalcemia (dose depends on clinical condition and serum calcium level):
Dose expressed in mg of **elemental calcium**:
Neonates: 50-150 mg/kg/day in 4-6 divided doses; not to exceed 1 g/day
Children: 45-65 mg/kg/day in 4 divided doses
Adults: 1-2 g or more per day in 3-4 divided doses
Dose expressed in mg of **calcium lactate**:
Neonates and Infants: 400-500 mg/kg/day divided every 4-6 hours
Children: 500 mg/kg/day divided every 6-8 hours; maximum daily dose: 9 g
Adults: 1.5-3 g/day divided every 8 hours; maximum daily dose: 9 g
Adjunctive prevention and treatment of osteoporosis: Adults: 500 mg elemental calcium 2-3 times/day; recommended dosage includes dietary intake and should be adjusted depending upon the patient's diet; to improve absorption do not administer more than 500 mg **elemental calcium**/dose

Dosage adjustment in renal impairment: Cl$_{cr}$ <25 mL/minute may require dosage adjustment depending upon serum calcium level

Administration Oral: Administer with plenty of fluids with or following meals

Monitoring Parameters See Calcium Supplements on page 239.

Reference Range See Calcium Supplements on page 239.

Additional Information 1 g calcium lactate = 130 mg elemental calcium = 6.5 mEq calcium. Due to a poor correlation between the serum ionized calcium (free) and total serum calcium, particularly in states of low albumin or acid/base imbalances, direct measurement of ionized calcium is recommended. If ionized calcium is unavailable, in low albumin states, the corrected **total** serum calcium may be estimated by this equation (assuming a normal albumin of 4 g/dL); corrected total calcium = total serum calcium + 0.8(4 - measured serum albumin)

Dosage Forms Excipient information presented when available (limited, particularly for generics); consult specific product labeling.
Tablet: 650 mg [equivalent to elemental calcium 84.5 mg]

◆ **Calcium Leucovorin** see Leucovorin Calcium on page 804

Calcium Phosphate (Tribasic)
(KAL see um FOS fate tri BAY sik)

U.S. Brand Names Posture® [OTC]

Therapeutic Category Calcium Salt; Electrolyte Supplement, Oral

Generic Available No

Use Prevention and treatment of calcium deficiency; dietary supplement; adjunctive prevention and treatment of osteoporosis

Contraindications See Calcium Supplements on page 239.

Warnings See Calcium Supplements on page 239. Avoid use of calcium phosphate, tribasic, in dialysis patients with hypercalcemia, or whose plasma PTH concentrations are <150 pg/mL on two consecutive measurements.

Precautions See Calcium Supplements on page 239.

Adverse Reactions See Calcium Supplements on page 239.

Drug Interactions

Avoid Concomitant Use There are no known interactions where it is recommended to avoid concomitant use.

Increased Effect/Toxicity
The levels/effects of Calcium Phosphate (Tribasic) may be increased by: Bisphosphonate Derivatives; Thiazide Diuretics

Decreased Effect
Calcium Phosphate (Tribasic) may decrease the levels/ effects of: Bisphosphonate Derivatives; Calcium Channel Blockers; DOBUTamine; Eltrombopag; Estramustine; Phosphate Supplements; Quinolone Antibiotics; Thyroid Products; Trientine

The levels/effects of Calcium Phosphate (Tribasic) may be decreased by: Antacids; Calcium Salts; Iron Salts; Magnesium Salts; Sucralfate; Trientine

Food Interactions See Calcium Supplements on page 239.

Stability Store at room temperature.

Mechanism of Action Calcium moderates nerve and muscle performance via action potential excitation threshold regulation; it is necessary for maintaining the functional integrity of nervous, muscular, and skeletal systems and cell-membrane and capillary permeability.

Pharmacokinetics (Adult data unless noted) See Calcium Supplements on page 239.

Usual Dosage Oral:
Recommended daily allowance (RDA) and adequate intake: See Calcium Supplements on page 239.
Hypocalcemia (dose depends on clinical condition and serum calcium level): Dose expressed in mg of **elemental calcium**:
Children: 45-65 mg/kg/day in 4 divided doses
Adults: 1-2 g or more per day in 3-4 divided doses
Adjunctive prevention and treatment of osteoporosis: Adults: 500 mg **elemental calcium** 2-3 times/day; recommended dosage includes dietary intake and should be adjusted depending upon the patient's diet; to improve absorption do not administer more than 500 mg **elemental calcium**/dose

Dosage adjustment in renal impairment: Cl$_{cr}$ <25 mL/minute may require dosage adjustment depending upon serum calcium level

Monitoring Parameters See Calcium Supplements on page 239.

Reference Range See Calcium Supplements on page 239.

Additional Information 1 g calcium phosphate, tribasic = 390 mg elemental calcium = 19.3 mEq calcium. Due to a poor correlation between the serum ionized calcium (free) and total serum calcium, particularly in states of low albumin or acid/base imbalances, direct measurement of ionized calcium is recommended. If ionized calcium is unavailable, in low albumin states, the corrected **total** serum calcium may be estimated by this equation (assuming a normal albumin of 4 g/dL); corrected total calcium = total serum calcium + 0.8(4 - measured serum albumin)

Dosage Forms Excipient information presented when available (limited, particularly for generics); consult specific product labeling.
Caplet:
Posture®: Calcium 600 mg and phosphorus 280 mg [as tricalcium phosphate]

Calcium Supplements (KAL see um SUP la ments)

Related Information
Calcium Acetate *on page 231*
Calcium Carbonate *on page 232*
Calcium Chloride *on page 233*
Calcium Citrate *on page 234*
Calcium Glubionate *on page 235*
Calcium Gluconate *on page 236*
Calcium Lactate *on page 237*
Calcium Phosphate (Tribasic) *on page 238*

U.S. Brand Names Alcalak [OTC]; Alka-Mints® [OTC]; Amitone® [OTC] [DSC]; Cal-Citrate® 250 [OTC]; Cal-Gest [OTC]; Cal-Mint [OTC]; Calcarb 600 [OTC]; Cal-Chew® [OTC]; Calci-Mix® [OTC]; Caltrate® 600 [OTC]; Children's Pepto [OTC]; Chooz® [OTC]; Citracal® [OTC]; Florical® [OTC]; Maalox® Quick Dissolve [OTC]; Mylanta® Children's [OTC]; Nephro-Calci® [OTC]; Nutralox® [OTC]; Os-Cal® 500 [OTC]; Oysco® 500 [OTC]; Oyst-Cal 500 [OTC]; PhosLo®; Posture®; Rolaids® Softchews [OTC]; Titralac® Extra Strength [OTC]; Titralac® [OTC]; Tums® E-X [OTC]; Tums® Extra Strength Sugar Free [OTC]; Tums® Smoothies™ [OTC]; Tums® Ultra® [OTC]; Tums® [OTC]

Therapeutic Category Antacid; Antidote, Hydrofluoric Acid; Calcium Salt; Electrolyte Supplement, Oral; Electrolyte Supplement, Parenteral

Generic Available Yes

Use
Treatment and prevention of calcium depletion:

Injection: See Calcium Acetate on page 231, Calcium Chloride on page 233, and Calcium Gluconate on page 236

Oral: See Calcium Glubionate on page 235, Calcium Citrate on page 234, Calcium Carbonate on page 232, and Calcium Lactate on page 237

Relief of acid indigestion, heartburn: See Calcium Carbonate on page 232

Treatment of hypocalcemic tetany; hypermagnesemia, cardiac disturbances of hyperkalemia, hypocalcemia, or calcium channel blocking agent toxicity: See Calcium Chloride on page 233 and Calcium Gluconate on page 236

Treatment and prevention of hyperphosphatemia in chronic renal failure: See Calcium Acetate on page 231, Calcium Carbonate on page 232, and Calcium Citrate on page 234

Adjunctive prevention and treatment of osteoporosis: See Calcium Carbonate on page 232, Calcium Citrate on page 234, Calcium Glubionate on page 235, Calcium Gluconate on page 236, and Calcium Lactate on page 237

Topical treatment of hydrofluoric acid burns: See Calcium Carbonate on page 232 and Calcium Gluconate on page 236

Pregnancy Risk Factor C

Contraindications Hypersensitivity to calcium formulation (see Warnings); hypercalcemia, renal calculi, ventricular fibrillation

Warnings Multiple salt forms of calcium exist; close attention must be paid to the salt form when ordering and administering calcium; incorrect selection or substitution of one salt for another without proper dosage adjustment may result in serious over- or under-dosing. Some products may contain tartrazine which may cause allergic reactions in susceptible individuals. Avoid use of calcium-containing phosphate binders (calcium acetate or phosphate) in dialysis patients with hypercalcemia or whose plasma PTH concentrations are <150 pg/mL on two consecutive measurements. Milk-Alkali syndrome (hypercalcemia, metabolic alkalosis, and rarely, renal insufficiency) has been associated with ingestion of large quantities of milk concomitantly with calcium carbonate; patients with renal impairment or dehydration and electrolyte imbalance are at increased risk for developing this syndrome; monitor calcium serum levels periodically

Precautions Use cautiously in patients with sarcoidosis, respiratory failure, acidosis, renal or cardiac disease; avoid too rapid I.V. administration; avoid extravasation; use with caution in digitalized patients; some products may contain aspartame which is metabolized to phenylalanine and must be avoided in patients with phenylketonuria

Adverse Reactions
Cardiovascular: Vasodilation, hypotension, bradycardia, cardiac arrhythmias, ventricular fibrillation, syncope
Central nervous system: Headache, mental confusion, dizziness, lethargy, coma
Dermatologic: Erythema
Endocrine & metabolic: Hypercalcemia, milk-alkali syndrome (calcium carbonate), hypophosphatemia, hypercalciuria, hypomagnesemia
Gastrointestinal: Constipation, nausea, vomiting, xerostomia, serum amylase elevated
Local: Tissue necrosis (I.V. administration)
Neuromuscular & skeletal: Muscle weakness

Food Interactions Do not give orally with bran, foods high in oxalates (spinach, sweet potatoes, rhubarb, beans), or phytic acid (unleavened bread, raw beans, seeds, nuts, grains, soy isolates) which may decrease calcium absorption; minimize administration with dairy products (when treating deficiency state) as this will reduce absorption

Stability Store at room temperature; parenteral solutions are incompatible with bicarbonates, phosphates, and sulfate formulations; mixing will result in precipitation. TPN solutions containing phosphate and calcium are compatible depending upon the parenteral amino-acid formulation and its concentration.

Mechanism of Action Calcium moderates nerve and muscle performance via action potential excitation threshold regulation; it is necessary for maintaining the functional integrity of nervous, muscular, and skeletal systems and cell-membrane and capillary permeability. Calcium acetate and carbonate combines with dietary phosphate to form insoluble calcium phosphate which is excreted in feces and reduces phosphate absorption. Neutralizes acidity of stomach (carbonate salt).

Pharmacokinetics (Adult data unless noted)
Absorption: 25% to 35%; varies with age (infants 60%, prepubertal children 28%, pubertal children 34%, young adults 25%); decreased absorption occurs in patients with achlorhydria, renal osteodystrophy, steatorrhea, or uremia
Protein binding: 45%
Elimination: Primarily in the feces as unabsorbed calcium

Usual Dosage See individual calcium monographs.

Recommended daily allowance (RDA): Dosage is in terms of elemental calcium:
<6 months: 400 mg/day
6-12 months: 600 mg/day
1-10 years: 800 mg/day
11-24 years: 1200 mg/day
Adults >24 years: 800 mg/day

Adequate intake (1997 National Academy of Science Recommendations): **Dosage is in terms of elemental calcium:**
0-6 months: 210 mg/day
7-12 months: 270 mg/day
1-3 years: 500 mg/day
4-8 years: 800 mg/day
9-18 years: 1300 mg/day
19-50 years: 1000 mg/day
>50 years: 1200 mg/day

◄ Oral: **Note:** For comparison information of calcium salts, see table.

Elemental Calcium Content of Calcium Salts

Calcium Salt	Elemental Calcium (mg/1 g of salt form)	Calcium (mEq/g)	Approximate Equivalent Doses (mg of calcium salt)
Calcium acetate	250	12.7	354
Calcium carbonate	400	20	225
Calcium chloride	270	13.5	330
Calcium citrate	211	10.6	425
Calcium glubionate	64	3.2	1400
Calcium gluconate	90	4.5	1000
Calcium lactate	130	6.5	700
Calcium phosphate, tribasic	390	19.3	233

Administration See individual calcium monographs.

Monitoring Parameters Serum calcium (ionized calcium preferred if available, see Additional Information), phosphate, magnesium, heart rate, ECG

Reference Range
Calcium: Newborns: 7-12 mg/dL; 0-2 years: 8.8-11.2 mg/dL; 2 years to adults: 9-11 mg/dL
Calcium, ionized, whole blood: 4.4-5.4 mg/dL

Patient Information May cause dry mouth

Additional Information Due to a poor correlation between the serum ionized calcium (free) and total serum calcium, particularly in states of low albumin or acid/base imbalances, direct measurement of ionized calcium is recommended. If ionized calcium is unavailable, in low albumin states, the corrected **total** serum calcium may be estimated by this equation (assuming a normal albumin of 4 g/dL); corrected total calcium = total serum calcium + 0.8 (4 - measured serum albumin)

Dosage Forms See individual monographs.

Extemporaneous Preparations
Calcium gluconate gel: Crush 3.5 g calcium gluconate tablets into a fine powder; add to 5 oz tube of water-soluble surgical lubricant (eg, K-Y® Jelly) or add 3.5 g calcium gluconate injection to 5 oz of water-soluble surgical lubricant (calcium carbonate may be substituted; do not use calcium chloride due to potential for irritation)
Calcium carbonate slurry: 32.5% slurry can be prepared by triturating ten 650 mg tablets into a fine powder and adding 20 mL of water-soluble lubricant gel (eg, K-Y® Jelly)

References
"2005 American Heart Association (AHA) Guidelines for Cardiopulmonary Resuscitation (CPR) and Emergency Cardiovascular Care (ECC) of Pediatric and Neonatal Patients: Pediatric Advanced Life Support," Pediatrics, 2006, 117(5):1005-28.
Baker SS, Cochran WJ, Flores CA, et al, "American Academy of Pediatrics. Committee on Nutrition: Calcium Requirements of Infants, Children, and Adolescents," Pediatrics, 1999, 104(5):1152-7.
"Dietary Reference Intakes for Calcium, Phosphorus, Magnesium, Vitamin D, and Fluoride. Standing Committee on the Scientific Evaluation of Dietary Reference Intakes, Food and Nutrition Board, Institute of Medicine," National Academy of Sciences, Washington, DC: National Academy Press, 1997.
NIH Consensus Conference, "Optimal Calcium Intake," JAMA, 1994, 272(24):1942-8.

♦ **Caldecort® [OTC]** see Hydrocortisone on page 685
♦ **Caldolor™** see Ibuprofen on page 702

Calfactant (cal FAC tant)

U.S. Brand Names Infasurf®

Therapeutic Category Lung Surfactant

Generic Available No

Use Prevention and treatment of respiratory distress syndrome (RDS) in premature infants
Prophylactic therapy: Infants <29 weeks at significant risk for RDS
Treatment: Infants ≤72 hours of age with RDS (confirmed by clinical and radiologic findings and requiring endotracheal intubation)

Warnings Rapidly affects oxygenation and lung compliance and should be restricted to a highly supervised use in a clinical setting with immediate availability of clinicians experienced with intubation and ventilatory management of premature infants; if transient episodes of bradycardia and decreased oxygen saturation occur, discontinue the dosing procedure and initiate measures to alleviate the condition; produces rapid improvement in lung oxygenation and compliance that may require immediate reductions in ventilator settings and FiO_2; for intratracheal administration only

Precautions Transient episodes of reflux of calfactant into the endotracheal tube, cyanosis, bradycardia, or airway obstruction have occurred during dosing procedures; such episodes may require stopping administration and taking appropriate measures to alleviate the condition before resuming therapy

Adverse Reactions Most adverse reactions occur during the dosing procedure
Cardiovascular: Bradycardia, cyanosis
Respiratory: Airway obstruction, pneumothorax, pulmonary hemorrhage, apnea

Drug Interactions

Avoid Concomitant Use There are no known interactions where it is recommended to avoid concomitant use.

Increased Effect/Toxicity There are no known significant interactions involving an increase in effect.

Decreased Effect There are no known significant interactions involving a decrease in effect.

Stability Refrigerate; protect from light; unopened, unused warmed vials of calfactant may be returned to refrigerator within 24 hours for future use; repeated warming to room temperature should be avoided

Mechanism of Action Replaces deficient or ineffective endogenous lung surfactant in neonates with RDS or in neonates at risk of developing RDS; surfactant prevents the alveoli from collapsing during expiration by lowering surface tension between air and alveolar surfaces

Usual Dosage Intratracheal: Neonates: 3 mL/kg every 12 hours up to a total of 3 doses; repeat doses have been administered as early as 6 hours after the previous dose for a total of up to four doses (if the infant was still intubated and required at least 30% inspired oxygen to maintain a PaO_2 ≤80 torr)

Administration Intratracheal: Gently swirl to redisperse suspension; do not shake; administer dosage divided into two aliquots of 1.5 mL/kg each into the endotracheal tube; after each instillation, reposition the infant with either the right or left side dependent; administration is made while ventilation is continued over 20-30 breaths for each aliquot, with small bursts timed only during the inspiratory cycles; a pause followed by evaluation of the respiratory status and repositioning should separate the two aliquots; calfactant dosage has also been divided into four equal aliquots and administered with repositioning in four different positions (prone, supine, right and left lateral)

Monitoring Parameters Continuous heart rate and transcutaneous O_2 saturation should be monitored during administration; frequent ABG sampling is necessary to prevent postdosing hyperoxia and hypocarbia

Dosage Forms Excipient information presented when available (limited, particularly for generics); consult specific product labeling.

Suspension, intratracheal [preservative free; calf lung derived]:

Infasurf®: 35 mg/mL (3 mL, 6 mL)

References

Hudak ML, Martin DJ, Egan EA, et al, "A Multicenter Randomized Masked Comparison Trail of Synthetic Surfactant Versus Calf Lung Surfactant Extract in the Prevention of Neonatal Respiratory Distress Syndrome," Pediatrics, 1997, 100(1):39-50.

Bloom BT, Kattwinkel J, Hall RT, et al, "Comparison of Infasurf® (Calf Lung Surfactant Extract) to Survanta® (Beractant) in the Treatment and Prevention of Respiratory Distress Syndrome," Pediatrics, 1997, 100(1):31-8.

Capsaicin (kap SAY sin)

Medication Safety Issues
Sound-alike/look-alike issues:
Zostrix® may be confused with Zestril®, Zovirax®

U.S. Brand Names Capzasin-HP® [OTC]; Capzasin-P® [OTC]; DiabetAid Pain and Tingling Relief [OTC]; Qutenza™; Salonpas® Hot [OTC]; Zostrix® Neuropathy [OTC]; Zostrix® [OTC]; Zostrix®-HP [OTC]

Canadian Brand Names Zostrix®; Zostrix® H.P.

Therapeutic Category Analgesic, Topical; Topical Skin Product

Generic Available Yes: Cream

Use Topical treatment of pain associated with postherpetic neuralgia, rheumatoid arthritis, osteoarthritis, diabetic neuropathy, and postsurgical pain; also used for treatment of pain associated with psoriasis, chronic neuralgias unresponsive to other forms of therapy, and intractable pruritus

Pregnancy Risk Factor C

Contraindications Hypersensitivity to capsaicin or any component

Warnings Avoid contact with eyes, mucous membrane, or with damaged or irritated skin

Precautions Since warm water or excessive sweating may intensify the localized burning sensation after capsaicin application, the affected area should not be tightly bandaged or exposed to direct sunlight or a heat lamp

Adverse Reactions
Dermatologic: Erythema
Local: Itching, burning, or stinging sensation
Respiratory: Cough

Drug Interactions
Metabolism/Transport Effects Substrate of CYP2E1 (minor)
Avoid Concomitant Use There are no known interactions where it is recommended to avoid concomitant use.
Increased Effect/Toxicity There are no known significant interactions involving an increase in effect.
Decreased Effect There are no known significant interactions involving a decrease in effect.

Mechanism of Action Induces release of substance P, the principal chemomediator of pain impulses from the periphery to the CNS, from peripheral sensory neurons. After repeated application, capsaicin depletes the neuron of substance P and prevents reaccumulation.

Pharmacodynamics
Onset of action: Pain relief is usually seen within 14-28 days of regular topical application; maximal response may require 4-6 weeks of continuous therapy
Duration: Several hours

Usual Dosage Children ≥2 years and Adults: Topical: Apply to affected area at least 3-4 times/day; application frequency less than 3-4 times/day prevents the total depletion, inhibition of synthesis, and transport of substance P resulting in decreased clinical efficacy and increased local discomfort

Administration Topical: Should not be applied to wounds or damaged skin; avoid eye and mucous membrane exposure

Patient Information For external use only. Avoid washing treated areas for 30 minutes after application

Nursing Implications Wash hands with soap and water after applying to avoid spreading cream to eyes or other sensitive areas of the body

Additional Information In patients with severe and persistent local discomfort, pretreatment with topical lidocaine 5% ointment or concurrent oral analgesics for the first 2 weeks of therapy have been effective in alleviating the initial burning sensation and enabling continuation of topical capsaicin

Product Availability
Qutenza™: FDA approved in November 2009; availability anticipated first half of 2010
Qutenza™ is a high-concentration capsaicin (8%) patch indicated for the management of neuropathic pain associated with postherpetic neuralgia.

Dosage Forms Excipient information presented when available (limited, particularly for generics); consult specific product labeling. [DSC] = Discontinued product

Cream, topical: 0.025% (60 g); 0.075% (60 g)
 Capzasin-P®: 0.025% (45 g)
 Capzasin-HP®: 0.075% (45 g)
 Zostrix®: 0.025% (60 g)
 Zostrix®-HP: 0.075% (60 g)
 Zostrix® Neuropathy: 0.25% (60 g) [in Lidocare™
 vehicle]
Lotion, topical:
 DiabetAid Pain and Tingling Relief: 0.025% (120 mL)
Patch, topical:
 Salonpas® Hot: 0.025% (1s) [contains natural rubber/
 natural latex in packaging]

References
Bernstein JE, Korman NJ, Bickers DR, et al, "Topical Capsaicin Treatment of Chronic Postherpetic Neuralgia," *J Am Acad Dermatol*, 1989, 21(2 Pt 1):265-70.

Captopril (KAP toe pril)

Medication Safety Issues
Sound-alike/look-alike issues:
 Captopril may be confused with calcitriol, Capitrol®,
 carvedilol

International issues:
 Acepril [Great Britain] may be confused with Accupril®
 which is a brand name for quinapril in the U.S.
 Acepril: Brand name for captopril [Great Britain], but also
 the brand name for enalapril [Hungary, Switzerland];
 lisinopril [Malaysia]

Related Information
Antihypertensive Agents by Class *on page 1481*

U.S. Brand Names Capoten® [DSC]
Canadian Brand Names Alti-Captopril; Apo-Capto®;
 Capoten®; Gen-Captopril; Mylan-Captopril; Novo-Capto-
 pril; Nu-Capto; PMS-Captopril
Therapeutic Category Angiotensin-Converting Enzyme
 (ACE) Inhibitor; Antihypertensive Agent
Generic Available Yes
Use Management of hypertension; treatment of CHF; in
 post-MI patients, improves survival in clinically stable
 patients with left-ventricular dysfunction
Pregnancy Risk Factor C (1st trimester); D (2nd and 3rd
 trimesters)
Pregnancy Considerations Due to adverse events
 observed in some animal studies, captopril is considered
 pregnancy category C during the first trimester. Based on
 human data, captopril is considered pregnancy category D
 if used during the second and third trimesters (per the
 manufacturer); however, one study suggests that fetal
 injury may occur at anytime during pregnancy. Captopril
 crosses the placenta and may affect ACE activity in the
 fetus. First trimester exposure to ACE inhibitors may cause
 major congenital malformations. An increased risk of
 cardiovascular and/or central nervous system malformations was observed in one study; however, an increased
 risk of teratogenic events was not observed in other
 studies. Second and third trimester use of an ACE inhibitor
 is associated with oligohydramnios. Oligohydramnios due
 to decreased fetal renal function may lead to fetal limb
 contractures, craniofacial deformation, and hypoplastic
 lung development. The use of ACE inhibitors during the
 second and third trimesters is also associated with anuria,
 hypotension, renal failure (reversible or irreversible), skull
 hypoplasia, and death in the fetus/neonate. Chronic
 maternal hypertension itself is also associated with
 adverse events in the fetus/infant. ACE inhibitors are not
 recommended during pregnancy to treat maternal hypertension or heart failure. Those who are planning a
 pregnancy should be considered for other medication
 options if an ACE inhibitor is currently prescribed or the
 ACE inhibitor should be discontinued as soon as possible
 once pregnancy is detected. The exposed fetus should be
 monitored for fetal growth, amniotic fluid volume, and
 organ formation. Infants exposed to an ACE inhibitor *in
 utero*, especially during the second and third trimester,
 should be monitored for hyperkalemia, hypotension, and
 oliguria.

**[U.S. Boxed Warning]: Based on human data, ACE
inhibitors can cause injury and death to the developing fetus when used in the second and third
trimesters. ACE inhibitors should be discontinued as
soon as possible once pregnancy is detected.**

Lactation Enters breast milk/not recommended (AAP rates
 "compatible")

Breast-Feeding Considerations Captopril is excreted in
 breast milk. Breast-feeding is not recommended by the
 manufacturer. The American Academy of Pediatrics
 considers captopril to be "usually compatible with breast-
 feeding."

Contraindications Hypersensitivity to captopril, any
 component, or other ACE inhibitors; patients with
 idiopathic or hereditary angioedema or a history of
 angioedema with previous ACE inhibitor use

Warnings Serious adverse effects including angioedema,
 anaphylactoid reactions, neutropenia, agranulocytosis,
 proteinuria, hypotension, and hepatic failure may occur
 (see Adverse Reactions). Angioedema can occur at any
 time during treatment (especially following first dose).
 Angioedema may occur in the head, neck, extremities, or
 intestines; angioedema of the larynx, glottis, or tongue may
 cause airway obstruction, especially in patients with a
 history of airway surgery; prolonged monitoring may be
 required, even in patients with swelling of only the tongue
 (ie, without respiratory distress) because treatment with
 corticosteroids and antihistamines may not be sufficient;
 very rare fatalities have occurred with angioedema of the
 larynx or tongue; appropriate treatment (eg, establishing
 patent airway and/or SubQ epinephrine) should be readily
 available for patients with angioedema of larynx, glottis, or
 tongue, in whom airway obstruction is likely to occur. Risk
 of neutropenia is increased 15 fold to 1 per 500 in patients
 with renal dysfunction, and increased to 3.7% in patients
 with both collagen vascular disease and renal dysfunction.

ACE inhibitors can cause injury and death to the
developing fetus when used during pregnancy. ACE
inhibitors should be discontinued as soon as possible
once pregnancy is detected **[U.S. Boxed Warning]**.
Neonatal hypotension, skull hypoplasia, anuria, renal
failure, death, oligohydramnios (associated with fetal limb
contractures, craniofacial deformities, hypoplastic lung
development), prematurity, intrauterine growth retardation,
patent ductus arteriosus, and death have been reported
with the use of ACE inhibitors, primarily in the second and
third trimesters. The risk of neonatal toxicity has been
considered less when ACE inhibitors are used in the first
trimester; however, major congenital malformations have
been reported. The cardiovascular and/or central nervous
systems are most commonly affected.

Precautions Use with caution and modify dosage in
 patients with renal impairment, especially those with
 severe renal artery stenosis; elevated BUN and serum
 creatinine may occur in these patients after decrease in
 blood pressure with captopril; dosage reduction of
 captopril or discontinuation of concurrent diuretic may be
 needed; control of blood pressure while maintaining
 adequate renal perfusion may not be possible in some of
 these patients. Use with caution in patients with collagen
 vascular disease and in patients with volume depletion.

Adverse Reactions
Cardiovascular: Hypotension, tachycardia

Central nervous system: Headache, dizziness, fatigue,
 insomnia, fever

Dermatologic: Rash, angioedema (see Warnings). **Note:** The relative risk of angioedema with ACE inhibitors is higher within the first 30 days of use (compared to >1 year of use), for Black Americans (compared to Whites), for lisinopril or enalapril (compared to captopril), and for patients previously hospitalized within 30 days (Brown, 1996).

Endocrine & metabolic: Hyperkalemia

Gastrointestinal: Ageusia

Hematologic: Neutropenia, agranulocytosis, eosinophilia

Hepatic: Cholestatic jaundice, fulminant hepatic necrosis (rare, but potentially fatal)

Renal: BUN and serum creatinine elevated, proteinuria, oliguria

Respiratory: Cough, dyspnea; **Note:** An isolated dry cough lasting >3 weeks was reported in 7 of 42 pediatric patients (17%) receiving ACE inhibitors (see von Vigier, 2000)

Miscellaneous: Anaphylactoid reactions

Drug Interactions

Metabolism/Transport Effects Substrate of CYP2D6 (major)

Avoid Concomitant Use There are no known interactions where it is recommended to avoid concomitant use.

Increased Effect/Toxicity

Captopril may increase the levels/effects of: Allopurinol; Amifostine; Antihypertensives; AzaTHIOprine; CycloSPORINE; CycloSPORINE (Systemic); Ferric Gluconate; Gold Sodium Thiomalate; Hypotensive Agents; Iron Dextran Complex; Lithium; RiTUXimab

The levels/effects of Captopril may be increased by: Angiotensin II Receptor Blockers; CYP2D6 Inhibitors (Moderate); CYP2D6 Inhibitors (Strong); Darunavir; Diazoxide; DPP-IV Inhibitors; Eplerenone; Everolimus; Herbs (Hypotensive Properties); Loop Diuretics; MAO Inhibitors; Pentoxifylline; Phosphodiesterase 5 Inhibitors; Potassium Salts; Potassium-Sparing Diuretics; Prostacyclin Analogues; Sirolimus; Temsirolimus; Thiazide Diuretics; Tolvaptan; Trimethoprim

Decreased Effect

The levels/effects of Captopril may be decreased by: Antacids; Aprotinin; Herbs (Hypertensive Properties); Methylphenidate; Nonsteroidal Anti-Inflammatory Agents; Peginterferon Alfa-2b; Salicylates; Yohimbine

Food Interactions Absorption of captopril may be reduced by food. Long-term use of captopril may result in a zinc deficiency which can result in a decrease in taste perception; zinc supplements may be used. Limit salt substitutes or potassium-rich diet. Avoid natural licorice (causes sodium and water retention and increases potassium loss)

Stability Unstable in aqueous solutions

Mechanism of Action Competitive inhibitor of angiotensin-converting enzyme (ACE); prevents conversion of angiotensin I to angiotensin II, a potent vasoconstrictor; results in lower levels of angiotensin II which causes an increase in plasma renin activity and a reduction in aldosterone secretion; a CNS mechanism may also be involved in hypotensive effect as angiotensin II increases adrenergic outflow from CNS; vasoactive kallikreins may be decreased in conversion to active hormones by ACE inhibitors, thus reducing blood pressure

Pharmacodynamics

Onset of action: Decrease in blood pressure within 15 minutes

Maximum effect: 60-90 minutes; may require several weeks of therapy before full hypotensive effect is seen

Duration: Dose-related

Pharmacokinetics (Adult data unless noted)

Absorption: 60% to 75%

Distribution: 7 L/kg

Protein binding: 25% to 30%

Metabolism: 50% metabolized

Half-life:

Infants with CHF: 3.3 hours; range: 1.2-12.4 hours

Children: 1.5 hours; range: 0.98-2.3 hours

Normal adults (dependent upon renal and cardiac function): 1.9 hours

Adults with CHF: 2.1 hours

Anuria: 20-40 hours

Time to peak serum concentration: Within 1-2 hours

Elimination: 95% excreted in urine in 24 hours

Usual Dosage Note: Dosage must be titrated according to patient's response; use lowest effective dose; lower doses (~1/2 of those listed) should be used in patients who are sodium and water depleted due to diuretic therapy; Oral:

Newborns and premature Neonates: Initial: 0.01 mg/kg/dose every 8-12 hours; titrate dose

Neonates: Initial: 0.05-0.1 mg/kg/dose every 8-24 hours; titrate dose up to 0.5 mg/kg/dose given every 6-24 hours

Infants: Initial: 0.15-0.3 mg/kg/dose; titrate dose upward to maximum of 6 mg/kg/day in 1-4 divided doses; usual required dose: 2.5-6 mg/kg/day

Children: Initial: 0.3-0.5 mg/kg/dose; titrate upward to maximum of 6 mg/kg/day in 2-4 divided doses

Older Children: Initial: 6.25-12.5 mg/dose every 12-24 hours; titrate upward to maximum of 6 mg/kg/day in 2-4 divided doses

Adolescents and Adults: Initial: 12.5-25 mg/dose given every 8-12 hours; increase by 25 mg/dose at 1-2 week intervals based on patient response; maximum dose: 450 mg/day; usual dosage range for hypertension (JNC 7): Adolescents ≥ 18 years and Adults: 25-100 mg/day in 2 divided doses

Dosing adjustment in renal impairment:

Cl_{cr} 10-50 mL/minute: Administer 75% of dose

Cl_{cr} <10 mL/minute: Administer 50% of dose

Administration Oral: Administer on an empty stomach 1 hour before meals or 2 hours after meals

Monitoring Parameters Blood pressure, BUN, serum creatinine, renal function, urine dipstick for protein, WBC with differential, serum potassium; monitor for angioedema and anaphylactoid reactions (see Warnings)

Patient Information Limit alcohol. Notify physician immediately if swelling of face, lips, tongue, or difficulty in breathing occurs; if these occur, do not take any more doses until a physician can be consulted. Notify physician if vomiting, diarrhea, excessive perspiration, dehydration, or persistent cough occurs. Do not use salt substitute (potassium-containing) without physician advice. May cause dizziness, fainting, and lightheadedness, especially in first week of therapy; sit and stand up slowly. May cause rash. Report sore throat, fever, other signs of infection, or other side effects. This medication may cause injury and death to the developing fetus when used during pregnancy; women of childbearing potential should be informed of potential risk; consult prescriber for appropriate contraceptive measures; this medication should be discontinued as soon as possible once pregnancy is detected (see Warnings).

Nursing Implications Discontinue if angioedema occurs; monitor blood pressure for hypotension within 1-3 hours after first dose or after a new higher dose

Additional Information Severe hypotension may occur in patients who are sodium and/or volume depleted

Dosage Forms Excipient information presented when available (limited, particularly for generics); consult specific product labeling. [DSC] = Discontinued product

Tablet, oral: 12.5 mg, 25 mg, 50 mg, 100 mg

Capoten® [DSC]: 12.5 mg, 25 mg, 50 mg [scored], 100 mg

Extemporaneous Preparations

Captopril has limited stability in aqueous preparations. The addition of an antioxidant [sodium ascorbate (using an injectable product) or ascorbic acid (using tablets)] has been shown to increase the stability of captopril in solution; captopril (1 mg/mL) in syrup with methylcellulose is stable for 7 days stored either at 4°C or 22°C. Captopril (1 mg/mL) in distilled water (no additives) is stable for 14 days if stored at 4°C and 7 days if stored at 22°C; captopril (1 mg/mL) with sodium ascorbate (5 mg/mL) in distilled water is stable for 56 days at 4°C and 14 days at 22°C (Nahata, 1994); captopril (1 mg/mL) with ascorbic acid (5 mg/mL) in distilled water is stable for 56 days at 4°C and 28 days at 22°C (Nahata, 1994a); captopril (1 mg/mL) in an undiluted syrup containing preservatives is stable for 30 days at 5°C in amber glass containers (Lye, 1997).

Captopril (0.75 mg/mL) in cherry syrup is stable for only 2 days in amber clear plastic containers stored at room temperature or under refrigeration; captopril (0.75 mg/mL) in either a 1:1 mixture of Ora-Sweet® and Ora-Plus® or a 1:1 mixture of Ora-Sweet® SF and Ora-Plus® is stable for 10 days or less depending on the storage temperature (see Allen, 1996).

Powder papers can also be made; powder papers are stable for 12 weeks when stored at room temperature (Taketomo, 1990).

Allen LV and Erickson MA, "Stability of Baclofen, Captopril, Diltiazem Hydrochloride, Dipyridamole, and Flecainide Acetate in Extemporaneously Compounded Oral Liquids," *Am J Health Sys Pharm*, 1996, 53 (18):2179-84.

Lye MY, Yow KL, Lim LY, et al, "Effects of Ingredients on Stability of Captopril in Extemporaneously Prepared Oral Liquids," *Am J Health Syst Pharm*, 1997, 54 (21):2483-7.

Nahata MC, Morosco RS, and Hipple TF, "Stability of Captopril in Three Liquid Dosage Forms," *Am J Hosp Pharm*, 1994, 51(1):95-6.

Nahata MC, Morosco RS, and Hipple TF, "Stability of Captopril in Liquid Containing Ascorbic Acid or Sodium Ascorbate," *Am J Hosp Pharm*, 1994a, 51(13):1707-8.

Taketomo CK, Chu SA, Cheng MH, et al, "Stability of Captopril in Powder Papers Under Three Storage Conditions," *Am J Hosp Pharm*, 1990, 47(8):1799-801.

References

Brown NJ, Ray WA, Snowden M, et al, "Black Americans Have an Increased Rate of Angiotensin-Converting Enzyme Inhibitor-Associated Angioedema," *Clin Pharmacol Ther*, 1996, 60(1):8-13.

Chobanian AV, Bakris GL, Black HR, et al, "The Seventh Report of the Joint National Committee on Prevention, Detection, Evaluation, and Treatment of High Blood Pressure: The JNC 7 Report," *JAMA*, 2003, 289(19):2560-72.

Friedman WF and George BL, "New Concepts and Drugs in the Treatment of Congestive Heart Failure," *Pediatr Clin North Am*, 1984, 31(6):1197-227.

Levy M, Koren G, Klein J, et al, "Captopril Pharmacokinetics, Blood Pressure Response and Plasma Renin Activity in Normotensive Children With Renal Scarring," *Dev Pharmacol Ther*, 1991, 16 (4):185-93.

Mirkin BL and Newman TJ, "Efficacy and Safety of Captopril in the Treatment of Severe Childhood Hypertension: Report of the International Collaborative Study Group," *Pediatrics*, 1985, 75(6):1091-100.

National High Blood Pressure Education Program Working Group on High Blood Pressure in Children and Adolescents, "The Fourth Report on the Diagnosis, Evaluation, and Treatment of High Blood Pressure in Children and Adolescents," *Pediatrics*, 2004, 114(2 Suppl):555-76.

Pereira CM, Tam YK, Collins-Nakai RL, "The Pharmacokinetics of Captopril in Infants With Congestive Heart Failure," *Ther Drug Monit*, 1991, 13(3):209-14.

von Vigier RO, Mozzettini S, Truttmann AC, et al, "Cough is Common in Children Prescribed Converting Enzyme Inhibitors," *Nephron*, 2000, 84(1):98.

◆ **Capzasin-HP® [OTC]** *see* Capsaicin *on page 241*

◆ **Capzasin-P® [OTC]** *see* Capsaicin *on page 241*

◆ **Carac®** *see* Fluorouracil *on page 598*

◆ **Carafate®** *see* Sucralfate *on page 1296*

◆ **Carapres® (Can)** *see* CloNIDine *on page 338*

CarBAMazepine (kar ba MAZ e peen)

Medication Safety Issues

Sound-alike/look-alike issues:

CarBAMazepine may be confused with OXcarbazepine
Carbatrol® may be confused with Cartrol®
Epitol® may be confused with Epinal®
Tegretol®, Tegretol®-XR may be confused with Mebaral®, Toprol-XL®, Toradol®, Trental®

Related Information

Antiepileptic Drugs *on page 1693*
Serotonin Syndrome *on page 1695*
Therapeutic Drug Monitoring: Blood Sampling Time Guidelines *on page 1704*

U.S. Brand Names Carbatrol®; Epitol®; Equetro®; Tegretol®; Tegretol®-XR

Canadian Brand Names Apo-Carbamazepine®; Bio-Carbamazepine; Carbamazepine; Dom-Carbamazepine; Gen-Carbamazepine CR; Mapezine®; Mylan-Carbamazepine CR; Novo-Carbamaz; Nu-Carbamazepine; PHL-Carbamazepine; PMS-Carbamazepine; Sandoz-Carbamazepine; Taro-Carbamazepine Chewable; Tegretol®

Therapeutic Category Anticonvulsant, Miscellaneous

Generic Available Yes: Excludes capsule (extended release)

Use Treatment of generalized tonic-clonic, partial (especially complex partial), and mixed partial or generalized seizure disorder; to relieve pain in trigeminal neuralgia or diabetic neuropathy; treatment of bipolar disorders (Equetro™ is approved for this use)

Pregnancy Risk Factor D

Pregnancy Considerations Crosses the placenta. Dysmorphic facial features, cranial defects, cardiac defects, spina bifida, IUGR, and multiple other malformations reported. Epilepsy itself, number of medications, genetic factors, or a combination of these probably influences the teratogenicity of anticonvulsant therapy. Benefit:risk ratio usually favors continued use during pregnancy and breast-feeding. Contraceptives may be rendered less effective by the coadministration of carbamazepine; alternative methods of contraception should be considered.

Patients exposed to carbamazepine during pregnancy are encouraged to enroll themselves into the AED Pregnancy Registry by calling 1-888-233-2334. Additional information is available at www.aedpregnancyregistry.org.

Lactation Enters breast milk/not recommended (AAP rates "compatible")

Breast-Feeding Considerations Carbamazepine and its metabolites are found in breast milk. The manufacturer does not recommend use while breast-feeding. However, AAP rates this medication "compatible" in breast-feeding.

Contraindications Hypersensitivity to carbamazepine, tricyclic antidepressants, or any component; patients with a history of bone marrow suppression; concomitant use or use within 14 days of MAO inhibitors; concurrent use with nefazodone

Warnings Potentially fatal blood cell abnormalities (aplastic anemia and agranulocytosis) have been reported in association with carbamazepine treatment **[U.S. Boxed Warning]**; history of adverse hematologic reaction to any drug may place patient at increased risk; early detection of hematologic change is important; baseline and periodic hematologic testing is recommended; advise patients of early signs and symptoms which are fever, sore throat, mouth ulcers, infections, easy bruising, petechial or purpuric hemorrhage; discontinue carbamazepine if evidence of significant bone marrow depression occurs.

Potentially fatal, severe dermatologic reactions (including Stevens-Johnson syndrome and toxic epidermal necrolysis) may occur **[U.S. Boxed Warning]**; over 90% of patients who experience these reactions do so within the first few months of treatment; patients of Asian descent are at higher risk for toxic dermatologic reactions (see Additional Information) and should be screened for the variant *HLA-B*1502* allele (genetic marker) prior to initiating therapy; this genetic variant has been associated with a significantly increased risk of developing toxic dermatologic reactions; patients with a positive result should not be started on carbamazepine, unless the benefit exceeds the risks; toxic dermatologic reactions can still occur infrequently in patients of any ethnicity who test negative for *HLA-B*1502*. Hepatic failure (rare) and multi-organ hypersensitivity reactions may occur (see Adverse Reactions); consider discontinuation of carbamazepine if any evidence of hypersensitivity occurs. Do not abruptly discontinue in patients being treated for seizures (precipitation of status epilepticus may occur). Carbamazepine may activate latent psychosis.

Avoid the use of carbamazepine in patients with hepatic porphyria (eg, variegate porphyria, acute intermittent porphyria, porphyria cutanea tarda); acute attacks of porphyria may occur. Substitution of Tegretol® with generic carbamazepine has resulted in decreased carbamazepine levels and increased seizure activity, as well as increased carbamazepine levels and toxicity. Monitoring of carbamazepine serum concentrations is mandatory when patients are switched from any product to another.

Antiepileptic drugs (AEDs) increase the risk of suicidal behavior and ideation in patients receiving these medications for any indication. Pooled analyses of placebo-controlled trials involving 11 different AEDs (regardless of indication) showed a twofold increased risk of suicidal thoughts or behavior (estimated incidence rate: 0.43% in AED treated patients compared to 0.24% of patients receiving placebo); increased risk was observed as early as 1 week after initiation of AED and continued through duration of trials (most trials ≤24 weeks); risk did not vary significantly by age (age range: 5-100 years). Consider risks and benefits of AEDs before prescribing. Monitor all patients receiving an AED for emergence of suicidal thoughts or behavior, thoughts of self-harm, any unusual changes in behavior or mood, or the emergence or worsening of depressive symptoms; notify heathcare provider immediately if symptoms or concerning behavior occur. **Note:** The FDA is requiring that a Medication Guide be developed for all antiepileptic drugs informing patients of this risk.

Precautions Use with caution and only after benefit-to-risk assessment in patients with history of cardiac disease, hepatic disease, renal failure, adverse hematologic reactions to other drugs, or history of hypersensitivity reactions to other anticonvulsants (eg, phenobarbital, phenytoin). Use with caution in patients with increased IOP (carbamazepine has mild anticholinergic effects). Use with caution when treating patients with a mixed seizure disorder that includes atypical absence seizures (carbamazepine may increase frequency of generalized convulsions in these patients). Higher peak concentrations occur with the suspension, so treatment is initiated with lower amounts per dose and increased slowly to avoid adverse effects.

Long-term risks and benefits of carbamazepine in the treatment of bipolar disorder have not been evaluated; periodic assessment of risks and benefits should be conducted for individual patient. For bipolar disorder, use the smallest effective dose to reduce the risk of overdose/suicide; high-risk patients should be monitored for suicidal ideations; to reduce risk of intentional overdose, write prescriptions for the smallest quantity consistent with good patient care.

Adverse Reactions

Cardiovascular: Edema, CHF, syncope, dysrhythmias, heart block

Central nervous system: Sedation, dizziness, drowsiness, somnolence, fatigue, slurred speech, ataxia, confusion; suicidal thinking and behavior (see Warnings)

Dermatologic: Rash, Stevens-Johnson syndrome, toxic epidermal necrolysis, photosensitivity, pruritus

Endocrine & metabolic: SIADH, hyponatremia

Gastrointestinal: Nausea, diarrhea, vomiting, abdominal cramps, pancreatitis, xerostomia

Genitourinary: Urinary retention

Hematologic: Neutropenia (can be transient), aplastic anemia, agranulocytosis, thrombocytopenia

Hepatic: Liver enzymes elevated, jaundice, hepatitis; hepatic failure (very rare)

Ocular: Nystagmus, diplopia, blurred vision

Miscellaneous: Multi-organ hypersensitivity reactions (rare): Reactions may include vasculitis, lymphadenopathy, fever, rash, lymphoma-like symptoms, arthralgia, eosinophilia, leukopenia, liver enzymes elevated, hepatosplenomegaly

Drug Interactions

Metabolism/Transport Effects Substrate of CYP2C8 (minor), 3A4 (major); **Induces** CYP1A2 (strong), 2B6 (strong), 2C8 (strong), 2C9 (strong), 2C19 (strong), 3A4 (strong), P-glycoprotein

Avoid Concomitant Use

Avoid concomitant use of CarBAMazepine with any of the following: Dronedarone; Etravirine; Everolimus; MAO Inhibitors; Nefazodone; Nilotinib; Pazopanib; Ranolazine; Romidepsin; Tolvaptan; Voriconazole

Increased Effect/Toxicity

CarBAMazepine may increase the levels/effects of: Adenosine; Alcohol (Ethyl); ClomiPRAMINE; CNS Depressants; Desmopressin; Lithium; MAO Inhibitors; Methotrimeprazine; Phenytoin

The levels/effects of CarBAMazepine may be increased by: Allopurinol; Antifungal Agents (Azole Derivatives, Systemic); Calcium Channel Blockers (Nondihydropyridine); Carbonic Anhydrase Inhibitors; Cimetidine; CYP3A4 Inhibitors (Moderate); CYP3A4 Inhibitors (Strong); Danazol; Darunavir; Dasatinib; Fluconazole; Grapefruit Juice; Isoniazid; LamoTRIgine; Macrolide Antibiotics; Methotrimeprazine; Nefazodone; Propoxyphene; Protease Inhibitors; Selective Serotonin Reuptake Inhibitors; Thiazide Diuretics

Decreased Effect

CarBAMazepine may decrease the levels/effects of: Acetaminophen; Aripiprazole; Bendamustine; Benzodiazepines (metabolized by oxidation); Calcium Channel Blockers (Dihydropyridine); Calcium Channel Blockers (Nondihydropyridine); Caspofungin; Clozapine; Contraceptives (Estrogens); Contraceptives (Progestins); CycloSPORINE; CycloSPORINE (Systemic); CYP1A2 Substrates; CYP2B6 Substrates; CYP2C19 Substrates; CYP2C8 Substrates (High risk); CYP2C9 Substrates (High risk); CYP3A4 Substrates; Dabigatran Etexilate; Divalproex; Doxycycline; Dronedarone; Etravirine; Everolimus; Flunarizine; GuanFACINE; Haloperidol; Irinotecan; Lacosamide; LamoTRIgine; Maraviroc; Mebendazole; Methadone; Nefazodone; Nilotinib; Paliperidone; Pazopanib; P-Glycoprotein Substrates; Phenytoin; Protease Inhibitors; Ranolazine; Risperidone; Romidepsin; Rufinamide; Saxagliptin; Selective Serotonin Reuptake Inhibitors; Sorafenib; Temsirolimus; Theophylline Derivatives; Thyroid Products; Tolvaptan; Topiramate; Treprostinil; Tricyclic Antidepressants; Valproic Acid; Vecuronium; Vitamin K Antagonists; Voriconazole; Ziprasidone

◄

The levels/effects of CarBAMazepine may be decreased by: CYP3A4 Inducers (Strong); Deferasirox; Divalproex; Herbs (CYP3A4 Inducers); Ketorolac; Ketorolac (Systemic); Mefloquine; Methylfolate; Phenytoin; Rufinamide; Valproic Acid

Food Interactions Extended release capsules (Carbatrol®, Equetro™): A high fat meal may increase the rate of absorption, reduce time to peak concentration (from 24 hours to 14 hours), and increase peak concentrations, but does not effect extent of absorption (AUC)

Grapefruit juice increases the oral bioavailability of carbamazepine by an average of 40%

Stability Store at room temperature, below 30°C (86°F).

Tablets, chewable: Protect from moisture and light; dispense in tight, light-resistant container

Tablets and extended release tablets: Protect from moisture; dispense in tightly closed container

Suspension: Dispense in tight, light-resistant container

Capsules, extended release: Protect from light and moisture

Mechanism of Action

Epilepsy: May depress activity in the nucleus ventralis of the thalamus or decrease synaptic transmission or decrease summation of temporal stimulation leading to neural discharge, by limiting influx of sodium ions across cell membrane; other unknown mechanisms.

Bipolar disorder: Mechanism of action is unknown.

Carbamazepine also stimulates the release of ADH and potentiates its action in promoting reabsorption of water; chemically related to tricyclic antidepressants; in addition to anticonvulsant effects, carbamazepine has anticholinergic, antineuralgic, antidiuretic, muscle relaxant and antiarrhythmic properties

Pharmacokinetics (Adult data unless noted)

Absorption: Slowly from the GI tract

Distribution: Carbamazepine and its active epoxide metabolite distribute into breast milk

V_d:

Neonates: 1.5 L/kg

Children: 1.9 L/kg

Adults: 0.59-2 L/kg

Protein binding: Carbamazepine: 75% to 90%, bound to alpha$_1$-acid glycoprotein and nonspecific binding sites on albumin; protein binding may be decreased in newborns

Epoxide metabolite: 50% protein bound

Metabolism: Induces liver enzymes to increase metabolism and shorten half-life over time; metabolized in the liver by cytochrome P450 3A4 to active epoxide metabolite; epoxide metabolite is metabolized by epoxide hydrolase to the trans-diol metabolite; ratio of serum epoxide to carbamazepine concentrations may be higher in patients receiving polytherapy (vs monotherapy) and in infants (vs older children); boys may have faster carbamazepine clearances and may, therefore, require higher mg/kg/day doses of carbamazepine compared to girls of similar age and weight

Bioavailability, oral: 75% to 85%; relative bioavailability of extended release tablet to suspension: 89%

Half-life:

Carbamazepine:

Initial: 25-65 hours

Multiple dosing:

Children: 8-14 hours

Adults: 12-17 hours

Epoxide metabolite: 34 ± 9 hours

Time to peak serum concentration: Unpredictable, within 4-8 hours

Chronic administration:

Suspension: 1.5 hours

Tablet: 4-5 hours

Extended release tablet: 3-12 hours

Elimination: 1% to 3% excreted unchanged in urine

Usual Dosage Dosage must be adjusted according to patient's response and serum concentrations. Administer tablets (chewable or conventional) in 2-3 divided doses daily and suspension in 4 divided doses daily. (See Additional Information for investigational oral loading dose and rectal maintenance dose information.) Oral:

Epilepsy:

Children:

<6 years: Initial: 10-20 mg/kg/day divided twice or 3 times daily as tablets or 4 times/day as suspension; increase dose every week until optimal response and therapeutic levels are achieved; maintenance dose: Divide into 3-4 doses daily (tablets or suspension); maximum recommended dose: 35 mg/kg/day

6-12 years: Initial: 100 mg twice daily (tablets or extended release tablets) or 50 mg of suspension 4 times/day (200 mg/day); increase by up to 100 mg/day at weekly intervals using a twice daily regimen of extended release tablets or 3-4 times daily regimen of other formulations until optimal response and therapeutic levels are achieved; usual maintenance: 400-800 mg/day; maximum recommended dose: 1000 mg/day

Note: Children <12 years who receive ≥400 mg/day of carbamazepine may be converted to extended release capsules (Carbatrol®) using the same total daily dosage divided twice daily

Children >12 years and Adults: Initial: 200 mg twice daily (tablets, extended release tablets, or extended release capsules) or 100 mg of suspension 4 times/day (400 mg daily); increase by up to 200 mg/day at weekly intervals using a twice daily regimen of extended release tablets or capsules, or a 3-4 times/day regimen of other formulations until optimal response and therapeutic levels are achieved; usual dose: 800-1200 mg/day

Maximum recommended doses:

Children 12-15 years: 1000 mg/day

Children >15 years: 1200 mg/day

Adults: 1600 mg/day; however, some patients have required up to 1.6-2.4 g/day

Bipolar disorder (Equetro™): Adults: Initial: 200 mg twice daily; adjust dose by 200 mg/day increments until optimal response is achieved; maximum dose: 1600 mg/day

Dosing adjustment in renal impairment: Cl_{cr} <10 mL/minute: Administer 75% of recommended dose; monitor serum levels

Administration

Oral: Administer with food to decrease GI upset; avoid administration with grapefruit juice; extended release capsules (Carbatrol®, Equetro™) may be taken without regard to meals; suspension dosage should be administered on a 3-4 times/day schedule vs tablet (conventional or chewable) which can be administered 2-4 times/day; extended release (XR) tablets should be dosed twice daily; do not crush or chew XR tablets; examine XR tablets for cracks or chips; do not use damaged XR tablets or XR tablets without a release portal; chewable tablet should be chewed well and swallowed. Swallow extended release capsules whole or open and sprinkle contents on small amount of soft food (eg, 1 teaspoonful of applesauce); swallow sprinkle/food mixture immediately; do not chew; do not store for later use; drink fluids after dose to make sure mixture is completely swallowed

Suspension: Tegretol® should not be administered with diluents or other liquid medicines due to the possibility of a component interaction (see Drug Interactions); shake suspension well before use

Monitoring Parameters *HLA-B*1502* genotype screening prior to therapy initiation in patients of Asian descent (see Warnings); CBC with platelet count, reticulocytes, serum iron, liver function tests, ophthalmic examinations (including slit-lamp, fundoscopy, and tonometry), urinalysis, BUN, lipid panel, serum drug concentrations, thyroid function tests, serum sodium; pregnancy test; observe patient for excessive sedation especially when instituting or increasing therapy; signs of edema, skin rash, and hypersensitivity reactions; signs and symptoms of suicidality (eg, anxiety, depression, behavior changes) (see Warnings).

Reference Range Therapeutic: 4-12 mcg/mL (SI: 17-51 micromoles/L). Patients who require higher levels [8-12 mcg/mL (SI: 34-51 micromoles/L)] should be carefully monitored. Side effects (especially CNS) occur commonly at higher levels. If other anticonvulsants (enzyme inducers) are given, therapeutic range is 4-8 mcg/mL (SI: 17-34 micromoles/L) due to increase in unmeasured active epoxide metabolite.

Test Interactions Carbamazepine may interfere with a serum immunoassay for tricyclic antidepressants; false-positive qualitative serum tricyclic antidepressant drug screen results have been reported in patients with carbamazepine intoxication (see Matos, 2000). Carbamazepine may interfere with some pregnancy tests.

Patient Information Avoid alcohol and grapefruit juice. May cause drowsiness and impair ability to perform activities requiring mental alertness or physical coordination. May cause dry mouth. Antiepileptic agents may increase the risk of suicidal thoughts and behavior; notify physician if you feel more depressed or have thoughts of suicide or self harm (see Warnings). Report fever, sore throat, infection, mouth ulcers, easy bruising, bleeding, loss of appetite, nausea, vomiting, yellow skin or eyes, changes in mentation or cognition, rash or skin irritations, worsening of seizure activity, or loss of seizure control to physician. Report the use of other medications, nonprescription medications, and herbal or natural products to your physician and pharmacist. The tablet coating of Tegretol®-XR tablet is not absorbed and may appear in the stool. May cause photosensitivity reactions (eg, exposure to sunlight may cause severe sunburn, skin rash, redness, or itching); avoid exposure to sunlight and artificial light sources (sunlamps, tanning booth/bed); wear protective clothing, wide-brimmed hats, sunglasses, and lip sunscreen (SPF ≥15); use a sunscreen [broad-spectrum sunscreen or physical sunscreen (preferred) or sunblock with SPF ≥15]; contact physician if reaction occurs.

Additional Information Carbamazepine is not effective in absence, myoclonic, akinetic, or febrile seizures; exacerbation of certain seizure types have been seen after initiation of carbamazepine therapy in children with mixed seizure disorders

Investigationally, loading doses of the suspension (10 mg/kg for children <12 years of age and 8 mg/kg for children >12 years) were given (via NG or ND tubes followed by 5-10 mL of water to flush through tube) to PICU patients with frequent seizures/status; 5 of 6 patients attained mean plasma concentrations of 4.3 mcg/mL and 7.3 mcg/mL at 1 and 2 hours postload; concurrent enteral feeding or ileus may delay absorption of loading dose (Miles, 1990)

Carbamazepine suspension may be administered rectally as maintenance doses, if oral therapy is not possible (**Note:** Rectally administered carbamazepine is not useful in status epilepticus due to its slow absorption); when using carbamazepine suspension rectally, administer the same total daily dose, but give in small, diluted, multiple doses; dilute the oral suspension with an equal volume of water; if defecation occurs within the first 2 hours, repeat the dose (see Graves, 1987)

Extended release capsule (Cabatrol®, Equetro™) contain three different types of beads: Immediate-, extended-, and enteric-release; the combination of the ratio of bead types allows for twice daily dosing.

A recent study (Relling, 2000) demonstrated that enzyme-inducing antiepileptic drugs (AEDs) (carbamazepine, phenobarbital, and phenytoin) increased systemic clearance of antileukemic drugs (teniposide and methotrexate) and were associated with a worse event-free survival, CNS relapse, and hematologic relapse, (ie, lower efficacy), in B-lineage ALL children receiving chemotherapy; the authors recommend using nonenzyme-inducing AEDs in patients receiving chemotherapy for ALL.

Individuals who possess a genetic susceptibility marker known as the *HLA-B*1502* allele have an increased risk of developing carbamazepine-associated Stevens-Johnson syndrome (SJS) and/or toxic epidermal necrolysis (TEN) compared to persons without this genotype. The presence of this genetic variant exists in up to 15% of people of Asian descent, varying from <1% in Japanese and Koreans, to 2% to 4% of South Asians and Indians, to 10% to 15% of populations from China, Taiwan, Malaysia, and the Philippines. This variant is virtually absent in those of Caucasian, African-American, Hispanic, Native American, or European ancestry. Risk assessments have suggested that incidence of SJS/TEN in Asians could be ~60 cases/10,000 new users depending on the country of origin (a nearly 10-fold higher incidence than in predominantly Caucasian populations). Patients of Asian descent should be screened for the variant *HLA-B*1502* allele (genetic marker) prior to initiating therapy. Those who test positive should not be started on carbamazepine, unless the benefit exceeds the risks. Presence of the *HLA-B*1502* allele may signify greater risk of developing SJS/TEN with other antiepileptic agents for which this degree of dermatologic reactions has been documented (see Warnings).

Dosage Forms Excipient information presented when available (limited, particularly for generics); consult specific product labeling.

Capsule, extended release:
  Carbatrol®, Equetro®: 100 mg, 200 mg, 300 mg
Suspension, oral: 100 mg/5 mL (5 mL, 10 mL, 450 mL)
  Tegretol®: 100 mg/5 mL (450 mL) [contains propylene glycol; citrus vanilla flavor]
Tablet: 200 mg
  Epitol®, Tegretol®: 200 mg
Tablet, chewable: 100 mg
  Tegretol®: 100 mg
Tablet, extended release: 200 mg, 400 mg
  Tegretol®-XR: 100 mg, 200 mg, 400 mg

References

Gilman JT, "Carbamazepine Dosing for Pediatric Seizure Disorders: The Highs and Lows," *DICP*, 1991, 25(10):1109-12.

Graves NM and Kriel RL, "Rectal Administration of Antiepileptic Drugs in Children," *Pediatr Neurol*, 1987, 3(6):321-6.

Koritenberg R, Haug C, and Hannak D, "The Metabolization of Carbamazepine to CBZ-10,11 Epoxide in Children From the Newborn Age to Adolescence," *Neuropediatrics*, 1994, 25(4):214-6.

Liu H and Delgado MR, "Influence of Sex, Age, Weight, and Carbamazepine Dose on Serum Concentrations, Concentration Ratios, and Level/Dose Ratios of Carbamazepine and Its Metabolites," *Ther Drug Monit*, 1994, 16(5):469-76.

Matos ME, Burns MM, and Shannon MW, "False-Positive Tricyclic Antidepressant Drug Screen Results Leading to the Diagnosis of Carbamazepine Intoxication," *Pediatrics*, 2000, 105(5), http://www.pediatrics.org/cgi/content/full/105/5/e66.

Miles MV, Lawless ST, Tennison MB, et al, "Rapid Loading of Critically Ill Patients With Carbamazepine Suspension," *Pediatrics*, 1990, 86 (2):263-6.

Relling MV, Pui CH, Sandlund JT, et al, "Adverse Effect of Anticonvulsants on Efficacy of Chemotherapy for Acute Lymphoblastic Leukaemia," *Lancet*, 2000, 356(9226):285-90.

◆ **Carbamazepine (Can)** *see* CarBAMazepine *on page 244*

Carbamide Peroxide (KAR ba mide per OKS ide)

U.S. Brand Names Auraphene® B [OTC]; Auro® [OTC]; Cankaid® [OTC]; Debrox® [OTC]; E•R•O [OTC]; Gly-Oxide® [OTC]; Murine® Ear Wax Removal System [OTC]; Otix® [OTC]

Therapeutic Category Otic Agent, Cerumenolytic

Generic Available Yes

Use

Oral: Relief of minor inflammation of gums, oral mucosal surfaces and lips including canker sores and dental irritation; adjunct in oral hygiene

Otic: Emulsify and disperse ear wax

Contraindications Hypersensitivity to carbamide peroxide or any component; otic preparation should not be used in patients with a perforated tympanic membrane or following otic surgery; ear drainage, ear pain, or rash in the ear; dizziness; oral preparation should not be used for self medication in children <3 years of age

Warnings With prolonged use of oral carbamide peroxide, there is a potential for overgrowth of opportunistic organisms, damage to periodontal tissues, delayed wound healing

Adverse Reactions

Central nervous system: Dizziness

Dermatologic: Rash

Local: Irritation, tenderness, pain, redness

Drug Interactions

Avoid Concomitant Use There are no known interactions where it is recommended to avoid concomitant use.

Increased Effect/Toxicity There are no known significant interactions involving an increase in effect.

Decreased Effect There are no known significant interactions involving a decrease in effect.

Stability Protect from heat and direct light

Mechanism of Action Carbamide peroxide releases hydrogen peroxide which serves as a source of nascent oxygen upon contact with catalase; deodorant action is probably due to inhibition of odor-causing bacteria; softens impacted cerumen due to its foaming action

Pharmacodynamics Onset of action: Otic: Slight disintegration of hard ear wax in 24 hours

Usual Dosage

Oral: Children and Adults: Solution: Apply several drops undiluted to affected area of the mouth 4 times/day after meals and at bedtime for up to 7 days, expectorate after 2-3 minutes; as an adjunct to oral hygiene after brushing, swish 10 drops for 2-3 minutes, then expectorate

Otic: Solution:

Children <12 years: Individualize the dose according to patient size; 3 drops (range: 1-5 drops) twice daily for up to 4 days

Children ≥12 years and Adults: Instill 5-10 drops twice daily for up to 4 days

Administration

Oral: Apply undiluted solution with an applicator or cotton swab to the affected area after meals and at bedtime; or place drops on the tongue, mix with saliva, swish in the mouth for several minutes, then expectorate. Patient should not rinse mouth or drink fluids for 5 minutes after oral administration.

Otic: Instill drops into the external ear canal; keep drops in ear for several minutes by keeping head tilted or placing cotton in ear. Gently irrigate ear canal with warm water to remove loosened cerumen.

Patient Information Contact physician if dizziness or otic redness, rash, irritation, tenderness, pain, drainage or discharge develop; do not use in the eye

Nursing Implications Drops foam on contact with ear wax

Dosage Forms Excipient information presented when available (limited, particularly for generics); consult specific product labeling.

Liquid, oral: 10% (60 mL)

Cankaid®: 10% (22 mL)

Gly-Oxide®: 10% (15 mL, 60 mL)

Solution, otic [drops]: 6.5% (15 mL)

Auraphene® B, Otix®: 6.5% (15 mL)

Auro®: 6.5% (22.2 mL)

Debrox®: 6.5% (15 mL, 30 mL)

E•R•O: 6.5% (15 mL) [alcohol free]

Murine® Ear Wax Removal System: 6.5% (15 mL) [contains alcohol 6.3%]

◆ **Carbatrol®** *see* CarBAMazepine *on page 244*

◆ **Carbaxefed RF [DSC]** *see* Carbinoxamine and Pseudoephedrine *on page 249*

Carbinoxamine (kar bi NOKS a meen)

U.S. Brand Names Palgic®

Therapeutic Category Antihistamine

Generic Available No

Use Relief of symptoms of seasonal and perennial allergic rhinitis, vasomotor rhinitis, allergic conjunctivitis, urticaria, angioedema, and dermatographism

Pregnancy Risk Factor C

Pregnancy Considerations Animal reproduction studies have not been conducted.

Lactation Excretion in breast milk unknown/contraindicated

Breast-Feeding Considerations It is not known if carbinoxamine is found in breast milk; prolonged or large doses may cause drowsiness in breast-feeding infants. Use while breast-feeding is contraindicated by the manufacturer.

Contraindications Hypersensitivity to carbinoxamine or any component of the formulation; use with or within 14 days of MAO inhibitor therapy; children <2 years of age

Warnings Safety and efficacy for the use of cough and cold products in children <2 years of age is limited. Serious adverse effects including death have been reported. The FDA notes that there are no approved OTC uses for these products in children <2 years of age. Healthcare providers are reminded to ask caregivers about the use of OTC cough and cold products in order to avoid exposure to multiple medications containing the same ingredient.

Precautions Use with caution in patients with mild to moderate hypertension, cardiovascular disease, diabetes, asthma, thyroid disease, increased intraocular pressure, GU or GI obstruction or symptomatic prostatic hypertrophy

Adverse Reactions

Cardiovascular: Hypotension, palpitations, tachycardia, extrasystoles, chills

Central nervous system: Dizziness, paradoxical excitability (children), headache, nervousness, sedation, fatigue, confusion, seizures, hysteria, euphoria, insomnia, irritability, vertigo

Dermatologic: Urticaria, rash, photosensitivity

Gastrointestinal: Anorexia, diarrhea, heartburn, nausea, vomiting, xerostomia

Hematologic: Hemolytic anemia (rare), thrombocytopenia (rare), agranulocytosis (rare)

Neuromuscular & skeletal: Weakness, tremor, paresthesia, neuritis

Ocular: Diplopia, blurred vision

Otic: Tinnitus, acute labyrinthitis

Renal: Polyuria

Respiratory: Thickening of bronchial secretions, chest tightness, wheezing

Miscellaneous: Excessive perspiration, anaphylactic shock

Drug Interactions

Avoid Concomitant Use There are no known interactions where it is recommended to avoid concomitant use.

Increased Effect/Toxicity

Carbinoxamine may increase the levels/effects of: Alcohol (Ethyl); Anticholinergics; CNS Depressants

The levels/effects of Carbinoxamine may be increased by: Pramlintide

Decreased Effect

Carbinoxamine may decrease the levels/effects of: Acetylcholinesterase Inhibitors (Central); Betahistine

The levels/effects of Carbinoxamine may be decreased by: Acetylcholinesterase Inhibitors (Central); Amphetamines

Stability Store at controlled room temperature of 15°C to 30°C (59°F to 86°F).

Mechanism of Action Carbinoxamine competes with histamine for H_1-receptor sites on effector cells in the gastrointestinal tract, blood vessels, and respiratory tract.

Pharmacodynamics Duration: 3-6 hours

Pharmacokinetics (Adult data unless noted) Half-life: Adults: 10-20 hours

Usual Dosage Oral:

Children >2 years: 0.2-0.4 mg/kg/day divided 3-4 times/day

Alternate dosing (manufacturer's recommendation); **Note:** When using this recommendation, be sure to compare with the weight-based dosage listed above as the age-based dosage may exceed 0.4 mg/kg/day in some individuals):

Palgic®:

2-3 years: 2 mg (2.5 mL) 3-4 times/day

3-6 years: 2-4 mg (2.5-5 mL) 3-4 times/day

>6 years: 4-6 mg (5-7.5 mL) 3-4 times/day

Adults: 4-8 mg 3-4 times/day

Administration Oral: Administer without regard to food

Patient Information May cause drowsiness or impair ability to perform activities requiring mental alertness or physical coordination; may cause blurred vision; may also cause CNS excitation and difficulty sleeping; may cause dry mouth; avoid alcohol; may rarely cause photosensitivity reactions (eg, exposure to sunlight may cause severe sunburn, skin rash, redness, or itching); avoid direct exposure to sunlight

Dosage Forms Excipient information presented when available (limited, particularly for generics); consult specific product labeling.

Solution, as maleate:

Palgic®: 4 mg/5 mL (480 mL) [bubble gum flavor]

Tablet, as maleate [scored]:

Palgic®: 4 mg

Carbinoxamine and Pseudoephedrine

(kar bi NOKS a meen & soo doe e FED rin)

U.S. Brand Names Andehist NR Drops [DSC]; Carbaxefed RF [DSC]; Carboxine-PSE [DSC]; Cordron-D NR [DSC]; Hydro-Tussin™-CBX [DSC]; Palgic®-D [DSC]; Palgic®-DS [DSC]; Pediatex™-D [DSC]; Sildec [DSC]

Therapeutic Category Antihistamine/Decongestant Combination

Generic Available Yes

Use Temporary relief of nasal congestion, running nose, sneezing, itching of nose or throat, and itchy, watery eyes due to the common cold, hay fever, or other respiratory allergies

Pregnancy Risk Factor C

Pregnancy Considerations Animal reproduction studies have not been conducted.

Lactation Enters breast milk/contraindicated

Breast-Feeding Considerations Small amounts of antihistamines and pseudoephedrine are excreted in breast milk. Premature infants and newborns have a higher risk of intolerance to antihistamines. Antihistamines may inhibit lactation.

Contraindications Hypersensitivity to carbinoxamine, pseudoephedrine, or any component; severe hypertension or coronary artery disease, MAO inhibitor therapy, GI or GU obstruction, narrow-angle glaucoma

Warnings Safety and efficacy for the use of cough and cold products in children <2 years of age is limited. Serious adverse effects including death have been reported in children <2 years of age (in some cases, high blood concentrations of pseudoephedrine were found). In addition, due to an association with the use of carbinoxamine and increased fatalities in children <2 years of age, the FDA is specifically not recommending the use of carbinoxamine in this age group. The FDA notes that there are no approved OTC uses for these products in children <2 years of age. Healthcare providers are reminded to ask caregivers about the use of OTC cough and cold products in order to avoid exposure to multiple medications containing the same ingredient.

Some products contains sodium benzoate; benzoic acid (benzoate) is a metabolite of benzyl alcohol; large amounts of benzyl alcohol (≥99 mg/kg/day) have been associated with a potentially fatal toxicity ("gasping syndrome") in neonates; the "gasping syndrome" consists of metabolic acidosis, respiratory distress, gasping respirations, CNS dysfunction (including convulsions, intracranial hemorrhage), hypotension and cardiovascular collapse; avoid use in neonates; *in vitro* and animal studies have shown that benzoate displaces bilirubin from protein binding sites

Precautions Use with caution in patients with mild to moderate hypertension, heart disease, diabetes, asthma, thyroid disease, or prostatic hypertrophy

Adverse Reactions

Cardiovascular: Hypertension, tachycardia, arrhythmias, edema, palpitations

Central nervous system: Sedation, CNS stimulation, headache, seizures, drowsiness, fatigue, nervousness, depression

Dermatologic: Angioedema, photosensitivity, rash

Gastrointestinal: Nausea, vomiting, xerostomia, anorexia, diarrhea, heart burn

Genitourinary: Dysuria

Hepatic: Hepatitis

Neuromuscular & skeletal: Weakness, myalgia, paresthesia

Ocular: Diplopia

Respiratory: Bronchospasm, epistaxis

Renal: Polyuria

Drug Interactions

Avoid Concomitant Use

Avoid concomitant use of Carbinoxamine and Pseudoephedrine with any of the following: Iobenguane I 123; MAO Inhibitors

Increased Effect/Toxicity

Carbinoxamine and Pseudoephedrine may increase the levels/effects of: Alcohol (Ethyl); Anticholinergics; Bromocriptine; CNS Depressants; Sympathomimetics

The levels/effects of Carbinoxamine and Pseudoephedrine may be increased by: Antacids; Atomoxetine; Cannabinoids; Carbonic Anhydrase Inhibitors; MAO Inhibitors; Pramlintide; Serotonin/Norepinephrine Reuptake Inhibitors

Decreased Effect

Carbinoxamine and Pseudoephedrine may decrease the levels/effects of: Acetylcholinesterase Inhibitors (Central); Betahistine; Iobenguane I 123

The levels/effects of Carbinoxamine and Pseudoephedrine may be decreased by: Acetylcholinesterase Inhibitors (Central); Amphetamines; Spironolactone

Mechanism of Action Carbinoxamine competes with histamine for H_1-receptor sites on effector cells in the GI tract, blood vessels, and respiratory tract; pseudoephedrine directly stimulates alpha-adrenergic receptors of respiratory mucosa causing vasoconstriction; directly stimulates beta-adrenergic receptors causing bronchial relaxation, increased heart rate and contractility

Usual Dosage Oral:

Children >2 years: May dose according to pseudoephedrine component: 4 mg/kg/day **or** the carbinoxamine component: 0.2-0.4 mg/kg/day

Administration Oral: Do not crush or chew extended release tablets

Patient Information May cause drowsiness or impair ability to perform activities requiring mental alertness or physical coordination; may cause blurred vision; may also cause CNS excitation and difficulty sleeping; may cause dry mouth; avoid alcohol. May rarely cause photosensitivity reactions (eg, exposure to sunlight may cause severe sunburn, skin rash, redness, or itching); avoid direct exposure to sunlight

Dosage Forms Excipient information presented when available (limited, particularly for generics); consult specific product labeling. [DSC] = Discontinued product

Liquid:

Cordron-D NR: Carbinoxamine maleate 2 mg and pseudoephedrine hydrochloride 12.5 mg per 5 mL (480 mL) [cotton candy flavor] [DSC]

Pediatex™-D: Carbinoxamine maleate 2 mg and pseudoephedrine hydrochloride 20 mg per 5 mL (480 mL) [alcohol free, dye free, sugar free; cotton candy flavor] [DSC]

Solution: Carbinoxamine maleate 2 mg and pseudoephedrine hydrochloride 25 mg per 5 mL (480 mL) [DSC]

Carboxine-PSE: Carbinoxamine maleate 2 mg and pseudoephedrine hydrochloride 20 mg per 5 mL (480 mL) [peach flavor] [DSC]

Solution, oral drops:

Andehist NR: Carbinoxamine maleate 1 mg and pseudoephedrine hydrochloride 15 mg per mL (30 mL) [alcohol free, sugar free; raspberry flavor] [DSC]

Carbaxefed RF: Carbinoxamine maleate 1 mg and pseudoephedrine hydrochloride 15 mg per mL (30 mL) [alcohol free; contains sodium benzoate; cherry flavor] [DSC]

Sildec: Carbinoxamine maleate 1 mg and pseudoephedrine hydrochloride 15 mg per mL (30 mL) [raspberry flavor] [DSC]

Syrup: Carbinoxamine maleate 2 mg and pseudoephedrine hydrochloride 25 mg per 5 mL (480 mL)

Hydro-Tussin™-CBX [DSC], Palgic®-DS [DSC]: Carbinoxamine maleate 2 mg and pseudoephedrine hydrochloride 25 mg per 5 mL (480 mL) [alcohol free, dye free, sugar free; strawberry/pineapple flavor] [DSC]

Tablet, timed release:

Palgic®-D: Carbinoxamine maleate 8 mg and pseudoephedrine hydrochloride 80 mg [dye free] [DSC]

◆ **Carbinoxamine Maleate** *see* Carbinoxamine *on page 248*

◆ **Carbocaine®** *see* Mepivacaine *on page 883*

◆ **Carbolith™ (Can)** *see* Lithium *on page 834*

CARBOplatin (KAR boe pla tin)

Medication Safety Issues

Sound-alike/look-alike issues:

CARBOplatin may be confused with CISplatin, oxaliplatin

Paraplatin® may be confused with Platinol®

High alert medication: The Institute for Safe Medication Practices (ISMP) includes this medication among its list of drugs which have a heightened risk of causing significant patient harm when used in error.

Related Information

Compatibility of Chemotherapy and Related Supportive Care Medications *on page 1580*

Emetogenic Potential of Antineoplastic Agents *on page 1579*

Canadian Brand Names Paraplatin-AQ

Therapeutic Category Antineoplastic Agent, Alkylating Agent

Generic Available Yes

Use Treatment of ovarian carcinoma; treatment of small cell lung cancer, squamous cell carcinoma of the esophagus; solid tumors of the bladder, cervix and testes; pediatric brain tumor, neuroblastoma, bony and soft tissue sarcomas, germ cell tumors, and high-dose therapy with stem cell/bone marrow transplants

Pregnancy Risk Factor D

Lactation Excretion in breast milk unknown/contraindicated

Breast-Feeding Considerations Due to the potential for toxicity in nursing infants, breast-feeding is contraindicated.

Contraindications Hypersensitivity to carboplatin, cisplatin, any component, other platinum-containing compounds, or mannitol; severe bone marrow suppression or excessive bleeding

Warnings Hazardous agent; use appropriate precautions for handling and disposal. When carboplatin is dosed using AUC as the endpoint, note that the calculated dose is the dose administered, not the dose based on body surface area; anaphylactic-like reactions can occur within minutes of administration **[U.S. Boxed Warning]**; risk for reaction increased in patients previously exposed to platinum therapy.

Precautions May cause severe, dose-limiting, dose-related bone marrow suppression **[U.S. Boxed Warning]**; anemia may be cumulative and require transfusion; may cause severe vomiting **[U.S. Boxed Warning]**; vomiting is dose-related and can be more severe in patients who previously received emetogenic therapy; high doses have also resulted in severe abnormalities of liver function; reduce dosage in patients with bone marrow suppression and impaired renal function (creatinine clearance values <60 mL/minute)

Adverse Reactions

Cardiovascular: Hypotension

Central nervous system: Pain

Dermatologic: Urticaria, rash, alopecia, pruritus, erythema

Endocrine & metabolic: Electrolyte abnormalities such as hypocalcemia, hypokalemia, hypomagnesemia

Gastrointestinal: Nausea, vomiting, diarrhea, anorexia, hemorrhagic colitis, mucositis, constipation, metallic taste

Hematologic: Neutropenia, leukopenia, thrombocytopenia (platelet count reaches a nadir between 14-21 days), anemia

Hepatic: Abnormal liver function tests

Neuromuscular & skeletal: Peripheral neuropathy, weakness

Otic: Tinnitus, hearing loss at high tones

Renal: Nephrotoxicity, BUN and serum creatinine elevated, hematuria

Respiratory: Bronchospasm, interstitial pneumonia

Miscellaneous: Anaphylactic-like reactions

Drug Interactions

Avoid Concomitant Use

Avoid concomitant use of CARBOplatin with any of the following: BCG; Natalizumab; Pimecrolimus; Tacrolimus (Topical); Vaccines (Live)

Increased Effect/Toxicity

CARBOplatin may increase the levels/effects of: Leflunomide; Natalizumab; Taxane Derivatives; Topotecan; Vaccines (Live)

The levels/effects of CARBOplatin may be increased by: Aminoglycosides; Denosumab; Pimecrolimus; Tacrolimus (Topical); Trastuzumab

Decreased Effect

CARBOplatin may decrease the levels/effects of: BCG; Sipuleucel-T; Vaccines (Inactivated); Vaccines (Live)

The levels/effects of CARBOplatin may be decreased by: Echinacea

Stability Store unopened vials at room temperature; protect from light; after reconstitution, solutions are stable for 8 hours; 2 mg/mL solutions diluted in D_5W for infusion are stable for 24 hours; 7 mg/mL solutions diluted in NS for infusion are stable for 24 hours; aluminum reacts with carboplatin resulting in a precipitate and loss of potency

Mechanism of Action Platination of DNA results in possible cross-linking and interference with the function of DNA

Pharmacokinetics (Adult data unless noted)

Distribution: V_d: 16 L/kg

Protein binding: 0%; however, platinum is 30% protein bound

Half-life: Patients with Cl_{cr} >60 mL/minute: 2.5-5.9 hours

Elimination: ~60% to 80% is excreted renally

Usual Dosage I.V. (refer to individual protocols):

Infants and Children <3 years or ≤12 kg: Various protocols calculate dosage on the basis of body weight rather than body surface area

Children:

Solid tumor: 560 mg/m^2 once every 4 weeks

Sarcoma (bony/soft tissue): 400 mg/m^2/day for 2 days

Brain tumor: 175 mg/m^2 once weekly for 4 weeks with a 2-week recovery period between courses; dose is then adjusted on platelet count and neutrophil count values; courses should not be repeated until the platelet count is ≥100,000/mm^3 and the neutrophil count is ≥2000/mm^3

Bone marrow transplant preparative regimen: 500 mg/m^2/day for 3 days

Retinoblastoma: Subconjunctival injection of carboplatin for intraocular retinoblastoma has been administered using 1-2 mL of a 10 mg/mL solution per dose to affected eye(s)

Alternative carboplatin dosing: Some investigators calculate pediatric carboplatin doses using a modified Calvert formula: Dosing based on target AUC (modified Calvert formula for use in children): Total dose (mg) = [Target AUC (mg/mL/minute)] x [GFR (mL/minute) + (0.36 x body weight in kilograms)]

Note: Calvert formula was based on using chromic edetate (^{51}Cr-EDTA) plasma clearance to establish GFR. Some clinicians have recommended that methods for estimating Cl_{cr} not be substituted for GFR since carboplatin dosing based on such estimates may not be predictive.

Note: The dose of carboplatin calculated is TOTAL mg DOSE not mg/m^2

Adults:

Single agent: 360 mg/m^2 once every 4 weeks; dose is then adjusted on platelet count and neutrophil count values; courses should not be repeated until the platelet count is ≥100,000/mm^3 and the neutrophil count is ≥2000/mm^3

Calvert formula: See table

Calvert Formula for Carboplatin Dosing in Adults

Total dose (mg) = target AUC (mg/mL/minute) x (GFR [mL/minute] + 25)

Single agent carboplatin/no prior chemotherapy	Total dose (mg): 6-8 (GFR + 25)
Single agent carboplatin/prior chemotherapy	Total dose (mg): 4-6 (GFR + 25)
Combination chemotherapy/ no prior chemotherapy	Total dose (mg): 4.5-6 (GFR + 25)
Combination chemotherapy/ prior chemotherapy	Use a target AUC value <5 for the initial cycle

Dosing adjustment in renal impairment: Adults: Calvert formula (dosing adjustment for renal impairment is implied with this formula):

Total dose (mg) = [Target AUC (mg/mL/minute)] x [GFR (mL/minute) + 25]

Note: The dose of carboplatin calculated is TOTAL mg DOSE not mg/m^2; target AUC will vary depending upon: Number of agents in the regimen and treatment status (ie, previously untreated or treated)

Administration Parenteral: Administer by I.V. intermittent infusion over 15 minutes to 1 hour, or by continuous infusion (continuous infusion regimens may be less toxic than the bolus route); reconstituted carboplatin 10 mg/mL should be further diluted to a final concentration of 0.5-2 mg/mL with D_5W or NS for administration

Monitoring Parameters CBC with differential and platelet count, serum electrolytes, urinalysis, creatinine clearance, liver function tests

Nursing Implications Needle or intravenous administration sets containing aluminum parts should not be used in the administration or preparation of carboplatin (aluminum can interact with carboplatin resulting in precipitate formation and loss of potency)

Dosage Forms Excipient information presented when available (limited, particularly for generics); consult specific product labeling.

Injection, powder for reconstitution: 50 mg, 150 mg, 450 mg

Injection, solution: 10 mg/mL (5 mL, 15 mL, 45 mL, 60 mL)

Injection, solution [preservative free]: 10 mg/mL (5 mL, 15 mL, 45 mL)

References

Abramson DH, Frank CM, and Dunkel IJ, "A Phase I/II Study of Subconjunctival Carboplatin for Intraocular Retinoblastoma," *Ophthalmology*, 1999, 106(10):1947-50.

Cairo MS, "The Use of Ifosfamide, Carboplatin, and Etoposide in Children With Solid Tumors," *Semin Oncol*, 1995, 22(3 Suppl 7):23-7.

Lovett D, Kelsen D, Eisenberger M, et al, "A Phase II Trial of Carboplatin and Vinblastine in the Treatment of Advanced Squamous Cell Carcinoma of the Esophagus," *Cancer*, 1991, 67(2):354-6.

Newell DR, Pearson AD, Balmanno K, et al, "Carboplatin Pharmacokinetics in Children: The Development of a Pediatric Dosing Formula. The United Kingdom Children's Cancer Study Group," *J Clin Oncol*, 1993, 11(12):2314-23.

Zeltzer PM, Epport K, Nelson MD Jr, et al, "Prolonged Response to Carboplatin in an Infant With Brain Stem Glioma," *Cancer*, 1991, 67 (1):43-7.

◆ **Carboxine-PSE [DSC]** *see* Carbinoxamine and Pseudoephedrine *on page 249*

◆ **Cardene®** *see* NiCARdipine *on page 988*

◆ **Cardene® I.V.** *see* NiCARdipine *on page 988*

◆ **Cardene® SR** *see* NiCARdipine *on page 988*

◆ **Cardizem®** *see* Diltiazem *on page 443*

◆ **Cardizem® CD** *see* Diltiazem *on page 443*

◆ **Cardizem® LA** *see* Diltiazem *on page 443*

◆ **Carimune® NF** *see* Immune Globulin (Intravenous) *on page 719*

◆ **Carmol® Scalp Treatment** *see* Sulfacetamide *on page 1298*

Carmustine (kar MUS teen)

Medication Safety Issues
Sound-alike/look-alike issues:
Carmustine may be confused with bendamustine, lomustine

High alert medication: The Institute for Safe Medication Practices (ISMP) includes this medication among its list of drugs which have a heightened risk of causing significant patient harm when used in error.

Related Information
Compatibility of Chemotherapy and Related Supportive Care Medications *on page 1580*
Emetogenic Potential of Antineoplastic Agents *on page 1579*

U.S. Brand Names BiCNU®; Gliadel®

Canadian Brand Names BiCNU®; Gliadel Wafer®

Therapeutic Category Antineoplastic Agent, Alkylating Agent (Nitrosourea)

Generic Available No

Use
Injection: Treatment of brain tumors (glioblastoma, brainstem glioma, medulloblastoma, astrocytoma, ependymoma, and metastatic brain tumor); multiple myeloma, Hodgkin's disease, and non-Hodgkin's lymphomas (relapsed or refractory) (FDA approved in adults); has also been used in the treatment of malignant melanoma

Wafer (implant): Adjunct to surgery in patients with recurrent glioblastoma multiforme; adjunct to surgery and radiation in patients with newly diagnosed high grade malignant glioma (FDA approved in adults)

Pregnancy Risk Factor D

Pregnancy Considerations Teratogenicity and embryotoxicity have been demonstrated in animal studies. Carmustine can cause fetal harm if administered to a pregnant woman. There are no adequate and well-controlled studies in pregnant women. Women of child-bearing potential should avoid becoming pregnant while on treatment.

Lactation Excretion in breast milk unknown/not recommended

Breast-Feeding Considerations Due to the potential for serious adverse reactions in the nursing infant, breast-feeding should be discontinued.

Contraindications Hypersensitivity to carmustine or any component

Warnings Hazardous agent; use appropriate precautions for handling and disposal. Bone marrow suppression, notably thrombocytopenia and leukopenia, may lead to bleeding and overwhelming infection in an already compromised patient **[U.S. Boxed Warning]**; myelosuppressive effects will last for at least 6 weeks after a dose, do not give courses more frequently than every 6 weeks because the toxicity is cumulative; delayed-onset pulmonary fibrosis (sometimes fatal) has occurred up to 17 years after carmustine treatment in children and adolescents who received cumulative doses ranging from 770-1800 mg/m²combined with cranial radiotherapy for intracranial tumors. Acute leukemia has been reported in patients receiving long-term carmustine. May cause fetal harm when administered to a pregnant woman; carmustine is potentially carcinogenic.

Cases of intracerebral mass effect unresponsive to corticosteroids, including one case leading to brain herniation, have been reported. Monitor patients receiving Gliadel® implant for seizures, intracranial infections, abnormal wound healing, and brain edema. Carmustine injection diluent contains absolute alcohol which can cause an "alcohol flushing syndrome" in susceptible patients; use with caution in patients with aldehyde dehydrogenase-2 deficiency.

Precautions Administer with caution to patients with depressed platelet, leukocyte or erythrocyte counts and in patients with renal or hepatic impairment; dosage reduction is recommended in patients with compromised bone marrow function (decreased leukocyte and platelet counts)

Adverse Reactions
Cardiovascular: Flushing; high dose (≥300 mg/m²) can produce chest pain, hypotension
Central nervous system: Ataxia, confusion, dizziness, encephalopathy, fever, headache, seizures
Dermatologic: Alopecia, hyperpigmentation, rash
Gastrointestinal: Anorexia, constipation, diarrhea, esophagitis, metallic taste, mucositis, nausea, vomiting
Hematologic: Anemia, myelosuppression (leukopenia, thrombocytopenia) with nadir at 28 days
Hepatic: Alkaline phosphatase and serum bilirubin increased, hepatotoxicity, jaundice, liver enzymes increased, veno-occlusive disease with high doses
Local: Burning sensation, pain and thrombophlebitis at injection site
Ocular: Blurred vision, conjunctival flushing, optic neuritis, retinitis
Respiratory: Cough, dyspnea, pulmonary fibrosis, pulmonary infiltrates, tachypnea
Miscellaneous: Secondary malignancies
Wafer:
Cardiovascular: Deep thrombophlebitis, facial edema, hypertension, peripheral edema
Central nervous system: Amnesia, anxiety, aphasia, ataxia, brain abscess, confusion, convulsion, CSF leaks, depression, diplopia, dizziness, facial paralysis, headache, hemiplegia, hydrocephalus, insomnia, intracranial hypertension, meningitis, somnolence
<1%, postmarketing, and/or case reports: Allergic reaction, azotemia (progressive), cerebral hemorrhage infarction (wafer), cyst formation (wafer), dermatitis, hepatic coma, kidney size decreased, neuroretinitis, renal failure, subacute hepatitis, tachycardia, thrombosis

Drug Interactions
Avoid Concomitant Use
Avoid concomitant use of Carmustine with any of the following: BCG; Natalizumab; Pimecrolimus; Tacrolimus (Topical); Vaccines (Live)

Increased Effect/Toxicity
Carmustine may increase the levels/effects of: Leflunomide; Natalizumab; Vaccines (Live)

The levels/effects of Carmustine may be increased by: Cimetidine; Denosumab; Melphalan; Pimecrolimus; Tacrolimus (Topical); Trastuzumab

Decreased Effect
Carmustine may decrease the levels/effects of: BCG; Cardiac Glycosides; Sipuleucel-T; Vaccines (Inactivated); Vaccines (Live)

The levels/effects of Carmustine may be decreased by: Echinacea

Stability Store vial at 2°C to 8°C (36°F to 46°F); protect from light and heat; discard vial if oily film is found on the bottom of the vial; reconstituted solution is stable for 8 hours at room temperature, 24 hours when refrigerated, or 48 hours when refrigerated after further dilution in D₅W in a glass bottle to a concentration of 0.1 mg/mL (defined in the study as <10% loss of potency) (Favier, 2001);

incompatible with sodium bicarbonate; adsorption of carmustine to plastics and polyvinyl chloride-based infusion containers has been documented. Store Gliadel® wafers at or below -20°C (-4°F). Unopened foil pouches may be kept at room temperature for a maximum of 6 hours.

Mechanism of Action Inhibits key enzymatic reactions involved with DNA synthesis; carbamoylation of amino acids in proteins; interferes with the normal function of DNA and RNA by alkylation and forms DNA-protein cross-links

Pharmacokinetics (Adult data unless noted)
Distribution: Readily crosses the blood-brain barrier since it is highly lipid soluble; CSF:plasma ratio >90%; distributes into breast milk
Protein binding: 75%
Metabolism: Denitrosation through action of microsomal enzymes; some enterohepatic circulation occurs
Half-life, terminal: 20-70 minutes (active metabolites may persist for days)
Elimination: ~60% to 70% excreted as metabolites in the urine and 6% to 10% excreted as CO_2 by the lungs

Usual Dosage
I.V. infusion (refer to individual protocols):
Children: 200-250 mg/m^2 every 4-6 weeks as a single dose; next dose is to be determined based on clinical and hematologic response to the previous dose (a repeat course should not be given until platelets are >100,000/mm^3 and leukocytes are >4000/mm^3)
BMT-conditioning agent: 300-600 mg/m^2 over at least 2 hours or may be divided into 2 doses administered 12 hours apart or 100 mg/m^2 every 12 hours for 6 doses
Adults: 150-200 mg/m^2 every 6 weeks as a single dose or divided into 75-100 mg/m^2/dose on 2 successive days; next dose is to be determined based on clinical and hematologic response to the previous dose (a repeat course should not be given until platelets are >100,000/mm^3 and leukocytes are >4000/mm^3)
Intracranial implant (wafer): Adults: Place 8 wafers (total dose: 61.6 mg) in the resection cavity; should the size and shape not accommodate 8 wafers, the maximum number of wafers as allowed should be placed

Administration Parenteral: Reconstitute 100 mg vial with 3 mL sterile dehydrated (absolute) alcohol followed by addition of 27 mL SWI. Further dilute the 3.3 mg of carmustine per mL solution with D_5W in a glass or polyolefin container to a final concentration of 0.2-1 mg/mL and administer by I.V. infusion over 1-2 hours to prevent vein irritation; rapid I.V. carmustine infusion may result in flushing, suffusion of the conjunctiva, hypotension, and agitation; carmustine has also been administered over 15-45 minutes diluted in 100-250 mL D_5W with monitoring for vein irritation; burning sensation and pain at I.V. site can be decreased with reduction of infusion rate and further dilution of solution or placing ice pack on I.V. site; flush line before and after carmustine administration to ensure vein patency. Maximum rate of infusion for high-dose carmustine: ≤3 mg/m^2/minute.

Monitoring Parameters CBC with differential and platelet count; baseline pulmonary function tests and tests during treatment (forced vital capacity; carbon monoxide diffusing capacity); liver function and renal function tests; monitor blood pressure and infusion site during administration

Patient Information Report occurrence of fever, sore throat, unusual bleeding or bruising to physician; may discolor skin brown; women of childbearing potential should avoid becoming pregnant while on carmustine therapy

Nursing Implications Must administer in glass containers; do not mix or administer with solutions containing sodium bicarbonate. Accidental skin contact may cause transient burning and brown discoloration of the skin; immediately wash skin with soap and water. To minimize risk of exposure to carmustine, wear impervious gloves when handling this agent. Care should be taken to avoid extravasation. If extravasation occurs, apply a cold pack within 30-60 minutes, then 4 times/day for 1 day.

Additional Information Myelosuppressive effects:
WBC: Moderate (nadir: 5-6 weeks)
Platelets: Severe (nadir: 4-5 weeks)

Dosage Forms Excipient information presented when available (limited, particularly for generics); consult specific product labeling.
Implant:
Gliadel®: 7.7 mg (8s)
Injection, powder for reconstitution:
BiCNU®: 100 mg [packaged with 3 mL of absolute alcohol as diluent]

References

Aronin PA, Mahaley MS Jr, Rudnick SA, et al, "Prediction of BCNU Pulmonary Toxicity in Patients With Malignant Gliomas," *N Engl J Med*, 1980, 303(4):183-8.
Colvin M, Hartner J, and Summerfield M, "Stability of Carmustine in the Presence of Sodium Bicarbonate," *Am J Hosp Pharm*, 1980, 37 (5):677-8.
Dunkel IJ, Garvin JH Jr, Goldman S, et al, "High Dose Chemotherapy With Autologous Bone Marrow Rescue for Children With Diffuse Pontine Brain Stem Tumors. Children's Cancer Group," *J Neurooncol*, 1998, 37(1):67-73.
Favier M, De Cazanove F, Coste A, et al, "Stability of Carmustine in Polyvinyl Chloride Bags and Polyethylene-Lined Trilayer Plastic Containers," *Am J Health Syst Pharm*, 2001, 58(3):238-41.
O'Driscoll BR, Hasleton PS, Taylor PM, et al, "Active Lung Fibrosis Up to 17 Years After Chemotherapy With Carmustine (BCNU) in Childhood," *N Engl J Med*, 1990, 323(6):378-82.
Papadakis V, Dunkel IJ, Cramer LD, et al, "High-Dose Carmustine, Thiotepa and Etoposide Followed by Autologous Bone Marrow Rescue for the Treatment of High Risk Central Nervous System Tumors," *Bone Marrow Transplant*, 2000, 26(2):153-60.

◆ **Carmustinum** *see* Carmustine *on page 252*

Carnitine (KAR ni teen)

Medication Safety Issues
Sound-alike/look-alike issues:
Levocarnitine may be confused with levetiracetam, levocabastine

U.S. Brand Names Carnitine-300 [OTC]; Carnitor®; Carnitor® SF; L-Carnitine® [OTC]

Canadian Brand Names Carnitor®

Therapeutic Category Nutritional Supplement

Generic Available Yes

Use Treatment of primary or secondary carnitine deficiency; prevention and treatment of carnitine deficiency (injection) in patients undergoing dialysis for end-stage renal disease (ESRD)

Pregnancy Risk Factor B

Pregnancy Considerations Teratogenic effects were not observed in animal studies. There are no adequate and well-controlled studies in pregnant women. However, carnitine is a naturally occurring substance in mammalian metabolism.

Lactation Excretion in breast milk unknown/use caution

Breast-Feeding Considerations In breast-feeding women, use must be weighed against the potential exposure of the infant to increased carnitine intake.

Contraindications Hypersensitivity to carnitine or any component

Precautions Use with caution in patients with seizure disorders; both new onset seizure activity and increased frequency of seizures have been reported. Safety and efficacy of oral carnitine has not been established in ESRD. Chronic administration of high doses of oral carnitine in patients with severely compromised renal function or ESRD on dialysis may result in accumulation of potentially toxic metabolites, trimethylamine and trimethylamine-N-oxide.

Adverse Reactions

Cardiovascular: I.V. use: Hypertension (18% to 21%), chest pain (6% to 15%), tachycardia (5% to 9%), palpitation, atrial fibrillation, ECG abnormality

Central nervous system: Myasthenia (in uremic patients on D,L-carnitine not L-carnitine), dizziness, fever, depression, seizures, headache, vertigo

Dermatologic: Rash

Endocrine & metabolic: Parathyroid disorder

Gastrointestinal: Nausea, vomiting, abdominal cramps, diarrhea, gastritis, taste perversion, anorexia

Neuromuscular & skeletal: Weakness, paresthesia, myasthenia (mild)

Respiratory: Cough, rhinitis, bronchitis

Miscellaneous: Body odor (dose-related), allergic reactions

Drug Interactions

Avoid Concomitant Use There are no known interactions where it is recommended to avoid concomitant use.

Increased Effect/Toxicity There are no known significant interactions involving an increase in effect.

Decreased Effect There are no known significant interactions involving a decrease in effect.

Stability Store at room temperature; protect from light

Mechanism of Action Endogenous substance required in energy metabolism; facilitates long chain fatty acid entry into the mitochondria; modulates intracellular coenzyme A homeostasis; carnitine deficiency exists when there is insufficient carnitine to buffer toxic acyl-Co A compounds; secondary carnitine deficiency may be a consequence of inborn errors of metabolism

Pharmacokinetics (Adult data unless noted)

Metabolism: Major metabolites: Trimethylamine, trimethylamine-N-oxide and acylcarnitine

Half-life, terminal: Adults: 17.4 hours

Bioavailability:

Tablet: 15.1% ± 5.3%

Solution: 15.9% ± 4.9%

Time to peak serum concentration: Oral: 3.3 hours

Elimination: Renal excretion of free and conjugated metabolites (acylcarnitine)

Clearance: 4 L/hour

Excretion: Urine 76% with 4% to 9% as unchanged drug; feces <1%

Usual Dosage

Primary carnitine deficiency:

Oral:

Children: 50-100 mg/kg/day divided 2-3 times/day, maximum 3 g/day; dosage must be individualized based upon patient response; higher dosages have been used

Adults: 330-990 mg/dose 2-3 times/day; maximum: 3 g/day

I.V.: Children and Adults: 50 mg/kg as a loading dose, followed (in severe cases) by 50 mg/kg/day infusion; maintenance: 50 mg/kg/day divided every 4-6 hours, increase as needed to a maximum of 300 mg/kg/day

ESRD patients on hemodialysis: Adults: I.V.: Predialysis carnitine levels below normal (30-60 micromoles): 10-20 mg/kg after each dialysis session; maintenance doses as low as 5 mg/kg may be used after 3-4 weeks of therapy depending upon response (carnitine level); National Kidney Foundation guidelines recommend basing treatment on clinical signs and symptoms; evaluate response at 3-month intervals and discontinue if no clinical improvement noted within 9-12 months.

Supplement to parenteral nutrition: I.V.: Neonates: 10-20 mg/kg/day in parenteral nutrition solution

Administration

Oral: Dilute in beverages or liquid food; administer with meals; consume slowly

Parenteral: May be administered by direct I.V. infusion over 2-3 minutes or as a continuous infusion diluted to 0.5-8 mg/mL in LR or NS

Monitoring Parameters Serum triglycerides, fatty acids, and carnitine levels

Reference Range Plasma free carnitine level: >20 micromoles/L; plasma total carnitine level 30-60 micromoles/L; to evaluate for carnitine deficiency determine the plasma acylcarnitine/free carnitine ratio (A/F ratio)

A/F ratio = [plasma total carnitine - free carnitine] divided by free carnitine

Normal plasma A/F ratio = 0.25; in carnitine deficiency A/F ratio >0.4

Additional Information Routine prophylactic use of carnitine in children receiving valproic acid to avoid carnitine deficiency and hepatotoxicity is probably not indicated

Dosage Forms Excipient information presented when available (limited, particularly for generics); consult specific product labeling.

Capsule, oral:

Carnitine-300: 300 mg

L-Carnitine®: 250 mg

Injection, solution [preservative free]: 200 mg/mL (5 mL, 12.5 mL)

Carnitor®: 200 mg/mL (5 mL)

Solution, oral: 100 mg/mL (118 mL)

Carnitor®: 100 mg/mL (118 mL) [cherry flavor]

Carnitor® SF: 100 mg/mL (118 mL) [sugar free; cherry flavor]

Tablet, oral: 330 mg

Carnitor®: 330 mg

L-Carnitine®: 500 mg

References

Bonner CM, De Brie KL, Hug G, et al, "Effects of Parenteral L-Carnitine Supplementation on Fat Metabolism and Nutrition in Premature Neonates," *J Pediatr*, 1995, 126(2):287-92.

Borum PR, "Carnitine in Neonatal Nutrition," *J Child Neurol*, 1995, 10 (Suppl 2):S25-31.

Eknoyan G, Latos DL, and Lindberg J, "Practice Recommendations for the Use of L-carnitine in Dialysis-Related Carnitine Disorder. National Kidney Foundation Carnitine Consensus Conference," *Am J Kidney Dis*, 2003, 41(4):868-76.

Helms RA, Mauer EC, and Hay WW Jr, "Effect of Intravenous L-Carnitine on Growth Parameters and Fat Metabolism During Parenteral Nutrition in Neonates," *JPEN J Parenter Enteral Nutr*, 1990, 14(5):448-53.

♦ **Carnitine-300 [OTC]** see Carnitine on page 253

♦ **Carnitor®** see Carnitine on page 253

♦ **Carnitor® SF** see Carnitine on page 253

♦ **Carrington Antifungal [OTC]** see Miconazole on page 927

♦ **Carter's Little Pills® (Can)** see Bisacodyl on page 194

♦ **Cartia XT®** see Diltiazem on page 443

Carvedilol (KAR ve dil ole)

Medication Safety Issues

Sound-alike/look-alike issues:

Carvedilol may be confused with atenolol, captopril, carbidopa, carteolol

Coreg® may be confused with Corgard®, Cortef®, Cozaar®

International issues:

Talliton® [Hungary] may be confused with Talacen® which is a brand name for pentazocine/acetaminophen combination in the U.S.

Related Information

Antihypertensive Agents by Class on page 1481

U.S. Brand Names Coreg CR®; Coreg®

Canadian Brand Names Apo-Carvedilol®; Coreg®; Dom-Carvedilol; Mylan-Carvedilol; Novo-Carvedilol; PHL-Carvedilol; PMS-Carvedilol; RAN™-Carvedilol; ratio-Carvedilol; ZYM-Carvedilol

Therapeutic Category Antihypertensive Agent; Beta-Adrenergic Blocker, Nonselective With Alpha-Blocking Activity

Generic Available Yes: Tablet

Use Treatment of mild to severe chronic heart failure of cardiomyopathic or ischemic origin (usually in addition to standard therapy) (FDA approved in adults); management of hypertension, alone or in combination with other agents (FDA approved in adults); reduction of cardiovascular mortality in patients with left ventricular dysfunction following MI (FDA approved in adults)

Pregnancy Risk Factor C

Pregnancy Considerations Because adverse events were not observed in animal reproduction studies, carvedilol is classified as pregnancy category C. It is not known if carvedilol crosses the human placenta. Information related to the use of carvedilol in pregnancy is limited. In a cohort study, an increased risk of cardiovascular defects was observed following maternal use of beta-blockers during pregnancy. Nonteratogenic adverse events, including bradycardia, hypoglycemia, hypotension, and respiratory depression, have been observed in the infant following maternal use of another beta-blocker with alpha-blocking activity during pregnancy. Refer to the Labetalol monograph for additional information. Untreated chronic maternal hypertension and pre-eclampsia are associated with adverse events in the fetus/infant and mother. Carvedilol is not currently recommended for the initial treatment of maternal hypertension during pregnancy.

Lactation Excretion in breast milk unknown/not recommended

Breast-Feeding Considerations It is not known if carvedilol is excreted into human milk. The manufacturer suggests that a decision should be made to either discontinue nursing or discontinue the medication.

Contraindications Hypersensitivity to carvedilol or any component; bronchial asthma or related bronchospastic conditions; sick sinus syndrome, second or third degree heart block, or severe bradycardia (except in patients with a functioning artificial pacemaker); cardiogenic shock; decompensated cardiac failure requiring intravenous inotropic therapy; severe hepatic impairment

Warnings May cause bradycardia, hypotension, postural hypotension, or syncope; to decrease risk of significant hypotension or syncope, initiate carvedilol cautiously at a low dose, administer with food (to slow the rate of absorption), and monitor closely while slowly titrating dose upwards; worsening of CHF or fluid retention may occur; adjustment of dose or other medications (eg, diuretics) may be required. Due to risk of syncope, avoid driving or hazardous tasks during initiation of therapy.

Beta blockers may block hypoglycemia-induced tachycardia and blood pressure changes; nonselective beta blockers may augment the insulin-induced hypoglycemia and delay the recovery of serum glucose concentrations; use with caution in patients with diabetes mellitus; worsening hyperglycemia may occur (monitor serum glucose). Use with caution in patients with peripheral vascular disease (may aggravate arterial insufficiency); use caution with anesthetic agents that decrease myocardial function. May mask signs of hyperthyroidism (eg, tachycardia); exacerbation of hyperthyroidism or thyroid storm may occur if beta blockers are abruptly discontinued. Exacerbation of angina, arrhythmias, and in some cases MI may occur following abrupt discontinuation of beta blockers; avoid abrupt discontinuation, wean

carvedilol slowly over 1-2 weeks, monitor for signs and symptoms of ischemia.

Deterioration of renal function may rarely occur in patients with CHF receiving carvedilol; patients with underlying renal dysfunction, diffuse vascular disease, ischemic heart disease or low blood pressure (eg, adults with systolic blood pressure <100 mm Hg) may be at risk; monitor renal function closely in these patients; decrease carvedilol dose or discontinue drug if renal function worsens. Beta-blocker use has been associated with induction or exacerbation of psoriasis, but cause and effect have not been firmly established.

Precautions Use with caution in patients with pheochromocytoma or Prinzmetal's variant angina. Beta-blockers should be avoided in patients with bronchospastic disease (see Contraindications); if administered to patients, use the lowest possible dose and monitor patients carefully. Patients who have a history of severe anaphylactic hypersensitivity reactions to various substances may be more reactive while receiving beta blockers; these patients may not be responsive to the normal doses of epinephrine used to treat hypersensitivity reactions. Use caution with concurrent use of verapamil or diltiazem (bradycardia or heart block can occur). Safety and efficacy in children <18 years of age have not been established.

Adverse Reactions

Cardiovascular: Angina, AV block, bradycardia, edema, hypertension, hypotension, palpitations, postural hypotension, syncope

Central nervous system: Dizziness, fatigue, fever, headache, insomnia, malaise, paresthesia, somnolence

Dermatologic: Psoriasiform rash, rash

Endocrine & metabolic: Hypercholesterolemia, hyperglycemia, hypertriglyceridemia, weight gain

Gastrointestinal: Diarrhea, nausea, vomiting

Hematologic: Thrombocytopenia

Hepatic: Liver enzymes elevated

Neuromuscular & skeletal: Arthralgia, asthenia, paresthesia

Ocular: Blurred vision

Renal: BUN elevated, renal function decreased (rare; see Warnings)

Respiratory: Cough increased, nasal congestion, nasopharyngitis, rhinitis, sinus congestion

Miscellaneous: Hypersensitivity reactions (rare, including anaphylactic reaction, angioedema, urticaria)

Drug Interactions

Metabolism/Transport Effects Substrate of CYP1A2 (minor), CYP2C9 (major), CYP2D6 (major), CYP2E1 (minor), CYP3A4 (minor), P-glycoprotein; **Inhibits** P-glycoprotein

Avoid Concomitant Use

Avoid concomitant use of Carvedilol with any of the following: Dabigatran Etexilate; Methacholine; Topotecan

Increased Effect/Toxicity

Carvedilol may increase the levels/effects of: Alpha-/Beta-Agonists (Direct-Acting); Alpha1-Blockers; Alpha2-Agonists; Amifostine; Antihypertensives; Antipsychotic Agents (Phenothiazines); Bupivacaine; Cardiac Glycosides; Colchicine; CycloSPORINE; CycloSPORINE (Systemic); Dabigatran Etexilate; Digoxin; Hypotensive Agents; Insulin; Lidocaine; Lidocaine (Systemic); Lidocaine (Topical); Mepivacaine; Methacholine; Midodrine; P-Glycoprotein Substrates; RiTUXimab; Rivaroxaban; Sulfonylureas; Topotecan

The levels/effects of Carvedilol may be increased by: Acetylcholinesterase Inhibitors; Aminoquinolines (Antimalarial); Amiodarone; Anilidopiperidine Opioids; Antipsychotic Agents (Phenothiazines); Calcium Channel Blockers (Nondihydropyridine); Cimetidine; CYP2C9 Inhibitors (Moderate); CYP2C9 Inhibitors (Strong); CYP2D6 Inhibitors (Moderate); CYP2D6 Inhibitors

(Strong); Darunavir; Diazoxide; Dipyridamole; Disopyramide; Dronedarone; Herbs (Hypotensive Properties); MAO Inhibitors; Pentoxifylline; P-Glycoprotein Inhibitors; Phosphodiesterase 5 Inhibitors; Propafenone; Propoxyphene; Prostacyclin Analogues; QuiNIDine; Reserpine; Selective Serotonin Reuptake Inhibitors

Decreased Effect

Carvedilol may decrease the levels/effects of: Beta2-Agonists; Theophylline Derivatives

The levels/effects of Carvedilol may be decreased by: Barbiturates; Herbs (Hypertensive Properties); Methylphenidate; Nonsteroidal Anti-Inflammatory Agents; Peginterferon Alfa-2b; P-Glycoprotein Inducers; Rifamycin Derivatives; Yohimbine

Food Interactions

Immediate release tablets: Food decreases the rate, but not the extent of absorption.

Extended release capsules: Compared with a standard meal, a high fat meal increases AUC and peak serum concentrations by ~20%; administration on an empty stomach decreases AUC by 27% and peak serum concentrations by 43%. In adults, administration of capsule contents on applesauce decreases the rate, but not the extent of absorption.

Stability

Immediate release tablets: Store below 30°C (86°F); protect from moisture; dispense in tightly closed, light resistant container

Extended release capsules: Store at controlled room temperature; dispense in tightly closed, light resistant container

Mechanism of Action Nonselective beta-adrenergic blocker with alpha-adrenergic blocking activity. Available as a racemic mixture; the S(-) enantiomer possesses the nonselective beta-adrenoreceptor blocking activity, while the alpha-adrenergic blocking activity is present in both R(+) and S(-) enantiomers at equal potency. Does not possess intrinsic sympathomimetic activity.

Associated effects in hypertensive patients include reduction of cardiac output, reduction of exercise- or beta agonist-induced tachycardia, reduction of reflex orthostatic tachycardia, vasodilation, decreased peripheral vascular resistance (especially in standing position), decreased renal vascular resistance, reduced plasma renin activity, and increased levels of atrial natriuretic peptide. In CHF patient, associated effects include decreased systemic blood pressure, decreased pulmonary capillary wedge pressure, decreased pulmonary artery pressure, decreased heart rate, decreased systemic vascular resistance, decreased right arterial pressure, increased stroke volume index, and increased left ventricular ejection fraction.

Pharmacodynamics Oral:

Onset of action:

Alpha-blockade: Within 30 minutes

Beta-blockade: Within 1 hour

Maximum effect: Antihypertensive effect, multiple dosing: 7-14 days

Pharmacokinetics (Adult data unless noted)

Absorption: Oral: Rapid and extensive, but with large first pass effect; first pass effect is stereoselective with R(+) enantiomer achieving plasma concentrations 2-3 times higher than S(-) enantiomer

Distribution: Distributes into extravascular tissues

V_d: Adults: 115 L

Protein binding: >98%, primarily to albumin

Metabolism: Extensively metabolized in the liver, primarily via cytochrome P450 isoenzymes CYP2D6 and CYP2C9 and to a lesser extent via CYP3A4, CYP2C19, CYP1A2 and CYP2E1; metabolized predominantly by aromatic ring oxidation and glucuronidation; oxidative metabolites undergo conjugation via glucuronidation and sulfation;

three active metabolites (4'-hydroxyphenyl metabolite is 13 times more potent than parent drug for beta blocking activity; however, active metabolites achieve plasma concentrations of only 1/10 of those for carvedilol). Metabolism is subject to genetic polymorphism; CYP2D6 poor metabolizers have a 2-3 fold higher plasma concentration of the R(+) enantiomer and a 20% to 25% increase in the S(-) enantiomer compared to extensive metabolizers.

Bioavailability: Immediate release tablets: 25% to 35%; extended release capsules: 85% of immediate release; bioavailability is increased in patients with CHF

Half-life:

(Laer, 2002):

Infants and children 6 weeks of age to 3.5 years (n=8): 2.2 hours

Children 5.5-19 years (n=7): 3.6 hours

Adults 24-37 years (n=9): 5.2 hours

(Manufacturer):

Adults (in general): 7-10 hours

R(+)-carvedilol: 5-9 hours

S(-)-carvedilol: 7-11 hours

Time to peak serum concentration: Extended release capsules: 5 hours

Elimination: <2% excreted unchanged in urine; metabolites are excreted via bile, into the feces

Dialysis: Hemodialysis does not significantly clear carvedilol

Usual Dosage Oral: **Note:** Individualize dosage for each patient; monitor patients closely during initiation and upwards titration of dose; reduce dosage if bradycardia or hypotension occurs

Infants and Children: **Heart Failure:** Immediate release tablets: Dose not established. Several case series and smaller studies have used a wide range of initial and target maintenance doses.

Although retrospective, the largest pediatric study to date (n=46; age range 3 months to 19 years) used mean initial doses of 0.08 mg/kg given twice daily. Doses were increased as tolerated by doubling the dose every 2 weeks. The dose was increased over a mean of 11 weeks to a mean maintenance dose of 0.46 mg/kg/dose given twice daily (see Bruns, 2001). Another retrospective study of 24 patients (mean age: 7.2 ± 6.4 years) used mean initial doses of 0.075 mg/kg/dose given twice daily. Doses were increased by 50% to 100% every 1-2 weeks with a target dose of 0.5 mg/kg/dose given twice daily. The mean maintenance dose achieved (after a median of 14 weeks of titration) was 0.98 mg/kg/day given in 2 divided doses per day (see Rusconi, 2004).

A large prospective randomized placebo controlled trial of 150 pediatric patients ranging in age from birth to 17 years will compare two doses of carvedilol. The following doses will be used: Initial: 0.05 mg/kg/dose given twice daily; maximum initial dose: 3.125 mg twice daily. Doses will be increased as tolerated by doubling the dose every 2 weeks until the target dose is attained. The "low dose" target dose will be 0.2 mg/kg/dose given twice daily; maximum: 12.5 mg twice daily. The "high dose" target dose will be 0.4 mg/kg/dose given twice daily; maximum: 25 mg twice daily (See Shady, 2002).

Note: Due to faster carvedilol elimination, 3 times daily dosing and a higher target dose per kg may be needed in young children (eg, <3.5 years) (see Laer, 2002). Further studies are needed to establish the optimal pediatric dose.

Adults:

CHF: Note: Prior to initiating therapy, other CHF medications should be stabilized and fluid retention minimized.

Immediate release tablets: Initial: 3.125 mg twice daily for 2 weeks; if tolerated, may increase to 6.25 mg twice daily. May double the dose every 2 weeks to the highest dose tolerated by patient.

Maximum recommended dose:

Mild to moderate heart failure:

<85 kg: 25 mg twice daily

>85 kg: 50 mg twice daily

Severe heart failure: 25 mg twice daily

Extended release capsules: Initial: 10 mg once daily for 2 weeks; if tolerated, may double the dose every 2 weeks up to 80 mg once daily; maintain on lower dose if higher dose is not tolerated.

Hypertension: Note: Use standing systolic blood pressure measured ~1 hour after dose as a guide for tolerance and trough blood pressure as a guide for efficacy.

Immediate release tablets: Initial: 6.25 mg twice daily; if tolerated, dose should be maintained for 1-2 weeks, then increased to 12.5 mg twice daily as needed. Dosage may be increased after 1-2 weeks if tolerated, to a maximum of 25 mg twice daily; maximum dose: 50 mg/day

Extended release capsules: Initial: 20 mg once daily; if tolerated, dose should be maintained for 1-2 weeks, then increased to 40 mg once daily as needed. Dosage may be increased after 1-2 weeks if tolerated, to 80 mg once daily; maximum dose: 80 mg once daily.

Left ventricular dysfunction following MI: Note: Initiate only after patient is hemodynamically stable and fluid retention has been minimized.

Immediate release tablets: Initial: 3.125-6.25 mg twice daily; use lower dose listed in patients with low blood pressure, low heart rate, or fluid retention; increase dosage incrementally (eg, from 6.25 to 12.5 mg twice daily) at intervals of 3-10 days, as tolerated, to a target dose of 25 mg twice daily.

Extended release capsules: Initial: 20 mg once daily; increase dosage incrementally (eg, from 20 mg to 40 mg once daily) at intervals of 3-10 days, as tolerated, to a target dose of 80 mg once daily; maintain on lower dose if higher dose is not tolerated.

Dosing adjustment in renal impairment: None recommended. **Note:** Mean AUCs were 40% to 50% higher in patients with moderate to severe renal dysfunction who received immediate release carvedilol, but the ranges of AUCs were similar to patients with normal renal function

Dosing adjustment in hepatic impairment: Use is contraindicated in patients with severe liver dysfunction, as drug is extensively metabolized by the liver. **Note:** Patients with severe cirrhotic liver disease achieved carvedilol serum concentrations 4-7 fold higher than normal patients following a single dose of immediate release carvedilol

Administration

Immediate release tablets: Administer with food to decrease the risk of orthostatic hypotension.

Extended release capsules: Administer with food, preferably in the morning; do not crush or chew capsule; swallow whole; do not take in divided doses. Capsule may be opened and contents sprinkled on a spoonful of applesauce; swallow applesauce/medication mixture immediately; do not chew; do not store for later use; do not use warm applesauce; do not sprinkle capsule contents on food other than applesauce; drink fluids after dose to make sure mixture is completely swallowed.

Monitoring Parameters Heart rate, blood pressure (seated and standing base); weight, BUN, serum creatinine, liver function, serum glucose, cholesterol, and triglycerides

Patient Information May cause fatigue, dizziness, low blood pressure (especially when standing), or fainting; rise slowly from sitting or lying position; may impair ability to perform activities requiring mental alertness or physical coordination; report unresolved swelling of extremities, weight gain, dizziness, fatigue, or fainting to healthcare provider; if diabetic, monitor serum glucose closely (drug may alter glucose tolerance or mask signs of hypoglycemia).

Nursing Implications Due to its alpha-blocking effects, carvedilol decreases blood pressure more in the standing position than in the supine position; be aware that postural hypotension and syncope may occur (see Warnings)

Additional Information Cytochrome P450 isoenzyme CYP2D6 poor metabolizers may have a higher rate of dizziness during initiation and upwards titration of carvedilol, perhaps due to the higher serum concentrations of the alpha blocking R(+) enantiomer and resulting vasodilation.

CHF: Carvedilol is a nonselective beta blocker with alpha-blocking and antioxidant properties. It is the only beta blocker approved in adults for the treatment of heart failure. Beta blocker therapy, without intrinsic sympathomimetic activity, should be initiated in adult patients with **stable** CHF (NYHA Class II-IV). To date, carvedilol, sustained release metoprolol, and bisoprolol have demonstrated a beneficial effect on morbidity and mortality. It is important that beta blocker therapy be instituted initially at very low doses with gradual and very careful titration. Because carvedilol has alpha-adrenergic blocking effects, it may lower blood pressure to a greater extent. The definitive clinical benefits of the antioxidant property are not known at this time.

Coreg CR® extended release capsules are hard gelatin capsules filled with immediate-release and controlled-release microparticles containing carvedilol phosphate; the microparticles are drug-layered and coated with methacrylic acid copolymers.

Dosage Forms Excipient information presented when available (limited, particularly for generics); consult specific product labeling.

Capsule, extended release; as phosphate:

Coreg CR®: 10 mg, 20 mg, 40 mg, 80 mg

Tablet: 3.125 mg, 6.25 mg, 12.5 mg, 25 mg

Coreg®: 3.125 mg, 6.25 mg, 12.5 mg, 25 mg

Extemporaneous Preparations Stability information of liquid carvedilol preparations has not been published, but is available from the manufacturer (see below). Two studies have used aqueous preparations. One study used a liquid suspension by dissolving one 3.125 mg tablet in 3 mL of water (see Bruns, 2001). A second study briefly mentions making a 1 mg/mL solution in water, details were not provided (see Rusconi, 2004).

Carvedilol oral liquid suspensions (0.1 mg/mL and 1.67 mg/mL) made from tablets, water, Ora-Plus®, and Ora-Sweet® were stable for 12 weeks when stored in glass amber bottles at room temperature (25°C); use one 3.125 mg tablet for the 0.1 mg/mL suspension or two 25 mg tablets for the 1.67 mg/mL suspension; grind the tablet(s) and compound a mixture with 5 mL of water, 15 mL Ora-Plus®, and 10 mL Ora-Sweet®; final volume of each suspension: 30 mL; label "shake well"; microbial testing at 5 and 12 weeks showed <10 colony forming units/mL for both aerobic count and the total combined mold and yeast count (data on file, GlaxoSmithKline, Philadelphia, PA: DOF #132).

References

Azeka E, Franchini Ramires JA, Valler C, et al, "Delisting of Infants and Children From the Heart Transplantation Waiting List After Carvedilol Treatment," *J Am Coll Cardiol*, 2002, 40(11):2034-8.

Brauchli YB, Jick SS, Curtin F, et al, "Association Between Beta-Blockers, Other Antihypertensive Drugs and Psoriasis: Population-Based Case-Control Study," *Br J Dermatol*, 2008, 158(6):1299-307.

Bruns LA and Canter CE, "Should Beta-Blockers be Used for the Treatment of Pediatric Patients With Chronic Heart Failure?" *Paediatr Drugs*, 2002, 4(12):771-8.

Bruns LA, Chrisant MK, Lamour JM, et al, "Carvedilol as Therapy in Pediatric Heart Failure: An Initial Multicenter Experience," *J Pediatr*, 2001, 138(4):505-11.

Gachara N, Prabhakaran S, Srinivas S, et al, "Efficacy and Safety of Carvedilol in Infants With Dilated Cardiomyopathy: A Preliminary Report," *Indian Heart J*, 2001, 53(1):74-8.

Giardini A, Formigari R, Bronzetti G, et al, "Modulation of Neurohormonal Activity After Treatment of Children in Heart Failure With Carvedilol," *Cardiol Young*, 2003, 13(4):333-6.

Gold MH, Holy AK, and Roenigk HH Jr, "Beta-Blocking Drugs and Psoriasis. A Review of Cutaneous Side Effects and Retrospective Analysis of Their Effects on Psoriasis," *J Am Acad Dermatol*, 1988, 19 (5 Pt 1):837-41.

Laer S, Mir TS, Behn F, et al, "Carvedilol Therapy in Pediatric Patients With Congestive Heart Failure: A Study Investigating Clinical and Pharmacokinetic Parameters," *Am Heart J*, 2002, 143(5):916-22.

Ratnapalan S, Griffiths K, Costei AM, et al, "Digoxin-Carvedilol Interactions in Children," *J Pediatr*, 2003, 142(5):572-4.

Rusconi P, Gomez-Marin O, Rossique-Gonzalez M, et al, "Carvedilol in Children With Cardiomyopathy: 3-Year Experience at a Single Institution," *J Heart Lung Transplant*, 2004, 23(7):832-8.

Schön MP and Boehncke WH, "Psoriasis," *N Engl J Med*, 2005, 352 (18):1899-912.

Shaddy RE, Curtin EL, Sower B, et al, "The Pediatric Randomized Carvedilol Trial in Children With Heart Failure: Rationale and Design," *Am Heart J*, 2002, 144(3):383-9.

Cascara (kas KAR a)

Therapeutic Category Laxative, Stimulant

Generic Available Yes

Use Temporary relief of constipation; sometimes used with milk of magnesia ("black and white" mixture)

Pregnancy Risk Factor C

Contraindications Nausea, vomiting, abdominal pain, fecal impaction, intestinal obstruction, GI bleeding, appendicitis, CHF

Warnings Long-term use may result in laxative dependence

Adverse Reactions

Cardiovascular: Faintness

Endocrine & metabolic: Electrolyte and fluid imbalance

Gastrointestinal: Abdominal cramps, nausea, diarrhea, benign pigmentation of the colonic mucosa (with prolonged use)

Genitourinary: Discoloration of urine (reddish, pink, or brown)

Stability Protect from light and heat

Mechanism of Action Direct chemical irritation of the intestinal mucosa resulting in an increased rate of colonic motility and change in fluid and electrolyte secretion

Pharmacodynamics Onset of action: 6-10 hours

Pharmacokinetics (Adult data unless noted)

Absorption: Oral: Small amount from small intestine

Metabolism: In the liver

Usual Dosage Oral (**aromatic** fluid extract):

Infants: 1.25 mL/day as a single dose (range: 0.5-2 mL) as needed

Children 2-11 years: 2.5 mL/day as a single dose (range: 1-3 mL) as needed

Children ≥12 years and Adults: 5 mL/day (range: 2-6 mL) as needed at bedtime

Administration Oral: Administer on an empty stomach at bedtime; drink plenty of fluids

Patient Information Should not be used regularly for more than 1 week; may discolor urine reddish, pink, or brown

Additional Information Cascara sagrada fluid extract is 5 times more potent than cascara sagrada aromatic fluid extract

Dosage Forms Excipient information presented when available (limited, particularly for generics); consult specific product labeling.

Aromatic fluid extract: 120 mL, 473 mL

Tablet: 325 mg

◆ **Cascara Sagrada** *see* Cascara *on page* 258

Caspofungin (kas poe FUN jin)

U.S. Brand Names Cancidas®

Canadian Brand Names Cancidas®

Therapeutic Category Antifungal Agent, Echinocandin; Antifungal Agent, Systemic

Generic Available No

Use Treatment of invasive aspergillosis in patients who are refractory to or intolerant of other therapies (ie, amphotericin B, lipid formulations of amphotericin B, and/or itraconazole); candidemia, intra-abdominal abscess, peritonitis, and pleural space infection caused by susceptible *Candida* species; esophageal candidiasis; empiric therapy of presumed fungal infection in febrile neutropenic patients (FDA approved in ages ≥3 months and adults)

Pregnancy Risk Factor C

Pregnancy Considerations Adverse events have been observed in animal studies. There are no adequate and well-controlled studies in pregnant women. Should be used during pregnancy only if potential benefit justifies the potential risk to the fetus.

Lactation Excretion in breast milk unknown/use caution

Contraindications Hypersensitivity to caspofungin or any component

Warnings Transient increases of alanine transaminase (ALT) and aspartate transaminase (AST) have been reported both with and without concomitant use of cyclosporine; limit use in patients receiving cyclosporine to those in whom the potential benefit outweighs the risk

Precautions Use with caution and modify dose in patients with moderate hepatic impairment; safety and efficacy have not been established in children with any degree of hepatic impairment and adults with severe hepatic impairment; use with caution and modify dose in patients on concurrent drugs which induce drug clearance such as efavirenz, nevirapine, phenytoin, dexamethasone, carbamazepine, or rifampin (see Drug Interactions)

Adverse Reactions

Cardiovascular: Hypertension, hypotension, peripheral edema, tachycardia

Central nervous system: Chills, fever, headache

Dermatologic: Erythema, pruritus, rash

Endocrine & metabolic: Hyperkalemia, hypokalemia

Gastrointestinal: Abdominal pain, diarrhea, mucosal inflammation, nausea, vomiting

Hematologic: Anemia, hemoglobin decreased

Hepatic: Alkaline phosphatase increased; ALT, AST, and serum bilirubin increased; hepatic impairment

Neuromuscular & skeletal: Back pain

Renal: Creatinine increased, hematuria, proteinuria

Respiratory: Bronchospasm, dyspnea

Miscellaneous: Anaphylaxis, ARDS, cough, GVHD, pneumonia

Drug Interactions

Avoid Concomitant Use There are no known interactions where it is recommended to avoid concomitant use.

Increased Effect/Toxicity

The levels/effects of Caspofungin may be increased by: CycloSPORINE; CycloSPORINE (Systemic)

Decreased Effect

Caspofungin may decrease the levels/effects of: Saccharomyces boulardii; Tacrolimus; Tacrolimus (Systemic)

The levels/effects of Caspofungin may be decreased by: Inducers of Drug Clearance; Rifampin

Stability Store lyophilized vial in refrigerator at 2°C to 8°C (36°F to 46°F); reconstitute 50 mg or 70 mg vial with 10.8 mL of NS (consult manufacturer's prescribing information for details); reconstituted solution may be stored at room temperature (≤25°C or ≤77°F) for 1 hour prior to preparation of the infusion solution; final infusion solution may be stored at room temperature (≤25°C or ≤77°F) for 24 hours or for 48 hours in the refrigerator; caspofungin is not stable in dextrose-containing solutions

Mechanism of Action Inhibits synthesis of beta (1,3)-D-glucan, an essential cell wall component of susceptible fungi

Pharmacokinetics (Adult data unless noted)

Distribution: CSF concentrations: Nondetectable [<10 ng/mL (n=1)] (see Sáez-Llorens, 2009)

Protein binding: 97% to albumin

Metabolism: Via hydrolysis and N-acetylation in the liver; undergoes spontaneous chemical degradation to an open-ring peptide and hydrolysis to amino acids

Half-life: Beta (distribution): 9-11 hours (~8 hours in children <12 years); terminal: 40-50 hours; beta phase half-life is 32% to 43% lower in pediatric patients than in adult patients

Elimination: 35% of dose excreted in feces primarily as metabolites; 41% of dose excreted in urine primarily as metabolites; 1.4% of dose excreted unchanged in urine

Dialysis: Not dialyzable

Usual Dosage I.V.: **Note:** Caspofungin treatment duration should be based on patient status and clinical response. Empiric therapy should be given until neutropenia resolves. In neutropenic patients, continue treatment for at least 7 days after both signs and symptoms of infection and neutropenia resolve. In patients with positive cultures, continue treatment for at least 14 days after the last positive culture.

Preterm neonates to infants <3 months: 25 mg/m²/dose once daily; dosing based on a neonatal pharmacokinetic study of 18 patients that showed similar serum concentrations to standard adult doses (50 mg/day). Reported trough concentrations were slightly elevated and not correlated with increased adverse events (see Sáez-Llorens, 2009)

Infants and Children 3 months to 17 years: Initial dose: 70 mg/m²/dose on day 1, subsequent dosing: 50 mg/m²/dose once daily; may increase to 70 mg/m²/dose once daily if clinical response inadequate (maximum dose: 70 mg). Patients receiving carbamazepine, dexamethasone, efavirenz, nevirapine, phenytoin, or rifampin (and possibly other enzyme inducers): Consider 70 mg/m²/dose once daily (maximum: 70 mg/day).

Adults: Loading dose: 70 mg on day 1, followed by 50 mg once daily thereafter; 70 mg daily dose has been administered and well tolerated in patients not clinically responding to the daily 50 mg dose; may need to adjust dose in patients receiving a concomitant enzyme inducer. Doses greater than the standard adult dosing regimen (ie, 150 mg once daily) have not demonstrated increased benefit or toxicity in patients with invasive candidiasis (see Betts, 2009).

Esophageal candidiasis: 50 mg once daily with no loading dose

Patients receiving concomitant enzyme inducer:

Patients receiving rifampin: 70 mg caspofungin once daily

Patients receiving carbamazepine, dexamethasone, phenytoin, nevirapine, or efavirenz: May require an increase in caspofungin dose to 70 mg once daily

Dosing adjustment in renal impairment: No adjustment needed

Dosing adjustment in hepatic impairment (based on adult data):

Mild hepatic impairment (Child-Pugh score 5 to 6): No dosage adjustment necessary

Moderate hepatic impairment (Child-Pugh score 7 to 9): Decrease daily dose by 30%

Administration Administer by slow I.V. infusion over 1 hour (manufacturer); higher doses (eg, 150 mg) have been infused over ~2 hours (see Betts, 2009); maximum concentration of 0.5 mg/mL diluted in NS, LR, 0.45% sodium chloride. Do not mix or coinfuse with other medications. Do not use diluents containing dextrose.

Monitoring Parameters Periodic liver function tests, serum potassium, CBC, hemoglobin

Nursing Implications Infuse slowly over 1 hour; possible histamine-related reactions have been reported (monitor during infusion)

Dosage Forms Excipient information presented when available (limited, particularly for generics); consult specific product labeling.

Injection, powder for reconstitution, as acetate:

Cancidas®: 50 mg [contains sucrose 39 mg], 70 mg [contains sucrose 54 mg]

References

Betts RF, Nucci M, Talwar D, et al, "A Multicenter, Double-Blind Trial of a High-Dose Caspofungin Treatment Regimen Versus a Standard Caspofungin Treatment Regimen for Adult Patients With Invasive Candidiasis," Clin Infect Dis, 2009, 48(12):1676-84.

Pappas PG, Kauffman CA, Andes D, et al, "Clinical Practice Guidelines for the Management of Candidiasis: 2009 Update by the Infectious Diseases Society of America," Clin Infect Dis, 2009, 48(5):503-35.

Sáez-Llorens X, Macias M, Maiya P, et al, "Pharmacokinetics and Safety of Caspofungin in Neonates and Infants Less Than 3 Months of Age," Antimicrob Agents Chemother, 2009, 53(3):869-75.

Walsh TJ, Adamson PC, Seibel NL, et al, "Pharmacokinetics (PK) of Caspofungin (CAS) in Pediatric Patients (#M-896)," 42nd Interscience Conference on Antimicrobial Agents and Chemotherapy, San Diego, CA, Sept 27-30, 2002.

Walsh TJ, Adamson PC, Seibel NL, et al, "Pharmacokinetics, Safety, and Tolerability of Caspofungin in Children and Adolescents," Antimicrob Agents Chemother, 2005, 49(11):4536-45.

Walsh TJ, Teppler H, Donowitz GR, et al, "Caspofungin Versus Liposomal Amphotericin B for Empirical Antifungal Therapy in Patients With Persistent Fever and Neutropenia," N Engl J Med, 2004, 351(14):1391-402.

◆ **Caspofungin Acetate** see Caspofungin on page 258

Castor Oil (KAS tor oyl)

Therapeutic Category Laxative, Stimulant

Generic Available Yes: Oil

Use Preparation for rectal or bowel examination or surgery; rarely used to relieve constipation; also applied to skin as emollient and protectant

Contraindications Hypersensitivity to castor oil; nausea, vomiting, abdominal pain, fecal impaction, GI bleeding, appendicitis, CHF, menstruation, dehydration

Warnings Long-term use may result in laxative dependence

Adverse Reactions

Central nervous system: Dizziness

Endocrine & metabolic: Electrolyte disturbance, dehydration

Gastrointestinal: Abdominal cramps, nausea, diarrhea

Drug Interactions

Avoid Concomitant Use There are no known interactions where it is recommended to avoid concomitant use.

Increased Effect/Toxicity There are no known significant interactions involving an increase in effect.

Decreased Effect There are no known significant interactions involving a decrease in effect.

Stability Protect from heat (emulsion should be protected from freezing)

Mechanism of Action Acts primarily in the small intestine; hydrolyzed to ricinoleic acid which reduces net absorption of fluid and electrolytes and stimulates peristalsis

◀ **Pharmacodynamics** Onset of action: Oral: Within 2-6 hours

Usual Dosage Oral:

Castor oil:

Infants <2 years: 1-5 mL or 15 mL/m^2/dose as a single dose

Children 2-11 years: 5-15 mL as a single dose

Children ≥12 years and Adults: 15-60 mL as a single dose

Emulsified castor oil:

Infants: 2.5-7.5 mL/dose

Children:

<2 years: 5-15 mL/dose

2-11 years: 7.5-30 mL/dose

Children ≥12 years and Adults: 30-60 mL/dose

Administration Oral: Do not administer at bedtime because of rapid onset of action; chill or administer with milk, juice, or carbonated beverage to improve palatability; administer on an empty stomach; castor oil emulsions should be shaken well before use

Monitoring Parameters I & O, serum electrolytes, stool frequency

Dosage Forms Excipient information presented when available (limited, particularly for generics); consult specific product labeling.

Oil, oral: 100% (60 mL, 120 mL, 180 mL, 480 mL, 3840 mL)

◆ **Cataflam®** see Diclofenac on page 429

◆ **Catapres®** see CloNIDine on page 338

◆ **Catapres-TTS®** see CloNIDine on page 338

◆ **Cathflo® Activase®** see Alteplase on page 71

◆ **Caverject®** see Alprostadil on page 69

◆ **Caverject Impulse®** see Alprostadil on page 69

◆ **CaviRinse™** see Fluoride on page 595

◆ **Cayston®** see Aztreonam on page 167

◆ **CB-1348** see Chlorambucil on page 287

◆ **CBDCA** see CARBOplatin on page 250

◆ **CBZ** see CarBAMazepine on page 244

◆ **CCNU** see Lomustine on page 837

◆ **CD271** see Adapalene on page 50

◆ **2-CdA** see Cladribine on page 323

◆ **CDDP** see CISplatin on page 318

◆ **CE** see Estrogens (Conjugated/Equine) on page 539

◆ **Ceclor® (Can)** see Cefaclor on page 260

◆ **Cecon® [OTC] [DSC]** see Ascorbic Acid on page 138

◆ **Cedax®** see Ceftibuten on page 273

◆ **CEE** see Estrogens (Conjugated/Equine) on page 539

◆ **CeeNU®** see Lomustine on page 837

Cefaclor (SEF a klor)

Medication Safety Issues

Sound-alike/look-alike issues:

Cefaclor may be confused with cephalexin

U.S. Brand Names Raniclor™

Canadian Brand Names Apo-Cefaclor®; Ceclor®; Novo-Cefaclor; Nu-Cefaclor; PMS-Cefaclor

Therapeutic Category Antibiotic, Cephalosporin (Second Generation)

Generic Available Yes: Excludes chewable tablet

Use Infections caused by susceptible bacteria including Staph aureus, S. pneumoniae, S. pyogenes, and H. influenzae (excluding β-lactamase negative, ampicillin-resistant strains); treatment of otitis media, sinusitis, and infections involving the respiratory tract, skin and skin structure, bone and joint; treatment of urinary tract infections caused by E. coli, Klebsiella, and Proteus mirabilis

Pregnancy Risk Factor B

Pregnancy Considerations Adverse events were not observed in animal reproduction studies; therefore, cefaclor is classified as pregnancy category B. It is not known if cefaclor crosses the placenta; other cephalosporins cross the placenta and are considered safe for use during pregnancy. An increased risk of teratogenic effects has not been observed following maternal use of cefaclor.

Lactation Enters breast milk/use caution

Breast-Feeding Considerations Small amounts of cefaclor are excreted in breast milk. The manufacturer recommends that caution be exercised when administering cefaclor to nursing women. Nondose-related effects could include modification of bowel flora.

Contraindications Hypersensitivity to cefaclor, any component, or cephalosporins

Warnings Prolonged use may result in superinfection; do not use in patients with immediate-type hypersensitivity reactions to penicillin

Precautions Use with caution in patients with impaired renal function, history of colitis, or history of penicillin hypersensitivity; modify dosage in patients with severe renal impairment. Chewable tablets contain aspartame which is metabolized to phenylalanine and must be avoided (or used with caution) in patients with phenylketonuria.

Adverse Reactions

Central nervous system: Dizziness, agitation, insomnia, confusion, fever

Dermatologic: Rash, urticaria, pruritus, erythema multiforme, Stevens-Johnson syndrome, toxic epidermal necrolysis, angioedema

Gastrointestinal: Nausea, vomiting, diarrhea, pseudomembranous colitis

Genitourinary: Genital moniliasis, vaginitis

Hematologic: Eosinophilia, neutropenia, aplastic anemia, agranulocytosis, thrombocytopenia

Hepatic: Liver enzymes elevated, cholestatic jaundice

Renal: Interstitial nephritis

Miscellaneous: Anaphylaxis (rare); serum sickness-like reaction (estimated incidence ranges from 0.024% to 0.2% per drug course); majority of reactions have occurred in children <5 years of age with symptoms of fever, rash, erythema multiforme, and arthralgia, often occurring during the second or third exposure

Drug Interactions

Avoid Concomitant Use

Avoid concomitant use of Cefaclor with any of the following: BCG

Increased Effect/Toxicity

The levels/effects of Cefaclor may be increased by: Probenecid

Decreased Effect

Cefaclor may decrease the levels/effects of: BCG; Typhoid Vaccine

Food Interactions Capsules and suspension: Food or milk delays and decreases peak concentration

Stability Store capsule, chewable tablet, and unreconstituted powder for oral suspension at room temperature. Refrigerate suspension after reconstitution; discard after 14 days.

Mechanism of Action Inhibits bacterial cell wall synthesis by binding to one or more of the penicillin-binding proteins and interfering with the final transpeptidation step of peptidoglycan synthesis resulting in cell wall death

Pharmacokinetics (Adult data unless noted)

Absorption: Oral: Well absorbed; acid stable

Distribution: Distributes into tissues and fluids including bone, pleural and synovial fluid; crosses the placenta; appears in breast milk

Protein binding: 25%

Half-life: 30-60 minutes (prolonged with renal impairment)

Time to peak serum concentration:

Capsule: 60 minutes

Suspension and chewable tablet: 45-60 minutes

Elimination: Most of dose (80%) excreted unchanged in urine by glomerular filtration and tubular secretion

Dialysis: Moderately dialyzable (20% to 50%)

Usual Dosage Oral:

Children >1 month: 20-40 mg/kg/day divided every 8-12 hours; maximum dose: 2 g/day (twice daily option is for treatment of otitis media or pharyngitis)

Otitis media: 40 mg/kg/day divided every 12 hours

Pharyngitis: 20 mg/kg/day divided every 12 hours

Adults: 250-500 mg every 8 hours

Dosing adjustment in renal impairment: Cl_{cr} <10 mL/minute: Administer 50% of dose

Administration Oral:

Capsule, suspension: Administer 1 hour before or 2 hours after a meal; shake suspension well before use

Tablet, chewable: Administer 1 hour before or 2 hours after a meal; chew tablet before swallowing

Monitoring Parameters With prolonged therapy, monitor CBC and stool frequency periodically

Test Interactions Positive Coombs' [direct], false-positive urine glucose (Clinitest®), false ↑ of serum or urine creatinine

Patient Information Counsel patient that cefaclor should only be used to treat bacterial infections. Entire course of medication should be taken even if patient feels better early in the course. Report persistent diarrhea to physician.

Dosage Forms Excipient information presented when available (limited, particularly for generics); consult specific product labeling.

Capsule: 250 mg, 500 mg

Powder for oral suspension: 125 mg/5 mL (75 mL, 150 mL); 250 mg/5 mL (75 mL, 150 mL); 375 mg/5 mL (50 mL, 100 mL)

Tablet, chewable:

Raniclor™: 250 mg [contains phenylalanine 5.6 mg/tablet and tartrazine; fruity flavor]; 375 mg [contains phenylalanine 8.4 mg/tablet and tartrazine; fruity flavor]

Tablet, extended release: 500 mg

References

Boguniewicz M and Leung DYM, "Hypersensitivity Reactions to Antibiotics Commonly Used in Children," *Pediatr Infect Dis J*, 1995, 14(3):221-31.

Hyslop DL, "Cefaclor Safety Profile: A Ten Year Review," *Clin Ther*, 1988, 11(Suppl A):83-94.

Levine LR, "Quantitative Comparison of Adverse Reactions to Cefaclor vs Amoxicillin in a Surveillance Study," *Pediatr Infect Dis*, 1985, 4 (4):358-61.

Cefadroxil (sef a DROKS il mon o HYE drate)

Canadian Brand Names Apo-Cefadroxil®; Novo-Cefadroxil; PRO-Cefadroxil

Therapeutic Category Antibiotic, Cephalosporin (First Generation)

Generic Available Yes

Use Treatment of susceptible bacterial infections including group A beta-hemolytic streptococcal pharyngitis or tonsillitis; skin and soft tissue infections caused by streptococci or staphylococci; urinary tract infections caused by *Klebsiella*, *E. coli*, and *Proteus mirabilis*

Pregnancy Risk Factor B

Pregnancy Considerations Adverse events were not observed in animal reproduction studies; therefore, cefadroxil is classified as pregnancy category B. Cefadroxil crosses the placenta. Limited data is available concerning the use of cefadroxil in pregnancy; however, adverse fetal effects were not noted in a small clinical trial. Adequate and well-controlled studies have been not completed in pregnant women.

Lactation Enters breast milk (small amounts)/use caution (AAP rates "compatible")

Breast-Feeding Considerations Very small amounts of cefadroxil are excreted in breast milk. The manufacturer recommends that caution be exercised when administering cefadroxil to nursing women. The American Academy of Pediatrics considers cefadroxil to be "usually compatible with breast-feeding." Nondose-related effects could include modification of bowel flora.

Contraindications Hypersensitivity to cefadroxil, any component, or cephalosporins

Warnings Prolonged use may result in superinfection; do not use in patients with immediate-type hypersensitivity reaction to penicillin

Oral suspension contains sodium benzoate; benzoic acid (benzoate) is a metabolite of benzyl alcohol; large amounts of benzyl alcohol (≥99 mg/kg/day) have been associated with a potentially fatal toxicity ("gasping syndrome") in neonates; the "gasping syndrome" consists of metabolic acidosis, respiratory distress, gasping respirations, CNS dysfunction (including convulsions, intracranial hemorrhage), hypotension and cardiovascular collapse; use cefadroxil oral suspensions containing sodium benzoate with caution in neonates; *in vitro* and animal studies have shown that benzoate displaces bilirubin from protein binding sites

Precautions Use with caution in patients who are hypersensitive to penicillin; modify dosage in patients with renal impairment

Adverse Reactions

Dermatologic: Rash

Gastrointestinal: Nausea, vomiting, diarrhea, pseudomembranous colitis

Genitourinary: Vaginitis

Hematologic: Transient neutropenia

Drug Interactions

Avoid Concomitant Use

Avoid concomitant use of Cefadroxil with any of the following: BCG

Increased Effect/Toxicity

The levels/effects of Cefadroxil may be increased by: Probenecid

Decreased Effect

Cefadroxil may decrease the levels/effects of: BCG; Typhoid Vaccine

Food Interactions Concomitant administration with food, infant formula, or cow's milk does **not** significantly affect absorption

Stability Refrigerate suspension after reconstitution; discard after 14 days

Mechanism of Action Interferes with bacterial cell wall synthesis during active replication, causing cell wall death and resultant bactericidal activity against susceptible bacteria

Pharmacokinetics (Adult data unless noted)

Absorption: Oral: Rapid; well absorbed from GI tract

Distribution: V_d: 0.31 L/kg; crosses the placenta; appears in breast milk

Protein binding: 20%

Half-life: 1-2 hours; 20-24 hours in renal failure

Time to peak serum concentration: Within 70-90 minutes

Elimination: >90% of dose excreted unchanged in urine within 24 hours

Usual Dosage Oral:

Infants and Children: 30 mg/kg/day divided twice daily up to a maximum of 2 g/day

Adolescents and Adults: 1-2 g/day in 1-2 divided doses; maximum dose for adults: 4 g/day

Dosing interval in renal impairment:

Cl_{cr} 10-25 mL/minute: Administer every 24 hours

Cl_{cr} <10 mL/minute: Administer every 36 hours

Administration Oral: May be administered without regard to food; administration with food may decrease nausea or vomiting; shake suspension well before use

Monitoring Parameters Stool frequency, resolution of infection

Test Interactions Positive Coombs' [direct], false-positive with urinary glucose tests using cupric sulfate (Clinitest®, Benedict's solution)

Patient Information Report persistent diarrhea; entire course of medication (eg, 10-14 days) should be taken to ensure eradication of organism

Dosage Forms Excipient information presented when available (limited, particularly for generics); consult specific product labeling.

Note: Strength is expressed as base

Capsule, as hemihydrate: 500 mg

Capsule, as monohydrate: 500 mg

Powder for oral suspension, as monohydrate: 250 mg/ 5 mL (100 mL); 500 mg/5 mL (75 mL, 100 mL)

Tablet, as hemihydrate: 1 g

Tablet, as monohydrate: 1 g

◆ **Cefadroxil Monohydrate** see Cefadroxil on page 261

CeFAZolin (sef A zoe lin)

Medication Safety Issues

Sound-alike/look-alike issues:

CeFAZolin may be confused with cefprozil, cefTRIAXone, cephalexin, cephalothin

Kefzol® may be confused with Cefzil®

Related Information

Endocarditis Prophylaxis on page 1610

Therapeutic Category Antibiotic, Cephalosporin (First Generation)

Generic Available Yes

Use Treatment of respiratory tract, skin and skin structure, urinary tract, biliary tract, bone and joint infections, genital infections, and septicemia due to susceptible gram-positive cocci (except enterococcus); some gram-negative bacilli including E. coli, Proteus, and Klebsiella may be susceptible; perioperative prophylaxis; bacterial endocarditis prophylaxis for dental and upper respiratory procedures

Pregnancy Risk Factor B

Pregnancy Considerations Adverse effects were not observed in animal reproduction studies; therefore, cefazolin is classified as pregnancy category B. Cefazolin crosses the placenta. Adverse events have not been reported in the fetus following administration of cefazolin prior to caesarean section. Cefazolin is recommended for group B streptococcus prophylaxis in pregnant patients with a nonanaphylactic penicillin allergy.

Due to pregnancy-induced physiologic changes, the pharmacokinetics of cefazolin are altered. The half-life is shorter and the AUC is smaller. The volume of distribution is unchanged.

Lactation Enters breast milk (small amounts)/use caution (AAP rates "compatible")

Breast-Feeding Considerations Small amounts of cefazolin are excreted in breast milk. The manufacturer recommends that caution be exercised when administering cefazolin to nursing women. The American Academy of Pediatrics considers cefazolin to be "usually compatible with breast-feeding." Nondose-related effects could include modification of bowel flora.

Contraindications Hypersensitivity to cefazolin sodium, any component, or cephalosporins

Warnings Prolonged use may result in superinfection; may cause pseudomembranous colitis or antibiotic-associated colitis; do not use in patients with immediate-type hypersensitivity reactions to penicillin

Precautions Use with caution in patients with a history of colitis, renal or hepatic impairment, poor nutritional state, patients previously stabilized on anticoagulant therapy, or in patients with a history of hypersensitivity to penicillins; modify dosage in patients with renal impairment

Adverse Reactions

Central nervous system: CNS irritation, fever, seizures

Dermatologic: Pruritus, rash, Stevens-Johnson syndrome, urticaria

Gastrointestinal: Diarrhea, nausea, vomiting, oral candidiasis, pseudomembranous colitis

Hematologic: Eosinophilia, leukopenia, neutropenia, thrombocytopenia

Hepatic: Transient elevation of ALT, AST, and alkaline phosphatase; hepatitis

Local: Pain at injection site, phlebitis

Renal: BUN and serum creatinine elevated; renal failure

Miscellaneous: Anaphylaxis

Drug Interactions

Avoid Concomitant Use

Avoid concomitant use of CeFAZolin with any of the following: BCG

Increased Effect/Toxicity

CeFAZolin may increase the levels/effects of: Vitamin K Antagonists

The levels/effects of CeFAZolin may be increased by: Probenecid

Decreased Effect

CeFAZolin may decrease the levels/effects of: BCG; Typhoid Vaccine

Stability Store intact vials at room temperature; protect from light. Reconstituted solution is stable for 24 hours at room temperature or 10 days when refrigerated; thawed solutions of the commercially available frozen cefazolin injections are stable for 48 hours at room temperature or 30 days when refrigerated

Mechanism of Action Inhibits bacterial cell wall synthesis by binding to one or more of the penicillin-binding proteins and interfering with the final transpeptidation step of peptidoglycan synthesis resulting in cell wall death

Pharmacokinetics (Adult data unless noted)

Distribution: Crosses the placenta; small amounts appear in breast milk; CSF penetration is poor; penetrates bone and synovial fluid well; distributes into bile

Protein binding: 74% to 86%

Metabolism: Minimally hepatic

Half-life:

Neonates: 3-5 hours

Adults: 90-150 minutes (prolonged with renal impairment)

Time to peak serum concentration:

I.M.: Within 0.5-2 hours

I.V.: Within 5 minutes

Elimination: 80% to 100% excreted unchanged in urine

Dialysis: Moderately dialyzable (20% to 50%)

Usual Dosage I.M., I.V.:

Neonates:

Postnatal age ≤7 days: 40 mg/kg/day divided every 12 hours

Postnatal age >7 days:

≤2000 g: 40 mg/kg/day divided every 12 hours

>2000 g: 60 mg/kg/day divided every 8 hours

Infants and Children: 25-100 mg/kg/day divided every 6-8 hours; maximum dose: 6 g/day

Mild-to-moderately-severe infections: 25-50 mg/kg/day divided every 6-8 hours

Severe infections: 100 mg/kg/day divided every 6-8 hours

Bacterial endocarditis prophylaxis for dental and upper respiratory procedures in penicillin allergic patients (see Precautions): 50 mg/kg 30-60 minutes before procedure; maximum dose: 1 g

Adults:

Mild infections: 250-500 mg every 8 hours

Pneumococcal pneumonia: 500 mg every 12 hours

Moderate-to-severe infections: 500 mg to 1 g every 6-8 hours

Severe, life-threatening infections (eg, endocarditis, septicemia): 1-1.5 g every 6 hours; maximum dose: 12 g/day

UTI: 1 g every 12 hours

Bacterial endocarditis prophylaxis for dental and upper respiratory procedures in penicillin allergic patients (see Precautions): 1 g 30-60 minutes before procedure

Perioperative prophylaxis: 1 g 30-60 minutes prior to surgery; 0.5-1 g every 8 hours for 24 hours post-operatively depending on the procedure

Dosing interval in renal impairment:

Children >1 month: After initial loading dose is adminis-tered, modify dose based on the degree of renal impairment:

Cl_{cr} 40-70 mL/minute: Administer 60% of usual dose every 12 hours

Cl_{cr} 20-40 mL/minute: Administer 25% of usual dose every 12 hours

Cl_{cr} 5-20 mL/minute: Administer 10% of usual dose every 24 hours

Adults:

Cl_{cr} 35-54 mL/minute: Administer full dose ≥every 8 hours

Cl_{cr} 11-34 mL/minute: Administer 50% of usual dose every 12 hours

Cl_{cr} ≤10 mL/minute: Administer 50% of usual dose every 18-24 hours

Administration Parenteral:

I.V.: Cefazolin may be administered IVP over 3-5 minutes at a maximum concentration of 100 mg/mL or I.V. intermittent infusion over 10-60 minutes at a final concentration for I.V. administration of 20 mg/mL. In fluid-restricted patients, a concentration of 138 mg/mL has been administered IVP.

I.M.: Deep I.M. injection into a large muscle mass. May dilute vial using SWI to a final concentration between 225-330 mg/mL (see package insert). Shake well before use.

Monitoring Parameters Renal function periodically when used in combination with other nephrotoxic drugs, hepatic function tests, and CBC; prothrombin time in patients at risk; number and type of stools/day for diarrhea

Test Interactions False-positive urine glucose using Clinitest®, positive Coombs' [direct], false increase serum or urine creatinine

Additional Information Sodium content of 1 g: 46 mg (2 mEq)

Dosage Forms Excipient information presented when available (limited, particularly for generics); consult specific product labeling.

Infusion [iso-osmotic dextrose solution]: 1 g (50 mL) [contains sodium 46 mg/g]

Injection, powder for reconstitution: 500 mg, 1 g, 10 g, 20 g [contains sodium 48 mg (2 mEq)/g]

References
Pickering LK, O'Connor DM, Anderson D, et al, "Clinical and Pharmacologic Evaluation of Cefazolin in Children," *J Infect Dis* 1973, 128(Suppl):S407-1.

Robinson DC, Cookson TL, and Grisafe JA, "Concentration Guidelines for Parenteral Antibiotics in Fluid-Restricted Patients," *Drug Intell Clin Pharm*, 1987, 21(12):985-9.

Wilson W, Taubert KA, Gewitz M, et al, "Prevention of Infective Endocarditis: Guidelines from the American Heart Association: A Gguideline from the American Heart Association Rheumatic Fever, Endocarditis, and Kawasaki Disease Committee, Council on Cardiovascular Disease in the Young, and the Council on Clinical Cardiology, Council on Cardiovascular Surgery and Anesthesia, and the Quality of Care and Outcomes Research Interdisciplinary Working Group," *Circulation*, 2007, 116(15):1736-54.

◆ **Cefazolin Sodium** *see* CeFAZolin *on page 262*

Cefdinir (SEF di ner)

U.S. Brand Names Omnicef®

Canadian Brand Names Omnicef®

Therapeutic Category Antibiotic, Cephalosporin (Third Generation)

Generic Available Yes

Use Infections caused by susceptible organisms including *S. pneumoniae* (penicillin-susceptible strains only; inad-equate activity against resistant pneumococcus), *H. influenzae* (including beta-lactamase-producing strains), *H. parainfluenzae* (including beta-lactamase-producing strains), *M. catarrhalis* (including beta-lactamase-produc-ing strains), *S. aureus* (inactive against methicillin-resistant staphylococci), and *S. pyogenes.*

FDA approved in Infants and Children ≥6 months: Treatment of acute bacterial otitis media, acute maxillary sinusitis, pharyngitis/tonsillitis, and uncomplicated skin and skin structure infection

FDA approved in Adolescents and Adults: Treatment of community-acquired pneumonia, acute exacerbations of chronic bronchitis, acute maxillary sinusitis, pharyngitis/ tonsillitis, and uncomplicated skin and skin structure infections

Pregnancy Risk Factor B

Pregnancy Considerations Teratogenic events have not been observed in animal studies; therefore, cefdinir is classified as pregnancy category B. It is not known if cefdinir crosses the human placenta.

Lactation Excretion in breast milk unknown

Breast-Feeding Considerations Cefdinir is not detect-able in breast milk following a single cefdinir 600 mg dose. It is not known if it would be detectable after multiple doses. If present in breast milk, nondose-related effects could include modification of bowel flora.

Contraindications Hypersensitivity to cefdinir, any com-ponent, or cephalosporins

Warnings Pseudomembranous colitis has been reported with cefdinir; prolonged use may result in superinfection; serum sickness-like reactions have been reported with signs and symptoms occurring after a few days of therapy and resolving a few days after drug discontinuation. Do not use in patients with immediate-type hypersensitivity reactions to penicillin. If an allergic reaction occurs, discontinue cefdinir. Powder for oral suspension contains sodium benzoate; benzoic acid (benzoate) is a metabolite of benzyl alcohol; large amounts of benzyl alcohol (≥99 mg/kg/day) have been associated with a potentially fatal toxicity ("gasping syndrome") in neonates; avoid use of cefdinir products containing sodium benzoate in neo-nates; *in vitro* and animal studies have shown that benzoate displaces bilirubin from protein binding sites

Precautions Use with caution in patients with impaired renal function, history of colitis, or in penicillin-sensitive patients; modify dosage in patients with severe renal impairment

Adverse Reactions

Central nervous system: Headache, hyperactivity, insom-nia, somnolence, seizures, dizziness

Dermatologic: Rash, pruritus, diaper rash, Stevens-Johnson syndrome, erythema multiforme, toxic epider-mal necrolysis

Gastrointestinal: Diarrhea, nausea, vomiting, abdominal pain, pseudomembranous colitis, dyspepsia, discolora-tion of stools (red), anorexia, constipation, upper GI bleed

Genitourinary: Vaginitis, microhematuria, vaginal moniliasis

Hematologic: Leukopenia, neutropenia, hemolytic anemia, eosinophilia, thrombocytopenia

◀ Hepatic: AST, ALT, alkaline phosphatase elevated; cholestatic jaundice, prolonged PT, hepatitis

Renal: BUN/serum creatinine elevated, acute renal failure

Respiratory: Acute respiratory failure, eosinophilic pneumonia

Miscellaneous: Serum sickness-like reactions, anaphylaxis

Drug Interactions

Avoid Concomitant Use

Avoid concomitant use of Cefdinir with any of the following: BCG

Increased Effect/Toxicity

The levels/effects of Cefdinir may be increased by: Probenecid

Decreased Effect

Cefdinir may decrease the levels/effects of: BCG; Typhoid Vaccine

The levels/effects of Cefdinir may be decreased by: Iron Salts

Food Interactions Total absorption is not affected by food. Iron-fortified infant formula has no significant effect on cefdinir absorption (cefdinir can be administered with iron-fortified infant formula)

Stability Store at room temperature; reconstituted suspension stable for 10 days at room temperature

Mechanism of Action Inhibits bacterial cell wall synthesis by binding to one or more of the penicillin-binding proteins resulting in disruption of cell wall synthesis and cell lysis

Pharmacokinetics (Adult data unless noted)

Absorption: High-fat meal decreases extent of absorption by 10%

Distribution: Penetrates into blister fluid, middle ear fluid, tonsils, sinus, and lung tissues

V_d:

Children 6 months to 12 years: 0.67 L/kg

Adults: 0.35 L/kg

Protein binding: 60% to 70%

Bioavailability:

Capsules: 16% to 21%

Suspension: 25%

Half-life, elimination: 1.7 (± 0.6) hours with normal renal function

Time to peak serum concentration: 2-4 hours

Elimination: 11.6% to 18.4% of a dose is excreted unchanged in urine

Dialysis: ~63% is removed by hemodialysis (4 hours duration)

Usual Dosage Oral:

Infants and Children (≥6 months to 12 years):

Otitis media or pharyngitis/tonsillitis: 14 mg/kg/day divided every 12 hours for 5-10 days or 14 mg/kg/day once daily for 10 days; maximum: 600 mg/day

Skin and skin structure infection: 14 mg/kg/day divided twice daily for 10 days; maximum: 600 mg/day

Acute maxillary sinusitis: 14 mg/kg/day divided every 12 hours for 10 days or 14 mg/kg/day once daily for 10 days; maximum: 600 mg/day

Children >12 years and Adults:

Acute exacerbations of chronic bronchitis or pharyngitis/tonsillitis: 600 mg once daily for 10 days or 300 mg every 12 hours for 5-10 days

Skin and skin structure infection or community-acquired pneumonia: 300 mg every 12 hours for 10 days

Acute maxillary sinusitis: 600 mg once daily for 10 days or 300 mg every 12 hours for 10 days

Dosing adjustment in renal impairment:

Cl_{cr} <30 mL/minute:

Children ≥6 months to 12 years: 7 mg/kg/dose once daily; maximum: 300 mg/dose

Adults: 300 mg once daily

Patients receiving hemodialysis: 300 mg or 7 mg/kg/dose starting at the conclusion of each hemodialysis session with subsequent doses every other day

Administration Oral: May administer with or without food; administer with food if stomach upset occurs; administer cefdinir at least 2 hours before or after antacids or iron supplements; shake suspension well before use

Monitoring Parameters Evaluate renal function before and during therapy; with prolonged therapy, monitor coagulation tests, CBC, liver function test periodically, and number and type of stools/day for diarrhea

Test Interactions Positive Coombs' [direct]; may produce false-positive reaction to urine glucose with Clinitest®; may produce false-positive reaction for ketones in the urine with tests using nitroprusside

Patient Information Report persistent diarrhea to physician; may discolor stools red if taken with iron

Additional Information Oral suspension contains 2.86 g of sucrose per teaspoon.

Dosage Forms Excipient information presented when available (limited, particularly for generics); consult specific product labeling.

Capsule: 300 mg

Omnicef®: 300 mg

Powder for oral suspension: 125 mg/5 mL (60 mL, 100 mL); 250 mg/5 mL (60 mL, 100 mL)

Omnicef®: 125 mg/5 mL (60 mL, 100 mL) [contains sodium benzoate and sucrose 2.86 g/5 mL; strawberry flavor]; 250 mg/5 mL (60 mL, 100 mL) [contains sodium benzoate and sucrose 2.86 g/5 mL; strawberry flavor]

References

Klein JO and McCracken GH Jr, "Summary: Role of a New Oral Cephalosporin, Cefdinir, for Therapy of Infections of Infants and Children," *Pediatr Infect Dis J*, 2000, 19(12 Suppl):S181-3.

Perry CM and Scott LJ, "Cefdinir: A Review of Its Use in the Management of Mild-to-Moderate Bacterial Infections," *Drugs*, 2004, 64(13):1433-64.

Cefepime (SEF e pim)

Medication Safety Issues

Sound-alike/look-alike issues:

Cefepime may be confused with cefixime, ceftazidime

U.S. Brand Names Maxipime®

Canadian Brand Names Maxipime®

Therapeutic Category Antibiotic, Cephalosporin (Fourth Generation)

Generic Available Yes

Use Treatment of pneumonia, uncomplicated skin and soft tissue infections, urinary tract infections (including pyelonephritis), and as empiric therapy for febrile neutropenic patients (FDA approved in ages 2 months to 16 years and adults); used in combination with metronidazole for complicated intra-abdominal infections (FDA approved in adults). Cefepime is a fourth generation cephalosporin with activity against gram-negative bacteria, including *Pseudomonas aeruginosa*, *E. coli*, *H. influenzae*, *M. catarrhalis*, *M morganii*, *P. mirabilis*, and strains of *Acinetobacter*, *Citrobacter*, *Enterobacter*, *Klebsiella*, *Providencia*, and *Serratia*; active against gram-positive bacteria, such as *Staphylococcus aureus*, *S. pyogenes*, and *S. pneumoniae*

Pregnancy Risk Factor B

Pregnancy Considerations Teratogenic effects were not observed in animal studies; therefore, cefepime is classified as pregnancy category B. It is not known if cefepime crosses the human placenta.

Lactation Enters breast milk/use caution

Breast-Feeding Considerations Small amounts of cefepime are excreted in breast milk. The manufacturer recommends that caution be exercised when administering cefepime to nursing women. Nondose-related effects could include modification of bowel flora.

Contraindications Hypersensitivity to cefepime, any component, or other cephalosporins, penicillins, or beta-lactam antibiotics

Warnings Modify dosage in patients with severe renal impairment; *C. difficile*-associated diarrhea has been reported with the use of cefepime; prolonged use may result in superinfection; use with caution in patients with penicillin hypersensitivity; do not use in patients with immediate-type hypersensitivity reactions to penicillin. CNS adverse events, including encephalopathy, confusion, hallucinations, stupor, coma, myoclonus, and seizures, have been reported, most commonly in patients with renal impairment.

Precautions The manufacturer does not recommend the use of cefepime in pediatric patients for the treatment of serious infections due to *Haemophilus influenzae* type b, for suspected meningitis, or for meningeal seeding from a distant infection site. However, limited data suggest that cefepime may be a valuable alternative for treating bacterial meningitis in children in conjunction with other agents like vancomycin in areas with cephalosporin nonsusceptible pneumococci. Use with caution in patients with a history of GI disease or seizures. May be associated with increased INR, especially in patients who are nutritionally-deficient, have prolonged treatment, or who have hepatic or renal disease.

Adverse Reactions

Central nervous system: Coma, confusion, encephalopathy, fever, hallucinations, headache, seizure, stupor

Dermatologic: Maculopapular rash, pruritus

Endocrine & metabolic: Hypophosphatemia

Gastrointestinal: Diarrhea, nausea, pseudomembranous colitis, vomiting

Hematologic: Eosinophilia, leukopenia, neutropenia, positive Coombs' test without hemolysis, thrombocytopenia

Hepatic: ALT increased, AST increased, PT abnormal, PTT abnormal

Local: Inflammation, pain, phlebitis

<1%, postmarketing, and/or case reports: Agranulocytosis, alkaline phosphatase increased, anaphylactic shock, anaphylaxis, bilirubin increased, BUN increased, colitis, creatinine increased, hematocrit decreased, hypercalcemia, hyperkalemia, hyperphosphatemia, hypocalcemia, myoclonus, oral moniliasis, urticaria, vaginitis

Drug Interactions

Avoid Concomitant Use

Avoid concomitant use of Cefepime with any of the following: BCG

Increased Effect/Toxicity

The levels/effects of Cefepime may be increased by: Probenecid

Decreased Effect

Cefepime may decrease the levels/effects of: BCG; Typhoid Vaccine

Stability Store vial at 2°C to 25°C (36°F to 77°F); protect from light; incompatible with metronidazole, vancomycin, aminoglycosides, and aminophylline. Cefepime diluted with NS, D_5W, $D_{10}W$, and D_5NS is stable for 24 hours at 20°C to 25°C (68°F to 77°F) or for 7 days at 2°C to 8°C (36°F to 46°F).

Mechanism of Action Inhibits bacterial cell wall synthesis by binding to one or more of the penicillin-binding proteins; inhibits the final transpeptidation step of peptidoglycan synthesis in bacterial cell walls

Pharmacokinetics (Adult data unless noted)

Distribution: V_d:

Infants (PCA <30 weeks): 0.51 L/kg

Children 2 months to 6 years: 0.32-0.35 L/kg

Adults: 16-20 L; penetrates into inflammatory fluid at concentrations ~80% of serum levels and into bronchial mucosa at levels ~60% of plasma levels; excreted in breast milk at very low concentrations

Protein binding: ~20%

Metabolism: Very little

Half-life:

Children 2 months to 6 years: 1.77-1.96 hours

Adults: 2 hours

Elimination: At least 85% eliminated as unchanged drug in urine

Dialysis: 45% to 68% removed by hemodialysis

Usual Dosage I.M., I.V.:

Neonates <14 days of age: 30 mg/kg/dose every 12 hours should provide antibiotic exposure equivalent to or greater than 50 mg/kg/dose every 8 hours used in older infants and children

Children 2 months to 16 years, ≤40 kg in weight: 50 mg/kg/dose (maximum dose: 2 g) every 12 hours

Febrile neutropenic patients: 50 mg/kg/dose (maximum dose: 2 g) every 8 hours for 7 days or until neutropenia resolves

Cefepime has been studied in 12 cystic fibrosis patients (ages 4-41 years) with bronchopulmonary infection at a dose of 50 mg/kg/dose every 8 hours (maximum dose: 2 g/dose every 8 hours); cefepime was as effective as cefotaxime in 90 children <15 years of age who were randomized to receive cefepime 50 mg/kg/dose every 8 hours (n=43) or cefotaxime 50 mg/kg/dose every 6 hours (n=47) for the treatment of bacterial meningitis

Adults: 1-2 g every 12 hours; high doses or more frequent administration may be required in pseudomonal infections

UTIs: 0.5-2 g every 12 hours for 7-10 days

Empiric monotherapy in febrile neutropenia: 2 g every 8 hours for 7 days or until neutropenia resolves

Intra-abdominal infection, complicated: 2 g every 12 hours with metronidazole for 7-10 days

Dosing Adjustment in Renal Impairment, Adults

Cl_{cr} (mL/min)	Infection		
	Mild to Moderate	Moderate to Severe	Severe
30-60	0.5-1 g I.M./I.V. every 24 h	1-2 g I.V. every 24 h	2 g I.V. every 24 h
11-29	0.5 g I.M./I.V. every 24 h	0.5-1 g I.V. every 24 h	1 g I.V. every 24 h
≤10	0.25 g I.M./I.V. every 24 h	0.25-0.5 g I.V. every 24 h	0.5 g I.V. every 24 h

Administration Parenteral:

I.V.: Cefepime may be administered by I.V. intermittent infusion over 20-30 minutes; final concentration for I.V. administration should not exceed 40 mg/mL in D_5W, NS, $D_{10}W$, D_5/NS, or D_5/LR; in clinical trials, cefepime was administered by direct I.V. injection over 3-5 minutes at a final concentration of 100 mg/mL for mild to moderate infections

I.M.: Deep I.M. injection. May dilute vial using SWI, NS, D_5W, or 0.5% or 1% lidocaine to a final concentration of 280 mg/mL (see package insert)

Monitoring Parameters With prolonged therapy, monitor renal and hepatic function periodically; number and type of stools/day for diarrhea; CBC with differential

Test Interactions Positive Coombs' [direct]; may falsely elevate creatinine values when Jaffé reaction is used; may cause false-positive results in urine glucose tests when using Clinitest®; false-positive urinary proteins and steroids

Patient Information Report side effects such as diarrhea, dyspepsia, headache, blurred vision, and lightheadedness to your physician

Nursing Implications Do not admix with aminoglycosides ▶

◀ **Dosage Forms** Excipient information presented when available (limited, particularly for generics); consult specific product labeling.

Infusion, premixed iso-osmotic dextrose solution: 1 g (50 mL); 2 g (100 mL)

Injection, powder for reconstitution, as hydrochloride: 500 mg, 1 g, 2 g

Maxipime®: 500 mg, 1 g, 2 g

References

Arguedas AG, Stutman HR, Zaleska M, et al, "Cefepime. Pharmacokinetics and Clinical Response in Patients With Cystic Fibrosis," *Am J Dis Child*, 1992, 146(7):797-802.

Blumer JL, Reed MD, Lemon E, et al, "Pharmacokinetics (PK) of Cefepime in Pediatric Patients Administered Single and Multiple 50 mg/kg Doses Every 8 Hours by the Intravenous (I.V.) or Intramuscular (I.M.) Route," 34th Interscience Conference on Antimicrobial Agents and Chemotherapy, 1994, Orlando, Fl. Abs. A69.

Capparelli E, Hochwald C, Rasmussen M, et al, "Population Pharmacokinetics of Cefepime in the Neonate," *Antimicrob Agents Chemother*, 2005, 49(7):2760-6.

Haase MR, "Acute Bacterial Meningitis in Children," *J Pharm Pract*, 2004, 17:392.

Saez-Llorens X, Castano E, Garcia R, et al, "Prospective Randomized Comparison of Cefepime and Cefotaxime for Treatment of Bacterial Meningitis in Infants and Children," *Antimicrob Agents Chemother*, 1995, 39(4):937-40.

Wynd MA and Paladino JA, "Cefepime: A Fourth-Generation Parenteral Cephalosporin," *Ann Pharmacother*, 1996, 30(12):1414-24.

♦ **Cefepime Hydrochloride** *see* Cefepime *on page 264*

Cefixime (sef IKS eem)

Medication Safety Issues

Sound-alike/look-alike issues:

Cefixime may be confused with cefepime

Suprax® may be confused with Sporanox®, Surbex®

International issues:

Cefiton® [Portugal] may be confused with Cefotan® which is a brand name for cefotetan in the U.S.

Cefiton® [Portugal] may be confused with Ceftim® which is a brand name for ceftazidime in Italy

Cefiton® [Portugal] may be confused with Ceftin® which is a brand name for cefuroxime in the U.S.

Cefiton® [Portugal] may be confused with Lexotan® which is a brand name for bromazepam in multiple international markets

U.S. Brand Names Suprax®

Canadian Brand Names Suprax®

Therapeutic Category Antibiotic, Cephalosporin (Third Generation)

Generic Available No

Use Treatment of urinary tract infections, otitis media, respiratory infections due to susceptible organisms including *S. pneumoniae* and *pyogenes*, *H. influenzae*, *M. catarrhalis*, and many *Enterobacteriaceae*; documented poor compliance with other oral antimicrobials; outpatient therapy of serious soft tissue or skeletal infections due to susceptible organisms; single-dose oral treatment of uncomplicated cervical/urethral gonorrhea due to *N. gonorrhoeae*; treatment of shigellosis in areas with a high rate of resistance to TMP-SMX

Pregnancy Risk Factor B

Pregnancy Considerations Teratogenic effects were not observed in animal studies; therefore cefixime is classified as pregnancy category B. It is not known if cefixime crosses the human placenta; other cephalosporins cross the placenta and are considered safe in pregnancy. Congenital anomalies have not been associated with cefixime use during pregnancy (limited data). Cefixime is recommended for use in pregnant women for the treatment of gonococcal infections.

Lactation Excretion in breast milk unknown

Breast-Feeding Considerations It is not known if cefixime is excreted in breast milk. The manufacturer recommends that consideration be given to discontinuing nursing temporarily during treatment. Other cephalosporins are considered safe during breast-feeding. If present in breast milk, nondose-related effects could include modification of bowel flora.

Contraindications Hypersensitivity to cefixime, any component, or cephalosporins

Warnings Prolonged use may result in superinfection; do not use in patients with immediate-type hypersensitivity reactions to penicillin

Suspension contains sodium benzoate; benzoic acid (benzoate) is a metabolite of benzyl alcohol; large amounts of benzyl alcohol (≥99 mg/kg/day) have been associated with a potentially fatal toxicity ("gasping syndrome") in neonates; the "gasping syndrome" consists of metabolic acidosis, respiratory distress, gasping respirations, CNS dysfunction (including convulsions, intracranial hemorrhage), hypotension and cardiovascular collapse; use suspension containing sodium benzoate with caution in neonates; *in vitro* and animal studies have shown that benzoate displaces bilirubin from protein binding sites

Precautions Use with caution in patients hypersensitive to penicillin, patients with impaired renal function, and patients with a history of colitis; modify dosage in patients with renal impairment

Adverse Reactions

Central nervous system: Headache, fever, dizziness, fatigue, nervousness, insomnia, seizures, somnolence

Dermatologic: Skin rash, urticaria, pruritus, angioedema, Stevens-Johnson syndrome, erythema multiforme, toxic epidermal necrolysis

Gastrointestinal: Nausea, diarrhea (up to 15% of children), abdominal pain, pseudomembranous colitis

Genitourinary: Vaginitis, dysuria

Hematologic: Eosinophilia, thrombocytopenia, leukopenia

Hepatic: Transient elevation of liver enzymes, hepatitis, jaundice

Neuromuscular & skeletal: Arthralgia

Renal: Transient elevation of BUN and serum creatinine, acute renal failure

Miscellaneous: Anaphylaxis

Drug Interactions

Avoid Concomitant Use

Avoid concomitant use of Cefixime with any of the following: BCG

Increased Effect/Toxicity

The levels/effects of Cefixime may be increased by: Probenecid

Decreased Effect

Cefixime may decrease the levels/effects of: BCG; Typhoid Vaccine

Food Interactions Food delays the time to reach peak concentrations

Stability After reconstitution, suspension may be stored for 14 days at room temperature or under refrigeration

Mechanism of Action Inhibits bacterial cell wall synthesis by binding to one or more of the penicillin-binding proteins; inhibits the final transpeptidation step of peptidoglycan synthesis resulting in cell wall death

Pharmacokinetics (Adult data unless noted)

Absorption: Oral: 40% to 50%

Distribution: Into bile, sputum, middle ear fluid; crosses the placenta

Protein binding: 65%

Half-life:

Normal renal function: 3-4 hours

Renal failure: Up to 11.5 hours

Time to peak serum concentration: Within 2-6 hours; peak serum concentrations are 25% to 50% higher for the oral suspension versus tablets (tablets are no longer commercially available in the U.S.)

Elimination: 50% of absorbed dose excreted as active drug in urine and 10% in bile

Dialysis: 10% removed by hemodialysis

Usual Dosage Oral:

Infants and Children: 8 mg/kg/day divided every 12-24 hours; maximum dose: 400 mg/day

Treatment of acute UTI: 16 mg/kg/day divided every 12 hours on day 1, then 8 mg/kg/day every 24 hours for 13 days

Prophylaxis after sexual victimization: 8 mg/kg in a single dose (maximum dose: 400 mg) **plus** azithromycin 20 mg/kg in a single dose (maximum dose: 1 g); also begin or complete hepatitis B virus immunization and consider prophylaxis for trichomoniasis and bacterial vaginosis

Adolescents and Adults: 400 mg/day divided every 12-24 hours

Uncomplicated cervical/urethral gonorrhea due to *N. gonorrhoeae*: 400 mg as a single dose plus azithromycin 1 g orally in a single dose **or** doxycycline 100 mg orally twice daily for 7 days

Prophylaxis after sexual victimization: 400 mg in a single dose **plus** azithromycin 1 g orally in a single dose **or** doxycycline 100 mg orally twice daily for 7 days **plus** metronidazole 2 g orally in a single dose **plus** hepatitis B virus immunization if not fully immunized plus consider prophylaxis for HIV depending on circumstances

Dosing adjustment in renal impairment:

Cl_{cr} 21-60 mL/minute: Administer 75% of the standard dose

Cl_{cr} <20 mL/minute: Administer 50% of the standard dose

Administration Oral: May be administered with or without food; administer with food to decrease GI distress; shake suspension well before use

Monitoring Parameters With prolonged therapy, monitor renal and hepatic function periodically; number and type of stools/day for diarrhea

Test Interactions False-positive reaction for urine glucose using Clinitest®; false-positive urine ketones using tests with nitroprusside

Patient Information Report problems with diarrhea

Dosage Forms Excipient information presented when available (limited, particularly for generics); consult specific product labeling. [DSC] = Discontinued product

Powder for oral suspension, as trihydrate:

Suprax®: 100 mg/5 mL (50 mL, 75 mL [DSC], 100 mL) [contains sodium benzoate; strawberry flavor]; 200 mg/5 mL (50 mL, 75 mL) [contains sodium benzoate; strawberry flavor]

Tablet, oral, as trihydrate:

Suprax®: 400 mg

References

Ashkenazi S, Amir J, Waisman Y, et al, "A Randomized, Double-Blind Study Comparing Cefixime and Trimethoprim-Sulfamethoxazole in the Treatment of Childhood Shigellosis," *J Pediatr*, 1993, 123 (5):817-21.

"2002 Guidelines for the Treatment of Sexually Transmitted Diseases. Centers for Disease Control and Prevention," *MMWR Morb Mortal Wkly Rep*, 2002, 51(RR-6):1-80.

Hoberman A, Wald ER, Hickey RW, et al, "Oral Versus Initial Intravenous Therapy for Urinary Tract Infections in Young Febrile Children," *Pediatrics*, 1999, 104(1 Pt 1):79-86.

Johnson CE, Carlin SA, Super DM, et al, "Cefixime Compared With Amoxicillin for Treatment of Acute Otitis Media," *J Pediatr*, 1991, 119 (1):117-22.

◆ **Cefixime Trihydrate** see Cefixime on page 266

◆ **Cefizox®** see Ceftizoxime on page 274

Cefotaxime (sef oh TAKS eem)

Medication Safety Issues

Sound-alike/look-alike issues:

Cefotaxime may be confused with cefoxitin, ceftizoxime, cefuroxime

International issues:

Spectrocef® [Italy] may be confused with Spectracef® which is a brand name for cefditoren in the U.S.

U.S. Brand Names Claforan®

Canadian Brand Names Claforan®

Therapeutic Category Antibiotic, Cephalosporin (Third Generation)

Generic Available Yes: Powder

Use Treatment of susceptible lower respiratory tract, skin and skin structure, bone and joint, intra-abdominal and genitourinary tract infections; treatment of a documented or suspected meningitis due to susceptible organisms such as *H. influenzae* and *N. meningitidis*; indicated for *Neisseria gonorrhoeae* infections (including uncomplicated cervical and urethral gonorrhea and gonorrhea pelvic inflammatory disease); nonpseudomonal gram-negative rod infection in a patient at risk of developing aminoglycoside-induced nephrotoxicity and/or ototoxicity; infection due to an organism whose susceptibilities clearly favor cefotaxime over cefuroxime or an aminoglycoside

Pregnancy Risk Factor B

Pregnancy Considerations Teratogenic effects were not observed in animal studies; therefore, cefotaxime is classified as pregnancy category B. Cefotaxime crosses the placenta and can be found in fetal tissue. An increased risk of teratogenic effects has not been observed following maternal use. During pregnancy, peak cefotaxime serum concentrations are decreased and the serum half-life is shorter.

Lactation Enters breast milk/use caution (AAP rates "compatible")

Breast-Feeding Considerations Very small amounts of cefotaxime are excreted in breast milk. The manufacturer recommends that caution be exercised when administering cefotaxime to nursing women. The American Academy of Pediatrics considers cefotaxime to be "usually compatible with breast-feeding." Nondose-related effects could include modification of bowel flora. The pregnancy-related changes in cefotaxime pharmacokinetics continue into the early postpartum period.

Contraindications Hypersensitivity to cefotaxime, any component, or cephalosporins

Warnings Prolonged use may result in superinfection; do not use in patients with immediate-type hypersensitivity reactions to penicillin; cefotaxime rapid bolus injection (over <1 minute through a central venous catheter) has been associated with potentially life-threatening arrhythmias

Precautions Use with caution in patients with history of penicillin hypersensitivity, impaired renal function, or history of colitis; modify dosage in patients with Cl_{cr} <20 mL/minute

Adverse Reactions

Cardiovascular: Arrhythmias

Central nervous system: Fever, headache

Dermatologic: Rash, pruritus

Gastrointestinal: Antibiotic-associated pseudomembranous colitis, diarrhea, nausea, vomiting

Hematologic: Transient neutropenia, thrombocytopenia, eosinophilia, leukopenia

Hepatic: Transient elevation of liver enzymes

Local: Phlebitis, pain at injection site

Renal: Transient elevation of BUN and serum creatinine

Drug Interactions

Avoid Concomitant Use
Avoid concomitant use of Cefotaxime with any of the following: BCG

Increased Effect/Toxicity
The levels/effects of Cefotaxime may be increased by: Probenecid

Decreased Effect
Cefotaxime may decrease the levels/effects of: BCG; Typhoid Vaccine

Stability Reconstituted solution is stable for 24 hours at room temperature and 10 days when refrigerated

Mechanism of Action Inhibits bacterial cell wall synthesis by binding to one or more of the penicillin-binding proteins; inhibits the final transpeptidation step of peptidoglycan synthesis resulting in cell wall death

Pharmacokinetics (Adult data unless noted)
Distribution: Into bronchial secretions, middle ear effusions, bone, bile; penetration into CSF when meninges are inflamed; crosses the placenta; appears in breast milk

Protein binding: 31% to 50%

Metabolism: Partially metabolized in the liver to active metabolite, desacetylcefotaxime

Half-life:

Cefotaxime:

Neonates, premature: <1 week: 5-6 hours

Neonates, full-term: <1 week: 2-3.4 hours; 1-4 weeks: 2 hours

Children: 1.5 hours

Adults: 1-1.5 hours (prolonged with renal and/or hepatic impairment)

Desacetylcefotaxime: Adults: 1.5-1.9 hours (prolonged with renal impairment)

Time to peak serum concentration: I.M.: Within 30 minutes

Elimination: 40% to 60% of a dose excreted as unchanged drug and 24% excreted as desacetylcefotaxime in the urine

Dialysis: Moderately dialyzable (20% to 50%)

Usual Dosage I.M., I.V.:
Neonates: 0-4 weeks: <1200 g: 100 mg/kg/day divided every 12 hours

Postnatal age ≤7 days:

1200-2000 g: 100 mg/kg/day divided every 12 hours

>2000 g: 100-150 mg/kg/day divided every 8-12 hours

Postnatal age >7 days:

1200-2000 g: 150 mg/kg/day divided every 8 hours

>2000 g: 150-200 mg/kg/day divided every 6-8 hours

Infants and Children 1 month to 12 years:

<50 kg: 100-200 mg/kg/day divided every 6-8 hours

Meningitis: 200 mg/kg/day divided every 6 hours; 225-300 mg/kg/day divided every 6-8 hours has been used to treat invasive pneumococcal meningitis

≥50 kg: Moderate to severe infection: 1-2 g every 6-8 hours; life-threatening infection: 2 g/dose every 4 hours; maximum dose: 12 g/day

Children >12 years and Adults: 1-2 g every 6-8 hours (up to 12 g/day)

Dosing adjustment in renal impairment: Cl_{cr} <20 mL/minute: Reduce dose by 50%

Administration Parenteral:
I.V.: Cefotaxime may be administered IVP over 3-5 minutes at a maximum concentration of 100 mg/mL or I.V. intermittent infusion over 15-30 minutes at a final concentration of 20-60 mg/mL; in fluid-restricted patients, a concentration of 150 mg/mL may be administered IVP; rapid IVP over <1 minute may cause arrhythmias (see Warnings)

I.M.: Deep I.M. injection into a large muscle mass such as the upper outer quadrant of the gluteus maximus. Doses as large as 2 g should be divided and administered at 2 different sites. May dilute vial using SWI to a final concentration between 230-330 mg/mL (see package insert).

Monitoring Parameters With prolonged therapy, monitor renal, hepatic, and hematologic function periodically; number and type of stools/day for diarrhea

Test Interactions Positive Coombs' [direct]

Additional Information Sodium content of 1 g: 2.2 mEq

Dosage Forms Excipient information presented when available (limited, particularly for generics); consult specific product labeling.

Infusion [premixed iso-osmotic solution]:

Claforan®: 1 g (50 mL); 2 g (50 mL) [contains sodium 50.5 mg (2.2 mEq) per cefotaxime 1 g]

Injection, powder for reconstitution: 500 mg, 1 g, 2 g, 10 g, 20 g

Claforan®: 500 mg, 1 g, 2 g, 10 g [contains sodium 50.5 mg (2.2 mEq) per cefotaxime 1 g]

References
Spritzer R, Kamp HJ, Dzoljic G, et al, "Five Years of Cefotaxime Use in a Neonatal Intensive Care Unit," Pediatr Infect Dis J, 1990, 9(2):92-6.

♦ **Cefotaxime Sodium** see Cefotaxime on page 267

Cefotetan (SEF oh tee tan)

Medication Safety Issues
Sound-alike/look-alike issues:

Cefotetan may be confused with cefoxitin, Ceftin®

Cefotan® may be confused with Ceftin®

International issues:

Cefotan® may be confused with Lexotan® which is a brand name for bromazepam in multiple international markets

Cefotan® may be confused with Cefiton® which is a brand name for cefixime in Portugal

Therapeutic Category Antibiotic, Cephalosporin (Second Generation)

Generic Available Yes

Use Treatment of susceptible lower respiratory tract, skin and skin structure, bone and joint, urinary tract, sepsis, gynecologic, and intra-abdominal infections; active against anaerobes including Bacteroides species of GI tract, gram-negative enteric bacilli including E. coli, Klebsiella, and Proteus; active against many strains of N. gonorrhoeae; inactive against Enterobacter sp.; less active against staphylococci and streptococci than first generation cephalosporins; preoperative prophylaxis

Pregnancy Risk Factor B

Pregnancy Considerations Adverse events have not been observed in animal reproduction studies; therefore, the manufacturer classifies cefotetan as pregnancy category B. Cefotetan crosses the placenta and produces therapeutic concentrations in the amniotic fluid and cord serum.

Lactation Enters breast milk (small amounts)/use caution

Breast-Feeding Considerations Very small amounts of cefotetan are excreted in human milk. The manufacturer recommends caution when giving cefotetan to a breast-feeding mother. Nondose-related effects could include modification of bowel flora.

Contraindications Hypersensitivity to cefotetan, cephalosporins, any component, or patients who have experienced a cephalosporin-associated hemolytic anemia

Warnings Prolonged use may result in superinfection; do not use in patients with immediate-type hypersensitivity reactions to penicillin. May cause pseudomembranous colitis or secondary antibiotic-associated colitis. Severe cases of immune mediated hemolytic anemia have been reported with cefotetan administration. Risk of developing cefotetan-induced hemolytic anemia is 3-fold higher relative to other cephalosporins. Monitor hematologic parameters; blood transfusion may be needed.

Precautions Use with caution and modify dosage in patients with renal impairment; use with caution in patients with history of colitis or penicillin hypersensitivity

Adverse Reactions

Central nervous system: Seizures, fever

Dermatologic: Rash, pruritus, urticaria

Gastrointestinal: Diarrhea, nausea, vomiting, pseudomem-branous colitis

Hematologic: Neutropenia, leukopenia, thrombocytopenia, eosinophilia, hemolytic anemia, bleeding, prolongation of PT

Hepatic: Serum AST, ALT, alkaline phosphatase, LDH elevated

Local: Phlebitis, pain at the injection site, edema

Renal: BUN elevated, serum creatinine elevated, neph-rotoxicity (rare)

Miscellaneous: Anaphylaxis

Drug Interactions

Avoid Concomitant Use

Avoid concomitant use of Cefotetan with any of the following: BCG

Increased Effect/Toxicity

Cefotetan may increase the levels/effects of: Alcohol (Ethyl); Vitamin K Antagonists

The levels/effects of Cefotetan may be increased by: Probenecid

Decreased Effect

Cefotetan may decrease the levels/effects of: BCG; Typhoid Vaccine

Stability Thawed solutions of the commercially available frozen cefotetan injections are stable for 48 hours at room temperature or 21 days when refrigerated; do not refreeze; incompatible with aminoglycosides, heparin, and tetracycline

Mechanism of Action Inhibits bacterial cell wall synthesis by binding to one or more of the penicillin-binding proteins; inhibits the final transpeptidation step of peptidoglycan synthesis resulting in cell wall death

Pharmacokinetics (Adult data unless noted)

Absorption: I.M.: Completely absorbed

Distribution: Distributes into tissues and fluids including gallbladder, kidney, skin, tonsils, uterus, sputum, pro-static and peritoneal fluids; poor penetration into CSF; crosses the placenta; small amounts appear in breast milk

Protein binding: 76% to 91%

Half-life: Adults: 3.5 hours, prolonged in patients with impaired renal function (up to 10 hours)

Time to peak serum concentration: I.M.: Within 1.5-3 hours

Elimination: 49% to 81% excreted as unchanged drug in urine, 20% of dose is excreted in bile

Dialysis: <10% removed by hemodialysis

Usual Dosage I.V.: Safety and efficacy in children have not been established

Children: 40-80 mg/kg/day divided every 12 hours; maximum dose: 6 g/day

Preoperative prophylaxis: 40 mg/kg 30-60 minutes prior to procedure; **Note:** May add gentamicin 2 mg/kg for cases of ruptured viscus

Adolescents and Adults: 2-4 g/day divided every 12 hours; maximum dose: 6 g/day

Urinary tract infections: 1-2 g/day divided every 12-24 hours

Preoperative prophylaxis: 1-2 g 30-60 minutes prior to procedure

Pelvic inflammatory disease: 2 g every 12 hours continued for 24-48 hours after significant clinical improvement is demonstrated **plus** doxycycline 100 mg I.V. or orally every 12 hours for 14 days

Dosing interval in renal impairment:

Cl$_{cr}$ 10-30 mL/minute: Administer every 24 hours

Cl$_{cr}$ <10 mL/minute: Administer every 48 hours

Administration Parenteral: I.V. intermittent: Infuse over 20-60 minutes at a concentration of 10-40 mg/mL

Monitoring Parameters CBC, prothrombin time, renal function tests; number and type of stools/day for diarrhea; signs and symptoms of hemolytic anemia

Test Interactions Positive Coombs' [direct], false-positive urine glucose (Clinitest®), falsely elevated serum or urinary creatinine (Jaffé reaction)

Patient Information Avoid alcohol during and for at least 72 hours after the last cefotetan dose.

Additional Information Sodium content of 1 g: 3.5 mEq; chemical structure contains a methyltetrazolethiol side chain which may be responsible for the disulfiram-like reaction with alcohol and increased risk of bleeding

Dosage Forms Excipient information presented when available (limited, particularly for generics); consult specific product labeling.

Injection, powder for reconstitution: 1 g, 2 g, 10 g [contains sodium 80 mg/g (3.5 mEq/g)]

References

Martin C, Thomachot L, and Albanese J, "Clinical Pharmacokinetics of Cefotetan," *Clin Pharmacokinet*, 1994, 26(4):248-58.

♦ **Cefotetan Disodium** *see* Cefotetan *on page 268*

Cefoxitin (se FOKS i tin)

Medication Safety Issues

Sound-alike/look-alike issues:

Cefoxitin may be confused with cefotaxime, cefotetan, Cytoxan

Mefoxin® may be confused with Lanoxin®

Canadian Brand Names Apo-Cefoxitin®

Therapeutic Category Antibiotic, Cephalosporin (Second Generation)

Generic Available Yes

Use Treatment of susceptible lower respiratory tract, skin and skin structure, bone and joint, genitourinary tract, sepsis, gynecologic, and intra-abdominal infections; active against anaerobes including *Bacteroides* species of the GI tract, gram-negative enteric bacilli including *E. coli*, *Klebsiella*, and *Proteus*; active against many strains of *N. gonorrhoeae*; inactive against *Enterobacter* sp.; perioper-ative prophylaxis

Pregnancy Risk Factor B

Pregnancy Considerations Adverse events have not been observed in animal reproduction studies; therefore, cefoxitin is classified as pregnancy category B. Cefoxitin crosses the placenta and reaches the cord serum and amniotic fluid. Adequate well-controlled studies are not available in pregnant women.

Peak serum concentrations of cefoxitin during pregnancy may be similar to or decreased compared to nonpregnant values. Maternal half-life may be shorter at term. Pregnancy-induced hypertension increases trough con-centrations in the immediate postpartum period.

Lactation Enters breast milk (small amounts)/use caution (AAP rates "compatible")

Breast-Feeding Considerations Very small amounts of cefoxitin are excreted in breast milk. The manufacturer recommends that caution be exercised when administer-ing cefoxitin to nursing women. The American Academy of Pediatrics considers cefoxitin to be "usually compatible with breast-feeding." Nondose-related effects could include modification of bowel flora. Cefoxitin pharmacoki-netics may be altered immediately postpartum.

◀ **Contraindications** Hypersensitivity to cefoxitin, any component, or cephalosporins

Warnings Prolonged use may result in superinfection; high doses in children have been associated with an increased incidence of eosinophilia and elevation of serum AST; safety and efficacy in infants <3 months have not been established; do not use in patients with immediate-type hypersensitivity reactions to penicillin

Precautions Use with caution and modify dosage in patients with renal impairment; use with caution in patients with history of colitis or penicillin hypersensitivity

Adverse Reactions

Central nervous system: Fever, headache

Dermatologic: Rash, pruritus, exfoliative dermatitis

Gastrointestinal: Pseudomembranous colitis, diarrhea, nausea, vomiting

Hematologic: Transient leukopenia, thrombocytopenia, neutropenia, anemia, eosinophilia

Hepatic: Transient elevation of liver enzymes, AST, ALT, and alkaline phosphatase

Local: Thrombophlebitis, pain at injection site

Renal: Transient elevation of BUN and serum creatinine

Drug Interactions

Avoid Concomitant Use

Avoid concomitant use of Cefoxitin with any of the following: BCG

Increased Effect/Toxicity

Cefoxitin may increase the levels/effects of: Vitamin K Antagonists

The levels/effects of Cefoxitin may be increased by: Probenecid

Decreased Effect

Cefoxitin may decrease the levels/effects of: BCG; Typhoid Vaccine

Stability Reconstituted solution is stable for 24 hours at room temperature and for 1 week under refrigeration; thawed solutions of the commercially available frozen cefoxitin injections are stable for 24 hours at room temperature or 5 days when refrigerated

Mechanism of Action Inhibits bacterial cell wall synthesis by binding to one or more of the penicillin-binding proteins; inhibits the final transpeptidation step of peptidoglycan synthesis resulting in cell wall death

Pharmacokinetics (Adult data unless noted)

Distribution: Distributes into tissues and fluids including ascitic, pleural, bile, and synovial fluids; poor penetration into CSF even with inflamed meninges; crosses the placenta; small amounts appear in breast milk

Protein binding: 65% to 79%

Half-life:

Infants (10-53 days of age): 1.4 hours

Adults: 45-60 minutes, increases significantly with renal insufficiency

Time to peak serum concentration: I.M.: Within 20-30 minutes

Elimination: Rapidly excreted as unchanged drug (85%) in the urine

Dialysis: Moderately dialyzable (20% to 50%)

Usual Dosage I.M., I.V.:

Neonates: 90-100 mg/kg/day divided every 8 hours

Infants ≥3 months and Children:

Mild-moderate infection: 80-100 mg/kg/day divided every 6-8 hours

Severe infection: 100-160 mg/kg/day divided every 4-6 hours; maximum dose: 12 g/day

Perioperative prophylaxis: 30-40 mg/kg 30-60 minutes prior to surgery followed by 30-40 mg/kg/dose every 6 hours for no more than 24 hours after surgery depending on the procedure

Adolescents and Adults: 1-2 g every 6-8 hours (I.M. injection is painful); maximum dose: 12 g/day

Pelvic inflammatory disease: I.V.: 2 g every 6 hours continued for 24-48 hours after significant clinical improvement is demonstrated **plus** doxycycline 100 mg I.V. or orally every 12 hours for 14 days

Perioperative prophylaxis: 1-2 g 30-60 minutes prior to surgery followed by 1-2 g every 6-8 hours for no more than 24 hours after surgery depending on the procedure

Dosing interval in renal impairment:

Cl_{cr} 30-50 mL/minute: Administer every 8-12 hours

Cl_{cr} 10-30 mL/minute: Administer every 12-24 hours

Cl_{cr} <10 mL/minute: Administer every 24-48 hours

Administration Parenteral:

IVP: Administer over 3-5 minutes at a maximum concentration of 200 mg/mL

I.V. intermittent infusion: Administer over 10-60 minutes at a final concentration not to exceed 40 mg/mL

I.M.: Deep I.M. injection into a large muscle mass such as the upper outer quadrant of the gluteus maximus. May dilute vial using SWI or 0.5% or 1% lidocaine to a final concentration of 400 mg/mL (see package insert)

Monitoring Parameters Renal function periodically when used in combination with other nephrotoxic drugs; liver function and hematologic function tests; number and type of stools/day for diarrhea

Test Interactions Positive Coombs' [direct]; false-positive urine glucose (Clinitest®), false ↑ in serum or urine creatinine

Additional Information Sodium content of 1 g: 53 mg (2.3 mEq)

Dosage Forms Excipient information presented when available (limited, particularly for generics); consult specific product labeling.

Injection, powder for reconstitution: 1 g, 2 g, 10 g [contains sodium 53.8 mg/g (2.3 mEq/g)]

Powder for prescription compounding: 100 g

References

Feldman WE, Moffitt S, and Sprow N, "Clinical and Pharmacokinetic Evaluation of Parenteral Cefoxitin in Infants and Children," *Antimicrob Agents Chemother*, 1980, 17(4):669-74.

Regazzi MB, Chirico G, Cristiani D, et al, "Cefoxitin in Newborn Infants. A Clinical and Pharmacokinetic Study," *Eur J Clin Pharmacol*, 1983, 25(4):507-9.

◆ **Cefoxitin Sodium** see Cefoxitin on page 269

Cefpodoxime (sef pode OKS eem)

Medication Safety Issues

Sound-alike/look-alike issues:

Vantin may be confused with Ventolin®

Therapeutic Category Antibiotic, Cephalosporin (Third Generation)

Generic Available Yes

Use Treatment of susceptible acute, community-acquired pneumonia caused by *S. pneumoniae* or nonbeta-lactamase producing *H. influenzae*; alternative regimen for acute uncomplicated gonorrhea caused by *N. gonorrhoeae*; uncomplicated skin and skin structure infections caused by *S. aureus* or *S. pyogenes*; acute otitis media caused by *S. pneumoniae, H. influenzae,* or *M. catarrhalis*; pharyngitis or tonsillitis; and uncomplicated urinary tract infections caused by *E. coli, Klebsiella,* and *Proteus*; inactive against *Pseudomonas* and *Enterobacter* spp.

Pregnancy Risk Factor B

Pregnancy Considerations Teratogenic events were not observed in animal studies; therefore, cefpodoxime is classified as pregnancy category B. It is not known if cefpodoxime crosses the human placenta. Other cephalosporins cross the placenta and are considered safe in pregnancy.

Lactation Enters breast milk (small amounts)/not recommended

Breast-Feeding Considerations Very small amounts of cefpodoxime are excreted in breast milk. Breast-feeding is not recommended by the manufacturer. Other cephalosporins are considered safe during breast-feeding. Non-dose-related effects could include modification of bowel flora.

Contraindications Hypersensitivity to cefpodoxime, any component, or cephalosporins

Warnings Prolonged use may result in superinfection; do not use in patients with immediate-type hypersensitivity reactions to penicillin

Suspension contains sodium benzoate; benzoic acid (benzoate) is a metabolite of benzyl alcohol; large amounts of benzyl alcohol (≥99 mg/kg/day) have been associated with a potentially fatal toxicity ("gasping syndrome") in neonates; the "gasping syndrome" consists of metabolic acidosis, respiratory distress, gasping respirations, CNS dysfunction (including convulsions, intracranial hemorrhage), hypotension and cardiovascular collapse; use suspension containing sodium benzoate with caution in neonates; *in vitro* and animal studies have shown that benzoate displaces bilirubin from protein binding sites

Precautions Use with caution in patients with history of penicillin hypersensitivity, impaired renal function, and patients with a history of colitis; modify dosage in patients with renal impairment

Adverse Reactions
Central nervous system: Headache
Dermatologic: Rash
Gastrointestinal: Nausea (3.8%), vomiting, abdominal pain, diarrhea (7.1%), pseudomembranous colitis
Genitourinary: Vaginal fungal infections (3.3%)
Hematologic: Eosinophilia, leukocytosis, thrombocytosis, decrease in hemoglobin or hematocrit, leukopenia, prolonged PT and PTT
Hepatic: Transient elevation in AST, ALT, bilirubin
Renal: BUN elevated, serum creatinine elevated

Drug Interactions

Avoid Concomitant Use
Avoid concomitant use of Cefpodoxime with any of the following: BCG

Increased Effect/Toxicity
The levels/effects of Cefpodoxime may be increased by: Probenecid

Decreased Effect
Cefpodoxime may decrease the levels/effects of: BCG; Typhoid Vaccine

The levels/effects of Cefpodoxime may be decreased by: Antacids; H2-Antagonists

Food Interactions Food increases oral bioavailability

Stability After reconstitution, suspension may be stored in refrigerator for 14 days

Mechanism of Action Inhibits bacterial cell wall synthesis by binding to one or more of the penicillin-binding proteins; inhibits the final transpeptidation step of peptidoglycan synthesis resulting in cell wall death

Pharmacokinetics (Adult data unless noted)
Absorption: Enhanced in the presence of food or low gastric pH
Distribution: Good tissue penetration, including lung and tonsils; penetrates into pleural fluid; poor penetration into CSF; small amounts appear in breast milk
Protein binding: 18% to 23%
Metabolism: Following oral administration, cefpodoxime proxetil is de-esterified in the GI tract to the active metabolite, cefpodoxime
Bioavailability: Oral: 50%
Half-life: 2.2 hours (prolonged with renal impairment)
Time to peak serum concentration: Within 2-3 hours
Elimination: Primarily by the kidney with 80% of absorbed dose excreted unchanged in urine in 24 hours

Usual Dosage Oral:
Infants >6 months and Children to 12 years: 10 mg/kg/day divided every 12 hours; maximum dose: 800 mg/day
Adolescents and Adults: 100-400 mg/dose every 12 hours
Uncomplicated gonorrhea: 200 mg as a single dose
Dosing adjustment in renal impairment: Cl$_{cr}$ <30 mL/minute: Administer every 24 hours; patients on hemodialysis, administer dose 3 times/week
Dosing adjustment in hepatic impairment: Not necessary in patient with cirrhosis

Administration Oral:
Tablet: Administer with food
Suspension: May administer with or without food; shake suspension well before use

Monitoring Parameters Observe patient for diarrhea; with prolonged therapy, monitor renal function periodically

Test Interactions Positive Coombs' [direct]

Dosage Forms Excipient information presented when available (limited, particularly for generics); consult specific product labeling.
Granules for suspension, oral: 50 mg/5 mL (50 mL, 75 mL, 100 mL); 100 mg/5 mL (50 mL, 75 mL, 100 mL)
Tablet: 100 mg, 200 mg

References
Borin MT, "A Review of the Pharmacokinetics of Cefpodoxime Proxetil," *Drugs,* 1991, 42(Suppl 3):13-21.
Fujii R, "Clinical Trials of Cefpodoxime Proxetil Suspension in Pediatrics," *Drugs,* 1991, 42(Suppl 3):57-60.
Mendelman PM, Del-Beccaro MA, McLinn SE, et al, "Cefpodoxime Proxetil Compared With Amoxicillin-Clavulanate for the Treatment of Otitis Media," *J Pediatr,* 1992, 121(3):459-65.

◆ **Cefpodoxime Proxetil** *see* Cefpodoxime *on page 270*

Cefprozil (sef PROE zil)

Medication Safety Issues
Sound-alike/look-alike issues:
Cefprozil may be confused with ceFAZolin, cefuroxime
Cefzil® may be confused with Cefol®, Ceftin®, Kefzol®

Canadian Brand Names Apo-Cefprozil®; Cefzil®; Mint-Cefprozil; RAN™-Cefprozil; Sandoz-Cefprozil

Therapeutic Category Antibiotic, Cephalosporin (Second Generation)

Generic Available Yes

Use Infections caused by susceptible organisms including *S. pneumoniae, H. influenzae, M. catarrhalis, S. aureus, S. pyogenes;* treatment of infections involving the respiratory tract, skin and skin structure, and otitis media

Pregnancy Risk Factor B

Pregnancy Considerations Adverse events were not observed in animal reproduction studies; therefore, cefprozil is classified as pregnancy category B. It is not known if cefprozil crosses the human placenta. Other cephalosporins cross the placenta and are considered safe for use during pregnancy.

Lactation Enters breast milk/use caution (AAP rates "compatible")

Breast-Feeding Considerations Small amounts of cefprozil are excreted in breast milk. The manufacturer recommends that caution be exercised when administering cefprozil to nursing women. The American Academy of Pediatrics considers cefprozil to be "usually compatible with breast-feeding." Nondose-related effects could include modification of bowel flora.

Contraindications Hypersensitivity to cefprozil, any component, or cephalosporins

Warnings Prolonged use may result in superinfection; do not use in patients with immediate-type hypersensitivity reactions to penicillin

◀ Oral suspension contains sodium benzoate; benzoic acid (benzoate) is a metabolite of benzyl alcohol; large amounts of benzyl alcohol (≥99 mg/kg/day) have been associated with a potentially fatal toxicity ("gasping syndrome") in neonates; the "gasping syndrome" consists of metabolic acidosis, respiratory distress, gasping respirations, CNS dysfunction (including convulsions, intracranial hemorrhage), hypotension and cardiovascular collapse; use oral suspension containing sodium benzoate with caution in neonates; *in vitro* and animal studies have shown that benzoate displaces bilirubin from protein binding sites

Precautions Use with caution in patients with impaired renal function, history of colitis, or in penicillin-sensitive patients; modify dosage in patients with severe renal impairment; some products (eg, oral suspension) contain aspartame which is metabolized to phenylalanine and must be used with caution in patients with phenylketonuria.

Adverse Reactions

Central nervous system: Headache, hyperactivity, insomnia, confusion, dizziness

Dermatologic: Rash, pruritus, diaper rash

Gastrointestinal: Diarrhea, nausea, vomiting, abdominal pain

Genitourinary: Vaginitis

Hematologic: Decrease in leukocyte and platelet count, eosinophilia

Hepatic: AST, ALT, and alkaline phosphatase elevated; cholestatic jaundice; prolonged PT

Renal: BUN and serum creatinine elevated

Miscellaneous: Serum sickness-like reactions

Drug Interactions

Avoid Concomitant Use

Avoid concomitant use of Cefprozil with any of the following: BCG

Increased Effect/Toxicity

The levels/effects of Cefprozil may be increased by: Probenecid

Decreased Effect

Cefprozil may decrease the levels/effects of: BCG; Typhoid Vaccine

Food Interactions Total absorption is not affected by food

Stability Refrigerate suspension after reconstitution; discard after 14 days

Mechanism of Action Inhibits bacterial cell wall synthesis by binding to one or more of the penicillin-binding proteins resulting in disruption of cell wall synthesis and cell lysis

Pharmacokinetics (Adult data unless noted)

Absorption: Oral: Well absorbed (95%)

Distribution: Low excretion into breast milk

Protein binding: 35% to 45%

Bioavailability: 94%

Half-life, elimination: 1.3 hours (normal renal function)

Time to peak serum concentration: 1.5 hours (fasting state)

Elimination: 61% excreted unchanged in urine

Dialysis: ~55% is removed by hemodialysis

Usual Dosage Oral:

Infants >6 months and Children to 12 years:

Otitis media: 30 mg/kg/day divided every 12 hours; maximum dose: 1 g/day

Children 2-12 years:

Pharyngitis/tonsillitis: 15 mg/kg/day divided every 12 hours; maximum dose: 1 g/day

Skin and skin structure infection: 20 mg/kg once daily

Children >12 years and Adults: 250-500 mg every 12 hours or 500 mg every 24 hours

Dosing adjustment in renal impairment: Cl_{cr} <30 mL/minute: Reduce dose by 50%

Administration Oral: May administer with or without food; administer with food if stomach upset occurs; chilling improves flavor of suspension (do not freeze); shake suspension well before use

Monitoring Parameters Evaluate renal function before and during therapy; with prolonged therapy, monitor coagulation tests, CBC, and liver function tests periodically

Test Interactions Positive Coombs' [direct]; may produce false-positive reaction for urine glucose with Clinitest®

Patient Information Report persistent diarrhea to physician

Additional Information Suspension also contains FD&C red No. 3, glycine, carboxymethylcellulose, and sucrose

Dosage Forms Excipient information presented when available (limited, particularly for generics); consult specific product labeling.

Powder for oral suspension: 125 mg/5 mL (50 mL, 75 mL, 100 mL); 250 mg/5 mL (50 mL, 75 mL, 100 mL)

Tablet: 250 mg, 500 mg

References

Arguedas AG, Zaleska M, Stutman HR, et al, "Comparative Trial of Cefprozil vs Amoxicillin Clavulanate Potassium in the Treatment of Children With Acute Otitis Media With Effusion," *Pediatr Infect Dis J*, 1991, 10(5):375-80.

Barriere SL, "Review of *In Vitro* Activity, Pharmacokinetic Characteristics, Safety, and Clinical Efficacy of Cefprozil, a New Oral Cephalosporin," *Ann Pharmacother*, 1993, 27(9):1082-9.

Lowery N, Kearns GL, Young RA, et al, "Serum Sickness-Like Reactions Associated With Cefprozil Therapy," *J Pediatr*, 1994, 125 (2):325-8.

Ceftazidime (SEF tay zi deem)

Medication Safety Issues

Sound-alike/look-alike issues:

Ceftazidime may be confused with cefepime, ceftizoxime

Ceptaz® may be confused with Septra®

Tazicef® may be confused with Tazidime®

Tazidime® may be confused with Tazicef®

International issues:

Ceftim® [Italy] may be confused with Ceftin® which is a brand name for cefuroxime in the U.S.

Ceftim® [Italy] may be confused with Cefiton® which is a brand name for cefixime in Portugal

Ceftim® [Italy] may be confused with Ceftina® which is a brand name for cefalotin in Mexico

U.S. Brand Names Fortaz®; Tazicef®

Canadian Brand Names Fortaz®

Therapeutic Category Antibiotic, Cephalosporin (Third Generation)

Generic Available Yes: Injection

Use Treatment of infections of the respiratory tract, urinary tract, skin and skin structure, intra-abdominal, osteomyelitis, sepsis, and meningitis caused by susceptible gram-negative aerobic organisms such as Enterobacteriaceae and *Pseudomonas*; pseudomonal infection in patient at risk of developing aminoglycoside-induced nephrotoxicity and/or ototoxicity; empiric therapy for febrile, granulocytopenic patients

Pregnancy Risk Factor B

Pregnancy Considerations Teratogenic effects were not observed in animal studies; therefore, ceftazidime is classified as pregnancy category B. Ceftazidime crosses the placenta and reaches the cord serum and amniotic fluid. Maternal peak serum concentration is unchanged in the first trimester. After the first trimester, serum concentrations decrease by approximately 50% of those in nonpregnant patients. Renal clearance is increased during pregnancy.

Lactation Enters breast milk (small amounts)/use caution (AAP rates "compatible")

Breast-Feeding Considerations Very small amounts of ceftazidime are excreted in breast milk. The manufacturer recommends that caution be exercised when administering ceftazidime to nursing women. The American Academy of Pediatrics considers ceftazidime to be "usually compatible with breast-feeding." Ceftazidime in not absorbed when given orally; therefore, any medication that is distributed to human milk should not result in systemic concentrations in the nursing infant. Nondose-related effects could include modification of bowel flora.

Contraindications Hypersensitivity to ceftazidime, any component, or cephalosporins

Warnings Prolonged use may result in superinfection; do not use in patients with immediate-type hypersensitivity reactions to penicillin

Precautions Use with caution and modify dosage in patients with impaired renal function; use with caution in patients with history of colitis or patients with penicillin hypersensitivity

Adverse Reactions

Central nervous system: Fever, headache, dizziness, coma

Dermatologic: Rash, pruritus, urticaria

Gastrointestinal: Pseudomembranous colitis, diarrhea, nausea, vomiting, candidiasis

Hematologic: Transient leukopenia, thrombocytopenia, eosinophilia, thrombocytosis, hemolytic anemia

Hepatic: Transient elevation of liver enzymes, jaundice, hyperbilirubinemia

Local: Phlebitis, pain at injection site

Neuromuscular & skeletal: Myoclonia

Renal: Transient elevation of BUN and serum creatinine, renal impairment

Miscellaneous: Anaphylaxis

Drug Interactions

Avoid Concomitant Use

Avoid concomitant use of Ceftazidime with any of the following: BCG

Increased Effect/Toxicity

The levels/effects of Ceftazidime may be increased by: Probenecid

Decreased Effect

Ceftazidime may decrease the levels/effects of: BCG; Typhoid Vaccine

Stability Reconstituted solution is stable for 24 hours at room temperature and 10 days when refrigerated; incompatible with sodium bicarbonate; potentially incompatible with aminoglycosides

Mechanism of Action Bactericidal antibiotic with a mechanism similar to that of penicillins by binding to one or more of the penicillin-binding proteins; inhibits mucopeptide synthesis in the bacterial cell wall

Pharmacokinetics (Adult data unless noted)

Distribution: Widely distributed throughout the body including bone, bile, skin, CSF (diffuses into CSF at higher concentrations when the meninges are inflamed), endometrium, heart, pleural and lymphatic fluids; distributes into breast milk

Protein binding: 17%

Half-life:

Neonates <23 days: 2.2-4.7 hours

Adults: 1-2 hours (prolonged with renal impairment)

Time to peak serum concentration: I.M.: Within 60 minutes

Elimination: By glomerular filtration with 80% to 90% of the dose excreted as unchanged drug in urine within 24 hours

Dialysis: Dialyzable (50% to 100%)

Usual Dosage I.M., I.V.:

Neonates: 0-4 weeks: <1200 g: 100 mg/kg/day divided every 12 hours

Postnatal age ≤7 days:

1200-2000 g: 100 mg/kg/day divided every 12 hours

>2000 g: 100-150 mg/kg/day divided every 8-12 hours

Postnatal age >7 days: ≥1200 g: 150 mg/kg/day divided every 8 hours

Infants and Children 1 month to 12 years: 100-150 mg/kg/day divided every 8 hours; maximum dose: 6 g/day

Meningitis: 150 mg/kg/day divided every 8 hours; maximum dose: 6 g/day

Adults: 1-2 g every 8-12 hours

Urinary tract infections: 250-500 mg every 12 hours

Dosing interval in renal impairment:

Cl_{cr} 30-50 mL/minute: Administer every 12 hours

Cl_{cr} 10-30 mL/minute: Administer every 24 hours

Cl_{cr} <10 mL/minute: Administer every 24-48 hours

Administration Parenteral: Any carbon dioxide bubbles that may be present in the withdrawn solution should be expelled prior to injection

IVP: Administer over 3-5 minutes at a maximum concentration of 180 mg/mL

I.V. intermittent infusion: Administer over 15-30 minutes at a final concentration ≤40 mg/mL

I.M.: Deep I.M. injection into a large muscle mass such as the upper outer quadrant of the gluteus maximus or lateral part of the thigh. May dilute vial using SWI or 0.5% or 1% lidocaine to a final concentration of 280 mg/mL (see package insert)

Monitoring Parameters Renal function periodically when used in combination with aminoglycosides; with prolonged therapy also monitor hepatic and hematologic function periodically; number and type of stools/day for diarrhea

Test Interactions Positive Coombs' [direct], false-positive urine glucose (Clinitest®)

Additional Information Sodium content of 1 g: 2.3 mEq

Dosage Forms Excipient information presented when available (limited, particularly for generics); consult specific product labeling.

Infusion, premixed iso-osmotic solution, as sodium [strength expressed as base]:

Fortaz®: 1 g (50 mL), 2 g (50 mL) [contains sodium ~54 mg (2.3 mEq)/g]

Injection, powder for reconstitution: 1 g, 2 g, 6 g

Fortaz®: 500 mg, 1 g, 2 g, 6 g [contains sodium ~54 mg (2.3 mEq)/g]

Tazicef®: 1 g, 2 g, 6 g [contains sodium ~54 mg (2.3 mEq)/g]

References

McCracken GH Jr, Threlkeld N, and Thomas ML, "Pharmacokinetics of Ceftazidime in Newborn Infants," *Antimicrob Agents Chemother*, 1984, 26(4):583-4.

Robinson DC, Cookson TL, and Grisafe JA, "Concentration Guidelines for Parenteral Antibiotics in Fluid-Restricted Patients," *Drug Intell Clin Pharm*, 1987, 21(12):985-9.

Ceftibuten (sef TYE byoo ten)

Medication Safety Issues

Sound-alike/look-alike issues:

Cedax® may be confused with Cidex®

International issues:

Cedax® may be confused with Codex which is a brand name for *Saccharomyces boulardii* in Italy

U.S. Brand Names Cedax®

Therapeutic Category Antibiotic, Cephalosporin (Third Generation)

Generic Available No

Use Treatment of acute exacerbations of chronic bronchitis, acute bacterial otitis media, pharyngitis/tonsillitis due to *H. influenzae* and *M. catarrhalis* (both beta-lactamase-producing and nonproducing strains), *S. pneumoniae* (penicillin-susceptible strains only), and *S. pyogenes*

Pregnancy Risk Factor B

Pregnancy Considerations Teratogenic effects were not observed in animal studies; therefore, ceftibuten is classified as pregnancy category B. It is not know if ceftibuten crosses the placenta; other cephalosporins cross the placenta and are considered safe for use during pregnancy. Adequate and well-controlled studies have not been completed in pregnant women.

273

Lactation Excretion in breast milk unknown/use caution

Breast-Feeding Considerations Ceftibuten was not detectable in milk after a single 200 mg dose (limit of detection: 1 mcg/mL). It is not known if it would be detectable after a 400 mg dose or multiple doses. The manufacturer recommends that caution be exercised when administering ceftibuten to nursing women. If ceftibuten does reach the human milk, nondose-related effects could include modification of bowel flora.

Contraindications Hypersensitivity to ceftibuten, any component, or cephalosporins

Warnings Prolonged use may result in superinfection. Pseudomembranous colitis has been reported with ceftibuten. Do not use in patients with immediate-type hypersensitivity reactions to penicillin. Cross hypersensitivity among beta-lactam antibiotics may occur in up to 10% of patients with penicillin allergy history.

Suspension contains sodium benzoate; benzoic acid (benzoate) is a metabolite of benzyl alcohol; large amounts of benzyl alcohol (≥99 mg/kg/day) have been associated with a potentially fatal toxicity ("gasping syndrome") in neonates; the "gasping syndrome" consists of metabolic acidosis, respiratory distress, gasping respirations, CNS dysfunction (including convulsions, intracranial hemorrhage), hypotension and cardiovascular collapse; use suspension containing sodium benzoate with caution in neonates; *in vitro* and animal studies have shown that benzoate displaces bilirubin from protein binding sites

Precautions Use with caution in patients with renal impairment, history of colitis, or in penicillin-sensitive patients; modify dosage in patients with moderate-to-severe renal impairment

Adverse Reactions
Central nervous system: Headache, dizziness, agitation, insomnia, irritability, somnolence, fever, psychosis
Dermatologic: Diaper rash, rash, urticaria, pruritus, Stevens-Johnson syndrome, toxic epidermal necrolysis
Gastrointestinal: Nausea, diarrhea (8% in patients ≤2 years; 2% in patients >2 years), dyspepsia, vomiting, abdominal pain, anorexia, constipation, melena, xerostomia, pseudomembranous colitis
Genitourinary: Dysuria
Hematologic: Eosinophils elevated, hemoglobin decreased, thrombocytosis, leukopenia
Hepatic: AST and ALT elevated, hyperbilirubinemia, alkaline phosphatase elevated, jaundice
Neuromuscular & skeletal: Paresthesia, rigors
Renal: BUN and serum creatinine elevated
Respiratory: Dyspnea, nasal congestion, stridor
Miscellaneous: Serum sickness-like reactions, anaphylaxis

Drug Interactions
Avoid Concomitant Use
Avoid concomitant use of Ceftibuten with any of the following: BCG
Increased Effect/Toxicity
The levels/effects of Ceftibuten may be increased by: Probenecid
Decreased Effect
Ceftibuten may decrease the levels/effects of: BCG; Typhoid Vaccine

Food Interactions Food decreases rate and extent of absorption

Stability Store capsules and powder for oral suspension at room temperature; reconstituted suspension is stable for 14 days if refrigerated

Mechanism of Action Inhibits bacterial cell wall synthesis by binding to one or more of the penicillin-binding proteins resulting in disruption of cell wall synthesis and cell lysis

Pharmacokinetics (Adult data unless noted)
Absorption: Rapid; food decreases peak concentration and lowers AUC

Distribution: Distributes into middle ear fluid, bronchial secretions, sputum, tonsillar tissue, and blister fluid:
V_d:
Children: 0.5 L/kg
Adults: 0.21 L/kg
Protein binding: 65%
Bioavailability: 75% to 90%
Half-life:
Children: 1.9-2.5 hours
Adults: 2-3 hours; Cl_{cr} 30-49 mL/minute: 7 hours; Cl_{cr} 5-29 mL/minute: 13 hours; Cl_{cr} <5 mL/minute: 22 hours
Time to peak serum concentration: 2-3 hours
Elimination: 60% to 70% excreted unchanged in urine
Dialysis: 39% to 65% removed by a 2-4 hour hemodialysis

Usual Dosage Oral:
Children <12 years: 9 mg/kg/day once daily for 10 days (maximum dose: 400 mg)
Children ≥12 years, Adolescents, and Adults: 400 mg once daily for 10 days
Dosing adjustment in renal impairment:
Cl_{cr} ≥50 mL/minute: No adjustment needed
Cl_{cr} 30-49 mL/minute: 4.5 mg/kg or 200 mg every 24 hours
Cl_{cr} 5-29 mL/minute: 2.25 mg/kg or 100 mg every 24 hours
Hemodialysis: Administer 9 mg/kg (maximum dose: 400 mg) after hemodialysis

Administration
Capsule: Administer without regard to food
Suspension: Shake suspension well before use. Administer 2 hours before or 1 hour after meals.

Monitoring Parameters Observe for signs and symptoms of anaphylaxis during first dose; with prolonged therapy, monitor renal, hepatic, and hematologic function periodically; number and type of stools/day for diarrhea

Test Interactions Positive direct Coombs'; false-positive urinary glucose test using cupric sulfate (Benedict's solution, Clinitest®, Fehling's solution); false-positive serum or urine creatinine with Jaffe reaction

Patient Information Report persistent diarrhea to physician

Dosage Forms Excipient information presented when available (limited, particularly for generics); consult specific product labeling.
Capsule:
Cedax®: 400 mg
Powder for oral suspension:
Cedax®: 90 mg/5 mL (60 mL, 90 mL, 120 mL) [contains sucrose 1g/5 mL and sodium benzoate; cherry flavor]

References
Barr WH, Affrime M, Lin CC, et al, "Pharmacokinetics of Ceftibuten in Children," *Pediatr Infect Dis J*, 1995, 14(7 Suppl):S93-101.
Guay DR, "Ceftibuten: A New Expanded-Spectrum Oral Cephalosporin," *Ann Pharmacother*, 1997, 31(9):1022-33.

◆ **Ceftin®** *see* Cefuroxime *on page 277*

Ceftizoxime (sef ti ZOKS eem)

Medication Safety Issues
Sound-alike/look-alike issues:
Ceftizoxime may be confused with cefotaxime, ceftazidime, cefuroxime

U.S. Brand Names Cefizox®
Canadian Brand Names Cefizox®
Therapeutic Category Antibiotic, Cephalosporin (Third Generation)
Generic Available No

Use Treatment of susceptible bacterial infections, mainly respiratory tract, skin and skin structure, bone and joint, urinary tract and sepsis; as a third generation cephalosporin, ceftizoxime has activity against gram-negative enteric bacilli (eg, *E. coli*, *Klebsiella*), and cocci (eg, *Neisseria*), and variable activity against gram-positive cocci (*Staphylococcus* and *Streptococcus*); ceftizoxime has some anaerobic coverage but is less active against *B. fragilis* than cefoxitin; also indicated for *Neisseria gonorrhoeae* infections (including uncomplicated cervical and urethral gonorrhea and gonorrhea pelvic inflammatory disease), and *Haemophilus influenzae* meningitis

Pregnancy Risk Factor B

Pregnancy Considerations Teratogenic effects have not been observed in animal studies; therefore, ceftizoxime is classified as pregnancy category B. Ceftizoxime crosses the placenta and is found in the cord blood and amniotic fluid in amounts that are higher than the maternal serum. The maternal peak concentrations at term are similar to those in nonpregnant volunteers.

Lactation Enters breast milk (small amounts)/use caution

Breast-Feeding Considerations Very small amounts of ceftizoxime are excreted in breast milk. The manufacturer recommends that caution be exercised when administering ceftizoxime to nursing women. Nondose-related effects could include modification of bowel flora.

Contraindications Hypersensitivity to ceftizoxime, any component, or cephalosporins

Warnings Prolonged use may result in superinfection; do not use in patients with immediate-type hypersensitivity reaction to penicillin

Precautions Use with caution in patients who are hypersensitive to penicillins; use with caution and modify dosage in patients with renal impairment

Adverse Reactions

Central nervous system: Fever

Dermatologic: Rash, pruritus

Gastrointestinal: Diarrhea, occasionally nausea and vomiting

Genitourinary: Vaginitis (rare)

Hematologic: Positive Coombs' test, eosinophilia, thrombocytosis (transient); rarely: anemia, leukopenia, neutropenia, thrombocytopenia

Hepatic: Bilirubin elevated; transient elevation of AST, ALT, alkaline phosphatase

Local: Pain, burning at injection site

Neuromuscular & skeletal: Numbness

Renal: Transient elevations of BUN and serum creatinine

Drug Interactions

Avoid Concomitant Use

Avoid concomitant use of Ceftizoxime with any of the following: BCG

Increased Effect/Toxicity

The levels/effects of Ceftizoxime may be increased by: Probenecid

Decreased Effect

Ceftizoxime may decrease the levels/effects of: BCG; Typhoid Vaccine

Stability Reconstituted solution is stable for 24 hours at room temperature and 96 hours when refrigerated; for I.V. infusion in NS or D_5W solution is stable for 24 hours at room temperature, 96 hours when refrigerated or 12 weeks when frozen; after freezing, thawed solution is stable for 24 hours at room temperature or 10 days when refrigerated; do not refreeze; do not mix with aminoglycosides

Mechanism of Action Interferes with bacterial cell wall synthesis during active replication, causing cell wall death and resultant bactericidal activity against susceptible bacteria

Pharmacokinetics (Adult data unless noted)

Distribution: V_d: 0.35-0.5 L/kg; penetrates CSF

Protein binding: 30%

Half-life: 1.6 hours, increases to 25 hours when Cl_{cr} falls to <10 mL/minute

Time to peak serum concentration: I.M.: Within 0.5-1 hour

Elimination: Excreted unchanged in urine

Dialysis: Moderately dialyzable (20% to 50%)

Usual Dosage I.M., I.V.:

Infants ≥6 months and Children: 150-200 mg/kg/day divided every 6-8 hours; maximum dose: 12 g/24 hours

Adults: 1-2 g every 8-12 hours

Life-threatening infections: Up to 2 g every 4 hours or 4 g every 8 hours

Uncomplicated gonorrhea: I.M.: 1 g (single dose)

Dosing interval in renal impairment:

Cl_{cr} 50-80 mL/minute: Administer every 8-12 hours

Cl_{cr} 10-50 mL/minute: Administer every 36-48 hours

Cl_{cr} <10 mL/minute: Administer every 48-72 hours

Administration Parenteral:

I.V. intermittent infusion: Administer over 30 minutes; usual dilution: 1 g/50 mL, doses >1 g are usually diluted to 100 mL

I.V. direct (bolus) injection: Administer slowly over 3-5 minutes at a concentration of 95 mg/mL

Test Interactions May falsely elevate creatine values when Jaffé reaction is used; may cause false-positive urinary glucose tests using cupric sulfate (Clinitest®, Benedict's solution)

Additional Information Sodium content of 1 g ceftizoxime: 60 mg (2.6 mEq); ceftizoxime does not cover *Chlamydia trachomatis* infections and must, therefore, be used with appropriate antichlamydial agents when treating pelvic inflammatory disease if *C. trachomatis* is suspected

Dosage Forms Excipient information presented when available (limited, particularly for generics); consult specific product labeling.

Infusion [premixed iso-osmotic solution]:

Cefizox®: 1 g (50 mL); 2 g (50 mL)

Injection, powder for reconstitution:

Cefizox®: 1 g, 2 g, 10 g [DSC]

◆ **Ceftizoxime Sodium** *see* Ceftizoxime *on page 274*

CefTRIAXone (sef trye AKS one)

Medication Safety Issues

Sound-alike/look-alike issues:

CefTRIAXone may be confused with CeFAZolin, Cetraxal®

Rocephin® may be confused with Roferon®

Related Information

Endocarditis Prophylaxis *on page 1610*

U.S. Brand Names Rocephin®

Canadian Brand Names Rocephin®

Therapeutic Category Antibiotic, Cephalosporin (Third Generation)

Generic Available Yes

Use Treatment of sepsis, meningitis, infections of the lower respiratory tract, acute bacterial otitis media, skin and skin structure, bone and joint, intra-abdominal and urinary tract due to susceptible organisms (FDA approved in children and adults; see Warnings and Contraindications); surgical prophylaxis (FDA approved in adults); documented or suspected gonococcal infection or chancroid (FDA approved for children and adults); documented or suspected infection due to susceptible organisms in home care patients and patients without I.V. line access; treatment of emergency room management of patients at high risk for bacteremia, periorbital or buccal cellulitis; salmonellosis or shigellosis, and pneumonia of unestablished etiology (<5 years of age); treatment of resistant acute otitis media; in children with acute otitis media who are unable to take oral antibiotics.

As a third generation cephalosporin, ceftriaxone has activity against gram-negative aerobic bacteria (ie, *H. influenzae*, Enterobacteriaceae, *Neisseria*), and activity against gram-positive cocci (ie, methicillin susceptible *staphylococcal sp.* and *streptococcous sp.*). Inactive against *Pseudomonas aeruginosa*, *C. trachomatis*, methicillin resistant *staphylococcus sp.* and *Enterococcus sp.*).

Pregnancy Risk Factor B

Pregnancy Considerations Teratogenic effects have not been observed in animal studies; therefore, ceftriaxone is classified as pregnancy category B. The pharmacokinetics of ceftriaxone in the third trimester are similar to those of nonpregnant patients, with the possible exception of lower peak concentrations during labor. Ceftriaxone crosses the placenta and distributes to amniotic fluid. Ceftriaxone is recommended for use in pregnant women for the treatment of gonococcal infections.

Lactation Enters breast milk/use caution (AAP rates "compatible")

Breast-Feeding Considerations Small amounts of ceftriaxone are excreted in breast milk. The manufacturer recommends that caution be exercised when administering ceftriaxone to nursing women. The American Academy of Pediatrics considers ceftriaxone to be "usually compatible with breast-feeding." Nondose-related effects could include modification of bowel flora.

Contraindications Hypersensitivity to ceftriaxone sodium, any component, or cephalosporins; do not use in hyperbilirubinemic neonates, particularly those who are premature since ceftriaxone is reported to displace bilirubin from albumin binding sites increasing the risk for kernicterus; do not use in neonates if they require or may require calcium-containing I.V. solutions

Warnings Prolonged use may result in superinfection with yeasts, enterococci, *B. fragilis*, or *P. aeruginosa*. Do not use in patients with immediate-type hypersensitivity reactions to penicillin. Fatal reactions involving calcium-ceftriaxone precipitates in the lungs and kidneys of neonates have been reported, even when calcium-containing solutions or products were administered through separate sites and/or at different times. Ceftriaxone is incompatible with calcium-containing solutions and should not be reconstituted or admixed with these solutions. Neonates are at an increased risk of having calcium-ceftriaxone precipitates. Do not administer ceftriaxone simultaneously with calcium-containing I.V. solutions (including Y-site infusions); may administer sequentially if patient is not a neonate and line is flushed thoroughly between infusions. Severe cases (including some fatalities) of immune-related hemolytic anemia have been reported in patients receiving cephalosporins, including ceftriaxone; if hemolytic anemia develops, ceftriaxone should be discontinued until the etiology is identified.

Precautions Use with caution in patients with gallbladder, biliary tract, liver, or pancreatic disease; or in patients with history of colitis or penicillin hypersensitivity

Adverse Reactions

Dermatologic: Rash

Gastrointestinal: Cholelithiasis, diarrhea, pseudomembranous colitis, sludging in the gallbladder

Hematologic: Bleeding, eosinophilia, hemolytic anemia, leukopenia, PT prolongation, thrombocytosis

Hepatic: Liver enzymes increased, jaundice, serum bilirubin increased

Local: Induration, pain at injection site

Renal: BUN and serum creatinine increased

<1% and/or postmarketing: Abdominal pain, agranulocytosis, allergic dermatitis, anaphylaxis, anemia, basophilia, biliary lithiasis, chills, diaphoriesis, dizziness, epistaxis, erythema multiforme, fever, flushing, glossitis, headache, leukocytosis, lymphocytosis, lymphopenia, monocytosis, nausea, nephrolithiasis, neutropenia, oliguria, palpitations, phlebitis, pruritus, seizure, Stevens-Johnson syndrome, stomatisis, thrombocytopenia, toxic epidermal necrolysis, urine casts, urticaria, vaginitis, vomiting

Drug Interactions

Avoid Concomitant Use

Avoid concomitant use of CefTRIAXone with any of the following: BCG

Increased Effect/Toxicity

CefTRIAXone may increase the levels/effects of: Vitamin K Antagonists

The levels/effects of CefTRIAXone may be increased by: Calcium Salts (Intravenous); Probenecid; Ringer's Injection (Lactated)

Decreased Effect

CefTRIAXone may decrease the levels/effects of: BCG; Typhoid Vaccine

Stability Reconstituted solution (100 mg/mL) is stable for 3 days at room temperature and 10 days when refrigerated; reconstituted injectable solution (250 mg/mL) is stable for 24 hours at room temperature and 3 days when refrigerated. Calcium-containing solutions or products (including Ringer's solution or Hartmann's solution) are incompatible with ceftriaxone; do not mix or administer ceftriaxone simultaneously with calcium-containing solutions, even via different infusion lines. Flush lines thoroughly if used sequentially.

Mechanism of Action Inhibits bacterial cell wall synthesis by binding to one or more of the penicillin-binding proteins; inhibits the final transpeptidation step of peptidoglycan synthesis resulting in cell wall death

Pharmacokinetics (Adult data unless noted)

Distribution: Widely distributed throughout the body including gallbladder, lungs, bone, bile, CSF (diffuses into the CSF at higher concentrations when the meninges are inflamed); crosses the placenta

Protein binding: 85% to 95%

Half-life:

Neonates:

1-4 days: 16 hours

9-30 days: 9 hours

Adults: 5-9 hours (with normal renal and hepatic function)

Time to peak serum concentration: I.M.: Within 1-2 hours

Elimination: Unchanged in the urine (33% to 65%) by glomerular filtration and in feces via bile

Dialysis: Not dialyzable (0% to 5%)

Usual Dosage I.M., I.V.:

Neonates:

Postnatal age ≤7 days: 50 mg/kg/day given every 24 hours

Postnatal age >7 days:

≤2000 g: 50 mg/kg/day given every 24 hours

>2000 g: 50-75 mg/kg/day given every 24 hours

Gonococcal prophylaxis: 25-50 mg/kg as a single dose (dose not to exceed 125 mg)

Gonococcal infection: 25-50 mg/kg/day (maximum dose: 125 mg) given every 24 hours for 7 days, up to 10-14 days if meningitis is documented

Note: Use cefotaxime in place of ceftriaxone in hyperbilirubinemic neonates.

Infants and Children: 50-75 mg/kg/day divided every 12-24 hours

Acute bacterial otitis media: 50 mg/kg in a single dose (maximum dose: 1 g)

Persistent or relapsing acute otitis media: 50 mg/kg once daily for 3 days (maximum dose: 1 g/day)

Meningitis: 100 mg/kg/day divided every 12-24 hours; loading dose of 100 mg/kg may be administered at the start of therapy; maximum dose: 4 g/day

Chemoprophylaxis for high-risk contacts of patients with invasive meningococcal disease:
≤12 years: I.M.: 125 mg in a single dose
>12 years: I.M.: 250 mg in a single dose
Epiglottis: 50-100 mg/kg once daily; reported duration of treatment ranged from 2-14 days
Skin/skin structure infections: 50-75 mg/kg/day in 1-2 divided doses (maximum: 2 g/day)
Typhoid fever: I.V.: 75-80 mg/kg once daily for 5-14 days
Lyme disease (persistent arthritis, meningitis, encephalitis): 75-100 mg/kg (maximum: 2 g) for 2-4 weeks
Uncomplicated gonococcal infections, sexual assault, and STD prophylaxis: I.M.: 125 mg in a single dose
Complicated gonococcal infections: I.M., I.V.:
<45 kg:
Peritonitis, arthritis, or bacteremia: 50 mg/kg/day once daily for 7 days; maximum dose: 1 g/day
Conjunctivitis: 50 mg/kg (maximum dose: 1 g) in a single dose
Meningitis or endocarditis: 50 mg/kg/day divided every 12 hours for 10-14 days (meningitis), for 28 days (endocarditis); maximum dose: 2 g/day
>45 kg:
Disseminated gonococcal infections: 1 g/day once daily for 7 days
Meningitis: 1-2 g/dose every 12 hours for 10-14 days
Endocarditis: 1-2 g/dose every 12 hours for 28 days
Conjunctivitis: I.M.: 1 g in a single dose
Chancroid: I.M.: 50 mg/kg as a single dose (maximum dose: 250 mg)
Acute epididymitis: I.M.: 250 mg in a single dose
Adults: 1-2 g every 12-24 hours depending on the type and severity of the infection; maximum dose: 4 g/day
Dosage adjustment in renal impairment: No change necessary with dose ≤2 g/day
Dosage adjustment in hepatic impairment: No adjustment necessary unless there is concurrent renal dysfunction, then dose should be a maximum of 2 g/day.
Administration Parenteral:
IVP: Administer over 2-4 minutes at a maximum concentration of 40 mg/mL. Rapid IVP injection over 5 minutes of a 2 g dose resulted in tachycardia, restlessness, diaphoresis, and palpitations in an adult patient
I.V. intermittent infusion: Administer over 10-30 minutes; final concentration for I.V. administration should not exceed 40 mg/mL
I.M. injection: May be diluted with SWI or 1% lidocaine to a final concentration of 250 mg/mL or may be concentrated by using the manufacturer's recommended diluent volume of 1% lidocaine with a resultant concentration of 350 mg/mL; administer I.M. injections deep into a large muscle mass
Monitoring Parameters CBC with differential, platelet count, PT, renal and hepatic function tests periodically; number and type of stools/day for diarrhea
Test Interactions False-positive urine glucose with Clinitest®; may falsely elevate serum or urinary creatinine values when a manual Jaffé method is used
Additional Information Sodium content of 1 g: 3.6 mEq
Dosage Forms Excipient information presented when available (limited, particularly for generics); consult specific product labeling. [DSC] = Discontinued product
Infusion [premixed in dextrose]: 1 g (50 mL); 2 g (50 mL)
Injection, powder for reconstitution: 250 mg, 500 mg, 1 g, 2 g, 10 g
Rocephin®: 250 mg [DSC], 500 mg, 1 g, 2 g [DSC], 10 g [contains sodium ~83 mg (3.6 mEq) per ceftriaxone 1 g] [DSC]
References
American Academy of Pediatrics Subcommittee on Management of Acute Otitis Media, "Diagnosis and Management of Acute Otitis Media," Pediatrics, 2004, 113(5):1451-65.

Bradley JS, Compogiannis LS, Murray WE, et al, "Pharmacokinetics and Safety of Intramuscular Injection of Concentrated Ceftriaxone in Children," Clin Pharm, 1992, 11(11):961-4.
Centers for Disease Control and Prevention, "2002 Guidelines for Treatment of Sexually Transmitted Diseases," MMWR Morb Mortal Wkly Rep, 2002, 51(RR-6):1-80.
Committee on Adolescence, American Academy of Pediatrics, "Sexual Assault and the Adolescent," Pediatrics, 1994, 94(5):761-5.
Dowell SF, Butler JC, Giebink GS, et al, "Acute Otitis Media: Management and Surveillance in an Era of Pneumococcal Resistance - A Report From the Drug-Resistant Streptococcus pneumoniae Therapeutic Working Group," Pediatr Infect Dis J, 1999, 18(1):1-9.
Frenck RW Jr, Nakhla I, Sultan Y, et al, "Azithromycin Versus Ceftriaxone for the Treatment of Uncomplicated Typhoid Fever in Children," Clin Infect Dis, 2000, 31(5):1134-8.
Frenkel LD, "Once-Daily Administration of Ceftriaxone for the Treatment of Selected Serious Bacterial Infections in Children," Pediatrics, 1988, 82(3 Pt 2):486-91.
Low YM, Leong JL, and Tan HK, "Paediatric Acute Epiglottitis Revisited," Singapore Med J, 2003, 44(10):539-41
Red Book: 2006 Report of the Committee on Infectious Diseases, 27th ed, Pickering LK, Baker CJ, Long SS, et al, eds, Elk Grove Village, IL: American Academy of Pediatrics, 2006, 306, 431.
Richards DM, Heel RC, Brogden RN, et al, "Ceftriaxone: A Review of Its Antibacterial Activity, Pharmacological Properties and Therapeutic Use," Drugs, 1984, 27(6):469-527.
Sawyer SM, Johnson PD, Hogg GG, et al, "Successful Treatment of Epiglottitis With Two Doses of Ceftriaxone," Arch Dis Child, 1994, 70 (2):129-32
Stephens I and Levine MM, "Management of Typhoid Fever in Children," Pediatr Infect Dis J, 2002, 21(2):157-8.

◆ **Ceftriaxone Sodium** see CefTRIAXone on page 275

Cefuroxime (se fyoor OKS eem)

Medication Safety Issues
Sound-alike/look-alike issues:
Cefuroxime may be confused with cefotaxime, cefprozil, ceftizoxime, deferoxamine
Ceftin® may be confused with Cefzil®, Cipro®
Zinacef® may be confused with Zithromax®

International issues:
Ceftin® may be confused with Cefiton® which is a brand name for cefixime in Portugal
Ceftin® may be confused with Ceftina® which is a brand name for cefalotin in Mexico
Ceftin® may be confused with Ceftim® which is a brand name for ceftazidime in Italy
U.S. Brand Names Ceftin®; Zinacef®
Canadian Brand Names Apo-Cefuroxime®; Ceftin®; Cefuroxime For Injection; PRO-Cefuroxime; ratio-Cefuroxime
Therapeutic Category Antibiotic, Cephalosporin (Second Generation)
Generic Available Yes
Use A second generation cephalosporin useful in infections caused by susceptible staphylococci, group B streptococci, pneumococci, H. influenzae (type A and B), E. coli, Enterobacter, and Klebsiella; treatment of susceptible infections of the upper and lower respiratory tract, otitis media, acute bacterial maxillary sinusitis, urinary tract, skin and soft tissue, bone and joint, and sepsis
Pregnancy Risk Factor B
Pregnancy Considerations Adverse events were not observed in animal studies; therefore, cefuroxime is classified as pregnancy category B. Cefuroxime crosses the placenta and reaches the cord serum and amniotic fluid. Placental transfer is decreased in the presence of oligohydramnios. Several studies have failed to identify a teratogenic risk to the fetus from maternal cefuroxime use.

During pregnancy, mean plasma concentrations of cefuroxime are 50% lower, the AUC is 25% lower, and the plasma half-life is shorter than nonpregnant values. At term, plasma half-life is similar to nonpregnant values and peak maternal concentrations after I.M. administration are

◀ slightly decreased. Pregnancy does not alter the volume of distribution.

Lactation Enters breast milk/use caution

Breast-Feeding Considerations Cefuroxime is excreted in breast milk. Manufacturer recommendations vary; caution is recommended if cefuroxime I.V. is given to a nursing woman and it is recommended to consider discontinuing nursing temporarily during treatment following oral cefuroxime. Nondose-related effects could include modification of bowel flora.

Contraindications Hypersensitivity to cefuroxime, any component, or cephalosporins

Warnings Prolonged use may result in superinfection; patients with renal or hepatic impairment, poor nutritional state, patients previously stabilized on anticoagulant therapy, or who have received a prolonged course of antimicrobial therapy are at risk for developing a fall in prothrombin activity. Monitor prothrombin time and consider administering vitamin K if indicated. Safety and efficacy in infants <3 months of age have not been established; do not use in patients with immediate-type hypersensitivity reactions to penicillin

Precautions Use with caution and modify dosage in patients with renal impairment; use with caution in patients with history of colitis or history of penicillin hypersensitivity

Adverse Reactions

Central nervous system: Fever, headache, dizziness, vertigo, seizures

Dermatologic: Rash, pruritus, erythema multiforme, diaper rash, urticaria

Gastrointestinal: Nausea, vomiting, diarrhea, stomach cramps, GI bleeding, antibiotic-associated colitis, stomatitis

Genitourinary: Vaginitis

Hematologic: Hemolytic anemia, transient neutropenia and leukopenia, hemoglobin and hematocrit decreased, eosinophilia, prothrombin time increased

Hepatic: Transient elevation in liver enzymes, hepatitis, cholestasis

Local: Pain at injection site, thrombophlebitis

Renal: BUN and serum creatinine elevated

Miscellaneous: Anaphylaxis

Drug Interactions

Avoid Concomitant Use

Avoid concomitant use of Cefuroxime with any of the following: BCG

Increased Effect/Toxicity

The levels/effects of Cefuroxime may be increased by: Probenecid

Decreased Effect

Cefuroxime may decrease the levels/effects of: BCG; Typhoid Vaccine

The levels/effects of Cefuroxime may be decreased by: Antacids; H2-Antagonists

Food Interactions Food and milk increase bioavailability and peak levels

Stability Reconstituted injectable solution (100 mg/mL) or injectable suspension (200-220 mg/mL) is stable for 24 hours at room temperature or 48 hours when refrigerated; reconstituted oral suspension can be stored in the refrigerator or at room temperature; discard after 10 days

Mechanism of Action Inhibits bacterial cell wall synthesis by binding to one or more of the penicillin-binding proteins; inhibits the final transpeptidation step of peptidoglycan synthesis resulting in cell wall death

Pharmacokinetics (Adult data unless noted)

Absorption: Oral: Increased when given with or shortly after food or infant formula

Distribution: Into bronchial secretions, synovial and pericardial fluid, kidneys, heart, liver, bone and bile; penetrates into CSF with inflamed meninges; crosses the placenta; excreted into breast milk

Protein binding: 33% to 50%

Bioavailability: Oral cefuroxime axetil tablets: 37% to 52%; cefuroxime axetil suspension is less bioavailable than the tablet (91% of the AUC for tablets)

Half-life:

Neonates:

≤3 days: 5.1-5.8 hours

6-14 days: 2-4.2 hours

3-4 weeks: 1-1.5 hours

Adults: 1-2 hours (prolonged in renal impairment)

Time to peak serum concentration:

Oral: 2-3 hours

I.M.: Within 15-60 minutes

Elimination: Primarily 66% to 100% as unchanged drug in urine by both glomerular filtration and tubular secretion

Dialysis: Dialyzable

Usual Dosage

I.M., I.V.:

Neonates: 50-100 mg/kg/day divided every 12 hours

Children: 75-150 mg/kg/day divided every 8 hours; maximum dose: 6 g/day

Meningitis: Not recommended due to reports of treatment failures and slower bacteriologic response time (doses of 200-240 mg/kg/day divided every 6-8 hours have been used); maximum dose: 9 g/day

Adults: 750 mg to 1.5 g/dose every 8 hours

Oral: **Cefuroxime axetil film-coated tablets and oral suspension are not bioequivalent and are not substitutable on a mg/mg basis**

Infants ≥3 months to Children 12 years:

Pharyngitis, tonsillitis: Suspension: 20 mg/kg/day (maximum dose: 500 mg/day) in 2 divided doses

Acute otitis media, acute bacterial maxillary sinusitis, impetigo:

Suspension: 30 mg/kg/day (maximum dose: 1 g/day) in 2 divided doses

Tablet: 250 mg every 12 hours

Adolescents and Adults: 250-500 mg twice daily

Uncomplicated urinary tract infection: 125-250 mg every 12 hours

Uncomplicated gonorrhea: Single 1 g dose

Early Lyme disease: 500 mg twice daily for 20 days

Dosing interval in renal impairment:

Cl_{cr} 10-20 mL/minute: Administer every 12 hours

Cl_{cr} <10 mL/minute: Administer every 24 hours

Administration

Oral: Cefuroxime axetil suspension must be administered with food; shake suspension well before use; tablets may be administered with or without food; administer with food to decrease GI upset; avoid crushing the tablet due to its bitter taste

Parenteral:

IVP: Administer over 3-5 minutes at a maximum concentration of 100 mg/mL

I.V. intermittent infusion: Administer over 15-30 minutes at a final concentration for administration ≤30 mg/mL; in fluid restricted patients, a concentration of 137 mg/mL may be administered

I.M.: I.M. injection is less painful when administered as an injectable suspension rather than a solution (see Stability), and is less painful when administered into the buttock rather than the thigh

Monitoring Parameters With prolonged therapy, monitor renal, hepatic, and hematologic function periodically; number and type of stools/day for diarrhea; and prothrombin time

Test Interactions Positive Coombs' [direct]; false-positive urine glucose with Clinitest®

Dosage Forms Excipient information presented when available (limited, particularly for generics); consult specific product labeling.

Note: Strength expressed as base

Infusion, as sodium [premixed]: 750 mg (50 mL); 1.5 g (50 mL)

Zinacef®: 750 mg (50 mL); 1.5 g (50 mL) [contains sodium 4.8 mEq (111 mg) per 750 mg]

Injection, powder for reconstitution, as sodium: 750 mg, 1.5 g, 7.5 g, 75 g, 225 g

Zinacef®: 750 mg, 1.5 g, 7.5 g [contains sodium 1.8 mEq (41 mg) per 750 mg]

Powder for suspension, oral, as axetil: 125 mg/5 mL (100 mL); 250 mg/5 mL (50 mL, 100 mL)

Ceftin®: 125 mg/5 mL (100 mL) [contains phenylalanine 11.8 mg/5 mL; tutti-frutti flavor]; 250 mg/5 mL (50 mL, 100 mL) [contains phenylalanine 25.2 mg/5 mL; tutti-frutti flavor]

Tablet, as axetil: 250 mg, 500 mg

Ceftin®: 250 mg, 500 mg

References

de Louvois J, Mulhall A, and Hurley R, "Cefuroxime in the Treatment of Neonates," *Arch Dis Child*, 1982, 57(1):59-62.

Gooch WM 3rd, Blair E, Puopolo A, et al, "Effectiveness of Five Days of Therapy With Cefuroxime Axetil Suspension for Treatment of Acute Otitis Media," *Pediatr Infect Dis J*, 1996, 15(2):157-64.

Nelson JD, "Cefuroxime: A Cephalosporin With Unique Applicability to Pediatric Practice," *Pediatr Infect Dis*, 1983, 2(5):394-6.

Thoene DE and Johnson CE, "Pharmacotherapy of Otitis Media," *Pharmacotherapy*, 1991, 11(3):212-21.

◆ **Cefuroxime Axetil** *see* Cefuroxime *on page 277*

◆ **Cefuroxime For Injection (Can)** *see* Cefuroxime *on page 277*

◆ **Cefuroxime Sodium** *see* Cefuroxime *on page 277*

◆ **Cefzil® (Can)** *see* Cefprozil *on page 271*

◆ **Celebrex®** *see* Celecoxib *on page 279*

Celecoxib (se le KOKS ib)

Medication Safety Issues

Sound-alike/look-alike issues:

Celebrex® may be confused with Celexa®, cerebra, Cerebyx®, Cervarix®, Clarinex®

U.S. Brand Names Celebrex®

Canadian Brand Names Celebrex®

Therapeutic Category Nonsteroidal Anti-inflammatory Drug (NSAID), COX-2 Selective

Generic Available No

Use Relief of signs and symptoms of osteoarthritis, adult rheumatoid arthritis, juvenile rheumatoid arthritis (juvenile idiopathic arthritis) (FDA approved in ages ≥2 years), and ankylosing spondylitis; management of acute pain; treatment of primary dysmenorrhea; to reduce the number of intestinal polyps in familial adenomatous polyposis (FAP). **Note:** Celecoxib does not affect platelet aggregation and thus, should not be used as a substitute for aspirin for cardiovascular prophylaxis.

Medication Guide An FDA-approved patient medication guide, which is available with the product information and at http://www.fda.gov/downloads/Drugs/DrugSafety/ ucm088567.pdf, must be dispensed with this medication for each new outpatient prescription and refill.

Pregnancy Risk Factor C (prior to 30 weeks gestation)/D (≥30 weeks gestation)

Pregnancy Considerations Teratogenic effects have been observed in some animal studies; therefore, celecoxib is classified as pregnancy category C. Celecoxib is a NSAID that primarily inhibits COX-2 whereas other currently available NSAIDs are nonselective for COX-1 and COX-2. The effects of this selective inhibition to the fetus have not been well studied and limited information is available specific to celecoxib. NSAID exposure during the first trimester is not strongly associated with congenital malformations; however, cardiovascular anomalies and cleft palate have been observed following NSAID exposure in some studies. The use of a NSAID close to conception may be associated with an increased risk of miscarriage. Nonteratogenic effects have been observed following NSAID administration during the third trimester including: Myocardial degenerative changes, prenatal constriction of the ductus arteriosus, fetal tricuspid regurgitation, failure of the ductus arteriosus to close postnatally; renal dysfunction or failure, oligohydramnios; gastrointestinal bleeding or perforation, increased risk of necrotizing enterocolitis; intracranial bleeding (including intraventricular hemorrhage), platelet dysfunction with resultant bleeding; pulmonary hypertension. Because it may cause premature closure of the ductus arteriosus, the use of celecoxib is not recommended ≥30 weeks gestation. The chronic use of NSAIDs in women of reproductive age may be associated with infertility that is reversible upon discontinuation of the medication. A registry is available for pregnant women exposed to autoimmune medications including celecoxib. For additional information contact the Organization of Teratology Information Specialists, OTIS Autoimmune Diseases Study, at 877-311-8972.

Lactation Enters breast milk/use caution

Breast-Feeding Considerations Small amounts of celecoxib are found in breast milk. The manufacturer recommends that caution be exercised when administering celecoxib to nursing women.

Contraindications Hypersensitivity to celecoxib, any component, sulfonamides (celecoxib is a sulfonamide), aspirin, or other NSAIDs; patients with the "aspirin triad" [asthma, rhinitis (with or without nasal polyps) and aspirin intolerance] (fatal asthmatic and anaphylactoid reactions may occur in these patients); perioperative pain in the setting of coronary artery bypass surgery (CABG)

Warnings NSAIDs are associated with an increased risk of adverse cardiovascular thrombotic events, including potentially fatal MI and stroke **[U.S. Boxed Warning]**; risk may be increased with duration of use or pre-existing cardiovascular risk factors or disease; carefully evaluate cardiovascular risk profile prior to prescribing; use the lowest effective dose for the shortest duration of time, taking into consideration individual patient treatment goals; alternate therapies should be considered for patients at high risk. Use is contraindicated for treatment of perioperative pain in the setting of CABG surgery **[U.S. Boxed Warning]**; an increased incidence of MI and stroke was found in patients receiving COX-2 selective NSAIDs for the treatment of pain within the first 10-14 days after CABG surgery. NSAIDs may cause fluid retention, edema, and new onset or worsening of pre-existing hypertension; use with caution in patients with hypertension, CHF, or fluid retention.

NSAIDs may increase the risk of gastrointestinal inflammation, ulceration, bleeding, and perforation **[U.S. Boxed Warning]**. These events, which can be potentially fatal, may occur at any time during therapy, and without warning. Avoid the use of NSAIDs in patients with active GI bleeding or ulcer disease. Use NSAIDs with extreme caution in patients with a history of GI bleeding or ulcers (these patients have a 10-fold increased risk for developing a GI bleed). Use NSAIDs with caution in patients with other risk factors which may increase GI bleeding (eg, concurrent therapy with aspirin, anticoagulants, and/or corticosteroids, longer duration of NSAID use, smoking, use of alcohol, and poor general health). Use the lowest effective dose for the shortest duration of time, taking into consideration individual patient treatment goals; alternate therapies should be considered for patients at high risk.

NSAIDs may compromise existing renal function. Renal toxicity may occur in patients with impaired renal function, dehydration, heart failure, liver dysfunction, those taking diuretics and ACE inhibitors; use with caution in these patients; monitor renal function closely. NSAIDs are not recommended for use in patients with advanced renal disease. Long-term use of NSAIDs may cause renal papillary necrosis and other renal injury.

Fatal asthmatic and anaphylactoid reactions may occur in patients with the "aspirin triad" who receive NSAIDs (see Contraindications). NSAIDs may cause serious dermatologic adverse reactions including exfoliative dermatitis, Stevens-Johnson syndrome, and toxic epidermal necrolysis; discontinue use at first sign of skin rash or any other sign of hypersensitivity reaction. Avoid use of NSAIDs in late pregnancy (≥30 weeks gestation) as they may cause premature closure of the ductus arteriosus. When used for the treatment of FAP, routine monitoring and care should be continued (ie, do **not** decrease frequency of routine endoscopic examinations or delay prophylactic colectomy or other FAP-related surgeries; use of celecoxib has **not** been shown to decrease risk of GI cancer in patients with FAP).

Precautions Use with caution and decrease the dose in patients with mild or moderate hepatic impairment; use in patients with severe hepatic impairment (Child-Pugh Class C) is not recommended. Closely monitor patients with abnormal LFTs; severe hepatic reactions (eg, fulminant hepatitis, hepatic necrosis, jaundice, liver failure) have occurred with NSAID use, rarely; discontinue if signs or symptoms of liver disease develop, or if systemic manifestations occur.

Use with caution in patients with asthma; asthmatic patients may have aspirin-sensitive asthma which may be associated with severe and potentially fatal bronchospasm when aspirin or NSAIDs are administered (see Contraindications). Anemia may sometimes occur; monitor hemoglobin and hematocrit in patients receiving long term therapy.

Use with caution in pediatric patients with systemic-onset JRA; serious adverse reactions, including disseminated intravascular coagulation, may occur. Celecoxib is FDA-approved for use in children with JRA who are ≥2 years of age and ≥10 kg; safety and efficacy of use in children with JRA for >6 months have not been evaluated; long-term cardiovascular toxicity in children has not been studied. Consider alternate therapy in JRA patients who are CYP2C9 poor metabolizers (see next paragraph). Safety and efficacy have not been established for use in children for indications other than JRA.

Use with caution and consider dosage reduction in patients who are known or suspected poor metabolizers of cytochrome P450 isoenzyme 2C9 substrates; these patients may have unusually high plasma levels due to reduced clearance. Consider alternate therapy in JRA patients who are identified to be CYP2C9 poor metabolizers. In a small pediatric study (n=4), the AUC of celecoxib was ~10 times higher in a child who was homozygous for CYP2C9*3, compared to children who were homozygous for the *1 allele (n=2) or who had the CYP2C9*1/*2 genotype; further studies are needed to determine if carriers of the CYP2C9*3 allele are at increased risk for cardiovascular toxicity or dose-related adverse effects of celecoxib, especially with long-term, high-dose use of the drug (see Stempak, 2005). Adult subjects who were homozygous for CYP2C9*3/*3 displayed celecoxib serum concentrations 3-7 times higher than subjects with CYP2C9*1/*1 or CYP2C9*1/*3 genotypes. The frequency of CYP2C9*3/*3 genotype is estimated to be 0.3% to 1% in various ethnic groups. Celecoxib should not be used as a substitute for corticosteroid therapy or to treat corticosteroid insufficiency. Avoid concomitant use of celecoxib and other NSAIDs.

Adverse Reactions

Cardiovascular: Peripheral edema, hypertension; cardiovascular thrombotic events, including potentially fatal MI and stroke (see Warnings)

Central nervous system: Headache, fever, insomnia, dizziness

Dermatologic: Skin rash

Endocrine & metabolic: Fluid retention

Gastrointestinal: Abdominal pain, nausea, diarrhea, vomiting, dyspepsia, gastroesophageal reflux, flatulence; peptic ulcer, GI bleeding, GI perforation (see Warnings)

Hepatic: ALT or AST elevated, hepatitis, jaundice

Neuromuscular & skeletal: Arthralgia, back pain

Renal: Renal impairment (see Warnings)

Respiratory: Cough, dyspnea, pharyngitis, nasopharyngitis, rhinitis, sinusitis, upper respiratory tract infection

Miscellaneous: Anaphylactoid reactions

Drug Interactions

Metabolism/Transport Effects Substrate of CYP2C9 (major), 3A4 (minor); **Inhibits** CYP2C8 (moderate), 2D6 (weak)

Avoid Concomitant Use

Avoid concomitant use of Celecoxib with any of the following: Ketorolac; Ketorolac (Systemic); Thioridazine

Increased Effect/Toxicity

Celecoxib may increase the levels/effects of: Aminoglycosides; Anticoagulants; Antiplatelet Agents; Bisphosphonate Derivatives; CycloSPORINE; CycloSPORINE (Systemic); CYP2C8 Substrates (High risk); CYP2D6 Substrates; Desmopressin; Digoxin; Eplerenone; Fesoterodine; Haloperidol; Lithium; Methotrexate; Nebivolol; Nonsteroidal Anti-Inflammatory Agents; Potassium-Sparing Diuretics; Pralatrexate; Quinolone Antibiotics; Tamoxifen; Thioridazine; Thrombolytic Agents; Vancomycin; Vitamin K Antagonists

The levels/effects of Celecoxib may be increased by: Antidepressants (Tricyclic, Tertiary Amine); Corticosteroids (Systemic); CYP2C9 Inhibitors (Moderate); CYP2C9 Inhibitors (Strong); Herbs (Anticoagulant/Antiplatelet Properties); Ketorolac; Ketorolac (Systemic); Probenecid; Selective Serotonin Reuptake Inhibitors; Treprostinil

Decreased Effect

Celecoxib may decrease the levels/effects of: ACE Inhibitors; Angiotensin II Receptor Blockers; Antiplatelet Agents; Beta-Blockers; Codeine; Eplerenone; HydrALAZINE; Loop Diuretics; Potassium-Sparing Diuretics; Thiazide Diuretics; TraMADol

The levels/effects of Celecoxib may be decreased by: Bile Acid Sequestrants; CYP2C9 Inducers (Highly Effective); Peginterferon Alfa-2b

Food Interactions

Adults: A high-fat meal delays the time to peak concentrations by 1-2 hours and increases AUC by 10% to 20%

Pediatric cancer patients: In a nonrandomized, noncrossover study, a high-fat meal or snack increased AUC by 60% (single-dose) and increased AUC by 75% at steady-state (Stempak, 2005a).

Stability Store at controlled room temperature of 25°C (77°F); excursions permitted to 15°C to 30°C (59°F to 86°F).

Mechanism of Action Inhibits prostaglandin synthesis by decreasing the activity of the enzyme, cyclooxygenase-2 (COX-2), which results in decreased formation of prostaglandin precursors. Celecoxib does not inhibit cyclooxygenase-1 (COX-1) at therapeutic concentrations. Celecoxib does not affect platelet aggregation. In FAP, celecoxib reduces the number of colorectal polyps.

Pharmacokinetics (Adult data unless noted)

Absorption: Prolonged due to low solubility

Distribution: Distributes into breast milk; V_d (apparent):

Children (steady-state): 8.3 ± 5.8 L/kg

Adults: ~400 L

Protein binding: ~97%; primarily to albumin; binds to alpha 1-acid glycoprotein to a lesser extent

Metabolism: Hepatic via CYP2C9; forms 3 inactive metabolites (a primary alcohol, corresponding carboxylic acid, and its glucuronide conjugate) **Note:** Meta-analysis suggests the AUC is 40% higher in Blacks compared to Caucasians (clinical significance unknown)

Bioavailability: Absolute: Unknown.

Half-life elimination:

Children (steady-state): 6 ± 2.7 hours (range: 3-10 hours)

Adults: ~11 hours (fasted)

Time to peak serum concentration:

Children: Median: 3 hours (range: 3-6.2 hours)

Adults: ~3 hours

Elimination: Feces (57% as metabolites, <3% as unchanged drug); urine (27% as metabolites, <3% as unchanged drug); primary metabolites in feces and urine: Carboxylic acid metabolite (73% of dose); low amounts of glucuronide metabolite appear in urine

Usual Dosage Note: Use the lowest effective dose for the shortest duration of time, consistent with individual patient goals. Oral:

Children ≥2 years: JRA

≥10 kg to ≤25 kg: 50 mg twice daily

>25 kg: 100 mg twice daily

Adults:

Acute pain or primary dysmenorrhea: Initial dose: 400 mg, followed by an additional 200 mg if needed on day 1; maintenance dose: 200 mg twice daily as needed

Ankylosing spondylitis: 200 mg/day as a single dose or in divided doses twice daily; if no effect after 6 weeks, may increase to 400 mg/day. If no response following 6 weeks of treatment with 400 mg/day, consider discontinuation and alternative treatment.

Familial adenomatous polyposis: 400 mg twice daily

Osteoarthritis: 200 mg/day as a single dose or in divided doses twice daily

Rheumatoid arthritis: 100-200 mg twice daily

Dosing adjustment in renal impairment: No specific dosage adjustment is recommended; not recommended in patients with severe renal dysfunction

Dosing adjustment in hepatic impairment:

Mild hepatic impairment: AUC is increased by 40%; monitor closely; reduce dose

Moderate hepatic impatient (Child-Pugh Class B): AUC is increased by 180%; monitor closely; decrease daily recommended dose by 50%

Severe hepatic impairment (Child-Pugh Class C): Has not been studied; use is not recommended

Dosing adjustment in poor metabolizers of CYP2C9 substrates: Use with caution in patients who are known or suspected poor metabolizers of cytochrome P450 isoenzyme 2C9 substrates. In poor metabolizers, consider initiation at 50% of the lowest recommended dose. Consider alternate therapy in JRA patients who are poor metabolizers.

Administration Lower doses (up to 200 mg twice daily) may be administered without regard to meals (may administer with food to reduce GI upset); larger doses should be administered with food to improve absorption.

Do not administer with antacids. Capsules may be swallowed whole or the entire contents emptied onto a teaspoon of cool or room temperature applesauce; the contents of the capsule sprinkled onto applesauce may be stored under refrigeration for up to 6 hours.

Monitoring Parameters CBC; blood chemistry profile; occult blood loss; periodic liver function tests; renal function (urine output, serum BUN and creatinine); monitor efficacy (eg, in arthritic conditions: Pain, range of motion, grip strength, mobility), inflammation; observe for weight gain, edema; observe for bleeding, bruising; evaluate GI effects (abdominal pain, bleeding, dyspepsia); blood pressure

Patient Information Celecoxib is a nonsteroidal anti-inflammatory drug (NSAID); NSAIDs may cause serious adverse reactions, especially with overuse; use exactly as directed; do not increase dose or frequency. NSAIDs may increase the risk for heart attack, stroke, or ulcers and bleeding in stomach or intestines; GI bleeding, ulceration, or perforation can occur with or without pain; it is unclear whether celecoxib has rates of these events which are similar to nonselective NSAIDs. Notify physician before use if you have hypertension; heart failure; heart, liver, or kidney disease; history of stomach ulcers or bleeding in stomach or intestines; asthma; aspirin-sensitive asthma; or other medical problems. Read the patient Medication Guide that you receive with each prescription and refill of celecoxib.

Avoid alcohol, aspirin, and OTC medication unless approved by prescriber. May cause dizziness and impair ability to perform activities requiring mental alertness or physical coordination (avoid driving or engaging in tasks requiring alertness until response to drug is known). Stop taking medication and report immediately stomach pain or cramping; unusual bleeding or bruising (blood in vomitus, stool, or urine); chest pain; shortness of breath; swelling of face or throat; weakness of extremities; slurring of speech or skin rash. Report persistent insomnia; unusual fatigue or flu-like symptoms; jaundice; muscle pain, tremors, or weakness; sudden weight gain or edema; changes in hearing (ringing in ears) or vision; changes in urination pattern; or respiratory difficulty.

Dosage Forms Excipient information presented when available (limited, particularly for generics); consult specific product labeling.

Capsule:

Celebrex®: 50 mg, 100 mg, 200 mg, 400 mg

References

Knoppert DC, Stempak D, Baruchel S, et al, "Celecoxib in Human Milk: A Case Report," *Pharmacotherapy*, 2003, 23(1):97-100.

Stempak D, Bukaveckas BL, Linder M, et al, "Cytochrome P450 2C9 Genotype: Impact on Celecoxib Safety and Pharmacokinetics in a Pediatric Patient," *Clin Pharmacol Ther*, 2005, 78(3):309-10.

Stempak D, Gammon J, Halton J, et al, "Modulation of Celecoxib Pharmacokinetics by Food in Pediatric Patients," *Clin Pharmacol Ther*, 2005a, 77(3):226-8.

Stempak D, Gammon J, Klein J, et al, "Single-Dose and Steady-State Pharmacokinetics of Celecoxib in Children," *Clin Pharmacol Ther*, 2002, 72(5):490-7.

◆ **Celestone®** *see* Betamethasone *on page 189*

◆ **Celestone® Soluspan®** *see* Betamethasone *on page 189*

◆ **Celexa®** *see* Citalopram *on page 319*

◆ **CellCept®** *see* Mycophenolate *on page 956*

◆ **Celontin®** *see* Methsuximide *on page 904*

◆ **Cemill [OTC]** *see* Ascorbic Acid *on page 138*

◆ **Cenolate® [DSC]** *see* Ascorbic Acid *on page 138*

◆ **Cepacol® Fizzlers™ [OTC]** *see* Benzocaine *on page 182*

◆ **Cepacol® Sore Throat [OTC]** *see* Benzocaine *on page 182*

Cephalexin (sef a LEKS in)

Medication Safety Issues
Sound-alike/look-alike issues:
Cephalexin may be confused with cefaclor, ceFAZolin, cephalothin, ciprofloxacin
Keflex® may be confused with Keppra®, Valtrex®

Related Information
Endocarditis Prophylaxis *on page 1610*

U.S. Brand Names Keflex®

Canadian Brand Names Apo-Cephalex®; Dom-Cephalexin; Keflex®; Keftab®; Novo-Lexin; Nu-Cephalex; PMS-Cephalexin

Therapeutic Category Antibiotic, Cephalosporin (First Generation)

Generic Available Yes

Use Treatment of susceptible bacterial infections, including those caused by group A beta-hemolytic *Streptococcus*, *Staphylococcus*, *Klebsiella pneumoniae*, *E. coli*, and *Proteus mirabilis*; not active against enterococci or methicillin-resistant staphylococci; used to treat susceptible infections of the respiratory tract, skin and skin structure, bone, genitourinary tract, and otitis media; alternative therapy for endocarditis prophylaxis

Pregnancy Risk Factor B

Pregnancy Considerations Adverse events were not observed in animal reproduction studies; therefore, cephalexin is classified as pregnancy category B. Cephalexin crosses the placenta and produces therapeutic concentrations in the fetal circulation and amniotic fluid. An increased risk of teratogenic effects has not been observed following maternal use of cephalexin; however, adequate and well-controlled studies have not been completed in pregnant women. Peak concentrations in pregnant patients are similar to those in nonpregnant patients. Prolonged labor may decrease oral absorption.

Lactation Enters breast milk (small amounts)/use caution

Breast-Feeding Considerations Small amounts of cephalexin are excreted in breast milk. The manufacturer recommends that caution be exercised when administering cephalexin to nursing women. Maximum milk concentration occurs ~4 hours after a single oral dose and gradually disappears by 8 hours after administration. Nondose-related effects could include modification of bowel flora.

Contraindications Hypersensitivity to cephalexin, any component, or cephalosporins

Warnings Prolonged use may result in GI or genitourinary superinfection; do not use in patients with immediate-type hypersensitivity reactions to penicillin

Precautions Use with caution and modify dosage in patients with renal impairment; use with caution in patients with history of colitis or history of penicillin hypersensitivity. Tablets for oral suspension contain aspartame which is metabolized to phenylalanine and must be avoided (or used with caution) in patients with phenylketonuria.

Adverse Reactions
Central nervous system: Dizziness, headache, fatigue, fever, confusion

Dermatologic: Rash, urticaria, angioedema; erythema multiforme, Stevens-Johnson syndrome, toxic epidermal necrolysis (rare)

Gastrointestinal: Nausea, vomiting, pseudomembranous colitis, diarrhea, cramps, gastritis

Genitourinary: Vaginal moniliasis, vaginitis

Hematologic: Transient neutropenia, thrombocytopenia, anemia, eosinophilia

Hepatic: Transient elevation in liver enzymes, hepatitis, cholestatic jaundice

Neuromuscular & skeletal: Arthralgia, arthritis

Renal: Interstitial nephritis (rare)

Miscellaneous: Anaphylaxis

Drug Interactions
Avoid Concomitant Use
Avoid concomitant use of Cephalexin with any of the following: BCG

Increased Effect/Toxicity
Cephalexin may increase the levels/effects of: MetFORMIN

The levels/effects of Cephalexin may be increased by: Probenecid

Decreased Effect
Cephalexin may decrease the levels/effects of: BCG; Typhoid Vaccine

Food Interactions Food may delay absorption

Stability Refrigerate suspension after reconstitution; discard after 14 days; tablets for oral suspension should be used immediately after dissolving

Mechanism of Action Inhibits bacterial cell wall synthesis by binding to one or more of the penicillin-binding proteins; inhibits the final transpeptidation step of peptidoglycan synthesis resulting in cell wall death

Pharmacokinetics (Adult data unless noted)
Absorption: Rapid (90%); delayed in young children and may be decreased up to 50% in neonates

Distribution: Into tissues and fluids including bone, pleural and synovial fluid; crosses the placenta; appears in breast milk

Protein binding: 6% to 15%

Half-life:
Neonates: 5 hours
Children 3-12 months: 2.5 hours
Adults: 0.5-1.2 hours (prolonged with renal impairment)

Time to peak serum concentration: Oral: Within 60 minutes

Elimination: 80% to 100% of dose excreted as unchanged drug in urine within 8 hours

Dialysis: Moderately dialyzable (20% to 50%)

Usual Dosage Oral:
Children: 25-50 mg/kg/day divided every 6-8 hours; severe infections: 50-100 mg/kg/day divided every 6-8 hours; maximum dose: 4 g/day

Otitis media: 75-100 mg/kg/day divided every 6 hours

Streptococcal pharyngitis, skin and skin structure infections: 25-50 mg/kg/day divided every 12 hours

Endocarditis prophylaxis: 50 mg/kg 1 hour prior to procedure (maximum: 2 g)

Uncomplicated cystitis: Children >15 years: 500 mg every 12 hours for 7-14 days

Adults: 250-500 mg every 6 hours; maximum dose: 4 g/day

Streptococcal pharyngitis, skin and skin structure infections: 500 mg every 12 hours

Endocarditis prophylaxis: 2 g 1 hour prior to procedure

Uncomplicated cystitis: 500 mg every 12 hours for 7-14 days

Dosing interval in renal impairment:
Cl_{cr} 10-40 mL/minute: Administer every 8-12 hours
Cl_{cr} <10 mL/minute: Administer every 12-24 hours

Administration Oral: Administer on an empty stomach (ie, 1 hour prior to, or 2 hours after meals); administer with food if GI upset occurs; shake suspension well before use

Tablet for oral suspension: Mix tablet in a small amount of water (~10 mL); stir until thoroughly mixed; entire mixture should be administered immediately after mixing; rinse container with an additional small amount of water and drink contents to assure the whole dose is taken. **Do not** chew or swallow tablets. **Do not** mix with liquids other than water.

Monitoring Parameters With prolonged therapy, monitor renal, hepatic, and hematologic function periodically; number and type of stools/day for diarrhea

Test Interactions False-positive urine glucose with Clinitest®; positive Coombs' [direct]; false ↑ serum or urine creatinine

Patient Information Counsel patient that cephalexin should only be used to treat bacterial infections. Entire course of medication should be taken even if patient feels better early in the course. Report prolonged diarrhea.

Dosage Forms Excipient information presented when available (limited, particularly for generics); consult specific product labeling.

Capsule: 250 mg, 500 mg
Keflex®: 250 mg, 500 mg, 750 mg
Powder for oral suspension: 125 mg/5 mL (100 mL, 200 mL); 250 mg/5 mL (100 mL, 200 mL)
Tablet: 250 mg, 500 mg

References

Bergan T, "Pharmacokinetic Properties of Cephalosporins," *Drugs*, 1987, 34 (Suppl 2):89-104.

◆ **Cephalexin Monohydrate** *see* Cephalexin *on page 282*

◆ **Cerebyx®** *see* Fosphenytoin *on page 630*

◆ **Ceredase®** *see* Alglucerase *on page 64*

◆ **Cerezyme®** *see* Imiglucerase *on page 713*

◆ **Cerubidine®** *see* DAUNOrubicin *on page 394*

◆ **Cervarix®** *see* Papillomavirus (Types 16, 18) Vaccine (Human, Recombinant) *on page 1058*

◆ **C.E.S.** *see* Estrogens (Conjugated/Equine) *on page 539*

◆ **C.E.S.® (Can)** *see* Estrogens (Conjugated/Equine) *on page 539*

◆ **Cesamet®** *see* Nabilone *on page 960*

◆ **Cetacort® [DSC]** *see* Hydrocortisone *on page 685*

◆ **Cetafen® [OTC]** *see* Acetaminophen *on page 36*

◆ **Cetafen® Extra [OTC]** *see* Acetaminophen *on page 36*

Cetirizine (se TI ra zeen)

Medication Safety Issues
Sound-alike/look-alike issues:
Zyrtec® may be confused with Lipitor©, Serax®, Xanax®, Zantac®, Zerit®, Zocor®, Zyprexa®, Zyrtec-D®
Zyrtec® (cetirizine) may be confused with Zyrtec® Itchy Eye (ketotifen)

U.S. Brand Names All Day Allergy; Zyrtec® Allergy [OTC]; Zyrtec® Children's Allergy [OTC]; Zyrtec® Children's Hives Relief [OTC]

Canadian Brand Names Apo-Cetirizine®; PMS-Cetirizine; Reactine™

Therapeutic Category Antihistamine

Generic Available Yes

Use Relief of symptoms associated with perennial and seasonal allergic rhinitis; treatment of the uncomplicated skin manifestations of chronic idiopathic urticaria

Pregnancy Risk Factor B

Pregnancy Considerations Cetirizine was not shown to be teratogenic in animal studies; however, adequate studies have not been conducted in pregnant women. Use during pregnancy only if clearly needed.

Lactation Enters breast milk/not recommended

Contraindications Hypersensitivity to cetirizine, hydroxyzine, or any component

Warnings Safety and efficacy for the use of cough and cold products in children <2 years of age is limited. Serious adverse effects including death have been reported. The FDA notes that there are no approved OTC uses for these products in children <2 years of age. Healthcare providers are reminded to ask caregivers about the use of OTC cough and cold products in order to avoid exposure to multiple medications containing the same ingredient. Doses >10 mg/day may cause significant drowsiness.

Precautions Use with caution in patients with hepatic or renal dysfunction

Adverse Reactions
Cardiovascular: Palpitations, tachycardia, hypertension, hypotension
Central nervous system: Headache, drowsiness, somnolence, fatigue, dizziness, depression, confusion, vertigo, ataxia, syncope, hallucinations, convulsions (rare), aggressive reactions (rare), suicidal ideation (rare)
Dermatologic: Rash, photosensitivity, pruritus
Gastrointestinal: Diarrhea, flatulence, constipation, xerostomia, dyspepsia, abdominal pain, pharyngitis, taste loss, taste perversion, anorexia
Genitourinary: Dysuria, cystitis, polyuria, urinary incontinence, dysmenorrhea, vaginitis
Hematologic: Hemolytic anemia (rare), thrombocytopenia (rare)
Hepatic: Transient hepatic enzyme elevation, cholestasis, hepatitis (rare)
Neuromuscular & skeletal: Paresthesias, hyperkinesia, hypertonia, tremor, leg cramps
Otic: Tinnitus, ototoxicity, earache (<2%)
Renal: Glomerulonephritis (rare)
Respiratory: Cough, epistaxis, bronchospasm
Miscellaneous: Anaphylaxis (rare)

Drug Interactions
Metabolism/Transport Effects Substrate of CYP3A4 (minor), P-glycoprotein

Avoid Concomitant Use There are no known interactions where it is recommended to avoid concomitant use.

Increased Effect/Toxicity
Cetirizine may increase the levels/effects of: Alcohol (Ethyl); Anticholinergics; CNS Depressants

The levels/effects of Cetirizine may be increased by: P-Glycoprotein Inhibitors; Pramlintide

Decreased Effect
Cetirizine may decrease the levels/effects of: Acetylcholinesterase Inhibitors (Central); Betahistine

The levels/effects of Cetirizine may be decreased by: Acetylcholinesterase Inhibitors (Central); Amphetamines; P-Glycoprotein Inducers

Stability Store at room temperature; protect syrup from light

Mechanism of Action Cetirizine, a metabolite of hydroxyzine, competes with histamine for H_1-receptor sites on effector cells in the GI tract, blood vessels, and respiratory tract

Pharmacodynamics
Onset of action: 20-60 minutes
Duration: 24 hours

Pharmacokinetics (Adult data unless noted)
Absorption: Well absorbed from the GI tract
Distribution: V_d:
Children: 0.7 L/kg
Adults: 0.5-0.8 L/kg
Protein binding: 93%
Metabolism: Exact fate is unknown, limited hepatic metabolism
Half-life:
Children: 6.2 hours
Adults: 7.4-9 hours
Adults with mild-moderate renal failure: 19-21 hours
Time to peak serum concentration: 1 hour
Elimination: 60% to 70% excreted unchanged in urine
Dialysis: <10% removed during hemodialysis

Usual Dosage Oral:
Children 6-12 months: 2.5 mg once daily
Children 12-23 months: Initial: 2.5 mg once daily; dosage may be increased to 2.5 mg twice daily

◀

Children 2-5 years: 2.5 mg/day; may be increased to a maximum of 5 mg/day given either as a single dose or divided into 2 doses

Children ≥6 years to Adults: 5-10 mg/day as a single dose or divided into 2 doses

Dosage adjustment in renal or hepatic impairment:
Children <6 years: Cetirizine use not recommended
Children 6-11 years: <2.5 mg once daily
Children ≥12 and Adults:
Cl$_{cr}$ 11-31 mL/minute, hemodialysis, or hepatic impairment: 5 mg once daily
Cl$_{cr}$ <11 mL/minute, not on dialysis: Cetirizine use not recommended

Administration Oral: Administer without regard to food

Patient Information May cause drowsiness and impair ability to perform activities requiring mental alertness or physical coordination; may cause dry mouth. May cause photosensitivity reactions (eg, exposure to sunlight may cause severe sunburn, skin rash, redness, or itching); avoid exposure to sunlight and artificial light sources (sunlamps, tanning booth/bed); wear protective clothing, wide-brimmed hats, sunglasses, and lip sunscreen (SPF ≥15); use a sunscreen [broad-spectrum sunscreen or physical sunscreen (preferred) or sunblock with SPF ≥15]; contact physician if reaction occurs.

Dosage Forms Excipient information presented when available (limited, particularly for generics); consult specific product labeling. [DSC] = Discontinued product
Capsule, liquid gel, as hydrochloride:
Zyrtec® Allergy: 10 mg
Syrup, oral, as hydrochloride: 5 mg/5 mL (118 mL, 120 mL, 473 mL, 480 mL)
Zyrtec® Children's Allergy: 5 mg/5 mL (15 mL [DSC]; 118 mL) [contains propylene glycol; grape flavor]
Zyrtec® Children's Allergy: 5 mg/5 mL (118 mL) [dye free, sugar free; contains propylene glycol, sodium benzoate; bubblegum flavor]
Zyrtec® Children's Hives Relief: 5 mg/5 mL (118 mL) [contains propylene glycol; grape flavor]
Tablet, oral, as hydrochloride: 5 mg, 10 mg
All Day Allergy: 10 mg
Zyrtec® Allergy: 10 mg
Tablet, chewable, as hydrochloride: 5 mg, 10 mg
Zyrtec® Children's Allergy: 5 mg, 10 mg [grape flavor]

♦ **Cetirizine Hydrochloride** see Cetirizine on page 283

♦ **Cetraxal®** see Ciprofloxacin on page 310

♦ **CFDN** see Cefdinir on page 263

♦ **CG** see Chorionic Gonadotropin on page 305

♦ **C-Gel [OTC]** see Ascorbic Acid on page 138

♦ **CGP-57148B** see Imatinib on page 710

♦ **C-Gram [OTC]** see Ascorbic Acid on page 138

♦ **Charcadole® (Can)** see Charcoal, Activated on page 284

♦ **Charcadole®, Aqueous (Can)** see Charcoal, Activated on page 284

♦ **Charcadole® TFS (Can)** see Charcoal, Activated on page 284

♦ **Char-Caps [OTC]** see Charcoal, Activated on page 284

Charcoal, Activated (CHAR kole AK tiv ay ted)

Medication Safety Issues
Sound-alike/look-alike issues:
Actidose® may be confused with Actos®

U.S. Brand Names Actidose-Aqua® [OTC]; Actidose® with Sorbitol [OTC]; Char-Caps [OTC]; Charcoal Plus® DS [OTC]; CharcoCaps® [OTC]; EZ-Char™ [OTC]; Kerr Insta-Char® [OTC]; Requa® Activated Charcoal [OTC]

Canadian Brand Names Charcadole®; Charcadole® TFS; Charcadole®, Aqueous

Therapeutic Category Antidiarrheal; Antidote; Adsorbent; Antiflatulent

Generic Available Yes: Powder

Use Emergency treatment in poisoning by drugs and chemicals (see Additional Information) (FDA approved in all ages); repetitive doses for GI dialysis in drug overdose to enhance the elimination of certain drugs (eg, theophylline, phenobarbital, carbamazepine, dapsone, quinine) (FDA approved in all ages); has also been used in uremia to adsorb various waste products; dietary supplement (digestive aid)

Pregnancy Risk Factor C

Lactation Does not enter breast milk/compatible

Contraindications Patients with an unprotected airway (eg, depressed CNS state without endotracheal intubation); patients at increased risk and severity of aspiration (eg, ingestion of hydrocarbon with a high potential for aspiration); patients at risk of GI perforation or hemorrhage due to medical conditions, recent surgery, or other pathology; **Note**: Ingestion of a corrosive (caustic) substance is **not** a contraindication if charcoal is used for coingested systemic toxin. Charcoal is not effective for cyanide, mineral acids, caustic alkalis, organic solvents, iron, ethanol, methanol, or lithium poisonings; do not use charcoal with sorbitol in patients with fructose intolerance; charcoal with sorbitol is not recommended in children <1 year of age

Warnings If charcoal in sorbitol is administered, doses should be limited to prevent excessive fluid and electrolyte losses. Some suspensions (eg, Kerr Insta-Char®) contain sodium benzoate; benzoic acid (benzoate) is a metabolite of benzyl alcohol; large amounts of benzyl alcohol (≥99 mg/kg/day) have been associated with a potentially fatal toxicity ("gasping syndrome") in neonates; the "gasping syndrome" consists of metabolic acidosis, respiratory distress, gasping respirations, CNS dysfunction (including convulsions, intracranial hemorrhage), hypotension, and cardiovascular collapse; use activated charcoal products containing sodium benzoate with caution in neonates; *in vitro* and animal studies have shown that benzoate displaces bilirubin from protein binding sites.

Precautions When using ipecac with charcoal, induce vomiting with ipecac before administering activated charcoal since charcoal adsorbs ipecac syrup; charcoal may cause vomiting which is hazardous in petroleum distillate and caustic ingestions; charcoal (especially in multiple doses) may adsorb maintenance medications and place the patient at risk for exacerbation of concomitant disorders

Adverse Reactions
Endocrine & metabolic: Excessive amounts of activated charcoal with sorbitol may cause hypernatremic dehydration in pediatric patients
Gastrointestinal: Vomiting (**Note:** Use of charcoal with sorbitol may increase rate of emesis), constipation, intestinal obstruction, black stools; diarrhea if product contains sorbitol
Ocular: Corneal abrasions if spilled into eyes
Miscellaneous: Aspiration may cause tracheal obstruction in infants, but usually not a major problem in adults; aspiration pneumonitis, bronchiolitis obliterans, and ARDS have been reported following aspiration of charcoal; however, these problems may be due to the aspiration of gastric contents and not charcoal per se

Drug Interactions
Avoid Concomitant Use There are no known interactions where it is recommended to avoid concomitant use.
Increased Effect/Toxicity There are no known significant interactions involving an increase in effect.

Decreased Effect

Charcoal, Activated may decrease the levels/effects of:
Leflunomide

Food Interactions Certain flavoring agents (eg, milk, ice cream, sherbet, marmalade) reduce the adsorptive capacity of activated charcoal and should be avoided (use of activated charcoal-water slurries is preferred). **Note:** These flavoring agents do not completely compromise the effectiveness of activated charcoal and may be required in select cases to enhance compliance; some experts recommend increasing the dose of activated charcoal if using with ice cream or sherbet (see Cooney, 1995; Dagnone, 2002). Chocolate or fruit syrup do not appear to reduce efficacy.

Stability Adsorbs gases from air; store in closed container

Mechanism of Action Adsorbs toxic substances or irritants, thus inhibiting GI absorption; for select drugs, increases drug clearance by interfering with enterohepatic recycling or causing dialysis across intestinal membrane; adsorbs intestinal gas; the addition of sorbitol results in hyperosmotic laxative action causing catharsis

Pharmacodynamics In studies using adult human volunteers: Mean **reduction** in drug absorption following a single dose of activated charcoal:

All size doses of activated charcoal:
Given within 30 minutes after ingestion: 69.1% reduction
Given at 60 minutes after ingestion: 34.4% reduction
50 g activated charcoal:
Given within 30 minutes after ingestion: 88.6% reduction
Given at 60 minutes after ingestion: 37.3% reduction

Pharmacokinetics (Adult data unless noted)

Absorption: Not absorbed from the GI tract
Metabolism: Not metabolized
Elimination: Excreted as charcoal in feces

Usual Dosage Oral:

Acute poisoning:
Single dose: Charcoal with sorbitol (**Note:** The use of repeated oral charcoal with sorbitol doses is not recommended):
Infants <1 year: Not recommended
Children 1-12 years: 1-2 g/kg or 25-50 g or approximately 5-10 times the weight of the ingested poison on a gram-to-gram basis; 1 g adsorbs 100-1000 mg of poison; in young children sorbitol should be repeated **no more** than 1-2 times/day
Adolescents and Adults: 30-100 g
Single dose: Charcoal in water (a cathartic such as sorbitol should be added in appropriate doses):
Infants <1 year: 1 g/kg
Children 1-12 years: 1-2 g/kg or 25-50 g
Adolescents and Adults: 30-100 g or 1-2 g/kg
Multiple dose: Charcoal in water (doses are repeated until clinical observations of toxicity subside and serum drug concentrations have returned to a subtherapeutic range or until the development of absent bowel sounds or ileus; use only one dose of cathartic daily):
Infants <1 year: 1 g/kg every 4-6 hours
Children 1-12 years: 1-2 g/kg or 15-30 g every 2-6 hours
Adolescents and Adults: 25-60 g or 1-2 g/kg every 2-6 hours
Gastric dialysis: Adults: 20-50 g every 6 hours for 1-2 days

Administration Oral: Administer as soon as possible after ingestion, preferably within 1 hour for greatest effect. Shake well before use; do not mix with milk, ice cream, sherbet, or marmalade (see Food Interactions); may be mixed with chocolate or fruit syrup to increase palatability. Instruct patient to drink slowly, rapid administration may increase frequency of vomiting; if patient has persistent vomiting, multiple doses may be administered as a continuous enteral infusion

Monitoring Parameters Fluid status, sorbitol intake, number of stools, electrolytes if increase in stools or diarrhea occurs; continually assess for active bowel sounds in patients receiving multiple dose activated charcoal

Patient Information Charcoal causes the stools to turn black

Nursing Implications Charcoal slurries that are too concentrated may clog airways, if aspirated

Additional Information 5-6 tablespoonfuls of activated charcoal powder is approximately equal to 30 g; minimum dilution of 240 mL water per 20-30 g activated charcoal should be mixed as an aqueous slurry; multiple dose activated charcoal has been shown to be effective in increasing the elimination of certain drugs (carbamazepine, theophylline, phenobarbital) even after these drugs have been absorbed

The Position Paper on single dose activated charcoal by The American Academy of Clinical Toxicology and The European Association of Poisons Centres and Clinical Toxicologists (see Chyka, 2005) does not advocate **routine** use of single dose activated charcoal in the treatment of poisoned patients. Scientific literature supports the use of activated charcoal within 1 hour of toxin ingestion, when it will be more likely to produce benefit. Studies in volunteers demonstrate that the effectiveness of activated charcoal decreases as the time of administration after toxin ingestion increases. Therefore, this publication states that activated charcoal may be considered up to 1 hour following ingestion of a potentially toxic amount of poison. In addition, the use of activated charcoal may be considered greater than 1 hour following ingestion, since the potential benefit cannot be excluded. Furthermore, based on current literature, the routine administration of a cathartic with activated charcoal is not recommended; when cathartics are used, only a single dose should be administered so as to decrease adverse effects (see Position Paper: Cathartics, 2004).

A policy statement by the American Academy of Pediatrics states that it is currently premature to recommend the **routine** administration of activated charcoal as a home treatment strategy for poisonings (see AAP, 2003).

Dosage Forms Excipient information presented when available (limited, particularly for generics); consult specific product labeling.

Capsule:
Char-Caps, CharcoCaps®: 260 mg
Pellets, for suspension:
EZ-Char™: 25 g
Powder for suspension, oral: USP: 100% (30 g, 240 g)
Suspension:
Actidose-Aqua®: 15 g (72 mL); 25 g (120 mL); 50 g (240 mL)
Kerr Insta-Char®: 25 g (120 mL) [contains sodium benzoate; packaged with cherry flavor (cherry flavor contains propylene glycol and sodium benzoate)]; 50 g (240 mL) [contains sodium benzoate; unflavored or packaged with cherry flavor (cherry flavor contains propylene glycol and sodium benzoate)]
Suspension [with sorbitol]:
Actidose® with Sorbitol: 25 g (120 mL); 50 g (240 mL)
Kerr Insta-Char®: 25 g (120 mL) [contains sodium benzoate; packaged with cherry flavor (cherry flavor contains propylene glycol and sodium benzoate)]; 50 g (240 mL) [contains sodium benzoate; packaged with cherry flavor (cherry flavor contains propylene glycol and sodium benzoate)]
Tablet:
Requa® Activated Charcoal: 250 mg
Tablet, enteric coated:
Charcoal Plus® DS: 250 mg

References

American Academy of Pediatrics Committee on Injury, Violence, and Poison Prevention, "Poison Treatment in the Home," *Pediatrics*, 2003, 112(5):1182-5.

Burns MM, "Activated Charcoal as the Sole Intervention for Treatment After Childhood Poisoning," *Curr Opin Pediatr*, 2000, 12(2):166-71.

Chyka PA, Seger D, Krenzelok EP, et al, "Position Paper: Single-Dose Activated Charcoal," *Clin Toxicol (Phila)*, 2005, 43(2):61-87.

Cooney DO, *Development of Palatable Formulations, Activated Charcoal in Medical Applications*, Cooney DO, ed, New York, NY: Marcel Dekker, Inc, 1995, 397-417.

Dagnone D, Matsui D, and Rieder MJ, "Assessment of the Palatability of Vehicles for Activated Charcoal in Pediatric Volunteers," *Pediatr Emerg Care*, 2002, 18(1):19-21.

Farley TA, "Severe Hypernatremic Dehydration After Use of an Activated Charcoal-Sorbitol Suspension," *J Pediatr*, 1986, 109 (4):719-22.

"Position Statement and Practice Guidelines on the Use of Multi-dose Activated Charcoal in the Treatment of Acute Poisoning," American Academy of Clinical Toxicology; European Association of Poisons Centres and Clinical Toxicologists," *J Toxicol Clin Toxicol*, 1999, 37 (6):731-51.

"Position Paper: Cathartics," *J Toxicol Clin Toxicol*, 2004, 42(3):243-53.

Shannon M, "Ingestion of Toxic Substances by Children," *N Engl J Med*, 2000, 342(3):186-91.

◆ **Charcoal Plus® DS [OTC]** *see* Charcoal, Activated *on page 284*

◆ **CharcoCaps® [OTC]** *see* Charcoal, Activated *on page 284*

◆ **Chemet®** *see* Succimer *on page 1294*

◆ **Cheracol® [DSC]** *see* Guaifenesin and Codeine *on page 657*

◆ **Cheracol® D [OTC]** *see* Guaifenesin and Dextromethorphan *on page 658*

◆ **Cheracol® Plus [OTC]** *see* Guaifenesin and Dextromethorphan *on page 658*

◆ **Chew-C [OTC]** *see* Ascorbic Acid *on page 138*

◆ **CHG** *see* Chlorhexidine Gluconate *on page 291*

◆ **Chickenpox Vaccine** *see* Varicella Virus Vaccine *on page 1407*

◆ **Chiggerex® [OTC]** *see* Benzocaine *on page 182*

◆ **Chiggerex® Plus** *see* Benzocaine *on page 182*

◆ **Chiggertox® [OTC]** *see* Benzocaine *on page 182*

◆ **Children's Advil® Cold (Can)** *see* Pseudoephedrine and Ibuprofen *on page 1184*

◆ **Children's Pepto [OTC]** *see* Calcium Carbonate *on page 232*

◆ **Children's Pepto [OTC]** *see* Calcium Supplements *on page 239*

◆ **Children's Motion Sickness Liquid (Can)** *see* Dimenhy-DRINATE *on page 446*

◆ **ChiRhoStim®** *see* Secretin *on page 1251*

◆ **Chloral** *see* Chloral Hydrate *on page 286*

Chloral Hydrate (KLOR al HYE drate)

Medication Safety Issues

High alert medication: The Institute for Safe Medication Practices (ISMP) includes this medication among its list of drugs which have a heightened risk of causing significant patient harm when used in error.

Related Information

Preprocedure Sedatives in Children *on page 1688*

U.S. Brand Names Aquachloral® Supprettes® [DSC]; Somnote®

Canadian Brand Names PMS-Chloral Hydrate

Therapeutic Category Hypnotic; Sedative

Generic Available Yes: Syrup and suppositories

Use Short-term sedative and hypnotic (<2 weeks), sedative/hypnotic prior to nonpainful therapeutic or diagnostic procedures (eg, EEG, CT scan, MRI, ophthalmic exam, dental procedure)

Restrictions C-IV

Pregnancy Risk Factor C

Lactation Enters breast milk/compatible

Contraindications Hypersensitivity to chloral hydrate or any component (see Warnings); hepatic or renal impairment; severe cardiac disease. Oral forms are also contraindicated in patients with gastritis, esophagitis, or gastric or duodenal ulcers.

Warnings Deaths and permanent neurologic injury from respiratory compromise have been reported in children sedated with chloral hydrate; respiratory obstruction may occur in children with tonsillar and adenoidal hypertrophy, obstructive sleep apnea, and Leigh's encephalopathy, and in ASA class III children; depressed levels of consciousness may occur; chloral hydrate should **not** be administered for sedation by nonmedical personnel or in a nonsupervised medical environment; sedation with chloral hydrate requires careful patient monitoring (see Monitoring Parameters) (Cote, 2000); animal studies suggest that chloral hydrate may depress the genioglossus muscle and other airway-maintaining muscles in patients who are already at risk for life-threatening airway obstruction (eg, obstructive sleep apnea); alternative sedative agents should be considered for these patients (see Hershenson, 1984).

Trichloroethanol (TCE), an active metabolite of chloral hydrate, is a carcinogen in mice; there is no data in humans. The 325 mg suppositories contain tartrazine which may cause allergic reactions in susceptible individuals. Syrup may contain sodium benzoate; benzoic acid (benzoate) is a metabolite of benzyl alcohol; large amounts of benzyl alcohol (≥99 mg/kg/day) have been associated with a potentially fatal toxicity ("gasping syndrome") in neonates; the "gasping syndrome" consists of metabolic acidosis, respiratory distress, gasping respirations, CNS dysfunction (including convulsions, intracranial hemorrhage), hypotension and cardiovascular collapse; use chloral hydrate products containing sodium benzoate with caution in neonates; *in vitro* and animal studies have shown that benzoate displaces bilirubin from protein binding sites

Precautions Use with caution in neonates, drug and metabolites may accumulate with repeated use; prolonged use in neonates is associated with direct hyperbilirubinemia [active metabolite (TCE) competes with bilirubin for glucuronide conjugation in the liver]; use with caution in patients with porphyria. Tolerance to hypnotic effect develops, therefore, not recommended for use >2 weeks; taper dosage to avoid withdrawal with prolonged use. Avoid use in patients with moderate to severe renal failure (Cl$_{cr}$ <50 mL/minute).

Adverse Reactions

Central nervous system: Disorientation, sedation, excitement (paradoxical), dizziness, fever, headache, ataxia

Dermatologic: Rash, urticaria

Gastrointestinal: Gastric irritation, nausea, vomiting, diarrhea, flatulence

Hematologic: Leukopenia, eosinophilia

Respiratory: Respiratory depression when combined with other sedatives or narcotics

Miscellaneous: Physical and psychological dependence with prolonged use

Drug Interactions

Avoid Concomitant Use There are no known interactions where it is recommended to avoid concomitant use.

Increased Effect/Toxicity
Chloral Hydrate may increase the levels/effects of: Alcohol (Ethyl); CNS Depressants; Methotrimeprazine

The levels/effects of Chloral Hydrate may be increased by: Methotrimeprazine

Decreased Effect
The levels/effects of Chloral Hydrate may be decreased by: Flumazenil

Stability Sensitive to light; exposure to air causes volatilization; store in light-resistant, airtight container at room temperature; do not refrigerate

Mechanism of Action Central nervous system depressant effects are primarily due to its active metabolite trichloroethanol, mechanism unknown; in neonates, chloral hydrate itself may play a role in the immediate sedative effects; **Note:** Chloral hydrate does not interfere with EEG results (unlike barbiturates and benzodiazepines)

Pharmacodynamics
Onset of action: 10-20 minutes
Maximum effect: Within 30-60 minutes
Duration: 4-8 hours

Pharmacokinetics (Adult data unless noted)
Absorption: Oral, rectal: Well absorbed

Distribution: Crosses the placenta; distributes to breast milk

Protein binding: Trichloroethanol: 35% to 40%; trichloroacetic acid: ~94% (may compete with bilirubin for albumin binding sites)

Metabolism: Rapidly metabolized by alcohol dehydrogenase to trichloroethanol (active metabolite); trichloroethanol undergoes glucuronidation in the liver; variable amounts of chloral hydrate and trichloroethanol are metabolized in liver and kidney to trichloroacetic acid (inactive)

Half-life:

Chloral hydrate: Infants: 1 hour

Trichloroethanol (active metabolite):

Neonates: Range: 8.5-66 hours

Half-life decreases with increasing postconceptional age (PCA):

Preterm infants (PCA 31-37 weeks): Mean half-life: 40 hours

Term infants (PCA 38-42 weeks): Mean half-life: 28 hours

Older children (PCA 57-708 weeks): Mean half-life: 10 hours

Adults: 8-11 hours

Trichloroacetic acid: Adults: 67.2 hours

Elimination: Metabolites excreted in urine; small amounts excreted in feces via bile

Dialysis: Dialyzable (50% to 100%)

Usual Dosage Oral, rectal:

Neonates: 25 mg/kg/dose for sedation prior to a procedure; **Note:** Repeat doses should be used with great caution, as drug and metabolites accumulate with repeated use; toxicity has been reported after 3 days in a preterm neonate and after 7 days in a term neonate receiving chloral hydrate 40-50 mg/kg every 6 hours

Infants and Children:

Sedation, anxiety: 25-50 mg/kg/day divided every 6-8 hours, maximum dose: 500 mg/dose

Prior to EEG: 25-50 mg/kg/dose 30-60 minutes prior to EEG; may repeat in 30 minutes to a total maximum of 100 mg/kg or 1 g total for infants and 2 g total for children

Sedation, nonpainful procedure: 50-75 mg/kg/dose 30-60 minutes prior to procedure; may repeat 30 minutes after initial dose if needed, to a total maximum dose of 120 mg/kg or 1 g total for infants and 2 g total for children

Hypnotic: 50 mg/kg/dose at bedtime; maximum dose: 1 g/dose; total maximum: 1 g/day for infants and 2 g/day for children

Adults:

Sedation, anxiety: 250 mg 3 times/day

Hypnotic: 500-1000 mg at bedtime or 30 minutes prior to procedure, not to exceed 2 g/24 hours

Dosing adjustment in renal impairment:
$Cl_{cr} \geq 50$ mL/minute: No dosage adjustment needed
$Cl_{cr} < 50$ mL/minute: Avoid use

Administration Oral: Minimize unpleasant taste and gastric irritation by administering with water, infant formula, fruit juice, or ginger ale; do not crush capsule, contains drug in liquid form with unpleasant taste

Monitoring Parameters Level of sedation; vital signs and O_2 saturation with doses used for sedation prior to procedure

Test Interactions False-positive urine glucose using Clinitest® method; may interfere with fluorometric urine catecholamine and urinary 17-hydroxycorticosteroid tests

Patient Information May cause drowsiness and impair ability to perform activities requiring mental alertness or physical coordination; avoid alcohol and other CNS depressants; may be habit-forming; avoid abrupt discontinuation after prolonged use

Nursing Implications May cause irritation of skin and mucous membranes

Additional Information Not an analgesic; osmolality of 500 mg/5 mL syrup is approximately 3500 mOsm/kg

Dosage Forms Excipient information presented when available (limited, particularly for generics); consult specific product labeling. [DSC] = Discontinued product

Capsule:

Somnote®: 500 mg

Suppository, rectal: 500 mg

Aquachloral® Supprettes®: 325 mg [contains tartrazine] [DSC]

Syrup: 500 mg/5 mL (5 mL, 480 mL)

References
American Academy of Pediatrics, Committee on Drugs and Committee on Environmental Health, "Use of Chloral Hydrate for Sedation in Children," *Pediatrics*, 1993, 92(3):471-3.

Buck ML, "Chloral Hydrate Use During Infancy," *Neonatal Pharmacology Quarterly*, 1992, 1(1):31-7.

Cote CJ, Karl HW, Notterman DA, et al, "Adverse Sedation Events in Pediatrics: Analysis of Medications Used for Sedation," *Pediatrics*, 2000, 106(4):633-44.

Hershenson M, Brouillette RT, Olsen E, et al, "The Effect of Chloral Hydrate on Genioglossus and Diaphragmatic Activity," *Pediatr Res*, 1984, 18(6):516-9.

Mayers DJ, Hindmarsh KW, Gorecki DK, et al, "Sedative/Hypnotic Effects of Chloral Hydrate in the Neonate: Trichloroethanol or Parent Drug?" *Dev Pharmacol Ther*, 1992, 19(2-3):141-6.

Mayers DJ, Hindmarsh KW, Sankaran K, et al, "Chloral Hydrate Disposition Following Single-Dose Administration to Critically Ill Neonates and Children," *Dev Pharmacol Ther*, 1991, 16(2):71-7.

Steinberg AD, "Should Chloral Hydrate be Banned?" *Pediatrics*, 1993, 92(3)442-6.

Chlorambucil (klor AM byoo sil)

Medication Safety Issues
Sound-alike/look-alike issues:

Chlorambucil may be confused with Chloromycetin®

Leukeran® may be confused with Alkeran®, leucovorin, Leukine®, Myleran®

High alert medication: The Institute for Safe Medication Practices (ISMP) includes this medication among its list of drugs which have a heightened risk of causing significant patient harm when used in error.

Related Information
Emetogenic Potential of Antineoplastic Agents *on page 1579*

U.S. Brand Names Leukeran®

◀ **Canadian Brand Names** Leukeran®

Therapeutic Category Antineoplastic Agent, Alkylating Agent (Nitrogen Mustard)

Generic Available No

Use Treatment of chronic lymphocytic leukemia (CLL), Hodgkin's and non-Hodgkin's lymphoma (FDA approved in adults); has also been used in the treatment of nephrotic syndrome (unresponsive to conventional therapy) and Waldenström's macroglobulinemia

Pregnancy Risk Factor D

Pregnancy Considerations Animal studies have demonstrated teratogenicity. Chlorambucil crosses the human placenta. Following exposure during the first trimester, case reports have noted adverse renal effects (unilateral agenesis). There are no adequate and well-controlled studies in pregnant women. Women of childbearing potential should avoid becoming pregnant while receiving treatment. **[U.S. Boxed Warning]: Affects human fertility; probably mutagenic and teratogenic as well**; chromosomal damage has been documented. Fertility effects (reversible and irreversible sterility) include azoospermia (when administered to prepubertal and pubertal males) and amenorrhea.

Lactation Excretion in breast milk unknown/not recommended

Breast-Feeding Considerations Due to the potential for serious adverse reactions in the nursing infant, breast-feeding is not recommended.

Contraindications Hypersensitivity to chlorambucil or any component; cross hypersensitivity (skin rash) may occur with other alkylating agents; previous resistance

Warnings Hazardous agent; use appropriate precautions for handling and disposal. Chlorambucil can severely suppress bone marrow function **[U.S. Boxed Warning]**; lymphopenia and neutropenia can develop during therapy; adversely affects human fertility **[U.S. Boxed Warning]**; both reversible and permanent sterility have been observed in males and females; possibly mutagenic and teratogenic **[U.S. Boxed Warning]**; carcinogenic in humans **[U.S. Boxed Warning]**; there are reports of acute leukemia following chlorambucil therapy; chromosomal damage has been documented; secondary AML may be associated with chronic therapy and large cumulative doses. Convulsions and severe skin reactions (eg, erythema multiforme, Stevens-Johnson syndrome and toxic epidermal necrolysis) have been reported.

Precautions Use with caution in patients with seizure disorder, head trauma, patients receiving epileptogenic drugs, and in patients with bone marrow suppression; avoid administration of live vaccines to immunocompromised patients; children with nephrotic syndrome may have an increased risk of seizures; reduce initial dosage if patient has received radiation therapy, myelosuppressive drugs, or has a depressed baseline leukocyte or platelet count within the previous 4 weeks. Chlorambucil dose should not exceed 0.1 mg/kg/day if bone marrow is hypoplastic.

Adverse Reactions

Central nervous system: Agitation, ataxia, confusion, fatigue, fever, hallucinations, hyperactivity, irritability, seizures (rare)

Dermatologic: Angioneurotic edema, erythema multiforme, pruritus, rash, Stevens-Johnson syndrome, toxic epidermal necrolysis, urticaria

Endocrine & metabolic: Amenorrhea, hyperuricemia, infertility, menstrual cramps

Gastrointestinal: Abdominal pain, anorexia, diarrhea, nausea, stomatitis, vomiting

Genitourinary: Azoospermia, cystitis, oligospermia

Hematologic: Anemia, leukopenia, lymphocytopenia, neutropenia (risk of irreversible bone marrow damage occurs as total chlorambucil dose approaches 6.5 mg/kg), pancytopenia, thrombocytopenia

Hepatic: AST increased, hepatotoxicity, jaundice

Neuromuscular & skeletal: Muscular twitching, myoclonia, peripheral neuropathy, tremor, weakness

Respiratory: Interstitial pneumonia, pulmonary fibrosis

Miscellaneous: Secondary malignancies

Drug Interactions

Avoid Concomitant Use

Avoid concomitant use of Chlorambucil with any of the following: BCG; Natalizumab; Pimecrolimus; Tacrolimus (Topical); Vaccines (Live)

Increased Effect/Toxicity

Chlorambucil may increase the levels/effects of: Leflunomide; Natalizumab; Vaccines (Live)

The levels/effects of Chlorambucil may be increased by: Denosumab; Pimecrolimus; Tacrolimus (Topical); Trastuzumab

Decreased Effect

Chlorambucil may decrease the levels/effects of: BCG; Sipuleucel-T; Vaccines (Inactivated); Vaccines (Live)

The levels/effects of Chlorambucil may be decreased by: Echinacea

Food Interactions Avoid acidic foods, hot foods, and spices; delayed absorption when administered with food

Stability Store in refrigerator; protect from light

Mechanism of Action Interferes with DNA replication and RNA transcription by alkylation and cross-linking the strands of DNA; immunosuppressive activity due to suppression of lymphocytes

Pharmacokinetics (Adult data unless noted)

Absorption: Oral: Rapid and almost completely absorbed from GI tract

Distribution: To liver, ascitic fluid, fat; extensively bound to plasma and tissue proteins; crosses the placenta

Protein binding: ~99%

Metabolism: In the liver to an active metabolite, phenylacetic acid mustard

Bioavailability: 56% to 100%

Half-life: Chlorambucil: 1.5 hours; phenylacetic acid mustard: 2.5 hours

Time to peak serum concentration: Chlorambucil: Within 1 hour; phenylacetic acid mustard: Within 2-4 hours

Elimination: 60% excreted in urine within 24 hours principally as metabolites; <1% excreted as unchanged drug or phenylacetic acid mustard in urine

Dialysis: Probably not dialyzable

Usual Dosage Oral (refer to individual protocols):

Children:

General short courses: 0.1-0.2 mg/kg/day or 4.5 mg/m^2/day once daily for 3-6 weeks for remission induction (usual: 4-10 mg/day); maintenance therapy: 0.03-0.1 mg/kg/day (usual: 2-4 mg/day)

Relapsing steroid-sensitive nephrotic syndrome: 0.2 mg/kg/day once daily for 8 weeks

CLL:

Biweekly regimen: Initial: 0.4 mg/kg/dose every 2 weeks; increase dose by 0.1 mg/kg every 2 weeks until a response occurs and/or myelosuppression occurs

Monthly regimen: Initial: 0.4 mg/kg every 4 weeks, increase dose by 0.2 mg/kg every 4 weeks until a response occurs and/or myelosuppression occurs

Malignant lymphomas:

Non-Hodgkin's lymphoma: 0.1 mg/kg/day

Hodgkin's: 0.2 mg/kg/day

Adults: 0.1-0.2 mg/kg/day or 3-6 mg/m^2/day once daily for 3-6 weeks, then adjust dose on basis of blood counts

Administration Oral: Administer 30-60 minutes before food; do not administer with acidic foods, hot foods, and spices

Monitoring Parameters Liver function tests, CBC with differential, hemoglobin, leukocyte and platelet counts, serum uric acid

Patient Information Notify physician if fever, sore throat, persistent cough, nausea, vomiting, jaundice, skin rash, seizures, amenorrhea, unusual lumps/masses, or bleeding occurs; discontinue chlorambucil if skin reaction occurs. Women of childbearing potential should avoid becoming pregnant while on chlorambucil. Avoid acidic foods, hot foods, and spices.

Additional Information Myelosuppressive effects:
WBC: Moderate
Platelets: Moderate
Onset (days): 7
Nadir (days): 14-21

Dosage Forms Excipient information presented when available (limited, particularly for generics); consult specific product labeling.
Tablet:
Leukeran®: 2 mg

Extemporaneous Preparations A 2 mg/mL suspension was stable for 7 days when refrigerated and compounded as follows: Pulverize sixty 2 mg tablets; levigate with a small amount of glycerin; add 20 mL Cologel® [DSC] and levigate until a uniform mixture is obtained; add a 2:1 simple syrup/cherry syrup mixture to make a total volume of 60 mL; label "refrigerate" and "shake well before use"
Dressman JB and Poust RI, "Stability of Allopurinol and of Five Antineoplastics in Suspension," *Am J Hosp Pharm*, 1983, 40(4):616-8.

References
Baluarte HJ, Hiner L, and Gruskin AB, "Chlorambucil Dosage in Frequently Relapsing Nephrotic Syndrome: A Controlled Clinical Trial," *J Pediatr*, 1978, 92(2):295-8.
Durkan A, Hodson EM, Willis NS, et al, "Non-corticosteroid Treatment for Nephrotic Syndrome in Children," *Cochrane Database Syst Rev*, 2005, 18(2):CD002290.
Singh BN and Malhotra BK, "Effects of Food on the Clinical Pharmacokinetics of Anticancer Agents: Underlying Mechanisms and Implications for Oral Chemotherapy," *Clin Pharmacokinet*, 2004, 43(15):1127-56.
Williams SA, Makker SP, and Grupe WE, "Seizures: A Significant Side Effect of Chlorambucil Therapy in Children," *J Pediatr*, 1978, 93(3):516-8.

◆ **Chlorambucilum** see Chlorambucil *on page 287*

◆ **Chloraminophene** see Chlorambucil *on page 287*

Chloramphenicol (klor am FEN i kole)

Medication Safety Issues
Sound-alike/look-alike issues:
Chloromycetin® may be confused with chlorambucil, Chlor-Trimeton®

Related Information
Therapeutic Drug Monitoring: Blood Sampling Time Guidelines *on page 1704*

Canadian Brand Names Chloromycetin®; Chloromycetin® Succinate; Diochloram®; Pentamycetin®

Therapeutic Category Antibiotic, Miscellaneous

Generic Available Yes

Use Treatment of serious infections due to organisms resistant to other less toxic antibiotics or when its penetrability into the site of infection is clinically superior to other antibiotics to which the organism is sensitive; useful in infections caused by *Bacteroides*, *H. influenzae*, *Neisseria meningitidis*, *S. pneumoniae*, *Salmonella*, and *Rickettsia*; active against many vancomycin-resistant enterococci

Pregnancy Considerations Chloramphenicol crosses the placenta producing cord concentrations approaching maternal serum concentrations. An increased risk of teratogenic effects has not been identified for chloramphenicol and there have been no reports of fetal harm related to use of chloramphenicol in pregnancy. "Gray Syndrome" has occurred in premature infants and newborns receiving chloramphenicol. In most cases, chloramphenicol was started during the first 48 hours of life, but it has also occurred in older patients after high doses. Symptoms began after 3-4 days of therapy, starting with abdominal distention and continuing to progressive pallid cyanosis, vasomotor collapse, irregular respiration, and death within a few hours of symptom onset. Stopping therapy can reverse the process and allow complete recovery. There is one case report of an infant with gray baby syndrome after *in utero* exposure to a single maternal dose during labor, followed by a 10-fold overdose of chloramphenicol in the first day of life. The extent of the contribution of the single dose given during labor is unknown. The manufacturer recommends caution if used in a pregnant patient near term or during labor.

Lactation Enters breast milk/use with caution (AAP rates "of concern")

Breast-Feeding Considerations Chloramphenicol is excreted in human milk in both the active form and as inactive metabolites. Chloramphenicol is well absorbed following oral administration; however, metabolism and excretion are highly variable in infants and children. The half-life is also significantly prolonged in low birth weight infants. There have been documented toxicities in neonates and preterm infants when chloramphenicol has been used at therapeutic doses. The manufacturer recommends caution if using chloramphenicol in a breast-feeding infant. The AAP considers chloramphenicol to be a drug "for which the effect on nursing infants is unknown but may be of concern." Nondose-related effects could include modification of bowel flora.

Contraindications Hypersensitivity to chloramphenicol or any component; treatment of trivial or viral infections; bacterial prophylaxis

Warnings Serious and fatal blood dyscrasias (aplastic anemia, hypoplastic anemia, thrombocytopenia, and granulocytopenia) have occurred after both short-term and prolonged therapy **[U.S. Boxed Warning]**; monitor CBC with platelets frequently in all patients; **[U.S. Boxed Warning]** discontinue if evidence of myelosuppression. Irreversible bone marrow suppression may occur weeks or months after therapy. Avoid repeated courses of treatment. Should not be used when less potentially toxic agents are effective; prolonged use may result in superinfection, including *C. difficile*-associated diarrhea (CDAD) and pseudomembranous colitis; breast-feeding is not recommended

Precautions Use with caution in patients with G-6-PD deficiency, impaired renal or hepatic function; reduce dose in patients with hepatic and renal impairment. Use in neonates and premature infants has resulted in "gray baby syndrome" due to immature metabolic system leading to excessive blood levels (see Additional Information); use a reduced dose.

Adverse Reactions
Cardiovascular: Cardiotoxicity (left ventricular dysfunction)
Central nervous system: Confusion, delirium, depression, fever, headache, nightmares
Dermatologic: Angioedema, rash, urticaria
Gastrointestinal: Diarrhea, enterocolitis, glossitis, nausea, stomatitis, vomiting
Hematologic: Aplastic anemia, bone marrow suppression, granulocytopenia, hemolysis in patients with G-6-PD deficiency hypoplastic anemia, pancytopenia, thrombocytopenia (see Additional Information)
Hepatic: Hepatitis-pancytopenia syndrome

Neuromuscular & skeletal: Peripheral neuropathy

Ocular: Optic neuritis

Miscellaneous: Anaphylaxis, gray baby syndrome, hypersensitivity

Drug Interactions

Metabolism/Transport Effects Inhibits CYP2C9 (weak), 3A4 (weak)

Avoid Concomitant Use

Avoid concomitant use of Chloramphenicol with any of the following: BCG

Increased Effect/Toxicity

Chloramphenicol may increase the levels/effects of: Anticonvulsants (Hydantoin); Barbiturates; Sulfonylureas

Decreased Effect

Chloramphenicol may decrease the levels/effects of: BCG; Cyanocobalamin; Typhoid Vaccine

The levels/effects of Chloramphenicol may be decreased by: Anticonvulsants (Hydantoin); Barbiturates; Rifampin

Food Interactions May decrease intestinal absorption of vitamin B_{12} (cobalamin); may have increased dietary need for riboflavin, pyridoxine (vitamin B_6), and vitamin B_{12}

Stability Reconstituted parenteral solution (100 mg/mL) is stable for 30 days at room temperature; frozen solutions remain stable for 6 months

Mechanism of Action Reversibly binds to 50S ribosomal subunits of susceptible organisms preventing amino acids from being transferred to growing peptide chains thus inhibiting protein synthesis

Pharmacokinetics (Adult data unless noted)

Distribution: Readily crosses the placenta; appears in breast milk; distributes to most tissues and body fluids; good CSF and brain penetration

CSF concentration with uninflamed meninges: 21% to 50% of plasma concentration

CSF concentration with inflamed meninges: 45% to 89% of plasma concentration

V_d:

Chloramphenicol: 0.5-1 L/kg

Chloramphenicol succinate: 0.2-3.1 L/kg; decreased with hepatic or renal dysfunction

Protein binding: Chloramphenicol: 60% decreased with hepatic or renal dysfunction and 30% to 40% in newborn infants

Metabolism:

Chloramphenicol succinate: Hydrolized in the liver, kidney, and lungs to chloramphenicol (active)

Chloramphenicol: Hepatic to metabolites (inactive)

Bioavailability:

Chloramphenicol: Oral: ~80%

Chloramphenicol succinate: I.V.: ~70%; highly variable, dependant upon rate and extent of metabolism to chloramphenicol

Half-life:

Neonates:

1-2 days: 24 hours

10-16 days: 10 hours

Children: 4-6 hours

Adults:

Normal renal function: ~4 hours

Chloramphenicol succinate: ~3 hours

End-stage renal disease: 3-7 hours

Hepatic disease: Prolonged

Elimination: ~30% as unchanged chloramphenicol succinate in urine; in infants and young children, 6% to 80% of the dose may be excreted unchanged in urine; 5% to 15% as chloramphenicol

Dialysis: Slightly dialyzable (5% to 20%)

Usual Dosage I.V.:

Neonates: Initial loading dose: 20 mg/kg (the first maintenance dose should be given 12 hours after the loading dose)

Maintenance dose: Postnatal age:

≤7 days: 25 mg/kg/day once every 24 hours

>7 days, ≤2000 g: 25 mg/kg/day once every 24 hours

>7 days, >2000 g: 50 mg/kg/day divided every 12 hours

Infants and Children:

Meningitis: Maintenance dose: 75-100 mg/kg/day divided every 6 hours

Other infections: 50-75 mg/kg/day divided every 6 hours; maximum daily dose: 4 g/day

Adults: 50-100 mg/kg/day in divided doses every 6 hours; maximum daily dose: 4 g/day

Dosing adjustment in renal and/or hepatic impairment: Dose reduction should be based upon serum chloramphenicol concentrations

Administration Do not administer I.M. Can administer I.V. push over 5 minutes at a maximum concentration of 100 mg/mL, or I.V. intermittent infusion over 15-30 minutes at a final concentration for administration ≤20 mg/mL

Monitoring Parameters CBC with reticulocyte and platelet counts, hematocrit, serum iron level, iron-binding capacity, periodic liver and renal function tests, serum drug concentration

Reference Range

Meningitis:

Peak: 15-25 mcg/mL

Trough: 5-15 mcg/mL

Other infections:

Peak: 10-20 mcg/mL

Trough: 5-10 mcg/mL

Nursing Implications Draw peak levels 90 minutes after completion of I.V. dose; trough levels should be drawn just prior to the next dose

Additional Information Sodium content of 1 g injection: 2.25 mEq

Three major toxicities associated with chloramphenicol include:

Aplastic anemia, an idiosyncratic reaction which can occur with any route of administration; usually occurs 3 weeks to 12 months after initial exposure to chloramphenicol; incidence: 1 in 40,000 cases

Bone marrow suppression is thought to be dose-related with serum concentrations >25 mcg/mL and reversible once chloramphenicol is discontinued; anemia and neutropenia may occur during the first week of therapy

Gray baby syndrome is characterized by circulatory collapse, hypothermia, cyanosis, acidosis, abdominal distention, myocardial depression, coma, and death; reaction appears to be associated with serum levels ≥50 mcg/mL; may result from drug accumulation in patients with impaired hepatic or renal function; may occur after 3-4 days of therapy or within hours of initiating therapy

Dosage Forms Excipient information presented when available (limited, particularly for generics); consult specific product labeling.

Injection, powder for reconstitution: 1 g [contains sodium ~52 mg/g (2.25 mEq/g)]

References

Ambrose PJ, "Clinical Pharmacokinetics of Chloramphenicol and Chloramphenicol Succinate," Clin Pharmacokinet, 1984, 9(3):222-38.

Aronoff GR, Bennett WM, Berns JS, et al, Drug Prescribing in Renal Failure: Dosing Guidelines for Adults and Children, 5th ed. Philadelphia, PA: American College of Physicians, 2007.

Powell DA and Nahata MC, "Chloramphenicol: New Perspectives on an Old Drug," Drug Intell Clin Pharm, 1982, 16(4):295-300.

Vozeh S, Schmidlin O, and Taeschner W, "Pharmacokinetic Drug Data," Clin Pharmacokinet, 1988, 15(4):254-82.

◆ **ChloraPrep® [OTC]** see Chlorhexidine Gluconate on page 291

◆ **ChloraPrep® Frepp® [OTC]** see Chlorhexidine Gluconate on page 291

◆ **ChloraPrep® Sepp® [OTC]** see Chlorhexidine Gluconate on page 291

♦ **Chlorascrub™ [OTC]** *see* Chlorhexidine Gluconate *on page 291*

♦ **Chlorascrub™ Maxi [OTC]** *see* Chlorhexidine Gluconate *on page 291*

♦ **Chlorbutinum** *see* Chlorambucil *on page 287*

♦ **Chlorethazine** *see* Mechlorethamine *on page 868*

♦ **Chlorethazine Mustard** *see* Mechlorethamine *on page 868*

Chlorhexidine Gluconate
(klor HEKS i deen GLOO koe nate)

Medication Safety Issues
Sound-alike/look-alike issues:
Peridex® may be confused with Precedex™

U.S. Brand Names Avagard™ [OTC]; BactoShield® CHG [OTC]; Betasept® [OTC]; ChloraPrep® Frepp® [OTC]; ChloraPrep® Sepp® [OTC]; ChloraPrep® [OTC]; Chlorascrub™ Maxi [OTC]; Chlorascrub™ [OTC]; Dyna-Hex® [OTC]; Hibiclens® [OTC]; Hibistat® [OTC]; Operand® Chlorhexidine Gluconate [OTC]; Peridex®; PerioChip®; PerioGard®

Canadian Brand Names Hibidil® 1:2000; ORO-Clense; Peridex® Oral Rinse

Therapeutic Category Antibacterial, Topical; Antibiotic, Oral Rinse

Generic Available Yes: Oral liquid

Use Skin cleanser for surgical scrub; cleanser for skin wounds; germicidal hand rinse; antibacterial dental rinse to reduce plaque formation and control gingivitis; prophylactic dental rinse to prevent oral infections in immunocompromised patients, particularly bone marrow transplant patients receiving cytotoxic therapy; and short-term substitute for toothbrushing in situations where the patient is unable to tolerate mechanical stimulation of the gums

Pregnancy Risk Factor B

Contraindications Hypersensitivity to chlorhexidine gluconate or any component; do not use as a preoperative skin preparation of the face or head (except Hibiclens® liquid) as serious, permanent eye injury has occurred when chlorhexidine gluconate enters and remains in the eye during surgery.

Warnings For topical use only; there have been several case reports of anaphylaxis following disinfection with chlorhexidine; a case of bradycardic episodes after breast-feeding in a 2 day old infant whose mother used chlorhexidine gluconate topically on her breasts to prevent mastitis has been reported

Precautions Staining of oral surfaces, teeth, restorations, and dorsum of tongue may occur and may be visible as soon as 1 week after therapy begins; staining is more pronounced when there is a heavy accumulation of unremoved plaque and when teeth fillings have rough surfaces; stain does not have clinically adverse effect, but because removal may not be possible, patients with frontal restoration should be advised of the potential permanency of the stain; avoid contact with meninges; corneal injury has been associated with direct eye contact (see Contraindications); deafness has been associated with direct instillation into the middle ear through a perforated eardrum

Adverse Reactions
Dermatologic: Skin irritation
Gastrointestinal: Tongue irritation, minor irritation and superficial desquamation of oral mucosa (particularly among children), tartar on teeth increased, staining of oral surfaces (mucosa, teeth, and dorsum of tongue; see Warnings), dysgeusia, transient parotiditis; toothache (chip)
Ocular: Corneal damage (see Precautions)
Otic: Deafness (see Precautions)

Respiratory: Nasal congestion, shortness of breath
Miscellaneous: Edema of face, anaphylactoid reactions

Drug Interactions
Avoid Concomitant Use There are no known interactions where it is recommended to avoid concomitant use.

Increased Effect/Toxicity There are no known significant interactions involving an increase in effect.

Decreased Effect There are no known significant interactions involving a decrease in effect.

Stability Store away from heat and direct light; do not freeze

Mechanism of Action The bactericidal effect of chlorhexidine is a result of the binding of this cationic molecule to negatively charged bacterial cell walls and extramicrobial complexes. At low concentrations, this causes an alteration of bacterial cell osmotic equilibrium and leakage of potassium and phosphorous resulting in a bacteriostatic effect. At high concentrations of chlorhexidine, the cytoplasmic contents of the bacterial cell precipitate and result in cell death. Chlorhexidine is active against gram-positive and gram-negative organisms, facultative anaerobes, anaerobes, and yeast.

Pharmacokinetics (Adult data unless noted)
Absorption: ~30% of chlorhexidine is retained in the oral cavity following rinsing and is slowly released into the oral fluids; chlorhexidine is poorly absorbed from the GI tract and is not absorbed topically through intact skin
Serum concentrations: Detectable levels are not present in the plasma 12 hours after administration
Elimination: Primarily through the feces (~90%); <1% excreted in the urine

Usual Dosage
Oral rinse (Peridex® or PerioGard®) (see Administration):
Children and Adults: 15 mL twice daily
Immunocompromised patient: 10-15 mL, 2-3 times/day
Cleanser: Children and Adults: Apply 5 mL per scrub or hand wash; apply 25 mL per body wash or hair wash

Administration
Oral rinse: Precede use of solution by flossing and brushing teeth, completely rinse toothpaste from mouth; swish undiluted oral rinse around in mouth for 30 seconds, then expectorate; caution patient not to swallow the medicine; avoid eating for 2-3 hours after treatment.
Topical:
Surgical scrub: Scrub 3 minutes and rinse thoroughly, wash for an additional 3 minutes
Hand wash: Wash for 15 seconds and rinse
Hand rinse: Rub vigorously for 15 seconds
Body wash: Wet body and/or hair, apply, rinse thoroughly, repeat.

Monitoring Parameters Improvement in gingival inflammation and bleeding; development of teeth or denture discoloration; dental prophylaxis to remove stains at regular intervals of no greater than 6 months.

Test Interactions If chlorhexidine is used as a disinfectant before midstream urine collection, a false-positive urine protein may result (when using dipstick method based upon a pH indicator color change).

Patient Information
Oral rinse: Use after tooth brushing; do not swallow, do not rinse after use; may cause reduced taste perception which is reversible; may cause discoloration of teeth which may be removed with professional dental cleaning; notify dentist or physician if difficulty breathing or flushing or swelling of face occurs
Topical administration is for external use only; if accidentally enters eyes or ears, rinse out promptly and thoroughly with water

Dosage Forms Excipient information presented when available (limited, particularly for generics); consult specific product labeling.

Chip, for periodontal pocket insertion:
PerioChip®: 2.5 mg
Liquid, topical [surgical scrub]:
BactoShield® CHG: 2% (120 mL, 480 mL, 750 mL, 960 mL, 3840 mL); 4% (120 mL, 480 mL, 960 mL, 3840 mL) [contains isopropyl alcohol]
Betasept®: 4% (120 mL, 240 mL, 480 mL, 960 mL, 3840 mL) [contains isopropyl alcohol]
ChloraPrep®: 2% (0.67 mL, 1.5 mL, 3 mL, 10.5 mL, 26 mL) [contains isopropyl alcohol 70%; prefilled applicator]
Dyna-Hex®: 2% (120 mL, 480 mL, 960 mL, 3840 mL) [contains isopropyl alcohol]; 4% (120 mL, 480 mL, 960 mL, 3840 mL) [contains isopropyl alcohol]
Hibiclens®: 4% (15 mL, 120 mL, 240 mL, 480 mL, 960 mL, 3840 mL) [contains isopropyl alcohol]
Operand® Chlorhexidine Gluconate: 2% (120 mL); 4% (120 mL, 240 mL, 480 mL, 960 mL, 3840 mL) [contains isopropyl alcohol]
Liquid, oral [rinse]: 0.12% (480 mL)
Peridex®: 0.12% (120 mL, 480 mL, 1920 mL) [contains alcohol 11.6%; mint flavor]
PerioGard®: 0.12% (480 mL) [contains alcohol 11.6%; mint flavor]
Lotion, topical [surgical scrub]:
Avagard™: 1% (500 mL) [contains ethyl alcohol and moisturizers]
Sponge/Brush, topical:
BactoShield® CHG): 4% [contains isopropyl alcohol]
Sponge, topical [surgical scrub]:
ChloraPrep® 3 mL: 2% (25s) [contains isopropyl alcohol; available in clear or Hi-Lite Orange™]
ChloraPrep® 10.5 mL: 2% (25s) [contains isopropyl alcohol; available in clear, Hi-Lite Orange™, and Scrub Teal™]
ChloraPrep® 26 mL: 2% (25s) [contains isopropyl alcohol; available in clear, Hi-Lite Orange™, and Scrub Teal™]
ChloraPrep® Frepp® 1.5 mL: 2% (20s) [contains isopropyl alcohol]
ChloraPrep® Sepp® 0.67 mL: 2% (200s) [contains isopropyl alcohol]
Swab, topical [prep pad]:
Chlorascrub™: 3.15% (100s) [contains isopropyl alcohol]
Swabstick, topical [surgical scrub]:
ChloraPrep® 1.75 mL: 2% (48s) [contains isopropyl alcohol]
ChloraPrep® 5.25 mL: 2% (40s) [contains isopropyl alcohol]
Chlorascrub™ 1.6 mL: 3.15% (50s) [contains isopropyl alcohol]
Chlorascrub™ Maxi 5.1 mL: 3.15% (30s) [contains isopropyl alcohol]
Wipe, topical [towelette]:
Hibistat®: 0.5% (50s) [contains isopropyl alcohol]

References
Quinn MW and Bini RM, "Bradycardia Associated With Chlorhexidine Spray," *Arch Dis Child*, 1989, 64(6):892-3.
Yong D, Parker FC, and Foran SM, "Severe Allergic Reactions and Intra-Urethral Chlorhexidine Gluconate," *Med J Aust*, 1995, 162 (5):257-8.

◆ **Chlormeprazine** *see* Prochlorperazine *on page 1161*

◆ **2-Chlorodeoxyadenosine** *see* Cladribine *on page 323*

◆ **Chloromag®** *see* Magnesium Chloride *on page 853*

◆ **Chloromag®** *see* Magnesium Supplements *on page 859*

◆ **Chloromycetin® (Can)** *see* Chloramphenicol *on page 289*

◆ **Chloromycetin® Succinate (Can)** *see* Chloramphenicol *on page 289*

Chloroprocaine (klor oh PROE kane)

Medication Safety Issues
Sound-alike/look-alike issues:
Nesacaine® may be confused with Neptazane®

High alert medication: The Institute for Safe Medication Practices (ISMP) includes this medication (epidural administration) among its list of drug classes which have a heightened risk of causing significant patient harm when used in error.

U.S. Brand Names Nesacaine®; Nesacaine®-MPF
Canadian Brand Names Nesacaine®-CE
Therapeutic Category Local Anesthetic, Injectable
Generic Available Yes
Use Production of local or regional analgesia and anesthesia by local infiltration and peripheral nerve block techniques
Pregnancy Risk Factor C
Pregnancy Considerations Animal reproduction studies have not been conducted. Local anesthetics rapidly cross the placenta and may cause varying degrees of maternal, fetal, and neonatal toxicity. Close maternal and fetal monitoring (heart rate and electronic fetal monitoring advised) are required during obstetrical use. Maternal hypotension has resulted from regional anesthesia. Positioning the patient on her left side and elevating the legs may help. Epidural, paracervical, or pudendal anesthesia may alter the forces of parturition through changes in uterine contractility or maternal expulsive efforts. The use of some local anesthetic drugs during labor and delivery may diminish muscle strength and tone for the first day or two of life. Administration as a paracervical block is not recommended with toxemia of pregnancy, fetal distress, or prematurity. Administration of a paracervical block early in pregnancy has resulted in maternal seizures and cardiovascular collapse. Fetal bradycardia and acidosis also have been reported. Fetal depression has occurred following unintended fetal intracranial injection while administering a paracervical and/or pudendal block.

Lactation Excretion in breast milk unknown/use caution
Contraindications Hypersensitivity to chloroprocaine, PABA, any anesthetic of the ester type, or any component of the formulation; cerebrospinal diseases such as meningitis or syphilis, and septicemia (spinal anesthetic use)

Warnings Convulsions and cardiac arrhythmias resulting in cardiac arrest have been reported, presumably due to systemic toxicity following unintentional I.V. injection; should be administered in small incremental doses. Chloroprocaine solutions containing preservatives (methylparaben) are not to be used for lumbar or caudal anesthesia. When using for obstetrical anesthesia, 5% to 10% of cases where initial total doses of 120-400 mg were administered, have been associated with fetal bradycardia. Chondrolysis has been reported following continuous intra-articular infusion; intra-articular administration of local anesthetics is not an FDA-approved route of administration.

Precautions Use with extreme caution as lumbar or caudal anesthesia in patients with existing neurologic disease, spinal deformities, or severe hypertension; use with caution in patients with hypotension, cardiac disease, and hepatic or renal disease. Use caution in debilitated, elderly, or acutely-ill patients; dose reduction may be required.

Adverse Reactions Degree of adverse effects in the CNS and cardiovascular system is directly related to the blood level of procaine, route of administration, and physical status of the patient. The effects below are more likely to occur after systemic administration rather than infiltration.

Cardiovascular: Bradycardia, cardiac arrest, cardiac output decreased, heart block, hypertension, hypotension, myocardial depression, syncope, tachycardia, ventricular arrhythmias

Central nervous system: Anxiety, chills, depression, dizziness, excitation, fever, headache, restlessness, seizures, tremors

Dermatologic: Angioneurotic edema, erythema, pruritus, urticaria

Gastrointestinal: Fecal incontinence, nausea, vomiting

Genitourinary: Incontinence, urinary retention

Neuromuscular & skeletal: Chondrolysis (continuous intra-articular administration), paralysis, paresthesia, tremors, weakness

Ocular: Blurred vision, pupil constriction

Otic: Tinnitus

Respiratory: Apnea, hypoventilation, sneezing, laryngeal edema

Miscellaneous: Allergic reaction, anaphylactoid reaction, diaphoresis

Drug Interactions

Avoid Concomitant Use There are no known interactions where it is recommended to avoid concomitant use.

Increased Effect/Toxicity There are no known significant interactions involving an increase in effect.

Decreased Effect There are no known significant interactions involving a decrease in effect.

Stability Store at controlled room temperature of 15°C to 30°C (59°F to 86°F); protect from light. Solutions may not be resterilized by autoclaving.

Mechanism of Action Blocks both the initiation and conduction of nerve impulses by decreasing the neuronal membrane's permeability to sodium ions, which results in inhibition of depolarization with resultant blockade of conduction

Pharmacodynamics

Onset of action: 6-12 minutes

Duration (patient, type of block, concentration, and method of anesthesia dependent): Up to 1 hour

Pharmacokinetics (Adult data unless noted)

Metabolism: Rapidly hydrolyzed by plasma enzymes to 2-chloro-4-aminobenzoic acid and 8-diethylaminoethanol (80% conjugated before elimination)

Half-life (*in vitro*):

Neonates: 43 ± 2 seconds

Adult males: 21 ± 2 seconds

Adult females: 25 ± 1 second

Elimination: Very little excreted as unchanged drug in urine; metabolites: Cloro-aminobenzoic acid and diethylaminoethanol primarily excreted unchanged in urine

Usual Dosage Dose varies with procedure, desired depth, and duration of anesthesia, desired muscle relaxation, vascularity of tissues, physical condition, and age of patient. The smallest dose and concentration required to produce the desired effect should be used.

Children >3 years: Maximum dose without epinephrine: 11 mg/kg

Adults: Maximum dose: 11 mg/kg; not to exceed 800 mg per treatment; with epinephrine: 14 mg/kg; not to exceed 1000 mg per treatment

Infiltration and peripheral nerve block:

Mandibular: 2-3 mL (40-60 mg) using 2%

Infraorbital: 0.5-1 mL (10-20 mg) using 2%

Brachial plexus: 30-40 mL (600-800 mg) using 2%

Digital (without epinephrine): 3-4 mL (30-40 mg) using 1%

Pudendal: 10 mL (200 mg) into each side (2 sites) using 2%

Paracervical: 3 mL (30 mg) per each of four sites using 1%

Caudal and lumbar epidural block:

Caudal: 15-25 mL using 2% to 3% solution; may repeat dose at 40- to 60-minute intervals

Lumbar: 2-2.5 mL per segment using 2% to 3% solution; usual total volume 15-25 mL; repeated doses 2-6 mL less than the original dose may be given at 40- to 50-minutes intervals

Administration Parenteral: Administer in small incremental doses; when using continuous intermittent catheter techniques, use frequent aspirations before and during the injection to avoid intravascular injection

Monitoring Parameters Blood pressure, heart rate, respiration, signs of CNS toxicity (lightheadedness, dizziness, tinnitus, restlessness, tremors, twitching, drowsiness, circumoral paresthesia)

Patient Information You will experience decreased sensation to pain, heat, or cold in the area and/or decreased muscle strength (depending on area of application) until effects wear off; use necessary caution to reduce incidence of possible injury until full sensation returns. Report irritation, pain, burning at injection site; chest pain or palpitations; or respiratory difficulty.

Dosage Forms Excipient information presented when available (limited, particularly for generics); consult specific product labeling.

Injection, solution, as hydrochloride:

Nesacaine®: 1% (30 mL); 2% (30 mL) [contains disodium EDTA and methylparaben]

Injection, solution, as hydrochloride [preservative free]: 2% (20 mL); 3% (20 mL)

Nesacaine®-MPF: 2% (20 mL); 3% (20 mL)

◆ **Chloroprocaine Hydrochloride** *see* Chloroprocaine *on page 292*

Chloroquine (KLOR oh kwin)

Medication Safety Issues

International issues:

Aralen® may be confused with Oralon® which is a brand name for povidone-iodine in Japan

Aralen® may be confused with Paralen® which is a brand name for acetaminophen in the Czech Republic

Related Information

Malaria *on page 1652*

Medications for Which A Single Dose May Be Fatal When Ingested By A Toddler *on page 1709*

U.S. Brand Names Aralen®

Canadian Brand Names Aralen®; Novo-Chloroquine

Therapeutic Category Amebicide; Antimalarial Agent

Generic Available Yes

Use Suppression or chemoprophylaxis of malaria in chloroquine-sensitive areas [FDA approved in pediatric patients (age not specified) and adults]; treatment of uncomplicated acute attacks of malaria due to susceptible *Plasmodium* species, except chloroquine-resistant *Plasmodium falciparum* [FDA approved in pediatric patients (age not specified) and adults]; extraintestinal amebiasis (FDA approved in adults); has been used for treatment of rheumatoid arthritis, discoid lupus erythematosus, scleroderma, pemphigus

Pregnancy Considerations There are no adequate and well-controlled studies using chloroquine during pregnancy. However, based on clinical experience and because malaria infection in pregnant women may be more severe than in nonpregnant women, chloroquine prophylaxis may be considered in areas of chloroquine-sensitive *P. falciparum* malaria. Pregnant women should be advised not to travel to areas of *P. falciparum* resistance to chloroquine. Consult current CDC guidelines for the treatment of malaria during pregnancy.

◀ **Lactation** Enters breast milk/not recommended (AAP considers "compatible")

Contraindications Hypersensitivity to 4-aminoquinoline compounds (eg, chloroquine, hydroxychloroquine) or any component; retinal or visual field changes

Warnings Physicians should be familiar with chloroquine before prescribing **[U.S. Boxed Warning]**. Resistance of *Plasmodium falciparum* to chloroquine is widespread, including everywhere that *P. falciparum* malaria is transmitted, except for areas of Central America (northwest of the Panama Canal), Haiti, the Dominican Republic, and most areas of the Middle East; cases of *Plasmodium vivax* resistance have been reported. Irreversible retinal damage has been reported in patients who received long-term or high-dose therapy; baseline and periodic ophthalmic exams should be performed. Periodically examine patients for evidence of muscular weakness; discontinue chloroquine if weakness occurs. Chloroquine may precipitate a severe attack of psoriasis in patients with psoriasis; may exacerbate porphyria in patients with porphyria.

Precautions Use with caution in patients with liver disease, G-6-PD deficiency, severe blood disorders, seizure disorders, pre-existing auditory damage, or in conjunction with hepatotoxic drugs; use in pregnancy should be avoided, except for the suppression or treatment of malaria when, in the judgement of the prescriber, the potential benefit outweighs the potential risks to the fetus.

Adverse Reactions

Cardiovascular: Cardiomyopathy, ECG changes (inversion or depression of T-wave with widening of the QRS complex), hypotension, torsade de pointes

Central nervous system: Agitation, anxiety, confusion, delirium, depression, dizziness, fatigue, hallucinations, headache, insomnia, personality changes, polyneuritis, psychotic episodes, seizures

Dermatologic: Alopecia, angioedema, erythema multiforme, exfoliative dermatitis, hair bleaching, hair loss, lichen planus eruptions, photosensitivity, pleomorphic skin eruptions, pruritus, skin/mucosal changes (blue-black), Stevens-Johnson syndrome, toxic epidermal necrolysis, urticaria

Gastrointestinal: Abdominal cramps, anorexia, diarrhea, nausea, vomiting

Hematologic: Blood dyscrasias (aplastic anemia, neutropenia, pancytopenia, thrombocytopenia)

Hepatic: Hepatitis, liver enzymes increased

Neuromuscular & skeletal: Depression of tendon reflexes, myopathy, neuromyopathy, proximal muscle atrophy, weakness

Ocular: Accommodation disturbances, blurred vision, corneal opacity, nyctalopia, retinopathy, visual field defects

Otic: Deafness, reduced hearing, tinnitus

Miscellaneous: Anaphylaxis

Drug Interactions

Metabolism/Transport Effects Substrate (major) of CYP2D6, 3A4; **Inhibits** CYP2D6 (moderate)

Avoid Concomitant Use

Avoid concomitant use of Chloroquine with any of the following: Agalsidase Beta; Artemether; Lumefantrine; Mefloquine

Increased Effect/Toxicity

Chloroquine may increase the levels/effects of: Antipsychotic Agents (Phenothiazines); Beta-Blockers; Cardiac Glycosides; CYP2D6 Substrates; Dapsone; Dapsone (Systemic); Dapsone (Topical); Fesoterodine; Lumefantrine; Mefloquine; QTc-Prolonging Agents; Tamoxifen

The levels/effects of Chloroquine may be increased by: Artemether; CYP2D6 Inhibitors (Moderate); CYP2D6 Inhibitors (Strong); CYP3A4 Inhibitors (Moderate); CYP3A4 Inhibitors (Strong); Dapsone; Dapsone (Systemic); Darunavir; Mefloquine

Decreased Effect

Chloroquine may decrease the levels/effects of: Agalsidase Beta; Ampicillin; Anthelmintics; Codeine; Rabies Vaccine; TraMADol

The levels/effects of Chloroquine may be decreased by: Antacids; CYP3A4 Inducers (Strong); Deferasirox; Herbs (CYP3A4 Inducers); Kaolin; Peginterferon Alfa-2b

Stability Protect from light. Store tablets at 25°C (77°F); excursions permitted to 15°C to 30°C (59°F to 86°F).

Mechanism of Action Binds to and inhibits DNA and RNA polymerase; interferes with metabolism and hemoglobin utilization by parasites; inhibits prostaglandin effects

Pharmacokinetics (Adult data unless noted)

Absorption: Oral: Rapid

Distribution: Widely distributed in body tissues including eyes, heart, kidneys, liver, leukocytes, and lungs where retention is prolonged; crosses the placenta; appears in breast milk

Protein binding: 50% to 65%

Metabolism: Partially hepatic; main metabolite is desethylchloroquine

Half-life: 3-5 days

Time to peak serum concentration: Oral: Within 1-2 hours

Elimination: ~70% of dose excreted in urine (~35% unchanged); acidification of the urine increases elimination of drug; small amounts of drug may be present in urine months following discontinuation of therapy

Dialysis: Minimally removed by hemodialysis

Usual Dosage (Dosage expressed in terms of base):

Oral:

Suppression or prophylaxis of malaria:

Infants and Children: Administer 5 mg base/kg/week on the same day each week (not to exceed 300 mg base/dose); begin 1-2 weeks prior to exposure; continue for 4 weeks after leaving endemic area; if suppressive therapy is not begun prior to exposure, double the initial loading dose to 10 mg base/kg and give in 2 divided doses 6 hours apart, followed by the usual dosage regimen

Adults: 300 mg/week (base) on the same day each week; begin 1-2 weeks prior to exposure; continue for 4 weeks after leaving endemic area; if suppressive therapy is not begun prior to exposure, double the initial loading dose to 600 mg base and give in 2 divided doses 6 hours apart, followed by the usual dosage regimen

Acute attack:

Infants and Children: 10 mg base/kg (maximum dose: 600 mg base) stat, then 5 mg base/kg 6, 24, and 48 hours after first dose (maximum dose: 300 mg base/dose) (see CDC Guideline Table, 2009)

Adults: 600 mg base/dose one time, then 300 mg base/dose 6, 24, and 48 hours after the first dose

Extraintestinal amebiasis:

Children: 10 mg base/kg once daily for 21 days (up to 600 mg base/day) (see Seidel, 1984)

Adults: 600 mg base/day for 2 days followed by 300 mg base/day for at least 2-3 weeks

Rheumatoid arthritis, lupus erythematosus: Adults: 150 mg base once daily

Dosing adjustment in renal impairment: Cl_{cr} <10 mL/minute: Administer 50% of dose (see Arnoff, 2007)

Administration Oral: Administer with meals to decrease GI upset; chloroquine phosphate tablets have also been mixed with chocolate syrup or enclosed in gelatin capsules to mask the bitter taste

Monitoring Parameters Periodic CBC, examination for muscular weakness, and ophthalmologic examination (visual acuity, slit-lamp, fundoscopic, and visual field tests) in patients receiving prolonged therapy

Patient Information Report any visual disturbances, muscular weakness, or difficulty in hearing or ringing in the ears; tablets are bitter tasting. May cause photosensitivity reactions (eg, exposure to sunlight may cause severe sunburn, skin rash, redness, or itching); avoid exposure to sunlight and artificial light sources (sunlamps, tanning booth/bed); wear protective clothing, wide-brimmed hats, sunglasses, and lip sunscreen (SPF ≥15); use a sunscreen [broad-spectrum sunscreen or physical sunscreen (preferred) or sunblock with SPF ≥15]; contact physician if reaction occurs.

Additional Information *P. vivax* and *P. ovale* infections treated with chloroquine only can relapse due to hypnozoites; add primaquine to eradicate hypnozoites

Dosage Forms Excipient information presented when available (limited, particularly for generics); consult specific product labeling.

Tablet, as phosphate: 250 mg [equivalent to 150 mg base]; 500 mg [equivalent to 300 mg base]

Aralen®: 500 mg [equivalent to 300 mg base]

Extemporaneous Preparations A 15 mg chloroquine phosphate/mL suspension (equivalent to 9 mg chloroquine base/mL) is made by pulverizing three Aralen® 500 mg phosphate = 300 mg base/tablet, levigating with 15 mL of a 1:1 vehicle of Ora-Sweet® and Ora-Plus®, and adding vehicle by geometric proportion, levigating until a uniform mixture is obtained; qsad to 100 mL with vehicle, stable for up to 60 days when stored at 5°C or 25°C and protected from light. Label "shake well before using" and "protect from light."

Allen LV Jr and Erickson MA, "Stability of Alprazolam, Chloroquine Phosphate, Cisapride, Enalapril Maleate, and Hydralazine Hydrochloride in Extemporaneously Compounded Oral Liquids," *Am J Health Syst Pharm*, 1998, 55(18):1915-20.

References

American Academy of Pediatrics, "Amebiasis," In: Pickering LK, ed. *Red Book: 2009 Report of the Committee on Infectious Diseases*, 28th ed, Elk Grove Village, IL: American Academy of Pediatrics, 2009, 206-8.

Aronoff GR, Bennett WM, Berns JS, et al, *Drug Prescribing in Renal Failure: Dosing Guidelines for Adults and Children*, 5th ed, Philadelphia, PA: American College of Physicians, 2007, 73.

Centers for Disease Control and Prevention, "Guidelines for Treatment of Malaria in the United States." Available at http://www.cdc.gov/malaria/pdf/treatmenttable.pdf.

Centers for Disease Control and Prevention, "Malaria Prescription Drug Information for Healthcare Providers." Available at http://www.cdc.gov/malaria/travel/drugs_hcp.htm.

Centers for Disease Control and Prevention, "Treatment of Malaria (Guidelines for Clinicians)." Available at http://www.cdc.gov/malaria/pdf/clinicalguidance.pdf.

Seidel J, "Diagnosis and Management of Amebic Liver Abscess in Children," *West J Med*, 1984, 140(6):932-3.

Wyler DJ, "Malaria Chemoprophylaxis for the Traveler," *N Engl J Med*, 1993, 329(1):31-7.

♦ **Chloroquine Phosphate** *see* Chloroquine *on page 293*

Chlorothiazide (klor oh THYE a zide)

Medication Safety Issues

International issues:

Diuril® may be confused with Duorol® which is a brand name for acetaminophen in Spain

Related Information

Antihypertensive Agents by Class *on page 1481*

U.S. Brand Names Diuril®; Sodium Diuril®

Canadian Brand Names Diuril®

Therapeutic Category Antihypertensive Agent; Diuretic, Thiazide

Generic Available Yes: Excludes oral suspension

Use Management of mild to moderate hypertension; edema associated with CHF, pregnancy, or nephrotic syndrome

Pregnancy Risk Factor C (manufacturer); D (expert analysis)

Pregnancy Considerations Crosses the placenta. Hypoglycemia, thrombocytopenia, hemolytic anemia, electrolyte disturbances reported. May exhibit a tocolytic effect. Generally, use of diuretics during pregnancy is avoided for pregnancy-induced hypertension due to risk of decreased placental perfusion. Use may be considered in select patients with heart disease or chronic hypertension if started prior to gestation.

Lactation Enters breast milk/not recommended (AAP rates "compatible")

Breast-Feeding Considerations Crosses into breast milk; may suppress lactation with high doses. AAP considers **compatible** with breast-feeding.

Contraindications Hypersensitivity to chlorothiazide or any component; cross-sensitivity with other thiazides or sulfonamides; do not use in anuric patients

Warnings Hypokalemia may occur, particularly with aggressive diuresis, when severe cirrhosis is present, or after prolonged therapy. Other electrolyte disorders including hyponatremia, hypomagnesemia, and hypochloremic metabolic alkalosis may occur; monitor electrolytes. Has been reported to activate or exacerbate SLE. The injection must not be administered subcutaneously or I.M.

Precautions Use with caution in patients with severe renal disease (ineffective) and may precipitate azotemia; use with caution in patients with impaired hepatic function, moderate-high cholesterol concentrations, and in patients with high triglycerides. Chemical similarities are present among sulfonamides, sulfonylureas, carbonic anhydrase inhibitors, thiazides, and loop diuretics (except ethacrynic acid). A risk of cross-reactivity exists in patients with allergies to any of these compounds.

Adverse Reactions

Cardiovascular: Hypotension, arrhythmia, weak pulse, necrotizing angiitis

Central nervous system: Dizziness, vertigo, headache, fever

Dermatologic: Rash, photosensitivity, alopecia, erythema multiforme, exfoliative dermatitis, purpura, Stevens-Johnson syndrome, toxic epidermal necrolysis, urticaria

Endocrine & metabolic: Hypokalemia, hypochloremic alkalosis, hyperglycemia, hyperlipidemia, hyperuricemia, hypomagnesemia

Gastrointestinal: Anorexia, nausea, vomiting, cramping, diarrhea, pancreatitis, constipation, gastric irritation

Genitourinary: Impotence, hematuria

Hematologic: Rarely blood dyscrasias (aplastic anemia, agranulocytosis, leukopenia, hemolytic anemia, thrombocytopenia)

Hepatic: Intrahepatic cholestatic jaundice

Neuromuscular & skeletal: Muscle weakness, paresthesia

Ocular: Transient blurred vision, xanthopsia

Renal: Prerenal azotemia, interstitial nephritis, renal failure

Respiratory: Pneumonitis, pulmonary edema

Miscellaneous: Hypersensitivity reactions including anaphylactic reactions

Drug Interactions

Avoid Concomitant Use

Avoid concomitant use of Chlorothiazide with any of the following: Dofetilide

Increased Effect/Toxicity

Chlorothiazide may increase the levels/effects of: ACE Inhibitors; Allopurinol; Amifostine; Antihypertensives; Calcitriol; Calcium Salts; CarBAMazepine; Dofetilide; Hypotensive Agents; Lithium; OXcarbazepine; RiTUXimab

The levels/effects of Chlorothiazide may be increased by: Alcohol (Ethyl); Analgesics (Opioid); Barbiturates; Corticosteroids (Orally Inhaled); Corticosteroids (Systemic); Herbs (Hypotensive Properties); MAO Inhibitors; Pentoxifylline; Phosphodiesterase 5 Inhibitors; Prostacyclin Analogues

Decreased Effect

Chlorothiazide may decrease the levels/effects of: Antidiabetic Agents

The levels/effects of Chlorothiazide may be decreased by: Bile Acid Sequestrants; Herbs (Hypertensive Properties); Methylphenidate; Nonsteroidal Anti-Inflammatory Agents; Yohimbine

Food Interactions Avoid natural licorice (causes sodium and water retention and increases potassium loss); may need to decrease sodium and calcium, may need to increase potassium, zinc, magnesium, and riboflavin in diet

Stability Store at room temperature; reconstituted injection is stable for 24 hours at room temperature

Mechanism of Action Inhibits sodium reabsorption in the distal tubules causing increased excretion of sodium, chloride, potassium, bicarbonate, magnesium, phosphate, calcium (transiently) and water

Pharmacodynamics

Diuresis: Onset of action: Oral: Within 2 hours

Duration:

Oral: ~6-12 hours

I.V.: 2 hours

Pharmacokinetics (Adult data unless noted)

Absorption: Oral: Poor (~10% to 20%); dose dependent

Distribution: Breast milk to plasma ratio: 0.05

Half-life: Adults: 45-120 minutes

Time to peak serum concentration: Within 4 hours

Elimination: Excreted unchanged in urine

Usual Dosage I.V. dosage in infants and children has not been established. The following I.V. dosages in infants and children are based upon anecdotal reports. Lower I.V. dosing regimens have been extrapolated from oral dosing recommendations, as 10% to 20% of an oral dose is absorbed.

Neonates and Infants <6 months:

Oral: 20-40 mg/kg/day in 2 divided doses; maximum: 375 mg/day

I.V.: 2-8 mg/kg/day in 2 divided doses; doses up to 20 mg/kg/day have been used

Infants >6 months and Children:

Oral: 20 mg/kg/day in 2 divided doses; maximum: 1 g/day

I.V.: 4 mg/kg/day divided in 1-2 doses; doses up to 20 mg/kg/day have been used

Adults:

Hypertension: Oral: 500-2000 mg/day divided in 1-2 doses (manufacturer labeling); doses of 125-500 mg/day have also been recommended (JNC 7)

Edema: Oral, I.V.: 500-1000 mg once or twice daily; intermittent treatment (eg, therapy on alternative days) may be appropriate for some patients

Dosage adjustment in renal impairment: Cl_{cr} <10 mL/minute: Avoid use. Ineffective with Cl_{cr} <30 mL/minute unless in combination with a loop diuretic

Note: ACC/AHA 2005 Heart Failure guidelines suggest that thiazides lose their efficacy when Cl_{cr} <40 mL/minute.

Administration

Oral: Administer with food; shake suspension well before use

Parenteral: Dilute 500 mg vial with 18 mL SWI (resulting in 27.8 mg/mL concentration); administer by direct I.V. infusion over 3-5 minutes or infusion over 30 minutes in dextrose or NS; avoid extravasation of parenteral solution since it is extremely irritating to tissues

Monitoring Parameters Serum electrolytes (sodium, potassium, chloride, and bicarbonate), glucose, uric acid, triglycerides; body weight; blood pressure

Patient Information May cause photosensitivity reactions (eg, exposure to sunlight may cause severe sunburn, skin rash, redness, or itching); avoid exposure to sunlight and artificial light sources (sunlamps, tanning booth/bed); wear protective clothing, wide-brimmed hats, sunglasses, and lip sunscreen (SPF ≥15); use a sunscreen [broad-spectrum sunscreen or physical sunscreen (preferred) or sunblock with SPF ≥15]; contact physician if reaction occurs.

Dosage Forms Excipient information presented when available (limited, particularly for generics); consult specific product labeling.

Injection, powder for reconstitution, as sodium [strength expressed as base]: 500 mg

Sodium Diuril®: 500 mg

Suspension, oral:

Diuril®: 250 mg/5 mL (237 mL) [contains alcohol 0.5% and benzoic acid]

Tablet: 250 mg, 500 mg

Extemporaneous Preparations A 50 mg/mL oral suspension may be made by crushing ten 500 mg chlorothiazide tablets; levigate with glycerin to form a uniform paste. Add 2 grams carboxymethylcellulose gel (2 g carboxymethylcellulose is mixed with 5-10 mL water to form paste, additional 40 mL water is added and heated to 60°C with moderate stirring until dissolution occurs; this is cooled and allowed to stand for 1-2 hours to form a clear gel). Dissolve 500 mg citric acid in 5 mL water; add to chlorothiazide carboxymethylcellulose mixture with 0.1% parabens; qs to 100 mL with water (Nahata, 2004).

Nahata, MC, Pai VB, and Hipple TF, Pediatric Drug Formulations, 5th ed, Cincinnati, OH: Harvey Whitney Books Co, 2004.

References

Chobanian AV, Bakris GL, Black HR, et al, "The Seventh Report of the Joint National Committee on Prevention, Detection, Evaluation, and Treatment of High Blood Pressure: The JNC 7 Report," JAMA, 2003, 289(19):2560-72.

Hunt SA, Abraham WT, Chin MH, et al, "ACC/AHA 2005 Guideline Update for the Diagnosis and Management of Chronic Heart Failure in the Adult: A Report of the American College of Cardiology/American Heart Association Task Force on Practice Guidelines (Writing Committee to Update the 2001 Guidelines for the Evaluation and Management of Heart Failure): Developed in Collaboration With the American College of Chest Physicians and the International Society for Heart and Lung Transplantation: Endorsed by the Heart Rhythm Society," Circulation, 2005, 112(12):e154-235.

◆ Chlorphen [OTC] see Chlorpheniramine on page 296

Chlorpheniramine (klor fen IR a meen)

Medication Safety Issues

Sound-alike/look-alike issues:

Chlor-Trimeton® may be confused with Chloromycetin®

Beers Criteria medication: This drug may be inappropriate for use in geriatric patients (high severity risk).

U.S. Brand Names Ahist™; Aller-Chlor® [OTC]; Chlor-Trimeton® Allergy [OTC]; Chlorphen [OTC]; CPM-12 [DSC]; Diabetic Tussin® Allergy Relief [OTC]; Ed Chlorped; Ed-Chlor-Tan; P-Tann; PediaTan™; Teldrin® HBP [OTC]

Canadian Brand Names Chlor-Tripolon®; Novo-Pheniram

Therapeutic Category Antihistamine

Generic Available Yes: Syrup, tablet

Use Perennial and seasonal allergic rhinitis and other allergic symptoms including urticaria

Pregnancy Risk Factor C

Pregnancy Considerations Reproduction studies have not been conducted with chlorpheniramine maleate.

Lactation Excretion in breast milk unknown/not recommended

Contraindications Hypersensitivity to chlorpheniramine maleate or any component; narrow-angle glaucoma, bladder neck obstruction, symptomatic prostatic hypertrophy, stenosing peptic ulcer, pyloroduodenal obstruction

Warnings Safety and efficacy for the use of cough and cold products in children <2 years of age is limited. Serious adverse effects including death have been reported. The FDA notes that there are no approved OTC uses for these products in children <2 years of age. Healthcare providers are reminded to ask caregivers about the use of OTC cough and cold products in order to avoid exposure to multiple medications containing the same ingredient.

The oral suspension (PediaTan™) contains sodium benzoate; *in vitro* and animal studies have shown that benzoate, a metabolite of benzyl alcohol, displaces bilirubin from protein binding sites; avoid use in neonates.

Precautions Use with caution in patients with asthma; young children may be more susceptible to side effects and CNS stimulation

Adverse Reactions

Cardiovascular: Palpitations

Central nervous system: Drowsiness, vertigo, headache, excitability (children may be at increased risk for developing CNS stimulation), nervousness, fatigue, dizziness, depression

Dermatologic: Dermatitis, photosensitivity, angioedema

Endocrine & metabolic: Weight gain

Gastrointestinal: Nausea, xerostomia, diarrhea, abdominal pain, appetite increase

Genitourinary: Urinary retention

Neuromuscular & skeletal: Weakness, arthralgia, paresthesia

Ocular: Diplopia, blurred vision

Renal: Polyuria

Respiratory: Thickening of bronchial secretions, pharyngitis, epistaxis

Drug Interactions

Metabolism/Transport Effects Substrate of CYP2D6 (minor), 3A4 (major); **Inhibits** CYP2D6 (weak)

Avoid Concomitant Use There are no known interactions where it is recommended to avoid concomitant use.

Increased Effect/Toxicity

Chlorpheniramine may increase the levels/effects of: Alcohol (Ethyl); Anticholinergics; CNS Depressants

The levels/effects of Chlorpheniramine may be increased by: CYP3A4 Inhibitors (Moderate); CYP3A4 Inhibitors (Strong); Dasatinib; Pramlintide

Decreased Effect

Chlorpheniramine may decrease the levels/effects of: Acetylcholinesterase Inhibitors (Central); Betahistine

The levels/effects of Chlorpheniramine may be decreased by: Acetylcholinesterase Inhibitors (Central); Amphetamines; Peginterferon Alfa-2b

Mechanism of Action Competes with histamine for H_1-receptor sites on effector cells in the GI tract, blood vessels, and respiratory tract

Pharmacodynamics

Onset of action: Oral: 6 hours

Duration: Oral: 24 hours

Pharmacokinetics (Adult data unless noted) (Data from chlorpheniramine maleate)

Distribution: V_d:

Children: 3.8 L/kg

Adults: 2.5-3.2 L/kg

Protein binding: 69% to 72%

Metabolism: Substantial metabolism in GI mucosa and on first pass through liver

Bioavailability: Chlorpheniramine:

Solution: 35% to 60%

Tablet: 25% to 45%

Half-life:

Children: Average: 9.6-13.1 hours (range: 5.2-23.1 hours)

Adults: 12-43 hours

Time to peak serum concentration: Oral (solution and conventional tablets): 2-6 hours

Elimination: 35% excreted in 48 hours

Usual Dosage Oral:

Chlorpheniramine maleate:

Children <12 years: 0.35 mg/kg/day in divided doses every 4-6 hours or as an alternative

2-5 years: 1 mg every 4-6 hours

6-11 years: 2 mg every 4-6 hours, not to exceed 12 mg/day or timed release 8 mg every 12 hours

Children ≥12 years and Adults: 4 mg every 4-6 hours, not to exceed 24 mg/day or timed release 8-12 mg every 12 hours

Chlorpheniramine tannate:

Children 2 to <6 years: 2 mg (1.25 mL) twice daily; not to exceed 8 mg (5 mL) in a 24-hour period

Children 6 to <12 years: 4-8 mg (2.5-5 mL) twice daily; not to exceed 16 mg (10mL) in a 24-hour period

Children ≥12 years and Adults: 8-16 mg (5-10 mL) twice daily; not to exceed 32 mg (20 mL) in a 24-hour period

Dexchlorpheniramine maleate:

Children 2-5 years: 0.5 mg every 4-6 hours, not to exceed 3 mg/day

Children 6-11 years: 1 mg every 4-6 hours, not to exceed 6 mg/day

Children ≥12 years and Adults: 2 mg every 4-6 hours; not to exceed 12 mg/day

Administration Oral: Administer with food to decrease GI distress; do not crush or chew timed release tablets; shake suspension well before use

Patient Information May cause drowsiness and impair ability to perform activities requiring mental alertness or physical coordination; may cause dry mouth. May cause photosensitivity reactions (eg, exposure to sunlight may cause severe sunburn, skin rash, redness, or itching); avoid direct exposure to sunlight

Dosage Forms Excipient information presented when available (limited, particularly for generics); consult specific product labeling. [DSC] = Discontinued product

Capsule, extended release, oral, as maleate: 8 mg, 12 mg

CPM-12: 12 mg [DSC]

Suspension, oral, as tannate:

PediaTan™: 8 mg/5 mL (480 mL) [sugar free; contains sodium benzoate; bubble gum flavor]

P-Tann: 8 mg/5 mL (473 mL) [sugar free; contains sodium benzoate; bubblegum flavor]

Suspension, oral, as tannate [drops]:

Ed Chlorped: 2 mg/mL (60 mL)

Syrup, as maleate:

Aller-Chlor®: 2 mg/5 mL (120 mL) [contains alcohol 5%]

Diabetic Tussin® Allergy Relief: 2 mg/5 mL (120 mL) [alcohol free, dye free, sugar free]

Tablet, as maleate: 4 mg

Aller-Chlor®: 4 mg

Chlor-Trimeton® Allergy: 4 mg

Chlorphen: 4 mg

Teldrin® HBP: 4 mg

Tablet, extended release, oral, as maleate:
Chlor-Trimeton® Allergy: 12 mg
Tablet, extended release, oral, as tannate:
Ed-Chlor-Tan: 8 mg
Tablet, long acting, as tannate [scored]:
Ahist™: 12 mg

♦ **Chlorpheniramine Maleate** *see* Chlorpheniramine
on page 296

ChlorproMAZINE (klor PROE ma zeen)

Medication Safety Issues
Sound-alike/look-alike issues:
ChlorproMAZINE may be confused with chlordiazeP-
OXIDE, chlorproPAMIDE, clomiPRAMINE, prochlorper-
azine, promethazine
Thorazine® may be confused with thiamine, thioridazine

Related Information
Compatibility of Medications Mixed in a Syringe *on page
1713*
Medications for Which A Single Dose May Be Fatal
When Ingested By A Toddler *on page 1709*
Prochlorperazine *on page 1161*

Canadian Brand Names Largactil®; Novo-
Chlorpromazine

Therapeutic Category Antiemetic; Antipsychotic Agent,
Typical, Phenothiazine; Phenothiazine Derivative

Generic Available Yes

Use Treatment of nausea and vomiting (FDA approved in
ages 6 months to 12 years and adults), restlessness and
apprehension prior to surgery (FDA approved in ages 6
months to 12 years and adults), severe behavioral
problems in children displayed by combativeness and/or
explosive hyperexcitable behavior and in short-term
treatment of hyperactive children (FDA approved in ages
1-12 years); schizophrenia (FDA approved in adults),
psychotic disorders (FDA approved in adults), mania (FDA
approved in adults), acute intermittent porphyria (FDA
approved in adults), intractable hiccups (FDA approved in
adults), adjunct in the treatment of tetanus (FDA approved
in adults); has also been used in Tourette's syndrome

Pregnancy Risk Factor C

Lactation Enters breast milk/not recommended (AAP rates
"of concern")

Breast-Feeding Considerations Drowsiness and lethargy have been reported in nursing infants; galactorrhea
has been reported in mother.

Contraindications Hypersensitivity to chlorpromazine
hydrochloride or any component (see Warnings); cross-
sensitivity with other phenothiazines may exist; avoid use
in patients with narrow-angle glaucoma, bone marrow
suppression, severe liver or cardiac disease

Warnings May alter cardiac conduction; life-threatening
arrhythmias have occurred with therapeutic doses of
neuroleptics. Significant hypotension may occur, particularly with parenteral administration. May be sedating; use
with caution in disorders in which CNS depression is a
feature; patients must be cautioned about performing tasks
which require mental alertness (eg, operating machinery or
driving). Impaired core body temperature regulation may
occur; use with caution with strenuous exercise, heat
exposure, dehydration, and concomitant medication possessing anticholinergic effects. Relative to other neuroleptics, chlorpromazine has a moderate potency of
cholinergic blockade. May mask toxicity of other drugs or
conditions (eg, intestinal obstruction, Reye's syndrome,
brain tumor) due to antiemetic effects. Elevates prolactin
levels; use with caution in patients with breast cancer or
other prolactin-dependent tumors.

May cause extrapyramidal symptoms (EPS), including
pseudoparkinsonism, acute dystonic reactions, akathisia,

and tardive dyskinesia (risk of these reactions is low-
moderate relative to other neuroleptics, and is dose-
dependent; to decrease risk of tardive dyskinesia: Use
smallest dose and shortest duration possible; evaluate
continued need periodically; risk of dystonia is increased
with the use of high potency and higher doses of
conventional antipsychotics and in males and younger
patients). Use may be associated with neuroleptic
malignant syndrome (NMS); monitor for mental status
changes, fever, muscle rigidity, and/or autonomic instability; risk may be increased in patients with Parkinson's
disease or Lewy body dementia. May cause pigmentary
retinopathy and lenticular and corneal deposits, particularly with prolonged therapy.

Leukopenia, neutropenia, and agranulocytosis (sometimes
fatal) have been reported in clinical trials and postmarketing reports with antipsychotic use; presence of risk factors
(eg, pre-existing low WBC or history of drug-induced leuko/
neutropenia) should prompt periodic blood count assessment. Discontinue therapy at first signs of blood dyscrasias
or if absolute neutrophil count <1000/mm^3.

An increased risk of death has been reported with the use
of antipsychotics in elderly patients with dementia-related
psychosis **[U.S. Boxed Warning]**; most deaths seemed to
be cardiovascular (eg, sudden death, heart failure) or
infectious (eg, pneumonia) in nature; chlorpromazine is not
approved for this indication.

Tablets may contain benzoic acid; benzoic acid (benzoate)
is a metabolite of benzyl alcohol; large amounts of benzyl
alcohol (≥99 mg/kg/day) have been associated with a
potentially fatal toxicity ("gasping syndrome") in neonates;
the "gasping syndrome" consists of metabolic acidosis,
respiratory distress, gasping respirations, CNS dysfunction
(including convulsions, intracranial hemorrhage), hypotension, and cardiovascular collapse; use chlorpromazine
products containing benzoic acid with caution in neonates;
in vitro and animal studies have shown that benzoate
displaces bilirubin from protein binding sites. Injection
contains sulfites which may cause allergic reactions in
susceptible individuals.

Precautions Use with caution in patients with cardiovascular, renal, or hepatic disease; chronic respiratory
diseases (especially in children); seizures; significant
medical disorders or children with acute illnesses

Adverse Reactions
Cardiovascular: Arrhythmias, hypotension (especially with
I.V. use), orthostatic hypotension, tachycardia
Central nervous system: Altered central temperature
regulation, anxiety, drowsiness, extrapyramidal reactions,
neuroleptic malignant syndrome, pseudoparkinsonian
signs and symptoms, restlessness, sedation, seizures,
tardive dyskinesia
Dermatologic: Hyperpigmentation, photosensitivity, pruri-
tus, rash; oral solution or injection may cause contact
dermatitis (avoid contact with skin)
Endocrine & metabolic: Amenorrhea, galactorrhea, gyne-
comastia, weight gain
Gastrointestinal: Constipation, GI upset, xerostomia
Genitourinary: Impotence, urinary retention
Hematologic: Agranulocytosis, eosinophilia, hemolytic
anemia, leukopenia (usually in patients with large doses
for prolonged periods), neutropenia, thrombocytopenia
Hepatic: Cholestatic jaundice (rare)
Local: Thrombophlebitis
Ocular: Blurred vision, retinal pigmentation
Miscellaneous: Anaphylactoid reactions

Drug Interactions
Metabolism/Transport Effects Substrate of CYP1A2
(minor), 2D6 (major), 3A4 (minor); **Inhibits** CYP2D6
(strong), 2E1 (weak)

Avoid Concomitant Use

Avoid concomitant use of ChlorproMAZINE with any of the following: Artemether; Dronedarone; Lumefantrine; Metoclopramide; Nilotinib; Pimozide; QuiNINE; Tetrabenazine; Thioridazine; Ziprasidone

Increased Effect/Toxicity

ChlorproMAZINE may increase the levels/effects of: Alcohol (Ethyl); Analgesics (Opioid); Anticholinergics; Anti-Parkinson's Agents (Dopamine Agonist); Beta-Blockers; CNS Depressants; CYP2D6 Substrates; Desmopressin; Divalproex; Dronedarone; Fesoterodine; Haloperidol; Pimozide; QTc-Prolonging Agents; QuiNINE; Tamoxifen; Tetrabenazine; Thioridazine; Valproic Acid; Ziprasidone

The levels/effects of ChlorproMAZINE may be increased by: Acetylcholinesterase Inhibitors (Central); Alfuzosin; Antimalarial Agents; Artemether; Beta-Blockers; Chloroquine; Ciprofloxacin; Ciprofloxacin (Systemic); CYP2D6 Inhibitors (Moderate); CYP2D6 Inhibitors (Strong); Darunavir; Gadobutrol; Haloperidol; Lithium formulations; Lumefantrine; Metoclopramide; Nilotinib; Pramlintide; QuiNINE; Tetrabenazine

Decreased Effect

ChlorproMAZINE may decrease the levels/effects of: Amphetamines; Quinagolide; TraMADol

The levels/effects of ChlorproMAZINE may be decreased by: Antacids; Anti-Parkinson's Agents (Dopamine Agonist); Lithium formulations; Peginterferon Alfa-2b

Food Interactions Increases riboflavin elimination and may induce depletion; some may recommend increasing riboflavin in diet; may also decrease absorption of vitamin B_{12}; brown precipitate may occur when chlorpromazine is mixed with caffeine-containing liquids

Stability Protect oral dosage forms from light; diluted injection (1 mg/mL) with NS stored in 5 mL vials remains stable for 30 days

Mechanism of Action Chlorpromazine is an aliphatic phenothiazine antipsychotic which blocks postsynaptic mesolimbic dopaminergic receptors in the brain; exhibits a strong alpha-adrenergic blocking effect and depresses the release of hypothalamic and hypophyseal hormones; believed to depress the reticular activating system, thus affecting basal metabolism, body temperature, wakefulness, vasomotor tone, and emesis

Pharmacodynamics

Onset of action:

Oral: 30-60 minutes

Antipsychotic effects: Gradual, may take up to several weeks

Maximum antipsychotic effect: 6 weeks to 6 months

Duration: Oral: 4-6 hours

Pharmacokinetics (Adult data unless noted)

Absorption: Oral: Rapid and virtually complete; large first-pass effect due to metabolism during absorption in the GI mucosa

Distribution: Widely distributed into most body tissues and fluids; crosses blood-brain barrier and placenta; appears in breast milk; V_d: 8-160 L/kg (adults)

Protein binding: 90% to 99%

Metabolism: Extensively in the liver by demethylation (followed by glucuronide conjugation) and amine oxidation

Bioavailability: Oral: ~32%

Half-life, biphasic:

Initial:

Children: 1.1 hours

Adults: ~2 hours

Terminal:

Children: 7.7 hours

Adults: ~30 hours

Elimination: <1% excreted in urine as unchanged drug within 24 hours

Dialysis: Not dialyzable (0% to 5%)

Usual Dosage

Neonates: Neonatal abstinence syndrome (withdrawal from maternal opioid use): I.M. and Oral: Initial: I.M.: 0.5-0.7 mg/kg/dose given every 6 hours; change to oral after ~4 days, decrease dose gradually over 2-3 weeks. **Note:** Chlorpromazine is rarely used for neonatal abstinence syndrome due to adverse effects such as hypothermia and eosinophilia. Other agents (eg, phenobarbital or a 25-fold dilution of tincture of opium) are preferred.

Infants ≥6 months and Children:

Schizophrenia/psychoses:

Oral: 0.5-1 mg/kg/dose every 4-6 hours; older children may require 200 mg/day or higher

I.M., I.V.: 0.5-1 mg/kg/dose every 6-8 hours

Maximum recommended doses:

Children <5 years (<22.7 kg): 40 mg/day

Children 5-12 years (22.7-45.5 kg): 75 mg/day

Nausea and vomiting:

Oral: 0.5-1 mg/kg/dose every 4-6 hours as needed

I.M., I.V.: 0.5-1 mg/kg/dose every 6-8 hours; maximum recommended doses:

Children <5 years (<22.7 kg): 40 mg/day

Children 5-12 years (22.7-45.5 kg): 75 mg/day

Adults:

Schizophrenia/psychoses:

Oral: Range: 30-800 mg/day in 1-4 divided doses, initiate at lower doses and titrate as needed; usual dose is 200 mg/day; some patients may require 1-2 g/day

I.M., I.V.: 25 mg initially, may repeat (25-50 mg) in 1-4 hours, gradually increase to a maximum of 400 mg/dose every 4-6 hours until patient controlled; usual dose 300-800 mg/day

Nausea and vomiting:

Oral: 10-25 mg every 4-6 hours

I.M., I.V.: 25-50 mg every 4-6 hours

Administration

Oral: Administer with water, food, or milk to decrease GI upset. Do not administer chlorpromazine liquid preparations simultaneously with carbamazepine suspension (see Drug Interactions).

Parenteral: Do not administer SubQ (tissue damage and irritation may occur); for direct I.V. injection: Dilute with NS to a maximum concentration of 1 mg/mL, administer slow I.V. at a rate not to exceed 0.5 mg/minute in children and 1 mg/minute in adults

Monitoring Parameters Periodic eye exam with prolonged therapy; blood pressure with parenteral administration; CBC with differential

Reference Range Relationship of plasma concentration to clinical response is not well established

Therapeutic: 50-300 ng/mL (SI: 157-942 nmol/L)

Toxic: >750 ng/mL (SI: >2355 nmol/L)

Test Interactions False-positives for phenylketonuria, amylase, uroporphyrins, urobilinogen; possible false-negative pregnancy urinary test

Patient Information May cause drowsiness and impair ability to perform activities requiring mental alertness or physical coordination; may cause dry mouth; avoid alcohol. May cause photosensitivity reactions (eg, exposure to sunlight may cause severe sunburn, skin rash, redness, or itching); avoid exposure to sunlight and artificial light sources (sunlamps, tanning booth/bed); wear protective clothing, wide-brimmed hats, sunglasses, and lip sunscreen (SPF ≥15); use a sunscreen [broad-spectrum sunscreen or physical sunscreen (preferred) or sunblock with SPF ≥15]; contact physician if reaction occurs.

◄| **Nursing Implications** Avoid contact of injection with skin (may cause contact dermatitis; use of rubber gloves is recommended)

Additional Information Although chlorpromazine has been used in combination with meperidine and promethazine as a premedication ("lytic cocktail"), this combination may have a higher rate of adverse effects compared to alternative sedatives/analgesics (see AAP, 1995). Use decreased doses in elderly or debilitated patients; dystonic reactions may be more common in patients with hypocalcemia; extrapyramidal reactions may be more common in pediatric patients, especially those with dehydration or acute illnesses (viral or CNS infections).

Dosage Forms Excipient information presented when available (limited, particularly for generics); consult specific product labeling.

Injection, solution, as hydrochloride: 25 mg/mL (1 mL, 2 mL)

Tablet, as hydrochloride: 10 mg, 25 mg, 50 mg, 100 mg, 200 mg

References

American Academy of Pediatrics Committee on Drugs, "Reappraisal of Lytic Cocktail/Demerol®, Phenergan®, and Thorazine® (DPT) for the Sedation of Children," *Pediatrics*, 1995, 95(4):598-602.

Furlanut M, Benetello P, Baraldo M, et al, "Chlorpromazine Disposition in Relation to Age in Children," *Clin Pharmacokinet*, 1990, 18 (4):329-31.

◆ **Chlorpromazine Hydrochloride** *see* ChlorproMAZINE *on page 298*

◆ **Chlor-Trimeton® Allergy [OTC]** *see* Chlorpheniramine *on page 296*

◆ **Chlor-Tripolon® (Can)** *see* Chlorpheniramine *on page 296*

◆ **Chlor-Tripolon ND® (Can)** *see* Loratadine and Pseudoephedrine *on page 844*

Chlorzoxazone (klor ZOKS a zone)

Medication Safety Issues

Sound-alike/look-alike issues:

Parafon Forte® may be confused with Fam-Pren Forte

Beers Criteria medication: This drug may be inappropriate for use in geriatric patients (high severity risk).

U.S. Brand Names Parafon Forte® DSC

Canadian Brand Names Parafon Forte®; Strifon Forte®

Therapeutic Category Skeletal Muscle Relaxant, Nonparalytic

Generic Available Yes

Use Symptomatic treatment of muscle spasm and pain associated with acute musculoskeletal conditions

Pregnancy Risk Factor C

Lactation Excretion in breast milk unknown/not recommended

Contraindications Hypersensitivity to chlorzoxazone or any component; impaired liver function

Warnings Serious (including fatal) hepatocellular toxicity has been reported rarely

Adverse Reactions

Cardiovascular: Tachycardia, tightness in chest, flushing of face, syncope

Central nervous system: Drowsiness, dizziness, lightheadedness, headache, paradoxical stimulation, ataxia

Dermatologic: Rash, urticaria, petechiae, angioneurotic edema, erythema multiforme

Gastrointestinal: Nausea, vomiting, diarrhea, GI bleeding (rare), stomach cramps

Genitourinary: Discoloration of urine (orange or purple-red)

Hematologic: Anemia, granulocytopenia, eosinophilia

Hepatic: Hepatitis

Neuromuscular & skeletal: Paresthesia, trembling

Ocular: Burning of eyes

Respiratory: Shortness of breath

Miscellaneous: Hiccups

Drug Interactions

Metabolism/Transport Effects Substrate of CYP1A2 (minor), 2A6 (minor), 2D6 (minor), 2E1 (major), 3A4 (minor); **Inhibits** CYP2E1 (weak), 3A4 (weak)

Avoid Concomitant Use There are no known interactions where it is recommended to avoid concomitant use.

Increased Effect/Toxicity

Chlorzoxazone may increase the levels/effects of: Alcohol (Ethyl); CNS Depressants; Methotrimeprazine

The levels/effects of Chlorzoxazone may be increased by: Disulfiram; Isoniazid; Methotrimeprazine

Decreased Effect

The levels/effects of Chlorzoxazone may be decreased by: Peginterferon Alfa-2b

Food Interactions Watercress may decrease chlorzoxazone clearance

Mechanism of Action Acts on the spinal cord and subcortical levels of the brain to inhibit multisynaptic reflex arcs involved in producing and maintaining skeletal muscle spasms

Pharmacodynamics

Onset of action: Within 60 minutes

Duration: 3-4 hours

Pharmacokinetics (Adult data unless noted)

Absorption: Oral: Readily

Metabolism: Extensive in the liver by glucuronidation

Half-life: ~60 minutes

Time to peak serum concentration: Adults: 1-2 hours

Elimination: In urine as conjugates; <1% excreted unchanged in urine

Usual Dosage Oral:

Children: 20 mg/kg/day or 600 mg/m^2/day in 3-4 divided doses

Adults: 250-750 mg 3-4 times/day

Administration Oral: Administer with food

Monitoring Parameters Periodic liver function tests

Patient Information May color urine orange or purple-red; may cause drowsiness and impair ability to perform activities requiring mental alertness or physical coordination; notify physician if experiencing fever, rash, anorexia, right upper quadrant pain, dark urine, or jaundice

Dosage Forms Excipient information presented when available (limited, particularly for generics); consult specific product labeling.

Caplet (Parafon Forte® DSC): 500 mg

Tablet: 250 mg, 500 mg

Cholecalciferol (kole e kal SI fer ole)

Medication Safety Issues

Sound-alike/look-alike issues:

Cholecalciferol may be confused with ergocalciferol

Potential for medication errors: Liquid vitamin D preparations have the potential for dosing errors when administered to infants. Droppers should be clearly marked to easily provide 400 international units. For products intended for infants, the FDA recommends that accompanying droppers deliver no more than 400 international units per dose.

U.S. Brand Names D-3 [OTC]; D3-50™ [OTC]; D3-5™ [OTC]; Delta® D3 [OTC]; Enfamil® D-Vi-Sol™ [OTC]; Maximum D3® [OTC]; Vitamin D3 [OTC]

Canadian Brand Names D-Vi-Sol®

Therapeutic Category Nutritional Supplement; Vitamin D Analog; Vitamin, Fat Soluble

Generic Available Yes

Use Prevention and treatment of vitamin D deficiency and/or rickets; dietary supplement (FDA approved in all ages)

Pregnancy Risk Factor C

Lactation Enters breast milk/use caution

Breast-Feeding Considerations Small quantities of vitamin D are found in breast milk following normal maternal exposure via sunlight and diet. The amount in breast milk does not correlate with serum levels in the infant. Therefore, vitamin D supplementation is recommended in all infants who are partially or exclusively breast fed. Hypercalcemia has been noted in a breast-feeding infant following maternal use of large doses of ergocalciferol; high doses should be avoided in lactating women.

Contraindications Hypersensitivity to cholecalciferol or any component; hypercalcemia

Precautions Adequate calcium intake is necessary for clinical response to cholecalciferol therapy; maintain adequate fluid intake

Adverse Reactions Note: Adverse effects are results of hypercalcemia induced by hypervitaminosis D.

Cardiovascular: Arrhythmia (QT shortening, sinus tachycardia)

Central nervous system: Confusion, headache, lethargy, sluggishness

Gastrointestinal: Abdominal pain, nausea, vomiting

Neuromuscular & skeletal: Soft tissue calcification

Renal: Calciuria, nephrocalcinosis

Drug Interactions

Metabolism/Transport Effects Inhibits CYP2C8/9 (weak), 2C19 (weak), 2D6 (weak)

Avoid Concomitant Use There are no known interactions where it is recommended to avoid concomitant use.

Increased Effect/Toxicity There are no known significant interactions involving an increase in effect.

Decreased Effect There are no known significant interactions involving a decrease in effect.

Stability Store at room temperature; protect from light

Mechanism of Action Vitamin D stimulates calcium and phosphate absorption from the small intestine, promotes secretion of calcium from bone to blood, promotes renal tubule phosphate resorption, acts directly on bone cells (osteoblasts) to stimulate skeletal growth and on the parathyroid glands to suppress parathyroid hormone synthesis and secretion. Cholecalciferol (vitamin D_3) is synthesized in the skin and also found in other animal sources.

Pharmacokinetics (Adult data unless noted)

Protein binding: Extensively to vitamin D-binding protein

Metabolism: Hydroxylated in liver to calcifidiol (25-OH-D3) then in kidney to the active form, calcitriol (1α,2-[OH]2 vitamin D_3)

Half-life: 19-25 hours

Elimination: As metabolites, urine and feces

Usual Dosage Oral:

Children:

Prevention of Vitamin D Deficiency:

Neonates, infants, and children: 200 international units/day; from Dietary Supplementation for Prevention of Vitamin D Deficiency: Dietary Intake Reference (DIR) (1997 National Academy of Science Recommendations): **Note:** DIR is under review as of March 2009.

Alternate dosing (see Greer 2000; Wagner, 2008):

Premature infants: 400-800 international units/day or 150-400 international units/**kg**/day

Breast-fed infants (fully or partially): 400 international units/day beginning in the first few days of life. Continue supplementation until infant is weaned to ≥1000 mL/day or 1 qt/day of vitamin D-fortified formula or whole milk (after 12 months of age)

Formula-fed infants ingesting <1000 mL of vitamin D-fortified formula: 400 international units/day

Children ingesting <1000 mL of vitamin D-fortified milk: 400 international units/day

Children with increased risk of vitamin D deficiency (chronic fat malabsorption, maintained on chronic antiseizure medications): Higher doses may be required; use laboratory testing [25(OH)D, PTH, bone mineral status] to evaluate

Adolescents without adequate intake: 400 international units/day

Treatment Vitamin D deficiency and/or rickets: In addition to calcium and phosphorus supplementation (see Gordon, 2008; Misra, 2008):

Infants <1 month: 1000 international units/day for 2-3 months; once radiologic evidence of healing is observed, dose should be decreased to 400 international units/day

Infants 1-12 months: 1000-5000 international units/day for 2-3 months; once radiologic evidence of healing is observed, dose should be decreased to 400 international units/day

Children >12 months: 5000-10,000 international units/day for 2-3 months; once radiologic evidence of healing is observed, dose should be decreased to 400 international units/day

Children with increased risk of vitamin D deficiency (chronic fat malabsorption, maintained on chronic antiseizure medications): Higher doses may be required; use laboratory testing [25(OH)D, PTH, bone mineral status] to evaluate

Note: If poor compliance, single high dose may be used or repeated periodically

Treatment of Vitamin D insufficiency or deficiency associated with CKD (stages 2-5, 5D): (see KDOQI Guidelines, 2009); serum 25 hydroxyvitamin D [25(OH)D] level ≤30 ng/mL:

Serum 25(OH)D level 16-30 ng/mL: Children: 2000 international units/day for 3 months or 50,000 international units every month for 3 months

Serum 25(OH)D level 5-15 ng/mL: Children: 4000 international units/day for 12 weeks or 50,000 international units every other week for 12 weeks

Serum 25(OH)D level <5 ng/mL: Children: 8000 international units/day for 4 weeks then 4000 international units/day for 2 months for total therapy of 3 months or 50,000 international units/week for 4 weeks followed by 50,000 international units 2 times/month for a total therapy of 3 months

Maintenance dose [once repletion accomplished; serum 25(OH)D level >30 ng/mL]: 200-1000 international units/day

Dosage adjustment: Monitor serum 25(OH)D, corrected total calcium and phosphorus levels 1 month following initiation of therapy, every 3 months during therapy and with any Vitamin D dose change.

Prevention and treatment Vitamin D Deficiency in cystic fibrosis:

Recommended daily intake (see Borowitz, 2002):

Infants <1 year: 400 international units/day

Children >1 year: 400-800 international units/day

Alternate dosing (see Hall, 2010):

Infants <1 year: 8000 international units/**week**

Children >1 year: 800 international units/day

Note: If serum 25 hydroxyvitamin D [25(OH)D] level remains ≤30 ng/mL (75 nmol/L) and patient compliance established; then medium dose regimen may be used:

Medium Dose Regimen:

Patient <5 years: 12,000 international units/week for 12 weeks

Patient ≥5 years: 50,000 international units/week for 12 weeks

Note: If repeat 25 hydroxyvitamin D [25(OH)D] level remains ≤30 ng/mL (75 nmol/L) and patient compliance established; then high dose regimen may be used:

High Dose Regimen:

Patient <5 years: 12,000 international units twice weekly for 12 weeks

Patient ≥5 years: 50,000 international units twice weekly for 12 weeks

Adults:

Dietary Intake Reference ([DIR] 1997): **Note:** DIR is currently being reviewed (March 2009): 200-600 international units/day

Osteoporosis prevention and treatment: 800-1000 international units/day

Administration May be administered without regard to meals; for oral liquid, use accompanying dropper for dosage measurements

Monitoring Parameters Children at increased risk of vitamin D deficiency (chronic fat malabsorption, chronic antiseizure medication use) require serum 25(OH)D, PTH, and bone-mineral status to evaluate. If vitamin D supplement is required, then 25(OH)D levels should be repeated at 3-month intervals until normal. PTH and bone mineral-status should be monitored every 6 months until normal.

Chronic kidney disease: Serum calcium and phosphorus levels (in CKD: After 1 month and then at least every 3 months); alkaline phosphatase, BUN; 25(OH)D (in CKD: After 3 months of treatment and as needed thereafter)

Reference Range Vitamin D status may be determined by serum 25(OH) D levels (see Misra, 2008):

Severe deficiency: ≤5 ng/mL (12.5 nmol/L)

Deficiency: 15 ng/mL (37.5 nmol/L)

Insufficiency: 15-20 ng/mL (37.5-50 nmol/L)

Sufficiency: 20-100 ng/mL (50-250 nmol/L)*

Excess: >100 ng/mL (250 nmol/L) **

Intoxication: 150 ng/mL (375 nmol/L)

* Based on adult data a level of >32 ng/mL (80 nmol/L) is desirable

** Arbitrary designation

Chronic kidney disease (CKD) is defined either as kidney damage or GFR <60 mL/minute/1.73 m^2 for ≥3 months); stages of CKD are described below:

CKD Stage 1: Kidney damage with normal or increased GFR; GFR >90 mL/minute/1.73m^2

CKD Stage 2: Kidney damage with mild decrease in GFR; GFR 60-89 mL/minute/1.73 m^2

CKD Stage 3: Moderate decrease in GFR; GFR 30-59 mL/minute/1.73 m^2

CKD Stage 4: Severe decrease in GFR; GFR 15-29 mL/minute/1.73 m^2

CKD Stage 5, 5D: Kidney failure; GFR <15 mL/minute/1.73 m^2 or dialysis (5D)

Target serum 25(OH)D level in CKD: >30 ng/mL

Patient Information Take as directed; do not increase dosage without consulting healthcare provider. Adhere to diet as recommended; do not take any other phosphate or vitamin D-related compounds while taking cholecalciferol. You may experience nausea, vomiting, dry mouth; small frequent meals, frequent mouth care, chewing gum, or sucking lozenges may help.

Additional Information 1 mcg cholecalciferol provides 40 international units of vitamin D activity

Biological potency may be greater with cholecalciferol (vitamin D$_3$) compared to ergocalciferol (vitamin D$_2$).

Maternal Supplementation of High Dose Vitamin D: Data has shown maternal doses of 2000 international units/day will raise the antirachitic activity of breast milk and the serum 25(OH)D levels in exclusively breast-fed infants. Higher maternal doses of 4000-6400 international units/day have been shown to produce significant satisfactory increases in these outcome measures without evidence of maternal vitamin D toxicity (see Hollis 2004; Misra 2008; Taylor, 2008; Wagner, 2008). In geographical areas where rickets is frequently seen and baseline maternal and infant serum 25(OH)D levels are very low (eg, Middle East), concurrent maternal high dose supplementation (2000 international units/day or 60,000 units/month) with infant supplementation (400 international units/day) has been shown to produce a 64% reduction in prevalence of vitamin D deficiency in the study population (see Saadi, 2009). Due to recent increase in number of reported cases of rickets, Canada has increased vitamin D recommendations for all full-term infants (400-800 international units/day depending on month) and 2000 international units/day maternal supplementation if lactating.

Dosage Forms Excipient information presented when available (limited, particularly for generics); consult specific product labeling.

Capsule, oral:

D-3: 1000 int. units

D3-5™: 5000 int. units

D3-50™: 50,000 int. units

Maximum D3®: 10,000 int. units [contains soybean lecithin]

Capsule, softgel, oral:

D-3: 2000 int. units

Solution, oral [drops]:

Enfamil® D-Vi-Sol™: 400 int. units/mL (150 mL) [gluten free, sugar free; citrus flavor]

Tablet, oral:

Delta® D3: 400 int. units [sugar-free]

Vitamin D3: 100 int. units [sugar-free]

References

Borowitz D, Baker RD, and Stallings V, "Consensus Report on Nutrition for Pediatric Patients With Cystic Fibrosis," *J Pediatr Gastroenterol Nutr*, 2002, 35(3):246-59.

"Dietary Reference Intakes for Calcium, Phosphorus, Magnesium, Vitamin D, and Fluoride. Standing Committee on the Scientific Evaluation of Dietary Reference Intakes, Food and Nutrition Board, Institute of Medicine," National Academy of Sciences, Washington, DC: National Academy Press, 1997.

Gordon CM, Williams AL, Feldman HA, et al, "Treatment of Hypovitaminosis D in Infants and Toddlers," *J Clin Endocrinol Metab*, 2008, 93:2716-21.

Greer FR, "Vitamin Metabolism and Requirements in the Micropremie," *Clin Perinatol*, 2000, 27(1):95-118.

KDOQI Work Group, "KDOQI Clinical Practice Guideline for Nutrition in Children with CKD: 2008 Update. Executive Summary," *Am J Kidney Dis*, 2009, 53(3 Suppl 2):S11-104.

Hall WB, Sparks AA, and Aris RM, "Vitamin D Deficiency in Cystic Fibrosis," *Int J Endocrinol*, 2010, 218691.

Hollis BW and Wagner CL, "Vitamin D Requirements During Lactation: High-Dose Maternal Supplementation as Therapy to Prevent Hypovitaminosis D for Both the Mother and the Nursing Infant," *Am J Clin Nutr*, 2004, 80(6 Suppl):1752S-8S.

Misra M, Pacaud D, Petryk A, et al, "Vitamin D Deficiency in Children and Its Management: Review of Current Knowledge and Recommendations," *Pediatrics*, 2008, 122(2):398-417.

Saadi HF, Dawodu A, Afandi B, et al, "Effect of Combined Maternal and Infant Vitamin D Supplementation on Vitamin D Status of Exclusively Breastfed Infants," *Matern Child Nutr*, 2009, 5(1):25-32.

Taylor SN, Wagner CL, and Hollis BW, "Vitamin D Supplementation During Lactation to Support Infant and Mother," *J Am Coll Nutr*, 2008, 27(6):690-701.

Wagner CL, Greer FR, American Academy of Pediatrics Section on Breastfeeding, et al, "Prevention of Rickets and Vitamin D Deficiency in Infants, Children, and Adolescents," *Pediatrics*, 2008, 122 (5):1142-52.

Cholestyramine Resin (koe LES tir a meen REZ in)

Related Information

Normal Laboratory Values for Children *on page 1672*

U.S. Brand Names Prevalite®; Questran®; Questran® Light

Canadian Brand Names Novo-Cholamine; Novo-Cholamine Light; PMS-Cholestyramine; Questran®; Questran® Light Sugar Free; ZYM-Cholestyramine-Light; ZYM-Cholestyramine-Regular

Therapeutic Category Antilipemic Agent

Generic Available Yes

Use Adjunct in the management of primary hypercholesterolemia (FDA approved in adults) (see Additional Information for recommendations on initiating hypercholesterolemia pharmacologic treatment in children ≥8 years); pruritus associated with elevated levels of bile acids (FDA approved in adults); diarrhea associated with excess fecal bile acids; pseudomembraneous colitis

Pregnancy Risk Factor C

Pregnancy Considerations Cholestyramine is not absorbed systemically, but may interfere with vitamin absorption; therefore, regular prenatal supplementation may not be adequate. There are no studies in pregnant women; use with caution.

Lactation Does not enter breast milk/use caution

Contraindications Hypersensitivity to cholestyramine or any component; avoid using in complete biliary obstruction or biliary atresia

Precautions Use with caution in patients with constipation or recent abdominal surgery (see Additional Information); some products (eg, Prevalite® and Questran® Light) contain aspartame which is metabolized to phenylalanine and must be avoided (or used with caution) in patients with phenylketonuria.

Adverse Reactions

Dermatologic: Rash

Endocrine & metabolic: Hyperchloremic acidosis

Gastrointestinal: Constipation, nausea, vomiting, abdominal distention and pain, steatorrhea, malabsorption of fat-soluble vitamins

Genitourinary: Urinary calcium excretion increased

Hematologic: Hypoprothrombinemia

Local: Irritation of perianal area, skin, or tongue

Drug Interactions

Avoid Concomitant Use

Avoid concomitant use of Cholestyramine Resin with any of the following: Mycophenolate

Increased Effect/Toxicity There are no known significant interactions involving an increase in effect.

Decreased Effect

Cholestyramine Resin may decrease the levels/effects of: Acetaminophen; Amiodarone; Antidiabetic Agents (Thiazolidinedione); Calcitriol; Cardiac Glycosides; Contraceptives (Estrogens); Contraceptives (Progestins); Corticosteroids (Oral); Deferasirox; Ezetimibe; Fibric Acid Derivatives; Fluvastatin; Leflunomide; Loop Diuretics; Methotrexate; Methylfolate; Mycophenolate; Niacin; Nonsteroidal Anti-Inflammatory Agents; PHENobarbital; Pravastatin; Propranolol; Raloxifene; Tetracycline Derivatives; Thiazide Diuretics; Thyroid Products; Ursodiol; Vitamin K Antagonists

Food Interactions Cholestyramine (especially high doses or long-term therapy) may decrease the absorption of fat-soluble vitamins (vitamins A, D, E, and K), folic acid, calcium, iron, zinc, and magnesium; deficiencies may occur including hypoprothrombinemia and increased bleeding from vitamin K deficiency; supplementation of vitamins A, D, E, and K, folic acid, and iron may be required with high-dose, long-term therapy (administer vitamins or mineral supplements at least 1 hour before or at least 4-6 hours after cholestyramine)

Mechanism of Action Forms a nonabsorbable complex with bile acids in the intestine, releasing chloride ions in the process; inhibits enterohepatic reuptake of intestinal bile salts and thereby increases the fecal loss of bile salt-bound low density lipoprotein cholesterol

Pharmacodynamics

Maximum effect on serum cholesterol levels: Within 4 weeks

Pharmacokinetics (Adult data unless noted)

Absorption: Not absorbed from the GI tract

Elimination: Forms an insoluble complex with bile acids which is excreted in feces

Usual Dosage Oral (dosages are expressed in terms of anhydrous resin):

Children: 240 mg/kg/day in 3 divided doses; need to titrate dose depending on indication

Hypercholesterolemia (**Note:** Doses >8 g/day may not provide additional significant cholesterol-lowering effects, but may increase adverse effects): Some centers use the following doses (see Sprecher, 1996):

Children ≤10 years: Initial: 2 g/day; titrate dose based on efficacy and tolerance; range: 1-4 g/day

Children >10 years and Adolescents: Initial: 2 g/day; titrate dose based on efficacy and tolerance, up to 8 g/day

Note: Lipid-lowering effects are better if dose is administered as a single daily dose with the evening meal (single daily morning doses are less effective); if patients cannot tolerate once daily dosing, the dose/day may be divided into 2 doses and administered with the morning and evening meals; may also be administered in 3 divided doses/day (Daniels, 2002)

Adults: 3-4 g 3-4 times/day to a maximum of 16-32 g/day in 2-4 divided doses

Administration Oral: Administer at mealtime; do not administer the powder in its dry form; just prior to administration, mix with 2-6 ounces of water, noncarbonated liquid, or applesauce; to minimize binding of concomitant medications, administer other drugs including vitamins or mineral supplements at least 1 hour before or at least 4-6 hours after cholestyramine

Monitoring Parameters Serum cholesterol, serum triglycerides; with prolonged use, prothrombin time, liver enzymes, CBC, electrolytes; number of stools/day

Reference Range See Related Information for age- and gender-specific serum cholesterol, LDL-C, TG, and HDL concentrations.

Nursing Implications Maintain adequate oral fluid intake to avoid constipation; with high-dose, long-term therapy, use of daily multivitamin with iron and folic acid is recommended

Additional Information The current recommendation for pharmacologic treatment of hypercholesterolemia in children is limited to children ≥8 years of age and is based on LDL-C concentrations and the presence of coronary vascular disease (CVD) risk factors (see table and Daniels, 2008). In adults, for each 1% lowering in LDL-C, the relative risk for major cardiovascular events is reduced by ~1%. For more specific risk assessment and treatment recommendations for adults, see NCEP ATPIII, 2001.

Recommendations for Initiating Pharmacologic Treatment in Children ≥8 Years[1]

No risk factors for CVD	LDL ≥190 mg/dL despite 6-month to 1-year diet therapy
Family history of premature CVD or ≥2 CVD risk factors present, including obesity, hypertension, or cigarette smoking	LDL ≥160 mg/dL despite 6-month to 1-year diet therapy
Diabetes mellitus present	LDL ≥130 mg/dL

[1]Adapted from Daniels SR, Greer FR, and Committee on Nutrition, "Lipid Screening and Cardiovascular Health in Childhood," *Pediatrics*, 2008, 122(1):198-208.

Dosage Forms Excipient information presented when available (limited, particularly for generics); consult specific product labeling.

Powder for oral suspension: Cholestyramine resin 4 g/5 g packet (60s); cholestyramine resin 4 g/5 g of powder (210 g); cholestyramine resin 4 g/5.7 g packet (60s); cholestyramine resin 4 g/5.7 g of powder (240 g can); cholestyramine resin 4 g/9 g packet (60s); cholestyramine resin 4 g of resin/9 g of powder (378 g)

Prevalite®: Cholestyramine resin 4 g/5.5 g packet (42s, 60s) [contains phenylalanine 14.1 mg/5.5 g; orange flavor]; cholestyramine resin 4 g/5.5 g of powder (231 g) [contains phenylalanine 14.1 mg/5.5 g; orange flavor]

Questran®: Cholestyramine resin 4 g/9 g packet (60s); cholestyramine resin 4 g/9 g of powder (378 g)

Questran® Light: Cholestyramine resin 4 g/5 g packet (60s) [contains phenylalanine 14 mg/5 g]; cholestyramine resin 4 g/5 g of powder (210 g) [contains phenylalanine 14 mg/5 g]

References

Daniels SR, Greer FR, and Committee on Nutrition, "Lipid Screening and Cardiovascular Health in Childhood," *Pediatrics*, 2008, 122 (1):198-208.

Daniels SR, personal communication, May 2002.

McCrindle BW, O'Neill MB, Cullen-Dean G, et al, "Acceptability and Compliance With Two Forms of Cholestyramine in the Treatment of Hypercholesterolemia in Children: A Randomized, Crossover Trial," *J Pediatr*, 1997, 130(2):266-73.

McCrindle BW, Urbina EM, Dennison BA, et al, "Drug Therapy of High-Risk Lipid Abnormalities in Children and Adolescents: A Scientific Statement from the American Heart Association Atherosclerosis, Hypertension, and Obesity in Youth Committee, Council of Cardiovascular Disease in the Young, With the Council on Cardiovascular Nursing," *Circulation*, 2007, 115(14):1948-67.

Sprecher DL and Daniels SR, "Rational Approach to Pharmacologic Reduction of Cholesterol Levels in Children," *J Pediatr*, 1996, 129 (1):4-7.

"Third Report of the National Cholesterol Education Program Expert Panel on Detection, Evaluation, and Treatment of High Blood Cholesterol in Adults (Adult Treatment Panel III)," May 2001. Available at http://www.nhlbi.nih.gov/guidelines/cholesterol.

Tonstad S, Knudtzon J, Sivertsen M, et al, "Efficacy and Safety of Cholestyramine Therapy in Peripubertal and Prepubertal Children With Familial Hypercholesterolemia," *J Pediatr*, 1996, 129(1):42-9.

Choline Magnesium Trisalicylate

(KOE leen mag NEE zhum trye sa LIS i late)

Therapeutic Category Analgesic, Non-narcotic; Anti-inflammatory Agent; Antipyretic; Nonsteroidal Anti-inflammatory Drug (NSAID), Oral; Salicylate

Generic Available Yes

Use Management of osteoarthritis, rheumatoid arthritis, and other arthritides; treatment of acute painful shoulder, mild to moderate pain, and fever

Pregnancy Risk Factor C/D (3rd trimester)

Pregnancy Considerations Animal reproduction studies have not been conducted. Due to the known effects of other salicylates (closure of ductus arteriosus), use during late pregnancy should be avoided.

Lactation Enters breast milk/use caution

Breast-Feeding Considerations Excreted in breast milk; peak levels occur 9-12 hours after dose. Use caution if used during breast-feeding.

Contraindications Hypersensitivity to salicylates, any component, or other nonacetylated salicylates; history of asthma, urticaria, or allergic-type reaction to aspirin, or other NSAIDs; patients with the "aspirin triad" [asthma, rhinitis (with or without nasal polyps), and aspirin intolerance] (fatal asthmatic and anaphylactoid reactions may occur in these patients)

Warnings Do not use salicylates in children and teenagers who have or who are recovering from chickenpox or flu symptoms (due to the association with Reye's syndrome); when using salicylates, changes in behavior (along with nausea and vomiting) may be an early sign of Reye's syndrome; instruct patients and caregivers to contact their healthcare provider if these symptoms occur.

Precautions Use with extreme caution in patients with impaired renal function, erosive gastritis or peptic ulcer

Adverse Reactions

Dermatologic: Rash, pruritus, urticaria

Gastrointestinal: Nausea, vomiting, GI distress, ulceration

Hepatic: Hepatotoxicity

Otic: Tinnitus

Respiratory: Pulmonary edema

Drug Interactions

Avoid Concomitant Use There are no known interactions where it is recommended to avoid concomitant use.

Increased Effect/Toxicity

Choline Magnesium Trisalicylate may increase the levels/effects of: Anticoagulants; Carbonic Anhydrase Inhibitors; Corticosteroids (Systemic); Divalproex; Drotrecogin Alfa; Methotrexate; Pralatrexate; Salicylates; Sulfonylureas; Thrombolytic Agents; Valproic Acid; Varicella Virus-Containing Vaccines; Vitamin K Antagonists

The levels/effects of Choline Magnesium Trisalicylate may be increased by: Antiplatelet Agents; Calcium Channel Blockers (Nondihydropyridine); Ginkgo Biloba; Herbs (Anticoagulant/Antiplatelet Properties); Loop Diuretics; Treprostinil

Decreased Effect

Choline Magnesium Trisalicylate may decrease the levels/effects of: ACE Inhibitors; Loop Diuretics; Probenecid

The levels/effects of Choline Magnesium Trisalicylate may be decreased by: Corticosteroids (Systemic)

Mechanism of Action Inhibits prostaglandin synthesis; acts on the hypothalamus heat-regulating center to reduce fever; blocks the generation of pain impulses

Pharmacokinetics (Adult data unless noted)

Absorption: From stomach and small intestine

Distribution: Readily distributes into most body fluids and tissues; crosses the placenta; appears in breast milk

Protein binding: 90% to 95%

Metabolism: Hepatic microsomal enzyme system

Half-life: Dose-dependent, ranging from 2-3 hours at low doses to 30 hours at high doses

Time to peak serum concentration:

Solution: 20-35 minutes

Tablet: Within ~2 hours

Elimination: 10% excreted as unchanged drug

Usual Dosage Oral (based on **total salicylate content**):

Children: 30-60 mg/kg/day given in 3-4 divided doses

Adults: 500 mg to 1.5 g 1-3 times/day

Administration Oral: Administer with food or milk to decrease GI upset; liquid may be mixed with fruit juice just before drinking; do not administer with antacids

Monitoring Parameters Serum salicylate levels; serum magnesium with high doses or in patients with decreased renal function

Reference Range

Salicylate blood levels for anti-inflammatory effect: 150-300 mcg/mL

Analgesia and antipyretic effect: 30-50 mcg/mL

Test Interactions False-negative results for Clinistix® urine test; false-positive results with Clinitest®

Patient Information Avoid alcohol; notify physician if ringing in ears, persistent GI pain, GI bleeding, or changes in behavior (along with nausea and vomiting) occur (see Warnings)

Additional Information Salicylate salts do not inhibit platelet aggregation and, therefore, should not be substituted for aspirin in the prophylaxis of thrombosis (ie, for aspirin's antiplatelet effects)

Dosage Forms Excipient information presented when available (limited, particularly for generics); consult specific product labeling.

Liquid: 500 mg/5 mL (240 mL) [choline salicylate 293 mg and magnesium salicylate 362 mg per 5 mL; cherry cordial flavor]

Tablet: 500 mg [choline salicylate 293 mg and magnesium salicylate 362 mg]; 750 mg [choline salicylate 440 mg and magnesium salicylate 544 mg]; 1000 mg [choline salicylate 587 mg and magnesium salicylate 725 mg]

References

Berde C, Ablin A, Glazer J, et al, "American Academy of Pediatrics Report of the Subcommittee on Disease-Related Pain in Childhood Cancer," *Pediatrics*, 1990, 86(5 Pt 2):818-25.

♦ **Chooz® [OTC]** *see* Calcium Carbonate *on page 232*
♦ **Chooz® [OTC]** *see* Calcium Supplements *on page 239*

Chorionic Gonadotropin

(kor ee ON ik goe NAD oh troe pin)

U.S. Brand Names Novarel®; Pregnyl®
Canadian Brand Names Chorionic Gonadotropin for Injection; Pregnyl®
Therapeutic Category Gonadotropin; Ovulation Stimulator
Generic Available Yes
Use Treatment of hypogonadotropic hypogonadism, prepubertal cryptorchidism; induce ovulation and pregnancy in anovulatory, infertile women
Pregnancy Risk Factor X
Pregnancy Considerations Teratogenic effects (forelimb, CNS) have been noted in animal studies at doses intended to induce superovulation (used in combination with gonadotropin). Testicular tumors in otherwise healthy men have been reported when treating secondary infertility.
Lactation Excretion in breast milk unknown/use caution
Contraindications Hypersensitivity to chorionic gonadotropin or any component (see Warnings); precocious puberty, prostatic carcinoma or other androgen-dependent neoplasms; pregnancy
Warnings hCG is **not** effective in the treatment of obesity. hCG should only be used by clinicians who are experienced in the management of fertility disorders. May cause ovarian hyperstimulation syndrome (OHSS); if severe, treatment should be discontinued and patient should be hospitalized. OHSS results in a rapid (<24 hours to 7 days) accumulation of fluid in the peritoneal cavity, thorax, and possibly, the pericardium, which may become more severe if pregnancy occurs; monitor for ovarian enlargement. Use may lead to multiple births, arterial thromboembolism, enlargement or rupture of pre-existing ovarian cysts with resultant hemoperitoneum.

Pregnyl® contains benzyl alcohol which may cause allergic reactions in susceptible individuals; large amounts of benzyl alcohol (≥99 mg/kg/day) have been associated with a potentially fatal toxicity ("gasping syndrome") in neonates; the "gasping syndrome" consists of metabolic acidosis, respiratory distress, gasping respirations, CNS dysfunction (including convulsions, intracranial hemorrhage), hypotension and cardiovascular collapse; avoid use of Pregnyl® in neonates. *In vitro* and animal studies have shown that benzoate, a metabolite of benzyl alcohol, displaces bilirubin from protein-binding sites.

Precautions Use with caution in patients with asthma, seizure disorders, migraine, cardiac or renal disease; may induce precocious puberty in children being treated for cryptorchidism; discontinue if signs of precocious puberty occur; safety and efficacy in children <4 years of age has not been established

Adverse Reactions

Cardiovascular: Edema, arterial thromboembolism
Central nervous system: Irritability, restlessness, depression, fatigue, headache, aggressive behavior

Endocrine & metabolic: Gynecomastia, precocious puberty, ovarian hyperstimulation (see Warnings), enlargement of preexisting ovarian cysts or rupture of ovarian cysts
Local: Pain at the injection site
Neuromuscular & skeletal: Premature closure of epiphyses
Respiratory: Shortness of breath, dyspnea
Miscellaneous: Hypersensitivity reactions

Drug Interactions
Avoid Concomitant Use There are no known interactions where it is recommended to avoid concomitant use.
Increased Effect/Toxicity There are no known significant interactions involving an increase in effect.
Decreased Effect There are no known significant interactions involving a decrease in effect.

Stability Following reconstitution with provided diluent, stable for 30-90 days (depending upon preparation) when stored at 2°C to 15°C

Mechanism of Action Stimulates production of gonadal steroid hormones by causing production of androgen by the testis; as a substitute for luteinizing hormone (LH) to stimulate ovulation

Pharmacokinetics (Adult data unless noted)
Distribution: Distributes mainly into the testes in males and into the ovaries in females
Half-life, biphasic:
Initial: 11 hours
Terminal: 23 hours
Time to peak serum concentration: 6 hours
Elimination: Approximately 10% to 12% excreted unchanged in urine within 24 hours; detectable amounts may continue to be excreted in the urine for up to 3-4 days

Usual Dosage
Children: I.M. (many regimens have been described):
Prepubertal cryptorchidism:
1000-2000 units/m²/dose 3 times/week for 3 weeks or 4000 units 3 times/week for 3 weeks
or
5000 units every second day for 4 injections
or
500 units 3 times/week for 4-6 weeks
Hypogonadotropic hypogonadism:
500-1000 units 3 times/week for 3 weeks, followed by the same dose twice weekly for 3 weeks
or
1000-2000 units 3 times/week
or
4000 units 3 times/week for 6-9 months; reduce dosage to 2000 units 3 times/week for additional 3 months
Adults:
Induction of ovulation: Females: 5000-10,000 units the day following the last dose of menotropins
Spermatogenesis induction associated with hypogonadotropic hypogonadism: Male: Treatment regimens vary (range: 1000-2000 units 2-3 times a week). Administer hCG until serum testosterone levels are normal (may require 2-3 months of therapy), then add follitropin alfa or menopausal gonadotropin if needed to induce spermatogenesis; continue hCG at the dose required to maintain testosterone levels.

Administration Parenteral: Administer I.M. only
Monitoring Parameters
Male: Serum testosterone levels, semen analysis
Female: Ultrasound and/or estradiol levels to assess follicle development; ultrasound to assess number and size of follicles; ovulation (basal body temperature, serum progestin level, menstruation, sonography)
Reference Range Depends on application and methodology; <3 milli international units/mL (SI: <3 units/L) usually normal (nonpregnant)

Test Interactions Cross reacts with radioimmunoassay of gonadotropins, especially LH

Dosage Forms Excipient information presented when available (limited, particularly for generics); consult specific product labeling.

Injection, powder for reconstitution: 10,000 units [packaged with diluent; diluent contains benzyl alcohol and mannitol]

Novarel®: 10,000 units [packaged with diluent; diluent contains benzyl alcohol and mannitol]

Pregnyl®: 10,000 units [packaged with diluent; diluent contains benzyl alcohol]

◆ **Chorionic Gonadotropin for Injection (Can)** see Chorionic Gonadotropin on page 305

◆ **Chromium Chloride** see Trace Metals on page 1366

◆ **Chronovera® (Can)** see Verapamil on page 1416

Ciclopirox (sye kloe PEER oks)

Medication Safety Issues
Sound-alike/look-alike issues:
Loprox® may be confused with Lonox®

U.S. Brand Names Loprox®; Penlac®

Canadian Brand Names Loprox®; Penlac®; Stieprox®

Therapeutic Category Antifungal Agent, Topical

Generic Available Yes

Use
Cream/lotion: Treatment of tinea pedis, tinea cruris, and tinea corporis caused by *Trichophyton mentagrophytes*, *T. rubrum*, *Epidermophyton floccosum*, or *Microsporum canis*; treatment of pityriasis versicolor caused by *Malassezia* species; treatment of cutaneous candidiasis caused by *Candida albicans*

Gel: Treatment of tinea corporis and interdigital tinea pedis; treatment of seborrheic dermatitis of the scalp

Shampoo: Treatment of seborrheic dermatitis of the scalp

Solution (lacquer): Treatment of mild to moderate onychomycosis of fingernails and toenails (not involving the lunula) and the immediately adjacent skin caused by *T. rubrum*

Pregnancy Risk Factor B

Pregnancy Considerations Teratogenic effects were not observed in animal studies, however, there are no adequate and well-controlled studies in pregnant women. Use during pregnancy only if clearly needed.

Lactation Excretion in breast milk unknown/use caution

Contraindications Hypersensitivity to ciclopirox or any component

Precautions Use with caution in immunocompromised patients and diabetics.

Adverse Reactions
Cardiovascular: Facial edema
Dermatologic: Irritant dermatitis, pruritus, burning sensation, pain, erythema, dry skin, acne, rash, alopecia, ingrown toenails, nail discoloration
Ocular: Ocular pain

Drug Interactions
Avoid Concomitant Use There are no known interactions where it is recommended to avoid concomitant use.
Increased Effect/Toxicity There are no known significant interactions involving an increase in effect.
Decreased Effect There are no known significant interactions involving a decrease in effect.

Stability Store at room temperature; protect from light. Store ciclopirox topical solution (nail lacquer) in a tight container, protected from heat; the solution's solvent is flammable.

Mechanism of Action Causes intracellular depletion of essential substrates and/or ions by inhibiting transmembrane transport of these substances into cells decreasing protein, RNA, and DNA synthesis. May chelate polyvalent cations (ie, iron, aluminum) which can result in inhibition of metal-dependent enzymes for the degradation of peroxides within the fungal cell.

Pharmacokinetics (Adult data unless noted)
Absorption: Topical: Rapid but minimal with intact skin
Distribution: Present in stratum corneum, dermis, sebaceous glands, nails
Protein binding: 94% to 98%
Metabolism: Conjugated with glucuronic acid
Half-life:
Ciclopirox olamine: 1.7 hours
Ciclopirox gel: 5.5 hours
Elimination: Urine

Usual Dosage Topical:
Children >10 years, Adolescents, and Adults: Tinea pedis, tinea cruris, tinea corporis, tinea versicolor, and cutaneous candidiasis: Cream/suspension: Apply twice daily for 4 weeks (4-6 weeks for tinea cruris; 2 weeks for tinea versicolor if response is adequate). If no improvement after 4 weeks of treatment, re-evaluate diagnosis.

Children ≥12 years, Adolescents, and Adults: Solution (lacquer): Apply daily as part of a comprehensive management program for onychomycosis; remove with alcohol every 7 days; 48 weeks of continuous therapy may be needed to achieve clear nails

Children >16 years, Adolescents, and Adults:
Tinea pedis, tinea corporis: Gel: Apply twice daily. If no improvement after 4 weeks of treatment, re-evaluate diagnosis.
Seborrheic dermatitis of the scalp:
Gel: Apply twice daily. If no improvement after 4 weeks of treatment, re-evaluate diagnosis.
Shampoo: Apply ~5 mL to wet hair; may use up to 10 mL for longer hair; repeat twice weekly for 4 weeks; allow a minimum of 3 days between applications. If no improvement after 4 weeks of treatment, re-evaluate diagnosis.

Administration Topical:
Cream, gel, suspension: Gently massage into affected areas and surrounding skin.
Lotion: Shake lotion vigorously before application.
Shampoo: Apply to wet hair and scalp, lather, and leave in place ~3 minutes; rinse thoroughly.
Solution (lacquer): Apply evenly over the entire nail plate and 5 mm of surrounding skin using the applicator brush; allow to dry for 30 seconds. Solution can be reapplied daily over previous applications; remove with alcohol every 7 days. Avoid contact with eyes and mucous membranes; do not administer orally or intravaginally. Do not occlude affected area with dressings or wrappings.

Monitoring Parameters Resolution of skin or nail infection

Patient Information Contact physician if skin condition does not improve, if skin irritation develops, or if infection worsens after 4 weeks of treatment. Nail polish should not be applied on treated nails. Insulin-dependent diabetic patients or those with diabetic neuropathy should use caution when trimming infected nails.

Nursing Implications Once daily application of topical solution (nail lacquer) to infected nail(s) should occur at bedtime or 8 hours before bathing.

Dosage Forms Excipient information presented when available (limited, particularly for generics); consult specific product labeling. [DSC] = Discontinued product
Cream, topical, as olamine: 0.77% (15 g, 30 g, 90 g)
Loprox®: 0.77% (15 g, 30 g, 90 g) [contains benzyl alcohol] [DSC]

Gel, topical: 0.77% (30 g, 45 g, 100 g)
Loprox®: 0.77% (30 g, 45 g, 100 g) [contains isopropyl alcohol]
Shampoo, topical: 1% (120 mL)
Loprox®: 1% (120 mL)
Solution, topical [nail lacquer]: 8% (6.6 mL)
Penlac®: 8% (6.6 mL) [contains isopropyl alcohol]
Suspension, topical, as olamine: 0.77% (30 mL, 60 mL)
Loprox®: 0.77% (30 mL, 60 mL) [contains benzyl alcohol] [DSC]

References

Barber K, Claveau J, and Thomas R, "Review of Treatment for Onychomycosis: Consideration for Special Populations," *J Cutan Med Surg*, 2006, 10(Suppl 2):S48-53.

Gallup E, Plott T, and Ciclopirox TS Investigators, "A Multicenter, Open-Label Study to Assess the Safety and Efficacy of Ciclopirox Topical Suspension 0.77% in the Treatment of Diaper Dermatitis Due to *Candida albicans*," *J Drugs Dermatol*, 2005, 4(1):29-34.

◆ **Ciclopirox Ethanolamine** *see* Ciclopirox *on page 306*
◆ **Ciclopirox Olamine** *see* Ciclopirox *on page 306*
◆ **Cidecin** *see* DAPTOmycin *on page 389*

Cidofovir (si DOF o veer)

U.S. Brand Names Vistide®
Therapeutic Category Antiviral Agent, Parenteral
Generic Available No
Use Treatment of cytomegalovirus (CMV) retinitis in patients with acquired immunodeficiency syndrome (FDA approved in adults). Has also been used for treatment of ganciclovir-resistant CMV, foscarnet-resistant CMV, acyclovir-resistant HSV or VZV, and adenovirus infections in immunocompromised patients; treatment of recurrent respiratory papillomatosis
Pregnancy Risk Factor C
Pregnancy Considerations [U.S. Boxed Warning]: Possibly carcinogenic and teratogenic based on animal data. May cause hypospermia. Cidofovir was shown to be teratogenic and embryotoxic in animal studies, some at doses which also produced maternal toxicity. Reduced testes weight and hypospermia were also noted in animal studies. There are no adequate and well-controlled studies in pregnant women; use during pregnancy only if the potential benefit to the mother outweighs the possible risk to the fetus. Women of childbearing potential should use effective contraception during therapy and for 1 month following treatment. Males should use a barrier contraceptive during therapy and for 3 months following treatment.
Lactation Excretion in breast milk unknown/contraindicated
Breast-Feeding Considerations The CDC recommends **not** to breast-feed if diagnosed with HIV to avoid postnatal transmission of the virus.
Contraindications Hypersensitivity to cidofovir or any component; history of clinically severe hypersensitivity to probenecid or other sulfa-containing medications; patients with a serum creatinine >1.5 mg/dL, creatinine clearance ≤55 mL/minute, urine protein ≥100 mg/dL (≥2 plus proteinuria); patients who are receiving other nephrotoxic agents; direct intraocular injection
Warnings Hazardous agent; use appropriate precautions for handling and disposal. Administration in children warrants extreme caution due to risk of long-term toxicity. Possibly carcinogenic and teratogenic based on animal data, and may cause hypospermia **[U.S. Boxed Warning]**; contraceptive precautions for female patients need to be used during and for 1 month following therapy; male patients should practice barrier contraceptive methods during and for 3 months following treatment. Prepare admixture in a Class II laminar flow hood; administer and dispose according to guidelines issued for cytotoxic drugs.

May cause severe renal impairment **[U.S. Boxed Warning]**; acute renal failure resulting in dialysis and/or contributing to death has been reported to occur after as few as one or two cidofovir doses. Dose-dependent nephrotoxicity requires dose adjustment or discontinuation if changes in renal function occur during therapy (eg, proteinuria, glycosuria, decreased serum phosphate, uric acid or bicarbonate, and elevated creatinine). Decreased serum bicarbonate associated with proximal tubule injury and renal wasting syndrome (including Fanconi's syndrome) has also been reported. Cidofovir administration must be accompanied by oral probenecid and NS I.V. prehydration to reduce possible nephrotoxicity. Probencid may decrease the metabolic clearance of zidovudine; patients on concurrent zidovudine therapy should decrease dose by 50% or hold dose on days of cidofovir treatment.

May cause neutropenia **[U.S. Boxed Warning]**; ocular hypotony, iritis, and permanent impairment of vision have been reported in association with cidofovir treatment. Intraocular pressure may be decreased during therapy and has been associated with decreased visual acuity; fatal cases of metabolic acidosis associated with liver dysfunction and pancreatitis have been reported.

Adverse Reactions
Cardiovascular: Cardiomyopathy, edema, hypertension, hypotension, pallor, syncope, tachycardia
Central nervous system: Agitation, amnesia, anxiety, chills, confusion, dizziness, fever, hallucinations, headache, insomnia, malaise, personality/mood disorder, seizures, somnolence
Dermatologic: Acne, alopecia, pruritus, rash, skin discoloration, urticaria
Endocrine & metabolic: Dehydration, hyperglycemia, hyperlipidemia, hypocalcemia, hypokalemia, hypomagnesemia, hyponatremia, hypophosphatemia, metabolic acidosis, serum bicarbonate decreased
Gastrointestinal: Abdominal pain, abnormal taste, anorexia, cholangitis, colitis, constipation, diarrhea, dyspepsia, dysphagia, gastritis, nausea, oral moniliasis, pancreatitis, stomatitis, vomiting
Genitourinary: Glycosuria, hematuria, proteinuria, urinary incontinence
Hematologic: Anemia, neutropenia (not dose-related; occurs in up to 24% of AIDS patients; see Warnings), thrombocytopenia
Hepatic: AST and ALT increased, hepatomegaly
Neuromuscular & skeletal: Paresthesia, peripheral neuropathy, skeletal pain, weakness
Ocular: Amblyopia, conjunctivitis, intraocular pressure decreased, iritis (see Warnings), ocular hypotony, retinal detachment, uveitis
Renal: BUN and serum creatinine increased (see Warnings), Fanconi-like syndrome, tubular damage (dose-dependent)
Respiratory: Asthma, bronchitis, coughing, dyspnea, pharyngitis, pneumonia, rhinitis, sinusitis
Miscellaneous: Allergic reactions, diaphoresis
<1%, postmarketing, and/or case reports: Hepatic failure

Drug Interactions
Avoid Concomitant Use There are no known interactions where it is recommended to avoid concomitant use.
Increased Effect/Toxicity There are no known significant interactions involving an increase in effect.
Decreased Effect There are no known significant interactions involving a decrease in effect.
Stability Store at controlled room temperature 20°C to 25°C (68°F to 77°F); cidofovir admixture is stable for 24 hours under refrigeration.

◄ **Mechanism of Action** Cidofovir is converted to cidofovir diphosphate which is the active intracellular metabolite; suppresses CMV replication by selective inhibition of viral DNA polymerase; incorporation of cidofovir into the growing viral DNA chain results in reduction in the rate of viral DNA synthesis

Pharmacokinetics (Adult data unless noted)

Distribution: V_d: 0.54 L/kg; does not cross significantly into the CSF

Protein binding: <6%

Metabolism: Cidofovir is phosphorylated intracellularly to the active metabolite cidofovir diphosphate

Half-life: ~2.6 hours (cidofovir); 17 hours (cidofovir diphosphate)

Elimination: Renal tubular secretion and glomerular filtration

Renal clearance without probenecid: 130-170 mL/minute/ 1.73 m²

Renal clearance with probenecid: 70-125 mL/minute/ 1.73 m²

Usual Dosage

I.V.:

Children: **Note:** Administration of cidofovir should be accompanied by concomitant oral probenecid and I.V. NS hydration; various regimens have been reported (see Anderson, 2008; Bhadri, 2009; Cesaro, 2005; Doan, 2007; Williams, 2009)

Hydration: 20 mL/kg of 0.9% sodium chloride (maximum: 1000 mL) administered for 1 hour before cidofovir infusion and 20 mL/kg of 0.9% sodium chloride (maximum: 1000 mL) over 1 hour during cidofovir infusion, followed by 2 hours of maintenance fluids **or** increase the maintenance fluid infusion rate to 3 times the maintenance rate for 1 hour before cidofovir infusion and 1 hour after, then decrease to 2 times the maintenance fluid rate for the subsequent 2 hours

Probenecid: 25-40 mg/kg/dose (maximum dose: 2000 mg) administered 3 hours before cidofovir infusion and 10-20 mg/kg/dose (maximum dose: 1000 mg) at 2-3 hours and 8-9 hours after cidofovir infusion **or** 1-2 g/m²/dose administered 3 hours prior to cidofovir, followed by 0.5-1.25 g/m²/dose 1-2 hours and 8 hours after completion

Treatment of adenovirus infection posthematopoietic stem cell: Limited data available; specific regimens may vary (see Legrand, 2001; Ljungman, 2003; Yusuf, 2006)

Induction: 5 mg/kg/dose once weekly for 2 consecutive weeks (with hydration and probenecid)

Maintenance: 5 mg/kg/dose once every 2 weeks (with hydration and probenecid) until consecutive negative adenovirus samples. **Note:** Patients requiring longer treatment courses have been switched to 1 mg/kg/ dose given 3 times/week (see Bhadri, 2009)

Treatment of adenovirus infection postlung transplant: Available data limited to case series (see Doan, 2007): 1 mg/kg/dose every other day or 3 times/week for 4 consecutive weeks (with hydration and probenecid)

Treatment of cytomegalovirus (CMV) infection: Limited data available. Dosing based on reported experience in 30 pediatric patients (2-14 years) as second-line therapy following allogeneic stem cell transplantation (see Cesaro, 2005).

Induction: 5 mg/kg/dose once weekly for 2 consecutive weeks (with hydration, probenecid and antiemetic)

Maintenance: 3-5 mg/kg/dose once every 2 weeks for 2-4 doses (with hydration, probenecid and antiemetic)

BK virus allograft nephropathy: Limited data available. Dosing based on reported experience in eight renal transplant pediatric patients [1-18 doses (mean: 8)]: Initial dose: 0.25 mg/kg/dose every 2-3 weeks; dose may be increased if BK virus PCR counts do not decrease 1 log fold to a maximum dose of 1 mg/kg/ dose. The reported hydration was $D_5^1/_2NS$ or $D_5^1/_4NS$ for 2 hours before cidofovir and for 2 hours following the infusion; cidofovir was infused over 2 hours and no probenecid was used (see Araya, 2008).

BK virus hemorrhagic cystitis: Limited data available. Dosing based on experience in seven pediatric posthematopoietic stem cell transplant patients: 1 mg/kg/dose once weekly without probenecid for 3-12 weeks (mean duration: 6.5 weeks) (see Faraci, 2009)

Intralesional: Recurrent respiratory papillomatosis: 7.5 mg/mL every 2 weeks until complete remission (see Naiman, 2006).

Adults:

Cytomegalovirus (CMV) retinitis: Administer 2 g probenecid orally 3 hours prior to each cidofovir dose and 1 g at 2 and 8 hours after completion of the cidofovir infusion (total probenecid dose: 4 g); infuse one liter NS over 1-2 hours prior to the cidofovir infusion; may administer second liter of NS over 1-3 hours with or immediately after the cidofovir infusion if tolerated

Induction: 5 mg/kg/dose once weekly for 2 consecutive weeks

Maintenance: 5 mg/kg/dose once every other week

Intralesional: Recurrent respiratory papillomatosis: Injection volume is adapted case by case according to lesion extension and so not to cause airway obstruction. Injection is administered once monthly for 3-4 doses (see Naiman, 2003)

Dosing adjustment in renal impairment:

Children: If the serum Cl_{Cr} >1.5 mg/dL, Cl_{Cr} <90 mL/ minute/1.73 m², >2+ proteinuria, the following dosing has been used for treatment of adenovirus post-transplant (see Yusuf, 2006):

Induction: 1 mg/kg/dose 3 times/week on alternate days for 2 consecutive weeks

Maintenance: 1 mg/kg/dose every other week

Adults: If the serum creatinine increases by 0.3-0.4 mg/dL above baseline, reduce the cidofovir dose to 3 mg/kg; discontinue cidofovir therapy for increases ≥0.5 mg/dL above baseline or development of ≥3+ proteinuria.

Administration Do **not** administer by direct intraocular injection due to risk of iritis, ocular hypotony, and permanent visual impairment.

Parenteral: Administer by I.V. infusion over 1 hour. Dilute in 100 mL NS or D_5W or to a final concentration not to exceed 8 mg/mL.

Intralesional: May administer a solution with final concentration of 5-10 mg/mL

Monitoring Parameters Monitor renal function (BUN, serum creatinine), urinalysis (urine glucose and protein), CBC with differential (neutrophil count), electrolytes (calcium, magnesium, phosphorus, uric acid), liver function tests (SGOT/SGPT), intraocular pressure and visual acuity

Patient Information Cidofovir is not a cure for CMV retinitis; regular follow-up ophthalmologic exams and careful monitoring of renal function are necessary; report any rash immediately to your physician; use contraception during and for 3 months following treatment

Nursing Implications Administration of probenecid with a meal may decrease associated nausea; acetaminophen and antihistamines may ameliorate hypersensitivity reactions. Handle and dispose of cidofovir according to guidelines issued for cytotoxic drugs. Maintain adequate patient hydration.

Dosage Forms Excipient information presented when available (limited, particularly for generics); consult specific product labeling.

Injection, solution [preservative free]: 75 mg/mL (5 mL)

References

Anderson EJ, Guzman-Cottrill JA, Kletzel M, et al, "High-Risk Adenovirus-Infected Pediatric Allogeneic Hematopoietic Progenitor Cell Transplant Recipients and Preemptive Cidofovir Therapy," *Pediatr Transplant*, 2008, 12(2):219-27.

Araya CE, Lew JF, Fennell RS, et al, "Intermediate Dose Cidofovir Does Not Cause Additive Nephrotoxicity in BK Virus Allograft Nephropathy," *Pediatr Transplant*, 2008, 12(7):790-5.

Bhadri VA, Lee-Horn L, and Shaw PJ, "Safety and Tolerability of Cidofovir in High-Risk Pediatric Patients," *Transpl Infect Dis*, 2009, 11 (4):373-9.

Cesaro S, Zhou X, Manzardo C, et al, "Cidofovir for Cytomegalovirus Reactivation in Pediatric Patients After Hematopoietic Stem Cell Transplantation," *J Clin Virol*, 2005, 34(2):129-32.

Doan ML, Mallory GB, Kaplan SL, et al, "Treatment of Adenovirus Pneumonia With Cidofovir in Pediatric Lung Transplant Recipients," *J Heart Lung Transplant*, 2007, 26(9):883-9.

Faraci M, Cuzzubbo D, Lanino E, et al, "Low Dosage Cidofovir Without Probenecid as Treatment for BK Virus Hamorrhagic Cystitis After Hemopoietic Stem Cell Transplant," *Pediatr Infect Dis J*, 2009, 28 (1):55-7.

Izadifar-Legrand F, Berrebi D, Faye A, et al, "Early Diagnosis of Adenovirus Infection and Treatment With Cidofovir After Bone Marrow Transplantation in Children," *Blood*, 1999, 94:341a.

Lalezari JP, Holland GN, Kramer F, et al, "Randomized, Controlled Study of the Safety and Efficacy of Intravenous Cidofovir for the Treatment of Relapsing Cytomegalovirus Retinitis in Patients With AIDS," *J Acquir Immune Defic Syndr Hum Retrovirol*, 1998, 17 (4):339-44.

Legrand F, Berrebi D, Houhou N, et al, "Early Diagnosis of Adenovirus Infection and Treatment With Cidofovir After Bone Marrow Transplantation in Children," *Bone Marrow Transplant*, 2001, 27(6):621-6.

Ljungman P, Ribaud P, Eyrich M, et al, "Cidofovir for Adenovirus Infections After Allogeneic Hematopoietic Stem Cell Transplantation: A Survey by the Infectious Diseases Working Party of the European Group for Blood and Marrow Transplantation," *Bone Marrow Transplant*, 2003, 31(6):481-6.

Naiman AN, Ayari S, Nicollas R, et al, "Intermediate-Term and Long-Term Results After Treatment by Cidofovir and Excision in Juvenile Laryngeal Papillomatosis," *Ann Otol Rhinol Laryngol*, 2006, 115 (9):667-72.

Naiman AN, Ceruse P, Coulombeau B, et al, "Intralesional Cidofovir and Surgical Excision for Laryngeal Papillomatosis," *Laryngoscope*, 2003, 113(12):2174-81.

Ribaud P, Scieux C, Freymuth F, et al, "Successful Treatment of Adenovirus Disease With Intravenous Cidofovir in an Unrelated Stem-Cell Transplant Recipient," *Clinical Infectious Diseases*, 1999, 28 (3):690-1.

Williams KM, Agwu AL, Dabb AA, et al, "A Clinical Algorithm Identifies High Risk Pediatric Oncology and Bone Marrow Transplant Patients Likely to Benefit From Treatment of Adenoviral Infection," *J Pediatr Hematol Oncol*, 2009, 31(11):825-31.

Yusuf U, Hale GA, Carr J, et al, "Cidofovir for the Treatment of Adenoviral Infection in Pediatric Hematopoietic Stem Cell Transplant Patients," *Transplantation*, 2006, 81(10):1398-404.

◆ **Cilastatin and Imipenem** *see* Imipenem and Cilastatin *on page 714*

◆ **Ciloxan®** *see* Ciprofloxacin *on page 310*

Cimetidine (sye MET i deen)

Medication Safety Issues

Sound-alike/look-alike issues:

Cimetidine may be confused with simethicone

Beers Criteria medication: This drug may be inappropriate for use in geriatric patients (low severity risk).

U.S. Brand Names Tagamet® HB 200 [OTC]

Canadian Brand Names Apo-Cimetidine®; Dom-Cimetidine; Mylan-Cimetidine; Novo-Cimetidine; Nu-Cimet; PMS-Cimetidine; Tagamet® HB

Therapeutic Category Gastrointestinal Agent, Gastric or Duodenal Ulcer Treatment; Histamine H_2 Antagonist

Generic Available Yes

Use Short-term treatment of active duodenal ulcers and benign gastric ulcers; long-term prophylaxis of duodenal ulcer; gastric hypersecretory states; gastroesophageal reflux (GERD); prevention of upper GI bleeding in critically ill patients; over-the-counter (OTC) formulation for relief of acid indigestion, heartburn, or sour stomach

Pregnancy Risk Factor B

Pregnancy Considerations Teratogenic events were not observed in animal studies.

Lactation Enters breast milk/not recommended

Contraindications Hypersensitivity to cimetidine or any component (see Warnings)

Warnings Rapid I.V. administration may cause hypotension or cardiac arrhythmias. Use of gastric acid inhibitors including proton pump inhibitors and H_2 blockers has been associated with an increased risk for development of acute gastroenteritis and community-acquired pneumonia (Canani, 2006). A large epidemiological study has suggested an increased risk for developing pneumonia in patients receiving H_2 receptor antagonists; however, a causal relationship with cimetidine has not been demonstrated.

Precautions Modify dosage in patients with renal and/or hepatic impairment; multiple drug interactions exist requiring dose modifications of other medications or cimetidine (see Drug Interactions)

Adverse Reactions

Cardiovascular: Bradycardia, hypotension, cardiac arrhythmias (after rapid I.V. administration), tachycardia

Central nervous system: Dizziness, mental confusion, agitation, headache, psychosis, drowsiness, fever

Dermatologic: Rash

Endocrine & metabolic: Gynecomastia

Gastrointestinal: Mild diarrhea, nausea, vomiting

Hematologic: Neutropenia, agranulocytosis, thrombocytopenia

Hepatic: AST and ALT elevated

Neuromuscular & skeletal: Myalgia

Renal: Serum creatinine elevated

Respiratory: Pneumonia (causal relationship has not been established; see Warnings)

Drug Interactions

Metabolism/Transport Effects Substrate of P-glycoprotein; **Inhibits** CYP1A2 (moderate), 2C9 (weak), 2C19 (moderate), 2D6 (moderate), 2E1 (weak), 3A4 (moderate)

Avoid Concomitant Use

Avoid concomitant use of Cimetidine with any of the following: Clopidogrel; Delavirdine; Dofetilide; Erlotinib; Thioridazine; Tolvaptan

Increased Effect/Toxicity

Cimetidine may increase the levels/effects of: Alfentanil; Amiodarone; Anticonvulsants (Hydantoin); Benzodiazepines (metabolized by oxidation); Calcium Channel Blockers; CarBAMazepine; Carmustine; Carvedilol; Cisapride; Clozapine; Colchicine; CYP1A2 Substrates; CYP2C19 Substrates; CYP2D6 Substrates; CYP3A4 Substrates; Dofetilide; Eplerenone; Everolimus; FentaNYL; Fesoterodine; Halofantrine; MetFORMIN; Moclobemide; Nebivolol; Nicotine; Pentoxifylline; Pimecrolimus; Pramipexole; Praziquantel; Procainamide; Propafenone; QuiNIDine; QuiNINE; Ranolazine; Salmeterol; Saquinavir; Saxagliptin; Selective Serotonin Reuptake Inhibitors; Sulfonylureas; Tamoxifen; Theophylline Derivatives; Thioridazine; Tolvaptan; Tricyclic Antidepressants; Vitamin K Antagonists; Zaleplon; Zolmitriptan

The levels/effects of Cimetidine may be increased by: P-Glycoprotein Inhibitors

Decreased Effect

Cimetidine may decrease the levels/effects of: Antifungal Agents (Azole Derivatives, Systemic); Atazanavir; Cefditoren; Cefpodoxime; Cefuroxime; Clopidogrel; Codeine; Dasatinib; Delavirdine; Erlotinib; Fosamprenavir; Indinavir; Iron Salts; Mesalamine; Nelfinavir; TraMADol

The levels/effects of Cimetidine may be decreased by: P-Glycoprotein Inducers

Food Interactions Limit xanthine-containing foods and beverages

Stability Protect from light; store at room temperature; do not refrigerate the injection since precipitation may occur (can be redissolved by warming without degradation); stable in parenteral nutrition solutions for up to 7 days when protected from light

Mechanism of Action Competitive inhibition of histamine at H_2-receptors of the gastric parietal cells resulting in reduced gastric acid secretion

Pharmacokinetics (Adult data unless noted)

Distribution: Crosses the placenta; breast milk to plasma ratio: 4.6-11.76

Protein binding: 13% to 25%

Metabolism: Hepatic with a sulfoxide as the major metabolite

Bioavailability: 60% to 70%

Half-life:

Neonates: 3.6 hours

Children: 1.4 hours

Adults with normal renal function: 2 hours

Time to peak serum concentration: Oral: 45-90 minutes

Elimination: Primarily in urine (48% unchanged drug); some excretion in bile and feces

Usual Dosage

Neonates: Oral, I.M., I.V.: 5-10 mg/kg/day in divided doses every 8-12 hours

Infants: Oral, I.M., I.V.: 10-20 mg/kg/day divided every 6-12 hours

Children: Oral, I.M., I.V.: 20-40 mg/kg/day in divided doses every 6 hours

Adults:

Short-term treatment of active ulcers:

Oral: 300 mg 4 times/day or 800 mg at bedtime or 400 mg twice daily for up to 8 weeks

I.M., I.V.: 300 mg every 6 hours or 150 mg single dose followed by 37.5 mg/hour by continuous infusion; adjust dosage to maintain an intragastric pH ≥5 or acid secretory rate of <10 mEq/hour; (average dose 160 mg/hour; range: 40-600 mg/hour)

Duodenal ulcer prophylaxis: Oral: 400-800 mg at bedtime

Gastric hypersecretory conditions: Oral, I.M., I.V.: 300-600 mg every 6 hours; dosage not to exceed 2.4 g/day

GERD: Oral: 800 mg twice daily or 400 mg 4 times/day for 12 weeks

Acid indigestion, heartburn, sour stomach relief (OTC use): Oral: 100 mg right before or up to 30 minutes before a meal; no more than 2 tablets per day

Prevention of upper GI bleeding: Continuous I.V. infusion of 50 mg/hour

Dosing interval in renal impairment using 5-10 mg/kg/ dose in children or 300 mg in adults (titrate dose to gastric pH and Cl_{cr}):

Cl_{cr} >40 mL/minute: Administer every 6 hours

Cl_{cr} 20-40 mL/minute: Administer every 8 hours or reduce dose by 25%

Cl_{cr} <20 mL/minute: Administer every 12 hours or reduce dose by 50%

Hemodialysis: Administer after dialysis and every 12 hours during the interdialysis period

Dosing adjustment in hepatic impairment: Reduce dosage in severe liver disease

Administration

Oral: Administer with food; do not administer with antacids

Parenteral: Can be administered as a slow I.V. push over 15 minutes (minimum 5 minutes; rapid administration has been associated with hypotension and cardiac arrhythmias) at a concentration not to exceed 15 mg/mL; or preferably as an I.V. intermittent or I.V. continuous infusion. Intermittent infusions are administered over 15-30 minutes at a final concentration not to exceed 6 mg/mL; for patients with an active bleed, preferred method of administration is continuous infusion; may be administered intramuscularly

Monitoring Parameters Blood pressure and heart rate with I.V. push administration; CBC; gastric pH

Patient Information Avoid excessive amount of coffee and aspirin; when self medicating, if symptoms of heartburn, acid indigestion, or sour stomach persist after 2 weeks of continuous use of the drug, consult a clinician; notify your physician if taking other medications (multiple drug interactions exist)

Dosage Forms Excipient information presented when available (limited, particularly for generics); consult specific product labeling. [DSC] = Discontinued product

Note: Strength is expressed as base

Infusion, as hydrochloride [premixed in NS]: 300 mg (50 mL) [DSC]

Injection, solution, as hydrochloride: 150 mg/mL (2 mL, 8 mL) [DSC]

Solution, oral, as hydrochloride: 300 mg/5 mL (240 mL, 480 mL)

Tablet: 200 mg [OTC], 300 mg, 400 mg, 800 mg

Tagamet® HB 200: 200 mg

References

Canani RB, Cirillo P, Roggero P, et al, "Therapy With Gastric Acidity Inhibitors Increases the Risk of Acute Gastroenteritis and Community-Acquired Pneumonia in Children," *Pediatrics*, 2006, 117(5):e817-20.

Lambert J, Mobassaleh M, and Grand RJ, "Efficacy of Cimetidine for Gastric Acid Suppression in Pediatric Patients," *J Pediatr*, 1992, 120 (3):474-8.

Lloyd CW, Martin WJ, Taylor BD, et al, "Pharmacokinetics and Pharmacodynamics of Cimetidine and Metabolites in Critically Ill Children," *J Pediatr*, 1985, 107(2):295-300.

Lloyd CW, Martin WJ, and Taylor BD, "The Pharmacokinetics of Cimetidine and Metabolites in a Neonate," *Drug Intell Clin Pharm*, 1985, 19(3):203-5.

Somogyi A and Gugler R, "Clinical Pharmacokinetics of Cimetidine," *Clin Pharmacokinet*, 1983, 8(6):463-95.

◆ **Cipralex® (Can)** *see* Escitalopram *on page 529*

◆ **Cipro®** *see* Ciprofloxacin *on page 310*

◆ **Cipro® XL (Can)** *see* Ciprofloxacin *on page 310*

◆ **Ciprodex®** *see* Ciprofloxacin and Dexamethasone *on page 314*

Ciprofloxacin (sip roe FLOKS a sin)

Medication Safety Issues

Sound-alike/look-alike issues:

Cetraxal® may be confused with cefTRIAXone

Ciprofloxacin may be confused with cephalexin

Ciloxan® may be confused with cinoxacin, Cytoxan

Cipro® may be confused with Ceftin®

U.S. Brand Names Cetraxal®; Ciloxan®; Cipro®; Cipro® I.V.; Cipro® XR; Proquin® XR

Canadian Brand Names Apo-Ciproflox®; Ciloxan®; Cipro®; Cipro® XL; CO Ciprofloxacin; Dom-Ciprofloxacin; Mint-Ciprofloxacin; Mylan-Ciprofloxacin; Novo-Ciprofloxacin; PHL-Ciprofloxacin; PMS-Ciprofloxacin; PRO-Ciprofloxacin; RAN™-Ciprofloxacin; ratio-Ciprofloxacin; Riva-Ciprofloxacin; Sandoz-Ciprofloxacin; Taro-Ciprofloxacin

Therapeutic Category Antibiotic, Ophthalmic; Antibiotic, Otic; Antibiotic, Quinolone

Generic Available Yes: Excludes ointment, otic solution, suspension

Use Treatment of documented or suspected pseudomonal infection of the respiratory or urinary tract, skin and soft tissue, bone and joint (FDA approved in adults); treatment of complicated UTIs and pyelonephritis due to *E. coli* (FDA approved in ages 1-17); documented multidrug-resistant, aerobic gram-negative bacilli, some gram-positive staphylococci, and *Mycobacterium tuberculosis*; documented infectious diarrhea due to *Campylobacter jejuni*, *Shigella*, or *E. coli*; typhoid fever caused by *Salmonella typhi*; osteomyelitis caused by susceptible organisms in which parenteral therapy is not feasible; uncomplicated cervical and urethral gonorrhea due to *N. gonorrhoeae*; chronic bacterial prostatitis caused by *E. coli* or *Proteus mirabilis* (FDA approved in adults); pulmonary exacerbation of cystic fibrosis; empiric therapy for febrile neutropenia in combination with piperacillin (FDA approved in adults); initial therapy or postexposure prophylaxis for inhalational anthrax (FDA approved in children and adults); used ophthalmically for treatment of corneal ulcers and conjunctivitis due to susceptible organisms (topical ointment FDA approved in ages >2 years to adults); extended release tablet is used for the treatment of UTI and acute uncomplicated pyelonephritis caused by susceptible *E. coli* and *Klebsiella pneumoniae*; treatment of acute otitis externa caused by susceptible *Pseudomonas aeruginosa* or *Staphylococcus aureus* [otic solution (FDA approved in ages >1 year to adults)]

Medication Guide An FDA-approved patient medication guide, which is available with the product information and as follows, must be dispensed with this medication for each new outpatient prescription and refill.

    Cipro®: http://www.accessdata.fda.gov/drugsatfda_docs/label/2009/019537s7019847444198575120780282147325L.pdf

    Proquin® XR: http://www.accessdata.fda.gov/drugsatfda_docs/label/2009/021744s012lbl.pdf

Pregnancy Risk Factor C

Pregnancy Considerations Adverse events have been observed in some animal studies; therefore, the manufacturer classifies ciprofloxacin as pregnancy category C. Ciprofloxacin crosses the placenta and produces measurable concentrations in the amniotic fluid and cord serum. An increased risk of teratogenic effects has not been observed in animals or humans following ciprofloxacin use during pregnancy; however, because of concerns of cartilage damage in immature animals, ciprofloxacin should only be used during pregnancy if a safer option is not available. Ciprofloxacin is recommended for prophylaxis and treatment of pregnant women exposed to anthrax. Serum concentrations of ciprofloxacin may be lower during pregnancy than in nonpregnant patients.

Lactation Enters breast milk/not recommended (AAP rates "compatible")

Breast-Feeding Considerations Ciprofloxacin is excreted in breast milk. Breast-feeding is not recommended by the manufacturer. The AAP considers ciprofloxacin to be "usually compatible with breast-feeding." Due to the low concentrations in human milk, minimal toxicity would be expected in the nursing infant and infant serum levels were undetectable in one report. Nondose-related effects could include modification of bowel flora. There has been a single case report of perforated pseudomembranous colitis in a breast-feeding infant whose mother was taking ciprofloxacin.

Contraindications Hypersensitivity to ciprofloxacin, any component, or other quinolones; concomitant administration with tizanidine; not recommended for use in pregnant women or during breast-feeding

Warnings Ciprofloxacin is not a drug of first choice in the pediatric population due to reported adverse events related to joints and/or surrounding tissues. Ciprofloxacin has caused arthropathy with erosions of the cartilage in weight bearing joints of immature animals; green

discoloration of teeth in newborns has been reported; Achilles tendonitis and tendon rupture have been reported with fluoroquinolones in patients of all ages **[U.S. Boxed Warning]**; risk increased in patients taking concomitant corticosteroids, patients >60 years of age, and in patients with kidney, heart, or lung transplants. Prolonged use may result in superinfection, including *C. difficile*-associated diarrhea and pseudomembranous colitis; CNS stimulation, increased intracranial pressure, and toxic psychosis may occur resulting in tremors, restlessness, confusion, and very rarely hallucinations, depression, nightmares, suicidal ideation, or convulsive seizures. If these reactions occur, discontinue ciprofloxacin. Rare cases of polyneuropathy affecting small and/or large axons resulting in paresthesias, hypoesthesias, dysesthesias, and weakness have been reported in patients receiving ciprofloxacin. Discontinue ciprofloxacin if patient experiences pain, burning, tingling, numbness, weakness, or is found to have deficits in light touch, pain, temperature, position sense, vibrating sensation, or motor strength.

Coadministration of ciprofloxacin with drugs metabolized by CYP1A2 (eg, theophylline, caffeine, tizanidine) may result in increased plasma concentrations of the coadministered drug with corresponding side effects. Serious and fatal reactions including cardiac arrest, seizure, status epilepticus, and respiratory failure have been reported in patients receiving ciprofloxacin and theophylline concurrently. Serum theophylline levels should be monitored and dosage adjustments made when concomitant use cannot be avoided. Hypotension and oversedation have been reported when ciprofloxacin and tizanidine were given concomitantly (concomitant administration of tizanidine and ciprofloxacin is contraindicated). Severe hypersensitivity reactions, including life-threatening anaphylactic shock, have been reported in patients receiving quinolones. If an allergic reaction occurs, discontinue drug immediately.

Precautions Use with caution in patients with known or suspected CNS disorders, seizure disorders, severe cerebral arteriosclerosis, or renal impairment; modify dosage in patients with renal impairment. Avoid excessive sunlight and take precautions to limit exposure (eg, loose-fitting clothing, sunscreen); may rarely cause moderate-to-severe phototoxicity reactions. Discontinue use if phototoxicity occurs.

Adverse Reactions

Cardiovascular: Angina pectoris, arrhythmia, atrial flutter, flushing, hypertension, hypotension, migraine, palpitations, syncope, tachycardia, torsade de pointes, vasculitis

Central nervous system: Agitation, confusion, depression, dizziness, fever, hallucinations, headache, insomnia, nervousness, nightmares, paranoia, restlessness, somnolence, seizures

Dermatologic: Angioedema, erythema multiforme, exfoliative dermatitis, Lyell's syndrome, photosensitivity, pruritus, rash, Stevens-Johnson syndrome, urticaria

Endocrine & metabolic: Cholesterol increased, hyperglycemia, lipase increased, serum triglyceride increased

Gastrointestinal: Abdominal pain, anorexia, constipation, diarrhea, GI bleeding, nausea, pseudomembranous colitis, pancreatitis, vomiting

Genitourinary: Crystalluria

Hematologic: Agranulocytosis, anemia, eosinophilia, neutropenia

Hepatic: Cholestatic jaundice, hepatitis, liver enzymes increased

Local: I.V.: Burning, erythema, pain, phlebitis, swelling (occurs more frequently with infusion time <30 minutes)

Neuromuscular & skeletal: Arthralgia, arthritis, back pain, dysesthesias, hypoesthesias, joint pain, joint stiffness, myalgia, myoclonus, paresthesias, peripheral neuropathy, tendon rupture, tendonitis, tremor, weakness

Ocular: Blurred vision, nystagmus; Ophthalmic ointment: Dry eye, eye pain, keratoconjunctivitis, photophobia, retardation of corneal healing, visual blurring

Otic: Hearing loss; Otic solution: Application site pain, fungal superinfection, pruritus

Renal: Acute renal failure, BUN and serum creatinine increased, hematuria, interstitial nephritis

Respiratory: Bronchospasm, dyspnea, pulmonary edema

Miscellaneous: Anaphylaxis, diaphoresis, serum sickness

Drug Interactions

Metabolism/Transport Effects Substrate of P-glycoprotein; **Inhibits** CYP1A2 (strong), 3A4 (weak)

Avoid Concomitant Use

Avoid concomitant use of Ciprofloxacin with any of the following: BCG; TiZANidine

Increased Effect/Toxicity

Ciprofloxacin may increase the levels/effects of: Bendamustine; Caffeine; Corticosteroids (Systemic); CYP1A2 Substrates; Erlotinib; Methotrexate; Pentoxifylline; QTc-Prolonging Agents; Ropinirole; Ropivacaine; Sulfonylureas; Theophylline Derivatives; TiZANidine; Vitamin K Antagonists

The levels/effects of Ciprofloxacin may be increased by: Insulin; Nonsteroidal Anti-Inflammatory Agents; P-Glycoprotein Inhibitors; Probenecid

Decreased Effect

Ciprofloxacin may decrease the levels/effects of: BCG; Mycophenolate; Phenytoin; Sulfonylureas; Typhoid Vaccine

The levels/effects of Ciprofloxacin may be decreased by: Antacids; Calcium Salts; Didanosine; Iron Salts; Magnesium Salts; P-Glycoprotein Inducers; Quinapril; Sevelamer; Sucralfate; Zinc Salts

Food Interactions Dairy foods (milk, yogurt) and mineral supplements decrease ciprofloxacin concentrations; avoid concomitant administration with dairy products, enteral feedings (enteral feeds need to be discontinued for 1-2 hours prior to and after ciprofloxacin administration), mineral supplements, iron, zinc, or with calcium-fortified juices; ciprofloxacin increases caffeine concentrations; use caution with xanthine-containing foods and beverages

Stability Premixed bags: Out of overwrap stability: 14 days at room temperature; reconstituted oral suspension: Stable for 14 days when stored at room temperature or refrigerated; store tablets, intact injection vial, ophthalmic solution/ointment, and oral suspension prior to reconstitution at room temperature; protect from intense light; protect from freezing

Mechanism of Action Inhibits DNA-gyrase and topoisomerase IV in susceptible organisms; inhibits relaxation of supercoiled DNA and promotes breakage of double-stranded DNA

Pharmacokinetics (Adult data unless noted)

Absorption: Oral: Well absorbed. 500 mg orally every 12 hours produces an equivalent AUC to that produced by 400 mg I.V. over 60 minutes every 12 hours.

Distribution: Widely distributed into body tissues and fluids with high concentration in bile, saliva, urine, sputum, stool, lungs, liver, skin, muscle, prostate, genital tissue, and bone; low concentration in CSF; crosses the placenta; appears in breast milk

Protein binding: 16% to 43%

Metabolism: Partially in the liver to four active metabolites

Bioavailability: Oral: 50% to 85%; younger CF patients have a lower bioavailability of 68% versus CF patients >13 years of age with bioavailability of 95%

Half-life:
Children: 4-5 hours
Adults with normal renal function: 3-5 hours

Time to peak serum concentration: Oral: Immediate release tablet: Within 0.5-2 hours; Extended release tablet: Cipro® XR: 1-4 hours; Proquin® XR: 3.5-8.7 hours

Elimination: 30% to 50% excreted as unchanged drug in urine via glomerular filtration and active tubular secretion; 20% to 40% excreted in feces primarily from biliary excretion; <1% excreted in bile as unchanged drug

Clearance: After I.V.:
CF child: 0.84 L/hour/kg
Adult: 0.5-0.6 L/hour/kg

Dialysis: Only small amounts of ciprofloxacin are removed by dialysis (<10%)

Usual Dosage Note: Extended release tablets and immediate release formulations are not interchangeable. Unless otherwise specified, oral dosing reflects the use of immediate release formulation.

Neonates: I.V. ciprofloxacin has been used in 23 neonates at doses ranging from 7-40 mg/kg/day divided every 12 hours (Schaad, 1995)

Children:
Oral: 20-30 mg/kg/day in 2 divided doses; maximum dose: 1.5 g/day
I.V.: 20-30 mg/kg/day divided every 12 hours; maximum dose: 800 mg/day

Inhalational anthrax (postexposure): Initial treatment:
I.V.: 20 mg/kg/day divided every 12 hours for 60 days; maximum dose: 800 mg/day (substitute oral antibiotics for I.V. antibiotics as soon as clinical condition improves)
Oral: 30 mg/kg/day divided every 12 hours for 60 days; maximum dose: 1000 mg/day

Complicated UTI or pyelonephritis:
I.V.: 18-30 mg/kg/day divided every 8 hours for 10-21 days; maximum dose: 1200 mg/day
Oral: 20-40 mg/kg/day divided every 12 hours for 10-21 days; maximum dose: 1500 mg/day

Cystic fibrosis:
Oral: 40 mg/kg/day divided every 12 hours; maximum dose: 2 g/day
I.V.: 30 mg/kg/day divided every 8-12 hours; maximum dose: 1.2 g/day

Adults:
Oral: 250-750 mg every 12 hours, depending on severity of infection and susceptibility

Acute sinusitis: Mild/moderate: 500 mg every 12 hours for 10 days

Uncomplicated UTI/acute cystitis:
Extended release tablet: 500 mg every 24 hours for 3 days
Immediate release formulation: Acute uncomplicated: 250 mg every 12 hours for 3 days; 250 mg every 12 hours for 7-14 days for mild to moderate UTI

Complicated UTI or acute uncomplicated pyelonephritis:
Extended release tablet: 1000 mg every 24 hours for 7-14 days
Immediate release formulation: 500 mg every 12 hours for 7-14 days

Bone and joint infections:
Mild/moderate: 500 mg every 12 hours for ≥4 to 6 weeks
Severe/complicated: 750 mg every 12 hours for ≥4 to 6 weeks

Chemoprophylaxis regimen for high-risk contacts of invasive meningococcal disease: 500 mg as a single dose

Chronic bacterial prostatitis: 500 mg every 12 hours for 28 days

Infectious diarrhea: 500 mg every 12 hours for 5-7 days

Skin and skin structure infections:

Mild/moderate: 500 mg every 12 hours for 7-14 days

Severe/complicated: 750 mg every 12 hours for 7-14 days

Uncomplicated gonorrhea: 500 mg as a single dose

Chancroid: 500 mg twice daily for 3 days

Lower respiratory tract infection:

Mild/moderate: 500 mg every 12 hours for 7-14 days

Severe/complicated: 750 mg every 12 hours for 7-14 days

Typhoid fever: 500 mg every 12 hours for 10 days

Inhalational anthrax (postexposure prophylaxis): 500 mg every 12 hours for 60 days

I.V.: 200-400 mg every 8-12 hours depending on severity of infection

Lower respiratory tract, skin and skin structure infection:

Mild/moderate: 400 mg every 12 hours for 7-14 days

Severe/complicated: 400 mg every 8 hours for 7-14 days

Treatment of anthrax infection: 400 mg every 12 hours for 60 days (substitute oral antibiotics for I.V. antibiotics as soon as clinical condition improves)

Empiric therapy in febrile neutropenic patients: 400 mg every 8 hours in combination with piperacillin for 7-14 days

Ophthalmic:

Children ≥1 year and Adults: Solution: Instill 1-2 drops into the affected eye(s) every 2 hours while awake for 2 days, then 1-2 drops every 4 hours while awake for the next 5 days

Treatment of corneal ulcers: Instill 2 drops every 15 minutes for the first 6 hours, then 2 drops every 30 minutes for the remainder of the first day; on the second day, 2 drops every hour; then 2 drops every 4 hours thereafter

Children ≥2 years and Adults: Ointment: Instill 0.5" ointment ribbon 3 times/day for 2 days, then twice daily for the next 5 days

Otic: Children ≥1 year and Adults: Acute otitis externa: Instill 0.25 mL (contents of 1 single dose container) into affected ear(s) twice daily for 7 days

Dosing interval in renal impairment: Adults:

Cl$_{cr}$ 30-50 mL/minute: Oral: 250-500 mg every 12 hours

Cl$_{cr}$ <30 mL/minute:

Immediate release formulations: 250-500 mg every 18 hours

Extended release tablet: Complicated UTI or acute uncomplicated pyelonephritis: 500 mg every 24 hours

Patients on hemodialysis or peritoneal dialysis: Immediate release formulations: 250-500 mg every 24 hours after dialysis

Administration

Oral: Administer immediate release tablets 2 hours after a meal; may administer with food to minimize GI upset; extended release tablet and oral suspension may be administered with or without food; Proquin® XR should be administered with a main meal (evening meal preferred); do not administer oral suspension through a feeding tube (suspension will adhere to the feeding tube); to prepare oral suspension, pour the microcapsules (small bottle) completely into the large bottle of diluent - DO NOT ADD WATER TO THE SUSPENSION. Shake suspension vigorously for 15 seconds before use. Avoid antacid use. Drink plenty of fluids to maintain proper hydration and urine output

Nasogastric/orogastric tube: Crush immediate release tablet and mix with water. Flush feeding tube before and after ciprofloxacin administration with water. Hold tube feeding at least 1 hour before and 2 hours after administration.

Parenteral: Administer by slow I.V. infusion over 60 minutes to reduce the risk of venous irritation (burning, pain, erythema, and swelling); final concentration for administration should not exceed 2 mg/mL

Ophthalmic: For topical ophthalmic use only. Avoid contacting tip with skin or eye.

Ointment: Instill ointment in the lower conjunctival sac

Solution: Apply finger pressure to lacrimal sac during and for 1-2 minutes after instillation to decrease risk of absorption and systemic effects

Otic: For otic use only. Prior to use, warm solution by holding container in hands for at least 1 minute. Patient should lie down with affected ear upward and medication instilled. Patients should remain in the position for at least 1 minute to allow penetration of solution.

Monitoring Parameters Monitor renal, hepatic, and hematopoietic function periodically; number and type of stools/day for diarrhea. Patients receiving concurrent ciprofloxacin and theophylline should have serum levels of theophylline monitored; monitor INR in patients receiving warfarin; patients receiving concurrent ciprofloxacin and cyclosporine should have cyclosporine levels monitored

Reference Range Avoid peak serum concentrations >5 mcg/mL

Patient Information Do not chew microcapsules of the oral suspension; do not split, crush, or chew extended release tablet; avoid caffeine; may cause dizziness or lightheadedness and impair ability to perform activities requiring mental alertness or physical coordination. Notify physician if tendon pain or swelling occurs, signs of allergy; burning, tingling, numbness, or weakness develops or persistent diarrhea occurs. Remove contact lenses prior to administration of ophthalmic solution and ointment. May cause photosensitivity reactions (eg, exposure to sunlight may cause severe sunburn, skin rash, redness, or itching); avoid exposure to sunlight and artificial light sources (sunlamps, tanning booth/bed); wear protective clothing, wide-brimmed hats, sunglasses, and lip sunscreen (SPF ≥15); use a sunscreen [broad-spectrum sunscreen or physical sunscreen (preferred) or sunblock with SPF ≥15]; contact physician if reaction occurs.

Nursing Implications Administer immediate release ciprofloxacin and Cipro® XR at least 2 hours before or 6 hours after, and Proquin® XR at least 4 hours before or 2 hours after antacids or other products containing calcium, iron, or zinc (including dairy products or calcium-fortified juices), sucralfate, or highly buffered drugs; ensure adequate patient hydration to prevent crystalluria. Cipro® XR and Proquin® XR are not interchangeable with ciprofloxacin immediate-release tablets.

Additional Information Although fluoroquinolones are only FDA approved for use in children for complicated UTI, pyelonephritis, and postexposure treatment for inhalational anthrax, the AAP has provided a list of other possible uses for fluoroquinolones once risks and benefits have been assessed to justify its use:

• UTI caused by *Pseudomonas aeruginosa* or other multidrug-resistant, gram-negative bacteria susceptible to fluoroquinolones

• Chronic suppurative otitis media or otitis externa caused by *P. aeruginosa*

• Chronic or acute osteomyelitis or osteochondritis caused by *P. aeruginosa*

• Mycobacterial infections caused by isolates sensitive to fluoroquinolones

• Gram-negative bacterial infections in immunocompromised hosts in which oral therapy is desired or resistance to alternative agents is present

Dosage Forms Excipient information presented when available (limited, particularly for generics); consult specific product labeling. [DSC] = Discontinued product

Infusion [premixed in D$_5$W]: 200 mg (100 mL); 400 mg (200 mL)

Cipro® I.V.: 200 mg (100 mL); 400 mg (200 mL)

Injection, solution [concentrate]: 10 mg/mL (20 mL, 40 mL, 120 mL)

Cipro® I.V.: 10 mg/mL (20 mL, 40 mL) [DSC]

Microcapsules for suspension, oral:

Cipro®: 250 mg/5 mL (100 mL); 500 mg/5 mL (100 mL) [strawberry flavor]

Ointment, ophthalmic, as hydrochloride:

Ciloxan®: 3.33 mg/g (3.5 g) [equivalent to ciprofloxacin base 0.3%]

Solution, ophthalmic, as hydrochloride: 3.5 mg/mL (2.5 mL, 5mL, 10 mL) [equivalent to ciprofloxacin base 0.3%]

Ciloxan®: 3.5 mg/mL (5 mL) [0.3% base; contains benzalkonium chloride]

Solution, otic, as hydrochloride [preservative free]:

Cetraxal®: 0.5 mg/0.25 mL (14s) [equivalent to ciprofloxacin base 0.2%]

Tablet, as hydrochloride: 100 mg [strength expressed as base], 250 mg [strength expressed as base], 500 mg [strength expressed as base], 750 mg [strength expressed as base]

Cipro®: 250 mg [strength expressed as base], 500 mg [strength expressed as base], 750 mg [strength expressed as base]

Tablet, extended release, as base and hydrochloride: 500 mg [strength expressed as base], 1000 mg [strength expressed as base]

Cipro® XR: 500 mg [strength expressed as base], 1000 mg [strength expressed as base]

Tablet, extended release, as hydrochloride:

Proquin® XR: 500 mg [strength expressed as base]

Tablet, extended release, as hydrochloride [dose pack]:

Proquin® XR: 500 mg (3s) [strength expressed as base]

References

Campoli-Richards DM, Monk JP, Price A, et al, "Ciprofloxacin: A Review of Its Antibacterial Activity, Pharmacokinetic Properties and Therapeutic Use," Drugs, 1988, 35(4):373-447.

Inglesby TV, Henderson DA, Bartlett JG, et al, "Anthrax as a Biological Weapon: Medical and Public Health Management. Working Group on Civilian Biodefense," JAMA, 1999, 281(18):1735-45.

Rodriguez WJ, and Wiedermann BL, "The Role of Newer Oral Cephalosporins, Fluoroquinolones, and Macrolides in the Treatment of Pediatric Infections," Adv Pediatr Infect Dis, 1994, 9:125-59.

Rubio TT, Miles MV, Lettieri JT, et al, "Pharmacokinetic Disposition of Sequential Intravenous/Oral Ciprofloxacin in Pediatric Cystic Fibrosis Patients with Acute Pulmonary Exacerbation," Pediatr Infect Dis J, 1997, 16:112-7.

Schaad UB, abdus Salam M, Aujard Y, et al, "Use of Fluoroquinolones in Pediatrics: Consensus Report of an International Society of Chemotherapy Commission," Pediatr Infect Dis J, 1995, 14(1):1-9.

Ciprofloxacin and Dexamethasone
(sip roe FLOKS a sin & deks a METH a sone)

U.S. Brand Names Ciprodex®

Canadian Brand Names Ciprodex®

Therapeutic Category Antibiotic/Corticosteroid, Otic

Generic Available No

Use Treatment of acute otitis media in pediatric patients with tympanostomy tubes due to *S. aureus, S. pneumoniae, H. influenzae, M. catarrhalis,* or *P. aeruginosa*; acute otitis externa in children and adults due to *S. aureus* or *P. aeruginosa*

Pregnancy Risk Factor C

Pregnancy Considerations Refer to individual agents. Reproduction studies have not been conducted with the otic preparation. Ciprofloxacin is detectable in the serum following otic administration.

Lactation Excretion in breast milk unknown/not recommended

Breast-Feeding Considerations It is not known if serum levels of ciprofloxacin or dexamethasone are high enough following otic administration to produce detectable quantities in breast milk.

Contraindications Hypersensitivity to ciprofloxacin, other quinolones, dexamethasone, or any component; herpes simplex or other viral infections of the external ear canal

Warnings For otic use only; do not administer parenterally or ophthalmically

Adverse Reactions

Central nervous system: Irritability, dizziness

Dermatologic: Rash

Gastrointestinal: Taste perversion

Otic: Ear discomfort (3%), ear pain (2.3%), ear precipitate (residue) (0.5%), tinnitus, ear pruritus and erythema

Drug Interactions

Avoid Concomitant Use

Avoid concomitant use of Ciprofloxacin and Dexamethasone with any of the following: Aldesleukin; BCG; Everolimus; Natalizumab; Nisoldipine; Pimecrolimus; Tacrolimus (Topical); TiZANidine; Tolvaptan; Vaccines (Live)

Increased Effect/Toxicity

Ciprofloxacin and Dexamethasone may increase the levels/effects of: Acetylcholinesterase Inhibitors; Amphotericin B; Bendamustine; Caffeine; Corticosteroids (Systemic); CYP1A2 Substrates; Erlotinib; Leflunomide; Lenalidomide; Loop Diuretics; Methotrexate; Natalizumab; NSAID (COX-2 Inhibitor); NSAID (Nonselective); Pentoxifylline; QTc-Prolonging Agents; Ropinirole; Ropivacaine; Sulfonylureas; Thalidomide; Theophylline Derivatives; Thiazide Diuretics; TiZANidine; Vaccines (Live); Vitamin K Antagonists; Warfarin

The levels/effects of Ciprofloxacin and Dexamethasone may be increased by: Antifungal Agents (Azole Derivatives, Systemic); Aprepitant; Asparaginase; Calcium Channel Blockers (Nondihydropyridine); CYP3A4 Inhibitors (Moderate); CYP3A4 Inhibitors (Strong); Denosumab; Estrogen Derivatives; Fluconazole; Fosaprepitant; Insulin; Macrolide Antibiotics; Neuromuscular-Blocking Agents (Nondepolarizing); P-Glycoprotein Inhibitors; Pimecrolimus; Probenecid; Quinolone Antibiotics; Salicylates; Tacrolimus (Topical); Trastuzumab

Decreased Effect

Ciprofloxacin and Dexamethasone may decrease the levels/effects of: Aldesleukin; Antidiabetic Agents; BCG; Calcitriol; Caspofungin; Corticorelin; CYP3A4 Substrates; Dabigatran Etexilate; Everolimus; GuanFACINE; Isoniazid; Maraviroc; Mycophenolate; NIFEdipine; Nisoldipine; P-Glycoprotein Substrates; Phenytoin; Salicylates; Sipuleucel-T; Sorafenib; Sulfonylureas; Tadalafil; Tolvaptan; Typhoid Vaccine; Vaccines (Inactivated); Vaccines (Live)

The levels/effects of Ciprofloxacin and Dexamethasone may be decreased by: Aminoglutethimide; Antacids; Barbiturates; Bile Acid Sequestrants; Calcium Salts; CYP3A4 Inducers (Strong); Deferasirox; Didanosine; Echinacea; Herbs (CYP3A4 Inducers); Iron Salts; Magnesium Salts; Mitotane; P-Glycoprotein Inducers; Primidone; Quinapril; Rifamycin Derivatives; Sevelamer; Sucralfate; Zinc Salts

Stability Store at room temperature; avoid freezing; protect from light

Pharmacokinetics (Adult data unless noted) Time to peak serum concentration: 15 minutes to 2 hours post dose application

Usual Dosage Otic: Children ≥6 months and Adults: Acute otitis media in patients with tympanostomy tubes or acute otitis externa: Instill 4 drops into affected ear(s) twice daily for 7 days

Administration To avoid dizziness which may result from the instillation of a cold solution, warm bottle in hand for 1-2 minutes. Shake suspension well before using; avoid contamination the tip of the bottle to fingers, ear, or any surfaces. Patient should lie with affected ear upward and maintain position for 60 seconds after suspension is instilled.

Acute otitis media with tympanostomy tubes: Instill drops then gently press the tragus 5 times in a pumping motion to allow the drops to pass through the tube into the middle ear.

Acute otitis externa: Gently pull the outer ear lobe upward and backward to allow the drops to flow down into the ear canal.

Patient Information Keep infected ear(s) clean and dry. Avoid swimming unless otherwise instructed by physician. Discontinue otic suspension and notify physician immediately if rash or an allergic reaction occurs.

Dosage Forms Excipient information presented when available (limited, particularly for generics); consult specific product labeling.

Suspension, otic: Ciprofloxacin 0.3% and dexamethasone 0.1% (7.5 mL) [contains benzalkonium chloride]

References

Roland PS, Dohar JE, Lanier BJ, et al, "Topical Ciprofloxacin/Dexamethasone Otic Suspension is Superior to Ofloxacin Otic Solution in the Treatment of Granulation Tissue in Children With Acute Otitis Media With Otorrhea Through Tympanostomy Tubes," *Otolaryngol Head Neck Surg*, 2004, 130(6):736-41.

Ciprofloxacin and Hydrocortisone
(sip roe FLOKS a sin & hye droe KOR ti sone)

Related Information
Ciprofloxacin *on page 310*
Hydrocortisone *on page 685*
U.S. Brand Names Cipro® HC
Canadian Brand Names Cipro® HC
Therapeutic Category Antibiotic/Corticosteroid, Otic
Generic Available No
Use Treatment of acute bacterial otitis externa due to susceptible strains of *S. aureus*, *P. aeruginosa*, or *Proteus mirabilis*
Pregnancy Risk Factor C
Contraindications Hypersensitivity to ciprofloxacin, hydrocortisone, any component, or other quinolones; patients with perforated tympanic membrane; patients with viral infections of the external ear canal
Adverse Reactions
Central nervous system: Headache
Dermatologic: Pruritus, fungal dermatitis, rash, urticaria, alopecia
Neuromuscular & skeletal: Paresthesia, hypoesthesia
Respiratory: Cough
Drug Interactions
Metabolism/Transport Effects Hydrocortisone: **Substrate** of CYP3A4 (minor), P-glycoprotein; **Induces** CYP3A4 (weak)
Avoid Concomitant Use
Avoid concomitant use of Ciprofloxacin and Hydrocortisone with any of the following: Aldesleukin; BCG; Natalizumab; Pimecrolimus; Tacrolimus (Topical); TiZANidine; Vaccines (Live)
Increased Effect/Toxicity
Ciprofloxacin and Hydrocortisone may increase the levels/effects of: Acetylcholinesterase Inhibitors; Amphotericin B; Bendamustine; Caffeine; Corticosteroids (Systemic); CYP1A2 Substrates; Erlotinib; Leflunomide; Loop Diuretics; Methotrexate; Natalizumab; NSAID (COX-2 Inhibitor); NSAID (Nonselective); Pentoxifylline; QTc-Prolonging Agents; Ropinirole; Ropivacaine; Sulfonylureas; Theophylline Derivatives; Thiazide Diuretics; TiZANidine; Vaccines (Live); Vitamin K Antagonists; Warfarin

The levels/effects of Ciprofloxacin and Hydrocortisone may be increased by: Antifungal Agents (Azole Derivatives, Systemic); Aprepitant; Calcium Channel Blockers (Nondihydropyridine); Denosumab; Estrogen Derivatives; Fluconazole; Fosaprepitant; Insulin; Macrolide Antibiotics; Neuromuscular-Blocking Agents (Nondepolarizing); P-Glycoprotein Inhibitors; Pimecrolimus; Probenecid; Quinolone Antibiotics; Salicylates; Tacrolimus (Topical); Trastuzumab

Decreased Effect
Ciprofloxacin and Hydrocortisone may decrease the levels/effects of: Aldesleukin; Antidiabetic Agents; BCG; Calcitriol; Corticorelin; Isoniazid; Mycophenolate; Phenytoin; Salicylates; Sipuleucel-T; Sulfonylureas; Typhoid Vaccine; Vaccines (Inactivated); Vaccines (Live)

The levels/effects of Ciprofloxacin and Hydrocortisone may be decreased by: Aminoglutethimide; Antacids; Barbiturates; Bile Acid Sequestrants; Calcium Salts; Didanosine; Echinacea; Iron Salts; Magnesium Salts; Mitotane; P-Glycoprotein Inducers; Primidone; Quinapril; Rifamycin Derivatives; Sevelamer; Sucralfate; Zinc Salts

Usual Dosage Children ≥1 year and Adults: Otic: Instill 3 drops into the affected ear(s) twice daily for 7 days
Administration Otic: Warm suspension by holding bottle in hand prior to instillation; shake well before use; patient should lie with affected ear upward and maintain position for 30-60 seconds after suspension is instilled into the ear canal
Dosage Forms Excipient information presented when available (limited, particularly for generics); consult specific product labeling.
Suspension, otic: Ciprofloxacin hydrochloride 0.2% and hydrocortisone 1% (10 mL) [contains benzyl alcohol]

◆ **Ciprofloxacin Hydrochloride** *see* Ciprofloxacin *on page 310*

◆ **Ciprofloxacin Hydrochloride and Dexamethasone** *see* Ciprofloxacin and Dexamethasone *on page 314*

◆ **Ciprofloxacin Hydrochloride and Hydrocortisone** *see* Ciprofloxacin and Hydrocortisone *on page 315*

◆ **Cipro® HC** *see* Ciprofloxacin and Hydrocortisone *on page 315*

◆ **Cipro® I.V.** *see* Ciprofloxacin *on page 310*

◆ **Cipro® XR** *see* Ciprofloxacin *on page 310*

Cisapride *U.S. - Available Via Limited-Access Protocol Only* (SIS a pride)

Medication Safety Issues
Sound-alike/look-alike issues:
Propulsid® may be confused with propranolol
U.S. Brand Names Propulsid®
Therapeutic Category Gastrointestinal Agent, Prokinetic
Generic Available No
Use Treatment of nocturnal symptoms of gastroesophageal reflux disease (GERD), also demonstrated effectiveness for gastroparesis, refractory constipation, and nonulcer dyspepsia in patients failing other therapies (see Warnings)
Medication Guide An FDA-approved patient medication guide, which is available with the product information and at http://www.fda.gov/downloads/Drugs/DrugSafety/ucm088994.pdf, must be dispensed with this medication for each new outpatient prescription and refill.
Pregnancy Risk Factor C
Lactation Enters breast milk/use caution (AAP rates "compatible")
Contraindications Hypersensitivity to cisapride or any component; GI hemorrhage, mechanical obstruction, GI perforation, or other situations when GI motility stimulation

is dangerous; patients with CHF, renal failure, multisystem organ failure, and COPD; patients at risk for developing or who have hypokalemia, hypocalcemia, or hypomagnesemia (eg, severe dehydration, vomiting, diarrhea, malnutrition, or receiving chronic diuretic therapy); patients with a known family history of congenital long-QT syndrome; prolonged QT intervals (QT_c >450), ventricular arrhythmias, ischemic heart disease, sinus node dysfunction, clinically significant bradycardia, and second or third degree AV block; patients receiving medications known to prolong the QT interval such as quinidine, procainamide, sotalol, amitriptyline (and other tricyclic antidepressants), maprotiline, phenothiazines, sertindole, astemizole, bepridil, or sparfloxacin (see Warnings and Drug Interactions); serious cardiac arrhythmias including ventricular tachycardia, ventricular fibrillation, torsade de pointes, and QT prolongations have been reported in patients taking medications which inhibit cytochrome P450 3A4; some of these events have been fatal; do not coadminister with ketoconazole, itraconazole, fluconazole, miconazole, erythromycin, clarithromycin, nefazodone, delavirdine, indinavir, nelfinavir, ritonavir, saquinavir, or troleandomycin; do not coadminister with grapefruit juice

Warnings Serious cardiac arrhythmias including ventricular tachycardia, ventricular fibrillation, torsade de pointes, and QT prolongation have been reported in patients receiving cisapride **[U.S. Boxed Warning]**; more than 270 cases have been reported including 70 fatalities; 85% of these cases occurred in patients with known risk factors (see Contraindications); for this reason, cisapride is available only for use in patients with severely debilitating conditions who meet specific criteria for a limited-access program directly through PRA International; for more information contact them at 877-795-4247

Precautions Use with caution in neonates, particularly if premature due to a potential increased risk of serious cardiac arrhythmias; decreased cisapride clearance found in neonates may result in increased serum levels; a 12-lead ECG (measuring QT intervals) should be done in all patients before beginning therapy

Adverse Reactions

Cardiovascular: Sinus tachycardia, QT interval prolongation, serious cardiac arrhythmias (see Warnings and Contraindications)

Central nervous system: Headache, insomnia, anxiety, nervousness, confusion

Dermatologic: Rash, pruritus

Endocrine & metabolic: Hypoglycemia with acidosis, hyperglycemia

Gastrointestinal: Diarrhea, abdominal pain, nausea, flatulence, dyspepsia, constipation, xerostomia

Genitourinary: Vaginitis (rare), urinary frequency

Hematologic: Thrombocytopenia, leukopenia, aplastic anemia, pancytopenia, hemolytic anemia, methemoglobinemia

Hepatic: Hepatitis, liver enzymes elevated

Neuromuscular & skeletal: Arthralgia, tremor

Respiratory: Rhinitis, sinusitis, cough, apnea

Miscellaneous: Positive ANA

Drug Interactions

Metabolism/Transport Effects Substrate of CYP1A2 (minor), 2A6 (minor), 2B6 (minor), 2C9 (minor), 2C19 (minor), 3A4 (major); **Inhibits** CYP2D6 (weak), 3A4 (weak)

Avoid Concomitant Use

Avoid concomitant use of Cisapride with any of the following: Amitriptyline; Antifungal Agents (Azole Derivatives, Systemic); Aprepitant; Artemether; Dronedarone; Efavirenz; Fosaprepitant; Lumefantrine; Macrolide Antibiotics; Nefazodone; Nilotinib; Pimozide; Protease Inhibitors; Protriptyline; QuiNINE; Tetrabenazine; Thioridazine; Ziprasidone

Increased Effect/Toxicity

Cisapride may increase the levels/effects of: Dronedarone; NIFEdipine; Pimozide; QTc-Prolonging Agents; QuiNINE; Tetrabenazine; Thioridazine; Ziprasidone

The levels/effects of Cisapride may be increased by: Alfuzosin; Amitriptyline; Antifungal Agents (Azole Derivatives, Systemic); Aprepitant; Artemether; Chloroquine; Cimetidine; Ciprofloxacin; Ciprofloxacin (Systemic); CYP3A4 Inhibitors (Moderate); CYP3A4 Inhibitors (Strong); Efavirenz; Fosaprepitant; Gadobutrol; Grapefruit Juice; Lumefantrine; Macrolide Antibiotics; Nefazodone; Nilotinib; Protease Inhibitors; Protriptyline; QuiNINE

Decreased Effect There are no known significant interactions involving a decrease in effect.

Food Interactions Do not use grapefruit juice which increases cisapride bioavailability

Mechanism of Action A GI prokinetic agent which enhances the release of acetylcholine at the myenteric plexus. In vitro studies have shown cisapride to have serotonin-4 receptor agonistic properties; it has no dopamine receptor blocking activity and, therefore, no extrapyramidal side effects or central antiemetic activity. It increases lower esophageal sphincter pressure, increases the amplitude of peristalsis, accelerates gastric emptying, improves antroduodenal coordination, increases colonic motility, and enhances cecal and ascending colonic emptying.

Pharmacodynamics Onset of action: 0.5-1 hour

Pharmacokinetics (Adult data unless noted)

Distribution: Breast milk to plasma ratio: 0.045

Protein binding: 98%

Metabolism: Extensive in liver via cytochrome P450 isoenzyme CYP 3A3/4 to norcisapride, which is eliminated in urine and feces

Bioavailability: 40% to 50%

Half-life: 7-10 hours

Elimination: <10% of dose excreted into feces and urine

Usual Dosage Oral:

Neonates: 0.15-0.2 mg/kg/dose 3-4 times/day; maximum dose: 0.8 mg/kg/day

Infants and Children: 0.15-0.3 mg/kg/dose 3-4 times/day; maximum dose: 10 mg/dose

Adults: Initial: 10 mg 4 times/day at least 15 minutes before meals and at bedtime; in some patients the dosage will need to be increased to 20 mg to obtain a satisfactory result

Dosage adjustment in liver dysfunction: Reduce daily dosage by 50%

Administration Oral: Administer 15 minutes before meals or feeding

Monitoring Parameters ECG (prior to beginning therapy), serum electrolytes in patients on diuretic therapy (prior to beginning therapy and periodically thereafter); see Contraindications

Patient Information May cause dry mouth.

References

Cucchiara S, Staiano A, Boccieri A, et al, "Effects of Cisapride on Parameters of Oesophageal Motility and on the Prolonged Intra-oesophageal pH Test in Infants With Gastro-Oesophageal Reflux Disease," Gut, 1990, 31(1):21-5.

Hill SL, Evangelista KJ, Pizzi AM, et al, "Proarrhythmia Associated With Cisapride in Children," Pediatrics, 1998, 101(6):1053-6.

Khongphatthanayothin A, Lane J, Thomas D, et al, "Effects of Cisapride on QT Interval in Children," J Pediatr, 1998, 133(1):51-6.

Lander A, "The Risks and Benefits of Cisapride in Premature Neonates, Infants and Children," Arch Dis Child, 1998, 79:469-71.

Lewin MB, Bryant RM, Fenrich AL, et al, "Cisapride-Induced QT Interval," J Pediatr, 1996, 128(2):279-81.

Tolia V, "Long-Term Use of Cisapride in Premature Neonates of <34 Weeks Gestational Age," J Pediatr Gastroenterol Nutr, 1990, 11:420-2.

Van Eygen M and Van Ravensteyn H, "Effect of Cisapride on Excessive Regurgitation in Infants," Clin Ther, 1989, 11(5):669-77.

Cisatracurium (sis a tra KYOO ree um)

Medication Safety Issues

Sound-alike/look-alike issues:

Nimbex® may be confused with Revex®

High alert medication: The Institute for Safe Medication Practices (ISMP) includes this medication among its list of drugs which have a heightened risk of causing significant patient harm when used in error.

United States Pharmacopeia (USP) 2006: The Interdisciplinary Safe Medication Use Expert Committee of the USP has recommended the following:

- Hospitals, clinics, and other practice sites should institute special safeguards in the storage, labeling, and use of these agents and should include these safeguards in staff orientation and competency training.
- Healthcare professionals should be on high alert (especially vigilant) whenever a neuromuscular-blocking agent (NMBA) is stocked, ordered, prepared, or administered.

U.S. Brand Names Nimbex®

Canadian Brand Names Nimbex®

Therapeutic Category Neuromuscular Blocker Agent, Nondepolarizing; Skeletal Muscle Relaxant, Paralytic

Generic Available No

Use Eases endotracheal intubation as an adjunct to general anesthesia and relaxes skeletal muscle during surgery or mechanical ventilation

Pregnancy Risk Factor B

Lactation Excretion in breast milk unknown/use caution

Contraindications Hypersensitivity to cisatracurium or any component (see Warnings)

Warnings Maintenance of an adequate airway and respiratory support is critical. Due to its intermediate onset of action, cisatracurium is not recommended for rapid sequence intubation; certain clinical conditions may result in potentiation or antagonism of neuromuscular blockade, see table.

10 mL multiple use vials contain benzyl alcohol as a preservative; benzyl alcohol may cause allergic reactions in susceptible individuals; large amounts of benzyl alcohol (≥99 mg/kg/day) have been associated with a potentially fatal toxicity ("gasping syndrome") in neonates; the "gasping syndrome" consists of metabolic acidosis, respiratory distress, gasping respirations, CNS dysfunction (including convulsions, intracranial hemorrhage), hypotension and cardiovascular collapse; avoid use of vials containing benzyl alcohol in neonates; in vitro and animal studies have shown that benzoate, a metabolite of benzyl alcohol, displaces bilirubin from protein-binding sites

Increased sensitivity in patients with myasthenia gravis, Eaton-Lambert syndrome, resistance to neuromuscular blockade in burn patients (>30% of body) for period of 5-70 days postinjury; resistance to neuromuscular blockade in patients with muscle trauma, denervation, immobilization, infection

Precautions Certain clinical conditions may result in potentiation or antagonism of neuromuscular blockade, see table.

Clinical Conditions Affecting Neuromuscular Blockade

Potentiation	Antagonism
Electrolyte abnormalities	Alkalosis
Severe hyponatremia	Hypercalcemia
Severe hypocalcemia	Demyelinating lesions
Severe hypokalemia	Peripheral neuropathies
Hypermagnesemia	Diabetes mellitus
Neuromuscular diseases	
Acidosis	
Acute intermittent porphyria	
Renal failure	
Hepatic failure	

Adverse Reactions

Cardiovascular: Rarely mild histamine release, cardiovascular effects are minimal and transient

Dermatologic: Rash, pruritus

Respiratory: Wheezing, bronchospasm, laryngospasm (rare)

Miscellaneous: Hypersensitivity reactions including anaphylaxis

Drug Interactions

Avoid Concomitant Use

Avoid concomitant use of Cisatracurium with any of the following: QuiNINE

Increased Effect/Toxicity

Cisatracurium may increase the levels/effects of: Cardiac Glycosides; Corticosteroids (Systemic); OnabotulinumtoxinA; RimabotulinumtoxinB

The levels/effects of Cisatracurium may be increased by: AbobotulinumtoxinA; Aminoglycosides; Calcium Channel Blockers; Capreomycin; Colistimethate; Inhalational Anesthetics; Ketorolac; Ketorolac (Systemic); Lincosamide Antibiotics; Lithium; Loop Diuretics; Magnesium Salts; Polymyxin B; Procainamide; QuiNIDine; QuiNINE; Spironolactone; Tetracycline Derivatives; Vancomycin

Decreased Effect

The levels/effects of Cisatracurium may be decreased by: Acetylcholinesterase Inhibitors; Loop Diuretics

Stability Protect from light; refrigerate; once removed from refrigerator, stable 21 days even if re-refrigerated; unstable in alkaline solutions; **compatible** with D$_5$W, D$_5$NS, and NS; do not dilute in LR; **incompatible** for Y-site administration with propofol or ketorolac; **compatible** for Y-site administration with sufentanil, alfentanil, fentanyl, midazolam, and droperidol.

Mechanism of Action Blocks neural transmission at the myoneural junction by binding with cholinergic receptor sites

Pharmacodynamics

Onset of action: I.V.: Within 2-3 minutes

Maximum effect: Within 3-5 minutes

Duration: Dose dependent, 35-45 minutes after a single 0.1 mg/kg dose; recovery begins in 20-35 minutes when anesthesia is balanced; recovery is attained in 90% of patients in 25-93 minutes

Pharmacokinetics (Adult data unless noted)

Distribution: V$_d$: Adults: 0.16 L/kg

Metabolism: Some metabolites are active; 80% of drug clearance is via a rapid nonenzymatic degradation (Hofmann elimination) in the bloodstream; additional metabolism occurs via ester hydrolysis

Half-life: 22-31 minutes

Elimination: <10% of dose excreted as unchanged drug in urine

Clearance:
  Children: 5.9 mL/kg/minute
  Adults: 5.1 mL/kg/minute

Usual Dosage I.V.:

Children 2-12 years: Initial: 0.1 mg/kg followed by maintenance dose of 0.03 mg/kg as needed to maintain neuromuscular blockade

Children >12 years to Adults: Initial: 0.15-0.2 mg/kg followed by maintenance dose of 0.03 mg/kg 40-65 minutes later or as needed to maintain neuromuscular blockade

Continuous infusion:

Children ≥2 years: 1-4 mcg/kg/minute (0.06-0.24 mg/kg/hour)

Note: Mean dosage of cisatracurium in 19 children ages 3 months to 16 years (median age: 4 years) to maintain neuromuscular blockade was 3.9 ± 1.3 mcg/kg/minute (0.23 ± 0.08 mg/kg/hour); (Burmester, 2005)

Adults: 1-3 mcg/kg/minute (0.06-0.18 mg/kg/hour)

Note: There may be wide interpatient variability in dosage (range 0.5-10 mcg/kg/minute in adults) which may increase and decrease over time; optimize patient dosage by utilizing a peripheral nerve stimulator

Administration Parenteral: May be administered without further dilution by rapid I.V. injection over 5-10 seconds; for continuous infusions, dilute to a concentration of 0.1-0.4 mg/mL in D_5W or NS; not for I.M. injection due to tissue irritation

Monitoring Parameters Muscle twitch response to peripheral nerve stimulation, heart rate, blood pressure

Additional Information Neuromuscular blocking potency is 3 times that of atracurium; maximum block is up to 2 minutes longer than for equipotent doses of atracurium; laudanosine, a metabolite without neuromuscular blocking activity has been associated with hypotension and seizure activity in animal studies.

Dosage Forms Excipient information presented when available (limited, particularly for generics); consult specific product labeling.

Injection, solution: 2 mg/mL (5 mL); 10 mg/mL (20 mL)

Injection, solution: 2 mg/mL (10 mL) [contains benzyl alcohol]

References

Burmester M and Mok Q, "Randomised Controlled Trial Comparing Cisatracurium and Vecuronium Infusions in a Paediatric Intensive Care Unit," *Intensive Care Med*, 2005, 31(5):686-92.

Martin LD, Bratton SL, and O'Rourke PP, "Clinical Uses and Controversies of Neuromuscular Blocking Agents in Infants and Children," *Crit Care Med*, 1999, 27(7):1358-68.

♦ **Cisatracurium Besylate** *see* Cisatracurium *on page 317*

CISplatin (SIS pla tin)

Medication Safety Issues

Sound-alike/look-alike issues:

CISplatin may be confused with CARBOplatin, oxaliplatin

High alert medication: This medication is in a class the Institute for Safe Medication Practices (ISMP) includes among its list of drugs which have a heightened risk of causing significant patient harm when used in error.

Doses >100 mg/m^2 once every 3-4 weeks are rarely used and should be verified with the prescriber.

Related Information

Compatibility of Chemotherapy and Related Supportive Care Medications *on page 1580*

Emetogenic Potential of Antineoplastic Agents *on page 1579*

Extravasation Treatment *on page 1522*

Therapeutic Category Antineoplastic Agent, Alkylating Agent

Generic Available Yes

Use Treatment of testicular, bladder, and ovarian cancers (FDA approved in adults); has also been used in the treatment of breast cancer; osteosarcoma, Hodgkin's and non-Hodgkin's lymphoma, head and neck cancer, gastric cancer, esophageal cancer, cervical cancer, nonsmall cell lung cancer, small cell lung cancer, neuroblastoma, prostate cancer, sarcomas, myeloma, melanoma, mesothelioma

Pregnancy Risk Factor D

Pregnancy Considerations Animal studies have demonstrated teratogenicity and embryotoxicity. There are no adequate and well-controlled studies in pregnant women. Women of childbearing potential should be advised to avoid pregnancy. If used in pregnancy, or if patient becomes pregnant during treatment, the patient should be apprised of potential hazard to the fetus.

Lactation Enters breast milk/not recommended

Contraindications Hypersensitivity to cisplatin, platinum-containing agents, or any component; pre-existing renal impairment, hearing impairment, and myelosuppression

Warnings Hazardous agent; use appropriate precautions for handling and disposal. Anaphylactic reactions have been reported **[U.S. Boxed Warning]**; facial edema, bronchoconstriction, tachycardia, and hypotension may occur within minutes of administration. Epinephrine, corticosteroids, and antihistamines may be used to treat reactions. Cumulative renal toxicity may be severe **[U.S. Boxed Warning]**; dose-related toxicities include myelosuppression, nausea and vomiting; renal toxicity is potentiated by aminoglycosides; ototoxicity, especially pronounced in children, is manifested by tinnitus or loss of high frequency hearing and occasionally, deafness **[U.S. Boxed Warning]**. May cause severe and potentially irreversible neuropathies with higher doses or more frequent dosing. Cisplatin may cause fetal harm; avoid pregnancy during use.

Precautions All patients should receive adequate hydration prior to and for 24 hours after cisplatin administration with a sodium chloride-containing I.V. solution to promote chloruresis, with or without mannitol and/or furosemide, to ensure good urine output and decrease the chance of nephrotoxicity; reduce dosage in renal impairment and in infants <6 months of age due to their decreased renal function and renal tubular secretion; serum magnesium, as well as electrolytes, should be monitored before and within 48 hours after cisplatin therapy. Patients who are magnesium-depleted should receive replacement therapy before the start of cisplatin. The development of acute leukemia has been reported when given in combination with other leukemogenic agents.

Adverse Reactions

Cardiovascular: Arrhythmias, bradycardia, Raynaud's phenomenon

Central nervous system: Encephalopathy, seizures

Endocrine & metabolic: Hyperuricemia, hypocalcemia, hypokalemia, hypomagnesemia, hypophosphatemia, SIADH

Gastrointestinal: Dysgeusia, nausea and vomiting occur in 76% to 100% of patients and is dose-related

Hematologic: Hemolytic anemia (Coombs +), leukopenia, myelosuppression, thrombocytopenia

Hepatic: Liver enzymes increased

Neuromuscular & skeletal: Muscle cramps, peripheral neuropathy (related to cumulative doses >200 mg/m^2)

Ocular: Blurred vision (reported with high dose), cerebellar blindness, optic neuritis, papilledema

Otic: Ototoxicity [especially pronounced in children; hearing loss in the high-frequency range is related to a cumulative dose of cisplatin >400 mg/m^2 (see Warnings)], vestibular toxicity

Renal: Azotemia, BUN and serum creatinine elevated, nephrotoxicity [damage to the proximal tubules (see Warnings)]

Miscellaneous: Anaphylactoid reactions (bronchoconstriction, facial edema, hypotension, tachycardia)

<1%, postmarketing, and/or case reports: Alopecia, asthenia, cerebrovascular accident, hiccups, local reactions (phlebitis, tissue sloughing, and necrosis, if infiltrated), malaise, MI, rash, Raynaud's phenomenon, thrombocytic microangiopathy

Drug Interactions

Avoid Concomitant Use
Avoid concomitant use of CISplatin with any of the following: BCG; Natalizumab; Pimecrolimus; Tacrolimus (Topical); Vaccines (Live)

Increased Effect/Toxicity
CISplatin may increase the levels/effects of: Aminoglycosides; Leflunomide; Natalizumab; Taxane Derivatives; Topotecan; Vaccines (Live); Vinorelbine

The levels/effects of CISplatin may be increased by: Denosumab; Loop Diuretics; Pimecrolimus; Tacrolimus (Topical); Trastuzumab

Decreased Effect
CISplatin may decrease the levels/effects of: BCG; Phenytoin; Sipuleucel-T; Vaccines (Inactivated); Vaccines (Live)

The levels/effects of CISplatin may be decreased by: Echinacea

Stability Reconstituted powder for injection is stable for 20 hours at room temperature; do not refrigerate reconstituted solution since precipitation may occur; protect from light; incompatible with sodium bicarbonate; do not infuse in solutions containing <0.2% sodium chloride; stable when combined with mannitol (12.5-50 g mannitol/L)

Mechanism of Action Platination of DNA leads to reactive intermediates that bind to DNA and form intrastrand and interstrand DNA cross-links

Pharmacokinetics (Adult data unless noted)
Distribution: I.V.: Rapid tissue distribution; CSF unbound platinum concentration: 40% of the plasma concentration
Protein binding: >90%; only the free (unbound) platinum and parent drug are cytotoxic
Metabolism: Undergoes nonenzymatic metabolism
Half-life, terminal: Children:
Free drug: 1.3 hours
Total platinum: 44 hours
Elimination: ~50% of dose excreted in urine within 5 days in an inactive form
Dialysis: Minimally removed by hemodialysis

Usual Dosage Children and Adults: I.V. (refer to individual protocols): **TO PREVENT POSSIBLE OVERDOSE, VERIFY ANY CISPLATIN DOSE EXCEEDING 120 mg/m² PER COURSE:**
Intermittent dosing schedule: 37-75 mg/m² once every 2-3 weeks or 50-100 mg/m² over 4-6 hours, once every 21-28 days
Daily dosing schedule: 15-20 mg/m²/day for 5 days every 3-4 weeks
Osteogenic sarcoma or neuroblastoma: 60-100 mg/m² on day 1 every 3-4 weeks
Recurrent brain tumors: 60 mg/m² once daily for 2 consecutive days every 3-4 weeks
Bone marrow/blood cell transplantation: Continuous infusion: High dose: 55 mg/m²/day for 72 hours; total dose = 165 mg/m²

Dosing adjustment in renal impairment:
Cl_{cr} 10-50 mL/minute: Administer 75% of dose
Cl_{cr} <10 mL/minute: Administer 50% of dose

Administration Parenteral: I.V.: Administer according to protocol; rate of administration has varied from a 15- to 20-minute infusion, 1 mg/minute infusion, 6- to 8-hour infusion or 24-hour infusion; rapid I.V. injection may be associated with increased nephrotoxicity or ototoxicity compared to a slower I.V. infusion

Monitoring Parameters Renal function tests (serum creatinine, BUN, Cl_{cr}), electrolytes (particularly magnesium, calcium, potassium), hearing test, neurologic exam (with high dose), liver function tests periodically, CBC with differential and platelet count, urine output, urinalysis

Nursing Implications Needles, syringes, catheters, or I.V. administration sets that contain aluminum parts should not be used for administration of drug; methods to prevent nephrotoxicity include prehydration, diuresis with mannitol, and administration of sodium chloride containing I.V. solutions to promote chloruresis. Adequate hydration and urinary output should be maintained for 24 hours after administration. Extravasation may cause tissue sloughing and necrosis; care should be taken to avoid extravasation. Infiltration of cisplatin infusions with concentrations >0.5 mg/mL may result in a more severe tissue toxicity.

Additional Information Myelosuppressive effects:
WBC: Mild
Platelets: Mild
Onset (days): 10
Nadir (days): 18-23
Recovery (days): 21-40

Dosage Forms Excipient information presented when available (limited, particularly for generics); consult specific product labeling.
Injection, solution [preservative free]: 1 mg/mL (50 mL, 100 mL, 200 mL)

References
Costello MA, Dominick C, and Clerico A, "A Pilot Study of 5-Day Continuous Infusion of High-Dose Cisplatin and Pulsed Etoposide in Childhood Solid Tumors," *Am J Pediatr Hematol Oncol*, 1988, 10:103-8.

Reece PA, Stafford I, Abbott RL, et al, "Two-Versus 24-Hour Infusion of Cisplatin: Pharmacokinetic Considerations," *J Clin Oncol*, 1989, 7 (2):270-5.

◆ **13-*cis*-Retinoic Acid** *see* Isotretinoin *on page 769*

Citalopram (sye TAL oh pram)

Medication Safety Issues
Sound-alike/look-alike issues:
Celexa® may be confused with Celebrex®, Cerebra®, Cerebyx®, Ranexa™, Zyprexa®

Related Information
Antidepressant Agents *on page 1484*
Serotonin Syndrome *on page 1695*

U.S. Brand Names Celexa®

Canadian Brand Names Apo-Citalopram®; Celexa®; Citalopram-Odan; CO Citalopram; CTP 30; Dom-Citalopram; JAMP-Citalopram; Mint-Citalopram; Mylan-Citalopram; NG-Citalopram; Novo-Citalopram; PHL-Citalopram; PMS-Citalopram; RAN™-Citalopram; ratio-Citalopram; Riva-Citalopram; Sandoz-Citalopram

Therapeutic Category Antidepressant, Selective Serotonin Reuptake Inhibitor (SSRI)

Generic Available Yes

Use Treatment of depression; obsessive-compulsive disorder (OCD) in children

Medication Guide An FDA-approved patient medication guide, which is available with the product information and at http://www.fda.gov/downloads/Drugs/DrugSafety/ucm088568.pdf, must be dispensed with this medication for each new outpatient prescription and refill.

Pregnancy Risk Factor C

Pregnancy Considerations Due to adverse effects observed in animal studies, citalopram is classified as pregnancy category C. Citalopram and its metabolites cross the human placenta. Nonteratogenic effects in the newborn following SSRI exposure late in the third trimester include respiratory distress, cyanosis, apnea, seizures, temperature instability, feeding difficulty, vomiting, hypoglycemia, hypo- or hypertonia, hyper-reflexia, jitteriness, irritability, constant crying, and tremor. An increased risk of low birth weight and lower Apgar scores have also been reported. Exposure to SSRIs after the twentieth week of gestation has been associated with persistent pulmonary hypertension of the newborn (PPHN). Adverse effects may be due to toxic effects of the SSRI or drug withdrawal without a taper. The long-term effects of *in utero* SSRI exposure on infant development and behavior are not known.

Due to pregnancy-induced physiologic changes, women who are pregnant may require increased doses of citalopram to achieve euthymia. Women treated for major depression and who are euthymic prior to pregnancy are more likely to experience a relapse when medication is discontinued as compared to pregnant women who continue taking antidepressant medications. The ACOG recommends that therapy with SSRIs or SNRIs during pregnancy be individualized; treatment of depression during pregnancy should incorporate the clinical expertise of the mental health clinician, obstetrician, primary health-care provider, and pediatrician. If treatment during pregnancy is required, consider tapering therapy during the third trimester in order to prevent withdrawal symptoms in the infant. If this is done and the woman is considered to be at risk of relapse from her major depressive disorder, the medication can be restarted following delivery, although the dose should be readjusted to that required before pregnancy. Treatment algorithms have been developed by the ACOG and the APA for the management of depression in women prior to conception and during pregnancy (Yonkers, 2009).

Lactation Enters breast milk/consider risk:benefit

Breast-Feeding Considerations Citalopram and its metabolites are excreted in human milk. According to the manufacturer, the decision to continue or discontinue breast-feeding during therapy should take into account the risk of exposure to the infant and the benefits of treatment to the mother. Excessive somnolence, decreased feeding, colic, irritability, restlessness, and weight loss have been reported in breast-fed infants. The long-term effects on development and behavior have not been studied; therefore, citalopram should be prescribed to a mother who is breast-feeding only when the benefits outweigh the potential risks.

Contraindications Hypersensitivity to citalopram or any component; use with MAO inhibitors within 14 days (potentially fatal reactions may occur, see Drug Inter-actions); concurrent use of pimozide

Warnings Citalopram is not approved for use in pediatric patients. Clinical worsening of depression or suicidal ideation and behavior may occur in children and adults with major depressive disorder **[U.S. Boxed Warning]**. In clinical trials, antidepressants increased the risk of suicidal thinking and behavior (suicidality) in children, adolescents, and young adults (18-24 years of age) with major depressive disorder and other psychiatric disorders. This risk must be considered before prescribing antidepressants for any clinical use. Short-term studies did **not** show an increased risk of suicidality with antidepressant use in patients >24 years of age and showed a decreased risk in patients ≥65 years.

Patients of all ages who are treated with antidepressants for any indication require appropriate monitoring and close observation for clinical worsening of depression, suicidality, and unusual changes in behavior, especially during the first few months after antidepressant initiation or when the dose is adjusted. Family members and caregivers should be instructed to closely observe the patient (ie, daily) and communicate condition with healthcare provider. Patients should also be monitored for associated behaviors (eg, anxiety, agitation, panic attacks, insomnia, irritability, hostility, aggressiveness, impulsivity, akathisia,

hypomania, mania) which may increase the risk for worsening depression or suicidality. Worsening depression or emergence of suicidality (or associated behaviors listed above) that is abrupt in onset, severe, or not part of the presenting symptoms, may require discontinuation or modification of drug therapy.

Avoid abrupt discontinuation; withdrawal syndrome with discontinuation symptoms (including agitation, dysphoria, anxiety, confusion, dizziness, hypomania, nightmares, irritability, sensory disturbances, headache, lethargy, emo-tional lability, insomnia, tinnitus, and seizures) may occur if therapy is abruptly discontinued or dose reduced; taper the dose to minimize risks of discontinuation symptoms. If intolerable symptoms occur following a decrease in dosage or upon discontinuation of therapy, consider resuming the previous dose with a more gradual taper. To reduce risk of intentional overdose, write prescriptions for the smallest quantity consistent with good patient care.

May worsen psychosis in some patients or precipitate a shift to mania or hypomania in patients with bipolar disorder. Monotherapy in patients with bipolar disorder should be avoided. Patients presenting with depressive symptoms should be screened for bipolar disorder. Citalopram is not FDA approved for the treatment of bipolar depression.

Potentially fatal serotonin syndrome may occur when SSRIs are used in combination with serotonergic drugs (eg, triptans) or drugs that impair the metabolism of serotonin (eg, MAO inhibitors); see Drug Interactions

Precautions Citalopram may impair platelet aggregation and cause abnormal bleeding (eg, ecchymosis, purpura, upper GI bleeding); risk may be increased in patients with impaired platelet aggregation and with concurrent use of aspirin, NSAIDs, warfarin, or other drugs that affect coagulation; bleeding related to SSRI or SNRI use has been reported to range from relatively minor bruising and epistaxis to life-threatening hemorrhage. Citalopram may impair cognitive or motor performance. Use with caution in patients with seizure disorders, concomitant illnesses that may effect hepatic metabolism or hemodynamic responses (eg, unstable cardiac disease, recent MI), and in suicidal patients; use with caution and decrease dose in patients with hepatic dysfunction; use with caution in patients with severe renal impairment.

Use with caution during third trimester of pregnancy [newborns may experience adverse effects or withdrawal symptoms (consider risk and benefits), see Additional Information; exposure to SSRIs late in pregnancy may also be associated with an increased risk for persistent pulmonary hypertension of the newborn (see Chambers, 2006)]; high doses of citalopram have been associated with teratogenicity in animals. Use with caution in patients receiving diuretics or those who are volume depleted (may cause hyponatremia or SIADH). No clinical studies have assessed the combined use of citalopram and electro-convulsive therapy; however, use with caution in patients receiving electroconvulsive therapy; may increase the risks associated with electroconvulsive therapy, consider discontinuing, when possible, prior to electroconvulsive therapy treatment.

Adverse Reactions Predominant adverse effects are CNS and GI.

Central nervous system: Somnolence, dizziness, insom-nia, anxiety, anorexia, agitation, yawning, apathy, fatigue, fever; suicidal thinking and behavior (see Warnings)

Note: SSRI-associated behavioral activation (ie, rest-lessness, hyperkinesis, hyperactivity, agitation) is 2- to 3-fold more prevalent in children compared to adoles-cents; it is more prevalent in adolescents compared to adults. Somnolence (including sedation and drowsiness) is more common in adults compared to children and adolescents (see Safer, 2006).

Dermatologic: Rash, pruritus

Endocrine & metabolic: Hyponatremia, SIADH (usually in volume-depleted patients); sexual dysfunction, dysmenorrhea, weight loss

Gastrointestinal: Nausea, xerostomia, diarrhea, dyspepsia, vomiting, abdominal pain

Note: SSRI-associated vomiting is 2- to 3-fold more prevalent in children compared to adolescents; it is more prevalent in adolescents compared to adults.

Hematologic: Altered platelet function (rare), bleeding increased, bruising

Neuromuscular & skeletal: Tremor, arthralgia, myalgia, asthenia

Respiratory: Cough, rhinitis, sinusitis

Miscellaneous: Diaphoresis; withdrawal symptoms following abrupt discontinuation (see Warnings)

Drug Interactions

Metabolism/Transport Effects Substrate of CYP2C19 (major), 2D6 (minor), 3A4 (major); **Inhibits** CYP1A2 (weak), 2B6 (weak), 2C19 (weak), 2D6 (weak)

Avoid Concomitant Use

Avoid concomitant use of Citalopram with any of the following: Artemether; Dronedarone; Iobenguane I 123; Lumefantrine; MAO Inhibitors; Metoclopramide; Nilotinib; Pimozide; QuiNINE; Sibutramine; Tetrabenazine; Thioridazine; Ziprasidone

Increased Effect/Toxicity

Citalopram may increase the levels/effects of: Alcohol (Ethyl); Alpha-/Beta-Blockers; Anticoagulants; Antidepressants (Serotonin Reuptake Inhibitor/Antagonist); Antiplatelet Agents; Aspirin; Beta-Blockers; BusPIRone; CarBAMazepine; Clozapine; CNS Depressants; Collagenase (Systemic); Desmopressin; Dextromethorphan; Dronedarone; Drotrecogin Alfa; Haloperidol; Ibritumomab; Lithium; Methadone; Mexiletine; NSAID (COX-2 Inhibitor); NSAID (Nonselective); Phenytoin; Pimozide; QTc-Prolonging Agents; QuiNINE; Risperidone; Salicylates; Serotonin Modulators; Tetrabenazine; Thioridazine; Thrombolytic Agents; Tositumomab and Iodine I 131 Tositumomab; TraMADol; Tricyclic Antidepressants; Vitamin K Antagonists; Ziprasidone

The levels/effects of Citalopram may be increased by: Alfuzosin; Analgesics (Opioid); Artemether; BusPIRone; Chloroquine; Cimetidine; Ciprofloxacin; Ciprofloxacin (Systemic); CYP2C19 Inhibitors (Moderate); CYP2C19 Inhibitors (Strong); CYP3A4 Inhibitors (Moderate); CYP3A4 Inhibitors (Strong); Fluconazole; Gadobutrol; Glucosamine; Herbs (Anticoagulant/Antiplatelet Properties); Lumefantrine; Macrolide Antibiotics; MAO Inhibitors; Metoclopramide; Nilotinib; Omega-3-Acid Ethyl Esters; Pentosan Polysulfate Sodium; Pentoxifylline; Prostacyclin Analogues; QuiNINE; Sibutramine; TraMADol; Tryptophan

Decreased Effect

Citalopram may decrease the levels/effects of: Iobenguane I 123

The levels/effects of Citalopram may be decreased by: CarBAMazepine; CYP2C19 Inducers (Strong); CYP3A4 Inducers (Strong); Cyproheptadine; Deferasirox; Peginterferon Alfa-2b

Food Interactions Absorption is not affected by food.

Tryptophan supplements may increase serious side effects; its use is **not recommended**

Stability Store at 25°C (77°F); excursions permitted to 15°C to 30°C (59°F to 86°F).

Mechanism of Action A racemic bicyclic phthalane derivative, citalopram selectively inhibits serotonin reuptake in the presynaptic neurons and has minimal effects on norepinephrine or dopamine. Uptake inhibition of serotonin

is primarily due to the S-enantiomer of citalopram. Displays little to no affinity for serotonin, dopamine, adrenergic, histamine, GABA, or muscarinic receptor subtypes.

Pharmacodynamics

Onset of action: 1-2 weeks

Maximum effect: 8-12 weeks

Duration: 1-2 days

Pharmacokinetics (Adult data unless noted)

Distribution: V_d: Adults: 12 L/kg

Protein binding, plasma: ~80%

Metabolism: Extensively hepatic, primarily via CYP3A4 and CYP2C19; metabolized to N-demethylated, N-oxide, and deaminated metabolites

Bioavailability: 80%; tablets and oral solution are bioequivalent

Half-life elimination: Adults: Range: 24-48 hours; mean: 35 hours (doubled with hepatic impairment)

Time to peak serum concentration: 1 to 6 hours, average within 4 hours

Elimination: Urine (10% as unchanged drug)

Clearance: Hepatic impairment: Decreased by 37%; Mild to moderate renal impairment: Decreased by 17%; Severe renal impairment (Cl_{cr} <20 mL/minute): No information available

Usual Dosage

Children and Adolescents: **Note:** Slower titration of dose every 2-4 weeks may minimize risk of SSRI associated behavioral activation, which has been shown to increase risk of suicidal behavior.

Depression: **Note:** Not FDA approved; see Warnings. Limited information is available; only one randomized, placebo controlled trial has shown citalopram to be effective for the treatment of depression in pediatric patients (see Wagner, 2004); other controlled pediatric trials have **not** shown benefit (see Sharp, 2006; von Knorring, 2006; and Wagner, 2005). Some experts recommend the following doses (see Dopheide, 2006):

Children ≤11 years: Initial: 10 mg/day given once daily; increase dose slowly by 5 mg/day every 2 weeks as clinically needed; dosage range: 20-60 mg/day

Children and Adolescents ≥12 years: Initial: 20 mg/day given once daily; increase dose slowly by 10 mg/day every 2 weeks as clinically needed; dosage range: 20-60 mg/day

Obsessive-compulsive disorder: **Note:** Not FDA approved; see Warnings. Limited information is available; several open label trials have been published (see Thomsen, 1997; Thomsen, 2001; Mukaddes, 2003). Some experts recommend the following doses:

Children ≤11 years: Initial: 5-10 mg/day given once daily; increase dose slowly by 5 mg/day every 2 weeks as clinically needed; dosage range: 10-40 mg/day.

Children and Adolescents ≥12 years: Initial: 10-20 mg/day given once daily; increase dose slowly by 10 mg/day every 2 weeks as clinically needed; dosage range: 10-40 mg/day.

Note: Higher mg/kg doses are needed in children compared to adolescents.

Adults: Depression: Initial: 20 mg/day given once daily; may increase daily dose in 20 mg increments at intervals of ≥1 week; usual dose: 40 mg/day; doses >40 mg are not usually necessary and may not increase effectiveness; maximum dose: 60 mg/day

Dosage adjustment in hepatic impairment: Adults: Initial: 20 mg/day; usual dose: 20 mg/day; in nonresponsive patients, may titrate to maximum dose of 40 mg/day

Dosage adjustment in renal impairment: Adults: Mild or moderate renal impairment: No dosage adjustment needed; Severe renal impairment (Cl_{cr} <20 mL/minute): Use with caution

◀ **Administration** May be administered without regard to meals

Monitoring Parameters Monitor patient periodically for symptom resolution; monitor for worsening depression, suicidality, and associated behaviors (especially at the beginning of therapy or when doses are increased or decreased; see Warnings). Monitor for anxiety, social functioning, mania, panic attacks; akathisia

Patient Information Read the patient Medication Guide that you receive with each prescription and refill of citalopram. An increased risk of suicidal thinking and behavior has been reported with the use of antidepressants in children, adolescents, and young adults (18-24 years of age). Notify physician if you feel more depressed, have thoughts of suicide, or become more agitated or irritable (see Warnings). Avoid alcohol, caffeine, CNS stimulants, tryptophan supplements, and the herbal medicine St John's wort; avoid aspirin, NSAIDs, or other drugs that affect coagulation (may increase risks of bleeding); may cause dizziness or drowsiness and impair ability to perform activities requiring mental alertness or physical coordination; may cause dry mouth. Some medicines should not be taken with citalopram or should not be taken for a while after citalopram has been discontinued; report the use of other medications, nonprescription medications, and herbal or natural products to your physician and pharmacist. It may take up to 4 weeks to see therapeutic effects from this medication. Take as directed; do not alter dose or frequency without consulting prescriber; avoid abrupt discontinuation.

Nursing Implications Assess other medications patient may be taking for possible interaction (especially MAO inhibitors, P450 inhibitors, and other CNS active agents). Assess mental status for depression, suicidal ideation, anxiety, social functioning, mania, or panic attack.

Additional Information If used for an extended period of time, long-term usefulness of citalopram should be periodically re-evaluated for the individual patient. A recent report describes 5 children (age: 8-15 years) who developed epistaxis (n=4) or bruising (n=1) while receiving SSRI therapy (sertraline) (Lake, 2000).

Neonates born to women receiving SSRIs later during the third trimester may experience respiratory distress, apnea, cyanosis, temperature instability, vomiting, feeding difficulty, hypoglycemia, constant crying, irritability, hypotonia, hypertonia, hyper-reflexia, tremor, jitteriness, and seizures; these symptoms may be due to a direct toxic effect, withdrawal syndrome, or (in some cases) serotonin syndrome. Withdrawal symptoms occur in 30% of neonates exposed to SSRIs *in utero*; monitor newborns for at least 48 hours after birth; long-term effects of *in utero* exposure to SSRIs are unknown (see Levinson-Castiel, 2006).

Dosage Forms Excipient information presented when available (limited, particularly for generics); consult specific product labeling. [DSC] = Discontinued product

Solution, oral: 10 mg/5 mL (240 mL)

Celexa®: 10 mg/5 mL (240 mL) [ethanol free, sugar free; contains propylene glycol; peppermint flavor] [DSC]

Tablet: 10 mg, 20 mg, 40 mg

Celexa®: 10 mg

Celexa®: 20 mg, 40 mg [scored]

References

Bernard L, Stern R, Lew D, et al, "Serotonin Syndrome After Concomitant Treatment With Linezolid and Citalopram," *Clin Infect Dis*, 2003, 36(9):1197.

Chambers CD, Hernandez-Diaz S, Van Marter LJ, et al, "Selective Serotonin-Reuptake Inhibitors and Risk of Persistent Pulmonary Hypertension of the Newborn," *N Engl J Med*, 2006, 354(6):579-87.

Dopheide JA, "Recognizing and Treating Depression in Children and Adolescents," *Am J Health Syst Pharm*, 2006, 63(3):233-43.

Lake MB, Birmaher B, Wassick S, et al, "Bleeding and Selective Serotonin Reuptake Inhibitors in Childhood and Adolescence," *J Child Adolesc Psychopharmacol*, 2000, 10(1):35-8.

Levinson-Castiel R, Merlob P, Linder N, et al, "Neonatal Abstinence Syndrome After *in utero* Exposure to Selective Serotonin Reuptake Inhibitors in Term Infants," *Arch Pediatr Adolesc Med*, 2006, 160 (2):173-6.

Mahlberg R, Kunz D, Sasse J, et al, "Serotonin Syndrome With Tramadol and Citalopram," *Am J Psychiatry*, 2004, 161(6):1129.

Mukaddes NM, Abali O, and Kaynak N, "Citalopram Treatment of Children and Adolescents With Obsessive-Compulsive Disorder: A Preliminary Report," *Psychiatry Clin Neurosci*, 2003, 57(4):405-8.

Pass SE and Simpson RW, "Discontinuation and Reinstitution of Medications During the Perioperative Period," *Am J Health Syst Pharm*, 2004, 61(9):899-912.

Reinblatt SP and Riddle MA, "Selective Serotonin Reuptake Inhibitors-Induced Apathy: A Pediatric Case Series," *J Child Adolesc Psychopharmacol*, 2006, 6(1/2):227-33.

Safer DJ and Zito JM, "Treatment Emergent Adverse Effects of Selective Serotonin Reuptake Inhibitors by Age Group: Children vs. Adolescents," *J Child Adolesc Psychopharmacol*, 2006, 16(1/2):159-69.

Sharp SC and Hellings JA, "Efficacy and Safety of Selective Serotonin Reuptake Inhibitors in the Treatment of Depression in Children and Adolescents: Practitioner Review," *Clin Drug Investig*, 2006, 26 (5):247-55.

Tahir N, "Serotonin Syndrome as a Consequence of Drug-Resistant Infections: An Interaction Between Linezolid and Citalopram," *J Am Med Dir Assoc*, 2004, 5(2):111-3.

Thomsen PH, "Child and Adolescent Obsessive-Compulsive Disorder Treated With Citalopram: Findings From an Open Trial of 23 Cases," *J Child Adolesc Psychopharmacol*, 1997, 7(3):157-66.

Thomsen PH, Ebbesen C, and Persson C, "Long-Term Experience With Citalopram in the Treatment of Adolescent OCD," *J Am Acad Child Adolesc Psychiatry*, 2001, 40(8):895-902.

von Knorring AL, Olsson GI, Thomsen PH, et al, "A Randomized, Double-Blind, Placebo-Controlled Study of Citalopram in Adolescents With Major Depressive Disorder," *J Clin Psychopharmacol*, 2006, 26 (3):311-5.

Wagner KD, "Pharmacotherapy for Major Depression in Children and Adolescents," *Prog Neuropsychopharmacol Biol Psychiatry*, 2005, 29 (5):819-26.

Wagner KD, Robb AS, Findling RL, et al, "A Randomized, Placebo-Controlled Trial of Citalopram for the Treatment of Major Depression in Children and Adolescents," *Am J Psych*, 2004, 161(6):1079-83.

♦ **Citalopram Hydrobromide** see Citalopram *on page 319*

♦ **Citalopram-Odan (Can)** see Citalopram *on page 319*

♦ **Citracal® [OTC]** see Calcium Supplements *on page 239*

♦ **Citracal® Kosher [OTC] [DSC]** see Calcium Citrate *on page 234*

Citrate and Citric Acid (SIT rate & SIT rik AS id)

Therapeutic Category Alkalinizing Agent, Oral

Use Treatment of metabolic acidosis; alkalinizing agent in conditions where long-term maintenance of an alkaline urine is desirable

Potassium citrate: Prevention of uric acid nephrolithiasis, prevention of calcium renal stones in patients with hypocitraturia; urinary alkalizer when sodium citrate is contraindicated

Pregnancy Risk Factor C

Contraindications Hypersensitivity to citrate, citric acid, or any component; patients receiving sodium-restricted diet (sodium salts); severe renal impairment with oliguria, azotemia, or anuria; untreated Addison's disease, acute dehydration, heat cramps, severe myocardial damage, hyperkalemia (potassium salts); Urocit®-K (wax matrix tablet) is contraindicated in patients with delayed gastric emptying, intestinal obstruction, or stricture, patients receiving anticholinergic medications and in patients with peptic ulcer disease

Warnings Conversion to bicarbonate may be impaired in patients with hepatic failure, in shock, or who are severely ill. Some products contain sodium benzoate; benzoic acid (benzoate) is a metabolite of benzyl alcohol; large amounts of benzyl alcohol (≥99 mg/kg/day) have been associated with a potentially fatal toxicity ("gasping syndrome") in neonates; the "gasping syndrome" consists of metabolic acidosis, respiratory distress, gasping respirations, CNS dysfunction (including convulsions, intracranial hemor-rhage), hypotension and cardiovascular collapse; avoid use of sodium benzoate containing products in neonates; *in vitro* and animal studies have shown that benzoate displaces bilirubin from protein binding sites

Precautions Use sodium salts with caution in patients with CHF, hypertension, pulmonary edema; may predispose patient to urolithiasis

Adverse Reactions
Central nervous system: Tetany

Endocrine & metabolic: Metabolic alkalosis, hypernatremia (if sodium salt used), hypocalcemia, hyperkalemia (if potassium salt used)

Gastrointestinal: Diarrhea, nausea, vomiting, stenotic or ulcerative lesions (wax matrix tablets)

Mechanism of Action Citrate salts are oxidized in the body to form bicarbonate

Usual Dosage Oral (dilute in water or juice):

Infants and Children: 2-3 mEq/kg/day in divided doses 3-4 times/day **or** 5-15 mL with water after meals and at bedtime

Adults:

Solution: 15-30 mL with water after meals and at bedtime

Wax matrix tablet (Urocit®-K): 30-60 mEq/day in divided doses 3-4 times/day

Administration Oral: Dilute with water or juice and administer after meals; do not crush or chew wax matrix tablets (Urocit®-K)

Monitoring Parameters Serum sodium, bicarbonate, potassium, urine pH

Dosage Forms
Crystals (Polycitra®-K): Potassium citrate monohydrate 1100 mg and citric acid monohydrate 334 mg per 5 mL when reconstituted [potassium 2 mEq and is equivalent to bicarbonate 2 mEq per mL] (unit dose packets)

Solution, oral:

Modified Shohl's, Bicitra® (alcohol free): Sodium citrate dihydrate 500 mg and citric acid monohydrate 334 mg per 5 mL [sodium 1 mEq and is equivalent to bicarbonate 1 mEq per mL] (15 mL, 30 mL, 120 mL, 473 mL)

Oracit®: Sodium citrate 490 mg and citric acid 640 mg per 5 mL [sodium 1 mEq and is equivalent to bicarbonate 1 mEq per mL] (15 mL, 30 mL, 500 mL)

Polycitra®-K (alcohol free): Potassium citrate monohy-drate 1100 mg and citric acid monohydrate 334 mg per 5 mL [potassium 2 mEq, and is equivalent to bicarbonate 2 mEq per mL] (473 mL)

Syrup, alcohol and sugar free (Polycitra®-LC): Potassium citrate monohydrate 550 mg, sodium citrate dihydrate 500 mg, and citric acid monohydrate 334 mg per 5 mL [potassium 1 mEq, sodium 1 mEq, and is equivalent to bicarbonate 2 mEq per mL] (473 mL)

Syrup, alcohol free (Polycitra®): Potassium citrate mono-hydrate 550 mg, sodium citrate dihydrate 500 mg, and citric acid monohydrate 334 mg per 5 mL [potassium 1 mEq, sodium 1 mEq, and is equivalent to bicarbonate 2 mEq per mL] (473 mL)

- ◆ **Citrate of Magnesia** *see* Magnesium Citrate *on page 854*
- ◆ **Citrate of Magnesia (Magnesium Citrate)** *see* Magne-sium Supplements *on page 859*
- ◆ **Citroma® [OTC]** *see* Magnesium Citrate *on page 854*
- ◆ **Citro-Mag® (Can)** *see* Magnesium Citrate *on page 854*
- ◆ **Citrovorum Factor** *see* Leucovorin Calcium *on page 804*
- ◆ **CL-65336** *see* Tranexamic Acid *on page 1369*
- ◆ **CL-232315** *see* Mitoxantrone *on page 938*

Cladribine (KLA dri been)

Medication Safety Issues
Sound-alike/look-alike issues:

Cladribine may be confused with clevidipine, clofarabine, fludarabine

Leustatin® may be confused with lovastatin

High alert medication: The Institute for Safe Medication Practices (ISMP) includes this medication among its list of drugs which have a heightened risk of causing significant patient harm when used in error.

Related Information
Compatibility of Chemotherapy and Related Supportive Care Medications *on page 1580*

Emetogenic Potential of Antineoplastic Agents *on page 1579*

U.S. Brand Names Leustatin®

Canadian Brand Names Leustatin®

Therapeutic Category Antineoplastic Agent, Antimetabo-lite (Purine)

Generic Available Yes

Use Treatment of hairy cell leukemia, chronic myeloid leukemia, and chronic lymphocytic leukemia; cladribine has activity in the treatment of Langerhans cell histiocy-tosis (LCH), non-Hodgkin's lymphomas, T-cell lymphomas, relapsed acute lymphocytic leukemia and relapsed acute myeloid leukemia

Pregnancy Risk Factor D

Pregnancy Considerations Teratogenic effects and fetal mortality were observed in animal studies. There are no adequate and well-controlled studies in pregnant women. Women of childbearing potential should avoid becoming pregnant.

Lactation Excretion in breast milk unknown/not recommended

Breast-Feeding Considerations Due to the potential for serious adverse reactions in the nursing infant, breast-feeding is not recommended.

Contraindications Hypersensitivity to cladribine or any component

Warnings Hazardous agent; use appropriate precautions for handling and disposal. Serious neurological toxicity has been reported in patients who received cladribine by continuous infusion at high doses (0.4-0.8 mg/kg/day or >16 mg/m^2/day) **[U.S. Boxed Warning]**; neurologic tox-icity appears to be dose-related. Severe neurologic toxicity has been reported rarely with standard dosing regimens. Acute nephrotoxicity has been observed with cladribine doses of 0.4-0.8 mg/kg/day, especially in patients con-currently receiving other nephrotoxic agents **[U.S. Boxed Warning]**.

Precautions Dose-limiting toxicity is myelosuppression **[U.S. Boxed Warning]**; myelosuppression is usually reversible; use with caution in patients with pre-existing hematologic or immunologic abnormalities; prophylactic administration of allopurinol should be considered in patients receiving cladribine due to the potential for hyperuricemia secondary to tumor lysis; appropriate antibiotic therapy should be administered promptly in patients exhibiting signs and symptoms of neutropenia and infection.

Adverse Reactions
Cardiovascular: Edema, tachycardia

Central nervous system: Fever (69%), fatigue (45%), headache, dizziness, insomnia, malaise, irreversible neurologic toxicity (paraparesis/quadriparesis) at high doses (0.4-0.8 mg/kg/day or >16 mg/m^2/day)

Dermatologic: Pruritus, erythema, rash

Gastrointestinal: Constipation, abdominal pain, nausea, vomiting, appetite decreased, diarrhea

Hematologic: Myelosuppression (prolonged pancytopenia), thrombocytopenia, aplastic anemia, hemolytic anemia

Hepatic: Reversible, mild elevations of bilirubin and transaminase levels

Local: Injection site reactions, pain

Neuromuscular & skeletal: Myalgia, trunk pain

Renal: Acute nephrotoxicity reported at high doses (rare)

Respiratory: Abnormal breath sounds, cough, shortness of breath

Drug Interactions

Avoid Concomitant Use

Avoid concomitant use of Cladribine with any of the following: BCG; Natalizumab; Pimecrolimus; Tacrolimus (Topical); Vaccines (Live)

Increased Effect/Toxicity

Cladribine may increase the levels/effects of: Leflunomide; Natalizumab; Vaccines (Live)

The levels/effects of Cladribine may be increased by: Denosumab; Pimecrolimus; Tacrolimus (Topical); Trastuzumab

Decreased Effect

Cladribine may decrease the levels/effects of: BCG; Sipuleucel-T; Vaccines (Inactivated); Vaccines (Live)

The levels/effects of Cladribine may be decreased by: Echinacea

Stability Refrigerate unopened vials (2°C to 8°C/36°F to 46°F); protect from light. Solutions should be administered immediately after the initial dilution or stored in the refrigerator (2°C to 8°C) for ≤8 hours. **The use of D$_5$W as a diluent is not recommended due to increased degradation of cladribine;** should not be mixed with other intravenous drugs or additives or infused simultaneously via a common intravenous line. Diluted solution of cladribine in NS is stable for 24 hours at room temperature under normal room light in polyvinyl chloride infusion containers.

Mechanism of Action A purine nucleoside analogue; prodrug which enters the cells through a transport system and is activated via phosphorylation by deoxycytidine kinase to a 5'-triphosphate derivative. This active form incorporates into DNA resulting in inhibition of DNA synthesis and early chain termination. The induction of strand breaks results in a drop in the cofactor nicotinamide adenine dinucleotide and disruption of cell metabolism. ATP is depleted to deprive cells of an important source of energy. Cladribine kills both resting as well as dividing cells.

Pharmacokinetics (Adult data unless noted)

Distribution: V$_d$:

Children: 305 L/m^2

Adults: 0.5-9 L/kg (53-160 L/m^2)

CSF: Plasma concentration ratio: 18.2%

Protein binding: 20%

Bioavailability: SubQ: 100%

Half-life: 19.7 hours ± 3.4 hours

Elimination: 21% to 44% renally excreted

Usual Dosage I.V.: (refer to individual protocols):

Children:

Hairy cell leukemia: 0.09 mg/kg/day continuous infusion for 7 days

AML:

<3 years: 0.3 mg/kg/day over 2 hours daily for 5 days

≥3 years: 9 mg/m^2/day over 2 hours daily for 5 days or 8.9 mg/m^2/day over 24 hours for 5 days

Langerhans cell histiocytosis: 5-7 mg/m^2/day for 5 days; repeat every 21-28 days; do not administer if platelet count <100,000

Adults: 0.09-0.1 mg/kg/day continuous infusion for 7 consecutive days

Administration Parenteral: I.V.: **Single daily infusion:** May administer diluted in NS as an intermittent infusion or continuous infusion; solutions for 7-day infusion should be prepared in bacteriostatic NS; the manufacturer recommends filtering with a 0.22 micron filter when preparing 7-day infusions

Monitoring Parameters CBC with differential and platelet count; creatinine clearance before initial dose; periodic renal and hepatic function tests

Nursing Implications Cladribine I.V. solution for administration should be inspected visually for particulates. A precipitate may occur at low temperatures and may be resolubilized at room temperature or by shaking the solution vigorously.

Dosage Forms Excipient information presented when available (limited, particularly for generics); consult specific product labeling.

Injection, solution [preservative free]: 1 mg/mL (10 mL)

References

Kearns CM, Biakley RL, Santane VM, et al, "Pharmacokinetics of Cladribine (2-Chlorodeoxyadenosine) in Children with Acute Leukemia," *Cancer Research*, 1994, 54:1235-39.

Larson RA, et al, "Dose Escalation Trial of Cladribine Using 5 Daily I.V. Infusions in Patients with Advanced Hematologic Malignancies," *J Clin Oncol*, 1996, 14(1):188-95.

Liliemark J, "The Clinical Pharmacokinetics of Cladribine," *Clin Pharmacokinet*, 1997, 32:120-131.

Rodriguez-Galindo C, Kelly P, Jeng M, et al, "Treatment of Children With Langerhans Cell Histiocytosis With 2-Chlorodeoxyadenosine," *Am J Hematol*, 2002, 69(3):179-84.

Stine KC, Saylors RL, Williams LL, et al, "2-Chlorodeoxyadenosine (2-CDA) for the Treatment of Refractory or Recurrent Langerhans Cell Histiocytosis (LCH) in Pediatric Patients," *Med Pediatr Oncol*, 1997, 29:288-92.

♦ **Claforan®** *see* Cefotaxime *on page 267*

♦ **Claravis™** *see* Isotretinoin *on page 769*

♦ **Clarinex®** *see* Desloratadine *on page 403*

Clarithromycin (kla RITH roe mye sin)

Medication Safety Issues

Sound-alike/look-alike issues:

Clarithromycin may be confused with Claritin®, clindamycin, erythromycin

Related Information

Endocarditis Prophylaxis *on page 1610*

U.S. Brand Names Biaxin®; Biaxin® XL

Canadian Brand Names Apo-Clarithromycin®; Biaxin®; Biaxin® XL; Mylan-Clarithromycin; PMS-Clarithromycin; ratio-Clarithromycin; Sandoz-Clarithromycin

Therapeutic Category Antibiotic, Macrolide

Generic Available Yes

Use Treatment of upper and lower respiratory tract infections, community-acquired pneumonia, acute otitis media, and infections of the skin and skin structure due to susceptible strains of *S. aureus*, *S. pyogenes*, *S. pneumoniae*, *H. influenzae*, *M. catarrhalis*, *Mycoplasma pneumoniae*, *C. trachomatis*, and *Legionella* species (FDA approved in ages ≥6 months and adults); prophylaxis and treatment of *Mycobacterium avium* complex (MAC) disease in patients with advanced HIV infection (FDA approved in ages ≥20 months and adults); treatment of *Helicobacter pylori* infection (FDA approved in adults); infective endocarditis prophylaxis for dental procedures in penicillin-allergic patients; postexposure prophylaxis and treatment of pertussis

Pregnancy Risk Factor C

Pregnancy Considerations Adverse fetal effects have been documented in some animal studies; therefore, clarithromycin is classified as pregnancy category C. Clarithromycin crosses the placenta. The manufacturer recommends that clarithromycin not be used in a pregnant woman unless there are no alternative therapies. An increased risk of teratogenic events has not been observed following maternal use of clarithromycin.

Lactation Excretion in breast milk unknown/use caution

Breast-Feeding Considerations It is not known if clarithromycin is excreted in human breast milk. The manufacturer recommends that caution be exercised when administering clarithromycin to breast-feeding women.

Other macrolides are considered compatible with breast-feeding and clarithromycin is used therapeutically in infants. Nondose-related effects could include modification of bowel flora.

Contraindications Hypersensitivity to clarithromycin, any component, erythromycin, or any macrolide antibiotics; concomitant administration of pimozide or cisapride with clarithromycin may result in QT interval prolongation, ventricular tachycardia, ventricular fibrillation, hypotension, palpitations, cardiac arrest, and death; coadministration of clarithromycin with ergot derivatives

Warnings Pseudomembranous colitis has been reported with use of clarithromycin. Colchicine toxicity with death has been reported with concomitant use of clarithromycin (some events occurred in patients with hepatic or renal impairment).

Precautions Use with caution in patients with hepatic or renal impairment; reduce dosage or prolong dosing interval in patients with severe renal impairment with or without coexisting hepatic impairment. Use caution in patients with myasthenia gravis; may exacerbate symptoms. When clarithromycin and colchicine are coadministered together, inhibition of CYP3A and p-glycoprotein may lead to increased exposure to colchicine (monitor for symptoms of colchicine toxicity).

Adverse Reactions

Central nervous system: Headache

Dermatologic: Rash

Gastrointestinal: Abdominal pain, diarrhea, dysgeusia, dyspepsia, nausea, pseudomembranous colitis, vomiting; incidence of adverse GI effects (diarrhea, nausea, vomiting, dyspepsia, abdominal pain) is lower (13%) compared to erythromycin treated patients (32%)

Hematologic: Prothrombin time elevated

Otic: Tinnitus

Renal: BUN increased

<1%, postmarketing, and/or case reports: Alkaline phosphatase increased, ALT increased, anaphylaxis, anorexia, anxiety, AST increased, behavioral changes, bilirubin increased, cholestatic hepatitis, confusion, depersonalization, depression, disorientation, dizziness, GGT increased, glossitis, hallucinations, hearing loss (reversible), hepatic dysfunction, hepatic failure, hepatitis, hypoglycemia, insomnia, interstitial nephritis, jaundice, leukopenia, LDH increased, manic behavior, neutropenia, nightmares, oral moniliasis, pancreatitis, psychosis, QT prolongation, seizure, serum creatinine increased, smell loss, Stevens-Johnson syndrome, stomatitis, thrombocytopenia, tinnitus, tongue discoloration, tooth discoloration (reversible), torsade de pointes, toxic epidermal necrolysis, tremor, urticaria, ventricular tachycardia, ventricular arrhythmia, vertigo, white blood cell count decreased

Drug Interactions

Metabolism/Transport Effects Substrate of CYP3A4 (major); **Inhibits** CYP1A2 (weak), CYP3A4 (strong), P-glycoprotein

Avoid Concomitant Use

Avoid concomitant use of Clarithromycin with any of the following: Alfuzosin; Artemether; BCG; Cisapride; Dabigatran Etexilate; Dihydroergotamine; Disopyramide; Dronedarone; Eplerenone; Ergotamine; Everolimus; Halofantrine; Lumefantrine; Nilotinib; Nisoldipine; Pimozide; QuiNINE; Ranolazine; Rivaroxaban; Romidepsin; Salmeterol; Silodosin; Tamsulosin; Tetrabenazine; Thioridazine; Tolvaptan; Topotecan; Ziprasidone

Increased Effect/Toxicity

Clarithromycin may increase the levels/effects of: Alfentanil; Alfuzosin; Almotriptan; Alosetron; Antifungal Agents (Azole Derivatives, Systemic); Antineoplastic Agents (Vinca Alkaloids); Benzodiazepines (metabolized by oxidation); Bortezomib; Brinzolamide; BusPIRone; Calcium Channel Blockers; CarBAMazepine; Cardiac Glycosides; Ciclesonide; Cilostazol; Cisapride; Clozapine; Colchicine; Corticosteroids (Systemic); Cyclo-SPORINE; CycloSPORINE (Systemic); CYP3A4 Substrates; Dabigatran Etexilate; Dienogest; Dihydroergotamine; Disopyramide; Dronedarone; Dutasteride; Eletriptan; Eplerenone; Ergot Derivatives; Ergotamine; Everolimus; FentaNYL; Fesoterodine; GlipiZIDE; GlyBURIDE; GuanFACINE; Halofantrine; HMG-CoA Reductase Inhibitors; Ixabepilone; Lumefantrine; Maraviroc; MethylPREDNISolone; Nilotinib; Nisoldipine; Paricalcitol; Pazopanib; P-Glycoprotein Substrates; Phosphodiesterase 5 Inhibitors; Pimecrolimus; Pimozide; Protease Inhibitors; QTc-Prolonging Agents; QuiNIDine; QuiNINE; Ranolazine; Repaglinide; Rifamycin Derivatives; Rivaroxaban; Romidepsin; Salmeterol; Saxagliptin; Selective Serotonin Reuptake Inhibitors; Silodosin; Sirolimus; Sorafenib; Tacrolimus; Tacrolimus (Systemic); Tacrolimus (Topical); Tadalafil; Tamsulosin; Temsirolimus; Tetrabenazine; Theophylline Derivatives; Thioridazine; Tolvaptan; Topotecan; Vitamin K Antagonists; Zidovudine; Ziprasidone; Zopiclone

The levels/effects of Clarithromycin may be increased by: Alfuzosin; Antifungal Agents (Azole Derivatives, Systemic); Artemether; Chloroquine; Ciprofloxacin; Ciprofloxacin (Systemic); CYP3A4 Inhibitors (Moderate); CYP3A4 Inhibitors (Strong); Gadobutrol; Lumefantrine; Nilotinib; Protease Inhibitors; QuiNINE

Decreased Effect

Clarithromycin may decrease the levels/effects of: BCG; Clopidogrel; Prasugrel; Typhoid Vaccine; Zidovudine

The levels/effects of Clarithromycin may be decreased by: CYP3A4 Inducers (Strong); Deferasirox; Etravirine; Herbs (CYP3A4 Inducers); Protease Inhibitors

Food Interactions

Immediate release formulations: Food may delay the rate but not the extent of oral absorption

Extended release formulations: Food increases AUC by 30% relative to fasting conditions

Stability Reconstituted oral suspension should **not** be refrigerated because it might gel; microencapsulated particles of clarithromycin in suspension are stable for 14 days when stored at room temperature

Mechanism of Action Inhibits bacterial RNA-dependent protein synthesis by binding to the 50S ribosomal subunit; the 14-hydroxy metabolite of clarithromycin is twice as active as the parent compound

Pharmacokinetics (Adult data unless noted)

Absorption: Rapid from the GI tract; food delays onset of absorption and formation of active metabolite, but does not affect the extent of tablet absorption; in pediatric patients, coadministration of the suspension with food did not significantly alter the extent of clarithromycin absorption or formation of the 14-OH metabolite (active)

Distribution: Widely distributed throughout the body with tissue concentrations higher than serum concentrations

Protein binding: 65% to 70%

Metabolism: In the liver to active and inactive metabolites; undergoes extensive first-pass metabolism

Bioavailability: 50% to 68%

Half-life: Dose-dependent, prolonged with renal dysfunction

Clarithromycin:
- 250 mg dose: 3-4 hours
- 500 mg dose: 5-7 hours

14-hydroxy metabolite:
- 250 mg dose: 5-6 hours
- 500 mg dose: 7-9 hours

Time to peak serum concentration: Immediate release formulations: 2-3 hours

Elimination: After a 250 mg tablet dose, 20% is excreted unchanged in urine, 10% to 15% is excreted as active metabolite 14-OH clarithromycin, and 4% is excreted in feces

Usual Dosage Oral:

Infants and Children:

Acute otitis media: 15 mg/kg/day divided every 12 hours for 10 days

Respiratory, skin and skin structure infections: 15 mg/kg/day divided every 12 hours for 7-14 days

Infective endocarditis prophylaxis for dental procedures in patients allergic to penicillins or ampicillin: 15 mg/kg 30-60 minutes before procedure; maximum dose: 500 mg

Prophylaxis for first episode of MAC with the following CD4[+] T-lymphocyte counts (see below): 15 mg/kg/day divided every 12 hours; maximum dose: 1 g/day

Children <12 months: <750 cells/microliter
1-2 years: <500 cells/microliter
2-6 years: <75 cells/microliter
≥6 years: <50 cells/microliter

Prophylaxis for recurrence of MAC: 15 mg/kg/day divided every 12 hours; maximum dose: 1 g/day (use in combination with ethambutol and with or without rifabutin)

Pertussis: Infants and Children ≥1 month: 15 mg/kg/day divided every 12 hours for 7 days; maximum dose: 1 g/day; **Note:** Use azithromycin in infants <1 month

Adolescents and Adults: Immediate-release tablet: 250 mg every 12 hours for 7-14 days for all indications except sinusitis and chronic bronchitis due to H. influenzae; for these indications, 500 mg every 12 hours for 7-14 days

Infective endocarditis prophylaxis for dental procedures in patients allergic to penicillins or ampicillin: 500 mg 30-60 minutes before procedure

Prophylaxis for first episode of MAC in patients with CD4[+] T-lymphocyte count <50 cells/microliter: 500 mg twice daily

Prophylaxis for recurrence of MAC: 500 mg twice daily in combination with ethambutol and with or without rifabutin

Helicobacter pylori (combination therapy): 500 mg twice daily with lansoprazole 30 mg twice daily and amoxicillin 1 g twice daily for 10-14 days (lansoprazole can be substituted with omeprazole 20 mg twice daily or esomeprazole 40 mg once daily)

Pertussis: 500 mg twice daily for 7 days

Adolescents and Adults: Extended-release tablet: Two 500 mg tablets every 24 hours for 7 days for chronic bronchitis and community-acquired pneumonia; two 500 mg tablets every 24 hours for 14 days for sinusitis

Dosing adjustment in renal impairment: Cl$_{cr}$ <30 mL/minute: Decrease dose by 50% and administer once or twice daily

Administration Oral: May administer immediate-release tablet or oral suspension with or without meals; extended-release tablet must be administered with food; do not crush or chew extended-release tablet; may administer with milk; shake suspension well before use

Monitoring Parameters Monitor serum concentration of drugs whose concentrations may be affected in patients receiving concomitant clarithromycin (ie, theophylline, carbamazepine, quinidine, digoxin, anticoagulants, triazolam); liver function tests; hearing (in patients receiving long-term treatment with clarithromycin); observe for changes in bowel frequency

Dosage Forms Excipient information presented when available (limited, particularly for generics); consult specific product labeling.

Granules for oral suspension: 125 mg/5 mL (50 mL, 100 mL); 250 mg/5 mL (50 mL, 100 mL)

Biaxin®: 125 mg/5 mL (50 mL, 100 mL); 250 mg/5 mL (50 mL, 100 mL) [fruit punch flavor]

Tablet: 250 mg, 500 mg

Biaxin®: 250 mg, 500 mg

Tablet, extended release: 500 mg

Biaxin® XL: 500 mg

References

Aspin MM, Hoberman A, McCarty J, et al, "Comparative Study of the Safety and Efficacy of Clarithromycin and Amoxicillin-Clavulanate in the Treatment of Acute Otitis Media in Children," J Pediatr, 1994, 125 (1):136-41.

Chey WD, Wong BC, and Practice Parameters Committee of the American College of Gastroenterology, "American College of Gastroenterology Guideline on the Management of Helicobacter pylori Infection," Am J Gastroenterol, 2007, 102(8):1808-25.

Guay DR and Craft JC, "Overview of the Pharmacology of Clarithromycin Suspension in Children and a Comparison With That in Adults," Pediatr Infect Dis J, 1993, 12(12 Suppl 3):S106-11.

Husson RN, Ross LA, Sandelli S, et al, "Orally Administered Clarithromycin for the Treatment of Systemic Mycobacterium avium Complex Infection in Children With Acquired Immunodeficiency Syndrome," J Pediatr, 1994, 124(5 Pt 1):807-14.

Kaplan JE, Masur H, and Holmes KK, "Guidelines for Preventing Opportunistic Infections Among HIV-Infected Persons - 2002 Recommendations of the USPHS and IDSA," MMWR, 2002, 51 (RR-8):1-46.

Neu HC, "The Development of Macrolides: Clarithromycin in Perspective," J Antimicrob Chemother, 1991, 27(Suppl A):1-9.

Tiwari T, Murphy TV, and Moran J, "Recommended Antimicrobial Agents for the Treatment and Postexposure Prophylaxis of Pertussis: 2005 CDC Guidelines," MMWR Recomm Rep, 2005, 54(RR-14):1-16.

Wilson W, Taubert KA, Gewitz M, et al, "Prevention of Infective Endocarditis. Guidelines From the American Heart Association," Circulation, 2007, 115:1-20.

♦ **Claritin® (Can)** see Loratadine on page 842

♦ **Claritin® 24 Hour Allergy [OTC]** see Loratadine on page 842

♦ **Claritin-D® 12 Hour Allergy & Congestion [OTC]** see Loratadine and Pseudoephedrine on page 844

♦ **Claritin-D® 24 Hour Allergy & Congestion [OTC]** see Loratadine and Pseudoephedrine on page 844

♦ **Claritin® Allergic Decongestant (Can)** see Oxymetazoline on page 1043

♦ **Claritin® Children's Allergy [OTC]** see Loratadine on page 842

♦ **Claritin® Extra (Can)** see Loratadine and Pseudoephedrine on page 844

♦ **Claritin™ Eye [OTC]** see Ketotifen on page 785

♦ **Claritin® Hives Relief [OTC] [DSC]** see Loratadine on page 842

♦ **Claritin® Kids (Can)** see Loratadine on page 842

♦ **Claritin® Liberator (Can)** see Loratadine and Pseudoephedrine on page 844

♦ **Claritin® Liqui-Gels® 24 Hour Allergy [OTC]** see Loratadine on page 842

♦ **Claritin® RediTabs® 24 Hour Allergy [OTC]** see Loratadine on page 842

♦ **Clarus™ (Can)** see Isotretinoin on page 769

♦ **Clavulanic Acid and Amoxicillin** see Amoxicillin and Clavulanic Acid on page 98

◆ **Clavulin® (Can)** *see* Amoxicillin and Clavulanic Acid *on page 98*

◆ **Clear eyes® for Dry Eyes and ACR Relief [OTC]** *see* Naphazoline *on page 966*

◆ **Clear eyes® for Dry Eyes and Redness Relief [OTC]** *see* Naphazoline *on page 966*

◆ **Clear eyes® Redness Relief [OTC]** *see* Naphazoline *on page 966*

◆ **Clear eyes® Seasonal Relief [OTC]** *see* Naphazoline *on page 966*

◆ **Clearskin [OTC]** *see* Benzoyl Peroxide *on page 184*

Clemastine (KLEM as teen)

U.S. Brand Names Dayhist® Allergy [OTC] [DSC]; Tavist® Allergy [OTC]

Therapeutic Category Antihistamine

Generic Available Yes

Use Perennial and seasonal allergic rhinitis and other allergic symptoms including urticaria

Pregnancy Risk Factor B

Lactation Enters breast milk/not recommended

Contraindications Hypersensitivity to clemastine or any component; narrow-angle glaucoma; patients receiving MAO inhibitors

Precautions Use with caution in patients with stenosing peptic ulcer, GI or GU obstruction, asthma, or prostatic hypertrophy

Adverse Reactions

Cardiovascular: Bradycardia, edema, palpitations

Central nervous system: Drowsiness, fatigue, headache, dizziness, vertigo, ataxia, CNS stimulation (more common in children)

Dermatologic: Rash, angioedema, photosensitivity

Endocrine & metabolic: Weight gain

Gastrointestinal: Nausea, vomiting, xerostomia, gastritis, appetite increase, diarrhea, abdominal pain

Hepatic: Hepatitis

Neuromuscular & skeletal: Arthralgia, myalgia, paresthesia

Respiratory: Shortness of breath, pharyngitis, bronchospasm, epistaxis

Drug Interactions

Metabolism/Transport Effects Inhibits CYP2D6 (weak), 3A4 (weak)

Avoid Concomitant Use There are no known interactions where it is recommended to avoid concomitant use.

Increased Effect/Toxicity

Clemastine may increase the levels/effects of: Alcohol (Ethyl); Anticholinergics; CNS Depressants

The levels/effects of Clemastine may be increased by: Pramlintide

Decreased Effect

Clemastine may decrease the levels/effects of: Acetylcholinesterase Inhibitors (Central); Betahistine

The levels/effects of Clemastine may be decreased by: Acetylcholinesterase Inhibitors (Central); Amphetamines

Mechanism of Action Competes with histamine for H_1-receptor sites on effector cells in the GI tract, blood vessels, and respiratory tract

Pharmacodynamics

Onset of action: 2 hours after administration

Maximum effect: 5-7 hours

Duration: 10-12 hours

Pharmacokinetics (Adult data unless noted)

Absorption: Oral: Well absorbed

Distribution: Breast milk to plasma ratio: 0.25-0.5

Metabolism: In the liver

Time to peak serum concentration: 2-4 hours

Elimination: Majority of an oral dose eliminated in the urine

Usual Dosage Oral:

Infants and Children <6 years: 0.05 mg/kg/day as **clemastine base** or 0.335-0.67 mg/day clemastine fumarate (0.25-0.5 mg base/day) divided into 2 or 3 doses; maximum daily dosage: 1.34 mg (1 mg base)

Children 6-12 years: 0.67-1.34 mg clemastine fumarate (0.5-1 mg base) twice daily; do not exceed 4.02 mg/day (3 mg/day base)

Children ≥12 years and Adults: 1.34 mg clemastine fumarate (1 mg base) twice daily to 2.68 mg (2 mg base) 3 times/day; do not exceed 8.04 mg/day (6 mg base)

Administration Oral: Administer with food

Monitoring Parameters Look for a reduction of rhinitis, urticaria, eczema, pruritus, or other allergic symptoms

Patient Information Avoid alcohol; may cause drowsiness and impair ability to perform activities requiring mental alertness or physical coordination; may cause dry mouth. May rarely cause photosensitivity reactions (eg, exposure to sunlight may cause severe sunburn, skin rash, redness, or itching); avoid direct exposure to sunlight

Dosage Forms Excipient information presented when available (limited, particularly for generics); consult specific product labeling. [DSC] = Discontinued product

Syrup, as fumarate: 0.67 mg/5 mL (120 mL, 480 mL) [prescription formulation; 0.5 mg base/5 mL]

Tablet, as fumarate: 1.34 mg [1 mg base; OTC], 2.68 mg [2 mg base; prescription formulation]

Dayhist® Allergy [DSC], Tavist® Allergy: 1.34 mg [1 mg base]

◆ **Clemastine Fumarate** *see* Clemastine *on page 327*

◆ **Cleocin®** *see* Clindamycin *on page 327*

◆ **Cleocin HCl®** *see* Clindamycin *on page 327*

◆ **Cleocin Pediatric®** *see* Clindamycin *on page 327*

◆ **Cleocin Phosphate®** *see* Clindamycin *on page 327*

◆ **Cleocin T®** *see* Clindamycin *on page 327*

◆ **Cleocin® Vaginal Ovule** *see* Clindamycin *on page 327*

◆ **Climara®** *see* Estradiol *on page 536*

◆ **Clindagel®** *see* Clindamycin *on page 327*

◆ **ClindaMax®** *see* Clindamycin *on page 327*

Clindamycin (klin da MYE sin)

Medication Safety Issues

Sound-alike/look-alike issues:

Cleocin® may be confused with bleomycin, Clinoril®, Cubicin®, Lincocin®

Clindamycin may be confused with clarithromycin, Claritin®, vancomycin

Related Information

Endocarditis Prophylaxis *on page 1610*

Malaria *on page 1652*

U.S. Brand Names Cleocin HCl®; Cleocin Pediatric®; Cleocin Phosphate®; Cleocin T®; Cleocin®; Cleocin® Vaginal Ovule; Clindagel®; ClindaMax®; ClindaReach®; Clindesse®; Evoclin®

Canadian Brand Names Apo-Clindamycin®; Clinda-T; Clindamycin Injection, USP; Clindamycine; Clindasol™; Clindets; Clindoxyl; Dalacin® C; Dalacin® T; Dalacin® Vaginal; Mylan-Clindamycin; Novo-Clindamycin; PMS-Clindamycin; ratio-Clindamycin; Riva-Clindamycin; Taro-Clindamycin

Therapeutic Category Acne Products; Antibiotic, Anaerobic; Antibiotic, Miscellaneous

Generic Available Yes: Excludes foam, granules, vaginal suppositories

Use Active against most aerobic gram-positive staphylococci and streptococci (except enterococci); useful against *Fusobacterium*, *Bacteroides* species, *Actinomyces*, and certain anaerobic gram-positive organisms. Use for treatment of infections of the respiratory tract, skin and soft tissue, and female pelvis and genital tract; sepsis and intra-abdominal infections due to susceptible organisms (FDA approved in children and adults); bacterial endocarditis prophylaxis for dental and upper respiratory procedures in penicillin-allergic patients; perioperative prophylaxis for head and neck surgery (incision through oral mucosa), colorectal surgery, appendectomy, or surgery for ruptured viscus; treatment of babesiosis; used topically in treatment of acne vulgaris (FDA approved in ages >12 years and adults); used intravaginally for treatment of bacterial vaginosis (FDA approved in adults)

Pregnancy Risk Factor B

Pregnancy Considerations Because adverse effects were not observed in animals, clindamycin is classified as pregnancy category B. Clindamycin crosses the placenta throughout pregnancy and at term, but use during pregnancy has not been shown to cause adverse fetal effects. Clindamycin pharmacokinetics are not affected by pregnancy. Clindamycin therapy is recommended in certain pregnant patients for prophylaxis of group B streptococcal disease in newborns, prophylaxis and treatment of *Toxoplasma gondii* encephalitis, or for the treatment of *Pneumocystis* pneumonia (PCP), bacterial vaginosis, or malaria.

Lactation Enters breast milk/not recommended

Breast-Feeding Considerations Small amounts of clindamycin transfer to human milk. Although the manufacturer does not recommend the use of clindamycin during breast-feeding, the American Academy of Pediatrics considers clindamycin to be "usually compatible with breast-feeding." Nondose-related effects could include modification of bowel flora. There has been one published case of bloody stools in a nursing infant, but a causal relationship was not proven.

Contraindications Hypersensitivity to clindamycin, lincomycin, or any component (see Warnings)

Warnings Use of topical and systemic clindamycin can cause severe and possibly fatal colitis **[U.S. Boxed Warning]** characterized by severe persistent diarrhea, severe abdominal cramps and possibly, the passage of blood and mucus; discontinue drug if significant diarrhea occurs. Antiperistaltic agents such as opiates or diphenoxylate with atropine may prolong and worsen the condition.

Capsule contains tartrazine which may cause allergic reactions in susceptible individuals. Injection contains benzyl alcohol which may cause allergic reactions in susceptible individuals; large amounts of benzyl alcohol (≥99 mg/kg/day) have been associated with a potentially fatal toxicity ("gasping syndrome") in neonates; the "gasping syndrome" consists of metabolic acidosis, respiratory distress, gasping respirations, CNS dysfunction (including convulsions, intracranial hemorrhage), hypotension and cardiovascular collapse; use clindamycin injection products containing benzyl alcohol with caution in neonates; *in vitro* and animal studies have shown that benzoate, a metabolite of benzyl alcohol, displaces bilirubin from protein binding sites

Precautions Use with caution and modify dosage in patients with severe renal and/or hepatic impairment; use with caution in atopic patients; use with caution in patients with previous pseudomembranous colitis, regional enteritis, or ulcerative colitis

Adverse Reactions

Cardiovascular: Arrhythmia due to QT_c prolongation,; cardiac arrest (with rapid I.V. administration), hypotension

Central nervous system: Dizziness, headache

Dermatologic: Dry skin, erythema, pruritus, rash, Stevens-Johnson syndrome, urticaria

Gastrointestinal: Abdominal pain, diarrhea, esophagitis, nausea, pseudomembranous colitis (see Warnings), vomiting

Genitourinary: Vaginal candidiasis, vaginitis

Hematologic: Eosinophilia, granulocytopenia, neutropenia, thrombocytopenia

Hepatic: Liver enzymes increased

Local: Application site burning, dryness, pruritus; erythema, pain, swelling, thrombophlebitis; sterile abscess at I.M. injection site

Neuromuscular & skeletal: Polyarthritis (rare)

Renal: Renal dysfunction (rare)

Miscellaneous: Hypersensitivity reactions

Drug Interactions

Avoid Concomitant Use

Avoid concomitant use of Clindamycin with any of the following: BCG; Erythromycin; Erythromycin (Systemic)

Increased Effect/Toxicity

Clindamycin may increase the levels/effects of: Neuromuscular-Blocking Agents

Decreased Effect

Clindamycin may decrease the levels/effects of: BCG; Erythromycin (Systemic); Typhoid Vaccine

The levels/effects of Clindamycin may be decreased by: Erythromycin; Kaolin

Stability Store foam at room temperature (Flammable: Do not expose to heat, fire, or flame). Do **not** refrigerate the reconstituted oral solution because it will thicken; oral solution stable for 2 weeks at room temperature following reconstitution

Mechanism of Action Reversibly binds to 50S ribosomal subunits preventing peptide bond formation thus inhibiting bacterial protein synthesis; bacteriostatic or bactericidal depending on drug concentration, infection site, and organism

Pharmacokinetics (Adult data unless noted)

Absorption:

Oral: 90% of clindamycin hydrochloride is rapidly absorbed; clindamycin palmitate must be hydrolyzed in the GI tract before it is active

Topical: ~10% absorbed systemically

Distribution: No significant levels are seen in CSF, even with inflamed meninges; crosses the placenta; distributes into breast milk, saliva, ascites fluid, pleural fluid, bone, and bile

Protein binding: 94%

Bioavailability: Oral: ~90%

Half-life:

Neonates:

Premature: 8.7 hours

Full-term: 3.6 hours

Infants 1 month to 1 year: 3 hours

Children and Adults with normal renal function: 2-3 hours

Time to peak serum concentration:

Oral: Within 60 minutes

I.M.: Within 1-3 hours

Elimination: Most of the drug is eliminated by hepatic metabolism; 10% of an oral dose excreted in urine and 3.6% excreted in feces as active drug and metabolites

Dialysis: Not dialyzable (0% to 5%)

Usual Dosage

Neonates: I.M., I.V.:

Postnatal age ≤7 days:

≤2000 g: 10 mg/kg/day divided every 12 hours

>2000 g: 15 mg/kg/day divided every 8 hours

Postnatal age >7 days:

<1200 g: 10 mg/kg/day divided every 12 hours

1200-2000 g: 15 mg/kg/day divided every 8 hours

>2000 g: 20-30 mg/kg/day divided every 6-8 hours

Infants and Children:
Oral: 10-30 mg/kg/day divided every 6-8 hours; maximum dose: 1.8 g/day
Primary prevention of rheumatic fever (treatment of streptococcal tonsillopharyngitis) in penicillin-allergic patients (>3 years): 20 mg/kg/day divided every 8 hours; maximum dose: 1.8 g/day
Bacterial endocarditis prophylaxis for dental and upper respiratory procedures in penicillin allergic patients: 20 mg/kg 1 hour before procedure
Babesiosis: 20-40 mg/kg/day divided every 8 hours for 7 days plus quinine
I.M., I.V.: 25-40 mg/kg/day divided every 6-8 hours; doses as high as 4.8 g/day I.V. have been given in life-threatening situations. Bacterial endocarditis prophylaxis for dental and upper respiratory procedures in penicillin allergic patients: I.V.: 20 mg/kg 30 minutes before procedure; maximum dose: 600 mg
Children >12 years and Adults: Topical:
Gel, pledget, lotion, solution: Apply a thin film twice daily
Foam: Apply once daily in an amount that will cover the affected area
Adolescents and Adults:
Oral: 150-450 mg/dose every 6-8 hours; maximum dose: 1.8 g/day
I.M., I.V.: 1.2-2.7 g/day in 2-4 divided doses; doses as high as 4.8 g/day have been given I.V. in life-threatening situations
Vaginal:
Cream: One full applicator (100 mg) inserted intravaginally once daily before bedtime for 3 or 7 consecutive days
Suppository: Insert one ovule (100 mg) intravaginally once daily before bedtime for 3 days
Bacterial endocarditis prophylaxis for dental and upper respiratory procedures in penicillin allergic patients:
Oral: 600 mg 1 hour before procedure **or** I.V.: 600 mg 30 minutes before procedure
Pelvic inflammatory disease: 900 mg I.V. every 8 hours for 24-48 hours after significant clinical improvement, followed by 600 mg orally 3 times/day to complete a 14-day course
Babesiosis:
I.V.: 1.2 g twice daily plus quinine
or
Oral: 600 mg 3 times/day for 7 days plus quinine
Dosing interval in renal/hepatic impairment: Reduce dosage in patients with severe renal or hepatic impairment

Administration

Intravaginal: Do not use for topical therapy, instillation in the eye, or oral administration. Wash hands; insert applicator into vagina and expel suppository or cream. Remain lying down for 30 minutes following administration. Wash applicator with soap and water following suppository use; if administering the cream, use each disposable applicator only once
Oral: Capsule should be taken with a full glass of water to avoid esophageal irritation; shake oral solution well before use; may administer with or without meals
Parenteral: Administer by I.V. intermittent infusion over at least 10-60 minutes, at a rate **not** to exceed 30 mg/minute; hypotension and cardiopulmonary arrest have been reported following rapid I.V. administration; final concentration for administration should not exceed 18 mg/mL
Topical: Do not use intravaginally, instill in the eye, or administer orally
Foam: Before applying foam, wash affected area with mild soap, then dry. Do not dispense foam directly onto hands or face. Remove cap, hold can at an upright angle and dispense foam directly into the cap or onto a cool surface. If can is warm or foam is runny, run can

under cold water. Use fingertips to pick up small amounts of foam and gently massage into affected area until foam disappears. Avoid fire, flame, or smoking during or immediately following application.
Lotion: Shake well before use
Monitoring Parameters Observe for changes in bowel frequency; during prolonged therapy monitor CBC with differential, platelet count, hepatic and renal function tests periodically
Patient Information Report any severe diarrhea immediately; clindamycin vaginal cream (oil-based) may weaken latex condoms for up to 72 hours after completing therapy
Dosage Forms Excipient information presented when available (limited, particularly for generics); consult specific product labeling. [DSC] = Discontinued product
Note: Strength is expressed as base
Aerosol, topical, as phosphate [foam]:
Evoclin®: 1% (50 g, 100 g) [contains ethanol 58%]
Capsule, as hydrochloride: 75 mg, 150 mg, 300 mg
Cleocin HCl®: 75 mg [contains tartrazine], 150 mg [contains tartrazine], 300 mg
Cream, vaginal, as phosphate: 2% (40 g)
Cleocin®: 2% (40 g) [contains benzyl alcohol and mineral oil; packaged with 7 disposable applicators]
ClindaMax®: 2% (40 g) [contains benzyl alcohol and mineral oil; packaged with 7 disposable applicators] [DSC]
Clindesse®: 2% (5 g) [contains mineral oil; prefilled single disposable applicator]
Gel, topical, as phosphate: 1% (30 g, 60 g)
Cleocin T®: 1% (30 g, 60 g)
Clindagel®: 1% (40 mL, 75 mL)
ClindaMax®: 1% (30 g, 60 g)
Granules for oral solution, as palmitate hydrochloride:
Cleocin Pediatric®: 75 mg/5 mL (100 mL) [cherry flavor]
Infusion, as phosphate [premixed in D_5W]:
Cleocin Phosphate®: 300 mg (50 mL), 600 mg (50 mL), 900 mg (50 mL) [contains edetate disodium]
Injection, solution, as phosphate: 150 mg/mL (2 mL, 4 mL, 6 mL, 60 mL)
Cleocin Phosphate®: 150 mg/mL (2 mL, 4 mL, 6 mL, 60 mL) [contains benzyl alcohol and edetate disodium]
Lotion, as phosphate: 1% (60 mL)
Cleocin T®, ClindaMax®: 1% (60 mL)
Pledgets, topical: 1% (60s, 69s)
Cleocin T®: 1% (60s) [contains isopropyl alcohol 50%]
ClindaReach®: 1% (120s) [contains isopropyl alcohol 50%; packaged as a kit containing 1 collapsible applicator, 64 appliques, and 64 unmedicated pads]
Solution, topical, as phosphate: 1% (30 mL, 60 mL)
Cleocin T®: 1% (30 mL, 60 mL) [contains isopropyl alcohol 50%]
Suppository, vaginal, as phosphate:
Cleocin® Vaginal Ovule: 100 mg (3s) [contains oleaginous base; single reusable applicator]

References

Gerber MA, Baltimore RS, Eaton CB, et al, "Prevention of Rheumatic Fever and Diagnosis and Treatment of Acute *Streptococcal pharyngitis*: A Scientific Statement from the American Heart Association Rheumatic Fever, Endocarditis, and Kawasaki Disease Committee of the Council on Cardiovascular Disease in the Young, the Interdisciplinary Council on Functional Genomics and Translational Biology, and the Interdisciplinary Council on Quality of Care and Outcomes Research: Endorsed by the American Academy of Pediatrics," *Circulation*, 2009, 119(11):1541-51.
Wilson W, Taubert KA, Gewitz M, et al, "Prevention of Infective Endocarditis. Guidelines From the American Heart Association," *Circulation*, 2007, 115:1-20.

Clindamycin and Benzoyl Peroxide
(klin da MYE sin & BEN zoe il peer OKS ide)

U.S. Brand Names Acanya™; BenzaClin®; Duac® CS
Canadian Brand Names BenzaClin®; Clindoxyl

◀ **Therapeutic Category** Acne Products; Topical Skin Product

Generic Available Yes

Use Topical treatment of acne vulgaris (FDA approved in ages ≥12 years and adults)

Pregnancy Risk Factor C

Pregnancy Considerations Reproduction studies have not been conducted; use during pregnancy only if clearly needed.

Lactation Excretion in breast milk unknown/not recommended

Breast-Feeding Considerations Clindamycin is excreted in breast milk following oral and parenteral administration; the extent of excretion, if any, following topical use, in this combination is not known.

Contraindications Hypersensitivity to benzoyl peroxide, clindamycin, lincomycin, or any component; history of regional enteritis, ulcerative colitis, pseudomembranous colitis, or antibiotic-associated colitis

Warnings Use of topical clindamycin results in absorption from the skin surface; diarrhea, bloody diarrhea, and colitis (including pseudomembranous colitis) have been reported with the use of topical and systemic clindamycin; the colitis is usually characterized by severe persistent diarrhea and severe abdominal cramps and may be associated with the passage of blood and mucus; discontinue drug if significant diarrhea occurs. Antiperistaltic agents such as opiates or diphenoxylate with atropine may prolong and worsen the condition. May bleach hair or clothing. Concomitant use with topical or oral erythromycin-containing products is not recommended.

Precautions Avoid contact with eyes and mucous membranes; use of antibiotic agents may be associated with the overgrowth of nonsusceptible organisms including fungi; if this occurs, discontinue use; concomitant topical acne therapy should be used with caution because a possible cumulative irritancy effect may occur, especially with the use of peeling, desquamating, or abrasive agents. Inform patients to use skin protection and minimize prolonged exposure to sun or tanning beds.

Adverse Reactions

Dermatologic: Dry skin, pruritus, peeling, scaling, erythema, photosensitivity

Gastrointestinal: Colitis, diarrhea, AAPC

Local: Burning, pain, stinging, irritation

Miscellaneous: Anaphylaxis

Drug Interactions

Avoid Concomitant Use

Avoid concomitant use of Clindamycin and Benzoyl Peroxide with any of the following: BCG; Erythromycin; Erythromycin (Systemic)

Increased Effect/Toxicity

Clindamycin and Benzoyl Peroxide may increase the levels/effects of: Neuromuscular-Blocking Agents

Decreased Effect

Clindamycin and Benzoyl Peroxide may decrease the levels/effects of: BCG; Erythromycin (Systemic); Typhoid Vaccine

The levels/effects of Clindamycin and Benzoyl Peroxide may be decreased by: Erythromycin; Kaolin

Stability

Acanya™: Store at room temperature; protect from freezing; stable at room temperature for 2 months after admixture

BenzaClin®: Store at room temperature; protect from freezing; stable at room temperature for 3 months after reconstitution with purified water for 3 months

Duac® CS: Store in refrigerator until dispensed; protect from freezing; stable at room temperature for 60 days

Mechanism of Action Clindamycin and benzoyl peroxide have activity against *Propionibacterium acnes in vitro*. This organism has been associated with acne vulgaris. Benzoyl peroxide releases free-radical oxygen which oxidizes bacterial proteins in the sebaceous follicles decreasing the number of anaerobic bacteria and decreasing irritating-type free fatty acids. Clindamycin reversibly binds to 50S ribosomal subunits preventing peptide bond formation thus inhibiting bacterial protein synthesis; bacteriostatic or bactericidal depending on the drug concentration, infection site, and organism.

Pharmacodynamics See individual agents.

Pharmacokinetics (Adult data unless noted) See individual agents.

Usual Dosage Topical: Children ≥12 years and Adults:
Acanya™: Apply pea-sized amount of gel once daily; use >12 weeks has not been studied.
BenzaClin®: Apply twice daily (morning and evening)
Duac® CS: Apply once daily in the evening

Administration

FOR EXTERNAL USE ONLY. Not for oral, ophthalmic, or intravaginal use.

Topical: Skin should be clean and dry before applying. Apply thin layer to affected areas avoiding contact with eyes, lips, inside of nose, mouth, and all mucous membranes.

Acanya™: Add clindamycin solution in the bottle to the benzoyl peroxide gel and stir 1 ½ minutes with spatula until homogenous.

BenzaClin®: Add indicated amount of purified water to the mark on the vial; immediately shake to dissolve clindamycin. Add clindamycin solution to the gel and stir 1 ½ minutes until homogenous.

Patient Information Avoid contact with eyes, inside of nose, mouth, and all mucous membranes; do not apply on cuts or open wounds; may bleach hair and clothing; notify physician if severe diarrhea, dryness, redness, peeling, or photosensitivity reaction occurs.

May cause photosensitivity reactions (eg, exposure to sunlight may cause severe sunburn, skin rash, redness, or itching); avoid exposure to sunlight and artificial light sources (sunlamps, tanning booth/bed); wear protective clothing, wide-brimmed hats, sunglasses, and lip sunscreen (SPF ≥15); use a sunscreen [broad-spectrum sunscreen or physical sunscreen (preferred) or sunblock with SPF ≥15].

Dosage Forms Excipient information presented when available (limited, particularly for generics); consult specific product labeling.

Gel, topical: Clindamycin phosphate 1% and benzoyl peroxide 5% (50 g)
Acanya™: Clindamycin phosphate 1% and benzoyl peroxide 2.5% (50 g)
BenzaClin®: Clindamycin phosphate 1% and benzoyl peroxide 5% (25 g, 50 g)
Duac® CS: Clindamycin phosphate 1% and benzoyl peroxide 5% (45 g) [packaged with SFC™ lotion 107 mL]

♦ **Clindoxyl (Can)** *see* Clindamycin *on page 327*

♦ **Clindoxyl (Can)** *see* Clindamycin and Benzoyl Peroxide *on page 329*

♦ **Clinic BPO** *see* Benzoyl Peroxide *on page 184*

♦ **Clinoril®** *see* Sulindac *on page 1307*

Clobetasol (kloe BAY ta sol)

Medication Safety Issues
International issues:
Clobex®: Brand name for clobetasol [U.S., Canada] may be confused with Codex® which is a brand name for *Saccharomyces boulardii* in Italy
Cloderm: Brand name for clobetasol [China, India, Malaysia, Singapore, Thailand], but also brand name for alclometasone [Indonesia]; clocortolone [U.S., Canada]; clotrimazole [Germany]

Related Information
Corticosteroids *on page 1487*

U.S. Brand Names Clobex®; Cormax®; Olux-E™; Olux®; Olux®/Olux-E™ CP; Temovate E®; Temovate®

Canadian Brand Names Clobex®; Dermovate®; Gen-Clobetasol; Mylan-Clobetasol Cream; Mylan-Clobetasol Ointment; Mylan-Clobetasol Scalp Application; Novo-Clobetasol; PMS-Clobetasol; ratio-Clobetasol; Taro-Clobetasol

Therapeutic Category Adrenal Corticosteroid; Anti-inflammatory Agent; Corticosteroid, Topical; Glucocorticoid

Generic Available Yes: Excludes lotion, shampoo, spray

Use Short-term relief of inflammation and pruritus associated with corticosteroid-responsive dermatoses

Pregnancy Risk Factor C

Pregnancy Considerations Extensive use in pregnant women is not recommended. There are no adequate and well-controlled studies in pregnant women, however, teratogenic effects were observed in animal studies.

Lactation Excretion in breast milk unknown/use caution

Breast-Feeding Considerations It is not known if topical application will result in detectable quantities in breast milk.

Contraindications Hypersensitivity to clobetasol propionate, other corticosteroids, or any component; the solution for scalp application is also contraindicated for use in patients with primary scalp infections

Warnings Hypothalamic-pituitary-adrenal (HPA) axis suppression may occur with topical clobetasol use, even at low doses; acute adrenal insufficiency may occur with abrupt withdrawal after long-term use or with stress; withdrawal or discontinuation should be done carefully; patients with HPA axis suppression may require increased doses of systemic glucocorticosteroids prior to, during, and after unusual stress (eg, surgery). Adverse systemic effects (including HPA axis suppression) may occur when topical steroids are used on large areas of the body, denuded areas, for prolonged periods of time, with an occlusive dressing, and/or in pediatric patients; infants and small children may be more susceptible to HPA axis suppression or other systemic toxicities due to a larger skin surface area to body mass ratio; use with caution in pediatric patients; due to the increased risk of HPA axis suppression and other systemic toxicities, the use of any clobetasol product for the treatment of steroid-responsive dermatoses is not recommended in children <12 years of age; use of clobetasol lotion or spray for moderate to severe plaque-type psoriasis in children <18 years is not recommended.

Do not use topical clobetasol for the treatment of rosacea or perioral dermatitis; do not apply to the face, groin, or axillae. Do not exceed maximum recommended dose or duration of therapy due to the potential development of HPA axis suppression.

Precautions Avoid using higher than recommended doses; suppression of HPA axis, suppression of linear growth (ie, reduction of growth velocity), reduced bone mineral, or hypercorticism (Cushing's syndrome) may occur. Discontinue treatment if local irritation develops. Use appropriate antibacterial or antifungal agents to treat concomitant skin infections; discontinue clobetasol treatment if infection does not resolve promptly.

Adverse Reactions
Central nervous system: Intracranial hypertension (systemic effect reported in children treated with topical corticosteroids); headache (with scalp application)
Dermatologic: Burning, stinging, cracking and fissuring of the skin, local pain, pigmentation change, dryness, erythema, folliculitis, irritation, pruritus, skin atrophy, telangiectasia. **Note:** Other dermatologic effects reported with scalp application: Scalp pustules, tightness of the scalp, dermatitis, tenderness, and hair loss. Other effects reported with other high-potency topical steroids: Acne eruptions, allergic contact dermatitis, hypertrichosis, hypopigmentation, maceration of the skin, miliaria, striae, perioral dermatitis, secondary infection.
Endocrine & metabolic: Hyperglycemia, HPA axis suppression, Cushing's syndrome, growth retardation
Neuromuscular & skeletal: Numbness of the fingers
Ocular: Eye irritation (with scalp application)
Renal: Glycosuria

Drug Interactions
Avoid Concomitant Use
Avoid concomitant use of Clobetasol with any of the following: Aldesleukin

Increased Effect/Toxicity There are no known significant interactions involving an increase in effect.

Decreased Effect
Clobetasol may decrease the levels/effects of: Aldesleukin; Corticorelin

Stability
Cream, emollient cream, ointment: Store at room temperature, between 15°C to 30°C (59°F to 86°F). Do not refrigerate.
Foam: Store at room temperature of 20°C to 25°C (68°F to 77°F); do not expose to heat or temperatures >49°C (120°F). Can be pressurized; do not puncture or incinerate. Contents are flammable; avoid flame, fire, or smoking during and immediately after application.
Gel: Store between 2°C to 30°C (36°F to 86°F)
Lotion: Store at room temperature of 20°C to 25°C (68°F to 77°F). Do not freeze.
Solution: Do not use near open flame.
Cormax® scalp application: Store at room temperature between 15°C to 30°C (59°F to 86°F); do not refrigerate.
Temovate® scalp application: Store between 4°C to 25°C (39°F to 77°F).
Spray: Store at controlled room temperature; do not refrigerate or freeze; do not store at >30°C; spray is flammable; avoid heat, do not use near open flame

Mechanism of Action Not well defined topically; possesses anti-inflammatory, antipruritic, antiproliferative, vasoconstrictive, and immunosuppressive properties

Pharmacokinetics (Adult data unless noted)
Absorption: Percutaneous absorption varies and depends on many factors including vehicle used, integrity of epidermis, dose, and use of occlusive dressing; absorption is increased by occlusive dressings or with decreased integrity of skin (eg, inflammation or skin disease); gel has greater absorption than cream
Metabolism: Hepatic
Elimination: Drug and metabolites are excreted in urine and bile

◀ **Usual Dosage** Topical: Use the smallest amount for the shortest period of time to avoid HPA suppression; discontinue therapy when control is achieved; reassess diagnosis if no improvement is seen within 2 weeks.

Children <12 years: Use not recommended (high risk of systemic adverse effects, eg, HPA axis suppression, Cushing's syndrome)

Children ≥12 years and Adults:

Steroid-responsive dermatoses:

Cream, emollient cream, gel, lotion, ointment: Apply sparingly twice daily for up to 2 weeks; maximum dose: 50 g/week or 50 mL/week

Foam, solution: Apply sparingly to affected area of scalp twice daily for up to 2 weeks; maximum dose: 50 g/week or 50 mL/week

Mild to moderate plaque-type psoriasis of nonscalp areas: Foam: Apply sparingly to affected area twice daily for up to 2 weeks; maximum dose: 50 g/week; do not apply to face or intertriginous areas

Moderate to severe plaque-type psoriasis: Emollient cream: Apply sparingly twice daily for up to 2 weeks; if response is not adequate, may be used for up to 2 more weeks if application is <10% of body surface area; use with caution; maximum dose: 50 g/week

Children ≥18 years and Adults: Moderate to severe plaque-type psoriasis:

Lotion: Apply sparingly twice daily for up to 2 weeks; if response is not adequate, may be used for up to 2 more weeks if application is <10% of body surface area; use with caution; maximum dose: 50 mL/week (see Additional Information)

Spray: Apply sparingly twice daily for up to 2 weeks; if response is not adequate, may be used for up to 2 more weeks, but use should be limited to skin lesions that have not sufficiently improved; maximum dose: 50 g (59 mL) per week

Administration

Topical: All products: Apply sparingly to clean dry skin of affected area, gently rub in until disappears; do not use on open skin; do not apply to face, underarms, or groin area; avoid contact with eyes and lips; do not occlude affected area; wash hands after applying

Foam: Turn can upside down and spray a small amount (maximum: 1 ½ capful or about the size of a golf ball) of foam into the cap, other cool surface, or to affected area. If the can is warm or foam is runny, place can under cold, running water. If fingers are warm, rinse with cool water and dry prior to handling (foam will melt on contact with warm skin). Massage foam into affected area.

Monitoring Parameters Assess HPA axis suppression in patients using potent topical steroids applied to a large surface area or to areas under occlusion (eg, ACTH stimulation test, morning plasma cortisol test, urinary free cortisol test)

Patient Information Avoid contact with eyes and lips; do not apply to face, underarms, or groin area; do not bandage, cover, or wrap affected area unless directed by physician; wash hands after applying. Use only as prescribed and for the minimum amount of time required; do not use for longer than directed; notify physician if condition being treated persists or worsens; inform physician of use if surgery is to be considered.

Additional Information Considered to be a super high potency topical corticosteroid; clobetasol is a prednisolone analog with a high level of glucocorticoid activity and slight degree of mineralocorticoid activity. Nine of 14 pediatric patients (12-17 years of age) with moderate to severe atopic dermatitis (involving ≥20% BSA), who were treated with clobetasol lotion 0.05% twice daily for 2 weeks, developed adrenal suppression (versus 2 of 10 patients treated with the cream). Due to this high incidence of adrenal suppression, the lotion is not approved for this indication in children <18 years of age.

Dosage Forms Excipient information presented when available (limited, particularly for generics); consult specific product labeling. [DSC] = Discontinued product

Aerosol, topical, as propionate [foam]: 0.05% (50 g, 100 g)

Olux-E™: 0.05% (50 g, 100 g) [ethanol free]

Olux®: 0.05% (50 g, 100 g) [contains ethanol 60%; for scalp application]

Combination package, topical, as propionate:

Olux®/Olux-E™ CP: Aerosol, topical [foam]:

Olux-E™: 0.05% (50 g)

Olux®: 0.05% (50 g) [contains ethanol 60%]

Olux®/Olux-E™ CP: Aerosol, topical [foam]:

Olux-E™: 0.05% (10 g)

Olux®: 0.05% (100 g) [contains ethanol 60%]

Cream, topical, as propionate: 0.05% (15 g, 30 g, 45 g, 60 g, 60s)

Cormax®: 0.05% (15 g, 30 g, 45 g) [DSC]

Temovate®: 0.05% (30 g, 60 g)

Cream, topical, as propionate [emulsion-based]: 0.05% (15 g, 30 g, 60 g)

Cream, topical, as propionate [in emollient base]: 0.05% (15 g, 30 g, 60 g)

Temovate E®: 0.05% (60 g)

Gel, topical, as propionate: 0.05% (15 g, 30 g, 60 g)

Temovate®: 0.05% (60 g)

Lotion, topical, as propionate:

Clobex®: 0.05% (30 mL, 59 mL, 118 mL)

Ointment, topical, as propionate: 0.05% (15 g, 30 g, 45 g, 60 g)

Cormax®: 0.05% (15 g, 45 g)

Temovate®: 0.05% (15 g, 30 g)

Shampoo, topical, as propionate:

Clobex®: 0.05% (118 mL) [contains ethanol]

Solution, topical, as propionate [for scalp application]: 0.05% (25 mL, 50 mL)·

Cormax®: 0.05% (25 mL, 50 mL) [contains isopropyl alcohol 40%]

Temovate®: 0.05% (50 mL) [contains isopropyl alcohol 39.3%]

Solution, topical, as propionate [spray]:

Clobex®: 0.05% (59 mL, 125 mL) [contains ethanol]

◆ **Clobetasol Propionate** see Clobetasol on page 331

◆ **Clobex®** see Clobetasol on page 331

Clofarabine (klo FARE a been)

Medication Safety Issues

Sound-alike/look-alike issues:

Clofarabine may be confused with cladribine, clevidipine

High alert medication: The Institute for Safe Medication Practices (ISMP) includes this medication among its list of drug classes which have a heightened risk of causing significant patient harm when used in error.

Related Information

Emetogenic Potential of Antineoplastic Agents on page 1579

U.S. Brand Names Clolar®

Therapeutic Category Antineoplastic Agent, Antimetabolite (Purine Antagonist)

Generic Available No

Use Treatment of relapsed or refractory acute lymphoblastic leukemia (ALL) after at least two prior treatment regimens (FDA approved in ages 1-21 years). Has been used for the treatment of acute myelogenous leukemia (AML) and myelodysplastic syndrome (MDS)

Pregnancy Risk Factor D

Pregnancy Considerations Teratogenic effects were observed in animal studies. There are no adequate or well-controlled studies in pregnant women. Women of childbearing potential should be advised to use effective contraception and avoid becoming pregnant during therapy.

Lactation Excretion in breast milk unknown/not recommended

Breast-Feeding Considerations Due to the potential for serious adverse reactions in the nursing infant, breast-feeding is not recommended.

Contraindications Hypersensitivity to clofarabine or any component

Warnings Hazardous agent; use appropriate precautions for handling and disposal. May cause fetal harm when administered to a pregnant woman (women of childbearing potential should be advised to avoid becoming pregnant while on clofarabine). Bone marrow suppression (appears to be dose dependent and reversible) increases the risk of infection. Tumor lysis syndrome/hyperuricemia may occur as a result of leukemia treatment with clofarabine, usually occurring in the first treatment cycle; may lead to life-threatening acute renal failure; adequate hydration and prophylactic allopurinol throughout the 5 days of clofar-abine treatment will reduce the risk/effects of tumor lysis syndrome; monitor closely. Cytokine release may develop into systemic inflammatory response syndrome (SIRS)/capillary leak syndrome and organ dysfunction. Prophy-lactic corticosteroids may prevent the signs/symptoms of cytokine release. Discontinue clofarabine (and consider use of diuretics, corticosteroids, and albumin) if SIRS, capillary leak syndrome, or hypotension occurs. If hypotension resolves without pharmacological interven-tion, clofarabine can be restarted at a lower dose. Transaminases and bilirubin may be increased during treatment; may require dosage modification or discontin-uation of clofarabine. The risk for hepatotoxicity, including hepatic veno-occlusive disease (VOD), is increased in patients who have previously undergone a hematopoietic stem cell transplant.

Precautions Safety and efficacy have not been estab-lished with renal or hepatic impairment; use with caution. Avoid concomitant use of nephrotoxic or hepatotoxic drugs.

Adverse Reactions

Cardiovascular: Hypotension, capillary leak syndrome (respiratory distress, hypotension, pleural and pericardial effusion, multi-organ failure), tachycardia, flushing, edema, left ventricular systolic function decreased, right ventricular pressure increased

Central nervous system: Dizziness, lightheadedness, fainting spells, fatigue, fever, headache, chills, anxiety, pain, irritability, lethargy, somnolence, agitation, mental status change, hallucination

Dermatologic: Rash, erythema, pruritus, palmar-plantar erythrodysesthesia syndrome, petechiae, cellulitis, der-matitis, Stevens-Johnson syndrome, toxic epidermal necrolysis

Endocrine & metabolic: Tumor lysis syndrome, hyper-uricemia, hypokalemia, hypophosphatemia

Gastrointestinal: Vomiting, diarrhea, nausea, abdominal pain, anorexia, mucosal inflammation, gingival bleeding, oral candidiasis, proctalgia, clostridium colitis, stomatitis, mouth hemorrhage, oral mucosal petechiae, cecitis, pancreatitis

Hematologic: Neutropenia, anemia, thrombocytopenia, lymphopenia, leukopenia, febrile neutropenia, bone marrow failure

Hepatic: Hyperbilirubinemia, elevated liver enzymes, jaundice, hepatomegaly, hepatic veno-occlusive disease

Neuromuscular & skeletal: Limb pain, myalgia, back pain, bone pain, asthenia, arthralgia

Renal: Hematuria, serum creatinine elevated, acute renal failure

Respiratory: Tachypnea, respiratory distress, pulmonary edema, cough, epistaxis, dyspnea, pleural effusion, pneumonia, upper respiratory infection, pulmonary edema

Miscellaneous: Sepsis, SIRS, infection (bacterial, fungal, viral), septic shock, hypersensitivity

Drug Interactions

Avoid Concomitant Use

Avoid concomitant use of Clofarabine with any of the following: BCG; Natalizumab; Pimecrolimus; Tacrolimus (Topical); Vaccines (Live)

Increased Effect/Toxicity

Clofarabine may increase the levels/effects of: Lefluno-mide; Natalizumab; Vaccines (Live); Vitamin K Antagonists

The levels/effects of Clofarabine may be increased by: Denosumab; Pimecrolimus; Tacrolimus (Topical); Trastuzumab

Decreased Effect

Clofarabine may decrease the levels/effects of: BCG; Cardiac Glycosides; Sipuleucel-T; Vaccines (Inactivated); Vaccines (Live); Vitamin K Antagonists

The levels/effects of Clofarabine may be decreased by: Echinacea

Stability Store undiluted drug at 15°C to 30°C (59°F to 86°F); diluted solution is stable for 24 hours at room temperature 15°C to 30°C (59°F to 86°F). To prevent drug incompatibilities, do not mix with other medications.

Mechanism of Action Clofarabine, a purine nucleoside analog is metabolized to clofarabine 5'-triphosphate which competes with deoxyadenosine triphosphate for binding to ribonucleotide reductase and DNA polymerase. Clofar-abine inhibits DNA synthesis, terminates DNA chain elongation, and inhibits DNA repair resulting in decreased cell replication and repair. Clofarabine disrupts the mitochondrial membrane which results in the release of proteins, cytochrome C and apoptosis-inducing factor leading to cell death.

Pharmacokinetics (Adult data unless noted)

Distribution: V_d: Children: 172 L/m^2

Protein binding: 47%, primarily to albumin

Metabolism: Intracellularly by deoxycytidine kinase and mono- and di-phosphokinases to active metabolite clofarabine 5'-triphosphate; limited hepatic metabolism (0.2%)

Half-life: Children: 5.2 hours

Elimination: 49% to 60% excreted in urine as unchanged drug

Clearance: 28.8 L/hour/m^2

Usual Dosage I.V. infusion (refer to individual protocols):

Note: Consider prophylactic corticosteroids (hydrocorti-sone 100 mg/m^2 on days 1-3 to prevent signs/symptoms of capillary leak syndrome or SIRS); provide I.V. hydration, allopurinol, and alkalinize urine (to reduce the risk of tumor lysis syndrome/hyperuricemia); consider prophylactic antiemetics.

Children 1-21 years of age: 52 mg/m^2/day once daily for 5 days of a 28 day cycle; repeat cycle every 2-6 weeks following recovery or return to baseline organ function; subsequent cycles should begin no sooner than 14 days from the start of the previous cycle (subsequent cycles may be administered when ANC ≥750/mm^3)

Children and Adults: Refractory and/or relapsed hemato-logic malignancy (ALL, AML, MDS) in combination therapy: 40 mg/m^2/day for 5 days every 28 days

Dosage adjustment for toxicity:

Hematologic toxicity: ANC <500/mm^3 lasting ≥4 weeks: Reduce clofarabine dose by 25% for next cycle

Nonhematologic toxicity:

Clinically significant infection: Withhold treatment until infection is under control, then restart clofarabine at full dose

Grade 3 toxicity, excluding infection, nausea, and vomiting, and transient elevations in transaminases and bilirubin: Withhold treatment; may reinitiate clofarabine with a 25% dose reduction with resolution or return to baseline

Grade ≥3 increase in creatinine or bilirubin: Discontinue clofarabine; may reinitiate with 25% dosage reduction when creatinine or bilirubin return to baseline and patient is stable; administer allopurinol for hyperuricemia.

Grade 4 toxicity (noninfectious): Discontinue clofarabine treatment

Capillary leak or systemic inflammatory response syndrome (SIRS) signs/symptoms (eg, hypotension, tachycardia, tachypnea, pulmonary edema): Discontinue clofarabine; institute supportive measures

Administration Parenteral: I.V. infusion: Filter clofarabine through a 0.2 μm syringe filter and then further dilute dose with D_5W or NS to a final concentration of 0.15-0.4 mg/mL; administer by I.V. infusion over 2 hours. Use appropriate precautions for handling and disposal of hazardous drugs.

Monitoring Parameters Renal and hepatic function tests, blood pressure, cardiac function, respiratory status, CBC with differential, platelet count, uric acid, urine output, signs and symptoms of infection

Patient Information Female patients of childbearing potential should avoid pregnancy during clofarabine therapy by using effective forms of contraception; avoid breast-feeding during treatment. Notify physician of signs of weakness, fatigue, pallor, shortness of breath, easy bruising, petechiae, purpura, fever, tachycardia, tachypnea, dyspnea, or hypotension.

Nursing Implications Ensure adequate hydration by giving continuous I.V. fluids throughout the 5 days of clofarabine administration to prevent tumor lysis and other adverse effects.

Dosage Forms Excipient information presented when available (limited, particularly for generics); consult specific product labeling.

Injection, solution [preservative free]:

Clolar®: 1 mg/mL (20 mL)

References

Faderl S, Ravandi F, Huang X, et al, "A Randomized Study of Clofarabine Versus Clofarabine Plus Low-Dose Cytarabine as Front-Line Therapy for Patients Aged 60 Years and Older With Acute Myeloid Leukemia and High-Risk Myelodysplastic Syndrome," *Blood*, 2008, 112(5):1638-45.

Jeha S, Gandhi V, Chan KW, et al, "Clofarabine, a Novel Nucleoside Analog, Is Active in Pediatric Patients With Advanced Leukemia," *Blood*, 2004, 103(3):784-9.

Jeha S, Gaynor PS, Razzouk BI, et al, "Phase II Study of Clofarabine in Pediatric Patients With Refractory or Relapsed Acute Lymphoblastic Leukemia," *J Clin Oncol*, 2006, 24(12):1917-23.

Kantarjian H, Gandhi V, Cortes J, et al, "Phase 2 Clinical and Pharmacologic Study of Clofarabine in Patients With Refractory or Relapsed Acute Leukemia," *Blood*, 2003, 102(7):2379-86.

◆ **Clofarex** *see* Clofarabine *on page 332*

◆ **Clolar®** *see* Clofarabine *on page 332*

ClomiPRAMINE (kloe MI pra meen)

Medication Safety Issues

Sound-alike/look-alike issues:

ClomiPRAMINE may be confused with chlorproMAZINE, clevidipine, clomiPHENE, desipramine, Norpramin®

Anafranil® may be confused with alfentanil, enalapril, nafarelin

Related Information

Antidepressant Agents *on page 1484*

U.S. Brand Names Anafranil®

Canadian Brand Names Anafranil®; Apo-Clomipramine®; CO Clomipramine; Gen-Clomipramine

Therapeutic Category Antidepressant, Tricyclic (Tertiary Amine)

Generic Available Yes

Use Treatment of obsessive-compulsive disorder (OCD)

Medication Guide An FDA-approved patient medication guide, which is available with the product information and at http://www.fda.gov/downloads/Drugs/DrugSafety/ucm085910.pdf, must be dispensed with this medication for each new outpatient prescription and refill.

Pregnancy Risk Factor C

Pregnancy Considerations There are no adequate and well-controlled studies in pregnant women. Withdrawal symptoms (including dizziness, nausea, vomiting, headache, malaise, sleep disturbance, hyperthermia, and/or irritability) have been observed in neonates whose mothers took clomipramine up to delivery. Use in pregnancy only if the benefits to the mother outweigh the potential risks to the fetus.

Lactation Enters breast milk/not recommended (AAP rates "of concern")

Breast-Feeding Considerations Generally, it is not recommended to breast-feed if taking antidepressants because of the long half-life, active metabolites, and potential for side effects in the infant.

Contraindications Hypersensitivity to clomipramine, other tricyclic agents, or any component; use of MAO inhibitors within 14 days (potentially fatal reactions may occur, see Drug Interactions); use in a patient during the acute recovery phase of MI

Warnings Clomipramine is FDA-approved for the treatment of obsessive compulsive disorder in children ≥10 years of age. Clomipramine is not approved for the treatment of depression in pediatric patients. Clinical worsening of depression or suicidal ideation and behavior may occur in children and adults with major depressive disorder **[U.S. Boxed Warning]**. In clinical trials, antidepressants increased the risk of suicidal thinking and behavior (suicidality) in children, adolescents, and young adults (18-24 years of age) with major depressive disorder and other psychiatric disorders. This risk must be considered before prescribing antidepressants for any clinical use. Short-term studies did not show an increased risk of suicidality with antidepressant use in patients >24 years of age and showed a decreased risk in patients ≥65 years.

Patients of all ages who are treated with antidepressants for any indication require appropriate monitoring and close observation for clinical worsening of depression, suicidality, and unusual changes in behavior, especially during the first few months after antidepressant initiation or when the dose is adjusted. Family members and caregivers should be instructed to closely observe the patient (ie, daily) and communicate condition with healthcare provider. Patients should also be monitored for associated behaviors (eg, anxiety, agitation, panic attacks, insomnia, irritability, hostility, aggressiveness, impulsivity, akathisia, hypomania, mania) which may increase the risk for worsening depression or suicidality. Worsening depression or emergence of suicidality (or associated behaviors listed above) that is abrupt in onset, severe, or not part of the presenting symptoms, may require discontinuation or modification of drug therapy.

Do not discontinue abruptly in patients receiving high doses chronically (withdrawal symptoms may occur; see Adverse Reactions). To reduce risk of intentional overdose, write prescriptions for the smallest quantity consistent with good patient care. Screen individuals for bipolar disorder prior to treatment (using antidepressants alone may induce manic episodes in patients with this condition). May worsen psychosis in some patients. Clomipramine is not FDA approved for the treatment of bipolar depression.

Clomipramine may cause seizures (direct relationship to dose and/or duration of therapy); do not exceed maximum doses. Use with caution in patients with a previous seizure disorder or condition predisposing to seizures such as brain damage, alcoholism, or concurrent therapy with other drugs which lower the seizure threshold.

Precautions May cause sedation, resulting in impaired performance of tasks requiring alertness (eg, operating machinery or driving). Sedative effects may be additive with other CNS depressants and/or ethanol. The degree of sedation is very high relative to other antidepressants. Weight gain may occur. May increase the risks associated with electroconvulsive therapy; limit such treatment to patients in whom it is essential. Consider discontinuing, when possible, prior to elective surgery. Therapy should not be abruptly discontinued in patients receiving high doses for prolonged periods.

May cause tachycardia and orthostatic hypotension (risk is moderate to high relative to other antidepressants); use with caution in patients at risk of hypotension or in patients where transient tachycardia and hypotensive episodes would be poorly tolerated (cardiovascular disease or cerebrovascular disease). The degree of anticholinergic blockade produced by this agent is very high relative to other cyclic antidepressants; use with caution in patients with urinary retention, benign prostatic hyperplasia, narrow-angle glaucoma, increased IOP, xerostomia, visual problems, constipation, or history of bowel obstruction.

Use with caution in patients with a history of cardiovascular disease (including previous MI, stroke, tachycardia, or conduction abnormalities). The risk of conduction abnormalities with this agent is high relative to other antidepressants. Use with caution in hyperthyroid patients or those receiving thyroid supplementation. Use with caution in patients with tumors of the adrenal medulla (hypertensive crisis may result). Use with caution in patients with hepatic or renal dysfunction.

Adverse Reactions Note: The adverse reaction profile in children 10-17 years of age is similar to that in adults; however, it is unknown what (if any) effects that long-term clomipramine treatment may have on growth and development in children.

Cardiovascular: Hypotension, palpitation, tachycardia

Central nervous system: Dizziness, drowsiness, headache, insomnia, nervousness, confusion, hypertonia, sleep disorder, yawning, speech disorder, abnormal dreaming, paresthesia, memory impairment, anxiety, twitching, coordination impaired, agitation, migraine, depersonalization, emotional lability, flushing, fever

Note: Activation is 2- to 3-fold more prevalent in children compared to adolescents; it is more prevalent in adolescents compared to adults. Somnolence or insomnia is more common in adults compared to children and adolescents.

Dermatologic: Rash, pruritus, dermatitis

Endocrine & metabolic: Libido changes, weight gain

Gastrointestinal: Xerostomia, constipation, appetite increased, nausea, dyspepsia, anorexia, abdominal pain, diarrhea, vomiting

Note: Vomiting is 2- to 3-fold more prevalent in children compared to adolescents; it is more prevalent in adolescents compared to adults. Divide the dose and give with food initially to minimize nausea and vomiting. Can consolidate to once daily dosing at bedtime during maintenance therapy. Cholinergic rebound upon abrupt discontinuation (nausea, vomiting, diarrhea, salivation,

lacrimation) is more problematic in youth compared to adults.

Genitourinary: Difficult urination

Neuromuscular & skeletal: Fatigue, tremors, myoclonus

Ocular: Blurred vision, eye pain

Miscellaneous: Diaphoresis increased; withdrawal symptoms following abrupt discontinuation (headache, nausea, malaise)

Drug Interactions

Metabolism/Transport Effects Substrate of CYP1A2 (major), 2C19 (major), 2D6 (major), 3A4 (minor); **Inhibits** CYP2D6 (moderate)

Avoid Concomitant Use

Avoid concomitant use of ClomiPRAMINE with any of the following: Artemether; Dronedarone; Iobenguane I 123; Lumefantrine; MAO Inhibitors; Metoclopramide; Nilotinib; Pimozide; QuiNINE; Sibutramine; Tetrabenazine; Thioridazine; Ziprasidone

Increased Effect/Toxicity

ClomiPRAMINE may increase the levels/effects of: Alcohol (Ethyl); Alpha-/Beta-Agonists (Direct-Acting); Alpha1-Agonists; Amphetamines; Anticholinergics; Aspirin; Beta2-Agonists; CNS Depressants; CYP2D6 Substrates; Desmopressin; Dronedarone; Fesoterodine; Milnacipran; Nebivolol; NSAID (COX-2 Inhibitor); NSAID (Nonselective); Pimozide; QTc-Prolonging Agents; QuiNIDine; QuiNINE; Serotonin Modulators; Sulfonylureas; Tamoxifen; Tetrabenazine; Thioridazine; TraMADol; Vitamin K Antagonists; Yohimbine; Ziprasidone

The levels/effects of ClomiPRAMINE may be increased by: Alfuzosin; Altretamine; Artemether; BuPROPion; CarBAMazepine; Chloroquine; Cimetidine; Cinacalcet; Ciprofloxacin; Ciprofloxacin (Systemic); CYP1A2 Inhibitors (Moderate); CYP1A2 Inhibitors (Strong); CYP2C19 Inhibitors (Moderate); CYP2C19 Inhibitors (Strong); CYP2D6 Inhibitors (Moderate); CYP2D6 Inhibitors (Strong); Dexmethylphenidate; Divalproex; DULoxetine; Gadobutrol; Grapefruit Juice; Lithium; Lumefantrine; MAO Inhibitors; Methylphenidate; Metoclopramide; Nilotinib; Pramlintide; Propoxyphene; Protease Inhibitors; QuiNIDine; QuiNINE; Selective Serotonin Reuptake Inhibitors; Sibutramine; Terbinafine; Terbinafine (Systemic); Valproic Acid

Decreased Effect

ClomiPRAMINE may decrease the levels/effects of: Acetylcholinesterase Inhibitors (Central); Alpha2-Agonists; Codeine; Iobenguane I 123

The levels/effects of ClomiPRAMINE may be decreased by: Acetylcholinesterase Inhibitors (Central); Barbiturates; CYP1A2 Inducers (Strong); CYP2C19 Inducers (Strong); Peginterferon Alfa-2b; St Johns Wort

Food Interactions Food does not affect bioavailability. Grapefruit juice may increase serum concentrations or toxicity.

Stability Store at controlled room temperature at 20°C to 25°C (68°F to 77°F). Dispense in tightly closed container; protect from moisture.

Mechanism of Action Tricyclic antidepressants increase the synaptic concentration of serotonin and/or norepinephrine in the CNS by inhibition of their reuptake by the presynaptic neuronal membrane. Clomipramine appears to affect serotonin uptake while its active metabolite, desmethylclomipramine, affects norepinephrine uptake.

Pharmacodynamics

Onset of action: 1-2 weeks

Maximum effect: 8-12 weeks

Duration: 1-2 days

CLOMIPRAMINE

Pharmacokinetics (Adult data unless noted)

◄ Absorption: Rapid

Distribution: Distributes into CSF, brain, and breast milk; active metabolite (desmethylclomipramine) also distributes into CSF with average CSF to plasma ratio: 2.6

Protein binding: 97%; primarily to albumin

Metabolism: Hepatic to desmethylclomipramine (DMI; active) and other metabolites; extensive first-pass effect; metabolites undergo glucuronide conjugation; metabolism of clomipramine and DMI may be capacity limited (ie, may display nonlinear pharmacokinetics); with multiple dosing, plasma concentrations of DMI are greater than clomipramine

Half-life: Adults (following a 150 mg dose): Clomipramine 19-37 hours (mean: 32 hours); DMI: 54-77 hours (mean: 69 hours)

Elimination: 50% to 60% of dose is excreted in the urine and 24% to 32% in feces; only 0.8% to 1.3% is excreted in urine as parent drug and active metabolite (combined amount)

Usual Dosage Note: During initial dose titration, divide the dose and give with meals to minimize nausea and vomiting. During maintenance therapy, may administer total daily dose once daily at bedtime to minimize daytime sedation.

Children: **Note:** Controlled clinical trials have not shown tricyclic antidepressants to be superior to placebo for the treatment of depression in children and adolescents (see Dopheide, 2006 and Wagner, 2005).

<10 years: Safety and efficacy have not been established; specific recommendations cannot be made for use in this age group

≥10 years: OCD: Initial: 25 mg/day; gradually increase, as tolerated, to a maximum of 3 mg/kg/day or 100 mg/day (whichever is smaller) during the first 2 weeks; may then gradually increase, if needed, over the next several weeks to a maximum of 3 mg/kg/day or 200 mg/day (whichever is smaller)

Adults: OCD: Initial: 25 mg/day; gradually increase, as tolerated, to 100 mg/day during the first 2 weeks; may then gradually increase, if needed, over the next several weeks to a total of 250 mg/day maximum

Administration Oral: May administer with food to decrease GI upset; see Note in Usual Dosage

Monitoring Parameters Monitor patient periodically for symptom resolution; monitor for worsening depression, suicidality, and associated behaviors (especially at the beginning of therapy or when doses are increased or decreased; see Warnings).

Monitor weight, pulse rate and blood pressure prior to and during therapy; ECG and cardiac status in patients with cardiac disease; periodic liver enzymes in patients with liver disease; CBC with differential in patients who develop fever and sore throat during treatment.

Patient Information Read the patient Medication Guide that you receive with each prescription and refill of clomipramine. An increased risk of suicidal thinking and behavior has been reported with the use of antidepressants in children, adolescents, and young adults (18-24 years of age). Notify physician if you feel more depressed, have thoughts of suicide, or become more agitated or irritable (see Warnings). Avoid alcohol, grapefruit juice, and the herbal medicine St John's wort; limit caffeine intake. This medication may cause drowsiness, lightheadedness, impaired coordination, dizziness, or blurred vision and impair ability to perform activities requiring mental alertness or physical coordination. May cause dry mouth or unpleasant aftertaste (sucking lozenges and frequent mouth care may help). Do not discontinue abruptly (withdrawal symptoms may occur).

If multiple doses are prescribed per day, take with meals to reduce side effects. Take single daily dose at bedtime to reduce daytime sedation. Do not take any new medication during therapy unless approved by prescriber. Take exactly as directed; do not increase dose or frequency; may take 2-3 weeks to achieve desired results. May cause headache, seizures, constipation, or orthostatic hypotension (use caution when rising from lying or sitting to standing position or when climbing stairs). Report unresolved constipation or GI upset, blurred vision or eye pain, difficulty in urination, unusual muscle weakness, chest pain, palpitations, rapid heart beat, or persistent CNS disturbances (hallucinations, suicidality, seizures, delirium, insomnia, or impaired gait).

Nursing Implications Assess other medications patient may be taking for possible interactions (especially MAO inhibitors, P450 inhibitors, and other CNS active agents). Assess mental status for depression, suicidal ideation, and associated behaviors (see Warnings). If history of cardiac problems, monitor cardiac status closely. Be alert to the potential of new or increased seizure activity. Periodically evaluate need for continued use. Taper dosage slowly when discontinuing (allow 3-4 weeks between discontinuing this medication and starting another antidepressant).

Additional Information If used for an extended period of time, long-term usefulness of clomipramine should be periodically re-evaluated for the individual patient.

Dosage Forms Excipient information presented when available (limited, particularly for generics); consult specific product labeling.

Capsule, as hydrochloride: 25 mg, 50 mg, 75 mg

Anafranil®: 25 mg, 50 mg, 75 mg

References

Braconnier A, LeCoent R, Cohen D, et al, "Paroxetine Versus Clomipramine in Adolescents With Severe Major Depression: A Double-Blind, Randomized, Multicenter Trial," *J Am Acad Child Adolesc Psychiatry*, 2003, 42(1):22-9.

Cano-Munoz JL, Montejo-Iglesias ML, Yanez-Saez RM, et al, "Possible Serotonin Syndrome Following the Combined Administration of Clomipramine and Alprazolam," *J Clin Psychiatry*, 1995, 56(3):122.

Dale O and Hole A, "Biphasic Time-Course of Serum Concentrations of Clomipramine and Desmethylclomipramine After a Near-Fatal Overdose," *Vet Hum Toxicol*, 1994, 36(4):309-10.

Dopheide JA, "Recognizing and Treating Depression in Children and Adolescents," *Am J Health Syst Pharm*, 2006, 63(3):233-43.

Geller DA, "Obsessive Compulsive and Spectrum Disorders in Children and Adolescents," *Psychiatr Clin North Am*, 2006, 29(2):353-70.

Hernandez AF, Montero MN, Pla A, et al, "Fatal Moclobemide Overdose or Death Caused by Serotonin Syndrome?" *J Forensic Sci*, 1995, 40 (1):128-30.

Kuisma MJ, "Fatal Serotonin Syndrome With Trismus," *Ann Emerg Med*, 1995, 26(1):108.

Larochelle P, Hamet P, and Enjalbert M, "Responses to Tyramine and Norepinephrine After Imipramine and Trazodone," *Clin Pharmacol Ther*, 1979, 26(1):24-30.

Larrey D, Rueff B, Pessayre D, et al, "Cross Hepatotoxicity Between Tricyclic Antidepressants," *Gut*, 1986, 27(6):726-7.

Lejoyeux M, et al, "Serotonin Syndrome: Incidence, Symptoms, and Treatment," *CNS Drugs*, 1994, 2:132-43.

Ljungren B and Bojs G, "A Case of Photosensitivity and Contact Allergy to Systemic Tricyclic Drugs, With Unusual Features," *Contact Dermatitis*, 1991, 24(4):259-65.

Pass SE and Simpson RW, "Discontinuation and Reinstitution of Medications During the Perioperative Period," *Am J Health Syst Pharm*, 2004, 61(9):899-912.

Roberge RJ, Martin TG, Hodgman M, et al, "Acute Chemical Pancreatitis Associated With a Tricyclic Antidepressant (Clomipramine) Overdose," *J Toxicol Clin Toxicol*, 1994, 32(4):425-9.

Safer DJ and Zito JM, "Treatment-Emergent Adverse Events From Selective Serotonin Reuptake Inhibitors by Age Group: Children vs Adolescents," *J Child and Adolesc Psychopharmacol*, 2006, 16(1/2):159-69.

Sternbach H, "Fluoxetine-Clomipramine Interaction," *J Clin Psychiatry*, 1995, 56(4):171-2.

Svedmyr N, "The Influence of a Tricyclic Antidepressive Agent (Protriptyline) on Some of the Circulatory Effects of Noradrenaline and Adrenalin® in Man," *Life Sci*, 1968, 7(1):77-84.

Swanson-Biearman B, Goetz CM, Dean BS, et al, "Anafranil® Overdose: A Fatal Outcome," *Vet Hum Toxicol*, 1989, 31:378.

Tueth MJ, "The Serotonin Syndrome in the Emergency Department," *Ann Emerg Med*, 1993, 22(8):1369.

Wagner KD, "Pharmacotherapy for Major Depression in Children and Adolescents," *Prog Neuropsychopharmacol Biol Psychiatry*, 2005, 29 (5):819-26.

Walsh KH and McDougle CJ, "Pharmacological Strategies for Trichotillomania," *Expert Opin Pharmacother*, 2005, 6(6):975-84.

◆ **Clomipramine Hydrochloride** *see* ClomiPRAMINE *on page 334*

◆ **Clonapam (Can)** *see* ClonazePAM *on page 337*

ClonazePAM (kloe NA ze pam)

Medication Safety Issues
Sound-alike/look-alike issues:
ClonazePAM may be confused with clofazimine, cloNI-Dine, clorazepate, clozapine, LORazepam
Klonopin® may be confused with clofazimine, cloNIDine, clorazepate, clozapine, LORazepam

Related Information
Antiepileptic Drugs *on page 1693*

U.S. Brand Names Klonopin®; Klonopin® Wafers [DSC]
Canadian Brand Names Alti-Clonazepam; Apo-Clonazepam®; Clonapam; CO Clonazepam; Gen-Clonazepam; Klonopin®; Mylan-Clonazepam; Novo-Clonazepam; Nu-Clonazepam; PMS-Clonazepam; PRO-Clonazepam; Rho®-Clonazepam; Rivotril®; Sandoz-Clonazepam; ZYM-Clonazepam

Therapeutic Category Anticonvulsant, Benzodiazepine; Benzodiazepine
Generic Available Yes
Use Alone or as an adjunct in the treatment of absence (petit mal), petit mal variant (Lennox-Gastaut), infantile spasms, akinetic, and myoclonic seizures; panic disorder with or without agoraphobia
Restrictions C-IV
Pregnancy Risk Factor D
Pregnancy Considerations Clonazepam was shown to be teratogenic in some animal studies. Clonazepam crosses the placenta. Benzodiazepine use during pregnancy is associated with increased risk of congenital malformations. Nonteratogenic effects (including neonatal flaccidity, respiratory and feeding problems, and withdrawal symptoms) during the postnatal period have also been reported with benzodiazepine use. Epilepsy itself, number of medications, genetic factors, or a combination of these probably influence the teratogenicity of anticonvulsant therapy.

Patients exposed to clonazepam during pregnancy are encouraged to enroll themselves into the AED Pregnancy Registry by calling 1-888-233-2334. Additional information is available at www.aedpregnancyregistry.org.

Lactation Enters breast milk/not recommended
Breast-Feeding Considerations Clonazepam enters breast milk; clinical effects on the infant include CNS depression, respiratory depression reported (no recommendation from the AAP).
Contraindications Hypersensitivity to clonazepam, any component, or other benzodiazepines; severe liver disease, acute narrow-angle glaucoma
Warnings Antiepileptic drugs (AEDs) increase the risk of suicidal behavior and ideation in patients receiving these medications for any indication. Pooled analyses of placebo-controlled trials involving 11 different AEDs (regardless of indication) showed a twofold increased risk of suicidal thoughts or behavior (estimated incidence rate: 0.43% in AED treated patients compared to 0.24% of patients receiving placebo); increased risk was observed as early as 1 week after initiation of AED and continued through duration of trials (most trials ≤24 weeks); risk did not vary significantly by age (age range: 5-100 years). Consider risks and benefits of AEDs before prescribing. Monitor all patients receiving an AED for emergence of suicidal thoughts or behavior, thoughts of self-harm, any unusual changes in behavior or mood, or the emergence or worsening of depressive symptoms; notify heathcare provider immediately if symptoms or concerning behavior occur. **Note:** The FDA is requiring that a Medication Guide be developed for all antiepileptic drugs informing patients of this risk.
Precautions Use with caution in patients with chronic respiratory disease, hepatic disease, or impaired renal function; abrupt discontinuance may precipitate withdrawal symptoms, status epilepticus or seizures (withdraw gradually when discontinuing therapy; see Additional Information); worsening of seizures may occur when clonazepam is added to patients with multiple seizure types
Adverse Reactions
Cardiovascular: Hypotension
Central nervous system: Drowsiness, changes in behavior or personality, aggression, vertigo, confusion, depression, memory impairment, concentration decreased, headache, ataxia, hypotonia; suicidal thinking and behavior (see Warnings)
Dermatologic: Rash
Gastrointestinal: Nausea, xerostomia, vomiting, diarrhea, constipation, anorexia, hypersalivation
Hematologic: Thrombocytopenia, anemia, leukopenia, eosinophilia
Neuromuscular & skeletal: Tremor, choreiform movements
Ocular: Nystagmus, blurred vision
Respiratory: Bronchial hypersecretion, respiratory depression
Miscellaneous: Physical and psychological dependence
Drug Interactions
Metabolism/Transport Effects Substrate of CYP3A4 (major)
Avoid Concomitant Use There are no known interactions where it is recommended to avoid concomitant use.
Increased Effect/Toxicity
ClonazePAM may increase the levels/effects of: Alcohol (Ethyl); Clozapine; CNS Depressants; Methotrimeprazine; Phenytoin

The levels/effects of ClonazePAM may be increased by: Antifungal Agents (Azole Derivatives, Systemic); Aprepitant; Calcium Channel Blockers (Nondihydropyridine); Cimetidine; Contraceptives (Estrogens); Contraceptives (Progestins); CYP3A4 Inhibitors (Moderate); CYP3A4 Inhibitors (Strong); Dasatinib; Fluconazole; Fosaprepitant; Grapefruit Juice; Isoniazid; Macrolide Antibiotics; Methotrimeprazine; Nefazodone; Proton Pump Inhibitors; Selective Serotonin Reuptake Inhibitors
Decreased Effect
The levels/effects of ClonazePAM may be decreased by: CarBAMazepine; CYP3A4 Inducers (Strong); Deferasirox; Rifamycin Derivatives; St Johns Wort; Theophylline Derivatives; Yohimbine
Stability Store at 25°C (77°F); excursions permitted to 15°C to 30°C (59°F to 80°F)
Mechanism of Action Suppresses the spike-and-wave discharge in absence seizures by depressing nerve transmission in the motor cortex; depresses all levels of the CNS, including the limbic and reticular formation, by binding to the benzodiazepine site on the gamma-aminobutyric acid (GABA) receptor complex and modulating GABA, which is a major inhibitory neurotransmitter in the brain
Pharmacodynamics
Onset of action: 20-60 minutes
Duration:
Infants and young children: Up to 6-8 hours
Adults: Up to 12 hours

Pharmacokinetics (Adult data unless noted)

Absorption: Oral: Well absorbed

Distribution: V_d: Adults: 1.5-4.4 L/kg

Protein binding: 85%

Metabolism: Extensively metabolized in the liver; undergoes nitroreduction to 7-aminoclonazepam, followed by acetylation to 7-acetamidoclonazepam; nitroreduction and acetylation are via cytochrome P450 enzyme system; metabolites undergo glucuronide and sulfate conjugation

Bioavailability: 90%

Half-life:

Children: 22-33 hours

Adults: Usual: 30-40 hours; range: 19-50 hours

Elimination: Metabolites excreted as glucuronide or sulfate conjugates; <2% excreted unchanged in urine

Usual Dosage Oral:

Seizure disorders:

Infants and Children <10 years or 30 kg:

Initial daily dose: 0.01-0.03 mg/kg/day (maximum initial dose: 0.05 mg/kg/day) given in 2-3 divided doses; increase by no more than 0.5 mg every third day until seizures are controlled or adverse effects seen

Maintenance dose: 0.1-0.2 mg/kg/day divided 3 times/day; not to exceed 0.2 mg/kg/day

Children ≥10 years (>30 kg) and Adults:

Initial daily dose not to exceed 1.5 mg given in 3 divided doses; may increase by 0.5-1 mg every third day until seizures are controlled or adverse effects seen

Maintenance dose: 0.05-0.2 mg/kg/day; do not exceed 20 mg/day

Panic disorder: Adolescents ≥18 years and Adults: Initial: 0.25 mg twice daily; increase in increments of 0.125-0.25 mg twice daily every 3 days; target dose: 1 mg/day; maximum dose: 4 mg/day

Administration

Oral: May administer with food or water to decrease GI distress

Orally-disintegrating tablet: Open pouch and peel back foil on the blister; do not push tablet through foil. Use dry hands to remove tablet and place in mouth. May be swallowed with or without water. Use immediately after removing from package.

Monitoring Parameters Signs and symptoms of suicidality (eg, anxiety, depression, behavior changes) (see Warnings). Long-term use: CBC with differential, platelets, liver enzymes

Reference Range Relationship between serum concentration and seizure control is not well established; measurement at random times postdose may contribute to this problem; predose concentrations are recommended

Proposed therapeutic levels: 20-80 ng/mL

Potentially toxic concentration: >80 ng/mL

Patient Information Avoid alcohol; limit caffeine. May cause drowsiness and impair ability to perform activities requiring mental alertness or physical coordination. May be habit-forming; avoid abrupt discontinuation after prolonged use (withdrawal symptoms or an increase in seizure activity may occur). May cause dry mouth. Antiepileptic agents may increase the risk of suicidal thoughts and behavior; notify physician if you feel more depressed or have thoughts of suicide or self harm (see Warnings). Report excessive drowsiness, CNS changes (eg, confusion, depression, headache) or changes in cognition; respiratory difficulty or shortness of breath; muscle tremors; visual disturbances; excessive GI symptoms (constipation, vomiting, anorexia); worsening of seizure activity, or loss of seizure control.

Additional Information Ethosuximide or valproic acid may be preferred for treatment of absence (petit mal) seizures. Clonazepam-induced behavioral disturbances may be more frequent in mentally handicapped patients. When discontinuing therapy in children, the clonazepam dose may be safely reduced by ≤0.04 mg/kg/week and discontinued when the daily dose is ≤0.04 mg/kg/day. When discontinuing therapy in adults treated for panic disorder, the clonazepam dose may be decreased by 0.125 mg twice daily every 3 days, until the drug is completely withdrawn. Treatment of panic disorder for >9 weeks has not been studied; long-term usefulness of clonazepam for the treatment of panic disorder should be re-evaluated periodically.

Dosage Forms Excipient information presented when available (limited, particularly for generics); consult specific product labeling. [DSC] = Discontinued product

Tablet: 0.5 mg, 1 mg, 2 mg

Klonopin®: 0.5 mg, 1 mg, 2 mg

Tablet, orally disintegrating: 0.125 mg, 0.25 mg, 0.5 mg, 1 mg, 2 mg

Klonopin® Wafers: 0.125 mg, 0.25 mg, 0.5 mg, 1 mg, 2 mg [DSC]

Extemporaneous Preparations A 0.1 mg/mL oral liquid can be made using 3 different vehicles (cherry syrup; a 1:1 mixture of Ora-Sweet® and Ora-Plus®; or a 1:1 mixture of Ora-Sweet® SF and Ora-Plus®); crush six 2 mg tablets into a fine powder in a mortar; add 10 mL of the vehicle and mix to make a uniform paste; mix while adding the vehicle in geometric portions to **almost** 120 mL; transfer to a calibrated bottle and qsad with vehicle to 120 mL; preparation is stable for 60 days when stored in amber prescription bottles in the dark at room temperature (25°C) or under refrigeration (5°C); label "shake well" and "protect from light"

Allen LV and Erickson MA, "Stability of Acetazolamide, Allopurinol, Azathioprine, Clonazepam, and Flucytosine in Extemporaneously Compounded Oral Liquids," *Am J Health Syst Pharm*, 1996, 53(16):1944-9.

References

Sugai K, "Seizures With Clonazepam: Discontinuation and Suggestions for Safe Discontinuation Rates in Children," *Epilepsia*, 1993, 34 (6):1089-97.

Walson PD and Edge JH, "Clonazepam Disposition in Pediatric Patients," *Ther Drug Monit*, 1996, 18(1):1-5.

CloNIDine (KLOE ni deen)

Medication Safety Issues

Sound-alike/look-alike issues:

CloNIDine may be confused with Clomid®, clomiPHENE, clonazePAM, clozapine, Klonopin®, quiNIDine

Catapres® may be confused with Cataflam®, Cetapred®, Combipres

High alert medication: The Institute for Safe Medication Practices (ISMP) includes this medication (epidural administration) among its list of drug classes which have a heightened risk of causing significant patient harm when used in error.

Beers Criteria medication: This drug may be inappropriate for use in geriatric patients (low severity risk).

Transdermal patch may contain conducting metal (eg, aluminum); remove patch prior to MRI.

Related Information

Antihypertensive Agents by Class *on page 1481*

U.S. Brand Names Catapres-TTS®; Catapres®; Duraclon®

Canadian Brand Names Apo-Clonidine®; Carapres®; Dixarit®; Dom-Clonidine; Novo-Clonidine; Nu-Clonidine

Therapeutic Category Adrenergic Agonist Agent; Alpha-Adrenergic Agonist; Analgesic, Non-narcotic (Epidural); Antihypertensive Agent ·

Generic Available Yes: Excludes epidural formulation

Use Management of hypertension; aid in the diagnosis of pheochromocytoma and growth hormone deficiency; used for heroin withdrawal and smoking cessation therapy in adults; alternate agent for the treatment of attention-deficit/ hyperactivity disorder (ADHD); adjunct in the treatment of neuropathic pain; epidural form is used in combination with opiates for relief of severe pain in cancer patients whose pain was not relieved by opiates alone

Pregnancy Risk Factor C

Pregnancy Considerations Clonidine crosses the placenta. Caution should be used with this drug due to the potential of rebound hypertension with abrupt discontinuation.

Lactation Enters breast milk/not recommended

Breast-Feeding Considerations Enters breast milk; AAP has no recommendation

Contraindications Hypersensitivity to clonidine hydrochloride or any component; epidural injection is contraindicated in patients receiving anticoagulation therapy and in patients with a bleeding diathesis or an infection at the injection site. Administration of epidural clonidine above the C_4 dermatome is contraindicated.

Warnings Do not abruptly discontinue as rapid increase in blood pressure and symptoms of sympathetic overactivity (such as increased heart rate, tremors, agitation, anxiety, insomnia, sweating, palpitations) may occur. If need to discontinue clonidine, taper oral dose gradually over more than 1 week; taper epidural dose gradually over 2-4 days. In patients receiving both a beta-blocker and clonidine, withdraw the beta-blocker several days before the gradual tapering of clonidine.

The American Heart Association recommends that all children diagnosed with ADHD who may be candidates for medication, such as clonidine, should have a thorough cardiovascular assessment prior to initiation of therapy. These recommendations are based upon reports of serious cardiovascular adverse events (including sudden death) in patients (both children and adults) taking usual doses of stimulant medications. Most of these patients were found to have underlying structural heart disease (eg, hypertrophic obstructive cardiomyopathy). This assessment should include a combination of thorough medical history, family history, and physical examination. An ECG is not mandatory but should be considered. **Note:** ECG abnormalities and 4 cases of sudden cardiac death have been reported in children receiving clonidine with methylphenidate; reduce dose of methylphenidate by 40% when used concurrently with clonidine; consider ECG monitoring.

Epidural clonidine is not recommended for perioperative, obstetrical, or postpartum pain [due to the risk of hemodynamic instability (hypotension, bradycardia)] **[U.S. Boxed Warning]**, in patients with severe cardiovascular disease, or those who are hemodynamically unstable.

Precautions Dosage modification is required in patients with renal impairment; use with caution in cerebrovascular disease, coronary insufficiency, recent MI, renal impairment, sinus node dysfunction, conduction disturbances. Monitor patients for signs of depression (especially those with a history of affective disorders). Epidural clonidine may result in bradycardia (symptomatic bradycardia may be treated with atropine); sedation, respiratory depression, and ventilatory abnormalities may occur with high epidural doses. Transdermal patch may contain conducting metal (eg, aluminum) which may cause a burn to the skin during an MRI scan; remove patch prior to MRI; reapply patch after scan is completed. Due to the potential for altered electrical conductivity, remove transdermal patch before cardioversion or defibrillation. Safety and efficacy of tablet and transdermal product have not been established in children <12 years of age. In pediatric patients, epidural clonidine should be reserved for cancer patients with severe intractable pain, unresponsive to other analgesics, or epidural or spinal opiates.

Adverse Reactions

Cardiovascular: Raynaud's phenomenon, hypotension, bradycardia, palpitations, tachycardia, CHF, rebound hypertension if discontinued abruptly

Central nervous system: Drowsiness, sedation, headache, dizziness, fatigue, insomnia, anxiety, depression

Dermatologic: Rash, local skin reactions with patch

Endocrine & metabolic: Sodium and water retention, parotid pain

Gastrointestinal: Constipation, anorexia, xerostomia

Respiratory: Respiratory depression and ventilatory abnormalities with high epidural doses

Drug Interactions

Avoid Concomitant Use

Avoid concomitant use of CloNIDine with any of the following: Iobenguane I 123

Increased Effect/Toxicity

CloNIDine may increase the levels/effects of: Amifostine; Antihypertensives; Hypotensive Agents; RiTUXimab

The levels/effects of CloNIDine may be increased by: Beta-Blockers; Diazoxide; Herbs (Hypotensive Properties); MAO Inhibitors; Methylphenidate; Pentoxifylline; Phosphodiesterase 5 Inhibitors; Prostacyclin Analogues

Decreased Effect

CloNIDine may decrease the levels/effects of: Iobenguane I 123

The levels/effects of CloNIDine may be decreased by: Antidepressants (Alpha2-Antagonist); Herbs (Hypertensive Properties); Serotonin/Norepinephrine Reuptake Inhibitors; Tricyclic Antidepressants; Yohimbine

Food Interactions Avoid natural licorice (causes sodium and water retention and increases potassium loss)

Stability

Tablets: Store at controlled room temperature at 25°C (77°F); dispense in tightly closed, light-resistant container

Transdermal product: Store below 86°F (30°C)

Epidural injection: Discard unused portion of vial (injection is preservative free); do not use with preservative

Mechanism of Action Stimulates alpha₂-adrenoreceptors in the brain stem, thus activating an inhibitory neuron, resulting in reduced sympathetic outflow, producing a decrease in vasomotor tone and heart rate. Clonidine also acutely stimulates the release of growth hormone in children and adults; however, with long-term use, it does not cause chronic elevation of growth hormone.

Epidural use: Prevents pain signal transmission to the brain and produces analgesia at presynaptic and postjunctional alpha₂-adrenoreceptors in the spinal cord

Pharmacodynamics Antihypertensive effects: Oral:

Onset of action: 30-60 minutes

Maximum effect: Within 2-4 hours

Duration: 6-10 hours

Pharmacokinetics (Adult data unless noted)

Distribution: V_d: Adults: 2.1 L/kg; distributes into breast milk

Protein binding: 20% to 40%

Metabolism: Hepatic to inactive metabolites

Bioavailability, oral: 75% to 95%

Half-life, serum:

Neonates: 44-72 hours

Children: 8-12 hours

Adults:

Normal renal function: 6-20 hours

Renal impairment: 18-41 hours

Half-life, CSF: Adults: 1.3 ± 0.5 hours

Elimination: 65% excreted in urine (32% unchanged) and 22% excreted in feces via enterohepatic recirculation

Dialysis: Not dialyzable (0% to 5%)

Usual Dosage

Children:

Hypertension: Oral:

Limited information exists in the literature; some centers use the following doses: Initial: 5-10 mcg/kg/day in divided doses every 8-12 hours; increase gradually, if needed, to 5-25 mcg/kg/day in divided doses every 6 hours; maximum dose: 0.9 mg/day (see Rocchini, 1984)

Manufacturer's recommendations: Adolescents ≥12 years: Initial dose: 0.1 mg twice daily; increase gradually, if needed, by 0.1 mg per day at weekly intervals; usual maintenance dose: 0.2-0.6 mg/day in divided doses; maximum recommended dose: 2.4 mg/day (rarely required)

ADHD: Oral: Initial: 0.05 mg/day, increase every 3-7 days by 0.05 mg/day to 3-5 mcg/kg/day given in divided doses 3-4 times/day; usual maximum dose: 0.3-0.4 mg/day. **Note:** Some centers use doses as high as 8 mcg/kg/day or 0.5 mg/day (see Hunt, 1990).

Clonidine tolerance test (test of growth hormone release from the pituitary): Oral: 0.15 mg/m^2 or 4 mcg/kg as a single dose

Analgesia: Epidural (continuous infusion): Reserved for cancer patients with severe intractable pain, unresponsive to other analgesics or epidural or spinal opiates: Initial: 0.5 mcg/kg/hour; adjust with caution, based on clinical effect; usual range: 0.5-2 mcg/kg/hour; do not exceed adult doses

Neuropathic pain: Oral: Some centers use the following doses (see Galloway, 2000): Initial: 2 mcg/kg/dose every 4-6 hours; increase incrementally over several days; range: 2-4 mcg/kg/dose every 4-6 hours; may also be given as transdermal (see Transdermal)

Transdermal: Children may be switched to the transdermal delivery system after oral therapy is titrated to an optimal and stable dose; a transdermal dose approximately equivalent to the total oral daily dose may be used (see Hunt, 1990; see Administration)

Adults:

Hypertension:

Oral: Initial dose: 0.1 mg twice daily, usual maintenance dose: 0.2-1.2 mg/day in 2-4 divided doses; maximum recommended dose: 2.4 mg/day; usual dosage range (JNC 7): 0.1-0.8 mg/day in 2 divided doses

Transdermal: Applied once weekly as transdermal delivery system; begin therapy with 0.1 mg/day patch applied once every 7 days; increase by 0.1 mg/day at 1-2 week intervals based on response; hypotensive action may not begin until 2-3 days after initial application; doses >0.6 mg/day do not improve efficacy; usual dosage range (JNC 7): 0.1-0.3 mg/day patch applied once weekly

Analgesia: Epidural (continuous infusion): Initial: 30 mcg/hour; titrate to clinical effect; usual maximum dose: 40 mcg/hour

Dosing adjustment in renal impairment: Adjust dosage according to degree of renal impairment; bradycardia may be more likely to occur in patients with renal failure; consider using doses at the lower end of the dosage range; monitor patients closely. Supplemental dose following hemodialysis is not necessary; unclear how much is removed via peritoneal dialysis (K/DOQI, 2005). Oral antihypertensive drugs given preferentially at night may reduce the nocturnal surge of blood pressure and minimize the intradialytic hypotension that may occur when taken the morning before a dialysis session.

Administration

Epidural: Dilute the 500 mcg/mL product with preservative free NS to a final concentration of 100 mcg/mL prior to use; visually inspect for particulate matter and discoloration prior to administration (whenever permitted by container and solution)

Oral: May be administered without regard to meals

Transdermal: Patches should be applied at bedtime to a clean, hairless area of the upper arm or chest; rotate patch sites weekly in adults; in children, the patch may need to be changed more frequently (eg, every 3-5 days); **Note:** Transdermal patch is a membrane-controlled system; do **not** cut the patch to deliver partial doses; rate of drug delivery, reservoir contents, and adhesion may be affected if cut; if partial dose is needed, surface area of patch can be blocked proportionally using adhesive bandage (see Lee, 1997)

Monitoring Parameters Blood pressure, heart rate; consider ECG monitoring in patients with history of heart disease or concurrent use of medications affecting cardiac conduction; with epidural administration: Blood pressure, heart rate; pulse oximetry with large bolus doses; monitor infusion pump and catheter tubing for obstruction or dislodgment throughout the course of therapy to decrease risk of inadvertent abrupt discontinuation

ADHD: Evaluate patients for cardiac disease prior to initiation of therapy for ADHD with thorough medical history, family history, and physical exam; consider ECG (see Warnings); perform ECG and echocardiogram if findings suggest cardiac disease; promptly conduct cardiac evaluation in patients who develop chest pain, unexplained syncope, or any other symptom of cardiac disease during treatment.

Patient Information Avoid alcohol; may cause drowsiness and impair ability to perform activities requiring mental alertness or physical coordination; do not stop drug abruptly; may cause dry mouth

Nursing Implications Counsel patient/parent about compliance and danger of withdrawal reaction if doses are missed or drug is discontinued

Additional Information Epidural clonidine may be more effective in the treatment of neuropathic pain compared to somatic or visceral pain. Clonidine-induced symptomatic bradycardia may be treated with atropine. Clonidine hydrochloride 0.1 mg is equal to 0.087 mg of the free base.

Dosage Forms Excipient information presented when available (limited, particularly for generics); consult specific product labeling.

Injection, solution, as hydrochloride [epidural; preservative free]: 100 mcg/mL (10 mL); 500 mcg/mL (10 mL)

Duraclon®: 100 mcg/mL (10 mL); 500 mcg/mL (10 mL)

Patch, transdermal [once-weekly patch]: 0.1 mg/24 hours (4s); 0.2 mg/24 hours (4s); 0.3 mg/24 hours (4s)

Catapres-TTS®-1: 0.1 mg/24 hours (4s)

Catapres-TTS®-2: 0.2 mg/24 hours (4s)

Catapres-TTS®-3: 0.3 mg/24 hours (4s)

Tablet, as hydrochloride: 0.1 mg, 0.2 mg, 0.3 mg

Catapres®: 0.1 mg, 0.2 mg, 0.3 mg

Extemporaneous Preparations A 0.1 mg/mL oral suspension compounded from tablets is stable for 28 days when stored in amber glass bottles and refrigerated (4°C); thirty 0.2 mg tablets are crushed in a glass mortar and ground to a fine powder; 2 mL Purified Water USP is slowly added, and triturated to make a fine paste; Simple Syrup, NF is slowly added in 15 mL increments and triturated; qsad 60 mL; shake well before use

Levinson ML and Johnson CE, "Stability of an Extemporaneously Compounded Clonidine Hydrochloride Oral Liquid," *Am J Hosp Pharm*, 1992, 49(1):122-5.

References

American Academy of Pediatrics/American Heart Association Clarification of Statement on Cardiovascular Evaluation and Monitoring of Children and Adolescents With Heart Disease Receiving Medications for ADHD; available at: http://americanheart.mediaroon.com/index.php?s=43&item=422.

Chobanian AV, Bakris GL, Black HR, et al, "The Seventh Report of the Joint National Committee on Prevention, Detection, Evaluation, and Treatment of High Blood Pressure: The JNC 7 report," *JAMA*, 2003, 289(19):2560-72.

Chafin CC, Hovinga CA,and Phelps SJ, "Clonidine in the Treatment of Attention Deficit Hyperactivity Disorder," *Journal of Pediatric Pharmacy Practice*, 1999, 4(6):308-15.

Galloway KS and Yaster M, "Pain and Symptom Control in Terminally Ill Children," *Pediatr Clin North Am*, 2000, 47(3):711-46.

Hart-Santora D and Hart LL, "Clonidine in Attention Deficit Hyperactivity Disorder," *Ann Pharmacother*, 1992, 26(1):37-9.

Hunt RD, Capper L, and O'Connell P, "Clonidine in Child and Adolescent Psychiatry," *J Child Adol Psychpharm*, 1990, 1(1):87-102.

Hunt RD, Minderaa RB, and Cohen DJ, "The Therapeutic Effect of Clonidine in Attention Deficit Disorder With Hyperactivity: A Comparison With Placebo and Methylphenidate," *Psychopharmacol Bull*, 1986, 22(1):229-35.

K/DOQI Workgroup, "K/DOQI Clinical Practice Guidelines for Cardiovascular Disease in Dialysis Patients," *Am J Kidney Dis*, 2005, 45(4 Suppl 3)`S46-57.

Lee HA and Anderson PO, "Giving Partial Doses of Transdermal Patches," *Am J Health Syst Pharm*, 1997, 54(15):1759-60.

Rocchini AP, "Childhood Hypertension: Etiology, Diagnosis, and Treatment," *Pediatr Clin North Am*, 1984, 31(6):1259-73.

Sinaiko AR, "Pharmacologic Management of Childhood Hypertension," *Pediatr Clin North Am*, 1993, 40(1):195-212.

Vetter VL, Elia J, Erickson C, et al, "Cardiovascular Monitoring of Children and Adolescents With Heart Disease Receiving Stimulant Drugs: A Scientific Statement From the American Heart Association Council on Cardiovascular Disease in the Young Congenital Cardiac Defects Committee and the Council on Cardiovascular Nursing," *Circulation*, 2008, 117(18):2407-23.

◆ **Clonidine Hydrochloride** *see* CloNIDine *on page 338*

Clopidogrel (kloh PID oh grel)

Medication Safety Issues
Sound-alike/look-alike issues:
Plavix® may be confused with Elavil®, Paxil®

U.S. Brand Names Plavix®

Canadian Brand Names Plavix®

Therapeutic Category Antiplatelet Agent

Generic Available No

Use Reduction of atherothrombotic events (MI, stroke, and vascular deaths) in patients with recent MI, stroke, or established peripheral arterial disease (FDA approved in adults); reduction of atherothrombotic events in patients with non-ST-segment elevation acute coronary syndrome (unstable angina and non-Q-wave MI) managed medically and through percutaneous coronary intervention (with or without stent) or CABG (FDA approved in adults); reduction of death rate and atherothrombotic events in patients with ST-segment elevation acute MI (STEMI) managed medically (FDA approved in adults).

Pregnancy Risk Factor B

Pregnancy Considerations Teratogenic effects were not observed in animal studies. Use during pregnancy only if clearly needed.

Lactation Excretion in breast milk unknown/not recommended

Contraindications Hypersensitivity to clopidogrel or any component; active pathological bleeding such as PUD or intracranial hemorrhage

Warnings Rare cases of thrombotic thrombocytopenic purpura (TTP) have been reported, sometimes with exposure of <2 weeks; fatalities have occurred; urgent treatment including plasmapheresis (plasma exchange) is required

Clopidogrel is a prodrug requiring hepatic conversion to its active metabolite, in part via cytochrome P450 isoenzyme CYP2C19. Impaired clopidogrel conversion to its active metabolite (due to either genetic variations in CYP2C19 or concomitant medications that interfere with CYP2C19) will result in suboptimal antiplatelet activity. Avoid the use of clopidogrel in patients with impaired CYP2C19 function due to known genetic variation or due to concomitant drugs that inhibit CYP2C19 activity.

Patients with one or more copies of the variant CYP2C19*2 and/or CYP2C19*3 alleles (and potentially other reduced-function variants) may have reduced conversion of clopidogrel to its active thiol metabolite. Lower active metabolite exposure may result in reduced platelet inhibition and thus, a higher rate of cardiovascular events following myocardial infarction or stent thrombosis following percutaneous coronary intervention. The optimal dose for these patients has yet to be determined. **Note:** Patients of Chinese ancestry have a higher incidence of CYP2C19*2 and CYP2C19*3 alleles (which results in a higher incidence of CYP2C19 intermediate and poor metabolism and an increased risk of inadequate platelet inhibition with clopidogrel) compared to Caucasian or African-American patients.

Concurrent use with omeprazole, a proton pump inhibitor known to inhibit CYP2C19, significantly reduces concentrations of the active metabolite of clopidogrel and subsequently reduces clinical efficacy; this reduction in pharmacologic activity of clopidogrel occurs if omeprazole is given concomitantly with clopidogrel or 12 hours apart. No evidence exists that other drugs that decrease stomach acid, such as most Histamine-2 blockers (except cimetidine, which is a CYP2C19 inhibitor) or antacids, interfere with the antiplatelet activity of clopidogrel. Avoid concurrent use of clopidogrel with CYP2C19 inhibitors, including omeprazole, esomeprazole, cimetidine, fluconazole, ketoconazole, voriconazole, etravirine, felbamate, fluoxetine, fluvoxamine, and ticlopidine (see Drug Interactions).

Precautions Use with caution in patients with platelet disorders, bleeding disorders, or an increased risk for bleeding (eg, peptic ulcer disease, intraocular conditions, trauma, surgery, or patients receiving medications associated with ulcers or bleeding). Use with caution in patients receiving other platelet aggregation inhibitors; risk of bleeding may be increased. Use with caution in patients with impaired renal or hepatic function (experience is limited). Discontinue clopidogrel in patients 5 days prior to elective surgery **only** if antiplatelet effect is **not** required; patient-specific situations need to be discussed with cardiologist. Safety and efficacy have not been established in pediatric patients.

Adverse Reactions Note: Bleeding is associated with clopidogrel use. Hemorrhage may occur at virtually any site. Risk is dependent on multiple variables, including the concurrent use of multiple agents which alter hemostasis and patient susceptibility.

Cardiovascular: Edema, hypertension

Central nervous system: Depression, dizziness, fatigue, headache, intracranial hemorrhage, pain

Dermatologic: Pruritus, rash

Endocrine & metabolic: Hypercholesterolemia

Gastrointestinal: Abdominal pain, diarrhea, dyspepsia, GI bleed, nausea

Genitourinary: Urinary tract infection

Hematologic: Anemia, bleeding, epistaxis, purpura, thrombotic thrombocytopenic purpura (TTP; rare)

Neuromuscular & skeletal: Arthralgia, arthrosis, back pain, hypoesthesia

Respiratory: Bronchitis, cough, dyspnea, pneumonia, rhinitis, sinusitis, upper respiratory tract infection

Miscellaneous: Anaphylactoid reaction, flu-like syndrome

<1% and/or postmarketing: Acute liver failure, acute renal failure, agranulocytosis, allergic reaction, anaphylactoid reaction, angioedema, aplastic anemia, bilirubinemia, bronchospasm, bullous eruption, colitis (including ulcerative, lymphocytic), confusion, creatinine increased, erythema multiforme, fatty liver, gastric ulcer perforation, gastritis, glomerulopathy, granulocytopenia, hallucination, hematuria, hemoptysis, hemorrhagic stroke, hemothorax, hepatitis, hypersensitivity, hypochromic anemia, interstitial pneumonitis, ischemic necrosis, leukopenia, lichen planus, menorrhagia, neutropenia, ocular

hemorrhage, pancreatitis, pancytopenia, paresthenia, peptic ulcer, pulmonary hemorrhage, rash (erythematous, maculopapular), renal function abnormal, retinal bleeding, retroperitoneal bleeding, Stevens-Johnson syndrome, stomatitis, taste disorder, thrombocytopenia, toxic epidermal necrolysis, urticaria, vasculitis

Drug Interactions

Metabolism/Transport Effects Substrate of CYP2C19, 3A4, 1A2 (minor); **Inhibits** CYP2B6 (moderate), 2C9 (weak)

Avoid Concomitant Use

Avoid concomitant use of Clopidogrel with any of the following: CYP2C19 Inhibitors (Moderate); CYP2C19 Inhibitors (Strong)

Increased Effect/Toxicity

Clopidogrel may increase the levels/effects of: Anticoagulants; Antiplatelet Agents; Collagenase (Systemic); CYP2B6 Substrates; Drotrecogin Alfa; Ibritumomab; Proton Pump Inhibitors; Salicylates; Thrombolytic Agents; Tositumomab and Iodine I 131 Tositumomab; Warfarin

The levels/effects of Clopidogrel may be increased by: Dasatinib; Glucosamine; Herbs (Anticoagulant/Antiplatelet Properties); Nonsteroidal Anti-Inflammatory Agents; Omega-3-Acid Ethyl Esters; Pentosan Polysulfate Sodium; Pentoxifylline; Prostacyclin Analogues; Rifamycin Derivatives

Decreased Effect

The levels/effects of Clopidogrel may be decreased by: Calcium Channel Blockers; CYP2C19 Inhibitors (Moderate); CYP2C19 Inhibitors (Strong); Macrolide Antibiotics; Nonsteroidal Anti-Inflammatory Agents; Proton Pump Inhibitors

Food Interactions Effects of food on bioavailability of clopidogrel or its active metabolite are unknown.

Stability Store at controlled room temperature of 25°C (77°F).

Mechanism of Action Clopidogrel is a prodrug; its active metabolite inhibits platelet aggregation. Clopidogrel requires *in vivo* biotransformation via cytochrome P450 enzymes to an active thiol metabolite. The active metabolite irreversibly modifies the P2Y12 platelet receptor, inhibiting the binding of ADP. This prevents the ADP activation of the GPIIb/IIIa receptor complex, thereby reducing platelet aggregation. Platelets blocked by clopidogrel's active metabolite are affected for the remainder of their lifespan (~7-10 days). **Note:** Not all patients who receive clopidrogrel will have adequate platelet inhibition. This is due to the fact that the formation of the active metabolite requires cytochrome P450 enzymes and some of these enzymes are polymorphic or may be inhibited by other medications (see Precautions).

Pharmacodynamics

Onset of action: Inhibition of platelet aggregation: Detected 2 hours after single oral dose

Maximum effect: Inhibition of platelet aggregation: 3-7 days; average inhibition level at steady-state in adults after receiving 75 mg/day: 40% to 60%.

Duration: Platelet aggregation and bleeding time gradually return to baseline after ~5 days after discontinuation.

Pharmacokinetics (Adult data unless noted)

Absorption: Rapid

Protein binding: Clopidogrel: 98%; main circulating metabolite (carboxylic acid derivative; inactive): 94%

Metabolism: Extensively hepatic via esterase-mediated hydrolysis to a carboxylic acid derivative (inactive) and via CYP450-mediated oxidation with a subsequent metabolism to a thiol metabolite (active).

Half-life: Parent drug: ~6 hours; carboxylic acid derivative (inactive; main circulating metabolite): ~8 hours; **Note:** A clopidogrel radiolabeled study has shown that covalent

binding to platelets accounts for 2% of radiolabel and has a half-life of 11 days

Time to peak serum concentration: ~0.75 hours

Elimination: Urine (50%) and feces (46%)

Usual Dosage Oral: **Note:** Safety and efficacy have not been established in pediatric patients; optimal dose is not known; limited dosing information is available; further pediatric studies are needed.

Neonates and Infants ≤24 months: In the PICOLO trial, a dose of 0.2 mg/kg once daily was found to achieve a mean inhibition of platelet aggregation similar to adults receiving the recommended dose; **Note:** This study included pediatric patients with a systemic-to-pulmonary artery shunt, intracardiac or intravascular stent, Kawasaki disease, or arterial graft; 79% of patients received concomitant aspirin; patients <2 kg and those born at <35 weeks gestational age were excluded (see Li, 2008).

Children >2 years of age: Optimal dose is not established; some centers use the following: Initial dose: 1 mg/kg once daily; titrate to response (see Monitoring Parameters); in general, do not exceed adult dose (see Finkelstein, 2005; Soman, 2006).

Adults:

Recent MI, recent stroke, or established peripheral arterial disease: 75 mg once daily

Acute coronary syndrome (also see Additional Information):

Unstable angina, non-ST-segment elevation myocardial infarction (UA/NSTEMI): Initial: 300 mg loading dose, followed by 75 mg once daily (in combination with aspirin 75-325 mg once daily). **Note:** A loading dose of 600 mg has been used in some investigations; limited research exists comparing the two doses

ST-segment elevation acute myocardial infarction (STEMI): 75 mg once daily (with or without loading dose; use in combination with aspirin 75-162 mg/day; with or without thrombolytics). The CLARITY study used a 300 mg loading dose of clopidogrel (with thrombolysis). The duration of therapy was <28 days (usually until hospital discharge).

Dosing adjustment in renal impairment: No dosage adjustment is required; use with caution; experience is limited; **Note:** Plasma concentrations of the main circulating metabolite were lower in adult patients with Cl_{cr} 5-15 mL/minute versus patients with Cl_{cr} 30-60 mL/minute or healthy adults. Inhibition of ADP-induced platelet aggregation was 25% lower compared to healthy adults; however, prolongation of bleeding time was similar.

Dosing adjustment in hepatic impairment: Use with caution; experience is limited; **Note:** Inhibition of ADP-induced platelet aggregation and mean bleeding time prolongation were similar in adult patients with severe hepatic impairment compared to healthy subjects after repeated doses of 75 mg once daily for 10 days.

Dosing adjustment in patients with CYP2C19 poor metabolizer status: Optimal dose is not established; CYP2C19 poor metabolizer status is associated with decreased response to clopidogrel (see Precautions)

Administration May be administered without regard to food.

Monitoring Parameters Signs of bleeding; hemoglobin and hematocrit periodically. Monitor mean inhibition of platelet aggregation: Goal of 30% to 50% inhibition (similar to adults receiving 75 mg/day)

Patient Information May cause dizziness and impair ability to perform activities requiring mental alertness or physical coordination. It may take longer than usual to stop bleeding. Inform prescribers and dentists that you are taking this medication prior to scheduling any surgery or dental procedure. Report any signs of bleeding to physician at once (eg, nosebleeds, bleeding gums, prolonged bleeding from a cut, heavier than normal menstrual or vaginal bleeding, coughing up blood, vomiting blood or coffee ground-like material, pink or dark brown urine, red or black tar-like stools, unusual bruising, headaches, dizziness, weakness, pain, swelling, or discomfort). Report the use of other medications, non-prescription medications, and herbal or natural products to your physician and pharmacist.

Additional Information Duration of therapy for patients with drug-eluting stents: Duration of clopidogrel (in combination with aspirin): Ideally 12 months following drug-eluting stent placement in patients not at high risk for bleeding; at a minimum, 1, 3, and 6 months for bare metal, sirolimus, and paclitaxel stents, respectively, for uninterrupted therapy. Interruption of therapy may result in stent thrombosis with subsequent fatal and nonfatal myocardial infarction.

Overdose may lead to prolonged bleeding time with resultant bleeding complications; platelet transfusions may be an appropriate treatment when attempting to rapidly reverse the effects of clopidogrel

Dosage Forms Excipient information presented when available (limited, particularly for generics); consult specific product labeling.

Tablet:

Plavix®: 75 mg, 300 mg

References

Angiolillo DJ, Fernandez-Ortiz A, Bernardo E, et al, "Contribution of Gene Sequence Variations of the Hepatic Cytochrome P450 3A4 Enzyme to Variability in Individual Responsiveness to Clopidogrel," *Arterioscler Thromb Vasc Biol*, 2006, 26(8):1895-900.

Clarke TA and Waskell LA, "The Metabolism of Clopidogrel Is Catalyzed by Human Cytochrome P450 3A and Is Inhibited by Atorvastatin," *Drug Metab Dispos*, 2003, 31(1):53-9.

Finkelstein Y, Nurmohamed L, Avner M, et al, "Clopidogrel Use in Children," *J Pediatr*, 2005, 147(5):657.

Lau WC, Gurbel PA, Watkins PB, et al, "Contribution of Hepatic Cytochrome P450 3A4 Metabolic Activity to the Phenomenon of Clopidogrel Resistance," *Circulation*, 2004, 109(2):166-71.

Li JS, Yow E, Berezny KY, et al, "Dosing of Clopidogrel for Platelet Inhibition in Infants and Young Children: Primary Results of the Platelet Inhibition in Children On cLOpidogrel (PICOLO) Trial," *Circulation*, 2008, 117(4):553-9.

Maltz LA, Gauvreau K, Connor JA, et al, "Clopidogrel in a Pediatric Population: Prescribing Practice and Outcomes From a Single Center," *J Pediatr Cardiol*, 2009, 30(2):99-105.

Savi P, Pereillo JM, Uzabiaga MF, et al, "Identification and Biological Activity of the Active Metabolite of Clopidogrel," *Thromb Haemost*, 2000, 84(5):891-6.

Scirica BM, Sabatine MS, Morrow DA, et al, "The Role of Clopidogrel in Early and Sustained Arterial Patency After Fibrinolysis for ST-Segment Elevation Myocardial Infarction: The ECG CLARITY-TIMI 28 Study," *J Am Coll Cardiol*, 2006, 48(1):37-42.

Soman T, Rafay MF, Hune S, et al, "The Risks and Safety of Clopidogrel in Pediatric Arterial Ischemic Stroke," *Stroke*, 2006, 37(4):1120-2.

Stanek EJ, Aubert RE, Flockhart DA, et al, "A National Study of the Effect of Individual Proton Pump Inhibitors on Cardiovascular Outcomes in Patients Treated With Clopidogrel Following Coronary Stenting: The Clopidogrel Medco Outcomes Study," Society for Cardiovascular Angiography and Interventions 2009 Scientific Sessions, Las Vegas, NV, May 6, 2009.

◆ **Clopidogrel Bisulfate** see Clopidogrel on page 341

Clorazepate (klor AZ e pate)

Medication Safety Issues

Sound-alike/look-alike issues:

Clorazepate may be confused with clofibrate, clonazepam

Beers Criteria medication: This drug may be inappropriate for use in geriatric patients (high severity risk).

U.S. Brand Names Tranxene® T-Tab®

Canadian Brand Names Apo-Clorazepate®; Novo-Clopate

Therapeutic Category Anticonvulsant, Benzodiazepine; Benzodiazepine; Sedative

Generic Available Yes

Use Adjunct anticonvulsant in the management of partial seizures (FDA approved in ages ≥9 years and adults); treatment of anxiety disorders (FDA approved in adults); management of alcohol withdrawal (FDA approved in adults)

Restrictions C-IV

Pregnancy Considerations Nordiazepam, the active metabolite of clorazepate, crosses the placenta and is measurable in cord blood and amniotic fluid. Congenital malformations have been noted in a case report following maternal use during the first trimester of pregnancy, and also with the use of similar agents.

Patients exposed to clorazepate during pregnancy are encouraged to enroll themselves into the AED Pregnancy Registry by calling 1-888-233-2334. Additional information is available at www.aedpregnancyregistry.org.

Lactation Enters breast milk/not recommended

Breast-Feeding Considerations Nordiazepam, the active metabolite of clorazepate, is found in breast milk and is measurable in the serum of breast-feeding infants.

Contraindications Hypersensitivity to clorazepate dipotassium or any component; cross-sensitivity with other benzodiazepines may exist; narrow-angle glaucoma; avoid using in patients with pre-existing CNS depression or severe uncontrolled pain

Warnings Physical and psychological dependence may occur; abrupt discontinuation may cause withdrawal symptoms or seizures; use with caution in patients with a psychological predisposition for drug dependence. Clorazepate is not recommended for use in depressive neuroses or psychotic reactions.

Antiepileptic drugs (AEDs) increase the risk of suicidal behavior and ideation in patients receiving these medications for any indication. Pooled analyses of placebo-controlled trials involving 11 different AEDs (regardless of indication) showed a twofold increased risk of suicidal thoughts or behavior (estimated incidence rate: 0.43% in AED treated patients compared to 0.24% of patients receiving placebo); increased risk was observed as early as 1 week after initiation of AED and continued through duration of trials (most trials ≤24 weeks); risk did not vary significantly by age (age range: 5-100 years). Consider risks and benefits of AEDs before prescribing. Monitor all patients receiving an AED for emergence of suicidal thoughts or behavior, thoughts of self-harm, any unusual changes in behavior or mood, or the emergence or worsening of depressive symptoms; notify heathcare provider immediately if symptoms or concerning behavior occur. **Note:** The FDA is requiring that a Medication Guide be developed for all antiepileptic drugs informing patients of this risk.

Precautions Use with caution in patients with hepatic or renal disease. Clorazepate may cause CNS depression which may impair physical or mental abilities; patients must be cautioned about performing tasks which require mental alertness (eg, operating machinery or driving). Use with caution in patients receiving other CNS depressants or psychoactive medication (effects with other sedative drugs or ethanol may be potentiated) and in patients with depression (see Warnings).

Adverse Reactions

Cardiovascular: Hypotension

Central nervous system: Amnesia, ataxia, confusion, depression, dizziness, drowsiness, fatigue, headache, insomnia, irritability, nervousness, slurred speech; suicidal thinking and behavior (see Warnings)

Dermatologic: Rash

Gastrointestinal: Nausea, xerostomia

Hematologic: Reduced hematocrit (with long-term use)

Hepatic: Hepatic function abnormalities

Neuromuscular & skeletal: Tremor

◀ Ocular: Blurred vision, diplopia

Renal: Renal function abnormalities

Miscellaneous: Long-term use may also be associated with renal or hepatic injury; physical and psychological dependence with long-term use

Drug Interactions

Metabolism/Transport Effects Substrate of CYP3A4 (major)

Avoid Concomitant Use There are no known interactions where it is recommended to avoid concomitant use.

Increased Effect/Toxicity

Clorazepate may increase the levels/effects of: Alcohol (Ethyl); Clozapine; CNS Depressants; Methotrimeprazine; Phenytoin

The levels/effects of Clorazepate may be increased by: Antifungal Agents (Azole Derivatives, Systemic); Aprepitant; Calcium Channel Blockers (Nondihydropyridine); Cimetidine; Contraceptives (Estrogens); Contraceptives (Progestins); CYP3A4 Inhibitors (Moderate); CYP3A4 Inhibitors (Strong); Dasatinib; Fluconazole; Fosamprenavir; Fosaprepitant; Grapefruit Juice; Isoniazid; Macrolide Antibiotics; MAO Inhibitors; Methotrimeprazine; Nefazodone; Proton Pump Inhibitors; Ritonavir; Saquinavir; Selective Serotonin Reuptake Inhibitors

Decreased Effect

The levels/effects of Clorazepate may be decreased by: CarBAMazepine; CYP3A4 Inducers (Strong); Deferasirox; Rifamycin Derivatives; St Johns Wort; Theophylline Derivatives; Yohimbine

Stability Unstable in water. Store at controlled room temperature at 20°C to 25°C (68°F to 77°F); protect from moisture; keep bottle tightly closed; dispense in tightly closed, light-resistant container

Mechanism of Action Depresses all levels of the CNS, including the limbic and reticular formation, by binding to the benzodiazepine site on the gamma-aminobutyric acid (GABA) receptor complex and modulating GABA, which is a major inhibitory neurotransmitter in the brain

Pharmacokinetics (Adult data unless noted)

Distribution: Crosses the placenta

Protein binding: Nordiazepam: 97% to 98%

Metabolism: Rapidly decarboxylated to desmethyldiazepam (nordiazepam; primary metabolite; active) in acidic stomach prior to absorption; hepatically to oxazepam (active)

Half-life:

Nordiazepam: 40-50 hours

Oxazepam: 6-8 hours

Time to peak serum concentration: Oral: Within 1 hour

Elimination: Primarily in urine (62% to 67% of dose); feces (15% to 19%); found in urine as conjugated oxazepam (3-hydroxynordiazepam) (major urinary metabolite) and conjugated p-hydroxynordiazepam and nordiazepam (smaller amounts)

Usual Dosage Oral:

Anticonvulsant:

Children: Initial dose: 0.3 mg/kg/day; maintenance dose: 0.5-3 mg/kg/day divided 2-4 times/day

or

Children 9-12 years: Initial: 3.75-7.5 mg/dose twice daily; increase dose by 3.75 mg at weekly intervals, not to exceed 60 mg/day in 2-3 divided doses

Children >12 years and Adults: Initial: Up to 7.5 mg/dose 2-3 times/day; increase dose by 7.5 mg at weekly intervals; usual dose: 0.5-1 mg/kg/day; not to exceed 90 mg/day

Anxiety: Adults: 7.5-15 mg 2-4 times/day; usual daily dose: 30 mg/day in divided doses; range: 15-60 mg/day; may be given as single dose of 15 mg at bedtime, with subsequent dosage adjustments based on patient response

Alcohol withdrawal: Adults: Initial: 30 mg, then 15 mg 2-4 times/day on first day; maximum daily dose: 90 mg; gradually decrease dose over subsequent days

Administration Oral: May administer with food or water to decrease GI upset

Monitoring Parameters Excessive CNS depression, respiratory rate, and cardiovascular status; with prolonged use: CBC, liver enzymes, renal function; signs and symptoms of suicidality (eg, anxiety, depression, behavior changes) (see Warnings)

Reference Range Therapeutic: 0.12-1 mcg/mL (SI: 0.36-3.01 micromoles/L)

Patient Information Avoid alcohol. May cause drowsiness and impair ability to perform activities requiring mental alertness or physical coordination. May be habit-forming; avoid abrupt discontinuation after prolonged use (withdrawal symptoms or an increase in seizure activity may occur). May cause dry mouth. Antiepileptic agents may increase the risk of suicidal thoughts and behavior; notify physician if you feel more depressed or have thoughts of suicide or self harm (see Warnings). Report persistent CNS effects (eg, confusion, depression, headache, dizziness, fatigue, changes in cognition); muscle tremor; visual disturbances; worsening of seizure activity, or loss of seizure control.

Dosage Forms Excipient information presented when available (limited, particularly for generics); consult specific product labeling.

Tablet, as dipotassium: 3.75 mg, 7.5 mg, 15 mg

Tranxene® T-Tab®: 3.75 mg, 7.5 mg, 15 mg

References

Fenichel GM, *Clinical Pediatric Neurology: A Signs and Symptoms Approach*, 2nd ed, Philadelphia, PA: WB Saunders Co, 1993.

Fujii T, Okuno T, Go T, et al, "Clorazepate Therapy for Intractable Epilepsy," *Brain Dev*, 1987, 9(3):288-91.

Mimaki T, Tagawa T, Ono J, et al, "Antiepileptic Effect and Serum Levels of Clorazepate on Children With Refractory Seizures," *Brain Dev*, 1984, 6(6):539-44.

◆ **Clorazepate Dipotassium** see Clorazepate *on page 343*

◆ **Clotrimaderm (Can)** see Clotrimazole *on page 344*

Clotrimazole (kloe TRIM a zole)

Medication Safety Issues

Sound-alike/look-alike issues:

Clotrimazole may be confused with co-trimoxazole

Lotrimin® may be confused with Lotrisone®, Otrivin®

Mycelex® may be confused with Myoflex®

International issues:

Cloderm: Brand name for clotrimazole [Germany], but also brand name for alclomethasone [Indonesia]; clobetasol [China, India, Malaysia, Singapore, Thailand]; clocortolone [U.S., Canada]

Canesten: Brand name for clotrimazole [multiple international markets] may be confused with Canesten Bifonazol Comp brand name for bifonazole/urea [Austria]; Canesten Extra brand name for bifonazole [China, Germany]; Canesten Extra Nagelset brand name for bifonazole/urea [Denmark]; Canesten Fluconazole brand name for fluconazole [New Zealand]; Canesten Oasis brand name for sodium citrate [Great Britain]; Canesten Once Daily brand name for bifonazole [Australia]; Canesten Oral brand name for fluconazole [United Kingdom]; Cenestin® brand name for estrogens (conjugated A/synthetic) [U.S., Canada]

Mycelex®: Brand name for clotrimazole [U.S.] may be confused with Mucolex brand name for carbocysteine [Ireland, Portugal, Thailand]; guaifenesin [China]

U.S. Brand Names Anti-Fungal™ [OTC]; Cruex® Cream [OTC]; Gyne-Lotrimin® 3 [OTC]; Gyne-Lotrimin® 7 [OTC]; Lotrimin® AF Athlete's Foot Cream [OTC]; Lotrimin® AF for Her [OTC]; Lotrimin® AF Jock Itch Cream [OTC]; Mycelex®

Canadian Brand Names Canesten® Topical; Canesten® Vaginal; Clotrimaderm; Trivagizole-3®

Therapeutic Category Antifungal Agent, Oral Non-absorbed; Antifungal Agent, Topical; Antifungal Agent, Vaginal

Generic Available Yes: Cream, solution, troche

Use Treatment of susceptible fungal infections, including oropharyngeal candidiasis, dermatophytoses, superficial mycoses, cutaneous candidiasis, as well as vulvovaginal candidiasis; limited data suggests that the use of clotrimazole troches may be effective for prophylaxis against oropharyngeal candidiasis in neutropenic patients

Pregnancy Risk Factor B (topical); C (troches)

Pregnancy Considerations In animal reproduction studies, adverse events were observed with oral, but not vaginal, administration of clotrimazole. Following topical and vaginal administration, clotrimazole is poorly absorbed systemically. Adverse events have not been reported following vaginal use during the second and third trimesters of pregnancy.

Lactation Excretion in breast milk unknown/use caution

Breast-Feeding Considerations Following topical and vaginal administration, clotrimazole is poorly absorbed systemically.

Contraindications Hypersensitivity to clotrimazole or any component

Warnings Clotrimazole troches should not be used for treatment of systemic fungal infection

Precautions Safety and effectiveness of clotrimazole lozenges (troches) in children <3 years of age have not been established

Adverse Reactions
Dermatologic: Erythema, pruritus, urticaria, skin fissures, blistering
Gastrointestinal: Nausea and vomiting may occur in patients on clotrimazole troches; lower abdominal cramps may occur in patients receiving clotrimazole vaginal tablets
Hepatic: Abnormal liver function tests (causal relationship between troches and elevated LFTs not clearly established)
Local: Mild burning, irritation, stinging of skin or vaginal area

Drug Interactions
Metabolism/Transport Effects Inhibits CYP1A2 (weak), 2A6 (weak), 2B6 (weak), 2C8 (weak), 2C9 (weak), 2C19 (weak), 2D6 (weak), 2E1 (weak), 3A4 (moderate)
Avoid Concomitant Use
Avoid concomitant use of Clotrimazole with any of the following: Tolvaptan
Increased Effect/Toxicity
Clotrimazole may increase the levels/effects of: Colchicine; CYP3A4 Substrates; Eplerenone; Everolimus; FentaNYL; Halofantrine; Pimecrolimus; Ranolazine; Salmeterol; Saxagliptin; Tolvaptan
Decreased Effect
Clotrimazole may decrease the levels/effects of: Saccharomyces boulardii

Mechanism of Action Binds to phospholipids in the fungal cell membrane altering cell wall permeability resulting in loss of essential intracellular elements

Pharmacokinetics (Adult data unless noted)
Absorption: Negligible through intact skin when administered topically; 3% to 10% of an intravaginal dose is absorbed

Distribution: Following oral/topical administration, clotrimazole is present in saliva for up to 3 hours following 30 minutes of dissolution time in the mouth

Usual Dosage
Children >3 years and Adults:
Topical/Oral: 10 mg troche dissolved slowly 5 times/day
Topical: Apply twice daily
Children >12 years and Adults: Vaginal: 100 mg/day at bedtime for 7 days or 200 mg/day at bedtime for 3 days or 500 mg single dose; or 5 g (= 1 applicatorful) of 1% vaginal cream daily at bedtime for 7-14 days

Administration
Oral: Dissolve lozenge (troche) in mouth over 15-30 minutes
Topical: Apply sparingly and rub gently into the cleansed, affected area and surrounding skin; do not apply to the eye
Vaginal: Wash hands before using. Insert full applicator into vagina gently and expel cream, or insert tablet into vagina. Wash applicator with soap and water following use. Remain lying down for 30 minutes following administration.

Monitoring Parameters Periodic liver function tests during oral therapy with clotrimazole lozenges

Patient Information Vaginal cream and tablet are oil-based and may weaken latex condoms and diaphragms; avoid intercourse during therapy. Do not use tampons until therapy is complete.

Dosage Forms Excipient information presented when available (limited, particularly for generics); consult specific product labeling. [DSC] = Discontinued product
Cream, topical: 1% (15 g, 30 g, 45 g)
Anti-Fungal™: 1% (113 g)
Cruex®: 1% (15 g) [contains benzyl alcohol]
Lotrimin® AF Athlete's Foot: 1% (12 g) [contains benzyl alcohol]
Lotrimin® AF Jock Itch: 1% (12 g) [contains benzyl alcohol]
Lotrimin® AF for Her: 1% (24 g) [contains benzyl alcohol]
Cream, topical/vaginal: 1% (45 g)
Gyne-Lotrimin® 7: 1% (45 g) [contains benzyl alcohol; packaged with refillable applicator]
Cream, vaginal: 2% (21 g)
Gyne-Lotrimin® 3: 2% (21 g) [contains benzyl alcohol; packaged with 3 disposable applicators]
Solution, topical: 1% (10 mL, 30 mL)
Tablet, vaginal:
Gyne-Lotrimin® 3: 200 mg (3s) [DSC]
Troche, oral: 10 mg
Mycelex®: 10 mg

Clozapine (KLOE za peen)

Medication Safety Issues
Sound-alike/look-alike issues:
Clozapine may be confused with clofazimine, clonidine, Klonopin®
Clozaril® may be confused with Clinoril®, Colazal®

U.S. Brand Names Clozaril®; FazaClo®

Canadian Brand Names Apo-Clozapine®; Clozaril®; Gen-Clozapine; PMS-Clozapine

Therapeutic Category Antipsychotic Agent; Antipsychotic Agent, Atypical

Generic Available Yes

Use Treatment of refractory schizophrenia (FDA approved in adults); to reduce the risk of recurrent suicidal behavior in schizophrenia or schizoaffective disorder (FDA approved in adults)

Restrictions Patient-specific registration is required to dispense clozapine to ensure that appropriate monitoring of WBC and ANC occur according to the recommended schedule. Monitoring systems for individual clozapine manufacturers are independent. If a patient is switched from one brand/manufacturer of clozapine to another, the patient must be entered into a new registry (must be completed by the prescriber and delivered to the dispensing pharmacy). Healthcare providers, including pharmacists dispensing clozapine, should verify the patient's hematological status and qualification to receive clozapine with all existing registries. The pharmacist may not dispense clozapine without verification of a safe WBC and ANC within 7 days of dispensing. Healthcare providers should submit all WBC/ANC values following discontinuation of therapy to the Clozaril National Registry for all nonrechallengable patients until WBC is ≥3500/mm^3 and ANC is ≥2000/mm^3.

Pregnancy Risk Factor B

Pregnancy Considerations Teratogenic effects were not seen in animal studies; however, there are no adequate and well-controlled studies in pregnant women. Use during pregnancy only if clearly needed. Healthcare providers are encouraged to enroll women 18-45 years of age exposed to clozapine during pregnancy in the Atypical Antipsychotics Pregnancy Registry (1-866-961-2388).

Lactation Enters breast milk/not recommended (AAP rates "of concern")

Contraindications Hypersensitivity to clozapine or any component; history of agranulocytosis or granulocytopenia with clozapine; uncontrolled epilepsy; severe CNS depression or comatose state; paralytic ileus; myeloproliferative disorders; use with other agents which have a well-known risk of agranulocytosis or bone marrow suppression

Warnings Potentially life-threatening agranulocytosis may occur **[U.S. Boxed Warning]**. Clozapine therapy should not be initiated in patients with WBC <3500 cells/mm^3 or ANC <2000 cells/mm^3 or history of myeloproliferative disorder. WBC testing should occur periodically on an on-going basis (see prescribing information for monitoring details) to ensure that acceptable WBC/ANC counts are maintained. Initial episodes of moderate leukopenia or granulopoietic suppression confer up to a 12-fold increased risk for subsequent episodes of agranulocytosis. WBCs must be monitored weekly for at least 4 weeks after therapy discontinuation or until WBC is ≥3500/mm^3 and ANC is ≥2000/mm^3. Use with caution in patients receiving other marrow suppressive agents. Eosinophilia has been reported to occur with clozapine and may require temporary or permanent interruption of therapy. Due to the significant risk of agranulocytosis, it is strongly recommended that a patient must fail at least two trials of other primary medications for the treatment of schizophrenia (of adequate dose and duration) before initiating therapy with clozapine. Safety and efficacy have not been established in children.

Myocarditis, pericarditis, pericardial effusion, cardiomyopathy, CHF, ECG changes, arrhythmias, MI, and sudden death have also been reported with clozapine. Use clozapine with caution in patients with known cardiovascular or respiratory disease; carefully follow gradual dosage titration in these patients. Fatalities due to myocarditis have been reported; the highest incidence of fatal myocarditis occurs in the first month of therapy; however, later cases have also been reported **[U.S. Boxed Warning]**. Myocarditis or cardiomyopathy should be considered in patients who present with signs/symptoms of heart failure (dyspnea, fatigue, orthopnea, paroxysmal nocturnal dyspnea, peripheral edema), chest pain, palpitations, new ECG abnormalities (arrhythmias, ST-T wave abnormalities), or unexplained fever. Patients with tachycardia during the first month of therapy should be closely monitored for other signs of myocarditis. Discontinue clozapine if myocarditis is suspected; do not rechallenge in patients with clozapine-related myocarditis. The reported rate of myocarditis in clozapine-treated patients appears to be 17-322 times greater than in the general population.

May cause orthostatic hypotension (with or without syncope) and tachycardia **[U.S. Boxed Warning]**; collapse may rarely be profound and accompanied by respiratory and/or cardiac arrest; use with caution in patients at risk of this effect or in those who would not tolerate transient hypotensive episodes (eg, patients with cerebrovascular disease, cardiovascular disease, hypovolemia, or concurrent medication use which may predispose to hypotension/bradycardia). Collapse, respiratory arrest, and cardiac arrest during initiation of therapy have been reported in patients concurrently receiving benzodiazepines or other psychotropic drugs.

Seizures have been associated with clozapine use in a dose-dependent manner **[U.S. Boxed Warning]**; use with caution in patients at risk of seizures, including those with a history of seizures, head trauma, brain damage, alcoholism, or concurrent therapy with medications which may lower seizure threshold.

Note: All of the above serious adverse effects have been reported in children and adolescents.

An increased risk of death has been reported with the use of antipsychotics in elderly patients with dementia-related psychosis **[U.S. Boxed Warning]**; most deaths seemed to be cardiovascular (eg, sudden death, heart failure) or infectious (eg, pneumonia) in nature. An increased incidence of cerebrovascular adverse events (eg, transient ischemic attack, stroke), including fatalities, has been reported with the use of atypical antipsychotics in elderly patients with dementia-related psychosis. Clozapine is not approved for the treatment of patients with dementia-related psychosis.

Precautions The possibility of a suicide attempt is inherent in psychotic illness or bipolar disorder; use with caution in high-risk patients during initiation of therapy. Prescriptions should be written for the smallest quantity consistent with good patient care.

May cause anticholinergic effects (constipation, xerostomia, blurred vision, urinary retention); use with caution in patients with decreased GI motility, paralytic ileus, urinary retention, benign prostatic hyperplasia, or visual problems. Use with caution in patients with narrow-angle glaucoma; condition may be exacerbated by cholinergic blockade; screening is recommended. Use with caution in patients with myasthenia gravis; condition may be exacerbated by cholinergic blockade. Impaired core body temperature regulation may occur; use with caution with strenuous exercise, heat exposure, dehydration, and concomitant medication possessing anticholinergic effects.

May cause extrapyramidal symptoms, including pseudoparkinsonism, acute dystonic reactions, akathisia, and tardive dyskinesia (risk of these reactions is generally much lower relative to typical/conventional antipsychotics, and is dose-dependent; risk of dystonia is increased with the use of high potency and higher doses of conventional antipsychotics and in males and younger patients). Atypical antipsychotics have been associated with development of hyperglycemia; in some cases, this may be extreme and associated with ketoacidosis, hyperosmolar coma, or death. Use with caution in patients with diabetes or other disorders of glucose regulation; monitor for worsening of glucose control. Significant weight gain has been observed with clozapine; individual weight gain varies.

Clozapine has been associated with benign, self-limiting fever (<100.4°F, usually within first 3 weeks). However, clozapine may also be associated with severe febrile reactions, including neuroleptic malignant syndrome (NMS); monitor for mental status changes, fever, muscle rigidity, and/or autonomic instability. May be moderate to highly sedating; use with caution in disorders where CNS depression is a feature; patients must be cautioned about performing tasks which require mental alertness (eg, operating machinery or driving). Use with caution in patients receiving general anesthesia (due to CNS effects). Rare cases of thromboembolism, including pulmonary embolism and stroke resulting in fatalities, have been associated with clozapine in patients with cardiovascular disease.

Concurrent use with benzodiazepines may increase the risk of severe cardiopulmonary reactions. Cigarette smoking may enhance the metabolism of clozapine. Use with caution in patients with hepatic disease or impairment; hepatitis has been reported as a consequence of therapy. Use with caution in patients with renal impairment.

Medication should not be stopped abruptly; taper off over 1-2 weeks. If conditions warrant abrupt discontinuation (leukopenia, myocarditis, cardiomyopathy), monitor patient for psychosis and cholinergic rebound (headache, nausea, vomiting, diarrhea).

Orally disintegrating tablets contain aspartame which is metabolized to phenylalanine and must be avoided (or used with caution) in patients with phenylketonuria. **Note:** The allowable intake for aspartame in adults is 50 mg/kg/day.

Adverse Reactions Note: Children and adolescents may be more sensitive to neutropenia compared to adults (see Sporn, 2007); patients should be carefully monitored and counseled to report mouth sores, flu-like symptoms, weakness; percents listed are reported for adults

Cardiovascular: Angina, ECG changes, hypertension, hypotension, myocarditis (see Warnings), orthostatic hypotension, syncope, tachycardia (25%)
Central nervous system: Agitation, akathisia (may be as high as 15% in children and adolescents; see Sporn, 2007), akinesia, anxiety, ataxia, confusion, depression, dizziness (19% to 27%), drowsiness/sedation (39% to 46%), dystonia, fatigue, headache, insomnia (2% to 20%), lethargy, myoclonic jerks, neuroleptic malignant syndrome (see Warnings), nightmares, restlessness, seizure (see Warnings), slurred speech, tardive dyskinesia (see Warnings)
Dermatologic: Rash
Endocrine & metabolic: Hyperglycemia (see Warnings), hypertriglyceridemia, metabolic syndrome (see Lamberti, 2006), serum cholesterol increased, weight gain (4% to 31%)
Gastrointestinal: Abdominal discomfort/heartburn (4% to 14%), anorexia, constipation (14% to 25%), diarrhea, nausea/vomiting (3% to 17%), sialorrhea (31% to 48%), throat discomfort, xerostomia
Genitourinary: Urinary abnormalities (eg, abnormal ejaculation, retention, urgency, incontinence)
Hematologic: Agranulocytosis (see Warnings), eosinophilia, granulocytopenia, leukocytosis, leukopenia
Hepatic: Liver function tests increased
Neuromuscular & skeletal: Hyperkinesia, hypokinesia, pain, rigidity, spasm, tremor, weakness
Ocular: Visual disturbances
Respiratory: Dyspnea, nasal congestion
Miscellaneous: Diaphoresis increased, fever, tongue numbness
1%, postmarketing, and/or case reports (limited to important or life-threatening): Amentia, amnesia, anemia, arrhythmia (atrial or ventricular), aspiration, bradycardia, breast pain, bronchitis, cardiomyopathy (usually dilated), cataplexy, CHF, cholestasis, coordination impaired, CPK increased, cyanosis, delirium, delusions, dermatitis, diabetes mellitus, DVT, dysarthria, dysmenorrhea, dysphagia, ear disorder, eczema, edema, epistaxis, eructation, erythema multiforme, ESR increased, fecal impaction, gastric ulcer, gastroenteritis, hallucinations, hematemesis, hepatitis, hemoglobin/hematocrit increased, histrionic movement, hyperuricemia, hyperventilation, hyponatremia, hypothermia, impotence, interstitial nephritis (acute), intestinal obstruction, jaundice, loss of speech, libido changes, malaise, MI, myasthenia syndrome, mydriasis, narrow-angle glaucoma, obsessive compulsive symptoms, pallor, palpitations, pancreatitis (acute), paralytic ileus, paranoia, Parkinsonism, PE, pericardial effusion, pericarditis, periorbital edema, petechiae, phlebitis, photosensitivity, pleural effusion, pneumonia, priapism, pruritus, PVC, rhabdomyolysis, rectal bleeding, salivary gland swelling, sepsis, shakiness, status epilepticus, stuttering, stroke, Stevens-Johnson syndrome, thrombocytopenia, thrombocytosis, thromboembolism, thrombophlebitis, tics, urticaria, vaginal itching/infection, vasculitis, weight loss, wheezing

Drug Interactions

Metabolism/Transport Effects Substrate of CYP1A2 (major), 2A6 (minor), 2C9 (minor), 2C19 (minor), 2D6 (minor), 3A4 (minor); **Inhibits** CYP1A2 (weak), 2C9 (weak), 2C19 (weak), 2D6 (moderate), 2E1 (weak), 3A4 (weak)

Avoid Concomitant Use
Avoid concomitant use of Clozapine with any of the following: Metoclopramide; Thioridazine

Increased Effect/Toxicity
Clozapine may increase the levels/effects of: Alcohol (Ethyl); Anticholinergics; CNS Depressants; CYP2D6 Substrates; Fesoterodine; Methotrimeprazine; Nebivolol; Tamoxifen; Thioridazine

The levels/effects of Clozapine may be increased by: Acetylcholinesterase Inhibitors (Central); Benzodiazepines; Cimetidine; CYP1A2 Inhibitors (Moderate); CYP1A2 Inhibitors (Strong); Lithium formulations; Macrolide Antibiotics; MAO Inhibitors; Methotrimeprazine; Metoclopramide; Nefazodone; Omeprazole; Pramlintide; Selective Serotonin Reuptake Inhibitors; Tetrabenazine

Decreased Effect
Clozapine may decrease the levels/effects of: Amphetamines; Anti-Parkinson's Agents (Dopamine Agonist); Codeine; Quinagolide; TraMADol

The levels/effects of Clozapine may be decreased by: CarBAMazepine; CYP1A2 Inducers (Strong); Lithium formulations; Omeprazole; Peginterferon Alfa-2b; Phenytoin

Food Interactions Food does not affect bioavailability.

Stability Clozaril®: Store at temperatures ≤30°C (86°F).
FazaClo®: Store at controlled room temperature at 25°C (77°F); excursions permitted to 15°C to 30°C (59°F to 86°F); protect from moisture; do not remove from package until ready to use
Dispensed in "clozapine patient system" packaging. **Note:** Drug is usually dispensed in a 1-week supply, unless patient is eligible for WBC and ANC testing at greater intervals (eg, every 2 or 4 weeks). Dispensing is contingent on WBC and ANC test results (see Restrictions).

Mechanism of Action Clozapine (dibenzodiazepine antipsychotic) exhibits weak antagonism of D_1, D_2, D_3, and D_5 dopamine receptor subtypes, but shows high affinity for D_4 receptors; in addition, it blocks the serotonin ($5HT_2$), alpha-adrenergic, histamine H_1, and cholinergic receptors

◄ **Pharmacodynamics**

Onset of action: Within 1 week for sedation, improvement in sleep; 6-12 weeks for antipsychotic effects

Adequate trial: 6-12 weeks at a therapeutic dose and blood level

Maximum effect: 6-12 months; improvement may continue 6-12 months after clozapine initiation (see Meltzer, 2003)

Duration: Variable

Pharmacokinetics (Adult data unless noted)

Protein binding: 97% to serum proteins

Metabolism: Extensively hepatic; forms metabolites with limited (desmethyl metabolite) or no activity (hydroxylated and N-oxide derivative derivatives). **Note:** A pediatric pharmacokinetic study (n=6; age: 9-16 years) found higher concentrations of the desmethyl metabolite in comparison to clozapine (especially in females) when compared to data from adult studies; the authors suggest that both the parent drug and desmethyl metabolite contribute to the efficacy and adverse effect profile in children and adolescents (see Frazier, 2003).

Bioavailability: 12% to 81% (not affected by food); orally disintegrating tablets are bioequivalent to the regular tablets

Half-life: Adults: Steady state: 12 hours (range: 4-66 hours)

Time to peak serum concentration: Tablets: 2.5 hours (range: 1-6 hours); orally disintegrating tablets: 2.3 hours (range: 1-6 hours)

Elimination: Urine (~50% of dose) and feces (30%); trace amounts of unchanged drug excreted in urine and feces

Usual Dosage Oral:

Children and Adolescents: Treatment of refractory childhood-onset schizophrenia or schizoaffective disorder: Initial: 12.5 mg once or twice daily; increase daily dose as tolerated every 3-5 days (usually by 25 mg increments) to a target dose of 125-475 mg/day in divided doses (based on patient's age, size, and tolerability). Mean dose in most pediatric studies: 175-200 mg/day (see Findling, 2007)

Adults:

Refractory schizophrenia or schizoaffective disorder: Initial: 12.5 mg once or twice daily; increase as tolerated, in increments of 25-50 mg/day to a target dose of 300-450 mg/day after 2-4 weeks; may increase further if needed, but no more than once or twice weekly, in increments ≤100 mg/day; some patients may require doses as high as 600-900 mg/day in divided doses. Do not exceed 900 mg/day. **Note:** Due to significant adverse effects, patients who fail to adequately respond clinically, should not be normally continued on therapy for an extended period of time; responding patients should be maintained on the lowest effective dose; patients should be periodically assessed to determine if maintenance treatment is still required.

Reduction of the risk of suicidal behavior in schizophrenia or schizoaffective disorder: Initial: 12.5 mg once or twice daily; increased, as tolerated, in increments of 25-50 mg/day to a target dose of 300-450 mg/day after 2-4-weeks; may increase further if needed, but no more than once or twice weekly, in increments ≤100 mg/day; mean effective dose is ~300 mg/day (range: 12.5-900 mg). **Note:** A treatment course of at least 2 years is recommended to maintain the decreased risk for suicidal behavior; patients should be reassessed after 2 years for risk of suicidal behavior and periodically thereafter.

Termination of therapy: If dosing is interrupted for ≥48 hours, therapy must be reinitiated at 12.5-25 mg/day; if tolerated, the dose may be increased more rapidly than with initial titration, unless cardiopulmonary arrest occurred during initial titration.

In the event of planned termination of clozapine, gradual reduction in dose over a 1- to 2-week period is recommended. If conditions warrant abrupt discontinuation (eg, leukopenia), monitor patient for psychosis and cholinergic rebound (headache, nausea, vomiting, diarrhea).

Note: Patients discontinued on clozapine therapy due to WBC <2000/mm^3 or ANC <1000/mm^3 should **not** be restarted on clozapine.

Administration May be administered without regard to food.

Orally-disintegrating tablet: Should be removed from foil blister by peeling apart (do not push tablet through the foil). Remove immediately prior to use. Place tablet in mouth and allow to dissolve; swallow with saliva (no water is needed to take the dose). If dosing requires splitting tablet, throw unused portion away.

Monitoring Parameters Mental status, ECG, WBC (see below), vital signs, fasting lipid profile, and fasting blood glucose/Hgb A$_{1c}$ (prior to treatment, at 3 months, then annually, or as symptoms warrant); height, weight, BMI, personal/family history of obesity, waist circumference (weight should be assessed prior to treatment, at 4 weeks, 8 weeks, 12 weeks, and then at quarterly intervals; consider titrating to a different antipsychotic agent for a weight gain ≥5% of the initial weight); blood pressure, pulse, abnormal involuntary movement scale (AIMS).

WBC and ANC should be obtained at baseline and at least weekly for the first 6 months of continuous treatment. If counts remain acceptable (WBC ≥3500/mm^3, ANC ≥2000/mm^3) during this time period, then they may be monitored every other week for the next 6 months. If WBC/ANC continue to remain within these acceptable limits after the second 6 months of therapy, monitoring can be decreased to every 4 weeks. (**Note:** The decrease in monitoring to every 4 weeks is applicable in the United States. Blood monitoring requirements related to the use of clozapine have not changed in Canada.) If clozapine is discontinued, a weekly WBC should be conducted for an additional 4 weeks or until WBC is ≥3500/mm^3 and ANC is ≥2000/mm^3. If clozapine therapy is interrupted due to moderate leukopenia, weekly WBC/ANC monitoring is required for 12 months in patients restarted on clozapine treatment. If therapy is interrupted for reasons other than leukopenia/granulocytopenia, the 6-month time period for initiation of biweekly WBCs may need to be reset. This determination depends upon the treatment duration, the length of the break in therapy, and whether or not an abnormal blood event occurred.

Consult full prescribing information for determination of appropriate WBC/ANC monitoring interval (http://www.clozaril.com/index.jsp or http://www.fazaclo.com).

Patient Information Use exactly as directed; do not increase dose or frequency. Do not discontinue this medication without consulting prescriber. If more than 2 days of medication are missed, do not restart at same dosage; contact physician for dosing instructions. Avoid alcohol, caffeine, other prescription, and nonprescription medications not approved by prescriber. Maintain adequate hydration unless instructed to restrict fluid intake. If you have diabetes, monitor blood glucose levels frequently. This medication may cause headache, excess drowsiness, dizziness, or blurred vision (use caution driving or when engaging in tasks requiring alertness until response to drug is known); constipation, diarrhea, dry mouth, nausea, vomiting, or postural hypotension (use caution climbing stairs or when changing position from lying or sitting to standing). This medication may decrease your white blood cell count (WBC); frequent blood tests are required to avoid serious adverse effects; due to low WBC, you may be prone to infections; report fever, sore throat, or other possible signs of infection. Report persistent CNS effects (insomnia, depression, altered consciousness), palpitations, rapid heartbeat, severe dizziness, vision change, hypersalivation, tearing, sweating, respiratory difficulty, or worsening of condition. Report seizures, flu-like symptoms, chest pain, shortness of breath, or excessive fatigue.

Additional Information Clozapine produces little or no prolactin elevation; this is in contrast to other more typical antipsychotic drugs

Dosage Forms Excipient information presented when available (limited, particularly for generics); consult specific product labeling.

Tablet: 25 mg, 50 mg, 100 mg, 200 mg

Clozaril®: 25 mg [scored], 100 mg [scored]

Tablet, orally disintegrating:

FazaClo®: 12.5 mg [contains phenylalanine 0.87 mg/tablet; mint flavor], 25 mg [contains phenylalanine 1.74 mg/tablet; mint flavor], 100 mg [contains phenylalanine 6.96 mg/tablet; mint flavor]

References

Alfaro CL, Wudarsky M, Nicolson R, et al, "Correlation of Antipsychotic and Prolactin Concentrations in Children and Adolescents Acutely Treated With Haloperidol, Clozapine or Olanzapine," J Child Adolesc Psychopharmacol, 2002, 12(2):83-91.

American Diabetes Association; American Psychiatric Association; American Association of Clinical Endocrinologists; North American Association for the Study of Obesity, "Consensus Development Conference on Antipsychotic Drugs and Obesity and Diabetes," Diabetes Care, 2004, 27(2):596-601.

Campellone JV, McCluskey LF, and Greenspan D, "Fatal Outcome From Neuroleptic Malignant Syndrome Associated With Clozapine," Neuropsychiatry, Neuropsychology, and Behavioral Neurology, 1995, 8:70-3.

Correll CU, Penzner JB, Parikh UH, et al, "Recognizing and Monitoring Adverse Events of Second-Generation Antipsychotics in Children and Adolescents," Child Adolesc Psych Clin N Am, 2006, 15(1):177-206.

Findling RL, Frazier JA, Gerbino-Rosen B, et al, "Is There a Role for Clozapine in the Treatment of Children and Adolescents?" J Am Acad Child Adolesc Psych, 2007, 46(3):423-8.

Frazier JA, Cohen LG, Jacobsen L, et al, "Clozapine Pharmacokinetics in Children and Adolescents With Childhood-Onset Schizophrenia," J Clin Psychopharmacol, 2003, 23(1):87-91.

Funderberg LG, Vertrees JE, True JE, et al, "Seizure Following Addition of Erythromycin to Clozapine Treatment," Am J Psychiatry, 1994, 151 (12):1840-1.

Gerbino-Rosen G, Roofeh D, Tompkins DA, et al, "Hematological Adverse Events in Clozapine-Treated Children and Adolescents," J Am Acad Child Adolesc Psychiatry, 2005, 44(10):1024-31.

Gerson SL and Meltzer H, "Mechanisms of Clozapine-Induced Agranulocytosis," Drug Saf, 1992, 7(Suppl 1):17-25.

Hagg S, Spigset O, and Soderstrom TG, "Association of Venous Thromboembolism and Clozapine," Lancet, 2000, 355(9210):1155-6.

Kane J, Honigfeld G, Singer J, et al, "Clozapine for the Treatment-Resistant Schizophrenic. A Double-Blind Comparison With Chlorpromazine," Arch Gen Psychiatry, 1988, 45(9):789-96.

Kant R, Chalansani R, Chengappa KN, et al, "The Off-Label Use of Clozapine in Adolescents With Bipolar Disorder, Intermittent Explosive Disorder, or Posttraumatic Stress Disorder," J Child Adolesc Psychopharmacol, 2004, 14(1):57-63.

Kranzler HN, Kester HM, Gerbino-Rosen G, et al, "Treatment-Refractory Schizophrenia in Children and Adolescents: An Update on Clozapine and Other Pharmacologic Interventions," Child Adolesc Psychiatr Clin N Am, 2006, 15(1):135-59.

Kranzler H, Roofeh D, Gerbino-Rosen G, et al, "Clozapine: Its Impact on Aggressive Behavior Among Children and Adolescents With Schizophrenia," J Am Acad Child Adolesc Psychiatry, 2005, 44 (1):55-63.

Kumra S, Frazier JA, Jacobsen LK, et al, "Childhood-Onset Schizophrenia. A Double-Blind Clozapine-Haloperidol Comparison," Arch Gen Psychiatry, 1996, 53(12):1090-7.

Lamberti JS, Olson D, Crilly JF, et al, "Prevalence of the Metabolic Syndrome Among Patients Receiving Clozapine," Am J Psychiatry, 2006, 163(7):1273-6.

Mady SP and Wax P, "Clozapine Intoxication in a Young Child," Vet Hum Toxicol, 1993, 35(4):338.

Meltzer HY, Alphs L, Green AI, et al, "Clozapine Treatment for Suicidality in Schizophrenia: International Suicide Prevention Trial (InterSePT)," Arch Gen Psychiatry, 2003, 60(1):82-91.

Pacia SV and Devinsky O, "Clozapine-Related Seizures: Experience With 5629 Patients," Neurology, 1994, 44(12):2247-9.

Radford JM, Brown TM, and Borison RL, "Unexpected Dystonia While Changing From Clozapine to Risperidone," J Clin Psychopharmacol, 1995, 15(3):225-6.

Shaw P, Sporn A, Gogtay N, et al, "Childhood-Onset Schizophrenia: A Double-Blind, Randomized, Clozapine-Olanzapine Comparison," Arch Gen Psych, 2006, 63(7):721-30.

Sporn AL, Vermani A, Greenstein DK, et al, "Clozapine Treatment of Childhood-Onset Schizophrenia: Evaluation of Effectiveness, Adverse Effects, and Long-Term Outcome," J Am Acad Child Adolesc Psychiatry, 2007, 46(10):1349-56.

Testani M, "Clozapine-Induced Orthostatic Hypotension Treated With Fludrocortisone," J Clin Psychiatry, 1994, 55(11):497-8.

Wheatley M, Plant J, Reader H, et al, "Clozapine Treatment of Adolescents With Posttraumatic Stress Disorder and Psychotic Symptoms," J Clin Psychopharmacol, 2004, 24(2):167-73.

Wilson WH and Claussen AM, "Seizures Associated With Clozapine Treatment in a State Hospital," J Clin Psychiatry, 1994, 55(5):184-8.

◆ **Clozaril®** see Clozapine on page 345

◆ **CMA-676** see Gemtuzumab Ozogamicin on page 640

◆ **CMV-IGIV** see Cytomegalovirus Immune Globulin (Intravenous-Human) on page 379

◆ **Coagulant Complex Inhibitor** see Anti-inhibitor Coagulant Complex on page 117

◆ **Coagulation Factor VIIa** see Factor VIIa (Recombinant) on page 556

Coal Tar (KOLE tar)

Medication Safety Issues

Sound-alike/look-alike issues:

Pentrax® may be confused with Permax®

U.S. Brand Names Balnetar® [OTC]; Betatar® Gel [OTC]; Cutar® [OTC]; Denorex® Original Therapeutic Strength [OTC]; DHS™ Tar [OTC]; DHS™ Targel [OTC]; Doak® Tar [OTC]; Exorex®; Fototar® [OTC] [DSC]; Ionil T® Plus [OTC] [DSC]; MG 217® Medicated Tar [OTC]; MG 217® [OTC]; Neutrogena® T/Gel Extra Strength [OTC]; Neutrogena® T/Gel Stubborn Itch Control [OTC]; Neutrogena® T/Gel [OTC]; Oxipor® VHC [OTC]; Polytar® [OTC] [DSC]; Reme-T™ [OTC]; Scytera™ [OTC]; Tera-Gel™ [OTC]; Zetar® [OTC]

Canadian Brand Names Balnetar®; Estar®; Targel®

Therapeutic Category Antipsoriatic Agent, Topical; Antiseborrheic Agent, Topical

Generic Available No

Use Topically for controlling dandruff, seborrheic dermatitis, or psoriasis

Pregnancy Risk Factor C

Contraindications Hypersensitivity to coal tar or any ingredient in the formulation

Warnings Due to a potential carcinogenic risk, do not use around the rectum or in the genital area or groin

Precautions Do not apply to acutely inflamed skin; avoid exposure to sunlight for at least 24 hours

Adverse Reactions Dermatologic: Dermatitis, folliculitis, irritation, acneiform eruption, photosensitivity

Drug Interactions

Avoid Concomitant Use There are no known interactions where it is recommended to avoid concomitant use.

Increased Effect/Toxicity There are no known significant interactions involving an increase in effect.

Decreased Effect There are no known significant interactions involving a decrease in effect.

Mechanism of Action Reduces the number and size of epidermal cells produced

Usual Dosage Children and Adults: Topical:

Bath: 60-90 mL of a 5% to 20% solution or 15-25 mL of 30% lotion is added to bath water; soak 5-20 minutes, then pat dry; use once daily to once every 3 days

Shampoo: Apply twice weekly for the first 2 weeks then once weekly or more often if needed

Skin: Apply to the affected area 1-4 times/day; decrease frequency to 2-3 times/week once condition has been controlled

Atopic dermatitis: 2% to 5% coal tar cream may be applied once daily or every other day to reduce inflammation

Scalp psoriasis: Tar oil bath or coal tar solution may be painted sparingly to the lesions 3-12 hours before each shampoo

Psoriasis of the body, arms, legs: Apply at bedtime; if thick scales are present, use product with salicylic acid and apply several times during the day

Administration Topical:

Bath: Add appropriate amount of coal tar to lukewarm bath water and mix thoroughly

Shampoo: Rub shampoo onto wet hair and scalp, rinse thoroughly; repeat; leave on 5 minutes; rinse thoroughly

Patient Information Avoid contact with eyes, genital, or rectal area; coal tar preparations frequently stain the skin and hair; shake suspension well before use. May cause photosensitivity reactions (eg, exposure to sunlight may cause severe sunburn, skin rash, redness, or itching); avoid exposure to sunlight and artificial light sources (sunlamps, tanning booth/bed); wear protective clothing, wide-brimmed hats, sunglasses, and lip sunscreen (SPF ≥15); use a sunscreen [broad-spectrum sunscreen or physical sunscreen (preferred) or sunblock with SPF ≥15]; contact physician if reaction occurs.

Dosage Forms Excipient information presented when available (limited, particularly for generics); consult specific product labeling. [DSC] = Discontinued product

Aerosol, topical [foam]:

Scytera™: Coal tar solution 10% (100 g) [equivalent to coal tar 2%]

Cream:

Fototar®: Coal tar 2% (85 g, 454 g) [DSC]

Emulsion, topical:

Cutar®: Coal tar solution 7.5% (180 mL, 3840 mL)

Exorex®: Coal tar 1% (240 mL)

Gel, shampoo:

DHS™ Targel: Coal tar solution 2.9% (240 mL) [equivalent to coal tar 0.5%]

Liquid:

Doak® Tar Distillate: Coal tar 40% (60 mL) [for compounding use only]

Lotion, topical:

MG 217®: Coal tar solution 5% (120 mL) [equivalent to coal tar 1%; contains jojoba]

Oxipor® VHC: Coal tar solution 25% (60 mL, 120 mL) [equivalent to coal tar 5%; contains alcohol 79%]

Oil, topical:

Balnetar®: Coal tar 2.5% (225 mL) [for use in bath]

Doak® Tar: Coal tar distillate 2% (240 mL) [equivalent to coal tar 0.8%; for use in bath]

Ointment, topical:

MG 217®: Coal tar solution 10% (107 g, 430 g) [equivalent to coal tar 2%]

Shampoo, topical:

Betatar Gel®: Coal tar solution 5% (240 mL) [equivalent to coal tar 2.5%; green apple scent]

Denorex® Original Therapeutic Strength: Coal tar solution 12.5% (120 mL, 240 mL, 360 mL) [equivalent to coal tar 2.5%; available with or without conditioner]

DHS™ Tar: Coal tar solution 2.9% (120 mL, 240 mL, 480 mL) [equivalent to coal tar 0.5%]

Doak® Tar: Coal tar distillate 3% (240 mL) [equivalent to coal tar 1.2%]

Ionil T® Plus: Coal tar 2% (240 mL) [DSC]

MG 217® Medicated Tar: Coal tar solution 15% (120 mL, 240 mL) [equivalent to coal tar 3%]

Neutrogena® T/Gel: Coal tar 0.5% (132 mL, 255 mL, 480 mL)

Neutrogena® T/Gel Extra Strength: Coal tar extract 4% (132 mL) [coal tar 1%]

Neutrogena® T/Gel Stubborn Itch Control: Coal tar extract 2% (132 mL) [coal tar 0.5%]

Polytar®: Coal tar 0.5% (177 mL) [DSC]

Reme-T™: Coal tar 5% (236 mL)

Tera-Gel™: Solubilized coal tar 0.5% (120 mL, 240 mL)

Zetar®: Coal tar 1% (180 mL)

Soap, topical:

Polytar®: Coal tar 0.5% (113 g) [DSC]

References

Greaves MW, Weinstein GD, "Treatment of Psoriasis," *N Engl J Med*, 1995, 332(9):581-8.

Hanifin JM, "Atopic Dermatitis in Infants and Children," *Pediatr Clin North Am*, 1991, 38(4):763-89.

◆ **CO Amlodipine (Can)** *see* AmLODIPine *on page 91*

◆ **Coartem®** *see* Artemether and Lumefantrine *on page 136*

◆ **CO Atenolol (Can)** *see* Atenolol *on page 147*

◆ **CO Atorvastatin (Can)** *see* Atorvastatin *on page 151*

◆ **CO Azithromycin (Can)** *see* Azithromycin *on page 164*

◆ **CO Buspirone (Can)** *see* BusPIRone *on page 222*

Cocaine (koe KANE)

Related Information

Laboratory Detection of Drugs in Urine *on page 1706*

Therapeutic Category Analgesic, Topical; Local Anesthetic, Topical

Generic Available Yes

Use Topical anesthesia for mucous membranes

Restrictions C-II

Pregnancy Risk Factor C/X (nonmedicinal use)

Lactation Enters breast milk/contraindicated

Breast-Feeding Considerations Irritability, vomiting, diarrhea, tremors, and seizures have been reported in nursing infants.

Contraindications Hypersensitivity to cocaine or any component; systemic use

Precautions Use with caution in patients with hypertension, severe cardiovascular disease, thyrotoxicosis, and in infants; use with caution in patients with severely traumatized mucosa in the region of intended application

Adverse Reactions

Cardiovascular: Hypertension, tachycardia, cardiac arrhythmias

Central nervous system: Restlessness, nervousness, euphoria, excitement, hallucinations, seizures

Gastrointestinal: Vomiting

Neuromuscular & skeletal: Tremor

Ocular: Topical: Sloughing of the corneal epithelium, ulceration of the cornea

Respiratory: Tachypnea

Drug Interactions

Metabolism/Transport Effects Substrate of CYP3A4 (major); **Inhibits** CYP2D6 (strong), 3A4 (weak)

Avoid Concomitant Use

Avoid concomitant use of Cocaine with any of the following: Iobenguane I 123; Tamoxifen; Thioridazine

Increased Effect/Toxicity

Cocaine may increase the levels/effects of: Atomoxetine; Cannabinoids; CYP2D6 Substrates; Fesoterodine; Nebivolol; Tamoxifen; Tetrabenazine; Thioridazine

The levels/effects of Cocaine may be increased by: CYP3A4 Inhibitors (Moderate); CYP3A4 Inhibitors (Strong); Dasatinib

Decreased Effect

Cocaine may decrease the levels/effects of: Codeine; Iobenguane I 123; TraMADol

Stability Store in well closed, light-resistant containers

Mechanism of Action Blocks both the initiation and conduction of nerve impulses by decreasing the neuronal membrane's permeability to sodium ions. This results in inhibition of depolarization with resultant blockade of conduction; interferes with the uptake of norepinephrine by adrenergic nerve terminals producing vasoconstriction.

Pharmacodynamics Following topical administration to mucosa:

Onset of action: Within 1 minute

Maximum effect: Within 5 minutes

Duration: ≥30 minutes, depending upon route and dosage administered

Pharmacokinetics (Adult data unless noted)

Absorption: Well absorbed through mucous membranes; absorption is limited by drug-induced vasoconstriction and enhanced by inflammation

Distribution: V_d: ~2 L/kg; appears in breast milk (see Additional Information)

Metabolism: In the liver; major metabolites are ecgonine methyl ester and benzoyl ecgonine

Half-life: 75 minutes

Elimination: Primarily in urine as metabolites and unchanged drug (<10%); cocaine metabolites may appear in the urine of neonates for up to 5 days after birth due to maternal cocaine use shortly before birth

Usual Dosage Topical application (ear, nose, throat, bronchoscopy): Concentrations of 1% to 4% are used; use lowest effective dose; do not exceed 1 mg/kg; patient tolerance, anesthetic technique, vascularity of tissue, and area to be anesthetized will determine dose needed. Solutions >4% are not recommended due to increased risk and severity of systemic toxicities.

Administration Topical: Use only on mucous membranes of the oral, laryngeal, and nasal cavities; do not use on extensive areas of broken skin; do not apply commercially available products to the eye (an extemporaneously prepared ophthalmic product must be made)

Monitoring Parameters Heart rate, blood pressure, respiratory rate, temperature

Additional Information Repeated ophthalmic applications to the eye may cause cornea to become clouded or pitted, therefore, NS should be used to irrigate and protect cornea during surgery; not for injection; cocaine intoxication of infants who are receiving breast milk from their mothers abusing cocaine has been reported

Dosage Forms Excipient information presented when available (limited, particularly for generics); consult specific product labeling.

Powder, for prescription compounding, as hydrochloride: USP: 100% (1 g, 5 g, 25 g)

Solution, topical, as hydrochloride: 4% (4 mL, 10 mL); 10% (4 mL, 10 mL)

References

Chasnoff IJ, Lewis DE, and Squires L, "Cocaine Intoxication in Breast-Fed Infants," *Pediatrics*, 1987, 80(6):836-8.

Greenglass EJ, "The Adverse Effects of Cocaine on the Developing Human," Yaffe SJ and Arana JV, eds, *Pediatric Pharmacology: Therapeutic Principles in Practice*, 2nd ed, Philadelphia, PA: WB Saunders Co, 1992, 598-604.

◆ **Cocaine Hydrochloride** *see* Cocaine *on page 350*

◆ **CO Ciprofloxacin (Can)** *see* Ciprofloxacin *on page 310*

◆ **CO Citalopram (Can)** *see* Citalopram *on page 319*

◆ **CO Clomipramine (Can)** *see* ClomiPRAMINE *on page 334*

◆ **CO Clonazepam (Can)** *see* ClonazePAM *on page 337*

Codeine (KOE deen)

Medication Safety Issues

Sound-alike/look-alike issues:

Codeine may be confused with Cardene®, Cophene®, Cordran®, iodine, Lodine®

High alert medication: The Institute for Safe Medication Practices (ISMP) includes this medication among its list of drug classes which have a heightened risk of causing significant patient harm when used in error.

Related Information

Compatibility of Medications Mixed in a Syringe *on page 1713*

Laboratory Detection of Drugs in Urine *on page 1706*

Opioid Analgesics Comparison *on page 1510*

Canadian Brand Names Codeine Contin®

Therapeutic Category Analgesic, Narcotic; Antitussive; Cough Preparation

Generic Available Yes

Use Treatment of mild to moderate pain; antitussive in lower doses (for nonproductive cough)

Restrictions C-II

Pregnancy Risk Factor C

Pregnancy Considerations Animal reproduction studies have not been conducted. Neonatal abstinence syndrome (NAS) has been observed in the newborn following maternal use of codeine during pregnancy. Symptoms of opiate withdrawal may include excessive crying, diarrhea, fever, hyper-reflexia, irritability, tremors, or vomiting. Perinatal stroke has also been reported.

Lactation Enters breast milk/use caution (AAP rates "compatible")

Breast-Feeding Considerations Codeine and its metabolite (morphine) are found in breast milk and can be detected in the serum of nursing infants. The relative dose to a nursing infant has been calculated to be ~1% of the weight-adjusted maternal dose. Higher levels of morphine may be found in the breast milk of lactating mothers who are "ultra-rapid metabolizers" of codeine; patients with two or more copies of the variant CYP2D6*2 allele may have extensive conversion to morphine and thus increased opioid-mediated effects. In one case, excessively high serum concentrations of morphine were reported in a breast-fed infant following maternal use of acetaminophen with codeine. The mother was later found to be an "ultra-rapid metabolizer" of codeine; symptoms in the infant included feeding difficulty and lethargy, followed by death. Because exposure to the nursing infant is generally low, the AAP considers codeine to be "usually compatible with breast-feeding." However, caution should be used since most persons are not aware if they have the genotype resulting in "ultra-rapid metabolizer" status. When codeine is used in breast-feeding women, it is recommended to use the lowest dose for the shortest duration of time and observe the infant for increased sleepiness, difficulty in feeding or breathing, or limpness.

Contraindications Hypersensitivity to codeine or any component (see Warnings)

Warnings May cause CNS depression, which may impair physical or mental abilities; patients must be cautioned about performing tasks which require mental alertness (eg, operating machinery or driving). Respiratory depression may occur even at therapeutic dosages; use with extreme caution in patients with respiratory diseases including asthma, emphysema, COPD, cor pulmonale, hypoxia, hypercapnia, pre-existing respiratory depression, significantly decreased respiratory reserve, other obstructive pulmonary disease, kyphoscoliosis, or other skeletal disorder which may alter respiratory function. Use with extreme caution in patients with head injury, intracranial lesions, or elevated intracranial pressure; exaggerated elevation of ICP may occur. May cause hypotension; use with caution in patients with circulatory shock, hypovolemia, impaired myocardial function, or those receiving drugs which may exaggerate hypotensive effects (including phenothiazines or general anesthetics). Codeine may obscure diagnosis or clinical course of patients with acute abdominal conditions.

Physical and psychological dependence may occur; abrupt discontinuation after prolonged use may result in withdrawal symptoms or seizures. Concurrent use of agonist/antagonist analgesics may precipitate withdrawal symptoms and/or reduce analgesic efficacy in patients following prolonged therapy with mu opioid agonists. Interactions with other CNS drugs may occur (see Drug Interactions). Healthcare provider should be alert to problems of abuse, misuse, and diversion. Infants born to women physically dependent on opioids will also be physically dependent and may experience respiratory difficulties or opioid withdrawal symptoms (neonatal abstinence syndrome). Symptoms of opiate withdrawal may include excessive crying, diarrhea, fever, hyperreflexia, irritability, tremors, or vomiting. Some preparations contain sulfites which may cause allergic reactions in susceptible individuals.

Precautions Use with caution in patients with hypersensitivity reactions to other phenanthrene derivative opioid agonists (morphine, hydrocodone, hydromorphone, levorphanol, oxycodone, oxymorphone), adrenal insufficiency, biliary tract impairment, CNS depression/coma, morbid obesity, prostatic hyperplasia, urinary stricture, thyroid dysfunction, or severe liver or renal insufficiency. Use with caution in patients with two or more copies of the variant CYP2D6*2 allele (ie, CYP2D6 "ultra-rapid metabolizers"); these patients may have extensive conversion of codeine to morphine with resultant increased opioid-mediated effects.

Not recommended for use for cough control in patients with a productive cough; not recommended as an antitussive for children <2 years of age. Debilitated patients may be particularly susceptible to adverse effects of narcotics.

Use codeine with caution in lactating women. Codeine and its metabolite (morphine) are found in breast milk and can be detected in the serum of nursing infants. Exposure to the nursing infant is generally considered to be low; the relative dose to a nursing infant has been calculated to be ~1% of the weight-adjusted maternal dose. Higher levels of morphine may be found in the breast milk of lactating mothers who are "ultra-rapid metabolizers" of codeine; patients with two or more copies of the variant CYP2D6*2 allele may have extensive conversion to morphine and thus increased opioid-mediated effects. In one case, excessively high serum concentrations of morphine were reported in a breast-fed infant following maternal use of acetaminophen with codeine (see Koren, 2006). The mother was later found to be an "ultra-rapid metabolizer" of codeine; symptoms in the infant included feeding difficulty and lethargy, followed by death. Because exposure to the nursing infant is generally low, the AAP considers codeine to be "usually compatible with breast-feeding." However, caution should be used since most persons are not aware if they have the genotype resulting in "ultra-rapid metabolizer" status. When codeine is used in breast-feeding women, it is recommended to use the lowest dose for the shortest duration of time and observe the infant for increased sleepiness, difficulty in feeding or breathing, or limpness. Medical attention should be sought immediately if the infant develops these symptoms.

Adverse Reactions
Cardiovascular: Palpitations, bradycardia, peripheral vasodilation, hypotension due to vasodilation from histamine release

Central nervous system: CNS depression, intracranial pressure elevated, dizziness, drowsiness, sedation

Dermatologic: Pruritus from histamine release

Endocrine & metabolic: Antidiuretic hormone release

Gastrointestinal: Nausea, vomiting, constipation, biliary tract spasm

Genitourinary: Urinary tract spasm

Hepatic: Transaminases elevated

Ocular: Miosis

Respiratory: Respiratory depression

Miscellaneous: Physical and psychological dependence, histamine release

Drug Interactions
Metabolism/Transport Effects Substrate of CYP2D6 (major), 3A4 (minor); **Inhibits** CYP2D6 (weak)

Avoid Concomitant Use There are no known interactions where it is recommended to avoid concomitant use.

Increased Effect/Toxicity
Codeine may increase the levels/effects of: Alcohol (Ethyl); Alvimopan; CNS Depressants; Desmopressin; Selective Serotonin Reuptake Inhibitors; Thiazide Diuretics

The levels/effects of Codeine may be increased by: Amphetamines; Antipsychotic Agents (Phenothiazines); Somatostatin Analogs; Succinylcholine

Decreased Effect
Codeine may decrease the levels/effects of: Pegvisomant

The levels/effects of Codeine may be decreased by: Ammonium Chloride; CYP2D6 Inhibitors (Moderate); CYP2D6 Inhibitors (Strong); Mixed Agonist / Antagonist Opioids

Stability Store injection between 15°C to 30°C; avoid freezing. Do not use if injection is discolored or contains a precipitate. Protect injection from light.

Mechanism of Action Binds to opiate receptors in the CNS, causing inhibition of ascending pain pathways, altering the perception of and response to pain; causes cough suppression by direct central action in the medulla; produces generalized CNS depression

Pharmacodynamics
Onset of action:
  Oral: 30-60 minutes
  I.M.: 10-30 minutes
Maximum effect:
  Oral: 60-90 minutes
  I.M.: 30-60 minutes
Duration: 4-6 hours

Pharmacokinetics (Adult data unless noted)
Absorption: Oral: Adequate

Distribution: Crosses the placenta; appears in breast milk

Protein binding: 7%

Metabolism: Hepatic to morphine (active); undergoes hydroxylation and O-demethylation via cytochrome P450 isoenzyme CYP2D6 and demethylation via CYP3A3/4

Bioavailability: 60% to 70%

Half-life: 2.5-3.5 hours

Elimination: 3% to 16% in urine as unchanged drug, norcodeine, and free and conjugated morphine

Usual Dosage Doses should be titrated to appropriate analgesic effect; when changing routes of administration, note that oral dose is $2/3$ as effective as parenteral dose

Analgesic: Oral, I.M., SubQ:
  Children: 0.5-1 mg/kg/dose every 4-6 hours as needed; maximum dose: 60 mg/dose
  Adults: Usual: 30 mg/dose; range: 15-60 mg every 4-6 hours as needed

Antitussive: Oral (for nonproductive cough):
Infants and Children <2 years: Not recommended
Children ≥2 years: 1-1.5 mg/kg/day in divided doses every 4-6 hours as needed
Alternatively dose according to age:
2-5 years: 2.5-5 mg every 4-6 hours as needed; maximum dose: 30 mg/day
6-12 years: 5-10 mg every 4-6 hours as needed; maximum dose: 60 mg/day
Children >12 years and Adults: 10-20 mg/dose every 4-6 hours as needed; maximum dose: 120 mg/day
Dosing adjustment in renal impairment:
Cl$_{cr}$ 10-50 mL/minute: Administer 75% of dose
Cl$_{cr}$ <10 mL/minute: Administer 50% of dose
Administration
Oral: Administer with food or water to decrease nausea and GI upset
Parenteral: I.M., SubQ: Not intended for I.V. use due to large histamine release and cardiovascular effects
Monitoring Parameters Respiratory rate, heart rate, blood pressure, pain relief, CNS status
Patient Information Increase fluid and fiber intake to avoid constipation. Avoid alcohol. May cause drowsiness and impair ability to perform activities requiring mental alertness or physical coordination. May be habit-forming; avoid abrupt discontinuation after prolonged use.
Nursing Implications Observe patient for excessive sedation and respiratory depression; implement safety measures; may need to assist with ambulation
Additional Information Not recommended for use for cough control in patients with a productive cough; equianalgesic doses: 120 mg codeine phosphate I.M. approximately equals morphine 10 mg I.M.
Dosage Forms Excipient information presented when available (limited, particularly for generics); consult specific product labeling. [DSC] = Discontinued product; [CAN] = Canadian brand name [not available in U.S.]
Injection, as phosphate: 15 mg/mL (2 mL); 30 mg/mL (2 mL) [contains sodium metabisulfite] [DSC]
Powder, for prescription compounding: USP: 100% (10 g, 25 g)
Tablet, as phosphate: 30 mg, 60 mg
Tablet, as sulfate: 15 mg, 30 mg, 60 mg
Tablet, controlled release: 50 mg, 100 mg, 150 mg, 200 mg
Codeine Contin® [CAN]: 50 mg, 100 mg, 150 mg, 200 mg

References
Khan K and Chang J, "Neonatal Abstinence Syndrome Due to Codeine," *Arch Dis Child Fetal Neonatal Ed*, 1997, 76(1):F59-60.
Koren G, Cairns J, Chitayat D, et al, "Pharmacogenetics of Morphine Poisoning in a Breastfed Neonate of a Codeine-Prescribed Mother," Lancet, 2006, 368(9536):704.
Reynolds EW, Riel-Romero RM, and Bada HS, "Neonatal Abstinence Syndrome and Cerebral Infarction Following Maternal Codeine Use During Pregnancy," *Clin Pediatr (Phila)*, 2007, 46(7):639-45.
Spigset O and Hägg S, "Analgesics and Breast-Feeding: Safety Considerations," *Paediatr Drugs*, 2000, 2(3):223-38.
U.S. Food and Drug Administration Center for Drug Evaluation and Research, "FDA Public Health Advisory: Use of Codeine By Some Breastfeeding Mothers May Lead to Life-Threatening Side Effects in Nursing Babies," available at: http://www.fda.gov/cder/drug/advisory/codeine.htm.

◆ **Codeine and Acetaminophen** *see* Acetaminophen and Codeine *on page 39*
◆ **Codeine and Guaifenesin** *see* Guaifenesin and Codeine *on page 657*
◆ **Codeine and Promethazine** *see* Promethazine and Codeine *on page 1165*
◆ **Codeine Contin® (Can)** *see* Codeine *on page 351*
◆ **Codeine, Phenylephrine, and Promethazine** *see* Promethazine, Phenylephrine, and Codeine *on page 1167*
◆ **Codeine Phosphate** *see* Codeine *on page 351*

◆ **Codeine Sulfate** *see* Codeine *on page 351*
◆ **CO Enalapril (Can)** *see* Enalapril/Enalaprilat *on page 499*
◆ **Coenzyme R** *see* Biotin *on page 194*
◆ **Co-Etidronate (Can)** *see* Etidronate Disodium *on page 549*
◆ **CO Famciclovir (Can)** *see* Famciclovir *on page 560*
◆ **CO Fluconazole (Can)** *see* Fluconazole *on page 584*
◆ **CO Fluoxetine (Can)** *see* FLUoxetine *on page 600*
◆ **CO Gabapentin (Can)** *see* Gabapentin *on page 634*
◆ **Cogentin®** *see* Benztropine *on page 185*
◆ **Co-Gesic® [DSC]** *see* Hydrocodone and Acetaminophen *on page 684*
◆ **Colace® [OTC]** *see* Docusate *on page 468*
◆ **Colace® (Can)** *see* Docusate *on page 468*
◆ **Colace® Adult/Children Suppositories [OTC]** *see* Glycerin *on page 650*
◆ **Colace® Infant/Children Suppositories [OTC]** *see* Glycerin *on page 650*
◆ **Colax-C® (Can)** *see* Docusate *on page 468*
◆ **Colazal®** *see* Balsalazide *on page 172*

Colchicine (KOL chi seen)

Medication Safety Issues
Sound-alike/look-alike issues:
Colchicine may be confused with Cortrosyn®
U.S. Brand Names Colcrys®
Therapeutic Category Anti-inflammatory Agent; Antigout Agent
Generic Available Yes
Use Treatment of familial Mediterranean fever (FMF) (FDA approved in ages ≥4 years and adults); prevention and treatment of acute gout flares (FDA approved in adults); has also been used for prophylaxis of pseudogout, management of Behçet's disease
Medication Guide An FDA-approved patient medication guide, which is available with the product information and at http://www.fda.gov/downloads/Drugs/DrugSafety/UCM176363.pdf, must be dispensed with this medication for each new outpatient prescription and refill.
Pregnancy Risk Factor C
Lactation Enters breast milk/use caution (AAP rates "compatible")
Contraindications Hypersensitivity to colchicine or any component; fatal toxicity has been reported with concomitant use of colchicine with a P-glycoprotein (P-gp) inhibitor (eg, cyclosporine, ranolazine) or strong CYP3A4 inhibitor (eg, atazanavir, clarithromycin, indinavir, itraconazole, ketoconazole, nefazodone, nelfinavir, ritonavir, saquinavir, telithromycin) in presence of renal or hepatic impairment; concurrent use of colchicine and P-gp or strong CYP3A4 inhibitors is contraindicated in renal or hepatic impairment
Warnings Patients who become pregnant while receiving colchicine therapy may be at greater risk of producing trisomic offspring. Myelosuppression (eg, thrombocytopenia, leukopenia, granulocytopenia, pancytopenia) and aplastic anemia have been reported in patients receiving therapeutic doses. Myotoxicity (including rhabdomyolysis) has been reported in patients receiving therapeutic doses. Patients with renal dysfunction and elderly patients are at increased risk. Concomitant use of cyclosporine, diltiazem, verapamil, fibrates, and statins may increase the risk of myopathy.
Precautions Use with caution and consider dose modification if colchicine is given with a P-gp or strong CYP3A4 inhibitor in patients with normal renal and hepatic function.

Adverse Reactions

Central nervous system: Fatigue

Endocrine & metabolic: Hypothyroidism, metabolic acidosis

Gastrointestinal: Abdominal pain, diarrhea, nausea, paralytic ileus, vomiting

Hematologic: (See Warnings): Aplastic anemia, granulocytopenia, leukopenia, pancytopenia, thrombocytopenia

Neuromuscular & skeletal: Muscle weakness, peripheral neuropathy, rhabdomyolysis (see Warnings)

Renal: Hematuria, renal failure

Respiratory: Pharyngolaryngeal pain

<1%, postmarketing, and/or case reports: Abdominal cramping, alopecia, azoospermia, CPK increased, lactose intolerance, liver enzymes increased, maculopapular rash, muscle pain, myalgia, myopathy, myotonia, oligospermia, purpura, rash, sensory motor neuropathy

Drug Interactions

Metabolism/Transport Effects Substrate of CYP3A4 (major), P-glycoprotein; **Induces** CYP2C8 (weak), 2C9 (weak), 2E1 (weak), 3A4 (weak)

Avoid Concomitant Use There are no known interactions where it is recommended to avoid concomitant use.

Increased Effect/Toxicity

Colchicine may increase the levels/effects of: HMG-CoA Reductase Inhibitors

The levels/effects of Colchicine may be increased by: CYP3A4 Inhibitors (Moderate); CYP3A4 Inhibitors (Strong); Dasatinib; Digoxin; Fibric Acid Derivatives; P-Glycoprotein Inhibitors

Decreased Effect

Colchicine may decrease the levels/effects of: Cyanocobalamin; Saxagliptin

The levels/effects of Colchicine may be decreased by: P-Glycoprotein Inducers

Food Interactions May need low purine diet during acute gouty attack. Avoid grapefruit and grapefruit juice; may increase colchicine concentrations

Stability Store at controlled room temperature; protect from light

Mechanism of Action Disrupts cytoskeletal functions by inhibiting β-tubulin polymerization into microtubules, preventing activation, degranulation, and migration of neutrophils associated with mediating some gout symptoms; decreases phagocytosis in joints and lactic acid production, thereby reducing the deposition of urate crystals that perpetuates the inflammatory response; inhibits secretion of serum amyloid A protein. In FMF, may interfere with intracellular assembly of the inflammasome complex present in neutrophils and monocytes that mediate activation of interleukin-1β.

Pharmacodynamics Onset of action: Oral: Relief of pain and inflammation occurs after 18-24 hours

Pharmacokinetics (Adult data unless noted)

Bioavailability: <50%

Distribution: Concentrates in leukocytes, kidney, spleen, and liver; distributes into breast milk; crosses the placenta; does not distribute in heart, skeletal muscle, and brain; V_d: 5-8 L/kg

Protein binding: 39%

Metabolism: Hepatic via CYP3A4; three metabolites (2 primary, 1 minor); partially deacetylated and demethylated

Half-life, elimination: 27-31 hours

Time to peak serum concentration: Oral: 1-2 hours (range: 0.5-3 hours)

Excretion: Urine (40% to 65% as unchanged drug), enterohepatic recirculation and biliary excretion also possible

Dialysis: Not dialyzable (0% to 5%)

Usual Dosage Oral:

Prophylaxis of familial Mediterranean fever (FMF):

Children:

4-6 years: 0.3-1.8 mg/day in 1-2 divided doses

6-12 years: 0.9-1.8 mg/day in 1-2 divided doses

Adolescents >12 years and Adults: 1.2-2.4 mg/day in 1-2 divided doses; titration: Increase or decrease dose in 0.3 mg/day increments based on efficacy or adverse effects; maximum dose: 2.4 mg/day

Gout: Children >16 years and Adults:

Flare treatment: Initial: 1.2 mg at the first sign of flare, followed in 1 hour with a single dose of 0.6 mg (maximum dose: 1.8 mg over 1 hour); **Note:** Current FDA approved dose for gout flare is substantially lower than what has been used historically. Doses larger than the currently recommended dosage for gout flare have not been proven to be more effective. **Note:** Patients receiving prophylaxis treatment may receive treatment dosing; wait 12 hours before resuming prophylactic dose

Prophylaxis: 0.6 mg once or twice daily; maximum dose: 1.2 mg/day

Dosage adjustment for concomitant therapy with CYP3A4 or P-gp inhibitors: Dosage adjustment also required in patients receiving CYP3A4 or P-gp inhibitors up to 14 days prior to initiation of colchicine. **Note:** Treatment of gout flare with colchicine is not recommended in patients receiving prophylactic colchicine and CYP3A4 inhibitors. **Note:** Dosage adjustments may also apply to patients 12-18 years of age with FMF.

Coadministration of **strong** CYP3A4 inhibitor (eg, atazanavir, clarithromycin, indinavir, itraconazole, ketoconazole, nefazodone, nelfinavir, ritonavir, saquinavir, telithromycin):

FMF: Maximum dose: 0.6 mg/day **or** 0.3 mg twice daily

Gout prophylaxis:

If original dose is 0.6 mg twice daily, adjust dose to 0.3 mg once daily

If original dose is 0.6 mg once daily, adjust dose to 0.3 mg every other day

Gout flare treatment: Initial: 0.6 mg, followed in 1 hour by a single dose of 0.3 mg; wait at least 3 days to repeat

Coadministration of **moderate** CYP3A4 inhibitor (eg, amprenavir, aprepitant, diltiazem, erythromycin, fluconazole, fosamprenavir, grapefruit juice, verapamil):

FMF: Maximum dose: 1.2 mg/day **or** 0.6 mg twice daily

Gout prophylaxis:

If original dose is 0.6 mg twice daily, adjust dose to 0.3 mg twice daily **or** 0.6 mg once daily

If original dose is 0.6 mg once daily, adjust dose to 0.3 mg once daily

Gout flare treatment: 1.2 mg as a single dose; wait at least 3 days to repeat days

Coadministration of P-gp inhibitor (eg, cyclosporine, ranolazine):

FMF: Maximum dose: 0.6 mg/day **or** 0.3 mg twice daily

Gout prophylaxis:

If original dose is 0.6 mg twice daily, adjust dose to 0.3 mg once daily

If original dose is 0.6 mg once daily, adjust dose to 0.3 mg every other day

Gout flare treatment: Initial: 0.6 mg as a single dose; wait at least 3 days to repeat

Dosing adjustment in renal impairment: Concurrent use of colchicine and P-gp or strong CYP3A4 inhibitors is **contraindicated** in renal impairment. Treatment of gout flares is not recommended in patients with renal impairment receiving prophylatic colchicine.

Children (see Kallinich, 2007):

Moderate impairment (Cl_{cr} 10-50 mL/minute): Consider dose reduction

Severe impairment (Cl_{cr} <10 mL/minute): Reduce dose by 50% or consider discontinuation of therapy; maximum dose: 1 mg/day

Adults:

FMF:

Cl_{cr} 30-80 mL/minute: Monitor closely for adverse effects; dose adjustment may be necessary

Cl_{cr} <30 mL/minute: Initial dose: 0.3 mg/day; use caution if dose titrated; monitor for adverse effects

Dialysis: Initial dose: 0.3 mg/day; dosing can be increased with close monitoring; monitor for adverse effects. Not removed by dialysis.

Gout prophylaxis:

Cl_{cr} 30-80 mL/minute: Dosage adjustment not required; monitor closely for adverse effects

Cl_{cr} <30 mL/minute: Initial dose: 0.3 mg/day; use caution if dose titrated; monitor for adverse effects

Dialysis: 0.3 mg twice weekly; monitor closely for adverse effects

Gout flare treatment:

Cl_{cr} 30-80 mL/minute: Dosage adjustment not required; monitor closely for adverse effects

Cl_{cr} <30 mL/minute: Dosage adjustment may be considered; treatment course should not be repeated more frequently than every 14 days

Dialysis: 0.6 mg as a single dose; wait at least 14 days to repeat

Administration Oral: Administer without regard to meals and maintain adequate fluid intake

Monitoring Parameters CBC with differential, urinalysis, and renal and hepatic function tests

Test Interactions May cause false-positive results in urine tests for erythrocytes or hemoglobin

Patient Information If taking for acute gouty attacks, discontinue if pain is relieved or if nausea, vomiting, or diarrhea occur; avoid alcohol. Report any signs of muscle pain or weakness or tingling or numbness in fingers or toes. This medication may cause bone marrow depression with agranulocytosis, aplastic anemia, and thrombocytopenia.

Dosage Forms Excipient information presented when available (limited, particularly for generics); consult specific product labeling.

Tablet: 0.6 mg

Colcrys®: 0.6 mg

References

Kallinich T, Haffner D, Niehues T, et al, "Colchicine Use in Children and Adolescents With Familial Mediterranean Fever: Literature Review and Consensus Statement," *Pediatrics*, 2007, 119(2):e474-83.

Levy M, Spino M, and Read SE, "Colchicine: A State-of-the-Art Review," *Pharmacotherapy*, 1991, 11(3):196-211.

Majeed HA, Carroll JE, Khuffash FA, et al, "Long-term Colchicine Prophylaxis in Children With Familial Mediterranean Fever (Recurrent Hereditary Polyserositis)," *J Pediatr*, 1990, 116(6):997-9.

Terkeltaub RA, "Colchicine Update: 2008," *Semin Arthritis Rheum*, 2009, 38(6):411-9.

◆ **Colcrys®** *see* Colchicine *on page 353*

◆ **Cold-Eeze® [OTC** *see* Zinc Supplements *on page 1445*

Colesevelam (koh le SEV a lam)

Related Information

Normal Laboratory Values for Children *on page 1672*

U.S. Brand Names Welchol®

Canadian Brand Names Welchol®

Therapeutic Category Antilipemic Agent, Bile Acid Sequestrant

Generic Available No

Use Management of heterozygous familial hypercholesterolemia in children and adolescent patients [FDA approved in ages 10-17 years (girls ≥1 year postmenarche)] (see Additional Information for recommendations for initiating treatment in children ≥8 years); management of elevated LDL in primary hypercholesterolemia (Fredrickson type IIa) when used alone or in combination with an HMG-CoA reductase inhibitor (FDA approved in adults); improve glycemic control in type 2 diabetes mellitus (noninsulin dependent, NIDDM) in conjunction with diet, exercise, and insulin or oral antidiabetic agents (FDA approved in adults)

Pregnancy Risk Factor B

Pregnancy Considerations There are no adequate and well-controlled studies in pregnant women; use only in pregnancy if clearly needed.

Lactation Excretion in breast milk unknown

Contraindications Hypersensitivity to bile acid sequestering resins or any component; history bowel obstruction; serum triglyceride concentration >500 mg/dL; history of hypertriglyceridemia-induced pancreatitis

Warnings Use in patients with gastroparesis, other severe GI motility disorders, or a history of major GI tract surgery is not recommended due to constipating effects of colesevelam. Patients with dysphagia or swallowing disorders should use the oral suspension form of colesevelam due to large tablet size and risk for esophageal obstruction. Avoid accidental inhalation or esophageal distress with colesevelam granules; always mix with other fluids prior to ingestion. May increase serum triglyceride concentrations (median increase 5% vs placebo in clinical trials); use caution if serum triglyceride levels are >300 mg/dL; discontinue if triglyceride concentrations exceed 500 mg/dL or hypertriglyceridemia-induced pancreatitis occurs. May interfere with fat-soluble vitamins (A, D, E, K). Chronic use may be associated with bleeding problems due to hypoprothrombinemia from vitamin K deficiency.

Precautions Granules for suspension contain phenylalanine which must be avoided in patients with phenylketonuria. May decrease absorption of many orally administered medications (see Drug Interactions); avoid concomitant administration with other orally administered medications; separate administration of drug with known interaction by ≥4 hours. Colesevelam should not be used for glycemic control in type I diabetes mellitus or to treat diabetic ketoacidosis; also not indicated in type 2 diabetes mellitus as monotherapy or in combination with dipeptidyl peptidase 4 inhibitors or thiazolidinediones. Colesevelam has not been studied in Fredrickson Type I, III, IV, or V dyslipidemias or in children <10 years of age.

Adverse Reactions

Cardiovascular: Hypertension

Central nervous system: Fatigue (pediatric patients), headache (pediatric patients)

Endocrine & metabolic: CPK increased (pediatric patients), hypertriglyceridemia (see Warnings), hypoglycemia

Gastrointestinal: Abdominal pain, constipation, dyspepsia, nausea, pancreatitis (see Warnings), vomiting

Neuromuscular & skeletal: Myalgia, weakness

Respiratory: Nasopharyngitis, pharyngitis, rhinitis, upper respiratory tract infection

Miscellaneous: Accidental injury, flu syndrome, influenza

<2%, postmarketing, and/or case reports: Abdominal distention, bowel obstruction, dysphagia, esophageal obstruction, fecal impaction, hemorrhoid exacerbation, hypersensitivity reaction, INR decreased, oral blisters, rash, seizure activity increased, transaminases increased, TSH increased

Drug Interactions

Avoid Concomitant Use There are no known interactions where it is recommended to avoid concomitant use.

◀ **Increased Effect/Toxicity** Refer to Decreased Effect.

Decreased Effect Sustained-release verapamil AUC and C_{max} were reduced. Clinical significance unknown.

Digoxin, lovastatin, metoprolol, quinidine, valproic acid, or warfarin absorption was not significantly affected with concurrent administration.

Clinical effects of atorvastatin, lovastatin, and simvastatin were not changed by concurrent administration.

Stability Store at 25°C (77°F); excursions permitted to 15°C to 30°C (59°F to 86°F). Protect from moisture.

Mechanism of Action Cholesterol is the major precursor of bile acid. Colesevelam binds with bile acids in the intestine to form an insoluble complex that is eliminated in feces. This increased excretion of bile acids results in an increased oxidation of cholesterol to bile acid and a lowering of the serum cholesterol. Serum triglyceride levels may increase or remain unchanged with colesevelam treatment. Colesevelam is an exchange resin and may have a higher affinity for anions other than bile acids (see Drug Interactions).

Pharmacodynamics

Onset of action:

Lipid-lowering: Within 2 weeks (maximum effect)

Reduction HgA1C (Type II diabetes): 4-6 weeks initial onset, 12-18 weeks maximal effect

Pharmacokinetics (Adult data unless noted)

Absorption: Insignificant

Elimination: Urine (0.05%) after 1 month of chronic dosing

Usual Dosage Oral: Children and Adolescents 10-17 years and Adults:

Once-daily dosing: 3.75 g (6 x 625 mg tablets or 1 packet)

Twice-daily dosing: 1.875 g (3 x 625 mg tablets)

Note: Due to large tablet size, oral suspension is recommended in pediatric patients. Do not administer granules in the dry form (to avoid GI distress).

Administration

Granules for oral suspension: Empty granules into glass, add ½-1 cup (4-8 ounces) of water; mix well. Administer with meals. Do not take in dry form (to avoid GI distress).

Tablets: Due to tablet size, it is recommended that any patient who has trouble swallowing tablets should use the oral suspension form. Administer with meal(s) and a liquid.

Monitoring Parameters Serum cholesterol, LDL, and triglyceride levels should be obtained before initiating treatment and periodically thereafter (in accordance with NCEP guidelines)

Reference Range See Related Information for age- and gender-specific serum cholesterol, LDL-C, TG, and HDL concentrations.

Patient Information Take medication exactly as directed; do not alter dosage without consulting prescriber. Other medications should be taken 1 hour before or 4 hours after colesevelam. You may experience constipation (increased exercise, fluids, fruit, fiber, or stool softener may help). Report persistent GI upset, severe abdominal pain, skeletal or muscle pain or weakness, or respiratory difficulties.

Additional Information The current recommendation for pharmacologic treatment of hypercholesterolemia in children is limited to children ≥8 years of age and is based on LDL-C concentrations and the presence of coronary vascular disease (CVD) risk factors (see table and Daniels, 2008). In adults, for each 1% lowering in LDL-C, the relative risk for major cardiovascular events is reduced by ~1%. For more specific risk assessment and treatment recommendations for adults, see NCEP ATPIII, 2001

Recommendations for Initiating Pharmacologic Treatment in Children ≥8 Years[1]

No risk factors for CVD	LDL ≥190 mg/dL despite 6-month to 1-year diet therapy
Family history of premature CVD or equal to CVD risk factors present, including obesity, hypertension, or cigarette smoking	LDL ≥160 mg/dL despite 6-month to 1-year diet therapy
Diabetes mellitus present	LDL ≥130 mg/dL

[1]Adapted from Daniels SR, Greer FR, and Committee on Nutrition, "Lipid Screening and Cardiovascular Health in Childhood," *Pediatrics*, 2008, 122(1):198-208.

Dosage Forms Excipient information presented when available (limited, particularly for generics); consult specific product labeling.

Granules for suspension, oral, as hydrochloride:
Welchol®: 3.75 g/packet (30s) [contains phenylalanine 48 mg/packet; citrus flavored]

Tablet, oral, as hydrochloride:
Welchol®: 625 mg

References
Daniels SR, Greer FR, and Committee on Nutrition, "Lipid Screening and Cardiovascular Health in Childhood," *Pediatrics*, 2008, 122 (1):198-208.

"Executive Summary of The Third Report of The National Cholesterol Education Program (NCEP) Expert Panel on Detection, Evaluation, And Treatment of High Blood Cholesterol In Adults (Adult Treatment Panel III)," *JAMA*, 2001, 285(19):2486-97.

Stein EA, Marais AD, Szamosi T, et al, "Colesevelam Hydrochloride: Efficacy and Safety in Pediatric Subjects With Heterozygous Familial Hypercholesterolemia," *J Pediatr*, 2010, 156(2):231-6.e1-3.

◆ **Colestid®** see Colestipol *on page 356*

Colestipol (koe LES ti pole)

Medication Safety Issues
Sound-alike/look-alike issues:
Colestipol may be confused with calcitriol

Related Information
Normal Laboratory Values for Children *on page 1672*

U.S. Brand Names Colestid®

Canadian Brand Names Colestid®

Therapeutic Category Antilipemic Agent, Bile Acid Sequestrant

Generic Available Yes

Use Adjunct to dietary therapy to decrease elevated serum total and low density lipoprotein cholesterol (LDL-C) in patients with primary hypercholesterolemia; primary prevention of cardiovascular disease in high risk patients; risk factors include: Age ≥55 years, smoking, hypertension, low HDL-C, or family history of early coronary heart disease; relief of pruritus associated with elevated levels of bile acids

Pregnancy Risk Factor C

Lactation Not recommended

Contraindications Hypersensitivity to bile acid sequestering resins or any component; bowel obstruction

Warnings May interfere with fat-soluble vitamins (A, D, E, K) and folate absorption. Chronic use may be associated with bleeding problems due to hypoprothrombinemia from vitamin K deficiency. May produce or severely exacerbate constipation and fecal impaction may occur. This may be lessened by a gradual increase in dosage, an increased intake of fluids and fiber, or addition of a stool softener. Avoid accidental inhalation or esophageal distress with colestipol powder and granules; always mix with other fluids prior to ingestion.

Precautions Some formulations contain phenylalanine; use with caution in patients with phenylketonuria; may decrease absorption of many orally administered medications (see Drug Interactions); avoid concomitant administration with other orally administered medications

Adverse Reactions

Cardiovascular: Chest pain, angina, tachycardia (very infrequent)

Central nervous system: Headache, dizziness, anxiety, vertigo, drowsiness, fatigue

Dermatologic: Rash, urticaria, dermatitis (rare)

Endocrine & metabolic: Hyperchloremic acidosis

Gastrointestinal: Constipation (>10%), abdominal pain and distention, belching, flatulence, nausea, vomiting, diarrhea, peptic ulceration, gallstones, GI irritation, anorexia, steatorrhea or malabsorption syndrome, cholelithiasis, cholecystitis, GI bleeding, bleeding hemorrhoids, difficulty swallowing, transient esophageal obstruction (rare)

Hepatic: Transient elevations of hepatic enzymes

Neuromuscular & skeletal: Joint pain, arthritis, back pain

Respiratory: Dyspnea

Miscellaneous: Swelling of hands and feet

Drug Interactions

Avoid Concomitant Use There are no known interactions where it is recommended to avoid concomitant use.

Increased Effect/Toxicity There are no known significant interactions involving an increase in effect.

Decreased Effect

Colestipol may decrease the levels/effects of: Amiodarone; Antidiabetic Agents (Thiazolidinedione); Calcitriol; Cardiac Glycosides; Contraceptives (Estrogens); Contraceptives (Progestins); Corticosteroids (Oral); Diltiazem; Ezetimibe; Fibric Acid Derivatives; Leflunomide; Loop Diuretics; Methotrexate; Methylfolate; Niacin; Nonsteroidal Anti-Inflammatory Agents; Pravastatin; Propranolol; Raloxifene; Tetracycline Derivatives; Thiazide Diuretics; Thyroid Products; Ursodiol; Vitamin K Antagonists

Stability Store at room temperature.

Mechanism of Action Cholesterol is the major precursor of bile acid. Colestipol binds with bile acids in the intestine to form an insoluble complex that is eliminated in feces. This increased excretion of bile acids results in an increased oxidation of cholesterol to bile acid and a lowering of the serum cholesterol. Serum triglyceride levels may increase or remain unchanged with colestipol treatment. Colestipol is an anion exchange resin and may have a higher affinity for anions other than bile acids (see Drug Interactions).

Pharmacodynamics

Lowering of serum cholesterol: ~1 month

LDL-C reduction: ~19%

Pharmacokinetics (Adult data unless noted)

Absorption: None

Elimination: Feces

Usual Dosage Oral:

Children >10 years: Limited studies with doses ranging between 2-12 g/day; the most recent study produced significant lowering of serum cholesterol utilizing either 10 g once daily or 5 g twice daily (Tonstad, 1996)

Adults:

Granules: 5-30 g/day given once or in divided doses 2-4 times/day; initial dose: 5 g 1-2 times/day; increase by 5 g at 1- to 2-month intervals

Tablets: 2-16 g/day; initial dose: 2 g 1-2 times/day; increase by 2 g at 1- to 2-month intervals

Administration Tablets should be administered one at a time, swallowed whole, with plenty of liquid. Do not cut, crush, or chew tablets. Dry powder or granules should be added to at least 3 ounces (90 mL) of liquid and stirred until completely mixed. Other drugs should be administered at least 1 hour before or 4 hours after colestipol.

Monitoring Parameters Serum cholesterol (total and fractionated), annual serum levels of fat-soluble vitamins A, D, E, K, and folic acid

Reference Range Hypercholesterolemia as defined by serum cholesterol, LDL-C, TG, and HDL concentration

Patient Information Take granules with 3-4 oz of water or fruit juice. Rinse glass with small amount of water to ensure full dose is taken. Take tablets one at a time. Other medications should be taken 1 hour before or 4 hours after colestipol. You may experience constipation (increased exercise, fluids, fruit, fiber, or stool softener may help). Report acute gastric pain, tarry stools, or respiratory difficulty.

Dosage Forms Excipient information presented when available (limited, particularly for generics); consult specific product labeling.

Granules for suspension, as hydrochloride, oral: 5 g/packet (30s, 90s); 5 g/scoopful (500 g)

Colestid®: 5 g/packet (30s, 90s); 5 g/teaspoon (300 g, 500 g) [unflavored]

Colestid®, flavored: 5 g/packet (60s) [contains phenylalanine (18.2 mg/packet); orange flavor]

Colestid®, flavored: 5 g/scoopful (450 g) [contains phenylalanine (18.2 mg/scoopful); orange flavor]

Tablet, as hydrochloride: 1 g

Tablet, as hydrochloride, oral [micronized]:

Colestid®: 1 g

References
American Academy of Pediatrics Committee on Nutrition, "Cholesterol in Childhood," *Pediatrics*, 1998, 101(1 Pt 1):141-7.

American Academy of Pediatrics, "National Cholesterol Education Program: Report of the Expert Panel on Blood Cholesterol Levels in Children and Adolescents," *Pediatrics*, 1992, 89(3 Pt 2):525-84.

"Executive Summary of The Third Report of The National Cholesterol Education Program (NCEP) Expert Panel on Detection, Evaluation, And Treatment of High Blood Cholesterol In Adults (Adult Treatment Panel III)," *JAMA*, 2001, 285(19):2486-97.

Groot PH, Dijkhuis-Stoffelsma R, Grose WF, et al, "The Effects of Colestipol Hydrochloride on Serum Lipoprotein Lipid and Apolipoprotein B and A-I Concentrations in Children Heterozygous for Familial Hypercholesterolemia," *Acta Paediatr Scand*, 1983, 72(1):81-5.

Grundy SM, Cleeman JI, Merz CN, et al, "Implications of Recent Clinical Trials for the National Cholesterol Education Program Adult Treatment Panel III Guidelines," *J Am Coll Cardiol*, 2004, 44(3):720-32.

Schwarz KB, Goldstein PD, Witztum JL, et al, "Fat-Soluble Vitamin Concentrations in Hypercholesterolemic Children Treated With Colestipol," *Pediatrics*, 1980, 65(2):243-50.

Tonstad S, Sivertsen M, Aksnes L, et al, "Low Dose Colestipol in Adolescents With Familial Hypercholesterolaemia," *Arch Dis Child*, 1996, 74(2):157-60.

Tonstad S and Ose L, "Colestipol Tablets in Adolescents With Familial Hypercholesterolaemia," *Acta Paediatr*, 1996, 85(9):1080-2.

◆ **Colestipol Hydrochloride** *see* Colestipol *on page 356*

◆ **CO Levetiracetam (Can)** *see* Levetiracetam *on page 808*

◆ **CO Levofloxacin (Can)** *see* Levofloxacin *on page 813*

◆ **CO Lisinopril (Can)** *see* Lisinopril *on page 832*

Colistimethate (koe lis ti METH ate)

U.S. Brand Names Coly-Mycin® M

Canadian Brand Names Coly-Mycin® M

Therapeutic Category Antibiotic, Miscellaneous

Generic Available Yes

Use Treatment of gram-negative infections due to susceptible *Pseudomonas aeruginosa, Enterobacter aerogenes, Escherichia coli,* and *Klebsiella pneumoniae*; not indicated for infections due to *Proteus* or *Neisseria* species. Parenteral use of colistimethate has mainly been replaced by less toxic antibiotics. Reserved for life-threatening infections caused by organisms resistant to the preferred drugs. Used as inhalation therapy in cystic fibrosis patients for treatment of initial colonization and management of chronic colonization with *P. aeruginosa*

Pregnancy Risk Factor C

Pregnancy Considerations Adverse events have been observed in animal reproduction studies; therefore, the manufacturer classifies colistimethate as pregnancy category C. Colistimethate crosses the placenta in humans. There are no adequate and well-controlled studies in pregnant women.

Lactation Excretion in breast milk unknown/use caution

Breast-Feeding Considerations It is not known if colistimethate sodium is excreted in human milk, but colistin sulphate (another form of colistin) is excreted in human milk. The manufacturer recommends caution if giving colistimethate sodium to a breast-feeding woman. If colistimethate sodium reaches the breast milk, nondose-related effects could include modification of bowel flora.

Contraindications Hypersensitivity to colistimethate or any component

Warnings Colistimethate can cause serious nephrotoxicity and or neurotoxicity; neurotoxic reactions may be manifested by circumoral paresthesia, numbness, tingling of the extremities, pruritus, vertigo, dizziness, and slurring of speech. Dosage reduction may alleviate symptoms. Nephrotoxicity is dose-dependent and reversible if the antibiotic is discontinued. Avoid concurrent or sequential use of other nephrotoxic and neurotoxic drugs, particularly bacitracin, kanamycin, streptomycin, paromomycin, polymyxin B, tobramycin, neomycin, gentamicin, and amikacin. Neuromuscular blockade resulting in respiratory arrest has been reported in patients with neuromuscular disease (ie, myasthenia gravis) and patients receiving neuromuscular blocking agents [see Drug Interactions]; impaired renal function increases the possibility of apnea and neuromuscular blockade. Pseudomembranous colitis has been reported with colistimethate.

Precautions Use with caution and modify dosage in patients with impaired renal function

Adverse Reactions

Central nervous system: Slurred speech, dizziness, vertigo, fever, ataxia, mental confusion, seizures

Dermatologic: Pruritus, urticaria, rash

Gastrointestinal: GI upset

Local: Pain at injection site

Neuromuscular & skeletal: Paresthesia, muscle weakness, peripheral neuropathy

Renal: BUN, creatinine elevated; urine output decreased; hematuria; albuminuria; nephrotoxicity

Respiratory: Apnea; respiratory distress; bronchospasm, cough (with inhaled colistimethate)

Drug Interactions

Avoid Concomitant Use

Avoid concomitant use of Colistimethate with any of the following: BCG

Increased Effect/Toxicity

Colistimethate may increase the levels/effects of: Neuromuscular-Blocking Agents

The levels/effects of Colistimethate may be increased by: Aminoglycosides; Amphotericin B; Capreomycin; Polymyxin B; Vancomycin

Decreased Effect

Colistimethate may decrease the levels/effects of: BCG; Typhoid Vaccine

Stability Store vial at room temperature; reconstituted solution for injection is stable for 7 days when stored in the refrigerator or at room temperature. For inhalation, use reconstituted solution immediately after preparation.

Mechanism of Action Hydrolyzed to colistin which acts as a cationic detergent damaging the bacterial cytoplasmic membrane of gram-negative organisms causing leakage of intracellular substances and cell death

Pharmacokinetics (Adult data unless noted)

Absorption: Not absorbed from the GI tract, mucous membranes, or intact skin

Distribution: Widely distributed to body tissues; does not penetrate into CSF, synovial, pleural, or pericardial fluids; crosses the placenta

V_d: Adults: 0.09 ± 0.03 L/kg

Protein binding: 50%

Half-life:

Children: 2-3 hours

Adolescents and adults with cystic fibrosis: 3.5 ± 1 hour

Time to peak serum concentration: I.M.: ~2 hours

Elimination: Primarily in urine as unchanged drug

Usual Dosage Children, Adolescents, and Adults: Dosage should be based on an estimate of ideal body weight: dosage expressed in terms of colistin:

I.M., I.V.: 2.5-5 mg/kg/day divided every 6-12 hours

I.V.: Cystic fibrosis: 5-8 mg/kg/day divided every 8 hours; maximum dose: 160 mg/dose

Inhalation: 75 mg in NS (4 mL total volume) via nebulizer twice daily

Dosing adjustment in renal impairment: Parenteral: Adults:

S_{cr} 1.3-1.5 mg/dL: 2.5-3.8 mg/kg/day divided every 12 hours

S_{cr} 1.6-2.5 mg/dL: 2.5 mg/kg/day divided every 12-24 hours

S_{cr} 2.6-4 mg/dL: 1.5 mg/kg/dose every 36 hours

Administration

Parenteral: Reconstitute vial with 2 mL SWI resulting in a concentration of 75 mg colistin/mL; swirl gently to avoid frothing. Administer by I.M., direct I.V. injection over 3-10 minutes, intermittent infusion over 30 minutes, or by continuous I.V. infusion. For continuous I.V. infusion, one-half of the total daily dose is administered by direct I.V. injection over 3-10 minutes followed 1-2 hours later by the remaining one-half of the total daily dose diluted in a compatible I.V. solution infused over 22-23 hours. The final concentration for administration should be based on the patient's fluid needs.

Inhalation: Reconstitute vial with 2 mL SWI resulting in a concentration of 75 mg colistin/mL. Further dilute dose to a total volume of 4 mL in NS and administer solution via nebulizer promptly following preparation of solution.

Monitoring Parameters Renal function tests, urine output; for inhalation therapy: Pre- and post-treatment spirometry

Patient Information May impair ability to perform activities requiring mental alertness or physical coordination

Nursing Implications May premedicate with a bronchodilator to reduce the potential of bronchospasm when administering inhaled colistimethate

Dosage Forms Excipient information presented when available (limited, particularly for generics); consult specific product labeling.

Injection, powder for reconstitution, as colistin base: 150 mg

Coly-Mycin® M: 150 mg

References

Beringer P, "The Clinical Use of Colistin in Patients With Cystic Fibrosis," *Curr Opin Pulm Med*, 2001, 7(6):434-40.

Cunningham S, Prasad A, Collyer L, et al, "Bronchoconstriction Following Nebulised Colistin in Cystic Fibrosis," *Arch Dis Child*, 2001, 84(5):432-3.

Reed MD, Stern RC, O'Riordan MA, et al, "The Pharmacokinetics of Colistin in Patients With Cystic Fibrosis," *J Clin Pharmacol*, 2001, 41 (6):645-54.

◆ **Colistimethate Sodium** *see* Colistimethate *on page 357*

◆ **Colistin Methanesulfonate** *see* Colistimethate *on page 357*

◆ **Colistin Sulfomethate** *see* Colistimethate *on page 357*

◆ **Colocort®** *see* Hydrocortisone *on page 685*

◆ **CO Lovastatin (Can)** *see* Lovastatin *on page 850*

◆ **Coly-Mycin® M** *see* Colistimethate *on page 357*

◆ **Colyte®** *see* Polyethylene Glycol-Electrolyte Solution *on page 1129*

◆ **Colyte™ (Can)** *see* Polyethylene Glycol-Electrolyte Solution *on page 1129*

◆ **Combantrin™ (Can)** *see* Pyrantel Pamoate *on page 1187*

◆ **Combivir®** *see* Lamivudine and Zidovudine *on page 794*

◆ **CO Metformin (Can)** *see* MetFORMIN *on page 891*

◆ **Compazine** *see* Prochlorperazine *on page 1161*

◆ **Compound E** *see* Cortisone *on page 360*

◆ **Compound F** *see* Hydrocortisone *on page 685*

◆ **Compound S** *see* Zidovudine *on page 1442*

◆ **Compound S, Abacavir, and Lamivudine** *see* Abacavir, Lamivudine, and Zidovudine *on page 31*

◆ **Compound W® [OTC]** *see* Salicylic Acid *on page 1241*

◆ **Compound W® One-Step Wart Remover [OTC]** *see* Salicylic Acid *on page 1241*

◆ **Compound W® One-Step Wart Remover for Feet [OTC]** *see* Salicylic Acid *on page 1241*

◆ **Compound W® One-Step Wart Remover for Kids [OTC]** *see* Salicylic Acid *on page 1241*

◆ **Compoz® Nighttime Sleep Aid [OTC]** *see* DiphenhydrAMINE *on page 448*

◆ **Compro™** *see* Prochlorperazine *on page 1161*

◆ **Comvax®** *see Haemophilus* b Conjugate and Hepatitis B Vaccine *on page 663*

◆ **Concerta®** *see* Methylphenidate *on page 908*

◆ **Conjugated Estrogen** *see* Estrogens (Conjugated/Equine) *on page 539*

◆ **Constulose** *see* Lactulose *on page 791*

◆ **Contac® Cold 12 Hour Relief Non Drowsy (Can)** *see* Pseudoephedrine *on page 1183*

◆ **ControlRx®** *see* Fluoride *on page 595*

◆ **CO Ondansetron (Can)** *see* Ondansetron *on page 1022*

◆ **CO Pantoprazole (Can)** *see* Pantoprazole *on page 1054*

◆ **CO Paroxetine (Can)** *see* PARoxetine *on page 1064*

◆ **Copegus®** *see* Ribavirin *on page 1210*

◆ **Copper Sulfate** *see* Trace Metals *on page 1366*

◆ **CO Pravastatin (Can)** *see* Pravastatin *on page 1145*

◆ **CO Ranitidine (Can)** *see* Ranitidine *on page 1200*

◆ **Cordarone®** *see* Amiodarone *on page 84*

◆ **Cordron-D NR [DSC]** *see* Carbinoxamine and Pseudoephedrine *on page 249*

◆ **Coreg®** *see* Carvedilol *on page 254*

◆ **Coreg CR®** *see* Carvedilol *on page 254*

◆ **Corgard®** *see* Nadolol *on page 961*

◆ **Coricidin HBP® Chest Congestion and Cough [OTC]** *see* Guaifenesin and Dextromethorphan *on page 658*

◆ **CO Risperidone (Can)** *see* Risperidone *on page 1218*

◆ **Cormax®** *see* Clobetasol *on page 331*

◆ **Correctol® [OTC]** *see* Docusate *on page 468*

◆ **Correctol® Tablets [OTC]** *see* Bisacodyl *on page 194*

◆ **Cortaid® Intensive Therapy [OTC]** *see* Hydrocortisone *on page 685*

◆ **Cortaid® Maximum Strength [OTC]** *see* Hydrocortisone *on page 685*

◆ **Cortaid® Sensitive Skin [OTC]** *see* Hydrocortisone *on page 685*

◆ **Cortamed® (Can)** *see* Hydrocortisone *on page 685*

◆ **Cortef®** *see* Hydrocortisone *on page 685*

◆ **Cortenema®** *see* Hydrocortisone *on page 685*

◆ **Corticool® [OTC]** *see* Hydrocortisone *on page 685*

Corticotropin (kor ti koe TROE pin)

Medication Safety Issues
Sound-alike/look-alike issues:
Corticotropin may be confused with corticorelin

U.S. Brand Names H.P. Acthar® Gel

Therapeutic Category Adrenal Corticosteroid; Diagnostic Agent, Adrenocortical Insufficiency; Infantile Spasms, Treatment

Generic Available No

Use Infantile spasms; diagnostic aid in adrenocortical insufficiency; acute exacerbations of multiple sclerosis; severe muscle weakness in myasthenia gravis

Pregnancy Risk Factor C

Pregnancy Considerations Embryocidal effects may be observed following corticotropin use during pregnancy. Endogenous ACTH levels are increased during pregnancy. Some studies have shown an association between first trimester systemic corticosteroid use and oral clefts; adverse events in the fetus/neonate have been noted in case reports following large doses of systemic corticosteroids during pregnancy.

Lactation Excretion in breast milk unknown/use caution

Breast-Feeding Considerations Corticosteroids are excreted in human milk; information specific to corticotropin has not been located.

Contraindications Hypersensitivity to corticotropin, porcine proteins, or any component; scleroderma, osteoporosis, systemic fungal infections, ocular herpes simplex, peptic ulcer, hypertension, CHF; I.V. route of administration

Warnings May mask signs of infection; do not administer live vaccines; long-term therapy in children may retard bone growth; acute adrenal insufficiency may occur with abrupt withdrawal after chronic use or with stress

Precautions Use with caution in patients with hypothyroidism, cirrhosis, thromboembolic disorders, seizure disorders or renal insufficiency

Adverse Reactions
Cardiovascular: Hypertension

Central nervous system: Seizures, mood swings, headache, pseudotumor cerebri

Dermatologic: Skin atrophy, bruising, hyperpigmentation, acne, hirsutism

Endocrine & metabolic: Amenorrhea, sodium and water retention, Cushing's syndrome, hyperglycemia, bone growth suppression, hypokalemia

Gastrointestinal: Abdominal distention, ulcerative esophagitis, pancreatitis

Neuromuscular & skeletal: Muscle wasting

Miscellaneous: Hypersensitivity reactions, including anaphylaxis

Drug Interactions
Avoid Concomitant Use
Avoid concomitant use of Corticotropin with any of the following: Aldesleukin; BCG; Natalizumab; Pimecrolimus; Tacrolimus (Topical); Vaccines (Live)

Increased Effect/Toxicity

Corticotropin may increase the levels/effects of: Acetylcholinesterase Inhibitors; Amphotericin B; Leflunomide; Loop Diuretics; Natalizumab; NSAID (COX-2 Inhibitor); NSAID (Nonselective); Thiazide Diuretics; Vaccines (Live); Warfarin

The levels/effects of Corticotropin may be increased by: Antifungal Agents (Azole Derivatives, Systemic); Aprepitant; Calcium Channel Blockers (Nondihydropyridine); Denosumab; Estrogen Derivatives; Fluconazole; Fosaprepitant; Macrolide Antibiotics; Neuromuscular-Blocking Agents (Nondepolarizing); Pimecrolimus; Quinolone Antibiotics; Salicylates; Tacrolimus (Topical); Trastuzumab

Decreased Effect

Corticotropin may decrease the levels/effects of: Aldesleukin; Antidiabetic Agents; BCG; Calcitriol; Corticorelin; Isoniazid; Salicylates; Sipuleucel-T; Vaccines (Inactivated); Vaccines (Live)

The levels/effects of Corticotropin may be decreased by: Aminoglutethimide; Barbiturates; Echinacea; Mitotane; Primidone; Rifamycin Derivatives

Food Interactions May increase renal loss of potassium, calcium, zinc, and vitamin C; may need to increase dietary intake or give supplements

Stability Store repository injection (gel) in the refrigerator; warm gel before administration

Mechanism of Action Stimulates the adrenal cortex to secrete adrenal steroids (including hydrocortisone, cortisone), androgenic substances, and a small amount of aldosterone. Exact mechanism of action for treatment of infantile spasms is unknown, but may be an independent antiepileptic effect (unrelated to stimulation of release of adrenocorticosteroids). One theory is that ACTH suppresses corticotropin-releasing hormone (CRH). CRH is an excitatory neuropeptide that has a greater potency in infants. Infants with infantile spasms may have increased CRH activity. ACTH may decrease CRH release and, therefore, decrease infantile spasms.

Pharmacodynamics

Maximum effect on cortisol levels: I.M., SubQ (gel): 3-12 hours

Duration: Repository (gel): 10-25 hours, up to 3 days

Pharmacokinetics (Adult data unless noted)

Absorption: I.M. (repository): Over 8-16 hours

Half-life: 15 minutes

Elimination: In urine

Usual Dosage

Children: I.M.: Gel (repository) formulation:

Anti-inflammatory/immunosuppressant: 0.8 units/kg/day or 25 units/m^2/day divided every 12-24 hours

Infantile spasms: Various regimens have been used. Some neurologists recommend low-dose ACTH (5-40 units/day) for short periods (1-6 weeks), while others recommend larger doses of ACTH (40-160 units/day) for long periods of treatment (3-12 months)

A prospective, single-blind study (Hrachovy, 1994) found no major difference in effectiveness between high-dose long-duration versus low-dose short-duration ACTH therapy. Hypertension, however, occurred more frequently in the high-dose group. Further studies comparing long-term outcomes are needed. Low-dose regimen used in this study:

Initial: 20 units/day for 2 weeks, if patient responds, taper and discontinue over a 1-week period; if patient does not respond, increase dose to 30 units/day for 4 weeks then taper and discontinue over a 1-week period

Usual dose: 20-40 units/day or 5-8 units/kg/day in 1-2 divided doses; range: 5-160 units/day

Adults: I.M.: Gel (repository) formulation:

Acute exacerbation of multiple sclerosis: 80-120 units/day in divided doses for 2-3 weeks

Diagnostic purposes: 25 units

Anti-inflammatory/immunosuppressant: 40-80 units every 24-72 hours

Administration Parenteral: Do **not** administer I.V.; may be administered I.M. or SubQ; I.M. route is recommended for the treatment of infantile spasms and multiple sclerosis; **Note:** Studies assessing use for infantile spasms used the I.M. route of administration

Monitoring Parameters Electrolytes, glucose, blood pressure, height, and weight; for infantile spasms, monitor seizure frequency, type, and duration

Test Interactions Skin tests

Patient Information Do not abruptly discontinue the medication; tell your physician you are using this drug if you are going to have skin tests, immunizations, surgery, emergency treatment, or if you have a serious infection or injury

Additional Information Cosyntropin is preferred over corticotropin for diagnostic test of adrenocortical insufficiency (cosyntropin is less allergenic and test is shorter in duration); oral prednisone (2 mg/kg/day) was as effective as I.M. ACTH gel (20 units/day) in controlling infantile spasms; corticotropin zinc hydroxide (Cortrophin® Zinc) and corticotropin aqueous (Acthar®) have been discontinued by the manufacturer

Dosage Forms Excipient information presented when available (limited, particularly for generics); consult specific product labeling.

Injection, gelatin: 80 units/mL (5 mL)

References

Haines ST and Casto DT, "Treatment of Infantile Spasms," *Ann Pharmacother*, 1994, 28(6):779-91.

Hrachovy RA and Frost JD Jr, "Infantile Spasms," *Pediatr Clin North Am*, 1989, 36(2):311-29.

Hrachovy RA, Frost JD Jr, and Glaze DG, "High-Dose, Long-Duration Versus Low-Dose, Short-Duration Corticotropin Therapy for Infantile Spasms," *J Pediatr*, 1994, 124(5 Pt 1):803-6.

Hrachovy RA, Frost JD Jr, Kellaway P, et al, "Double-Blind Study of ACTH vs Prednisone Therapy in Infantile Spasms," *J Pediatr*, 1983, 103(5):641-5.

♦ **Corticotropin, Repository** *see* Corticotropin *on page 359*

♦ **Cortifoam®** *see* Hydrocortisone *on page 685*

♦ **Cortifoam™ (Can)** *see* Hydrocortisone *on page 685*

♦ **Cortimyxin® (Can)** *see* Neomycin, (Bacitracin) Polymyxin B, and Hydrocortisone *on page 980*

♦ **Cortisol** *see* Hydrocortisone *on page 685*

Cortisone (KOR ti sone)

Medication Safety Issues

Sound-alike/look-alike issues:

Cortisone may be confused with Cardizem®, Cortizone®

Related Information

Corticosteroids *on page 1487*

Therapeutic Category Adrenal Corticosteroid; Anti-inflammatory Agent; Corticosteroid, Systemic; Glucocorticoid

Generic Available Yes

Use Management of adrenocortical insufficiency

Pregnancy Considerations Adverse events have been observed with corticosteroids in animal reproduction studies. Cortisone is found in cord blood; endogenous maternal cortisol (active) is metabolized by placental enzymes to cortisone (inactive), regulating the amount of maternal glucocorticoids reaching the fetus. Some studies have shown an association between first trimester systemic corticosteroid use and oral clefts; adverse events in the fetus/neonate have been noted in case reports following large doses of systemic corticosteroids during pregnancy. Women exposed to cortisone during pregnancy for the treatment of an autoimmune disease may contact the OTIS Autoimmune Diseases Study at 877-311-8972.

Lactation Excretion in breast milk unknown/use caution

Contraindications Hypersensitivity to cortisone, any component, or corticosteroids; serious infections, except septic shock or tuberculous meningitis; systemic fungal or viral infections

Warnings Hypothalamic-pituitary-adrenal (HPA) suppression may occur; acute adrenal insufficiency (adrenal crisis) may occur with abrupt withdrawal after long term therapy or with stress; withdrawal or discontinuation of corticosteroids should be done carefully; patients with HPA axis suppression may require increased doses of systemic glucocorticosteroids prior to, during, and after unusual stress (eg, surgery). Immunosuppression may occur; patients may be more susceptible to infections; avoid exposure to chickenpox and measles. Corticosteroids may mask signs of infection. Corticosteroids may activate latent opportunistic infections or exacerbate systemic fungal infections. May cause osteoporosis (at any age) or inhibition of bone growth in pediatric patients. Acute myopathy may occur with high doses, elevated IOP may occur (especially with prolonged use), CNS effects (ranging from euphoria to psychosis) may occur. Rare cases of anaphylactoid reactions have been reported with corticosteroids.

Precautions Avoid using higher than recommended doses; suppression of HPA axis, suppression of linear growth (ie, reduction of growth velocity), reduced bone mineral density, hypercorticism (Cushing's syndrome), hyperglycemia, or glucosuria may occur; titrate to lowest effective dose. Reduction in growth velocity may occur when corticosteroids are administered to pediatric patients by any route (monitor growth). Use with extreme caution in patients with respiratory tuberculosis, untreated systemic infections, or ocular herpes simplex; use with caution in patients with thyroid dysfunction, cirrhosis, nonspecific ulcerative colitis, hypertension, renal impairment, osteoporosis, thromboembolic tendencies, CHF, recent MI, convulsive disorders, myasthenia gravis, thrombophlebitis, peptic ulcer, diabetes, glaucoma, cataracts, or hepatic impairment. Prolonged use may result in cataracts or glaucoma.

Adverse Reactions

Cardiovascular: Edema, hypertension, CHF

Central nervous system: Vertigo, seizures, headache, psychoses, pseudotumor cerebri, euphoria, insomnia, intracranial hypertension, nervousness

Dermatologic: Acne, skin atrophy, impaired wound healing, petechiae, bruising

Endocrine & metabolic: HPA suppression, Cushing's syndrome, growth suppression, glucose intolerance, hypokalemia, alkalosis, weight gain

Gastrointestinal: Peptic ulcer, nausea, vomiting

Genitourinary: Menstrual irregularities

Neuromuscular & skeletal: Muscle weakness, osteoporosis, fractures, bone mineral density decreased

Ocular: Cataracts, IOP elevated, glaucoma

Miscellaneous: Immunosuppression, anaphylactoid reactions (rare)

Drug Interactions

Avoid Concomitant Use

Avoid concomitant use of Cortisone with any of the following: Aldesleukin; BCG; Natalizumab; Pimecrolimus; Tacrolimus (Topical); Vaccines (Live)

Increased Effect/Toxicity

Cortisone may increase the levels/effects of: Acetylcholinesterase Inhibitors; Amphotericin B; Leflunomide; Loop Diuretics; Natalizumab; NSAID (COX-2 Inhibitor); NSAID (Nonselective); Thiazide Diuretics; Vaccines (Live); Warfarin

The levels/effects of Cortisone may be increased by: Antifungal Agents (Azole Derivatives, Systemic); Aprepitant; Calcium Channel Blockers (Nondihydropyridine); Denosumab; Estrogen Derivatives; Fluconazole; Fosaprepitant; Macrolide Antibiotics; Neuromuscular-Blocking Agents (Nondepolarizing); Pimecrolimus; Quinolone Antibiotics; Salicylates; Tacrolimus (Topical); Trastuzumab

Decreased Effect

Cortisone may decrease the levels/effects of: Aldesleukin; Antidiabetic Agents; BCG; Calcitriol; Corticorelin; Isoniazid; Salicylates; Sipuleucel-T; Vaccines (Inactivated); Vaccines (Live)

The levels/effects of Cortisone may be decreased by: Aminoglutethimide; Antacids; Barbiturates; Bile Acid Sequestrants; Echinacea; Mitotane; Primidone; Rifamycin Derivatives; Somatropin

Food Interactions Systemic use of corticosteroids may require a diet with increased potassium, vitamins A, B$_6$, C, D, folate, calcium, zinc, phosphorus, and decreased sodium

Mechanism of Action Controls the rate of protein synthesis, depresses the migration of polymorphonuclear leukocytes and fibroblasts, reverses capillary permeability, and stabilizes lysosomal membranes at the cellular level to prevent or control inflammation

Pharmacodynamics

Maximum effect: Oral: Within 2 hours

Duration: 30-36 hours

Pharmacokinetics (Adult data unless noted)

Distribution: Crosses the placenta; appears in breast milk; distributes to muscles, liver, skin, intestines, and kidneys

Metabolism: In the liver to inactive metabolites

Half-life: 30 minutes

Elimination: In bile and urine

Usual Dosage Depends upon the condition being treated and the response of the patient. Supplemental doses may be warranted during times of stress in the course of withdrawing therapy. Oral:

Children:

Anti-inflammatory or immunosuppressive: 2.5-10 mg/kg/day or 20-300 mg/m^2/day in divided doses every 6-8 hours

Physiologic replacement: 0.5-0.75 mg/kg/day or 20-25 mg/m^2/day in divided doses every 8 hours

Adults: 20-300 mg/day divided every 12-24 hours

Administration Oral: Administer with meals, food, or milk to decrease GI effects

Monitoring Parameters Long-term use: Electrolytes, glucose, blood pressure, height, weight

Test Interactions Skin tests

Patient Information Do not discontinue or reduce dose without physician's approval; limit caffeine; avoid alcohol

Nursing Implications Taper dose gradually with long-term use

Additional Information Insoluble in water

Dosage Forms Excipient information presented when available (limited, particularly for generics); consult specific product labeling.

Tablet, as acetate: 25 mg

◆ **Cortisone Acetate** *see* Cortisone *on page 360*

◆ **Cortisporin® Cream** *see* Neomycin, (Bacitracin) Polymyxin B, and Hydrocortisone *on page 980*

◆ **Cortisporin® Ophthalmic [DSC]** *see* Neomycin, (Bacitracin) Polymyxin B, and Hydrocortisone *on page 980*

◆ **Cortisporin® Otic** *see* Neomycin, (Bacitracin) Polymyxin B, and Hydrocortisone *on page 980*

◆ **Cortizone-10® Maximum Strength [OTC]** *see* Hydrocortisone *on page 685*

◆ **Cortizone-10® Maximum Strength Cooling Relief [OTC]** see Hydrocortisone on page 685

◆ **Cortizone-10® Maximum Strength Easy Relief [OTC]** see Hydrocortisone on page 685

◆ **Cortizone-10® Maximum Strength Intensive Healing Formula [OTC]** see Hydrocortisone on page 685

◆ **Cortizone-10® Plus Maximum Strength [OTC]** see Hydrocortisone on page 685

◆ **Cortizone-10® Quick Shot [OTC] [DSC]** see Hydrocortisone on page 685

◆ **Cortrosyn®** see Cosyntropin on page 362

◆ **CO Sertraline (Can)** see Sertraline on page 1254

◆ **CO Simvastatin (Can)** see Simvastatin on page 1263

◆ **Cosmegen®** see DACTINomycin on page 383

◆ **CO Sotalol (Can)** see Sotalol on page 1284

◆ **CO Sumatriptan (Can)** see SUMAtriptan on page 1308

Cosyntropin (koe sin TROE pin)

Medication Safety Issues
Sound-alike/look-alike issues:
   Cortrosyn® may be confused with colchicine, Cotazym®

U.S. Brand Names Cortrosyn®

Canadian Brand Names Cortrosyn®

Therapeutic Category Adrenal Corticosteroid; Diagnostic Agent, Adrenocortical Insufficiency

Generic Available Yes

Use Diagnostic test to differentiate primary adrenal from secondary (pituitary) adrenocortical insufficiency; used in the diagnosis of congenital adrenal hyperplasia

Pregnancy Risk Factor C

Lactation Excretion in breast milk unknown/use caution

Contraindications Hypersensitivity to cosyntropin or any component

Precautions Use with caution in patients with pre-existing allergic disease or a history of allergic reactions to corticotropin

Adverse Reactions
Cardiovascular: Bradycardia, tachycardia, hypertension, peripheral edema

Dermatologic: Pruritus, flushing, rash

Miscellaneous: Hypersensitivity reactions, including anaphylaxis

Drug Interactions
Avoid Concomitant Use There are no known interactions where it is recommended to avoid concomitant use.

Increased Effect/Toxicity There are no known significant interactions involving an increase in effect.

Decreased Effect There are no known significant interactions involving a decrease in effect.

Stability Store unreconstituted vials at 15°C to 30°C (59°F to 86°F); reconstituted solution is stable for 24 hours at room temperature and 21 days when refrigerated; when diluted in NS or D_5W, I.V. infusion is stable for 12 hours at room temperature; do not add to plasma or blood infusions (inactivation by enzymes may occur)

Mechanism of Action Stimulates the adrenal cortex to secrete adrenal steroids (including hydrocortisone, cortisone), androgenic substances, and a small amount of aldosterone

Pharmacodynamics I.M., I.V.:
Onset of action: Plasma cortisol levels rise in healthy individuals in 5 minutes

Maximum effect: Plasma cortisol levels usually peak at 45-60 minutes after the cosyntropin dose

Pharmacokinetics (Adult data unless noted) Metabolism: Unknown

Usual Dosage Diagnostic test doses:
Adrenocortical insufficiency: I.M., I.V.:
   Preterm neonates: Dose not well defined; Korte 1996 used physiologic doses of cosyntropin (0.1 mcg/kg) to test adrenal function in VLBW infants [mean weight 900 g; mean gestational age 27 weeks (range: 23-32 weeks)]; only 36% of infants responded; increasing the dose to 0.2 mcg/kg resulted in 67% of the infants responding, but sensitivity of the test was decreased. Cole,1999 used cosyntropin doses of 3.5 mcg/kg to test adrenal function in 44 preterm infants [mean birthweight 823 g; mean gestational age 26.2 weeks; mean postmenstrual age 30.1 weeks] during inhaled beclomethasone therapy.
   Neonates: 0.015 mcg/kg/dose
   Children ≤2 years: 0.125 mg
   Children >2 years and Adults: 0.25 mg
When greater cortisol stimulation is needed, an I.V. infusion may be used: Children >2 years and Adults: 0.25 mg administered over 4-8 hours (usually 6 hours)
Congenital adrenal hyperplasia evaluation: 1 mg/m^2/dose up to a maximum of 1 mg

Administration Parenteral: Reconstitute vial with 1 mL NS; visually inspect solution for discoloration and particulate matter prior to injection
I.M.: Administer as 0.25 mg/mL concentration
I.V. push: Administer in 2-5 mL of NS over 2 minutes
I.V. infusion (Children >2 years and Adults): Dose may be added to dextrose or NS solution and administered over 4-8 hours (at a rate of approximately 0.04 mg/hour for 6 hours)

Reference Range Plasma cortisol concentrations should be measured immediately before and exactly 30 minutes after the dose; dose should be given in the early morning; normal morning baseline cortisol >5 mcg/dL (SI: >138 nmol/L); normal response 30 minutes after cosyntropin injection: an increase in serum cortisol concentration of ≥7 mcg/dL (SI: ≥193 nmol/L) or peak response >18 mcg/dL (SI: >497 nmol/L).

Nursing Implications Patient should not receive corticosteroids or spironolactone the day prior to and the day of the test

Additional Information Each 0.25 mg of cosyntropin is equivalent to 25 units of corticotropin.

Dosage Forms Excipient information presented when available (limited, particularly for generics); consult specific product labeling.
Injection, powder for reconstitution: 0.25 mg
   Cortrosyn®: 0.25 mg

References
Cole CH, Shah B, Abbasi S, et al, "Adrenal Function in Premature Infants During Inhaled Beclomethasone Therapy," J Pediatr, 1999, 135(1):65-70.

Korte C, Styne D, Merritt TA, et al, "Adrenocortical Function in the Very Low Birth Weight Infant: Improved Testing Sensitivity and Association With Neonatal Outcome," J Pediatr, 1996, 128(2):257-63.

◆ **Cotazym® (Can)** see Pancrelipase on page 1051

◆ **CO Terbinafine (Can)** see Terbinafine on page 1322

◆ **CO Topiramate (Can)** see Topiramate on page 1360

◆ **Co-Trimoxazole** see Sulfamethoxazole and Trimethoprim on page 1302

◆ **Coumadin®** see Warfarin on page 1432

◆ **CO Venlafaxine XR (Can)** see Venlafaxine on page 1412

◆ **Covera® (Can)** see Verapamil on page 1416

◆ **Covera-HS®** see Verapamil on page 1416

◆ **Co-Vidarabine** see Pentostatin on page 1088

◆ **Coviracil** see Emtricitabine on page 496

◆ **Cozaar®** see Losartan on page 847

◆ **CPM** see Cyclophosphamide on page 369

◆ **CPM-12 [DSC]** see Chlorpheniramine on page 296

- ◆ **CPT-11** *see* Irinotecan *on page* 760
- ◆ **CPZ** *see* ChlorproMAZINE *on page* 298
- ◆ **Creomulsion® Adult Formula [OTC]** *see* Dextromethorphan *on page* 421
- ◆ **Creomulsion® for Children [OTC]** *see* Dextromethorphan *on page* 421
- ◆ **Creon®** *see* Pancrelipase *on page* 1051
- ◆ **Creo-Terpin® [OTC]** *see* Dextromethorphan *on page* 421
- ◆ **Crestor®** *see* Rosuvastatin *on page* 1235
- ◆ **Critic-Aid® Clear AF [OTC]** *see* Miconazole *on page* 927
- ◆ **Critic-Aid Skin Care® [OTC]** *see* Zinc Oxide *on page* 1445
- ◆ **Crixivan®** *see* Indinavir *on page* 723
- ◆ **Crolom®** *see* Cromolyn *on page* 363
- ◆ **Cromoglycic Acid** *see* Cromolyn *on page* 363

Cromolyn (KROE moe lin)

Medication Safety Issues
Sound-alike/look-alike issues:
NasalCrom® may be confused with Nasacort®, Nasalide®

Related Information
Asthma *on page* 1697

U.S. Brand Names Crolom®; Gastrocrom®; Intal® [DSC]; NasalCrom® [OTC]

Canadian Brand Names Apo-Cromolyn®; Intal®; Nalcrom®; Nu-Cromolyn; Opticrom®; Rhinaris-CS Anti-Allergic Nasal Mist

Therapeutic Category Antiasthmatic; Inhalation, Miscellaneous

Generic Available Yes: Excludes aerosol, oral solution

Use
Oral inhalation and nebulization: Prophylactic agent used for long-term (chronic) control of persistent asthma (see Additional Information); **NOT** indicated for the relief of acute bronchospasm; also used for the prevention of allergen- or exercise-induced bronchospasm (**Note:** Cromolyn is not as effective as inhaled short acting beta₂-agonists for exercise-induced bronchospasm; see NAEPP, 2007).

Intranasal: Management of seasonal or perennial allergic rhinitis

Ophthalmologic: Vernal conjunctivitis, vernal keratoconjunctivitis, and vernal keratitis

Systemic: Mastocytosis, food allergy, and treatment of inflammatory bowel disease

Pregnancy Risk Factor B

Pregnancy Considerations Adverse events were not observed in animal reproduction studies. No data available on whether cromolyn crosses the placenta or clinical effects on the fetus. Available evidence suggests safe use during pregnancy.

Lactation Excretion in breast milk unknown/use caution

Breast-Feeding Considerations No data available on whether cromolyn enters into breast milk or clinical effects on the infant. Use of cromolyn is not considered a contraindication to breast-feeding.

Contraindications Hypersensitivity to cromolyn or any component; primary treatment of status asthmaticus

Warnings Cromolyn is a prophylactic drug with no benefit for acute situations; rare but severe anaphylactic reactions can occur; discontinue if eosinophilic pneumonia occurs

Precautions Use with caution and decrease dose in patients with renal and hepatic impairment; use inhalation aerosol with caution in patients with coronary artery disease or history of cardiac arrhythmias (due to propellants); use with caution when tapering the dose or withdrawing the drug since symptoms may reoccur; patients should not wear contact lenses during treatment with ophthalmic solution.

Oral cromolyn increased mortality in neonatal rats when administered at ~9 times the maximum recommended daily dose for infants, but not at ~3 times the maximum recommended daily dose; use of oral cromolyn in infants and children <2 years is not recommended and should be reserved for patients with severe mastocytosis in whom potential benefits clearly outweigh the risks.

Adverse Reactions
Central nervous system: Dizziness, headache
Dermatologic: Rash, urticaria, angioedema
Gastrointestinal: Nausea, vomiting, diarrhea, xerostomia, unpleasant taste (inhalation aerosol)
Local: Nasal burning
Neuromuscular & skeletal: Arthralgia
Ocular (topical): Ocular stinging, lacrimation
Respiratory: Coughing, wheezing, sneezing, nasal congestion, throat irritation, eosinophilic pneumonia, pulmonary infiltrates, hoarseness, laryngeal edema (rare)
Miscellaneous: Anaphylaxis (rare)

Drug Interactions
Avoid Concomitant Use There are no known interactions where it is recommended to avoid concomitant use.
Increased Effect/Toxicity There are no known significant interactions involving an increase in effect.
Decreased Effect There are no known significant interactions involving a decrease in effect.

Stability Protect from direct light and heat; nebulization solution is compatible with beta agonists, anticholinergic solutions, acetylcysteine and NS; incompatible with alkaline solutions, calcium and magnesium salts; store oral concentrate ampuls in foil pouch until ready for use

Mechanism of Action Prevents the mast cell release of histamine, leukotrienes and slow-reacting substance of anaphylaxis by inhibiting degranulation after contact with antigens

Pharmacodynamics Not effective for immediate relief of symptoms in acute asthmatic attacks; must be used at regular intervals for 2-4 weeks to be effective; **Note:** Therapeutic response may occur within 2 weeks; however, a trial of 4-6 weeks may be needed to determine maximum benefits.

Pharmacokinetics (Adult data unless noted)
Absorption:
Oral: 0.5% to 2%
Inhalation: ~8% of dose reaches the lungs upon inhalation of the powder and is well absorbed
Half-life: 80-90 minutes
Time to peak serum concentration: Within 15 minutes after inhalation
Elimination: Equally excreted unchanged in urine and feces (via bile); small amounts after inhalation are exhaled

Usual Dosage
Inhalation:
For chronic control of asthma; **Note:** Once control is achieved, taper frequency to the lowest effective dose (ie, 4 times/day to 3 times/day to twice daily):
Nebulization solution: Children ≥2 years and Adults: Initial: 20 mg 4 times/day; usual dose: 20 mg 3-4 times/day
Metered spray:
Children 5-12 years: Initial: 2 inhalations 4 times/day; usual dose: 1-2 inhalations 3-4 times/day
Children ≥12 years and Adults: Initial: 2 inhalations 4 times/day; usual dose: 2-4 inhalations 3-4 times/day

Prevention of allergen- or exercise-induced broncho-spasm: Administer 10-15 minutes prior to exercise or allergen exposure but no longer than 1 hour before:

Nebulization solution: Children ≥2 years and Adults: Single dose of 20 mg

Metered spray: Children >5 years and Adults: Single dose of 2 inhalations

NIH Asthma Guidelines (NAEPP, 2007):

Nebulization solution: Children ≥2 years and Adults: 20 mg 4 times/day

Metered spray: Children ≥5 years and Adults: 2 inhalations 4 times/day

Intranasal: Children ≥2 years and Adults: 1 spray in each nostril 3-4 times/day; maximum dose: 1 spray in each nostril 6 times/day

Ophthalmic: Children >4 years and Adults: Instill 1-2 drops 4-6 times/day

Oral:

Systemic mastocytosis:

Neonates and Preterm Infants: Not recommended

Infants and Children <2 years: Not recommended; reserve use for patients with severe disease in whom potential benefits outweigh risks (see Precautions); 20 mg/kg/day in 4 divided doses; may increase in patients 6 months to 2 years of age if benefits not seen after 2-3 weeks; do not exceed 30 mg/kg/day

Children 2-12 years: 100 mg 4 times/day; not to exceed 40 mg/kg/day

Children >12 years and Adults: 200 mg 4 times/day

Food allergy and inflammatory bowel disease:

Infants and Children <2 years: Not recommended

Children 2-12 years: Initial dose: 100 mg 4 times/day; may double the dose if effect is not satisfactory within 2-3 weeks; not to exceed 40 mg/kg/day

Children >12 years and Adults: Initial dose: 200 mg 4 times/day; may double the dose if effect is not satisfactory within 2-3 weeks; up to 400 mg 4 times/day

Once desired effect is achieved, dose may be tapered to lowest effective dose

Administration

Oral concentrate: Open ampul and squeeze contents into glass of water; stir well; administer at least 30 minutes before meals and at bedtime; do not mix with juice, milk, or food

Oral inhalation: Shake canister gently before use; do not immerse canister in water

Nasal inhalation: Clear nasal passages by blowing nose prior to use

Monitoring Parameters Asthma: Periodic pulmonary function tests; signs and symptoms of disease state when tapering dose

Patient Information May cause dry mouth. Cromolyn is not effective for the immediate relief of symptoms in acute asthmatic attacks; must be used at regular intervals for 2-4 weeks to be effective for asthma control. Cromolyn nasal spray is not effective for the immediate relief of nasal allergies; must be used at regular intervals for 1-2 weeks for optimal control of nasal allergies; to prevent nasal allergy symptoms, start using product 1-2 weeks before contact with the cause of allergies.

Additional Information The 2007 Expert Panel Report of the National Asthma Education and Prevention Program (NAEPP, 2007) does not recommend cromolyn for initial treatment of persistent asthma in children; inhaled corticosteroids are the preferred agents; cromolyn is considered an alternative medication for the treatment of mild persistent asthma in children. Inhalation aerosol contains fluorocarbon propellants. Reserve systemic use in children <2 years of age for severe disease; avoid systemic use in premature infants.

Dosage Forms Excipient information presented when available (limited, particularly for generics); consult specific product labeling. [DSC] = Discontinued product

Aerosol, for oral inhalation, as sodium:

Intal®: 800 mcg/inhalation (8.1 g) [112 metered inhalations; 56 doses] [DSC], (14.2 g) [200 metered inhalations; 100 doses]

Solution for nebulization, as sodium: 20 mg/2 mL (60s, 120s)

Intal®: 20 mg/2 mL (60s, 120s) [DSC]

Solution, intranasal, as sodium [spray]:

NasalCrom®: 40 mg/mL (13 mL, 26 mL) [5.2 mg/inhalation; contains benzalkonium chloride]

Solution, ophthalmic, as sodium: 4% (10 mL)

Crolom®: 4% (10 mL) [contains benzalkonium chloride]

Solution, oral, as sodium [concentrate]:

Gastrocrom®: 100 mg/5 mL (96s)

References

National Asthma Education and Prevention Program (NAEPP), "Expert Panel Report 3 (EPR-3): Guidelines for the Diagnosis and Management of Asthma," Clinical Practice Guidelines, National Institutes of Health, National Heart, Lung, and Blood Institute, NIH Publication No. 08-4051, prepublication 2007; available at http://www.nhlbi.nih.gov/guidelines/asthma/asthgdln.htm.

◆ **Cromolyn Sodium** see Cromolyn on page 363

Crotamiton (kroe TAM i tonn)

Medication Safety Issues

Sound-alike/look-alike issues:

Eurax® may be confused with Efudex®, Eulexin®, Evoxac™, Serax®, Urex®

International issues:

Eurax® may be confused with Urex® which is a brand name for furosemide in Australia

U.S. Brand Names Eurax®

Therapeutic Category Scabicidal Agent

Generic Available No

Use Treatment of scabies (Sarcoptes scabiei) in infants and children; symptomatic treatment of pruritic skin

Pregnancy Risk Factor C

Pregnancy Considerations Animal reproduction studies have not been conducted; use during pregnancy only if clearly needed.

Lactation Excretion in breast milk unknown

Contraindications Hypersensitivity to crotamiton or any component; patients who manifest a primary irritation response to topical medications

Precautions Avoid contact with face, eyes, mucous membranes, and urethral meatus; do not apply to acutely inflamed or raw skin

Adverse Reactions

Dermatologic: Pruritus, contact dermatitis, rash

Local: Irritation

Miscellaneous: Allergic sensitivity reaction

Drug Interactions

Avoid Concomitant Use There are no known interactions where it is recommended to avoid concomitant use.

Increased Effect/Toxicity There are no known significant interactions involving an increase in effect.

Decreased Effect There are no known significant interactions involving a decrease in effect.

Stability Store at room temperature.

Mechanism of Action Mechanism for scabicidal activity is unknown

Pharmacokinetics (Adult data unless noted) Absorption: Amount of systemic absorption following topical use has not been determined

Usual Dosage Topical: Infants, Children, and Adults:
Scabicide: Apply over entire body below the head; apply once daily for 2 days followed by a cleansing bath 48 hours after the last application; treatment may be repeated after 7-10 days if mites appear
Pruritus: Massage into affected areas until medication is completely absorbed; may repeat as necessary

Administration Topical: Wash thoroughly and scrub away loose scales, then towel dry; apply a thin layer and gently massage drug onto skin of the entire body from the neck to the toes (with special attention to skin folds, creases, and interdigital spaces); also apply cream or lotion under fingernails after trimming nails short; since scabies can affect the head, scalp, and neck in infants and young children, apply to scalp, neck, and body of this age group; do not apply to the face, eyes, mouth, mucous membranes, or urethral meatus; shake lotion well before use

Patient Information For topical use only. Not for ophthalmic, oral, or intravaginal use. All contaminated clothing and bed linen should be washed to avoid reinfestation.

Additional Information Treatment may be repeated after 7-10 days if live mites are still present

Dosage Forms Excipient information presented when available (limited, particularly for generics); consult specific product labeling.
Cream: 10% (60 g)
Lotion: 10% (60 mL, 480 mL)

References
Eichenfield LF, Honig PJ, "Blistering Disorders in Childhood," *Pediatr Clin North Am*, 1991, 38(4):959-76.
Hogan DJ, Schachner L, Tanglertsampan C, "Diagnosis and Treatment of Childhood Scabies and Pediculosis," *Pediatr Clin North Am*, 1991, 38(4):941-57.

◆ **Crude Coal Tar** *see* Coal Tar *on page 349*
◆ **Cruex® Cream [OTC]** *see* Clotrimazole *on page 344*
◆ **Crystalline Penicillin** *see* Penicillin G (Parenteral/Aqueous) *on page 1080*
◆ **Crystal Violet** *see* Gentian Violet *on page 645*
◆ **Crystapen® (Can)** *see* Penicillin G (Parenteral/Aqueous) *on page 1080*
◆ **CsA** *see* CycloSPORINE *on page 372*
◆ **C-Time [OTC]** *see* Ascorbic Acid *on page 138*
◆ **CTLA-4lg** *see* Abatacept *on page 34*
◆ **CTM** *see* Chlorpheniramine *on page 296*
◆ **CTP 30 (Can)** *see* Citalopram *on page 319*
◆ **CTX** *see* Cyclophosphamide *on page 369*
◆ **Cubicin®** *see* DAPTOmycin *on page 389*
◆ **Culturelle® [OTC]** *see* Lactobacillus *on page 790*
◆ **Cupric Chloride** *see* Trace Metals *on page 1366*
◆ **Cuprimine®** *see* Penicillamine *on page 1076*
◆ **Curosurf® [DSC]** *see* Poractant Alfa *on page 1131*
◆ **Curosurf® (Can)** *see* Poractant Alfa *on page 1131*
◆ **Cutar® [OTC]** *see* Coal Tar *on page 349*
◆ **Cutivate®** *see* Fluticasone *on page 607*
◆ **Cutivate™ (Can)** *see* Fluticasone *on page 607*
◆ **CyA** *see* CycloSPORINE *on page 372*
◆ **Cyanide Antidote Kit** *see* Sodium Nitrite, Sodium Thiosulfate, and Amyl Nitrite *on page 1273*
◆ **Cyanide Antidote Package** *see* Sodium Nitrite, Sodium Thiosulfate, and Amyl Nitrite *on page 1273*

Cyanocobalamin (sye an oh koe BAL a min)

U.S. Brand Names CaloMist™; Nascobal®; Twelve Resin-K [OTC]

Therapeutic Category Nutritional Supplement; Vitamin, Water Soluble

Generic Available Yes: Excludes nasal spray

Use Treatment of pernicious anemia; vitamin B_{12} deficiency due to dietary deficiencies or malabsorption diseases; inadequate secretion of intrinsic factor, inadequate utilization of B_{12} (eg, during neoplastic treatment); increased B_{12} requirements due to pregnancy, thyrotoxicosis, hemorrhage, malignancy, liver or kidney disease; nutritional supplement

CaloMist™: Maintenance of vitamin B_{12} concentrations after initial correction in patients with B_{12} deficiency without CNS involvement

Pregnancy Risk Factor A/C (dose exceeding RDA recommendation); C (intranasal)

Lactation Enters breast milk/compatible

Breast-Feeding Considerations Vegetarian diets which contain no animal products do not supply any vitamin B_{12}. Deficiency recognized in infants of vegetarian mothers who were breast-fed; consider supplementation during breast-feeding.

Contraindications Hypersensitivity to cyanocobalamin, any component (see Warnings), or cobalt; patients with hereditary optic nerve atrophy (Leber's disease)

Warnings Only I.M./SubQ routes are used to treat pernicious anemia; oral and intranasal administration are not indicated until hematologic remission and there are no signs of nervous system involvement. Avoid the I.V. route as it has been associated with anaphylaxis. Vitamin B_{12} deficiency for >3 months results in irreversible degenerative CNS lesions; neurologic manifestations will not be prevented with folic acid unless vitamin B_{12} is also given; spinal cord degeneration might also occur when folic acid is used as a substitute for vitamin B_{12} in anemia prevention. Vegetarian diets may result in vitamin B_{12} deficiency.

Injection may contain benzyl alcohol which may cause allergic reactions in susceptible individuals; large amounts of benzyl alcohol (≥99 mg/kg/day) have been associated with a potentially fatal toxicity ("gasping syndrome") in neonates; the "gasping syndrome" consists of metabolic acidosis, respiratory distress, gasping respirations, CNS dysfunction (including convulsions, intracranial hemorrhage), hypotension and cardiovascular collapse; avoid use of benzyl alcohol containing injections in neonates; *in vitro* and animal studies have shown that benzoate, a metabolite of benzyl alcohol, displaces bilirubin from protein-binding sites.

Intranasal therapy is only for use in patients who are in remission following injectable treatment. Efficacy of intranasal treatment in patients with nasal pathology or with other concomitant intranasal therapy has not been determined. Patients with early Leber's disease (hereditary optic nerve atrophy) who were treated with vitamin B_{12} suffered severe and swift optic atrophy. These patients should not receive cyanocobalamin therapy.

Precautions Serum potassium concentrations and platelet counts should be monitored early as severe hypokalemia (sometimes fatal) and thrombocytosis have occurred after the conversion of megaloblastic anemia to normal erythropoiesis; an intradermal test dose of parenteral cyanocobalamin is recommended before initiating the nasal spray in patients suspected to be sensitive to cyanocobalamin. Vitamin B_{12} deficiency masks signs of polycythemia vera; use caution in other conditions where folic acid or vitamin B_{12} administration alone might mask true diagnosis despite hematologic response. Some parenteral products contain aluminum; use caution in neonates and patients with impaired renal function.

Adverse Reactions

Cardiovascular: Peripheral vascular thrombosis (parenteral route)

Central nervous system: Headache, dizziness

Dermatologic: Itching, urticaria, exanthema

Endocrine & metabolic: Hypokalemia

Gastrointestinal: Diarrhea (mild)

Respiratory: Rhinitis (nasal gel), pulmonary edema (parenteral route), rhinorrhea and nasal discomfort (nasal spray)

Miscellaneous: Anaphylactic reactions, infection

Drug Interactions

Avoid Concomitant Use There are no known interactions where it is recommended to avoid concomitant use.

Increased Effect/Toxicity There are no known significant interactions involving an increase in effect.

Decreased Effect

The levels/effects of Cyanocobalamin may be decreased by: Chloramphenicol; Colchicine

Stability Store at room temperature; protect from light; injection is **incompatible** with chlorpromazine, phytonadione, prochlorperazine, warfarin, ascorbic acid, dextrose, heavy metals, oxidizing or reducing agents

Mechanism of Action Coenzyme for various metabolic functions, including fat and carbohydrate metabolism and protein synthesis, used in cell replication and hematopoiesis

Pharmacodynamics Onset of action:

Megaloblastic anemia: I.M.:

Conversion of megaloblastic to normoblastic erythroid hyperplasia within bone marrow: 8 hours

Increased reticulocytes: 2-5 days

Complicated vitamin B_{12} deficiency: I.M., SubQ: Resolution of:

Psychiatric sequelae: 24 hours

Thrombocytopenia: 10 days

Granulocytopenia: 2 weeks

Pharmacokinetics (Adult data unless noted)

Absorption: Oral: Drug is absorbed from the terminal ileum in the presence of calcium; for absorption to occur, gastric "intrinsic factor" must be present to transfer the compound across the intestinal mucosa

Distribution: Principally stored in the liver, also stored in the kidneys and adrenals

Protein binding: Bound to transcobalamin II

Metabolism: Converted in the tissues to active coenzymes methylcobalamin and deoxyadenosylcobalamin

Bioavailability:

Oral: Pernicious anemia: 1.2%

Intranasal gel: 8.9% (relative to I.M. formulation)

Intranasal spray: Nascobal®: 6.1% (relative to I.M. formulation)

Time to peak serum concentration:

I.M., SubQ: 30 minutes to 2 hours

Intranasal: 1.6 hours

Elimination: 50% to 98% unchanged in the urine

Usual Dosage

Adequate intake (AI): Oral, sublingual: **Note:** Infants born to vegan mothers should be supplemented with the AI for vitamin B_{12} from birth as their vitamin B_{12} stores at birth are low and their mother's milk may supply very small amounts of the vitamin.

Infants 0-6 months: 0.4 mcg/day (0.06 mcg/kg/day)

Children 7-12 months: 0.5 mcg/day (0.06 mcg/kg/day)

Recommended daily allowance (RDA): Oral, Sublingual:

Children:

1-3 years: 0.9 mcg/day

4-8 years: 1.2 mcg/day

9-13 years: 1.8 mcg/day

Children >14 years and Adults: 2.4 mcg/day

Adults, pregnancy: 2.6 mcg/day

Adults, lactation: 2. mcg/day

Pernicious anemia: **Note:** Initial low dosage recommended due to potential hypokalemia observed during initial treatment of adults with severe anemia (Rasmussen, 2001)

Neonates and infants (congenital; if evidence of neurologic involvement): I.M., SubQ: 0.2 mcg/kg for 2 days, followed by 1000 mcg/day for 2-7 days; maintenance: 100 mcg/month

Children: I.M., SubQ: 30-50 mcg/day for 2 or more weeks (to a total dose of 1000 mcg); maintenance: 100 mcg/month

Adults: I.M., SubQ: Initial treatment: 100 mcg/day for 6-7 days; if improvement, give same dose on alternate days for 7 doses; then every 3-4 days for 2-3 weeks or as an alternative, 1000 mcg/day for 7 days followed by 1000 mcg/week for 4 weeks; follow initial therapy with maintenance treatment (see below) for life.

Maintenance:

I.M., SubQ: 100-1000 mcg/month

Intranasal: Nascobal®: 500 mcg (1 spray) in one nostril once weekly

Oral, Sublingual: 1000-2000 mcg/day; recommended only as a option for use in patients who are very compliant; avoid use of timed release formulations

Vitamin B_{12} deficiency:

Children (dosage in children not well established): I.M., SubQ: Initial: 0.2 mcg/kg for 2 days followed by 1000 mcg/day for 2-7 days followed by 100 mcg/week for a month; for malabsorptive causes of B_{12} deficiency, monthly maintenance doses of 100 mcg have been recommended or as an alternative 100 mcg/day for 10-15 days (total dose of 1-1.5 mg), then once or twice weekly for several months; may taper to 60 mcg every month

Adults:

Uncomplicated: Initial:

Oral, Sublingual: 1000-2500 mcg/day

I.M. or deep SubQ: 100 mcg/day for 5-10 days, followed by 100-200 mcg monthly until remission is complete **or** as an alternative: 100 mcg/day for 7 days, followed by 100 mcg every other day for 2 weeks, followed by 100 mcg every 3-4 days until remission is complete

Complicated (severe anemia, CHF, thrombocytopenia with bleeding, severe neurologic damage or granulocytopenia with infection): Initial: I.M. or deep SubQ: 1000 mcg with I.M. or I.V. folic acid 15 mg as single doses, followed by 1000 mcg/day plus oral folic acid 5 mg/day for 1 week; **Note:** Oral cyanocobalamin therapy is **not** indicated for treatment of complicated deficiency due to potential poor compliance

Maintenance:

I.M., deep SubQ: 100-200 mcg monthly

Oral, Sublingual: 1000-2500 mcg/day

Intranasal:

Nascobal®: 500 mcg (1 spray) once weekly

CaloMist™: 25 mcg (1 spray) each nostril daily; may increase to twice daily for patients not responding to daily therapy

Note: Low initial B_{12} doses combined with potassium supplementation (as needed) may prevent a hypokalemia seen in patients with severe deficiency.

Dosage adjustment in renal impairment: Increased dosage may be required in vitamin B$_{12}$-deficient patients

Administration

Oral: Not generally recommended for treatment of severe vitamin B$_{12}$ deficiency due to poor oral absorption (lack of intrinsic factor); oral administration may be used in less severe deficiencies and maintenance therapy; may be administered without regard to food

Sublingual: Place under the tongue and allow to dissolve; do not swallow whole, chew, or crush

Parenteral: I.M. or deep SubQ: Avoid I.V. administration due to a more rapid system elimination with resulting decreased utilization

Intranasal:

Nascobal® nasal spray: Prior to initial dose, activate (prime) spray nozzle by pumping unit quickly and firmly until first appearance of spray, then prime twice more. The unit must be reprimed once immediately before each use. Administer at least one hour before or after ingestion of hot foods or liquids; hot foods can cause nasal secretions and a resulting loss of medication

CaloMist™ nasal spray: Prime unit by spraying 7 times. If >5 days have elapsed since use, reprime with 2 sprays. Separate from other intranasal medications by several hours.

Monitoring Parameters Serum potassium (particularly during initial treatment of deficiency), erythrocyte and reticulocyte count, hemoglobin, hematocrit, platelets, serum cyanocobalamin and folate concentrations; methylmalonate (MMA) and total homocysteine (elevated in Vitamin B$_{12}$ deficiency)

Reference Range Serum vitamin B$_{12}$ levels: Normal: >300 pg/mL; vitamin B$_{12}$ deficiency: <200 pg/mL (200-300 pg/mL borderline result, possible deficiency); megaloblastic anemia: <100 pg/mL

Dosage Forms Excipient information presented when available (limited, particularly for generics); consult specific product labeling.

Injection, solution: 1000 mcg/mL (1 mL, 10 mL, 30 mL) [may contain benzyl alcohol]

Lozenge: 50 mcg, 100 mcg, 250 mcg, 500 mcg

Lozenge, sublingual: 500 mcg

Solution, intranasal [spray]:

CaloMist™: 25 mcg/spray (10.7 mL) [contains benzyl alcohol, benzalkonium chloride; 60 metered sprays]

Nascobal®: 500 mcg/spray (2.3 mL) [contains benzalkonium chloride; delivers 8 sprays]

Tablet: 50 mcg, 100 mcg, 250 mcg, 500 mcg, 1000 mcg

Twelve Resin-K: 1000 mcg [may be used as oral, sublingual, or buccal]

Tablet, timed release: 1000 mcg, 1500 mcg

Tablet, sublingual: 1000 mcg, 2500 mcg, 5000 mcg

References

"Dietary Reference Intakes for Thiamin, Riboflavin, Niacin, Vitamin B$_6$, Folate, Vitamin B$_{12}$, Pantothenic Acid, Biotin, and Choline," (Chapter 9) available at http://books.nap.edu/openbook/0309065542/html/306.html. Last accessed February 22, 2005.

Lane LA and Rojas-Fernandez C, "Treatment of Vitamin B(12)-Deficiency Anemia: Oral Versus Parenteral Therapy," *Ann Pharmacother*, 2002, 36(7):1268-72.

Rasmussen SA, Fernhoff PM, and Scanlon KS, "Vitamin B$_{12}$ Deficiency in Children and Adolescents," *J Pediatr*, 2001, 138(1):10-7.

◆ **Cyanokit®** *see* Hydroxocobalamin *on page 692*

Cyclobenzaprine (sye kloe BEN za preen)

Medication Safety Issues

Sound-alike/look-alike issues:

Cyclobenzaprine may be confused with cycloSERINE, cyproheptadine

Flexeril® may be confused with Floxin®

Beers Criteria medication: This drug may be inappropriate for use in geriatric patients (high severity risk).

U.S. Brand Names Amrix®; Fexmid®; Flexeril®

Canadian Brand Names Apo-Cyclobenzaprine®; Dom-Cyclobenzaprine; Flexeril®; Flexitec; Gen-Cyclobenzaprine; Mylan-Cyclobenzaprine; Novo-Cycloprine; Nu-Cyclobenzaprine; PHL-Cyclobenzaprine; PMS-Cyclobenzaprine; ratio-Cyclobenzaprine; Riva-Cycloprine

Therapeutic Category Skeletal Muscle Relaxant, Nonparalytic

Generic Available Yes: Excludes capsule

Use Treatment of muscle spasm associated with acute painful musculoskeletal conditions; treatment of muscle spasm associated with acute temporomandibular joint pain (TMJ)

Pregnancy Risk Factor B

Pregnancy Considerations Teratogenic effects were not observed in animal studies. There are no adequate and well-controlled studies in pregnant women. Use during pregnancy only if clearly needed.

Lactation Excretion in breast milk unknown/use caution

Contraindications Hypersensitivity to cyclobenzaprine or any component; hyperthyroidism; acute recovery phase of MI, CHF, arrhythmias, heart block; do not use concomitantly or within 14 days of MAO inhibitors

Warnings Not effective in the treatment of spasticity due to cerebral or spinal cord disease or in children with cerebral palsy; shares the toxic potentials of the tricyclic antidepressants, including prolongation of conduction time, arrhythmias, and tachycardia; the usual precautions of tricyclic antidepressant therapy should be observed

Precautions Use with caution in patients with urinary retention, angle-closure glaucoma, increased intraocular pressure, and patients receiving anticholinergic medications; use with caution and reduce dosage in patients with mildly impaired liver function; avoid use in patients with moderate to severe hepatic dysfunction; may cause CNS depression which may impair physical or mental abilities; patients must be cautioned about performing tasks which require mental alertness

Adverse Reactions

Cardiovascular: Tachycardia, hypotension, arrhythmias, edema of face/lips, syncope, palpitations

Central nervous system: Drowsiness (39%), somnolence, headache, dizziness (11%), fatigue, malaise, nervousness, confusion, seizures, ataxia, vertigo, insomnia, psychosis, anxiety, agitation, hallucinations, abnormal dreams, depression

Dermatologic: Rash, pruritus, urticaria

Gastrointestinal: Dyspepsia, nausea, constipation, xerostomia (27%), vomiting, diarrhea, paralytic ileus, dysgeusia, stomach cramps, flatulence, tongue edema, ageusia, anorexia, GI pain, gastritis

Genitourinary: Urinary frequency or retention

Hepatic: Hepatitis (rare), cholestasis, jaundice, abnormal liver function tests

Neuromuscular & skeletal: Weakness, muscle twitching, tremors, paresthesia, hypertonia

Ocular: Diplopia, blurred vision

Otic: Tinnitus

Respiratory: Upper respiratory infection

Miscellaneous: Hypersensitivity reactions, angioedema, diaphoresis

Drug Interactions

Metabolism/Transport Effects Substrate of CYP1A2 (major), 2D6 (minor), 3A4 (minor)

Avoid Concomitant Use

Avoid concomitant use of Cyclobenzaprine with any of the following: MAO Inhibitors

Increased Effect/Toxicity

Cyclobenzaprine may increase the levels/effects of: Alcohol (Ethyl); Anticholinergics; CNS Depressants; MAO Inhibitors; Methotrimeprazine

◀

The levels/effects of Cyclobenzaprine may be increased by: CYP1A2 Inhibitors (Moderate); CYP1A2 Inhibitors (Strong); Methotrimeprazine; Pramlintide

Decreased Effect

Cyclobenzaprine may decrease the levels/effects of: Acetylcholinesterase Inhibitors (Central)

The levels/effects of Cyclobenzaprine may be decreased by: Acetylcholinesterase Inhibitors (Central); Peginterferon Alfa-2b

Food Interactions Food increases bioavailability (peak plasma concentrations increased by 35% and AUC by 20%) of the extended release capsule; avoid ethanol; avoid valerian, kava kava, gotu kola

Stability Store at room temperature

Mechanism of Action Centrally-acting skeletal muscle relaxant pharmacologically related to tricyclic antidepressants; reduces tonic somatic motor activity influencing both alpha and gamma motor neurons

Pharmacodynamics

Onset of action: Immediate release tablet: Within 1 hour
Duration: Immediate release tablet: 12-24 hours

Pharmacokinetics (Adult data unless noted)

Absorption: Oral: Complete
Metabolism: Hepatic via CYP3A4, 1A2, and 2D6; may undergo enterohepatic recirculation
Bioavailability: 33% to 55%
Half-life: Adults: Range: 8-37 hours; immediate release tablet: 18 hours; extended release capsule: 32 hours
Time to peak serum concentration: Immediate release tablet: 3-8 hours; extended release capsule: 7-8 hours
Elimination: Primarily renal as inactive metabolites and in the feces (via bile) as unchanged drug
Clearance: Adults: 0.7 L/minute

Usual Dosage Oral: **Note:** Do not use longer than 2-3 weeks

Children: Dosage has not been established
Adolescents and Adults: Immediate release tablet: 5 mg 3 times/day; may increase to 7.5-10 mg 3 times/day; or extended release capsule: 15 mg once daily; may increase to 30 mg once daily

Dosage adjustment in hepatic impairment:

Immediate release tablet:
Mild: 5 mg 3 times/day
Moderate to severe: Use not recommended
Extended release capsule: Mild to severe impairment: Use not recommended

Administration Oral:

Immediate release tablet: May be administered without regard to meals
Extended release capsule: Administer at the same time daily; do not crush or chew

Monitoring Parameters Relief of muscle spasms and pain; improvement in physical activities

Patient Information Avoid alcohol; do not use prescriptive or OTC antidepressants, sedatives, or pain medications without consulting healthcare provider; may cause drowsiness and impair ability to perform activities requiring mental alertness or physical coordination; may cause dry mouth

Dosage Forms Excipient information presented when available (limited, particularly for generics); consult specific product labeling.

Capsule, extended release, as hydrochloride:
Amrix®: 15 mg, 30 mg
Tablet, as hydrochloride: 5 mg, 10 mg
Fexmid®: 7.5 mg
Flexeril®: 5 mg, 10 mg

◆ **Cyclobenzaprine Hydrochloride** see Cyclobenzaprine on page 367

◆ **Cyclogyl®** see Cyclopentolate on page 368

◆ **Cyclomen® (Can)** see Danazol on page 384

◆ **Cyclomydril®** see Cyclopentolate and Phenylephrine on page 369

Cyclopentolate (sye kloe PEN toe late)

U.S. Brand Names AK-Pentolate™; Cyclogyl®; Cylate™

Canadian Brand Names Cyclogyl®; Diopentolate®

Therapeutic Category Anticholinergic Agent, Ophthalmic; Ophthalmic Agent, Mydriatic

Generic Available Yes

Use Diagnostic procedures requiring mydriasis and cycloplegia

Pregnancy Risk Factor C

Contraindications Hypersensitivity to cyclopentolate or any component; narrow-angle glaucoma

Warnings Use of cyclopentolate has been associated with psychotic reactions and behavioral disturbances in pediatric patients; increased susceptibility to these effects has been reported in young infants, young children, and in children with spastic paralysis or brain damage, particularly with concentrations >1%; observe neonates and infants closely for at least 30 minutes after administration; may cause transient elevation of intraocular pressure

Adverse Reactions Central nervous system and cardiovascular reactions most commonly seen in children after receiving 2% solution:

Cardiovascular: Tachycardia, hypertension
Central nervous system: Psychotic and behavioral disturbances manifested by ataxia, restlessness, hallucinations, psychosis, hyperactivity, seizures, incoherent speech
Local: Burning sensation
Ocular: Intraocular pressure elevated, loss of visual accommodation
Miscellaneous: Allergic reactions

Drug Interactions

Avoid Concomitant Use There are no known interactions where it is recommended to avoid concomitant use.

Increased Effect/Toxicity

Cyclopentolate may increase the levels/effects of: AbobotulinumtoxinA; Anticholinergics; Cannabinoids; OnabotulinumtoxinA; Potassium Chloride; RimabotulinumtoxinB

The levels/effects of Cyclopentolate may be increased by: Pramlintide

Decreased Effect

Cyclopentolate may decrease the levels/effects of: Acetylcholinesterase Inhibitors (Central); Secretin

The levels/effects of Cyclopentolate may be decreased by: Acetylcholinesterase Inhibitors (Central)

Mechanism of Action Prevents the muscle of the ciliary body and the sphincter muscle of the iris from responding to cholinergic stimulation, causing mydriasis and cycloplegia

Pharmacodynamics

Maximum effect:
Cycloplegia: 15-60 minutes
Mydriasis: Within 15-60 minutes, with recovery taking up to 24 hours

Usual Dosage Ophthalmic:

Neonates and Infants: See Cyclopentolate and Phenylephrine on page 369 (preferred agent for use in neonates and infants due to lower cyclopentolate concentration and reduced risk for systemic reactions)
Children: 1 drop of 0.5% or 1% in eye followed by 1 drop of 0.5% or 1% in 5 minutes, if necessary, approximately 40-50 minutes before procedure
Adults: 1 drop of 1% followed by another drop in 5 minutes; approximately 40-50 minutes prior to the procedure, may use 2% solution in heavily pigmented iris

Administration Ophthalmic: Instill drops into conjunctival sac of affected eye(s); avoid contact of bottle tip with skin or eye; to avoid excessive systemic absorption, finger pressure should be applied on the lacrimal sac during and for 1-2 minutes following application

Patient Information May cause blurred vision and increased sensitivity to light

Additional Information Pilocarpine ophthalmic drops applied after the examination may reduce recovery time to 3-6 hours

Dosage Forms Excipient information presented when available (limited, particularly for generics); consult specific product labeling.

Solution, ophthalmic, as hydrochloride: 1% (2 mL, 15 mL)
AK-Pentolate™, Cylate™: 1% (2 mL, 15 mL) [contains benzalkonium chloride]
Cyclogyl®: 0.5% (15 mL); 1% (2 mL, 5 mL, 15 mL); 2% (2 mL, 5 mL, 15 mL) [contains benzalkonium chloride]

Cyclopentolate and Phenylephrine
(sye kloe PEN toe late & fen il EF rin)

U.S. Brand Names Cyclomydril®

Therapeutic Category Adrenergic Agonist Agent, Ophthalmic; Anticholinergic Agent, Ophthalmic; Ophthalmic Agent, Mydriatic

Generic Available No

Use Diagnostic procedures requiring mydriasis and cycloplegia; preferred agent for use in neonates and infants

Pregnancy Risk Factor C

Contraindications Hypersensitivity to cyclopentolate, phenylephrine, or any component; narrow-angle glaucoma or untreated anatomically narrow angles

Warnings Use of cyclopentolate has been associated with psychotic reactions and behavioral disturbances in pediatric patients; increased susceptibility to these effects has been reported in young infants, young children, and in children with spastic paralysis or brain damage, particularly with concentrations >1%; observe neonates and infants closely for at least 30 minutes after administration; may cause transient elevation of intraocular pressure. The preservative, benzalkonium chloride, may be absorbed by soft contact lenses. Wait at least 10 minutes after instillation before reinserting lenses.

Precautions Use with caution in patient's with Down's syndrome, cardiovascular disease, hypertension, and hyperthyroidism; feeding intolerance may follow ophthalmic use of this product in neonates and infants; withhold feedings for 4 hours after examination

Adverse Reactions

Cardiovascular: Tachycardia, hypertension

Central nervous system: Psychotic and behavioral disturbances manifested by ataxia, restlessness, hallucinations, psychosis, hyperactivity, seizures, incoherent speech, hyperpyrexia

Gastrointestinal: Feeding intolerance, gastric motility decreased

Genitourinary: Urinary retention

Local: Burning sensation

Ocular: Intraocular pressure elevated, loss of visual accommodation, transient stinging, browache, photophobia, lacrimation, superficial punctate keratitis

Miscellaneous: Allergic reactions

Drug Interactions

Avoid Concomitant Use

Avoid concomitant use of Cyclopentolate and Phenylephrine with any of the following: Iobenguane I 123; MAO Inhibitors

Increased Effect/Toxicity

Cyclopentolate and Phenylephrine may increase the levels/effects of: AbobotulinumtoxinA; Anticholinergics; Cannabinoids; OnabotulinumtoxinA; Potassium Chloride; RimabotulinumtoxinB; Sympathomimetics

The levels/effects of Cyclopentolate and Phenylephrine may be increased by: Atomoxetine; MAO Inhibitors; Pramlintide; Tricyclic Antidepressants

Decreased Effect

Cyclopentolate and Phenylephrine may decrease the levels/effects of: Acetylcholinesterase Inhibitors (Central); Iobenguane I 123; Secretin

The levels/effects of Cyclopentolate and Phenylephrine may be decreased by: Acetylcholinesterase Inhibitors (Central)

Stability Store at room temperature

Mechanism of Action See individual agents.

Pharmacodynamics Onset of action and duration of effect are partially dependent upon eye pigment; dark eyes have a prolonged onset of action and shorter duration than blue eyes

Onset of action: 15-60 minutes

Duration: 4-12 hours

Usual Dosage Ophthalmic:

Neonates, Infants, Children, and Adults: Instill 1 drop into the eye every 5-10 minutes, for up to 3 doses, approximately 40-50 minutes before the examination

Administration Ophthalmic: Instill drops into conjunctival sac of affected eye(s); avoid contact of bottle tip with skin or eye; to avoid excessive systemic absorption, finger pressure should be applied on the lacrimal sac during and for 1-2 minutes following application; preservative absorbed by soft contact lenses; wait at least 10 minutes before reinserting

Patient Information May cause blurred vision and increased sensitivity to light; preservative is absorbed by soft contact lenses (see Warnings)

Nursing Implications Do not repeat dosage within at least 4 hours, but preferably 24 hours, after initial treatment to prevent drug accumulation and potential systemic toxicity; see Warnings

Additional Information Cyclomydril® is the preferred agent for use in neonates and infants because lower concentrations of both cyclopentolate and phenylephrine provide optimal dilation while minimizing the systemic side effects noted with a higher concentration of each agent used alone

Dosage Forms Excipient information presented when available (limited, particularly for generics); consult specific product labeling.

Solution, ophthalmic: Cyclopentolate hydrochloride 0.2% and phenylephrine hydrochloride 1% (2 mL, 5 mL) [contains benzalkonium chloride]

◆ **Cyclopentolate Hydrochloride** see Cyclopentolate on page 368

Cyclophosphamide (sye kloe FOS fa mide)

Medication Safety Issues

Sound-alike/look-alike issues:

Cyclophosphamide may be confused with cycloSPORINE, ifosfamide

Cytoxan may be confused with cefoxitin, Centoxin®, Ciloxan®, cytarabine, CytoGam®, Cytosar®, Cytosar-U®, Cytotec®

High alert medication: This medication is in a class the Institute for Safe Medication Practices (ISMP) includes among its list of drugs which have a heightened risk of causing significant patient harm when used in error.

Related Information

Compatibility of Chemotherapy and Related Supportive Care Medications *on page 1580*

Emetogenic Potential of Antineoplastic Agents *on page 1579*

Canadian Brand Names Procytox®

Therapeutic Category Antineoplastic Agent, Alkylating Agent (Nitrogen Mustard)

Generic Available Yes

Use

Oncology: Treatment of Hodgkin's lymphoma, non-Hodgkin's lymphoma (including Burkitt's lymphoma), chronic lymphocytic leukemia (CLL), chronic myelocytic leukemia (CML), acute myelocytic leukemia (AML), acute lymphocytic leukemia (ALL), mycosis fungoides, multiple myeloma, neuroblastoma, retinoblastoma, breast cancer, ovarian adenocarcinoma [FDA approved in pediatrics (age not specified) and adults]; has also been used for Ewing's sarcoma, rhabdomyosarcoma, Wilms tumor, ovarian germ cell tumors, small cell lung cancer, testicular cancer, pheochromocytoma, bone marrow transplantation conditioning regimen

Nononcology: Treatment of nephrotic syndrome in children [FDA approved in pediatrics (age not specified) and adults]; has also been used for severe rheumatoid disorders, Wegener's granulomatosis, myasthenia gravis, multiple sclerosis, systemic lupus erythematosus, lupus nephritis, autoimmune hemolytic anemia, idiopathic thrombocytic purpura (ITP), and antibody-induced pure red cell aplasia

Pregnancy Risk Factor D

Lactation Enters breast milk/contraindicated

Contraindications Hypersensitivity to cyclophosphamide or any component

Warnings Hazardous agent; use appropriate precautions for handling and disposal; cyclophosphamide is potentially carcinogenic and mutagenic; it may impair fertility or cause sterility and birth defects

Precautions Use with caution in patients with bone marrow suppression and impaired renal or hepatic function; modify dosage in patients with renal impairment or compromised bone marrow function. Patients with compromised bone marrow function may require a 33% to 50% reduction in initial dose.

Adverse Reactions

Cardiovascular: Pericardial effusion

Dermatologic: Alopecia, rash

Endocrine & metabolic: Amenorrhea, hyperkalemia, hyperuricemia, hyponatremia, oligospermia, SIADH, sterility (interferes with oogenesis and spermatogenesis) which may be irreversible

Gastrointestinal: Anorexia, diarrhea, dysgeusia, mucositis, nausea, vomiting

Genitourinary: Hemorrhagic cystitis (5% to 10%)

Hematologic: Hemolytic anemia, hypothrombinemia, leukopenia nadir at 8-15 days, thrombocytopenia

Hepatic: Dose-related hepatotoxicity

Renal: Nephrotoxicity

Respiratory: Nasal stuffiness

<1%, postmarketing, and/or case reports: High-dose therapy may cause cardiac dysfunction manifested as heart failure; cardiac necrosis or hemorrhagic myocarditis has occurred rarely, but may be fatal. Interstitial pneumonitis and pulmonary fibrosis are occasionally seen with high doses. Cyclophosphamide may also potentiate the cardiac toxicity of anthracyclines. Other adverse reactions include anaphylactic reactions, darkening of skin/fingernails, dizziness, hemorrhagic colitis, hemorrhagic ureteritis, hepatotoxicity, hyperuricemia, hypokalemia,

jaundice, malaise, neutrophilic eccrine hidradenitis, radiation recall, renal tubular necrosis, secondary malignancy (eg, bladder carcinoma), SIADH, Stevens-Johnson syndrome, toxic epidermal necrolysis, weakness

Drug Interactions

Metabolism/Transport Effects Substrate of CYP2A6 (minor), 2B6 (major), 2C9 (minor), 2C19 (minor), 3A4 (minor); **Inhibits** CYP3A4 (weak); **Induces** CYP2B6 (weak), 2C8 (weak), 2C9 (weak)

Avoid Concomitant Use

Avoid concomitant use of Cyclophosphamide with any of the following: BCG; Etanercept; Natalizumab; Pimecrolimus; Tacrolimus (Topical); Vaccines (Live)

Increased Effect/Toxicity

Cyclophosphamide may increase the levels/effects of: Leflunomide; Natalizumab; Succinylcholine; Vaccines (Live); Vitamin K Antagonists

The levels/effects of Cyclophosphamide may be increased by: Allopurinol; CYP2B6 Inhibitors (Moderate); CYP2B6 Inhibitors (Strong); Denosumab; Etanercept; Pentostatin; Pimecrolimus; Quazepam; Tacrolimus (Topical); Trastuzumab

Decreased Effect

Cyclophosphamide may decrease the levels/effects of: BCG; Cardiac Glycosides; Sipuleucel-T; Vaccines (Inactivated); Vaccines (Live); Vitamin K Antagonists

The levels/effects of Cyclophosphamide may be decreased by: CYP2B6 Inducers (Strong); Echinacea

Stability Reconstituted I.V. solution is stable for 24 hours at room temperature or 6 days if refrigerated

Mechanism of Action Interferes with the normal function of DNA by alkylation and cross-linking the strands of DNA, and by possible protein modification

Pharmacokinetics (Adult data unless noted)

Absorption: 75% to 95% with low doses

Distribution: Crosses the placenta; appears in breast milk; distributes throughout the body including the brain and CSF, but not in concentrations high enough to treat meningeal leukemia

Protein binding: 20%; metabolite: 60%

Metabolism: Inactive prodrug must undergo hydroxylation to form active alkylating mustards; further oxidation leads to formation of inactive metabolites

Half-life: Range 3-12 hours

Children: 4 hours

Adults: 6-8 hours

Time to peak serum concentration: Oral: Within 1 hour

Elimination: In urine as unchanged drug (<20%) and as metabolites (85% to 90%)

Dialysis: Moderately dialyzable (20% to 50%)

Usual Dosage Refer to individual protocols

Children and Adults with no hematologic problems:

Induction:

Oral, I.V.: Children: 2-8 mg/kg or 60-250 mg/m^2/day

I.V.: 40-50 mg/kg (1.5-1.8 g/m^2) in divided doses over 2-5 days

Maintenance:

Oral: Children: 2-5 mg/kg or 50-150 mg/m^2 twice weekly

Oral: Adults: 1-5 mg/kg/day

I.V.: 10-15 mg/kg (350-550 mg/m^2) every 7-10 days or 3-5 mg/kg (110-185 mg/m^2) twice weekly

Children:

SLE: I.V.: 500-750 mg/m^2 every month; maximum dose: 1 g/m^2

JRA/vasculitis: I.V.: 10 mg/kg every 2 weeks

BMT conditioning regimen: I.V.: 50 mg/kg/day once daily for 3-4 days

Nephrotic syndrome: Oral: 2-3 mg/kg/day every day for up to 12 weeks when corticosteroids are unsuccessful

Dosing adjustment in renal impairment:
Cl_{cr} >10 mL/minute: Administer 100% of normal dose
Cl_{cr} ≤10 mL/minute: Administer 75% of normal dose

Administration

Oral: Administer with food only if GI distress occurs
Parenteral: May administer IVP, I.V. intermittent, or continuous infusion at a final maximum concentration for administration of 20-25 mg/mL; usually administered as a single bolus dose or in fractionated doses over 2-3 days. Most protocols use a 30-60 minute infusion time; doses >1800 mg/m^2 need to be infused over a longer period (ie, 4- or 6-hour infusions)

Monitoring Parameters CBC with differential and platelet count, ESR, BUN, urinalysis, serum electrolytes, serum creatinine, urine specific gravity, urine output

Test Interactions Positive Coombs' [direct]

Patient Information Maintain high fluid intake and urine output. Report any difficulty or pain with urination, unusual bleeding or bruising, persistent fever or sore throat, blood in urine or stool, skin rash, or yellowing of skin or eyes. You may be more susceptible to infection; avoid crowds and unnecessary exposure to infection.

Nursing Implications Encourage adequate hydration and frequent voiding to help prevent hemorrhagic cystitis; before initiating cyclophosphamide therapy, verify that urine specific gravity is <1.010 and that urine output is >100 mL/m^2/hour (or 3 mL/kg/hour)

Additional Information Aggressive hydration using fluid containing at least 0.45% sodium chloride at 125 mL/m^2/hour, frequent emptying of the bladder, and concurrent administration of mesna are used to reduce the potential of hemorrhagic cystitis (use mesna with cyclophosphamide doses >1 g/m^2/day; doses ≤1 g/m^2/day may not require use of mesna)

Myelosuppressive effects:
WBC: Moderate
Platelets: Moderate
Onset (days): 7
Nadir (days): 8-14
Recovery (days): 21

Dosage Forms Excipient information presented when available (limited, particularly for generics); consult specific product labeling. [DSC] = Discontinued product
Injection, powder for reconstitution: 500 mg, 1 g, 2 g
Cytoxan®: 500 mg, 1 g, 2 g [DSC]
Tablet: 25 mg, 50 mg
Cytoxan®: 25 mg, 50 mg [DSC]

Extemporaneous Preparations To make a 2 mg/mL oral elixir, reconstitute a 200 mg vial with aromatic elixir, withdraw the solution, and add sufficient aromatic elixir to make a final volume of 100 mL in a graduate; store in amber glass; stable for 14 days in the refrigerator
Brook D, Davis RE, and Bequette RJ, "Chemical Stability of Cyclophosphamide in Aromatic Elixir USP," *Am J Hosp Pharm*, 1973, 30:618-20.

References

Bostrom BC, Weisdorf DJ, Kim TH, et al, "Bone Marrow Transplantation for Advanced Acute Leukemia: A Pilot Study of High-Energy Total Body Irradiation, Cyclophosphamide and Continuous Infusion Etoposide," *Bone Marrow Transplant*, 1990, 5(2):83-9.

McCune WJ, Golbus J, Zeldes W, et al, "Clinical and Immunologic Effects of Monthly Administration of Intravenous Cyclophosphamide in Severe Systemic Lupus Erythematosus," *N Engl J Med*, 1988, 318 (22):1423-31.

CycloSERINE (sye kloe SER een)

Medication Safety Issues

Sound-alike/look-alike issues:
CycloSERINE may be confused with cyclobenzaprine, cycloSPORINE

U.S. Brand Names Seromycin®

Therapeutic Category Antibiotic, Miscellaneous; Antitubercular Agent

Generic Available No

Use Adjunctive treatment in pulmonary or extrapulmonary tuberculosis; treatment of acute urinary tract infections caused by *E. coli* or *Enterobacter* species when less toxic conventional therapy has failed or is contraindicated

Pregnancy Risk Factor C

Lactation Enters breast milk/compatible

Contraindications Hypersensitivity to cycloserine or any component; epilepsy, depression, severe anxiety or psychosis, severe renal insufficiency, chronic alcoholism

Precautions Dosage must be adjusted in patients with renal impairment

Adverse Reactions
Cardiovascular: Cardiac arrhythmias, CHF
Central nervous system: Drowsiness, headache, dizziness, vertigo, seizures, confusion, psychosis, paresis, coma, anxiety, nervousness, depression, personality changes
Dermatologic: Rash, photosensitivity
Endocrine & metabolic: Vitamin B_{12} deficiency, folate deficiency
Hepatic: Liver enzymes elevated
Neuromuscular & skeletal: Tremor, dysarthria

Drug Interactions
Avoid Concomitant Use
Avoid concomitant use of CycloSERINE with any of the following: Alcohol (Ethyl); BCG
Increased Effect/Toxicity
The levels/effects of CycloSERINE may be increased by: Alcohol (Ethyl); Isoniazid
Decreased Effect
CycloSERINE may decrease the levels/effects of: BCG; Typhoid Vaccine

Food Interactions May increase vitamin B_{12} and folic acid dietary requirements

Mechanism of Action Inhibits bacterial cell wall synthesis by competing with amino acid (D-alanine) for incorporation into the bacterial cell wall

Pharmacokinetics (Adult data unless noted)
Absorption: ~70% to 90% from the GI tract
Distribution: Crosses the placenta; appears in breast milk, bile, sputum, synovial fluid and CSF
Protein binding: Not plasma protein bound
Half-life: Patients with normal renal function: 10 hours
Time to peak serum concentration: Within 3-4 hours
Elimination: 60% to 70% of an oral dose excreted unchanged in urine by glomerular filtration within 72 hours, small amounts excreted in feces, remainder is metabolized

Usual Dosage Oral:
Tuberculosis:
Children: 10-20 mg/kg/day divided every 12 hours up to 1000 mg/day
Adults: Initial: 250 mg every 12 hours for 14 days, then give 500 mg to 1 g/day in 2 divided doses
Urinary tract infection: Adults: 250 mg every 12 hours for 14 days

Dosing adjustment in renal impairment:
Cl_{cr} 10-50 mL/minute: Administer every 24 hours
Cl_{cr} <10 mL/minute: Administer every 36-48 hours

Administration Oral: May administer without regard to meals

Monitoring Parameters Periodic renal, hepatic, hematological tests, and plasma cycloserine concentrations

Reference Range Adjust dosage to maintain blood cycloserine concentrations <30 mcg/mL

Patient Information May cause drowsiness and impair ability to perform activities requiring mental alertness or physical coordination; avoid alcohol. May cause photosensitivity reactions (eg, exposure to sunlight may cause severe sunburn, skin rash, redness, or itching); avoid exposure to sunlight and artificial light sources (sunlamps, tanning booth/bed); wear protective clothing, wide-brimmed hats, sunglasses, and lip sunscreen (SPF ≥15); use a sunscreen [broad-spectrum sunscreen or physical sunscreen (preferred) or sunblock with SPF ≥15]; contact physician if reaction occurs.

Nursing Implications Some of the neurotoxic effects may be relieved or prevented by the concomitant administration of pyridoxine; sedatives may be effective in reducing anxiety or tremor

Dosage Forms Excipient information presented when available (limited, particularly for generics); consult specific product labeling.
Capsule: 250 mg

♦ **Cycloset®** see Bromocriptine *on page 203*
♦ **Cyclosporin A** see CycloSPORINE *on page 372*

CycloSPORINE (SYE kloe spor een)

Medication Safety Issues
Sound-alike/look-alike issues:
CycloSPORINE may be confused with cyclophospha-mide, Cyklokapron®, cycloSERINE
CycloSPORINE modified (Neoral®, Gengraf®) may be confused with cycloSPORINE non-modified (Sandimmne®)
Gengraf® may be confused with Prograf®
Neoral® may be confused with Neurontin®, Nizoral®
Sandimmune® may be confused with Sandostatin®

Related Information
Therapeutic Drug Monitoring: Blood Sampling Time Guidelines *on page 1704*

U.S. Brand Names Gengraf®; Neoral®; Restasis®; Sandimmune®

Canadian Brand Names Apo-Cyclosporine®; Neoral®; Rhoxal-cyclosporine; Sandimmune® I.V.; Sandoz-Cyclosporine

Therapeutic Category Immunosuppressant Agent

Generic Available Yes: Excludes ophthalmic emulsion

Use Immunosuppressant used with corticosteroids to prevent organ rejection in patients with kidney, liver, lung, heart, and bone marrow transplants; treatment of nephrotic syndrome in patients with documented focal glomerulo-sclerosis when corticosteroids and cyclophosphamide are unsuccessful; severe psoriasis; severe rheumatoid arthritis not responsive to methotrexate alone; severe autoimmune disease that is resistant to corticosteroids and other therapy; prevention and treatment of graft-versus-host disease in bone marrow transplant patients
Ophthalmic emulsion: Increase tear production in patients with moderate to severe keratoconjunctivitis sicca-associated ocular inflammation

Pregnancy Risk Factor C

Pregnancy Considerations Reproductive toxicity has been observed in animal studies; mutagenic and terato-genic effects were not observed in the standard test systems following oral administration. In humans, cyclo-sporine crosses the placenta. Based on clinical use, premature births and low birth weight were consistently observed. Use only if the benefit to the mother outweighs the possible risks to the fetus.

A pregnancy registry has been established for pregnant women taking immunosuppressants following any solid organ transplant (National Transplantation Pregnancy Registry, Temple University, 877-955-6877).

Lactation Enters breast milk/not recommended

Breast-Feeding Considerations The AAP does not recommend breast-feeding during therapy due to possible immune suppression in the infant as well as the unknown effects on growth or association with carcinogenesis.

Contraindications Hypersensitivity to cyclosporine or any component (ie, polyoxyl 35 castor oil is an ingredient of the parenteral formulation and polyoxyl 40 hydrogenated castor oil is an ingredient of the cyclosporine capsules and solution for microemulsion). AAP considers cyclo-sporine to be contraindicated during breast-feeding. Concurrent therapy with PUVA or UVB, methotrexate, coal tar, or radiation therapy for use in patients with psoriasis; presence of uncontrolled hypertension, abnor-mal renal function, or malignancies in treatment of psoriasis or rheumatoid arthritis. Ophthalmic emulsion is contraindicated in patients with active ocular infections.

Warnings Immunosuppression with cyclosporine may result in an increased susceptibility to infection **[U.S. Boxed Warning]**; fatal infections have been reported. May increase the risk of malignancy (lymphomas, lymphopro-liferative disorders, and squamous cell carcinoma) **[U.S. Boxed Warning]**; closely monitor and be prepared to treat anaphylaxis in patients receiving I.V. cyclosporine. Renal impairment, including structural kidney damage, has occurred (when used at high doses) **[U.S. Boxed Warning]**; serious nephrotoxicity, hepatotoxicity, hyper-tension, and/or seizures may occur in children receiving cyclosporine; **monitor renal function and adjust dosage to avoid toxicity or possible organ rejection via cyclosporine blood or plasma concentration monitor-ing.** Use caution when using with other nephrotoxic drugs.

Transplant patients: Cyclosporine may cause significant hyperkalemia and hyperuricemia. May cause seizures, particularly if used with high-dose corticosteroids. Predis-posing factors associated with neurological disorders include hypertension, hypomagnesemia, hypocholestero-lemia, high-dose corticosteroids, high cyclosporine serum concentration, and graft-versus-host disease. Risk of skin cancer may be increased in psoriasis patients with a history of PUVA and possibly methotrexate or other immunosuppressants, UVB, coal tar, or radiation **[U.S. Boxed Warning]**.

Precautions Close monitoring and dosage adjustment is required in patients with renal and hepatic impairment. Cyclosporine (modified) has increased bioavailability as compared to cyclosporine (non-modified) and cannot be used interchangeably without close monitoring **[U.S. Boxed Warning]**; use caution when changing dosage forms since products cannot be used interchangeably.

Adverse Reactions
Cardiovascular: Hypertension, flushing, edema, arrhythmia

Central nervous system: Seizures, headache, confusion, fever, anxiety, lethargy, dizziness, depression

Dermatologic: Hirsutism, gingival hyperplasia, acne, hypertrichosis, pruritus

Endocrine & metabolic: Hyperkalemia, hypomagnesemia, hyperuricemia, hyperchloremic metabolic acidosis, gyne-comastia, hyperlipidemia (in patients receiving I.V. cyclo-sporine), weight loss

Gastrointestinal: Abdominal discomfort, diarrhea, nausea, vomiting, anorexia, pancreatitis, hiccups, peptic ulcer, stomatitis

Hematologic: Leukopenia, anemia, thrombocytopenia

Hepatic: Hepatotoxicity (liver enzymes elevated, hyperbilirubinemia)

Neuromuscular & skeletal: Myositis, tremor, paresthesia, leg cramps, weakness

Ocular: Ophthalmic preparation: Ocular burning, hyper-emia, eye pain, pruritus, stinging

Otic: Tinnitus, hearing loss

Renal: Nephrotoxicity (BUN and serum creatinine elevated)

Respiratory: Sinusitis, cough, dyspnea

Miscellaneous: Lymphoproliferative disorder, susceptibility to infection increased, sensitivity to temperature extremes, anaphylaxis in patients receiving I.V. cyclosporine (reaction includes flushing of the face, respiratory distress with dyspnea and wheezing, hypotension, tachycardia), flu-like symptoms

Drug Interactions

Metabolism/Transport Effects Substrate of CYP3A4 (major), P-glycoprotein; **Inhibits** CYP2C9 (weak), CYP3A4 (moderate), P-glycoprotein

Avoid Concomitant Use

Avoid concomitant use of CycloSPORINE with any of the following: Aliskiren; BCG; Bosentan; Dabigatran Etexilate; Dronedarone; Natalizumab; Pimecrolimus; Pitavastatin; Silodosin; Sitaxsentan; Tacrolimus; Tacrolimus (Topical); Tolvaptan; Topotecan; Vaccines (Live)

Increased Effect/Toxicity

CycloSPORINE may increase the levels/effects of: Aliskiren; Ambrisentan; Bosentan; Calcium Channel Blockers (Dihydropyridine); Calcium Channel Blockers (Nondihydropyridine); Cardiac Glycosides; Caspofungin; Colchicine; CYP3A4 Substrates; Dabigatran Etexilate; DOXOrubicin; Dronedarone; Eplerenone; Etoposide; Etoposide Phosphate; Everolimus; Ezetimibe; FentaNYL; Fibric Acid Derivatives; Halofantrine; HMG-CoA Reductase Inhibitors; Imipenem; Leflunomide; Methotrexate; Minoxidil; Minoxidil (Systemic); Minoxidil (Topical); Natalizumab; P-Glycoprotein Substrates; Pitavastatin; PrednisoLONE; PrednisoLONE (Systemic); PredniSONE; Protease Inhibitors; Ranolazine; Repaglinide; Rivaroxaban; Salmeterol; Saxagliptin; Silodosin; Sirolimus; Sitaxsentan; Tacrolimus; Tacrolimus (Topical); Tolvaptan; Topotecan; Vaccines (Live)

The levels/effects of CycloSPORINE may be increased by: ACE Inhibitors; Aminoglycosides; Amiodarone; Amphotericin B; Androgens; Antifungal Agents (Azole Derivatives, Systemic); Bromocriptine; Calcium Channel Blockers (Nondihydropyridine); Carvedilol; CYP3A4 Inhibitors (Moderate); CYP3A4 Inhibitors (Strong); Dasatinib; Denosumab; Ezetimibe; Fluconazole; Grapefruit Juice; Imatinib; Imipenem; Macrolide Antibiotics; Melphalan; Methotrexate; MethylPREDNISolone; Metoclopramide; MetroNIDAZOLE; MetroNIDAZOLE (Systemic); Nonsteroidal Anti-Inflammatory Agents; Norfloxacin; Omeprazole; P-Glycoprotein Inhibitors; Pimecrolimus; PrednisoLONE; PrednisoLONE (Systemic); PredniSONE; Protease Inhibitors; Quinupristin; Sirolimus; Sulfonamide Derivatives; Sulfonylureas; Tacrolimus; Tacrolimus (Topical); Temsirolimus; Trastuzumab

Decreased Effect

CycloSPORINE may decrease the levels/effects of: BCG; Mycophenolate; Sipuleucel-T; Vaccines (Inactivated); Vaccines (Live)

The levels/effects of CycloSPORINE may be decreased by: Barbiturates; Bosentan; CarBAMazepine; CYP3A4 Inducers (Strong); Deferasirox; Echinacea; Efavirenz; Fibric Acid Derivatives; Griseofulvin; Imipenem; Nafcillin; Orlistat; P-Glycoprotein Inducers; Phenytoin; Probucol; Pyrazinamide; Rifamycin Derivatives; Somatostatin Analogs; St Johns Wort; Sulfinpyrazone [Off Market]; Sulfonamide Derivatives; Terbinafine; Terbinafine (Systemic)

Food Interactions Grapefruit and grapefruit juice may affect cyclosporine metabolism resulting in increased cyclosporine concentrations

Stability Do **not** store oral solution or oral solution for emulsion in the refrigerator; store oral solutions in original container only and use contents within 2 months after opening; store ampuls and ophthalmic emulsion-containing vials at room temperature; protect from light; I.V. cyclosporine prepared in NS is stable 6 hours in a polyvinyl chloride container or 12 hours in a glass container; I.V. cyclosporine diluted in D_5W to a final concentration of 2 mg/mL is stable for 24 hours in glass or polyvinyl chloride containers; I.V. cyclosporine may bind to the plastic tubing in I.V. administration sets and to polyvinyl chloride bags. Polyoxyethylated castor oil (Cremophor EI®) surfactant in cyclosporine injection may leach phthalate from polyvinyl chloride containers such as bags and tubing.

Mechanism of Action Inhibition of production and release of interleukin II and inhibits interleukin II-induced activation of resting T lymphocytes

Pharmacokinetics (Adult data unless noted)

Absorption: Oral:

Cyclosporine (non-modified) solution or soft gelatin capsule: Erratically and incompletely absorbed; dependent on the presence of food, bile acids, and GI motility; larger oral doses of cyclosporine are needed in pediatric patients vs adults due to a shorter bowel length resulting in limited intestinal absorption

Cyclosporine (modified) solution in a microemulsion or soft gelatin capsule in a microemulsion: Erratically and incompletely absorbed; increased absorption, up to 30% when compared to cyclosporine (non-modified); absorption is less dependent on food intake, bile, or GI motility when compared to cyclosporine (non-modified)

Distribution: Widely distributed in tissues and body fluids including the liver, pancreas, and lungs; crosses the placenta; excreted into breast milk

V_{dss}: 4-6 L/kg in renal, liver, and marrow transplant recipients (slightly lower values in cardiac transplant patients; children <10 years of age have higher values)

Protein binding: 90% to 98% of dose binds to blood lipoproteins

Metabolism: Undergoes extensive first-pass metabolism following oral administration; extensively metabolized by the cytochrome P450 system in the liver; forms at least 25 metabolites

Bioavailability:

Cyclosporine (non-modified): Dependent on patient population and transplant type (<10% in adult liver transplant patients and as high as 89% in renal patients). The bioavailability of Sandimmune® capsules and oral solution are equivalent; bioavailability of oral solution is ~30% of the I.V. solution.

Children: 28% (range: 17% to 42%); with gut dysfunction commonly seen in BMT recipients, oral bioavailability is further reduced

Cyclosporine (modified): Bioavailability of Neoral® capsules and oral solution are equivalent:

Children: 43% (range: 30% to 68%)

Adults: 23% greater than with Sandimmune® in renal transplant patients, 50% greater in liver transplant patients

Half-life: May be prolonged in patients with hepatic impairment and lower in pediatric patients due to a higher metabolic rate

Cyclosporine (non-modified): Biphasic

Alpha phase: 1.4 hours

Terminal phase: 6-24 hours

Cyclosporine (modified): 8.4 hours (range: 5-18 hours)

Time to peak serum concentration:

Cyclosporine (non-modified): 2-6 hours; some patients have a second peak at 5-6 hours

Cyclosporine (modified): 1.5-2 hours (in renal transplant patients)

Elimination: Primarily biliary with 6% of the dose excreted in urine as unchanged drug (0.1%) and metabolites; clearance is more rapid in pediatric patients than in adults

Usual Dosage Children and Adults (oral dosage is ~3 times the I.V. dosage):

Transplantations:

I.V.: Cyclosporine (non-modified):

Initial: 5-6 mg/kg/dose ($^1/_3$ the oral dose) administered 4-12 hours prior to organ transplantation

Maintenance: 2-10 mg/kg/day in divided doses every 8-24 hours; patients should be switched to oral cyclosporine as soon as possible; cyclosporine doses should be adjusted to maintain whole blood HPLC trough concentrations in the reference range

Oral: Cyclosporine (non-modified):

Initial: 14-18 mg/kg/dose administered 4-12 hours prior to organ transplantation; lower initial doses of 10-14 mg/kg/day have been used for renal transplants

Maintenance, postoperative: 5-15 mg/kg/day divided every 12-24 hours; maintenance dose is usually tapered to 3-10 mg/kg/day

When using non-modified formulation, cyclosporine levels may increase in liver transplant patients when the T-tube is closed; may need to decrease dose

Oral: Cyclosporine (modified): Based on the organ transplant population:

Initial: Same as the initial dose for solution or soft gelatin capsule

or

Renal: 9 mg/kg/day (range: 6-12 mg/kg/day) divided every 12 hours

Liver: 8 mg/kg/day (range: 4-12 mg/kg/day) divided every 12 hours

Heart: 7 mg/kg/day (range: 4-10 mg/kg/day) divided every 12 hours

Note: A 1:1 ratio conversion from Sandimmune® to Neoral® has been recommended initially; however, lower doses of Neoral® may be required after conversion to prevent overdose. Total daily doses should be adjusted based on the cyclosporine trough blood concentration and clinical assessment of organ rejection. Cyclosporine blood trough levels should be determined prior to conversion. After conversion to Neoral®, cyclosporine trough levels should be monitored every 4-7 days. **Neoral® and Sandimmune® are not bioequivalent and cannot be used interchangeably.**

Focal segmental glomerulosclerosis: Oral: Initial: 3 mg/kg/day divided every 12 hours

Rheumatoid arthritis: Oral: Cyclosporine (modified): Initial: 2.5 mg/kg/day divided every 12 hours; may increase dose by 0.5-0.75 mg/kg/day if insufficient response is seen after 8 weeks of treatment; maximum dose: 4 mg/kg/day

Psoriasis: Oral: Cyclosporine (modified): Initial: 2.5 mg/kg/day divided every 12 hours; may increase dose by 0.5 mg/kg/day if insufficient response is seen after 4 weeks of treatment; maximum dose: 4 mg/kg/day

Autoimmune diseases: Oral: 1-3 mg/kg/day

Ophthalmic: Children ≥16 years and Adults: Instill one drop in affected eye(s) every 12 hours

Administration

Oral: Administer consistently at the same time twice daily; use oral syringe, glass dropper, or glass container (not plastic or styrofoam cup); to improve palatability, oral solution may be mixed with milk, chocolate milk, orange juice, or apple juice that is at room temperature; dilution of Neoral® with milk can be unpalatable; stir well and drink at once; do not allow to stand before drinking; rinse with more diluent to ensure that the total dose is taken; after use, dry outside of glass dropper, do not rinse with water or other cleaning agents

Parenteral: May administer by I.V. intermittent infusion or continuous infusion; for intermittent infusion, administer over 2-6 hours at a final concentration not to exceed 2.5 mg/mL. Anaphylaxis has been reported with I.V. use.

Patients should be continuously monitored for at least the first 30 minutes of the infusion, and should be monitored frequently thereafter

Ophthalmic: Invert vial prior to use to obtain a uniform emulsion. Avoid contact of vial tip with skin or eye; remove contact lenses prior to administration; lenses may be inserted 15 minutes after instillation. May be used with artificial tears; separate administration by at least 15 minutes.

Monitoring Parameters Blood/serum drug concentration (trough), renal and hepatic function tests, serum electrolytes, lipid profile, blood pressure, heart rate

Reference Range Reference ranges are method dependent and specimen dependent; use the same analytical method consistently; trough levels should be obtained immediately prior to next dose

Therapeutic: Not well defined, dependent on organ transplanted, time after transplant, organ function, and cyclosporine toxicity. Empiric therapeutic concentration ranges for trough cyclosporine concentrations:

Kidney: 100-200 ng/mL (serum, RIA)

BMT: 100-250 ng/mL (serum, RIA)

Heart: 100-200 ng/mL (serum, RIA)

Liver: 100-400 ng/mL (blood, HPLC)

Method dependent (optimum cyclosporine trough concentrations):

Serum, RIA: 150-300 ng/mL; 50-150 ng/mL (late post-transplant period)

Whole blood, RIA: 250-800 ng/mL; 150-450 ng/mL (late post-transplant period)

Whole blood, HPLC: 100-500 ng/mL

Test Interactions Cyclosporine adsorbs to silicone; specific whole blood assay for cyclosporine may be falsely elevated if sample is drawn from the same central venous line through which dose was administered (even if flush has been administered and/or dose was given hours before); cyclosporine metabolites cross-react with radioimmunoassay and fluorescence polarization immunoassay

Patient Information Avoid the herbal medicine St John's wort; take dose at the same time each day; do not allow diluted oral solution to stand before drinking; do not change brands of cyclosporine unless directed by your physician. Patients with psoriasis should avoid excessive sun exposure. Notify physician of severe headache; persistent nausea, vomiting; muscle pain or cramping; unusual swelling of extremities; chest pain or rapid heartbeat.

Nursing Implications Adequate airway, supportive measures, epinephrine and I.V. steroids for treating anaphylaxis should be present when I.V. cyclosporine is administered

Additional Information Diltiazem has been used to prevent cyclosporine nephrotoxicity, reduce the frequency of delayed graft function when administered before and after surgery, and used to treat the mild hypertension that occurs in most patients after transplantation; diltiazem increases cyclosporine blood concentration by delaying its clearance resulting in decreased dosage requirements for cyclosporine

Dosage Forms Excipient information presented when available (limited, particularly for generics); consult specific product labeling.

Capsule [modified]:

Gengraf®: 25 mg [contains alcohol 12.8%]; 100 mg [contains alcohol 12.8%]

Capsule [non-modified]: 25 mg, 100 mg

Capsule, soft gel [modified]: 25 mg, 50 mg, 100 mg

Neoral®: 25 mg [contains alcohol 11.9% and corn oil]; 100 mg [contains alcohol 11.9% and corn oil]

Capsule, soft gel [non-modified]:
Sandimmune®: 25 mg [contains alcohol 12.7% and corn oil]; 100 mg [contains alcohol 12.7% and corn oil]
Emulsion, ophthalmic [preservative free]:
Restasis®: 0.05% (0.4 mL) [contains 30 single-use vials/box]
Injection, solution [non-modified]: 50 mg/mL (5 mL)
Sandimmune®: 50 mg/mL (5 mL) [contains Cremophor® EL (polyoxyethylated castor oil) and alcohol 32.9%]
Solution, oral [modified]: 100 mg/mL (50 mL)
Gengraf®: 100 mg/mL (50 mL) [contains propylene glycol]
Neoral®: 100 mg/mL (50 mL) [contains alcohol 11.9%, corn oil, and propylene glycol]
Solution, oral [non-modified]: 100 mg/mL (50 mL)
Sandimmune®: 100 mg/mL (50 mL) [contains alcohol 12.5%]

References

Burckart GJ, Canafax DM, and Yee GC, "Cyclosporine Monitoring," *Drug Intell Clin Pharm*, 1986, 20(9):649-52.

Holt DW, Mueller EA, Kovarik JM, et al, "Sandimmune® Neoral® Pharmacokinetics: Impact of the New Oral Formulation," *Transplant Proc*, 1995, 27(1):1434-7.

Lin CY and Lee SF, "Comparison of Pharmacokinetics Between CsA Capsules and Sandimmune® Neoral® in Pediatric Patients," *Transplant Proc*, 1994, 26(5):2973-4.

Niese D, "A Double-Blind Randomized Study of Sandimmune® Neoral® vs Sandimmune® in New Renal Transplant Recipients: Results After 12 Months," *Transplant Proc*, 1995, 27(2):1849-56.

Taesch S, Niese D, and Mueller EA, "Sandimmune® Neoral®, A New Oral Formulation of Cyclosporine With Improved Pharmacokinetic Characteristics: Safety and Tolerability in Renal Transplant Patients," *Transplant Proc*, 1994, 26(6):3147-9.

Wandstrat TL, Schroeder TJ, and Myre SA, "Cyclosporine Pharmacokinetics in Pediatric Transplant Recipients," *Ther Drug Monit*, 1989, 11(5):493-6.

Yee GC, "Recent Advances in Cyclosporine Pharmacokinetics," *Pharmacotherapy*, 1991, 11(5):130S-134S.

◆ **Cyklokapron®** *see* Tranexamic Acid *on page 1369*

◆ **Cylate™** *see* Cyclopentolate *on page 368*

◆ **Cylex® [OTC] [DSC]** *see* Benzocaine *on page 182*

Cyproheptadine (si proe HEP ta deen)

Medication Safety Issues
Sound-alike/look-alike issues:
Cyproheptadine may be confused with cyclobenzaprine
Periactin may be confused with Perative®, Percodan®, Persantine®

Beers Criteria medication: This drug may be inappropriate for use in geriatric patients (high severity risk).

Therapeutic Category Antihistamine

Generic Available Yes

Use
Perennial and seasonal allergic rhinitis and other allergic symptoms including urticaria; appetite stimulant (useful in the management of anorexia nervosa); prophylactic treatment of cluster and migraine headaches; spinal cord damage associated with spasticity

Pregnancy Risk Factor B

Lactation
Excretion in breast milk unknown/contraindicated

Contraindications
Hypersensitivity to cyproheptadine or any component; narrow-angle glaucoma, bladder neck obstruction, acute asthmatic attack, stenosing peptic ulcer, GI tract obstruction, those on MAO inhibitors

Adverse Reactions
Cardiovascular: Tachycardia, palpitations, edema
Central nervous system: Sedation, CNS stimulation, seizures, fatigue, headache, nervousness, depression
Dermatologic: Photosensitivity, rash, angioedema
Gastrointestinal: Appetite stimulation, xerostomia, nausea, diarrhea, abdominal pain
Hematologic: Hemolytic anemia, leukopenia, thrombocytopenia
Hepatic: Hepatitis
Neuromuscular & skeletal: Myalgia, paresthesia, arthralgia
Respiratory: Bronchospasm, epistaxis, pharyngitis
Miscellaneous: Allergic reactions

Drug Interactions
Avoid Concomitant Use There are no known interactions where it is recommended to avoid concomitant use.

Increased Effect/Toxicity
Cyproheptadine may increase the levels/effects of: Alcohol (Ethyl); Anticholinergics; CNS Depressants

The levels/effects of Cyproheptadine may be increased by: Pramlintide

Decreased Effect
Cyproheptadine may decrease the levels/effects of: Acetylcholinesterase Inhibitors (Central); Betahistine; Selective Serotonin Reuptake Inhibitors

The levels/effects of Cyproheptadine may be decreased by: Acetylcholinesterase Inhibitors (Central); Amphetamines

Mechanism of Action
A potent antihistamine and serotonin antagonist, competes with histamine for H_1-receptor sites on effector cells in the GI tract, blood vessels, and respiratory tract

Pharmacokinetics (Adult data unless noted)
Absorption: Well absorbed
Metabolism: Extensively by conjugation
Elimination: >50% excreted in urine (primarily as metabolites); approximately 25% excreted in feces

Usual Dosage Oral:
Allergic conditions:
Children: 0.25 mg/kg/day or 8 mg/m^2/day in 2-3 divided doses **or**
2-6 years: 2 mg every 8-12 hours (not to exceed 12 mg/day)
7-14 years: 4 mg every 8-12 hours (not to exceed 16 mg/day)
Adults: 4-20 mg/day divided every 8 hours (not to exceed 0.5 mg/kg/day)
Appetite stimulation (anorexia nervosa): Children >13 years and Adults: 2 mg 4 times/day; may be increased gradually over a 3-week period to 8 mg 4 times/day
Cluster headaches: Adults: 4 mg 4 times/day
Migraine headaches:
Children: 4 mg 2-3 times/day
Adults: 4-8 mg 3 times/day
Spasticity associated with spinal cord damage: Children ≥12 years and Adults: 4 mg at bedtime; increase by a 4 mg dose every 3-4 days; average daily dose: 16 mg in divided doses; not to exceed 36 mg/day

Dosage adjustment in hepatic impairment:
Reduce dosage in patients with significant hepatic dysfunction

Administration Oral:
Administer with food or milk

Test Interactions
Diagnostic antigen skin tests; ↑ amylase (S); ↓ fasting glucose (S)

Patient Information
May cause drowsiness and impair ability to perform activities requiring mental alertness or physical coordination; may cause dry mouth. May rarely cause photosensitivity reactions (eg, exposure to sunlight may cause severe sunburn, skin rash, redness, or itching); avoid direct exposure to sunlight

Dosage Forms
Excipient information presented when available (limited, particularly for generics); consult specific product labeling.
Syrup, as hydrochloride: 2 mg/5 mL (473 mL) [contains alcohol 5%; mint flavor]
Tablet, as hydrochloride: 4 mg

References

Gracies JM, Nance P, Elovic E, et al, "Traditional Pharmacological Treatments for Spasticity. Part II: General and Regional Treatments," *Muscle Nerve Suppl*, 1997, 6:S92-120.

◆ **Cyproheptadine Hydrochloride** *see* Cyproheptadine *on page 375*

◆ **Cystadane®** *see* Betaine *on page 188*

◆ **Cystagon®** *see* Cysteamine *on page 376*

Cysteamine (sis TEE a meen)

U.S. Brand Names Cystagon®
Therapeutic Category Cystinosis, Treatment Agent
Generic Available No
Use Management of nephropathic cystinosis
Pregnancy Risk Factor C
Pregnancy Considerations Use only when the potential benefits outweigh the potential hazards to the fetus; in animal studies, cysteamine is teratogenic and fetotoxic. There are no adequate and well-controlled studies in pregnant women.
Lactation Excretion in breast milk unknown/not recommended
Breast-Feeding Considerations It is unknown whether cysteamine is excreted in breast milk. Discontinue nursing or discontinue drug during lactation.
Contraindications Hypersensitivity to cysteamine, penicillamine, or any component
Warnings Leukocyte cystine levels should be monitored during oral cysteamine therapy (at least every 3 months); cysteamine should be given in the lowest dose possible to achieve adequate leukocyte cystine depletion; toxicity may be reduced by initiating therapy with a slowly increasing dose schedule (see Usual Dosage); if skin rash develops, discontinue treatment until rash clears; may then resume treatment at a lower dose with a slow titration to the therapeutic dose; if severe rash develops (eg, erythema multiforme bullosa or toxic epidermal necrolysis), immediately discontinue and do not resume therapy. High doses of cysteamine salts have been associated with purplish hemorrhagic lesions over the elbow area on both arms and have been described as molluscoid pseudotumors. Skin striae, bone lesions (described as osteopenia, compression fractures, scoliosis, and genu valgum) along with leg pain and joint hyperextension may also be present. Reduce dosage if this reaction occurs. Routine monitoring of skin and bones is recommended.

CNS symptoms such as seizures, lethargy, somnolence, depression, and encephalopathy have been associated with cysteamine therapy; patients who develop these symptoms should be carefully evaluated and the dosage adjusted as necessary. Benign intracranial hypertension (or pseudotumor cerebri) and/or papilledema with cysteamine therapy has resolved with diuretic therapy.

Precautions Use with caution in patients with a history of blood dyscrasias, gastric or duodenal ulcer, or neurologic disorder

Adverse Reactions
Cardiovascular: Hypertension
Central nervous system: Somnolence, encephalopathy, headache, seizures, ataxia, confusion, dizziness, jitteriness, nervousness, impaired cognition, emotional changes, hallucinations, nightmares, fever (22%), lethargy (11%), depression, hyperthermia, abnormal thinking, benign intracranial hypertension (or pseudotumor cerebri)
Dermatologic: Urticaria, rash (7%), molluscoid pseudotumors, skin striae, skin fragility (see Warnings)
Endocrine & metabolic: Dehydration
Gastrointestinal: Bad breath, abdominal pain, dyspepsia, constipation, gastroenteritis, duodenitis, duodenal ulceration and bleeding, vomiting (35%), anorexia (31%), diarrhea (16%), nausea
Hematologic: Anemia, leukopenia (reversible)
Hepatic: Abnormal liver enzymes

Neuromuscular & skeletal: Tremor, hyperkinesias, joint hyperextension, leg pain, osteopenia, compression fracture, scoliosis
Ocular: Papilledema
Otic: Hearing decreased
Renal: Interstitial nephritis, renal failure
Drug Interactions
Avoid Concomitant Use There are no known interactions where it is recommended to avoid concomitant use.
Increased Effect/Toxicity There are no known significant interactions involving an increase in effect.
Decreased Effect There are no known significant interactions involving a decrease in effect.
Stability Store at room temperature; protect from light
Mechanism of Action Reacts with cystine in the lysosome to convert it to cysteine and to a cysteine-cysteamine mixed disulfide, both of which can then exit the lysosome in patients with cystinosis, an inherited defect of cystine transport. Patients with untreated cystinosis develop renal tubular Fanconi syndrome leading to progressive glomerular failure and end-stage renal failure in addition to growth failure, rickets, and photophobia due to cystine deposits in the cornea.
Pharmacodynamics
Peak effect: 1.8 hours
Duration: 6 hours
Pharmacokinetics (Adult data unless noted)
Absorption: Rapid
Distribution: V_d: Children: 156 L
Protein binding: Mean: 52%
Half-life: 1 hour
Time to peak serum concentration: 1.4 hours
Elimination: Clearance: Children: 1.2 L/minute
Usual Dosage Dose-related side effects resulting in withdrawal from research studies occurred more frequently in those patients receiving 1.95 g/m^2/day as compared to 1.3 g/m^2/day; start at the lowest dose and titrate gradually to prevent intolerance.
Oral: Initiate therapy with 1/4 to 1/6 of maintenance dose and titrate slowly over 4-6 weeks:
Children <12 years: Initial: 1.3 g/m^2/day in 4 divided doses; may increase gradually to a maximum of 1.95 g/m^2/day
Children ≥12 years (>110 lbs) and Adults (>110 lbs): 2 g/day in 4 divided doses; dosage may be increased gradually to 1.95 g/m^2/day

Approximate Cysteamine Initial Dose
(to achieve ~1.3 g/m^2/day)

Weight (lbs)	Dose (mg every 6 h)
≤10	100
11-20	150
21-30	200
31-40	250
41-50	300
51-70	350
71-90	400
91-110	450
>110	500

Administration Oral: Contents of capsule may be sprinkled over food; if a dose is missed, take it as soon as possible then return to normal dosing schedule; if identified within 2 hours of next scheduled dose, skip dose; do **not** double the next dose

Monitoring Parameters Blood counts and liver enzymes during therapy; blood pressure; monitor leukocyte cystine measurements to determine adequate dosage and compliance (measure 5-6 hours after administration); monitor skin and bone (see Warnings)

Reference Range Leukocyte cystine level goal (measured 5-6 hours after cysteamine dose): <1 nmol of half-cystine/mg protein (some measurable benefits have been seen with levels <2); routine measurements are recommended every 3 months

Patient Information May cause drowsiness or impair ability to perform activities requiring mental alertness or physical coordination; notify healthcare provider if skin rash, changes to skin, stomach pain, nausea, vomiting, loss of appetite, severe headache, or a change in vision occurs.

Dosage Forms Excipient information presented when available (limited, particularly for generics); consult specific product labeling.
Capsule:
Cystagon®: 50 mg, 150 mg

◆ **Cysteamine Bitartrate** see Cysteamine on page 376

Cysteine (SIS teen)

U.S. Brand Names Cysteine-500
Therapeutic Category Nutritional Supplement
Generic Available Yes
Use Supplement to crystalline amino acid solutions, in particular the specialized pediatric formulas (eg, Aminosyn® PF, TrophAmine®) to meet the intravenous amino acid nutritional requirements of infants receiving parenteral nutrition (PN)

Contraindications Hypersensitivity to cysteine or any component; patients with hepatic coma or metabolic disorders involving impaired nitrogen utilization

Warnings Metabolic acidosis has occurred in infants related to the "hydrochloride" component of cysteine; each 1 mmol cysteine (175 mg) delivers 1 mEq chloride and 1 mEq hydrogen ion; to balance the extra hydrochloride ions and prevent acidosis, addition to the PN solution of a 1 mEq acetate electrolyte salt for each mmol (175 mg) of cysteine may be needed; each 40 mg cysteine (equal to every 1 g amino acid when used in the recommended ratio) adds 0.228 mEq chloride and hydrogen

Precautions Use with caution in patients with renal dysfunction and hepatic insufficiency

Adverse Reactions
Central nervous system: Fever
Endocrine & metabolic: Metabolic acidosis (see Warnings)
Gastrointestinal: Nausea
Renal: BUN elevated, azotemia

Stability Avoid excessive heat, do not freeze; when combined with parenteral amino acid solutions, cysteine is relatively unstable; it is intended to be added immediately prior to administration to the patient; infusion of the admixture should begin within 1 hour of mixing or refrigerated until use; stable 24 hours in PN solution; opened vials must be used within 4 hours of entry

Mechanism of Action Cysteine is a sulfur-containing amino acid synthesized from methionine via the transulfuration pathway. It is a precursor of the tripeptide glutathione and also of taurine. Newborn infants have a relative deficiency of the enzyme necessary to affect this conversion. Cysteine may be considered an essential amino acid in infants.

Usual Dosage I.V.: Neonates and Infants: Added as a fixed ratio to crystalline amino acid solution: 40 mg cysteine per g of amino acids; dosage will vary with the daily amino acid dosage (eg, 0.5-2.5 g/kg/day amino acids would result in 20-100 mg/kg/day cysteine); individual doses of cysteine of 0.8-1 mmol/kg/day have also been added directly to the daily PN solution; the duration of treatment relates to the need for PN; patients on chronic PN therapy have received cysteine until 6 months of age and in some cases until 2 years of age

Administration Parenteral: Use only after dilution into PN solution; dilute with amino acid solution in a ratio of 40 mg cysteine to 1 g amino acid: eg, 500 mg cysteine is added to 12.5 g (250 mL) of 5% amino acid solution

Monitoring Parameters BUN, ammonia, electrolytes, pH, acid-base balance, serum creatinine, liver function tests, growth curve

Additional Information Addition of cysteine to PN solutions enhances the solubility of calcium and phosphate by lowering the overall pH of the solution

Dosage Forms Excipient information presented when available (limited, particularly for generics); consult specific product labeling.
Capsule:
Cysteine-500: 500 mg
Injection, solution, as hydrochloride: 50 mg/mL (10 mL, 50 mL)

◆ **Cysteine-500** see Cysteine on page 377
◆ **Cysteine Hydrochloride** see Cysteine on page 377
◆ **CYT** see Cyclophosphamide on page 369

Cytarabine (sye TARE a been)

Medication Safety Issues
Sound-alike/look-alike issues:
Cytarabine may be confused with Cytadren®, Cytosar®, Cytoxan, vidarabine
Cytarabine (conventional) may be confused with cytarabine liposomal
Cytosar-U may be confused with cytarabine, Cytovene®, Cytoxan, Neosar®

High alert medication: This medication is in a class the Institute for Safe Medication Practices (ISMP) includes among its list of drugs which have a heightened risk of causing significant patient harm when used in error.

Intrathecal medication safety: The American Society of Clinical Oncology (ASCO)/Oncology Nursing Society (ONS) chemotherapy administration safety standards (Jacobson, 2009) encourage the following safety measures for intrathecal chemotherapy:
• Intrathecal medication should not be prepared during the preparation of any other agents
• After preparation, store in an isolated location or container clearly marked with a label identifying as "intrathecal" use only
• Delivery to the patient should only be with other medications intended for administration into the central nervous system

Related Information
Compatibility of Chemotherapy and Related Supportive Care Medications on page 1580
Emetogenic Potential of Antineoplastic Agents on page 1579

Canadian Brand Names Cytosar®
Therapeutic Category Antineoplastic Agent, Antimetabolite
Generic Available Yes
Use Used in combination regimens for the treatment of leukemias, meningeal leukemia, Hodgkin's lymphoma, and non-Hodgkin's lymphoma

Pregnancy Risk Factor D
Pregnancy Considerations Cytarabine is teratogenic in animal studies. Limb and ear defects have been noted in case reports when cytarabine has been used during pregnancy. The following have also been noted in the

neonate: Pancytopenia, WBC depression, electrolyte abnormalities, prematurity, low birth weight, decreased hematocrit or platelets. Risk to the fetus is decreased if therapy is avoided during the 1st trimester; however, women of childbearing potential should be advised of the potential risks.

Lactation Excretion in breast milk unknown/not recommended

Breast-Feeding Considerations Due to the potential for serious adverse reactions in the nursing infant, breast-feeding is not recommended.

Contraindications Hypersensitivity to cytarabine or any component

Warnings Hazardous agent; use appropriate precautions for handling and disposal. Causes significant bone marrow depression (leukopenia, thrombocytopenia, and anemia) **[U.S. Boxed Warning]**; use with caution in patients with prior bone marrow suppression; monitor for signs of febrile neutropenia. Must monitor for drug toxicity; high dose regimens have been associated with GI, CNS, pulmonary, ocular (prophylaxis with ophthalmic corticosteroids is recommended) toxicities, and cardiomyopathy. Neurotoxicity associated with high-dose treatment may present as acute cerebellar toxicity or may be severe with seizure and/or coma; may be delayed, occurring up to 3-8 days after treatment has begun; possibly irreversible. Risk factors for neurotoxicity include cumulative cytarabine dose, prior CNS disease, and renal impairment (incidence may be up to 55% in patients with renal impairment). May cause nausea, vomiting, diarrhea, abdominal pain, oral ulceration, and hepatic dysfunction; irreversible cerebellar toxicity may occur. There have been reports of acute pancreatitis in patients receiving continuous infusion and in patients previously treated with L-asparaginase.

When used for intrathecal administration, should not be prepared during the preparation of any other agents; after preparation, store intrathecal medications in an isolated location or container clearly marked with a label identifying as "intrathecal" use only; delivery of intrathecal medications to the patient should only be with other medications intended for administration into the central nervous system (see Jacobson, 2009).

Precautions Marked bone marrow suppression necessitates dosage reduction or a reduction in the number of days of administration; with severe hepatic dysfunction, dosage may need to be reduced; with high dose therapy, tumor lysis syndrome and subsequent hyperuricemia may occur; consider allopurinol and hydrate accordingly

Adverse Reactions
Cardiovascular: Cardiomegaly, chest pain, pericarditis
Central nervous system: Headache, malaise, confusion, seizures, fever, irritability, cerebral and cerebellar dysfunction (somnolence, personality changes, coma, ataxia)
Dermatologic: Alopecia, rash
Endocrine & metabolic: Hyperuricemia
Gastrointestinal: Nausea, vomiting, oral and anal inflammation with ulceration, anorexia, diarrhea, GI hemorrhage, mucositis
Hematologic: Myelosuppression (leukopenia, thrombocytopenia, anemia)
Hepatic: Hepatic dysfunction, jaundice, serum bilirubin and liver enzymes elevated
Local: Thrombophlebitis
Neuromuscular & skeletal: Myalgia, bone pain, peripheral neuropathy, weakness, gait disturbances
Ocular: Conjunctivitis, hemorrhagic conjunctivitis, corneal toxicity, photophobia, blurred vision
Respiratory: Syndrome of sudden respiratory distress progressing to pulmonary edema and diffuse interstitial pneumonitis have been reported with high-dose regimens

Miscellaneous: Ara-C syndrome (fever, myalgia, bone pain, rash, conjunctivitis, malaise occurring 6-12 hours after administration); headache and vomiting with I.T. administration; anaphylactoid reaction

Drug Interactions
Avoid Concomitant Use
Avoid concomitant use of Cytarabine with any of the following: BCG; Natalizumab; Pimecrolimus; Tacrolimus (Topical); Vaccines (Live)
Increased Effect/Toxicity
Cytarabine may increase the levels/effects of: Leflunomide; Natalizumab; Vaccines (Live)

The levels/effects of Cytarabine may be increased by: Denosumab; Pimecrolimus; Tacrolimus (Topical); Trastuzumab
Decreased Effect
Cytarabine may decrease the levels/effects of: BCG; Cardiac Glycosides; Flucytosine; Sipuleucel-T; Vaccines (Inactivated); Vaccines (Live)

The levels/effects of Cytarabine may be decreased by: Echinacea

Stability Reconstituted solutions containing 20-100 mg/mL cytarabine are stable for 48 hours at room temperature; I.T. Ara-C is compatible with methotrexate and hydrocortisone mixed in the same syringe; physically incompatible with fluorouracil, heparin

Intrathecal mediations should not be prepared during the preparation of any other agents. After preparation, store intrathecal medications in an isolated location or container clearly marked with a label identifying as "intrathecal" use only.

Mechanism of Action Converted intracellularly to the active metabolite cytarabine triphosphate; inhibits DNA polymerase by competing with deoxycytidine triphosphate resulting in inhibition of DNA synthesis; incorporated into DNA chain resulting in termination of chain elongation; cell cycle-specific for the S-phase of cell division

Pharmacokinetics (Adult data unless noted)
Distribution: Penetrates the CSF in limited amounts, crosses the placenta
Protein binding: 13%
Metabolism: Deactivated by cytidine deaminase primarily in the liver, but also in kidneys, GI mucosa, and granulocytes
Half-life, terminal: 1-3 hours
Elimination: ~80% of dose excreted in urine as metabolites within 24 hours; 10% excreted in urine as unchanged drug

Usual Dosage Children and Adults (refer to individual protocols):
Induction remission:
I.V.: 200 mg/m^2/day for 5 days at 2-week intervals as a single agent; in combination chemotherapy, 100-200 mg/m^2/day for 5- to 10-day therapy course every 2-4 weeks, or every day until remission, given as an I.V. continuous drip or in 2 divided doses/day
I.T.: 5-75 mg/m^2 every 2-7 days until CNS findings normalize
Maintenance remission:
I.V.: 70-200 mg/m^2/day for 2-5 days at monthly intervals
I.M., SubQ: 1-1.5 mg/kg single dose for maintenance at 1- to 4-week intervals
I.T.: 5-75 mg/m^2 every 2-7 days until CNS findings normalize **or**
<1 year: 20 mg
1-2 years: 30 mg
2-3 years: 50 mg
>3 years: 70 mg
High-dose regimen: Refractory leukemias or refractory non-Hodgkin's lymphoma: I.V. infusion: 3 g/m^2/dose every 12 hours for up to 12 doses

Administration Parenteral: May administer SubQ, I.M., IVP, I.V. infusion, or I.T. at a concentration not to exceed 100 mg/mL

High-dose regimens or for use in neonates: Diluents containing benzyl alcohol should not be used to reconstitute the drug; high-dose regimens (dose >1 g/m^2) are usually administered by I.V. infusion over 2 hours or longer, or as an I.V. continuous infusion

IVP: May administer over 15 minutes; rapid administration is associated with greater neurotoxicity

I.T. administration: Reconstitute with preservative free NS, Elliotts B solution, or preservative free LR solution; use preservative free injection formulation for I.T. use; filter through a 0.22 micron filter; the volume to be given I.T. is in the range of 3-10 mL and should correspond to an equivalent volume of CSF removed; antiemetic therapy should be administered prior to intrathecal doses of cytarabine

SubQ administration: Rotate injection sites to thigh, abdomen, and flank regions; avoid repeated administration to a single site

Monitoring Parameters Liver function tests, CBC with differential and platelet count, serum creatinine, BUN, serum uric acid; signs of neurotoxicity

Patient Information Notify physician of any fever, sore throat, bleeding, or bruising

Nursing Implications Administer corticosteroid eye drops for prophylaxis of conjunctivitis around-the-clock prior to, during, and for 2-7 days after high-dose Ara-C; pyridoxine has been administered on days of high-dose Ara-C therapy for prophylaxis of CNS toxicity.

Additional Information Myelosuppressive effects:
WBC: Severe
Platelets: Severe
Onset (days): 4-7
Nadir (days): 14-18
Recovery (days): 21-28

Dosage Forms Excipient information presented when available (limited, particularly for generics); consult specific product labeling.

Injection, powder for reconstitution: 100 mg, 500 mg, 1 g, 2 g [contains benzyl alcohol (in diluent)]

Injection, solution: 100 mg/mL (20 mL)

Injection, solution: 20 mg/mL (25 mL) [contains benzyl alcohol]

Injection, solution [preservative free]: 20 mg/mL (5 mL, 50 mL); 100 mg/mL (20 mL)

References
Baker WJ, Royer GL, and Weiss RB, "Cytarabine and Neurologic Toxicity," *J Clinical Oncology*, 1991, 9(4):679-93.

Grossman L, Baker MA, Sutton DM, et al, "Central Nervous System Toxicity of High-Dose Cytosine Arabinoside," *Med Pediatr Oncol*, 1983, 11(4):246-50.

Jacobson JO, Polovich M, McNiff KK, et al, "American Society of Clinical Oncology/Oncology Nursing Society Chemotherapy Administration Safety Standards," *J Clin Oncol*, 2009, 27(32):5469-75.

◆ **Cytarabine (Conventional)** *see* Cytarabine *on page 377*

◆ **Cytarabine Hydrochloride** *see* Cytarabine *on page 377*

◆ **CytoGam®** *see* Cytomegalovirus Immune Globulin (Intravenous-Human) *on page 379*

Cytomegalovirus Immune Globulin (Intravenous-Human)
(sye toe meg a low VYE rus i MYUN GLOB yoo lin in tra VEE nus HYU man)

Medication Safety Issues
Sound-alike/look-alike issues:
CytoGam® may be confused with Cytoxan, Gamimune® N

U.S. Brand Names CytoGam®
Canadian Brand Names CytoGam®

Therapeutic Category Immune Globulin

Generic Available No

Use Prophylaxis of cytomegalovirus disease associated with kidney, lung, liver, pancreas, heart, or bone marrow transplantation; concomitant use with ganciclovir should be considered in organ transplants other than kidney from CMV seropositive donors to CMV seronegative recipients; adjunctive treatment of CMV disease in immunocompromised patients

Pregnancy Risk Factor C

Pregnancy Considerations Reproduction studies have not been conducted.

Lactation Excretion in breast milk unknown

Contraindications Hypersensitivity to CMV immune globulin, other immune globulin preparations, blood products, or any component; IgA deficiency

Warnings Renal dysfunction and/or acute renal failure has been reported with the administration of IVIG; 88% of the cases were associated with the administration of sucrose-containing IVIG products. CytoGam® contains sucrose as a stabilizing agent. May theoretically transmit blood-borne viruses and the Creutzfeldt-Jakob disease agent.

Precautions Use with caution in patients with a history of cardiovascular disease or thrombotic episodes. Rapid infusion may be a possible risk factor for vascular occlusive events. Do not exceed manufacturer's recommended initial infusion rate and advance slowly in patients at risk. Use with caution in patients at increased risk for developing acute renal failure (patients with pre-existing renal insufficiency, diabetes mellitus, volume depletion, sepsis, paraproteinemia, and concomitant nephrotoxic drugs). Assure that patients are not volume depleted prior to the initiation of a CMV-IGIV infusion.

Adverse Reactions

Cardiovascular: Flushing, hypotension, thrombosis

Central nervous system: Fever, chills, dizziness, headache, aseptic meningitis syndrome

Dermatologic: Angioneurotic edema

Gastrointestinal: Nausea, vomiting

Hematologic: Hemolysis

Neuromuscular & skeletal: Arthralgia, back pain, muscle cramps

Renal: Acute renal failure, acute tubular necrosis, BUN and serum creatinine elevated, oliguria

Respiratory: Wheezing, tightness in chest, transfusion-related acute lung injury (respiratory distress, pulmonary edema, hypoxemia)

Miscellaneous: Anaphylaxis, diaphoresis

Drug Interactions

Avoid Concomitant Use There are no known interactions where it is recommended to avoid concomitant use.

Increased Effect/Toxicity There are no known significant interactions involving an increase in effect.

Decreased Effect

Cytomegalovirus Immune Globulin (Intravenous-Human) may decrease the levels/effects of: Vaccines (Live)

Stability Refrigerate; do not freeze; do not shake vials; do not admix or dilute with other medications prior to I.V. infusion; may piggyback into existing infusions of NS, D$_{2.5}$W, D$_5$W, D$_{10}$W, or D$_{20}$W at no greater than a 1:2 dilution

Mechanism of Action CMV-IGIV contains a high titer of CMV-specific antibodies which can neutralize the CMV virus; may exert immunomodulating effects

Pharmacokinetics (Adult data unless noted) Half-life: 8-24 days

Usual Dosage I.V.: Children and Adults:

Prophylaxis:

Kidney transplant: 150 mg/kg within 72 hours prior to transplant; 100 mg/kg at weeks 2, 4, 6, and 8 after transplant and 50 mg/kg at weeks 12 and 16 after transplant

Liver, lung, pancreas, or heart transplant (CMV (+) donor and CMV (-) recipient): 150 mg/kg within 72 hours prior to transplant, 150 mg/kg at weeks 2, 4, 6, and 8 after transplant; 100 mg/kg at weeks 12 and 16 after transplant

Bone marrow transplant: 200 mg/kg given 6 and 8 days prior to transplant and on days 1, 7, 14, 21, 28, 42, 56, and 70 after transplant

Treatment: 100 mg/kg every other day for 3 doses, then once every week based upon CMV antigenemia assay (pp65) or EBV PCR

Severe CMV pneumonia: 400 mg/kg in combination with ganciclovir on days 1, 2, 7, or 8, followed by 200 mg/kg on days 14 and 21

Dosage adjustment in renal impairment: Use with caution and infuse at the minimum rate possible. Specific dosage adjustment recommendations are not available.

Administration Parenteral: I.V. infusion: Initial infusion is started at 15 mg/kg/hour; if there are no infusion-related reactions after 30 minutes, increase to 30 mg/kg/hour; if no infusion-related reactions after 30 minutes, increase to 60 mg/kg/hour and maintain this rate until completion of dose. Subsequent doses can be initiated at an infusion rate of 15 mg/kg/hour for the first 15 minutes, if no infusion-related reactions, increase to 30 mg/kg/hour for the next 15 minutes; if rate is tolerated, increase to 60 mg/kg/hour and maintain this rate until completion of dose; maximum infusion rate: 60 mg/kg/hour or not to exceed 75 mL/hour at a maximum concentration of 50 mg/mL. Infuse through a 0.2-15 micron in-line filter.

Monitoring Parameters Vital signs during infusion, urine output, renal function

Additional Information

IgA content: Trace

Plasma Source: 2000-5000 donors (5% with top CMV titers)

IgG subclass (%):

IgG$_1$: 65

IgG$_2$: 28

IgG$_3$: 5.2

IgG$_4$: 1.7

Monomers + dimer (%): ≥95 monomers + dimers

Gamma globulin (%): 99

Albumin: 10 mg/mL

Sodium content: 20-30 mEq/L

Sugar content: 5% sucrose

Osmolality: >200 mOsm/L

Dosage Forms Excipient information presented when available (limited, particularly for generics); consult specific product labeling.

Injection, solution [preservative free]:

CytoGam®: 50 mg ± 10 mg/mL (50 mL) [contains sodium 20-30 mEq/L, human albumin, and sucrose]

References

Bowden RA, Fisher LD, Rogers K, et al, "Cytomegalovirus (CMV)-Specific Intravenous Immunoglobulin for the Prevention of Primary CMV Infection and Disease After Marrow Transplant," *J Infect Dis*, 1991, 164(3):483-7.

Snydman DR, Werner BG, Dougherty NN, et al, "Cytomegalovirus Immune Globulin Prophylaxis in Liver Transplantation. A Randomized, Double-Blind, Placebo-Controlled Trial," *Ann Intern Med*, 1993, 119(10):984-91.

Valantine HA, Luikart H, Doyle R, et al, "Impact of Cytomegalovirus Hyperimmune Globulin on Outcome After Cardiothoracic Transplantation: A Comparative Study of Combined Prophylaxis With CMV Hyperimmune Globulin Plus Ganciclovir Versus Ganciclovir Alone," *Transplantation*, 2001, 72(10):1647-52.

◆ **Cytomel®** see Liothyronine *on page 828*

◆ **Cytosar® (Can)** see Cytarabine *on page 377*

◆ **Cytosar-U** see Cytarabine *on page 377*

◆ **Cytosine Arabinosine Hydrochloride** see Cytarabine *on page 377*

◆ **Cytotec®** see Misoprostol *on page 937*

◆ **Cytovene® (Can)** see Ganciclovir *on page 636*

◆ **Cytovene®-IV** see Ganciclovir *on page 636*

◆ **Cytoxan** see Cyclophosphamide *on page 369*

◆ **Cēpacol® Dual Action Maximum Strength [OTC]** see Dyclonine *on page 486*

◆ **D2** see Ergocalciferol *on page 519*

◆ **D2E7** see Adalimumab *on page 48*

◆ **D3** see Cholecalciferol *on page 300*

◆ **D-3 [OTC]** see Cholecalciferol *on page 300*

◆ **D3-5™ [OTC]** see Cholecalciferol *on page 300*

◆ **D3-50™ [OTC]** see Cholecalciferol *on page 300*

◆ **D-3-Mercaptovaline** see Penicillamine *on page 1076*

◆ **d4T** see Stavudine *on page 1290*

◆ **D$_5$W** see Dextrose *on page 422*

◆ **D$_{10}$W** see Dextrose *on page 422*

◆ **D$_{25}$W** see Dextrose *on page 422*

◆ **D$_{30}$W** see Dextrose *on page 422*

◆ **D$_{40}$W** see Dextrose *on page 422*

◆ **D$_{50}$W** see Dextrose *on page 422*

◆ **D$_{60}$W** see Dextrose *on page 422*

◆ **D$_{70}$W** see Dextrose *on page 422*

Dacarbazine (da KAR ba zeen)

Medication Safety Issues

Sound-alike/look-alike issues:

Dacarbazine may be confused with Dicarbosil®, procarbazine

High alert medication: This medication is in a class the Institute for Safe Medication Practices (ISMP) includes among its list of drugs which have a heightened risk of causing significant patient harm when used in error.

Related Information

Compatibility of Chemotherapy and Related Supportive Care Medications *on page 1580*

Emetogenic Potential of Antineoplastic Agents *on page 1579*

Canadian Brand Names Dacarbazine for Injection

Therapeutic Category Antineoplastic Agent, Miscellaneous

Generic Available Yes

Use Treatment of malignant melanoma, Hodgkin's disease (FDA approved in adults); has also been used in the treatment of soft tissue sarcomas (fibrosarcomas, rhabdomyosarcoma), islet cell carcinoma, pheochromocytoma, and medullary carcinoma of the thyroid

Pregnancy Risk Factor C

Pregnancy Considerations [U.S. Boxed Warning]: This agent is carcinogenic and/or teratogenic when used in animals; adverse effects have been observed in animal studies. There are no adequate and well-controlled trials in pregnant women; use in pregnancy only if the potential benefit outweighs the potential risk to the fetus.

Lactation Excretion in breast milk unknown/not recommended

Breast-Feeding Considerations Due to the potential for serious adverse reactions in the nursing infant, breast-feeding is not recommended.

Contraindications Hypersensitivity to dacarbazine or any component

Warnings Hazardous agent; use appropriate precautions for handling and disposal. Hematopoietic depression is common **[U.S. Boxed Warning]**. Leukopenia and thrombocytopenia may be life-threatening; temporary cessation of drug may be required with bone marrow suppression. Hepatotoxicity with hepatocellular necrosis and hepatic vein thrombosis has been reported **[U.S. Boxed Warning]**; hepatotoxicity usually occurs with combination chemotherapy, but may occur with dacarbazine alone; may be carcinogenic and/or teratogenic **[U.S. Boxed Warning]**; dacarbazine has been reported to cause sterility and is mutagenic and teratogenic in rats.

Precautions Use with caution in patients with bone marrow suppression, renal and/or hepatic impairment; dosage reduction may be necessary in patients with renal or hepatic insufficiency; avoid extravasation of the drug; extravasation may result in tissue damage and severe pain

Adverse Reactions

Cardiovascular: Facial flushing, hypotension

Central nervous system: Confusion, fever, malaise, seizure

Dermatologic: Alopecia, photosensitivity, rash

Gastrointestinal: Anorexia, metallic taste, nausea, vomiting

Hematologic: Myelosuppression (nadir: 2-4 weeks): Leukopenia, thrombocytopenia (see Warnings)

Hepatic: Hepatic vein thrombosis, hepatocellular necrosis, hepatotoxicity (see Warnings)

Local: Pain and burning at infusion site, thrombophlebitis

Neuromuscular & skeletal: Myalgia, paresthesia

Ocular: Blurred vision

Respiratory: Sinus congestion

Miscellaneous: Anaphylactic reactions, flu-like syndrome

<1%, postmarketing, and/or case reports: BUN increased, diarrhea (following high-dose bolus injection), eosinophilia, headache, hepatic necrosis, hepatic vein occlusion, liver enzymes increased (transient), paresthesia

Drug Interactions

Metabolism/Transport Effects Substrate (major) of CYP1A2, 2E1

Avoid Concomitant Use

Avoid concomitant use of Dacarbazine with any of the following: BCG; Natalizumab; Pimecrolimus; Tacrolimus (Topical); Vaccines (Live)

Increased Effect/Toxicity

Dacarbazine may increase the levels/effects of: Leflunomide; Natalizumab; Vaccines (Live)

The levels/effects of Dacarbazine may be increased by: CYP1A2 Inhibitors (Moderate); CYP1A2 Inhibitors (Strong); CYP2E1 Inhibitors (Moderate); CYP2E1 Inhibitors (Strong); Denosumab; MAO Inhibitors; Pimecrolimus; Tacrolimus (Topical); Trastuzumab

Decreased Effect

Dacarbazine may decrease the levels/effects of: BCG; Sipuleucel-T; Vaccines (Inactivated); Vaccines (Live)

The levels/effects of Dacarbazine may be decreased by: CYP1A2 Inducers (Strong); Echinacea; Sorafenib

Stability Store intact vials at 2°C to 8°C (36°F to 46°F); protect from light; reconstituted dacarbazine solution 10 mg/mL is stable for 72 hours when refrigerated or 8 hours at room temperature; dacarbazine solution further diluted in D₅W or NS is stable for 24 hours when refrigerated or 8 hours at room temperature; drug decomposition has occurred if the solution turns pink; dacarbazine is incompatible with hydrocortisone sodium succinate

Mechanism of Action Alkylating agent which forms methyldiazonium ions that attack nucleophilic groups in DNA; inhibits DNA, RNA, and protein synthesis by cross-linking DNA strands

Pharmacokinetics (Adult data unless noted)

Distribution: Distributes to the liver; very little distribution into CSF with CSF concentrations ~14% of plasma concentrations

V_{dss}: Adults: 17 L/m^2

Protein binding: Minimal, 5%

Metabolism: N-demethylated in the liver by microsomal enzymes; metabolites may also have an antineoplastic effect

Half-life, biphasic: Initial: 20-40 minutes; terminal: 5 hours (in patients with normal renal/hepatic function)

Elimination: ~30% to 50% of dose excreted in urine by tubular secretion, 15% to 25% is excreted in urine as unchanged drug

Usual Dosage I.V. (refer to individual protocols):

Children:

Pediatric solid tumors: 200-470 mg/m^2/day over 5 days every 21-28 days

Hodgkin's disease: 375 mg/m^2 on days 1 and 15 of treatment course, repeat every 28 days

Adults:

Malignant melanoma: 2-4.5 mg/kg/day for 10 days, repeat in 4 weeks or may use 250 mg/m^2/day for 5 days, repeat in 3 weeks

Hodgkin's disease: 150 mg/m^2/day for 5 days, repeat every 4 weeks **or** 375 mg/m^2 on day 1, repeat in 15 days of each 28-day cycle in combination with other agents

Administration Parenteral: Reconstitute 100 mg vial with 9.9 mL SWI or 200 mg vial with 19.7 mL SWI, resulting in a concentration of 10 mg/mL; may further dilute in D₅W or NS and administer by slow IVP over 2-3 minutes or by I.V. infusion over 15-120 minutes at a concentration not to exceed 10 mg/mL

Monitoring Parameters CBC with differential, erythrocytes and platelet count; liver function tests

Patient Information Restrict intake of food for 4-6 hours prior to dacarbazine dose to decrease vomiting; flu-like symptoms (ie, malaise, fever, myalgia) may occur 1 week after infusion. May cause photosensitivity reactions (eg, exposure to sunlight may cause severe sunburn, skin rash, redness, or itching); avoid exposure to sunlight and artificial light sources (sunlamps, tanning booth/bed); wear protective clothing, wide-brimmed hats, sunglasses, and lip sunscreen (SPF ≥15); use a sunscreen [broadspectrum sunscreen or physical sunscreen (preferred) or sunblock with SPF ≥15]; contact physician if reaction occurs. Women of childbearing age should be advised to avoid becoming pregnant.

Nursing Implications Avoid extravasation; use a D₅W or NS flush before and after a dacarbazine infusion; local pain, burning sensation, and irritation at the injection site may be relieved by local application of hot packs, slowing the I.V. rate and further dilution in I.V. fluid

Dosage Forms Excipient information presented when available (limited, particularly for generics); consult specific product labeling.

Injection, powder for reconstitution: 100 mg, 200 mg

References

Berg SL, Grisell DL, DeLaney TF, et al, "Principles of Treatment of Pediatric Solid Tumors," *Pediatr Clin North Am*, 1991, 38(2):249-67.

Finklestein JZ, Albo V, Ertel I, et al, "5-(3,3-Dimethyl-I-triazeno) imidazole-4-carboxamide (NSC-45388) in the Treatment of Solid Tumors in Children," *Cancer Chemother Rep*, 1975, 59(2 Pt 1):351-7.

Mutz ID and Urban CE, "Dimethyl-triazeno-imidazole-carboxamide (DTIC) in Combination Chemotherapy for Childhood Neuroblastoma," *Wien Klin Wochenschr*, 1978, 90(24):867-70.

◆ **Dacarbazine for Injection (Can)** *see* Dacarbazine *on page 380*

◆ **Dacliximab** *see* Daclizumab *on page 382*

Daclizumab (da CLI zoo mab)

U.S. Brand Names Zenapax® [DSC]

Canadian Brand Names Zenapax®

Therapeutic Category Immunosuppressant Agent

Generic Available No

Use In combination with an immunosuppressive regimen, including cyclosporine and corticosteroids, for prophylaxis of acute organ rejection in patients receiving renal transplants; daclizumab has also been studied in pediatric bone marrow patients; steroid-refractory graft-versus-host disease

Pregnancy Risk Factor C

Pregnancy Considerations An increased risk of fetal loss was observed in animal reproduction studies. Generally, IgG molecules cross the placenta. Use during pregnancy only if the potential benefit to the mother outweighs the possible risk to the fetus. Women of childbearing potential should use effective contraception before, during, and for 4 months following daclizumab treatment.

Lactation Excretion in breast milk unknown/not recommended

Contraindications Hypersensitivity to daclizumab or any component

Warnings May result in an increased susceptibility to infection or an increased risk for developing lymphoproliferative disorders. Severe, acute hypersensitivity reactions, including anaphylaxis have been reported following initial exposure or following re-exposure to daclizumab. If a severe hypersensitivity reaction occurs, daclizumab should be permanently discontinued. Medications for the management of severe allergic reactions should be available for immediate use. The combined use of daclizumab, cyclosporine, mycophenolate mofetil, and corticosteroids has been associated with an increased mortality in cardiac transplant patients. Higher mortality may be associated with the use of antilymphocyte globulin and a higher incidence of severe infections.

Adverse Reactions

Cardiovascular: Edema, hypertension (48% in pediatric patients), hypotension, tachycardia, thrombosis, chest pain, cardiac arrest

Central nervous system: Headache, dizziness, insomnia, depression, anxiety, fever, chills

Dermatologic: Impaired wound healing, acne, pruritus, rash, hirsutism

Endocrine & metabolic: Dehydration (frequency may be higher for pediatric patients than for adults), diabetes mellitus

Gastrointestinal: Constipation, nausea, diarrhea (36%), vomiting (32%), abdominal pain, abdominal distention

Genitourinary: Oliguria, dysuria

Hematologic: Bleeding

Neuromuscular & skeletal: Tremors, back pain, arthralgia, myalgia

Ocular: Blurred vision

Renal: Renal tubular necrosis, hematuria

Respiratory: Atelectasis, congestion, hypoxia, pharyngitis, pleural effusion, respiratory arrest

Miscellaneous: Anaphylaxis, diaphoresis; incidence of anti-daclizumab antibodies (children: 34%)

Drug Interactions

Avoid Concomitant Use

Avoid concomitant use of Daclizumab with any of the following: BCG; Natalizumab; Pimecrolimus; Tacrolimus (Topical); Vaccines (Live)

Increased Effect/Toxicity

Daclizumab may increase the levels/effects of: Leflunomide; Natalizumab; Vaccines (Live)

The levels/effects of Daclizumab may be increased by: Denosumab; Pimecrolimus; Tacrolimus (Topical); Trastuzumab

Decreased Effect

Daclizumab may decrease the levels/effects of: BCG; Sipuleucel-T; Vaccines (Inactivated); Vaccines (Live)

The levels/effects of Daclizumab may be decreased by: Echinacea

Stability Refrigerate; do not shake or freeze; protect from direct light; diluted daclizumab solution is stable for 24 hours if refrigerated or for 4 hours at room temperature; discard solution if colored or if particulate matter is present

Mechanism of Action A humanized IgG1 monoclonal antibody produced by recombinant DNA technology that binds specifically to the alpha subunit (p55 alpha, CD25, or Tac subunit) of the human high affinity interleukin-2 receptor (IL-2R) on the surface of activated lymphocytes inhibiting IL-2 binding; inhibits IL-2 mediated activation of lymphocytes which is involved in allograft rejection

Pharmacokinetics (Adult data unless noted) Daclizumab serum levels appeared to be somewhat lower in pediatric renal transplant patients than in adult transplant patients administered the same 1 mg/kg dosing regimen

Distribution: V_d: Adults: ~6 L

Half-life:

Children: 13 days

Adults: 20 days

Usual Dosage I.V. (refer to individual protocols): Children and Adults:

Initial dose: 1 mg/kg given no more than 24 hours before transplantation, followed by 1 mg/kg/dose administered every 14 days for a total of 5 doses; maximum dose: 100 mg

Steroid-refractory graft-versus-host disease: 0.5-1.5 mg/kg as a single dose administered for transient response (repeat doses have been given 11-48 days following the initial dose)

Dosing interval in renal impairment: No dosage adjustment necessary

Administration Parenteral: Daclizumab dose should be diluted in 50 mL NS solution. In fluid-restricted patients, a final concentration of 1 mg/mL can be administered over 15 minutes. When mixing the solution, gently invert the bag to avoid foaming; do not shake. Daclizumab solution should be administered within 4 hours of preparation if stored at room temperature; infuse over a 15-minute period via a peripheral or central vein. Do not mix or infuse other medications through the same I.V. line.

Monitoring Parameters CBC with differential, vital signs, immunologic monitoring of T cells, renal function tests, serum glucose

Reference Range Serum trough levels: 5-10 mcg/mL

Patient Information Women of childbearing potential should avoid becoming pregnant while on daclizumab. Use an effective form of contraception before beginning therapy, during therapy, and for 4 months following daclizumab treatment.

Product Availability Zenapax®: Due to diminishing market demand, the manufacturer of daclizumab has discontinued production; it is anticipated that available supplies will be depleted in January 2010; all remaining lots will expire in 2011.

Dosage Forms Excipient information presented when available (limited, particularly for generics); consult specific product labeling. [DSC] = Discontinued product

Injection, solution [concentrate; preservative free]:

Zenapax®: 5 mg/mL (5 mL) [contains polysorbate 80] [DSC]

References

Vincenti F, Kirkman R, Light S, et al, "Interleukin-2-Receptor Blockade With Daclizumab to Prevent Acute Rejection in Renal Transplantation. Daclizumab Triple Therapy Study Group," *N Engl J Med*, 1998, 338(3):161-5.

◆ **Dacodyl™ [OTC]** *see* Bisacodyl *on page 194*

◆ **DACT** *see* DACTINomycin *on page 383*

DACTINomycin (dak ti noe MYE sin)

Medication Safety Issues

Sound-alike/look-alike issues:

DACTINomycin may be confused with DAPTOmycin, DAUNOrubicin

Actinomycin may be confused with achromycin

High alert medication: The Institute for Safe Medication Practices (ISMP) includes this medication among its list of drug classes which have a heightened risk of causing significant patient harm when used in error.

Related Information

Compatibility of Chemotherapy and Related Supportive Care Medications *on page 1580*

Emetogenic Potential of Antineoplastic Agents *on page 1579*

Extravasation Treatment *on page 1522*

U.S. Brand Names Cosmegen®

Canadian Brand Names Cosmegen®

Therapeutic Category Antineoplastic Agent, Antibiotic

Generic Available No

Use Management (either alone or in combination with other treatment modalities) of Wilms' tumor, childhood rhabdomyosarcoma, Ewing's sarcoma, gestational trophoblastic neoplasms, and metastatic nonseminomatous testicular tumors (FDA approved in ages >6 months and adults); used in regional perfusion (palliative or adjunctive) of locally recurrent or locoregional solid tumors (sarcomas, carcinomas, and adenocarcinomas). Has also been used for treatment of soft tissue sarcoma (other than rhabdomyosarcoma).

Pregnancy Risk Factor D

Pregnancy Considerations Animal studies have demonstrated teratogenic effects and fetal loss. There are no adequate and well-controlled studies in pregnant women. Women of childbearing potential are advised not to become pregnant. Use only when potential benefit justifies potential risk to the fetus. **[U.S. Boxed Warning]: Avoid exposure during pregnancy.**

Lactation Excretion in breast milk unknown/not recommended

Breast-Feeding Considerations It is not known if dactinomycin is excreted in human breast milk. Due to the potential for serious adverse reactions in the nursing infant, breast-feeding is not recommended.

Contraindications Hypersensitivity to dactinomycin or any component; patients with chickenpox or herpes zoster; avoid in infants <6 months of age since the incidence of adverse effects is increased in infants

Warnings Hazardous agent; use appropriate precautions for handling and disposal.

Dactinomycin is extremely toxic; avoid inhalation of vapors or contact with skin, mucous membrane, or eyes **[U.S. Boxed Warning]**; in case of accidental exposure to eyes or mucous membranes, irrigate area with water, normal saline, or balanced salt ophthalmic irrigating solution for at least 15 minutes. Avoid exposure during pregnancy **[U.S. Boxed Warning]**; dactinomycin may cause fetal harm when administered to pregnant women. Women of childbearing potential must be warned to avoid becoming pregnant. Dactinomycin is extremely irritating to tissues **[U.S. Boxed Warning]**. If extravasation occurs during I.V.

use, severe damage to soft tissue will occur leading to pain, swelling, ulceration, and necrosis. Extravasation leading to contracture of the arms has also been reported.

Reports of secondary malignancies (including leukemia) following treatment with radiation and dactinomycin have occurred; long-term observation of cancer survivors is recommended. May cause potentially fatal hepatic veno-occlusive disease (VOD); reported incidence of veno-occlusive disease across different clinical studies is 2% to 13.5% with increased risk in children <4 years of age. Monitor for signs or symptoms of hepatic VOD, including biliribin >1.4 mg/dL, unexplained weight gain, ascites, hepatomegaly, or unexplained right upper quadrant pain (Arndt, 2004).

Precautions Use with caution and reduce dosage in patients with hepatobiliary dysfunction or in patients receiving radiation therapy; patients receiving radiation therapy are at increased risk for gastrointestinal and myelosuppresive effects; avoid administering live virus vaccinations during therapy with dactinomycin. Erythema from prior radiation therapy may be reactivated by dactinomycin. Avoid dactinomycin use within 2 months of radiation treatment for right-sided Wilms' tumor; may increase the risk of hepatotoxicity. Regional perfusion therapy may result in local limb edema, soft tissue damage, and possible venous thrombosis; dactinomycin leakage into systemic circulation may result in hematologic toxicity, infection, impaired wound healing, and mucositis.

Adverse Reactions

Central nervous system: Chills, fatigue, fever, lethargy, malaise

Dermatologic: Acne, alopecia, cheilitis, desquamation, erythema, hyperpigmentation of skin, maculopapular rash, sloughing/erythema of previously irradiated skin, urticaria

Endocrine & metabolic: Growth retardation, hyperuricemia, hypocalcemia

Gastrointestinal: Abdominal pain, anorexia, diarrhea, dysphagia, esophagitis, GI ulceration, nausea, proctitis, stomatitis, vomiting

Hematologic: Agranulocytosis, anemia, aplastic anemia, febrile neutropenia, leukopenia, myelosuppression (nadir: 2-3 weeks), neutropenia, pancytopenia, reticulocytopenia, thrombocytopenia

Hepatic: Ascites, bilirubin increased, hepatic veno-occlusive disease, hepatitis, hepatomegaly, hepatopathy thrombocytopenia syndrome, liver enzymes elevated

Local: Erythema, pain, soft tissue damage with extravasation

Neuromuscular & skeletal: Myalgia

Renal: Renal function abnormality

Respiratory: Pharyngitis, pneumonitis

Miscellaneous: Anaphylactoid reaction, immunosuppression, second primary tumors

Drug Interactions

Avoid Concomitant Use

Avoid concomitant use of DACTINomycin with any of the following: BCG; Natalizumab; Pimecrolimus; Tacrolimus (Topical); Vaccines (Live)

Increased Effect/Toxicity

DACTINomycin may increase the levels/effects of: Leflunomide; Natalizumab; Vaccines (Live)

The levels/effects of DACTINomycin may be increased by: Denosumab; Pimecrolimus; Tacrolimus (Topical); Trastuzumab

Decreased Effect

DACTINomycin may decrease the levels/effects of: BCG; Sipuleucel-T; Vaccines (Inactivated); Vaccines (Live)

The levels/effects of DACTINomycin may be decreased by: Echinacea

Stability Store at 25°C (77°F); excursions permitted to 15°C to 30°C (59°F to 86°F); protect from light and humidity. Binds to cellulose filters, therefore, avoid in-line filtration; use of a diluent containing preservatives for reconstitution may result in a precipitate; any unused portion of the reconstituted 0.5 mg/mL solution should be discarded after 24 hours

Mechanism of Action Binds to the guanine portion of DNA intercalating between guanine and cytosine base pairs blocking replication and transcription of the DNA template inhibiting RNA synthesis; causes topoisomerase-mediated single-strand breaks in DNA

Pharmacokinetics (Adult data unless noted)

Distribution: Extensive extravascular distribution with high concentration in nucleated cells and bone marrow; does not penetrate blood brain barrier; crosses the placenta

Metabolism: Minimal

Half-life, terminal:

Children: 14-43 hours

Adults: 36 hours

Elimination: ~10% of dose excreted as unchanged drug in urine; 15% recovered in feces; 50% appears in bile

Usual Dosage Dosage should be based on body surface area in obese or edematous patients. Details concerning dosing in combination regimens should also be consulted. **Note:** Medication orders for dactinomycin are commonly written in MICROgrams (eg, 150 mcg) although many regimens state the dose in MILLIgrams (eg, mg/kg or mg/m^2). The dose intensity per 2-week cycle for adults and children should not exceed 15 mcg/kg/day for 5 days or 400-600 mcg/m^2/day for 5 days.

Children >6 months: I.V.: Usual dose: 15 mcg/kg/day for 5 days every 3-6 weeks or 400-600 mcg/m^2/day for 5 days every 3-6 weeks

Wilms' tumor, rhabdomyosarcoma, Ewing's sarcoma: 15 mcg/kg/day for 5 days (in various combination regimens and schedules)

Osteosarcoma: 600 mcg/m^2/day days 1, 2, and 3 as part of a combination chemotherapy regimen (see Goorin, 2003)

Adults: I.V.: Usual doses: 15 mcg/kg/day for 5 days every 3-6 weeks or 400-600 mcg/m^2/day for 5 days every 3-6 weeks **or** 1000 mcg/m^2 on day 1 or 12 mcg/kg/day for 5 days (monotherapy) **or** 500 mcg/dose days 1 and 2 (as part of a combination chemotherapy regimen)

Testicular cancer: 1000 mcg/m^2 on day 1 (as part of a combination chemotherapy regimen)

Gestational trophoblastic neoplasm: 12 mcg/kg/day for 5 days (monotherapy) **or** 500 mcg/dose days 1 and 2 (as part of a combination chemotherapy regimen)

Wilms' tumor, Ewing's sarcoma, rhabdomyosarcoma: 15 mcg/kg/day for 5 days (in various combination regimens and schedules)

Osteosarcoma: 600 mcg/m^2/day days 1, 2, and 3 as part of a combination chemotherapy regimen (see Goorin, 2003)

Ovarian (germ cell) tumor: 500 mcg/day for 5 days every 4 weeks (see Gershenson, 1985) or 300 mcg/m^2/day for 5 days every 4 weeks (see Slayton, 1985)

Regional Perfusion (dosages and techniques may vary by institution; obese patients and patients with prior chemotherapy or radiation therapy may require lower doses): Lower extremity or pelvis: 50 mcg/kg; upper extremity: 35 mcg/kg

Administration Parenteral: I.V.: For I.V. administration only; since drug is extremely irritating to tissues, **do not give I.M. or SubQ**; avoid extravasation; use a D$_5$W or NS flush before and after a dactinomycin dose to ensure venous patency; administer by slow IVP over a few minutes at a concentration not to exceed 500 mcg/mL into the side-port of a freely flowing I.V. infusion. Cellulose ester membrane filters may partially remove dactinomycin from solution and should not be used during preparation or administration.

Monitoring Parameters CBC with differential and platelet count, liver function tests and renal function tests; monitor for signs/symptoms of hepatic VOD, including unexplained weight gain, ascites, hepatomegaly, or unexplained right upper quadrant pain (Arndt, 2004); monitor serum beta-hCG (management of gestational trophoblastic neoplasms)

Test Interactions May interfere with bioassays of antibacterial drug concentrations

Patient Information Notify physician if fever, sore throat, bleeding, or bruising occurs; report immediately any pain, burning, or swelling at the infusion site. Advise women of childbearing potential to avoid becoming pregnant while receiving dactinomycin.

Nursing Implications Dactinomycin is corrosive to soft tissue. Avoid inhalation of drug particles or vapors and contact with skin or mucous membranes, especially those of the eyes. Avoid extravasation; if extravasation occurs, apply ice to the site for 15 minutes 4 times/day for 3 days; close observation with plastic surgery consultation is recommended

Dosage Forms Excipient information presented when available (limited, particularly for generics); consult specific product labeling.

Injection, powder for reconstitution:

Cosmegen®: 0.5 mg [contains mannitol 20 mg]

References

Arndt C, Hawkins D, Anderson JR, et al, "Age Is a Risk Factor for Chemotherapy-Induced Hepatopathy With Vincristine, Dactinomycin, and Cyclophosphamide," *J Clin Oncol*, 2004, 22(10):1894-90.

Bagshawe KD, "High-Risk Metastatic Trophoblastic Disease," *Obstet Gynecol Clin North Am*, 1988, 15(3):531-43.

Berg SL, Grisell DL, DeLaney TF, et al, "Principles of Treatment of Pediatric Solid Tumors," *Pediatr Clin North Am*, 1991, 38(2):249-67.

Berkowitz RS and Goldstein DP, "Gestational Trophoblastic Disease," *Cancer*, 1995, 76(10 Suppl):2079-85.

Carli M, Pastore G, Perilongo G, et al, "Tumor Response and Toxicity After Single High-Dose Versus Standard Five-Day Divided Dose Dactinomycin in Childhood Rhabdomyosarcoma," *J Clin Oncol*, 1988, 6(4):654-8.

Gershenson DM, Copeland LJ, Kavanagh JJ, et al, "Treatment of Malignant Nondysgerminomatous Germ Cell Tumors of the Ovary With Vincristine, Dactinomycin, and Cyclophosphamide," *Cancer*, 1985, 56(12):2756-6.

Goorin AM, Schwartzentruber DJ, Devidas M, et al, "Presurgical Chemotherapy Compared With Immediate Surgery and Adjuvant Chemotherapy for Nonmetastatic Osteosarcoma: Pediatric Oncology Group Study POG-8651," *J Clin Oncol*, 2003, 21(8):1574-80.

Slayton RE, Park RC, Silverberg SG, et al, "Vincristine, Dactinomycin, and Cyclophosphamide in the Treatment of Malignant Germ Cell Tumors of the Ovary. A Gynecologic Oncology Group Study (A Final Report)," *Cancer*, 1985, 56(2):243-8.

Veal GJ, Cole M, Errington J, et al, "Pharmacokinetics of Dactinomycin in a Pediatric Patient Population: A United Kingdom Children's Cancer Study Group Study," *Clin Cancer Res*, 2005, 11(16):5893-9.

◆ **Dalacin® C (Can)** see Clindamycin on page 327

◆ **Dalacin® T (Can)** see Clindamycin on page 327

◆ **Dalacin® Vaginal (Can)** see Clindamycin on page 327

◆ **Dalfopristin and Quinupristin** see Quinupristin/Dalfopristin on page 1196

◆ **Dalmane® (Can)** see Flurazepam on page 604

◆ **d-Alpha-Gems™ [OTC]** see Vitamin E on page 1427

◆ **d-Alpha Tocopherol** see Vitamin E on page 1427

Danazol (DA na zole)

Medication Safety Issues

Sound-alike/look-alike issues:

Danazol may be confused with Dantrium®

Danocrine may be confused with Dacriose®

Canadian Brand Names Cyclomen®

Therapeutic Category Androgen

Generic Available Yes

Use Treatment of endometriosis amenable to hormonal management; fibrocystic breast disease; hereditary angioedema (see also Additional Information)

Pregnancy Risk Factor X

Pregnancy Considerations [U.S. Boxed Warning]: Pregnancy should be ruled out prior to treatment using a sensitive test (beta subunit test, if available). Nonhormonal contraception should be used during therapy. May cause androgenic effects to the female fetus; clitoral hypertrophy, labial fusion, urogenital sinus defect, vaginal atresia, and ambiguous genitalia have been reported.

Lactation Enters breast milk/contraindicated

Contraindications Hypersensitivity to danazol or any component; pregnancy; undiagnosed abnormal genital bleeding; breast-feeding; porphyria; markedly impaired renal, hepatic, or cardiac function

Warnings Use of danazol in pregnancy is contraindicated **[U.S. Boxed Warning]**; exposure to danazol *in utero* may result in androgenic effects on the female fetus; clitoral hypertrophy, labial fusion, urogenital sinus defect, vaginal atresia, and ambiguous genitalia have been reported; a sensitive test capable of determining early pregnancy is recommended immediately prior to initiation of therapy; nonhormonal method of contraception should be used during treatment if indicated. Thromboembolism, thrombotic, and thrombophlebitic events have been reported (including life-threatening or fatal stroke) **[U.S. Boxed Warning]**. Long-term use has been associated with peliosis hepatis and hepatic adenoma **[U.S. Boxed Warning]**; these conditions may be complicated by acute, potentially life-threatening intra-abdominal hemorrhage; monitor liver function. Danazol has been associated with benign intracranial hypertension (pseudotumor cerebri) **[U.S. Boxed Warning]**; monitor for early signs and symptoms including papilledema, headache, nausea, vomiting, and visual disturbances. May increase risk of atherosclerosis and CAD due to decreased HDL and possible increase LDL. May cause nonreversible androgenic effects; patients should be watched closely for signs of androgenic effects.

Precautions Use with caution in patients with seizure disorders, migraine headaches, or conditions influenced by edema

Adverse Reactions

Cardiovascular: Edema, benign intracranial hypertension (rare), flushing, hypertension, diaphoresis, thromboembolism

Central nervous system: Nervousness, emotional lability, depression, dizziness, fainting, fever (rare), headache, sleep disorders, anxiety (rare), chills (rare), seizures (rare), stroke, Guillain-Barré syndrome

Dermatologic: Acne, seborrhea, mild hirsutism, hair loss, rashes (maculopapular, vestibular, papular, purpuric, and petechial), erythema multiforme, pruritus, urticaria, photosensitivity (rare)

Endocrine & metabolic: Weight gain, menstrual irregularities (spotting, altered timing of cycle), amenorrhea, clitoral hypertrophy (rare), breast size reduction, nipple discharge, semen abnormalities (changes in volume, viscosity, sperm count, and motility), libido changes, glucose intolerance, HDL decreased, LDL increased

Gastrointestinal: Nausea, vomiting, gastroenteritis, pancreatitis (rare), appetite changes (rare), bleeding gums (rare), constipation

Genitourinary: Vaginal dryness, vaginal irritation, pelvic pain

Hematologic: Eosinophilia, erythrocytosis (reversible), leukocytosis, leukopenia, thrombocytosis, polycythemia, thrombocytopenia

Hepatic: Peliosis hepatis, hepatic adenoma, cholestatic jaundice, liver enzymes elevated

Neuromuscular & skeletal: Back pain, carpal tunnel syndrome (rare), extremity pain, joint pain, joint swelling, muscle cramps, neck pain, paresthesias, spasms, weakness, tremor

Ocular: Cataracts (rare), visual disturbances

Renal: Hematuria

Respiratory: Nasal congestion (rare)

Miscellaneous: Voice alterations (hoarseness, sore throat, instability, deepening of pitch)

Drug Interactions

Metabolism/Transport Effects Inhibits CYP3A4 (weak)

Avoid Concomitant Use There are no known interactions where it is recommended to avoid concomitant use.

Increased Effect/Toxicity

Danazol may increase the levels/effects of: CarBAMazepine; CycloSPORINE; CycloSPORINE (Systemic); HMG-CoA Reductase Inhibitors; Vitamin K Antagonists

Decreased Effect There are no known significant interactions involving a decrease in effect.

Food Interactions Food delays time to peak serum level; high-fat meal increases plasma concentration

Stability Store at room temperature.

Mechanism of Action Danazol, a synthetic steroid analog, has strong antigonadotropic properties. It inhibits the mid-cycle surge of LH and FSH from the pituitary resulting in suppression of ovarian steroidogenesis. Danazol does not have any progestational or estrogenic properties but does exhibit weak anabolic and androgenic effects. Through its inactivation of the pituitary-ovarian axis, regression and atrophy of normal and ectopic endometrial tissue occurs. Danazol decreases the rate of growth of abnormal breast tissue and reduces attacks associated with hereditary angioedema by increasing levels of C4 component of complement.

Pharmacodynamics

Endometriosis:
Onset of action: 3 weeks

Fibrocystic breast disease:
Onset of action: 1 month
Maximum effect: 4-6 months
Duration: Symptoms recur in 50% of patients within one year after discontinuation of treatment

Pharmacokinetics (Adult data unless noted)

Absorption: Well absorbed

Metabolism: Extensive hepatic metabolism to inactive metabolites

Half-life: Adults: 4.5 hours

Time to peak serum concentration: 2 hours

Usual Dosage Adolescents and Adults: Oral: **Note:** Begin treatment during menstruation or obtain appropriate tests to ensure patient is not pregnant:

Endometriosis:
Mild case: 100-200 mg twice daily for 3-6 months; may be continued up to 9 months if necessary

Moderate to severe case: 400 mg twice daily for 3-6 months; may be continued up to 9 months if necessary

Note: A gradual downward titration to a dose sufficient to maintain amenorrhea may be considered depending upon the patient's response

Fibrocystic breast disease: 50-200 mg twice daily

Hereditary angioedema: Initial: 200 mg 2-3 times/day depending upon the patient's response; after a favorable response is obtained, decrease the dosage by 50% or less at intervals of 1-3 months or longer. If an attack occurs, the daily dosage may be increased by up to 200 mg.

Administration Oral: Avoid administration with fatty meals.

Monitoring Parameters Liver function tests, symptomatology and site of disease; serum glucose (if diabetic); HDL and LDL cholesterol; signs and symptoms of pseudotumor cerebri; androgenic effects

Test Interactions Danazol may interfere with laboratory determinations for testosterone, androstenedione, and dehydroepiandrosterone.

Patient Information Do not discontinue without consulting prescriber; therapy may take up to several months for full benefit depending upon the purpose of treatment. Report any prodromal symptoms of hepatitis (fatigue, weakness, nausea, vomiting, dark urine, or yellowing of eyes); avoid becoming pregnant while taking this medicine and for several months after stopping; use an effective form of birth control. This medication may alter hypoglycemic requirements; diabetics should monitor serum glucose closely. May cause photosensitivity reactions (eg, exposure to sunlight may cause severe sunburn, skin rash, redness, or itching); avoid direct exposure to sunlight.

Additional Information Danazol has seen limited use for treatment of ITP in children refractory to steroids. Ten children, 2.5-17 years of age were treated with 20-30 mg/kg/day in divided doses (maximum: 800 mg/day). Treatment was tapered off after patients responded to therapy (Weinblatt, 1988). Danazol has also been evaluated in hemophilia A in a randomized, double-blind placebo-controlled crossover trial in 19 children. Children <15 years received 150 mg/day and >15 years received 300 mg/day for 3 months. Factor VIII:C levels were increased (Mehta, 1992).

Dosage Forms Excipient information presented when available (limited, particularly for generics); consult specific product labeling.
Capsule: 50 mg, 100 mg, 200 mg

References
Mehta J, Singhal S, Kamath MV, et al, "A Randomized Placebo-Controlled Double-Blind Study of Danazol in Hemophilia A," *Acta Haematol*, 1992, 88(1):14-6.
Weinblatt ME, Kochen J, and Ortega J, "Danazol for Children With Immune Thrombocytopenic Purpura," *Am J Dis Child*, 1988, 142 (12):1317-9.

◆ **Dandrex [OTC]** *see* Selenium Sulfide *on page 1252*
◆ **Danocrine** *see* Danazol *on page 384*
◆ **Dantrium®** *see* Dantrolene *on page 386*

Dantrolene (DAN troe leen)

Medication Safety Issues
Sound-alike/look-alike issues:
Dantrium® may be confused with danazol, Daraprim®

U.S. Brand Names Dantrium®

Canadian Brand Names Dantrium®

Therapeutic Category Antidote, Malignant Hyperthermia; Hyperthermia, Treatment; Skeletal Muscle Relaxant, Nonparalytic

Generic Available Yes: Capsule

Use Treatment of spasticity associated with upper motor neuron disorders such as spinal cord injury, stroke, cerebral palsy, or multiple sclerosis; treatment of malignant hyperthermia

Pregnancy Risk Factor C

Lactation Enters breast milk/not recommended

Contraindications Hypersensitivity to dantrolene or any component; active hepatic disease such as hepatitis and cirrhosis; should not be administered where spasticity is used to maintain posture or balance

Warnings May cause hepatotoxicity **[U.S. Boxed Warning]**; overt hepatitis has been most frequently observed between the third and twelfth month of therapy and with doses ≥800 mg/day; hepatic injury appears to be greater in females and in patients >35 years of age; monitor LFTs, use lowest effective dose and discontinue if no benefit is observed after a total of 45 days of therapy. Injection is extremely irritating to peripheral veins and may cause severe tissue necrosis if extravasation occurs; administer in a fast moving I.V. solution into a large vein or into a central line.

Precautions Use with caution in patients with impaired cardiac or pulmonary function or history of previous liver disease; crosses placenta with fetal whole blood levels up to 65% of maternal at delivery

Adverse Reactions
Cardiovascular: Pericarditis (with pleural effusion), tachycardia
Central nervous system: Seizures, drowsiness, dizziness, lightheadedness, confusion, headache, fatigue, speech disturbances, mental depression, chills, fever
Dermatologic: Rash, acne-like rash, pruritus, urticaria, abnormal hair growth
Gastrointestinal: Diarrhea, nausea, vomiting, severe constipation, gastric irritation, GI bleeding, abdominal cramps, dysphagia, anorexia, swallowing difficulty, drooling
Genitourinary: Urinary retention or frequency, urinary incontinence
Hematologic: Aplastic anemia, anemia, leucopenia, lymphocytic lymphoma, thrombocytopenia
Hepatic: Hepatitis (see Warnings)
Local: Phlebitis, tissue necrosis
Neuromuscular & skeletal: Muscle weakness, myalgia, backache
Ocular: Visual disturbances, excessive tearing
Renal: Hematuria
Respiratory: Respiratory depression, pleural effusion (with pericarditis)

Drug Interactions
Metabolism/Transport Effects Substrate of CYP3A4 (major)
Avoid Concomitant Use There are no known interactions where it is recommended to avoid concomitant use.

Increased Effect/Toxicity
Dantrolene may increase the levels/effects of: Alcohol (Ethyl); CNS Depressants; Methotrimeprazine

The levels/effects of Dantrolene may be increased by: CYP3A4 Inhibitors (Moderate); CYP3A4 Inhibitors (Strong); Dasatinib; Methotrimeprazine

Decreased Effect
The levels/effects of Dantrolene may be decreased by: CYP3A4 Inducers (Strong); Deferasirox; Herbs (CYP3A4 Inducers)

Stability Protect from light; use reconstituted injection within 6 hours; incompatible with dextrose, NS, or bacteriostatic water for injection; precipitates when placed in glass containers for infusion

Mechanism of Action Acts directly on skeletal muscle by interfering with release of calcium ion from the sarcoplasmic reticulum; prevents or reduces the increase in myoplasmic calcium ion concentration that activates the acute catabolic processes associated with malignant hyperthermia

Pharmacokinetics (Adult data unless noted)
Absorption: Oral: 70%
Metabolism: Extensive; metabolized to active metabolite: 5-hydroxydantrolene
Half-life:
Neonates (at birth): ~20 hours
Children: 10 ± 2.6 hours
Adults: 12 hours (range: 4-21 hours)
Elimination: 25% excreted in urine as metabolites and unchanged drug; 45% to 50% excreted in feces via bile

Usual Dosage

Spasticity: Oral: **Note:** Titrate to desired effect; if no further benefit is observed at a higher dosage, decrease dose to previous lower dose.

Children: Initial: 0.5 mg/kg/dose once daily for 7 days, increase to 0.5 mg/kg/dose 3 times/day for 7 days, increase to 1 mg/kg/dose 3 times/day for 7 days, and then increase to 2 mg/kg/dose 3 times/day; not to exceed 400 mg/day

Adults: 25 mg once daily for 7 days, increase to 25 mg 3 times/day for 7 days, increase to 50 mg 3 times/day for 7 days, and then increase to 100 mg 3 times/day; not to exceed 400 mg/day

Malignant hyperthermia: Children and Adults:

Preoperative prophylaxis: No longer recommended providing that there is immediate availability of dantrolene and adequate perioperative patient management (eg, avoiding known trigger agents in susceptible patients; see Additional Information)

Oral: 4-8 mg/kg/day in 3-4 divided doses for 1-2 days prior to surgery with the last dose administered approximately 3-4 hours before scheduled surgery

I.V.: 2.5 mg/kg administered approximately 1.25 hours prior to surgery (infuse over 1 hour)

Crisis: I.V.: Malignant Hyperthermia Association of the U.S. (MHAUS) and European recommendation: 2.5 mg/kg; may repeat as often as necessary until normalization of the hypermetabolic state and the disappearance of all symptoms (typically 1-4 doses; if >20 mg/kg is used without benefit, consider other potential diagnoses)

Postcrisis: MHAUS and European recommendations differ slightly in the postcrisis treatment regimen. Both are described below.

MHAUS recommendation: I.V.: Continue therapy with 1 mg/kg/dose every 6 hours for at least 24 hours after control of symptoms

European recommendation: I.V.: Continue therapy with a continuous infusion of 10 mg/kg/day for at least 36 hours

Manufacturer's recommendation: Oral: 4-8 mg/kg/day in 4 divided doses for 1-3 days following crisis

Administration

Oral: Contents of capsule may be mixed with juice or liquid

Parenteral: Reconstitute by adding 60 mL SWI (**not bacteriostatic water for injection**), resultant concentration 0.333 mg/mL; administer by rapid I.V. injection; for infusion, do **not** further dilute with NS or dextrose; place solution in plastic container for continuous infusion

Monitoring Parameters Baseline and periodic liver function tests; temperature (hyperthermia use)

Patient Information Avoid alcohol; may cause drowsiness and impair ability to perform activities requiring mental alertness or physical coordination

Nursing Implications Avoid extravasation since dantrolene is a tissue irritant

Additional Information MHAUS provides educational and technical information to patients and healthcare providers; contact at 607-674-7901 or email to info@mhaus.org; on-call anesthesiologists available to consult in MH emergencies may be obtained 24 hours/day at 1-(800)-MH-HYPER or 1-(800)-644-9737. Triggers for the development of malignant hyperthermia in susceptible individuals include: All volatile inhalation anesthetics (desflurane, sevoflurane, isoflurane, halothane, enflurane, ether, methoxyflurane, and cyclopropane) and succinylcholine.

Dantrolene has been used successfully to treat neuroleptic malignant syndrome associated with antipsychotic agents such as prochlorperazine, promethazine, clozapine, and risperidone and also non-neuroleptic agents such as metoclopramide, amoxapine, and lithium. The recommended dose for this indication has not been established. Published case reports have used doses ranging from 1-10 mg/kg/day in divided doses both I.V. and orally.

Dosage Forms Excipient information presented when available (limited, particularly for generics); consult specific product labeling.

Capsule, as sodium: 25 mg, 50 mg, 100 mg
Dantrium®: 25 mg, 50 mg, 100 mg

Injection, powder for reconstitution, as sodium:
Dantrium®: 20 mg [contains mannitol 3 g]

Extemporaneous Preparations A 5 mg/mL suspension may be made by adding five 100 mg capsules to a citric acid solution (150 mg citric acid powder in 10 mL water) and then adding syrup to a total volume of 100 mL; shake well; stable 2 days in refrigerator. Stability is improved when syrup BP (containing 0.5% w/v methylhydroxybenzoate) is used. This solution is stable 30 days refrigerated.

Nahata, MC, Pai VB, and Hipple TF, *Pediatric Drug Formulations*, 5th ed, Cincinnati, OH: Harvey Whitney Books Co, 2004.

References

Ali SZ, Taguchi A, and Rosenberg H, "Malignant Hyperthermia," *Best Pract Res Clin Anaesthesiol*, 2003, 17(4):519-33.

Allen GC, Cattran CB, Peterson RG, et al, "Plasma Levels of Dantrolene Following Oral Administration in Malignant Hyperthermia-Susceptible Patients," *Anesthesiology*, 1988, 69(6):900-4.

Guze BH and Baxter LR Jr, "Current Concepts. Neuroleptic Malignant Syndrome," *N Engl J Med*, 1985, 313(3):163-6.

Krause T, Gerbershagen MU, Fiege M, et al, "Dantrolene - A Review of Its Pharmacology, Therapeutic Use and New Developments," *Anaesthesia*, 2004, 59(4):364-73.

Lerman J, McLeod ME, and Strong HA, "Pharmacokinetics of Intravenous Dantrolene in Children," *Anesthesiology*, 1989, 70 (4):625-9.

Podranski T, Bouillon T, Schumacher PM, et al, "Compartmental Pharmacokinetics of Dantrolene in Adults: Do Malignant Hyperthermia Association Dosing Guidelines Work?" *Anesth Analg*, 2005, 101(6):1695-9.

Shime J, Gare D, Andrews J, et al, "Dantrolene in Pregnancy: Lack of Adverse Effects on the Fetus and Newborn Infant," *Am J Obstet Gynecol*, 1988, 159(4):831-4.

Susman VL, " Clinical Management of Neuroleptic Malignant Syndrome," *Psychiatr Q*, 2001, 72(4):325-36.

◆ **Dantrolene Sodium** see Dantrolene on page 386
◆ **Dapcin** see DAPTOmycin on page 389

Dapsone (DAP sone)

Medication Safety Issues
Sound-alike/look-alike issues:
Dapsone may be confused with Diprosone®

U.S. Brand Names Aczone®

Therapeutic Category Antibiotic, Sulfone; Leprostatic Agent

Generic Available Yes: Tablet

Use Treatment of leprosy due to susceptible strains of *M. leprae*; treatment of dermatitis herpetiformis; prophylaxis against *Pneumocystis jiroveci* pneumonia (PCP) in patients who cannot tolerate sulfamethoxazole and trimethoprim or aerosolized pentamidine; prophylaxis against toxoplasmic encephalitis in patients who cannot tolerate sulfamethoxazole and trimethoprim; topical treatment of acne vulgaris

Pregnancy Risk Factor C

Pregnancy Considerations Because of adverse events observed in some animal studies, dapsone is classified as pregnancy category C. Per the manufacturer, dapsone has not shown an increased risk of congenital anomalies when given during all trimesters of pregnancy. Several reports have described adverse effects in the newborn after *in utero* exposure to dapsone, including neonatal hemolytic disease, methemoglobinemia, and hyperbilirubinemia. Dapsone is an alternative for prophylaxis and treatment of *Pneumocystis jiroveci* pneumonia (PCP) in pregnant,

◀ HIV-infected patients. Dapsone is also recommended for pregnant women requiring maintenance therapy of either leprosy or dermatitis herpetiformis

Lactation Enters breast milk/not recommended (AAP rates "compatible")

Breast-Feeding Considerations Dapsone is excreted in breast milk and can be detected in the serum of nursing infants. Hemolytic anemia has been reported in a breast-fed infant. The AAP considers dapsone to be "usually compatible with breast-feeding"; however, breast-feeding is not recommended by the manufacturer due to the potential for carcinogenicity observed in animal studies and the potential for hemolysis in the neonate, especially if there is a family history of G6PD deficiency.

Contraindications Hypersensitivity to dapsone or any component; patients with severe anemia

Precautions Use with caution in patients with G-6-PD deficiency, methemoglobin reductase deficiency or hemoglobin M; in patients receiving drugs capable of inducing hemolysis and in patients with severe cardiopulmonary disease; hypersensitivity to other sulfonamides; obtain G6PD levels prior to initiating dapsone therapy

Adverse Reactions

Cardiovascular: Tachycardia

Central nervous system: Psychotic episodes, hallucinations, insomnia, vertigo, irritability, depression, headache, fever, uncoordinated speech, suicidal behavior

Dermatologic: Rash, exfoliative dermatitis, erythema multiforme, toxic epidermal necrolysis, urticaria, morbilliform reactions, erythema nodosum, photosensitivity (oral)

Topical: erythema, skin peeling

Endocrine & metabolic: Hyperkalemia, hypoalbuminemia

Gastrointestinal: Nausea, vomiting, abdominal pain, anorexia, pancreatitis

Hematologic: Hemolytic anemia, methemoglobinemia, leukopenia, agranulocytosis, aplastic anemia, neutropenia

Hepatic: Hepatitis, cholestatic jaundice; alkaline phosphatase, AST, bilirubin, and LDH elevated

Neuromuscular & skeletal: Muscle weakness, peripheral neuropathy, tonic clonic movements

Ocular: Blurred vision

Otic: Tinnitus

Renal: Acute tubular necrosis, nephrotic syndrome, albuminuria

Respiratory: Pharyngitis

Miscellaneous: Lupus erythematosus, mononucleosis-like syndrome

Drug Interactions

Metabolism/Transport Effects Substrate of CYP2C8 (minor), 2C9 (major), 2C19 (minor), 2E1 (minor), 3A4 (major)

Avoid Concomitant Use

Avoid concomitant use of Dapsone with any of the following: BCG

Increased Effect/Toxicity

Dapsone may increase the levels/effects of: Antimalarial Agents; Trimethoprim

The levels/effects of Dapsone may be increased by: Antimalarial Agents; CYP2C9 Inhibitors (Moderate); CYP2C9 Inhibitors (Strong); CYP3A4 Inhibitors (Moderate); CYP3A4 Inhibitors (Strong); Dasatinib; Probenecid; Trimethoprim

Decreased Effect

Dapsone may decrease the levels/effects of: BCG; Typhoid Vaccine

The levels/effects of Dapsone may be decreased by: CYP2C9 Inducers (Highly Effective); CYP3A4 Inducers (Strong); Deferasirox; Didanosine; Herbs (CYP3A4 Inducers); Peginterferon Alfa-2b; Rifamycin Derivatives

Food Interactions Do not administer with antacids, alkaline foods, or alkaline drugs (may decrease dapsone absorption)

Stability Protect from freezing and light. Store at room temperature. Store gel in original box after use.

Mechanism of Action Dapsone is a sulfone antimicrobial. The mechanism of action of the sulfones is similar to that of the sulfonamides. Sulfonamides are competitive antagonists of para-aminobenzoic acid (PABA) and inhibit folic acid synthesis in susceptible organisms.

Pharmacokinetics (Adult data unless noted)

Absorption: Oral: 86% to 100%

Distribution: Distributes into skin, muscle, kidneys, liver, sweat, sputum, saliva, tears, and bile; distributes into breast milk; crosses the placenta

V_d: Adults: 1.5-2.5 L/kg

Protein binding: 50% to 90%

Metabolism: Acetylated and hydroxylated in the liver

Half-life:

Children: 15.1 hours

Adults: 13-83 hours (mean: 20-30 hours)

Time to peak serum concentration: Within 2-8 hours

Elimination: 5% to 20% of dose excreted in urine as unchanged drug; 70% to 85% excreted in urine as metabolites; small amount excreted in feces

Usual Dosage

Oral:

Children ≥1 month of age:

Prophylaxis for first episode of opportunistic disease due to *Toxoplasma gondii*: 2 mg/kg or 15 mg/m^2 (maximum dose: 25 mg) once daily in combination with pyrimethamine 1 mg/kg once daily and leucovorin calcium 5 mg every 3 days

Primary and secondary PCP prophylaxis (see **Note** in Additional Information): 2 mg/kg/day once daily (maximum dose: 100 mg/day), or 4 mg/kg/dose once weekly (maximum dose: 200 mg)

Children:

Leprosy: 1-2 mg/kg/day given once daily in combination therapy; maximum dose: 100 mg/day

Adults:

Leprosy: 50-100 mg once daily; combination therapy with one or more antileprosy drugs is recommended to avoid dapsone resistance

Dermatitis herpetiformis: Initial: 50 mg once daily; maintenance dosage range: 25-400 mg/day

PCP treatment: 100 mg once daily in combination with trimethoprim

Primary and secondary PCP prophylaxis: 50 mg twice daily; or dapsone 50 mg once daily plus pyrimethamine 50 mg orally every week plus leucovorin calcium 25 mg orally every week; or dapsone 200 mg orally plus pyrimethamine 75 mg orally plus leucovorin calcium 25 mg orally every week

Toxoplasma gondii prophylaxis: 50 mg once daily plus pyrimethamine 50 mg orally every week, plus leucovorin calcium 25 mg orally every week

Topical: Children ≥12 years, Adolescents, and Adults: Apply a pea-sized amount of gel to the acne-affected areas twice daily

Administration

Oral: Administer with water. Separate buffered didanosine administration from dapsone by at least 2 hours.

Topical: Wash skin and pat dry then rub in thin layer of gel gently and completely. Wash hands after application.

Monitoring Parameters CBC with differential, platelet count, hemoglobin, reticulocyte count, hematocrit, liver function tests, and urinalysis; check G6PD levels prior to initiation of dapsone

Patient Information Notify physician if fever, sore throat, pallor, fatigue, muscle weakness, rash, purpura, or jaundice occurs. May cause photosensitivity reactions (eg, exposure to sunlight may cause severe sunburn, skin rash, redness, or itching); avoid exposure to sunlight and artificial light sources (sunlamps, tanning booth/bed); wear protective clothing, wide-brimmed hats, sunglasses, and lip sunscreen (SPF ≥15); use a sunscreen [broad-spectrum sunscreen or physical sunscreen (preferred) or sunblock with SPF ≥15]; contact physician if reaction occurs. Dapsone distributes into breast milk and may harm your baby. A decision should be made to discontinue breast-feeding or the drug.

Additional Information Note: Guidelines for prophylaxis of *Pneumocystis jiroveci* pneumonia: Initiate PCP prophylaxis in the following patients: In all HIV-exposed children at 4-6 weeks of age and continue through the first year of life or until HIV infection has been reasonably excluded; children 1-5 years of age with CD4+ count <500 or CD4+ percentage <15%; children 6-12 years of age with CD4+ count <200 or CD4+ percentage <15%; adolescents and adults with CD4+ count <200 or oropharyngeal candidiasis. Leucovorin calcium should be given if bone marrow suppression occurs.

Dosage Forms Excipient information presented when available (limited, particularly for generics); consult specific product labeling.

Gel, topical:

Aczone®: 5% (30 g, 60 g)

Tablet: 25 mg, 100 mg

Extemporaneous Preparations A 2 mg/mL oral suspension can be made using a 1:1 mixture of Ora-Sweet® and Ora-Plus®; crush eight 25 mg tablets into a fine powder in a mortar; add a small amount of vehicle and mix to make a uniform paste; mix while adding the vehicle in geometric portions to almost 100 mL; transfer to a calibrated bottle and qsad with vehicle to 100 mL; preparation is stable for 90 days when stored at room temperature or under refrigeration; label "shake well"

Jacobus Pharmaceutical Company (609) 921-7447 makes a 2 mg/mL proprietary liquid formulation available under an IND for the prophylaxis of *Pneumocystis jiroveci* pneumonia

Nahata MC, Morosco RS, and Trowbridge JM, "Stability of Dapsone in Two Oral Liquid Dosage Forms," *Ann Pharmacother*, 2000, 34(7-8):848-50.

References

Barnett ED, Pelton SI, Mirochnick M, et al, "Dapsone for Prevention of *Pneumocystis* Pneumonia in Children With Acquired Immunodeficiency Syndrome," *Pediatr Infect Dis J*, 1994, 13(1):72-4.

Kaplan JE, Masur H, and Holmes KK, "Guidelines for Preventing Opportunistic Infections Among HIV-Infected Persons - 2002 Recommendations of the USPHS and IDSA," *MMWR*, 2002, 51 (RR-8):1-46.

Mirochnick M, Michaels M, Clarke D, et al, "Pharmacokinetics of Dapsone in Children," *J Pediatr*, 1993, 122(5 Pt 1):806-9.

Stavola JJ and Noel GJ, "Efficacy and Safety of Dapsone Prophylaxis Against *Pneumocystis carinii* Pneumonia in Human Immunodeficiency Virus-Infected Children," *Pediatr Infect Dis J*, 1993, 12 (8):644-7.

♦ **Daptacel®** *see* Diphtheria, Tetanus Toxoids, and Acellular Pertussis Vaccine *on page* 458

DAPTOmycin (DAP toe mye sin)

Medication Safety Issues

Sound-alike/look-alike issues:

Cubicin® may be confused with Cleocin®

DAPTOmycin may be confused with DACTINomycin

U.S. Brand Names Cubicin®

Canadian Brand Names Cubicin®

Therapeutic Category Antibiotic, Cyclic Lipopeptide

Generic Available No

Use Treatment of complicated skin and skin structure infections caused by susceptible aerobic gram-positive organisms including *S. aureus* [methicillin-sensitive *Staph. aureus* (MSSA) and methicillin-resistant *Staph. aureus* (MRSA)], *S. pyogenes*, *S. agalactiae*, *S. dysgalactiae*, and *E. faecalis*. Treatment of *S. aureus* bacteremia, including right-sided infective endocarditis caused by MSSA or MRSA (FDA approved in ages ≥18 years). Daptomycin is active against bacteria resistant to methicillin, vancomycin, and linezolid.

Pregnancy Risk Factor B

Pregnancy Considerations Because adverse events were not observed in animal reproduction studies, daptomycin is classified as pregnancy category B. There are no adequate and well-controlled studies in pregnant women

Lactation Excretion in breast milk unknown/use caution

Breast-Feeding Considerations It is not known if daptomycin is excreted in breast milk. The manufacturer recommends caution if daptomycin is used during breast-feeding. The high molecular weight of daptomycin may limit the transfer to the maternal milk. If daptomycin reaches the breast milk, nondose-related effects could include modification of bowel flora.

Contraindications Hypersensitivity to daptomycin or any component

Warnings May be associated with an increased incidence of myopathy; discontinue daptomycin in patients with unexplained signs and symptoms of myopathy in conjunction with CPK elevation >5 times ULN or >1000 units/L or in asymptomatic patients who have CPK elevations ≥10 x ULN. Myopathy may occur more frequently when daptomycin dose and/or frequency exceeds the recommended dose. Symptoms suggestive of peripheral neuropathy have been observed with treatment; monitor for new-onset or worsening neuropathy. Prolonged use may result in superinfection, including *C. difficile*-associated diarrhea and pseudomembranous colitis. Daptomycin is not indicated for treatment of pneumonia due to its inactivation by pulmonary surfactant and its poor lung penetration.

Precautions Use with caution in patients receiving other drugs associated with myopathy (eg, HMG-CoA reductase inhibitors); consider temporarily suspending the use of HMG-CoA reductase inhibitors in patients receiving daptomycin. Use caution and adjust dosage in patients with severe renal impairment (Cl_{cr} <30 mL/minute).

Adverse Reactions

Cardiovascular: Peripheral edema, hypotension, hypertension, chest pain, atrial fibrillation, supraventricular arrhythmia

Central nervous system: Headache, insomnia, fever, dizziness, anxiety, hallucination, jitteriness, vertigo

Dermatologic: Rash, pruritus, erythema

Endocrine & metabolic: Hypokalemia, hyperkalemia, hyperphosphatemia, hypomagnesemia

Gastrointestinal: Constipation, diarrhea, nausea, vomiting, dyspepsia, abdominal pain, GI hemorrhage, stomatitis, pseudomembranous colitis, *C. difficile*-associated diarrhea

Hematologic: Anemia, thrombocytopenia, INR elevated, eosinophilia

Hepatic: Transaminases and alkaline phosphatase elevated, jaundice

Local: Injection site reaction

Neuromuscular & skeletal: Myopathy, arthralgia, limb pain, CPK elevated, back pain, weakness, arthralgia, myalgia, muscle cramps, paresthesia, rhabdomyolysis

Ocular: Blurred vision

Otic: Tinnitus

Renal: Renal failure, proteinuria

Respiratory: Dyspnea, pharyngolaryngeal pain, pleural effusion, cough, pneumonia, pulmonary eosinophilic infiltrate, shortness of breath

◀

Miscellaneous: Sepsis, infection (fungal), diaphoresis, anaphylaxis

Drug Interactions

Avoid Concomitant Use There are no known interactions where it is recommended to avoid concomitant use.

Increased Effect/Toxicity
The levels/effects of DAPTOmycin may be increased by: HMG-CoA Reductase Inhibitors

Decreased Effect There are no known significant interactions involving a decrease in effect.

Stability Refrigerate vial containing lyophilized powder for injection. Reconstitute vial with 10 mL NS by gently rotating vial to wet powder; allow vial to stand for 10 minutes, then gently swirl to obtain completely reconstituted solution. Do not shake or agitate vial vigorously. Further dilute reconstituted solution in an appropriate volume of NS. Reconstituted vial or infusion solution is stable for 12 hours at room temperature or 48 hours if refrigerated. Daptomycin is incompatible with dextrose-containing solutions.

Mechanism of Action Daptomycin binds to cell membrane components of susceptible organisms causing rapid depolarization by calcium-dependent insertion, inhibiting intracellular synthesis of DNA, RNA, and protein resulting in bacterial cell death.

Pharmacokinetics (Adult data unless noted)
Distribution: V_d:
Children 2-6 years: 0.14 ± 0.02 L/kg
Children 7-17 years: 0.11 ± 0.02 L/kg
Adults: 0.1 L/kg
Protein binding: 90% to 93%; 84% to 88% in patients with Cl_{cr}<30 mL/minute
Metabolism: Minor amounts of oxidative metabolites have been detected; does not induce or inhibit cytochrome P450 enzymes
Half-life:
Children 2-6 years: 5.3 ± 1.9 hours
Children 7-11 years: 5.6 ± 2.2 hours
Children 12-17 years: 6.7 ± 2.2 hours
Adults: 8-9 hours (prolonged with renal impairment)
Elimination: 78% of the dose excreted in urine primarily as unchanged drug; feces (6%)
Dialysis: 15% removed by hemodialysis (4 hour duration)

Usual Dosage I.V.:
Children 2-17 years: **Note:** Not FDA approved in children; limited information is available.
Retrospective review of 16 children who received daptomycin for treatment of invasive infections caused by gram-positive bacteria (median age: 6.5 years; 10 male); daptomycin was added to the antimicrobial regimen of 15 patients in a dose of 4-6 mg/kg/dose given intravenously once daily; one patient received daptomycin monotherapy in a dose of 4 mg/kg/dose every 48 hours due to a creatinine clearance <30 mL/minute. Fourteen patients improved after addition of daptomycin and were discharged home; 2 patients died of complications of their underlying medical condition. No adverse events were attributed to daptomycin (Ardura, 2007). Further studies are needed.
Adults:
Complicated skin and skin structure infections: 4 mg/kg once daily for 7-14 days
S. aureus bacteremia or right-sided endocarditis: 6 mg/kg once daily for 2-6 weeks

Dosage adjustment in renal impairment: Adults:
Cl_{cr} <30 mL/minute: 4 mg/kg once every 48 hours for complicated skin infections; 6 mg/kg once every 48 hours for S. aureus bacteremia
Hemodialysis and/or CAPD: Dose as in Cl_{cr} <30 mL/minute and administer after dialysis
Continuous renal replacement therapy (CRRT): Dose as in Cl_{cr} <30 mL/minute

Dosage adjustment in hepatic impairment: No adjustment required for mild-to-moderate impairment (Child-Pugh Class A or B); not evaluated in severe hepatic impairment

Administration I.V.: Infuse over 30 minutes at a final concentration not to exceed 20 mg/mL. Do not use in conjunction with ReadyMED® elastomeric infusion pumps (Cardinal Health, Inc) due to an impurity (2-mercaptobenzothiazole) which leaches from the pump system into the daptomycin solution.

Monitoring Parameters Signs and symptoms of myopathy (muscle pain or weakness, particularly of the distal extremities), weekly CPK levels during therapy (more frequent monitoring if history of current or prior statin therapy and/or renal impairment), signs of peripheral neuropathy; observe for changes in bowel frequency; monitor renal function periodically

Reference Range
Trough concentrations at steady-state:
4 mg/kg once daily: 5.9 ± 1.6 mcg/mL
6 mg/kg once daily: 6.7 ± 1.6 mcg/mL
Note: Trough concentrations are not predictive of efficacy or toxicity. Daptomycin exhibits concentration-dependent bactericidal activity, so C_{max}:MIC ratios may be a more useful parameter.

Test Interactions Daptomycin may cause false prolongation of the PT and elevate the INR with certain reagents. Test interaction may be minimized by obtaining blood samples for PT/INR immediately prior to next daptomycin dose (trough level).

Patient Information Report immediately any burning, pain, or redness at infusion site; any throat tightness, respiratory difficulty, or chest tightness. Inform physician if muscle pain, weakness, peripheral neuropathy, or persistent diarrhea occur.

Dosage Forms Excipient information presented when available (limited, particularly for generics); consult specific product labeling.

Injection, powder for reconstitution:
Cubicin®: 500 mg

References
Abdel-Rahman SM, Benziger DP, Jacobs RF, et al, "Single-Dose Pharmacokinetics of Daptomycin in Children With Suspected or Proved Gram-Positive Infections," Pediatr Infect Dis J, 2008, 27 (4):330-4.
Ardura MI, Mejías A, Katz KS, et al, "Daptomycin Therapy for Invasive Gram-Positive Bacterial Infections in Children," Pediatr Infect Dis J, 2007, 26(12):1128-32.

◆ **Daraprim®** see Pyrimethamine on page 1191

Darbepoetin Alfa (dar be POE e tin AL fa)

Medication Safety Issues
Sound-alike/look-alike issues:
Aranesp® may be confused with Aralast, Aricept®
Darbepoetin alfa may be confused with dalteparin, epoetin alfa, epoetin beta

U.S. Brand Names Aranesp®

Canadian Brand Names Aranesp®

Therapeutic Category Colony-Stimulating Factor; Erythropoiesis Stimulating Protein

Generic Available No

Use Treatment of anemia associated with chronic renal failure (requiring dialysis or not) (FDA approved in ages >1 year and adults) or anemia associated with concurrent chemotherapy for nonmyeloid malignancies (FDA approved in adults)

Restrictions Healthcare providers and hospitals must be enrolled in the ESA APPRISE (Assisting Providers and Cancer Patients with Risk Information for the Safe use of ESAs) Oncology Program (866-284-8089; http://www.esa-apprise.com) to prescribe or dispense ESAs (ie, darbepoetin alfa, epoetin alfa) to patients with cancer.

Medication Guide An FDA-approved patient medication guide, which is available with the product information and at http://www.fda.gov/downloads/Drugs/DrugSafety/UCM085918.pdf, must be dispensed with this medication for each new outpatient prescription and refill.

Pregnancy Risk Factor C

Pregnancy Considerations There are no adequate and well-controlled studies in pregnant women. Darbepoetin alfa should be used in a pregnant woman only if potential benefit justifies the potential risk to the fetus.

Lactation Excretion in breast milk unknown/use caution

Contraindications Hypersensitivity to darbepoetin alfa or any component; uncontrolled hypertension

Warnings Patients with chronic renal failure are at greater risk for death, serious cardiovascular events, and stroke when using erthryopoiesis-stimulating agents (ESAs) to target higher hemoglobin concentrations (≥13 g/dL) in clinical trials; dosing should be individualized to achieve and maintain hemoglobin concentrations within 10-12 g/dL range **[U.S. Boxed Warning]**. Increased thrombotic events have also been documented in cancer patients. Due to an increased risk of cardiac arrest, neurologic events (including seizures and stroke), exacerbations of hypertension, CHF, vascular thrombosis/ischemia/infarction, acute MI, and fluid overdose/edema in patients whose Hgb increased >12 g/dL, hemoglobin should be monitored twice weekly for 2-6 weeks following initiation and dosage adjustments. The darbepoetin alfa dosage should be decreased if the the Hgb exccode 12 g/dL or the rate of rise of hemoglobin exceeds 1 g/dL in any 2-week period. In clinical trials, ~40% of CRF patients required initiation or intensification of antihypertensive therapy; blood pressure should be controlled adequately before initiation of darbepoetin alfa therapy; close blood pressure monitoring is recommended. ESA therapy may reduce dialysis efficacy (due to increase in red blood cells and decrease in plasma volume); adjustments in dialysis parameters may be needed.

ESAs shortened survival and/or time-to-tumor progression in studies of advanced breast, head and neck, lymphoid, and nonsmall cell lung cancer in patients receiving ESAs dosed to target a hemoglobin of ≥12 g/dL **[U.S. Boxed Warning]**. This risk has not been excluded when a lower target hemoglobin is used. Because of the risks of decreased survival and increased risk of tumor growth or progression, all healthcare providers and hospitals are required to enroll and comply with the ESA APPRISE (Assisting Providers and Cancer Patients with Risk Information for the Safe use of ESAs) Oncology Program prior to prescribing or dispensing ESAs to cancer patients, ESA APPRISE Oncology Program **[U.S. Boxed Warning]**. Prescribers and patients will have to provide written documentation of discussed risks. For patients with cancer, use only for the treatment of anemia due to concomitant myelosuppressive chemotherapy, use the lowest dose needed to avoid transfusions, and discontinue following completion of chemotherapy course **[U.S. Boxed Warning]**. Darbepoetin alfa is not approved for use in patients with myeloid malignancies or in patients with cancer-related anemia who are not receiving concurrent chemotherapy.

The risk of thrombotic events (eg, pulmonary emboli, thrombophlebitis, thrombosis) is increased with ESA therapy. Increased mortality was observed in patients undergoing coronary artery bypass surgery who received ESAs; these deaths were associated with thrombotic events. An increased risk of DVT has been observed in patients treated with ESAs undergoing surgical orthopedic procedures. Darbepoetin alfa is not approved for reduction in allogeneic RBC transfusions in patients scheduled for surgical procedures.

Cases of pure red cell aplasia (PRCA) and severe anemia with or without other cytopenias associated with neutralizing antibodies to erythropoietin have been reported in CRF patients and patients receiving other ESAs. Cases have also been reported in patients with hepatitis C who were receiving ESAs, interferon, and ribavirin. Patients who develop a sudden loss of responsiveness to darbepoetin therapy along with a severe anemia and low reticulocyte count should be evaluated for the presence of these antibodies. Withhold darbepoetin until the etiology is confirmed. Amgen can perform assays for binding and neutralizing antibodies. Safety and efficacy in patients with underlying hematologic diseases (eg, porphyria, thalassemia, hemolytic anemia, and sickle cell disease) have not been established.

Precautions Use with caution in patients with a history of seizures or hypertension; an excessive rate of rise of hematocrit may possibly be associated with the exacerbation of hypertension or seizures. Decrease the darbepoetin alfa dosage if the hemoglobin increase exceeds 1 g/dL in any 2-week period. Blood pressure should be controlled prior to the start of therapy and monitored closely throughout treatment. Hypertensive encephalopathy has been reported with patients receiving erythropoietic therapy. Seizures have occurred during ESA therapy; monitor closely for premonitory neurologic symptoms during the first several months of therapy. Potentially serious allergic reactions have been reported (rarely). Discontinue immediately (and permanently) in patients who experience serious allergic/anaphylactic reactions.

Darbepoetin alfa is not intended for patients who require acute corrections of anemia and is not a substitute for emergency blood transfusion. Allow sufficient time (an interval of 4-6 weeks) to determine the patient's response to a particular dosage (see Warnings regarding rapid responsiveness); patients with CRF not yet requiring dialysis may require lower maintenance doses. Assessment of iron stores and therapeutic iron supplementation is essential for optimal therapy. Iron supplementation is necessary to provide for increased requirements during expansion of the red cell mass secondary to marrow stimulation unless iron stores are already in excess. Optimal iron stores are demonstrated by a transferrin saturation of 20% or more and a serum ferritin of 100-150 mcg/L. Some products contain albumin, which confers a theoretical risk of transmission of viral disease or Creutzfeldt-Jakob disease.

Factors Limiting Response to Darbepoetin Alfa

Factor	Mechanism
Iron deficiency	Limits hemoglobin synthesis
Blood loss/hemolysis	Counteracts darbepoetin alfa-stimulated erythropoiesis
Infection/inflammation	Inhibits iron transfer from storage to bone marrow
	Suppresses erythropoiesis through activated macrophages
Aluminum overload	Inhibits iron incorporation into heme protein
Bone marrow replacement Hyperparathyroidism Metastatic, neoplastic disease	Limits bone marrow volume
Folic acid/vitamin B_{12} deficiency	Limits hemoglobin synthesis
Patient compliance	Self administered darbepoetin alfa or iron therapy

Adverse Reactions

Cardiovascular: Cardiac arrest, cardiac arrhythmia, chest pain, CHF, edema, hypertension, hypotension, MI, tachycardia, thrombophlebitis, TIA/CVA (see Warnings), venous thrombosis

Central nervous system: Dizziness, fatigue, fever, headache, seizure

Dermatologic: Pruritus, rash

Gastrointestinal: Abdominal pain, constipation, diarrhea, nausea, vomiting

Hematologic: Neutropenia, pure red cell aplasia, severe anemia (see Warnings)

Local: Irritation at injection site (SubQ injection), pain

Neuromuscular & skeletal: Arthralgia, back pain, limb pain, myalgia

Respiratory: Bronchitis, cough, dyspnea, pulmonary embolism, upper respiratory infection

Miscellaneous: Allergic reaction, flu-like symptoms, tumor progression (cancer patients) (see Warnings)

<1%, postmarketing, and/or case reports: Abscess, bacteremia, deep vein thrombosis, GI hemorrhage, hypertensive encephalopathy, peritonitis, sepsis, thromboembolism, thrombophlebitis

Drug Interactions

Avoid Concomitant Use There are no known interactions where it is recommended to avoid concomitant use.

Increased Effect/Toxicity There are no known significant interactions involving an increase in effect.

Decreased Effect There are no known significant interactions involving a decrease in effect.

Stability Store at 2°C to 8°C (36°F to 46°F); protect from light; contains no preservatives; discard after entry

Mechanism of Action Darbepoetin alfa, manufactured by recombinant DNA technology, has the same effects as endogenous erythropoietin (EPO). It differs slightly from recombinant human erythropoietin in containing 5 N-linked oligosaccharide chains instead of 3. EPO induces erythropoiesis by stimulating the division and differentiation of committed erythroid progenitor cells. It induces the release of reticulocytes from the bone marrow into the bloodstream, where they mature to erythrocytes (dose response relationship) resulting in an increase in reticulocyte counts followed by a rise in hematocrit and hemoglobin concentrations. There is normally an inverse correlation between the plasma EPO concentration and the hemoglobin concentration (only when the hemoglobin concentration is <10.5 g/dL).

Pharmacodynamics

Onset of action: Several days

Maximum effect: 4-6 weeks

Pharmacokinetics (Adult data unless noted)

Absorption: SubQ: Slow and rate-limiting

Distribution: V_d:

Children: 51.6 mL/kg (range: 21-73 mL/kg)

Adults: 52.4 ± 6.6 mL/kg

Bioavailability: SubQ: CRF:

Children: 54% (range:32% to 70%)

Adults: ~37% (range: 30% to 50%)

Half-life:

Children:

I.V.: Terminal: 22.1 hours (range: 12-30 hours)

SubQ: Terminal: 42.8 hours (range: 16-86 hours); Children with cancer: 49.4 hours

Adults: CRF:

I.V.: Terminal: 21 hours

SubQ: Terminal: 49 ± 12.7 hours

Time to peak serum concentration: SubQ:

CRF patients: 34 hours (range: 24-72 hours)

Cancer patients:

Children: 71.4 hours (median time)

Adults: 90 hours (range: 71-123 hours)

Elimination:

Clearance: I.V.:

Children: 2.29 mL/hour/kg (range: 1.6-3.5 mL/hour/kg)

Adults: 1.6 ± 1.0 mL/hour/kg

Usual Dosage Dosing schedules need to be individualized by treatment indication and patient response. Careful monitoring of hemoglobin in patients receiving the drug is recommended. The Hgb should not exceed 12 g/dL or increase by >1 g/dL in any 2-week period. Darbepoetin alfa may be ineffective if other factors such as iron or B_{12}/folate deficiency limit marrow response.

Anemia in chronic renal failure: Children >1 year and Adults: I.V., SubQ: 0.45 mcg/kg/dose once weekly; alternative dose for nondialysis patients: 0.75 mcg/kg once every 2 weeks (studied in adults but due to similar pharmacokinetics, may be applicable to children). See "Darbepoetin Alfa Dosage Adjustments in CRF" table on next page.

Note: Allow at least 4 weeks to determine full effects of the new regimen. For many patients, the appropriate maintenance dose may be less than the initial dose. Patients not receiving hemodialysis may be particularly sensitive and require lower doses. SubQ dosing every two weeks has been effective in some patients.

Darbepoetin Alfa Dosage Adjustments in CRF

Target hemoglobin range[1]	10-12 g/dL; not to exceed 12 g/dL
Increase dose (not more frequently than once monthly)	By 25% when hemoglobin does not increase by 1 g/dL after 4 weeks of therapy and hemoglobin is below target range
Reduce dose	By 25% when hemoglobin increases >1 g/dL in any 2-week period or when hemoglobin >12 g/dL
Stop therapy	When hemoglobin continues to increase after dosage reduction; reinstate therapy at a 25% lower dose after the hemoglobin begins to decrease
Inadequate response (patient does not attain target hemoglobin range or 10-12 g/dL after appropriate dose titrations over 12 weeks)	Do not continue to increase dose but use the minimum effective dose that will maintain a hemoglobin concentration sufficient to avoid RBC transfusions and evaluate patient for other causes of anemia Monitor hemoglobin closely, if responsiveness improves, may resume making dosage adjustments as recommended above. If responsiveness does not improve and recurrent RBC transfusions continue to be needed, discontinue therapy

[1]The National Kidney Foundation Clinical Practice Guideline for Anemia in CKD: 2007 Update of Hemoglobin Target (September, 2007) recommend hemoglobin concentrations in the range of 11-12 g/dL for dialysis and nondialysis patients receiving ESAs; hemoglobin concentrations should not be >13 g/dL

Anemia associated with chemotherapy in patients with nonmyeloid malignancies: Titrate dosage to use the minimum effective dose that will maintain a hemoglobin concentration sufficient to avoid RBC transfusions and not to exceed a hemoglobin concentration of 12 g/dL. **Note:** Use in patients with pretreatment serum EPO concentrations >200 mIU/ML is not recommended.

Children and Adults: SubQ: 2.25 mcg/kg/dose once weekly or as an alternative in adults: 500 mcg once every 3 weeks. Adjust dosage depending upon response; if indicated dosage may be increased to a maximum of 4.5 mcg/kg/dose; allow at least 6 weeks of therapy before increasing the dosage. Discontinue treatment when chemotherapy course has been completed. See "Darbepoetin Alfa Dosage Adjustments in Anemia Associated with Chemotherapy" table.

Darbepoetin Alfa Dosage Adjustments in Anemia Associated With Chemotherapy

Target hemoglobin	Not to exceed 12 g/dL
Increase dose	When hemoglobin does not increase by 1 g/dL after 6 weeks of therapy and hemoglobin is below target range
Reduce dose	By 40% when hemoglobin increases >1 g/dL in any 2-week period or when hemoglobin reaches a concentration sufficient to avoid RBC transfusions
Withhold dose	When hemoglobin exceeds 12 g/dL; resume treatment with a dose 40% below the previous dose when hemoglobin approaches a concentration where transfusions may be required

Conversion From Epoetin Alfa to Darbepoetin Alfa (I.V. or SubQ)[1]

(maintain the same route of administration for the conversion)

Previous Weekly Epoetin Alfa Dose (units/wk)	Weekly Darbepoetin Alfa Dosage[2]		
	Pediatric (mcg/wk)	Adults (mcg/wk)	Adults (mcg every 2 wks)
<1500	Not established	6.25	12.5
1500-2499	6.25	6.25	12.5
2500-4999	10	12.5	25
5000-10,999	20	25	50
11,000-17,999	40	40	80
18,000-33,999	60	60	120
34,000-89,999	100	100	200
≥90,000	200	200	400

[1]1 mcg darbepoetin alfa is equivalent to 200 units epoetin alfa.

[2]Due to the longer serum half-life of darbepoetin alfa, when converting from epoetin alfa, administer darbepoetin alfa once weekly if the patient was receiving epoetin alfa 2-3 times weekly and administer darbepoetin alfa once every two weeks if the patient was receiving epoetin alfa once weekly.

Administration May be administered I.V. or SubQ. Do not shake as this may denature the glycoprotein rendering the drug biologically inactive; only use SureClick™ auto-injectors if administering the full dose. Autoinjectors are for subcutaneous administration only. I.V.: Infuse over 1-3 minutes; I.V. route preferred for hemodialysis patients.

Monitoring Parameters
Careful monitoring of blood pressure is indicated; problems with hypertension have been noted especially in renal failure patients treated with darbepoetin alfa. See table.

Test	Initial Phase Frequency	Maintenance Phase Frequency
Hemoglobin	Once weekly until stabilized	2-4 times/mo
Blood pressure	3 times/week	3 times/wk
Serum ferritin	Monthly	Quarterly
Transferrin saturation	Monthly	Quarterly
Serum chemistries[1]	Regularly per routine	Regularly per routine
Reticulocyte count	Baseline prior to starting therapy	After 10 days of therapy

[1]Including CBC with differential, creatinine, BUN, potassium, phosphorus

Patient Information Frequent blood tests are needed to determine the correct dose; notify physician if any signs of edema (swollen extremities, respiratory difficulty), sudden onset of severe headache, back pain, chest pain, muscle tremors or weakness, fever, cough or signs of respiratory infection, dizziness or loss of consciousness, extreme tiredness, or blood clots in hemodialysis vascular access ports (CRF patients) develops. Due to an increased risk of seizure activity in CRF patients during the first 90 days of therapy, avoid potentially hazardous activities (eg, driving) during this period.

Additional Information Optimal response is achieved when iron stores are maintained with supplemental iron if necessary; evaluate iron stores prior to and during therapy. Use of ESAs in anemic patients with HIV who have been treated with zidovudine has not been demonstrated in controlled clinical trails to improve the symptoms of anemia, quality of life, fatigue, or well-being.

393

Dosage Forms Excipient information presented when available (limited, particularly for generics); consult specific product labeling.

Injection, solution [preservative free]:

Aranesp®: 25 mcg/0.42 mL (0.42 mL); 40 mcg/ 0.4 mL (0.4 mL); 60 mcg/0.3 mL (0.3 mL); 100 mcg/0.5 mL (0.5 mL); 150 mcg/0.3 mL (0.3 mL); 200 mcg/0.4 mL (0.4 mL); 300 mcg/0.6 mL (0.6 mL); 500 mcg/mL (1 mL) [contains polysorbate 80; prefilled syringe; needle cover contains latex]

Aranesp®: 25 mcg/mL (1 mL); 40 mcg/mL (1 mL); 60 mcg/mL (1 mL); 100 mcg/mL (1 mL); 150 mcg/0.75 mL (0.75 mL); 200 mcg/mL (1 mL); 300 mcg/mL (1 mL) [contains polysorbate 80; single-dose vial]

References

André JL, Deschênes G, Boudailliez B, et al, "Darbepoetin, Effective Treatment of Anaemia in Paediatric Patients With Chronic Renal Failure," *Pediatr Nephrol*, 2007, 22(5):708-14.

Blumer J, Berg S, Adamson PC, et al, "Pharmacokinetic Evaluation of Darbepoetin Alfa for the Treatment of Pediatric Patients With Chemotherapy-Induced Anemia," *Pediatr Blood Cancer*, 2007, 49 (5):687-93.

Joy MS, "Darbepoetin Alfa: A Novel Erythropoiesis-Stimulating Protein," *Ann Pharmacother*, 2002, 36(7):1183-92.

KDOQI, "KDOQI Clinical Practice Guideline and Clinical Practice Recommendations for Anemia in Chronic Kidney Disease: 2007 Update of Hemoglobin Target," *Am J Kidney Dis*, 2007, 50 (3):471-530.

Lerner J, Kale AS, Warady BA, et al, "Pharmacokinetics of Darbepoetin Alfa in Pediatric Patients With Chronic Kidney Disease," *Pediatr Nephrol*, 2002, 17(11):933-7.

Rizzo JD, Somerfield MR, Hagerty KL, et al, "Use of Epoetin and Darbepoetin in Patients With Cancer: 2007 American Society of Hematology/American Society of Clinical Oncology Clinical Practice Guideline Update," *Blood*, 2008, 111(1):25-41.

◆ **Darvocet A500®** *see* Propoxyphene and Acetaminophen *on page 1173*

◆ **Darvocet-N® 50** *see* Propoxyphene and Acetaminophen *on page 1173*

◆ **Darvocet-N® 100** *see* Propoxyphene and Acetaminophen *on page 1173*

◆ **Darvon®** *see* Propoxyphene *on page 1171*

◆ **Darvon-N®** *see* Propoxyphene *on page 1171*

◆ **Daunomycin** *see* DAUNOrubicin *on page 394*

DAUNOrubicin (daw noe ROO bi sin)

Medication Safety Issues

Sound-alike/look-alike issues:

DAUNOrubicin may be confused with DACTINomycin, DOXOrubicin, DOXOrubicin liposomal, epirubicin, IDArubicin, valrubicin

Conventional formulation (Cerubidine®, DAUNOrubicin hydrochloride) may be confused with the liposomal formulation (DaunoXome®)

High alert medication: The Institute for Safe Medication Practices (ISMP) includes this medication among its list of drug classes which have a heightened risk of causing significant patient harm when used in error.

Related Information

Emetogenic Potential of Antineoplastic Agents *on page 1579*

Extravasation Treatment *on page 1522*

U.S. Brand Names Cerubidine®

Canadian Brand Names Cerubidine®

Therapeutic Category Antineoplastic Agent, Anthracycline; Antineoplastic Agent, Antibiotic

Generic Available Yes

Use In combination with other agents in the treatment of leukemias (ALL, AML)

Pregnancy Risk Factor D

Pregnancy Considerations May cause fetal harm when administered to a pregnant woman. Animal studies have shown an increased incidence of fetal abnormalities.

Lactation Excretion in breast milk unknown/not recommended

Contraindications Hypersensitivity to daunorubicin or any component; CHF, left ventricular ejection fraction <30% to 40%, or arrhythmias; pre-existing bone marrow suppression

Warnings Hazardous agent; use appropriate precautions for handling and disposal; I.V. use only; severe local tissue necrosis will result if extravasation occurs **[U.S. Boxed Warning]**. May cause severe myelosuppression, dose-limiting, primarily leukopenia and neutropenia **[U.S. Boxed Warning]**; irreversible myocardial toxicity may occur as total dosage approaches 550 mg/m^2 in adults, 400 mg/m^2 in patients receiving chest radiation, 300 mg/m^2 in children ≥2 years of age, or 10 mg/kg in children <2 years **[U.S. Boxed Warning]**; this may occur during therapy or several months after therapy; total cumulative dose should take into account previous or concomitant treatment with cardiotoxic agents or irradiation of chest; infants and children may be more susceptible to anthracycline-induced cardiotoxicity than adults; monitor left ventricular (LV) function (baseline and periodic) with ECHO or MUGA scan; monitor ECG. Secondary leukemias may occur when used with combination chemotherapy or radiation therapy.

Precautions Reduce dosage in patients with hepatic, or renal impairment **[U.S. Boxed Warning]**, or in patients with biliary impairment. Should be administered under the supervision of an experienced cancer chemotherapy physician **[U.S. Boxed Warning]**.

Adverse Reactions

Cardiovascular: Cardiotoxicity, CHF (dose-related, may occur 7-8 years after treatment), arrhythmias, ECG abnormalities

Central nervous system: Fever, chills

Dermatologic: Alopecia, hyperpigmentation of skin and nail beds, urticaria, pruritus

Endocrine & metabolic: Hyperuricemia, infertility, sterility

Gastrointestinal: Stomatitis, esophagitis, nausea, vomiting, diarrhea

Genitourinary: Discoloration of urine (red-orange)

Hematologic: Myelosuppression (thrombocytopenia, leukopenia)

Hepatic: Serum bilirubin elevated, AST, and alkaline phosphatase

Local: Severe tissue necrosis with extravasation

Drug Interactions

Metabolism/Transport Effects Substrate of P-glycoprotein

Avoid Concomitant Use

Avoid concomitant use of DAUNOrubicin Hydrochloride with any of the following: BCG; Natalizumab; Pimecrolimus; Tacrolimus (Topical); Vaccines (Live)

Increased Effect/Toxicity

DAUNOrubicin Hydrochloride may increase the levels/ effects of: Leflunomide; Natalizumab; Vaccines (Live)

The levels/effects of DAUNOrubicin Hydrochloride may be increased by: Bevacizumab; Denosumab; P-Glycoprotein Inhibitors; Pimecrolimus; Tacrolimus (Topical); Taxane Derivatives; Trastuzumab

Decreased Effect

DAUNOrubicin Hydrochloride may decrease the levels/ effects of: BCG; Cardiac Glycosides; Sipuleucel-T; Vaccines (Inactivated); Vaccines (Live)

The levels/effects of DAUNOrubicin Hydrochloride may be decreased by: Cardiac Glycosides; Echinacea; P-Glycoprotein Inducers

Stability Protect from light; reconstituted solution is stable for 48 hours when refrigerated and 24 hours at room temperature; a color change from red to blue/purple indicates decomposition of the drug; unstable in solutions with a pH >8; incompatible with heparin, sodium bicarbonate, fluorouracil, and dexamethasone

Mechanism of Action Inhibition of DNA and RNA synthesis by intercalating between DNA base pairs, uncoiling of the helix, and by steric obstruction; not cell cycle-specific for the S-phase of cell division; may cause free radical damage to DNA

Pharmacokinetics (Adult data unless noted)

Distribution: Widely distributed in tissues such as spleen, heart, kidneys, liver, and lungs; does not cross the blood-brain barrier; crosses the placenta

Metabolism: To daunorubicinol (active)

Half-life, terminal: 14-18.5 hours

Daunorubicinol, active metabolite: 26.7 hours

Elimination: 40% of dose excreted in bile; ~14% to 23% excreted in urine as metabolite and unchanged drug

Usual Dosage I.V. (refer to individual protocols):

Children <2 years or <0.5 m^2: Dosage should be calculated on the basis of body weight rather than body surface area: 1 mg/kg or per protocol with frequency dependent on regimen employed

Children:

ALL combination therapy: Remission induction: 25-45 mg/m^2 on days 1 and 8 of cycle, or 30-45 mg/m^2/day for 3 days every 3-4 weeks, or 25 mg/m^2 every week for 4 weeks

AML combination therapy: Induction: I.V. continuous infusion: 30-60 mg/m^2/day on days 1-3 of cycle, or 20 mg/m^2/day for 4 days every 14 days

Adults: 30-60 mg/m^2/day for 3-5 days, repeat dose in 3-4 weeks; total cumulative dose should not exceed 400-600 mg/m^2

AML: Single agent induction: 60 mg/m^2/day for 3 days; repeat every 3-4 weeks

AML: Combination therapy induction: 45 mg/m^2/day for 3 days of the first course of induction therapy; subsequent courses: Every day for 2 days

ALL: Combination therapy: Remission induction: 45 mg/m^2 on days 1, 2, and 3 of induction course

Dosing adjustment in hepatic or renal impairment: Reduce dose by 25% in patients with serum bilirubin of 1.2-3 mg/dL; reduce dose by 50% in patients with serum bilirubin and/or creatinine >3 mg/dL

Administration Parenteral: Drug is very irritating, do not inject I.M. or SubQ; administer IVP diluting the reconstituted dose in 10-15 mL NS and administering over 2-3 minutes into the tubing of a rapidly infusing I.V. solution of D$_5$W or NS; daunorubicin has also been diluted in 100 mL of D$_5$W or NS and infused over 30-45 minutes or as a continuous 24-hour infusion

Monitoring Parameters CBC with differential and platelet count, serum bilirubin, serum uric acid, liver function test, ECG, ventricular ejection fraction, renal function test; patency of I.V. line

Patient Information Transient red-orange discoloration of urine can occur for up to 48 hours after a dose; notify physician if fever, sore throat, bleeding, bruising, chills, signs of infection, abdominal pain, blood in stools, excessive fatigue, yellowing of eyes or skin, or difficulty breathing occurs

Nursing Implications Leukemic patients should receive prophylactic allopurinol to prevent acute urate nephropathy; avoid extravasation; if extravasation occurs, apply a cold compress immediately for 30-60 minutes, then alternate off/on every 15 minutes for 1 day; apply 1.5 mL of dimethylsulfoxide 99% (w/v) solution to the site every 6 hours for 14 days; allow to air-dry; do not cover

Additional Information Myelosuppressive effects:

WBC: Severe

Platelets: Severe

Onset (days): 7

Nadir (days): 10-14

Recovery (days): 21-28

Dosage Forms Excipient information presented when available (limited, particularly for generics); consult specific product labeling. **Note: Strength expressed as base**

Injection, powder for reconstitution: 20 mg

Cerubidine®: 20 mg [contains mannitol 100 mg]

Injection, solution: 5 mg/mL (4 mL, 10 mL)

References

Crom WR, Glynn-Barnhart AM, Rodman JH, et al, "Pharmacokinetics of Anticancer Drugs in Children," *Clin Pharmacokinet*, 1987, 12 (3):168-213.

♦ **Dayhist® Allergy [OTC] [DSC]** *see* Clemastine *on page 327*

♦ **Daypro®** *see* Oxaprozin *on page 1033*

♦ **Daytrana™** *see* Methylphenidate *on page 908*

♦ **dCF** *see* Pentostatin *on page 1088*

♦ **DDAVP®** *see* Desmopressin *on page 404*

♦ **DDAVP® Melt (Can)** *see* Desmopressin *on page 404*

♦ **ddl** *see* Didanosine *on page 434*

♦ **1-Deamino-8-D-Arginine Vasopressin** *see* Desmopressin *on page 404*

♦ **Debrox® [OTC]** *see* Carbamide Peroxide *on page 248*

♦ **Decadron** *see* Dexamethasone *on page 406*

♦ **Decavac®** *see* Diphtheria and Tetanus Toxoid *on page 452*

♦ **Declomycin® [DSC]** *see* Demeclocycline *on page 399*

♦ **Declomycin® (Can)** *see* Demeclocycline *on page 399*

♦ **Deep Sea [OTC]** *see* Sodium Chloride *on page 1270*

Deferasirox (de FER a sir ox)

Medication Safety Issues

Sound-alike/look-alike issues:

Deferasirox may be confused with deferoxamine

International issues:

Deferasirox may be confused with deferiprone [Great Britain]

U.S. Brand Names Exjade®

Canadian Brand Names Exjade®

Therapeutic Category Chelating Agent, Oral

Generic Available No

Use Treatment of chronic iron overload due to blood transfusions (FDA approved in children ≥2 years and adults)

Pregnancy Risk Factor C

Pregnancy Considerations Teratogenic effects were observed in animal studies. There are no adequate and well-controlled studies in pregnant women. Use during pregnancy only if clearly needed.

Lactation Excretion in breast milk unknown/not recommended

Contraindications Hypersensitivity to deferasirox or any component; platelet counts (<50,000/mm^3); poor performance status and high-risk MDS or advanced malignancies; creatinine clearance <40 mL/minute or serum creatinine >2 x age-appropriate ULN

Warnings Serious and sometimes fatal acute renal failure has been reported **[U.S. Boxed Warning]**. Most of these events occurred in patients with multiple comorbidities who were in advanced stages of their hematological disorders. Dose-related elevations in serum creatinine have been reported; monitor and consider dose reduction, interruption, or discontinuation. Monitor serum creatinine and/or creatinine clearance in all patients; monitor patients at risk for renal complications (eg, pre-existing renal conditions, elderly, comorbid conditions, and/or with concurrent medications that may affect renal function) more closely. Dose reduction, interruption, or discontinuation may be required for serum creatinine elevations. May cause intermittent proteinuria; monitor closely. Renal tubulopathy has also been reported, primarily in pediatric patients with β-thalassemia and serum ferritin levels <1500 mcg/L.

Serious and sometimes fatal hepatic injury including hepatic failure has been reported **[U.S. Boxed Warning]**; most of these cases occurred in patients >55 years of age and in patients with significant comorbidities including liver cirrhosis and multiple organ failure. Hepatitis and elevated transaminases have been reported; monitor transaminases and bilirubin closely, and consider dose modifications. Gastrointestinal hemorrhage, including fatalities, has occurred with use **[U.S. Boxed Warning]**; more common in elderly patients with advanced hematologic malignancies and/or low platelets). Other GI effects including irritation and upper GI ulceration have been reported; monitor patients closely for signs and symptoms of GI effects and bleeding. Use caution when combining with anticoagulants, NSAIDs, and corticosteroids. Auditory or ocular disturbances have been reported; monitor and consider dose reduction or treatment interruption. Do not combine with other iron chelation therapies; safety of combinations has not been established. Rare cases of peripheral cytopenias including agranulocytosis, neutropenia, and thrombocytopenia have been reported postmarketing; some of these patients died; most patients had pre-existing hematologic disorders that are frequently associated with bone marrow failure; monitor CBC closely.

May cause skin rash (dose-related), including erythema multiforme; mild-to-moderate rashes may resolve without treatment interruption; for severe rash, interrupt treatment and consider restarting at a lower dose with dose escalation in combination with a short period of oral steroid administration.

Potent UDP-glucuronosyltransferase (UGT) inducers (eg, rifampin) or cholestyramine may decrease the efficacy of deferasirox; avoid concomitant use. If coadministration necessary, dosage modifications may be needed; monitor serum ferritin and clinical response.

Adverse Reactions
Central nervous system: Fatigue

Dermatologic: Erythema multiforme, rash (dose-related)

Gastrointestinal: Abdominal pain, cholelithiasis, diarrhea, gastritis, gastrointestinal hemorrhage (see Warnings), gastrointestinal ulceration, nausea, vomiting

Hematologic: Cytopenia including agranulocytosis, Henoch-Schönlein purpura, neutropenia, thrombocytopenia (see Warnings)

Hepatic: Hepatic failure (see Warnings), hepatitis, serum transaminases increased

Neuromuscular & skeletal: Arthralgia, back pain

Ocular: Cataract, IOP increase, lens opacities, visual disturbance

Otic: Ear infection, hearing loss (including high frequency)

Renal: Acute renal failure (rare; see Warnings), interstitial nephritis, proteinuria (intermittent), serum creatinine increased (dose-related)

Respiratory: Acute tonsillitis, bronchitis, cough, nasopharyngitis, pharyngitis, respiratory tract infection, rhinitis

Miscellaneous: Influenza, serious hypersensitivity reactions including anaphylaxis and angioedema

<1%, postmarketing, and/or case reports: Alopecia, anxiety, ascites, bilirubin increased, dizziness, drug fever, duodenal ulcer, edema, esophagitis, glucosuria, headache, hyperactivity, hypocalcemia, insomnia, jaundice, leukocytoclastic vasculitis, maculopathy, optic neuritis, pigment disorder, purpurarenal tubulopathy, sleep disorder, urticaria

Drug Interactions
Metabolism/Transport Effects Substrate of UGT1A1 (major), 1A3; **Inhibits** CYP2C8 (moderate); **Induces** 3A4 (weak)

Avoid Concomitant Use There are no known interactions where it is recommended to avoid concomitant use.

Increased Effect/Toxicity
Deferasirox may increase the levels/effects of: CYP2C8 Substrates (High risk)

Decreased Effect
Deferasirox may decrease the levels/effects of: CYP3A4 Substrates

The levels/effects of Deferasirox may be decreased by: Aluminum Hydroxide; Cholestyramine Resin; PHENobarbital; Phenytoin; Rifampin; Ritonavir

Food Interactions Bioavailability increased variably when taken with food; administer on empty stomach

Stability Store at room temperature between 15°C and 30°C (59°F and 86°F). Protect from moisture.

Mechanism of Action Selectively binds iron with a high affinity in a 2:1 ratio, forming a complex which is excreted primarily through the feces.

Pharmacokinetics (Adult data unless noted)
Distribution: Adults: 14 L

Protein binding: 99% to serum albumin

Metabolism: Hepatic via glucuronidation by UGT1A1 and UGT1A3; minor oxidation by CYP450; undergoes enterohepatic recirculation

Bioavailability: 70%

Half-life: 8-16 hours

Time to peak serum concentration: 1.5-4 hours (median times)

Elimination: Feces (84%), urine (6% to 8%)

Clearance: Females have moderately lower clearance than males (17.5% lower)

Usual Dosage Note: Baseline serum ferritin and iron levels should be obtained prior to therapy; toxicity may be increased in patients with low iron burden or with only slightly elevated serum ferritin.

Oral: Children ≥2 years and Adults: Initiate therapy when patient has evidence of chronic iron overload (eg, transfusion of approximately 100 mL/kg of packed RBCs and serum ferritin consistently >1000 mcg/L)

Initial: 20 mg/kg daily (calculate dose to nearest whole tablet)

Maintenance: Adjust dose every 3-6 months based on serum ferritin levels; increase by 5 or 10 mg/kg/day (calculate dose to nearest whole tablet); titrate. Usual range: 20-30 mg/kg/day; doses up to 40 mg/kg/day may be considered for serum ferritin levels persistently >2500 mcg/L (doses above 40 mg/kg/day are not recommended). **Note:** Consider holding dose for serum ferritin <500 mcg/L. Consider dose reduction or interruption for hearing loss or visual disturbances.

Dosage adjustment with concomitant cholestyramine or potent UGT inducers (eg, rifampin, phenytoin, phenobarbital, ritonavir): Avoid concomitant use; if coadministration necessary, consider increasing the initial deferasirox dose to 30 mg/kg; monitor serum ferritin and clinical response. Doses >40 mg/kg are not recommended.

Dosage adjustment in renal impairment: Adults:

Cl_{cr} ≥40 to <60 mL/minute: Use caution; monitor renal function closely, particularly in patients at increased risk for further renal impairment (eg, concomitant therapy, dehydration, severe infection)

Cl_{cr} <40 mL/minute or serum creatinine >2 times age-appropriate ULN: Use is contraindicated

Progressive increase in serum creatinine: Consider dose reduction, interruption, or discontinuation. Interrupt treatment for progressive increase in serum creatinine above the age-appropriate upper limits of normal; once serum creatinine recovers to within the normal range, reinitiate treatment at a reduced dose; gradually escalate the dose if the clinical benefit outweighs potential risk.

Children: For increase in serum creatinine above the age-appropriate upper limits of normal for two consecutive levels, reduce daily dose by 10 mg/kg

Adults: For increase in serum creatinine >33% above the average pretreatment level at two consecutive levels (and cannot be attributed to other causes), reduce daily dose by 10 mg/kg

Dosage adjustment in hepatic impairment: Consider dose adjustment or discontinuation for severe elevations in liver function tests.

Administration Oral: **Do not chew or swallow whole tablets.** Disperse tablets in water, orange juice, or apple juice (use 3.5 ounces for total doses <1 g; 7 ounces for doses ≥1 g); stir to form suspension and drink entire contents. Rinse remaining residue with more fluid; drink. Administer at same time each day on an empty stomach, 30 minutes before food. Do not administer simultaneously with aluminum-containing antacids or cholestyramine.

Monitoring Parameters Serum ferritin (baseline, then monthly), serum creatinine, and/or creatinine clearance [two baseline assessments, then monthly thereafter in patients who are at increased risk of complications (eg, pre-existing renal conditions, elderly, comorbid conditions, or receiving other potentially nephrotoxic medications); weekly for the first month then monthly thereafter]; urine protein, CBC, serum transaminases, and bilirubin (baseline, every 2 weeks for 1 month, then monthly); baseline and annual auditory and ophthalmic function (including slit lamp examinations and dilated fundoscopy); number of RBC units received

Patient Information You may experience a fever, headache, abdominal pain, nausea, diarrhea, cough, sore throat, or dizziness; may impair ability to perform activities requiring physical coordination; use caution when driving or operating machinery. Report severe skin rashes, changes in vision or hearing, swelling of extremities, decrease in urine output, shortness of breath, unusual bleeding or bruising, change in color of urine or stool, yellowing of skin or eyes, or unusual fatigue.

Additional Information Deferasirox has a low affinity for binding with zinc and copper; may cause variable decreases in the serum concentration of these trace minerals. Deferasirox available via EPASS™ (Exjade® Patient Assistance & Support Services) network; contact at 888-903-7277.

Dosage Forms Excipient information presented when available (limited, particularly for generics); consult specific product labeling.

Tablet, for oral suspension:

Exjade®: 125 mg, 250 mg, 500 mg

References

Cappellini MD, "Long-Term Efficacy and Safety of Deferasirox," *Blood Rev*, 2008, (22 Suppl)2:35-41.

Galanello R, Piga A, Alberti D, et al, "Safety, Tolerability, and Pharmacokinetics of ICL670, a New Orally Active Iron-Chelating Agent in Patients With Transfusion-Dependent Iron Overload Due to Beta-Thalassaemia," *J Clin Pharmacol*, 2003, 43(6):565-72.

Nisbet-Brown E, Oliveri NF, Giardina PJ, et al, "Effectiveness and Safety of ICL670 in Iron-Loaded Patients With Thalassaemia: A Randomised, Double-Blind, Placebo-Controlled, Dose-Escalation Trial," *Lancet*, 2003, 361(9369):1597-602.

Raphael JL, Bernhardt MB, Mahoney DH, et al, "Oral Iron Chelation and the Treatment of Iron Overload in a Pediatric Hematology Center," *Pediatr Blood Cancer*, 2009, 52(5):616-20.

Rund D and Rachmilewitz E, "Beta-Thalassemia," *N Engl J Med*, 2005, 353(11):1135-46.

Yusuf B, McPhedran P, and Brewster UC, "Hypocalcemia in a Dialysis Patient Treated With Deferasirox for Iron Overload," *Am J Kidney Dis*, 2008, 52(3):587-90.

Deferoxamine (de fer OKS a meen)

Medication Safety Issues
Sound-alike/look-alike issues:

Deferoxamine may be confused with cefuroxime, deferasirox

Desferal® may be confused with desflurane, Dexferrum®, Disophrol®

International issues:

Desferal® may be confused with Deseril® which is a brand name for methysergide in multiple international markets

U.S. Brand Names Desferal®

Canadian Brand Names Desferal®; PMS-Deferoxamine

Therapeutic Category Antidote, Aluminum Toxicity; Antidote, Iron Toxicity; Chelating Agent, Parenteral

Generic Available Yes

Use Acute iron intoxication; chronic iron overload secondary to multiple transfusions; diagnostic test for iron overload; the diagnosis and treatment of aluminum accumulation in renal failure

Pregnancy Risk Factor C

Pregnancy Considerations Skeletal anomalies and delayed ossification were observed in some but not all animal studies. Toxic amounts of iron or deferoxamine have not been noted to cross the placenta. In case of acute toxicity, treatment during pregnancy should not be withheld.

Lactation Excretion in breast milk unknown/use caution

Contraindications Hypersensitivity to deferoxamine or any component; patients with severe renal disease, anuria, or primary hemochromatosis

Warnings Cataracts, decreased visual acuity, impaired peripheral and color vision, impaired night vision, and retinal pigmentary abnormalities have been reported after usage for prolonged periods at high dosages or in patients with low ferritin levels; periodic eye exams are recommended while on chronic therapy; neurotoxicity-related auditory abnormalities have been reported including high frequency sensorineural hearing loss; periodic auditory exams are recommended. ARDS has been reported following treatment of acute iron intoxication or thalassemia with high doses of deferoxamine; flushing of the skin, urticaria, hypotension, and shock have been reported after rapid I.V. administration. High doses (>60 mg/kg), especially in patients ≤3 years of age, with resulting low ferritin levels have been associated with growth retardation; a reduction in deferoxamine dosage may partially improve growth velocity; monitor growth in children receiving chronic therapy closely.

In patients with aluminum-related encephalopathy, deferoxamine may exacerbate neurologic dysfunction (seizures) possibly due to an acute increase in circulating aluminum and also may decrease serum calcium aggravating hyperparathyroidism. Deferoxamine may precipitate the onset of dialysis dementia. Avoid deferoxamine use in patients with serum aluminium levels >200 mcg/L. Fatal mucormycosis has been reported in chronic renal failure patients receiving deferoxamine for aluminium toxicity. Ferrioxamine (chelated form of iron with deferoxamine) enhances the growth and pathogenicity of certain species of *Mucor*.

Patients with severe chronic iron overload treated with deferoxamine and high dose vitamin C have been reported to develop impaired cardiac function which is reversed after discontinuation of vitamin C; vitamin C increases the availability of iron for chelation with deferoxamine. To decrease the risk of impaired cardiac function, the manufacturer recommends: Avoiding vitamin C in patients with pre-existing cardiac failure; start vitamin C supplementation only after the first month of deferoxamine therapy; use vitamin C only if the patient is regularly receiving deferoxamine; do not exceed vitamin C doses of 50 mg/day in children <10 years, 100 mg/day in older children, and 200 mg/day in adults; monitor cardiac function.

Precautions Use with caution in patients with pyelonephritis; may increase susceptibility to *Yersinia enterocolitica* infections

Adverse Reactions

Cardiovascular: Flushing, hypotension with rapid I.V. injection, tachycardia, shock, edema, impaired cardiac function (see Warnings)

Central nervous system: Fever, seizures, dialysis dementia, headache, dizziness

Dermatologic: Erythema, urticaria, pruritus, rash, cutaneous wheal formation

Endocrine & Metabolic: Growth impairment (dose related; see Warnings)

Gastrointestinal: Abdominal discomfort, diarrhea, nausea, vomiting

Genitourinary: Discoloration of urine (reddish color), dysuria

Hematologic: Thrombocytopenia (rare), leukopenia (rare)

Local: Pain, induration at injection site

Neuromuscular & skeletal: Leg cramps, metaphyseal dysplasia, arthralgia, myalgia, paresthesia

Ocular: Blurred vision; visual acuity decreased, dichromatopsia, maculopathy; cataracts; impaired peripheral and night vision, scotoma, visual field defects, color and night blindness; retinal pigmentary abnormalities

Otic: High frequency sensorineural hearing loss, tinnitus

Respiratory: ARDS (see Warnings), asthma

Miscellaneous: Anaphylaxis, possible increased risk of infections particularly with *Y. enterocolitica*; rare cases of mucormycosis

Drug Interactions

Avoid Concomitant Use There are no known interactions where it is recommended to avoid concomitant use.

Increased Effect/Toxicity

The levels/effects of Deferoxamine may be increased by:
Ascorbic Acid

Decreased Effect There are no known significant interactions involving a decrease in effect.

Stability Do not store vials above 25°C (77°F). Following reconstitution, solutions may be stored for 24 hours at room temperature; do not refrigerate solutions as they will precipitate. Due to a lack of preservative, the manufacturer recommends immediate use after reconstitution.

Mechanism of Action Complexes with trivalent ions (ferric ions) to form ferrioxamine, which is removed by the kidneys

Pharmacokinetics (Adult data unless noted)

Absorption: Oral: <15%

Metabolism: By plasma enzymes to ferrioxamine

Half-life:

Deferoxamine: 6.1 hours

Ferrioxamine: 5.8 hours

Elimination: Renal excretion of the metabolite iron chelate and unchanged drug

Dialysis: Dialyzable

Usual Dosage

Acute iron intoxication: **Note:** I.V. route is used when severe toxicity is evidenced by systemic symptoms (coma, shock, metabolic acidosis, or severe GI bleeding) or potentially severe intoxications (serum iron level >500 mcg/dL). When severe symptoms are not present, the I.M. route may be preferred (per manufacturer); however,

the use of I.V. deferoxamine in situations where the serum iron concentration is <500 mcg/dL or when severe toxicity is not evident is a subject of some clinical debate.

Children:

I.M.: 50 mg/kg/dose every 6 hours; maximum dose: 6 g/day or as an alternative, 90 mg/kg/dose every 8 hours; not to exceed 1 g/dose or 6 g/day

I.V.: 15 mg/kg/hour; maximum dose: 6 g/day

Alternative dosing I.M. or I.V.: 20 mg/kg or 600 mg/m^2 (not to exceed 1000 mg) initially followed by 10 mg/kg or 300 mg/m^2 (not to exceed 500 mg) at 4-hour intervals for 2 doses; subsequent doses of 10 mg/kg or 300 mg/m^2 (not to exceed 500 mg) every 4-12 hours may be repeated depending upon the clinical response; maximum dose: 6 g/day

Chronic iron overload:

I.V.: 15 mg/kg/hour; maximum dose: 12 g/day

SubQ infusion via a portable, controlled infusion device: 20-50 mg/kg/day over 8-12 hours; maximum dose: 2 g/day

Adults:

Acute iron intoxication:

I.M.: 1 g stat, then 0.5 g every 4 hours for two doses; additional doses of 0.5 g every 4-12 hours up to 6 g/day may be needed depending upon the clinical response

I.V.: 15 mg/kg/hour; maximum dose: 6 g/day

Chronic iron overload:

I.M.: 0.5-1 g/day

I.V.: 15 mg/kg/hour; maximum dose: 12 g/day

Manufacturer's recommendations: 2 g per each unit of blood transfused; maximum dose: 6 g/day if transfused or 1 g/day without transfusion

SubQ infusion via a portable, controlled infusion device: 1-2 g/day over 8-24 hours

Aluminum-induced bone disease in chronic renal failure (serum aluminium 60-200 mcg/L; do not use if baseline serum aluminium >200 mcg/L; see Warnings): Children and Adults:

Test (diagnostic) dose: 5 mg/kg as a single dose infused over the last hour of dialysis. Measure serum aluminum 2 days later. Depending upon the change in serum aluminum, treatment with deferoxamine may be indicated (see National Kidney Foundation, 2003)

Treatment of aluminum toxicity in chronic renal failure: 5-10 mg/kg as a single dose. Repeat every 7-10 days with 3-4 dialysis procedures between doses. Monitor serum aluminum levels closely. See National Kidney Foundation reference for more detailed treatment algorithms.

Administration Parenteral: Add 2 mL SWI to 500 mg vial, resulting in a 210 mg/mL solution, or 8 mL SWI to each 2 g vial, resulting in a 213 mg/mL solution; for I.M. or SubQ administration, no further dilution is required; for I.V. infusion, may reconstitute 500 mg vial with 5 mL SWI or 2 g vial with 20 mL, resulting in 95 mg/mL concentration, then further dilute in dextrose, NS, 0.45% sodium chloride, LR 10 mg/mL (maximum concentration: 250 mg/mL); maximum rate of infusion: 15 mg/kg/hour; the manufacturer recommends using a reduced rate of infusion (not to exceed 125 mg/hour) after the first 1000 mg has been infused; local reactions at the site of subcutaneous infusion may be minimized by diluting the deferoxamine in 5-10 mL SWI and adding 1 mg hydrocortisone to each mL of deferoxamine solution (Kirking, 1991)

Monitoring Parameters Serum ferritin, iron, total iron binding capacity; body weight, growth, ophthalmologic exam, and audiometry (with chronic use); blood pressure (with I.V. infusions); aluminum level (if applicable)

Reference Range Effective plasma concentration: 3-15 mcg/mL

Test Interactions Gallium-67 imaging results may be distorted due to rapid urinary excretion of deferoxamine-bound gallium-67; discontinue deferoxamine at least 48 hours prior to imaging

Patient Information May cause dizziness or impairment of vision or hearing; report any hearing loss, night blindness, decreased visual acuity, impaired peripheral vision, or loss of color vision; may cause the urine to turn a reddish color

Nursing Implications Local injection site reactions may be minimized by daily rotation of subcutaneous injection sites and by applying topical corticosteroids; painful lumps formed under the skin may indicate that the rate of SubQ administration exceeds the rate of absorption from the injection site or the needle is inserted too close to the dermis

Dosage Forms Excipient information presented when available (limited, particularly for generics); consult specific product labeling.

Injection, powder for reconstitution, as mesylate: 500 mg, 2 g

Desferal®: 500 mg, 2 g

References
Bentur Y, McGuigan M, and Koren G, "Deferoxamine (Desferrioxamine): New Toxicities for an Old Drug," *Drug Saf*, 1991, 6(1):37-46.
Cohen AR, Mizanin J, and Schwartz E, "Rapid Removal of Excessive Iron With Daily, High-Dose Intravenous Chelation Therapy," *J Pediatr*, 1989, 115(1):151-5.
Freedman MH, Olivieri N, Benson L, et al, "Clinical Studies on Iron Chelation in Patients With Thalassemia Major," *Haematologica*, 1990, 75(Suppl 5):74-83.
Giardina PJ, Grady RW, Ehlers KH, et al, "Current Therapy of Cooley's Anemia: A Decade of Experience With Subcutaneous Desferrioxamine," *Ann N Y Acad Sci*, 1990, 612:275-85.
Kirking MH, "Treatment of Chronic Iron Overload," *Clin Pharm*, 1991, 10(10):775-83.
National Kidney Foundation, "K/DOQI Clinical Practice Guidelines for Bone Metabolism and Disease in Chronic Kidney Failure," *Am J Kidney Dis*, 2003, 42(4 Suppl 3):1-201.
Pippard MJ, "Iron Metabolism and Iron Chelation in the Thalassemia Disorders," *Haematologica*, 1990, 75(Suppl 5):66-71.

◆ **Deferoxamine Mesylate** *see* Deferoxamine *on page 397*
◆ **Dehydral® (Can)** *see* Methenamine *on page 896*
◆ **Dehydrobenzperidol** *see* Droperidol *on page 483*
◆ **Delatestryl®** *see* Testosterone *on page 1325*
◆ **Delestrogen®** *see* Estradiol *on page 536*
◆ **Delsym® [OTC]** *see* Dextromethorphan *on page 421*
◆ **Delta-9-tetrahydro-cannabinol** *see* Dronabinol *on page 482*
◆ **Delta-9 THC** *see* Dronabinol *on page 482*
◆ **Deltacortisone** *see* PredniSONE *on page 1151*
◆ **Delta® D3 [OTC]** *see* Cholecalciferol *on page 300*
◆ **Deltadehydrocortisone** *see* PredniSONE *on page 1151*
◆ **Deltahydrocortisone** *see* PrednisoLONE *on page 1148*
◆ **Demadex®** *see* Torsemide *on page 1365*

Demeclocycline (dem e kloe SYE kleen)

U.S. Brand Names Declomycin® [DSC]
Canadian Brand Names Declomycin®
Therapeutic Category Antibiotic, Tetracycline Derivative
Generic Available Yes
Use Treatment of susceptible bacterial infections (acne, gonorrhea, pertussis, chronic bronchitis, and urinary tract infections) caused by both gram-negative and gram-positive organisms; treatment of chronic syndrome of inappropriate antidiuretic hormone (SIADH) secretion
Pregnancy Risk Factor D
Pregnancy Considerations Demeclocycline has been shown to cross the placenta in rats and other tetracyclines cross the placenta in humans causing permanent discoloration of teeth if used during the second or third trimester. Because use during pregnancy may cause fetal harm, demeclocyline is classified as pregnancy category D.

Lactation Enters breast milk/not recommended

Breast-Feeding Considerations Demeclocycline has been shown to cause tooth discolorations in newborn rats when exposed to high doses, but not low doses via breast milk. Other tetracyclines are excreted in breast milk. There is no data on the amount of demeclocycline that is excreted in human breast milk. Breast-feeding is not recommended by the manufacturer.

Tetracyclines, including demeclocycline, bind to calcium. The calcium in maternal milk will significantly decrease the amount of demeclocycline absorbed by the breast-feeding infant. Nondose-related effects could include modification of bowel flora.

Contraindications Hypersensitivity to demeclocycline, tetracyclines, or any component; pregnancy

Warnings Photosensitivity reactions, characterized as severe burns of exposed surfaces, occur frequently with this drug; avoid prolonged exposure to sunlight; do not use tanning equipment. Do not administer to children ≤8 years of age; use of tetracyclines during tooth development (last half of pregnancy, infancy, and children ≤8 years of age) may cause permanent discoloration of the teeth and enamel hypoplasia; do not administer to pregnant women; use of tetracyclines in pregnant women may result in retardation of bone growth and skeletal development of the fetus; prolonged use may result in superinfection. Avoid use when possible in patients with hepatic disease. Demeclocycline may cause a reversible, dose-related diabetes insipidus syndrome. Use of outdated tetracyclines has caused a Fanconi-like syndrome.

Precautions Use with caution in patients with impaired renal or hepatic function; modify dose in patients with renal impairment

Adverse Reactions
Central nervous system: Intracranial pressure elevated, bulging fontanels in infants, headache, dizziness, vertigo
Dermatologic: Rash, pruritus, photosensitivity, exfoliative dermatitis, erythema multiforme, urticaria, discoloration of nails, Stevens-Johnson syndrome
Endocrine & metabolic: Diabetes insipidus syndrome, hyperphosphatemia
Gastrointestinal: Nausea, vomiting, diarrhea, anorexia, pancreatitis, enterocolitis
Hematologic: Leukopenia, neutropenia, thrombocytopenia, hemolytic anemia, eosinophilia
Hepatic: Hepatotoxicity, liver enzymes elevated
Neuromuscular & skeletal: Paresthesia, weakness, polyarthralgia
Ocular: Blurred vision
Renal: Azotemia, acute renal failure, nephrogenic diabetes insipidus
Miscellaneous: Anaphylaxis, lupus-like syndrome, superinfections

Drug Interactions
Avoid Concomitant Use
Avoid concomitant use of Demeclocycline with any of the following: BCG; Retinoic Acid Derivatives
Increased Effect/Toxicity
Demeclocycline may increase the levels/effects of: Neuromuscular-Blocking Agents; Retinoic Acid Derivatives; Vitamin K Antagonists
Decreased Effect
Demeclocycline may decrease the levels/effects of: BCG; Desmopressin; Penicillins; Typhoid Vaccine

The levels/effects of Demeclocycline may be decreased by: Antacids; Bile Acid Sequestrants; Bismuth; Bismuth Subsalicylate; Iron Salts; Magnesium Salts; Quinapril; Sucralfate; Zinc Salts

Food Interactions Food, milk, milk formulas, dairy products, and iron decrease absorption of demeclocycline

Mechanism of Action Inhibits protein synthesis by binding with the 30S ribosomal subunits and preventing the binding of transfer RNA to those ribosomes of susceptible bacteria; may also cause alterations in the cytoplasmic membrane

Pharmacodynamics Onset of action for diuresis in SIADH: Within 5 days

Pharmacokinetics (Adult data unless noted)

Absorption: ~60% to 80% of dose absorbed from the GI tract; food and dairy products reduce absorption by 50% or more

Distribution: Distributes into pleural fluid, bronchial secretions, sputum, prostatic and seminal fluids, and to body tissues; crosses into breast milk

Protein binding: 36% to 91%

Metabolism: Small amounts metabolized in the liver to inactive metabolites; enterohepatically recycled

Half-life: Adults: 10-17 hours (prolonged with reduced renal function)

Time to peak serum concentration: Oral: Within 3-4 hours

Elimination: Excreted as unchanged drug (42% to 50%) in urine and 31% in feces

Usual Dosage Oral:

Children >8 years: 8-12 mg/kg/day divided every 6-12 hours

Adults: 150 mg 4 times/day or 300 mg twice daily

Uncomplicated gonorrhea: 600 mg stat, 300 mg every 12 hours for 4 days (3 g total)

SIADH: Initial: 600-1200 mg/day or 13-15 mg/kg/day divided every 6-8 hours; then decrease to 600-900 mg/day

Dosing adjustment in renal impairment: Dose and/or frequency should be modified in response to the degree of renal impairment

Dosing adjustment in hepatic impairment: Not recommended for use

Administration Oral: Administer 1 hour before or 2 hours after food or milk with plenty of fluids; do not administer with food, milk, dairy products, antacids, zinc, or iron supplements

Monitoring Parameters CBC, renal and hepatic function tests, I & O, urine output, serum sodium

Test Interactions May interfere with tests for urinary glucose (false-negative urine glucose using Clinistix®, Tes-Tape®)

Patient Information May cause photosensitivity reactions (eg, exposure to sunlight may cause severe sunburn, skin rash, redness, or itching); avoid exposure to sunlight and artificial light sources (sunlamps, tanning booth/bed); wear protective clothing, wide-brimmed hats, sunglasses, and lip sunscreen (SPF ≥15); use a sunscreen [broad-spectrum sunscreen or physical sunscreen (preferred) or sunblock with SPF ≥15]; contact physician if reaction occurs. May cause dizziness, vertigo, lightheadedness, blurred vision and impair ability to perform activities requiring mental alertness or physical coordination; may discolor fingernails. Avoid taking dosages at bedtime to reduce risk of esophageal ulceration

Dosage Forms Excipient information presented when available (limited, particularly for generics); consult specific product labeling. [DSC] = Discontinued product

Tablet, as hydrochloride: 150 mg, 300 mg

Declomycin® [DSC]: 150 mg, 300 mg

References

Abdi EA and Bishop S, "The Syndrome of Inappropriate Antidiuretic Hormone Secretion With Carcinoma of the Tongue," *Med Pediatr Oncol*, 1988, 16(3):210-5.

De Troyer AD, "Demeclocycline. Treatment for Syndrome of Inappropriate Antidiuretic Hormone Secretion," *JAMA*, 1977, 237(25):2723-6.

◆ **Demeclocycline Hydrochloride** *see* Demeclocycline *on page 399*

◆ **Demerol®** *see* Meperidine *on page 880*

◆ **4-Demethoxydaunorubicin** *see* IDArubicin *on page 707*

◆ **Demethylchlortetracycline** *see* Demeclocycline *on page 399*

◆ **Denavir®** *see* Penciclovir *on page 1076*

◆ **Denorex® Original Therapeutic Strength [OTC]** *see* Coal Tar *on page 349*

◆ **Denta 5000 Plus** *see* Fluoride *on page 595*

◆ **DentaGel** *see* Fluoride *on page 595*

◆ **Dentapaine [OTC]** *see* Benzocaine *on page 182*

◆ **Dent's Extra Strength Toothache [OTC]** *see* Benzocaine *on page 182*

◆ **2'-Deoxycoformycin** *see* Pentostatin *on page 1088*

◆ **2'-Deoxy-3'-Thiacytidine** *see* LamiVUDine *on page 791*

◆ **Deoxycoformycin** *see* Pentostatin *on page 1088*

◆ **Depacon®** *see* Valproic Acid and Derivatives *on page 1398*

◆ **Depakene®** *see* Valproic Acid and Derivatives *on page 1398*

◆ **Depakote®** *see* Valproic Acid and Derivatives *on page 1398*

◆ **Depakote® ER** *see* Valproic Acid and Derivatives *on page 1398*

◆ **Depakote® Sprinkle** *see* Valproic Acid and Derivatives *on page 1398*

◆ **Depen®** *see* Penicillamine *on page 1076*

◆ **DepoDur®** *see* Morphine Sulfate *on page 946*

◆ **Depo®-Estradiol** *see* Estradiol *on page 536*

◆ **Depo-Medrol®** *see* MethylPREDNISolone *on page 912*

◆ **Depo-Prevera® (Can)** *see* MedroxyPROGESTERone *on page 870*

◆ **Depo-Provera®** *see* MedroxyPROGESTERone *on page 870*

◆ **Depo-Provera® Contraceptive** *see* MedroxyPROGESTERone *on page 870*

◆ **depo-subQ provera 104™** *see* MedroxyPROGESTERone *on page 870*

◆ **Depotest® 100 (Can)** *see* Testosterone *on page 1325*

◆ **Depo®-Testosterone** *see* Testosterone *on page 1325*

◆ **DermaFungal [OTC]** *see* Miconazole *on page 927*

◆ **Dermagran® [OTC]** *see* Aluminum Hydroxide *on page 75*

◆ **Dermagran® AF [OTC]** *see* Miconazole *on page 927*

◆ **Dermamycin® [OTC]** *see* DiphenhydrAMINE *on page 448*

◆ **Dermarest® Dricort® [OTC]** *see* Hydrocortisone *on page 685*

◆ **Dermarest® Psoriasis Medicated Moisturizer [OTC]** *see* Salicylic Acid *on page 1241*

◆ **Dermarest® Psoriasis Medicated Scalp Treatment [OTC]** *see* Salicylic Acid *on page 1241*

◆ **Dermarest® Psoriasis Medicated Shampoo/Conditioner [OTC]** *see* Salicylic Acid *on page 1241*

◆ **Dermarest® Psoriasis Medicated Skin Treatment [OTC]** *see* Salicylic Acid *on page 1241*

◆ **Dermarest® Psoriasis Overnight Treatment [OTC]** *see* Salicylic Acid *on page 1241*

♦ **Dermarest® Psoriasis Scalp Treatment Mousse [OTC] [DSC]** *see* Salicylic Acid *on page 1241*

♦ **Derma-Smoothe/FS®** *see* Fluocinolone *on page 593*

♦ **Dermazole (Can)** *see* Miconazole *on page 927*

♦ **Dermoplast® Antibacterial [OTC]** *see* Benzocaine *on page 182*

♦ **Dermoplast® Pain Relieving [OTC]** *see* Benzocaine *on page 182*

♦ **DermOtic®** *see* Fluocinolone *on page 593*

♦ **Dermovate® (Can)** *see* Clobetasol *on page 331*

♦ **Dermtex® HC [OTC]** *see* Hydrocortisone *on page 685*

♦ **Desferal®** *see* Deferoxamine *on page 397*

♦ **Desferrioxamine** *see* Deferoxamine *on page 397*

Desipramine (des IP ra meen)

Medication Safety Issues

Sound-alike/look-alike issues:

Desipramine may be confused with clomiPRAMINE, dalfampridine, deserpidine, diphenhydrAMINE, disopyramide, imipramine, nortriptyline

Norpramin® may be confused with clomiPRAMINE, imipramine, Normodyne®, Norpace®, nortriptyline, Tenormin®

International issues:

Norpramin®: Brand name for nortriptyline [U.S., Canada], but also the brand name for enalapril/hydrochlorothiazide [Portugal]; omeprazole [Spain]

Related Information

Antidepressant Agents *on page 1484*

Medications for Which A Single Dose May Be Fatal When Ingested By A Toddler *on page 1709*

U.S. Brand Names Norpramin®

Canadian Brand Names Alti-Desipramine; Apo-Desipramine®; Norpramin®; Nu-Desipramine; PMS-Desipramine

Therapeutic Category Antidepressant, Tricyclic (Secondary Amine)

Generic Available Yes

Use Treatment of depression (FDA approved in adults); has also been used as an analgesic in chronic pain; treatment of peripheral neuropathies

Medication Guide An FDA-approved patient medication guide, which is available with the product information and at http://www.fda.gov/downloads/Drugs/DrugSafety/ucm088665.pdf, must be dispensed with this medication for each new outpatient prescription and refill.

Pregnancy Risk Factor C

Lactation Enters breast milk/not recommended (AAP rates "of concern")

Breast-Feeding Considerations Generally, it is not recommended to breast-feed if taking antidepressants because of the long half-life, active metabolites, and the potential for side effects in the infant.

Contraindications Hypersensitivity to desipramine (cross-sensitivity with other tricyclic antidepressants may occur) or any component; use of MAO inhibitors within 14 days (potentially fatal reactions may occur, see Drug Interactions); use in patients during the acute recovery phase following MI; narrow-angle glaucoma

Warnings Desipramine is not approved for use in pediatric patients. Clinical worsening of depression or suicidal ideation and behavior may occur in children and adults with major depressive disorder **[U.S. Boxed Warning]**. In clinical trials, antidepressants increased the risk of suicidal thinking and behavior (suicidality) in children, adolescents, and young adults (18-24 years of age) with major depressive disorder and other psychiatric disorders. This risk must be considered before prescribing antidepressants for any clinical use. Short-term studies did **not** show an increased risk of suicidality with antidepressant use in patients >24 years of age and showed a decreased risk in patients ≥65 years.

Patients of all ages who are treated with antidepressants for any indication require appropriate monitoring and close observation for clinical worsening of depression, suicidality, and unusual changes in behavior, especially during the first few months after antidepressant initiation or when the dose is adjusted. Family members and caregivers should be instructed to closely observe the patient (ie, daily) and communicate condition with healthcare provider. Patients should also be monitored for associated behaviors (eg, anxiety, agitation, panic attacks, insomnia, irritability, hostility, aggressiveness, impulsivity, akathisia, hypomania, mania) which may increase the risk for worsening depression or suicidality. Worsening depression or emergence of suicidality (or associated behaviors listed above) that is abrupt in onset, severe, or not part of the presenting symptoms, may require discontinuation or modification of drug therapy.

Do not discontinue abruptly in patients receiving high doses chronically (withdrawal symptoms may occur). To reduce risk of intentional overdose, write prescriptions for the smallest quantity consistent with good patient care. Screen individuals for bipolar disorder prior to treatment (using antidepressants alone may induce manic episodes in patients with this condition). Hypertensive episodes have been reported during surgery in patients receiving desipramine (discontinue desipramine use as soon as possible prior to elective surgery).

The American Heart Association recommends that all children diagnosed with ADHD who may be candidates for medication, such as desipramine, should have a thorough cardiovascular assessment prior to initiation of therapy. These recommendations are based upon reports of serious cardiovascular adverse events (including sudden death) in patients (both children and adults) taking usual doses of stimulant medications. Most of these patients were found to have underlying structural heart disease (eg, hypertrophic obstructive cardiomyopathy). This assessment should include a combination of thorough medical history, family history, and physical examination. An ECG is not mandatory but should be considered.

Precautions Use with extreme caution in the following patients: Patients with cardiovascular disease (due to the possibility of conduction defects, arrhythmias, tachycardias, strokes, and acute MI); patients who have a family history of sudden death, dysrhythmias, or conduction abnormalities; patients with thyroid disease or taking thyroid medications (due to the possibility of cardiovascular toxicity and arrhythmias); patients with a history of seizure disorders (desipramine may lower the seizure threshold; in some patients, seizures may precede cardiac dysrhythmias and death); patients with a history of urinary retention or glaucoma (due to the anticholinergic effects of the medication). It should be noted that overdose of desipramine has resulted in a higher death rate compared to other tricyclic antidepressants.

Adverse Reactions Less sedation and anticholinergic adverse effects than amitriptyline or imipramine

Cardiovascular: Arrhythmias, edema, flushing, heart block, hypertension, hypotension, MI, palpitations, stroke, tachycardia; asymptomatic ECG changes and minor increases in diastolic blood pressure and heart rate have been noted in children receiving >3.5 mg/kg/day; **Note:** Four cases of sudden death have been reported in children 5-14 years of age; an association between desipramine and sudden death was not shown to be significant in one retrospective study; further studies are needed

Central nervous system: Agitation, anxiety, ataxia, confusion, dizziness, drowsiness, drug fever, exacerbation of psychosis, extrapyramidal symptoms, fatigue, hallucinations, headache, hypomania, incoordination, insomnia, nervousness, nightmares, restlessness, sedation, seizure, suicidal thinking and behavior (see Warnings)

Dermatologic: Itching, petechiae, photosensitivity, skin rash, urticaria

Endocrine & metabolic: Breast enlargement, galactorrhea, hyperglycemia, hypoglycemia, sexual dysfunction, SIADH, weight gain or weight loss

Gastrointestinal: Abdominal cramps, anorexia, black tongue, constipation, diarrhea, heartburn, lower esophageal sphincter tone decreased (may cause GE reflux), nausea, paralytic ileus, stomatitis, unpleasant taste, vomiting, xerostomia

Genitourinary: Discoloration of urine (blue-green), urinary retention

Hematologic: Agranulocytosis, eosinophilia, purpura, thrombocytopenia

Hepatic: Cholestatic jaundice, hepatitis, liver enzymes increased

Neuromuscular & skeletal: Numbness, paresthesias of extremities, peripheral neuropathy, tingling, tremor, weakness

Ocular: Blurred vision, disturbances of accommodation, intraocular pressure elevated, mydriasis

Otic: Tinnitus

Miscellaneous: Diaphoresis, hypersensitivity reactions, withdrawal symptoms following abrupt discontinuation (see Warnings)

Drug Interactions

Metabolism/Transport Effects Substrate of CYP1A2 (minor), 2D6 (major); **Inhibits** CYP2A6 (moderate), 2B6 (moderate), 2D6 (moderate), 2E1 (weak), 3A4 (moderate)

Avoid Concomitant Use

Avoid concomitant use of Desipramine with any of the following: Artemether; Dronedarone; Iobenguane I 123; Lumefantrine; MAO Inhibitors; Metoclopramide; Nilotinib; Pimozide; QuiNINE; Sibutramine; Tetrabenazine; Thioridazine; Tolvaptan; Ziprasidone

Increased Effect/Toxicity

Desipramine may increase the levels/effects of: Alcohol (Ethyl); Alpha-/Beta-Agonists (Direct-Acting); Alpha1-Agonists; Amphetamines; Anticholinergics; Beta2-Agonists; CNS Depressants; Colchicine; CYP2A6 Substrates; CYP2B6 Substrates; CYP2D6 Substrates; CYP3A4 Substrates; Desmopressin; Dronedarone; Eplerenone; Everolimus; FentaNYL; Fesoterodine; Nebivolol; Pimecrolimus; Pimozide; QTc-Prolonging Agents; QuiNIDine; QuiNINE; Saxagliptin; Serotonin Modulators; Sulfonylureas; Tamoxifen; Tetrabenazine; Thioridazine; Tolvaptan; TraMADol; Vitamin K Antagonists; Yohimbine; Ziprasidone

The levels/effects of Desipramine may be increased by: Alfuzosin; Altretamine; Artemether; BuPROPion; Chloroquine; Cimetidine; Cinacalcet; Ciprofloxacin; Ciprofloxacin (Systemic); CYP2D6 Inhibitors (Moderate); CYP2D6 Inhibitors (Strong); Dexmethylphenidate; Divalproex; DULoxetine; Gadobutrol; Lithium; Lumefantrine; MAO Inhibitors; Methylphenidate; Metoclopramide; Nilotinib; Pramlintide; Propoxyphene; Protease Inhibitors; QuiNIDine; QuiNINE; Selective Serotonin Reuptake Inhibitors; Sibutramine; Terbinafine; Terbinafine (Systemic); Valproic Acid

Decreased Effect

Desipramine may decrease the levels/effects of: Acetylcholinesterase Inhibitors (Central); Alpha2-Agonists; Codeine; Iobenguane I 123

The levels/effects of Desipramine may be decreased by: Acetylcholinesterase Inhibitors (Central); Barbiturates; CarBAMazepine; Peginterferon Alfa-2b; St Johns Wort

Food Interactions May increase riboflavin dietary requirements

Mechanism of Action Increases the synaptic concentration of serotonin and/or norepinephrine in the CNS by inhibition of their reuptake by the presynaptic neuronal membrane

Pharmacodynamics Antidepressant effects:
Onset of action: Occasionally seen in 2-5 days
Maximum effect: After more than 2 weeks

Pharmacokinetics (Adult data unless noted)
Absorption: Rapidly and well absorbed from the GI tract
Distribution: V_d: 21 L/kg; distributes into breast milk (concentrations approximately equal to maternal plasma)
Protein binding: 90%
Metabolism: In the liver
Half-life: 12-57 hours
Elimination: 70% in urine

Usual Dosage Oral: Depression: **Note:** Not FDA approved for use in pediatric patients; controlled clinical trials have not shown tricyclic antidepressants to be superior to placebo for the treatment of depression in children and adolescents (see Dopheide, 2006 and Wagner, 2005).
Children 6-12 years: 1-3 mg/kg/day in divided doses; monitor carefully with doses >3 mg/kg/day; maximum dose: 5 mg/kg/day
Adolescents: Initial: 25-50 mg/day; gradually increase to 100 mg/day in single or divided doses; maximum dose: 150 mg/day
Adults: Initial: 75 mg/day in divided doses; increase gradually to 150-200 mg/day in divided or single dose; maximum dose: 300 mg/day

Administration Oral: Administer with food to decrease GI upset

Monitoring Parameters Blood pressure, heart rate, ECG, mental status, weight. Monitor patient periodically for symptom resolution; monitor for worsening of depression, suicidality, and associated behaviors (especially at the beginning of therapy or when doses are increased or decreased; see Warnings)

ADHD: Evaluate patients for cardiac disease prior to initiation of therapy for ADHD with thorough medical history, family history, and physical exam; consider ECG (see Warnings); perform ECG and echocardiogram if findings suggest cardiac disease; promptly conduct cardiac evaluation in patients who develop chest pain, unexplained syncope, or any other symptom of cardiac disease during treatment.

Long-term use: Also monitor CBC with differential, liver enzymes, serum concentrations

Reference Range Plasma concentrations do not always correlate with clinical effectiveness.
Timing of serum samples: Draw trough just before next dose
Therapeutic: 50-300 ng/mL (SI: 188-1125 nmol/L)
Possible toxicity: >300 ng/mL (SI: >1070 nmol/L)
Toxic: >1000 ng/mL (SI: >3750 nmol/L)

Patient Information Before starting treatment notify physician if you have any of the following: Cardiovascular disease; family history of sudden death, cardiac dysrhythmias, or cardiac disturbances; thyroid disease or are taking thyroid medication; history of seizure disorder; urinary retention; or glaucoma. Read the patient Medication Guide that you receive with each prescription and refill of desipramine. An increased risk of suicidal thinking and behavior has been reported with the use of antidepressants in children, adolescents, and young adults (18-24 years of age). Notify physician if you feel more depressed, have thoughts of suicide, or become more agitated or irritable (see Warnings). May cause drowsiness and impair ability to perform activities requiring mental alertness or physical coordination; may cause dry mouth; avoid alcohol and the herbal medicine St John's wort; limit caffeine; may discolor urine to blue-green color; do not discontinue medication abruptly; may increase appetite. May cause photosensitivity reactions (eg, exposure to sunlight may cause severe sunburn, skin rash, redness, or itching); avoid exposure to sunlight and artificial light sources (sunlamps, tanning booth/bed); wear protective clothing, wide-brimmed hats, sunglasses, and lip sunscreen (SPF ≥15); use a sunscreen [broad-spectrum sunscreen or physical sunscreen (preferred) or sunblock with SPF ≥15]; contact physician if reaction occurs.

Dosage Forms Excipient information presented when available (limited, particularly for generics); consult specific product labeling.

Tablet, as hydrochloride: 10 mg, 25 mg, 50 mg, 75 mg, 100 mg, 150 mg

Norpramin®: 10 mg, 25 mg, 50 mg, 75 mg, 100 mg, 150 mg [contains soy oil]

References

American Academy of Pediatrics/American Heart Association Clarification of Statement on Cardiovascular Evaluation and Monitoring of Children and Adolescents With Heart Disease Receiving Medications for ADHD; available at: http://americanheart.mediaroon.com/index.php?s=43&item=422.

Biederman J, Thisted RA, Greenhill LL, et al, "Estimation of the Association Between Desipramine and the Risk for Sudden Death in 5-14 Year-Old Children," *J Clin Psychiatry,* 1995, 56(3):87-93.

Dopheide JA, "Recognizing and Treating Depression in Children and Adolescents," *Am J Health Syst Pharm,* 2006, 63(3):233-43.

Levy HB, Harper CR, and Weinberg WA, "A Practical Approach to Children Failing in School," *Pediatr Clin North Am,* 1992, 39 (4):895-928.

Vetter VL, Elia J, Erickson C, et al, "Cardiovascular Monitoring of Children and Adolescents With Heart Disease Receiving Stimulant Drugs: A Scientific Statement From the American Heart Association Council on Cardiovascular Disease in the Young Congenital Cardiac Defects Committee and the Council on Cardiovascular Nursing," *Circulation,* 2008, 117(18):2407-23.

Wagner KD, "Pharmacotherapy for Major Depression in Children and Adolescents," *Prog Neuropsychopharmacol Biol Psychiatry,* 2005, 29 (5):819-20.

♦ **Desipramine Hydrochloride** *see* Desipramine *on page 401*

♦ **Desitin® [OTC]** *see* Zinc Oxide *on page 1445*

♦ **Desitin® Creamy [OTC]** *see* Zinc Oxide *on page 1445*

Desloratadine (des lor AT a deen)

Medication Safety Issues
Sound-alike/look-alike issues:
Clarinex® may be confused with Celebrex®

U.S. Brand Names Clarinex®

Canadian Brand Names Aerius®

Therapeutic Category Antihistamine

Generic Available No

Use Symptomatic relief of nasal and non-nasal symptoms of allergic rhinitis; chronic idiopathic urticaria

Pregnancy Risk Factor C

Pregnancy Considerations There are no adequate and well-controlled studies in pregnant women. Use during pregnancy only if clearly needed.

Lactation Enters breast milk/not recommended

Contraindications Hypersensitivity to desloratadine, loratadine, or any component

Warnings Use with caution and adjust dosage in patients with liver or renal impairment. Syrup contains sodium benzoate; benzoic acid (benzoate) is a metabolite of benzyl alcohol; large amounts of benzyl alcohol (≥99 mg/kg/day) have been associated with a potentially fatal toxicity ("gasping syndrome") in neonates; the "gasping syndrome" consists of metabolic acidosis, respiratory distress, gasping respirations, CNS dysfunction (including convulsions, intracranial hemorrhage), hypotension and cardiovascular collapse; avoid use in neonates; *in vitro* and animal studies have shown that benzoate displaces bilirubin from protein binding sites

Precautions A subset of the general population (7% in clinical trials) are slow metabolizers of desloratadine; the frequency of slow metabolism appears to be higher in African Americans; patients who are slow metabolizers may be more susceptible to dose-related side effects; use with caution in "slow metabolizers." Use cautiously in patients who are also taking ketoconazole, itraconazole, fluconazole, erythromycin, clarithromycin, or other drugs which may impair desloratadine's hepatic metabolism; although increased plasma levels of desloratadine have been observed, no adverse effects with concomitant administration have been reported, including QT interval prolongation which has occurred when similar antihistamines, terfenadine and astemizole, were combined with these agents. While less sedating than other antihistamines, desloratadine may cause drowsiness and impair ability to perform hazardous activities requiring mental alertness. Use cautiously in breast-feeding women as desloratadine passes into breast milk. RediTabs® contain aspartame which is metabolized to phenylalanine and must be used with caution in patients with phenylketonuria.

Adverse Reactions
Cardiovascular: Tachycardia, edema

Central nervous system: Somnolence, fatigue, dizziness

Dermatologic: Pruritus, urticaria

Gastrointestinal: Xerostomia, nausea, dry throat

Hepatic: Liver enzymes elevated, bilirubin elevated

Neuromuscular & skeletal: Myalgia

Respiratory: Pharyngitis, dyspnea

Miscellaneous: Hypersensitivity reactions, flu-like symptoms

Drug Interactions
Metabolism/Transport Effects Substrate of P-glycoprotein

Avoid Concomitant Use There are no known interactions where it is recommended to avoid concomitant use.

Increased Effect/Toxicity

Desloratadine may increase the levels/effects of: Alcohol (Ethyl); Anticholinergics; CNS Depressants

The levels/effects of Desloratadine may be increased by: P-Glycoprotein Inhibitors; Pramlintide

Decreased Effect

Desloratadine may decrease the levels/effects of: Acetylcholinesterase Inhibitors (Central); Betahistine

The levels/effects of Desloratadine may be decreased by: Acetylcholinesterase Inhibitors (Central); Amphetamines; P-Glycoprotein Inducers

Food Interactions Administration with food has no effect on desloratadine's bioavailability

Stability Store at room temperature; avoid excessive heat and moisture; RediTabs® must be used immediately after removal from blister pack

Mechanism of Action Long-acting tricyclic antihistamine with selective peripheral histamine H_1-receptor antagonistic properties; active metabolite of loratadine

Pharmacodynamics
Onset of action: 1 hour

Duration: 24 hours

Pharmacokinetics (Adult data unless noted)
Distribution: Distributes into breast milk

Protein binding: 82% to 87% (desloratadine), 85% to 89% (metabolite)

Metabolism: Metabolized to an active metabolite (3-hydroxydesloratadine); subset of population are slow metabolizers of desloratadine (7% of patients in clinical trials were slow-metabolizers; see Precautions)

Half-life: 27 hours (both desloratadine and active metabolite)

Time to peak serum concentration: 3 hours

Elimination: 87% eliminated via urine and feces as metabolic products

Usual Dosage Oral:

Children 6-11 months: 1 mg once daily

Children 1-5 years: 1.25 mg once daily

Children 6-11 years: 2.5 mg once daily

Children ≥12 years and Adults: 5 mg once daily

Dosage adjustment in renal/hepatic impairment: Administer dosage every other day

Administration Oral: May administer without regard to food. Place RediTabs® directly on the tongue; tablet will disintegrate immediately; may be taken with or without water

Monitoring Parameters Improvement in signs and symptoms of allergic rhinitis

Reference Range Therapeutic serum levels (not used clinically): Desloratadine: 2.5-4 ng/mL

Test Interactions Antigen skin testing

Patient Information Drink plenty of water; may cause dry mouth; may cause drowsiness and impair ability to perform activities requiring mental alertness or physical coordination; avoid alcohol

Dosage Forms Excipient information presented when available (limited, particularly for generics); consult specific product labeling.

Syrup:

Clarinex®: 0.5 mg/mL (480 mL) [contains propylene glycol, sodium benzoate; bubble gum flavor]

Tablet:

Clarinex®: 5 mg

Tablet, orally disintegrating:

Clarinex® RediTabs®: 2.5 mg [contains phenylalanine 1.4 mg/tablet; tutti-frutti flavor]; 5 mg [contains phenylalanine 2.9 mg/tablet; tutti-frutti flavor]

References

Murdoch D, Goa KL, and Keam SJ, "Desloratadine: An Update of Its Efficacy in the Management of Allergic Disorders," *Drugs*, 2003, 63 (19):2051-77.

◆ **Desmethylimipramine Hydrochloride** *see* Desipramine *on page 401*

Desmopressin (des moe PRES in)

U.S. Brand Names DDAVP®; Stimate®

Canadian Brand Names Apo-Desmopressin®; DDAVP®; DDAVP® Melt; Minirin®; Novo-Desmopressin; Octostim®; PMS-Desmopressin

Therapeutic Category Antihemophilic Agent; Hemostatic Agent; Vasopressin Analog, Synthetic

Generic Available Yes

Use Treatment of diabetes insipidus (tablets: FDA approved in ages ≥4 years and adults; injection: FDA approved in ages >12 years and adults); control of bleeding in hemophilia A (with factor VIII levels >5%), mild to moderate type I von Willebrand disease (injection: FDA approved in ages >3 months and adults; nasal spray: FDA approved in ages >12 months and adults), and thrombocytopenia; primary nocturnal enuresis (tablets only: FDA approved in ages ≥6 years)

Pregnancy Risk Factor B

Pregnancy Considerations Adverse events were not observed in animal reproductive studies. There are no adequate and well-controlled studies in pregnant women. Anecdotal reports suggest congenital anomalies and low birth weight. However, causal relationship has not been established. Desmopressin has been used safely during pregnancy.

Lactation Excretion in breast milk unknown/use caution

Contraindications Hypersensitivity to desmopressin or any component; avoid using in patients with severe type I, type IIB, or platelet-type (pseudo) von Willebrand disease, hemophilia A with factor VIII levels ≤5% or hemophilia B; moderate-to-severe renal impairment (Cl_{cr} <50 mL/minute); patients with hyponatremia or history of hyponatremia

Warnings Desmopressin in combination with excessive fluid consumption can result in hyponatremia, an imbalance between intracellular and extracellular sodium. This imbalance can lead to seizures, brain swelling, coma, and death. The FDA has reviewed 61 postmarketing cases of hyponatremia-related seizures associated with the use of desmopressin acetate. Intranasal desmopressin was used in the majority of cases. Many of the patients were children being treated for primary nocturnal enuresis (PNE). An association with at least one concomitant drug or disease that also may cause hyponatremia and/or seizures was noted. As a result, **intranasal** desmopressin is no longer indicated for the treatment of PNE. In addition, **intranasal** desmopressin should not be used in patients with hyponatremia or a history of hyponatremia. Desmopressin acetate **tablets** may be used for the treatment of PNE; however, treatment should be interrupted if the patient experiences an acute illness (eg, fever, recurrent vomiting, diarrhea), vigorous exercise, or any condition associated with an increase in water consumption. Patients and caregivers should also be instructed to restrict fluid intake 1 hour prior to dose until the next morning, or for at least 8 hours after administration.

Avoid intranasal use in patients with nasal mucosa changes (scarring, edema, discharge, obstruction, or severe atopic rhinitis)

Precautions Use with caution in patients with predisposition to thrombus formation, conditions associated with fluid and electrolyte imbalance (eg, cystic fibrosis, CHF, renal disorders), in patients with habitual or psychogenic polydipsia or using medications known to either increase thirst or cause syndrome of inappropriate antidiuretic hormone secretion (SIADH) (eg, carbamazepine, SSRIs), and in patients with coronary artery disease and/or hypertensive cardiovascular disease; fluid intake may need to be reduced to decrease potential for development of water intoxication

Adverse Reactions

Cardiovascular: Blood pressure increased, facial flushing, tachycardia

Central nervous system: Cerebral edema (see Warnings), headache

Endocrine & metabolic: Hyponatremia, water intoxication (see Warnings)

Gastrointestinal: Abdominal cramps, dyspepsia, nausea, sore throat

Genitourinary: Vulval pain

Local: Pain at the injection site

Respiratory: Epistaxis, nasal congestion, rhinitis, upper respiratory infections

Miscellaneous: Anaphylaxis

<1%, postmarketing, and/or case reports: Abnormal thinking, agitation, balanitis, chest pain, chills, diarrhea, dizziness, edema, hyponatremic seizure, insomnia, itchy or light-sensitive eyes, MI, palpitations, somnolence, vomiting

Drug Interactions

Avoid Concomitant Use There are no known interactions where it is recommended to avoid concomitant use.

Increased Effect/Toxicity

Desmopressin may increase the levels/effects of: Lithium

The levels/effects of Desmopressin may be increased by: Analgesics (Opioid); CarBAMazepine; ChlorproMAZINE; LamoTRIgine; Nonsteroidal Anti-Inflammatory Agents; Selective Serotonin Reuptake Inhibitors; Tricyclic Antidepressants

Decreased Effect

The levels/effects of Desmopressin may be decreased by: Demeclocycline; Lithium

Stability Refrigerate injection, nasal solution and Stimate® nasal spray; nasal solution and Stimate® nasal spray are stable for 3 weeks when stored at room temperature if unopened; injection is stable for 2 weeks at room temperature; DDAVP® nasal spray is stable at room temperature

Mechanism of Action Enhances reabsorption of water in the kidneys by increasing cellular permeability of the collecting ducts; possibly causes smooth muscle constriction with resultant vasoconstriction; dose-dependent increase in plasma factor VIII and plasminogen activator

Pharmacodynamics

Oral administration:
Onset of ADH action: 1 hour
Maximum effect: 2-7 hours
Duration: 6-8 hours; **Note:** 0.4 mcg doses have had antidiuretic effects for up to 12 hours

Intranasal administration:
Onset of ADH action: Within 1 hour
Maximum effect: Within 1.5 hours
Duration: 5-21 hours

I.V. infusion:
Onset of increased factor VIII activity: Within 15-30 minutes
Maximum effect: 90 minutes to 3 hours

Pharmacokinetics (Adult data unless noted) Note:

Due to large differences in bioavailability between product formulations and patient variability in response, dosage conversions between product formulations should be done conservatively titrating to clinical improvement.

Absorption:
Oral tablets: 0.08% to 0.16%; **Note:** Bioavailability of tablet is ~5% of nasal spray.
Nasal solution: 10% to 20%
Nasal spray (1.5 mg/mL concentration): 3.3% to 4.1%

Metabolism: Unknown

Half-life:
Oral: 1.5-2.5 hours
I.V.:
Initial: 7.8 minutes
Terminal: 75.5 minutes (range: 0.4-4 hours); severe renal impairment: 9 hours
Intranasal: 3.3-3.5 hours

Time to peak serum concentration:
Oral: 0.9 hours
Intranasal: 1.5 hours

Excretion: Primarily in urine

Usual Dosage

Diabetes insipidus:

Oral:
Children ≤12 years: Initial: 0.05 mg twice daily; titrate to desired response (range: 0.1-0.8 mg daily)
Children >12 years and Adults: 0.05 mg twice daily; titrate to desired response (range: 0.1-1.2 mg divided 2-3 times/day)

Intranasal: **Note:** Use nasal solution in patients whose dosage needs are <10 mcg or are not met with 10 mcg per spray increments in spray formulation.
Children 3 months to ≤12 years: Initial: 5 mcg/day (0.05 mL/day nasal solution) divided 1-2 times/day; range: 5-30 mcg/day (0.05-0.3 mL/day nasal solution); adjust morning and evening doses separately for an adequate diurnal rhythm of water turnover

Children >12 years and Adults: Initial: 5-40 mcg (0.05-0.4 mL nasal solution) divided 1-3 times/day; most patients require 0.2 mL daily in 2 divided doses; adjust morning and evening doses separately for an adequate diurnal rhythm of water turnover

I.V., SubQ: Children <12 years: No definitive dosing available. Adult dosing should not be used in this age group; adverse events such as hyponatremia-induced seizures may occur. Dose should be reduced. Some have suggested an initial dosage range of 0.1-1 mcg in 1 or 2 divided doses (Cheetham, 2002). Initiate at low dose and increase as necessary. Closely monitor serum sodium levels and urine output; fluid restriction is recommended.

I.V., SubQ: Children ≥12 years and Adults: 2-4 mcg/day in 2 divided doses or 1/10 of the maintenance intranasal dose; adjust morning and evening doses separately for an adequate diurnal rhythm of water turnover

Hemophilia:

I.V.: Children ≥3 months and Adults: 0.3 mcg/kg beginning 30 minutes before procedure; may repeat dose if needed. **Note:** Adverse events such as hyponatremia-induced seizures have been reported especially in young children using this dosing regimen (Das, 2005; Molnár, 2005; Smith, 1989; Thumfart, 2005; Weinstein, 1989). Fluid restriction and careful monitoring of serum sodium levels and urine output are necessary.

Intranasal: Children >12 years and Adults: Using high concentration Stimate® nasal spray:
≤50 kg: 150 mcg (1 spray)
>50 kg: 300 mcg (1 spray each nostril)
Repeat use is determined by the patient's clinical condition and laboratory work; if using preoperatively, administer 2 hours before surgery

Nocturnal enuresis (short-term treatment, 4-8 weeks); intranasal formulations are not recommended for nocturnal enuresis treatment; see Warnings:
Oral: Children ≥6 years: Initial dose: 0.2 mg once before bedtime; titrate as needed to a maximum of 0.6 mg; fluid intake should be limited to a minimum from 1 hour before desmopressin administration until the next morning, or at least 8 hours after administration

Administration

Intranasal: Using rhinal tube delivery system, draw solution into flexible, calibrated rhinal tube; insert one end into nostril; blow on the other end to deposit the solution deep into the nasal cavity. The Stimate® spray pump must be primed prior to first use; to prime pump, press down 4 times. Avoid spray use in children <6 years of age due to difficulty in titrating dosage; discard any solution remaining after 25 or 50 doses (2.5 or 5 mL vials, respectively) because the amount delivered may be substantially less than prescribed

Parenteral: I.V.: Dilute to a maximum concentration of 0.5 mcg/mL in NS (recommended: Children <10 kg: 10 mL diluent; Children >10 kg and Adults: 50 mL diluent); infuse over 15-30 minutes; if desmopressin I.V. is given preoperatively, administer 30 minutes prior to surgery

Monitoring Parameters Note: For all indications, fluid intake, urine volume, and signs and symptoms of hyponatremia should be closely monitored especially in high risk patient subgroups (eg, young children, elderly, patients with heart failure).
I.V. infusion: Blood pressure and pulse should be monitored
Diabetes insipidus: Urine specific gravity, plasma and urine osmolality, serum electrolytes
Hemophilia: Factor VIII antigen levels, APTT, Factor VIII activity level

◀ **Patient Information** Avoid overhydration; blow nose before using nasal solution or spray; notify physician if headache, shortness of breath, heartburn, nausea, abdominal cramps, or vulval pain occur; when treating nocturnal enuresis, restrict fluid intake 1 hour prior to dose until the next morning, or for at least 8 hours after administration

Additional Information 1 mcg of desmopressin acetate injection is approximately equal to 4 international units of antidiuretic activity; desmopressin acetate injection has an antidiuretic effect about ten times that of an equivalent dose administered intranasally

Dosage Forms Excipient information presented when available (limited, particularly for generics); consult specific product labeling. [DSC] = Discontinued product; [CAN] = Canadian product [not available in U.S]

Injection, solution, as acetate: 4 mcg/mL (1 mL, 10 mL)
DDAVP®: 4 mcg/mL (1 mL, 10 mL)

Solution, intranasal, as acetate: 100 mcg/mL (2.5 mL)
DDAVP®: 100 mcg/mL (2.5 mL) [contains benzalkonium chloride; with rhinal tube]

Solution, intranasal, as acetate [spray]: 0.1 mg/mL (5 mL)
DDAVP®: 0.1 mg/mL (5 mL) [contains benzalkonium chloride; delivers 10 mcg/spray]

Stimate®: 1.5 mg/mL (2.5 mL) [delivers 150 mcg/spray] [DSC]

Stimate®: 1.5 mg/mL (2.5 mL) [contains benzalkonium chloride; delivers 150 mcg/spray]

Tablet, as acetate, oral: 0.1 mg, 0.2 mg
DDAVP®: 0.1 mg, 0.2 mg [scored]

Tablet, as acetate, sublingual:
DDAVP® Melt [CAN]: 60 mcg, 120 mcg, 240 mcg

References

Cheetham T and Baylis PH, "Diabetes Insipidus in Children: Pathophysiology, Diagnosis and Management," *Paediatr Drugs*, 2002, 4(12):785-96.

Das P, Carcao M, and Hitzler J, "DDAVP-Induced Hyponatremia in Young Children," *J Pediatr Hematol Oncol*, 2005, 27(6):330-2.

Eller N, Kollenz CJ, Bauer P, et al, "The Duration of Antidiuretic Response of Two Desmopressin Nasal Sprays," *Int J Clin Pharmacol Ther*, 1998, 36(9):494-500.

Eller N, Kollenz CJ, and Hitzenberger G, "A Comparative Study of Pharmacodynamics and Bioavailability of 2 Different Desmopressin Nasal Sprays," *Int J Clin Pharmacol Ther*, 1998, 36(3):139-45.

Molnár Z, Farkas V, Nemes L, et al, "Hyponatraemic Seizures Resulting From Inadequate Post-Operative Fluid Intake Following a Single Dose of Desmopressin," *Nephrol Dial Transplant*, 2005, 20 (10):2265-7.

Robson WL, Leung AK, and Norgaard JP, "The Comparative Safety of Oral Versus Intranasal Desmopressin for the Treatment of Children With Nocturnal Enuresis," *J Urol*, 2007, 178(1):24-30.

Smith TJ, Gill JC, Ambruso DR, et al, "Hyponatremia and Seizures in Young Children Given DDAVP," *Am J Hematol*, 1989, 31(3):199-202.

Stenberg A and Läckgren G, "Desmopressin Tablets in the Treatment of Severe Nocturnal Enuresis in Adolescents," *Pediatrics*, 1994, 94(6 Pt 1):841-46.

Thumfart J, Roehr CC, Kapelari K, et al, "Desmopressin Associated Symptomatic Hyponatremic Hypervolemia in Children. Are There Predictive Factors?" *J Urol*, 2005, 174(1):294-8.

Weinstein RE, Bona RD, Altman AJ, et al, "Severe Hyponatremia After Repeated Intravenous Administration of Desmopressin," *Am J Hematol*, 1989, 32(4):258-61.

◆ **Desmopressin Acetate** see Desmopressin on page 404
◆ **Desoxyphenobarbital** see Primidone on page 1154
◆ **Desquam-X®** see Benzoyl Peroxide on page 184
◆ **Desquam-E™ [DSC]** see Benzoyl Peroxide on page 184
◆ **Desyrel® (Can)** see TraZODone on page 1371
◆ **Detane® [OTC]** see Benzocaine on page 182
◆ **Detemir Insulin** see Insulin Detemir on page 740
◆ **Detrol®** see Tolterodine on page 1359
◆ **Detrol® LA** see Tolterodine on page 1359
◆ **Dex4® [OTC]** see Dextrose on page 422

Dexamethasone (deks a METH a sone)

Medication Safety Issues
Sound-alike/look-alike issues:
Dexamethasone may be confused with desoximetasone, dextroamphetamine
Decadron® may be confused with Percodan®
Maxidex® may be confused with Maxzide®

Related Information
Corticosteroids on page 1487

U.S. Brand Names Baycadron™; Dexamethasone Intensol™; DexPak® 10 Day TaperPak®; DexPak® 13 Day TaperPak®; DexPak® 6 Day TaperPak®; DexPak® TaperPak® [DSC]; Maxidex®; Ozurdex™

Canadian Brand Names Apo-Dexamethasone®; Dexasone®; Diodex®; Maxidex®; PMS-Dexamethasone

Therapeutic Category Adrenal Corticosteroid; Anti-inflammatory Agent; Anti-inflammatory Agent, Ophthalmic; Antiemetic; Corticosteroid, Ophthalmic; Corticosteroid, Systemic; Glucocorticoid

Generic Available Yes: Excludes ophthalmic suspension, intravitreal implant

Use Treatment of chronic inflammation, allergic, hematologic, dermatologic, neoplastic, rheumatic, and autoimmune diseases; may be used in management of cerebral edema, septic shock, and as a diagnostic agent; adjunctive antiemetic agent in the treatment of chemotherapy-induced emesis; treatment of airway edema prior to extubation; used in neonates with bronchopulmonary dysplasia to facilitate ventilator weaning

Pregnancy Risk Factor C

Pregnancy Considerations Adverse events have been observed with corticosteroids in animal reproduction studies. Dexamethasone crosses the placenta; and is partially metabolized to an inactive metabolite by placental enzymes. Due to its positive effect on stimulating fetal lung maturation, the injection is often used in patients with premature labor (24-34 weeks gestation). Some studies have shown an association between first trimester systemic corticosteroid use and oral clefts; adverse events in the fetus/neonate have been noted in case reports following large doses of systemic corticosteroids during pregnancy. Women exposed to dexamethasone during pregnancy for the treatment of an autoimmune disease may contact the OTIS Autoimmune Diseases Study at 877-311-8972.

Lactation Excretion in breast milk unknown/use caution

Breast-Feeding Considerations Corticosteroids are excreted in human milk; information specific to dexamethasone has not been located.

Contraindications Hypersensitivity to dexamethasone or any component (see Warnings); active untreated infections; systemic fungal infections; cerebral malaria; viral, fungal, or tuberculous diseases of the eye

Warnings Hypothalamic-pituitary-adrenal (HPA) suppression may occur; acute adrenal insufficiency (adrenal crisis) may occur with abrupt withdrawal after long term therapy or with stress; withdrawal and discontinuation of corticosteroids should be done carefully; patients with HPA axis suppression may require doses of systemic glucocorticosteroids prior to, during, and after unusual stress (eg, surgery). Immunosuppression may occur; patients may be more susceptible to infections; avoid exposure to chickenpox and measles. Corticosteroids may activate latent opportunistic infections or exacerbate systemic fungal infections. May cause osteoporosis (at any age) or inhibition of bone growth in pediatric patients. Acute myopathy may occur with high doses, elevated IOP may occur (especially with prolonged use), CNS effects (ranging from euphoria to psychosis) may occur. Rare cases of anaphylactoid reactions have been reported with corticosteroids.

Injection may contain sulfites and 0.5 mg tablet may contain tartrazine, either may cause allergic reactions in susceptible individuals. Concentrated oral solution (Intensol™) contains 30% ethanol and propylene glycol. Elixir may contain benzoic acid; benzoic acid (benzoate) is a metabolite of benzyl alcohol; large amounts of benzyl alcohol (≥99 mg/kg/day) have been associated with a potentially fatal toxicity ("gasping syndrome") in neonates; the "gasping syndrome" consists of metabolic acidosis, respiratory distress, gasping respirations, CNS dysfunction (including convulsions, intracranial hemorrhage), hypotension and cardiovascular collapse; use dexamethasone products containing benzoic acid with caution in neonates; *in vitro* and animal studies have shown that benzoate displaces bilirubin from protein binding sites

Precautions Avoid using higher than recommended doses; suppression of HPA function, suppression of linear growth (ie, reduction of growth velocity), reduced bone mineral density, hypercorticism (Cushing's syndrome), hyperglycemia, or glucosuria may occur; titrate to lowest effective dose. Reduction in growth velocity may occur when corticosteroids are administered to pediatric patients by any route (monitor growth). Use with extreme caution in patients with respiratory tuberculosis, untreated systemic infections, or ocular herpes simplex; use with caution in patients with thyroid dysfunction, cirrhosis, ulcerative colitis, hypertension, renal impairment, osteoporosis, thromboembolic tendencies, CHF, recent MI, convulsive disorders, myasthenia gravis, thrombophlebitis, peptic ulcer, diabetes; prolonged use may result in cataracts or glaucoma

Adverse Reactions

Cardiovascular: Edema, hypertension

Central nervous system: Headache, vertigo, seizures, euphoria, psychosis, pseudotumor cerebri, insomnia, nervousness

Dermatologic: Acne, skin atrophy

Endocrine & metabolic: HPA suppression, growth suppression, glucose intolerance, hypokalemia, alkalosis, Cushing's syndrome

Gastrointestinal: Peptic ulcer, nausea, vomiting

Neuromuscular & skeletal: Muscle weakness, osteoporosis, bone mineral density decreased, fractures

Ocular: Cataracts, IOP increased, glaucoma

Miscellaneous: Immunosuppression, anaphylactoid reactions (rare)

Drug Interactions

Metabolism/Transport Effects Substrate of CYP3A4 (major), P-glycoprotein; **Induces** CYP2A6 (weak), CYP2B6 (weak), CYP2C8 (weak), CYP2C9 (weak), CYP3A4 (strong), P-glycoprotein

Avoid Concomitant Use

Avoid concomitant use of Dexamethasone with any of the following: Aldesleukin; BCG; Dronedarone; Everolimus; Natalizumab; Nilotinib; Nisoldipine; Pazopanib; Pimecrolimus; Ranolazine; Romidepsin; Tacrolimus (Topical); Tolvaptan; Vaccines (Live)

Increased Effect/Toxicity

Dexamethasone may increase the levels/effects of: Acetylcholinesterase Inhibitors; Amphotericin B; Leflunomide; Lenalidomide; Loop Diuretics; Natalizumab; NSAID (COX-2 Inhibitor); NSAID (Nonselective); Thalidomide; Thiazide Diuretics; Vaccines (Live); Warfarin

The levels/effects of Dexamethasone may be increased by: Antifungal Agents (Azole Derivatives, Systemic); Aprepitant; Asparaginase; Calcium Channel Blockers (Nondihydropyridine); CYP3A4 Inhibitors (Moderate); CYP3A4 Inhibitors (Strong); Dasatinib; Denosumab; Estrogen Derivatives; Fluconazole; Fosaprepitant; Macrolide Antibiotics; Neuromuscular-Blocking Agents (Nondepolarizing); P-Glycoprotein Inhibitors; Pimecrolimus;

Quinolone Antibiotics; Salicylates; Tacrolimus (Topical); Trastuzumab

Decreased Effect

Dexamethasone may decrease the levels/effects of: Aldesleukin; Antidiabetic Agents; BCG; Calcitriol; Caspofungin; Corticorelin; CYP3A4 Substrates; Dabigatran Etexilate; Dronedarone; Everolimus; GuanFACINE; Isoniazid; Maraviroc; NIFEdipine; Nilotinib; Nisoldipine; Pazopanib; P-Glycoprotein Substrates; Ranolazine; Romidepsin; Salicylates; Sipuleucel-T; Sorafenib; Tadalafil; Tolvaptan; Vaccines (Inactivated); Vaccines (Live)

The levels/effects of Dexamethasone may be decreased by: Aminoglutethimide; Antacids; Barbiturates; Bile Acid Sequestrants; CYP3A4 Inducers (Strong); Deferasirox; Echinacea; Herbs (CYP3A4 Inducers); Mitotane; P-Glycoprotein Inducers; Primidone; Rifamycin Derivatives

Food Interactions Systemic use of corticosteroids may require a diet with increased potassium, vitamins A, B_6, C, D, folate, calcium, zinc, and phosphorus and decreased sodium

Stability Dilution of dexamethasone sodium phosphate injection with D_5W or NS is stable for at least 24 hours

Mechanism of Action Decreases inflammation by suppression of migration of polymorphonuclear leukocytes and reversal of increased capillary permeability; suppresses normal immune response

Pharmacodynamics Duration: Metabolic effects can last for 72 hours

Pharmacokinetics (Adult data unless noted)

Metabolism: In the liver

Half-life: Terminal:

Extremely low birth weight infants with BPD: 9.3 hours

Children 3 months to 16 years: 4.3 hours

Healthy adults: 3 hours

Time to peak serum concentration:

Oral: Within 1-2 hours

I.M.: Within 8 hours

Elimination: In urine and bile

Usual Dosage

Neonates:

Airway edema or extubation: I.V.: Usual: 0.25 mg/kg/dose given ~4 hours prior to scheduled extubation and then every 8 hours for 3 doses total; range: 0.25-1 mg/kg/dose for 1-3 doses; maximum dose: 1 mg/kg/day. **Note:** A longer duration of therapy may be needed in more severe cases.

Bronchopulmonary dysplasia (to facilitate ventilator weaning): Oral, I.V.: Numerous dosing schedules have been proposed; range: 0.5-0.6 mg/kg/day given in divided doses every 12 hours for 3-7 days, then taper over 1-6 weeks

Children:

Airway edema or extubation: Oral, I.M., I.V.: 0.5-2 mg/kg/day in divided doses every 6 hours; begin 24 hours prior to extubation and continue for 4-6 doses after extubation

Antiemetic (chemotherapy induced): I.V.: Initial: 10 mg/m²/dose (maximum dose: 20 mg) then 5 mg/m²/dose every 6 hours

Anti-inflammatory: Oral, I.M., I.V.: 0.08-0.3 mg/kg/day or 2.5-10 mg/m²/day in divided doses every 6-12 hours

Bacterial meningitis: Infants and Children >2 months: I.V.: 0.6 mg/kg/day divided every 6 hours for the first 4 days of antibiotic treatment; start dexamethasone at the time of the first dose of antibiotic

Cerebral edema: Oral, I.M., I.V.: Loading dose: 1-2 mg/kg/dose as a single dose; maintenance: 1-1.5 mg/kg/day (maximum dose: 16 mg/day) in divided doses every 4-6 hours

Physiologic replacement: Oral, I.M., I.V.: 0.03-0.15 mg/kg/day or 0.6-0.75 mg/m²/day in divided doses every 6-12 hours

Children and Adults: Ophthalmic:

Suspension: Instill 2 drops every hour during the day and every other hour during the night; gradually reduce dose to every 3-4 hours, then to 3-4 times/day

Adults:

Acute nonlymphoblastic leukemia (ANLL) protocol: I.V.: 2 mg/m^2/dose every 8 hours for 12 doses

Anti-inflammatory: Oral, I.M., I.V.: 0.75-9 mg/day in divided doses every 6-12 hours

Cerebral edema: I.V.: Initial: 10 mg then 4 mg I.M./I.V. every 6 hours

Diagnosis for Cushing's syndrome: Oral: 1 mg at 11 PM, draw blood at 8 AM

Administration

Ophthalmic: Avoid contact of container tip with skin or eye; remove soft contact lenses prior to using solutions containing benzalkonium chloride

Solution and suspension: Apply finger pressure to lacrimal sac during and for 1-2 minutes after instillation to decrease risk of absorption and systemic effects

Oral: May administer with food or milk to decrease GI adverse effects

Parenteral: I.V.: Administer undiluted solution (4 mg/mL) I.V. push over 1-4 minutes if dose is <10 mg; high-dose therapy must be diluted in D$_5$W or NS and administered by I.V. intermittent infusion over 15-30 minutes

Monitoring Parameters Hemoglobin, occult blood loss, blood pressure, serum potassium and glucose; IOP with systemic use >6 weeks; weight and height in children

Reference Range Dexamethasone suppression test: 8 AM cortisol <6 mcg/100 mL in adults given dexamethasone 1 mg at 11 PM the previous night

Test Interactions Skin tests

Patient Information Avoid alcohol; limit caffeine; do not decrease dose or discontinue drug without physician's approval; avoid exposure to measles or chicken pox; advise physician immediately if exposed; notify physician if acute illness including fever or other signs of infection occurs. Inform physician you are taking corticosteroid prior to any surgery or with any injury

Additional Information Due to the long duration of effect (36-54 hours), alternate day dosing does not allow time for adrenal recovery between doses.

Dosage Forms Excipient information presented when available (limited, particularly for generics); consult specific product labeling. [DSC] = Discontinued product

Elixir: 0.5 mg/5 mL (240 mL)

Baycadron™: 0.5 mg/5 mL (237 mL) [contains benzoic acid; ethanol 5.1%; propylene glycol; raspberry flavor]

Implant, intravitreal:

Ozurdex™: 0.7 mg (1s)

Injection, solution, as sodium phosphate: 4 mg/mL (1 mL, 5 mL, 30 mL); 10 mg/mL (10 mL)

Injection, solution, as sodium phosphate [preservative free]: 10 mg/mL (1 mL)

Solution, ophthalmic, as sodium phosphate [drops]: 0.1% (5 mL)

Solution, oral: 0.5 mg/5 mL (500 mL)

Solution, oral [concentrate]:

Dexamethasone Intensol™: 1 mg/mL (30 mL) [dye free, sugar free; contains alcohol 30% and propylene glycol]

Suspension, ophthalmic [drops]:

Maxidex®: 0.1% (5 mL) [contains benzalkonium chloride]

Tablet [scored]: 0.5 mg, 0.75 mg, 1 mg, 1.5 mg, 2 mg, 4 mg, 6 mg

DexPak® 10 Day TaperPak®: 1.5 mg [35 tablets on taper dose card]

DexPak® 13 Day TaperPak®: 1.5 mg [51 tablets on taper dose card]

DexPak® 6 Day TaperPak®: 1.5 mg [21 tablets on taper dose card]

DexPak® TaperPak®: 1.5 mg [51 tablets on taper dose card] [DSC]

References

American Academy of Pediatrics Committee on Infectious Diseases, "Dexamethasone Therapy for Bacterial Meningitis in Infants and Children," *Pediatrics*, 1990, 86(1):130-3.

Bahal N and Nahata MC, "The Role of Corticosteroids in Infants and Children With Bacterial Meningitis," *DICP*, 1991, 25(5):542-5.

Couser RJ, Ferrara TB, Falde B, et al, "Effectiveness of Dexamethasone in Preventing Extubation Failure in Preterm Infants at Increased Risk for Airway Edema," *J Pediatr*, 1992, 121(4):591-6.

Durand M, Sardesai S, and McEvoy C, "Effects of Early Dexamethasone Therapy on Pulmonary Mechanics and Chronic Lung Disease in Very Low Birth Weight Infants: A Randomized, Controlled Trial," *Pediatrics*, 1995, 95(4):584-90.

Ng PC, "The Effectiveness and Side Effects of Dexamethasone in Preterm Infants With Bronchopulmonary Dysplasia," *Arch Dis Child*, 1993, 68(3 Spec No):330-6.

◆ **Dexamethasone and Ciprofloxacin** *see* Ciprofloxacin and Dexamethasone *on page 314*

◆ **Dexamethasone Intensol™** *see* Dexamethasone *on page 406*

Dexamethasone, Neomycin, and Polymyxin B

(deks a METH a sone, nee oh MYE sin, & pol i MIKS in bee)

U.S. Brand Names Maxitrol®; Poly-Dex™

Canadian Brand Names Dioptrol®; Maxitrol®

Therapeutic Category Antibiotic, Ophthalmic; Corticosteroid, Ophthalmic

Generic Available Yes

Use Steroid-responsive inflammatory ocular conditions in which a corticosteroid is indicated and where bacterial infection or a risk of bacterial infection exists

Pregnancy Risk Factor C

Pregnancy Considerations See individual agents.

Lactation Excretion in breast milk unknown/use caution

Breast-Feeding Considerations It is unknown if topical use results in sufficient absorption to produce detectable quantities in breast milk.

Contraindications Hypersensitivity to dexamethasone, polymyxin, neomycin, or any component; viral diseases of the cornea and conjunctiva; mycobacterial infection of the eye; fungal disease of ocular structures; dendritic keratitis; use after uncomplicated removal of a corneal foreign body

Warnings Prolonged use may result in glaucoma, defects in visual acuity, posterior subcapsular cataract formation, and secondary ocular infections

Adverse Reactions

Dermatologic: Contact dermatitis, cutaneous sensitization (sensitivity to topical neomycin has been reported to occur in 5% to 15% of patients)

Local: Pain, stinging

Ocular: Development of glaucoma, cataract, intraocular pressure elevated, optic nerve damage, visual defects, blurred vision

Miscellaneous: Delayed wound healing, secondary infections

Drug Interactions

Avoid Concomitant Use

Avoid concomitant use of Neomycin, Polymyxin B, and Dexamethasone with any of the following: Aldesleukin; BCG; Dronedarone; Everolimus; Gallium Nitrate; Natalizumab; Nilotinib; Nisoldipine; Pazopanib; Pimecrolimus; Ranolazine; Romidepsin; Tacrolimus (Topical); Tolvaptan; Vaccines (Live)

Increased Effect/Toxicity

Neomycin, Polymyxin B, and Dexamethasone may increase the levels/effects of: AbobotulinumtoxinA; Acetylcholinesterase Inhibitors; Amphotericin B; Bisphosphonate Derivatives; CARBOplatin; Colistimethate; CycloSPORINE; CycloSPORINE (Systemic); Gallium Nitrate; Leflunomide; Lenalidomide; Loop Diuretics;

Natalizumab; Neuromuscular-Blocking Agents; NSAID (COX-2 Inhibitor); NSAID (Nonselective); Onabotulinum-toxinA; RimabotulinumtoxinB; Thalidomide; Thiazide Diuretics; Vaccines (Live); Warfarin

The levels/effects of Neomycin, Polymyxin B, and Dexamethasone may be increased by: Amphotericin B; Antifungal Agents (Azole Derivatives, Systemic); Aprepitant; Asparaginase; Calcium Channel Blockers (Non-dihydropyridine); Capreomycin; CISplatin; CYP3A4 Inhibitors (Moderate); CYP3A4 Inhibitors (Strong); Dasatinib; Denosumab; Estrogen Derivatives; Fluconazole; Fosaprepitant; Loop Diuretics; Macrolide Antibiotics; Neuromuscular-Blocking Agents (Nondepolarizing); P-Glycoprotein Inhibitors; Pimecrolimus; Quinolone Antibiotics; Salicylates; Tacrolimus (Topical); Trastuzumab; Vancomycin

Decreased Effect

Neomycin, Polymyxin B, and Dexamethasone may decrease the levels/effects of: Aldesleukin; Antidiabetic Agents; BCG; Calcitriol; Cardiac Glycosides; Caspofungin; Corticorelin; CYP3A4 Substrates; Dabigatran Etexilate; Dronedarone; Everolimus; GuanFACINE; Isoniazid; Maraviroc; NIFEdipine; Nilotinib; Nisoldipine; Pazopanib; P-Glycoprotein Substrates; Ranolazine; Romidepsin; Salicylates; Sipuleucel-T; Sorafenib; Tadalafil; Tolvaptan; Vaccines (Inactivated); Vaccines (Live)

The levels/effects of Neomycin, Polymyxin B, and Dexamethasone may be decreased by: Aminoglutethimide; Antacids; Barbiturates; Bile Acid Sequestrants; CYP3A4 Inducers (Strong); Deferasirox; Echinacea; Herbs (CYP3A4 Inducers); Mitotane; Penicillins; P-Glycoprotein Inducers; Primidone; Rifamycin Derivatives

Usual Dosage Children and Adults: Ophthalmic:

Ointment: Apply a small amount (~1/2") in the affected eye 3-4 times/day or apply at bedtime as an adjunct with drops

Suspension: Instill 1-2 drops into affected eye(s) every 4-6 hours; in severe disease, drops may be used hourly and tapered to discontinuation

Administration Ophthalmic: Shake suspension well before using; instill drop into affected eye; avoid contacting bottle tip with skin or eye; apply finger pressure to lacrimal sac during and for 1-2 minutes after instillation to decrease risk of absorption and systemic effects

Monitoring Parameters Intraocular pressure with use >10 days

Patient Information May cause temporary blurring of vision or stinging following administration

Dosage Forms Excipient information presented when available (limited, particularly for generics); consult specific product labeling.

Ointment, ophthalmic (Maxitrol®, Poly-Dex™): Neomycin 3.5 mg, polymyxin B sulfate 10,000 units, and dexamethasone 0.1% per g (3.5 g)

Suspension, ophthalmic (Maxitrol®, Poly-Dex™): Neomycin 3.5 mg, polymyxin B sulfate 10,000 units, and dexamethasone 0.1% per mL (5 mL) [contains benzalkonium chloride]

◆ **Dexamethasone, Neomycin, and Polymyxin B** *see* Dexamethasone, Neomycin, and Polymyxin B *on page 408*

◆ **Dexamethasone Sodium Phosphate** *see* Dexamethasone *on page 406*

◆ **Dexasone® (Can)** *see* Dexamethasone *on page 406*

◆ **Dexedrine®** *see* Dextroamphetamine *on page 416*

◆ **Dexferrum®** *see* Iron Dextran Complex *on page 762*

◆ **Dexiron™ (Can)** *see* Iron Dextran Complex *on page 762*

Dexmedetomidine (deks MED e toe mi deen)

Medication Safety Issues

Sound-alike/look-alike issues:

Precedex® may be confused with Peridex®

U.S. Brand Names Precedex®

Canadian Brand Names Precedex®

Therapeutic Category Adrenergic Agonist Agent; Alpha-Adrenergic Agonist; Sedative

Generic Available No

Use Sedation of initially intubated and mechanically ventilated patients during treatment in an intensive care setting; sedation prior to and/or during surgical or other procedures of nonintubated patients; duration of infusion should not exceed 24 hours. Other uses include premedication prior to anesthesia induction with thiopental; relief of pain and reduction of opioid dose following laparoscopic tubal ligation; as an adjunct anesthetic in ophthalmic surgery; treatment of shivering; premedication to attenuate the cardiostimulatory and postanesthetic delirium of ketamine. FDA approved in ages ≥18 years.

Pregnancy Risk Factor C

Pregnancy Considerations Teratogenic effects were not observed in animal studies. There are no adequate and well-controlled studies in pregnant women.

Lactation Excretion in breast milk unknown/use caution

Contraindications Hypersensitivity to dexmedetomidine or any component; use outside of an intensive care setting

Warnings Should be administered only by persons skilled in management of patients in intensive care setting or operating room. Patients should be continuously monitored. Episodes of bradycardia and sinus arrest have been associated with dexmedetomidine when administered rapidly I.V. (eg, bolus administration) or to patients with high vagal tone. Hypotension and bradycardia have been associated with dexmedetomidine infusion; treatment may include the use of atropine or glycopyrrolate, stopping or decreasing the infusion, increasing the rate of I.V. fluid administration, use of pressor agents, and elevation of the lower extremities. Transient hypertension has been primarily observed during the loading dose in association with the initial peripheral vasoconstrictive effects of dexmedetomidine. Treatment is usually unnecessary; however, reduction of infusion rate may be required.

Usage for >24 hours is not recommended; abrupt discontinuation, if used for prolonged periods may result in withdrawal symptoms similar to those reported for another alpha$_2$ adrenergic agent, clonidine.

Precautions Use with caution in patients with advanced heart block, severe ventricular dysfunction, hypovolemia, diabetes mellitus, and chronic hypertension. Use with caution in patients receiving vasodilators or drugs which decrease heart rate. Patients may be arousable and alert when stimulated. This alone should not be considered as lack of efficacy in the absence of other clinical signs/symptoms.

Adverse Reactions

Cardiovascular: Hypotension (28%), hypertension (16%), bradycardia, atrial fibrillation, tachycardia, hypovolemia

Central nervous system: Pain, fever, agitation, dizziness, headache, speech disorder

Endocrine & metabolic: Hyperglycemia, acidosis, hyperkalemia, hypocalcemia

Gastrointestinal: Nausea (11%), xerostomia, abdominal pain, diarrhea, vomiting

Hematologic: Anemia, hemorrhage, leukocytosis

Hepatic: Liver enzymes elevated

Neuromuscular & skeletal: Pain, rigors

Ocular: Abnormal vision, photopsia

Renal: Urine output decreased

Respiratory: Hypoxia, pulmonary edema, pleural effusion, respiratory acidosis, apnea, bronchospasm, dyspnea, hypercapnia, hypoventilation, pulmonary congestion

Miscellaneous: Infection, thirst, diaphoresis

Drug Interactions

Metabolism/Transport Effects Substrate of CYP2A6 (major); **Inhibits** CYP1A2 (weak), 2C9 (weak), 2D6 (strong), 3A4 (weak)

Avoid Concomitant Use

Avoid concomitant use of Dexmedetomidine with any of the following: lobenguane I 123

Increased Effect/Toxicity

Dexmedetomidine may increase the levels/effects of: Hypotensive Agents

The levels/effects of Dexmedetomidine may be increased by: Beta-Blockers; CYP2A6 Inhibitors (Moderate); CYP2A6 Inhibitors (Strong); MAO Inhibitors

Decreased Effect

Dexmedetomidine may decrease the levels/effects of: lobenguane I 123

The levels/effects of Dexmedetomidine may be decreased by: Antidepressants (Alpha2-Antagonist); Serotonin/Norepinephrine Reuptake Inhibitors; Tricyclic Antidepressants

Stability Store at room temperature; compatible when administered with LR, D_5W, NS, 20% mannitol, thiopental, etomidate, vecuronium, pancuronium, succinylcholine, atracurium, mivacurium, glycopyrrolate, phenylephrine, atropine, midazolam, morphine, and fentanyl (see manufacturer's information for more extensive compatibility listings). Incompatible when administered with amphotericin B and diazepam.

May adsorb to certain types of natural rubber; use components made with synthetic or coated natural rubber gaskets whenever possible.

Mechanism of Action Selective alpha₂-adrenoceptor agonist similar to clonidine, but with a much higher affinity for alpha₂-receptors over alpha₁-receptors; alpha₁ activity was observed at high doses or after rapid infusions; produces "arousable sedation" in which patients experience clinically effective sedation yet are easily arousable. The sedative response exhibits properties similar to natural sleep specifically simulating NREM sleep. The sedative properties result primarily from its activity in the locus ceruleus of the brain stem. Analgesic effects are produced by stimulation of the alpha₂-receptors in the dorsal horn of the spinal cord.

Pharmacokinetics (Adult data unless noted)

Distribution: V_{dss}: Approximately 118 L

Bioavailability: I.M.: 73%

Protein binding: 94%

Metabolism: Hepatic via N-glucuronidation, N-methylation, and CYP2A6

Half-life: Distribution: 6 minutes; Terminal: 2 hours

Elimination: Urine (95%); feces (4%)

Clearance: Adults: 39 L/hour; hepatic impairment (Child-Pugh Class A, B, or C): mean clearance values were 74%, 64%, and 53% respectively, of those observed in healthy adults; clearance at birth is approximately 30% of adults, reaching adult values between 6-12 months of age

Usual Dosage Individualize and titrate to desired clinical effect: I.V.:

Children (limited data): Loading dose: 0.5-1 mcg/kg; followed by a maintenance infusion of 0.2-0.7 mcg/kg/hour; children <1 year may require higher infusion rates; average infusion range: 0.4 mcg/kg/hour vs 0.29 mcg/kg/hour in children >1 year; doses as high as 0.75 mcg/kg/hour were used (Chrysostomou, 2006). Other studies have used maintenance doses as high as 1 mcg/kg/hour (Munro, 2007; Nichols, 2005).

Adults:

ICU sedation: Initial: Loading dose: 1 mcg/kg, followed by a maintenance infusion of 0.2-0.7 mcg/kg/hour; adjust rate to desired level of sedation

Procedural sedation: Initial: Loading infusion of 1 mcg/kg [or 0.5 mcg/kg for less invasive procedures (eg, ophthalmic)] over 10 minutes, followed by a maintenance infusion of 0.6 mcg/kg/hour, titrate to desired effect; usual range: 0.2-1 mcg/kg/hour

Fiberoptic intubation (awake): Initial: Loading infusion of 1 mcg/kg over 10 minutes, followed by a maintenance infusion of 0.7 mcg/kg/hour until endotracheal tube is secured

Note: The manufacturer does not recommend that the duration of infusion exceed 24 hours; however, there have been a few studies in adults demonstrating that dexmedetomidine was well tolerated in treatment periods >24 hours; titrate infusion rate so patient awakens slowly; abrupt discontinuation, particularly after prolonged infusions may result in withdrawal symptoms.

Dosage adjustment in hepatic impairment: Dosage reduction may need to be considered. No specific guidelines available.

Administration I.V.: Administer using a controlled infusion device. Dilute 200 mcg (2 mL) in 48 mL NS to achieve a final concentration of 4 mcg/mL. Infuse loading dose over 10 minutes; rapid infusions are associated with severe side effects (see Warnings). Dexmedetomidine may adhere to natural rubber; use administration components made with synthetic or coated natural rubber gaskets.

Monitoring Parameters Level of sedation, heart rate, respiration, ECG, blood pressure, pain control

Nursing Implications Continuous monitoring of vital signs, cardiac and respiratory status, and level of sedation during infusion and until full consciousness is regained. Do not discontinue abruptly (may result in rapid awakening associated with anxiety, agitation, and resistance to mechanical ventilation).

Additional Information As an adjunct to anesthesia, dexmedetomidine has been administered I.M. 0.5-1.5 mcg/kg/dose, 60 minutes prior to anesthesia.

Dosage Forms Excipient information presented when available (limited, particularly for generics); consult specific product labeling.

Injection, solution [preservative free]:

Precedex®: 100 mcg/mL (2 mL)

References

Berkenbosch JW, Wankum PC, and Tobias JD, "Prospective Evaluation of Dexmedetomidine for Noninvasive Procedural Sedation in Children," *Pediatr Crit Care Med*, 2005, 6(4):435-9.

Buck ML, "Dexmedetomidine for Sedation in the Pediatric Intensive Care Setting," *Pediatr Pharm*, 2006, 12(1).

Chrysostomou C, Di Filippo S, Manrique AM, et al, "Use of Dexmedetomidine in Children After Cardiac and Thoracic Surgery," *Pediatr Crit Care Med*, 2006, 7(2):126-31.

Munro HM, Tirotta CF, Felix DE, et al, "Initial Experience With Dexmedetomidine for Diagnostic and Interventional Cardiac Catheterization in Children," *Paediatr Anaesth*, 2007, 17(2):109-12.

Nichols DP, Berkenbosch JW, and Tobias JD, "Rescue Sedation With Dexmedetomidine for Diagnostic Imaging: A Preliminary Report," *Paediatr Anaesth*, 2005, 15(3):199-203.

Phan H and Nahata MC, "Clinical Uses of Dexmedetomidine in Pediatric Patients," *Paediatr Drugs*, 2008, 10(1):49-69.

Walker J, Maccalum M, Fischer C, et al, "Sedation Using Dexmedetomidine in Pediatric Burn Patients," *J Burn Care Res*, 2006, 27(2):206-10.

♦ **Dexmedetomidine Hydrochloride** see Dexmedetomidine *on page 409*

Dexmethylphenidate (dex meth il FEN i date)

Medication Safety Issues

Sound-alike/look-alike issues:

Dexmethylphenidate may be confused with methadone

Focalin® may be confused with Folotyn™

U.S. Brand Names Focalin®; Focalin® XR

Therapeutic Category Central Nervous System Stimulant

Generic Available Yes: Tablet

Use Treatment of attention-deficit/hyperactivity disorder (ADHD) (FDA approved in ages ≥6 years and adults)

Restrictions C-II

Medication Guide An FDA-approved patient medication guide, which is available with the product information and as follows, must be dispensed with this medication for each new outpatient prescription and refill.

Focalin®: http://www.fda.gov/downloads/Drugs/DrugSafety/ucm088600.pdf

Focalin® XR: http://www.fda.gov/downloads/Drugs/DrugSafety/ucm088601.pdf

Pregnancy Risk Factor C

Pregnancy Considerations Teratogenic effects were noted in animal studies. There are no adequate and well-controlled studies in pregnant women. Use only if the potential benefit to the mother outweighs the possible risks to the fetus.

Lactation Excretion in breast milk unknown/use caution

Breast-Feeding Considerations It is not known if dexmethylphenidate is excreted into breast milk. Dexmethylphenidate is the more active *d-threo*-enantiomer of racemic methylphenidate, and methylphenidate is excreted into breast milk. Refer to Methylphenidate monograph for additional information.

Contraindications Hypersensitivity to dexmethylphenidate, methylphenidate, or any component; glaucoma; motor tics; Tourette's syndrome (diagnosis or family history); patients with marked agitation, tension, and anxiety; use with or within 14 days following MAO inhibitor therapy (hypertensive crisis may occur)

Warnings Serious cardiovascular events including sudden death may occur in patients with pre-existing structural cardiac abnormalities or other serious heart problems. Sudden death has been reported in children and adolescents; sudden death, stroke, and MI have been reported in adults. Avoid the use of CNS stimulants in patients with known serious structural cardiac abnormalities, cardiomyopathy, serious heart rhythm abnormalities, coronary artery disease, or other serious cardiac problems that could place patients at an increased risk to the sympathomimetic effects of a stimulant drug. Patients should be carefully evaluated for cardiac disease prior to initiation of therapy (see Monitoring Parameters). The American Heart Association recommends that all children diagnosed with ADHD who may be candidates for medication, such as dexmethylphenidate, should have a thorough cardiovascular assessment prior to initiation of therapy. This assessment should include a combination of medical history, family history, and physical examination focusing on cardiovascular disease risk factors. An ECG is not mandatory but should be considered. **Note:** ECG abnormalities and 4 cases of sudden cardiac death have been reported in children receiving clonidine with methylphenidate; this problem may potentially occur with dexmethylphenidate; consider ECG monitoring and reduction of dexmethylphenidate dose when used concurrently with clonidine.

Stimulant medications may increase blood pressure (average increase 2-4 mm Hg) and heart rate (average increase 3-6 bpm); some patients may experience greater increases; use stimulant medications with caution in patients with hypertension and other cardiovascular conditions that may be exacerbated by increases in blood pressure or heart rate. Psychiatric adverse events may occur. Stimulants may exacerbate symptoms of behavior disturbance and thought disorder in patients with pre-existing psychosis. New-onset psychosis or mania may occur with stimulant use. May induce mixed/manic episode in patients with bipolar disorder. May be associated with aggressive behavior or hostility (monitor for development or worsening of these behaviors).

Safety and efficacy have not been established in children <6 years of age (use is **not** recommended in children <6 years of age). Long-term effects in pediatric patients have not been determined. Use of stimulants in children has been associated with growth suppression (monitor growth; treatment interruption may be needed). Appetite suppression may occur; monitor weight during therapy, particularly in children. Stimulants may lower seizure threshold leading to new onset or breakthrough seizure activity (use with caution in patients with a history of seizure disorder). Visual disturbances (difficulty in accommodation and blurred vision) have been reported.

CNS stimulants possess a high potential for abuse **[U.S. Boxed Warning]**; misuse may cause sudden death and serious cardiovascular adverse events; prolonged administration may lead to drug dependence; abrupt discontinuation following high doses or for prolonged periods may result in symptoms of withdrawal; avoid abrupt discontinuation in patients who have received dexmethylphenidate for prolonged periods; use with caution in patients with history of ethanol or drug abuse. Do not use for severe depression or normal fatigue states.

Precautions Use with caution in patients with heart failure, recent MI, hyperthyroidism, seizures, acute stress reactions, emotional instability. Hematological monitoring is advised with long term use (see Monitoring Parameters). Stimulants like dexmethylphenidate have a demonstrated value as part of a comprehensive treatment program for ADHD.

Adverse Reactions Note: See Methylphenidate for adverse reactions observed with other methylphenidate products.

Cardiovascular: Hypertension; serious cardiovascular events, including sudden death in patients with pre-existing structural cardiac abnormalities or other serious heart problems (see Warnings); tachycardia

Central nervous system: Anxiety, depression, dizziness, feeling jittery, fever, headache, insomnia, irritability, mood swings, motor tics, restlessness, vocal tics

Dermatologic: Pruritus

Endocrine & metabolic: Potential growth suppression, weight loss

Gastrointestinal: Abdominal pain, anorexia, appetite decreased, dyspepsia, nausea, pharyngolaryngeal pain, vomiting, xerostomia

Ocular: Accommodation difficulties, blurred vision

Respiratory: Nasal congestion

<1%, postmarketing, and/or case reports (limited to important or life-threatening): Hallucinations, seizures

Drug Interactions

Avoid Concomitant Use

Avoid concomitant use of Dexmethylphenidate with any of the following: Iobenguane I 123; MAO Inhibitors

Increased Effect/Toxicity

Dexmethylphenidate may increase the levels/effects of: Phenytoin; Sympathomimetics; Tricyclic Antidepressants

The levels/effects of Dexmethylphenidate may be increased by: Atomoxetine; Cannabinoids; MAO Inhibitors

Decreased Effect

Dexmethylphenidate may decrease the levels/effects of: Iobenguane I 123

Food Interactions

Immediate release tablets: A high-fat meal delays the time to peak concentration, but not the extent of absorption

Extended release capsules: Effect of food has not been studied. Based on studies of the same type of extended release formulation of racemic methylphenidate, a high-fat meal may decrease the time to peak concentration, but not the extent of absorption. Administration with applesauce should not affect the plasma concentration-time profile.

Stability

Immediate release tablets: Store at controlled room temperature at 25°C (77°F); excursions permitted to 15°C to 30°C (59°F to 86°F). Protect from light and moisture.

Extended release capsule: Store at controlled room temperature at 25°C (77°F); excursions permitted to 15°C to 30°C (59°F to 86°F). Dispense in tight container.

Mechanism of Action Dexmethylphenidate is the more active, *d-threo*-enantiomer, of racemic methylphenidate. It is a CNS stimulant; blocks the reuptake of norepinephrine and dopamine into presynaptic neurons, thus increasing the concentrations of these neurotransmitters in the extraneuronal space. It also inhibits monoamine oxidase which is responsible for the breakdown of neurotransmitters norepinephrine and dopamine.

Pharmacodynamics

Onset of action: Rapid, within 1-2 hours of an effective dose

Maximum effect: Variable

Duration: Immediate release: 3-5 hours; extended release: Capsule: 8-12 hours

Pharmacokinetics (Adult data unless noted)

Absorption: Oral: Tablet: Rapid; Extended release capsule: Bimodal (with 2 peak concentrations ~4 hours apart)

Distribution: V_d: Adults: 2.65 ± 1.11 L/kg

Protein binding: Unknown; racemic methylphenidate: 12% to 15%

Metabolism: Via de-esterification to inactive metabolite, *d*-α-phenyl-piperidine acetate (*d*-ritalinic acid)

Bioavailability: 22% to 25%

Half-life: Immediate release:
Children: Mean: 2-3 hours
Adults: Mean: 2-4.5 hours; **Note:** A few subjects displayed a half-life between 5-7 hours

Time to peak serum concentration: Fasting:
Immediate release tablet: 1-1.5 hours
Extended release capsule: First peak: 1.5 hours (range: 1-4 hours); second peak: 6.5 hours (range: 4.5-7 hours)

Elimination: 90% of dose is eliminated in the urine, primarily as inactive metabolite (ie, 80% of dose is eliminated in urine as ritalinic acid). **Note:** 0.5% of an I.V. dose was found in the urine as unchanged drug.

Usual Dosage Treatment of ADHD: Oral:

Patients not currently taking methylphenidate:
Children ≥6 years:
Immediate release: Initial: 2.5 mg twice daily; dosage may be adjusted in increments of 2.5-5 mg at weekly intervals (maximum dose: 20 mg/day); doses should be taken at least 4 hours apart
Extended release: Initial: 5 mg once daily; dosage may be adjusted in increments of 5 mg/day at weekly intervals (maximum dose: 30 mg/day)
Adults:
Immediate release: Initial: 2.5 mg twice daily; dosage may be adjusted in increments of 2.5-5 mg at weekly intervals (maximum dose: 20 mg/day); doses should be taken at least 4 hours apart
Extended release: Initial: 10 mg once daily; dosage may be adjusted in increments of 10 mg/day at weekly intervals (maximum dose: 40 mg/day)

Conversion to dexmethylphenidate from methyl-phenidate:
Immediate release: Initial: Half the total daily dose of racemic methylphenidate; maximum dexmethylpheni-date dose: Children ≥6 years and Adults: 20 mg/day

Extended release: Initial: Half the total daily dose of racemic methylphenidate; maximum dexmethylpheni-date dose: Children ≥6 years: 30 mg/day; Adults: 40 mg/day

Conversion from dexmethylphenidate immediate release to dexmethylphenidate extended release: When changing from Focalin® tablets to Focalin® XR capsules, patients may be switched to the same daily dose using Focalin® XR; maximum dose: Children ≥6 years: 30 mg/day; Adults: 40 mg/day

Dose reductions and discontinuation: Children ≥6 years and Adults: Reduce dose or discontinue in patients with paradoxical aggravation of symptoms. Discontinue if no improvement is seen after one month of treatment.

Dosage adjustment/comments in renal impairment: No information is available; **Note:** Since very little unchanged drug is eliminated in the urine, dosage adjustment in renal impairment is not expected to be required.

Dosage adjustment/comments in hepatic impairment: No information is available; use with caution

Administration

Capsule: Administer once daily in the morning. Do not crush, chew, or divide capsule; swallow whole. Capsule may be opened and contents sprinkled over a spoonful of applesauce; consume immediately and entirely; do not store for future use.

Tablet: Twice daily dosing should be administered at least 4 hours apart; may be taken with or without food.

Monitoring Parameters Evaluate patients for cardiac disease prior to initiation of therapy with thorough medical history, family history, and physical exam; consider ECG (see Warnings); perform ECG and echocardiogram if findings suggest cardiac disease; promptly conduct cardiac evaluation in patients who develop chest pain, unexplained syncope, or any other symptom of cardiac disease during treatment. Monitor CBC with differential, platelet count, blood pressure, heart rate, height, weight, sleep, appetite, abnormal movements, growth in children. Patients should be re-evaluated at appropriate intervals to assess continued need of the medication. Observe for signs/symptoms of aggression or hostility, or depression.

Patient Information Read the patient Medication Guide that you receive with each prescription and refill of dexmethylphenidate. Serious cardiac effects or psychiatric adverse effects may occur; notify your physician of any heart problems, high blood pressure, or psychiatric conditions before starting therapy. May reduce the growth rate in children and has been associated with worsening of aggressive behavior; notify your physician if your child displays aggression or hostility; make sure your physician monitors your child's weight and height. Avoid caffeine and the herbal medicine St John's wort. May be habit-forming; avoid abrupt discontinuation after prolonged use. May cause dizziness or drowsiness and impair ability to perform activities requiring mental alertness or physical coordination. Notify physician if blurred vision occurs. Report the use of other medications and herbal or natural products to your physician and pharmacist.

Additional Information Treatment with dexmethylpheni-date should include "drug holidays" or periodic discontin-uation in order to assess the patient's requirements, decrease tolerance, and limit suppression of linear growth and weight. Medications used to treat ADHD should be part of a total treatment program that may include other components such as psychological, educational, and social measures. Long-term use of the immediate release tablets (ie, >6 weeks) and extended release capsules (>7 weeks) has not been studied; long-term usefulness should be periodically re-evaluated for the individual patient.

Focalin® XR capsules use a bimodal release where $1/2$ the dose is provided in immediate release beads and $1/2$ the dose is provided in delayed release beads. A single, once-daily dose of a capsule provides the same amount of dexmethylphenidate as two tablets given 4 hours apart. **Note:** The modified release properties of Focalin® XR capsules are pH dependent; thus, concomitant administration of antacids or acid suppressants might alter the release of dexmethylphenidate.

Dosage Forms Excipient information presented when available (limited, particularly for generics); consult specific product labeling.

Capsule, extended release:
Focalin® XR: 5 mg, 10 mg, 15 mg, 20 mg, 30 mg [bimodal release]

Tablet, as hydrochloride: 2.5 mg, 5 mg, 10 mg
Focalin®: 2.5 mg, 5 mg; 10 mg [dye free]

References

American Academy of Pediatrics/American Heart Association Clarification of Statement on Cardiovascular Evaluation and Monitoring of Children and Adolescents With Heart Disease Receiving Medications for ADHD; available at: http://americanheart.mediaroon.com/index.-php?s=43&item=422.

American Academy of Pediatrics, "Clinical Practice Guideline: Treatment of the School-Aged Child With Attention-Deficit/Hyperactivity Disorder," *Pediatrics*, 2001, 108(4):1033-44.

Gelperin K, "Cardiovascular Risk With Drug Treatments of ADHD," available at: http://www.fda.gov/ohrms/dockets/ac/06/slides/2006-4210s-index.htm. Accessed May 25, 2006.

Gelperin K, "Psychiatric Adverse Events With Drug Treatments of ADHD," available at: http://www.fda.gov/ohrms/dockets/ac/06/slides/2006-4210s-index.htm. Accessed May 25, 2006.

Greenhill LL, Muniz R, Ball RR, et al, "Efficacy and Safety of Dexmethylphenidate Extended-Release Capsules in Children With Attention-Deficit/Hyperactivity Disorder," *J Am Acad Child Adolesc Psychiatry*, 2006, 45(7):817-23.

"National Institute of Mental Health Multimodal Treatment Study of ADHD Follow-Up: Changes in Effectiveness and Growth After the End of Treatment," *Pediatrics*, 2004, 113(4):762-9.

Nissen SE, "ADHD Drugs and Cardiovascular Risk," *New Eng J Med*, 2006, 354(14):1445-8.

Poulton A, "Growth on Stimulant Medication; Clarifying the Confusion: A Review," *Arch Dis Child*, 2005, 00(8):801-6.

Prince JB, "Pharmacotherapy of Attention-Deficit Hyperactivity Disorder in Children and Adolescents: Update on New Stimulant Preparations, Atomoxetine, and Novel Treatments," *Child Adolesc Psych Clin N Am*, 2006, 15(1):13-50.

Robinson DM and Keating GM, "Dexmethylphenidate Extended Release: In Attention-Deficit Hyperactivity Disorder," *Drugs*, 2006, 66(5):661-8.

Silva RR, Muniz R, Pestreich L, et al, "Dexmethylphenidate Extended-Release Capsules in Children With Attention-Deficit/Hyperactivity Disorder," *J Am Acad Child Adolesc Psychiatry*, 2008, 47(2):199-208.

Silva RR, Muniz R, Pestreich L, et al, "Efficacy and Duration of Effect of Extended-Release Dexmethylphenidate Versus Placebo in Schoolchildren With Attention-Deficit/Hyperactivity Disorder," *J Child Adolesc Psychopharmacol*, 2006, 16(3):239-51.

Vetter VL, Elia J, Erickson C, et al, "Cardiovascular Monitoring of Children and Adolescents With Heart Disease Receiving Stimulant Drugs: A Scientific Statement From the American Heart Association Council on Cardiovascular Disease in the Young Congenital Cardiac Defects Committee and the Council on Cardiovascular Nursing," *Circulation*, 2008, 117(18):2407-23.

Wilens TE, "Mechanism of Action of Agents Used in Attention-deficit Hyperactivity Disorder," *J Clin Psychiatry*, 2006, 67(suppl 8):32-8.

◆ **Dexmethylphenidate Hydrochloride** *see* Dexmethylphenidate *on page 410*

◆ **DexPak® 6 Day TaperPak®** *see* Dexamethasone *on page 406*

◆ **DexPak® 10 Day TaperPak®** *see* Dexamethasone *on page 406*

◆ **DexPak® 13 Day TaperPak®** *see* Dexamethasone *on page 406*

◆ **DexPak® TaperPak® [DSC]** *see* Dexamethasone *on page 406*

Dexrazoxane (deks ray ZOKS ane)

Medication Safety Issues
Sound-alike/look-alike issues:
Zinecard® may be confused with Gemzar®

Related Information
Compatibility of Chemotherapy and Related Supportive Care Medications *on page 1580*
Emetogenic Potential of Antineoplastic Agents *on page 1579*

U.S. Brand Names Totect®; Zinecard®

Canadian Brand Names Zinecard®

Therapeutic Category Antidote; Cardioprotective Agent; Chelating Agent

Generic Available Yes

Use
Zinecard®: Reduction of anthracycline-induced (ie, doxorubicin-induced) cardiotoxicity in women with metastatic breast cancer (FDA approved in adults). Not generally recommended for use with the initiation of anthracycline therapy. Most dexrazoxane studies have been done in women with metastatic breast cancer who had received a cumulative doxorubicin dose of 300 mg/m^2.

Totect®: Treatment of anthracycline extravasation (FDA approved in adults)

Pregnancy Risk Factor C (Zinecard®) / D (Totect®)

Pregnancy Considerations Embryotoxicity and teratogenicity were observed in animal studies; maternal toxicity was also noted. There are no adequate and well-controlled studies in pregnant women. Avoid use in pregnant women unless the potential benefit justifies the potential risk to the fetus.

Lactation Excretion in breast milk unknown/not recommended

Breast-Feeding Considerations Due to the potential for serious adverse reactions in the nursing infant, discontinue nursing during dexrazoxane therapy.

Contraindications Hypersensitivity to dexrazoxane or any component; should only be used with chemotherapy regimens containing an anthracycline

Warnings Due to limited experience, the possibility of dexrazoxane interference with antineoplastic efficacy may exist; use Zinecard® only in those patients who have received a cumulative doxorubicin dose of 300 mg/m^2 and are continuing with doxorubicin therapy. Dose-limiting toxicity is myelosuppression; dexrazoxane may add to the myelosuppression caused by chemotherapeutic agents. Hazardous agent; use appropriate precautions for handling and disposal (see prescribing information). Secondary malignancies have been reported with razoxane use [racemic mixture of which dexrazoxane is the S(+) enantiomer]

Precautions Do not give doxorubicin prior to dexrazoxane administration. Doxorubicin should be given within 30 minutes after the beginning of a dexrazoxane infusion. For I.V. administration; not for local infiltration into extravasation site. Do not use dimethylsulfoxide (DMSO) in patients receiving dexrazoxane for anthracycline-induced extravasation. Use with caution in patients with renal impairment; dosage adjustment required for Cl$_{cr}$ <40 mL/minute.

Adverse Reactions
Cardiovascular: Peripheral edema

Central nervous system: Depression, dizziness, fatigue, headache, insomnia, low grade fever, malaise

Dermatologic: Alopecia (possibly dose-related), streaking/erythema

Endocrine & metabolic: Calcium total increased, hyponatremia, serum iron and serum triglyceride levels increased, serum zinc decreased

Gastrointestinal: Abdominal pain, anorexia, constipation, diarrhea, mild nausea and vomiting, serum amylase levels increased, stomatitis

Hematologic: Anemia, **dose-limiting, additive myelosuppression** (leukopenia, neutropenia, and thrombocytopenia at high doses >1000 mg/m^2), hemorrhage, neutropenic fever

Hepatic: Alkaline phosphatase increased, bilirubin increased, LDH increased, transient elevation of serum transaminase levels

Local: Discomfort, pain at injection site (13%), phlebitis (6% to 8%)

Neuromuscular & skeletal: Neurotoxicity

Renal: Creatinine increased

Respiratory: Cough, dyspnea, pneumonia

Miscellaneous: Infection, sepsis

Drug Interactions

Avoid Concomitant Use

Avoid concomitant use of Dexrazoxane with any of the following: Dimethyl Sulfoxide

Increased Effect/Toxicity There are no known significant interactions involving an increase in effect.

Decreased Effect

The levels/effects of Dexrazoxane may be decreased by: Dimethyl Sulfoxide

Stability Store vials at room temperature; protect from light. Reconstituted and diluted Zinecard® solution is stable for 6 hours at room temperature or under refrigeration. Dexrazoxane degrades rapidly at pH >7. Reconstituted and diluted Totect® infusion solution in NS is stable for 4 hours (begin infusion within 2 hours of preparation) at temperatures <25°C (<77°F).

Mechanism of Action Dexrazoxane is a cyclic derivative of ethylenediaminetetraacetic acid (EDTA) that rapidly penetrates the myocardial cell membrane. It binds intracellular iron and prevents generation of oxygen free radicals by anthracyclines. Dexrazoxane is hydrolyzed intracellularly to an open-ring chelating agent which is responsible for chelating heavy metals and preventing formation of superhydroxide free radicals believed to be responsible for anthracycline-induced cardiomyopathy. Dexrazoxane may also have antitumor activity and have synergistic activity with certain cytotoxic agents. In the management of anthracycline-induced extravasation, dexrazoxane may act by reversibly inhibiting topoisomerase II, protecting tissue from anthracycline cytotoxicity, thereby decreasing tissue damage.

Pharmacokinetics (Adult data unless noted)

Distribution: Distributes to heart, liver, and kidneys

V_d:

Children: 0.96 L/kg

Adults: 22-25 L/m^2

Protein binding: Insignificant

Metabolism: Hydrolyzed by dihydropyrimidine aminohydrolase and dihydrocrotase

Half-life: Biphasic: Adults:

Distribution half-life: 8-21 minutes

Elimination half-life: 2-3 hours

Elimination: 40% to 60% of dose excreted renally within 24 hours

Usual Dosage I.V.:

Prevention of anthracycline cardiomyopathy: **Note:** Cardiac monitoring should continue during dexrazoxane therapy; anthracycline/dexrazoxane should be discontinued in patients who develop a decline in LVEF or clinical CHF.

Children: 10:1 dose ratio with doxorubicin for acute lymphoblastic leukemia (example: 300 mg/m^2 dexrazoxane: 30 mg/m^2 doxorubicin) was used in patients with high-risk acute lymphoblastic leukemia (see Moghrabi, 2007)

Adults: 10:1 ratio with doxorubicin (example: 500 mg/m^2 dexrazoxane; 50 mg/m^2 doxorubicin); administer 30 minutes before doxorubicin

Treatment of extravasation: Adolescents ≥18 years and Adults: 1000 mg/m^2/dose on days 1 and 2 (maximum dose: 2000 mg), followed by 500 mg/m^2/dose on day 3 (maximum dose: 1000 mg); begin the first infusion as soon as possible, within 6 hours of extravasation. Subsequent doses on days 2 and 3 should start at the same hour as on the first day.

Dosage adjustment in renal impairment: Adults: Moderate-to-severe (Cl_{cr}<40 mL/minute):

Prevention of cardiomyopathy: Reduce dose by 50%, using a 5:1 dexrazoxane:doxorubicin ratio (Example: 250 mg/m^2 dexrazoxane: 50 mg/m^2 doxorubicin)

Anthracycline-induced extravasation: Reduce dose by 50%

Dosage adjustment in hepatic impairment:

Prevention of cardiomyopathy: Since doxorubicin dosage is reduced in hepatic impairment, a proportional reduction in dexrazoxane dosage is recommended (maintain a 10:1 ratio of dexrazoxane:doxorubicin).

Anthracycline-induced extravasation: Use has not been evaluated in patients with hepatic impairment

Administration I.V.:

Prevention of anthracycline-induced cardiotoxicity: Reconstitute Zinecard® with 0.167 Molar sodium lactate injection to a concentration of 10 mg/mL. Administer slow I.V. push or further dilute in NS or D$_5$W to a final concentration of 1.3-5 mg/mL and give as a rapid I.V. infusion over 15-30 minutes

Treatment of anthracycline extravasation: **Note:** Not for local infiltration into extravasation site. Reconstitute Totect® with 0.167 Molar solution lactate injection to a concentration of 10 mg/mL. The mixed dose volume should be further diluted in 1 liter NS. Do not mix or administer with any other drug during infusion. Infuse over 1-2 hours in a large caliber vein in an area other than the one affected by extravasation. Infusion solution should be at room temperature prior to administration.

Monitoring Parameters CBC with differential and platelet count; cardiac function tests; serum triglycerides, iron, calcium, and zinc levels; liver function tests, serum creatinine; monitor extravasation site

Patient Information Women of childbearing potential should be advised that Totect® may cause fetal harm; consult prescriber for appropriate contraceptive measures. Notify physician of bleeding or bruising problems.

Nursing Implications To ensure optimal cardioprotectant effect, do not allow chemotherapy to be delayed following completion of dexrazoxane. To ensure optimal management of anthracycline-induced extravasation, cooling procedures (eg, ice packs), if used, should be removed from the area at least 15 minutes before Totect™ administration to allow sufficient blood flow to the area of extravasation. Protective gloves should be used during the handling of dexrazoxane injection. If contact occurs with skin or mucous membranes, immediately and thoroughly wash the affected area with water. Use appropriate procedures for handling and disposing of cytotoxic drugs.

Dosage Forms Excipient information presented when available (limited, particularly for generics); consult specific product labeling.

Injection, powder for reconstitution: 250 mg, 500 mg

Totect®: 500 mg [provided with 0.167 Molar sodium lactate injection, USP]

Zinecard®: 250 mg, 500 mg [provided with 0.167 Molar sodium lactate injection, USP]

References

Hensley ML, Hagerty KL, Kewalramani T, et al, "American Society of Clinical Oncology 2008 Clinical Practice Guideline Update: Use of Chemotherapy and Radiation Therapy Protectants," *J Clin Oncol*, 2009, 27(1):127-45.

Holcenberg JS, Tutsch KD, Earhart RH, et al, "Phase I Study of ICRF-187 in Pediatric Cancer Patients and Comparison of Its Pharmaco-kinetics in Children and Adults," *Cancer Treat Rep*, 1986, 70(6):703-9.

Lipshultz SE, Rifai N, Dalton VM, et al, "The Effect of Dexrazoxane on Myocardial Injury in Doxorubicin-Treated Children With Acute Lymphoblastic Leukemia," *N Engl J Med*, 2004, 351(2):145-53.

Moghrabi A, Levy DE, Asselin B, et al, "Results of the Dana-Farber Cancer Institute ALL Consortium Protocol 95-01 for Children With Acute Lymphoblastic Leukemia," *Blood*, 2007, 109(3):896-904.

Sehested M, Holm B, and Jensen PB, "Dexrazoxane for Protection Against Cardiotoxic Effects of Anthracyclines," *J Clin Oncol*, 1996, 14:2884.

Swain SM, Whaley FS, Gerber MC, et al, "Cardioprotection With Dexrazoxane for Doxorubicin-Containing Therapy in Advanced Breast Cancer," *J Clin Oncol*, 1997, 15:1318-32.

Swain SM, Whaley FS, Gerber MC, et al, "Delayed Administration of Dexrazoxane Provides Cardioprotection for Patients With Advanced Breast Cancer Treated With Doxorubicin-Containing Therapy," *J Clin Oncol*, 1997, 15:1333-40.

Wexler LH, Andrich MP, Venzon D, et al, "Randomized Trial of the Cardioprotective Agent ICRF-187 in Pediatric Sarcoma Patients Treated With Doxorubicin," *J Clin Oncol*, 1996, 14:362-72.

Dextran (DEKS tran)

Medication Safety Issues
Sound-alike/look-alike issues:
Dextran may be confused with Dexatrim®, Dexedrine®

U.S. Brand Names LMD®

Therapeutic Category Plasma Volume Expander

Generic Available No

Use
Fluid replacement and blood volume expander used in the treatment of hypovolemia, shock, or near shock states; dextran 40 is also indicated for use as a priming fluid in pump oxygenators during extracorporeal circulation and for venous thrombosis and pulmonary embolism prophylaxis in patients undergoing surgery associated with a high incidence of thromboembolic complications (eg, hip surgery)

Pregnancy Risk Factor C

Lactation Excretion in breast milk unknown

Contraindications
Hypersensitivity to dextrans or any component; severe CHF, renal failure, severe thrombocytopenia; hypervolemia; hypofibrinogenemia; severe bleeding disorders

Warnings
Use with caution in patients with CHF, pulmonary edema, renal insufficiency, thrombocytopenia, or active hemorrhage; watch for anaphylactoid reactions, have epinephrine and diphenhydramine at bedside

Precautions
Use with caution in patients with extreme dehydration (renal failure may occur) and in patients with chronic liver disease

Adverse Reactions
Cardiovascular: Hypotension
Central nervous system: Fever
Dermatologic: Urticaria
Gastrointestinal: Nausea, vomiting
Hematologic: Prolongation of bleeding time with higher doses (may interfere with platelet function)
Neuromuscular & skeletal: Arthralgia
Respiratory: Wheezing, pulmonary edema with high doses, tightness of chest, dyspnea, nasal congestion
Miscellaneous: Anaphylaxis

Drug Interactions
Avoid Concomitant Use
Avoid concomitant use of Dextran with any of the following: Abciximab
Increased Effect/Toxicity
Dextran may increase the levels/effects of: Abciximab
Decreased Effect
There are no known significant interactions involving a decrease in effect.

Stability
Store at room temperature; do not freeze; do not use if crystallization has occurred; discard partially used containers

Mechanism of Action
Produces plasma volume expansion due to high colloidal osmotic effect (similar to albumin); draws interstitial fluid into the intravascular space; dextran 40 may also increase blood flow in microcirculation

Pharmacodynamics
Maximum effect on plasma volume:
Dextran 40: Within several minutes
Dextran 70 and dextran 75: ~1 hour

Pharmacokinetics (Adult data unless noted)
Metabolism: Molecules with molecular weight ≥50,000 are metabolized to glucose
Elimination:
Molecules with molecular weight ≤15,000: Rapidly eliminated in the kidney
Dextran 40: ~70% excreted in urine (unchanged) within 24 hours
Dextran 70 & 75: ~50% excreted in urine within 24 hours

Usual Dosage
I.V. (dose and infusion rate are dependent upon the patient's fluid status and must be individualized):

Volume expansion/shock:
Children: Total dose should not be >20 mL/kg during first 24 hours and not >10 mL/kg/day thereafter; do not treat for >5 days
Adults: 500-1000 mL at rate of 20-40 mL/minute
Maximum daily dose: First 24 hours: 20 mL/kg and 10 mL/kg/day thereafter; therapy should not continue beyond 5 days

Administration
Parenteral: I.V. infusion only; usual maximum infusion rate (adults): 4 mL/minute; maximum infusion rate in emergency situations (adults): 20-40 mL/minute

Monitoring Parameters
Vital signs, signs of allergic/anaphylactoid reaction especially for 30 minutes after starting infusions; signs of circulatory overload (ie, heart rate, blood pressure, central venous pressure, hematocrit), urine output; urine specific gravity; platelets

Test Interactions
Falsely elevated serum glucose when determined by methods that use high concentrations of acid (eg, sulfuric acid, acetic acid); may interfere with bilirubin assays that use alcohol and total protein assays using biuret reagents; dextran 70 may produce erythrocyte aggregation and interfere with blood typing and cross matching of blood

Nursing Implications
Be prepared to treat anaphylaxis with epinephrine, antihistamines, supportive therapy, and alternative agents to dextran to maintain circulation; do not administer if cloudy or if solution contains dextran flakes; discontinue dextran if urine specific gravity is low, if oliguria or anuria occur, or if there is a rapid acute rise in central venous pressure or other signs of circulatory overload

Additional Information
Dextran in sodium chloride 0.9% contains sodium chloride 154 mEq/L

Dosage Forms
Excipient information presented when available (limited, particularly for generics); consult specific product labeling.
Infusion [premixed in D$_5$W; low molecular weight]:
LMD®: 10% Dextran 40 (500 mL)
Infusion [premixed in NS; low molecular weight]:
LMD®: 10% Dextran (500 mL)

◆ **Dextran 40** see Dextran on page 415

◆ **Dextran 70** see Dextran on page 415

◆ **Dextran, High Molecular Weight** see Dextran on page 415

◆ **Dextran, Low Molecular Weight** see Dextran on page 415

Dextroamphetamine (deks troe am FET a meen)

Medication Safety Issues
Sound-alike/look-alike issues:
Dexedrine® may be confused with dextran, Excedrin®
Dextroamphetamine may be confused with dexamethasone

Beers Criteria medication: This drug may be inappropriate for use in geriatric patients (high severity risk).

Related Information
Laboratory Detection of Drugs in Urine *on page 1706*

U.S. Brand Names Dexedrine®; DextroStat®; Liquadd™ [DSC]

Canadian Brand Names Dexedrine®

Therapeutic Category Amphetamine; Anorexiant; Central Nervous System Stimulant

Generic Available Yes: Excludes oral suspension

Use Adjunct in treatment of attention-deficit/hyperactivity disorder (ADHD) in children, narcolepsy, exogenous obesity

Restrictions C-II

Medication Guide An FDA-approved patient medication guide, which is available with the product information and at http://www.fda.gov/downloads/Drugs/DrugSafety/ucm088583.pdf, must be dispensed with this medication for each new outpatient prescription and refill.

Pregnancy Risk Factor C

Pregnancy Considerations Teratogenic and embryocidal effects have been observed in animal studies. There are no adequate and well-controlled studies in pregnant women. Use only if potential benefit justifies the potential risk to the fetus.

Lactation Enters breast milk/not recommended

Contraindications Hypersensitivity or idiosyncrasy to dextroamphetamine, other sympathomimetic amines, or any component (see Warnings); advanced arteriosclerosis, symptomatic cardiovascular disease, moderate to severe hypertension, hyperthyroidism, glaucoma, agitated states, patients with a history of drug abuse; concurrent use or use within 14 days of MAO inhibitors (hypertensive crisis may occur)

Warnings Serious cardiovascular events including sudden death may occur in patients with pre-existing structural cardiac abnormalities or other serious heart problems. Sudden death has been reported in children and adolescents; sudden death, stroke, and MI have been reported in adults. Avoid the use of amphetamines in patients with known serious structural cardiac abnormalities, cardiomyopathy, serious heart rhythm abnormalities, coronary artery disease, or other serious cardiac problems that could place patients at an increased risk to the sympathomimetic effects of amphetamines. Patients should be carefully evaluated for cardiac disease prior to initiation of therapy. **Note:** The American Heart Association recommends that all children diagnosed with ADHD who may be candidates for medication, such as dextroamphetamine, should have a thorough cardiovascular assessment prior to initiation of therapy. This assessment should include a combination of medical history, family history, and physical examination focusing on cardiovascular disease risk factors. An ECG is not mandatory but should be considered.

Stimulant medications may increase blood pressure (average increase 2-4 mm Hg) and heart rate (average increase 3-6 bpm); some patients may experience greater increases; use stimulant medications with caution in patients with hypertension and other cardiovascular conditions that may be exacerbated by increases in blood pressure or heart rate; use is contraindicated in patients with moderate to severe hypertension. Psychiatric adverse events may occur. Stimulants may exacerbate symptoms of behavior disturbance and thought disorder in patients with pre-existing psychosis. New-onset psychosis or mania may occur with stimulant use. May induce mixed/manic episode in patients with bipolar disorder. May be associated with aggressive behavior or hostility (monitor for development or worsening of these behaviors).

Safety and efficacy have not been established in children <3 years of age; long-term effects in pediatric patients have not been determined. Use of stimulants in children has been associated with growth suppression (monitor growth; treatment interruption may be needed). Appetite suppression may occur; monitor weight during therapy, particularly in children. Stimulants may lower seizure threshold leading to new onset or breakthrough seizure activity (use with caution in patients with a history of seizure disorder). Visual disturbances (difficulty in accommodation and blurred vision) have been reported.

Amphetamines possess a high potential for abuse **[U.S. Boxed Warning]**; misuse may cause sudden death and serious cardiovascular adverse events **[U.S. Boxed Warning]**; use in weight reduction programs only when alternative therapy has been ineffective; prolonged administration may lead to drug dependence; abrupt discontinuation following high doses or for prolonged periods may result in symptoms of withdrawal; avoid abrupt discontinuation in patients who have received amphetamines for prolonged periods; use is contraindicated in patients with history of ethanol or drug abuse. Amphetamines may impair the ability to engage in potentially hazardous activities. May exacerbate motor and phonic tics and Tourette's syndrome.

DextroStat® tablets contain and generic tablets may contain tartrazine which may cause allergic reactions in susceptible individuals. Oral solution contains benzoic acid; benzoic acid (benzoate) is a metabolite of benzyl alcohol; large amounts of benzyl alcohol (≥99 mg/kg/day) have been associated with a potentially fatal toxicity ("gasping syndrome") in neonates; avoid use of dextroamphetamine products containing benzoic acid in neonates; *in vitro* and animal studies have shown that benzoate displaces bilirubin from protein binding sites.

Precautions Prescriptions should be written for the smallest quantity consistent with good patient care to minimize possibility of overdose.

Adverse Reactions
Cardiovascular: Hypertension, tachycardia, palpitations, cardiac arrhythmias; cardiomyopathy with chronic use (case reports); serious cardiovascular events including sudden death in patients with pre-existing structural cardiac abnormalities or other serious heart problems (see Warnings)

Central nervous system: Insomnia, headache, nervousness, dizziness, irritability, aggression, overstimulation, restlessness, euphoria, dyskinesia, dysphoria, depression, exacerbation of phonic and motor tics, Tourette's syndrome, seizures, psychotic episodes (rare with recommended doses); psychiatric adverse effects (see Warnings)

Dermatologic: Rash, urticaria

Endocrine & metabolic: Growth suppression, weight loss, libido changes

Gastrointestinal: Anorexia, nausea, vomiting, diarrhea, abdominal cramps, metallic taste, xerostomia, constipation

Genitourinary: Impotence

Neuromuscular & skeletal: Movement disorders, tremor

Ocular: Mydriasis, difficulty in accommodation, blurred vision

Miscellaneous: Physical and psychologic dependence with long-term use

Drug Interactions

Avoid Concomitant Use
Avoid concomitant use of Dextroamphetamine with any of the following: Iobenguane I 123; MAO Inhibitors

Increased Effect/Toxicity
Dextroamphetamine may increase the levels/effects of: Analgesics (Opioid); Sympathomimetics

The levels/effects of Dextroamphetamine may be increased by: Alkalinizing Agents; Antacids; Atomoxetine; Cannabinoids; Carbonic Anhydrase Inhibitors; MAO Inhibitors; Tricyclic Antidepressants

Decreased Effect
Dextroamphetamine may decrease the levels/effects of: Antihistamines; Ethosuximide; Iobenguane I 123; PHENobarbital; Phenytoin

The levels/effects of Dextroamphetamine may be decreased by: Ammonium Chloride; Antipsychotics; Gastrointestinal Acidifying Agents; Lithium; Methenamine; Peginterferon Alfa-2b

Food Interactions Acidic foods, juices, or vitamin C may decrease GI absorption. Food does not affect the rate or extent of absorption of the sustained release capsules.

Stability Store at controlled room temperature; protect from light; dispense in tightly closed container

Mechanism of Action Amphetamines are noncatecholamine, sympathomimetic amines that promote the release of catecholamines (primarily dopamine and norepinephrine) from their storage sites in the presynaptic nerve terminals, thus increasing the amounts of circulating dopamine and norepinephrine in the cerebral cortex and reticular activating system. A less significant mechanism may include their ability to block the reuptake of catecholamines by competitive inhibition. Amphetamines also weakly inhibit the action of monoamine oxidase. They peripherally increase blood pressure and act as a respiratory stimulant and weak bronchodilator.

Pharmacodynamics Onset of action: Oral: 60-90 minutes

Pharmacokinetics (Adult data unless noted)
Distribution: V_d: Adults: 3.5-4.6 L/kg; distributes into CNS; mean CSF concentrations are 80% of plasma; enters breast milk

Metabolism: Hepatic via CYP monooxygenase and glucuronidation

Half-life: Adults: 12 hours (pH dependent)

Time to peak serum concentration: Oral: Immediate release: 3 hours; sustained release: 8 hours

Elimination: In urine as unchanged drug and inactive metabolites; urinary excretion is pH dependent and is increased with acid urine (low pH)

Usual Dosage Oral: **Note:** Use lowest effective individualized dose; administer first dose as soon as awake

ADHD: Children:

<3 years: Not recommended

3-5 years: Initial: 2.5 mg/day given every morning; increase by 2.5 mg/day at weekly intervals until optimal response is obtained, usual range is 0.1-0.5 mg/kg/dose every morning with maximum of 40 mg/day given in 1-3 divided doses per day

≥6 years: 5 mg once or twice daily; increase in increments of 5 mg/day at weekly intervals until optimal response is reached, usual range is 0.1-0.5 mg/kg/dose every morning (5-20 mg/day) with maximum of 40 mg/day given in 1-3 divided doses per day

Note: Tablets are usually dosed 2-3 times/day with first dose on awakening and additional doses (1 or 2) at intervals of 4-6 hours. Sustained release capsules are usually given 1-2 times/day.

Narcolepsy:

Children 6-12 years: Initial: 5 mg/day, may increase at 5 mg increments at weekly intervals until optimal response is obtained; maximum dose: 60 mg/day

Children >12 and Adults: Initial: 10 mg/day, may increase at 10 mg increments at weekly intervals until optimal response is obtained; maximum dose: 60 mg/day

Exogenous obesity: Children >12 years and Adults: 5-30 mg/day in divided doses of 5-10 mg given 30-60 minutes before meals

Administration Oral: Sustained release preparations should be used for once daily dosing; do not crush or chew sustained release preparations; to avoid insomnia, last daily dose should be administered no less than 6 hours before retiring

Monitoring Parameters Evaluate patients for cardiac disease prior to initiation of therapy with thorough medical history, family history, and physical exam; consider ECG (see Warnings); perform ECG and echocardiogram if findings suggest cardiac disease; promptly conduct cardiac evaluation in patients who develop chest pain, unexplained syncope, or any other symptom of cardiac disease during treatment. Monitor CNS activity, blood pressure, heart rate, height, weight, sleep, appetite, abnormal movements, growth in children. Patients should be re-evaluated at appropriate intervals to assess continued need of the medication. Observe for signs/symptoms of aggression or hostility, or depression.

Test Interactions Amphetamines may interfere with urinary steroid measurements; may cause significant increase in plasma corticosteroid levels

Patient Information Read the patient Medication Guide that you receive with each prescription and refill of dextroamphetamine. Serious cardiac effects or psychiatric adverse effects may occur; notify your physician of any heart problems, high blood pressure, or psychiatric conditions before starting therapy. May reduce the growth rate in children and has been associated with worsening of aggressive behavior; notify your physician if your child displays aggression or hostility; make sure your physician monitors your child's weight and height. May impair ability to perform activities requiring mental alertness or physical coordination. May be habit-forming; avoid abrupt discontinuation after prolonged use. Limit caffeine; avoid alcohol and the herbal medicine St. John's wort. May cause dry mouth.

Additional Information Treatment for ADHD should include "drug holiday" or periodic discontinuation in order to assess the patient's requirements, decrease tolerance, and limit suppression of linear growth and weight. Medications used to treat ADHD should be part of a total treatment program that may include other components such as psychological, educational, and social measures. Sustained release capsule (Dexedrine® Spansule®) is formulated to release an initial dose promptly with the remaining medication gradually released over a prolonged time.

Dosage Forms Excipient information presented when available (limited, particularly for generics); consult specific product labeling. [DSC] = Discontinued product

Capsule, extended release, as sulfate: 5 mg, 10 mg, 15 mg

Capsule, sustained release, as sulfate:

Dexedrine® Spansule®: 5 mg, 10 mg, 15 mg

Tablet, as sulfate: 5 mg, 10 mg

DextroStat®: 5 mg, 10 mg [contains tartrazine]

Solution, oral, as sulfate:

Liquadd™: 5 mg/5 mL (480 mL) [contains benzoic acid; bubblegum flavor] [DSC]

◀ ## References

American Academy of Pediatrics/American Heart Association Clarification of Statement on Cardiovascular Evaluation and Monitoring of Children and Adolescents With Heart Disease Receiving Medications for ADHD; available at: http://americanheart.mediaroon.com/index.php?s=43&item=422.

American Academy of Pediatrics, "Clinical Practice Guideline: Treatment of the School-Aged Child With Attention-Deficit/Hyperactivity Disorder," *Pediatrics*, 2001, 108(4):1033-44.

Chiang WK, "Amphetamines," *Goldfrank's Toxicologic Emergencies*, 8th ed, Flomenbaum NE, Goldfrank LR, Hoffman RS, eds, New York, NY: The McGraw-Hill Companies, 2006, 1119.

Greenhill LL, Pliszka S, Dulcan MK, et al, "Practice Parameter for the Use of Stimulant Medications in the Treatment of Children, Adolescents, and Adults," *J Am Acad Child Adolesc Psychiatry*, 2002, 41(2 Suppl):26S-49S.

Vetter VL, Elia J, Erickson C, et al, "Cardiovascular Monitoring of Children and Adolescents With Heart Disease Receiving Stimulant Drugs: A Scientific Statement From the American Heart Association Council on Cardiovascular Disease in the Young Congenital Cardiac Defects Committee and the Council on Cardiovascular Nursing," *Circulation*, 2008, 117(18):2407-23.

Westfall TC and Westfall DP, "Adrenergic Agonists and Antagonists," *Goodman and Gilman's the Pharmacological Basis of Therapeutics*, 11th ed, Brunton LL, ed, New York, NY: McGraw-Hill, 2006, 257-8.

Dextroamphetamine and Amphetamine
(deks troe am FET a meen & am FET a meen)

Medication Safety Issues
Sound-alike/look-alike issues:
Adderall® may be confused with Inderal®

Beers Criteria medication: This drug may be inappropriate for use in geriatric patients (high severity risk).

Related Information
Dextroamphetamine *on page 416*
Laboratory Detection of Drugs in Urine *on page 1706*

U.S. Brand Names Adderall XR®; Adderall®

Canadian Brand Names Adderall XR®

Therapeutic Category Amphetamine; Anorexiant; Central Nervous System Stimulant

Generic Available Yes

Use Attention-deficit/hyperactivity disorder (ADHD); narcolepsy

Restrictions C-II

Medication Guide An FDA-approved patient medication guide, which is available with the product information and at http://www.fda.gov/downloads/Drugs/DrugSafety/ucm085819.pdf, must be dispensed with this medication for each new outpatient prescription and refill.

Pregnancy Risk Factor C

Pregnancy Considerations Use during pregnancy may lead to increased risk of premature delivery and low birth weight. Infants may experience symptoms of withdrawal. Teratogenic effects were reported when taken during the 1st trimester.

Lactation Enters breast milk/contraindicated

Contraindications Hypersensitivity or idiosyncrasy to dextroamphetamine, amphetamine, sympathomimetic amines, or any component; advanced arteriosclerosis, moderate to severe hypertension, symptomatic cardiovascular disease, hyperthyroidism, glaucoma, agitated states, history of drug abuse; concurrent use or use within 14 days of MAO inhibitors (hypertensive crisis may occur)

Warnings Serious cardiovascular events including sudden death may occur in patients with pre-existing structural cardiac abnormalities or other serious heart problems. Sudden death has been reported in children and adolescents; sudden death, stroke, and MI have been reported in adults. Avoid the use of amphetamines in patients with known serious structural cardiac abnormalities, cardiomyopathy, serious heart rhythm abnormalities, coronary artery disease, or other serious cardiac problems that could place patients at an increased risk to the sympathomimetic effects of amphetamines. Patients should be carefully evaluated for cardiac disease prior to initiation of therapy. **Note:** The American Heart Association recommends that all children diagnosed with ADHD who may be candidates for medication, such as dextroamphetamine and amphetamine, should have a thorough cardiovascular assessment prior to initiation of therapy. This assessment should include a combination of medical history, family history, and physical examination focusing on cardiovascular disease risk factors. An ECG is not mandatory but should be considered.

Stimulant medications may increase blood pressure (average increase 2-4 mm Hg) and heart rate (average increase 3-6 bpm); some patients may experience greater increases; use stimulant medications with caution in patients with hypertension and other cardiovascular conditions that may be exacerbated by increases in blood pressure or heart rate; use is contraindicated in patients with moderate to severe hypertension. Psychiatric adverse events may occur. Stimulants may exacerbate symptoms of behavior disturbance and thought disorder in patients with pre-existing psychosis. New-onset psychosis or mania may occur with stimulant use. May induce mixed/manic episode in patients with bipolar disorder. May be associated with aggressive behavior or hostility (monitor for development or worsening of these behaviors).

Safety and efficacy have not been established in children <3 years of age (use in children <3 years is **not** recommended); effects of extended-release capsule have not been studied in children 3-5 years old; long-term effects in pediatric patients have not been determined. Use of stimulants in children has been associated with growth suppression (monitor growth; treatment interruption may be needed). Appetite suppression may occur; monitor weight during therapy, particularly in children. Stimulants may lower seizure threshold leading to new onset or breakthrough seizure activity (use with caution in patients with a history of seizure disorder). Visual disturbances (difficulty in accommodation and blurred vision) have been reported.

Amphetamines possess a high potential for abuse **[U.S. Boxed Warning]**; misuse may cause sudden death and serious cardiovascular adverse events **[U.S. Boxed Warning]**; prolonged administration may lead to drug dependence; abrupt discontinuation following high doses or for prolonged periods may result in symptoms of withdrawal; avoid abrupt discontinuation in patients who have received amphetamines for prolonged periods; use is contraindicated in patients with history of ethanol or drug abuse. Amphetamines may impair the ability to engage in potentially hazardous activities. May exacerbate motor and phonic tics and Tourette's syndrome.

Precautions Use with caution in patients with mild hypertension (use is contraindicated in patients with moderate to severe hypertension) and in those receiving other sympathomimetic agents. Prescribe or dispense least amount feasible to minimize chance of overdose.

Adverse Reactions
Cardiovascular system: Hypertension, tachycardia, palpitations, chest pain; cardiomyopathy with chronic use (case reports); serious cardiovascular events including sudden death in patients with pre-existing structural cardiac abnormalities or other serious heart problems (see Warnings)

Central nervous system: Insomnia, headache, nervousness, overstimulation, dizziness, lightheadedness, euphoria, dysphoria, dyskinesia, exacerbation of phonic and motor tics, Tourette's syndrome, seizures, psychotic episodes (rare at recommended doses), emotional lability, depression, anxiety, irritability, somnolence, agitation, fever

Dermatologic: Rash, urticaria, Stevens-Johnson syndrome, toxic epidermal necrolysis

Endocrine and metabolic: Growth suppression, weight loss, libido changes

Gastrointestinal: Anorexia, diarrhea, constipation, xerostomia, unpleasant taste, abdominal pain, dyspepsia, nausea, vomiting

Genitourinary: Impotence

Hepatic: Transaminases elevated

Neuromuscular and skeletal: Tremor, asthenia

Ocular: Mydriasis, difficulty in accommodation, blurred vision

Miscellaneous: Hypersensitivity reactions, angioedema, anaphylaxis, physical and psychological dependence with long-term use

Drug Interactions

Metabolism/Transport Effects Amphetamine: **Inhibits** CYP2D6 (weak)

Avoid Concomitant Use

Avoid concomitant use of Dextroamphetamine and Amphetamine with any of the following: Iobenguane I 123; MAO Inhibitors

Increased Effect/Toxicity

Dextroamphetamine and Amphetamine may increase the levels/effects of: Analgesics (Opioid); Sympathomimetics

The levels/effects of Dextroamphetamine and Amphetamine may be increased by: Alkalinizing Agents; Antacids; Atomoxetine; Cannabinoids; Carbonic Anhydrase Inhibitors; MAO Inhibitors; Tricyclic Antidepressants

Decreased Effect

Dextroamphetamine and Amphetamine may decrease the levels/effects of: Antihistamines; Ethosuximide; Iobenguane I 123; PHENobarbital; Phenytoin

The levels/effects of Dextroamphetamine and Amphetamine may be decreased by: Ammonium Chloride; Antipsychotics; Gastrointestinal Acidifying Agents; Lithium; Methenamine; Peginterferon Alfa-2b

Food Interactions Acidic foods, juices, or vitamin C may decrease oral absorption; extended release capsules: Food does not affect the extent of absorption; a high-fat meal delays the time to peak concentration of d-amphetamine by 2.5 hours and l-amphetamine by 2.1 hours; similar absorption occurs if capsule is opened and contents sprinkled on applesauce versus swallowing intact capsule on an empty stomach

Stability Store at controlled room temperature; dispense in tight, light-resistant container

Mechanism of Action Amphetamines are noncatecholamine, sympathomimetic amines that promote the release of catecholamines (primarily dopamine and norepinephrine) from their storage sites in the presynaptic nerve terminals, thus increasing the amounts of circulating dopamine and norepinephrine in the cerebral cortex and reticular activating system. A less significant mechanism may include their ability to block the reuptake of catecholamines by competitive inhibition. Amphetamines also weakly inhibit the action of monoamine oxidase. They peripherally increase blood pressure and act as a respiratory stimulant and weak bronchodilator.

Pharmacodynamics Oral:

Onset of action: Tablet: 30-60 minutes

Duration: Tablet: 4-6 hours

Pharmacokinetics (Adult data unless noted)

Absorption: Oral: Well-absorbed

Distribution: V_d: Adults: 3.5-4.6 L/kg; concentrates in breast milk (avoid breast-feeding); distributes into CNS, mean CSF concentrations are 80% of plasma

Metabolism: In the liver by cytochrome P450 monooxygenase and glucuronidation; two active metabolites (norephedrine and 4-hydroxyamphetamine) are formed via oxidation

Half-life:

d-amphetamine:

Children 6-12 years: 9 hours

Adolescents 13-17 years: 11 hours

Adults: 10 hours

l-amphetamine:

Children 6-12 years: 11 hours

Adolescents 13-17 years: 13-14 hours

Adults: 13 hours

Time to peak serum concentration:

Tablet (immediate release): 3 hours

Capsule (extended release): 7 hours

Elimination: 70% of a single dose is eliminated within 24 hours; excreted as unchanged amphetamine (30%), benzoic acid, hydroxyamphetamine, hippuric acid, norephedrine and p-hydroxynorephedrine; **Note:** Urinary recovery of amphetamine is highly dependent on urine flow rates and urinary pH; urinary recovery of amphetamine may range from 1% in alkaline urine to 75% in acidic urine

Clearance: Children have a higher clearance (on a mg/kg basis) than adolescents and adults

Usual Dosage Oral: **Note:** Use lowest effective individualized dose; administer first dose as soon as awake

Tablet: **Note:** Use intervals of 4-6 hours between additional doses; tablets are usually doses 1-2 times/day

ADHD:

Children <3 years: Not recommended

Children 3-5 years: Initial: 2.5 mg/day given every morning; increase daily dose by 2.5 mg at weekly intervals until optimal response is obtained; maximum dose: 40 mg/day given in 1-3 divided doses per day

Children ≥6 years: Initial: 5 mg once or twice daily; increase daily dose by 5 mg at weekly intervals until optimal response is obtained; usual maximum dose: 40 mg/day given in 1-3 divided doses per day

Narcolepsy:

Children 6-12 years: Initial: 5 mg/day; increase daily dose by 5 mg at weekly intervals until optimal response is obtained; maximum dose: 60 mg/day given in 1-3 divided doses per day

Children >12 years and Adults: Initial: 10 mg/day; increase daily dose by 10 mg at weekly intervals until optimal response is obtained; maximum dose: 60 mg/day given in 1-3 divided doses per day

Extended release capsule (Adderall XR®):

ADHD:

Children <3 years: Not recommended

Children 3-5 years: Has not been studied

Children ≥6 years: Initial: 10 mg/day given every morning (may initiate with 5 mg/day given every morning if lower dose is clinically needed); increase daily dose by 5 mg or 10 mg at weekly intervals until optimal response is obtained; maximum dose: 30 mg once daily; doses >30 mg/day have not been studied; **Note:** Patients taking divided doses of immediate release tablets may be switched to extended release capsule using the same total daily dose (taken once daily); titrate dose at weekly intervals to achieve optimal response

Adolescents 13-17 years: Initial: 10 mg/day given every morning; may increase to 20 mg/day after one week if symptoms are not controlled; **Note:** Although higher doses (up to 60 mg once daily) have been studied, there is not adequate evidence that doses >20 mg/day provide additional benefit

Adults: Initial: 20 mg/day given every morning; **Note:** Although higher doses (up to 60 mg once daily) have been studied, there is not adequate evidence that doses >20 mg/day provide additional benefit

◄ **Administration** Oral:

Tablet: To avoid insomnia, last daily dose should be administered no less than 6 hours before retiring

Extended release capsule: Avoid afternoon doses to prevent insomnia. Swallow capsule whole; do not chew or divide. May be administered with or without food. May open capsule and sprinkle contents on applesauce; consume applesauce/medication mixture immediately; do not store; do not chew sprinkled beads from capsule

Monitoring Parameters Evaluate patients for cardiac disease prior to initiation of therapy with thorough medical history, family history, and physical exam; consider ECG (see Warnings); perform ECG and echocardiogram if findings suggest cardiac disease; promptly conduct cardiac evaluation in patients who develop chest pain, unexplained syncope, or any other symptom of cardiac disease during treatment. Monitor CNS activity, blood pressure, heart rate, height, weight, sleep, appetite, abnormal movements, growth in children. Patients should be re-evaluated at appropriate intervals to assess continued need of the medication. Observe for signs/symptoms of aggression or hostility, or depression.

Test Interactions Amphetamines may interfere with urinary steroid measurements; may cause significant increase in plasma corticosteroid levels

Patient Information Read the patient Medication Guide that you receive with each prescription and refill of dextroamphetamine and amphetamine. Serious cardiac effects or psychiatric adverse effects may occur; notify your physician of any heart problems, high blood pressure, or psychiatric conditions before starting therapy. May reduce the growth rate in children and has been associated with worsening of aggressive behavior; notify your physician if your child displays aggression or hostility; make sure your physician monitors your child's weight and height. May impair ability to perform activities requiring mental alertness or physical coordination. May be habit-forming; avoid abrupt discontinuation after prolonged use. Limit caffeine; avoid alcohol and the herbal medicine St John's wort. May cause dry mouth.

Additional Information Treatment of ADHD should include "drug holidays" or periodic discontinuation of medication in order to assess the patient's requirments, decrease tolerance, and limit suppression of linear growth and weight. Medications used to treat ADHD should be part of a total treatment program that may include other components such as psychological, educational, and social measures. The combination of equal parts of d, l-amphetamine aspartate, d, l-amphetamine sulfate, dextroamphetamine saccharate and dextroamphetamine sulfate results in a 3:1 ratio of the dextro- and levo-isomers of amphetamine.

The duration of action of Adderall® is longer than methylphenidate; behavioral effects of a single morning dose of Adderall® may last throughout the school day; a single morning dose of Adderall® has been shown in several studies to be as effective as twice daily dosing of methylphenidate for the treatment of ADHD (see Manos, 1999; Pelham, 1999a; Pliszka, 2000).

A recent randomized, double-blind, placebo-controlled crossover trial of Adderall® in children with ADHD demonstrated efficacy rates of 82% based on parent response, 77% based on teacher response, and 59% based on concurrence between parent and teacher response; reported side effects included decreased appetite, stomach aches, insomnia, and headaches; decreased appetite and insomnia were more problematic on the high dose (0.3 mg/kg/dose twice daily) versus the low dose (0.15 mg/kg/dose twice daily); headaches occurred more frequently on the high dose, suggesting a dose-dependency (Ahmann, 2001).

Long term use of Adderall XR® (ie, >3 weeks) has not been studied; long term usefulness should be periodically re-evaluated for the individual patient

Dosage Forms Excipient information presented when available (limited, particularly for generics); consult specific product labeling.

Capsule, extended release:

5 mg [dextroamphetamine sulfate 1.25 mg, dextroamphetamine saccharate 1.25 mg, amphetamine aspartate monohydrate 1.25 mg, amphetamine sulfate 1.25 mg (equivalent to amphetamine base 3.1 mg)]

10 mg [dextroamphetamine sulfate 2.5 mg, dextroamphetamine saccharate 2.5 mg, amphetamine aspartate monohydrate 2.5 mg, amphetamine sulfate 2.5 mg (equivalent to amphetamine base 6.3 mg)]

15 mg [dextroamphetamine sulfate 3.75 mg, dextroamphetamine saccharate 3.75 mg, amphetamine aspartate monohydrate 3.75 mg, amphetamine sulfate 3.75 mg (equivalent to amphetamine base 9.4 mg)]

20 mg [dextroamphetamine sulfate 5 mg, dextroamphetamine saccharate 5 mg, amphetamine aspartate monohydrate 5 mg, amphetamine sulfate 5 mg (equivalent to amphetamine base 12.5 mg)]

25 mg [dextroamphetamine sulfate 6.25 mg, dextroamphetamine saccharate 6.25 mg, amphetamine aspartate monohydrate 6.25 mg, amphetamine sulfate 6.25 mg (equivalent to amphetamine base 15.6 mg)]

30 mg [dextroamphetamine sulfate 7.5 mg, dextroamphetamine saccharate 7.5 mg, amphetamine aspartate monohydrate 7.5 mg, amphetamine sulfate 7.5 mg (equivalent to amphetamine base 18.8 mg)]

Adderall XR®

5 mg [dextroamphetamine sulfate 1.25 mg, dextroamphetamine saccharate 1.25 mg, amphetamine aspartate monohydrate 1.25 mg, amphetamine sulfate 1.25 mg (equivalent to amphetamine base 3.1 mg)]

10 mg [dextroamphetamine sulfate 2.5 mg, dextroamphetamine saccharate 2.5 mg, amphetamine aspartate monohydrate 2.5 mg, amphetamine sulfate 2.5 mg (equivalent to amphetamine base 6.3 mg)]

15 mg [dextroamphetamine sulfate 3.75 mg, dextroamphetamine saccharate 3.75 mg, amphetamine aspartate monohydrate 3.75 mg, amphetamine sulfate 3.75 mg (equivalent to amphetamine base 9.4 mg)]

20 mg [dextroamphetamine sulfate 5 mg, dextroamphetamine saccharate 5 mg, amphetamine aspartate monohydrate 5 mg, amphetamine sulfate 5 mg (equivalent to amphetamine base 12.5 mg)]

25 mg [dextroamphetamine sulfate 6.25 mg, dextroamphetamine saccharate 6.25 mg, amphetamine aspartate monohydrate 6.25 mg, amphetamine sulfate 6.25 mg (equivalent to amphetamine base 15.6 mg)]

30 mg [dextroamphetamine sulfate 7.5 mg, dextroamphetamine saccharate 7.5 mg, amphetamine aspartate monohydrate 7.5 mg, amphetamine sulfate 7.5 mg (equivalent to amphetamine base 18.8 mg)]

Tablet:

5 mg [dextroamphetamine sulfate 1.25 mg, dextroamphetamine saccharate 1.25 mg, amphetamine aspartate monohydrate 1.25 mg, amphetamine sulfate 1.25 mg (equivalent to amphetamine base 3.13 mg)]

7.5 mg [dextroamphetamine 1.875 mg, dextroamphetamine saccharate 1.875 mg, amphetamine aspartate monohydrate 1.875 mg, amphetamine sulfate 1.875 mg (equivalent to amphetamine base 4.7 mg)]

10 mg [dextroamphetamine sulfate 2.5 mg, dextroamphetamine saccharate 2.5 mg, amphetamine aspartate monohydrate 2.5 mg, amphetamine sulfate 2.5 mg (equivalent to amphetamine base 6.3 mg)]

12.5 mg [dextroamphetamine sulfate 3.125 mg, dextro-amphetamine saccharate 3.125 mg, amphetamine aspartate monohydrate 3.125 mg, amphetamine sulfate 3.125 mg (equivalent to amphetamine base 7.8 mg)]

15 mg [dextroamphetamine sulfate 3.75 mg, dextro-amphetamine saccharate 3.75 mg, amphetamine aspartate monohydrate 3.75 mg, amphetamine sulfate 3.75 mg (equivalent to amphetamine base 9.4 mg)]

20 mg [dextroamphetamine sulfate 5 mg, dextroamphet-amine saccharate 5 mg, amphetamine aspartate mono-hydrate 5 mg, amphetamine sulfate 5 mg (equivalent to amphetamine base 12.6 mg)]

30 mg [dextroamphetamine sulfate 7.5 mg, dextroam-phetamine saccharate 7.5 mg, amphetamine aspartate monohydrate 7.5 mg, amphetamine sulfate 7.5 mg (equivalent to amphetamine base 18.8 mg)]

Adderall®:

5 mg [dextroamphetamine sulfate 1.25 mg, dextro-amphetamine saccharate 1.25 mg, amphetamine aspartate monohydrate 1.25 mg, amphetamine sul-fate 1.25 mg (equivalent to amphetamine base 3.13 mg)]

7.5 mg [dextroamphetamine sulfate 1.875 mg, dextro-amphetamine saccharate 1.875 mg, amphetamine aspartate monohydrate 1.875 mg, amphetamine sul-fate 1.875 mg (equivalent to amphetamine base 4.7 mg)]

10 mg [dextroamphetamine sulfate 2.5 mg, dextro-amphetamine saccharate 2.5 mg, amphetamine aspartate monohydrate 2.5 mg, amphetamine sulfate 2.5 mg (equivalent to amphetamine base 6.3 mg)]

12.5 mg [dextroamphetamine sulfate 3.125 mg, dextro-amphetamine saccharate 3.125 mg, amphetamine aspartate monohydrate 3.125 mg, amphetamine sul-fate 3.125 mg (equivalent to amphetamine base 7.8 mg)]

15 mg [dextroamphetamine sulfate 3.75 mg, dextro-amphetamine saccharate 3.75 mg, amphetamine aspartate monohydrate 3.75 mg, amphetamine sul-fate 3.75 mg (equivalent to amphetamine base 9.4 mg)]

20 mg [dextroamphetamine sulfate 5 mg, dextroam-phetamine saccharate 5 mg, amphetamine aspartate monohydrate 5 mg, amphetamine sulfate 5 mg (equivalent to amphetamine base 12.6 mg)]

30 mg [dextroamphetamine sulfate 7.5 mg, dextro-amphetamine saccharate 7.5 mg, amphetamine aspartate monohydrate 7.5 mg, amphetamine sulfate 7.5 mg (equivalent to amphetamine base 18.8 mg)]

Extemporaneous Preparations A 1 mg/mL oral for-mulation of Adderall® in 3 different vehicles (Ora-Sweet®, Ora-Plus®, and a 1:1 mixture of Ora-Sweet® and Ora-Plus®) was found to be stable for 30 days when stored in glass bottles in the dark at 25°C and 60% relative humidity; ten 10 mg Adderall® tablets were crushed in a mortar into a fine powder; approximately 20 mL of vehicle was added to the mortar and triturated well; the contents were transferred to a 4 ounce glass prescription bottle; the mortar was rinsed with approximately 20 mL of vehicle and transferred to the bottle (this was repeated until the final volume was qsad to 100 mL); label "shake well" and "protect from light"

Justice J, Kupiec TC, Matthews P, et al, "Stability of Adderall® in Extemporaneously Compounded Oral Liquids," *Am J Health Syst Pharm*, 2001, 58 (15):1418-21.

References
Ahmann PA, Theye FW, Berg R, et al, "Placebo-Controlled Evaluation of Amphetamine Mixture - Dextroamphetamine Salts and Amphet-amine Salts (Adderall): Efficacy Rate and Side Effects," *Pediatrics*, 2001, 107(1), http://www.pediatrics.org/cgi/content/full/107/1/e10.

American Academy of Pediatrics/American Heart Association Clar-ification of Statement on Cardiovascular Evaluation and Monitoring of Children and Adolescents With Heart Disease Receiving Medications for ADHD; available at: http://americanheart.mediaroon.com/index.-php?s=43&item=422.

American Academy of Pediatrics, "Clinical Practice Guideline: Treat-ment of the School-Aged Child With Attention-Deficit/Hyperactivity Disorder," *Pediatrics*, 2001, 108(4):1033-44.

Chiang WK, "Amphetamines," *Goldfrank's Toxicologic Emergencies*, 8th ed, Flomenbaum NE, Goldfrank LR, Hoffman RS, eds, New York, NY: The McGraw-Hill Companies, 2006, 1119.

Greenhill LL, Pliszka S, Dulcan MK, et al, "Practice Parameter for the Use of Stimulant Medications in the Treatment of Children, Adolescents, and Adults," *J Am Acad Child Adolesc Psychiatry*, 2002, 41(2 Suppl):26S-49S.

Manos MJ, Short EJ, and Findling RL, "Differential Effectiveness of Methylphenidate and Adderall® in School-Age Youths With Attention-Deficit/Hyperactivity Disorder," *J Am Acad Child Adolesc Psychiatry*, 1999, 38(7):813-9.

Pelham WE, Aronoff HR, Midlam JK, et al, "A Comparison of Ritalin® and Adderall®: Efficacy and Time-Course in Children With Attention-Deficit/Hyperactivity Disorder," *Pediatrics*, 1999, 103(4):e43. URL: http://www.pediatrics.org/cgi/content/full/103/4/e43

Pelham WE, Gnagy EM, Chronis AM, et al, "A Comparison of Morning-Only and Morning/Late Afternoon Adderall® to Morning-Only, Twice-Daily, and Three Times-Daily Methylphenidate in Children With Attention-Deficit/Hyperactivity Disorder," *Pediatrics*, 1999a, 104 (6):1300-11.

Pliszka SR, Browne RG, Olvera RL, et al, "A Double-Blind, Placebo-Controlled Study of Adderall® and Methylphenidate in the Treatment of Attention-Deficit/Hyperactivity Disorder," *J Am Acad Child Adolesc Psychiatry*, 2000, 39(5):619-26.

Swanson JM, Wigal S, Greenhill LL, et al, "Analog Classroom Assessment of Adderall® in Children With ADHD," *J Am Acad Child Adolesc Psychiatry*, 1998, 37(5):519-26.

Vetter VL, Elia J, Erickson C, et al, "Cardiovascular Monitoring of Children and Adolescents With Heart Disease Receiving Stimulant Drugs: A Scientific Statement From the American Heart Association Council on Cardiovascular Disease in the Young Congenital Cardiac Defects Committee and the Council on Cardiovascular Nursing," *Circulation*, 2008, 117(18):2407-23.

Westfall TC and Westfall DP, "Adrenergic Agonists and Antagonists," *Goodman and Gilman's the Pharmacological Basis of Therapeutics*, 11th ed, Brunton LL, ed, New York, NY: McGraw-Hill, 2006, 257-8.

◆ **Dextroamphetamine Sulfate** *see* Dextroamphetamine *on page 416*

Dextromethorphan (deks troe meth OR fan)

Medication Safety Issues
Sound-alike/look-alike issues:
Benylin® may be confused with Benadryl®, Ventolin®
Delsym® may be confused with Delfen®, Desyrel®

U.S. Brand Names Creo-Terpin® [OTC]; Creomulsion® Adult Formula [OTC]; Creomulsion® for Children [OTC]; Delsym® [OTC]; Father John's® [OTC]; Hold® DM [OTC]; Nycoff [OTC]; PediaCare® Children's Long-Acting Cough [OTC]; Robafen Cough [OTC]; Robitussin® Children's Cough Long Acting [OTC]; Robitussin® Cough Long-Acting [OTC]; Robitussin® CoughGels™ [OTC]; Robitus-sin® Pediatric Cough [OTC] [DSC]; Scot-Tussin® Dia-betes [OTC]; Silphen DM® [OTC]; Triaminic® Children's Cough Long Acting [OTC]; Triaminic® Thin Strips® Children's Long Acting Cough [OTC]; Trocal® [OTC]; Vicks® 44® Cough Relief [OTC]; Vicks® DayQuil® Cough [OTC]

Therapeutic Category Antitussive; Cough Preparation

Generic Available Yes: Excludes strip, liquid freezer pop

Use Symptomatic relief of coughs caused by minor viral upper respiratory tract infections or inhaled irritants

Contraindications Hypersensitivity to dextromethorphan or any component (see Warnings); concurrent adminis-tration with or within 14 days of discontinuing an MAO inhibitor

Warnings Do not use for persistent or chronic cough, or for cough accompanied by excessive secretions; Creo-Terpin® contains tartrazine which may cause allergic reactions in susceptible individuals; some products may contain sodium benzoate which may cause allergic reactions in susceptible individuals; sodium benzoate has been associated with a potentially fatal toxicity ("gasping syndrome") in neonates; *in vitro* and animal studies have shown that benzoate, a metabolite of benzyl alcohol, displaces bilirubin from protein binding sites; avoid use of products containing sodium benzoate in neonates. Serotonin syndrome may occur when administered with concomitant proserotonergic drugs (ie, SSRIs/SNRIs or triptans); especially with higher dextromethorphan doses.

Precautions Anecdotal reports of abuse of dextromethorphan-containing cough/cold products have increased, especially among teenagers. Healthcare providers should be alert to problems of abuse or misuse as abuse can cause death, brain damage, seizure, loss of consciousness, and irregular heartbeat.

Adverse Reactions
Central nervous system: Drowsiness, dizziness
Gastrointestinal: Nausea

Drug Interactions

Metabolism/Transport Effects Substrate of CYP2B6 (minor), 2C9 (minor), 2C19 (minor), 2D6 (major), 2E1 (minor), 3A4 (minor); **Inhibits** CYP2D6 (weak)

Avoid Concomitant Use
Avoid concomitant use of Dextromethorphan with any of the following: MAO Inhibitors; Sibutramine

Increased Effect/Toxicity
Dextromethorphan may increase the levels/effects of: Serotonin Modulators

The levels/effects of Dextromethorphan may be increased by: CYP2D6 Inhibitors (Moderate); CYP2D6 Inhibitors (Strong); Darunavir; MAO Inhibitors; QuiNIDine; Selective Serotonin Reuptake Inhibitors; Sibutramine

Decreased Effect
The levels/effects of Dextromethorphan may be decreased by: Peginterferon Alfa-2b

Mechanism of Action Non-narcotic chemical relative of morphine; controls cough by depressing the medullary cough center

Pharmacodynamics
Onset of antitussive action: Within 15-30 minutes
Duration: Up to 6 hours

Pharmacokinetics (Adult data unless noted)
Metabolism: In the liver
Half-Life: 1.4-3.9 hours
Time to peak serum concentration: 2-2.5 hours
Elimination: Principally in urine

Usual Dosage Dosage in children <4 years of age is not well established
Oral:
Children:
1-3 months: 0.5-1 mg every 6-8 hours
3-6 months: 1-2 mg every 6-8 hours
7 months to 1 year: 2-4 mg every 6-8 hours
≥2-6 years: 2.5-7.5 mg every 4-8 hours; extended release formulation: 15 mg twice daily (maximum: 30 mg/24 hours)
7-12 years: 5-10 mg every 4 hours or 15 mg every 6-8 hours; extended release formulation: 30 mg twice daily (maximum: 60 mg/24 hours)
Children >12 years and Adults: 10-30 mg every 4-8 hours or extended release formulation: 60 mg twice daily (maximum: 120 mg/24 hours)

Administration Oral: May administer without regard to meals

Monitoring Parameters Cough, mental status

Test Interactions Can give a false-positive on phencyclidine qualitative immunoassay screen, opiate, opioid, and heroin urine screen

Patient Information If cough lasts more than 1 week or is accompanied by fever or headache, notify physician

Additional Information Dextromethorphan 15-30 mg equals 8-15 mg codeine as an antitussive

Dosage Forms Excipient information presented when available (limited, particularly for generics); consult specific product labeling. [DSC] = Discontinued product
Capsule, liquid filled, oral, as hydrobromide:
  Robafen Cough: 15 mg
  Robitussin® CoughGels™: 15 mg
Liquid, oral, as hydrobromide:
  Creo-Terpin®: 10 mg/15 mL (120 mL) [contains ethanol 25% and tartrazine]
  Scot-Tussin® Diabetes: 10 mg/5 mL (118 mL) [ethanol free, gluten free, sugar free; contains propylene glycol; cherry-strawberry flavor]
  Vicks® 44® Cough Relief: 10 mg/5 mL (120 mL) [contains ethanol, propylene glycol, sodium 10 mg/5 mL, sodium benzoate]
Lozenge, oral, as hydrobromide:
  Hold® DM: 5 mg (10s) [cherry or original flavor]
  Trocal®: 7.5 mg (50s, 300s) [cherry flavor]
Solution, oral, as hydrochloride:
  PediaCare® Children's Long-Acting Cough: 7.5 mg/5 mL (118 mL) [ethanol free; contains sodium 15 mg/5 mL, sodium benzoate; grape flavor]
  Vicks® DayQuil® Cough: 15 mg/15 mL (177 mL, 295 mL) [ethanol free; contains propylene glycol, sodium 15 mg/15 mL; citrus flavor]
Strip, orally disintegrating, as hydrobromide:
  Triaminic® Thin Strips™ Children's Long Acting Cough: 7.5 mg (14s, 16s) [equivalent to dextromethorphan 5.5 mg; contains ethanol; cherry flavor]
Suspension, extended release, oral:
  Delsym®: Dextromethorphan polistirex [equivalent to dextromethorphan hydrobromide 30 mg/5 mL] (78 mL, 148 mL) [ethanol free; contains propylene glycol, sodium 7 mg/5 mL; grape and orange flavors]
Syrup, oral, as hydrobromide:
  Creomulsion® Adult Formula: 20 mg/15 mL (120 mL) [ethanol free; contains sodium benzoate]
  Creomulsion® for Children: 5 mg/5 mL (120 mL) [ethanol free; contains sodium benzoate; cherry flavor]
  Father John's®: 10 mg/5 mL (118 mL, 236 mL) [ethanol free]
  Robitussin® Children's Cough Long Acting: 7.5 mg/5 mL (118 mL) [ethanol free; contains propylene glycol, sodium 5 mg/5 mL, sodium benzoate, fruit punch flavor]
  Robitussin® Cough Long-Acting: 15 mg/5 mL (120 mL, 240 mL) [contains ethanol, sodium benzoate]
  Robitussin® Pediatric Cough: 7.5 mg/5 mL (120 mL) [ethanol free; contains propylene glycol, sodium 5 mg/5 mL, sodium benzoate; fruit punch flavor] [DSC]
  Silphen DM®: 10 mg/5 mL (120 mL) [strawberry flavor]
  Triaminic® Children's Cough Long Acting: 7.5 mg/5 mL (118 mL) [contains benzoic acid, propylene glycol, sodium 7 mg/5 mL]
Tablet, oral, as hydrobromide:
  Nycoff: 15 mg

♦ **Dextromethorphan and Guaifenesin** see Guaifenesin and Dextromethorphan *on page 658*

♦ **Dextropropoxyphene** see Propoxyphene *on page 1171*

Dextrose (DEKS trose)

Medication Safety Issues
Sound-alike/look-alike issues:
  Glutose™ may be confused with Glutofac®

High alert medication: The Institute for Safe Medication Practices (ISMP) includes this medication (hypertonic solutions ≥20%) among its list of drugs which have a heightened risk of causing significant patient harm when used in error.

Inappropriate use of low sodium or sodium-free intravenous fluids (eg D_5W, hypotonic saline) in pediatric patients can lead to significant morbidity and mortality due to hyponatremia (ISMP, 2009).

Related Information

CPR Pediatric Drug Dosages *on page 1455*

Fluid and Electrolyte Requirements in Children *on page 1556*

Parenteral Nutrition (PN) *on page 1559*

U.S. Brand Names
BD™ Glucose [OTC]; Dex4® [OTC]; Enfamil® Glucose; GlucoBurst® [OTC]; Glutol™ [OTC]; Glutose 15™ [OTC]; Glutose 45™ [OTC]; Insta-Glucose® [OTC]; Similac® Glucose

Therapeutic Category
Antidote, Insulin; Antidote, Oral Hypoglycemic; Fluid Replacement, Enteral; Fluid Replacement, Parenteral; Hyperglycemic Agent; Hyperkalemia, Adjunctive Treatment Agent; Intravenous Nutritional Therapy

Generic Available
Yes

Use

5% and 10% solutions: Peripheral infusion to provide calories and fluid replacement

10% solution: Treatment of hypoglycemia in premature neonates

25% (hypertonic) solution: Treatment of acute symptomatic episodes of hypoglycemia in infants and children to restore depressed blood glucose levels; adjunctive treatment of hyperkalemia when combined with insulin

50% (hypertonic) solution: Treatment of insulin-induced hypoglycemia (hyperinsulinemia or insulin shock) and adjunctive treatment of hyperkalemia in adolescents and adults

≥10% solutions: Infusion after admixture with amino acids for nutritional support

Pregnancy Risk Factor
C/A (oral)

Contraindications
Hypersensitivity to corn or corn products; diabetic coma with hyperglycemia; hypertonic solutions in patients with intracranial or intraspinal hemorrhage; patients with delirium tremens and dehydration; patients with anuria, hepatic coma, or glucose-galactose malabsorption syndrome

Warnings
Hypertonic solutions (>10%) may cause thrombosis if infused via peripheral veins; administer hypertonic solutions via a central venous catheter; rapid administration of hypertonic solutions may produce significant hyperglycemia, glycosuria, and shifts in electrolytes; this may result in dehydration, hyperosmolar syndrome, coma, and death especially in patients with chronic uremia or carbohydrate intolerance; excessive or rapid dextrose administration in very low birth weight infants has been associated with increased serum osmolality and possible intracerebral hemorrhage; hyperglycemia and glycosuria may be functions of the rate of administration of dextrose; to minimize these effects, reduce the rate of infusion; addition of insulin may be necessary; administration of potassium free I.V. dextrose solutions may result in significant hypokalemia, particularly if highly concentrated dextrose solutions are used; add potassium to dextrose solutions for patients with adequate renal function; administration of low sodium or sodium free I.V. dextrose solutions may result in significant hyponatremia or water intoxication in pediatric patients; monitor serum sodium concentration; abrupt withdrawal of dextrose solution may be associated with rebound hypoglycemia; an unexpected rise in blood glucose level in an otherwise stable patient may be an early symptom of infection; glucose is not absorbed from the buccal cavity; it must be swallowed to be effective; do not use oral forms in unconscious patients

Parenteral dextrose solutions contain aluminum which may accumulate to toxic levels with prolonged administration particularly in patients with impaired renal function. Patients with impaired renal function including premature neonates who receive aluminum at >4-5 mcg/kg/day accumulate aluminum at levels associated with CNS and bone toxicity.

Precautions
Use with caution in premature infants, especially very low birth weight infants, as rapid changes is osmolality may produce profound effects on the brain, including intraventricular hemorrhage; small incremental changes in infusion rates are necessary in these patients; use with caution also in patients with diabetes mellitus

Adverse Reactions Note:
Most adverse effects are associated with excessive dosage or rate of infusion

Cardiovascular: Venous thrombosis, phlebitis, hypovolemia, hypervolemia, dehydration, edema

Central nervous system: Fever, mental confusion, unconsciousness, hyperosmolar syndrome

Endocrine & metabolic: Hyperglycemia, hypokalemia, acidosis, hypophosphatemia, hypomagnesemia

Local: Pain, vein irritation, tissue necrosis

Genitourinary: Polyuria, glycosuria, ketonuria

Gastrointestinal: Polydipsia, nausea

Respiratory: Tachypnea, pulmonary edema

Drug Interactions

Avoid Concomitant Use There are no known interactions where it is recommended to avoid concomitant use.

Increased Effect/Toxicity There are no known significant interactions involving an increase in effect.

Decreased Effect There are no known significant interactions involving a decrease in effect.

Stability Stable at room temperature; protect from freezing and extreme heat; store oral dextrose in airtight containers

Mechanism of Action Dextrose, a monosaccharide, is a source of calories and fluid for patients unable to obtain an adequate oral intake; may decrease body protein and nitrogen losses; promotes glycogen deposition in the liver; for the treatment of hyperkalemia, when combined with insulin, dextrose stimulates the uptake of potassium by cells, especially in muscle tissue

Pharmacodynamics

Onset of action: Treatment of hypoglycemia: Oral: 10 minutes

Maximum effect: Treatment of hyperkalemia: I.V.: 30 minutes

Pharmacokinetics (Adult data unless noted)

Absorption: Rapidly from the small intestine by an active mechanism

Metabolism: Metabolized to carbon dioxide and water

Time to peak serum concentration: Oral: 40 minutes

Usual Dosage

Hypoglycemia: Doses may be repeated in severe cases I.V.:

Premature neonates: 0.1-0.2 g/kg/dose (1-2 mL/kg/dose of 10% solution); followed by continuous infusion at a rate of 4-6 mg/kg/minute

Infants ≤6 months: 0.25-0.5 g/kg/dose (1-2 mL/kg/dose of 25% solution; 2.5-5 mL/kg of 10% solution; 0.5-1 mL/kg of 50% solution); maximum: 25 g/dose

Infants >6 months and Children: 0.5-1 g/kg/dose (2-4 mL/kg/dose of 25% solution; 5-10 mL/kg of 10% solution; 1-2 mL/kg of 50% solution); maximum: 25 g/dose

Adolescents and Adults: 10-25 g (40-100 mL of 25% solution or 20-50 mL of 50% solution)

Oral:

Children >2 years and Adults: 10-20 g as single dose; repeat in 10 minutes if necessary

Treatment of Hyperkalemia: I.V. (in combination with insulin):

Infants and Children: 0.5-1 g/kg (using 25% or 50% solution) combined with regular insulin 1 unit for every 4-5 g dextrose given; infuse over 2 hours (infusions as short as 30 minutes have been recommended); repeat as needed

Adolescents and Adults: 25-50 g dextrose (250-500 mL $D_{10}W$) combined with 10 units regular insulin administered over 30-60 minutes; repeat as needed or as an alternative 25 g dextrose (50 mL $D_{50}W$) combined with 5-10 units regular insulin infused over 5 minutes; repeat as needed

Note: More rapid infusions (<30 minutes) may be associated with hyperglycemia and hyperosmolality and will exacerbate hyperkalemia; avoid use in patients who are already hyperglycemic

Fluid therapy: See Fluid and Electrolyte Requirements in Children on page 1556

Nutrition: See Parenteral Nutrition (PN) on page 1559

Administration

Oral: Must be swallowed to be absorbed (see Warnings)

Parenteral: Not for SubQ or I.M. administration; dilute concentrated dextrose solutions for peripheral venous administration to a maximum concentration of 12.5%; in emergency situations, 25% dextrose has been used peripherally; for direct I.V. infusion, infuse at a maximum rate of 200 mg/kg over 1 minute; continuous infusion rates very with tolerance (see Parenteral Nutrition (PN) on page 1559) and range from 4.5-15 mg/kg/minute; hyperinsulinemic neonates may require up to 15-25 mg/kg/minute infusion rates

Monitoring Parameters Blood and urine sugar, serum electrolytes, I & O, caloric intake

Additional Information Each g of I.V. dextrose contains 3.4 kcal; glucose monohydrate 1 g is equal to 1 g anhydrous dextrose; osmolarity of 10% dextrose is 505 mOsm/L and 25% dextrose is 1330 mOsm/L. Normal body fluid osmolarity is 310 mOsm/L.

Dosage Forms Excipient information presented when available (limited, particularly for generics); consult specific product labeling. [DSC] = Discontinued product

Gel, oral:
Glutose™: 40% (15 g, 45 g)
Insta-Glucose®: 40% (30 g)

Infusion:
2.5% (1000 mL)
5% (25 mL, 50 mL, 100 mL, 150 mL, 250 mL, 500 mL, 1000 mL)
10% (250 mL, 500 mL, 1000 mL)
20% (500 mL)
30% (500 mL)
40% (500 mL)
50% (500 mL, 1000 mL, 2000 mL)
60% (500 mL, 1000 mL)
70% (500 mL, 1000 mL, 2000 mL)

Injection, solution: 10% (5 mL); 25% (10 mL); 50% (50 mL)

Solution, oral:
Glutol™: 55% (180 mL) [provides dextrose 100 g/180 mL]

Tablet, chewable:
B-D™ Glucose: 5 g
Dex4 Glucose: 4 g

References

Institute for Safe Medication Practice, "Plain D5W or Hypotonic Saline Solutions Post-Op Could Result in Acute Hyponatremia and Death in Healthy Children," ISMP Medication Safety Alert, August 13, 2009. Available online at http://www.ismp.org/Newsletters/acutecare/articles/20090813.asp.

♦ **Dextrose Monohydrate** see Dextrose on page 422

♦ **DextroStat®** see Dextroamphetamine on page 416

♦ **Dex-Tuss** see Guaifenesin and Codeine on page 657

♦ **DHAD** see Mitoxantrone on page 938

♦ **DHAQ** see Mitoxantrone on page 938

♦ **DHE** see Dihydroergotamine on page 442

♦ **D.H.E. 45®** see Dihydroergotamine on page 442

♦ **DHPG Sodium** see Ganciclovir on page 636

♦ **DHS™ Sal [OTC]** see Salicylic Acid on page 1241

♦ **DHS™ Tar [OTC]** see Coal Tar on page 349

♦ **DHS™ Targel [OTC]** see Coal Tar on page 349

♦ **Diabeta** see GlyBURIDE on page 648

♦ **DiabetAid™ Antifungal Foot Bath [OTC]** see Miconazole on page 927

♦ **DiabetAid Pain and Tingling Relief [OTC]** see Capsaicin on page 241

♦ **Diabetic Tussin® Allergy Relief [OTC]** see Chlorpheniramine on page 296

♦ **Diabetic Tussin® DM [OTC]** see Guaifenesin and Dextromethorphan on page 658

♦ **Diabetic Tussin® DM Maximum Strength [OTC]** see Guaifenesin and Dextromethorphan on page 658

♦ **Diabetic Tussin® EX [OTC]** see GuaiFENesin on page 656

♦ **Diaβeta®** see GlyBURIDE on page 648

♦ **Diaminocyclohexane Oxalatoplatinum** see Oxaliplatin on page 1030

♦ **Diaminodiphenylsulfone** see Dapsone on page 387

♦ **Diamode [OTC]** see Loperamide on page 838

♦ **Diamox® (Can)** see AcetaZOLAMIDE on page 41

♦ **Diamox® Sequels®** see AcetaZOLAMIDE on page 41

♦ **Diarr-Eze (Can)** see Loperamide on page 838

♦ **Diastat®** see Diazepam on page 424

♦ **Diastat® AcuDial™** see Diazepam on page 424

♦ **Diastat® Rectal Delivery System (Can)** see Diazepam on page 424

♦ **Diazemuls® (Can)** see Diazepam on page 424

Diazepam (dye AZ e pam)

Medication Safety Issues

Sound-alike/look-alike issues:
Diazepam may be confused with diazoxide, diltiazem, Ditropan®, LORazepam
Valium® may be confused with Valcyte®

Beers Criteria medication: This drug may be inappropriate for use in geriatric patients (high severity risk).

Related Information

Febrile Seizures on page 1690
Laboratory Detection of Drugs in Urine on page 1706
Preprocedure Sedatives in Children on page 1688

U.S. Brand Names Diastat®; Diastat® AcuDial™; Diazepam Intensol™; Valium®

Canadian Brand Names Apo-Diazepam®; Diastat®; Diastat® Rectal Delivery System; Diazemuls®; Novo-Dipam; Valium®

Therapeutic Category Antianxiety Agent; Anticonvulsant; Benzodiazepine; Benzodiazepine; Hypnotic; Sedative

Generic Available Yes: Injection, tablet, solution only

Use Management of general anxiety disorders, panic disorders, ethanol withdrawal symptoms, relief of skeletal muscle spasms, muscle spasticity, and tetany; to provide preoperative or preprocedural sedation and amnesia; adjunct in the treatment of convulsive disorders; treatment of status epilepticus and severe recurrent convulsive seizures; rectal gel formulation indicated for the management of intermittent bouts of increased seizure activity in refractory epilepsy patients on stable AED therapy

Restrictions C-IV

Pregnancy Risk Factor D

Pregnancy Considerations Teratogenic effects have been reported in animal studies. In humans, diazepam crosses the placenta. An increased risk of congenital malformations and other developmental abnormalities have been associated with diazepam; epilepsy itself may also increase the risk. Hypotonia, hypothermia, withdrawal symptoms, respiratory and feeding difficulties have been reported in the infant following maternal use of benzodiazepines near time of delivery.

Lactation Enters breast milk/contraindicated (AAP rates "of concern")

Breast-Feeding Considerations Clinical effects on the infant include sedation; AAP reports that USE MAY BE OF CONCERN.

Contraindications Hypersensitivity to diazepam or any component (see Warnings); possible cross-sensitivity with other benzodiazepines; do not use in a comatose patient, in those with pre-existing CNS depression, respiratory depression, acute narrow-angle glaucoma, severe uncontrolled pain, myasthenia gravis, severe respiratory insufficiency, severe hepatic insufficiency, or sleep apnea syndrome; oral dosage forms are listed by manufacturer as being contraindicated in patients <6 months of age (due to lack of adequate clinical experience).

Warnings Abrupt discontinuation may cause withdrawal symptoms or seizures. Rapid I.V. push may cause sudden respiratory depression, apnea, hypotension, or cardiac arrest. Appropriate resuscitative equipment and qualified personnel should be available during parenteral administration with appropriate monitoring. Do not administer injection to patients in coma, shock, or acute ethanol intoxication with depression of vital signs. Tonic status epilepticus may occur in patients with petit mal status or petit mal variant status who are treated with diazepam. Administration of rectal gel should only be performed by individuals trained to recognize characteristic seizure activity for which the product is indicated and who are capable of monitoring patient's response to determine need for additional medical intervention.

Psychiatric and paradoxical reactions, including hyperactive or aggressive behavior, hallucinations, and psychoses, have been reported with benzodiazepines, particularly in adolescent/pediatric or elderly patients; discontinue diazepam if such reactions occur. Diazepam is not recommended for the treatment of psychotic patients, in place of appropriate therapy. Teratogenic effects have been reported in animal studies. In humans, diazepam crosses the placenta. An increased risk of congenital malformations and other developmental abnormalities have been associated with diazepam; epilepsy itself may also increase the risk. Hypotonia, hypothermia, withdrawal symptoms, and respiratory and feeding difficulties have been reported in the infant following maternal use of benzodiazepines near time of delivery.

Injection and rectal gel contain benzoic acid, benzyl alcohol, and sodium benzoate; benzyl alcohol may cause allergic reactions in susceptible individuals; benzoic acid (benzoate) is a metabolite of benzyl alcohol; large amounts of benzyl alcohol (≥99 mg/kg/day) have been associated with a potentially fatal toxicity ("gasping syndrome") in neonates; the "gasping syndrome" consists of metabolic acidosis, respiratory distress, gasping respirations, CNS dysfunction (including convulsions, intracranial hemorrhage), hypotension and cardiovascular collapse; use diazepam products containing benzoic acid, benzyl alcohol, or sodium benzoate with caution in neonates; *in vitro* and animal studies have shown that benzoate displaces bilirubin from protein binding sites. Parenteral formulation contains propylene glycol (40%) and alcohol (10%) which have been associated with toxicities when administered in high dosages or at rapid rates of infusion. Oral liquid products contain polyethylene glycol and propylene glycol which may have adverse effects (see Additional Information).

Precautions Use with caution in patients receiving other CNS depressants or psychoactive medication (effects with other sedative drugs or ethanol may be potentiated) and in patients with depression. Use with caution in patients with hypoalbuminemia, renal or hepatic dysfunction, and in neonates and young infants; neonates have decreased metabolism of diazepam and desmethyldiazepam (active metabolite), both can accumulate with repeated use and cause increased toxicity. Modify dosage in patients with hepatic impairment or chronic respiratory insufficiency, and in debilitated patients. Use with extreme caution in patients with a history of drug or alcohol abuse. Safety and efficacy have not been established in neonates (≤30 days) for parenteral product; in infants <6 months of age for oral products; or in children <2 years of age for rectal gel.

Adverse Reactions

Cardiovascular: Bradycardia, hypotension, cardiovascular collapse, cardiac arrest

Central nervous system: Amnesia, ataxia, confusion, depression, dizziness, drowsiness, fatigue, headache, hypoactivity, incoordination, paradoxical reactions (eg, acute hyperexcited states, anxiety, hallucinations, increased muscle spasms, insomnia, rage, sleep disturbances, stimulation), slurred speech, somnolence, syncope, vertigo

Dermatologic: Dermatitis, rash, urticaria

Gastrointestinal: Constipation, diarrhea, GI disturbances, nausea, salivation changes

Genitourinary: Incontinence, urinary retention

Hematological: Neutropenia (rare)

Hepatic: Liver enzymes elevated, jaundice

Local: Pain with injection, thrombophlebitis, tissue necrosis may occur following extravasation

Neuromuscular & skeletal: Dysarthria, tremor, weakness

Ocular: Blurred vision, diplopia, nystagmus

Respiratory: Apnea, decrease in respiratory rate, laryngospasm

Miscellaneous: Physical and psychological dependence with prolonged use; hiccups

Drug Interactions

Metabolism/Transport Effects Substrate of CYP1A2 (minor), 2B6 (minor), 2C9 (minor), 2C19 (major), 3A4 (major); **Inhibits** CYP2C19 (weak), 3A4 (weak)

Avoid Concomitant Use There are no known interactions where it is recommended to avoid concomitant use.

Increased Effect/Toxicity

Diazepam may increase the levels/effects of: Alcohol (Ethyl); Clozapine; CNS Depressants; Methotrimeprazine; Phenytoin

The levels/effects of Diazepam may be increased by: Antifungal Agents (Azole Derivatives, Systemic); Aprepitant; Calcium Channel Blockers (Nondihydropyridine); Cimetidine; Contraceptives (Estrogens); Contraceptives (Progestins); CYP2C19 Inhibitors (Moderate); CYP2C19 Inhibitors (Strong); CYP3A4 Inhibitors (Moderate); CYP3A4 Inhibitors (Strong); Dasatinib; Disulfiram; Fluconazole; Fosamprenavir; Fosaprepitant; Grapefruit Juice; Isoniazid; Macrolide Antibiotics; Methotrimeprazine; Nefazodone; Proton Pump Inhibitors; Ritonavir; Saquinavir; Selective Serotonin Reuptake Inhibitors

Decreased Effect

The levels/effects of Diazepam may be decreased by: CarBAMazepine; CYP2C19 Inducers (Strong); CYP3A4 Inducers (Strong); Deferasirox; Rifamycin Derivatives; St Johns Wort; Theophylline Derivatives; Yohimbine

425

Food Interactions Grapefruit juice significantly increases oral bioavailability of diazepam. Food may delay and decrease oral absorption.

Stability Store all products at controlled room temperature. Do not mix injection with other medications; protect from light. Dispense tablets and oral solution in tightly-closed, light-resistant container. Protect oral concentrated solution (Intensol®) from light; discard opened bottle after 90 days.

Mechanism of Action Depresses all levels of the CNS, including the limbic and reticular formation by binding to the benzodiazepine site on the gamma-aminobutyric acid (GABA) receptor complex and modulating GABA, which is a major inhibitory neurotransmitter in the brain

Pharmacodynamics Status epilepticus:

Onset of action:

I.V.: 1-3 minutes

Rectal: 2-10 minutes

Duration: 15-30 minutes

Pharmacokinetics (Adult data unless noted)

Absorption:

Oral: 85% to 100%

I.M.: Poor

Rectal (gel): Well absorbed

Distribution: Widely distributed; crosses blood-brain barrier and placenta; distributes into breast milk; V_d: Adults: 0.8-1 L/kg

Protein binding:

Neonates: 84% to 86%

Adults: 98%

Metabolism: In the liver to desmethyldiazepam (active metabolite) and N-methyloxazepam (active metabolite); these are metabolized to oxazepam (active) which undergoes glucuronide conjugation before being excreted

Bioavailability: Rectal (gel): 90%

Half-life:

Diazepam:

Neonates: 50-95 hours

Infants 1 month to 2 years: 40-50 hours

Children 2-12 years: 15-21 hours

Children 12-16 years: 18-20 hours

Adults: 20-50 hours

Increased half-life in those with severe hepatic disorders

Desmethyldiazepam (active metabolite): Adults: 50-100 hours; may be further prolonged in neonates

Time to peak serum concentration:

Oral: Mean: 1-1.5 hours; range: 0.25-2.5 hours

Rectal (gel): 1.5 hours

Elimination: In urine, primarily as conjugated oxazepam (75%), desmethyldiazepam, and N-methyloxazepam

Dialysis: Not dialyzable (0% to 5%)

Usual Dosage

Children:

Status epilepticus: I.V:

Neonates: (Not recommended as first-line agent; injection contains benzoic acid, benzyl alcohol, and sodium benzoate; see Warnings): 0.1-0.3 mg/kg/dose given over 3-5 minutes, every 15-30 minutes to a maximum total dose of 2 mg

Infants >30 days and Children: 0.1-0.3 mg/kg/dose given over 3-5 minutes, every 5–10 minutes (maximum: 10 mg/dose) (see Hegenbarth, 2008)

Manufacturer's recommendations:

Infants >30 days and Children <5 years: 0.2-0.5 mg slow I.V. every 2-5 minutes up to a maximum total dose of 5 mg; repeat in 2-4 hours if needed

Children ≥5 years: 1 mg slow I.V. every 2-5 minutes up to a maximum of 10 mg; repeat in 2-4 hours if needed

Anticonvulsant: Acute treatment:

Rectal gel formulation:

Infants <6 months: Not recommended

Children <2 years: Safety and efficacy not established

Children 2-5 years: 0.5 mg/kg

Children 6-11 years: 0.3 mg/kg

Children ≥12 years and Adults: 0.2 mg/kg

Note: Round dose to 2.5, 5, 7.5, 10, 12.5, 15, 17.5, and 20 mg/dose; dose may be repeated in 4-12 hours if needed; do not use more than 5 times per month or more than once every 5 days

Rectal: Undiluted 5 mg/mL parenteral formulation (filter if using ampul): 0.5 mg/kg/dose then 0.25 mg/kg/dose in 10 minutes if needed

Febrile seizure prophylaxis: Oral: 1 mg/kg/day divided every 8 hours; initiate therapy at first sign of fever and continue for 24 hours after fever resolves (Rosman, 1993; Steering Committee, 2008)

Moderate sedation for procedures:

Oral: 0.2-0.3 mg/kg (maximum dose: 10 mg) 45-60 minutes prior to procedure

I.V.: Initial: 0.05-0.1 mg/kg over 3-5 minutes, titrate slowly to effect (maximum total dose: 0.25 mg/kg) (see Krauss, 2006)

Sedation or muscle relaxation or anxiety:

Oral: 0.12-0.8 mg/kg/day in divided doses every 6-8 hours

I.M., I.V.: 0.04-0.3 mg/kg/dose every 2-4 hours to a maximum of 0.6 mg/kg within an 8-hour period, if needed

Muscle spasm associated with tetanus: I.V., I.M.:

Infants >30 days: 1-2 mg/dose every 3-4 hours as needed

Children ≥5 years: 5-10 mg/dose every 3-4 hours as needed

Adolescents: Moderate sedation for procedures:

Oral: 10 mg

I.V.: 5 mg; may repeat with 2.5 mg if needed

Adults:

Anxiety:

Oral: 2-10 mg 2-4 times/day

I.M., I.V.: 2-10 mg, may repeat in 3-4 hours if needed

Skeletal muscle relaxation:

Oral: 2-10 mg 3-4 times/day

I.M., I.V.: 5-10 mg, may repeat in 2-4 hours; larger doses may be required to treat tetanus

Status epilepticus: I.V.: Initial: 5-10 mg; may repeat every 10-15 minutes up to a maximum dose of 30 mg; may repeat in 2-4 hours if needed, but residual active metabolites may still be present

Adjunct in convulsive disorders: Oral: 2-10 mg 2-4 times/day

Preoperative medication: I.M.: 10 mg before surgery

Administration

Oral: Administer with food or water; do not administer with grapefruit juice. Oral concentrate solution (5 mg/mL): Measure dose only with calibrated dropper provided; dose should be diluted or mixed with water, juice, soda, applesauce, or pudding before use

Parenteral: I.V.: Rapid injection may cause respiratory depression or hypotension; infants and children: Do not exceed 1-2 mg/minute I.V. push; adults: Maximum infusion rate: 5 mg/minute; maximum concentration for administration: 5 mg/mL

Rectal: Diastat® AcuDial™: Prior to administration, confirm that the syringe is properly set to the correct dose and that the green "ready" band is visible.

Diastat® AcuDial™ and Diastat®: Place patient on side (facing person responsible for monitoring), with top leg bent forward. Insert rectal tip (lubricated) gently into rectum until rim fits snug against rectal opening; push plunger gently over 3 seconds. After additional 3 seconds, remove syringe; hold buttocks together while slowly counting to 3 to prevent leakage; keep patient on side, facing towards you and continue to observe patient; discard any unused medication, syringe, and all used materials safely away from children; do not reuse; see Administration and Disposal Instructions that come with product.

Monitoring Parameters Heart rate, respiratory rate, blood pressure, mental status; with long-term therapy: Liver enzymes, CBC

Reference Range Effective therapeutic range not well established

Proposed therapeutic:

Diazepam: 0.2-1.5 mcg/mL (SI: 0.7-5.3 micromoles/L)
N-desmethyldiazepam (nordiazepam): 0.1-0.5 mcg/mL (SI: 0.35-1.8 micromoles/L)

Test Interactions False-negative urinary glucose determinations with Clinistix® or Diastix®

Patient Information Avoid alcohol and grapefruit juice; limit caffeine. May cause drowsiness and impair ability to perform activities requiring mental alertness or physical coordination. May be habit-forming; avoid abrupt discontinuation after prolonged use

Nursing Implications Avoid extravasation (tissue necrosis may occur); infuse I.V. into secure line using larger veins

Additional Information Diazepam does not have any analgesic effects. Diarrhea in a 9 month old infant receiving high-dose oral diazepam was attributed to the diazepam oral solution that contained polyethylene glycol and propylene glycol (both are osmotically active); diarrhea resolved when crushed tablets were substituted for the oral solution (see Marshall, 1995).

Diastat® AcuDial™: Prescribed dose must be "dialed in" and locked before dispensing; consult package insert for directions on setting prescribed dose; confirm green "ready" band is visible prior to dispensing product.

Dosage Forms Excipient information presented when available (limited, particularly for generics); consult specific product labeling.

Gel, rectal [adult rectal tip (6 cm)]:
Diastat® AcuDial™: 20 mg (4 mL) [contains benzoic acid, benzyl alcohol, ethanol 10%, propylene glycol, sodium benzoate; delivers set doses of 12.5 mg, 15 mg, 17.5 mg, and 20 mg]
Gel, rectal [pediatric rectal tip (4.4 cm)]:
Diastat®: 5 mg/mL (0.5 mL) [contains benzoic acid, benzyl alcohol, ethanol 10%, propylene glycol, sodium benzoate]
Gel, rectal [pediatric/adult rectal tip (4.4 cm)]:
Diastat® AcuDial™: 10 mg (2 mL) [contains benzoic acid, benzyl alcohol, ethanol 10%, propylene glycol, sodium benzoate; delivers set doses of 5 mg, 7.5 mg, and 10 mg]
Injection, solution: 5 mg/mL (2 mL, 10 mL)
Solution, oral: 5 mg/5 mL (5 mL, 500 mL)
Solution, oral [concentrate]:
Diazepam Intensol™: 5 mg/mL (30 mL) [contains ethanol 19%, propylene glycol]
Tablet: 2 mg, 5 mg, 10 mg
Valium®: 2 mg, 5 mg, 10 mg

References

American Academy of Pediatrics; American Academy of Pediatric Dentistry, Coté CJ, et al, "Guidelines for Monitoring and Management of Pediatric Patients During and After Sedation for Diagnostic and Therapeutic Procedures: An Update," *Pediatrics*, 2006, 118 (6):2587-602.

Dreifuss FE, Rosman NP, Cloyd JC, et al, "A Comparison of Rectal Diazepam Gel and Placebo for Acute Repetitive Seizures," *N Engl J Med*, 1998, 338(26):1869-75.

Hegenbarth MA and American Academy of Pediatrics Committee on Drugs, "Preparing for Pediatric Emergencies: Drugs to Consider," *Pediatrics*, 2008, 121(2):433-43.

Krauss B and Green SM, "Procedural Sedation and Analgesia in Children," *Lancet*, 2006, 367(9512):766-80.

Marshall JD, Farrar HC, and Kearns GL, "Diarrhea Associated With Enteral Benzodiazepine Solutions," *J Pediatr*, 1995, 126(4):657-9.

Rosman NP, Colton T, Labazzo J, et al, "A Controlled Trial of Diazepam Administered During Febrile Illnesses to Prevent Recurrence of Febrile Seizures," *N Engl J Med*, 1993, 329(2):79-84.

Steering Committee on Quality Improvement and Management, Subcommittee on Febrile Seizures American Academy of Pediatrics, "Febrile Seizures: Clinical Practice Guideline for the Long-Term Management of the Child With Simple Febrile Seizures," *Pediatrics*, 2008, 121(6):1281-6.

Zeltzer LK, Altman A, Cohen D, et al, "Report of the Subcommittee on the Management of Pain Associated With Procedures in Children With Cancer," *Pediatrics*, 1990, 86(5 Pt 2):826-31.

◆ **Diazepam Intensol™** *see* Diazepam *on page 424*

Diazoxide (dye az OKS ide)

Medication Safety Issues
Sound-alike/look-alike issues:
Diazoxide may be confused with diazepam, Dyazide®

Related Information
Antihypertensive Agents by Class *on page 1481*

U.S. Brand Names Proglycem®

Canadian Brand Names Proglycem®

Therapeutic Category Antihypertensive Agent; Antihypoglycemic Agent; Vasodilator

Generic Available No

Use Oral: Management of hypoglycemia related to hyperinsulinism secondary to: Islet cell adenoma, carcinoma, or hyperplasia; adenomatosis; nesidioblastosis (persistent hyperinsulinemic hypoglycemia of infancy); leucine sensitivity, or extrapancreatic malignancy

Pregnancy Risk Factor C

Pregnancy Considerations Adverse events have been observed in animal studies. Diazoxide crosses the human placenta. Altered carbohydrate metabolism, hyperbilirubinemia, or thrombocytopenia have been reported in the fetus or neonate. Alopecia and hypertrichosis lanuginosa have also been reported in infants following maternal use of diazoxide during the last 19-60 days of pregnancy.

Lactation Excretion in breast milk unknown/not recommended

Contraindications Hypersensitivity to diazoxide, any component, thiazides, or other sulfonamide derivatives; functional hypoglycemia

Warnings Diazoxide use may lead to increased fluid retention and precipitate CHF in patients with compromised cardiac reserve; used with caution in patients with heart failure; diuretics may be used to treat fluid retention. Ketoacidosis or nonketotic hyperosmolar coma may occur during treatment, usually in patients with concomitant illness; prompt recognition and treatment are essential (especially due to the long half-life of the drug). Transient cataracts have been reported in an infant in association with hyperosmolar coma; cataracts subsided following correction of hyperosmolarity. Abnormal facial features have been reported in four children who received diazoxide for >4 years for the treatment of hypoglycemia hyperinsulinism.

Solution contains propylene glycol and sodium benzoate; benzoic acid (benzoate) is a metabolite of benzyl alcohol; large amounts of benzyl alcohol (≥99 mg/kg/day) have been associated with a potentially fatal toxicity ("gasping syndrome") in neonates; the "gasping syndrome" consists of metabolic acidosis, respiratory distress, gasping respirations, CNS dysfunction (including convulsions, intracranial hemorrhage), hypotension, and cardiovascular collapse; use solution containing sodium benzoate with caution in neonates; *in vitro* and animal studies have shown that benzoate displaces bilirubin from protein binding sites.

Precautions Use with caution and consider dosage reduction in patients with renal impairment. Use with caution in patients with diabetes mellitus, hepatic impairment, hyperuricemia, or history of gout. May displace bilirubin from albumin; use caution in newborns with hyperbilirubinemia.

Initiate treatment with diazoxide under close clinical supervision; carefully monitor blood glucose and clinical response until patient's condition becomes stable (usually several days); discontinue diazoxide if drug is not effective after 2-3 weeks of therapy. Regular monitoring of urine for glucose and ketones (especially under conditions of stress) are required with prolonged therapy; abnormal results should be reported to physician promptly. Periodic monitoring of blood glucose is required for dosage adjustment.

Adverse Reactions

Cardiovascular: Hypotension, tachycardia, palpitations, CHF (due to sodium and water retention), chest pain (rarely)

Central nervous system: Dizziness, seizure, headache, anxiety, fever, insomnia, malaise, polyneuritis

Dermatologic: Rash, hirsutism (mainly on forehead, back, and limbs; most commonly in children and women; may be cosmetically unacceptable; reversible after discontinuation of drug), pruritus, purpura, scalp hair loss

Endocrine & metabolic: Hyperglycemia, diabetic ketoacidosis, hyperosmolar nonketotic coma, hyperuricemia, gout, sodium and water retention, serum free fatty acids elevated, breast lump enlargement, galactorrhea

Gastrointestinal: Nausea, vomiting, anorexia, constipation, abdominal pain, diarrhea, ileus, pancreatitis, pancreatic necrosis, taste loss (transient)

Hematologic: Neutropenia, thrombocytopenia, bleeding (excessive), eosinophilia, anemia

Hepatic: Alkaline phosphatase elevated, AST elevated

Neuromuscular & skeletal: Weakness, paresthesia

Ocular: Blurred vision, cataracts (transient), diplopia, lacrimation, ring scotoma, subconjunctival hemorrhage

Renal: Albuminuria, azotemia, creatinine clearance decreased, glucosuria, hematuria, nephrotic syndrome (reversible), uric acid increased, urinary output decreased

Miscellaneous: Extrapyramidal symptoms and development of abnormal facies with chronic oral use; IgG decreased, lymphadenopathy

Drug Interactions

Avoid Concomitant Use There are no known interactions where it is recommended to avoid concomitant use.

Increased Effect/Toxicity

Diazoxide may increase the levels/effects of: Antihypertensives

The levels/effects of Diazoxide may be increased by: MAO Inhibitors

Decreased Effect

Diazoxide may decrease the levels/effects of: Phenytoin

Stability Suspension: Store at controlled room temperature of 25°C (77°F). Protect from light. Store in carton until ready to use.

Mechanism of Action Inhibits insulin release from the pancreas, resulting in a dose-related increase in blood glucose; also possesses an extra-pancreatic effect to increase blood glucose

Pharmacodynamics

Hyperglycemic effects (oral):

Onset of action: Within 1 hour

Duration (normal renal function): 8 hours

Pharmacokinetics (Adult data unless noted)

Protein binding: >90%

Half-life:

Children: 9-24 hours

Adults: 24-36 hours

Elimination: 50% excreted unchanged in urine

Usual Dosage

Oral: Hyperinsulinemic hypoglycemia:

Newborns and Infants: Initial: 10 mg/kg/day in divided doses every 8 hours; usual range: 8-15 mg/kg/day in divided doses every 8-12 hours

Children and Adults: Initial: 3 mg/kg/day in divided doses every 8 hours; usual range: 3-8 mg/kg/day in divided doses every 8-12 hours. **Note:** In certain instances, patients with refractory hypoglycemia may require higher doses.

Dosing adjustment in renal impairment: Half-life may be prolonged with renal impairment; a reduced dose should be considered.

Administration Oral: Administer on an empty stomach 1 hour before or 1 hour after meals; shake suspension well before use; suspension comes with calibrated dropper (to deliver dose of 10-50 mg, in 10 mg increments).

Monitoring Parameters Blood glucose, serum uric acid, electrolytes, BUN; renal function; AST, CBC with differential, platelets; urine glucose and ketones; blood pressure, heart rate

Test Interactions False-negative insulin response to glucagon (diazoxide inhibits glucagon-stimulated insulin release)

Additional Information The injectable form of diazoxide, which was used for the emergency treatment of hypertension, is no longer available.

Dosage Forms Excipient information presented when available (limited, particularly for generics); consult specific product labeling.

Capsule, oral:

Proglycem®: 50 mg [not available in the U.S.]

Suspension, oral:

Proglycem®: 50 mg/mL (30 mL) [contains ethanol 7.25%, sodium benzoate, propylene glycol; chocolate-mint flavor]

◆ **Dibenzyline®** *see* Phenoxybenzamine *on page 1100*

Dibucaine (DYE byoo kane)

U.S. Brand Names Nupercainal® [OTC]

Therapeutic Category Analgesic, Topical; Local Anesthetic, Topical

Generic Available Yes

Use Fast, temporary relief of pain and itching due to hemorrhoids, minor burns, other minor skin conditions

Breast-Feeding Considerations No data reported; however, topical administration is probably compatible.

Contraindications Hypersensitivity to dibucaine, other amide-type anesthetics, or any component (see Warnings)

Warnings Some products may contain sulfites which may cause allergic reactions in susceptible individuals

Adverse Reactions

Cardiovascular: Edema

Dermatologic: Urticaria, cutaneous lesions, contact dermatitis

Local: Burning, tenderness, irritation, inflammation

Drug Interactions

Avoid Concomitant Use There are no known interactions where it is recommended to avoid concomitant use.

Increased Effect/Toxicity There are no known significant interactions involving an increase in effect.

Decreased Effect There are no known significant interactions involving a decrease in effect.

Mechanism of Action Blocks both the initiation and conduction of nerve impulses by decreasing the neuronal membrane's permeability to sodium ions, which results in inhibition of depolarization with resultant blockade of conduction

Pharmacodynamics
Onset of action: Within 15 minutes
Duration: 2-4 hours

Pharmacokinetics (Adult data unless noted) Absorption: Poor through intact skin, but well absorbed through mucous membranes and excoriated skin

Usual Dosage Children and Adults:
Rectal: Hemorrhoids: Administer each morning, evening, and after each bowel movement
Topical: Apply gently to the affected areas; no more than 30 g for adults or 7.5 g for children should be used in any 24-hour period

Administration
Rectal: Insert ointment into rectum using a rectal applicator
Topical: Apply gently to affected areas; do not use near the eyes or over denuded surfaces or blistered areas

Dosage Forms Excipient information presented when available (limited, particularly for generics); consult specific product labeling.
Ointment, topical: 1% (30 g)
Nupercainal®: 1% (30 g, 60g) [contains sodium bisulfite]

♦ **DIC** see Dacarbazine on page 380

Diclofenac (dye KLOE fen ak)

Medication Safety Issues
Sound-alike/look-alike issues:
Diclofenac may be confused with Diflucan®, Duphalac® Cataflam® may be confused with Catapres®
Voltaren® may be confused with traMADol, Ultram®, Verelan®

Transdermal patch (Flector®) contains conducting metal (eg, aluminum); remove patch prior to MRI.

U.S. Brand Names Cataflam®; Flector®; Pennsaid®; Solaraze®; Voltaren Ophthalmic®; Voltaren® Gel; Voltaren® [DSC]; Voltaren®-XR; Zipsor™

Canadian Brand Names Apo-Diclo Rapide®; Apo-Diclo SR®; Apo-Diclo®; Cataflam®; Diclofenac ECT; Diclofenac SR; Dom-Diclofenac; Dom-Diclofenac SR; Novo-Difenac ECT; Novo-Difenac K; Novo-Difenac Suppositories; Novo-Difenac-SR; Nu-Diclo; Nu-Diclo-SR; Pennsaid®; PMS-Diclofenac; PMS-Diclofenac SR; PMS-Diclofenac-K; PRO-Diclo-Rapide; Sandoz-Diclofenac; Sandoz-Diclofenac Rapide; Sandoz-Diclofenac SR; Voltaren Ophtha®; Voltaren Rapide®; Voltaren SR®; Voltaren®; Voltaren® Emulgel™

Therapeutic Category Analgesic, Non-narcotic; Anti-inflammatory Agent; Nonsteroidal Anti-inflammatory Drug (NSAID), Ophthalmic; Nonsteroidal Anti-inflammatory Drug (NSAID), Oral

Generic Available Yes: Excludes gel, patch

Use
Oral: Acute treatment of mild to moderate pain (FDA approved in adults); acute and chronic treatment of rheumatoid arthritis, ankylosing spondylitis, and osteoarthritis (FDA approved in adults); treatment of primary dysmenorrhea (FDA approved in adults); also used for juvenile rheumatoid arthritis, gout
Ophthalmic solution: Treatment of postoperative inflammation after cataract extraction (FDA approved in adults); temporary relief of pain and photophobia in patients undergoing corneal refractive surgery (FDA approved in adults)
Topical gel 1%: Relief of osteoarthritis pain in joints amenable to topical therapy (eg, ankle, elbow, foot, hand, knee, wrist) (FDA approved in adults)

Topical gel 3%: Treatment of actinic keratosis (in conjunction with sun avoidance) (FDA approved in adults)
Topical patch: Acute pain due to minor strains, sprains, and contusions (FDA approved in adults)

Medication Guide An FDA-approved patient medication guide, which is available with the product information and as follows, must be dispensed with this medication for each new outpatient prescription and refill.
Cataflam®: http://www.fda.gov/downloads/Drugs/DrugSafety/UCM135935.pdf
Flector®: http://www.fda.gov/downloads/Drugs/DrugSafety/ucm088598.pdf
Voltaren®: http://www.fda.gov/downloads/Drugs/DrugSafety/ucm089822.pdf
Zipsor™: http://zipsor.com/patient/html_pages/medication_guide.html

Pregnancy Risk Factor B (topical gel 3%); C (ophthalmic, oral, topical gel 1%, topical patch); D (≥30 weeks gestation [oral])

Pregnancy Considerations Adverse events were not observed in the initial animal reproduction studies; therefore, manufacturers classify most dosage forms of diclofenac as pregnancy category C (oral: category D ≥30 weeks gestation). Diclofenac crosses the placenta and can be detected in fetal tissue and amniotic fluid. NSAID exposure during the first trimester is not strongly associated with congenital malformations; however, cardiovascular anomalies and cleft palate have been observed following NSAID exposure in some studies. The use of a NSAID close to conception may be associated with an increased risk of miscarriage. Nonteratogenic effects have been observed following NSAID administration during the third trimester including: Myocardial degenerative changes, prenatal constriction of the ductus arteriosus, fetal tricuspid regurgitation, failure of the ductus arteriosus to close postnatally; renal dysfunction or failure, oligohydramnios; gastrointestinal bleeding or perforation, increased risk of necrotizing enterocolitis; intracranial bleeding (including intraventricular hemorrhage), platelet dysfunction with resultant bleeding; pulmonary hypertension. Because they may cause premature closure of the ductus arteriosus, use of NSAIDs late in pregnancy should be avoided (use after 31 or 32 weeks gestation is not recommended by some clinicians). Product labeling for Zipsor™ specifically notes that use at ≥30 weeks gestation should be avoided and, therefore, classifies diclofenac as pregnancy category D at this time. Use in the third trimester is contraindicated in the Canadian labeling. The chronic use of NSAIDs in women of reproductive age may be associated with infertility that is reversible upon discontinuation of the medication. A registry is available for pregnant women exposed to autoimmune medications including diclofenac. For additional information contact the Organization of Teratology Information Specialists, OTIS Autoimmune Diseases Study, at 877-311-8972

Lactation Excreted in breast milk/not recommended

Breast-Feeding Considerations Low concentrations of diclofenac can be found in breast milk. Breast-feeding is not recommended by the manufacturer. Use while breast-feeding is contraindicated in Canadian labeling.

Contraindications Hypersensitivity to diclofenac or any component (see Warnings); history of asthma, urticaria, or allergic-type reaction to aspirin, or other NSAIDs; patients with the "aspirin triad" [asthma, rhinitis (with or without nasal polyps), and aspirin intolerance] (fatal asthmatic and anaphylactoid reactions may occur in these patients); perioperative pain in the setting of coronary artery bypass graft (CABG)

Topical patch (additional contraindication to above): Do not apply to nonintact or damaged skin (eg, exudative dermatitis, eczema, infected lesions, burns, or wounds)

Warnings NSAIDs are associated with an increased risk of adverse cardiovascular thrombotic events, including potentially fatal MI and stroke **[U.S. Boxed Warning]**; risk may be increased with duration of use or pre-existing cardiovascular risk factors or disease; carefully evaluate cardiovascular risk profile prior to prescribing; use the lowest effective dose for the shortest duration of time, taking into consideration individual patient treatment goals; alternate therapies should be considered for patients at high risk. Use is contraindicated for treatment of perioperative pain in the setting of CABG surgery **[U.S. Boxed Warning]**; an increased incidence of MI and stroke was found in patients receiving COX-2 selective NSAIDs for the treatment of pain within the first 10-14 days after CABG surgery. NSAIDs may cause fluid retention, edema, and new onset or worsening of pre-existing hypertension; use with caution in patients with hypertension, CHF, or fluid retention. Concurrent administration of ibuprofen, and potentially other nonselective NSAIDs, may interfere with aspirin's cardioprotective effect.

Oral use: NSAIDs may increase the risk of gastrointestinal inflammation, ulceration, bleeding, and perforation **[U.S. Boxed Warning]**. These events, which can be potentially fatal, may occur at any time during therapy, and without warning. Avoid the use of NSAIDs in patients with active GI bleeding or ulcer disease. Use NSAIDs with extreme caution in patients with a history of GI bleeding or ulcers (these patients have a 10-fold increased risk for developing a GI bleed). Use NSAIDs with caution in patients with other risk factors which may increase GI bleeding (eg, concurrent therapy with aspirin, anticoagulants, and/or corticosteroids, longer duration of NSAID use, smoking, use of alcohol, and poor general health). Use the lowest effective dose for the shortest duration of time, taking into consideration individual patient treatment goals; alternate therapies should be considered for patients at high risk.

NSAIDs may compromise existing renal function. Renal toxicity may occur in patients with impaired renal function, dehydration, heart failure, liver dysfunction, those taking diuretics and ACE inhibitors; use with caution in these patients; monitor renal function closely. NSAIDs are not recommended for use in patients with advanced renal disease. Long-term use of NSAIDs may cause renal papillary necrosis and other renal injury.

Fatal asthmatic and anaphylactoid reactions may occur in patients with the "aspirin triad" who receive NSAIDs (see Contraindications). NSAIDs may cause serious dermatologic adverse reactions including exfoliative dermatitis, Stevens-Johnson syndrome, and toxic epidermal necrolysis. Avoid use of NSAIDs in late pregnancy as they may cause premature closure of the ductus arteriosus. Avoid the use of diclofenac in patients with hepatic porphyria (eg, variegate porphyria, acute intermittent porphyria, porphyria cutanea tarda); acute attacks of porphyria may occur.

Cases of drug-induced hepatotoxicity, including hepatic failure resulting in death or requiring transplantation, have been reported. A potential for liver function test elevation exists with use of any diclofenac-containing product. Transaminase elevations generally occur within the first 2 months of therapy but may occur at any time; initiate monitoring after 4-8 weeks of therapy. Discontinue therapy immediately if abnormal liver tests persist or worsen, if clinical signs and/or symptoms consistent with liver disease develop, or if systemic manifestations occur (eg, eosinophilia, rash, abdominal pain, diarrhea, dark urine).

Transdermal patch (used and unused) contains a large amount of medication which can cause serious adverse effects in children or pets if patch is chewed or ingested; fold used patches so the adhesive side sticks to itself; store and dispose used patches properly and out of the reach of children and pets. Transdermal patch contains conducting metal (aluminum) which may cause a burn to the skin during an MRI scan; remove patch prior to MRI; reapply patch after scan is completed. Due to the potential for altered electrical conductivity, remove transdermal patch before cardioversion or defibrillation. Apply transdermal patch only to intact skin. Do not apply topical patch to the eyes, mucous membranes, open wounds, infected areas, or to exudative dermatitis. Patch should not be worn during bathing or showering.

Topical gel 3% contains benzyl alcohol which may cause allergic reactions in susceptible individuals; large amounts of benzyl alcohol (≥99 mg/kg/day) have been associated with a potentially fatal toxicity ("gasping syndrome") in neonates; avoid use of diclofenac products containing benzyl alcohol in neonates; in vitro and animal studies have shown that benzoate, a metabolite of benzyl alcohol, displaces bilirubin from protein binding sites. Topical gel 1% and transdermal patch contain propylene glycol.

Precautions Use with caution and decrease the dose in patients with decreased hepatic function; closely monitor patients with abnormal LFTs; severe hepatic reactions (eg, fulminant hepatitis, liver failure) have occurred (see Warnings). Use with caution in patients with asthma; asthmatic patients may have aspirin-sensitive asthma which may be associated with severe and potentially fatal bronchospasm when aspirin or NSAIDs are administered (see Contraindications). Anemia (due to occult or gross blood loss from the GI tract, fluid retention, or other effect on erythropoiesis) may occur; monitor hemoglobin and hematocrit in patients receiving long term therapy. Use with caution and monitor carefully in patients with coagulation disorders or those receiving anticoagulants; NSAIDs inhibit platelet aggregation and may prolong bleeding time.

Patients should not wear soft contact lenses while using ophthalmic solution; do not apply topical gel to open skin wounds, infections, or exfoliative dermatitis; do not allow gel to come in contact with eyes; do not use topical gel in neonates, infants, or children

Adverse Reactions

Central nervous system: Dizziness, headache

Dermatologic: Pruritus, rash; topical use: Contact dermatitis, dry skin, rash, skin exfoliation (scaling), skin irritation

Endocrine & metabolic: Fluid retention

Gastrointestinal: Abdominal pain, constipation, diarrhea, GI bleeding, GI perforation, indigestion, peptic ulcer

Hematologic: Agranulocytosis, aplastic anemia (rare), inhibition of platelet aggregation

Hepatic: ALT or AST increased, hepatic failure, hepatitis, jaundice

Ocular: With ophthalmic use: Burning, irritation, itching, ocular irritation with use of hydrogel redness, soft contact lenses, tearing (allergic reaction)

Otic: Tinnitus

Renal: Nephrotic-like syndrome, renal impairment

Drug Interactions

Metabolism/Transport Effects Substrate (minor) of CYP1A2, 2B6, 2C8, 2C9, 2C19, 2D6, 3A4; **Inhibits** CYP1A2 (moderate), 2C9 (weak), 2E1 (weak), 3A4 (weak)

Avoid Concomitant Use

Avoid concomitant use of Diclofenac with any of the following: Ketorolac; Ketorolac (Systemic)

Increased Effect/Toxicity

Diclofenac may increase the levels/effects of: Amino-glycosides; Anticoagulants; Antiplatelet Agents; Bisphosphonate Derivatives; Collagenase (Systemic); CycloSPORINE; CycloSPORINE (Systemic); CYP1A2 Substrates; Desmopressin; Digoxin; Drotrecogin Alfa; Eplerenone; Haloperidol; Ibritumomab; Lithium; Metho-trexate; Nonsteroidal Anti-Inflammatory Agents; Peme-trexed; Potassium-Sparing Diuretics; Pralatrexate; Quinolone Antibiotics; Salicylates; Thrombolytic Agents; Tositumomab and Iodine I 131 Tositumomab; Vancomy-cin; Vitamin K Antagonists

The levels/effects of Diclofenac may be increased by: Antidepressants (Tricyclic, Tertiary Amine); Corticoste-roids (Systemic); Dasatinib; Glucosamine; Herbs (Anti-coagulant/Antiplatelet Properties); Ketorolac; Ketorolac (Systemic); Nonsteroidal Anti-Inflammatory Agents; Omega-3-Acid Ethyl Esters; Pentosan Polysulfate Sodium; Pentoxifylline; Probenecid; Prostacyclin Ana-logues; Selective Serotonin Reuptake Inhibitors; Seroto-nin/Norepinephrine Reuptake Inhibitors; Treprostinil; Voriconazole

Decreased Effect

Diclofenac may decrease the levels/effects of: ACE Inhibitors; Angiotensin II Receptor Blockers; Antiplatelet Agents; Beta-Blockers; Eplerenone; HydrALAZINE; Lata-noprost; Loop Diuretics; Potassium-Sparing Diuretics; Thiazide Diuretics

The levels/effects of Diclofenac may be decreased by: Bile Acid Sequestrants; Nonsteroidal Anti-Inflammatory Agents; Peginterferon Alfa-2b

Food Interactions Delayed oral absorption has been reported with food for single doses but not with chronic multiple-dose administration

Stability

Ophthalmic solution: Store at room temperature; protect from light

Tablets: Store at ≤30°C (86°F); protect from moisture; dispense in tight container

Topical gel: Store at room temperature; protect from heat; do not freeze

Transdermal patch: Store at controlled room temperature 25°C (77°F); excursions permitted to 15°C to 30°C (59°F to 86°F). Keep envelope sealed when not being used.

Mechanism of Action Inhibits prostaglandin synthesis by decreasing the activity of the enzyme, cyclooxygenase, which results in decreased formation of prostaglandin precursors

Pharmacokinetics (Adult data unless noted)

Absorption: Topical gel: 10%

Distribution: V_d: 1.4 L/kg

Protein binding: >99%

Metabolism: In the liver; undergoes hydroxylation then glucuronide and sulfate conjugation

Bioavailability: Oral: 50%

Half-life: 2.3 hours

Time to peak serum concentration:

Cataflam®: 1 hour

Voltaren®: 2.22 hours

Voltaren®-XR: 5.25 hours

Elimination: About 65% of the dose is eliminated in the urine and ~35% in the bile (primarily as conjugated forms); little or no unchanged drug is excreted in urine or bile

Usual Dosage Note: Cataflam® tablets are immediate release and is the formulation which should be used when prompt onset of pain relief is desired; Voltaren®-XR should not be used for acute pain relief due to its extended release

Oral:

Children: 2-3 mg/kg/day divided 2-4 times/day; maximum dose: 200 mg/day

Adults:

Rheumatoid arthritis:

Cataflam® or Voltaren®: 100-200 mg/day in 2-4 divided doses; maximum dose: 225 mg/day

Voltaren®-XR: 100 mg/day; dose may be increased to 100 mg twice daily; maximum dose: 200 mg/day

Osteoarthritis:

Cataflam® or Voltaren®: 100-150 mg/day in 2-3 divided doses

Voltaren®-XR: 100 mg/day

Ankylosing spondylitis: Voltaren®: 100-125 mg/day in 4-5 divided doses

Analgesia and primary dysmenorrhea: Cataflam®: 50 mg given 3 times/day; some patients may have better relief with an initial dose of 100 mg

Ophthalmic: Adults:

Cataract surgery: Instill 1 drop into affected eye 4 times/day beginning 24 hours after cataract surgery and continuing for 2 weeks

Corneal refractive surgery: Instill 1-2 drops into operative eye within the hour prior to surgery, within 15 minutes after surgery, and continuing 4 times/day for up to 3 days

Topical: Adults:

Actinic keratosis: (Solaraze® Gel): Apply 3% gel to affected area twice daily; recommended duration of therapy: 60-90 days

Acute pain (strains, sprains, contusions): Topical (patch): Apply 1 patch twice daily to most painful area of skin

Osteoarthritis: (Voltaren® Gel): **Note:** Maximum total body dose of 1% gel should not exceed 32 g per day

Lower extremities: Apply 4 g of 1% gel to affected area 4 times daily (maximum: 16 g per joint per day)

Upper extremities: Apply 2 g of 1% gel to affected area 4 times daily (maximum: 8 g per joint per day)

Dosing adjustment in renal impairment: Not recom-mended in patients with advanced renal disease or significant renal impairment.

Dosing adjustment in hepatic impairment: Dosage adjustment may be required

Administration

Ophthalmic: Avoid contact of bottle tip with skin or eye; apply finger pressure to lacrimal sac during and for 1-2 minutes after instillation to decrease risk of absorption and systemic effects. Wait at least 5 minutes before administering other types of eye drops.

Oral: Administer with milk or food to decrease GI upset; do not chew or crush delayed release or extended release tablets, swallow whole

Topical gel: Do not apply topical gel to the eyes, mucous membranes, open wounds, infected areas, or to exfoliative dermatitis. Avoid sunlight exposure to treated areas.

1% formulation: Use dosing card supplied with product to measure correct amount of medication. Apply gel to affected joint and rub into skin gently, making sure to apply to entire joint. Do not cover area with occlusive dressings or apply sunscreens, cosmetics, other medications, or external heat to affected area. Do not wash area for 1 hour following application. Wash hands immediately after application (unless hands are treated joint). Avoid wearing clothes or gloves for at least 10 minutes after applying gel.

3% formulation: Apply a small amount of gel to affected area; smooth gently over lesion; usually 0.5 g of gel is used per 5 x 5 cm lesion site. Do not cover lesion with occlusive dressings or apply sunscreens, cosmetics, or other medications to affected area.

Transdermal patch: Apply to intact, nondamaged skin. Remove transparent liner prior to applying to skin. Wash hands after applying, handling, or removal of patch. Avoid contact with eyes. May tape down edges of patch, if peeling occurs. Should not be worn while bathing or showering. Fold used patches so the adhesive side sticks to itself; dispose of used patches out of reach of children and pets (see Warnings).

Monitoring Parameters CBC, liver enzymes (periodically during chronic therapy starting 4-8 weeks after initiation); monitor urine output, BUN, serum creatinine in patients receiving diuretics

Patient Information
Oral use: Avoid alcohol; report any signs of blood in stool, GI bleeding, weight gain, edema, skin rash, yellow skin

Ophthalmic use: Do not use hydrogel soft contact lenses during ophthalmic diclofenac therapy

Topical use: Avoid exposure to sunlight or sunlamps; notify physician if rash occurs

Additional Information Vomiting, drowsiness, and acute renal failure have been reported with overdoses; the safety of concurrent use of cosmetics, sunscreens, or other topical agents with diclofenac gel is not known

Dosage Forms Excipient information presented when available (limited, particularly for generics); consult specific product labeling. [DSC] = Discontinued product; [CAN] = Canadian product [not available in U.S]
Capsule, liquid filled, oral, as potassium:
Zipsor™: 25 mg [contains gelatin]
Gel, topical, as diethylamine:
Voltaren® Emulgel™ [CAN]: 1.16% (20 g, 50 g, 100 g)
Gel, topical, as sodium:
Solaraze®: 3% (50 g, 100 g) [contains benzyl alcohol]
Voltaren® Gel: 1% (100 g) [contains isopropyl alcohol]
Patch, transdermal, as epolamine:
Flector®: 1.3% (30s) [180 mg]
Solution, ophthalmic, as sodium [drops]: 0.1% (2.5 mL, 5 mL)
Voltaren Ophthalmic®: 0.1% (2.5 mL, 5 mL) [contains sorbic acid]
Solution, topical, as sodium:
Pennsaid®: 1.5% (150 mL)
Suppository, rectal, as sodium [CAN]:
Voltaren®: 50 mg, 100 mg
Tablet, oral, as potassium: 50 mg
Cataflam®: 50 mg
Tablet, delayed release, enteric coated, oral, as sodium: 50 mg, 75 mg
Voltaren®: 75 mg [DSC]
Tablet, extended release, oral, as sodium: 100 mg
Voltaren®-XR: 100 mg

References
Brogden RN, Heel RC, Pakes GE, et al, "Diclofenac Sodium: A Review of Its Pharmacological Properties and Therapeutic Use in Rheumatic Diseases and Pain of Varying Origin," Drugs, 1980, 20(1):24-48.
Haapasaari J, Wuolijoki E, and Ylijoki H, "Treatment of Juvenile Rheumatoid Arthritis With Diclofenac Sodium" Scand J Rheumatol, 1983, 12(4):325-30.

♦ **Diclofenac Diethylamine [CAN]** see Diclofenac on page 429

♦ **Diclofenac ECT (Can)** see Diclofenac on page 429

♦ **Diclofenac Epolamine** see Diclofenac on page 429

♦ **Diclofenac Potassium** see Diclofenac on page 429

♦ **Diclofenac Sodium** see Diclofenac on page 429

♦ **Diclofenac SR (Can)** see Diclofenac on page 429

Dicloxacillin (dye kloks a SIL in)

Canadian Brand Names Dycill®; Pathocil®
Therapeutic Category Antibiotic, Penicillin (Antistaphylococcal)
Generic Available Yes
Use Treatment of skin and soft tissue infections, pneumonia and follow-up therapy of osteomyelitis caused by susceptible penicillinase-producing staphylococci
Pregnancy Risk Factor B

Pregnancy Considerations Adverse events have not been observed in animal studies; therefore, dicloxacillin is classified as pregnancy category B. Dicloxacillin crosses the placenta. Teratogenic effects have not been reported with dicloxacillin, but adequate and well-controlled studies of dicloxacillin have not been completed in pregnant women. Other penicillins are considered safe for use in pregnancy.

Lactation Excretion in breast milk unknown/use caution

Breast-Feeding Considerations It is not known if dicloxacillin crosses into human milk. The manufacturer recommends that caution be exercised when administering dicloxacillin to nursing women. Other penicillins distribute into human milk and are considered safe for use during breast-feeding. Nondose-related effects could include modification of bowel flora.

Contraindications Hypersensitivity to dicloxacillin, penicillin, or any component

Warnings Elimination is prolonged in neonates

Adverse Reactions
Central nervous system: Fever
Dermatologic: Rash
Gastrointestinal: Nausea, vomiting, diarrhea, C. difficile colitis
Hematologic: Eosinophilia, neutropenia, leukopenia, thrombocytopenia
Hepatic: Liver enzymes elevated
Miscellaneous: Serum sickness-like reaction

Drug Interactions
Metabolism/Transport Effects Induces CYP3A4 (weak)

Avoid Concomitant Use
Avoid concomitant use of Dicloxacillin with any of the following: BCG

Increased Effect/Toxicity
Dicloxacillin may increase the levels/effects of: Methotrexate

The levels/effects of Dicloxacillin may be increased by: Probenecid

Decreased Effect
Dicloxacillin may decrease the levels/effects of: BCG; Mycophenolate; Saxagliptin; Typhoid Vaccine; Vitamin K Antagonists

The levels/effects of Dicloxacillin may be decreased by: Fusidic Acid; Tetracycline Derivatives

Food Interactions Food decreases the rate and extent of absorption

Mechanism of Action Inhibits bacterial cell wall synthesis by binding to one or more of the penicillin-binding proteins and interfering with the final transpeptidation step of peptidoglycan synthesis

Pharmacokinetics (Adult data unless noted)
Absorption: 35% to 76% absorbed from the GI tract
Distribution: Into bone, bile, pleural fluid, synovial fluid, and amniotic fluid; appears in breast milk
Protein binding: 96% to 98%
Half-life: Adults: 0.6-0.8 hours; slightly prolonged in patients with renal impairment
Time to peak serum concentration: Within 0.5-2 hours
Elimination: Partially eliminated by the liver and excreted in bile; 31% to 65% eliminated in urine as unchanged drug and active metabolite
Neonates: Prolonged
CF patients: More rapid elimination than healthy patients
Dialysis: Not dialyzable (0% to 5%)

Usual Dosage Oral:

Children <40 kg: 25-50 mg/kg/day divided every 6 hours; doses of 50-100 mg/kg/day in divided doses every 6 hours have been used for follow-up therapy of osteomyelitis; maximum dose: 2 g/day

Children >40 kg and Adults: 125-500 mg every 6 hours; maximum dose: 2 g/day

Administration Oral: Administer with water 1 hour before or 2 hours after meals on an empty stomach

Monitoring Parameters Periodic monitoring of CBC, platelet count, BUN, serum creatinine, urinalysis, and liver enzymes during prolonged therapy

Additional Information Sodium content of 250 mg capsule: 0.6 mEq

Dosage Forms Excipient information presented when available (limited, particularly for generics); consult specific product labeling.

Capsule: 250 mg, 500 mg

◆ **Dicloxacillin Sodium** see Dicloxacillin on page 432

Dicyclomine (dye SYE kloe meen)

Medication Safety Issues

Sound-alike/look-alike issues:

Dicyclomine may be confused with diphenhydrAMINE, doxycycline, dyclonine

Bentyl® may be confused with Aventyl®, Benadryl®, Bontril®, Cantil®, Proventil®, Trental®

Beers Criteria medication: This drug may be inappropriate for use in geriatric patients (high severity risk).

U.S. Brand Names Bentyl®

Canadian Brand Names Bentylol®; Formulex®; Lomine; Riva-Dicyclomine

Therapeutic Category Anticholinergic Agent; Antispasmodic Agent, Gastrointestinal

Generic Available Yes: Excludes syrup

Use Treatment of functional bowel/irritable bowel syndrome

Pregnancy Risk Factor B

Pregnancy Considerations Teratogenic effects have not been observed in animal studies.

Lactation Enters breast milk/contraindicated

Contraindications Hypersensitivity to dicyclomine or any component; narrow-angle glaucoma, tachycardia, GI obstruction, obstruction of the urinary tract, severe ulcerative colitis, myasthenia gravis; should not be used in infants <6 months of age (due to reports of respiratory distress, seizures, syncope, asphyxia, pulse rate fluctuations, muscular hypotonia, and coma), nursing mothers

Warnings Heat prostration may occur in the presence of increased environmental temperature; use caution in hot weather and/or exercise. Psychosis has been reported in patients with an extreme sensitivity to anticholinergic effects.

Precautions Use with caution in patients with hepatic or renal disease, mild-moderate ulcerative colitis, hyperthyroidism, coronary heart disease, CHF, cardiac tachyarrhythmias, hypertension, hiatal hernia, autonomic neuropathy

Adverse Reactions Children with Down's syndrome, spastic paralysis, or brain damage are more sensitive to toxic effects than adults

Cardiovascular: Tachycardia, palpitations, orthostatic hypotension

Central nervous system: Seizures, coma, nervousness, excitement, confusion, insomnia, headache, dizziness, lightheadedness, drowsiness, lethargy, speech disturbance, syncope

Dermatologic: Urticaria, pruritus, dry skin, rash

Gastrointestinal: Nausea, vomiting, constipation, xerostomia, dry throat, dysphagia, taste loss, anorexia

Genitourinary: Urinary retention

Local: Injection site reactions (I.M. injection)

Neuromuscular & skeletal: Muscular hypotonia, weakness, tingling, numbness

Ocular: Blurred vision, diplopia, mydriasis, cycloplegia, ocular tension increased, photophobia

Respiratory: Respiratory distress, asphyxia, dry nose, nasal stuffiness, apnea, sneezing

Miscellaneous: Diaphoresis decreased

Drug Interactions

Avoid Concomitant Use There are no known interactions where it is recommended to avoid concomitant use.

Increased Effect/Toxicity

Dicyclomine may increase the levels/effects of: AbobotulinumtoxinA; Anticholinergics; Cannabinoids; OnabotulinumtoxinA; Potassium Chloride; RimabotulinumtoxinB

The levels/effects of Dicyclomine may be increased by: Pramlintide

Decreased Effect

Dicyclomine may decrease the levels/effects of: Acetylcholinesterase Inhibitors (Central); Secretin

The levels/effects of Dicyclomine may be decreased by: Acetylcholinesterase Inhibitors (Central)

Stability Protect from light

Mechanism of Action Blocks the action of acetylcholine at parasympathetic sites in smooth muscle, secretory glands and the CNS

Pharmacodynamics

Onset of action: 1-2 hours

Duration: Up to 4 hours

Pharmacokinetics (Adult data unless noted)

Absorption: Oral: Well absorbed

Distribution: V_d: 3.65 L/kg

Bioavailability: 67%

Half-life:

Initial phase: 1.8 hours

Terminal phase: 9-10 hours

Time to peak serum concentration: Oral: 1-1.5 hours

Elimination: 80% in urine; 10% in feces

Usual Dosage

Infants >6 months: Oral: 5 mg/dose 3-4 times/day

Children: Oral: 10 mg/dose 3-4 times/day

Adults:

Oral: Initial: 20 mg 4 times/day, then increase up to 40 mg 4 times/day

I.M.: 20 mg/dose 4 times/day; oral therapy should replace I.M. therapy as soon as possible

Administration

Oral: Administer 30 minutes before eating

Parenteral: I.M. only; not for I.V. use

Patient Information Limit alcohol; may cause dry mouth; may cause drowsiness and impair ability to perform activities requiring mental alertness or physical coordination

Dosage Forms Excipient information presented when available (limited, particularly for generics); consult specific product labeling.

Capsule, as hydrochloride: 10 mg

Bentyl®: 10 mg

Injection, solution, as hydrochloride: 10 mg/mL (2 mL)

Bentyl®: 10 mg/mL (2 mL)

Syrup, as hydrochloride:

Bentyl®: 10 mg/5 mL (480 mL) [contains propylene glycol]

Tablet, as hydrochloride: 20 mg

Bentyl®: 20 mg

◆ **Dicyclomine Hydrochloride** see Dicyclomine on page 433

♦ **Dicycloverine Hydrochloride** *see* Dicyclomine *on page 433*

Didanosine (dye DAN oh seen)

Medication Safety Issues
Sound-alike/look-alike issues:
Videx® may be confused with Lidex®

Related Information
Adult and Adolescent HIV *on page 1620*
Management of Healthcare Worker Exposures to HBV, HCV, and HIV *on page 1661*
Pediatric HIV *on page 1613*
Perinatal HIV *on page 1628*

U.S. Brand Names Videx®; Videx® EC

Canadian Brand Names Videx®; Videx® EC

Therapeutic Category Antiretroviral Agent; HIV Agents (Anti-HIV Agents); Nucleoside Reverse Transcriptase Inhibitor (NRTI)

Generic Available Yes: Delayed release capsule

Use Treatment of HIV infection in combination with other antiretroviral agents (FDA approved in ages ≥2 weeks and adults); (**Note:** HIV regimens consisting of **three** antiretroviral agents are strongly recommended)

Medication Guide An FDA-approved patient medication guide, which is available with the product information and as follows, must be dispensed with this medication for each new outpatient prescription and refill.

Videx®: http://www.fda.gov/downloads/Drugs/DrugSafety/UCM199211.pdf

Videx® EC: http://www.fda.gov/downloads/Drug-Safety/UCM199212.pdf

Pregnancy Risk Factor B

Pregnancy Considerations Adverse events have not been observed in animal reproduction studies. Cases of fatal and nonfatal lactic acidosis, with or without pancreatitis, have been reported in pregnant women. It is not known if pregnancy itself potentiates this known side effect; however, pregnant women may be at increased risk of lactic acidosis and liver damage. Hepatic enzymes and electrolytes should be monitored frequently during the 3rd trimester of pregnancy. Use during pregnancy only if the potential benefit to the mother outweighs the potential risk of this complication. Didanosine has been shown to cross the placenta. Pharmacokinetics are not significantly altered during pregnancy; dose adjustments are not needed. The Perinatal HIV Guidelines Working Group considers didanosine to be an alternative NRTI in dual nucleoside combination regimens; use with stavudine only if no other alternatives are available. Health professionals are encouraged to contact the antiretroviral pregnancy registry to monitor outcomes of pregnant women exposed to antiretroviral medications (1-800-258-4263 or www.APRegistry.com).

Lactation Excretion in breast milk unknown/contraindicated

Breast-Feeding Considerations In infants born to mothers who are HIV positive, HAART while breast-feeding may decrease postnatal infection. However, maternal or infant antiretroviral therapy does not completely eliminate the risk of postnatal HIV transmission.

In the United States where formula is accessible, affordable, safe, and sustainable, complete avoidance of breast-feeding by HIV-infected women is recommended to decrease potential transmission of HIV.

Contraindications Hypersensitivity to didanosine or any component; concurrent therapy with allopurinol or ribavirin

Warnings Fatal and nonfatal pancreatitis have been reported during therapy **[U.S. Boxed Warning]**; risk factors for developing pancreatitis include a previous history of the condition, higher doses (eg, >10 mg/kg/day), renal impairment without dose adjustment, concurrent CMV or MAC infection, advanced HIV infection, and concomitant use of stavudine with or without hydroxyurea (see Drug Interactions); use didanosine with extreme caution and only if clearly indicated in patients with risk factors for pancreatitis; discontinue didanosine if clinical signs of pancreatitis occur; only after pancreatitis has been ruled out should dosing be resumed. Dose-related (treatment-limiting) peripheral neuropathy occurs most often after 2-6 months of continuous didanosine administration; may occur more frequently in patients with a history of neuropathy, advanced HIV disease, or concurrent treatment with neurotoxic drugs, including stavudine or hydroxyurea; consider discontinuation of didanosine in patients who develop peripheral neuropathy. Retinal depigmentation in children receiving doses >300 mg/m^2/day may occur; retinal changes and optic neuritis have been reported in pediatric and adult patients; perform periodic retinal examinations (see Monitoring Parameters).

Cases of lactic acidosis, severe hepatomegaly with steatosis, and death have been reported in patients receiving nucleoside analogs **[U.S. Boxed Warning]**; most of these cases have been in women; prolonged nucleoside use, obesity, and prior liver disease may be risk factors; use with extreme caution in patients with other risk factors for liver disease; discontinue therapy in patients who develop laboratory or clinical evidence of lactic acidosis or pronounced hepatotoxicity. Fatal lactic acidosis has occurred in pregnant women who received didanosine plus stavudine with other antiretroviral agents; use didanosine plus stavudine with caution during pregnancy and only if benefit outweighs risks.

Didanosine-associated noncirrhotic portal hypertension may occur; cases leading to liver transplantation or death have been reported. Onset of signs and symptoms of portal hypertension occurred within months to years of initiating didanosine. Patients may present with increased liver enzymes, hematemesis, esophageal varices, splenomegaly, and ascites. Monitor patients for early signs of portal hypertension (eg, splenomegaly, thrombocytopenia); consider appropriate laboratory testing (see Monitoring Parameters); discontinue didanosine in patients with evidence of noncirrhotic portal hypertension.

Precautions Use with caution in patients with renal or hepatic impairment. Adjust dosage in patients with renal impairment. Monitor patients with hepatic impairment closely; these patients may be at risk for didanosine-associated liver function abnormalities, including severe and potentially fatal hepatic adverse events. Avoid using the combination of didanosine, stavudine, and hydroxyurea; fatal hepatic events were reported most often in HIV patients receiving this combination. Due to an increased risk of serious toxicities, the combined use of stavudine and didanosine is **not** recommended, unless the potential benefit clearly outweighs the risks (see Panel on Antiretroviral Guidelines for Adults and Adolescents, 2009 and Working Group on Antiretroviral Therapy and Medical Management of HIV-Infected Children, 2009).

Fat redistribution and accumulation [ie, central obesity, peripheral wasting, facial wasting, breast enlargement, dorsocervical fat enlargement (buffalo hump), and cushingoid appearance] have been observed in patients receiving antiretroviral agents (causal relationship not established). Immune reconstitution syndrome (an acute inflammatory response to residual or indolent opportunistic infections) may occur in HIV patients during initial treatment with combination antiretroviral agents, including didanosine; this syndrome may require further patient assessment and therapy.

Safety and efficacy of didanosine delayed-release capsules have not been established in pediatric patients <20 kg. **Note:** Oral chewable buffered tablets are no longer available.

Adverse Reactions

Central nervous system: CNS depression, headache, insomnia, malaise

Dermatologic: Pruritus, rash

Endocrine & metabolic: Fat redistribution and accumulation (see Precautions), hyperuricemia, hypokalemia, lactic acidosis, triglycerides increased

Gastrointestinal: Abdominal pain, amylase increased, diarrhea, nausea, pancreatitis [Adults: 1% to 7%; dose-related, less common in children (up to 3% with normal doses) than adults], stomatitis, vomiting

Hepatic: Hepatic failure, liver enzymes increased, portal hypertension (noncirrhotic; see Warnings), severe hepatomegaly with steatosis

Neuromuscular & skeletal: Arthritis, peripheral neuropathy (dose-related), weakness

Ocular: Optic neuritis, retinal depigmentation

Respiratory: Cough, dyspnea

Miscellaneous: Immune reconstitution syndrome (see Precautions)

<1%, postmarketing, and/or case reports: Acute renal impairment, alopecia, anaphylactoid reaction, anemia, anorexia, arthralgia, chills/fever, diabetes mellitus, dry eyes, dyspepsia, flatulence, granulocytopenia, hepatic steatosis, hepatitis, hyper-/hypoglycemia, hyperlactatemia (symptomatic), hypersensitivity, leukopenia, myalgia, myopathy, pain, parotid gland enlargement, rhabdomyolysis, sialoadenitis, thrombocytopenia, weakness, xerostomia

Drug Interactions

Avoid Concomitant Use

Avoid concomitant use of Didanosine with any of the following: Alcohol (Ethyl); Allopurinol; Febuxostat; Hydroxyurea; Ribavirin

Increased Effect/Toxicity

Didanosine may increase the levels/effects of: Hydroxyurea

The levels/effects of Didanosine may be increased by: Alcohol (Ethyl); Allopurinol; Febuxostat; Ganciclovir-Valganciclovir; Hydroxyurea; Ribavirin; Stavudine; Tenofovir

Decreased Effect

Didanosine may decrease the levels/effects of: Antifungal Agents (Azole Derivatives, Systemic); Atazanavir; Dapsone; Dapsone (Systemic); Indinavir; Quinolone Antibiotics

The levels/effects of Didanosine may be decreased by: Atazanavir; Darunavir; Lopinavir; Methadone; Tenofovir; Tipranavir

Food Interactions Food significantly decreases bioavailability. Food decreases the bioavailability of the delayed release capsules by 19%. Do not mix with fruit juice or other acid-containing liquid since didanosine is unstable in acidic solutions

Stability Undergoes rapid degradation when exposed to an acidic environment; 10% of the drug decomposes to hypoxanthine in <2 minutes at pH <3 at 37°C.

Delayed release capsules: Store in tightly closed bottles at 25°C (77°F); excursions permitted to 15°C to 30°C (59°F to 86°F).

Powder for oral solution: Unreconstituted powder should be stored at 15°C to 30°C (59°F to 86°F). Powder for oral solution is unbuffered and must be reconstituted with water and mixed with an equal volume of double-strength antacid at time of preparation. Reconstituted solution (10 mg/mL) is stable for 30 days if refrigerated; discard unused portion after 30 days. When unbuffered powder for oral solution is reconstituted and admixed with a double-strength antacid to make a 20 mg/mL solution for adult once-daily dosing, the admixture is stable for 24 hours at room temperature and for 30 days if refrigerated

Mechanism of Action A purine dideoxynucleoside analog converted within the cell to an active metabolite, dideoxyadenosine triphosphate which serves as a substrate and inhibitor of viral RNA-directed DNA polymerase resulting in premature termination of viral DNA synthesis

Pharmacokinetics (Adult data unless noted)

Absorption: Subject to degradation by acidic pH of stomach; some formulations are buffered to resist acidic pH. Delayed release capsules contain enteric-coated beadlets which dissolve in the small intestine.

Distribution: Extensive intracellular distribution; crosses the placenta

CSF/plasma ratio:

Infants 8 months to Adolescents 19 years: 46% (range: 12% to 85%)

Adults: 21%

V_d:

Infants 8 months to Adolescents 19 years: 28 ± 15 L/m^2

Adults: 43.7 ± 8.9 L/m^2

V_d (apparent):

Children 20 kg to <25 kg: 98 ± 30 L

Children 25 kg to <60 kg: 155 ± 55 L

Children ≥60 kg: 363 ± 138 L

Adults ≥60 kg: 308 ± 164 L

Protein binding: <5%

Metabolism: Converted intracellularly to active triphosphate form; presumed to be metabolized via the same metabolic pathway as endogenous purines

Bioavailability: Variable and affected by the presence of food in the GI tract, gastric pH, and the dosage form administered

Infants 8 months to Adolescents 19 years: 25% ± 20%

Adults: 42% ± 12%

Half-life:

Plasma:

Newborns (1 day old): 2 ± 0.7 hours

Infants 2 weeks to 4 months: 1.2 ± 0.3 hours

Infants 8 months to Adolescents 19 years: 0.8 ± 0.3 hours

Adults with normal renal function: 1.5 ± 0.4 hours

Intracellular: Adults: 25-40 hours

Elimination:

Children 20 kg to <25 kg: 0.75 ± 0.13 hours

Children 25 kg to <60 kg: 0.92 ± 0.09 hours

Children ≥60 kg: 1.26 ± 0.19 hours

Adults ≥60 kg: 1.19 ± 21 hours

Time to peak serum concentration: Delayed release capsules: 2 hours; Oral solution: 0.25-1.5 hours

Elimination: Unchanged drug excreted in urine

Infants 8 months to Adolescents 19 years: 18% ± 10%

Adults: 18% ± 8%

Usual Dosage Oral: (Use in combination with other antiretroviral agents):

Neonates and Infants 2 weeks to 8 months: Oral solution: 100 mg/m^2/dose every 12 hours

Infants >8 months and Children:

Oral solution: 120 mg/m^2/dose every 12 hours; do not exceed adult dose; **Note:** Pediatric clinical studies used doses of 90-150 mg/m^2/dose every 12 hours; once-daily dosing of the oral solution is **not** FDA approved in children; limited data is available; (see Additional Information)

◀ Children 6-18 years:
Delayed-release capsule (see also Additional Information):
20 kg to <25 kg: 200 mg once daily
25 kg to <60 kg: 250 mg once daily
≥60 kg: 400 mg once daily
Adolescents and Adults:
Oral solution: **Note:** Although once-daily dosing is available, it should only be considered for adolescent/adult patients whose management requires once-daily administration (eg, to enhance compliance); the preferred dosing frequency of didanosine oral solution is twice daily because there is more evidence to support the effectiveness of this dosing frequency
<60 kg: 125 mg every 12 hours **or** 250 mg once daily
≥60 kg: 200 mg every 12 hours **or** 400 mg once daily using a special Videx® solution in double-strength antacid which provides 400 mg/20 mL for once-daily dosing
Delayed-release capsule:
20 kg to <25 kg: 200 mg once daily
25 kg to <60 kg: 250 mg once daily
≥60 kg: 400 mg once daily
Adults: **Coadministration with tenofovir:** Reduce the dose of didanosine when used in combination with tenofovir; **Note:** Dose of didanosine with concomitant tenofovir in patients with Cl_{cr} < 60 mL/minute or in patients <18 years has not been established
Adults <60 kg: Didanosine 200 mg once daily with tenofovir 300 mg once daily
Adults ≥60 kg: Didanosine 250 mg once daily with tenofovir 300 mg once daily
Dosing adjustment in renal impairment:
Neonates, Infants, and Children: Insufficient data exists to recommend a specific dosage adjustment; however, a decrease in the dose should be considered in pediatric patients with renal impairment
Adults: Dosing based on patient weight, creatinine clearance, and dosage form:
Dosing for patients <60 kg:
Cl_{cr} 30-59 mL/minute:
Oral solution: 75 mg twice daily or 150 mg once daily
Delayed-release capsule: 125 mg once daily
Cl_{cr} 10-29 mL/minute:
Oral solution: 100 mg once daily
Delayed-release capsule: 125 mg once daily
Cl_{cr} <10 mL/minute:
Oral solution: 75 mg once daily
Delayed-release capsule: Use alternate formulation
Dosing for patients ≥60 kg:
Cl_{cr} 30-59 mL/minute:
Oral solution: 100 mg twice daily or 200 mg once daily
Delayed-release capsule: 200 mg once daily
Cl_{cr} 10-29 mL/minute:
Oral solution: 150 mg once daily
Delayed-release capsule: 125 mg once daily
Cl_{cr} <10 mL/minute:
Oral solution: 100 mg once daily
Delayed-release capsule: 125 mg once daily
Dosage adjustment in patients requiring continuous ambulatory peritoneal dialysis (CAPD) or hemodialysis: Adults: Use dosing recommendations for patients with Cl_{cr} <10 mL/minute; supplemental doses following hemodialysis are not needed
Dosing adjustment in hepatic impairment: Adults: In a single-dose study, mean AUC and peak serum concentrations of didanosine were 13% and 19% higher, respectively, in adults with moderate-to-severe hepatic impairment (Child-Pugh Class B or C). However, since a similar range and distribution of AUC and peak concentrations were observed, no dose adjustment is recommended. It is important to monitor patients with hepatic impairment closely for didanosine toxicity.

Patients with hepatic impairment may be at increased risk for didanosine toxicities (see Warnings and Precautions).
Administration Oral: Administer oral solution and delayed release capsule on an empty stomach 30 minutes before or at least 2 hours after a meal. Swallow capsule whole; do not break open or chew. If administered with tenofovir, the delayed release capsule may be administered with a light meal or in the fasted state. Administer didanosine at least 1 hour apart from indinavir. Administer didanosine at least 2 hours apart from ritonavir or atazanavir. Didanosine should be given at least 1 hour before or 2 hours after lopinavir/ritonavir. Nelfinavir should be administered 2 hours before or 1 hour after didanosine. Administer buffered formulations of didanosine at least 1 hour apart from fosamprenavir.

Unbuffered pediatric powder should be reconstituted with water and admixed in equal parts with a double-strength antacid to provide a final concentration of 10 mg/mL; unbuffered pediatric powder has also been reconstituted and admixed with a double-strength antacid to provide a final concentration of 20 mg/mL to be used for once-daily dosing in adults; shake oral solution well before use.
Monitoring Parameters Serum potassium, glucose, uric acid, lactic acid, creatinine; hemoglobin, CBC with neutrophil and platelet count, CD4 cells; HIV RNA plasma level; liver function tests, serum amylase and triglyceride levels; weight gain; perform dilated retinal exam every 6 months; signs and symptoms of peripheral neuropathy

To monitor for portal hypertension: CBC with platelet count, splenomegaly on physical exam, liver enzymes, serum bilirubin, albumin, INR, ultrasound
Patient Information Read the patient Medication Guide that you receive with each prescription and refill of didanosine. Avoid alcohol. Shake oral solution well before use and keep refrigerated; discard solution after 30 days and obtain new supply. The buffered powder vehicle may contribute to the development of diarrhea.

Inform physician if numbness, tingling, or pain in hands or feet; persistent severe abdominal pain, nausea, or vomiting; or changes in vision occur. Didanosine may cause serious and potentially fatal problems of the pancreas and liver. Serious eye problems have also been reported. Frequent blood tests and periodic eye examinations may be required. HIV medications may cause changes in body fat, including an increase in fat in the upper back and neck, breasts, and trunk; a loss of fat from the face, arms, and legs may also occur.

Didanosine is not a cure for HIV. Take didanosine every day as prescribed; do not change dose or discontinue without physician's advice. If a dose is missed, take it as soon as possible, then return to normal dosing schedule; if a dose is skipped, do **not** double the next dose.
Additional Information Once daily, didanosine delayed-release capsules have recently been approved for use in children 6-18 years of age who are ≥20 kg. This approval was based on pharmacokinetic studies; however, limited published literature exists. In a single-dose pharmacokinetic study in children 4-11.5 years of age (n=10; median age: 7.6 years), a dose of 240 mg/m^2 was shown to have a similar plasma AUC as compared to the buffered formulation. However, two patients were excluded from data analysis, one due to extremely low didanosine serum concentrations throughout the dosing interval (see King, 2002). Doses of 240 mg/m^2 once daily, with a maximum of 400 mg once daily, are being studied in pediatric clinical trials. **Note:** In PACTG 1021, treatment-naïve children (3-21 years of age) received 240 mg/m^2/dose once daily (maximum: 400 mg/dose) with good viral suppression (Working Group, 2009). Children with a surface area ≥0.45 m^2 who could swallow capsules received the

delayed-release capsule; the oral suspension was used for smaller children (see McKinney, 2007).

The relative bioavailability of didanosine suspension administered once daily versus twice daily was studied in 24 children, 4.8 ± 2.9 years of age. Didanosine was administered in doses of 90 mg/m^2/dose every 12 hours and 180 mg/m^2/dose once daily. The relative bioavailability of once-daily dosing compared to twice daily dosing was 0.95 ± 0.49 (range: 0.22-1.97). The authors suggest these results support the potential clinical use of once-daily dosing in pediatric patients. However, due to the large inter- and intrasubject variability, these 2 regimens would **not** be considered to be bioequivalent based on FDA criteria (see Abreu, 2000). Further studies are needed.

A high rate of early virologic failure in therapy-naive adult HIV patients has been observed with the once-daily three-drug combination therapy of didanosine enteric-coated beadlets (Videx® EC), lamivudine, and tenofovir and the once-daily three-drug combination therapy of abacavir, lamivudine, and tenofovir. These combinations should not be used or offered at any time. Any patient currently receiving either of these regimens should be closely monitored for virologic failure and considered for treatment modification. Early virologic failure was also observed in therapy-naive adult HIV patients treated with tenofovir, didanosine enteric-coated beadlets (Videx® EC), and either efavirenz or nevirapine; rapid emergence of resistant mutations has also been reported with this combination; the combination of tenofovir, didanosine, and any non-nucleoside reverse transcriptase inhibitor is **not** recommended as initial antiretroviral therapy. **Note:** Didanosine plus tenofovir is **not** recommended as a component to any initial antiretroviral therapy regimen.

One major study found an increased risk of MI in patients receiving didanosine; however, a subsequent study did not find an increased cardiovascular risk (see Panel on Antiretroviral Guidelines, 2008).

Dosage Forms Excipient information presented when available (limited, particularly for generics); consult specific product labeling.

Capsule, delayed release, enteric coated pellets: 200 mg, 250 mg, 400 mg

Capsule, delayed release, enteric coated beadlets:
Videx® EC: 125 mg, 200 mg, 250 mg, 400 mg

Powder for oral solution, pediatric:
Videx®: 2 g, 4 g [makes 10 mg/mL solution after final mixing]

References

Abreu T, Plaisance K, Rexroad V, et al, "Bioavailability of Once- and Twice-Daily Regimens of Didanosine in Human Immunodeficiency Virus-Infected Children," *Antimicrob Agents Chemother*, 2000, 44 (5):1375-6.

Balis FM, Pizzo PA, Butler KM, et al, "Clinical Pharmacology of 2', 3'-Dideoxyinosine in Human Immunodeficiency Virus-Infected Children," *J Infect Dis*, 1992, 165(1):99-104.

Briars LA, Hilao JJ, and Kraus DM, "A Review of Pediatric Human Immunodeficiency Virus Infection," *Journal of Pharmacy Practice*, 2004, 17(6):407-31.

Butler KM, Husson RN, Balis FM, et al, "Dideoxyinosine in Children With Symptomatic Human Immunodeficiency Virus Infection," *N Engl J Med*, 1991, 324(3):137-44.

King JR, Nachman S, Yogev R, et al, "Single-Dose Pharmacokinetics of Enteric-Coated Didanosine in HIV-Infected Children," *Antivir Ther*, 2002, 7(4):267-70.

Kovari H, Ledergerber B, Peter U, et al, "Association of Noncirrhotic Portal Hypertension in HIV-Infected Persons and Antiretroviral Therapy With Didanosine: A Nested Case-Control Study," *Clin Infect Dis*, 2009, 49(4):626-35.

McKinney RE Jr, Rodman J, Hu C, et al, "Long-Term Safety and Efficacy of a Once-Daily Regimen of Emtricitabine, Didanosine, and Efavirenz in HIV-Infected, Therapy-Naive Children and Adolescents: Pediatric AIDS Clinical Trials Group Protocol P1021," *Pediatrics*, 2007, 120(2):e416-23.

Panel on Antiretroviral Guidelines for Adults and Adolescents, "Guidelines for the Use of Antiretroviral Agents in HIV-Infected Adults and Adolescents," December 1, 2009. Available at: http://www.aidsinfo.nih.gov.

Working Group on Antiretroviral Therapy and Medical Management of HIV-Infected Children, "Guidelines for the Use of Antiretroviral Agents in Pediatric HIV Infection," February 23, 2009. Available at http://www.aidsinfo.nih.gov.

♦ **2',3'-didehydro-3'-deoxythymidine** see Stavudine on page 1290

♦ **Dideoxyinosine** see Didanosine on page 434

♦ **Didronel®** see Etidronate Disodium on page 549

♦ **Differin®** see Adapalene on page 50

♦ **Differin® XP (Can)** see Adapalene on page 50

♦ **Diflucan®** see Fluconazole on page 584

♦ **Digibind®** see Digoxin Immune Fab on page 440

♦ **DigiFab™** see Digoxin Immune Fab on page 440

♦ **Digitalis** see Digoxin on page 437

Digoxin (di JOKS in)

Medication Safety Issues
Sound-alike/look-alike issues:
Digoxin may be confused with Desoxyn®, doxepin
Lanoxin® may be confused with Lasix®, levothyroxine, Levoxyl®, Levsinex®, Lomotil®, Lonox®, Mefoxin®, naloxone, Xanax®

High alert medication: The Institute for Safe Medication Practices (ISMP) includes this medication among its list of drugs which have a heightened risk of causing significant patient harm when used in error.

Beers Criteria medication: This drug may be inappropriate for use in geriatric patients (low severity risk).

International issues:
Dilacor®: Brand name for digoxin in Belgium and Serbia, brand name for diltiazem in the U.S.; brand name for verapamil in Brazil; brand name for barnidipine in Argentina
Lanoxin® may be confused with Lemoxin® which is a brand name for cefuroxime in Mexico
Lanoxin® may be confused with Limoxin® which is a brand name for amoxicillin in Mexico

Related Information
Therapeutic Drug Monitoring: Blood Sampling Time Guidelines on page 1704

U.S. Brand Names Lanoxin®

Canadian Brand Names Apo-Digoxin®; Digoxin CSD; Lanoxin®; Pediatric Digoxin CSD; PMS-Digoxin; Toloxin®

Therapeutic Category Antiarrhythmic Agent, Miscellaneous; Cardiac Glycoside

Generic Available Yes

Use Treatment of mild to moderate heart failure (HF) (FDA approved in all ages); chronic atrial fibrillation (rate-control) (FDA approved in adults). Has also been used for fetal tachycardia with or without hydrops; to slow ventricular rate in supraventricular tachyarrhythmias such as supraventricular tachycardias (SVT), excluding atrioventricular reciprocating tachycardia (AVRT)

Pregnancy Risk Factor C

Pregnancy Considerations Animal reproduction studies have not been conducted. Digoxin crosses the placenta and can be detected in the fetus. Digoxin is recommended as first-line in the treatment of fetal tachycardia determined to be SVT. In pregnant women with atrial fibrillation or SVT, use of digoxin is recommended (Class I recommendation; Blomström-Lundqvist, 2003; Fuster, 2006).

Lactation Enters breast milk/use caution (AAP rates "compatible")

Breast-Feeding Considerations Digoxin is excreted into breast milk and similar concentrations are found within mother's serum and milk. Although the manufacturer recommends that caution be used in nursing women, the AAP considers digoxin to be usually compatible with breast-feeding.

Contraindications Hypersensitivity to digoxin (rare), other forms of digitalis, or any component; ventricular fibrillation

Warnings Use with extreme caution in patients with hypoxia, hypothyroidism, acute myocarditis, electrolyte disorders, acute MI. Correct electrolyte disturbances, especially hypokalemia or hypomagnesemia, prior to use and throughout therapy. Hypercalcemia may increase the risk of digoxin toxicity; maintain normocalcemia. Monitor for proarrhythmic effects (especially with toxicity); monitor and adjust dose to prevent QT$_c$ prolongation.

Precautions Use with caution and reduce dosage in patients with renal impairment. Use with caution in patients with sinus nodal disease (may worsen condition). Withdrawal of digoxin in patients with heart failure may lead to recurrence of heart failure symptoms (monitor carefully). Atrial arrhythmias associated with hypermetabolic states are difficult to treat (use with caution). Use with caution in patients with an acute MI (within 6 months); may increase myocardial oxygen demand. During the immediate post-MI period, digoxin administered I.V. may be used in the acute treatment of refractory atrial fibrillation/flutter (especially when HF or LV dysfunction coexists) or refractory re-entrant PSVT (see Antman, 2004).

During an episode of atrial fibrillation or flutter in patients with an accessory bypass tract, digoxin use has been associated with increased anterograde conduction down the accessory pathway leading to ventricular fibrillation; avoid use in such patients. Avoid use in patients with second- or third-degree heart block (except in patients with a functioning artificial pacemaker); incomplete AV block (eg, Stokes-Adams attacks) may progress to complete block with digoxin administration.

HF patients with preserved left ventricular function, including patients with restrictive cardiomyopathy, constrictive pericarditis, and amyloid heart disease, may be susceptible to digoxin toxicity; avoid use unless used to control ventricular response with atrial fibrillation. Digoxin should not be used in patients with low ejection fraction, sinus rhythm, and no HF symptoms since the risk of harm may be greater than clinical benefit (see Hunt, 2009). Outflow obstruction may worsen due to the positive inotropic effects of digoxin; avoid use unless used to control ventricular response with atrial fibrillation.

Use with caution in patients with hypothyroidism; higher digoxin concentrations may result. Use with caution in patients with hyperthyroidism; lower digoxin concentrations may result due to decreased absorption. **Note:** New-onset atrial fibrillation or exacerbation of ventricular arrhythmias should prompt evaluation of thyroid status. Avoid rapid I.V. administration of calcium in digitalized patients; may produce serious arrhythmias. Use with caution in patients taking strong inducers or inhibitors of P-glycoprotein (eg, cyclosporine). Upon initiation of amiodarone, propafenone, quinidine, or verapamil, the need for digoxin should be evaluated and the digoxin dose should be reduced (eg, by 50%) to avoid toxicity.

Adverse Reactions Note: Children are more likely to experience cardiac arrhythmia as a sign of excessive dosing. The most common are conduction disturbances or tachyarrhythmia (atrial tachycardia with or without block) and junctional tachycardia. Ventricular tachyarrhythmias are less common. In infants, sinus bradycardia may be a sign of digoxin toxicity. Any arrhythmia seen in a child on digoxin should be considered as digoxin toxicity. The gastrointestinal and central nervous system symptoms are not frequently seen in children.

Cardiovascular: Accelerated junctional rhythm, asystole, atrial or nodal ectopic beats, atrial tachycardia with or without A-V block, A-V block, AV dissociation, bigeminy, facial edema, PR prolongation, S-A block, sinus bradycardia, ST segment depression, trigeminy, ventricular arrhythmias, ventricular tachycardia or ventricular fibrillation; first-, second- (Wenckebach), or third-degree heart block

Central nervous system: Anxiety, apathy, confusion, delirium, depression, disorientation, dizziness (6%), drowsiness, fatigue, fever, hallucinations, headache (4%), lethargy, mental disturbances (5%), vertigo

Dermatologic: Angioneurotic edema, pruritus, rash [erythematous, maculopapular (most common), papular, scarlatiniform, vesicular, or bullous], urticaria

Endocrine & metabolic: Hyperkalemia with acute toxicity

Gastrointestinal: Abdominal pain, diarrhea, feeding intolerance, nausea, vomiting

Neuromuscular & skeletal: Neuralgia, weakness

Ocular: Blurred vision, diplopia, flashing lights, halos, photophobia, yellow or green vision

Respiratory: Laryngeal edema

<1%, postmarketing, and/or case reports: Asymmetric chorea, diaphoresis, eosinophilia, gynecomastia, hemorrhagic necrosis of the intestines, intestinal ischemia, palpitation, sexual dysfunction, thrombocytopenia, vaginal cornification

Drug Interactions

Metabolism/Transport Effects Substrate of CYP3A4 (minor), P-glycoprotein

Avoid Concomitant Use There are no known interactions where it is recommended to avoid concomitant use.

Increased Effect/Toxicity

Digoxin may increase the levels/effects of: Colchicine; Dronedarone; Midodrine

The levels/effects of Digoxin may be increased by: Aminoquinolines (Antimalarial); Amiodarone; Atorvastatin; Beta-Blockers; Calcitriol; Calcium Channel Blockers (Nondihydropyridine); Carvedilol; Conivaptan; CycloSPORINE; CycloSPORINE (Systemic); Dronedarone; Itraconazole; Macrolide Antibiotics; Milnacipran; Nefazodone; Neuromuscular-Blocking Agents; Nonsteroidal Anti-Inflammatory Agents; P-Glycoprotein Inhibitors; Posaconazole; Potassium-Sparing Diuretics; Propafenone; Protease Inhibitors; QuiNIDine; QuiNINE; Ranolazine; SitaGLIPtin; Sodium Polystyrene Sulfonate; Spironolactone; Telmisartan

Decreased Effect

Digoxin may decrease the levels/effects of: Antineoplastic Agents (Anthracycline)

The levels/effects of Digoxin may be decreased by: 5-ASA Derivatives; Acarbose; Aminoglycosides; Antineoplastic Agents; Antineoplastic Agents (Anthracycline); Bile Acid Sequestrants; Kaolin; Penicillamine; P-Glycoprotein Inducers; Potassium-Sparing Diuretics; St Johns Wort; Sucralfate

Food Interactions Meals containing increased fiber (bran) or foods high in pectin, may decrease oral absorption of digoxin; avoid natural licorice (causes sodium and water retention and increases potassium loss); maintain adequate amounts of potassium in diet to decrease risk of hypokalemia (hypokalemia may increase risk of digoxin toxicity)

Stability I.V.: Store at 25°C (77°F); excursions permitted to 15°C to 30°C (59°F to 86°F); protect from light. Compatible with D$_5$W, D$_{10}$W, NS, SWI (when diluted fourfold or greater); do not mix with other drugs

Mechanism of Action Increases the influx of calcium ions, from extracellular to intracellular cytoplasm by inhibition of sodium and potassium ion movement across the myocardial membranes; this increase in calcium ions results in a potentiation of the activity of the contractile heart muscle fibers and an increase in the force of myocardial contraction (positive inotropic effect); inhibits adenosine triphosphatase (ATPase); decreases conduction through the S-A and A-V nodes

Pharmacodynamics

Onset of action (heart rate control):

Oral: 1-2 hours

I.V.: 5-60 minutes

Maximum effect (heart rate control):

Oral: 2-8 hours

I.V.: 1-6 hours; **Note:** In adult patients with atrial fibrillation, median time to ventricular rate control in one study was 6 hours (range: 3-15 hours) (Siu, 2009)

Duration (adults): 3-4 days

Pharmacokinetics (Adult data unless noted)

Absorption: By passive nonsaturable diffusion in the upper small intestine; food may delay but does not affect extent of absorption

Distribution: Distribution phase: 6-8 hours

V_d: Extensive to peripheral tissues; concentrates in heart, liver, kidney, skeletal muscle, and intestines. Heart/ serum concentration is 70:1. Pharmacologic effects are delayed and do not correlate well with serum concentrations during distribution phase

Neonates, full-term: 7.5-10 L/kg

Children: 16 L/kg

Adults: 7 L/kg

Renal disease: Decreased V_d

Hyperthyroidism: Increased V_d

Hyperkalemia, hyponatremia: Decreased digoxin distribution to heart and muscle

Hypokalemia: Increased digoxin distribution to heart and muscles

Concomitant quinidine therapy: Decreased V_d

Chronic renal failure: Adults: 4-6 L/kg

Decreased sodium/potassium ATPase activity: Decreased tissue binding

Protein binding: ~25%; in uremic patients, digoxin is displaced from plasma protein binding sites

Metabolism: Via sequential sugar hydrolysis in the stomach or by reduction of lactone ring by intestinal bacteria (in ~10% of population, gut bacteria may metabolize up to 40% of digoxin dose); once absorbed, only ~16% is metabolized to 3-beta-digoxigenin, 3-keto-digoxigenin, and glucuronide and sulfate conjugates; metabolites may contribute to therapeutic and toxic effects of digoxin; metabolism is reduced with decompensated heart failure

Bioavailability (dependent upon formulation):

Elixir: 70% to 85%

Tablets: 60% to 80%

Half-life, elimination (dependent upon age, renal and cardiac function):

Premature: 61-170 hours

Neonates, full-term: 35-45 hours

Infants: 18-25 hours

Children: 35 hours

Adults: 36-48 hours

Anephric adults: >4.5 days

Anuric adults: 3.5-5 days

Metabolites: Adults: Digoxigenin: 4 hours; Monodigitoxoside: 3-12 hours

Elimination: 50% to 70% excreted unchanged in urine

Dialysis: Nondialyzable (0% to 5%)

Usual Dosage

Neonates, Infants, Children, and Adolescents: Dosage must be individualized due to substantial individual variation; table lists dosage recommendations based on average patient response.

Note: Total digitalizing dose should be divided (see below).

Dosage Recommendations for Digoxin[1,2]

Age	Total Digitalizing Dose[3] (mcg/kg)		Daily Maintenance Dose[4] (mcg/kg)	
	Oral	I.V. or I.M.[5]	Oral	I.V. or I.M.[5]
Neonates				
Preterm	20-30	15-25	5-7.5	4-6
Full-term	25-35	20-30	6-10	5-8
Infants and children				
1 mo - 2 y	35-60	30-50	10-15	7.5-12
2-5 y	30-40	25-35	7.5-10	6-9
5-10 y	20-35	15-30	5-10	4-8
>10 y	10-15	8-12	2.5-5	2-3

[1] **Heart failure:** A lower serum digoxin concentration may be adequate to treat heart failure (compared to cardiac arrhythmias); consider doses at the lower end of the recommended range for treatment of heart failure; a digitalizing dose (loading dose) may not be necessary when treating heart failure (see Ross, 2001).

[2] Based on lean body weight and normal renal function for age. Decrease maintenance dose in patients with decreased renal function and decrease total digitalizing dose by 50% in end-stage renal disease.

[3] **Do not give full total digitalizing dose (TDD) at once.** Give one-half of the total digitalizing dose (TDD) for the initial dose, then give one-quarter of the TDD for each of two subsequent doses at 6- to 12-hour intervals. Obtain ECG 6 hours after each dose to assess potential toxicity.

[4] Divided every 12 hours in infants and children ≤10 years of age. Given once daily to children >10 years of age and adults.

[5] I.M. route not usually recommended (see Administration).

Adults:

Atrial fibrillation (rate control) in patients with heart failure (Fuster, 2006): Loading dose: I.V.: 0.25 mg every 2 hours, up to 1.5 mg within 24 hours; for nonacute situations, may administer 0.5 mg orally once daily for 2 days, followed by oral maintenance dose. Maintenance dose: I.V., Oral: 0.125-0.375 mg once daily

Heart failure: Note: Loading dose not recommended; Daily maintenance dose: Oral: 0.125-0.25 mg once daily; higher daily doses (up to 0.5 mg/day) are rarely necessary. If patient is >70 years old, has impaired renal function, or has a low lean body mass, low doses (eg, 0.125 mg daily or every other day) should be used (Hunt, 2009).

Supraventricular tachyarrhythmias (rate control):

Initial: Total digitalizing dose:

Oral: 0.75-1.5 mg

I.V., I.M.: 0.5-1 mg (**Note:** I.M. not preferred due to severe injection site pain.)

Give $\frac{1}{2}$ of the total digitalizing dose (TDD) as the initial dose, then give $\frac{1}{4}$ of the TDD in each of two subsequent doses at 6- to 8-hour intervals. Obtain ECG 6 hours after each dose to assess potential toxicity.

Daily maintenance dose:

Oral: 0.125-0.5 mg once daily

I.V., I.M.: 0.1-0.4 mg once daily (**Note:** I.M. not preferred due to severe injection site pain.)

Dosing adjustment in renal impairment: (Monitor patient closely):

Total digitalizing dose: Reduce by 50% in end-stage renal disease

Maintenance dose:

Cl_{cr} 10-50 mL/minute: Administer 25% to 75% of normal daily dose (divided and given at normal intervals) or administer normal dose every 36 hours

Cl_{cr} <10 mL/minute: Administer 10% to 25% of normal daily dose (divided and given at normal intervals) or give normal dose every 48 hours

Administration

Oral: Administer consistently with relationship to meals; avoid concurrent administration (ie, administer digoxin 1 hour before or 2 hours after) with meals high in fiber or pectin and with drugs that decrease oral absorption of digoxin

Parenteral: Administer I.V. doses (undiluted or diluted at least fourfold in D_5W, $D_{10}W$, NS, or SWI) slowly over 5-10 minutes; avoid rapid I.V. infusion since this may result in systemic and coronary arteriolar vasoconstriction; I.M. route not usually recommended due to local irritation, pain, and tissue damage.

Monitoring Parameters Heart rate and rhythm, periodic ECG; follow serum potassium, magnesium, and calcium closely (especially in patients receiving diuretics or amphotericin); decreased serum potassium and magnesium, or increased serum magnesium and calcium may increase digoxin toxicity; assess renal function (serum BUN, S_{cr}) in order to adjust dose; obtain serum drug concentrations at least 8-12 hours after a dose, preferably prior to next scheduled dose

Reference Range Digoxin therapeutic serum concentrations:

Heart failure: 0.5-0.8 ng/mL

Adults: <0.5 ng/mL (SI: <0.6 nmol/L); probably indicates underdigitalization unless there are special circumstances

Toxic: >2 ng/mL; (SI: >2.6 nmol/L). **Note:** Serum concentration must be used in conjunction with clinical symptoms and ECG to confirm diagnosis of digoxin intoxication.

Digoxin-like immunoreactive substance (DLIS) may cross-react with digoxin immunoassay and falsely increase serum concentrations. DLIS has been found in patients with renal and liver disease, heart failure, neonates, and pregnant women (3rd trimester).

Test Interactions Spironolactone may interfere with digoxin radioimmunoassay

Patient Information Notify physician if decreased appetite, nausea, vomiting, diarrhea, or visual changes occur; avoid the herbal medicine St John's wort

Dosage Forms Excipient information presented when available (limited, particularly for generics); consult specific product labeling. [CAN] = Canadian brand name; [DSC] = Discontinued product

Injection, solution: 250 mcg/mL (1 mL [DSC], 2 mL)

Lanoxin®: 250 mcg/mL (2 mL) [contains ethanol 10%, propylene glycol 40%]

Injection, solution [pediatric]:

Lanoxin®: 100 mcg/mL (1 mL) [contains ethanol 10%, propylene glycol 40%]

Solution, oral: 50 mcg/mL (2.5 mL, 5 mL [DSC], 60 mL)

Tablet, oral: 125 mcg, 250 mcg

Apo-Digoxin® [CAN]: 62.5 mcg, 125 mcg, 250 mcg

Lanoxin®: 125 mcg, 250 mcg [scored]

References

American Academy of Pediatrics Committee on Drugs, "Transfer of Drugs and Other Chemicals Into Human Milk," *Pediatrics*, 2001, 108 (3):776-89.

Antman EM, Anbe DT, Armstrong PW, et al, "ACC/AHA Guidelines for the Management of Patients With ST-Elevation Myocardial Infarction: A Report of the American College of Cardiology/American Heart Association Task Force on Practice Guidelines (Committee to Revise the 1999 Guidelines for the Management of Patients With Acute Myocardial Infarction)," *Circulation*, 2004, 110(9):e82-292.

Bakir M and Bilgic A, "Single Daily Dose of Digoxin for Maintenance Therapy of Infants and Children With Cardiac Disease: Is It Reliable?" *Pediatr Cardiol*, 1994, 15(5):229-32.

Bendayan R and McKenzie MW, "Digoxin Pharmacokinetics and Dosage Requirements in Pediatric Patients," *Clin Pharm*, 1983, 2 (3):224-35.

Blomström-Lundqvist C, Scheinman MM, Aliot EM, et al, "ACC/AHA/ESC Guidelines for the Management of Patients With Supraventricular Arrhythmias – Executive Summary. A Report of the American College of Cardiology/American Heart Association Task Force on Practice Guidelines and the European Society of Cardiology Committee for Practice Guidelines (Writing Committee to Develop Guidelines for the Management of Patients With Supraventricular Arrhythmias) Developed in Collaboration With NASPE-Heart Rhythm Society," *J Am Coll Cardiol*, 2003, 42(8):1493-531.

European Heart Rhythm Association; Heart Rhythm Society, Fuster V, et al, "ACC/AHA/ESC 2006 Guidelines for the Management of Patients With Atrial Fibrillation – Executive Summary: A Report of the American College of Cardiology/American Heart Association Task Force on Practice Guidelines and the European Society of Cardiology Committee for Practice Guidelines (Writing Committee to Revise the 2001 Guidelines for the Management of Patients With Atrial Fibrillation)," *J Am Coll Cardiol*, 2006, 48(4):854-906.

Hunt SA, Abraham WT, Chin MH, et al, "2009 Focused Update Incorporated Into the ACC/AHA 2005 Guidelines for the Diagnosis and Management of Heart Failure in Adults: A Report of the American College of Cardiology Foundation/American Heart Association Task Force on Practice Guidelines Developed in Collaboration With the International Society for Heart and Lung Transplantation," *J Am Coll Cardiol*, 2009, 53(15):e1-e90.

Johne A, Brockmöller J, Bauer S, et al, "Pharmacokinetic Interaction of Digoxin With an Herbal Extract From St John's Wort (*Hypericum perforatum*)," *Clin Pharmacol Ther*, 1999, 66(4):338-45.

Packer M, Gheorghiade M, Young JB, et al, "Withdrawal of Digoxin From Patients With Chronic Heart Failure Treated With Angiotensin-Converting-Enzyme Inhibitors. RADIANCE Study," *N Engl J Med*, 1993, 329(1):1-7.

Park MK, "Use of Digoxin in Infants and Children With Specific Emphasis on Dosage," *J Pediatr*, 1986, 108(6):871-7.

Ross RD, "Medical Management of Chronic Heart Failure in Children," *Am J Cardiovasc Drugs*, 2001, 1(1):37-44.

Siu CW, Lau CP, Lee WL, et al, "Intravenous Diltiazem Is Superior to Intravenous Amiodarone or Digoxin for Achieving Ventricular Rate Control in Patients With Acute Uncomplicated Atrial Fibrillation," *Crit Care Med*, 2009, 37(7):2174-9.

◆ **Digoxin CSD (Can)** *see* Digoxin *on page 437*

Digoxin Immune Fab (di JOKS in i MYUN fab)

U.S. Brand Names Digibind®; DigiFab™

Canadian Brand Names Digibind®

Therapeutic Category Antidote, Digoxin

Generic Available No

Use Treatment of potentially life-threatening digoxin or digitoxin intoxication in carefully selected patients; use in life-threatening ventricular arrhythmias secondary to digoxin, acute digoxin ingestion (ie, >10 mg in adults or >4 mg in children), hyperkalemia (serum potassium >5 mEq/L) in the setting of digoxin toxicity

Pregnancy Risk Factor C

Pregnancy Considerations Animal reproduction studies have not been conducted. Safety and efficacy in pregnant women have not been established. Use during pregnancy only if clearly needed.

Lactation Excretion in breast milk unknown/use caution

Contraindications Hypersensitivity to digoxin immune fab, ovine (sheep) proteins, or (DigiFab™ only) papain, chymopapain, other papaya extracts, or the pineapple enzyme bromelain

Warnings Hypokalemia has been reported to occur following reversal of digitalis intoxication; monitor serum potassium levels closely; Fab fragments may be eliminated more slowly in patients with renal failure; heart failure may be exacerbated as digoxin level is reduced; total serum digoxin concentration may rise precipitously following administration of digoxin immune Fab, but this will be almost entirely bound to the Fab fragment and not able to react with receptors in the body; digoxin immune Fab will interfere with digitalis immunoassay measurements - this will result in clinically misleading serum digoxin concentrations until the Fab fragment is eliminated from the body (several days to >1 week after digoxin immune Fab administration); serum digoxin levels drawn prior to therapy may be difficult to evaluate if 6-8 hours have not elapsed after the last dose of digoxin (time to equilibration between serum and tissue); redigitalization should not be initiated until Fab fragments have been eliminated from the body, which may occur over several days or greater than a week in patients with impaired renal function

Precautions Use with caution in renal or cardiac failure; allergic reactions possible; epinephrine should be immediately available; patients may deteriorate due to withdrawal of digoxin and may require I.V. inotropic support (eg, dobutamine) or vasodilators

Adverse Reactions

Cardiovascular: Worsening of low cardiac output or CHF, rapid ventricular response in patients with atrial fibrillation as digoxin is withdrawn

Dermatologic: Urticarial rash

Endocrine & metabolic: Hypokalemia

Miscellaneous: Facial edema and redness, allergic reactions

Drug Interactions

Avoid Concomitant Use There are no known interactions where it is recommended to avoid concomitant use.

Increased Effect/Toxicity There are no known significant interactions involving an increase in effect.

Decreased Effect There are no known significant interactions involving a decrease in effect.

Stability Store in refrigerator; reconstituted solutions are stable 4 hours at 2°C to 8°C

Mechanism of Action Binds with molecules of free (unbound) digoxin or digitoxin and then is removed from the body by renal excretion

Pharmacodynamics Onset of action: Improvement in signs and symptoms occurs within 2-30 minutes following I.V. infusion

Pharmacokinetics (Adult data unless noted)

Distribution: V_d:

Digibind®: 0.3 L/kg

DigiFab™: 0.4 L/kg

Half-life: Renal impairment prolongs the half-life of both agents:

Digibind®: 15-20 hours

DigiFab™: 15 hours

Elimination: Renal with levels declining to undetectable amounts within 5-7 days

Usual Dosage To determine the dose of digoxin immune Fab, first determine the total body load of digoxin (TBL) or digitoxin (depending upon which product was ingested) as follows [using either an approximation of the amount ingested or a postdistribution serum digoxin/digitoxin concentration (C)]:

TBL of **digoxin** (in mg) = C (in ng/mL) x 5.6 x body weight (in kg)/1000

or

TBL = mg of **digoxin** ingested (as tablets or elixir) x 0.8

TBL of **digitoxin** (mg) = C (in ng/mL) x 0.56 x body weight (in kg)/1000

or

TBL of **digitoxin** (in mg) = mg digitoxin ingested

Dose of Digibind® **(in mg)** I.V. = TBL x 76

Dose of DigiFab™ **(in mg)** I.V. = TBL x 80

Dose of digoxin immune Fab (Digibind® or DigiFab™) **(# vials)** I.V. = TBL/0.5

See tables.

Infants and Children Dose Estimates of Digoxin Immune Fab (in mg)[1] From Serum Digoxin Concentration

Patient Weight (kg)	Serum Digoxin Concentration (ng/mL)						
	1	2	4	8	12	16	20
1	0.4 mg[2]	1 mg[2]	1.5 mg[2]	3 mg	5 mg	6-6.5 mg	8 mg
3	1 mg[2]	2-2.5 mg[2]	5 mg	9-10 mg	14 mg	18-19 mg	23-24 mg
5	2 mg[2]	4 mg	8 mg	15-16 mg	23-24 mg	30-32 mg	38-40 mg
10	4 mg	8 mg	15-16 mg	30-32 mg	46-48 mg	61-64 mg	76-80 mg
20	8 mg	15-16 mg	30-32 mg	61-64 mg	91-96 mg	122-128 mg	152-160 mg

[1]When a range in dose is listed, the lower number represents the Digibind® dose and the higher number represents the Digifab™ dose. A single dose is the same for both products.

[2]Dilution of reconstituted vial to 1 mg/mL may be desirable.

Adult Dose Estimate of Digoxin Immune Fab (in # of Vials) From Serum Digoxin Concentration

Patient Weight (kg)	Serum Digoxin Concentration (ng/mL)						
	1	2	4	8	12	16	20
40	0.5 v	1 v	2 v	3 v	5 v	7 v	8 v
60	0.5 v	1 v	3 v	5 v	7 v	10 v	12 v
70	1 v	2 v	3 v	6 v	9 v	11 v	14 v
80	1 v	2 v	3 v	7 v	10 v	13 v	16 v
100	1 v	2 v	4 v	8 v	12 v	16 v	20 v

v = vials.

Administration Parenteral: I.V.: Digibind® is reconstituted by adding 4 mL SWI, resulting in a 9.5 mg/mL concentration for I.V. infusion; DigiFab™ is reconstituted with 4 mL SWI, resulting in an 10 mg/mL concentration for I.V. infusion; both formulations may be further diluted with NS to a convenient volume (eg, 1 mg/mL); infuse over 15-30 minutes; to remove protein aggregates, 0.22 micron in-line filter is needed (Digibind® only)

Monitoring Parameters Serum potassium; serum digoxin/digitoxin level prior to first dose of digoxin immune Fab; (digoxin levels will greatly increase with digoxin immune Fab use and are not an accurate determination of body stores); continuous ECG monitoring

Additional Information Each 38 mg vial (Digibind®) or 40 mg vial (DigiFab™) will bind approximately 0.5 mg digoxin or digitoxin; for individuals at increased risk of sensitivity (see Contraindications) an intradermal or scratch technique skin test using a 1:100 dilution of reconstituted digoxin immune Fab diluted in NS has been used. Skin test volume is 0.1 mL of 1:100 dilution; evaluate after 20 minutes.

Dosage Forms Excipient information presented when available (limited, particularly for generics); consult specific product labeling.

Injection, powder for reconstitution [ovine derived]:

Digibind®: 38 mg [derived from or manufactured using papain]

DigiFab™: 40 mg [derived from or manufactured using papain]

References

Hickey AR, Wenger TL, Carpenter VP, et al, "Digoxin Immune Fab Therapy in the Management of Digitalis Intoxication: Safety and Efficacy Results of an Observational Surveillance Study," *J Am Coll Cardiol*, 1991, 17(3):590-8.

Dihydroergotamine (dye hye droe er GOT a meen)

U.S. Brand Names D.H.E. 45®; Migranal®
Canadian Brand Names Migranal®
Therapeutic Category Alpha-Adrenergic Blocking Agent, Intranasal; Alpha-Adrenergic Blocking Agent, Parenteral; Antimigraine Agent; Ergot Alkaloid and Derivative
Generic Available Yes: Injection
Use Treatment of migraine headache with or without aura; injection also indicated for treatment of cluster headaches
Pregnancy Risk Factor X
Pregnancy Considerations Dihydroergotamine is oxytocic and should not be used during pregnancy.
Lactation May be excreted in breast milk/contraindicated
Breast-Feeding Considerations Ergot derivatives inhibit prolactin and it is known that ergotamine is excreted in breast milk (vomiting, diarrhea, weak pulse, and unstable blood pressure have been reported in nursing infants). It is not known if dihydroergotamine would also cause these effects, however, it is likely that it is excreted in human breast milk. Do not use in nursing women.
Contraindications Hypersensitivity to dihydroergotamine, other ergot alkaloids, caffeine (nasal spray only), or any component; pregnancy; patients with uncontrolled hypertension, ischemic heart disease, angina pectoris, history of MI, silent ischemia, or coronary artery vasospasm including Prinzmetal's angina; patients with hemiplegic or basilar migraine; patients with peripheral vascular disease, sepsis, severe hepatic or renal dysfunction, and following vascular surgery; concurrent therapy with potent CYP3A4 inhibitors (eg, protease inhibitors and macrolide antibiotics); do not use within 24 hours of sumatriptan, zolmitriptan, other serotonin agonists, or ergot-like agents; do not use during or within 2 weeks of discontinuing MAO inhibitors (see Drug Interactions)
Warnings May cause vasospastic reactions; persistent vasospasm may lead to gangrene or death in patients with compromised circulation; discontinue if signs of vasoconstriction develop; rare reports of increased blood pressure in patients without history of hypertension; rare reports of adverse cardiac events (acute MI, life-threatening arrhythmias, death) have been reported following use of the injection; cerebral hemorrhage, subarachnoid hemorrhage, and stroke have also occurred following use of the injection; concomitant use with potent inhibitors of CYP3A4 (including protease inhibitors and macrolide antibiotics) has been associated with acute ergot toxicity characterized by serious and/or life-threatening cerebral and peripheral ischemia **[U.S. Boxed Warning]**; some cases have resulted in amputation (see Contraindications); less potent CYP3A4 inhibitors (eg, metronidazole, fluoxetine, nefazodone, zileuton, and azole antifungals) may carry the same risk (see Contraindications and Drug Interactions).
Precautions Prolonged use has been associated with fibrotic changes to heart and pulmonary valves (see Adverse Reactions); use with caution and only after a satisfactory cardiovascular evaluation has been performed in patients with risk factors for CAD; it is also recommended in these patients that the healthcare provider should administer the first dose; cardiovascular status should be periodically evaluated
Adverse Reactions
Cardiovascular: Cerebral hemorrhage, coronary artery vasospasm, edema, flushing, hypertension, MI, myocardial ischemia, palpitations, subarachnoid hemorrhage, transient ventricular tachycardia, ventricular fibrillation, tachycardia, bradycardia; fibrotic thickening of the aortic, mitral, tricuspid, and/or pulmonary valves (rare)
Central nervous system: Dizziness, somnolence, anxiety, headache, stroke
Dermatologic: Rash, pruritus

Endocrine & metabolic: Hot flashes
Gastrointestinal: Nausea, taste disturbance, vomiting, diarrhea, abdominal pain, cramps, diarrhea, xerostomia
Local: Application site reaction
Neuromuscular & skeletal: Asthenia, stiffness, hyperkinesis, muscular weakness, myalgia, paresthesia, tremor
Respiratory:
Nasal spray: Pharyngitis, rhinitis, nasal congestion, rhinorrhea, sneezing, nasal edema
Injection: Pleuropulmonary fibrosis
Miscellaneous: Retroperitoneal fibrosis (injection), sweating increased
Drug Interactions
Metabolism/Transport Effects Substrate of CYP3A4 (major); **Inhibits** CYP3A4 (weak)
Avoid Concomitant Use
Avoid concomitant use of Dihydroergotamine with any of the following: Clarithromycin; Efavirenz; Itraconazole; Posaconazole; Protease Inhibitors; Serotonin 5-HT1D Receptor Agonists; Sibutramine; Voriconazole
Increased Effect/Toxicity
Dihydroergotamine may increase the levels/effects of: Serotonin 5-HT1D Receptor Agonists; Serotonin Modulators

The levels/effects of Dihydroergotamine may be increased by: Clarithromycin; CYP3A4 Inhibitors (Moderate); CYP3A4 Inhibitors (Strong); Dasatinib; Efavirenz; Itraconazole; Macrolide Antibiotics; Posaconazole; Protease Inhibitors; Serotonin 5-HT1D Receptor Agonists; Sibutramine; Voriconazole
Decreased Effect There are no known significant interactions involving a decrease in effect.
Stability Store below 25°C (77°F); do not refrigerate or freeze; protect from heat and light; once the nasal spray applicator has been prepared, use within 8 hours; discard any unused nasal solution
Mechanism of Action Ergot alkaloid alpha-adrenergic blocker which aborts vascular headaches by direct vasoconstriction of vascular smooth muscle, particularly of the carotid artery bed but also peripheral and cerebral vessels, which reduces the amplitude of pulsation in the cranial arteries; it also has partial agonist or antagonist activity against tryptaminergic and dopaminergic receptors; it is less active than ergotamine
Pharmacodynamics
Onset of action:
I.M.: 15-30 minutes
Intranasal: 30 minutes
I.V.: Immediate
Duration: I.M.: 3-4 hours
Pharmacokinetics (Adult data unless noted)
Distribution: V_d: 14.5 L/kg (~800 L)
Bioavailability: Intranasal: 32%
Protein binding: 93%
Metabolism: Extensively in the liver; one active metabolite
Half-life: Distribution phase: 0.9-2.1 hours; terminal elimination phase: 7-32 hours
Time to peak serum concentration: I.M.: Within 15-30 minutes; intranasal: 0.5-1 hour; I.V.: 15 minutes; SubQ: 15-45 minutes
Elimination: Predominately into bile and feces and 10% excreted in urine, mostly as metabolites
Clearance: 1.5 L/minute
Usual Dosage Adolescents and Adults: Treatment should be initiated at the first symptom or sign of an attack; nasal spray may be used at any stage of a migraine attack:
I.M., SubQ: 1 mg at first sign of headache; repeat hourly to a maximum total dose of 3 mg/day; do not exceed 6 mg/week

I.V.: 1 mg at first sign of headache; repeat hourly up to a maximum total dose of 2 mg/day; do not exceed 6 mg/week

Intranasal: 1 spray (0.5 mg) of nasal spray into each nostril (total: 1 mg); repeat if needed within 15 minutes; maximum: 4 sprays (2 mg/day); do not exceed 8 sprays (4 mg)/week

Dosing adjustment in renal impairment: Contraindicated in severe renal impairment

Dosing adjustment in hepatic impairment: Dosage reductions are probably necessary but specific guidelines are not available; contraindicated in severe hepatic dysfunction

Administration

Intranasal (For complete directions, see patient instruction booklet): Prior to administration, the nasal spray applicator must be primed (pumped 4 times); spray once into each nostril; avoid deep inhalation through the nose while spraying or immediately after spraying; do not tilt head back

I.M., SubQ: Administer without dilution

I.V.: Administer without dilution slowly over 2-3 minutes

Patient Information Take this drug as rapidly as possible when first symptoms occur; may cause dry mouth; may cause drowsiness and impair ability to perform activities requiring mental alertness or physical coordination; report heart palpitations, severe nausea or vomiting, or severe numbness of fingers or toes; do not assemble nasal spray until needed for use

Dosage Forms Excipient information presented when available (limited, particularly for generics); consult specific product labeling.

Injection, solution, as mesylate: 1 mg/mL (1 mL) [contains ethanol 6.2%]

D.H.E. 45®: 1 mg/mL (1 mL) [contains ethanol 6.2%]

Solution, intranasal spray, as mesylate (Migranal®): 4 mg/mL [0.5 mg/spray] (1 mL) [contains caffeine 10 mg/mL]

- ◆ **Dihydroergotamine Mesylate** *see* Dihydroergotamine *on page 442*

- ◆ **Dihydrohydroxycodeinone** *see* OxyCODONE *on page 1038*

- ◆ **Dihydromorphinone** *see* HYDROmorphone *on page 689*

- ◆ **Dihydroxyanthracenedione** *see* Mitoxantrone *on page 938*

- ◆ **Dihydroxyanthracenedione Dihydrochloride** *see* Mitoxantrone *on page 938*

- ◆ **1,25 Dihydroxycholecalciferol** *see* Calcitriol *on page 229*

- ◆ **Diiodohydroxyquin** *see* Iodoquinol *on page 755*

- ◆ **Dilacor XR®** *see* Diltiazem *on page 443*

- ◆ **Dilantin®** *see* Phenytoin *on page 1104*

- ◆ **Dilaudid®** *see* HYDROmorphone *on page 689*

- ◆ **Dilaudid-HP®** *see* HYDROmorphone *on page 689*

- ◆ **Dilaudid-HP-Plus® (Can)** *see* HYDROmorphone *on page 689*

- ◆ **Dilaudid® Sterile Powder (Can)** *see* HYDROmorphone *on page 689*

- ◆ **Dilaudid-XP® (Can)** *see* HYDROmorphone *on page 689*

- ◆ **Dilt-CD** *see* Diltiazem *on page 443*

- ◆ **Diltia XT®** *see* Diltiazem *on page 443*

Diltiazem (dil TYE a zem)

Medication Safety Issues

Sound-alike/look-alike issues:

Cardizem® may be confused with Cardene®, Cardene SR®, Cardizem CD®, Cardizem SR®, cardiem, cortisone

Cartia XT® may be confused with Procardia XL®

Diltiazem may be confused with Calan®, diazepam, Dilantin®

Tiazac® may be confused with Tigan®, Tiazac® XC [CAN], Ziac®

High alert medication: The Institute for Safe Medication Practices (ISMP) includes this medication (I.V. formulation) among its list of drug classes which have a heightened risk of causing significant patient harm when used in error.

Significant differences exist between oral and I.V. dosing. Use caution when converting from one route of administration to another.

International issues:

Cardizem® may be confused with Cardem® which is a brand name for celiprolol in Spain

Cartia XT® may be confused with Cartia® which is a brand name for aspirin in multiple international markets

Dilacor®: Brand name for digoxin in Belgium and Serbia; brand name for verapamil in Brazil; brand name for barnidipine in Argentina

Tiazac® may be confused with Tazac® which is a brand name for nizatidine in Australia

Tiazac® may be confused with Tiazac® XC which is a brand name for diltiazem available in Canada (not available in U.S.)

Related Information

Adult ACLS Algorithms *on page 1463*
Antihypertensive Agents by Class *on page 1481*
Medications for Which A Single Dose May Be Fatal When Ingested By A Toddler *on page 1709*

U.S. Brand Names Cardizem®; Cardizem® CD; Cardizem® LA; Cartia XT®; Dilacor XR®; Dilt-CD; Dilt-XR; Diltia XT®; Diltzac; Taztia XT®; Tiazac®

Canadian Brand Names Apo-Diltiaz CD®; Apo-Diltiaz SR®; Apo-Diltiaz TZ®; Apo-Diltiaz®; Apo-Diltiaz® Injectable; Cardizem® CD; Diltiazem HCl ER®; Diltiazem Hydrochloride Injection; Diltiazem TZ; Med-Diltiazem; Novo-Diltazem; Novo-Diltiazem-CD; Novo-Diltiazem HCl ER; Nu-Diltiaz; Nu-Diltiaz-CD; ratio-Diltiazem CD; Sandoz-Diltiazem CD; Sandoz-Diltiazem T; Tiazac®; Tiazac® XC

Therapeutic Category Antianginal Agent; Antihypertensive Agent; Calcium Channel Blocker; Calcium Channel Blocker, Nondihydropyridine

Generic Available Yes: Excludes extended release tablet

Use

Oral: Treatment of chronic stable angina or angina from coronary artery spasm; hypertension (**Note:** Only extended release products are FDA approved for the treatment of hypertension) (FDA approved in adults)

Injection: Management of atrial fibrillation or atrial flutter; paroxysmal supraventricular tachycardias (PSVT) (FDA approved in adults)

Pregnancy Risk Factor C

Pregnancy Considerations Teratogenic and embryotoxic effects have been demonstrated in small animals. There are no adequate and well-controlled studies in pregnant women.

Lactation Enters breast milk/not recommended (AAP considers "compatible")

Breast-Feeding Considerations Freely diffuses into breast milk; however, the AAP considers diltiazem to be **compatible** with breast-feeding. Available evidence suggests safe use during breast-feeding.

Contraindications Hypersensitivity to diltiazem or any component; severe hypotension; second or third degree heart block (except in patients with a functioning artificial pacemaker); sick-sinus syndrome (except in patients with a functioning artificial pacemaker); acute MI with pulmonary congestion; cardiogenic shock; I.V. administration concomitantly or within a few hours of the administration of I.V. beta-blockers; atrial fibrillation or flutter associated with accessory bypass tract (eg, Wolff-Parkinson-White syndrome or short PR syndrome); ventricular tachycardia (with wide-complex tachycardia, must determine whether origin is supraventricular or ventricular)

Warnings May cause bradycardia, second or third degree heart block, hypotension, or rarely, acute hepatic injury (with significant elevations in hepatic transaminases); may worsen CHF; use with certain medications may result in additive effects on cardiac condition (see Drug Interactions)

Precautions Use with caution in patients with CHF or impaired renal or hepatic function. Dermatologic reactions may occur; these may be transient or disappear with continued therapy; however, erythema multiforme or exfoliative dermatitis have been reported; discontinue diltiazem if skin rash persists or is severe.

Adverse Reactions Note: Patients with impaired ventricular function or cardiac conduction abnormalities may have higher incidence of serious adverse reactions

Cardiovascular: Arrhythmia, atrial fibrillation, A-V block, bradycardia, flushing, hypotension, palpitations, peripheral edema, vasodilation

Central nervous system: Dizziness, fatigue, headache, nervousness

Dermatologic: Erythema multiforme (rare), exfoliative dermatitis (rare), injection site reactions (I.V. form), rash, pruritus

Gastrointestinal: Abdominal pain, diarrhea, dyspepsia, nausea

Hepatic: ALT, AST, LDH, and alkaline phosphatase increased (rare)

Neuromuscular & skeletal: Asthenia, myalgia, weakness

Respiratory: Cough, dyspnea, pharyngitis, rhinitis

<1% and postmarketing events: Abnormal dreams, albuminuria, allergic reactions, amnesia, amblyopia, angina, angioedema, anorexia, asystole, atrial flutter, bleeding time increased, chest pain, CHF, constipation, CPK elevation, depression, dysgeusia, epistaxis, extrapyramidal symptoms, eye irritation, gait abnormality, gingival hyperplasia, hallucinations, hemolytic anemia, hyperglycemia, hyperuricemia, impotence, insomnia, leukopenia, muscle cramps, myopathy, nocturia, osteoarticular pain, paresthesia, petechiae, photosensitivity, polyuria, pruritus, purpura, retinopathy, sinus node dysfunction, sinus pause, somnolence, sweating, syncope, tachycardia, taste abnormality, thirst, thrombocytopenia, tinnitus, tremor, urticaria, weight increase, ventricular arrhythmia, ventricular extrasystoles, ventricular fibrillation, ventricular tachycardia, vertigo, vomiting, xerostomia

Drug Interactions

Metabolism/Transport Effects Substrate of CYP2C9 (minor), 2D6 (minor), 3A4 (major), P-glycoprotein; **Inhibits** CYP2C9 (weak), 2D6 (weak), 3A4 (moderate)

Avoid Concomitant Use

Avoid concomitant use of Diltiazem with any of the following: Tolvaptan

Increased Effect/Toxicity

Diltiazem may increase the levels/effects of: Alfentanil; Amifostine; Amiodarone; Antihypertensives; Aprepitant; Atorvastatin; Benzodiazepines (metabolized by oxidation); Beta-Blockers; BusPIRone; Calcium Channel Blockers (Dihydropyridine); CarBAMazepine; Cardiac Glycosides; Colchicine; Corticosteroids (Systemic); CycloSPORINE; CycloSPORINE (Systemic); CYP3A4 Substrates; Dronedarone; Eletriptan; Eplerenone; Everolimus; Fosaprepitant; Halofantrine; Hypotensive Agents; Lithium; Lovastatin; Magnesium Salts; Midodrine; Neuromuscular-Blocking Agents (Nondepolarizing); Nitroprusside; Phenytoin; Pimecrolimus; QuiNIDine; Ranolazine; Red Yeast Rice; RiTUXimab; Salicylates; Salmeterol; Saxagliptin; Simvastatin; Tacrolimus; Tacrolimus (Systemic); Tacrolimus (Topical); Tolvaptan

The levels/effects of Diltiazem may be increased by: Alpha1-Blockers; Anilidopiperidine Opioids; Antifungal Agents (Azole Derivatives, Systemic); Aprepitant; Atorvastatin; Calcium Channel Blockers (Dihydropyridine); Cimetidine; CycloSPORINE; CycloSPORINE (Systemic); CYP3A4 Inhibitors (Moderate); CYP3A4 Inhibitors (Strong); Dasatinib; Diazoxide; Dronedarone; Fluconazole; Fosaprepitant; Grapefruit Juice; Herbs (Hypotensive Properties); Lovastatin; Macrolide Antibiotics; Magnesium Salts; MAO Inhibitors; Pentoxifylline; P-Glycoprotein Inhibitors; Phosphodiesterase 5 Inhibitors; Prostacyclin Analogues; Protease Inhibitors; Quinupristin; Simvastatin

Decreased Effect

Diltiazem may decrease the levels/effects of: Clopidogrel

The levels/effects of Diltiazem may be decreased by: Barbiturates; Calcium Salts; CarBAMazepine; Colestipol; CYP3A4 Inducers (Strong); Deferasirox; Herbs (CYP3A4 Inducers); Herbs (Hypertensive Properties); Methylphenidate; Nafcillin; Peginterferon Alfa-2b; P-Glycoprotein Inducers; Rifamycin Derivatives; Yohimbine

Food Interactions A high fat meal does not effect extent of absorption of Cardizem® CD, Cardizem® LA, Cartia XT®, Taztia XT®, or Tiazac®, but peak serum concentrations for Taztia XT® and Tiazac® may occur slightly earlier. Administration of Diltia XT® with a high fat meal may increase extent of absorption and peak concentration. Avoid natural licorice (causes sodium and water retention and increases potassium loss).

Stability

Capsule, tablet: Store at controlled room temperature; avoid excessive humidity; dispense in a tight, light resistant container

Injection: Refrigerate vials; do not freeze; may store at room temperature for up to 1 month; compatible in D_5W, NS, and $D_5^{1}/_2NS$ at a maximum concentration of 1 mg/mL for 24 hours when stored at room temperature or under refrigeration. Do not mix with other drugs in the same container; do not coinfuse with other drugs in the same I.V. line; **not** physically compatible with acetazolamide, acyclovir, aminophylline, ampicillin, ampicillin and sulbactam, cefamandole, cefoperazone, diazepam, furosemide, hydrocortisone, insulin, methylprednisolone, mezlocillin, nafcillin, phenytoin, rifampin, and sodium bicarbonate.

Mechanism of Action Inhibits calcium ions from entering the "slow channels" or select voltage-sensitive areas of vascular smooth muscle and myocardium during depolarization; produces a relaxation of coronary vascular smooth muscle and coronary vasodilation; increases myocardial oxygen delivery in patients with vasospastic angina

Pharmacodynamics

Onset of action:

Oral: Tablet: Immediate release: 30-60 minutes

Parenteral: I.V. (bolus): Within 3 minutes

Maximum effect:

Antiarrhythmic (I.V. bolus): 2-7 minutes

Antihypertensive (Oral; multiple dosing): Within 2 weeks

Pharmacokinetics (Adult data unless noted)

Absorption: 80%

Distribution: V_d: 1.7 L/kg; appears in breast milk

Protein binding: 70% to 80%

Metabolism: Extensive first-pass effect; metabolized in the liver; desacetyldiltiazem is an active metabolite (25% to 50% as potent as diltiazem based on coronary vasodilation effects); desacetyldiltiazem may accumulate with plasma concentrations 10% to 20% of diltiazem levels

Bioavailability: Oral: ~40%

Half-life: 3-4.5 hours, up to 8 hours with chronic high dosing

Time to peak serum concentration:
Tablet: Immediate release: 2-4 hours
Cardizem® CD: 10-14 hours
Cardizem® LA: 11-18 hours
Cardizem® SR: 6-11 hours

Elimination: In urine and bile mostly as metabolites; 2% to 4% excreted as unchanged drug in urine

Dialysis: Not dialyzable

Usual Dosage

Children: Minimal information available; some centers use the following:

Hypertension: Oral: Initial: 1.5-2 mg/kg/day in 3-4 divided doses (extended release formulations may be dosed once or twice daily); maximum dose: 3.5 mg/kg/day; some centers use a maximum dose of 6 mg/kg/day up to 360 mg/day (see Flynn, 2000)

Note: Doses up to 8 mg/kg/day given in 4 divided doses have been used for investigational therapy of Duchenne muscular dystrophy

Adolescents and Adults:

Hypertension: Oral:

Capsule, extended release (once-daily dosing): **Note:** Usual dosage range: Adolescents ≥18 years and Adults (JNC 7): 180-420 mg once daily

Cardizem® CD, Cartia XT®, Dilt-CD: Initial: 180-240 mg once daily; may increase dose after 14 days; usual: 240-360 mg once daily; maximum: 480 mg once daily

Dilacor® XR, Diltia XT®, Dilt-XR: Initial: 180-240 mg once daily; may increase after 14 days; usual: 180-480 mg once daily; maximum: 540 mg once daily

Taztia XT® Tiazac®: Initial: 120-240 mg once daily; may increase dose after 14 days; maximum: 540 mg once daily

Capsule, extended release (twice-daily dosing): Initial: 60-120 mg twice daily; may increase dose after 14 days; usual: 240-360 mg/day

Note: Diltiazem is available as a generic intended for either once- or twice-daily dosing, depending on the formulation; verify appropriate extended release capsule formulation is administered.

Tablet, extended release: Cardizem® LA: Initial: 180-240 mg once daily; may increase dose after 14 days; limited clinical experience with doses >360 mg/day; maximum dose: 540 mg once daily; usual dosage range for Adolescents ≥18 years and Adults (JNC 7): 120-540 mg once daily

Tablet, immediate release: 30-120 mg 3-4 times/day; dosage should be increased gradually, at 1- to 2-day intervals until optimum response is obtained; usual maintenance dose: 180-360 mg/day (see Use)

Atrial fibrillation, atrial flutter, PSVT:

I.V.: Initial: 0.25 mg/kg as a bolus over 2 minutes, if response is inadequate a second bolus dose (0.35 mg/kg) may be administered after 15 minutes; further bolus doses should be individualized; **Note:** Some patients may respond to an initial bolus dose of 0.15 mg/kg; however, duration of action may be shorted and experience with this dose is limited.

I.V. continuous infusion (start after I.V. bolus doses): **Note:** Infusions >24 hours or infusion rated >15 mg/hour are not recommended: Initial infusion rate of 10 mg/hour; rate may be increased in 5 mg/hour increments up to 15 mg/hour as needed; some patients may respond to an initial rate of 5 mg/hour.

Conversion from I.V. diltiazem to oral diltiazem: Start first oral dose approximately 3 hours after bolus dose

Oral dose (mg/day) is approximately equal to [(rate in mg/hour x 3) + 3] x 10; Note: Dose per day may need to be divided depending on formulation used (see Usual Dosage)

3 mg/hour = 120 mg/day
5 mg/hour = 180 mg/day
7 mg/hour = 240 mg/day
11 mg/hour = 360 mg/day (maximum recommended dose)

Administration

Oral:

Tablet, immediate release (Cardizem®): Administer before meals and at bedtime

Extended release preparations (CD, LA, XR, XT, Tiazac): Swallow whole; do not chew, break, or crush.

Dilacor XR®, Dilt-XR, Diltia XT®: Take on an empty stomach

Cardizem® CD, Cardizem® LA, Cartia XT®, Dilt-CD: May be administered with or without food, but should be administered consistently with relation to meals; administer with a full glass of water

Taztia XT® and Tiazac® capsules (extended release) may be opened and sprinkled on applesauce; swallow applesauce immediately, do not chew; follow with some cool water (adults: 1 glass) to ensure complete swallowing; do not use hot applesauce; do not divide capsule contents (ie, do not administer partial doses); do not store mixture of applesauce and capsule contents, use immediately

Parenteral:

I.V. bolus: Adults: Infuse over 2 minutes

I.V. continuous infusion: May dilute with NS, D_5W, or $D_5^{1}/_2NS$; maximum final concentration: 1 mg/mL

Monitoring Parameters Blood pressure, heart rate, renal function, liver enzymes; ECG with I.V. therapy

Patient Information Do not discontinue abruptly; report any dizziness, shortness of breath, palpitations, or edema; avoid alcohol. May cause photosensitivity reactions (eg, exposure to sunlight may cause severe sunburn, skin rash, redness, or itching); avoid exposure to sunlight and artificial light sources (sunlamps, tanning booth/bed); wear protective clothing, wide-brimmed hats, sunglasses, and lip sunscreen (SPF ≥15); use a sunscreen [broad-spectrum sunscreen or physical sunscreen (preferred) or sunblock with SPF ≥15]; contact physician if reaction occurs.

Nursing Implications Do not crush extended release preparations (CD, LA, XR, XT, Tiazac)

Additional Information Cartia XT® and Dilt CD are the generic versions of Cardizem® CD; Diltia XT® and Dilt-XR are the generic versions of Dilacor XR®; Taztia XT® is the generic version of Tiazac®

Dosage Forms Excipient information presented when available (limited, particularly for generics); consult specific product labeling. [CAN] = Canadian brand name

Capsule, extended release, as hydrochloride [once-daily dosing]: 120 mg, 180 mg, 240 mg, 300 mg, 360 mg, 420 mg

Cardizem® CD: 120 mg, 180 mg, 240 mg, 300 mg, 360 mg

Cartia XT®: 120 mg, 180 mg, 240 mg, 300 mg

Dilacor XR®: 120 mg, 180 mg, 240 mg

Dilt-CD: 120 mg, 180 mg, 240 mg, 300 mg

Dilt-XR: 120 mg, 180 mg, 240 mg

Diltia XT®: 120 mg, 180 mg, 240 mg

Diltzac: 120 mg, 180 mg, 240 mg, 300 mg, 360 mg
Taztia XT®: 120 mg, 180 mg, 240 mg, 300 mg, 360 mg
Tiazac®: 120 mg, 180 mg, 240 mg, 300 mg, 360 mg, 420 mg
Capsule, extended release, as hydrochloride [twice-daily dosing]: 60 mg, 90 mg, 120 mg
Injection, solution, as hydrochloride: 5 mg/mL (5 mL, 10 mL, 25 mL)
Injection, powder for reconstitution, as hydrochloride: 100 mg
Tablet, as hydrochloride: 30 mg, 60 mg, 90 mg, 120 mg
Cardizem®: 30 mg, 60 mg, 90 mg, 120 mg
Tablet, extended release, as hydrochloride:
Cardizem® LA: 120 mg, 180 mg, 240 mg, 300 mg, 360 mg, 420 mg
Tiazac® XC [CAN; not available in U.S.]: 120 mg, 180 mg, 240 mg, 300 mg, 360 mg
Extemporaneous Preparations A 12 mg/mL oral liquid preparation made from tablets (regular, not extended release) and 3 different vehicles (cherry syrup, a 1:1 mixture of Ora-Sweet® and Ora-Plus®, or a 1:1 mixture of Ora-Sweet® SF and Ora-Plus®) was stable for 60 days when stored in amber plastic prescription bottles in the dark at room temperature (25°C) or under refrigeration (5°C); grind sixteen 90 mg tablets in a mortar into a fine powder; add 10 mL of the vehicle and mix well to form a uniform paste; mix while adding the vehicle in geometric proportions to **almost** 120 mL; transfer to a calibrated bottle and qsad with vehicle to 120 mL; label "shake well" and "protect from light"

Allen LV and Erickson MA, "Stability of Baclofen, Captopril, Diltiazem Hydrochloride, Dipyridamole, and Flecainide Acetate in Extemporaneously Compounded Oral Liquids," *Am J Health Sys Pharm*, 1996, 53 (18):2179-84.

References

Bertorini TE, Palmieri GMA, Griffin JW, et al, "Effect of Chronic Treatment With the Calcium Antagonist Diltiazem in Duchenne Muscular Dystrophy," *Neurology*, 1988, 38(4):609-13.

Chobanian AV, Bakris GL, Black HR, et al, "The Seventh Report of the Joint National Committee on Prevention, Detection, Evaluation, and Treatment of High Blood Pressure: The JNC 7 report," *JAMA*, 2003, 289(19):2560-72.

Flynn JT and Pasko DA, "Calcium Channel Blockers: Pharmacology and Place in Therapy of Pediatric Hypertension," *Pediatr Nephrol*, 2000, 15(3-4):302-16.

Pass RH, Liberman L, Al-Fayaddh M, et al, "Continuous Intravenous Diltiazem Infusion for Short-Term Ventricular Rate Control in Children," *Am J Cardiol*, 2000, 86(5):559-62, A9.

◆ **Diltiazem HCl ER® (Can)** see Diltiazem on page 443
◆ **Diltiazem Hydrochloride** see Diltiazem on page 443
◆ **Diltiazem Hydrochloride Injection (Can)** see Diltiazem on page 443
◆ **Diltiazem TZ (Can)** see Diltiazem on page 443
◆ **Dilt-XR** see Diltiazem on page 443
◆ **Diltzac** see Diltiazem on page 443

DimenhyDRINATE (dye men HYE dri nate)

Medication Safety Issues
Sound-alike/look-alike issues:
DimenhyDRINATE may be confused with diphenhydrAMINE
U.S. Brand Names Dramamine® [OTC]; Driminate® [OTC]; TripTone® [OTC]
Canadian Brand Names Apo-Dimenhydrinate®; Children's Motion Sickness Liquid; Dimenhydrinate Injection; Dinate®; Gravol®; Nauseatol; Novo-Dimenate; PMS-Dimenhydrinate; Sandoz-Dimenhydrinate
Therapeutic Category Antiemetic; Antihistamine
Generic Available Yes

Use Treatment and prevention of nausea, vertigo, and vomiting associated with motion sickness (oral tablets: FDA approved in children ≥2 years and adults; I.V. product: FDA approved in infants, children, and adults)
Pregnancy Risk Factor B
Lactation Enters breast milk/not recommended
Contraindications Hypersensitivity to dimenhydrinate or any component (see Warnings), neonates (injection contains benzyl alcohol)
Warnings Chewable tablets contain tartrazine which may cause allergic reactions in susceptible individuals
Precautions Use with caution in patients with a history of seizure disorder; may produce excitation in the young child; use with caution in any condition which may be aggravated by anticholinergic symptoms such as prostatic hypertrophy, asthma, bladder neck obstruction, narrow-angle glaucoma, etc; chewable tablets contain aspartame which is metabolized to phenylalanine and must be used with caution in patients with phenylketonuria; use caution if used in conjunction with antibiotics that have the potential to cause ototoxicity (dimenhydrinate may mask symptoms of ototoxicity); do not inject intra-arterially; vials contain benzyl alcohol as a preservative; benzyl alcohol may cause allergic reactions in susceptible individuals; large amounts of benzyl alcohol (≥99 mg/kg/day) have been associated with a potentially fatal toxicity ("gasping syndrome") in neonates; the "gasping syndrome" consists of metabolic acidosis, respiratory distress, gasping respirations, CNS dysfunction (including convulsions, intracranial hemorrhage), hypotension, and cardiovascular collapse; avoid use of vials containing benzyl alcohol in neonates
Adverse Reactions
Cardiovascular: Hypotension, palpitations, tachycardia
Central nervous system: Drowsiness, headache, paradoxical CNS stimulation (excitation, nervousness, restlessness, insomnia), dizziness, lassitude
Dermatologic: Photosensitivity, urticaria, rash
Gastrointestinal: Anorexia, xerostomia, dry mucous membranes, constipation, nausea, epigastric distress
Genitourinary: Urinary frequency, dysuria
Hematologic: Hemolytic anemia
Ocular: Blurred vision, diplopia
Otic: Tinnitus
Respiratory: Chest tightness, wheezing, thickened secretions
Drug Interactions
Avoid Concomitant Use There are no known interactions where it is recommended to avoid concomitant use.
Increased Effect/Toxicity
DimenhyDRINATE may increase the levels/effects of: Alcohol (Ethyl); Anticholinergics; CNS Depressants

The levels/effects of DimenhyDRINATE may be increased by: Pramlintide
Decreased Effect
DimenhyDRINATE may decrease the levels/effects of: Acetylcholinesterase Inhibitors (Central); Betahistine

The levels/effects of DimenhyDRINATE may be decreased by: Acetylcholinesterase Inhibitors (Central); Amphetamines
Mechanism of Action Competes with histamine for H$_1$-receptor sites on effector cells in the GI tract, blood vessels, and respiratory tract; diminishes vestibular stimulation and depresses labyrinthine function through its central anticholinergic activity; consists of equimolar proportions of diphenhydramine and chlorotheophylline
Pharmacodynamics
Onset of action: Oral: Within 15-30 minutes
Duration: ~3-6 hours

Pharmacokinetics (Adult data unless noted)
Absorption: Well absorbed from the GI tract
Metabolism: Extensive in the liver
Usual Dosage
Children 2-5 years:
Oral:
12.5-25 mg every 6-8 hours; maximum dose: 75 mg/day
or
5 mg/kg/day or 150 mg/m^2/day in 4 divided doses, not to exceed 75 mg/day
I.M.:
1.25 mg/kg
or
37.5 mg/m^2 4 times/day; maximum: 75 mg/day
Children: 6-12 years:
Oral:
25-50 mg every 6-8 hours; maximum dose: 150 mg/day
or
5 mg/kg/day or 150 mg/m^2/day in 4 divided doses, not to exceed 150 mg/day
I.M.:
1.25 mg /kg
or
37.5 mg/m^2 4 times/day; maximum: 150 mg/day
Children ≥12 years and Adults:
Oral: 50-100 mg every 4-6 hours, not to exceed 400 mg/day
I.M., I.V.: 50-100 mg every 4 hours
Administration
Oral: Administer with food or water
Parenteral: Using the I.V. route in children is not recommended by the manufacturer; administer I.M. Do not inject intra-arterially. Must dilute each 50 mg in 10 mL of NS for I.V. administration.
Patient Information
May cause drowsiness and impair ability to perform activities requiring mental alertness or physical coordination; may cause dry mouth. May rarely cause photosensitivity reactions (eg, exposure to sunlight may cause severe sunburn, skin rash, redness, or itching); avoid direct exposure to sunlight.
Dosage Forms
Excipient information presented when available (limited, particularly for generics); consult specific product labeling.
Injection, solution: 50 mg/mL (1 mL, 10 mL) [contains benzyl alcohol]
Tablet, oral:
Dramamine®: 50 mg
Driminate®: 50 mg [scored]
TripTone®: 50 mg
Tablet, chewable:
Dramamine®: 50 mg [contains phenylalanine 0.84 mg/tablet; orange flavor]

◆ **Dimenhydrinate Injection (Can)** *see* DimenhyDRINATE *on page 446*

Dimercaprol (dye mer KAP role)

U.S. Brand Names BAL in Oil®
Therapeutic Category
Antidote, Arsenic Toxicity; Antidote, Gold Toxicity; Antidote, Lead Toxicity; Antidote, Mercury Toxicity; Chelating Agent, Parenteral
Generic Available No
Use
Antidote to gold, arsenic (except arsine), and mercury poisoning (except nonalkyl mercury); adjunct to edetate calcium disodium in lead poisoning
Pregnancy Risk Factor C
Pregnancy Considerations
Animal reproduction studies have not been conducted. There are no adequate and well-controlled studies in pregnant women.

Lead poisoning: Following maternal occupational exposure, lead was found to cross the placenta in amounts related to maternal plasma levels. Possible outcomes of maternal lead exposure >10 mcg/dL include spontaneous abortion, postnatal developmental delay, and reduced birth weight. Chelation therapy during pregnancy is for maternal benefit only and should be limited to the treatment of severe, symptomatic lead poisoning.
Lactation Excretion in breast milk unknown/use caution
Breast-Feeding Considerations
It is not known if dimercaprol is excreted in breast milk; however, it is not absorbed orally, which would limit the exposure to a nursing infant. When used for the treatment of lead poisoning, the amount of lead in breast milk may range from 0.6% to 3% of the maternal serum concentration. Calcium supplementation may reduce the amount of lead in breast milk.
Contraindications
Hypersensitivity to dimercaprol, peanuts (injection in peanut oil), or any component; hepatic insufficiency; do not use in iron, cadmium, or selenium poisoning (produces complexes more toxic to the kidney than the metal alone); do not use iron supplements during therapy
Precautions
Use with caution in patients with renal impairment or hypertension; produces hemolysis in persons with G-6-PD deficiency, especially in the presence of infection or other stressful situations; due to increased frequency of histamine-release related side effects, pretreatment with antihistamines is recommended; urine should be kept alkaline to prevent dissociation of chelate; fevers may occur in up to 30% of children and may persist for the duration of therapy
Adverse Reactions
Cardiovascular: Hypertension (dose-related), tachycardia (dose-related), chest pain
Central nervous system: Nervousness, seizures, fever (30% of children), headache, anxiety
Dermatologic: Abscess
Gastrointestinal: Vomiting, nausea, salivation, abdominal pain, throat constriction
Hematologic: Transient neutropenia
Local: Pain at the injection site, sterile abscesses
Neuromuscular & skeletal: Paresthesia of hands, weakness
Ocular: Blepharospasm, conjunctivitis, lacrimation, burning eyes
Renal: Nephrotoxicity
Respiratory: Rhinorrhea
Miscellaneous: Burning sensation of the lips, mouth, throat, and penis; diaphoresis
Drug Interactions
Avoid Concomitant Use
Avoid concomitant use of Dimercaprol with any of the following: Iron Salts
Increased Effect/Toxicity
Dimercaprol may increase the levels/effects of: Iron Salts
Decreased Effect
There are no known significant interactions involving a decrease in effect.
Stability
Store at room temperature 20°C to 25°C (68°F to 77°F); do not mix in the same syringe with edetate calcium disodium
Mechanism of Action
Sulfhydryl group combines with ions of various heavy metals (arsenic, gold, mercury, lead) to form relatively stable, nontoxic, soluble chelates which are excreted in the urine
Pharmacokinetics (Adult data unless noted)
Distribution: To all tissues including the brain
Metabolism: Rapid to inactive products
Time to peak serum concentration: 30-60 minutes
Elimination: In urine and feces via bile

Usual Dosage Children and Adults: I.M.:

Mild arsenic and gold poisoning: 2.5 mg/kg/dose every 6 hours for 2 days, then every 12 hours on the third day, and once daily thereafter for 10 days

Severe arsenic and gold poisoning: 3 mg/kg/dose every 4 hours for 2 days then every 6 hours on the third day, then every 12 hours thereafter for 10 days

Mercury poisoning: 5 mg/kg initially followed by 2.5 mg/kg/dose 1-2 times/day for 10 days

Lead poisoning: (use with edetate calcium disodium):

Mild: 4 mg/kg/dose for one dose then 3 mg/kg/dose every 4 hours for 2-7 days

Severe and acute encephalopathy: (**blood lead levels** >70 mcg/dL): 4 mg/kg/dose every 4 hours in combination with edetate calcium disodium (see Administration) for at least 72 hours; may use for up to 5 days; if additional days of therapy (>5 days) are indicated, a minimum of 2 days without treatment should elapse before considering another treatment course

Administration Parenteral: Administer undiluted, deep I.M.; when used with calcium EDTA for lead poisoning, do not administer calcium EDTA with first dimercaprol dose; begin with second dimercaprol dose

Monitoring Parameters Specific heavy metal levels, urine pH, renal function, infusion-related reactions

Dosage Forms Excipient information presented when available (limited, particularly for generics); consult specific product labeling.

Injection, oil:

BAL in Oil®: 100 mg/mL (3 mL) [contains benzyl benzoate and peanut oil]

References

Gracia RC and Snodgrass WR, "Lead Toxicity and Chelation Therapy," Am J Health Syst Pharm, 2007, 64(1):45-53.
"Treatment Guidelines for Lead Exposure in Children. American Academy of Pediatrics Committee on Drugs," Pediatrics, 1995, 96(1 Pt 1):155-60.

◆ **Dimetapp® ND Children's [OTC] [DSC]** see Loratadine on page 842

◆ **Dimethyl Triazeno Imidazole Carboxamide** see Dacarbazine on page 380

◆ **Dinate® (Can)** see DimenhyDRINATE on page 446

◆ **Diocaine® (Can)** see Proparacaine on page 1168

◆ **Diocarpine (Can)** see Pilocarpine on page 1110

◆ **Diochloram® (Can)** see Chloramphenicol on page 289

◆ **Diocto® [OTC]** see Docusate on page 468

◆ **Dioctyl Calcium Sulfosuccinate** see Docusate on page 468

◆ **Dioctyl Sodium Sulfosuccinate** see Docusate on page 468

◆ **Diodex® (Can)** see Dexamethasone on page 406

◆ **Diodoquin® (Can)** see Iodoquinol on page 755

◆ **Diogent® (Can)** see Gentamicin on page 642

◆ **Diomycin® (Can)** see Erythromycin on page 525

◆ **Dionephrine® (Can)** see Phenylephrine on page 1102

◆ **Diopentolate® (Can)** see Cyclopentolate on page 368

◆ **Diopred® (Can)** see PrednisoLONE on page 1148

◆ **Dioptic's Atropine Solution (Can)** see Atropine on page 157

◆ **Dioptrol® (Can)** see Dexamethasone, Neomycin, and Polymyxin B on page 408

◆ **Diosulf™ (Can)** see Sulfacetamide on page 1298

◆ **Diotame® [OTC]** see Bismuth on page 195

◆ **Diotrope® (Can)** see Tropicamide on page 1390

◆ **Diovan®** see Valsartan on page 1402

◆ **Diovol® (Can)** see Aluminum Hydroxide and Magnesium Hydroxide on page 76

◆ **Diovol® Ex (Can)** see Aluminum Hydroxide and Magnesium Hydroxide on page 76

◆ **Dipentum®** see Olsalazine on page 1013

◆ **Diphen [OTC]** see DiphenhydrAMINE on page 448

◆ **Diphenhist® [OTC]** see DiphenhydrAMINE on page 448

DiphenhydrAMINE (dye fen HYE dra meen)

Medication Safety Issues

Institute for Safe Medication Practices (ISMP) has reported cases of patients mistakenly *swallowing* Benadryl® Itch Stopping [OTC] gel intended for topical application. Unclear labeling and similar packaging of the topical gel in containers resembling an oral liquid are factors believed to be contributing to the administration errors. The topical gel contains camphor which can be toxic if swallowed. ISMP has requested the manufacturer to make the necessary changes to prevent further confusion.

Sound-alike/look-alike issues:

DiphenhydrAMINE may be confused with desipramine, dicyclomine, dimenhyDRINATE

Benadryl® may be confused with benazepril, Bentyl®, Benylin®, Caladryl®

Beers Criteria medication: This drug may be inappropriate for use in geriatric patients (high severity risk).

International issues:

Sominex®: Brand name for promethazine in Great Britain

Related Information

Compatibility of Chemotherapy and Related Supportive Care Medications on page 1580

Compatibility of Medications Mixed in a Syringe on page 1713

U.S. Brand Names Aler-Cap [OTC]; Aler-Dryl [OTC]; Aler-Tab [OTC]; AllerMax® [OTC]; Altaryl [OTC]; Anti-Hist [OTC]; Banophen™ Anti-Itch [OTC]; Banophen™ [OTC]; Ben-Tann [DSC]; Benadryl® Allergy Quick Dissolve [OTC]; Benadryl® Allergy [OTC]; Benadryl® Children's Allergy Fastmelt® [OTC]; Benadryl® Children's Allergy Perfect Measure™; Benadryl® Children's Allergy [OTC]; Benadryl® Children's Dye-Free Allergy [OTC]; Benadryl® Children's Allergy Quick Dissolve [OTC] [DSC]; Benadryl® Dye-Free Allergy [OTC]; Benadryl® Itch Relief Extra Strength [OTC]; Benadryl® Itch Stopping Extra Strength [OTC]; Benadryl® Itch Stopping [OTC]; Compoz® Nighttime Sleep Aid [OTC]; Dermamycin® [OTC]; Diphen [OTC]; Diphenhist® [OTC]; Dytan™; Genahist™ [OTC]; Histaprin [OTC]; Hydramine [OTC] [DSC]; Nytol® Quick Caps [OTC]; Nytol® Quick Gels [OTC]; PediaCare® Children's Allergy [OTC]; PediaCare® Children's Night-Time Cough [OTC]; Siladryl Allergy [OTC]; Silphen Cough [OTC]; Simply Sleep™ [OTC]; Sleep-ettes D [OTC]; Sleep-Tabs [OTC]; Sleepinal® [OTC]; Sominex® Maximum Strength [OTC]; Sominex® [OTC]; Theraflu® Thin Strips® Multi Symptom [OTC]; Triaminic Thin Strips® Children's Cough and Runny Nose [OTC]; Twilite® [OTC]; Unisom® SleepGels® Maximum Strength [OTC]; Unisom® Sleep-Melts™ [OTC]

Canadian Brand Names Allerdryl®; Allernix; Benadryl®; Nytol®; Nytol® Extra Strength; PMS-Diphenhydramine; Simply Sleep®

Therapeutic Category Antidote, Drug-induced Dystonic Reactions; Antidote, Hypersensitivity Reactions; Antihistamine; Sedative

Generic Available Yes: Excludes chewable tablet, gel, liquid stick, orally-disintegrating tablet, strip

Use Symptomatic relief of allergic symptoms caused by histamine release which include nasal allergies and allergic dermatosis; mild nighttime sedation, prevention of motion sickness, as an antitussive; treatment of phenothiazine-induced dystonic reactions; adjunct to epinephrine in the treatment of anaphylaxis; topically for relief of pain and itching associated with insect bites, minor cuts and burns, or rashes

Pregnancy Risk Factor B

Pregnancy Considerations Teratogenic effects were not observed in animal studies. Diphenhydramine crosses the human placenta. One retrospective study showed an increased risk of cleft palate formation following maternal use of diphenhydramine during the 1st trimester of pregnancy; however, later studies have not confirmed this finding. Signs of toxicity and symptoms of withdrawal have been reported in infants following high doses or chronic maternal use close to term. Diphenhydramine has been evaluated for the treatment of hyperemesis gravidarum. It is generally not considered the antihistamine of choice for treating allergic rhinitis or nausea and vomiting during pregnancy.

Lactation Enters breast milk/contraindicated

Breast-Feeding Considerations Infants may be more sensitive to the effects of antihistamines. Use while breast-feeding is contraindicated by the manufacturer.

Contraindications Hypersensitivity to diphenhydramine or any component; should not be used in acute attacks of asthma; breast-feeding (infants may be more sensitive to the effects of antihistamines)

Warnings Safety and efficacy for the use of cough and cold products in children <2 years of age is limited. Serious adverse effects including death have been reported. The FDA notes that there are no approved OTC uses for these products in children <2 years of age. Healthcare providers are reminded to ask caregivers about the use of OTC cough and cold products in order to avoid exposure to multiple medications containing the same ingredient.

Topical diphenhydramine should not be used to treat chickenpox, poison ivy, or sunburn, on large areas of the body, or on blistered or oozing skin, due to potential for causing toxic psychosis, particularly in children.

Precautions Use with caution in patients with angle-closure glaucoma, peptic ulcer, urinary tract obstruction, hyperthyroidism; may cause paradoxical excitation in young children; toxicity can result in hallucinations, coma, and death; chewable tablets contain phenylalanine and must be used with caution in patients with phenylketonuria

Adverse Reactions

Cardiovascular: Hypotension, palpitations, tachycardia

Central nervous system: Sedation, dizziness, paradoxical excitement, fatigue, insomnia

Dermatologic: Photosensitivity, rash, urticaria

Gastrointestinal: Nausea, vomiting, xerostomia, dry mucous membranes, anorexia, constipation, epigastric distress

Genitourinary: Urinary retention, dysuria

Hematologic: Rare: Hemolytic anemia, aplastic anemia, thrombocytopenia

Neuromuscular & skeletal: Paresthesia of hands, tremor

Ocular: Blurred vision

Respiratory: Chest tightness, thickened bronchial secretions, wheezing

Drug Interactions

Metabolism/Transport Effects Inhibits CYP2D6 (moderate)

Avoid Concomitant Use There are no known interactions where it is recommended to avoid concomitant use.

Increased Effect/Toxicity

DiphenhydrAMINE may increase the levels/effects of: Alcohol (Ethyl); Anticholinergics; CNS Depressants; CYP2D6 Substrates; Fesoterodine; Nebivolol; Tamoxifen

The levels/effects of DiphenhydrAMINE may be increased by: Pramlintide

Decreased Effect

DiphenhydrAMINE may decrease the levels/effects of: Acetylcholinesterase Inhibitors (Central); Betahistine; Codeine; TraMADol

The levels/effects of DiphenhydrAMINE may be decreased by: Acetylcholinesterase Inhibitors (Central); Amphetamines

Stability Compatible when mixed in the same syringe: atropine, chlorpromazine, cimetidine, droperidol, fentanyl, glycopyrrolate, hydromorphone, meperidine, metoclopramide, midazolam, morphine, promethazine, and ranitidine

Mechanism of Action Competes with histamine for H_1-receptor sites on effector cells in the GI tract, blood vessels, and respiratory tract

Pharmacodynamics

Maximum sedative effect: 1-3 hours after administration

Duration: 4-7 hours

Pharmacokinetics (Adult data unless noted)

Absorption: Oral: Well absorbed but 40% to 60% of an oral dose reaches the systemic circulation due to first-pass metabolism

Distribution: Adults: V_d: 3-22 L/kg

Protein-binding: 78%

Metabolism: Extensive hepatic n-demethylation via CYP2D6; minor demethylation via CYP1A2, 2C9, and 2C19; significant first-pass effect

Bioavailability: ~40% to 70%

Half-life: 2-8 hours

Time to peak serum concentration: 2-4 hours

Elimination: Urine (as unchanged drug)

Usual Dosage

Oral, I.M., I.V.:

Treatment of phenothiazine dystonic reactions and moderate to severe allergic reactions:

Children: 5 mg/kg/day or 150 mg/m²/day in divided doses every 6-8 hours, not to exceed 300 mg/day

Adults: 25-50 mg every 4 hours, not to exceed 400 mg/day

Minor allergic rhinitis or motion sickness:

Children 2 to <6 years: 6.25 mg every 4-6 hours; maximum: 37.5 mg/day

Children 6 to <12 years: 12.5-25 mg [equivalent to 19-38 mg diphenhydramine citrate (Children's Benadryl® Allergy Fastmelt® 1-2 tablets)] every 4-6 hours; maximum: 150 mg/day (228 mg diphenhydramine citrate)

Children ≥12 years and Adults: 25-50 mg [equivalent to 38-76 mg diphenhydramine citrate (Children's Benadryl® Allergy Fastmelt® 2-4 tablets)] every 4-6 hours; maximum: 300 mg/day (456 mg diphenhydramine citrate)

Antitussive: Oral:

Children 2 to <6 years: 6.25 mg every 4 hours; maximum: 37.5 mg/day

Children 6 to <12 years: 12.5 mg every 4 hours; maximum: 75 mg/day

Children ≥12 years and Adults: 25 mg every 4 hours; maximum: 150 mg/day

Night-time sleep aid: 30 minutes before bedtime:

Children 2 to <12 years: 1 mg/kg/dose; maximum: 50 mg/dose

Children ≥12 years and Adults: 50 mg

Topical cream, gel, spray, or stick:

Children ≥2 to 12 years: Apply 1% concentration not more than 3-4 times/day

Children ≥12 years and Adults: Apply 1% or 2% concentration not more than 3-4 times/day

Administration

Oral: Administer with food to avoid GI distress

Parenteral:

I.V.: Dilute with compatible I.V. fluid to a maximum concentration of 25 mg/mL and infuse over 10-15 minutes (maximum rate of infusion: 25 mg/minute)

I.M.: 50 mg/mL concentration by deep I.M. injection

Topical: Shake well (gel); apply thin coat to affected area (see Warnings)

Test Interactions May suppress the wheal and flare reactions to skin test antigens; discontinue 4 days prior to skin testing procedures

Patient Information May cause drowsiness and impair ability to perform activities requiring mental alertness or physical coordination; may cause dry mouth. May rarely cause photosensitivity reactions (eg, exposure to sunlight may cause severe sunburn, skin rash, redness, or itching); avoid direct exposure to sunlight.

Additional Information Diphenhydramine citrate 19 mg is equivalent to diphenhydramine hydrochloride 12.5 mg

Dosage Forms Excipient information presented when available (limited, particularly for generics); consult specific product labeling. [DSC] = Discontinued product

Caplet, as hydrochloride: 25 mg, 50 mg
  Aler-Dryl, AllerMax®, Compoz® Nighttime Sleep Aid, Sleep-ettes D, Sominex® Maximum Strength, Twilite®: 50 mg
  Anti-Hist, Histaprin, Nytol® Quick Caps: 25 mg
  Simply Sleep™: 25 mg [contains calcium 20 mg/caplet]

Capsule, as hydrochloride: 25 mg, 50 mg
  Aler-Cap, Banophen™, Diphen, Diphenhist®, Genah-ist™: 25 mg
  Benadryl® Allergy: 25 mg [contains calcium 35 mg/capsule]
  Sleepinal®: 50 mg

Capsule, softgel, as hydrochloride: 50 mg
  Benadryl® Dye-Free Allergy: 25 mg [dye-free]
  Compoz® Nighttime Sleep Aid, Nytol® Quick Gels, Unisom® SleepGels® Maximum Strength: 50 mg

Captab, as hydrochloride:
  Diphenhist®: 25 mg

Cream, as hydrochloride: 2% (30 g)
  Banophen™ Anti-Itch: 2% (30 g) [contains zinc acetate 0.1%]
  Benadryl® Itch Stopping: 1% (15 g, 30 g) [contains zinc acetate 0.1%]
  Benadryl® Itch Stopping Extra Strength: 2% (15 g, 30 g) [contains zinc acetate 0.1%]
  Diphenhist®: 2% (30 g) [contains zinc acetate 0.1%]

Elixir, as hydrochloride: 12.5 mg/5 mL
  Altaryl: 12.5 mg/5 mL (120 mL, 480 mL, 3840 mL) [ethanol free; cherry flavor]
  Banophen™: 12.5 mg/5 mL (120 mL)

Gel, topical, as hydrochloride:
  Benadryl® Itch Stopping Extra Strength: 2% (120 mL)

Injection, solution, as hydrochloride: 50 mg/mL (1 mL, 10 mL)

Liquid, oral, as hydrochloride:
  AllerMax®: 12.5 mg/5 mL (120 mL)
  Benadryl® Children's Allergy: 12.5 mg/5 mL (120 mL, 240 mL) [ethanol free; contains sodium 14 mg/5 mL, sodium benzoate; cherry flavor]
  Benadryl® Children's Allergy Perfect Measure™: 12.5 mg/5 mL (5 mL) [ethanol free; contains sodium 14 mg/5 mL, sodium benzoate; cherry flavor]
  Benadryl® Children's Dye-Free Allergy: 12.5 mg/5 mL (120 mL) [ethanol free, dye free, sugar free; contains sodium 11 mg/5 mL, sodium benzoate; bubble gum flavor]
  Genahist™: 12.5 mg/5 mL (120 mL) [ethanol free, sugar free; contains sodium benzoate; cherry flavor]
  Hydramine: 12.5 mg/5 mL (120 mL, 480 mL) [ethanol free] [DSC]

Siladryl Allergy: 12.5 mg/5 mL (120 mL, 240 mL, 480 mL) [ethanol free, sugar free; black cherry flavor]

Liquid, topical, as hydrochloride [spray]:
  Benadryl® Itch Stopping Extra Strength: 2% (60 mL) [contains zinc acetate 0.1% and ethanol]
  Dermamycin®: 2% (60 mL) [contains menthol 1%]

Liquid, topical, as hydrochloride [stick]:
  Benadryl® Itch Relief Extra Strength: 2% (14 mL) [contains zinc acetate 0.1% and ethanol]

Solution, oral, as hydrochloride:
  Diphenhist®: 12.5 mg/5 mL (120 mL, 480 mL) [ethanol free; contains sodium benzoate]

Strips, orally disintegrating, as hydrochloride:
  Benadryl® Allergy Quick Dissolve: 25 mg (10s) [contains sodium 4 mg/strip; vanilla mint flavor]
  Benadryl® Children's Allergy Quick Dissolve: 12.5 mg (10s) [vanilla mint flavor] [DSC]
  Theraflu® Thin Strips® Multi Symptom: 25 mg (12s) [contains ethanol; vanilla mint flavor]
  Triaminic Thin Strips® Children's Cough and Runny Nose: 12.5 mg (14s) [contains ethanol; grape flavor]

Suspension, as tannate:
  Ben-Tann: 25 mg/5 mL (120 ml) [contains sodium benzoate; strawberry flavor] [DSC]

Syrup, as hydrochloride:
  PediaCare® Children's Allergy: 12.5 mg/5 mL (120 mL) [contains sodium 14 mg/5 mL, sodium benzoate; cherry flavor]
  PediaCare® Children's NightTime Cough: 12.5 mg/5 mL (120 mL) [ethanol free; contains sodium 15 mg/5 mL, sodium benzoate; cherry flavor]
  Silphen Cough: 12.5 mg/5 mL (120 mL, 240 mL, 480 mL) [contains ethanol 5%; strawberry flavor]

Tablet, as hydrochloride: 25 mg, 50 mg
  Aler-Tab, Banophen™, Benadryl® Allergy, Genahist™, Sominex®, Sleep-Tabs: 25 mg

Tablet, chewable, as hydrochloride:
  Benadryl® Children's Allergy: 12.5 mg [contains phenylalanine 4.2 mg, magnesium 15 mg, and sodium 2 mg per tablet; grape flavor] [DSC]

Tablet, chewable, as tannate:
  Dytan™: 25 mg [contains phenylalanine; strawberry flavor]

Tablet, orally disintegrating, as citrate:
  Benadryl® Children's Allergy Fastmelt®: 19 mg [equivalent to diphenhydramine hydrochloride 12.5 mg; contains phenylalanine 4.5 mg/tablet and soy protein isolate; cherry flavor] [DSC]

Tablet, orally dissolving, as hydrochloride:
  Benadryl® Children's Allergy Fastmelt®: 12.5 mg [cherry and grape flavors]
  Unisom® SleepMelts™: 25 mg [cherry flavor]

♦ **Diphenhydramine Citrate** *see* DiphenhydrAMINE *on page 448*

♦ **Diphenhydramine Hydrochloride** *see* Diphenhydr-AMINE *on page 448*

♦ **Diphenhydramine Tannate** *see* DiphenhydrAMINE *on page 448*

Diphenoxylate and Atropine
(dye fen OKS i late & A troe peen)

Medication Safety Issues

Sound-alike/look-alike issues:

Lomotil® may be confused with Lamictal®, Lamisil®, lamoTRIgine, Lanoxin®, Lasix®, ludiomil

Lonox® may be confused with Lanoxin®, Loprox®

International issues:

Lomotil® may be confused with Lemesil® which is a brand name for nimesulide in Greece

Lonox® may be confused with Flomox® which is a brand of cefcapene in Japan

U.S. Brand Names Lomotil®

Canadian Brand Names Lomotil®

Therapeutic Category Antidiarrheal

Generic Available Yes

Use Treatment of diarrhea

Restrictions C-V

Pregnancy Risk Factor C

Pregnancy Considerations Teratogenic effects were not noted in animal studies; decreased maternal weight, fertility and litter sizes were observed. There are no adequate and well-controlled studies in pregnant women.

Lactation Enters breast milk/use caution

Breast-Feeding Considerations Atropine is excreted in breast milk (refer to Atropine monograph); the manufacturer states that diphenoxylic acid may be excreted in breast milk.

Contraindications Hypersensitivity to diphenoxylate, atropine, or any component; severe liver disease, obstructive jaundice, dehydration, narrow-angle glaucoma, diarrhea associated with pseudomembranous enterocolitis or enterotoxin-producing bacteria. Do not use in children <2 years of age.

Warnings Use in conjunction with fluid and electrolyte therapy in children and in adults when appropriate. In case of severe dehydration or electrolyte imbalance, withhold diphenoxylate/atropine treatment until corrective therapy has been initiated. Inhibiting peristalsis may lead to fluid retention in the intestine aggravating dehydration and electrolyte imbalance. Reduction of intestinal motility may be deleterious in diarrhea resulting from *Shigella*, *Salmonella*, toxigenic strains of *E. coli* and from pseudomembranous enterocolitis associated with broad spectrum antibiotics; use is not recommended.

Use with caution in children. Younger children (especially those with Down syndrome) may develop signs of atropinism (dry skin and mucous membranes, thirst, hyperthermia, tachycardia, urinary retention, flushing) even at the recommended dosages. Overdose in children may result in severe respiratory depression, coma, and possibly permanent brain damage.

If acute diarrhea does not clinically improve within 48 hours, this medication is unlikely to be effective and should be discontinued; if chronic diarrhea is not improved symptomatically within 10 days at maximum dosage, control is unlikely with further use. Prolonged use may result in tolerance to antidiarrheal effects and physical or psychological dependence; abrupt discontinuation may cause withdrawal symptoms.

Precautions Use with extreme caution in patients with dehydration, cirrhosis, hepatorenal disease, renal dysfunction, and acute ulcerative colitis

Adverse Reactions

Cardiovascular: Tachycardia

Central nervous system: Sedation, dizziness, euphoria, headache, depression, lethargy, confusion, restlessness, hyperthermia, flushing

Dermatologic: Pruritus, urticaria, angioneurotic edema, dry skin and mucous membranes

Gastrointestinal: Nausea, vomiting, abdominal discomfort, anorexia, paralytic ileus, pancreatitis, toxic megacolon, xerostomia, gum swelling

Genitourinary: Urinary retention

Neuromuscular & skeletal: Weakness, numbness of extremities

Ocular: Blurred vision

Respiratory: Respiratory depression (young children may be at greater risk)

Miscellaneous: Anaphylaxis; physical and psychological dependence with prolonged use

Drug Interactions

Avoid Concomitant Use There are no known interactions where it is recommended to avoid concomitant use.

Increased Effect/Toxicity

Diphenoxylate and Atropine may increase the levels/ effects of: AbobotulinumtoxinA; Alcohol (Ethyl); Anticholinergics; Cannabinoids; CNS Depressants; Methotrimeprazine; OnabotulinumtoxinA; Potassium Chloride; RimabotulinumtoxinB

The levels/effects of Diphenoxylate and Atropine may be increased by: Methotrimeprazine; Pramlintide

Decreased Effect

Diphenoxylate and Atropine may decrease the levels/ effects of: Acetylcholinesterase Inhibitors (Central); Secretin

The levels/effects of Diphenoxylate and Atropine may be decreased by: Acetylcholinesterase Inhibitors (Central)

Stability Protect from light; dispense liquid only in original container

Mechanism of Action Diphenoxylate inhibits excessive GI motility and GI propulsion; commercial preparations contain a subtherapeutic amount of atropine to discourage abuse

Pharmacodynamics Antidiarrheal effects:

Onset of action: Within 45-60 minutes

Maximum effect: Within 2 hours

Duration: 3-4 hours

Tolerance to antidiarrheal effects may occur with prolonged use

Pharmacokinetics (Adult data unless noted)

Atropine: See Atropine

Diphenoxylate:

Absorption: Oral: Well absorbed

Distribution: Major metabolite (diphenoxylic acid) may be excreted in breast milk

Metabolism: Extensive in the liver via ester hydrolysis to diphenoxylic acid (active)

Half-life:

Diphenoxylate: 2.5 hours

Diphenoxylic acid: 12-24 hours

Time to peak serum concentration: ~2 hours

Elimination: Primarily (49%) in feces (via bile); ~14% is excreted in urine; <1% excreted unchanged in urine

Usual Dosage Oral (as diphenoxylate):

Children 2-12 years: **Liquid: Note:** Only the liquid product is recommended for children under 13 years of age; do not exceed recommended doses; reduce dose as soon as symptoms are initially controlled; maintenance doses may be as low as 25% of initial dose; if no improvement within 48 hours of therapy, diphenoxylate is not likely to be effective

Initial: 0.3-0.4 mg/kg/day in 4 divided doses (maximum: 10 mg/day) **or**

Manufacturer's recommendations: Initial:

<2 years: Not recommended

2 years (11-14 kg): 1.5-3 mL 4 times/day

3 years (12-16 kg): 2-3 mL 4 times/day

4 years (14-20 kg): 2-4 mL 4 times/day

5 years (16-23 kg): 2.5-4.5 mL 4 times/day

6-8 years (17-32 kg): 2.5-5 mL 4 times/day

9-12 years (23-55 kg): 3.5-5 mL 4 times/day

Alternative pediatric dosing: Initial:

<2 years: Not recommended

2-5 years: 2 mg 3 times/day

5-8 years: 2 mg 4 times/day

8-12 years: 2 mg 5 times/day

Adults: Initial: 5 mg (2 tablets or 10 mL) 4 times/day until control achieved (maximum: 20 mg/day); then reduced dose as needed; maintenance: 5-15 mg/day in 2-3 divided doses; some patients may be controlled on doses as low as 5 mg/day

Note: Do not exceed recommended doses; reduce dose once symptoms are initially controlled; acute diarrhea usually improves within 48 hours; if chronic diarrhea dose not improve within 10 days at maximum daily doses of 20 mg, diphenoxylate is not likely to be effective.

Administration Oral: May be administered with food to decrease GI upset; use plastic dropper provided when measuring liquid; **Note:** Dropper has a 2 mL (1 mg) capacity and is calibrated in increments of ½ mL (0.25 mg)

Monitoring Parameters Bowel frequency, signs and symptoms of atropinism, fluid and electrolytes

Patient Information Take as directed; do not exceed recommended dosage. If diarrhea does not improve within 48 hours, notify prescriber. Avoid alcohol and the herbal medicine St John's wort; may cause dizziness or drowsiness and impair ability to perform activities requiring mental alertness or physical coordination; may cause dry mouth; may be habit-forming; avoid abrupt discontinuation after prolonged use

Additional Information Naloxone reverses toxicity due to diphenoxylate; Lomotil® solution also contains sorbitol

Dosage Forms Excipient information presented when available (limited, particularly for generics); consult specific product labeling. [DSC] = Discontinued product

Solution, oral: Diphenoxylate hydrochloride 2.5 mg and atropine sulfate 0.025 mg per 5 mL (5 mL, 10 mL, 60 mL)

Lomotil®: Diphenoxylate hydrochloride 2.5 mg and atropine sulfate 0.025 mg per 5 mL (60 mL) [contains alcohol 15%; cherry flavor] [DSC]

Tablet: Diphenoxylate hydrochloride 2.5 mg and atropine sulfate 0.025 mg

Lomotil®: Diphenoxylate hydrochloride 2.5 mg and atropine sulfate 0.025 mg

♦ **Diphenylhydantoin** *see* Phenytoin *on page 1104*

Diphtheria and Tetanus Toxoid
(dif THEER ee a & TET a nus TOKS oyd)

Medication Safety Issues
Sound-alike/look-alike issues:
Diphtheria and Tetanus Toxoids (Td) may be confused with tuberculin purified protein derivative (PPD)

Related Information
Immunization Guidelines *on page 1636*

U.S. Brand Names Decavac®

Canadian Brand Names Td Adsorbed

Therapeutic Category Vaccine

Generic Available Yes

Use
Diphtheria and tetanus toxoids adsorbed for pediatric use (DT): Infants and Children through 6 years of age: Active immunity against diphtheria and tetanus and tetanus prophylaxis in wound management when pertussis vaccine is contraindicated

Tetanus and diphtheria toxoids adsorbed for adult use (Td) (Decavac™): Children ≥7 years of age and Adults: Active immunity against diphtheria and tetanus; tetanus prophylaxis in wound management

Pregnancy Risk Factor C

Pregnancy Considerations Reproduction studies have not been conducted. DT is not recommended for use in persons ≥7 years of age. The Advisory Committee on Immunization Practices (ACIP) recommends booster injections for previously vaccinated pregnant women who have not had Td vaccination within the past 10 years.

Pregnant women who are not immunized or are only partially immunized should complete the primary series. Vaccination may be deferred until the postpartum period in women who are likely to have sufficient diphtheria and tetanus protection until delivery; Tdap may be substituted for Td after delivery to add extra protection against pertussis. Td should be administered during pregnancy to women who do not have sufficient tetanus immunity to protect against maternal and neonatal tetanus, and if booster protection for diphtheria is required (eg, travel to where diphtheria is endemic). Tetanus immune globulin and a tetanus toxoid containing vaccine are recommended by the ACIP as part of the standard wound management to prevent tetanus in pregnant women; the use of Td during pregnancy is recommended for wound management if ≥5 years have passed since the last Td vaccination.

Lactation Excretion in breast milk unknown/use caution

Contraindications Hypersensitivity to diphtheria, tetanus toxoid, or any component of the formulation

Warnings Diphtheria and tetanus toxoid is available in two formulations which contain different amounts of the diphtheria toxoid; DT or "pediatric" formulation has twice the diphtheria toxoid as Td or "adult" toxoid; use of DT in children >7 years and adults is associated with more severe adverse reactions to the diphtheria toxoid than in infants and younger children. Immediate treatment for anaphylactic/anaphylactoid reaction should be available during administration of these vaccines. Patients with a history of severe local reaction (Arthus-type) or temperature of >39.4°C (103°F) following a previous dose should not be given further routine or emergency doses of Td more frequently than every 10 years. Defer administration during moderate or severe illness (with or without fever). Immune response may be decreased in immunocompromised patients. Guillain-Barré syndrome, occurring within 6 weeks of tetanus toxoid vaccination, has been reported.

Precautions Administer with caution to patients with thrombocytopenia or any coagulation disorder that would be compromised by I.M. injection; if the patient receives antihemophilia or other similar therapy, I.M. injection can be scheduled shortly after such therapy is administered. Routine prophylactic administration of acetaminophen to prevent fever due to vaccines has been shown to decrease the immune response of some vaccines; the clinical significance of this reduction in immune response has not been established (see Prymula, 2009).

Adverse Reactions All serious adverse reactions must be reported to the U.S. Department of Health and Human Services (DHHS) Vaccine Adverse Event Reporting System (VAERS) 1-800-822-7967.

Central nervous system: Brachial neuritis, Guillain-Barré syndrome (rare), dizziness, paresthesia, seizures, fever, malaise, EEG disturbances, encephalopathy (rare)

Dermatologic: Rash, urticaria

Gastrointestinal: Nausea, vomiting

Local: Tenderness, erythema, swelling, or pain at injection site; sterile abscess; palpable nodule at injection site

Neuromuscular & skeletal: Arthralgia, myalgia

Miscellaneous: Allergic/anaphylactic reactions, Arthus-type hypersensitivity reaction

Drug Interactions
Avoid Concomitant Use There are no known interactions where it is recommended to avoid concomitant use.

Increased Effect/Toxicity There are no known significant interactions involving an increase in effect.

Decreased Effect
The levels/effects of Diphtheria and Tetanus Toxoids may be decreased by: Immunosuppressants

Stability Refrigerate; do not freeze

Usual Dosage I.M.: 0.5 mL/dose; preterm infants should be vaccinated according to their chronological age from birth

Infants and Children up to 6 years (prior to 7th birthday) with contraindication to immunization containing pertussis: Pediatric formulation (DT):

Recommended schedule: A series of 5 doses administered at 2 months, 4 months, 6 months, 15-18 months, and 4-6 years of age; the 4th dose may be administered as early as 12 months if there has been at least 6 months between the 3rd and 4th doses and the child is unlikely to return at age 15-18 months.

Catch-up schedule: Age at onset of immunization series: Children 4 months through 6 years (prior to 7th birthday): 3 doses at least 4 weeks apart followed 6 months later with dose 4; a 5th dose may be given 6 months later (the 5th dose is not necessary if the child received the 4th dose after 4 years of age)

Children ≥7 years and Adults: Adult formulation (Td):

Primary immunization: 3 total doses; 2 given at intervals of 4-6 weeks; the third 6-12 months later

Booster immunization:

Children 11-12 years: A single dose when at least 5 years have elapsed since last dose of toxoid containing vaccine

Adults: A single dose every 10 years

Tetanus prophylaxis in wound management: Use of tetanus toxoid (DT or Td) and/or tetanus immune globulin (TIG) depends upon the number of prior tetanus toxoid (TT) doses and type of wound: A single 0.5 mL dose; see table.

Tetanus Prophylaxis in Wound Management

Number of Prior Tetanus Toxoid Doses	Clean, Minor Wounds		All Other Wounds	
	DT or Td[1] or Tdap[2]	TIG[3]	DT or Td[1] or Tdap[2]	TIG[3]
Unknown or <3	Yes	No	Yes	Yes
≥3[4]	No[5]	No	No[6]	No

[1]Use of combined antigen immunization (DT, Td, or DTaP) is preferred. Use tetanus and diphtheria toxoids formulation based upon age; use pediatric preparations (DT or DTaP) if the patient is <7 years old and Td if ≥7 years.

[2]Tdap is preferred in adolescents ≥10 years and adults who have never received Tdap. Td is preferred to TT in adolescents ≥10 years and adults who received Tdap previously or when Tdap is not available. If TT and TIG are both used, tetanus toxoid (adsorbed) rather than tetanus toxoid (fluid) should be used.

[3]Tetanus immune globulin.

[4]If only three doses of fluid tetanus toxoid have been received, a fourth dose of toxoid, preferably an adsorbed toxoid, should be given.

[5]Yes, if >10 years since last dose.

[6]Yes, if >5 years since last dose.

Adapted from *MMWR*, 1991, 40(RR-10):1-28; *MMWR*, 2009, 58 (14):374-5; *MMWR*, 2006, 55(RR-3):1-34; *MMWR Recomm Rep*, 2006, 55(RR-17)1-37

Administration I.M. Prior to use, shake suspension well; **not for I.V. or SubQ administration**

Td: Administer in the deltoid muscle; do not inject in the gluteal area

DT: Administer in either the anterolateral aspect of the thigh or arm; do not inject in the gluteal area

Patient Information May experience mild fever or soreness, swelling, and redness/knot at the injection site usually lasting 1-2 days

Nursing Implications Federal law requires that the date of administration, the vaccine manufacturer, lot number of vaccine, and the administering person's name, title, and address be entered into the patient's permanent medical record.

Additional Information In order to maximize vaccination rates, the ACIP recommends simultaneous administration of all age-appropriate vaccines (live or inactivated) for which a person is eligible at a single visit, unless contraindications exist. The use of combination vaccines is generally preferred over separate infections, taking into consideration provider assessment, patient preference, and potential adverse events.

For additional information, please refer to the following website: http://www.cdc.gov/vaccines/vpd-vac/.

Dosage Forms Excipient information presented when available (limited, particularly for generics); consult specific product labeling. [DSC] = Discontinued product

Injection, suspension [Td, adult]: Diphtheria 2 Lf units and tetanus 2 Lf units per 0.5 mL (7.5 mL) [DSC]; Diphtheria 2 Lf units and tetanus 5 Lf units per 0.5 mL (5 mL) [DSC]

Injection, suspension [Td, adult; preservative free]: Diphtheria 2 Lf units and tetanus 2 Lf units per 0.5 mL (0.5 mL)

Decavac®: Diphtheria 2 Lf units and tetanus 5 Lf units per 0.5 mL (0.5 mL) [contains aluminum, thimerosal (may have trace amounts)]

Injection, suspension [DT, pediatric; preservative free]: Diphtheria 6.7 Lf units and tetanus 5 Lf units per 0.5 mL (0.5 mL)

References

American Academy of Pediatrics Committee on Infectious Diseases, "Recommended Immunization Schedules for Children and Adolescents - United States, 2007," *Pediatrics*, 2007, 119(1):207-8.

Atkinson WL, Pickering LK, Schwartz B, et al, "General Recommendations on Immunization. Recommendations of the Advisory Committee on Immunization Practices (ACIP) and the American Academy of Family Physicians (AAFP)," *MMWR Recomm Rep*, 2002, 51(RR-2):18.

Broder KR, Cortese MM, Iskander JK, et al, "Preventing Tetanus, Diphtheria, and Pertussis Among Adolescents: Use of Tetanus Toxoid, Reduced Diphtheria Toxoid and Acellular Pertussis Vaccines Recommendations of the Advisory Committee on Immunization Practices (ACIP)," *MMWR Recomm Rep*, 2006, 55(RR-3):1-34.

Centers for Disease Control and Prevention (CDC), "FDA Approval of Expanded Age Indication for a Tetanus Toxoid, Reduced Diphtheria Toxoid and Acellular Pertussis Vaccine," *MMWR Morb Mortal Wkly Rep*, 2009, 58(14):374-5.

Centers for Disease Control and Prevention (CDC), "General Recommendations on Immunization. Recommendations of the Advisory Committee on Immunization Practices (ACIP)," *MMWR Recomm Rep*, 2006, 55(RR-15):1-48. Available at: http://www.cdc.gov/mmwr/preview/mmwrhtml/rr5515a1.htm.

Centers for Disease Control, "Recommended Adult Immunization Schedule, October 2004-September 2005," available at www.cdc.gov.

"Diphtheria, Tetanus, and Pertussis: Recommendations for Vaccine Use and Other Preventive Measures. Recommendations of the Immunization Practices Advisory committee (ACIP)," *MMWR Recomm Rep*, 1991, 40(RR-10):1-28.

Kretsinger K, Broder KR, Cortese MM, et al, "Preventing Tetanus, Diphtheria, and Pertussis Among Adults: Use of Tetanus Toxoid, Reduced Diphtheria Toxoid and Acellular Pertussis Vaccine Recommendations of the Advisory Committee on Immunization Practices (ACIP) and Recommendation of ACIP, Supported by the Healthcare Infection Control Practices Advisory Committee (HICPAC), for Use of Tdap Among Health-Care Personnel," *MMWR Recomm Rep*, 2006, 55(RR-17):1-37.

Prymula R, Siegrist CA, Chlibek R, et al, "Effect of Prophylactic Paracetamol Administration at Time of Vaccination on Febrile Reactions and Antibody Responses in Children: Two Open-Label, Randomised Controlled Trials," *Lancet*, 2009, 374(9698):1339-50.

Diphtheria and Tetanus Toxoids, Acellular Pertussis, and Poliovirus Vaccine

(dif THEER ee a & TET a nus TOKS oyds, ay CEL yoo lar per TUS sis & POE lee oh VYE rus vak SEEN)

Related Information

Immunization Guidelines *on page 1636*

U.S. Brand Names Kinrix™

Therapeutic Category Vaccine

Generic Available No

Use Active immunization in children 4-6 years of age against diphtheria, tetanus, pertussis, and poliomyelitis; used as the 5th dose in the DTaP series and the 4th dose in the IPV series (FDA approved in ages 4-6 years)

The Advisory Committee on Immunization Practices (ACIP) recommends this as routine vaccination for use as the fifth dose in the DTaP series and the fourth dose in the IPV series in children who received DTaP (Infanrix®) and/or DTaP-Hepatitis B-IPV (Pediarix®) as the first 3 doses and DTaP (Infanrix®) as the fourth dose. Whenever feasible, the same manufacturer should be used to provide the pertussis component; however, vaccination should not be deferred if a specific brand is not known or is not available.

Pregnancy Risk Factor C

Pregnancy Considerations Reproduction studies have not been conducted; not indicated for women of child-bearing age.

Breast-Feeding Considerations Not indicated for use by patients ≥7 years of age

Contraindications Hypersensitivity to any component including neomycin and polymyxin B; encephalopathy occurring within 7 days of administration of a previous dose of a pertussis-containing vaccine that is not attributable to another cause; progressive neurological disorder, including infantile spasms, uncontrolled epilepsy, or progressive encephalopathy (pertussis vaccine should be withheld until the clinical condition has stabilized)

Warnings Subsequent vaccination with a pertussis-containing vaccine should be carefully considered if the following reactions occur with a temporal relationship to a previous dose of DTaP: Temperature ≥40.5°C (105°F) within 48 hours, not attributable to another identifiable cause; collapse or shock-like state (hypotonic-hyporesponsive episode) within 48 hours; persistent crying lasting ≥3 hours within 48 hours; or convulsions with or without fever, occurring within 3 days. Guillain Barré syndrome occurring within 6 weeks of vaccines containing tetanus toxoid has been reported. Tetanus toxoid containing vaccine (including emergency doses) should not be given more frequently than every 10 years in patients who have experienced a serious Arthus-type hypersensitivity reaction following a prior use of tetanus toxoid; these patients generally have high serum antitoxin levels. Patients with latex allergy should not handle the needle cover or plunger of the prefilled syringes since they contain latex.

Precautions Defer vaccination for persons with acute febrile illness until recovery. A family history of seizures is not a contraindication to use of DTaP. Routine prophylactic administration of acetaminophen to prevent fever due to vaccines has been shown to decrease the immune response of some vaccines; the clinical significance of this reduction in immune response has not been established (see Prymula, 2009). Immediate treatment for anaphylactoid or acute hypersensitivity reactions should be available during vaccine use; administer with caution to patients with thrombocytopenia or any coagulation disorder that would be compromised by I.M. injection; if the patient receives antihemophilia or other similar therapy, I.M. injection can be scheduled shortly after such therapy is administered.

Adverse Reactions All serious adverse reactions must be reported to the U.S. Department of Health and Human Services (DHHS) Vaccine Adverse Event Reporting System (VAERS) 1-800-822-7967. See individual agents.

Central nervous system: Drowsiness, fever

Gastrointestinal: Loss of appetite

Local: Injection site: Arm circumference increase, pain, redness, swelling

<1%, postmarketing, and/or case reports: Cellulitis, cerebrovascular accident, constipation, dehydration, gastroenteritis, hypernatremia, injection site vesicles, pruritus. Additional postmarketing events associated with Infanrix®: Allergic reactions, anaphylactoid reactions, anaphylaxis, angioedema, apnea, hypotonic-hyporesponsive episode, lymphadenopathy, seizures, thrombocytopenia, urticaria

Drug Interactions

Avoid Concomitant Use There are no known interactions where it is recommended to avoid concomitant use.

Increased Effect/Toxicity There are no known significant interactions involving an increase in effect.

Decreased Effect

The levels/effects of Diphtheria and Tetanus Toxoids, Acellular Pertussis, and Poliovirus Vaccine may be decreased by: Immunosuppressants

Stability Store under refrigeration of 2°C to 8°C (36°F to 46°F); do not freeze. Discard if frozen.

Mechanism of Action Promotes active immunity to diphtheria, tetanus, pertussis, and poliovirus (types 1, 2, and 3) by inducing production of specific antibodies and antitoxins

Usual Dosage I.M.: Children 4-6 years: 0.5 mL; **Note:** For use as the 5th dose in the DTaP series and the 4th dose in the IPV series

Administration Shake well; do not use unless a homogeneous, turbid, white suspension forms; administer I.M. the deltoid muscle of the upper arm; **not for I.V. or SubQ administration**

Administration with other vaccines:

Multiple inactivated vaccines: May be given simultaneously or at any interval between doses.

Inactivated and live vaccines: May be given simultaneously or at any interval between doses.

Patient Information May cause increased sleeping, restlessness, fussiness, decreased appetite, or fever (use antipyretic if directed by healthcare provider). May cause some redness, pain, or swelling at injection site; consult healthcare provider if excessive or persistent. Notify healthcare provider immediately of any excessive or persistent reactions (eg, fever >105°F within 48 hours, inconsolable crying that occurs within 48 hours and lasts 3 hours, seizures that occur within 3 days).

Nursing Implications Federal law requires that the date of administration, name of the vaccine manufacturer, lot number of vaccine, and the administering person's name, title, and address be entered into the patient's permanent medical record.

Additional Information Contains the following three pertussis antigens: Inactivated pertussis toxin (PT), filamentous hemagglutinin (FHA), and pertactin. Contains the same diphtheria, tetanus toxoids, and pertussis antigens found in Infanrix® and Pediarix®. Contains the same poliovirus antigens found in Infanrix®.

In order to maximize vaccination rates, the ACIP recommends simultaneous administration of all age-appropriate vaccines (live or inactivated) for which a person is eligible at a single visit, unless contraindications exist. The use of combination vaccines is generally preferred over separate infections, taking into consideration provider assessment, patient preference, and potential adverse events.

For additional information, please refer to the following website: http://www.cdc.gov/vaccines/vpd-vac/.

Dosage Forms Excipient information presented when available (limited, particularly for generics); consult specific product labeling.

Injection, suspension [preservative free]:

Kinrix™: Diphtheria toxoid 25 Lf, tetanus toxoid 10 Lf, acellular pertussis antigens [inactivated pertussis toxin 25 mcg, filamentous hemagglutinin 25 mcg, pertactin 8 mcg], type 1 poliovirus 40 D-antigen units, type 2 poliovirus 8 D-antigen units, and type 3 poliovirus 32 D-antigen units per 0.5 mL (0.5 mL) [contains aluminum, neomycin sulfate, polymyxin B, polysorbate 80, natural rubber/natural latex in packaging]

References

Centers for Disease Control and Prevention (CDC), "General Recommendations on Immunization. Recommendations of the Advisory Committee on Immunization Practices (ACIP)," *MMWR Recomm Rep*, 2006, 55(RR-15):1-48. Available at: http://www.cdc.gov/mmwr/preview/mmwrhtml/rr5515a1.htm.

Centers for Disease Control and Prevention (CDC), "Recommended Immunization Schedules for Persons Aged 0 Through 18 years – United States, 2009," *MMWR Morb Mortal Wkly Rep*, 2009, 57(51):Q1-4.

Centers for Disease Control and Prevention (CDC), "Licensure of a Diphtheria and Tetanus Toxoids and Acellular Pertussis Adsorbed and Inactivated Poliovirus Vaccine and Guidance for Use as a Booster Dose," *MMWR Morb Mortal Wkly Rep*, 2008, 57(39):1078-9.

Prymula R, Siegrist CA, Chlibek R, et al, "Effect of Prophylactic Paracetamol Administration at Time of Vaccination on Febrile Reactions and Antibody Responses in Children: Two Open-Label, Randomised Controlled Trials," *Lancet*, 2009, 374(9698):1339-50.

Diphtheria and Tetanus Toxoids, Acellular Pertussis, Poliovirus and *Haemophilus* b Conjugate Vaccine

(dif THEER ee a & TET a nus TOKS oyds ay CEL yoo lar per TUS sis POE lee oh VYE rus & hem OF fi lus in floo EN za bee KON joo gate vak SEEN)

Medication Safety Issues

Pentacel® is supplied in two vials, one containing DTaP-IPV liquid and one containing Hib powder, which must be mixed together in order to administer the recommended vaccine components.

Related Information

Immunization Guidelines *on page 1636*

U.S. Brand Names Pentacel®

Canadian Brand Names Pediacel®; Pentacel®

Therapeutic Category Vaccine

Generic Available No

Use Active immunization against diphtheria, tetanus, pertussis, poliomyelitis, and invasive disease caused by *H. influenzae* type b in infants (at least 6 weeks of age) and children (prior to fifth birthday) (FDA approved in ages 6 weeks through 4 years)

Advisory Committee on Immunization Practices (ACIP) states that Pentacel® (DTaP-IPV/Hib) may be used to provide the recommended DTaP, IPV, and Hib immunization in children <5 years of age. Whenever feasible, the same manufacturer should be used to provide the pertussis component; however, vaccination should not be deferred if a specific brand is not known or is not available.

Pregnancy Risk Factor C

Pregnancy Considerations Reproduction studies have not been conducted for this combination product. This product is not indicated for use in women of childbearing age.

Breast-Feeding Considerations Not indicated for use by patients ≥5 years of age

Contraindications Hypersensitivity to any component including neomycin, polymyxin B; encephalopathy occurring within 7 days of administration of a previous dose of a pertussis-containing vaccine that is not attributable to another cause; progressive neurological disorder, including infantile spasms, uncontrolled epilepsy, or progressive encephalopathy (pertussis vaccine should be withheld until the clinical condition has stabilized)

Warnings Subsequent vaccination with a pertussis-containing vaccine should be carefully considered if the following reactions occur with a temporal relationship to a previous dose of DTaP: Temperature ≥40.5°C (105°F) within 48 hours, not attributable to another identifiable cause; collapse or shock-like state (hypotonic-hyporesponsive episode) within 48 hours; persistent crying lasting ≥3 hours within 48 hours; or convulsions with or without fever, occurring within 3 days. Guillain-Barré syndrome occurring within 6 weeks of vaccines containing tetanus toxoid has been reported. Tetanus toxoid containing vaccine (including emergency doses) should not be given more frequently than every 10 years in patients who have experienced a serious arthus-type hypersensitivity reaction following a prior use of tetanus toxoid; these patients generally have high serum antitoxin levels.

Precautions Defer vaccination in persons with moderate to severe illness until recovery. A family history of seizures is not a contraindication to use of DTaP; immediate treatment for anaphylactoid or acute hypersensitivity reactions should be available during vaccine use; administer with caution to patients with thrombocytopenia or any coagulation disorder that would be compromised by I.M. injection; if the patient receives antihemophilia or other similar therapy, I.M. injection can be scheduled shortly after such therapy is administered. Routine prophylactic administration of acetaminophen to prevent fever due to vaccines has been shown to decrease the immune response of some vaccines; the clinical significance of this reduction in immune response has not been established (see Prymula, 2009). Contains polysorbate 80; use caution in patients who may be sensitive.

Immunocompromised patients may have impaired response to vaccination. Examples include those with HIV infection, immunoglobulin deficiency, anatomic or functional asplenia, and sickle cell disease, as well as recipients of bone marrow transplants and recipients of chemotherapy for malignancy.

Adverse Reactions All serious adverse reactions must be reported to the U.S. Department of Health and Human Services (DHHS) Vaccine Adverse Event Reporting System (VAERS) 1-800-822-7967.

Central nervous system: Activity deceased, crying (inconsolable), fever (see Warnings), fussiness, hypotonic-hyporesponsive episodes (see Warnings), irritability, lethargy

Local: Injection site: Arm circumference increased, redness, swelling, tenderness

Miscellaneous: Hypersensitivity reactions (see Warnings)

<1%, postmarketing, and/or case reports: Apnea, appetite decreased, asthma, bronchiolitis, consciousness decreased, cough, cyanosis, dehydration, diarrhea, encephalopathy, erythema, gastroenteritis, hypotonia, injection site reactions (abscess, inflammation, mass), pallor, pneumonia, screaming, seizure, skin discoloration, somnolence, vomiting

Drug Interactions

Avoid Concomitant Use There are no known interactions where it is recommended to avoid concomitant use.

Increased Effect/Toxicity There are no known significant interactions involving an increase in effect.

Decreased Effect

The levels/effects of Diphtheria and Tetanus Toxoids, Acellular Pertussis, Poliovirus and Haemophilus b Conjugate Vaccine may be decreased by: Immunosuppressants

Stability Store under refrigeration of 2°C to 8°C (35°F to 46°F); do not freeze. Discard if frozen. Use immediately after reconstitution.

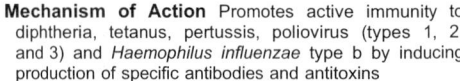

Mechanism of Action Promotes active immunity to diphtheria, tetanus, pertussis, poliovirus (types 1, 2, and 3) and *Haemophilus influenzae* type b by inducing production of specific antibodies and antitoxins

Usual Dosage

Children 6 weeks to ≤4 years: I.M.: 0.5 mL/dose administered at 2, 4, 6, and 15-18 months of age (total of 4 doses). The first dose may be administered as early as 6 weeks of age. Following completion of the 4-dose series, children should receive a dose of DTaP vaccine at 4-6 years of age (Daptacel® recommended due to same pertussis antigen used in both products).

Note: Per the ACIP, polio vaccine should not be administered more frequently than 4 weeks apart. Use of the minimum age and minimum intervals during the first 6 months of life should only be done when the vaccine recipient is at risk for imminent exposure to circulating poliovirus (shorter intervals and earlier start dates may lead to lower seroconversion). Pentacel® is not indicated for the polio booster dose given at 4-6 years of age; Kinrix® or IPV should be used.

Children previously vaccinated with ≥1 dose of Daptacel® or IPV vaccines: Pentacel® may be used to complete the first 4 doses of the DTaP or IPV series in children scheduled to receive the other components in the vaccine.

Children previously vaccinated with ≥1 dose of *Haemophilus b* Conjugate vaccine: Pentacel® may be used to complete the series in children scheduled to receive the other components in the vaccine; however, if different brands of *Haemophilus b* Conjugate vaccine are administered to complete the series, 3 primary immunizing doses are needed, followed by a booster dose.

Note: Completion of 3 doses of Pentacel® provides primary immunization against diphtheria, tetanus, *H. influenzae* type B, and poliomyelitis. Completion of the 4-dose series with Pentacel® provides primary immunization against pertussis. It also provides a booster vaccination against diphtheria, tetanus, *H. influenzae* type B, and poliomyelitis.

Administration Pentacel® is supplied in two vials, one containing DTaP-IPV liquid and one containing Hib powder. First, gently shake vial containing DTaP-IPV component; withdraw liquid contents, and inject into vial containing Hib powder; shake until uniform, cloudy suspension results.

Administer I.M. in the anterolateral aspect of thigh in children <1 year of age or deltoid muscle of upper arm in older children. Do not administer to gluteal area or areas near a major nerve trunk; **not for I.V. or SubQ administration**. Do not administer additional vaccines or immunoglobulins at the same site or using the same syringe.

Administration with other vaccines:
- Multiple inactivated vaccines: May be given simultaneously or at any interval between doses
- Inactivated and live vaccines: May be given simultaneously or at any interval between doses
- Vaccine administration with antibody-containing products: DTaP-IPV/Hib may be given simultaneously at different sites or at any interval between doses. Examples of antibody-containing products include I.M. and I.V. immune globulin, hepatitis B immune globulin, tetanus immune globulin, varicella zoster immune globulin, rabies immune globulin, whole blood, packed red cells, plasma, and platelet products.

Patient Information May cause increased sleeping, restlessness, fussiness, decreased appetite, or fever; use antipyretic if directed by healthcare provider. May cause some redness, pain, or swelling at injection site; consult healthcare provider if excessive or persistent. Notify healthcare provider immediately of any excessive or persistent reactions (eg, fever >105°F within 48 hours, inconsolable crying that occurs within 48 hours and lasts 3 hours, seizures that occur within 3 days).

Nursing Implications Federal law requires that the date of administration, name of the vaccine manufacturer, lot number of vaccine, and the administering person's name, title, and address be entered into the patient's permanent medical record.

Additional Information Contains the following three pertussis antigens: Inactivated pertussis toxin (PT), filamentous hemagglutinin (FHA), and pertactin. Contains the same diphtheria, tetanus toxoids, and pertussis antigens found in Daptacel®; the same poliovirus antigens found in IPOL®; the same Hib-PRP found in ActHIB®.

In order to maximize vaccination rates, the ACIP recommends simultaneous administration of all age-appropriate vaccines (live or inactivated) for which a person is eligible at a single visit, unless contraindications exist. The use of combination vaccines is generally preferred over separate infections, taking into consideration provider assessment, patient preference, and potential adverse events.

For additional information, please refer to the following website: http://www.cdc.gov/vaccines/vpd-vac/.

Dosage Forms Excipient information presented when available (limited, particularly for generics); consult specific product labeling.

Injection, suspension:

Pentacel®: Diphtheria toxoid 15 Lf, tetanus toxoid 5 Lf, acellular pertussis antigens (pertussis toxin detoxified 20 mcg, filamentous hemagglutinin 20 mcg, pertactin 3 mcg, fimbriae [types 2 and 3] 5 mcg), poliovirus (type 1: 40 D-antigen units; type 2: 8 D antigen units; type 3: 32 D-antigen units), and *Haemophilus* b capsular polysaccharide 10 mcg (bound to tetanus toxoid 24 mcg) per 0.5 mL (0.5 mL) [contains albumin, aluminum, neomycin, polymyxin B sulfate, and polysorbate 80; supplied in two vials, one containing DTaP-IPV liquid and one containing Hib powder]

References

Centers for Disease Control and Prevention (CDC), "General Recommendations on Immunization. Recommendations of the Advisory Committee on Immunization Practices (ACIP)," *MMWR Recomm Rep*, 2006, 55(RR-15):1-48. Available at: http://www.cdc.gov/mmwr/preview/mmwrhtml/rr5515a1.htm.

Centers for Disease Control and Prevention (CDC), "Licensure of a Diphtheria and Tetanus Toxoids and Acellular Pertussis Adsorbed, Inactivated Poliovirus, and *Haemophilus* B Conjugate Vaccine and Guidance for Use in Infants and Children," *MMWR Morb Mortal Wkly Rep*, 2008, 57(39):1079-80.

Centers for Disease Control and Prevention (CDC), "Updated Recommendations of the Advisory Committee on Immunization Practices (ACIP) Regarding Routine Poliovirus Vaccination," *MMWR Morb Mortal Wkly Rep*, 2009, 58(30):829-30.

Prymula R, Siegrist CA, Chlibek R, et al, "Effect of Prophylactic Paracetamol Administration at Time of Vaccination on Febrile Reactions and Antibody Responses in Children: Two Open-Label, Randomised Controlled Trials," *Lancet*, 2009, 374(9698):1339-50.

◆ **Diphtheria and Tetanus Toxoids and Acellular Pertussis Adsorbed, and Inactivated Poliovirus Vaccine Combined** *see* Diphtheria and Tetanus Toxoids, Acellular Pertussis, and Poliovirus Vaccine *on page 453*

◆ **Diphtheria and Tetanus Toxoids and Acellular Pertussis Adsorbed, Hepatitis B (Recombinant) and Inactivated Poliovirus Vaccine Combined** *see* Diphtheria, Tetanus Toxoids, Acellular Pertussis, Hepatitis B (Recombinant), and Poliovirus (Inactivated) Vaccine *on page 457*

◆ **Diphtheria CRM$_{197}$ Protein** *see* Pneumococcal Conjugate Vaccine (7-Valent) *on page 1121*

◆ **Diphtheria CRM$_{197}$ Protein** *see* Pneumococcal Conjugate Vaccine (13-Valent) *on page 1123*

◆ **Diphtheria, Tetanus Toxoids, Acellular Pertussis (DTaP)** *see* Diphtheria and Tetanus Toxoids, Acellular Pertussis, and Poliovirus Vaccine *on page 453*

◆ **Diphtheria, Tetanus Toxoids, Acellular Pertussis (DTaP)** *see* Diphtheria and Tetanus Toxoids, Acellular Pertussis, Poliovirus and *Haemophilus* b Conjugate Vaccine *on page 455*

Diphtheria, Tetanus Toxoids, Acellular Pertussis, Hepatitis B (Recombinant), and Poliovirus (Inactivated) Vaccine

(dif THEER ee a, TET a nus TOKS oyds, ay CEL yoo lar per TUS sis, hep a TYE tis bee ree KOM be nant, & POE lee oh VYE rus in ak ti VAY ted vak SEEN)

Related Information
Immunization Guidelines *on page 1636*

U.S. Brand Names Pediarix®

Canadian Brand Names Pediarix®

Therapeutic Category Vaccine

Generic Available No

Use Combination vaccine for the active immunization against diphtheria, tetanus, pertussis, hepatitis B virus (all known subtypes), and poliomyelitis (caused by poliovirus types 1, 2, and 3) (FDA approved in ages 6 weeks through 6 years)

Pregnancy Risk Factor C

Pregnancy Considerations Reproduction studies have not been conducted; not indicated for women of childbearing age.

Breast-Feeding Considerations Not indicated for women of childbearing age.

Contraindications Hypersensitivity to any component including yeast, neomycin, and polymyxin B; encephalopathy occurring within 7 days of administration of a previous dose of a pertussis-containing vaccine that is not attributable to another cause; progressive neurological disorder, including infantile spasms, uncontrolled epilepsy, or progressive encephalopathy (pertussis vaccine should be withheld until the clinical condition has stabilized); defer vaccination for persons with acute febrile illness until recovery; children ≥7 years and adults (formulation without pertussis is indicated for use in these patients)

Warnings Immediate treatment for anaphylactic/anaphylactoid reaction should be available during vaccine use. Subsequent vaccination with a pertussis containing vaccine should be carefully considered if the following reactions occur with a temporal relationship to a previous dose: Temperature ≥40.5°C (105°F) within 48 hours, not attributable to another identifiable cause; collapse, or shock-like state (hypotonic-hyporesponsive episode) within 48 hours, persistent crying lasting ≥3 hours within 48 hours, or convulsions with or without fever, occurring within 3 days. Guillain-Barré syndrome occurring within 6 weeks of vaccines containing tetanus toxoid has been reported; due to a higher rate of fever with this combination formulation than with individual vaccines, antipyretic prophylaxis at the time of and following vaccination may be considered for patients at high risk for seizures. Apnea has occurred following intramuscular vaccine administration in premature infants; consider clinical status implications.

Precautions Use with caution in patients with coagulation disorders including thrombocytopenia, due to an increased risk for bleeding following I.M. administration; if the patient receives antihemophilia or other similar therapy, I.M. injection can be scheduled shortly after such therapy is administered. Routine prophylactic administration of acetaminophen to prevent fever due to vaccines has been shown to decrease the immune response of some vaccines; the clinical significance of this reduction in

immune response has not been established (see Prymula, 2009).

Adverse Reactions All serious adverse reactions must be reported to the U.S. Department of Health and Human Services (DHHS) Vaccine Adverse Event Reporting System (VAERS) 1-800-822-7967. See individual agents.

Drug Interactions

Avoid Concomitant Use There are no known interactions where it is recommended to avoid concomitant use.

Increased Effect/Toxicity There are no known significant interactions involving an increase in effect.

Decreased Effect
The levels/effects of Diphtheria, Tetanus Toxoids, Acellular Pertussis, Hepatitis B (Recombinant), and Poliovirus Vaccine may be decreased by: Immunosuppressants

Stability Store under refrigeration at 2°C to 8°C (36°F to 46°F); do not freeze. Discard if frozen.

Mechanism of Action Promotes active immunity to diphtheria, tetanus, pertussis, hepatitis B and poliovirus (types 1, 2, and 3) by inducing production of specific antibodies and antitoxins.

Usual Dosage I.M.: Infants ≥6 weeks and Children <7 years: 0.5 mL per dose; preterm infants should be vaccinated according to their chronological age from birth Recommended schedule: 3 doses repeated in 6- to 8-week intervals (preferably 8-week intervals); vaccination usually begins at 2 months, but may be started as early as 6 weeks of age.

Note: Infants ≥6 weeks and children previously vaccinated with one or more components of this combination vaccine, and who are also scheduled to receive all vaccine components, may use Pediarix™ to complete the series.

Administration Shake well; administer I.M. in either the anterolateral aspect of the thigh or arm; **not for I.V. or SubQ administration**

Monitoring Parameters Monitor for syncope for ≥15 minutes following vaccination.

Patient Information May cause increased sleeping, restlessness, fussiness, decreased appetite, or fever (use antipyretic if directed by healthcare provider). May cause some redness, pain, or swelling at injection site; consult healthcare provider if excessive or persistent. Notify healthcare provider immediately if any excessive or persistent reactions (eg, fever >105°F within 48 hours, inconsolable crying that occurs within 48 hours and lasts 3 hours, seizures that occur within 3 days).

Nursing Implications Federal law requires that the date of administration, name of the vaccine manufacturer, lot number of vaccine, and the administering person's name, title, and address be entered into the patient's permanent medical record.

Additional Information Contains the following three pertussis antigens: Inactivated pertussis toxin (PT), filamentous hemagglutinin (FHA), and pertactin. Contains the same diphtheria and tetanus toxoids and pertussis antigens found in Infanrix®. Contains the same hepatitis B surface antigen (HB_sAg) found in Engerix-B® (recombinant vaccine). Thimerosal is used during manufacturing, but removed to less than detectable levels in the final suspension.

In order to maximize vaccination rates, the ACIP recommends simultaneous administration of all age-appropriate vaccines (live or inactivated) for which a person is eligible at a single visit, unless contraindications exist. The use of combination vaccines is generally preferred over separate infections, taking into consideration provider assessment, patient preference, and potential adverse events.

For additional information, please refer to the following website: http://www.cdc.gov/vaccines/vpd-vac/.

Dosage Forms Excipient information presented when available (limited, particularly for generics); consult specific product labeling.

Injection, suspension [preservative free]:

Pediarix®: Diphtheria toxoid 25 Lf, tetanus toxoid 10 Lf, acellular pertussis antigens [inactivated pertussis toxin 25 mcg, filamentous hemagglutin 25 mcg, pertactin 8 mcg, HBsAg 10 mcg, type 1 poliovirus 40 D antigen units, type 2 poliovirus 8 D antigen units and type 3 poliovirus 32 D antigen units] per 0.5 mL (0.5 mL) [contains aluminum, neomycin sulfate (trace amounts), polymyxin B (trace amounts), polysorbate 80, and yeast protein ≤5%; prefilled syringes contain natural rubber/natural latex]

References

Centers for Disease Control and Prevention (CDC), "General Recommendations on Immunization. Recommendations of the Advisory Committee on Immunization Practices (ACIP)," *MMWR Recomm Rep*, 2006, 55(RR-15):1-48. Available at: http://www.cdc.gov/mmwr/preview/mmwrhtml/rr5515a1.htm.

Centers for Disease Control and Prevention (CDC), "Syncope After Vaccination – United States, January 2005-July 2007," *MMWR Morb Mortal Wkly Rep*, 2008, 57(17):457-60.

Prymula R, Siegrist CA, Chlibek R, et al, "Effect of Prophylactic Paracetamol Administration at Time of Vaccination on Febrile Reactions and Antibody Responses in Children: Two Open-Label, Randomised Controlled Trials," *Lancet*, 2009, 374(9698):1339-50.

Diphtheria, Tetanus Toxoids, and Acellular Pertussis Vaccine

(dif THEER ee a, TET a nus TOKS oyds & ay CEL yoo lar per TUS sis vak SEEN)

Medication Safety Issues

Sound-alike/look-alike issues:

Adacel® (Tdap) may be confused with Daptacel® (DTap)

Carefully review product labeling to prevent inadvertent administration of Tdap when DTaP is indicated. Tdap contains lower amounts of diphtheria toxoid and some pertussis antigens than DTaP.

Tdap is not indicated for use in children <10 years of age
DTaP is not indicated for use in persons ≥7 years of age

Guidelines are available in case of inadvertent administration of these products; refer to ACIP recommendations, February 2006 available at http://www.cdc.gov/mmwr/preview/mmwrhtml/rr55e223a1.htm

Note:

DTaP: Diphtheria and tetanus toxoids and acellular pertussis vaccine

DTP: Diphtheria and tetanus toxoids and pertussis vaccine (unspecified pertussis antigens)

DTwP: Diphtheria and tetanus toxoids and whole-cell pertussis vaccine (no longer available on U.S. market)

Tdap: Tetanus toxoid, reduced diphtheria toxoid, and acellular pertussis vaccine

Related Information

Immunization Guidelines *on page 1636*

U.S. Brand Names Adacel®; Boostrix®; Daptacel®; Infanrix®; Tripedia®

Canadian Brand Names Adacel®; Boostrix®

Therapeutic Category Vaccine

Generic Available No

Use

Daptacel®, Infanrix®, Tripedia®: Active immunization for prevention of diphtheria, tetanus, and pertussis (FDA approved in ages 6 weeks through 6 years)

Adacel®: Active booster immunization for prevention of diphtheria, tetanus, and pertussis (FDA approved in ages 11-64 years); the Advisory Committee on Immunization Practices (ACIP) recommends a single dose for adults 19-64 years [this vaccine replaces tetanus and diphtheria

toxoids (Td) vaccine if the individual has received the last dose of Td ≥10 years earlier and has not previously received Tdap], adults who have or who anticipate having close contact with an infant <12 months, healthcare personnel who have direct patient contact, and persons wounded in bombings or similar mass casualty events who cannot confirm receipt of a tetanus booster within the last 5 years and who have penetrating injuries or nonintact skin exposure

Boostrix®: Active booster immunization for prevention of diphtheria, tetanus, and pertussis (FDA approved in ages 10-64 years)

Pregnancy Risk Factor C

Pregnancy Considerations Animal reproduction studies have not been conducted. It is not known whether the vaccine can cause fetal harm when administered to a pregnant woman or can affect reproductive capacity. Daptacel®, Infanrix®, and Tripedia® are not recommended for use in a pregnant woman or any patient ≥7 years of age. Although pregnancy itself is generally not considered a contraindication to Tdap (Adacel®, Boostrix®) vaccination, Td is preferred to Tdap when vaccination cannot be delayed during pregnancy. In order to help prevent pertussis exposure among infants, the use of Tdap, is recommended in women of childbearing potential prior to pregnancy. Due to lack of information with Tdap, a pregnancy registry has been established for women who may become exposed to Boostrix® (888-825-5249) or Adacel® (800-822-2463) while pregnant.

Lactation Excretion in breast milk unknown/use caution

Breast-Feeding Considerations Breast-feeding is not a contraindication to vaccine administration. Women who have not previously had a dose of Tdap should receive a dose postpartum to help prevent pertussis in infants <12 months of age.

Contraindications Hypersensitivity to any component; encephalopathy occurring within 7 days of administration of a previous dose of a pertussis-containing vaccine that is not attributable to another cause; progressive neurological disorder, including infantile spasms, uncontrolled epilepsy, or progressive encephalopathy; (pertussis vaccine should be withheld until the clinical condition has stabilized)

Warnings Subsequent vaccination with a pertussis containing vaccine should be carefully considered if the following reactions occur with a temporal relationship to a previous dose of DTaP: Temperature ≥40.5°C (105°F) within 48 hours, not attributable to another identifiable cause, collapse or shock-like state (hypotonic-hyporesponsive episode) within 48 hours, persistent crying lasting ≥3 hours within 48 hours, or convulsions with or without fever occurring within 3 days. Guillain Barré syndrome occurring within 6 weeks of vaccines containing tetanus toxoid has been reported. Tetanus toxoid containing vaccine (including emergency doses) should not be given more frequently than every 10 years in patients who have experienced a serious Arthus-type hypersensitivity reaction following a prior use of tetanus toxoid; these patients generally have high serum antitoxin concentrations. Boostrix® and Adacel® contain reduced antigens and are not indicated for use in the primary vaccine series (ages 6 weeks to 6 years). Apnea has occurred following intramuscular vaccine administration in premature infants; consider clinical status implications.

Precautions Defer vaccination for persons with acute febrile illness until recovery. A family history of seizures is not a contraindication to use of DTaP. Routine prophylactic administration of acetaminophen to prevent fever due to vaccines has been shown to decrease the immune response of some vaccines; the clinical significance of this reduction in immune response has not been established (see Prymula, 2009). Immediate treatment for anaphylactoid or acute hypersensitivity reactions should be available during vaccine use; administer with caution to patients with thrombocytopenia or any coagulation disorder that would be compromised by I.M. injection; if the patient receives antihemophilia or other similar therapy, I.M. injection can be scheduled shortly after such therapy is administered. Persons sensitive to latex should avoid contact with Infanrix® tip cap and plunger of needleless prefilled syringes.

Adverse Reactions All serious adverse reactions must be reported to the U.S. Department of Health and Human Services (DHHS) Vaccine Adverse Event Reporting System (VAERS) 1-800-822-7967.

Daptacel®, Infanrix®, Tripedia®:

Central nervous system: Fatigue, febrile seizures, fever, fussiness, Guillain-Barré (see Warnings), high-pitched cry, irritability, persistent crying, sleepiness

Gastrointestinal: Anorexia, vomiting

Local: Erythema, pain, swelling, or tenderness at injection site

Respiratory: Apnea (premature neonate) (see Warnings)

Miscellaneous: Hypersensitivity reactions including anaphylaxis or arthus type (see Warnings)

<1%, postmarketing, and/or case reports: Angioedema, autism, bronchitis, cellulitis, cough, cyanosis, diarrhea, ear pain, encephalopathy, erythema, fatigue, headache, hypersensitivity, hypotonia, hypotonic-hyporesponsive episode, idiopathic thrombocytopenic purpura, infantile spasm, injection site reaction (abscess, cellulitis, induration, mass, nodule, rash), intussusception, irritability, limb swelling, lymphadenopathy, nausea, pruritus, rash, respiratory tract infection, seizure, screaming, somnolence, SIDS (causal relationship has not been demonstrated), thrombocytopenia, urticaria

Boostrix® and Adacel®:

Central nervous system: Chills, fatigue, fever, Guillain-Barré (see Warnings), headache, tiredness

Dermatologic: Rash

Local: Erythema, pain, swelling, or tenderness at injection sit

Gastrointestinal: Abdominal pain, diarrhea, nausea, vomiting

Neuromuscular: Body aches/muscle weakness, sore/swollen joints

Miscellaneous: Anaphylaxis, arthus hypersensitivity (see Warnings), lymph node swelling

<1%, postmarketing and/or case reports: Arthralgia, back pain, brachial neuritis, bruising, diabetes mellitus, encephalitis, exanthema, facial palsy, Henoch-Schönlein purpura, injection site reaction (induration, inflammation, mass, nodule, warmth), limb swelling (extensive), lymphadenitis, lymphadenopathy, myalgia, myocarditis, nerve compression, paresthesia, pruritus, seizure, sterile abscess, urticaria, peripheral/central mononeuropathies

Drug Interactions

Avoid Concomitant Use There are no known interactions where it is recommended to avoid concomitant use.

Increased Effect/Toxicity There are no known significant interactions involving an increase in effect.

Decreased Effect

The levels/effects of Diphtheria and Tetanus Toxoids, and Acellular Pertussis Vaccine may be decreased by: Immunosuppressants

Stability Refrigerate; Tripedia® may be used to reconstitute ActHIB® for children ≥15 months of age

Usual Dosage I.M.: 0.5 mL per dose; preterm infants should be vaccinated according to their chronological age from birth

Recommended schedule: Children 6 weeks through 6 years (prior to 7th birthday): A series of five doses administered at 2 months, 4 months, 6 months, 15-20 months, and 4-6 years of age; the 4th dose may be administered as early as 12 months if there has been at least 6 months between the 3rd and 4th doses and the child is unlikely to return at age 15-20 months.

Catch-up schedule: Children 4 months through 6 years (prior to 7th birthday): 3 doses at least 4 weeks apart followed 6 months later with dose 4; a 5th dose may be given 6 months later (the 5th dose is not necessary if the child received the 4th dose after 4 years of age)

Booster immunization: Adacel® (children and adults: 11-64 years), Boostrix® (children and adults: 10-64 years): A single dose; do not administer within 5 years of the previous dose of DTaP; may be administered within 2 years of last Td; when possible, women should receive prior to becoming pregnant or in the immediate postpartum period (ACIP Recommendation)

Administration Shake vial well before withdrawing the dose; administer I.M. in either the anterolateral aspect of the thigh (Daptacel®, Infanrix®, Tripedia®) or deltoid muscle of the arm (Boostrix®, Adacel®); **not for I.V., intradermal, or SubQ administration**

Administration with other vaccines:*Multiple inactivated vaccines:* May be given simultaneously or at any interval between doses*Inactivated and live vaccines:* May be given simultaneously or at any interval between doses

Monitoring Parameters Monitor for syncope for ≥15 minutes following vaccination

Nursing Implications Federal law requires that the date of administration, the vaccine manufacturer, lot number of vaccine, and the administering person's name, title, and address be entered into the patient's permanent medical record.

Additional Information Adacel® is formulated with the same antigens found in Daptacel® but with reduced quantities of tetanus and pertussis; Boostrix® is formulated with the same antigens found in Infanrix® but in reduced quantities. Use of Adacel® or Boostrix® in the primary immunization series or to complete the primary series has not been evaluated. The ACIP considers Adacel® and Boostrix® to be interchangeable when administered to adolescents for childhood vaccination according to the Child and Adolescent Immunization Schedule.

In order to maximize vaccination rates, the ACIP recommends simultaneous administration of all age-appropriate vaccines (live or inactivated) for which a person is eligible at a single visit, unless contraindications exist. The use of combination vaccines is generally preferred over separate infections, taking into consideration provider assessment, patient preference, and potential adverse events.

For additional information, please refer to the following website: http://www.cdc.gov/vaccines/vpd-vac/.

Dosage Forms Excipient information presented when available (limited, particularly for generics); consult specific product labeling.

Injection, suspension [Tdap, booster formulation]:

Adacel®: Diphtheria 2 Lf units, tetanus 5 Lf units, and acellular pertussis antigens (detoxified pertussis toxin 2.5 mcg, filamentous hemagglutinin 5 mcg, pertactin 3 mcg, fimbriae [types 2 and 3] 5 mcg) per 0.5 mL (0.5 mL) [contains aluminum]

Boostrix®: Diphtheria 2.5 Lf units, tetanus 5 Lf units, and acellular pertussis antigens (inactivated pertussis toxin 8 mcg, filamentous hemagglutinin 8 mcg, pertactin 2.5 mcg) per 0.5 mL (0.5 mL) [preservative free; contains aluminum and polysorbate 80; prefilled syringes contain natural rubber/natural latex]

Injection, suspension [DTaP, active immunization formulation]:

Daptacel®: Diphtheria 15 Lf units, tetanus 5 Lf units, and acellular pertussis antigens (detoxified pertussis toxin 10 mcg, filamentous hemagglutinin 5 mcg, pertactin 3 mcg, fimbriae [types 2 and 3] 5 mcg) per 0.5 mL (0.5 mL) [contains aluminum; contains natural rubber/natural latex in packaging]

Infanrix®: Diphtheria 25 Lf units, tetanus 10 Lf units, and acellular pertussis antigens (inactivated pertussis toxin 25 mcg, filamentous hemagglutinin 25 mcg, pertactin 8 mcg) per 0.5 mL (0.5 mL) [contains aluminum and polysorbate 80; prefilled syringes contain natural rubber/natural latex]

Tripedia®: Diphtheria 6.7 Lf units, tetanus 5 Lf units, and acellular pertussis antigens (inactivated pertussis toxin 23.4 mcg, filamentous hemagglutinin 23.4 mcg) per 0.5 mL (0.5 mL) [contains aluminum, natural rubber/natural latex in packaging, polysorbate 80, and thimerosal (trace amounts)]

Note: Tripedia® vaccine is also used to reconstitute ActHIB® to prepare TriHIBit® vaccine (diphtheria, tetanus toxoids, and acellular pertussis and *Haemophilus influenzae* b conjugate vaccine combination)

References

Broder KR, Cortese MM, Iskander JK, et al, "Preventing Tetanus, Diphtheria, and Pertussis Among Adolescents: Use of Tetanus Toxoid, Reduced Diphtheria Toxoid and Acellular Pertussis Vaccines Recommendations of the Advisory Committee on Immunization Practices (ACIP)," *MMWR Recomm Rep*, 2006, 55(RR-3):1-34.

Centers for Disease Control and Prevention (CDC), "General Recommendations on Immunization. Recommendations of the Advisory Committee on Immunization Practices (ACIP)," *MMWR Recomm Rep*, 2006, 55(RR-15):1-48. Available at: http://www.cdc.gov/mmwr/preview/mmwrhtml/rr5515a1.htm.

Chapman LE, Sullivent EE, Grohskopf LA, et al, "Recommendations for Postexposure Interventions to Prevent Infection With Hepatitis B Virus, Hepatitis C Virus, or Human Immunodeficiency Virus, and Tetanus in Persons Wounded During Bombings and Other Mass-Casualty Events--United States, 2008: Recommendations of the Centers for Disease Control and Prevention (CDC)," *MMWR Recomm Rep*, 2008, 57(RR-6):1-21.

Kretsinger K, Broder KR, Cortese MM, et al, "Preventing Tetanus, Diphtheria, and Pertussis Among Adults: Use of Tetanus Toxoid, Reduced Diphtheria Toxoid and Acellular Pertussis Vaccine," *MMWR Recomm Rep*, 2006, 55(RR-17):1-37.

Murphy TV, Slade BA, Broder KR, "Prevention of Pertussis, Tetanus, and Diphtheria Among Pregnant and Postpartum Women and Their Infants," *MMWR*, 2008, 57(Early Release);1-47; available at http://www.cdc.gov/mmwr/preview/mmwrhtml/rr57e0514a1.htm?s_cid=rr57e0514a1_e.

Prymula R, Siegrist CA, Chlibek R, et al, "Effect of Prophylactic Paracetamol Administration at Time of Vaccination on Febrile Reactions and Antibody Responses in Children: Two Open-Label, Randomised Controlled Trials," *Lancet*, 2009, 374(9698):1339-50.

Diphtheria, Tetanus Toxoids, and Acellular Pertussis Vaccine and *Haemophilus influenzae* b Conjugate Vaccine

(dif THEER ee a, TET a nus TOKS oyds & ay CEL yoo lar per TUS sis vak SEEN & hem OF fi lus in floo EN za bee KON joo gate vak SEEN)

Related Information

Immunization Guidelines *on page 1636*

U.S. Brand Names TriHIBit®

Therapeutic Category Vaccine

Generic Available No

Use Active immunization of children 15-18 months of age for prevention of diphtheria, tetanus, pertussis, and invasive disease caused by *H. influenzae* type b.

Contraindications Hypersensitivity to any component

Warnings See individual agents.

Precautions Routine prophylactic administration of acetaminophen to prevent fever due to vaccines has been shown to decrease the immune response of some vaccines; the clinical significance of this reduction in immune response has not been established (see Prymula, 2009).

Adverse Reactions See individual agents.

Drug Interactions

Avoid Concomitant Use There are no known interactions where it is recommended to avoid concomitant use.

Increased Effect/Toxicity There are no known significant interactions involving an increase in effect.

Decreased Effect

The levels/effects of Diphtheria and Tetanus Toxoids, Acellular Pertussis and Haemophilus influenzae b Conjugate Vaccine may be decreased by: Immunosuppressants

Usual Dosage The combination can be used for the DTaP dose given at 15-18 months when a primary series of HIB vaccine has been given.

Children >15 months of age: I.M.: 0.5 mL (**Note:** 2008 immunization schedule states that this may be used as a booster in children as young as 12 months as long as 6 months have elapsed since the third dose.)

Administration Reconstitute by adding Tripedia® vaccine to ActHIB® vaccine; shake well; administer I.M. in either the anterolateral aspect of the thigh or deltoid muscle of the arm; **not for I.V. or SubQ administration**

Nursing Implications Federal law requires that the date of administration, the vaccine manufacturer, lot number of vaccine, and the administering person's name, title, and address be entered into the patient's permanent medical record.

Additional Information In order to maximize vaccination rates, the ACIP recommends simultaneous administration of all age-appropriate vaccines (live or inactivated) for which a person is eligible at a single visit, unless contraindications exist. The use of combination vaccines is generally preferred over separate infections, taking into consideration provider assessment, patient preference, and potential adverse events.

For additional information, please refer to the following website: http://www.cdc.gov/vaccines/vpd-vac/.

Dosage Forms Excipient information presented when available (limited, particularly for generics); consult specific product labeling.

Injection, suspension [preservative free]:

TriHIBit®: Diphtheria 6.7 Lf units, tetanus 5 Lf units, acellular pertussis antigens [inactivated pertussis toxin 23.4 mcg, filamentous hemagglutinin 23.4 mcg], and *Haemophilus* b capsular polysaccharide 10 mcg [bound to tetanus toxoid 24 mcg] per 0.5 mL (0.5 mL) [contains aluminum, natural rubber/natural latex in packaging, polysorbate 80, sucrose, and trace amounts of thimerosal; Tripedia® vaccine used to reconstitute ActHIB® forms TriHIBit®]

References

Centers for Disease Control and Prevention (CDC), "General Recommendations on Immunization. Recommendations of the Advisory Committee on Immunization Practices (ACIP)," *MMWR Recomm Rep*, 2006, 55(RR-15):1-48. Available at: http://www.cdc.gov/mmwr/preview/mmwrhtml/rr5515a1.htm.

Centers for Disease Control and Prevention, "Recommended Immunization Schedules for Persons Aged 0-18 Years − United States, 2008," *MMWR*, 2008, 57(1):Q1-4.

Prymula R, Siegrist CA, Chlibek R, et al, "Effect of Prophylactic Paracetamol Administration at Time of Vaccination on Febrile Reactions and Antibody Responses in Children: Two Open-Label, Randomised Controlled Trials," *Lancet*, 2009, 374(9698):1339-50.

♦ **Diphtheria Toxoid** see Diphtheria and Tetanus Toxoids, Acellular Pertussis, Poliovirus and *Haemophilus* b Conjugate Vaccine *on page 455*

◆ **Diphtheria Toxoid Conjugate** *see Haemophilus* b Conjugate Vaccine *on page 664*

◆ **Dipivalyl Epinephrine** *see* Dipivefrin *on page 461*

Dipivefrin (dye PI ve frin)

U.S. Brand Names Propine® [DSC]
Canadian Brand Names Ophtho-Dipivefrin™; PMS-Dipivefrin; Propine®
Therapeutic Category Adrenergic Agonist Agent, Ophthalmic; Ophthalmic Agent, Vasoconstrictor
Generic Available No
Use Reduces elevated IOP in chronic open-angle glaucoma; treatment of ocular hypertension
Pregnancy Risk Factor B
Contraindications Hypersensitivity to dipivefrin, any component (see Warnings), or epinephrine; contraindicated in patients with angle-closure glaucoma
Warnings Commercial preparation contains sodium metabisulfite which may cause allergic reactions in susceptible individuals
Precautions Use with caution in patients with vascular hypertension or cardiac disorders and in aphakic patients (dipivefrin may cause cystoid macular edema in aphakic patients)
Adverse Reactions
Central nervous system: Headache
Local: Burning, stinging
Ocular: Ocular congestion, photophobia, mydriasis, blurred vision, ocular pain, bulbar conjunctival follicles, blepharoconjunctivitis, cystoid macular edema
Drug Interactions
Avoid Concomitant Use
Avoid concomitant use of Dipivefrin with any of the following: Iobenguane I 123
Increased Effect/Toxicity
Dipivefrin may increase the levels/effects of: Sympathomimetics

The levels/effects of Dipivefrin may be increased by: Atomoxetine; Cannabinoids; Serotonin/Norepinephrine Reuptake Inhibitors
Decreased Effect
Dipivefrin may decrease the levels/effects of: Iobenguane I 123

The levels/effects of Dipivefrin may be decreased by: Spironolactone
Stability Protect from light and avoid exposure to air; discolored or darkened solutions indicate loss of potency
Mechanism of Action Dipivefrin is a prodrug of epinephrine which is the active agent that stimulates alpha- and/or beta-adrenergic receptors increasing aqueous humor outflow
Pharmacodynamics
Onset of action:
Ocular pressure effects: Within 30 minutes
Mydriasis: Within 30 minutes
Maximum effect: Ocular pressure effects: Within 1 hour
Duration:
Ocular pressure effects: 12 hours or longer
Mydriasis: Several hours
Pharmacokinetics (Adult data unless noted) Absorption: Rapid into the aqueous humor; converted to epinephrine
Usual Dosage Children and Adults: Ophthalmic: Initial: Instill 1 drop every 12 hours
Administration Ophthalmic: Instill drop into eye; apply finger pressure to lacrimal sac during and for 1-2 minutes after instillation to decrease risk of absorption and systemic effects; avoid contacting bottle tip with skin or eye
Monitoring Parameters IOP

Patient Information Discolored solutions should be discarded; may cause burning or stinging, blurred vision, and sensitivity to light
Dosage Forms Excipient information presented when available (limited, particularly for generics); consult specific product labeling. [DSC] = Discontinued product
Solution, ophthalmic, as hydrochloride:
Propine®: 0.1% (10 mL [DSC]) [contains benzalkonium chloride]

◆ **Dipivefrin Hydrochloride** *see* Dipivefrin *on page 461*

◆ **Diprivan®** *see* Propofol *on page 1169*

◆ **Diprolene®** *see* Betamethasone *on page 189*

◆ **Diprolene® AF** *see* Betamethasone *on page 189*

◆ **Diprolene® Glycol (Can)** *see* Betamethasone *on page 189*

◆ **Dipropylacetic Acid** *see* Valproic Acid and Derivatives *on page 1398*

◆ **Diprosone® (Can)** *see* Betamethasone *on page 189*

Dipyridamole (dye peer ID a mole)

Medication Safety Issues
Sound-alike/look-alike issues:
Dipyridamole may be confused with disopyramide
Persantine® may be confused with Periactin®, Permitil®

Beers Criteria medication: This drug may be inappropriate for use in geriatric patients (low severity risk).
Related Information
Antithrombotic Therapy in Neonates and Children *on page 1602*
U.S. Brand Names Persantine®
Canadian Brand Names Apo-Dipyridamole FC®; Dipyridamole For Injection; Persantine®
Therapeutic Category Antiplatelet Agent; Vasodilator, Coronary
Generic Available Yes
Use Maintain patency after surgical grafting procedures including coronary artery bypass; with warfarin to decrease thrombosis in patients after artificial heart valve replacement; for chronic management of angina pectoris; with aspirin to prevent coronary artery thrombosis; in combination with aspirin or warfarin to prevent other thromboembolic disorders; dipyridamole may also be given 2 days prior to open heart surgery to prevent platelet activation by extracorporeal bypass pump; diagnostic agent I.V. (dipyridamole stress test) for coronary artery disease
Pregnancy Risk Factor B
Pregnancy Considerations Teratogenic effects were not observed in animal studies.
Lactation Enters breast milk/use caution
Breast-Feeding Considerations Excretion in breast milk is reported to be minimal.
Contraindications Hypersensitivity to dipyridamole or any component
Precautions Use with caution in patients with hypotension (may further decrease blood pressure due to peripheral vasodilation); use with caution in patients with CAD (may aggravate chest pain)
Adverse Reactions
Cardiovascular: Vasodilatation, flushing, syncope
Central nervous system: Dizziness, headache (dose-related)
Dermatologic: Rash, pruritus
Gastrointestinal: Abdominal distress, nausea, vomiting, diarrhea
Hepatic: Liver enzymes elevated, hepatic failure (rare)
Neuromuscular & skeletal: Weakness

461

Drug Interactions

Metabolism/Transport Effects Inhibits ABCG2, P-glycoprotein

Avoid Concomitant Use

Avoid concomitant use of Dipyridamole with any of the following: Dabigatran Etexilate; Silodosin

Increased Effect/Toxicity

Dipyridamole may increase the levels/effects of: Adenosine; Anticoagulants; Antiplatelet Agents; Beta-Blockers; Colchicine; Collagenase (Systemic); Dabigatran Etexilate; Drotrecogin Alfa; Hypotensive Agents; Ibritumomab; P-Glycoprotein Substrates; Regadenoson; Rivaroxaban; Salicylates; Silodosin; Thrombolytic Agents; Topotecan; Tositumomab and Iodine I 131 Tositumomab

The levels/effects of Dipyridamole may be increased by: Dasatinib; Glucosamine; Herbs (Anticoagulant/Antiplatelet Properties); Nonsteroidal Anti-Inflammatory Agents; Omega-3-Acid Ethyl Esters; Pentosan Polysulfate Sodium; Pentoxifylline; Prostacyclin Analogues

Decreased Effect

The levels/effects of Dipyridamole may be decreased by: Nonsteroidal Anti-Inflammatory Agents

Stability Do not freeze; protect I.V. preparation from light

Mechanism of Action Inhibits the activity of adenosine deaminase and phosphodiesterase, which causes an accumulation of adenosine, adenine nucleotides, and cyclic AMP; these mediators then inhibit platelet aggregation and may cause vasodilation; may also stimulate release of prostacyclin or PGD_2; causes coronary vasodilation

Pharmacokinetics (Adult data unless noted) Oral:

Absorption: Slow and variable

Distribution: Distributes to breast milk

V_d: Adults: 2-3 L/kg

Protein binding: 91% to 99%

Metabolism: In the liver to glucuronide conjugate

Bioavailability: 27% to 66%

Half-life, terminal: 10-12 hours

Time to peak serum concentration: Oral: 75 minutes

Elimination: In feces via bile as glucuronide conjugates and unchanged drug

Usual Dosage

Children:

Oral: 3-6 mg/kg/day in 3 divided doses

Doses of 4-10 mg/kg/day have been used investigationally to treat proteinuria in pediatric renal disease

Mechanical prosthetic heart valves: 2-5 mg/kg/day [used in combination with an oral anticoagulant in children who have systemic embolism despite adequate oral anticoagulant therapy (INR 2.5-3.5), and used in combination with low-dose oral anticoagulation (INR 2-3) plus aspirin in children in whom full-dose oral anticoagulation is contraindicated] (see Monagle, 2001). Note: The Chest guidelines (Monagle, 2004) do not mention the use of dipyridamole for prophylaxis for mechanical prosthetic heart valves in children; an oral anticoagulant plus aspirin is recommended for the patient groups mentioned above.

Adults:

Prophylaxis of thromboembolism after cardiac valve replacement (adjunctive use): Oral: 75-100 mg 4 times/day

Dipyridamole stress test (for evaluation of myocardial perfusion): I.V.: 0.142 mg/kg/minute for a total of 4 minutes (0.57 mg/kg total); maximum dose: 60 mg; inject thallium 201 within 5 minutes after end of injection of dipyridamole

Administration

Oral: Administer with water on an empty stomach 1 hour before or 2 hours after meals; may take with milk or food to decrease GI upset

Parenteral: I.V.: Dilute in at least a 1:2 ratio with NS, 1/2NS, or D_5W; infusion of undiluted dipyridamole may cause local irritation; see Usual Dosage for infusion rates

Monitoring Parameters Blood pressure, heart rate

Test Interactions Patients on theophylline may show false-negative thallium scan result on dipyridamole stress test

Patient Information Notify physician or pharmacist if taking other medications that affect bleeding, such as warfarin or NSAIDs; avoid alcohol

Dosage Forms Excipient information presented when available (limited, particularly for generics); consult specific product labeling.

Injection, solution: 5 mg/mL (2 mL, 10 mL)

Tablet: 25 mg, 50 mg, 75 mg

Persantine®: 25 mg, 50 mg, 75 mg

Extemporaneous Preparations A 10 mg/mL oral liquid preparation made from tablets and 3 different vehicles (cherry syrup, a 1:1 mixture of Ora-Sweet® and Ora-Plus®, or a 1:1 mixture of Ora-Sweet® SF and Ora-Plus®) was stable for 60 days when stored in amber plastic prescription bottles in the dark, at room temperature (25°C) or under refrigeration (5°C); grind twenty-four 50 mg tablets in a mortar into a fine powder; add 20 mL of the vehicle and mix well to form a uniform paste; mix while adding the vehicle in geometric proportions to almost 120 mL; transfer to a calibrated bottle and qsad with vehicle to 120 mL; label "shake well" and "protect from light"

Allen LV and Erickson MA, "Stability of Baclofen, Captopril, Diltiazem Hydrochloride, Dipyridamole, and Flecainide Acetate in Extemporaneously Compounded Oral Liquids," Am J Health Sys Pharm, 1996, 53(18):2179-84.

References

Monagle P, Chan A, Massicotte P, et al, "Antithrombotic Therapy in Children: The Seventh ACCP Conference on Antithrombotic and Thrombolytic Therapy," Chest, 2004, 126(3 Suppl):645S-687S.

Monagle P, Michelson AD, Bovill E, et al, "Antithrombotic Therapy in Children," Chest, 2001, 119(1 Suppl):344S-370S.

Rao PS, Solymar L, Mardini MK, et al, "Anticoagulant Therapy in Children With Prosthetic Valves," Ann Thorac Surg, 1989, 47 (4):589-92.

Ueda N, Kawaguchi S, Niinomi Y, et al, "Effect of Dipyridamole Treatment on Proteinuria in Pediatric Renal Disease," Nephron, 1986, 44(3):174-9.

♦ **Dipyridamole For Injection (Can)** see Dipyridamole on page 461

♦ **Disodium Cromoglycate** see Cromolyn on page 363

♦ **Disodium Thiosulfate Pentahydrate** see Sodium Thiosulfate on page 1280

♦ **d-Isoephedrine Hydrochloride** see Pseudoephedrine on page 1183

Disopyramide (dye soe PEER a mide)

Medication Safety Issues

Sound-alike/look-alike issues:

Disopyramide may be confused with desipramine, dipyridamole

Norpace® may be confused with Norpramin®

Beers Criteria medication: This drug may be inappropriate for use in geriatric patients (high severity risk).

Related Information

Medications for Which A Single Dose May Be Fatal When Ingested By A Toddler on page 1709

U.S. Brand Names Norpace®; Norpace® CR

Canadian Brand Names Norpace®; Rythmodan®; Rythmodan®-LA

Therapeutic Category Antiarrhythmic Agent, Class I-A

Generic Available Yes

Use Treatment of life-threatening ventricular arrhythmias; suppression and prevention of unifocal and multifocal ventricular premature complexes, coupled ventricular premature complexes, and/or paroxysmal ventricular tachycardia; also effective in the conversion and prevention of recurrence of atrial fibrillation, atrial flutter, and paroxysmal atrial tachycardia

Pregnancy Risk Factor C

Lactation Enters breast milk/compatible

Contraindications Hypersensitivity to disopyramide or any component; pre-existing second or third degree A-V block (except in patients with a functioning artificial pacemaker); congenital QT prolongation; cardiogenic shock

Warnings Antiarrhythmic agents should be reserved for patients with life-threatening ventricular arrhythmias **[U.S. Boxed Warning]**. In the Cardiac Arrhythmia Suppression Trial (CAST), recent (>6 days but <2 years ago) myocardial infarction patients with asymptomatic, nonlife-threatening ventricular arrhythmias did not benefit and may have been harmed by attempts to suppress the arrhythmia with flecainide or encainide. An increased mortality or nonfatal cardiac arrest rate (7.7%) was seen in the active treatment group compared with patients in the placebo group (3%). The applicability of the CAST results to other populations is unknown.

May cause or worsen CHF; may cause severe hypotension; not recommended for use in patients with uncompensated or marginally compensated CHF or hypotension unless caused by an arrhythmia. May cause significant widening (>25%) of QRS complex; discontinue disopyramide if this occurs. Lengthening of QT interval and worsening of arrhythmia (including ventricular tachycardia or ventricular fibrillation) may occur; patients with quinidine-associated QT prolongation may be at higher risk; torsade de pointes may occur. Monitor patients carefully and consider discontinuation of disopyramide if QT prolongation is >25% and ectopy continues. May cause heart block; reduce dosage if first-degree heart block develops; discontinue drug if second or third degree AV block or unifascicular, bifascicular, or trifascicular block develops (unless pacemaker is present).

Disopyramide may cause hypoglycemia. Significant anticholinergic activity occurs; avoid use in patients with glaucoma, myasthenia gravis, or urinary retention unless appropriate overriding measures are taken.

Serious and potentially fatal drug interactions may occur. Avoid concurrent use with other drugs known to prolong QT$_c$ interval or decrease myocardial contractibility. Life-threatening interactions have been reported with concomitant use of disopyramide with clarithromycin and erythromycin. Disopyramide is not recommended for use 48 hours before or 24 hours after verapamil (see Drug Interactions).

Precautions Use with caution in patients with sick sinus syndrome, Wolf Parkinson White syndrome (WPW) or bundle-branch block. May increase ventricular rate in patients with atrial fibrillation or flutter who have not received digoxin. Use with caution and do not give loading dose in patients with myocarditis or other cardiomyopathy; may cause significant hypotension. Use with caution and decrease dose in patients with renal or hepatic impairment; extended release form is not recommended for patients with severe renal impairment (Cl$_{Cr}$ <40 mL/minute). Correct electrolyte disturbances, especially hypokalemia or hypomagnesemia, prior to use and throughout therapy.

Adverse Reactions

Cardiovascular: CHF, edema, chest pain, syncope and hypotension, conduction disturbances including A-V block, widening QRS complex and lengthening of QT interval

Central nervous system: Fatigue, headache, malaise, nervousness, acute psychosis, depression, dizziness

Dermatologic: Generalized rashes

Endocrine & metabolic: Hypoglycemia, weight gain, cholesterol and triglycerides elevated; may initiate contractions of pregnant uterus; hyperkalemia may enhance toxicities

Gastrointestinal: Xerostomia, dry throat, constipation, nausea, vomiting, diarrhea, pain, gas, anorexia

Genitourinary: Urinary retention/hesitancy

Hepatic: Liver enzymes elevated, hepatic cholestasis

Neuromuscular & skeletal: Weakness

Ocular: Blurred vision, dry eyes

Respiratory: Dyspnea (<1%), dry nasal membranes

Drug Interactions

Metabolism/Transport Effects Substrate of CYP3A4 (major)

Avoid Concomitant Use

Avoid concomitant use of Disopyramide with any of the following: Artemether; Dronedarone; Lumefantrine; Macrolide Antibiotics; Nilotinib; Pimozide; QuiNINE; Tetrabenazine; Thioridazine; Verapamil; Ziprasidone

Increased Effect/Toxicity

Disopyramide may increase the levels/effects of: AbobotulinumtoxinA; Anticholinergics; Beta-Blockers; Cannabinoids; Dronedarone; Lidocaine; Lidocaine (Systemic); OnabotulinumtoxinA; Pimozide; Potassium Chloride; QTc-Prolonging Agents; QuiNINE; RimabotulinumtoxinB; Tetrabenazine; Thioridazine; Ziprasidone

The levels/effects of Disopyramide may be increased by: Alfuzosin; Amiodarone; Artemether; Chloroquine; Ciprofloxacin; Ciprofloxacin (Systemic); CYP3A4 Inhibitors (Moderate); CYP3A4 Inhibitors (Strong); Gadobutrol; Lumefantrine; Macrolide Antibiotics; Nilotinib; Pramlintide; QuiNINE; Verapamil

Decreased Effect

Disopyramide may decrease the levels/effects of: Acetylcholinesterase Inhibitors (Central); Secretin

The levels/effects of Disopyramide may be decreased by: Acetylcholinesterase Inhibitors (Central); Barbiturates; CYP3A4 Inducers (Strong); Deferasirox; Herbs (CYP3A4 Inducers); Phenytoin; Rifamycin Derivatives

Mechanism of Action Class IA antiarrhythmic: Decreases myocardial excitability and conduction velocity; reduces disparity in refractory period between normal and infarcted myocardium; possesses anticholinergic, peripheral vasoconstrictive and negative inotropic effects

Pharmacodynamics

Capsules, regular:

Onset of action: 30-210 minutes

Duration: 1.5-8.5 hours

Pharmacokinetics (Adult data unless noted)

Protein binding: Concentration dependent, stereoselective, and ranges from 20% to 60%

Distribution: V$_d$: Children: 1 L/kg

Metabolism: In the liver; major metabolite has anticholinergic and antiarrhythmic effects

Bioavailability: 60% to 83%

Half-life:

Children: 3.15 hours

Adults: 4-10 hours (mean: 6.7 hours), increased half-life with hepatic or renal disease

Elimination: 40% to 60% excreted unchanged in urine and 10% to 15% in feces

Clearance is greater and half-life shorter in children vs adults; clearance (children): 3.76 mL/minute/kg

Usual Dosage Oral:
Children (start with lower dose listed):
<1 year: 10-30 mg/kg/day in 4 divided doses
1-4 years: 10-20 mg/kg/day in 4 divided doses
4-12 years: 10-15 mg/kg/day in 4 divided doses
12-18 years: 6-15 mg/kg/day in 4 divided doses
Adults: **Note:** Some patients may require initial loading dose; see product information for details
<50 kg: 100 mg every 6 hours **or** 200 mg every 12 hours (controlled release)
>50 kg: 150 mg every 6 hours **or** 300 mg every 12 hours (controlled release); if no response, may increase to 200 mg every 6 hours; maximum dose required for patients with severe refractory ventricular tachycardia is 400 mg every 6 hours. **Note:** Use lower doses (100 mg of nonsustained release every 6-8 hours) in adults with cardiomyopathy or cardiac decompensation.

Adult dosing adjustment in renal impairment: 100 mg (nonsustained release) given at the following intervals: See table

Creatinine Clearance (mL/min)	Dosage Interval
30-40	Every 8 h
15-30	Every 12 h
<15	Every 24 h

Administration Oral: Administer on an empty stomach; do not crush, break, or chew controlled release capsules, swallow whole

Monitoring Parameters Blood pressure, ECG, drug level; serum potassium, glucose, cholesterol, triglycerides, and liver enzymes; especially important to monitor ECG in patients with hepatic or renal disease, heart disease, or others with increased risk of adverse effects

Reference Range Therapeutic:
Atrial arrhythmias: 2.8-3.2 mcg/mL (SI: 8.3-9.4 micromoles/L)
Ventricular arrhythmias: 3.3-7.5 mcg/mL (SI: 9.7-22 micromoles/L)
Toxic: >7 mcg/mL (SI: >20.7 micromoles/L)

Patient Information Avoid alcohol; notify physician if urinary retention or worsening of CHF occurs; may cause dry mouth

Dosage Forms Excipient information presented when available (limited, particularly for generics); consult specific product labeling.
Capsule (Norpace®): 100 mg, 150 mg
Capsule, controlled release (Norpace® CR): 100 mg, 150 mg

Extemporaneous Preparations Extemporaneous suspensions in cherry syrup (1 mg/mL and 10 mg/mL) are stable for 4 weeks in amber glass bottles stored at 5°C, 30°C, or at room temperature; shake well before use; do not use extended release capsules for this suspension
Mathur LK, Lai PK, and Shively CD, "Stability of Disopyramide Phosphate in Cherry Syrup," *J Hosp Pharm*, 1982, 39(2):309-10.

References
Chiba K, Koike K, Nakamoto M, et al, "Steady-State Pharmacokinetics and Bioavailability of Total and Unbound Disopyramide in Children With Cardiac Arrhythmias," *Ther Drug Monit*, 1992, 14(2):112-8.
Echizen H, Takahashi H, Nakamura H, et al, "Stereoselective Disposition and Metabolism of Disopyramide in Pediatric Patients," *J Pharmacol Exp Ther*, 1991, 259(3):953-60.

◆ **Disopyramide Phosphate** *see* Disopyramide *on page 462*

◆ **Dithioglycerol** *see* Dimercaprol *on page 447*

◆ **Ditropan®** *see* Oxybutynin *on page 1037*

◆ **Ditropan XL®** *see* Oxybutynin *on page 1037*

◆ **Diuril®** *see* Chlorothiazide *on page 295*

◆ **Divalproex Sodium** *see* Valproic Acid and Derivatives *on page 1398*

◆ **Divigel®** *see* Estradiol *on page 536*

◆ **Dixarit® (Can)** *see* CloNIDine *on page 338*

◆ **5071-1DL(6)** *see* Megestrol *on page 874*

◆ **dl-Alpha Tocopherol** *see* Vitamin E *on page 1427*

◆ **DM** *see* Dextromethorphan *on page 421*

◆ **D-Mannitol** *see* Mannitol *on page 861*

◆ **4-DMDR** *see* IDArubicin *on page 707*

◆ **DMSA** *see* Succimer *on page 1294*

◆ **Doak® Tar [OTC]** *see* Coal Tar *on page 349*

DOBUTamine (doe BYOO ta meen)

Medication Safety Issues
Sound-alike/look-alike issues:
DOBUTamine may be confused with DOPamine

High alert medication: The Institute for Safe Medication Practices (ISMP) includes this medication among its list of drugs which have a heightened risk of causing significant patient harm when used in error.

Related Information
CPR Pediatric Drug Dosages *on page 1455*
Emergency Pediatric Drip Calculations *on page 1457*
Extravasation Treatment *on page 1522*

Canadian Brand Names Dobutamine Injection, USP; Dobutrex®

Therapeutic Category Adrenergic Agonist Agent; Sympathomimetic

Generic Available Yes

Use Short-term management of patients with cardiac decompensation

Pregnancy Risk Factor B

Lactation Excretion in breast milk unknown

Contraindications Hypersensitivity to dobutamine or any component (see Warnings); patients with idiopathic hypertrophic subaortic stenosis (IHSS)

Warnings Potent drug; must be diluted prior to use; patient's hemodynamic status should be monitored; contains sulfites which may cause allergic reactions in susceptible individuals

Precautions Hypovolemia should be corrected prior to use; infiltration causes local inflammatory changes, extravasation may cause dermal necrosis

Adverse Reactions
Cardiovascular: Ectopic heartbeats, heart rate elevated, chest pain, palpitations, elevation in blood pressure; in higher doses ventricular tachycardia or arrhythmias may be seen; patients with atrial fibrillation or flutter are at risk of developing a rapid ventricular response
Central nervous system: Headache
Gastrointestinal: Nausea, vomiting
Local: Phlebitis
Neuromuscular & skeletal: Mild leg cramps, paresthesia
Respiratory: Dyspnea

Drug Interactions
Avoid Concomitant Use
Avoid concomitant use of DOBUTamine with any of the following: Iobenguane I 123

Increased Effect/Toxicity
DOBUTamine may increase the levels/effects of: Sympathomimetics

The levels/effects of DOBUTamine may be increased by: Atomoxetine; Cannabinoids; COMT Inhibitors

Decreased Effect

DOBUTamine may decrease the levels/effects of:
Iobenguane I 123

The levels/effects of DOBUTamine may be decreased by:
Calcium Salts

Stability Stable in various parenteral solutions for 24 hours; incompatible with alkaline solutions, do not give through same I.V. line as heparin, sodium bicarbonate, ethacrynic acid, cefazolin, or penicillin; compatible when coadministered with dopamine, nitroprusside, potassium chloride, protamine sulfate, tobramycin, epinephrine, atracurium, vecuronium, isoproterenol, and lidocaine; pink discoloration of dobutamine hydrochloride indicates slight oxidation, but no significant loss of potency if administered within the recommended time period

Mechanism of Action Stimulates $beta_1$-adrenergic receptors, causing increased contractility and heart rate, with little effect on $beta_2$- or alpha-receptors

Pharmacodynamics

Onset of action: I.V.: 1-10 minutes
Maximum effect: Within 10-20 minutes

Pharmacokinetics (Adult data unless noted)

Metabolism: In tissues and the liver to inactive metabolites
Half-life: 2 minutes

Usual Dosage I.V. continuous infusion:
Neonates: 2-15 mcg/kg/minute, titrate to desired response
Children and Adults: 2.5-15 mcg/kg/minute, titrate to desired response; maximum dose: 40 mcg/kg/minute

Administration Parenteral: Dilute in dextrose or NS; maximum recommended concentration: 5000 mcg/mL (5 mg/mL); rate of infusion (mL/hour) = dose (mcg/kg/minute) x weight (kg) x 60 minutes/hour divided by the concentration (mcg/mL); administer into large vein; use infusion device to control rate of flow

Monitoring Parameters ECG, heart rate, CVP, MAP, urine output; if pulmonary artery catheter is in place, monitor CI, PCWP, RAP, and SVR. Dobutamine lowers central venous pressure and wedge pressure but has little effect on pulmonary vascular resistance.

Dosage Forms Excipient information presented when available (limited, particularly for generics); consult specific product labeling.
Infusion, as hydrochloride [premixed in dextrose]: 1 mg/mL (250 mL, 500 mL); 2 mg/mL (250 mL); 4 mg/mL (250 mL)
Injection, solution, as hydrochloride: 12.5 mg/mL (20 mL, 40 mL, 100 mL) [contains sodium bisulfite]

◆ **Dobutamine Hydrochloride** *see* DOBUTamine *on page 464*

◆ **Dobutamine Injection, USP (Can)** *see* DOBUTamine *on page 464*

◆ **Dobutrex® (Can)** *see* DOBUTamine *on page 464*

Docetaxel (doe se TAKS el)

Medication Safety Issues

Sound-alike/look-alike issues:
Taxotere® may be confused with Taxol®

High alert medication: The Institute for Safe Medication Practices (ISMP) includes this medication among its list of drug classes which have a heightened risk of causing significant patient harm when used in error.

Related Information

Emetogenic Potential of Antineoplastic Agents *on page 1579*

U.S. Brand Names Taxotere®
Canadian Brand Names Taxotere®
Therapeutic Category Antineoplastic Agent, Antimicrotubular; Antineoplastic Agent, Natural Source (Plant) Derivative; Antineoplastic Agent, Taxane Derivative
Generic Available No

Use Treatment of breast cancer; locally-advanced or metastatic nonsmall cell lung cancer (NSCLC); hormone refractory, metastatic prostate cancer; advanced gastric adenocarcinoma; locally-advanced squamous cell head and neck cancer; other uses include treatment of bladder cancer, ovarian cancer, small cell lung cancer, and soft tissue sarcoma; recurrent solid tumors in children

Pregnancy Risk Factor D

Pregnancy Considerations Animal studies have demonstrated embryotoxicity, fetal toxicity, and maternal toxicity. There are no adequate and well-controlled studies in pregnant women; however, fetal harm may occur. Women of childbearing potential should avoid becoming pregnant. A pregnancy registry is available for all cancers diagnosed during pregnancy at Cooper Health (856-757-7876).

Lactation Excretion in breast milk unknown/not recommended

Breast-Feeding Considerations Due to the potential for serious adverse reactions in nursing the infant, breast-feeding is not recommended.

Contraindications Hypersensitivity to docetaxel or any component; prior hypersensitivity to medications containing polysorbate 80; pre-existing bone marrow suppression (neutrophils <1500 cells/mm^3)

Warnings Hazardous agent; use appropriate precautions for handling and disposal; should be administered under the supervision of an experienced cancer chemotherapy physician. Safety and efficacy have not been established in children.

Fluid retention syndrome characterized by pleural effusions, ascites, edema, and weight gain (2-15 kg) has been reported **[U.S. Boxed Warning]**. The incidence and severity of the syndrome increase sharply at cumulative doses ≥400 mg/m^2. Patients should be premedicated with a corticosteroid to prevent fluid retention; severity is reduced with dexamethasone premedication starting one day prior to docetaxel administration.

Severe hypersensitivity reactions characterized by rash/erythema, hypotension, bronchospasms, or anaphylaxis may occur **[U.S. Boxed Warning]**; minor reactions including flushing or localized skin reactions may also occur. Patients should be premedicated with a corticosteroid to prevent hypersensitivity reactions; severity is reduced with dexamethasone premedication starting 1 day prior to docetaxel administration; however, severe reactions may still occur. Patients should be observed closely for hypersensitivity reactions, especially during the first and second infusions. Do not administer to patients who have a history of severe hypersensitivity reactions to docetaxel or polysorbate 80.

The dose-limiting toxicity is neutropenia and frequent WBCs should be monitored. Patients with an absolute neutrophil count <1500 cells/mm^3 should not receive docetaxel **[U.S. Boxed Warning]**. When administered as sequential infusions, taxane derivatives (docetaxel, paclitaxel) should be administered before platinum derivatives (carboplatin, cisplatin) to limit myelosuppression and to enhance efficacy.

Patients with abnormal liver function, those receiving higher doses, and patients with nonsmall cell lung cancer and a history of prior treatment with platinum derivatives who receive docetaxel doses >100 mg/m^2 are at higher risk for treatment-related mortality **[U.S. Boxed Warning]**.

Avoid use in patients with bilirubin exceeding upper limit of normal (ULN) or AST and/or ALT >1.5 times ULN in conjunction with alkaline phosphatase >2.5 times ULN **[U.S. Boxed Warning]**; patients with abnormal liver function are at increased risk for the development of grade 4 neutropenia, febrile neutropenia, infections, severe thrombocytopenia, severe stomatitis, severe skin toxicity, and toxic death.

Cutaneous reactions including erythema and desquamation have been reported; may require dose reduction. Dosage adjustment is recommended with severe neurosensory symptoms (paresthesia, dysesthesia, pain); persistent symptoms may require discontinuation

Precautions Should be administered under the supervision of an experienced cancer chemotherapy physician.

Adverse Reactions Percentages reported for docetaxel monotherapy; frequency may vary depending on diagnosis, dose, liver function, prior treatment, and premedication. The incidence of adverse events was usually higher in patients with elevated liver function tests.

Cardiovascular: Fluid retention (13% to 60%; dose dependent), left ventricular ejection fraction decreased (prostate cancer: 10%; metastatic breast cancer: 8%), hypotension (3%), CHF, hypertension, angina, atrial fibrillation, atrial flutter, cardiac tamponade, chest pain, chest tightness, dysrhythmia, ECG abnormalities, MI, deep vein thrombosis, sinus tachycardia

Central nervous system: Neurosensory events (20% to 58%; including neuropathy), fever (31% to 35%), neuromotor events (16%), syncope, loss of consciousness (transient), seizure

Dermatologic: Alopecia (56% to 76%), cutaneous events (20% to 48%), nail disorder (11% to 41%), rash/erythema (2%), cutaneous lupus erythematosus, erythema multiforme, Stevens-Johnson syndrome, toxic epidermal necrolysis, pruritus

Gastrointestinal: Stomatitis (19% to 53%; severe 1% to 8%), diarrhea (23% to 43%; severe: 5% to 6%), nausea (34% to 42%), vomiting (22% to 23%), taste perversion (6%), esophagitis, gastrointestinal hemorrhage, gastrointestinal obstruction, gastrointestinal perforation, ileus, colitis, constipation, duodenal ulcer, neutropenic enterocolitis

Hematologic: Neutropenia (84% to 99%; grade 4: 75% to 86%; onset: 4-7 days, nadir: 5-9 days, recovery: 21 days; dose dependent), leukopenia (84% to 99%; grade 4: 32% to 44%), anemia (65% to 94%; dose dependent; grades 3/4: 8% to 9%), thrombocytopenia (8% to 14%; grade 4: 1%; dose dependent), febrile neutropenia (6% to 12%; dose dependent), acute myeloid leukemia (AML), myelodysplastic syndrome, disseminated intravascular coagulation (DIC)

Hepatic: Transaminases elevated (4% to 19%), bilirubin elevated (9%), alkaline phosphatase elevated (4% to 7%), hepatitis

Local: Infusion-site reactions (4%, including hyperpigmentation, inflammation, redness, dryness, phlebitis, extravasation, swelling of the vein)

Neuromuscular & skeletal: Weakness (53% to 66%; severe 13% to 18%), myalgia (3% to 23%), arthralgia (3% to 9%)

Ocular: Epiphora associated with canalicular stenosis (≤77% with weekly administration; ≤1% with every-3-week administration), visual disturbances (transient), lacrimal duct obstruction, conjunctivitis

Otic: Hearing loss, ototoxicity

Renal: Renal insufficiency

Respiratory: Pulmonary events (41%), acute respiratory distress syndrome (ARDS), bronchospasm, interstitial pneumonia, pleural effusion, pulmonary edema, pulmonary embolism, pulmonary fibrosis, radiation pneumonitis, dyspnea

Miscellaneous: Infection (1% to 34%; dose dependent), hypersensitivity (1% to 21%; with premedication 15%) including anaphylactic shock, drug fever, hand and foot syndrome, multiorgan failure

Drug Interactions

Metabolism/Transport Effects Substrate of CYP3A4 (major), P-glycoprotein; **Inhibits** CYP3A4 (weak)

Avoid Concomitant Use

Avoid concomitant use of Docetaxel with any of the following: BCG; Natalizumab; Pimecrolimus; Tacrolimus (Topical); Vaccines (Live)

Increased Effect/Toxicity

Docetaxel may increase the levels/effects of: Antineoplastic Agents (Anthracycline); Leflunomide; Natalizumab; Vaccines (Live)

The levels/effects of Docetaxel may be increased by: Antifungal Agents (Azole Derivatives, Systemic); CYP3A4 Inhibitors (Moderate); CYP3A4 Inhibitors (Strong); Dasatinib; Denosumab; P-Glycoprotein Inhibitors; Pimecrolimus; Platinum Derivatives; Tacrolimus (Topical); Trastuzumab

Decreased Effect

Docetaxel may decrease the levels/effects of: BCG; Sipuleucel-T; Vaccines (Inactivated); Vaccines (Live)

The levels/effects of Docetaxel may be decreased by: CYP3A4 Inducers (Strong); Deferasirox; Echinacea; Herbs (CYP3A4 Inducers); P-Glycoprotein Inducers

Food Interactions Avoid ethanol due to GI irritation. Avoid the herbal St John's wort as it may decrease docetaxel levels.

Stability Intact vials should be stored at 2°C to 25°C (36°F to 77°F) and protected from light. Freezing does not adversely affect the product. If refrigerated, vials should be stored at room temperature for approximately 5 minutes before using. Diluted solutions in the vial are stable for 8 hours at room temperature or under refrigeration. Solutions diluted for infusion in D_5W or NS are stable for up to 4 weeks at room temperature of 15°C to 25°C (59°F to 77°F) in polyolefin containers; however, the manufacturer recommends use within 4 hours.

Mechanism of Action Docetaxel promotes the assembly of microtubules from tubulin dimers and inhibits the depolymerization of tubulin which stabilizes microtubules in the cell. This results in inhibition of DNA, RNA, and protein synthesis. Most activity occurs during the M phase of the cell cycle.

Pharmacokinetics (Adult data unless noted) Exhibits linear pharmacokinetics at the recommended dosage range

Distribution: Extensive extravascular distribution and/or tissue binding; V_d: 80-90 L/m^2, V_{dss}: 113 L (mean steady state)

Protein binding: ~94% to 97%, primarily to $alpha_1$-acid glycoprotein, albumin, and lipoproteins

Metabolism: Hepatic; oxidation via CYP3A4 to metabolites

Half-life: Terminal: 11 hours

Excretion: Feces (75%, <8% as unchanged drug); urine (6%); ~80% within 48 hours

Clearance: Total body: Mean: 21 $L/hour/m^2$

Usual Dosage I.V. infusion: Refer to individual protocols:

Note: Premedicate with corticosteroids, beginning the day before docetaxel administration, (administer for 1-5 days) to reduce the severity of hypersensitivity reactions and pulmonary/peripheral edema

Children (Investigational for recurrent solid tumors): 125 mg/m^2 every 21 days

Adults:

Breast cancer:

Locally-advanced or metastatic: 60-100 mg/m^2 every 3 weeks; patients initially started at 60 mg/m^2 who do not develop toxicity may tolerate higher doses

Operable, node-positive (adjuvant treatment): 75 mg/m^2 every 3 weeks for 6 courses (in combination with doxorubicin and cyclophosphamide)

Nonsmall cell lung cancer: 75 mg/m^2 every 3 weeks (as monotherapy or in combination with cisplatin)

Prostate cancer: 75 mg/m^2 every 3 weeks (in combination with prednisone)

Gastric adenocarcinoma: 75 mg/m^2 every 3 weeks (in combination with cisplatin and fluorouracil)

Head and neck cancer: 75 mg/m^2 every 3 weeks (in combination with cisplatin and fluorouracil) for 3 or 4 cycles, followed by radiation therapy

Dosing adjustment for toxicity: Note: Toxicity includes febrile neutropenia, neutrophils ≤500/mm^3 for >1 week, severe or cumulative cutaneous reactions; in nonsmall cell lung cancer, this may also include platelets <25,000/mm^3 and other grade 3/4 nonhematologic toxicities.

Breast cancer: Patients dosed initially at 100 mg/m^2; reduce dose to 75 mg/m^2; **Note:** If the patient continues to experience these adverse reactions, the dosage should be reduced to 55 mg/m^2 or therapy should be discontinued; discontinue for peripheral neuropathy ≥grade 3

Breast cancer, adjuvant treatment: TAC regimen should be administered when neutrophils are ≥1500 cells/mm^3. Patients experiencing febrile neutropenia should receive G-CSF in all subsequent cycles. Patients continuing to experience febrile neutropenia or patients experiencing severe/cumulative cutaneous reactions or moderate neurosensory effects (signs/symptoms) should receive a reduced dose (60 mg/m^2) of docetaxel. Patients who experience grade 3 or 4 stomatitis should also receive a reduced dose (60 mg/m^2) of docetaxel. Discontinue therapy in patients continuing to experience these reactions after dosage reduction.

Nonsmall cell lung cancer:

Monotherapy: Patients dosed initially at 75 mg/m^2 should have dose held until toxicity is resolved, then resume at 55 mg/m^2; discontinue patients who develop ≥grade 3 peripheral neuropathy.

Combination therapy (with cisplatin): Patients dosed initially at 75 mg/m^2 should have the docetaxel dosage reduced to 65 mg/m^2 in subsequent cycles; if further adjustment is required, dosage may be reduced to 50 mg/m^2

Prostate cancer: Reduce dose to 60 mg/m^2; discontinue therapy if adverse reactions persist at lower dose.

Gastric cancer, head and neck cancer: **Note:** Cisplatin may require dose reductions/therapy delays for peripheral neuropathy, ototoxicity, and/or nephrotoxicity. Patients experiencing febrile neutropenia, documented infection with neutropenia or neutropenia >7 days should receive G-CSF in all subsequent cycles. For neutropenic complications despite G-CSF use, further reduce dose to 60 mg/m^2. Neutropenic complications in subsequent cycles should be further dose reduced to 45 mg/m^2. Patients who experience grade 4 thrombocytopenia should receive a dose reduction from 75 mg/m^2 to 60 mg/m^2. Discontinue therapy for persistent toxicities.

Gastrointestinal toxicity for docetaxel in combination with cisplatin and fluorouracil for treatment of gastric cancer or head and neck cancer:

Diarrhea, grade 3:

First episode: Reduce fluorouracil dose by 20%

Second episode: Reduce docetaxel dose by 20%

Diarrhea, grade 4:

First episode: Reduce fluorouracil and docetaxel doses by 20%

Second episode: Discontinue treatment

Stomatitis, grade 3:

First episode: Reduce fluorouracil dose by 20%

Second episode: Discontinue fluorouracil for all subsequent cycles

Third episode: Reduce docetaxel dose by 20%

Stomatitis, grade 4:

First episode: Discontinue fluorouracil for all subsequent cycles

Second episode: Reduce docetaxel dose by 20%

Dosing adjustment in renal impairment: Docetaxel has minimal renal excretion; dosage adjustments for renal dysfunction may not be needed.

Dosing adjustment in hepatic impairment: The FDA-approved labeling recommends the following adjustments:

Total bilirubin greater than the ULN, or AST/ALT >1.5 times ULN concomitant with alkaline phosphatase >2.5 times ULN: Docetaxel generally should not be administered.

Hepatic impairment dosing adjustment specific for gastric adenocarcinoma:

AST/ALT >2.5 to ≤5 times ULN and alkaline phosphatase ≤2.5 times ULN: Administer 80% of dose

AST/ALT >1.5 to ≤5 times ULN and alkaline phosphatase >2.5 to ≤5 times ULN: Administer 80% of dose

AST/ALT >5 times ULN and /or alkaline phosphatase >5 times ULN: Discontinue docetaxel

The following guidelines have been used by some clinicians (Floyd, 2006):

AST/ALT 1.6-6 times ULN: Administer 75% of dose

AST/ALT >6 times ULN: Use clinical judgment

Administration Dilute vial with 13% (w/w) ethanol/water (provided with the drug) to a final concentration of 10 mg/mL. Do not shake. The solution should be further diluted in 250-1000 mL of NS or D$_5$W to a final concentration of 0.3-0.9 mg/mL (although the manufacturer recommends a final concentration of 0.3-0.74 mg/mL) and dispensed in a non-DEHP container (eg, glass, polypropylene, polyolefin).

Administer as an I.V. infusion over 1 hour through nonsorbing polyethylene lined (non-DEHP) tubing; in-line filter is not necessary. **Note:** Premedication with corticosteroids for 1-5 days, beginning the day before docetaxel administration, is recommended to prevent hypersensitivity reactions and pulmonary/peripheral edema (see Additional Information).

Monitoring Parameters CBC with differential, liver function tests, bilirubin, alkaline phosphatase, renal function; monitor for hypersensitivity reactions, fluid retention, epiphora, and canalicular stenosis

Patient Information Do not take any new medication during therapy unless approved by healthcare provider. This medication can only be administered by infusion; report immediately any pain, burning, swelling, or redness at infusion site, difficulty breathing or swallowing, chest pain, or sudden chills. It is important to maintain adequate hydration (unless instructed to restrict fluid intake and adequate nutrition (small frequent meals may help). You will be more susceptible to infection (avoid crowds and exposure to infection and do not have any vaccinations without consulting prescriber). May cause nausea or vomiting (small frequent meals, frequent mouth care, sucking lozenges, or chewing gum may help); loss of hair (reversible); or diarrhea. Report immediately swelling of extremities, respiratory difficulty, unusual weight gain, abdominal distention, chest pain, palpitations, fever, chills, unusual bruising or bleeding, signs of infection, excessive fatigue, or rash.

Additional Information Premedication with oral corticosteroids is recommended to decrease the incidence and severity of fluid retention and severity of hypersensitivity reactions. Dexamethasone 8-10 mg (3 mg/m^2 used in

◄ pediatric clinical trials) orally twice daily for 3-5 days, starting the day before docetaxel administration, is usually recommended. When prednisone is part of the antineoplastic regimen (eg, prostate cancer), the prednisone is sometimes withheld on the days dexamethasone is administered.

Dosage Forms Excipient information presented when available (limited, particularly for generics); consult specific product labeling.

Injection, solution [concentrate]:
Taxotere®: 20 mg/0.5 mL (0.5 mL, 2 mL) [contains Polysorbate 80®; diluent contains ethanol 13%]

References

Ajani JA, Fodor MB, Tjulandin SA, et al, "Phase II Multi-Institutional Randomized Trial of Docetaxel Plus Cisplatin With or Without Fluorouracil in Patients With Untreated, Advanced Gastric, or Gastroesophageal Adenocarcinoma," *J Clin Oncol*, 2005, 23 (24):5660-7.

Bruno R and Sanderink GJ, "Pharmacokinetics and Metabolism of Taxotere® (Docetaxel)," *Cancer Surv*, 1993, 17:305-13.

Clarke SJ and Rivory LP, "Clinical Pharmacokinetics of Docetaxel," *Clin Pharmacokinet*, 1999, 36(2):99-114.

Cortes JE and Pazdur R, "Docetaxel," *J Clin Oncol*, 1995, 13 (10):2643-55.

Floyd J, Mirza I, Sachs B, et al, "Hepatotoxicity of Chemotherapy," *Semin Oncol*, 2006, 33(1):50-67.

Fulton B and Spencer CM, "Docetaxel. A Review of Its Pharmacodynamic and Pharmacokinetic Properties and Therapeutic Efficacy in the Management of Metastatic Breast Cancer," *Drugs*, 1996, 51 (6):1075-92.

Posner MR, Glisson B, Frenette G, et al "Multicenter Phase I-II Trial of Docetaxel, Cisplatin, and Fluorouracil Induction Chemotherapy for Patients With Locally Advanced Squamous Cell Cancer of the Head and Neck," *J Clin Oncol*, 2001, 19(4):1096-104.

Posner MR, Hershock DM, Blajman CR, et al, "Cisplatin and Fluorouracil Alone or With Docetaxel in Head and Neck Cancer," *N Engl J Med*, 2007, 357(17):1705-15.

Ravdin PM, "The International Experience With Docetaxel in the Treatment of Breast Cancer," *Oncology*, 1997, 11(3 Suppl 2):38-42.

Schrijvers D, Van Herpen C, Kerger J, et al, "Docetaxel, Cisplatin and 5-Fluorouracil in Patients With Locally Advanced Unresectable Head and Neck Cancer: A Phase I-II Feasibility Study," *Ann Oncol*, 2004, 15 (4):638-45.

Thiesen J and Kramer I, "Physico-Chemical Stability of Docetaxel Premix Solution and Docetaxel Infusion Solutions in PVC Bags and Polyolefine Containers," *Pharm World Sci*, 1999, 21(3):137-41.

Trudeau ME, "Docetaxel: A Review of Its Pharmacology and Clinical Activity," *Can J Oncol*, 1996, 6(1):443-57.

Vermorken JB, Remenar E, van Herpen C, et al, "Cisplatin, Fluorouracil, and Docetaxel in Unresectable Head and Neck Cancer," *N Engl J Med*, 2007, 357(17):1695-704.

Zwerdling T, Krailo M, Monteleone P, et al, "Phase II Investigation of Docetaxel in Pediatric Patients With Recurrent Solid Tumors: A Report From the Children's Oncology Group," *Cancer*, 2006, 106 (8):1821-8.

Docusate (DOK yoo sate)

Medication Safety Issues

Sound-alike/look-alike issues:

Colace® may be confused with Calan®, Cozaar®

Docusate may be confused with Doxinate®

Dulcolax® (docusate) may be confused with Dulcolax® (bisacodyl)

Surfak® may be confused with Surbex®

U.S. Brand Names Colace® [OTC]; Correctol® [OTC]; D-S-S® [OTC]; Diocto® [OTC]; Docu-Soft [OTC]; Docusoft-S™ [OTC]; DOK™ [OTC]; DOS® [OTC]; Dulcolax® Stool Softener [OTC]; Enemeez® Plus [OTC]; Enemeez® [OTC]; Fleet® Pedia-Lax™ Liquid Stool Softener [OTC]; Fleet® Sof-Lax® [OTC]; Genasoft® [OTC]; Phillips'® Stool Softener Laxative [OTC]; Silace [OTC]; Surfak® [OTC]

Canadian Brand Names Apo-Docusate-Sodium®; Colace®; Colax-C®; Novo-Docusate Calcium; Novo-Docusate Sodium; PMS-Docusate Calcium; PMS-Docusate Sodium; Regulex®; Selax®; Soflax™

Therapeutic Category Laxative, Surfactant; Stool Softener

Generic Available Yes: Excludes enema, gelcap, tablet

Use Stool softener in patients who should avoid straining during defecation; constipation associated with hard, dry stools; ceruminolytic

Pregnancy Risk Factor C

Lactation Excretion in breast milk unknown/compatible

Contraindications Hypersensitivity to docusate or any component; concomitant use of mineral oil; intestinal obstruction, acute abdominal pain, nausea, vomiting

Adverse Reactions

Dermatologic: Rash

Gastrointestinal: Intestinal obstruction, diarrhea, abdominal cramping

Local: Throat irritation

Drug Interactions

Avoid Concomitant Use There are no known interactions where it is recommended to avoid concomitant use.

Increased Effect/Toxicity There are no known significant interactions involving an increase in effect.

Decreased Effect There are no known significant interactions involving a decrease in effect.

Mechanism of Action Reduces surface tension of the oil-water interface of the stool resulting in enhanced incorporation of water and fat allowing for stool softening

Pharmacodynamics Onset of action: 12-72 hours

Usual Dosage

Infants and Children: Oral: 5 mg/kg/day in 1-4 divided doses **or** dose by age:

<3 years: 10-40 mg/day in 1-4 divided doses

3-6 years: 20-60 mg/day in 1-4 divided doses

6-12 years: 40-150 mg/day in 1-4 divided doses

Adolescents and Adults: Oral: 50-400 mg/day in 1-4 divided doses

Older Children and Adults: Rectal: Add 50-100 mg of docusate liquid (not syrup) to enema fluid (NS or water)

Administration

Oral: Administer docusate liquid (not syrup) with milk, fruit juice, or infant formula to mask the bitter taste; ensure adequate fluid intake

Rectal: Administer as a retention or flushing enema

Additional Information Docusate sodium 5-10 mg/mL liquid instilled in the ear as a ceruminolytic produces substantial ear wax disintegration within 15 minutes and complete disintegration after 24 hours

Dosage Forms Excipient information presented when available (limited, particularly for generics); consult specific product labeling. [DSC] = Discontinued product

Capsule, oral, as calcium: 240 mg

Capsule, oral, as sodium: 100 mg, 250 mg [DSC]
Colace®: 50 mg [contains sodium 3 mg/capsule]; 100 mg [contains sodium 5 mg/capsule]

Capsule, liquid, oral, as calcium:
Surfak®: 240 mg

Capsule, liquid, oral, as sodium:
Docusoft-S™: 100 mg [contains sodium 5 mg/capsule]

Capsule, softgel, oral, as calcium: 240 mg

Capsule, softgel, oral, as sodium: 100 mg, 250 mg
Correctol®: 100 mg
Docu-Soft: 100 mg
DOK™: 100 mg, 250 mg
Dulcolax® Stool Softener: 100 mg [contains sodium 5 mg/softgel]
Fleet® Sof-Lax®: 100 mg [contains sodium 5 mg/softgel]
DOS®, D-S-S®: 100 mg, 250 mg
Genasoft®: 100 mg
Phillips'® Stool Softener Laxative: 100 mg [contains sodium 5.2 mg/softgel]

Liquid, oral, as sodium: 150 mg/15 mL (480 mL)
Colace®: 150 mg/15 mL (30 mL) [contains propylene glycol, sodium 1 mg/mL]
Diocto®: 150 mg/15 mL (480 mL)

Fleet® Pedia-Lax™ Liquid Stool Softener: 50 mg/15 mL (120 mL) [contains propylene glycol, sodium 13 mg/15 mL; fruit punch flavor]

Silace: 150 mg/15 mL (480 mL) [lemon-vanilla flavor]

Solution, rectal, as sodium [enema]:

Enemeez®: 283 mg/5 mL

Enemeez® Plus: 283 mg/5 mL [contains benzocaine]

Syrup, oral, as sodium: 60 mg/15 mL (480 mL)

Colace®: 60 mg/15 mL (480 mL) [alcohol free, sugar free; contains sodium 36 mg/5 mL]

Diocto®: 60 mg/15 mL (480 mL)

Silace: 20 mg/5 mL (480 mL) [peppermint flavor]

Tablet, oral, as sodium:

DOK™: 100 mg

References

Chen DA and Caparosa RJ, "A Nonprescription Cerumenolytic," *Am J Otol*, 1991, 12(6):475-6.

Docusate and Senna (DOK yoo sate & SEN na)

Medication Safety Issues

Sound-alike/look-alike issues:

Senokot® may be confused with Depakote®

U.S. Brand Names Dok™ Plus [OTC]; Peri-Colace® [OTC]; Senokot-S® [OTC]; SenoSol™-SS [OTC]

Therapeutic Category Laxative, Stimulant; Laxative, Surfactant; Stool Softener

Generic Available Yes

Use Treatment of constipation generally associated with dry, hard stools and decreased intestinal motility; prevention of opiate-induced constipation

Contraindications Hypersensitivity to docusate, senna, or any component; concomitant use of mineral oil; undiagnosed abdominal pain; appendicitis, intestinal obstruction or perforation; acute abdominal pain; nausea, vomiting

Warnings Do not use when abdominal pain, rectal bleeding, nausea, or vomiting are present

Precautions Avoid prolonged use (>1 week); chronic use may lead to dependency, fluid and electrolyte imbalance, vitamin and mineral deficiencies

Adverse Reactions

Dermatologic: Rash

Endocrine & metabolic: Electrolyte and fluid imbalance

Gastrointestinal: Nausea, vomiting, diarrhea, abdominal cramps, perianal irritation, discoloration of feces, melanosis coli

Genitourinary: Discoloration of urine

Hepatic: Idiosyncratic hepatitis

Mechanism of Action Senna's active metabolite (aglycone) acts as a local irritant on the colon and stimulates the myenteric plexus to produce peristalsis; docusate reduces surface tension of the oil-water interface of the stool resulting in enhanced incorporation of water and fat allowing for stool softening

Pharmacodynamics Onset of action: Within 6-12 hours

Pharmacokinetics (Adult data unless noted) Senna:

Metabolism: Senna is metabolized in the liver

Elimination: In the feces (via bile) and in urine

Usual Dosage Oral:

Children 2 to <6 years: 1/2 tablet once daily at bedtime; maximum: 1 tablet twice daily

Children 6 to <12 years: 1 tablet once daily at bedtime; maximum: 2 tablets twice daily

Children ≥12 years, Adolescents, and Adults: 2 tablets once daily at bedtime; maximum: 4 tablets twice daily

Administration Administer with water, preferably in the evening

Monitoring Parameters I & O, frequency of bowel movements, serum electrolytes if severe diarrhea develops

Patient Information May discolor urine or feces; drink plenty of fluids

Dosage Forms Excipient information presented when available (limited, particularly for generics); consult specific product labeling.

Tablet, oral: Docusate sodium 50 mg and sennosides 8.6 mg

Dok™ Plus: Docusate sodium 50 mg and sennosides 8.6 mg

Peri-Colace®: Docusate sodium 50 mg and sennosides 8.6 mg

Senokot-S®: Docusate sodium 50 mg and sennosides 8.6 mg [sugar free; contains sodium 4 mg/tablet]

SenoSol™-SS: Docusate sodium 50 mg and sennosides 8.6 mg [contains sodium 3 mg/tablet]

References

Baker SS, Liptak GS, Colletti RB, et al, "Constipation in Infants and Children: Evaluation and Treatment. A Medical Position Statement of the North American Society for Pediatric Gastroenterology and Nutrition," *J Pediatr Gastroenterol Nutr*, 1999, 29(5):612-26.

Herndon CM, Jackson KC II, and Hallin PA, "Management of Opioid-Induced Gastrointestinal Effects in Patients Receiving Palliative Care," *Pharmacotherapy*, 2002, 22(2):240-50.

♦ **Docusate Calcium** *see* Docusate *on page 468*

♦ **Docusate Potassium** *see* Docusate *on page 468*

♦ **Docusate Sodium** *see* Docusate *on page 468*

♦ **Docu-Soft [OTC]** *see* Docusate *on page 468*

♦ **Docusoft-S™ [OTC]** *see* Docusate *on page 468*

♦ **Dofus [OTC]** *see* Lactobacillus *on page 790*

♦ **DOK™ [OTC]** *see* Docusate *on page 468*

♦ **Dok™ Plus [OTC]** *see* Docusate and Senna *on page 469*

Dolasetron (dol A se tron)

Medication Safety Issues

Sound-alike/look-alike issues:

Anzemet® may be confused with Aldomet®, Antivert®, Avandamet®

Dolasetron may be confused with granisetron, ondansetron, palonosetron

U.S. Brand Names Anzemet®

Canadian Brand Names Anzemet®

Therapeutic Category 5-HT$_3$ Receptor Antagonist; Antiemetic

Generic Available No

Use Prevention of nausea and vomiting associated with emetogenic cancer chemotherapy (initial and repeat courses); prevention of postoperative nausea and vomiting; treatment (injectable form only) of postoperative nausea and vomiting (FDA approved in ages 2-16 years and adults); has also been used in adults for breakthrough treatment of nausea and vomiting associated with chemotherapy

Pregnancy Risk Factor B

Pregnancy Considerations Teratogenic effects were not observed in animal studies. There are no adequate and well-controlled studies in pregnant women.

Lactation Excretion in breast milk unknown/use caution

Contraindications Hypersensitivity to dolasetron or any component

Warnings Dolasetron may cause ECG interval changes (PR, QT/QT$_c$, JT prolongation, and QRS widening) related in magnitude and frequency to blood concentrations of the active metabolite, hydrodolasetron; usually occurring 1-2 hours after I.V. administration and usually lasting 6-8 hours; however, may last ≥24 hours; interval prolongation could (rarely) lead to cardiovascular consequences such as heart block or cardiac arrhythmias. Use with caution in children and adolescents who have or may develop QT$_c$ prolongation due to rare reports of arrhythmias, MI, and cardiac arrest in pediatric and adolescent patients;

Canadian healthcare officials have deemed dolasetron contraindicated for the treatment of children and adolescents <18 years of age, and in addition, its use in adults for the treatment of postoperative nausea and vomiting (it has never been indicated for use in children in Canada).

Precautions Use with caution in patients with, or who may develop, prolongation of cardiac conduction intervals, particularly QT_c; conditions include hypokalemia, hypomagnesemia, or congenital QT syndrome; use with caution in patients receiving antiarrhythmic or other medications known to prolong the QT interval (eg, class I or III antiarrhythmic agents) or medications known to reduce potassium or magnesium concentrations (eg, diuretics) and cumulative high-dose anthracycline therapy. Clinically relevant QT interval prolongation may occur resulting in torsade de pointes, when used in conjunction with other agents that prolong the QT interval (eg, Class I and III antiarrhythmics). Use with caution in patients allergic to other 5-HT$_3$ receptor antagonists; cross reactivity has been reported with other 5-HT$_3$ receptor antagonists. For chemotherapy associated nausea and vomiting, should be used on a scheduled basis, not on an "as needed" (PRN) basis, since data support the use of this drug only in the prevention of nausea and vomiting (due to antineoplastic therapy) and not in the rescue of nausea and vomiting. Not intended for treatment of nausea and vomiting or for chronic continuous therapy.

Adverse Reactions

Cardiovascular: Arrhythmias, bradycardia, cardiac arrest (see Warnings), hypertension, hypotension, MI, prolonged QT interval and other ECG changes, tachycardia

Central nervous system: Agitation, anxiety, chills, dizziness, fatigue, fever, headache, pain, shivering, sleep disorder

Dermatologic: Rash

Gastrointestinal: Abdominal pain, anorexia, diarrhea, dyspepsia, taste perversion

Genitourinary: Acute renal failure (rarely), dysuria (rarely), polyuria (rarely), urinary retention

Hepatic: Transient elevations in liver enzymes

Local: Venous irritation

Neuromuscular & skeletal: Arthralgia, myalgia

Ocular: Photophobia (rarely)

Otic: Tinnitus (rarely)

Renal: Oliguria

Miscellaneous: Hypersensitivity reactions

<1%, postmarketing, and/or case reports (limited to important or life-threatening): Abnormal dreams, abnormal vision, alkaline phosphatase increased, ALT increased, anaphylactic reaction, anemia, AST increased, ataxia, bronchospasm, cardiac conduction abnormalities (including arrhythmia [sinus, supraventricular, and ventricular], atrial flutter/fibrillation, AV block, bundle branch block, extrasystoles, poor R wave progression, prolonged PR, QRS, JT, and QT_c intervals, ST, T, and U wave changes, ventricular tachycardia, wide complex tachycardia and ventricular fibrillation); chest pain, confusion, constipation, diaphoresis, dyspnea, edema, epistaxis, facial edema, flushing, GGT increased, hematuria, hyperbilirubinemia, ischemia (peripheral), local injection site reaction (pain, burning), myocardial ischemia, orthostatic hypotension, palpitation, pancreatitis, paresthesia, peripheral edema, prothrombin time increased, PTT increased, purpura/hematoma, rash, syncope, thrombocytopenia, thrombophlebitis/phlebitis, tremor, twitching, urticaria, vertigo

Drug Interactions

Metabolism/Transport Effects Substrate (minor) of CYP2C9, 3A4; **Inhibits** CYP2D6 (weak)

Avoid Concomitant Use

Avoid concomitant use of Dolasetron with any of the following: Apomorphine; Artemether; Dronedarone; Lumefantrine; Nilotinib; Pimozide; QuiNINE; Tetrabenazine; Thioridazine; Ziprasidone

Increased Effect/Toxicity

Dolasetron may increase the levels/effects of: Apomorphine; Dronedarone; Pimozide; QTc-Prolonging Agents; QuiNINE; Tetrabenazine; Thioridazine; Ziprasidone

The levels/effects of Dolasetron may be increased by: Alfuzosin; Artemether; Chloroquine; Ciprofloxacin; Ciprofloxacin (Systemic); Gadobutrol; Lumefantrine; Nilotinib; QuiNINE

Decreased Effect There are no known significant interactions involving a decrease in effect.

Stability Store intact vials and tablets at 20°C to 25°C (68°F to 77°F) with vial excursions permitted to 15°C to 30°C (59°F to 86°F); protect from light. Injection is stable after dilution in NS, D$_5$W, D$_5$1/2NS, D$_5$LR, LR, and 10% mannitol injection under normal lighting conditions for 24 hours at room temperature and 48 hours under refrigeration

Mechanism of Action Dolasetron and its major metabolite, hydrodolasetron, are selective 5-HT$_3$ receptor antagonists, blocking serotonin, both peripherally on vagal nerve terminals and centrally in the chemoreceptor trigger zone

Pharmacokinetics (Adult data unless noted) Due to the rapid metabolism of dolasetron to hydrodolasetron (primary active metabolite), the majority of the following pharmacokinetic parameters relate to hydrodolasetron:

Absorption: Oral: Rapid and complete

Distribution:

Children: 5.9-7.4 L/kg

Adults: 4.15-5.5 L/kg

Metabolism: Hepatic; rapidly converted by carbonyl reductase to active major metabolite, hydrodolasetron; hydrodolasetron is metabolized by the cytochrome P450 CYP2D6 and CYP3A enzyme systems and flavin monooxygenase

Bioavailability: Oral: Children: 59% (formulation not specified), adults: 70% to 80% (not affected by food)

Protein binding: 69% to 77% (active metabolite)

Half-life, elimination:

Dolasetron: <10 minutes

Hydrodolasetron:

Oral: Children: 5.7 hours, adults: 8.1 hours (range: 5-10 hours)

I.V.: Children: 4.8 hours, adults: 7.3 hours (range: 4-8 hours)

Time to peak serum concentration:

Oral: 1-1.5 hours

I.V.: 0.6 hours

Elimination: Dolasetron: <1% excreted unchanged in urine; hydrodolasetron: 53% to 61% of total dose excreted unchanged in urine within 36 hours

Usual Dosage

Prevention of chemotherapy-induced nausea and vomiting: **Oral:** Administered within 1 hour before chemotherapy; or **I.V.:** Administered ~30 minutes before chemotherapy:

Children 2-16 years:

Oral, I.V.: 1.8 mg/kg as a single dose (maximum: 100 mg)

Adults:

Oral: 100 mg as a single dose

I.V.: 1.8 mg/kg or 100 mg as a single dose

Postoperative nausea and vomiting:
Children 2-16 years:
Prevention:
Oral: 1.2 mg/kg within 2 hours before surgery; maximum: 100 mg/dose
I.V.: 0.35 mg/kg ~15 minutes before cessation of anesthesia; maximum: 12.5 mg/dose
Treatment: I.V. (only): 0.35 mg/kg as soon as nausea or vomiting present; maximum: 12.5 mg/dose
Adults:
Prevention:
Oral: 100 mg within 2 hours before surgery (doses of 25-200 mg have been used)
I.V.: 12.5 mg ~15 minutes before cessation of anesthesia
Treatment: I.V. (only): 12.5 mg as soon as nausea or vomiting present
Dosage adjustment in hepatic or renal impairment: No dosage adjustment is necessary
Administration
Oral: May be administered with or without food; injection may be administered orally, diluted in apple or apple-grape juice; stable for 2 hours at room temperature
Parenteral: I.V.: Infuse undiluted over 30 seconds or dilute in 50 mL compatible I.V. fluid and infuse over ≤15 minutes; do not mix with other medications; flush line before and after dolasetron administration
Monitoring Parameters Baseline ECG and electrolytes in high-risk patients (see Warnings and Precautions), emesis episodes
Dosage Forms Excipient information presented when available (limited, particularly for generics); consult specific product labeling.
Injection, solution, as mesylate:
Anzemet®: 20 mg/mL (0.625 mL) [single-use Carpuject® or vial; contains mannitol 38.2 mg/mL]; 20 mg/mL (5 mL) [single-use vial; contains mannitol 38.2 mg/mL]; 20 mg/mL (25 mL) [multidose vial; contains mannitol 29 mg/mL]
Tablet, as mesylate:
Anzemet®: 50 mg, 100 mg
Extemporaneous Preparations A 10 mg/mL suspension may be made by crushing twelve 50 mg tablets; slowly add a 1:1 mixture of Ora-Plus® and Ora-Sweet® SF (or 1:1 mixture of strawberry syrup and Ora-Plus®) to a final volume of 60 mL; stable for 90 days refrigerated
Johnson CE, Wagner DS, and Bussard WE, "Stability of Dolasetron in Two Oral Liquid Vehicles," *Am J Health Syst Pharm*, 2003, 60(21):2242-4.

References
American Society of Clinical Oncology, Kris MG, Hesketh PJ, et al, "American Society of Clinical Oncology Guideline for Antiemetics in Oncology: Update 2006," *J Clin Oncol*, 2006, 24(18):2932-47.
"ASHP Therapeutic Guidelines on the Pharmacologic Management of Nausea and Vomiting in Adult and Pediatric Patients Receiving Chemotherapy or Radiation Therapy or Undergoing Surgery," *Am J Health Syst Pharm*, 1999, 56(8):729-64.
National Comprehensive Cancer Network® (NCCN), "Clinical Practice Guidelines in Oncology™: Antiemesis," Version 4.2009. Available at: http://www.nccn.org/professionals/physician_gls/PDF/antiemesis.pdf.
Olutoye O, Jantzen EC, Alexis R, et al, "A Comparison of the Costs and Efficacy of Ondansetron and Dolasetron in the Prophylaxis of Postoperative Vomiting in Pediatric Patients Undergoing Ambulatory Surgery," *Anesth Analg*, 2003, 97(2):390-6.

◆ **Dolasetron Mesylate** *see* Dolasetron *on page 469*
◆ **Dolophine®** *see* Methadone *on page 893*
◆ **Doloral (Can)** *see* Morphine Sulfate *on page 946*
◆ **Dom-Amiodarone (Can)** *see* Amiodarone *on page 84*
◆ **Dom-Amitriptyline (Can)** *see* Amitriptyline *on page 89*
◆ **Dom-Amlodipine (Can)** *see* AmLODIPine *on page 91*
◆ **Dom-Atenolol (Can)** *see* Atenolol *on page 147*
◆ **Dom-Azithromycin (Can)** *see* Azithromycin *on page 164*

◆ **Dom-Baclofen (Can)** *see* Baclofen *on page 171*
◆ **Dom-Buspirone (Can)** *see* BusPIRone *on page 222*
◆ **Dom-Carbamazepine (Can)** *see* CarBAMazepine *on page 244*
◆ **Dom-Carvedilol (Can)** *see* Carvedilol *on page 254*
◆ **Dom-Cephalexin (Can)** *see* Cephalexin *on page 282*
◆ **Dom-Cimetidine (Can)** *see* Cimetidine *on page 309*
◆ **Dom-Ciprofloxacin (Can)** *see* Ciprofloxacin *on page 310*
◆ **Dom-Citalopram (Can)** *see* Citalopram *on page 319*
◆ **Dom-Clonidine (Can)** *see* CloNIDine *on page 338*
◆ **Dom-Cyclobenzaprine (Can)** *see* Cyclobenzaprine *on page 367*
◆ **Dom-Diclofenac (Can)** *see* Diclofenac *on page 429*
◆ **Dom-Diclofenac SR (Can)** *see* Diclofenac *on page 429*
◆ **Dom-Divalproex (Can)** *see* Valproic Acid and Derivatives *on page 1398*
◆ **Dom-Doxycycline (Can)** *see* Doxycycline *on page 479*
◆ **Domeboro®** *see* Aluminum Acetate *on page 74*
◆ **Dom-Fluconazole (Can)** *see* Fluconazole *on page 584*
◆ **Dom-Fluoxetine (Can)** *see* FLUoxetine *on page 600*
◆ **Dom-Furosemide (Can)** *see* Furosemide *on page 632*
◆ **Dom-Gabapentin (Can)** *see* Gabapentin *on page 634*
◆ **Dom-Glyburide (Can)** *see* GlyBURIDE *on page 648*
◆ **Dom-Hydrochlorothiazide (Can)** *see* Hydrochlorothiazide *on page 682*
◆ **Dom-Levetiracetam (Can)** *see* Levetiracetam *on page 808*
◆ **Dom-Lisinopril (Can)** *see* Lisinopril *on page 832*
◆ **Dom-Loperamide (Can)** *see* Loperamide *on page 838*
◆ **Dom-Lorazepam (Can)** *see* LORazepam *on page 845*
◆ **Dom-Lovastatin (Can)** *see* Lovastatin *on page 850*
◆ **Dom-Metformin (Can)** *see* MetFORMIN *on page 891*
◆ **Dom-Methimazole (Can)** *see* Methimazole *on page 897*
◆ **Dom-Metoprolol (Can)** *see* Metoprolol *on page 918*
◆ **Dom-Minocycline (Can)** *see* Minocycline *on page 933*
◆ **Dom-Ondansetron (Can)** *see* Ondansetron *on page 1022*
◆ **Dom-Oxybutynin (Can)** *see* Oxybutynin *on page 1037*
◆ **Dom-Paroxetine (Can)** *see* PARoxetine *on page 1064*
◆ **Dom-Piroxicam (Can)** *see* Piroxicam *on page 1118*
◆ **Dom-Pravastatin (Can)** *see* Pravastatin *on page 1145*
◆ **Dom-Propranolol (Can)** *see* Propranolol *on page 1175*
◆ **Dom-Ranitidine (Can)** *see* Ranitidine *on page 1200*
◆ **Dom-Risperidone (Can)** *see* Risperidone *on page 1218*
◆ **Dom-Sertraline (Can)** *see* Sertraline *on page 1254*
◆ **Dom-Simvastatin (Can)** *see* Simvastatin *on page 1263*
◆ **Dom-Sotalol (Can)** *see* Sotalol *on page 1284*
◆ **Dom-Sumatriptan (Can)** *see* SUMAtriptan *on page 1308*
◆ **Dom-Topiramate (Can)** *see* Topiramate *on page 1360*
◆ **Dom-Trazodone (Can)** *see* TraZODone *on page 1371*
◆ **Dom-Ursodiol C (Can)** *see* Ursodiol *on page 1393*
◆ **Dom-Verapamil SR (Can)** *see* Verapamil *on page 1416*
◆ **Donnatal®** *see* Hyoscyamine, Atropine, Scopolamine, and Phenobarbital *on page 700*
◆ **Donnatal Extentabs®** *see* Hyoscyamine, Atropine, Scopolamine, and Phenobarbital *on page 700*

DOPamine (DOE pa meen)

Medication Safety Issues
Sound-alike/look-alike issues:
DOPamine may be confused with DOBUTamine, Dopram®

High alert medication: The Institute for Safe Medication Practices (ISMP) includes this medication among its list of drugs which have a heightened risk of causing significant patient harm when used in error.

Related Information
Adult ACLS Algorithms *on page 1463*
CPR Pediatric Drug Dosages *on page 1455*
Emergency Pediatric Drip Calculations *on page 1457*
Extravasation Treatment *on page 1522*

Therapeutic Category Adrenergic Agonist Agent;
Sympathomimetic

Generic Available Yes

Use Increase cardiac output, blood pressure, and urine flow as an adjunct in the treatment of shock or hypotension which persists after adequate fluid volume replacement; in low dosage to increase renal perfusion

Pregnancy Risk Factor C

Lactation Excretion in breast milk unknown

Contraindications Hypersensitivity to dopamine or any component (see Warnings); pheochromocytoma, or ventricular fibrillation

Warnings Potent drug; must be diluted prior to use; patient's hemodynamic status should be monitored; injection solution contains sulfites which may cause allergic reactions in susceptible individuals

Precautions Blood volume depletion should be corrected, if possible, before starting dopamine therapy. Dopamine must not be used as sole therapy in hypovolemic patients. Extravasation may cause tissue necrosis (treat extravasation with phentolamine; see Extravasation Treatment on page 1522) **[U.S. Boxed Warning]**; due to potential gangrene of extremities, use with caution in patients with occlusive vascular disease.

Adverse Reactions
Cardiovascular: Ectopic heartbeats, tachycardia, vasoconstriction, cardiac conduction abnormalities, widened QRS complex, hypertension, ventricular arrhythmias, gangrene of the extremities (with high doses for prolonged periods or even with low doses in patients with occlusive vascular disease), anginal pain, palpitations
Central nervous system: Anxiety, headache
Gastrointestinal: Nausea, vomiting
Genitourinary: Urine output decreased (high dose)
Neuromuscular & skeletal: Piloerection
Ocular: Dilated pupils
Renal: Azotemia
Respiratory: Dyspnea

Drug Interactions
Avoid Concomitant Use
Avoid concomitant use of DOPamine with any of the following: Inhalational Anesthetics; Iobenguane I 123

Increased Effect/Toxicity
DOPamine may increase the levels/effects of: Sympathomimetics

The levels/effects of DOPamine may be increased by: Atomoxetine; Cannabinoids; COMT Inhibitors; Inhalational Anesthetics

Decreased Effect
DOPamine may decrease the levels/effects of: Iobenguane I 123

Stability Protect from light; solutions that are darker than slightly yellow should not be used; incompatible with alkaline solutions or iron salts; compatible when coadministered with dobutamine, epinephrine, isoproterenol, lidocaine, atracurium, vecuronium

Mechanism of Action Stimulates both adrenergic and dopaminergic receptors; low doses are mainly dopaminergic which stimulate and produce renal and mesenteric vasodilation; intermediate doses stimulate both dopaminergic and beta$_1$-adrenergic receptors and produce cardiac stimulation (increased heart rate and cardiac index) and increased renal blood flow; high doses stimulate alpha-adrenergic receptors primarily (vasoconstriction and increased blood pressure)

Pharmacodynamics
Onset of action: Adults: 5 minutes
Duration: Due to its short duration of action (<10 minutes) a continuous infusion must be used

Pharmacokinetics (Adult data unless noted)
Metabolism: In plasma, kidneys, and liver; 75% to inactive metabolites by monoamine oxidase and catechol-o-methyltransferase and 25% to norepinephrine (active)
Half-life: 2 minutes
Clearance: Neonatal clearance varies and appears to be age related. Clearance is more prolonged with combined hepatic and renal dysfunction. Dopamine has exhibited nonlinear kinetics in children; dose changes in children may not achieve steady-state for approximately 1 hour rather than 20 minutes seen in adults.

Usual Dosage I.V. infusion:
The hemodynamic effects of dopamine are dose-dependent:
Low dosage: 1-5 mcg/kg/minute, increased renal blood flow and urine output
Intermediate dosage: 5-15 mcg/kg/minute, increased renal blood flow, heart rate, cardiac contractility, cardiac output, and blood pressure
High dosage: >15 mcg/kg/minute, alpha-adrenergic effects begin to predominate, vasoconstriction, increased blood pressure
Neonates: 1-20 mcg/kg/minute continuous infusion, titrate to desired response
Infants and Children: 1-20 mcg/kg/minute, maximum dose: 50 mcg/kg/minute continuous infusion, titrate to desired response
Adults: 1 mcg/kg/minute up to 50 mcg/kg/minute, titrate to desired response
If dosages >20-30 mcg/kg/minute are needed, a more direct-acting pressor may be beneficial (ie, epinephrine, norepinephrine)

Administration Parenteral: Must be diluted prior to administration; maximum concentration: 3200 mcg/mL (3.2 mg/mL); (concentrations as high as 6000 mcg/mL have been infused into large veins, safely and with efficacy, in cases of extreme fluid restriction); rate of infusion (mL/hour) = dose (mcg/kg/minute) x weight (kg) x 60 minutes/hour divided by concentration (mcg/mL); administer into large vein to prevent the possibility of extravasation; use infusion device to control rate of flow; administration into an umbilical arterial catheter is **not** recommended

Monitoring Parameters ECG, heart rate, CVP, MAP, urine output; if pulmonary artery catheter is in place, monitor CI, PWCP, SVR, RAP, and PVR

Dosage Forms Excipient information presented when available (limited, particularly for generics); consult specific product labeling.
Infusion, as hydrochloride [premixed in D$_5$W]: 0.8 mg/mL (250 mL, 500 mL); 1.6 mg/mL (250 mL, 500 mL); 3.2 mg/mL (250 mL)
Injection, solution, as hydrochloride: 40 mg/mL (5 mL, 10 mL); 80 mg/mL (5 mL); 160 mg/mL (5 mL) [contains sodium metabisulfite]

References

Banner W, Jr, Vernon DD, Dean JM, et al, "Nonlinear Dopamine Pharmacokinetics in Pediatric Patients," *J Pharmacol Exp Ther*, 1989, 249(1):131-3.

◆ **Dopamine Hydrochloride** *see* DOPamine *on page 472*

◆ **Dopram®** *see* Doxapram *on page 474*

Dornase Alfa (DOOR nase AL fa)

U.S. Brand Names Pulmozyme®
Canadian Brand Names Pulmozyme®
Therapeutic Category Enzyme, Inhalant; Mucolytic Agent
Generic Available No
Use Management of cystic fibrosis patients to reduce the frequency of respiratory infections and to improve pulmonary function
Pregnancy Risk Factor B
Pregnancy Considerations Teratogenic effects were not observed in animal studies. There are no adequate and well-controlled studies in pregnant women.
Lactation Excretion in breast milk unknown/use caution
Breast-Feeding Considerations Measurable amounts would not be expected in breast milk following inhalation; however, it is not known if dornase alfa is excreted in human milk.
Contraindications Hypersensitivity to dornase alfa, Chinese hamster ovary cell products (eg, epoetin alfa), or any component
Warnings Safety and efficacy has not been established in children <5 years of age or in patients with forced vital capacity <40% of normal; no data exists regarding safety during lactation
Adverse Reactions
Cardiovascular: Chest pain
Central nervous system: Fever (32% in patients with FVC <40%), headache, malaise
Dermatologic: Skin rash, urticaria
Gastrointestinal: Sore throat, dyspepsia
Hepatic: Liver disease
Ocular: Conjunctivitis
Respiratory: Cough increased (higher incidence in younger patients (<3 months -5 years) 45% vs 30% (5-10 years), dyspnea, hemoptysis, wheezing, laryngitis, rhinitis (higher incidence in younger patients (<3 months-5 years) 35% vs 27% (5-10 years), pharyngitis
Miscellaneous: Voice alteration, hoarseness, serum antibodies to dornase (2% to 4%)
Drug Interactions
Avoid Concomitant Use There are no known interactions where it is recommended to avoid concomitant use.
Increased Effect/Toxicity There are no known significant interactions involving an increase in effect.
Decreased Effect There are no known significant interactions involving a decrease in effect.
Stability Must be stored in the refrigerator at 2°C to 8°C (36°F to 46°F) and protected from strong light; unopened vials left at room temperature for a total time of 24 hours should be discarded; discard solution if cloudy or discolored
Mechanism of Action Dornase alfa is a deoxyribonuclease (DNA) enzyme produced by recombinant gene technology. Dornase selectively cleaves DNA, thus reducing mucous viscosity seen in the pulmonary secretions of cystic fibrosis patients. As a result, airflow in the lung is improved and the risk of bacterial infection may be decreased.
Pharmacodynamics Onset of improved pulmonary function tests (PFTs): 3-8 days; PFTs will return to baseline 2-3 weeks after discontinuation of therapy

Pharmacokinetics (Adult data unless noted) Following nebulization, enzyme levels are measurable in the sputum within 15 minutes and decline rapidly thereafter
Usual Dosage
Infants and Children ≤5 years: Not approved for use, however studies using this therapy in small numbers of children as young as 3 months of age have reported efficacy and similar side effects. See References.
Children >5 years and Adults: Inhalation: 2.5 mg/day through selected nebulizers in conjunction with a Pulmo-Aide®, Pari-Proneb®, Mobilaire™, Porta-Neb®, or Pari Baby™ compressor system
Note: While some patients, especially older than 21 years of age or with forced vital capacity (FVC) >85%, may benefit from twice daily administration, another study (Fuchs, 1994) reported no difference between once or twice daily therapy; in a randomized crossover trial involving 48 children, alternate day treatment was as effective as daily treatment over a 12-week period (Suri, 2001).
Administration Nebulization: Should not be diluted or mixed with any other drugs in the nebulizer, this may inactivate the drug
Dosage Forms Excipient information presented when available (limited, particularly for generics); consult specific product labeling.
Solution for nebulization [preservative free]:
Pulmozyme®: 1 mg/mL (2.5 mL) [derived from Chinese hamster cells]

References

Fuchs HJ, Borowitz DS, Christiansen DH, et al, "Effect of Aerosolized Recombinant Human DNase on Exacerbations of Respiratory Symptoms and on Pulmonary Function in Patients With Cystic Fibrosis," *N Engl J Med*, 1994, 331(10):637-42.

Mueller GA, Rubins G, Wessel D, et al, "Effects of Dornase Alfa on Pulmonary Function Tests in Infants with Cystic Fibrosis," *Am J Respir Crit Care Med*, 1996, 153:A70.

Rock M, Kirchner K, McCubbin M, et al, "Aerosol Delivery and Safety of rhDNASE in Young Children With Cystic Fibrosis: A Bronchoscopic Study." *Pediatr Pulmonol*, 1996, 13(Suppl):A268.

Suri R, Metcalfe C, Lees B, et al, "Comparison of Hypertonic Saline and Alternate-Day or Daily Recombinant Human Deoxyribonuclease in Children With Cystic Fibrosis: A Randomised Trial," *Lancet*, 2001, 358 (9290):1316-21.

Suri R, "The Use of Human Deoxyribonuclease (rhDNase) in the Management of Cystic Fibrosis," *BioDrugs*, 2005, 19(3):135-44.

Wagener JS, Rock MJ, McCubbin MM, et al, "Aerosol Delivery and Safety of Recombinant Human Deoxyribonuclease in Young Children With Cystic Fibrosis: A Bronchoscopic Study. Pulmozyme Pediatric Broncoscopy Study Group," *J Pediatr*, 1998, 133(4):486-91.

◆ **Doryx®** *see* Doxycycline *on page 479*

Dorzolamide (dor ZOLE a mide)

U.S. Brand Names Trusopt®
Canadian Brand Names Trusopt®
Therapeutic Category Carbonic Anhydrase Inhibitor, Ophthalmic
Generic Available Yes
Use Treatment of elevated intraocular pressure in patients with ocular hypertension or open-angle glaucoma
Pregnancy Risk Factor C
Lactation Excretion in breast milk unknown/not recommended
Contraindications Hypersensitivity to dorzolamide, sulfonamides, or any component
Warnings Dorzolamide, a sulfonamide, is absorbed systemically and may produce the same adverse effects seen with other sulfonamides; avoid use in patients with severe renal dysfunction (Cl$_{cr}$ <30 mL/minute); contains the preservative benzalkonium chloride which may be absorbed by soft contact lenses; contact lenses should be removed prior to administration of the solution and may be reinserted 15 minutes following administration;

concomitant use with other carbonic anhydrase inhibitors is not recommended; avoid use in patients receiving high-dose salicylate therapy (see Drug Interactions)

Precautions Use with caution in patients with hepatic impairment

Adverse Reactions

Central nervous system: Headache, fatigue, dizziness, vertigo

Dermatologic: Rash, pruritus, urticaria

Gastrointestinal: Bitter taste, nausea, throat irritation

Genitourinary: Urolithiasis

Neuromuscular & skeletal: Paresthesia

Ocular: Burning, stinging, discomfort, and pain, punctate keratitis, conjunctivitis, blurred vision, eye redness, tearing, dryness, photophobia, transient myopia, eyelid crusting, corneal fibrosis increased, iridocyclitis

Respiratory: Dyspnea

Drug Interactions

Metabolism/Transport Effects Substrate (minor) of CYP2C9, 3A4

Avoid Concomitant Use

Avoid concomitant use of Dorzolamide with any of the following: Brinzolamide

Increased Effect/Toxicity

Dorzolamide may increase the levels/effects of: Brinzolamide

Decreased Effect There are no known significant interactions involving a decrease in effect.

Stability Store at room temperature.

Mechanism of Action Competitive, reversible inhibition of the enzyme carbonic anhydrase in the ciliary processes of the eye resulting in decreased secretion of aqueous humor

Pharmacodynamics

Peak effect: 2 hours

Duration: 8-12 hours

Average lowering of intraoptic pressure: 3-5 mm Hg or at least 15% decrease from unmedicated baseline value

Pharmacokinetics (Adult data unless noted)

Absorption: Topical: Reaches systemic circulation

Distribution: Accumulates in RBCs during chronic administration

Protein binding: 33%

Metabolism: In liver to active but less potent metabolite, N-desethyl dorzolamide

Half-life: Terminal RBC half-life: 147 days

Elimination: Primarily unchanged in the urine

Usual Dosage Glaucoma: Children and Adults: 1 drop into the affected eye(s) 3 times/day

Administration Ophthalmic: Apply gentle pressure to lacrimal sac during and immediately following instillation (1 minute) or instruct patient to gently close eyelid after administration to decrease systemic absorption of ophthalmic drops; avoid contact of bottle tip with skin or eye; remove contact lenses prior to administration (see Warnings); lenses may be inserted 15 minutes after instillation; if more than one topical ophthalmic drug is being used, separate administration by at least 10 minutes

Monitoring Parameters Intraoptic pressure

Patient Information Avoid contact of bottle tip with skin or eye to prevent contamination by bacteria which may cause ocular infections; report any ocular reactions, particularly conjunctivitis and lid reactions to your physician promptly

Dosage Forms Excipient information presented when available (limited, particularly for generics); consult specific product labeling

Solution, ophthalmic: 2% (10 mL)

Trusopt®: 2% (10 mL) [contains benzalkonium chloride]

References

Portellos M, Buckley EG, and Freedman SF, "Topical Versus Oral Carbonic Anhydrase Inhibitor Therapy for Pediatric Glaucoma," *J AAPOS*, 1998, 2(1):43-7.

◆ **Dorzolamide Hydrochloride** *see* Dorzolamide *on page 473*

◆ **DOS® [OTC]** *see* Docusate *on page 468*

◆ **DOSS** *see* Docusate *on page 468*

◆ **Double Tussin DM [OTC]** *see* Guaifenesin and Dextromethorphan *on page 658*

Doxapram (DOKS a pram)

Medication Safety Issues

Sound-alike/look-alike issues:

Doxapram may be confused with doxacurium, doxazosin, doxepin, Doxinate®, DOXOrubicin

Dopram® may be confused with DOPamine

U.S. Brand Names Dopram®

Therapeutic Category Central Nervous System Stimulant; Respiratory Stimulant

Generic Available Yes

Use Respiratory and CNS stimulant for treatment of respiratory depression secondary to anesthesia, drug-induced CNS depression, idiopathic apnea of prematurity refractory to xanthines, and acute hypercapnia secondary to COPD (see Contraindications)

Pregnancy Risk Factor B

Pregnancy Considerations Teratogenic effects were not observed in animal studies.

Lactation Excretion in breast milk unknown/use caution

Contraindications Hypersensitivity to doxapram or any component (see Warnings); epilepsy, cerebral edema, head injury, suspected or proven pulmonary embolism, pheochromocytoma, cardiovascular or coronary artery disease, severe hypertension, hyperthyroidism, cardiac arrhythmias; concomitant use with mechanical ventilation in COPD patients; patients with mechanical disorders of ventilation such as bronchial obstruction, muscle paresis (including NM blockade), flail chest, pneumothorax, pulmonary fibrosis, asthma, or other conditions resulting in restriction of chest wall muscles of respiration or alveolar expansion

Warnings Doxapram contains benzyl alcohol which may cause allergic reactions in susceptible individuals; large amounts of benzyl alcohol (≥99 mg/kg/day) have been associated with a potentially fatal toxicity ("gasping syndrome") in neonates; the "gasping syndrome" consists of metabolic acidosis, respiratory distress, gasping respirations, CNS dysfunction (including convulsions, intracranial hemorrhage), hypotension and cardiovascular collapse. Recommended doses of doxapram for treatment of neonatal apnea will deliver 5.4-27 mg/kg/day of benzyl alcohol; the use of doxapram should be reserved for neonates who are unresponsive to the treatment of apnea with therapeutic serum concentrations of theophylline or caffeine. *In vitro* and animal studies have shown that benzoate, a metabolite of benzyl alcohol, displaces bilirubin from protein-binding sites.

Doxapram is not an antagonist to muscle relaxant drugs nor a specific narcotic antagonist; doxapram alone may not stimulate adequate spontaneous breathing or provide sufficient arousal in patients who are severely depressed; use as an adjunct to establish supportive measures; since respiratory depression may recur after stimulation with doxapram, monitor closely until the patient has been fully alert for 30-60 minutes; to reduce the potential for arrhythmias, including VT and VF, in patients who have received general anesthesia with a volatile agent known to sensitize the myocardium to catecholamines, administration of doxapram should be delayed until the complete excretion of anesthetic has occurred.

Precautions Oxygen, resuscitative equipment, and anticonvulsants should be readily available to manage excessive CNS stimulation. Frequent arterial blood gas measurements are recommended to identify and prevent the development of CO_2 retention and acidosis in COPD patients with acute hypercapnia; infusion of doxapram in premature infants has been associated with a statistically significant but moderate lengthening of QT_c interval; cardiac monitoring during treatment is suggested (Maillard, 2001); use caution in patients with impaired hepatic or renal function or receiving MAOIs or sympathomimetic drugs (see Drug Interactions)

Adverse Reactions

Cardiovascular: Hypertension* (dose-related), tachycardia, arrhythmias, hypotension, flushing, chest pain, QT prolongation with heartblock*

Central nervous system: CNS stimulation, restlessness, apprehension, disorientation, lightheadedness, jitters*, hallucinations, irritability*, seizures*, headache, fever, hypothermia, excessive crying*, sleep disturbances*

Gastrointestinal: Abdominal distension*, nausea, vomiting*, retching, gastric residuals increased*, bloody stools*, necrotising enterocolitis*

Genitourinary: Urinary retention, burning sensation in genital area or perineum, spontaneous voiding

Hematologic: Hemolysis (associated with rapid infusion)

Local: Phlebitis

Metabolic: Hyperglycemia*

Neuromuscular & skeletal: Tremor, hyper-reflexia, paresthesia, involuntary movements, muscle spasticity and fasciculations, clonus, bilateral Babinski

Ocular: Lacrimation, mydriasis

Renal: Glucosuria*, albuminuria, BUN elevated

Respiratory: Coughing, laryngospasm, dyspnea, hiccups, bronchospasm, rebound hypoventilation

Miscellaneous: Diaphoresis

*Reported with infusions in premature infants

Drug Interactions

Avoid Concomitant Use

Avoid concomitant use of Doxapram with any of the following: Iobenguane I 123

Increased Effect/Toxicity

Doxapram may increase the levels/effects of: Sympathomimetics

The levels/effects of Doxapram may be increased by: Atomoxetine; Cannabinoids

Decreased Effect

Doxapram may decrease the levels/effects of: Iobenguane I 123

Stability Stable at room temperature; incompatible with aminophylline, sodium bicarbonate, thiopental sodium, and other alkaline solutions

Mechanism of Action Stimulates respiration through action on respiratory center in medulla or through reflex stimulation of carotid, aortic, or other peripheral chemoreceptors; antagonizes opiate-induced respiratory depression, but does not affect analgesia

Pharmacodynamics Following a single I.V. injection:

Onset of respiratory stimulation: Within 20-40 seconds

Maximum effect: Within 1-2 minutes

Duration: 5-12 minutes

Pharmacokinetics (Adult data unless noted)

Metabolism: Extensive in the liver to active metabolite (keto-doxapram)

Distribution: V_d: Neonates: 4-7.3 L/kg

Half-life:

Neonates, premature: 6.6-12 hours

Adults: Mean: 3.4 hours (range: 2.4-4.1 hours)

Clearance: Neonates, premature: 0.44-0.7 L/hour/kg

Usual Dosage I.V.:

Neonatal apnea (apnea of prematurity): Initial loading dose: 2.5-3 mg/kg followed by a continuous infusion of 1 mg/kg/hour; titrate to the lowest rate at which apnea is controlled (maximum dose: 2.5 mg/kg/hour)

Respiratory depression following anesthesia: Adults: Titrate to sustain the desired level of respiratory stimulation with a minimum of side effects:

Initial: 0.5-1 mg/kg; may repeat at 5-minute intervals; maximum total dose: 2 mg/kg

I.V. infusion: Initial: 5 mg/minute until adequate response or adverse effects seen; decrease to 1-3 mg/minute; usual total infusion dose: 0.5-4 mg/kg or 300 mg

Drug-induced CNS depression: Adults: Mild to moderate depression: Initial: 1-2 mg/kg; may repeat in 5 minutes; may repeat at 1-2 hour intervals (until sustained consciousness); maximum dose: 3 g/day; if depression recurs, may repeat in 24 hours. As an alternative, after the initial doses, a continuous infusion of 1-3 mg/minute may be used. Discontinue if patient begins to waken; do not infuse for more than 2 hours.

Hypercapnia associated with COPD: Adults: Continuous infusion of 1-2 mg/minute for 2 hours; may increase to 3 mg/minute if needed. Do not infuse for more than 2 hours. Monitor arterial blood gases closely (in a minimum of 30-minute intervals)

Administration Parenteral: I.V. use only: Dilute loading dose to a maximum concentration of 2 mg/mL and infuse over 15-30 minutes; for infusion, dilute in NS or dextrose (D_5W or $D_{10}W$) to 1 mg/mL (maximum concentration: 2 mg/mL); irritating to tissues; avoid extravasation

Monitoring Parameters Pulse oximetry, blood pressure, heart rate, arterial blood gases, deep tendon reflexes; for apnea: number, duration, and severity of apneic episodes

Reference Range Initial studies suggest a therapeutic serum level of at least 1.5 mg/L; toxicity becomes frequent at serum levels >5 mg/L

Nursing Implications Doxapram is an extravasant; monitor injection site closely; rapid infusion may result in hemolysis

Dosage Forms Excipient information presented when available (limited, particularly for generics); consult specific product labeling.

Injection, solution, as hydrochloride: 20 mg/mL (20 mL) [contains benzyl alcohol]

References

Barrington KJ, Finer NN, Torok-Both G, et al, "Dose-Response Relationship of Doxapram in the Therapy for Refractory Idiopathic Apnea of Prematurity," Pediatrics, 1987, 80(1):22-7.

Bhatt-Mehta V and Schumacher RE, "Treatment of Apnea of Prematurity," Paediatr Drugs, 2003, 5(3):195-210.

Maillard C, Boutroy MJ, Fresson J, et al, "QT Interval Lengthening in Premature Infants Treated With Doxapram," Clin Pharmacol Ther, 2001, 70(6):540-5.

♦ **Doxapram Hydrochloride** see Doxapram on page 474

Doxepin (DOKS e pin)

Medication Safety Issues

Sound-alike/look-alike issues:

Doxepin may be confused with digoxin, doxapram, doxazosin, Doxidan®, doxycycline

Sinequan® may be confused with saquinavir, Serentil®, Seroquel®, Singulair®, Zonegran®

Zonalon® may be confused with Zone-A Forte®

Beers Criteria medication: This drug may be inappropriate for use in geriatric patients (high severity risk).

International issues:

Doxal® [Finland] may be confused with Doxil® which is a brand name for doxorubicin in the U.S.

Doxal® [Finland]: Brand name for doxycycline in Austria; brand name for pyridoxine/thiamine in Brazil

Related Information

Antidepressant Agents on page 1484

U.S. Brand Names Prudoxin™; Sinequan® [DSC]; Zonalon®

Canadian Brand Names Apo-Doxepin®; Doxepine; Novo-Doxepin; Sinequan®; Zonalon®

Therapeutic Category Antianxiety Agent; Antidepressant, Tricyclic (Tertiary Amine)

Generic Available Yes: Capsule, solution

Use

Oral: Treatment of various forms of depression, usually in conjunction with psychotherapy; treatment of anxiety disorders; analgesic for certain chronic and neuropathic pain

Topical: Adults: Short-term (<8 days) therapy of moderate pruritus due to atopic dermatitis or lichen simplex chronicus

Medication Guide An FDA-approved patient medication guide, which is available with the product information and at http://www.fda.gov/downloads/Drugs/DrugSafety/ ucm089129.pdf, must be dispensed with this medication for each new outpatient prescription and refill.

Pregnancy Risk Factor B (cream)

Pregnancy Considerations Teratogenic effects were not observed in animal studies.

Lactation Enters breast milk/not recommended (AAP rates "of concern")

Breast-Feeding Considerations Drowsiness and apnea have been reported in a nursing infant following maternal use of doxepin.

Contraindications Hypersensitivity to doxepin or any component (see Warnings); cross-sensitivity with other tricyclic antidepressants may occur; narrow-angle glaucoma; patients with urinary retention

Warnings Doxepin is not approved for use in pediatric patients; use is not recommended in children <12 years old. Clinical worsening of depression or suicidal ideation and behavior may occur in children and adults with major depressive disorder **[U.S. Boxed Warning]**. In clinical trials, antidepressants increased the risk of suicidal thinking and behavior (suicidality) in children, adolescents, and young adults (18-24 years of age) with major depressive disorder and other psychiatric disorders. This risk must be considered before prescribing antidepressants for any clinical use. Short-term studies did **not** show an increased risk of suicidality with antidepressant use in patients >24 years of age and showed a decreased risk in patients ≥65 years.

Patients of all ages who are treated with antidepressants for any indication require appropriate monitoring and close observation for clinical worsening of depression, suicidality, and unusual changes in behavior, especially during the first few months after antidepressant initiation or when the dose is adjusted. Family members and caregivers should be instructed to closely observe the patient (ie, daily) and communicate condition with healthcare provider. Patients should also be monitored for associated behaviors (eg, anxiety, agitation, panic attacks, insomnia, irritability, hostility, aggressiveness, impulsivity, akathisia, hypomania, mania) which may increase the risk for worsening depression or suicidality. Worsening depression or emergence of suicidality (or associated behaviors listed above) that is abrupt in onset, severe, or not part of the presenting symptoms, may require discontinuation or modification of drug therapy.

Avoid abrupt discontinuation; discontinuation symptoms (including headache, nausea, malaise) may occur if therapy is abruptly discontinued or dose reduced; taper the dose to minimize risks of discontinuation symptoms. To reduce risk of intentional overdose, write prescriptions for the smallest quantity consistent with good patient care. Screen individuals for bipolar disorder prior to treatment (using antidepressants alone may induce manic episodes in patients with this condition).

Doxepin causes a high degree of sedation (relative to other antidepressants); may cause orthostatic hypotension and anticholinergic side effects; may worsen psychosis or precipitate mania or hypomania in patients with bipolar disease; may increase the risks associated with electroconvulsive therapy. Discontinue therapy, when possible, prior to elective surgery (do not discontinue abruptly); cream contains benzyl alcohol which may cause allergic reactions in susceptible individuals; large amounts of benzyl alcohol (≥99 mg/kg/day) have been associated with a potentially fatal toxicity ("gasping syndrome") in neonates; avoid use of doxepin products containing benzyl alcohol in neonates; *in vitro* and animal studies have shown that benzoate, a metabolite of benzyl alcohol, displaces bilirubin from protein binding sites

Precautions Use with caution in patients with cardiovascular disease, conduction disturbances, seizure disorders, urinary retention, hyperthyroidism or those receiving thyroid replacement; avoid use during lactation; use with caution in pregnancy

Drowsiness and other systemic effects may occur with topical use; occlusive dressings may increase absorption of doxepin; allergic contact dermatitis may occur with topical use, risk may be increased with use >8 days. **Note:** Cream is not recommended for use in pediatric patients; overdoses from topical administration in children have been reported.

Adverse Reactions Pronounced sedation and anticholinergic adverse effects may occur

Cardiovascular: Hypotension, arrhythmias

Central nervous system: Sedation, confusion, dizziness, headache; suicidal thinking and behavior (see Warnings); drowsiness occurs in 22% of patients receiving topical cream especially if applied to >10% of body surface area; reduction in area treated, number of applications per day, amount of cream used, or discontinuation of cream may be needed if excessive drowsiness occurs

Dermatologic: Photosensitivity

Endocrine & metabolic: SIADH (rare), weight gain

Gastrointestinal: Constipation, nausea, vomiting, xerostomia, appetite increased

Genitourinary: Urinary retention

Hematologic: Blood dyscrasias (rare)

Hepatic: Hepatitis

Local: Stinging and burning at application site; exacerbation of pruritus or eczema; allergic contact dermatitis

Neuromuscular & skeletal: Fine tremor

Ocular: Blurred vision

Otic: Tinnitus

Miscellaneous: Hypersensitivity reactions; withdrawal symptoms following abrupt discontinuation (headache, nausea, malaise)

Drug Interactions

Metabolism/Transport Effects Substrate of CYP2D6 (major), 1A2 (minor), 2C19 (minor), 3A4 (minor)

Avoid Concomitant Use

Avoid concomitant use of Doxepin with any of the following: Artemether; Dronedarone; Iobenguane I 123; Lumefantrine; MAO Inhibitors; Metoclopramide; Nilotinib; Pimozide; QuiNINE; Sibutramine; Tetrabenazine; Thioridazine; Ziprasidone

Increased Effect/Toxicity

Doxepin may increase the levels/effects of: Alcohol (Ethyl); Alpha-/Beta-Agonists (Direct-Acting); Alpha1-Agonists; Amphetamines; Anticholinergics; Aspirin; Beta2-Agonists; CNS Depressants; Desmopressin; Dronedarone; NSAID (COX-2 Inhibitor); NSAID (Nonselective); Pimozide; QTc-Prolonging Agents; QuiNIDine; QuiNINE; Serotonin Modulators; Sulfonylureas; Tetrabenazine; Thioridazine; TraMADol; Vitamin K Antagonists; Yohimbine; Ziprasidone

The levels/effects of Doxepin may be increased by: Alfuzosin; Altretamine; Artemether; BuPROPion; Chloroquine; Cimetidine; Cinacalcet; Ciprofloxacin; Ciprofloxacin (Systemic); CYP2D6 Inhibitors (Moderate); CYP2D6 Inhibitors (Strong); Dexmethylphenidate; Divalproex; DULoxetine; Gadobutrol; Lithium; Lumefantrine; MAO Inhibitors; Methylphenidate; Metoclopramide; Nilotinib; Pramlintide; Propoxyphene; Protease Inhibitors; QuiNIDine; QuiNINE; Selective Serotonin Reuptake Inhibitors; Sibutramine; Terbinafine; Terbinafine (Systemic); Valproic Acid

Decreased Effect

Doxepin may decrease the levels/effects of: Acetylcholinesterase Inhibitors (Central); Alpha2-Agonists; Iobenguane I 123

The levels/effects of Doxepin may be decreased by: Acetylcholinesterase Inhibitors (Central); Barbiturates; CarBAMazepine; Peginterferon Alfa-2b; St Johns Wort

Food Interactions Oral solution is physically incompatible with carbonated beverages and grape juice; diets rich in fiber may decrease drug effects

Stability Protect from light; store cream at ≤80°F (27°C)

Mechanism of Action Increases the synaptic concentration of serotonin and/or norepinephrine in the CNS by inhibition of their reuptake by the presynaptic neuronal membrane

Pharmacodynamics Maximum antidepressant effects: Usually occur after >2 weeks; anxiolytic effects may occur sooner

Pharmacokinetics (Adult data unless noted)

Distribution: Crosses the placenta; appears in breast milk

Protein binding: 80% to 85%

Metabolism: Hepatic to metabolites, including desmethyldoxepin (active)

Half-life, adults: 6-8 hours

Elimination: Renal

Usual Dosage

Oral: **Note:** Not FDA approved for use in pediatric patients; controlled clinical trials have not shown tricyclic antidepressants to be superior to placebo for the treatment of depression in children and adolescents (see Dopheide, 2006; Wagner, 2005). Manufacturer does not recommend use in children <12 years of age; some centers use the following doses for children and adolescents:

Children: 1-3 mg/kg/day in single or divided doses

Adolescents: Initial: 25-50 mg/day in single or divided doses; gradually increase to 100 mg/day

Adults: Initial: 30-150 mg/day at bedtime or in 2-3 divided doses; may increase up to 300 mg/day; single dose should not exceed 150 mg; select patients may respond to 25-50 mg/day

Topical: Adults: Apply to affected area 4 times/day

Administration

Oral: Administer with food to decrease GI upset; oral concentrate should be diluted in water, milk, or juice (but not grape juice) prior to administration (use 120 mL for adults); do not mix with carbonated beverages

Topical: Apply thin film of cream to affected area with at least 3-4 hours between applications; do not use occlusive dressings; do not use for >8 days; avoid contact with eyes

Monitoring Parameters Blood pressure, heart rate, mental status, weight, liver enzymes, CBC with differential. Monitor patient periodically for symptom resolution; monitor for worsening depression, suicidality, and associated behaviors (especially at the beginning of therapy or when doses are increased or decreased; see Warnings).

Reference Range Utility of serum level monitoring controversial

Doxepin plus desmethyldoxepin:

Proposed therapeutic concentration: 110-250 ng/mL (394-895 nmol/L)

Toxic concentration: >500 ng/mL (>1790 nmol/L) (toxicities may be seen at lower concentrations in some patients)

Patient Information Read the patient Medication Guide that you receive with each prescription and refill of doxepin. An increased risk of suicidal thinking and behavior has been reported with the use of antidepressants in children, adolescents, and young adults (18-24 years of age). Notify physician if you feel more depressed, have thoughts of suicide, or become more agitated or irritable (see Warnings). May cause drowsiness and impair ability to perform activities requiring mental alertness or physical coordination; may cause dry mouth; avoid alcohol and the herbal medicine St John's wort; limit caffeine; may increase appetite; do not discontinue abruptly. May cause photosensitivity reactions (eg, exposure to sunlight may cause severe sunburn, skin rash, redness, or itching); avoid exposure to sunlight and artificial light sources (sunlamps, tanning booth/bed); wear protective clothing, wide-brimmed hats, sunglasses, and lip sunscreen (SPF ≥15); use a sunscreen [broad-spectrum sunscreen or physical sunscreen (preferred) or sunblock with SPF ≥15]; contact physician if reaction occurs.

Nursing Implications Do not use occlusive dressings with cream (increases dermal absorption)

Additional Information Safety and effectiveness of topical cream when used for >8 days has not been established; use >8 days may result in an increase in serum concentrations and systemic effects

Dosage Forms Excipient information presented when available (limited, particularly for generics); consult specific product labeling. [DSC] = Discontinued product

Capsule, as hydrochloride: 10 mg, 25 mg, 50 mg, 75 mg, 100 mg, 150 mg

Sinequan®: 10 mg, 25 mg, 50 mg, 75 mg, 100 mg, 150 mg [DSC]

Cream, as hydrochloride:

Prudoxin™: 5% (45 g) [contains benzyl alcohol]

Zonalon®: 5% (30 g, 45 g) [contains benzyl alcohol]

Solution, oral concentrate, as hydrochloride: 10 mg/mL (120 mL)

Sinequan®: 10 mg/mL (120 mL) [DSC]

References

Dopheide JA, "Recognizing and Treating Depression in Children and Adolescents," *Am J Health Syst Pharm*, 2006, 63(3):233-43.

Levy HB, Harper CR, and Weinberg WA, "A Practical Approach to Children Failing in School," *Pediatr Clin North Am*, 1992, 39 (4):895-928.

Wagner KD, "Pharmacotherapy for Major Depression in Children and Adolescents," *Prog Neuropsychopharmacol Biol Psychiatry*, 2005, 29 (5):819-26.

♦ **Doxepine (Can)** *see* Doxepin *on page* 475

♦ **Doxepin Hydrochloride** *see* Doxepin *on page* 475

♦ **Doxidan® [OTC]** *see* Bisacodyl *on page* 194

DOXOrubicin (doks oh ROO bi sin)

Medication Safety Issues

Sound-alike/look-alike issues:

DOXOrubicin may be confused with DACTINomycin, DAUNOrubicin, DAUNOrubicin liposomal, doxacurium, doxapram, doxazosin, DOXOrubicin liposomal, epirubicin, IDArubicin, valrubicin

Adriamycin PFS® may be confused with achromycin, Aredia®, Idamycin®

Conventional formulation (Adriamycin PFS®, Adriamycin RDF®) may be confused with the liposomal formulation (Doxil®)

Use caution when selecting product for preparation and dispensing; indications, dosages and adverse event profiles differ between conventional DOXOrubicin hydrochloride solution and DOXOrubicin liposomal. Both formulations are the same concentration. As a result, serious errors have occurred.

High alert medication: The Institute for Safe Medication Practices (ISMP) includes this medication among its list of drug classes which have a heightened risk of causing significant patient harm when used in error.

ADR is an error-prone abbreviation

International issues:
Doxil® may be confused with Doxal® which is a brand name for doxepin in Finland, a brand name for doxycycline in Austria, and a brand name for pyridoxine/thiamine combination in Brazil
Rubex, a discontinued brand name for DOXOrubicin in the U.S, is a brand name for ascorbic acid in Ireland

Related Information
Compatibility of Chemotherapy and Related Supportive Care Medications *on page 1580*
Emetogenic Potential of Antineoplastic Agents *on page 1579*
Extravasation Treatment *on page 1522*

U.S. Brand Names Adriamycin®
Canadian Brand Names Adriamycin®
Therapeutic Category Antineoplastic Agent, Anthracycline; Antineoplastic Agent, Antibiotic
Generic Available Yes
Use Treatment of acute lymphocytic leukemia (ALL), acute myeloid leukemia (AML), Hodgkin's disease, malignant lymphoma, soft tissue and bone sarcomas, thyroid cancer, small cell lung cancer, breast cancer, gastric cancer, ovarian cancer, bladder cancer, neuroblastoma, and Wilms' tumor [FDA approved in pediatrics (age not specified) and adults]; has also been used for the treatment of multiple myeloma, endometrial carcinoma, uterine sarcoma, head and neck cancer, liver cancer, and kidney cancer
Pregnancy Risk Factor D
Pregnancy Considerations Teratogenicity and embryotoxicity were observed in animal studies. There are no adequate and well-controlled studies in pregnant women. Advise patients to avoid becoming pregnant (females) and to avoid causing pregnancy (males) during treatment. According to the National Comprehensive Cancer Network (NCCN) breast cancer guidelines, doxorubicin, if indicated, may be administered to pregnant women with breast cancer as part of a combination chemotherapy regimen, although chemotherapy should not be administered during the first trimester or after 35 weeks gestation.
Lactation Enters breast milk/not recommended
Breast-Feeding Considerations Doxorubicin and its metabolites are found in breast milk. Due to the potential for serious adverse reactions in the nursing infant, breast-feeding should be discontinued during treatment.
Contraindications Hypersensitivity to doxorubicin or any component; severe CHF, cardiomyopathy, pre-existing myelosuppression; patients who have received a total dose of 550 mg/m² of doxorubicin or 400 mg/m² in patients with previous or concomitant treatment with daunorubicin, idarubicin, mitoxantrone, cyclophosphamide, or irradiation of the cardiac region; patients who have received previous treatment with complete cumulative doses of daunorubicin, idarubicin, or other anthracycline derivatives; pregnancy
Warnings Hazardous agent; use appropriate precautions for handling and disposal. **I.V. use only**, severe local tissue necrosis will result if extravasation occurs **[U.S. Boxed Warning]**. May cause severe myelosuppression; dose-limiting, primarily leukopenia and neutropenia **[U.S. Boxed**

Warning]; irreversible myocardial toxicity, including potentially fatal CHF, may occur during therapy or months to years after therapy termination **[U.S. Boxed Warning]**. The probability of developing myocardial toxicity is estimated to be 1% to 2% at a total cumulative dose of 300 mg/m² of doxorubicin, 3% to 5% at a total cumulative dose of 400 mg/m², 5% to 8% at a total cumulative dose of 450 mg/m², and 6% to 20% at 500 mg/m². Myocardial toxicity may occur at lower cumulative doses in patients with prior mediastinal irradiation, concurrent cyclophosphamide therapy, or pre-existing heart disease. Pediatric patients are at increased risk for developing delayed cardiac toxicity and CHF during early adulthood due to an increasing census of long-term survivors; periodic long-term monitoring of cardiac function is recommended. Doxorubicin may contribute to prepubertal growth failure in pediatric patients. Secondary acute myelogenous leukemia and myelodysplastic syndrome have been reported following treatment **[U.S. Boxed Warning]**.
Precautions Use with caution and modify dosage in patients with impaired hepatic function **[U.S. Boxed Warning]**
Adverse Reactions
Cardiovascular: Cardiomyopathy, cardiorespiratory decompensation, cardiotoxicity (transient type with abnormal ECG and arrhythmias, or a chronic, cumulative, dose-dependent type which progresses to CHF), CHF, facial flushing
Central nervous system: Fever
Dermatologic: Alopecia, photosensitivity
Endocrine & metabolic: Hyperuricemia, infertility, prepubertal growth failure
Gastrointestinal: Anorexia, diarrhea, esophagitis, mucositis, nausea, stomatitis, vomiting, ulceration and necrosis of the colon
Genitourinary: Cystitis, discoloration of urine (red/orange), hematuria, urinary frequency
Hematologic: Anemia, leukopenia (nadir: 10-14 days), myelodysplastic syndrome, secondary acute myelogenous leukemia, thrombocytopenia
Local: Erythematous streaking along the vein if administered too rapidly, phlebitis, tissue necrosis upon extravasation
Ocular: Lacrimation
1%, postmarketing, and/or case reports: Anaphylaxis, azoospermia, bilirubin increased, chills, coma (when in combination with cisplatin or vincristine), conjunctivitis, fever, gonadal impairment (children), hepatitis, hyperpigmentation (nail, skin & oral mucosa), infection, keratitis, lacrimation, neutropenic fever, oligospermia, onycholysis, peripheral neurotoxicity (with intra-arterial doxorubicin), phlebosclerosis, radiation recall pneumonitis (children), seizure (when in combination with cisplatin or vincristine), sepsis, shock, systemic hypersensitivity (including urticaria, pruritus, angioedema, dysphagia, and dyspnea), transaminases increased, urticaria
Drug Interactions
Metabolism/Transport Effects Substrate of CYP2D6 (major), CYP3A4 (major), P-glycoprotein; **Inhibits** CYP2B6 (moderate), 2D6 (weak), 3A4 (weak); **Induces** P-glycoprotein
Avoid Concomitant Use
Avoid concomitant use of DOXOrubicin with any of the following: BCG; Natalizumab; Pimecrolimus; Tacrolimus (Topical); Vaccines (Live)
Increased Effect/Toxicity
DOXOrubicin may increase the levels/effects of: CYP2B6 Substrates; Leflunomide; Natalizumab; Vaccines (Live); Vitamin K Antagonists; Zidovudine

The levels/effects of DOXOrubicin may be increased by: Bevacizumab; CycloSPORINE; CycloSPORINE

(Systemic); CYP2D6 Inhibitors (Moderate); CYP2D6 Inhibitors (Strong); CYP3A4 Inhibitors (Moderate); CYP3A4 Inhibitors (Strong); Darunavir; Dasatinib; Denosumab; P-Glycoprotein Inhibitors; Pimecrolimus; Sorafenib; Tacrolimus (Topical); Taxane Derivatives; Trastuzumab

Decreased Effect

DOXOrubicin may decrease the levels/effects of: BCG; Cardiac Glycosides; Dabigatran Etexilate; P-Glycoprotein Substrates; Sipuleucel-T; Stavudine; Vaccines (Inactivated); Vaccines (Live); Vitamin K Antagonists; Zidovudine

The levels/effects of DOXOrubicin may be decreased by: Cardiac Glycosides; CYP3A4 Inducers (Strong); Deferasirox; Echinacea; Herbs (CYP3A4 Inducers); Peginterferon Alfa-2b; P-Glycoprotein Inducers

Stability Protect from light; store vials containing powder at room temperature, refrigerate vials containing liquid; reconstituted vials stable for 7 days at room temperature and 15 days if refrigerated and protected from light. Discard unused portion of preservative free injection vial. Incompatible with hydrocortisone, fluorouracil, furosemide, sodium bicarbonate, aminophylline, heparin, cephalothin, dexamethasone; unstable in solutions with a pH <3 or >7. Color change from red to purple indicates decomposition of drug.

Mechanism of Action Inhibits DNA and RNA synthesis by intercalating between DNA base pairs and by steric obstruction inducing DNA breaks; produces oxygen-free radicals which cause DNA denaturation

Pharmacokinetics (Adult data unless noted)

Distribution: Into breast milk; does not penetrate into CSF; distributes into cells rapidly with high concentrations in lung, kidney, muscle, spleen, and liver

Protein binding: 75%

Metabolism: In both the liver and in plasma to both active and inactive metabolites

Half-life, triphasic:

Primary: 30 minutes

Secondary: 3-3.5 hours for its metabolites

Terminal: 17-30 hours for doxorubicin and its metabolites

Elimination: Undergoes triphasic elimination; 40% to 60% eventually excreted in bile and feces; <5% excreted in urine, primarily as unchanged drug and metabolites

Clearance:

Infants <2 years: 813 mL/minute/m^2

Children >2 years: 1540 mL/minute/m^2

Usual Dosage Patient's ideal weight should be used to calculate body surface area. Lower dose regimens should be given to patients with decreased bone marrow reserve, prior radiation therapy, or marrow infiltration with malignant cells.

I.V. (refer to individual protocols):

Children: 35-75 mg/m^2 as a single dose, repeat every 21 days; or 20-30 mg/m^2 once weekly; or 60-90 mg/m^2 given as a continuous infusion over 96 hours every 3-4 weeks

Adults: 60-75 mg/m^2 as a single dose, repeat every 21 days; or 20-30 mg/m^2/day for 2-3 days, repeat in 4 weeks or 20 mg/m^2 once weekly

Dosing adjustment in hepatic impairment:

Bilirubin 1.2-3 mg/dL: Reduce dose by 50%

Bilirubin >3 mg/dL: Reduce dose by 75%

Administration Parenteral: I.V. use only; reconstitute IVP doses with D$_5$W or NS to ensure isotonicity of the final solution; administer slow IVP at a rate no faster than over 3-5 minutes or by I.V. infusion over 1-4 hours at a concentration not to exceed 2 mg/mL, or by I.V. continuous infusion

Monitoring Parameters CBC with differential, erythrocyte and platelet count; serum uric acid, echocardiogram, radionuclide left ventricular ejection fraction, liver enzymes, and bilirubin; observe I.V. injection site for infiltration and vein irritation

Patient Information Transient red-orange discoloration of urine can occur for up to 48 hours after a dose; notify physician if fever, sore throat, bleeding, or bruising occurs; report any stinging sensation at the injection site during infusion. May cause photosensitivity reactions (eg, exposure to sunlight may cause severe sunburn, skin rash, redness, or itching); avoid exposure to sunlight and artificial light sources (sunlamps, tanning booth/bed); wear protective clothing, wide-brimmed hats, sunglasses, and lip sunscreen (SPF ≥15); use a sunscreen [broad-spectrum sunscreen or physical sunscreen (preferred) or sunblock with SPF ≥15]; contact physician if reaction occurs.

Nursing Implications Local erythematous streaking along the vein and/or facial flushing may indicate too rapid a rate of administration; drug is very irritating; avoid extravasation; if extravasation occurs, apply cold packs immediately for 30-60 minutes, then alternate off/on every 15 minutes for 1 day; apply 1.5 mL of dimethylsulfoxide 99% (w/v) solution to the site every 6 hours for 14 days; allow to air-dry; do not cover. Take precautions to prevent contact with the patient's urine and other body fluids for at least 5 days after each treatment.

Additional Information Myelosuppressive effects:

WBC: Moderate

Platelets: Moderate

Onset (days): 7

Nadir (days): 10-14

Recovery (days): 21-28

Dosage Forms Excipient information presented when available (limited, particularly for generics); consult specific product labeling.

Injection, powder for reconstitution, as hydrochloride: 10 mg, 50 mg

Adriamycin®: 10 mg, 20 mg, 50 mg, [contains lactose]

Injection, solution, as hydrochloride: 2 mg/mL (5 mL, 10 mL, 25 mL, 100 mL)

Adriamycin®: 2 mg/mL (5 mL, 10 mL, 25 mL, 100 mL)

References

Berg SL, Grisell DL, DeLaney TF, et al, "Principles of Treatment of Pediatric Solid Tumors," *Pediatr Clin North Am*, 1991, 38(2):249-67.

Ishii E, Hara T, Ohkubo K, et al, "Treatment of Childhood Acute Lymphoblastic Leukemia With Intermediate Dose Cytosine Arabinoside and Adriamycin," *Med Pediatr Oncol*, 1986, 14(2):73-7.

Legha SS, Benjamin RS, Mackay B, et al, "Reduction of Doxorubicin Cardiotoxicity by Prolonged Continuous Intravenous Infusion," *Ann Intern Med*, 1982, 96(2):133-9.

◆ **Doxorubicin Hydrochloride** *see* DOXOrubicin *on page 477*

◆ **Doxy100™** *see* Doxycycline *on page 479*

◆ **Doxycin (Can)** *see* Doxycycline *on page 479*

Doxycycline (doks i SYE kleen)

Medication Safety Issues

Sound-alike/look-alike issues:

Doxycycline may be confused with dicyclomine, doxepin, doxylamine

Doxy100™ may be confused with Doxil®

Monodox® may be confused with Maalox®

Oracea™ may be confused with Orencia®

Vibramycin® may be confused with vancomycin, Vibativ™

Related Information

Malaria *on page 1652*

U.S. Brand Names Adoxa®; Alodox™; Doryx®; Doxy100™; Monodox®; Oracea™; Oraxyl™; Periostat®; Vibramycin®

Canadian Brand Names Apo-Doxy Tabs®; Apo-Doxy®; Dom-Doxycycline; Doxycin; Doxytab; Novo-Doxylin; Nu-Doxycycline; Periostat®; PHL-Doxycycline; PMS-Doxycycline; Vibra-Tabs®; Vibramycin®

Therapeutic Category Antibiotic, Tetracycline Derivative

Generic Available Yes: Excludes capsule (variable release), syrup, tablet (delayed release)

Use Treatment of infections caused by susceptible *Rickettsia, Chlamydia,* and *Mycoplasma;* alternative to mefloquine for malaria prophylaxis; treatment for syphilis, uncomplicated *Neisseria gonorrhoeae, Listeria, Actinomyces israelii, Fusobacterium fusiforme,* and *Clostridium* infections in penicillin-allergic patients; used for community-acquired pneumonia and other common infections due to susceptible organisms; anthrax due to *Bacillus anthracis,* including inhalational anthrax (postexposure); treatment of infections caused by uncommon susceptible gram-negative and gram-positive organisms, including *Borrelia recurrentis, Ureaplasma urealyticum, Haemophilus ducreyi, Yersinia pestis, Francisella tularensis, Vibrio cholerae, Campylobacter fetus, Brucella* spp, *Bartonella bacilliformis,* and *Calymmatobacterium granulomatis,* Q fever, Lyme disease; treatment of inflammatory lesions associated with rosacea; adjunct to amebicides for intestinal amebiasis; adjunct for treatment of severe acne. (FDA approved in ages ≥8 years and adults). Has also been used in ehrlichiosis and management of malignant pleural effusions with intrapleural administration.

Pregnancy Risk Factor D

Pregnancy Considerations Because use during pregnancy may cause fetal harm, doxycycline is classified as pregnancy category D. Exposure to tetracyclines during the second or third trimester may cause permanent discoloration of the teeth. Most reports do not show an increase risk for teratogenicity with the exception of a potential small increased risk for cleft palate or esophageal atresia/stenosis. When considering treatment for life-threatening infection and/or prolonged duration of therapy (such as in anthrax), the potential risk to the fetus must be balanced against the severity of the potential illness.

Lactation Enters breast milk/not recommended

Breast-Feeding Considerations Tetracyclines, including doxycycline, are excreted in breast milk and therefore, breast-feeding is not recommended by the manufacturer.

Doxycycline is less bound to the calcium in maternal milk which may lead to increased absorption compared to other tetracyclines. Only minimal amounts of doxycycline are excreted in human milk and the relative amount of tooth staining has been reported to be lower when compared to other tetracycline analogs. Nondose-related effects could include modification of bowel flora.

Contraindications Hypersensitivity to doxycycline, tetracycline, or any component (see Warnings); children <8 years (except in treatment of anthrax exposure); severe hepatic dysfunction

Warnings Syrup contains sodium metabisulfite which may cause allergic reactions in susceptible individuals. Photosensitivity reaction may occur with this drug; avoid prolonged exposure to sunlight or tanning equipment. Do not administer to children <8 years of age (except in treatment of anthrax exposure, tickborne rickettsial diseases, or ehrlichiosis); administration of tetracycline 25 mg/kg/day was associated with decreased fibular growth rate in premature infants (reversible with discontinuation of drug); retardation of skeletal development has been observed in fetal animal studies. Use of tetracyclines during tooth development may cause permanent discoloration of the teeth and enamel hypoplasia; staining of teeth is dose-related so that duration of therapy should be minimized; doxycycline may be less likely to stain developing teeth than tetracycline since it binds less strongly to calcium (see Additional Information); pseudomembranous colitis has been reported with doxycycline; prolonged use may result in superinfection.

Adverse Reactions

Central nervous system: Bulging fontanels in infants, intracranial pressure increased

Dermatologic: Angioneurotic edema, discoloration of nails, exfoliative dermatitis, photosensitivity (see Warnings), rash, Stevens-Johnson syndrome, toxic epidermal necrolysis, urticaria

Gastrointestinal: Anorexia, diarrhea, dysphagia, enterocolitis, esophagitis and esophageal ulceration with the hyclate salt formulation, glossitis, nausea, oral candidiasis, pseudomembranous colitis, vomiting

Hematologic: Eosinophilia, hemolytic anemia, neutropenia, thrombocytopenia

Hepatic: Hepatotoxicity

Local: Pain at the injection site, phlebitis

Neuromuscular & skeletal: Retardation of skeletal development in premature infants (see Warnings)

Renal: BUN increased

Miscellaneous: Anaphylaxis, exacerbation of SLE, serum sickness. May cause discoloration of teeth in children <8 years of age (see Additional Information).

Drug Interactions

Metabolism/Transport Effects Inhibits CYP3A4 (moderate)

Avoid Concomitant Use

Avoid concomitant use of Doxycycline with any of the following: BCG; Retinoic Acid Derivatives

Increased Effect/Toxicity

Doxycycline may increase the levels/effects of: Neuromuscular-Blocking Agents; Retinoic Acid Derivatives; Vitamin K Antagonists

Decreased Effect

Doxycycline may decrease the levels/effects of: BCG; Penicillins; Typhoid Vaccine

The levels/effects of Doxycycline may be decreased by: Antacids; Barbiturates; Bile Acid Sequestrants; Bismuth; Bismuth Subsalicylate; CarBAMazepine; Iron Salts; Magnesium Salts; Phenytoin; Quinapril; Sucralfate

Food Interactions Administration with iron, calcium, milk, or dairy products may decrease doxycycline absorption; may decrease absorption of calcium, iron, magnesium, zinc, and amino acids

Stability Store below 30°C (86°F); protect from light. Reconstituted oral doxycycline suspension is stable for 2 weeks at room temperature; I.V. doxycycline solutions must be protected from direct sunlight

Mechanism of Action Inhibits protein synthesis by binding to the 30S and possibly the 50S ribosomal subunit(s) of susceptible bacteria preventing additions of amino acids to the growing peptide chain; may also cause alterations in the cytoplasmic membrane

Pharmacokinetics (Adult data unless noted)

Absorption: Almost completely from the GI tract; absorption can be reduced by food or milk by 20%

Distribution: Widely distributed into body tissues and fluids including synovial and pleural fluid, bile, bronchial secretions; poor penetration into the CSF; appears in breast milk

Protein binding: 80% to 85%

Metabolism: Not metabolized in the liver; partially inactivated in the GI tract by chelate formation

Bioavailability: 90% to 100%

Half-life: 12-15 hours (usually increases to 22-24 hours with multiple dosing)

Time to peak serum concentration: Oral: Within 1.5-4 hours

Elimination: In the urine (23%) and feces (30%)

Dialysis: Not dialyzable (0% to 5%)

Usual Dosage

Children <8 years:

Anthrax: **Note:** In the presence of systemic involvement, extensive edema, and/or lesions on head/neck, doxycycline should initially be administered I.V. Initial treatment should include two or more agents per CDC recommendations. Agents suggested for use in conjunction with doxycycline include rifampin, vancomycin, penicillin, ampicillin, chloramphenicol, imipenem, clindamycin, or clarithromycin. For bioterrorism postexposure, continue combined therapy for 60 days; if natural exposure, 7-10 days of therapy.

Treatment I.V.: 2.2 mg/kg every 12 hours (maximum: 100 mg/dose); may switch to oral therapy (same dosing) when clinically appropriate (see CDC, 2001)

Inhalation or cutaneous (postexposure prophylaxis): Oral: 2.2 mg/kg every 12 hours (maximum: 100 mg/dose) (see CDC, 2001; Red Book, 2009)

Ehrlichiosis: Oral, I.V.: 2 mg/kg every 12 hours (maximum: 100 mg/dose) for 3 days after defervescence and at least 7 days total (see Red Book, 2009)

Tickborne rickettsial disease: Oral, I.V.: 2.2 mg/kg every 12 hours (maximum: 100 mg/dose) for 5-7 days. Severe or complicated disease may require longer treatment; human granulocytotropic anaplasmosis (HGA) should be treated for 10-14 days (see CDC, 2006)

Children ≥8 years: Oral, I.V.: 2-4 mg/kg/day divided every 12-24 hours, not to exceed 200 mg/day

Lyme disease, Q fever, or Tularemia: Oral: 100 mg/dose twice daily for 14-21 days

Chlamydial infections, uncomplicated: Oral: 100 mg/dose twice daily for 7 days

Brucellosis: Oral: 1-2 mg/kg/dose twice daily for 6 weeks (maximum: 100 mg/dose); use in combination with rifampin

Tickborne rickettsial disease or Ehrlichiosis: >45 kg: Oral, I.V.: 100 mg every 12 hours. Severe or complicated disease may require longer treatment; HGA should be treated for 10-14 days

Anthrax (if strain is proven susceptible): **Note:** In the presence of systemic involvement, extensive edema, and/or lesions on head/neck, doxycycline should initially be administered I.V. Initial treatment should include two or more agents per CDC recommendations. Agents suggested for use in conjunction with doxycycline include rifampin, vancomycin, penicillin, ampicillin, chloramphenicol, imipenem, clindamycin, or clarithromycin. For bioterrorism postexposure, continue combined therapy for 60 days; if natural exposure, administer 7-10 days of therapy.

Treatment: I.V.: 2.2 mg/kg every 12 hours (maximum: 100 mg/dose); may switch to oral therapy (same dosing) when clinically appropriate

Inhalation or cutaneous (postexposure prophylaxis): Oral: 2.2 mg/kg every 12 hours (maximum: 100 mg/dose)

Prophylaxis of malaria: Oral: 2 mg/kg once daily; maximum dose: 100 mg/day starting 1-2 days before travel to the area with endemic infection, continuing daily during travel and for 4 weeks after leaving endemic area; maximum duration of prophylaxis: 4 months

Adolescents and Adults: Oral, I.V.: 100-200 mg/day in 1-2 divided doses

Anthrax (if strain is proven susceptible): Refer to Children's dosing for **"Note"** on route, combined therapy, and duration

Treatment: I.V.: 100 mg every 12 hours for 60 days (substitute oral antibiotics for I.V. antibiotics as soon as clinical condition improves)

Inhalation (postexposure prophylaxis): Oral: 100 mg every 12 hours for 60 days

Lyme disease, Q fever, or Tularemia: Oral: 100 mg/dose twice daily for 14-21 days

Pelvic inflammatory disease:

Hospitalized regimen: Oral, I.V.: 100 mg every 12 hours for 14 days administered with cefoxitin or cefotetan

Outpatient regimen: Oral: 100 mg every 12 hours for 14 days plus single dose ceftriaxone

Periodontitis: Oral (Periostat®): 20 mg twice daily as an adjunct following scaling and root planing; may be administered for up to 9 months

Prophylaxis of malaria: Oral: 100 mg/dose once daily starting 1-2 days before travel to the area with endemic infection, continuing daily during travel, and for 4 weeks after leaving endemic area; maximum duration of prophylaxis: 4 months

Tickborne rickettsial disease or ehrlichiosis: Oral, I.V.: 100 mg every 12 hours. Severe or complicated disease may require longer treatment; HGA should be treated for 10-14 days

Rosacea: Oral (Oracea™): 40 mg once daily in the morning

Chlamydial infections, uncomplicated: Oral: 100 mg/dose twice daily for 7 days

Nongonococcal urethritis caused by *C. trachomatis* or *U. urealyticum*: Oral: 100 mg/dose twice daily for 7 days

Sclerosing agent for pleural effusion: 500 mg in 25-30 mL of NS instilled into the pleural space to control pleural effusions associated with metastatic tumors; or for recurrent malignant pleural effusions: 500 mg in 250 mL NS

Dosing adjustment in renal impairment: No adjustment necessary

Administration

Oral: Administer capsules or tablets with adequate amounts of fluid; avoid antacids, infant formula, milk, dairy products, and iron for 1 hour before or 2 hours after administration of doxycycline (unless extemporaneously prepared in the instance of public health emergency when milk or pudding is appropriate); may be administered with food to decrease GI upset; shake suspension well before use

Doryx®: May break up the tablet and sprinkle the delayed release pellets on a spoonful of applesauce. Do **not** crush or damage the delayed release pellets; loss or damage of pellets prevents using the dose. Swallow the Doryx®/applesauce mixture immediately without chewing. Discard mixture if it cannot be used immediately.

Parenteral: For I.V. use only; administer by slow I.V. intermittent infusion over a minimum of 1-2 hours at a concentration not to exceed 1 mg/mL (may be infused over 1-4 hours); concentrations <0.1 mg/mL are not recommended

Sclerosing agent:

To control pleural effusions associated with metastatic tumors: Instill into the pleural space through a thoracostomy tube following drainage of the accumulated pleural fluid; clamp the tube then remove the fluid

For recurrent malignant pleural effusions: Administer via chest tube lavage, clamp tube for 24 hours then drain

Monitoring Parameters Periodic monitoring of renal, hematologic, and hepatic function tests; observe for changes in bowel frequency

Test Interactions False-negative urine glucose using Clinistix®, Tes-Tape®; false-positive urine glucose using Clinitest®; false elevations of urinary catecholamines with fluorescence test

Patient Information May discolor teeth if <8 years of age; may discolor fingernails. May cause photosensitivity reactions (eg, exposure to sunlight may cause severe sunburn, skin rash, redness, or itching); avoid exposure to sunlight and artificial light sources (sunlamps, tanning booth/bed); wear protective clothing, wide-brimmed hats, sunglasses, and lip sunscreen (SPF ≥15); use a sunscreen [broad-spectrum sunscreen or physical sunscreen (preferred) or sunblock with SPF ≥15]; contact physician if reaction occurs.

Nursing Implications Check for signs of phlebitis; I.V. doxycycline should not be given I.M. or SubQ; avoid extravasation. Encourage patient to drink plenty of fluids with doxycycline capsules or tablets to reduce the risk of esophageal ulceration.

Additional Information Injection contains ascorbic acid. According to the CDC, staining of the teeth is negligible with short courses of doxycycline and is of minimal consequence in children >6 or 7 years of age because visible tooth formation is complete by this age. Benefits outweigh the risks for rickettsial infections, ehrlichiosis, anthrax, and cholera (see CDC, 2006; Red Book, 2009).

Dosage Forms Excipient information presented when available (limited, particularly for generics); consult specific product labeling. [DSC] = Discontinued product

Note: Strength expressed as base.

Capsule, as hyclate: 50 mg, 100 mg
  Oraxyl™: 20 mg
  Vibramycin®: 100 mg
Capsule, as monohydrate: 50 mg, 100 mg
  Adoxa®: 150 mg
  Monodox®: 50 mg, 75 mg, 100 mg
Capsule, variable release:
  Oracea™: 40 mg [30 mg (immediate-release) and 10 mg (delayed-release)]
Injection, powder for reconstitution, as hyclate: 100 mg
  Doxy100™: 100 mg
Powder for oral suspension, as monohydrate: 25 mg/5 mL (60 mL)
  Vibramycin®: 25 mg/5 mL (60 mL) [raspberry flavor]
Syrup, as calcium:
  Vibramycin®: 50 mg/5 mL (480 mL) [contains propylene glycol, sodium metabisulfite; raspberry-apple flavor]
Tablet, as hyclate: 20 mg, 100 mg
  Alodox™: 20 mg [kit includes Alodox™ tablets (60s), Ocusoft® Lid Scrub™ pads, eyelid cleanser, and goggles]
  Periostat®: 20 mg
Tablet, as monohydrate: 50 mg, 75 mg, 100 mg, 150 mg
  Adoxa®: 50 mg, 75 mg, 100 mg, 150 mg
  Adoxa® Pak™ 1/75 [unit-dose pack]: 75 mg (31s)
  Adoxa® Pak™ 1/100 [unit-dose pack]: 100 mg (31s) [DSC]
  Adoxa® Pak™ 1/150 [unit-dose pack]: 150 mg (30s)
  Adoxa® Pak™ 2/100 [unit-dose pack]: 100 mg (60s) [DSC]
Tablet, delayed-release coated pellets, as hyclate:
  Doryx®: 75 mg [scored; contains sodium 4.5 mg (0.196 mEq); 100 mg [scored; contains sodium 6 mg (0.261 mEq)]; 150 mg [scored; contains sodium 9 mg (0.392 mEq)]

Extemporaneous Preparations If a public health emergency is declared and liquid doxycycline is unavailable for the treatment of anthrax, emergency doses may be prepared for children or adults who cannot swallow tablets.

Add 4 teaspoons of water to one 100 mg tablet. Allow tablet to soak in the water for 5 minutes to soften. Crush into a fine powder and stir until well mixed. Appropriate dose should be taken from this mixture. To increase palatability, mix with food or drink. If mixing with drink, add 3 teaspoons of apple juice to the appropriate dose of

mixture and 4 teaspoons of sugar. Doxycycline and water mixture may be stored at room temperature for up to 24 hours.

  U.S. Food and Drug Administration, Center for Drug Evaluation and Research, "Public Health Emergency Home Preparation Instructions for Doxycycline." Available at http://www.fda.gov/Drugs/EmergencyPreparedness/BioterrorismandDrugPreparedness/ucm130996.htm.

References

American Academy of Pediatrics, "*Ehrlichia* and *Anaplasma* Infections (Human Ehrlichiosis and Anaplasmosis)," *Red Book®, 2009 Report of the Committee on Infectious Diseases*, 28th ed, Pickering LK ed, Elk Grove Village, IL: American Academy of Pediatrics, 2009, 284-7. Available at: http://aapredbook.aappublications.org/cgi/content/full/2009/1/3.37.

American Academy of Pediatrics, "Tetracyclines," *Red Book®, 2009 Report of the Committee on Infectious Diseases*, 28th ed, Pickering LK, ed, Elk Grove Village, IL: American Academy of Pediatrics, 2009, 739. Available at: http://aapredbook.aappublications.org/cgi/content/full/2009/1/4.1.2..

Centers for Disease Control and Prevention, "Update: Investigation of Anthrax Associated with Intentional Exposure and Interim Public Health Guidelines, October 2001," *MMWR Morb Mortal Wkly Rep*, 2001, 50(41):889-93.

Centers for Disease Control and Prevention, Workowski KA, and Berman SM, "Sexually Transmitted Diseases Treatment Guidelines, 2006," *MMWR Recomm Rep*, 2006, 55(RR-11):1-94.

Chapman AS, Bakken JS, Folk SM, et al, "Diagnosis and Management of Tickborne Rickettsial Diseases: Rocky Mountain Spotted Fever, Ehrlichioses, and Anaplasmosis–United States: A Practical Guide for Physicians and Other Health-Care and Public Health Professionals," *MMWR Recomm Rep*, 2006, 55(RR-4):1-27.

Inglesby TV, Henderson DA, Bartlett JG, et al, "Anthrax as a Biological Weapon: Medical and Public Health Management. Working Group on Civilian Biodefense," *JAMA*, 1999, 281(18):1735-45.

◆ **Doxycycline Calcium** *see* Doxycycline *on page* 479
◆ **Doxycycline Hyclate** *see* Doxycycline *on page* 479
◆ **Doxycycline Monohydrate** *see* Doxycycline *on page* 479
◆ **Doxytab (Can)** *see* Doxycycline *on page* 479
◆ **DPA** *see* Valproic Acid and Derivatives *on page* 1398
◆ **DPE** *see* Dipivefrin *on page* 461
◆ **D-Penicillamine** *see* Penicillamine *on page* 1076
◆ **DPH** *see* Phenytoin *on page* 1104
◆ **Dramamine® [OTC]** *see* DimenhyDRINATE *on page* 446
◆ **Dramamine® Less Drowsy Formula [OTC]** *see* Meclizine *on page* 869
◆ **Driminate® [OTC]** *see* DimenhyDRINATE *on page* 446
◆ **Drisdol®** *see* Ergocalciferol *on page* 519
◆ **Dristan™ 12-Hour [OTC]** *see* Oxymetazoline *on page* 1043
◆ **Dristan® Long Lasting Nasal (Can)** *see* Oxymetazoline *on page* 1043
◆ **Drixoral® Nasal (Can)** *see* Oxymetazoline *on page* 1043
◆ **Drixoral® ND (Can)** *see* Pseudoephedrine *on page* 1183

Dronabinol (droe NAB i nol)

Medication Safety Issues
  Sound-alike/look-alike issues:
    Dronabinol may be confused with droperidol

U.S. Brand Names Marinol®

Canadian Brand Names Marinol®

Therapeutic Category Antiemetic

Generic Available Yes

Use Treatment of nausea and vomiting secondary to cancer chemotherapy in patients who have not responded to conventional antiemetics; treatment of anorexia associated with weight loss in AIDS patients

Restrictions C-III

Pregnancy Risk Factor C

Lactation Enters breast milk/contraindicated

Contraindications Hypersensitivity to dronabinol, sesame oil, or any component, marijuana, or cannabinoids; should not be used in patients with a history of schizophrenia

Warnings Dronabinol has a high potential for abuse; limit antiemetic therapy availability to current cycle of chemotherapy

Precautions Use with caution in patients with heart disease, history of substance abuse, hepatic disease, or seizure disorders (may lower seizure threshold); reduce dosage in patients with severe hepatic impairment; tolerance to CNS side effects usually occurs in 1-3 days of continued use; tachyphylaxis and tolerance does not appear to develop when used as an appetite stimulant as efficacy has been documented in clinical trials for up to 5 months of treatment. Use with caution in patients with mania or depression as dronabinol may exacerbate these conditions

Adverse Reactions

Cardiovascular: Orthostatic hypotension, tachycardia, palpitations, vasodilation, hypotension, flushing

Central nervous system: Drowsiness, dizziness, vertigo, difficulty in concentrating, mood change, euphoria, detachment, depression, anxiety, paranoia, hallucinations, nervousness, ataxia, headache, memory lapse, seizures, fatigue, nightmares

Gastrointestinal: Xerostomia, diarrhea, abdominal pain

Hepatic: Liver enzymes elevated

Neuromuscular & skeletal: Myalgia, tremor, paresthesia, weakness

Ocular: Vision difficulties, conjunctivitis

Otic: Tinnitus

Respiratory: Sinusitis, cough, rhinitis

Miscellaneous: Diaphoresis

Drug Interactions

Avoid Concomitant Use There are no known interactions where it is recommended to avoid concomitant use.

Increased Effect/Toxicity

Dronabinol may increase the levels/effects of: Alcohol (Ethyl); CNS Depressants; Methotrimeprazine; Sympathomimetics

The levels/effects of Dronabinol may be increased by: Anticholinergic Agents; Cocaine; MAO Inhibitors; Methotrimeprazine; Ritonavir

Decreased Effect There are no known significant interactions involving a decrease in effect.

Stability Store in a cool environment (46°F to 59°F); may be refrigerated; do not freeze

Mechanism of Action Dronabinol is the principal psychoactive substance found in *Cannabis sativa* (marijuana); its mechanism of action as an antiemetic is not well defined, it probably inhibits the vomiting center in the medulla oblongata; has complex effects on CNS including central sympathomimetic activity

Pharmacodynamics

Onset of action: 30 minutes to 1 hour

Maximum effect: 2-4 hours

Duration:

Psychoactive effects: 4-6 hours

Appetite stimulation: 24 hours

Pharmacokinetics (Adult data unless noted)

Absorption: Oral: 90% to 95%; first-pass metabolism results in low systemic bioavailability

Distribution: V_d: ~10L/kg

Protein binding: ~97%

Metabolism: Extensive first-pass; metabolized in the liver to several metabolites some of which are active

Bioavailability: 10% to 20%

Half-life:

Biphasic: Alpha: 4 hours

Terminal: 25-36 hours

Dronabinol metabolites: 44-59 hours

Time to peak serum concentration: Within 0.5-4 hours

Elimination: Biliary excretion is the major route of elimination; 50% excreted in feces within 72 hours; 10% to 15% excreted in urine within 72 hours

Clearance: Adults: Mean 0.2 L/kg/hour (highly variable)

Usual Dosage Oral:

Antiemetic: Children and Adults: 5 mg/m^2 1-3 hours before chemotherapy, then give 5 mg/m^2/dose every 2-4 hours after chemotherapy for a total of 4-6 doses/day; dose may be increased in 2.5 mg/m^2 increments to a maximum of 15 mg/m^2 per dose if needed

Alternative dosing: Adults: 5 mg 3-4 times/day; dosage may be escalated during a chemotherapy cycle or at subsequent cycles depending upon response

Appetite stimulant: Adults: 2.5 mg twice daily before lunch and dinner; if intolerant, a dosage of 2.5 mg once daily at night may be tried; maximum dosage (escalating): 10 mg twice daily

Administration May be administered without regard to meals; take before meals if used to stimulate appetite

Monitoring Parameters Heart rate, blood pressure

Patient Information May cause drowsiness and impair ability to perform activities requiring mental alertness or physical coordination; may cause dry mouth; avoid alcohol

Dosage Forms Excipient information presented when available (limited, particularly for generics); consult specific product labeling.

Capsule, soft gelatin: 2.5 mg, 5 mg, 10 mg

Marinol®: 2.5 mg, 5 mg, 10 mg [contains sesame oil]

References

Lane M, Smith FE, Sullivan RA, et al, "Dronabinol and Prochlorperazine Alone and in Combination as Antiemetic Agents for Cancer Chemotherapy," *Am J Clin Oncol*, 1990, 13(6):480-4.

Droperidol (droe PER i dole)

Medication Safety Issues

Sound-alike/look-alike issues:

Droperidol may be confused with dronabinol

Inapsine® may be confused with asenapine, Nebcin®

Related Information

Compatibility of Chemotherapy and Related Supportive Care Medications *on page 1580*

Compatibility of Medications Mixed in a Syringe *on page 1713*

U.S. Brand Names Inapsine® [DSC]

Canadian Brand Names Droperidol Injection, USP

Therapeutic Category Antiemetic; Antipsychotic Agent, Typical, Butyrophenone

Generic Available Yes

Use Treatment of nausea and vomiting associated with surgical and diagnostic procedures in patients for whom other treatments are ineffective or inappropriate

Pregnancy Risk Factor C

Pregnancy Considerations Crosses the placenta

Lactation Excretion in breast milk unknown

Contraindications Hypersensitivity to droperidol or any component; known or suspected QT prolongation; congenital long QT syndrome

Warnings Cases of QT prolongation and torsade de pointes in patients treated with droperidol in doses within or even below the approved dosage range have been reported **[U.S. Boxed Warning]**. Some cases occurred in patients with no underlying risk factors for QT prolongation; fatalities have occurred. Droperidol should be reserved for patients who fail other treatments. Prior to its use, all patients should undergo a 12-lead ECG. If the QT interval is prolonged, droperidol should not be used. Droperidol should be used with extreme caution in patients with risk factors for prolonged QT syndrome (ie, CHF; bradycardia; cardiac hypertrophy; any clinically significant cardiac disease; diuretic use; hypokalemia; hypomagnesemia; concomitant use of Class I or Class III antiarrhythmics, MAO inhibitors, or medications known to prolong the QT interval; age >65 years; alcohol abuse; and use of medications such as benzodiazepines, volatile anesthetics, and I.V. opiates).

The dosage of droperidol should be individualized; dosages should be started low and titrated upward. Continuous ECG monitoring should be done prior to treatment and for 2-3 hours after treatment to monitor for arrhythmias. I.V. fluids and other therapy to treat hypotension should be readily available; monitor patients carefully. Use reduced initial doses of opioids, if needed. Neuromalignant syndrome may rarely occur.

Precautions Use with caution in patients with impaired hepatic or renal function; severe hypertension and tachycardia may occur in patients with pheochromocytoma

Adverse Reactions
Cardiovascular: Hypotension (especially in hypovolemic patients), tachycardia; QT prolongation, torsade de pointes, cardiac arrest, ventricular tachycardia (see Warnings)
Central nervous system: Extrapyramidal reactions such as dystonic reactions, akathisia, and oculogyric crisis; anxiety, hyperactivity, drowsiness, dizziness, hallucinations, chills, dysphoria, restlessness
Respiratory: Laryngospasm, bronchospasm
Miscellaneous: Anaphylaxis; neuromalignant syndrome (rare)

Drug Interactions
Avoid Concomitant Use
Avoid concomitant use of Droperidol with any of the following: Artemether; Dronedarone; Lumefantrine; Metoclopramide; Nilotinib; Pimozide; QuiNINE; Tetrabenazine; Thioridazine; Ziprasidone
Increased Effect/Toxicity
Droperidol may increase the levels/effects of: Alcohol (Ethyl); Anticholinergics; Anti-Parkinson's Agents (Dopamine Agonist); CNS Depressants; Dronedarone; Metoclopramide; Pimozide; QTc-Prolonging Agents; QuiNINE; Tetrabenazine; Thioridazine; Ziprasidone

The levels/effects of Droperidol may be increased by: Acetylcholinesterase Inhibitors (Central); Alfuzosin; Artemether; Chloroquine; Ciprofloxacin; Ciprofloxacin (Systemic); Gadobutrol; Lithium formulations; Lumefantrine; MAO Inhibitors; Metoclopramide; Nilotinib; Pramlintide; QuiNINE; Tetrabenazine
Decreased Effect
Droperidol may decrease the levels/effects of: Amphetamines; Quinagolide

The levels/effects of Droperidol may be decreased by: Anti-Parkinson's Agents (Dopamine Agonist); Lithium formulations

Stability Store at room temperature; protect from light. Physically compatible and chemically stable with D_5W, LR, NS at a concentration of 20 mg/L

Mechanism of Action Alters the action of dopamine in the CNS, at subcortical levels, to produce sedation and a dissociative state; also possesses alpha-adrenergic blockade effects

Pharmacodynamics
Onset of action: 3-10 minutes
Maximum effect: Within 30 minutes
Duration: 2-4 hours (up to 12 hours)
Pharmacokinetics (Adult data unless noted)
Metabolism: In the liver
Half-life, adults: 2.3 hours
Elimination: In urine (75%) and feces (22%)

Usual Dosage Dosage must be individualized, based on age, body weight, underlying medical conditions, physical status, concomitant medications, type of anesthesia, and surgical procedure
Children 2-12 years:
Postoperative nausea and vomiting prophylaxis for high risk surgery: I.M., I.V.: Doses as low as 0.015 mg/kg/dose may be effective; usual: 0.05-0.06 mg/kg/dose administered once; maximum initial dose: 0.1 mg/kg; administer additional doses with caution and only if potential benefit outweighs risks (see Warnings); **Note:** A recent meta-analysis of 74 randomised controlled trials (29 pediatric trials) assessed droperidol use for the prevention of postoperative nausea and vomiting; the analysis suggested that 0.075 mg/kg/dose was likely to be the most effective prophylactic dose; it was also the most frequently used dose in the trials that were assessed; however, due to side effects associated with this dose, the study considered 0.05 mg/kg/dose to be the best prophylactic dose for children in cases where sedation and drowsiness should be prevented (eg, day surgery) (see Henzi, 2000)
Postoperative nausea and vomiting (treatment): I.V.: Doses as low as 0.01-0.03 mg/kg/dose may be effective for breakthrough nausea and vomiting; maximum initial dose: 0.1 mg/kg; administer additional doses with caution and only if potential benefit outweighs risks (see Warnings)
Adults: Nausea and vomiting: I.M., I.V.: Maximum initial dose: 2.5 mg; additional doses of 1.25 mg may be administered to achieve desired effect; administer additional doses with caution and only if potential benefit outweighs risks (see Warnings)

Administration Parenteral: Administer by slow I.V. injection over 2-5 minutes; maximum concentration: 2.5 mg/mL (I.M. or I.V.)

Monitoring Parameters Prior to use: 12-lead ECG to identify patients with QT prolongation (use is contraindicated); continuous ECG during and for 2-3 hours after dosage administration is recommended. Blood pressure, heart rate, respiratory rate; serum potassium and magnesium; observe for dystonias, extrapyramidal side effects; temperature

Additional Information Does not possess analgesic effects; has little or no amnesic properties. A dose-dependent prolongation of the QT interval has been observed in adults; significant QT prolongation was noted at doses of 0.1 mg/kg, 0.175 mg/kg, and 0.25 mg/kg with prolongation of median QT_c interval by 37, 44, and 59 msec, respectively (see package insert)

Dosage Forms Excipient information presented when available (limited, particularly for generics); consult specific product labeling. [DSC] = Discontinued product
Injection, solution [preservative free]: 2.5 mg/mL (1 mL, 2 mL)
Inapsine®: 2.5 mg/mL (1 mL, 2 mL) [DSC]

References
Henzi I, Sonderegger J, and Tramer MR, "Efficacy, Dose-Response, and Adverse Effects of Droperidol for Prevention of Postoperative Nausea and Vomiting," Can J Anaesth, 2000, 47(6):537-51.
Yaster M, Sola JE, Pegoli W Jr, et al, "The Night After Surgery: Postoperative Management of the Pediatric Outpatient - Surgical and Anesthetic Aspects," Pediatr Clin North Am, 1994, 41(1):199-220.

◆ **Droperidol Injection, USP (Can)** see Droperidol on page 483

Drotrecogin Alfa (Activated)
(dro TRE coe jin AL fa ak ti VAY ted)

U.S. Brand Names Xigris®
Canadian Brand Names Xigris®
Therapeutic Category Biological Response Modulator
Generic Available No

Use Reduction of mortality in adult patients with severe sepsis (sepsis associated with acute organ dysfunction) who have a high risk of death (ie, as determined by APACHE II score ≥25); purpura fulminans (compassionate use protocol)

Pregnancy Risk Factor C

Lactation Excretion in breast milk unknown/not recommended

Contraindications Hypersensitivity to drotrecogin alfa or any component; patients with active internal bleeding; recent (within 3 months) hemorrhagic stroke, recent (within 2 months) intracranial or intraspinal surgery, or severe head trauma; trauma with an increased risk of life-threatening bleeding; presence of an epidural catheter; intracranial neoplasm or mass lesion or evidence of cerebral herniation

Warnings Serious bleeding was observed in 3.5% of drotrecogin alfa-treated patients and is the most common adverse effect associated with this agent. Conditions which may increase the risk of bleeding with drotrecogin alfa include concurrent heparin administration (≥15 units/kg/hour), platelet count <30,000 x 10^6/L, INR >3, recent (within 6 weeks) gastrointestinal bleeding, recent administration (within 3 days) of thrombolytic therapy, recent administration (within 7 days) of oral anticoagulants or glycoprotein IIb/IIIa inhibitors, recent administration (within 7 days) of aspirin >650 mg/day, NSAIDs, clopidogrel, dipyridamole, or other platelet inhibitors, intracranial arteriovenous malformation or aneurysm, known bleeding diathesis, and chronic severe hepatic disease. If bleeding occurs, immediately stop the infusion. Once hemostasis has been achieved, restarting drotrecogin alfa may be considered. Stop drotrecogin alfa 2 hours prior to undergoing an invasive surgical procedure or procedure with an inherent risk of bleeding. Once hemostasis has been achieved, drotrecogin alfa may be restarted 12 hours after major invasive procedures or surgery or immediately after less invasive procedures.

Precautions Use with caution in patients at risk of bleeding, patients with chronic renal failure requiring dialysis, patients with hypercoagulable conditions (ie, hereditary deficiencies of protein C, protein S, or antithrombin III, suspected thromboembolism), or resistance to activated protein C

Adverse Reactions

Central nervous system: Intracranial hemorrhage
Gastrointestinal: GI hemorrhage
Genitourinary: GU hemorrhage
Hematologic: Bleeding, bruising

Drug Interactions

Avoid Concomitant Use There are no known interactions where it is recommended to avoid concomitant use.

Increased Effect/Toxicity

Drotrecogin Alfa may increase the levels/effects of: Anticoagulants; Collagenase (Systemic); Fondaparinux; Ibritumomab; Tositumomab and Iodine I 131 Tositumomab

The levels/effects of Drotrecogin Alfa may be increased by: Antiplatelet Agents; Antithrombin; Danaparoid; Dasatinib; Heparin; Heparin (Low Molecular Weight); Herbs (Anticoagulant/Antiplatelet Properties); Nonsteroidal Anti-Inflammatory Agents; Pentosan Polysulfate Sodium; Prostacyclin Analogues; Salicylates; Thrombolytic Agents; Vitamin K Antagonists

Decreased Effect There are no known significant interactions involving a decrease in effect.

Stability Refrigerate and protect unreconstituted vials from light. Do not freeze. Drotrecogin alfa for injection contains no preservatives. Reconstituted vial is stable for 3 hours at room temperature. Once reconstituted and further diluted with NS, infusion must be completed within 12 hours. If not used immediately, a prepared solution may be stored in the refrigerator for up to 12 hours. The maximum time limit for use of the drotrecogin alfa infusion solution, including dilution, refrigeration, and administration, is 24 hours. The only compatible solutions which can be administered through the same line as drotrecogin alfa are NS, LR, dextrose, or dextrose and saline mixtures. Avoid exposing drotrecogin alfa infusion solution to heat and/or direct sunlight.

Mechanism of Action Drotrecogin alfa, a serine protease with the same amino acid sequence as human plasma-derived activated protein C, possesses profibrinolytic, antithrombotic, and anti-inflammatory activities. Activated protein C inactivates factors Va and VIIIa decreasing generation of thrombin and ultimately decreasing fibrin/clot formation; binds to plasminogen activator type 1 enhancing the action of tissue plasminogen activator and stimulates fibrinolysis; inhibits cytokine production

Pharmacodynamics

Maximum effect on decreasing D-dimer levels: At the end of a 96-hour 24 mcg/kg/hour infusion

Duration: Nondetectable in plasma within 2 hours of discontinuation

Pharmacokinetics (Adult data unless noted) A phase 2 pharmacokinetic study has been performed in pediatric patients, but results from this trial are not yet available (communication with Lilly Research Laboratories, Jan 2002)

Metabolism: Plasma protease inhibitors inactivate drotrecogin alfa and endogenous activated protein C

Half-life: Children: 30 minutes

Clearance: Children: 0.45 L/hour/kg

Usual Dosage I.V.: Continuous infusion:

Infants, Children, and Adults: Purpura fulminans: In a compassionate use program, 42 patients (range: >3 kg to 135 kg; >1 year of age) received a dose of 24 mcg/kg/hour for 96 hours. If the patient had improved after 96 hours, but had laboratory evidence of an ongoing coagulopathy, or had tissue still deemed to be at risk for necrosis, the drotrecogin alfa infusion could be continued. The maximum allowed infusion time was 168 hours.

Adults: Severe sepsis: 24 mcg/kg/hour for 4 days. Infusion should be started within 24 hours of the onset of at least three signs of systemic inflammation and evidence of at least one organ/system dysfunction

Administration Parenteral: I.V.: May administer via a dedicated I.V. line or a dedicated lumen of a central venous catheter at a final concentration between 0.1-0.2 mg/mL in NS. When using low concentrations <200 mcg/mL at low flow rates <5 mL/hour, the infusion set must be primed for approximately 15 minutes at a flow rate of approximately 5 mL/hour.

Monitoring Parameters Hemoglobin, hematocrit, PT, coagulation panel, CBC with differential, platelet count, signs and symptoms of bleeding; for select patients: Plasma D-dimer levels, plasma interleukin-6 level, protein C and protein S activity; for purpura fulminans: Evaluate tissue for necrosis risk

Test Interactions Drotrecogin alfa may prolong the one-stage coagulation assay based on the APTT (such as factor VIII, IX, and XI assays) so that an apparent factor concentration appears lower than the true concentration.

Additional Information Human plasma derived protein C concentrate (an alternative, investigational product) has been used in infants and children with severe meningococcemia associated with purpura fulminans (see Ettingshausen, 1999).

Dosage Forms Excipient information presented when available (limited, particularly for generics); consult specific product labeling.

Injection, powder for reconstitution [preservative free]: 5 mg [contains sucrose 31.8 mg], 20 mg [contains sucrose 124.9 mg]

References

Alberio L, Lammle B, and Esmon CT, "Protein C Replacement in Severe Meningococcemia: Rationale and Clinical Experience," *Clin Infect Dis*, 2001, 32(9):1338-46.

Bachli EB, Vavricka SR, Walter RB, et al, "Drotrecogin Alfa (Activated) for the Treatment of Meningococcal Purpura Fulminans," *Intensive Care Med*, 2003, 29(2):337.

Barton P, Kalil AC, Nadel S, et al, "Safety, Pharmacokinetics, and Pharmacodynamics of Drotrecogin Alfa (Activated) in Children With Severe Sepsis," *Pediatrics*, 2004, 113(1 Pt 1):7-17.

Bernard GR, Vincent JL, Laterre PF, et al, "Efficacy and Safety of Recombinant Human Activated Protein C for Severe Sepsis," *N Engl J Med*, 2001, 344(10):699-709.

Ettingshausen CE, Veldmann A, Beeg T, et al, "Replacement Therapy With Protein C Concentrate in Infants and Adolescents With Meningococcal Sepsis and Purpura Fulminans," *Semin Thromb Hemost*, 1999, 25(6):537-41.

Faust SN, Levin M, Harrison OB, et al, "Dysfunction of Endothelial Protein C Activation in Severe Meningococcal Sepsis," *N Engl J Med*, 2001, 345(6):408-16.

◆ **Drotrecogin Alfa, Activated** *see* Drotrecogin Alfa (Activated) *on page 484*

◆ **Droxia®** *see* Hydroxyurea *on page 695*

◆ **DSCG** *see* Cromolyn *on page 363*

◆ **DSS** *see* Docusate *on page 468*

◆ **D-S-S® [OTC]** *see* Docusate *on page 468*

◆ **DT** *see* Diphtheria and Tetanus Toxoid *on page 452*

◆ **DTaP** *see* Diphtheria, Tetanus Toxoids, and Acellular Pertussis Vaccine *on page 458*

◆ **DTap-HepB-IPV** *see* Diphtheria, Tetanus Toxoids, Acellular Pertussis, Hepatitis B (Recombinant), and Poliovirus (Inactivated) Vaccine *on page 457*

◆ **DTaP/Hib** *see* Diphtheria, Tetanus Toxoids, and Acellular Pertussis Vaccine and *Haemophilus influenzae* b Conjugate Vaccine *on page 460*

◆ **DTaP-IPV** *see* Diphtheria and Tetanus Toxoids, Acellular Pertussis, and Poliovirus Vaccine *on page 453*

◆ **DTaP-IPV/Hib** *see* Diphtheria and Tetanus Toxoids, Acellular Pertussis, Poliovirus and *Haemophilus* b Conjugate Vaccine *on page 455*

◆ **DTIC** *see* Dacarbazine *on page 380*

◆ **DTIC-Dome** *see* Dacarbazine *on page 380*

◆ **DTO (error-prone abbreviation)** *see* Opium Tincture *on page 1024*

◆ **dTpa** *see* Diphtheria, Tetanus Toxoids, and Acellular Pertussis Vaccine *on page 458*

◆ **Duac® CS** *see* Clindamycin and Benzoyl Peroxide *on page 329*

◆ **Dulcolax® [OTC]** *see* Bisacodyl *on page 194*

◆ **Dulcolax® (Can)** *see* Bisacodyl *on page 194*

◆ **Dulcolax Balance® [OTC]** *see* Polyethylene Glycol 3350 *on page 1128*

◆ **Dulcolax® Milk of Magnesia [OTC]** *see* Magnesium Hydroxide *on page 855*

◆ **Dulcolax® Milk of Magnesia [OTC]** *see* Magnesium Supplements *on page 859*

◆ **Dulcolax® Stool Softener [OTC]** *see* Docusate *on page 468*

◆ **Dull-C® [OTC]** *see* Ascorbic Acid *on page 138*

◆ **Duofilm® (Can)** *see* Salicylic Acid *on page 1241*

◆ **Duoforte® 27 (Can)** *see* Salicylic Acid *on page 1241*

◆ **Duraclon®** *see* CloNIDine *on page 338*

◆ **Duragesic®** *see* FentaNYL *on page 567*

◆ **Duragesic MAT (Can)** *see* FentaNYL *on page 567*

◆ **Duralith® (Can)** *see* Lithium *on page 834*

◆ **Duramist® Plus [OTC]** *see* Oxymetazoline *on page 1043*

◆ **Duramorph®** *see* Morphine Sulfate *on page 946*

◆ **Durasal™** *see* Salicylic Acid *on page 1241*

◆ **Duratuss® DM [DSC]** *see* Guaifenesin and Dextromethorphan *on page 658*

◆ **Duricef** *see* Cefadroxil *on page 261*

◆ **Duvoid® (Can)** *see* Bethanechol *on page 191*

◆ **D-Vi-Sol® (Can)** *see* Cholecalciferol *on page 300*

◆ **Dycill® (Can)** *see* Dicloxacillin *on page 432*

Dyclonine (DYE kloe neen)

Medication Safety Issues

Sound-alike/look-alike issues:

Dyclonine may be confused with dicyclomine

U.S. Brand Names Cēpacol® Dual Action Maximum Strength [OTC]; Orajel® Maximum Strength Overnight Cold Sore [OTC]; Sucrets® [OTC]

Therapeutic Category Local Anesthetic, Oral

Generic Available No

Use As a local anesthetic prior to laryngoscopy, bronchoscopy, or endotracheal intubation; used topically for temporary relief of pain associated with oral mucosa, skin, episiotomy, or anogenital lesions; the 0.5% topical solution may be used to block the gag reflex, and to relieve the pain of oral ulcers or stomatitis; the lozenge is used for temporary relief of sore throat pain and gum irritation

Contraindications Hypersensitivity to chlorobutanol (preservative used in dyclonine), dyclonine, or any component

Warnings Resuscitative equipment, oxygen and resuscitative drugs should be immediately available when dyclonine topical solution is administered to mucous membranes; may impair swallowing and enhance the danger of aspiration

Precautions Use with caution in patients with infection present in the area of application or traumatized mucosa in the area of application to avoid rapid systemic absorption; use with caution in patients with shock or heart block

Adverse Reactions Excessive dosage and rapid absorption may result in adverse CNS and cardiovascular effects

Cardiovascular: Hypotension, bradycardia, cardiac arrest, edema

Central nervous system: Excitation, drowsiness, nervousness, dizziness, seizures

Dermatologic: Rash, urticaria

Local: Slight irritation and stinging may occur when applied

Ocular: Blurred vision

Respiratory: Respiratory arrest

Miscellaneous: Allergic reactions

Drug Interactions

Avoid Concomitant Use There are no known interactions where it is recommended to avoid concomitant use.

Increased Effect/Toxicity There are no known significant interactions involving an increase in effect.

Decreased Effect There are no known significant interactions involving a decrease in effect.

Stability Store in tight, light-resistant container; avoid freezing

Mechanism of Action Blocks impulses at peripheral nerve endings in skin and mucous membranes by altering cell membrane permeability to ionic transfer

Pharmacodynamics

Onset of action: Local anesthesia: 2-10 minutes

Duration: 30-60 minutes

Usual Dosage

Children and Adults:

Topical solution: Mouth sores: 5-10 mL of 0.5% or 1% to oral mucosa (swab or swish and then spit) 3-4 times/day as needed; maximum single dose: 200 mg (40 mL of 0.5% solution or 20 mL of 1% solution); solution may be diluted 1:1 with water

Bronchoscopy: Use 2 mL of the 1% solution or 4 mL of the 0.5% solution sprayed onto the larynx and trachea every 5 minutes for 2-3 applications until the reflex has been abolished

Children >3 years: Topical: Slowly dissolve 1 lozenge (1.2 mg) in mouth every 2 hours, if necessary

Children >12 years and Adults: Topical: Slowly dissolve 1 lozenge (3 mg) in mouth every 2 hours, if necessary

Administration Topical: Apply to mucous membranes of the mouth or throat area: food should not be ingested for 60 minutes following application in the mouth or throat area

Patient Information Do not chew lozenge; numbness of the tongue and buccal mucosa may result in increased risk of biting trauma; may impair swallowing

Nursing Implications Use the lowest dose needed to provide effective anesthesia; not for injection; do not apply nasally or to the eye

Dosage Forms Excipient information presented when available (limited, particularly for generics); consult specific product labeling.

Lozenge, as hydrochloride:

Sucrets®: 1.2 mg [children's cherry flavor]; 2 mg [wild cherry and assorted flavors]; 3 mg [vapor black cherry and wintergreen flavors]

Patch, topical, as hydrochloride:

Orajel® Maximum Strength Overnight Cold Sore: 3 mg (8s) [contains ethanol]

Spray, oral, as hydrochloride:

Cepacol® Dual Action Maximum Strength: 0.1% (120 mL) [contains glycerin 33%; cherry, honey lemon and cool menthol flavors]

References

Carnel SB, Blakeslee DB, Oswald SG, et al, "Treatment of Radiation- and Chemotherapy-Induced Stomatitis," *Otolaryngol Head Neck Surg*, 1990, 102(4):326-30.

◆ **Dyclonine Hydrochloride** *see* Dyclonine *on page 486*

◆ **Dygase [DSC]** *see* Pancreatin *on page 1050*

◆ **Dynacin®** *see* Minocycline *on page 933*

◆ **DynaCirc® (Can)** *see* Isradipine *on page 771*

◆ **DynaCirc® CR** *see* Isradipine *on page 771*

◆ **Dyna-Hex® [OTC]** *see* Chlorhexidine Gluconate *on page 291*

◆ **Dyrenium®** *see* Triamterene *on page 1380*

◆ **Dytan™** *see* DiphenhydrAMINE *on page 448*

◆ **EACA** *see* Aminocaproic Acid *on page 82*

◆ **Easprin®** *see* Aspirin *on page 141*

◆ **EC-Naprosyn®** *see* Naproxen *on page 967*

◆ ***E. coli* Asparaginase** *see* Asparaginase *on page 139*

Econazole (e KONE a zole)

Therapeutic Category Antifungal Agent, Topical
Generic Available Yes
Use Topical treatment of tinea pedis, tinea cruris, tinea corporis, tinea versicolor, and cutaneous candidiasis
Pregnancy Risk Factor C
Pregnancy Considerations Fetotoxic and embryotoxic events were observed in animal studies. The manufacturer does not recommend use during pregnancy.
Lactation Excretion in breast milk unknown/use caution
Contraindications Hypersensitivity to econazole or any component

Warnings Not for ophthalmic or intravaginal use

Precautions Discontinue the drug if sensitivity or chemical irritation occurs; cross-sensitization may occur with other imidazole derivatives (ie, clotrimazole, miconazole)

Adverse Reactions

Dermatologic: Pruritus, erythema, contact dermatitis

Local: Burning, stinging

Drug Interactions

Metabolism/Transport Effects Inhibits CYP2E1 (weak)

Avoid Concomitant Use There are no known interactions where it is recommended to avoid concomitant use.

Increased Effect/Toxicity There are no known significant interactions involving an increase in effect.

Decreased Effect There are no known significant interactions involving a decrease in effect.

Mechanism of Action Alters fungal cell wall membrane permeability; may interfere with RNA and protein synthesis, and lipid metabolism

Pharmacokinetics (Adult data unless noted)

Absorption: Following topical administration, <10% is percutaneously absorbed

Metabolism: In the liver to >20 metabolites

Elimination: <1% of an applied dose recovered in urine or feces

Usual Dosage Children and Adults: Topical:

Tinea cruris, corporis, pedis, and tinea versicolor: Apply once daily

Cutaneous candidiasis: Apply twice daily

Administration Topical: Apply a sufficient amount of cream to cover affected areas; do not apply to the eye or intravaginally

Patient Information For external use only. Notify physician if condition worsens or persists, or if irritation occurs.

Additional Information Candidal infections and tinea cruris, versicolor, and corporis should be treated for 2 weeks and tinea pedis for 1 month; occasionally, longer treatment periods may be required

Dosage Forms Excipient information presented when available (limited, particularly for generics); consult specific product labeling.

Cream, topical, as nitrate: 1% (15 g, 30 g, 85 g)

◆ **Econazole Nitrate** *see* Econazole *on page 487*

◆ **Econopred® Plus [DSC]** *see* PrednisoLONE *on page 1148*

◆ **Ecotrin® [OTC]** *see* Aspirin *on page 141*

◆ **Ecotrin® Low Strength [OTC]** *see* Aspirin *on page 141*

◆ **Ecotrin® Maximum Strength [OTC]** *see* Aspirin *on page 141*

◆ **Ectosone (Can)** *see* Betamethasone *on page 189*

◆ **Edathamil Disodium** *see* Edetate Disodium *on page 489*

◆ **Ed Chlorped** *see* Chlorpheniramine *on page 296*

◆ **Ed-Chlor-Tan** *see* Chlorpheniramine *on page 296*

◆ **Edecrin®** *see* Ethacrynic Acid *on page 543*

Edetate CALCIUM Disodium
(ED e tate KAL see um dye SOW dee um)

Medication Safety Issues

Sound-alike look-alike issues:

To avoid potentially serious errors, the abbreviation "EDTA" should **never** be used.

◀

Edetate CALCIUM disodium (CaEDTA) may be confused with edetate disodium (Na$_2$EDTA). CDC recommends that edetate disodium should **never** be used for chelation therapy in children. Fatal hypocalcemia may result if edetate disodium is used for chelation therapy instead of edetate calcium disodium. ISMP recommends confirming the diagnosis to help distinguish between the two drugs prior to dispensing and/or administering either drug.

Edetate CALCIUM disodium may be confused with etomidate

U.S. Brand Names Calcium Disodium Versenate®

Therapeutic Category Antidote, Lead Toxicity; Chelating Agent, Parenteral

Generic Available No

Use Treatment of acute and chronic lead poisoning; also used as an aid in the diagnosis of lead poisoning

Pregnancy Risk Factor B

Pregnancy Considerations Adverse events were observed in some animal reproduction studies; there are no well controlled studies of edetate CALCIUM disodium in pregnant women. Following maternal occupational exposure, lead was found to cross the placenta in amounts related to maternal plasma levels. Possible outcomes of maternal lead exposure >10 mcg/dL includes spontaneous abortion, postnatal developmental delay, and reduced birth weight. Chelation therapy during pregnancy is for maternal benefit only and should be limited to the treatment of severe, symptomatic lead poisoning.

Lactation Excretion in breast milk unknown/use caution

Breast-Feeding Considerations
If present in breast milk, oral absorption of edetate CALCIUM disodium is poor (<5%) which would limit exposure to a nursing infant. However, edetate CALCIUM disodium is not used orally because it may increase lead absorption from the GI tract. The amount of lead in breast milk may range from 0.6% to 3% of the maternal serum concentration. Calcium supplementation may reduce the amount of lead in breast milk.

Contraindications Hypersensitivity to edetate calcium disodium or any component; active renal disease, anuria, hepatitis

Warnings Patients with lead encephalopathy and cerebral edema may experience a lethal increase in intracranial pressure following I.V. infusion of edetate CALCIUM EDTA **[U.S. Boxed Warning]**; avoid rapid I.V. infusion, particularly in the management of lead encephalopathy; I.M. administration is the preferred route in these patients, if the I.V. route is necessary, infuse slowly (over at least 3 hours) **[U.S. Boxed Warning]**; do not exceed recommended daily dose **[U.S. Boxed Warning]**; if anuria, increasing proteinuria, or hematuria occurs during therapy, discontinue calcium EDTA.

Precautions Renal tubular necrosis and fatal nephrosis may occur, especially with high doses; establish urine flow prior to administration

Adverse Reactions

Cardiovascular: Hypotension, arrhythmias, ECG changes

Central nervous system: Fever, headache, chills

Dermatologic: Skin lesions, cheilosis

Endocrine & metabolic: Hypercalcemia, zinc deficiency

Gastrointestinal: GI upset, anorexia, nausea, vomiting

Hematologic: Transient marrow suppression, anemia

Hepatic: Mild elevation in liver function tests

Local: Pain at injection site following I.M. injection, thrombophlebitis following I.V. infusion (when concentration >5 mg/mL)

Neuromuscular & skeletal: Arthralgia, tremor, numbness, paresthesia

Ocular: Lacrimation

Renal: Renal tubular necrosis, proteinuria, microscopic hematuria

Respiratory: Sneezing, nasal congestion

Drug Interactions

Avoid Concomitant Use There are no known interactions where it is recommended to avoid concomitant use.

Increased Effect/Toxicity
Edetate CALCIUM Disodium may increase the levels/effects of: Insulin

Decreased Effect There are no known significant interactions involving a decrease in effect.

Stability Dilute with NS or D$_5$W; physically incompatible with D$_{10}$W, LR; do not mix in the same syringe with dimercaprol

Mechanism of Action Calcium is displaced by divalent and trivalent heavy metals, forming a nonionizing soluble complex that is excreted in the urine

Pharmacodynamics

Onset of chelation with I.V. administration: 1 hour

Maximum excretion of chelated lead with I.V. administration: 24-48 hours

Pharmacokinetics (Adult data unless noted)

Absorption: I.M., SubQ: Well absorbed

Distribution: Into extracellular fluid; minimal CSF penetration

Half-life, plasma:
I.M.: 1.5 hours
I.V.: 20 minutes

Elimination: Rapid in urine as metal chelates or unchanged drug

Usual Dosage Several regimens have been recommended:

Diagnosis of lead poisoning: Mobilization test (not recommended by AAP guidelines): I.M., I.V.:

Children: 500 mg/m^2/dose, (maximum dose: 1 g) as a single dose or divided into 2 doses

Adults: 500 mg/m^2/dose

Note: Urine is collected for 24 hours after first EDTA dose and analyzed for lead content; if the ratio of mcg of lead in urine to mg calcium EDTA given is >1, then test is considered positive; for convenience, an 8-hour urine collection may be done after a single 50 mg/kg I.M. (maximum dose: 1 g) or 500 mg/m^2 I.V. dose; a positive test occurs if the ratio of lead excretion to mg calcium EDTA >0.5-0.6.

Treatment of lead poisoning: Children and Adults (each regimen is specific for route):

Symptoms of lead encephalopathy and/or blood lead level >70 mcg/dL: Treat 5 days; give in conjunction with dimercaprol; wait a minimum of 2 days with no treatment before considering a repeat course:

I.M.: 250 mg/m^2/dose every 4 hours

I.V.: 50 mg/kg/day as 24-hour continuous I.V. infusion **or** 1-1.5 g/m^2 I.V. as either an 8- to 24-hour infusion or divided into 2 doses every 12 hours

Symptomatic lead poisoning **without** encephalopathy **or** asymptomatic with blood lead level >70 mcg/dL: Treat 3-5 days; treatment with dimercaprol is recommended until the blood lead level concentration <50 mcg/dL:

I.M.: 167 mg/m^2 every 4 hours

I.V.: 1 g/m^2 as an 8- to 24-hour infusion or divided every 12 hours

Asymptomatic **children** with blood lead level 45-69 mcg/dL: I.V.: 25 mg/kg/day for 5 days as an 8- to 24-hour infusion or divided into 2 doses every 12 hours

Depending upon the blood lead level, additional courses may be necessary; repeat at least 2-4 days and preferably 2-4 weeks apart

Adults with lead nephropathy: An alternative dosing regimen reflecting the reduction in renal clearance is based upon the serum creatinine (adapted from Morgan, 1975; see table):

Alternative Dosing I.V. Regimen for Adults With Lead Nephropathy

Serum Creatinine (mg/dL)	Ca EDTA Dosage
>2-3	Reduce recommended dosage by 50%
>3-4	Reduce recommended dosage by 50% and administer every other day
>4	Reduce recommended dosage by 50% and administer once weekly

Adapted from Morgan, 1975.

Repeat these regimens monthly until lead excretion is reduced toward normal.

Administration Parenteral:

Intermittent I.V. infusion: Administer the dose I.V. over at least 1 hour in asymptomatic patients, 2 hours in symptomatic patients

Single daily I.V. continuous infusion: Dilute to 2-4 mg/mL in D_5W or NS and infuse over at least 8 hours, usually over 12-24 hours

I.M. injection: To minimize pain at the injection site, 1.67 mL of 2% procaine may be added to 5 mL calcium EDTA, resulting in 150 mg/mL concentration with 0.5% procaine (stable 3 months; see Nahata, 1997)

Monitoring Parameters BUN, serum creatinine, urinalysis, fluid balance, ECG, blood and urine lead concentrations

Test Interactions If calcium EDTA is given as a continuous I.V. infusion, stop the infusion for at least 1 hour before blood is drawn for lead concentration to avoid a falsely elevated value

Dosage Forms Excipient information presented when available (limited, particularly for generics); consult specific product labeling.

Injection, solution: 200 mg/mL (2.5 mL)

References

American Academy of Pediatrics Committee on Drugs, "Treatment Guidelines for Lead Exposure in Children," *Pediatrics*, 1995, 96(1 Pt 1):155-60.

Gracia RC and Snodgrass WR, "Lead Toxicity and Chelation Therapy," *Am J Health Syst Pharm*, 2007, 64(1):45-53.

Morgan JM, "Chelation Therapy in Lead Nephropathy," *South Med J*, 1975, 68(8):1001-6.

Nahata MC and Hipple TF, *Pediatric Drug Formulations*, 3rd ed, Cincinnati, OH: Harvey Whitney Books Co, 1997.

Edetate Disodium (ED e tate dye SOW dee um)

Medication Safety Issues

Sound-alike look-alike issues:

To avoid potentially serious errors, the abbreviation "EDTA" should **never** be used.

Edetate disodium (Na_2EDTA) may be confused with edetate calcium disodium (CaEDTA). CDC recommends that edetate disodium should **never** be used for chelation therapy in children. Fatal hypocalcemia may result if edetate disodium is used for chelation therapy instead of edetate calcium disodium. ISMP recommends confirming the diagnosis to help distinguish between the two drugs prior to dispensing and/or administering either drug.

Edetate disodium may be confused with etomidate

U.S. Brand Names Endrate

Therapeutic Category Antidote, Hypercalcemia; Chelating Agent, Parenteral

Generic Available Yes

Use Emergency treatment of hypercalcemia; control digitalis-induced cardiac dysrhythmias (ventricular arrhythmias)

Pregnancy Risk Factor C

Contraindications Hypersensitivity to edetate disodium or any component; severe renal failure or anuria, hypocalcemia, patients with active tuberculosis or healed calcified tubercular lesions

Warnings The U.S. Food and Drug Administration (FDA) has issued a public health advisory alerting healthcare professionals, patients, and caregivers about the possibility of serious outcomes that may result from the improper use of edetate disodium. Edetate disodium (Na_2EDTA) may be confused with edetate CALCIUM disodium (CaEDTA). Fatalities have been reported in children and adults who were inadvertently given edetate disodium instead of edetate CALCIUM disodium or when edetate disodium was used for "chelation therapy" and other non-FDA-approved uses. **Edetate Disodium is not for use with chelation treatment.** Use with caution in patients with intracranial lesions, seizure disorders, coronary or peripheral vascular disease; cardiac function should be evaluated prior to therapy

Precautions Sudden, precipitous decreases of serum calcium may occur, a source of I.V. calcium replacement should be readily available; blood sugar and insulin requirements may be lower when used in insulin-dependent diabetics

Adverse Reactions

Cardiovascular: Arrhythmias, hypotension

Central nervous system: Seizures, headache, chills, fever

Dermatologic: Skin eruptions

Endocrine & metabolic: Hypomagnesemia, hypokalemia, hypocalcemia, hyperuricemia

Gastrointestinal: Vomiting, diarrhea, abdominal cramps

Genitourinary: Urinary urgency, dysuria

Hematologic: Anemia

Local: Thrombophlebitis, pain at injection site

Neuromuscular & skeletal: Back pain, muscle cramps, paresthesia, tetany

Renal: Nephrotoxicity, acute tubular necrosis, polyuria, oliguria, glucosuria

Respiratory: Respiratory arrest

Drug Interactions

Avoid Concomitant Use There are no known interactions where it is recommended to avoid concomitant use.

Increased Effect/Toxicity

Edetate Disodium may increase the levels/effects of: Insulin

Decreased Effect There are no known significant interactions involving a decrease in effect.

Stability Physically compatible with dextrose and saline I.V. solutions

Mechanism of Action Chelates with divalent or trivalent metals to form a soluble complex that is then eliminated in urine

Pharmacokinetics (Adult data unless noted)

Metabolism: Not metabolized

Half-life: 20-60 minutes

Elimination: Following chelation, 95% excreted in urine as chelates within 24-48 hours

Usual Dosage I.V.: Hypercalcemia:

Children: 40-70 mg/kg/day slow infusion over 3-4 hours or more to a maximum of 3 g/24 hours; administer for 5 days and allow 5 days between courses of therapy **or** 50 mg/kg **or** 1.5 g/m² as a single dose

Adults: 50 mg/kg/day over 3 or more hours to a maximum of 3 g/24 hours; administer for 5 days followed by 2 days without drug and repeat course up to 15 total doses

Administration Parenteral: I.V.: Must be diluted before I.V. use in D₅W or NS to a maximum concentration of 30 mg/mL (3%) and infused over at least 3 hours; avoid extravasation; **not for I.M. use**

Monitoring Parameters Serum and urine electrolytes (including calcium and magnesium), blood pressure (during infusion), renal function (before and during therapy), liver function, ECG

Test Interactions Colorimetric, oxalate, or other precipitation methods for measuring serum calcium

Nursing Implications Patient should remain supine for a short period after infusion

Additional Information Sodium content of 1 g: 5.4 mEq

Dosage Forms Excipient information presented when available (limited, particularly for generics); consult specific product labeling.

Injection, solution: 150 mg/mL (20 mL)

♦ **Edetate Disodium CALCIUM** see Edetate CALCIUM Disodium *on page 487*

♦ **Edex®** see Alprostadil *on page 69*

♦ **Edluar™** see Zolpidem *on page 1447*

Edrophonium (ed roe FOE nee um)

U.S. Brand Names Enlon®
Canadian Brand Names Enlon®; Tensilon®
Therapeutic Category Antidote, Neuromuscular Blocking Agent; Cholinergic Agent; Diagnostic Agent, Myasthenia Gravis
Generic Available No
Use Diagnosis of myasthenia gravis; differentiation of cholinergic crises from myasthenia crises; reversal of nondepolarizing neuromuscular blockers; treatment of paroxysmal atrial tachycardia
Pregnancy Risk Factor C
Lactation Excretion in breast milk unknown
Contraindications Hypersensitivity to edrophonium or any component; GI or GU mechanical obstruction
Warnings Overdosage can cause cholinergic crisis which may be fatal; I.V. atropine should be readily available for treatment of cholinergic reactions; injection contains sulfites which may cause allergic reactions in susceptible individuals
Precautions Use with caution in asthmatic patients, patients with cardiac dysrhythmias, and those receiving a cardiac glycoside

Adverse Reactions
Cardiovascular: Arrhythmias (especially bradycardia), hypotension, A-V block
Central nervous system: Seizures, drowsiness, headache, dysphoria
Gastrointestinal: Nausea, vomiting, diarrhea, excessive salivation, stomach cramps
Genitourinary: Urinary frequency
Local: Thrombophlebitis
Neuromuscular & skeletal: Weakness, muscle cramps, muscle spasms
Ocular: Diplopia, miosis, lacrimation, conjunctival hyperemia
Respiratory: Laryngospasm, bronchospasm, respiratory paralysis, bronchial secretions increased
Miscellaneous: Diaphoresis, hypersensitivity reactions

Drug Interactions
Avoid Concomitant Use There are no known interactions where it is recommended to avoid concomitant use.

Increased Effect/Toxicity
Edrophonium may increase the levels/effects of: Beta-Blockers; Cholinergic Agonists; Succinylcholine

The levels/effects of Edrophonium may be increased by: Corticosteroids (Systemic)

Decreased Effect
Edrophonium may decrease the levels/effects of: Neuromuscular-Blocking Agents (Nondepolarizing)

Mechanism of Action Inhibits destruction of acetylcholine by acetylcholinesterase. This facilitates transmission of impulses across myoneural junction and results in increased cholinergic responses such as miosis, increased tonus of intestinal and skeletal muscles, bronchial and ureteral constriction, bradycardia, and increased salivary and sweat gland secretions

Pharmacodynamics
Onset of action:
I.M.: 2-10 minutes
I.V.: 30-60 seconds
Duration:
I.M.: 5-30 minutes
I.V.: 5-10 minutes

Pharmacokinetics (Adult data unless noted)
Distribution: V_d:
Infants: 1.18 ± 0.2 L/kg
Children: 1.22 ± 0.74 L/kg
Adults: 0.9 ± 0.13 L/kg
Half-life:
Infants: 73 ± 30 minutes
Children: 99 ± 31 minutes
Adults: 126 ± 59 minutes
Elimination: Clearance:
Infants: 17.8 mL/kg/minute
Children: 14.2 mL/kg/minute
Adults: 8.3 ± 2.9 mL/kg/minute

Usual Dosage Usually administered I.V., however, if not possible, I.M. or SubQ may be used

Infants: Diagnosis of myasthenia gravis: Initial:
I.M., SubQ: 0.5-1 mg
I.V.: Initial: 0.1 mg, followed by 0.4 mg (if no response); total dose = 0.5 mg
Children:
Diagnosis of myasthenia gravis: Initial:
I.M., SubQ: ≤34 kg: 2 mg; >34 kg: 5 mg
I.V.: 0.04 mg/kg given over 1 minute followed by 0.16 mg/kg given within 45 seconds (if no response) (maximum dose: 10 mg total)
or
Alternative (manufacturer's recommendations):
≤34 kg: 1 mg; if no response after 45 seconds, it may be repeated in 1 mg increments every 30-45 seconds to a total of 5 mg
>34 kg: 2 mg; if no response after 45 seconds, it may be repeated in 1 mg increments every 30-45 seconds to a total of 10 mg
Titration of oral anticholinesterase therapy: I.V.: 0.04 mg/kg once given 1 hour after oral intake of the drug being used in treatment; if strength improves, an increase in neostigmine or pyridostigmine dose is indicated
Adults:
Diagnosis of myasthenia gravis: Initial:
I.M., SubQ: Initial: 10 mg; if no cholinergic reaction occurs, administer 2 mg 30 minutes later to rule out false-negative reaction
I.V.: 2 mg test dose administered over 15-30 seconds; 8 mg given 45 seconds later (if no response is seen); test dose may be repeated after 30 minutes.
Titration of oral anticholinesterase therapy: I.V.: 1-2 mg given 1 hour after oral dose of anticholinesterase; if strength improves, an increase in neostigmine or pyridostigmine dose is indicated
Differentiation of cholinergic from myasthenic crisis: I.V.: 1 mg, may repeat after 1 minute (**Note:** Intubation and controlled ventilation may be required if patient has cholinergic crises.)

Reversal of nondepolarizing neuromuscular blocking agents (neostigmine with atropine usually preferred): I.V.: 10 mg over 30-45 seconds, may repeat every 5-10 minutes up to 40 mg total dose

Termination of paroxysmal atrial tachycardia: I.V.: 5-10 mg

Dosing adjustment in renal impairment: Dose may need to be reduced in patients with chronic renal failure

Administration Parenteral: Edrophonium is administered by direct I.V. or I.M. injection; see Usual Dosage

Monitoring Parameters Pre- and postinjection strength (cranial musculature is most useful); heart rate, respiratory rate, blood pressure, changes in fasciculations

Dosage Forms Excipient information presented when available (limited, particularly for generics); consult specific product labeling.

Injection, solution, as chloride:

Enlon®: 10 mg/mL (15 mL) [contains natural rubber/natural latex in packaging; sodium sulfite]

◆ **Edrophonium Chloride** see Edrophonium on page 490

◆ **EDTA (CALCIUM Disodium) (error-prone abbreviation)** see Edetate CALCIUM Disodium on page 487

◆ **EDTA (Disodium) (error-prone abbreviation)** see Edetate Disodium on page 489

◆ **E.E.S.®** see Erythromycin on page 525

◆ **EES® (Can)** see Erythromycin on page 525

Efavirenz (eh FAH vih rehnz)

Related Information
Adult and Adolescent HIV on page 1620
Management of Healthcare Worker Exposures to HBV, HCV, and HIV on page 1661
Pediatric HIV on page 1613
Perinatal HIV on page 1628

U.S. Brand Names Sustiva®

Canadian Brand Names Sustiva®

Therapeutic Category Antiretroviral Agent; HIV Agents (Anti-HIV Agents); Non-nucleoside Reverse Transcriptase Inhibitor (NNRTI)

Generic Available No

Use Treatment of HIV-1 infection in combination with other antiretroviral agents (FDA approved in ages ≥3 years and adults). (**Note:** HIV regimens consisting of **three** antiretroviral agents are strongly recommended)

Pregnancy Risk Factor D

Pregnancy Considerations Teratogenic effects have been observed in Primates receiving efavirenz. Severe CNS defects have been reported in infants following efavirenz exposure in the first trimester. Pregnancy should be avoided and alternate therapy should be considered in women of childbearing potential. Women of childbearing potential should undergo pregnancy testing prior to initiation of efavirenz. Barrier contraception should be used in combination with other (hormonal) methods of contraception and for 12 weeks after efavirenz is discontinued. If therapy with efavirenz is administered during pregnancy, avoid use during the first trimester; use in the second and third trimesters only after considering other alternatives. Pharmacokinetic data from small study indicates that peak serum levels in the third trimester may be significantly increased. Health professionals are encouraged to contact the antiretroviral pregnancy registry to monitor outcomes of pregnant women exposed to antiretroviral medications (800-258-4263 or www.-APRegistry.com).

Lactation Excretion is breast milk unknown/contraindicated

Breast-Feeding Considerations In infants born to mothers who are HIV positive, HAART while breast-feeding may decrease postnatal infection. However, maternal or infant antiretroviral therapy does not completely eliminate the risk of postnatal HIV transmission.

In the United States where formula is accessible, affordable, safe, and sustainable, complete avoidance of breast-feeding by HIV-infected women is recommended to decrease potential transmission of HIV.

Contraindications Hypersensitivity (eg, Stevens-Johnson syndrome, erythema multiforme, or toxic skin eruptions) to efavirenz or any component; concurrent therapy with bepridil, cisapride, midazolam, pimozide, triazolam, ergot derivatives, or St John's wort

Warnings Efavirenz is a mixed inducer/inhibitor of CYP450 enzymes and numerous drug interactions occur. Due to potential serious and/or life-threatening drug interactions, certain drugs are contraindicated (see Contraindications and Drug Interactions). Other drug interactions require dosage adjustment; standard doses of efavirenz and voriconazole must **not** be coadministered (**Note:** Adjusted doses of efavirenz and voriconazole may be administered concurrently; see Drug Interactions and Usual Dosage).

Resistance emerges rapidly if administered as monotherapy; always use efavirenz in combination with at least two other antiretroviral agents; do not add efavirenz as a single agent to antiretroviral regimens that are failing; initiate in combination with at least one other antiretroviral agent to which the patient is naive. Immune reconstitution syndrome (an acute inflammatory response to residual or indolent opportunistic infections) may occur in HIV patients during initial treatment with combination antiretroviral agents, including efavirenz; this syndrome may require further patient assessment and therapy. Do not administer efavirenz with other efavirenz-containing products (eg, Atripla®).

Teratogenic effects have been observed in primates receiving efavirenz; human birth defects following efavirenz exposure in the first trimester have been reported, including cases of neural tube defects (including meningomyelocele and Dandy-Walker malformation) and one case of anophthalmia. Women of childbearing potential should be tested for pregnancy before starting efavirenz; women receiving efavirenz should avoid pregnancy while receiving this drug and for 12 weeks after discontinuation of this drug (due to long half-life of efavirenz); barrier contraception in combination with other (hormonal) methods of contraception should be used. Avoid use of efavirenz during the first trimester of pregnancy and in women with significant childbearing potential; women who use this drug during the first trimester or who become pregnant while taking this drug should be apprised of the potential harm to the fetus.

Precautions Use with caution in patients with a history of mental illness or substance abuse (delusions, inappropriate behavior, and severe acute depression may occur). Serious CNS and psychiatric symptoms may occur (see Adverse Reactions). Use with caution in patients with a history of seizures (convulsions may occur). Efavirenz may decrease the serum concentrations of antiepileptic agents that are metabolized by the liver (monitor anticonvulsant serum concentrations periodically; see Drug Interactions). Discontinue efavirenz if severe rash (involving blistering, desquamation, mucosal involvement, or fever) occurs; rash is more common and more severe in children versus adults, **consider prophylaxis with antihistamines in children.** Use with caution in patients with known or suspected hepatitis B or C, those receiving other hepatotoxic medications, and those with hepatic impairment; weigh risk versus benefit in patients with persistent elevations of serum transaminases (ie, >5 times normal). Cross resistance with other non-nucleoside reverse transcriptase inhibitors may occur. Elevations of serum cholesterol and triglyceride concentrations may occur (monitor during therapy). Fat redistribution and accumulation [ie, central obesity, peripheral wasting, facial wasting, breast enlargement, dorsocervical fat enlargement (buffalo hump), and cushingoid appearance] have been observed in patients receiving antiretroviral agents (causal relationship not established).

Adverse Reactions

Central nervous system (**Note:** Overall incidence of CNS adverse effects was 53% versus 25% in controls; nervous system symptoms in children have been reported to be 18%): Abnormal dreams, abnormal thinking, agitation, amnesia, anxiety, confusion, delusions, depersonalization, dizziness, drowsiness, euphoria, fatigue, fever (children 21%), hallucinations, headache (children 11%), hypoesthesia, impaired concentration, inappropriate behavior, insomnia, nervousness, somnolence; serious psychiatric adverse effects (patients with history of psychiatric disorders may be at greater risk): Aggressive behavior, manic reactions, paranoid reactions, severe acute depression, suicidal ideation/attempts; convulsions (rare)

Dermatologic: Rash, usually pruritic maculopapular skin eruptions (incidence: Children 46%, adults 26%; median onset, adults: 11 days, children: 9 days [range: 6-205 days], **Note:** Most rashes in children appeared within 14 days after starting therapy; median duration, adults: 16 days, children: 6 days [range: 2-37 days], **Note:** Median duration of rash in children who continued therapy was 9 days; rash may be treated with antihistamines and corticosteroids and usually resolves within one month while continuing therapy; **Note:** Blistering, desquamation, fever, mucosal involvement, or ulceration may occur and requires discontinuation of drug; see Precautions), pruritus, sweating increased

Endocrine & metabolic: Fat redistribution and accumulation (see Precautions), hypercholesterolemia, hyperglycemia, hypertriglyceridemia

Gastrointestinal: Abdominal pain, anorexia, diarrhea/loose stools (children: 39%), dyspepsia, nausea or vomiting (children: 12%), pancreatitis, serum amylase increased (asymptomatic)

Hematologic: Neutropenia

Hepatic: Liver enzymes increased (patients with hepatitis B or C may be at greater risk)

Respiratory: Cough (children 16%)

Miscellaneous: Alcohol intolerance, immune reconstitution syndrome (see Warnings)

<1%, postmarketing, and/or case reports: Allergic reaction, arthralgia, ataxia, balance disturbances, cerebellar coordination disturbances, constipation, coordination abnormal, dermatitis (photoallergic), dyspnea, emotional lability, erythema multiforme, flushing, gynecomastia, hepatic failure, hepatitis, malabsorption, mania, myalgia, myopathy, neuropathy, neurosis, palpitation, paresthesia, psychosis, Stevens-Johnson syndrome, tinnitus, tremor, visual abnormality, weakness

Drug Interactions

Metabolism/Transport Effects Substrate (major) of CYP2B6, 3A4; **Inhibits** CYP2C9 (moderate), 2C19 (moderate), 3A4 (moderate); **Induces** CYP2B6 (weak), 3A4 (strong)

Avoid Concomitant Use

Avoid concomitant use of Efavirenz with any of the following: Cisapride; Clopidogrel; Dienogest; Dronedarone; Ergot Derivatives; Etravirine; Midazolam; Nilotinib; Nisoldipine; Pazopanib; Pimozide; Posaconazole; Ranolazine; Romidepsin; St Johns Wort; Tolvaptan; Triazolam

Increased Effect/Toxicity

Efavirenz may increase the levels/effects of: Alcohol (Ethyl); Carvedilol; Cisapride; CNS Depressants; Colchicine; CYP2C19 Substrates; CYP2C9 Substrates (High risk); CYP3A4 Substrates; Eplerenone; Ergot Derivatives; Etravirine; FentaNYL; Halofantrine; Methotrimeprazine; Midazolam; Paclitaxel; Phenytoin; Pimecrolimus; Pimozide; Protease Inhibitors; Ranolazine; Salmeterol; Saxagliptin; Tolvaptan; Triazolam; Vitamin K Antagonists

The levels/effects of Efavirenz may be increased by: CYP2B6 Inhibitors (Moderate); CYP2B6 Inhibitors (Strong); Darunavir; Methotrimeprazine; Quazepam; Voriconazole

Decreased Effect

Efavirenz may decrease the levels/effects of: Atazanavir; Caspofungin; Clopidogrel; CycloSPORINE; CycloSPORINE (Systemic); CYP3A4 Substrates; Darunavir; Dienogest; Dronedarone; Etonogestrel; Etravirine; Everolimus; GuanFACINE; Itraconazole; Lopinavir; Maraviroc; Methadone; NIFEdipine; Nilotinib; Nisoldipine; Norgestimate; Pazopanib; Posaconazole; Protease Inhibitors; Raltegravir; Ranolazine; Rifabutin; Romidepsin; Saxagliptin; Sertraline; Sirolimus; Sorafenib; Tacrolimus; Tacrolimus (Systemic); Tadalafil; Tolvaptan; Voriconazole

The levels/effects of Efavirenz may be decreased by: CYP2B6 Inducers (Strong); CYP3A4 Inducers (Strong); Deferasirox; Phenytoin; Rifabutin; Rifampin; St Johns Wort

Food Interactions

Capsules: Compared to fasting conditions, high fat/high caloric meals increase efavirenz AUC by 22% and peak concentrations by 39%; reduced fat/normal caloric meals increase efavirenz AUC by 17% and peak concentrations by 51%

Tablets: Compared to fasting conditions, high fat/high caloric meals increase efavirenz AUC by 28% and peak concentrations by 79%

Stability Store at 25°C (77°F); with excursions permitted to 15°C to 30°C (59°F to 86°F)

Mechanism of Action A non-nucleoside reverse transcriptase inhibitor which specifically binds to HIV-1 reverse transcriptase and blocks RNA-dependent and DNA-dependent DNA polymerase activity including HIV-1 replication; does not require intracellular phosphorylation for antiviral activity

Pharmacokinetics (Adult data unless noted) Note: Pharmacokinetics in children ≥3 years of age are thought to be similar to adults

Distribution: CSF concentrations are 0.69% of plasma (range 0.26% to 1.2%); however, CSF:plasma concentration ratio is 3 times higher than free fraction in plasma

Protein binding: 99.5% to 99.8%, primarily to albumin

Metabolism: In the liver, primarily by cytochrome P450 enzymes (mainly isoenzymes CYP3A4 and CYP2B6) to hydroxylated metabolites which then undergo glucuronidation; induces P450 enzymes and its own metabolism

Bioavailability: 42% (increased with fatty meal)

Half-life:

Single dose: 52-76 hours

Multiple dose: 40-55 hours

Time to peak serum concentration: 3-5 hours

Elimination: <1% excreted unchanged in the urine; 14% to 34% excreted as metabolites in the urine and 16% to 61% in feces (primarily as unchanged drug)

Usual Dosage Oral: (use in combination with other antiretroviral agents)

Neonates, Infants, and Children <3 years: Not recommended for use; limited pharmacokinetic data demonstrate that target trough concentrations are difficult to achieve in children <3 years of age; additional studies are needed to determine the appropriate dosage

Children ≥3 years: Dose according to body weight:
10 kg to <15 kg: 200 mg once daily
15 kg to <20 kg: 250 mg once daily
20 kg to <25 kg: 300 mg once daily
25 kg to <32.5 kg: 350 mg once daily
32.5 kg to <40 kg: 400 mg once daily
≥40 kg: 600 mg once daily
Adults: 600 mg once daily

Dosage adjustment for concomitant voriconazole: Adults: Reduce efavirenz dose to 300 mg once daily (use capsule formulation) and increase voriconazole dose to 400 mg every 12 hours

Dosage adjustment in renal impairment: No adjustment required

Dosage comments in hepatic impairment: Use with caution; limited clinical experience; no dosing adjustments are currently available

Administration Administer dose at bedtime to decrease CNS adverse effects; administer with water on an empty stomach (administration with food may increase efavirenz concentrations and adverse effects; see Food Interactions). Capsules may be opened and added to small amount of food or liquid, but efavirenz tastes peppery (grape jelly may be used to improve taste). Tablets should not be broken.

Monitoring Parameters Signs and symptoms of rash; viral load; CD4 counts; serum amylase; liver enzymes in patients with known or suspected hepatitis B or C, those receiving concomitant ritonavir, and those receiving other hepatotoxic medications; serum cholesterol, triglycerides

Test Interactions False positive test for cannabinoids using the CEDIA DAU Multilevel THC assay. False-positive tests for benzodiazepines have been reported and are likely due to the 8-hydroxy-efavirenz major metabolite.

Patient Information May cause drowsiness and impair ability to perform activities requiring mental alertness or physical coordination; avoid alcohol; efavirenz is not a cure for HIV; notify physician immediately if rash develops; some medicines should not be taken with efavirenz; report the use of other medications, nonprescription medications and herbal or natural products to your physician and pharmacist; avoid the herbal medicine St John's wort; inform your physician if you have ever had seizures or if you now take seizure medications (blood samples to check the level of seizure medications may be needed more frequently when taking efavirenz); take efavirenz everyday as prescribed; do not change dose or discontinue without physician's advice; if a dose is missed, take it as soon as possible, then return to normal dosing schedule; if a dose is skipped, do **not** double the next dose. Do not take Sustiva® with other efavirenz-containing medications (eg, Atripla®).

HIV medications may cause changes in body fat, including an increase in fat in the upper back and neck, breasts, and trunk; a loss of fat from the face, arms, and legs may also occur. Due to possible teratogenic effects, female patients of childbearing potential should be tested for pregnancy prior to starting efavirenz and should avoid pregnancy while receiving this drug and for 12 weeks after discontinuation of this drug; barrier contraception with other (hormonal) methods of contraception should be used (see Precautions).

Additional Information An oral liquid formulation of efavirenz (strawberry/mint-flavored solution) is available on an investigational basis from Bristol-Myers Squibb Company as part of an expanded access program for HIV-infected children and adolescents 3-16 years of age; for further details call 877-372-7097. **Note:** The bioavailability of the investigational liquid was found to be 20% lower than that of the capsules in adult volunteers; a recent pediatric study used initial doses of the liquid formulation

that were 20% higher than pediatric capsule doses; these higher doses resulted in AUC values that were similar to AUCs achieved with the capsules (see Starr, 2002).

Early virologic failure and rapid emergence of resistant mutations have been observed in therapy-naive adult HIV patients treated with tenofovir, didanosine enteric-coated beadlets (Videx® EC), and either efavirenz or nevirapine; the combination of tenofovir, didanosine, and any non-nucleoside reverse transcriptase inhibitor is **not** recommended as initial antiretroviral therapy.

Dosage Forms Excipient information presented when available (limited, particularly for generics); consult specific product labeling. [DSC] = Discontinued product
Capsule:
Sustiva®: 50 mg; 100 mg [DSC]; 200 mg
Tablet:
Sustiva®: 600 mg

References
Adkins JC and Noble S, "Efavirenz," *Drugs,* 1998, 56(6):1055-64.

Briars LA, Hilao JJ, and Kraus DM, "A Review of Pediatric Human Immunodeficiency Virus Infection," *Journal of Pharmacy Practice,* 2004, 17(6):407-31.

Collura JM and Kraus DM, "New Pediatric Antiretroviral Agents," *J Pediatr Health Care,* 2000, 14(4):183-90.

Maddocks S and Dwyer D, "The Role of Non-Nucleoside Reverse Transcriptase Inhibitors in Children With HIV-1 Infection," *Paediatr Drugs,* 2001, 3(9):681-702.

Panel on Antiretroviral Guidelines for Adults and Adolescents, "Guidelines for the Use of Antiretroviral Agents in HIV-Infected Adults and Adolescents," December 1, 2009, http://www.aidsinfo.nih.gov.

Piscitelli SC, Burstein AH, Chaitt D, et al, "Indinavir Concentrations and St John's Wort," *Lancet,* 2000, 355(9203):547-8.

Starr SE, Fletcher CV, Spector SA, et al, "Combination Therapy With Efavirenz, Nelfinavir, and Nucleoside Reverse-transcriptase Inhibitors in Children Infected with Human Immunodeficiency Virus Type 1. Pediatric AIDS Clinical Trials Group 382 Team," *N Engl J Med,* 1999, 341(25):1874-81.

Starr SE, Fletcher CV, Spector SA, et al, "Efavirenz Liquid Formulation in Human Immunodeficiency Virus-Infected Children," *Pediatr Infect Dis J,* 2002, 21(7):659-63.

Working Group on Antiretroviral Therapy and Medical Management of HIV-Infected Children, "Guidelines for the Use of Antiretroviral Agents in Pediatric HIV Infection," February 23, 2009. Available at http://www.aidsinfo.nih.gov.

Efavirenz, Emtricitabine, and Tenofovir
(e FAV e renz, em trye SYE ta been, & te NOE fo veer)

Related Information
Adult and Adolescent HIV *on page 1620*
Management of Healthcare Worker Exposures to HBV, HCV, and HIV *on page 1661*
Pediatric HIV *on page 1613*
Perinatal HIV *on page 1628*

U.S. Brand Names Atripla®

Canadian Brand Names Atripla®

Therapeutic Category Antiretroviral Agent; HIV Agents (Anti-HIV Agents); Non-nucleoside Reverse Transcriptase Inhibitor (NNRTI); Nucleoside Reverse Transcriptase Inhibitor (NRTI); Nucleotide Reverse Transcriptase Inhibitor (NRTI)

Generic Available No

Use Treatment of HIV infection either alone or in combination with other antiretroviral agents (FDA approved in ages ≥18 years) (**Note:** HIV regimens consisting of **three** antiretroviral agents are strongly recommended)

Pregnancy Risk Factor D

Pregnancy Considerations See individual agents.

Lactation Excretion in breast milk unknown/contraindicated

Breast-Feeding Considerations HIV-infected mothers are discouraged from breast-feeding to decrease potential transmission of HIV.

Contraindications Hypersensitivity to efavirenz, emtricitabine, tenofovir, or any component; concurrent therapy with bepridil, cisapride, midazolam, pimozide, triazolam, ergot derivatives, voriconazole, or St John's wort

Warnings Cases of lactic acidosis, severe hepatomegaly with steatosis, and death have been reported in patients receiving nucleoside analogues **[U.S. Boxed Warning]**; most of these cases have been in women; prolonged nucleoside use, obesity, and prior liver disease may be risk factors; use with extreme caution in patients with other risk factors for liver disease; discontinue therapy in patients who develop laboratory or clinical evidence of lactic acidosis or pronounced hepatotoxicity. Testing for hepatitis B is recommended prior to the initiation of efavirenz, emtricitabine, and tenofovir therapy; HIV-infected patients who are coinfected with hepatitis B may experience severe acute exacerbations of hepatitis (ie, clinical symptoms or laboratory evidence of hepatitis) when emtricitabine or tenofovir is discontinued **[U.S. Boxed Warning]**; liver decompensation and hepatic failure have been associated with exacerbation of hepatitis B in patients treated with emtricitabine following discontinuation of emtricitabine; monitor patients closely for at least several months after discontinuation of emtricitabine and tenofovir; initiate anti-hepatitis B therapy if needed.

Efavirenz is a mixed inducer/inhibitor of CYP450 enzymes and numerous drug interactions occur. Due to potential serious and/or life-threatening drug interactions, certain drugs are contraindicated (see Contraindications and Drug Interactions; significant drug interactions may also occur with tenofovir). Emtricitabine and tenofovir are primarily eliminated by the kidney; while efavirenz is not; do not use this fixed dose combination of efavirenz, emtricitabine, and tenofovir in patients with moderate or severe renal impairment (Cl$_{cr}$ <50 mL/minute); monitor renal function closely; renal dysfunction, including acute renal failure and Fanconi syndrome (renal tubular injury with severe hypophosphatemia) has been reported with tenofovir use; this may occur especially in patients with renal disease, underlying systemic disease, or those taking nephrotoxic medications; adults with a low body weight and those taking medications that increase tenofovir serum concentration may also be at increased risk for tenofovir-associated nephrotoxicity; avoid tenofovir in patients with concomitant or recent use of nephrotoxic agents; cases of nephrotoxicity have been reported in adolescents receiving tenofovir-containing regimens; evaluate and monitor renal function in all patients receiving tenofovir (regardless of age).

Teratogenic effects have been observed in primates receiving efavirenz; human birth defects following efavirenz exposure in the first trimester have been reported, including cases of neural tube defects (including meningomyelocele and Dandy-Walker malformation); women of childbearing potential should be tested for pregnancy before starting efavirenz; women receiving efavirenz should avoid pregnancy while receiving this drug and for 12 weeks after discontinuation of this drug (due to long half-life of efavirenz); barrier contraception in combination with other (hormonal) methods of contraception should be used; avoid use of efavirenz during the first trimester of pregnancy and in women with significant childbearing potential; women who use this drug during the first trimester or who become pregnant while taking this drug should be apprised of the potential harm to the fetus.

Atripla® contains efavirenz, emtricitabine, and tenofovir as a fixed-dose combination; do not administer Atripla® with efavirenz, emtricitabine, tenofovir, or lamivudine-containing products.

Precautions Use efavirenz, emtricitabine, and tenofovir with caution in patients with hepatic impairment. Use efavirenz with caution in patients with a history of mental illness or substance abuse (delusions, inappropriate behavior, and severe acute depression may occur). Serious CNS and psychiatric symptoms may occur (see Adverse Reactions). Use with caution in patients with a history of seizures (convulsions may occur). Efavirenz may decrease the serum concentrations of antiepileptic agents that are metabolized by the liver (monitor anticonvulsant levels periodically; see Drug Interactions). Discontinue efavirenz-containing products if severe rash (involving blistering, desquamation, mucosal involvement, or fever) occurs. Use with caution in patients with known or suspected hepatitis B or C, those receiving other hepatotoxic medications, and those with hepatic impairment; weigh risk versus benefit in patients with persistent elevations of serum transaminases (ie, >5 times normal). Cross-resistance with other non-nucleoside reverse transcriptase inhibitors may occur. Elevations of serum cholesterol and triglycerides may occur (monitor during therapy).

Emtricitabine-associated hyperpigmentation may occur at a higher frequency in pediatric patients compared to adults (see Adverse Reactions of Emtricitabine). Tenofovir-associated bone toxicity (osteomalacia and reduced bone mineral density) may occur; long-term effects in humans are not known (see Adverse Reactions and Precautions of Tenofovir); monitor for potential bone toxicities during therapy; supplementation with calcium and vitamin D may be beneficial (but has not been studied).

Fat redistribution and accumulation [ie, central obesity, peripheral wasting, facial wasting, breast enlargement, dorsocervical fat enlargement (buffalo hump), and cushingoid appearance] have been observed in patients receiving antiretroviral agents (causal relationship not established). Immune reconstitution syndrome (an acute inflammatory response to residual or indolent opportunistic infection) may occur in HIV patients during initial treatment with combination antiretroviral agents, including efavirenz, emtricitabine, and tenofovir; this syndrome may require further patient assessment and therapy. Safety and efficacy have not been established in patients <18 years of age.

Adverse Reactions See individual agents.

Drug Interactions

Metabolism/Transport Effects

Efavirenz: **Substrate** (major) of CYP2B6, 3A4; **Inhibits** CYP2C9 (moderate), 2C19 (moderate), 3A4 (moderate); **Induces** CYP2B6 (weak), 3A4 (strong)

Tenofovir: **Inhibits** CYP1A2 (weak)

Avoid Concomitant Use

Avoid concomitant use of Efavirenz, Emtricitabine, and Tenofovir with any of the following: Cisapride; Clopidogrel; Dienogest; Dronedarone; Ergot Derivatives; Etravirine; LamiVUDine; Midazolam; Nilotinib; Nisoldipine; Pazopanib; Pimozide; Posaconazole; Ranolazine; Romidepsin; St Johns Wort; Tolvaptan; Triazolam

Increased Effect/Toxicity

Efavirenz, Emtricitabine, and Tenofovir may increase the levels/effects of: Adefovir; Alcohol (Ethyl); Carvedilol; Cisapride; CNS Depressants; Colchicine; CYP2C19 Substrates; CYP2C9 Substrates (High risk); CYP3A4 Substrates; Didanosine; Eplerenone; Ergot Derivatives; Etravirine; FentaNYL; Halofantrine; Methotrimeprazine; Midazolam; Paclitaxel; Phenytoin; Pimecrolimus; Pimozide; Protease Inhibitors; Ranolazine; Salmeterol; Saxagliptin; Tolvaptan; Triazolam; Vitamin K Antagonists

The levels/effects of Efavirenz, Emtricitabine, and Tenofovir may be increased by: Acyclovir-Valacyclovir; Atazanavir; CYP2B6 Inhibitors (Moderate); CYP2B6

494

Inhibitors (Strong); Darunavir; Ganciclovir-Valganciclovir; LamiVUDine; Lopinavir; Methotrimeprazine; Protease Inhibitors; Quazepam; Ribavirin; Voriconazole

Decreased Effect

Efavirenz, Emtricitabine, and Tenofovir may decrease the levels/effects of: Atazanavir; Caspofungin; Clopidogrel; CycloSPORINE; CycloSPORINE (Systemic); CYP3A4 Substrates; Darunavir; Didanosine; Dienogest; Dronedarone; Etonogestrel; Etravirine; Everolimus; GuanFACINE; Itraconazole; Lopinavir; Maraviroc; Methadone; NIFEdipine; Nilotinib; Nisoldipine; Norgestimate; Pazopanib; Posaconazole; Protease Inhibitors; Raltegravir; Ranolazine; Rifabutin; Romidepsin; Saxagliptin; Sertraline; Sirolimus; Sorafenib; Tacrolimus; Tacrolimus (Systemic); Tadalafil; Tolvaptan; Voriconazole

The levels/effects of Efavirenz, Emtricitabine, and Tenofovir may be decreased by: Adefovir; CYP2B6 Inducers (Strong); CYP3A4 Inducers (Strong); Deferasirox; Phenytoin; Rifabutin; Rifampin; St Johns Wort

Food Interactions Effect of food on absorption of Atripla® has not been evaluated. Compared to fasting conditions, high fat/high caloric meals increase efavirenz AUC by 28% and peak concentrations by 79%. Administration of tenofovir and emtricitabine with either a high fat meal or a light meal delayed the time to peak concentrations of tenofovir; mean tenofovir AUC increased by 30% and peak concentrations increased by 15%; emtricitabine AUC and peak concentrations were not affected.

Stability Store tablets at controlled room temperature at 25°C (77°F); excursions permitted to 15°C to 30°C (59°F to 86°F). Keep container tightly closed; do not use if seal on bottle is broken or missing. Dispense only in original container.

Mechanism of Action See individual agents.

Pharmacokinetics (Adult data unless noted) One Atripla® tablet is bioequivalent to one efavirenz 600 mg tablet plus one emtricitabine 200 mg capsule plus one tenofovir 300 mg tablet (single dose study); see individual agents

Usual Dosage Oral (use in combination with other antiretroviral agents):

Children and Adolescents <18 years: Not intended for pediatric use; product is a fixed-dose combination; safety and efficacy have not been established in pediatric patients; use in pediatric patients <40 kg would result in an excessive efavirenz dose

Adolescents ≥18 years and Adults: One tablet once daily

Dosage adjustment in renal impairment: Moderate-to-severe renal impairment (Cl_{cr} <50 mL/minute): Use not recommended

Dosage adjustment in hepatic impairment: Use with caution; very limited clinical experience; no dosing adjustments are currently available

Administration Administer dose at bedtime to decrease CNS adverse effects; administer with water on an empty stomach (administration with food may increase efavirenz concentrations and adverse effects; see Food Interactions).

Monitoring Parameters CBC with differential, hemoglobin, MCV, reticulocyte count, liver enzymes, serum cholesterol, triglycerides, amylase, bilirubin; renal function; signs and symptoms of rash, lactic acidosis, and pronounced hepatotoxicity; CD4 cell count, HIV RNA plasma levels; monitor for potential bone and renal abnormalities. Calculate creatinine clearance in all patients prior to starting therapy and as clinically needed; monitor for alterations in calculated creatinine clearance and serum phosphorus in patients at risk or with a history of renal dysfunction and patients receiving concurrent nephrotoxic agents. Test patients for hepatitis B (HBV) prior to starting therapy; in patients coinfected with HBV, monitor hepatic function closely (clinically and with

laboratory tests) for at least several months after discontinuing therapy (see Warnings).

Test Interactions Efavirenz: False positive test for cannabinoids using the CEDIA DAU Multilevel THC assay. False-positive results with other assays for cannabinoids have not been observed.

Patient Information Before starting efavirenz, emtricitabine, and tenofovir, inform your physician about your medical conditions, including any liver or kidney problems. Patients with HIV should be tested for hepatitis B before starting therapy. Due to possible teratogenic effects, female patients of childbearing potential should be tested for pregnancy prior to starting efavirenz-containing products and should avoid pregnancy while receiving this drug and for 12 weeks after discontinuation of this drug; barrier contraception with other (hormonal) methods of contraception should be used (see Warnings).

Efavirenz, emtricitabine, and tenofovir is not a cure for HIV; take efavirenz, emtricitabine, and tenofovir every day as prescribed; do not change dose or discontinue without physician's advice; if a dose is missed, take it as soon as possible, then return to normal dosing schedule; if a dose is skipped, do **not** double the next dose. Some medicines should not be taken with this product; report the use of other medications, nonprescription medications, and herbal or natural products to your physician and pharmacist; avoid alcohol and the herbal medicine St John's wort. Inform your physician if you have ever had seizures or if you now take seizure medications (blood samples to check the level of seizure medications may be needed more frequently when taking efavirenz-containing products).

Notify physician immediately if rash develops. Notify physician if persistent severe abdominal pain, nausea, vomiting, rash, numbness, or tingling occur. May cause dizziness or drowsiness and impair ability to perform activities requiring mental alertness or physical coordination. Long-term effects are not known. HIV medications may cause changes in body fat, including an increase in fat in the upper back and neck, breasts, and trunk; a loss of fat from the face, arms, and legs may also occur. Some HIV medications (including emtricitabine and tenofovir) may cause a serious, but rare, condition called lactic acidosis with an increase in liver size (hepatomegaly). Tenofovir may decrease bone mineral density; bone mineral density monitoring may be needed in patients at risk. Do not take Atripla® with other efavirenz, emtricitabine, or tenofovir-containing medications (eg, Emtriva®, Sustiva®, Truvada®, or Viread®) or with medications that contain lamivudine (eg, Epivir®, Epivir-HBV®, Combivir®, Epzicom®, or Trizivir®).

Dosage Forms Excipient information presented when available (limited, particularly for generics); consult specific product labeling.

Tablet:

Atripla®: Efavirenz 600 mg, emtricitabine 200 mg, and tenofovir disoproxil fumarate 300 mg

References

Panel on Antiretroviral Guidelines for Adults and Adolescents, "Guidelines for the Use of Antiretroviral Agents in HIV-Infected Adults and Adolescents," December 1, 2009, http://www.aidsinfo.nih.gov.

Working Group on Antiretroviral Therapy and Medical Management of HIV-Infected Children, "Guidelines for the Use of Antiretroviral Agents in Pediatric HIV Infection," February 23, 2009. Available at http://www.aidsinfo.nih.gov.

◆ **Efavirenz, FTC, and TDF** *see* Efavirenz, Emtricitabine, and Tenofovir *on page 493*

◆ **Efavirenz, TDF, and FTC** *see* Efavirenz, Emtricitabine, and Tenofovir *on page 493*

◆ **Efavirenz, Tenofovir, and Emtricitabine** *see* Efavirenz, Emtricitabine, and Tenofovir *on page 493*

- **Effexor®** *see* Venlafaxine *on page 1412*
- **Effexor XR®** *see* Venlafaxine *on page 1412*
- **Effexor® XR (Can)** *see* Venlafaxine *on page 1412*
- **Eformoterol and Budesonide** *see* Budesonide and Formoterol *on page 210*
- **Efudex®** *see* Fluorouracil *on page 598*
- **E-Gems® [OTC]** *see* Vitamin E *on page 1427*
- **E-Gems Elite® [OTC]** *see* Vitamin E *on page 1427*
- **E-Gems Plus® [OTC]** *see* Vitamin E *on page 1427*
- **EHDP** *see* Etidronate Disodium *on page 549*
- **Elavil** *see* Amitriptyline *on page 89*
- **Electrolyte Lavage Solution** *see* Polyethylene Glycol-Electrolyte Solution *on page 1129*
- **Elestat™** *see* Epinastine *on page 510*
- **Elestrin™** *see* Estradiol *on page 536*
- **Elidel®** *see* Pimecrolimus *on page 1111*
- **Eligard®** *see* Leuprolide *on page 805*
- **Elimite®** *see* Permethrin *on page 1094*
- **Elitek®** *see* Rasburicase *on page 1203*
- **Elixophyllin®** *see* Theophylline *on page 1335*
- **Elocom® (Can)** *see* Mometasone Furoate *on page 942*
- **Elocon®** *see* Mometasone Furoate *on page 942*
- **Eloxatin®** *see* Oxaliplatin *on page 1030*
- **Elspar®** *see* Asparaginase *on page 139*
- **Eltor® (Can)** *see* Pseudoephedrine *on page 1183*
- **Eltroxin® (Can)** *see* Levothyroxine *on page 816*
- **Emend®** *see* Aprepitant/Fosaprepitant *on page 125*
- **EMLA®** *see* Lidocaine and Prilocaine *on page 823*
- **Emo-Cort® (Can)** *see* Hydrocortisone *on page 685*

Emtricitabine (em trye SYE ta been)

Related Information
Adult and Adolescent HIV *on page 1620*
Management of Healthcare Worker Exposures to HBV, HCV, and HIV *on page 1661*
Pediatric HIV *on page 1613*
Perinatal HIV *on page 1628*
U.S. Brand Names Emtriva®
Canadian Brand Names Emtriva®
Therapeutic Category Antiretroviral Agent; HIV Agents (Anti-HIV Agents); Nucleoside Reverse Transcriptase Inhibitor (NRTI)
Generic Available No
Use Treatment of HIV infection in combination with other antiretroviral agents. (**Note:** HIV regimens consisting of **three** antiretroviral agents are strongly recommended); has been used investigationally for the treatment of chronic hepatitis B infection in adults
Pregnancy Risk Factor B
Pregnancy Considerations Adverse events were not observed in animal studies. No increased risk of overall birth defects has been observed according to data collected by the antiretroviral pregnancy registry. Cases of fatal and nonfatal lactic acidosis, with or without pancreatitis, have been reported in pregnant women receiving reverse transcriptase inhibitors. It is not known if pregnancy itself potentiates this known side effect; however, pregnant women may be at increased risk of lactic acidosis and liver damage. Hepatic enzymes and electrolytes should be monitored frequently during the third trimester of pregnancy. A pharmacokinetic study shows a slight decrease in emtricitabine serum levels during the third trimester; however, there is no clear need to adjust the dose. The Perinatal HIV Guidelines Working Group considers emtricitabine to be an alternative NRTI in dual nucleoside combination regimens. Health professionals are encouraged to contact the antiretroviral pregnancy registry to monitor outcomes of pregnant women exposed to antiretroviral medications (1-800-258-4263 or www.-APRegistry.com).

Lactation Excretion in breast milk unknown/contraindicated

Breast-Feeding Considerations In infants born to mothers who are HIV positive, HAART while breast-feeding may decrease postnatal infection. However, maternal or infant antiretroviral therapy does not completely eliminate the risk of postnatal HIV transmission.

In the United States where formula is accessible, affordable, safe, and sustainable, complete avoidance of breast-feeding by HIV-infected women is recommended to decrease potential transmission of HIV.

Contraindications Hypersensitivity to emtricitabine or any component

Warnings Cases of lactic acidosis, severe hepatomegaly with steatosis, and death have been reported in patients receiving nucleoside analogues **[U.S. Boxed Warning]**; most of these cases have been in women; prolonged nucleoside use, obesity, and prior liver disease may be risk factors; use with extreme caution in patients with other risk factors for liver disease; discontinue therapy in patients who develop laboratory or clinical evidence of lactic acidosis or pronounced hepatotoxicity. Testing for hepatitis B is recommended prior to the initiation of emtricitabine therapy; HIV-infected patients who are coinfected with hepatitis B may experience severe acute exacerbations of hepatitis (ie, clinical symptoms or laboratory evidence of hepatitis) when emtricitabine is discontinued **[U.S. Boxed Warning]**; monitor patients for at least several months after discontinuation of emtricitabine; initiate anti-hepatitis B therapy if needed

Precautions Use with caution and reduce dosage in patients with impaired renal function. Fat redistribution and accumulation [ie, central obesity, peripheral wasting, facial wasting, breast enlargement, dorsocervical fat enlargement (buffalo hump), and cushingoid appearance] have been observed in patients receiving antiretroviral agents (causal relationship not established). Immune reconstitution syndrome (an acute inflammatory response to residual or indolent opportunistic infection) may occur in HIV patients during initial treatment with combination antiretroviral agents, including emtricitabine; this syndrome may require further patient assessment and therapy. Hyperpigmentation may occur at a higher frequency in pediatric patients compared to adults (see Adverse Reactions). Do not administer with other emtricitabine or lamivudine-containing products (see Drug Interactions). Safety and efficacy have not been established in infants ≤3 months of age; recommended dosing is based on pharmacokinetic studies.

Adverse Reactions
Central nervous system: Headache, dizziness, insomnia, abnormal dreams, depression, fever
Dermatologic: Rash, pruritus, maculopapular rash, vesiculobullous rash, pustular rash; hyperpigmentation [incidence: Children: 32%; adults: 2% to 6% (may be higher in African Americans); hyperpigmentation occurs primarily of palms and/or soles but may include tongue, arms, lips, and nails; generally mild, asymptomatic, nonprogressive, and without associated local reactions such as pruritus or rash]
Endocrine & metabolic: Serum triglycerides elevated, lactic acidosis, hyperglycemia; fat redistribution and accumulation (see Precautions)
Gastrointestinal: Diarrhea, nausea, abdominal pain, dyspepsia, vomiting, gastroenteritis
Hematologic: Neutropenia, anemia

Hepatic: ALT, AST, CPK, bilirubin, lipase, and amylase elevated; hepatic steatosis, severe hepatomegaly

Neuromuscular & skeletal: Paresthesias, peripheral neuropathy, asthenia, myalgia, arthralgia, CPK elevated

Respiratory: Cough, rhinitis

Miscellaneous: Hypersensitivity reaction, immune reconstitution syndrome

Drug Interactions

Avoid Concomitant Use

Avoid concomitant use of Emtricitabine with any of the following: LamiVUDine

Increased Effect/Toxicity

The levels/effects of Emtricitabine may be increased by: Ganciclovir-Valganciclovir; LamiVUDine; Ribavirin

Decreased Effect There are no known significant interactions involving a decrease in effect.

Food Interactions

Capsules: A high fat meal decreases peak plasma concentrations, but not the extent of absorption (AUC not affected)

Oral solution: Neither a high-fat nor a low-fat meal affected peak plasma concentrations or AUC

Stability

Capsules: Store at 25°C (77°F); excursions permitted to 15°C to 30°C (59°F to 86°F).

Oral solution: Store refrigerated at 2°C to 8°C (36°F to 46°F); use within 3 months if stored at room temperature [25°C (77°F)]

Mechanism of Action A synthetic nucleoside analogue that is phosphorylated by intracellular kinases to the active triphosphate metabolite (emtricitabine 5'-triphosphate) which inhibits HIV-1 reverse transcription via viral DNA chain termination after incorporation of the nucleoside analogue. Emtricitabine triphosphate is a weak inhibitor of mammalian DNA polymerase alpha-, beta-, epsilon- and mitochondrial DNA polymerase gamma.

Pharmacokinetics (Adult data unless noted)

Absorption: Rapid, extensive

Distribution: Unknown if distributes into breast milk

Protein binding: <4%

Metabolism: Converted intracellularly to the active triphosphate form; undergoes minimal biotransformation via oxidation and glucuronide conjugation

Bioavailability:

Capsules: 93%

Oral solution: 75%

Note: Relative bioavailability of solution to capsule: 80%

Half-life: Normal renal function:

Children and Adolescents: Elimination half-life (emtricitabine):

Single dose: 11 hours

Multiple dose: 7.9-9.5 hours

Infants 0-3 months (n=20; median age: 26 days): 12.1 ± 3.1 hours

Infants 3-24 months (n=14): 8.9 ± 3.2 hours

Children 25 months to 6 years (n=19): 11.3 ± 6.4 hours

Children 7-12 years (n=17): 8.2 ± 3.2 hours

Adolescents 13-17 years (n=27): 8.9 ± 3.3 hours

Adults:

Elimination half-life (emtricitabine): 10 hours

Intracellular half-life (emtricitabine 5'-triphosphate): 39 hours

Time to peak serum concentration: 1-2 hours

Elimination: Urine (86% of dose, primarily as unchanged drug; 13% as metabolites; 9% of dose as oxidative metabolite; 4% as glucuronide metabolite); feces (14% of dose)

Clearance: Renal clearance is > creatinine clearance; thus, emtricitabine may be eliminated by both glomerular filtration and active tubular secretion

Dialysis: 30% of the dose is removed by hemodialysis (over 3 hours)

Usual Dosage Oral (use in combination with other antiretroviral agents):

Neonates and Infants 0-3 months: Oral solution: 3 mg/kg once daily

Infants ≥3 months, Children, and Adolescents <18 years: Oral solution: 6 mg/kg once daily (maximum dose: 240 mg once daily)

Children >33 kg who can swallow capsule intact: Capsule: 200 mg once daily

Adolescents ≥18 years and Adults:

Capsules: 200 mg once daily

Oral solution: 240 mg once daily

Dosage adjustment in renal impairment: Monitor clinical response and renal function closely:

Neonates, Infants, Children, and Adolescents <18 years: Specific dose adjustment not yet established; consider a reduction in the dose and/or an increase in the dosing interval similar to dosage adjustments for adults

Adolescents ≥18 years and Adults:

Cl_{cr} 30-49 mL/minute: Capsule: 200 mg every 48 hours; oral solution: 120 mg every 24 hours

Cl_{cr} 15-29 mL/minute: Capsule: 200 mg every 72 hours; oral solution: 80 mg every 24 hours

Cl_{cr} <15 mL/minute (including hemodialysis patients): **Note:** If dose is given on day of dialysis, administer dose after dialysis: Capsule: 200 mg every 96 hours; oral solution: 60 mg every 24 hours

Dosage adjustment in hepatic impairment: No adjustment required.

Administration May be administered without regard to food

Monitoring Parameters CBC with differential, ALT, AST, serum amylase, bilirubin; signs and symptoms of lactic acidosis, and pronounced hepatotoxicity; CD4 cell count, HIV RNA plasma levels; patients should be screened for hepatitis B infection before starting emtricitabine (see Warnings)

Patient Information Emtricitabine is not a cure for HIV. Notify physician if persistent severe abdominal pain, nausea, vomiting, rash, numbness, or tingling occur. May cause dizziness and impair ability to perform activities requiring mental alertness or physical coordination. Take emtricitabine every day as prescribed; do not change dose or discontinue without physician's advice; if a dose is missed, take it as soon as possible, then return to normal dosing schedule; if a dose is skipped, do **not** double the next dose.

HIV medications may cause changes in body fat, including an increase in fat in the upper back and neck, breasts, and trunk; a loss of fat from the face, arms, and legs may also occur. Some HIV medications (including emtricitabine) may cause a serious, but rare, condition called lactic acidosis with an increase in liver size (hepatomegaly). Before starting emtricitabine, inform your physician about your medical conditions, including any liver or kidney problems. Do not take Emtriva® with other emtricitabine-containing medications (eg, Atripla® or Truvada®) or with medications that contain lamivudine (eg, Epivir®, Epivir-HBV®, Combivir®, Epzicom®, or Trizivir®).

Additional Information Emtricitabine is the (-) enantiomer of 2', 3'-dideoxy-5-fluoro-3'-thiacytidine (FTC), a fluorinated derivative of lamivudine.

Mutation in the HIV reverse transcriptase gene at codon 184, M184V/I (ie, substitution of methionine by valine or isoleucine) is associated with resistance to emtricitabine. Emtricitabine-resistant isolates (M184V/I) are cross-resistant to lamivudine and zalcitabine. HIV-1 isolates containing the K65R mutation show reduced susceptibility to emtricitabine.

Dosage Forms Excipient information presented when available (limited, particularly for generics); consult specific product labeling.
Capsule:
Emtriva®: 200 mg
Solution:
Emtriva®: 10 mg/mL (170 mL) [contains propylene glycol; cotton candy flavor]

References

Bang LM and Scott LJ, "Emtricitabine: An Antiretroviral Agent for HIV Infection," *Drugs*, 2003, 63(22):2413-24.

Briars LA, Hilao JJ, and Kraus DM, "A Review of Pediatric Human Immunodeficiency Virus Infection," *Journal of Pharmacy Practice*, 2004, 17(6):407-31.

Frampton JE and Perry CM, "Emtricitabine: A Review of Its Use in the Management of HIV Infection," *Drugs*, 2005, 65(10):1427-48.

Morris JL and Kraus DM, "New Antiretroviral Therapies for Pediatric HIV Infection," *J Pediatr Pharmacol Ther*, 2005, 10:215-47.

Panel on Antiretroviral Guidelines for Adults and Adolescents, "Guidelines for the Use of Antiretroviral Agents in HIV-Infected Adults and Adolescents," December 1, 2009, http://www.aidsinfo.nih.gov.

Wang LH, Wiznia AA, Rathore MH, et al, "Pharmacokinetics and Safety of Single Oral Doses of Emtricitabine in Human Immunodeficiency Virus-Infected Children," *Antimicrob Agents Chemother*, 2004, 48 (1):183-91.

Working Group on Antiretroviral Therapy and Medical Management of HIV-Infected Children, "Guidelines for the Use of Antiretroviral Agents in Pediatric HIV Infection," February 23, 2009. Available at http://www.aidsinfo.nih.gov.

Emtricitabine and Tenofovir
(em trye SYE ta been & te NOE fo veer)

Related Information

Adult and Adolescent HIV *on page 1620*
Management of Healthcare Worker Exposures to HBV, HCV, and HIV *on page 1661*
Pediatric HIV *on page 1613*
Perinatal HIV *on page 1628*

U.S. Brand Names Truvada®

Canadian Brand Names Truvada®

Therapeutic Category Antiretroviral Agent; HIV Agents (Anti-HIV Agents); Nucleoside Reverse Transcriptase Inhibitor (NRTI); Nucleotide Reverse Transcriptase Inhibitor (NRTI)

Generic Available No

Use Treatment of HIV infection in combination with other antiretroviral agents (**Note:** HIV regimens consisting of **three** antiretroviral agents are strongly recommended)

Pregnancy Risk Factor B

Pregnancy Considerations Refer to individual agents.

Lactation Excretion in breast milk unknown/not recommended

Breast-Feeding Considerations HIV-infected women are discouraged from breast-feeding to decrease the potential transmission of HIV.

Contraindications Hypersensitivity to emtricitabine, tenofovir, or any component

Warnings Cases of lactic acidosis, severe hepatomegaly with steatosis, and death have been reported in patients receiving nucleoside analogues (including tenofovir) **[U.S. Boxed Warning]**; most of these cases have been in women; prolonged nucleoside use, obesity, and prior liver disease may be risk factors; use with extreme caution in patients with other risk factors for liver disease; discontinue therapy in patients who develop laboratory or clinical evidence of lactic acidosis or pronounced hepatotoxicity. Testing for hepatitis B is recommended prior to the initiation of emtricitabine and tenofovir therapy; HIV-infected patients who are coinfected with hepatitis B may experience severe acute exacerbations of hepatitis (ie, clinical symptoms or laboratory evidence of hepatitis) when emtricitabine and tenofovir is discontinued **[U.S. Boxed Warning]**; monitor patients closely for at least several months after discontinuation of emtricitabine and tenofovir; initiate anti-hepatitis B therapy if needed.

Both emtricitabine and tenofovir are primarily eliminated by the kidney; do not use in patients with severe renal impairment (Cl_{cr} < 30 mL/minute or patients requiring hemodialysis); use with caution and adjust dose in patients with Cl_{cr} 30-49 mL/minute; monitor renal function closely; renal dysfunction, including acute renal failure and Fanconi syndrome (renal tubular injury with severe hypophosphatemia) has been reported with tenofovir use; this may occur especially in patients with renal disease, underlying systemic disease, or those taking nephrotoxic medications; adults with a low body weight and those taking medications that increase tenofovir serum concentration may also be at increased risk for tenofovir-associated nephrotoxicity; avoid tenofovir in patients with concomitant or recent use of nephrotoxic agents; cases of nephrotoxicity have been reported in adolescents receiving tenofovir-containing regimens; evaluate and monitor renal function in all patients receiving tenofovir (regardless of age).

Truvada® is not recommended as a component of a triple nucleoside regimen; Truvada® contains emtricitabine and tenofovir as a fixed-dose combination; do not administer Truvada® with adefovir, emtricitabine, tenofovir, or lamivudine-containing products.

Precautions Use with caution in patients with hepatic impairment. Significant drug interactions may occur (see Drug Interactions). Fat redistribution and accumulation [ie, central obesity, peripheral wasting, facial wasting, breast enlargement, dorsocervical fat enlargement (buffalo hump), and cushingoid appearance] have been observed in patients receiving antiretroviral agents (causal relationship not established). Immune reconstitution syndrome (an acute inflammatory response to residual or indolent opportunistic infection) may occur in HIV patients during initial treatment with combination antiretroviral agents, including emtricitabine and tenofovir; this syndrome may require further patient assessment and therapy. Emtricitabine-associated hyperpigmentation may occur at a higher frequency in pediatric patients compared to adults (see Adverse Reactions of Emtricitabine). Tenofovir-associated bone toxicity (osteomalacia and reduced bone mineral density) may occur; long-term effects in humans are not known (see Adverse Reactions and Precautions of Tenofovir); monitor for potential bone toxicities during therapy; supplementation with calcium and vitamin D may be beneficial (but has not been studied). Safety and efficacy have not been established in patients <18 years of age.

The use of antiretroviral regimens that only contain triple nucleoside reverse transcriptase inhibitors (NRTIs) are generally less effective than regimens containing 2 NRTIs and either a non-nucleoside reverse transcriptase inhibitor or protease inhibitor; use triple NRTI-containing regimens with great caution; early virological failure and high rates of resistance may occur; closely monitor for virologic failure and consider treatment modification

Adverse Reactions See individual agents.

Drug Interactions

Avoid Concomitant Use

Avoid concomitant use of Emtricitabine and Tenofovir with any of the following: LamiVUDine

Increased Effect/Toxicity

Emtricitabine and Tenofovir may increase the levels/effects of: Adefovir; Didanosine

The levels/effects of Emtricitabine and Tenofovir may be increased by: Acyclovir-Valacyclovir; Atazanavir; Ganciclovir-Valganciclovir; LamiVUDine; Lopinavir; Protease Inhibitors; Ribavirin

Decreased Effect
Emtricitabine and Tenofovir may decrease the levels/ effects of: Atazanavir; Didanosine; Protease Inhibitors

The levels/effects of Emtricitabine and Tenofovir may be decreased by: Adefovir

Food Interactions Compared to the fasted state, a high fat or light meal delayed the time to peak concentrations of tenofovir; mean tenofovir AUC increased by 30% and peak concentrations increased by 15%; emtricitabine AUC and peak concentrations were not affected

Stability Store tablets at controlled room temperature at 25°C (77°F); excursions permitted to 15°C to 30°C (59°F to 86°F). Keep container tightly closed; do not use if seal on bottle is broken or missing. Dispense only in original container.

Mechanism of Action See individual agents.

Pharmacokinetics (Adult data unless noted) One Truvada® tablet is bioequivalent to one emtricitabine 200 mg capsule and one tenofovir 300 mg tablet (single dose study); see individual agents

Usual Dosage Oral (in combination with other antiretroviral agents):
Children and Adolescents <18 years: Not intended for pediatric use; product is a fixed-dose combination; safety and efficacy have not been established in pediatric patients
Adolescents ≥18 years and Adults: One tablet (emtricitabine 200 mg and tenofovir 300 mg) once daily
Dosage adjustment in renal impairment: Adolescents ≥18 years and Adults: **Note:** Closely monitor clinical response and renal function in these patients (clinical effectiveness and safety of these guidelines have not been evaluated)
Cl_{cr} 30-49 mL/minute: Increase dosing interval to every 48 hours.
Cl_{cr} <30 mL/minute or patients requiring hemodialysis: Use not recommended.
Dosage adjustment in hepatic impairment: No adjustment required; use with caution.

Administration May be administered without regard to food

Monitoring Parameters CBC with differential, hemoglobin, MCV, reticulocyte count, liver enzymes, serum amylase, bilirubin, renal function; signs and symptoms of lactic acidosis, and pronounced hepatotoxicity; CD4 cell count, HIV RNA plasma levels; monitor for potential bone and renal abnormalities. Calculate creatinine clearance in all patients prior to starting therapy and as clinically needed; monitor for alterations in calculated creatinine clearance and serum phosphorus in patients at risk or with a history of renal dysfunction and patients receiving concurrent nephrotoxic agents. Test patients for hepatitis B (HBV) prior to starting therapy; in patients coinfected with HBV, monitor hepatic function closely (clinically and with laboratory tests) for at least several months after discontinuing tenofovir therapy (see Warnings).

Patient Information Emtricitabine and tenofovir is not a cure for HIV; take emtricitabine and tenofovir every day as prescribed; do **not** change dose or discontinue without physician's advice; if a dose is missed, take it as soon as possible, then return to normal dosing schedule; if a dose is skipped, do not double the next dose. Report the use of other medications, nonprescription medications, and herbal or natural products to your physician and pharmacist. Long-term effects are not known. Notify physician if persistent severe abdominal pain, nausea, vomiting, rash, numbness, or tingling occur. May cause dizziness and impair ability to perform activities requiring mental alertness or physical coordination.

HIV medications may cause changes in body fat, including an increase in fat in the upper back and neck, breasts, and trunk; a loss of fat from the face, arms, and legs may also occur. Some HIV medications (including emtricitabine and tenofovir) may cause a serious, but rare, condition called lactic acidosis with an increase in liver size (hepatomegaly). Before starting emtricitabine and tenofovir, inform your physician about your medical conditions, including any liver or kidney problems. Do not take Truvada® with other emtricitabine or tenofovir-containing medications (eg, Atripla®, Emtriva®, or Viread®) or with medications that contain lamivudine (eg, Epivir®, Epivir-HBV®, Combivir®, Epzicom®, or Trizivir®). Do not take Truvada® with adefovir (Hepsera®).

Dosage Forms Excipient information presented when available (limited, particularly for generics); consult specific product labeling.
Tablet:
Truvada®: Emtricitabine 200 mg and tenofovir disoproxil fumarate 300 mg [equivalent to 245 mg tenofovir disoproxil]

References
Panel on Antiretroviral Guidelines for Adults and Adolescents, "Guidelines for the Use of Antiretroviral Agents in HIV-Infected Adults and Adolescents," December 1, 2009, http://www.aidsinfo.nih.gov.
Working Group on Antiretroviral Therapy and Medical Management of HIV-Infected Children, "Guidelines for the Use of Antiretroviral Agents in Pediatric HIV Infection," February 23, 2009. Available at http://www.aidsinfo.nih.gov.

◆ **Emtricitabine and Tenofovir Disoproxil Fumarate** *see* Emtricitabine and Tenofovir *on page 498*

◆ **Emtricitabine, Efavirenz, and Tenofovir** *see* Efavirenz, Emtricitabine, and Tenofovir *on page 493*

◆ **Emtricitabine, Efavirenz, and Tenofovir Disoproxil Fumarate** *see* Efavirenz, Emtricitabine, and Tenofovir *on page 493*

◆ **Emtricitabine, Tenofovir, and Efavirenz** *see* Efavirenz, Emtricitabine, and Tenofovir *on page 493*

◆ **Emtriva®** *see* Emtricitabine *on page 496*

◆ **Enalaprilat** *see* Enalapril/Enalaprilat *on page 499*

Enalapril/Enalaprilat (e NAL a pril/e NAL a pril at)

Medication Safety Issues
Sound-alike/look-alike issues:
Enalapril may be confused with Anafranil®, Elavil®, Eldepryl®, ramipril

Significant differences exist between oral and I.V. dosing. Use caution when converting from one route of administration to another.

International issues:
Acepril [Hungary, Switzerland] may be confused with Accupril® which is a brand name for quinapril [U.S.]
Acepril: Brand name for enalapril [Hungary, Switzerland], but also brand name for captopril [Great Britain]; lisinopril [Malaysia]

Related Information
Antihypertensive Agents by Class *on page 1481*

U.S. Brand Names Vasotec®

Canadian Brand Names Apo-Enalapril®; CO Enalapril; Mylan-Enalapril; Novo-Enalapril; PMS-Enalapril; PRO-Enalapril; ratio-Enalapril; Riva-Enalapril; Sandoz-Enalapril; Sig-Enalapril; Taro-Enalapril; Vasotec®; Vasotec® I.V.

Therapeutic Category Angiotensin-Converting Enzyme (ACE) Inhibitor; Antihypertensive Agent

Generic Available Yes

Use Management of mild to severe hypertension, CHF, and asymptomatic left ventricular dysfunction; has also been used to treat proteinuria in steroid-resistant nephrotic syndrome patients (see Additional Information)

Pregnancy Risk Factor C (1st trimester); D (2nd and 3rd trimesters)

Pregnancy Considerations Due to adverse events observed in some animal studies, enalapril is considered pregnancy category C during the first trimester. Based on human data, enalapril is considered pregnancy category D if used during the second and third trimesters (per the manufacturer; however, one study suggests that fetal injury may occur at anytime during pregnancy). Enalaprilat, the active metabolite of enalapril, crosses the placenta. First trimester exposure to ACE inhibitors may cause major congenital malformations. An increased risk of cardiovascular and/or central nervous system malformations was observed in one study; however, an increased risk of teratogenic events was not observed in other studies. Second and third trimester use of an ACE inhibitor is associated with oligohydramnios. Oligohydramnios due to decreased fetal renal function may lead to fetal limb contractures, craniofacial deformation, and hypoplastic lung development. The use of ACE inhibitors during the second and third trimesters is also associated with anuria, hypotension, renal failure (reversible or irreversible), skull hypoplasia, and death in the fetus/neonate. Chronic maternal hypertension itself is also associated with adverse events in the fetus/infant. ACE inhibitors are not recommended during pregnancy to treat maternal hypertension or heart failure. Those who are planning a pregnancy should be considered for other medication options if an ACE inhibitor is currently prescribed or the ACE inhibitor should be discontinued as soon as possible once pregnancy is detected. The exposed fetus should be monitored for fetal growth, amniotic fluid volume, and organ formation. Infants exposed to an ACE inhibitor *in utero*, especially during the second and third trimester, should be monitored for hyperkalemia, hypotension, and oliguria.

[U.S. Boxed Warning]: Based on human data, ACE inhibitors can cause injury and death to the developing fetus when used in the second and third trimesters. ACE inhibitors should be discontinued as soon as possible once pregnancy is detected.

Lactation Enters breast milk/not recommended (AAP rates "compatible")

Breast-Feeding Considerations Enalapril and enalaprilat are excreted in breast milk. Breast-feeding is not recommended by the manufacturer. The AAP considers enalapril to be "usually compatible with breast-feeding."

Contraindications Hypersensitivity to enalapril, enalaprilat, any component (see Warnings), or other ACE inhibitors; patients with idiopathic or hereditary angioedema or a history of angioedema with ACE inhibitors

Warnings Serious adverse effects including angioedema, anaphylactoid reactions, neutropenia, agranulocytosis, hypotension, and hepatic failure may occur (see Adverse Reactions). Angioedema can occur at any time during treatment (especially following first dose). Angioedema may occur in the head, neck, extremities, or intestines; angioedema of the larynx, glottis, or tongue may cause airway obstruction, especially in patients with a history of airway surgery; prolonged monitoring may be required, even in patients with swelling of only the tongue (ie, without respiratory distress) because treatment with corticosteroids and antihistamines may not be sufficient; very rare fatalities have occurred with angioedema of the larynx or tongue; appropriate treatment (eg, establishing patent airway and/or SubQ epinephrine) should be readily available for patients with angioedema of larynx, glottis, or tongue, in whom airway obstruction is likely to occur. Risk of neutropenia may be increased in patients with renal dysfunction and especially in patients with both collagen vascular disease and renal dysfunction.

ACE inhibitors can cause injury and death to the developing fetus when used during pregnancy. ACE inhibitors should be discontinued as soon as possible

once pregnancy is detected **[U.S. Boxed Warning]**. Neonatal hypotension, skull hypoplasia, anuria, renal failure, oligohydramnios (associated with fetal limb contractures, craniofacial deformities, hypoplastic lung development), prematurity, intrauterine growth retardation, patent ductus arteriosus, and death have been reported with the use of ACE inhibitors, primarily in the second and third trimesters. The risk of neonatal toxicity has been considered less when ACE inhibitors are used in the first trimester; however, major congenital malformations have been reported. The cardiovascular and/or central nervous systems are most commonly affected.

Injectable product contains benzyl alcohol (9 mg/mL) which may cause allergic reactions in susceptible individuals; large amounts of benzyl alcohol (≥99 mg/kg/day) have been associated with a potentially fatal toxicity ("gasping syndrome") in neonates; the "gasping syndrome" consists of metabolic acidosis, respiratory distress, gasping respirations, CNS dysfunction (including convulsions, intracranial hemorrhage), hypotension and cardiovascular collapse; use enalaprilat products containing benzyl alcohol with caution in neonates; *in vitro* and animal studies have shown that benzoate, a metabolite of benzyl alcohol, displaces bilirubin from protein binding sites

Precautions Use with caution and modify dosage in patients with renal impairment, especially renal artery stenosis; elevated BUN and S_{cr} may occur in these patients; dosage reduction or discontinuation of enalapril or discontinuation of concomitant diuretic may be needed; use with caution and modify dosage in patients with hyponatremia, hypovolemia, severe CHF, left ventricular outflow tract obstruction, or with coadministered diuretic therapy; experience in children is limited; severe hypotension may occur in patients who are sodium and/or volume depleted, initiate lower doses and monitor closely when starting therapy in these patients

Adverse Reactions

Cardiovascular: Hypotension, syncope

Central nervous system: Fatigue, vertigo, insomnia, dizziness, headache

Dermatologic: Rash, angioedema (see Warnings). **Note:** The relative risk of angioedema with ACE inhibitors is higher within the first 30 days of use (compared to >1 year of use), for Black Americans (compared to Whites), for lisinopril or enalapril (compared to captopril), and for patients previously hospitalized within 30 days (Brown, 1996).

Endocrine & metabolic: Hypoglycemia, hyperkalemia

Gastrointestinal: Nausea, diarrhea, ageusia

Genitourinary: Impotence

Hematologic: Agranulocytosis, neutropenia, anemia

Hepatic: Cholestatic jaundice, fulminant hepatic necrosis (rare, but potentially fatal)

Neuromuscular & skeletal: Muscle cramps

Renal: Deterioration in renal function

Respiratory: Cough, dyspnea, eosinophilic pneumonitis; **Note:** An isolated dry cough lasting >3 weeks reported in 7 of 42 pediatric patients (17%) receiving ACE inhibitors (see von Vigier, 2000)

Miscellaneous: Anaphylactoid reactions

Drug Interactions

Metabolism/Transport Effects Substrate of CYP3A4 (minor)

Avoid Concomitant Use There are no known interactions where it is recommended to avoid concomitant use.

Increased Effect/Toxicity

Enalapril may increase the levels/effects of: Allopurinol; Amifostine; Antihypertensives; AzaTHIOprine; Cyclo-SPORINE; CycloSPORINE (Systemic); Ferric Gluconate; Gold Sodium Thiomalate; Hypotensive Agents; Iron Dextran Complex; Lithium; RiTUXimab

The levels/effects of Enalapril may be increased by: Angiotensin II Receptor Blockers; Diazoxide; DPP-IV Inhibitors; Eplerenone; Everolimus; Herbs (Hypotensive Properties); Loop Diuretics; MAO Inhibitors; Pentoxifylline; Phosphodiesterase 5 Inhibitors; Potassium Salts; Potassium-Sparing Diuretics; Prostacyclin Analogues; Sirolimus; Temsirolimus; Thiazide Diuretics; Tolvaptan; Trimethoprim

Decreased Effect

The levels/effects of Enalapril may be decreased by: Antacids; Aprotinin; CYP3A4 Inducers (Strong); Deferasirox; Herbs (CYP3A4 Inducers); Herbs (Hypertensive Properties); Methylphenidate; Nonsteroidal Anti-Inflammatory Agents; Salicylates; Yohimbine

Food Interactions Food does not affect absorption. Limit salt substitutes or potassium-rich diet. Avoid natural licorice (causes sodium and water retention and increases potassium loss).

Stability Store vials below 86°F (30°C); solutions for I.V. infusion mixed in NS, D_5W, D_5NS, or D_5LR are stable for 24 hours at room temperature

Mechanism of Action Competitive inhibitor of angiotensin-converting enzyme (ACE); prevents conversion of angiotensin I to angiotensin II, a potent vasoconstrictor; results in lower levels of angiotensin II which causes an increase in plasma renin activity and a reduction in aldosterone secretion; a CNS mechanism may also be involved in hypotensive effect as angiotensin II increases adrenergic outflow from CNS; vasoactive kallikreins may be decreased in conversion to active hormones by ACE inhibitors, thus reducing blood pressure

Pharmacodynamics (Antihypertensive effect)

Onset of action:
Oral: Within 1 hour
I.V.: Within 15 minutes
Maximum effect:
Oral: Within 4-8 hours
I.V.: Within 1-4 hour
Duration:
Oral: 12-24 hours
I.V.: Dose dependent, usually 4-6 hours

Pharmacokinetics (Adult data unless noted)

Absorption: Oral: 55% to 75% (enalapril)
Protein binding: 50% to 60%
Metabolism: Enalapril is a prodrug (inactive) and undergoes biotransformation to enalaprilat (active) in the liver
Half-life:
Enalapril:
CHF neonates 10-19 days of age (n=3): 10.3 hours (range: 4.2-13.4 hours)
CHF: Infants >27 days and Children ≤6.5 years of age (n=11): 2.7 hours (range: 1.3-6.3 hours)
Healthy adults: 2 hours
CHF adults: 3.4-5.8 hours
Enalaprilat:
CHF neonates 10-19 days of age (n=3): 11.9 hours (range 5.9-15.6 hours)
CHF: Infants >27 days and Children ≤6.5 years of age (n=11): 11.1 hours (range: 5.1-20.8 hours)
Infants 6 weeks to 8 months: 6-10 hours
Adults: 35-38 hours
Time to peak serum concentration: Oral:
Enalapril: Within 0.5-1.5 hours
Enalaprilat (active): Within 3-4.5 hours
Elimination: Principally in urine (60% to 80%) with some fecal excretion

Usual Dosage Use lower listed initial dose in patients with hyponatremia, hypovolemia, severe CHF, decreased renal function, or in those receiving diuretics

Manufacturer's recommendations: Pediatric hypertensive patients: Oral: **Enalapril:** Initial: 0.08 mg/kg once daily (maximum dose: 5 mg); adjust dose according to blood pressure readings; doses >0.58 mg/kg (or >40 mg) have not been studied

Alternative pediatric dosing:
Neonates:
Oral: **Enalapril**: Initial: 0.1 mg/kg/day given every 24 hours; increase dose and interval as required every few days (see Additional Information)
I.V.: **Enalaprilat:** 5-10 mcg/kg/dose administered every 8-24 hours (as determined by blood pressure readings) has been used for the treatment of neonatal hypertension; monitor patients carefully; select patients may require higher doses
Infants and Children:
Oral: **Enalapril**: Initial: 0.1 mg/kg/day in 1-2 divided doses; increase as required over 2 weeks to maximum of 0.5 mg/kg/day; mean dose required for CHF improvement in 39 children (9 days to 17 years of age) was 0.36 mg/kg/day; investigationally, select individuals have been treated with doses up to 0.94 mg/kg/day (Leversha, 1994)
I.V.: **Enalaprilat:** 5-10 mcg/kg/dose administered every 8-24 hours (as determined by blood pressure readings); monitor patients carefully; select patients may require higher doses

Adolescents and Adults:
Oral: **Enalapril**: Initial: 2.5-5 mg/day then increase as required; usual dose for hypertension: 10-40 mg/day in 1-2 divided doses; usual dosage range for hypertension in Adolescents ≥18 years and Adults (JNC 7): 2.5-40 mg/day in 1-2 divided doses; usual dose for CHF: 5-20 mg/day in 2 divided doses; maximum dose: 40 mg/day
Asymptomatic left ventricular dysfunction: Initial: 2.5 mg twice daily; increase as tolerated; usual dose: 20 mg/day in 2 divided doses
I.V.: **Enalaprilat:** 0.625-1.25 mg/dose every 6 hours; doses as high as 5 mg/dose every 6 hours have been tolerated for up to 36 hours; little experience with doses >20 mg/day

Dosing adjustment in renal impairment: Note: Use in neonates and children ≤16 years of age with GFR <30 mL/min/1.73 m^2 is not recommended (no dosing data exists)
Cl_{cr} 10-50 mL/minute: Administer 75% to 100% of dose
Cl_{cr} <10 mL/minute: Administer 50% of dose

Administration

Oral: May administer without regard to food
Parenteral: I.V.: Administer as I.V. infusion (undiluted solution or further diluted) over 5 minutes; to deliver small I.V. doses, a dilution with NS to a final concentration of 25 mcg/mL can be made

Monitoring Parameters Blood pressure, renal function, WBC, serum potassium, serum glucose; monitor for angioedema and anaphylactoid reactions (see Warnings)

Patient Information Limit alcohol. Notify physician immediately if swelling of face, lips, tongue, or difficulty in breathing occurs; if these occur, do not take any more doses until a physician can be consulted. Notify physician if vomiting, diarrhea, excessive perspiration, dehydration, or persistent cough occurs. Do not use a salt substitute (potassium-containing) without physician advice. May cause dizziness, fainting, and lightheadedness, especially in first week of therapy; sit and stand up slowly. May cause rash. Report sore throat, fever, other signs of infection, or other side effects. This medication may cause injury and death to the developing fetus when used during pregnancy; women of childbearing potential should be informed of potential risk; consult prescriber for appropriate contraceptive measures; this medication should be discontinued as soon as possible once pregnancy is detected (see Warnings).

Nursing Implications Discontinue if angioedema occurs; observe closely for hypotension within 1-3 hours of first dose or with new higher dose

Additional Information Severe hypotension was reported in a **preterm** neonate (birth weight 835 g, gestational age 26 weeks, postnatal age 9 days) who was treated with enalapril 0.1 mg/kg orally; hypotension responded to I.V. plasma and dopamine; the authors suggest starting enalapril in preterm infants at 0.01 mg/kg and increasing upwards in a stepwise fashion with very close monitoring of blood pressure and urine output. However, in this case report, oral enalapril at doses of 0.01 mg/kg to 0.04 mg/kg did not adequately control blood pressure. Further studies are needed. (Schilder, 1995)

Over the years, several pediatric studies have examined the effects of ACE inhibitors on proteinuria. In a more recent retrospective study, enalapril (in doses of 2.5-5 mg/day) administered either as monotherapy (n=17; mean age: 13.7 years; range 8-17 years) or with prednisone (n=11; mean age: 12.6 years; range: 7-16 years), significantly decreased proteinuria in normotensive proteinuric children (with or without nephrotic syndrome); no significant change in blood pressure was observed (Sasinka, 1999). In a smaller study of children with persistent proteinuria (n=7; 6 with steroid resistant nephrotic syndrome; mean age: 13.5 years; range: 7-18 years), enalapril (at mean oral doses of 0.3 mg/kg/day) significantly reduced proteinuria in 5 of the 7 patients (Lama, 2000). Another recent study assessed the effects of enalapril on urinary protein electrophoretic patterns in 13 children (mean age: 8 years; range: 1.8-12 years) with steroid resistant nephrotic syndrome; oral enalapril was initially dosed at 0.2 mg/kg/day (with a maximum dose of 30 mg/day); doses were increased each month by 0.1 mg/kg/day until the patients' urinary protein decreased by 50% from baseline; prednisone was added after 2 months in 11 of the 13 children at doses of 30 mg/m^2 given every other day; four patients had a complete remission of proteinuria after 4-12 months; an 80% decrease in urinary total protein and a 70% decrease in urinary albumin was observed in the other patients; the pattern of urinary protein shifted from a nonselective to an albumin-selective urinary protein loss in all patients; significant increases in plasma total protein and albumin occurred; it is important to note that 3 of the 13 patients (23%) required interruption of enalapril during transient acute renal failure due to an infectious disease (Delucchi, 2000). Further pediatric studies are needed to identify optimal enalapril oral doses and to establish safety and efficacy for this use.

Dosage Forms Excipient information presented when available (limited, particularly for generics); consult specific product labeling.

Injection, solution, as enalaprilat: 1.25 mg/mL (1 mL, 2 mL) [contains benzyl alcohol]

Tablet, as maleate: 2.5 mg, 5 mg, 10 mg, 20 mg

Vasotec®: 2.5 mg, 5 mg, 10 mg, 20 mg

Extemporaneous Preparations

A 1 mg/mL oral suspension made from tablets, Bicitra®, and Ora-Sweet® SF is stable for 30 days when stored in a polyethylene terephthalate bottle under refrigeration (2°C to 8°C); place ten 20 mg tablets in a 200 mL polyethylene terephthalate bottle; add 50 mL of Bicitra®; shake well for at least 2 minutes; let stand for 1 hour than shake for one additional minute; add 150 mL of Ora-Sweet® SF and shake well; label "shake well" [Vasotec® tablets (package insert), 2001].

A 1 mg/mL oral liquid preparation made from tablets and 3 different vehicles (cherry syrup, a 1:1 mixture of Ora-Sweet® and Ora-Plus®, or a 1:1 mixture of Ora-Sweet® SF and Ora-Plus®) was stable for 60 days when stored in amber plastic prescription bottles in the dark at room temperature (25°C) or under refrigeration (5°C); grind six 20 mg tablets in a mortar into a fine powder; add 15 mL of the vehicle and mix well to form a uniform paste; mix while adding the vehicle in geometric proportions to almost 120 mL; transfer to a calibrated bottle and qsad with vehicle to 120 mL; label "shake well" and "protect from light" (Allen, 1998).

A 1 mg/mL oral liquid preparation made from tablets and 3 different vehicles (deionized water, citrate buffer solution at pH 5.0, or a 1:1 mixture of Ora-Sweet® and Ora-Plus®) was stable for 91 days when stored in plastic prescription bottles in the dark under refrigeration (4°C). When stored at room temperature (25°C), the preparations made in citrate buffer solution at pH 5.0 and the 1:1 mixture of Ora-Sweet® and Ora-Plus® were also stable for 91 days, but the preparation made in deionized water was stable for only 56 days. Grind twenty 10 mg tablets in a mortar; add a small amount of vehicle and mix well to form a smooth paste; mix while adding increasing amounts of the vehicle to make the mixture pourable; transfer to a graduated cylinder and qsad to 200 mL; **Note:** To prepare the isotonic citrate buffer solution (pH 5.0), see reference; label "shake well" and "protect from light" (Nahata, 1998).

A more dilute oral liquid preparation of 0.1 mg/mL made from tablets and an isotonic buffer solution at pH 5.0 was stable for 90 days when stored in amber, high density polyethylene bottles under refrigeration (5°C); grind one 20 mg tablet in a glass mortar into a fine powder; triturate with isotonic citrate buffer (pH 5.0) and filter; qsad to 200 mL with buffer solution; label "shake well" and "protect from light" (Boulton, 1994).

Allen LV and Erickson MA, "Stability of Alprazolam, Chloroquine Phosphate, Cisapride, Enalapril Maleate, and Hydralazine Hydrochloride in Extemporaneously Compounded Oral Liquids," *Am J Health Syst Pharm,* 1998, 55(18):1915-20.

Boulton DW, Woods DJ, Fawcett JP, et al, "The Stability of an Enalapril Maleate Oral Solution Prepared From Tablets," *Aust J Hosp Pharm,* 1994, 24(2):151-6.

Nahata MC, Morosco RS, and Hipple TF, "Stability of Enalapril Maleate in Three Extemporaneously Prepared Oral Liquids," *Am J Health Syst Pharm,* 1998, 55(11):1155-7.

Vasotec® (package insert), West Point, PA: Merck & Co., Inc; 2001.

References

Brown NJ, Ray WA, Snowden M, et al, "Black Americans Have an Increased Rate of Angiotensin-Converting Enzyme Inhibitor-Associated Angioedema," *Clin Pharmacol Ther,* 1996, 60(1):8-13.

Bult Y and van den Anker J, "Hypertension in a Preterm Infant Treated With Enalapril," *J Pediatr Pharm Pract,* 1997, 2(4):229-31.

Chobanian AV, Bakris GL, Black HR, et al, "The Seventh Report of the Joint National Committee on Prevention, Detection, Evaluation, and Treatment of High Blood Pressure: The JNC 7 Report," *JAMA,* 2003, 289(19):2560-72.

Delucchi A, Cano F, Rodriguez E, et al, "Enalapril and Prednisone in Children With Nephrotic-Range Proteinuria," *Pediatr Nephrol,* 2000, 14(12):1088-91.

Frenneaux M, Stewart RA, Newman CM, et al, "Enalapril for Severe Heart Failure in Infancy," *Arch Dis Child,* 1989, 64(2):219-23.

Lama G, Luongo I, Piscitelli A, et al, "Enalapril: Antiproteinuric Effect in Children With Nephrotic Syndrome," *Clin Nephrol,* 2000, 53(6):432-6.

Leversha AM, Wilson NJ, Clarkson PM, et al, "Efficacy and Dosage of Enalapril in Congenital and Acquired Heart Disease," *Arch Dis Child,* 1994, 70(1):35-9.

Lloyd TR, Mahoney LT, Knoedel D, et al, "Orally Administered Enalapril for Infants With Congestive Heart Failure: A Dose Finding Study," *J Pediatr,* 1989, 114(4 Pt 1):650-4.

Marcadis ML, Kraus DM, Hatzopoulos FK, et al, "Use of Enalaprilat for Neonatal Hypertension," *J Pediatr,* 1991, 119(3):505-6.

Nakamura H, Ishii M, Sugimura T, et al, "The Kinetic Profiles of Enalapril and Enalaprilat and Their Possible Developmental Changes in Pediatric Patients With Congestive Heart Failure," *Clin Pharmacol Ther*, 1994, 56(2):160-8.

National High Blood Pressure Education Program Working Group on High Blood Pressure in Children and Adolescents, "The Fourth Report on the Diagnosis, Evaluation, and Treatment of High Blood Pressure in Children and Adolescents," *Pediatrics*, 2004, 114(2 Suppl):555-76.

Sasinka MA, Podracka L, Boor A, et al, "Enalapril Treatment of Proteinuria in Normotensive Children," *Bratisl Lek Listy*, 1999, 100 (9):476-80.

Schilder JL and Van den Anker JN, "Use of Enalapril in Neonatal Hypertension," *Acta Paediatr*, 1995, 84(12):1426-8.

von Vigier RO, Mozzettini S, Truttmann AC, et al, "Cough is Common in Children Prescribed Converting Enzyme Inhibitors," *Nephron*, 2000, 84(1):98.

Wells T, Frame V, Soffer B, et al, "A Double-Blind, Placebo-Controlled, Dose-Response Study of the Effectiveness and Safety of Enalapril for Children With Hypertension," *J Clin Pharmacol*, 2002, 42(8):870-80.

Wells TG, Bunchman TE, Kearns GL, "Treatment of Neonatal Hypertension With Enalaprilat," *J Pediatr*, 1990, 117(4):664-7.

◆ **Enalapril Maleate** *see* Enalapril/Enalaprilat *on page 499*

◆ **Enbrel®** *see* Etanercept *on page 541*

◆ **Encort™** *see* Hydrocortisone *on page 685*

◆ **Endantadine® (Can)** *see* Amantadine *on page 77*

◆ **Endocet®** *see* Oxycodone and Acetaminophen *on page 1041*

◆ **Endodan®** *see* Oxycodone and Aspirin *on page 1042*

◆ **Endrate** *see* Edetate Disodium *on page 489*

◆ **Endrate** *see* Edetate Disodium *on page 489*

◆ **Enemeez® [OTC]** *see* Docusate *on page 468*

◆ **Enemeez® Plus [OTC]** *see* Docusate *on page 468*

◆ **Enerjets [OTC]** *see* Caffeine *on page 225*

◆ **Enfamil® D-Vi-Sol™ [OTC]** *see* Cholecalciferol *on page 300*

◆ **Enfamil® Glucose** *see* Dextrose *on page 422*

Enfuvirtide (en FY00 vir tide)

Related Information
Adult and Adolescent HIV *on page 1620*
Management of Healthcare Worker Exposures to HBV, HCV, and HIV *on page 1661*
Pediatric HIV *on page 1613*
Perinatal HIV *on page 1628*

U.S. Brand Names Fuzeon®

Canadian Brand Names Fuzeon®

Therapeutic Category Antiretroviral Agent; Fusion Inhibitor; HIV Agents (Anti-HIV Agents)

Generic Available No

Use Treatment of HIV-1 infection in combination with other antiretroviral agents in treatment-experienced patients who are failing current antiretroviral therapy. (**Note:** HIV regimens consisting of **three** antiretroviral agents are strongly recommended. However, in published studies, enfuvirtide was added onto a new optimized background regimen of 3-5 antiretroviral agents, in patients failing their current antiretroviral regimen. Selection of the new optimized regimen was based on medication history, genotyping, and phenotyping. Due to the lack of studies, enfuvirtide cannot be recommended as initial therapy in patients who are antiretroviral naïve.)

Pregnancy Risk Factor B

Pregnancy Considerations Teratogenic effects were not observed in animal studies; however, there are no adequate and well-controlled studies in pregnant women and data is insufficient to recommend use during pregnancy. An antiretroviral registry has been established to monitor maternal and fetal outcomes in women receiving antiretroviral drugs. Physicians are encouraged to register patients at 1-800-258-4263 or www.APRegistry.com.

Lactation Excretion in breast milk unknown/contraindicated

Breast-Feeding Considerations In infants born to mothers who are HIV positive, HAART while breast-feeding may decrease postnatal infection. However, maternal or infant antiretroviral therapy does not completely eliminate the risk of postnatal HIV transmission.

In the United States where formula is accessible, affordable, safe, and sustainable, complete avoidance of breast-feeding by HIV-infected women is recommended to decrease potential transmission of HIV.

Contraindications Hypersensitivity to enfuvirtide or any component

Warnings Local injection site reactions occur in the majority of patients (see Adverse Reactions); instruct patient or caregiver on proper injection method; monitor patients for local infection or cellulitis. Administration using a needle-free device (Biojector® 2000) has been associated with nerve pain (including neuralgia and/or paresthesia lasting up to 6 months) when administered at sites where large nerves are close to the skin, bruising, and hematomas; administer medication only in recommended sites. A higher risk of postinjection bleeding may occur in patients receiving anticoagulants and in those with hemophilia or other coagulation disorders.

Bacterial pneumonia was observed at a higher rate in patients receiving enfuvirtide during clinical trials; certain patients may be at greater risk (eg, those with a history of lung disease, low CD4 cell count, high initial viral load, I.V. drug use, or smoking); monitor patients closely for signs and symptoms of pneumonia. Systemic hypersensitivity reactions may occur (see Adverse Reactions); discontinue enfuvirtide and do not restart in patients with systemic hypersensitivity reactions.

Precautions Efficacy data is limited in pediatric patients ≥6 years of age; safety and pharmacokinetics in children <6 years is not established. Use of enfuvirtide may theoretically result in the production of anti-enfuvirtide antibodies, which may cross react with HIV-1 gp41; this could potentially result in a false positive ELISA test in noninfected HIV individuals; the western blot test would be expected to be negative; use of enfuvirtide in non-HIV infected individuals has not been studied.

Immune reconstitution syndrome (an acute inflammatory response to residual or indolent opportunistic infections) may occur in HIV patients during initial treatment with combination antiretroviral agents, including enfuvirtide; this syndrome may require further patient assessment and therapy.

Adverse Reactions Note: Adverse effects in pediatric patients 5-16 years of age were reported to be similar to those in adults; however, infections at injection site (cellulitis or abscess) were found to be more frequent in adolescent patients (11%) compared to adults (1.7%)

Central nervous system: Anxiety, depression, dizziness, insomnia

Dermatologic: Pruritus

Endocrine & metabolic: Triglycerides elevated, weight loss

Gastrointestinal: Abdominal pain, anorexia, constipation, pancreatitis, serum amylase elevated, serum lipase elevated, taste disturbance

Hematologic: Anemia, eosinophilia

Hepatic: Serum transaminases elevated

Local: Injection site reactions [98% incidence; most patients have first injection site reaction during initial week of therapy; reactions are usually mild to moderate in severity, but may be more severe; symptoms may include discomfort, ecchymosis, erythema, induration, pain, pruritus, and nodule or cyst formation; infection, including cellulitis or abscess, occurs in 1.7% of adults, but in 11% of adolescent patients; 11% of patients require ▶

analgesics or limitation of usual activities; reactions often occur at >1 injection site; 26% of patients have 6-14 injection site reactions and 1.3% have >14 injection site reactions at any given time; average duration of single injection site reaction is 3-7 days in 41% of patients and >7 days in 24%; 7% of patients discontinue therapy due to injection site reactions (4%) or problems with administering injections (3%)]. Nerve pain (including neuralgia and/or paresthesia lasting up to 6 months) when administered at sites where large nerves are close to the skin, bruising, and hematomas have been associated with the use of a needle-free device (Biojector® 2000).

Neuromuscular & skeletal: CPK elevated, myalgia, peripheral neuropathy, weakness

Ocular: Conjunctivitis

Respiratory: Cough, sinusitis; bacterial pneumonia (6.7 events per 100 patient years vs 0.6 events per 100 patient years in control group; about 50% of patients with pneumonia required hospitalization; see Warnings for risk factors)

Miscellaneous: Flu-like symptoms, infections, lymphadenopathy; hypersensitivity reactions (<1% incidence; symptoms may include chills, fever, hypotension, nausea, rash, rigors, serum transaminases elevated, and vomiting; other immune-mediated adverse reactions that have been reported include: Glomerulonephritis, Guillain-Barré syndrome, primary immune complex reaction, respiratory distress), immune reconstitution syndrome

Drug Interactions

Avoid Concomitant Use There are no known interactions where it is recommended to avoid concomitant use.

Increased Effect/Toxicity

Enfuvirtide may increase the levels/effects of: Protease Inhibitors

The levels/effects of Enfuvirtide may be increased by: Protease Inhibitors

Decreased Effect There are no known significant interactions involving a decrease in effect.

Stability Store unreconstituted vials at controlled room temperature, 25°C (77°F); excursions permitted to 15°C to 30°C (59°F to 86°F). Store reconstituted solution under refrigeration at 2°C to 8°C (36°F to 46°F); use within 24 hours.

Mechanism of Action Enfuvirtide is a synthetic protein consisting of a linear sequence of 36 amino acids. It mimics the amino acid sequence HR2 (heptad repeat 2) found in the C-terminal portion of gp41 (an HIV-1 transmembrane glycoprotein) and competitively binds with HR1 (sequence heptad repeat 1). Normally, the HR1 sequence interacts with HR2 to form a hairpin structure needed for gp41 to initiate the fusion between the HIV-1 viral membrane and host CD4 cell membrane. By mimicking HR2 and binding with HR1, enfuvirtide inhibits the fusion of viral and cellular membranes and interferes with the entry of HIV-1 into cells.

Pharmacokinetics (Adult data unless noted)

Absorption: SubQ: Absorption is comparable when injected into abdomen, arm, or thigh

Distribution: Adults: V_d (mean ± SD): 5.5 ± 1.1 L

CSF concentrations (2-18 hours after administration; n=4): Nondetectable (<0.025 mcg/mL)

Protein Binding: 92%; primarily to albumin, but also to alpha-1 acid glycoprotein (to a lesser extent); CNS penetration: Unknown (but expected to be minimal due to large molecule and high protein binding)

Metabolism: Expected to undergo catabolism via peptidases and proteinases in the liver and kidneys to amino acids; amino acids would then be recycled in the body pool. A deaminated metabolite (with 20% activity compared to parent drug) was formed via hydrolysis during *in vitro* human microsomal and hepatocyte studies.

Bioavailability:

Oral: Not bioavailable by this route

SubQ: Absolute: 84.3% ± 15.5%; **Note:** Bioequivalence was found to be similar in a study comparing standard administration using a needle versus a needle-free device.

Half-life: 3.8 ± 0.6 hours

Time to peak serum concentration: SubQ:

Single dose: Median: 8 hours (range: 3-12 hours)

Multiple dosing: Median: 4 hours (range: 4-8 hours)

Clearance:

Plasma clearance is decreased in adults with lower body weight and in females after adjusting for body weight (clearance in adults females is 20% lower compared to adults males). However, no adjustment in dose is recommended for gender or weight.

Compared to patients with normal renal function, enfuvirtide clearance is decreased by 38% in patients with severe renal impairment (Cl_{cr} 11-35 mL/minute) and by 14% to 28% in patients with end-stage renal disease who are maintained on dialysis. However, no adjustment in dose is recommended for patients with renal impairment.

Apparent clearance: Multiple dosing:

Children: 40 ± 17 mL/hour/kg

Adults: 30.6 ± 10.6 mL/hour/kg

Dialysis: Hemodialysis does not significantly affect clearance of enfuvirtide

Usual Dosage SubQ (use in combination with other antiretroviral agents):

Neonates, Infants, and Children <6 years: Not approved for use

Children 6-16 years: 2 mg/kg twice daily (maximum dose: 90 mg twice daily)

Adolescent >16 years and Adults: 90 mg twice daily

Dosage adjustment in renal impairment: Adults:

Cl_{cr} >35 mL/minute: Clearance of enfuvirtide is not affected; no dosage adjustment required.

Cl_{cr} ≤35 mL/minute: Limited data showed decreased clearance; however, no dosage adjustment recommended.

End-stage renal disease (on dialysis): Limited data showed decreased clearance; however, no dosage adjustment recommended.

Dosage adjustment in hepatic impairment: No dosage adjustment required.

Administration Reconstitute vial with 1.1 mL SWI to result in delivery of 90 per 1 mL; to avoid foaming, gently tap vial for 10 seconds and roll gently between hands to ensure contact of drug with liquid; allow vial to stand until lyophilized powder goes completely into solution; this may require up to 45 minutes; to reduce reconstitution time, may gently roll vial between hands until drug is completely dissolved; visually inspect vial to ensure complete dissolution of drug; solution should be clear, colorless, and without particulate matter or bubbles; do not use vials that contain particulate matter.

Vial does not contain preservatives; reconstituted solutions should be injected immediately or refrigerated and used within 24 hours; bring refrigerated reconstituted vials to room temperature before injection and visually inspect vial again as outlined above.

Inject SubQ into upper arm, abdomen, or anterior thigh. Do not inject I.M. (severity of reactions is increased). Do not inject into skin abnormalities including directly over a blood vessel, into moles, bruises, scar tissue, near the navel, surgical scars, burn sites, or tattoos. Do not inject in or near sites where large nerves are close to the skin including near the elbow, knee, groin, and inferior or medial sections of the buttocks. Rotate injection site (ie, give injections at a site different from the preceding injection site); do not inject into any site where an injection site reaction is present. After injection, apply heat or ice to injection site or gently massage area to better disperse the dose, to minimize local injection reactions; discard unused portion of the vial (vial is for single use only).

Monitoring Parameters Serum triglycerides, CBC, liver enzymes, CD4 cell count, HIV RNA plasma levels; local injection site reactions, local infection, cellulitis; signs and symptoms of pneumonia, especially in patients at risk (see Warnings)

Patient Information Enfuvirtide can only be administered by injection; follow exact injection instructions that come with your medication. Do not mix any other medications in the same syringe with enfuvirtide. Inject subcutaneously into the upper arm, abdomen, or anterior thigh. Do not inject in the same area you did the time before or where there is an injection site reaction. Do not inject into skin abnormalities including directly over a blood vessel, into moles, bruises, scar tissue, near the navel, surgical scars, burn sites, or tattoos. Do not inject in or near sites where large nerves are close to the skin including near the elbow, knee, groin, and inferior or medial sections of the buttocks. After injection, apply heat or ice to injection site or gently massage area to better disperse the dose, to minimize local injection reactions; discard unused portion of the vial (vial is for single use only).

Enfuvirtide may cause injection site reactions such as itching, swelling, redness, pain, hardened skin, or bumps (each local reaction usually lasts for <7 days); notify physician immediately if reaction is severe or if injection site becomes infected. Nerve pain and tingling up to 6 months (from injecting enfuvirtide too close to large nerves or near joints), bruising, and a collection of blood under the skin have occurred with the use of a needle-free injection device. The risk of bruising or bleeding may be increased in patients taking blood thinners and in those with hemophilia or other bleeding disorders. Patients receiving enfuvirtide may experience bacterial pneumonia or hypersensitivity reactions; notify physician if you experience cough, fever, rapid breathing, trouble breathing, vomiting, chills, rash, blood in the urine, or swelling of the feet. Enfuvirtide may cause dizziness and impair ability to perform activities requiring mental alertness or physical coordination.

Enfuvirtide is not a cure for HIV; take enfuvirtide everyday as prescribed; do not change dose or discontinue without physician's advice; if a dose is missed, take it as soon as possible, then return to normal dosing schedule; if a dose is skipped, do not double the next dose; make sure you have adequate supply of medication; do not allow supply to run out.

Nursing Implications Teach patient or caregiver proper reconstitution, aseptic injection technique, and proper needle and syringe disposal (see Stability and Administration specifics).

Additional Information Reconstituted injection has a pH ~9.0.

Dosage Forms Excipient information presented when available (limited, particularly for generics); consult specific product labeling.

Injection, powder for reconstitution [preservative free]:

Fuzeon®: 108 mg [90 mg/mL following reconstitution; available in convenience kit of 60 vials, SWFI, syringes, alcohol wipes, patient instructions]

References

Briars LA, Hilao JJ, and Kraus DM, "A Review of Pediatric Human Immunodeficiency Virus Infection," *Journal of Pharmacy Practice*, 2004, 17(6):407-31.

Church JA, Cunningham C, Hughes M, et al, "Safety and Antiretroviral Activity of Chronic Subcutaneous Administration of T-20 in Human Immunodeficiency Virus 1-Infected Children," *Pediatr Infect Dis J*, 2002, 21(7):653-9.

Hardy H and Skolnik PR, "Enfuvirtide, a New Fusion Inhibitor for Therapy of Human Immunodeficiency Virus Infection," *Pharmacotherapy*, 2004, 24(2):198-211.

Morris JL and Kraus DM, "New Antiretroviral Therapies for Pediatric HIV Infection," *J Pediatr Pharmacol Ther*, 2005, 10:215-47.

Panel on Antiretroviral Guidelines for Adults and Adolescents, "Guidelines for the Use of Antiretroviral Agents in HIV-Infected Adults and Adolescents," December 1, 2009, http://www.aidsinfo.nih.gov.

Soy D, Aweeka FT, Church JA, et al, "Population Pharmacokinetics of Enfuvirtide in Pediatric Patients With Human Immunodeficiency Virus: Searching for Exposure-Response Relationships," *Clin Pharmacol Ther*, 2003, 74(6):569-80.

Working Group on Antiretroviral Therapy and Medical Management of HIV-Infected Children, "Guidelines for the Use of Antiretroviral Agents in Pediatric HIV Infection," February 23, 2009. Available at http://www.aidsinfo.nih.gov.

◆ **Engerix-B®** *see* Hepatitis B Vaccine *on page 675*

◆ **Enhanced-Potency Inactivated Poliovirus Vaccine** *see* Poliovirus Vaccine (Inactivated) *on page 1127*

◆ **Enlon®** *see* Edrophonium *on page 490*

Enoxaparin (e noks ah PAIR in)

Medication Safety Issues

Sound-alike/look-alike issues:

Lovenox® may be confused with Lasix®, Levaquin®, Lotronex®, Protonix®

High alert medication: The Institute for Safe Medication Practices (ISMP) includes this medication among its list of drugs which have a heightened risk of causing significant patient harm when used in error.

International issues:

Lovenox® may be confused with Lotanax® which is a brand name for terfenadine in the Czech Republic

2009 National Patient Safety Goals: The Joint Commission (TJC) requires healthcare organizations that provide anticoagulant therapy to have a process in place to reduce the risk of anticoagulant-associated patient harm. Patients receiving anticoagulants should receive individualized care through a defined process that includes standardized ordering, dispensing, administration, monitoring and education. This does not apply to routine short-term use of anticoagulants for prevention of venous thromboembolism when the expectation is that the patient's laboratory values will remain within or close to normal values (NPSG.03.05.01).

Related Information

Antithrombotic Therapy in Neonates and Children *on page 1602*

U.S. Brand Names Lovenox®

Canadian Brand Names Enoxaparin Injection; Lovenox®; Lovenox® HP

Therapeutic Category Anticoagulant; Low Molecular Weight Heparin (LMWH)

Generic Available No

Use Prophylaxis and treatment of thromboembolic disorders, specifically prevention of DVT following hip or knee replacement surgery, abdominal surgery in patients at thromboembolic risk (ie, >40 years of age, obese, general anesthesia >30 minutes, malignancy, history of DVT, or pulmonary embolism), and in medical patients at thromboembolic risk due to severely restricted mobility during acute illness (FDA approved in adults). Administered with warfarin: For inpatient treatment of acute DVT (with or without pulmonary embolism) and outpatient treatment of ▶

acute DVT (without pulmonary embolism) (FDA approved in adults). Administered with aspirin: For prevention of ischemic complications of non-Q-wave MI and unstable angina and for the treatment of acute ST-segment elevation myocardial infarction (STEMI) (FDA approved in adults)

Pregnancy Risk Factor B

Pregnancy Considerations Animal studies have not shown teratogenic or fetotoxic effects. Pregnancy itself increases the risk of thromboembolism. Pregnant women with a history of thromboembolic disease are at increased risk of maternal and fetal complications. Enoxaparin does not cross the placenta. Use may be recommended in pregnant women for the management of VTE. Monitoring antifactor Xa levels is recommended. Risk of adverse events may be increased in pregnant women with mechanical heart valves; use is controversial and has not been adequately studied. Postmarketing reports include congenital abnormalities (cause and effect not established) and also fetal death when used in pregnant women. Multiple-dose vials contain benzyl alcohol; use caution in pregnant women.

Lactation Excretion in breast milk unknown/use caution

Breast-Feeding Considerations This drug has a high molecular weight that would minimize excretion in breast milk and is inactivated by the GI tract which further reduces the risk to the infant.

Contraindications Hypersensitivity to enoxaparin, heparin, any component (see Warnings), or pork products (enoxaparin is derived from porcine intestinal mucosa); active major bleeding; acute heparin-induced or low molecular weight heparin-induced thrombocytopenia

Warnings Bleeding or thrombocytopenia may occur; major hemorrhages (eg, intracranial and retroperitoneal bleeding) may be fatal; thrombocytopenia with thrombosis may occur and may be complicated by limb ischemia, organ infarction, or death; discontinue therapy and consider alternative treatment if platelets are <100,000/mm^3 and/or thrombosis develops. Use with extreme caution in patients with an increased risk of hemorrhage (eg, active GI ulceration or bleeding, angiodysplastic GI disease, bacterial endocarditis, bleeding disorders, hemorrhagic stroke); recent brain, spinal, or ophthalmic surgery; concomitant platelet inhibitor therapy (see Drug Interactions); or a history of heparin-induced thrombocytopenia. Do not use unit-for-unit in place of heparin or other low molecular weight heparins (units are not equivalent). Enoxaparin is **not** recommended for prophylaxis of thromboembolic disorders in patients with prosthetic heart valves, especially pregnant women (prosthetic heart valve thrombosis may occur; several cases occurred in pregnant women and resulted in maternal and fetal deaths; pregnant women with prosthetic heart valves may be at a higher risk for thromboembolism; use with extreme caution and monitor peak and trough anti-Factor Xa levels frequently in these patients; adjust dosage accordingly)

Epidural or spinal hematoma resulting in long-term or permanent paralysis may occur in patients receiving low molecular weight heparins or heparinoids during epidural/spinal anesthesia or spinal puncture **[U.S. Boxed Warning]**; these patients must be monitored frequently for neurological impairment and treated immediately if compromised. The risk of epidural/spinal hematoma is increased with the following: The use of indwelling epidural catheters for analgesia; concomitant use of platelet inhibitors, NSAIDs, or other anticoagulants; history of spinal deformity or spinal surgery; and repeated or traumatic epidural/spinal puncture. Potential benefits must be weighed against the risks. Enoxaparin should be withheld (at least 2 doses) and antifactor Xa activity should be determined (if possible), prior to lumbar or epidural procedures.

To minimize the risk of bleeding following percutaneous coronary revascularization procedures (eg, vascular instrumentation during treatment of unstable angina, non-Q-wave MI and acute STEMI), strictly adhere to the recommended dosing intervals. Hemostasis must be achieved at the puncture site after percutaneous coronary interventions (PCI). See product labeling for further information. Cases of hyperkalemia have been reported, usually in patients with risk factors for the development of hyperkalemia (eg, renal dysfunction, concomitant use of potassium-sparing diuretics or potassium supplements, hematoma in body tissues); monitor serum potassium.

Enoxaparin multidose vial contains benzyl alcohol which may cause allergic reactions in susceptible individuals; large amounts of benzyl alcohol (≥99 mg/kg/day) have been associated with a potentially fatal toxicity ("gasping syndrome") in neonates; the "gasping syndrome" consists of metabolic acidosis, respiratory distress, gasping respirations, CNS dysfunction (including convulsions, intracranial hemorrhage), hypotension and cardiovascular collapse; avoid use of enoxaparin products containing benzyl alcohol in neonates; use the preservative free injection; *in vitro* and animal studies have shown that benzoate, a metabolite of benzyl alcohol, displaces bilirubin from protein binding sites. Use multidose vial with caution in pregnant women and only if clearly needed (benzyl alcohol may cross the placenta).

Precautions Use with caution in patients with uncontrolled arterial hypertension, bleeding diathesis, pregnancy, history of recent GI ulceration, diabetic retinopathy, and hemorrhage. Use with caution in patients with renal impairment; decrease dose in patients with severe renal dysfunction (Cl$_{cr}$ <30 mL/minute). Use with caution and monitor carefully in low-weight patients (ie, women <45 kg and men <57 kg) receiving nonweight-adjusted doses (an increase in enoxaparin AUC has been reported). Institute appropriate therapy if thromboembolism occurs despite enoxaparin prophylaxis

Adverse Reactions

Cardiovascular: Edema

Central nervous system: Confusion, fever, intracranial hemorrhage (see Warnings)

Endocrine & metabolic: Hyperlipidemia (very rare), hyperkalemia (see Warnings)

Gastrointestinal: Diarrhea, nausea

Hematologic: Anemia, hemorrhage, prosthetic heart valve thrombosis (see Warnings), thrombocytopenia (with possible thrombosis; incidence of heparin-induced thrombocytopenia is less than with heparin therapy; see Warnings)

Hepatic: SGOT and SGPT increased (asymptomatic, fully reversible, rarely associated with elevated bilirubin levels)

Local: Cutaneous vasculitis (hypersensitive); ecchymosis, erythema, hematoma, irritation, and pain at SubQ injection site; epidural or spinal hematoma (see Warnings); skin necrosis (at or distant from injection site)

Renal: Hematuria

Miscellaneous: Allergic reactions

<1%, postmarketing, and/or case reports (limited to important or life-threatening): Anaphylactoid reaction, eczematous plaques, erythematous pruritic patches, hypertriglyceridemia, pruritus, purpura, retroperitoneal bleeding, thrombocytosis, urticaria, vesicobullous rash

Drug Interactions

Avoid Concomitant Use There are no known interactions where it is recommended to avoid concomitant use.

Increased Effect/Toxicity

Enoxaparin may increase the levels/effects of: Anticoagulants; Collagenase (Systemic); Drotrecogin Alfa; Ibritumomab; Tositumomab and Iodine I 131 Tositumomab

The levels/effects of Enoxaparin may be increased by: 5-ASA Derivatives; Antiplatelet Agents; Dasatinib; Herbs (Anticoagulant/Antiplatelet Properties); Nonsteroidal Anti-Inflammatory Agents; Pentosan Polysulfate Sodium; Pentoxifylline; Prostacyclin Analogues; Salicylates; Thrombolytic Agents

Decreased Effect There are no known significant interactions involving a decrease in effect.

Stability Store at 25°C (77°F); excursions permitted to 15°C to 30°C (59°F to 86°F). Prefilled syringes do not contain preservatives, discard unused portions; multidose vials should be discarded within 28 days after first use. For SubQ use, do not mix with other injections or infusions. For I.V. use (treatment of acute STEMI only), multidose vials may be mixed with NS or D_5W; do not mix with other drugs.

Mechanism of Action Potentiates the action of antithrombin III and inactivates coagulation factor Xa; also inactivates factor IIa (thrombin), but to a much lesser degree; ratio of antifactor Xa to antifactor IIa activity is ~4:1 (ratio for unfractionated heparin is 1:1)

Pharmacodynamics Antifactor Xa and antithrombin (antifactor IIa) activities:

Maximum effect: SubQ: 3-5 hours

Duration: ~12 hours following a 40 mg daily dose given SubQ

Pharmacokinetics (Adult data unless noted) Based on antifactor Xa activity

Distribution: Does not cross the placental barrier

Mean V_d: Adults: 4.3 L

Protein binding: Does not bind to most heparin binding proteins

Metabolism: Primarily in the liver via desulfation and depolymerization to lower molecular weight molecules with very low biological activity

Bioavailability: Adults: SubQ: ~100%

Half-life: SubQ: Adults: Single dose: 4.5 hours; repeat dosing: 7 hours

Elimination: 40% of I.V. dose is excreted in urine as active and inactive fragments; 10% of dose is excreted by kidneys as active enoxaparin fragments; 8% to 20% of antifactor Xa activity is recovered within 24 hours in the urine

Clearance: Decreased by 30% in patients with Cl_{cr} <30 mL/minute

Usual Dosage

Neonates, Infants, and Children:

Initial: SubQ:

Chest, 2008 Recommendations:

Infants <2 months:

Prophylaxis: 0.75 mg/kg/dose every 12 hours

Treatment: 1.5 mg/kg/dose every 12 hours

Infants ≥2 months and Children ≤18 years:

Prophylaxis: 0.5 mg/kg/dose every 12 hours

Treatment: 1 mg/kg/dose every 12 hours

Alternate dosing: Treatment: **Note:** Several recent studies suggest that doses higher than those recommended in the *Chest* guidelines are required in pediatric patients (especially in preterm neonates, neonates, and young infants) (see Bauman, 2009; Malowany, 2007; Malowany, 2008). Some centers are using the following; however, further studies are needed to validate these proposed higher initial doses.

Premature neonates: 2 mg/kg/dose every 12 hours

Full-term neonates: 1.7 mg/kg/dose every 12 hours

Infants <3 months: 1.8 mg/kg/dose every 12 hours

3-12 months: 1.5 mg/kg/dose every 12 hours

1-5 years: 1.2 mg/kg/dose every 12 hours

6-18 years: 1.1 mg/kg/dose every 12 hours

Maintenance: SubQ: *Chest*, 2008 Recommendations: See **Dosage Titration** table: **Note:** In a prospective study of 177 courses of enoxaparin in pediatric patients (146 treatment courses; 31 prophylactic courses) considerable variation in maintenance dosage requirements was observed (see Dix, 2000).

Enoxaparin Dosage Titration

Antifactor Xa	Dose Titration	Time to Repeat Antifactor Xa Level
<0.35 units/mL	Increase dose by 25%	4 h after next dose
0.35-0.49 units/mL	Increase dose by 10%	4 h after next dose
0.5-1 unit/mL	Keep same dosage	Next day, then 1 wk later, then monthly (4 h after dose)
1.1-1.5 units/mL	Decrease dose by 20%	Before next dose
1.6-2 units/mL	Hold dose for 3 h and decrease dose by 30%	Before next dose, then 4 h after next dose
>2 units/mL	Hold all doses until antifactor Xa is 0.5 units/mL, then decrease dose by 40%	Before next dose and every 12 h until antifactor Xa <0.5 units/mL

Modified from Monagle P, Michelson AD, Bovill E, et al, "Antithrombotic Therapy in Children," *Chest*, 2001, 119:344S-70S.

Adults: **Note:** Consider lower doses for patients <45 kg

Prevention of DVT: SubQ:

Knee replacement surgery: 30 mg every 12 hours; give first dose 12-24 hours after surgery (provided hemostasis has been established); average duration 7-10 days, up to 14 days

Hip replacement surgery: Initial phase: 30 mg every 12 hours with first dose 12-24 hours after surgery (provided hemostasis has been established) or consider 40 mg once daily with first dose given 12 ± 3 hours prior to surgery; average duration of initial phase: 7-10 days, up to 14 days; after initial phase, give 40 mg once daily for 3 weeks

Abdominal surgery in patients at risk: 40 mg once daily; give first dose 2 hours prior to surgery; average duration: 7-10 days, up to 12 days

Medical patients at risk due to severely restricted mobility during acute illness: 40 mg once daily; average duration: 6-11 days, up to 14 days

Treatment of acute DVT and pulmonary embolism: SubQ: **Note:** Initiate warfarin therapy on the same day of starting enoxaparin; continue enoxaparin for a minimum of 5 days (average 7 days) until INR is therapeutic (between 2 and 3) for 24 hours (see Kearon, 2008).

Inpatient treatment of acute DVT with or without pulmonary embolism: 1 mg/kg every 12 hours or 1.5 mg/kg once daily

Outpatient treatment of acute DVT without pulmonary embolism: 1 mg/kg every 12 hours

Prevention of ischemic complications of non-Q-wave MI or unstable angina: SubQ: 1 mg/kg every 12 hours in conjunction with oral aspirin (100-325 mg once daily); continue treatment for a minimum of 2 days until patient is clinically stabilized (usually 2-8 days; up to 12.5 days)

Treatment of acute ST-segment elevation myocardial infarction (STEMI): Note: Optimal duration is not defined; in the major clinical trial, therapy was continued for 8 days or until hospital discharge; optimal duration may be >8 days. All patients should receive aspirin (75-325 mg once daily) as soon as they are identified as having STEMI. In patients with STEMI receiving thrombolytics, initiate enoxaparin dosing between 15 minutes before and 30 minutes after fibrinolytic therapy. In patients undergoing percutaneous coronary intervention (PCI), if balloon inflation occurs ≤8 hours after the last SubQ enoxaparin dose, no additional dosing is needed. If balloon inflation occurs 8-12 hours after last SubQ enoxaparin dose, a single I.V. dose of 0.3 mg/kg should be administered (see Hirsh, 2008; King, 2007).

Adults <75 years of age: Initial: 30 mg single I.V. bolus **plus** 1 mg/kg (maximum: 100 mg/dose for the first 2 doses only) SubQ every 12 hours. The first SubQ dose should be administered with the I.V. bolus. Maintenance: After first 2 doses, administer 1 mg/kg SubQ every 12 hours.

Adults ≥75 years of age: Dosage adjustment required; see package insert

Dosage adjustment in renal impairment:

Cl_{cr} ≥30 mL/minute: No specific adjustment recommended; monitor patients closely for bleeding

Cl_{cr} <30 mL/minute: **Note:** Monitor antifactor Xa activity closely. Adults:

DVT prophylaxis in abdominal surgery, hip replacement, knee replacement, or in medical patients during acute illness: SubQ: 30 mg once daily

DVT treatment in conjunction with warfarin (in inpatients with or without pulmonary embolism and in outpatients without pulmonary embolism): SubQ: 1 mg/kg once daily

Prevention of ischemic complications of non-Q-wave MI or unstable angina (with aspirin): SubQ: 1 mg/kg once daily

Treatment of STEMI:

Adults <75 years: Initial: 30 mg single I.V. bolus **plus** 1 mg/kg SubQ (administered at the same time as the I.V. bolus); maintenance: SubQ: 1 mg/kg once daily
Adults ≥75 years: See package insert

Dosage adjustment in hepatic impairment: Dosage adjustment not established; use with caution in patients with hepatic impairment

Administration Parenteral: Do not administer I.M. For SubQ use, administer by deep SubQ injection; do not rub injection site after SubQ administration as bruising may occur. When administering 30 mg or 40 mg SubQ from a commercially prefilled syringe, do not expel the air bubble from the syringe prior to injection (in order to avoid loss of drug). I.V. administration is indicated as part of treatment of STEMI only; flush I.V. access with NS or D_5W before and after enoxaparin I.V. bolus administration (to clear drug from port)

Monitoring Parameters CBC with platelets, stool occult blood tests, serum creatinine and potassium; antifactor Xa activity in select patients (eg, neonates, infants, children, obese patients, and patients with significant renal impairment, active bleeding, or abnormal coagulation parameters); **Note:** Routine monitoring of PT and APTT is not warranted since PT and APTT are relatively insensitive measures of low molecular weight heparin activity; consider monitoring bone density in infants and children with long-term use

Reference Range Antifactor Xa: **Note:** No clear consensus exists; the following are suggested peak values of antifactor Xa for VTE in adults, measured 4-6 hours after SubQ administration (see Nutescu, 2009)

Therapeutic:

Twice daily dosing: 0.5-1.0 units/mL

Once daily dosing: 1.0-2.0 units/mL; **Note:** Once daily dosing in pediatric patients is not feasible due to faster enoxaparin clearance and lower drug exposure in pediatric patients compared to adults (see O'Brien, 2007).

Prophylactic: 0.2-0.45 units/mL

Patient Information Enoxaparin may increase the time it takes to stop bleeding; report any unusual bleeding or bruising to prescriber. Inform physicians and dentists you are taking enoxaparin, especially before any surgery is scheduled. Report the use of other medication, nonprescription medications, and herbal or natural products to your physician and pharmacist; do not take any new medications or products without consulting prescriber.

If you had an epidural or spinal anesthesia or spinal puncture (lumbar puncture), contact physician immediately if you develop tingling or numbness (especially in the lower limbs) or muscular weakness.

Nursing Implications Instruct patients on proper SubQ injection technique if patient will self-inject.

Additional Information Each 10 mg of enoxaparin sodium equals ~1000 international units of antifactor Xa activity.

Enoxaparin contains fragments of unfractionated heparin produced by alkaline degradation (depolymerization) of heparin benzyl ester; enoxaparin has mean molecular weights of 3500-5600 daltons, which are much lower than mean molecular weights of unfractionated heparin (12,000-15,000 daltons). Low molecular weight heparins (LMWH) have several advantages over unfractionated heparin: Better SubQ bioavailability, more convenient administration (SubQ versus I.V.), longer half-life (longer dosing interval), more predictable pharmacokinetics and pharmacodynamic (anticoagulant) effect, less intensive laboratory monitoring, reduced risk of heparin-induced thrombocytopenia, potential for outpatient use, and probable reduced risk of osteoporosis (further studies are needed).

Accidental overdosage of enoxaparin may be treated with protamine sulfate; 1 mg protamine sulfate neutralizes 1 mg enoxaparin; first dose of protamine sulfate should equal the dose of enoxaparin injected, if enoxaparin was given in the previous 8 hours; use 0.5 mg protamine sulfate per 1 mg enoxaparin if enoxaparin was given >8 hours prior to protamine or if a second dose of protamine is needed; a second dose of protamine sulfate (0.5 mg per 1 mg enoxaparin) may be given if APTT remains prolonged 2-4 hours after first dose; protamine may not be required ≥12 hours after enoxaparin administration; avoid overdosage with protamine (see Protamine on page 1180)

Some centers dispense pediatric doses in an insulin syringe for greater delivery accuracy and to avoid errors associated with dilutions. Each 1 unit on a 30, 50, or 100 unit graduated insulin syringe is 0.01 mL; using a **100 mg/mL** enoxaparin injection, each "1 unit" on the insulin syringe would provide 1 mg of enoxaparin (see Bauman, 2009a).

Dosage Forms Excipient information presented when available (limited, particularly for generics); consult specific product labeling.

Injection, solution, as sodium [graduated prefilled syringe; preservative free]:

Lovenox®: 60 mg/0.6 mL (0.6 mL); 80 mg/0.8 mL (0.8 mL); 100 mg/mL (1 mL); 120 mg/0.8 mL (0.8 mL); 150 mg/mL (1 mL)

Injection, solution, as sodium [multidose vial]:

Lovenox®: 100 mg/mL (3 mL) [contains benzyl alcohol]

Injection, solution, as sodium [prefilled syringe; preservative free]:

Lovenox®: 30 mg/0.3 mL (0.3 mL); 40 mg/0.4 mL (0.4 mL)

References

Bauman ME, Belletrutti MJ, Bajzar L, et al, "Evaluation of Enoxaparin Dosing Requirements in Infants and Children. Better Dosing to Achieve Therapeutic Levels," *Thromb Haemost*, 2009, 101(1):86-92.

Bauman ME, Black KL, Bauman ML, "Novel Uses of Insulin Syringes to Reduce Dosing Errors: A Retrospective Chart Review of Enoxaparin Whole Milligram Dosing," *Thromb Res*, 2009a, 123(6):845-7.

Bontadelli J, Moeller A, Schmugge M, et al, "Enoxaparin Therapy for Arterial Thrombosis in Infants With Congenital Heart Disease," *Intensive Care Med*, 2007, 33(11):1978-84.

deVeber G, Chan A, Monagle P, et al, "Anticoagulation Therapy in Pediatric Patients With Sinovenous Thrombosis: A Cohort Study," *Arch Neurol*, 1998, 55(12):1533-7.

Dix D, Andrew M, Marzinotto V, et al, "The Use of Low Molecular Weight Heparin in Pediatric Patients: A Prospective Cohort Study," *J Pediatr*, 2000, 136(4):439-45.

Dunaway KK, Gal P, and Ransom JL, "Use of Enoxaparin in a Preterm Infant," *Ann Pharmacother*, 2000, 34(12):1410-3.

Hirsh J, Guyatt G, Albers GW, et al, "Executive Summary: American College of Chest Physicians Evidence-Based Clinical Practice Guidelines (8th Edition)," *Chest*, 2008, 133(6 Suppl):71-109.

Hirsh J, Warkentin TE, Shaughnessy SG, et al, "Heparin and Low-Molecular-Weight Heparin: Mechanisms of Action, Pharmacokinetics, Dosing, Monitoring, Efficacy, and Safety," *Chest*, 2001, 119:64S-94S.

Kearon C, Kahn SR, Agnelli G, et al, "Antithrombotic Therapy for Venous Thromboembolic Disease: American College of Chest Physicians Evidence-Based Clinical Practice Guidelines (8th Edition)," *Chest*, 2008, 33(6 Suppl):454-545.

King SB 3rd, Smith SC Jr, Hirshfeld JW JR, et al, "2007 Focused Update of the ACC/AHA/SCAI 2005 Guideline Update for Percutaneous Coronary Intervention. A Report of the American College of Cardiology/American Heart Association Task Force on Practice Guidelines: 2007 Writing Group to Review New Evidence and Update the ACC/AHA/SCAI 2005 Guideline Update for Percutaneous Coronary Intervention, Writing on Behalf of the 2005 Writing Committee," *Circulation*, 2008, 117(2):261-95.

Malowany JI, Knoppert DC, Chan AK, et al, "Enoxaparin Use in the Neonatal Intensive Care Unit: Experience Over 8 Years," *Pharmacotherapy*, 2007, 27(9):1263-71.

Malowany JI, Monagle P, Knoppert DC, et al, "Enoxaparin for Neonatal Thrombosis: A Call for a Higher Dose for Neonates," *Thromb Res*, 2008, 122(6):826-30.

Martineau P and Tawil N, "Low-Molecular-Weight Heparins in the Treatment of Deep-Vein Thrombosis," *Ann Pharmacother*, 1998, 32 (5):588-98, 601.

Massicotte P, Adams M, Marzinotto V, et al, "Low-Molecular-Weight Heparin in Pediatric Patients With Thrombotic Disease: A Dose Finding Study," *J Pediatr*, 1996, 128(3):313-8.

Michaels LA, Gurian M, Hegyi T, et al, "Low Molecular Weight Heparin in the Treatment of Venous and Arterial Thromboses in the Premature Infant," *Pediatrics*, 2004, 114(3):703-7.

Monagle P, Chalmers E, Chan A, et al, "Antithrombotic Therapy in Neonates and Children: American College of Chest Physicians Evidence-Based Clinical Practice Guidelines (8th Edition)," *Chest*, 2008, 133(6 Suppl):887S-968S.

Monagle P, Michelson AD, Bovill E, et al, "Antithrombotic Therapy in Children," *Chest*, 2001, 119:344S-70S.

Nutescu EA, Spinler SA, Wittkowsky A, et al, "Low-Molecular-Weight Heparins in Renal Impairment and Obesity: Available Evidence and Clinical Practice Recommendations Across Medical and Surgical Settings," *Ann Pharmacother*, 2009, 43(6):1064-83.

O'Brien SH, Lee H, and Ritchey AK, "Once-Daily Enoxaparin in Pediatric Thromboembolism: A Dose Finding and Pharmacodynamics/Pharmacokinetics Study," *J Thromb Haemost*, 2007, 5(9):1985-91.

♦ **Enoxaparin Injection (Can)** *see* Enoxaparin *on page 505*

♦ **Enoxaparin Sodium** *see* Enoxaparin *on page 505*

♦ **Entocort® (Can)** *see* Budesonide *on page 206*

♦ **Entocort® EC** *see* Budesonide *on page 206*

♦ **Entrophen® (Can)** *see* Aspirin *on page 141*

♦ **Entsol® [OTC]** *see* Sodium Chloride *on page 1270*

♦ **Enulose** *see* Lactulose *on page 791*

EPHEDrine (e FED rin)

Medication Safety Issues
Sound-alike/look-alike issues:
EPHEDrine may be confused with Epifrin®, EPINEPHrine

Therapeutic Category Adrenergic Agonist Agent; Antiasthmatic; Bronchodilator; Sympathomimetic

Generic Available Yes

Use Treatment of mild asthma, nasal congestion, acute bronchospasm, idiopathic orthostatic hypotension; adjunctive agent for treatment of shock

Pregnancy Risk Factor C

Lactation Enters breast milk/not recommended

Contraindications Hypersensitivity to ephedrine or any component; patients with hypertension, cardiac arrhythmias, angle-closure glaucoma, and psychoneurosis; use during halothane or cyclopropane anesthesia (see Drug Interactions)

Warnings Use of ephedrine as a pressor is not a substitute for replacement of blood, plasma, fluids, and electrolytes; blood volume should be corrected as fully as possible before ephedrine therapy; must not be used as sole therapy in hypovolemic patients; hypoxia, hypercapnia, and acidosis may reduce the effectiveness and increase the incidence of side effects of ephedrine; may cause hypertension which may result in intracranial hemorrhage; long-term use may cause anxiety and symptoms of paranoid schizophrenia; the FDA has issued warnings concerning ephedrine-containing nonprescription products with claims of producing such effects as euphoria, increased sexual sensation, increased energy, and weight loss; healthcare professionals are urged to be aware of these products and counsel patients, when appropriate, about the potential adverse effects of ephedrine such as headache, dizziness, heart irregularities, seizures, and possibly death

Precautions Use with caution in patients with hyperthyroidism, diabetes mellitus, prostatic hypertrophy, coronary insufficiency, and angina

Adverse Reactions
Cardiovascular: Hypertension, precordial pain, edema, palpitations, tachycardia, arrhythmias

Central nervous system: Nervousness, anxiety, apprehension, fear, tension, agitation, excitation, restlessness, irritability, insomnia, dizziness, vertigo, confusion, delirium, hallucinations, euphoria, paranoid psychosis, headache

Dermatologic: Rash

Gastrointestinal: Nausea, vomiting, xerostomia, mild epigastric distress, anorexia

Genitourinary: Urinary retention

Neuromuscular & skeletal: Tremors, hyperactive reflexes, weakness

Drug Interactions
Avoid Concomitant Use
Avoid concomitant use of EPHEDrine with any of the following: Inhalational Anesthetics; Iobenguane I 123; MAO Inhibitors

Increased Effect/Toxicity
EPHEDrine may increase the levels/effects of: Bromocriptine; Inhalational Anesthetics; Sympathomimetics

The levels/effects of EPHEDrine may be increased by: Antacids; Atomoxetine; Cannabinoids; Carbonic Anhydrase Inhibitors; MAO Inhibitors; Serotonin/Norepinephrine Reuptake Inhibitors

Decreased Effect
EPHEDrine may decrease the levels/effects of: Iobenguane I 123

The levels/effects of EPHEDrine may be decreased by: Spironolactone

Stability Protect from light

Mechanism of Action Stimulates both alpha- and beta-adrenergic receptors and also stimulates the release of norepinephrine from storage sites resulting in bronchodilation, cardiac stimulation, and increased systolic and diastolic blood pressure; tachyphylaxis may occur

Pharmacodynamics
Bronchodilation:
Onset of action: Oral: 15-60 minutes
Duration: Oral: 2-4 hours
Pressor/cardiac effects: Duration:
Oral: 4 hours
I.M., SubQ: 1 hour

Pharmacokinetics (Adult data unless noted)
Absorption: Oral: Complete
Metabolism: Liver by oxidative deamination, demethylation, aromatic hydroxylation, and conjugation
Bioavailability: Oral: 85%
Half-life: 4.9-6.5 hours
Elimination: Dependent upon urinary pH with greatest excretion in acid pH; urine pH 5: 74% to 99% excreted unchanged; urine pH 8: 22% to 25% excreted unchanged

Usual Dosage
Bronchodilation and nasal decongestion:
Oral:
Children >2-6 years: 2-3 mg/kg/day or 100 mg/m^2/day in 4-6 divided doses
Children 7-11 years: 6.25-12.5 mg every 4 hours; not to exceed 75 mg/day
Children ≥12 years and Adults: 12.5-50 mg every 3-4 hours; not to exceed 150 mg/day
Spray:
Children 6-12 years: 1-2 sprays in each nostril not more than every 4 hours; do not exceed 3 days of therapy
Children >12 years and Adults: 2-3 sprays in each nostril not more than every 4 hours; do not exceed 3 days of therapy

Orthostatic hypotension: Oral: Adults: 25 mg 1-4 times/day

Adjunctive agent in the treatment of shock: Use the smallest effective dose for the shortest time:
Children <12 years: I.M., I.V., SubQ: 3 mg/kg/day in 4-6 divided doses
Children ≥12 years and Adults:
I.M., SubQ: 25-50 mg (range: 10-50 mg); may repeat with a second dose of 50 mg; not to exceed 150 mg/24 hours
I.V.: 10-25 mg; may repeat with a second dose in 5-10 minutes of 25 mg; not to exceed 150 mg/24 hours

Administration
Oral: May be administered without regard to food
Parenteral:
I.M., SubQ: May be administered undiluted
I.V.: May be administered by slow I.V. push
Spray: Spray into each nostril while gently occluding the other

Monitoring Parameters Vital signs, pulmonary function tests, respiratory rate (when applicable)

Test Interactions May cause a false-positive test for amphetamine (by EMIT assay)

Patient Information Use for self-medication for asthma only under physician's direction; see Warnings; contact your physician if nervousness, tremor, insomnia, nausea, or loss of appetite occur; may cause dry mouth

Additional Information Because ephedrine has been used to synthesize methamphetamine, restrictions are in place to reduce the potential for misuse (diversion) and abuse; 24 g of ephedrine (in terms of base) is the limit for a single transaction for drug products containing ephedrine regardless of the form in which these drugs are packaged

Dosage Forms Excipient information presented when available (limited, particularly for generics); consult specific product labeling.
Capsule, as sulfate: 25 mg
Injection, solution, as sulfate: 50 mg/mL (1 mL, 10 mL)

♦ **Ephedrine Sulfate** see EPHEDrine on page 509
♦ **EpiClenz™ [OTC]** see Ethyl Alcohol on page 547
♦ **Epiflur™** see Fluoride on page 595
♦ **Epiklor™** see Potassium Chloride on page 1136
♦ **Epiklor™/25** see Potassium Chloride on page 1136

Epinastine (ep i NAS teen)

U.S. Brand Names Elestat™
Therapeutic Category Antiallergic, Ophthalmic
Generic Available No
Use Treatment of allergic conjunctivitis
Pregnancy Risk Factor C
Pregnancy Considerations Teratogenic effects were not observed in animal studies. There are no adequate and well-controlled studies in pregnant women.
Lactation Excretion in breast milk unknown/use caution
Contraindications Hypersensitivity to epinastine or any component of the formulation
Warnings Not for the treatment of contact lens irritation; contains the preservative, benzalkonium chloride, which may be absorbed by soft contact lenses; wait at least 10 minutes after instillation before inserting soft contact lenses. Safety and efficacy in children <3 years of age have not been established.

Adverse Reactions
Central nervous system: Headache
Ocular: Burning sensation, folliculosis, hyperemia, pruritus
Respiratory: Cough, pharyngitis, rhinitis, sinusitis
Miscellaneous: Infection (defined as cold symptoms and upper respiratory infection)

Drug Interactions
Avoid Concomitant Use There are no known interactions where it is recommended to avoid concomitant use.

Increased Effect/Toxicity
Epinastine may increase the levels/effects of: Anticholinergics; CNS Depressants; Methotrimeprazine

The levels/effects of Epinastine may be increased by: Methotrimeprazine; Pramlintide

Decreased Effect
Epinastine may decrease the levels/effects of: Acetylcholinesterase Inhibitors (Central)

The levels/effects of Epinastine may be decreased by: Acetylcholinesterase Inhibitors (Central); Amphetamines

Stability Store at controlled room temperature of 15°C to 25°C (59°F to 77°F). Keep tightly closed.

Mechanism of Action Selective H$_1$-receptor antagonist; inhibits release of histamine from the mast cell

Pharmacodynamics
Onset of action: 3-5 minutes
Duration: 8 hours

Pharmacokinetics (Adult data unless noted)
Absorption: Low systemic absorption following topical application
Distribution: Does not cross blood-brain barrier
Protein binding: 64%
Metabolism: <10% metabolized
Half-life: 12 hours
Elimination: I.V.: Urine (55%); feces (30%)

Usual Dosage Ophthalmic: Children ≥3 years and Adults: Instill 1 drop into each eye twice daily; continue throughout period of exposure, even in the absence of symptoms

Administration For ophthalmic use only; avoid touching tip of applicator to eye or other surfaces. Contact lenses should be removed prior to application; may be reinserted after 10 minutes. Do not wear contact lenses if eyes are red.

Patient Information For ophthalmic use only. Wash hands before using. Remove contact lenses before application (may be reinserted after ten minutes). May cause blurred vision, temporary stinging or burning sensation. Do not wear contact lenses if eyes are red.

Dosage Forms Excipient information presented when available (limited, particularly for generics); consult specific product labeling.

Solution, ophthalmic, as hydrochloride: 0.05% (5 mL) [contains benzalkonium chloride]

◆ **Epinastine Hydrochloride** *see* Epinastine *on page 510*

EPINEPHrine (ep i NEF rin)

Medication Safety Issues
Sound-alike/look-alike issues:
EPINEPHrine may be confused with ePHEDrine
Epifrin® may be confused with ephedrine, EpiPen®
EpiPen® may be confused with Epifrin®

High alert medication: The Institute for Safe Medication Practices (ISMP) includes this medication among its list of drugs which have a heightened risk of causing significant patient harm when used in error.

Medication errors have occurred due to confusion with epinephrine products expressed as ratio strengths (eg, 1:1000 vs 1:10,000).
Epinephrine 1:1000 = 1 mg/mL and is most commonly used I.M.
Epinephrine 1:10,000 = 0.1 mg/mL and is used I.V.

Medication errors have occurred when topical epinephrine 1 mg/mL (1:1000) has been inadvertently injected. Vials of injectable and topical epinephrine look very similar. Epinephrine should always be appropriately labeled with the intended administration.

International issues:
EpiPen® may be confused with Epigen® which is a brand name for glycyrrhizinic acid in Mexico
EpiPen® may be confused with Epopen® which is a brand name for epoetin alfa in Spain

Related Information
Adult ACLS Algorithms *on page 1463*
Asthma *on page 1697*
CPR Pediatric Drug Dosages *on page 1455*
Emergency Pediatric Drip Calculations *on page 1457*
Extravasation Treatment *on page 1522*
Neonatal Resuscitation Algorithm *on page 1459*
Pediatric ALS Algorithms *on page 1460*

U.S. Brand Names Adrenaclick™; Adrenalin®; EpiPen®; EpiPen® Jr; Primatene® Mist [OTC]; S2® [OTC]; Twinject®

Canadian Brand Names Adrenalin®; EpiPen®; EpiPen® Jr; Twinject®

Therapeutic Category Adrenergic Agonist Agent; Antiasthmatic; Antidote; Hypersensitivity Reactions; Bronchodilator; Decongestant, Nasal; Sympathomimetic

Generic Available Yes: Solution for injection

Use Treatment of bronchospasm, anaphylactic reactions, and cardiac arrest; nasal decongestant (topical nasal formulation); upper airway obstruction and croup (racemic epinephrine)

Pregnancy Risk Factor C

Pregnancy Considerations Teratogenic effects have been observed in animal reproduction studies. Epinephrine crosses the placenta and may cause fetal anoxia. Use during pregnancy when the potential benefit to the mother outweighs the possible risk to the fetus.

Lactation Excretion in breast milk unknown

Contraindications Hypersensitivity to epinephrine or any component (see Warnings); cardiac arrhythmias, angleclosure glaucoma

Warnings Some products contain sulfites which may cause allergic reactions in susceptible individuals

Precautions Use with caution in patients with diabetes mellitus, cardiovascular disease (angina, tachycardia, MI), thyroid disease, or cerebral arteriosclerosis; rebound nasal congestion may occur after frequent nasal use

Adverse Reactions
Cardiovascular: Pallor, tachycardia, hypertension, myocardial oxygen consumption increased, cardiac arrhythmias, sudden death
Central nervous system: Anxiety, headache
Gastrointestinal: Nausea
Genitourinary: Acute urinary retention in patients with bladder outflow obstruction
Neuromuscular & skeletal: Weakness, tremor
Ocular: Precipitation of or exacerbation of narrow-angle glaucoma
Renal: Renal and splanchnic blood flow decreased

Drug Interactions
Avoid Concomitant Use
Avoid concomitant use of EPINEPHrine with any of the following: Iobenguane I 123

Increased Effect/Toxicity
EPINEPHrine may increase the levels/effects of: Bromocriptine; Sympathomimetics

The levels/effects of EPINEPHrine may be increased by: Antacids; Atomoxetine; Beta-Blockers; Cannabinoids; Carbonic Anhydrase Inhibitors; COMT Inhibitors; Inhalational Anesthetics; MAO Inhibitors; Serotonin/Norepinephrine Reuptake Inhibitors; Tricyclic Antidepressants

Decreased Effect
EPINEPHrine may decrease the levels/effects of: Iobenguane I 123

The levels/effects of EPINEPHrine may be decreased by: Spironolactone

Stability Protect from light; incompatible with alkaline solutions (sodium bicarbonate); compatible when coadministered with dopamine, dobutamine, inamrinone (amrinone), atracurium, pancuronium, and vecuronium

Mechanism of Action Stimulates alpha-, beta$_1$- and beta$_2$-adrenergic receptors resulting in relaxation of smooth muscle of the bronchial tree, cardiac stimulation, and dilation of skeletal muscle vasculature; small doses can cause vasodilation via beta$_2$-vascular receptors; large doses may produce constriction of skeletal and vascular smooth muscle; decreases production of aqueous humor and increases aqueous outflow; dilates the pupil by contracting the dilator muscle

Pharmacodynamics
Local vasoconstriction (topical):
Onset of action: 5 minutes
Duration: <1 hour
Onset of bronchodilation:
Inhalation: Within 1 minute
SubQ.: Within 5-10 minutes

Pharmacokinetics (Adult data unless noted)
Absorption: Orally ingested doses are rapidly metabolized in GI tract and liver; pharmacologically active concentrations are **not** achieved
Distribution: Crosses placenta but not blood-brain barrier
Metabolism: Extensive in the liver and other tissues by the enzymes catechol-o-methyltransferase and monoamine oxidase

Usual Dosage
Neonates: I.V., Intratracheal: 0.01-0.03 mg/kg (0.1-0.3 mL/kg of **1:10,000** solution) every 3-5 minutes as needed
Infants and Children:
Hypersensitivity reactions: **Note:** For self-administration following severe allergic reactions (eg, insect stings, food), the World Health Organization (WHO) and Anaphylaxis Canada recommend the availability of 1 dose for every 10-20 minutes of travel time to a medical emergency facility.
I.M.: EpiPen® and EpiPen® Jr: 0.01 mg/kg
or as alternative
<30 kg: 0.15 mg
≥30 kg: 0.3 mg

I.M., SubQ: Twinject™:
Children 15-30 kg: 0.15 mg
Children >30 kg: 0.3 mg
I.V.: 0.01 mg/kg (0.1 mL/kg of **1:10,000** solution) not to exceed 0.5 mg every 20 minutes; may use continuous infusion (0.1 mcg/kg/minute) to prevent frequent doses in more severe reactions
SubQ, I.M.: 0.01 mg/kg (0.01 mL/kg/dose of **1:1000** solution) not to exceed 0.5 mg every 20 minutes
Bradycardia:
I.V.: 0.01 mg/kg (0.1 mL/kg) of **1:10,000** solution (maximum dose: 1 mg or 10 mL); may repeat every 3-5 minutes as needed
Intratracheal: 0.1 mg/kg (0.1 mL/kg) of **1:1000** solution; doses as high as 0.2 mg/kg may be effective; may repeat every 3-5 minutes as needed
Asystole or pulseless arrest:
I.V. or I.O.: 0.01 mg/kg (0.1 mL/kg) of **1:10,000** solution; may repeat every 3-5 minutes as needed; if ineffective, may increase dosage to 0.1 mg/kg (0.1 mL/kg of **1:1000** solution; doses as high as 0.2 mg/kg may be effective); repeat every 3-5 minutes as needed [increased dosage no longer routinely recommended by the American Heart Association (see References)]
Intratracheal: 0.1 mg/kg (0.1 mL/kg) of **1:1000** solution (doses as high as 0.2 mg/kg may be effective); **Note:** Recent clinical studies suggest that lower epinephrine concentrations delivered by intrathecal administration may produce transient β-adrenergic effects which may be detrimental (eg, hypotension, lower coronary artery perfusion pressure). I.V. or I.O. are the preferred methods of administration (AHA, 2005).
Inotropic support: Continuous I.V. infusion rate: 0.1-1 mcg/kg/minute; titrate dosage to desired effect
Nebulization: 0.25-0.5 mL of 2.25% **racemic epinephrine** solution diluted in 3 mL NS, or L-epinephrine at an equivalent dose; racemic epinephrine 10 mg = 5 mg L-epinephrine; use lower end of dosing range for younger infants
Nasal: Children ≥6 years and Adults: Apply drops locally as needed; do not exceed 1 mL every 15 minutes
Adults:
Asystole/pulseless arrest bradycardia, VT/VF: I.V., I.O.: 1 mg every 3-5 minutes; if this approach fails, alternative regimens include:
Intermediate: 2-5 mg every 3-5 minutes
Escalating: 1 mg, 3 mg, 5 mg at 3-minute intervals
High: 0.1 mg/kg every 3-5 minutes
Intratracheal: 1 mg (although the optimal dose is unknown, doses of 2-2.5 times the I.V. dose may be needed)
Bradycardia (symptomatic) or hypotension (not responsive to atropine or pacing): I.V. infusion: 2-10 mcg/minute; titrate to desired effect
Bronchodilator:
SubQ: 0.3-0.5 mg every 20 minutes for 3 doses
Nebulization: S2® (racemic epinephrine, OTC labeling): 0.5 mL: Repeat no more frequently than every 3-4 hours as needed.
Inhalation: Primatene® Mist (OTC labeling): One inhalation, wait at least 1 minute; if relieved, may use once more. Do not use again for at least 3 hours.
Hypersensitivity reactions: **Note:** For self-administration following severe allergic reactions (eg, insect stings, food), the World Health Organization (WHO) and Anaphylaxis Canada recommend the availability of 1 dose for every 10-20 minutes of travel time to a medical emergency facility. More than 2 doses should only be administered under direct medical supervision.
I.M.: EpiPen®: 0.3 mg
I.M., SubQ: Twinject™: 0.3 mg

I.M., SubQ: 0.3-0.5 mg (**1:1000** formulation) may repeat every 15-20 minutes, if condition requires; I.M. route is preferred
I.V.: 0.1 mg (**1:10,000** formulation); may use continuous infusion (1-4 mcg/minute) to prevent the need to repeat injections

Administration

Inhalation: Nebulization: Dilute in 3 mL NS
Intratracheal: Administer and flush with a minimum of 5 mL NS, followed by 5 manual ventilations
Nasal: Apply as drops or with sterile swab
Oral inhalation: Shake well before use; use spacer in children <8 years of age
Parenteral:
Direct I.V. or I.O. administration: Dilute to a maximum concentration of 100 mcg/mL (if using 1:10,000 concentration, no dilution is necessary)
Continuous I.V. infusion: Rate of infusion (mL/hour) = dose (mcg/kg/minute) x weight (kg) x 60 minutes/hour divided by the concentration (mcg/mL); maximum concentration: 64 mcg/mL
I.M. (EpiPen®, EpiPen® Jr, and Twinject™): Intramuscularly into anterolateral aspect of thigh
SubQ: Use only 1:1000 solution or 1:200 suspension
Monitoring Parameters ECG, heart rate, blood pressure, site of infusion for excessive blanching/extravasation
Nursing Implications Tissue irritant; extravasation may be treated by local small injections of a diluted phentolamine solution (mix 5 mg with 9 mL NS)
Dosage Forms Excipient information presented when available (limited, particularly for generics); consult specific product labeling. [DSC] = Discontinued product
Aerosol for oral inhalation:
Primatene® Mist: 0.22 mg/inhalation (15 mL, 22.5 mL [DSC]) [contains CFCs]
Injection, solution [prefilled auto injector]:
Adrenaclick™: 0.15 mg/0.15 mL (1.1 mL) [1:1000 solution; delivers 0.15 mg per injection; contains chlorobutanol, sodium bisulfite; available as single unit or double-unit pack]; 0.3 mg/0.3 mL (1.1 mL) [1:1000 solution; delivers 0.3 mg per injection; contains chlorobutanol, sodium bisulfite; available as a single unit or in double-unit pack]
EpiPen®: 0.3 mg/0.3 mL (2 mL) [1:1000 solution; delivers 0.3 mg per injection; contains sodium metabisulfite; available as single unit or in double-unit pack with training unit]
EpiPen® Jr: 0.15 mg/0.3 mL (2 mL) [1:2000 solution; delivers 0.15 mg per injection; contains sodium metabisulfite; available as single unit or in double-unit pack with training unit]
Twinject®: 0.15 mg/0.15 mL (1.1 mL) [1:1000 solution; delivers 0.15 mg per injection; contains chlorobutanol, sodium bisulfite; two 0.15 mg doses per injector]; 0.3 mg/0.3 mL (1.1 mL) [1:1000 solution; delivers 0.3 mg per injection; contains chlorobutanol, sodium bisulfite; two 0.3 mg doses per injector]
Injection, solution, as hydrochloride: 0.1 mg/mL (10 mL) [1:10,000 solution]; 1 mg/mL (1 mL) [1:1000 solution]
Adrenalin®: 1 mg/mL (1 mL) [1:1000 solution; contains sodium bisulfite]
Adrenalin®: 1 mg/mL (30 mL) [1:1000 solution; contains chlorobutanol, sodium bisulfite]
Solution for oral inhalation [racepinephrine; preservative free]:
S2®: 2.25% (0.5 mL) [as d-epinephrine 1.125% and l-epinephrine 1.125%]
Solution, intranasal, as hydrochloride [drops, spray]:
Adrenalin®: 1 mg/mL (30 mL) [1:1000 solution; contains sodium bisulfite]

References

American College of Cardiology, American Heart Association Task Force, "Adult Advanced Cardiac Life Support" and "Pediatric Advanced Life Support Guidelines," *JAMA*, 1992, 268(16):2199-241 and 2262-75.

"2005 American Heart Association (AHA) Guidelines for Cardiopulmonary Resuscitation (CPR) and Emergency Cardiovascular Care (ECC) of Pediatric and Neonatal Patients: Pediatric Advanced Life Support," *Pediatrics*, 2006, 117(5):1005-28.

Waisman Y, Klein BL, Boenning DA, et al, "Prospective Randomized Double-Blind Study Comparing L-Epinephrine and Racemic Epinephrine Aerosols in the Treatment of Laryngotracheitis (Croup)," *Pediatrics*, 1992, 89(2):302-6.

♦ **Epinephrine and Lidocaine** *see* Lidocaine and Epinephrine *on page 821*

♦ **Epinephrine Bitartrate** *see* EPINEPHrine *on page 511*

♦ **Epinephrine Hydrochloride** *see* EPINEPHrine *on page 511*

♦ **EpiPen®** *see* EPINEPHrine *on page 511*

♦ **EpiPen® Jr** *see* EPINEPHrine *on page 511*

♦ **Epipodophyllotoxin** *see* Etoposide *on page 551*

♦ **Epitol®** *see* CarBAMazepine *on page 244*

♦ **Epival® I.V. (Can)** *see* Valproic Acid and Derivatives *on page 1398*

♦ **Epivir®** *see* LamiVUDine *on page 791*

♦ **Epivir-HBV®** *see* LamiVUDine *on page 791*

♦ **EPO** *see* Epoetin Alfa *on page 513*

Epoetin Alfa (e POE e tin AL fa)

Medication Safety Issues

Sound-alike/look-alike issues:

Epoetin alfa may be confused with darbepoetin alfa, epoetin beta

Epogen® may be confused with Neupogen®

International issues:

Epopen® [Spain] may be confused with EpiPen® which is a brand name for epinephrine in the U.S.

U.S. Brand Names Epogen®; Procrit®

Canadian Brand Names Eprex®

Therapeutic Category Colony-Stimulating Factor; Recombinant Human Erythropoietin

Generic Available No

Use Treatment of anemia associated with chronic renal failure (CRF) in patients on dialysis (FDA approved in ages 1 month to 16 years and adults); treatment of anemia associated with CRF without dialysis (FDA approved in ages ≥3 months and adults); anemia in cancer patients with nonmyeloid malignancies receiving chemotherapy [FDA approved in pediatrics (age not specified) and adults]; anemia related to HIV therapy with zidovudine (FDA approved in ages ≥8 months and adults); has also been used for anemia of prematurity and reduction of allogeneic blood transfusion for elective, noncardiac, or nonvascular surgery

Restrictions Healthcare providers and hospitals must be enrolled in the ESA APPRISE (Assisting Providers and Cancer Patients with Risk Information for the Safe use of ESAs) Oncology Program (866-284-8089; http://www.esa-apprise.com) to prescribe or dispense ESAs (darbepoetin; epoetin alfa) to patients with cancer.

Medication Guide An FDA-approved patient medication guide, which is available with the product information and as follows, must be dispensed with this medication for each new outpatient prescription and refill.

Epogen®: http://www.fda.gov/downloads/Drugs/DrugSafety/UCM088591.pdf

Procrit®: http://www.fda.gov/downloads/Drugs/DrugSafety/UCM088988.pdf

Pregnancy Risk Factor C

Pregnancy Considerations Epoetin alfa has been shown to have adverse effects (decreased weight gain, delayed development, delayed ossification) in animal studies. Studies suggest that rHuEPO-α does not cross the human placenta. Based on case reports, treatment with rHuEPO-α may be an option in pregnant women with ESRD on dialysis. Amenorrheic premenopausal women should be cautioned that menstruation may resume following treatment with rHuEPO-α and contraception should be considered if pregnancy is to be avoided.

Lactation Excretion in breast milk unknown/use caution

Breast-Feeding Considerations When administered enterally to neonates (mixed with human milk or infant formula), rHuEPO-α did not significantly increase serum EPO concentrations. If passage via breast milk does occur, risk to a nursing infant appears low.

Contraindications Hypersensitivity to epoetin alfa, albumin (human) or mammalian cell-derived products, or any component of epoetin alfa (see Warnings); uncontrolled hypertension; neutropenia in newborns

Warnings Patients with chronic renal failure are at greater risk for death, serious cardiovascular events, and stroke when using erthyropoiesis-stimulating agents (ESAs) to target higher hemoglobin concentrations (≥13 g/dL) in clinical trials; dosing should be individualized to achieve and maintain hemoglobin concentrations within 10-12 g/dL range **[U.S. Boxed Warning]**. Increased thrombotic events have also been documented in cancer patients. Due to an increased risk of cardiac arrest, neurologic events (including seizures and stroke), exacerbations of hypertension, CHF, vascular thrombosis/ischemia, infarction, acute MI, and fluid overdose/edema in patients whose Hgb increased >12 g/dL, hemoglobin should be monitored twice weekly for 2-6 weeks following initiation and the EPO dosage should be decreased if the Hgb exceeds 12 g/dL or the rate of rise of hemoglobin exceeds 1 g/dL in any 2-week period. Blood pressure should be controlled adequately before initiation of EPO therapy particularly in CRF patients; approximately 25% of CRF patients on dialysis may require increased antihypertensive medications while receiving epoetin; hypertensive encephalopathy and seizures have been observed in CRF patients treated with epoetin; close blood pressure monitoring is recommended. ESA therapy may reduce dialysis efficacy (due to increase in red blood cells and decrease in plasma volume); adjustments in dialysis parameters may be needed.

ESAs shortened survival and/or time-to-tumor progression in studies of advanced breast, cervical, head and neck, lymphoid, and nonsmall cell lung cancer in patients receiving ESAs when dosed to target a hemoglobin of ≥12 g/dL **[U.S. Boxed Warning]**. This risk has not been excluded when a lower target hemoglobin is used. Because of the risks of decreased survival and increased risk of tumor growth or progression, all healthcare providers and hospitals are required to enroll and comply with the ESA APPRISE (Assisting Providers and Cancer Patients with Risk Information for the Safe use of ESAs) Oncology Program prior to prescribing or dispensing ESAs to cancer patients **[U.S. Boxed Warning]**. Prescribers and patients will have to provide written documentation of discussed risks. For patients with cancer, use only for the treatment of anemia due to concomitant myelosuppressive chemotherapy, use the lowest dose needed to avoid RBC transfusions, and discontinue following completion of chemotherapy course **[U.S. Boxed Warning]**. EPO is not approved for use in patients with myeloid malignancies or in patients with cancer-related anemia who are not receiving concurrent chemotherapy.

An increased rate of DVT in surgical orthopedic procedures when EPO was used to reduce red blood cell infusions **[U.S. Boxed Warning]**. DVT prophylaxis should be strongly considered in these patients. Increased mortality in patients using EPO to prevent red blood cell infusions during cardiac surgery, EPO is not approved for this indication. **Seizures** have occurred during therapy; monitor closely for premonitory neurologic symptoms during the first several months of therapy. Pure red cell aplasia (PRCA) and severe anemia have been reported, predominantly in patients with CRF and patients receiving other ESAs. Should a sudden loss of responsiveness to epoetin alfa combined with a severe anemia and low reticulocyte count occur, temporarily discontinue epoetin and determine if anti-erythropoietin antibodies are present. Discontinue epoetin if these antibodies are detected. Prior to and during epoetin therapy, assess the patient's iron stores utilizing serum ferritin, TIBC; supplemental iron therapy is recommended to support erythropoiesis and avoid depletion of iron stores.

The multidose formulation contains benzyl alcohol which may cause allergic reactions in susceptible individuals; large amounts of benzyl alcohol ($\geq$99 mg/kg/day) have been associated with a potentially fatal toxicity ("gasping syndrome") in neonates; the "gasping syndrome" consists of metabolic acidosis, respiratory distress, gasping respirations, CNS dysfunction (including convulsions, intracranial hemorrhage), hypotension and cardiovascular collapse; avoid use of multidose formulation in neonates; *in vitro* and animal studies have shown that benzoate, a metabolite of benzyl alcohol, displaces bilirubin from protein-binding sites. Pooled use of unused portions of preservative-free EPO has resulted in microbial contamination, bacteremia, and pyrogenic reactions. Preservative-free formulations are intended for single use only.

Precautions Use with caution in patients with porphyria as exacerbations of porphyria have been reported in patients with CRF. Use with caution in patients with a history of seizures or hypertension; an excessive rate of rise of hematocrit may possibly be associated with the exacerbation of hypertension or seizures. Decrease the epoetin alfa dosage if the hemoglobin increase exceeds 1g/dL in any 2-week period. Blood pressure should be controlled prior to the start of therapy and monitored closely throughout treatment. Hypertensive encephalopathy has been reported with patients receiving erythropoietic therapy. Seizures have occurred during ESA therapy; monitor closely for premonitory neurologic symptoms during the first several months of therapy.

EPO is not intended for patients who require acute corrections of anemia and is not a substitute for emergency blood transfusion. EPO contains albumin, which confers a theoretical risk of transmission of viral disease or Creutzfeldt-Jakob disease.

Assessment of iron stores and therapeutic iron supplementation is essential to optimal EPO therapy. Iron supplementation is necessary to provide for increased requirements during expansion of the red cell mass secondary to marrow stimulation by EPO, unless iron stores are already in excess. Supplemental iron is recommended if serum ferritin <100 mcg/mL or serum transferrin saturation <20%.

Factors Limiting Response to Epoetin Alfa

Factor	Mechanism
Iron deficiency	Limits hemoglobin synthesis
Blood loss/hemolysis	Counteracts epoetin alfa-stimulated erythropoiesis
Infection/inflammation	Inhibits iron transfer from storage to bone marrow Suppresses erythropoiesis through activated macrophages
Aluminum overload	Inhibits iron incorporation into heme protein
Bone marrow replacement Hyperparathyroidism Metastatic, neoplastic disease	Limits bone marrow volume
Folic acid/vitamin B_{12} deficiency	Limits hemoglobin synthesis
Patient compliance	Self-administered epoetin alfa or iron therapy

Adverse Reactions

Cardiovascular: Chest pain, edema, hypertension, thrombophlebitis, thrombotic vascular events (eg, MI, CVA/TIA, DVT; see Warnings)

Central nervous system: Dizziness, fatigue, fever, headache, insomnia, seizure

Dermatologic: Pruritus, rash

Gastrointestinal: Constipation, diarrhea, dyspepsia, nausea, vomiting

Genitourinary: Urinary tract infection

Hematologic: Anemia (see Warnings), neutropenia, pure red cell aplasia (PRCA)

Local: Clotted vascular access, irritation at injection site (SubQ injection), pain

Neuromuscular & skeletal: Arthralgias, paresthesia, weakness

Respiratory: Congestion, cough, dyspnea, upper respiratory infection

Miscellaneous: Tumor progression (see Warnings)

<1%, postmarketing, and/or case reports: Allergic reaction, flu-like syndrome, hyperkalemia, hypertensive encephalopathy, microvascular thrombosis, myalgia, neutralizing antibodies, pulmonary embolism, renal vein thrombosis, retinal artery tachycardia, temporal vein thrombosis, thrombophlebitis, thrombosis, urticaria

Drug Interactions

Avoid Concomitant Use There are no known interactions where it is recommended to avoid concomitant use.

Increased Effect/Toxicity There are no known significant interactions involving an increase in effect.

Decreased Effect There are no known significant interactions involving a decrease in effect.

Stability Refrigerate; single-dose vials contain no preservatives; discard after entry (see Warnings). Multiple-dose vials contain benzyl alcohol preservative and may be used up to 21 days after initial entry when stored between 2°C to 8°C. Prefilled syringes containing the preservative formulation are stable for 6 weeks refrigerated (2°C to 8°C) (see Naughton, 2003). EPO is stable for 24 hours when diluted in dextrose I.V. fluid which contains at least 0.05% human albumin or parenteral nutrition solutions containing at least 0.5% amino acids.

Mechanism of Action Epoetin alfa, a glycoprotein manufactured by recombinant DNA technology, has the same effects as endogenous erythropoietin. EPO induces erythropoiesis by stimulating the division and differentiation of committed erythroid progenitor cells. It induces the release of reticulocytes from the bone marrow into the bloodstream, where they mature to erythrocytes (dose response relationship) resulting in an increase in reticulocyte counts followed by a rise in hematocrit and hemoglobin concentrations. There is normally an inverse correlation between the plasma EPO concentration and the hemoglobin concentration (only when the hemoglobin concentration is <10.5 g/dL).

Pharmacodynamics

Onset of action: Several days

Maximum effect: 2-6 weeks

Pharmacokinetics (Adult data unless noted)

Absorption: SubQ: 31.9%

Distribution: Adults: V_d: 9 L; rapid in the plasma compartment; majority of drug is taken up by the liver, kidneys, and bone marrow

Bioavailability: SubQ: ~21% to 31%

Half-life:

Neonates: SubQ: 17.6 hours on day 3 of therapy, 11.2 hours on day 10 of therapy

Children and Adults: I.V.: 4-13 hours in patients with chronic renal failure (CRF); half-life is 20% shorter in patients with normal renal function; Cancer: Adults: SubQ: 16-67 hours

Time to peak serum concentration: SubQ: 5-24 hours

Elimination: Some metabolic degradation does occur with small amounts recovered in the urine

Clearance: Neonates: SubQ or continuous I.V. infusion: 26-35 mL/hour/kg on day 3 of therapy and 65-87 mL/hour/kg on day 10 of therapy

Note: While a much higher peak plasma concentration is achieved after I.V. bolus administration, it declines at a more rapid rate (over 2-3 days) than after subcutaneous administration (plasma concentrations greater than endogenous are maintained for at least 4 days). Subcutaneous administration is associated with a 30% to 50% lower EPO dose requirement.

Usual Dosage Dosing schedules need to be individualized and careful monitoring of patients receiving the drug is recommended. EPO may be ineffective if other factors such as iron or B_{12}/folate deficiency limit marrow response. Dosage based upon SubQ administration; use of I.V. administration may result in the need to increase doses by as much as 30% to 50% to achieve the same outcome: I.V., SubQ:

Anemia of prematurity: Neonates: Variable regimens: 25-100 units/kg/dose 3 times/week **or** 100 units/kg/dose 5 times/week **or** 200 units/kg/dose every other day for 10 doses

Anemia in cancer patients: **Note:** Use in patients with pretreatment serum EPO concentrations >200 mIU/mL is **not** recommended; titrate dose to achieve and maintain the lowest hemoglobin concentration sufficient to avoid the need for blood transfusion and not to exceed 12 g/dL

Children 6 months to 18 years: Doses ranging from 25-300 units/kg 3-7 times/week have been reported

Manufacturer's recommendation: Based upon a randomized, double-blind, placebo controlled study of 222 children, 5-18 years, using I.V. administration only: 600 units/kg weekly (not to exceed 40,000 units/week); may increase to 900 units/kg weekly (not to exceed 60,000 units/week); use caution in considering this dosage for administration by the SubQ route as SubQ administration has been shown to produce effect at doses 30% to 50% lower than I.V. administration

Adults: 150 units/kg/dose 3 times/week; maximum 1200 units/kg/week; or as an alternative: 40,000 units once weekly; may increase to 60,000 units once weekly if hemoglobin is not increased by at least 1 g/dL after 4 weeks of treatment

Epoetin Alfa Dosage Adjustments in Cancer Patients

Target hemoglobin range	Achieve and maintain the lowest hemoglobin concentration sufficient to avoid the need for blood transfusion and not to exceed 12 g/dL
Reduce dose by 25% when	Hemoglobin reaches a concentration needed to avoid transfusion **or** increases >1 g/dL in any 2-week period
Increase dose when	Response is not satisfactory (no reduction in transfusion requirements or rise in hemoglobin) after 8 weeks to achieve and maintain the lowest hemoglobin concentration sufficient to avoid the need for RBC transfusion and not to exceed 12 g/dL
Stop therapy when	Hemoglobin >12 g/dL; reinstate therapy at a 25% lower dose after the hemoglobin approaches a concentration where transfusion may be required or chemotherapy regimen is completed

Anemia in chronic renal failure:

Initial dose:

Children: 50 units/kg/dose 3 times/week

Adults: 50-100 units/kg/dose 3 times/week

Maintenance dose: Children and Adults: Titrate dose to response (see Epoetin Alfa Dosage Adjustments in CRF table); increases should not be made more frequently than once every 4 weeks; median dose: Children (hemodialysis): 167 units/kg/week (range: 49-447 units/kg/week); children (peritoneal dialysis): 76 units/kg/week (range: 24-323 units/kg/week); adults (hemodialysis): 75 units/kg 3 times/week (range: 12.5-525 units/kg 3 times/week)

Note: Once weekly dosage has been studied in chronic renal failure patients. When transitioning from multiple doses/week to once weekly, begin with a weekly dosage equal to the current total dose per week. Allow at least 4 weeks to determine full effects of the new regimen.

Epoetin Alfa Dosage Adjustments in CRF

Target hemoglobin range[1]	10-12 g/dL
Reduce dose by 25% when	Target range is reached **or** hemoglobin increases >1 g/dL in any 2-week period
Increase dose by 25% when	Hemoglobin <10 g/dL **and** has not increased by 1 g/dL after 4 weeks of therapy
Stop therapy when	Hemoglobin continues to increase after dosage reduction; reinstate therapy at a 25% lower dose after the hemoglobin begins to decrease

[1]The National Kidney Foundation Clinical Practice Guideline for Anemia in CKD: 2007 Update of Hemoglobin Target (September, 2007) recommend hemoglobin concentrations in the range of 11-12 g/dL for dialysis and nondialysis patients receiving ESAs; hemoglobin concentrations should not be >13 g/dL

Zidovudine-treated, HIV-infected patients: Use has not been demonstrated in controlled clinical trials to improve symptoms of anemia, quality of life, fatigue, or patient well-being

Children 8 months to 17 years: Limited data available; doses ranging from 50-400 units/kg 2-3 times/week have been reported

Adults (pretreatment serum EPO concentrations ≤500 mUnits/mL and receiving zidovudine ≤4200 mg/week): Initial: 100 units/kg/dose 3 times/week for 8 weeks; after 8 weeks of therapy the dose may be adjusted by 50-100 units/kg increments 3 times/week to a maximum dose of 300 units/kg 3 times/week. Titrate dose to maintain the response based on factors such as variations in zidovudine dose and the presence of intercurrent infectious or inflammatory episodes. If hemoglobin >12 g/dL, discontinue until hemoglobin decreases to 11 g/dL, resume with 25% dosage reduction and continue to titrate.

Presurgery, autologous blood donation: Adults: Prior to initiating treatment, obtain a hemoglobin to establish that it is >10 g/dL or <13 g/dL: 300 units/kg/day for 10 days before surgery, the day of surgery, and 4 days after **or as an alternative**, 600 units/kg/week at 21-, 14-, and 7 days before surgery and on the day of surgery

Administration Parenteral: Do not shake as this may denature the glycoprotein rendering the drug biologically inactive

SubQ is the preferred route of administration; 1:1 dilution with bacteriostatic NS (containing benzyl alcohol) acts as a local anesthetic to reduce pain at the injection site. Multiple-dose vials already contain benzyl alcohol.

I.V.: Manufacturer recommends administering without dilution; some institutions may wish to dilutewith an equal volume of NS; infuse over 1-3 minutes; it may be administered into the venous line at the end of the dialysis procedure; may be infused in dextrose solution when diluted with albumin (see Stability)

Monitoring Parameters
Careful monitoring of blood pressure is indicated; problems with hypertension have been noted especially in renal failure patients treated with EPO. Other patients are less likely to develop this complication. See table.

Test	Initial Phase Frequency	Maintenance Phase Frequency
Hemoglobin	CRF: 2 times/week Cancer, HIV: Once weekly	2-4 times/month
Blood pressure	3 times/week	3 times/week
Serum ferritin	Monthly	Quarterly
Transferrin saturation	Monthly	Quarterly
Serum chemistries including CBC with differential, creatinine, BUN, potassium, phosphorous	Regularly per routine	Regularly per routine
Reticulocyte count	Baseline prior to starting therapy	After 10 days of therapy

Reference Range The decision to initiate EPO therapy may be made by utilizing an endogenous erythropoietin serum concentration measurement. Endogenous erythropoietin concentrations are inversely related to the hemoglobin (and hematocrit) concentration in anemias that are not attributed to impaired erythropoietin production (eg, iron deficiency anemia). A normal erythropoietin concentration, for subjects with normal hemoglobin and hematocrit, is 4.1-22.2 mIU/mL. Baseline erythropoietin concentrations in anemic patients may increase up to 100-1000 fold in untreated patients with a normal release of erythropoietin. The following table illustrates the "normal" response to anemia. EPO is indicated in patients who do not exhibit a normal response to anemia (eg, the measurement of endogenous erythropoietin is low relative to a normal response). If the patient has exhibited a normal response, addition of exogenous EPO may not be beneficial. Clinical studies involving the following disease states have established criteria for assessment of endogenous erythropoietin concentrations prior to initiating EPO therapy:

Zidovudine-treated HIV patients: Available evidence indicates patients with endogenous serum erythropoietin concentrations >500 mIU/mL are unlikely to respond

Cancer chemotherapy patients: Treatment of patients with endogenous serum erythropoietin concentrations >200 mIU/mL is not recommended.

Inverse Relationship of Endogenous Erythropoietin to Hemoglobin

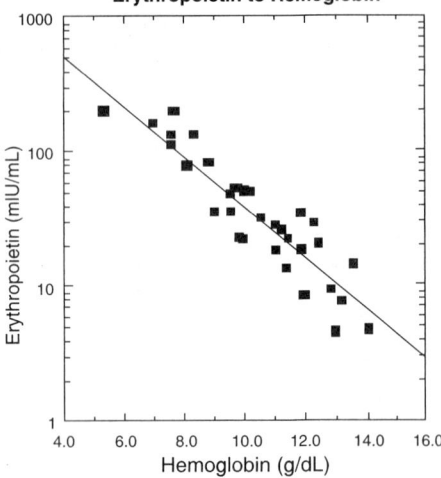

Patient Information Frequent blood tests are needed to determine the correct dose; notify physician if any signs of edema (swollen extremities, respiratory difficulty), sudden onset of severe headache, back pain, chest pain, muscle tremors or weakness, fever, cough or signs of respiratory infection, dizziness or loss of consciousness, extreme tiredness, or blood clots in hemodialysis vascular access ports (CRF patients) develops. Due to an increased risk of seizure activity in CRF patients during the first 90 days of therapy, avoid potentially hazardous activities (eg, driving) during this period.

Additional Information Optimal response is achieved when iron stores are maintained with supplemental iron if necessary; evaluate iron stores prior to and during therapy

Reimbursement Hotline (Epogen®): 1-800-272-9376
Professional Services [Amgen]: 1-800-77-AMGEN
Reimbursement Hotline (Procrit®): 1-800-553-3851
Professional Services [Ortho Biotech]: 1-800-325-7504

Dosage Forms Excipient information presented when available (limited, particularly for generics); consult specific product labeling.

Injection, solution [preservative free]:
   Epogen®, Procrit®: 2000 units/mL (1 mL); 3000 units/mL (1 mL); 4000 units/mL (1 mL); 10,000 units/mL (1 mL); 40,000 units/mL (1 mL) [contains human albumin]

Injection, solution [with preservative]:
   Epogen®, Procrit®: 10,000 units/mL (2 mL); 20,000 units/mL (1 mL) [contains human albumin and benzyl alcohol]

References
Blanche S, Caniglia M, Fischer A, et al, "Zidovudine Therapy in Children With Acquired Immunodeficiency Syndrome," Am J Med, 1988, 85 (2A):203-7.

Halperin DS, Wacker P, Lacourt G, et al, "Effects of Recombinant Human Erythropoietin in Infants With the Anemia of Prematurity: A Pilot Study," J Pediatr, 1990, 116(5):779-86.

KDOQI, "KDOQI Clinical Practice Guideline and Clinical Practice Recommendations for Anemia in Chronic Kidney Disease: 2007 Update of Hemoglobin Target," Am J Kidney Dis, 2007, 50 (3):471-530.

Naughton CA, Duppong LM, Forbes KD, et al, "Stability of Multidose, Preserved Formulation Epoetin Alfa in Syringes for Three and Six Weeks," Am J Health Syst Pharm, 2003, 60(5):464-8.

Ohls RK and Christensen, RD, "Stability of Human Recombinant Epoetin Alfa in Commonly Used Neonatal Intravenous Solutions," Ann Pharmacother, 1996, 30(5):466-468.

Ohls RK, Veerman MW, and Christensen RD, "Pharmacokinetics and Effectiveness of Recombinant Erythropoietin Administered to Preterm Infants by Continuous Infusion in Total Parenteral Nutrition Solution," *J Pediatr*, 1996, 128(4):518-23.

Rhondeau SM, Christensen RD, Ross MP, et al, "Responsiveness to Recombinant Human Erythropoietin of Marrow Erythroid Progenitors From Infants With the Anemia of Prematurity," *J Pediatr*, 1988, 112 (6):935-40.

Rizzo JD, Somerfield MR, Hagerty KL, et al, "Use of Epoetin and Darbepoetin in Patients With Cancer: 2007 American Society of Hematology/American Society of Clinical Oncology Clinical Practice Guideline Update," *Blood*, 2008, 111(1):25-41.

Shannon KM, Keith JF 3rd, Mentzer WC, et al, "Recombinant Human Erythropoietin Stimulates Erythropoiesis and Reduces Erythrocyte Transfusions in Very Low Birth Weight Preterm Infants," *Pediatrics*, 1995, 95(1):1-8.

Sinai-Trieman L, Salusky IB, and Fine RN, "Use of Subcutaneous Recombinant Human Erythropoietin in Children Undergoing Continuous Cycling Peritoneal Dialysis," *J Pediatr*, 1989, 114(4 Pt 1):550-4.

◆ **Epogen®** see Epoetin Alfa *on page 513*

Epoprostenol (e poe PROST en ole)

Medication Safety Issues

High alert medication: The Institute for Safe Medication Practices (ISMP) includes this medication among its list of drugs which have a heightened risk of causing significant patient harm when used in error.

Related Information

New York Heart Association (NYHA) Classification of Functional Capacity of Patients With Diseases of the Heart, 1994 Revisions *on page 1482*

U.S. Brand Names Flolan®

Canadian Brand Names Flolan®

Therapeutic Category Prostaglandin

Generic Available Yes

Use

Long-term I.V. treatment of primary pulmonary hypertension (PPH) and pulmonary hypertension secondary to the scleroderma spectrum of disease, in NYHA Class III and Class IV patients who are not fully responsive to other therapy.

Short-term I.V. infusion of epoprostenol in patients with pulmonary hypertension may be used diagnostically in the cardiac catheterization laboratory to screen for responsiveness to other oral vasodilating agents (eg, calcium channel blockers). **Note:** Responsiveness to short-term (acute) I.V. infusions of epoprostenol predicts responsiveness to long-term treatment with oral calcium channel blockers; however, it does not predict responsiveness to long-term I.V. epoprostenol therapy. Patients who do not respond acutely to epoprostenol, may respond to the drug when used chronically.

Other potential uses include treatment of secondary pulmonary hypertension associated with ARDS, SLE, congenital heart disease, congenital diaphragmatic hernia, neonatal pulmonary hypertension, cardiopulmonary bypass surgery, hemodialysis, peripheral vascular disorders, portal hypertension, and neonatal purpura fulminans.

Restrictions Orders for epoprostenol are distributed by two sources in the United States. Information on orders or reimbursement assistance may be obtained from either Accredo Health, Inc (1-800-935-6526) or TheraCom, Inc (1-877-356-5264).

Pregnancy Risk Factor B

Pregnancy Considerations Teratogenic effects were not reported in animal studies. There are no adequate and well-controlled studies in pregnant women. Women with IPAH are encouraged to avoid pregnancy.

Lactation Excretion in breast milk unknown/use caution

Contraindications Hypersensitivity to epoprostenol, any component, or structurally-related compounds; chronic use in patients with CHF due to severe left ventricular systolic dysfunction. **Note:** Do not use epoprostenol chronically in patients who develop pulmonary edema during dose initiation (see Warnings).

Warnings Epoprostenol **must** be reconstituted with the manufacturer-supplied sterile diluent only; do **not** reconstitute or mix with other I.V. fluids or I.V. medications prior to or during administration. Abrupt withdrawal, interruptions in drug delivery, or sudden reductions in epoprostenol dosage may result in symptoms associated with rebound pulmonary hypertension (eg, asthenia, dizziness, dyspnea) and can be potentially fatal; avoid abrupt withdrawal, interruptions in drug delivery, and sudden large reductions in dosage. Pulmonary edema, which may be associated with pulmonary veno-occlusive disease may develop in patients with pulmonary hypertension during epoprostenol dose initiation (do not use epoprostenol chronically in these patients).

Symptoms of overdose include headache, hypotension, tachycardia, nausea, vomiting, diarrhea, and flushing. Reduce the infusion rate to decrease symptoms. If symptoms do not subside or worsen, consider drug discontinuation. Fatalities due to hypoxemia, hypotension, and respiratory arrest have been reported following overdose with epoprostenol.

Precautions Use with caution and appropriately monitor patients; epoprostenol is a potent pulmonary and systemic vasodilator; it should be used only by clinicians who are experienced in the diagnosis and treatment of pulmonary hypertension; dose initiation must occur in a setting with adequately trained personnel and proper equipment for physiologic monitoring and emergency care. Asymptomatic increases in pulmonary artery pressure, associated with increases in cardiac output, may rarely occur during dose initiation; consider dosage reduction in these patients. During chronic use, unless contraindicated, anticoagulants should be coadministered in adult patients to reduce the risk of thromboembolism [**Note:** The use of anticoagulants in **adult** patients with primary pulmonary hypertension has been shown to improve survival. Although such efficacy has **not** been demonstrated in pediatric patients, some studies have reported the routine use of warfarin in pediatric patients receiving long-term (chronic) infusions of epoprosentol for pulmonary hypertension (see Barst, 1999 and Rosenzweig, 1999), while other studies have routinely discontinued anticoagulants prior to the initiation of epoprostenol therapy (see Higenbottam, 1993); further studies are needed to assess the risks and benefits of routine anticoagulation in pediatric patients treated with epoprostenol.]

Adverse Reactions Note: Some reported adverse reactions may be related to the underlying disease (eg, chest pain, dyspnea, edema, fatigue, hypoxia, pallor, and right heart failure).

Cardiovascular: Flushing (acute: 58%; chronic 42%), hypotension, chest pain, bradycardia (vagal effect), reflex tachycardia, palpitations, arrhythmia, supraventricular tachycardia, MI

Central nervous system: Headache (acute: 49%; chronic: 83%), anxiety, nervousness, agitation, dizziness, restlessness, depression, convulsions, CVA

Dermatologic: Rash, urticaria, eczema, pruritus, skin ulcer

Endocrine & metabolic: Hypokalemia, hyperkalemia, weight reduction, weight gain

Gastrointestinal: Nausea, vomiting, diarrhea, abdominal pain, dyspepsia, anorexia, constipation, abdominal enlargement

Hematologic: Hemorrhage, thrombocytopenia

Local: Injection-site reactions: Infection (21%), pain (13%), irritation, erythema, thrombophlebitis

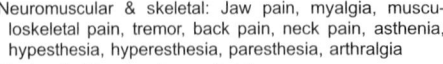

Neuromuscular & skeletal: Jaw pain, myalgia, musculoskeletal pain, tremor, back pain, neck pain, asthenia, hypesthesia, hyperesthesia, paresthesia, arthralgia

Ocular: Amblyopia, abnormal vision

Respiratory: Dyspnea, epistaxis, pleural effusion; pulmonary edema, which may be associated with pulmonary veno-occlusive disease (see Warnings)

Miscellaneous: Flu-like symptoms, diaphoresis, catheter-related sepsis

Drug Interactions

Avoid Concomitant Use There are no known interactions where it is recommended to avoid concomitant use.

Increased Effect/Toxicity

Epoprostenol may increase the levels/effects of: Anticoagulants; Antihypertensives; Antiplatelet Agents

Decreased Effect There are no known significant interactions involving a decrease in effect.

Stability Store unopened vials of drug and sterile diluent at room temperature 15°C to 25°C (59°F to 77°F); protect drug vials from light; do not freeze diluent. Following reconstitution, solution must be stored under refrigeration at 2°C to 8°C (36°F to 46°F) if not used immediately; reconstituted solution is stable for up to 48 hours when refrigerated; protect from light; do not freeze (discard if solution has been frozen). Reconstituted solution (pH 10.2-10.8) is increasingly unstable at a lower pH and drug is rapidly hydrolyzed at the pH of I.V. fluids.

During use, a single reservoir of solution may be used at room temperature for a total duration of 8 hours, or used with a cold pouch for administration up to 24 hours. **Note:** Reconstituted solutions may be refrigerated for ≤40 hours prior to administration at room temperature for up to 8 hours. Reconstituted solutions may be refrigerated for ≤24 hours prior to administration with a cold pouch for up to 24 hours. Cold pouch should be changed every 12 hours and must be capable of maintaining the reconstituted solution at a temperature between 2°C to 8°C for 12 hours.

Mechanism of Action Epoprostenol (also known as prostacyclin, PGI_2 and PGX), is a metabolite of arachidonic acid and a naturally-occurring prostaglandin. It is a potent, direct-acting, vasodilator of pulmonary and systemic arterial vascular beds. In addition, it inhibits platelet aggregation and vascular smooth muscle proliferation. The reduction in platelet aggregation results from epoprostenol's activation of intracellular adenylate cyclase and the resultant increase in cyclic adenosine monophosphate concentrations within the platelets (**Note:** Patients with PPH have an imbalance in the ratio of thromboxane to prostacyclin metabolites and have a decreased amount of prostacyclin synthase in the pulmonary arteries).

Clinically, the vasodilator effects decrease right ventricular and left ventricular afterload and increase cardiac output and stroke volume. Epoprostenol decreases pulmonary vascular resistance, mean pulmonary artery pressure, and mean systemic arterial pressure. Additionally, it is capable of decreasing thrombogenesis and platelet clumping in the lungs by inhibiting platelet aggregation. Studies have demonstrated an increase in exercise capacity and improvements in dyspnea and fatigue.

Pharmacokinetics (Adult data unless noted)

Metabolism: Rapidly hydrolyzed at a neutral pH in blood; also metabolized by enzymatic degradation; two primary metabolites with pharmacologic activity less than epoprostenol are formed: 6-keto-PGF_{1alpha} (via spontaneous degradation) and 6,15-diketo-13,14-dihydro-PGF_{1alpha} (via enzymatic degradation); 14 minor metabolites have also been isolated in the urine

Half-life: ≤6 minutes

Elimination: Urine (84% of dose); feces (4%)

Usual Dosage I.V.: Continuous infusion: **Note:** The need for increased doses should be expected with chronic use; incremental increases occur more frequently during the first few months after the drug is initiated. The optimal dose in children is not well defined. The mean chronic dose at 1 year of therapy is 20-40 ng/kg/minute in adults, but is 50-80 ng/kg/minute in children (particularly younger children); significant variability in optimal dose occurs in pediatric patients (see Barst, 1999; Rosenweig, 1999; and Widlitz, 2003).

Children and Adults:

Chronic infusion: Initial: 1-2 ng/kg/minute, increase dose in increments of 1-2 ng/kg/minute every 15 minutes or longer until dose-limiting side effects are noted or tolerance limit to epoprostenol is observed

Dose adjustment:

Increase dose in 1-2 ng/kg/minute increments at intervals of at least 15 minutes if symptoms of pulmonary hypertension persist or recur following improvement. In clinical trials, dosing increases occurred at intervals of 24-48 hours or longer.

Decrease dose in 2 ng/kg/minute decrements at intervals of at least 15 minutes in case of dose-limiting pharmacologic (adverse) events. Avoid abrupt withdrawal or sudden large dose reductions.

Lung transplant: In patients receiving lung transplants, epoprostenol was tapered after the initiation of cardiopulmonary bypass.

Administration Reconstitute with the manufacturer-supplied sterile diluent only; do **not** reconstitute or mix with other I.V. fluids or I.V. medications prior to or during administration (epoprostenol is very unstable in neutral or acidic pH solutions). To make a 100 mL solution (daily supply) with a final concentration of 3000 ng/mL, dilute one 0.5 mg vial of epoprostenol with 5 mL of supplied diluent; withdraw 3 mL and add to sufficient diluent to make a total of 100 mL. This 100 mL 24-hour supply may be divided into 3 equal parts; one portion can be used for up to 8 hours at room temperature, and the two other portions should be stored in the refrigerator and protected from light (see Stability). During use, a single reservoir of solution may be used at room temperature for a total duration of 8 hours, or used with a cold pouch for administration up to 24 hours (see Stability). The final concentration of epoprostenol solution is determined by the minimum and maximum flow rates of the infusion pump and desired duration of infusion from the specific reservoir volume. Concentrations >15,000 ng/mL may be required for patients receiving higher infusion rates. Maximum concentration for administration: 70,000 ng/mL.

I.V.: Continuous infusion: Chronic continuous I.V. infusions of epoprostenol must be administered through a permanent indwelling central venous catheter; use an ambulatory infusion pump for patients discharged home. Peripheral infusion may be used temporarily until central line is established. Epoprostenol should be infused in a dedicated lumen exclusive of any other drugs; consider a multilumen catheter if other I.V. medications are routinely administered. Avoid abrupt withdrawal, interruptions in delivery, or sudden large reductions in dosing (see Warnings). Patients should have access to a backup infusion pump and infusion sets.

Note: The ambulatory infusion pump should be small and lightweight; be able to adjust infusion rates in 2 ng/kg/minute increments; have occlusion, end of infusion, and low battery alarms; have ±6% accuracy of the programmed rate; and be positive continuous or pulsatile pressure-driven with intervals ≤3 minutes between pulses. The reservoir should be made of polypropylene, polyvinyl chloride, or glass. The infusion pump used in the most recent clinical trial was CADD-1 HFX 5100 (Pharmacia Deltec).

Monitoring Parameters Hemodynamic effects (pulmonary vascular resistance, pulmonary arterial pressure, systemic blood pressure, heart rate). Monitor blood pressure (standing and supine) and heart rate closely for several hours following dosage adjustments. Monitor for improvements in exercise capacity, exertional dyspnea, fatigue, syncope, chest pain, and quality of life. Monitor the infusion pump device and catheters to avoid drug delivery system related failures. Monitor weight; serum potassium.

Patient Information For most adult patients and some pediatric patients, therapy with this medication will probably be prolonged, possibly for years. This medication is infused through a permanent indwelling central venous catheter, on a continuous basis, by a small, portable infusion pump. Interruptions of the infusion (even for a brief time) may result in a rapid symptomatic deterioration of the patient. The patient or caregiver must become familiar with and perform a sterile technique to prepare and administer the medication and to care for the central venous catheter.

This medication may cause jaw pain, headache, diarrhea, nervousness, and muscular pains (use of a mild analgesia may be recommended by your prescriber); may cause dizziness and impair ability to perform activities requiring mental alertness or physical coordination. Report immediately any signs or symptoms of acute or severe headache; back pain; increased difficult breathing; flushing; fever or chills; any unusual bleeding or bruising; chest pain; palpitations; irregular, slow or fast pulse; flushing; loss of sensation; or any onset of unresolved diarrhea.

Nursing Implications Epoprostenol must be reconstituted with manufacturer-supplied sterile diluent only. When administered chronically, it must be infused through a permanent indwelling central venous catheter via a portable infusion pump. Avoid abrupt withdrawal, interruptions in drug delivery, and sudden large reductions in dosage (see Warnings); be alert for any infusion pump malfunction. Assess for signs of overdose (eg, hypotension, hypoxia, flushing, tachycardia, fever, chills, anxiety, acute headache, tremor, vomiting, diarrhea). Instruct the patient or caregiver about proper aseptic technique, appropriate catheter care, and proper drug reconstitution and administration. Instruct patient to report adverse reactions since dosage adjustments may be necessary.

Additional Information The primary role of epoprostenol is in the treatment of primary pulmonary hypertension in patients unresponsive to other therapy. Response to initial therapy is evaluated in a controlled setting before chronic therapy is administered. The role of epoprostenol in the treatment of heart failure confers a negative impact on cardiovascular morbidity and mortality. Clinical trials in adults showed improvement of heart failure symptoms and exercise tolerance, but an increase in mortality.

Dosage Forms Excipient information presented when available (limited, particularly for generics); consult specific product labeling.

Injection, powder for reconstitution: 0.5 mg, 1.5 mg [provided with 50 mL sterile diluent]

Flolan®: 0.5 mg, 1.5 mg

References
Barst RJ, "Pharmacologically Induced Pulmonary Vasodilatation in Children and Young Adults With Primary Pulmonary Hypertension," *Chest*, 1986, 89(4):497-503.

Barst RJ, Maislin G, and Fishman AP, "Vasodilator Therapy for Primary Pulmonary Hypertension in Children," *Circulation*, 1999, 99 (9):1197-208.

Barst RJ, Rubin LJ, Long WA, et al, "A Comparison of Continuous Intravenous Epoprostenol (Prostacyclin) With Conventional Therapy for Primary Pulmonary Hypertension. The Primary Pulmonary Hypertension Study Group," *N Engl J Med*, 1996, 334(5):296-302.

Higenbottam TW, Spiegelhalter D, Scott JP, et al, "Prostacyclin (Epoprostenol) and Heart-Lung Transplantation as Treatments for Severe Pulmonary Hypertension," Br Heart J, 1994, 70:366-70.

Kermode J, Butt W, and Shann F, "Comparison Between Prostaglandin E1 and Epoprostenol (Prostacyclin) in Infants After Heart Surgery," *Br Heart J*, 1991, 66(2):175-8.

Rosenzweig EB, Kerstein D, and Barst RJ, "Long-Term Prostacyclin for Pulmonary Hypertension With Associated Congenital Heart Defects," *Circulation*, 1999, 99(14):1858-65.

Widlitz A and Barst RJ, "Pulmonary Arterial Hypertension in Children," *Eur Respir J*, 2003, 21(1):155-76.

◆ **Epoprostenol Sodium** *see* Epoprostenol *on page 517*

◆ **Eprex® (Can)** *see* Epoetin Alfa *on page 513*

◆ **Epsilon Aminocaproic Acid** *see* Aminocaproic Acid *on page 82*

◆ **Epsom Salts** *see* Magnesium Sulfate *on page 858*

◆ **Epsom Salts (Magnesium Sulfate)** *see* Magnesium Supplements *on page 859*

◆ **EPT** *see* Teniposide *on page 1318*

◆ **Eptacog Alfa (Activated)** *see* Factor VIIa (Recombinant) *on page 556*

◆ **Epzicom®** *see* Abacavir and Lamivudine *on page 29*

◆ **Equalizer Gas Relief [OTC]** *see* Simethicone *on page 1262*

◆ **Equetro®** *see* CarBAMazepine *on page 244*

Ergocalciferol (er goe kal SIF e role)

Medication Safety Issues

Sound-alike/look-alike issues:

Calciferol™ may be confused with calcitriol

Drisdol® may be confused with Drysol™

Ergocalciferol may be confused with cholecalciferol

Potential for medication errors: Liquid vitamin D preparations have the potential for dosing errors when administered to infants. Droppers should be clearly marked to easily provide 400 international units. For products intended for infants, the FDA recommends that accompanying droppers deliver no more than 400 international units per dose.

U.S. Brand Names Calciferol™ [OTC]; Drisdol®; Drisdol® [OTC]

Canadian Brand Names Drisdol®; Ostoforte®

Therapeutic Category Nutritional Supplement; Vitamin D Analog; Vitamin, Fat Soluble

Generic Available Yes: Capsule (softgel), tablet

Use Prevention and treatment of vitamin D deficiency and/or rickets or osteomalacia (FDA approved in all ages); treatment of familial hypophosphatemia; treatment of hypoparathyroidism; prevention and treatment of vitamin D deficiency and insufficiency in patients with chronic kidney disease (CKD); dietary supplement

Pregnancy Risk Factor C (manufacturer); A/C (dose exceeding RDA recommendation; per expert analysis)

Pregnancy Considerations Abnormalities have been observed in animal studies with maternal doses causing hypervitaminosis D. Doses larger than the RDA should be avoided during pregnancy.

Lactation Enters breast milk/use caution

Breast-Feeding Considerations Small quantities of vitamin D are found in breast milk following normal maternal exposure via sunlight and diet. The amount in breast milk does not correlate with serum levels in the infant. Therefore, vitamin D supplementation is recommended in all infants who are partially or exclusively breast fed. Hypercalcemia has been noted in a breast-feeding infant following maternal use of large doses of ergocalciferol; high doses should be avoided in lactating women.

Contraindications Hypersensitivity to ergocalciferol or any component (see Warnings); hypercalcemia; malabsorption syndrome; evidence of vitamin D toxicity

Warnings Some products contain tartrazine which may cause allergic reactions in susceptible individuals. Oral solution contains propylene glycol. Serum calcium times phosphorus (Ca x P) should not exceed 65 mg^2/dL^2 for infants and children ≤12 years and 55 mg^2/dL^2 for children >12 years and adults.

Precautions Use with caution in patients with coronary artery disease, renal stones, and impaired renal function; adequate calcium intake is necessary for clinical response to ergocalciferol therapy; maintain adequate fluid intake; avoid hypercalcemia

Adverse Reactions Note: Adverse effects are results of hypercalcemia induced by hypervitaminosis D.

Cardiovascular: Arrhythmia (QT shortening, sinus tachycardia)

Central nervous system: Confusion, headache, lethargy, sluggishness

Gastrointestinal: Abdominal pain, nausea, vomiting

Neuromuscular & skeletal: Soft tissue calcification

Renal: Calciuria, nephrocalcinosis

Drug Interactions

Avoid Concomitant Use There are no known interactions where it is recommended to avoid concomitant use.

Increased Effect/Toxicity There are no known significant interactions involving an increase in effect.

Decreased Effect There are no known significant interactions involving a decrease in effect.

Stability Store at room temperature; protect from light

Mechanism of Action Vitamin D stimulates calcium and phosphate absorption from the small intestine; promotes secretion of calcium from bone to blood; promotes renal tubule phosphate resorption; acts directly on bone cells (osteoblasts) to stimulate skeletal growth and on the parathyroid glands to suppress parathyroid hormone synthesis and secretion

Pharmacodynamics Maximum effect occurs in ~1 month following daily doses

Pharmacokinetics (Adult data unless noted)

Absorption: Readily absorbed from GI tract; absorption requires intestinal presence of bile

Metabolism: Inactive until hydroxylated in the liver and the kidney to calcifediol and then to calcitriol (most active form)

Usual Dosage Oral: **Note:** 1 mcg = 40 USP international units

Infants and Children:

Prevention of Vitamin D Deficiency:

Neonates, infants, and children: 200 international units/day; Dietary Supplementation for Prevention of Vitamin D Deficiency: Dietary Intake Reference (DIR) (1997 National Academy of Science Recommendations); **Note:** DIR is under review as of March 2009.

Alternative dosing (see Greer, 2000; Wagner, 2008):

Premature infants: 10-20 mcg/day (400-800 international units), up to 750 mcg/day (30,000 international units)

Breast-fed infants (fully or partially): 10 mcg/day (400 international units/day) beginning in the first few days of life. Continue supplementation until infant is weaned to ≥1000 mL/day or 1 qt/day of vitamin D-fortified formula or whole milk (after 12 months of age)

Formula-fed infants ingesting <1000 mL of vitamin D-fortified formula or milk: 10 mcg/day (400 international units/day)

Children ingesting <1000 mL of vitamin D-fortified milk: 10 mcg/day (400 international units/day)

Children with increased risk of vitamin D deficiency (chronic fat malabsorption, maintained on chronic antiseizure medications): Higher doses may be

required. Use laboratory testing [25(OH)D, PTH, bone mineral status] to evaluate.

Adolescents without adequate intake: 10 mcg/day (400 international units/day)

Vitamin D insufficiency or deficiency associated with CKD (stages 2-5, 5D): (K/DOQI Guidelines, 2009); serum 25 hydroxyvitamin D (25[OH]D) level <30 ng/mL:

Serum 25(OH)D level 16-30 ng/mL: Children: 2000 international units/day for 3 months or 50,000 international units every month for 3 months

Serum 25(OH)D level 5-15 ng/mL: Children: 4000 international units/day or 50,000 international units every other week for 12 weeks

Serum 25(OH)D level <5 ng/mL: Children: 8000 international units/day for 4 weeks then 4000 international units/day for 2 months for total therapy of 3 months or 50,000 international units/week for 4 weeks followed by 50,000 international units 2 times/month for a total therapy of 3 months

Maintenance dose [once repletion accomplished; serum 25(OH)D level >30 ng/mL]: 200-1000 international units/day

Dosage adjustment: Monitor 25(OH)D, corrected total calcium and phosphorus levels 1 month following initiation of therapy, every 3 months during therapy and with any Vitamin D dose change.

Hypoparathyroidism: Children: 1.25-5 mg/day (50,000-200,000 international units) with calcium supplements

Vitamin D-dependent rickets: In addition to calcium supplementation:

Infants <1 month: 25 mcg/day (1000 international units) for 2-3 months; once radiologic evidence of healing is observed, dose should be decreased to 10 mcg/day (400 international units/day)

Infants 1-12 months: 25-125 mcg/day (1000-5000 international units) for 2-3 months; once radiologic evidence of healing is observed, dose should be decreased to 10 mcg/day (400 international units/day)

Infants and Children >12 months: 125-250 mcg/day (5000-10,000 international units) for 2-3 months; once radiologic evidence of healing is observed, dose should be decreased to 10 mcg/day (400 international units/day)

Prevention and treatment vitamin D Deficiency in cystic fibrosis: Recommended daily intake (see Borowitz 2002):

Infants <1 year: 400 international units/day

Children >1 year: 400-800 international units/day

Nutritional rickets and osteomalacia:

Children and Adults (with normal absorption): 25-125 mcg/day (1000-5000 international units) for 6-12 weeks

Children with malabsorption: 250-625 mcg/day (10,000-25,000 international units)

Familial hypophosphatemia: Children: Initial: 1000-2000 mcg/day (40,000-80,000 international units) with phosphate supplements; daily dosage is increased at 3- to 4-month intervals in 250-500 mcg (10,000-20,000 international units) increments

Adults:

Dietary Intake Reference (DIR), 1997: **Note:** DIR is currently being reviewed (March, 2009): Oral: 5-10 mcg/day (200-400 international units/day)

Osteoporosis prevention and treatment: 10 mcg/day (800-1000 international units/day)

Vitamin D deficiency/insufficiency in patients with CKD stages 3-4 (K/DOQI guidelines): Dose is based on 25-hydroxyvitamin D serum level [25(OH) D]: Treatment duration should be a total of 6 months:

Serum 25(OH)D 16-30 ng/mL: 50,000 international units/month

Serum 25(OH)D 5-15 ng/mL: 50,000 international units/week for 4 weeks, then 50,000 international units/month

Serum 25(OH)D <5 ng/mL: 50,000 international units/week for 12 weeks, then 50,000 international units/month

Hypoparathyroidism: 625 mcg to 5 mg/day (25,000-200,000 international units) and calcium supplements

Nutritional rickets and osteomalacia:

Adults with normal absorption: 25-125 mcg/day (1000-5000 international units)

Adults with malabsorption: 250-7500 mcg (10,000-300,000 international units)

Vitamin D-dependent rickets: 250 mcg to 1.5 mg/day (10,000-60,000 international units)

Vitamin D-resistant rickets: 12,000-500,000 international units/day

Familial hypophosphatemia: 10,000-60,000 international units plus phosphate supplements

Administration Oral: May be administered without regard to meals; for oral liquid, use accompanying dropper for dosage measurements

Monitoring Parameters Children at increased risk of vitamin D deficiency (chronic fat malabsorption, chronic antiseizure medication use) require serum 25(OH)D, PTH, and bone-mineral status to evaluate. If vitamin D supplement is required, then 25(OH)D levels should be repeated at 3-month intervals until normal. PTH and bone mineral-status should be monitored every 6 months until normal.

Chronic kidney disease: Serum calcium and phosphorus levels (in CKD: After 1 month and then at least every 3 months); alkaline phosphatase, BUN; bone x-ray (hypophosphatemia or hypoparathyroidism); 25(OH)D (in CKD: After 3 months of treatment and as needed thereafter)

Reference Range Vitamin D status may be determined by serum 25(OH) D levels (see Misra, 2008):

Severe deficiency: ≤5 ng/mL (12.5 nmol/L)

Deficiency: 15 ng/mL (37.5 nmol/L)

Insufficiency: 15-20 ng/mL (37.5-50 nmol/L)

Sufficiency: 20-100 ng/mL (50-250 nmol/L)*

Excess: >100 ng/mL (250 nmol/L) **

Intoxication: 150 ng/mL (375 nmol/L)

* Based on adult data a level of >32 ng/mL (80 nmol/L) is desirable

** Arbitrary designation

Chronic kidney disease (CKD) is defined either as kidney damage or GFR <60 mL/minute/1.73 m^2 for ≥3 months); stages of CKD are described below:

CKD Stage 1: Kidney damage with normal or increased GFR; GFR >90 mL/minute/1.73m^2

CKD Stage 2: Kidney damage with mild decrease in GFR; GFR 60-89 mL/minute/1.73 m^2

CKD Stage 3: Moderate decrease in GFR; GFR 30-59 mL/minute/1.73 m^2

CKD Stage 4: Severe decrease in GFR; GFR 15-29 mL/minute/1.73 m^2

CKD Stage 5: Kidney failure; GFR <15 mL/minute/1.73 m^2 or dialysis

Target serum 25(OH)D: >30 ng/mL

Patient Information Take as directed; do not increase dosage without consulting healthcare provider. Adhere to diet as recommended (do not take any other phosphate or vitamin D-related compounds while taking ergocalciferol). You may experience nausea, vomiting, dry mouth (small frequent meals, frequent mouth care, chewing gums, or sucking lozenges may help).

Additional Information 1.25 mg ergocalciferol provides 50,000 international units of vitamin D activity; 1 drop of 8000 international units/mL = 200 international units (40 drops = 1 mL)

Dosage Forms Excipient information presented when available (limited, particularly for generics); consult specific product labeling.

Capsule, oral:

Drisdol®: 50,000 int. units [1.25 mg; contains tartrazine and soybean oil]

Capsule, softgel, oral: 50,000 int. units

Solution, oral [drops]:

Calciferol™: 8000 int. units/mL (60 mL) [contains propylene glycol; 200 mcg/mL; OTC]

Drisdol®: 8000 int. units/mL (60 mL) [contains propylene glycol; 200 mcg/mL; OTC]

Tablet, oral: 400 int. units [10 mcg; OTC]

References

Borowitz D, Baker RD, and Stallings V, "Consensus Report on Nutrition for Pediatric Patients With Cystic Fibrosis," *J Pediatr Gastroenterol Nutr*, 2002, 35(3):246-59.

"Dietary Reference Intakes for Calcium, Phosphorus, Magnesium, Vitamin D, and Fluoride. Standing Committee on the Scientific Evaluation of Dietary Reference Intakes, Food and Nutrition Board, Institute of Medicine," National Academy of Sciences, Washington, DC: National Academy Press, 1997.

"K/DOQI Clinical Practice Guidelines for Chronic Kidney Disease: Evaluation, Classification, and Stratification, Part 4. Definition and Classification of Stages of Chronic Kidney Disease," *Am J Kidney Dis*, 2002, 39(2 Suppl 1):46-75.

KDOQI Work Group, "KDOQI Clinical Practice Guideline for Nutrition in Children with CKD: 2008 Update. Executive Summary," *Am J Kidney Dis*, 2009, 53(3 Suppl 2):S11-104.

Misra M, Pacaud D, Petryk A, et al, "Vitamin D Deficiency in Children and Its Management: Review of Current Knowledge and Recommendations," *Pediatrics*, 2008, 122(2):398-417.

Sanchez CP, "Secondary Hyperparathyroidism in Children With Chronic Renal Failure: Pathogenesis and Treatment," *Paediatr Drugs*, 2003, 5 (11): 763-76.

Wagner CL, Greer FR; American Academy of Pediatrics Section on Breastfeeding, et al, "Prevention of Rickets and Vitamin D Deficiency in Infants, Children, and Adolescents," *Pediatrics*, 2008, 122 (5):1142-52.

Ziolkowska H, "Minimizing Bone Abnormalities in Children With Renal Failure," *Paediatr Drugs*, 2006, 8(4):205-22.

◆ **Ergomar®** *see* Ergotamine *on page 521*

Ergotamine (er GOT a meen)

U.S. Brand Names Ergomar®

Therapeutic Category Alpha-Adrenergic Blocking Agent, Oral; Antimigraine Agent; Ergot Alkaloid

Generic Available No

Use Prevent or abort vascular headaches, such as migraine and migraine variants also known as "histaminic cephalalgia"

Pregnancy Risk Factor X

Pregnancy Considerations May cause prolonged constriction of the uterine vessels and/or increased myometrial tone leading to reduced placental blood flow. This has contributed to fetal growth retardation in animals.

Lactation Enters breast milk/not recommended

Breast-Feeding Considerations Ergotamine is excreted in breast milk and may cause vomiting, diarrhea, weak pulse, and unstable blood pressure in the nursing infant. Consider discontinuing the drug or discontinuing nursing.

Contraindications Hypersensitivity to ergotamine or any component; pregnancy; peripheral vascular disease, hepatic or renal disease, hypertension, peptic ulcer disease, sepsis, coronary heart disease; concurrent therapy with potent CYP3A4 inhibitors (eg, protease inhibitors and macrolide antibiotics) (see Drug Interactions).

Warnings Long-term use is associated with fibrotic changes to heart, pulmonary valves, and rare cases of retroperitoneal fibrosis; chronic usage may also be harmful due to a reduction in cerebral blood flow, ECG changes, and hypertension; sustained vasoconstriction may precipitate angina or MI, aggravate intermittent claudication, or lead to ischemic colitis. Concomitant use with potent inhibitors of CYP3A4 (including protease inhibitors and macrolide antibiotics) has been associated with acute ergot toxicity characterized by serious and/or life-threatening cerebral and peripheral ischemia **[U.S. Boxed Warning]**; some cases have resulted in amputation (see Contraindications); less potent CYP3A4 inhibitors (eg, metronidazole, nefazodone, fluoxetine, zileuton, and azole antifungals) may carry the same risk. Patients who take ergotamine for extended periods of time may become dependent on it and discontinuation may result in withdrawal symptoms (eg, rebound headache). Safety and efficacy have not been established in children.

Adverse Reactions

Cardiovascular: Angina-like precordial pain, transient tachycardia or bradycardia, vasospasm, vasoconstriction, claudication; fibrotic thickening of the aortic, pulmonary, mitral, and/or tricuspid valves (rare after long-term use)

Central nervous system: Rebound headaches (with abrupt withdrawal), drowsiness, dizziness

Dermatologic: Pruritus

Gastrointestinal: Nausea, vomiting, diarrhea, xerostomia, retroperitoneal fibrosis (rare)

Local: Edema

Neuromuscular & skeletal: Leg cramps, myalgia, weakness, paresthesia of the extremities

Respiratory: Pleuropulmonary fibrosis (rare)

Drug Interactions

Metabolism/Transport Effects Substrate of CYP3A4 (major); Inhibits CYP3A4 (weak)

Avoid Concomitant Use

Avoid concomitant use of Ergotamine with any of the following: Clarithromycin; Efavirenz; Itraconazole; Posaconazole; Protease Inhibitors; Serotonin 5-HT1D Receptor Agonists; Sibutramine; Voriconazole

Increased Effect/Toxicity

Ergotamine may increase the levels/effects of: Serotonin 5-HT1D Receptor Agonists; Serotonin Modulators

The levels/effects of Ergotamine may be increased by: Clarithromycin; CYP3A4 Inhibitors (Moderate); CYP3A4 Inhibitors (Strong); Dasatinib; Efavirenz; Itraconazole; Macrolide Antibiotics; Posaconazole; Protease Inhibitors; Serotonin 5-HT1D Receptor Agonists; Sibutramine; Voriconazole

Decreased Effect There are no known significant interactions involving a decrease in effect.

Food Interactions Avoid tea, cola, and coffee (caffeine may increase GI absorption of ergotamine). Avoid grapefruit juice; may cause increased blood levels of ergotamine, leading to increased toxicity

Mechanism of Action Has partial agonist and/or antagonist activity against tryptaminergic, dopaminergic and alpha-adrenergic receptors depending upon their site; is a highly active uterine stimulant; it causes constriction of peripheral and cranial blood vessels and produces depression of central vasomotor centers

Pharmacokinetics (Adult data unless noted)

Absorption: Oral, rectal: Erratic

Distribution: V_d: Adults: 1.85 L/kg

Metabolism: Extensive in the liver

Bioavailability: Poor overall (<5%)

Half-life: Adults: 2-2.5 hours

Time to peak serum concentration: Oral: Within 0.5-3 hours

Elimination: In bile as metabolites (90%)

Usual Dosage Adolescents and Adults: **Note:** Not for chronic daily administration: Sublingual: 1 tablet under tongue at first sign, then 1 tablet every 30 minutes; maximum: 3 tablets/24 hours, 5 tablets/week

Administration Sublingual: Place tablet under the tongue; do not crush; may administer without regard to meals

Patient Information Any symptoms such as nausea, vomiting, numbness or tingling, and chest, muscle, or abdominal pain should be reported to the physician at the first sign of an attack; do **not** exceed recommended dosage; avoid coffee, tea, cola, and grapefruit juice; may cause dry mouth

Dosage Forms Excipient information presented when available (limited, particularly for generics); consult specific product labeling.

Tablet, sublingual, as tartrate:

Ergomar®: 2 mg [peppermint flavor]

Ergotamine and Caffeine
(er GOT a meen & KAF een)

Medication Safety Issues

Sound-alike/look-alike issues:

Cafergot® may be confused with Carafate®

U.S. Brand Names Cafergot®; Migergot

Canadian Brand Names Cafergor®

Therapeutic Category Alpha-Adrenergic Blocking Agent, Oral; Antimigraine Agent; Ergot Alkaloid

Generic Available Yes

Use Prevent or abort vascular headaches, such as migraine and migraine variants also known as "histaminic cephalalgia"

Pregnancy Risk Factor X

Pregnancy Considerations May cause prolonged constriction of the uterine vessels and/or increased myometrial tone leading to reduced placental blood flow. This has contributed to fetal growth retardation in animals.

Lactation Enters breast milk/not recommended

Breast-Feeding Considerations Ergotamine is excreted in breast milk and may cause vomiting, diarrhea, weak pulse, and unstable blood pressure in the nursing infant. Consider discontinuing the drug or discontinuing nursing.

Contraindications Hypersensitivity to ergotamine, caffeine, or any component; pregnancy; peripheral vascular disease, hepatic or renal disease, hypertension, peptic ulcer disease, sepsis, coronary heart disease; concurrent therapy with potent CYP3A4 inhibitors (eg, protease inhibitors and macrolide antibiotics) (see Drug Interactions)

Warnings Long-term use is associated with fibrotic changes to heart, pulmonary valves, and rare cases of retroperitoneal fibrosis; chronic usage may also be harmful due to a reduction in cerebral blood flow, ECG changes, and hypertension; sustained vasoconstriction may precipitate angina or MI, aggravate intermittent claudication, or lead to ischemic colitis. Concomitant use with potent inhibitors of CYP3A4 (including protease inhibitors and macrolide antibiotics) has been associated with acute ergot toxicity characterized by serious and/or life-threatening cerebral and peripheral ischemia **[U.S. Boxed Warning]**; some cases have resulted in amputation (see Contraindications); less potent CYP3A4 inhibitors (eg, metronidazole, fluoxetine, nefazodone, zileuton, and azole antifungals) may carry the same risk. Patients who take ergotamine for extended periods of time may become dependent on it and discontinuation may result in withdrawal symptoms (eg, rebound headache). Safety and efficacy have not been established in children.

Adverse Reactions

Cardiovascular: Angina-like precordial pain, transient tachycardia or bradycardia, MI, vasospasm, vasoconstriction, claudication; fibrotic thickening of the aortic, pulmonary, mitral, and/or tricuspid valves (rare after long-term use)

Central nervous system: Rebound headaches (with abrupt withdrawal), drowsiness, dizziness

Dermatologic: Pruritus

Gastrointestinal: Nausea, vomiting, diarrhea, xerostomia, retroperitoneal fibrosis (rare), rectal or anal ulcers (suppository use)

Local: Edema

Neuromuscular & skeletal: Leg cramps, myalgia, weakness, paresthesia of the extremities

Respiratory: Pleuropulmonary fibrosis (rare)

Drug Interactions

Metabolism/Transport Effects

Ergotamine: **Substrate** of CYP3A4 (major); **Inhibits** CYP3A4 (weak)

Caffeine: **Substrate** of CYP1A2 (major), 2C9 (minor), 2D6 (minor), 2E1 (minor), 3A4 (minor); **Inhibits** CYP1A2 (weak), 3A4 (moderate)

Avoid Concomitant Use

Avoid concomitant use of Ergotamine and Caffeine with any of the following: Clarithromycin; Efavirenz; Iobenguane I 123; Itraconazole; Posaconazole; Protease Inhibitors; Serotonin 5-HT1D Receptor Agonists; Sibutramine; Voriconazole

Increased Effect/Toxicity

Ergotamine and Caffeine may increase the levels/effects of: Serotonin 5-HT1D Receptor Agonists; Serotonin Modulators; Sympathomimetics

The levels/effects of Ergotamine and Caffeine may be increased by: Atomoxetine; Cannabinoids; Clarithromycin; CYP1A2 Inhibitors (Moderate); CYP1A2 Inhibitors (Strong); CYP3A4 Inhibitors (Moderate); CYP3A4 Inhibitors (Strong); Dasatinib; Efavirenz; Itraconazole; Macrolide Antibiotics; Posaconazole; Protease Inhibitors; Quinolone Antibiotics; Serotonin 5-HT1D Receptor Agonists; Sibutramine; Voriconazole

Decreased Effect

Ergotamine and Caffeine may decrease the levels/effects of: Iobenguane I 123; Regadenoson

The levels/effects of Ergotamine and Caffeine may be decreased by: Peginterferon Alfa-2b

Food Interactions Avoid tea, cola, and coffee (caffeine may increase GI absorption of ergotamine). Avoid grapefruit juice; may cause increased blood levels of ergotamine, leading to increased toxicity

Mechanism of Action Has partial agonist and/or antagonist activity against tryptaminergic, dopaminergic and alpha-adrenergic receptors depending upon their site; is a highly active uterine stimulant; it causes constriction of peripheral and cranial blood vessels and produces depression of central vasomotor centers; caffeine is also a vasoconstrictor which was added to potentially enhance ergotamine's effects

Pharmacokinetics (Adult data unless noted)

Absorption: Oral, rectal: Erratic; absorption is enhanced by caffeine coadministration

Metabolism: Extensive in the liver

Bioavailability: Poor overall (<5%)

Half-life: 2-2.5 hours

Time to peak serum concentration: Oral: Within 0.5-3 hours

Elimination: In bile as metabolites (90%)

Usual Dosage Adolescents and Adults: **Note:** Not for chronic daily administration:

Oral: 2 mg at onset of attack; then 1-2 mg every 30 minutes as needed; maximum dose: 6 mg per attack; do not exceed 10 mg/week

Rectal, suppositories: 1 suppository at first sign of an attack; follow with second dose after 1 hour, if needed; maximum dose: 2 per attack; do not exceed 5/week

Administration Oral: Tablets may be taken without regard to meals

Patient Information Any symptoms such as nausea, vomiting, numbness or tingling, and chest, muscle, or abdominal pain should be reported to the physician at the first sign of an attack; do **not** exceed recommended dosage; not for chronic daily use; avoid coffee, tea, cola, and grapefruit juice; may cause dry mouth

Dosage Forms Excipient information presented when available (limited, particularly for generics); consult specific product labeling.

Suppository, rectal:

Migergot: Ergotamine tartrate 2 mg and caffeine 100 mg (12s)

Tablet: Ergotamine tartrate 1 mg and caffeine 100 mg

Cafergot®: Ergotamine tartrate 1 mg and caffeine 100 mg

♦ **Ergotamine Tartrate** *see* Ergotamine *on page 521*

♦ **Ergotamine Tartrate and Caffeine** *see* Ergotamine and Caffeine *on page 522*

♦ **Errin™** *see* Norethindrone *on page 1001*

Ertapenem (er ta PEN em)

Medication Safety Issues

Sound-alike/look-alike issues:

Ertapenem may be confused with imipenem, meropenem

Invanz® may be confused with Avinza™, I.V. vancomycin

U.S. Brand Names Invanz®

Canadian Brand Names Invanz®

Therapeutic Category Antibiotic, Carbapenem

Generic Available No

Use Treatment of moderate to severe, complicated intra-abdominal infections, acute pelvic infections, complicated skin and skin structure infections (including diabetic foot infections without osteomyelitis), community-acquired pneumonia, and complicated urinary tract infections caused by susceptible *S. aureus* (methicillin susceptible strains only), *S. pneumoniae* (penicillin-sensitive strains), *S. agalactiae*, *S. pyogenes*, *E. coli*, *B. fragilis*, *C. clostridioforme*, *Peptostreptococcus* species, *H. influenzae* (beta-lactamase negative strains), *K. pneumoniae*, and *M. catarrhalis* (FDA approved in ages ≥3 months and adults); prophylaxis of surgical site infection following colorectal surgery (FDA approved in adults); has also been used for documented or suspected infection due to susceptible organisms for outpatient parenteral therapy

Pregnancy Risk Factor B

Pregnancy Considerations With the exception of slightly decreased fetal weights in mice, teratogenic effects and fetal harm have not been shown in animal studies. Adequate and well-controlled studies have not been conducted in pregnant women and it is not known whether ertapenem can cause fetal harm.

Lactation Enters breast milk/use caution

Breast-Feeding Considerations Ertapenem is excreted in breast milk. The low concentrations in milk and low oral bioavailability suggest minimal exposure risk to the infant. Although the manufacturer recommends that caution be exercised when administering ertapenem to nursing women, most penicillins and carbapenems are safe for use in breast-feeding. Nondose-related effects could include modification of bowel flora.

Contraindications Hypersensitivity to ertapenem, carbapenems, or any component; patients who have had an anaphylactoid reaction to beta-lactams; hypersensitivity to local anesthetics of the amide type for patients receiving I.M. injections

Warnings Serious and occasionally fatal hypersensitivity reactions have been reported in patients receiving beta-lactam therapy; careful inquiry should be made concerning previous hypersensitivity reactions to penicillins, cephalosporins, or other beta-lactams before initiating ertapenem. Seizures have been reported with ertapenem therapy. Valproic acid (VPA) serum concentrations may be significantly decreased by concurrent carbapenem use leading to breakthrough seizures; VPA dosage adjustment may not adequately compensate for this interaction; concurrent use with valproic acid/divalproex sodium not recommended (see Drug Interactions). Pseudomembranous colitis has been reported in patients receiving ertapenem; prolonged use may result in superinfection.

Precautions Use with caution in patients with CNS disorders, history of seizures and/or compromised renal function; dosage adjustment required in patients with renal impairment

Adverse Reactions

Cardiovascular: Chest pain, edema, hypertension, hypotension, tachycardia

Central nervous system: Altered mental status, anxiety, dizziness, fatigue, fever, hallucinations, headache, insomnia, seizures (see Warnings), somnolence

Dermatologic: Pruritus, rash

Gastrointestinal: Abdominal pain, constipation, diarrhea, nausea, oral candidiasis, pancreatitis, pseudomembranous colitis (see Warnings), vomiting

Hematologic: Eosinophil count increased, neutrophil count decreased, platelet count increased

Hepatic: AST, ALT, and alkaline phosphatase increased

Local: Erythema and tenderness at injection site, induration, pain, phlebitis

Neuromuscular & skeletal: Arthralgia, paresthesia, tremor

Renal: Hematuria, renal insufficiency

Respiratory: Cough, dyspnea, respiratory distress, rhinitis, wheezing

Miscellaneous: Anaphylaxis, hypersensitivity reaction (see Warnings)

<1%, postmarketing, and/or case reports: Abdominal distention, aggressive behavior, anaphylactoid reactions, anorexia, arrhythmia, asthma, asystole, atrial fibrillation, bicarbonate (serum) decreased, bilirubin (direct and indirect) increased, bladder dysfunction, bradycardia, bronchoconstriction, BUN increased, *C. difficile*-associated diarrhea, cardiac arrest, chills, cholelithiasis, dehydration, depression, dermatitis, desquamation, diaphoresis, duodenitis, dysphagia, epistaxis, epithelial (urine) cells increased, esophagitis, facial edema, flank pain, flatulence, flushing, gastritis, gastrointestinal hemorrhage, gout, heart failure, heart murmur, hematoma, hemoptysis, hemorrhoids, hiccups, hypoesthesia, hypoxemia, ileus, jaundice, malaise, monocytes increased, mouth ulcer, muscle spasm, necrosis, nervousness, oliguria/anuria, pain, pharyngeal discomfort, pleural effusion, pleuritic pain, PTT increased, pyloric stenosis, septicemia, septic shock, sodium (serum) increased, stomatitis, subdural hemorrhage, syncope, taste perversion, urinary retention, urticaria, vaginal candidiasis, vaginal pruritus, ventricular tachycardia, vertigo, voice disturbance, vulvovaginitis, weight loss

Drug Interactions

Avoid Concomitant Use

Avoid concomitant use of Ertapenem with any of the following: BCG

Increased Effect/Toxicity

The levels/effects of Ertapenem may be increased by: Probenecid

Decreased Effect

Ertapenem may decrease the levels/effects of: BCG; Divalproex; Typhoid Vaccine; Valproic Acid

Stability Store lyophilized powder at room temperature not to exceed 25°C (77°F). Reconstituted I.V. ertapenem solution further diluted in NS or following activation of ertapenem in ADD-Vantage® vials with ADD-Vantage® diluent: Stable for 6 hours at room temperature or 24 hours if refrigerated and used within 4 hours after removal from refrigeration; do not freeze. Incompatible with dextrose-containing solutions. Reconstituted I.M. ertapenem solution should be used within 1 hour after preparation.

Mechanism of Action Inhibits cell wall synthesis by binding to penicillin-binding proteins

Pharmacokinetics (Adult data unless noted)

Distribution: Excreted in breast milk

V_d:

Children 3 months to 12 years: ~0.2 L/kg

Children 13-17 years: 0.16 L/kg

Adults: 0.12 L/kg

Protein binding: 85% to 95% (concentration-dependent plasma protein binding)

Metabolism: Renal metabolism to an open-ring metabolite

Bioavailability: I.M.: 90%

Half-life:

Children 3 months to 12 years: 2.5 hours

Children 13-17 years: 4 hours

Adults: 4 hours

Time to peak serum concentration: I.M.: 2.3 hours

Elimination: 80% of a dose is excreted in the urine (38% as unchanged drug) and 10% in feces; undergoes glomerular filtration and tubular secretion

Dialysis: 30% removed by hemodialysis

Usual Dosage I.M., I.V.:

Children 3 months to 12 years: 15 mg/kg/dose every 12 hours; maximum dose: 1 g/day

Adolescents and Adults: Treatment guidelines: 1 g once daily. Total antimicrobial treatment duration for pediatric and adult patients:

Complicated intra-abdominal infections: 5-14 days

Complicated skin and skin structure infections (including diabetic foot infections): 7-14 days

Community-acquired pneumonia: 10-14 days

Complicated UTI/pyelonephritis: 10-14 days

Acute pelvic infections: 3-10 days

Adults: Prophylaxis of surgical site infection following colorectal surgery: I.V.: Single 1 g dose administered 1 hour prior to surgical procedure

Dosage adjustment in renal impairment: Adults: Cl_{cr} ≤30 mL/minute/1.73 m^2: Decrease dose 50%

Hemodialysis: Adults: If daily dose is given within 6 hours prior to hemodialysis, a supplementary dose of 150 mg should be given following hemodialysis.

Administration Parenteral:

I.M. injection: Reconstitute 1 g vial with 3.2 mL of 1% lidocaine immediately prior to administration with a resultant concentration of 312.5 mg/mL. Shake vial well. Administer I.M. injection deep into a large muscle mass such as the gluteus maximus or lateral part of the thigh.

I.V. intermittent infusion: Reconstitute 1 g vial with 10 mL SWI or NS with a resultant concentration of 100 mg/mL. Further dilute dose with NS to a final maximum concentration of 20 mg/mL and administer over 30 minutes. Do not coinfuse with other medications. **Do not infuse with dextrose-containing solutions.**

Monitoring Parameters Periodic renal, hepatic, and hematologic function tests; neurological assessment

Patient Information Inform physician if you are taking valproic acid or divalproex sodium since an alternative treatment may be needed; inform physician of prolonged diarrhea, abdominal pain, or vomiting. Report any chest pain, respiratory difficulty, dizziness, or confusion.

Additional Information Sodium content 1 g: 6 mEq

Dosage Forms Excipient information presented when available (limited, particularly for generics); consult specific product labeling.

Injection, powder for reconstitution:

Invanz®: 1 g [contains sodium 137 mg/g (~6 mEq/g)]

References

Curran M, Simpson D, and Perry C, "Ertapenem: A Review of Its Use in the Management of Bacterial Infections," *Drugs*, 2003, 63 (17):1855-78.

Keating GM and Perry CM, "Ertapenem: A Review of Its Use in the Treatment of Bacterial Infections," *Drugs*, 2005, 65(15):2151-78.

Nix DE, Majumdar AK, and DiNubile MJ, "Pharmacokinetics and Pharmacodynamics of Ertapenem: An Overview for Clinicians," *J Antimicrob Chemother*, 2004, 53(Suppl 2):ii23-8.

◆ **Ertapenem Sodium** *see* Ertapenem *on page 523*

◆ **Erybid™ (Can)** *see* Erythromycin *on page 525*

◆ **Eryc® [DSC]** *see* Erythromycin *on page 525*

◆ **Eryc® (Can)** *see* Erythromycin *on page 525*

◆ **Eryderm® [DSC]** *see* Erythromycin *on page 525*

◆ **Erygel® [DSC]** *see* Erythromycin *on page 525*

◆ **EryPed®** *see* Erythromycin *on page 525*

◆ **Ery-Tab®** *see* Erythromycin *on page 525*

◆ **Erythrocin®** *see* Erythromycin *on page 525*

Erythromycin (er ith roe MYE sin)

Medication Safety Issues
Sound-alike/look-alike issues:
Erythromycin may be confused with azithromycin, clarithromycin, Ethmozine®
Akne-Mycin® may be confused with AK-Mycin®
E.E.S.® may be confused with DES®
Eryc® may be confused with Emcyt®, Ery-Tab®
Ery-Tab® may be confused with Eryc®
Erythrocin® may be confused with Ethmozine®

U.S. Brand Names Akne-Mycin®; E.E.S.®; Ery-Tab®; Eryc® [DSC]; Eryderm® [DSC]; Erygel® [DSC]; EryPed®; Erythro-RX; Erythrocin®; PCE®; Romycin® [DSC]

Canadian Brand Names Apo-Erythro Base®; Apo-Erythro E-C®; Apo-Erythro-ES®; Apo-Erythro-S®; Diomycin®; EES®; Erybid™; Eryc®; Novo-Rythro Estolate; Novo-Rythro Ethylsuccinate; Nu-Erythromycin-S; PCE®; PMS-Erythromycin; Sans Acne®

Therapeutic Category Antibiotic, Macrolide; Antibiotic, Ophthalmic

Generic Available Yes: Capsule, gel, ophthalmic ointment, topical solution, suspension (as ethylsuccinate), swab, tablet (as base, ethylsuccinate, and stearate)

Use Treatment of mild to moderately severe infections of the upper and lower respiratory tract and skin infections due to susceptible streptococci and staphylococci; other susceptible bacterial infections including *Mycoplasma pneumoniae*, *Legionella* pneumonia, nongonococcal urethritis, Lyme disease, diphtheria, pertussis, chancroid, *Chlamydia*, and *Campylobacter* gastroenteritis; used in conjunction with neomycin for decontaminating the bowel for surgery; prophylaxis of recurrent rheumatic fever in penicillin or sulfa-allergic patients

Ophthalmic: Treatment of superficial eye infections involving the conjunctiva or cornea; treatment of chlamydial ophthalmic infections; prevention of gonococcal ophthalmia neonatorum
Topical: Treatment of acne vulgaris

Pregnancy Risk Factor B

Pregnancy Considerations Adverse events were not observed in animal studies; therefore, erythromycin is classified as pregnancy category B. Erythromycin crosses the placenta and low concentrations are found in the fetal serum. No increased risk for congenital abnormalities has been documented, with the exception of a possible slight increase in risk for cardiovascular anomalies. Most studies do not support a link between prenatal exposure to erythromycin and pyloric stenosis in the neonate. In general, serum concentrations of erythromycin are lower in pregnant women. Erythromycin therapy in patients with preterm, premature rupture of membranes is associated with a range of health benefits to the neonate and long-term adverse events to the child have not been observed. However, maternal use of erythromycin in women with preterm labor, intact membranes, and no documented infection does not improve neonatal health and may have adverse effects in childhood (use is not recommended). Erythromycin is the antibiotic of choice for preterm premature rupture of membranes (with membrane rupture prior to 34 weeks gestation), the treatment of granuloma inguinale and lymphogranuloma venereum in pregnancy, and the treatment of or long-term suppression of *Bartonella* infection in HIV-infected pregnant patients. Erythromycin may be appropriate as an alternative agent for the prevention of group B streptococcal disease or the treatment of chlamydial infections in pregnant women (consult current guidelines).

Lactation Enters breast milk/use caution (AAP considers "compatible")

Breast-Feeding Considerations Erythromycin is excreted in breast milk; therefore, the manufacturer recommends that caution be exercised when administering erythromycin to breast-feeding women.

Due to the low concentrations in human milk, minimal toxicity would be expected in the nursing infant. One case report and a cohort study raise the possibility for a connection with pyloric stenosis in neonates exposed to erythromycin via breast milk and an alternative antibiotic may be preferred for breast-feeding mothers of infants in this age group. Nondose-related effects could include modification of bowel flora. The AAP considers erythromycin to be "usually compatible with breast-feeding."

Contraindications Hypersensitivity to erythromycin or any component (see Warnings); hepatic impairment; concomitant administration with pimozide, astemizole, terfenadine, or cisapride

Warnings Hepatic impairment with or without jaundice has occurred primarily in older children and adults; it may be accompanied by malaise, nausea, vomiting, abdominal colic, and fever; discontinue use if these occur; risk of serious cardiac arrhythmias exist in patients receiving erythromycin and pimozide, astemizole, terfenadine, or cisapride (do not use concurrently with erythromycin) Rhabdomyolysis has been reported in seriously ill patients receiving erythromycin and lovastatin concomitantly (monitor creatine kinase and serum transaminase levels). Infantile hypertrophic pyloric stenosis with symptoms of nonbilious vomiting or irritability with feeding has been reported in 5% of infants who received erythromycin for pertussis prophylaxis. Prolonged or repeated use may result in superinfection or antibiotic-associated pseudomembranous colitis. Erythromycin has been associated with rare QT_c prolongation and ventricular arrhythmias, including torsade de pointes.

Erythromycin lactobionate injection contains benzyl alcohol which may cause allergic reactions in susceptible individuals; large amounts of benzyl alcohol ($\geq$99 mg/kg/day) have been associated with a potentially fatal toxicity ("gasping syndrome") in neonates; the "gasping syndrome" consists of metabolic acidosis, respiratory distress, gasping respirations, CNS dysfunction (including convulsions, intracranial hemorrhage), hypotension and cardiovascular collapse; use erythromycin lactobionate injection products containing benzyl alcohol with caution in neonates; *in vitro* and animal studies have shown that benzoate, a metabolite of benzyl alcohol, displaces bilirubin from protein binding sites

Precautions Use with caution in patients with hepatic impairment; use caution in patients on concomitant drugs which inhibit CYP3A (eg, fluconazole, ketoconazole, itraconazole, diltiazem, verapamil) due to increased risk of sudden cardiac death

Adverse Reactions
Cardiovascular: Ventricular arrhythmias, prolongation of the QT interval, cardiac arrest; bradycardia, hypotension with I.V. administration

Central nervous system: Fever, dizziness, vertigo, seizures, hallucinations, confusion

Dermatologic: Skin rash, pruritus, Stevens-Johnson syndrome, urticaria

Gastrointestinal: Abdominal pain, cramping, nausea, vomiting, diarrhea, stomatitis, pseudomembraneous colitis, infantile hypertrophic pyloric stenosis

Hematologic: Eosinophilia

Hepatic: Cholestatic hepatitis, jaundice; (incidence of erythromycin-associated hepatotoxicity is ~0.1% in children and 0.25% in adults)

Local: Thrombophlebitis (I.V. form)

Otic: Ototoxicity (after I.V. use), tinnitus

Miscellaneous: Allergic reactions, anaphylaxis

Drug Interactions

Metabolism/Transport Effects Substrate of CYP2B6 (minor), CYP3A4 (major), P-glycoprotein; **Inhibits** CYP1A2 (weak), CYP3A4 (moderate), P-glycoprotein

Avoid Concomitant Use

Avoid concomitant use of Erythromycin with any of the following: Artemether; BCG; Cisapride; Dabigatran Etexilate; Disopyramide; Dronedarone; Lincosamide Antibiotics; Lumefantrine; Nilotinib; Pimozide; QuiNINE; Silodosin; Tetrabenazine; Thioridazine; Tolvaptan; Topotecan; Ziprasidone

Increased Effect/Toxicity

Erythromycin may increase the levels/effects of: Alfentanil; Antifungal Agents (Azole Derivatives, Systemic); Antineoplastic Agents (Vinca Alkaloids); Benzodiazepines (metabolized by oxidation); BusPIRone; Calcium Channel Blockers; CarBAMazepine; Cardiac Glycosides; Cilostazol; Cisapride; Clozapine; Colchicine; Corticosteroids (Systemic); CycloSPORINE; CycloSPORINE (Systemic); CYP3A4 Substrates; Dabigatran Etexilate; Disopyramide; Dronedarone; Eletriptan; Eplerenone; Ergot Derivatives; Everolimus; FentaNYL; Fexofenadine; HMG-CoA Reductase Inhibitors; P-Glycoprotein Substrates; Phosphodiesterase 5 Inhibitors; Pimecrolimus; Pimozide; QTc-Prolonging Agents; QuiNIDine; QuiNINE; Repaglinide; Rifamycin Derivatives; Rivaroxaban; Salmeterol; Saxagliptin; Selective Serotonin Reuptake Inhibitors; Silodosin; Sirolimus; Tacrolimus; Tacrolimus (Systemic); Tacrolimus (Topical); Temsirolimus; Tetrabenazine; Theophylline Derivatives; Thioridazine; Tolvaptan; Topotecan; Vitamin K Antagonists; Ziprasidone; Zopiclone

The levels/effects of Erythromycin may be increased by: Alfuzosin; Antifungal Agents (Azole Derivatives, Systemic); Artemether; Chloroquine; Ciprofloxacin; Ciprofloxacin (Systemic); CYP3A4 Inhibitors (Moderate); CYP3A4 Inhibitors (Strong); Gadobutrol; Lumefantrine; Nilotinib; P-Glycoprotein Inhibitors; QuiNINE

Decreased Effect

Erythromycin may decrease the levels/effects of: BCG; Clopidogrel; Lincosamide Antibiotics; Typhoid Vaccine; Zafirlukast

The levels/effects of Erythromycin may be decreased by: CYP3A4 Inducers (Strong); Deferasirox; Etravirine; Herbs (CYP3A4 Inducers); P-Glycoprotein Inducers

Stability Erythromycin lactobionate should be reconstituted with SWI without preservatives to avoid gel formation; the reconstituted solution is stable for 2 weeks when refrigerated or 24 hours at room temperature. Erythromycin I.V. infusion solution is stable at pH 6-8.

Mechanism of Action Inhibits bacterial RNA-dependent protein synthesis at the chain elongation step; binds to the 50S ribosomal subunit resulting in blockage of transpeptidation

Pharmacokinetics (Adult data unless noted)

Absorption: Variable, but better with salt forms than with base; 18% to 45% absorbed orally; ethylsuccinate may be better absorbed with food

Distribution: Crosses the placenta; distributes into body tissues, fluids, liver, bile, and breast milk with poor penetration into the CSF

V_d: 0.64 L/kg

Protein binding: 73% to 81%

Metabolism: In the liver by demethylation via CYP3A4

Half-life:

Neonates (≤15 days of age): 2.1 hours

Adults: 1.5-2 hours

Time to peak serum concentration: Oral:

Base: 4 hours

Stearate: 3 hours

Ethylsuccinate: 0.5-2.5 hours

Elimination: 2% to 5% unchanged drug excreted in urine, major excretion in feces (via bile)

Dialysis: Not removed by peritoneal dialysis or hemodialysis

Usual Dosage

Neonates:

Oral: Ethylsuccinate: Postnatal age:

≤7 days: 20 mg/kg/day in divided doses every 12 hours

>7 days, <1200 g: 20 mg/kg/day in divided doses every 12 hours

>7 days, 1200-2000 g: 30 mg/kg/day in divided doses every 8 hours

>7 days, >2000 g: 30-40 mg/kg/day in divided doses every 6-8 hours

Ophthalmic: Prophylaxis of neonatal gonococcal ophthalmia: 0.5-1 cm ribbon of ointment should be instilled into each conjunctival sac once

I.V.: One study (n=14, ≤15 days of age, birth weight ≤1500 g) used erythromycin lactobionate in doses of 25 or 40 mg/kg/day divided every 6 hours for treatment of *Ureaplasma urealyticum* infection

Chlamydial conjunctivitis and pneumonia: Oral: Ethylsuccinate: 50 mg/kg/day divided every 6 hours for 14 days

Infants and Children:

Oral:

Base and ethylsuccinate: 30-50 mg/kg/day divided every 6-8 hours; do not exceed 2 g/day (as base) or 3.2 g/day (as ethylsuccinate); (**Note:** Due to differences in absorption, 200 mg erythromycin ethylsuccinate produces the same serum levels as 125 mg erythromycin base)

Stearate: 30-50 mg/kg/day divided every 6 hours; do not exceed 2 g/day

Chlamydia trachomatis: Child <45 kg: Oral: 50 mg/kg/day divided every 6 hours for 14 days; maximum dose: 2 g/day

Pertussis: Oral: 40-50 mg/kg/day divided every 6 hours for 14 days; maximum dose: 2 g/day (not preferred agent for infants <1 month)

Preop bowel preparation: Oral: 20 mg/kg erythromycin base at 1, 2, and 11 PM on the day before surgery combined with mechanical cleansing of the large intestine and oral neomycin

I.V.: Lactobionate: 15-50 mg/kg/day divided every 6 hours, not to exceed 4 g/day

Children and Adults:

Ophthalmic: Instill ointment one or more times daily depending on the severity of the infection

Topical: Apply 2% solution over the affected area twice daily after the skin has been thoroughly washed and patted dry

Adults:

Oral:

Base, delayed release: 333 mg every 8 hours

Stearate or base: 250-500 mg every 6-12 hours

Ethylsuccinate: 400-800 mg every 6-12 hours

Chancroid: Oral: Base: 500 mg 4 times/day for 7 days

Chlamydia trachomatis: Oral:

Base: 500 mg 4 times/day for 7 days **or**

Ethylsuccinate: 800 mg 4 times/day for 7 days

Pertussis: Oral: 500 mg every 6 hours for 14 days

Preop bowel preparation: Oral: 1 g erythromycin base at 1, 2, and 11 PM on the day before surgery combined with mechanical cleansing of the large intestine and oral neomycin

I.V.: Lactobionate: 15-20 mg/kg/day divided every 6 hours or given as a continuous infusion over 24 hours, not to exceed 4 g/day

Prokinetic agent (to improve gastric emptying time and intestinal motility): **Note:** Oral route is preferred since all erythromycin-related, life-threatening, and fatal cardiac complications have been associated with I.V. erythromycin.

Infants: Oral: 10 mg/kg/dose every 8 hours (high antibacterial dose) was effective in improving gastric emptying time (*JPEN*, 2002, 34(1):23-5); a second study using low dose oral erythromycin (0.75-3 mg/kg) for two doses was not useful in very preterm infants, partially useful in older preterm infants, and useful in full-term infants in increasing duodenal contraction amplitude and amplitude/frequency of antral contractions (*JPEN*, 2002, 34(1):16-22). **Note:** Exposure to high antimicrobial doses (30-50 mg/kg/day) for ≥14 days in neonates up to 2 weeks old has been associated with a 10-fold increase in the risk of hypertrophic pyloric stenosis.

Children: Lactobionate: Initial: 1-3 mg/kg I.V. infused over 60 minutes followed by 10-20 mg/kg/day orally in 2-4 divided doses before meals, or before meals and at bedtime

Adults: Lactobionate: Initial: 200 mg I.V. followed by 250 mg orally 3 times/day 30 minutes before meals

Administration

Ophthalmic ointment for prevention of neonatal ophthalmia: Wipe each eyelid gently with sterile cotton; instill 0.5-1 cm ribbon of ointment in each lower conjunctival sac; massage eyelids gently to spread the ointment; after 1 minute, excess ointment can be wiped away with sterile cotton

Oral: Avoid milk and acidic beverages 1 hour before or after a dose; administer after food to decrease GI discomfort; ethylsuccinate chewable tablets should not be swallowed whole; do not chew or break delayed release capsule or enteric coated tablets, swallow whole

Parenteral: Administer by I.V. intermittent or continuous infusion diluted in either dextrose or saline solutions to a concentration of 1-2.5 mg/mL; maximum concentration: 5 mg/mL; I.V. intermittent infusions may be administered over 20-60 minutes; to decrease vein irritation, administer as a continuous infusion at a concentration ≤1 mg/mL; prolonging the infusion duration over 60 minutes or longer has been recommended to decrease the cardiotoxic effects of erythromycin

Topical: Apply thin film to the cleansed, affected area.

Monitoring Parameters Liver function tests; with I.V. use: Blood pressure, heart rate

Test Interactions False-positive urinary catecholamines, 17-hydroxycorticosteroids and 17-ketosteroids

Patient Information Notify physician if vomiting or irritability with feeding occurs when administered to infants.

Nursing Implications Do not crush enteric coated or delayed release drug products

Additional Information Treatment of erythromycin-associated cardiac toxicity with prolongation of the QT interval and ventricular tachydysrhythmias includes discontinuing erythromycin and administering magnesium.

Dosage Forms Excipient information presented when available (limited, particularly for generics); consult specific product labeling. [DSC] = Discontinued product; [CAN] = Canadian brand name

Note: Strength expressed as base

Capsule, delayed release, enteric-coated pellets, as base: 250 mg

Eryc®: 250 mg [DSC]

Gel, topical: 2% (30 g, 60 g)

Erygel®: 2% (30 g, 60 g) [DSC] [contains alcohol 92%]

Granules for oral suspension, as ethylsuccinate:

E.E.S.®: 200 mg/5 mL (100 mL, 200 mL) [contains sodium 25.9 mg (1.1 mEq)/5 mL; cherry flavor]

Injection, powder for reconstitution, as lactobionate:

Erythrocin®: 500 mg, 1 g

Ointment, ophthalmic: 0.5% (1 g, 3.5 g)

Romycin®: 0.5% (3.5 g) [DSC]

Ointment, topical:

Akne-Mycin®: 2% (25 g)

Powder for oral suspension, as ethylsuccinate:

EryPed®: 200 mg/5 mL (100 mL, 200 mL [DSC]) [contains sodium 117.5 mg (5.1 mEq)/5 mL; fruit flavor]; 400 mg/5 mL (100 mL, 200 mL [DSC]) [contains sodium 117.5 mg (5.1 mEq)/5 mL; banana flavor]

Powder for oral suspension, as ethylsuccinate [drops]:

EryPed®: 100 mg/2.5 mL (50 mL) [DSC] [contains sodium 58.8 mg (2.6 mEq)/dropperful; fruit flavor]

Powder, for prescription compounding:

Erythro-RX: USP: 100% (50 g)

Solution, topical: 2% (60 mL)

Eryderm®: 2% (60 mL) [contain alcohol] [DSC]

Sans acne [CAN]: 2% (60 mL) [contains ethyl alcohol 44%; not available in U.S.]

Suspension, oral, as ethylsuccinate: 200 mg/5 mL (480 mL) [DSC]; 400 mg/5 mL (480 mL) [DSC]

E.E.S.®: 200 mg/5 mL (100 mL, 480 mL) [fruit flavor] [DSC]; 400 mg/5 mL (100 mL, 480 mL) [orange flavor]

Tablet, as base: 250 mg, 500 mg

Tablet, as base [polymer-coated particles]:

PCE®: 333 mg, 500 mg

Tablet, as ethylsuccinate: 400 mg

E.E.S.®: 400 mg [DSC]

Tablet, as stearate: 250 mg, 500 mg

Erythrocin®: 250 mg, 500 mg

Tablet, delayed release, enteric coated, as base:

Ery-Tab®: 250 mg, 333 mg, 500 mg

References

Curry JI, Lander TD, and Stringer MD, "Review Article: Erythromycin as a Prokinetic Agent in Infants and Children," *Aliment Pharmacol Ther*, 2001, 15(5):595-603.

Di Lorenzo C, Lachman R, and Hyman PE, "Intravenous Erythromycin for Postpyloric Intubation," *J Pediatr Gastroenterol Nutr*, 1990, 11(1):45-7.

Patole S, Rao S, and Doherty D, "Erythromycin as a Prokinetic Agent in Preterm Neonates: A Systematic Review," *Arch Dis Child Fetal Neonatal Ed*, 2005, 90(4):F301-6.

Reid B, DiLorenzo C, Travis L, et al, "Diabetic Gastroparesis Due to Postprandial Antral Hypomotility in Childhood," *Pediatrics*, 1992, 90(1 Pt 1):43-6.

Tiwari T, Murphy TV, and Moran J, "Recommended Antimicrobial Agents for the Treatment and Postexposure Prophylaxis of Pertussis: 2005 CDC Guidelines," *MMWR Recomm Rep*, 2005, 54(RR-14):1-16.

Vanderhoof JA, Young R, Kaufman SS, et al, "Treatment of Cyclic Vomiting in Childhood With Erythromycin," *J Pediatr Gastroenterol Nutr*, 1995, 21 Suppl 1:S60-2.

Waites KB, Sims PJ, Crouse DT, et al, "Serum Concentrations of Erythromycin After Intravenous Infusion in Preterm Neonates Treated for *Ureaplasma urealyticum* Infection," *Pediatr Infect Dis J*, 1994, 13(4):287-93.

Erythromycin and Sulfisoxazole

(er ith roe MYE sin & sul fi SOKS a zole)

Medication Safety Issues

Sound-alike/look-alike issues:

Pediazole® may be confused with Pediapred®

U.S. Brand Names E.S.P.®

Canadian Brand Names Pediazole®

Therapeutic Category Antibiotic, Macrolide; Antibiotic, Sulfonamide Derivative

Generic Available Yes

Use Treatment of susceptible bacterial infections of the upper and lower respiratory tract; otitis media in children caused by susceptible strains of *Haemophilus influenzae*; other infections in patients allergic to penicillin

Pregnancy Risk Factor C

Pregnancy Considerations Animal reproduction studies have not been conducted with this combination; therefore, the manufacturer classifies erythromycin/sulfisoxazole as pregnancy category C. Erythromycin and sulfisoxazole cross the placenta. Sulfisoxazole is contraindicated in late pregnancy because sulfonamides may cause kernicterus in the newborn. Neonatal healthcare providers should be informed if maternal sulfonamide therapy is used near the time of delivery. See individual agents.

Lactation Enters breast milk

Breast-Feeding Considerations Erythromycin and sulfisoxazole are both transferred to breast milk. Per the manufacturer, sulfisoxazole is contraindicated in mothers nursing infants <2 months of age because sulfonamides cross into milk and may cause kernicterus in the newborn. The AAP considers use of sulfisoxazole during breast-feeding "compatible" in full-term neonates; however, breast-feeding is not recommended if the infant is ill, stressed, or premature or if the infant has G6PD deficiency or hyperbilirubinemia. The AAP considers erythromycin to be "usually compatible with breast-feeding." See individual agents.

Contraindications Hypersensitivity to erythromycin, any component, or sulfonamides; hepatic dysfunction; infants <2 months of age (sulfas compete with bilirubin for binding sites which may result in kernicterus in newborns); patients with porphyria; pregnant women at term; mothers nursing infants <2 months of age; concomitant administration of astemizole, terfenadine, or cisapride

Warnings Risk of serious cardiac arrhythmias exist in patients receiving erythromycin, astemizole, terfenadine, or cisapride (do not use concurrently); fatalities due to Stevens-Johnson syndrome, toxic epidermal necrolysis, fulminant hepatic necrosis, agranulocytosis, and aplastic anemia have occurred with the administration of sulfonamides; prolonged use may result in superinfection or pseudomembranous colitis

Precautions Use with caution in patients with impaired renal or hepatic function, G-6-PD deficiency (hemolysis may occur)

Adverse Reactions

Cardiovascular: Tachycardia, palpitations, syncope

Central nervous system: Headache, disorientation, fever, dizziness

Dermatologic: Rash, photosensitivity, Stevens-Johnson syndrome, toxic epidermal necrolysis, pruritus, urticaria

Gastrointestinal: Abdominal cramping, nausea, vomiting, diarrhea, pseudomembranous colitis, anorexia, stomatitis, pancreatitis

Genitourinary: Crystalluria, hematuria

Hematologic: Agranulocytosis, aplastic anemia, leukopenia, eosinophilia, thrombocytopenia

Hepatic: Hepatic necrosis, jaundice

Renal: Toxic nephrosis, BUN and serum creatinine elevated, acute renal failure

Respiratory: Cough, shortness of breath, pulmonary infiltrates

Miscellaneous: Anaphylaxis

Drug Interactions

Metabolism/Transport Effects

Erythromycin: **Substrate** of CYP2B6 (minor), CYP3A4 (major), P-glycoprotein; **Inhibits** CYP1A2 (weak), CYP3A4 (moderate), P-glycoprotein

Sulfisoxazole: **Substrate** of CYP2C9 (major); **Inhibits** CYP2C8/9 (strong)

Avoid Concomitant Use

Avoid concomitant use of Erythromycin and Sulfisoxazole with any of the following: Artemether; BCG; Cisapride; Dabigatran Etexilate; Disopyramide; Dronedarone; Lincosamide Antibiotics; Lumefantrine; Methenamine; Nilotinib; Pimozide; Procaine; QuiNINE; Silodosin; Tetrabenazine; Thioridazine; Tolvaptan; Topotecan; Ziprasidone

Increased Effect/Toxicity

Erythromycin and Sulfisoxazole may increase the levels/effects of: Alfentanil; Antifungal Agents (Azole Derivatives, Systemic); Antineoplastic Agents (Vinca Alkaloids); Benzodiazepines (metabolized by oxidation); BusPIRone; Calcium Channel Blockers; CarBAMazepine; Cardiac Glycosides; Carvedilol; Cilostazol; Cisapride; Clozapine; Colchicine; Corticosteroids (Systemic); CycloSPORINE; CycloSPORINE (Systemic); CYP2C9 Substrates (High risk); CYP3A4 Substrates; Dabigatran Etexilate; Disopyramide; Dronedarone; Eletriptan; Eplerenone; Ergot Derivatives; Everolimus; FentaNYL; Fexofenadine; HMG-CoA Reductase Inhibitors; Methotrexate; P-Glycoprotein Substrates; Phenytoin; Phosphodiesterase 5 Inhibitors; Pimecrolimus; Pimozide; QTc-Prolonging Agents; QuiNIDine; QuiNINE; Repaglinide; Rifamycin Derivatives; Rivaroxaban; Salmeterol; Saxagliptin; Selective Serotonin Reuptake Inhibitors; Silodosin; Sirolimus; Sulfonylureas; Tacrolimus; Tacrolimus (Systemic); Tacrolimus (Topical); Temsirolimus; Tetrabenazine; Theophylline Derivatives; Thioridazine; Tolvaptan; Topotecan; Vitamin K Antagonists; Ziprasidone; Zopiclone

The levels/effects of Erythromycin and Sulfisoxazole may be increased by: Alfuzosin; Antifungal Agents (Azole Derivatives, Systemic); Artemether; Chloroquine; Ciprofloxacin; Ciprofloxacin (Systemic); CYP2C9 Inhibitors (Moderate); CYP2C9 Inhibitors (Strong); CYP3A4 Inhibitors (Moderate); CYP3A4 Inhibitors (Strong); Gadobutrol; Lumefantrine; Methenamine; Nilotinib; P-Glycoprotein Inhibitors; QuiNINE

Decreased Effect

Erythromycin and Sulfisoxazole may decrease the levels/effects of: BCG; Clopidogrel; CycloSPORINE; CycloSPORINE (Systemic); Lincosamide Antibiotics; Typhoid Vaccine; Zafirlukast

The levels/effects of Erythromycin and Sulfisoxazole may be decreased by: CYP2C9 Inducers (Highly Effective); CYP3A4 Inducers (Strong); Deferasirox; Etravirine; Herbs (CYP3A4 Inducers); Peginterferon Alfa-2b; P-Glycoprotein Inducers; Procaine

Stability Reconstituted suspension is stable for 14 days when refrigerated

Mechanism of Action Erythromycin inhibits bacterial protein synthesis by binding to the 50S ribosomal subunit; sulfisoxazole competitively inhibits bacterial synthesis of folic acid from para-aminobenzoic acid

Pharmacokinetics (Adult data unless noted)

Erythromycin ethylsuccinate:

Absorption: Well absorbed from the GI tract

Distribution: Widely distributed into most body tissues and fluids; poor penetration into CSF; crosses the placenta; excreted in breast milk

Protein binding: 75% to 90%

Metabolism: In the liver by demethylation

Half-life: 1-1.5 hours

Elimination: Unchanged drug is excreted and concentrated in bile; <5% of dose eliminated in urine

Dialysis: Not removed by peritoneal dialysis or hemodialysis

Sulfisoxazole acetyl:

Absorption: Hydrolyzed in the GI tract to sulfisoxazole which is rapidly and completely absorbed; the small intestine is the major site of absorption

Distribution: Into extracellular space; CSF concentration ranges from 8% to 57% of blood concentration in patients with normal meninges; crosses the placenta, excreted in breast milk

Protein binding: 85%

Metabolism: Undergoes N-acetylation and N-glucuronide conjugation in the liver

Half-life: 4.6-7.8 hours, prolonged in renal impairment

Elimination: 50% in urine as unchanged drug

Dialysis: >50% removed by hemodialysis

Usual Dosage Oral (dosage recommendation is based on the product's erythromycin content):

Children ≥2 months: 40-50 mg/kg/day in divided doses every 6-8 hours; not to exceed 2 g erythromycin or 6 g sulfisoxazole/day

Adults: 400 mg erythromycin and 1200 mg sulfisoxazole every 6 hours

Administration Oral: Administer with or without food; shake suspension well before use; maintain adequate fluid intake to prevent crystalluria and kidney stone formation

Monitoring Parameters CBC with differential and platelet count, urinalysis; periodic liver function and renal function tests; observe patient for diarrhea

Test Interactions False-positive urinary protein; false-positive urinary catecholamines, 17-hydroxycorticosteroids and 17-ketosteroids

Patient Information May cause photosensitivity reactions (eg, exposure to sunlight may cause severe sunburn, skin rash, redness, or itching); avoid exposure to sunlight and artificial light sources (sunlamps, tanning booth/bed); wear protective clothing, wide-brimmed hats, sunglasses, and lip sunscreen (SPF ≥15); use a sunscreen [broad-spectrum sunscreen or physical sunscreen (preferred) or sunblock with SPF ≥15]; contact physician if reaction occurs.

Dosage Forms Excipient information presented when available (limited, particularly for generics); consult specific product labeling.

Powder for oral suspension: Erythromycin ethylsuccinate 200 mg and sulfisoxazole acetyl 600 mg per 5 mL (100 mL, 150 mL, 200 mL)

E.S.P.®: Erythromycin ethylsuccinate 200 mg and sulfisoxazole acetyl 600 mg per 5 mL (100 mL, 150 mL, 200 mL) [cheri beri flavor]

References

Rodriguez WJ, Schwartz RH, Sait T, et al, "Erythromycin-Sulfisoxazole vs Amoxicillin in the Treatment of Acute Otitis Media in Children," *Am J Dis Child*, 1985, 139(8):766-70.

◆ **Erythromycin Base** *see* Erythromycin *on page 525*

◆ **Erythromycin Ethylsuccinate** *see* Erythromycin *on page 525*

◆ **Erythromycin Lactobionate** *see* Erythromycin *on page 525*

◆ **Erythromycin Stearate** *see* Erythromycin *on page 525*

◆ **Erythropoiesis-Stimulating Agent (ESA)** *see* Darbepoetin Alfa *on page 390*

◆ **Erythropoiesis-Stimulating Agent (ESA)** *see* Epoetin Alfa *on page 513*

◆ **Erythropoiesis-Stimulating Protein** *see* Darbepoetin Alfa *on page 390*

◆ **Erythropoietin** *see* Epoetin Alfa *on page 513*

◆ **Erythro-RX** *see* Erythromycin *on page 525*

Escitalopram (es sye TAL oh pram)

Medication Safety Issues

Sound-alike/look-alike issues:

Lexapro® may be confused with Loxitane®

International issues:

Zavesca®: Brand name for escitalopram [in multiple international markets; ISMP April 21, 2010], but also brand name for miglustat [Canada, U.S., and multiple international markets]

Related Information

Antidepressant Agents *on page 1484*

Serotonin Syndrome *on page 1695*

U.S. Brand Names Lexapro®

Canadian Brand Names Cipralex®

Therapeutic Category Antidepressant, Selective Serotonin Reuptake Inhibitor (SSRI)

Generic Available No

Use Treatment of major depressive disorder (FDA approved in ages 12-17 years and adults); treatment of generalized anxiety disorders (GAD) (FDA approved in adults); has also been studied in children and adolescents with social anxiety disorders and pervasive developmental disorders (PDD) including autism

Medication Guide An FDA-approved patient medication guide, which is available with the product information and at http://www.fda.gov/downloads/Drugs/DrugSafety/ucm088620.pdf, must be dispensed with this medication for each new outpatient prescription and refill.

Pregnancy Risk Factor C

Pregnancy Considerations Due to adverse effects observed in animal studies, escitalopram is classified as pregnancy category C. Escitalopram is distributed into the amniotic fluid. Limited data is available concerning the use of escitalopram during pregnancy. Nonteratogenic effects in the newborn following SSRI exposure late in the third trimester include respiratory distress, cyanosis, apnea, seizures, temperature instability, feeding difficulty, vomiting, hypoglycemia, hypo- or hypertonia, hyper-reflexia, jitteriness, irritability, constant crying, and tremor. An increased risk of low birth weight and lower Apgar scores have also been reported. Exposure to SSRIs after the twentieth week of gestation has been associated with persistent pulmonary hypertension of the newborn (PPHN). Adverse effects may be due to toxic effects of the SSRI or drug withdrawal without a taper. The long-term effects of *in utero* SSRI exposure on infant development and behavior are not known. Escitalopram is the S-enantiomer of the racemic derivative citalopram; also refer to the Citalopram monograph.

Women treated for major depression and who are euthymic prior to pregnancy are more likely to experience a relapse when medication is discontinued as compared to pregnant women who continue taking antidepressant medications. The ACOG recommends that therapy with SSRIs or SNRIs during pregnancy be individualized; treatment of depression during pregnancy should incorporate the clinical expertise of the mental health clinician, obstetrician, primary healthcare provider, and pediatrician. If treatment during pregnancy is required, consider tapering therapy during the third trimester in order to prevent withdrawal symptoms in the infant. If this is done and the woman is considered to be at risk of relapse from her major depressive disorder, the medication can be restarted following delivery, although the dose should be readjusted to that required before pregnancy. Treatment algorithms have been developed by the ACOG and the APA for the management of depression in women prior to conception and during pregnancy (Yonkers, 2009).

Lactation Enters breast milk/consider risk:benefit

Breast-Feeding Considerations Escitalopram and its metabolite are excreted into breast milk. Limited data is available concerning the effects escitalopram may have in the nursing infant and the long-term effects on development and behavior have not been studied. According to the manufacturer, the decision to continue or discontinue breast-feeding during therapy should take into account the risk of exposure to the infant and the benefits of treatment to the mother. Escitalopram is the S-enantiomer of the racemic derivative citalopram; also refer to the Citalopram monograph.

Contraindications Hypersensitivity to escitalopram, citalopram, or any component; use with MAO inhibitors within 14 days (potentially fatal reactions may occur); concurrent use of pimozide

Warnings Escitalopram is not approved for use in pediatric patients <12 years of age. Clinical worsening of depression or suicidal ideation and behavior may occur in children and adults with major depressive disorder **[U.S. Boxed Warning]**. In clinical trials, antidepressants increased the risk of suicidal thinking and behavior (suicidality) in children, adolescents, and young adults (18-24 years of age) with major depressive disorder and other psychiatric disorders. This risk must be considered before prescribing antidepressants for any clinical use. Short-term studies did **not** show an increased risk of suicidality with antidepressant use in patients >24 years of age and showed a decreased risk in patients ≥65 years.

Patients of all ages who are treated with antidepressants for any indication require appropriate monitoring and close observation for clinical worsening of depression, suicidality, and unusual changes in behavior, especially during the first few months after antidepressant initiation or when the dose is adjusted. Family members and caregivers should be instructed to closely observe the patient (ie, daily) and communicate condition with healthcare provider. Patients should also be monitored for associated behaviors (eg, anxiety, agitation, panic attacks, insomnia, irritability, hostility, aggressiveness, impulsivity, akathisia, hypomania, mania) which may increase the risk for worsening depression or suicidality. Worsening depression or emergence of suicidality (or associated behaviors listed above) that is abrupt in onset, severe, or not part of the presenting symptoms may require discontinuation or modification of drug therapy.

Avoid abrupt discontinuation; withdrawal syndrome with discontinuation symptoms (including agitation, dysphoria, anxiety, confusion, dizziness, hypomania, nightmares, irritability, sensory disturbances, headache, lethargy, emotional lability, insomnia, tinnitus, and seizures) may occur if therapy is abruptly discontinued or dose is reduced; taper the dose to minimize risks of discontinuation symptoms. If intolerable symptoms occur following a decrease in dosage or upon discontinuation of therapy, consider resuming the previous dose with a more gradual taper. To reduce risk of intentional overdose, write prescriptions for the smallest quantity consistent with good patient care.

May worsen psychosis in some patients or precipitate a shift to mania or hypomania in patients with bipolar disorder. Monotherapy in patients with bipolar disorder should be avoided. Patients presenting with depressive symptoms should be screened for bipolar disorder. Use with caution in patients with a history of mania. Escitalopram is not FDA approved for the treatment of bipolar depression.

Potentially fatal serotonin syndrome (SS) or neuroleptic malignant syndrome (NMS)-like reactions have occurred with selective serotonin reuptake inhibitors (SSRIs) and serotonin/norepinephrine reuptake inhibitors (SNRIs) when used alone and particularly when used in combination with serotonergic drugs (eg, triptans), drugs that impair the metabolism of serotonin (eg, MAO inhibitors, linezolid), or antidopaminergic agents (eg, antipsychotics). Identification and differentiation of SS (eg, tremor, myoclonus, agitation) and more severe NMS-like reactions (eg, hyperthermia, muscle rigidity, autonomic instability, mental status changes) can be complex; monitor patients closely for either syndrome. Discontinue treatment (and any concomitant serotonergic and/or antidopaminergic agents) immediately if signs or symptoms arise and initiate supportive symptomatic therapy. Tryptophan (which can be metabolized to serotonin) and the herbal medicine St John's wort (*Hypericum perforatum*) may increase serious side effects (concomitant use of these agents with escitalopram is not recommended); see Drug Interactions.

Precautions Escitalopram may impair platelet aggregation and cause abnormal bleeding (eg, ecchymosis, purpura, upper GI bleeding); risk may be increased in patients with impaired platelet aggregation and with concurrent use of aspirin, NSAIDs, warfarin, or other drugs that affect coagulation; bleeding related to SSRI or SNRI use has been reported to range from relatively minor bruising and epistaxis to life-threatening hemorrhage. Escitalopram may impair cognitive or motor performance. Use with caution in patients with seizure disorders, concomitant illnesses that may affect hepatic metabolism or hemodynamic responses (eg, unstable cardiac disease, recent MI), and suicidal ideation; use with caution and decrease dose in patients with hepatic dysfunction; use with caution in patients with severe renal impairment.

Use with caution during third trimester of pregnancy [newborns may experience adverse effects or withdrawal symptoms (consider risk:benefits); see Additional Information; exposure to SSRIs late in pregnancy may also be associated with an increased risk for persistent pulmonary hypertension of the newborn (see Chambers, 2006)]; high doses of escitalopram have been associated with teratogenicity in animals. Use with caution in patients receiving diuretics or those who are volume-depleted (may cause hyponatremia or SIADH). No clinical studies have assessed the combined use of escitalopram and electroconvulsive therapy; however, use with caution in patients receiving electroconvulsive therapy; may increase the risks associated with electroconvulsive therapy; consider discontinuing, when possible, prior to electroconvulsive therapy treatment. Oral solution contains propylene glycol and sorbitol.

Adverse Reactions

Cardiovascular: Chest pain, hypertension, palpitation

Central nervous system: Headache, somnolence, insomnia, dizziness, fatigue, abnormal dreaming, impaired concentration, fever, irritability, lethargy, lightheadedness, migraine, vertigo, yawning; suicidal thinking and behavior (see Warnings)

> **Note:** SSRI-associated behavioral activation (eg, restlessness, hyperkinesis, hyperactivity, agitation) is two- to threefold more prevalent in children compared to adolescents; it is more prevalent in adolescents compared to adults. Somnolence (including sedation and drowsiness) is more common in adults compared to children and adolescents (Safer, 2006).

Dermatologic: Rash

Endocrine & metabolic: Hyponatremia, SIADH (usually in volume-depleted patients); sexual dysfunction, dysmenorrhea

Gastrointestinal: Nausea, diarrhea, xerostomia, appetite decreased, constipation, indigestion, abdominal pain, abdominal cramps, appetite increased, flatulence, gastroenteritis, gastroesophageal reflux, heartburn, toothache, vomiting

Note: SSRI-associated vomiting is two- to threefold more prevalent in children compared to adolescents; it is more prevalent in adolescents compared to adults (Safer, 2006).

Genitourinary: Urinary tract infection, urinary frequency

Neuromuscular & skeletal: Arthralgia, limb pain, muscle cramp, myalgia, neck/shoulder pain, paresthesia, tremor, back pain

Ocular: Blurred vision

Otic: Earache, tinnitus

Respiratory: Rhinitis, sinusitis, bronchitis, cough, nasal or sinus congestion, sinus headache

Miscellaneous: Diaphoresis, flu-like syndrome, allergy; withdrawal symptoms following abrupt discontinuation (see Warnings)

Drug Interactions

Metabolism/Transport Effects Substrate (major) of CYP2C19, 3A4; **Inhibits** CYP2D6 (weak)

Avoid Concomitant Use

Avoid concomitant use of Escitalopram with any of the following: Artemether; Dronedarone; Iobenguane I 123; Lumefantrine; MAO Inhibitors; Metoclopramide; Nilotinib; Pimozide; QuiNINE; Sibutramine; Tetrabenazine; Thioridazine; Ziprasidone

Increased Effect/Toxicity

Escitalopram may increase the levels/effects of: Alcohol (Ethyl); Alpha-/Beta-Blockers; Anticoagulants; Antidepressants (Serotonin Reuptake Inhibitor/Antagonist); Antiplatelet Agents; Aspirin; Beta-Blockers; BusPIRone; CarBAMazepine; Clozapine; CNS Depressants; Collagenase (Systemic); Desmopressin; Dextromethorphan; Dronedarone; Drotrecogin Alfa; Haloperidol; Ibritumomab; Lithium; Methadone; Mexiletine; NSAID (COX-2 Inhibitor); NSAID (Nonselective); Phenytoin; Pimozide; QTc-Prolonging Agents; QuiNINE; Risperidone; Salicylates; Serotonin Modulators; Tetrabenazine; Thioridazine; Thrombolytic Agents; Tositumomab and Iodine I 131 Tositumomab; TraMADol; Tricyclic Antidepressants; Vitamin K Antagonists; Ziprasidone

The levels/effects of Escitalopram may be increased by: Alfuzosin; Analgesics (Opioid); Artemether; BusPIRone; Chloroquine; Cimetidine; Ciprofloxacin; Ciprofloxacin (Systemic); CYP2C19 Inhibitors (Moderate); CYP2C19 Inhibitors (Strong); CYP3A4 Inhibitors (Moderate); CYP3A4 Inhibitors (Strong); Gadobutrol; Glucosamine; Herbs (Anticoagulant/Antiplatelet Properties); Lumefantrine; Macrolide Antibiotics; MAO Inhibitors; Metoclopramide; Nilotinib; Omega-3-Acid Ethyl Esters; Pentosan Polysulfate Sodium; Pentoxifylline; Prostacyclin Analogues; QuiNINE; Sibutramine; TraMADol; Tryptophan

Decreased Effect

Escitalopram may decrease the levels/effects of: Iobenguane I 123

The levels/effects of Escitalopram may be decreased by: CarBAMazepine; CYP2C19 Inducers (Strong); CYP3A4 Inducers (Strong); Cyproheptadine; Deferasirox

Food Interactions Absorption is not affected by food. Tryptophan supplements may increase serious side effects; its use is **not recommended**.

Stability Store at 25°C (77°F); excursions permitted to 15°C to 30°C (59°F to 86°F)

Mechanism of Action Escitalopram (the S-enantiomer of racemic citalopram) selectively inhibits the reuptake of serotonin in the presynaptic neuron and has minimal effects on norepinephrine or dopamine neuronal reuptake. Displays little to no affinity for serotonin, dopamine,

adrenergic, histamine, GABA, or muscarinic receptor subtypes.

Pharmacodynamics

Onset of action: 1-2 weeks

Maximum effect: 8-12 weeks

Pharmacokinetics (Adult data unless noted)

Distribution: V_d: Adults: 12 L/kg

Protein binding, plasma: ~56%

Metabolism: Extensively hepatic via CYP2C19 and 3A4 to S-demethylcitalopram (S-DCT; $1/7$ the activity of escitalopram); S-DCT is metabolized to S-didemethylcitalopram (S-DDCT; active; $1/27$ the activity of escitalopram) via CYP2D6

Bioavailability: 80%; tablets and oral solution are bioequivalent

Half-life elimination: Mean:

Adults: 27-32 hours

Adolescents: 19 hours

Time to peak serum concentration: Adults: 5 hours; Adolescents: 2.9 hours

Elimination: Urine (8% as unchanged drug)

Clearance (citalopram):

Hepatic impairment: Decreased by 37%

Mild-to-moderate renal impairment: Decreased by 17%

Severe renal impairment (Cl_{cr} <20 mL/minute): No information available

Usual Dosage Oral:

Children and Adolescents:

Depression:

Children <12 years: **Note:** Not FDA approved; see Warnings. Limited information is available; only one randomized, placebo-controlled trial has been published; efficacy was not demonstrated for children <12 years of age (see Wagner, 2006)

Adolescents ≥12 years: Initial: 10 mg once daily; may be increased to 20 mg/day after at least 3 weeks

Autism and PDD: **Note:** Not FDA approved; see Warnings. Information is limited and based on one published prospective, 10-week, open-labeled, forced dose-titration trial of 28 children and adolescents 6-17 years of age (mean age: 10.4 years) (Owley, 2005). Mean severity outcome scores showed significant improvement; mean final dose: 11.1 ± 6.5 mg/day (range: 0-20 mg/day); no significant correlation between final tolerated dose and weight was shown; 10 of 28 treated subjects could not tolerate a 10 mg/day dose; further studies are needed

Children and Adolescents 6-17 years: Initial: 2.5 mg once daily; may increase if needed to 5 mg/day after 1 week; may then increase at weekly intervals by 5 mg/day if needed and as tolerated; maximum dose: 20 mg/day

Social anxiety disorder: **Note:** Not FDA approved; see Warnings. Information is limited and based on one prospective, 12-week, open-labeled trial of 20 children and adolescents 10-17 years of age (mean age: 15 years) (Isolan, 2007). At the end of the 12 weeks, 65% of patients met overall response criteria and all symptomatic and quality of life outcome measures showed significant improvements; mean final dose: 13 ± 4.1 mg/day; further studies are needed

Children and Adolescents 10-17 years: Initial: 5 mg once daily for 7 days, then 10 mg/day for 7 days; may then increase at weekly intervals by 5 mg/day if needed, based on clinical response and tolerability; maximum dose: 20 mg/day

Adults: Depression, generalized anxiety disorder: Initial: 10 mg once daily; dose may be increased to 20 mg/day after at least 1 week

Dosage adjustment in renal impairment:
Mild-to-moderate impairment: No dosage adjustment needed
Severe impairment: Cl$_{cr}$ <20 mL/minute: Use with caution
Dosage adjustment in hepatic impairment: Adolescents >12 years and Adults: 10 mg/day
Administration Administer once daily (morning or evening); may be administered with or without food.
Monitoring Parameters Monitor patient periodically for symptom resolution; monitor for worsening depression, suicidality, and associated behaviors (especially at the beginning of therapy or when doses are increased or decreased; see Warnings). Monitor for anxiety, social functioning, mania, panic attacks; akathisia. Monitor for signs and symptoms of serotonin syndrome or neuroleptic malignant syndrome-like reactions.
Patient Information Read the patient Medication Guide that you receive with each prescription and refill of escitalopram. An increased risk of suicidal thinking and behavior has been reported with the use of antidepressants in children, adolescents, and young adults (18-24 years of age). Notify physician if you feel more depressed, have thoughts of suicide, or become more agitated or irritable (see Warnings). Avoid alcohol, caffeine, CNS stimulants, tryptophan supplements, and the herbal medicine St John's wort; avoid aspirin, NSAIDs, or other drugs that affect coagulation (may increase risks of bleeding); may cause dizziness or drowsiness and impair ability to perform activities requiring mental alertness or physical coordination; may cause dry mouth. Some medicines should not be taken with escitalopram or should not be taken for a while after escitalopram has been discontinued; report the use of other medications, nonprescription medications, and herbal or natural products to your physician and pharmacist. It may take up to 4 weeks to see therapeutic effects from this medication. Take as directed; do not alter dose or frequency without consulting prescriber; avoid abrupt discontinuation.
Nursing Implications
Assess other medications patient may be taking for possible interaction (especially MAO inhibitors, P450 inhibitors, and other CNS active agents). Assess mental status for depression, suicidal ideation, anxiety, social functioning, mania, or panic attack.
Additional Information If used for an extended period of time, long-term usefulness of escitalopram should be periodically re-evaluated for the individual patient. A recent report describes 5 children (age: 8-15 years) who developed epistaxis (n=4) or bruising (n=1) while receiving SSRI therapy (sertraline) (see Lake, 2000).

Neonates born to women receiving SSRIs later during the third trimester may experience respiratory distress, apnea, cyanosis, temperature instability, vomiting, feeding difficulty, hypoglycemia, constant crying, irritability, hypotonia, hypertonia, hyper-reflexia, tremor, jitteriness, and seizures; these symptoms may be due to a direct toxic effect, withdrawal syndrome, or (in some cases) serotonin syndrome. Withdrawal symptoms occur in 30% of neonates exposed to SSRIs *in utero*; monitor newborns for at least 48 hours after birth; long-term effects of *in utero* exposure to SSRIs are unknown (see Levinson-Castiel, 2006).

Dosage Forms Excipient information presented when available (limited, particularly for generics); consult specific product labeling.
Solution, oral:
Lexapro®: 1 mg/mL (240 mL) [contains propylene glycol; peppermint flavor]
Tablet:
Lexapro®: 5 mg, 10 mg, 20 mg
Note: Cipralex® [CAN] is available only in 10 mg and 20 mg strengths.

References
Boyer EW and Shannon M, "The Serotonin Syndrome," *New Engl J Med*, 2005, 352:1112-20.
Chambers CD, Hernandez-Diaz S, Van Marter LJ, et al, "Selective Serotonin-Reuptake Inhibitors and Risk of Persistent Pulmonary Hypertension of the Newborn," *N Engl J Med*, 2006, 354(6):579-87.
Isolan L, Pheula G, Salum GA Jr, et al, "An Open-Label Trial of Escitalopram in Children and Adolescents With Social Anxiety Disorder," *J Child Adolesc Psychopharmacol*, 2007, 17(6):751-60.
Lake MB, Birmaher B, Wassick S, et al, "Bleeding and Selective Serotonin Reuptake Inhibitors in Childhood and Adolescence," *J Child Adolesc Psychopharmacol*, 2000, 10(1):35-8.
Levinson-Castiel R, Merlob P, Linder N, et al, "Neonatal Abstinence Syndrome After *in utero* Exposure to Selective Serotonin Reuptake Inhibitors in Term Infants," *Arch Pediatr Adolesc Med*, 2006, 160 (2):173-6.
Murdoch D and Keam SJ, "Escitalopram: A Review of Its Use in the Management of Major Depressive Disorder," *Drugs*, 2005, 65 (16):2379-404.
Owley T, Walton L, Salt J, et al, "An Open-Label Trial of Escitalopram in Pervasive Developmental Disorders," *J Am Acad Child Adolesc Psychiatry*, 2005, 44(4):343-8.
Rao N, "The Clinical Pharmacokinetics of Escitalopram," *Clin Pharmacokinet*, 2007, 46(4):281-90.
Safer DJ and Zito JM, "Treatment Emergent Adverse Effects of Selective Serotonin Reuptake Inhibitors by Age Group: Children vs. Adolescents," *J Child Adolesc Psychopharmacol*, 2006, 16 (1-2):159-69.
Wagner KD, Jonas J, Findling RL, et al, "A Double-Blind, Randomized, Placebo-Controlled Trial of Escitalopram in the Treatment of Pediatric Depression," *J Am Acad Child Adolesc Psychiatry*, 2006, 45(3):280-8.

♦ **Escitalopram Oxalate** see Escitalopram on page 529
♦ **Eserine Salicylate** see Physostigmine on page 1108
♦ **Eskalith** see Lithium on page 834

Esmolol (ES moe lol)

Medication Safety Issues
Sound-alike/look-alike issues:
Esmolol may be confused with Osmitrol®
Brevibloc® may be confused with Brevital®, Bumex®, Buprenex®

High alert medication: The Institute for Safe Medication Practices (ISMP) includes this medication among its list of drugs which have a heightened risk of causing significant patient harm when used in error.
Related Information
Antihypertensive Agents by Class on page 1481
U.S. Brand Names Brevibloc®
Canadian Brand Names Brevibloc®
Therapeutic Category Antiarrhythmic Agent, Class II; Antihypertensive Agent; Beta-Adrenergic Blocker
Generic Available Yes: Excludes infusion
Use Treatment of supraventricular tachycardia (primarily to control ventricular rate in patients with atrial fibrillation or flutter) (FDA approved in adults); noncompensatory sinus tachycardia (FDA approved in adults); perioperative tachycardia and hypertension (FDA approved in adults)
Pregnancy Risk Factor C (manufacturer); D (2nd and 3rd trimesters - expert analysis)
Pregnancy Considerations Teratogenic effects are not noted in animal studies. There are no well-controlled studies in pregnant women; however, fetal bradycardia can occur when administered in the 3rd trimester of pregnancy or at delivery.
Lactation Excretion in breast milk unknown/use with caution
Contraindications Hypersensitivity to esmolol, any component, or other beta-blockers; sinus bradycardia or heart block, uncompensated CHF, cardiogenic shock
Warnings Caution should be exercised when discontinuing esmolol infusions to avoid withdrawal effects
Precautions Use with extreme caution in patients with hyper-reactive airway disease; use lowest dose possible and discontinue infusion if bronchospasm occurs; use with

caution in diabetes mellitus, hypoglycemia, renal failure; avoid extravasation; patients receiving beta blockers who have a history of anaphylactic reactions, may be more reactive to a repeated allergen challenge and may not be responsive to the usual epinephrine doses used to treat an allergic reaction

Adverse Reactions

Cardiovascular: Bradycardia, hypotension (especially with doses >200 mcg/kg/minute), peripheral ischemia, Raynaud's phenomena

Central nervous system: Agitation, confusion, depression, dizziness, headache, lethargy, somnolence

Gastrointestinal: Nausea, vomiting

Local: Induration, inflammation, phlebitis, skin necrosis after extravasation

Respiratory: Bronchoconstriction (less than propranolol, but more likely with higher doses)

Miscellaneous: Adverse reactions similar to other beta-blockers may occur, diaphoresis

Drug Interactions

Avoid Concomitant Use

Avoid concomitant use of Esmolol with any of the following: Methacholine

Increased Effect/Toxicity

Esmolol may increase the levels/effects of: Alpha-/Beta-Agonists (Direct-Acting); Alpha1-Blockers; Alpha2-Agonists; Amifostine; Antihypertensives; Antipsychotic Agents (Phenothiazines); Bupivacaine; Cardiac Glycosides; Hypotensive Agents; Insulin; Lidocaine; Lidocaine (Systemic); Lidocaine (Topical); Mepivacaine; Methacholine; Midodrine; RiTUXimab; Sulfonylureas

The levels/effects of Esmolol may be increased by: Acetylcholinesterase Inhibitors; Aminoquinolines (Antimalarial); Amiodarone; Anilidopiperidine Opioids; Antipsychotic Agents (Phenothiazines); Calcium Channel Blockers (Nondihydropyridine); Diazoxide; Dipyridamole; Disopyramide; Dronedarone; Herbs (Hypotensive Properties); MAO Inhibitors; Pentoxifylline; Phosphodiesterase 5 Inhibitors; Propafenone; Propoxyphene; Prostacyclin Analogues; QuiNIDine; Reserpine

Decreased Effect

Esmolol may decrease the levels/effects of: Beta2-Agonists; Theophylline Derivatives

The levels/effects of Esmolol may be decreased by: Barbiturates; Herbs (Hypertensive Properties); Methylphenidate; Nonsteroidal Anti-Inflammatory Agents; Rifamycin Derivatives; Yohimbine

Food Interactions Avoid xanthine-containing foods or beverages

Stability Store at controlled room temperature at 25°C (77°F); excursions permitted to 15°C to 30°C (59°F to 86°F); protect from freezing and excessive heat. Stable for at least 24 hours (under refrigeration or at controlled room temperature) at a final concentration of 10 mg/mL in the following solutions: D_5W, D_5LR, D_5 $^1/_2NS$, D_5NS, LR, NS, $^1/_2NS$, D_5W with KCl 40 mEq/L; **not** compatible with sodium bicarbonate 5%

Mechanism of Action Class II antiarrhythmic: Competitively blocks response to beta$_1$-adrenergic stimulation with little or no effect on beta$_2$-receptors except at high doses (ie, cardioselective at lower doses); no intrinsic sympathomimetic activity; no membrane-stabilizing activity; ultra-short-acting

Pharmacodynamics

Onset of action: I.V.: Beta blockade occurs within 2-10 minutes (onset of effects is quickest when loading doses are administered)

Duration: Short (10-30 minutes)

Pharmacokinetics (Adult data unless noted)

Protein binding: 55%

Distribution: V_d:

Children: 2 L/kg

Adults: 3.5 L/kg (range: 2-5 L/kg)

Metabolism: In blood by esterases

Half-life, elimination:

Children:

18 months to 14 years (n=12): 2.88 ± 2.67 minutes

2.5-16 years (n=20): 4.5 ± 2.1 minutes

Adults: 9 minutes

Elimination: ~69% of dose excreted in urine as metabolites and 2% as unchanged drug

Usual Dosage Must be adjusted to individual response and tolerance

Children: I.V.: Limited information available

Supraventricular tachycardia (SVT): Some centers have utilized initial doses of 100-500 mcg/kg given over 1 minute followed by a continuous infusion for control of SVT. One electrophysiologic study assessing esmolol-induced beta-blockade (n=20, 2-16 years of age) used an initial dose of 600 mcg/kg over 2 minutes followed by an infusion of 200 mcg/kg/minute; the infusion was titrated upward by 50-100 mcg/kg/minute every 5-10 minutes until a reduction >10% in heart rate or mean blood pressure occurred. Mean dose required: 550 mcg/kg/minute with a range of 300-1000 mcg/kg/minute (Trippel, 1991).

Postoperative hypertension: Loading doses of 500 mcg/kg/minute over 1 minute followed by a continuous infusion with doses of 50-250 mcg/kg/minute (mean: 173) have been used in addition to nitroprusside in a small number of patients (7 patients, 7-19 years of age, median age: 13 years) after coarctation of aorta repair (Vincent, 1990).

An open-label trial of 20 infants and children (1 month to 12 years of age; median age: 25.6 months) used the following dosing guidelines to treat postoperative hypertension following cardiac surgery: Age 0-7 days: Initial: 50 mcg/kg/minute; titrate dose by 25-50 mcg/kg/minute every 20 minutes; age 8 days to 1 month: Initial: 75 mcg/kg/minute; titrate dose by 50 mcg/kg/minute every 20 minutes; age >1 month to 1 year: Initial: 100 mcg/kg/minute; titrate dose by 50 mcg/kg/minute every 10 minutes; age >1 year to 12 years: Initial: 150 mcg/kg/minute; titrate dose by 50-100 mcg/kg/minute every 10 minutes; dose was titrated until blood pressure was ≤90th percentile for age or until maximum dose of 1000 mcg/kg/minute was reached; mean required dose: 700 mcg/kg/minute (range: 300-1000 mcg/kg/minute); final dose required was significantly higher in patients with aortic coarctation repair (mean ± SD: 830 ± 153 mcg/kg/minute) than in patients with repair of other congenital heart defects (mean ± SD: 570 ± 230 mcg/kg/minute) (Wiest, 1998)

Adults: I.V.:

Intraoperative tachycardia and/or hypertension (immediate control): Loading dose: 80 mg (~1 mg/kg) over 30 seconds; follow with a 150 mcg/kg/minute infusion, if necessary; adjust infusion rate as needed to maintain desired heart rate and/or blood pressure; maximum dose: 300 mcg/kg/minute.

Supraventricular tachycardia or gradual control of postoperative tachycardia and hypertension: Loading dose: 500 mcg/kg over 1 minute; follow with a 50 mcg/kg/minute infusion for 4 minutes; if response is inadequate, rebolus with another 500 mcg/kg loading dose over 1 minute, and increase the maintenance infusion to 100 mcg/kg/minute. Repeat this process until a therapeutic effect has been achieved or to a maximum recommended maintenance dose of 200 mcg/kg/minute. Usual dosage range: 50-200 mcg/kg/minute with average dose = 100 mcg/kg/minute.

Administration Parenteral: I.V.: Commercially available concentrations (10 mg/mL and 20 mg/mL) are iso-osmotic and can be used for direct I.V. use; infuse I.V. loading dose over 1-2 minutes. **Note:** Parenteral drug products are for single patient use only; products do **not** contain preservatives. Do not introduce additives into the premixed bags. Medication port of premixed bag should be used to withdraw only the initial bolus; do not use medication port to withdraw additional bolus doses (sterility cannot be assured).

Monitoring Parameters Blood pressure, ECG, heart rate, respiratory rate, I.V. site

Nursing Implications Decrease infusion rate or discontinue if hypotension, CHF, etc occur

Dosage Forms Excipient information presented when available (limited, particularly for generics); consult specific product labeling.

Infusion [premixed in sodium chloride; preservative free]:
Brevibloc®: 2000 mg (100 mL) [20 mg/mL; double strength]; 2500 mg (250 mL) [10 mg/mL]

Injection, solution, as hydrochloride: 10 mg/mL (10 mL)
Brevibloc®:
10 mg/mL (10 mL) [alcohol free; premixed in sodium chloride]
20 mg/mL (5 mL, 100 mL) [alcohol free; double strength; premixed in sodium chloride]

References

Cuneo BF, Zales VR, Blahunka PC, et al, "Pharmacodynamics and Pharmacokinetics of Esmolol, A Short-Acting Beta-Blocking Agent in Children," *Pediatr Cardiol*, 1994, 15(6):296-301.

Trippel DL, Wiest DB, and Gillette PC, "Cardiovascular and Antiarrhythmic Effects of Esmolol in Children," *J Pediatr*, 1991, 119 (1):142-7.

Vincent RN, Click LA, Williams HM, et al, "Esmolol As an Adjunct in the Treatment of Systemic Hypertension After Operative Repair of Coarctation of the Aorta," *Am J Cardiol*, 1990, 65(13):941-3.

Wiest DB, Garner SS, Uber WE, et al, "Esmolol for the Management of Pediatric Hypertension After Cardiac Operations," *J Thorac Cardiovasc Surg*, 1998, 115(4):890-7.

Wiest DB, Trippel DL, Gillette PC, et al, "Pharmacokinetics of Esmolol in Children," *Clin Pharmacol Ther*, 1991, 49(6):618-23.

◆ **Esmolol Hydrochloride** *see* Esmolol *on page 532*

Esomeprazole (es oh ME pray zol)

Medication Safety Issues
Sound-alike/look-alike issues:
Esomeprazole may be confused with aripiprazole
Nexium® may be confused with Nexavar®

U.S. Brand Names Nexium®

Canadian Brand Names Nexium®

Therapeutic Category Gastric Acid Secretion Inhibitor; Gastrointestinal Agent, Gastric or Duodenal Ulcer Treatment; Proton Pump Inhibitor

Generic Available No

Use
Oral formulation: Treatment and maintenance of healing of severe erosive esophagitis; treatment of symptomatic gastroesophageal reflux disease (GERD); adjunctive treatment of duodenal ulcers associated with *Helicobacter pylori*; prevention of gastric ulcers associated with continuous NSAID therapy; long term treatment of pathological hypersecretory conditions (eg, Zollinger-Ellison syndrome)

I.V. formulation: Short-term alternative treatment when oral therapy is not possible or appropriate

Pregnancy Risk Factor B

Pregnancy Considerations Teratogenic effects were not observed in animal studies. However, there are no adequate and well-controlled studies in pregnant women. Congenital abnormalities have been reported sporadically following omeprazole use during pregnancy.

Lactation Excretion in breast milk unknown/not recommended

Breast-Feeding Considerations Esomeprazole excretion into breast milk has not been studied. However, omeprazole is excreted in breast milk, and therefore considered likely that esomeprazole is similarly excreted; breast-feeding is not recommended.

Contraindications Hypersensitivity to esomeprazole, substituted benzimidazole proton pump inhibitors (eg, omeprazole, lansoprazole, pantoprazole), or any component

Warnings Esomeprazole is an enantiomer of omeprazole and may share the same potential long-term side effects as omeprazole; atrophic gastritis has been noted occasionally in gastric corpus biopsies from patients treated long-term with omeprazole; in long-term (2-year) studies in rats, omeprazole produced a dose-related increase in gastric carcinoid tumors. While available endoscopic evaluations and histologic examinations of biopsy specimens from human stomachs have not detected a risk from short-term exposure to omeprazole, further human data on the effect of sustained hypochlorhydria and hypergastrinemia are needed to rule out the possibility of an increased risk for the development of tumors in humans receiving long-term therapy. Symptomatic relief does not preclude the presence of a gastric malignancy. Use of gastric acid inhibitors including proton pump inhibitors and H_2 blockers has been associated with an increased risk for development of acute gastroenteritis and community-acquired pneumonia (Canani, 2006).

Precautions Modify dosage in patients with liver impairment.

Adverse Reactions

Cardiovascular: Chest pain, tachycardia, bradycardia, flushing, hypertension

Central nervous system: Headache (8.1%), dizziness, vertigo, insomnia, anxiety, nervousness, fever, anorexia, confusion, somnolence, depression, aggression, agitation, hallucination

Dermatologic: Rash, acne, angioedema, dermatitis, pruritus, urticaria, erythema multiforme, Stevens-Johnson syndrome, toxic epidermal necrolysis, alopecia, hyperhidrosis, photosensitivity

Endocrine & metabolic: Goiter, glycosuria, hyperuricemia, hyponatremia

Gastrointestinal: Diarrhea (2%), nausea (2%), abdominal pain (2.7%), vomiting, constipation, flatulence, dyspepsia, dysphagia, epigastric pain, eructation, gastroenteritis, GI hemorrhage, hiccup, melena, irritable colon, xerostomia, anorexia, dysgeusia, abdominal pain, taste loss, taste perversion, pancreatitis, stomatitis

Genitourinary: Dysmenorrhea, vaginitis, urinary frequency, dysuria, hematuria, gynecomastia

Hematologic: Leukopenia, pancytopenia, thrombocytopenia, anemia, leukocytosis, agranulocytosis (rare)

Hepatic: Liver function tests elevated, hepatitis (with or without jaundice)

Local: Mild erythema, pruritus (at injection site)

Neuromuscular & skeletal: Myalgia, arthralgia, back pain, arthropathy, cramps, fibromyalgia syndrome, polymyalgia rheumatica, paresthesia, weakness

Ocular: Conjunctivitis, abnormal vision

Otic: Tinnitus, earache

Renal: Hematuria, pyuria, proteinuria, interstitial nephritis (rare)

Respiratory: Cough, dyspnea, larynx edema, pharyngitis, rhinitis, sinusitis

Miscellaneous: Hypersensitivity reactions including anaphylaxis (rare), GI candidiasis

Drug Interactions

Metabolism/Transport Effects Substrate of CYP2C19 (major), 3A4 (major); **Inhibits** CYP2C19 (moderate)

Avoid Concomitant Use

Avoid concomitant use of Esomeprazole with any of the following: Delavirdine; Erlotinib; Nelfinavir; Posaconazole

Increased Effect/Toxicity

Esomeprazole may increase the levels/effects of: Benzodiazepines (metabolized by oxidation); Cilostazol; CYP2C19 Substrates; Methotrexate; Raltegravir; Saquinavir; Tacrolimus; Tacrolimus (Systemic); Vitamin K Antagonists; Voriconazole

The levels/effects of Esomeprazole may be increased by: Clopidogrel; Fluconazole; Ketoconazole; Ketoconazole (Systemic)

Decreased Effect

Esomeprazole may decrease the levels/effects of: Atazanavir; Cefditoren; Clopidogrel; Dabigatran Etexilate; Dasatinib; Delavirdine; Erlotinib; Indinavir; Iron Salts; Itraconazole; Ketoconazole; Ketoconazole (Systemic); Mesalamine; Mycophenolate; Nelfinavir; Posaconazole

The levels/effects of Esomeprazole may be decreased by: CYP2C19 Inducers (Strong); Tipranavir

Food Interactions Absorption is decreased by 43% to 53% when taken with food.

Stability Store at room temperature; protect from light. Esomeprazole stability is a function of pH; it is rapidly degraded in acidic media, but has acceptable stability under alkaline conditions. Each capsule of esomeprazole contains enteric coated granules to prevent esomeprazole degradation by gastric acidity. I.V. formulation is stable at room temperature after reconstitution with NS and LR 12 hours and with D_5W 6 hours.

Mechanism of Action Esomeprazole is the S-isomer of omeprazole. Esomeprazole suppresses gastric acid secretion by inhibiting the parietal cell membrane enzyme (H^+/K^+)-ATPase or proton pump; demonstrates antimicrobial activity against *Helicobacter pylori*.

Pharmacokinetics (Adult data unless noted)

Distribution: Adults: V_d: 0.22 L/kg

Protein binding: 97%

Metabolism: Hepatic via CYP2C19 and 3A3/4 isoenzymes to hydroxy, desmethyl, and sulfone metabolites (all inactive)

Bioavailability: 64% after a single dose; 90% with repeated administration

Half-life:

Children 1-11 years: 0.42-0.88 hours

Adults: 1.2-1.5 hours

Time to peak serum concentration: Oral: Children and Adults: 1.3-1.8 hours

Elimination: Urine (80%, primarily as inactive metabolites; <1% excreted as active drug); feces (20%)

Clearance: Children 1-11 years: 6-19.44 L/hour

Usual Dosage Oral, I.V.: **Note:** I.V. treatment should be discontinued as soon as the patient tolerates oral therapy.

Children 1-11 years: Safety and efficacy of doses >1 mg/kg/day and/or therapy beyond 8 weeks have not been established.

GERD:

<20 kg: 10 mg once daily for 8 weeks

>20 kg: 10 or 20 mg once daily for 8 weeks

Nonerosive Reflux disease (NERD): 10 mg once daily for up to 8 weeks

Adolescents 12-17 years: 20-40 mg once daily for up to 8 weeks

Adults:

Erosive esophagitis (healing): Initial: 20-40 mg once daily for 4-8 weeks; if incomplete, continue for an additional 4-8 weeks; maintenance: 20 mg once daily (controlled studies did not extend beyond 6 months)

Symptomatic GERD: 20 mg once daily for 4-8 weeks

Pathological hypersecretory conditions including Zollinger-Ellison syndrome: 40 mg twice daily; dosage may be increased depending upon the response to therapy; doses up to 240 mg/day have been used

Adjunctive therapy of duodenal ulcers associated with *Helicobacter pylori* (in combination with antibiotic therapy): 40 mg once daily for 10 days

Prevention of NSAID-induced gastric ulcers: 20-40 mg once daily for up to 6 months

Dosage adjustment in hepatic impairment:

Mild to moderate liver impairment (Child-Pugh Class A or B): No dosage adjustment needed

Severe liver impairment (Child-Pugh Class C): Not to exceed 20 mg daily

Administration

Oral: Administer at least 1 hour before food or meals

Capsule: Swallow whole, do not chew or crush; capsule may be opened and the enteric coated pellets may be mixed with applesauce (applesauce should not be hot) and swallowed immediately; do not store mixture for future use; esomeprazole pellets also remain intact when mixed with tap water, orange juice, apple juice, and yogurt; due to small pellet size, the entire contents of an opened capsule may be completely delivered via small caliber and standard NG tubes when mixed with 50 mL water (White, 2002); administer immediately; do not administer if the pellets have dissolved or disintegrated

Granules: Mix contents of packet with 15 mL water and leave for 2-3 minutes to thicken; stir and drink within 30 minutes. Granules may be administered by nasogastric or gastric tube: Add 15 mL of water to a syringe, add granules from packet. Shake the syringe, leave 2-3 minutes to thicken. Shake the syringe and administer through nasogastric or gastric tube (French size 6 or greater) within 30 minutes. Refill the syringe with 15 mL of water, shake and flush tube.

I.V.: Reconstitute vial (20 mg or 40 mg) with 5 mL D_5W, NS, or LR. May administer dosage without further dilution over at least 3 minutes. May also be diluted in 50 mL D_5W, NS, or LR (0.4-0.8 mg/mL) and infuse over 10-30 minutes.

Patient Information May cause dry mouth; do not chew or crush granules. May cause photosensitivity reactions (eg, exposure to sunlight may cause severe sunburn, skin rash, redness, or itching); avoid direct exposure to sunlight.

Dosage Forms Excipient information presented when available (limited, particularly for generics); consult specific product labeling. [CAN] = Canadian availability

Note: Strength expressed as base

Capsule, delayed release, as magnesium:

Nexium®: 20 mg, 40 mg

Granules, for oral suspension, delayed release, as magnesium:

Nexium®: 10 mg/packet (30s); 20 mg/packet (30s); 40 mg/packet (30s)

Nexium® [CAN]: 10 mg/packet (28s)

Injection, powder for reconstitution, as sodium:

Nexium®: 20 mg, 40 mg [contains edetate sodium]

Tablet, extended release, as magnesium:

Nexium® [CAN]: 20 mg, 40 mg [not available in U.S.]

References

Canani RB, Cirillo P, Roggero P, et al, "Therapy With Gastric Acidity Inhibitors Increases the Risk of Acute Gastroenteritis and Community-Acquired Pneumonia in Children," *Pediatrics*, 2006, 117(5):e817-20.

Dohil R, Fidler M, Barshop B, et al, "Esomeprazole Therapy for Gastric Acid Hypersecretion in Children With Cystinosis," *Pediatr Nephrol*, 2005, 20(12):1786-93.

Gibbons TE and Gold BD, "The Use of Proton Pump Inhibitors in Children: A Comprehensive Review," *Paediatr Drugs*, 2003, 5(1):25-40.

Li J, Zhao J, Hamer-Maansson JE, et al, "Pharmacokinetic Properties of Esomeprazole in Adolescent Patients Aged 12 to 17 Years With Symptoms of Gastroesophageal Reflux Disease: A Randomized, Open-Label Study," Clin Ther, 2006, 28(3):419-27.

White CM, Kalus JS, Quercia R, et al, "Delivery of Esomeprazole Magnesium Enteric-Coated Pellets Through Small Caliber and Standard Nasogastric Tubes and Gastrostomy Tubes In Vitro," Am J Health Syst Pharm, 2002, 59(21):2085-8.

◆ **Esomeprazole Magnesium** see Esomeprazole on page 534

◆ **Esomeprazole Sodium** see Esomeprazole on page 534

◆ **E.S.P.®** see Erythromycin and Sulfisoxazole on page 528

◆ **Estar® (Can)** see Coal Tar on page 349

◆ **Ester-E™ [OTC]** see Vitamin E on page 1427

◆ **Estrace®** see Estradiol on page 536

◆ **Estraderm®** see Estradiol on page 536

Estradiol (es tra DYE ole)

Medication Safety Issues

Sound-alike/look-alike issues:

Alora® may be confused with Aldara®

Elestrin™ may be confused with alosetron

Estraderm® may be confused with Testoderm®

Beers Criteria medication: This drug may be inappropriate for use in geriatric patients (low severity risk).

Transdermal patch may contain conducting metal (eg, aluminum); remove patch prior to MRI.

International issues:

Vivelle®: Brand name for ethinyl estradiol and norgestimate in Austria

Estring® may be confused with Estrena® [Finland]

U.S. Brand Names Alora®; Climara®; Delestrogen®; Depo®-Estradiol; Divigel®; Elestrin™; Estrace®; Estraderm®; Estrasorb™; Estring®; EstroGel®; Evamist™; Femring®; Femtrace®; Gynodiol® [DSC]; Menostar®; Vagifem®; Vivelle-Dot®; Vivelle® [DSC]

Canadian Brand Names Climara®; Depo®-Estradiol; Estrace®; Estraderm®; Estradot®; Estring®; EstroGel®; Menostar®; Oesclim®; Sandoz-Estradiol Derm 100; Sandoz-Estradiol Derm 50; Sandoz-Estradiol Derm 75; Vagifem®

Therapeutic Category Estrogen Derivative; Estrogen Derivative, Vaginal

Generic Available Yes: Oral tablet, patch, valerate oil for injection

Use Treatment of hypoestrogenism (due to hypogonadism, castration, or primary ovarian failure), moderate to severe vasomotor symptoms of menopause, moderate to severe symptoms of vulvar and vaginal atrophy due to menopause; palliative treatment of breast cancer in select patients; palliative treatment of androgen-dependent prostate cancer; prevention of osteoporosis in postmenopausal women; FDA approved in adults. See Warnings and Additional Information

Pregnancy Risk Factor X

Pregnancy Considerations Estrogens are not indicated for use during pregnancy or immediately postpartum. Increased risk of fetal reproductive tract disorders and other birth defects have been observed with diethylstilbestrol (DES). In general, the use of estrogen and progestin as in combination hormonal contraceptives have not been associated with teratogenic effects when inadvertently taken early in pregnancy. These products are not intended to be used during pregnancy.

Lactation Enters breast milk/use caution

Breast-Feeding Considerations The AAP considers ethinyl estradiol, an estrogen derivative, to be "usually compatible" with breast-feeding. Estrogen has been shown to decrease the quantity and quality of human milk; use only if clearly needed; monitor the growth of the infant closely.

Contraindications Hypersensitivity to estradiol or any component (see Warnings); history of or current DVT or PE; recent (eg, within past year) or current arterial thromboembolic disease (eg, MI, stroke); undiagnosed vaginal bleeding; pregnancy; known, suspected, or history of breast cancer (except in select patients being treated for metastatic disease); estrogen-dependent neoplasia; liver disease or dysfunction

Warnings Estrogens have been reported to increase the risk of endometrial carcinoma **[U.S. Boxed Warning]**; adequate diagnostic measures, including endometrial sampling, if indicated, should be performed to rule out malignancy in all cases of undiagnosed abnormal vaginal bleeding; the addition of a progestin has been shown to decrease the risk of estrogen-induced endometrial hyperplasia, a condition thought to be a precursor to endometrial cancer. Do not use estrogens (with or without progestins) for the prevention of cardiovascular disease **[U.S. Boxed Warning]**; a significantly increased risk of MI, stroke, PE, DVT, and invasive breast cancer was reported in postmenopausal women receiving conjugated equine estrogens combined with medroxyprogesterone acetate (see Rossouw, 2002); use of conjugated estrogens alone significantly increased the risk of stroke in postmenopausal women, but did not affect the risk of coronary heart disease (see Women's Health Initiative Steering Committee, 2004); due to these risks, use estrogens (with or without progestins) at the lowest effective doses and for the shortest duration possible that is consistent with an individual's treatment goals and risks **[U.S. Boxed Warning]**; periodic risk:benefit assessments should be conducted; discontinue estrogens immediately if MI, stroke, PE, or DVT occur; in order to minimize the risk of thromboembolism in patients receiving estrogens, other risk factors for venous thromboembolism (eg, obesity, SLE, personal or family history of venous thromboembolism) and arterial vascular disease (eg, diabetes mellitus, hypertension, tobacco use, obesity, and hypercholesterolemia) should be appropriately managed.

Consider topical vaginal products when estrogen is used solely for the treatment of vulvar and vaginal atrophy; if used solely for the prevention of osteoporosis in postmenopausal women, estrogens should only be considered for those at significant risk of osteoporosis and for whom nonestrogen treatment options are not considered to be appropriate. Do not use estrogens during pregnancy.

Since estrogens may increase the risk of venous thromboembolism, discontinue therapy, if possible, at least 4-6 weeks before surgery that is associated with an increased risk of thromboembolism, or during times of prolonged immobilization. Estrogens may increase the risk of breast cancer, gallbladder disease, hypercalcemia, and retinal vascular thrombosis (discontinue estrogen therapy in patients with sudden partial or complete loss of vision, sudden onset of diplopia, proptosis, or migraine, or if eye exam reveals retinal vascular lesions or papilledema). The combined use of conjugated equine estrogens and medroxyprogesterone acetate was reported to significantly increase the risk of probable dementia in postmenopausal women **[U.S. Boxed Warning]**; it is currently not known if these findings apply to younger women or to patients receiving estrogen alone.

Absorption of topical emulsion is significantly increased by application of sunscreen (do not apply both products within close proximity of each other); estradiol may be absorbed by others upon physical contact with topical emulsion application site. Topical gel is alcohol based and is flammable; patients should avoid fire, flame, or smoking until the gel has dried (gel dries in 2-5 minutes after application); photosensitivity after gel application and effects of concurrent application of sunscreen with gel have not been evaluated; estradiol was **not** absorbed by others after physical contact with topical gel application site 1 hour after application.

Transdermal patch may contain conducting metal (eg, aluminum) which may cause a burn to the skin during an MRI scan; remove patch prior to MRI; reapply patch after scan is completed. Due to the potential for altered electrical conductivity, remove transdermal patch before cardioversion or defibrillation. Injection may contain benzyl alcohol and oral tablet may contain tartrazine, both of which may cause allergic reactions in susceptible individuals; large amounts of benzyl alcohol (≥99 mg/kg/day) have been associated with a potentially fatal toxicity ("gasping syndrome") in neonates; avoid use of estradiol products containing benzyl alcohol in neonates; in vitro and animal studies have shown that benzoate, a metabolite of benzyl alcohol, displaces bilirubin from protein binding sites

Precautions Use with caution in patients with asthma, epilepsy, migraines, diabetes, hypothyroidism, hypocalcemia, hypercalcemia, endometriosis, porphyria, SLE, hepatic hemangioma, history of cholestatic jaundice due to past estrogen use or pregnancy, cardiac, liver, or renal dysfunction. Estrogens may cause premature closure of the epiphyses in young individuals; may cause premature breast development in prepubertal girls or gynecomastia in boys; may include vaginal bleeding or vaginal cornification in girls; may increase risk of ovarian cancer; may increase blood pressure; may cause fluid retention; may greatly increase triglycerides and lead to pancreatitis and other problems in patients with familial defects of lipoprotein metabolism; Femring™ may not be suitable for women that have conditions which make the vagina more susceptible to vaginal ulceration or irritation, or make expulsion of the ring more likely (eg, vaginal stenosis, cervical prolapse, etc)

Adverse Reactions

Cardiovascular: Edema, hypertension, thromboembolic disorders

Central nervous system: Dementia, depression, dizziness, exacerbation of epilepsy, headache, irritability, migraine, mood disturbances, nervousness

Dermatologic: Chloasma, melasma, urticaria

Endocrine & metabolic: Breast enlargement, breast pain, breast tenderness, changes in libido, folate deficiency, hypercalcemia, hypertriglyceridemia, impaired glucose tolerance, weight gain or weight loss; risk of endometrial hyperplasia increased

Gastrointestinal: Abdominal cramps, abdominal pain, bloating, gall bladder disease, nausea, pancreatitis, vomiting

Genitourinary: Changes in menstrual flow, dysmenorrhea, ring adherence to vaginal wall (vaginal ring), toxic shock syndrome (vaginal ring), vaginal hemorrhage

Hepatic: Cholestatic jaundice, enlargement of hepatic hemangiomas

Local: Pain at injection site; topical may cause burning, irritation, pruritus, rash, redness

Neuromuscular & skeletal: Premature closure of epiphyses in young patients (large and repeated doses over an extended period of time); arthralgia, chorea, leg cramps

Miscellaneous: Anaphylactoid reaction, angioedema, bowel obstruction (vaginal ring)

Drug Interactions

Metabolism/Transport Effects Substrate of CYP1A2 (major), CYP2A6 (minor), CYP2B6 (minor), CYP2C9 (minor), CYP2C19 (minor), CYP2D6 (minor), CYP2E1 (minor), CYP3A4 (major), P-glycoprotein; **Inhibits** CYP1A2 (weak), 2C8 (weak); **Induces** CYP3A4 (weak)

Avoid Concomitant Use

Avoid concomitant use of Estradiol with any of the following: Anastrozole

Increased Effect/Toxicity

Estradiol may increase the levels/effects of: Corticosteroids (Systemic); Ropinirole; Tipranavir

The levels/effects of Estradiol may be increased by: Herbs (Estrogenic Properties); P-Glycoprotein Inhibitors

Decreased Effect

Estradiol may decrease the levels/effects of: Anastrozole; Saxagliptin; Somatropin; Thyroid Products; Ursodiol

The levels/effects of Estradiol may be decreased by: CYP1A2 Inducers (Strong); CYP3A4 Inducers (Strong); Deferasirox; Herbs (CYP3A4 Inducers); Peginterferon Alfa-2b; P-Glycoprotein Inducers; Tipranavir

Food Interactions Larger doses of vitamin C (eg, 1 g/day in adults) may increase the serum concentrations and adverse effects of estradiol; vitamin C supplements are not recommended, but this effect may be decreased if vitamin C supplement is given 2-3 hours after estrogen; dietary intake of folate and pyridoxine may need to be increased; grapefruit juice may possibly increase estrogen plasma concentrations and effects

Mechanism of Action Increases the synthesis of DNA, RNA, and various proteins in target tissues; reduces the release of gonadotropin-releasing hormone from the hypothalamus; reduces FSH and LH release from the pituitary

Pharmacokinetics (Adult data unless noted)

Absorption: Oral, topical well absorbed

Topical emulsion: Absorption is significantly increased by application of sunscreen (see Warnings)

Distribution: Widely distributes throughout the body; sex hormone target organs contain higher concentrations; distributes into breast milk

Protein binding: Primarily bound to sex hormone-binding globulin and albumin

Metabolism: Hepatic, via cytochrome P450 isoenzyme CYP3A4; estradiol is converted to estrone and estriol; estrone is also converted to estriol and is converted to estradiol (**Note:** A dynamic equilibrium of metabolic interconversions between estrogens exists in the circulation); estrogens also undergo sulfate and glucuronide conjugation and enterohepatic recirculation

Elimination: Excreted in the urine as estradiol, estrone, and estriol and glucuronide and sulfate conjugates

Usual Dosage Adolescents and Adults: **Note:** Use lowest effective dose for shortest duration possible that is consistent with an individual's treatment goals and risks; all dosage needs to be adjusted based upon the patient's response

Female hypogonadism:

I.M.:

Cypionate: 1.5-2 mg given once each month

Valerate: 10-20 mg given once each month

Oral: 0.5-2 mg/day in a cyclic regimen (3 weeks on drug, 1 week off)

Transdermal:

Once-weekly patch (Climara®): Initial: 0.025 mg/day patch applied once weekly (titrate dosage to response)

Twice-weekly patch: Alora®, Esclim®, Estraderm®: Initial: 0.05 mg patch; Vivelle®, Vivelle Dot®: Initial: 0.0375 mg patch; titrate dosage to response; apply patch twice weekly in a cyclic regimen (3 weeks on drug, 1 week off) in patients with intact uterus and continuously in patients without a uterus

Vaginal and vulval atrophy: Intravaginal: Initial: 200-400 mcg of estradiol once daily for 1-2 weeks; taper dose gradually to 100-200 mcg of estradiol once daily for 1-2 weeks; maintenance, cyclic regimen (after vaginal mucosa restored): 100 mcg of estradiol 1-3 times/week for 3 weeks, then no drug for the 4th week per cycle

Vaginal ring:

Postmenopausal vaginal atrophy, urogenital symptoms: Estring®: 2 mg intravaginally; following insertion, ring should remain in place for 90 days

Moderate to severe vasomotor symptoms associated with menopause; vulvar/vaginal atrophy: Femring™: 0.05 mg intravaginally; following insertion, ring should remain in place for 3 months; dose may be increased to 0.1 mg if needed

Topical emulsion: Moderate to severe vasomotor symptoms associated with menopause: 3.84 g (contents of 2 pouches) applied once daily in the morning

Topical gel: Moderate to severe vasomotor symptoms associated with menopause or vulvar and vaginal atrophy: 1.25 g applied once daily at the same time each day

Administration

Oral: Administer with food or after a meal to reduce GI upset

Parenteral: Injection for I.M. use only

Transdermal: Apply to clean dry area; do not apply to breasts; do not apply to waistline (may loosen patch); rotate application sites

Vaginal ring: Exact positioning is not critical for efficacy, however, patient should not feel ring or discomfort once inserted. In case of discomfort, ring should be gently pushed further into vagina. If ring is expelled prior to 90 days, it may be rinsed off and reinserted. Ensure proper vaginal placement of the ring to avoid inadvertent urinary bladder insertion. If vaginal infection develops, Estring® should be removed; reinsert only after infection has been appropriately treated. Femring® may remain in place during local treatment of a vaginal infection.

Topical emulsion: Apply to clean dry skin on both legs while sitting. Apply contents of first pouch to top of left thigh, massage into skin of left thigh and calf until thoroughly absorbed (~3 minutes). Apply excess from hands to buttocks. Apply contents of second pouch to right thigh and calf in the same manner. Wash hands with soap and water. Allow skin to dry before covering legs with clothes. Do not apply to other areas of the body. Do not apply to red or irritated skin. Do not apply sunscreen at the same time.

Topical gel: Apply to clean, dry, unbroken skin at the same time each day. Apply gel to the arm, from the wrist to shoulder. Spread gel as thinly as possible over one arm. Allow to dry for 5 minutes prior to dressing. Wash hands with soap and water. Avoid fire, flame, or smoking until gel is dry (gel is flammable). Do not apply gel to breasts or red or irritated skin. Prior to the first use, pump must be primed by fully depressing pump twice (and discarding the gel); **Note:** Discard unused gel by rinsing down sink; avoid exposure to others and pets.

Monitoring Parameters Blood pressure, weight, serum calcium, glucose, liver enzymes; bone maturation and epiphyseal effects in young patients in whom bone growth is not complete; breast exam, mammogram, Papanicolaou smear, signs for endometrial cancer in female patients with a uterus; bone density measurement if used for prevention of osteoporosis

Test Interactions Thyroid function tests: Estrogens may increase thyroid binding globulin and circulating total thyroid hormone (when measured by T_4 RIA, T_4 by column, or by PBI); decreases free T_3 resin uptake; concentration of free T_4 is not altered; metyrapone test: Response may be reduced

Patient Information Limit alcohol, caffeine, and grapefruit juice; notify physician if sudden severe headache or vomiting, disturbance of vision or speech, numbness or weakness of extremity, sharp or crushing chest pain, calf pain, shortness of breath, severe abdominal pain or mass, mental depression, or unusual bleeding occurs

Additional Information See package insert for doses related to postmenopausal symptoms, prevention of osteoporosis in postmenopausal women, and palliative treatment of breast cancer or androgen-dependent prostate cancer in adults. Femring™ can remain in place during local treatment of vaginal infections.

Dosage Forms Excipient information presented when available (limited, particularly for generics); consult specific product labeling. [DSC] = Discontinued product

Cream, vaginal:
Estrace®: 0.1 mg/g (42.5 g)

Emulsion, topical, as hemihydrate:
Estrasorb™: 2.5 mg/g (56s) [each pouch contains 4.35 mg estradiol hemihydrate; contents of two pouches delivers estradiol 0.05 mg/day]

Gel, topical:
Divigel®: 0.1% (0.25 g) [delivers estradiol 0.25 mg/packet]; (0.5 g) [delivers 0.5 mg estradiol/packet]; (1 g) [delivers estradiol 1 mg/packet]
Elestrin™: 0.06% (144 g) [delivers estradiol 0.52 mg/0.87 g; 100 actuations]
EstroGel®: 0.06% (50 g) [delivers estradiol 0.75 mg/1.25 g; 32 actuations; contains ethanol]

Injection, oil, as cypionate:
Depo®-Estradiol: 5 mg/mL (5 mL) [contains chlorobutanol, cottonseed oil]

Injection, oil, as valerate: 10 mg/mL (5 mL); 20 mg/mL (5 mL); 40 mg/mL (5 mL)
Delestrogen®:
10 mg/mL (5 mL) [contains chlorobutanol, sesame oil]
20 mg/mL (5 mL) [contains benzyl alcohol, castor oil]
40 mg/mL (5 mL) [contains benzyl alcohol, castor oil]

Patch, transdermal: 0.025 mg/24 hours (4s) [once-weekly patch]; 0.0375 mg/24 hours (4s) [once-weekly patch]; 0.05 mg/24 hours (4s) [once-weekly patch]; 0.06 mg/24 hours (4s) [once-weekly patch]; 0.075 mg/24 hours [once-weekly patch]; 0.1 mg/24 hours (4s) [once-weekly patch]

Alora® [twice-weekly patch]:
0.025 mg/24 hours (8s) [9 cm^2, total estradiol 0.77 mg]
0.05 mg/24 hours (8s, 24s [DSC]) [18 cm^2, total estradiol 1.5 mg]
0.075 mg/24 hours (8s) [27 cm^2, total estradiol 2.3 mg]
0.1 mg/24 hours (8s) [36 cm^2, total estradiol 3.1 mg]

Climara® [once-weekly patch]:
0.025 mg/24 hours (4s) [6.5 cm^2, total estradiol 2.04 mg]
0.0375 mg/24 hours (4s) [9.375 cm^2, total estradiol 2.85 mg]
0.05 mg/24 hours (4s) [12.5 cm^2, total estradiol 3.8 mg]
0.06 mg/24 hours (4s) [15 cm^2, total estradiol 4.55 mg]
0.075 mg/24 hours (4s) [18.75 cm^2, total estradiol 5.7 mg]
0.1 mg/24 hours (4s) [25 cm^2, total estradiol 7.6 mg]

Estraderm® [twice-weekly patch]:
0.05 mg/24 hours (8s) [10 cm^2, total estradiol 4 mg]
0.1 mg/24 hours (8s) [20 cm^2, total estradiol 8 mg]

Menostar® [once-weekly patch]: 0.014 mg/24 hours (4s) [3.25 cm^2, total estradiol 1 mg]

Vivelle® [twice-weekly patch]:
0.05 mg/24 hours (8s) [14.5 cm^2, total estradiol 4.33 mg] [DSC]
0.1 mg/24 hours (8s) [29 cm^2, total estradiol 8.66 mg] [DSC]

Vivelle-Dot® [twice-weekly patch]:
0.025 mg/day (24s) [2.5 cm^2, total estradiol 0.39 mg]
0.0375 mg/day (24s) [3.75 cm^2, total estradiol 0.585 mg]
0.05 mg/day (24s) [5 cm^2, total estradiol 0.78 mg]
0.075 mg/day (24s) [7.5 cm^2, total estradiol 1.17 mg]
0.1 mg/day (24s) [10 cm^2, total estradiol 1.56 mg]

Ring, vaginal, as base:
Estring®: 2 mg (1s) [total estradiol 2 mg; releases 7.5 mcg/day over 90 days]

Ring, vaginal, as acetate:
Femring®: 0.05 mg/day (1s) [total estradiol 12.4 mg; releases 0.05 mg/day over 3 months]; 0.1 mg/day (1s) [total estradiol 24.8 mg; releases 0.1 mg/day over 3 months]

Solution, topical [spray]:
Evamist™: 1.53 mg/spray (8.1 mL) [contains 56 sprays after priming; contains ethanol]

Tablet, oral, as acetate:
Femtrace®: 0.45 mg, 0.9 mg, 1.8 mg

Tablet, oral, micronized: 0.5 mg, 1 mg, 2 mg
Estrace®: 0.5 mg, 1 mg, 2 mg [2 mg tablets contain tartrazine]
Gynodiol®: 0.5 mg [DSC], 1 mg [DSC], 1.5 mg [DSC], 2 mg [DSC]

Tablet, vaginal, as base:
Vagifem®: 10 mcg, 25 mcg

References

Rossouw JE, Anderson GL, Prentice RL, et al, "Risks and Benefits of Estrogen Plus Progestin in Healthy Postmenopausal Women: Principal Results From the Women's Health Initiative Randomized Controlled Trial," JAMA, 2002, 288(3):321-33.

Women's Health Initiative Steering Committee, "Effects of Conjugated Equine Estrogen in Postmenopausal Women With Hysterectomy: The Women's Health Initiative Randomized Controlled Trial," JAMA, 2004, 291(14):1701-12.

◆ **Estradiol Acetate** see Estradiol on page 536
◆ **Estradiol Cypionate** see Estradiol on page 536
◆ **Estradiol Hemihydrate** see Estradiol on page 536
◆ **Estradiol Transdermal** see Estradiol on page 536
◆ **Estradiol Valerate** see Estradiol on page 536
◆ **Estradot® (Can)** see Estradiol on page 536
◆ **Estrasorb™** see Estradiol on page 536
◆ **Estring®** see Estradiol on page 536
◆ **EstroGel®** see Estradiol on page 536
◆ **Estrogenic Substances, Conjugated** see Estrogens (Conjugated/Equine) on page 539

Estrogens (Conjugated/Equine)
(ES troe jenz KON joo gate ed/E kwine)

Medication Safety Issues
Sound-alike/look-alike issues:
Premarin® may be confused with Primaxin®, Provera®, Remeron®

Beers Criteria medication: This drug may be inappropriate for use in geriatric patients (low severity risk).

U.S. Brand Names Premarin®

Canadian Brand Names C.E.S.®; Premarin®

Therapeutic Category Estrogen Derivative; Estrogen Derivative, Vaginal

Generic Available No

Use Treatment of dysfunctional uterine bleeding, hypoestrogenism (due to hypogonadism, castration, or primary ovarian failure), moderate to severe vasomotor symptoms of menopause; moderate to severe symptoms of vulvar and vaginal atrophy due to menopause; palliative treatment of breast cancer in select patients; palliative treatment of androgen-dependent prostate cancer; prevention of osteoporosis in postmenopausal women; see Warnings and Additional Information; **Note:** Intravenous product is indicated for short-term use only

Pregnancy Considerations Estrogens are not indicated for use during pregnancy or immediately postpartum. In general, the use of estrogen and progestin as in combination hormonal contraceptives have not been associated with teratogenic effects when inadvertently taken early in pregnancy. These products are contraindicated for use during pregnancy. Use of the vaginal cream may weaken latex found in condoms, diaphragms or cervical caps.

Lactation Enters breast milk/use caution

Breast-Feeding Considerations Estrogens have been detected in breast milk following maternal use. The AAP considers ethinyl estradiol, an estrogen derivative, to be "usually compatible" with breast-feeding. Estrogen has been shown to decrease the quantity and quality of human milk. Use only if clearly needed. Monitor the growth of the infant closely.

Contraindications Hypersensitivity to estrogens or any component (see Warnings); history of or current DVT or PE; recent (eg, within past year) or current arterial thromboembolic disease (eg, MI, stroke); undiagnosed vaginal bleeding; pregnancy; known, suspected, or history of breast cancer (except in select patients being treated for metastatic disease); estrogen-dependent neoplasia; liver disease or dysfunction

Warnings Estrogens have been reported to increase the risk of endometrial carcinoma **[U.S. Boxed Warning]**; adequate diagnostic measures, including endometrial sampling, if indicated, should be performed to rule out malignancy in all cases of undiagnosed abnormal vaginal bleeding; the addition of a progestin has been shown to decrease the risk of estrogen-induced endometrial hyperplasia, a condition thought to be a precursor to endometrial cancer. Do not use estrogens (with or without progestins) for the prevention of cardiovascular disease **[U.S. Boxed Warning]**; a significantly increased risk of MI, stroke, PE, DVT, and invasive breast cancer was reported in postmenopausal women receiving conjugated equine estrogens combined with medroxyprogesterone acetate (see Rossouw, 2002); use of conjugated estrogens alone significantly increased the risk of stroke in postmenopausal women, but did not affect the risk of coronary heart disease (see Women's Health Initiative Steering Committee, 2004); due to these risks, use estrogens (with or without progestins) at the lowest effective dose and for the shortest duration possible that is consistent with an individual's treatment goals and risks; periodic risk:benefit assessments should be conducted; discontinue estrogens immediately if MI, stroke, PE, or DVT occur; in order to minimize the risk of thromboembolism in patients receiving estrogens, other risk factors for venous thromboembolism (eg, obesity, SLE, personal or family history of venous thromboembolism) and arterial vascular disease (eg, diabetes mellitus, hypertension, tobacco use, obesity, and hypercholesterolemia) should be appropriately managed.

Consider topical vaginal products when estrogen is used solely for the treatment of vulvar and vaginal atrophy; if used solely for the prevention of osteoporosis in postmenopausal women, estrogens should only be considered for those at significant risk of osteoporosis and for whom nonestrogen treatment options are not considered to be appropriate. Do not use estrogens during pregnancy.

Since estrogens may increase the risk of venous thromboembolism, discontinue therapy, if possible, at least 4-6 weeks before surgery that is associated with an increased risk of thromboembolism, or during times of prolonged immobilization. Estrogens may increase the risk of breast cancer, gallbladder disease, hypercalcemia, and retinal vascular thrombosis (discontinue estrogen therapy in patients with sudden partial or complete loss of vision, sudden onset of diplopia, proptosis, or migraine, or if eye exam reveals retinal vascular lesions or papilledema). The combined use of conjugated equine estrogens and medroxyprogesterone acetate was reported to significantly increase the risk of probable dementia in postmenopausal women; it is currently not known if these findings apply to younger women or to patients receiving estrogen alone.

Systemic absorption may occur with intravaginal or topical use. Diluent for injection contains benzyl alcohol which may cause allergic reactions in susceptible individuals; large amounts of benzyl alcohol (≥99 mg/kg/day) have been associated with a potentially fatal toxicity ("gasping syndrome") in neonates; avoid use of estrogen products containing benzyl alcohol in neonates; *in vitro* and animal studies have shown that benzoate, a metabolite of benzyl alcohol, displaces bilirubin from protein binding sites

Precautions Use with caution in patients with asthma, epilepsy, migraines, diabetes, hypothyroidism, hypocalcemia, hypercalcemia, endometriosis, porphyria, SLE, hepatic hemangioma, history of cholestatic jaundice due to past estrogen use or pregnancy, cardiac, liver, or renal dysfunction. Estrogens may cause premature closure of the epiphyses in young individuals; may cause premature breast development in prepubertal girls or gynecomastia in boys; may induce vaginal bleeding or vaginal cornification in girls; may increase risk of ovarian cancer. May increase blood pressure; may cause fluid retention; may greatly increase triglycerides and lead to pancreatitis and other problems in patients with familial defects of lipoprotein metabolism. Estrogen vaginal creams may contribute to the failure of barrier contraceptives by weakening condoms, diaphragms, or cervical caps made of latex or rubber.

Adverse Reactions

Cardiovascular: Hypertension, edema, thromboembolic disorder

Central nervous system: Depression, headache, dizziness, nervousness, migraine, irritability, mood disturbances, exacerbation of epilepsy, dementia

Dermatologic: Chloasma, melasma, urticaria

Endocrine & metabolic: Breast enlargement, breast tenderness, breast pain, changes in libido, impaired glucose tolerance, hypercalcemia, hypertriglyceridemia, folate deficiency, weight gain or weight loss; risk of endometrial hyperplasia increased

Gastrointestinal: Nausea, vomiting, bloating, abdominal cramps, abdominal pain, pancreatitis, gall bladder disease

Genitourinary: Changes in menstrual flow, vaginal hemorrhage, dysmenorrhea

Hepatic: Cholestatic jaundice, enlargement of hepatic hemangiomas

Local: Pain at injection site

Neuromuscular & skeletal: Premature closure of epiphyses in young patients; chorea, leg cramps, arthralgia

Miscellaneous: Angioedema, anaphylactoid reaction

Drug Interactions

Metabolism/Transport Effects

Based on estradiol and estrone: **Substrate** of CYP1A2 (major), 2A6 (minor), 2B6 (minor), 2C9 (minor), 2C19 (minor), 2D6 (minor), 2E1 (minor), 3A4 (major); Inhibits CYP1A2 (weak), 2C8 (weak); Induces CYP3A4 (weak)

Avoid Concomitant Use

Avoid concomitant use of Estrogens (Conjugated/ Equine) with any of the following: Anastrozole

Increased Effect/Toxicity

Estrogens (Conjugated/Equine) may increase the levels/ effects of: Corticosteroids (Systemic); Ropinirole; Tipranavir

The levels/effects of Estrogens (Conjugated/Equine) may be increased by: Herbs (Estrogenic Properties)

Decreased Effect

Estrogens (Conjugated/Equine) may decrease the levels/ effects of: Anastrozole; Saxagliptin; Somatropin; Thyroid Products; Ursodiol

The levels/effects of Estrogens (Conjugated/Equine) may be decreased by: CYP1A2 Inducers (Strong); CYP3A4 Inducers (Strong); Deferasirox; Herbs (CYP3A4 Inducers); Peginterferon Alfa-2b; Tipranavir

Food Interactions Larger doses of vitamin C (eg, 1 g/day in adults) may increase the serum concentrations and adverse effects of estrogens; vitamin C supplements are not recommended, but this effect may be decreased if vitamin C supplement is given 2-3 hours after estrogen; dietary intake of folate and pyridoxine may need to be increased; grapefruit juice may possibly increase estrogen plasma concentrations and effects

Stability Injection: Store unreconstituted vials in the refrigerator at 2°C to 8°C (36°F to 46°F); if reconstituted solution is not used within a few hours, store under refrigeration; reconstituted solution is stable for 60 days when stored under refrigeration; compatible with NS, dextrose, and invert sugar solutions; **not** compatible with ascorbic acid, protein hydrolysate, or acidic pH

Mechanism of Action Increases the synthesis of DNA, RNA, and various proteins in target tissues; reduces the release of gonadotropin-releasing hormone from the hypothalamus; reduces FSH and LH release from the pituitary

Pharmacokinetics (Adult data unless noted)

Absorption: Oral, transmucosal, transdermal: Well absorbed

Distribution: Widely distributes throughout the body; sex hormone target organs contain higher concentrations; distributes into breast milk

Protein binding: Primarily bound to sex hormone-binding globulin and albumin

Metabolism: Hepatic, via cytochrome P450 isoenzyme CYP3A4; estradiol is converted to estrone and estriol; estrone is also converted to estriol and is converted to estradiol (**Note:** A dynamic equilibrium of metabolic interconversions between estrogens exists in the circulation); estrogens also undergo hepatic sulfate and glucuronide conjugation and enterohepatic recirculation

Elimination: Excreted in the urine as estradiol, estrone, estriol (major urinary metabolite), and glucuronide and sulfate conjugates

Usual Dosage Adolescents and Adults: **Note:** Use lowest effective dose for the shortest duration possible that is consistent with an individual's treatment goals and risks:

Female castration or primary ovarian failure: Oral: Cyclic regimen: 1.25 mg/day for 3 weeks, then no drug for the 4th week per cycle; repeat; titrate dose to response; use lowest effective dose

Female hypogonadism: Oral:

Manufacturer's recommendation: Cyclic regimen: 0.3-0.625 mg/day for 3 weeks, then no drug for the 4th week per cycle; titrate dose to response; use lowest effective dose

Alternative dosing: 2.5-7.5 mg/day in divided doses for 20 days, off 10 days and repeat until menses occur

Dysfunctional uterine bleeding:

Stable hematocrit: Oral: 1.25 mg twice daily for 21 days; if bleeding persists after 48 hours, increase to 2.5 mg twice daily; if bleeding persists after 48 more hours, increase to 2.5 mg 4 times/day; some recommend starting at 2.5 mg 4 times/day (**Note:** Medroxyprogesterone acetate 10 mg/day is also given on days 17-21; see Neistein, 1991)

Alternatively: Oral: 2.5-5 mg/day for 7-10 days; then decrease to 1.25 mg/day for 2 weeks

Unstable hematocrit: Oral, I.V.: 5 mg 2-4 times/day; if bleeding is profuse, 20-40 mg every 4 hours up to 24 hours may be used; **Note:** A progestational-weighted contraception pill should also be given (eg, Ovral® 2 tablets stat and 1 tablet 4 times/day or medroxyprogesterone acetate 5-10 mg 4 times/day; see Neistein, 1991)

Alternatively: I.M., I.V.: 25 mg every 6-12 hours until bleeding stops

Vaginal and vulval atrophy: Intravaginal or topical (vaginal cream): Cyclic regimen: 0.5-2 g daily (0.3125-1.25 mg/day of conjugated estrogens) for 3 weeks, then no drug for the 4th week per cycle; repeat as clinically needed

Administration

Oral: Administer with food or after eating to reduce GI upset; administration of dose at bedtime may decrease adverse effects

Intravaginal: Use marked stopping points on applicator to measure prescribed dose; to administer, lay down on back and draw knees up; gently insert applicator into vagina and press plunger downward to deliver medication; wash plunger and barrel with mild soap and water after use; do not boil or use hot water

Parenteral: Add sterile diluent provided by manufacturer and shake gently; I.V.: Administer slow I.V. to avoid vascular flushing; I.M.: may be administered I.M. for dysfunctional uterine bleeding, but I.V. use is preferred (more rapid response)

Monitoring Parameters Blood pressure, weight, serum calcium, glucose, liver enzymes; dysfunctional uterine bleeding: Hematocrit, hemoglobin, PT; bone maturation and epiphyseal effects in young patients in whom bone growth is not complete; breast exam, mammogram, Papanicolaou smear, signs for endometrial cancer in female patients with a uterus; bone density measurement if used for prevention of osteoporosis

Test Interactions Thyroid function tests: Estrogens may increase thyroid binding globulin and circulating total thyroid hormone (when measured by T_4 RIA, T_4 by column, or by PBI); decreases free T_3 resin uptake; concentration of free T_4 is not altered; metyrapone test: Response may be reduced

Patient Information Limit caffeine and grapefruit juice; notify physician if sudden severe headache, vomiting, disturbance of vision or speech, numbness or weakness of extremity, sharp or crushing chest pain, calf pain, shortness of breath, severe abdominal pain or mass, mental depression, or unusual bleeding occurs

Additional Information See package insert for doses related to postmenopausal symptoms, prevention of osteoporosis in postmenopausal women, and palliative treatment of breast cancer or androgen-dependent prostate cancer in adults.

Dosage Forms Excipient information presented when available (limited, particularly for generics); consult specific product labeling.

Cream, vaginal:
Premarin®: 0.625 mg/g (42.5 g)
Injection, powder for reconstitution:
Premarin®: 25 mg [contains benzyl alcohol (in diluent), lactose 200 mg]
Tablet:
Premarin®: 0.3 mg, 0.45 mg, 0.625 mg, 0.9 mg, 1.25 mg

References

Minjarez DA and Bradshaw KD, "Abnormal Uterine Bleeding in Adolescents," *Obstet Gynecol Clin North Am*, 2000, 27(1):63-78.
Mitan LA and Slap GB, "Adolescent Menstrual Disorders. Update," *Med Clin North Am*, 2000, 84(4):851-68.
Neistein LS, *Adolescent Health Care - A Practical Guide*, 2nd ed, Baltimore: Urban & Schwarzenberg, 1991, 661-6.
Rossouw JE, Anderson GL, Prentice RL, et al, "Risks and Benefits of Estrogen Plus Progestin in Healthy Postmenopausal Women: Principal Results From the Women's Health Initiative Randomized Controlled Trial," *JAMA*, 2002, 288(3):321-33.
Women's Health Initiative Steering Committee, "Effects of Conjugated Equine Estrogen in Postmenopausal Women With Hysterectomy: The Women's Health Initiative Randomized Controlled Trial," *JAMA*, 2004, 291(14):1701-12.

Etanercept (et a NER cept)

Medication Safety Issues
Sound-alike/look-alike issues:
Enbrel® may be confused with Levbid®
U.S. Brand Names Enbrel®
Canadian Brand Names Enbrel®
Therapeutic Category Antirheumatic, Disease Modifying
Generic Available No
Use Treatment of moderately- to severely-active polyarticular juvenile idiopathic arthritis (FDA approved in ages ≥2 years). Treatment of signs and symptoms of moderately- to severely-active rheumatoid arthritis; psoriatic arthritis; active ankylosing spondylitis; treatment of chronic (moderate-to-severe) plaque psoriasis in patients who are candidates for systemic therapy or phototherapy (FDA approved in ages ≥18 years)
Medication Guide An FDA-approved patient medication guide, which is available with the product information and at http://www.fda.gov/downloads/Drugs/DrugSafety/ucm088590.pdf, must be dispensed with this medication for each new outpatient prescription and refill.
Pregnancy Risk Factor B
Pregnancy Considerations Developmental toxicity studies performed in animals have revealed no evidence of harm to the fetus. There are no studies in pregnant women; this drug should be used during pregnancy only if clearly needed. A pregnancy registry has been established to monitor outcomes of women exposed to etanercept during pregnancy (877-311-8972).
Lactation Excretion in breast milk unknown/not recommended
Breast-Feeding Considerations It is not known whether etanercept is excreted in human milk. Because many drugs and immunoglobulins are excreted in human milk and the potential for serious adverse reactions exists, a decision should be made whether to discontinue nursing or to discontinue the drug, taking into account the importance of the drug to the mother.
Contraindications Hypersensitivity to etanercept or any component (ie, mannitol, sucrose, tromethamine, and benzyl alcohol) (see Warnings); patients with sepsis
Warnings Serious and potentially fatal infections have been reported with use **[U.S. Boxed Warning]**. Patients were frequently taking concomitant immunosuppressants or corticosteroids. Discontinue administration if patient develops a serious infection or sepsis. Caution should be exercised when considering the use in patients with chronic infection, history of recurrent infection, or predisposition to infection (such as poorly-controlled diabetes). Do not give to patients with an active or localized infection. Closely monitor patients for signs and symptoms of infection while undergoing and after treatment. Tuberculosis (disseminated or extrapulmonary) has been reported in patients receiving etanercept **[U.S. Boxed Warning]**; both reactivation of latent infection and new infections have been reported. Patients should be evaluated for latent tuberculosis with a tuberculin skin test

prior to starting and periodically during therapy. Treatment of latent tuberculosis should be initiated before etanercept is used. Some patients who tested negative prior to therapy have developed active infection; monitor for signs and symptoms of tuberculosis in all patients. Rare reactivation of hepatitis B has occurred in chronic carriers of the virus; evaluate prior to etanercept initiation and during treatment in patients at risk for hepatitis B infection. Due to higher incidence of serious infections, should not be used in combination with anakinra unless no satisfactory alternatives exist, and then only with extreme caution.

Rare cases of CNS demyelinating disorders, such as multiple sclerosis, transverse myelitis, optic neuritis, and seizure disorders have been reported in patients undergoing etanercept therapy; cases may present with mental status changes and some may be associated with permanent disability.

A threefold higher incidence of lymphoma has been observed in patients receiving etanercept compared to that expected in the general population. Malignancies other than lymphoma have also been observed. Long-term carcinogenic potential or effect on fertility are unknown. Use is not recommended in patients with Wegener's granulomatosis receiving immunosuppressive therapy due to higher incidence of noncutaneous solid malignancies. Positive antinuclear antibody titers have been detected in patients (with negative baselines). Rare cases of autoimmune disorders, including lupus-like syndrome or autoimmune hepatitis, have been reported; monitor and discontinue if symptoms develop.

Diluent for etanercept injection contains benzyl alcohol which may cause allergic reactions in susceptible individuals; large amounts of benzyl alcohol (≥99 mg/kg/day) have been associated with a potentially fatal toxicity ("gasping syndrome") in neonates; avoid use of etanercept products containing benzyl alcohol in neonates; in vitro and animal studies have shown that benzoate, a metabolite of benzyl alcohol, displaces bilirubin from protein binding sites; patients with latex allergy should not handle the needle cap on the prefilled syringe and on the SureClick autoinjector since it contains latex.

Precautions Use with caution in patients with a history of hematologic abnormalities, heart failure, or in patients with a history of recurrent infections or illnesses such as poorly controlled diabetes which predisposes the patient to infection; discontinue etanercept in a child who develops varicella infection or who has a significant exposure to varicella virus and consider prophylactic treatment with varicella-zoster immune globulin.

Adverse Reactions

Cardiovascular: CHF, flushing, MI, peripheral edema, hypertension, chest pain

Central nervous system: Headache (19%), depression, personality disorder, dizziness, fever, mental status change, seizures, multiple sclerosis, myelitis, cerebral ischemia

Dermatologic: Rash, angioedema, cutaneous vasculitis, urticaria, pruritus, erythema multiforme, Stevens-Johnson syndrome, toxic epidermal necrolysis

Gastrointestinal: Nausea (9%), abdominal pain (17%), vomiting (13%), pancreatitis, anorexia, diarrhea, esophagitis/gastritis, GI bleeding

Hematologic: Pancytopenia, aplastic anemia, leukopenia, neutropenia, thrombocytopenia, coagulopathy

Hepatic: Autoimmune hepatitis

Local: Injection site reactions (erythema, discomfort, itching, swelling, bruising)

Neuromuscular & skeletal: Joint pain, paresthesia, polymyositis

Ocular: Optic neuritis

Respiratory: Respiratory tract infection, rhinitis, dyspnea, cough, interstitial lung disease

Miscellaneous: Allergic reaction (hives, difficulty breathing), positive antinuclear antibodies, lupus-like syndrome, positive antidouble-stranded DNA antibodies, sepsis, infections (viral, bacterial, fungal, and protozoal), malignancies (including lymphomas)

Drug Interactions

Avoid Concomitant Use

Avoid concomitant use of Etanercept with any of the following: Abatacept; Anakinra; BCG; Canakinumab; Certolizumab Pegol; Cyclophosphamide; Natalizumab; Pimecrolimus; Rilonacept; Tacrolimus (Topical); Vaccines (Live)

Increased Effect/Toxicity

Etanercept may increase the levels/effects of: Abatacept; Anakinra; Canakinumab; Certolizumab Pegol; Cyclophosphamide; Leflunomide; Natalizumab; Rilonacept; Vaccines (Live)

The levels/effects of Etanercept may be increased by: Denosumab; Pimecrolimus; Tacrolimus (Topical); Trastuzumab

Decreased Effect

Etanercept may decrease the levels/effects of: BCG; Sipuleucel-T; Vaccines (Inactivated); Vaccines (Live)

The levels/effects of Etanercept may be decreased by: Echinacea

Stability Store vial, single-use prefilled syringe, and prefilled SureClick autoinjector in the refrigerator 2°C to 8°C (36°F to 46°F); do not freeze; protect from light; reconstituted solution prepared with bacteriostatic water for injection is stable for 14 days if refrigerated; do not shake or agitate vigorously; do not use if discolored or cloudy or if particulate matter is present; do not filter reconstituted solution; do not add or mix with other medications

Mechanism of Action Binds to tumor necrosis factor (TNF) and blocks its interaction with cell surface TNF receptors rendering TNF biologically inactive; modulates biological responses that are induced or regulated by TNF

Pharmacodynamics

Onset of action: RA: 1-2 weeks

Maximum effect: Full effect is usually seen within 3 months

Pharmacokinetics (Adult data unless noted)

Absorption: Absorbed slowly after SubQ injection

Distribution: V_d: 1.78-3.39 L/m^2

Bioavailability: SubQ: 60%

Half-life: Adults: 102 ± 30 hours

Time to peak serum concentration: SubQ: 72 hours (range: 48-96 hours)

Elimination: Clearance:

Children 4-17 years: 46 mL/hour/m^2

Adults: 52 mL/hour/m^2

Usual Dosage SubQ:

Children 2-17 years: Juvenile idiopathic arthritis:

Twice-weekly dosing: 0.4 mg/kg/dose twice weekly given 72-96 hours apart; maximum dose: 25 mg

Alternative once-weekly dosing: 0.8 mg/kg/dose once weekly; maximum dose: 50 mg

Adults:

Rheumatoid arthritis, psoriatic arthritis, ankylosing spondylitis:

Once-weekly dosing: 50 mg once weekly

Twice weekly dosing: 25 mg given twice weekly (individual doses should be separated by 72-96 hours); maximum amount administered at a single injection site: 25 mg

Plaque psoriasis: Initial: 50 mg twice weekly (administered 3-4 days apart) for 3 months; **Note:** Initial doses of 25 mg or 50 mg per week were also shown to be efficacious; maintenance dose: 50 mg once weekly

Administration Parenteral: SubQ:

Multiple-use vial: To avoid foaming, add 1 mL of bacteriostatic water for injection slowly to 25 mg vial, resulting in 25 mg/mL solution.

Single-use prefilled syringe or prefilled SureClick auto-injector: Allow injection to reach room temperature (do not remove needle cover or needle shield during this period). Administer by SubQ injection into thigh, abdomen, or upper arm; injection sites should be rotated with subsequent doses given at least 1 inch from an old site; do not inject into areas where the skin is tender, bruised, red, or hard. Do not administer >25 mg at a single injection site if the multiple-use vial is used to prepare the dose.

Monitoring Parameters Assess for joint swelling, pain, and tenderness; ESR or C-reactive protein level; CBC with differential and platelet count; tuberculin skin test; signs and symptoms of infection; screen for hepatitis B in high risk patients

Patient Information Read the Medication Guide that you receive with this prescription and ask questions prior to therapy initiation. Notify physician if persistent fever, bruising, bleeding, or pallor occurs.

Dosage Forms Excipient information presented when available (limited, particularly for generics); consult specific product labeling.

Injection, powder for reconstitution:

Enbrel®: 25 mg [contains sucrose 10 mg; diluent contains benzyl alcohol]

Injection, solution [preservative free]:

Enbrel®: 50 mg/mL (0.51 mL, 0.98 mL) [contains sucrose 1%; natural rubber/natural latex in packaging]

References

Ilowite NT, "Current Treatment of Juvenile Rheumatoid Arthritis," *Pediatrics*, 2002, 109(1):109-15.

Lovell DJ, Reiff A, Jones OY, et al, "Long-Term Safety and Efficacy of Etanercept in Children With Polyarticular-Course Juvenile Rheumatoid Arthritis," *Arthritis Rheum*, 2006, 54(6):1087-04.

Moreland LW, Baumgartner SW, Schiff MH, et al, "Treatment of Rheumatoid Arthritis With a Recombinant Human Tumor Necrosis Factor Receptor (p75)-Fc Fusion Protein," *N Engl J Med*, 1997, 337 (3):141-7.

◆ **Ethacrynate Sodium** *see* Ethacrynic Acid *on page 543*

Ethacrynic Acid (eth a KRIN ik AS id)

Medication Safety Issues

Sound-alike/look-alike issues:

Edecrin® may be confused with Eulexin®, Ecotrin®

Beers Criteria medication: This drug may be inappropriate for use in geriatric patients (low severity risk).

Related Information

Antihypertensive Agents by Class *on page 1481*

U.S. Brand Names Edecrin®; Sodium Edecrin®

Canadian Brand Names Edecrin®

Therapeutic Category Antihypertensive Agent; Diuretic, Loop

Generic Available No

Use Management of edema secondary to CHF, hepatic or renal disease; hypertension

Pregnancy Risk Factor B

Pregnancy Considerations No data available. Generally, use of diuretics during pregnancy is avoided due to risk of decreased placental perfusion.

Lactation Contraindicated

Contraindications Hypersensitivity to ethacrynic acid or any component; hypotension, hyponatremic dehydration, metabolic alkalosis with hypokalemia, or anuria

Warnings Loop diuretics are potent diuretics; excess amounts can lead to profound diuresis with fluid and electrolyte loss; close medical supervision and dose evaluation is required; may increase risk of gastric hemorrhage associated with corticosteroid treatment

Precautions Avoid use in patients with severe renal dysfunction (Cl$_{cr}$ <10 mL/minute)

Adverse Reactions

Cardiovascular: Hypotension

Central nervous system: Headache, fatigue, mental confusion, vertigo

Dermatologic: Rash, photosensitivity

Endocrine & metabolic: Hyperglycemia, fluid and electrolyte imbalances (fluid depletion, hypokalemia, hyponatremia, hypomagnesemia, hypocalcemia), hyperuricemia

Gastrointestinal: GI irritation, diarrhea, anorexia, abdominal pain, dysphagia, GI bleed

Hematologic: Thrombocytopenia, neutropenia, agranulocytosis

Hepatic: Abnormal liver function tests, jaundice, hepatocellular damage

Local: Local irritation, pain at injection site

Otic: Ototoxicity, tinnitus

Renal: Renal injury, hematuria

Drug Interactions

Avoid Concomitant Use

Avoid concomitant use of Ethacrynic Acid with any of the following: Furosemide

Increased Effect/Toxicity

Ethacrynic Acid may increase the levels/effects of: ACE Inhibitors; Allopurinol; Amifostine; Aminoglycosides; Antihypertensives; CISplatin; Dofetilide; Hypotensive Agents; Lithium; Neuromuscular-Blocking Agents; RiTUXimab; Salicylates

The levels/effects of Ethacrynic Acid may be increased by: Corticosteroids (Orally Inhaled); Corticosteroids (Systemic); Diazoxide; Furosemide; Herbs (Hypotensive Properties); MAO Inhibitors; Pentoxifylline; Phosphodiesterase 5 Inhibitors; Probenecid; Prostacyclin Analogues

Decreased Effect

Ethacrynic Acid may decrease the levels/effects of: Lithium; Neuromuscular-Blocking Agents

The levels/effects of Ethacrynic Acid may be decreased by: Bile Acid Sequestrants; Herbs (Hypertensive Properties); Methylphenidate; Nonsteroidal Anti-Inflammatory Agents; Phenytoin; Probenecid; Salicylates; Yohimbine

Food Interactions Need diet rich in potassium and magnesium

Stability When reconstituted with 50 mL D$_5$W or NS, resultant solution (1 mg/mL) is stable for 24 hours at room temperature

Mechanism of Action Inhibits reabsorption of sodium and chloride in the ascending loop of Henle and distal renal tubule, interfering with the chloride-binding cotransport system, thus causing increased excretion of water, sodium, chloride, magnesium, and calcium

Pharmacodynamics

Onset of action:

Oral: Within 30 minutes

I.V.: 5 minutes

Peak effect:

Oral: 2 hours

I.V.: 15-30 minutes

Duration:

Oral: 6-8 hours

I.V.: 2 hours

Pharmacokinetics (Adult data unless noted)

Absorption: Oral: Rapid

Protein binding: >90%

Metabolism: In the liver to active cysteine conjugate (35% to 40%)

Elimination: In bile, 30% to 60% excreted unchanged in urine

Usual Dosage

Children:

Oral: 1 mg/kg/dose once daily, increase at intervals of 2-3 days to a maximum of 3 mg/kg/day

I.V.: 1 mg/kg/dose; repeat doses are not routinely recommended, however if indicated, repeat doses every 8-12 hours

Adults:

Oral: 25-400 mg/day in 1-2 divided doses

I.V.: 0.5-1 mg/kg/dose (maximum dose: 100 mg/dose); repeat doses not routinely recommended, however if indicated, repeat every 8-12 hours

Administration

Oral: Administer with food or milk

Parenteral: Dilute injection with 50 mL D_5W or NS (1 mg/mL concentration resulting); maximum concentration 2 mg/mL; may be injected without further dilution over a period of several minutes or infused over 20-30 minutes; tissue irritant; not to be administered I.M. or SubQ

Monitoring Parameters Serum electrolytes, blood pressure, renal function, hearing

Additional Information Injection contains thimerosal

Dosage Forms Excipient information presented when available (limited, particularly for generics); consult specific product labeling.

Injection, powder for reconstitution, as ethacrynate sodium:

Sodium Edecrin®: 50 mg

Tablet:

Edecrin®: 25 mg [scored]

Extemporaneous Preparations To make a 1 mg/mL suspension: Dissolve 120 mg ethacrynic acid powder in 13 mL alcohol, USP; add a small amount of methylparaben 0.005% and propylparaben 0.002% (final concentrations); adjust pH to 7 with 0.1N sodium hydroxide solution; add sufficient 50% sorbitol solution to make a final volume of 120 mL. Stable 220 days at room temperature. Shake well before use.

Das Gupta V, Gibbs CW Jr, and Ghanekar AG, "Stability of Pediatric Liquid Dosage Forms of Ethacrynic Acid, Indomethacin, Methyldopate Hydrochloride, Prednisone and Spironolactone," *Am J Hosp Pharm*, 1978, 35 (11):1382-5.

Ethambutol (e THAM byoo tole)

Medication Safety Issues

Sound-alike/look-alike issues:

Myambutol® may be confused with Nembutal®

U.S. Brand Names Myambutol®

Canadian Brand Names Etibi®

Therapeutic Category Antitubercular Agent

Generic Available Yes

Use Treatment of pulmonary tuberculosis (FDA approved in ages ≥13 years and adults) and other mycobacterial diseases in conjunction with other antimycobacterial agents

Pregnancy Risk Factor C

Pregnancy Considerations Teratogenic effects have been seen in animals. There are no adequate and well-controlled studies in pregnant women; there have been reports of ophthalmic abnormalities in infants born to women receiving ethambutol as a component of anti-tuberculous therapy. Use only during pregnancy if benefits outweigh risks.

Lactation Enters breast milk/use caution (AAP considers "compatible")

Breast-Feeding Considerations The manufacturer suggests use during breast-feeding only if benefits to the mother outweigh the possible risk to the infant. Some references suggest that exposure to the infant is low and does not produce toxicity, and breast-feeding should not be discouraged. Other references recommend if breast-feeding, monitor the infant for rash, malaise, nausea, or vomiting.

Contraindications Hypersensitivity to ethambutol or any component; optic neuritis, unless clinical judgment determines that it may be used; use in patients unable to discern and report visual changes (eg, very young, unconscious patients)

Warnings Optic neuropathy including optic neuritis or retrobulbar neuritis characterized by decreased visual acuity, scotoma, color blindness, and/or visual defect has been reported with ethambutol therapy and may be related to dose and treatment duration; irreversible blindness has also been reported. Loss of visual acuity is generally reversible when ethambutol is discontinued promptly, but reversal may require up to a year. Some patients have received ethambutol again after such recovery without recurrence of visual acuity loss. Use only in children whose visual acuity can accurately be determined and monitored; fatal hepatotoxicity has been reported; not recommended for use in children <13 years of age unless benefit outweighs risk of therapy

Precautions Use with caution in patients with ocular defects or impaired renal function; modify dose in patients with renal impairment

Adverse Reactions

Cardiovascular: Myocarditis, pericarditis

Central nervous system: Malaise, mental confusion, fever, headache, dizziness, hallucinations, disorientation

Dermatologic: Rash, pruritus, dermatitis, erythema multiforme

Endocrine & metabolic: Uric acid levels elevated, acute gout

Gastrointestinal: Nausea, vomiting, anorexia, abdominal pain, GI upset

Hematologic: Thrombocytopenia, leukopenia, eosinophilia, neutropenia

Hepatic: Abnormal liver function tests, hepatotoxicity, cholestatic jaundice

Neuromuscular & skeletal: Peripheral neuropathy, arthralgia, joint pain

Ocular: Optic neuritis, visual acuity decreased, red-green color discrimination decreased, irreversible blindness, retrobulbar neuritis

Respiratory: Pulmonary infiltrates

Miscellaneous: Anaphylaxis, hypersensitivity syndrome

Drug Interactions

Avoid Concomitant Use There are no known interactions where it is recommended to avoid concomitant use.

Increased Effect/Toxicity There are no known significant interactions involving an increase in effect.

Decreased Effect

The levels/effects of Ethambutol may be decreased by: Aluminum Hydroxide

Stability Store tablets at controlled room temperature 20°C to 25°C (68°F to 77°F)

Mechanism of Action Suppresses mycobacterial multiplication by interfering with RNA synthesis

Pharmacokinetics (Adult data unless noted)

Absorption: Oral: ~80%

Distribution: Well distributed throughout the body with high concentrations in kidneys, lungs, saliva, and red blood cells; concentrations in CSF are low; crosses the placenta; excreted into breast milk

Protein binding: 20% to 30%

Metabolism: 20% by the liver to inactive metabolite

Half-life: 2.5-3.6 hours (up to 7 hours or longer with renal impairment)

Time to peak serum concentration: Within 2-4 hours

Elimination: ~50% in urine and 20% excreted in feces as unchanged drug

Dialysis: Slightly dialyzable (5% to 20%)

Usual Dosage Oral:

Tuberculosis: Adolescents ≥13 years and Adults: 15-25 mg/kg/day once every 24 hours **or** 50 mg/kg/dose twice weekly, not to exceed 2.5 g/dose

WHO recommendations: Children: 20 mg/kg once daily (range: 15-25 mg/kg/day)

Nontuberculous mycobacterial infection: Children, Adolescents, and Adults: 15-25 mg/kg/day once daily, not to exceed 2.5 g/dose

Dosing interval in renal impairment:

Cl_{cr} 10-50 mL/minute: Administer every 24-36 hours

Cl_{cr} <10 mL/minute: Administer every 48 hours and/or reduce usual dose

Continuous arteriovenous or venovenous hemofiltration: Administer every 24-36 hours

Administration Oral: Administer with or without food; if GI upset occurs, administer with food. Tablet may be pulverized and mixed with apple juice or apple sauce. Do not mix with other juices or syrups since they do not mask ethambutol's bitter taste or are not stable. Administer ethambutol at least 4 hours before aluminum hydroxide.

Monitoring Parameters Monthly examination of visual acuity and color discrimination in patients receiving >15 mg/kg/day; periodic renal, hepatic, and hematologic function tests

Patient Information Report to physician any visual changes, numbness or tingling in hands or feet, rash, fever, and chills

Dosage Forms Excipient information presented when available (limited, particularly for generics); consult specific product labeling.

Tablet, as hydrochloride: 100 mg, 400 mg

Myambutol®: 100 mg, 400 mg

References

American Academy of Pediatrics, Committee on Infectious Diseases, "Chemotherapy for Tuberculosis in Infants and Children," Pediatrics, 1992, 89(1):161-5.

CDC, NIH, IDSA, et al, "Guidelines for Prevention and Treatment of Opportunistic Infections Among HIV-Exposed and HIV-Infected Children," June 20, 2008. Available at http://www.aidsinfo.nih.gov.

Graham SM, Bell DJ, Nyirongo S, et al, "Low Levels of Pyrazinamide and Ethambutol in Children With Tuberculosis and Impact of Age, Nutritional Status, and Human Immunodeficiency Virus Infection," Antimicrob Agents Chemother, 2006, 50(2):407-13.

Hill S, Regondi I, Grzemska M, et al, "Children and Tuberculosis Medicines: Bridging the Research Gap," Bull World Health Organ, 2008, 86(9):658.

Starke JR and Correa AG, "Management of Mycobacterial Infection and Disease in Children," Pediatr Infect Dis J, 1995, 14:455-70.

◆ **Ethambutol Hydrochloride** *see* Ethambutol *on page 544*

◆ **Ethanol** *see* Ethyl Alcohol *on page 547*

◆ **EtheDent™ [DSC]** *see* Fluoride *on page 595*

◆ **EthexDERM™ BPW-5 [DSC]** *see* Benzoyl Peroxide *on page 184*

◆ **EthexDERM™ BPW-10 [DSC]** *see* Benzoyl Peroxide *on page 184*

◆ **Ethiofos** *see* Amifostine *on page 78*

Ethionamide (e thye on AM ide)

U.S. Brand Names Trecator®

Canadian Brand Names Trecator®

Therapeutic Category Antitubercular Agent

Generic Available No

Use In conjunction with other antituberculosis agents in the treatment of tuberculosis and other mycobacterial diseases

Pregnancy Risk Factor C

Pregnancy Considerations Ethionamide crosses the placenta; teratogenic effects were observed in animal studies. Use during pregnancy is not recommended.

Lactation Excretion in breast milk unknown/use caution

Breast-Feeding Considerations If ethionamide is used while breast-feeding, monitor the infant for adverse effects.

Contraindications Hypersensitivity to ethionamide or any component; severe hepatic impairment

Precautions Use with caution in patients receiving cycloserine or isoniazid or in diabetic patients

Adverse Reactions

Cardiovascular: Postural hypotension

Central nervous system: Drowsiness, dizziness, seizures, headache, encephalopathy, depression, psychotic disturbances

Dermatologic: Rash

Endocrine & metabolic: Hypoglycemia, goiter, gynecomastia, weight loss

Gastrointestinal: Nausea, vomiting, abdominal pain, diarrhea, anorexia, stomatitis, metallic taste

Hematologic: Thrombocytopenia

Hepatic: Hepatitis; jaundice; AST, ALT, and serum bilirubin elevated

Neuromuscular & skeletal: Peripheral neuropathy, tremor

Ocular: Optic neuritis

Miscellaneous: Excessive salivation

Drug Interactions

Avoid Concomitant Use There are no known interactions where it is recommended to avoid concomitant use.

Increased Effect/Toxicity

The levels/effects of Ethionamide may be increased by: Alcohol (Ethyl)

Decreased Effect There are no known significant interactions involving a decrease in effect.

Food Interactions Increase dietary intake of pyridoxine to prevent neurotoxic effects of ethionamide

Mechanism of Action Inhibits peptide synthesis in susceptible organisms

Pharmacokinetics (Adult data unless noted)

Absorption: ~80% is rapidly absorbed from the GI tract

Distribution: Crosses the placenta; widely distributed into body tissues and fluids including liver, kidneys, and CSF

Protein binding: 10%

Metabolism: In the liver to active and inactive metabolites

Bioavailability: 80%

Half-life: 2-3 hours

Time to peak serum concentration: Oral: Within 3 hours

Elimination: As metabolites (active and inactive) and parent drug in the urine

Usual Dosage Oral:

Children: 15-20 mg/kg/day in 2-3 divided doses, not to exceed 1 g/day

Adults: 500-1000 mg/day in 1-3 divided doses

Administration Oral: Administer with meals to decrease GI distress

Monitoring Parameters Initial and periodic serum AST and ALT, blood glucose, thyroid function tests, periodic ophthalmologic exams

Nursing Implications Neurotoxic effects may be relieved by the administration of pyridoxine

Dosage Forms Excipient information presented when available (limited, particularly for generics); consult specific product labeling.

Tablet: 250 mg

References

Donald PR and Seifart HI,"Cerebrospinal Fluid Concentrations of Ethionamide in Children With Tuberculous Meningitis," J Pediatr, 1989, 115(3):483-6.

Starke JR and Correa AG, "Management of Mycobacterial Infection and Disease in Children," Pediatr Infect Dis J, 1995, 14(6):455-69.

Ethosuximide (eth oh SUKS i mide)

Medication Safety Issues

Sound-alike/look-alike issues:

Ethosuximide may be confused with methsuximide

Zarontin® may be confused with Neurontin®, Xalatan®, Zantac®, Zaroxolyn®

Related Information

Antiepileptic Drugs *on page 1693*

Therapeutic Drug Monitoring: Blood Sampling Time Guidelines *on page 1704*

U.S. Brand Names Zarontin®

Canadian Brand Names Zarontin®

Therapeutic Category Anticonvulsant, Succinimide

Generic Available Yes

Use Management of absence (petit mal) epilepsy (FDA approved in ages ≥3 years and adults); also used for management of myoclonic seizures and akinetic epilepsy

Pregnancy Considerations Ethosuximide crosses the placenta. Cases of birth defects have been reported in infants. Epilepsy itself, the number of medications, genetic factors, or a combination of these probably influence the teratogenicity of anticonvulsant therapy.

Patients exposed to ethosuximide during pregnancy are encouraged to enroll themselves into the NAAED Pregnancy Registry by calling 1-888-233-2334. Additional information is available at www.aedpregnancyregistry.org.

Lactation Enters breast milk/use caution (AAP rates "compatible")

Contraindications Hypersensitivity to ethosuximide, other succinimides, or any component

Warnings Blood dyscrasias (sometimes fatal) have been reported (monitor hematologic function periodically or if signs/symptoms of infection develop); SLE has been reported.

Antiepileptic drugs (AEDs) increase the risk of suicidal behavior and ideation in patients receiving these medications for any indication. Pooled analyses of placebo-controlled trials involving 11 different AEDs (regardless of indication) showed a two-fold increased risk of suicidal thoughts or behavior (estimated incidence rate: 0.43% in AED-treated patients compared to 0.24% in patients receiving placebo); increased risk was observed as early as one week after initiation of AED and continued through duration of trials (most trials ≤24 weeks); risk did not vary significantly by age (age range: 5–100 years). Consider risks and benefits of AEDs before prescribing. Monitor all patients receiving an AED for emergence of suicidal thoughts or behavior, thoughts of self-harm, any unusual changes in behavior or mood, or the emergence or worsening of depressive symptoms; notify heathcare provider immediately if symptoms or concerning behavior occur. **Note:** The FDA is requiring that a Medication Guide be developed for all antiepileptic drugs, informing patients of this risk.

Oral solution may contain sodium benzoate; benzoic acid (benzoate) is a metabolite of benzyl alcohol; large amounts of benzyl alcohol (≥99 mg/kg/day) have been associated with a potentially fatal toxicity ("gasping syndrome") in neonates; the "gasping syndrome" consists of metabolic acidosis, respiratory distress, gasping respirations, CNS dysfunction (including convulsions, intracranial hemorrhage), hypotension and cardiovascular collapse; use ethosuximide products containing sodium benzoate with caution in neonates; *in vitro* and animal studies have shown that benzoate displaces bilirubin from protein binding sites

Precautions Use with caution in patients with hepatic or renal disease. Avoid abrupt withdrawal (may precipitate absence status). When used alone, ethosuximide may increase tonic-clonic seizures in patients with mixed seizure disorders; ethosuximide must be used in combination with other anticonvulsants in patients with both absence and tonic-clonic seizures. May cause CNS depression, which may impair physical or mental abilities; patients must be cautioned about performing tasks which require mental alertness.

Adverse Reactions

Central nervous system: Aggressiveness, agitation, ataxia, behavioral changes, disturbance in sleep, dizziness, drowsiness, euphoria, fatigue, hallucinations, headache, hyperactivity, inability to concentrate, increase in tonic-clonic seizures (see Precautions), insomnia, irritability, lethargy, mental depression with cases of overt suicidal intentions (rare), night terrors, paranoid psychosis (rare), suicidal thinking and behavior (see Warnings)

Dermatologic: Hirsutism, pruritus, rash, Stevens-Johnson syndrome, urticaria

Endocrine & metabolic: Libido increased, weight loss

Gastrointestinal: Abdominal pain, anorexia, cramps, diarrhea, epigastric pain, gastric upset, gum hypertrophy, nausea, tongue swelling, vomiting

Genitourinary: Vaginal bleeding

Hematologic: Agranulocytosis, eosinophilia, leukopenia, pancytopenia (with and without bone marrow suppression) (see Warnings)

Ocular: Myopia

Renal: Microscopic hematuria

Miscellaneous: Allergic reactions, hiccups, rarely systemic lupus erythematosus

Drug Interactions

Metabolism/Transport Effects Substrate of CYP3A4 (major)

Avoid Concomitant Use There are no known interactions where it is recommended to avoid concomitant use.

Increased Effect/Toxicity

Ethosuximide may increase the levels/effects of: Alcohol (Ethyl); CNS Depressants; Methotrimeprazine

The levels/effects of Ethosuximide may be increased by: CYP3A4 Inhibitors (Moderate); CYP3A4 Inhibitors (Strong); Dasatinib; Divalproex; Methotrimeprazine; Valproic Acid

Decreased Effect

Ethosuximide may decrease the levels/effects of: Divalproex; Valproic Acid

The levels/effects of Ethosuximide may be decreased by: Amphetamines; CYP3A4 Inducers (Strong); Deferasirox; Herbs (CYP3A4 Inducers); Ketorolac; Ketorolac (Systemic); Mefloquine

Food Interactions Folate requirements may be increased

Stability

Capsules: Store at controlled room temperature

Solution: Store below 30°C (86°F) in tightly-closed container. Protect from light; do not freeze.

Mechanism of Action Increases the seizure threshold and suppresses paroxysmal spike-and-wave pattern in absence seizures; depresses nerve transmission in the motor cortex

Pharmacokinetics (Adult data unless noted)

Distribution: V_d: Adults: 0.62-0.72 L/kg; crosses the placenta; excreted in human breast milk

Protein binding: <10%

Metabolism: ~80% metabolized in the liver to three inactive metabolites

Half-life:

Children: 30 hours

Adults: 50-60 hours

Time to peak serum concentration:

Capsule: Within 2-4 hours

Solution: <2-4 hours

Elimination: Slow in urine as metabolites (50%) and as unchanged drug (10% to 20%); small amounts excreted in feces

Dialysis: Removed by hemodialysis and peritoneal dialysis

Usual Dosage Oral:

Children <6 years: Initial: 15 mg/kg/day in 2 divided doses (maximum dose: 250 mg/dose); increase every 4-7 days; usual maintenance dose: 15-40 mg/kg/day in 2 divided doses; maximum dose: 1.5 g/day

Children ≥6 years and Adults: Initial: 250 mg twice daily; increase by 250 mg/day as needed every 4-7 days up to 1.5 g/day in 2 divided doses; usual maintenance dose: 20-40 mg/kg/day in 2 divided doses

Administration Oral: Administer with food or milk to decrease GI upset

Monitoring Parameters Seizure frequency, trough serum concentrations; CBC with differential, platelets, liver enzymes, urinalysis, renal function; signs and symptoms of suicidality (eg, anxiety, depression, behavior changes) (see Warnings)

Reference Range

Therapeutic: 40-100 mcg/mL (SI: 280-710 micromoles/L)

Toxic: >150 mcg/mL (SI: >1062 micromoles/L)

Patient Information Avoid alcohol. May cause drowsiness and impair ability to perform activities requiring mental alertness or physical coordination. Do not discontinue abruptly (seizures may occur). Antiepileptic agents may increase the risk of suicidal thoughts and behavior; notify physician if you feel more depressed or have thoughts of suicide or self-harm (see Warnings). Notify physician if sore throat or fever occurs. Report worsening of seizure activity or loss of seizure control.

Additional Information Considered to be a drug of choice for simple absence seizures

Dosage Forms Excipient information presented when available (limited, particularly for generics); consult specific product labeling.

Capsule: 250 mg

Zarontin®: 250 mg

Solution, oral: 250 mg/5 mL (473 mL)

Zarontin®: 250 mg/5 mL [contains sodium benzoate; raspberry flavor]

Syrup: 250 mg/5 mL (473 mL)

References

Marquardt ED, Ishisaka DY, Batra KK, et al, "Removal of Ethosuximide and Phenobarbital by Peritoneal Dialysis in a Child," *Clin Pharm*, 1992, 11(12):1030-1.

♦ **Ethoxynaphthamido Penicillin Sodium** *see* Nacillin *on page 962*

Ethyl Alcohol (ETH il AL koe hol)

Medication Safety Issues

Sound-alike/look-alike issues:

Ethanol may be confused with Ethyol®, Ethamolin®

U.S. Brand Names EpiClenz™ [OTC]; Gel-Stat™ [OTC]; GelRite [OTC]; Isagel® [OTC]; Lavacol® [OTC]; Prevacare® [OTC]; Protection Plus® [OTC]; Purell® 2 in 1 [OTC]; Purell® Lasting Care [OTC]; Purell® Moisture Therapy [OTC]; Purell® with Aloe [OTC]; Purell® [OTC]

Canadian Brand Names Biobase-G™; Biobase™

Therapeutic Category Anti-infective Agent, Topical; Antidote, Ethylene Glycol Toxicity; Antidote, Methanol Toxicity; Fat Occlusion (Central Venous Catheter), Treatment Agent; Neurolytic

Generic Available Yes

Use Antidote for the treatment of methanol and ethylene glycol intoxication; neurolysis of nerves or ganglia for the relief of intractable, chronic pain in such conditions as inoperable cancer and trigeminal neuralgia (dehydrated alcohol injection); topical anti-infective; treatment of occluded central venous catheters due to lipid deposition from fat emulsion infusion (particularly 3-in-1 admixture)

Pregnancy Risk Factor C (injection)

Pregnancy Considerations Reproduction studies have not been conducted with alcohol injection. Ethanol crosses the placenta, enters the fetal circulation, and has teratogenic effects in humans. The following withdrawal symptoms have been noted in the neonate following maternal ethanol consumption during pregnancy: Crying, hyperactivity, irritability, poor suck, tremors, seizures, poor sleeping pattern, hyperphagia, and diaphoresis. Fetal alcohol syndrome (FAS) is a term referring to a combination of physical, behavioral, and cognitive abnormalities resulting from ethanol exposure during fetal development. Since a "safe" amount of ethanol consumption during pregnancy has not been determined, the AAP recommends those women who are pregnant or planning a pregnancy refrain from all ethanol intake. When used as an antidote during the second or third trimester, FAS is not likely to occur due to the short treatment period; use during the first trimester is controversial.

Lactation Enters breast milk/use caution (AAP rates "compatible")

Breast-Feeding Considerations Ethanol is found in breast milk. Drowsiness, diaphoresis, deep sleep, weakness, decreased linear growth, and abnormal weight gain have been reported in infants following large amounts of ethanol ingestion by the mother. Ingestion >1 g/kg/day decreases milk ejection reflex. The actual clearance of ethanol from breast milk is dependent upon the mother's weight and amount of ethanol consumed.

Contraindications Hypersensitivity to ethyl alcohol; seizure disorder and diabetic coma; subarachnoid injection of dehydrated alcohol in patients receiving anticoagulants

Warnings Ethyl alcohol is a flammable liquid and should be kept cool and away from any heat source; proper positioning of the patient for neurolytic administration is essential to control localization of the injection of dehydrated alcohol (which is hypobaric) into the subarachnoid space; avoid extravasation; not for SubQ administration; do not administer simultaneously with blood due to the possibility of pseudoagglutination or hemolysis; may potentiate severe hypoprothrombic bleeding; clinical evaluation and periodic lab determinations, including serum ethyl alcohol levels, are necessary to monitor effectiveness, changes in electrolyte concentrations, and acid-base balance (when used as an antidote)

Precautions Use with caution in diabetics (ethyl alcohol decreases blood sugar), hepatic impairment, patients with gout, shock, following cranial surgery, and in anticipated postpartum hemorrhage; monitor blood glucose closely, particularly in children as treatment of ingestions is associated with hypoglycemia; avoid extravasation during I.V. administration; ethyl alcohol passes freely into breast milk at a level approximately equivalent to maternal serum level; effects on the infant are insignificant until maternal blood level reaches 300 mg/dL; minimize dermal exposure of ethyl alcohol in infants as significant systemic absorption and toxicity can occur

Adverse Reactions

Cardiovascular: Tachycardia, hypertension, hypotension, arrhythmias, cardiomegaly, angina, CHF, vasodilation, flushing, hypothermia

Central nervous system: Ataxia, dementia, Wernicke-Korsakoff syndrome, amnesia, paranoia, hyperthermia, vertigo, lethargy, sedation, coma, seizures, hallucinations

Endocrine & metabolic: Hypoglycemia, acidosis, hypokalemia, hypomagnesemia, serum osmolality increased

Dermatologic: Dry skin, irritation

Gastrointestinal: Nausea, diarrhea, abdominal pain, dyspepsia, vomiting, GI hemorrhage, anorexia, pancreatitis, hiccups

Hematologic: Porphyria, megaloblastic anemia

Hepatic: Hepatic cirrhosis, fatty degeneration of liver, hepatic steatosis

Local: Phlebitis, nerve and tissue destruction (injection)

Neuromuscular & skeletal: Hypotonia, dysarthria, myopathy, neuropathy (peripheral); postinjection neuritis with persistent pain, hyperesthesia, and paresthesia (after neurolytic use)

Ocular: Eye stinging (from vapors)

Respiratory: Respiratory depression, tachypnea, bronchial irritation

Drug Interactions

Avoid Concomitant Use

Avoid concomitant use of Alcohol (Ethyl) with any of the following: Acitretin; CycloSERINE; Didanosine; Disulfiram

Increased Effect/Toxicity

Alcohol (Ethyl) may increase the levels/effects of: Acitretin; CycloSERINE; Didanosine; Ethionamide; Isotretinoin; NIFEdipine; Propranolol; Thiazide Diuretics

The levels/effects of Alcohol (Ethyl) may be increased by: Cefotetan; CNS Depressants; Disulfiram; Furazolidone; Griseofulvin; MetroNIDAZOLE; MetroNIDAZOLE (Systemic); MetroNIDAZOLE (Topical); Sulfonylureas; Tacrolimus; Tacrolimus (Topical); Verapamil

Decreased Effect

Alcohol (Ethyl) may decrease the levels/effects of: Propranolol

Stability Store at room temperature (see Warnings); do not use unless solution is clear and container is intact

Mechanism of Action Competitively inhibits the oxidation of methanol and ethylene oxide by alcohol dehydrogenase to their more toxic metabolites; as a neurolytic, ethyl alcohol produces injury to tissue cells by producing dehydration and precipitation of protoplasm; when injected in close proximity to nerve cells, it produces neuritis and nerve degeneration

Pharmacokinetics (Adult data unless noted)

Distribution: V_d: 0.6-0.7 L/kg

Metabolism: Hepatic to acetaldehyde or acetate by alcohol dehydrogenase

Clearance: Adults: 15-20 mg/dL/hour (range: 10-34 mg/dL/hour)

Dialysis: Hemodialysis clearance: 300-400 mL/minute with an ethanol removal rate of 280 mg/minute

Usual Dosage

Absolute ethanol/ethyl alcohol (EtOH):

Treatment of methanol or ethylene glycol ingestion: Children, Adolescents, and Adults:

Loading dose (LD):

Oral: 0.8-1 mL/kg of 95% EtOH or 2 mL/kg of 40% EtOH (equivalent to 80 proof undiluted liquor) or 1.8 mL/kg of 43% EtOH (equivalent to 86 proof undiluted liquor)

I.V.: 8-10 mL/kg of 10% EtOH solution (see Administration), not to exceed 200 mL

Modified loading dose (if ingestion consists of both EtOH **and** methanol or ethylene glycol): The loading dose is reduced in a proportional manner related to the measured EtOH blood level by multiplying the calculated loading dose described above by the following factor:

$$LD \times \left[\frac{100 - (\text{patient's serum ethanol level in mg/dL})}{100} \right]$$

Maintenance dose: See table

	Non-Drinker	Average Drinker	Chronic Drinker
EtOH dosage by weight	66 mg/kg/h	110 mg/kg/h	154 mg/kg/h
Oral: 43% EtOH (34 g EtOH/dL; 86 proof undiluted liquor)	0.2 mL/kg/h	0.3 mL/kg/h	0.46 mL/kg/h
Oral: 95% EtOH (75 g EtOH/dL)	0.1 mL/kg/h	0.15 mL/kg/h	0.2 mL/kg/h
I.V.: 10% EtOH (7.9 g EtOH/dL)	0.83 mL/kg/h	1.4 mL/kg/h	2 mL/kg/h

Note: Continue therapy until methanol or ethylene glycol blood level <10 mg/dL.

Dosage adjustment for hemodialysis: See table

Maintenance Dose Adjustment of Dialysis[1]:

	Non-Drinker	Chronic Drinker
EtOH dosage by weight	169 mg/kg/h	257 mg/kg/h
Oral: 43% EtOH (34 g EtOH/dL)	0.5 mL/kg/h	0.77 mL/kg/h
I.V.: 10% EtOH (7.9 g EtOH/dL)	2.13 mL/kg/h	3.26 mL/kg/h

[1]Due to considerable variability of EtOH clearance between patients, adjust dosage as needed based upon serum EtOH levels.

Treatment of fat occlusion of central venous catheters: Children and Adults: I.V. (see institutional-based protocol for catheter clearance assessment, the following assessment is a general methodology): Up to 3 mL of 70% ethanol (maximum: 0.55 mL/kg); instill a volume equal to the internal volume of the catheter; may repeat if patency not restored after 30- minute dwell time; if dose repeated, reassess after 4-hour dwell time

Dehydrated alcohol injection: Therapeutic neurolysis (nerve or ganglion block): Adults: Intraneural: Dosage variable depending upon the site of injection, eg, trigeminal neuralgia: 0.05-0.5 mL as a single injection per interspace vs subarachnoid injection: 0.5-1 mL as a single injection per interspace; single doses >1.5 mL are seldom required

Liquid denatured alcohol: Topical: Children and Adults: Apply as needed

Administration

Oral: Dilute ethanol in 6 ounces orange juice and give over 30 minutes

Parenteral: Not for SubQ administration; I.V.: Dilute absolute alcohol for I.V. administration to a final concentration of 5% to 10% v/v in D_5W or $D_{10}W$; infuse loading dose plus 1 hour of maintenance dosage over 60 minutes; for treatment of occluded central venous catheter, a 70% dilution of ethanol may be made by adding 0.8 mL SWI to 2 mL 98% ethanol; instill with a volume equal to the internal volume of the catheter; assess patency at 30 minutes (or per institutional protocol); may repeat (see Usual Dosage)

Intraneural: Separate needles should be used for each of multiple injections or sites to prevent residual alcohol deposition at sites not intended for tissue destruction; inject slowly after determining proper placement of needle; since dehydrated alcohol is hypobaric when compared with spinal fluid, proper positioning of the patient is essential to control localization of injections into the subarachnoid space

Monitoring Parameters Antidotal therapy: Blood ethanol levels (at the end of the loading dose, every hour until stabilized, and then every 8-12 hours thereafter); blood glucose, electrolytes (including serum magnesium), arterial pH, blood gases, methanol or ethylene glycol blood levels, heart rate, blood pressure

Reference Range

Symptoms associated with serum ethanol levels:
Nausea and vomiting: Serum level >100 mg/dL
Coma: Serum level >300 mg/dL
Antidote for methanol/ethylene glycol: Goal range: Blood ethanol level: 100-150 mg/dL (22-32 mmol/liter)

Patient Information May cause drowsiness and impair ability to perform activities requiring mental alertness or physical coordination

Additional Information Eighty-proof spirits contain 40% ethanol; 86 proof spirits contain 43% ethanol

Dosage Forms Excipient information presented when available (limited, particularly for generics); consult specific product labeling. [DSC] = Discontinued product

Foam, topical:
Epi-Clenz™: 62% (240 mL, 480 mL) [instant hand sanitizer; contains aloe vera and vitamin E]

Gel, topical:
Epi-Clenz™: 70% (45 mL, 120 mL, 480 mL) [instant hand sanitizer; contains aloe vera and vitamin E]
GelRite: 67% (120 mL, 480 mL, 800 mL) [instant hand sanitizer; contains vitamin E)
Gel-Stat™: 62% (120 mL, 480 mL) [instant hand sanitizer]
Isagel®: 60% (59 mL, 118 mL, 621 mL, 800 mL) [instant hand sanitizer]
Prevacare®: 60% (120 mL, 240 mL, 960 mL, 1200 mL, 1500 mL) [instant hand sanitizer]
Protection Plus®: 62% (800 mL) [instant hand sanitizer]
Purell®: 62% (15 mL, 30 mL, 59 mL, 120 mL, 236 mL, 250 mL, 360 mL, 500 mL, 800 mL, 1000 mL, 2000 mL) [instant hand sanitizer; contains moisturizers and vitamin E]
Purell® Lasting Care: 62% (120 mL, 240 mL, 1000 mL) [contains moisturizers]
Purell® Moisture Therapy: 62% (75 mL) [instant hand sanitizer]
Purell® with Aloe: 62% (15 mL, 59 mL, 236 mL, 360 mL, 800 mL, 1000 mL, 2000 mL) [instant hand sanitizer; contains aloe and tartrazine]
Infusion [in D₅W, dehydrated]: Alcohol 5% (1000 mL) [DSC]
Injection, solution [dehydrated]: 98% (1 mL, 5 mL)
Liquid, topical [denatured]: 70% (3840 mL)
Lavacol®: 70% (473 mL)
Lotion, topical:
Purell® 2 in 1: 62% (60 mL, 360 mL, 1000 mL) [instant hand sanitizer]
Towelettes, topical:
Isagel®: 60% (50s, 300s) [instant hand sanitizer]
Purell®: 62% (35s, 175s) [instant hand sanitizer]

References
Barceloux DG, Bond GR, Krenzelok EP, et al, "American Academy of Clinical Toxicology Practice Guidelines on the Treatment of Methanol Poisoning," *J Toxicol Clin Toxicol*, 2002, 40(4):415-46.
Chernow B, ed, "Poisoning", *Essentials of Critical Care Pharmacology*, 2nd ed, Baltimore: Williams & Wilkins, 1994, 501-29.
Pennington CR and Pithie AD, "Ethanol Lock in the Management of Catheter Occlusion," *JPEN J Parenter Enteral Nutr*, 1987, 11 (5):507-8.
Poisoning and Drug Overdose, 2nd ed, Olson KR, ed, Norwalk, Connecticut: Appleton and Lange, 1994, 339-40.
Werlin SL, Lausten T, Jessens, et al, "Treatment of Central Venous Catheter Occlusions With Ethanol and Hydrochloric Acid," *JPEN J Parenter Enteral Nutr*, 1995, 19(5):416-8.

◆ **Ethyl Alcohol** *see Ethyl Alcohol on page 547*
◆ **Ethyl Aminobenzoate** *see Benzocaine on page 182*
◆ **Ethyol®** *see Amifostine on page 78*
◆ **Etibi® (Can)** *see Ethambutol on page 544*

Etidronate Disodium
(e ti DROE nate dye SOW dee um)

Medication Safety Issues
Sound-alike/look-alike issues:
Etidronate may be confused with etidocaine, etomidate, etretinate

U.S. Brand Names Didronel®

Canadian Brand Names Co-Etidronate; Didronel®; Mylan-Etidronate

Therapeutic Category Antidote, Hypercalcemia; Bisphosphonate Derivative

Generic Available No

Use Symptomatic treatment of Paget's disease of bone and prevention and treatment of heterotopic ossification following spinal cord injury or total hip replacement

Pregnancy Risk Factor C

Pregnancy Considerations Teratogenic effects have been reported in some but not all animal studies. There are no adequate and well-controlled studies in pregnant women. Bisphosphonates are incorporated into the bone matrix and gradually released over time. Theoretically, there may be a risk of fetal harm when pregnancy follows the completion of therapy. Based on limited case reports with pamidronate, serum calcium levels in the newborn may be altered if administered during pregnancy.

Lactation Excretion in breast milk unknown/use caution

Contraindications Hypersensitivity to etidronate, biphosphonates or any component; clinically overt osteomalacia

Warnings Response to therapy in Paget's disease may be slow in onset and continue for months after therapy is discontinued; do not increase dosage rapidly; treatment >6 months or at doses >20 mg/kg/day have been associated with osteomalacia and increased risk of fracture; hyperphosphatemia may occur at doses of 10-20 mg/kg/day due to drug related increases in the tubular reabsorption of phosphate; serum phosphate levels usually return to normal 2-4 weeks after discontinuation of therapy; monitor serum phosphate closely

Precautions Use with caution in patients with restricted calcium and vitamin D intake; use with caution in patients with enterocolitis due to etidronate's potential to cause diarrhea particularly when using high dosages; dosage modification required in renal impairment

Adverse Reactions Generally dose-related and most significant when taking oral doses >5 mg/kg/day

Central nervous system: Fever, convulsions, pain, amnesia, confusion, depression, hallucinations
Dermatologic: Angioedema, rash, alopecia, follicular eruption
Endocrine & metabolic: Hyperphosphatemia, hypocalcemia, hypomagnesemia, fluid overload
Gastrointestinal: Diarrhea, nausea, vomiting, occult blood in stools, dysgeusia, esophagitis, glossitis
Hematologic: Agranulocytosis (rare), leukopenia (rare)
Neuromuscular & skeletal: Bone pain, risk of fractures increased, rachitic syndrome (found in children taking dosage >10 mg/kg/day over 1 year or longer); joint pain, muscle pain, paresthesia
Renal: Nephrotoxicity
Miscellaneous: Hypersensitivity reactions

Drug Interactions
Avoid Concomitant Use There are no known interactions where it is recommended to avoid concomitant use.

Increased Effect/Toxicity
Etidronate Disodium may increase the levels/effects of: Phosphate Supplements

The levels/effects of Etidronate Disodium may be increased by: Aminoglycosides; Nonsteroidal Anti-Inflammatory Agents

Decreased Effect

The levels/effects of Etidronate Disodium may be decreased by: Antacids; Calcium Salts; Iron Salts; Magnesium Salts

Food Interactions Avoid concurrent administration with food high in calcium (eg, milk or milk products) which may decrease absorption; separate administration by at least 2 hours

Stability Store at room temperature.

Mechanism of Action Decreases bone resorption by inhibiting osteocystic osteolysis; decreases mineral release and matrix or collagen breakdown in bone

Pharmacodynamics

Onset of therapeutic effects: Within 1-3 months of therapy

Duration: Persists for 12 months without continuous therapy

Pharmacokinetics (Adult data unless noted)

Absorption: ~3%

Half-life: 1-6 hours

Elimination: Primarily as unchanged drug in urine (50%) with unabsorbed drug eliminated in feces

Usual Dosage

Oral:

Heterotopic ossification: Children and Adults:

Spinal cord injury: 20 mg/kg once daily (or in divided doses if GI discomfort occurs) for 2 weeks, then 10 mg/kg/day for 10 weeks

Total hip replacement: 20 mg/kg/day 1 month before and 3 months after surgery

Note: This dosage when used in children for >1 year has been associated with a rachitic syndrome.

Paget's disease: Adults: 5-10 mg/kg once daily for no more than 6 months; may give 11-20 mg/kg/day for up to 3 months. Daily dose may be divided if adverse GI effects occur; courses of therapy should be separated by drug-free periods of at least 3 months.

Dosing adjustment in renal impairment:

S_{cr} 2.5-4.9 mg/dL: Use with caution

S_{cr} ≥5 mg/dL: **Not recommended**

Administration

Oral: Administer on an empty stomach, 2 hours before meals

Monitoring Parameters Serum calcium, phosphate, creatinine, BUN

Patient Information Maintain adequate intake of calcium and vitamin D

Dosage Forms Excipient information presented when available (limited, particularly for generics); consult specific product labeling. [DSC] = Discontinued product

Tablet:

Didronel®: 200 mg [DSC]; 400 mg

◆ **EtOH** see Ethyl Alcohol on page 547

Etomidate (e TOM i date)

Medication Safety Issues

Sound-alike/look-alike issues:

Etomidate may be confused with etidronate

High alert medication: The Institute for Safe Medication Practices (ISMP) includes this medication among its list of drugs which have a heightened risk of causing significant patient harm when used in error.

U.S. Brand Names Amidate®

Canadian Brand Names Amidate®

Therapeutic Category General Anesthetic

Generic Available Yes

Use Induction and maintenance of general anesthesia particularly in patients with diminished cardiovascular function; sedation for short procedures

Pregnancy Risk Factor C

Contraindications Hypersensitivity to etomidate or any component of the formulation

Warnings Etomidate inhibits 11-B-hydroxylase, an enzyme necessary for the production of cortisol, aldosterone, and corticosterone. A single induction dose blocks the normal stress-induced increase in adrenal cortisol production for 4-8 hours and up to 24 hours in elderly and debilitated patients. This suppression does not appear to be dose related and is unresponsive to ACTH stimulation. Since prolonged infusion of etomidate for sedation particularly in critically ill patients may prevent the response to stress, use of prolonged continuous infusions is not recommended. Consider exogenous corticosteroid replacement in patients undergoing severe stress. Etomidate does not possess analgesic activity; use in combination with narcotic analgesics to blunt the hemodynamic response to endotracheal intubation or for painful procedures.

Precautions Use with caution in patients with renal failure and hepatic cirrhosis as the duration of effect may be prolonged; use with caution in patients with seizure disorder due to its ability to increase EEG activation with epileptiform spikes; high doses of etomidate have been associated with EEG slowing and isoelectricity; involuntary muscles movements or myoclonus occur in up to 30% of patients; this may be minimized by pretreatment with benzodiazepines or fentanyl

Adverse Reactions

Cardiovascular: Bradycardia, tachycardia and other arrhythmias, hypertension, hypotension

Central nervous system: Apnea

Endocrine & metabolic: Adrenal suppression (cortisol and aldosterone levels decreased)

Gastrointestinal: Nausea, vomiting, hiccups (10%)

Local: Pain at injection site (30% to 80%), thrombophlebitis

Neuromuscular & skeletal: Myoclonus (33%), transient skeletal movements, uncontrolled eye movements

Respiratory: Laryngospasm, hyperventilation, hypoventilation

Drug Interactions

Avoid Concomitant Use There are no known interactions where it is recommended to avoid concomitant use.

Increased Effect/Toxicity There are no known significant interactions involving an increase in effect.

Decreased Effect There are no known significant interactions involving a decrease in effect.

Stability Store at room temperature. Compatible when administered by Y-site injection with: Alfentanil, atracurium, atropine, doxacurium, ephedrine, fentanyl, lidocaine, lorazepam, midazolam, mivacurium, morphine, pancuronium, phenylephrine, succinylcholine, sufentanil. Incompatible with ascorbic acid, vecuronium

Mechanism of Action A carboxylated imidazole, etomidate is an ultrashort-acting nonbarbiturate hypnotic which produces a rapid induction of anesthesia with minimal cardiovascular effects; produces EEG burst suppression at high doses; decreases intracranial pressure with no effect on cerebral perfusion or heart rate; decreases intraocular pressure; does not produce histamine release

Pharmacodynamics

Onset of action: 30-60 seconds

Maximum effect: 1 minute

Duration: Dose dependent: 2-3 minutes (0.15 mg/kg dose); 4-10 minutes (0.3 mg/kg dose); rapid recovery is due to rapid redistribution

Pharmacokinetics (Adult data unless noted)

Distribution: V_d: 3.6-4.5 L/kg

Protein binding: 76%; decreased protein binding resulting in an increased percentage of "free" etomidate in patients with renal failure or hepatic cirrhosis

Metabolism: Hepatic and plasma esterases

Half-life, elimination: Terminal: 2.6-3.5 hours

Time to peak serum concentration: 7 minutes

Excretion: 75% excreted in urine over 24 hours; 2% excreted unchanged

Usual Dosage I.V.:

Induction & maintenance of anesthesia: Children >10 years and Adults: Initial: 0.2-0.6 mg/kg over 30-60 seconds; maintenance: 10-20 mcg/kg/minute; smaller doses may be used to supplement subpotent anesthetic agents

Procedural sedation: Limited data in children; initial doses 0.1-0.3 mg/kg have been used (see References); repeat doses may be needed depending upon the duration of the procedure and the response of the patient

Administration I.V.: Administer I.V. push over 30-60 seconds; very irritating; avoid administration into small vessels on the dorsum of the head or hand; preadministration of lidocaine may be beneficial

Monitoring Parameters Cardiac monitoring, blood pressure, respiratory rate, sedation score (procedural sedation)

Dosage Forms Excipient information presented when available (limited, particularly for generics); consult specific product labeling.

Injection, solution: 2 mg/mL (10 mL, 20 mL) [contains propylene glycol 35% v/v]

References

Falk J and Zed PJ, "Etomidate for Procedural Sedation in the Emergency Department," *Ann Pharmacother*, 2004, 38(7-8):1272-7.

Kienstra AJ, Ward MA, Sasan F, et al, "Etomidate Versus Pentobarbital for Sedation of Children for Head and Neck CT Imaging," *Pediatr Emerg Care*, 2004, 20(8):499-506.

Tobias JD, "Etomidate: Applications in Pediatric Critical Care and Pediatric Aanesthesiology," *Pediatr Crit Care Med*, 2000, 1(2):100-6.

Etoposide (e toe POE side)

Medication Safety Issues

Sound-alike/look-alike issues:

Etoposide may be confused with teniposide

VePesid® may be confused with Versed

High alert medication: The Institute for Safe Medication Practices (ISMP) includes this medication among its list of drugs which have a heightened risk of causing significant patient harm when used in error.

Related Information

Compatibility of Chemotherapy and Related Supportive Care Medications *on page 1580*

Emetogenic Potential of Antineoplastic Agents *on page 1579*

U.S. Brand Names Toposar™

Therapeutic Category Antineoplastic Agent, Mitotic Inhibitor

Generic Available Yes

Use Treatment of testicular and lung carcinomas, malignant lymphoma, Hodgkin's disease, leukemias (ALL, ANLL, AML), neuroblastoma; treatment of Ewing's sarcoma, rhabdomyosarcoma, osteosarcoma, Wilms' tumor, brain tumors; conditioning regimen with hematopoietic stem cell support

Pregnancy Risk Factor D

Pregnancy Considerations Animal studies have demonstrated teratogenicity and fetal loss. There are no adequate and well-controlled studies in pregnant women. Women of childbearing potential should be advised to avoid pregnancy.

Lactation Enters breast milk/contraindicated

Contraindications Hypersensitivity to etoposide or any component (see Warnings); pregnancy

Warnings Hazardous agent; use appropriate precautions for handling and disposal. Etoposide is mutagenic, potentially carcinogenic, teratogenic, and embryotoxic. Severe myelosuppression with resulting infection or bleeding may occur **[U.S. Boxed Warning]**; treatment should be withheld for platelets <50,000/mm³ or absolute neutrophil count (ANC) <500/mm³ until counts recover; injectable etoposide contains polysorbate 80 (polysorbate 80 has caused thrombocytopenia, ascites, and renal, pulmonary, and hepatic failure in premature infants who received an injectable vitamin E product containing polysorbate 80). Higher rates of anaphylactoid reactions have been reported in children who received I.V. infusions of etoposide at higher than recommended concentrations.

Etoposide injection contains benzyl alcohol which may cause allergic reactions in susceptible individuals; large amounts of benzyl alcohol (≥99 mg/kg/day) have been associated with a potentially fatal toxicity ("gasping syndrome") in neonates; the "gasping syndrome" consists of metabolic acidosis, respiratory distress, gasping respirations, CNS dysfunction (including convulsions, intracranial hemorrhage), hypotension and cardiovascular collapse; use etoposide injection containing benzyl alcohol with caution in neonates; *in vitro* and animal studies have shown that benzoate, a metabolite of benzyl alcohol, displaces bilirubin from protein binding sites

Precautions Use with caution and consider dosage reduction in patients with hepatic impairment, bone marrow suppression, and renal impairment

Adverse Reactions

Cardiovascular: Hypotension, tachycardia, facial flushing

Central nervous system: Somnolence, fatigue, fever, headache, chills

Dermatologic: Alopecia, rash, urticaria, angioedema

Gastrointestinal: Nausea, vomiting, diarrhea, mucositis, anorexia, constipation

Hematologic: Myelosuppression, anemia (granulocyte nadir: ~7-14 days, platelet nadir: ~9-16 days)

Hepatic: Hepatotoxicity

Local: Thrombophlebitis

Neuromuscular & skeletal: Peripheral neuropathy, weakness

Respiratory: Bronchospasm

Miscellaneous: Anaphylactoid reactions

Drug Interactions

Metabolism/Transport Effects Substrate of CYP1A2 (minor), CYP2E1 (minor), CYP3A4 (major), P-glycoprotein; **Inhibits** CYP2C9 (weak), 3A4 (weak)

Avoid Concomitant Use

Avoid concomitant use of Etoposide with any of the following: BCG; Natalizumab; Pimecrolimus; Tacrolimus (Topical); Vaccines (Live)

Increased Effect/Toxicity

Etoposide may increase the levels/effects of: Leflunomide; Natalizumab; Vaccines (Live); Vitamin K Antagonists

The levels/effects of Etoposide may be increased by: Atovaquone; CycloSPORINE; CycloSPORINE (Systemic); CYP3A4 Inhibitors (Moderate); CYP3A4 Inhibitors (Strong); Dasatinib; Denosumab; P-Glycoprotein Inhibitors; Pimecrolimus; Tacrolimus (Topical); Trastuzumab

Decreased Effect

Etoposide may decrease the levels/effects of: BCG; Sipuleucel-T; Vaccines (Inactivated); Vaccines (Live); Vitamin K Antagonists

The levels/effects of Etoposide may be decreased by: Barbiturates; CYP3A4 Inducers (Strong); Deferasirox; Echinacea; Herbs (CYP3A4 Inducers); P-Glycoprotein Inducers; Phenytoin

Food Interactions Administration of food does not affect GI absorption with doses ≤200 mg

Stability Stability of diluted injection is concentration dependent when diluted in D_5W or NS (ie, 0.2 mg/mL: 96 hours; 0.4 mg/mL: 24 hours); at a concentration of 1 mg/mL in D_5W or NS, crystallization has occurred within 30 minutes; incidence of precipitation increases when final infusion concentration is >0.4 mg/mL; intact vials remain stable for 2 years at room temperature; refrigerate capsules.

Mechanism of Action Inhibits mitotic activity; inhibits DNA type II topoisomerase producing single- and double-strand DNA breaks

Pharmacokinetics (Adult data unless noted)
Absorption: Oral: Large variability
Distribution: CSF concentration is <5% of plasma concentration
Children: V_{dss}: 10 L/m^2
Adults: V_{dss}: 7-17 L/m^2
Protein binding: 94% to 97%
Metabolism: In the liver (with a biphasic decay)
Bioavailability: Averages 50% (range: 10% to 80%, dose-dependent)
Half-life, terminal:
Children: 6-8 hours
Adults: 4-15 hours with normal renal and hepatic function
Time to peak serum concentration: Oral: Within 1-1.5 hours
Elimination: Both unchanged drug and metabolites are excreted in urine and a small amount (2% to 16%) in feces; up to 55% of an I.V. dose is excreted unchanged in urine in children

Usual Dosage Refer to individual protocols
Children: I.V.: 60-150 mg/m^2/day for 2-5 days every 3-6 weeks
AML:
Remission induction: 150 mg/m^2/day for 2-3 days for 2-3 cycles
Intensification or consolidation: 250 mg/m^2/day for 3 days, on courses 2-5
Brain tumor: 150 mg/m^2/day on days 2 and 3 of treatment course
Neuroblastoma: 100 mg/m^2/day over 1 hour on days 1-5 of cycle; repeat cycle every 4 weeks
High-dose conditioning regimen for allogeneic BMT: 60 mg/kg/dose as a single dose
BMT conditioning regimen used in patients with rhabdomyosarcoma or neuroblastoma: I.V. continuous infusion: 160 mg/m^2/day for 4 days
Adults:
Testicular cancer: I.V.: 50-100 mg/m^2/day on days 1-5 or 100 mg/m^2/day on days 1, 3 and 5 every 3-4 weeks for 3-4 courses
Small cell lung cancer:
Oral: Twice the I.V. dose rounded to the nearest 50 mg given once daily if total dose ≤400 mg/day or in divided doses if >400 mg/day
I.V.: 35 mg/m^2/day for 4 days or 50 mg/m^2/day for 5 days every 3-4 weeks

Dosing adjustment in renal impairment:
Cl_{cr} 10-50 mL/minute: Administer 75% of normal dose
Cl_{cr} <10 mL/minute: Administer 50% of normal dose

Dosing adjustment in patients with elevated serum bilirubin: Reduce dose by 50% for bilirubin 1.5-3 mg/dL; reduce dose by 75% for bilirubin >3 mg/dL

Administration
Oral: If necessary, the injection may be used for oral administration. Mix with orange juice, apple juice, or lemonade at a final concentration not to exceed 0.4 mg/mL to prevent precipitation. Etoposide has been found to be stable with no loss of potency over 3 hours when administered in apple juice or lemonade at concentrations of 1 mg/mL.

Parenteral: I.V.: Do not administer by rapid I.V. injection or by intrathecal, intraperitoneal, or intrapleural routes due to possible severe toxicity. Administer by continuous I.V. infusion or I.V. intermittent infusion via an in-line 0.22 micron filter over at least 60 minutes at a rate not to exceed 100 mg/m^2/hour (or 3.3 mg/kg/hour) to minimize the risk of hypotensive reactions at a final concentration for administration of 0.2-0.4 mg/mL in NS or D_5W. More concentrated I.V. solutions (0.6-1 mg/mL) can be infused but have shorter stability times (see Stability). For high-dose etoposide infusions, undiluted etoposide (20 mg/mL) has been infused as a single dose from a glass syringe via syringe pump through a central venous catheter over 1-4 hours. Problems associated with higher than recommended concentrations of etoposide infusions include cracking of hard plastic in chemo venting pins and infusion lines; inspect infusion solution for particulate matter and plastic devices for cracks and leaks.

Monitoring Parameters CBC with differential and platelet count, hemoglobin, vital signs (blood pressure), bilirubin, liver and renal function tests; inspect solution and tubing for precipitation before and during infusion

Patient Information Notify physician if fever, sore throat, painful/burning urination, extreme fatigue, pain or numbness in extremities, yellowing of eyes or skin, bruising, bleeding or shortness of breath occurs

Nursing Implications Adequate airway and other supportive measures and agents for treating hypotension or anaphylactoid reactions should be present when I.V. etoposide is given

Dosage Forms Excipient information presented when available (limited, particularly for generics); consult specific product labeling.
Capsule, softgel: 50 mg
Injection, solution: 20 mg/mL (5 mL, 25 mL, 50 mL) [contains benzyl alcohol, ethanol 30.5%, polyethylene glycol 300, and polysorbate 80]
Toposar™: 20 mg/mL (5 mL, 25 mL, 50 mL) [contains dehydrated ethanol 33.2%, polyethylene glycol 300, and polysorbate 80]

References

Berg SL, Grisell DL, DeLaney TF, et al, "Principles of Treatment of Pediatric Solid Tumors," *Pediatr Clin North Am*, 1991, 38(2):249-67.

Boos J, Krümpelmann S, Schulze-Westhoff P, et al, "Steady-State Levels and Bone Marrow Toxicity of Etoposide in Children and Infants: Does Etoposide Require Age-Dependent Dose Calculation?" *J Clin Oncol*, 1995, 13(12):2954-60.

Clark PI and Slevin ML, "The Clinical Pharmacology of Etoposide and Teniposide," *Clin Pharmacokinet*, 1987, 12(4):223-52.

Lazarus HM, Creger RJ, and Diaz D, "Simple Method for the Administration of High-Dose Etoposide During Autologous Bone Marrow Transplantation," *Cancer Treat Rep*, 1986, 70(6):819-20.

Nishikawa A, Nakamura Y, Nobori U, et al, "Acute Monocytic Leukemia in Children. Response to VP-16-213 as a Single Agent," *Cancer*, 1987, 60(9):2146-9.

O'Dwyer PJ, Leyland-Jones B, Alonso MT, et al, "Etoposide (VP-16-213): Current Status of an Active Anticancer Drug," *N Engl J Med*, 1985, 312(11):692-700.

◆ **Euglucon® (Can)** *see* GlyBURIDE *on page 648*

◆ **Eurax®** *see* Crotamiton *on page 364*

◆ **Euro-Lithium (Can)** *see* Lithium *on page 834*

◆ **Eutectic Mixture of Lidocaine and Tetracaine** *see* Lidocaine and Tetracaine *on page 824*

◆ **Euthyrox (Can)** *see* Levothyroxine *on page 816*

◆ **Evac-U-Gen [OTC]** *see* Senna *on page 1253*

◆ **Evamist™** *see* Estradiol *on page 536*

◆ **Everone® 200 (Can)** *see* Testosterone *on page 1325*

◆ **Evithrom™** *see* Thrombin (Topical) *on page 1345*

◆ **Evoclin®** *see* Clindamycin *on page 327*

◆ **Exalgo™** *see* HYDROmorphone *on page 689*

◆ **Excedrin® Tension Headache [OTC]** *see* Acetaminophen *on page 36*

- **ExeClear-C** *see* Guaifenesin and Codeine *on page 657*
- **Exjade®** *see* Deferasirox *on page 395*
- **ex-lax® [OTC]** *see* Senna *on page 1253*
- **ex-lax® Maximum Strength [OTC]** *see* Senna *on page 1253*
- **ex-lax® Ultra [OTC]** *see* Bisacodyl *on page 194*
- **Exorex®** *see* Coal Tar *on page 349*
- **Extina®** *see* Ketoconazole *on page 780*
- **EZ-Char™ [OTC]** *see* Charcoal, Activated *on page 284*

Ezetimibe (ez ET i mibe)

Medication Safety Issues
Sound-alike/look-alike issues:
Zetia® may be confused with Zebeta®, Zestril®

Related Information
Normal Laboratory Values for Children *on page 1672*

U.S. Brand Names Zetia®

Canadian Brand Names Ezetrol®

Therapeutic Category Antilipemic Agent; Cholesterol Absorption Inhibitor

Generic Available No

Use Adjunct to dietary therapy or in combination with HMG-CoA reductase inhibitor (atorvastatin, simvastatin) to decrease elevated serum total and low density lipoprotein cholesterol (LDL-C), apolipoprotein B (apo-B), and triglyceride levels in patients with primary hypercholesterolemia (heterozygous, familial and nonfamilial); in combination with HMG-CoA reductase inhibitor (atorvastatin, simvastatin) in the treatment of homozygous familial hypercholesterolemia; in combination with fenofibrate in the treatment of mixed hyperlipidemia; adjunct to dietary therapy for the reduction of elevated sitosterol and campesterol levels in patients with homozygous familial sitosterolemia (FDA approved in ages ≥10 years and adults) (see Additional Information for recommendations on Initiating hypercholesterolemia pharmacologic treatment in children ≥8 years)

Pregnancy Risk Factor C

Pregnancy Considerations Safety and efficacy have not been established; use during pregnancy only if the potential benefit to the mother outweighs the possible risk to the fetus.

Lactation Excretion in breast milk unknown/not recommended

Contraindications Hypersensitivity to ezetimibe or any component; active liver disease; unexplained persistent elevations of serum transaminases

Warnings The incidence of rhabdomyolysis or myopathy in clinical trials with ezetimibe was no different than that of placebo; however, rhabdomyolysis and myopathy are known adverse effects of HMG-CoA reductase inhibitors which are often used in combination with ezetimibe; follow rhabdomyolysis and myopathy monitoring recommendations for HMG-CoA reductase inhibitors when used in combination; also when ezetimibe is used in combination with HMG-CoA reductase inhibitors, the incidence of elevated serum transaminases was higher than when the HMG-CoA reductase inhibitors were used alone; monitor serum transaminases when used in combination with HMG-CoA reductase inhibitors. When studied in combination with fenofibrate, an increase in cholecystectomy rate (0.6% vs 1.7%) when compared with monotherapy was observed; monitor for signs and symptoms of cholelithiasis when used with fenofibrate.

Precautions Use with caution in patients with renal or mild hepatic impairment

Adverse Reactions
Cardiovascular: Chest pain
Central nervous system: Fatigue

Gastrointestinal: Abdominal pain, cholelithiasis (when used in combination with fenofibrate; see Warnings), diarrhea

Hepatic: Serum transaminases elevated (0.5%; 1.3% when used in combination with HMG-CoA reductase inhibitors)

Neuromuscular & skeletal: Arthralgia, back pain

Respiratory: Cough, pharyngitis, sinusitis, URI

Miscellaneous: Viral infections

<1% and postmarketing/case reports: Abdominal pain, anaphylaxis, angioedema, autoimmune hepatitis (Stolk, 2006), cholecystitis, cholelithiasis, cholestatic hepatitis (Stolk, 2006), CPK increased, depression, dizziness, erythema multiforme, headache, hepatitis, hypersensitivity reactions, myalgia, myopathy, nausea, pancreatitis, paresthesia, rash, rhabdomyolysis, thrombocytopenia, urticaria

Drug Interactions
Metabolism/Transport Effects Substrate of SLCO1B1

Avoid Concomitant Use There are no known interactions where it is recommended to avoid concomitant use.

Increased Effect/Toxicity
Ezetimibe may increase the levels/effects of: CycloSPORINE; CycloSPORINE (Systemic)

The levels/effects of Ezetimibe may be increased by: CycloSPORINE; CycloSPORINE (Systemic); Eltrombopag; Fibric Acid Derivatives

Decreased Effect
The levels/effects of Ezetimibe may be decreased by: Bile Acid Sequestrants

Stability Store at controlled room temperature.

Mechanism of Action Ezetimibe reduces blood cholesterol by inhibiting the absorption of cholesterol by the small intestine

Pharmacodynamics
Onset of action: Within 1 week
Maximum effect: 2-4 weeks

Pharmacokinetics (Adult data unless noted)
Protein binding: >90%

Metabolism: Extensively conjugated in the liver and small intestine to a pharmacologically active metabolite; may undergo enterohepatic recycling

Bioavailability: Variable

Hepatic impairment: Child-Pugh score 7-9: AUC increased 3-4 times; Child-Pugh 10-15: AUC increased 5-6 times

Renal impairment: Severe renal dysfunction (Cl_{cr} <30 mL/minute/1.73 m^2): AUC increased 1.5 times

Half-life: Adults: 22 hours

Time to peak serum concentration: 4-12 hours (ezetimibe); 1-2 hours (active metabolite)

Elimination: Feces (78%, 69% as ezetimibe): urine (11%, 9% as metabolite)

Usual Dosage Oral: Adolescents ≥10 years and Adults: 10 mg once daily

Dosing adjustment in renal impairment: Bioavailability increased with severe impairment; no dosage adjustment is necessary

Dosing adjustment in hepatic impairment: Bioavailability increased with moderate to severe impairment
Mild hepatic impairment (Child-Pugh score 5-6): No dosing adjustment necessary
Moderate to severe impairment (Child-Pugh score 7-15): Use of ezetimibe not recommended due to increased bioavailability (see Pharmacokinetics)

Administration Oral: May be taken without regard to meals or time of day; may be administered with an HMG-CoA inhibitor (eg, atorvastatin, simvastatin)

Monitoring Parameters Serum cholesterol (total and fractionated), CPK; liver function tests (see Precautions)

Reference Range See Related Information for age- and gender-specific serum cholesterol, LDL-C, TG, and HDL concentrations.

Patient Information May cause dizziness or fatigue; may impair ability to perform activities requiring mental alertness or physical coordination

Additional Information The current recommendation for pharmacologic treatment of hypercholesterolemia in children is limited to children ≥8 years of age and is based on LDL-C concentrations and the presence of coronary vascular disease (CVD) risk factors (see table and Daniels, 2008). In adults, for each 1% lowering in LDL-C, the relative risk for major cardiovascular events is reduced by ~1%. For more specific risk assessment and treatment recommendations for adults, see NCEP ATPIII, 2001.

Recommendations for Initiating Pharmacologic Treatment in Children ≥8 Years[1]

No risk factors for CVD	LDL ≥190 mg/dL despite 6-month to 1-year diet therapy
Family history of premature CVD or ≥2 CVD risk factors present, including obesity, hypertension, or cigarette smoking	LDL ≥160 mg/dL despite 6-month to 1-year diet therapy
Diabetes mellitus present	LDL ≥130 mg/dL

[1]Adapted from Daniels SR, Greer FR, and Committee on Nutrition, "Lipid Screening and Cardiovascular Health in Childhood," *Pediatrics*, 2008, 122 (1):198-208.

Dosage Forms Excipient information presented when available (limited, particularly for generics); consult specific product labeling.
Tablet:
Zetia®: 10 mg

References

American Academy of Pediatrics Committee on Nutrition, "Cholesterol in Childhood," *Pediatrics*, 1998, 101(1 Pt 1):141-7.

American Academy of Pediatrics, "National Cholesterol Education Program: Report of the Expert Panel on Blood Cholesterol Levels in Children and Adolescents," *Pediatrics*, 1992, 89(3 Pt 2):525-84.

Daniels SR, Greer FR, and Committee on Nutrition, "Lipid Screening and Cardiovascular Health in Childhood," *Pediatrics*, 2008, 122 (1):198-208.

Gagne C, Gaudet D, Bruckert E, et al, "Efficacy and Safety of Ezetimibe Coadministered With Atorvastatin or Simvastatin in Patients With Homozygous Familial Hypercholesterolemia," *Circulation*, 2002, 105 (21):2469-75.

McCrindle BW, Urbina EM, Dennison BA, et al, "Drug Therapy of High-Risk Lipid Abnormalities in Children and Adolescents: A Scientific Statement from the American Heart Association Atherosclerosis, Hypertension, and Obesity in Youth Committee, Council of Cardiovascular Disease in the Young, With the Council on Cardiovascular Nursing," *Circulation*, 2007, 115(14):1948-67.

Stolk MF, Becx MC, Kuypers KC, et al, "Severe Hepatic Side Effects of Ezetimibe," *Clin Gastroenterol Hepatol*, 2006, 4(7):908-11.

"Third Report of the National Cholesterol Education Program Expert Panel on Detection, Evaluation, and Treatment of High Blood Cholesterol in Adults (Adult Treatment Panel III)," May 2001, www.nhlbi.nih.gov/guidelines/cholesterol.

Ezetimibe and Simvastatin
(ez ET i mibe & SIM va stat in)

Medication Safety Issues
Sound-alike/look-alike issues:
Vytorin® may be confused with Vyvanse™

Related Information
Normal Laboratory Values for Children *on page 1672*

U.S. Brand Names Vytorin®

Therapeutic Category Antilipemic Agent; Cholesterol Absorption Inhibitor; HMG-CoA Reductase Inhibitor

Generic Available No

Use
Hyperlipidemia: Adjunct to dietary therapy to decrease elevated serum total and low density lipoprotein cholesterol (LDL-C), apolipoprotein B (apo-B), and triglyceride levels, and to increase high density lipoprotein cholesterol (HDL-C) in patients with primary hypercholesterolemia (heterozygous, familial and nonfamilial) and mixed dyslipidemia (Fredrickson types IIa and IIb); treatment of homozygous familial hypercholesterolemia (see Additional Information for recommendations on initiating hypercholesterolemia pharmacologic treatment in children ≥8 years); treatment of isolated hypertriglyceridemia (Fredrickson type IV) and type III hyperlipoproteinemia

Primary prevention of cardiovascular disease in high risk patients; risk factors include: Age >55 years, smoking, hypertension, low HDL-C, or family history of early coronary heart disease

Pregnancy Risk Factor X

Pregnancy Considerations See individual agents.

Lactation Excretion in breast milk unknown/contraindicated

Breast-Feeding Considerations See individual agents.

Contraindications Hypersensitivity to simvastatin, ezetimibe, or any component; active liver disease; unexplained persistent elevations of serum transaminases; pregnancy

Warnings Rhabdomyolysis with or without acute renal failure secondary to myoglobinuria has occurred rarely. Risk is increased with increasing simvastatin doses (0.02% at 20 mg, 0.07% at 40 mg, and 0.3% at 80 mg) and with concurrent use of amiodarone, clarithromycin, danazol, diltiazem, fluvoxamine, indinavir, nefazodone, nelfinavir, ritonavir, verapamil, troleandomycin, cyclosporine, fibric acid derivatives, erythromycin, niacin, or azole antifungals. Avoid concomitant use with itraconazole, ketoconazole, erythromycin, clarithromycin, telithromycin, HIV protease inhibitors, and nefazodone. Assess the risk versus benefit before combining amiodarone, danazol, diltiazem, fluvoxamine, verapamil, cyclosporine, fibric acid derivatives, and niacin with simvastatin. A lowered dosage of simvastatin is recommended when used with some of these medications (see Usual Dosage). Discontinue Vytorin™ in any patient experiencing unexplained muscle pain, tenderness or weakness, and/or CPK level >10 times the normal range. Monitor CPK periodically in patients with complicated medical histories including renal insufficiency.

Precautions Persistent increases in serum transaminases have occurred; liver function must be monitored by laboratory assessment at the initiation of therapy and periodically thereafter for the first year of treatment or until one year after the last elevation in dose. Patients titrated to the 80 mg dose should receive an additional test at 3 months of therapy. Use with caution in patients with liver dysfunction, diabetes mellitus, and renal impairment (may be at increased risk for developing rhabdomyolysis)

Drug Interactions

Metabolism/Transport Effects
Ezetimibe: **Substrate** of SLCO1B1
Simvastatin: **Substrate** of CYP3A4 (major), SLCO1B1; **Inhibits** CYP2C8 (weak), 2C9 (weak), 2D6 (weak)

Avoid Concomitant Use
Avoid concomitant use of Ezetimibe and Simvastatin with any of the following: Protease Inhibitors

Increased Effect/Toxicity
Ezetimibe and Simvastatin may increase the levels/effects of: CycloSPORINE; CycloSPORINE (Systemic); DAPTOmycin; Diltiazem; Vitamin K Antagonists

The levels/effects of Ezetimibe and Simvastatin may be increased by: Amiodarone; Antifungal Agents (Azole Derivatives, Systemic); Colchicine; CycloSPORINE; CycloSPORINE (Systemic); CYP3A4 Inhibitors (Moderate); CYP3A4 Inhibitors (Strong); Danazol; Dasatinib; Diltiazem; Dronedarone; Eltrombopag; Fenofibrate; Fenofibric Acid; Fibric Acid Derivatives; Fluconazole; Fusidic Acid; Gemfibrozil; Grapefruit Juice; Imatinib; Macrolide Antibiotics; Nefazodone; Niacin; Niacinamide;

Protease Inhibitors; QuiNINE; Ranolazine; Rifamycin Derivatives; Sildenafil; Verapamil

Decreased Effect

The levels/effects of Ezetimibe and Simvastatin may be decreased by: Antacids; Bile Acid Sequestrants; Bosentan; CYP3A4 Inducers (Strong); Deferasirox; Etravirine; Phenytoin; Rifamycin Derivatives; St Johns Wort

Food Interactions Simvastatin serum concentration may be increased when taken with large quantities (>1 quart/ day) of grapefruit juice; avoid concurrent use

Stability Tablets should be stored in well closed containers at temperatures between 5°C to 30°C (41°F to 86°F)

Mechanism of Action Ezetimibe reduces blood cholesterol by inhibiting the absorption of cholesterol by the small intestine. Simvastatin is a methylated derivative of lovastatin that acts by competitively inhibiting 3-hydroxy-3-methylglutaryl-coenzyme A (HMG-CoA) reductase, the enzyme that catalyzes the rate-limiting step in cholesterol biosynthesis.

Pharmacodynamics

Onset of action: >3 days

Maximum effect: After 2-4 weeks

Pharmacokinetics (Adult data unless noted) See individual agents

Usual Dosage Oral:

Homozygous familial hypercholesterolemia: Children ≥10 years and Adults: Ezetimibe 10 mg/simvastatin 40 mg once daily in the evening; may increase to ezetimibe 10 mg/simvastatin 80 mg once daily as needed

Hyperlipidemia: Adults: Initial: 10 mg ezetimibe/20 mg simvastatin once daily in the evening; patients requiring less aggressive LDL-C reductions may be started on 10 mg ezetimibe/10 mg simvastatin; patients who require a reduction of >55% in LDL-C may be started at 10 mg ezetimibe/40 mg simvastatin once daily

Dosage adjustment in patients who are concomitantly receiving cyclosporine or danazol: Adults: Not for use unless the patient has tolerated simvastatin at a does of ≥5 mg; the daily dose should not to exceed 10 mg ezetimibe/10 mg simvastatin

Dosage adjustment in patients receiving concomitant amiodarone or verapamil: Adults: The daily dose should not exceed 10 mg ezetimibe/20 mg simvastatin

Dosage adjustment with gemfibrozil: Although concurrent use is not recommended by manufacturer, the daily dose should not exceed 10 mg ezetimibe/10 mg simvastatin

Dosing adjustment in renal impairment: Adults: Because simvastatin does not undergo significant renal excretion, modification of dose should only be necessary in patients with severe renal impairment: Cl_{cr}<10 mL/ minute: Not for use unless the patient has tolerated simvastatin at a dose of ≥5 mg, the daily dose should not to exceed 10 mg ezetimibe/10 mg simvastatin

Administration Oral: May be taken without regard to meals. Administration with the evening meal or at bedtime has been associated with somewhat greater LDL-C reduction.

Monitoring Parameters Serum cholesterol (total and fractionated), CPK; liver function tests (see Precautions)

Reference Range See Related Information for age- and gender-specific serum cholesterol, LDL-C, TG, and HDL concentrations.

Patient Information May rarely cause photosensitivity reactions (eg, exposure to sunlight may cause severe sunburn, skin rash, redness, or itching); avoid direct exposure to sunlight. Report severe and unresolved gastric upset, any vision changes, muscle pain and weakness, changes in color of urine or stool, yellowing of skin or eyes, and any unusual bruising. Female patients of childbearing age must be counseled to use 2 effective forms of contraception simultaneously, unless absolute abstinence is the chosen method; this drug may cause severe fetal defects.

Additional Information The current recommendation for pharmacologic treatment of hypercholesterolemia in children is limited to children ≥8 years of age and is based on LDL-C concentrations and the presence of coronary vascular disease (CVD) risk factors (see table and Daniels, 2008). In adults, for each 1% lowering in LDL-C, the relative risk for major cardiovascular events is reduced by ~1%. For more specific risk assessment and treatment recommendations for adults, see NCEP ATPIII, 2001.

Recommendations for Initiating Pharmacologic Treatment in Children ≥8 Years[1]

No risk factors for CVD	LDL ≥190 mg/dL despite 6-month to 1-year diet therapy
Family history of premature CVD or ≥2 CVD risk factors present, including obesity, hypertension, or cigarette smoking	LDL ≥160 mg/dL despite 6-month to 1-year diet therapy
Diabetes mellitus present	LDL ≥130 mg/dL

[1]Adapted from Daniels SR, Greer FR, and Committee on Nutrition, "Lipid Screening and Cardiovascular Health in Childhood," *Pediatrics*, 2008, 122 (1):198-208.

Dosage Forms Excipient information presented when available (limited, particularly for generics); consult specific product labeling.

Tablet:

Vytorin® 10/10: Ezetimibe 10 mg and simvastatin 10 mg

Vytorin® 10/20: Ezetimibe 10 mg and simvastatin 20 mg

Vytorin® 10/40: Ezetimibe 10 mg and simvastatin 40 mg

Vytorin® 10/80: Ezetimibe 10 mg and simvastatin 80 mg

References

American Academy of Pediatrics, Committee on Nutrition, "Cholesterol in Childhood," *Pediatrics*, 1998, 101(1 Pt 1):141-7.

"American Academy of Pediatrics, National Cholesterol Education Program: Report of the Expert Panel on Blood Cholesterol Levels in Children and Adolescents," *Pediatrics*, 1992, 89(3 Pt 2):525-84.

Daniels SR, Greer FR, and Committee on Nutrition, "Lipid Screening and Cardiovascular Health in Childhood," *Pediatrics*, 2008, 122 (1):198-208.

Dejongh S, Stalenhoef AF, Tuohy MB, et al, "Efficacy, Safety, and Tolerability of Simvastatin in Children With Familial Hypercholesterolemia: Rational, Design and Baseline Characterisitics," *Clin Drug Invest*, 2002, 23(8):533-40.

Ducobu J, Brasseur D, Chaudron JM, et al, "Simvastatin Use in Children," *Lancet*, 1992, 339(8807):1488.

Duplaga BA, "Treatment of Childhood Hypercholesterolemia With HMG-CoA Reductase Inhibitors," *Ann Pharmacother*, 1999, 33 (11):1224-7.

Gagne C, Gaudet D, Bruckert E, et al, "Efficacy and Safety of Ezetimibe Coadministered With Atorvastatin or Simvastatin in Patients With Homozygous Familial Hypercholesterolemia," *Circulation*, 2002, 105 (21):2469-75.

Grundy SM, Cleeman JI, Merz CN, et al, "Implications of Recent Clinical Trials for the National Cholesterol Education Program Adult Treatment Panel III Guidelines," *Circulation*, 2004, 110(2):227-39.

McCrindle BW, Urbina EM, Dennison BA, et al, "Drug Therapy of High-Risk Lipid Abnormalities in Children and Adolescents: A Scientific Statement from the American Heart Association Atherosclerosis, Hypertension, and Obesity in Youth Committee, Council of Cardiovascular Disease in the Young, With the Council on Cardiovascular Nursing," *Circulation*, 2007, 115(14):1948-67.

"Third Report of the National Cholesterol Education Program Expert Panel on Detection, Evaluation, and Treatment of High Blood Cholesterol in Adults (Adult Treatment Panel III)," May 2001, www.nhlbi.nih.gov/guidelines/cholesterol.

♦ **Ezetrol® (Can)** *see* Ezetimibe *on page 553*

♦ **E•R•O [OTC]** *see* Carbamide Peroxide *on page 248*

♦ **F₃T** *see* Trifluridine *on page 1384*

♦ **Fabrazyme®** *see* Agalsidase Beta *on page 53*

Factor VIIa (Recombinant)
(FAK ter SEV en ree KOM be nant)

Medication Safety Issues
Sound-alike/look-alike issues:
NovoSeven® RT may be confused with Novacet®

U.S. Brand Names NovoSeven® RT

Canadian Brand Names Niastase®

Therapeutic Category Antihemophilic Agent

Generic Available No

Use Treatment of bleeding episodes and prevention of bleeding in surgical interventions in patients with either hemophilia A or B when inhibitors to factor VIII or factor IX are present, acquired hemophilia, or congenital factor VII deficiency [FDA approved in pediatrics (age not specified) and adults]

Pregnancy Risk Factor C

Pregnancy Considerations Animal studies have demonstrated fetal loss, but no evidence of teratogenic effects. There are no adequate and well-controlled studies in pregnant women. Use only if the potential benefit justifies the potential risk to the fetus.

Lactation Excretion in breast milk unknown/not recommended

Contraindications Hypersensitivity to factor VII or any component

Warnings Serious and sometimes fatal thrombotic events have been associated with the use of factor VIIa outside labeled indications **[U.S. Boxed Warning]**. Arterial and venous thrombotic and thromboembolic events, some fatal, following administration of factor VIIa have been reported during postmarketing surveillance. Thrombotic events have also been reported when used within labeled indications; thrombotic events may be increased in patients with disseminated intravascular coagulation (DIC), advanced atherosclerotic disease, sepsis, crush injury, or concomitant treatment with prothrombin complex concentrates. All patients receiving factor VIIa should be monitored for signs and symptoms of activation of the coagulation system or thrombosis. Efficacy with prolonged infusions and data evaluating long-term adverse effects are limited.

Precautions Use with caution in patients with hypersensitivity to mouse, hamster, bovine proteins, or polysorbate 80. Monitor PT and factor VII coagulant activity in factor VII deficient patients; if no response, may consider testing for antibody formation.

Adverse Reactions
Cardiovascular: Angina, bradycardia, edema, hypertension, hypotension, MI, peripheral ischemia

Central nervous system: Ataxia, cerebral artery occlusion, cerebrovascular events, fever, headache, pain

Dermatologic: Pruritus, purpura, rash, urticaria

Gastrointestinal: Bowel infarction, nausea, vomiting

Hematologic: Arterial thrombosis (see Warnings), coagulation disorder, deep venous thrombosis, disseminated intravascular coagulation (DIC), fibrin degredation products increased, fibrinolysis increased, hemorrhage, hepatic artery thrombosis, plasma fibrinogen decreased, prothrombin decreased, renal artery thrombosis, retinal artery embolism, retinal artery thrombosis, thrombophlebitis

Local: Injection site reactions, I.V. site thrombosis

Neuromuscular & skeletal: Arthralgia, arthrosis, hemarthrosis

Renal: Abnormal renal function

Respiratory: Pneumonia, pulmonary embolism

Miscellaneous: Allergic reactions (including anaphylactic shock, angioedema, flushing, rash, and urticaria), antibody formation

Drug Interactions
Avoid Concomitant Use There are no known interactions where it is recommended to avoid concomitant use.

Increased Effect/Toxicity There are no known significant interactions involving an increase in effect.

Decreased Effect There are no known significant interactions involving a decrease in effect.

Stability NovoSeven® RT: Prior to reconstitution, store under refrigeration or between 2°C to 25°C (36°F to 77°F). Do not freeze. Protect from light. Reconstituted solutions may be stored at room temperature or under refrigeration but must be infused within 3 hours of reconstitution. Do not freeze reconstituted solutions. Do not store reconstituted solutions in syringes.

Mechanism of Action Recombinant factor VIIa, a vitamin K-dependent glycoprotein, promotes hemostasis by activating the extrinsic pathway of the coagulation cascade. It replaces deficient activated coagulation factor VII, which complexes with tissue factor and may activate coagulation factor X to Xa and factor IX to IXa. When complexed with other factors, coagulation factor Xa converts prothrombin to thrombin, a key step in the formation of a fibrin-platelet hemostatic plug.

Pharmacodynamics
Onset of action: 10-20 minutes

Maximum effect: 6 hours

Pharmacokinetics (Adult data unless noted)
Distribution: V_d: Children: 130 mL/kg; Adults: 103-105 mL/kg (range: 78-139 mL/kg)

Half-life: Elimination: Children: 1.32 hours; Adults: 2.3 hours (range: 1.7-2.7 hours)

Time to peak serum concentration: 15 minutes

Elimination: Clearance: Children: 67 mL/kg/hour; Adults: 30-36 mL/kg/hour (range: 27-49 mL/kg/hour)

Usual Dosage I.V.: Children and Adults:

Hemophilia A or B with inhibitors:

Bleeding episodes: 90 mcg/kg every 2 hours until hemostasis is achieved or until the treatment is judged ineffective. The dose and interval may be adjusted based upon the severity of bleeding and the degree of hemostasis achieved. Doses between 35-120 mcg/kg have been used successfully in clinical trials. The dose, interval, and duration of therapy may be adjusted based on severity of bleeding and the degree of hemostasis achieved. For patients treated for joint or muscle bleeds, a decision on the outcome of treatment was reached within 8 doses in the majority of patients, although more doses were required for severe bleeds; adverse effects were reported most commonly in patients treated with 12 or more doses. For patients experiencing severe bleeds to maintain the hemostatic plug, dosing should be continued at 3- to 6-hour intervals; the duration of posthemostatic dosing should be minimized.

Surgical interventions: 90 mcg/kg immediately before surgery; repeat at 2-hour intervals for the duration of surgery. Continue every 2 hours for 48 hours, then every 2-6 hours until healed for minor surgery; continue every 2 hours for 5 days, then every 4 hours until healed for major surgery

Congenital factor VII deficiency: Bleeding episodes and surgical interventions: 15-30 mcg/kg every 4-6 hours until hemostasis is achieved. Doses as low as 10 mcg/kg have been effective; individualized dosing is recommended.

Acquired hemophilia: 70-90 mcg/kg every 2-3 hours until hemostasis is achieved

Administration Parenteral: I.V.: NovoSeven® RT: Prior to reconstitution, bring to room temperature. Add recommended diluent along wall of vial; do not inject directly onto powder. Gently swirl until dissolved. Reconstitute each vial to a final concentration of 1 mg/mL using the provided histidine diluent as follows:

1 mg vial: 1.1 mL histidine diluent
2 mg vial: 2.1 mL histidine diluent
5 mg vial: 5.2 mL histidine diluent
Administer as a slow bolus over 2-5 minutes.

Monitoring Parameters Monitor for evidence of hemostasis; although the prothrombin time/INR, aPTT, and factor VII clotting activity have no correlation with achieving clinical hemostasis, these parameters may be useful as adjunct tests to evaluate efficacy and guide dose or interval adjustments

Patient Information This medication can only be administered I.V. Report swelling, pain, burning, or itching at infusion site. Report acute headache, visual changes, pain in joints or muscles, respiratory difficulty, chills, back pain, dizziness, nausea, or other unusual effects; inform healthcare provider if you are or intend to become pregnant.

Additional Information Each mg factor VIIa contains 0.4 mEq sodium and 0.01 mEq calcium; "off-label" uses in limited patient populations have been reported (primarily adult patients) including reversal of anticoagulant over dose and reduction in bleeding associated with thrombocytopenia, trauma, hepatic dysfunction, and cardiac bypass surgery; further randomized, blinded clinical trials are needed to determine efficacy, dosage, and safety for these indications (see Ghorashian, 2004; Tobias, 2004)

Dosage Forms Excipient information presented when available (limited, particularly for generics); consult specific product labeling.

Injection, powder for reconstitution [preservative free]:
NovoSeven® RT:
1 mg [contains polysorbate 80, sodium 0.4 mEq/mg rFVIIa, sucrose 10 mg/vial]
2 mg [contains polysorbate 80, sodium 0.4 mEq/mg rFVIIa, sucrose 20 mg/vial]
5 mg [contains polysorbate 80, sodium 0.4 mEq/mg rFVIIa, sucrose 50 mg/vial]

References

Ghorashian S and Hunt BJ, "'Off-License' Use of Recombinant Activated Factor VII," *Blood Rev*, 2004, 18(4):245-59.

Goodnough LT, Lublin DM, Zhang L, et al, "Transfusion Medicine Service Policies for Recombinant Factor VIIa Administration," *Transfusion*, 2004, 44(9):1325-31.

Tobias JD, Simsic JM, Weinstein S, et al, "Recombinant Factor VIIa to Control Excessive Bleeding Following Surgery for Congenital Heart Disease in Pediatric Patients," *J Intensive Care Med*, 2004, 19 (5):270-3.

◆ **Factor VIII** see Antihemophilic Factor (Human) on page 109

◆ **Factor VIII (Human)** see Antihemophilic Factor / von Willebrand Factor Complex (Human) on page 114

◆ **Factor VIII (Recombinant)** see Antihemophilic Factor (Recombinant) on page 112

Factor IX (FAK ter nyne)

U.S. Brand Names AlphaNine® SD; BeneFix®; Mononine®

Canadian Brand Names BeneFix®; Immunine® VH; Mononine®

Therapeutic Category Antihemophilic Agent; Blood Product Derivative

Generic Available No

Use Control bleeding in patients with factor IX deficiency (hemophilia B or Christmas disease)

Pregnancy Risk Factor C

Pregnancy Considerations Animal reproduction studies have not been conducted. Safety and efficacy in pregnant women have not been established. Use during pregnancy only if clearly needed. Parvovirus B19 or hepatitis A, which may be present in plasma-derived products, may affect a pregnant woman more seriously than a nonpregnant woman.

Contraindications Hypersensitivity to mouse protein (Mononine®), hamster protein (BeneFix®), or any component; DIC; fibrinolysis

Warnings Some products are prepared from pooled human plasma; such plasma may contain the causative agents of viral disease; risk of transmission is extremely rare; hypersensitivity reactions, including anaphylaxis, have been reported; these events have occurred in a close temporal relationship with the development of factor IX inhibitors; patients experiencing allergic reactions should be evaluated for the presence of inhibitors; there may be a direct relationship between the development of factor IX inhibitors and deletion mutations of the factor IX gene; patients with these deletion mutations should be observed closely for signs and symptoms of acute hypersensitivity reactions

To achieve the desired factor IX activity level, monitor factor IX activity assay; in the presence of an inhibitor, higher factor IX doses may be required

AlphaNine® SD, Mononine® contain **nondetectable levels of factors II, VII, and X** (<0.0025 units per factor IX unit using standard coagulation assays) and are **NOT INDICATED** for replacement therapy of any of these clotting factors.

BeneFix®, Mononine®, and AlphaNine® are **NOT INDICATED** in the treatment or reversal of coumarin-induced anticoagulation or in a hemorrhagic state caused by hepatitis-induced lack of production of liver dependent coagulation factors.

Precautions Due to the potential risk of thromboembolic complications, use with caution in patients with liver dysfunction, patients in the postoperative period, in neonates, or in patients at risk of thromboembolic phenomena or DIC

Adverse Reactions

Cardiovascular: Angioedema, cyanosis, flushing, hypotension, tightness in chest, thrombosis

Central nervous system: Fever, headache, chills, somnolence, dizziness, drowsiness, lightheadedness

Dermatologic: Urticaria, rash

Gastrointestinal: Nausea, vomiting, abnormal taste, diarrhea

Hematologic: DIC

Local: Injection site discomfort, phlebitis

Neuromuscular & skeletal: Tingling

Ocular: Visual disturbances

Respiratory: Dyspnea, laryngeal edema, allergic rhinitis, cough

Miscellaneous: Transient fever (following rapid administration), anaphylaxis, burning sensation in jaw/skull

Drug Interactions

Avoid Concomitant Use

Avoid concomitant use of Factor IX with any of the following: Aminocaproic Acid

Increased Effect/Toxicity

The levels/effects of Factor IX may be increased by: Aminocaproic Acid

Decreased Effect There are no known significant interactions involving a decrease in effect.

Stability Refrigerate 2°C to 8°C (36°F to 46°F); do not freeze

AlphaNine® SD: May also be stored at ≤30°C (≤86°F) for up to 3 months.

◄ BeneFix®: May also be stored at ≤25°C (≤77°F) for up to 6 months.

Mononine®: May also be stored at ≤30°C (≤86°F) for up to 1 month.

Mechanism of Action Hemophilia B, or Christmas disease, is an X-linked inherited disorder of blood coagulation characterized by insufficient or abnormal synthesis of the clotting protein factor IX. Factor IX is a vitamin K-dependent coagulation factor which is synthesized in the liver. Factor IX is activated by factor XIa in the intrinsic coagulation pathway. Activated factor IX (IXa), in combination with factor VII, activates factor X to Xa, resulting ultimately in the conversion of prothrombin to thrombin and the formation of a fibrin clot. The infusion of exogenous factor IX to replace the deficiency present in hemophilia B temporarily restores hemostasis.

Pharmacokinetics (Adult data unless noted) Elimination: Half-life: 17-22 hours (range: 10-37 hours)

Usual Dosage Dosage is expressed in units of factor IX activity and must be individualized related to formulation, severity, and clinical situation. I.V. only:

Formula for units required to raise blood level %:
AlphaNine® SD, Mononine®: Children and Adults:
Number of Factor IX International Units Required = body weight (in kg) x desired Factor IX level increase (% normal) x 1 international unit/kg
For example, for a 100% level a patient who has an actual level of 20%: Number of Factor IX International Units needed = 70 kg x 80% x 1 international unit/kg = 5600 international units
BeneFix®:
Children <15 years:
Number of Factor IX International Units Required = body weight (in kg) x desired Factor IX level increase (% normal) x 1.4 international units/kg
Adults:
Number of Factor IX International Units Required = body weight (in kg) x desired Factor IX level increase (% normal) x 1.2 international units/kg

Guidelines: As a general rule, the level of factor IX required for treatment of different conditions is listed below:
Minor spontaneous hemorrhage, prophylaxis:
Desired levels of factor IX for hemostasis: 15% to 25%
Initial loading dose to achieve desired level: Up to 20-30 international units/kg
Frequency of dosing: Every 12-24 hours
Duration of treatment: 1-2 days
Moderate hemorrhage:
Desired levels of factor IX for hemostasis: 25% to 50%
Initial loading dose to achieve desired level: 25-50 international units/kg
Frequency of dosing: Every 12-24 hours
Duration of treatment: 2-7 days
Major hemorrhage:
Desired levels of factor IX for hemostasis: >50%
Initial loading dose to achieve desired level: 30-50 international units/kg
Frequency of dosing: Every 12-24 hours, depending on half-life and measured factor IX levels (after 3-5 days, maintain at least 20% activity)
Duration of treatment: 7-10 days, depending upon nature of insult
Surgery:
Desired levels of factor IX for hemostasis: 50% to 100%
Initial loading dose to achieve desired level: 50-100 international units/kg
Frequency of dosing: Every 12-24 hours, depending on half-life and measured factor IX levels
Duration of treatment: 7-10 days, depending upon nature of insult

Administration I.V.: Solution should be infused at room temperature; reconstitute with SWI; use within 3 hours of reconstitution; infuse without further dilution **slowly**. The rate of administration should be determined by the response and comfort of the patient.
Mononine®: Infuse at 2 mL/minute
Alphanine® SD: Infuse at a rate not to exceed 10 mL/minute

Monitoring Parameters Factors IX level, PTT

Reference Range Average normal factor IX levels are 50% to 150%; patients with severe hemophilia will have levels <1%, often undetectable. Moderate forms of the disease have levels of 1% to 10% while some mild cases may have 11% to 49% of normal factor IX.

Maintain factor IX plasma level at least 20% until hemostasis achieved after acute joint or muscle bleeding
In preparation for and following surgery:
Level to prevent spontaneous hemorrhage: 5%
Minimum level for hemostasis following trauma and surgery: 30% to 50%
Severe hemorrhage: >60%
Major surgery: ≥50% prior to procedure, 30% to 50% for several days after surgery, and >20% for 10-14 days thereafter

Additional Information 1 international unit is equal to the amount of Factor IX activity present in 1 mL of pooled, normal human plasma

Dosage Forms Excipient information presented when available (limited, particularly for generics); consult specific product labeling.
Injection, powder for reconstitution [recombinant]:
BeneFix®: ~250 int. units, ~500 int. units, ~1000 int. units, ~2000 int. units [contains polysorbate 80 and sucrose 0.8%; exact potency labeled on each vial]
Injection, powder for reconstitution [human derived]:
AlphaNine® SD: ~500 int. units, ~1000 int. units, ~1500 int. units [contains polysorbate 80 and trace amounts of factors II, VII, and X; exact potency labeled on each vial; solvent detergent treated; virus filtered]
Mononine®: ~500 int. units, ~1000 int. units [contains polysorbate 80 and trace amounts of factors II, VII, and X; exact potency labeled on each vial; monoclonal antibody purified]

Factor IX Complex (Human)
(FAK ter nyne KOM pleks HYU man)

U.S. Brand Names Bebulin® VH; Profilnine® SD

Therapeutic Category Antihemophilic Agent; Blood Product Derivative

Generic Available No

Use Prevention and control of bleeding in patients with factor IX deficiency (hemophilia B or Christmas disease) (Profilnine® SD is FDA approved in ages >16 years; Bebulin® VH is FDA approved in adults)

Pregnancy Risk Factor C

Pregnancy Considerations Reproduction studies have not been conducted.

Contraindications Hypersensitivity to factor IX complex or any component

Warnings Human factor IX complex is prepared from human plasma and even with heat treated or other viral attenuated processes, the risk of viral transmission (ie, viral hepatitis, HIV, parvovirus B19, and theoretically, Creutzfeldt-Jacob disease agent) is not totally eradicated. Hepatitis B vaccination and hepatitis A vaccination are recommended for patients with hemophilia (at birth or at diagnosis). Serious and potentially fatal thrombosis or DIC may occur in patients with hepatic impairment and in patients undergoing surgery (risk is greater following surgery); use with caution in these patients; consider risk versus benefit before prescribing.

Precautions Products do not contain therapeutic levels of factor VII and should not be used for the treatment of factor VII deficiency. Some products (eg, Bebulin® VH) contain natural rubber latex (in certain components of the product packaging) which may cause allergic reactions in susceptible individuals; avoid use in patients with allergy to latex. Some products contain heparin; use with caution in patients with a history of heparin-induced thrombocytopenia type II.

Adverse Reactions
Cardiovascular: Flushing

Central nervous system: Somnolence, fever, headache, chills

Dermatologic: Urticaria

Gastrointestinal: Nausea, vomiting

Hematologic: Disseminated intravascular coagulation, thrombosis following high dosages in hemophilia B patients

Neuromuscular & skeletal: Paresthesia

Miscellaneous: Tightness in chest and neck, hypersensitivity reactions, anaphylactic shock

Drug Interactions
Avoid Concomitant Use
Avoid concomitant use of Factor IX Complex (Human) with any of the following: Aminocaproic Acid

Increased Effect/Toxicity
The levels/effects of Factor IX Complex (Human) may be increased by: Aminocaproic Acid

Decreased Effect There are no known significant interactions involving a decrease in effect.

Stability Store unopened vials in refrigerator; do not freeze. Profilnine® SD: May store unopened vials at room temperature (<30°C) for up to 3 months. Administer within 3 hours after reconstitution; **do not refrigerate after reconstitution**; discard unused portion.

Mechanism of Action Replaces deficient clotting factors including factor IX (antihemophilic factor B); also contains factor II (prothrombin), factor X, and low amounts of factor VII. Hemophilia B, or Christmas disease, is an X-linked recessively inherited disorder of blood coagulation characterized by insufficient or abnormal synthesis of the clotting protein factor IX. Factor IX is a vitamin K-dependent coagulation factor which is synthesized in the liver. Factor IX is activated by factor XIa in the intrinsic coagulation pathway. Activated factor IX (IXa), in combination with factor VII:C, activates factor X to Xa, resulting ultimately in the conversion of prothrombin to thrombin and the formation of a fibrin clot. The infusion of exogenous factor IX to replace the deficiency present in hemophilia B temporarily restores hemostasis.

Pharmacokinetics (Adult data unless noted) Cleared rapidly from the serum in two phases

Half-life:

First phase: 4-6 hours

Terminal: 22.5 hours

Usual Dosage Dosage is expressed in units of factor IX activity and must be individualized according to formulation, severity, and clinical situation.

Children and Adults: I.V.:

Formulas for units required to raise blood level %:

Bebulin® VH: In general, 1 international unit/kg of factor IX will increase the plasma factor IX level by 0.8%

Number of factor IX international units required = body weight (kg) x desired factor IX increase (% of normal) x 1.2 international units/kg

Profilnine® SD: In general, 1 international unit/kg of factor IX will increase the plasma factor IX level by 1%

Number of factor IX international units required = bodyweight (kg) x desired factor IX increase (% of normal) x 1 international unit/kg

Bebulin® VH (see also General Dosing Guidelines below):

Minor bleeding (factor IX level ~20% normal): 25-35 international units/kg

Moderate bleeding (factor IX level ~40% normal): 40-55 international units/kg

Major bleeding (factor IX level ~60% normal): 60-70 international units/kg; **Note:** Do not raise ≥50% in patients who may be predisposed to thrombosis.

Minor surgical procedures dental extraction: Day 1: 50-60 international units/kg; initial postoperative period (1-2 weeks): 55 international units/kg decreasing to 25 international units/kg

Major surgical procedures: Day 1: 70-95 international units/kg; initial postoperative period (1-2 weeks): 70 international units/kg decreasing to 35 international units/kg; late postoperative period (≥3 weeks): 35 international units/kg decreasing to 25 international units/kg

Long-term prophylactic treatment: 20-30 international units/kg 1-2 times/week may reduce frequency of spontaneous hemorrhage; dosing should be individualized.

General Dosing Guidelines: As a general rule, the level of factor IX required for treatment of different conditions is listed below:

Minor bleeding (early hemarthrosis, minor epistaxis, gingival bleeding, mild hematuria): Raise factor IX level to 20% of normal; generally a single dose required

Moderate bleeding (severe joint bleeding, early hematoma, major open bleeding, minor trauma, minor hemoptysis, hematemesis, melena, major hematuria): Raise factor IX level to 40% of normal; average duration of treatment is 2 days or until adequate wound healing.

Major bleeding (severe hematoma, major trauma, severe hemoptysis, hematemesis, melaena): Raise factor IX level to 50% to ≥60% of normal; average duration of treatment is 2-3 days or until adequate wound healing. Do not raise ≥50% in patients who may be predisposed to thrombosis.

Minor surgery: Raise factor IX level to 40% to 60% of normal on day of surgery; then decrease from 40% of normal to 20% of normal during initial postoperative period (1-2 weeks) or until adequate wound healing. The preoperative dose should be given 1 hour prior to surgery. The average dosing interval may be every 12 hours initially, then every 24 hours later in the postoperative period.

Dental surgery: Raise factor IX level to 40% to 60% of normal on day of surgery. One infusion is generally sufficient for the extraction of one tooth; for the extraction of multiple teeth replacement therapy may be required for up to 1 week; use same doses as for minor surgery (see dosing guidelines for Minor Surgery).

Major surgery: Raise factor IX level to ≥60% of normal on day of surgery; do not raise ≥50% in patients who may be predisposed to thrombosis. Decrease from 60% of normal to 20% of normal during initial postoperative period (1-2 weeks), continue at 20% of normal during the late postoperative period (≥3 weeks), continuing until adequate wound healing is achieved. The preoperative dose should be given 1 hour prior to surgery. The average dosing interval may be every 12 hours initially, then every 24 hours later in the postoperative period.

Administration Parenteral: I.V. administration only; infuse slowly; rate of administration should be individualized for patient's comfort; rapid I.V. administration may cause vasomotor reactions; maximum rates of administration: Bebulin® VH: 2 mL/minute; Profilnine® SD: 10 mL/minute; visually inspect for particulate matter and discoloration prior to administration whenever permitted by solution or container. **Note:** Slowing the rate of infusion, changing the lot of medication, or administering antihistamines may relieve some adverse reactions

Monitoring Parameters Levels of factors II, IX, and X; signs/symptoms of hypersensitivity reactions and bleeding; hemoglobin, hematocrit

Reference Range Patients with severe hemophilia will have factor IX levels <1%, often undetectable. Moderate forms of the disease have levels of 1% to 10% while some mild cases may have 11% to 49% of normal factor IX. Plasma concentration is about 4 mg/L.

Additional Information AlphaNine® SD and Mononine® contain only factor IX and should not be confused with factor IX **complex**

Dosage Forms Excipient information presented when available (limited, particularly for generics); consult specific product labeling. [DSC] = Discontinued product

Injection, powder for reconstitution:

Bebulin® VH: Exact potency labeled on each vial [vapor heated; contains heparin and natural rubber/natural latex in packaging]

Profilnine® SD: ~500 int. units, ~1000 int. units, ~1500 int. units [exact potency labeled on each vial; solvent detergent treated]

References

Lee JW, "Von Willebrand Disease, Hemophilia A and B, and Other Factor Deficiencies," *Int Anesthesiol Clin*, 2004, 42(3):59-76.

Lusher JM, "Thrombogenicity Associated With Factor IX Complex Concentrates," *Semin Hematol*, 1991, 28(3 Suppl 6):3-5.

Shord SS and Lindley CM, "Coagulation Products and Their Uses," *Am J Health Syst Pharm*, 2000, 57(15):1403-20.

◆ **Factor IX Concentrate** *see* Factor IX *on page 557*

Famciclovir (fam SYE kloe veer)

Medication Safety Issues

Sound-alike/look-alike issues:

Famvir® may be confused with Femara®

U.S. Brand Names Famvir®

Canadian Brand Names Apo-Famciclovir®; CO Famciclovir; Famvir®; PMS-Famciclovir; Sandoz-Famciclovir

Therapeutic Category Antiviral Agent, Oral

Generic Available Yes

Use Treatment of acute herpes zoster (shingles); treatment or suppression of recurrent episodes of genital herpes in immunocompetent patients; treatment of recurrent episodes of herpes labialis (cold sores) in immunocompetent patients; treatment of recurrent episodes of mucocutaneous herpes simplex infections in HIV patients (FDA approved in ages ≥18 years)

Pregnancy Risk Factor B

Pregnancy Considerations Teratogenic effects were not observed in animal studies. There are no adequate and well-controlled studies in pregnant women. Use only if benefit outweighs risk. A registry has been established for women exposed to famciclovir during pregnancy (888-669-6682).

Lactation Excretion in breast milk unknown/not recommended

Breast-Feeding Considerations There is no specific data describing the excretion of famciclovir in breast milk. Breast-feeding is not recommended by the manufacturer unless the potential benefits outweigh any possible risk. If herpes lesions are on breast, breast-feeding should be avoided in order to avoid transmission to infant.

Contraindications Hypersensitivity to famciclovir, penciclovir, or any component

Precautions Use with caution and decrease dose in patients with renal dysfunction; acute renal failure has been reported in patients with renal dysfunction who received inappropriately high doses of famciclovir for their

level of renal function. Dosage adjustment may be needed in patients with poorly compensated hepatic impairment. Tablets contain lactose; do not use in patients with galactose intolerance, severe lactase deficiency, or glucose-galactose malabsorption syndromes. Safety and efficacy have not been established in children <18 years of age. Efficacy has not been established in adults for treatment of initial episodes of genital herpes infection, ophthalmic zoster, disseminated zoster, or in immunocompromised patients with herpes zoster.

Adverse Reactions Note: Frequency of adverse effects vary with dose and duration; single-dose treatment of herpes labialis (cold sores) was associated with headache (10%), nausea (2%), diarrhea (2%), fatigue (1.3%), and dysmenorrhea (1%).

Central nervous system: Headache (14% to 39%), fatigue (1% to 5%), dizziness, fever, somnolence

Dermatologic: Pruritus (0 to 4%), rash (0 to 3%)

Endocrine & metabolic: Dysmenorrhea (0 to 8%)

Gastrointestinal: Nausea (2% to 13%), diarrhea (2% to 9%), vomiting (1% to 5%), abdominal pain (0% to 8%), flatulence (1% to 5%)

Hematologic: Neutropenia (3%), leukopenia (1%)

Hepatic: Liver enzymes elevated (2% to 3%), bilirubin elevated (2%)

Neuromuscular & skeletal: Paresthesia (0 to 3%)

Drug Interactions

Avoid Concomitant Use

Avoid concomitant use of Famciclovir with any of the following: Zoster Vaccine

Increased Effect/Toxicity There are no known significant interactions involving an increase in effect.

Decreased Effect

Famciclovir may decrease the levels/effects of: Zoster Vaccine

Food Interactions Rate of absorption and/or conversion to penciclovir and peak concentration are reduced with food, but bioavailability is not affected

Mechanism of Action Synthetic guanine derivative, prodrug for penciclovir; penciclovir has inhibitory activity against varicella zoster virus (VZV) and herpes simplex virus type 1 and 2 (HSV 1 and HSV 2); penciclovir is converted to penciclovir monophosphate (by viral thymidine kinase in VZV-, HSV 1-, and HSV 2-infected cells), then to penciclovir triphosphate which competes with deoxyguanosine triphosphate for viral DNA polymerase and incorporation into viral DNA; therefore, inhibits DNA synthesis and viral replication

Pharmacokinetics (Adult data unless noted)

Penciclovir:

Absorption: Rapid

Distribution: V_{dss}: Healthy adults: 1.08 ± 0.17 L/kg

Protein binding: <20%

Metabolism: Famciclovir is a prodrug which is metabolized via deacetylation and oxidation in the intestinal wall and liver to penciclovir (active) during extensive first-pass metabolism

Bioavailability: 77% ± 8%

Half-life:

Serum: Mean: 2-3 hours; increased with renal dysfunction

Mean half-life, terminal:

Cl_{cr} >80 mL/minute: 2.15 hours

Cl_{cr} 60-80 mL/minute: 2.47 hours

Cl_{cr} 30-59 mL/minute: 3.87 hours

Cl_{cr} <29 mL/minute: 9.85 hours

Intracellular penciclovir triphosphate: HSV 1: 10 hours; HSV 2: 20 hours; VZV: 7 hours

Time to peak serum concentration: ~1 hour

Elimination: Primarily excreted via the kidneys; after oral administration, 73% is excreted in the urine (predominantly as penciclovir) and 27% in feces; penciclovir undergoes tubular secretion; requires dosage adjustment with renal impairment

Dialysis: Hemodialysis: May enhance elimination of penciclovir

Usual Dosage Oral:

Children and Adolescents: Insufficient clinical data exists to identify an appropriate pediatric dose (AAP, 2006):

Adults:

Herpes zoster: 500 mg every 8 hours for 7 days; initiate as soon as diagnosed; initiation of therapy within 48 hours of rash onset may be more beneficial; no efficacy data available for treatment initiated >72 hours after onset of rash

Genital herpes: Treatment of initial clinical episode: 250 mg 3 times/day for 7-10 days; **Note:** Treatment may be continued if healing is not complete after 10 days of therapy (CDC, 2006)

Recurrent genital herpes in immunocompetent patients:

Treatment: 1000 mg twice daily for 1 day or 125 mg twice daily for 5 days (CDC, 2006); initiate at first sign or symptom; efficacy is not established if treatment is started >6 hours after onset of lesions or symptoms

Suppression: 250 mg twice daily for up to 1 year

Recurrent herpes labialis (cold sores): 1500 mg as a single dose; initiate at first sign or symptom such as tingling, burning, or itching; efficacy established for initiation of treatment within 1 hour of symptom onset

Recurrent orolabial or genital herpes in HIV patients: Treatment: 500 mg twice daily for 7 days

Recurrent genital herpes in HIV patients: Suppression: 500 mg twice daily (CDC, 2006)

Dosing interval in renal impairment: Adults:

Herpes zoster:

Cl_{cr} ≥60 mL/minute: Administer 500 mg every 8 hours

Cl_{cr} 40-59 mL/minute: Administer 500 mg every 12 hours

Cl_{cr} 20-39 mL/minute: Administer 500 mg every 24 hours

Cl_{cr} <20 mL/minute: Administer 250 mg every 24 hours

Patients on hemodialysis: Administer 250 mg after each dialysis session

Recurrent genital herpes: Treatment (single day regimen):

Cl_{cr} ≥60 mL/minute: Administer 1000 mg every 12 hours for 1 day

Cl_{cr} 40-59 mL/minute: Administer 500 mg every 12 hours for 1 day

Cl_{cr} 20-39 mL/minute: Administer 500 mg as a single dose

Cl_{cr} <20 mL/minute: Administer 250 mg as a single dose

Patients on hemodialysis: Administer 250 mg as a single dose after dialysis session

Recurrent genital herpes: Suppression:

Cl_{cr} ≥40 mL/minute: Administer 250 mg every 12 hours

Cl_{cr} 20-39 mL/minute: Administer 125 mg every 12 hours

Cl_{cr} <20 mL/minute: Administer 125 mg every 24 hours

Patients on hemodialysis: Administer 125 mg after each dialysis session

Recurrent herpes labialis: Treatment (single dose regimen):

Cl_{cr} ≥60 mL/minute: Administer 1500 mg as a single dose

Cl_{cr} 40-59 mL/minute: Administer 750 mg as a single dose

Cl_{cr} 20-39 mL/minute: Administer 500 mg as a single dose

Cl_{cr} <20 mL/minute: Administer 250 mg as a single dose

Patients on hemodialysis: Administer 250 mg as a single dose after dialysis session

Recurrent orolabial or genital herpes in HIV infected patients:

Cl_{cr} ≥40 mL/minute: Administer 500 mg every 12 hours

Cl_{cr} 20-39 mL/minute: Administer 500 mg every 24 hours

Cl_{cr} <20 mL/minute: Administer 250 mg every 24 hours

Patients on hemodialysis: Administer 250 mg after each dialysis session

Administration Oral: May be administered without regard to meals; may be administered with food to decrease GI upset

Monitoring Parameters Resolution of rash, renal function, WBC, liver enzymes

Patient Information Famciclovir is not a cure for genital herpes; may cause dizziness and impair ability to perform activities requiring mental alertness or physical coordination

Dosage Forms Excipient information presented when available (limited, particularly for generics); consult specific product labeling.

Tablet: 125 mg, 250 mg, 500 mg

Famvir®: 125 mg, 250 mg, 500 mg

References

Boike SC, Pue MA, and Freed MI, "Pharmacokinetics of Famciclovir in Subjects With Varying Degrees of Renal Impairment," *Clin Pharmacol Ther*, 1994, 55(4):418-26.

Centers for Disease Control and Prevention (CDC), "Sexually Transmitted Diseases Treatment Guidelines, 2006," *MMWR Recomm Rep*, 2006, 55(RR-11):1-94.

Pickering LK, ed, *2006 Red Book, Report of the Committee on Infectious Diseases*, 27th ed. Elk Grove Village IL: American Academy of Pediatrics, 2006, 787.

Spruance SL, Bodsworth N, Resnick H, et al, "Single-Dose, Patient-Initiated Famciclovir: A Randomized, Double-Blind, Placebo-Controlled Trial for Episodic Treatment of Herpes Labialis," *J Am Acad Dermatol*, 2006, 55(1):47-53.

Famotidine (fa MOE ti deen)

Medication Safety Issues

Sound-alike/look-alike issues:

Famotidine may be confused with FLUoxetine, furosemide

U.S. Brand Names Heartburn Relief Maximum Strength [OTC]; Heartburn Relief [OTC]; Pepcid®; Pepcid® AC Maximum Strength [OTC]; Pepcid® AC [OTC]

Canadian Brand Names Acid Control; Apo-Famotidine®; Apo-Famotidine® Injectable; Famotidine Omega; Mylan-Famotidine; Novo-Famotidine; Nu-Famotidine; Pepcid®; Pepcid® AC; Pepcid® I.V.; Ulcidine

Therapeutic Category Gastrointestinal Agent, Gastric or Duodenal Ulcer Treatment; Histamine H_2 Antagonist

Generic Available Yes: Injection, tablet

Use Short-term therapy and treatment of duodenal ulcer, gastric ulcer, control gastric pH in critically ill patients, symptomatic relief in gastritis, gastroesophageal reflux disease (GERD), active benign ulcer, and pathological hypersecretory conditions; over-the-counter (OTC) formulation for use in the relief of heartburn, acid indigestion, and sour stomach

Pregnancy Risk Factor B

Pregnancy Considerations Crosses the placenta. There are no adequate and well-controlled studies in pregnant women. Use only if clearly needed.

Lactation Enters breast milk/not recommended

Breast-Feeding Considerations Famotidine is concentrated in breast milk, but to a lesser degree than cimetidine or ranitidine; some sources prefer its use if one of these agents is needed.

Contraindications Hypersensitivity to famotidine, any component (see Warnings), or other H_2 antagonists

Warnings Use with caution and modify dose in patients with renal impairment. Use of gastric acid inhibitors including proton pump inhibitors and H_2 blockers has been associated with an increased risk for development of acute gastroenteritis and community-acquired pneumonia (Canani, 2006).

Multidose injection contains benzyl alcohol which may cause allergic reactions in susceptible individuals; large amounts of benzyl alcohol (≥99 mg/kg/day) have been associated with a potentially fatal toxicity ("gasping syndrome") in neonates; the "gasping syndrome" consists of metabolic acidosis, respiratory distress, gasping respirations, CNS dysfunction (including convulsions, intracranial hemorrhage), hypotension and cardiovascular collapse; avoid use of the multidose injection in neonates. The oral suspension contains sodium benzoate; *in vitro* and animal studies have shown that benzoate, a metabolite of benzyl alcohol, displaces bilirubin from protein binding sites; avoid use in neonates.

Precautions Pepcid® chewable tablets contain phenylalanine which should be used with caution in patients with phenylketonuria.

Adverse Reactions

Cardiovascular: Bradycardia, tachycardia, AV block, palpitations, hypertension, angioedema

Central nervous system: Headache, vertigo, anxiety, dizziness, seizures, depression, insomnia, drowsiness, confusion, fever, fatigue, seizures (in patients with impaired renal function), psychic disturbances including hallucinations, agitation

Dermatologic: Acne, pruritus, urticaria, dry skin, alopecia, rash, toxic epidermal necrolysis/Stevens-Johnson syndrome (rare)

Gastrointestinal: Constipation, nausea, vomiting, diarrhea, abdominal discomfort, flatulence, belching, dysgeusia, dry mouth, anorexia

Genitourinary: Impotence

Hematologic: Thrombocytopenia, pancytopenia, leukopenia (rare)

Hepatic: Liver enzymes elevated, hepatomegaly, cholestatic jaundice

Neuromuscular & skeletal: Weakness, arthralgias, paresthesia, muscle cramps

Ocular: Orbital edema, conjunctival injection

Otic: Ototoxicity, tinnitus

Renal: BUN and serum creatinine elevated, proteinuria

Respiratory: Bronchospasm, interstitial pneumonia

Miscellaneous: Hypersensitivity reactions including anaphylaxis

Drug Interactions

Avoid Concomitant Use

Avoid concomitant use of Famotidine with any of the following: Delavirdine; Erlotinib

Increased Effect/Toxicity

Famotidine may increase the levels/effects of: Saquinavir

Decreased Effect

Famotidine may decrease the levels/effects of: Antifungal Agents (Azole Derivatives, Systemic); Atazanavir; Cefditoren; Cefpodoxime; Cefuroxime; Dasatinib; Delavirdine; Erlotinib; Fosamprenavir; Indinavir; Iron Salts; Mesalamine; Nelfinavir

Food Interactions Limit xanthine-containing foods and beverages

Stability Concentrate for injection must be refrigerated but is stable for 48 hours at room temperature; if concentrated injection is diluted in D_5W or NS it is stable 48 hours at room temperature; commercially available diluted solution in NS is stable at room temperature for 15 months; injection is also compatible with $D_{10}W$, LR injection, 5% bicarbonate injection, and standard parenteral nutrition solutions with electrolytes, multivitamins, and trace minerals; reconstituted oral solution is stable for 30 days at room temperature

Mechanism of Action Competitive inhibition of histamine at H_2-receptors of the gastric parietal cells, which results in inhibition of gastric acid secretion

Pharmacodynamics

Onset of GI effect: Oral, I.V.: Within 1 hour

Maximum effect:
  Oral: 1-4 hours
  I.V.: 30 minutes to 3 hours
Duration: 10-12 hours

Pharmacokinetics (Adult data unless noted)

Distribution: V_d:
  Infants:
    0-3 months: 1.4-1.8 ± 0.3-0.4 L/kg
    >3 to 12 months: 2.3 ± 0.7 L/kg
  Children: 2 ± 1.5 L/kg
  Adults: 0.94-1.33 L/kg
Protein binding: 15% to 20%
Metabolism: 30% to 35% liver metabolism
Bioavailability: Oral: 40% to 45%
Half-life:
  Infants:
    0-3 months: 8.1-10.5 ± 3.5-5.4 hours
    >3 to 12 months: 4.5 ± 1.1 hours
  Children: 3.3 ± 2.5 hours
  Adults: Injection, oral suspension, tablet: 2.5-3.5 hours; orally-disintegrating tablet: 5 hours; increases with renal impairment; if Cl_{cr} <10 mL/minute, half-life ≥20 hours
  Anuria: 24 hours
Time to peak serum concentration: Orally-disintegrating tablet: 2.5 hours
Elimination: 65% to 70% unchanged drug in urine
Clearance:
  Infants:
    0-3 months: 0.13-0.21 ± 0.06 L/hour/kg
    >3-12 months: 0.49 ± 0.17 L/hour/kg
  Children 1-11 years: 0.54 ± 0.34 L/hour/kg
  Adults: 0.39 ± 0.14 L/hour/kg

Usual Dosage

Neonates and Infants <3 months: Oral: GERD: 0.5 mg/kg/dose once daily

Infants ≥3 months to 1 year: Oral: GERD: 0.5 mg/kg/dose twice daily

Children 1-12 years: Oral, I.V.:
  Peptic ulcer: 0.5 mg/kg/day at bedtime or divided twice daily (maximum: 40 mg/day)
  GERD: 1 mg/kg/day divided twice daily (maximum: 80 mg/day)

Children >12 years and Adults:
  Oral:
    Duodenal ulcer, gastric ulcer: 20 mg/day at bedtime for 4-8 weeks (a regimen of 10 mg twice daily is also effective); maximum: 40 mg/day
    Hypersecretory conditions: Initial: 20 mg every 6 hours, may increase up to 160 mg every 6 hours
    Esophagitis: 20-40 mg twice daily for up to 12 weeks
    GERD: 20 mg twice daily for 6 weeks
    Acid indigestion, heartburn, or sour stomach (OTC use): 10-20 mg 15-60 minutes before eating; not more than 2 tablets per day
  I.V.: 20 mg every 12 hours

Dosing adjustment in renal impairment:
  Cl_{cr} 10-50 mL/minute: Administer normal dose every 24 hours or 50% of dose at normal dosing interval
  Cl_{cr} <10 mL/minute: Administer normal dose every 36-48 hours

Administration

Oral: May administer with food and antacids; shake suspension vigorously for 10-15 seconds prior to each use; place orally-disintegrating tablet (Fluxid™) on the top of the tongue, wait until it dissolves than swallow with saliva; tablet disintegrates in <2 minutes; do not break or chew tablet

Parenteral: I.V.: Dilute to a maximum concentration of 4 mg/mL; may be administered I.V. push at 10 mg/minute over 2 minutes or as an infusion over 15-30 minutes

Patient Information Avoid excessive amounts of coffee and aspirin; when self medicating, if the symptoms of heartburn, acid indigestion, or sour stomach persist after 2 weeks of continuous use of the drug, consult a clinician.

Dosage Forms Excipient information presented when available (limited, particularly for generics); consult specific product labeling. [DSC] = Discontinued product

Gelcap, oral:
Pepcid® AC: 10 mg [DSC]

Infusion, premixed in NS [preservative free]: 20 mg (50 mL)

Injection, solution: 10 mg/mL (4 mL, 20 mL, 50 mL)

Injection, solution [preservative free]: 10 mg/mL (2 mL)

Powder for oral suspension:
Pepcid®: 40 mg/5 mL (50 mL) [contains sodium benzoate; cherry-banana-mint flavor]

Tablet, oral: 10 mg [OTC], 20 mg, 40 mg
Heartburn Relief: 10 mg
Heartburn Relief Maximum Strength: 20 mg
Pepcid®: 20 mg, 40 mg
Pepcid® AC: 10 mg
Pepcid® AC Maximum Strength: 20 mg

Tablet, chewable, oral:
Pepcid® AC Maximum Strength: 20 mg [berries 'n' cream flavor]
Pepcid® AC Maximum Strength: 20 mg [cool mint flavor]

Extemporaneous Preparations An 8 mg/mL suspension may be made by crushing seventy 40 mg tablets; work into a paste with a small amount of sterile water; add a 1:1 mixture of Ora-Plus® and Ora-Sweet® to a total volume of 350 mL; stable 95 days at 23°C to 35°C

Dentinger PJ, Swenson CF, and Anaizi NH, "Stability of Famotidine in an Extemporaneously Compounded Oral Liquid," *Am J Health Syst Pharm*, 2000, 57(14):1340-2.

References

Canani RB, Cirillo P, Roggero P, et al, "Therapy With Gastric Acidity Inhibitors Increases the Risk of Acute Gastroenteritis and Community-Acquired Pneumonia in Children," *Pediatrics*, 2006, 117(5):e817-20.

James LP and Kearns GL, "Pharmacokinetics and Pharmacodynamics of Famotidine in Paediatric Patients," *Clin Pharmacokinet*, 1996, 31 (2):103-10.

Treem WR, Davis PM, and Hyams JS, "Suppression of Gastric Acid Secretion by Intravenous Administration of Famotidine in Children," *J Pediatr*, 1991, 118(5):812-6.

◆ **Famotidine Omega (Can)** *see* Famotidine *on page 561*

◆ **FAMP** *see* Fludarabine *on page 587*

◆ **Famvir®** *see* Famciclovir *on page 560*

◆ **Fansidar® [DSC]** *see* Sulfadoxine and Pyrimethamine *on page 1301*

◆ **2F-ara-AMP** *see* Fludarabine *on page 587*

◆ **Fasturtec® (Can)** *see* Rasburicase *on page 1203*

Fat Emulsion (fat e MUL shun)

Related Information
Parenteral Nutrition (PN) *on page 1559*

U.S. Brand Names Intralipid®; Liposyn® II [DSC]; Liposyn® III

Canadian Brand Names Intralipid®; Liposyn® II

Therapeutic Category Caloric Agent; Intravenous Nutritional Therapy

Generic Available No

Use Source of calories and essential fatty acids for patients requiring parenteral nutrition of extended duration; prevention and treatment of **essential fatty acid deficiency (EFAD)**; treatment of local anesthetic-induced cardiac arrest unresponsive to conventional resuscitation

Pregnancy Risk Factor C

Pregnancy Considerations Reproductive studies have not been conducted. The A.S.P.E.N. guidelines for parenteral and enteral nutrition state that intravenous fat emulsion may be used safely in pregnant women to provide calories and prevent essential fatty acid deficiency.

Lactation Excretion in breast milk unknown/compatible

Contraindications Hypersensitivity to fat emulsion or any component; severe egg or legume (soybean) allergies; pathologic hyperlipidemia; lipoid nephrosis; pancreatitis with hyperlipemia

Warnings Deaths in preterm neonates after infusion of I.V. fat emulsions have been reported **[U.S. Boxed Warning]**. Autopsy findings included intravascular fat accumulation in the lungs. Use of I.V. fat emulsion in preterm neonates should be done carefully adhering to maximum daily dosages and infusing as slowly as possible (see Usual Dosage). Preterm infants have a decreased ability to eliminate infused fat and must be monitored closely using triglyceride or plasma free fatty acid levels. Frequent platelet counts (some advise daily) should also be done in neonatal patients receiving fat emulsion. Monitor liver function tests when using as long-term therapy.

Fat emulsions contain aluminum which may be toxic, particularly in patients with decreased renal function. Premature neonates are at increased risk for developing aluminum toxicity due to immature (decreased) renal function and the concomitant use of parenteral electrolytes, particularly calcium and phosphate, which also contain high amounts of aluminum. Administration of aluminum at >4-5 mcg/kg/day may result in accumulation and potential CNS and bone toxicity. Tissue loading with aluminum may occur at even lower rates of infusion

Fat emulsion in a 3-in-1 mixture may obscure the presence of a precipitate; follow compounding guidelines, especially for calcium and phosphate compatibility. 30% fat emulsions are not intended for direct I.V. infusion and dilution with another I.V. fluid (eg, NS or SWI) does not produce a dilution equivalent to 10% or 20% I.V. fat emulsion; such dilutions should not be administered by direct I.V. infusion (see Additional Information).

Precautions Use with caution in patients with severe liver damage, pulmonary disease, anemia, or blood coagulation disorders or when there is risk for fat embolism; use with caution in cholestatic patients or in those at risk for parenteral nutrition-associated cholestasis. When cholestatsis occurs, fat emulsion may be temporarily decreased or stopped.

Adverse Reactions

Cardiovascular: Cyanosis, flushing, chest pain

Central nervous system: Headache, fever, sleepiness, dizziness

Gastrointestinal: Nausea, vomiting

Hematologic: Hypercoagulability, thrombocytopenia (neonates), leukopenia

Hepatic: Hyperlipemia, hepatomegaly, jaundice, cholestasis, transient increases in liver enzymes

Local: Thrombophlebitis

Neuromuscular & skeletal: Back pain

Ocular: Slight pressure over the eyes

Respiratory: Dyspnea

Miscellaneous: Sepsis, hypersensitivity reactions, diaphoresis, splenomegaly, deposition of brown pigment in the reticuloendothelial system (clinical significance is unknown); overloading syndrome (focal seizures, fever, leukocytosis, hepatomegaly, spenlomegaly, and shock)

◀ **Stability** May be stored at room temperature; do note freeze; do not store in partly used containers; fat emulsion can support the growth of various organisms. Do not use if emulsion appears to be layering out; exposure to light, particularly phototherapy light, used in treatment or prevention of hyperbilirubinemia has been associated with increased lipid oxidation; the clinical significance remains to be established; do not mix other drugs with fat emulsion; only heparin at a concentration of 1-2 units/mL may be added to fat emulsion

Mechanism of Action Fatty acids are essential for normal structure and function of cell membranes; infusion of fatty acids as I.V. fat emulsion provides a source of calories and essential fatty acids normally obtained in the enteral diet

Usual Dosage

Nutrition: I.V. infusion: Fat emulsion should not exceed 60% of the total daily calories

Note: At the onset of therapy, the patient should be observed for any immediate allergic reactions such as dyspnea, cyanosis, and fever. Slower initial rates of infusion may be used for the first 10-15 minutes of the infusion (eg, 0.1 mL/minute of 10% or 0.05 mL/minute of 20% solution).

Premature infants: Initial dose: 0.25-0.5 g/kg/day, increase by 0.25-0.5 g/kg/day to a maximum of 3-4 g/kg/day depending upon the needs/nutritional goals; limit to 1 g/kg/day if on phototherapy; daily dose should be infused over 24 hours if possible (ASPEN Guidelines, 2002); maximum rate of infusion: 0.15 g/kg/hour (0.75 mL/kg/hour of 20% solution) (see Warnings)

Infants and Children: Initial dose: 0.5-1 g/kg/day, increase by 0.5 g/kg/day to a maximum of 3-4 g/kg/day depending upon the needs/nutritional goals; daily dose may be infused over 24 hours if possible (ASPEN Guidelines, 2002); maximum rate of infusion: 0.25 g/kg/hour (1.25 mL/kg/hour of 20% solution)

Adolescents and Adults: Initial dose: 1 g/kg/day; not to exceed 500 mL 20% fat emulsion on the first day of therapy, increase by 0.5-1 g/kg/day to a maximum of 2.5 g/kg/day; maximum rate of infusion: 0.25 g/kg/hour (1.25 mL/kg/hour of 20% solution); do not exceed 50 mL/hour (20%) or 100 mL/hour (10%)

Prevention of essential fatty acid deficiency (EFAD): Children and Adults: Administer 8% to 10% of total caloric intake as fat emulsion; infuse 2-3 times weekly. If EFAD occurs with stress, the dosage needed to correct EFAD may be increased.

Treatment of local anesthetic-induced cardiac arrest unresponsive to conventional resuscitation: Adults: Infuse 1.5 mL/kg (20% solution) over 1 minute; followed immediately by an infusion of 0.25 mL/kg/minute; continue chest compressions (lipid must circulate); repeat bolus every 3-5 minutes up to 3 mL/kg total dose until circulation restored. Continue infusion until hemodynamic stability is restored. Increase the infusion rate to 0.5 mL/kg/minute if BP declines. A maximum total dose of 8 mL/kg is recommended (see Corcoran, 2006; Foxall, 2007; Litz, 2006).

Administration Parenteral: 10% and 20% emulsions may be simultaneously infused with amino acid, dextrose mixtures by means of Y-connector located near infusion site into either central or peripheral line or administered in total nutrient mixtures (3-in-1) with amino acids, dextrose, and other nutrients; 30% emulsions must not be infused directly (see Warnings and Additional Information). Hang fat emulsion solution higher than other parenteral fluids (has low specific gravity and could run up into other I.V. lines). For Intralipid®, Liposyn® II: Do not use <1.2 micron filter; for Liposyn® III: Do not use a filter.

Monitoring Parameters Serum triglycerides, free fatty acids, platelets (neonates), liver enzymes

Additional Information 10% = 1.1 Kcal/mL, 20% = 2 Kcal/mL, 30% = 3 Kcal/mL; 10% and 20% solutions are isotonic and may be administered peripherally; 30% solution is not intended for direct infusion; it must be diluted to a final concentration not to exceed 20% when added to 3-in-1 or total nutrient admixture; avoid use of 10% fat emulsion in preterm infants as a greater accumulation of plasma lipids occurs with the greater phospholipid load of the 10% fat emulsion

Dosage Forms Excipient information presented when available (limited, particularly for generics); consult specific product labeling. [DSC] = Discontinued product

Injection, emulsion:

Intralipid®: 20% (100 mL, 250 mL, 500 mL, 1000 mL) [contains aluminum, egg yolk phospholipids, and soybean oil]; 30% (500 mL) [contains aluminum, egg yolk phospholipids, and soybean oil]

Liposyn® II: 10% (500 mL) [contains aluminum, egg yolk phospholipids, safflower oil, and soybean oil] [DSC]; 20% (500 mL) [contains aluminum, egg yolk phospholipids, safflower oil, and soybean oil] [DSC]

Liposyn® III: 10% (200 mL, 500 mL) [contains aluminum, egg yolk phospholipids, and soybean oil]; 20% (200 mL, 500 mL) [contains aluminum, egg yolk phospholipids, and soybean oil]; 30% (500 mL) [contains aluminum, egg yolk phospholipids, and soybean oil]

References

ASPEN Board of Directors and the Clinical Guidelines Task Force, "Guidelines for the Use of Parenteral and Enteral Nutrition in Adult and Pediatric Patients," *JPEN J Parenter Enteral Nutr*, 2002, 26(1 Suppl):1SA-138SA.

Colomb V, Jobert-Giraud A, Lacaille F, et al, "Role of Lipid Emulsions in Cholestasis Associated With Long-Term Parenteral Nutrition in Children," *JPEN J Parenter Enteral Nutr*, 2000, 24(6):345-50.

Corcoran W, Butterworth J, Weller RS, et al, "Local Anesthetic-Induced Cardiac Toxicity: A Survey of Contemporary Practice Strategies Among Academic Anesthesiology Departments," *Anesth Analg*, 2006, 103(5):1322-6.

Foxall G, McCahon R, Lamb J, et al, "Levobupivacaine-Induced Seizures and Cardiovascular Collapse Treated With Intralipid," *Anaesthesia*, 2007, 62(5):516-8.

Haumont D, Richelle M, Deckelbaum RJ, et al, "Effect of Liposomal Content of Lipid Emulsions of Plasma Lipid Concentrations in Low Birth Weight Infants Receiving Parenteral Nutrition," *J Pediatr*, 1992, 121(5 Pt 1):759-63.

Litz RJ, Popp M, Stehr SN, et al, "Successful Resuscitation of a Patient With Ropivacaine-Induced Asystole After Axillary Plexus Block Using Lipid Infusion," *Anaesthesia*, 2006, 61(8):800-1.

Neuzil J, Darlow BA, Inder TE, et al, "Oxidation of Parenteral Lipid Emulsion by Ambient and Phototherapy Lights: Potential Toxicity of Routine Parenteral Feeding," *J Pediatr*, 1995, 126(5 Pt 1):785-90.

Shin JI, Namgung R, Park MS, et al, "Could Lipid Infusion Be a Risk for Parenteral Nutrition-Associated Cholestasis in Low Birth Weight Neonates?" *Eur J Pediatr*, 2008, 167(2):197-202.

◆ **Father John's® [OTC]** *see* Dextromethorphan *on page 421*

◆ **FazaClo®** *see* Clozapine *on page 345*

◆ **5-FC** *see* Flucytosine *on page 586*

◆ **Feiba VH** *see* Anti-inhibitor Coagulant Complex *on page 117*

◆ **Feiba VH Immuno (Can)** *see* Anti-inhibitor Coagulant Complex *on page 117*

Felbamate (FEL ba mate)

Related Information

Antiepileptic Drugs *on page 1693*

U.S. Brand Names Felbatol®

Therapeutic Category Anticonvulsant, Miscellaneous

Generic Available No

Use Not a first-line agent, see Warnings; reserved for patients who do not adequately respond to alternative agents and whose epilepsy is so severe that the benefit outweighs the risk of liver failure or aplastic anemia; used as monotherapy and adjunctive therapy in patients with partial seizures with and without secondary generalization (FDA approved in ages ≥14 years and adults); adjunctive therapy in children who have partial and generalized seizures associated with Lennox-Gastaut syndrome (FDA approved in ages 2–14 years)

Pregnancy Risk Factor C

Pregnancy Considerations There are no adequate and well-controlled studies in pregnant women. Postmarketing case reports in humans include fetal death, genital malformation, anencephaly, encephalocele, and placental disorder.

Patients exposed to felbamate during pregnancy are encouraged to enroll themselves into the AED Pregnancy Registry by calling 1-888-233-2334. Additional information is available at www.aedpregnancyregistry.org.

Lactation Enters breast milk/not recommended

Breast-Feeding Considerations Rat studies show a decreased weight and increased death in nursing pups. Felbamate has been detected in human milk. Adverse effects in human infants is unknown.

Contraindications Hypersensitivity to felbamate, any component, or other carbamates (eg, meprobamate); history of or current blood dyscrasia or hepatic dysfunction

Warnings Felbamate is associated with a significant increased risk of aplastic anemia **[U.S. Boxed Warning]**. Risk may be more than 100-fold greater than in untreated population. Current estimates of aplastic anemia-related fatality are 20% to 30%, but higher rates (up to 70%) have been reported in the past. It is not known if dose, duration, or use of concomitant medications affects risk. Aplastic anemia can develop at any point during therapy. Routine blood monitoring is recommended to potentially allow for detection of hematologic changes, although aplastic anemia can occur without warning.

Use is associated with acute hepatic failure **[U.S. Boxed Warning]**. The overall postmarketing reported rate of hepatic failure leading to transplant or death is 6 cases per 75,000 patient years of use; this rate is underestimated due to under reporting (eg, the true rate could be as high as 1 case per 1250 patient years of use if the reporting rate is only 10%). Approximately 67% of the reported cases of hepatic failure led to liver transplantation or death, usually within 5 weeks of the onset of signs and symptoms of hepatic failure; the earliest onset of severe liver dysfunction was 3 weeks after starting felbamate; in some cases, dark urine and nonspecific prodromal symptoms (eg, malaise, anorexia, GI symptoms) preceded the onset of jaundice. It is not known if dose, duration, or use of concomitant medications affects risk of hepatic failure. Felbamate should not be used in any patient with a history of hepatic dysfunction.

All patients receiving felbamate must be monitored closely; in addition, a CBC with differential and platelet count should be taken before, during, and for a significant time after discontinuing felbamate therapy; liver enzyme tests and bilirubin should be obtained before initiation and periodically during therapy. Felbamate should be immediately withdrawn if abnormal liver function tests or bone marrow suppression occur. Do not restart felbamate in patients who experience hematologic or hepatic adverse reactions.

Felbamate should only be used in patients who have severe, refractory seizures that are unresponsive to other medications. The FDA and the manufacturer strongly recommend that physicians discuss the risks of felbamate with each patient and a written informed consent be obtained from the patient prior to starting therapy or before continuing therapy. A patient information consent form is included as part of the package insert and is available from the local Wallace representative or by calling 800-526-3840.

Antiepileptic drugs (AEDs) increase the risk of suicidal behavior and ideation in patients receiving these medications for any indication. Pooled analyses of placebo-controlled trials involving 11 different AEDs (regardless of indication) showed a twofold increased risk of suicidal thoughts or behavior (estimated incidence rate: 0.43% in AED treated patients compared to 0.24% of patients receiving placebo); increased risk was observed as early as 1 week after initiation of AED and continued through duration of trials (most trials ≤24 weeks); risk did not vary significantly by age (age range: 5–100 years). Consider risks and benefits of AEDs before prescribing. Monitor all patients receiving an AED for emergence of suicidal thoughts or behavior, thoughts of self-harm, any unusual changes in behavior or mood, or the emergence or worsening of depressive symptoms; notify heathcare provider immediately if symptoms or concerning behavior occur. **Note:** The FDA is requiring that a Medication Guide be developed for all antiepileptic drugs informing patients of this risk.

Precautions Use with caution in patients concurrently receiving other antiepileptic drugs due to the potential for drug interactions; felbamate may increase the serum concentrations of phenytoin, valproic acid, phenobarbital, and carbamazepine epoxide (active metabolite of carbamazepine; see Drug Interactions); a 20% to 33% reduction in the dose of these concomitant medications is recommended when felbamate is added to the regimen; further dosage reductions may be needed when felbamate doses are titrated upward; monitor serum levels of concomitant antiepileptic drug therapy.

Use with caution and reduce dose in patients with renal dysfunction. Anticonvulsants should not be discontinued abruptly because of the possibility of increasing seizure frequency; felbamate should be withdrawn gradually to minimize the potential of increased seizure frequency, unless safety concerns require a more rapid withdrawal.

Adverse Reactions

Cardiovascular: Tremor, palpitation, tachycardia

Central nervous system: Somnolence, fever, insomnia, nervousness, fatigue, abnormal gait, headache, ataxia, abnormal thinking, emotional lability, pain, depression, anxiety, behavior changes, drowsiness, agitation, dizziness; suicidal thinking and behavior (see Warnings)

Dermatologic: Rash, acne, pruritus

Endocrine & metabolic: Weight loss

Gastrointestinal: Anorexia, vomiting, constipation, hiccup, nausea, dyspepsia, diarrhea, abdominal pain, gum bleeding or hyperplasia

Hematologic: Purpura, leukopenia, thrombocytopenia, granulocytopenia, agranulocytosis, aplastic anemia (100-fold increase in risk; see Warnings)

Hepatic: Liver enzymes elevated, hepatitis, acute liver failure (may be associated with death; see Warnings)

Ocular: Miosis, diplopia

Drug Interactions

Metabolism/Transport Effects Substrate of CYP2E1 (minor), 3A4 (major); **Inhibits** CYP2C19 (weak); **Induces** CYP3A4 (weak)

Avoid Concomitant Use There are no known interactions where it is recommended to avoid concomitant use.

Increased Effect/Toxicity

Felbamate may increase the levels/effects of: Alcohol (Ethyl); Barbiturates; CNS Depressants; Divalproex; Methotrimeprazine; Phenytoin; Primidone; Valproic Acid

The levels/effects of Felbamate may be increased by: CYP3A4 Inhibitors (Moderate); CYP3A4 Inhibitors (Strong); Dasatinib; Methotrimeprazine

Decreased Effect

Felbamate may decrease the levels/effects of: Contraceptives (Estrogens); Contraceptives (Progestins); Saxagliptin

The levels/effects of Felbamate may be decreased by: CYP3A4 Inducers (Strong); Deferasirox; Herbs (CYP3A4 Inducers); Ketorolac; Ketorolac (Systemic); Mefloquine; Phenytoin

Food Interactions Food does **not** affect absorption

Stability Store in tightly closed container at room temperature of 20°C to 25°C (68°F to 77°F).

Mechanism of Action Mechanism of action is unknown but may be similar to other anticonvulsants; has weak inhibitory effects on GABA and benzodiazepine receptor binding; does not have activity at the MK-801 receptor binding site of the NMDA receptor-ionophore complex.

Pharmacokinetics (Adult data unless noted)

Absorption: Oral: Rapid and almost complete

Distribution: V_d: Adults: Mean: 0.75 L/kg; range: 0.7-1.1 L/kg

Protein binding: 20% to 25%, primarily to albumin

Metabolism: In the liver via hydroxylation and conjugation

Bioavailability: >90%

Half-life: Adults: Mean: 20-30 hours; shorter (ie, 14 hours) with concomitant enzyme-inducing drugs; half-life is prolonged (by 9-15 hours) in patients with renal dysfunction

Time to peak serum concentration: 1-4 hours

Elimination: 40% to 50% excreted as unchanged drug and 40% as inactive metabolites in urine

Clearance, apparent: Clearance is decreased (by 40% to 50%) in patients with renal impairment

Children 2-9 years: 61.3 ± 8.2 mL/kg/hour

Children 10-12 years: 34.3 ± 4.3 mL/kg/hour

Usual Dosage See Precautions regarding concomitant antiepileptic drugs

Children 2-14 years with Lennox-Gastaut: Adjunctive therapy: Initial: 15 mg/kg/day in 3-4 divided doses; increase dose by 15 mg/kg/day increments at weekly intervals; maximum dose: 45 mg/kg/day or 3600 mg/day (whichever is less). Decrease dose of concomitant anticonvulsants (ie, carbamazepine, phenytoin, phenobarbital, valproic acid) by 20% at initiation of felbamate; further dosage reductions of concurrent anticonvulsants may be needed.

Children ≥14 years and Adults:

Adjunctive therapy: Initial: 1200 mg/day in 3-4 divided doses; increase daily dose by 1200 mg increments every week to a maximum dose of 3600 mg/day. Decrease dose of concomitant anticonvulsants (ie, carbamazepine, phenytoin, phenobarbital, valproic acid) by 20% at initiation of felbamate; further dosage reductions of concurrent anticonvulsants may be needed.

Conversion to monotherapy: Initial: 1200 mg/day in 3 or 4 divided doses; at week 2, increase daily dose by 1200 mg increments every week up to a maximum dose of 3600 mg/day. Decrease dose of other anticonvulsants by ¹/₃ their original dose at initiation of felbamate, and when felbamate dose is increased at week 2; continue to reduce other anticonvulsants as clinically needed.

Monotherapy: Initial: 1200 mg/day in 3 or 4 divided doses; titrate dosage upward according to clinical response and monitor patients closely; increase daily dose in 600 mg increments every 2 weeks to 2400 mg/day; maximum dose: 3600 mg/day

Dosage adjustment in renal impairment: Use with caution; reduce initial and maintenance doses by 50%

Administration Oral: May be administered without regard to meals; shake suspension well before use

Monitoring Parameters Serum concentrations of concomitant anticonvulsant therapy; CBC with differential and platelet count before, during, and for a significant time after discontinuing felbamate therapy; liver enzyme tests and bilirubin before initiation and periodically during therapy; signs and symptoms of suicidality (eg, anxiety, depression, behavior changes) (see Warnings)

Reference Range Not necessary to routinely monitor serum drug levels; dose should be titrated to clinical response; therapeutic range not fully determined; proposed 30-100 mcg/mL

Patient Information Antiepileptic agents may increase the risk of suicidal thoughts and behavior; notify physician if you feel more depressed or have thoughts of suicide or self harm (see Warnings). Do not abruptly discontinue (an increase in seizure activity may result). Report any unusual symptoms, such as a rash, bruises, bleeding, sore throat, fever, yellow skin, GI complaints, loss of appetite, tiredness, and/or dark urine to physician immediately. Report worsening of seizure activity or loss of seizure control.

Additional Information Monotherapy has not been associated with gingival hyperplasia, impaired concentration, weight gain, or abnormal thinking; felbamate has also been used in a small number of patients with infantile spasms (see Pellock, 1999); an open-label study in children with refractory partial seizures (n=30; mean age: 9 years; range: 2-17 years) found that children >10 years of age had a more favorable response; this was thought to be related to the higher felbamate serum concentrations (and lower apparent clearance) in children >10 years of age compared to those <10 years; the faster apparent clearance in children <10 years of age should be considered when using this agent (Carmant, 1994)

Dosage Forms Excipient information presented when available (limited, particularly for generics); consult specific product labeling.

Suspension, oral:

Felbatol®: 600 mg/5 mL (240 mL, 960 mL)

Tablet:

Felbatol®: 400 mg; 600 mg

References

Carmant L, Holmes GL, Sawyer S, et al, "Efficacy of Felbamate in Therapy for Partial Epilepsy in Children," *J Pediatr*, 1994, 125 (3):481-6.

Dodson WE, "Felbamate in the Treatment of Lennox-Gastaut Syndrome: Results of a 12-Month Open-Label Study Following a Randomized Clinical Trial," *Epilepsia*, 1993, 34(Suppl 7):518-24.

French J, Smith M, Faught E, et al, "Practice Advisory: The Use of Felbamate in the Treatment of Patients With Intractable Epilepsy: Report of the Quality Standards Subcommittee of the American Academy of Neurology and the American Epilepsy Society," *Neurology*, 1999, 52(8):1540-5.

Kaufman DW, Kelly JP, Anderson T, et al, "Evaluation of Case Reports of Aplastic Anemia Among Patients Treated With Felbamate," *Epilepsia*, 1997, 38(12):1265-9.

Leppik IE, "Felbamate," *Epilepsia*, 1995, 36(Suppl 2):S66-72.

Pellock JM, "Felbamate in Epilepsy Therapy: Evaluating the Risks," *Drug Saf*, 1999, 21(3):225-39.

Pellock JM, "Managing Pediatric Epilepsy Syndromes With New Antiepileptic Drugs," *Pediatrics*, 1999, 104(5 Pt 1):1106-16.

Perucca E, "Clinically Relevant Drug Interactions With Antiepileptic Drugs," *Br J Clin Pharmacol*, 2006, 61(3):246-55.

The Felbamate Study Group in Lennox-Gastaut Syndrome, "Efficacy of Felbamate in Childhood Epileptic Encephalopathy (Lennox-Gastaut Syndrome)," *N Engl J Med*, 1993, 328(1):29-33.

◆ **Felbatol®** *see* Felbamate *on page 564*

◆ **Feldene®** *see* Piroxicam *on page 1118*

◆ **Femilax™ [OTC]** *see* Bisacodyl *on page 194*

◆ **Femiron® [OTC]** *see* Ferrous Fumarate *on page 576*

◆ **Femring®** *see* Estradiol *on page 536*

◆ **Femtrace®** *see* Estradiol *on page 536*

◆ **Fenesin DM IR** *see* Guaifenesin and Dextromethorphan *on page 658*

◆ **Fenesin IR [OTC]** *see* GuaiFENesin *on page 656*

FentaNYL (FEN ta nil)

Medication Safety Issues
Sound-alike/look-alike issues:

FentaNYL may be confused with alfentanil, SUFentanil

Dosing of transdermal fentanyl patches may be confusing. Transdermal fentanyl patches should always be prescribed in mcg/hour, not size. Patch dosage form of Duragesic®-12 actually delivers 12.5 mcg/hour of fentanyl. Use caution, as orders may be written as "Duragesic 12.5" which can be erroneously interpreted as a 125 mcg dose.

Fentora®, Onsolis™, and Actiq® are not interchangeable; do not substitute doses on a mcg-per-mcg basis.

High alert medication: The Institute for Safe Medication Practices (ISMP) includes this medication among its list of drug classes which have a heightened risk of causing significant patient harm when used in error.

Fentanyl transdermal system patches: Leakage of fentanyl gel from the patch has been reported; patch may be less effective; do not use. Thoroughly wash any skin surfaces coming into direct contact with gel with water (do not use soap).

Related Information
Adult ACLS Algorithms *on page 1463*
Compatibility of Medications Mixed in a Syringe *on page 1713*
Opioid Analgesics Comparison *on page 1510*
Preprocedure Sedatives in Children *on page 1688*
Serotonin Syndrome *on page 1695*

U.S. Brand Names Actiq®; Duragesic®; Fentora®; Onsolis™; Sublimaze® [DSC]

Canadian Brand Names Actiq®; Duragesic MAT; Duragesic®; Fentanyl Citrate Injection, USP; Novo-Fentanyl; PMS-Fentanyl MTX; RAN™-Fentanyl Transdermal System; ratio-Fentanyl

Therapeutic Category Analgesic, Narcotic; General Anesthetic

Generic Available Yes: Excludes buccal film, buccal tablet

Use
Injection: Sedation; relief of pain; preoperative medication; adjunct to general or regional anesthesia (FDA approved in ages ≥2 years and adults)

Transdermal patch (Duragesic®): Treatment of persistent, moderate-to-severe chronic pain in opioid-tolerant patients who are currently receiving opiates (FDA approved in ages ≥2 years and adults); see **Note**

Oral transmucosal lozenge (Actiq®): Breakthrough cancer pain in opioid-tolerant patients who are currently receiving around-the-clock opiates for persistent cancer pain (FDA approved in ages ≥16 years and adults); see **Note**

Buccal film (Onsolis™): Breakthrough cancer pain in opioid-tolerant patients who are currently receiving opiates for persistent cancer pain (FDA approved in adults); see **Note**

Buccal tablet (Fentora®): Breakthrough cancer pain in opioid-tolerant patients who are currently receiving opiates for persistent cancer pain (FDA approved in adults); see **Note**

Note: Patients are considered opioid-tolerant if they are receiving around-the-clock opioids at a dose of at least 60 mg/day of morphine, 25 mcg/hour of transdermal fentanyl, 30 mg/day of oral oxycodone, 8 mg/day of oral hydromorphone, or an equivalent dose of another opioid for 1 week or longer.

Restrictions C-II
Onsolis™ (fentanyl buccal film) is only available through the restricted distribution program (FOCUS™). Enrollment in the FOCUS™ program is required for prescribers, pharmacies, and patients. Further information may be obtained from the manufacturer, Meda Pharmaceuticals, Inc (877-466-7654).

Medication Guide An FDA-approved patient medication guide, which is available with the product information and as follows, must be dispensed with each new outpatient prescription and refill.

Actiq®: http://www.fda.gov/downloads/Drugs/DrugSafety/ucm085817.pdf

Duragesic®: http://www.fda.gov/downloads/Drugs/DrugSafety/ucm088584.pdf

Fentora®: http://www.fda.gov/downloads/Drugs/DrugSafety/ucm088597.pdf

Onsolis™ http://www.accessdata.fda.gov/drugsatfda_docs/label/2009/022266s000MedGuide.pdf

Pregnancy Risk Factor C

Pregnancy Considerations Teratogenic effects were not observed; however, embryo and fetotoxicity were noted in animal studies. Fentanyl crosses the placenta and the injectable formulation has been used safely during labor. Chronic use during pregnancy has shown detectable serum concentrations in the newborn with transient respiratory depression, behavioral changes, or seizures in the newborn infant characteristic of neonatal abstinence syndrome; transient neonatal muscular rigidity has also been observed. Transdermal patch, transmucosal lozenge, buccal tablet (Fentora®), and buccal film (Onsolis™) are not recommended for analgesia during labor and delivery.

Lactation Enters breast milk/not recommended (AAP rates "compatible")

Breast-Feeding Considerations Fentanyl is excreted in low concentrations into breast milk. Breast-feeding is considered acceptable following single doses to the mother; however, limited information is available when used long-term. **Note:** Transdermal patch, transmucosal lozenge, buccal tablet (Fentora®), and buccal film (Onsolis™) are not recommended in nursing women due to potential for sedation and/or respiratory depression. Symptoms of opioid withdrawal may occur in infants following the cessation of breast-feeding.

Contraindications Hypersensitivity or intolerance to fentanyl, other opioid agonists, or any component

Transdermal system: Severe respiratory disease or depression including acute asthma (unless patient is mechanically ventilated); paralytic ileus; patients requiring short-term therapy; management of pain following outpatient or day surgery, intermittent pain, or mild pain

Transmucosal buccal film (eg Onsolis™), buccal tablets (Fentora®), lozenges (eg, Actiq®), and transdermal patches (eg, Duragesic®) are also contraindicated in patients who are not opioid-tolerant (see **Note** in Use field) and in the management of acute or postoperative pain (including headache or migraine pain). Onsolis™ is also contraindicated in the management of dental pain or use in the emergency room.

Warnings High potential for abuse; physical and psychological dependence may occur with prolonged use **[U.S. Boxed Warning]**; abrupt discontinuation may result in withdrawal or seizures; potent opioids have a high risk of fatal overdose due to respiratory depression. Symptoms of opioid withdrawal may occur in patients after conversion of one dosage form to another or after dosage adjustment. Use with CYP3A4 inhibitors may result in increased effects and potentially fatal respiratory depression **[U.S. Boxed Warning]** (see Drug Interactions).

I.V. use: Rapid I.V. infusion may result in skeletal muscle and chest wall rigidity, impaired ventilation, respiratory distress, apnea, bronchoconstriction, laryngospasm; inject slowly over 3-5 minutes; nondepolarizing skeletal muscle relaxant may be required

Transdermal patch: Overdoses and deaths have occurred in patients using both the generic and brand name (Duragesic®) products **[U.S. Boxed Warning]**; the directions for use must be followed exactly for safe and effective therapy. Keep used and unused patches out of the reach of children; accidental or deliberate application or ingestion by an infant, child, or adolescent may cause respiratory depression which may result in death. Should be prescribed only by specialists who are knowledgeable in treating pain with potent opioids. Indicated for the management of persistent moderate-to-severe pain when around the clock pain control is needed for an extended time period **[U.S. Boxed Warning]**. Should only be used in patients who are already receiving opioid therapy, are opioid-tolerant, and who require a total daily dose equivalent to 25 mcg/h transdermal patch **[U.S. Boxed Warning]**. Use in patients who are not opioid-tolerant may result in fatal respiratory depression **[U.S. Boxed Warning]**. Use in pediatric patients **only** if they are opioid-tolerant, receiving at least 60 mg oral morphine equivalents per day, and ≥2 years of age **[U.S. Boxed Warning]**; safety has not been established in children <2 years. Serious or potential fatal respiratory depression may occur (even in opioid-tolerant individuals) during the initial application of the patch **[U.S. Boxed Warning]**; patients should be monitored carefully, especially 24-72 hours after initial patch application (when peak fentanyl serum levels occur) and following increases in dosage. Monitor patients who experience adverse reactions for at least 24 hours after removal of the patch (apparent transdermal half-life is 17 hours). Serum fentanyl concentrations may increase by ~1/3 in patients with a body temperature of 104°F (40°C) secondary to temperature-dependent increases in drug released from the transdermal system and an increase in skin permeability; thus, patients with fever should be monitored for opioid adverse effects. Do not expose transdermal patch application site to direct heat sources (eg, electric blankets, heating pads, heated water beds, heat lamps, tanning lamps, hot tubs, hot baths, saunas, sunbathing) **[U.S. Boxed Warning]**; temperature-dependent increases in drug released from patch may result in possible overdose or death. Possible overdose or death may also occur in people accidentally exposed to the transdermal system (eg, transfer of the patch from an adult to a child while hugging). Should be applied only to intact skin. Use of a patch that has been cut, damaged, or altered in any way may result in potentially fatal overdosage **[U.S. Boxed Warning]**. Do not place the patch in the mouth; do not chew, swallow, or use in ways that are not indicated; choking or overdose may occur and result in serious medical problems or death. Transdermal patch may contain conducting metal (eg, aluminum) which may cause a burn to the skin during an MRI scan; remove patch prior to MRI; reapply patch after scan is completed. Due to the potential for altered electrical conductivity, remove transdermal patch before cardioversion or defibrillation.

Oral transmucosal lozenge (Actiq®): Serious adverse events, including deaths, have been reported; deaths may occur due to improper dosing or improper patient selection (eg, use in patients who are not opioid-tolerant) **[U.S. Boxed Warning]**. Use only for the care of cancer patients who are opioid-tolerant to around-the-clock opioid therapy **[U.S. Boxed Warning]**; use in patients who are not opioid-tolerant at any dose may result in fatal respiratory depression **[U.S. Boxed Warning]**. Should be prescribed only by healthcare professionals who are knowledgeable

in treating cancer pain with potent opioids **[U.S. Boxed Warning]**. May cause potentially life-threatening hypoventilation, respiratory depression, and/or death **[U.S. Boxed Warning]**. Risk of respiratory depression increased in elderly patients, debilitated patients, and patients with conditions associated with hypoxia or hypercapnia; usually occurs after administration of initial dose in nontolerant patients or when given with other drugs that depress respiratory function. The substitution of Actiq® for any other fentanyl product may result in an fatal overdose. Do not convert patients on a mcg-per-mcg basis to Actiq® from other fentanyl products (products are not equivalent). Do not substitute Actiq® for any other fentanyl product. Substantial differences exist in the pharmacokinetic profile of Actiq® compared to other fentanyl products **[U.S. Boxed Warning]**. No safe conversion directions exist for patients on any other fentanyl products; opioid-tolerant patients should always receive an initial Actiq® dose of 200 mcg. Patients using Actiq® who experience breakthrough pain may only take one additional dose using the same strength and must wait 4 hours before taking another dose **[U.S. Boxed Warning]**. Keep out of the reach of children and discard any open units properly; contains an amount of medication that can be fatal to children; death has been reported in children who accidentally ingested Actiq® **[U.S. Boxed Warning]**. Safety and efficacy have not been established for patients <16 years of age; 15 opioid-tolerant pediatric patients (age: 5-15 years) with breakthrough pain were treated with Actiq® in a clinical study; 12 of the 15 patients received doses of 200 mcg to 600 mcg; no conclusions about safety and efficacy could be drawn due to the small sample size.

Buccal film (Onsolis™): Serious adverse events, including deaths, have been reported with other oral transmucosal fentanyl products; deaths may occur due to improper dosing or improper patient selection (eg, use in patients who are not opioid-tolerant) **[U.S. Boxed Warning]**. Use only for the care of opioid-tolerant cancer patients **[U.S. Boxed Warning]**; use in patients who are not opioid-tolerant at any dose may result in fatal respiratory depression **[U.S. Boxed Warning]**. Should be prescribed only by healthcare professionals who are knowledgeable in treating cancer pain with potent opioids **[U.S. Boxed Warning]**. May cause potentially life-threatening hypoventilation, respiratory depression, and/or death **[U.S. Boxed Warning]**. Due to the risk for misuse, abuse, and overdose, Onsolis™ is available only through a restricted distribution program, called the FOCUS Program (see Restrictions) **[U.S. Boxed Warning]**. If a breakthrough pain episode is not relieved, at least 2 hours should pass before taking another dose **[U.S. Boxed Warning]**. Onsolis™ is contraindicated in the management of acute or postoperative pain, including headache/migraine, dental pain, or use in the emergency room (see Contraindications) **[U.S. Boxed Warning]**. Do not substitute Onsolis™ for any other fentanyl product as substantial differences exist in the pharmacokinetic profile; substitution may result in fatal overdose. Do not convert patients on a mcg-per-mcg basis to Onsolis™ from other fentanyl products **[U.S. Boxed Warning]**. Keep out of the reach of children and discard any open units properly; contains an amount of medication that can be fatal to children **[U.S. Boxed Warning]**.

Buccal tablet (Fentora®): Use only for the care of opioid-tolerant cancer patients who are already receiving opioid therapy for persistent cancer pain **[U.S. Boxed Warning]**; use in patients who are not opioid-tolerant may result in fatal respiratory depression **[U.S. Boxed Warning]**; should be prescribed only by healthcare professionals who are knowledgeable in treating cancer pain with potent opioids. Keep out of the reach of children and discard any open units properly; contains an amount of medication that can be fatal to children **[U.S. Boxed Warning]**. Buccal tablets have a higher bioavailability than other oral fentanyl products (including oral transmucosal lozenge); do not substitute products on a mcg per mcg basis; substitution of buccal tablets for any other fentanyl product may result in fatal overdose; appropriate dosage adjustments must be made **[U.S. Boxed Warning]**; use caution and monitor closely when changing patients from one product to another. Fentora® is contraindicated in the management of acute or postoperative pain, including headache/migraine **[U.S. Boxed Warning]**; serious adverse events, including death, have been reported when used inappropriately (improper dose or patient selection) **[U.S. Boxed Warning]**. Patients using Fentora® who experience breakthrough pain may only take **one** additional dose (if pain not relieved after 30 minutes) using the same strength tablet and must wait 4 hours before taking another dose **[U.S. Boxed Warning]**. Safety and efficacy have not been established for patients <18 years of age.

Precautions Use with extreme caution in patients with bradycardia; hepatic, biliary tract, renal, or respiratory disease; acute pancreatitis; cor pulmonale; significant COPD; other chronic respiratory conditions; or those with increased ICP, head injuries, or impaired consciousness. Patients must be monitored until fully recovered; decrease dose in patients with hepatic and/or renal disease; not recommended if patient received MAO inhibitors within 14 days. Use transdermal patch with caution in cachectic or debilitated patients; these patients may have altered pharmacokinetics due to muscle wasting, poor fat stores, or altered clearance. Frequent use of Actiq® or generic lozenge may increase risk of dental caries; Actiq® and generic lozenge contain 2 g of sugar/unit, as hydrated dextrates; patients should maintain good oral hygiene; inform diabetic patients of sugar content. Use buccal tablets with caution in patients with mucositis (no dose adjustment is needed in patients with Grade I mucositis; safety and efficacy in patients with more severe mucositis have not been studied).

Fentanyl is not recommended for analgesia during labor and delivery; transient muscular rigidity has been observed in neonates born to women who were treated with I.V. fentanyl

Adverse Reactions

Cardiovascular: Bradycardia, cardiac arrhythmia, edema, flushing, hypertension, hypotension, orthostatic hypotension, syncope, tachycardia

Central nervous system: Abnormal dreams, abnormal thinking, agitation, amnesia, anxiety, CNS depression, confusion, dizziness, drowsiness, euphoria, fatigue, fever, hallucinations, headache, insomnia, nervousness, paranoid reaction, sedation, somnolence

Dermatologic: Erythema, pruritus, rash; facial pruritus with oral transmucosal product

Endocrine & metabolic: ADH release, dehydration, hypokalemia (6% with buccal tablets), weight loss

Gastrointestinal: Abdominal pain, anorexia, appetite decreased, biliary tract spasm, constipation, diarrhea, dyspepsia, flatulence, ileus, nausea, vomiting, xerostomia; dental caries, tooth loss, and gum line erosion have been reported with transmucosal lozenge containing sugar

Genitourinary: Urinary retention, urinary tract spasm

Hematologic: Anemia, neutropenia

Local:
Buccal tablet: Application-site reactions, bleeding, irritation, local paresthesia, pain, ulceration
Transdermal patch: Edema, erythema, pruritus
Transmucosal lozenge: Application-site reactions, irritation, pain, ulcer

Neuromuscular & skeletal: Abnormal coordination, abnormal gait, asthenia, back pain, paresthesia, rigors, tremor;

skeletal muscle and chest wall rigidity especially following rapid I.V. administration

Ocular: Miosis

Respiratory: Apnea, cough, dyspnea, hemoptysis, hypoxia, respiratory depression

Miscellaneous: Flu-like symptoms, rigors, sweating; physical and psychological dependence with prolonged use (**Note:** Neonates who receive a total fentanyl dose >1.6 mg/kg or continuous infusion duration >5 days are more likely to develop narcotic withdrawal symptoms; children 1 week to 22 months: Those who receive a total dose of 1.5 mg/kg or duration >5 days have a 50% chance of developing narcotic withdrawal and those receiving a total dose >2.5 mg/kg or duration of infusion >9 days have a 100% chance of developing withdrawal. Doses should be tapered to prevent withdrawal symptoms.)

Drug Interactions

Metabolism/Transport Effects Substrate of CYP3A4 (major); **Inhibits** CYP3A4 (weak)

Avoid Concomitant Use

Avoid concomitant use of FentaNYL with any of the following: MAO Inhibitors

Increased Effect/Toxicity

FentaNYL may increase the levels/effects of: Alcohol (Ethyl); Alvimopan; Beta-Blockers; Calcium Channel Blockers (Nondihydropyridine); CNS Depressants; Desmopressin; MAO Inhibitors; Selective Serotonin Reuptake Inhibitors; Thiazide Diuretics

The levels/effects of FentaNYL may be increased by: Amphetamines; Antipsychotic Agents (Phenothiazines); CYP3A4 Inhibitors (Moderate); CYP3A4 Inhibitors (Strong); Dasatinib; MAO Inhibitors; Succinylcholine

Decreased Effect

FentaNYL may decrease the levels/effects of: Pegvisomant

The levels/effects of FentaNYL may be decreased by: Ammonium Chloride; Mixed Agonist / Antagonist Opioids; Rifamycin Derivatives

Food Interactions Grapefruit juice may significantly increase fentanyl serum concentrations and adverse effects.

Stability

Injection formulation: Store at controlled room temperature of 15°C to 25°C (59°F to 86°F). Protect from light.

Transdermal patch: Do not store above 25°C (77°F). Store in protective pouch until ready to use.

Transmucosal lozenge, buccal film, and buccal tablets: Store at controlled room temperature of 20°C to 25°C (68°F to 77°F); excursions permitted to 15°C to 30°C (56°F to 86°F); protect from freezing and moisture. Store in original child-resistant blister packaging until ready to use. Do not use if foil package has been opened.

Mechanism of Action Binds with stereospecific opioid mu receptors at many sites within the CNS, increases pain threshold, alters pain reception, inhibits ascending pain pathways

Pharmacodynamics Respiratory depressant effect may last longer than analgesic effect

Onset of action: Analgesia:
I.M.: 7-15 minutes
I.V.: Almost immediate
Transdermal patch: 6-8 hours
Transmucosal lozenge: 5-15 minutes

Maximum effect:
Transdermal patch: 24 hours
Transmucosal lozenge: 20-30 minutes

Duration:
I.M.: 1-2 hours
I.V.: 30-60 minutes
Transdermal patch: 72 hours
Transmucosal lozenge: 1-2 hours

Pharmacokinetics (Adult data unless noted) Note: Fentanyl serum concentrations are ~twofold higher in children 1.5-5 years old who are not opioid-tolerant and are receiving the transdermal patch. Pharmacokinetic parameters in older pediatric patients are similar to adults. Pharmacokinetics of transdermal patch with or without Bioclusive™ overlay (polyurethane film dressing) were bioequivalent.

Absorption:
Transmucosal lozenge: Rapid; ~25% absorbed from buccal mucosa; 75% swallowed with saliva and slowly absorbed from GI tract
Buccal film and buccal tablet: Rapid; ~50% from the buccal mucosa; 50% swallowed with saliva and slowly absorbed from GI tract

Distribution: Highly lipophilic, redistributes into muscle and fat; crosses placenta; excreted in breast milk; **Note:** I.V. fentanyl exhibits a 3-compartment distribution model. Changes in blood pH may alter ionization of fentanyl and affect its distribution between plasma and CNS

V_{dss}: Children: 0.05-14 years of age (after long-term continuous infusion): ~15 L/kg (range: 5-30 L/kg)
V_{dss}: Adults: 4 L/kg

Protein binding: 80% to 85%, primarily to alpha-1-acid glycoprotein; also binds to albumin and erythrocytes; **Note:** Free fraction increases with acidosis

Metabolism: >90% metabolized in the liver via cytochrome P450 isoenzyme CYP3A4 by N-dealkylation (to norfentanyl) and hydroxylation to other inactive metabolites

Bioavailability: **Note:** Comparative studies have found the buccal film to have a 40% greater systemic exposure (ie, AUC) than the transmucosal lozenge, and the buccal tablet to have a 30% to 50% greater exposure than the transmucosal lozenge
Transmucosal lozenge: ~50% (range: 36% to 71%)
Buccal film: 71% (mucositis did not have a clinically significant effect on peak concentration and AUC; however, bioavailability is expected to decrease if film is inappropriately chewed and swallowed)
Buccal tablet: 65% ± 20%

Half-life:
Children 5 months to 4.5 years: Mean: 2.4 hours
Children 0.5-14 years (after long-term continuous infusion): ~21 hours (range: 11-36 hours)
Adults: I.V.: 2-4 hours; **Note:** Using a 3-compartment model, fentanyl displayed an initial distribution half-life of 6 minutes; second distribution half-life of 1 hour and terminal half-life of 16 hours
Transdermal patch: 17 hours (range: 13-22); apparent half-life increased with transdermal patch due to continued absorption
Transmucosal lozenge: 6.6 hours (range: 5-15 hours)
Buccal film: ~14 hours
Buccal tablet: 100-200 mcg: 3-4 hours; 400-800 mcg: 11-12 hours

Time to peak serum concentration:
Transdermal patch: 24-72 hours
Transmucosal lozenge: Median: 20-40 minutes (range: 20-480 minutes), measured after the start of dose administration
Buccal film: Median: 1 hour (range: 0.75-4 hours)
Buccal tablet: Median: 47 minutes (range: 20-240 minutes)

Elimination: In urine primarily as metabolites and <7% to 10% as unchanged drug
Clearance: Newborn infants: Clearance may be significantly correlated to gestational age and birth weight (see Saarenmaa, 2000)

Usual Dosage Doses should be titrated to appropriate effects; wide range of doses exist, dependent upon desired degree of analgesia/anesthesia, clinical environment, patient's status, and presence of opioid tolerance.

Neonates: Analgesia: International Evidence-Based Group for Neonatal Pain recommendations (Anand, 2001):
Intermittent doses: Slow I.V. push: 0.5-3 mcg/kg/dose
Continuous I.V. infusion: 0.5-2 mcg/kg/hour

Neonates and younger Infants:
Sedation/analgesia: Slow I.V. push: 1-4 mcg/kg/dose; may repeat every 2-4 hours
Continuous sedation/analgesia: Initial I.V. bolus: 1-2 mcg/kg, then 0.5-1 mcg/kg/hour; titrate upward
Mean required dose: Neonates with gestational age <34 weeks: 0.64 mcg/kg/hour; neonates with gestational age ≥34 weeks: 0.75 mcg/kg/hour
Continuous sedation/analgesia during ECMO: Initial I.V. bolus: 5-10 mcg/kg slow I.V. push over 10 minutes, then 1-5 mcg/kg/hour; titrate upward; tolerance may develop; higher doses (up to 20 mcg/kg/hour) may be needed by day 6 of ECMO

Older Infants and Children 1-12 years:
Sedation for minor procedures/analgesia: I.M., I.V.: 1-2 mcg/kg/dose; may repeat at 30- to 60-minute intervals. **Note:** Children 18-36 months of age may require 2-3 mcg/kg/dose.
Continuous sedation/analgesia: Initial I.V. bolus: 1-2 mcg/kg then 1 mcg/kg/hour; titrate upward; usual: 1-3 mcg/kg/hour; some require 5 mcg/kg/hour
Moderate to severe chronic pain: Transdermal patch: Opioid-tolerant children ≥2 years receiving at least 60 mg oral morphine equivalents per day: Initial: 25 mcg/hour system or higher, based on conversion to fentanyl equivalents and administration of equianalgesic dosage (see package insert for further information); use short-acting analgesics for first 24 hours with supplemental PRN doses thereafter (for breakthrough pain); dose may be increased after 3 days, based on the daily dose of supplementary PRN opioids required; use the ratio of 45 mg of oral morphine equivalents per day to a 12.5 mcg/hour increase in transdermal patch dosage; change patch every 72 hours; **Note:** Dosing intervals less than every 72 hours are **not** recommended for children and adolescents. Initiation of the transdermal patch in children taking <60 mg of oral morphine equivalents per day has not been studied in controlled clinical trials; in open-label trials, children 2-18 years of age who were receiving at least 45 mg of oral morphine equivalents per day were started with an initial transdermal dose of 25 mcg/hour (or higher, depending upon equianalgesic dose of opioid received).

Children ≥5 years and <50 kg:
Patient-controlled analgesia (PCA): I.V.: Opioid-naïve: **Note:** PCA has been used in children as young as 5 years of age; however, clinicians need to assess children 5-8 years of age to determine if they are able to use the PCA device correctly. All patients should receive an initial loading dose of an analgesic (to attain adequate control of pain) before starting PCA for maintenance. Adjust doses, lockouts, and limits based on required loading dose, age, state of health, and presence of opioid tolerance. Use lower end of dosing range for opioid-naïve. Assess patient and pain control at regular intervals and adjust settings if needed (see American Pain Society, 2008):
Usual concentration: Determined by weight; some centers use the following:
Children <12 kg: 10 mcg/mL
Children 12-30 kg: 25 mcg/mL
Children >30 kg: 50 mcg/mL

Demand dose: Usual initial: 0.5-1 mcg/kg/dose; usual range: 0.5-1 mcg/kg/dose

Lockout: Usual initial: 5 doses/hour

Lockout interval: Range: 6-8 minutes

Usual basal rate: 0-0.5 mcg/kg/hour

Children >12 years and Adults:

Sedation for minor procedures/analgesia: I.V.: 0.5-1 mcg/kg/dose; may repeat after 30-60 minutes; or 25-50 mcg, repeat full dose in 5 minutes if needed, may repeat 4-5 times with 25 mcg at 5-minute intervals if needed. **Note:** Higher doses are used for major procedures.

Continuous sedation/analgesia:

<50 kg: Initial I.V. bolus: 1-2 mcg/kg; continuous infusion rate: 1-2 mcg/kg/hour

>50 kg: Initial I.V. bolus: 1-2 mcg/kg **or** 25-100 mcg/dose; continuous infusion rate: 1-2 mcg/kg/hour **or** 25-200 mcg/hour

Patient-controlled analgesia (PCA): I.V.: Children >50 kg, Adolescents >50 kg, and Adults: **Note:** All patients should receive an initial loading dose of an analgesic (to attain adequate control of pain) before starting PCA for maintenance. Adjust doses, lockouts, and limits based on required loading dose, age, state of health, and presence of opioid tolerance. Use lower end of dosing range for opioid-naïve. Assess patient and pain control at regular intervals and adjust settings if needed (see American Pain Society, 2008):

Usual concentration: 50 mcg/mL

Demand dose: Usual initial: 20 mcg; usual range: 10-50 mcg

Lockout interval: Usual initial: 6 minutes; usual range: 5-8 minutes

Usual basal rate: ≤50 mcg/hour

Preoperative sedation, adjunct to regional anesthesia, postoperative pain: I.M., I.V.: 25-100 mcg/dose

Adjunct to general anesthesia: Slow I.V.:

Low dose: 0.5-2 mcg/kg/dose depending on the indication

Moderate dose: Initial: 2-20 mcg/kg/dose; Maintenance (bolus or infusion): 1-2 mcg/kg/hour. Discontinuing fentanyl infusion 30-60 minutes prior to the end of surgery will usually allow adequate ventilation upon emergence from anesthesia. For "fast-tracking" and early extubation following major surgery, total fentanyl doses are limited to 10-15 mcg/kg.

High dose: 20-50 mcg/kg/dose; **Note:** High dose fentanyl as an adjunct to general anesthesia is rarely used, but is still described in the manufacturer's label.

General anesthesia without additional anesthetic agents: I.V.: 50-100 mcg/kg with O_2 and skeletal muscle relaxant

Moderate to severe chronic pain: Transdermal patch: Opioid-tolerant patients receiving at least 60 mg oral morphine equivalents per day: Initial: 25 mcg/hour system or higher, based on conversion to fentanyl equivalents and administration of equianalgesic dosage (see package insert for further information); use short-acting analgesics for first 24 hours with supplemental PRN doses thereafter (for breakthrough pain); dose may be increased after 3 days based on the daily dose of supplementary PRN opioids required; use the ratio of 45 mg of oral morphine equivalents per day to a 12.5 mcg/hour increase in transdermal patch dosage; transdermal patch is usually administered every 72 hours but select **adult** patients may require every 48-hour administration; dosage increase administered every 72 hours should be tried before 48-hour schedule is used

Adolescents ≥16 years and Adults: Breakthrough cancer pain: Transmucosal lozenge (Actiq®): Opioid-tolerant patients: Titrate dose to provide adequate analgesia: Initial: 200 mcg; may repeat dose only once, 15 minutes after completion of first dose if needed. Do

not exceed a maximum of 2 doses per each breakthrough cancer pain episode; patient must wait at least 4 hours before treating another episode. Titrate dose up to next higher strength if treatment of several consecutive breakthrough episodes requires >1 Actiq® per episode; evaluate each new dose over several breakthrough cancer pain episodes (generally 1-2 days) to determine proper dose of analgesia with acceptable side effects. Once dose has been determined, consumption should be limited to ≤4 units/day. Re-evaluate maintenance (around-the-clock) opioid dose if patient requires >4 units/day. If signs of excessive opioid effects occur before a dose is complete, the unit should be removed from the mouth immediately, and subsequent doses decreased.

Adolescents ≥18 years and Adults:

Severe pain: I.M, I.V.: 50-100 mcg/dose every 1-2 hours as needed; patients with prior opioid exposure may tolerate higher initial doses

Intrathecal (American Pain Society, 2008): **Note: Must use preservative-free.** Doses must be adjusted for age, injection site, and patient's medical condition and degree of opioid tolerance.

Single dose: 5-25 mcg/dose; may provide adequate relief for up to 6 hours

Continuous infusion: Not recommended in acute pain management due to risk of excessive accumulation. For chronic cancer pain, infusion of very small doses may be practical (American Pain Society, 2008).

Epidural (American Pain Society, 2008): **Note: Must use preservative-free.** Doses must be adjusted for age, injection site, and patient's medical condition and degree of opioid tolerance.

Single dose: 25-100 mcg/dose; may provide adequate relief for up to 8 hours

Continuous infusion: 25-100 mcg/hour

Breakthrough cancer pain:

Buccal film (Onsolis™): Opioid-tolerant patients: Titrate dose to provide adequate analgesia: Initial dose: 200 mcg for all patients; **Note:** Patients previously using another transmucosal product should be initiated at doses of 200 mcg; do **not** switch patients using any other fentanyl product on a mcg-per-mcg basis.

Dose titration: If titration of dose is required, increase dose in 200 mcg increments once per episode using multiples of the 200 mcg film; do not redose within a single episode of breakthrough pain and separate single doses by ≥2 hours. During titration, do not exceed 4 simultaneous applications of the 200 mcg films (800 mcg). If >800 mcg required, treat next episode with one 1200 mcg film (maximum dose: 1200 mcg). Once maintenance dose is determined, all other unused films should be disposed of and that strength (using a single film) should be used. During any pain episode, if adequate relief is not achieved after 30 minutes following buccal film application, a rescue medication (as determined by healthcare provider) may be used.

Maintenance: Determined dose applied as a single film once per episode and separated by ≥2 hours (dose range: 200-1200 mcg); limit to 4 applications/day. Consider increasing the around-the-clock opioid therapy in patients experiencing >4 breakthrough pain episodes/day.

Buccal tablets (Fentora®): Opioid-tolerant patients not being converted from transmucosal lozenge: Initial dose: 100 mcg; if needed, a second 100 mcg dose may be administered 30 minutes after the start of the first dose; no further doses should be given until at least 4 hours later (ie, maximum: 2 doses per breakthrough pain episode every 4 hours)

If needed, dose titration should be done using multiples of the 100 mcg tablets. May increase dose, if needed, to two 100 mcg tablets (one on each side of mouth). If that dose is not successful, increase dose to four 100 mcg tablets (two on each side of mouth). If titration requires >400 mcg/dose, then use 200 mcg tablets. Do not use more than 4 tablets/dose.

Conversion from transmucosal lozenge to buccal tablet (Fentora®): Initial dose:

If lozenge dose 200-400 mcg, then use buccal tablet 100 mcg

If lozenge dose 600-800 mcg, then use buccal tablet 200 mcg

If lozenge dose 1200-1600 mcg, then use two 200 mcg buccal tablets (400 mcg/dose)

Note: Four 100 mcg buccal tablets deliver approximately 12% and 13% higher values of C_{max} and AUC, respectively, compared to one 400 mcg buccal tablet. To prevent confusion, patient should only have one strength of tablets available at a time. Using more than four buccal tablets at a time has not been studied. Re-evaluate maintenance (around-the-clock) opioid dose if patient requires >4 doses of buccal tablets/day. Once buccal tablet dose is titrated to an effective dose, patients should use only one tablet (of the appropriate strength) per episode of breakthrough pain. On occasion, if pain is not relieved after 30 minutes, a second dose may be administered; no further doses should be given until at least 4 hours later (ie, maximum: 2 doses per breakthrough pain episode every 4 hours).

Dosing adjustment in renal impairment:
Cl_{cr} 10-50 mL/minute: Administer 75% of dose
Cl_{cr} <10 mL/minute: Administer 50% of dose

Dosing adjustment in hepatic impairment: Use with caution; specific guidelines are not available; lower dose is recommended

Administration

Parenteral: I.V.: Administer by slow I.V. push over 3-5 minutes or by continuous infusion. Larger bolus doses (>5 mcg/kg) should be given slow I.V. push over 5-10 minutes (see Warnings)

Transdermal patch: Apply to nonhairy, clean, dry, non-irritated, intact skin of the flat area of front or back of upper torso, flank area, or upper arm; apply to upper back in young children or in people with cognitive impairment to decrease the potential of the patient removing the patch. Monitor the adhesion of the system closely in children. Clip hair prior to application, do **not** shave area; prior to application, skin may be cleaned with clear water (do not use soaps, lotions, alcohol, oils, or other substances which may irritate the skin); allow skin to dry thoroughly prior to application. Apply patch immediately after removing from package; firmly press in place and hold for at least 30 seconds; change patch every 72 hours; remove old patch before applying new patch; do not apply new patch to same place as old patch; wash hands after applying patch. If there is difficulty with patch adhesion, the edges of the system may be taped in place with first-aid tape; if difficulty with adhesion persists, an adhesive film dressing (eg, Bioclusive™, Tegaderm™) may be applied over the system. If patch falls off before 72 hours, a new patch may be applied to a different skin site.

Note: Transdermal patch is a membrane-controlled system; do **not** cut the patch to deliver partial doses; do **not** use patches that are cut, damaged, or leaking; do **not** use if seal of package is broken; rate of drug delivery may be significantly increased if patch is cut, damaged, or leaking and result in absorption of a potentially fatal dose; reservoir contents and adhesion may be affected if cut; if partial dose is needed, surface area of patch can be blocked proportionally using adhesive bandage (see Lee, 1997). Do **not** use soap, alcohol, or other solvents to remove transdermal gel if it

accidentally touches skin as they may increase transdermal absorption, use copious amounts of water. Avoid exposing application site to external heat sources (eg, electric blanket, heating pad, heat lamp, tanning lamp, sauna, heated water bed, hot tub, hot baths, sunbathing). Dispose of properly (see Patient Information).

Transmucosal lozenge (Actiq®): Oral: Do not use if blister package has been opened. Blister package should be opened with scissors just prior to administration; once removed, patient should place the lozenge in mouth and suck it; do not bite or chew lozenge. Place lozenge in mouth between cheek and lower gum; occasionally move lozenge from one side of the mouth to the other; consume lozenge over 15 minutes; remove lozenge from mouth if signs of excessive opioid effects appear before lozenge is totally consumed. Remove handle after lozenge is consumed or patient achieves adequate response.

Buccal film: Foil overwrap should be removed just prior to administration. Prior to placing film, wet inside of cheek using tongue or by rinsing with water. Place film inside mouth with the pink side of the unit against the inside of the moistened cheek. With finger, press the film against cheek and hold for 5 seconds. The film should stick to the inside of cheek after 5 seconds. The film should be left in place until it dissolves (usually within 15-30 minutes after application). Liquids may be consumed after 5 minutes of application. Food can be eaten after film dissolves. If using more than one film simultaneously (during titration period), apply films on either side of mouth (do not apply on top of each other). Do not chew or swallow film. Do not cut or tear the film.

Buccal tablet: Do not use if blister package has been opened or tampered with. Blister package should be opened just prior to administration. Peel back the blister backing to expose the tablet; do not push tablet through the blister (damage to the tablet may occur). Administer tablet immediately after removal from blister. Place entire tablet in the buccal cavity (above a rear molar, between the upper cheek and gum). Use alternate side of mouth for subsequent doses. Do not break, suck, chew, or swallow tablet (this will result in decreased effect). Tablet should dissolve in about 14-25 minutes when left between the cheek and the gum. If remnants remain after 30 minutes, they may be swallowed with a glass of water. If excessive opioid effects appear before tablet is completely dissolved (eg, dizziness, sedation, nausea), instruct patient to rinse mouth with water and spit remaining pieces of tablet into sink or toilet immediately; rinse the sink or flush toilet to dispose of tablet particles.

Monitoring Parameters Respiratory rate, blood pressure, heart rate, oxygen saturation, bowel sounds, abdominal distention; signs of misuse, abuse, or addiction

Transdermal patch: Monitor patient for at least 24 hours after application of first dose

Patient Information All products: Report the use of other medications, nonprescription medications, and herbal or natural products to your physician and pharmacist; avoid alcohol, other CNS depressants (eg, sleep medications, tranquilizers), grapefruit juice, and the herbal medicine St John's wort. Fentanyl may cause drowsiness and impair ability to perform activities requiring mental alertness or physical coordination; may be habit-forming; avoid abrupt discontinuation after prolonged use; may cause dry mouth and constipation. Notify physician immediately or seek emergency help if acute dizziness, chest pain, slow or rapid heartbeat, shortness of breath, respiratory difficulty, confusion, or unusual symptoms occur. Notify physician if acute headache, changes in mentation, changes in voiding frequency or amount, swelling of extremities, unusual weight gain, or vision changes occur.

Transdermal patch: Read the patient Medication Guide that you receive with each prescription and refill of this medication. Read this guide for details on proper storage, administration, and disposal of transdermal patch, as well as instructions about overdose management. Keep all transdermal patches (even if used) out of the reach of children; even used patches may be dangerous or even lethal to babies, children, pets, and other adults; discard used transdermal patches immediately after removal by folding in half (so the sticky side sticks to itself) and flushing down the toilet; discard unused patches that are no longer needed in the same manner; protective pouch and liner should be thrown in garbage. Notify physician if you develop a high fever while wearing the patch. Do **not** use patches that are cut, damaged, or leaking. Wash skin with clear water (not soap, alcohol, or other chemicals) if gel from patch accidentally comes into contact with skin. If patch accidentally sticks to the skin of another person, take patch off immediately, wash exposed skin with water, and seek medical attention for that person. Accidental exposure or misuse may lead to serious medical problems, even death. Do **not** adjust the dose or number of patches applied to the skin without the prescribing healthcare professional's instruction. If the patch is not sticking, the edges of the system may be taped in place with first-aid tape; if the patch continues to not stick to the skin, an adhesive film dressing (eg, Bioclusive™, Tegaderm™) may be applied over the system; do not cover the patch with any other bandage or tape. If patch falls off before 72 hours, a new patch may be applied to a different skin site.

Transmucosal lozenge: Do not allow other people to use this product (serious adverse effects and potentially fatal overdose may occur). An Actiq® Child Safety Kit and OTFC (Oral Transmucosal Fentanyl Citrate) Child Safety Kit, containing a child-resistant lock, portable locking pouch, and a child-resistant temporary storage bottle (to keep medication away from children), are available from the manufacturer; these kits can be obtained by calling 800-896-5855. Read the patient Medication Guide that you receive with each prescription and refill of this medication. Read this guide for details on proper storage, administration, and disposal of oral transmucosal lozenges, as well as instructions about overdose management. This product contains an amount of medication that can be fatal to children; death has been reported in children who accidentally ingested Actiq®; dispose of transmucosal products properly; keep all products (even if used) out of the reach of children and pets. After consumption of a complete unit, the handle may be disposed of in a trash container that is out of the reach of children and pets. For a partially consumed unit, or a unit that still has any drug matrix remaining on the handle, the handle should be placed under hot running tap water until the drug matrix has dissolved. Use the special child-resistant container available in the Child Safety Kit to temporarily store partially consumed units that cannot be disposed of immediately. Frequent use of oral transmucosal fentanyl lozenges may increase risk of dental caries; consult dentist for appropriate oral hygiene. Diabetic patients should note that oral transmucosal lozenge contains 2 g of sugar/unit (about 1/2 teaspoon of sugar).

Buccal film: Patients need to be enrolled in the FOCUS program in order to receive this product (Onsolis™); product will be delivered via a traceable courier. This product contains an amount of medication that can be fatal to people for whom it was not prescribed, those who are not tolerant to opioids, and children; keep film out of the reach of children. Do not use this product unless you have been regularly using other opioid medications around the clock for your constant cancer pain and your body is used to taking these medications. Read the patient Medication Guide that you receive with each prescription and refill of

fentanyl buccal film. Read this guide for details on proper storage, administration, and disposal of buccal film, as well as instructions about overdose management. Do not allow other people to use this product (serious adverse effects and potentially fatal overdose may occur). Discard unused film appropriately; remove foil overwraps from any unused, unneeded films and dispose by flushing down the toilet.

Buccal tablets: This product contains an amount of medication that can be fatal to children; keep tablets out of the reach of children. Do not use this product unless you have been regularly using other opioid medications around the clock for your constant cancer pain and your body is used to taking these medications. Read the patient Medication Guide that you receive with each prescription and refill of fentanyl buccal tablets. Read this guide for details on proper storage, administration, and disposal of buccal tablets, as well as instructions about overdose management. Do not allow other people to use this product (serious adverse effects and potentially fatal overdose may occur). Discard unused tablets appropriately; remove unusable tablets from blister package and flush tablets down the toilet; to dispose of excess unusable tablets call manufacturer at 1-800-896-5855.

Nursing Implications An opioid antagonist, resuscitative and intubation equipment, and oxygen should be available; rapid I.V. injection may result in apnea. Patients with elevated temperature may have increased fentanyl absorption transdermally from patch; observe for adverse effects, dosage adjustment may be needed. Pharmacologic and adverse effects can be seen after discontinuation of transdermal patch; observe patients for at least 24 hours after transdermal product is removed. Do **not** cut transdermal patch or use if cut, damaged, or leaking. Dispose of transdermal products properly (see Patient Information and Additional Information). Destroy unused portion of Actiq® according to hospital policy on controlled substances; partial unused doses of Actiq® can be dissolved under hot running tap water; dispose of handle properly. Keep all fentanyl products out of the reach of children; products contain an amount of medication that can be fatal to children. Assess other medications patient may be taking for additive or adverse interactions. Order safety precautions for inpatient use. Assess knowledge and teach patient appropriate use (if self-administered), adverse reactions to report, and appropriate interventions to reduce side effects.

Additional Information Fentanyl is 50-100 times as potent as morphine; morphine 10 mg I.M. = fentanyl 0.1-0.2 mg I.M. Fentanyl has less hypotensive effects than morphine or meperidine due to minimal or no histamine release. I.V. product has a pH of 4.0-7.5.

Buccal film (Onsolis™): Product is a buccal-soluble film which utilizes the BioErodible MucoAdhesive (BEMA™) bilayer delivery technology. The pink side contains the active ingredient in a water-soluble bioadhesive polymer; the white side is an inactive layer which lists the strength with an identifying number.

Buccal tablets (Fentora®): Product uses an effervescent reaction which may enhance the rate and extent of absorption of fentanyl through the buccal mucosa.

Transmucosal lozenge: Actiq is mounted on a plastic radiopaque handle; the generic oral transmucosal lozenge is formulated as a solid drug matrix and is mounted on a plastic fracture-resistant handle. Transmucosal lozenge contains sugar 2 g/unit.

Dosage Forms Excipient information presented when available (limited, particularly for generics); consult specific product labeling. [DSC] = Discontinued product

Note: Strengths expressed as base.

Film, for buccal application, as citrate:
Onsolis™: 200 mcg, 400 mcg, 600 mcg, 800 mcg, 1200 mcg
Injection, solution, as citrate [preservative free]: 0.05 mg/mL (2 mL, 5 mL, 10 mL, 20 mL; 30 mL [DSC]; 50 mL)
Sublimaze®: 0.05 mg/mL (2 mL, 5 mL, 10 mL, 20 mL) [DSC]
Lozenge, oral, as citrate [transmucosal]: 200 mcg, 400 mcg, 600 mcg, 800 mcg, 1200 mcg, 1600 mcg
Actiq®: 200 mcg, 400 mcg, 600 mcg, 800 mcg, 1200 mcg, 1600 mcg [contains sugar 2 g/lozenge; berry flavor]
Patch transdermal, topical, as base: 12 (5s) [delivers 12.5 mcg/hour; 3.13 cm^2]; 12 (5s) [delivers 12.5 mcg/hour; 5 cm^2]; 25 (5s) [delivers 25 mcg/hour; 10 cm^2]; 25 (5s) [delivers 25 mcg/hour; 6.25 cm^2]; 50 (5s) [delivers 50 mcg/hour; 12.5 cm^2]; 50 (5s) [delivers 50 mcg/hour; 20 cm^2]; 75 (5s) [delivers 75 mcg/hour; 18.75 cm^2]; 75 (5s) [delivers 75 mcg/hour; 30 cm^2]; 75 (5s) [delivers 75 mcg/hour; 32.1 cm^2]; 100 (5s) [delivers 100 mcg/hour; 25 cm^2]; 100 (5s) [delivers 100 mcg/hour; 40 cm^2]; 100 (5s) [delivers 100 mcg/hour; 42.8 cm^2]
Duragesic®: 12 (5s) [delivers 12.5 mcg/hour; 5 cm^2; contains ethanol 0.1 mL/10 cm^2]; 25 (5s) [delivers 25 mcg/hour; 10 cm^2; contains ethanol 0.1 mL/10 cm^2]; 50 (5s) [delivers 50 mcg/hour; 20 cm^2; contains ethanol 0.1 mL/10 cm^2]; 75 (5s) [delivers 75 mcg/hour; 30 cm^2; contains ethanol 0.1 mL/10 cm^2]; 100 (5s) [delivers 100 mcg/hour; 40 cm^2; contains ethanol 0.1 mL/10 cm^2]
Powder, for prescription compounding, as citrate: USP: 100% (1 g)
Tablet, for buccal application, as citrate:
Fentora®: 100 mcg, 200 mcg, 300 mcg [DSC], 400 mcg, 600 mcg, 800 mcg

References

Anand KJ and International Evidence-Based Group for Neonatal Pain, "Consensus Statement for the Prevention and Management of Pain in the Newborn," *Arch Pediatr Adolesc Med*, 2001, 155(2):173-80.

Billmire DA, Neale HW, and Gregory RO, "Use of I.V. Fentanyl in the Outpatient Treatment of Pediatric Facial Trauma," *J Trauma*, 1985, 25 (11):1079-80.

Katz R, Kelly HW, and Hsi A, "Prospective Study on the Occurrence of Withdrawal in Critically Ill Children Who Receive Fentanyl by Continuous Infusion," *Crit Care Med*, 1994, 22(5):763-7.

Lee HA and Anderson PO, "Giving Partial Doses of Transdermal Patches," *Am J Health Syst Pharm*, 1997, 54(15):1759-60.

Leuschen MP, Willett LD, Hoie EB, et al, "Plasma Fentanyl Levels in Infants Undergoing Extracorporeal Membrane Oxygenation," *J Thorac Cardiovasc Surg*, 1993, 105(5):885-91.

"Principles of Analgesic Use in the Treatment of Acute Pain and Cancer Pain," 6th ed, Glenview, IL: American Pain Society, 2008.

Roth B, Schlunder C, Houben F, et al, "Analgesia and Sedation in Neonatal Intensive Care Using Fentanyl by Continuous Infusion," *Dev Pharmacol Ther*, 1991, 17(3-4):121-7.

Saarenmaa E, Neuvonen PJ, and Fellman V, "Gestational Age and Birth Weight Effects on Plasma Clearance of Fentanyl in Newborn Infants," *J Pediatr*, 2000, 136(6):767-70.

Schechter NL, Weisman SJ, Rosenblum M, et al, "The Use of Oral Transmucosal Fentanyl Citrate for Painful Procedures in Children," *Pediatrics*, 1995, 95(3):335-9.

Zeltzer LK, Altman A, Cohen D, et al, "Report of the Subcommittee on the Management of Pain Associated With Procedures in Children With Cancer," *Pediatrics*, 1990, 86(5 Pt 2):826-31.

Ferric Gluconate (FER ik GLOO koe nate)

Medication Safety Issues
Sound-alike/look-alike issues:
Ferric gluconate may be confused with ferumoxytol
Ferrlecit® may be confused with Ferralet®

U.S. Brand Names Ferrlecit®

Canadian Brand Names Ferrlecit®

Therapeutic Category Iron Salt, Parenteral; Mineral, Parenteral

Generic Available No

Use Treatment of microcytic, hypochromic anemia resulting from iron deficiency in combination with erythropoietin in hemodialysis patients when iron administration is not feasible or ineffective

Pregnancy Risk Factor B

Pregnancy Considerations Adverse events were not observed in animal reproduction studies. There are no well-controlled studies available in pregnant women. It is recommended that pregnant women meet the dietary requirements of iron with diet and/or supplements in order to prevent adverse events associated with iron deficiency anemia in pregnancy. Treatment of iron deficiency anemia in pregnant women is the same as in nonpregnant women and in most cases, oral iron preparations may be used. Except in severe cases of maternal anemia, the fetus achieves normal iron stores regardless of maternal concentrations.

Lactation Excretion in breast milk unknown/use caution

Breast-Feeding Considerations Iron is normally found in breast milk. Breast milk or iron fortified formulas generally provide enough iron to meet the recommended dietary requirements of infants. The amount of iron in breast milk is generally not influenced by maternal iron status.

Contraindications Hypersensitivity to the iron formulation or any component (see Warnings); anemias that are not associated with iron deficiency; hemochromatosis; hemolytic anemia; iron overload

Warnings Deaths associated with parenteral iron administration following anaphylactic-type reactions have been reported; treatment agents for anaphylactic reactions (eg, epinephrine, steroids, diphenhydramine) should be immediately available; a test dose is recommended prior to initial therapy; rapid I.V. administration is associated with flushing, fatigue, weakness, hypotension, and chest, back, groin, or flank pain; use parenteral iron only in patients where the iron deficient state is not amenable to oral iron therapy; ferric gluconate is not approved for I.M. administration.

Ferric gluconate contains benzyl alcohol which may cause allergic reactions in susceptible individuals; large amounts of benzyl alcohol (≥99 mg/kg/day) have been associated with a potentially fatal toxicity ("gasping syndrome") in neonates; the "gasping syndrome" consists of metabolic acidosis, respiratory distress, gasping respirations, CNS dysfunction (including convulsions, intracranial hemorrhage), hypotension and cardiovascular collapse; *in vitro* and animal studies have shown that benzoate, a metabolite of benzyl alcohol, displaces bilirubin from protein-binding sites; avoid use of ferric gluconate formulation in neonates.

Precautions Use with caution in patients with histories of significant allergies, asthma, hepatic impairment, rheumatoid arthritis

Adverse Reactions

Anaphylactoid reactions: Respiratory difficulties and cardiovascular collapse have been reported and occur most frequently within the first several minutes of administration.

Cardiovascular: Cardiovascular collapse, hypotension, flushing, chest pain, syncope, tachycardia, MI, hypovolemia, hypertension, thrombosis

Central nervous system: Dizziness, fever, headache, chills, shivering, malaise, insomnia, agitation, somnolence

Dermatologic: Urticaria, pruritus, rash

Gastrointestinal: Nausea, vomiting, diarrhea, metallic taste, abdominal pain, dyspepsia, flatulence, eructation, melena, pharyngitis

Genitourinary: Discoloration of urine

Hematologic: Leukocytosis

Hepatic: Liver enzymes elevated

Local: Pain, phlebitis

Neuromuscular & skeletal: Arthralgia, arthritic reactivation in patients with quiescent arthritis, backache, paresthesia, leg cramps, weakness

Ocular: Blurred vision, conjunctivitis

Renal: Hematuria

Respiratory: Dyspnea, cough, rhinitis, upper respiratory infection, pulmonary edema, pneumonia

Miscellaneous: Lymphadenopathy, diaphoresis

Note: Sweating, urticaria, arthralgia, fever, chills, dizziness, headache, and nausea may be delayed 24-48 hours after I.V. administration.

Drug Interactions

Avoid Concomitant Use

Avoid concomitant use of Ferric Gluconate with any of the following: Dimercaprol

Increased Effect/Toxicity

The levels/effects of Ferric Gluconate may be increased by: ACE Inhibitors; Dimercaprol

Decreased Effect

Ferric Gluconate may decrease the levels/effects of: Cefdinir; Eltrombopag; Levothyroxine; Phosphate Supplements; Trientine

The levels/effects of Ferric Gluconate may be decreased by: Pancrelipase; Trientine

Stability Store at room temperature; do not freeze; use immediately after dilution in NS. Product literature states parenteral iron formulations should not be mixed with other medications or in parenteral nutrition solutions.

Mechanism of Action Replaces iron found in hemoglobin, myoglobin, and specific enzymes; allows transportation of oxygen via hemoglobin

Pharmacodynamics

Onset of action: Hematologic response to either oral or parenteral iron salts is essentially the same; red blood cell form and color changes within 3-10 days

Maximum effect: Peak reticulocytosis occurs in 5-10 days, and hemoglobin values increase within 2-4 weeks

Pharmacokinetics (Adult data unless noted)

Following I.V. doses, the uptake of iron by the reticuloendothelial system appears to be constant at about 40-60 mg/hour

Half-life: 1.31 hours

Elimination: By the reticuloendothelial system and excreted in urine and feces (via bile)

Dialysis: Not dialyzable

Usual Dosage Multiple forms for parenteral iron exist; close attention must be paid to the specific product when ordering and administering; incorrect selection or substitution of one form for another without proper dosage adjustment may result in serious over- or under-dosing; test doses are recommended before starting therapy. **Note:** Per National Kidney Foundation DOQI Guidelines, initiation of iron therapy, determination of dose, and duration of therapy should be guided by results of iron status tests combined with the Hb level and the dose of the erythropoietin stimulating agent. See Reference Range for target levels. There is insufficient evidence to recommend I.V. iron if ferritin level >500 ng/mL. Dosage expressed in mg **elemental** iron: I.V.:

Children ≥6 years: 1.5 mg/kg (0.12 mL/kg Ferrlecit®) repeated at each of 8 sequential dialysis sessions not to exceed 125 mg (10 mL) per dose

Adults: 125 mg (10 mL) during hemodialysis; most patients will require a cumulative dose of 1 g over ~8 sequential dialysis treatments to achieve a favorable response

Note: A test dose (25 mg in adult patients) previously recommended in product literature is no longer listed. No pediatric test dose has been recommended by the manufacturer.

Administration Parenteral: Avoid dilution in dextrose due to an increased incidence of local pain and phlebitis

I.V. infusion: If a test dose is used, dilute in 50 mL NS and infuse over 1 hour; dilute repletion dose in 25-100 mL NS and infuse over at least 1 hour; do not exceed 12.5 mg/minute; not for I.M. administration

Slow I.V. injection: 1 mL (12.5 mg iron) of undiluted solution per minute (5 minutes/vial)

Monitoring Parameters Vital signs and other symptoms of anaphylactoid reactions (during I.V. infusion); reticulocyte count, serum ferritin, hemoglobin, serum iron concentrations, and transferrin saturation (TSAT). Ferritin and TSAT may be inaccurate if measured within 14 days of receiving a large single dose (1000 mg in adults).

Reference Range

Serum iron:

Newborns: 110-270 mcg/dL

Infants: 30-70 mcg/dL

Children: 55-120 mcg/dL

Adults: Male: 75-175 mcg/dL; female: 65-165 mcg/dL

Total iron binding capacity:

Newborns: 59-175 mcg/dL

Infants: 100-400 mcg/dL

Children and Adults: 230-430 mcg/dL

Transferrin: 204-360 mg/dL

Percent transferrin saturation (TSAT): 20% to 50%

Iron levels >300 mcg/dL may be considered toxic; should be treated as an overdosage

Ferritin: 13-300 ng/mL

Chronic kidney disease (CKD): Targets for iron therapy (KDOQI Guidelines, 2007) to maintain Hgb 11-12 g/dL:

Children: Nondialysis CKD, hemodialysis, or peritoneal dialysis: Ferritin: >100 ng/mL and TSAT >20%

Adults: Nondialysis (CKD) or peritoneal dialysis: Ferritin: >100 ng/mL and TSAT >20%

Hemodialysis: Ferritin >200 ng/mL and TSAT >20% or CHr (content of hemoglobin in reticulocytes) >29 pg/cell

Test Interactions May cause falsely elevated values of serum bilirubin and falsely decreased values of serum calcium

Additional Information Iron storage may lag behind the appearance of normal red blood cell morphology; use periodic hematologic determination to assess therapy

Dosage Forms Excipient information presented when available (limited, particularly for generics); consult specific product labeling.

Injection, solution:

Ferrlecit®: Elemental iron 12.5 mg/mL (5 mL) [contains benzyl alcohol and sucrose 20%]

References

"KDOQI Clinical Practice Guideline and Clinical Practice Recommen-dations for Anemia in Chronic Kidney Disease: 2007 Update of Hemoglobin Target," *Am J Kidney Dis*, 2007, 50(3):471-530.

Seligman PA, Dahl NV, Strobos J, et al, "Single-Dose Pharmacokinetics of Sodium Ferric Gluconate Complex in Iron-Deficient Subjects," *Pharmacotherapy*, 2004, 24(5):574-83.

Warady BA, Zobrist RH, Wu J, et al, "Sodium Ferric Gluconate Complex Therapy in Anemic Children on Hemodialysis," *Pediatr Nephrol*, 2005, 20(9):1320-7.

◆ **Ferrlecit®** see Ferric Gluconate *on page 574*

◆ **Ferro-Sequels® [OTC]** *see* Ferrous Fumarate *on page 576*

Ferrous Fumarate (FER us FYOO ma rate)

U.S. Brand Names Femiron® [OTC]; Ferretts [OTC]; Ferro-Sequels® [OTC]; Hemocyte® [OTC]; Ircon® [OTC]; Nephro-Fer® [OTC] [DSC]

Canadian Brand Names Palafer®

Therapeutic Category Iron Salt; Mineral, Oral

Generic Available Yes: Tablet

Use Prevention and treatment of iron deficiency anemias; supplemental therapy for patients receiving epoetin alfa

Pregnancy Considerations It is recommended that pregnant women meet the dietary requirements of iron with diet and/or supplements in order to prevent adverse events associated with iron deficiency anemia in preg-nancy. Treatment of iron deficiency anemia in pregnant women is the same as in nonpregnant women and in most cases, oral iron preparations may be used. Except in severe cases of maternal anemia, the fetus achieves normal iron stores regardless of maternal concentrations.

Lactation Enters breast milk

Breast-Feeding Considerations Iron is normally found in breast milk. Breast milk or iron-fortified formulas generally provide enough iron to meet the recommended dietary requirements of infants. The amount of iron in breast milk is generally not influenced by maternal iron status.

Contraindications Hypersensitivity to iron salts or any component (see Warnings); hemochromatosis, hemolytic anemia

Warnings Some products contain tartrazine which may cause allergic reactions in susceptible individuals

Precautions Avoid using for longer than 6 months, except in patients with conditions that require prolonged therapy; avoid in patients with peptic ulcer, enteritis, or ulcerative colitis; avoid in patients receiving frequent blood trans-fusions. Severe iron toxicity may occur in overdose, particularly when ingested by children **[U.S. Boxed Warning]**; iron is a leading cause of fatal poisoning in children; store out of children's reach and in child-resistant containers.

Adverse Reactions

Gastrointestinal: GI irritation, epigastric pain, nausea, diarrhea, dark stools, constipation

Genitourinary: Discoloration of urine (black or dark)

Miscellaneous: Liquid preparations may temporarily stain the teeth

Drug Interactions

Avoid Concomitant Use

Avoid concomitant use of Ferrous Fumarate with any of the following: Dimercaprol

Increased Effect/Toxicity

The levels/effects of Ferrous Fumarate may be increased by: Dimercaprol

Decreased Effect

Ferrous Fumarate may decrease the levels/effects of: Bisphosphonate Derivatives; Cefdinir; Eltrombopag; Levodopa; Levothyroxine; Methyldopa; Penicillamine; Phosphate Supplements; Quinolone Antibiotics; Tetracy-cline Derivatives; Trientine

The levels/effects of Ferrous Fumarate may be decreased by: Antacids; H2-Antagonists; Pancrelipase; Proton Pump Inhibitors; Trientine

Food Interactions Milk, cereals, dietary fiber, tea, coffee, or eggs decrease absorption of iron.

Mechanism of Action Iron is released from the plasma and eventually replenishes the depleted iron stores in the bone marrow where it is incorporated into hemoglobin

Pharmacodynamics See Iron Supplements (Oral/Enteral) on page 766

Pharmacokinetics (Adult data unless noted) See Iron Supplements (Oral/Enteral) on page 766

Usual Dosage Oral (dose expressed in terms of **elemental** iron):

Recommended Daily Allowance: See Iron Supplements (Oral/Enteral) on page 766.

Treatment and prevention of iron deficiency:

Children:

Severe iron deficiency anemia: 4-6 mg elemental iron/kg/day in 3 divided doses

Mild to moderate iron deficiency anemia: 3 mg elemental iron/kg/day in 1-2 divided doses

Prophylaxis: 1-2 mg elemental iron/kg/day up to a maximum of 15 mg elemental iron/day

Adults:

Iron deficiency: 2-3 mg/kg/day or 60-100 mg elemental iron twice daily up to 60 mg elemental iron 4 times/day, or 50 mg elemental iron (extended release) 1-2 times/day

Prophylaxis: 60-100 mg elemental iron/day

Administration Oral: Do not chew or crush sustained release preparations; administer with water or juice between meals for maximum absorption; may administer with food if GI upset occurs; do not administer with milk or milk products

Monitoring Parameters See Iron Supplements (Oral/Enteral) on page 766

Reference Range See Iron Supplements (Oral/Enteral) on page 766

Test Interactions See Iron Supplements (Oral/Enteral) on page 766

Patient Information See Iron Supplements (Oral/Enteral) on page 766

Additional Information Elemental iron content of ferrous fumarate is 33% of salt content; see Iron Supplements (Oral/Enteral) on page 766 for comparison chart with other iron salt forms; when treating iron deficiency anemias, treat for 3-4 months after hemoglobin/hematocrit return to normal in order to replenish total body stores

Dosage Forms Excipient information presented when available (limited, particularly for generics); consult specific product labeling. [DSC] = Discontinued product

Tablet: 324 mg [elemental iron 106 mg]

Femiron®: 63 mg [elemental iron 20 mg]

Ferretts: 325 mg [elemental iron 106 mg]

Hemocyte®: 324 mg [elemental iron 106 mg]

Ircon®: 200 mg [elemental iron 66 mg]

Nephro-Fer®: 350 mg [elemental iron 115 mg; contains tartrazine] [DSC]

Tablet, timed release (Ferro-Sequels®): 150 mg [elemen-tal iron 50 mg; contains docusate sodium and sodium benzoate]

♦ **Ferrous Fumarate** *see* Iron Supplements (Oral/Enteral) *on page 766*

Ferrous Gluconate (FER us GLOO koe nate)

U.S. Brand Names Fergon® [OTC]
Canadian Brand Names Apo-Ferrous Gluconate®; Novo-Ferrogluc
Therapeutic Category Iron Salt; Mineral, Oral
Generic Available Yes
Use Prevention and treatment of iron deficiency anemias; supplemental therapy for patients receiving epoetin alfa
Pregnancy Considerations It is recommended that pregnant women meet the dietary requirements of iron with diet and/or supplements in order to prevent adverse events associated with iron deficiency anemia in pregnancy. Treatment of iron deficiency anemia in pregnant women is the same as in nonpregnant women and in most cases, oral iron preparations may be used. Except in severe cases of maternal anemia, the fetus achieves normal iron stores regardless of maternal concentrations.
Lactation Enters breast milk
Breast-Feeding Considerations Iron is normally found in breast milk. Breast milk or iron fortified formulas generally provide enough iron to meet the recommended dietary requirements of infants. The amount of iron in breast milk is generally not influenced by maternal iron status.
Contraindications Hypersensitivity to iron salts or any component (see Warnings); hemochromatosis, hemolytic anemia
Warnings Avoid use in premature infants until the vitamin E stores, deficient at birth, are replenished
Precautions Avoid using for longer than 6 months, except in patients with conditions that require prolonged therapy; avoid in patients with peptic ulcer, enteritis, or ulcerative colitis; avoid in patients receiving frequent blood transfusions. Severe iron toxicity may occur in overdose, particularly when ingested by children **[U.S. Boxed Warning]**; iron is a leading cause of fatal poisoning in children; store out of children's reach and in child-resistant containers.
Adverse Reactions
Gastrointestinal: GI irritation, epigastric pain, nausea, diarrhea, dark stools, constipation
Genitourinary: Discoloration of urine (black or dark)
Miscellaneous: Liquid preparations may temporarily stain the teeth
Drug Interactions
Avoid Concomitant Use
Avoid concomitant use of Ferrous Gluconate with any of the following: Dimercaprol
Increased Effect/Toxicity
The levels/effects of Ferrous Gluconate may be increased by: Dimercaprol
Decreased Effect
Ferrous Gluconate may decrease the levels/effects of: Bisphosphonate Derivatives; Cefdinir; Eltrombopag; Levodopa; Levothyroxine; Methyldopa; Penicillamine; Phosphate Supplements; Quinolone Antibiotics; Tetracycline Derivatives; Trientine

The levels/effects of Ferrous Gluconate may be decreased by: Antacids; H2-Antagonists; Pancrelipase; Proton Pump Inhibitors; Trientine
Food Interactions Milk, cereals, dietary fiber, tea, coffee, or eggs decrease absorption of iron.
Mechanism of Action Iron is released from the plasma and eventually replenishes the depleted iron stores in the bone marrow where it is incorporated into hemoglobin
Pharmacodynamics See Iron Supplements (Oral/Enteral) on page 766

Pharmacokinetics (Adult data unless noted) See Iron Supplements (Oral/Enteral) on page 766
Usual Dosage Oral (dose expressed in terms of **elemental** iron):
Recommended Daily Allowance: See Iron Supplements (Oral/Enteral) on page 766
Treatment and prevention of iron deficiency:
Children:
Severe iron deficiency anemia: 4-6 mg elemental iron/kg/day in 3 divided doses
Mild to moderate iron deficiency anemia: 3 mg elemental iron/kg/day in 1-2 divided doses
Prophylaxis: 1-2 mg elemental iron/kg/day up to a maximum of 15 mg elemental iron/day
Adults:
Iron deficiency: 2-3 mg/kg/day or 60-100 mg elemental iron twice daily up to 60 mg elemental iron 4 times/day, or 50 mg elemental iron (extended release) 1-2 times/day
Prophylaxis: 60-100 mg elemental iron/day
Administration Oral: Do not chew or crush sustained release preparations; administer with water or juice between meals for maximum absorption; may administer with food if GI upset occurs; do not administer with milk or milk products
Monitoring Parameters See Iron Supplements (Oral/Enteral) on page 766
Reference Range See Iron Supplements (Oral/Enteral) on page 766
Test Interactions See Iron Supplements (Oral/Enteral) on page 766
Patient Information See Iron Supplements (Oral/Enteral) on page 766
Additional Information Approximate elemental iron content of ferrous gluconate is 11.6% of salt form. See Iron Supplements (Oral/Enteral) for comparison chart with other iron salt forms; when treating iron deficiency anemias, treat for 3-4 months after hemoglobin/hematocrit return to normal in order to replenish total body stores
Dosage Forms Excipient information presented when available (limited, particularly for generics); consult specific product labeling. [DSC] = Discontinued product
Tablet: 246 mg [elemental iron 28 mg] [DSC]; 300 mg [elemental iron 34 mg] [DSC]; 325 mg [elemental iron 36 mg]
Fergon®: 240 mg [elemental iron 27 mg]

♦ **Ferrous Gluconate** *see* Iron Supplements (Oral/Enteral) *on page 766*

Ferrous Sulfate (FER us SUL fate)

Medication Safety Issues
Sound-alike/look-alike issues:
Feosol® may be confused with Fer-In-Sol®
Fer-In-Sol® may be confused with Feosol®
Slow FE® may be confused with Slow-K®

Potential for medication errors: Fer-In-Sol® (manufactured by Mead Johnson) is available at a concentration of 15 mg/mL. However, generics and other brand name products of ferrous sulfate oral liquid drops are available at a concentration of 15 mg/0.6 mL. Check concentration closely prior to dispensing. Prescriptions written in milliliters (mL) should be clarified.

Beers Criteria medication: This drug may be inappropriate for use in geriatric patients (dosage dependent, low severity risk).
U.S. Brand Names Feosol® [OTC]; Fer-Gen-Sol [OTC] [DSC]; Fer-In-Sol® [OTC]; Fer-iron® [OTC]; Feratab® [OTC] [DSC]; MyKidz Iron 10™ [OTC]; Slow FE® [OTC]

Canadian Brand Names Apo-Ferrous Sulfate®; Fer-In-Sol®; Ferodan™

Therapeutic Category Iron Salt; Mineral, Oral

Generic Available Yes

Use Prevention and treatment of iron deficiency anemias; supplemental therapy for patients receiving epoetin alfa

Pregnancy Considerations It is recommended that pregnant women meet the dietary requirements of iron with diet and/or supplements in order to prevent adverse events associated with iron deficiency anemia in pregnancy. Treatment of iron deficiency anemia in pregnant women is the same as in nonpregnant women and in most cases, oral iron preparations may be used. Except in severe cases of maternal anemia, the fetus achieves normal iron stores regardless of maternal concentrations.

Lactation Enters breast milk

Breast-Feeding Considerations Iron is normally found in breast milk. Breast milk or iron fortified formulas generally provide enough iron to meet the recommended dietary requirements of infants. The amount of iron in breast milk is generally not influenced by maternal iron status.

Contraindications Hypersensitivity to iron salts or any component (see Warnings); hemochromatosis, hemolytic anemia

Warnings Avoid use in premature infants until the vitamin E stores, deficient at birth, are replenished; some products contain sulfites which may cause allergic reactions in susceptible individuals

Precautions Avoid using for longer than 6 months, except in patients with conditions that require prolonged therapy; avoid in patients with peptic ulcer, enteritis, or ulcerative colitis; avoid in patients receiving frequent blood transfusions. Severe iron toxicity may occur in overdose, particularly when ingested by children **[U.S. Boxed Warning]**; iron is a leading cause of fatal poisoning in children; store out of children's reach and in child-resistant containers.

Adverse Reactions

Gastrointestinal: GI irritation, epigastric pain, nausea, diarrhea, dark stools, constipation

Genitourinary: Discoloration of urine (black or dark)

Miscellaneous: Liquid preparations may temporarily stain the teeth

Drug Interactions

Avoid Concomitant Use

Avoid concomitant use of Ferrous Sulfate with any of the following: Dimercaprol

Increased Effect/Toxicity

The levels/effects of Ferrous Sulfate may be increased by: Dimercaprol

Decreased Effect

Ferrous Sulfate may decrease the levels/effects of: Bisphosphonate Derivatives; Cefdinir; Eltrombopag; Levodopa; Levothyroxine; Methyldopa; Penicillamine; Phosphate Supplements; Quinolone Antibiotics; Tetracycline Derivatives; Trientine

The levels/effects of Ferrous Sulfate may be decreased by: Antacids; H2-Antagonists; Pancrelipase; Proton Pump Inhibitors; Trientine

Food Interactions Milk, cereals, dietary fiber, tea, coffee, or eggs decrease absorption of iron.

Mechanism of Action Iron is released from the plasma and eventually replenishes the depleted iron stores in the bone marrow where it is incorporated into hemoglobin

Pharmacodynamics

Onset of action: Hematologic response to either oral or parenteral iron salts is essentially the same; red blood cells form and color changes within 3-10 days

Maximum effect: Peak reticulocytosis occurs in 5-10 days, and hemoglobin values increase within 2-4 weeks

Pharmacokinetics (Adult data unless noted)

Absorption: Oral: Iron is absorbed in the duodenum and upper jejunum; in persons with normal iron stores 10% of an oral dose is absorbed, this is increased to 20% to 30% in persons with inadequate iron stores; food and achlorhydria will decrease absorption

Elimination: Iron is largely bound to serum transferrin and excreted in the urine, sweat, sloughing of intestinal mucosa, and by menses

Usual Dosage Note: Multiple concentrations of ferrous sulfate oral liquid exist; close attention must be paid to the concentration when ordering and administering ferrous sulfate; incorrect selection or substitution of one ferrous sulfate liquid for another without proper dosage volume adjustment may result in serious over- or underdosing. Oral (dose expressed in terms of elemental iron):

Recommended Daily Allowance: See table.

Recommended Daily Allowance of Iron

(Dosage expressed as elemental iron)

Age	RDA (mg)
<5 months	5
5 months to 10 years	10
Male	
11-18 years	12
>18 years	10
Female	
11-50 years	15
>50 years	10

Treatment and prevention of iron deficiency:

Premature neonates: 2-4 mg elemental iron/kg/day divided every 12-24 hours (maximum dose: 15 mg/day)

Infants and Children:

Severe iron deficiency anemia: 4-6 mg elemental iron/kg/day in 3 divided doses

Mild to moderate iron deficiency anemia: 3 mg elemental iron/kg/day in 1-2 divided doses

Prophylaxis: 1-2 mg elemental iron/kg/day up to a maximum of 15 mg elemental iron/day

Adults:

Iron deficiency: 2-3 mg/kg/day or 60-100 mg elemental iron twice daily up to 60 mg elemental iron 4 times/day, or 50 mg elemental iron (extended release) 1-2 times/day

Prophylaxis: 60-100 mg elemental iron/day; see table

Administration Oral: Do not chew or crush sustained release preparations; administer with water or juice between meals for maximum absorption; may administer with food if GI upset occurs; do not administer with milk or milk products

Monitoring Parameters Serum iron, total iron binding capacity, reticulocyte count, hemoglobin, ferritin

Reference Range

Serum iron:

Newborns: 110-270 mcg/dL

Infants: 30-70 mcg/dL

Children: 55-120 mcg/dL

Adults: Male: 75-175 mcg/dL; Female: 65-165 mcg/dL

Total iron binding capacity:

Newborns: 59-175 mcg/dL

Infants: 100-400 mcg/dL

Children and Adults: 230-430 mcg/dL

Transferrin: 204-360 mg/dL

Percent transferrin saturation: 20% to 50%

Note: Iron levels >300 mcg/dL may be considered toxic; should be treated as an overdosage

Ferritin: 13-300 ng/mL

Test Interactions False-positive for blood in stool by the guaiac test

Patient Information May color the stools and urine black; do not take within 2 hours of tetracyclines or fluoroquinolones; do not take with milk or antacids; keep out of reach of children

Additional Information Elemental iron content of ferrous sulfate is 20% of salt content and of exsiccated ferrous sulfate (Feosol®, Slow FE®) is 30%. See Iron Supplements (Oral/Enteral) on page 766 for comparison chart with other iron salt forms.

When treating iron deficiency anemias, treat for 3-4 months after hemoglobin/hematocrit return to normal in order to replenish total body stores; elemental iron dosages as high as 15 mg/kg/day have been used to supplement neonates receiving concomitant epoetin alpha in the treatment of anemia of prematurity

Dosage Forms Excipient information presented when available (limited, particularly for generics); consult specific product labeling. [DSC] = Discontinued product

Elixir, oral: 220 mg/5 mL (480 mL) [elemental iron 44 mg/ 5 mL; contains alcohol]

Liquid, oral: 300 mg/5 mL (5 mL) [elemental iron ~60 mg/ 5mL]

Liquid, oral [drops]: 75 mg/0.6 mL (50 mL) [elemental iron 15 mg/0.6 mL]; 75 mg/mL (50 mL) [elemental iron 15 mg/mL]

Fer-Gen-Sol: 75 mg/0.6 mL (50 mL) [elemental iron 15 mg/0.6 mL] [DSC]

Fer-In-Sol®: 75 mg/mL (50 mL) [elemental iron 15 mg/mL; contains ethanol 0.2% and sodium bisulfite]

Fer-iron®: 75 mg/mL (50 mL) [elemental iron 15 mg/mL; contains ethanol 0.2%; lemon flavor]

Suspension, oral [drops]:

MyKidz Iron 10™: 75 mg/1.5 mL (118 mL) [elemental iron 15 mg/1.5 mL; ethanol free, dye free; contains propylene glycol; strawberry-banana flavor]

Tablet, oral: 324 mg [elemental iron 65 mg]; 325 mg [elemental iron 65 mg]

Feratab®: 300 mg [elemental iron 60 mg] [DSC]

Tablet, oral [exsiccated]: 200 mg [elemental iron 65 mg]

Feosol®: 200 mg [elemental iron 65 mg]

Tablet, oral [exsiccated, timed release]: 160 mg [elemental iron 50 mg]

Slow FE®: 160 mg [elemental iron 50 mg]

Tablet, oral, slow release: 160 mg [elemental iron 50 mg]

◆ **Ferrous Sulfate** see Iron Supplements (Oral/Enteral) on page 766

◆ **FeSO₄** see Ferrous Sulfate on page 577

◆ **FeSO₄ (Ferrous Sulfate)** see Iron Supplements (Oral/ Enteral) on page 766

◆ **FeverALL® [OTC]** see Acetaminophen on page 36

◆ **Fexmid®** see Cyclobenzaprine on page 367

Fexofenadine (feks oh FEN a deen)

Medication Safety Issues

Sound-alike/look-alike issues:

Fexofenadine may be confused with fesoterodine

Allegra® may be confused with Viagra®

International issues:

Allegra® may be confused with Allegro® which is a brand name for frovatriptan in Germany; a brand name for fluticasone in Israel

U.S. Brand Names Allegra®; Allegra® ODT

Canadian Brand Names Allegra®

Therapeutic Category Antihistamine

Generic Available Yes: Excludes orally disintegrating tablet and suspension

Use Symptomatic relief of seasonal allergic rhinitis and chronic idiopathic urticaria

Pregnancy Risk Factor C

Pregnancy Considerations Decreased fetal weight gain and survival were observed in animal studies. There are no adequate and well-controlled studies in pregnant women; use during pregnancy only if potential benefit to mother outweighs possible risk to fetus.

Lactation Excretion in breast milk unknown/use caution (AAP rates "compatible")

Contraindications Hypersensitivity to fexofenadine, terfenadine, or any component

Warnings Adjust dosage in patients with decreased renal function

Precautions Use cautiously in patients who are also taking ketoconazole and erythromycin (see Drug Interactions); although increased plasma levels of fexofenadine have been observed, no adverse effects with concomitant administration have been reported including QT prolongation which occurred when terfenadine was combined with these agents; while less sedating than other antihistamines, fexofenadine may cause drowsiness and impair ability to perform hazardous activities requiring mental alertness

Adverse Reactions

Central nervous system: Headache, fever, drowsiness, fatigue, dizziness

Endocrine & metabolic: Dysmenorrhea

Gastrointestinal: Nausea, dyspepsia

Neuromuscular & skeletal: Back pain

Otic: Otitis media

Respiratory: Upper respiratory tract infection, cough, sinusitis

Miscellaneous: Hypersensitivity reactions, viral infections

Drug Interactions

Metabolism/Transport Effects Substrate of CYP3A4 (minor), P-glycoprotein, SLCO1B1; **Inhibits** CYP2D6 (weak)

Avoid Concomitant Use There are no known interactions where it is recommended to avoid concomitant use.

Increased Effect/Toxicity

Fexofenadine may increase the levels/effects of: Alcohol (Ethyl); Anticholinergics; CNS Depressants

The levels/effects of Fexofenadine may be increased by: Eltrombopag; Erythromycin; Erythromycin (Systemic); Itraconazole; Ketoconazole; Ketoconazole (Systemic); P-Glycoprotein Inhibitors; Pramlintide; Verapamil

Decreased Effect

Fexofenadine may decrease the levels/effects of: Acetylcholinesterase Inhibitors (Central); Betahistine

The levels/effects of Fexofenadine may be decreased by: Acetylcholinesterase Inhibitors (Central); Amphetamines; Antacids; Grapefruit Juice; P-Glycoprotein Inducers; Rifampin

Food Interactions Fruit juices may reduce the bioavailability of fexofenadine by 36%

Stability Store at controlled room temperature; protect from excessive moisture

Mechanism of Action Fexofenadine is an active metabolite of terfenadine; it competes with histamine for H_1 receptor sites on effector cells in the GI tract, blood vessels, and respiratory tract; it appears that fexofenadine does not cross the blood brain barrier to any appreciable degree, resulting in a reduced potential for sedation

Pharmacodynamics
Onset of action: 1 hour
Maximum effect: 2-3 hours
Duration: ≥12 hours

Pharmacokinetics (Adult data unless noted)
Absorption: Rapid
Distribution: V_d: Children: 5.4-5.8 L/kg
Protein binding: 60% to 70%
Metabolism: 5% in liver; 3.5% transformed into methylester metabolite found only in feces (possibly transformed by gut microflora)
Half-life: 14-18 hours
Time to peak serum concentration: Tablets: 2.6 hours; Suspension: 1 hour
Elimination: 11% excreted unchanged in urine; 80% excreted unchanged in feces
Clearance: Children: 14-18 mL/minute/kg
Dialysis: Not effectively removed by hemodialysis

Usual Dosage Oral:
Children 6 months to <2 years: 15 mg twice daily
Children 2-11 years: 30 mg twice daily
Children ≥12 years and Adults: 60 mg twice daily or 180 mg once daily

Dosing adjustment in renal impairment:
Children 6 months to <2 years: 15 mg once daily
Children 2-11 years: 30 mg once daily
Children ≥12 years and Adults: 60 mg once daily

Administration May administer without respect to food; avoid administration with fruit juices; shake suspension well before use

Monitoring Parameters Improvement in signs and symptoms of allergic rhinitis and chronic idiopathic urticaria

Test Interactions Antigen skin testing

Patient Information May cause drowsiness and impair ability to perform activities requiring mental alertness or physical coordination; avoid alcohol

Dosage Forms Excipient information presented when available (limited, particularly for generics); consult specific product labeling.
Suspension, oral, as hydrochloride:
Allegra®: 6 mg/mL (300 mL) [contains propylene glycol; raspberry cream]
Tablet, oral, as hydrochloride: 30 mg, 60 mg, 180 mg
Allegra®: 60 mg, 180 mg
Tablet, orally disintegrating, oral, as hydrochloride:
Allegra® ODT: 30 mg [contains phenylalanine 5.3 mg/tablet; orange cream flavor]

◆ **Fexofenadine Hydrochloride** see Fexofenadine on page 579

◆ **Fiberall®** see Psyllium on page 1185

◆ **Fibro-XL [OTC]** see Psyllium on page 1185

◆ **Fibro-Lax [OTC]** see Psyllium on page 1185

Filgrastim (fil GRA stim)

Medication Safety Issues
Sound-alike/look-alike issues:
Neupogen® may be confused with Epogen®, Neulasta®, Neumega®, Neupro®, Nutramigen®

Related Information
Compatibility of Chemotherapy and Related Supportive Care Medications on page 1580

U.S. Brand Names Neupogen®

Canadian Brand Names Neupogen®

Therapeutic Category Colony-Stimulating Factor

Generic Available No

Use Reduction of the duration of neutropenia and the associated risk of infection in patients with malignancies receiving myelosuppressive chemotherapeutic regimens associated with a significant incidence of severe neutropenia with fever; cancer patients receiving bone marrow transplant; severe chronic neutropenia which includes patients with congenital neutropenia, cyclic neutropenia, or idiopathic neutropenia; mobilization of peripheral blood progenitor cells into the peripheral blood for collection by leukapheresis; AIDS patients receiving zidovudine; neonatal neutropenia

Pregnancy Risk Factor C

Pregnancy Considerations Animal studies have demonstrated adverse effects and fetal loss. Filgrastim has been shown to cross the placenta in humans. There are no adequate and well-controlled studies in pregnant women. Use only if potential benefit to mother justifies risk to the fetus.

Lactation Excretion in breast milk unknown/use caution

Contraindications Hypersensitivity to E. coli-derived proteins, G-CSF, or any component; use in patients receiving concomitant chemotherapy and radiation therapy

Warnings Leukocytosis (white blood cell counts ≥100,000/mm^3) has been observed in approximately 2% of patients receiving G-CSF at doses >5 mcg/kg/day

Precautions Do not administer 24 hours prior to or within 24 hours following the administration of chemotherapy; use with caution in any malignancy with myeloid characteristics due to G-CSF's potential to act as a growth factor; use with caution in patients with gout, psoriasis; monitor patients with pre-existing cardiac conditions as cardiac events (MIs, arrhythmias) have been reported in premarketing clinical studies. Be alert to the possibility of ARDS in septic patients.

Premature discontinuation of G-CSF therapy prior to the time of recovery from the expected neutrophil nadir is generally not recommended. A transient increase in neutrophil counts is typically seen 1-2 days after initiation of therapy. For a sustained therapeutic response, G-CSF should be continued until the post nadir absolute neutrophil count (ANC) reaches:
10,000/mm^3 in chemotherapy treated patients, or
>1000/mm^3 for 3 consecutive days in bone marrow transplant patients

Most patients experience a 30% to 50% decrease in circulating leukocytes within 1-2 days following discontinuation of G-CSF

Adverse Reactions
Cardiovascular: Transient decrease in blood pressure, vasculitis, chest pain
Central nervous system: Fever, headache
Dermatologic: Exacerbation of pre-existing skin disorders, alopecia, rash, pruritus
Endocrine & metabolic: Reversible elevation in uric acid
Gastrointestinal: Splenomegaly, nausea, vomiting, diarrhea, mucositis
Hematologic: Thrombocytopenia, leukocytosis
Hepatic: Alkaline phosphatase elevated, lactate dehydrogenase
Neuromuscular & skeletal: Medullary bone pain (24% incidence) is generally dose-related, localized to the lower back, posterior iliac crests, and sternum; osteoporosis
Renal: Hematuria, proteinuria
Miscellaneous: Anaphylactoid reaction (rare)

Drug Interactions
Avoid Concomitant Use There are no known interactions where it is recommended to avoid concomitant use.

Increased Effect/Toxicity
Filgrastim may increase the levels/effects of: Bleomycin; Topotecan

Decreased Effect There are no known significant interactions involving a decrease in effect.

Stability Store in refrigerator; do not freeze; protect from direct sunlight; stable for 24 hours at room temperature; solutions with concentration ≥15 mcg/mL in D_5W are stable for 24 hours; incompatible with salt solutions

Mechanism of Action Stimulates the production, maturation, and activation of neutrophils; G-CSF activates neutrophils to increase both their migration and cytotoxicity

Pharmacodynamics

Onset of action: Immediate transient leukopenia with the nadir occurring 5-15 minutes after an I.V. dose or 30-60 minutes after a SubQ dose followed by a sustained elevation in neutrophil levels within the first 24 hours reaching a plateau in 3-5 days

Duration: Upon discontinuation of G-CSF, ANC decreases by 50% within 2 days and returns to pretreatment levels within 1 week; WBC counts return to normal range in 4-7 days

Pharmacokinetics (Adult data unless noted)

Distribution: V_d: 150 mL/kg

Bioavailability: Not bioavailable after oral administration

Half-life: Neonates: 4.4 hours; Adults: 1.8-3.5 hours

Time to peak serum concentration: SubQ: Within 2-6 hours

Elimination: No evidence of drug accumulation over a 11- to 20-day period

Usual Dosage I.V., SubQ (refer to individual protocols):

Neonates: 5-10 mcg/kg/day once daily for 3-5 days has been administered to neutropenic neonates with sepsis. There was a rapid and significant increase in peripheral neutrophil counts and the neutrophil storage pool.

Children and Adults: 5-10 mcg/kg/day (~150-300 mcg/m^2/day) once daily for up to 14 days until ANC = 10,000/mm^3; dose escalations at 5 mcg/kg/day may be required in some individuals when response at 5 mcg/kg/day is not adequate; in phase 3 trials, efficacy was observed at dosages of 4-8 mcg/kg/day with myelosuppressive chemotherapy

Peripheral blood progenitor cell (PBPC) mobilization: SubQ: 10 mcg/kg/day given for 4 days before the first leukapheresis procedure and continued until the last leukapheresis

Patients with congenital neutropenia: SubQ: Initial: 6 mcg/kg/dose twice daily; dosages of 2-60 mcg/kg/day individualized according to neutrophil count have been administered to children and adults

Patients with idiopathic or cyclic neutropenia: SubQ: 5 mcg/kg/day once daily

Cancer patients receiving bone marrow transplant: I.V. infusion, SubQ: 5-10 mcg/kg/day administered ≥24 hours after cytotoxic chemotherapy and ≥24 hours after bone marrow infusion

Dosage adjustment during neutrophil recovery period: see table

Filgrastim Dose Based on Neutrophil Response

Absolute Neutrophil Count (ANC)	Filgrastim Dose Adjustment
When ANC >1000/mm^3 for 3 consecutive days	Reduce to 5 mcg/kg/day
If ANC remains >1000/mm^3 for 3 more consecutive days	Discontinue filgrastim
If ANC decreases to <1000/mm^3	Resume at 5 mcg/kg/day

If ANC decreases <1000/mm^3 during the 5 mcg/kg/day dose, increase dose to 10 mcg/kg/day and follow the above steps in the table.

Administration Parenteral:

SubQ: Administer undiluted solution

SubQ continuous infusion: Dilute dose in 10 mL D_5W and infuse at a rate of 10 mL/24 hours

I.V. continuous infusion; Administer over 15-60 minutes or as a continuous I.V. infusion at a final concentration of at least 15 mcg/mL in D_5W. If the final concentration of G-CSF in D_5W is <15 mcg/mL, then add 2 mg albumin/mL to I.V. fluid; the solution is stable for 24 hours; albumin acts as a carrier molecule to prevent drug adsorption to the I.V. tubing. Albumin should be added to the D_5W prior to addition of G-CSF; final concentration of G-CSF for administration <5 mcg/mL is not recommended; do not shake solution to avoid foaming.

Monitoring Parameters Temperature, CBC with differential and platelet count, hematocrit, uric acid, urinalysis, liver function tests

Reference Range Blood samples for monitoring the hematologic effects of G-CSF should be drawn just before the next dose at least twice weekly

Patient Information Possible bone pain; notify physician of unusual fever or chills, severe bone pain, or chest pain and palpitations

Nursing Implications Bone pain management is usually successful with non-narcotic analgesic therapy

Additional Information Reimbursement hotline: 1-800-272-9376. Injection solution contains sodium 0.035 mg/mL.

Dosage Forms Excipient information presented when available (limited, particularly for generics); consult specific product labeling.

Injection, solution [preservative free]:

Neupogen®: 300 mcg/mL (1 mL, 1.6 mL) [vial; contains sodium 0.035 mg/mL and sorbitol]

Injection, solution [preservative free]:

Neupogen®: 600 mcg/mL (0.5 mL, 0.8 mL) [prefilled Singleject®·syringe; contains sodium 0.035 mg/mL and sorbitol; needle cover contains latex]

References

Bonilla MA, Gillio AP, Ruggeiro M, et al, "Effects of Recombinant Human Granulocyte Colony-Stimulating Factor on Neutropenia in Patients With Congenital Agranulocytosis," *N Engl J Med*, 1989, 320 (24):1574-80.

Gilmore MM, Stroncek DF, and Korones DN, "Treatment of Alloimmune Neonatal Neutropenia With Granulocyte Colony-Stimulating Factor," *J Pediatr*, 1994, 125(6 Pt 1):948-51

Hollingshead LM, Goa KL, "Recombinant Granulocyte Colony-Stimulating Factor (rG-CSF): A Review of Its Pharmacological Properties and Prospective Role in Neutropenic Conditions," *Drugs*, 1991, 42 (2):300-30.

Morstyn G, Campbell L, Lieschke G, et al, "Treatment of Chemotherapy-Induced Neutropenia by Subcutaneously Administered Granulocyte Colony-Stimulating Factor With Optimization of Dose and Duration of Therapy," *J Clin Oncol*, 1989, 7(10):1554-62.

"Update of Recommendations for the Use of Hematopoietic Colony-Stimulating Factors: Evidence-based Clinical Practice Guidelines. American Society of Clinical Oncology," *J Clin Oncol*, 1996, 14 (6):1957-60.

Wolach B, "Neonatal Sepsis: Pathogenesis and Supportive Therapy," *Semin Perinatol*, 1997, 21(1):28-38.

Flecainide (fle KAY nide)

Medication Safety Issues
Sound-alike/look-alike issues:
Flecainide may be confused with fluconazole
Tambocor™ may be confused with Pamelor®, Temodar®, tamoxifen, Tamiflu®

Related Information
Medications for Which A Single Dose May Be Fatal When Ingested By A Toddler on page 1709

U.S. Brand Names Tambocor™

Canadian Brand Names Apo-Flecainide®; Tambocor™

Therapeutic Category Antiarrhythmic Agent, Class I-C

Generic Available Yes

Use Prevention and suppression of documented life-threatening ventricular arrhythmias (ie, sustained ventricular tachycardia); prevention of symptomatic, disabling supraventricular tachycardias in patients without structural heart disease

Pregnancy Risk Factor C

Lactation Enters breast milk/compatible

Contraindications Hypersensitivity to flecainide or any component; pre-existing second or third degree A-V block; right bundle-branch block associated with left hemiblock (bifascicular block) or trifascicular block (unless a functioning pacemaker is present); cardiogenic shock; myocardial depression

Warnings Antiarrhythmic agents should be reserved for patients with life-threatening ventricular arrhythmias [U.S. Boxed Warning]. In the Cardiac Arrhythmia Suppression Trial (CAST), recent (>6 days but <2 years ago) myocardial infarction patients with asymptomatic, nonlife-threatening ventricular arrhythmias did not benefit and may have been harmed by attempts to suppress the arrhythmia with flecainide or encainide. An increased mortality or nonfatal cardiac arrest rate (7.7%) was seen in the active treatment group compared with patients in the placebo group (3%). The applicability of the CAST results to other populations is unknown. The risks of class IC agents and the lack of improved survival make use in patients without life-threatening arrhythmias generally unacceptable.

Use for symptomatic nonsustained ventricular tachycardia, frequent premature ventricular complexes (PVCs), uniform and multiform PVCs and/or coupled PVCs, or chronic atrial fibrillation is not recommended. Flecainide can worsen or cause arrhythmias with an associated risk of death [U.S. Boxed Warnings]. Proarrhythmic effects range from an increased number of PVCs to more severe ventricular tachycardias (ie, tachycardias that are more sustained or more resistant to conversion to sinus rhythm). Risk is reduced when lower doses were initiated; monitor and adjust dose to prevent QT$_c$ prolongation. Flecainide is not recommended for patients with chronic atrial fibrillation. When treating atrial flutter, 1:1 atrioventricular conduction may occur; pre-emptive negative chronotropic therapy (eg, digoxin, beta-blockers) may lower the risk [U.S. Boxed Warning].

Precautions Use with caution in patients with pacemakers, sick sinus syndrome, CHF, myocardial dysfunction, and renal and/or hepatic impairment; use decreased doses and cautiously titrate dose according to serum concentrations and clinical effects in patients with CHF, or myocardial, liver or renal dysfunction. Flecainide may cause increases in PR, QRS, and QT intervals and new first degree or bundle branch block; use with caution and consider dosing reduction when increases in such intervals occur.

Adverse Reactions
Cardiovascular: Bradycardia, heart block, worsening ventricular arrhythmias, CHF, palpitations, chest pain, edema; P-R interval and QRS duration increased

Central nervous system: Dizziness, fatigue, nervousness, hypoesthesia, headache
Dermatologic: Rash
Gastrointestinal: Nausea
Hematologic: Blood dyscrasias
Hepatic: Hepatic dysfunction
Neuromuscular & skeletal: Paresthesia, tremor
Ocular: Blurred vision
Respiratory: Dyspnea

Drug Interactions
Metabolism/Transport Effects Substrate of CYP1A2 (minor), 2D6 (major); Inhibits CYP2D6 (weak)

Avoid Concomitant Use
Avoid concomitant use of Flecainide with any of the following: Artemether; Dronedarone; Lumefantrine; Nilotinib; Pimozide; QuiNINE; Ritonavir; Tetrabenazine; Thioridazine; Tipranavir; Ziprasidone

Increased Effect/Toxicity
Flecainide may increase the levels/effects of: Dronedarone; Pimozide; QTc-Prolonging Agents; QuiNINE; Tetrabenazine; Thioridazine; Ziprasidone

The levels/effects of Flecainide may be increased by: Alfuzosin; Amiodarone; Artemether; Carbonic Anhydrase Inhibitors; Chloroquine; Ciprofloxacin; Ciprofloxacin (Systemic); CYP2D6 Inhibitors (Moderate); CYP2D6 Inhibitors (Strong); Darunavir; Gadobutrol; Lumefantrine; Nilotinib; QuiNINE; Ritonavir; Sodium Bicarbonate; Sodium Lactate; Tipranavir; Tromethamine; Verapamil

Decreased Effect
The levels/effects of Flecainide may be decreased by: Peginterferon Alfa-2b; Sodium Bicarbonate

Food Interactions Dairy products (milk, infant formula, yogurt) may interfere with the absorption of flecainide in infants; there is one case report of a neonate (GA 34 weeks PNA >6 days) who required extremely large doses of oral flecainide when administered every 8 hours with feedings ("milk feeds"); changing the feedings from "milk feeds" to 5% glucose feeds alone resulted in a doubling of the flecainide serum concentration and toxicity (see Russell, 1989); clearance of flecainide may be decreased in patients with strict vegetarian diets due to urinary pH ≥8

Mechanism of Action Class IC antiarrhythmic; slows conduction in cardiac tissue by altering transport of ions across cell membranes; causes slight prolongation of refractory periods; decreases the rate of rise of the action potential without affecting its duration; increases electrical stimulation threshold of ventricle, His-Purkinje system; possesses local anesthetic and moderate negative inotropic effects

Pharmacokinetics (Adult data unless noted)
Absorption: Oral: Rapid and nearly complete
Distribution: V$_d$: Adults: 5-13.4 L/kg
Protein binding: 40% to 50% (alpha$_1$ glycoprotein)
Metabolism: In the liver
Bioavailability: 85% to 90%
Half-life, elimination: Increased half-life with CHF or renal dysfunction
Newborns: ~29 hours
Infants: 11-12 hours
Children: 8 hours
Adults: ~20 hours (range: 12-27 hours)
Time to peak serum concentration: ~3 hours (range 1-6 hours)
Elimination: In urine as unchanged drug (10% to 50%) and metabolites
Dialysis: Not dialyzable

Usual Dosage Oral:
Children: Initial: 1-3 mg/kg/day or 50-100 mg/m^2/day in 3 divided doses; usual: 3-6 mg/kg/day or 100-150 mg/m^2/day in 3 divided doses; up to 8 mg/kg/day or 200 mg/m^2/day for uncontrolled patients with subtherapeutic levels; higher doses have been reported, however they may be

associated with an increased risk of proarrhythmias; a review of world literature reports the average effective dose to be 4 mg/kg/day or 140 mg/m^2/day

Adults:

Life-threatening ventricular arrhythmias: Initial: 100 mg every 12 hours, increase by 100 mg/day (given in 2 doses/day) every 4 days; usual: ≤300 mg/day; maximum: 400 mg/day; for patients receiving 400 mg/day who are not controlled and have trough concentrations <0.6 mcg/mL, dosage may be increased to 600 mg/day

Prevention of paroxysmal supraventricular arrhythmias in patients with disabling symptoms but no structural heart disease: Initial: 50 mg every 12 hours; increase by 50 mg twice daily at 4-day intervals; maximum dose: 300 mg/day

Paroxysmal atrial fibrillation: Outpatient: "Pill-in-the-pocket" dose (for selected patients; see Alboni, 2004 and EHRA, 2006): 200 mg (patient weight <70 kg), 300 mg (weight ≥70 kg). May not repeat in ≤24 hours. **Note:** An initial inpatient conversion trial should have been successful before sending patient home on this approach. Patient must be taking an AV nodal-blocking agent (eg, beta-blocker, nondihydropyridine calcium channel blocker) prior to initiation of antiarrhythmic.

Dosing adjustment in renal failure:

Manufacturer recommendations: Adults: Cl$_{cr}$ ≤35 mL/minute/1.73 m^2: Initial: 50 mg every 12 hours or 100 mg once daily; increase dose slowly at intervals >4 days; monitor plasma levels closely

Alternative adjustment: Children and Adults Cl$_{cr}$ ≤20 mL/minute: Decrease the usual dose by 25% to 50%

Administration Oral: May be administered in children and adults without regard to food; in infants receiving milk or milk based formulas, avoid concurrent administration with feedings; monitor serum concentrations and decrease the dose when the diet changes to a decreased consumption of milk

Monitoring Parameters ECG, serum concentrations [Note: Obtain serum trough concentrations at steady state (after at least 3 days when doses are started or changed) or when dietary changes due to maturation or concurrent illness occur], liver enzymes, CBC with differential

Reference Range Therapeutic: 0.2-1 mcg/mL (SI: 0.4-2 micromoles/L). **Note:** Pediatric patients may respond at the lower end of the recommended therapeutic range (0.2-0.5 mcg/mL) but up to 0.8 mcg/mL may be required.

Patient Information May cause dizziness; notify physician if chest pain, faintness, palpitations, dizziness or visual disturbances occur

Additional Information Single oral dose flecainide for termination of PSVT in children and young adults (n=25) and combination therapy of flecainide with amiodarone for refractory tachyarrhythmias in infancy (n=9) have been reported (see References)

Dosage Forms Excipient information presented when available (limited, particularly for generics); consult specific product labeling.

Tablet, as acetate: 50 mg, 100 mg, 150 mg

Extemporaneous Preparations

A 5 mg/mL suspension compounded from tablets and an oral flavored commercially available diluent (Roxane®) was stable for up to 45 days when stored at 5°C or 25°C in amber glass bottles (Wiest, 1992)

A 20 mg/mL oral liquid preparation made from tablets and 3 different vehicles (cherry syrup, a 1:1 mixture of Ora-Sweet® and Ora-Plus®, or a 1:1 mixture of Ora-Sweet® SF and Ora-Plus®) was stable for 60 days when stored in amber plastic prescription bottles in the dark at room temperature (25°C) or under refrigeration (5°C); grind twenty-four 100 mg tablets in a mortar into a fine powder; add 20 mL of the vehicle and mix well to form a uniform paste; mix while adding the vehicle in geometric proportions to **almost** 120 mL; transfer to a calibrated

bottle and qsad with vehicle to 120 mL; label "shake well" and "protect from light" (Allen, 1996).

Allen LV and Erickson MA, "Stability of Baclofen, Captopril, Diltiazem Hydrochloride, Dipyridamole, and Flecainide Acetate in Extemporaneously Compounded Oral Liquids," *Am J Health Syst Pharm*, 1996, 53 (18):2179-84.

Wiest DB, Garner SS, and Pagacz LR, "Stability of Flecainide Acetate in an Extemporaneously Compounded Oral Suspension," *Am J Hosp Pharm*, 1992, 49(6):1467-70.

References

Alboni P, Botto GL, Baldi N, et al, "Outpatient Treatment of Recent-Onset Atrial Fibrillation With the 'Pill-in-the-Pocket' Approach," *N Engl J Med*, 2004, 351(23):2384-91.

European Heart Rhythm Association, Heart Rhythm Society, Fuster V, et al, "ACC/AHA/ESC 2006 Guidelines for the Management of Patients With Atrial Fibrillation - Executive Summary: A Report of the American College of Cardiology/American Heart Association Task Force on Practice Guidelines and the European Society of Cardiology Committee for Practice Guidelines (Writing Committee to Revise the 2001 Guidelines for the Management of Patients With Atrial Fibrillation)," *J Am Coll Cardiol*, 2006, 48(4):854-906.

Fenrich AL Jr, Perry JC, and Friedman RA, "Flecainide and Amiodarone: Combined Therapy for Refractory Tachyarrhythmias in Infants," *J Am Coll Cardiol*, 1995, 25(5):1195-8.

Musto B, Cavallaro C, Musto A, et al, "Flecainide Single Oral Dose for Management of Paroxysmal Supraventricular Tachycardia in Children and Young Adults," *Am Heart J*, 1992, 124(1):110-5.

Perry JC and Garson A Jr, "Flecainide Acetate for Treatment of Tachyarrhythmias in Children: Review of World Literature on Efficacy, Safety, and Dosing," *Am Heart J*, 1992, 124(6):1614-21.

Perry JC, McQuinn RL, Smith RT Jr, et al, "Flecainide Acetate for Resistant Arrhythmias in the Young: Efficacy and Pharmacokinetics," *J Am Coll Cardiol*, 1989, 14(1):185-91.

Priestley KA, Ladusans EJ, Rosenthal E, et al, "Experience With Flecainide for the Treatment of Cardiac Arrhythmias in Children," *Eur Heart J*, 1988, 9(12):1284-90.

Russell GA and Martin RP, "Flecainide Toxicity," *Arch Dis Child*, 1989, 64(6):860-2.

Zeigler V, Gillette PC, Ross BA, et al, "Flecainide for Supraventricular and Ventricular Arrhythmias in Children and Young Adults," *Am J Cardiol*, 1988, 62(10 Pt 1):818-20.

♦ **Flecainide Acetate** *see* Flecainide *on page 582*

♦ **Flector®** *see* Diclofenac *on page 429*

♦ **Fleet® Babylax® [OTC] [DSC]** *see* Glycerin *on page 650*

♦ **Fleet® Bisacodyl [OTC]** *see* Bisacodyl *on page 194*

♦ **Fleet® Enema [OTC]** *see* Sodium Phosphate *on page 1276*

♦ **Fleet Enema® (Can)** *see* Sodium Phosphate *on page 1276*

♦ **Fleet® Enema Extra® [OTC]** *see* Sodium Phosphate *on page 1276*

♦ **Fleet® Glycerin Suppositories [OTC]** *see* Glycerin *on page 650*

♦ **Fleet® Glycerin Suppositories Maximum Strength [OTC]** *see* Glycerin *on page 650*

♦ **Fleet® Liquid Glycerin Suppositories [OTC]** *see* Glycerin *on page 650*

♦ **Fleet® Mineral Oil Enema [OTC]** *see* Mineral Oil *on page 933*

♦ **Fleet® Pedia-Lax™ Enema [OTC]** *see* Sodium Phosphate *on page 1276*

♦ **Fleet® Pedia-Lax™ Glycerin Suppositories [OTC]** *see* Glycerin *on page 650*

♦ **Fleet® Pedia-Lax™ Liquid Glycerin Suppositories [OTC]** *see* Glycerin *on page 650*

♦ **Fleet® Pedia-Lax™ Liquid Stool Softener [OTC]** *see* Docusate *on page 468*

♦ **Fleet® Pedia-Lax™ Quick Dissolve [OTC]** *see* Senna *on page 1253*

◆ **Fleet® Phospho-soda® [OTC] [DSC]** *see* Sodium Phosphate *on page 1276*

◆ **Fleet® Phospho-soda® EZ-Prep™ [OTC] [DSC]** *see* Sodium Phosphate *on page 1276*

◆ **Fleet® Sof-Lax® [OTC]** *see* Docusate *on page 468*

◆ **Fleet® Stimulant Laxative [OTC]** *see* Bisacodyl *on page 194*

◆ **Fletcher's® [OTC]** *see* Senna *on page 1253*

◆ **Flexbumin** *see* Albumin *on page 55*

◆ **Flexeril®** *see* Cyclobenzaprine *on page 367*

◆ **Flexitec (Can)** *see* Cyclobenzaprine *on page 367*

◆ **Flolan®** *see* Epoprostenol *on page 517*

◆ **Flonase®** *see* Fluticasone *on page 607*

◆ **Floranex™ [OTC]** *see* Lactobacillus *on page 790*

◆ **Flora-Q™ [OTC]** *see* Lactobacillus *on page 790*

◆ **Florazole® ER (Can)** *see* MetroNIDAZOLE *on page 921*

◆ **Florical® [OTC]** *see* Calcium Carbonate *on page 232*

◆ **Florical® [OTC]** *see* Calcium Supplements *on page 239*

◆ **Florinef** *see* Fludrocortisone *on page 589*

◆ **Florinef® (Can)** *see* Fludrocortisone *on page 589*

◆ **Flovent® Diskus®** *see* Fluticasone *on page 607*

◆ **Flovent® HFA** *see* Fluticasone *on page 607*

◆ **Floxin®** *see* Ofloxacin *on page 1011*

◆ **Floxin Otic Singles** *see* Ofloxacin *on page 1011*

◆ **Fluarix®** *see* Influenza Virus Vaccine (Inactivated) *on page 734*

◆ **Flubenisolone** *see* Betamethasone *on page 189*

Fluconazole (floo KOE na zole)

Medication Safety Issues

Sound-alike/look-alike issues:

Fluconazole may be confused with flecainide, FLUoxetine, furosemide, itraconazole

Diflucan® may be confused with diclofenac, Diprivan®, disulfiram

International issues:

Canesten® [Great Britain]: Brand name for clotrimazole in multiple international markets

U.S. Brand Names Diflucan®

Canadian Brand Names Apo-Fluconazole®; CanesOral®; CO Fluconazole; Diflucan®; Dom-Fluconazole; Fluconazole Injection; Fluconazole Omega; Mylan-Fluconazole; Novo-Fluconazole; PHL-Fluconazole; PMS-Fluconazole; PRO-Fluconazole; Riva-Fluconazole; Taro-Fluconazole; ZYM-Fluconazole

Therapeutic Category Antifungal Agent, Systemic

Generic Available Yes

Use Treatment of susceptible fungal infections including oropharyngeal, esophageal, and vaginal candidiasis; treatment of systemic candidal infections including urinary tract infection, peritonitis, cystitis, and pneumonia; strains of *Candida* with decreased *in vitro* susceptibility to fluconazole are being isolated with increasing frequency; fluconazole is more active against *C. albicans* than other candidal strains like *C. parapsilosis*, *C. glabrata*, and *C. tropicalis*; treatment and suppression of cryptococcal meningitis; prophylaxis of candidiasis in patients undergoing bone marrow transplantation; alternative to amphotericin B in patients with pre-existing renal impairment or when requiring concomitant therapy with other potentially nephrotoxic drugs

Pregnancy Risk Factor C

Pregnancy Considerations When used in high doses, fluconazole is teratogenic in animal studies. Following exposure during the first trimester, case reports have noted similar malformations in humans when used in higher doses (400 mg/day) over extended periods of time. Use of lower doses (150 mg as a single dose or 200 mg/day) may have less risk; however, additional data is needed. Use during pregnancy only if the potential benefit to the mother outweighs any potential risk to the fetus.

Lactation Enters breast/not recommended (AAP rates "compatible")

Breast-Feeding Considerations Fluconazole is found in breast milk at concentration similar to plasma.

Contraindications Hypersensitivity to fluconazole, other azoles, or any component; concurrent use with astemizole, cisapride, and terfenadine

Warnings Rare cases, including fatalities, due to fluconazole-associated hepatotoxicity have been reported. Patients who develop abnormal liver function tests during fluconazole therapy should be monitored closely for the development of more severe hepatic injury; if clinical signs and symptoms consistent with liver disease develop that may be attributable to fluconazole, fluconazole should be discontinued. Rare cases of exfoliative skin disorders have been reported. Closely monitor patients who develop rashes during fluconazole therapy.

Fluconazole oral suspension contains sodium benzoate; benzoic acid (benzoate) is a metabolite of benzyl alcohol; large amounts of benzyl alcohol (≥99 mg/kg/day) have been associated with a potentially fatal toxicity ("gasping syndrome") in neonates; the "gasping syndrome" consists of metabolic acidosis, respiratory distress, gasping respirations, CNS dysfunction (including convulsions, intracranial hemorrhage), hypotension and cardiovascular collapse; use fluconazole oral suspension containing sodium benzoate with caution in neonates; *in vitro* and animal studies have shown that benzoate displaces bilirubin from protein binding sites

Precautions Use with caution and modify dosage in patients with impaired renal function. Use with caution in patients with hepatic dysfunction or in patients with proarrhythmic conditions.

Adverse Reactions

Cardiovascular: Pallor, angioedema, QT prolongation, torsade de pointes

Central nervous system: Dizziness, headache (1.9%), seizures

Dermatologic: Skin rash (1.8%), exfoliative skin disorders, Stevens-Johnson syndrome, pruritus

Endocrine & metabolic: Hypokalemia, hypercholesterolemia, hypertriglyceridemia

Gastrointestinal: Nausea (2%), abdominal pain (3%), vomiting (5%), diarrhea (2%), dysgeusia, dyspepsia

Hematologic: Eosinophilia, leukopenia, thrombocytopenia, neutropenia, agranulocytosis

Hepatic: AST, ALT, or alkaline phosphatase elevated; hepatitis; cholestasis, jaundice

Miscellaneous: Anaphylaxis

Drug Interactions

Metabolism/Transport Effects Inhibits CYP1A2 (weak), 2C9 (strong), 2C19 (strong), 3A4 (moderate)

Avoid Concomitant Use

Avoid concomitant use of Fluconazole with any of the following: Artemether; Cisapride; Clopidogrel; Conivaptan; Dofetilide; Dronedarone; Lumefantrine; Nilotinib; Pimozide; QuiNIDine; QuiNINE; Ranolazine; Tetrabenazine; Thioridazine; Tolvaptan; Ziprasidone

Increased Effect/Toxicity

Fluconazole may increase the levels/effects of: Alfentanil; Aprepitant; Benzodiazepines (metabolized by oxidation); Bosentan; BusPIRone; Busulfan; Calcium Channel Blockers; CarBAMazepine; Carvedilol; Cilostazol; Cinacalcet; Cisapride; Citalopram; Colchicine; Conivaptan; Corticosteroids (Orally Inhaled); Corticosteroids (Systemic); CycloSPORINE; CycloSPORINE (Systemic);

CYP2C19 Substrates; CYP2C9 Substrates (High risk); CYP3A4 Substrates; Docetaxel; Dofetilide; Dronedarone; Eletriptan; Eplerenone; Erlotinib; Eszopiclone; Everolimus; FentaNYL; Fosaprepitant; Gefitinib; HMG-CoA Reductase Inhibitors; Imatinib; Irbesartan; Irinotecan; Losartan; Macrolide Antibiotics; Methadone; Phenytoin; Phosphodiesterase 5 Inhibitors; Pimecrolimus; Pimozide; Protease Inhibitors; Proton Pump Inhibitors; QTc-Prolonging Agents; QuiNIDine; QuiNINE; Ramelteon; Ranolazine; Repaglinide; Rifamycin Derivatives; Salmeterol; Saxagliptin; Sirolimus; Solifenacin; Sulfonylureas; Sunitinib; Tacrolimus; Tacrolimus (Systemic); Tacrolimus (Topical); Temsirolimus; Tetrabenazine; Thioridazine; Tolterodine; Tolvaptan; Vitamin K Antagonists; Zidovudine; Ziprasidone; Zolpidem

The levels/effects of Fluconazole may be increased by: Alfuzosin; Artemether; Chloroquine; Ciprofloxacin; Ciprofloxacin (Systemic); Gadobutrol; Grapefruit Juice; Lumefantrine; Macrolide Antibiotics; Nilotinib; Protease Inhibitors; QuiNINE

Decreased Effect
Fluconazole may decrease the levels/effects of: Amphotericin B; Clopidogrel; Saccharomyces boulardii

The levels/effects of Fluconazole may be decreased by: Didanosine; Phenytoin; Rifamycin Derivatives; Sucralfate

Food Interactions Food decreases the rate but not the extent of absorption

Stability Store tablets, powder for oral suspension, and premixed infusion at room temperature; do not freeze. Reconstituted oral suspension is stable for 14 days at room temperature or if refrigerated.
Fluconazole injection is incompatible with ampicillin, calcium gluconate, ceftazidime, cefotaxime, cefuroxime, ceftriaxone, clindamycin, furosemide, imipenem, ticarcillin, and piperacillin

Mechanism of Action Interferes with fungal cytochrome P450 sterol C-14 alpha-demethylation activity, decreasing ergosterol synthesis (principal sterol in fungal cell membrane) and inhibiting cell membrane formation

Pharmacokinetics (Adult data unless noted)
Absorption: Oral: Well absorbed; food does not affect extent of absorption
Distribution: Distributes widely into body tissues and fluids including the CSF, saliva, sputum, vaginal fluid, skin, eye; excreted in breast milk
Protein binding: 11% to 12%
Bioavailability: Oral: >90%
Half-life:
Premature newborns: 73.6 hours; 6 days PNA: 53.2 hours; 12 days PNA: 46.6 hours
Children:
9 months to 13 years: 19.5-25 hours (with oral dose)
5-15 years: 15.2-17.6 hours (with multiple I.V. dosing)
Adults: 25-30 hours with normal renal function
Time to peak serum concentration: Oral: Within 2-4 hours (1-2 hours in fasted patients)
Elimination: 80% of dose excreted unchanged in urine; 11% of dose excreted in urine as metabolites
Dialysis: Hemodialysis: 3-hour session decreases plasma concentration 50%

Usual Dosage Daily dose of fluconazole is the same for oral and I.V. administration:
Oral, I.V.:
Premature neonates:
≤29 weeks gestation:
Postnatal age 0-14 days: 5-6 mg/kg/dose every 72 hours
Postnatal age >14 days: 5-6 mg/kg/dose every 48 hours
30-36 weeks gestation: Postnatal age 0-14 days: 3-6 mg/kg/dose every 48 hours
Neonates >14 days, Infants, Children: Once daily.

Indication	Day 1	Daily Therapy	Minimum Duration of Therapy
Neonates 0-14 days: Same dosage as older children but administered every 24-72 h			
Neonates >14 days, infants, and children			
Oropharyngeal candidiasis	6 mg/kg	3 mg/kg	14 d
Esophageal candidiasis	6 mg/kg	3 mg/kg up to 12 mg/kg/d	21 d
Systemic candidiasis	6-12 mg/kg/d		28 d
Cryptococcal meningitis			
acute	12 mg/kg	6 mg/kg up to 12 mg/kg/d	10-12 wk after CSF culture becomes negative
relapse	6 mg/kg		

Safety profile of fluconazole has been studied in 577 children ages 1 day to 17 years. Doses as high as 12 mg/kg/day once daily (equivalent to adult doses of 400 mg/day) have been used to treat candidiasis in immunocompromised children; 10-12 mg/kg/day doses once daily have been used prophylactically against fungal infections in pediatric bone marrow transplantation patients. Do not exceed 600 mg/day.
Dose equivalency:
Pediatric patients 3 mg/kg = Adults 100 mg
Pediatric patients 6 mg/kg = Adults 200 mg
Pediatric patients 12 mg/kg = Adults 400 mg
Adults: 200-800 mg daily; duration and dosage depends on severity of infection

Indication	Day 1	Daily Therapy	Minimum Duration of Therapy
Oropharyngeal candidiasis	200 mg	100 mg	14 d
Esophageal candidiasis	200 mg	100-400 mg	21 d
Systemic candidiasis	400 mg	200-800 mg	28 d
Cryptococcal meningitis			
acute	400 mg	200-800 mg	10-12 wk after CSF culture becomes negative
relapse	200 mg	200 mg	
Vaginal candidiasis	150 mg		single dose
Prophylaxis against fungal infections in bone marrow transplantation patients	400 mg/d		28 d

Dosing adjustment in renal impairment: Adults:
Cl_{cr} ≤50 mL/minute (not on dialysis): Administer 50% of recommended dose
Patients receiving hemodialysis: Administer 100% of recommended dose after each dialysis treatment

Administration
Oral: Administer with or without food; shake suspension well before use
Parenteral: Fluconazole must be administered by I.V. infusion over approximately 1-2 hours at a rate not to exceed 200 mg/hour and a final concentration for administration of 2 mg/mL; for pediatric patients receiving doses ≥6 mg/kg/day, administer I.V. infusion over 2 hours

Monitoring Parameters Periodic liver function and renal function tests, serum potassium, CBC with differential, and platelet count

Patient Information Notify physician of unusual bleeding or bruising, yellowing of skin and eyes, or severe skin rash

Dosage Forms Excipient information presented when available (limited, particularly for generics); consult specific product labeling. [DSC] = Discontinued product

Infusion premixed iso-osmotic dextrose solution: 200 mg (100 mL); 400 mg (200 mL)

Diflucan®: 200 mg (100 mL) [DSC]; 400 mg (200 mL)

Infusion, premixed iso-osmotic sodium chloride solution: 100 mg (50 mL); 200 mg (100 mL); 400 mg (200 mL)

Diflucan®: 200 mg (100 mL); 400 mg (200 mL)

Infusion, premixed iso-osmotic sodium chloride solution [preservative free]: 200 mg (100 mL); 400 mg (200 mL)

Powder for oral suspension: 10 mg/mL (35 mL); 40 mg/mL (35 mL)

Diflucan®: 10 mg/mL (35 mL); 40 mg/mL (35 mL) [contains sodium benzoate; orange flavor]

Tablet: 50 mg, 100 mg, 150 mg, 200 mg

Diflucan®: 50 mg, 100 mg, 150 mg, 200 mg

References

Como JA and Dismukes WE, "Oral Azole Drugs as Systemic Antifungal Therapy," *N Engl J Med*, 1993, 330(4):263-72.

Goodman JL, Winston DJ, Greenfield RA, et al, "A Controlled Trial of Fluconazole to Prevent Fungal Infections in Patients Undergoing Bone Marrow Transplantation," *N Engl J Med*, 1992, 326(13):845-51.

Lee JW, Seibel NL, Amantea M, et al, "Safety and Pharmacokinetics of Fluconazole in Children With Neoplastic Diseases," *J Pediatr*, 1992, 120(6):987-93.

Moncino MD and Gutman LT, "Severe Systemic Cryptococcal Disease in a Child: Review of Prognostic Indicators Predicting Treatment Failure and an Approach to Maintenance Therapy With Oral Fluconazole," *Pediatr Infect Dis J*, 1990, 9(5):363-8.

Viscoli C, Castagnola E, Fioredda F, et al, "Fluconazole in the Treatment of Candidiasis in Immunocompromised Children," *Antimicrob Agents Chemother*, 1991, 35(2):365-7.

♦ **Fluconazole Injection (Can)** *see* Fluconazole *on page 584*

♦ **Fluconazole Omega (Can)** *see* Fluconazole *on page 584*

Flucytosine (floo SYE toe seen)

Medication Safety Issues

Sound-alike/look-alike issues:

Flucytosine may be confused with fluorouracil

Ancobon® may be confused with Oncovin®

High alert medication: The Institute for Safe Medication Practices (ISMP) includes this medication among its list of drugs which have a heightened risk of causing significant patient harm when used in error.

Related Information

Therapeutic Drug Monitoring: Blood Sampling Time Guidelines *on page 1704*

U.S. Brand Names Ancobon®

Canadian Brand Names Ancobon®

Therapeutic Category Antifungal Agent, Systemic

Generic Available No

Use In combination with amphotericin B in the treatment of serious Candidal or Cryptococcal pulmonary or urinary tract infections, sepsis, meningitis, or endocarditis (resistance emerges if flucytosine is used as a single agent); used in combination with another antifungal agent for treatment of chromomycosis and aspergillosis

Pregnancy Risk Factor C

Pregnancy Considerations Teratogenic in some animal studies, however, there are no adequate and well-controlled studies in pregnant women.

Lactation Excretion in breast milk unknown/not recommended

Contraindications Hypersensitivity to flucytosine or any component

Warnings Use with extreme caution in patients with renal impairment **[U.S. Boxed Warning]**; renal impairment may lead to accumulation; dosage modification required in patients with impaired renal function based on serum flucytosine concentrations; use with extreme caution in patients with bone marrow suppression, patients with AIDS, patients being treated with radiation or with drugs which depress bone marrow; closely monitor hematologic, renal, and hepatic function of all patients receiving flucytosine **[U.S. Boxed Warning]**; bone marrow toxicity can be irreversible and is potentially fatal; hepatotoxicity and bone marrow toxicity appear to be dose related; monitor levels closely and adjust dose accordingly.

Precautions Avoid monotherapy due to rapid emergence of resistance.

Adverse Reactions

Cardiovascular: Chest pain, myocardial toxicity, ventricular dysfunction, cardiac arrest

Central nervous system: Confusion, headache, sedation, hallucinations, psychosis, seizures, vertigo, ataxia, fever

Dermatologic: Rash, pruritus, urticaria, photosensitivity

Endocrine & metabolic: Temporary growth failure, hypokalemia, hypoglycemia, acidemia

Gastrointestinal: Nausea, vomiting, diarrhea, enterocolitis, anorexia, GI hemorrhage, dry mouth, duodenal ulcer, abdominal pain

Genitourinary: Crystalluria

Hematologic: Bone marrow suppression (often observed after 10-26 days of therapy and occurs more frequently with sustained concentrations >100 mcg/mL), anemia, leukopenia, thrombocytopenia, agranulocytosis, eosinophilia, aplastic anemia

Hepatic: Bilirubin and liver enzymes elevated; hepatitis, jaundice

Neuromuscular & skeletal: Neuropathy, paresthesia

Otic: Hearing loss

Renal: BUN and serum creatinine elevated, renal failure

Respiratory: Dyspnea, respiratory arrest

Miscellaneous: Anaphylaxis

Drug Interactions

Avoid Concomitant Use There are no known interactions where it is recommended to avoid concomitant use.

Increased Effect/Toxicity

The levels/effects of Flucytosine may be increased by: Amphotericin B

Decreased Effect

Flucytosine may decrease the levels/effects of: Saccharomyces boulardii

The levels/effects of Flucytosine may be decreased by: Cytarabine

Food Interactions Food decreases the rate, but not the extent of absorption

Stability Store at room temperature; protect from light

Mechanism of Action Penetrates fungal cells and is converted to fluorouracil which competes with uracil interfering with fungal RNA and protein synthesis

Pharmacokinetics (Adult data unless noted)

Absorption: Oral: Rapid; rate of absorption is delayed in patients with renal impairment

Distribution: Widely distributed into body tissues and fluids including CSF, aqueous humor, peritoneal fluid, bronchial secretions, liver, spleen, kidney, heart, and joints

V_d: Adults: 0.68 L/kg

Protein binding: 2.9% to 4%

Metabolism: Minimal hepatic metabolism; deaminated to 5-fluorouracil (probably by gut bacteria)

Bioavailability: 78% to 89%; decreased in neonates

Half-life:
Neonates: 4-34 hours
Infants: 7.4 hours
Adults: 2.5-6 hours (prolonged as high as 200 hours in anuria)

Time to peak serum concentration: Oral:
Children: 2.5 ± 1.3 hours
Adults: Within 2 hours

Elimination: 75% to 90% excreted unchanged in urine by glomerular filtration; small portion is excreted in the feces

Dialysis: Dialyzable (50% to 100%)

Usual Dosage Oral: **Note:** Should be used in combination with amphotericin B due to development of resistance.

Neonates: Initial: 25-100 mg/kg/day in divided doses every 12-24 hours

Infants, Children, and Adults: 50-150 mg/kg/day in divided doses every 6 hours

Dosing adjustment in renal impairment: Use lower initial dose:
Cl_{cr} 20-40 mL/minute: Administer usual individual dose every 12 hours
Cl_{cr} 10-20 mL/minute: Administer usual individual dose every 24 hours
Cl_{cr} <10 mL/minute: Administer usual individual dose every 24-48 hours

Patients receiving hemodialysis: Administer 20-50 mg/kg dose postdialysis

Administration Oral: Administer with food over a 15-minute period to decrease incidence and severity of nausea and vomiting

Monitoring Parameters Serum electrolytes, creatinine, BUN, alkaline phosphatase, AST, ALT, CBC, platelet count; serum flucytosine concentrations; *in vitro* susceptibility tests to flucytosine

Reference Range Therapeutic levels: 25-100 mcg/mL; with invasive candidiasis, maintain peak plasma concentration between 40-60 mcg/mL; increased bone marrow suppression with sustained serum flucytosine concentration >100 mcg/mL; obtain flucytosine concentration 60-120 minutes after an oral dose; obtain trough level immediately before the next dose; maintain trough ≥25 mcg/mL to prevent emergence of resistant strains

Test Interactions Flucytosine causes markedly false elevations in serum creatinine values when the Ektachem® analyzer is used. The Jaffé reaction is recommended for determining serum creatinine levels.

Patient Information May cause photosensitivity reactions (eg, exposure to sunlight may cause severe sunburn, skin rash, redness, or itching); avoid exposure to sunlight and artificial light sources (sunlamps, tanning booth/bed); wear protective clothing, wide-brimmed hats, sunglasses, and lip sunscreen (SPF ≥15); use a sunscreen [broad-spectrum sunscreen or physical sunscreen (preferred) or sunblock with SPF ≥15]; contact physician if reaction occurs.

Additional Information Resistance develops rapidly if used alone; more rapid emergence of fungal resistance may occur when lower doses are used

Dosage Forms Excipient information presented when available (limited, particularly for generics); consult specific product labeling.
Capsule: 250 mg, 500 mg

Extemporaneous Preparations Flucytosine oral liquid has been prepared by using the contents of ten 500 mg capsules triturated in a mortar and pestle with a small amount of distilled water; the mixture was transferred to a 500 mL volumetric flask; the mortar was rinsed several times with a small amount of distilled water and the fluid added to the flask; sufficient distilled water was added to make a total volume of 500 mL of a 10 mg/mL liquid; oral liquid was stable for 70 days when stored in glass or plastic prescription bottles at 4°C or for up to 14 days at room temperature.

Wintermeyer SM and Nahata MC, "Stability of Flucytosine in an Extemporaneously Compounded Oral Liquid," *Am J Health-Syst Pharm*, 1996, 53:407-9.

References

Baley JE, Meyers C, Kliegman RM, et al, "Pharmacokinetics, Outcome of Treatment, and Toxic Effects of Amphotericin B and 5-Fluorocytosine in Neonates," *J Pediatr*, 1990, 116(5):791-7.

Hope WW, Warn PA, Sharp A, et al, "Optimization of the Dosage of Flucytosine in Combination With Amphotericin B for Disseminated Candidiasis: A Pharmacodynamic Rationale for Reduced Dosing," *Antimicrob Agents Chemother*, 2007, 51(10):3760-2.

Soltani M, Tobin CM, Bowker KE, et al, "Evidence of Excessive Concentrations of 5-Flucytosine in Children Aged Below 12 Years: A 12-Year Review of Serum Concentrations From a UK Clinical Assay Reference Laboratory," *Int J Antimicrob Agents*, 2006, 28(6):574-7.

◆ **Fludara®** *see* Fludarabine *on page 587*

Fludarabine (floo DARE a been)

Medication Safety Issues
Sound-alike/look-alike issues:
Fludarabine may be confused with cladribine, floxuridine, Flumadine®
Fludara® may be confused with FUDR®

High alert medication: The Institute for Safe Medication Practices (ISMP) includes this medication among its list of drug classes which have a heightened risk of causing significant patient harm when used in error.

Related Information
Compatibility of Chemotherapy and Related Supportive Care Medications *on page 1580*
Emetogenic Potential of Antineoplastic Agents *on page 1579*

U.S. Brand Names Fludara®; Oforta™
Canadian Brand Names Fludara®
Therapeutic Category Antineoplastic Agent, Antimetabolite (Purine Antagonist)
Generic Available Yes
Use Treatment of B-cell chronic lymphocytic leukemia (CLL) unresponsive to previous therapy with an alkylating agent-containing regimen (FDA approved in ages ≥18 years). Treatment of acute leukemias and solid tumors in pediatric patients; non-Hodgkin's lymphoma; reduced intensity conditioning regimens prior to allogeneic hematopoietic stem-cell transplantation
Pregnancy Risk Factor D
Pregnancy Considerations Teratogenic effects were observed in animal studies. Based on the mechanism of action, fludarabine has the potential to cause fetal harm if administered during pregnancy. There are no adequate and well-controlled studies in pregnant women. Effective contraception is recommended during and for 6 months after treatment for women and men of reproductive potential.
Lactation Excretion in breast milk unknown/not recommended
Breast-Feeding Considerations Due to the potential for serious adverse reactions in the nursing infant, breast-feeding is not recommended.
Contraindications Hypersensitivity to fludarabine or any component
Warnings Hazardous agent; use appropriate precautions for handling and disposal; high doses have been associated with severe neurotoxicity **[U.S. Boxed Warning]**, including delayed blindness, coma, and death. Neurotoxicity from high doses can occur 21-60 days after completing a course of fludarabine and appears to be dose related. Similar neurotoxicity (agitation, coma, confusion, and seizure) has been reported with standard CLL doses (delay or discontinue therapy if neurotoxicity occurs). Possible neurotoxic effects of chronic administration are unknown. Severe bone marrow suppression (anemia,

thrombocytopenia, and neutropenia) has been observed at therapeutic doses **[U.S. Boxed Warning]**; may be cumulative; bone marrow hypoplasia or aplasia resulting in death has been reported; life-threatening and sometimes fatal autoimmune disorders, such as hemolytic anemia, autoimmune thrombocytopenia/thrombocytopenic purpura, Evan's syndrome, and acquired hemophilia, have been reported after one or more cycles of treatment **[U.S. Boxed Warning]**. Monitor closely for hemolysis; discontinue fludarabine if hemolysis occurs; hemolytic effects usually recur with fludarabine rechallenge. Concomitant therapy with pentostatin may be associated with severe and potentially fatal pulmonary toxicity **[U.S. Boxed Warning]**; concomitant use not recommended. Patients receiving blood products should only receive irradiated blood products due to the potential for transfusion-related GVHD. Fludarabine can cause fetal harm when administered to a pregnant women (advise women of childbearing potential to avoid becoming pregnant).

Precautions Use with caution in patients with pre-existing neurologic problems; patients with a fever, infection, immunodeficiency, history of opportunistic infection, or pre-existing hematological disorder; and in patients with renal insufficiency; dosage modification may be needed in patients with impaired renal function or bone marrow suppression. Prophylactic anti-infectives should be considered for patients with an increased risk for developing opportunistic infections. May cause tumor lysis syndrome; risk is increased in patients with large tumor burden prior to treatment. Avoid vaccination with live vaccines during and after fludarabine treatment.

Adverse Reactions
Cardiovascular: Edema, peripheral edema, CHF, pericardial effusion, chest pain, arrhythmia, cerebrovascular accident, MI, supraventricular tachycardia, deep vein thrombosis, phlebitis, aneurysm, transient ischemic attack

Central nervous system: Neurotoxicity (primarily progressive demyelinating encephalopathy with mental status deterioration), somnolence, seizures, fever, agitation, confusion, depression, chills, headache, coma, fatigue, pain, headache, malaise, sleep disorder, cerebellar syndrome, mentation impaired

Dermatologic: Pruritus, rash, alopecia, erythema multiforme, Stevens-Johnson syndrome, toxic epidermal necrolysis, pemphigus, seborrhea

Endocrine & metabolic: Metabolic acidosis, tumor lysis syndrome (hyperuricemia, hyperphosphatemia, hypocalcemia, hyperkalemia), hyperglycemia, LDH increased, dehydration, weight loss

Gastrointestinal: Nausea, vomiting, diarrhea, stomatitis, metallic taste, GI bleeding, anorexia, constipation, abdominal pain, esophagitis, mucositis

Genitourinary: Hemorrhagic cystitis (rare), urate crystalluria, urinary tract infection, dysuria, hesistancy

Hematologic: Leukopenia, neutropenia, thrombocytopenia, lymphocytopenia, autoimmune hemolytic anemia, anemia, pancytopenia, acquired hemophilia, myelodysplastic syndrome, hemorrhage

Hepatic: Transaminase levels elevated, cholelithiasis, liver failure

Neuromuscular & skeletal: Myalgia, peripheral neuropathy, weakness, arthralgia, back pain, osteoporosis, paresthesia

Ocular: Blindness, blurred vision, photophobia, optic neuritis, optic neuropathy, visual disturbance

Otic: Hearing loss

Renal: Hematuria, renal failure, renal function test abnormal, proteinuria

Respiratory: Interstitial pneumonitis, dyspnea, cough, ARDS, pulmonary hemorrhage, pulmonary fibrosis, respiratory failure, pharyngitis, allergic pneumonitis, hemoptysis, sinusitis, bronchitis, epistaxis, hypoxia, pneumonia, upper respiratory infection, rhinitis

Miscellaneous: Infections, acute myeloid leukemia, skin cancer, anaphylaxis, diaphoresis

Drug Interactions
Avoid Concomitant Use
Avoid concomitant use of Fludarabine with any of the following: BCG; Natalizumab; Pentostatin; Pimecrolimus; Tacrolimus (Topical); Vaccines (Live)

Increased Effect/Toxicity
Fludarabine may increase the levels/effects of: Leflunomide; Natalizumab; Pentostatin; Vaccines (Live)

The levels/effects of Fludarabine may be increased by: Denosumab; Pentostatin; Pimecrolimus; Tacrolimus (Topical); Trastuzumab

Decreased Effect
Fludarabine may decrease the levels/effects of: BCG; Sipuleucel-T; Vaccines (Inactivated); Vaccines (Live)

The levels/effects of Fludarabine may be decreased by: Echinacea; Imatinib

Stability
Vial: Store in refrigerator; reconstituted 25 mg/mL fludarabine solution should be used within 8 hours after preparation since it contains no preservatives. When fludarabine is diluted in D_5W or NS to a final concentration of 1 mg/mL, the solution is stable for 24 hours at room temperature. Discard solution if a slight haze develops.

Tablet: Store at room temperature; should be kept within packaging until use.

Mechanism of Action
F-ara-AMP is dephosphorylated to 2-fluoro-ara-A which enters the cell by a carrier-mediated transport process; it is phosphorylated intracellularly to the active metabolite F-ara-ATP. F-ara-ATP competes with deoxyadenosine triphosphate for incorporation into the A-sites of the DNA strand inhibiting DNA synthesis in the S-phase via inhibition of DNA polymerases, RNA reductase, DNA primase, and DNA ligase.

Pharmacokinetics (Adult data unless noted)
Distribution: Widely distributed with extensive tissue binding

Protein binding: 2-fluoro-ara-A: 19% to 29%

Metabolism: Fludarabine is dephosphorylated to 2-fluoro-ara-A which enters tumor cells and is phosphorylated to the active 2F-ara-ATP; active metabolite is dephosphorylated in the serum

Bioavailability: Oral: 2-fluoro-ara-A: 50% to 65%

Half-life: Terminal (2-fluoro-ara-A):
 Children: 12.4-19 hours
 Adults: 15-23 hours

Time to peak serum concentration: Oral: 1-2 hours

Elimination: Fludarabine clearance appears to be inversely correlated with serum creatinine; at a dose of 25 mg/m²/day for 5 days, 24% of dose excreted in urine; at higher doses, 41% to 60% of dose renally excreted

Usual Dosage
Not currently FDA approved for use in children (refer to individual protocols):
I.V.:
 Children:
  Acute leukemia: 10 mg/m² bolus over 15 minutes followed by a continuous infusion of 30.5 mg/m²/day for 5 days; or 10.5 mg/m² bolus over 15 minutes followed by a continuous infusion of 30.5 mg/m²/day over 48 hours followed by cytarabine has been used in clinical trials

  Reduced-intensity conditioning regimens prior to allogenic hematopoietic stem-cell transplantation: 30 mg/m²/day for 5 days

  Solid tumors: 7-9 mg/m² bolus followed by 20-27 mg/m²/day continuous infusion for 5 days. Maximum tolerated dose: Loading dose: 7 mg/m² followed by a continuous infusion of 20 mg/m²/day for 5 days.

Adults:

CLL: 25 mg/m^2/day for 5 days every 28 days

Non-Hodgkin's lymphoma: 25 mg/m^2/day for 5 days every 28 days

Oral: Adults: CLL: 40 mg/m^2 once daily for 5 days every 28 days

Dosing adjustment in renal impairment:

Cl$_{cr}$ 30-70 mL/minute/1.73 m^2: Reduce dose by 20% and monitor closely for toxicity

Cl$_{cr}$ <30 mL/minute/1.73 m^2:

I.V.: Not recommended

Oral (adults): Reduce dose by 50% and monitor closely for toxicity.

Dosing adjustment for toxicity:

Hematologic or nonhematologic toxicity (other than neurotoxicity): Consider treatment delay or dosage reduction

Hemolysis: Discontinue treatment

Neurotoxicity: Consider treatment delay or discontinuation

Administration

Parenteral: Fludarabine phosphate has been administered by intermittent I.V. infusion over 15-30 minutes and by continuous infusion; in clinical trials, the loading dose has been diluted in 20 mL D$_5$W and administered over 15 minutes and the continuous infusion diluted to 240 mL in D$_5$W and administered at a constant rate of 10 mL/hour; in other clinical studies, fludarabine has been diluted to a concentration of 0.25-1 mg/mL in D$_5$W or NS

Oral (adults): Tablet may be administered with or without food; should be swallowed whole with water; do not chew, break, or crush tablet

Monitoring Parameters CBC with differential, platelet count, hemoglobin, AST, ALT, creatinine, serum electrolytes, albumin, uric acid, and examination for visual changes; monitor for signs of infection and neurotoxicity

Patient Information Notify physician if fever, sore throat, bleeding, bruising, tachypnea, respiratory distress, or neurologic changes occur. Women of childbearing potential or fertile males must take contraceptive measures during and at least 6 months after discontinuing therapy. Fludarabine may cause fatigue, weakness, and visual disturbances which may impair ability to perform activities requiring mental alertness.

Nursing Implications Prophylactic allopurinol, adequate hydration, and urinary alkalinization should be considered for patients with large initial tumor burdens to avoid tumor lysis syndrome. Avoid exposure by inhalation or by direct contact of the skin or mucous membranes to fludarabine. If the solution contacts the skin or mucous membranes, wash thoroughly with soap and water; rinse eyes thoroughly with plain water. Use proper procedures for handling, preparation, and disposal of hazardous agents.

Additional Information Myelosuppressive effects:

Granulocyte nadir: 13 days (3-25)

Platelet nadir: 16 days (2-32)

Recovery: 5-7 weeks

Dosage Forms Excipient information presented when available (limited, particularly for generics); consult specific product labeling. [CAN] = Canadian brand name

Injection, powder for reconstitution, as phosphate: 50 mg
Fludara®: 50 mg

Injection, solution, as phosphate [preservative free]:
25 mg/mL (2 mL)

Tablet, as phosphate: 10 mg
Fludara® [CAN]: 10 mg
Oforta™: 10 mg

References

Avramis VI, Champagne J, Sato J, et al, "Pharmacology of Fludarabine Phosphate After a Phase I/II Trial by a Loading Bolus and Continuous Infusion in Pediatric Patients," *Cancer Res*, 1990, 50(22):7226-31.

Jacobsohn DA, Emerick KM, Scholl P, et al, "Nonmyeloablative Hematopoietic Stem Cell Transplant for X-Linked Hyper-Immunoglobulin M Syndrome With Cholangiopathy," *Pediatrics*, 2004, 113(2): e122-7.

Lange BJ, Smith FO, Feusner J, et al, "Outcomes in CCG-2961, a Children's Oncology Group Phase 3 Trial for Untreated Pediatric Acute Myeloid Leukemia: A Report From the Children's Oncology Group," *Blood*, 2008, 111(3):1044-53.

♦ **Fludarabine Phosphate** see Fludarabine on page 587

Fludrocortisone (floo droe KOR ti sone)

Medication Safety Issues

Sound-alike/look-alike issues:

Florinef® may be confused with Fioricet®, Fiorinal®

Related Information

Corticosteroids on page 1487

Canadian Brand Names Florinef®

Therapeutic Category Adrenal Corticosteroid; Corticosteroid, Systemic; Glucocorticoid; Mineralocorticoid

Generic Available Yes

Use Treatment of Addison's disease; partial replacement therapy for adrenal insufficiency; treatment of salt-losing forms of congenital adrenogenital syndrome; has been used in conjunction with an increased sodium intake for the treatment of idiopathic orthostatic hypotension

Pregnancy Risk Factor C

Pregnancy Considerations Animal reproduction studies have not been conducted with fludrocortisone; adverse events have been observed with corticosteroids in animal reproduction studies. Some studies have shown an association between first trimester systemic corticosteroid use and oral clefts; adverse events in the fetus/neonate have been noted in case reports following large doses of systemic corticosteroids during pregnancy.

Lactation Excretion in breast milk unknown/use caution

Breast-Feeding Considerations Corticosteroids are excreted in human milk; information specific to fludrocortisone has not been located.

Contraindications Hypersensitivity to fludrocortisone or any component; CHF, systemic fungal infections

Precautions Dosage should be tapered gradually if therapy is discontinued; use with caution in patients with hypertension, edema, or renal dysfunction

Adverse Reactions

Cardiovascular: Hypertension, edema, CHF

Central nervous system: Convulsions, headache

Dermatologic: Acne, rash, bruising

Endocrine & metabolic: Hypokalemic alkalosis, suppression of growth, hyperglycemia, hypothalamic-pituitary-adrenal suppression

Gastrointestinal: Peptic ulcer

Neuromuscular & skeletal: Muscle weakness

Ocular: Cataracts

Drug Interactions

Avoid Concomitant Use

Avoid concomitant use of Fludrocortisone with any of the following: Aldesleukin; BCG; Natalizumab; Pimecrolimus; Tacrolimus (Topical); Vaccines (Live)

Increased Effect/Toxicity

Fludrocortisone may increase the levels/effects of: Acetylcholinesterase Inhibitors; Amphotericin B; Leflunomide; Loop Diuretics; Natalizumab; NSAID (COX-2 Inhibitor); NSAID (Nonselective); Thiazide Diuretics; Vaccines (Live); Warfarin

The levels/effects of Fludrocortisone may be increased by: Antifungal Agents (Azole Derivatives, Systemic); Aprepitant; Calcium Channel Blockers (Nondihydropyridine); Denosumab; Estrogen Derivatives; Fluconazole; Fosaprepitant; Macrolide Antibiotics; Neuromuscular-Blocking Agents (Nondepolarizing); Pimecrolimus;

Quinolone Antibiotics; Salicylates; Tacrolimus (Topical); Trastuzumab

Decreased Effect

Fludrocortisone may decrease the levels/effects of: Aldesleukin; Antidiabetic Agents; BCG; Calcitriol; Corticorelin; Isoniazid; Salicylates; Sipuleucel-T; Vaccines (Inactivated); Vaccines (Live)

The levels/effects of Fludrocortisone may be decreased by: Aminoglutethimide; Antacids; Barbiturates; Bile Acid Sequestrants; Echinacea; Mitotane; Primidone; Rifamycin Derivatives

Food Interactions Systemic use of mineralocorticoids/corticosteroids may require a diet with increased potassium, vitamins A, B_6, C, D, folate, calcium, zinc, and phosphorus, and decreased sodium; with fludrocortisone a decrease in dietary sodium is often not required as the increased retention of sodium is usually the desired therapeutic effect

Mechanism of Action Potent mineralocorticoid with glucocorticoid activity; promotes increased reabsorption of sodium and loss of potassium from distal tubules

Pharmacodynamics Duration: 1-2 days

Pharmacokinetics (Adult data unless noted)

Absorption: Rapid and complete from GI tract

Protein binding: 42%

Metabolism: In the liver

Half-life:

Plasma: ~3.5 hours

Biological: 18-36 hours

Usual Dosage Oral:

Infants and Children: 0.05-0.1 mg/day

Congenital adrenal hyperplasia (salt losers): Maintenance: Range: 0.05-0.3 mg/day (AAP, 2000)

Adults: 0.05-0.2 mg/day

Administration Oral: May administer with food to decrease GI upset

Monitoring Parameters Serum electrolytes and glucose, blood pressure, serum renin

Patient Information Notify physician if dizziness, severe or continuing headache, swelling of feet or lower legs, or unusual weight gain occurs

Additional Information In patients with salt-losing forms of congenital adrenogenital syndrome, use along with cortisone or hydrocortisone; fludrocortisone 0.1 mg has sodium retention activity equal to DOCA® 1 mg

Dosage Forms Excipient information presented when available (limited, particularly for generics); consult specific product labeling.

Tablet, as acetate: 0.1 mg

References

American Academy of Pediatrics, Section on Endocrinology and Committee on Genetics, "Technical Report: Congenital Adrenal Hyperplasia," *Pediatrics*, 2000, 106(6):1511-8.

◆ **Fludrocortisone Acetate** *see* Fludrocortisone *on page 589*

◆ **FluLaval®** *see* Influenza Virus Vaccine (Inactivated) *on page 734*

◆ **Flumadine®** *see* Rimantadine *on page 1217*

Flumazenil (FLO may ze nil)

Medication Safety Issues

Sound-alike/look-alike issues:

Flumazenil may be confused with influenza virus vaccine

U.S. Brand Names Romazicon®

Canadian Brand Names Anexate®; Flumazenil Injection; Flumazenil Injection, USP; Romazicon®

Therapeutic Category Antidote, Benzodiazepine

Generic Available Yes

Use Benzodiazepine antagonist; reverses sedative effects of benzodiazepines used in general anesthesia or conscious sedation; management of benzodiazepine overdose; **not indicated** for ethanol, barbiturate, general anesthetic or narcotic overdose

Pregnancy Risk Factor C

Pregnancy Considerations Teratogenic effects were not seen in animal studies. Embryocidal effects were seen at large doses. There are no adequate or well-controlled studies in pregnant women. Use only if clearly needed.

Lactation Excretion in breast milk unknown/use caution

Contraindications Hypersensitivity to flumazenil, any component, or benzodiazepines; patients given benzodiazepines for control of potentially life-threatening conditions (eg, control of intracranial pressure or status epilepticus); patients with signs of serious cyclic-antidepressant overdosage

Warnings Flumazenil may precipitate seizures in high risk patients **[U.S. Boxed Warning]**; possible risk factors for seizures include patients physically dependent on benzodiazepines, patients treated with benzodiazepines for seizure disorders or other reasons, patients who received recent repeated doses of parenteral benzodiazepines, overdose patients with seizure activity prior to flumazenil, patients with serious cyclic antidepressant or mixed drug overdoses, patients with concurrent major sedative-hypnotic drug withdrawal, and patients with severe hepatic impairment. Higher than normal doses of benzodiazepines may be required to treat these seizures. Mixed drug overdose patients who have ingested drugs that increase the likelihood of seizures (eg, cocaine, lithium, cyclosporine, cyclic antidepressants, bupropion, methylxanthines, MAO inhibitors, isoniazid, or propoxyphene) are at extremely high risk for seizures (flumazenil may be contraindicated in these patients). Flumazenil is not recommended in epileptic patients receiving chronic benzodiazepine therapy or in cases of serious cyclic antidepressant overdoses. Dosage of flumazenil should be individualized; clinicians should be prepared to manage seizure activity.

Precautions Resedation may occur with flumazenil use (due to its short half-life in comparison to some benzodiazepines); pediatric patients (especially 1-5 years of age) may experience resedation; these patients may require repeat bolus doses or continuous infusion; monitor patients for return of sedation, respiratory depression, and other residual benzodiazepine effects. Flumazenil should be used with caution in the intensive care unit because of increased risk of unrecognized benzodiazepine dependence in such settings. Flumazenil may provoke panic attacks in patients with panic disorder. Do not use flumazenil until effects of neuromuscular blockers have been fully reversed. Use with caution in patients with liver disease and decrease the amount or frequency of repeat doses. Use with caution in patients with head injury due to possibility of precipitating convulsions or altering blood flow in patients receiving benzodiazepines. Use with caution in patients with alcoholism and other drug dependencies; these patients may also be dependent on benzodiazepines. Clinicians should not rely on flumazenil to reverse respiratory depression/hypoventilation; flumazenil is not a substitute for evaluation of oxygenation; establishing an airway and assisting ventilation, as necessary, is always the initial step in overdose management. Safety and efficacy of flumazenil have not been established in children <1 year of age.

Adverse Reactions

Cardiovascular: Arrhythmias, bradycardia, tachycardia, chest pain, hypertension, hypotension

Central nervous system: Seizures (more common in patients physically dependent on benzodiazepines or with cyclic antidepressant overdoses, see Warnings), fatigue, dizziness, headache, agitation, emotional lability, anxiety, euphoria, depression, abnormal crying

Endocrine & metabolic: Hot flashes

Gastrointestinal: Nausea, vomiting, xerostomia

Local: Pain at injection site

Ocular: Blurred vision

Miscellaneous: Diaphoresis increased, shivering, hiccups, sensation of coldness; can precipitate acute withdrawal symptoms in patients physically dependent on benzodiazepines

Drug Interactions

Avoid Concomitant Use There are no known interactions where it is recommended to avoid concomitant use.

Increased Effect/Toxicity There are no known significant interactions involving an increase in effect.

Decreased Effect

Flumazenil may decrease the levels/effects of: Hypnotics (Nonbenzodiazepine)

Stability Store at 25°C (77°F); compatible with D_5W, LR, or NS for 24 hours; discard any unused solution after 24 hours

Mechanism of Action Antagonizes the effect of benzodiazepines on the GABA/benzodiazepine receptor complex. Flumazenil is benzodiazepine specific and does not antagonize other nonbenzodiazepine GABA agonists (including ethanol, barbiturates, general anesthetics); does not reverse the effects of opiates.

Pharmacodynamics

Onset of action: Benzodiazepine reversal: Within 1-3 minutes

Maximum effect: 6-10 minutes

Duration: Usually <1 hour; duration is related to dose given and benzodiazepine plasma concentrations; reversal effects of flumazenil may wear off before effects of benzodiazepine and resedation may occur

Pharmacokinetics (Adult data unless noted) Follows a two compartment open model; **Note:** Clearance and V_d per kg are similar for children and adults, but children display more variability

Distribution: Distributes extensively in the extravascular space; Adults:

Initial V_d: 0.5 L/kg

V_{dss}: 0.9-1.1 L/kg

Protein binding: ~50%; primarily to albumin

Metabolism: In the liver to the de-ethylated free acid and its glucuronide conjugate

Half-life

Children: Terminal: 20-75 minutes (mean: 40 minutes)

Adults:

Alpha: 4-11 minutes

Terminal: 40-80 minutes

Elimination: 99% hepatically eliminated; <1% excreted unchanged in urine

Clearance: Dependent upon hepatic blood flow; Adults: 0.8-1 L/hour/kg

Usual Dosage I.V.:

Children:

Reversal of benzodiazepine when used in conscious sedation or general anesthesia: Initial dose: 0.01 mg/kg (maximum dose: 0.2 mg) given over 15 seconds; may repeat 0.01 mg/kg (maximum dose: 0.2 mg) after 45 seconds, and then every minute to a maximum total cumulative dose of 0.05 mg/kg or 1 mg, whichever is lower; usual total dose: 0.08-1 mg (mean: 0.65 mg)

Management of benzodiazepine overdose: Minimal information available; initial dose: 0.01 mg/kg (maximum dose: 0.2 mg) with repeat doses of 0.01 mg/kg (maximum dose: 0.2 mg) given every minute to a maximum total cumulative dose of 1 mg; as an alternative to repeat bolus doses, follow up continuous infusions of 0.005-0.01 mg/kg/hour have been used; further studies are needed

Adults:

Reversal of benzodiazepine when used in conscious sedation or general anesthesia: 0.2 mg given over 15 seconds; may repeat 0.2 mg after 45 seconds and then every 60 seconds up to a total of 1 mg, usual total dose: 0.6-1 mg. In event of resedation, may repeat doses at 20-minute intervals with maximum of 1 mg/dose (given at 0.2 mg/minute); maximum dose: 3 mg in 1 hour.

Management of benzodiazepine overdose: 0.2 mg over 30 seconds; may give 0.3 mg dose after 30 seconds if desired level of consciousness is not obtained; additional doses of 0.5 mg can be given over 30 seconds at 1-minute intervals up to a cumulative dose of 3 mg; usual cumulative dose: 1-3 mg; rarely, patients with partial response at 3 mg may require additional titration up to total dose of 5 mg; if patient has not responded 5 minutes after cumulative dose of 5 mg, the major cause of sedation is not likely due to benzodiazepines. In the event of resedation, may repeat doses at 20-minute intervals with maximum of 1 mg/dose (given at 0.5 mg/minute); maximum dose: 3 mg in 1 hour.

Dosing adjustment in hepatic impairment: Initial dose: Use normal dose; repeat doses should be decreased in size or frequency

Administration Parenteral: For I.V. use only; administer by rapid I.V. injection over 15-30 seconds via a freely running I.V. infusion into larger vein (to decrease chance of pain, phlebitis). Children: Do not exceed 0.2 mg/minute. Adults: Repeat doses: Do not exceed 0.2 mg/minute for reversal of general anesthesia and do not exceed 0.5 mg/minute for reversal of benzodiazepine overdose.

Monitoring Parameters Level of consciousness and resedation, blood pressure, heart rate, respiratory rate, continuous pulse oximetry; monitor for resedation for 1-2 hours after reversal of sedation in patients who receive benzodiazepine sedation

Patient Information Flumazenil does not consistently reverse amnesia; do not engage in activities requiring alertness for 24 hours after discharge; resedation may occur in patients on long-acting benzodiazepines (such as diazepam); avoid alcohol or OTC medications for 24 hours after flumazenil is used or if benzodiazepine effects persist; may cause dry mouth

Nursing Implications Flumazenil does not effectively reverse hypoventilation, even in alert patients

Additional Information Flumazenil is a weak lipophilic base. In one study of conscious sedation reversal in 107 pediatric patients (1-17 years of age), resedation occurred between 19-50 minutes after the start of flumazenil. Flumazenil has been used to successfully treat paradoxical reactions in children associated with midazolam use (eg, agitation, restlessness, combativeness) (see Massanari, 1997).

Dosage Forms Excipient information presented when available (limited, particularly for generics); consult specific product labeling.

Injection, solution: 0.1 mg/mL (5 mL, 10 mL)

Romazicon®: 0.1 mg/mL (5 mL, 10 mL) [contains edetate disodium]

References

Baktai G, Szekely E, Marialigeti T, et al, "Use of Midazolam (Dormicum) and Flumazenil (Anexate) in Paediatric Bronchology," *Curr Med Res Opin,* 1992, 12(9):552-9.

Clark RF, Sage TA, Tunget C, et al, "Delayed Onset Lorazepam Poisoning Successfully Reversed By Flumazenil in a Child: Case Report and Review of the Literature," *Pediatr Emerg Care,* 1995, 11 (1):32-4.

Jones RD, Lawson AD, Andrew LJ, et al, "Antagonism of the Hypnotic Effect of Midazolam in Children: A Randomized, Double Blind Study of Placebo and Flumazenil Administered After Midazolam-Induced Anaesthesia," *Br J Anaesth,* 1991, 66(6):660-6.

Massanari M, Novitsky J, and Reinstein LJ, "Paradoxical Reactions in Children Associated With Midazolam Use During Endoscopy," *Clin Pediatr,* 1997, 36(12):681-4.

Richard P, Autret E, Bardol J, et al, "The Use of Flumazenil in a Neonate," *J Toxicol Clin Toxicol*, 1991, 29(1):137-40.

Roald OK and Dahl V, "Flunitrazepam Intoxication in a Child Successfully Treated With the Benzodiazepine Antagonist Flumazenil," *Crit Care Med*, 1989, 17(12):1355-6.

Shannon M, Albers G, Burkhart K, et al, "Safety and Efficacy of Flumazenil in the Reversal of Benzodiazepine-Induced Conscious Sedation. The Flumazenil Pediatric Study Group," *J Pediatr*, 1997, 131(4):582-6.

Sugarman JM and Paul RI, "Flumazenil: A Review," *Pediatr Emerg Care*, 1994, 10(1):37-43.

◆ **Flumazenil Injection (Can)** *see* Flumazenil *on page 590*

◆ **Flumazenil Injection, USP (Can)** *see* Flumazenil *on page 590*

◆ **FluMist®** *see* Influenza Virus Vaccine (Live/Attenuated) *on page 736*

Flunisolide (floo NIS oh lide)

Medication Safety Issues
Sound-alike/look-alike issues:
Flunisolide may be confused with Flumadine®, fluocinonide
Nasarel® may be confused with Nizoral®

Related Information
Asthma *on page 1697*

U.S. Brand Names AeroBid®; AeroBid®-M

Canadian Brand Names Alti-Flunisolide; Apo-Flunisolide®; Nasalide®; PMS-Flunisolide; Rhinalar®

Therapeutic Category Adrenal Corticosteroid; Anti-inflammatory Agent; Antiasthmatic; Corticosteroid, Inhalant (Oral); Corticosteroid, Intranasal; Glucocorticoid

Generic Available Yes: Nasal spray

Use
Oral inhalation: Long-term (chronic) control of persistent bronchial asthma; **NOT** indicated for the relief of acute bronchospasm. Also used to help reduce or discontinue oral corticosteroid therapy for asthma (see Additional Information).

Intranasal: Management of seasonal or perennial rhinitis

Pregnancy Risk Factor C

Pregnancy Considerations Teratogenic effects were observed in animal studies. A decrease in fetal growth has not been observed with inhaled corticosteroid use during pregnancy. Inhaled corticosteroids are recommended for the treatment of asthma (most information available using budesonide) and allergic rhinitis during pregnancy.

Lactation Excretion in breast milk unknown/use caution

Breast-Feeding Considerations Other corticosteroids have been found in breast milk. It is not known if sufficient quantities of flunisolide are absorbed following inhalation to produce detectable amounts in breast milk. The use of inhaled corticosteroids is not considered a contraindication to breast-feeding.

Contraindications Hypersensitivity to flunisolide or any component; primary treatment of status asthmaticus; untreated nasal mucosa infection

Warnings Fatalities have occurred due to adrenal insufficiency in asthmatic patients during and after switching from systemic corticosteroids to aerosol steroids (see Additional Information); several months may be required for full recovery of hypothalamic-pituitary-adrenal (HPA) function; patients receiving higher doses of systemic corticosteroids (eg, adults receiving ≥20 mg of prednisone per day) may be at greater risk; during this period of HPA suppression, aerosol steroids do **not** provide the systemic glucocorticoid or mineralocorticoid activity needed to treat patients requiring stress doses (ie, patients with major stress such as trauma, surgery, infections, or other conditions associated with severe electrolyte loss). When used at high doses, HPA suppression may occur; use with inhaled or systemic corticosteroids (even alternate-day dosing) may increase risk of HPA suppression. Acute adrenal insufficiency may occur with abrupt withdrawal after long-term use or with stress; withdrawal or discontinuation of corticosteroids should be done carefully; patients with HPA axis suppression may require doses of systemic glucocorticosteroids prior to, during, and after unusual stress (eg, surgery). Immunosuppression may occur; patients may be more susceptible to infections; avoid exposure to chickenpox and measles. Switching patients from systemic corticosteroids to aerosol steroids may unmask allergic conditions previously treated by the systemic steroid. Bronchospasm may occur after use of inhaled asthma medications (see Additional Information).

Precautions Avoid using higher than recommended doses; suppression of HPA function, suppression of linear growth (ie, reduction of growth velocity), reduced bone mineral density, hypercorticism (Cushing's syndrome), hyperglycemia, or glucosuria may occur; use with extreme caution in patients with respiratory tuberculosis, untreated systemic infections, or ocular herpes simplex

Adverse Reactions
Cardiovascular: Oral inhalation: Palpitations, hypertension, chest pain, edema

Central nervous system: Dizziness, headache, fever, nervousness, insomnia, migraine

Dermatologic: Rash, itching, eczema

Endocrine & metabolic: HPA suppression, Cushing's syndrome, growth suppression

Gastrointestinal: Oral candidiasis (oral inhalation), nausea, vomiting, diarrhea, upset stomach, abdominal pain, sore throat, bitter taste, aftertaste

Genitourinary: Menstrual disturbances (oral inhalation)

Local: Nasal burning

Neuromuscular & skeletal: Muscular soreness, bone mineral density decreased

Ocular: Rarely: IOP increased, glaucoma, cataracts (oral inhalation)

Respiratory: Sneezing, nasal congestion, nasal dryness, pharyngitis, dysphonia, rhinitis, epistaxis, *Candida* infections of the nose or pharynx, atrophic rhinitis, upper respiratory infections

Drug Interactions

Metabolism/Transport Effects
Substrate of CYP3A4 (major)

Avoid Concomitant Use
Avoid concomitant use of Flunisolide with any of the following: Aldesleukin; BCG; Natalizumab; Pimecrolimus; Tacrolimus (Topical); Vaccines (Live)

Increased Effect/Toxicity
Flunisolide may increase the levels/effects of: Amphotericin B; Leflunomide; Loop Diuretics; Natalizumab; Thiazide Diuretics; Vaccines (Live)

The levels/effects of Flunisolide may be increased by: CYP3A4 Inhibitors (Moderate); CYP3A4 Inhibitors (Strong); Dasatinib; Denosumab; Pimecrolimus; Tacrolimus (Topical); Trastuzumab

Decreased Effect
Flunisolide may decrease the levels/effects of: Aldesleukin; Antidiabetic Agents; BCG; Corticorelin; Sipuleucel-T; Vaccines (Inactivated); Vaccines (Live)

The levels/effects of Flunisolide may be decreased by: Echinacea

Stability Intranasal solutions: Store at 59°F to 86°F

Mechanism of Action Controls the rate of protein synthesis, depresses the migration of polymorphonuclear leukocytes and fibroblasts, reverses capillary permeability, and stabilizes lysosomal membranes at the cellular level to prevent or control inflammation

Pharmacodynamics Clinical effects are due to a direct local effect rather than systemic absorption

Onset of action: Intranasal: Within a few days

Maximum effect: Intranasal: 1-2 weeks; oral inhalation: 2-4 weeks

Pharmacokinetics (Adult data unless noted)

Absorption: Rapid

Metabolism: Rapid in the liver via cytochrome P450 isoenzyme CYP3A4 to a less active metabolite (6 beta-OH flunisolide), followed by glucuronide and sulfate conjugation

Bioavailability:

Nasal inhalation: 50%

Oral: 20%

Oral inhalation: AeroBid®-M: 40%

Half-life: 1.8 hours

Elimination: Excreted in urine and feces

Usual Dosage

Intranasal: Manufacturer's recommendation:

Children 6-14 years: Initial: 1 spray to each nostril 3 times/day or 2 sprays to each nostril 2 times/day; maximum dose: 4 sprays to each nostril per day; after symptoms are controlled, dose should be reduced to lowest effective amount; maintenance: 1 spray each nostril once daily

Adults: Initial: 2 sprays to each nostril twice daily; may increase in 4-7 days if needed to 2 sprays to each nostril 3 times/day; maximum dose: 8 sprays to each nostril per day; after symptoms are controlled, dose should be reduced to lowest effective amount; maintenance: 1 spray to each nostril once daily

Oral inhalation: **Note:** Doses should be titrated to the lowest dose once asthma is controlled:

AeroBid® and AeroBid®-M:

Manufacturer's recommendation:

Children: 6-15 years: 2 inhalations twice daily; maximum dose: 4 inhalations/day

Children ≥16 years and Adults: 2 inhalations twice daily; maximum dose: 8 inhalations/day

NIH Asthma Guidelines (NAEPP, 2007) [give in divided doses twice daily]:

Children 5-11 years:

"Low" dose: 500-750 mcg/day (2-3 puffs/day)

"Medium" dose: 1000-1250 mcg/day (4-5 puffs/day)

"High" dose: >1250 mcg/day (>5 puffs/day)

Children ≥12 years and Adults:

"Low" dose: 500-1000 mcg/day (2-4 puffs/day)

"Medium" dose: >1000-2000 mcg/day (4-8 puffs/day)

"High" dose: >2000 mcg/day (>8 puffs/day)

Administration Shake well before use; do not spray in eyes

Oral inhalant: Rinse mouth after inhalation to decrease chance of oral candidiasis

Aerobid® and Aerobid®-M: Use a spacer for children <8 years of age

Intranasal: Clear nasal passages by blowing nose prior to use

Monitoring Parameters Check mucus membranes for signs of fungal infection; monitor growth in pediatric patients; monitor blood pressure with oral inhalation

Patient Information Notify physician if condition being treated persists or worsens; do not decrease dose or discontinue without physician approval. Avoid exposure to chicken pox or measles; if exposed, seek medical advice without delay.

Oral inhalation: Report sore mouth or mouth lesions to physician; carefully read and follow the patient instructions for use leaflet that accompanies the product

Additional Information AeroBid® and AeroBid®-M contain fluorocarbon propellants. The FDA, in accordance with the Montreal Protocol on Substances that Deplete the Ozone Layer, has issued a phase-out of seven metered-dose inhalers (MDIs) that contain ozone-depleting chlorofluorocarbons (CFCs). The CFC-propelled Aerobid® and Aero-Bid®-M inhaler systems (flunisolide) will not be manufactured, sold, or dispensed in the U.S. after June 30, 2011, and patients should be transitioned to another therapy.

When using flunisolide oral inhalation to help reduce or discontinue oral corticosteroid therapy, begin corticosteroid taper after at least 1 week of flunisolide inhalation therapy; reduce dose of oral corticosteroid gradually, with next decrease after 1-2 weeks depending on patient's response; do not decrease prednisone faster than 2.5 mg/day on a weekly basis; monitor patients for signs of asthma instability and adrenal insufficiency (see Warnings); decrease flunisolide to lowest effective dose **after** prednisone reduction is complete. If bronchospasm with wheezing occurs after use of oral inhalation, a fast-acting bronchodilator may be used; discontinue orally inhaled corticosteroid and initiate alternative chronic therapy.

Dosage Forms Excipient information presented when available (limited, particularly for generics); consult specific product labeling.

Aerosol for oral inhalation:

AeroBid®: 250 mcg/actuation (7 g) [100 metered inhalations; contains chlorofluorocarbon]

AeroBid®-M: 250 mcg/actuation (7 g) [100 metered inhalations; contains chlorofluorocarbon; menthol flavor]

Solution, intranasal [spray]: 25 mcg/actuation (25 mL); 29 mcg/actuation (25 mL) [200 sprays]

References

National Asthma Education and Prevention Program (NAEPP), "Expert Panel Report 3 (EPR-3): Guidelines for the Diagnosis and Management of Asthma," *Clinical Practice Guidelines*, National Institutes of Health, National Heart, Lung, and Blood Institute, NIH Publication No. 08-4051, prepublication 2007; available at http://www.nhlbi.nih.gov/guidelines/asthma/asthgdln.htm.

Fluocinolone (floo oh SIN oh lone)

Medication Safety Issues

Sound-alike/look-alike issues:

Fluocinolone may be confused with fluocinonide

Related Information

Corticosteroids *on page 1487*

U.S. Brand Names Capex®; Derma-Smoothe/FS®; DermOtic®; Retisert®

Canadian Brand Names Capex®; Derma-Smoothe/FS®; Synalar®

Therapeutic Category Adrenal Corticosteroid; Anti-inflammatory Agent; Corticosteroid, Ophthalmic; Corticosteroid, Topical; Glucocorticoid

Generic Available Yes: Excludes ocular implant, oil, otic, shampoo

Use Relief of susceptible inflammatory dermatosis

Capex™ shampoo: Adults: Treatment of seborrheic dermatitis of the scalp

Derma-Smoothe/FS®: Children ≥2 years: Moderate to severe atopic dermatitis (for use ≤4 weeks); Adults: Atopic dermatitis or psoriasis of the scalp

Retisert™ (ocular implant): Adults: treatment of chronic, noninfectious uveitis affecting the posterior segment of the eye

Pregnancy Risk Factor C

Pregnancy Considerations Adverse events have been observed with corticosteroids in animal reproduction studies. In general, the use of topical corticosteroids during pregnancy is not considered to have significant risk; however, intrauterine growth retardation in the infant has been reported (rare). The use of large amounts or for prolonged periods of time should be avoided.

Lactation Excretion in breast milk unknown/use caution

Breast-Feeding Considerations Systemic corticosteroids are excreted in human milk. It is not known if sufficient quantities of fluocinolone are absorbed following topical or ocular administration to produce detectable amounts in breast milk. Hypertension in the nursing infant has been reported following corticosteroid ointment applied to the nipples. Use with caution.

Contraindications Hypersensitivity to fluocinolone or any component (see Warnings); fungal infection; TB of skin; herpes (including varicella)

Ocular implant: Additional contraindications include viral, fungal, and mycobacterial ocular infections; hypersensitivity to other corticosteroids

Warnings

Topical: Infants and small children may be more susceptible to adrenal axis suppression from topical corticosteroid therapy; systemic effects may occur when used on large areas of the body, denuded areas, for prolonged periods of time, or with an occlusive dressing; Derma-Smoothe/FS® contains refined peanut oil, use with caution in patients with peanut hypersensitivity (see Additional Information). Hypothalamic pituitary adrenal (HPA) axis suppression may occur; acute adrenal insufficiency may occur with abrupt withdrawal after long term use or with stress; withdrawal or discontinuation should be done carefully; patients with HPA axis suppression may require doses of systemic glucocorticosteroids prior to, during, and after unusual stress (eg, surgery).

Ocular implant: Transient decrease in visual acuity of 1-4 weeks duration following implantation may occur. Increased IOP or glaucoma may occur; use with caution in glaucoma patients; routine monitoring of IOP is recommended; patients may require use of medications or other treatments to lower IOP. Prolonged use of ocular corticosteroids may also increase the risk of secondary occular infections, cataract formation, delayed wound healing, perforation of globe (if thinning of sclera occurs), or optic nerve damage. Unilateral implantation is recommended to minimize risk of postoperative infections in both eyes. Procedural complications with implantation may occur (eg, cataract formation, choroidal detachment, endophthalmitis, hypotony, retinal detachment, vitreous loss, or hemorrhage).

Precautions Ocular implant: Safety and efficacy have not been established in children <12 years of age

Adverse Reactions

Topical products:
Dermatologic: Acne, hypopigmentation, allergic dermatitis, maceration of the skin, skin atrophy, folliculitis, hypertrichosis, striae, miliaria
Endocrine & metabolic: Hypothalamic-pituitary-adrenal (HPA) axis suppression, Cushing's syndrome, growth retardation
Local: Burning, itching, irritation, dryness
Miscellaneous: Secondary infection
Ocular implant:
Central nervous system: Dizziness, headache, pain, pyrexia
Dermatologic: Rash
Gastrointestinal: Nausea, vomiting
Neuromuscular and skeletal: Arthralgia, back pain, limb pain
Ocular: Cataracts, IOP elevated, glaucoma, eye pain or irritation, postprocedural complications (cataract fragments, implant migration, wound complications), visual acuity decreased, blurred vision, conjunctival

hemorrhage or hyperemia, pruritus, hypotony, vitreous floaters or hemorrhage, ptosis, eye inflammation, eyelid edema, tearing, dry eye

Drug Interactions

Avoid Concomitant Use

Avoid concomitant use of Fluocinolone with any of the following: Aldesleukin

Increased Effect/Toxicity There are no known significant interactions involving an increase in effect.

Decreased Effect

Fluocinolone may decrease the levels/effects of: Aldesleukin; Corticorelin

Stability Store at controlled room temperature in tightly closed container

Ocular implant (Retisert™): Store in original container at 15°C to 25°C (59°F to 77°F); protect from freezing

Mechanism of Action Not well defined topically; possesses anti-inflammatory, antiproliferative, and immunosuppressive properties

Pharmacokinetics (Adult data unless noted)

Absorption:
Topical: Dependent on strength of preparation, amount applied, nature of skin at application site, vehicle, and use of occlusive dressing; increased in areas of skin damage, inflammation, or occlusion
Ocular implant: Systemic absorption is negligible
Duration: Ocular implant: Releases fluocinolone acetonide at a rate of 0.6 mcg/day, decreasing over 30 days to a steady-state release rate of 0.3-0.4 mcg/day for 30 months
Distribution:
Topical: Throughout local skin; absorbed drug is distributed rapidly into muscle, liver, skin, intestines, and kidneys
Ocular implant: Aqueous and vitreous humor
Metabolism: Primarily in skin; small amount absorbed into systemic circulation is primarily hepatic to inactive compounds
Excretion: Urine (primarily as glucuronide and sulfate, also as unconjugated products); feces (small amounts)

Usual Dosage

Children and Adults: Topical: Apply thin layer 2-4 times/day

Capex™ shampoo: Adults: Thoroughly wet hair and scalp; apply ≤1 ounce to scalp area; massage well; work into lather; allow to remain on scalp for 5 minutes; then rinse hair and scalp thoroughly; repeat daily until symptoms subside; **Note:** Once patient is symptom free, once weekly use usually keeps itching and flaking of dandruff from returning

Derma-Smoothe/FS®:
Children ≥2 years: Atopic dermatitis: Apply in a thin layer to moistened skin of affected area twice daily for ≤4 weeks
Adults:
Atopic dermatitis: Apply a thin layer to affected area 3 times/day
Scalp psoriasis: Thoroughly wet or dampen hair and scalp; apply to scalp in a thin layer, massage well, cover scalp with shower cap (supplied); leave for a minimum of 4 hours or overnight, then wash hair and rinse thoroughly

Retisert™ (ocular implant): Chronic uveitis: One silicone-encased tablet (0.59 mg) surgically implanted into the posterior segment of the eye is designed to release 0.6 mcg/day, decreasing over 30 days to a steady-state release rate of 0.3-0.4 mcg/day for 30 months. Recurrence of uveitis denotes depletion of tablet, requiring reimplantation.

Administration

Topical: Apply sparingly in a thin film; rub in lightly

Capex™ shampoo: Shake well before use; do not bandage, wrap, or cover treated scalp area unless directed by physician; discard shampoo after 3 months (**Note:** Pharmacist must empty the contents of the 12 mg fluocinolone acetonide capsule into the shampoo base before dispensing to patient)

Derma-Smoothe/FS®: Do not apply to face or diaper area; avoid application to intertriginous areas (may increase local adverse effects)

Ocular implant: Retisert™: Handle only by suture tab to avoid damaging the tablet integrity and adversely affecting release characteristics. Maintain strict adherence to aseptic handling of product; do not resterilize.

Patient Information Topical products: Avoid contact with eyes; do not use for longer than directed; do not overuse; notify physician if condition being treated persists or worsens

Nursing Implications Do not use tight fitting diapers or plastic pants on a child being treated in diaper area; Derma-Smoothe/FS® is not recommended for diaper dermatitis

Additional Information Considered a moderate-potency steroid (Derma-Smoothe/FS® and Capex™ shampoo are considered to be low to medium potency); Derma-Smoothe/FS® is made with 48% refined peanut oil, NF (peanut protein is not detectable at 2.5 ppm)

Dosage Forms Excipient information presented when available (limited, particularly for generics); consult specific product labeling.

Cream, as acetonide: 0.01% (15 g, 60 g); 0.025% (15 g, 60 g)

Implant, intravitreal, as acetonide:

Retisert®: 0.59 mg [enclosed in silicone elastomer]

Oil, as acetonide:

Derma-Smoothe/FS® [body oil]: 0.01% (120 mL) [contains peanut oil]

Derma-Smoothe/FS® [scalp oil]: 0.01% (120 mL) [contains peanut oil; packaged with shower caps]

DermOtic® [otic drops]: 0.01% (20 mL) [contains peanut oil; packaged with dropper]

Ointment, as acetonide: 0.025% (15 g, 60 g)

Shampoo, as acetonide:

Capex®: 0.01% (120 mL)

Solution, as acetonide: 0.01% (60 mL)

◆ **Fluocinolone Acetonide** *see* Fluocinolone *on page 593*

Fluocinonide (floo oh SIN oh nide)

Medication Safety Issues

Sound-alike/look-alike issues:

Fluocinonide may be confused with flunisolide, fluocinolone

Lidex® may be confused with Lasix®, Videx®, Wydase®

Related Information

Corticosteroids *on page 1487*

U.S. Brand Names Vanos™

Canadian Brand Names Lidemol®; Lidex®; Lyderm®; Tiamol®; Topactin; Topsyn®

Therapeutic Category Adrenal Corticosteroid; Anti-inflammatory Agent; Corticosteroid, Topical; Glucocorticoid

Generic Available Yes

Use Inflammation of corticosteroid-responsive dermatoses

Pregnancy Risk Factor C

Contraindications Hypersensitivity to fluocinonide or any component; viral, fungal, or tubercular skin lesions; herpes (including varicella)

Warnings Infants and small children may be more susceptible to adrenal axis suppression from topical corticosteroid therapy; systemic effects may occur when used on large areas of the body, denuded areas, for prolonged periods of time, or with occlusive dressings

Adverse Reactions

Dermatologic: Acne, hypopigmentation, allergic dermatitis, maceration of the skin, skin atrophy, folliculitis, hypertrichosis

Endocrine & metabolic: Hypothalamic-pituitary-adrenal suppression, Cushing's syndrome, growth retardation

Local: Burning, itching, irritation, dryness

Miscellaneous: Secondary infection

Drug Interactions

Avoid Concomitant Use

Avoid concomitant use of Fluocinonide with any of the following: Aldesleukin

Increased Effect/Toxicity There are no known significant interactions involving an increase in effect.

Decreased Effect

Fluocinonide may decrease the levels/effects of: Aldesleukin; Corticorelin

Mechanism of Action Not well defined topically; possesses anti-inflammatory, antiproliferative, and immunosuppressive properties

Usual Dosage Children and Adults: Topical: Apply thin layer to affected area 2-4 times/day depending on the severity of the condition

Administration Topical: Apply sparingly in a thin film; rub in lightly

Patient Information Do not overuse; avoid contact with eyes; do not use for longer than directed; avoid use on face; notify physician if condition being treated persists or worsens

Nursing Implications Do not use tight fitting diapers or plastic pants on a child being treated in diaper area

Additional Information Considered to be a high potency steroid

Dosage Forms Excipient information presented when available (limited, particularly for generics); consult specific product labeling.

Cream, anhydrous, emollient: 0.05% (15 g, 30 g, 60 g, 120 g)

Cream, aqueous, emollient: 0.05% (15 g, 30 g, 60 g)

Cream:

Vanos™: 0.1% (30 g, 60 g)

Gel: 0.05% (15 g, 30 g, 60 g)

Ointment: 0.05% (15 g, 30 g, 60 g)

Solution: 0.05% (20 mL, 60 mL)

◆ **Fluohydrisone Acetate** *see* Fludrocortisone *on page 589*

◆ **Fluohydrocortisone Acetate** *see* Fludrocortisone *on page 589*

◆ **Fluor-A-Day** *see* Fluoride *on page 595*

Fluoride (FLOR ide)

Medication Safety Issues

Sound-alike/look-alike issues:

EtheDent™ may be confused with Effient™

Luride® may be confused with Lortab®

Phos-Flur® may be confused with PhosLo®

Thera-Flur-N® may be confused with Thera-Flu®

International issues:

Fluorex® [France] may be confused with Flarex® which is a brand name for fluorometholone in the U.S.

U.S. Brand Names ACT® Plus [OTC]; ACT® x2™ [OTC]; ACT® [OTC]; CaviRinse™; ControlRx®; Denta 5000 Plus; DentaGel; Epiflur™; EtheDent™ [DSC]; Fluor-A-Day; Fluorigard® [OTC]; Fluorinse®; Flura-Drops®; Gel-Kam®

Rinse; Gel-Kam® [OTC]; Just for Kids™ [OTC]; Lozi-Flur™; Luride® Lozi-Tab®; Luride® [DSC]; NeutraCare®; NeutraGard® Advanced; NeutraGard® Plus; NeutraGard® [OTC]; Omnii Gel™ [OTC]; PerioMed™; Pharmaflur® 1.1 [DSC]; Pharmaflur® [DSC]; Phos-Flur®; Phos-Flur® Rinse [OTC]; PreviDent®; PreviDent® 5000 Plus®; StanGard®; StanGard® Perio; Stop®; Thera-Flur-N® [DSC]

Canadian Brand Names Fluor-A-Day

Therapeutic Category Mineral, Oral; Mineral, Oral Topical

Generic Available Yes: Excludes lozenge, gel drops

Use Prevention of dental caries

Pregnancy Risk Factor C

Contraindications Hypersensitivity to fluoride or any component (see Warnings); when fluoride content of drinking water exceeds 0.7 ppm; low sodium or sodium-free diets; do not use 1 mg tablets in children ≤3 years of age or when drinking water fluoride content is ≥0.3 ppm; do not use 1 mg/5 mL rinse (as supplement) in children <6 years of age

Warnings Some products may contain tartrazine which may cause allergic reactions in susceptible individuals

Precautions Prolonged ingestion with excessive doses may result in dental fluorosis and osseous changes; dosage should be adjusted in proportion to the amount of fluoride in the drinking water; do **not** exceed recommended dosage

Adverse Reactions

Central nervous system: Headache

Dermatologic: Rash, eczema, atopic dermatitis, urticaria

Gastrointestinal: GI upset, nausea, vomiting

Miscellaneous: Products containing stannous fluoride may stain the teeth

Drug Interactions

Avoid Concomitant Use There are no known interactions where it is recommended to avoid concomitant use.

Increased Effect/Toxicity There are no known significant interactions involving an increase in effect.

Decreased Effect There are no known significant interactions involving a decrease in effect.

Food Interactions Do not administer with milk

Stability Sodium fluoride solutions decompose in glass containers; store only in tightly closed plastic containers; aqueous solutions of stannous fluoride decompose within hours of preparation; prepare solutions immediately before use

Mechanism of Action Promotes remineralization of decalcified enamel; inhibits the cariogenic microbial process in dental plaque; increases tooth resistance to acid dissolution

Pharmacokinetics (Adult data unless noted)

Absorption: Via GI tract, lungs, and skin

Distribution: 50% of fluoride is deposited in teeth and bone after ingestion; crosses placenta; appears in breast milk; topical application works superficially on enamel and plaque

Elimination: In urine and feces

Usual Dosage Oral:

Adequate Intake (AI) (1997 National Academy of Science Recommendations):

Children:

0-6 months: 0.01 mg/day

7-12 months: 0.5 mg/day

1-3 years: 0.7 mg/day

4-8 years: 1 mg/day

9-13 years: 2 mg/day

14-18 years: 3 mg/day

Children >19 and Adults:

Males: 4 mg/day

Females: 3 mg/day

The recommended daily fluoride intake is adjusted in proportion to the fluoride content of available drinking water; see **Recommended Daily Fluoride Dose** table

Recommended Daily Fluoride Dose

Fluoride Content of Drinking Water	Daily Dose, Oral Fluoride (mg)
<0.3 ppm	
Birth - 6 mo	0
6 mo to 3 y	0.25
3-6 y	0.5
6-16 y	1
0.3-0.6 ppm	
Birth - 3 y	0
3-6 y	0.25
6-16 y	0.5
>0.6 ppm	
All ages	0

Adapted from *AAP News*, 1995, 11(2):18.

Dental rinse: See **Sodium Fluoride Dental Rinse Dosing** table

Sodium fluoride (dosage based upon concentration of solution):

Note: 2% concentrations are administered by dental personnel only

Sodium Fluoride Dental Rinse Dosing

Age	% Solution	Dosage
6 y	0.05%	10 mL daily
6-12 y	0.02%	10 mL twice daily
	0.2%	5 mL once weekly
>12 y	0.02%	10 mL twice daily
	0.2%	10 mL once weekly

Acidulated phosphate fluoride rinse: Children 6 years and Adults: 5-10 mL of 0.02% daily at bedtime

Gel:

Acidulated phosphate fluoride: Adults: 4-8 drops of 0.5% gel daily or for desensitizing exposed root surfaces, use a few drops of 0.5% to 1.2% gel applied and brushed onto affected area each night

Stannous fluoride: Children >6 years and Adults: Apply 0.4% gel to teeth once daily

Administration Oral:

Dental gel: Do **not** swallow; gel drops are placed in trough of applicator; applicator is applied over upper and lower teeth at same time; bite down for 6 minutes

Dental rinse: Swish or rinse in mouth then expectorate; do not swallow

Tablet: Dissolve in mouth, chew, swallow whole, or add to drinking water or fruit juice; administer with food (but not milk) to eliminate GI upset

Reference Range Total plasma fluoride: 0.14-0.19 mcg/mL

Dosage Forms Excipient information presented when available (limited, particularly for generics); consult specific product labeling. [DSC] = Discontinued product

Cream, oral, as sodium [toothpaste]: 1.1% (51 g) [equivalent to fluoride 2.5 mg/dose]

Denta 5000 Plus: 1.1% (51 g) [equivalent to fluoride 2.5 mg/dose; spearmint flavor]

EtheDent™: 1.1% (51 g) [equivalent to fluoride 2.5 mg/dose] [DSC]

PreviDent® 5000 Plus®: 1.1% (51 g) [equivalent to fluoride 2.5 mg/dose; contains sodium benzoate; Fruitastic™ flavor]

PreviDent® 5000 Plus®: 1.1% (51 g) [equivalent to fluoride 2.5 mg/dose; contains sodium benzoate; spearmint flavor]

Gel-drops, as sodium fluoride:

Thera-Flur-N®: 1.1% (24 mL) [equivalent to fluoride 0.5%; neutral pH; no artificial color or flavor] [DSC]

Gel, topical, as acidulated phosphate fluoride:

Phos-Flur®: 1.1% (60 g) [equivalent to fluoride 0.5%; cherry and mint flavors]

Gel, topical, as sodium fluoride: 1.1% (56 g) [equivalent to fluoride 2 mg/dose]

DentaGel, EtheDent™ [DSC]: 1.1% (56 g) [equivalent to fluoride 2 mg/dose; fresh mint flavor]

NeutraCare®: 1.1% (60 g) [neutral pH; grape and mint flavors]

NeutraGard® Advanced: 1.1% (60 g) [cinnamon and mint flavors]

PreviDent®: 1.1% (60 g) [equivalent to fluoride 2 mg/ dose; berry and mint flavors]

Gel, topical, as stannous fluoride:

Gel-Kam®: 0.4% (129 g) [cinnamon, fruit/berry, and mint flavors]

Just for Kids™: 0.4% (122 g) [bubble gum, fruit punch, and grapey grape flavors]

Omnii Gel™: 0.4% (122 g) [cinnamon, grape, natural, mint, and raspberry flavors]

StanGard®: 0.4% (122 g) [bubble gum, cherry, mint, and raspberry flavors]

Stop®: 0.4% (120 g) [bubble gum, cinnamon, grape, and mint flavors]

Lozenge, as sodium:

Lozi-Flur™: 2.21 mg [equivalent to fluoride 1 mg; cherry flavor]

Paste, oral, as sodium [toothpaste]:

ControlRx®: 1.1% (56 g) [vanilla mint flavor]

Solution, oral drops, as sodium: 1.1 mg/mL (50 mL) [equivalent to fluoride 0.5 mg/mL]

Flura-Drops®: 0.55 mg/drop (24 mL) [equivalent to fluoride 0.25 mg/drop; dye free, sugar free]

Luride®: 1.1 mg/mL (50 mL) [equivalent to fluoride 0.5 mg/mL; sugar free] [DSC]

Solution, oral rinse, as sodium:

ACT®: 0.05% (530 mL) [equivalent to fluoride 0.02%; bubble gum, cinnamon (contains tartrazine), and mint flavors]

ACT® Plus: 0.05% (530 mL) [equivalent to fluoride 0.02%; alcohol free; icy cool mint flavor]

ACT® x2™: 0.5% (530 mL) [equivalent to fluoride 0.02%; contains alcohol 11%; icy cool mint and spearmint flavors]

CaviRinse™: 0.2% (240 mL) [mint flavor]

Fluorigard®: 0.05% (480 mL) [alcohol free, sugar free; contains sodium benzoate and tartrazine; mint flavor]

Fluorinse®: 0.2% (480 mL) [alcohol free; cinnamon and mint flavors]

NeutraGard®: 0.05% (480 mL) [neutral pH; mint and tropical blast flavors]

NeutraGard® Plus: 0.2% (480 mL) [neutral pH; mint and tropical blast flavors]

Phos-Flur®: 0.044% (500 mL) [bubble gum, grape, and mint flavors]

PreviDent®: 0.2% (250 mL) [contains alcohol; mint flavor]

Solution, oral rinse concentrate, as stannous fluoride:

Gel-Kam®: 0.63% (300 mL) [cinnamon and mint flavors]

PerioMed™: 0.63% (284 mL) [equivalent to fluoride 7 mg/30 mL; alcohol free; cinnamon, mint and tropical fruit flavors]

StanGard® Perio: 0.63% (284 mL) [mint flavor]

Tablet, chewable, as sodium: 0.5 mg [equivalent to fluoride 0.25 mg]; 1.1 mg [fluoride 0.5 mg]; 2.2 mg [fluoride 1 mg]

Epiflur™:

0.55 mg [equivalent to fluoride 0.25 mg; sugar free; vanilla flavor]

1.1 mg [equivalent to fluoride 0.5 mg; sugar free; vanilla flavor]

2.2 mg [equivalent to fluoride 1 mg; sugar free; vanilla flavor]

EtheDent™:

0.55 mg [equivalent to fluoride 0.25 mg; sugar free; contains aspartame; vanilla flavor] [DSC]

1.1 mg [equivalent to fluoride 0.5 mg; sugar free; contains aspartame; grape flavor] [DSC]

2.2 mg [equivalent to fluoride 1 mg; sugar free; contains aspartame; cherry flavor] [DSC]

Fluor-A-Day:

0.56 mg [equivalent to fluoride 0.25 mg; raspberry flavor]

1.1 mg [equivalent to fluoride 0.5 mg; raspberry flavor]

2.21 mg [equivalent to fluoride 1 mg; raspberry flavor]

Luride® Lozi-Tab®:

0.55 mg [equivalent to fluoride 0.25 mg; sugar free; vanilla flavor]

1.1 mg [equivalent to fluoride 0.5 mg; sugar free; grape flavor]

2.2 mg [equivalent to fluoride 1 mg; sugar free; cherry flavor] [DSC]

Pharmaflur®: 2.2 mg [equivalent to fluoride 1 mg; dye free, sugar free; cherry flavor] [DSC]

Pharmaflur® 1.1: 1.1 mg [equivalent to fluoride 0.5 mg; dye free, sugar free; grape flavor] [DSC]

References

"Dietary Reference Intakes for Calcium, Phosphorus, Magnesium, Vitamin D, and Fluoride. Standing Committee on the Scientific Evaluation of Dietary Reference Intakes, Food and Nutrition Board, Institute of Medicine," National Academy of Sciences, Washington, DC: National Academy Press, 1997.

◆ **Fluorigard® [OTC]** see Fluoride on page 595

◆ **Fluorinse®** see Fluoride on page 595

◆ **2-Fluoro-ara-AMP** see Fludarabine on page 587

◆ **5-Fluorocytosine** see Flucytosine on page 586

◆ **9α-Fluorohydrocortisone Acetate** see Fludrocortisone on page 589

Fluorometholone (flure oh METH oh lone)

Medication Safety Issues

International issues:

Flarex® may be confused with Flurets® which is a brand name for sodium fluoride in Australia

Flarex® may be confused with Fluarix® which is a brand name for influenza virus vaccine in the U.S. and in numerous international markets

Flarex® may be confused with Fluorex® which is a brand name for sodium fluoride in France

Fluor-Op® may be confused with Fluoron® which is a brand name for fluorine in Canada

U.S. Brand Names Flarex®; FML®; FML® Forte

Canadian Brand Names Flarex®; FML Forte®; FML®; PMS-Fluorometholone

Therapeutic Category Adrenal Corticosteroid; Anti-inflammatory Agent, Ophthalmic; Corticosteroid, Ophthalmic; Glucocorticoid

Generic Available Yes: Suspension (as base)

Use Inflammatory conditions of the eye, including keratitis, iritis, cyclitis, and conjunctivitis

Pregnancy Risk Factor C

Pregnancy Considerations The extent of systemic absorption is not known. Use with caution in pregnant women.

Lactation Excretion in breast milk unknown/use caution

Contraindications Hypersensitivity to fluorometholone, other corticosteroids, or any component; herpes simplex keratitis, fungal diseases of ocular structures, mycobacterial infections of the eye, and most viral diseases of cornea and conjunctiva

Warnings Not recommended for children <2 years of age

Precautions Prolonged use may result in glaucoma, increased intraocular pressure, or other ocular damage

Adverse Reactions

Local: Stinging, burning

Ocular: Intraocular pressure elevated, open-angle glaucoma, defect in visual acuity and field of vision, cataracts, photosensitivity

Drug Interactions

Avoid Concomitant Use

Avoid concomitant use of Fluorometholone with any of the following: Aldesleukin

Increased Effect/Toxicity There are no known significant interactions involving an increase in effect.

Decreased Effect

Fluorometholone may decrease the levels/effects of: Aldesleukin; Corticorelin

Mechanism of Action Decreases inflammation by suppression of migration of polymorphonuclear leukocytes and reversal of increased capillary permeability

Pharmacokinetics (Adult data unless noted) Absorption: Into aqueous humor with slight systemic absorption

Usual Dosage Children >2 years and Adults: Ophthalmic:

Ointment: May be applied every 4 hours in severe cases or 1-3 times/day in mild to moderate cases.

Drops: Instill 1-2 drops into conjunctival sac every hour during day, every 2 hours at night until favorable response is obtained, then use 1 drop every 4 hours; in mild or moderate inflammation: 1-2 drops into conjunctival sac 2-4 times/day.

Administration Ophthalmic: Avoid contact of medication tube or bottle tip with skin or eye; suspension: Shake well before use; apply finger pressure to lacrimal sac during and for 1-2 minutes after instillation to decrease risk of absorption and systemic effects; the preservative (benzalkonium chloride) may be absorbed by soft contact lenses; wait at least 15 minutes after administration of suspension before inserting soft contact lenses

Monitoring Parameters Intraocular pressure (if used ≥10 days)

Patient Information May cause blurring of vision; do not discontinue without consulting physician; notify physician if improvement does not occur after 2 days

Dosage Forms Excipient information presented when available (limited, particularly for generics); consult specific product labeling. [DSC] = Discontinued product

Ointment, ophthalmic, as base:

FML®: 0.1% (3.5 g)

Suspension, ophthalmic, as base: 0.1% (5 mL, 10 mL, 15 mL)

FML®: 0.1% (5 mL, 10 mL, 15 mL) [contains benzalkonium chloride]

FML® Forte: 0.25% (2 mL, 5 mL, 10 mL, 15 mL) [contains benzalkonium chloride]

Suspension, ophthalmic, as acetate:

Flarex®: 0.1% (5 mL) [contains benzalkonium chloride]

◆ **Fluoroplex®** *see* Fluorouracil *on page 598*

Fluorouracil (flure oh YOOR a sil)

Medication Safety Issues

Sound-alike/look-alike issues:

Carac® may be confused with Kuric™

Fluorouracil may be confused with flucytosine

Efudex® may be confused with Efidac (Efidac 24®), Eurax®

High alert medication: This medication is in a class the Institute for Safe Medication Practices (ISMP) includes among its list of drugs which have a heightened risk of causing significant patient harm when used in error.

International issues:

Carac® may be confused with Carace® which is a brand name for lisinopril in Ireland and Great Britain

Related Information

Compatibility of Chemotherapy and Related Supportive Care Medications *on page 1580*

Emetogenic Potential of Antineoplastic Agents *on page 1579*

U.S. Brand Names Adrucil®; Carac®; Efudex®; Fluoroplex®; Fluorouracil® [DSC]

Canadian Brand Names Efudex®

Therapeutic Category Antineoplastic Agent, Antimetabolite

Generic Available Yes: Injection, topical solution

Use Treatment of carcinoma of stomach, colon, rectum, breast, and pancreas (FDA approved in adults); topically for management of multiple actinic or solar keratoses and superficial basal cell carcinomas (FDA approved in adults); has also been used for the treatment of head and neck cancer, bladder cancer, hepatoblastoma, and cervical cancer

Pregnancy Risk Factor D (injection); X (topical)

Pregnancy Considerations Teratogenic effects have been observed with parenteral administration in animal studies; fetal defects and miscarriages have been reported following use of topical and intravenous products in humans. Use of topical products is contraindicated during pregnancy.

Lactation Excretion in breast milk unknown/not recommended

Contraindications Hypersensitivity to fluorouracil or any component; patients with poor nutritional status, bone marrow suppression, or serious infections

Warnings Hazardous agent; use appropriate precautions for handling and disposal; if intractable vomiting, diarrhea, stomatitis, GI ulceration/bleeding, hemorrhage, or precipitous falls in leukocyte or platelet counts occur, discontinue fluorouracil immediately

Administration to patients with genetic dihydropyrimidine dehydrogenase (DPD) enzyme deficiency has been associated with increased toxicity following administration (diarrhea, stomatitis, neutropenia, and neurotoxicity). Absence of the DPD enzyme may result in prolonged fluorouracil clearance. Systemic toxicity normally associated with parenteral administration has also been associated with topical use, particularly in patients with DPD enzyme deficiency; discontinue if symptoms of DPD enzyme deficiency occur.

Topical: Avoid topical application to mucous membranes due to potential for local inflammation and ulceration. The use of occlusive dressings with topical preparations may increase the severity of inflammation in nearby skin areas. Avoid exposure to ultraviolet rays during and immediately following therapy.

Precautions Use with caution and modify dosage in patients with renal or hepatic impairment; use with caution in patients who have had high-dose pelvic radiation; palmar-plantar erythrodysesthesia (hand-foot) syndrome has been associated with use.

Adverse Reactions

Cardiovascular: Angina, chest pain, cardiac arrhythmias, heart failure, hypotension, myocardial ischemia

Central nervous system: Cerebellar ataxia (gait and speech abnormalities), confusion, disorientation, dizziness, euphoria, headache, somnolence

Dermatologic: Alopecia, dry skin, fissuring, partial loss of nails or hyperpigmentation of nail bed, photosensitivity, pruritic maculopapular rash, skin irritation, skin pigmentation

Gastrointestinal: Anorexia, diarrhea, esophagitis, GI hemorrhage, nausea, stomatitis, vomiting

Hematologic: Anemia, granulocytopenia, leukopenia, myelosuppression, thrombocytopenia

Hepatic: Hepatotoxicity

Local: Thrombophlebitis

Ocular: Conjunctivitis, lacrimation, nystagmus, photophobia, visual disturbances

Miscellaneous: Anaphylaxis, palmar-plantar erythrodysesthesia (erythematous, desquamative rash involving hands and feet accompanied by pain, tingling, and swollen palms; this adverse effect may be treated with oral pyridoxine)

Drug Interactions

Metabolism/Transport Effects Inhibits CYP2C9 (strong)

Avoid Concomitant Use

Avoid concomitant use of Fluorouracil with any of the following: BCG; Natalizumab; Pimecrolimus; Tacrolimus (Topical); Vaccines (Live)

Increased Effect/Toxicity

Fluorouracil may increase the levels/effects of: Carvedilol; CYP2C9 Substrates (High risk); Leflunomide; Natalizumab; Phenytoin; Vaccines (Live); Vitamin K Antagonists

The levels/effects of Fluorouracil may be increased by: Denosumab; Gemcitabine; Leucovorin Calcium-Levoleucovorin; Pimecrolimus; Sorafenib; Tacrolimus (Topical); Trastuzumab

Decreased Effect

Fluorouracil may decrease the levels/effects of: BCG; Sipuleucel-T; Vaccines (Inactivated); Vaccines (Live); Vitamin K Antagonists

The levels/effects of Fluorouracil may be decreased by: Echinacea; Sorafenib

Food Interactions Increase dietary intake of thiamine

Stability

Injection: Store at room temperature 15°C to 30°C (59°F to 86°F); protect from light; slight discoloration of injection during storage does not affect potency; if precipitate forms, redissolve drug by heating to 140°F, shake well; allow to cool to body temperature before administration; incompatible with ciprofloxacin, cytarabine, diazepam, droperidol, filgrastim, ondansetron, vinorelbine

Topical: Store at controlled room temperature 15°C to 30°C (59°F to 86°F)

Mechanism of Action A pyrimidine antimetabolite that inhibits thymidylate synthase leading to depletion of the DNA precursor thymidine; incorporated into RNA, DNA

Pharmacokinetics (Adult data unless noted)

Distribution: Into tumors, intestinal mucosa, liver, bone marrow, ascitic fluid, brain tissue, and CSF

Protein binding: <10%

Metabolism: Inactive metabolites are formed following metabolism in the liver

Bioavailability: 50% to 80%; variable due to saturable first-pass elimination process

Half-life, biphasic:

Alpha: 10-20 minutes

Terminal: 15-19 hours

Elimination: Biphasic elimination with <10% of dose excreted unchanged in the urine; 25% to 80% excreted as respiratory CO_2

Usual Dosage Children and Adults (refer to individual protocols with dose based on lean body weight):

I.V.:

Initial: 400-500 mg/m²/day (12 mg/kg/day; maximum dose: 800 mg/day) for 4-5 days every 4 weeks; **or** 500-600 mg/m²/dose every 3-4 weeks

Maintenance: 200-250 mg/m²/dose (6 mg/kg) every other day for 4 doses; repeat in 4 weeks

Single weekly bolus dose of 15 mg/kg or 500 mg/m² can be administered depending on the patient's reaction to the previous course of treatment; maintenance dose of 5-15 mg/kg/week as a single dose not to exceed 1 g/week

I.V. infusion: 15 mg/kg/day or 500 mg/m²/day (maximum daily dose: 1 g) has been given by I.V. infusion over 4 hours for 5 days; **or** 800-1200 mg/m² for continuous infusion over 24-120 hours; **or** 1000 mg/m²/day for 3 days

Topical:

Actinic keratoses:

Efudex® or Fluoroplex®: Apply twice daily

Carac™: Apply once daily

Basal cell carcinoma: Efudex®: Apply twice daily

Dosing adjustment in hepatic impairment: Bilirubin >5 mg/dL: Not recommended for use

Administration

Parenteral: Administer by direct I.V. injection (50 mg/mL solution needs no further dilution) over several minutes or by I.V. intermittent or continuous infusion diluted in saline or dextrose solutions; toxicity (eg, myelosuppression) may be reduced by giving the drug as a continuous infusion. Doses >750-800 mg/m² should be administered as a continuous infusion, **not** by bolus injection; dose-limiting toxicity with continuous infusion is mucous membrane toxicity (ie, stomatitis, diarrhea)

Topical: For external use only. Not for ophthalmic or intravaginal use. Cleanse affected area thoroughly and wait 10 minutes before applying. Apply with a nonmetallic applicator or gloved fingers in a sufficient amount to cover affected area. Avoid contact with eyes, eyelids, nostrils, and mouth. Do not cover area with an occlusive dressing

1% or 2%: Apply to lesions on the head and neck for the treatment of multiple actinic keratoses

5%: Use on lesions in areas other than the head and neck for multiple actinic keratoses; only 5% preparations are used for the treatment of superficial basal cell carcinoma

Monitoring Parameters CBC with differential and platelet count, renal function tests, liver function tests; observe for changes in bowel frequency

Patient Information Avoid alcohol; maintain adequate hydration; report signs and symptoms of infection, bleeding, bruising, vision changes, unremitting nausea, vomiting, or diarrhea, chest pain or palpitations, or CNS changes. May cause photosensitivity reactions (eg, exposure to sunlight may cause severe sunburn, skin rash, redness, or itching); avoid exposure to sunlight and artificial light sources (sunlamps, tanning booth/bed); wear protective clothing, wide-brimmed hats, sunglasses, and lip sunscreen (SPF ≥15); use a sunscreen [broad-spectrum sunscreen or physical sunscreen (preferred) or sunblock with SPF ≥15]; contact physician if reaction occurs. Women of childbearing age should be advised to avoid becoming pregnant.

Nursing Implications Wash hands immediately after topical application of the cream or solution. Care should be taken to avoid extravasation of I.V. fluorouracil.

◄ **Additional Information** Myelosuppressive effects:
WBC: Mild
Platelets: Mild
Onset (days): 7-10
Nadir (days): 9-14
Recovery (days): 21

Dosage Forms Excipient information presented when available (limited, particularly for generics); consult specific product labeling. [DSC] = Discontinued product

Cream, topical:
Carac®: 0.5% (30 g)
Efudex®: 5% (40 g)
Fluoroplex®: 1% (30 g) [contains benzyl alcohol]
Injection, solution: 50 mg/mL (10 mL, 20 mL, 50 mL, 100 mL)
Adrucil®: 50 mg/mL (10 mL, 50 mL, 100 mL)
Solution, topical: 2% (10 mL); 5% (10 mL)
Efudex®: 2% (10 mL, 25 mL) [DSC]; 5% (10 mL, 25 mL [DSC])
Fluorouracil®: 5% (10 mL) [DSC]

References

Balis FM, Holcenberg JS and Bleyer WA, "Clinical Pharmacokinetics of Commonly Used Anticancer Drugs," *Clin Pharmacokinet*, 1983, 8 (3):202-32.

Ortega JA, Douglass EC, Feusner JH, et al, "Randomized Comparison of Cisplatin/Vincristine/Fluorouracil and Cisplatin/Continuous Infusion Doxorubicin for Treatment of Pediatric Hepatoblastoma: A Report From the Children's Cancer Group and the Pediatric Oncology Group," *J Clin Oncol*, 2000, 18(14):2665-75.

Rodriguez-Galindo C, Wofford M, Castleberry RP, et al, "Preradiation Chemotherapy With Methotrexate, Cisplatin, 5-Fluorouracil, and Leucovorin for Pediatric Nasopharyngeal Carcinoma," *Cancer*, 2005, 103(4):850-7.

♦ **Fluorouracil® [DSC]** *see* Fluorouracil *on page 598*

♦ **5-Fluorouracil** *see* Fluorouracil *on page 598*

FLUoxetine (floo OKS e teen)

Medication Safety Issues

Sound-alike/look-alike issues:
FLUoxetine may be confused with DULoxetine, famotidine, Feldene®, fluconazole, fluvastatin, fluvoxamine, fosinopril, furosemide, PARoxetine, thiothixene
Prozac® may be confused with Paxil®, Prelone®, Prilosec®, Prograf®, Proscar®, ProSom®, ProStep®, Provera®
Sarafem® may be confused with Serophene®

Beers Criteria medication: This drug may be inappropriate for use in geriatric patients (high severity risk).

International issues:
Fluoxin® [Czech Republic and Romania] may be confused with Floxin® which is a brand name for ofloxacin in the U.S.
Prozac® may be confused with Prazac® a brand of prazosin in Denmark
Reneuron® [Spain] may be confused with Remeron® a brand of mirtazapine in the U.S.

Related Information

Antidepressant Agents *on page 1484*
Serotonin Syndrome *on page 1695*

U.S. Brand Names Prozac®; Prozac® Weekly™; Sarafem®; Selfemra®

Canadian Brand Names Apo-Fluoxetine®; CO Fluoxetine; Dom-Fluoxetine; Fluoxetine; FXT 40; Gen-Fluoxetine; Mylan-Fluoxetine; Novo-Fluoxetine; Nu-Fluoxetine; PHL-Fluoxetine; PMS-Fluoxetine; PRO-Fluoxetine; Prozac®; ratio-Fluoxetine; Riva-Fluoxetine; Sandoz-Fluoxetine; ZYM-Fluoxetine

Therapeutic Category Antidepressant, Selective Serotonin Reuptake Inhibitor (SSRI)

Generic Available Yes

Use Treatment of major depressive disorder, obsessive-compulsive disorder, bulimia nervosa, premenstrual dysphoric disorder (PMDD), panic disorder with or without agoraphobia

Medication Guide An FDA-approved patient medication guide, which is available with the product information and as follows, must be dispensed with this medication for each new outpatient prescription and refill.

Prozac® & Prozac® Weekly™: http://www.fda.gov/downloads/Drugs/DrugSafety/ucm088999.pdf

Sarafem®: http://www.fda.gov/downloads/Drugs/DrugSafety/ucm089119.pdf

Pregnancy Risk Factor C

Pregnancy Considerations Due to adverse effects observed in animal studies, fluoxetine is classified as pregnancy category C. Fluoxetine and its metabolite cross the human placenta. Nonteratogenic effects in the newborn following SSRIs exposure late in the third trimester include respiratory distress, cyanosis, apnea, seizures, temperature instability, feeding difficulty, vomiting, hypoglycemia, hypo- or hypertonia, hyper-reflexia, jitteriness, irritability, constant crying, and tremor. An increased risk of low birth weight, lower APGAR score, and blunted behavioral response to pain for a prolonged period after delivery have also been reported. Exposure to SSRIs after the twentieth week of gestation has been associated with persistent pulmonary hypertension of the newborn (PPHN). Adverse effects may be due to toxic effects of the SSRI or drug withdrawal without a taper. The long term effects of *in utero* SSRI exposure on infant development and behavior are not known.

Due to pregnancy-induced physiologic changes, women who are pregnant may require increased doses of fluoxetine to achieve euthymia. Women treated for major depression and who are euthymic prior to pregnancy are more likely to experience a relapse when medication is discontinued as compared to pregnant women who continue taking antidepressant medications. The ACOG recommends that therapy with SSRIs or SNRIs during pregnancy be individualized; treatment of depression during pregnancy should incorporate the clinical expertise of the mental health clinician, obstetrician, primary healthcare provider, and pediatrician. If treatment during pregnancy is required, consider tapering therapy during the third trimester in order to prevent withdrawal symptoms in the infant. If this is done and the woman is considered to be at risk of relapse from her major depressive disorder, the medication can be restarted following delivery, although the dose should be readjusted to that required before pregnancy. Treatment algorithms have been developed by the ACOG and the APA for the management of depression in women prior to conception and during pregnancy (Yonkers, 2009).

Lactation Enters breast milk/not recommended (AAP rates "of concern")

Breast-Feeding Considerations Fluoxetine and its metabolite are excreted into breast milk and can be detected in the serum of breast-feeding infants. Concentrations in breast milk are variable. Colic, irritability, slow weight gain, and feeding and sleep disorders have been reported in nursing infants. The AAP considers fluoxetine to be a "drug for which the effect on the nursing infant is unknown but may be of concern." Breast-feeding is not recommended by the manufacturer.

Because the long-term effects on development and behavior have not been studied and adverse effects have been noted in some infants exposed, one should prescribe fluoxetine to a mother who is breast-feeding only when the benefits outweigh the potential risks.

Contraindications Hypersensitivity to fluoxetine or any component; use of MAO inhibitors within 14 days (potentially fatal reactions may occur, see Drug Interactions; do not use MAO inhibitors for at least 5 weeks after fluoxetine is discontinued); concurrent use of thioridazine or use within 5 weeks after fluoxetine is discontinued (see Drug Interactions); concurrent use of pimozide

Warnings Fluoxetine is approved for use in pediatric patients only for the treatment of major depressive disorder and obsessive compulsive disorder. Clinical worsening of depression or suicidal ideation and behavior may occur in children and adults with major depressive disorder **[U.S. Boxed Warning]**. In clinical trials, antidepressants increased the risk of suicidal thinking and behavior (suicidality) in children, adolescents, and young adults (18-24 years of age) with major depressive disorder and other psychiatric disorders. This risk must be considered before prescribing antidepressants for any clinical use. Short-term studies did **not** show an increased risk of suicidality with antidepressant use in patients >24 years of age and showed a decreased risk in patients ≥65 years.

Patients of all ages who are treated with antidepressants for any indication require appropriate monitoring and close observation for clinical worsening of depression, suicidality, and unusual changes in behavior, especially during the first few months after antidepressant initiation or when the dose is adjusted. Family members and caregivers should be instructed to closely observe the patient (ie, daily) and communicate condition with healthcare provider. Patients should also be monitored for associated behaviors (eg, anxiety, agitation, panic attacks, insomnia, irritability, hostility, aggressiveness, impulsivity, akathisia, hypomania, mania) which may increase the risk for worsening depression or suicidality. Worsening depression or emergence of suicidality (or associated behaviors listed above) that is abrupt in onset, severe, or not part of the presenting symptoms, may require discontinuation or modification of drug therapy.

Avoid abrupt discontinuation; discontinuation symptoms (including agitation, dysphoria, anxiety, confusion, dizziness, hypomania, nightmares, and other symptoms) may occur if therapy is abruptly discontinued or dose reduced; taper the dose to minimize risks of discontinuation symptoms; if intolerable symptoms occur following a decrease in dosage or upon discontinuation of therapy, consider resuming the previous dose with a more gradual taper. To reduce risk of intentional overdose, write prescriptions for the smallest quantity consistent with good patient care. Screen individuals for bipolar disorder prior to treatment (using antidepressants alone may induce manic episodes in patients with this condition). Potentially fatal serotonin syndrome may occur when SSRIs are used in combination with serotonergic drugs (eg, triptans) or drugs that impair the metabolism of serotonin (eg, MAO inhibitors); see Drug Interactions.

Rash or urticaria may occur along with leukocytosis, fever, edema, arthralgia, lymphadenopathy, respiratory distress, and other symptoms; rare cases of vasculitis and lupus-like syndrome have been reported; anaphylactoid reactions including laryngospasm, bronchospasm, angioedema, and urticaria may occur; discontinue use if rash or other allergic reaction occurs

Oral solution contains benzoic acid; benzoic acid (benzoate) is a metabolite of benzyl alcohol; large amounts of benzyl alcohol (≥99 mg/kg/day) have been associated with a potentially fatal toxicity ("gasping syndrome") in neonates; avoid use of fluoxetine products containing benzoic acid in neonates; *in vitro* and animal studies have shown that benzoate displaces bilirubin from protein binding sites

Precautions May cause abnormal bleeding (eg, ecchymosis, purpura, upper GI bleeding); use with caution in patients with impaired platelet aggregation and with concurrent use of aspirin, NSAIDs, or other drugs that affect coagulation. May cause insomnia, anxiety, nervousness, anorexia, or weight loss. Use with caution in patients where weight loss is undesirable. May impair cognitive or motor performance. Use with caution in patients with renal or hepatic impairment, seizure disorders, cardiac dysfunction, diabetes mellitus; use with caution during third trimester of pregnancy [newborns may experience adverse effects or withdrawal symptoms (consider risk and benefits); see Additional Information; exposure to SSRIs late in pregnancy may also be associated with an increased risk for persistent pulmonary hypertension of the newborn (see Chambers, 2006)]. Use with caution in patients receiving diuretics or those who are volume-depleted (may cause hyponatremia or SIADH). Decrease dose in liver dysfunction; use with caution in patients at high risk for suicide; add or initiate other antidepressants with caution after 5 weeks or longer after stopping fluoxetine.

Fluoxetine may cause decreased growth (smaller increases in weight and height) in children and adolescent patients; currently, no studies directly evaluate fluoxetine's long term effects on growth, development, and maturation of pediatric patients; periodic monitoring of height and weight in pediatric patients is recommended **Note:** Case reports of decreased growth in children receiving fluoxetine or fluvoxamine (n=4; age: 11.6-13.7 years) for 6 months to 5 years suggest a suppression of growth hormone secretion during SSRI therapy (see Weintrob, 2002). Further studies are needed.

Significant toxicities have been observed after exposure to fluoxetine in juvenile animals (some occurring at clinically relevant doses). Toxicities included myotoxicity (eg, skeletal muscle damage and necrosis, elevated serum CPK), impaired bone development, and long-term neurobehavioral and reproductive toxicity. The clinical significance of these findings is uncertain.

Adverse Reactions Predominant adverse effects are CNS and GI:

Cardiovascular: Vasodilation

Central nervous system: Headache, nervousness, insomnia, drowsiness, anxiety, dizziness, fatigue, sedation, somnolence, mania, hypomania, irritability, extrapyramidal reactions (rare); difficulty concentrating, abnormal dreams; suicidal thinking and behavior (see Warnings)

> **Note:** SSRI-associated behavioral activation (ie, restlessness, hyperkinesis, hyperactivity, agitation) is 2- to 3-fold more prevalent in children compared to adolescents; it is more prevalent in adolescents compared to adults. Somnolence (including sedation and drowsiness) is more common in adults compared to children and adolescents (see Safer, 2006).

Dermatologic: Rash, urticaria, pruritus

Endocrine & metabolic: Hypoglycemia; hyponatremia, SIADH (usually in volume-depleted patients); sexual dysfunction, libido decreased, weight loss; growth in pediatric patients decreased

Gastrointestinal: Nausea, diarrhea, xerostomia, anorexia, dyspepsia, constipation

> **Note:** SSRI-associated vomiting is 2- to 3-fold more prevalent in children compared to adolescents; it is more prevalent in adolescents compared to adults.

Hematologic: Altered platelet function (rare)

Neuromuscular & skeletal: Tremor, asthenia, weakness

Ocular: Visual disturbances

Respiratory: Rhinitis, pharyngitis, yawn

Miscellaneous: Anaphylactoid reactions, allergies, diaphoresis, flu-like syndrome; withdrawal symptoms following abrupt discontinuation (see Warnings)

Drug Interactions

Metabolism/Transport Effects **Substrate** of CYP1A2 (minor), 2B6 (minor), 2C9 (major), 2C19 (minor), 2D6 (major), 2E1 (minor), 3A4 (minor); **Inhibits** CYP1A2 (moderate), 2B6 (weak), 2C9 (weak), 2C19 (moderate), 2D6 (strong), 3A4 (weak)

Avoid Concomitant Use

Avoid concomitant use of FLUoxetine with any of the following: Artemether; Clopidogrel; Dronedarone; Iobenguane I 123; Lumefantrine; MAO Inhibitors; Metoclopramide; Nilotinib; Pimozide; QuiNINE; Sibutramine; Tamoxifen; Tetrabenazine; Thioridazine; Ziprasidone

Increased Effect/Toxicity

FLUoxetine may increase the levels/effects of: Alcohol (Ethyl); Alpha-/Beta-Blockers; Anticoagulants; Antidepressants (Serotonin Reuptake Inhibitor/Antagonist); Antiplatelet Agents; Aspirin; Atomoxetine; Benzodiazepines (metabolized by oxidation); Beta-Blockers; BusPIRone; CarBAMazepine; Clozapine; CNS Depressants; Collagenase (Systemic); CYP1A2 Substrates; CYP2C19 Substrates; CYP2D6 Substrates; Desmopressin; Dextromethorphan; Dronedarone; Drotrecogin Alfa; Fesoterodine; Galantamine; Haloperidol; Ibritumomab; Lithium; Methadone; Mexiletine; NSAID (COX-2 Inhibitor); NSAID (Nonselective); Phenytoin; Pimozide; Propafenone; QTc-Prolonging Agents; QuiNIDine; QuiNINE; Risperidone; Salicylates; Serotonin Modulators; Tamoxifen; Tetrabenazine; Thioridazine; Thrombolytic Agents; Tositumomab and Iodine I 131 Tositumomab; TraMADol; Tricyclic Antidepressants; Vitamin K Antagonists; Ziprasidone

The levels/effects of FLUoxetine may be increased by: Alfuzosin; Analgesics (Opioid); Artemether; BusPIRone; Chloroquine; Cimetidine; Ciprofloxacin; Ciprofloxacin (Systemic); CYP2C9 Inhibitors (Moderate); CYP2C9 Inhibitors (Strong); CYP2D6 Inhibitors (Moderate); CYP2D6 Inhibitors (Strong); Darunavir; Gadobutrol; Glucosamine; Herbs (Anticoagulant/Antiplatelet Properties); Lumefantrine; Macrolide Antibiotics; MAO Inhibitors; Metoclopramide; Nilotinib; Omega-3-Acid Ethyl Esters; Pentosan Polysulfate Sodium; Pentoxifylline; Prostacyclin Analogues; QuiNINE; Sibutramine; TraMADol; Tryptophan

Decreased Effect

FLUoxetine may decrease the levels/effects of: Clopidogrel; Iobenguane I 123

The levels/effects of FLUoxetine may be decreased by: CarBAMazepine; CYP2C9 Inducers (Highly Effective); Cyproheptadine; Peginterferon Alfa-2b

Food Interactions Tryptophan supplements may increase CNS and GI adverse effects (eg, restlessness, agitation, GI problems); its use is **not recommended**. Food does not affect bioavailability, but may delay absorption by 1-2 hours

Stability Store at room temperature; protect tablets, immediate release capsules, and solution from light

Mechanism of Action Inhibits CNS neuron serotonin uptake; minimal or no effect on reuptake of norepinephrine or dopamine; does not significantly bind to alpha-adrenergic, histamine or cholinergic receptors; may therefore be useful in patients at risk from sedation, hypotension and anticholinergic effects of tricyclic antidepressants

Pharmacodynamics Maximum effect: Maximum antidepressant effects usually occur after >4 weeks; due to long half-life, resolution of adverse reactions after discontinuation may be slow

Pharmacokinetics (Adult data unless noted) Note: Average steady-state fluoxetine serum concentrations in children (n=10; 6 to <13 years of age) were 2-fold higher than in adolescents (n=11; 13 to <18 years of age); all patients received 20 mg/day; average steady-state norfluoxetine serum concentrations were 1.5-fold higher in the children compared with adolescents; differences in weight almost entirely explained the differences in serum concentrations

Absorption: Oral: Well absorbed; enteric-coated pellets contained in Prozac® Weekly™ resist dissolution until GI pH >5.5 and therefore delay onset of absorption 1-2 hours compared to immediate release formulations

Distribution: Adults: V_d: 20-45 L/kg; widely distributed

Protein binding: ~95% (albumin and alpha$_1$-glycoprotein)

Metabolism: In the liver to norfluoxetine (active) and other metabolites

Bioavailability: Capsules, tablets, solution, and weekly capsules are bioequivalent

Half-life: Adults:

Fluoxetine: Acute dosing: 1-3 days; chronic dosing: 4-6 days; cirrhosis: 7.6 days

Norfluoxetine: Acute and chronic dosing: 4-16 days; cirrhosis: 12 days

Time to peak serum concentration: Immediate release formulation: After 6-8 hours

Elimination: In urine as fluoxetine (2.5% to 5%) and norfluoxetine (10%)

Usual Dosage Oral:

Children and Adolescents:

Depression: 8-18 years of age: Manufacturer's recommendation: Initial: 10-20 mg/day; in patients started at 10 mg/day, may increase dose to 20 mg/day after 1 week. Lower weight children: Initial: 10 mg/day; usual: 10 mg/day; if needed, may increase dose to 20 mg/day after several weeks.

Note: Some experts recommend the following lower initial doses: Children ≤11 years: Initial: 5 mg/day; children ≥12 years: Initial: 10 mg/day; clinically, doses have been titrated up to 40 mg/day in pediatric patients (see Dopheide, 2006).

Obsessive-compulsive disorder: 7-18 years of age:

Lower weight children: Initial: 10 mg/day; if needed, may increase dose after several weeks; usual range: 20-30 mg/day; minimal experience with doses >20 mg/day; no experience with doses >60 mg/day

Higher weight children and Adolescents: Initial: 10 mg/day; may increase dose to 20 mg/day after 2 weeks; may increase dose after several more weeks, if needed; usual range: 20-60 mg/day

Elective mutism: 6 children 6-12 years of age with elective mutism were treated with initial doses of 0.2 mg/kg/day for 1 week, then 0.4 mg/kg/day for 1 week, then 0.6 mg/kg/day for 10 weeks (Black,1994); further studies are needed

Adults:

Depression or obsessive-compulsive disorder: Initial dose: 20 mg/day administered in the morning; may increase after several weeks by 20 mg/day increments; maximum dose: 80 mg/day; doses >20 mg/day can be given either once daily (in the morning) or divided into morning or noon doses

Depression: Weekly dosing: Patients maintained on 20 mg/day may be changed to Prozac® Weekly™ 90 mg/week, starting 7 days after the last 20 mg/day dose

Bulimia nervosa: 60 mg/day administered in the morning; may need to titrate up to this dose over several days in some patients; higher doses have not been well studied

Premenstrual dysphoric disorder: 20 mg/day; given continuously (every day), **or** 20 mg/day given intermittently (starting the daily dose 14 days prior to the expected onset of menstruation with administration of daily dose through the first full day of menses); repeat with each menstrual cycle; doses >60 mg/day have not been studied; maximum dose: 80 mg/day

Panic disorder: Initial: 10 mg/day; increase dose to 20 mg/day after 1 week; if needed, may increase dose further after several weeks; doses >60 mg/day have not been evaluated

Dosage adjustment in renal impairment: Adjustment not routinely needed

Dosage adjustment in hepatic impairment: Lower doses or less frequent administration are recommended

Administration Oral: May be administered without regard to food

Monitoring Parameters Liver function, weight, serum glucose; serum sodium (in volume depleted patients); monitor for rash and signs or symptoms of anaphylactoid reactions; monitor height and weight in pediatric patients periodically. Monitor patient periodically for symptom resolution; monitor for worsening depression, suicidality, and associated behaviors (especially at the beginning of therapy or when doses are increased or decreased; see Warnings)

Reference Range

Therapeutic: Fluoxetine 100-800 ng/mL (SI: 289-2314 nmol/L); norfluoxetine 100-600 ng/mL (SI: 289-1735 nmol/L)

Toxic: (Fluoxetine plus norfluoxetine): >2000 ng/mL (SI: >5784 nmol/L)

Patient Information Read the patient Medication Guide that you receive with each prescription and refill of fluoxetine. An increased risk of suicidal thinking and behavior has been reported with the use of antidepressants in children, adolescents, and young adults (18-24 years of age). Notify physician if you feel more depressed, have thoughts of suicide, or become more agitated or irritable (see Warnings). Avoid alcohol, tryptophan supplements, and the herbal medicine St John's wort; avoid aspirin, NSAIDs, or other drugs that affect coagulation (may increase risks of bleeding); may cause dizziness or drowsiness and impair ability to perform activities requiring mental alertness or physical coordination; may cause dry mouth; inform physician immediately if hives or rash develops. Some medicines should not be taken with fluoxetine or should not be taken for a while after fluoxetine has been discontinued; report the use of other medications, nonprescription medications, and herbal or natural products to your physician and pharmacist. Take as directed; do not alter dose or frequency without consulting prescriber, avoid abrupt discontinuation.

Nursing Implications Last dose of the day should be given before 4 PM (to avoid insomnia). Assess other medications patient may be taking for possible interaction (especially MAO inhibitors, P450 inhibitors, and other CNS active agents). Assess mental status for depression, suicidal ideation, anxiety, social functioning, mania, or panic attack.

Additional Information If used for an extended period of time, long-term usefulness of fluoxetine should be periodically re-evaluated for the individual patient. A recent report describes 5 children (age: 8-15 years) who developed epistaxis (n=4) or bruising (n=1) while receiving SSRI therapy (sertraline) (Lake, 2000).

Neonates born to women receiving SSRIs later during the third trimester may experience respiratory distress, apnea, cyanosis, temperature instability, vomiting, feeding difficulty, hypoglycemia, constant crying, irritability, hypotonia, hypertonia, hyper-reflexia, tremor, jitteriness, and seizures; these symptoms may be due to a direct toxic effect, withdrawal syndrome, or (in some cases) serotonin syndrome. Withdrawal symptoms occur in 30% of neonates exposed to SSRIs *in utero*; monitor newborns for at least 48 hours after birth; long-term effects of *in utero* exposure to SSRIs are unknown (see Levinson-Castiel, 2006).

Dosage Forms Excipient information presented when available (limited, particularly for generics); consult specific product labeling. [DSC] = Discontinued product

Capsule, oral: 10 mg, 20 mg, 40 mg

Prozac®: 10 mg, 20 mg, 40 mg

Sarafem®: 10 mg, 20 mg [DSC]

Selfemra®: 10 mg, 20 mg [contains soya lecithin]

Capsule, delayed release, enteric coated pellets, oral: 90 mg

Prozac® Weekly™: 90 mg

Solution, oral: 20 mg/5 mL (5 mL, 120 mL)

Prozac®: 20 mg/5 mL (120 mL) [contains ethanol 0.23% and benzoic acid; mint flavor] [DSC]

Tablet, oral: 10 mg, 20 mg

Sarafem®: 10 mg, 20 mg

Extemporaneous Preparations Dilutions of the commercially available oral solution may be made; 1 mg/mL and 2 mg/mL dilutions in Simple Syrup USP, Simple Syrup - British Pharmacopoeia, Aromatic Elixir USP, grape-cranberry drink (Ocean Spray® Cran-Grape), and deionized water were stable for 8 weeks when stored in amber glass bottles at 5°C and 30°C (Peterson, 1994).

Peterson JA, Risley DS, Anderson PN, et al, "Stability of Fluoxetine Hydrochloride in Fluoxetine Solution Diluted With Common Pharmaceutical Diluents," *Am J Hosp Pharm*, 1994, 51(10):1342-5.

References

Black B and Uhde TW, "Treatment of Elective Mutism With Fluoxetine: A Double Blind, Placebo-Controlled Study," *J Am Acad Child Adolesc Psychiatry*, 1994, 33(7):1000-6.

Chambers CD, Hernandez-Diaz S, Van Marter LJ, et al, "Selective Serotonin-Reuptake Inhibitors and Risk of Persistent Pulmonary Hypertension of the Newborn," *N Engl J Med*, 2006, 354(6):579-87.

Como PG and Kurlan R, "An Open-Label Trial of Fluoxetine for Obsessive-Compulsive Disorder in Gilles de la Tourette's Syndrome," *Neurology*, 1991, 41(6):872-4.

DeSilva KE, Le Flore DB, Marston BJ, et al, "Serotonin Syndrome in HIV-Infected Individuals Receiving Antiretroviral Therapy and Fluoxetine," *AIDS*, 2001, 15(10):1281-5.

Dopheide JA, "Recognizing and Treating Depression in Children and Adolescents," *Am J Health Syst Pharm*, 2006, 63(3):233-43.

Emslie GJ, Rush AJ, Weinberg WA, et al, "A Double-Blind, Randomized, Placebo-Controlled Trial of Fluoxetine in Children and Adolescents With Depression," *Arch Gen Psychiatry*, 1997, 54(11):1031-7.

Findling RL, Reed MD, and Blumer JL, "Pharmacological Treatment of Depression in Children and Adolescents," *Paediatr Drugs*, 1999, 1(3):161-82.

Kurlan R, Como PG, Deeley C, et al, "A Pilot Controlled Study of Fluoxetine for Obsessive-Compulsive Symptoms in Children With Tourette's Syndrome," *Clin Neuropharmacol*, 1993, 16(2):167-72.

Lake MB, Birmaher B, Wassick S, et al, "Bleeding and Selective Serotonin Reuptake Inhibitors in Childhood and Adolescence," *J Child Adolesc Psychopharmacol*, 2000, 10(1):35-8.

Levinson-Castiel R, Merlob P, Linder N, et al, "Neonatal Abstinence Syndrome After *in utero* Exposure to Selective Serotonin Reuptake Inhibitors in Term Infants," *Arch Pediatr Adolesc Med*, 2006, 160(2):173-6.

Riddle MA, Hardin MT, King R, et al, "Fluoxetine Treatment of Children and Adolescents With Tourette's and Obsessive-Compulsive Disorders: Preliminary Clinical Experience," *J Am Acad Child Adolesc Psychiatry*, 1990, 29(1):45-8.

Riddle MA, Scahill L, King RA, et al, "Double-Blind, Crossover Trial of Fluoxetine and Placebo in Children and Adolescents With Obsessive-Compulsive Disorder," *J Am Acad Child Adolesc Psychiatry*, 1992, 31(6):1062-9.

Safer DJ and Zito JM, "Treatment Emergent Adverse Effects of Selective Serotonin Reuptake Inhibitors by Age Group: Children vs. Adolescents," *J Child Adolesc Psychopharmacol*, 2006, 16(1/2):159-69.

Sharp SC and Hellings JA, "Efficacy and Safety of Selective Serotonin Reuptake Inhibitors in the Treatment of Depression in Children and Adolescents: Practitioner Review," *Clin Drug Investig*, 2006, 26(5):247-55.

Thomsen PH, "Obsessive-Compulsive Disorder: Pharmacological Treatment," *Eur Child Adolesc Psychiatry*, 2000, 9(Suppl 1):I76-84.

Wagner KD, "Pharmacotherapy for Major Depression in Children and Adolescents," *Prog Neuropsychopharmacol Biol Psychiatry*, 2005, 29(5):819-26.

Weintrob N, Cohen D, Klipper-Aurbach Y, et al, "Decreased Growth During Therapy With Selective Serotonin Reuptake Inhibitors," *Arch Pediatr Adolesc Med*, 2002, 156(7):696-701.

◆ **Fluoxetine (Can)** *see* FLUoxetine *on page 600*

◆ **Fluoxetine Hydrochloride** *see* FLUoxetine *on page 600*

Fluoxymesterone (floo oks i MES te rone)

Medication Safety Issues
Sound-alike/look-alike issues:
Halotestin® may be confused with Haldol®, haloperidol

U.S. Brand Names Androxy™

Therapeutic Category Androgen

Generic Available Yes

Use Replacement of endogenous testicular hormone; in females used as palliative treatment of breast cancer, postpartum breast engorgement

Restrictions C-III

Pregnancy Risk Factor X

Lactation Excretion in breast milk unknown/contraindicated

Contraindications Hypersensitivity to fluoxymesterone or any component (see Warnings); serious cardiac disease, liver or kidney disease

Warnings Some tablets (brand name) contain tartrazine which may cause allergic reactions in susceptible individuals

Precautions May accelerate bone maturation without producing compensatory gain in linear growth; in prepubertal children perform radiographic examination of the hand and wrist every 6 months to determine the rate of bone maturation and to assess the effect of treatment on the epiphyseal centers

Adverse Reactions
Cardiovascular: Edema
Central nervous system: Anxiety, mental depression, headache
Dermatologic: Acne, hirsutism
Endocrine & metabolic: Gynecomastia, amenorrhea, hypercalcemia, female virilization
Gastrointestinal: Nausea
Genitourinary: Priapism
Hematologic: Polycythemia, suppression of clotting factors II, VII, IX, X
Hepatic: Cholestatic hepatitis
Neuromuscular & skeletal: Paresthesia
Miscellaneous: Hypersensitivity reactions

Drug Interactions
Avoid Concomitant Use There are no known interactions where it is recommended to avoid concomitant use.

Increased Effect/Toxicity
Fluoxymesterone may increase the levels/effects of: CycloSPORINE; CycloSPORINE (Systemic); Vitamin K Antagonists

Decreased Effect There are no known significant interactions involving a decrease in effect.

Mechanism of Action Synthetic androgenic anabolic steroid hormone responsible for the normal growth and development of male sex organs and maintenance of secondary sex characteristics; synthetic testosterone derivative with significant androgen activity; stimulates RNA polymerase activity resulting in an increase in protein production; increases bone development

Pharmacokinetics (Adult data unless noted)
Absorption: Oral: Rapid
Protein binding: 98%
Metabolism: In the liver
Half-life: 10-100 minutes
Elimination: Enterohepatic circulation and urinary excretion (90%)

Halogenated derivative of testosterone with up to 5 times the activity of methyltestosterone

Usual Dosage Adults: Oral:
Male:
Hypogonadism: 5-20 mg/day
Delayed puberty: 2.5-20 mg/day for 4-6 months
Female:
Inoperable breast carcinoma: 10-40 mg/day in divided doses for 1-3 months
Breast engorgement: 2.5 mg after delivery, 5-10 mg/day in divided doses for 4-5 days

Monitoring Parameters Periodic radiographic exams of hand and wrist (when used in children); hemoglobin, hematocrit (if receiving high dosages or long-term therapy)

Dosage Forms Excipient information presented when available (limited, particularly for generics); consult specific product labeling.
Tablet: 10 mg
Androxy™: 10 mg

◆ **Flura-Drops®** *see* Fluoride *on page 595*

Flurazepam (flure AZ e pam)

Medication Safety Issues
Sound-alike/look-alike issues:
Flurazepam may be confused with temazepam
Dalmane® may be confused with Demulen®, Dialume®

Beers Criteria medication: This drug may be inappropriate for use in geriatric patients (high severity risk).

Canadian Brand Names Apo-Flurazepam®; Dalmane®; Som Pam

Therapeutic Category Benzodiazepine; Hypnotic; Sedative

Generic Available Yes

Use Short-term treatment of insomnia (FDA approved in ages ≥15 years)

Restrictions C-IV

Medication Guide An FDA-approved patient medication guide, which is available with the product information and at http://www.accessdata.fda.gov/drugsatfda_docs/label/2009/016721s077lbl.pdf, must be dispensed with this medication for each new outpatient prescription and refill.

Pregnancy Risk Factor X

Pregnancy Considerations An increased risk of fetal malformations has been associated with maternal use of other benzodiazepines during the 1st trimester of pregnancy. Neonatal depression has been observed, specifically following exposure to flurazepam when used maternally for 10 consecutive days prior to delivery. Serum levels of N-desalkylflurazepam were measurable in the infant during the first 4 days of life. Use of flurazepam during pregnancy is contraindicated.

Lactation Excretion in breast milk unknown/not recommended

Contraindications Hypersensitivity to flurazepam or any component (there may be cross-sensitivity with other benzodiazepines), pregnancy, pre-existing CNS depression, respiratory depression, narrow-angle glaucoma

Warnings Evaluate patient carefully for medical or psychiatric causes of insomnia prior to initiation of drug treatment; failure of flurazepam to treat insomnia (after 7-10 days of therapy), a worsening of insomnia, the emergence of behavioral changes, or thinking abnormalities may indicate a medical or psychiatric illness requiring evaluation; these effects also have been reported with flurazepam use. Due to possible adverse effects, use lowest effective dose. Abrupt discontinuation after prolonged use may result in withdrawal symptoms or rebound insomnia.

Hypersensitivity reactions including anaphylaxis and angioedema may occur. Hazardous sleep-related activities, such as sleep-driving (driving while not fully awake without any recollection of driving), preparing and eating food, and making phone calls while asleep have also been reported. Effects with other sedative drugs or ethanol may be potentiated.

Precautions Use with caution in patients with depression, chronic pulmonary insufficiency, impaired renal or hepatic function, or low albumin. May cause CNS depression impairing physical and mental capabilities; patients should be cautioned about performing tasks which require mental alertness (operating machinery or driving). Use with caution in patients receiving other CNS depressants or in patients with a history of drug dependence.

Adverse Reactions

Cardiovascular: Chest pain, palpitation, rarely: flushing, hypotension

Central nervous system: Drowsiness, dizziness, lightheadedness, headache, nervousness, talkativeness, irritability, apprehension, ataxia, falling, staggering; residual daytime sedation; rarely: paradoxical reactions (hyperactivity, stimulation, excitement), confusion, depression, euphoria, faintness, hallucinations, hangover effect, memory impairment, restlessness, slurred speech

Dermatologic: Pruritus, rash (rare)

Gastrointestinal: Heartburn, upset stomach, nausea, vomiting, diarrhea, constipation, GI pain; rarely: anorexia, bitter taste, salivation increased/excessive, xerostomia

Hematologic: Rarely: granulocytopenia, leukopenia

Hepatic: Rarely: alkaline phosphatase increased, ALT increased, AST increased, total and direct bilirubin increased

Neuromuscular & skeletal: Body and joint pain, weakness

Ocular: Rarely: blurred vision, burning eyes, difficulty focusing

Respiratory: Rarely: shortness of breath

Miscellaneous: Physical and psychological dependence with prolonged use; hypersensitivity reactions, anaphylaxis, angioedema; hazardous sleep-related activities (see Warnings); diaphoresis (rare)

Drug Interactions

Metabolism/Transport Effects Substrate of CYP3A4 (major); **Inhibits** CYP2E1 (weak)

Avoid Concomitant Use There are no known interactions where it is recommended to avoid concomitant use.

Increased Effect/Toxicity

Flurazepam may increase the levels/effects of: Alcohol (Ethyl); Clozapine; CNS Depressants; Methotrimeprazine; Phenytoin

The levels/effects of Flurazepam may be increased by: Antifungal Agents (Azole Derivatives, Systemic); Aprepitant; Calcium Channel Blockers (Nondihydropyridine); Cimetidine; Contraceptives (Estrogens); Contraceptives (Progestins); CYP3A4 Inhibitors (Moderate); CYP3A4 Inhibitors (Strong); Dasatinib; Fluconazole; Fosamprenavir; Fosaprepitant; Grapefruit Juice; Isoniazid; Macrolide Antibiotics; Methotrimeprazine; Nefazodone; Proton Pump Inhibitors; Ritonavir; Saquinavir; Selective Serotonin Reuptake Inhibitors

Decreased Effect

The levels/effects of Flurazepam may be decreased by: CarBAMazepine; CYP3A4 Inducers (Strong); Deferasirox; Rifamycin Derivatives; St Johns Wort; Theophylline Derivatives; Yohimbine

Stability Dalmane®: Store at controlled room temperature at 25°C (77°F); excursions permitted to 15°C to 30°C (59°F to 86°F)

Generic: Store at controlled room temperature at 20°C to 25°C (68°F to 77°F); protect from light and moisture; dispense in tightly closed, light-resistant container

Mechanism of Action Depresses all levels of the CNS, including the limbic and reticular formation, by binding to the benzodiazepine site on the gamma-aminobutyric acid (GABA) receptor complex and modulating GABA, which is a major inhibitory neurotransmitter in the brain

Pharmacodynamics Hypnotic effects:
Onset of action: 15-20 minutes
Maximum effect: 3-6 hours
Duration: 7-8 hours

Pharmacokinetics (Adult data unless noted)
Absorption: Rapid
Distribution: V_d: Adults: 3.4 L/kg
Protein binding: ~97%
Metabolism: Hepatic to N-desalkylflurazepam (active) and N-hydroxyethylflurazepam
Half-life: Adults:
Flurazepam: Mean: 2.3 hours
N-desalkylflurazepam: Single dose: 74-90 hours; multiple doses: 111-113 hours
Time to peak serum concentration:
Flurazepam: 30–60 minutes
N-desalkylflurazepam: 10.6 hours (range: 7.6-13.6 hours)
N-hydroxyethylflurazepam: ~1 hour
Elimination: Urine: N-hydroxyethylflurazepam (22% to 55%); N-desalkylflurazepam (<1%)

Usual Dosage Oral:
Children:
<15 years: Dose not established; use not recommended by manufacturer
≥15 years: 15 mg at bedtime
Adults: 15-30 mg at bedtime

Administration May be administered without regard to meals; administer dose at bedtime

Patient Information Read the patient Medication Guide that you receive with each prescription and refill of flurazepam. Avoid alcohol and other CNS depressants. May be habit-forming; avoid abrupt discontinuation after prolonged use. May cause dizziness or drowsiness and impair ability to perform activities requiring mental alertness or physical coordination. Take dose immediately before bedtime (not sooner). May also cause daytime drowsiness. May cause dry mouth. May cause hypersensitivity reactions. May cause hazardous sleep-related activities (ie, driving, preparing and eating foods, and making phone calls while not fully awake).

Dosage Forms Excipient information presented when available (limited, particularly for generics); consult specific product labeling.
Capsule, as hydrochloride: 15 mg, 30 mg

References

Cooper SF and Drolet D, "Protein Binding of Flurazepam and Its Major Metabolites in Plasma," *Curr Ther Res*, 1982, 32(5):757-60.
Greenblatt DJ, Harmatz JS, Engelhardt N, et al, "Pharmacokinetic Determinants of Dynamic Differences Among Three Benzodiazepine Hypnotics. Flurazepam, Temazepam, and Triazolam," *Arch Gen Psychiatry*, 1989, 46(4):326-32.
Vozeh S, Schmidlin O, and Taeschner W, "Pharmacokinetic Drug Data," *Clin Pharmacokinet*, 1988, 15(4):254-82.

◆ **Flurazepam Hydrochloride** *see* Flurazepam *on page 604*

Flurbiprofen (flure BI proe fen)

Medication Safety Issues
Sound-alike/look-alike issues:
Flurbiprofen may be confused with fenoprofen
Ansaid® may be confused with Asacol®, Axid®
Ocufen® may be confused with Ocuflox®, Ocupress®
U.S. Brand Names Ocufen®

Canadian Brand Names Alti-Flurbiprofen; Ansaid®; Apo-Flurbiprofen®; Froben-SR®; Froben®; Novo-Flurprofen; Nu-Flurprofen; Ocufen®

Therapeutic Category Analgesic, Non-narcotic; Anti-inflammatory Agent; Anti-inflammatory Agent, Ophthalmic; Nonsteroidal Anti-inflammatory Drug (NSAID), Ophthalmic; Nonsteroidal Anti-inflammatory Drug (NSAID), Oral

Generic Available Yes

Use

Ophthalmic: For inhibition of intraoperative trauma-induced miosis; the value of flurbiprofen for the prevention and management of postoperative ocular inflammation and postoperative cystoid macular edema remains to be determined

Systemic: Management of inflammatory disease and rheumatoid disorders; dysmenorrhea; pain

Medication Guide An FDA-approved patient medication guide, which is available with the product information and at http://www.fda.gov/downloads/Drugs/DrugSafety/ucm085913.pdf, must be dispensed with this medication for each new outpatient prescription and refill.

Pregnancy Risk Factor C

Pregnancy Considerations Adverse events were not observed in the initial animal reproduction studies; therefore, the manufacturer classifies flurbiprofen as pregnancy category C. NSAID exposure during the first trimester is not strongly associated with congenital malformations; however, cardiovascular anomalies and cleft palate have been observed following NSAID exposure in some studies. The use of an NSAID close to conception may be associated with an increased risk of miscarriage. Non-teratogenic effects have been observed following NSAID administration during the third trimester including myocardial degenerative changes, prenatal constriction of the ductus arteriosus, fetal tricuspid regurgitation, failure of the ductus arteriosus to close postnatally; renal dysfunction or failure, oligohydramnios; gastrointestinal bleeding or perforation, increased risk of necrotizing enterocolitis; intracranial bleeding (including intraventricular hemorrhage), platelet dysfunction with resultant bleeding; pulmonary hypertension. Because they may cause premature closure of the ductus arteriosus, use of NSAIDs late in pregnancy should be avoided (use after 31 or 32 weeks gestation is not recommended by some clinicians). The chronic use of NSAIDs in women of reproductive age may be associated with infertility that is reversible upon discontinuation of the medication.

Lactation Enters breast milk/not recommended

Breast-Feeding Considerations Low levels of flurbiprofen are found in breast milk. Breast-feeding is not recommended by the manufacturer. The pharmacokinetics of flurbiprofen immediately postpartum are similar to healthy volunteers.

Contraindications Hypersensitivity to flurbiprofen or any component; history of asthma, urticaria, or allergic-type reaction to aspirin, or other NSAIDs; patients with the "aspirin triad" [asthma, rhinitis (with or without nasal polyps), and aspirin intolerance] (fatal asthmatic and anaphylactoid reactions may occur in these patients); perioperative pain in the setting of coronary artery bypass graft (CABG)

Warnings NSAIDs are associated with an increased risk of adverse cardiovascular thrombotic events, including potentially fatal MI and stroke **[U.S. Boxed Warning]**; risk may be increased with duration of use or pre-existing cardiovascular risk factors or disease; carefully evaluate cardiovascular risk profile prior to prescribing; use the lowest effective dose for the shortest duration of time, taking into consideration individual patient treatment goals; alternate therapies should be considered for patients at high risk. Use is contraindicated for treatment of perioperative pain in the setting of CABG surgery **[U.S.**

Boxed Warning]; an increased incidence of MI and stroke was found in patients receiving COX-2 selective NSAIDs for the treatment of pain within the first 10-14 days after CABG surgery. NSAIDs may cause fluid retention, edema, and new-onset or worsening of pre-existing hypertension; use with caution in patients with hypertension, CHF, or fluid retention. Concurrent administration of ibuprofen, and potentially other nonselective NSAIDs, may interfere with aspirin's cardioprotective effect.

Oral use: NSAIDs may increase the risk of gastrointestinal inflammation, ulceration, bleeding, and perforation **[U.S. Boxed Warning]**. These events, which can be potentially fatal, may occur at any time during therapy, and without warning. Avoid the use of NSAIDs in patients with active GI bleeding or ulcer disease. Use NSAIDs with extreme caution in patients with a history of GI bleeding or ulcers (these patients have a 10-fold increased risk for developing a GI bleed). Use NSAIDs with caution in patients with other risk factors which may increase GI bleeding (eg, concurrent therapy with aspirin, anticoagulants, and/or corticosteroids, longer duration of NSAID use, smoking, use of alcohol, and poor general health). Use the lowest effective dose for the shortest duration of time, taking into consideration individual patient treatment goals; alternate therapies should be considered for patients at high risk.

NSAIDs may compromise existing renal function. Renal toxicity may occur in patients with impaired renal function, dehydration, heart failure, liver dysfunction, those taking diuretics and ACE inhibitors; use with caution in these patients; monitor renal function closely. NSAIDs are not recommended for use in patients with advanced renal disease. Long-term use of NSAIDs may cause renal papillary necrosis and other renal injury.

Fatal asthmatic and anaphylactoid reactions may occur in patients with the "aspirin triad" who receive NSAIDs (see Contraindications). NSAIDs may cause serious dermatologic adverse reactions including exfoliative dermatitis, Stevens-Johnson syndrome, and toxic epidermal necrolysis. Avoid use of NSAIDs in late pregnancy as they may cause premature closure of the ductus arteriosus.

Ocular use: An increased bleeding of ocular tissues may occur in conjunction with ocular surgery

Precautions Use oral form with caution in renal or hepatic impairment, GI disease, cardiac disease, and patients receiving anticoagulants

Adverse Reactions

Cardiovascular: Edema

Central nervous system: Headache, fatigue, drowsiness, vertigo

Dermatologic: Pruritus, rash

Gastrointestinal: Abdominal discomfort, nausea, heartburn, constipation, vomiting, GI bleeding, ulcers, perforation

Hematologic: Thrombocytopenia, inhibits platelet aggregation; prolongs bleeding time; agranulocytosis; bleeding of ocular tissues with ocular surgery increased (ophthalmic use)

Hepatic: Hepatitis

Ocular: Slowing of corneal wound healing, mild ocular stinging, itching, burning, ocular irritation

Otic: Tinnitus

Renal: Renal dysfunction

Drug Interactions

Metabolism/Transport Effects Substrate of CYP2C9 (minor); **Inhibits** CYP2C9 (strong)

Avoid Concomitant Use

Avoid concomitant use of Flurbiprofen with any of the following: Ketorolac; Ketorolac (Systemic)

Increased Effect/Toxicity

Flurbiprofen may increase the levels/effects of: Aminoglycosides; Anticoagulants; Antiplatelet Agents; Bisphosphonate Derivatives; Collagenase (Systemic); CycloSPORINE; CycloSPORINE (Systemic); Desmopressin; Digoxin; Drotrecogin Alfa; Eplerenone; Haloperidol; Ibritumomab; Lithium; Methotrexate; Nonsteroidal Anti-Inflammatory Agents; Pemetrexed; Potassium-Sparing Diuretics; Pralatrexate; Quinolone Antibiotics; Salicylates; Thrombolytic Agents; Tositumomab and Iodine I 131 Tositumomab; Vancomycin; Vitamin K Antagonists

The levels/effects of Flurbiprofen may be increased by: Antidepressants (Tricyclic, Tertiary Amine); Corticosteroids (Systemic); Dasatinib; Glucosamine; Herbs (Anticoagulant/Antiplatelet Properties); Ketorolac; Ketorolac (Systemic); Nonsteroidal Anti-Inflammatory Agents; Omega-3-Acid Ethyl Esters; Pentosan Polysulfate Sodium; Pentoxifylline; Probenecid; Prostacyclin Analogues; Selective Serotonin Reuptake Inhibitors; Serotonin/Norepinephrine Reuptake Inhibitors; Treprostinil

Decreased Effect

Flurbiprofen may decrease the levels/effects of: ACE Inhibitors; Angiotensin II Receptor Blockers; Antiplatelet Agents; Beta-Blockers; Eplerenone; HydrALAZINE; Latanoprost; Loop Diuretics; Potassium-Sparing Diuretics; Salicylates; Thiazide Diuretics

The levels/effects of Flurbiprofen may be decreased by: Bile Acid Sequestrants; Nonsteroidal Anti-Inflammatory Agents; Salicylates

Food Interactions Food may decrease the rate but not the extent of absorption

Mechanism of Action Inhibits prostaglandin synthesis by decreasing the activity of the enzyme, cyclooxygenase, which results in decreased formation of prostaglandin precursors

Pharmacokinetics (Adult data unless noted) Oral:
Time to peak serum concentration: Within 1.5-2 hours
Elimination: 95% in urine

Usual Dosage

Children and Adults: Ophthalmic: Instill 1 drop every 30 minutes starting 2 hours prior to surgery (total of 4 drops to each affected eye)

Adults: Oral:
Arthritis: 200-300 mg/day in 2-4 divided doses; maximum dose: 100 mg/dose; maximum: 300 mg/day
Dysmenorrhea: 50 mg 4 times/day

Administration

Oral: Administer with food, milk, or antacid to decrease GI effects

Ophthalmic: Instill drops into affected eye(s); avoid contact of container tip with skin or eye; apply finger pressure to lacrimal sac during and for 1-2 minutes after instillation to decrease risk of absorption and systemic effects

Monitoring Parameters Systemic use: CBC, platelets, BUN, serum creatinine, liver enzymes, occult blood loss; ocular use: Periodic eye exams

Patient Information Ophthalmic solution may cause mild burning or stinging, notify physician if this becomes severe or is persistent

Dosage Forms Excipient information presented when available (limited, particularly for generics); consult specific product labeling.
Solution, ophthalmic, as sodium: 0.03% (2.5 mL)
Ocufen®: 0.03% (2.5 mL)
Tablet: 50 mg, 100 mg

♦ **Flurbiprofen Sodium** *see* Flurbiprofen *on page 605*

♦ **5-Flurocytosine** *see* Flucytosine *on page 586*

Fluticasone (floo TIK a sone)

Medication Safety Issues

Sound-alike/look-alike issues:
Cutivate® may be confused with Ultravate®
Flonase® may be confused with Flovent®
Flovent® may be confused with Flonase®

International issues:
Allegro® [Israel] may be confused with Allegra® which is a brand name for fexofenadine in the U.S.
Allegro®: Brand name for frovatriptan in Germany
Flovent® may be confused with Flogen® which is a brand name for naproxen in Mexico

Related Information

Asthma *on page 1697*
Corticosteroids *on page 1487*

U.S. Brand Names Cutivate®; Flonase®; Flovent® Diskus®; Flovent® HFA; Veramyst®

Canadian Brand Names Apo-Fluticasone®; Avamys®; Cutivate™; Flonase®; Flovent® Diskus®; Flovent® HFA; ratio-Fluticasone

Therapeutic Category Adrenal Corticosteroid; Anti-inflammatory Agent; Antiasthmatic; Corticosteroid, Inhalant (Oral); Corticosteroid, Intranasal; Corticosteroid, Topical; Glucocorticoid

Generic Available Yes: Cream, nasal spray, ointment

Use

Oral inhalation: Long-term (chronic) control of persistent bronchial asthma; **NOT** indicated for the relief of acute bronchospasm. Also used to help reduce or discontinue oral corticosteroid therapy for asthma (FDA approved in ages ≥4 years and adults; see Additional Information)

Intranasal:
Flonase®: Management of seasonal and perennial allergic rhinitis and nonallergic rhinitis (FDA approved in ages ≥4 years and adults)
Veramyst®: Management of seasonal and perennial allergic rhinitis (FDA approved in ages ≥2 years and adults)

Topical:
Cream: Relief of inflammation and pruritus associated with corticosteroid-responsive dermatoses (eg, atopic dermatitis) [medium potency topical corticosteroid] (FDA approved in ages ≥3 months and adults)
Lotion: Relief of inflammation and pruritus associated with atopic dermatitis (FDA approved in ages ≥1 year and adults)
Ointment: Relief of inflammation and pruritus associated with corticosteroid-responsive dermatoses [medium potency topical corticosteroid] (FDA approved in adults)

Oral (swallowed; using metered dose inhaler): Has been used for eosinophilic esophagitis

Pregnancy Risk Factor C

Pregnancy Considerations Adverse events have been observed with systemic corticosteroids in animal reproduction studies; teratogenic effects were not observed following administration of fluticasone furoate via inhalation to pregnant rats or rabbits. A decrease in fetal growth has not been observed with inhaled corticosteroid use during pregnancy. Inhaled corticosteroids are recommended for the treatment of asthma (most information available using budesonide) and allergic rhinitis during pregnancy. In general, the use of topical corticosteroids during pregnancy is not considered to have significant risk; however, intrauterine growth retardation in the infant has been reported (rare). The use of large amounts or for prolonged periods of time should be avoided.

Lactation Excretion in breast milk unknown/use caution

Breast-Feeding Considerations Systemic corticosteroids are excreted in human milk. It is not known if sufficient quantities of fluticasone are absorbed following topical administration or inhalation to produce detectable amounts in breast milk. Hypertension in the nursing infant has been reported following corticosteroid ointment applied to the nipples. Use with caution. The use of inhaled corticosteroids is not considered a contraindication to breast-feeding.

Contraindications Hypersensitivity to fluticasone or any component (see Warnings); primary treatment of status asthmaticus

Warnings Fatalities have occurred due to adrenal insufficiency in asthmatic patients during and after switching from systemic corticosteroids to aerosol steroids (see Additional Information); several months may be required for full recovery of hypothalamic-pituitary-adrenal (HPA) axis function; patients receiving higher doses of systemic corticosteroids (eg, adults receiving ≥20 mg of prednisone per day) may be at greater risk; during this period of HPA axis suppression, aerosol steroids do **not** provide the systemic glucocorticoid or mineralocorticoid activity needed to treat patients requiring stress doses (ie, patients with major stress such as trauma, surgery, or infections, or other conditions associated with severe electrolyte loss). When used at high doses or for a prolonged time, hypercorticism and HPA axis suppression (including adrenal crisis) may occur; use with inhaled or systemic corticosteroids (even alternate-day dosing) may increase risk of HPA axis suppression. Acute adrenal insufficiency may occur with abrupt withdrawal after long-term use or with stress; withdrawal and discontinuation of corticosteroids should be done carefully; patients with HPA axis suppression may require doses of systemic glucocorticosteroids prior to, during, and after unusual stress (eg, surgery). Immunosuppression may occur; patients may be more susceptible to infections; avoid exposure to chickenpox and measles. Switching patients from systemic corticosteroids to aerosol steroids may unmask allergic conditions previously treated by the systemic steroid. Bronchospasm may occur after use of inhaled asthma medications (see Additional Information).

Potent inhibitors of cytochrome P450 isoenzyme CYP3A4 (eg, ritonavir) may significantly increase fluticasone serum concentrations and result in systemic corticosteroid effects (see Drug Interactions). Powder for oral inhalation (Flovent® Diskus®) contains lactose (milk proteins) which may cause allergic reactions in patients with severe milk protein allergy.

Topical use: Adverse systemic effects may occur when topical steroids are used on large areas of the body, denuded areas, for prolonged periods of time, with an occlusive dressing, and/or in infants or small children; infants and small children may be more susceptible to HPA axis suppression or other systemic toxicities due to a larger skin surface area to body mass ratio; use with caution in pediatric patients; do not use for the treatment of rosacea, perioral dermatitis, or in the presence of skin atrophy or infection at treatment site. Cutivate® lotion contains imidurea, an excipient; imidurea releases trace amounts of formaldehyde which may cause irritation or allergic sensitization upon contact with skin. Discontinue lotion if irritation occurs and institute appropriate therapy.

Intranasal use: Hypersensitivity reactions, including anaphylaxis, angioedema, rash, and urticaria, may occur; discontinue use if hypersensitivity reaction occurs.

Precautions Avoid using higher than recommended doses; suppression of HPA function, suppression of linear growth (ie, reduction of growth velocity), reduced bone mineral density, hypercorticism (Cushing's syndrome), hyperglycemia, or glucosuria may occur; these adverse effects (as well as intracranial hypertension) may occur with topical use and have been reported in pediatric patients (see also Additional Information). Use with extreme caution in patients with respiratory tuberculosis, untreated systemic infections, or ocular herpes simplex. Use with caution and monitor patients closely with hepatic dysfunction. Eosinophilic conditions (eosinophilia, vasculitic rash, cardiac complications, worsening pulmonary symptoms, and/or neuropathy) may occur and are usually associated with withdrawal or decrease of oral corticosteroids after the initiation of fluticasone (oral inhalation); a causal relationship by fluticasone has not been established. Increased IOP, glaucoma, and cataracts may occur with long-term use of inhaled corticosteroids.

Epistaxis and nasal ulceration may occur with intranasal use. Nasal septum perforation has been reported with intranasal use of corticosteroids. Corticosteroids impair wound healing; do not use intranasal fluticasone in patients with recent nasal ulcers, nasal surgery, or nasal trauma; allow healing to occur before use.

Adverse Reactions
Central nervous system: Dizziness, fatigue, fever, headache, insomnia, malaise, migraines, mood disorders

Dermatologic:

Intranasal use: Angioedema, facial edema, rash, urticaria

Inhalational use: Dermatitis, facial edema, rash

Topical use: Acne, allergic dermatitis, dry skin, excoriation, folliculitis, hypertrichosis, hypopigmentation, itching, maceration of the skin, numbness of fingers, pruritus, skin atrophy, stinging at application site, striae, telanglectasia

Endocrine & metabolic: Cushing's syndrome, growth suppression, HPA axis suppression, hyperglycemia, reduction of growth velocity, weight gain

Gastrointestinal: Diarrhea, dyspepsia, nausea, vomiting

Local: Burning, irritation; growth of *Candida* in the mouth, nares, or throat

Neuromuscular & skeletal: Bone mineral density decreased, muscular soreness, osteoporosis

Ocular: Cataracts, eye pain, glaucoma, IOP increased

Respiratory: Nasal congestion, nasal discharge, oropharyngeal edema, pharyngitis, respiratory infection, rhinitis, sinus infection, sinusitis, throat irritation, upper respiratory inflammation

Oral inhalation: Bronchitis, bronchospasm, cough, dysphonia, hoarseness

Intranasal: Epistaxis, nasal burning, nasal irritation, nasal ulceration

Miscellaneous: Anaphylactic reaction (very rare), eosinophilic conditions (see Precautions), secondary infection

<1%, postmarketing, and/or case reports: Aggression, agitation, anxiety, aphonia, asthma exacerbation, behavioral changes (eg, hyperactivity and irritability in children; rare), chest tightness, Churg-Strauss syndrome, contusion, cutaneous hypersensitivity, depression, dyspnea, ecchymoses, eosinophilia, hypersensitivity reactions (immediate and delayed), oropharyngeal edema, restlessness, throat soreness, vasculitis, wheeze

Drug Interactions
Metabolism/Transport Effects Substrate of CYP3A4 (major)

Avoid Concomitant Use

Avoid concomitant use of Fluticasone with any of the following: Aldesleukin; BCG; Natalizumab; Pimecrolimus; Tacrolimus (Topical); Vaccines (Live)

Increased Effect/Toxicity

Fluticasone may increase the levels/effects of: Amphotericin B; Leflunomide; Loop Diuretics; Natalizumab; Thiazide Diuretics; Vaccines (Live)

The levels/effects of Fluticasone may be increased by: Antifungal Agents (Azole Derivatives, Systemic); CYP3A4 Inhibitors (Moderate); CYP3A4 Inhibitors (Strong); Dasatinib; Denosumab; Pimecrolimus; Protease Inhibitors; Tacrolimus (Topical); Trastuzumab

Decreased Effect

Fluticasone may decrease the levels/effects of: Aldesleukin; Antidiabetic Agents; BCG; Corticorelin; Sipuleucel-T; Vaccines (Inactivated); Vaccines (Live)

The levels/effects of Fluticasone may be decreased by: Echinacea

Stability

Oral inhalation:

Flovent® HFA: Store at controlled room temperature of 25°C (77°F) with mouthpiece down. Do not use or store near heat or open flame. Do not expose to temperatures >120°F. Do not puncture or incinerate. Discard device when the dose counter reads "000."

Diskus®: Store at controlled room temperature; keep dry; protect from direct heat or sunlight; discard Diskus® 6 weeks (for 50 mcg strength) or 2 months (for 100 mcg and 250 mcg strengths) after opening moistureproof foil overwrap or when dose indicator reads "0" (whichever comes first); **Note:** Diskus® device is not reusable.

Intranasal:

Flonase®: Store between 4°C to 30°C (39°F to 86°F)

Veramyst®: Store between 15°C to 30°C (59°F to 86°F) in upright position. Do not refrigerate or freeze.

Topical:

Cream, ointment: Store at 2°C to 30°C (36°F to 86°F)

Lotion: Store at 15°C to 30°C (59°F to 86°F); do not refrigerate; keep tightly closed

Mechanism of Action Controls the rate of protein synthesis, depresses the migration of polymorphonuclear leukocytes and fibroblasts, reverses capillary permeability, and stabilizes lysosomal membranes at the cellular level to prevent or control inflammation

Pharmacodynamics

Oral inhalation: Clinical effects are due to direct local effect rather than systemic absorption

Onset of action: Variable; may occur within 24 hours

Maximum effect: 1-2 weeks or more

Duration after discontinuation: Several days or more

Pharmacokinetics (Adult data unless noted)

Distribution: V_d: Adults: 4.2 L/kg

Protein binding: 91% to 99%

Metabolism: Via cytochrome P450 3A4 pathway to 17β-carboxylic acid (inactive)

Bioavailability: Oral inhalation: Flovent®: 30% of dose delivered from actuator; Flovent® HFA: 30% lower than Flovent®; Diskus®: 18%

Half-life: 7.8 hours

Usual Dosage

Intranasal: Note: For optimal effects, nasal spray should be used at regular intervals (eg, once or twice daily); however, some adolescent patients ≥12 years of age and adults with seasonal allergic rhinitis may have effective control of symptoms with prn (as needed) use

Flonase®:

Children <4 years: Not recommended

Children ≥4 years and Adolescents: Initial: 1 spray (50 mcg/spray) to each nostril daily (100 mcg/day); if response is inadequate, give 2 sprays to each nostril daily (200 mcg/day); once symptoms are controlled, reduce dose to 100 mcg/day (1 spray to each nostril daily); maximum dose: 200 mcg/day (4 sprays/day)

Adults: Initial: 200 mcg/day given as 2 sprays (50 mcg/ spray) to each nostril daily or 1 spray to each nostril twice daily; dosage may be reduced to 100 mcg/day (1 spray to each nostril daily) after the first few days if symptoms are controlled; maximum dose: 200 mcg/ day (4 sprays/day)

Veramyst®:

Children <2 years: Not recommended

Children 2-11 years: Initial: 1 spray (27.5 mcg/spray) to each nostril daily (55 mcg/day); if response is inadequate, give 2 sprays to each nostril daily (110 mcg/day); once symptoms have been controlled, the dosage may be reduced to 55 mcg/day (1 spray to each nostril daily); maximum dose: 110 mcg/day (4 sprays/day)

Children >11 years and Adults: Initial: 2 sprays (27.5 mcg/spray) to each nostril daily (110 mcg/day); once symptoms are controlled, dosage may be reduced to 55 mcg/day (1 spray to each nostril daily); maximum dose: 110 mcg/day (4 sprays/day)

Oral inhalation: If adequate response is not seen after 2 weeks of initial dosage, increase dosage; doses should be titrated to the lowest effective dose once asthma is controlled:

Inhalation aerosol (Flovent® HFA): Manufacturer's recommendations:

Children 4-11 years: Initial: 88 mcg twice daily; maximum dose: 88 mcg twice daily

Children ≥12 years and Adults:

Patients previously treated with bronchodilators only: Initial: 88 mcg twice daily; maximum dose: 440 mcg twice daily

Patients treated with an inhaled corticosteroid: Initial: 88-220 mcg twice daily; maximum dose: 440 mcg twice daily; may start doses above 88 mcg twice daily in poorly controlled patients or in those who previously required higher doses of inhaled corticosteroids

Patients previously treated with oral corticosteroids: 440 mcg twice daily; maximum dose: 880 mcg twice daily

NIH Asthma Guidelines (NAEPP, 2007) [give in divided doses twice daily]:

Children <12 years:

"Low" dose: 88-176 mcg/day (44 mcg/puff: 2-4 puffs/ day)

"Medium" dose: >176-352 mcg/day (44 mcg/puff: 4-8 puffs/day or 110 mcg/puff: 2-3 puffs/day)

"High" dose: >352 mcg/day (110 mcg/puff: >3 puffs/ day or 220 mcg/puff: >1 puff/day)

Children ≥12 years and Adults:

"Low" dose: 88-264 mcg/day (44 mcg/puff: 2-6 puffs/ day or 110 mcg/puff: 2 puffs/day)

"Medium" dose: >264-440 mcg/day (110 mcg/puff: 2-4 puffs/day)

"High" dose: >440 mcg/day (110 mcg/puff: >4 puffs/ day or 220 mcg/puff: >2 puffs/day)

Inhalation powder (Flovent® Diskus®): Manufacturer's recommendations:

Children 4-11 years: Patients previously treated with bronchodilators alone or inhaled corticosteroids: Initial: 50 mcg twice daily; maximum dose: 100 mcg twice daily; may start higher initial dose in poorly controlled patients or in those who previously required higher doses of inhaled corticosteroids

Adolescents and Adults:

Patients previously treated with bronchodilators alone: Initial: 100 mcg twice daily; maximum dose: 500 mcg twice daily

Patients previously treated with inhaled corticosteroids: Initial: 100-250 mcg twice daily; maximum dose: 500 mcg twice daily; may start doses above 100 mcg twice daily in poorly controlled patients or in those who previously required higher doses of inhaled corticosteroids

Patients previously treated with oral corticosteroids: Initial: 500-1000 mcg twice daily (select dose based on assessment of individual patient); maximum dose: 1000 mcg twice daily; **Note:** Inability to reduce oral corticosteroid therapy (see Additional Information) may indicate need for maximum fluticasone dose.

NIH Asthma Guidelines (NAEPP, 2007) [give in divided doses twice daily]:

Children 5-11 years:

"Low" dose: 100-200 mcg/day (50 mcg/puff: 2-4 puffs/day or 100 mcg/puff: 1-2 puffs/day)

"Medium" dose: >200-400 mcg/day (50 mcg/puff: 4-8 puffs/day or 100 mcg/puff: 2-4 puffs/day)

"High" dose: >400 mcg/day (50 mcg/puff: >8 puffs/day or 100 mcg/puff: >4 puffs/day)

Children ≥12 years and Adults:

"Low" dose: 100-300 mcg/day (50 mcg/puff: 2-6 puffs/day or 100 mcg/puff: 1-3 puffs/day)

"Medium" dose: >300-500 mcg/day (50 mcg/puff: 6-10 puffs/day or 100 mcg/puff: 3-5 puffs/day)

"High" dose: >500 mcg/day (50 mcg/puff: >10 puffs/day or 100 mcg/puff: >5 puffs/day)

Oral (swallowed): Note: Patients use an oral inhaler without a spacer and swallow the medication.

Children: Eosinophilic esophagitis: Optimal dose and dosing regimen are **not** established. Dosing from two more recent studies is presented.

A randomized, double-blind, placebo-controlled trial (n=31) demonstrated efficacy by assessment of histologic remission (see Konikoff, 2006): Children: 3-16 years: 440 mcg twice daily for 3 months

A prospective, randomized trial (n=80) compared swallowed fluticasone to oral prednisone; a greater degree of improvement in histologic response was seen in the prednisone group; however, no difference in clinical response was observed between the two groups (see Additional Information and Schaffer, 2008):

Children: 1-10 years: 220 mcg 4 times daily for 4 weeks, 220 mcg 3 times daily for 3 weeks, 220 mcg twice daily for 3 weeks, 220 mcg daily for 2 weeks

Children and Adolescents: 11-18 years: 440 mcg 4 times daily for 4 weeks, 440 mcg 3 times daily for 3 weeks, 440 mcg twice daily for 3 weeks, 440 mcg daily for 2 weeks

Topical:

Cream:

Infants <3 months: Not approved for use; safety and efficacy not established

Infants ≥3 months, Children, and Adults: **Note:** Safety and efficacy of use >4 weeks in pediatric patients have not been established:

Atopic dermatitis: Apply a thin film to affected area once or twice daily

Other dermatoses: Apply a thin film to affected area twice daily

Lotion:

Infants <1 year: Not approved for use; safety and efficacy not established

Children ≥1 year and Adults: **Note:** Safety and efficacy of use >4 weeks has not been established:

Atopic dermatitis: Apply a thin film to affected area once daily

Ointment:

Pediatric patients: Not approved for use (due to potential for adrenal suppression)

Adults: Apply sparingly in a thin film twice daily

Dosage adjustment in hepatic impairment: Use with caution; monitor patients closely; **Note:** Fluticasone is primarily eliminated via hepatic metabolism and serum concentrations may be elevated in patients with hepatic disease.

Administration

Intranasal spray: Shake bottle gently before use; clear nasal passages by blowing nose prior to use. Insert applicator into nostril, keeping bottle upright, and close off the other nostril; breathe in through nose; while inhaling,

press pump to release spray. Avoid spraying into eyes. Discard after labeled number of doses has been used, even if bottle is not completely empty.

Flonase®: Prime pump (press 6 times until fine spray appears) prior to first use or if spray unused for ≥7 days.

Veramyst®: Prime pump (press 6 times until fine spray appears) prior to first use, if spray unused for >30 days, or if cap left off bottle for ≥5 days.

Oral inhalation: Rinse mouth with water (without swallowing) after inhalation to decrease chance of oral candidiasis

Aerosol inhalation: Shake canister well for 5 seconds before each spray; use at room temperature. Inhaler must be primed before first use with four test sprays (spray into air away from face, shake well for 5 seconds between sprays) and primed again with one test spray if not used for >7 days or if dropped. Use a spacer device for children <8 years of age. Patient should contact pharmacy for refill when the dose counter reads "020." Discard device when the dose counter reads "000." Do not try to alter numbers on counter or remove the counter from the metal canister. Do not immerse canister into water (ie, do not use "float test" to determine contents).

Powder for oral inhalation: Flovent® Diskus®: Do not use with spacer device; do not exhale into Diskus®; do not wash or take apart; activate and use Diskus® in horizontal position

Oral (swallowed): **Note:** This method of administration is for treatment of eosinophilic esophagitis only. Use metered dose inhaler. Do not use a spacer. Shake canister well for 5 seconds before each spray. Prime inhaler as outlined above. Actuate inhaler and spray medication into pharynx; swallow the medication (rather than inhale). Do not eat, drink, or rinse mouth for 30 minutes following administration (see Konikoff, 2006 and Schaefer, 2008).

Topical: Apply sparingly to affected area, gently rub in until disappears; do not use on open skin; avoid application on face, underarms, or groin area unless directed by physician; avoid contact with eyes; do not occlude area unless directed; do not apply to diaper area

Monitoring Parameters Oral inhalation: Check mucus membranes for signs of fungal infection; monitor growth in pediatric patients; monitor IOP with therapy >6 weeks. Monitor for symptoms of asthma, FEV$_1$, peak flow, and/or other pulmonary function tests. Assess HPA suppression in patients using potent topical steroids applied to a large surface area or to areas under occlusion.

Patient Information Notify physician if condition being treated persists or worsens; do not decrease dose or discontinue without physician approval. Avoid exposure to chicken pox or measles; if exposed, seek medical advice without delay. May cause headache. Notify physician immediately if allergic symptoms develop. Report signs of infection or change in vision to prescriber.

Oral inhalation: Report sore mouth or mouth lesions to physician; carefully read and follow the Patient's Instructions for Use leaflet that accompanies the product

Additional Information Flovent® HFA does **not** contain CFCs as the propellant; Flovent® HFA is packaged in a plastic-coated, moisture-protective foil pouch that also contains a desiccant; the desiccant should be discarded when the pouch is opened.

When using fluticasone oral inhalation to help reduce or discontinue oral corticosteroid therapy, begin prednisone taper after at least 1 week of fluticasone inhalation therapy; do not decrease prednisone faster than 2.5 mg/day on a weekly basis; monitor patients for signs of asthma instability and adrenal insufficiency (see Warnings); decrease fluticasone to lowest effective dose **after** prednisone reduction is complete. If bronchospasm with wheezing occurs after oral inhalation use, a fast-acting bronchodilator may be used; discontinue orally inhaled corticosteroid and initiate alternative chronic therapy.

Topical: HPA axis suppression occurred in 2 children (2 and 5 years old) of 43 pediatric patients treated topically with fluticasone cream for 4 weeks; application covered at least 35% of body surface area

Nasal spray: In a small pediatric study conducted over 1 year, no statistically significant effect on growth velocity or clinically relevant changes in bone mineral density or HPA axis function were observed in children 3-9 years of age receiving fluticasone nasal spray (200 mcg/day; n=56) versus placebo (n=52); effects at higher doses or in susceptible pediatric patients cannot be ruled out

Oral (swallowed) use: In the study by Schaffer that compared swallowed fluticasone to oral prednisone, systemic adverse effects occurred more frequently in the oral prednisone group; esophageal candidiasis occurred in 15% of patients using swallowed fluticasone (see Schaffer, 2008).

Dosage Forms Excipient information presented when available (limited, particularly for generics); consult specific product labeling. [CAN] = Canadian brand name
Aerosol for oral inhalation, as propionate:
Flovent® HFA: 44 mcg/inhalation (10.6 g) [chlorofluorocarbon free; 120 metered actuations]
Flovent® HFA: 110 mcg/inhalation (12 g) [chlorofluorocarbon free; 120 metered actuations]
Flovent® HFA: 220 mcg/inhalation (12 g) [chlorofluorocarbon free; 120 metered actuations]
Cream, topical, as propionate: 0.05% (15 g, 30 g, 60 g)
Cutivate®: 0.05% (30 g, 60 g)
Lotion, topical, as propionate:
Cutivate®: 0.05% (120 mL)
Ointment, topical, as propionate: 0.005% (15 g, 30 g, 60 g)
Cutivate®: 0.005% (30 g, 60 g)
Powder, for oral inhalation, as propionate:
Flovent® Diskus® [U.S.]: 50 mcg (60s) [contains lactose; prefilled blister pack]
Flovent® Diskus® [U.S.]: 100 mcg (60s) [contains lactose; prefilled blister pack]
Flovent® Diskus® [U.S.]: 250 mcg (60s) [contains lactose; prefilled blister pack]
Flovent® Diskus® [CAN]: 50 mcg (28s, 60s) [contains lactose; prefilled blister pack] [not available in the U.S.]
Flovent® Diskus® [CAN]: 100 mcg (28s, 60s) [contains lactose; prefilled blister pack] [not available in the U.S.]
Flovent® Diskus® [CAN]: 250 mcg (28s, 60s) [contains lactose; prefilled blister pack] [not available in the U.S.]
Flovent® Diskus® [CAN]: 500 mcg (28s, 60s) [contains lactose; prefilled blister pack] [not available in the U.S.]
Suspension, intranasal, as furoate [spray]:
Avamys® [CAN]: 27.5 mcg/inhalation (4.5 g) [30 metered actuations; contains benzalkonium chloride]; (10 g) [120 metered actuations; contains benzalkonium chloride] [not available in the U.S.]
Veramyst®: 27.5 mcg/inhalation (10 g) [120 metered actuations; contains benzalkonium chloride]
Suspension, intranasal, as propionate [spray]: 50 mcg/inhalation (16 g)
Flonase®: 50 mcg/inhalation (16 g) [120 metered actuations; contains benzalkonium chloride]

References

Konikoff MR, Noel RJ, Blanchard C, et al, "A Randomized, Double-Blind, Placebo-Controlled Trial of Fluticasone Propionate for Pediatric Eosinophilic Esophagitis," *Gastroenterology*, 2006, 131(5):1381-91.
National Asthma Education and Prevention Program (NAEPP), "Expert Panel Report 3 (EPR-3): Guidelines for the Diagnosis and Management of Asthma," *Clinical Practice Guidelines*, National Institutes of Health, National Heart, Lung, and Blood Institute, NIH Publication No. 08-4051, prepublication 2007; available at http://www.nhlbi.nih.gov/guidelines/asthma/asthgdln.htm.
Schaffer ET, Fitzgerald JF, Molleston JP, et al, "Comparison of Oral Prednisone and Topical Fluticasone in the Treatment of Eosinophilic Esophagitis: A Randomized Trial in Children," *Clin Gastroenterol Hepatol*, 2008, 6(2):165-73.

Fluticasone and Salmeterol
(floo TIK a sone & sal ME te role)

Medication Safety Issues
Sound-alike/look-alike issues:
Advair® may be confused with Adcirca™, Advicor®
Related Information
Asthma *on page 1697*
U.S. Brand Names Advair Diskus®; Advair® HFA
Canadian Brand Names Advair Diskus®; Advair®
Therapeutic Category Adrenal Corticosteroid; Adrenergic Agonist Agent; Anti-inflammatory Agent; Antiasthmatic; Beta$_2$-Adrenergic Agonist Agent; Bronchodilator; Corticosteroid, Inhalant (Oral); Glucocorticoid
Generic Available No
Use
Advair Diskus®, Advair® HFA: Maintenance treatment of asthma
Advair Diskus®: Maintenance treatment of airflow obstruction in patients with COPD associated with chronic bronchitis
Medication Guide An FDA-approved patient medication guide, which is available with the product information and as follows, must be dispensed with this medication for each new outpatient prescription and refill.
Advair Diskus®: http://www.fda.gov/downloads/Drugs/DrugSafety/ucm111326.pdf
Advair® HFA: http://www.fda.gov/downloads/Drugs/DrugSafety/ucm111333.pdf
Pregnancy Risk Factor C
Pregnancy Considerations See individual agents.
Lactation
Fluticasone: Excretion in breast milk unknown/use caution
Salmeterol: Enters breast milk/use caution
Contraindications Hypersensitivity to salmeterol, adrenergic amines, fluticasone, or any component; primary treatment of status asthmaticus or other acute episodes of asthma or COPD
Warnings Fatalities have occurred due to adrenal insufficiency in asthmatic patients during and after switching from systemic corticosteroids to aerosol steroids; several months may be required for full recovery of the adrenal glands; patients receiving higher doses of systemic corticosteroids (eg, adults receiving ≥20 mg of prednisone per day) may be at greater risk; during this period of adrenal suppression, aerosol steroids do not provide the systemic corticosteroid needed to treat patients requiring stress doses (ie, patients with major stress such as trauma, surgery, or infections); when used at high doses or for a prolonged time, hypercorticism and hypothalamic-pituitary-adrenal (HPA) suppression (including adrenal crisis) may occur; withdrawal and discontinuation of corticosteroid therapy should be done carefully. Immunosuppression may occur. Prolonged use of corticosteroids may also increase the incidence of secondary infection, mask acute infection (including pneumonia and fungal infection), prolong or exacerbate viral infection, or limit response to vaccines; lower respiratory tract infections, including pneumonia, have been reported in patients with COPD using the oral inhalation with an even higher incidence in the elderly. Advair® should not be used for transferring patients from systemic corticosteroid therapy.

Long-acting beta$_2$ adrenergic agents (eg, salmeterol) have been associated with an increased risk of asthma-related death **[U.S. Boxed Warning]**. Salmeterol should only be prescribed in patients not adequately controlled on other asthma-controller medications or whose disease severity clearly warrants treatment with two maintenance therapies. A medication guide is available to provide information to patients covering the risk of use. Advair® should not be used in conjunction with other inhaled, long-acting beta$_2$ agonists.

Fluticasone/salmeterol is not intended to relieve acute asthmatic symptoms. Acute episodes should be treated with short-acting beta$_2$ agonist. Do not increase the frequency of fluticasone/salmeterol use. Paroxysmal bronchospasm (which can be fatal) has been reported with this and other inhaled beta$_2$-agonist agents. If paroxysmal bronchospasm occurs, discontinue treatment; symptoms of laryngeal spasm, irritation, or swelling, such as stridor and choking, have been reported in patients receiving fluticasone/salmeterol; if occurs, discontinue treatment.

Precautions Use with caution in patients with cardiovascular disorders, convulsive disorders, thyrotoxicosis, or others who are sensitive to the effects of sympathomimetic amines; avoid using higher than recommended doses; suppression of HPA function, suppression of linear growth, or hypercorticism (Cushing's syndrome) may occur; use with extreme caution in patients with respiratory tuberculosis, untreated systemic infections, or ocular herpes simplex; use with caution and monitor patients closely with hepatic dysfunction; eosinophilic conditions (eosinophilia, vasculitic rash, cardiac complications, worsening pulmonary symptoms, and/or neuropathy) may occur and are usually associated with withdrawal or decrease of oral corticosteroids after the initiation of fluticasone oral inhalation; a causal relationship by fluticasone has not been established.

Adverse Reactions See individual agents.

Drug Interactions

Metabolism/Transport Effects Fluticasone: **Substrate** of CYP3A4 (major); Salmeterol: **Substrate** of CYP3A4 (major)

Avoid Concomitant Use
Avoid concomitant use of Fluticasone and Salmeterol with any of the following: Aldesleukin; BCG; CYP3A4 Inhibitors (Strong); Iobenguane I 123; Natalizumab; Pimecrolimus; Tacrolimus (Topical); Vaccines (Live)

Increased Effect/Toxicity
Fluticasone and Salmeterol may increase the levels/ effects of: Amphotericin B; Leflunomide; Loop Diuretics; Natalizumab; Sympathomimetics; Thiazide Diuretics; Vaccines (Live)

The levels/effects of Fluticasone and Salmeterol may be increased by: Antifungal Agents (Azole Derivatives, Systemic); Atomoxetine; Cannabinoids; CYP3A4 Inhibitors (Moderate); CYP3A4 Inhibitors (Strong); Dasatinib; Denosumab; MAO Inhibitors; Pimecrolimus; Protease Inhibitors; Tacrolimus (Topical); Trastuzumab; Tricyclic Antidepressants

Decreased Effect
Fluticasone and Salmeterol may decrease the levels/ effects of: Aldesleukin; Antidiabetic Agents; BCG; Corticorelin; Iobenguane I 123; Sipuleucel-T; Vaccines (Inactivated); Vaccines (Live)

The levels/effects of Fluticasone and Salmeterol may be decreased by: Alpha-/Beta-Blockers; Beta-Blockers (Beta1 Selective); Beta-Blockers (Nonselective); Betahistine; Echinacea

Stability Store at controlled room temperature; avoid direct heat or sunlight. Advair Diskus®: Discard device 1 month after removal from the moisture-protective foil overwrap pouch or after every blister has been used (when the dose indicator reads "0") whichever comes first. Advair® HFA: Store with mouthpiece down. When the counter reads "000," discard device.

Mechanism of Action
Fluticasone: Controls the rate of protein synthesis, depresses the migration of polymorphonuclear leukocytes and fibroblasts, reverses capillary permeability, and stabilizes lysosomal membranes at the cellular level to prevent or control inflammation.

Salmeterol: Relaxes bronchial smooth muscle by selective action on beta$_2$-receptors with little effect on heart rate

Pharmacodynamics See individual agents.

Pharmacokinetics (Adult data unless noted) See individual agents.

Usual Dosage
Oral powder for inhalation: Advair Diskus®:

Maintenance treatment of asthma: **Note:** Titrate dosage to the lowest effective strength which maintains control of asthma. Dose may be increased after 2 weeks if patient does not respond adequately.

Children 4-11 years without prior inhaled corticosteroid: Fluticasone 100 mcg/salmeterol 50 mcg (Advair™ Diskus® 100/50) 1 inhalation twice daily

Children ≥12 years and Adults without prior inhaled corticosteroid: Fluticasone 100 mcg/salmeterol 50 mcg (Advair™ Diskus® 100/50) 1 inhalation twice daily

Children ≥12 years and Adults currently receiving an inhaled corticosteroid: The starting dose is dependent upon the current steroid therapy, see table on next page.

Maintenance treatment of COPD with chronic bronchitis: Adults: Fluticasone 250 mcg/salmeterol 50 mcg (Advair Diskus® 250/50) 1 inhalation twice daily

Oral inhalation: Metered dose inhaler: Advair® HFA: Maintenance treatment of asthma:

Children ≥12 years and Adults without prior inhaled corticosteroid: 2 inhalations twice daily of either fluticasone 45 mcg/salmeterol 21 mcg (Advair® HFA 45/21) or fluticasone 115 mcg/salmeterol 21 mcg (Advair® HFA 115/21); not to exceed 2 inhalations twice daily of fluticasone 230 mcg/salmeterol 21 mcg (Advair® HFA 230/21)

Children ≥12 years and Adults currently receiving an inhaled corticosteroid: The starting dose is dependent upon the current steroid therapy; see table on next page. Not to exceed 2 inhalations twice daily of fluticasone 230 mcg/salmeterol 21 mcg (Advair® HFA 230/21)

Recommended Starting Dose of Fluticasone / Salmeterol (Advair Diskus®) for Patients Currently Taking Inhaled Corticosteroids

Current Daily Dose of Inhaled Corticosteroid[1]		Advair Diskus® 1 inhalation twice daily
Beclomethasone dipropionate HFA inhalation aerosol	160 mcg	100/50
	320 mcg	250/50
	640 mcg	500/50
Budesonide inhalation aerosol	≤400 mcg	100/50
	800-1200 mcg	250/50
	1600 mcg	500/50
Flunisolide inhalation aerosol	≤1000 mcg	100/50
	1250-2000 mcg	250/50
Flunisolide HFA inhalation aerosol	≤320 mcg	100/50
	640 mcg	250/50
Fluticasone propionate HFA inhalation aerosol	≤176 mcg	100/50
	440 mcg	250/50
	660-880 mcg	500/50
Fluticasone propionate inhalation powder	≤200 mcg	100/50
	500 mcg	250/50
	1000 mcg	500/50
Mometasone furoate inhalation powder	220 mcg	100/50
	440 mcg	250/50
	880 mcg	500/50
Triamcinolone acetate inhalation aerosol	≤1000 mcg	100/50
	1100-1600 mcg	250/50

[1]Not for use in patients transferring from systemic corticosteroid therapy

Recommended Starting Dose of Fluticasone / Salmeterol (Advair® HFA) for Patients Currently Taking Inhaled Corticosteroids

Current Daily Dose of Inhaled Corticosteroid[1]		Advair® HFA 2 inhalations twice daily
Beclomethasone dipropionate HFA inhalation aerosol	≤160 mcg	45/21
	320 mcg	115/21
	640 mcg	230/21
Budesonide inhalation powder	≤400 mcg	45/21
	800-1200 mcg	115/21
	1600 mcg	230/21
Flunisolide CFC inhalation aerosol	≤1000 mcg	45/21
	1250-2000 mcg	115/21
Flunisolide HFA inhalation aerosol	≤320 mcg	45/21
	640 mcg	115/21
Fluticasone propionate HFA inhalation aerosol	≤176 mcg	45/21
	440 mcg	115/21
	660-880 mcg	230/21
Fluticasone propionate inhalation powder	≤200 mcg	45/21
	500 mcg	115/21
	1000 mcg	230/21
Mometasone furoate inhalation powder	220 mcg	45/21
	440 mcg	115/21
	880 mcg	230/21
Triamcinolone acetonide inhalation aerosol	≤1000 mcg	45/21
	1100-1600 mcg	115/21

[1]Not for use in patients transferring from systemic corticosteroid therapy

Administration Oral inhalation:

Advair Diskus®, powder for oral inhalation: A device containing a double-foil blister of a powder formulation for oral inhalation; each blister contains 1 complete dose of both medications; the medication is opened by activating the device, dispersed into the airstream created by the patient inhaling through the mouthpiece; it may not be used with a spacer. Follow the patient directions for use which are provided with each device; do not exhale into the Diskus® or attempt to take it apart. Always activate and use the Diskus® in a level, horizontal position. Do not wash the mouthpiece or any part of the Diskus®; it must be kept dry.

Advair® HFA, metered dose inhalation: Prime before using the first time by releasing 4 test sprays into the air away from the face, shaking well for 5 seconds before each spray. Reprime with 2 test sprays if the inhaler has been dropped or not used for more than 4 weeks; discard after 120 actuations. Never immerse canister into water. Shake well for 5 seconds before using.

Monitoring Parameters Pulmonary function tests, check mucous membranes for signs of fungal infection; monitor growth in pediatric patients

Patient Information Do not use to treat acute symptoms; do not exceed the prescribed dose of fluticasone/salmeterol; report sore mouth or mouth lesions to physician; avoid exposure to chickenpox or measles; if exposed, seek medical advice without delay; do not use with spacer (see Administration)

Additional Information When fluticasone/salmeterol is initiated in patients previously receiving a short-acting beta agonist, instruct the patient to discontinue regular use of the short-acting beta agonist and to utilize the shorter-acting agent for symptomatic acute episodes only.

Dosage Forms Excipient information presented when available (limited, particularly for generics); consult specific product labeling. [DSC] = Discontinued product; [CAN] = Canadian brand name/formulation

Aerosol, for oral inhalation:

Advair® HFA:

45/21: Fluticasone propionate 45 mcg and salmeterol 21 mcg per inhalation (8 g) [chlorofluorocarbon free; 60 metered actuations]

45/21: Fluticasone propionate 45 mcg and salmeterol 21 mcg per inhalation (12 g) [chlorofluorocarbon free; 120 metered actuations]

115/21: Fluticasone propionate 115 mcg and salmeterol 21 mcg per inhalation (8 g) [chlorofluorocarbon free; 60 metered actuations]

115/21: Fluticasone propionate 115 mcg and salmeterol 21 mcg per inhalation (12 g) [chlorofluorocarbon free; 120 metered actuations]

230/21: Fluticasone propionate 230 mcg and salmeterol 21 mcg per inhalation (8 g) [chlorofluorocarbon free; 60 metered actuations]

230/21: Fluticasone propionate 230 mcg and salmeterol 21 mcg per inhalation (12 g) [chlorofluorocarbon free; 120 metered actuations]

Advair® [CAN]:

125/25: Fluticasone propionate 125 mcg and salmeterol 25 mcg per inhalation (12 g) [120 metered actuations] [not available in the U.S.]

250/25: Fluticasone propionate 250 mcg and salmeterol 25 mcg per inhalation (12 g) [120 metered actuations] [not available in the U.S.]

Powder, for oral inhalation:
Advair Diskus®:
100/50: Fluticasone propionate 100 mcg and salmeterol 50 mcg (14s, 28s [DSC], 60s) [contains lactose]
250/50: Fluticasone propionate 250 mcg and salmeterol 50 mcg (14s [DSC], 60s) [contains lactose]
500/50: Fluticasone propionate 500 mcg and salmeterol 50 mcg (14s [DSC], 60s) [contains lactose]

References
National Asthma Education and Prevention Program (NAEPP), "Expert Panel Report 3 (EPR-3): Guidelines for the Diagnosis and Management of Asthma," *Clinical Practice Guidelines*, National Institutes of Health, National Heart, Lung, and Blood Institute, NIH Publication No. 08-4051, prepublication 2007; available at http://www.nhlbi.nih.gov/guidelines/asthma/asthgdln.htm.

◆ **Fluticasone Furoate** *see* Fluticasone *on page 607*

◆ **Fluticasone Propionate** *see* Fluticasone *on page 607*

◆ **Fluticasone Propionate and Salmeterol Xinafoate** *see* Fluticasone and Salmeterol *on page 611*

Fluvastatin (FLOO va sta tin)

Medication Safety Issues
Sound-alike/look-alike issues:
Fluvastatin may be confused with fluoxetine, nystatin, pitavastatin

Related Information
Normal Laboratory Values for Children *on page 1672*

U.S. Brand Names Lescol®; Lescol® XL

Canadian Brand Names Lescol®; Lescol® XL

Therapeutic Category Antilipemic Agent; HMG-CoA Reductase Inhibitor

Generic Available No

Use Adjunct to dietary therapy to reduce elevated total-C, LDL-C, and apo-B levels in patients with heterozygous familial hypercholesterolemia (HFH) [FDA approved in ages 10-16 years (girls ≥1 year postmenarche)] (see Additional Information for recommendations on initiating hypercholesterolemia pharmacologic treatment in children ≥8 years). Adjunct to dietary therapy to reduce elevated total cholesterol (total-C), LDL-C, triglyceride, and apolipoprotein B (apo-B) levels and to increase HDL-C in primary hypercholesterolemia, and mixed dyslipidemia (Fredrickson types IIa and IIb) (FDA approved in adults); to slow the progression of coronary atherosclerosis in patients with coronary heart disease (FDA approved in adults); to reduce risk of coronary revascularization procedures in patients with coronary heart disease (FDA approved in adults)

Pregnancy Risk Factor X

Pregnancy Considerations Cholesterol biosynthesis may be important in fetal development. Contraindicated in pregnancy. Administer to women of childbearing potential only when conception is highly unlikely and patients have been informed of potential hazards.

Lactation Enters breast milk/contraindicated

Breast-Feeding Considerations Fluvastatin is excreted in human breast milk (milk plasma ratio 2:1); do not use in breast-feeding women.

Contraindications Hypersensitivity to fluvastatin or any component of the formulation; active liver disease; unexplained persistent elevations of serum transaminases; pregnancy; breast-feeding

Warnings Persistent, dose-associated elevations of liver transaminase levels to >3 times the upper limit of normal have been reported; liver function must be monitored by laboratory assessment at the initiation of therapy and at 12 weeks following initiation or any dose increases. Therapy discontinuation is recommended if AST or ALT remain ≥3 times the upper limit of normal on 2 consecutive occasions.

Rhabdomyolysis (with or without acute renal failure) secondary to myoglobinuria and/or myopathy has occurred rarely. Increased risk associated with concurrent use of amiodarone, clarithromycin, danazol, diltiazem, fluvoxamine, indinavir, nefazodone, nelfinavir, ritonavir, verapamil, troleandomycin, cyclosporine, fibric acid derivatives, erythromycin, niacin, or azole antifungals. Assess the risk versus benefit before combining any of these medications with fluvastatin. Advise patients to promptly report any unexplained muscle pain, tenderness, or weakness. Temporarily discontinue fluvastatin for any patient experiencing an acute or serious condition predisposing to renal failure due to the potential risk of developing rhabdomyolysis.

Precautions Use with caution in patients with a history of liver disease or heavy alcohol ingestion. Use caution in patients with conditions or on medications that reduce steroidogenesis (eg, ketoconazole, spironolactone, cimetidine).

Adverse Reactions As reported with fluvastatin capsules; in general, adverse reactions reported with fluvastatin extended release tablet were similar, but the incidence was less.

Central nervous system: Anxiety, depression, dizziness, dysfunction certain cranial nerves (eg, alteration taste, impairment of extraocular movement, facial paresis), fatigue, headache, insomnia, memory loss, paresthesia, peripheral nerve palsy, peripheral neuropathy, psychic disturbances, tremor, vertigo

Dermatologic: Alopecia, pruritus, variety skin changes (eg, nodules, discoloration, skin/mucous membrane dryness, hair/nail changes)

Endocrine & metabolic: Gynecomastia

Gastrointestinal: Abdominal pain, anorexia, diarrhea, dyspepsia, nausea, vomiting, hepatitis (including chronic active hepatitis, cholestatic jaundice, fatty liver changes, cirrhosis, fulminant hepatic necrosis, hepatoma)

Genitourinary: Erectile dysfunction, loss of libido, urinary tract infection

Neuromuscular & skeletal: Arthritis, arthralgias, muscle cramps, myalgia, myopathy

Ocular: Cataracts progression, ophthalmoplegia

Respiratory: Bronchitis, sinusitis

Miscellaneous: Hypersensitivity syndrome including anaphylaxis, infections, influenza

Drug Interactions

Metabolism/Transport Effects Substrate of CYP2C9 (major), CYP2C8 (minor), CYP2D6 (minor), CYP3A4 (minor), SLCO1B1; **Inhibits** CYP1A2 (weak), 2C8 (weak), 2C9 (moderate), 2D6 (weak), 3A4 (weak)

Avoid Concomitant Use There are no known interactions where it is recommended to avoid concomitant use.

Increased Effect/Toxicity
Fluvastatin may increase the levels/effects of: Carvedilol; CYP2C9 Substrates (High risk); DAPTOmycin; Vitamin K Antagonists

The levels/effects of Fluvastatin may be increased by: Amiodarone; Colchicine; Eltrombopag; Fenofibrate; Fenofibric Acid; Fluconazole; Gemfibrozil; Niacin; Niacinamide; Rifamycin Derivatives

Decreased Effect
The levels/effects of Fluvastatin may be decreased by: Antacids; Cholestyramine Resin; Etravirine; Peginterferon Alfa-2b; Phenytoin; Rifamycin Derivatives

Food Interactions Food reduces rate of absorption but not extent. Excessive ethanol consumption should be avoided.

Stability Store at 15°C to 30°C (59°F to 86°F). Protect from light.

Mechanism of Action Acts as a selective, competitive inhibitor of 3-hydroxy-3-methylglutaryl-coenzyme A (HMG-CoA) reductase, the enzyme that catalyzes the rate-limiting step in cholesterol biosynthesis

Pharmacodynamics

Onset of action: Peak effect: Maximal LDL-C reductions achieved within 4 weeks

Pharmacokinetics (Adult data unless noted)

Distribution: Adults: V_d: 0.35 L/kg

Protein binding: >98%

Metabolism: To inactive and active metabolites (oxidative metabolism via CYP2C9 [75%], 2C8 [~5%], and 3A4 [~20%] isoenzymes); active forms do not circulate systemically; extensive (saturable) first-pass hepatic extraction

Bioavailability: Absolute: Capsule: 24%; Extended release tablet: 29%

Half-life: Capsule: <3 hours; Extended release tablet: 9 hours

Time to peak serum concentration: Capsule: 1 hour; Extended release tablet: 3 hours

Elimination: Feces (90%); urine (5%)

Usual Dosage

Oral:

Adolescents (10-16 years): Initial: 20 mg once daily (immediate release capsule); may increase every 6 weeks based on tolerability and response to a maximum recommended dose of 80 mg/day, given as 40 mg twice daily (immediate release capsule) or as 80 mg single daily dose (extended release tablet)

Adults:

Patients requiring ≥25% decrease in LDL-C: 40 mg capsule once daily in the evening, 80 mg extended release tablet once daily (anytime), or 40 mg capsule twice daily

Patients requiring <25% decrease in LDL-C: Initial: 20 mg capsule once daily in the evening; may increase based on tolerability and response to a maximum recommended dose of 80 mg/day, given in 2 divided doses (immediate release capsule) or as a single daily dose (extended release tablet)

Elderly: No dosage adjustment necessary based on age

Dosage adjustment in renal impairment: Less than 6% excreted renally; no dosage adjustment needed with mild-to-moderate renal impairment; use with caution in severe impairment

Dosage adjustment in hepatic impairment: Levels may accumulate in patients with liver disease (increased AUC and C_{max}); use caution with severe hepatic impairment or heavy ethanol ingestion; contraindicated in active liver disease or unexplained transaminase elevations; decrease dose and monitor effects carefully in patients with hepatic insufficiency

Administration Fluvastatin may be taken without regard to meals. Do not break, chew, or crush extended release tablets; do not open capsules.

Monitoring Parameters Serum cholesterol (total and fractionated); CPK; liver function tests

Baseline cholesterol (total and fractionated), LFTs, and CPK. With initiation or dose increase, repeat tests at 4 weeks, 8 weeks, and 3 months of therapy and periodically thereafter at a minimum of every 3-6 months.

Reference Range See Related Information for age- and gender-specific serum cholesterol, LDL-C, TG, and HDL concentrations.

Patient Information May rarely cause photosensitivity reactions (eg, exposure to sunlight may cause severe sunburn, skin rash, redness, or itching); avoid direct exposure to sunlight. Report severe and unresolved gastric upset, any vision changes, muscle pain and weakness, changes in color of urine or stool, yellowing of skin or eyes, and any unusual bruising. Female patients of childbearing age must be counseled to use two effective forms of contraception simultaneously, unless absolute abstinence is the chosen method; this drug may cause severe fetal defects.

Additional Information The current recommendation for pharmacologic treatment of hypercholesterolemia in children is limited to children ≥8 years of age and is based on LDL-C concentrations and the presence of coronary vascular disease (CVD) risk factors (see table and Daniels, 2008). In adults, for each 1% lowering in LDL-C, the relative risk for major cardiovascular events is reduced by ~1%. For more specific risk assessment and treatment recommendations for adults, see NCEP ATPIII, 2001.

Recommendations for Initiating Pharmacologic Treatment in Children ≥8 Years[1]

No risk factors for CVD	LDL ≥190 mg/dL despite 6-month to 1-year diet therapy
Family history of premature CVD or ≥2 CVD risk factors present, including obesity, hypertension, or cigarette smoking	LDL ≥160 mg/dL despite 6-month to 1-year diet therapy
Diabetes mellitus present	LDL ≥130 mg/dL

[1]Adapted from Daniels SR, Greer FR, and Committee on Nutrition, "Lipid Screening and Cardiovascular Health in Childhood," *Pediatrics*, 2008, 122(1):198-208.

Dosage Forms Excipient information presented when available (limited, particularly for generics); consult specific product labeling.

Capsule (Lescol®): 20 mg, 40 mg

Tablet, extended release (Lescol® XL): 80 mg

References

American Academy of Pediatrics Committee on Nutrition, "Cholesterol in Childhood," *Pediatrics*, 1998, 101(1 Pt 1):141-7.

American Academy of Pediatrics, "National Cholesterol Education Program: Report of the Expert Panel on Blood Cholesterol Levels in Children and Adolescents," *Pediatrics*, 1992, 89(3 Pt 2):525-84.

Daniels SR, Greer FR, and Committee on Nutrition, "Lipid Screening and Cardiovascular Health in Childhood," *Pediatrics*, 2008, 122 (1):198-208.

"Executive Summary of the Third Report of the National Cholesterol Education Program (NCEP) Expert Panel on Detection, Evaluation, and Treatment of High Blood Cholesterol in Adults (Adult Treatment Panel III)," *JAMA*, 2001, 285(19):2486-97.

Grundy SM, Cleeman JI, Merz CN, et al, "Implications of Recent Clinical Trials for the National Cholesterol Education Program Adult Treatment Panel III Guidelines," *Circulation*, 2004, 110(2):227-39.

McCrindle BW, Urbina EM, Dennison BA, et al, "Drug Therapy of High-Risk Lipid Abnormalities in Children and Adolescents: A Scientific Statement from the American Heart Association Atherosclerosis, Hypertension, and Obesity in Youth Committee, Council of Cardiovascular Disease in the Young, With the Council on Cardiovascular Nursing," *Circulation*, 2007, 115(14):1948-67.

van der Graaf A, Nierman MC, Firth JC, et al, "Efficacy and Safety of Fluvastatin in Children and Adolescents With Heterozygous Familial Hypercholesterolaemia," *Acta Paediatr*, 2006, 95(11):1461-6

♦ **Fluviral S/F® (Can)** see Influenza Virus Vaccine (Inactivated) *on page 734*

♦ **Fluvirin®** see Influenza Virus Vaccine (Inactivated) *on page 734*

Fluvoxamine (floo VOKS a meen)

Medication Safety Issues

Sound-alike/look-alike issues:

Fluvoxamine may be confused with flavoxate, fluoxetine

Luvox may be confused with Lasix®, Levoxyl®, Lovenox®

Related Information

Antidepressant Agents *on page 1484*

Serotonin Syndrome *on page 1695*

U.S. Brand Names Luvox® CR

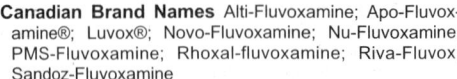

Canadian Brand Names Alti-Fluvoxamine; Apo-Fluvox-amine®; Luvox®; Novo-Fluvoxamine; Nu-Fluvoxamine; PMS-Fluvoxamine; Rhoxal-fluvoxamine; Riva-Fluvox; Sandoz-Fluvoxamine

Therapeutic Category Antidepressant, Selective Seroto-nin Reuptake Inhibitor (SSRI)

Generic Available Yes: Excludes extended release capsule

Use

Tablets: Treatment of obsessive-compulsive disorder (OCD) (FDA approved in ages ≥8 years and adults)

Extended-release capsules: Treatment of obsessive-compulsive disorder (OCD) (FDA approved in adults); treatment of social anxiety disorder (FDA approved in adults)

Medication Guide An FDA-approved patient medication guide, which is available with the product information and at http://www.fda.gov/downloads/Drugs/DrugSafety/ucm088625.pdf, must be dispensed with this medication for each new outpatient prescription and refill.

Pregnancy Risk Factor C

Pregnancy Considerations Due to adverse effects observed in animal studies, fluvoxamine is classified as pregnancy category C. Fluvoxamine crosses the human placenta. Nonteratogenic effects in the newborn following SSRI exposure late in the third trimester include respiratory distress, cyanosis, apnea, seizures, temper-ature instability, feeding difficulty, vomiting, hypoglycemia, hypo- or hypertonia, hyper-reflexia, jitteriness, irritability, constant crying, and tremor. An increased risk of low birth weight and low Apgar scores has also been reported. Exposure to SSRIs after the twentieth week of gestation has been associated with persistent pulmonary hyper-tension of the newborn (PPHN). Adverse effects may be due to toxic effects of the SSRI or drug withdrawal due to discontinuation. The long-term effects of *in utero* SSRI exposure on infant development and behavior are not known.

Women treated for major depression and who are euthymic prior to pregnancy are more likely to experience a relapse when medication is discontinued as compared to pregnant women who continue taking antidepressant medications. The ACOG recommends that therapy with SSRIs or SNRIs during pregnancy be individualized; treatment of depression during pregnancy should incorpo-rate the clinical expertise of the mental health clinician, obstetrician, primary healthcare provider, and pediatrician. If treatment during pregnancy is required, consider tapering therapy during the third trimester in order to prevent withdrawal symptoms in the infant. If this is done and the woman is considered to be at risk of relapse from her major depressive disorder, the medication can be restarted following delivery, although the dose should be readjusted to that required before pregnancy. Treatment algorithms have been developed by the ACOG and the APA for the management of depression in women prior to conception and during pregnancy (Yonkers, 2009).

Lactation Enters breast milk/not recommended (AAP rates "of concern")

Breast-Feeding Considerations Fluvoxamine is excreted in breast milk. Based on case reports, the dose the infant receives is relatively small and adverse events have not been observed. According to the manufacturer, the decision to continue or discontinue breast-feeding during therapy should take into account the risk of exposure to the infant and the benefits of treatment to the mother. The AAP considers fluvoxamine to be a "drug for which the effect on the nursing infant is unknown, but may be of concern."

The long-term effects on development and behavior have not been studied; therefore, fluvoxamine should be prescribed to a mother who is breast-feeding only when the benefits outweigh the potential risks.

Contraindications Hypersensitivity to fluvoxamine or any component; concurrent use with thioridazine, pimozide, alosetron, or tizanidine; use of MAO inhibitors within 14 days (potentially fatal reactions may occur; see Drug Interactions)

Warnings Safety and efficacy in pediatric patients ≥8 years of age have been established only for the treatment of obsessive compulsive disorder using the immediate-release tablets; extended-release capsules have not been evaluated in pediatric patients; **fluvoxamine is not FDA approved for the treatment of depression in pediatric or adult patients.** Clinical worsening of depression or suicidal ideation and behavior may occur in children and adults with major depressive disorder **[U.S. Boxed Warning]**. In clinical trials, antidepressants increased the risk of suicidal thinking and behavior (suicidality) in children, adolescents, and young adults (18-24 years of age) with major depressive disorder and other psychiatric disorders. This risk must be considered before prescribing antidepressants for any clinical use. Short-term studies did **not** show an increased risk of suicidality with antidepres-sant use in patients >24 years of age and showed a decreased risk in patients ≥65 years.

Patients of all ages who are treated with antidepressants for any indication require appropriate monitoring and close observation for clinical worsening of depression, suicidal-ity, and unusual changes in behavior, especially during the first few months after antidepressant initiation or when the dose is adjusted. Family members and caregivers should be instructed to closely observe the patient (ie, daily) and communicate condition with healthcare provider. Patients should also be monitored for associated behaviors (eg, anxiety, agitation, panic attacks, insomnia, irritability, hostility, aggressiveness, impulsivity, akathisia, hypoma-nia, mania) which may increase the risk for worsening depression or suicidality. Worsening depression or emergence of suicidality (or associated behaviors listed above) that is abrupt in onset, severe, or not part of the presenting symptoms, may require discontinuation or modification of drug therapy.

Avoid abrupt discontinuation; withdrawal syndrome with discontinuation symptoms (including agitation, dysphoria, anxiety, confusion, dizziness, hypomania, nightmares, irritability, sensory disturbances, headache, lethargy, emo-tional lability, insomnia, tinnitus, and seizures) may occur if therapy is abruptly discontinued or dose reduced; taper the dose to minimize risks of discontinuation symptoms. If intolerable symptoms occur following a decrease in dosage or upon discontinuation of therapy, consider resuming the previous dose with a more gradual taper. To reduce risk of intentional overdose, write prescriptions for the smallest quantity consistent with good patient care.

May worsen psychosis in some patients or precipitate a shift to mania or hypomania in patients with bipolar disorder. Monotherapy in patients with bipolar disorder should be avoided. Patients presenting with depressive symptoms should be screened for bipolar disorder. **Fluvoxamine is not FDA approved for the treatment of bipolar depression.**

Potentially fatal serotonin syndrome (SS) or neuroleptic malignant syndrome (NMS)-like reactions have occurred with selective serotonin reuptake inhibitors (SSRIs) and serotonin/norepinephrine reuptake inhibitors (SNRIs) when used alone, and particularly when used in combination with serotonergic drugs (eg, triptans), drugs that impair the metabolism of serotonin (eg, MAO inhibitors), or antidopaminergic agents (eg, antipsychotics). Identification and differentiation of SS (eg, tremor, myoclonus, agitation) and more severe NMS-like reactions (eg, hyperthermia, muscle rigidity, autonomic instability, mental status changes) can be complex; monitor patients closely for either syndrome. Discontinue treatment (and any concomitant serotonergic and/or antidopaminergic agents) immediately if signs or symptoms arise and initiate supportive symptomatic therapy. Tryptophan (which can be metabolized to serotonin) and the herbal medicine St John's wort (*Hypericum perforatum*) may increase serious side effects (concomitant use of these agents with fluvoxamine is not recommended).

Precautions Fluvoxamine may cause abnormal bleeding (eg, ecchymosis, purpura, upper GI bleeding); use with caution in patients with impaired platelet aggregation and with concurrent use of aspirin, NSAIDs, or other drugs that affect coagulation. May impair cognitive or motor performance. Use with caution in patients with seizure disorders (monitor closely; avoid use in patients with unstable epilepsy), concomitant illnesses that may effect hepatic metabolism or hemodynamic responses (eg, unstable cardiac disease, recent MI), and in suicidal patients; use with caution and decrease dose in patients with hepatic dysfunction; use with caution in patients with severe renal impairment. Use with caution in patients receiving diuretics or those who are volume depleted (may cause hyponatremia or SIADH). No clinical studies have assessed the combined use of fluvoxamine and electroconvulsive therapy; however, use with caution in patients receiving electroconvulsive therapy; may increase the risks associated with electroconvulsive therapy, consider discontinuing, when possible, prior to electroconvulsive therapy treatment.

Use with caution during third trimester of pregnancy [newborns may experience adverse effects or withdrawal symptoms (consider risk and benefits), see Additional Information; exposure to SSRIs late in pregnancy may also be associated with an increased risk for persistent pulmonary hypertension of the newborn (see Chambers, 2006)].

Adverse Reactions

Cardiovascular: Palpitations

Central nervous system: Headache, somnolence, insomnia, nervousness, dizziness, mania, hypomania, vertigo, abnormal thinking, agitation, anxiety, malaise, amnesia, yawning, hypertonia, CNS stimulation, depression, apathy, emotional lability, hyperkinesia; suicidal thinking and behavior (see Warnings)

Note: SSRI-associated behavioral activation (ie, restlessness, hyperkinesis, hyperactivity, agitation) is 2- to 3-fold more prevalent in children compared to adolescents; it is more prevalent in adolescents compared to adults. Somnolence (including sedation and drowsiness) is more common in adults compared to children and adolescents (see Safer, 2006).

Dermatologic: Rash

Endocrine & metabolic: Libido decreased, sexual dysfunction, dysmenorrhea, weight loss

Gastrointestinal: Nausea, diarrhea, xerostomia, abdominal pain, vomiting, dyspepsia, constipation, abnormal taste, anorexia, flatulence

Note: SSRI-associated vomiting is 2- to 3-fold more prevalent in children compared to adolescents; it is more prevalent in adolescents compared to adults

Genitourinary: Urinary frequency, urinary retention

Hematologic: Altered platelet function (rare), bleeding increased, bruising

Neuromuscular & skeletal: Tremors, weakness (14%)

Ocular: Blurred vision

Respiratory: Dyspnea, cough

Miscellaneous: Diaphoresis, allergic reactions (infrequent); withdrawal symptoms following abrupt discontinuation (see Warnings)

Drug Interactions

Metabolism/Transport Effects Substrate (major) of CYP1A2, 2D6; **Inhibits** CYP1A2 (strong), 2B6 (weak), 2C9 (weak), 2C19 (strong), 2D6 (weak), 3A4 (weak)

Avoid Concomitant Use

Avoid concomitant use of Fluvoxamine with any of the following: Alosetron; Clopidogrel; Iobenguane I 123; MAO Inhibitors; Metoclopramide; Pimozide; Ramelteon; Sibutramine; Thioridazine; TiZANidine

Increased Effect/Toxicity

Fluvoxamine may increase the levels/effects of: Alcohol (Ethyl); Alosetron; Anticoagulants; Antidepressants (Serotonin Reuptake Inhibitor/Antagonist); Antiplatelet Agents; Asenapine; Aspirin; Bendamustine; Benzodiazepines (metabolized by oxidation); BusPIRone; CarBAMazepine; Clozapine; CNS Depressants; Collagenase (Systemic); CYP1A2 Substrates; CYP2C19 Substrates; Desmopressin; Drotrecogin Alfa; DULoxetine; Erlotinib; Haloperidol; Ibritumomab; Lithium; Methadone; Methotrimeprazine; Mexiletine; NSAID (COX-2 Inhibitor); NSAID (Nonselective); OLANZapine; Phenytoin; Pimozide; Propafenone; Propranolol; QuiNIDine; Ramelteon; Ropivacaine; Salicylates; Serotonin Modulators; Theophylline Derivatives; Thioridazine; Thrombolytic Agents; TiZANidine; Tositumomab and Iodine I 131 Tositumomab; TraMADol; Tricyclic Antidepressants; Vitamin K Antagonists

The levels/effects of Fluvoxamine may be increased by: Analgesics (Opioid); BusPIRone; Cimetidine; CYP1A2 Inhibitors (Moderate); CYP1A2 Inhibitors (Strong); CYP2D6 Inhibitors (Moderate); CYP2D6 Inhibitors (Strong); Darunavir; Dasatinib; Glucosamine; Herbs (Anticoagulant/Antiplatelet Properties); MAO Inhibitors; Methotrimeprazine; Metoclopramide; Omega-3-Acid Ethyl Esters; Pentosan Polysulfate Sodium; Pentoxifylline; Prostacyclin Analogues; Sibutramine; TraMADol; Tryptophan

Decreased Effect

Fluvoxamine may decrease the levels/effects of: Clopidogrel; Iobenguane I 123

The levels/effects of Fluvoxamine may be decreased by: CarBAMazepine; CYP1A2 Inducers (Strong); Cyproheptadine; Peginterferon Alfa-2b

Food Interactions Food does not significantly affect bioavailability.

Stability Protect from high humidity and store at controlled room temperature of 25°C (77°F). Dispense in tight containers. Avoid exposing extended-release capsules to temperatures >30°C (86°F).

Mechanism of Action Inhibits CNS neuron serotonin uptake; minimal or no effect on reuptake of norepinephrine or dopamine; does not significantly bind to alpha-adrenergic, histamine or cholinergic receptors

Pharmacodynamics

Onset of action: 1-2 weeks

Maximum effect: 8-12 weeks

Duration: 1-2 days

Pharmacokinetics (Adult data unless noted) Note: Steady-state plasma concentrations (following administration of the immediate-release product) have been noted to be 2-3 times higher in children than those in adolescents; female children demonstrated a significantly higher AUC and peak concentration than males.

Distribution: V_d, apparent: Adults: ~25 L/kg

Protein binding: ~80%, primarily to albumin

Metabolism: Extensive via the liver; major metabolic routes are oxidative demethylation and deamination; dose-dependent (nonlinear) pharmacokinetics

◄ Bioavailability: Immediate release: 53%; extended release: 84% (compared to immediate release); bioavailability is not significantly affected by food for either formulation

Half-life: Adults: 15.6 hours

Time to peak serum concentration: 3-8 hours

Elimination: 94% of the dose is excreted in the urine, primarily as metabolites; 2% as unchanged drug

Clearance: Hepatic dysfunction: Decreased by 30%

Usual Dosage Oral:

Obsessive compulsive disorder:

Children 8-17 years: Immediate release: Initial: 25 mg once daily at bedtime; adjust in 25 mg increments at 7- to 14-day intervals, as tolerated, to maximum therapeutic benefit; usual dosage range: 50-200 mg/day; daily doses >50 mg should be divided into 2 doses; administer larger portion at bedtime

Maximum: Children: 8-11 years: 200 mg/day; Adolescents: 300 mg/day; lower doses may be effective in female versus male patients

Note: Slower titration of dose every 2-4 weeks may minimize the risk of behavioral activation; behavioral activation associated with SSRI use increases the risk of suicidal behavior. Higher mg/kg doses are needed in children compared to adolescents.

Adults:

Immediate release: Initial: 50 mg once daily at bedtime; adjust in 50 mg increments at 4- to 7-day intervals; usual dosage range: 100-300 mg/day; daily doses >100 mg should be divided into 2 doses; administer larger portion at bedtime; maximum dose: 300 mg/day

Extended release: Initial: 100 mg once daily at bedtime; may be increased in 50 mg increments at intervals of at least 1 week; usual dosage range: 100-300 mg/day; maximum dose: 300 mg/day

Social anxiety disorder: Adults: Extended release: Initial: 100 mg once daily at bedtime; may be increased in 50 mg increments at intervals of at least 1 week; usual dosage range: 100-300 mg/day; maximum dose: 300 mg/day

Dosage adjustment in hepatic impairment: Decrease initial dose and dose titration; titrate slowly

Administration May be administered without regard to meals. Do not chew or crush extended-release capsule; swallow whole.

Monitoring Parameters Monitor patient periodically for symptom resolution; monitor for worsening depression, suicidality, and associated behaviors (especially at the beginning of therapy or when doses are increased or decreased; see Warnings). Monitor for anxiety, social functioning, mania, panic attacks; akathisia, weight gain or loss, nutritional intake, sleep. Monitor for signs and symptoms of serotonin syndrome or neuroleptic malignant syndrome-like reactions.

Patient Information Read the patient Medication Guide that you receive with each prescription and refill of fluvoxamine. An increased risk of suicidal thinking and behavior has been reported with the use of antidepressants in children, adolescents, and young adults (18-24 years of age). Notify physician if you feel more depressed, have thoughts of suicide, or become more agitated or irritable (see Warnings). Notify physician if you experience rash, hives, or other allergic reactions. Avoid alcohol, caffeine, CNS stimulants, tryptophan supplements, and the herbal medicine St John's wort; avoid aspirin, NSAIDs, or other drugs that affect coagulation (may increase risks of bleeding); may cause dizziness or drowsiness and impair ability to perform activities requiring mental alertness or physical coordination; may cause dry mouth. Some medicines should not be taken with fluvoxamine or should not be taken for a while after fluvoxamine has been discontinued; report the use of other medications, nonprescription medications, and herbal or natural products to your physician and pharmacist. It may take 2-3 weeks to see therapeutic effects from this medication. Take as directed; do not alter dose or frequency without consulting prescriber; avoid abrupt discontinuation.

Nursing Implications Taper dosage slowly when discontinuing. Assess mental status for depression, suicidal ideation, anxiety, social functioning, mania, or panic attack.

Additional Information A recent report (Lake, 2000) describes 5 children (age 8-15 years) who developed epistaxis (n=4) or bruising (n=1) while receiving sertraline therapy. Another recent report describes the SSRI discontinuation syndrome in 6 children; the syndrome was similar to that reported in adults (see Diler, 2002). Due to limited long-term studies, the clinical usefulness of fluvoxamine should be periodically re-evaluated in patients receiving the drug for extended intervals; effects of long term use of fluvoxamine on pediatric growth, development, and maturation have not been directly assessed. **Note:** Case reports of decreased growth in children receiving fluoxetine or fluvoxamine (n=4; age: 11.6-13.7 years) for 6 months to 5 years suggest a suppression of growth hormone secretion during SSRI therapy (see Weintrob, 2002). Further studies are needed.

Neonates born to women receiving SSRIs late during the third trimester may experience respiratory distress, apnea, cyanosis, temperature instability, vomiting, feeding difficulty, hypoglycemia, constant crying, irritability, hypotonia, hypertonia, hyper-reflexia, tremor, jitteriness, and seizures; these symptoms may be due to a direct toxic effect, withdrawal syndrome, or (in some cases) serotonin syndrome. Withdrawal symptoms occur in 30% of neonates exposed to SSRIs *in utero*; monitor newborns for at least 48 hours after birth; long-term effects of *in utero* exposure to SSRIs are unknown (see Levinson-Castiel, 2006).

Dosage Forms Excipient information presented when available (limited, particularly for generics); consult specific product labeling.

Tablet, as maleate: 25 mg, 50 mg, 100 mg

Capsule, extended release, as maleate:

Luvox® CR: 100 mg, 150 mg [gluten free]

References

Chambers CD, Hernandez-Diaz S, Van Marter LJ, et al, "Selective Serotonin-Reuptake Inhibitors and Risk of Persistent Pulmonary Hypertension of the Newborn," *N Engl J Med*, 2006, 354(6):579-87.

Cheer SM and Figgitt DP, "Fluvoxamine: A Review of Its Therapeutic Potential in the Management of Anxiety Disorders in Children and Adolescents," *Paediatr Drugs*, 2001, 3(10):763-81.

Cheer SM and Figgitt DP, "Spotlight on Fluvoxamine in Anxiety Disorders in Children and Adolescents," *CNS Drugs*, 2002, 16 (2):139-44.

de Vries MH, Raghoebar M, Mathlener IS, et al, "Single and Multiple Oral Dose Fluvoxamine Kinetics in Young and Elderly Subjects," *Ther Drug Monit*, 1992, 14(6):493-8.

Diler R and Avci A, "Selective Serotonin Reuptake Inhibitor Discontinuation Syndrome in Children: Six Case Reports," *Current Therapeutic Research*, 2002, 63(3):188-97.

Dopheide JA, "Recognizing and Treating Depression in Children and Adolescents," *Am J of Health Syst Pharm*, 2006, 63(3):233-43.

"Fluvoxamine for the Treatment of Anxiety Disorders in Children and Adolescents. The Research Unit on Pediatric Psychopharmacology Anxiety Study Group," *N Engl J Med*, 2001, 344(17):1279-85.

Grimsley SR and Jann MW, "Paroxetine, Sertraline, and Fluvoxamine: New Selective Serotonin Reuptake Inhibitors," *Clin Pharm*, 1992, 11 (11):930-57.

Lake MB, Birmaher B, Wassick S, et al, "Bleeding and Selective Serotonin Reuptake Inhibitors in Childhood and Adolescence," *J Child Adolesc Psychopharmacol*, 2000, 10(1):35-8.

Levinson-Castiel R, Merlob P, Linder N, et al, "Neonatal Abstinence Syndrome After *in utero* Exposure to Selective Serotonin Reuptake Inhibitors in Term Infants," *Arch Pediatr Adolesc Med*, 2006, 160 (2):173-6.

Pass SE and Simpson RW, "Discontinuation and Reinstitution of Medications During the Perioperative Period," *Am J Health Syst Pharm*, 2004, 61(9):899-912.

Reinblatt SP and Riddle MA, "Selective Serotonin Reuptake Inhibitor-Induced Apathy: A Pediatric Case Series," *J Child Adolesc Psychopharmacol*, 2006, 16(1/2):227-33.

Riddle MA, Reeve EA, Yaryura-Tobias JA, et al, "Fluvoxamine for Children and Adolescents With Obsessive-Compulsive Disorder: A Randomized, Controlled, Multicenter Trial," *J Am Acad Child Adolesc Psychiatry*, 2001, 40(2):222-9.

Roose SP, Glassman AH, Attia E, et al, "Comparative Efficacy of Selective Serotonin Reuptake Inhibitors and Tricyclics in the Treatment of Melancholia," *Am J Psychiatry*, 1994, 151(12):1735-9.

Safer DJ and Zito JM, "Treatment Emergent Adverse Effects of Selective Serotonin Reuptake Inhibitors by Age Group: Children vs. Adolescents," *J Child Adolesc Psychopharmacol*, 2006, 16(1/2):159-69.

Weintrob N, Cohen D, Klipper-Aurbach Y, et al, "Decreased Growth During Therapy With Selective Serotonin Reuptake Inhibitors," *Arch Pediatr Adolesc Med*, 2002, 156(7):696-701.

◆ **Fluzone®** *see* Influenza Virus Vaccine (Inactivated) *on page 734*

◆ **FML®** *see* Fluorometholone *on page 597*

◆ **FML® Forte** *see* Fluorometholone *on page 597*

◆ **FML Forte® (Can)** *see* Fluorometholone *on page 597*

◆ **Focalin®** *see* Dexmethylphenidate *on page 410*

◆ **Focalin® XR** *see* Dexmethylphenidate *on page 410*

◆ **Foille® [OTC]** *see* Benzocaine *on page 182*

◆ **Folacin** *see* Folic Acid *on page 619*

◆ **Folacin-800 [OTC]** *see* Folic Acid *on page 619*

◆ **Folate** *see* Folic Acid *on page 619*

Folic Acid (FOE lik AS id)

Medication Safety Issues
Sound-alike/look-alike issues:
Folic acid may be confused with folinic acid

U.S. Brand Names Folacin-800 [OTC]

Canadian Brand Names Apo-Folic®

Therapeutic Category Nutritional Supplement; Vitamin, Water Soluble

Generic Available Yes

Use Treatment of megaloblastic and macrocytic anemias due to folate deficiency; dietary supplement to prevent neural tube defects

Pregnancy Risk Factor A

Pregnancy Considerations Folic acid requirements are increased during pregnancy; a deficiency may result in fetal harm.

Lactation Enters breast milk/compatible

Contraindications Hypersensitivity to folic acid or any component (see Warnings); pernicious, aplastic, or normocytic anemias

Warnings Large doses may mask the hematologic effects of B_{12} deficiency, thus obscuring the diagnosis of pernicious anemia while allowing the neurologic complications due to B_{12} deficiency to progress. Folic acid injection contains benzyl alcohol (1.5%) as preservative, which may cause allergic reactions in susceptible individuals; large amounts of benzyl alcohol (≥99 mg/kg/day) have been associated with a potentially fatal toxicity ("gasping syndrome") in neonates; the "gasping syndrome" consists of metabolic acidosis, respiratory distress, gasping respirations, CNS dysfunction (including convulsions, intracranial hemorrhage), hypotension and cardiovascular collapse; avoid use of injection in neonates; *in vitro* and animal studies have shown that benzoate, a metabolite of benzyl alcohol, displaces bilirubin from protein-binding sites

Adverse Reactions
Cardiovascular: Slight flushing
Central nervous system: At high doses (15 mg/day): Irritability, difficulty sleeping, difficulty concentrating, confusion, overactivity, excitement, depression, impaired judgment
Dermatologic: Pruritus, rash

Gastrointestinal: GI upset; at high doses (15 mg/day): Anorexia, nausea, abdominal distention, flatulence, bitter or bad taste
Miscellaneous: Hypersensitivity reactions

Drug Interactions
Avoid Concomitant Use
Avoid concomitant use of Folic Acid with any of the following: Raltitrexed
Increased Effect/Toxicity There are no known significant interactions involving an increase in effect.
Decreased Effect
Folic Acid may decrease the levels/effects of: PHENobarbital; Phenytoin; Primidone; Raltitrexed

Mechanism of Action Folic acid is necessary for formation of a number of coenzymes in many metabolic systems, particularly for purine and pyrimidine synthesis; required for nucleoprotein synthesis and maintenance in erythropoiesis; stimulates WBC and platelet production in folate deficiency anemia

Pharmacodynamics Maximum effect: Oral: Within 30-60 minutes

Pharmacokinetics (Adult data unless noted)
Absorption: In the proximal part of the small intestine
Bioavailability: ~100%; in presence of food: 85%
Time to peak serum concentration: Oral: 1 hour
Elimination: Primarily via liver metabolism

Usual Dosage Recommended daily allowance (RDA): Oral:
Infants:
Premature neonates: 50 mcg/day (~15 mcg/kg/day)
Neonates to 6 months: 25-35 mcg/day
Children: Expressed as dietary folate equivalents (DFE):
1-3 years: 150 mcg/day
4-8 years: 200 mcg/day
9-13 years: 300 mcg/day
Children ≥14 years: 400 mcg/day
Adults: 400 mcg/day
Folic acid deficiency: Oral, I.M., I.V., SubQ:
Infants: 0.1 mg/day
Children <4 years: Up to 0.3 mg/day
Children >4 years and Adults: 0.4 mg/day
Pregnant and lactating women: 0.8 mg/day
Prevention of neural tube defects:
Females of childbearing potential: 400-800 mcg/day
Females at high risk or with family history of neural tube defects: 4 mg/day

Administration
Oral: May be administered without regard to meals
Parenteral: I.V.: Dilute with SWI, dextrose or saline solution to 0.1 mg/mL; if I.M. route used, administer deep I.M.; may also administer SubQ

Monitoring Parameters CBC with differential

Reference Range Total folate: Normal: 5-15 ng/mL; folate deficiency: <5 ng/mL; megaloblastic anemia: <2 ng/mL

Additional Information Dietary folate equivalents (DFE) is used to adjust for ~50% decreased bioavailability of food folate compared with that of folic acid supplement:
1 mcg DFE = 0.6 mcg folic acid from fortified food or as a supplement taken with meals, or
1 mcg DFE of food folate = 0.5 mcg of a supplement taken on an empty stomach.

Dosage Forms Excipient information presented when available (limited, particularly for generics); consult specific product labeling.
Injection, solution, as sodium folate: 5 mg/mL (10 mL) [contains benzyl alcohol, edetate disodium]
Tablet: 0.4 mg, 0.8 mg, 1 mg
Folacin-800: 0.8 mg

Extemporaneous Preparations A 50 mcg/mL oral solution may be made by mixing 1 mL (5 mg) folic acid injection in 90 mL purified water; adjust pH to 9 with sodium hydroxide 0.1 N (approximately 2.8 mL), then add purified water to make a total volume of 100 mL; stable 30 days at room temperature

Smith SG, "A Folic Acid Solution for Oral Use," *Pharm J*, 1976, 216:108.

References
ACOG Committee on Practice Bulletins, "Clinical Management Guidelines for Obstetrician-Gynecologists. Number 44, July 2003 (Replaces Committee Opinion Number 252, March 2001)," *Obstet Gynecol*, 2003, 102(1):203-13.

Standing Committee on the Scientific Evaluation of Dietary Reference Intakes, Food and Nutrition Board, Institute of Medicine, "Dietary Reference Intakes for Thiamin, Riboflavin, Niacin, Vitamin B$_6$, Folate, Vitamin B$_{12}$, Pantothenic Acid, Biotin and Choline," National Academy of Sciences, Washington, DC: National Academy Press, 1999. Available at: http://www.nap.edu.

U.S. Preventive Services Task Force (USPSTF), "Folic Acid for the Prevention of Neural Tube Defects: U.S. Preventive Services Task Force Recommendation Statement," *Ann Intern Med*, 2009, 150 (9):626-31.

◆ **Folinic Acid (error prone synonym)** *see* Leucovorin Calcium *on page 804*

Fomepizole (foe ME pi zole)

Medication Safety Issues
Sound-alike/look-alike issues:
Fomepizole may be confused with omeprazole

U.S. Brand Names Antizol®

Therapeutic Category Antidote, Ethylene Glycol Toxicity; Antidote, Methanol Toxicity

Generic Available Yes

Use Antidote for ethylene glycol (antifreeze) or methanol toxicity; may be useful in propylene glycol toxicity; FDA approved in ages ≥18 years

Pregnancy Risk Factor C

Pregnancy Considerations Reproduction studies have not been conducted; use in pregnant women only if the benefits clearly outweigh the risks.

Lactation Excretion in breast milk unknown/not recommended

Contraindications Hypersensitivity to fomepizole, other pyrazoles, or any component

Warnings By inhibiting the action of alcohol dehydrogenase, fomepizole reduces the elimination of alcohol; this must be considered when using fomepizole, as alcohol is often ingested concomitantly by patients with ethylene glycol intoxication; likewise, alcohol may reduce the elimination of fomepizole by the same mechanism. Pediatric administration is not FDA approved; however, safe and efficacious use in this patient population for ethylene glycol and methanol intoxication has been reported (Baum, 2000; Benitez, 2000; Boyer, 2001; Brown, 2001; De Brabander, 2005; Detaille, 2004; Fisher, 1998). Consider consultation with a clinical toxicologist or poison control center.

Precautions Management of ethylene glycol ingestion may require treatment of metabolic acidosis, acute renal failure, adult respiratory distress syndrome, and hypocalcemia; dialysis should be considered, in addition to fomepizole therapy, in patients with acute renal failure, severe metabolic acidosis, or a serum ethylene glycol concentration >50 mg/dL; adjust dosage for renal dysfunction (see Usual Dosage)

Adverse Reactions
Cardiovascular: Bradycardia, tachycardia, hypotension
Central nervous system: Headache, dizziness, seizure, slurred speech, fever, somnolence
Dermatologic: Rash
Gastrointestinal: Nausea, vomiting, diarrhea, anorexia, heartburn, metallic taste, abdominal pain
Hematologic: Eosinophilia, anemia
Hepatic: Transient elevations in transaminase levels
Local: Phlebosclerosis, vein irritation
Ocular: Nystagmus, blurred vision

Respiratory: Pharyngitis, hiccups
Miscellaneous: Hypersensitivity reactions

Drug Interactions

Avoid Concomitant Use There are no known interactions where it is recommended to avoid concomitant use.

Increased Effect/Toxicity There are no known significant interactions involving an increase in effect.

Decreased Effect There are no known significant interactions involving a decrease in effect.

Stability Store at room temperature; fomepizole solidifies at temperatures <25°C (77°F); if solidification occurs, liquefy by running the vial under warm water or by holding in the hand; solidification does not affect the efficacy, safety, or stability of fomepizole; stabile diluted in NS or D$_5$W for 48 hours; does not contain a preservative; use within 24 hours of dilution

Mechanism of Action A competitive alcohol dehydrogenase inhibitor, fomepizole complexes and inactivates alcohol dehydrogenase thus preventing formation of the toxic metabolites of the alcohols

Pharmacokinetics (Adult data unless noted)
Distribution: V$_d$: 0.6-1.02 L/kg; rapidly distributes into total body water

Protein binding: Negligible

Metabolism: Liver; primarily to 4-carboxypyrazole; after single doses, exhibits saturable, Michaelis-Menton kinetics; with multiple dosing, fomepizole induces its own metabolism via the cytochrome P450 system; after enzyme induction elimination follows first order kinetics

Elimination: 1% to 3.5% excreted unchanged in the urine

Dialysis: Dialyzable

Usual Dosage I.V.:
Children and Adults **not requiring** hemodialysis: Initial: 15 mg/kg loading dose; followed by 10 mg/kg every 12 hours for 4 doses; then 15 mg/kg every 12 hours until ethylene glycol or methanol levels have been reduced to <20 mg/dL

Children and Adults **requiring** hemodialysis: Since fomepizole is dialyzable, follow the above dose recommendations at intervals related to institution of hemodialysis and its duration:

Dose at the beginning of hemodialysis:
If <6 hours since last fomepizole dose: Do **not** administer dose
If ≥6 hours since last fomepizole dose: Administer next scheduled dose

Dose during hemodialysis: Administer every 4 hours or as continuous infusion 1-1.5 mg/kg/hour

Dose at the time hemodialysis is completed (dependent upon the time between the last dose and the end of hemodialysis):
<1 hour: Do **not** administer at the end of hemodialysis
1-3 hours: Administer 1/2 of the next scheduled dose
>3 hours: Administer the next scheduled dose

Maintenance dose off hemodialysis: Give next scheduled dose 12 hours from last dose administered

Dosage adjustment in renal impairment: Fomepizole is substantially excreted by the kidney and the risk of toxic reactions to this drug may be increased in patients with impaired renal function; no dosage recommendations for patients with impaired renal function have been established

Administration Parenteral: I.V. Dilute in at least 100 mL NS or D$_5$W (<25 mg/mL); infuse over 30 minutes; rapid infusion of concentrations ≥25 mg/mL has been associated with vein irritation and phlebosclerosis

Monitoring Parameters Vital signs, arterial blood gases, acid-base status, urinary oxalate, anion and osmolar gaps, clinical signs and symptoms of toxicity (arrhythmias, seizures, coma); serum and urinary ethylene glycol or serum methanol level depending upon the agent ingested; formic acid level (methanol ingestion)

Reference Range Ethylene glycol or methanol serum concentration: Goal: <20 mg/dL; therapeutic plasma fomepizole level: 0.8 mcg/mL

Additional Information If ethylene glycol poisoning is left untreated, the natural progression of the poisoning leads to accumulation of toxic metabolites, including glycolic and oxalic acids; these metabolites can induce metabolic acidosis, seizures, stupor, coma, calcium oxaluria, acute tubular necrosis and death; as ethylene glycol levels diminish in the blood when metabolized to glycolate, the diagnosis of this poisoning may be difficult

Dosage Forms Excipient information presented when available (limited, particularly for generics); consult specific product labeling.

Injection, solution [preservative free]: 1 g/mL (1.5 mL)
Antizol®: 1 g/mL (1.5 mL)

References

Baum CR, Langman CB, Oker EE, et al, "Fomepizole Treatment of Ethylene Glycol Poisoning in an Infant," *Pediatrics*, 2000, 106 (6):1489-91.

Benitez JG, Swanson-Biearman B, and Krenzelok EP, "Nystagmus Secondary to Fomepizole Administration in a Pediatric Patient," *J Toxicol Clin Toxicol*, 2000, 38(7):795-8.

Boyer EW, Mejia M, Woolf A, et al, "Severe Ethylene Glycol Ingestion Treated Without Hemodialysis," *Pediatrics*, 2001, 107(1):172-3.

Brown MJ, Shannon MW, Woolf A, et al, "Childhood Methanol Ingestion Treated With Fomepizole and Hemodialysis," *Pediatrics*, 2001, 108 (4):e77-9.

De Brabander N, Wojciechowski M, De Decker K, et al, "Fomepizole as a Therapeutic Strategy in Paediatric Methanol Poisoning: A Case Report and Review of the Literature," *Eur J Pediatr*, 2005, 164 (3):158-61.

Detaille T, Wallemacq P, Clement de Clety S, et al, "Fomepizole Alone for Severe Infant Ethylene Glycol Poisoning," *Pediatr Crit Care Med*, 2004, 5(5):490-1.

Druteika DP, Zed PJ, and Ensom MH, "Role of Fomepizole in the Management of Ethylene Glycol Toxicity," *Pharmacotherapy*, 2002, 22 (3):365-72.

Fisher DM and Diaz JE, "Pediatric Methanol Poisoning Treated With Fomepizole (Antizol®)," *J Toxicol Clin Toxicol*, 1998, 36:512.

◆ **Foradil® (Can)** *see* Formoterol *on page 621*

◆ **Foradil® Aerolizer®** *see* Formoterol *on page 621*

Formoterol (for MOH te rol)

Medication Safety Issues
Sound-alike/look-alike issues:
Foradil® may be confused with Toradol®
Foradil® capsules for inhalation are for administration via Aerolizer™ inhaler and are **not** for oral use.

International issues:
Foradil® may be confused with Theradol® which is a brand name for tramadol in the Netherlands.

Related Information
Asthma *on page 1697*

U.S. Brand Names Foradil® Aerolizer®; Perforomist™

Canadian Brand Names Foradil®; Oxeze® Turbuhaler®

Therapeutic Category Adrenergic Agonist Agent; Anti-asthmatic; Beta$_2$-Adrenergic Agonist Agent; Bronchodilator; Sympathomimetic

Generic Available No

Use
Foradil® Aerolizer™: Maintenance treatment of asthma and prevention of bronchospasm in patients with reversible obstructive airway disease (FDA approved in >5 years and adults); prevention of exercise-induced bronchospasm (FDA approved in >5 years and adults)

Foradil® Aerolizer™, Perforomist™: Maintenance treatment of bronchoconstriction in COPD

Medication Guide An FDA-approved patient medication guide, which is available with the product information and at http://www.fda.gov/downloads/Drugs/DrugSafety/ ucm088602.pdf, must be dispensed with this medication for each new outpatient prescription and refill.

Pregnancy Risk Factor C

Pregnancy Considerations When given orally to rats throughout organogenesis, formoterol caused delayed ossification and decreased fetal weight, but no malformations. There were no adverse events when given to pregnant rats in late pregnancy. Doses used were ≥70 times the recommended daily inhalation dose in humans. There are no adequate and well-controlled studies in pregnant women. Use only if benefit outweighs risk to the fetus. Beta-agonists interfere with uterine contractility so use during labor only if benefit outweighs risk to the fetus.

Lactation Excretion in breast milk unknown/use caution

Contraindications Hypersensitivity to formoterol, adrenergic amines, or any component

Warnings Long-acting beta$_2$-adrenergic agents (eg, formoterol) have been associated with an increased risk of serious asthma exacerbations and asthma-related death **[U.S. Boxed Warning]**. Formoterol should only be prescribed in patients not adequately controlled on other asthma-controller medications, such as inhaled corticosteroids or patients whose disease severity clearly warrants treatment with two maintenance therapies; formoterol should not be used as monotherapy. Formoterol is not indicated to relieve acute asthma symptoms or for those patients who are successfully maintained with occasional use of beta$_2$-agonists. Acute asthma episodes should be treated with short-acting beta$_2$-agonists. Do not increase the frequency of formoterol use. Paroxysmal bronchospasm (which can be fatal) has been reported with this and other inhaled beta$_2$-agonists. If this occurs, discontinue treatment. A medication guide is available to provide information to patients covering the risk of use. Because long-acting beta$_2$-agonists (LABAs) may disguise poorly-controlled persistent asthma, frequent or chronic use of LABAs for exercise-induced bronchospasm is discouraged by the NIH Asthma Guidelines (NIH, 2007).

The safety and efficacy of Perforomist™ in the treatment of asthma or in children <18 years of age have not been established. Foradil® Aerolizer™ and Perforomist™ should not be used for the treatment of rapidly deteriorating COPD or for acute symptomatic COPD; increased use and/or ineffectiveness of short-acting beta$_2$-agonists may indicate rapidly deteriorating disease and should prompt re-evaluation of the patient's condition. Foradil® capsules should **only** be used with the Aerolizer™ inhaler and should **not** be taken orally.

Precautions Use with caution in patients with cardiovascular disorders (especially coronary insufficiency, arrhythmias, hypertension, heart failure), although uncommon at recommended doses, beta-agonists may cause elevation in BP and HR and result in CNS stimulation and excitation. Caution should also be used in patients with thyrotoxicosis, convulsive disorders, glaucoma, or conditions that are unusually sensitive to sympathomimetic amines. Transient hypokalemia from intracellular shunting may occur and produce adverse cardiovascular effects. Use with caution in patients with diabetes mellitus (DM); beta$_2$-agonists can increase serum glucose aggravating pre-existing DM and ketoacidosis. Use caution in patients with hepatic impairment. Foradil® aerolizer contains lactose; very rare anaphylactic reactions have been reported in patients with severe milk protein allergy.

Adverse Reactions

Cardiovascular: Chest pain, palpitations

Central nervous system: Dizziness, insomnia, fever, anxiety, dysphonia

Dermatologic: Rash, pruritus

Gastrointestinal: Diarrhea, nausea, vomiting, xerostomia, tonsillitis, gastroenteritis, abdominal pain, dyspepsia

Neuromuscular & skeletal: Back pain, tremors, muscle cramps

Respiratory: Upper/lower respiratory tract infection, asthma, pharyngitis, bronchitis, rhinitis, sinusitis, dyspnea, paradoxical bronchospasm (see Warnings)

Miscellaneous: Hypersensitivity reactions, tachyphylaxis, viral infection

Drug Interactions

Metabolism/Transport Effects Substrate (minor) of CYP2A6, 2C9, 2C19, 2D6

Avoid Concomitant Use

Avoid concomitant use of Formoterol with any of the following: Iobenguane I 123

Increased Effect/Toxicity

Formoterol may increase the levels/effects of: Sympathomimetics

The levels/effects of Formoterol may be increased by: Atomoxetine; Cannabinoids; MAO Inhibitors; Tricyclic Antidepressants

Decreased Effect

Formoterol may decrease the levels/effects of: Iobenguane I 123

The levels/effects of Formoterol may be decreased by: Alpha-/Beta-Blockers; Beta-Blockers (Beta1 Selective); Beta-Blockers (Nonselective); Betahistine

Stability

Foradil® Aerolizer™: Prior to dispensing, store in refrigerator at 2°C to 8°C (36°F to 46°F); after dispensing, store at controlled room temperature at 20°C to 25°C (68°F to 77°F); protect from heat and moisture. Capsules should always be stored in the blister pack and only removed immediately before use. Use within 4 months of purchase date or product expiration date, whichever comes first.

Performist™: Prior to dispensing, store in refrigerator at 2°C to 8°C (36°F to 46°F); after dispensing, store at controlled room temperature at 20°C to 25°C (68°F to 77°F) for up to 3 months. Protect from heat. Unit-dose vials should always be stored in the foil pouch and only removed immediately before use.

Mechanism of Action Formoterol is a long-acting selective beta$_2$-adrenergic receptor agonist. It relaxes bronchial smooth muscle by selective action on beta$_2$-receptors with little effect on heart rate

Pharmacodynamics

Onset of action: 1-3 minutes

Peak effect: 80% of peak effect within 15 minutes

Duration: Improvement in FEV$_1$ observed for 12 hours in most patients

Pharmacokinetics (Adult data unless noted)

Protein binding: 61% to 64%

Metabolism: Extensive via glucuronidation and o-demethylation

Half-life: Adults:

Powder for oral inhalation: ~10-14 hours

Solution for nebulization: ~7 hours

Time to peak serum concentration: Inhalation: 5 minutes

Elimination:

Children 5-12 years: 7% to 9% eliminated in urine as direct glucuronide metabolites, 6% as unchanged drug

Adults: 15% to 18% eliminated in urine as direct glucuronide metabolites, 2% to 10% as unchanged drug

Usual Dosage

Asthma maintenance treatment: Children ≥5 years and Adults: Inhalation: Foradil® Aerolizer™: 12 mcg (contents of 1 capsule aerosolized) twice daily, 12 hours apart; **Note:** For long-term asthma control, long-acting beta$_2$-agonists should be used in combination with inhaled corticosteroids and **not** as monotherapy

Prevention of exercise-induced asthma: Children ≥5 years and Adults: Inhalation: Foradil® Aerolizer™: 12 mcg (contents of 1 capsule aerosolized) 15 minutes prior to exercise; additional doses should not be used for 12 hours; patients who are using formoterol twice daily should **not** use an additional formoterol dose prior to exercise; if twice daily use is not effective during exercise, consider other appropriate therapy; **Note:** Because long-acting beta$_2$-agonists (LABAs) may disguise poorly-controlled persistent asthma, frequent or chronic use of LABAs for exercise-induced bronchospasm is discouraged by the NIH Asthma Guidelines (NIH, 2007).

COPD maintenance treatment: Adults: Inhalation:

Foradil® Aerolizer™: 12 mcg (contents of 1 capsule aerosolized) twice daily, 12 hours apart

Performist™: 20 mcg (2 mL) twice daily (maximum dose: 40 mcg/day) by nebulization

Administration

Foradil® Aerolizer™: Remove capsule from foil blister immediately before use. The contents of a capsule are aerosolized via a device called an Aerolizer™. Place the capsule into the Aerolizer™. The capsule is pierced by pressing and releasing the buttons on the side of the Aerolizer™. The formoterol formulation is dispersed into the air stream when the patient inhales rapidly and deeply through the mouthpiece. The patient should not exhale into the device. May not be used with spacer device.

Performist™: Remove unit-dose vial from foil pouch immediately before use. Solution does not require dilution prior to administration; do not mix other medications with Performist™ solution. Place contents of vial into the reservoir of a standard jet nebulizer connected to an air compressor; nebulize until all of the medication has been inhaled. Discard any unused medication immediately. Not for oral ingestion.

Monitoring Parameters Pulmonary function tests, vital signs, CNS stimulation, serum glucose, serum potassium

Patient Information Do not use to treat acute symptoms; do not exceed the prescribed dose of formoterol; do not stop using inhaled or oral corticosteroids without medical advice even if feeling better; may cause dry mouth; the capsule is not to be taken by mouth

Additional Information When formoterol is initiated in patients previously receiving a short-acting beta agonist, instruct the patient to discontinue the regular use of the short-acting beta agonist and to utilize the shorter-acting agent for symptomatic or acute episodes only.

Dosage Forms Excipient information presented when available (limited, particularly for generics); consult specific product labeling. [CAN] = Canadian brand name

Powder for oral inhalation, as fumarate:

Foradil® Aerolizer™ [capsule]: 12 mcg (12s, 60s) [contains lactose 25 mg]

Oxeze® Turbuhaler® [CAN]: 6 mcg/inhalation [delivers 60 metered doses; contains lactose 600 mcg/dose]; 12 mcg/inhalation [delivers 60 metered doses; contains lactose 600 mcg/dose] [not available in the U.S.]

Solution for nebulization, as fumarate dihydrate:

Performist™: 20 mcg/2 mL (2 mL)

References

Bisgaard H, "Long-acting Beta$_2$-Agonists in Management of Childhood Asthma: A Critical Review of the Literature," *Pediatr Pulmonol*, 2000, 29(3):221-34

"Guidelines for the Diagnosis and Management of Asthma. NAEPP Expert Panel Report 3," August 2007, www.nhlbi.nih.gov/guidelines/asthma/asthgdln.pdf.
"National Asthma Education and Prevention Program. Expert Panel Report: Guidelines for the Diagnosis and Management of Asthma Update on Selected Topics–2002," *J Allergy Clin Immunol*, 2002, 110 (5 Suppl):S141-219.

♦ **Formoterol Fumarate** *see* Formoterol *on page 621*

♦ **Formoterol Fumarate Dehydrate and Budesonide** *see* Budesonide and Formoterol *on page 210*

♦ **Formoterol Fumarate Dihydrate** *see* Formoterol *on page 621*

♦ **Formulex® (Can)** *see* Dicyclomine *on page 433*

♦ **5-Formyl Tetrahydrofolate** *see* Leucovorin Calcium *on page 804*

♦ **Fortamet®** *see* MetFORMIN *on page 891*

♦ **Fortaz®** *see* Ceftazidime *on page 272*

♦ **Fortical®** *see* Calcitonin *on page 227*

Fosamprenavir (FOS am pren a veer)

Medication Safety Issues
Sound-alike/look-alike issues:
Lexiva® may be confused with Levitra®

Related Information
Adult and Adolescent HIV *on page 1620*
Management of Healthcare Worker Exposures to HBV, HCV, and HIV *on page 1661*
Pediatric HIV *on page 1613*
Perinatal HIV *on page 1628*

U.S. Brand Names Lexiva®
Canadian Brand Names Telzir®
Therapeutic Category Antiretroviral Agent; HIV Agents (Anti-HIV Agents); Protease Inhibitor
Generic Available No
Use Treatment of HIV infection in combination with other antiretroviral agents (FDA approved in therapy-naïve patients ages ≥2 years and adults and in therapy-experienced patients ages ≥6 years and adults) (**Note:** HIV regimens consisting of **three** antiretroviral agents are strongly recommended)
Pregnancy Risk Factor C
Pregnancy Considerations Animal data showed some abortifacient and minor skeletal abnormalities with amprenavir. It is not known if amprenavir crosses the human placenta. There are no adequate and well-controlled studies in pregnant women. Pregnancy and protease inhibitors are both associated with an increased risk of hyperglycemia. Glucose levels should be closely monitored. The Perinatal HIV Guidelines Working Group notes there is insufficient data to recommend use during pregnancy; however, if used, they recommend that fosamprenavir be given with low-dose ritonavir boosting. Health professionals are encouraged to contact the antiretroviral pregnancy registry to monitor outcomes of pregnant women exposed to antiretroviral medications (1-800-258-4263 or www.APRegistry.com).
Lactation Excretion in breast milk unknown/contraindicated
Breast-Feeding Considerations In infants born to mothers who are HIV positive, HAART while breast-feeding may decrease postnatal infection. However, maternal or infant antiretroviral therapy does not completely eliminate the risk of postnatal HIV transmission.

In the United States where formula is accessible, affordable, safe, and sustainable, complete avoidance of breast-feeding by HIV-infected women is recommended to decrease potential transmission of HIV.
Contraindications Hypersensitivity to fosamprenavir, amprenavir, or any component; concurrent therapy with CYP3A4 substrates with a narrow therapeutic window; concomitant therapy with cisapride, delavirdine, dihydroergotamine, ergonovine, ergotamine, methylergonovine, lovastatin, midazolam, pimozide, rifampin, simvastatin, St John's wort, and triazolam; if fosamprenavir is administered with ritonavir, flecainide and propafenone are also contraindicated.

Warnings Fosamprenavir (a prodrug of amprenavir) is a potent CYP3A4 isoenzyme inhibitor that interacts with numerous drugs. Due to potential serious and/or life-threatening drug interactions, some drugs are contraindicated (see Contraindications and Drug Interactions) and the following drugs require serum concentration monitoring if coadministered with fosamprenavir: Amiodarone, systemic lidocaine, tricyclic antidepressants, and quinidine. Concurrent use with rifampin, St John's wort, certain cholesterol-lowering agents (lovastatin, simvastatin), and delavirdine are contraindicated.

Severe and life-threatening skin reactions (including Stevens-Johnson syndrome) may occur; discontinue fosamprenavir in patients who develop severe or life-threatening rashes or in patients with moderate rashes and systemic symptoms. Acute hemolytic anemia has been reported. Spontaneous bleeding episodes have been reported in patients with hemophilia type A and B receiving protease inhibitors. New-onset diabetes mellitus, exacerbations of diabetes, and hyperglycemia have been reported in HIV-infected patients receiving protease inhibitors. Higher than recommended combination doses of fosamprenavir and ritonavir may result in increased risk of transaminase elevations. Cases of nephrolithiasis have been reported with fosamprenavir use; consider temporary or permanent discontinuation of therapy if symptoms develop.

Significant elevations of serum triglycerides and cholesterol may occur; obtain serum triglyceride and cholesterol prior to initiation of therapy and periodically thereafter; manage lipid elevations appropriately. Modifiable risk factors for cardiovascular disease (eg, smoking, diabetes, hypertension) should also be monitored and managed appropriately. A possible increased risk of MI may occur in adult patients with HIV receiving fosamprenavir. Data recently reported from a nested case-control study linked cumulative fosamprenavir exposure to an increased risk of MI [OR = 1.52 per additional year of exposure (95% CI: 1.19-1.95)]. Previously, the Data Collection on Adverse Events of Anti-HIV Drugs (DAD) study identified a possible association between MI and the use of protease inhibitors.

Precautions Use with caution in patients with diabetes mellitus, sulfonamide allergy (fosamprenavir is a sulfonamide), or hemophilia. Use with caution and decrease the dose in patients with hepatic impairment; patients coinfected with hepatitis B or C and those with baseline liver enzyme elevation may be at risk for elevated liver enzymes with fosamprenavir therapy. Fat redistribution and accumulation [ie, central obesity, peripheral wasting, facial wasting, breast enlargement, dorsocervical fat enlargement (buffalo hump), and cushingoid appearance] have been observed in patients receiving antiretroviral agents (causal relationship not established). Immune reconstitution syndrome (an acute inflammatory response to residual or indolent opportunistic infections) may occur in HIV patients during initial treatment with combination antiretroviral agents; this syndrome may require further patient assessment and therapy. Safety and efficacy have not been established in children <2 years of age.

Animal studies indicate that fosamprenavir may be carcinogenic and may possess abortifacient properties; minor skeletal abnormalities have been observed in the offspring when amprenavir was administered to pregnant rabbits; the relevance for humans of these animal studies is uncertain.

Adverse Reactions Note: With the exception of vomiting, the incidence of adverse reactions is similar in pediatric patients and adults (higher incidence of vomiting in pediatric patients).

Central nervous system: Depression or mood disorders, fatigue (moderate-to-severe; 2% to 4%), headache (moderate-to-severe; 2% to 4%)

Dermatologic: Pruritus (7%); rash (~19% incidence; usually mild-to-moderate, maculopapular, some pruritic; median onset: 11 days, median duration: 13 days); severe or life-threatening rash, including Stevens-Johnson syndrome (<1% of patients; see Warnings)

Endocrine & metabolic: Exacerbation of diabetes mellitus, fat redistribution and accumulation (see Precautions), hypercholesterolemia, hyperglycemia (>251 mg/dL: <1% to 2%), hypertriglyceridemia (>750 mg/dL: 0% to 6%; up to 11% when used with ritonavir), ketoacidosis, new-onset diabetes, serum creatine phosphokinase increased, serum lipase increased (>2 times upper limit of normal: 5% to 8%)

Gastrointestinal: Abdominal pain (moderate-to-severe; 1% to 2%), diarrhea (moderate-to-severe; 5% to 13%), nausea (moderate-to-severe; 3% to 7%), vomiting [adults: Moderate-to-severe; 2% to 6%; **Note:** Vomiting (regardless of causality) occurred in 30% of pediatric patients receiving fosamprenavir twice daily with ritonavir (compared to 10% of adults) and occurred in 56% of children 2-5 years of age receiving twice daily fosamprenavir without ritonavir (compared to 16% of adults)]

Hematologic: Hemolytic anemia, neutropenia (<750 cells/mm^3: 3%), spontaneous bleeding in hemophiliacs (see Warnings)

Hepatic: Serum transaminases increased (>5 times upper limit of normal: 4% to 8%)

Neuromuscular & skeletal: Perioral paresthesia (2%)

Renal: Nephrolithiasis

Miscellaneous: Immune reconstitution syndrome (see Precautions)

<1%, postmarketing, and/or case reports: Angioedema, MI

Drug Interactions

Metabolism/Transport Effects As amprenavir: **Substrate** of CYP2C9 (minor), 3A4 (major), P-glycoprotein; **Inhibits** CYP2C19 (weak), 3A4 (strong)

Avoid Concomitant Use

Avoid concomitant use of Fosamprenavir with any of the following: Alfuzosin; Amiodarone; Cisapride; Delavirdine; Dronedarone; Eplerenone; Ergot Derivatives; Etravirine; Everolimus; Halofantrine; Lovastatin; Midazolam; Nilotinib; Nisoldipine; Pimozide; QuiNIDine; Ranolazine; Rivaroxaban; Romidepsin; Salmeterol; Silodosin; Simvastatin; St Johns Wort; Tamsulosin; Tolvaptan; Triazolam

Increased Effect/Toxicity

Fosamprenavir may increase the levels/effects of: Alfuzosin; Almotriptan; Alosetron; ALPRAZolam; Amiodarone; Antifungal Agents (Azole Derivatives, Systemic); Bortezomib; Brinzolamide; Calcium Channel Blockers (Dihydropyridine); Calcium Channel Blockers (Nondihydropyridine); CarBAMazepine; Ciclesonide; Cisapride; Clarithromycin; Clorazepate; Colchicine; Corticosteroids (Orally Inhaled); CycloSPORINE; CycloSPORINE (Systemic); CYP3A4 Substrates; Diazepam; Dienogest; Digoxin; Dronedarone; Dutasteride; Enfuvirtide; Eplerenone; Ergot Derivatives; Everolimus; FentaNYL; Fesoterodine; Flurazepam; Fusidic Acid; GuanFACINE; Halofantrine; HMG-CoA Reductase Inhibitors; Ixabepilone; Lovastatin; Lumefantrine; Maraviroc; Meperidine; MethylPREDNISolone; Midazolam; Nefazodone; Nilotinib; Nisoldipine; Paricalcitol; Pazopanib; Pimecrolimus; Pimozide; Protease Inhibitors; QuiNIDine; Ranolazine;

Rifamycin Derivatives; Rivaroxaban; Romidepsin; Salmeterol; Saxagliptin; Sildenafil; Silodosin; Simvastatin; Sirolimus; Sorafenib; Tacrolimus; Tacrolimus (Systemic); Tacrolimus (Topical); Tadalafil; Tamsulosin; Temsirolimus; Tenofovir; Tolvaptan; TraZODone; Triazolam; Tricyclic Antidepressants; Vardenafil; Warfarin

The levels/effects of Fosamprenavir may be increased by: Antifungal Agents (Azole Derivatives, Systemic); Clarithromycin; CycloSPORINE; CycloSPORINE (Systemic); Delavirdine; Efavirenz; Enfuvirtide; Etravirine; Fusidic Acid; P-Glycoprotein Inhibitors; Phenytoin

Decreased Effect

Fosamprenavir may decrease the levels/effects of: Abacavir; Clarithromycin; Contraceptives (Estrogens); Delavirdine; Divalproex; Meperidine; Methadone; PARoxetine; Phenytoin; Prasugrel; Valproic Acid; Zidovudine

The levels/effects of Fosamprenavir may be decreased by: Antacids; CarBAMazepine; Contraceptives (Estrogens); CYP3A4 Inducers (Strong); Deferasirox; Efavirenz; Garlic; H2-Antagonists; Nevirapine; Peginterferon Alfa-2b; P-Glycoprotein Inducers; Rifamycin Derivatives; St Johns Wort; Tenofovir

Food Interactions

Oral suspension: In adults, a standardized high-fat meal decreased the peak concentration by 46%, delayed the time to peak by 0.72 hours, and decreased the amprenavir AUC by 28% compared with the fasted state.

Tablets: Food does not significantly affect absorption.

Stability

Oral suspension: Store at 5°C to 30°C (41°F to 86°F). Do not freeze. Refrigeration is not required, but it may improve the taste of the suspension for some patients.

Tablets: Store at controlled room temperature of 25°C (77°F) in tightly closed container; excursions permitted to 15°C to 30°C (59°F to 86°F)

Mechanism of Action Fosamprenavir is rapidly converted to amprenavir *in vivo.* Amprenavir is a protease inhibitor which acts on an enzyme (protease) late in the HIV replication process after the virus has entered into the cell's nucleus; amprenavir binds to the protease activity site and inhibits the activity of the enzyme, thus preventing cleavage of viral polyprotein precursors (gag-pol protein precursors) into individual functional proteins found in infectious HIV; this results in the formation of immature, noninfectious viral particles

Pharmacokinetics (Adult data unless noted)

Protein binding: 90%; primarily to alpha$_1$ acid glycoprotein; concentration-dependent binding; protein binding is decreased in patients with hepatic impairment

Metabolism: Fosamprenavir is the prodrug of amprenavir; fosamprenavir is rapidly hydrolyzed to amprenavir and inorganic phosphate by cellular phosphatases in the gut epithelium as it is absorbed; amprenavir is metabolized in the liver via cytochrome P450 CYP3A4 isoenzyme system; glucuronide conjugation of oxidized metabolites also occurs

Bioavailability: Absolute oral bioavailability is not established. Similar amprenavir AUCs occurred in adults when single doses of the oral suspension versus tablets were administered in the fasted state; however, the suspension provided a 14.5% higher peak concentration (see also Food Interactions)

Half-life: Amprenavir: Adults: 7.7 hours

Time to peak serum concentration: Amprenavir (single dose of fosamprenavir): Median: 2.5 hours; range: 1.5-4 hours

Elimination: Minimal excretion of unchanged drug in urine (1%) and feces; 75% of dose excreted as metabolites via biliary tract into feces and 14% excreted as metabolites in urine

Dialysis: Peritoneal or hemodialysis: Amount removed is not known

Usual Dosage Oral (use in combination with other antiretroviral agents); **Note:** Dosing is based on whether patient is antiretroviral therapy-naïve or experienced and on concomitant therapy

Neonates, Infants, and Children <2 years: Not approved for use; appropriate dose is unknown

Children 2-18 years: Do not exceed adult dose; **Note:** Once-daily dosing of fosamprenavir is **not** recommended in pediatric patients (data from a pediatric once-daily dosing study of fosamprenavir plus ritonavir were insufficient to support once-daily dosing in any pediatric patient population).

Antiretroviral therapy-naïve pediatric patients:
Children 2-5 years: Unboosted regimen (ie, regimen without ritonavir): Fosamprenavir 30 mg/kg/dose twice daily; maximum dose: 1400 mg twice daily

Children ≥6 years and Adolescents:
Unboosted regimen (ie, regimen without ritonavir): Fosamprenavir 30 mg/kg/dose twice daily; maximum dose: 1400 mg twice daily

Ritonavir boosted regimen: Fosamprenavir 18 mg/kg/dose (maximum dose: 700 mg) twice daily plus ritonavir 3 mg/kg/dose (maximum dose: 100 mg) twice daily

Protease inhibitor-experienced pediatric patients:
Children 2-5 years: Not approved for use; appropriate dose is unknown

Children ≥6 years and Adolescents: Ritonavir boosted regimen: Fosamprenavir 18 mg/kg/dose (maximum dose: 700 mg) twice daily plus ritonavir 3 mg/kg/dose (maximum dose: 100 mg) twice daily

Note: The unboosted adult regimen of 1400 mg twice daily may be used for pediatric patients who weigh ≥47 kg. When combined with ritonavir, fosamprenavir tablets may be administered to children who weigh ≥39 kg; ritonavir capsules may be used for pediatric patients who weigh ≥33 kg.

Adults:
Antiretroviral therapy-naïve adult patients:
Unboosted regimen (ie, regimen without ritonavir): Fosamprenavir 1400 mg twice daily

Ritonavir boosted regimens:
Once-daily regimens:
Fosamprenavir 1400 mg once daily plus ritonavir 200 mg once daily

Fosamprenavir 1400 mg once daily plus ritonavir 100 mg once daily

Twice-daily regimen: Fosamprenavir 700 mg twice daily plus ritonavir 100 mg twice daily

Protease inhibitor-experienced adult patients:
Fosamprenavir 700 mg twice daily plus ritonavir 100 mg twice daily. **Note:** Once-daily dosing of fosamprenavir is not recommended in protease inhibitor-experienced patients.

Concomitant therapy with efavirenz: Note: Only ritonavir-boosted regimens should be used when efavirenz is used in combination with fosamprenavir.

Once-daily regimen: Fosamprenavir 1400 mg once daily plus ritonavir 300 mg once daily

Twice-daily regimen: Fosamprenavir 700 mg twice daily plus ritonavir 100 mg twice daily. **Note:** No change in ritonavir dosage is required when patients receive efavirenz with twice-daily dosing of fosamprenavir with ritonavir.

Concomitant therapy with nevirapine: Note: Only ritonavir-boosted regimens should be used when nevirapine is used in combination with fosamprenavir.

Once-daily regimen: Not studied

Twice-daily regimen: Fosamprenavir 700 mg twice daily plus ritonavir 100 mg twice daily.

Dosage adjustment in renal impairment: No dosage adjustment required

Dosage adjustment in hepatic impairment: Use with caution: Adults:

Mild impairment (Child-Pugh score 5-6): Reduce dosage of fosamprenavir to 700 mg twice daily without concurrent ritonavir (therapy-naïve) or fosamprenavir 700 mg twice daily plus ritonavir 100 mg once daily (therapy-naïve or PI-experienced)

Moderate impairment (Child-Pugh score 7-9): Reduce dosage of fosamprenavir to 700 mg twice daily without concurrent ritonavir (therapy-naïve) or fosamprenavir 450 mg twice daily plus ritonavir 100 mg once daily (therapy-naïve or PI-experienced)

Severe impairment (Child-Pugh score 10-15): Reduce dosage of fosamprenavir to 350 mg twice daily without concurrent ritonavir (therapy naïve) or use fosamprenavir 300 mg twice daily plus ritonavir 100 mg once daily (therapy naïve or protease inhibitor experienced).

Administration Do not administer concurrently with antacids or buffered formulations of other medications (separate administration by 1 hour).

Oral suspension: Administer **with** food to pediatric patients; administer **without** food to adults. Readminister dose of suspension if emesis occurs within 30 minutes after dosing. Shake suspension vigorously prior to use.

Tablets: May be administered without regard to meals.

Monitoring Parameters Signs and symptoms of rash or adverse effects; serum glucose, triglycerides, cholesterol (see Warnings), liver enzymes, CBC with differential, CD4 cell count, viral load

Patient Information Inform your physician if you have a sulfa allergy. Notify physician immediately if rash develops. Some medicines should not be taken with fosamprenavir; report the use of other medications, nonprescription medications, and herbal or natural products to your physician and pharmacist. Avoid the herbal medicine St John's wort; use alternate contraceptive measures instead of hormonal contraception (ie, the birth control pill) during therapy with fosamprenavir (hormonal contraceptives may not be effective if taken with fosamprenavir and liver enzymes may increase if hormonal contraceptives are taken with fosamprenavir plus ritonavir). Fosamprenavir is not a cure for HIV. Take fosamprenavir every day as prescribed; do not change dose or discontinue without physician's advice; if a dose is missed, take it as soon as possible, then return to normal dosing schedule; if a dose is skipped, do not double the next dose.

Kidney stones may occur in some patients; notify physician immediately if you develop pain in your side or when you urinate, or blood in your urine. HIV medications may cause changes in body fat, including an increase in fat in the upper back and neck, breasts, and trunk; a loss of fat from the face, arms, and legs may also occur.

Additional Information Oral suspension contains 50 mg/mL of fosamprenavir as fosamprenavir calcium and is equivalent to amprenavir 43 mg/mL. Fosamprenavir calcium 700 mg (1 tablet) is approximately equal to amprenavir 600 mg.

Dosage Forms Excipient information presented when available (limited, particularly for generics); consult specific product labeling. [CAN] = Canadian brand name

Tablet, as calcium:
Lexiva®: 700 mg [equivalent to amprenavir ~600 mg)
Telzir® [CAN]: 700 mg [not available in the U.S.]

Suspension, oral, as calcium:
Lexiva®: 50 mg/mL (225 mL) [equivalent to amprenavir ~43 mg/mL; contains propylene glycol; grape-bubble-gum-peppermint flavored]

Telzir® [CAN]: 50 mg/mL (225 mL) [not available in the U.S.]

References

Briars LA, Hilao JJ, and Kraus DM, "A Review of Pediatric Human Immunodeficiency Virus Infection," *Journal of Pharmacy Practice*, 2004, 17(6):407-31.

Chapman TM, Plosker GL, and Perry CM, "Fosamprenavir: A Review of Its Use in the Management of Antiretroviral Therapy-Naive Patients With HIV Infection," *Drugs*, 2004, 64(18):2101-24.

Morris JL and Kraus DM, "New Antiretroviral Therapies for Pediatric HIV Infection," *J Pediatr Pharmacol Ther*, 2005, 10:215-47.

Panel on Antiretroviral Guidelines for Adults and Adolescents, "Guidelines for the Use of Antiretroviral Agents in HIV-Infected Adults and Adolescents," December 1, 2009, http://www.aidsinfo.nih.gov.

Wire MB, Shelton MJ, and Studenberg S, "Fosamprenavir: Clinical Pharmacokinetics and Drug Interactions of the Amprenavir Prodrug," *Clin Pharmacokinet*, 2006, 45(2):137-68.

Working Group on Antiretroviral Therapy and Medical Management of HIV-Infected Children, "Guidelines for the Use of Antiretroviral Agents in Pediatric HIV Infection," February 23, 2009. Available at http://www.aidsinfo.nih.gov.

♦ **Fosamprenavir Calcium** *see* Fosamprenavir *on page 623*

♦ **Fosaprepitant Dimeglumine** *see* Aprepitant/Fosaprepitant *on page 125*

Foscarnet (fos KAR net)

U.S. Brand Names Foscavir® [DSC]
Canadian Brand Names Foscavir®
Therapeutic Category Antiviral Agent, Parenteral
Generic Available Yes
Use Alternative to ganciclovir for treatment of CMV infections; treatment of CMV retinitis in patients with acquired immunodeficiency syndrome (FDA approved in adults); treatment of acyclovir-resistant mucocutaneous herpes simplex virus infections in immunocompromised patients and acyclovir-resistant herpes zoster infections (FDA approved in adults)
Pregnancy Risk Factor C
Pregnancy Considerations Associated with an increase in skeletal anomalies in animal studies at approximately the equivalent of 13% to 33% of the maximal daily human dose. There are no adequate and well controlled studies in pregnant women. A single case report of use during the third trimester with normal infant outcome was observed. Monitoring of amniotic fluid volumes by ultrasound is recommended weekly after 20 weeks of gestation to detect oligohydramnios.
Lactation Excretion in breast milk unknown/contraindicated
Breast-Feeding Considerations The CDC recommends **not** to breast-feed if diagnosed with HIV to avoid postnatal transmission of the virus.
Contraindications Hypersensitivity to foscarnet or any component
Warnings Renal impairment occurs to some degree in the majority of patients treated with foscarnet **[U.S. Boxed Warning]**; renal impairment may occur at any time and is usually reversible within 1 week following dose adjustment or discontinuation of therapy; however, several patients have died with renal failure within 4 weeks of stopping foscarnet. To reduce the risk of nephrotoxicity and the potential to administer a relative overdose, always calculate the Cl_{cr} even if serum creatinine is within the normal range. Dosage adjustments are recommended for renal dysfunction; safety and efficacy in patients with a baseline S_{cr} >2.8 mg/dL or Cl_{cr} <50 mL/minute are limited. Adequate hydration may reduce the risk of nephrotoxicity and prehydration is recommended; foscarnet use is not recommended in patients with a Cl_{cr} <0.4 mL/kg/minute.

Foscarnet is deposited in teeth and bone of young, growing animals; it has adversely affected tooth enamel development in rats; deposition in human bone has also

been demonstrated; safety and effectiveness in children has not been fully evaluated.

Serum electrolyte imbalance occurs in 6% to 48% of patients (hypocalcemia, low ionized calcium, hypo- or hyperphosphatemia, hypokalemia, or hypomagnesemia). Patients with a low ionized calcium may experience perioral tingling, numbness, parasthesia, tetany, and seizures.

Seizures related to electrolyte/mineral imbalance may occur **[U.S. Boxed Warning]**; incidence has been reported in up to 10% of HIV patients. Risk factors for seizures include impaired baseline renal function, low total serum calcium, and underlying CNS condition. Some patients who have experienced seizures have been able to continue or resume foscarnet treatment after their mineral or electrolyte abnormality has been corrected, their underlying disease state treated, or their dose decreased.
Precautions Use with caution in patients with renal impairment, patients with altered electrolyte levels, and patients with neurologic or cardiac abnormalities; adjust dose for patients with impaired renal function; discontinue treatment in adults if serum creatinine ≥2.9 mg/dL; therapy can be restarted if serum creatinine ≤2 mg/dL; anemia and granulocytopenia have been reported; monitor CBC; foscarnet is a venous irritant, infuse only into veins with adequate blood flow
Adverse Reactions
Cardiovascular: Arrhythmias, chest pain, ECG abnormalities, flushing, hypertension, hypotension, palpitations
Central nervous system: Agitation, amnesia, depression, dizziness, fatigue, fever, hallucinations, headache, seizures
Dermatologic: Pruritus, rash
Endocrine & metabolic: Hypocalcemia, hypokalemia, hypomagnesemia, hypo- or hyperphosphatemia, weight loss
Gastrointestinal: Anorexia, constipation, diarrhea, dyspepsia, nausea, pancreatitis, stomatitis, vomiting
Genitourinary: Dysuria, penile epithelium ulceration, urethral disorder, vulvovaginal ulceration
Hematologic: Hemoglobin and hematocrit decreased, leukopenia
Hepatic: Cholecystitis, hepatitis, liver enzymes increased
Local: Thrombophlebitis
Neuromuscular & skeletal: Paresthesia, peripheral neuropathy, tremor
Ocular: Conjunctivitis, ocular pain
Renal: BUN and serum creatinine increased, oliguria, polyuria, proteinuria, renal failure
Respiratory: Bronchospasm, coughing, dyspnea
<1%, postmarketing, and/or case reports: Diabetes insipidus (usually nephrogenic), erythema multiforme, gamma GT increased, myopathy, myositis, muscle weakness, renal calculus, rhabdomyolysis, QT interval prolongation, Stevens-Johnson syndrome, toxic epidermal necrolysis, ventricular arrhythmia
Drug Interactions
Avoid Concomitant Use
Avoid concomitant use of Foscarnet with any of the following: Artemether; Dronedarone; Lumefantrine; Nilotinib; Pimozide; QuiNINE; Tetrabenazine; Thioridazine; Ziprasidone
Increased Effect/Toxicity
Foscarnet may increase the levels/effects of: Dronedarone; Pimozide; QTc-Prolonging Agents; QuiNINE; Tetrabenazine; Thioridazine; Ziprasidone

The levels/effects of Foscarnet may be increased by: Alfuzosin; Artemether; Chloroquine; Ciprofloxacin; Ciprofloxacin (Systemic); Gadobutrol; Lumefantrine; Nilotinib; QuiNINE

Decreased Effect There are no known significant interactions involving a decrease in effect.

Stability Store at room temperature; refrigeration may result in crystallization of the drug; incompatible with dextrose ≥30%, I.V. solutions containing calcium, magnesium, vancomycin, TPN; use within 24 hours of mixing

Mechanism of Action Pyrophosphate analog which inhibits DNA synthesis by interfering with viral DNA polymerase and reverse transcriptase

Pharmacokinetics (Adult data unless noted)
Distribution: V_d: Adults: 0.6 L/kg; up to 20% of cumulative I.V. dose may be deposited in bone
Protein binding: 14% to 17%
Half-life, plasma: Adults: 2-4.5 hours
Elimination: 80% to 90% excreted unchanged in urine

Usual Dosage Children and Adults: I.V.:
CMV retinitis: Induction treatment: 180 mg/kg/day divided every 8-12 hours for 14-21 days
Maintenance therapy: 90-120 mg/kg/day as a single infusion once daily
Acyclovir-resistant herpes simplex virus infection: 40 mg/kg/dose every 8-12 hours for up to 3 weeks or until lesions heal; repeat treatment may lead to the development of resistance

Dosing interval in renal impairment: Adults:
CMV Induction (equivalent to 60 mg/kg every 8 hours):
Cl_{cr} >1.4 mL/minute/kg: 60 mg/kg every 8 hours
Cl_{cr} >1-1.4 mL/minute/kg: 45 mg/kg every 8 hours
Cl_{cr} >0.8-1 mL/minute/kg: 50 mg/kg every 12 hours
Cl_{cr} >0.6-0.8 mL/minute/kg: 40 mg/kg every 12 hours
Cl_{cr} >0.5-0.6 mL/minute/kg: 60 mg/kg every 24 hours
Cl_{cr} ≥0.4-0.5 mL/minute/kg: 50 mg/kg every 24 hours
Cl_{cr} <0.4 mL/minute/kg: Not recommended
CMV Induction (equivalent to 90 mg/kg every 12 hours):
Cl_{cr} >1.4 mL/minute/kg: 90 mg/kg every 12 hours
Cl_{cr} >1-1.4 mL/minute/kg: 70 mg/kg every 12 hours
Cl_{cr} >0.8-1 mL/minute/kg: 50 mg/kg every 12 hours
Cl_{cr} >0.6-0.8 mL/minute/kg: 80 mg/kg every 24 hours
Cl_{cr} >0.5-0.6 mL/minute/kg: 60 mg/kg every 24 hours
Cl_{cr} ≥0.4-0.5 mL/minute/kg: 50 mg/kg every 24 hours
Cl_{cr} <0.4 mL/minute/kg: Not recommended
CMV Maintenance:
Cl_{cr} >1.4 mL/minute/kg: 90-120 mg/kg every 24 hours
Cl_{cr} >1-1.4 mL/minute/kg: 70-90 mg/kg every 24 hours
Cl_{cr} >0.8-1 mL/minute/kg: 50-65 mg/kg every 24 hours
Cl_{cr} >0.6-0.8 mL/minute/kg: 80-105 mg/kg every 48 hours
Cl_{cr} >0.5-0.6 mL/minute/kg: 60-80 mg/kg every 48 hours
Cl_{cr} ≥0.4-0.5 mL/minute/kg: 50-65 mg/kg every 48 hours
Cl_{cr} <0.4 mL/minute/kg: Not recommended
HSV Infection (equivalent to 40 mg/kg every 8 hours):
Cl_{cr} >1.4 mL/minute/kg: 40 mg/kg every 8 hours
Cl_{cr} >1-1.4 mL/minute/kg: 30 mg/kg every 8 hours
Cl_{cr} >0.8-1 mL/minute/kg: 35 mg/kg every 12 hours
Cl_{cr} >0.6-0.8 mL/minute/kg: 25 mg/kg every 12 hours
Cl_{cr} >0.5-0.6 mL/minute/kg: 40 mg/kg every 24 hours
Cl_{cr} ≥0.4-0.5 mL/minute/kg: 35 mg/kg every 24 hours
Cl_{cr} <0.4 mL/minute/kg: Not recommended
HSV Infection (equivalent to 40 mg/kg every 12 hours):
Cl_{cr} >1.4 mL/minute/kg: 40 mg/kg every 12 hours
Cl_{cr} >1-1.4 mL/minute/kg: 30 mg/kg every 12 hours
Cl_{cr} >0.8-1 mL/minute/kg: 20 mg/kg every 12 hours
Cl_{cr} >0.6-0.8 mL/minute/kg: 35 mg/kg every 24 hours
Cl_{cr} >0.5-0.6 mL/minute/kg: 25 mg/kg every 24 hours
Cl_{cr} ≥0.4-0.5 mL/minute/kg: 20 mg/kg every 24 hours
Cl_{cr} <0.4 mL/minute/kg: Not recommended

Administration Parenteral: 24 mg/mL solution may be administered without further dilution when using a central venous catheter for infusion; for peripheral vein administration, the solution **must** be diluted to a final concentration **not to exceed** 12 mg/mL with either NS or D_5W; administer by I.V. infusion at a rate **not to exceed** 60 mg/kg/dose over 1 hour or 120 mg/kg/dose over 2 hours (1 mg/kg/minute); prior to initial infusion, prehydrate children with 10-20 mL/kg (maximum: 1000 mL) of age-appropriate fluid (usually NS) or adults with 750-1000 mL NS or D_5W; for subsequent infusions, hydrate children concurrently with 10-20 mL/kg (maximum: 1000 mL) of age-appropriate fluid or adults with 500-1000 mL NS or D_5W; concurrent hydration volume is dependant on foscarnet dose

Monitoring Parameters Serum creatinine, calcium, phosphorus, potassium, magnesium, CBC, ophthalmologic exams

Reference Range Therapeutic serum concentration for CMV: 150 mcg/mL

Patient Information Report any numbness in the extremities, paresthesias, perioral tingling, or seizures

Nursing Implications Provide adequate hydration with I.V. NS or D_5W prior to and during treatment to minimize nephrotoxicity

Dosage Forms Excipient information presented when available (limited, particularly for generics); consult specific product labeling. [DSC] = Discontinued product
Injection, solution, as sodium [preservative-free]: 24 mg/mL (250 mL, 500 mL)
Foscavir®: 24 mg/mL (500 mL) [DSC]

References
Aweeka FT, Jacobson MA, Martin-Munley S, et al, "Effect of Renal Disease and Hemodialysis on Foscarnet Pharmacokinetics and Dosing Recommendations," *J Acquir Immune Defic Syndr Hum Retrovirol*, 1999, 20(4):350-7.
Butler KM, DeSmet MD, Husson RN, et al, "Treatment of Aggressive Cytomegalovirus Retinitis With Ganciclovir in Combination With Foscarnet in a Child Infected With Human Immunodeficiency Virus," *J Pediatr*, 1992, 120(3):483-6.
Kaplan JE, Masur H, and Holmes KK, "Guidelines for Preventing Opportunistic Infections Among HIV-Infected Persons - 2002. Recommendations of the USPHS and IDSA," *MMWR*, 2002, 51 (RR-8):1-27, 29-46.

◆ **Foscavir® [DSC]** *see* Foscarnet *on page 626*

◆ **Foscavir® (Can)** *see* Foscarnet *on page 626*

Fosinopril (foe SIN oh pril)

Medication Safety Issues
Sound-alike/look-alike issues:
Fosinopril may be confused with FLUoxetine, Fosamax®, furosemide, lisinopril
Monopril® may be confused with Accupril®, minoxidil, moexipril, Monoket®, Monurol®, ramipril

Related Information
Antihypertensive Agents by Class *on page 1481*

U.S. Brand Names Monopril® [DSC]

Canadian Brand Names Apo-Fosinopril®; Monopril®; Mylan-Fosinopril; PMS-Fosinopril; RAN™-Fosinopril; Riva-Fosinopril; Teva-Fosinopril

Therapeutic Category Angiotensin-Converting Enzyme (ACE) Inhibitor; Antihypertensive Agent

Generic Available Yes

Use Treatment of hypertension, either alone or in combination with other antihypertensive agents; adjunctive treatment of CHF; management of left ventricular dysfunction after MI; has also been used for the treatment of diabetic nephropathy

Pregnancy Risk Factor C (1st trimester); D (2nd and 3rd trimesters)

Pregnancy Considerations Due to adverse events observed in some animal studies, fosinopril is considered pregnancy category C during the first trimester. Based on human data, fosinopril is considered pregnancy category D if used during the second and third trimesters (per the manufacturer; however, one study suggests that fetal injury may occur at anytime during pregnancy). First trimester exposure to ACE inhibitors may cause major congenital malformations. An increased risk of cardiovascular and/or central nervous system malformations was observed in one study; however, an increased risk of teratogenic events was not observed in other studies. Second and third trimester use of an ACE inhibitor is associated with oligohydramnios. Oligohydramnios due to decreased fetal renal function may lead to fetal limb contractures, craniofacial deformation, and hypoplastic lung development. The use of ACE inhibitors during the second and third trimesters is also associated with anuria, hypotension, renal failure (reversible or irreversible), skull hypoplasia, and death in the fetus/neonate. Chronic maternal hypertension itself is also associated with adverse events in the fetus/infant. ACE inhibitors are not recommended during pregnancy to treat maternal hypertension or heart failure. Those who are planning a pregnancy should be considered for other medication options if an ACE inhibitor is currently prescribed or the ACE inhibitor should be discontinued as soon as possible once pregnancy is detected. The exposed fetus should be monitored for fetal growth, amniotic fluid volume, and organ formation. Infants exposed to an ACE inhibitor *in utero*, especially during the second and third trimester, should be monitored for hyperkalemia, hypotension, and oliguria.

[U.S. Boxed Warning]: Based on human data, ACE inhibitors can cause injury and death to the developing fetus when used in the second and third trimesters. ACE inhibitors should be discontinued as soon as possible once pregnancy is detected.

Lactation Enters breast milk/not recommended

Breast-Feeding Considerations Fosinoprilat is excreted in breast milk. Breast-feeding is not recommended by the manufacturer.

Contraindications Hypersensitivity to fosinopril, any component, or other ACE inhibitors; patients with idiopathic or hereditary angioedema or a history of angioedema with previous ACE inhibitor use

Warnings Serious adverse effects including angioedema, anaphylactoid reactions, neutropenia, agranulocytosis, hypotension, and hepatic failure may occur (see Adverse Reactions). Angioedema can occur at any time during treatment (especially following first dose). Angioedema may occur in the head, neck, extremities, or intestines; angioedema of the larynx, glottis, or tongue may cause airway obstruction, especially in patients with a history of airway surgery; prolonged monitoring may be required, even in patients with swelling of only the tongue (ie, without respiratory distress) because treatment with corticosteroids and antihistamines may not be sufficient; very rare fatalities have occurred with angioedema of the larynx or tongue; appropriate treatment (eg, establishing patent airway and/or SubQ epinephrine) should be readily available for patients with angioedema of larynx, glottis, or tongue, in whom airway obstruction is likely to occur. Risk of neutropenia may be increased in patients with renal dysfunction and especially in patients with both collagen vascular disease and renal dysfunction.

ACE inhibitors can cause injury and death to the developing fetus when used during pregnancy. ACE inhibitors should be discontinued as soon as possible once pregnancy is detected **[U.S. Boxed Warning]**. Neonatal hypotension, skull hypoplasia, anuria, renal failure, oligohydramnios (associated with fetal limb contractures, craniofacial deformities, hypoplastic lung development), prematurity, intrauterine growth retardation, patent ductus arteriosus, and death have been reported with the use of ACE inhibitors, primarily in the second and third trimesters. The risk of neonatal toxicity has been considered less when ACE inhibitors are used in the first

trimester; however, major congenital malformations have been reported. The cardiovascular and/or central nervous systems are most commonly affected.

Precautions Careful blood pressure monitoring is required (hypotension can occur especially in volume-depleted patients). Use with caution in patients with hypovolemia, collagen vascular diseases, valvular stenosis (particularly aortic stenosis), hyperkalemia, or before, during, or immediately after anesthesia. Avoid rapid dosage escalation which may lead to renal insufficiency. Rare toxicities associated with ACE inhibitors include cholestatic jaundice (which may progress to hepatic necrosis) and neutropenia/agranulocytosis with myeloid hyperplasia. Hyperkalemia may rarely occur. ACE inhibitors may be associated with deterioration of renal function and/or increases in serum creatinine, particularly in patients dependent on renin-angiotensin-aldosterone system (eg, those with severe CHF). Use with caution in patients with renal artery stenosis or pre-existing renal insufficiency; if patient has renal impairment then a baseline WBC with differential and serum creatinine should be evaluated and monitored closely during the first 3 months of therapy. Hypersensitivity reactions may be seen during hemodialysis with high-flux dialysis membranes (eg, AN69). Safety and efficacy have not been established in children <6 years of age; long-term effects of fosinopril on growth and development have not been evaluated.

Adverse Reactions Note: Higher rates of adverse reactions have generally been noted in patients with CHF; however, the frequency of adverse effects associated with placebo is also increased in this population. The adverse reaction profile for pediatric patients is similar to that observed in adults with hypertension.

Cardiovascular: Hypotension, syncope, palpitation

Central nervous system: Dizziness, fatigue, headache

Dermatologic: Rash, angioedema (see Warnings); **Note:** The relative risk of angioedema with ACE inhibitors is higher within the first 30 days of use (compared to >1 year of use), for Black Americans (compared to Whites), for lisinopril or enalapril (compared to captopril), and for patients hospitalized within 30 days (Brown, 1996).

Endocrine & metabolic: Hyperkalemia

Gastrointestinal: Diarrhea, nausea, vomiting

Hematologic: Neutropenia, agranulocytosis

Hepatic: Transaminases increased, cholestatic jaundice, hepatitis, fulminant hepatic necrosis (rare, but potentially fatal)

Neuromuscular & skeletal: Musculoskeletal pain, noncardiac chest pain, weakness

Renal: BUN and serum creatinine elevated, worsening of renal function (in patients with bilateral renal artery stenosis or hypovolemia)

Respiratory: Cough; **Note:** An isolated dry cough lasting >3 weeks was reported in 7 of 42 pediatric patients (17%) receiving ACE inhibitors (von Vigier, 2000).

Miscellaneous: Anaphylactoid reactions

Drug Interactions

Avoid Concomitant Use There are no known interactions where it is recommended to avoid concomitant use.

Increased Effect/Toxicity

Fosinopril may increase the levels/effects of: Allopurinol; Amifostine; Antihypertensives; AzaTHIOprine; CycloSPORINE; CycloSPORINE (Systemic); Ferric Gluconate; Gold Sodium Thiomalate; Hypotensive Agents; Iron Dextran Complex; Lithium; RiTUXimab

The levels/effects of Fosinopril may be increased by: Angiotensin II Receptor Blockers; Diazoxide; DPP-IV Inhibitors; Eplerenone; Everolimus; Herbs (Hypotensive Properties); Loop Diuretics; MAO Inhibitors; Pentoxifylline; Phosphodiesterase 5 Inhibitors; Potassium Salts; Potassium-Sparing Diuretics; Prostacyclin Analogues;

Sirolimus; Temsirolimus; Thiazide Diuretics; Tolvaptan; Trimethoprim

Decreased Effect

The levels/effects of Fosinopril may be decreased by: Antacids; Aprotinin; Herbs (Hypertensive Properties); Methylphenidate; Nonsteroidal Anti-Inflammatory Agents; Salicylates; Yohimbine

Food Interactions Food decreases the rate, but not the extent of absorption. Limit salt substitutes or potassium-rich diet. Avoid natural licorice (causes sodium and water retention and increases potassium loss).

Stability Store at 25°C (77°F); excursions permitted to 15°C to 30°C (59°F to 86°F). Protect from moisture; keep bottle tightly closed.

Mechanism of Action Competitive inhibitor of angiotensin-converting enzyme (ACE); prevents conversion of angiotensin I to angiotensin II, a potent vasoconstrictor; results in lower levels of angiotensin II which causes an increase in plasma renin activity and a reduction in aldosterone secretion; a CNS mechanism may also be involved in hypotensive effect as angiotensin II increases adrenergic outflow from CNS; vasoactive kallikreins may be decreased in conversion to active hormones by ACE inhibitors, thus reducing blood pressure

Pharmacodynamics

Reduction in blood pressure:
Onset of action: 1 hour
Maximum effect: 2-6 hours postdose
Duration: 24 hours

Pharmacokinetics (Adult data unless noted)

Absorption: Oral: 30% to 36% (fosinopril)

Protein binding: 95%

Metabolism: Fosinopril is a prodrug (inactive) and is hydrolyzed to fosinoprilat (active) by intestinal wall and hepatic esterases; fosinopril is also metabolized to a glucuronide conjugate and a p-hydroxy metabolite of fosinoprilat

Bioavailability: 36%

Half-life: Fosinoprilat:
Children 6-16 years: 11-13 hours
Adults: 12 hours
Adults with CHF: 14 hours

Time to peak serum concentration: ~3 hours

Elimination: Urine and feces (as fosinoprilat and other metabolites in roughly equal proportions, 45% to 50%)

Usual Dosage Note: Dosage must be titrated according to patient's response; use lowest effective dose

Oral: Manufacturer's recommendations: **Note:** Doses of 0.1-0.6 mg/kg have been studied in children 6-16 years of age.

Children ≤50 kg: Dosage not established; appropriate dosage strength is not available

Children >50 kg: Hypertension: Initial: 5-10 mg once daily, as monotherapy (maximum: 40 mg/day)

Adults:

Hypertension: Initial: 10 mg once daily; usual maintenance: 20-40 mg/day. May need to divide the dose into two if trough effect is inadequate; discontinue the diuretic, if possible 2-3 days before initiation of therapy; resume diuretic therapy carefully, if needed.

Heart failure: Initial: 10 mg once daily (5 mg once daily if renal dysfunction present or if patient has been vigorously diuresed); increase dose, as needed, to a maximum of 40 mg once daily over several weeks; usual dose: 20-40 mg/day. If hypotension, orthostasis, or azotemia occurs during titration, consider decreasing concomitant diuretic dose, if any.

Dosing adjustment/comments in renal impairment: In general, no dosage adjustments are needed since hepatobiliary elimination compensates adequately for diminished renal elimination. **Note:** Patients with heart failure and severely decrease renal function may be more sensitive to the hemodynamic effects (ie, hypotension) of ACE inhibitors.

Administration Oral: May be administered without regard to food.

Monitoring Parameters Blood pressure (supervise for at least 2 hours after the initial dose or any dosage increase for significant orthostasis); renal function, WBC, serum potassium; monitor for angioedema and anaphylactoid reactions (see Warnings)

Test Interactions Positive Coombs' (direct); may cause false-positive results in urine acetone determinations using sodium nitroprusside reagent; may cause false low serum digoxin levels with the Digi-Tab RIA kit for digoxin

Patient Information Notify physician immediately if swelling of face, lips, tongue, or difficulty in breathing occurs; if these occur, do not take any more doses until a physician can be consulted. Notify physician if vomiting, diarrhea, excessive perspiration, dehydration, or persistent cough occurs. Do not add a salt substitute (potassium-containing) without physician advice. May cause dizziness, fainting, and lightheadedness, especially in first week of therapy; sit and stand up slowly. May cause rash. Report sore throat, fever, other signs of infection or other side effects. This medication may cause injury and death to the developing fetus when used during pregnancy; women of childbearing potential should be informed of potential risk; consult prescriber for appropriate contraceptive measures; this medication should be discontinued as soon as possible once pregnancy is detected (see Warnings).

Nursing Implications Discontinue if angioedema occurs; observe closely for hypotension after the first dose or initiation of a new higher dose (keep in mind that maximum effect on blood pressure occurs at 2-6 hours after dose)

Additional Information Racial differences were identified in a multicentered, prospective, double-blind, placebo-controlled trial that investigated the dose-response of fosinopril in 253 children 6-16 years of age. This study found that black children required a higher dose of fosinopril (per kg body weight) in order to adequately control blood pressure (Menon, 2006). The findings of this study are consistent with adult studies assessing ACE inhibitors.

Dosage Forms Excipient information presented when available (limited, particularly for generics); consult specific product labeling. [DSC] = Discontinued product

Tablet, as sodium: 10 mg, 20 mg, 40 mg
Monopril®: 10 mg, 20 mg, 40 mg [DSC]

References

ALLHAT Officers and Coordinators for the ALLHAT Collaborative Research Group, "Major Outcomes in High-Risk Hypertensive Patients Randomized to Angiotensin-Converting Enzyme Inhibitor or Calcium Channel Blocker vs Diuretic: The Antihypertensive and Lipid-Lowering Treatment to Prevent Heart Attack Trial (ALLHAT)," *JAMA*, 2002, 288(23):2981-97.

Antman EM, Anbe DT, Armstrong PW, et al, "ACC/AHA Guidelines for the Management of Patients With ST-Elevation Myocardial Infarction - Executive Summary: A Report of the American College of Cardiology/American Heart Association Task Force on Practice Guidelines (Writing Committee to Revise the 1999 Guidelines for the Management of Patients With Acute Myocardial Infarction)," *Circulation*, 2004, 110:588-636.

Brown NJ, Ray WA, Snowden M, et al, "Black Americans Have an Increased Rate of Angiotensin-Converting Enzyme Inhibitor-Associated Angioedema," *Clin Pharmacol Ther*, 1996, 60(1):8-13.

Chase MP, Fiarman GS, Scholz FJ, et al, "Angioedema of the Small Bowel Due to an Angiotensin-Converting Enzyme Inhibitor," *J Clin Gastroenterol*, 2000, 31(3):254-7.

Chobanian AV, Bakris GL, Black HR, et al, "The Seventh Report of the Joint National Committee on Prevention, Detection, Evaluation, and Treatment of High Blood Pressure: The JNC 7 Report," *JAMA*, 2003, 289(19):2560-72.

"Consensus Recommendations for the Management of Chronic Heart Failure. On Behalf of the Membership of the Advisory Council to Improve Outcomes Nationwide in Heart Failure," *Am J Cardiol*, 1999, 83(2A):1A-38A.

Cooper WO, Hernandez-Diaz S, Arbogast PG, et al, "Major Congenital Malformations After First-Trimester Exposure to ACE Inhibitors," *N Engl J Med*, 2006, 354(23):2443-51.

"Guidelines for the Evaluation and Management of Heart Failure. Report of the American College of Cardiology/American Heart Association Task Force on Practice Guidelines (Committee on Evaluation and Management of Heart Failure)," *Circulation*, 1995, 92(9):2764-84.

"K/DOQI Clinical Practice Guidelines for Chronic Kidney Disease: Evaluation, Classification, and Stratification. Kidney Disease Outcome Quality Initiative," *Am J Kidney Dis*, 2002, 39(2 Suppl 2):1-246.

Konstam MA, Dracup K, Baker DW, et al, "Heart Failure Evaluation and Care of Patients With Left Ventricular Systolic Dysfunction," *J Card Fail*, 1995, 1(2):183-7.

Li JS, Berezny K, Kilaru R, et al, "Is the Extrapolated Adult Dose of Fosinopril Safe and Effective in Treating Hypertensive Children?" *Hypertension*, 2004, 44(3):289-93.

Mastrobattista JM, "Angiotensin Converting Enzyme Inhibitors in Pregnancy," *Semin Perinatol*, 1997, 21(2):124-34.

Menon S, Berezny KY, Kilaru R, et al, "Racial Differences are Seen in Blood Pressure Response to Fosinopril in Hypertensive Children," *Am Heart J*, 2006,152(2):394-9.

National High Blood Pressure Education Program Working Group on High Blood Pressure in Children and Adolescents, "The Fourth Report on the Diagnosis, Evaluation, and Treatment of High Blood Pressure in Children and Adolescents," *Pediatrics*, 2004, 114(2 Suppl):555-76.

Packer M, Poole-Wilson PA, Armstrong PW, et al, "Comparative Effects of Low and High Doses of the Angiotensin-Converting Enzyme Inhibitor, Lisinopril, on Morbidity and Mortality in Chronic Heart Failure," *Circulation*, 1999, 100(23):2312-8.

Quan A, "Fetopathy Associated With Exposure to Angiotensin Converting Enzyme Inhibitors and Angiotensin Receptor Antagonists," *Early Hum Dev*, 2006, 82(1):23-8.

Smoger SH and Sayed MA, "Simultaneous Mucosal and Small Bowel Angioedema Due to Captopril," *South Med J*, 1998, 91(11):1060-3.

von Vigier RO, Mozzettini S, Truttmann AC, et al, "Cough is Common in Children Prescribed Converting Enzyme Inhibitors," *Nephron*, 2000, 84(1):98.

Yi Z, Li Z, Wu XC, et al, "Effect of Fosinopril in Children With Steroid-Resistant Idiopathic Nephrotic Syndrome," *Pediatr Nephrol*, 2006, 21 (7):967-72.

◆ **Fosinopril Sodium** *see* Fosinopril *on page 627*

Fosphenytoin (FOS fen i toyn)

Medication Safety Issues
Sound-alike/look-alike issues:
Cerebyx® may be confused with Celebrex®, Celexa™, Cerezyme®, Cervarix®
Fosphenytoin may be confused with fospropofol

Overdoses have occurred due to confusion between the **mg per mL concentration** of fosphenytoin (50 mg PE/mL) and **total drug content per vial** (either 100 mg PE/2 mL vial or 500 mg PE/10 mL vial). ISMP recommends that the total drug content per container is identified instead of the concentration in mg per mL to avoid confusion and potential overdosages. Additionally, since most errors have occurred with overdoses in children, they recommend that pediatric hospitals should consider stocking only the 2 mL vial.

Related Information
Phenytoin *on page 1104*
Therapeutic Drug Monitoring: Blood Sampling Time Guidelines *on page 1704*

U.S. Brand Names Cerebyx®
Canadian Brand Names Cerebyx®
Therapeutic Category Anticonvulsant, Hydantoin
Generic Available Yes
Use Management of generalized convulsive status epilepticus; used for short-term parenteral administration of phenytoin; prevention and management of seizures responsive to phenytoin
Pregnancy Risk Factor D
Pregnancy Considerations Fosphenytoin is the prodrug of phenytoin. Refer to Phenytoin *on page 1104* for additional information.

Lactation Excretion in breast milk unknown/not recommended
Breast-Feeding Considerations Fosphenytoin is the prodrug of phenytoin. It is not known if fosphenytoin is excreted in breast milk prior to conversion to phenytoin. Refer to Phenytoin monograph for additional information.
Contraindications Hypersensitivity to fosphenytoin, phenytoin, other hydantoins, or any other component; second and third degree heart block, sinoatrial block, sinus bradycardia, Adams-Stokes syndrome
Warnings Monitor blood pressure and ECG with I.V. loading doses. Use with caution in patients with severe myocardial insufficiency and hypotension. Discontinue if acute hepatotoxicity occurs. Hematologic toxicities and lymphadenopathy have been reported with phenytoin use. Abrupt withdrawal of fosphenytoin may precipitate status epilepticus in epileptic patients; do not discontinue abruptly; fosphenytoin should be withdrawn gradually, unless safety concerns (eg, allergic or hypersensitivity reaction) require a more rapid withdrawal. Serious skin reactions, including toxic epidermal necrolysis (TEN) and Stevens-Johnson syndrome (SJS), although rarely reported (with phenytoin), have resulted in fatalities; fosphenytoin should be discontinued if there are any signs of rash; do not resume drug if rash is exfoliative, purpuric, bullous, or if SLE, SJS, or TEN is suspected. Preliminary data suggests that patients testing positive for the human leukocyte antigen (HLA) allele *HLA-B*1502* have an increased risk of developing SJS and/or TEN. The risk appears to be highest in the early months of therapy initiation. The presence of this genetic variant exists in up to 15% of people of Asian descent in China, Thailand, Malaysia, Indonesia, Taiwan, and the Philippines, and may vary from <1% in Japanese and Koreans to 2% to 4% of South Asians and Indians. This variant is virtually absent in those of Caucasian, African-American, Hispanic, or European ancestry. Of note, carbamazepine, another antiepileptic with a chemical structure similar to phenytoin, updated its prescribing information (December 2007) to include a warning of an increased risk of SJS and TEN in patients carrying the *HLA-B*1502* allele and a recommendation to screen patients of Asian descent for the allele prior to initiating therapy. In contrast to carbamazepine, the FDA is not recommending testing for the presence of *HLA-B*1502* prior to initiating phenytoin therapy until more information is available. In the interim, the FDA is advising that prescribers avoid phenytoin or fosphenytoin as alternatives to carbamazepine therapy in patients positive for *HLA-B*1502*.
Precautions Use with caution in patients with porphyria; consider the amount of phosphate delivered by fosphenytoin in patients who require phosphate restriction; sensory disturbances (burning, pruritus, tingling, paresthesia) may occur especially at higher doses (≥15 mg PE/kg) and at maximum I.V. infusion rates (see Adverse Reactions); use with caution and modify dosage in patients with hepatic or renal dysfunction. Safety of fosphenytoin in pediatric patients has not been established.

Adverse Reactions
Cardiovascular: Hypotension (with rapid I.V. administration), vasodilation, tachycardia, bradycardia
Central nervous system: Slurred speech, dizziness, drowsiness, headache, somnolence, ataxia, fever
Dermatologic: Rash, exfoliative dermatitis, facial edema
Endocrine & metabolic: Folic acid depletion, hyperglycemia
Gastrointestinal: Nausea, vomiting, taste perversion
Genitourinary: Pelvic pain
Hematologic: Neutropenia, thrombocytopenia, anemia (megaloblastic)

Local: Pain on injection; since fosphenytoin is water soluble and has a lower pH (8.8) than phenytoin (12), irritation at injection site or phlebitis is reduced; I.M.: Local itching

Neuromuscular & skeletal: Osteomalacia

Ocular: Nystagmus, blurred vision, diplopia

Otic: Tinnitus

Miscellaneous: Lymphadenopathy; sensory disturbances (burning, pruritus, tingling, paresthesia) occur predominately in the groin area, but may occur in the lower back, abdomen, head or neck (these effects may be related to the phosphate load); paresthesia and pruritus are more common with I.V. vs I.M. administration and are dose and infusion rate related

Drug Interactions

Metabolism/Transport Effects As phenytoin: **Substrate** of CYP2C9 (major), 2C19 (major), 3A4 (minor); **Induces** CYP2B6 (strong), 2C8 (strong), 2C9 (strong), 2C19 (strong), 3A4 (strong)

Avoid Concomitant Use

Avoid concomitant use of Fosphenytoin with any of the following: Dienogest; Dronedarone; Everolimus; Nilotinib; Nisoldipine; Pazopanib; Ranolazine; Romidepsin; Tolvaptan

Increased Effect/Toxicity

Fosphenytoin may increase the levels/effects of: Alcohol (Ethyl); CNS Depressants; Methotrimeprazine

The levels/effects of Fosphenytoin may be increased by: Allopurinol; Carbonic Anhydrase Inhibitors; Chloramphenicol; Cimetidine; CYP2C19 Inhibitors (Moderate); CYP2C19 Inhibitors (Strong); CYP2C9 Inhibitors (Moderate); CYP2C9 Inhibitors (Strong); Methotrimeprazine

Decreased Effect

Fosphenytoin may decrease the levels/effects of: Acetaminophen; Chloramphenicol; CYP2B6 Substrates; CYP2C19 Substrates; CYP2C8 Substrates (High risk); CYP2C9 Substrates (High risk); CYP3A4 Substrates; Dienogest; Dronedarone; Everolimus; GuanFACINE; Maraviroc; NIFEdipine; Nilotinib; Nisoldipine; Pazopanib; Ranolazine; Romidepsin; Saxagliptin; Sorafenib; Tadalafil; Tolvaptan; Treprostinil

The levels/effects of Fosphenytoin may be decreased by: Antacids; CYP2C19 Inducers (Strong); CYP2C9 Inducers (Highly Effective); Ketorolac; Ketorolac (Systemic); Mefloquine; Peginterferon Alfa-2b

Stability Store unopened vials in the refrigerator; do not store unopened vials at room temperature for >48 hours; do not use vials containing particulate matter. Fosphenytoin at concentrations of 1, 8, and 20 mg phenytoin sodium equivalents **(PE)**/mL in D_5W or NS is stable for 30 days when stored at 25°C or 4°C in glass bottles or polyvinyl chloride infusion bags, and when frozen at -20°C in polyvinyl chloride infusion bags. After removal from the freezer, these solutions are stable for 7 days at 25°C or 4°C.

Undiluted fosphenytoin injection (50 mg **PE**/mL) is stable in polypropylene syringes for 30 days at 25°C, 4°C, or frozen at -20°C.

Fosphenytoin at concentrations of 1, 8, and 20 mg **PE**/mL prepared in $D_5/^1/_2$NS, $D_5/^1/_2$NS with KCl 20 mEq/L, $D_5/^1/_2$NS with 40 mEq/L, LR, D_5/LR, $D_{10}W$, amino acid 10%, mannitol 20%, hetastarch 6% in NS or Plasma-Lyte® A injection is stable in polyvinyl chloride bags for 7 days when stored at 25°C (room temperature).

Mechanism of Action Diphosphate ester salt of phenytoin which acts as a water soluble prodrug of phenytoin; after administration, plasma and tissue esterases convert fosphenytoin to phosphate, formaldehyde and phenytoin (as the active moiety); phenytoin works by stabilizing neuronal membranes and decreasing seizure activity by increasing efflux or decreasing influx of sodium ions across cell membranes in the motor cortex during generation of nerve impulses

Pharmacokinetics (Adult data unless noted) The pharmacokinetics of fosphenytoin-derived phenytoin are the same as those for phenytoin (see Phenytoin on page 1104). Parameters listed below are for fosphenytoin (the prodrug) unless otherwise noted. **Note:** The pharmacokinetics of fosphenytoin have been studied in a limited number of children 5-18 years of age and have been found to be similar to the pharmacokinetics observed in young adults (see Pellock, 1996).

Bioavailability: I.M., I.V.: 100%

Distribution: Adults: V_d: 4.3-10.8 L; V_d of fosphenytoin increases with dose and rate of administration

Protein binding: 95% to 99% primarily to albumin; binding of fosphenytoin to protein is saturable (the percent bound decreases as total concentration increases); fosphenytoin displaces phenytoin from protein binding sites; during the time fosphenytoin is being converted to phenytoin, fosphenytoin may temporarily increase the free fraction of phenytoin up to 30% unbound

Metabolism: Each millimole of fosphenytoin is metabolized to 1 millimole of phenytoin, phosphate, and formaldehyde; formaldehyde is converted to formate, which is then metabolized by a folate-dependent mechanism; conversion of fosphenytoin to phenytoin increases with increasing dose and infusion rate, most likely due to a decrease in fosphenytoin protein binding

Conversion of fosphenytoin to phenytoin: Half-life: 15 minutes

Time for complete conversion to phenytoin:

I.M.: 4 hours after injection

I.V.: 2 hours after the end of infusion

Time to peak serum concentration (phenytoin): I.M.: 3 hours

Elimination: 0% fosphenytoin excreted in urine

Usual Dosage

The dose, concentration in solutions, and infusion rates for fosphenytoin are expressed as PHENYTOIN SODIUM EQUIVALENTS (PE)

Fosphenytoin should ALWAYS be prescribed and dispensed in mg of PE; otherwise significant medication errors may occur

Neonates, Infants, and Children: I.V.: **Note:** Not FDA approved for use. A limited number of clinical studies have been conducted in pediatric patients; based on pharmacokinetic studies, experts recommend the following (see Fischer, 2003): Use the pediatric I.V. phenytoin dosing guidelines to dose fosphenytoin using doses in **PE** equal to the phenytoin doses (ie, phenytoin 1 mg = fosphenytoin 1 mg **PE**). Further pediatric studies are needed.

Adults:

Loading dose:

Status epilepticus: I.V.: 15-20 mg **PE**/kg

Nonemergent loading: I.M., I.V.: 10-20 mg **PE**/kg

Initial daily maintenance dose: I.M., I.V.: 4-6 mg **PE**/kg; I.M. dose may be administered as a single daily dose using 1 or 2 injection sites; some patients may require more frequent dosing

I.M. or I.V. substitution for oral phenytoin: Initial: Use the same total daily dose in **PE** of fosphenytoin (ie, phenytoin 1 mg = fosphenytoin 1 mg **PE**); plasma concentrations may increase slightly with this method because oral phenytoin sodium is 90% bioavailable and phenytoin derived from I.M. or I.V. fosphenytoin is 100% bioavailable. Monitor clinical response and phenytoin concentrations to further guide dosage adjustments after 3-4 days

Dosing adjustments in renal/hepatic impairment:

Cirrhosis: Phenytoin clearance may be substantially reduced and monitoring of plasma concentrations with dosage adjustments is advisable

Renal or hepatic disease and patients with hypoalbuminemia: Fosphenytoin conversion to phenytoin may be increased (due to lower protein binding) without a similar increase in phenytoin clearance, leading to a potential increase in the frequency and severity of adverse effects

Administration Dilute with D_5W or NS to 1.5-25 mg **PE**/mL

Children 5-18 years: An administration rate of 3 mg **PE**/kg/minute with a maximum of 150 mg **PE**/minute was used in 7 patients (see Pellock, 1996)

Adults: Administer at a rate of 100-150 mg **PE**/minute with a maximum infusion rate of 150 mg **PE**/minute

Monitoring Parameters Serum phenytoin concentrations, CBC with differential, platelets, serum glucose, liver enzymes; blood pressure, continuous ECG, respiratory function with I.V. loading doses; free (unbound) and total serum phenytoin concentrations in patients with hyperbilirubinemia, hypoalbuminemia, renal dysfunction, uremia, or hepatic disease

Reference Range Monitor **phenytoin** serum concentrations; obtain phenytoin concentrations 2 hours after the end of an I.V. infusion or 4 hours after an I.M. injection of fosphenytoin; see Phenytoin on page 1104 for phenytoin reference range

Test Interactions Falsely high plasma phenytoin concentrations (due to cross-reactivity with fosphenytoin) when measured by immunoanalytical techniques (eg, TD_x®, TD_xFL_x™, Emit® 2000) prior to complete conversion of fosphenytoin to phenytoin; see Reference Range for proper times to measure phenytoin concentrations. Phenytoin may produce falsely low results for dexamethasone or metyrapone tests.

Additional Information Dosing equivalency: Fosphenytoin sodium 1.5 mg is equivalent to phenytoin sodium 1 mg which is equivalent to fosphenytoin 1 mg **PE**

Phosphate load: Each mg **PE** of fosphenytoin delivers 0.0037 mmol of phosphate

Formaldehyde production from fosphenytoin is not expected to be clinically significant in adults with short-term use (eg, 1 week); potentially harmful amounts of phosphate and formaldehyde could occur with an overdose of fosphenytoin; fosphenytoin is more water soluble than phenytoin and, therefore, the injection does not contain propylene glycol; antiarrhythmic effects should be similar to phenytoin

Overdose may result in: Lethargy, nausea, vomiting, hypotension, syncope, tachycardia, bradycardia, asystole, cardiac arrest, hypocalcemia, and metabolic acidosis; fatalities have also been reported

Dosage Forms Excipient information presented when available (limited, particularly for generics); consult specific product labeling. [DSC] = Discontinued product
Injection, solution, as sodium: 75 mg/mL (2 mL, 10 mL) [equivalent to phenytoin sodium 50 mg/mL]
Cerebyx®: 75 mg/mL (2 mL, 10 mL [DSC]) [equivalent to phenytoin sodium 50 mg/mL]

References

Adams BD, Buckley NH, Kim JY, et al, "Fosphenytoin May Cause Hemodynamically Unstable Bradydysrhythmias," *J Emerg Med*, 2006, 30(1):75-9.

Fischer JH, Cwik MS, Luer MS, et al, "Stability of Fosphenytoin Sodium With Intravenous Solutions in Glass Bottles, Polyvinyl Chloride Bags, and Polypropylene Syringes," *Ann Pharmacother*, 1997, 31(5):553-9.

Koul R and Deleu D, "Subtherapeutic Free Phenytoin Levels Following Fosphenytoin Therapy in Status Epilepticus," *Neurology*, 2002, 58 (1):147-8.

Kriel RL and Cifuentes RF, "Fosphenytoin in Infants of Extremely Low Birth Weight," *Pediatr Neurol*, 2001, 24(3):219-21.

McBryde KD, Wilcox J, and Kher KK, "Hyperphosphatemia Due to Fosphenytoin in a Pediatric ESRD Patient," *Pediatr Nephrol*, 2005, 20 (8):1182-5.

Morton LD, "Clinical Experience With Fosphenytoin in Children," *J Child Neurol*, 1998, 13(Suppl 1):S19-22.

Ogutu BR, Newton CR, Muchohi SN, et al, "Pharmacokinetics and Clinical Effects of Phenytoin and Fosphenytoin in Children With Severe Malaria and Status Epilepticus," *Br J Clin Pharmacol*, 2003, 56(1):112-9.

Ogutu BR, Newton CR, Muchohi SN, et al, "Phenytoin Pharmacokinetics and Clinical Effects in African Children Following Fosphenytoin and Chloramphenicol Coadministration," *Br J Clin Pharmacol*, 2002, 54(6):635-42.

Pellock JM, "Fosphenytoin Use in Children," *Neurology*, 1996, 46(6 Suppl 1):S14-6.

Takeoka M, Krishnamoorthy KS, Soman TB, et al, "Fosphenytoin in Infants," *J Child Neurol*, 1998, 13(11):537-40.

◆ **Fosphenytoin Sodium** see Fosphenytoin on page 630

◆ **Fototar® [OTC] [DSC]** see Coal Tar on page 349

◆ **Freezone® [OTC]** see Salicylic Acid on page 1241

◆ **Froben® (Can)** see Flurbiprofen on page 605

◆ **Froben-SR® (Can)** see Flurbiprofen on page 605

◆ **Frusemide** see Furosemide on page 632

◆ **FTC** see Emtricitabine on page 496

◆ **FTC and TDF** see Emtricitabine and Tenofovir on page 498

◆ **FTC, Efavirenz, and TDF** see Efavirenz, Emtricitabine, and Tenofovir on page 493

◆ **FTC, TDF, and Efavirenz** see Efavirenz, Emtricitabine, and Tenofovir on page 493

◆ **FU** see Fluorouracil on page 598

◆ **5-FU** see Fluorouracil on page 598

◆ **FungiGuard [OTC]** see Tolnaftate on page 1358

◆ **Fungi-Nail® [OTC]** see Undecylenic Acid and Derivatives on page 1392

◆ **Fungizone® (Can)** see Amphotericin B (Conventional) on page 100

◆ **Fung-O® [OTC]** see Salicylic Acid on page 1241

◆ **Fungoid® [OTC]** see Miconazole on page 927

◆ **Furadantin®** see Nitrofurantoin on page 995

◆ **Furazosin** see Prazosin on page 1147

Furosemide (fyoor OH se mide)

Medication Safety Issues

Sound-alike/look-alike issues:

Furosemide may be confused with famotidine, finasteride, fluconazole, FLUoxetine, fosinopril, loperamide, torsemide

Lasix® may be confused with Esidrix®, Lanoxin®, Lidex®, Lomotil®, Lovenox®, Luvox®, Luxiq®

International issues:

Urex [Australia] may be confused with Eurax® which is a brand name for crotamiton [U.S.]

Urex: Brand name for furosemide [Australia], but is also the brand name for methenamine [U.S., Canada]

Related Information

Antihypertensive Agents by Class on page 1481

Tumor Lysis Syndrome on page 1599

U.S. Brand Names Lasix®

Canadian Brand Names Apo-Furosemide®; Dom-Furosemide; Furosemide Injection, USP; Furosemide Special; Lasix®; Lasix® Special; Novo-Semide; Nu-Furosemide; PMS-Furosemide

Therapeutic Category Antihypertensive Agent; Diuretic, Loop

Generic Available Yes

Use Management of edema associated with heart failure and hepatic or renal disease; used alone or in combination with antihypertensives in treatment of hypertension

Pregnancy Risk Factor C

Pregnancy Considerations Animal studies have demonstrated maternal death, fetal toxicity, and fetal loss. There are no adequate and well-controlled studies in pregnant women. Crosses the placenta. Increased fetal urine production, electrolyte disturbances reported. Generally, use of diuretics during pregnancy is avoided due to risk of decreased placental perfusion.

Lactation Enters breast milk/use caution

Breast-Feeding Considerations Crosses into breast milk; may suppress lactation. AAP has NO RECOMMENDATION.

Contraindications Hypersensitivity to furosemide or any component of the formulation; anuria

Warnings Loop diuretics are potent diuretics; excess amounts can lead to profound diuresis with fluid and electrolyte loss **[U.S. Boxed Warning]**; monitor for and correct electrolyte disturbances; adjust dose to avoid dehydration

Precautions Hepatic cirrhosis (rapid alterations in fluid/electrolytes may precipitate coma)

Adverse Reactions

Cardiovascular: Orthostatic hypotension

Central nervous system: Dizziness, vertigo, headache

Dermatologic: Urticaria, photosensitivity

Endocrine & metabolic: Hypokalemia, hyponatremia, hypomagnesemia, hypocalcemia, hyperglycemia, hypochloremia, alkalosis, dehydration, hyperuricemia

Gastrointestinal: Pancreatitis, nausea; oral solutions may cause diarrhea due to sorbitol content; anorexia, vomiting, constipation, abdominal cramping

Hematologic: Agranulocytosis, anemia, thrombocytopenia

Hepatic: Ischemic hepatitis, jaundice

Otic: Potential ototoxicity

Renal: Nephrocalcinosis, prerenal azotemia, interstitial nephritis, hypercalciuria

Drug Interactions

Avoid Concomitant Use

Avoid concomitant use of Furosemide with any of the following: Ethacrynic Acid

Increased Effect/Toxicity

Furosemide may increase the levels/effects of: ACE Inhibitors; Allopurinol; Amifostine; Aminoglycosides; Antihypertensives; CISplatin; Dofetilide; Ethacrynic Acid; Hypotensive Agents; Lithium; Neuromuscular-Blocking Agents; RiTUXimab; Salicylates

The levels/effects of Furosemide may be increased by: Corticosteroids (Orally Inhaled); Corticosteroids (Systemic); Diazoxide; Herbs (Hypotensive Properties); MAO Inhibitors; Pentoxifylline; Phosphodiesterase 5 Inhibitors; Probenecid; Prostacyclin Analogues

Decreased Effect

Furosemide may decrease the levels/effects of: Lithium; Neuromuscular-Blocking Agents

The levels/effects of Furosemide may be decreased by: Aliskiren; Bile Acid Sequestrants; Herbs (Hypertensive Properties); Methylphenidate; Nonsteroidal Anti-Inflammatory Agents; Phenytoin; Probenecid; Salicylates; Yohimbine

Food Interactions Do not mix with acidic solutions; limit intake of natural licorice (causes sodium and water retention and increases potassium loss)

Stability Furosemide injection should be stored at controlled room temperature and protected from light; exposure to light may cause discoloration; do not use furosemide solutions if they have a yellow color; refrigeration may result in precipitation or crystallization, however, resolubilization at room temperature or warming may be performed without affecting the stability; furosemide solutions are unstable in acidic media but very stable in basic media; I.V. infusion solution mixed in NS or D_5W solution is stable for 24 hours at room temperature

Tablets: Store at 25°C (77°F); excursions permitted to 15°C to 30°C (59°F to 89°F)

Mechanism of Action Inhibits reabsorption of sodium and chloride in the ascending loop of Henle and distal renal tubule, interfering with the chloride-binding cotransport system, thus causing increased excretion of water, potassium, sodium, chloride, magnesium, and calcium

Pharmacodynamics

Onset of action:

Oral: Within 30-60 minutes

I.M.: 30 minutes

I.V.: 5 minutes

Maximum effect: Oral: Within 1-2 hours

Duration:

Oral: 6-8 hours

I.V.: 2 hours

Pharmacokinetics (Adult data unless noted)

Absorption: 65% in patients with normal renal function, decreases to 45% in patients with renal failure

Protein binding: 98%

Half-life: Adults:

Normal renal function: 30 minutes

Renal failure: 9 hours

Elimination: 50% of oral dose and 80% of I.V. dose excreted unchanged in the urine within 24 hours; the remainder is eliminated by other nonrenal pathways including liver metabolism and excretion of unchanged drug in feces

Usual Dosage

Neonates, premature: (see Additional Information)

Oral: Bioavailability is poor by this route; doses of 1-4 mg/kg/dose 1-2 times/day have been used

I.M., I.V.: 1-2 mg/kg/dose given every 12-24 hours

Infants and Children:

Oral: 2 mg/kg once daily; if ineffective, may increase in increments of 1-2 mg/kg/dose every 6-8 hours; not to exceed 6 mg/kg/dose. In most cases, it is not necessary to exceed individual doses of 4 mg/kg or a dosing frequency of once or twice daily

I.M., I.V.: 1-2 mg/kg/dose every 6-12 hours

Continuous infusion: 0.05 mg/kg/hour; titrate dosage to clinical effect

Adults:

Edema, heart failure:

Oral: Initial: 20-80 mg/dose with the same dose repeated or increased in increments of 20-40 mg/dose at intervals of 6-8 hours; usual maintenance dose interval is once or twice daily; may be titrated up to 600 mg/day with severe edematous states. **Note:** May also be given on 2-4 consecutive days every week

I.M., I.V.: 20-40 mg/dose; repeat in 1-2 hours as needed and increase by 20 mg/dose until the desired effect has been obtained; usual dosing interval: 6-12 hours

Continuous I.V. infusion: Initial I.V. bolus dose of 20-40 mg over 1-2 minutes, followed by continuous I.V. infusion doses of 10-40 mg/hour. If urine output is <1 mL/kg/hour, increase as necessary to a maximum of 80-160 mg/hour. The risk associated with higher infusion rates (80-160 mg/hour) must be weighed against alternative strategies. **Note:** ACC/AHA 2005 guidelines for chronic HF recommend 40 mg I.V. dose followed by 10-40 mg/hour infusion.

Acute pulmonary edema: I.V.: 40 mg over 1-2 minutes; if response not adequate within 1 hour, may increase dose to 80 mg; **Note:** ACC/AHA 2005 guidelines for chronic HF recommend a maximum single dose of 160-200 mg.

Hypertension, resistant (JNC 7): Oral: 20-80 mg/day in 2 divided doses

Refractory CHF: Oral, I.V.: Doses up to 8 g/day have been used

Dosing adjustment in renal impairment: Adults: Acute renal failure: High doses (up to 1-3 g/day - oral/I.V.) have been used to initiate desired response; avoid use in oliguric states

Dialysis: Not removed by hemo- or peritoneal dialysis; supplemental dose is not necessary

Dosing adjustment in hepatic disease: Diminished natriuretic effect with increased sensitivity to hypokalemia and volume depletion in cirrhosis; monitor effects, particularly with high doses

Administration

Oral: May administer with food or milk to decrease GI distress

Parenteral: I.V.: May be administered undiluted direct I.V. at a maximum rate of 0.5 mg/kg/minute for doses <120 mg and 4 mg/minute for doses >120 mg; may also be diluted for infusion 1-2 mg/mL (maximum concentration: 10 mg/mL) over 10-15 minutes (following maximum rate as above)

Monitoring Parameters Serum electrolytes, renal function, blood pressure, hearing (if high dosages used)

Patient Information May cause photosensitivity reactions (eg, exposure to sunlight may cause severe sunburn, skin rash, redness, or itching); avoid exposure to sunlight and artificial light sources (sunlamps, tanning booth/bed); wear protective clothing, wide-brimmed hats, sunglasses, and lip sunscreen (SPF ≥15); use a sunscreen [broad-spectrum sunscreen or physical sunscreen (preferred) or sunblock with SPF ≥15]; contact physician if reaction occurs.

Additional Information Single dose studies utilizing nebulized furosemide at 1-2 mg/kg/dose (diluted to a final volume of 2 mL with NS) have been shown to be effective in improving pulmonary function in preterm infants with bronchopulmonary dysplasia undergoing mechanical ventilation; no diuresis or systemic side effects were noted

Dosage Forms Excipient information presented when available (limited, particularly for generics); consult specific product labeling.

Injection, solution: 10 mg/mL (2 mL)

Injection, solution [preservative free]: 10 mg/mL (2 mL, 4 mL, 10 mL)

Solution, oral: 10 mg/mL (60 mL, 120 mL) [orange flavor]; 40 mg/5 mL (5 mL, 500 mL) [pineapple-peach flavor]

Tablet, oral: 20 mg, 40 mg, 80 mg

Lasix®: 20 mg

Lasix®: 40 mg, 80 mg [scored]

References

Chobanian AV, Bakris GL, Black HR, et al, "The Seventh Report of the Joint National Committee on Prevention, Detection, Evaluation, and Treatment of High Blood Pressure: The JNC 7 Report," *JAMA*, 2003, 289(19):2560-72.

Copeland JG, Campbell DW, Plachetka JR, et al, "Diuresis With Continuous Infusion of Furosemide After Cardiac Surgery," *Am J Surg*, 1983, 146(6):796-9.

Hunt SA, Abraham WT, Chin MH, et al, "ACC/AHA 2005 Guideline Update for the Diagnosis and Management of Chronic Heart Failure in the Adult-Summary Article: A Report of the American College of Cardiology/American Heart Association Task Force on Practice Guidelines (Writing Committee to Update the 2001 Guidelines for the Evaluation and Management of Heart Failure)," *J Am Coll Cardiol*, 2005, 46(6):1116-43.

Pai VB and Nahata MC, "Aerosolized Furosemide in the Treatment of Acute Respiratory Distress and Possible Bronchopulmonary Dysplasia in Preterm Neonates," *Ann Pharmacother*, 2000, 34(3):386-92.

Rastogi A, Luayon M, Ajayi OA, et al, "Nebulized Furosemide in Infants With Bronchopulmonary Dysplasia," *J Pediatr*, 1994, 125(6 Pt 1):976-9.

Rudy DW, Voelker JR, Greene PK, et al, "Loop Diuretics for Chronic Renal Insufficiency: A Continuous Infusion Is More Efficacious Than Bolus Therapy," *Ann Intern Med*, 1991, 115(5):360-6.

◆ **Furosemide Injection, USP (Can)** *see* Furosemide *on page 632*

◆ **Furosemide Special (Can)** *see* Furosemide *on page 632*

◆ **Fuzeon®** *see* Enfuvirtide *on page 503*

◆ **FVIII/vWF** *see* Antihemophilic Factor / von Willebrand Factor Complex (Human) *on page 114*

◆ **FXT 40 (Can)** *see* FLUoxetine *on page 600*

◆ **GAA** *see* Alglucosidase Alfa *on page 64*

Gabapentin (GA ba pen tin)

Medication Safety Issues

Sound-alike/look-alike issues:

Neurontin® may be confused with Motrin®, Neoral®, nitrofurantoin, Noroxin®, Zarontin®

Related Information

Antiepileptic Drugs *on page 1693*

U.S. Brand Names Neurontin®

Canadian Brand Names Apo-Gabapentin®; CO Gabapentin; Dom-Gabapentin; Mylan-Gabapentin; Neurontin®; PHL-Gabapentin; PMS-Gabapentin; PRO-Gabapentin; RAN™-Gabapentin; ratio-Gabapentin; Riva-Gabapentin; Teva-Gabapentin

Therapeutic Category Anticonvulsant, Miscellaneous

Generic Available Yes: Capsule, tablet

Use Adjunct for treatment of partial seizures with or without secondary generalized seizures (FDA approved in ages >12 years and adults); adjunct for treatment of partial seizures in children (FDA approved in ages 3-12 years); management of post-herpetic neuralgia (FDA approved in adults); also used as adjunct in the treatment of neuropathic pain

Pregnancy Risk Factor C

Pregnancy Considerations Animal studies have documented teratogenic effects. There are no adequate and well-controlled studies in pregnant women. Use during pregnancy only if the potential benefit to the mother outweighs the potential risk to the fetus.

Patients exposed to gabapentin during pregnancy are encouraged to enroll themselves into the AED Pregnancy Registry by calling 1-888-233-2334. Additional information is available at www.aedpregnancyregistry.org.

Lactation Enters breast milk/use caution

Breast-Feeding Considerations Gabapentin is excreted in human breast milk. A nursed infant could be exposed to ~1 mg/kg/day of gabapentin; the effect on the child is not known. Use in breast-feeding women only if the benefits to the mother outweigh the potential risk to the infant.

Contraindications Hypersensitivity to gabapentin or any component

Warnings Neuropsychiatric adverse events, such as emotional lability (eg, behavioral problems), hostility, aggressive behaviors, thought disorder (eg, problems with concentration and school performance) and hyperkinesia (eg, hyperactivity and restlessness), have been reported in pediatric patients (see Adverse Reactions); abrupt withdrawal may precipitate status epilepticus or increase in seizures; decrease dose gradually over at least 1 week

Antiepileptic drugs (AEDs) increase the risk of suicidal behavior and ideation in patients receiving these medications for any indication. Pooled analyses of placebo-controlled trials involving 11 different AEDs (regardless of indication) showed a twofold increased risk of suicidal thoughts or behavior (estimated incidence rate: 0.43% in AED treated patients compared to 0.24% of patients receiving placebo); increased risk was observed as early as 1 week after initiation of AED and continued through duration of trials (most trials ≤24 weeks); risk did not vary significantly by age (age range: 5-100 years). Consider risks and benefits of AEDs before prescribing. Monitor all patients receiving an AED for emergence of suicidal thoughts or behavior, thoughts of self-harm, any unusual changes in behavior or mood, or the emergence or worsening of depressive symptoms; notify heathcare provider immediately if symptoms or concerning behavior occur. **Note:** The FDA is requiring that a Medication Guide be developed for all antiepileptic drugs informing patients of this risk.

Precautions Use with caution and decrease the dose in patients with renal dysfunction; in male (but not female) rats receiving gabapentin, a high incidence of pancreatic acinar adenocarcinoma was noted, the clinical significance in humans is unknown; effectiveness in children <3 years is not established

Adverse Reactions

Cardiovascular: Peripheral edema

Central nervous system: Somnolence, dizziness, ataxia, fatigue, depression, nervousness, fever; suicidal thinking and behavior (see Warnings); neuropsychiatric adverse events in children 3-12 years of age: Emotional lability (behavioral problems): 6% incidence; hostility (including aggressive behaviors): 5.2%; hyperkinesia (hyperactivity, restlessness): 4.7%; thought disorder (problems with concentration and school performance): 1.7%; **Note:** Most of these pediatric neuropsychiatric adverse events are mild to moderate in terms of intensity but discontinuation of gabapentin may be required; children with mental retardation and attention deficit disorders may be at increased risk for behavioral side effects

Dermatologic: Pruritus

Endocrine & metabolic: Weight gain

Gastrointestinal: Dyspepsia, constipation, nausea, vomiting

Genitourinary: Impotence

Hematologic: Leukopenia

Neuromuscular & skeletal: Back pain, dysarthria, tremor, myalgia

Ocular: Nystagmus, diplopia

Drug Interactions

Avoid Concomitant Use There are no known interactions where it is recommended to avoid concomitant use.

Increased Effect/Toxicity

Gabapentin may increase the levels/effects of: Alcohol (Ethyl); CNS Depressants; Methotrimeprazine

The levels/effects of Gabapentin may be increased by: Methotrimeprazine

Decreased Effect

The levels/effects of Gabapentin may be decreased by: Ketorolac; Ketorolac (Systemic); Mefloquine

Food Interactions Food slightly increases rate and extent of absorption (AUC and peak increase by 14%)

Stability Refrigerate oral solution; store capsules and tablets at room temperature

Mechanism of Action Not fully elucidated, most likely binds to an undefined neuroreceptor in the brain that is possibly linked with, or identical to a site resembling the L-system amino acid carrier protein; although structurally similar to the inhibitory neurotransmitter, gamma-amino-butyric acid (GABA), gabapentin does not significantly affect the GABA system; it does **not** bind to GABA receptors, affect GABA neuronal uptake nor mimic GABA effects

Pharmacokinetics (Adult data unless noted)

Absorption: Very rapid; via an active (ie, facilitated transport) saturable process; dose-dependent

Distribution: V_d: Adults: 50-60 L or 0.65-1.04 L/kg; CSF concentrations are ~20% of plasma concentrations; distributes to breast milk

Protein binding: <3% (not clinically significant)

Metabolism: Not metabolized

Bioavailability: ~60% (300 mg dose given 3 times/day); bioavailability decreases with increasing doses; bioavailability is 27% with 1600 mg dose given 3 times/day

Time to peak serum concentration: Infants 1 month to Children 12 years and Adults: 2-3 hours

Half-life, elimination:

Infants 1 month to Children 12 years: 4.7 hours

Adults, normal: 5.3 hours (range: 5-9); increased half-life with decreased renal function; anuric adult patients: 132 hours; adults during hemodialysis: 3.8 hours

Elimination: Excreted unchanged in the urine (75% to 80%) and feces (10% to 20%)

Clearance: (**Note:** Apparent oral clearance is directly proportional to Cl_{cr}): Clearance in infants is highly variable; oral clearance (per kg) in children <5 years of age is higher than in children ≥5 years of age

Usual Dosage Oral: **Note:** Do not exceed 12 hours between doses with 3 times/day dosing:

Anticonvulsant:

Children 3-12 years: Initial: 10-15 mg/kg/day divided into 3 doses/day; titrate dose upward over ~3 days; usual dose: Children 3-4 years: 40 mg/kg/day divided into 3 doses/day; children ≥5 to 12 years: 25-35 mg/kg/day divided into 3 doses/day; doses up to 50 mg/kg/day were well tolerated in one long-term study

Children >12 years and Adults: Initial: 300 mg 3 times/day; titrate dose upward if needed; usual dose: 900-1800 mg/day divided into 3 doses/day; doses up to 2400 mg/day divided into 3 doses/day are well tolerated long-term; maximum dose: 3600 mg/day

Neuropathic pain:

Children: Limited information is available; some centers use the following doses: Initial: 5 mg/kg/dose at bedtime; day 2: Increase to 5 mg/kg/dose twice daily; day 3: Increase to 5 mg/kg/dose 3 times/day; titrate to effect; usual dosage range: 8-35 mg/kg/day divided into 3 doses/day (Galloway, 2000)

Adults: Initial: 100 mg 3 times/day; titrate to effect; doses can be increased by 300 mg/day at weekly intervals; doses of at least 900 mg/day appear to be more effective; usual dosage range: 1800-2400 mg/day divided into 3 doses/day; maximum dose: 3600 mg/day (see Laird, 2000)

Post-herpetic neuralgia: Adults: Initial: Day 1: 300 mg/day; day 2: 300 mg twice daily; day 3: 300 mg 3 times/day; titrate dose as needed for relief of pain to 600 mg 3 times/day; doses of 1800-3600 mg/day have been studied; doses >1800 mg/day did not show additional benefit

Dosing adjustment in renal impairment:

Children <12 years: Dosing in renal impairment has not been studied

Children ≥12 years and Adults: See table on next page

◄

Gabapentin Dosing Adjustments in Renal Impairment

Creatinine Clearance (mL/min)	Total Daily Dose Range (mg/day)	Dosage Regimens (Maintenance Doses) (mg)				
≥60	900-3600	300 3 times/ day	400 3 times/ day	600 3 times/ day	800 3 times/ day	1200 tid
>30-59	400-1400	200 twice daily	300 twice daily	400 twice daily	500 twice daily	700 twice daily
>15-29	200-700	200 daily	300 daily	400 daily	500 daily	700 daily
15[1]	100-300	100 daily	125 daily	150 daily	200 daily	300 daily
Hemodialysis[2]	**Posthemodialysis Supplemental Dose**					
	125 mg	150 mg	200 mg	250 mg	350 mg	

[1]Cl$_{cr}$ <15 mL/minute: Reduce daily dose in proportion to creatinine clearance.

[2]Supplemental dose should be administered after each 4 hours of hemodialysis (patients on hemodialysis should also receive maintenance doses based on renal function as listed in the upper portion of the table).

Administration Oral: May be administered without regard to meals; administration with meals may decrease adverse GI effects; dose may be administered as combination of dosage forms; do not administer within 2 hours of magnesium- or aluminum-containing antacids

One pediatric study (Khurana, 1996) mixed the contents of the capsule in drinks (eg, orange juice) or food (eg, applesauce) for patients who could not swallow the capsule; oral solution is now available

Monitoring Parameters Seizure frequency and duration; renal function; weight; behavior in children; signs and symptoms of suicidality (eg, anxiety, depression, behavior changes) (see Warnings)

Reference Range Minimum effective serum concentration may be 2 mcg/mL; **routine monitoring of drug levels is not required**

Test Interactions False positive urinary protein with N-Multistix SG® test

Patient Information Take only as prescribed. May cause dizziness or drowsiness and impair ability to perform activities requiring mental alertness or physical coordination; may cause somnolence, and other symptoms and signs of CNS depression; do not operate machinery or drive a car until you have experience with the drug. Do not discontinue abruptly (an increase in seizure activity may result). Antiepileptic agents may increase the risk of suicidal thoughts and behavior; notify physician if you feel more depressed or have thoughts of suicide or self-harm (see Warnings). Report persistent side effects, worsening of seizure activity, or loss of seizure control.

Nursing Implications Doses should be titrated based on clinical response; content of capsule is bitter tasting

Additional Information Gabapentin is not effective for absence seizures; gabapentin does not induce liver enzymes

Dosage Forms Excipient information presented when available (limited, particularly for generics); consult specific product labeling.

Capsule, oral: 100 mg, 300 mg, 400 mg
Neurontin®: 100 mg, 300 mg, 400 mg
Solution, oral:
Neurontin®: 250 mg/5 mL (480 mL) [cool strawberry anise flavor]
Tablet, oral: 600 mg, 800 mg
Neurontin®: 600 mg, 800 mg [scored]

References

Andrews CO and Fischer JH, "Gabapentin: A New Agent for the Management of Epilepsy," *Ann Pharmacother*, 1994, 28(10):1188-96.

Bourgeois BF, "Antiepileptic Drugs in Pediatric Practice," *Epilepsia*, 1995, 36(Suppl 2):S34-45.

Galloway KS and Yaster M, "Pain and Symptom Control in Terminally Ill Children," *Pediatr Clin North Am*, 2000, 47(3):711-46.

Khurana DS, Riviello J, Helmers S, et al, "Efficacy of Gabapentin Therapy in Children With Refractory Partial Seizures," *J Pediatr*, 1996, 128(6):829-33.

Laird MA and Gidal BE, "Use of Gabapentin in the Treatment of Neuropathic Pain," *Ann Pharmacother*, 2000, 34(6):802-7.

Lee DO, Steingard RJ, Cesena M, et al, "Behavioral Side Effects of Gabapentin in Children," *Epilepsia*, 1996, 37(1):87-90.

Leiderman D, Garofalo E, and LaMoreaux L, "Gabapentin Patients With Absence Seizures: Two Double-Blind, Placebo Controlled Studies," *Epilepsia*, 1993, 34(Suppl 6):45 (abstract).

Pellock JM, "Managing Pediatric Epilepsy Syndromes With New Antiepileptic Drugs," *Pediatrics*, 1999, 104(5 Pt 1):1106-16.

Pressler KL, Jabbour JT, Rose DF, et al, "Gabapentin and Aggression in Pediatric Patients: A Review of the Literature," *Journal of Pediatric Pharmacy Practice*, 1998, 3(2):100-5.

◆ **Gabitril®** *see* TiaGABine *on page 1346*

◆ **Galzin™** *see* Zinc Supplements *on page 1445*

◆ **GamaSTAN™ S/D** *see* Immune Globulin (Intramuscular) *on page 718*

◆ **Gamimune® N (Can)** *see* Immune Globulin (Intravenous) *on page 719*

◆ **Gamma Benzene Hexachloride** *see* Lindane *on page 825*

◆ **Gamma E-Gems® [OTC]** *see* Vitamin E *on page 1427*

◆ **Gamma-E Plus [OTC]** *see* Vitamin E *on page 1427*

◆ **Gammagard Liquid** *see* Immune Globulin (Intravenous) *on page 719*

◆ **Gammagard S/D** *see* Immune Globulin (Intravenous) *on page 719*

◆ **Gamma Globulin** *see* Immune Globulin (Intramuscular) *on page 718*

◆ **Gammaphos** *see* Amifostine *on page 78*

◆ **Gamunex®** *see* Immune Globulin (Intravenous) *on page 719*

Ganciclovir (gan SYE kloe veer)

Medication Safety Issues
Sound-alike/look-alike issues:
Cytovene® may be confused with Cytosar®, Cytosar-U®
Ganciclovir may be confused with acyclovir

U.S. Brand Names Cytovene®-IV; Vitrasert®; Zirgan™

Canadian Brand Names Cytovene®; Vitrasert®

Therapeutic Category Antiviral Agent, Oral; Antiviral Agent, Parenteral

Generic Available No

Use Treatment of cytomegalovirus (CMV) retinitis in immunocompromised patients, as well as CMV GI infections and pneumonitis; prevention of CMV disease in transplant patients who have been diagnosed with latent or active CMV; ganciclovir also has antiviral activity against herpes simplex virus types 1 and 2

Pregnancy Risk Factor C

Pregnancy Considerations
Parenteral: **[U.S. Boxed Warning]: Animal studies have demonstrated carcinogenic and teratogenic effects, and inhibition of spermatogenesis.** Female patients should use effective contraception during therapy; male patients should use a barrier contraceptive during and for at least 90 days after therapy.

Ophthalmic: Adverse events were observed in animal reproduction studies conducted with systemic ganciclovir. Based on animal studies, a U.S. Boxed Warning has been added to the labeling of the systemic product and effective contraception is recommended in males and females using systemic therapy. The amount of ganciclovir available systemically following topical application of the Zirgan™ ophthalmic gel is significantly less in comparison to I.V. doses (0.1%). Vitrasert® intravitreal implant contains only 4.5-6.4 mg of ganciclovir and is released locally in the vitreous from the implant. Ophthalmic formulations should be used only if potential benefit justifies the risk to the fetus.

Lactation Excretion in breast milk unknown/not recommended

Breast-Feeding Considerations

Parenteral: Due to the carcinogenic and teratogenic effects observed in animal studies, the possibility of adverse events in a nursing infant is considered likely. Therefore, nursing should be discontinued during therapy. In addition, the CDC recommends **not** to breast-feed if diagnosed with HIV to avoid postnatal transmission of the virus.

Ophthalmic: The amount of ganciclovir available systemically following ophthalmic application is not known. Caution should be used with administration of the ophthalmic gel. Due to adverse events in nursing animals, the manufacturer of the intravitreal implant recommends that breast feeding be discontinued during therapy; in addition, the CDC recommends **not** to breast-feed if diagnosed with HIV to avoid postnatal transmission of the virus.

Contraindications Hypersensitivity to ganciclovir, acyclovir, or any component; absolute neutrophil count <500/mm³; platelet count <25,000/mm³

Warnings Granulocytopenia (neutropenia), anemia, and thrombocytopenia may occur **[U.S. Boxed Warning]**. Dosage adjustment or interruption of therapy may be necessary in patients with neutropenia, anemia, and/or thrombocytopenia; ganciclovir should not be administered if ANC <500/mm³ or if platelet count <25,000/mm³.

Animal studies have demonstrated carcinogenic and teratogenic effects, and inhibition of spermatogenesis **[U.S. Boxed Warning]**; due to its mutagenic potential, contraceptive precautions for female and male patients need to be followed during and for at least 90 days after therapy with the drug; phlebitis may occur at site of infusion, infuse only into veins with adequate blood flow.

Precautions Use with caution in patients with renal impairment. Use with extreme caution in children since long-term safety has not been determined and due to ganciclovir's potential for long-term carcinogenic and adverse reproductive effects.

Adverse Reactions

Cardiovascular: Edema, arrhythmias, hypertension, chest pain, cardiac arrest

Central nervous system: Headaches, seizure, confusion, nervousness, dizziness, chills, hallucinations, coma, fever, encephalopathy, malaise, insomnia

Dermatologic: Rash, pruritus, urticaria, acne, Stevens-Johnson syndrome

Endocrine & metabolic: Hypokalemia, hypercalcemia, hyponatremia, SIADH

Gastrointestinal: Nausea, vomiting, diarrhea, pancreatitis, anorexia, GI perforation

Hematologic: Neutropenia (oral ganciclovir is associated with less neutropenia and fewer bacterial infections than I.V. ganciclovir), thrombocytopenia, leukopenia, anemia, eosinophilia

Hepatic: Liver enzymes elevated, cholestasis, hepatic failure

Local: Phlebitis

Neuromuscular & skeletal: Neuropathy, arthralgia, myalgia, paresthesia

Ocular: Retinal detachment, photophobia, abnormal vision, loss of vision

Otic: Tinnitus

Renal: Hematuria, BUN and serum creatinine elevated, renal failure

Respiratory: Dyspnea, pneumonia, bronchospasm

Miscellaneous: Sepsis, anaphylactic reaction

Drug Interactions

Avoid Concomitant Use

Avoid concomitant use of Ganciclovir with any of the following: Imipenem

Increased Effect/Toxicity

Ganciclovir may increase the levels/effects of: Imipenem; Mycophenolate; Reverse Transcriptase Inhibitors (Nucleoside); Tenofovir

The levels/effects of Ganciclovir may be increased by: Mycophenolate; Probenecid

Decreased Effect There are no known significant interactions involving a decrease in effect.

Food Interactions High fat meal may increase AUC by 22%

Stability Reconstituted solution is stable for 12 hours at room temperature; **do not refrigerate**; reconstitute with SWI **not** bacteriostatic water because parabens may cause precipitation; diluted I.V. ganciclovir solutions in D_5W or NS with a concentration <10 mg/mL are stable for 24 hours

Mechanism of Action Ganciclovir is phosphorylated to a substrate which competitively inhibits the binding of deoxyguanosine triphosphate to DNA polymerase; ganciclovir triphosphate competes with deoxyguanosine triphosphate for incorporation into viral DNA and interferes with viral DNA chain elongation resulting in inhibition of viral replication

Pharmacokinetics (Adult data unless noted)

Absorption: Oral: Poor

Distribution: Distributes to most body fluids, tissues, and organs including the eyes and brain

V_d:

Children 9 months to 12 years: 0.64 ± 0.22 L/kg

Adults: 0.74 ± 0.15 L/kg

Protein binding: 1% to 2%

Bioavailability: Fasting: 5%; following food: 6% to 9%

Half-life (prolonged with impaired renal function):

Neonates 2-49 days of age: 2.4 hours

Children 9 months to 12 years: 2.4 ± 0.7 hours

Adults: Mean: 2.5-3.6 hours (range: 1.7-5.8 hours)

Time to peak serum concentration: Oral: 2-2.5 hours

Elimination: Majority (80% to 99%) excreted as unchanged drug in the urine

Dialysis: 40% to 50% removed by a 4-hour hemodialysis

Usual Dosage

Slow I.V. infusion:

Congenital CMV infection: Neonates and Infants: 12 mg/kg/day divided every 12 hours for 6 weeks

Retinitis: Children >3 months and Adults:

Induction therapy: 10 mg/kg/day divided every 12 hours as a 1 hour infusion for 14-21 days

Maintenance therapy: 5 mg/kg/day as a single daily dose for 7 days/week or 6 mg/kg/day for 5 days/week

Prevention of CMV disease in transplant recipients: Children and Adults:

Initial: 10 mg/kg/day divided every 12 hours for 1-2 weeks, followed by 5 mg/kg/day once daily 7 days/week or 6 mg/kg/day once daily 5 days/week for 100 days

Lung/heart-lung transplant patients (CMV-positive donor with CMV-positive recipient): 6 mg/kg/day once daily for 28 days

Other CMV infections: Children and Adults: Initial: 10 mg/kg/day divided every 12 hours for 14-21 days or 7.5 mg/kg/day divided every 8 hours; maintenance therapy: 5 mg/kg/day as a single daily dose for 7 days/week or 6 mg/kg/day for 5 days/week

Oral (following induction treatment with I.V. ganciclovir):

Children: Maintenance dose, prophylaxis of CMV disease: In a study of 36 children 6 months to 16 years of age, 30 mg/kg/dose every 8 hours with food produced serum levels similar to the 1000 mg 3 times/day regimen that is effective for maintenance treatment of CMV retinitis in adults (see Frenkel, 2000).

Adults: Maintenance: 1000 mg 3 times/day **or** 500 mg 6 times/day every 3 hours during waking hours

Sustained release intravitreal implant: CMV retinitis:

Children ≥9 years: One implant every 5-8 months plus ganciclovir 30 mg/kg/dose orally 3 times/day

Adults: One implant every 5-8 months plus ganciclovir 1-1.5 g orally 3 times/day

Dosing interval in renal impairment:

Oral: Adults:

Cl_{cr} 50-69 mL/minute: Administer 1500 mg/day or 500 mg 3 times/day

Cl_{cr} 25-49 mL/minute: Administer 1000 mg/day or 500 mg twice daily

Cl_{cr} 10-24 mL/minute: Administer 500 mg/day

Cl_{cr} <10 mL/minute: Administer 500 mg 3 times/week following hemodialysis

I.V. induction:

Cl_{cr} 50-69 mL/minute: Administer 2.5 mg/kg every 12 hours

Cl_{cr} 25-49 mL/minute: Administer 2.5 mg/kg every 24 hours

Cl_{cr} 10-24 mL/minute: Administer 1.25 mg/kg every 24 hours

Cl_{cr} <10 mL/minute: Administer 1.25 mg/kg/dose 3 times/week following hemodialysis

I.V. maintenance:

Cl_{cr} 50-69 mL/minute: Administer 2.5 mg/kg/dose every 24 hours

Cl_{cr} 25-49 mL/minute: Administer 1.25 mg/kg/dose every 24 hours

Cl_{cr} 10-24 mL/minute: Administer 0.625 mg/kg/dose every 24 hours

Cl_{cr} <10 mL/minute: Administer 0.625 mg/kg/dose 3 times/week following hemodialysis

Administration Follow same precautions utilized with antineoplastic agents when preparing and administering ganciclovir

Oral: Do not open or crush ganciclovir capsules; administer with food

Parenteral: Do not administer I.M. or SubQ since the reconstituted ganciclovir injection may cause severe tissue irritation due to its high pH; administer by slow I.V. infusion over at least 1 hour at a final concentration for administration not to exceed 10 mg/mL

Monitoring Parameters CBC with differential and platelet count, urine output, serum creatinine, ophthalmologic exams, liver enzyme tests, blood pressure, urinalysis

Patient Information Women of childbearing potential should be advised to use effective contraception during treatment. Men should be advised to practice barrier contraception during and for at least 90 days following treatment with ganciclovir. Mothers should discontinue breast-feeding while on ganciclovir therapy. Ganciclovir is not a cure for CMV retinitis. Regular follow-up ophthalmologic exams are necessary.

Nursing Implications Handle and dispose according to guidelines issued for cytotoxic drugs; avoid direct contact of skin or mucous membranes with the powder contained in capsules or the I.V. solution; to minimize the risk of phlebitis, infuse through a large vein with adequate blood flow; maintain adequate patient hydration

Additional Information Sodium content of 1 g: 4 mEq

Dosage Forms Excipient information presented when available (limited, particularly for generics); consult specific product labeling.

Gel, ophthalmic:

Zirgan™: 0.15% (5 g) [contains benzalkonium chloride]

Implant, intravitreal:

Vitrasert®: 4.5 mg [released gradually over 5-8 months]

Injection, powder for reconstitution:

Cytovene®-IV: 500 mg

Extemporaneous Preparations A 100 mg/mL oral suspension can be prepared in a vertical flow hood by emptying eighty 250 mg capsules of ganciclovir into a glass mortar wetted and triturated with Ora-Sweet® to a smooth paste. Add 50 mL of Ora-Sweet® to the paste, mix, and transfer contents to an amber polyethylene terephthate bottle. Rinse the mortar with 50 mL of Ora-Sweet® and transfer contents to the bottle. Rinse the mortar with the last third of the vehicle and transfer contents to the bottle. Add enough vehicle to make a final volume of 200 mL. The suspension is stable for 123 days when stored at 23°C to 25°C.

Anaizi NH, Swenson CF, and Dentinger PJ, "Stability of Ganciclovir in Extemporaneously Compounded Oral Liquids," *Am J Health Syst Pharm*, 1999, 56 (17):1738-41.

References

Fletcher C, Sawchuk R, Chinnock B, et al, "Human Pharmacokinetics of the Antiviral Drug DHPG," *Clin Pharmacol Ther*, 1986, 40(3):281-6.

Frenkel LM, Capparelli EV, Dankner WM, et al, "Oral Ganciclovir in Children: Pharmacokinetics, Safety, Tolerance, and Antiviral Effects," *J Infect Dis*, 2000, 182(6):1616-24.

Goodrich JM, Bowden RA, Fisher L, et al, "Ganciclovir Prophylaxis to Prevent Cytomegalovirus Disease After Allogeneic Marrow Transplant," *Ann Intern Med*, 1993, 118(3):173-8.

Gudnason T, Belani KK, and Balfour HH Jr, "Ganciclovir Treatment of Cytomegalovirus Disease in Immunocompromised Children," *Pediatr Infect Dis J*, 1989, 8(7):436-40.

Kaplan JE, Masur H, and Holmes KK, "Guidelines for Preventing Opportunistic Infections Among HIV-Infected Persons - 2002 Recommendations of the USPHS and IDSA," *MMWR*, 2002, 51 (RR-8):1-46.

Merigan TC, Renlund DG, Keay S, et al, "A Controlled Trial of Ganciclovir to Prevent Cytomegalovirus Disease After Heart Transplantation," *N Engl J Med*, 1992, 326(18):1182-6.

Schleiss MR, "Antiviral Therapy of Congenital Cytomegalovirus Infection," *Semin Pediatr Infect Dis*, 2005, 16(1):50-9.

◆ **Gel-Kam® [OTC]** *see* Fluoride *on page 595*

◆ **Gel-Kam® Rinse** *see* Fluoride *on page 595*

◆ **Gelnique™** *see* Oxybutynin *on page 1037*

◆ **GelRite [OTC]** *see* Ethyl Alcohol *on page 547*

◆ **Gel-Stat™ [OTC]** *see* Ethyl Alcohol *on page 547*

◆ **Gelusil® Extra Strength (Can)** *see* Aluminum Hydroxide and Magnesium Hydroxide *on page 76*

Gemcitabine (jem SITE a been)

Medication Safety Issues
Sound-alike/look-alike issues:
Gemcitabine may be confused with gemtuzumab
Gemzar® may be confused with Zinecard®

High alert medication: This medication is in a class the Institute for Safe Medication Practices (ISMP) includes among its list of drugs which have a heightened risk of causing significant patient harm when used in error.

U.S. Brand Names Gemzar®

Canadian Brand Names Gemcitabine For Injection, USP; Gemzar®

Therapeutic Category Antineoplastic Agent, Antimetabolite (Pyrimidine Antagonist)

Generic Available No

Use Treatment of locally-advanced, inoperable (stage IIIA or IIIB), or metastatic (stage IV) nonsmall cell lung cancer (NSCLC); locally advanced or metastatic pancreatic cancer; metastatic breast cancer; advanced relapsed ovarian cancer (FDA approved in adults); has also been used in the treatment of bladder cancer, cervical cancer, Hodgkin's disease, non-Hodgkin's lymphomas, small cell lung cancer, hepatobiliary cancers and in children for the treatment of refractory solid tumors (including brain tumors), refractory Hodgkin's disease, recurrent germ cell tumors, and hepatocellular carcinomas

Pregnancy Risk Factor D

Pregnancy Considerations Embryotoxicity and fetal malformations (cleft palate, incomplete ossification, fused pulmonary artery, absence of gallbladder) have been reported in animal studies. There are no adequate and well-controlled studies in pregnant women. If patient becomes pregnant, she should be informed of risks.

Lactation Excretion in breast milk unknown/contraindicated

Contraindications Hypersensitivity to gemcitabine or any component; pregnancy

Warnings The FDA currently recommends that procedures for proper handling and disposal of antineoplastic agents be considered. Prolongation of the infusion time >60 minutes and more frequent than once weekly dosing have been shown to increase toxicity, including myelosuppression. Myelosuppression is usually the dose-limiting toxicity (CBC with differential and platelet count should be monitored prior to each dose of gemcitabine; reduce or withhold dose depending on the degree of hematologic toxicity). Gemcitabine has been reported to cause pulmonary toxicity, hemolytic uremic syndrome, and/or renal failure requiring dialysis or leading to death, and hepatotoxicity (including liver failure and death); discontinue gemcitabine if severe lung, renal or hepatotoxicity occurs. Gemcitabine may cause fever in the absence of clinical infection.

Precautions Use with caution in patients with renal or hepatic impairment

Adverse Reactions
Cardiovascular: Arrhythmias, peripheral edema
Central nervous system: Asthenia, fatigue, fever, lethargy, somnolence
Dermatologic: Alopecia, pruritus, rash

Gastrointestinal: Constipation, diarrhea, nausea, stomatitis, vomiting
Genitourinary: Hematuria, proteinuria
Hematologic: Anemia, hemorrhage, leukopenia, neutropenia, thrombocytopenia
Hepatic: AST, ALT, bilirubin, and alkaline phosphatase increased; hepatotoxicity; liver failure (rare)
Neuromuscular & skeletal: Paresthesias, peripheral neuropathy
Renal: BUN and serum creatinine increased, hemolytic uremic syndrome, renal failure
Respiratory: Bronchospasm, dyspnea, interstitial pneumonitis, pulmonary edema, pulmonary fibrosis
Miscellaneous: Anaphylactoid reaction, flu-like symptoms, infection
<1%, postmarketing, and/or case reports (reported with single-agent use or with combination therapy, all reported rarely): Adult respiratory distress syndrome, anorexia, bullous skin eruptions, cellulitis, cerebrovascular accident, chills, cough, desquamation, diaphoresis, gangrene, GGT increased, headache, heart failure, hepatotoxic reaction (rare), hypertension, insomnia, malaise, MI, peripheral vasculitis, petechiae, radiation recall, respiratory failure, rhinitis, sepsis, supraventricular arrhythmia, weakness

Drug Interactions

Avoid Concomitant Use
Avoid concomitant use of Gemcitabine with any of the following: BCG; Natalizumab; Pimecrolimus; Tacrolimus (Topical); Vaccines (Live)

Increased Effect/Toxicity
Gemcitabine may increase the levels/effects of: Bleomycin; Fluorouracil; Fluorouracil (Systemic); Fluorouracil (Topical); Leflunomide; Natalizumab; Vaccines (Live); Vitamin K Antagonists

The levels/effects of Gemcitabine may be increased by: Denosumab; Pimecrolimus; Tacrolimus (Topical); Trastuzumab

Decreased Effect
Gemcitabine may decrease the levels/effects of: BCG; Sipuleucel-T; Vaccines (Inactivated); Vaccines (Live); Vitamin K Antagonists

The levels/effects of Gemcitabine may be decreased by: Echinacea

Stability Store vial at room temperature; reconstituted vials and infusion solutions diluted in NS are stable up to 24 hours; do not refrigerate reconstituted and/or diluted solutions as crystallization may occur. Incompatible with acyclovir, cefotaxime, furosemide, ganciclovir, imipenem/cilastatin, irinotecan, methotrexate, methylprednisolone sodium succinate, piperacillin/tazobactam, and prochlorperazine

Mechanism of Action Gemcitabine undergoes intracellular phosphorylation to its corresponding diphosphate and triphosphate nucleosides which inhibit DNA polymerase and ribonucleotide reductase; results in inhibition of DNA synthesis; specific for the S-phase of the cell cycle.

Pharmacokinetics (Adult data unless noted)
Distribution: Widely distributed into tissues; present in ascitic fluid
V_d: Adults:
I.V. infusion <70 minutes: 50 L/m^2
I.V. infusion 70-285 minutes: 370 L/m^2
Protein binding: <10%
Metabolism: Intracellularly by nucleoside kinases to active di- and triphosphate metabolites; metabolized by cytidine deaminase to an inactive metabolite
Half-life: Adults:
I.V. infusion <70 minutes: 0.7-1.6 hours
I.V. infusion 70-285 minutes: 4.1-10.6 hours
Elimination: 92% to 98% excreted in the urine

◀ **Usual Dosage** Refer to individual protocols: I.V.:
Children:
Refractory solid tumor, including Hodgkin's disease: 1000-1250 mg/m²/dose on days 1 and 8 of a 4-week cycle; maximum single dose: 2500 mg
Refractory solid tumor in combination with docetaxel: 900 mg/m²/dose over 60 minutes on days 1 and 8
Patients with pelvic radiation (decrease dose by 25%): 675 mg/m²/dose over 60 minutes on days 1 and 8
Recurrent germ cell tumor: 800 mg/m²/dose over 90 minutes on day 1
Hepatocellular carcinoma: 1000 mg/m²/dose over 90 minutes on day 1
Dose modification for hematologic toxicity: 800 mg/m²/dose on day 1
Adults:
Pancreatic cancer: 1000 mg/m² once weekly for up to 7 weeks
Nonsmall cell lung cancer: 1000 mg/m² on days 1,8, and 15 every 28 days in combination with cisplatin; or 1250 mg/m² on day 1 and 8 every 21 days in combination with cisplatin
Breast cancer: 1250 mg/m² on days 1 and 8 every 21 days in combination with paclitaxel
Ovarian cancer: 1000 mg/m² days 1 and 8; repeat cycle every 21 days
Dosing adjustment for hematologic toxicity: Adults:
Absolute granulocyte count (AGC) 500-999/mm³ or platelet count 50,000-99,000/mm³: Administer 75% of the full dose
AGC <500/mm³ or platelet count <50,000/mm³: Hold dose
Dosing adjustment in renal and/or hepatic impairment: No dosing information available
Administration I.V.: Reconstitute 200 mg vial of gemcitabine by adding 5 mL NS without preservatives or add 25 mL NS without preservatives to 1 g vial; resulting concentration is 38 mg/mL. Maximum concentration for administration: 38 mg/mL; gemcitabine can be further diluted with 50-500 mL NS to concentrations as low as 0.1 mg/mL. Infuse over 30-90 minutes based on the protocol. **Note:** Prolongation of the infusion time >60 minutes has been shown to prolong gemcitabine's half-life and increase toxicity in adults.
Monitoring Parameters CBC with differential and platelet count prior to each dose; monitor renal and hepatic function, bilirubin, LDH, and reticulocyte count
Patient Information Notify physician if extreme fatigue, severe GI upset or diarrhea, bleeding or bruising, fever, chills, sore throat, vaginal discharge, signs of fluid retention, yellowing of the skin or eyes, change in color of urine or stool, muscle or skeletal pain/weakness occur. Advise women of childbearing potential to avoid becoming pregnant while receiving gemcitabine.
Nursing Implications Maintain adequate hydration unless instructed to restrict fluid intake. If gemcitabine solution comes in contact with skin or mucosa, immediately wash the skin thoroughly with soap and water or rinse the mucosa with large amounts of water.
Dosage Forms Excipient information presented when available (limited, particularly for generics); consult specific product labeling.
Injection, powder for reconstitution:
Gemzar®: 200 mg, 1 g

References
Reid JM, Qu W, Safgren SL, et al, "Phase I Trial and Pharmacokinetics of Gemcitabine in Children With Advanced Solid Tumors," *J Clin Oncol*, 2004, 22(12):2445-51.

◆ **Gemcitabine For Injection, USP (Can)** *see* Gemcitabine *on page 639*

◆ **Gemcitabine Hydrochloride** *see* Gemcitabine *on page 639*

Gemtuzumab Ozogamicin
(gem TOO zoo mab oh zog a MY sin)

Medication Safety Issues
Sound-alike/look-alike issues:
Gemtuzumab may be confused with gemcitabine

High alert medication: The Institute for Safe Medication Practices (ISMP) includes this medication among its list of drug classes which have a heightened risk of causing significant patient harm when used in error.
Related Information
Emetogenic Potential of Antineoplastic Agents *on page 1579*
U.S. Brand Names Mylotarg®
Canadian Brand Names Mylotarg®
Therapeutic Category Antineoplastic Agent, Monoclonal Antibody
Generic Available No
Use Treatment of relapsed or *de novo* CD33-positive acute myeloid leukemia (AML)
Pregnancy Risk Factor D
Pregnancy Considerations Animal studies have demonstrated teratogenic effects, fetal loss, and maternal toxicity. There are no adequate and well-controlled studies in pregnant women. May cause fetal harm when administered to a pregnant woman. Women of childbearing potential should avoid becoming pregnant while receiving treatment.
Lactation Excretion in breast milk unknown/not recommended
Breast-Feeding Considerations Due to the potential for serious adverse reactions in the nursing infant, breast-feeding is not recommended.
Contraindications Hypersensitivity to gemtuzumab ozogamicin, calicheamicin derivatives, or any component; patients with anti-CD33 antibody
Warnings Hazardous agent; use appropriate precautions for handling and disposal. Severe myelosuppression may occur at recommended doses **[U.S. Boxed Warning]**.

Severe hypersensitivity reactions (including anaphylaxis) and other infusion-related reactions may occur **[U.S. Boxed Warning]**. Infusion-related events are common and generally occur with the first dose at the end of a 2-hour infusion. Infusion-related symptoms usually resolve after 2-4 hours with supportive therapy (acetaminophen, diphenhydramine, I.V. fluids). Postinfusion reactions, which include fever, chills, hypotension, and dyspnea, may occur during the first 24 hours after gemtuzumab administration. Infusion-related reactions may be severe (including anaphylaxis, pulmonary edema, or acute respiratory distress syndrome); do not administer via I.V. push or by rapid I.V. injection. Symptomatic intrinsic lung disease or high peripheral blast counts may increase the risk of severe reactions; consider discontinuing therapy in patients who develop severe infusion-related reactions. In addition to infusion related pulmonary events, gemtuzumab therapy is also associated with pulmonary infiltrates, pleural effusion, noncardiogenic pulmonary edema, and pulmonary insufficiency.

Gemtuzumab has been associated with severe hepatotoxicity, including hepatic veno-occlusive disease (VOD) **[U.S. Boxed Warning]**; symptoms of VOD include right upper quadrant pain, rapid weight gain, ascites, hepatomegaly, and bilirubin/transaminase elevations. Risk may be increased by combination chemotherapy, underlying hepatic disease, or hematopoietic stem cell transplant.
Precautions Use with caution in patients with pulmonary disease and renal or hepatic impairment. Tumor lysis syndrome may occur as a consequence of leukemia treatment; adequate hydration and prophylactic allopurinol

must be initiated prior to starting gemtuzumab therapy. Other methods to reduce WBC <30,000 cells/mm^3 (hydroxyurea or leukapheresis) may be considered to minimize tumor lysis syndrome and/or severe infusion reactions. May cause fetal harm when administered to pregnant women; women should be advised to avoid becoming pregnant.

Adverse Reactions

Cardiovascular: Peripheral edema, hypertension, hypotension, tachycardia, bradycardia

Central nervous system: Chills, fever, headache, pain, dizziness, insomnia, depression, anxiety, cerebral hemorrhage, intracranial hemorrhage

Dermatologic: Rash, petechiae, ecchymosis, pruritus

Endocrine & metabolic: Hypokalemia, hypomagnesemia, hyperglycemia, hyperuricemia, hypocalcemia, hypophosphatemia

Gastrointestinal: Nausea, vomiting, diarrhea, anorexia, abdominal pain, constipation, stomatitis, mucositis, abdominal distention, dyspepsia, gingival hemorrhage, melena

Genitourinary: Hematuria, vaginal hemorrhage

Hematologic: Neutropenia, thrombocytopenia, anemia, leukopenia, bleeding, lymphopenia, disseminated intravascular coagulation, PT and PTT elevated, neutropenic fever, neutropenic sepsis

Hepatic: Hyperbilirubinemia, LDH, ALT, AST, and alkaline phosphatase elevated; veno-occlusive disease (higher incidence in patients with prior history of hematopoietic stem cell transplant), hepatic failure, jaundice, ascites, hepatosplenomegaly, portal vein thrombosis

Neuromuscular & skeletal: Weakness, back pain, arthralgia, myalgia

Renal: Renal failure secondary to tumor lysis syndrome, creatinine increased, renal impairment

Respiratory: Dyspnea, epistaxis, cough, pharyngitis, rhinitis, hypoxia, acute respiratory distress syndrome, pneumonia, pulmonary edema, pulmonary hemorrhage

Miscellaneous: Infection, sepsis, anaphylaxis, hypersensitivity, herpes simplex

Drug Interactions

Avoid Concomitant Use

Avoid concomitant use of Gemtuzumab Ozogamicin with any of the following: BCG; Natalizumab; Pimecrolimus; Tacrolimus (Topical); Vaccines (Live)

Increased Effect/Toxicity

Gemtuzumab Ozogamicin may increase the levels/effects of: Leflunomide; Natalizumab; Vaccines (Live)

The levels/effects of Gemtuzumab Ozogamicin may be increased by: Abciximab; Denosumab; Pimecrolimus; Tacrolimus (Topical); Trastuzumab

Decreased Effect

Gemtuzumab Ozogamicin may decrease the levels/effects of: BCG; Sipuleucel-T; Vaccines (Inactivated); Vaccines (Live)

The levels/effects of Gemtuzumab Ozogamicin may be decreased by: Echinacea

Food Interactions Alcohol (avoid alcohol due to GI irritation)

Stability Protect from light (including direct and indirect sunlight, and unshielded fluorescent light) during storage, dispensing, and administration. Refrigerate vials. Reconstituted solutions may be stored for up to 2 hours at room temperature or under refrigeration. Following dilution for infusion, solutions are stable for up to 16 hours at room temperature. Administration requires 2 hours; therefore, the maximum elapsed time from initial reconstitution to completion of infusion should be 20 hours.

Mechanism of Action Antibody to CD33 antigen which is expressed on leukemic blasts in >80% of AML patients, as well as normal myeloid cells. Binding results in internalization of the antibody-antigen complex, leading to the release of the calicheamicin derivative inside the myeloid cell. The calicheamicin derivative binds to DNA resulting in double strand breaks and cell death. Pluripotent stem cells and nonhematopoietic cells are not affected.

Pharmacokinetics (Adult data unless noted)

Half-life: Adults:

Calicheamicin derivative: 45 hours (with repeat dose: 60 hours)

Unconjugated derivative: 100 hours

Usual Dosage Refer to individual protocols: I.V.:

Children: Combination therapy:

Relapsed/refractory AML:

Children <3 years: 0.07-0.1 mg/kg/dose

Children ≥3 years: 2-3 mg/m^2/dose

Newly diagnosed childhood AML: 3 mg/m^2/dose (no dose adjustment for age or body surface area <0.6 m^2)

Children: Monotherapy: Phase I (MTD):

Children <3 years: 0.2 mg/kg/dose for a total of 2 doses separated by 14 days

Children >3 years: 6 mg/m^2/dose for a total of 2 doses separated by 14 days

Adults: AML in first relapse: 9 mg/m^2; full treatment course consists of a total of 2 doses separated by 14 days; maximum dose: 15 mg

Dosage adjustment in renal impairment: No recommendation (not studied)

Dosage adjustment in hepatic impairment: Use extra caution (not studied in patients with bilirubin >2 mg/dL)

Dosage adjustment with recent hematopoietic stem cell transplant (HSCT): Gemtuzumab use within 3-4 months of HSCT is associated with an increased risk of hepatic veno-occlusive disease, the National Comprehensive Cancer Network (NCCN) guidelines (AML, v.1, 2009) recommend a 30% to 50% dosage reduction in this situation)

Dosage adjustment for toxicity:

Dyspnea or significant hypotension: Interrupt infusion; monitor

Anaphylaxis, pulmonary edema, acute respiratory distress syndrome: Strongly consider discontinuing treatment

Administration Prepare dose in a biologic safety hood with the fluorescent light turned off. Allow vial to warm to room temperature prior to reconstitution. Reconstitute vial with 5 mL SWI to a concentration of 1 mg/mL; reconstituted solutions may be stored for up to 2 hours at room temperature or under refrigeration. Further dilute dose in 100 mL NS; place infusion container in a UV protectant bag immediately after preparation. Following dilution for infusion, solutions are stable for up to 16 hours at room temperature. Administration requires 2 hours; therefore, the maximum elapsed time from initial reconstitution to completion of infusion should be 20 hours.

DO NOT ADMINISTER I.V. PUSH or by RAPID I.V. INJECTION; Administer via I.V. infusion over 2 hours through a dedicated line with a filter (low protein binding 0.2-1.2 micron in-line filter is recommended). May administer through a peripheral or central line. Cover dose with UV protective bag during infusion.

Monitoring Parameters Vital signs during infusion and for 4 hours following the infusion; signs and symptoms of postinfusion reaction; electrolytes, CBC with differential, platelet count, LFTs. Monitor for signs and symptoms of hepatic veno-occlusive disease (weight gain, abdominal girth, right upper quadrant abdominal pain, hepatomegaly, ascites).

Patient Information Notify physician if fever, chills, unusual bruising or bleeding, signs of infection, dizziness, lightheadedness, difficulty breathing, or yellowing of the eyes or skin occurs. Advise women of childbearing potential to avoid becoming pregnant while receiving gemtuzumab.

Nursing Implications Handle and dispose according to guidelines issued for cytotoxic drugs. Administer diphenhydramine and acetaminophen prior to each infusion. Acetaminophen should be repeated every 4 hours for 2 additional doses as needed. Pretreatment with methylprednisolone may ameliorate infusion-related symptoms.

Dosage Forms Excipient information presented when available (limited, particularly for generics); consult specific product labeling.

Injection, powder for reconstitution [preservative free]:
Mylotarg®: 5 mg

References

Aplenc R, Alonzo TA, Gerbing RB, et al, "Safety and Efficacy of Gemtuzumab Ozogamicin in Combination With Chemotherapy for Pediatric Acute Myeloid Leukemia: A Report From the Children's Oncology Group," *J Clin Oncol*, 2008, 26(14):2390-3295.

Arceci RJ, Sande J, Lange B, et al, "Safety and Efficacy of Gemtuzumab Ozogamicin in Pediatric Patients With Advanced CD33+ Acute Myeloid Leukemia," *Blood*, 2005, 106(4):1183-8.

Buckwalter M, Dowell JA, Korth-Bradley J, et al, "Pharmacokinetics of Gemtuzumab Ozogamicin as a Single-Agent Treatment of Pediatric Patients With Refractory or Relapsed Acute Myeloid Leukemia," *J Clin Pharmacol*, 2004, 44(8):873-80.

Zwaan CM, Reinhardt D, Corbacioglu S, et al, "Gemtuzumab Ozogamicin: First Clinical Experiences in Children With Relapsed/Refractory Acute Myeloid Leukemia Treated on Compassionate-Use Basis," *Blood*, 2003, 101(10):3868-71.

◆ **Gemzar®** see Gemcitabine *on page 639*

◆ **Genac™ [OTC]** see Triprolidine and Pseudoephedrine *on page 1388*

◆ **Genacote™ [OTC] [DSC]** see Aspirin *on page 141*

◆ **Genahist™ [OTC]** see DiphenhydrAMINE *on page 448*

◆ **Gen-Amoxicillin (Can)** see Amoxicillin *on page 96*

◆ **Genapap™ [OTC] [DSC]** see Acetaminophen *on page 36*

◆ **Genapap™ Extra Strength [OTC] [DSC]** see Acetaminophen *on page 36*

◆ **Genapap™ Infant [OTC] [DSC]** see Acetaminophen *on page 36*

◆ **Genaphed® [OTC]** see Pseudoephedrine *on page 1183*

◆ **Genasal [OTC]** see Oxymetazoline *on page 1043*

◆ **Genasoft® [OTC]** see Docusate *on page 468*

◆ **Genasyme® [OTC] [DSC]** see Simethicone *on page 1262*

◆ **Genatuss DM® [OTC] [DSC]** see Guaifenesin and Dextromethorphan *on page 658*

◆ **Gen-Beclo (Can)** see Beclomethasone *on page 176*

◆ **Gen-Budesonide AQ (Can)** see Budesonide *on page 206*

◆ **Gen-Buspirone (Can)** see BusPIRone *on page 222*

◆ **Gen-Captopril (Can)** see Captopril *on page 242*

◆ **Gen-Carbamazepine CR (Can)** see CarBAMazepine *on page 244*

◆ **Gen-Clobetasol (Can)** see Clobetasol *on page 331*

◆ **Gen-Clomipramine (Can)** see ClomiPRAMINE *on page 334*

◆ **Gen-Clonazepam (Can)** see ClonazePAM *on page 337*

◆ **Gen-Clozapine (Can)** see Clozapine *on page 345*

◆ **Gen-Cyclobenzaprine (Can)** see Cyclobenzaprine *on page 367*

◆ **Gen-Divalproex (Can)** see Valproic Acid and Derivatives *on page 1398*

◆ **Genebs [OTC] [DSC]** see Acetaminophen *on page 36*

◆ **Genebs Extra Strength [OTC]** see Acetaminophen *on page 36*

◆ **Generlac** see Lactulose *on page 791*

◆ **Genfiber™ [OTC]** see Psyllium *on page 1185*

◆ **Gen-Fluoxetine (Can)** see FLUoxetine *on page 600*

◆ **Gengraf®** see CycloSPORINE *on page 372*

◆ **Gen-Hydroxychloroquine (Can)** see Hydroxychloroquine *on page 694*

◆ **Gen-Hydroxyurea (Can)** see Hydroxyurea *on page 695*

◆ **Gen-Ipratropium (Can)** see Ipratropium *on page 757*

◆ **Gen-Lovastatin (Can)** see Lovastatin *on page 850*

◆ **Gen-Medroxy (Can)** see MedroxyPROGESTERone *on page 870*

◆ **Gen-Metoprolol (Can)** see Metoprolol *on page 918*

◆ **Gen-Nifedipine XL (Can)** see NIFEdipine *on page 991*

◆ **Gen-Nitro (Can)** see Nitroglycerin *on page 996*

◆ **Gen-Nizatidine (Can)** see Nizatidine *on page 999*

◆ **Gen-Nortriptyline (Can)** see Nortriptyline *on page 1002*

◆ **Genotropin®** see Somatropin *on page 1281*

◆ **Genotropin Miniquick®** see Somatropin *on page 1281*

◆ **Gen-Piroxicam (Can)** see Piroxicam *on page 1118*

◆ **Genpril® [OTC] [DSC]** see Ibuprofen *on page 702*

◆ **Gen-Risperidone (Can)** see Risperidone *on page 1218*

◆ **Gen-Sumatriptan (Can)** see SUMAtriptan *on page 1308*

◆ **Gentak®** see Gentamicin *on page 642*

Gentamicin (jen ta MYE sin)

Medication Safety Issues
Sound-alike/look-alike issues:
Garamycin® may be confused with kanamycin, Terramycin®
Gentamicin may be confused with gentian violet, kanamycin, vancomycin

High alert medication: The Institute for Safe Medication Practices (ISMP) includes this medication (intrathecal administration) among its list of drug classes which have a heightened risk of causing significant patient harm when used in error.

Related Information
Therapeutic Drug Monitoring: Blood Sampling Time Guidelines *on page 1704*

U.S. Brand Names Gentak®; Gentasol™

Canadian Brand Names Alcomicin®; Diogent®; Garamycin®; Gentamicin Injection, USP

Therapeutic Category Antibiotic, Aminoglycoside; Antibiotic, Ophthalmic; Antibiotic, Topical

Generic Available Yes

Use Treatment of susceptible bacterial infections, normally gram-negative organisms including *Pseudomonas*, *E. coli*, *Proteus*, *Serratia*, and gram-positive *Staphylococcus*; treatment of bone infections, CNS infections, respiratory tract infections, skin and soft tissue infections, as well as abdominal and urinary tract infections, endocarditis, and septicemia; used in combination with ampicillin as empiric therapy for sepsis in newborns; prevention of bacterial endocarditis prior to surgical procedures in high risk patients; used topically to treat superficial infections of the skin or ophthalmic infections caused by susceptible bacteria

Pregnancy Risk Factor C (ophthalmic); D (injection)

Pregnancy Considerations Gentamicin crosses the placenta and produces detectable serum levels in the fetus. Renal toxicity has been described in two case reports following first trimester exposure. There are several reports of total irreversible bilateral congenital deafness in children whose mothers received streptomycin during pregnancy; therefore, the manufacturer classifies gentamicin as pregnancy category D. Although ototoxicity has not been reported following maternal use of gentamicin, a potential for harm exists. **[U.S. Boxed Warning]: Aminoglycosides may cause fetal harm if administered to a pregnant woman.**

Due to pregnancy induced physiologic changes, some pharmacokinetic parameters of gentamicin may be altered. Pregnant women have an average-to-larger volume of distribution which may result in lower serum peak levels than for the same dose in nonpregnant women. Serum half-life is also shorter.

Lactation Enters breast milk/use caution (AAP rates "compatible")

Breast-Feeding Considerations Gentamicin is excreted into breast milk; however, it is not well absorbed when taken orally. This limited oral absorption may minimize exposure to the nursing infant. Nondose-related effects could include modification of bowel flora. The AAP considers gentamicin to be "usually compatible with breast-feeding."

Contraindications Hypersensitivity to gentamicin, any component (see Warnings), or other aminoglycosides

Warnings Aminoglycosides are associated with significant nephrotoxicity **[U.S. Boxed Warning]**; vestibular and permanent bilateral auditory ototoxicity can occur **[U.S. Boxed Warning]**; tinnitus or vertigo are indications of vestibular injury and impending bilateral irreversible deafness. Risk of nephrotoxicity and ototoxicity is increased in patients with impaired renal function, high dose therapy, or prolonged therapy. Risk of nephrotoxicity increases when used concurrently with other potentially nephrotoxic drugs **[U.S. Boxed Warning]**; renal damage is usually reversible. Risk of ototoxicity increases with use of potent diuretics **[U.S. Boxed Warning]**; once-daily gentamicin administration has been associated with a pyrogenic endotoxin-like reaction (fever, chills, hypotension, tachycardia); some products contain sulfites which may cause allergic reactions in susceptible individuals. Aminoglycosides can cause fetal harm when administered to a pregnant woman **[U.S. Boxed Warning]**; aminoglycosides have been associated with several reports of total irreversible bilateral congenital deafness in pediatric patients exposed *in utero*.

Precautions Use with caution in neonates due to renal immaturity that results in a prolonged gentamicin half-life and in patients with pre-existing renal impairment, auditory or vestibular impairment, hypocalcemia, myasthenia gravis, and in conditions which depress neuromuscular transmission; may cause neuromuscular blockade and respiratory paralysis; risk increased with concomitant use of anesthesia or muscle relaxants; modify dosage in patients with renal impairment and in neonates on extracorporeal membrane oxygenation (ECMO); monitor renal and eigth-nerve function in patients with known or suspected renal impairment **[U.S. Boxed Warning]**; cross-allergenicity with other aminoglycosides has been observed

Adverse Reactions
Central nervous system: Vertigo, ataxia, gait instability, dizziness, headache, fever
Dermatologic: Rash, pruritus, erythema
Endocrine & metabolic: Hypomagnesemia
Gastrointestinal: Nausea, vomiting, anorexia
Genitourinary: Decrease in urine specific gravity, casts in urine, possible electrolyte wasting
Hematologic: Granulocytopenia, thrombocytopenia, eosinophilia
Hepatic: AST and ALT elevated
Local: Thrombophlebitis

Neuromuscular & skeletal: Neuromuscular blockade, muscle cramps, tremor, weakness
Ocular: Optic neuritis; ophthalmic use: burning, stinging, redness, lacrimation
Otic: Ototoxicity (may be associated with high serum aminoglycoside concentrations persisting for prolonged periods) with tinnitus, hearing loss; early toxicity usually affects high-pitched sound
Renal: Nephrotoxicity (high trough levels) with proteinuria, reduction in glomerular filtration rate, serum creatinine elevated

Drug Interactions
Avoid Concomitant Use
Avoid concomitant use of Gentamicin with any of the following: Agalsidase Beta; BCG; Gallium Nitrate
Increased Effect/Toxicity
Gentamicin may increase the levels/effects of: AbobotulinumtoxinA; Bisphosphonate Derivatives; CARBOplatin; Colistimethate; CycloSPORINE; CycloSPORINE (Systemic); Gallium Nitrate; Neuromuscular-Blocking Agents; OnabotulinumtoxinA; RimabotulinumtoxinB

The levels/effects of Gentamicin may be increased by: Amphotericin B; Capreomycin; CISplatin; Loop Diuretics; Nonsteroidal Anti-Inflammatory Agents; Vancomycin
Decreased Effect
Gentamicin may decrease the levels/effects of: Agalsidase Beta; BCG; Typhoid Vaccine

The levels/effects of Gentamicin may be decreased by: Penicillins
Stability Incompatible with penicillins, cephalosporins, heparin
Mechanism of Action Inhibits cellular initiation of bacterial protein synthesis by binding to 30S and 50S ribosomal subunits resulting in a defective bacterial cell membrane
Pharmacokinetics (Adult data unless noted)
Absorption: Oral: Poorly absorbed (<2%)
Distribution: Crosses the placenta; distributes primarily in the extracellular fluid volume and in most tissues; poor penetration into CSF; drug accumulates in the renal cortex; small amounts distribute into bile, sputum, saliva, tears, and breast milk
V_d: Increased in neonates and with fever, edema, ascites, fluid overload; V_d is decreased in patients with dehydration:
Neonates: 0.45 ± 0.1 L/kg
Infants: 0.4 ± 0.1 L/kg
Children: 0.35 ± 0.15 L/kg
Adolescents: 0.3 ± 0.1 L/kg
Adults: 0.2-0.3 L/kg
Protein binding: <30%
Half-life:
Neonates:
<1 week: 3-11.5 hours
1 week to 1 month: 3-6 hours
Infants: 4 ± 1 hour
Children: 2 ± 1 hour
Adolescents: 1.5 ± 1 hour
Adults with normal renal function: 1.5-3 hours
Anuria: 36-70 hours
Time to peak serum concentration:
I.M.: Within 30-90 minutes
I.V.: 30 minutes after 30-minute infusion
Elimination: Clearance is directly related to renal function; eliminated almost completely by glomerular filtration of unchanged drug with excretion into urine
Clearance:
Neonates: 0.045 ± 0.01 L/hour/kg
Infants: 0.1 ± 0.05 L/hour/kg
Children: 0.1 ± 0.03 L/hour/kg
Adolescents: 0.09 ± 0.03 L/hour/kg
Dialysis: Dialyzable (50% to 100%)

◀ **Usual Dosage** Dosage should be based on an estimate of ideal body weight, except in neonates (neonatal dosage should be based on actual weight unless the patient has hydrocephalus or hydrops fetalis):

Neonates: I.M., I.V.:

Premature neonate, <1000 g: 3.5 mg/kg/dose every 24 hours

0-4 weeks, <1200 g: 2.5 mg/kg/dose every 18-24 hours

Postnatal age ≤7 days: 2.5 mg/kg/dose every 12 hours

Postnatal age >7 days:

1200-2000 g: 2.5 mg/kg/dose every 8-12 hours

>2000 g: 2.5 mg/kg/dose every 8 hours

Initial dose for term neonates receiving ECMO: I.V.: 2.5 mg/kg/dose every 18 hours; subsequent doses should be individualized by monitoring serum drug concentrations; when ECMO is discontinued, dosage may require readjustment due to large shifts in body water

Once daily dosing:

Premature neonates with normal renal function: 3.5-4 mg/kg/dose every 24 hours

Term neonates with normal renal function: 3.5-5 mg/kg/dose every 24 hours

Infants and Children <5 years: I.M., I.V.: 2.5 mg/kg/dose every 8 hours*

Once daily dosing in patients with normal renal function: 5-7.5 mg/kg/dose every 24 hours

Endocarditis prophylaxis (high-risk patients): 1.5 mg/kg (maximum: 120 mg) within 30 minutes of starting the procedure plus ampicillin or vancomycin (in patients allergic to ampicillin)

Pulmonary infection in cystic fibrosis: 2.5-3.3 mg/kg/dose every 6-8 hours

Patients on hemodialysis: 1.25-1.75 mg/kg/dose postdialysis

Children ≥5 years: I.M., I.V.: 2-2.5 mg/kg/dose every 8 hours*

Once daily dosing in children with normal renal function: 5-7.5 mg/kg/dose every 24 hours

Endocarditis prophylaxis (high-risk patients): 1.5 mg/kg (maximum: 120 mg) within 30 minutes of starting the procedure plus ampicillin or vancomycin (in patients allergic to ampicillin)

Pulmonary infection in cystic fibrosis: 2.5-3.3 mg/kg/dose every 6-8 hours

Patients on hemodialysis: 1.25-1.75 mg/kg/dose postdialysis

*Some patients may require larger or more frequent doses (eg, every 6 hours) if serum levels document the need (ie, cystic fibrosis, patients with major burns, or febrile granulocytopenic patients); modify dose based on individual patient requirements as determined by renal function, serum drug concentrations, and patient-specific clinical parameters

Intraventricular/intrathecal (use a preservative free preparation):

Newborns: 1 mg/day

Infants >3 months and Children: 1-2 mg/day

Adults: 4-8 mg/day

Infants, Children, and Adults:

Topical: Apply 3-4 times/day

Ophthalmic:

Ointment: Apply 2-3 times/day

Solution: Instill 1-2 drops every 2-4 hours, up to 2 drops every hour for severe infections

Adults: I.M., I.V.: 3-6 mg/kg/day in divided doses every 8 hours; studies of once daily dosing have used I.V. doses of 4-6.6 mg/kg once daily

Endocarditis prophylaxis (high-risk patients): 1.5 mg/kg (maximum: 120 mg) within 30 minutes of starting the procedure plus ampicillin or vancomycin (in patients allergic to ampicillin)

Patients on hemodialysis: 0.5-0.7 mg/kg/dose postdialysis

Dosing adjustment in renal impairment: I.M., I.V.: 2.5 mg/kg** (Cl_{cr} <60 mL/minute/1.73 m^2) or

Cl_{cr} 40-60 mL/minute: Administer every 12 hours

Cl_{cr} 20-40 mL/minute: Administer every 24 hours

Cl_{cr} <20 mL/minute: Administer normal dose, then monitor levels

**2-3 serum level measurements should be obtained after the initial dose to measure the patient's pharmacokinetic parameters (eg, half-life, V_d) in order to determine the frequency and amount of subsequent doses

Administration

Ophthalmic: Gentamicin solution is not for subconjunctival injection. Solution may be instilled into the affected eye or a small amount of ointment may be placed into the conjunctival sac. Avoid contaminating tip of the solution bottle or ointment tube. Solution: Apply finger pressure to lacrimal sac during and for 1-2 minutes after instillation to decrease risk of absorption and systemic effects.

Parenteral: Administer by I.M., I.V. slow intermittent infusion over 30-60 minutes or by direct injection over 15 minutes; final concentration for I.V. administration should not exceed 10 mg/mL; administer other antibiotics, such as penicillins and cephalosporins, at least 1 hour before or after gentamicin

Topical: Apply a small amount gently to the cleansed affected area

Monitoring Parameters Urinalysis, urine output, BUN, serum creatinine, peak and trough serum gentamicin concentrations, hearing test, CBC with differential

Not all infants and children who receive aminoglycosides require monitoring of serum aminoglycoside concentrations. Indications for use of aminoglycoside serum concentration monitoring include:

Treatment course >5 days

Patients with decreased or changing renal function

Patients with poor therapeutic response

Infants <3 months of age

Atypical body constituency (obesity, expanded extracellular fluid volume)

Clinical need for higher doses or shorter intervals (eg, cystic fibrosis, burns, endocarditis, meningitis, critically ill patients, relatively resistant organism)

Patients on hemodialysis or chronic ambulatory peritoneal dialysis

Signs of nephrotoxicity or ototoxicity

Concomitant use of other nephrotoxic agents

Reference Range

Peak: 4-12 mcg/mL; peak values are 2-3 times greater with once daily dosing regimens

Trough: 0.5-2 mcg/mL

Test Interactions Aminoglycoside levels measured in blood taken from Silastic® central line catheters can sometimes give falsely high readings

Patient Information Report any dizziness or sensations of ringing or fullness in ears to the physician

Nursing Implications Obtain drug levels after the third or fourth dose except in neonates and patients with rapidly changing renal function in whom levels need to be measured sooner; peak gentamicin serum concentrations are drawn 30 minutes after the end of a 30-minute I.V. infusion, immediately on completion of a 1-hour I.V. infusion, or 1 hour after an intramuscular injection; trough levels are drawn within 30 minutes before the next dose; provide adequate patient hydration and perfusion

Dosage Forms Excipient information presented when available (limited, particularly for generics); consult specific product labeling. [DSC] = Discontinued product

Cream, topical: 0.1% (15 g, 30 g)

Infusion [premixed in NS]: 40 mg (50 mL); 60 mg (50 mL, 100 mL); 70 mg (50 mL); 80 mg (50 mL, 100 mL); 90 mg (100 mL); 100 mg (50 mL, 100 mL); 120 mg (100 mL)

Injection, solution: 10 mg/mL (6 mL, 8 mL, 10 mL)

Injection, solution: 40 mg/mL (2 mL, 20 mL)

Injection, solution [pediatric]: 10 mg/mL (2 mL)

Injection, solution [pediatric] [preservative free]: 10 mg/mL (2 mL)

Ointment, ophthalmic: 0.3% (3.5 g)

Gentak®: 0.3% (3.5 g)

Ointment, topical: 0.1% (15 g, 30 g)

Solution, ophthalmic: 0.3% (5 mL, 15 mL) [contains benzalkonium chloride]

Gentak®: 0.3% (5 mL; 15 mL [DSC]) [contains benzalkonium chloride]

Gentasol™: 0.3% (5 mL) [contains benzalkonium chloride]

References

Bhatt-Mehta V, Johnson CE and Schumacher RE, "Gentamicin Pharmacokinetics in Term Neonates Receiving Extracorporeal Membrane Oxygenation," *Pharmacotherapy*, 1992, 12(1):28-32.

Gilbert DN, "Once-Daily Aminoglycoside Therapy," *Antimicrob Agents Chemother*, 1991, 35(3):399-405.

Kraus DM, Pai MP, and Rodvold KA, "Efficacy and Tolerability of Extended-Interval Aminoglycoside Administration in Pediatric Patients," *Paediatr Drugs*, 2002, 4(7):469-84.

Reimche LD, Rooney, ME, Hindmarsh KW, et al, "An Evaluation of Gentamicin Dosing According to Renal Function in Neonates With Suspected Sepsis," *Am J Perinatol*, 1987, 4(3):262-5.

Shevchuk YM and Taylor DM, "Aminoglycoside Volume of Distribution in Pediatric Patients," *DICP*, 1990, 24(3):273-6.

◆ **Gentamicin and Prednisolone** see Prednisolone and Gentamicin *on page 1150*

◆ **Gentamicin Injection, USP (Can)** see Gentamicin *on page 642*

◆ **Gentamicin Sulfate** see Gentamicin *on page 642*

◆ **Gentasol™** see Gentamicin *on page 642*

◆ **Gen-Terbinafine (Can)** see Terbinafine *on page 1322*

Gentian Violet (JEN shun VYE oh let)

Medication Safety Issues

Sound-alike/look-alike issues:

Gentian violet may be confused with gentamicin

Therapeutic Category Antibacterial, Topical; Antifungal Agent, Topical

Generic Available Yes

Use Treatment of cutaneous or mucocutaneous infections caused by *Candida albicans* and other superficial skin infections refractory to topical nystatin, clotrimazole, miconazole, or econazole

Pregnancy Risk Factor C

Contraindications Hypersensitivity to gentian violet; ulcerated areas; patients with porphyria

Warnings May result in tattooing of the skin when applied to granulation tissue

Adverse Reactions

Dermatological: Staining of skin (purple), vesicle formation

Gastrointestinal: Esophagitis

Local: Burning, irritation, vesicle formation, sensitivity reactions, ulceration of mucous membranes

Respiratory: Laryngitis, tracheitis may result from swallowing gentian violet solution, laryngeal obstruction following frequent or prolonged use

Drug Interactions

Avoid Concomitant Use

Avoid concomitant use of Gentian Violet with any of the following: BCG

Increased Effect/Toxicity There are no known significant interactions involving an increase in effect.

Decreased Effect

Gentian Violet may decrease the levels/effects of: BCG

Mechanism of Action Topical antiseptic/germicide effective against some vegetative gram-positive bacteria, particularly *Staphylococcus* species, and some yeast; it is much less effective against gram-negative bacteria and is ineffective against acid-fast bacteria

Usual Dosage Topical:

Infants: Apply 3-4 drops of a 0.5% solution under the tongue or on lesion after feedings

Children and Adults: Apply 1% to 2% solution to lesion 2-3 times/day for 3 days, do not swallow

Administration Topical: Apply to lesions with cotton; do not apply to ulcerative lesions on the face

Patient Information Drug stains skin and clothing purple; proper hygiene and skin care need to be used to prevent spread of infection and reinfection

Nursing Implications Keep affected area dry and exposed to air

Additional Information 0.25% or 0.5% solution is less irritating than a 1% to 2% solution and is reported to be as effective

Dosage Forms Excipient information presented when available (limited, particularly for generics); consult specific product labeling.

Solution, topical: 1% (59 mL); 2% (60 mL)

◆ **Gen-Timolol (Can)** see Timolol *on page 1351*

◆ **Gentlax® (Can)** see Bisacodyl *on page 194*

◆ **Gen-Triazolam (Can)** see Triazolam *on page 1381*

◆ **Gen-Verapamil (Can)** see Verapamil *on page 1416*

◆ **Gen-Verapamil SR (Can)** see Verapamil *on page 1416*

◆ **Geri-Hydrolac™ [OTC]** see Lactic Acid and Ammonium Hydroxide *on page 789*

◆ **Geri-Hydrolac™-12 [OTC]** see Lactic Acid and Ammonium Hydroxide *on page 789*

◆ **German Measles Vaccine** see Rubella Virus Vaccine (Live) *on page 1238*

◆ **GG** see GuaiFENesin *on page 656*

◆ **GI87084B** see Remifentanil *on page 1205*

◆ **Glargine Insulin** see Insulin Glargine *on page 741*

◆ **Gleevec®** see Imatinib *on page 710*

◆ **Gliadel®** see Carmustine *on page 252*

◆ **Gliadel Wafer® (Can)** see Carmustine *on page 252*

◆ **Glibenclamide** see GlyBURIDE *on page 648*

GlipiZIDE (GLIP i zide)

Medication Safety Issues

Sound-alike/look-alike issues:

GlipiZIDE may be confused with glimepiride, glyBURIDE

Glucotrol® may be confused with Glucophage®, Glucotrol® XL, glyBURIDE

Glucotrol XL® may be confused with Glucotrol®

High alert medication: The Institute for Safe Medication Practices (ISMP) includes this medication among its list of drugs which have a heightened risk of causing significant patient harm when used in error.

Related Information

Medications for Which A Single Dose May Be Fatal When Ingested By A Toddler *on page 1709*

U.S. Brand Names Glucotrol XL®; Glucotrol®

Therapeutic Category Antidiabetic Agent, Oral; Antidiabetic Agent, Sulfonylurea; Hypoglycemic Agent, Oral

Generic Available Yes

Use Management of type II diabetes mellitus (noninsulin-dependent, NIDDM) when hyperglycemia cannot be managed by diet alone; may be used concomitantly with metformin or insulin to improve glycemic control

Pregnancy Risk Factor C

Pregnancy Considerations Adverse events have been observed in animal studies; therefore, glipizide is classified as pregnancy category C. Glipizide crosses the placenta. Severe hypoglycemia lasting 4-10 days has been noted in infants born to mothers taking a sulfonylurea at the time of delivery. Maternal hyperglycemia can be associated with adverse effects in the fetus, including macrosomia, neonatal hyperglycemia, and hyperbilirubinemia; the risk of congenital malformations is increased when the Hb A_{1c} is above the normal range. Diabetes can also be associated with adverse effects in the mother. Poorly-treated diabetes may cause end-organ damage that may in turn negatively affect obstetric outcomes. Physiologic glucose levels should be maintained prior to and during pregnancy to decrease the risk of adverse events in the mother and the fetus. Until additional safety and efficacy data are obtained, the use of oral agents is generally not recommended as routine management of GDM or type 2 diabetes mellitus during pregnancy. The manufacturer recommends if glipizide is used during pregnancy it should be discontinued at least 1 month before the expected delivery date. Insulin is the drug of choice for the control of diabetes mellitus during pregnancy.

Lactation Excretion in breast milk unknown/not recommended

Breast-Feeding Considerations Data from initial studies note that glipizide was not detected in breast milk. Breast-feeding is not recommended by the manufacturer. Potentially, hypoglycemia may occur in a nursing infant exposed to a sulfonylurea via breast milk.

Contraindications Hypersensitivity to glipizide, any component, or other sulfonamides; type 1 diabetes mellitus (insulin-dependent, IDDM), diabetic ketoacidosis with or without coma

Warnings Chemical similarities are present among sulfonamides, sulfonylureas, carbonic anhydrase inhibitors, thiazides, and loop diuretics (except ethacrynic acid), and although only glipizide use in patients with sulfonamide allergy is specifically contraindicated in product labeling, there is a risk of cross-reaction in patients with allergies to any of these compounds; avoid use when the previous reaction has been severe; product labeling states oral hypoglycemic drugs may be associated with an increased cardiovascular mortality as compared to treatment with diet alone or diet plus insulin; data to support this association are limited, and several studies, including a large prospective trial (UKPDS) have not supported an association

Precautions Use with caution in patients with adrenal or pituitary insufficiency; hypoglycemic reactions are more prevalent in debilitated, malnourished patients, patients with mild disease or impaired hepatic or renal function; hypoglycemia may also occur with inadequate caloric intake, strenuous exercise, or concurrent use with other hypoglycemic drugs; use of extended release formulation in patients with markedly reduced GI retention time eg, short-bowel syndrome, may potentially result in lower plasma levels and decreased effect

Adverse Reactions

Cardiovascular: Edema, flushing, hypertension, arrhythmias, syncope

Central nervous system: Headache, dizziness, drowsiness, insomnia, anxiety, depression, migraine, nervousness, confusion, somnolence, vertigo

Dermatologic: Rash, urticaria, photosensitivity, pruritus

Endocrine & metabolic: Hypoglycemia, hyponatremia, weight gain

Gastrointestinal: Anorexia, nausea, vomiting, diarrhea, epigastric fullness, flatulence, constipation, heartburn, abdominal pain

Genitourinary: Dysuria, polyuria

Hematologic: Blood dyscrasias, aplastic anemia, hemolytic anemia, bone marrow suppression, thrombocytopenia, agranulocytosis

Hepatic: Cholestatic jaundice, liver enzymes elevated

Neuromuscular & skeletal: Arthralgia, leg cramps, myalgia, tremor, hypertonia

Ocular: Blurred vision, ocular pain, conjunctivitis, retinal hemorrhage

Renal: Diuretic effect (mild), SIADH, urolithiasis

Respiratory: Rhinitis, dyspnea, pharyngitis

Miscellaneous: Diaphoresis

Drug Interactions

Metabolism/Transport Effects Substrate of 2C9 (major)

Avoid Concomitant Use There are no known interactions where it is recommended to avoid concomitant use.

Increased Effect/Toxicity

GlipiZIDE may increase the levels/effects of: Alcohol (Ethyl); CycloSPORINE; CycloSPORINE (Systemic); Hypoglycemic Agents

The levels/effects of GlipiZIDE may be increased by: Beta-Blockers; Chloramphenicol; Cimetidine; Clarithromycin; Cyclic Antidepressants; CYP2C9 Inhibitors (Moderate); CYP2C9 Inhibitors (Strong); Fibric Acid Derivatives; Fluconazole; GLP-1 Agonists; Herbs (Hypoglycemic Properties); Pegvisomant; Quinolone Antibiotics; Ranitidine; Salicylates; Sulfonamide Derivatives

Decreased Effect

The levels/effects of GlipiZIDE may be decreased by: Corticosteroids (Orally Inhaled); Corticosteroids (Systemic); CYP2C9 Inducers (Highly Effective); Luteinizing Hormone-Releasing Hormone Analogs; Peginterferon Alfa-2b; Quinolone Antibiotics; Rifampin; Somatropin; Thiazide Diuretics

Food Interactions Food delays absorption but does not affect the extent of absorption or peak levels achieved

Stability Store at room temperature; protect from light

Mechanism of Action Stimulates insulin release from the pancreatic beta cells, reduces glucose output from the liver, and increases insulin sensitivity at peripheral target sites

Pharmacodynamics

Onset of action: Immediate release formulation: 15-30 minutes; extended release formulation: 2-3 hours

Maximum effect: Immediate release formulation: Within 2-3 hours; extended release formulation: 6-12 hours

Duration: Immediate release formulation: 12-24 hours; extended release formulation: 24 hours

Average decrease in fasting blood glucose (when used as monotherapy): 60-70 mg/dL

Pharmacokinetics (Adult data unless noted)

Absorption: Rapid and complete

Distribution: V_d: Adults: 10 L

Protein binding: 98% to 99%

Metabolism: Extensive liver metabolism to inactive metabolites

Bioavailability: 80% to 100%

Half-life: Adults: 2-5 hours

Time to peak serum concentration:

Immediate release formulation: 1-3 hours

Extended release formulation: 6-12 hours

Elimination: <10% of drug excreted into urine as unchanged drug; 90% of drug excreted as metabolites in urine and 10% excreted in feces

Usual Dosage Adults: Oral:

Management of noninsulin-dependent diabetes mellitus in patients **previously untreated:** Initial: 5 mg/day immediate release or extended release tablets; adjust dosage in 2.5-5 mg daily increments in intervals of 3-7 days for immediate release tablets or 5 mg daily increments in intervals of at least 7 days for extended release tablets; if total daily dose for immediate release tablets is >15 mg, divide into twice daily dosage; maximum daily dose for immediate release tablets: 40 mg; maximum daily dose for extended release tablets: 20 mg

Note: Patients may be converted from immediate release tablets to extended release tablets by giving the nearest equivalent total daily dose once daily

Management of noninsulin-dependent diabetes mellitus in patients **previously maintained on insulin:**

Insulin dosage ≤20 units/day: Use recommended initial dose and abruptly discontinue insulin

Insulin dosage >20 units/day: Use recommended initial dose and reduce daily insulin dosage by 50%; continue to withdraw daily insulin dosage gradually over several days as tolerated with incremental increases of glipizide

Dosing adjustment/comments in renal impairment: Cl_{cr} <10 mL/minute: Some investigators recommend not using

Dosing adjustment in hepatic impairment: Reduce initial dosage to 2.5 mg/day

Administration Oral: Administer immediate release tablets 30 minutes before a meal; extended release tablets should be swallowed whole and administered with breakfast; do not cut, crush, or chew

Monitoring Parameters Signs and symptoms of hypoglycemia, fasting blood glucose, glycosylated hemoglobin (hemoglobin A_{1c})

Reference Range Target range:

Blood glucose: Fasting and preprandial: 80-120 mg/dL; bedtime: 100-140 mg/dL

Glycosylated hemoglobin (hemoglobin A_{1c}): <7%

Patient Information Do not change dose or discontinue without consulting prescriber; avoid alcohol while taking this medication, may cause severe reaction; maintain regular dietary intake and exercise routine; always carry quick source of sugar; if experiencing a hypoglycemic reaction, contact prescriber immediately; report severe or persistent side effects, extended vomiting or flu-like symptoms, skin rash, easy bruising or bleeding, or change in color of urine or stool; when taking extended release tablets, it is not unusual to observe a tablet in the stool; this is the nonabsorbable shell containing the active drug which has been released. May rarely cause photosensitivity reactions (eg, exposure to sunlight may cause severe sunburn, skin rash, redness, or itching); avoid direct exposure to sunlight

Additional Information When transferring from other sulfonylurea antidiabetic agents to glyburide, with the exception of chlorpropamide, the administration of the other agent may be abruptly discontinued; due to the prolonged elimination half-life of chlorpropamide, a 2- to 3-day drug-free interval may be advisable before glipizide therapy is begun

Dosage Forms Excipient information presented when available (limited, particularly for generics); consult specific product labeling.

Tablet, oral: 5 mg, 10 mg

Glucotrol®: 5 mg, 10 mg [scored; dye free]

Tablet, extended release, oral: 2.5 mg, 5 mg, 10 mg

Glucotrol XL®: 2.5 mg, 5 mg, 10 mg

References

DeFronzo RA, "Pharmacologic Therapy for Type 2 Diabetes Mellitus," *Ann Intern Med*, 1999, 131(4):281-303.

"Intensive Blood-Glucose Control With Sulphonylureas or Insulin Compared With Conventional Treatment and Risk of Complications in Patients With Type 2 Diabetes (UKPDS 33) UK Prospective Diabetes Study (UKPDS) Group," *Lancet*, 1998, 352(9131):837-53.

◆ **Glivec** *see* Imatinib *on page 710*

◆ **GlucaGen®** *see* Glucagon (rDNA Origin) *on page 647*

◆ **GlucaGen® Diagnostic Kit** *see* Glucagon (rDNA Origin) *on page 647*

◆ **GlucaGen® HypoKit™** *see* Glucagon (rDNA Origin) *on page 647*

◆ **Glucagon Emergency Kit** *see* Glucagon (rDNA Origin) *on page 647*

◆ **Glucagon Hydrochloride** *see* Glucagon (rDNA Origin) *on page 647*

Glucagon (rDNA Origin) (GLOO ka gon)

Medication Safety Issues

Sound-alike/look-alike issues:

Glucagon may be confused with Glaucon®

U.S. Brand Names GlucaGen®; GlucaGen® Diagnostic Kit; GlucaGen® HypoKit™; Glucagon Emergency Kit

Therapeutic Category Antihypoglycemic Agent

Generic Available No

Use Management of hypoglycemia; diagnostic aid in the radiologic examination of GI tract when a hypotonic state is needed; used with some success as a cardiac stimulant in management of severe cases of beta-adrenergic blocking agent overdosage

Pregnancy Risk Factor B

Lactation Excretion in breast milk unknown/compatible

Contraindications Hypersensitivity to glucagon or any component

Warnings Use with caution in patients with a history of insulinoma and/or pheochromocytoma; because glucagon depletes glycogen stores, the patient should be given supplemental carbohydrates as soon as physically possible

Adverse Reactions

Frequency not defined.

Cardiovascular: Hypertension, hypotension (up to 2 hours after GI procedures), tachycardia

Gastrointestinal: Nausea, vomiting (high incidence with rapid administration of high doses)

Hematologic: Hyponatremia, platelet count decreased

Miscellaneous: Anaphylaxis, hypersensitivity reactions

Drug Interactions

Avoid Concomitant Use There are no known interactions where it is recommended to avoid concomitant use.

Increased Effect/Toxicity

Glucagon may increase the levels/effects of: Vitamin K Antagonists

Decreased Effect There are no known significant interactions involving a decrease in effect.

Stability Glucagon (rDNA origin) for injection (Lilly) should be stored at controlled room temperature; glucagon (rDNA origin) for injection (GlucaGen®) should be refrigerated; both injections should be used immediately after reconstitution

Mechanism of Action Glucagon (rDNA origin) is genetically engineered and identical to human glucagon. It stimulates adenylate cyclase to produce increased cyclic AMP. It promotes hepatic glycogenolysis and gluconeogenesis, causing an increase in blood glucose levels; produces both positive inotropic and chronotropic effects.

Pharmacodynamics

Blood glucose effect (after 1 mg dosage):

Onset of action: I.M.: 8-10 minutes; I.V.: 1 minute

Duration: I.M.: 12-27 minutes; I.V.: 9-17 minutes

GI tract effect:
Onset of action: Within 1-10 minutes
Duration: 12-30 minutes
Pharmacokinetics (Adult data unless noted)
Distribution: V_d: 0.25 L/kg
Metabolism: Extensively degraded in liver and kidneys
Half-life, plasma: 8-18 minutes
Clearance: 13.5 mL/minute/kg
Usual Dosage Hypoglycemia, persistent:
I.M., I.V., SubQ (may repeat in 20 minutes as needed):
Neonates: 0.02-0.2 mg/kg (maximum dose: 1 mg) (Hawdon, 1993; Mehta, 1987); **Note:** Wide variance in doses exists between manufacturer's labeling and published case reports.
Infants and Children ≤20 kg (manufacturer's dosing): 0.02-0.03 mg/kg or 0.5 mg
Children >20 kg and Adults: 1 mg
I.V. continuous infusion:
Neonates: 1 mg infused over 24 hours; doses >0.02 mg/kg/hour did not produce additional benefit (Miralles, 2002)
Administration Parenteral: Dilute with manufacturer provided diluent resulting in 1 mg/mL; administer by direct I.V. injection, I.M., or SubQ
Monitoring Parameters Blood glucose, blood pressure, ECG, heart rate, mentation, platelet count, serum sodium
Additional Information 1 unit = 1 mg
Dosage Forms Excipient information presented when available (limited, particularly for generics); consult specific product labeling.
Injection, powder for reconstitution, as hydrochloride:
GlucaGen®: 1 mg [equivalent to 1 unit; contains lactose 107 mg]
GlucaGen® Diagnostic Kit: 1 mg [equivalent to 1 unit; contains lactose 107 mg; packaged with sterile water]
GlucaGen® HypoKit™: 1 mg [equivalent to 1 unit; contains lactose 107 mg; packaged with prefilled syringe containing sterile water]
Glucagon Emergency Kit: 1 mg [equivalent to 1 unit; contains lactose 49 mg; packaged with diluent syringe containing glycerin 12 mg/mL and water for injection]
References

Hawdon JM, Aynsley-Green A, and Ward Platt MP, "Neonatal Blood Glucose Concentrations: Metabolic Effects of Intravenous Glucagon and Intragastric Medium Chain Triglyceride," *Arch Dis Child*, 1993, 68 (3 Spec No):255-61.

Mehta A, Wootton R, Cheng KN, et al, "Effect of Diazoxide or Glucagon on Hepatic Glucose Production Rate During Extreme Neonatal Hypoglycaemia," *Arch Dis Child*, 1987, 62(9):924-30.

Miralles RE, Lodha A, Perlman M, et al, "Experience With Intravenous Glucagon Infusions as a Treatment for Resistant Neonatal Hypoglycemia," *Arch Pediatr Adolesc Med*, 2002, 156(10):999-1004.

◆ **Glucobay™ (Can)** *see* Acarbose *on page 35*

◆ **GlucoBurst® [OTC]** *see* Dextrose *on page 422*

◆ **Glucocerebrosidase** *see* Alglucerase *on page 64*

◆ **Glucophage®** *see* MetFORMIN *on page 891*

◆ **Glucophage® XR** *see* MetFORMIN *on page 891*

◆ **Glucose** *see* Dextrose *on page 422*

◆ **Glucose Monohydrate** *see* Dextrose *on page 422*

◆ **Glucotrol®** *see* GlipiZIDE *on page 645*

◆ **Glucotrol XL®** *see* GlipiZIDE *on page 645*

◆ **Glulisine Insulin** *see* Insulin Glulisine *on page 742*

◆ **Glumetza®** *see* MetFORMIN *on page 891*

◆ **Glutol™ [OTC]** *see* Dextrose *on page 422*

◆ **Glutose 15™ [OTC]** *see* Dextrose *on page 422*

◆ **Glutose 45™ [OTC]** *see* Dextrose *on page 422*

◆ **Glybenclamide** *see* GlyBURIDE *on page 648*

◆ **Glybenzcyclamide** *see* GlyBURIDE *on page 648*

GlyBURIDE (GLYE byoor ide)

Medication Safety Issues
Sound-alike/look-alike issues:
GlyBURIDE may be confused with glipiZIDE, Glucotrol®
Diaβeta® may be confused with Diabinese®, Zebeta®
Micronase® may be confused with microK®, miconazole, Micronor®, Microzide™

High alert medication: The Institute for Safe Medication Practices (ISMP) includes this medication among its list of drugs which have a heightened risk of causing significant patient harm when used in error.
U.S. Brand Names Diaβeta®; Glynase® PresTab®; Micronase® [DSC]
Canadian Brand Names Apo-Glyburide®; Diaβeta®; Dom-Glyburide; Euglucon®; Med-Glybe; Mylan-Glybe; Novo-Glyburide; Nu-Glyburide; PMS-Glyburide; PRO-Glyburide; ratio-Glyburide; Riva-Glyburide; Sandoz-Glyburide
Therapeutic Category Antidiabetic Agent, Oral; Antidiabetic Agent, Sulfonylurea; Hypoglycemic Agent, Oral
Generic Available Yes
Use Adjunct to diet and exercise for the management of type II diabetes mellitus (noninsulin-dependent, NIDDM); may be used concomitantly with metformin or insulin to improve glycemic control
Pregnancy Risk Factor B/C (manufacturer dependent)
Pregnancy Considerations Reproduction studies differ by manufacturer labeling. Because adverse events were not observed in animal reproduction studies, one manufacturer classifies glyburide as pregnancy category B. Because adverse events were noted in animal studies during the period of lactation, another manufacturer classifies glyburide as pregnancy category C.

Glyburide was not found to significantly cross the placenta *in vitro* and was not found in the cord serum infants of mothers taking glyburide for gestational diabetes mellitus (GDM). Nonteratogenic effects such as hypoglycemia in the neonate have been associated with maternal glyburide use. Maternal hyperglycemia can be associated with adverse effects in the fetus, including macrosomia, neonatal hyperglycemia, and hyperbilirubinemia; the risk of congenital malformations is increased when the Hb A_{1c} is above the normal range. Diabetes can also be associated with adverse effects in the mother. Poorly-treated diabetes may cause end-organ damage that may in turn negatively affect obstetric outcomes. Physiologic glucose levels should be maintained prior to and during pregnancy to decrease the risk of adverse events in the mother and the fetus. The manufacturer recommends that if glyburide is used during pregnancy, it should be discontinued at least 2 weeks before the expected delivery date. Although studies have shown positive outcomes using glyburide for the treatment of GDM, use may not be appropriate for all women. Until additional safety and efficacy data are obtained, the use of oral agents is generally not recommended as routine management of type 2 diabetes mellitus during pregnancy. Insulin is considered the drug of choice for the control of diabetes mellitus during pregnancy.

Lactation Does not enter breast milk/use caution
Breast-Feeding Considerations Data from initial studies note that glyburide was not detected in breast milk. Breast-feeding is not recommended by the manufacturer. Potentially, hypoglycemia may occur in a nursing infant exposed to a sulfonylurea via breast milk.
Contraindications Hypersensitivity to glyburide, any component, or other sulfonamides; type 1 diabetes mellitus (insulin-dependent, IDDM), diabetic ketoacidosis with or without coma; concomitant use with bosentan

Warnings Chemical similarities are present among sulfonamides, sulfonylureas, carbonic anhydrase inhibitors, thiazides, and loop diuretics (except ethacrynic acid). Use in patients with sulfonamide allergy is not specifically contraindicated in product labeling; however, there is a risk of cross-reaction in patients with allergies to any of these compounds; avoid use when the previous reaction has been severe; product labeling states oral hypoglycemic drugs may be associated with an increased cardiovascular mortality as compared to treatment with diet alone or diet plus insulin; data to support this association are limited, and several studies, including a large prospective trial (UKPDS) have not supported an association. Formulations of micronized glyburide (Glynase® Prestab®) are not bioequivalent with conventional formulations (Diaβeta®, Micronase®) and dosage should be retitrated when transferring patients from one formulation to the other.

Precautions Use with caution in patients with adrenal or pituitary insufficiency; hypoglycemic reactions are more prevalent in debilitated, malnourished patients, patients with mild disease or impaired hepatic or renal function; hypoglycemia may also occur with inadequate caloric intake, strenuous exercise, or concurrent use with other hypoglycemic drugs; patients with G6PD deficiency may be at an increased risk of sulfonylurea-induced hemolytic anemia; however, cases have also been described in patients without G6PD deficiency during postmarketing surveillance. Use with caution and consider a non-sulfonylurea alternative in patients with G6PD deficiency.

Adverse Reactions

Central nervous system: Headache, dizziness

Dermatologic: Pruritus, rash, urticaria, photosensitivity

Endocrine & metabolic: Hypoglycemia, weight gain

Gastrointestinal: Nausea, epigastric fullness, heartburn, constipation, diarrhea, anorexia

Genitourinary: Nocturia

Hematologic: Leukopenia, thrombocytopenia, hemolytic anemia, aplastic anemia, bone marrow suppression, agranulocytosis

Hepatic: Cholestatic jaundice, liver enzymes elevated

Neuromuscular & skeletal: Arthralgia, paresthesia

Ocular: Blurred vision

Renal: Diuretic effect (minor), urolithiasis

Drug Interactions

Metabolism/Transport Effects Inhibits CYP2C8 (weak), 3A4 (weak)

Avoid Concomitant Use

Avoid concomitant use of GlyBURIDE with any of the following: Bosentan

Increased Effect/Toxicity

GlyBURIDE may increase the levels/effects of: Alcohol (Ethyl); Bosentan; CycloSPORINE; CycloSPORINE (Systemic); Hypoglycemic Agents

The levels/effects of GlyBURIDE may be increased by: Beta-Blockers; Chloramphenicol; Cimetidine; Clarithromycin; Cyclic Antidepressants; Fibric Acid Derivatives; Fluconazole; GLP-1 Agonists; Herbs (Hypoglycemic Properties); Pegvisomant; Quinolone Antibiotics; Ranitidine; Salicylates; Sulfonamide Derivatives

Decreased Effect

GlyBURIDE may decrease the levels/effects of: Bosentan

The levels/effects of GlyBURIDE may be decreased by: Bosentan; Colesevelam; Corticosteroids (Orally Inhaled); Corticosteroids (Systemic); Luteinizing Hormone-Releasing Hormone Analogs; Quinolone Antibiotics; Rifampin; Somatropin; Thiazide Diuretics

Food Interactions Food does not affect absorption.

Mechanism of Action Stimulates insulin release from the pancreatic beta cells, reduces glucose output from the liver, and increases insulin sensitivity at peripheral target sites

Pharmacodynamics

Onset of action: 45-60 minutes

Maximum effect: 1.5-3 hours

Duration: Conventional formulations: 16-24 hours; micronized formulations: 12-24 hours

Average decrease in fasting blood glucose (when used as monotherapy): 60-70 mg/dL

Pharmacokinetics (Adult data unless noted)

Absorption: Reliably and almost completely absorbed

Distribution: V_d: 0.125 L/kg

Metabolism: Completely metabolized to one moderately active and several inactive metabolites

Protein binding: High (>99%)

Half-life: Biphasic: Terminal elimination half-life: Average: 1.4-1.8 hours (range: 0.7-3 hours); may be prolonged with renal or hepatic insufficiency

Time to peak serum concentration: Conventional formulation: 4 hours; micronized formulation: 2-3 hours

Elimination: 30% to 50% of dose excreted in the urine as metabolites in first 24 hours; the remainder of the metabolite via biliary excretion

Dialysis: Not dialyzable

Usual Dosage Adults: Oral: Formulations of micronized glyburide (Glynase® Prestab®) are **not** bioequivalent with conventional formulations (Diaβeta®, Micronase®) and dosage should be retitrated when transferring patients from one formulation to the other

Management of noninsulin-dependent diabetes mellitus in patients **previously untreated**:

Tablet (Diaβeta®, Micronase®):

Initial: 2.5-5 mg/day; in patients who are more sensitive to hypoglycemic drugs (see Precautions), start at 1.25 mg/day; increase in increments of no more than 2.5 mg/day at weekly intervals

Maintenance: 1.25-20 mg/day given as single or divided doses; maximum: 20 mg/day; doses >10 mg should be divided into twice daily doses

Micronized tablets (Glynase® Prestab®):

Initial: 1.5-3 mg/day; in patients who are more sensitive to hypoglycemic drugs (see Precautions), start at 0.75 mg/day; increase in increments of no more than 1.5 mg/day at weekly intervals

Maintenance: 0.75-12 mg/day given as a single dose or in divided doses; maximum: 12 mg/day; doses >6 mg/day should be divided into twice daily doses

Management of noninsulin-dependent diabetes mellitus in patients **previously maintained on insulin:** Initial dosage dependent upon previous insulin dosage, see table

Previous Daily Insulin Dosage (units)	Initial Glyburide Dosage (mg conventional formulation)	Initial Glyburide Dosage (mg micronized formulation)	Insulin Dosage Change (after glyburide started)
<20	2.5-5	1.5-3	Discontinue
20-40	5	3	Discontinue
>40	5 (increase in increments of 1.25-2.5 mg every 2-10 days)	3 (increase in increments of 0.75-1.5 mg every 2-10 days)	Reduce insulin dosage by 50% (gradually taper off insulin as glyburide dosage increased)

Dosing adjustment in renal impairment: Cl_{cr} <50 mL/minute: Not recommended

Dosing adjustment in hepatic impairment: Use conservative initial and maintenance doses and avoid use in severe disease

Administration Oral: May administer with food every morning 30 minutes before breakfast or the first main meal

Monitoring Parameters Signs and symptoms of hypoglycemia, fasting blood glucose, hemoglobin A_{1c}

Reference Range Target range:

Blood glucose: Fasting and preprandial: 80-120 mg/dL; bedtime: 100-140 mg/dL

Glycosylated hemoglobin (hemoglobin A_{1c}): <7%

Patient Information Do not change dose or discontinue without consulting prescriber; avoid alcohol while taking this medication, may cause severe reaction; maintain regular dietary intake and exercise routine; always carry quick source of sugar; if experiencing a hypoglycemic reaction, contact prescriber immediately; report severe or persistent side effects, extended vomiting or flu-like symptoms, skin rash, easy bruising or bleeding, or change in color of urine or stool. May rarely cause photosensitivity reactions (eg, exposure to sunlight may cause severe sunburn, skin rash, redness, or itching); avoid direct exposure to sunlight

Additional Information When transferring from other sulfonylurea antidiabetic agents to glyburide, with the exception of chlorpropamide, the administration of the other agent may be abruptly discontinued; due to the prolonged elimination half-life of chlorpropamide, a 2- to 3-day drug-free interval may be advisable before glyburide therapy is begun

Dosage Forms Excipient information presented when available (limited, particularly for generics); consult specific product labeling. [DSC] = Discontinued product

Tablet: 1.25 mg, 2.5 mg, 5 mg

DiaβBeta®: 1.25 mg, 2.5 mg, 5 mg

Micronase® [DSC]: 1.25 mg, 2.5 mg, 5 mg

Tablet, micronized: 1.5 mg, 3 mg, 6 mg

Glynase® PresTab®: 1.5 mg, 3 mg, 6 mg

References

DeFronzo RA, "Pharmacologic Therapy for Type 2 Diabetes Mellitus," *Ann Intern Med*, 1999, 131(4):281-303.

"Intensive Blood-Glucose Control With Sulphonylureas or Insulin Compared With Conventional Treatment and Risk of Complications in Patients With Type 2 Diabetes (UKPDS 33) UK Prospective Diabetes Study (UKPDS) Group," *Lancet*, 1998, 352(9131):837-53.

Glycerin (GLIS er in)

U.S. Brand Names Bausch & Lomb® Computer Eye Drops [OTC]; Colace® Adult/Children Suppositories [OTC]; Colace® Infant/Children Suppositories [OTC]; Fleet® Babylax® [OTC] [DSC]; Fleet® Glycerin Suppositories Maximum Strength [OTC]; Fleet® Glycerin Suppositories [OTC]; Fleet® Liquid Glycerin Suppositories [OTC]; Fleet® Pedia-Lax™ Glycerin Suppositories [OTC]; Fleet® Pedia-Lax™ Liquid Glycerin Suppositories [OTC]; Orajel® Dry Mouth [OTC]; Sani-Supp® [OTC]

Therapeutic Category Laxative, Osmotic

Generic Available Yes: Suppositories

Use Treatment of constipation; reduction of intraocular pressure; reduction of corneal edema; glycerin has been administered orally to reduce intracranial pressure; laxative used in newborns to promote bilirubin excretion by reducing enterohepatic circulation, decreasing GI transit time, and stimulating passage of meconium

Pregnancy Risk Factor C

Contraindications Hypersensitivity to glycerin or any component; severe dehydration, anuria

Precautions Use oral glycerin with caution in patients with cardiac, renal or hepatic disease and in diabetics

Adverse Reactions

Central nervous system: Dizziness, headache, confusion, disorientation

Endocrine & metabolic: Hyperglycemia, dehydration

Gastrointestinal: Diarrhea, nausea, tenesmus, thirst, cramping pain, vomiting, rectal irritation

Local: Pain/irritation with ophthalmic solution (may need to apply a topical ophthalmic anesthetic before glycerin administration)

Drug Interactions

Avoid Concomitant Use There are no known interactions where it is recommended to avoid concomitant use.

Increased Effect/Toxicity There are no known significant interactions involving an increase in effect.

Decreased Effect There are no known significant interactions involving a decrease in effect.

Stability Protect from heat; freezing should be avoided

Mechanism of Action

Rectal: Osmotic dehydrating agent which increases osmotic pressure; draws fluid into colon and thus stimulates evacuation

Ophthalmic: Osmotic action reduces edema and causes clearing of corneal haze

Oral: Glycerin increases osmotic pressure of the plasma drawing water from the extravascular spaces into the blood producing a decrease in intraocular and intracranial pressure

Pharmacodynamics

Onset of action for glycerin suppository or enema: 15-30 minutes

Onset of action in decreasing intraocular pressure: Within 10-30 minutes

Duration: 4-8 hours

Increased intracranial pressure decreases within 10-60 minutes following an oral dose

Duration: ~2-3 hours

Pharmacokinetics (Adult data unless noted)

Absorption:

Oral: Well absorbed

Rectal: Poorly absorbed

Metabolism: Primarily in the liver with 20% metabolized in the kidney

Half-life: 30-45 minutes

Time to peak serum concentration: Oral: Within 60-90 minutes

Elimination: Only a small percentage of drug is excreted unchanged in urine

Usual Dosage

Constipation: Rectal: Administered in single doses only at infrequent intervals

Neonates: 0.5 mL/kg/dose of rectal solution as an enema

Children <6 years: 1 infant suppository as needed or 2-5 mL of rectal solution as an enema

Children ≥6 years and Adults: 1 adult suppository as needed or 5-15 mL of rectal solution as an enema

Children and Adults:

Reduction of intraocular pressure: Oral: 1-1.8 g/kg administered 1-1^1/$_2$ hours preoperatively; additional doses may be administered at 5-hour intervals

Reduction of intracranial pressure: Oral: 1.5 g/kg/day divided every 4 hours; 1 g/kg/dose every 6 hours has also been used

Reduction of corneal edema: Ophthalmic: Instill 1-2 drops in eye(s) every 3-4 hours

Administration

Oral: Orange or lemon juice may be added to unflavored 50% oral solution; pour solution over crushed ice and drink through a straw to improve palatability

Ophthalmic: Instill drops onto the eye; avoid contaminating tip of the solution bottle

Rectal: Insert suppository in the rectum and retain 15 minutes

Monitoring Parameters Blood glucose, intraocular pressure, evacuation of stool

Patient Information Do not use if experiencing abdominal pain, nausea, or vomiting

Nursing Implications Use caution during insertion of suppository to avoid intestinal perforation, especially in neonates; instruct patient to lie down after oral glycerin administration to prevent or relieve headaches

Dosage Forms Excipient information presented when available (limited, particularly for generics); consult specific product labeling. [DSC] = Discontinued product

Gel, oral:

Orajel® Dry Mouth: 18% (42 g) [contains benzalkonium chloride]

Liquid, for prescription compounding: USP: 100% (3840 mL)

Solution, ophthalmic, sterile:

Bausch & Lomb® Computer Eye Drops: 1% (15 mL) [contains benzalkonium chloride]

Solution, oral:

Osmoglyn®: 50% (220 mL) [lime flavor] [DSC]

Solution, rectal:

Fleet® Babylax®: 2.3 g/2.3 mL (4 mL) [6 units per box] [DSC]

Fleet® Liquid Glycerin Suppositories: 5.6 g/5.5 mL (7.5 mL) [4 units per box]

Fleet® Pedia-Lax™ Liquid Glycerin Suppositories: 2.3 mg/2.3 mL (4 mL) [6 units per box]

Suppository, rectal [adult]: 82.5% (12s, 24s, 25s, 50s, 100s)

Colace® Adult/Children: 2.1 g (12s, 24s, 48s, 100s)

Fleet® Glycerin Suppositories: 2 g (12s, 24s, 50s)

Fleet® Glycerin Suppositories Maximum Strength: 3 g (18s)

Sani-Supp®: 82.5% (10s, 25s, 50s)

Suppository, rectal [pediatric]: 82.5% (12s, 25s)

Colace® Infant/Children: 1.2 g (12s, 24s)

Fleet® Glycerin Suppositories: 1 g (12s) [DSC]

Fleet® Pedia-Lax™ Glycerin Suppositories: 1 g (12s)

Sani-Supp®: 82.5% (10s, 25s)

References

Heinemeyer G, "Clinical Pharmacokinetic Considerations in the Treatment of Increased Intracranial Pressure," Clin Pharmacokinet, 1987, 13(1):1-25.

Rottenberg DA, Hurwitz BJ, and Posner JB, "The Effect of Oral Glycerol on Intraventricular Pressure in Man," Neurology, 1977, 27(7):600-8.

Zenk KE, Koeppel RM, and Liem LA, "Comparative Efficacy of Glycerin Enemas and Suppository Chips in Neonates," Clin Pharm, 1993, 12 (11):846-8.

♦ **Glycerol** see Glycerin *on page 650*

♦ **Glycerol Guaiacolate** see GuaiFENesin *on page 656*

♦ **Glyceryl Trinitrate** see Nitroglycerin *on page 996*

♦ **Glycon (Can)** see MetFORMIN *on page 891*

Glycopyrrolate (glye koe PYE roe late)

Medication Safety Issues

Sound-alike/look-alike issues:

Robinul® may be confused with Reminyl®

Related Information

Compatibility of Medications Mixed in a Syringe *on page 1713*

U.S. Brand Names Robinul®; Robinul® Forte

Canadian Brand Names Glycopyrrolate Injection, USP

Therapeutic Category Anticholinergic Agent; Antispasmodic Agent, Gastrointestinal

Generic Available Yes

Use Adjunct in treatment of peptic ulcer disease; inhibition of salivation and excessive secretions of the respiratory tract; reversal of the muscarinic effects of cholinergic agents such as neostigmine and pyridostigmine during reversal of neuromuscular blockade

Pregnancy Risk Factor B

Pregnancy Considerations Teratogenic effects were not observed in animal studies. Small amounts of glycopyrrolate cross the human placenta.

Lactation Excretion in breast milk unknown/use caution

Breast-Feeding Considerations May suppress lactation

Contraindications Hypersensitivity to glycopyrrolate or any component (see Warnings); narrow-angle glaucoma; acute hemorrhage; tachycardia; severe ulcerative colitis; obstructive uropathy; paralytic ileus; myasthenia gravis; intestinal atony; obstructive disease of GI tract; toxic megacolon complicating ulcerative colitis

Warnings Infants, patients with Down syndrome, and children with spastic paralysis or brain damage may be hypersensitive to antimuscarinic effects. Monitor closely in patients with renal impairment as clearance is prolonged. Paradoxical excitation may occur in infants and young children.

Precautions Use with caution in patients with fever, hyperthyroidism, hepatic or renal disease, hypertension, CHF, GI infections, diarrhea, reflux esophagitis

Adverse Reactions

Cardiovascular: Tachycardia, orthostatic hypotension, ventricular fibrillation, palpitations

Central nervous system: Drowsiness, nervousness, headache, insomnia, confusion, loss of memory, fatigue, ataxia, paradoxical excitation (infants and young children)

Dermatologic: Rash, dry skin

Gastrointestinal: Xerostomia, constipation, nausea, vomiting, dry throat, dysphagia

Genitourinary: Urinary retention, dysuria

Local: Irritation at injection site

Neuromuscular & skeletal: Weakness

Ocular: Blurred vision, light sensitivity

Respiratory: Dry nose

Miscellaneous: Diaphoresis decreased

Drug Interactions

Avoid Concomitant Use There are no known interactions where it is recommended to avoid concomitant use.

Increased Effect/Toxicity

Glycopyrrolate may increase the levels/effects of: AbobotulinumtoxinA; Anticholinergics; Cannabinoids; OnabotulinumtoxinA; Potassium Chloride; RimabotulinumtoxinB

The levels/effects of Glycopyrrolate may be increased by: MAO Inhibitors; Pramlintide

Decreased Effect

Glycopyrrolate may decrease the levels/effects of: Acetylcholinesterase Inhibitors (Central); Secretin

The levels/effects of Glycopyrrolate may be decreased by: Acetylcholinesterase Inhibitors (Central)

Stability Unstable at pH >6; compatible in the same syringe with atropine, benzquinamide, chlorpromazine, codeine, diphenhydramine, droperidol, fentanyl, hydromorphone, hydroxyzine, lidocaine, meperidine, promethazine, morphine, neostigmine, oxymorphone, procaine, prochlorperazine, promazine, pyridostigmine, scopolamine, triflupromazine, and trimethobenzamide

Mechanism of Action Inhibits the muscarinic action of acetylcholine at postganglionic parasympathetic neuroeffector sites in smooth muscle, secretory glands, and CNS

Pharmacodynamics

Onset of action:

Oral: Within 1 hour

I.M., SubQ: 15-30 minutes

I.V.: 1-10 minutes

Maximum effect: I.M., SubQ: 30-45 minutes

Duration (anticholinergic effects):

Oral: 8-12 hours

Parenteral: 7 hours

Pharmacokinetics (Adult data unless noted)

Absorption: Oral: Poor and erratic; 10% absorption

Distribution: Does not adequately penetrate into CNS

V_d: Adults: 0.42 ± 0.22 L/kg

Half-life:
Infants: 21.6-130 minutes
Children: 19.2-99.2 minutes
Adults: 0.83 ± 0.13 hours
Elimination: Primarily unchanged via biliary elimination (70% to 90%)
Clearance: Adults: 0.54 ± 0.14 L/kg/hour

Usual Dosage

Children:
Control of secretions:
Oral: 40-100 mcg/kg/dose 3-4 times/day
I.M., I.V.: 4-10 mcg/kg/dose every 3-4 hours
Preoperative: I.M.:
≤2 years: 4-9 mcg/kg 30-60 minutes before procedure; may repeat intraoperatively 4 mcg/kg not to exceed 0.1 mg/day in intervals of 2-3 minutes
>2 years: 4 mcg/kg 30-60 minutes before procedure; may repeat intraoperatively 4 mcg/kg not to exceed 0.1 mg/day in intervals of 2-3 minutes
Children and Adults: Reversal of muscarinic effects of cholinergic agents: I.V.: 0.2 mg for each 1 mg of neostigmine or 5 mg of pyridostigmine administered
Adults:
Peptic ulcer:
Oral: 1-2 mg 2-3 times/day
I.M., I.V.: 0.1-0.2 mg 3-4 times/day; may increase to 0.4 mg 3-4 times/day
Preoperative: I.M.: 4 mcg/kg 30-60 minutes before procedure; may repeat intraoperatively in single doses of 0.1 mg as needed in intervals of 2-3 minutes

Administration

Oral: May be administered without regard to meals
Parenteral: Dilute to a concentration of 2 mcg/mL (maximum concentration: 200 mcg/mL); infuse over 15-20 minutes; may be administered direct I.V. at a maximum rate of 20 mcg/minute; may be administered I.M.

Monitoring Parameters Heart rate

Patient Information May cause dry mouth; may cause drowsiness and blurred vision and impair ability to perform activities requiring mental alertness or physical coordination; use caution during exercise or hot weather as overheating may result in heat stroke

Dosage Forms Excipient information presented when available (limited, particularly for generics); consult specific product labeling. [DSC] = Discontinued product
Injection, solution: 0.2 mg/mL (1 mL, 2 mL, 5 mL, 20 mL)
Robinul®: 0.2 mg/mL (1 mL, 2 mL, 5 mL; 20 mL [DSC]) [contains benzyl alcohol]
Tablet: 1 mg, 2 mg
Robinul®: 1 mg
Robinul® Forte: 2 mg

♦ **Glycopyrrolate Injection, USP (Can)** see Glycopyrrolate on page 651

♦ **Glycopyrronium Bromide** see Glycopyrrolate on page 651

♦ **Glycosum** see Dextrose on page 422

♦ **Glydiazinamide** see GlipiZIDE on page 645

♦ **Glynase® PresTab®** see GlyBURIDE on page 648

♦ **Gly-Oxide® [OTC]** see Carbamide Peroxide on page 248

♦ **GM-CSF** see Sargramostim on page 1247

Gold Sodium Thiomalate
(gold SOW dee um thye oh MAL ate)

U.S. Brand Names Myochrysine®
Canadian Brand Names Myochrysine®
Therapeutic Category Gold Compound
Generic Available No

Use Treatment of progressive rheumatoid arthritis
Pregnancy Risk Factor C
Lactation Enters breast milk/not recommended
Contraindications Hypersensitivity to gold compounds, any component (see Warnings); systemic lupus erythematosus; avoid concomitant use of antimalarials, immunosuppressive agents, penicillamine, or phenylbutazone; severe toxicity from previous exposure or from other heavy metals; severe debilitation

Warnings Use may be associated with significant toxicity involving dermatologic, GI, hematologic, pulmonary, renal, and hepatic systems; patient education is required **[U.S. Boxed Warning]**. Signs of gold toxicity include decrease in hemoglobin, leukocytes, granulocytes and platelets, proteinuria, hematuria, or persistent diarrhea, rash, metallic taste; dermatitis (urticaria or eczema) and lesions of the mucous membranes are common and may be serious; pruritus may precede the early development of a skin reaction; advise patient to report any symptoms of toxicity; prior to each injection, the patient should be fully evaluated for any signs of adverse reactions.

Injection contains benzyl alcohol which may cause allergic reactions in susceptible individuals; large amounts of benzyl alcohol (≥99 mg/kg/day) have been associated with a potentially fatal toxicity ("gasping syndrome") in neonates; the "gasping syndrome" consists of metabolic acidosis, respiratory distress, gasping respirations, CNS dysfunction (including convulsions, intracranial hemorrhage), hypotension and cardiovascular collapse; *in vitro* and animal studies have shown that benzoate displaces bilirubin from protein binding sites; avoid use of gold sodium thiomalate in neonates

Precautions Frequent monitoring of patients for signs and symptoms of toxicity will prevent serious adverse reactions; NSAIDs and corticosteroids may be discontinued after initiating gold therapy; must not be injected I.V. Use with caution in patients with a history of blood dyscrasia, allergy or hypersensitivity to drugs, skin rash, history of hepatic or renal disease, marked hypertension, or compromised cerebral or cardiovascular circulation; ensure that CHF and diabetes are well controlled prior to starting therapy.

Adverse Reactions
Cardiovascular: Flushing
Central nervous system: Seizures, headache
Dermatologic: Exfoliative urticaria, eczema, dermatitis, erythema nodosum, alopecia, shedding of nails, pruritus, gray-to-blue pigmentation of skin and mucous membranes
Gastrointestinal: Stomatitis, nausea, diarrhea, abdominal cramps, metallic taste, gingivitis, glossitis, ulcerative enterocolitis, GI hemorrhage, dysphagia
Genitourinary: Vaginitis
Hematologic: Eosinophilia, leukopenia, agranulocytosis, aplastic anemia, thrombocytopenia
Hepatic: Hepatitis, cholestatic jaundice
Neuromuscular & skeletal: Arthralgias, peripheral neuropathy
Ocular: Blurred vision, conjunctivitis, corneal ulcers, iritis
Renal: Hematuria, proteinuria, nephrotic syndrome
Respiratory: Interstitial pneumonitis and fibrosis
Miscellaneous: Hypersensitivity reactions including anaphylaxis (rare)

Drug Interactions
Avoid Concomitant Use There are no known interactions where it is recommended to avoid concomitant use.
Increased Effect/Toxicity
The levels/effects of Gold Sodium Thiomalate may be increased by: ACE Inhibitors
Decreased Effect There are no known significant interactions involving a decrease in effect.

Mechanism of Action Unknown, may decrease prostaglandin synthesis or may alter cellular mechanisms by inhibiting sulfhydryl systems

Pharmacodynamics

Onset of action: Delayed; may require up to 3 months of therapy

Pharmacokinetics (Adult data unless noted)

Distribution: Breast milk to plasma ratio: 0.02-0.3

Half-life: 5 days (range: 3-27 days); may lengthen with multiple doses

Time to peak serum concentration: I.M.: Within 3-6 hours

Elimination: Majority (50% to 90%) excreted in urine with smaller amounts (10% to 50%) excreted in feces (via bile)

Usual Dosage I.M.:

Children: Initial: Test dose of 10 mg I.M. is recommended, followed by 1 mg/kg I.M. weekly for 20 weeks (maximum dose: 50 mg); maintenance: 1 mg/kg/dose at 2- to 4-week intervals thereafter for as long as therapy is clinically beneficial and toxicity does not develop. Administration for 2-4 months is usually required before clinical improvement is observed.

Adults: 10 mg first week; 25 mg second week; then 25-50 mg/week until clinical improvement or a 1 g cumulative dose has been given. If improvement occurs without adverse reactions, give 25-50 mg every 2 weeks for 2-20 weeks; if continues stable, give 25-50 mg every 3-4 weeks indefinitely.

Dosage adjustment in renal impairment:

Cl_{cr} 50-80 mL/minute: Administer 50% of dose

Cl_{cr} <50 mL/minute: Avoid use

Administration Parenteral: Administer I.M. only, preferably intraglutaneally; addition of 0.1 mL of 1% lidocaine to each injection may reduce the discomfort associated with I.M. administration; patients should be recumbent during injection and for 10 minutes afterwards; observe closely for 15 minutes after injection

Monitoring Parameters CBC with differential, platelets, hemoglobin, urinalysis for protein, white cells, red cells, and casts at baseline and prior to each injection. Skin and oral mucosa should be inspected for skin rash, bruising, or oral ulceration/stomatitis. Treatment should be withheld in patients with significant GI, renal, dermatologic, or hematologic effects (eg, platelets <100,000/mm^3, WBC <4000, granulocytes <1500/mm^3)

Reference Range Gold: Normal: 0-0.1 mcg/mL (SI: 0-0.0064 micromoles/L); Therapeutic: 1-3 mcg/mL (SI: 0.06-0.18 micromoles/L); Urine <0.1 mcg/24 hours

Dosage Forms Excipient information presented when available (limited, particularly for generics); consult specific product labeling.

Injection, solution:

Myochrysine®: 50 mg/mL (1 mL, 10 mL) [contains benzyl alcohol]

♦ **GoLYTELY®** see Polyethylene Glycol-Electrolyte Solution on page 1129

♦ **Gordofilm® [OTC]** see Salicylic Acid on page 1241

♦ **GP 47680** see OXcarbazepine on page 1035

♦ **GR38032R** see Ondansetron on page 1022

Granisetron (gra NI se tron)

Medication Safety Issues

Sound-alike/look-alike issues:

Granisetron may be confused with dolasetron, ondansetron, palonosetron

U.S. Brand Names Granisol™; Kytril®; Sancuso®

Canadian Brand Names Apo-Granisetron®; Kytril®

Therapeutic Category 5-HT$_3$ Receptor Antagonist; Antiemetic

Generic Available Yes

Use Prophylaxis and treatment of chemotherapy- and radiation-related nausea and emesis (FDA approved in ages 2-16 and adults); prophylaxis and treatment of postoperative nausea and vomiting (FDA approved in adults)

Transdermal patch: Prophylaxis of nausea and vomiting associated with moderate-to-high emetogenic chemotherapy regimens ≤5 days consecutive duration (FDA approved in adults)

Pregnancy Risk Factor B

Pregnancy Considerations There are no adequate or well-controlled studies in pregnant women. Teratogenic effects were not observed in animal studies. Injection (1 mg/mL strength) contains benzyl alcohol which may cross the placenta. Use only if benefit exceeds the risk.

Lactation Excretion in breast milk unknown/use caution

Contraindications Hypersensitivity to granisetron or any component (see Warnings)

Warnings Selective 5-HT$_3$ antagonists, including granisetron, have been associated with a number of dose-dependent increases in ECG intervals (eg, PR, QRS duration, QT/QT$_c$, JT), usually occurring 1-2 hours after I.V. administration. In general, these changes are not clinically relevant; however, when used in conjunction with other agents that prolong these intervals, arrhythmia may occur. When used with agents that prolong the QT interval (eg, Class I and III antiarrhythmics), clinically relevant QT interval prolongation may occur resulting in torsade de pointes. A number of trials have shown that 5-HT$_3$ antagonists produce QT interval prolongation to variable degrees. Reduction in heart rate may also occur with the 5-HT$_3$ antagonists. I.V. formulations of 5-HT$_3$ antagonists have more association with ECG interval changes compared to oral formulations. Some injectable products contain benzyl alcohol which may cause allergic reactions in susceptible individuals; large amounts of benzyl alcohol (≥99 mg/day) have been associated with a potentially fatal toxicity ("gasping syndrome") in neonates; the "gasping syndrome" consists of metabolic acidosis, respiratory distress, gasping respirations, CNS dysfunction (including convulsions, intracranial hemorrhage), hypotension and cardiovascular collapse; avoid use of products containing benzyl alcohol in neonates. *In vitro* and animal studies have shown that benzoate, a metabolite of benzyl alcohol, displaces bilirubin from protein-binding sites

Precautions Use with caution in patients with liver disease or in pregnant patients. Use with caution in patients following abdominal surgery; may mask progressive ileus or gastric distension. Application site reactions, generally mild, have occurred with transdermal patch use; if skin reaction is severe or generalized, remove patch. Cover patch application site with clothing to protect from natural or artificial sunlight exposure while patch is applied and for 10 days following removal; granisetron may potentially be affected by natural or artificial sunlight. Do not apply patch to red, irritated, or damaged skin.

Adverse Reactions

Cardiovascular: A-V block, hypertension, hypotension, syncope

Central nervous system: Anxiety, CNS stimulation, dizziness, fever, headache, insomnia, somnolence

Dermatologic: Skin rashes

Gastrointestinal: Abdominal pain, constipation, diarrhea, dysgeusia

Hepatic: Liver enzymes increased

Neuromuscular & skeletal: Asthenia, weakness

Local: Application site reactions with transdermal patch

Miscellaneous: Anaphylaxis (including dyspnea, hypotension, urticaria)

<1%, postmarking, and/or case reports: Agitation, allergic reactions, angina, arrhythmias, atrial fibrillation, bradycardia, extrapyramidal syndrome, hot flashes, hypersensitivity, syncope

Drug Interactions

Metabolism/Transport Effects Substrate of CYP3A4 (minor)

Avoid Concomitant Use

Avoid concomitant use of Granisetron with any of the following: Apomorphine

Increased Effect/Toxicity

Granisetron may increase the levels/effects of: Apomorphine

Decreased Effect There are no known significant interactions involving a decrease in effect.

Stability Tablets and injections: Store at room temperature, protect from light; injection stable when mixed in NS, D_5W for at least 24 hours; multi-use vial (with preservative) stable for 30 days after opening

Mechanism of Action Selective 5-HT$_3$ receptor antagonist, blocking serotonin, both peripherally on vagal nerve terminals and centrally in the chemoreceptor trigger zone

Pharmacodynamics

Onset of action: I.V.: 1-3 minutes

Duration: I.V.: ≤24 hours

Pharmacokinetics (Adult data unless noted)

Distribution: V_d: 2-3 L/kg; widely distributed throughout the body

Protein binding: 65%

Metabolism: Hepatic via N-demethylation, oxidation, and conjugation; some metabolites may have 5-HT$_3$ antagonist activity

Half-life:

Cancer patients: 10-12 hours

Healthy volunteers: 3-4 hours

Elimination: Primarily nonrenal, 8% to 15% of dose excreted unchanged in urine

Usual Dosage

Treatment of chemotherapy-induced emesis: Initial dose given just prior to chemotherapy (15-60 minutes before)

Children ≥2 years and Adults: I.V.: Manufacturer's recommendation: 10 mcg/kg; or as an alternative based on clinical research: 20-40 mcg/kg/day divided once or twice daily; maximum: 3 mg/dose or 9 mg/day

As intervention therapy for breakthrough nausea and vomiting, during the first 24 hours following chemotherapy, 2 or 3 repeat infusions (same dose) have been administered

Adults: Oral: 2 mg once daily or 1 mg twice daily

Prevention and treatment of postoperative nausea and vomiting, before induction of surgery, immediately before reversal of anesthesia, or postoperatively: I.V.:

Children ≥4 years: 20-40 mcg/kg given as a single dose; not to exceed 1 mg

Adults: 0.1 mg given as a single dose; this dosage is not yet approved by the FDA; trends in randomized, double-blind, multicenter, dose-ranging studies have shown doses of 0.1 mg, 0.2 mg, and 0.3 mg to be more effective than placebo for postoperative nausea and vomiting (Gan, 2005; Shillington, 2005; Taylor, 1997); 1 mg is the FDA approved dosage

Transdermal patch: Adults: Prophylaxis of chemotherapy-related emesis: Apply 1 patch at least 24 hours prior to chemotherapy; do not apply ≥48 hours before chemotherapy. Remove patch a minimum of 24 hours after chemotherapy completion. Maximum duration: Patch may be worn up to 7 days, depending on chemotherapy regimen duration.

Administration

Oral: Given at least 1 hour prior to chemotherapy and then 12 hours later; shake oral suspension well before use

Parenteral: I.V.: Infuse over 30 seconds undiluted **or** dilute in small volume NS or D_5W and administer over 5 minutes **or** dilute in 20-50 mL of NS or D_5W and infuse over 30 minutes to 1 hour

Transdermal (Sancuso®): Apply patch to clean, dry, intact skin on upper outer arm. Do not use on red, irritated, or damaged skin. Remove patch from pouch immediately before application. Do not cut patch.

Dosage Forms Excipient information presented when available (limited, particularly for generics); consult specific product labeling. [DSC] = Discontinued product

Injection, solution: 1 mg/mL (1 mL, 4 mL)

Kytril®: 1 mg/mL (1 mL [DSC], 4 mL) [contains benzyl alcohol]

Injection, solution [preservative free]: 0.1 mg/mL (1 mL); 1 mg/mL (1 mL)

Kytril®: 0.1 mg/mL (1 mL) [DSC]

Patch, transdermal:

Sancuso®: 3.1 mg/24 hours (1s) [52 cm^2, total granisetron 34.3 mg]

Solution, oral:

Granisol™: 2 mg/10 mL (30 mL) [contains sodium benzoate; orange flavor]

Kytril®: 2 mg/10 mL (30 mL) [contains sodium benzoate; orange flavor] [DSC]

Tablet, oral: 1 mg

Kytril®: 1 mg

Extemporaneous Preparations

A 0.2 mg/mL suspension may be made by crushing twelve 1 mg tablets. Add 30 mL distilled water, mix well, and transfer to a bottle. Rinse the mortar with 10 mL cherry syrup and add to bottle. Add enough cherry syrup to make a final volume of 60 mL. Label "shake well"; stable 14 days at room temperature or refrigerated (Quercia, 1997).

A 50 mcg/mL suspension may be made by crushing one 1 mg tablet. Add 1% methylcellulose and syrup NF to a total volume of 20 mL (may also use Ora-Sweet® or Ora-Plus® instead of methylcellulose and syrup); shake well; stable 91 days refrigerated (Nahata, 1998).

Nahata MC, Morosco RS, and Hipple TF, "Stability of Granisetron Hydrochloride in Two Oral Suspensions," *Am J Health Syst Pharm*, 1998, 55(23):2511-3.

Quercia RA, Zhang J, Fan C, et al, "Stability of Granisetron Hydrochloride in an Extemporaneously Prepared Oral Liquid," *Am J Health-Syst Pharm*, 1997, 54(12):1404-6.

References

"ASHP Therapeutic Guidelines on the Pharmacologic Management of Nausea and Vomiting in Adult and Pediatric Patients Receiving Chemotherapy or Radiation Therapy or Undergoing Surgery," *Am J Health Syst Pharm*, 1999, 56(8):729-64.

Gan TJ, Coop A, and Philip BK, "A Randomized, Double-Blind Study of Granisetron Plus Dexamethasone Versus Ondansetron Plus Dexamethasone to Prevent Postoperative Nausea and Vomiting in Patients Undergoing Abdominal Hysterectomy," *Aneth Analg*, 2005, 101(5):1323-9.

Hahlen K, Quintana E, Pinkerton CR, et al, "A Randomized Comparison of Intravenously Administered Granisetron Versus Chlorpromazine Plus Dexamethasone in the Prevention of Ifosfamide-Induced Emesis in Children," *J Pediatr*, 1995, 126(2):309-13.

Lemerle J, Amaral D, Southall DP, et al, "Efficacy and Safety of Granisetron in the Prevention of Chemotherapy-Induced Emesis in Paediatric Patients," *Eur J Cancer*, 1991, 27(9):1081-3.

Shillington A, et al, "Retrospective Cohort Study of Granisetron Administration for Postoperative Nausea and Vomiting Prophylaxis and Treatment," *Hosp Pharm*, 2005, 40(7): 592-8.

Taylor AM, Rosen M, Diemunsch PA, et al, "A Double-Blind, Parallel-Group, Placebo-Controlled, Dose-Ranging, Multicenter Study of Intravenous Granisetron in the Treatment of Postoperative Nausea and Vomiting in Patients Undergoing Surgery With General Anesthesia," *J Clin Anesth*, 1997, 9(8); 658-63.

◆ **Granisol™** *see* Granisetron *on page 653*

◆ **Granulocyte Colony Stimulating Factor** *see* Filgrastim *on page 580*

◆ **Granulocyte Colony Stimulating Factor (PEG Conjugate)** *see* Pegfilgrastim *on page 1070*

- ◆ **Granulocyte-Macrophage Colony Stimulating Factor** see Sargramostim *on page 1247*
- ◆ **Gravol® (Can)** *see* DimenhyDRINATE *on page 446*
- ◆ **Grifulvin® V** *see* Griseofulvin *on page 655*

Griseofulvin (gri see oh FUL vin)

Medication Safety Issues
Sound-alike/look-alike issues:
International issues: Fulvicin® (brand name used in international markets) may be confused with Furacin®

U.S. Brand Names Grifulvin® V; Gris-PEG®

Therapeutic Category Antifungal Agent, Systemic

Generic Available Yes: Suspension, ultramicrosized product

Use Treatment of tinea infections of the skin and hair caused by susceptible species of *Microsporum*, *Epidermophyton*, or *Trichophyton*. **Note:** Griseofulvin is no longer recommended for the treatment of onychomycosis.

Pregnancy Risk Factor C

Pregnancy Considerations Animal studies have shown decreased spermatogenesis, as well as embryotoxic and teratogenic effects with griseofulvin. There are no adequate and well-controlled studies in pregnant women. Use during pregnancy is contraindicated.

Lactation Excretion in breast milk unknown/use caution

Contraindications Hypersensitivity to griseofulvin or any component; severe liver disease, porphyria (interferes with porphyrin metabolism); pregnant women (may cause fetal harm)

Warnings Lupus erythematosus or lupus-like syndromes have been reported in patients receiving griseofulvin.

Precautions Avoid exposure to intense sunlight to prevent photosensitivity reactions; use with caution in patients with penicillin hypersensitivity since cross-reactivity with griseofulvin is possible

Adverse Reactions
Central nervous system: Fatigue, confusion, impaired judgment, insomnia, headache, incoordination, dizziness
Dermatologic: Rash, urticaria, photosensitivity, erythema multiforme-like drug reaction, angioneurotic edema (rare)
Endocrine & metabolic: Estrogen-like effects in children
Gastrointestinal: Nausea, vomiting, diarrhea, oral thrush
Hematologic: Leukopenia, granulocytopenia
Hepatic: Hepatotoxicity
Neuromuscular & skeletal: Paresthesia of the hand and feet (with extended therapy)
Renal: Proteinuria
Miscellaneous: Lupus-like syndrome

Drug Interactions
Metabolism/Transport Effects Induces CYP1A2 (weak), 2C8 (weak), 2C9 (weak), 3A4 (weak)

Avoid Concomitant Use
Avoid concomitant use of Griseofulvin with any of the following: Contraceptives (Progestins)

Increased Effect/Toxicity
Griseofulvin may increase the levels/effects of: Alcohol (Ethyl)

Decreased Effect
Griseofulvin may decrease the levels/effects of: Contraceptives (Estrogens); Contraceptives (Progestins); CycloSPORINE; CycloSPORINE (Systemic); Saccharomyces boulardii; Saxagliptin; Vitamin K Antagonists

The levels/effects of Griseofulvin may be decreased by: Barbiturates

Food Interactions Fatty meal will increase griseofulvin absorption

Stability Store at room temperature; protect from light

Mechanism of Action Inhibits fungal cell mitosis at metaphase by disrupting the cell's mitotic spindle structure; binds to human keratin making it resistant to fungal invasion

Pharmacokinetics (Adult data unless noted)
Absorption: Ultramicrosize griseofulvin absorption is almost complete; absorption of microsize griseofulvin is variable (25% to 70% of an oral dose); absorbed from the duodenum
Distribution: Deposited in the keratin layer of skin, hair, and nails; concentrates in liver, fat, and skeletal muscles; crosses the placenta
Metabolism: Extensive in the liver
Half-life: 9-22 hours
Elimination: <1% excreted unchanged in urine; also excreted in feces and perspiration

Usual Dosage Oral:
Children >2 years:
Microsize: 10-20 mg/kg/day in single or 2 divided doses. **Note:** Some references recommend high-dose griseofulvin (20-25 mg/kg/day) for 6-8 weeks for the treatment of tinea capitis.
Ultramicrosize: 5-15 mg/kg/day once daily or in 2 divided doses; maximum dose: 750 mg/day in 2 divided doses for fungal infections like tinea pedis or tinea unguium which are more difficult to eradicate
Adults:
Microsize: 500-1000 mg/day in single or divided doses
Ultramicrosize: 330-375 mg/day in single or divided doses; doses up to 750 mg/day have been used for infections more difficult to eradicate such as tinea pedis and tinea unguium
Duration of therapy depends on the site of infection:
Tinea corporis: 2-4 weeks
Tinea capitis: 4-6 weeks or longer (AAP Red Book® recommends continuing treatment for 2 weeks after clinical resolution of symptoms)
Tinea pedis: 4-8 weeks
Tinea unguium: 4-6 months or longer

Administration Oral: Administer with a fatty meal (peanut butter or ice cream to increase absorption), or with food or milk to avoid GI upset; shake suspension well before use. Ultramicrosize tablets may be swallowed whole or crushed and sprinkled onto 1 tablespoonful of applesauce and taken immediately without chewing.

Monitoring Parameters Periodic renal, hepatic, and hematopoietic function tests

Test Interactions False-positive urinary VMA levels

Patient Information Avoid alcohol. May cause photosensitivity reactions (eg, exposure to sunlight may cause severe sunburn, skin rash, redness, or itching); avoid exposure to sunlight and artificial light sources (sunlamps, tanning booth/bed); wear protective clothing, wide-brimmed hats, sunglasses, and lip sunscreen (SPF ≥15); use a sunscreen [broad-spectrum sunscreen or physical sunscreen (preferred) or sunblock with SPF ≥15]; notify physician if skin rash occurs

Dosage Forms Excipient information presented when available (limited, particularly for generics); consult specific product labeling. [DSC] = Discontinued product
Suspension, oral [microsize]: 125 mg/5mL (120 mL)
Grifulvin® V: 125 mg/5 mL (120 mL) [contains alcohol 0.2%] [DSC]
Tablet, oral [microsize]:
Grifulvin® V: 500 mg
Tablet, oral [ultramicrosize]:
Gris-PEG®: 125 mg, 250 mg

References
Ali S, Graham TA, and Forgie SE, "The Assessment and Management of Tinea Capitis in Children," *Pediatr Emerg Care*, 2007, 23(9):662-5.
American Academy of Pediatrics, *Red Book®, 2006 Report of the Committee on Infectious Diseases*, 27th ed, Pickering LK ed, Elk Grove Village, IL: American Academy of Pediatrics, 2006, 654-5.

Fleece D, Gaughan JP, and Aronoff SC, "Griseofulvin Versus Terbinafine in the Treatment of Tinea Capitis: A Meta-Analysis of Randomized, Clinical Trials," *Pediatrics*, 2004, 114(5):1312-5.

Ginsburg CM, McCracken GH Jr, Petruska M, et al, "Effect of Feeding on Bioavailability of Griseofulvin in Children," *J Pediatr*, 1983, 102 (2):309-11.

Gupta AK, Adam P, Dlova N, et al, "Therapeutic Options for the Treatment of Tinea Capitis Caused by Trichophyton Species: Griseofulvin Versus the New Oral Antifungal Agents, Terbinafine, Itraconazole, and Fluconazole," *Pediatr Dermatol*, 2001, 18(5):433-8.

Gupta AK, Ryder JE, Nicol K, et al, "Superficial Fungal Infections: An Update on Pityriasis Versicolor, Seborrheic Dermatitis, Tinea Capitis, and Onychomycosis," *Clin Dermatol*, 2003, 21(5):417-25.

Higgins EM, Fuller LC, and Smith CH, "Guidelines for the Management of Tinea Capitis. British Association of Dermatologists," *Br J Dermatol*, 2000, 143(1):53-8.

Lipozencic J, Skerlev M, Orofino-Costa R, et al, "A Randomized, Double-Blind, Parallel-Group, Duration-Finding Study of Oral Terbinafine and Open-Label, High-Dose Griseofulvin in Children With Tinea Capitis Due to Microsporum Species," *Br J Dermatol*, 2002, 146 (5):816-23.

Sethi A and Antaya R, "Systemic Antifungal Therapy for Cutaneous Infections in Children," *Pediatr Infect Dis J*, 2006, 25(7):643-4.

♦ **Griseofulvin Microsize** *see* Griseofulvin *on page 655*

♦ **Griseofulvin Ultramicrosize** *see* Griseofulvin *on page 655*

♦ **Gris-PEG®** *see* Griseofulvin *on page 655*

♦ **Growth Hormone, Human** *see* Somatropin *on page 1281*

♦ **Guaicon DM [OTC]** *see* Guaifenesin and Dextromethorphan *on page 658*

♦ **Guaicon DMS [OTC]** *see* Guaifenesin and Dextromethorphan *on page 658*

GuaiFENesin (gwye FEN e sin)

Medication Safety Issues

Sound-alike/look-alike issues:

GuaiFENesin may be confused with guanFACINE

Mucinex® may be confused with Mucomyst®

Naldecon® may be confused with Nalfon®

International issues:

Mucolex® [Hong Kong] may be confused with Mycelex® which is a brand name for clotrimazole in the U.S.

U.S. Brand Names Allfen [OTC]; Diabetic Tussin® EX [OTC]; Fenesin IR [OTC]; Ganidin® NR; Guiatuss [OTC] [DSC]; Humibid® Maximum Strength [OTC]; Mucinex® Children's [OTC] [DSC]; Mucinex® Kid's Mini-Melts™ [OTC]; Mucinex® Kid's [OTC]; Mucinex® Maximum Strength [OTC]; Mucinex® Mini-Melts™ Junior Strength [OTC] [DSC]; Mucinex® Mini-Melts™ [OTC] [DSC]; Mucinex® [OTC]; Muco-Fen® 1200 [DSC]; Muco-Fen® [DSC]; Organidin® NR [OTC]; Phanasin® Diabetic Choice® [OTC] [DSC]; Phanasin® [OTC] [DSC]; Q-Tussin [OTC]; Refenesen™ 400 [OTC]; Refenesen™ [OTC]; Robitussin® Chest Congestion [OTC]; Scot-Tussin® Expectorant [OTC]; Siltussin DAS [OTC]; Siltussin SA [OTC]; Vicks® Casero™ Chest Congestion Relief [OTC]; Xpect™ [OTC]

Canadian Brand Names Balminil Expectorant; Benylin® E Extra Strength; Koffex Expectorant; Robitussin®

Therapeutic Category Expectorant

Generic Available Yes: Excludes extended release and granules

Use Expectorant used for the symptomatic treatment of coughs

Pregnancy Risk Factor C

Pregnancy Considerations Reproduction studies have not been conducted.

Lactation Excretion in breast milk unknown/use caution

Contraindications Hypersensitivity to guaifenesin or any component (see Warnings)

Warnings Safety and efficacy for the use of cough and cold products in children <2 years of age is limited. Serious adverse effects including death have been reported. The FDA notes that there are no approved OTC uses for these products in children <2 years of age. Healthcare providers are reminded to ask caregivers about the use of OTC cough and cold products in order to avoid exposure to multiple medications containing the same ingredient.

Some products contain sodium benzoate; benzoic acid (benzoate) is a metabolite of benzyl alcohol; large amounts of benzyl alcohol (≥99 mg/kg/day) have been associated with a potentially fatal toxicity ("gasping syndrome") in neonates; *in vitro* and animal studies have shown that benzoate displaces bilirubin from protein binding sites; avoid use of products containing sodium benzoate in neonates

Precautions Some products contain phenylalanine which must be used with caution in patients with phenylketonuria.

Adverse Reactions

Central nervous system: Drowsiness, headache, dizziness

Dermatologic: Rash

Gastrointestinal: Nausea, vomiting, stomach pain

Drug Interactions

Avoid Concomitant Use There are no known interactions where it is recommended to avoid concomitant use.

Increased Effect/Toxicity There are no known significant interactions involving an increase in effect.

Decreased Effect There are no known significant interactions involving a decrease in effect.

Mechanism of Action Thought to act as an expectorant by irritating the gastric mucosa and stimulating respiratory tract secretions, thereby increasing respiratory fluid volumes and decreasing phlegm viscosity

Pharmacokinetics (Adult data unless noted) Absorption: Well absorbed

Usual Dosage Oral:

Children:

≥2 years: 12 mg/kg/day in 6 divided doses or as an alternative:

2-5 years: 50-100 mg every 4 hours, not to exceed 600 mg/day

6-11 years: 100-200 mg every 4 hours or as extended release product 600 mg every 12 hours; not to exceed 1.2 g/day

Children >12 years and Adults: 200-400 mg every 4 hours or as extended release product 600-1200 mg every 12 hours; not to exceed 2.4 g/day

Administration Oral: Administer with a large quantity of fluid to ensure proper action; do not crush or chew extended release tablet

Test Interactions May cause a colorimetric interference with certain laboratory determinations of 5-hydroxyindole-acetic acid (5-HIAA) and vanillylmandelic acid (VMA)

Dosage Forms Excipient information presented when available (limited, particularly for generics); consult specific product labeling. [DSC] = Discontinued product

Caplet, oral:

Fenesin IR: 400 mg

Refenesen™ 400: 400 mg [dye free]

Granules, oral:

Mucinex® Kid's Mini-Melts™:

50 mg/packet (12s) [contains magnesium 6 mg/packet, phenylalanine 0.6 mg/packet, and sodium 2 mg/packet; grape flavor]

100 mg/packet (12s) [contains magnesium 6 mg/packet, phenylalanine 1 mg/packet, and sodium 3 mg/packet; bubblegum flavor]

Mucinex® Mini-Melts™: 50 mg/packet (12s) [contains magnesium 6 mg/packet and phenylalanine 0.6 mg/packet; grape flavor] [DSC]

Mucinex® Mini-Melts™ Junior Strength: 100 mg/packet (12s) [bubblegum flavor] [DSC]

Liquid, oral:

Diabetic Tussin® EX: 100 mg/5 mL (118 mL) [dye free, ethanol free, sugar free; contains phenylalanine 8.4 mg/5 mL]

Ganidin® NR: 100 mg/5 mL (473 mL) [raspberry flavor]

Mucinex® Children's: 100 mg/5 mL (118 mL) [ethanol free; contains sodium 3 mg/5 mL; grape flavor] [DSC]

Mucinex® Kid's: 100 mg/5 mL (118 mL) [contains propylene glycol, sodium 3 mg/5 mL; grape flavor]

Organidin® NR: 100 mg/5 mL (480 mL) [contains sodium benzoate; raspberry flavor] [DSC]

Q-Tussin: 100 mg/5 mL (120 mL, 240 mL, 480 mL, 3840 mL) [ethanol free; cherry flavor]

Scot-Tussin® Expectorant: 100 mg/5 mL (120 mL) [dye free, ethanol free, sugar free; contains benzoic acid; grape flavor]

Siltussin DAS: 100 mg/5 mL (120 mL) [dye free, ethanol free, sugar free; strawberry flavor]

Vicks® Casero™ Chest Congestion Relief: 100 mg/6.25 mL (120 mL) [contains phenylalanine 5.5 mg/12.5 mL, sodium 32 mg/12.5 mL, sodium benzoate; honey-menthol flavor]

Syrup, oral: 100 mg/5 mL (5 mL, 10 mL, 15 mL, 118 mL, 120 mL, 473 mL, 480 mL)

Guiatuss: 100 mg/5 mL (120 mL, 480 mL) [DSC]

Phanasin®: 100 mg/5 mL (118 mL, 236 mL) [ethanol free, sugar free; mint flavor] [DSC]

Phanasin® Diabetic Choice®: 100 mg/5 mL (118 mL) [ethanol free, sugar free; mint flavor] [DSC]

Robitussin® Chest Congestion: 100 mg/5 mL (118 mL, 240 mL) [ethanol free; contains propylene glycol, sodium 2 mg/5 mL, sodium benzoate]

Siltussin SA: 100 mg/5 mL (120 mL, 240 mL, 480 mL) [ethanol free, sugar free; strawberry flavor]

Vicks® Casero™ Chest Congestion Relief: 100 mg/6.25 mL (240 mL) [contains phenylalanine 5.5 mg/12.5 mL, sodium 32 mg/12.5 mL, sodium benzoate; honey-menthol flavor]

Tablet, oral: 200 mg

Allfen: 400 mg [scored]

Organidin® NR: 200 mg [scored]

Refenesen™: 200 mg

Xpect™: 400 mg [sugar free]

Tablet, extended release, oral:

Humibid® Maximum Strength: 1200 mg

Mucinex®: 600 mg

Mucinex® Maximum Strength: 1200 mg

Tablet, sustained release, oral:

Muco-Fen®: 1000 mg [DSC]

Muco-Fen® 1200: 1200 mg [scored] [DSC]

Guaifenesin and Codeine
(gwye FEN e sin & KOE deen)

U.S. Brand Names Brontex® [DSC]; Cheracol® [DSC]; Dex-Tuss; ExeClear-C; Gani-Tuss® NR; Mar-Cof® CG; Robafen AC; Romilar® AC [DSC]; Tussi-Organidin® NR [DSC]; Tussi-Organidin® S-NR [DSC]; Tusso-C™

Therapeutic Category Antitussive; Cough Preparation; Expectorant

Generic Available Yes

Use Temporary control of cough due to minor throat and bronchial irritation

Restrictions C-V

Pregnancy Risk Factor C

Pregnancy Considerations Reproduction studies have not been conducted with this combination. Also see individual agents.

Lactation Excretion in breast milk unknown/use caution

Breast-Feeding Considerations Codeine is excreted in breast milk. Excretion of guaifenesin is not known. Also refer to Codeine monograph.

Contraindications Hypersensitivity to guaifenesin, codeine, or any component

Warnings Some products contain sodium benzoate; benzoic acid (benzoate) is a metabolite of benzyl alcohol; large amounts of benzyl alcohol (≥99 mg/kg/day) have been associated with a potentially fatal toxicity ("gasping syndrome") in neonates; in vitro and animal studies have shown that benzoate displaces bilirubin from protein binding sites; avoid use of sodium benzoate products in neonates

Precautions Use with caution in patients with hypersensitivity reactions to other phenanthrene derivative opioid agonists (morphine, hydrocodone, hydromorphone, levorphanol, oxycodone, oxymorphone). Some products contain phenylalanine which must be used with caution in patients with phenylketonuria.

Adverse Reactions

Codeine:

Cardiovascular: Palpitations, bradycardia, peripheral vasodilation

Central nervous system: CNS depression, dizziness, drowsiness, sedation, intracranial pressure elevated

Dermatologic: Pruritus from histamine release

Endocrine & metabolic: Antidiuretic hormone release

Gastrointestinal: Nausea, vomiting, constipation, biliary tract spasm

Genitourinary: Urinary tract spasm

Ocular: Miosis

Respiratory: Respiratory depression

Miscellaneous: Histamine release, physical and psychological dependence with prolonged use

Guaifenesin:

Central nervous system: Drowsiness, headache

Dermatologic: Rash

Gastrointestinal: Nausea, vomiting

Drug Interactions

Avoid Concomitant Use There are no known interactions where it is recommended to avoid concomitant use.

Increased Effect/Toxicity

Guaifenesin and Codeine may increase the levels/effects of: Alcohol (Ethyl); Alvimopan; CNS Depressants; Desmopressin; Selective Serotonin Reuptake Inhibitors; Thiazide Diuretics

The levels/effects of Guaifenesin and Codeine may be increased by: Amphetamines; Antipsychotic Agents (Phenothiazines); Somatostatin Analogs; Succinylcholine

Decreased Effect

Guaifenesin and Codeine may decrease the levels/effects of: Pegvisomant

The levels/effects of Guaifenesin and Codeine may be decreased by: Ammonium Chloride; CYP2D6 Inhibitors (Moderate); CYP2D6 Inhibitors (Strong); Mixed Agonist / Antagonist Opioids

Mechanism of Action See individual agents.

Usual Dosage Oral:

Children:

2-6 years: 1-1.5 mg/kg codeine/day divided into 4 doses administered every 4-6 hours (maximum dose: 30 mg/24 hours)

6-12 years: 5 mL every 4 hours, not to exceed 30 mL/24 hours

>12 years: 10 mL every 4 hours, up to 60 mL/24 hours

Adults: 5-10 mL or 1 tablet every 4-6 hours; not to exceed 120 mg (60 mL) codeine/day or 6 tablets/day

Administration Oral: Administer with a large quantity of fluid to ensure proper action; may administer with food to decrease nausea and GI upset from codeine

◀ **Test Interactions** May cause a colorimetric interference with certain laboratory determinations of 5-hydroxy indole-acetic acid (5-HIAA) and vanillylmandelic acid (VMA)

Patient Information May be habit-forming; do not discontinue abruptly

Dosage Forms Excipient information presented when available (limited, particularly for generics); consult specific product labeling. [DSC] = Discontinued product

Liquid: Guaifenesin 300 mg and codeine phosphate 10 mg per 5 mL (120 mL, 480 mL) [DSC]

Brontex®: Guaifenesin 75 mg and codeine phosphate 2.5 mg per 5 mL (480 mL) [ethanol free; strawberry mint flavor] [DSC]

Dex-Tuss: Guaifenesin 300 mg and codeine phosphate 10 mg per 5 mL (473 mL) [ethanol free, gluten free, sugar free; contains propylene glycol; grape flavor]

Gani-Tuss® NR: Guaifenesin 100 mg and codeine phosphate 10 mg per 5 mL (480 mL) [raspberry flavor]

Tussi-Organidin® NR: Guaifenesin 300 mg and codeine phosphate 10 mg per 5 mL (480 mL) [ethanol free, sugar free; contains sodium benzoate; raspberry flavor] [DSC]

Tussi-Organidin® S-NR: Guaifenesin 300 mg and codeine phosphate 10 mg per 5 mL (120 mL) [ethanol free, sugar free; contains sodium benzoate; raspberry flavor] [DSC]

Solution, oral: Guaifenesin 100 mg and codeine phosphate 10 mg per 5 mL (5 mL, 10 mL, 118 mL, 473 mL)

Mar-Cof® CG: Guaifenesin 225 mg and codeine phosphate 7.5 mg per 5 mL (473 ml) [ethanol free, sugar free; contains propylene glycol, sodium benzoate; sodium 6 mg/5 mL]

Syrup:

Cheracol®: Guaifenesin 100 mg and codeine phosphate 10 mg per 5 mL (120 mL) [contains ethanol 4.75% and benzoic acid] [DSC]

ExeClear-C: Guaifenesin 200 mg and codeine phosphate 10 mg per 5 mL (473 mL) [dye free, ethanol free, sugar free; contains prolylene glycol, sodium benzoate; fruit flavor]

Robafen AC: Guaifenesin 100 mg and codeine phosphate 10 mg per 5 mL (120 mL, 480 mL) [contains ethanol 3.5%, sodium 4 mg/5 mL, sodium benzoate; cherry flavor]

Romilar® AC: Guaifenesin 100 mg and codeine phosphate 10 mg per 5 mL (480 mL) [ethanol free, sugar free, dye free; contains benzoic acid and phenylalanine; grape flavor] [DSC]

Tusso-C™: Guaifenesin 200 mg and codeine phosphate 10 mg per 5 mL (480 mL) [ethanol free, dye free, sugar free; contains menthol, phenylalanine 0.03 mcg/5 mL; cherry vanilla flavor]

Tablet: Guaifenesin 300 mg and codeine phosphate 10 mg [DSC]

Brontex®: Guaifenesin 300 mg and codeine phosphate 10 mg [DSC]

Guaifenesin and Dextromethorphan
(gwye FEN e sin & deks troe meth OR fan)

Medication Safety Issues
Sound-alike/look-alike issues:
Benylin® may be confused with Benadryl®, Ventolin®

U.S. Brand Names Allfen DM [OTC]; Cheracol® D [OTC]; Cheracol® Plus [OTC]; Coricidin HBP® Chest Congestion and Cough [OTC]; Diabetic Tussin® DM Maximum Strength [OTC]; Diabetic Tussin® DM [OTC]; Double Tussin DM [OTC]; Duratuss® DM [DSC]; Fenesin DM IR; Gani-Tuss DM NR; Genatuss DM® [OTC] [DSC]; Guaicon DM [OTC]; Guaicon DMS [OTC]; Guaifenex® DM [DSC]; Guia-D; Guiatuss-DM® [OTC] [DSC]; Hydro-Tussin™ DM [DSC]; Kolephrin® GG/DM [OTC]; Mintab DM; Mucinex® Children's Cough [OTC] [DSC]; Mucinex® DM Maximum

Strength [OTC]; Mucinex® DM [OTC]; Mucinex® Kid's Cough Mini-Melts™ [OTC]; Mucinex® Kid's Cough [OTC]; Phanatuss® DM [OTC] [DSC]; Phlemex; Refenesen™ DM [OTC]; Respa-DM®; Robafen DM Clear [OTC]; Robafen DM [OTC]; Robitussin® Cough and Congestion [OTC]; Robitussin® DM Infant [OTC] [DSC]; Robitussin® DM [OTC]; Robitussin® Sugar Free Cough [OTC]; Safe Tussin® DM [OTC]; Scot-Tussin® Senior [OTC]; Silexin [OTC]; Siltussin DM DAS [OTC]; Siltussin DM [OTC]; Simuc-DM; Su-Tuss DM [DSC]; Tussi-Bid®; Tussi-Organidin® DM NR [DSC]; Tussi-Organidin® DM-S NR [DSC]; Vicks® 44E [OTC]; Vicks® DayQuil® Mucus Control DM [OTC]; Vicks® Pediatric Formula 44E [OTC]; Z-Cof LA™

Canadian Brand Names Balminil DM E; Benylin® DM-E; Koffex DM-Expectorant; Robitussin® DM

Therapeutic Category Antitussive; Cough Preparation; Expectorant

Generic Available Yes

Use Temporary control of cough due to minor throat and bronchial irritation

Pregnancy Risk Factor C

Pregnancy Considerations Reproduction studies have not been conducted with this combination. Refer to individual agents.

Lactation Excretion in breast milk unknown/use caution

Contraindications Hypersensitivity to guaifenesin, dextromethorphan, or any component; use within 14 days of MAO inhibitor therapy

Warnings Some products contain sodium benzoate; benzoic acid (benzoate) is a metabolite of benzyl alcohol; large amounts of benzyl alcohol (≥99 mg/kg/day) have been associated with a potentially fatal toxicity ("gasping syndrome") in neonates; in vitro and animal studies have shown that benzoate displaces bilirubin from protein binding sites; avoid use of sodium benzoate products in neonates

Precautions Some products contain phenylalanine which must be used with caution in patients with phenylketonuria.

Adverse Reactions

Central nervous system: Drowsiness, dizziness, headache

Dermatologic: Rash

Gastrointestinal: Nausea

Drug Interactions

Metabolism/Transport Effects Dextromethorphan: **Substrate** of CYP2B6 (minor), 2C9 (minor), 2C19 (minor), 2D6 (major), 2E1 (minor), 3A4 (minor); **Inhibits** CYP2D6 (weak)

Avoid Concomitant Use

Avoid concomitant use of Guaifenesin and Dextromethorphan with any of the following: MAO Inhibitors; Sibutramine

Increased Effect/Toxicity

Guaifenesin and Dextromethorphan may increase the levels/effects of: Serotonin Modulators

The levels/effects of Guaifenesin and Dextromethorphan may be increased by: CYP2D6 Inhibitors (Moderate); CYP2D6 Inhibitors (Strong); Darunavir; MAO Inhibitors; QuiNIDine; Selective Serotonin Reuptake Inhibitors; Sibutramine

Decreased Effect

The levels/effects of Guaifenesin and Dextromethorphan may be decreased by: Peginterferon Alfa-2b

Mechanism of Action See individual agents.

Pharmacodynamics Onset of action: Antitussive effect: Oral (rapid release formulation): 15-30 minutes

Pharmacokinetics (Adult data unless noted) Absorption: Dextromethorphan is rapidly absorbed from the GI tract

Usual Dosage Oral (dose expressed in mg of **dextromethorphan**):

Children: 1-2 mg/kg/day every 6-8 hours

Children >12 years and Adults: 60-120 mg/day divided every 6-8 hours or as extended release product 30-60 mg every 12 hours; not to exceed 120 mg/day

Administration Oral: Administer without regard to meals, with a large quantity of fluid to ensure proper effect; do not crush, chew, or break extended release tablets

Test Interactions May cause a colorimetric interference with certain laboratory determinations of 5-hydroxy indole-acetic acid (5-HIAA) and vanillylmandelic acid (VMA)

Patient Information Notify healthcare provider if cough persists for greater than 7 days or if cough is associated with a fever, rash, or persistent headache

Dosage Forms Excipient information presented when available (limited, particularly for generics); consult specific product labeling. [DSC] = Discontinued product

Caplet, oral:

Fenesin DM IR: Guaifenesin 400 mg and dextromethorphan hydrobromide 15 mg

Refenesen™ DM: Guaifenesin 400 mg and dextromethorphan hydrobromide 20 mg

Capsule, softgel, oral:

Coricidin HBP® Chest Congestion and Cough: Guaifenesin 200 mg and dextromethorphan hydrobromide 10 mg

Elixir, oral:

Duratuss® DM: Guaifenesin 225 mg and dextromethorphan hydrobromide 25 mg per 5 mL (480 mL) [contains sodium benzoate; grape flavor] [DSC]

Simuc-DM: Guaifenesin 225 mg and dextromethorphan hydrobromide 25 mg per 5 mL (480 mL) [grape flavor]

Su-Tuss DM: Guaifenesin 200 mg and dextromethorphan hydrobromide 20 mg per 5 mL (480 mL) [fruit flavor] [DSC]

Granules, oral:

Mucinex® Kid's Cough Mini-Melts™: Guaifenesin 100 mg and dextromethorphan hydrobromide 5 mg per packet (12s) [contains magnesium 6 mg/pack, phenylalanine 2 mg/packet, sodium 3 mg/packet; orange crème flavor]

Liquid, oral: Guaifenesin 100 mg and dextromethorphan hydrobromide 10 mg per 5 mL (480 mL); guaifenesin 300 mg and dextromethorphan hydrobromide 10 mg per 5 mL (120 mL, 480 mL)

Diabetic Tussin® DM: Guaifenesin 100 mg and dextromethorphan hydrobromide 10 mg per 5 mL (120 mL) [alcohol free, sugar free, dye free; contains phenylalanine 8.4 mg/5 mL]

Diabetic Tussin® DM Maximum Strength: Guaifenesin 200 mg and dextromethorphan hydrobromide 10 mg per 5 mL (120 mL) [alcohol free, sugar free, dye free; contains phenylalanine 8.4 mg/5 mL]

Double Tussin DM: Guaifenesin 300 mg and dextromethorphan hydrobromide 20 mg per 5 mL (120 mL, 480 mL) [alcohol free, dye free, sugar free]

Gani-Tuss DM NR: Guaifenesin 100 mg and dextromethorphan hydrobromide 10 mg per 5 mL (480 mL) [raspberry flavor]

Hydro-Tussin™ DM: Guaifenesin 200 mg and dextromethorphan hydrobromide 20 mg per 5 mL (480 mL) [alcohol free, sugar free; contains sodium benzoate] [DSC]

Kolephrin® GG/DM: Guaifenesin 150 mg and dextromethorphan hydrobromide 10 mg per 5 mL (120 mL) [alcohol free; cherry flavor]

Mucinex® Children's Cough: Guaifenesin 100 mg and dextromethorphan hydrobromide 5 mg per 5 mL (120 mL) [contains sodium 3 mg/5 mL; cherry flavor] [DSC]

Mucinex® Kid's Cough: Guaifenesin 100 mg and dextromethorphan hydrobromide 5 mg per 5 mL (120 mL)

[contains propylene glycol, sodium 3 mg/5 mL; cherry flavor]

Safe Tussin® DM: Guaifenesin 100 mg and dextromethorphan hydrobromide 15 mg per 5 mL (120 mL) [contains phenylalanine 4.2 mg/5 mL, benzoic acid, and propylene glycol; orange and mint flavors]

Scot-Tussin® Senior: Guaifenesin 200 mg and dextromethorphan hydrobromide 15 mg per 5 mL (120 mL) [alcohol free, sodium free, sugar free]

Tussi-Organidin® DM NR: Guaifenesin 300 mg and dextromethorphan hydrobromide 10 mg per 5 mL (480 mL) [alcohol free, sugar free; contains sodium benzoate; grape flavor] [DSC]

Tussi-Organidin® DM-S NR: Guaifenesin 300 mg and dextromethorphan hydrobromide 10 mg per 5 mL (120 mL) [alcohol free, sugar free; contains sodium benzoate; grape flavor] [DSC]

Vicks® 44E: Guaifenesin 200 mg and dextromethorphan hydrobromide 20 mg per 15 mL (120 mL, 235 mL) [contains sodium 31 mg/15 mL, alcohol, sodium benzoate]

Vicks® DayQuil® Mucus Control DM: Guaifenesin 200 mg and dextromethorphan hydrobromide 10 mg per 15 mL (295 mL) [contains propylene glycol, sodium 25 mg/15 mL, sodium benzoate; citrus blend flavor]

Vicks® Pediatric Formula 44E: Guaifenesin 100 mg and dextromethorphan hydrobromide 10 mg per 15 mL (120 mL) [alcohol free; contains sodium 30 mg/15 mL, sodium benzoate; cherry flavor]

Liquid, oral [drops]:

Robitussin® DM Infant: Guaifenesin 100 mg and dextromethorphan hydrobromide 5 mg per 2.5 mL (30 mL) [alcohol free; contains sodium benzoate; fruit punch flavor] [DSC]

Syrup, oral: Guaifenesin 100 mg and dextromethorphan hydrobromide 10 mg per 5 mL (120 mL, 480 mL)

Cheracol® D: Guaifenesin 100 mg and dextromethorphan hydrobromide 10 mg per 5 mL (120 mL, 180 mL) [contains alcohol 4.75%, benzoic acid]

Cheracol® Plus: Guaifenesin 100 mg and dextromethorphan hydrobromide 10 mg per 5 mL (120 mL) [contains alcohol 4.75%, benzoic acid]

Genatuss DM®: Guaifenesin 100 mg and dextromethorphan hydrobromide 10 mg per 5 mL (120 mL) [DSC]

Guiatuss® DM: Guaifenesin 100 mg and dextromethorphan hydrobromide 10 mg per 5 mL (120 mL, 480 mL, 3840 mL) [alcohol free; contains sodium benzoate] [DSC]

Guaicon DM®: Guaifenesin 100 mg and dextromethorphan hydrobromide 10 mg per 5 mL (10 mL) [alcohol free]

Guaicon DMS®: Guaifenesin 100 mg and dextromethorphan hydrobromide 10 mg per 5 mL (10 mL) [alcohol free, sugar free]

Mintab DM: Guaifenesin 200 mg and dextromethorphan hydrobromide 10 mg per 5 mL (480 mL) [alcohol free, dye free; cherry vanilla flavor]

Phanatuss® DM: Guaifenesin 100 mg and dextromethorphan hydrobromide 10 mg per 5 mL (120 mL) [alcohol free, sugar free] [DSC]

Robafen DM: Guaifenesin 100 mg and dextromethorphan hydrobromide 10 mg per 5 mL (120 mL, 240 mL, 480 mL) [cherry flavor]

Robafen DM Clear: Guaifenesin 100 mg and dextromethorphan hydrobromide 10 mg per 5 mL (120 mL)

Robitussin® Cough and Congestion: Guaifenesin 100 mg and dextromethorphan hydrobromide 10 mg per 5 mL (120 mL) [alcohol free; contains sodium benzoate]

Robitussin® DM: Guaifenesin 100 mg and dextromethorphan hydrobromide 10 mg per 5 mL (5 mL, 120 mL, 340 mL, 360 mL) [alcohol free; contains sodium benzoate]

◀

Robitussin® Sugar Free Cough: Guaifenesin 100 mg and dextromethorphan hydrobromide 10 mg per 5 mL (120 mL) [alcohol free, sugar free; contains sodium benzoate]

Silexin: Guaifenesin 100 mg and dextromethorphan hydrobromide 10 mg per 5 mL (45 mL) [alcohol free, sugar free)]

Siltussin DM: Guaifenesin 100 mg and dextromethorphan hydrobromide 10 mg per 5 mL (120 mL, 240 mL, 480 mL) [strawberry flavor]

Siltussin DM DAS: Guaifenesin 100 mg and dextromethorphan hydrobromide 10 mg per 5 mL (120 mL) [alcohol free, dye free, sugar free; strawberry flavor]

Tablet, oral: Guaifenesin 1000 mg and dextromethorphan hydrobromide 60 mg; guaifenesin 1200 mg and dextromethorphan hydrobromide 60 mg

Allfen DM: Guaifenesin 400 mg and dextromethorphan hydrobromide 20 mg

Silexin: Guaifenesin 100 mg and dextromethorphan hydrobromide 10 mg

Tablet, extended release, oral: 800/30: Guaifenesin 800 mg and dextromethorphan hydrobromide 30 mg; 1200/20: Guaifenesin 1200 mg and dextromethorphan hydrobromide 20 mg

Guaifenex® DM: Guaifenesin 600 mg and dextromethorphan hydrobromide 30 mg [DSC]

Mucinex® DM, Respa-DM®: Guaifenesin 600 mg and dextromethorphan hydrobromide 30 mg

Mucinex® DM Maximum Strength: Guaifenesin 1200 mg and dextromethorphan hydrobromide 60 mg

Phlemex: Guaifenesin 1200 mg and dextromethorphan hydrobromide 20 mg

Tablet, long-acting, oral: Guaifenesin 1000 mg and dextromethorphan hydrobromide 60 mg

Z-Cof LA™ [scored]: Guaifenesin 650 mg and dextromethorphan hydrobromide 30 mg

Tablet, sustained release, oral

Tussi-Bid®: Guaifenesin 1200 mg and dextromethorphan hydrobromide 60 mg

Tablet, timed release, oral [scored]: Guaifenesin 1200 mg and dextromethorphan hydrobromide 60 mg

Guia-D: Guaifenesin 1000 mg and dextromethorphan hydrobromide 60 mg [dye free]

◆ Guaifenex® DM [DSC] see Guaifenesin and Dextromethorphan on page 658

GuanFACINE (GWAHN fa seen)

Medication Safety Issues

Sound-alike/look-alike issues:

GuanFACINE may be confused with guaiFENesin, guanabenz, guanidine

Tenex® may be confused with Entex®, Ten-K®, Xanax®

International issues:

Tenex® may be confused with Kinex® which is a brand name for biperiden in Mexico

Related Information

Antihypertensive Agents by Class on page 1481

U.S. Brand Names Intuniv™; Tenex®

Canadian Brand Names Tenex®

Therapeutic Category Alpha$_2$-Adrenergic Agonist

Generic Available Yes: Excludes extended release tablet

Use

Immediate release: Management of hypertension (FDA approved ages ≥12 years and adults); has also been used in attention-deficit/hyperactivity disorder (ADHD), including ADHD with tic disorder (or Tourette's syndrome) and ADHD with autism or pervasive developmental disorders (PDD) comorbidities

Extended release: Short-term treatment (≤9 weeks) of ADHD (FDA approved in ages 6-17 years); has also

been used for long-term treatment (24 months) of ADHD (see Biederman, 2008; Sallee, 2009) and as adjunct treatment with psychostimulants for ADHD (see Sallee, 2009; Spencer, 2009)

Pregnancy Risk Factor B

Pregnancy Considerations Animal studies indicate decreased fetal survival when administered at higher doses than recommended in humans. There are no adequate and well-controlled studies in pregnant women. Use during pregnancy only if the benefits justify the risk to the fetus.

Lactation Excretion in breast milk unknown/use caution

Contraindications Hypersensitivity to guanfacine or any component

Warnings May cause bradycardia, hypotension, orthostatic hypotension, and syncope; these effects may be more pronounced during the first month of therapy. Modest, dose-dependent decreases in blood pressure and heart rate (typically asymptomatic) have also been reported. Do not abruptly discontinue; abrupt discontinuation can result in nervousness, anxiety, and rebound hypertension; dose should be tapered by no more than 1 mg every 3-7 days.

The American Heart Association recommends that all children diagnosed with ADHD who may be candidates for medication, such as guanfacine, should have a thorough cardiovascular assessment prior to initiation of therapy. These recommendations are based upon reports of serious cardiovascular adverse events (including sudden death) in patients (both children and adults) taking usual doses of stimulant medications. Most of these patients were found to have underlying structural heart disease (eg, hypertrophic obstructive cardiomyopathy). This assessment should include a combination of thorough medical history, family history, and physical examination. An ECG is not mandatory but should be considered. **Note:** ECG abnormalities and four cases of sudden cardiac death have been reported in children receiving clonidine (a less selective alpha$_2$-agonist) with methylphenidate; reduce dose of methylphenidate by 40% when used concurrently with clonidine; consider ECG monitoring. The effect of the addition of extended release guanfacine therapy at usual doses (mean: 3.1 mg/day) to existing psychostimulant therapy was studied in children and adolescents (n=75; mean age: 11.4 years; age range: 6-17 years) with previous suboptimal responses to methylphenidate or amphetamine treatment for ADHD. During the 9-week study period, no subjects had ECG findings that were of clinical interest or that met outlier criteria; clinical adverse effects due to heart rate changes were infrequent, but the percentage of patients with bradycardia (heart rate ≤50 bpm) was higher with treatment (10.3%) versus baseline (1.3%) (see Spencer, 2009). Fifty-three patients from this study population were further evaluated as part of an open-label, long-term (2 years) study of extended release guanfacine alone or in combination with concurrent psychostimulant therapy; safety analysis findings were similar to short-term studies with no exceptional safety issues identified; however, the vast majority of patients received guanfacine monotherapy (see Sallee, 2009). Further studies are needed to examine the long-term safety and efficacy of guanfacine in combination with psychostimulants.

Several cases of skin rash with exfoliation have been reported; however, a clear causal relationship could not be established. Discontinue guanfacine and monitor patients who develop a rash. Formulations of guanfacine (immediate release vs extended release) are not interchangeable on a mg-per-mg basis (due to differences in bioavailability).

Precautions Use with caution in patients with renal or hepatic impairment; dose reduction may be required if impairment is clinically significant. Use with caution in patients with a history of hypotension, heart block, bradycardia, cardiovascular disease, severe coronary insufficiency, recent MI, cerebrovascular disease, syncope, or a condition that predisposes patient to syncope. Use with caution with other agents that may reduce blood pressure or heart rate or increase risk of syncope. May cause drowsiness, sedation, and somnolence; use with caution with other agents that may cause CNS depression (eg, phenothiazines, barbituates, benzodiazepines). Warn patient of possible impairment of alertness or physical coordination (see Patient Information) and to avoid alcohol.

Adverse Reactions

Cardiovascular: Bradycardia, hypotension, orthostatic hypotension, syncopal events (see Warnings)

Central nervous system: Depression, dizziness, fatigue, headache, insomnia, irritability, lethargy, pyrexia (see Biederman, 2008), somnolence

Dermatologic: Skin rash with exfoliation (see Warnings)

Endocrine & metabolic: Impotence, weight increased

Gastrointestinal: Abdominal pain, appetite decreased, constipation, diarrhea, nausea, stomach discomfort, vomiting, xerostomia

Neuromuscular & skeletal: Weakness

≤3%, postmarketing, and/or case reports: Agitation, alopecia, ALT increased, amnesia, anxiety, arthralgia, asthma, AV block, blurred vision, chest pain, confusion, conjunctivitis, dermatitis, dyspepsia, dysphagia, dyspnea, edema, enuresis, hypertension, hypokinesia, iritis, leg cramps/pain, libido decrease, liver function tests abnormal, malaise, myalgia, nausea, nervousness, nocturia, pallor, palpitations, paresis, paresthesia, postural dizziness, pruritus, purpura, rash, rhinitis, sinus arrhythmias, substernal pain, sweating, tachycardia, taste perversion, tinnitus, testicular disorder, tremor, urinary frequency increased, urinary incontinence, vertigo, vision disturbance

Drug Interactions

Metabolism/Transport Effects Substrate of CYP3A4 (major)

Avoid Concomitant Use

Avoid concomitant use of GuanFACINE with any of the following: Iobenguane I 123

Increased Effect/Toxicity Nitroprusside and guanfacine have additive hypotensive effects. Noncardioselective beta-blockers (nadolol, propranolol, timolol) may exacerbate rebound hypertension when guanfacine is withdrawn. The beta-blocker should be withdrawn first. The gradual withdrawal of guanfacine or a cardioselective beta-blocker could be substituted.

Decreased Effect TCAs decrease the hypotensive effect of guanfacine.

Food Interactions Extended release formulation: A high-fat meal increases peak concentration by 75% and AUC by 40% compared to the fasted state

Stability

Immediate release: Store at room temperature between 20°C to 25°C (68°F to 77°F). Dispense in tightly closed, light-resistant container.

Extended release: Store at 25°C (77°F); excursions permitted to 15°C to 30°C (59°F to 86°F).

Mechanism of Action Selectively stimulates alpha$_{2A}$-adrenoreceptors in the brain stem, thus activating an inhibitory neuron, resulting in reduced sympathetic outflow, producing a decrease in vasomotor tone and heart rate. The exact mechanism in ADHD is not known. It has been proposed that postsynaptic alpha$_{2A}$-agonist stimulation regulates subcortical activity in the prefrontal cortex, the area of the brain responsible for emotions, attentions, and behaviors and causes reduced hyperactivity, impulsiveness, and distractibility. Guanfacine also acutely stimulates the release of growth hormone; however, with long-term use, it has no effect on growth hormone serum concentrations.

Pharmacodynamics Antihypertensive effect: Duration: 24 hours following single dose

Pharmacokinetics (Adult data unless noted) Note: When dosed at same mg dose, the extended-release product has a lower peak serum concentration (60% lower) and AUC (43% lower) compared to the immediate release formulation.

Distribution:

Immediate release: V$_d$: 6.3 L/kg

Extended release: V$_d$ (apparent): Children: 23.7 L/kg; Adolescent: 19.9 L/kg (see Boellner, 2007)

Protein binding: ~70%

Metabolism: Hepatic via CYP3A4

Bioavailability: Oral:

Immediate release: ~80%

Extended release (relative to immediate release): 58%

Half-life:

Immediate release: ~17 hours (range: 10-30 hours)

Extended release: Children: 14.4 hours; Adolescents: 18 hours (see Boellner, 2007)

Time to peak serum concentration:

Immediate release: 2.6 hours (range: 1-4 hours)

Extended release: Children and Adolescents: 5 hours (see Boellner, 2007); Adults: 4-8 hours

Elimination: ~50% (40% to 75% of dose) excreted as unchanged drug in urine; tubular secretion of the drug may occur

Dialysis: Not dialyzable in clinically significant amounts (2.4%)

Usual Dosage Oral: **Note:** Immediate release and extended release products should not be interchanged on a mg-per-mg basis due to differences in pharmacokinetic profiles.

ADHD:

Immediate release product: Children ≥6 years and Adolescents: Limited information exists in the literature [see Pliszka, 2007 (AACAP Practice Parameters)]

≤45 kg: Initial dose: 0.5 mg once daily at bedtime; may titrate in 0.5 mg/day increments every 3-4 days to two, three, or four times daily dosing; maximum dose: Patient weight 27-40.5 kg: 2 mg/day; 40.5-45 kg: 3 mg/day

>45 kg: Initial dose: 1 mg once daily at bedtime; may titrate in 1 mg/day increments every 3-4 days to two, three, or four times daily dosing; maximum dose: 4 mg/day

Extended release product (Intuniv™): Children and Adolescents 6-17 years: Initial dose: 1 mg once daily administered in the morning; may titrate dose by no more than 1 mg/week increments, as tolerated. Usual maintenance dose: 1-4 mg/day; maximum dose: 4 mg/day. If patient misses two or more consecutive doses, repeat titration of dose should be considered.

Note: In clinical trials, initial clinical response was associated with doses of 0.05-0.08 mg/kg once daily; increased efficacy was seen with increasing mg/kg doses; doses up to 0.12 mg/kg once daily have shown benefit when tolerated; however, doses >4 mg/day have not been evaluated.

Conversion from immediate release guanfacine to the extended release product: Discontinue the immediate release product; initiate the extended release product at the doses recommended above.

Discontinuation of therapy: Taper dose by no more than 1 mg every 3-7 days.

Note: See Additional Information for dosing information from pediatric studies of patients with ADHD and other comorbidities (eg, tic disorder or PDD)

Hypertension:

Children and Adolescents ≥12 years: Immediate release product: 1 mg usually at bedtime; may increase, if needed, at 3- to 4-week intervals; usual dose range (see JNC 7): 0.5-2 mg once daily

Adults: Immediate release: 1 mg usually at bedtime; may increase, if needed, at 3- to 4-week intervals; usual dose range (see JNC 7): 0.5-2 mg once daily

Dosing adjustment in renal impairment: No specific dosage adjustments are recommended by the manufacturer; use low end of the dosing range; consider dosage reduction in patients with clinically significant renal impairment.

Dosing adjustment in hepatic impairment: No specific dosage adjustments are recommended by the manufacturer; consider dosage reduction in patients with clinically significant hepatic impairment.

Administration Swallow extended release tablet whole with water, milk, or other liquid; do not crush, break, or chew; do not administer with high-fat meal.

Monitoring Parameters Heart rate, blood pressure, consider ECG monitoring in patients with history of heart disease or concurrent use of medications affecting cardiac conduction

ADHD: Evaluate patients for cardiac disease prior to initiation of therapy for ADHD with thorough medical history, family history, and physical exam; consider ECG (see Warnings); perform ECG and echocardiogram if findings suggest cardiac disease; promptly conduct cardiac evaluation in patients who develop chest pain, unexplained syncope, or any other symptom of cardiac disease during treatment.

Patient Information Avoid alcohol; may cause drowsiness and impair ability to perform activities requiring mental alertness or physical coordination; do not stop drug abruptly; may cause dry mouth; avoid becoming dehydrated or overheated. Do not take Intuniv™ with other guanfacine-containing medications (eg, Tenex®).

Nursing Implications Monitor blood pressure, standing and sitting/supine; observe for orthostasis

Additional Information More selective alpha$_2$-agonist than clonidine; withdrawal effects less commonly occur due to its longer half-life.

Medications used to treat ADHD should be part of a total treatment program that may include other components, such as psychological, educational, and social measures. Long-term usefulness of guanfacine for the treatment of ADHD should be periodically re-evaluated in patients receiving the drug for extended periods of time.

Additional dosing information for use in children and adolescents with ADHD and tic disorder or PDD comorbities.

ADHD and tic disorder: Immediate release product: Children and Adolescents 7-16 years: Limited information exists in the literature. One double-blind, placebo-controlled study in patients with ADHD and mild to moderate tics (n=34; mean age: 10.4 years; age range: 7-14 years) used an initial guanfacine dose of 0.5 mg once daily at bedtime for 3 days, then 0.5 mg twice daily for 4 days, then 0.5 mg 3 times daily for 7 days; upward titration was then made on the basis of clinical response and side effects; final dose range: 1.5-3 mg/day in 3 divided doses per day. An improvement in teacher-rated ADHD scores and tic scores after 8 weeks was reported (see Scahill, 2001). A small open-label trial (n=10; age range: 8-16 years) used similar initial doses with dose titration; final dose range: 0.75-3 mg/day in divided doses; 7 of 10 patients required a final dose of 1.5 mg/day in divided doses (see Chappell, 1995). Further studies are needed.

ADHD and pervasive developmental disorders (PDD): Immediate release product: Children and Adolescents 5-14 years: Limited information exists in the literature. A small double-blind, placebo-controlled, crossover 6-week trial conducted in children with ADHD and autism or intellectual disabilities (n=11; age: 5-9 years) used initial doses of 0.5 mg once daily; doses were increased by 0.5 mg/day increments every 4 days until a maximum of 3 mg/day (given in 3 divided doses) or adverse effects forced a dosage decrease; 8 of 11 patients were able to tolerate the maximum dose; three patients received doses of 1-2.5 mg/day; only 5 of 11 patients showed improvement in hyperactivity scores at final doses of 2.5-3 mg/day; other patient assessment parameters did not show improvements (see Handen, 2008). An open-label 8-week pilot study in children with ADHD and PDD (n=25; mean age: 9 years; range: 5-14 years) used the following doses: Patients <25 kg: Initial 0.25 mg once daily at bedtime; doses were increased as tolerated in 0.25 mg/day increments every fourth day and given in 3 divided doses per day; patients ≥25 kg: Initial 0.5 mg once daily at bedtime; doses were increased as tolerated in 0.5 mg/day increments every fourth day and given in 3 divided doses per day. Final doses ranged from 1-3 mg/day given in 2-3 divided doses per day. Patients showed improvement in parent- and teacher-rated hyperactivity subscale scores; increased irritability occurred in seven patients; the authors note that patients with PDD may be more sensitive to irritability-type adverse effects (see Scahill, 2006). Further studies are needed.

Dosage Forms Excipient information presented when available (limited, particularly for generics); consult specific product labeling.

Tablet: 1 mg, 2 mg

Tenex®: 1 mg, 2 mg

Tablet, extended release:

Intuniv™: 1 mg, 2 mg, 3 mg, 4 mg

References

American Academy of Pediatrics/American Heart Association Clarification of Statement on Cardiovascular Evaluation and Monitoring of Children and Adolescents With Heart Disease Receiving Medications for ADHD; available at: http://americanheart.mediaroom.com/index.php?s=43&item=422.

Biederman J, Melmed RD, Patel A, et al, "A Randomized, Double-Blind, Placebo-Controlled Study of Guanfacine Extended Release in Children and Adolescents With Attention-Deficit/Hyperactivity Disorder," *Pediatrics*, 2008, 121(1):e73-84.

Biederman J, Melmed RD, Patel A, et al, "Long-Term, Open-Label Extension Study of Guanfacine Extended Release in Children and Adolescents With ADHD," *CNS Spectr*, 2008, 13(12):1047-55.

Boellner SW, Pennick M, Fiske K, et al, "Pharmacokinetics of a Guanfacine Extended-Release Formulation in Children and Adolescents With Attention-Deficit-Hyperactivity Disorder," *Pharmacotherapy*, 2007, 27(9):1253-62.

Chappell PB, Riddle MA, Scahill L, et al, "Guanfacine Treatment of Comorbid Attention-Deficit Hyperactivity Disorder and Tourette's Syndrome: Preliminary Clinical Experience," *J Am Acad Child Adolesc Psychiatry*, 1995, 34(9):1140-6.

Chobanian AV, Bakris GL, Black HR, et al, "The Seventh Report of the Joint National Committee on Prevention, Detection, Evaluation, and Treatment of High Blood Pressure: The JNC 7 Report," *JAMA*, 2003, 289(19):2560-71.

Dopheide JA and Pliszka SR, "Attention-Deficit-Hyperactivity Disorder: An Update," *Pharmacotherapy*, 2009, 29(6):656-79.

Handen BL, Sahl R, and Hardan AY, "Guanfacine in Children With Autism and/or Intellectual Disabilities," *J Dev Behav Pediatr*, 2008, 29(4):303-8.

Pliszka S and AACAP Work Group on Quality Issues, "Practice Parameter for the Assessment and Treatment of Children and Adolescents With Attention-Deficit/Hyperactivity Disorder," *Am Acad Child Adolesc Psychiatry*, 2007, 46(7):894-921.

Sallee FR, Lyne A, Wigal T, et al, "Long-Term Safety and Efficacy of Guanfacine Extended Release in Children and Adolescents With Attention-Deficit/Hyperactivity Disorder," *J Child Adolesc Psychopharmacol*, 2009, 19(3):215-26.

Sallee FR, McGough J, Wigal T, et al, "Guanfacine Extended Release in Children and Adolescents With Attention-Deficit/Hyperactivity Disorder: A Placebo-Controlled Trial," *J Am Acad Child Adolesc Psychiatry*, 2009, 48(2):155-65.

Scahill L, Aman MG, McDougle CJ, et al, "A Prospective Open Trial of Guanfacine in Children With Pervasive Developmental Disorders," *J Child Adolesc Psychopharmacol*, 2006, 16(5):589-98.

Scahill L, Chappell PB, Kim YS, et al, "A Placebo-Controlled Study of Guanfacine in the Treatment of Children With Tic Disorders and Attention Deficit Hyperactivity Disorder," *Am J Psychiatry*, 2001, 158(7):1067-74.

Scahill L, "Alpha-2 Adrenergic Agonists in Attention Deficit Hyperactivity Disorder," *J Pediatr,* 2009, 154:S32-7.

Spencer TJ, Greenbaum M, Ginsberg LD, et al, "Safety and Effectiveness of Coadministration of Guanfacine Extended Release and Psychostimulants in Children and Adolescents With Attention-Deficit/Hyperactivity Disorder," *J Child Adolesc Psychopharmacol,* 2009, 19(5):501-10.

Vetter VL, Elia J, Erickson C, et al, "Cardiovascular Monitoring of Children and Adolescents With Heart Disease Receiving Medications for Attention Deficit/Hyperactivity Disorder [Corrected]: A Scientific Statement From the American Heart Association Council on Cardiovascular Disease in the Young Congenital Cardiac Defects Committee and the Council on Cardiovascular Nursing," *Circulation,* 2008, 117(18):2407-23.

◆ **Guanfacine Hydrochloride** *see* GuanFACINE *on page 660*

◆ **Guia-D** *see* Guaifenesin and Dextromethorphan *on page 658*

◆ **Guiatuss [OTC] [DSC]** *see* GuaiFENesin *on page 656*

◆ **Guiatuss-DM® [OTC] [DSC]** *see* Guaifenesin and Dextromethorphan *on page 658*

◆ **GW506U78** *see* Nelarabine *on page 974*

◆ **GW433908G** *see* Fosamprenavir *on page 623*

◆ **Gyne-Lotrimin® 3 [OTC]** *see* Clotrimazole *on page 344*

◆ **Gyne-Lotrimin® 7 [OTC]** *see* Clotrimazole *on page 344*

◆ **Gynodiol® [DSC]** *see* Estradiol *on page 536*

◆ **H1N1 Influenza Vaccine** *see* Influenza Virus Vaccine (H1N1, Inactivated) *on page 731*

◆ **H1N1 Influenza Vaccine** *see* Influenza Virus Vaccine (H1N1, Live/Attenuated) *on page 733*

◆ **H₂O₂** *see* Hydrogen Peroxide *on page 689*

Haemophilus b Conjugate and Hepatitis B Vaccine

(he MOF i lus bee KON joo gate & hep a TYE tis bee vak SEEN)

Medication Safety Issues
Sound-alike/look-alike issues:
Comvax® may be confused with Recombivax [Recombivax HB®]

Related Information
Immunization Guidelines *on page 1636*

U.S. Brand Names Comvax®

Therapeutic Category Vaccine

Generic Available No

Use Immunization against invasive disease caused by *H. influenzae* type b and against infection caused by all known subtypes of hepatitis B virus in infants 6 weeks to 15 months of age born of HB₅Ag-negative mothers

Infants born of HB₅Ag-positive mothers or mothers of unknown HB₅Ag status should receive hepatitis B immune globulin and monovalent hepatitis B vaccine (recombinant) at birth and should complete the hepatitis B vaccination series

Pregnancy Risk Factor C

Pregnancy Considerations Reproduction studies have not been conducted. This product is not indicated for use in women of childbearing age.

Contraindications Hypersensitivity to hepatitis vaccine, *Haemophilus* b vaccine, yeast, or any component of the formulation

Warnings Immediate treatment for anaphylactic/anaphylactoid reactions should be available during vaccine use; defer vaccination during the course of a moderate or severely febrile illness; children with chronic illness associated with increased risk of *Haemophilus influenzae* type b disease may have impaired anti-PRP antibody responses to conjugate vaccination. Examples include those with HIV infection, immunoglobulin deficiency, anatomic or functional asplenia, and sickle cell disease,

as well as recipients of bone marrow transplants and recipients of chemotherapy for malignancy.

Precautions Administer with caution to patients with thrombocytopenia or any coagulation disorder that would be compromised by I.M. injection; if the patient receives antihemophilia or other similar therapy, I.M. injection can be scheduled shortly after such therapy is administered; use with caution in patients with decreased cardiopulmonary function. Routine prophylactic administration of acetaminophen to prevent fever due to vaccines has been shown to decrease the immune response of some vaccines; the clinical significance of this reduction in immune response has not been established (see Prymula, 2009).

Adverse Reactions All serious adverse reactions must be reported to the U.S. Department of Health and Human Services (DHHS) Vaccine Adverse Event Reporting System (VAERS) 1-800-822-7967. For specific adverse reactions, see individual agents.

Drug Interactions

Avoid Concomitant Use There are no known interactions where it is recommended to avoid concomitant use.

Increased Effect/Toxicity There are no known significant interactions involving an increase in effect.

Decreased Effect
The levels/effects of *Haemophilus b Conjugate and Hepatitis B Vaccine* may be decreased by: Immunosuppressants

Stability Refrigerate; do not freeze

Mechanism of Action See individual agents.

Usual Dosage Infants and Children 6 weeks through 15 months: I.M.: 0.5 mL per dose
Recommended schedule: 3 doses repeated at 2, 4, and 12-15 months of age

Administration Shake well and administer I.M. in either the anterolateral aspect of the thigh or deltoid muscle of the arm; **not for I.V. or SubQ administration**

Patient Information May use antipyretics for postdose fever

Nursing Implications Federal law requires that the date of administration, the vaccine manufacturer, lot number of vaccine, and the administering person's name, title, and address be entered into the patient's permanent medical record.

Additional Information In order to maximize vaccination rates, the ACIP recommends simultaneous administration of all age-appropriate vaccines (live or inactivated) for which a person is eligible at a single visit, unless contraindications exist. The use of combination vaccines is generally preferred over separate infections, taking into consideration provider assessment, patient preference, and potential adverse events.

For additional information, please refer to the following website: http://www.cdc.gov/vaccines/vpd-vac/.

Dosage Forms Excipient information presented when available (limited, particularly for generics); consult specific product labeling.

Injection, suspension [preservative free]:
Comvax®: *Haemophilus* b capsular polysaccharide 7.5 mcg (bound to *Neisseria meningitides* OMPC 125 mcg) and hepatitis B surface antigen 5 mcg per 0.5 mL (0.5 mL) [contains aluminum; contains natural rubber/natural latex in packaging]

References
American Academy of Pediatrics Committee on Infectious Diseases, "Recommended Immunization Schedules for Children and Adolescents - United States, 2007," *Pediatrics,* 2007, 119(1):207-8.

◀ Centers for Disease Control and Prevention (CDC), "General Recommendations on Immunization. Recommendations of the Advisory Committee on Immunization Practices (ACIP)," *MMWR Recomm Rep*, 2006, 55(RR-15):1-48. Available at: http://www.cdc.gov/mmwr/preview/mmwrhtml/rr5515a1.htm.

Centers for Disease Control and Prevention, "Recommended Childhood and Adolescent Immunization Schedule – United States, July-December 2004," *MMWR Morb Mortal Wkly Rep*, 2004, 53(1):Q1-4.

Prymula R, Siegrist CA, Chlibek R, et al, "Effect of Prophylactic Paracetamol Administration at Time of Vaccination on Febrile Reactions and Antibody Responses in Children: Two Open-Label, Randomised Controlled Trials," *Lancet*, 2009, 374(9698):1339-50.

◆ *Haemophilus* B Conjugate (Hib) *see* Diphtheria and Tetanus Toxoids, Acellular Pertussis, Poliovirus and *Haemophilus* b Conjugate Vaccine *on page 455*

Haemophilus b Conjugate Vaccine
(he MOF fi lus bee KON joo gate vak SEEN)

Medication Safety Issues
Sound-alike/look-alike issues:
International issues:
Hiberix is also a brand name for influenza virus vaccine in multiple international markets

Related Information
Immunization Guidelines *on page 1636*

U.S. Brand Names ActHIB®; Hiberix®; PedvaxHIB®

Canadian Brand Names ActHIB®; PedvaxHIB®

Therapeutic Category Vaccine

Generic Available No

Use
Routine, full series immunization of children 2 months to 5 years of age against invasive disease caused by *H. influenzae* (ActHIB®: FDA approved in ages 2-18 months; PedvaxHIB®: FDA approved in ages 2-71 months)

Routine booster only immunization of children (FDA approval: Hiberix® in ages 15 months to 4 years)

Unimmunized children ≥5 years of age with a chronic illness known to be associated with increased risk of *Haemophilus influenzae* type b disease, specifically, persons with anatomic or functional asplenia or sickle cell anemia or those who have undergone splenectomy, should receive Hib vaccine.

Adolescents and adults with specific dysfunction or certain complement deficiencies who are at especially high risk of *H. influenzae* type b infection (HIV-infected adults); patients with Hodgkin's disease (vaccinated at least 2 weeks before the initiation of chemotherapy or 3 months after the end of chemotherapy)

Pregnancy Risk Factor C

Pregnancy Considerations Reproduction studies have not been conducted.

Contraindications Hypersensitivity to any component including tetanus toxoid (ActHIB®, Hiberix®)

Warnings Immediate treatment for anaphylactic/anaphylactoid reactions should be available during vaccine use; defer vaccination during the course of a moderate or severely febrile illness; the carrier proteins used in Haemophilus b polyribosylribitol phosphate-outer membrane polysaccharide conjugate (PRP-T, ActHIB®, Hiberix®) are chemically and immunologically related to toxoids contained in DTaP vaccine. Earlier or simultaneous vaccination with tetanus toxoids may be required to elicit an optimal anti-PRP antibody response. In contrast, the immunogenicity of PedvaxHIB® is not affected by vaccination with DTP. In infants in whom DTaP or DT vaccination is deferred, PedvaxHIB® may be advantageous for *Haemophilus influenzae* type b vaccination. Immunization with ActHIB® and Hiberix® is not a substitute for routine tetanus immunization.

Children with chronic illness associated with increased risk of *Haemophilus influenzae* type b disease may have impaired anti-PRP antibody responses to conjugate vaccination. Examples include those with HIV infection, immunoglobulin deficiency, anatomic or functional asplenia, and sickle cell disease, as well as recipients of bone marrow transplants and recipients of chemotherapy for malignancy. Some children with immunologic impairment may benefit from more doses of conjugate vaccine than normally indicated.

Precautions Administer with caution to patients with thrombocytopenia or any coagulation disorder that would be compromised by I.M. injection; if the patient receives antihemophilia or other similar therapy, I.M. injection can be scheduled shortly after such therapy is administered. In order to maximize vaccination rates, the ACIP recommends simultaneous administration of all age-appropriate vaccines (live or inactivated) for which a person is eligible at a single clinic visit, unless contraindications exist. Routine prophylactic administration of acetaminophen to prevent fever due to vaccines has been shown to decrease the immune response of some vaccines; the clinical significance of this reduction in immune response has not been established (see Prymula, 2009). Use caution in patients with history of Guillain-Barré syndrome (GBS) especially if it occurred within 6 weeks following a prior *Haemophilus* b vaccine. Some products may contain lactose; some packaging may contain natural latex rubber.

Adverse Reactions All serious adverse reactions must be reported to the U.S. Department of Health and Human Services (DHHS) Vaccine Adverse Event Reporting System (VAERS) 1-800-822-7967.
Central nervous system: Crying [high pitched and/or prolonged (>4 hours)], drowsiness, fatigue, fever, fussiness, irritability, lethargy, restlessnes

Dermatologic: Rash

Gastrointestinal: Anorexia, diarrhea, vomiting

Local: Erythema, induration, pain, swelling, tenderness

Otic: Otitis media

Respiratory: Upper respiratory infection

Miscellaneous: Risk of *Haemophilus* b infections increased first week following vaccination

<1%, postmarketing, and/or case reports: Allergic reactions, anaphylactoid reactions, angioedema, apnea, convulsions, erythema multiforme, facial edema, febrile seizures, Guillain-Barré syndrome, headache, hives, hypersensitivity, hyporesponsive episodes, hypotonia, inflammation, injection site abscess, lymphadenopathy, renal failure, seizures, swelling (extensive) of the injected limb, urticaria

Drug Interactions

Avoid Concomitant Use There are no known interactions where it is recommended to avoid concomitant use.

Increased Effect/Toxicity There are no known significant interactions involving an increase in effect.

Decreased Effect
The levels/effects of Haemophilus b Conjugate Vaccine may be decreased by: Immunosuppressants

Stability Store under refrigeration at 2°C to 8°C (36°F to 46°F); do not freeze; protect from light (Hiberix®). Once reconstituted with saline, store under refrigeration and use within 24 hours. ActHIB® reconstituted with Tripedia® should be administered within 30 minutes. Hiberix® saline diluent may be stored under refrigeration or at room temperature; do not freeze, discard diluent if frozen. Shake well before use. Discard any unused portion.

Mechanism of Action Stimulates production of anticapsular antibodies to provide active immunity to *Haemophilus influenzae*

Usual Dosage Children: I.M.: 0.5 mL as a single dose; administer according to "brand-specific" schedules (see table); preterm infants should be vaccinated based on chronological age (see table). ActHIB® and PedvaxHIB® are approved for a complete vaccine series; Hiberix® is approved only as a booster dose (15-59 months) in children who have received primary immunization

Vaccination Schedule for *Haemophilus* b Conjugate Vaccines

Age at 1st Dose (mo)	ActHIB® Primary Series	ActHIB® Booster	PedvaxHIB® Primary Series	PedvaxHIB® Booster
2-6	3 doses, 2 months aparts	1 dose[1,2]	2 doses, 2 months apart	1 dose[1,2]
7-11	2 doses, 2 months apart	1 dose[1,2]	2 doses, 2 months apart	1 dose[1,2]
12-14	1 dose	1 dose[1,2]	1 dose	1 dose[1,2]
15-71[2]	1 dose	—	1 dose	—

Note: Some combination vaccines containing Hib should not be used in infants <6 months; consult product specific information prior to administration.

[1]At least 2 months after previous dose and ≥12 months of age.

[2]Hiberix® may be used as a booster dose at 15-59 months (prior to 5 years of age)

Administration Shake well; administer I.M. in either the anterolateral aspect of the thigh or deltoid muscle of the arm; **not for I.V. or SubQ administration**

Nursing Implications Federal law requires that the date of administration, the vaccine manufacturer, lot number of vaccine, and the administering person's name, title, and address be entered into the patient's permanent medical record

Additional Information If Hiberix® is inadvertently administered during the primary vaccination series, the dose can be counted as a valid PRP-T dose that does not need repeated if administered according to schedule. In this case, a total of 3 doses completes the primary series.

In order to maximize vaccination rates, the ACIP recommends simultaneous administration of all age-appropriate vaccines (live or inactivated) for which a person is eligible at a single visit, unless contraindications exist. The use of combination vaccines is generally preferred over separate infections, taking into consideration provider assessment, patient preference, and potential adverse events.

For additional information, please refer to the following website: http://www.cdc.gov/vaccines/vpd-vac/.

Dosage Forms Excipient information presented when available (limited, particularly for generics); consult specific product labeling.

Injection, powder for reconstitution [preservative free]:

ActHIB® *Haemophilus* b capsular polysaccharide 10 mcg [bound to tetanus toxoid 24 mcg] per 0.5 mL [contains sucrose; may be reconstituted with provided diluent (forms solution; contains natural rubber/natural latex in packaging) or Tripedia® (forms suspension)]

Hiberix®: *Haemophilus* b capsular polysaccharide 10 mcg [bound to tetanus toxoid 25 mcg] per 0.5 mL (0.5 mL) [contains lactose 12.6 mg]

Injection, suspension:

PedvaxHIB®: *Haemophilus* b capsular polysaccharide 7.5 mcg [bound to *Neisseria meningitidis* OMPC 125 mcg] per 0.5 mL (0.5 mL) [contains aluminum]

References

CDC Licensure of a Haemophilus influenzae Type b (Hib) Vaccine (Hiberix) and Updated Recommendations for Use of Hib Vaccine. Available at: http://www.cdc.gov/mmwr/preview/mmwrhtml/mm5836a5.htm?s_cid=mm5836a5_e.

Centers for Disease Control and Prevention (CDC), "General Recommendations on Immunization. Recommendations of the Advisory Committee on Immunization Practices (ACIP)," *MMWR Recomm Rep*, 2006, 55(RR-15):1-48. Available at: http://www.cdc.gov/mmwr/preview/mmwrhtml/rr5515a1.htm.

Prymula R, Siegrist CA, Chlibek R, et al, "Effect of Prophylactic Paracetamol Administration at Time of Vaccination on Febrile Reactions and Antibody Responses in Children: Two Open-Label, Randomised Controlled Trials," *Lancet*, 2009, 374(9698):1339-50.

"Recommended Immunization Schedules for Persons Aged 0-18 Years – United States, 2009," *MMWR*, 2008, 57(51&52):Q1-4.

◆ *Haemophilus* **b (meningococcal protein conjugate) Conjugate Vaccine** see *Haemophilus* b Conjugate and Hepatitis B Vaccine *on page 663*

◆ *Haemophilus* **b Oligosaccharide Conjugate Vaccine** see *Haemophilus* b Conjugate Vaccine *on page 664*

◆ *Haemophilus* **B Polysaccharide** see Diphtheria and Tetanus Toxoids, Acellular Pertussis, Poliovirus and *Haemophilus* b Conjugate Vaccine *on page 455*

◆ *Haemophilus* **b Polysaccharide Vaccine** see *Haemophilus* b Conjugate Vaccine *on page 664*

◆ *Haemophilus* **influenzae b Conjugate Vaccine and Diphtheria, Tetanus Toxoids, and Acellular Pertussis Vaccine** see Diphtheria, Tetanus Toxoids, and Acellular Pertussis Vaccine and *Haemophilus influenzae* b Conjugate Vaccine *on page 460*

◆ **Halcion®** see Triazolam *on page 1381*

◆ **Haldol®** see Haloperidol *on page 666*

◆ **Haldol® Decanoate** see Haloperidol *on page 666*

◆ **Halfprin® [OTC]** see Aspirin *on page 141*

Halobetasol (hal oh BAY ta sol)

Medication Safety Issues
Sound-alike/look-alike issues:
Ultravate® may be confused with Cutivate®

Related Information
Corticosteroids *on page 1487*

U.S. Brand Names Ultravate®

Canadian Brand Names Ultravate®

Therapeutic Category Adrenal Corticosteroid; Anti-inflammatory Agent; Corticosteroid, Topical; Glucocorticoid

Generic Available Yes

Use Relief of inflammation and pruritus associated with corticosteroid-response dermatoses

Pregnancy Risk Factor C

Pregnancy Considerations There are no adequate and well-controlled studies in pregnant women, however, halobetasol is teratogenic in animals; use during pregnancy with caution. Increased incidence of cleft palate, neonatal adrenal suppression, low birth weight, and cataracts in the infant have been reported following corticosteroid use during pregnancy. In general, the use of large amounts, or prolonged use, of topical corticosteroids during pregnancy should be avoided.

Lactation Excretion in breast milk unknown/use caution

Breast-Feeding Considerations Systemically administered corticosteroids appear in human milk and may cause adverse effects in a nursing infant. It is not known if the systemic absorption of topical halobetasol results in detectable quantities in human milk.

Contraindications Hypersensitivity to halobetasol propionate, other corticosteroids, or any component

Warnings Hypothalamic-pituitary-adrenal (HPA) axis suppression may occur with topical corticosteroid use; acute adrenal insufficiency may occur with abrupt withdrawal after long-term use or with stress; withdrawal or discontinuation should be done carefully; patients with HPA axis suppression may require increased doses of systemic glucocorticosteroids prior to, during, and after unusual stress (eg, surgery). Adverse systemic effects (including HPA axis suppression) may occur when topical steroids are used on large areas of the body, denuded areas, for prolonged periods of time, with an occlusive dressing, and/or in infants or small children; infants and small children may be more susceptible to HPA axis suppression or other systemic toxicities due to a larger skin surface area to body mass ratio; use with caution in pediatric patients; safety and efficacy have not been established in children <12 years of age (use is not recommended)

Do not use topical halobetasol for the treatment of rosacea or perioral dermatitis; do not apply to the face, groin, or axillae. Do not exceed maximum recommended dose or duration of therapy due to the potential development of HPA axis suppression.

Precautions Avoid using higher than recommended doses; suppression of HPA axis, suppression of linear growth (ie, reduction of growth velocity), reduced bone mineral, or hypercorticism (Cushing's syndrome) may occur. Discontinue treatment if local irritation develops. Use appropriate antibacterial or antifungal agents to treat concomitant skin infections; discontinue halobetasol treatment if infection does not resolve promptly.

Adverse Reactions

Central nervous system: Intracranial hypertension (systemic effect reported in children treated with topical corticosteroids)

Dermatologic: Burning, itching, stinging, acne, dry skin, erythema, skin atrophy, leukoderma, pustulation, rash, secondary infection, striae, vesicles, telangiectasia, urticaria, miliaria, paresthesia, allergic contact dermatitis, hypopigmentation, perioral dermatitis, folliculitis, hypertrichosis

Endocrine & metabolic: Hyperglycemia, HPA axis suppression, Cushing's syndrome, growth retardation

Renal: Glycosuria

Drug Interactions

Avoid Concomitant Use

Avoid concomitant use of Halobetasol with any of the following: Aldesleukin

Increased Effect/Toxicity There are no known significant interactions involving an increase in effect.

Decreased Effect

Halobetasol may decrease the levels/effects of: Aldesleukin; Corticorelin

Stability Store between 59°F to 86°F (15°C to 30°C)

Mechanism of Action Not well defined topically; possesses anti-inflammatory, antipruritic, antiproliferative, vasoconstrictive, and immunosuppressive properties

Pharmacokinetics (Adult data unless noted)

Absorption: Percutaneous absorption varies and depends on many factors including vehicle used, integrity of epidermis, dose, and use of occlusive dressing; absorption is increased by occlusive dressings or with decreased integrity of skin (eg, inflammation or skin disease)

Cream: <6% of topically applied dose enters circulation within 96 hours following application

Metabolism: Hepatic

Elimination: Renal

Usual Dosage

Children <12 years: Use not recommended (high risk of systemic adverse effects, eg, HPA axis suppression, Cushing's syndrome)

Children ≥12 years and Adults: Topical: Steroid-responsive dermatoses: Apply sparingly once or twice daily; maximum dose: 50 g/week; do not treat for >2 weeks. **Note:** To decrease risk of systemic effects, only treat small areas at any one time; discontinue therapy when control is achieved; reassess diagnosis if no improvement is seen in 2 weeks.

Administration Topical: Apply sparingly to affected area, gently rub in until disappears; do not use on open skin; do not apply to face, underarms, or groin area; avoid contact with eyes; do not occlude affected area.

Monitoring Parameters Assess HPA axis suppression in patients using potent topical steroids applied to a large surface area or to areas under occlusion (eg, ACTH stimulation test, morning plasma cortisol test, urinary free cortisol test)

Patient Information Avoid contact with eyes; do not apply to face, underarms, or groin area; do not bandage, cover, or wrap affected area unless directed by physician; do not use for longer than directed; notify physician if condition being treated persists or worsens. Do not use tight-fitting diapers or plastic pants on a child being treated in diaper area. Wash hands after applying.

Additional Information Considered to be a super high potency topical corticosteroid; patients with psoriasis who were treated with halobetasol cream or ointment in divided doses of 7 g/day for one week developed HPA axis suppression

Dosage Forms Excipient information presented when available (limited, particularly for generics); consult specific product labeling.

Cream, as propionate: 0.05% (15 g, 50 g)

Ointment, as propionate: 0.05% (15 g, 50 g)

♦ **Halobetasol Propionate** *see* Halobetasol *on page 665*

Haloperidol (ha loe PER i dole)

Medication Safety Issues

Sound-alike/look-alike issues:

Haloperidol may be confused Halotestin®

Haldol® may be confused with Halcion®, Halenol®, Halog®, Halotestin®, Stadol®

Related Information

Compatibility of Chemotherapy and Related Supportive Care Medications *on page 1580*

U.S. Brand Names Haldol®; Haldol® Decanoate

Canadian Brand Names Apo-Haloperidol LA®; Apo-Haloperidol®; Haloperidol Injection, USP; Haloperidol Long Acting; Haloperidol-LA; Haloperidol-LA Omega; Novo-Peridol; Peridol; PMS-Haloperidol LA

Therapeutic Category Antipsychotic Agent, Typical, Butyrophenone

Generic Available Yes

Use

Injection, immediate release (lactate): Management of schizophrenia (FDA approved in adults); control of tics and vocal utterances of Tourette's disorder (FDA approved in adults); emergency sedation of severely agitated or delirious patients

Injection, extended release (decanoate): Management of schizophrenia in patients requiring prolonged parenteral antipsychotic treatment (FDA approved in adults)

Tablet and solution: Management of psychotic disorders (FDA approved in ages ≥3 years and adults), control of tics and vocal utterances of Tourette's disorder (FDA approved in ages ≥3 years and adults), treatment of severe behavioral problems in children displayed by combativeness and/or explosive hyperexcitable behavior and in short-term treatment of hyperactive children (FDA approved in ages 3-12 years); emergency sedation of severely agitated or delirious patients

Pregnancy Risk Factor C

Lactation Enters breast milk/not recommended (AAP rates "of concern")

Breast-Feeding Considerations Decline in developmental scores may be seen in nursing infants.

Contraindications Hypersensitivity to haloperidol or any component (see Warnings); narrow-angle glaucoma, bone marrow suppression, CNS depression, coma, severe liver or cardiac disease, parkinsonism

Warnings Cases of sudden death, QT prolongation and torsade de pointes have occurred; risk of QT prolongation and torsade de pointes may be increased with the use of any formulation in amounts exceeding the recommended dose and with the use of I.V. administration of haloperidol lactate (not an FDA-approved route of administration). Use haloperidol with caution or avoid use in patients with electrolyte abnormalities (eg, hypokalemia, hypomagnesemia), hypothyroidism, familial long QT syndrome, concomitant medications which may augment QT prolongation, or any underlying cardiac abnormality which may also potentiate risk. If haloperidol lactate is administered I.V., monitor ECG closely for QT effects and arrhythmias. Do **not** administer haloperidol decanoate I.V.

May cause extrapyramidal symptoms, including pseudoparkinsonism, acute dystonic reactions, akathisia, and tardive dyskinesia (risk of these reactions is high relative to other neuroleptics, and is dose-dependent; to decrease risk of tardive dyskinesia: Use smallest dose and shortest duration possible; evaluate continued need periodically; risk of dystonia is increased with the use of high potency and higher doses of conventional antipsychotics and in males and younger patients). Use may be associated with neuroleptic malignant syndrome. May be sedating; use with caution in disorders where CNS depression is a feature; patients must be cautioned about performing tasks which require mental alertness (eg, operating machinery or driving). Impaired core body temperature regulation may occur; use with caution with strenuous exercise, heat exposure, dehydration, and concomitant medication possessing anticholinergic effects. Safety and efficacy have not been established in children <3 years of age.

Leukopenia, neutropenia, and agranulocytosis (sometimes fatal) have been reported in clinical trials and postmarketing reports with antipsychotic use; presence of risk factors (eg, pre-existing low WBC or history of drug-induced leuko/neutropenia) should prompt periodic blood count assessment. Discontinue therapy at first signs of blood dyscrasias or if absolute neutrophil count <1000/mm^3. Use is contraindicated in patients with bone marrow suppression.

An increased risk of death has been reported with the use of antipsychotics in elderly patients with dementia-related psychosis **[U.S. Boxed Warning]**; most deaths seemed to be cardiovascular (eg, sudden death, heart failure) or infectious (eg, pneumonia) in nature; haloperidol is not approved for this indication.

Injection as deconate contains benzyl alcohol which may cause allergic reactions in susceptible individuals; large amounts of benzyl alcohol (≥99 mg/kg/day) have been associated with a potentially fatal toxicity ("gasping syndrome") in neonates; avoid use of haloperidol products containing benzyl alcohol in neonates; *in vitro* and animal studies have shown that benzoate, a metabolite of benzyl alcohol, displaces bilirubin from protein binding sites

Precautions Use with caution in patients with renal or hepatic dysfunction, respiratory disease, thyrotoxicosis, cardiovascular disease, history of seizures, or EEG abnormalities; haloperidol may cause hypotension (particularly with parenteral administration), precipitation of anginal pain, anticholinergic effects (low incidence relative to other neuroleptics), elevation of prolactin levels

Adverse Reactions

Cardiovascular: ECG changes (eg, prolongation of QT interval, torsade de pointes), hypertension, hypotension, sudden death, tachycardia, ventricular arrhythmias

Central nervous system: Agitation, anxiety, confusion, depression, drowsiness, euphoria, exacerbation of psychotic symptoms, extrapyramidal reactions, headache, heat stroke, hyperpyrexia, insomnia, lethargy, neuroleptic malignant syndrome, restlessness, seizures, tardive dyskinesia, vertigo

Dermatologic: Contact dermatitis, photosensitivity (rare), rash

Endocrine & metabolic: Galactorrhea, gynecomastia, hyperglycemia, hypoglycemia, hypomagnesemia, hyponatremia, menstrual irregularities, prolactin levels elevated, sexual dysfunction

Gastrointestinal: Constipation, diarrhea, dyspepsia, hypersalivation, nausea, vomiting, xerostomia

Genitourinary: Priapism, urinary retention

Hematologic: Agranulocytosis (rare), leukopenia, leukocytosis, neutropenia, anemia, lymphomonocytosis

Hepatic: Hepatotoxicity (rare)

Ocular: Blurred vision, retinopathy, visual disturbances

Respiratory: Bronchospasm, depth of respiration increased, laryngospasm

Miscellaneous: Diaphoresis

Drug Interactions

Metabolism/Transport Effects Substrate of CYP1A2 (minor), 2D6 (major), 3A4 (major); **Inhibits** CYP2D6 (moderate), 3A4 (moderate)

Avoid Concomitant Use

Avoid concomitant use of Haloperidol with any of the following: Artemether; Dronedarone; Lumefantrine; Metoclopramide; Nilotinib; Pimozide; QuiNINE; Tetrabenazine; Thioridazine; Tolvaptan; Ziprasidone

Increased Effect/Toxicity

Haloperidol may increase the levels/effects of: Alcohol (Ethyl); Anticholinergics; Anti-Parkinson's Agents (Dopamine Agonist); ChlorproMAZINE; CNS Depressants; Colchicine; CYP2D6 Substrates; CYP3A4 Substrates; Dronedarone; Eplerenone; Everolimus; FentaNYL; Fesoterodine; Nebivolol; Pimecrolimus; Pimozide; QTc-Prolonging Agents; QuiNINE; Salmeterol; Saxagliptin; Tamoxifen; Tetrabenazine; Thioridazine; Tolvaptan; Ziprasidone

The levels/effects of Haloperidol may be increased by: Acetylcholinesterase Inhibitors (Central); Alfuzosin; Artemether; Chloroquine; ChlorproMAZINE; Ciprofloxacin; Ciprofloxacin (Systemic); CYP2D6 Inhibitors (Moderate); CYP2D6 Inhibitors (Strong); CYP3A4 Inhibitors (Moderate); CYP3A4 Inhibitors (Strong); Darunavir; Gadobutrol; Lithium formulations; Lumefantrine; Metoclopramide; Nilotinib; Nonsteroidal Anti-Inflammatory Agents; Pramlintide; QuiNIDine; QuiNINE; Selective Serotonin Reuptake Inhibitors; Tetrabenazine

Decreased Effect

Haloperidol may decrease the levels/effects of: Amphetamines; Codeine; Quinagolide; TraMADol

The levels/effects of Haloperidol may be decreased by: Anti-Parkinson's Agents (Dopamine Agonist); CarBAMazepine; CYP3A4 Inducers (Strong); Deferasirox; Herbs (CYP3A4 Inducers); Lithium formulations; Peginterferon Alfa-2b

Food Interactions Drug may precipitate if oral concentrate is mixed with coffee or tea

Stability All dosage forms: Store at controlled room temperature; protect from light

Oral concentrate and injection, as lactate: Do not freeze

Injection, as deconate: Do not refrigerate or freeze

Mechanism of Action Competitive blockade of post-synaptic dopamine receptors in the mesolimbic dopaminergic system; depresses cerebral cortex and hypothalamus; exhibits a strong alpha-adrenergic and anticholinergic blocking activity

Pharmacokinetics (Adult data unless noted)

Absorption: Oral: Well absorbed, undergoes first-pass metabolism in the liver

Distribution: Crosses the placenta; appears in breast milk

Protein binding: 92%

Metabolism: In the liver, hydroxy-metabolite is active

Bioavailability: Oral: 60%

Half-life: Adults: 20 hours; range: 13-35 hours

Elimination: Excreted in urine and feces as drug and metabolites

Usual Dosage Note: Gradually decrease dose to the lowest effective maintenance dosage once a satisfactory therapeutic response is obtained

Children:

3-12 years (15-40 kg): Oral: Initial: 0.25-0.5 mg/day given in 2-3 divided doses; increase by 0.25-0.5 mg every 5-7 days; maximum dose: 0.15 mg/kg/day; usual maintenance:

Agitation or hyperkinesia: 0.01-0.03 mg/kg/day once daily

Tourette's disorder or nonpsychotic behavior disorders: 0.05-0.075 mg/kg/day in 2-3 divided doses

Psychotic disorders: 0.05-0.15 mg/kg/day in 2-3 divided doses

Note: Maximum effective dosage has not been established; doses >6 mg/day have not been shown to further enhance behavior improvement. Preliminary findings of a double-blind, placebo controlled study reported the mean optimal dose in 12 schizophrenic children 5-12 years to be ~2 mg/day (range: 0.5-3.5 mg/day or 0.02-0.12 mg/kg/day) given in 3 divided doses

6-12 years: I.M. **(as lactate):** 1-3 mg/dose every 4-8 hours to a maximum of 0.15 mg/kg/day; switch to oral therapy as soon as able

Adults:

Oral: 0.5-5 mg 2-3 times/day; usual maximum dose: 30 mg/day; some patients may require 100 mg/day

I.M.:

As **lactate:** 2-5 mg every 4-8 hours as needed

As **decanoate:** Initial: 10-15 times the individual patients' stabilized oral dose, given at 3- to 4-week intervals

Administration

Oral: Administer with food or milk to decrease GI distress; prior to administration, dilute oral concentrate with ≥2 ounces of water or acidic beverage; do not mix oral concentrate with coffee or tea. Avoid skin contact with oral suspension or solution; may cause contact dermatitis.

Parenteral: **Decanoate** product is for I.M. use only, **do not administer decanoate I.V.** Although not FDA-approved, haloperidol **lactate** has been administered I.V.; however, this may increase the risk of altered cardiac conduction (see Warnings).

Monitoring Parameters Blood pressure, heart rate, CBC with differential, liver enzymes with long-term use; serum glucose, sodium, magnesium; ECG (with non-FDA approved intravenous administration; mental status, abnormal involuntary movement scale (AIMS), extrapyramidal symptoms (EPS)

Patient Information Avoid alcohol; may cause drowsiness and impair ability to perform activities requiring mental alertness or physical coordination; may cause dry mouth. May rarely cause photosensitivity reactions; avoid exposure to sunlight and artificial light sources (sunlamps, tanning booth/bed); use a sunscreen; contact physician if reaction occurs

Nursing Implications Observe for extrapyramidal effects

Dosage Forms Excipient information presented when available (limited, particularly for generics); consult specific product labeling. [DSC] = Discontinued product

Note: Strength expressed as base.

Injection, oil, as decanoate: 50 mg/mL (1 mL, 5 mL); 100 mg/mL (1 mL, 5 mL)

Haldol® Decanoate: 50 mg/mL (1 mL; 5 mL [DSC]); 100 mg/mL (1 mL; 5 mL [DSC]) [contains benzyl alcohol, sesame oil]

Injection, solution, as lactate: 5 mg/mL (1 mL, 10 mL)

Haldol®: 5 mg/mL (1 mL)

Solution, oral concentrate, as lactate: 2 mg/mL (15 mL, 120 mL)

Tablet: 0.5 mg, 1 mg, 2 mg, 5 mg, 10 mg, 20 mg

References

Serrano AC, "Haloperidol - Its Use in Children," *J Clin Psychiatry*, 1981, 42(4):154-6.

Spencer EK, Kafantaris V, Padron-Gayol MV, et al, "Haloperidol in Schizophrenic Children: Early Findings From a Study in Progress," *Psychopharmacol Bull*, 1992, 28(2):183-6.

◆ **Haloperidol Decanoate** *see* Haloperidol *on page 666*

◆ **Haloperidol Injection, USP (Can)** *see* Haloperidol *on page 666*

◆ **Haloperidol-LA (Can)** *see* Haloperidol *on page 666*

◆ **Haloperidol Lactate** *see* Haloperidol *on page 666*

◆ **Haloperidol-LA Omega (Can)** *see* Haloperidol *on page 666*

◆ **Haloperidol Long Acting (Can)** *see* Haloperidol *on page 666*

◆ **HAVRIX®** *see* Hepatitis A Vaccine *on page 672*

◆ **HbCV** *see Haemophilus* b Conjugate Vaccine *on page 664*

◆ **HBIG** *see* Hepatitis B Immune Globulin *on page 673*

◆ **hCG** *see* Chorionic Gonadotropin *on page 305*

◆ **HCTZ (error-prone abbreviation)** *see* Hydrochlorothiazide *on page 682*

◆ **HDA® Toothache [OTC]** *see* Benzocaine *on page 182*

◆ **HDCV** *see* Rabies Virus Vaccine *on page 1199*

◆ **Head & Shoulders® Intensive Treatment [OTC]** *see* Selenium Sulfide *on page 1252*

◆ **Heartburn Relief [OTC]** *see* Famotidine *on page 561*

◆ **Heartburn Relief Maximum Strength [OTC]** *see* Famotidine *on page 561*

◆ **Heavy Mineral Oil** *see* Mineral Oil *on page 933*

◆ **Helixate® FS** *see* Antihemophilic Factor (Recombinant) *on page 112*

◆ **Hemocyte® [OTC]** *see* Ferrous Fumarate *on page 576*

◆ **Hemofil M** *see* Antihemophilic Factor (Human) *on page 109*

◆ **Hemorrhoidal HC** *see* Hydrocortisone *on page 685*

Hemorrhoidal Preparations

(HEM or oyd al prep a RAY shuns)

Therapeutic Category Hemorrhoidal Treatment Agent; Topical Skin Product

Use Symptomatic relief of pain and discomfort in external and internal hemorrhoids, proctitis, papillitis, cryptitis, anal fissures, incomplete fistulas and relief of local pain following anorectal surgery

Pregnancy Risk Factor C

Contraindications Hypersensitivity to any component (see Warnings)

Warnings Some preparations contain sulfites which may cause allergic reactions in susceptible individuals

Adverse Reactions
Dermatologic: Rash
Local: Irritation, burning, itching

Mechanism of Action
Dibucaine, benzocaine, pramoxine: Temporarily relieves pain, itching, and irritation by blocking nerve impulses at the sensory nerve endings in the skin and mucous membranes
Emollient/protectant (glycerin, lanolin, mineral oil, petrolatum, zinc oxide, cocoa butter, shark liver oil): Form a physical barrier and lubricate tissues preventing irritation of the anorectal area and water loss

Pharmacodynamics Onset of action: Topical:
Pramoxine: 3-5 minutes
Dibucaine: <15 minutes
Benzocaine: 1 minute

Usual Dosage
Children and Adults: Topical: Apply ointment as a thin layer to the perianal area and the anal canal 3-6 times/day
Benzocaine-containing preparations: Apply up to 6 times/day
Dibucaine-containing preparations: Apply ointment into the rectum each morning and evening and after each bowel movement; ointment may be applied topically to anal tissues; apply up to 3-4 times/day
Children: No more than 7.5 g in a 24-hour period
Adults: No more than 30 g in a 24-hour period
Pramoxine-containing preparations: Apply up to 5 times/day (2-3 times/day and after bowel movements)
Adults: Rectal: Insert 1 suppository in the morning and at bedtime and after each bowel movement

Administration
Rectal: Foam, ointment, and cream for rectal use are instilled using a rectal applicator. The aerosol should not be inserted into the anus.
Topical: Apply cream or ointment to affected areas and rub in gently. A small amount of foam may be applied to the affected area using a cleansing tissue or pad.

Patient Information
If anorectal symptoms do not improve in 7 days, or if bleeding, protrusion or seepage occurs, consult physician; avoid contact of topical preparations to the eyes

Dosage Forms
Excipient information presented when available (limited, particularly for generics); consult specific product labeling.
Foam (Perifoam®, proctoFoam®): 15 g, 45 g
Ointment:
A-Caine® Rectal, Hemocaine®, Hemet® Rectal: 30 g, 60 g
Anusol®: 30 g, 60 g
Posterisan®: 25 g
Preparation H®: 30 g, 60 g
Suppository, rectal:
Anocaine®, Hemet®
Anumed®, Anusol®, CPI®
Calmol 4®
Hem-Prep®
Pazo® Hemorrhoid
Posterisan®
Preparation H®
Rectal Medicone®

◆ Hemril®-30 *see* Hydrocortisone *on page 685*
◆ HepA *see* Hepatitis A Vaccine *on page 672*
◆ HepaGam B™ *see* Hepatitis B Immune Globulin *on page 673*
◆ Hepalean® (Can) *see* Heparin *on page 669*
◆ Hepalean® Leo (Can) *see* Heparin *on page 669*
◆ Hepalean®-LOK (Can) *see* Heparin *on page 669*

Heparin (HEP a rin)

Medication Safety Issues
Sound-alike/look-alike issues:
Heparin may be confused with Hespan®

High alert medication: The Institute for Safe Medication Practices (ISMP) includes this medication among its list of drugs which have a heightened risk of causing significant patient harm when used in error.

Heparin sodium injection 10,000 units/mL and Hep-Lock U/P 10 units/mL have been confused with each other. Fatal medication errors have occurred between the two whose labels are both blue. **Never rely on color as a sole indicator to differentiate product identity.**

Heparin lock flush solution is intended only to maintain patency of I.V. devices and is **not** to be used for anticoagulant therapy.

Note: The 100 unit/mL concentration should not be used in neonates or infants <10 kg. The 10 unit/mL concentration may cause systemic anticoagulation in infants <1 kg who receive frequent flushes.

2009 National Patient Safety Goals: The Joint Commission (TJC) requires healthcare organizations that provide anticoagulant therapy to have a process in place to reduce the risk of anticoagulant-associated patient harm. Patients receiving anticoagulants should receive individualized care through a defined process that includes standardized ordering, dispensing, administration, monitoring and education. This does not apply to routine short-term use of anticoagulants for prevention of venous thromboembolism when the expectation is that the patient's laboratory values will remain within or close to normal values (NPSG.03.05.01).

Related Information
Antithrombotic Therapy in Neonates and Children *on page 1602*
Compatibility of Chemotherapy and Related Supportive Care Medications *on page 1580*

U.S. Brand Names Hep-Lock U/P; Hep-Lock®; Hep-Flush®-10
Canadian Brand Names Hepalean®; Hepalean® Leo; Hepalean®-LOK
Therapeutic Category Anticoagulant
Generic Available Yes
Use Prophylaxis and treatment of thromboembolic disorders
Pregnancy Risk Factor C
Pregnancy Considerations Animal reproduction studies have not been conducted. Heparin does not cross the placenta.
Lactation Does not enter breast milk/compatible
Contraindications Hypersensitivity to heparin or any component (see Warnings); severe thrombocytopenia, subacute bacterial endocarditis, suspected intracranial hemorrhage, shock, severe hypotension, uncontrollable bleeding (unless secondary to disseminated intravascular coagulation)
Warnings Updates to the United States Pharmacopeia (USP) heparin monograph were recently made in response to over 200 deaths linked to contaminated heparin products in 2007-2008. Serious adverse effects (including hypersensitivity reactions) were associated with a heparin-like contaminant (oversulfated chondroitin sulfate). At the time, the available quality assurance tests did not test for oversulfated chondroitin sulfate. Effective October 1, 2009, a new reference standard for heparin and a new test to determine potency (the chromogenic antifactor IIa test) were established by USP. The updated USP heparin monograph also harmonized the USP unit

with the WHO international standard (IS) unit (ie, international unit). The new standard may result in a 10% reduction in potency for heparin marketed in the United States. For therapeutic use, practitioners may or may not notice that larger doses of heparin are required to achieve "therapeutic" activity of anticoagulation. The impact of this change in potency should be less significant when heparin is administered by subcutaneous injection due to low and variable bioavailability.

Heparin manufactured by the "old" and "new" USP standards is currently available. These products have differences in potency. The FDA cautions healthcare practitioners to consider not using the "old" and "new" heparin products interchangeably, separating supplies, and/or exhausting any "old" heparin supplies prior to transitioning to the "new" product. The reduction in potency should be considered when utilizing heparin in situations when aggressive anticoagulation is necessary to treat or prevent life-threatening thrombosis. Special consideration should be given to pediatric patients requiring ECMO, patients of any age requiring cardiopulmonary bypass, and patients with potentially fatal thromboses. More frequent or intensive aPTT or ACT monitoring may be required. It should be noted that the FDA-approved labeling (including dosing) for heparin has not changed. Heparin dosing should always be individualized according to the patient-specific clinical situation. Appropriate clinical judgment is essential in determining heparin dosage (see Additional Information and Smythe, 2010).

Some preparations contain sulfites or benzyl alcohol both of which may cause allergic reactions in susceptible individuals; large amounts of benzyl alcohol (≥99 mg/kg/day) have been associated with a potentially fatal toxicity ("gasping syndrome") in neonates; the "gasping syndrome" consists of metabolic acidosis, respiratory distress, gasping respirations, CNS dysfunction (including convulsions, intracranial hemorrhage), hypotension and cardiovascular collapse; avoid use of heparin products containing benzyl alcohol in neonates (use preservative free heparin); *in vitro* and animal studies have shown that benzoate, a metabolite of benzyl alcohol, displaces bilirubin from protein binding sites

Precautions Use with caution as hemorrhage may occur; risk factors for hemorrhage include: I.M. injections; peptic ulcer disease; intermittent I.V. injections (vs continuous I.V. infusion); increased capillary permeability; menstruation; recent surgery or invasive procedures; severe renal, hepatic, or biliary disease; and indwelling catheters

Heparin does not possess fibrinolytic activity and, therefore, cannot lyse established thrombi; discontinue heparin if hemorrhage occurs; severe hemorrhage or overdosage may require protamine

Adverse Reactions
Central nervous system: Fever, headache, chills

Dermatologic: Urticaria, alopecia

Gastrointestinal: Nausea, vomiting

Hematologic: Hemorrhage, thrombocytopenia (may be more common with bovine lung heparin vs porcine mucosa heparin; however, if a patient receiving bovine lung heparin experiences severe thrombocytopenia it is **not** recommended to switch to porcine mucosa heparin because a similar reaction may occur)

Hepatic: Liver enzymes elevated

Local: Irritation, ulceration, cutaneous necrosis has been rarely reported with deep SubQ injections

Neuromuscular & skeletal: Osteoporosis (with long-term use)

Drug Interactions
Avoid Concomitant Use
Avoid concomitant use of Heparin with any of the following: Corticorelin

Increased Effect/Toxicity
Heparin may increase the levels/effects of: Anticoagulants; Collagenase (Systemic); Corticorelin; Drotrecogin Alfa; Ibritumomab; Tositumomab and Iodine I 131 Tositumomab

The levels/effects of Heparin may be increased by: 5-ASA Derivatives; Antiplatelet Agents; Aspirin; Dasatinib; Herbs (Anticoagulant/Antiplatelet Properties); Nonsteroidal Anti-Inflammatory Agents; Pentosan Polysulfate Sodium; Pentoxifylline; Prostacyclin Analogues; Salicylates; Thrombolytic Agents

Decreased Effect
The levels/effects of Heparin may be decreased by: Nitroglycerin

Mechanism of Action Potentiates the action of antithrombin III and thereby inactivates thrombin (as well as activated coagulation factors IX, X, XI, XII, and plasmin) and prevents the conversion of fibrinogen to fibrin; heparin also stimulates release of lipoprotein lipase (lipoprotein lipase hydrolyzes triglycerides to glycerol and free fatty acids)

Pharmacodynamics Anticoagulation effect: Onset of action:

SubQ: 20-60 minutes

I.V.: Immediate

Pharmacokinetics (Adult data unless noted)
Absorption: SubQ, I.M.: Erratic

Distribution: Does not cross the placenta; does not appear in breast milk

Metabolism: Believed to be partially metabolized in the reticuloendothelial system

Half-life: Mean: 90 minutes (range: 1-2 hours); affected by obesity, renal function, hepatic function, malignancy, presence of pulmonary embolism, and infections

Elimination: Renal; small amount excreted unchanged in urine

Usual Dosage
Note: Many concentrations of heparin are available and range from 1 unit/mL to 20,000 units/mL. Carefully examine each prefilled syringe, bag, or vial prior to use to ensure that the correct concentration is chosen. Heparin lock flush solution is intended only to maintain patency of I.V. devices and is not to be used for anticoagulant therapy.

Line flushing: When using daily flushes of heparin to maintain patency of single and double lumen central catheters, 10 units/mL is commonly used for younger infants (eg, <10 kg) while 100 units/mL is used for older infants, children, and adults. Capped polyvinyl chloride catheters and peripheral heparin locks require flushing more frequently (eg, every 6-8 hours). Volume of heparin flush is usually similar to volume of catheter (or slightly greater) or may be standardized according to specific hospital's policy (eg, 2-5 mL/flush). Dose of heparin flush used should not approach therapeutic unit per kg dose. Additional flushes should be given when stagnant blood is observed in catheter, after catheter is used for drug or blood administration, and after blood withdrawal from catheter.

TPN: Heparin 1 unit/mL (final concentration) may be added to TPN solutions, both central and peripheral. (Addition of heparin to peripheral TPN has been shown to increase duration of line patency.) The final concentration of heparin used for TPN solutions may need to be decreased to 0.5 units/mL in small infants receiving larger TPN volumes in order to avoid approaching therapeutic amounts.

Arterial lines: Heparinize with a usual final concentration of 1 unit/mL; range: 0.5-2 units/mL; in order to avoid large total doses and systemic effects, use 0.5 unit/mL in low birth weight/premature newborns and in other patients receiving multiple lines containing heparin

Peripheral arterial catheters *in situ*: Neonates and Children: Continuous I.V. infusion of heparin at a final concentration of 5 units/mL at 1 mL/hour (see Monagle, 2008)

Umbilical artery catheter (UAC) prophylaxis: Neonates: Low-dose heparin continuous I.V. infusion via the UAC with a heparin concentration of 0.25–1 unit/mL (see Monagle, 2008)

Prophylaxis for cardiac catheterization via an artery: Neonates and Children: I.V.: Bolus: 100-150 units/kg; for prolonged procedures, further doses may be required (see Monagle, 2008)

Systemic heparinization:

Neonates and Infants <1 year: I.V. infusion: Initial loading dose: 75 units/kg given over 10 minutes; then initial maintenance dose: 28 units/kg/hour; adjust dose to maintain APTT of 60-85 seconds (assuming this reflects an antifactor Xa level of 0.35-0.7 units/mL); see table.

Children >1 year:

Intermittent I.V.: Initial: 50-100 units/kg, then 50-100 units/kg every 4 hours (**Note:** Continuous I.V. infusion is preferred):

I.V. infusion: Initial loading dose: 75 units/kg given over 10 minutes, then initial maintenance dose: 20 units/kg/hour; adjust dose to maintain APTT of 60-85 seconds (assuming this reflects an antifactor Xa level of 0.35-0.7 units/mL); see table.

PEDIATRIC PROTOCOL FOR SYSTEMIC HEPARIN ADJUSTMENT

To be used after initial loading dose and maintenance I.V. infusion dose (see Usual Dosage) to maintain APTT of 60-85 seconds (assuming this reflects antifactor Xa level of 0.35-0.7 units/mL)

Obtain blood for APTT 4 hours after heparin loading dose and 4 hours after every infusion rate change

Obtain daily CBC and APTT after APTT is therapeutic

APTT* (seconds)	Dosage Adjustment	Time to Repeat APTT
<50	Give 50 units/kg bolus and increase infusion rate by 10%	4 h after rate change
50-59	Increase infusion rate by 10%	4 h after rate change
60-85	Keep rate the same	Next day
86-95	Decrease infusion rate by 10%	4 h after rate change
96-120	Hold infusion for 30 minutes and decrease infusion rate by 10%	4 h after rate change
>120	Hold infusion for 60 minutes and decrease infusion rate by 15%	4 h after rate change

* Adjust heparin rate to maintain APTT of 60-85 seconds, assuming this reflects antifactor-Xa level of 0.35-0.7 units/mL (reagent specific)

Modified from Monagle P, Chalmers E, Chan A, et al, "Antithrombotic Therapy in Neonates and Children," *Chest*, 2008, 133 (6):887S-968S.

Adults:

Prophylaxis (low dose heparin): SubQ: 5000 units every 8-12 hours

Intermittent I.V.: Initial: 10,000 units, then 50-70 units/kg/dose (5000-10,000 units) every 4-6 hours (**Note:** Continuous I.V. infusion is preferred)

I.V. infusion: Initial loading dose: 80 units/kg; initial maintenance dose: 18 units/kg/hour with dose adjusted according to APTT; usual range: 10-30 units/kg/hour

Adults: *Chest*, 2008 Recommendations (see Goodman, 2008; Harrington, 2008; Kearon, 2008):

Prophylaxis of DVT and PE: SubQ: 5000 units every 8 or 12 hours or adjusted low-dose heparin

Treatment of DVT and PE:

I.V.: Initial (loading dose): I.V. bolus: 80 units/kg (or 5000 units); follow with continuous I.V. infusion of 18 units/kg/hour (or 1300 units/hour). Adjust dosage to achieve and maintain therapeutic APTT as determined by correlating APPT results with a therapeutic range of heparin levels as measured by antifactor Xa assay (0.3-0.7 units/mL).

SubQ:

Monitored dosing regimen: Initial: 17,500 units (or 250 units/kg) then 250 units/kg/dose every 12 hours. Adjust dosage to achieve and maintain therapeutic APTT as determined by correlating APPT results with a therapeutic range of heparin levels as measured by antifactor Xa assay (0.3-0.7 units/mL) when measured 6 hours after injection.

Unmonitored dosing regimen: Initial: 333 units/kg; followed by 250 units/kg/dose every 12 hours

Unstable angina or Non-ST-elevation myocardial infarction (NSTEMI): Initial loading dose: I.V. bolus: 60-70 units/kg (maximum: 5000 units), then initial maintenance dose: I.V. infusion: 12-15 units/kg/hour (maximum: 1000 units/hour); adjust dose to maintain therapeutic APTT of 50-75s

STEMI after thrombolytic therapy (full dose alteplase, tenecteplase, or reteplase): Initial loading dose: I.V. bolus: 60 units/kg (maximum: 4000 units), then initial maintenance dose: I.V. infusion: 12 units/kg/hour (maximum: 1000 units/hour); adjust dose to maintain therapeutic APTT of 50-70s for 48 hours

Administration Parenteral: Continuous I.V. infusion is preferred vs I.V. intermittent injections; I.V. bolus should be administered over 10 minutes; heparin lock flush solutions are intended only to maintain patency of I.V. devices and are **not** for systemic anticoagulation

Monitoring Parameters Platelet counts, signs of bleeding, hemoglobin, hematocrit, APTT; for full-dose heparin (ie, nonlow dose), the dose should be titrated according to APTT (see table). For intermittent I.V. injections, APTT is measured 3.5-4 hours after I.V. injection.

Reference Range Treatment of venous thrombotic disease: Recommended APTT should reflect a heparin level by protamine titration of 0.2-0.4 units/mL or an antifactor Xa level of 0.35-0.7 units/mL; this usually reflects an APTT of 60-85 seconds or a ratio (patient/control APTT) of 1.5-2.5; a lower therapeutic range (corresponding to antifactor Xa level of 0.14-0.34 units/mL) is recommended for patients with acute MI who received thrombolytic therapy

Test Interactions ↑ thyroxine (S) (competitive protein binding methods)

Patient Information Limit alcohol

Nursing Implications Do not administer I.M. due to pain, irritation, and hematoma formation

Additional Information To reverse the effects of heparin, use protamine (see Protamine on page 1180 for specifics); heparin is available from bovine lung and from porcine intestinal mucosa sources

Duration of heparin therapy (pediatric):

DVT and PE: At least 5-10 days

Note: Oral anticoagulation should be started on day 1 of heparin; oral anticoagulation should be overlapped with heparin for 5 days (or more, if INR is not >2)

Effective October 1, 2009, a new reference standard for heparin and a new test to determine potency have been established by USP (see Warnings). The FDA has requested that all manufacturers differentiate (from "old" heparin products) heparin products manufactured by the new standards. The labels of products manufactured according to the new standard will have an "N" in the lot number or following the expiration date. Additionally, products manufactured by Hospira may be identified by the number "82" or higher (eg, 83, 84) at the beginning of their lot numbers.

Dosage Forms Excipient information presented when available (limited, particularly for generics); consult specific product labeling.

Infusion, as sodium [premixed in NaCl 0.45%; porcine intestinal mucosa source]: 12,500 units (250 mL); 25,000 units (250 mL, 500 mL)

Infusion, as sodium [preservative free; premixed in D_5W; porcine intestinal mucosa source]: 10,000 units (100 mL) [contains sodium metabisulfite]; 12,500 units (250 mL) [contains sodium metabisulfite]; 20,000 units (500 mL) [contains sodium metabisulfite]; 25,000 units (250 mL, 500 mL) [contains sodium metabisulfite]

Infusion, as sodium [preservative free; premixed in NaCl 0.9%; porcine intestinal mucosa source]: 1000 units (500 mL); 2000 units (1000 mL)

Injection, solution, as sodium [lock flush preparation; porcine intestinal mucosa source; multidose vial]: 10 units/mL (1 mL, 10 mL, 30 mL) [contains parabens]; 100 units/mL (1 mL, 5 mL) [contains parabens]

Injection, solution, as sodium [lock flush preparation; porcine intestinal mucosa source; multidose vial]: 10 units/mL (10 mL, 30 mL); 100 units/mL (10 mL, 30 mL) [contains benzyl alcohol]

Hep-Lock®: 10 units/mL (1 mL, 2 mL, 10 mL, 30 mL); 100 units/mL (1 mL, 2 mL, 10 mL, 30 mL) [contains benzyl alcohol]

Injection, solution, as sodium [lock flush preparation; porcine intestinal mucosa source; prefilled syringe]: 10 units/mL (1 mL, 2 mL, 3 mL, 5 mL); 100 units/mL (1 mL, 2 mL, 3 mL, 5 mL) [contains benzyl alcohol]

Injection, solution, as sodium [preservative free; lock flush preparation; porcine intestinal mucosa source; prefilled syringe]: 1 unit/mL (2 mL, 3 mL, 5 mL); 2 units/mL (3 mL); 10 units/mL (2.5 mL, 3 mL, 5 mL, 10 mL); 100 units/mL (3 mL, 5 mL, 10 mL)

Injection, solution, as sodium [preservative free; lock flush preparation; porcine intestinal mucosa source; vial]:

HepFlush®-10: 10 units/mL (10 mL)

Hep-Lock U/P: 10 units/mL (1 mL); 100 units/mL (1 mL)

Injection, solution, as sodium [porcine intestinal mucosa source; multidose vial]: 1000 units/mL (1 mL, 10 mL, 30 mL) [contains benzyl alcohol]; 1000 units/mL (1 mL, 10 mL, 30 mL) [contains methylparabens]; 5000 units/mL (1 mL, 10 mL) [contains benzyl alcohol]; 5000 units/mL (1 mL) [contains methylparabens]; 10,000 units/mL (1 mL, 4 mL) [contains benzyl alcohol]; 10,000 units/mL (1 mL, 5 mL) [contains methylparabens]; 20,000 units/mL (1 mL) [contains methylparabens]

Injection, solution, as sodium [porcine intestinal mucosa source; prefilled syringe]: 5000 units/mL (1 mL) [contains benzyl alcohol]

Injection, solution, as sodium [preservative free; porcine intestinal mucosa source; prefilled syringe]: 10,000 units/mL (0.5 mL)

Injection, solution, as sodium [preservative free; porcine intestinal mucosa source; vial]: 1000 units/mL (2 mL); 2000 units/mL (5 mL); 2500 units/mL (10 mL)

References

Andrew M, Marzinotto V, Massicotte P, et al, "Heparin Therapy in Pediatric Patients: A Prospective Cohort Study," *Pediatr Res*, 1994, 35(1):78-83.

Goodman SG, Menon V, Cannon CP, et al, "Acute ST-Segment Elevation Myocardial Infarction: American College of Chest Physicians Evidence-Based Clinical Practice Guidelines (8th Edition)," *Chest*, 2008, 133(6 Suppl):708S-775S.

Harrington RA, Becker RC, Cannon CP, et al, "Antithrombotic Therapy for Non-ST-Segment Elevation Acute Coronary Syndromes: American College of Chest Physicians Evidence-Based Clinical Practice Guidelines (8th Edition)," *Chest*, 2008, 133(6 Suppl):670S-707S.

Hirsh J, Bauer KA, Donati MB, et al, "Parenteral Anticoagulants: American College of Chest Physicians Evidence-Based Clinical Practice Guidelines (8th Edition)," *Chest*, 2008,133(6 Suppl):141S-159S.

Kearon C, Kahn SR, Agnelli G, et al, "Antithrombotic Therapy for Venous Thromboembolic Disease: American College of Chest Physicians Evidence-Based Clinical Practice Guidelines (8th Edition)," *Chest*, 2008, 133(6 Suppl):454S-545S.

Monagle P, Chalmers E, Chan A, et al, "Antithrombotic Therapy in Neonates and Children: American College of Chest Physicians Evidence-Based Clinical Practice Guidelines (8th Edition)," *Chest*, 2008, 133(6 Suppl):887S-968S.

Newall F, Johnston L, Ignjatovic V, et al, "Unfractionated Heparin Therapy in Infants and Children," *Pediatrics*, 2009, 123(3):e510-8.

Smythe MA, Nutescu EA, and Wittkowsky AK, "Changes in the USP Heparin Monograph and Implications for Clinicians," *Pharmacotherapy*, 2010, 30(5):428-31.

◆ **Heparin Calcium** *see* Heparin *on page* 669

◆ **Heparin Lock Flush** *see* Heparin *on page* 669

◆ **Heparin Sodium** *see* Heparin *on page* 669

Hepatitis A Vaccine (hep a TYE tis aye vak SEEN)

Medication Safety Issues

International issues:

Avaxim® [Canada and multiple international markets] may be confused with Avastin® brand name for bevacizumab [U.S., Canada, and multiple international markets]

Related Information

Immunization Guidelines *on page* 1636

U.S. Brand Names HAVRIX®; VAQTA®

Canadian Brand Names Avaxim®; Avaxim®-Pediatric; HAVRIX®; VAQTA®

Therapeutic Category Vaccine

Generic Available No

Use Active immunization for children ≥12 months to adults against disease caused by hepatitis A virus; populations desiring protection against hepatitis A or at high risk of exposure to hepatitis A virus include: Residents and travelers to areas of high endemicity, household and sexual contacts of persons infected with hepatitis A, child daycare employees, patients with chronic liver disease, illicit drug users, male homosexuals, institutional workers (eg, institutions for the mentally and physically handicapped persons, prisons), healthcare workers who may be exposed to hepatitis A virus (eg, laboratory employees) and persons who anticipate close personal contact with international adoptee from a country of intermediate to high endemicity of HAV, during their first 60 days of arrival into the United States (eg, household contacts, babysitters) (FDA approved in ages >12 months and adults)

Pregnancy Risk Factor C

Pregnancy Considerations Reproduction studies have not been conducted. The safety of vaccination during pregnancy has not been determined, however, the theoretical risk to the infant is expected to be low.

Lactation Excretion in breast milk unknown/use caution

Contraindications Hypersensitivity to hepatitis A vaccine or any component such as aluminum hydroxide and phenoxyethanol

Warnings Treatment for anaphylactic reactions should be immediately available; primary immunization series should be completed at least 2 weeks prior to travel to an area of high endemicity; defer vaccination during the course of a moderate or severely febrile illness

Precautions Use caution in patients with serious active infection, cardiovascular disease, or pulmonary disorders; administer with caution to patients with thrombocytopenia or any coagulation disorder that would be compromised by I.M. injection; if the patient receives antihemophilia or other similar therapy, I.M. injection can be scheduled shortly after such therapy is administered. In order to maximize vaccination rates, the ACIP recommends simultaneous administration of all age-appropriate vaccines (live or inactivated) for which a person is eligible at a single clinic visit, unless contraindications exist. Packaging may contain natural latex rubber; some products may contain neomycin. Routine prophylactic administration of acetaminophen to prevent fever due to vaccines has been shown to decrease the immune response of some vaccines; the clinical significance of this reduction in immune response has not been established (see Prymula, 2009).

Adverse Reactions All serious adverse reactions must be reported to the U.S. Department of Health and Human Services (DHHS) Vaccine Adverse Event Reporting System (VAERS) 1-800-822-7967.

Cardiovascular: Syncope

Central nervous system: Dizziness, encephalopathy (rare), fatigue, fever (rare), headache, insomnia, seizures, vertigo

Dermatologic: Erythema multiforme (rare), rash, urticaria

Gastrointestinal: Abdominal pain, anorexia, diarrhea, dysgeusia, nausea, pharyngitis, vomiting

Hepatic: Hepatitis, jaundice, LFTs increased

Local: Erythema, pain, pruritus, swelling and tenderness at the injection site

Neuromuscular & skeletal: Arthralgia, Guillain-Barré syndrome (rare), myalgia, myelitis, neuropathy, paresthesia

Ophthalmic: Photophobia

Respiratory: Dyspnea

Miscellaneous: Anaphylaxis, hypersensitivity reactions

<1% and/or postmarketing: Conjunctivitis, cough, crying, ecchymosis, irritability, nasal congestion, respiratory congestion, rhinorrhea, viral exanthema

Drug Interactions

Avoid Concomitant Use There are no known interactions where it is recommended to avoid concomitant use.

Increased Effect/Toxicity There are no known significant interactions involving an increase in effect.

Decreased Effect

The levels/effects of Hepatitis A Vaccine may be decreased by: Immunosuppressants

Stability Refrigerate; do not freeze

Mechanism of Action As an inactivated virus vaccine, hepatitis A vaccine offers active immunization against hepatitis A virus infection at an effective immune response rate in up to 99% of subjects

Pharmacodynamics Onset of protective immunity: Within 1 month of first dose: Children and Adults: 95%; after second dose: Children and Adults: 100%

Usual Dosage I.M.: **Note:** When used for primary immunization, the vaccine should be given at least 2 weeks prior to expected HAV exposure. When used prior to an international adoption, the vaccination series should begin when adoption is being planned, but at least ≥2 weeks prior to expected arrival of adoptee. When used for postexposure prophylaxis, the vaccine should be given as soon as possible.

Havrix®:

Children 12 months to 18 years: 2 dose series of 0.5 mL (720 ELISA units)/dose given 6-12 months apart.

Adolescents ≥19 years and Adults: 2 dose series of 1 mL (1440 ELISA units)/dose given 6-12 months apart

VAQTA®:

Children 12 months to 18 years: 2 dose series of 0.5 mL (25 units)/dose given 6-12 months apart

Adolescents ≥19 years and Adults: 2 dose series of 1 mL (50 units)/dose given 6-12 months apart

Administration Shake well and administer I.M. in either the anterolateral aspect of the thigh or deltoid muscle of the arm; **not for I.V., intradermal, or SubQ administration**.

Nursing Implications Federal law requires that the date of administration, the vaccine manufacturer, lot number of vaccine, and the administering person's name, title, and address be entered into the patient's permanent medical record.

Additional Information In order to maximize vaccination rates, the ACIP recommends simultaneous administration of all age-appropriate vaccines (live or inactivated) for which a person is eligible at a single visit, unless contraindications exist. The use of combination vaccines is generally preferred over separate infections, taking into consideration provider assessment, patient preference, and potential adverse events.

For additional information, please refer to the following website: http://www.cdc.gov/vaccines/vpd-vac/.

Dosage Forms Excipient information presented when available (limited, particularly for generics); consult specific product labeling.

Injection, suspension [adult formulation; preservative free]:
HAVRIX®: Hepatitis A virus antigen 1440 ELISA units/mL (1 mL) [contains aluminum, trace amounts of neomycin; prefilled syringe contains natural rubber/natural latex]
VAQTA®: Hepatitis A virus antigen 50 units/mL (1 mL) [contains aluminum, natural rubber/natural latex in packaging]

Injection, suspension [pediatric formulation; preservative free]:
HAVRIX®: Hepatitis A virus antigen 720 ELISA units/ 0.5 mL (0.5 mL) [contains aluminum, trace amounts of neomycin; prefilled syringe contains natural rubber/ natural latex]

Injection, suspension [pediatric/adolescent formulation; preservative free]:
VAQTA®: Hepatitis A virus antigen 25 units/0.5 mL (0.5 mL) [contains aluminum, natural rubber/natural latex in packaging]

References

American Academy of Pediatrics Committee on Infectious Diseases, "Hepatitis A Vaccine Recommendations," *Pediatrics*, 2007, 120 (1):189-99.

Bancroft WH, "Hepatitis A Vaccine," *N Engl J Med*, 1992, 327 (7):488-90.

Centers for Disease Control and Prevention (CDC), "General Recommendations on Immunization. Recommendations of the Advisory Committee on Immunization Practices (ACIP)," *MMWR Recomm Rep*, 2006, 55(RR-15):1-48. Available at: http://www.cdc.gov/mmwr/preview/mmwrhtml/rr5515a1.htm.

Centers for Disease Control, "Updated Recommendations from the Advisory Committee on Immunization Practices (ACIP) for Use of Hepatitis A Vaccine in Close Contacts of Newly Arriving International Adoptees." Available at http://www.cdc.gov/mmwr/preview/mmwrhtml/mm5836a4.htm?s_cid=mm5836a4_e.

Koff RS, "Hepatitis A," *Lancet*, 1998, 351(9116):1643-9.

Lemon SM, "Inactivated Hepatitis A Vaccines," *JAMA*, 1994, 271 (17):1363-4.

Niu MT, Salive M, Krueger C, et al, "Two-Year Review of Hepatitis A Vaccine Safety: Data From the Vaccine Adverse Event Reporting System (VAERS)," *Clin Infect Dis*, 1998, 26(6):1475-6.

Prymula R, Siegrist CA, Chlibek R, et al, "Effect of Prophylactic Paracetamol Administration at Time of Vaccination on Febrile Reactions and Antibody Responses in Children: Two Open-Label, Randomised Controlled Trials," *Lancet*, 2009, 374(9698):1339-50.

Hepatitis B Immune Globulin
(hep a TYE tis bee i MYUN GLOB yoo lin)

Medication Safety Issues
Sound-alike/look-alike issues:
HBIG may be confused with BabyBIG

Related Information
Immunization Guidelines *on page 1636*
Management of Healthcare Worker Exposures to HBV, HCV, and HIV *on page 1661*

U.S. Brand Names HepaGam B™; HyperHEP B™ S/D; Nabi-HB®

Canadian Brand Names HepaGam B™; HyperHep B®

◄ **Therapeutic Category** Immune Globulin
Generic Available No
Use Provide prophylactic passive immunity to hepatitis B infection for those individuals exposed either by direct contact with hepatitis B surface antigen positive (HB$_s$Ag-positive) materials (blood, plasma, or serum), sexual exposure to an individual who is HB$_s$Ag-positive, or an infant <12 months of age with close "household contact" with an individual who is HB$_s$Ag-positive; newborns of mothers known to be HB$_s$Ag-positive. Prevention of hepatitis B virus recurrence after liver transplantation in HB$_s$Ag-positive transplant patients.

Note: Hepatitis B immune globulin is not indicated for treatment of active hepatitis B infection and is ineffective in the treatment of chronic active hepatitis B infection.

Pregnancy Risk Factor C
Pregnancy Considerations Reproduction studies have not been conducted.
Lactation Excretion in breast milk unknown/use caution
Breast-Feeding Considerations Infants born to HBsAg-positive mothers may be breast fed.
Contraindications Hypersensitivity to hepatitis B immune globulin or any component; severe allergy to gamma globulin or anti-immunoglobulin therapies
Warnings As a product of human plasma, this product may potentially transmit infectious agents such as viruses; screening of donors, as well as testing and/or inactivation of certain viruses, has reduced this risk. Not for intravenous administration. Although extremely rare, severe hypersensitivity reactions including anaphylaxis may occur; epinephrine and other anaphylactic treatment agents should be readily available.
Precautions Administer with caution to patients with thrombocytopenia or any coagulation disorder that would be compromised by I.M. injection; administer with caution in patients with IgA deficiency or a prior history of systemic allergic reactions following the administration of human immunoglobulin preparations
Adverse Reactions Adverse events reported in liver transplant patients included tremor and hypotension, were associated with a single infusion during the first week of treatment, and did not recur with additional infusions.
Cardiovascular: Hypotension, hypertension
Central nervous system: Dizziness, malaise, fever, lethargy, chills, headache
Dermatologic: Urticaria, angioedema, rash, erythema
Gastrointestinal: Vomiting, nausea
Genitourinary: Nephrotic syndrome
Local: Pain, tenderness, and muscular stiffness at I.M. injection site
Neuromuscular & skeletal: Arthralgia, myalgia, tremor, moderate low back pain
Miscellaneous: Anaphylaxis

Drug Interactions
Avoid Concomitant Use There are no known interactions where it is recommended to avoid concomitant use.
Increased Effect/Toxicity There are no known significant interactions involving an increase in effect.
Decreased Effect
Hepatitis B Immune Globulin (Human) may decrease the levels/effects of: Vaccines (Live)

Stability Refrigerate at 2°C to 8°C (36°F to 46°F); do not freeze; use within 6 hours of puncturing the vial
Mechanism of Action Passive immunity toward hepatitis B virus
Pharmacodynamics Duration: Postexposure prophylaxis: 3-6 months
Pharmacokinetics (Adult data unless noted)
Absorption: I.M.: Slow
Half-life: 17-25 days
Time to peak serum concentration: I.M.: 2-10 days

Usual Dosage
Newborns of HB$_s$Ag-positive mothers: I.M.: Hepatitis B: 0.5 mL as soon after birth as possible (within 12 hours; efficacy decreases significantly if treatment is delayed >48 hours); hepatitis B vaccine series to begin at the same time; if this series is delayed for as long as 3 months, the HBIG dose may be repeated; see Hepatitis B Vaccine on page 675.

Postexposure prophylaxis: I.M.:
Children <12 months: 0.5 mL; initiate hepatitis vaccine series
Children ≥12 months and Adults: 0.06 mL/kg as soon as possible after exposure (ie, within 24 hours of needle-stick, ocular, or mucosal exposure or within 14 days of sexual exposure); usual dose: 3-5 mL; repeat at 28-30 days after exposure

Prevention of hepatitis B recurrence in liver transplant patients: Adults: I.V.: HepaGam B™: 20,000 int. units/dose according to the following schedule:
Anhepatic phase (initial dose): One dose given with the liver transplant
Week 1 postop: One dose daily for 7 days (days 1-7)
Weeks 2-12 postop: One dose every 2 weeks starting on day 14
Month 4 onward: One dose monthly starting on month 4
Dose adjustment: Adjust dose to reach anti-HB$_s$ levels of 500 int. units/L within the first week after transplantation. In patients with surgical bleeding, abdominal fluid drainage >500 mL or those undergoing plasmapheresis, administer 10,000 int. units/dose every 6 hours until target anti-HB$_s$ levels are reached.

Administration
I.M.: Inject only in the anterolateral aspects of the upper thigh or the deltoid muscle; multiple injections may be necessary when the dosage is a large volume (postexposure prophylaxis). Do not administer hepatitis vaccine and HBIG in same syringe (vaccine will be neutralized); hepatitis vaccine may be administered at the same time at a separate site
I.V.: HepaGam B™: Administer at 2 mL/minute. Decrease infusion to <1 mL/minute for patient discomfort or infusion-related adverse events. Actual volume of dosage is dependent upon potency labeled on each individual vial.

Monitoring Parameters Liver transplant patients: anti-HB levels; infusion-related adverse events
Test Interactions Maltose contained in HepaGam B™ may interfere with some types of blood glucose monitoring systems [eg, those based on the glucose dehydrogenase pyrroloquinequinone (GDH-PQQ) method]. This may result in falsely elevated glucose results.

Dosage Forms Excipient information presented when available (limited, particularly for generics); consult specific product labeling.
Note: Potency expressed in international units (as compared to the WHO standard) is noted by individual lot on the vial label.
Injection, solution [preservative free]:
HyperHEP B™ S/D: Anti-HBs ≥220 int. units/mL (0.5 mL, 1 mL, 5 mL)
Nabi-HB®: Anti-HBs >312 int. units/mL (1 mL, 5 mL) [contains polysorbate 80]
HepaGam B™: Anti-HBs 312 int. units/mL (1 mL, 5 mL) [contains maltose and polysorbate 80]

◆ **Hepatitis B Inactivated Virus Vaccine (recombinant DNA)** *see* Hepatitis B Vaccine *on page 675*

Hepatitis B Vaccine (hep a TYE tis bee vak SEEN)

Medication Safety Issues
Sound-alike/look-alike issues:
Engerix-B® adult may be confused with Engerix-B® pediatric/adolescent
Recombivax HB® may be confused with Comvax®

Related Information
Immunization Guidelines *on page 1636*
Management of Healthcare Worker Exposures to HBV, HCV, and HIV *on page 1661*

U.S. Brand Names Engerix-B®; Recombivax HB®

Canadian Brand Names Engerix-B®; Recombivax HB®

Therapeutic Category Vaccine

Generic Available No

Use Immunization against infection caused by all known subtypes of hepatitis B virus, in individuals considered at high risk of potential exposure to hepatitis B virus or HB$_s$Ag-positive materials: See table.

Pre-exposure Prophylaxis for Hepatitis B
Healthcare workers with blood exposure
Special patient groups (eg, adolescents, infants born to HB$_s$Ag-positive mothers, children born after 11/21/91, military personnel, Alaskan natives, Pacific Islanders)
Hemodialysis patients
Recipients of certain blood products
Lifestyle factors
Homosexual and bisexual men
Intravenous drug abusers
Heterosexually-active persons with multiple sexual partners or recently acquired sexually-transmitted diseases
Environmental factors
Household and sexual contacts of HBV carriers
Prison inmates
Clients and staff of institutions for the mentally handicapped
Residents, immigrants, and refugees from areas with endemic HBV infection
International travelers at increased risk of acquiring HBV infection

In addition, the Advisory Committee on Immunization Practices (ACIP) recommends vaccination for any persons who are wounded in bombings or similar mass casualty events who have penetrating injuries or nonintact skin exposure, or who have contact with mucous membranes (exception: superficial contact with intact skin) and who cannot confirm receipt of a hepatitis B vaccination.

Pregnancy Risk Factor C

Pregnancy Considerations Reproduction studies have not been conducted. The ACIP recommends HBsAg testing for all pregnant women. Based on limited data, there is no apparent risk to the fetus when the hepatitis B vaccine is administered during pregnancy. Pregnancy itself is not a contraindication to vaccination; vaccination should be considered if otherwise indicated.

Lactation Excretion in breast milk unknown/use caution

Breast-Feeding Considerations Studies suggest that infants born to HBsAg-positive mothers do not incur an increased risk of HBV infection through breast-feeding.

Contraindications Hypersensitivity to hepatitis vaccine, yeast, or any component of the formulation

Warnings Immediate treatment for anaphylactic reactions should be available during vaccine use; defer vaccination for persons with acute febrile illness until recovery

Precautions Use with caution in patients with coagulation disorders including thrombocytopenia, due to an increased risk for bleeding following I.M. administration; if the patient receives antihemophilia or other similar therapy, I.M. injection can be scheduled shortly after such therapy is administered; use with caution in patients with decreased

cardiopulmonary function. Routine prophylactic administration of acetaminophen to prevent fever due to vaccines has been shown to decrease the immune response of some vaccines; the clinical significance of this reduction in immune response has not been established (see Prymula, 2009).

Adverse Reactions All serious adverse reactions must be reported to the U.S. Department of Health and Human Services (DHHS) Vaccine Adverse Event Reporting System (VAERS) 1-800-822-7967.

Cardiovascular: Hypotension, syncope, tachycardia, palpitations

Central nervous system: Agitation, chills, dizziness, fatigue, fever, flushing, headache, insomnia, irritability, lightheadedness, malaise, vertigo, encephalitis, migraine, seizures, vertigo

Dermatologic: Angioedema, petechiae, pruritus, rash, urticaria, alopecia, eczema, erythema nodosum, erythema multiforme, Stevens-Johnson syndrome, purpura, keratitis

Gastrointestinal: Abdominal pain, appetite decreased, cramps, diarrhea, dyspepsia, nausea, vomiting, constipation

Genitourinary: Dysuria

Hematologic: Thrombocytopenia

Hepatic: Liver enzymes elevated

Local: Injection site reactions: Ecchymosis, erythema, induration, pain, nodule formation, soreness, swelling, tenderness, warmth

Neuromuscular & skeletal: Achiness, arthralgia, back pain, myalgia, neck pain, neck stiffness, paresthesia, shoulder pain, weakness, arthritis, Bell's palsy, Guillain-Barré syndrome, transverse myelitis, paresthesia, hypoesthesia

Ophthalmic: Conjunctivitis, optic neuritis, visual disturbances,

Otic: Earache

Respiratory: Cough, pharyngitis, rhinitis, upper respiratory tract infection, bronchospasm

Miscellaneous: Hypersensitivity reactions, lymphadenopathy, diaphoresis, serum-sickness like syndrome (may be delayed days to weeks)

Drug Interactions
Avoid Concomitant Use There are no known interactions where it is recommended to avoid concomitant use.

Increased Effect/Toxicity There are no known significant interactions involving an increase in effect.

Decreased Effect
The levels/effects of Hepatitis B Vaccine (Recombinant) may be decreased by: Immunosuppressants

Stability Refrigerate; do not freeze

Mechanism of Action Recombinant hepatitis B vaccine is a noninfectious subunit viral vaccine. The vaccine is derived from hepatitis B surface antigen (HB$_s$Ag) produced through recombinant DNA techniques from yeast cells. The portion of the hepatitis B gene which codes for HB$_s$Ag is cloned into yeast which is then cultured to produce hepatitis B vaccine. Promotes immunity to hepatitis B virus by inducing the production of specific antibodies to the virus.

Usual Dosage I.M.: The strengths for each brand hepatitis B vaccine are different; however, the equivalent dose by volume is the same. Combination vaccines (eg, also containing DTaP, HIB) should not be used for the "birth" dose but may be used to complete the course beginning after the infant is 6 weeks of age.
Recommended schedule: 0.5 mL/dose in 3 total doses; special circumstances for at risk infants are described below
Infants born of HB$_s$Ag **positive** mothers: First dose should be given within the first 12 hours of life, even if premature and regardless of birth weight (hepatitis

immune globulin should also be administered at the same time/different site); the second dose is administered at 1-2 months of age and the third dose at 6 months of age; anti-HB$_s$ and HB$_s$Ag should be checked at 9-15 months of age. If anti-HB$_s$ and HB$_s$Ag are negative, reimmunize with 3 doses 2 months apart and reassess. **Note:** Premature infants <2000 g should receive 4 total doses at 0, 1, 2-3, and 6-7 months of chronological age

Infants born of HB$_s$Ag **negative** mothers: First dose should be given prior to leaving the hospital; however, the first dose may be given at 1-2 months of age; another dose is given 1-2 months later and a final dose at 6 months of age; 4 total doses of vaccine may be given if a "birth dose" is administered and a combination vaccine is used to complete the series. **Note:** Premature infants <2000 g may have the initial dose deferred up to 30 days of chronological age.

Infants born of mothers whose HB$_s$Ag status is unknown at birth: First dose given within 12 hours of birth even if premature regardless of birth weight, second dose following 1-2 months later; the third dose at 6 months of age; if the mother's blood HB$_s$Ag test is positive, the infant should receive hepatitis immune globulin as soon as possible (no later than age 1 week)

Children and Adolescents ≤18 years: 0.5 mL/dose in 3 total doses; first dose given on the elected date, second dose given 1 month later, third dose given 8 weeks later and at least 16 weeks after the first dose

Adults >19 years: 1 mL/dose in 3 total doses; first dose given on the elected date, second dose given 1-2 months later, third dose given 4-6 months later

Dialysis patients: <20 years: 20 mcg/dose and >20 years: 40 mcg/dose; given at 0, 1-2, and 4-6 months; repeat dose depending upon annual assessment of hepatitis B surface antigen (anti-HB) level; if anti-HB <10 milli-international units/mL administer an additional dose

Note: When used for immediate prophylactic intervention (eg, administration to persons who are wounded in bombings or similar mass casualty events), vaccination should begin within 24 hours and no later than 7 days following the event.

Alternative schedules per manufacturer's recommendations:

Children 0-10 years with recent exposure to the virus or certain travelers to high-risk areas: Engerix-B®: 0.5 mL/dose for 4 doses given at 0, 1, 2, and 12 months

Children 5-10 years: Engerix-B®: 0.5 mL for 3 doses given 12 months apart

Adolescents ≥11 years and Adults with recent exposure to the virus or certain travelers to high-risk areas: Engerix-B®: 1 mL for 4 doses given at 0, 1, 2, and 12 months

Adolescents 11-15 years: Recombivax HB®: 1 mL/dose initially and repeated 4-6 months later

Administration Shake well; administer I.M. in either the anterolateral aspect of the thigh or arm; **not for I.V. or SubQ administration**

It is possible to interchange the vaccines for completion of a series or for booster doses; the antibody produced in response to each type of vaccine is comparable

Monitoring Parameters HB$_s$Ag and antibodies to HB$_s$Ag (anti-HB$_s$) should be tested in infants born to mothers positive for HB$_s$Ag when they are 9-15 months of age; annual anti-HB in dialysis patients. Vaccination at the time of HBsAg testing: For persons in whom vaccination is recommended, the first dose of hepatitis B vaccine can be given after blood is drawn to test for HG$_s$Ag.

Nursing Implications Federal law requires that the date of administration, the vaccine manufacturer, lot number of vaccine, and the administering person's name, title, and address be entered into the patient's permanent medical record.

Additional Information In order to maximize vaccination rates, the ACIP recommends simultaneous administration of all age-appropriate vaccines (live or inactivated) for which a person is eligible at a single visit, unless contraindications exist. The use of combination vaccines is generally preferred over separate infections, taking into consideration provider assessment, patient preference, and potential adverse events.

For additional information, please refer to the following website: http://www.cdc.gov/vaccines/vpd-vac/.

Dosage Forms Excipient information presented when available (limited, particularly for generics); consult specific product labeling.

Injection, suspension [adult; preservative free]:
Engerix-B®: Hepatitis B surface antigen 20 mcg/mL (1 mL) [contains aluminum; prefilled syringes contain natural rubber/natural latex]
Recombivax HB®: Hepatitis B surface antigen 10 mcg/mL (1 mL, 3 mL) [contains aluminum and yeast protein]

Injection, suspension [pediatric/adolescent; preservative free]:
Engerix-B®: Hepatitis B surface antigen 10 mcg/0.5 mL (0.5 mL) [contains aluminum; prefilled syringes contain natural rubber/natural latex]
Recombivax HB®: Hepatitis B surface antigen 5 mcg/ 0.5 mL (0.5 mL) [contains aluminum and yeast protein]

Injection, suspension [dialysis formulation; preservative free]:
Recombivax HB®: Hepatitis B surface antigen 40 mcg/mL (1 mL) [contains aluminum and yeast protein]

References

American Academy of Pediatrics Committee on Infectious Diseases, "Recommended Immunization Schedules for Children and Adolescents - United States, 2007," *Pediatrics,* 2007, 119(1):207-8.

Centers for Disease Control and Prevention (CDC), "General Recommendations on Immunization. Recommendations of the Advisory Committee on Immunization Practices (ACIP)," *MMWR Recomm Rep,* 2006, 55(RR-15):1-48. Available at: http://www.cdc.gov/mmwr/preview/mmwrhtml/rr5515a1.htm.

Center for Disease Control and Prevention, "Recommended Adult Immunization Schedule – United States, October 2007-September 2008," *MMWR,* 2007, 56:Q1-4.

Center for Disease Control and Prevention, "Recommended Immunization Schedules for Persons Aged 0-18 Years – United States, 2008," *MMWR,* 2008, 57(01)Q1-4.

Chapman LE, Sullivent EE, Grohskopf LA, et al, "Recommendations for Postexposure Interventions to Prevent Infection With Hepatitis B Virus, Hepatitis C Virus, or Human Immunodeficiency Virus, and Tetanus in Persons Wounded During Bombings and Other Mass-Casualty Events – United States, 2008: Recommendations of the Centers for Disease Control and Prevention (CDC)," *MMWR Recomm Rep,* 2008, 57(RR-6):1-21.

"Prevention of Hepatitis A Through Active or Passive Immunization: Recommendations of the Advisory Committee on Immunization Practices (ACIP)," *MMWR Recomm Rep,* 1999, 48(RR-12):1-37.

Prymula R, Siegrist CA, Chlibek R, et al, "Effect of Prophylactic Paracetamol Administration at Time of Vaccination on Febrile Reactions and Antibody Responses in Children: Two Open-Label, Randomised Controlled Trials," *Lancet,* 2009, 374(9698):1339-50.

Hetastarch (HET a starch)

Medication Safety Issues
Sound-alike/look-alike issues:
Hespan® may be confused with heparin

U.S. Brand Names Hespan®; Hextend®

Canadian Brand Names Hextend®

Therapeutic Category Plasma Volume Expander

Generic Available Yes: Sodium chloride infusion

Use Blood volume expander used in treatment of shock or impending shock when blood or blood products are not available; does not have oxygen-carrying capacity and is not a substitute for blood or plasma

Pregnancy Risk Factor C

Lactation Excretion in breast milk unknown/use caution

Contraindications Hypersensitivity to hetastarch or any component; severe bleeding disorders, renal failure with oliguria or anuria, or severe CHF; management of cerebral vasospasm associated with subarachnoid hemorrhage or for conditions other than leukapheresis which necessitate repeated use of the drug over several days; per manufacturer, Hextend® is contraindicated in the treatment of lactic acidosis and in leukapheresis

Warnings Anaphylactoid reactions have occurred; use with caution in patients with thrombocytopenia (may interfere with platelet function); large volume may cause drops in hemoglobin concentrations; use with caution in patients at risk from overexpansion of blood volume, including the very young or aged patients, those with CHF or pulmonary edema; large volumes (>1500 mL) may interfere with platelet function and prolong PT and PTT times; use with caution in patients with a history of liver disease

Precautions Use with caution in patients allergic to corn (may have cross allergy to hetastarch). Note electrolyte content of Hextend® including calcium, lactate, and potassium (see Additional Information); use with caution in situations where electrolyte and/or acid-base disturbances may be exacerbated (renal impairment, respiratory alkalosis).

Adverse Reactions
Cardiovascular: Heart failure, circulatory overload, peripheral edema

Central nervous system: Headache, fever, chills, intracranial bleeding

Dermatologic: Urticaria, pruritus, rash

Endocrine & metabolic: Parotid gland enlargement, hyperchloremic metabolic acidosis, hypernatremia

Gastrointestinal: Vomiting, amylase levels elevated

Hematologic: Thrombocytopenia, transient prolongation of PT, PTT, clotting time, and bleeding time, anemia, DIC (rare), hemolysis (rare)

Hepatic: Indirect bilirubin elevated

Neuromuscular & skeletal: Myalgia

Ocular: Periorbital edema

Respiratory: Wheezing

Miscellaneous: Anaphylactoid reactions, flu-like symptoms

Drug Interactions
Avoid Concomitant Use There are no known interactions where it is recommended to avoid concomitant use.

Increased Effect/Toxicity There are no known significant interactions involving an increase in effect.

Decreased Effect There are no known significant interactions involving a decrease in effect.

Stability Store at room temperature; do not freeze; do not use if crystalline precipitate forms or is turbid deep brown

Mechanism of Action Hetastarch. a synthetic polymer, produces plasma volume expansion by virtue of its highly colloidal starch structure

Pharmacodynamics
Onset of volume expansion: I.V.: Within 30 minutes

Duration: 24-36 hours

Pharmacokinetics (Adult data unless noted)
Metabolism: Molecules >50,000 daltons require enzymatic degradation by the reticuloendothelial system or amylases in the blood prior to urinary and fecal excretion

Elimination: Smaller molecular weight molecules are readily excreted in urine; approximately 40% of dose excreted in first 24 hours in patients with normal renal function

Usual Dosage I.V. infusion:
Children: 10 mL/kg/dose; the total daily dose should not exceed 20 mL/kg

Adults: 500-1000 mL (30-60 g) per dose; the total daily dose should not exceed 1.2 g/kg or 90 g (1500 mL).

Dosing adjustment in renal impairment: Cl_{cr} <10 mL/minute: Initial dose is the same but subsequent doses should be reduced by 20% to 50% of normal

Administration Parenteral: I.V.: Maximum rate of infusion: 1.2 g/kg/hour (20 mL/kg/hour)

Monitoring Parameters Volume expansion: capillary refill time, CVP, RAP, MAP, urine output, heart rate, if pulmonary artery catheter in place, monitor PWCP, SVR, and PVR; hemoglobin, hematocrit; for leukapheresis, monitor CBC, total leukocyte and platelet counts, leukocyte differential count, hemoglobin, hematocrit, prothrombin time, and partial thromboplastin time

Additional Information Hetastarch is a synthetic polymer derived from a waxy starch composed of amylopectin, average molecular weight = 450,000; each liter of Hespan® provides 154 mEq sodium chloride; each liter of Hextend® contains the following electrolytes: Sodium 143 mEq, chloride 124 mEq, lactate 28 mEq, calcium 5 mEq, magnesium 0.9 mEq, potassium 3 mEq, and dextrose 0.99 g

Dosage Forms Excipient information presented when available (limited, particularly for generics); consult specific product labeling.

Infusion [premixed in lactated electrolyte injection]:
Hextend®: 6% (500 mL)

Infusion, solution [premixed in NaCl 0.9%]: 6% (500 mL)
Hespan®: 6% (500 mL)

References
Brutocao D, Bratton SL, Thomas JR, et al, "Comparison of Hetastarch With Albumin for Postoperative Volume Expansion in Children After Cardiopulmonary Bypass," *J Cardiothoracic Vasc Anesth*, 1996, 10 (3):348-51.

♦ **Hexachlorocyclohexane** see Lindane on page 825

Hexachlorophene (heks a KLOR oh feen)

Medication Safety Issues
Sound-alike/look-alike issues:
pHisoHex® may be confused with Fostex®, pHisoDerm®

U.S. Brand Names pHisoHex®

Canadian Brand Names pHisoHex®

Therapeutic Category Antibacterial, Topical; Soap

Generic Available No

Use Surgical scrub and as a bacteriostatic skin cleanser; to control an outbreak of gram-positive staphylococcal infection when other infection control procedures have been unsuccessful

Pregnancy Risk Factor C

Contraindications Hypersensitivity to halogenated phenol derivatives or hexachlorophene; use in premature infants; use on burned or denuded skin; use with an occlusive dressing; application to mucous membranes

Warnings Do not use for bathing infants; do not apply to mucous membranes; premature and low birth weight infants are particularly susceptible to hexachlorophene topical absorption; irritability, generalized clonic muscular contractions, decerebrate rigidity, and brain lesions in the white matter have occurred in infants following topical use of 6% hexachlorophene; exposure of preterm infants or patients with extensive burns has been associated with apnea, convulsions, agitation, and coma

Adverse Reactions
Central nervous system: CNS injury, seizures, irritability
Dermatologic: Dermatitis, erythema, dry skin, photo-sensitivity

Drug Interactions
Avoid Concomitant Use
Avoid concomitant use of Hexachlorophene with any of the following: BCG
Increased Effect/Toxicity There are no known significant interactions involving an increase in effect.
Decreased Effect
Hexachlorophene may decrease the levels/effects of: BCG

Stability Store in nonmetallic container (incompatible with many metals); protect from light

Mechanism of Action Bacteriostatic polychlorinated biphenol which inhibits membrane-bound enzymes and disrupts the cell membrane

Pharmacokinetics (Adult data unless noted)
Absorption: Percutaneously through inflamed, excoriated and intact skin
Distribution: Crosses the placenta
Half-life, infants: 6.1-44.2 hours

Usual Dosage Children and Adults: Topical: Apply 5 mL cleanser and water to area to be cleansed; lather and rinse thoroughly under running water; for use as a surgical scrub, a second application of 5 mL cleanser should be made and the hands and forearms scrubbed for an additional 3 minutes, rinsed thoroughly with running water and dried

Administration Topical: For external use only; rinse thoroughly after each use

Patient Information Avoid prolonged contact with skin. May cause photosensitivity reactions (eg, exposure to sunlight may cause severe sunburn, skin rash, redness, or itching); avoid exposure to sunlight and artificial light sources (sunlamps, tanning booth/bed); wear protective clothing, wide-brimmed hats, sunglasses, and lip sunscreen (SPF ≥15); use a sunscreen [broad-spectrum sunscreen or physical sunscreen (preferred) or sunblock with SPF ≥15]; contact physician if reaction occurs.

Dosage Forms Excipient information presented when available (limited, particularly for generics); consult specific product labeling. [DSC] = Discontinued product
Liquid, topical: 3% (150 mL, 500 mL, 3840 mL [DSC])

References
Lester RS, "Topical Formulary for the Pediatrician," *Pediatr Clin North Am*, 1983, 30(4):749-65.

Homatropine (hoe MA troe peen)

Medication Safety Issues
Sound-alike/look-alike issues:
Homatropine may be confused with Humatrope®, somatropin

U.S. Brand Names Isopto® Homatropine

Therapeutic Category Anticholinergic Agent, Ophthalmic; Ophthalmic Agent, Mydriatic

Generic Available No

Use Producing cycloplegia and mydriasis for refraction; treatment of acute inflammatory conditions of the uveal tract

Pregnancy Risk Factor C

Pregnancy Considerations Reproduction studies have not been conducted.

Lactation Excretion in breast milk unknown/use caution

Contraindications Hypersensitivity to homatropine or any component; narrow-angle glaucoma, acute hemorrhage

Precautions Use with caution in patients with hypertension, cardiac disease, increased intraocular pressure, obstructive uropathy, paralytic ileus, or ulcerative colitis

Adverse Reactions
Cardiovascular: Vascular congestion, edema
Central nervous system: Drowsiness
Dermatologic: Eczematoid dermatitis
Ocular: Follicular conjunctivitis, blurred vision, intraocular pressure elevated, stinging, exudate

Drug Interactions
Avoid Concomitant Use There are no known interactions where it is recommended to avoid concomitant use.

Increased Effect/Toxicity
Homatropine may increase the levels/effects of: AbobotulinumtoxinA; Anticholinergics; Cannabinoids; OnabotulinumtoxinA; Potassium Chloride; RimabotulinumtoxinB

The levels/effects of Homatropine may be increased by: Pramlintide

Decreased Effect
Homatropine may decrease the levels/effects of: Acetylcholinesterase Inhibitors (Central); Secretin

The levels/effects of Homatropine may be decreased by: Acetylcholinesterase Inhibitors (Central)

Mechanism of Action Blocks response of iris sphincter muscle and the accommodative muscle of the ciliary body to cholinergic stimulation resulting in dilation and loss of accommodation

Pharmacodynamics Ophthalmic:
Onset of accommodation and pupil action:
Maximum mydriatic effect: Within 10-30 minutes
Maximum cycloplegic effect: Within 30-90 minutes
Duration:
Mydriasis: Persists for 6 hours to 4 days
Cycloplegia: 10-48 hours
Usual Dosage Ophthalmic:
Children:
Mydriasis and cycloplegia for refraction: Instill 1 drop of 2% solution immediately before the procedure; repeat at 10-minute intervals as needed
Uveitis: Instill 1 drop of 2% solution 2-3 times/day
Adults:
Mydriasis and cycloplegia for refraction: Instill 1-2 drops of 2% solution or 1 drop of 5% solution before the procedure; repeat at 5- to 10-minute intervals as needed
Uveitis: Instill 1-2 drops of either 2% or 5% solution 2-3 times/day up to every 3-4 hours as needed
Administration Ophthalmic: Finger pressure should be applied to lacrimal sac for 1-2 minutes after instillation to decrease risk of absorption and systemic effects
Dosage Forms Excipient information presented when available (limited, particularly for generics); consult specific product labeling.
Solution, ophthalmic, as hydrobromide:
Isopto® Homatropine: 2% (5 mL); 5% (5 mL, 15 mL) [contains benzalkonium chloride]

◆ **Homatropine Hydrobromide** see Homatropine on page 678

◆ **Horse Antihuman Thymocyte Gamma Globulin** see Antithymocyte Globulin (Equine) on page 118

◆ **H.P. Acthar® Gel** see Corticotropin on page 359

◆ **HPMPC** see Cidofovir on page 307

◆ **HPV2** see Papillomavirus (Types 16, 18) Vaccine (Human, Recombinant) on page 1058

◆ **HPV4** see Papillomavirus (Types 6, 11, 16, 18) Recombinant Vaccine on page 1057

◆ **HPV Vaccine** see Papillomavirus (Types 6, 11, 16, 18) Recombinant Vaccine on page 1057

◆ **HPV Vaccine** see Papillomavirus (Types 16, 18) Vaccine (Human, Recombinant) on page 1058

◆ **HRIG** see Rabies Immune Globulin (Human) on page 1198

◆ **Humalog®** see Insulin Lispro on page 744

◆ **Humalog® Mix 25 (Can)** see Insulin Lispro Protamine and Insulin Lispro on page 745

◆ **Humalog® Mix 50/50™** see Insulin Lispro Protamine and Insulin Lispro on page 745

◆ **Humalog® Mix 75/25™** see Insulin Lispro Protamine and Insulin Lispro on page 745

◆ **Human Albumin Grifols®** see Albumin on page 55

◆ **Human Antitumor Necrosis Factor Alpha** see Adalimumab on page 48

◆ **Human Diploid Cell Cultures Rabies Vaccine** see Rabies Virus Vaccine on page 1199

◆ **Human Growth Hormone** see Somatropin on page 1281

◆ **Human Papillomavirus Vaccine** see Papillomavirus (Types 6, 11, 16, 18) Recombinant Vaccine on page 1057

◆ **Human Papillomavirus Vaccine** see Papillomavirus (Types 16, 18) Vaccine (Human, Recombinant) on page 1058

◆ **Human Rotavirus Vaccine, Attenuated (HRV)** see Rotavirus Vaccine on page 1237

◆ **Humate-P®** see Antihemophilic Factor / von Willebrand Factor Complex (Human) on page 114

◆ **Humatin® [DSC]** see Paromomycin on page 1063

◆ **Humatin® (Can)** see Paromomycin on page 1063

◆ **Humatrope®** see Somatropin on page 1281

◆ **Humibid® Maximum Strength [OTC]** see GuaiFENesin on page 656

◆ **Humira®** see Adalimumab on page 48

◆ **Humist® [OTC]** see Sodium Chloride on page 1270

◆ **Humist® for Kids [OTC]** see Sodium Chloride on page 1270

◆ **Humulin® 20/80 (Can)** see Insulin NPH and Insulin Regular on page 747

◆ **Humulin® 50/50 [DSC]** see Insulin NPH and Insulin Regular on page 747

◆ **Humulin® 70/30** see Insulin NPH and Insulin Regular on page 747

◆ **Humulin® N** see Insulin NPH on page 746

◆ **Humulin® R** see Insulin Regular on page 748

◆ **Humulin® R U-500** see Insulin Regular on page 748

◆ **Hurricaine® [OTC]** see Benzocaine on page 182

Hyaluronidase (hye al yoor ON i dase)

Medication Safety Issues
Sound-alike/look-alike issues:
Wydase may be confused with Lidex®, Wyamine®
Related Information
Extravasation Treatment on page 1522
U.S. Brand Names Amphadase™; Hydase™ [DSC]; Hylenex™; Vitrase®
Therapeutic Category Antidote, Extravasation
Generic Available No
Use Increase the dispersion and absorption of other drugs; increase rate of absorption of parenteral fluids given by hypodermoclysis; adjunct in subcutaneous urography for improving resorption of radiopaque agents; management of I.V. extravasations
Pregnancy Risk Factor C
Pregnancy Considerations There are no adequate or well-controlled studies in pregnant women; use only if clearly needed. Administration during labor did not cause any increase in blood loss or differences in cervical trauma. It is not known whether it affects the fetus if used during labor.
Lactation Excretion in breast milk unknown/use caution
Contraindications Hypersensitivity to hyaluronidase or any component; do not inject in or around infected, inflamed, or cancerous areas; do not use to reduce the swelling of bites or stings; do not apply directly to the cornea; do not administer intravenously (enzyme is rapidly inactivated)
Warnings Drug infiltrates in which hyaluronidase is **not** the extravasation management of choice include dopamine and alpha agonists
Precautions Hypersensitivity reactions may occur; a preliminary intradermal skin test should be performed utilizing 0.02 mL of a 150 units/mL solution. Discontinue hyaluronidase if sensitization occurs.
Adverse Reactions
Cardiovascular: Tachycardia, hypotension
Central nervous system: Dizziness, chills
Dermatologic: Urticaria, erythema, angioedema
Gastrointestinal: Nausea, vomiting
Local: Edema
Miscellaneous: Anaphylactic-like reaction (rare)

◄ **Drug Interactions**

Avoid Concomitant Use There are no known interactions where it is recommended to avoid concomitant use.

Increased Effect/Toxicity There are no known significant interactions involving an increase in effect.

Decreased Effect There are no known significant interactions involving a decrease in effect.

Stability Hyaluronidase is incompatible with furosemide, benzodiazepines and phenytoin.
Amphadase™, Hydase™, Hylenex™: Store in refrigerator; do not freeze
Vitrase®: Store unopened vial in refrigerator; after reconstitution, stable for 6 hours at room temperature.

Mechanism of Action Modifies the permeability of connective tissue through hydrolysis of hyaluronic acid, one of the chief ingredients of tissue cement which offers resistance to diffusion of liquids through tissues; hyaluronidase increases both the distribution and absorption of locally injected substances

Pharmacodynamics

Onset of action by the SubQ or intradermal routes for the treatment of extravasation: Immediate
Duration: 24-48 hours

Usual Dosage

Management of I.V. extravasation: SubQ, intradermal (see Administration): Infants and Children: Inject five 0.2 mL injections of a solution (made by diluting 0.1 mL of the 150 unit/mL solution in 0.9 mL NS to yield 15 units/mL) into the extravasation site at the leading edge. **Note:** Some centers utilize a 150 units/mL hyaluronidase solution and, without further dilution, administer 0.2 mL injections subcutaneously or intradermally into the extravasation site at the leading edge as soon as possible (within 1 hour) after extravasation is recognized.

Absorption and dispersion of drugs: I.M., SubQ: Adults: 150 units is added to the vehicle containing the drug

Subcutaneous urography: Children and Adults: SubQ: 75 units over each scapula followed by injection of contrast medium at the same site; patient should be in the prone position during drug administration

Subcutaneous fluid administration: Hypodermoclysis: Infants and Children: SubQ: 15 units is added to each 100 mL of I.V. fluid to be administered or 150 units is injected under skin, followed by subcutaneous isotonic fluid administration at a rate appropriate for age, weight, and clinical condition of the patient; 150 units facilitates absorption of >1000 mL of solution

Premature Infants and Neonates: Volume of a single clysis should not exceed 25 mL/kg and the rate of administration should not exceed 2 mL/minute

Children <3 years (Amphadase™; Hydase™; Vitrase®): Volume of a single clysis should not exceed 200 mL

Children ≥3 years and Adults: Rate and volume of a single clysis should not exceed those used for infusion of I.V. fluids

Administration Parenteral: Treatment of extravasation: Infiltrate area of extravasation with multiple small injections of a diluted solution (see Usual Dosage); use 27- or 30-gauge needles and change needle between each skin entry to prevent bacterial contamination and minimize pain; do not administer I.V.

Monitoring Parameters Observe appearance of lesion for induration, swelling, discoloration, blanching, and blister formation every 15 minutes for ~2 hours

Patient Information Notify physician if pain, redness, swelling, unusual skin rash at or around injection site, swelling of mouth or lips; difficulty breathing or sudden dizziness occurs.

Dosage Forms Excipient information presented when available (limited, particularly for generics); consult specific product labeling. [DSC] = Discontinued product

Injection, powder for reconstitution:
Vitrase®: 6200 units [ovine derived; contains lactose]
Injection, solution:
Amphadase™: 150 units/mL (1 mL) [bovine derived; contains edetate disodium 1 mg, thimerosal ≤0.1 mg]
Injection, solution [preservative free]:
Hydase™: 150 units/mL (1 mL) [bovine derived; contains edetate disodium 1 mg] [DSC]
Hylenex™: 150 units/mL (1 mL, 2 mL) [recombinant; contains human albumin and edetate disodium]
Vitrase®: 200 units/mL (2 mL) [ovine derived; contains lactose]

References

Flemmer L and Chan JS, "A Pediatric Protocol for Management of Extravasation Injuries," Pediatr Nurs, 1993, 19(4):355-8, 424.
MacCara ME, "Extravasation: A Hazard of Intravenous Therapy," Drug Intell Clin Pharm, 1983, 17(10):713-7.
Raszka WV, Keuser TK, Smith FR, et al, "The Use of Hyaluronidase in the Treatment of Intravenous Extravasation Injuries," J Perinatol, 1990, 10(2):146-9.
Zenk KE, Dungy CI, and Greene GR, "Nafcillin Extravasation Injury: Use of Hyaluronidase as an Antidote," Am J Dis Child, 1981, 135 (12):1113-4.
Zenk KE, "Hyaluronidase: An Antidote for Intravenous Extravasations," CSHP Voice, 1981, 66-8.
Zenk KE, "Management of Intravenous Extravasations," Infusion, 1981, 5:77-9.

♦ **Hycamptamine** see Topotecan on page 1363

♦ **Hycamtin®** see Topotecan on page 1363

♦ **hycet™** see Hydrocodone and Acetaminophen on page 684

♦ **Hycort™ (Can)** see Hydrocortisone on page 685

♦ **Hydase™ [DSC]** see Hyaluronidase on page 679

♦ **Hydeltra T.B.A.® (Can)** see PrednisoLONE on page 1148

♦ **Hyderm (Can)** see Hydrocortisone on page 685

HydrALAZINE (hye DRAL a zeen)

Medication Safety Issues
Sound-alike/look-alike issues:
HydrALAZINE may be confused with hydrOXYzine

Related Information
Antihypertensive Agents by Class on page 1481

Canadian Brand Names Apo-Hydralazine®; Apresoline®; Novo-Hylazin; Nu-Hydral

Therapeutic Category Antihypertensive Agent; Vasodilator

Generic Available Yes

Use Management of moderate to severe hypertension, CHF, hypertension secondary to pre-eclampsia/eclampsia, primary pulmonary hypertension

Pregnancy Risk Factor C

Pregnancy Considerations Crosses the placenta. One report of fetal arrhythmia; transient neonatal thrombocytopenia and fetal distress reported following late 3rd trimester use. A large amount of clinical experience in the use of this drug for management of hypertension during pregnancy is available. Available evidence suggests safe use during pregnancy.

Lactation Enters breast milk/compatible

Breast-Feeding Considerations Crosses into breast milk in extremely small amounts. Available evidence suggests safe use during breast-feeding. AAP considers **compatible** with breast-feeding.

Contraindications Hypersensitivity to hydralazine or any component; dissecting aortic aneurysm, mitral valve rheumatic heart disease, coronary artery disease

Warnings Monitor blood pressure closely with I.V. use; modify dosage in patients with severe renal impairment

Precautions Discontinue hydralazine in patients who develop SLE-like syndrome or positive ANA; use with caution in patients with severe renal disease or cerebral vascular accidents

Adverse Reactions

Cardiovascular: Palpitations, flushing, tachycardia, edema, orthostatic hypotension (rare)

Central nervous system: Malaise, fever, headache, dizziness

Dermatologic: Rash

Gastrointestinal: Anorexia, nausea, vomiting, diarrhea

Neuromuscular & skeletal: Arthralgias, weakness, pyridoxine deficiency-induced peripheral neuropathy (paresthesia, numbness)

Miscellaneous: Positive ANA, positive LE cells, SLE-like syndrome

Drug Interactions

Metabolism/Transport Effects Inhibits CYP3A4 (weak)

Avoid Concomitant Use There are no known interactions where it is recommended to avoid concomitant use.

Increased Effect/Toxicity

HydrALAZINE may increase the levels/effects of: Amifostine; Antihypertensives; Hypotensive Agents; RiTUXimab

The levels/effects of HydrALAZINE may be increased by: Diazoxide; Herbs (Hypotensive Properties); MAO Inhibitors; Pentoxifylline; Phosphodiesterase 5 Inhibitors; Prostacyclin Analogues

Decreased Effect

The levels/effects of HydrALAZINE may be decreased by: Herbs (Hypertensive Properties); Methylphenidate; Nonsteroidal Anti-Inflammatory Agents; Yohimbine

Food Interactions Avoid natural licorice (causes sodium and water retention and increases potassium loss); long-term use of hydralazine may cause pyridoxine deficiency resulting in numbness, tingling, and paresthesias; if symptoms develop, pyridoxine supplements may be needed

Stability Changes color after contact with a metal filter; do not store intact ampuls in refrigerator

Mechanism of Action Direct vasodilation of arterioles (with little effect on veins) which results in decreased systemic resistance

Pharmacodynamics

Onset of action:

Oral: 20-30 minutes

I.V.: 5-20 minutes

Duration:

Oral: 2-4 hours

I.V.: 2-6 hours

Pharmacokinetics (Adult data unless noted)

Distribution: Crosses placenta; appears in breast milk

Protein-binding: 85% to 90%

Metabolism: Acetylated in the liver

Bioavailability: 30% to 50%; large first-pass effect orally

Half-life, adults: 2-8 hours; half-life varies with genetically determined acetylation rates

Elimination: 14% excreted unchanged in urine

Usual Dosage

Infants and Children:

Oral: Initial: 0.75-1 mg/kg/day in 2-4 divided doses, not to exceed 25 mg/dose; increase over 3-4 weeks to maximum of 5 mg/kg/day in infants and 7.5 mg/kg/day in children, given in 2-4 divided doses; maximum daily dose: 200 mg/day

I.M., I.V.: Initial: 0.1-0.2 mg/kg/dose (not to exceed 20 mg) every 4-6 hours as needed; up to 1.7-3.5 mg/kg/day divided in 4-6 doses

Adults:

Oral: Initial: 10 mg 4 times/day, increase by 10-25 mg/dose every 2-5 days to maximum of 300 mg/day; usual dosage range for hypertension (JNC 7): 25-100 mg/day in 2 divided doses

I.M., I.V.: Hypertension: Initial: 10-20 mg/dose every 4-6 hours as needed, may increase to 40 mg/dose

I.M., I.V.: Pre-eclampsia/eclampsia: 5 mg/dose then 5-10 mg every 20-30 minutes as needed

Dosing interval in renal impairment:

Cl_{cr} 10-50 mL/minute: Administer every 8 hours

Cl_{cr} <10 mL/minute: Administer every 8-16 hours in fast acetylators and every 12-24 hours in slow acetylators

Administration

Oral: Administer with food

Parenteral: I.V.: Do not exceed rate of 0.2 mg/kg/minute; maximum concentration for I.V. use: 20 mg/mL

Monitoring Parameters Heart rate, blood pressure, ANA titer

Patient Information Limit alcohol; notify physician if flu-like symptoms occur

Nursing Implications I.V. use: Monitor blood pressure closely

Additional Information Slow acetylators, patients with decreased renal function and patients receiving >200 mg/day (chronically) are at higher risk for SLE. Titrate dosage to patient's response. Usually administered with diuretic and a beta-blocker to counteract hydralazine's side effects of sodium and water retention and reflex tachycardia.

Dosage Forms Excipient information presented when available (limited, particularly for generics); consult specific product labeling.

Injection, solution, as hydrochloride: 20 mg/mL (1 mL)

Tablet, as hydrochloride: 10 mg, 25 mg, 50 mg, 100 mg

Extemporaneous Preparations

A flavored syrup (1.25 mg/mL) has been made using seventy-five hydralazine hydrochloride 50 mg tablets, dissolved in 250 mL of distilled water with 2250 g of Lycasin® (75% w/w maltitol syrup vehicle); edetate disodium 3 g and sodium saccharin 3 g dissolved in 50 mL distilled water was added; solution was preserved with 30 mL of a solution containing methylparaben 10% (w/v) and propylparaben 2% (w/v) in propylene glycol; flavored with 3 mL orange flavoring; qsad to 3 L with distilled water and then pH adjusted to pH of 3.7 using glacial acetic acid; measured stability was 5 days at room temperature (25°C); less than 2% loss of hydralazine occurred at 2 weeks when syrup was stored at 5°C (Alexander, 1993)

A 4 mg/mL oral liquid preparation made from tablets was **not** stable for very long; preparation made in cherry syrup was not even stable for 1 day; preparation made in a 1:1 mixture of Ora-Sweet® and Ora-Plus® was stable for only 1 day under refrigeration (5°C) and not even 1 day at room temperature (25°C); preparation made in a 1:1 mixture of Ora-Sweet® SF and Ora-Plus® was stable for only 2 days under refrigeration (5°C), but not even 1 day at room temperature (25°C) (Allen, 1998).

Alexander KS, Pudipeddi M, and Parker GA, "Stability of Hydralazine Hydrochloride Syrup Compounded From Tablets," *Am J Hosp Pharm*, 1993, 50(4):683-6.

Allen LV and Erickson MA, "Stability of Alprazolam, Chloroquine Phosphate, Cisapride, Enalapril Maleate, and Hydralazine Hydrochloride in Extemporaneously Compounded Oral Liquids," *Am J Health Syst Pharm*, 1998, 55(18):1915-20.

References

Chobanian AV, Bakris GL, Black HR, et al, "The Seventh Report of the Joint National Committee on Prevention, Detection, Evaluation, and Treatment of High Blood Pressure: The JNC 7 report," *JAMA*, 2003, 289(19):2560-72.

◆ **Hydralazine Hydrochloride** *see* HydrALAZINE
on page 680

◆ **Hydramine [OTC] [DSC]** *see* DiphenhydrAMINE *on page 448*

◆ **Hydrated Chloral** *see* Chloral Hydrate *on page 286*

◆ **Hydrea®** *see* Hydroxyurea *on page 695*

◆ **Hydrisalic™ [OTC]** *see* Salicylic Acid *on page 1241*

Hydrochlorothiazide (hye droe klor oh THYE a zide)

Medication Safety Issues
Sound-alike/look-alike issues:
Esidrix may be confused with Lasix®
HCTZ is an error-prone abbreviation (mistaken as hydrocortisone)
Hydrochlorothiazide may be confused with hydrocortisone, hydroflumethiazide, Viskazide®
Microzide™ may be confused with Maxzide®, Micronase®

International issues:
Microzide™ may be confused with Nitrobide® which is a brand name for isosorbide dinitrate in Japan
Microzide™ may be confused with Mikrozid® which is a brand name for ethanol/propanol combination in Great Britain

Related Information
Antihypertensive Agents by Class *on page 1481*

U.S. Brand Names Microzide®

Canadian Brand Names Apo-Hydro®; Bio-Hydrochlorothiazide; Dom-Hydrochlorothiazide; Novo-Hydrazide; Nu-Hydro; PMS-Hydrochlorothiazide

Therapeutic Category Antihypertensive Agent; Diuretic, Thiazide

Generic Available Yes

Use Management of mild to moderate hypertension; treatment of edema in CHF and nephrotic syndrome

Pregnancy Risk Factor B

Pregnancy Considerations Although there are no adequate and well-controlled studies using hydrochlorothiazide in pregnancy, thiazide diuretics may cause an increased risk of congenital defects. Hypoglycemia, hypokalemia, hyponatremia, jaundice, and thrombocytopenia are also reported as possible complications in the fetus or newborn.

Lactation Enters breast milk/use caution (AAP rates "compatible")

Contraindications Hypersensitivity to hydrochlorothiazide or any component; cross-sensitivity with other thiazides or sulfonamides; anuria

Warnings Hypokalemia may occur, particularly with aggressive diuresis, when severe cirrhosis is present, or after prolonged therapy. Other electrolyte disorders including hyponatremia, hypomagnesemia, and hypochloremic metabolic alkalosis may occur; monitor electrolytes. Has been reported to activate or exacerbate SLE.

Oral solution contains sodium benzoate; benzoic acid (benzoate) is a metabolite of benzyl alcohol; large amounts of benzyl alcohol (≥99 mg/kg/day) have been associated with a potentially fatal toxicity ("gasping syndrome") in neonates; *in vitro* and animal studies have shown that benzoate displaces bilirubin from protein binding sites; avoid use in neonates

Precautions Use with caution in patients with severe renal disease (ineffective) and may precipitate azotemia; use with caution in patients with impaired hepatic function, moderate-to-high cholesterol concentrations, and in patients with high triglycerides. Chemical similarities are present among sulfonamides, sulfonylureas, carbonic anhydrase inhibitors, thiazides, and loop diuretics (except ethacrynic acid). A risk of cross-reactivity exists in patients with allergies to any of these compounds

Adverse Reactions
Cardiovascular: Hypotension
Central nervous system: Drowsiness, vertigo, headache
Dermatologic: Photosensitivity
Endocrine & metabolic: Hypokalemia, hyperglycemia, hypochloremic metabolic alkalosis, hyperlipidemia, hyperuricemia
Gastrointestinal: Nausea, vomiting, anorexia, diarrhea, cramping, pancreatitis
Hematologic: Aplastic anemia, hemolytic anemia, leukopenia, agranulocytosis, thrombocytopenia
Hepatic: Hepatitis, intrahepatic cholestasis
Neuromuscular & skeletal: Muscle weakness, paresthesia
Renal: Polyuria, prerenal azotemia

Drug Interactions
Avoid Concomitant Use
Avoid concomitant use of Hydrochlorothiazide with any of the following: Dofetilide

Increased Effect/Toxicity
Hydrochlorothiazide may increase the levels/effects of: ACE Inhibitors; Allopurinol; Amifostine; Antihypertensives; Calcitriol; Calcium Salts; CarBAMazepine; Dofetilide; Hypotensive Agents; Lithium; OXcarbazepine; RiTUXimab

The levels/effects of Hydrochlorothiazide may be increased by: Alcohol (Ethyl); Analgesics (Opioid); Barbiturates; Corticosteroids (Orally Inhaled); Corticosteroids (Systemic); Herbs (Hypotensive Properties); MAO Inhibitors; Pentoxifylline; Phosphodiesterase 5 Inhibitors; Prostacyclin Analogues

Decreased Effect
Hydrochlorothiazide may decrease the levels/effects of: Antidiabetic Agents

The levels/effects of Hydrochlorothiazide may be decreased by: Bile Acid Sequestrants; Herbs (Hypertensive Properties); Methylphenidate; Nonsteroidal Anti-Inflammatory Agents; Yohimbine

Food Interactions Avoid natural licorice (causes sodium and water retention and increases potassium loss); may need to decrease sodium and calcium and increase potassium, zinc, magnesium, and riboflavin in diet

Mechanism of Action Inhibits sodium reabsorption in the distal tubules causing increased excretion of sodium and water as well as potassium, hydrogen, magnesium, phosphate, calcium, and bicarbonate ions

Pharmacodynamics
Onset of diuretic action: Oral: Within 2 hours
Maximum effect: Within 3-6 hours
Duration: 6-12 hours

Pharmacokinetics (Adult data unless noted)
Absorption: Oral: ~60% to 80%
Distribution: Breast milk to plasma ratio: 0.25
Half-life: 5.6-14.8 hours
Elimination: Unchanged in urine

Usual Dosage Oral:
Edema:
Neonates and Infants <6 months: 2-3.3 mg/kg/day in 2 divided doses; maximum dose: 37.5 mg/day
Infants >6 months and Children: 2 mg/kg/day in 2 divided doses; maximum dose: 200 mg/day
Adults: 25-100 mg/day in 1-2 doses; maximum dose: 200 mg/day
Hypertension:
Infants and Children: Initial: 1 mg/kg/day once daily; may increase to maximum 3 mg/kg/day; not to exceed 50 mg/day
Adults: 12.5-50 mg once daily; minimal increase in response and more electrolyte disturbances are seen with doses >50 mg/day

Dosage adjustment in renal impairment:
Cl$_{cr}$ <25-50 mL/minute: Usually not effective
Cl$_{cr}$ <10 mL/minute: Avoid use

Administration Oral: Administer with food or milk

Monitoring Parameters Serum electrolytes, BUN, creatinine, blood pressure, fluid balance, body weight

Patient Information May cause photosensitivity reactions (eg, exposure to sunlight may cause severe sunburn, skin rash, redness, or itching); avoid exposure to sunlight and artificial light sources (sunlamps, tanning booth/bed); wear protective clothing, wide-brimmed hats, sunglasses, and lip sunscreen (SPF ≥15); use a sunscreen [broad-spectrum sunscreen or physical sunscreen (preferred) or sunblock with SPF ≥15]; contact physician if reaction occurs.

Dosage Forms Excipient information presented when available (limited, particularly for generics); consult specific product labeling.
Capsule, oral: 12.5 mg
Microzide®: 12.5 mg
Tablet, oral: 12.5 mg, 25 mg, 50 mg

References
Chobanian AV, Bakris GL, Black HR, et al, "The Seventh Report of the Joint National Committee on Prevention, Detection, Evaluation, and Treatment of High Blood Pressure: The JNC 7 Report," *JAMA*, 2003, 289(19):2560-72.
National High Blood Pressure Education Program Working Group on High Blood Pressure in Children and Adolescents, "The Fourth Report on the Diagnosis, Evaluation, and Treatment of High Blood Pressure in Children and Adolescents," *Pediatrics*, 2004, 114(2 Suppl):555-76.
van der Vorst MM, Kist JE, van der Heijden AJ, et al, "Diuretics in Pediatrics: Current Knowledge and Future Prospects," *Paediatr Drugs*, 2006, 8(4):245-64.

Hydrochlorothiazide and Spironolactone
(hye droe klor oh THYE a zide & speer on oh LAK tone)

Medication Safety Issues
Sound-alike/look-alike issues:
Aldactazide® may be confused with Aldactone®

U.S. Brand Names Aldactazide®

Canadian Brand Names Aldactazide 25®; Aldactazide 50®; Novo-Spirozine

Therapeutic Category Antihypertensive Agent, Combination; Diuretic, Combination

Generic Available Yes

Use Management of mild to moderate hypertension; treatment of edema in CHF and nephrotic syndrome

Pregnancy Risk Factor C

Pregnancy Considerations See individual agents.

Lactation Enters breast milk/use caution

Contraindications Hypersensitivity to hydrochlorothiazide, spironolactone, or any component; cross-sensitivity with other thiazides or sulfonamides; anuria, hyperkalemia, acute or significant renal impairment, acute or severe hepatic failure

Warnings This fixed combination is not indicated for initial therapy of hypertension or edema **[U.S. Boxed Warning]**; therapy requires titration to the individual patient; if dosage so determined represents this fixed combination, its use may be more convenient; use with caution in impaired hepatic function, electrolyte changes may precipitate hepatic encephalopathy; spironolactone has been shown to be a tumorigen in chronic toxicity animal studies **[U.S. Boxed Warning]**. May exacerbation systemic lupus erythematosus.

Precautions Concomitant administration of potassium-sparing diuretics (eg, amiloride and triamterene) and ACE inhibitors or NSAIDs has been associated with severe hyperkalemia; may cause transient elevation of BUN, possibly due to a concentration effect; sustained elevations should be evaluated; thiazides may cause hyperuricemia or precipitate acute gout; use thiazides with caution in patients with prediabetes or diabetes mellitus; may see a change in glucose control

Adverse Reactions See individual agents.

Drug Interactions

Avoid Concomitant Use
Avoid concomitant use of Hydrochlorothiazide and Spironolactone with any of the following: Dofetilide

Increased Effect/Toxicity
Hydrochlorothiazide and Spironolactone may increase the levels/effects of: ACE Inhibitors; Allopurinol; Amifostine; Ammonium Chloride; Antihypertensives; Calcitriol; Calcium Salts; CarBAMazepine; Cardiac Glycosides; Digoxin; Dofetilide; Hypotensive Agents; Lithium; Neuromuscular-Blocking Agents (Nondepolarizing); OXcarbazepine; RiTUXimab

The levels/effects of Hydrochlorothiazide and Spironolactone may be increased by: Alcohol (Ethyl); Analgesics (Opioid); Angiotensin II Receptor Blockers; Barbiturates; Corticosteroids (Orally Inhaled); Corticosteroids (Systemic); Drospirenone; Eplerenone; Herbs (Hypotensive Properties); MAO Inhibitors; Nonsteroidal Anti-Inflammatory Agents; Pentoxifylline; Phosphodiesterase 5 Inhibitors; Potassium Salts; Prostacyclin Analogues; Tolvaptan

Decreased Effect
Hydrochlorothiazide and Spironolactone may decrease the levels/effects of: Alpha-/Beta-Agonists; Antidiabetic Agents; Cardiac Glycosides; Mitotane; QuiNIDine

The levels/effects of Hydrochlorothiazide and Spironolactone may be decreased by: Bile Acid Sequestrants; Herbs (Hypertensive Properties); Methylphenidate; Nonsteroidal Anti-Inflammatory Agents; Yohimbine

Food Interactions Avoid food with high potassium content, natural licorice (causes sodium and water retention and increases potassium loss), and salt substitutes

Usual Dosage Oral: As the product is in a fixed combination of equal mg doses, the following dosages represent mg of either spironolactone **or** hydrochlorothiazide

Children: 1.5-3 mg/kg/day in 2-4 divided doses; maximum daily dosage: 200 mg

Adults: 12.5-200 mg in 1-2 divided doses

Administration Oral: Administer in the morning; administer the last dose of multiple doses before 6 PM unless instructed otherwise; administer with food or milk

Monitoring Parameters Blood pressure, serum electrolytes, renal function

Test Interactions Spironolactone may interfere with plasma and urinary cortisol levels and the radioimmunoassay for digoxin

Dosage Forms Excipient information presented when available (limited, particularly for generics); consult specific product labeling.
Tablet: Hydrochlorothiazide 25 mg and spironolactone 25 mg
Aldactazide®:
25/25: Hydrochlorothiazide 25 mg and spironolactone 25 mg
50/50: Hydrochlorothiazide 50 mg and spironolactone 50 mg

Extemporaneous Preparations A 5 mg/mL oral suspension may be compounded by crushing twenty-four 25 mg (spironolactone/HCTZ) Aldactazide® tablets; add geometric amounts of a 1:1 mixture of Ora-Sweet® and Ora-Plus®, or Ora-Sweet® SF and Ora-Plus®, or cherry syrup alone to a final volume of 120 mL; shake well, refrigerate; stable 60 days
Allen LV and Erickson MA, "Stability of Labetalol Hydrochloride, Metoprolol Tartrate, Verapamil Hydrochloride, and Spironolactone With Hydrochlorothiazide in Extemporaneously Compounded Oral Liquids," *Am J Health Syst Pharm*, 1996, 53(19):2304-9.

◆ **Hydrocil® Instant [OTC]** *see* Psyllium *on page 1185*

Hydrocodone and Acetaminophen
(hye droe KOE done & a seet a MIN oh fen)

Medication Safety Issues
Sound-alike/look-alike issues:
Lorcet® may be confused with Fioricet®
Lortab® may be confused with Cortef®, Lorabid®, Luride®
Vicodin® may be confused with Hycodan®, Hycomine®, Indocin®, Uridon®
Zydone® may be confused with Vytone®

High alert medication: The Institute for Safe Medication Practices (ISMP) includes this medication among its list of drug classes which have a heightened risk of causing significant patient harm when used in error.

Duplicate therapy issues: This product contains acetaminophen, which may be a component of other combination products. Do not exceed the maximum recommended daily dose of acetaminophen.

Related Information
Opioid Analgesics Comparison *on page 1510*

U.S. Brand Names Co-Gesic® [DSC]; hycet™; Lorcet® 10/650; Lorcet® Plus; Lortab®; Margesic® H; Maxidone®; Norco®; Stagesic™; Vicodin®; Vicodin® ES; Vicodin® HP; Xodol® 10/300; Xodol® 5/300; Xodol® 7.5/300; Zamicet™; Zydone®

Therapeutic Category Analgesic, Narcotic; Antitussive; Cough Preparation

Generic Available Yes

Use Relief of moderate to severe pain; antitussive (hydrocodone)

Restrictions C-III

Pregnancy Risk Factor C

Pregnancy Considerations Animal reproduction studies have not been conducted with this combination product. Use of opioids during pregnancy may produce physical dependence in the neonate; respiratory depression may occur in the newborn if opioids are used prior to delivery (especially high doses).

Lactation Enters breast milk/not recommended

Breast-Feeding Considerations Acetaminophen and hydrocodone are excreted in breast milk. The manufacturers recommend discontinuing the medication or to discontinue nursing during therapy. Also refer to Acetaminophen monograph.

Contraindications Hypersensitivity to hydrocodone, acetaminophen, or any component; CNS depression; severe respiratory depression

Warnings Abrupt discontinuation after prolonged use may result in withdrawal symptoms or seizures

Precautions Use with caution in patients with hypersensitivity reactions to other phenanthrene derivative opioid agonists (morphine, codeine, hydromorphone, oxycodone, oxymorphone, levorphanol)

Adverse Reactions
Cardiovascular: Hypotension, bradycardia, peripheral vasodilation
Central nervous system: CNS depression, drowsiness, dizziness, sedation, intracranial pressure elevated
Endocrine & metabolic: Antidiuretic hormone release
Gastrointestinal: Nausea, vomiting, constipation, biliary tract spasm
Genitourinary: Urinary tract spasm
Ocular: Miosis
Respiratory: Respiratory depression

Miscellaneous: Histamine release, physical and psychological dependence with prolonged use

Drug Interactions
Metabolism/Transport Effects
Hydrocodone: **Substrate** (minor) of CYP2D6, 3A
Acetaminophen: **Substrate** (minor) of CYP1A2, 2A6, 2C9, 2D6, 2E1, 3A4; **Inhibits** CYP3A4 (weak)

Avoid Concomitant Use There are no known interactions where it is recommended to avoid concomitant use.

Increased Effect/Toxicity
Hydrocodone and Acetaminophen may increase the levels/effects of: Alcohol (Ethyl); Alvimopan; CNS Depressants; Desmopressin; Selective Serotonin Reuptake Inhibitors; Thiazide Diuretics; Vitamin K Antagonists

The levels/effects of Hydrocodone and Acetaminophen may be increased by: Amphetamines; Antipsychotic Agents (Phenothiazines); Imatinib; Isoniazid; MAO Inhibitors; Succinylcholine

Decreased Effect
Hydrocodone and Acetaminophen may decrease the levels/effects of: Pegvisomant

The levels/effects of Hydrocodone and Acetaminophen may be decreased by: Ammonium Chloride; Anticonvulsants (Hydantoin); Barbiturates; CarBAMazepine; Cholestyramine Resin; Mixed Agonist / Antagonist Opioids; Peginterferon Alfa-2b; QuiNIDine

Food Interactions Rate of absorption of acetaminophen may be decreased when given with food high in carbohydrates

Mechanism of Action Inhibits the synthesis of prostaglandins in the CNS and peripherally blocks pain impulse generation; produces antipyresis from inhibition of hypothalamic heat-regulating center

Pharmacodynamics Narcotic analgesia: Oral:
Onset of action: Within 10-20 minutes
Duration: 3-6 hours

Usual Dosage Oral:
Antitussive (doses based on hydrocodone):
Children: 0.6 mg/kg/day or 20 mg/m^2/day divided in 3-4 doses/day
<2 years: Do not exceed 1.25 mg/single dose
2-12 years: Do not exceed 5 mg/single dose
>12 years: Do not exceed 10 mg/single dose

Analgesic: **Doses should be titrated to appropriate analgesic effect**
Children: Dose has not been well established
Adults: 1-2 tablets or capsules every 4-6 hours as needed
AHCPR dosing guidelines (doses based on hydrocodone): Opioid naive patients: (See Carr, 1992 and Jacox, 1994)
Children and Adults <50 kg: Moderate to severe pain: Usual initial dose: 0.2 mg/kg every 3-4 hours
Children and Adults ≥50 kg: Moderate to severe pain: Usual initial dose: 10 mg every 3-4 hours

Administration Oral: May administer with food or milk to decrease GI distress

Monitoring Parameters Pain relief, respiratory rate, blood pressure

Patient Information Avoid alcohol; may cause drowsiness and impair ability to perform activities requiring mental alertness or physical coordination; may be habit-forming; avoid abrupt discontinuation after prolonged use

Dosage Forms Excipient information presented when available (limited, particularly for generics); consult specific product labeling. [DSC] = Discontinued product

Capsule:

Margesic® H, Stagesic™: Hydrocodone bitartrate 5 mg and acetaminophen 500 mg

Elixir: Hydrocodone bitartrate 7.5 mg and acetaminophen 500 mg per 15 mL (480 mL)

Lortab®: Hydrocodone bitartrate 7.5 mg and acetaminophen 500 mg per 15 mL (480 mL) [contains ethanol 7%, propylene glycol; tropical fruit punch flavor]

Solution, oral: Hydrocodone bitartrate 7.5 mg and acetaminophen 500 mg per 15 mL (5 mL, 10 mL, 15 mL, 118 mL, 473 mL)

hycet™: Hydrocodone bitartrate 7.5 mg and acetaminophen 325 mg per 15 mL (473 mL) [contains ethanol 6.7%, propylene glycol; fruit flavor]

Zamicet™: Hydrocodone bitartrate 10 mg and acetaminophen 325 mg per 15 mL (473 mL) [contains ethanol 6.7%, propylene glycol; fruit flavor]

Tablet:

Hydrocodone bitartrate 2.5 mg and acetaminophen 500 mg

Hydrocodone bitartrate 5 mg and acetaminophen 325 mg

Hydrocodone bitartrate 5 mg and acetaminophen 500 mg

Hydrocodone bitartrate 7.5 mg and acetaminophen 325 mg

Hydrocodone bitartrate 7.5 mg and acetaminophen 500 mg

Hydrocodone bitartrate 7.5 mg and acetaminophen 650 mg

Hydrocodone bitartrate 7.5 mg and acetaminophen 750 mg

Hydrocodone bitartrate 10 mg and acetaminophen 325 mg

Hydrocodone bitartrate 10 mg and acetaminophen 500 mg

Hydrocodone bitartrate 10 mg and acetaminophen 650 mg

Hydrocodone bitartrate 10 mg and acetaminophen 660 mg

Hydrocodone bitartrate 10 mg and acetaminophen 750 mg

Co-Gesic® 5/500: Hydrocodone bitartrate 5 mg and acetaminophen 500 mg [DSC]

Lorcet® 10/650: Hydrocodone bitartrate 10 mg and acetaminophen 650 mg

Lorcet® Plus: Hydrocodone bitartrate 7.5 mg and acetaminophen 650 mg

Lortab®:

5/500: Hydrocodone bitartrate 5 mg and acetaminophen 500 mg

7.5/500: Hydrocodone bitartrate 7.5 mg and acetaminophen 500 mg

10/500: Hydrocodone bitartrate 10 mg and acetaminophen 500 mg

Maxidone®: Hydrocodone bitartrate 10 mg and acetaminophen 750 mg

Norco®:

Hydrocodone bitartrate 5 mg and acetaminophen 325 mg

Hydrocodone bitartrate 7.5 mg and acetaminophen 325 mg

Hydrocodone bitartrate 10 mg and acetaminophen 325 mg

Vicodin®: Hydrocodone bitartrate 5 mg and acetaminophen 500 mg

Vicodin® ES: Hydrocodone bitartrate 7.5 mg and acetaminophen 750 mg

Vicodin® HP: Hydrocodone bitartrate 10 mg and acetaminophen 660 mg

Xodol®:

5/300: Hydrocodone bitartrate 5 mg and acetaminophen 300 mg

7.5/300: Hydrocodone bitartrate 7.5 mg and acetaminophen 300 mg

10/300: Hydrocodone bitartrate 10 mg and acetaminophen 300 mg

Zydone®:

Hydrocodone bitartrate 5 mg and acetaminophen 400 mg

Hydrocodone bitartrate 7.5 mg and acetaminophen 400 mg

Hydrocodone bitartrate 10 mg and acetaminophen 400 mg

References

Carr D, Jacox A, Chapman CR, et al, "Clinical Practice Guideline Number 1: Acute Pain Management: Operative or Medical Procedures and Trauma," Rockville, Maryland: U.S. Department of Health and Human Services, Public Health Service, Agency for Health Care Policy and Research, AHCPR Publication No 92-0032, 1992.

Jacox A, Carr D, Payne R, et al, "Clinical Practice Guideline Number 9: Management of Cancer Pain," Rockville, Maryland: U.S. Department of Health and Human Services, Public Health Service, Agency for Health Care Policy and Research, AHCPR Publication No. 94-0592, 1994.

Hydrocortisone (hye droe KOR ti sone)

Medication Safety Issues

Sound-alike/look-alike issues:

Hydrocortisone may be confused with hydrocodone, hydroxychloroquine, hydrochlorothiazide

Anusol® may be confused with Anusol-HC®, Aplisol®, Aquasol®

Anusol-HC® may be confused with Anusol®

Cortef® may be confused with Coreg®, Lortab®

Cortizone® may be confused with cortisone

HCT (occasional abbreviation for hydrocortisone) is an error-prone abbreviation (mistaken as hydrochlorothiazide)

Hytone® may be confused with Vytone®

Proctocort® may be confused with ProctoCream®

ProctoCream® may be confused with Proctocort®

Solu-Cortef® may be confused with Solu-Medrol®

International issues:

Hytone® may be confused with Hysone® [Australia]

Nutracort® may be confused with Nitrocor® which is a brand name of nitroglycerin in Chile and Italy

Related Information

Corticosteroids *on page 1487*

U.S. Brand Names A-Hydrocort®; Anucort-HC®; Anusol-HC®; Anusol® HC-1 [OTC]; Aquanil™ HC [OTC]; Beta-HC®; Caldecort® [OTC]; Cetacort® [DSC]; Colocort®; Cortaid® Intensive Therapy [OTC]; Cortaid® Maximum Strength [OTC]; Cortaid® Sensitive Skin [OTC]; Cortef®; Cortenema®; Corticool® [OTC]; Cortifoam®; Cortizone-10® Maximum Strength Cooling Relief [OTC]; Cortizone-10® Maximum Strength Easy Relief [OTC]; Cortizone-10® Maximum Strength Intensive Healing Formula [OTC]; Cortizone-10® Maximum Strength [OTC]; Cortizone-10® Plus Maximum Strength [OTC]; Cortizone-10® Quick Shot [OTC] [DSC]; Dermarest® Dricort® [OTC]; Dermtex® HC [OTC]; Encort™; Hemril®-30; HYDRO-Rx; HydroZone Plus [OTC] [DSC]; Hytone® [DSC]; IvySoothe® [OTC]; Locoid Lipocream®; Locoid®; Nupercainal® Hydrocortisone Cream [OTC]; Nutracort®; Pandel®; Post Peel Healing Balm [OTC]; Preparation H® Hydrocortisone [OTC]; Procto-Kit™; Procto-Pak™; Proctocort®; ProctoCream® HC; Proctosert; Proctosol-HC®; Proctozone-HC™; Sarnol®-HC [OTC]; Solu-Cortef®; Summer's Eve® SpecialCare™ Medicated Anti-Itch Cream [OTC] [DSC]; Texacort®; Tucks® Anti-Itch [OTC]; U-Cort™; Westcort®

Canadian Brand Names Aquacort®; Cortamed®; Cortef®; Cortenema®; Cortifoam™; Emo-Cort®; Hycort™; Hyderm; HydroVal®; Locoid®; Prevex® HC; Sarna® HC; Solu-Cortef®; Westcort®

Therapeutic Category Adrenal Corticosteroid; Anti-inflammatory Agent; Anti-inflammatory Agent, Rectal; Antiasthmatic; Corticosteroid, Rectal; Corticosteroid, Systemic; Corticosteroid, Topical; Glucocorticoid

Generic Available Yes: Excludes acetate foam, gel as base, otic drops as base, probutate cream, sodium succinate injection

Use Management of adrenocortical insufficiency; relief of inflammation and pruritus associated with corticosteroid-responsive dermatoses; adjunctive treatment of ulcerative colitis; septic shock

Pregnancy Risk Factor C

Pregnancy Considerations Adverse events have been observed with corticosteroids in animal reproduction studies. Hydrocortisone crosses the placenta. Some studies have shown an association between first trimester systemic corticosteroid use and oral clefts; adverse events in the fetus/neonate have been noted in case reports following large doses of systemic corticosteroids during pregnancy. Topical products are not recommended for extensive use, in large quantities, or for long periods of time in pregnant women.

Lactation Enters breast milk/use caution

Breast-Feeding Considerations Corticosteroids are excreted in breast milk and endogenous hydrocortisone is also found in human milk; the effect of maternal hydrocortisone intake is not known.

Contraindications Hypersensitivity to hydrocortisone or any component (see Warnings); serious infections, except septic shock or tuberculous meningitis; viral, fungal, or tubercular skin lesions

Warnings Hypothalamic-pituitary-adrenal (HPA) suppression may occur; acute adrenal insufficiency (adrenal crisis) may occur with abrupt withdrawal after long-term therapy or with stress; withdrawal and discontinuation of corticosteroids should be done carefully; patients with HPA axis suppression may require doses of systemic glucocorticosteroids prior to, during, and after unusual stress (eg, surgery). Immunosuppression may occur; patients may be more susceptible to infections; avoid exposure to chickenpox and measles. Corticosteroids may activate latent opportunistic infections or exacerbate systemic fungal infections. May cause osteoporosis (at any age) or inhibition of bone growth in pediatric patients. Acute myopathy may occur with high doses, elevated IOP may occur (especially with prolonged use), and CNS effects (ranging from euphoria to psychosis) may occur. Rare cases of anaphylactoid reactions have been reported with corticosteroids.

Topical: Adverse systemic effects may occur when topical steroids are used in large areas of the body, denuded areas, for prolonged periods of time, with an occlusive dressing, and/or in infants and small children; infants and small children may be more susceptible to HPA axis suppression or other systemic toxicities due to larger skin surface area to body mass ratio; use with caution in pediatric patients.

Manufacturer supplied diluents for injection (eg, Solu-Cortef®) contain benzyl alcohol and topical aerosol spray and topical cream may contain benzyl alcohol which may cause allergic reactions in susceptible individuals; otic solution contains benzyl benzoate and oral suspension (see Additional Information) contains benzoic acid; benzoic acid (benzoate) is a metabolite of benzyl alcohol; large amounts of benzyl alcohol (≥99 mg/kg/day) have been associated with a potentially fatal toxicity ("gasping syndrome") in neonates; the "gasping syndrome" consists of metabolic acidosis, respiratory distress, gasping respirations, CNS dysfunction (including convulsions, intracranial hemorrhage), hypotension and cardiovascular collapse; avoid use of hydrocortisone products containing benzoic acid, benzyl alcohol, or benzyl benzoate in neonates; *in vitro* and animal studies have shown that benzoate displaces bilirubin from protein binding sites

Precautions Avoid using higher than recommended doses; suppression of HPA function, suppression of linear growth (ie, reduction of growth velocity), reduced bone mineral density, hypercorticism (Cushing's syndrome), hyperglycemia, or glucosuria may occur; titrate to lowest effective dose; these adverse effects (as well as intra-cranial hypertension) may also occur with topical use and have been reported in pediatric patients. Reduction in growth velocity may occur when corticosteroids are administered to pediatric patients by any route (monitor growth). Use with extreme caution in patients with respiratory tuberculosis, untreated systemic infections, or ocular herpes simplex; use with caution in patients with thyroid dysfunction, cirrhosis, nonspecific ulcerative colitis, hypertension, renal impairment, osteoporosis, thromboembolic tendencies, CHF, recent MI, convulsive disorders, myasthenia gravis, thrombophlebitis, peptic ulcer, diabetes, glaucoma, cataracts, or hepatic impairment. Prolonged use may result in cataracts or glaucoma.

Adverse Reactions

Cardiovascular: Hypertension, edema, CHF

Central nervous system: Euphoria, insomnia, headache, intracranial hypertension, vertigo, seizures, psychosis, pseudotumor cerebri, nervousness

Dermatologic: Acne, dermatitis, skin atrophy; topical use: eczema, folliculitis, pruritus, stinging, burning, dry skin, irritation, redness, hypertrichosis, hypopigmentation, maceration of the skin, striae, miliaria

Endocrine & metabolic: HPA suppression, hypokalemia, hyperglycemia, Cushing's syndrome, growth suppression, sodium and water retention

Gastrointestinal: Peptic ulcer, nausea, vomiting

Neuromuscular & skeletal: Muscle weakness, osteoporosis, bone mineral density decreased, fractures

Ocular: Cataracts, IOP increased, glaucoma

Miscellaneous: Immunosuppression, anaphylactoid reactions (rare)

Drug Interactions

Metabolism/Transport Effects Substrate of CYP3A4 (minor), P-glycoprotein; **Induces** CYP3A4 (weak)

Avoid Concomitant Use

Avoid concomitant use of Hydrocortisone with any of the following: Aldesleukin; BCG; Natalizumab; Pimecrolimus; Tacrolimus (Topical); Vaccines (Live)

Increased Effect/Toxicity

Hydrocortisone may increase the levels/effects of: Acetylcholinesterase Inhibitors; Amphotericin B; Leflunomide; Loop Diuretics; Natalizumab; NSAID (COX-2 Inhibitor); NSAID (Nonselective); Thiazide Diuretics; Vaccines (Live); Warfarin

The levels/effects of Hydrocortisone may be increased by: Antifungal Agents (Azole Derivatives, Systemic); Aprepitant; Calcium Channel Blockers (Nondihydropyridine); Denosumab; Estrogen Derivatives; Fluconazole; Fosaprepitant; Macrolide Antibiotics; Neuromuscular-Blocking Agents (Nondepolarizing); P-Glycoprotein Inhibitors; Pimecrolimus; Quinolone Antibiotics; Salicylates; Tacrolimus (Topical); Trastuzumab

Decreased Effect

Hydrocortisone may decrease the levels/effects of: Aldesleukin; Antidiabetic Agents; BCG; Calcitriol; Corticorelin; Isoniazid; Salicylates; Sipuleucel-T; Vaccines (Inactivated); Vaccines (Live)

The levels/effects of Hydrocortisone may be decreased by: Aminoglutethimide; Antacids; Barbiturates; Bile Acid Sequestrants; Echinacea; Mitotane; P-Glycoprotein Inducers; Primidone; Rifamycin Derivatives

Food Interactions Systemic use of corticosteroids may require a diet with increased potassium, vitamins A, B_6, C, D, folate, calcium, zinc, phosphorus, and decreased sodium

Stability Injection: Store at controlled room temperature 20°C to 25°C (59°F to 86°F). Reconstituted solution is clear, light yellow and heat labile.

After initial reconstitution, hydrocortisone sodium succinate solutions are stable for 3 days at room temperature or under refrigeration when protected from light. Stability of parenteral admixture (Solu-Cortef®) at room temperature (25°C) and at refrigeration temperature (4°C) is concentration-dependent:

Stability of concentration 1 mg/mL: 24 hours

Stability of concentration 2 mg/mL to 60 mg/mL: At least 4 hours

Solutions for I.V. infusion: Reconstituted solutions may be added to an appropriate volume of compatible solution for infusion. Concentration should generally not exceed 1 mg/mL. However, in adult cases where administration of a small volume of fluid is desirable, 100-3000 mg may be added to 50 mL of D_5W or NS (stability limited to 4 hours).

Mechanism of Action Decreases inflammation by suppression of migration of polymorphonuclear leukocytes and reversal of increased capillary permeability

Pharmacodynamics Anti-inflammatory effects:
Maximum effect:
Oral: 12-24 hours
I.V.: 4-6 hours
Duration: 8-12 hours

Pharmacokinetics (Adult data unless noted)
Absorption: Rapid by all routes, except rectally
Metabolism: In the liver
Half-life, biologic: 8-12 hours
Elimination: Renally, mainly as 17-hydroxysteroids and 17-ketosteroids

Usual Dosage Dose should be based on severity of disease and patient response; **Note:** A variety of salt forms are available and can lead to confusion in prescribing, dispensing, and administration; use the appropriate salt/dosage form for the following indications:

Acetate: For intra-articular, intrasynovial, intrabursal, intralesional, or soft tissue injection only

Cypionate: Oral suspension (see Additional Information)

Sodium succinate: For general I.V. use, I.V. use in patients allergic to sodium phosphate salt, I.V. for shock and for intrathecal use (must reconstitute with a preservative free diluent or use a preservative free product)

Acute adrenal insufficiency: I.M., I.V.:
Infants and young Children: 1-2 mg/kg/dose I.V. bolus, then 25-150 mg/day in divided doses every 6-8 hours
Older Children: 1-2 mg/kg I.V. bolus, then 150-250 mg/day in divided doses every 6-8 hours
Adults: 100 mg I.V. bolus, then 300 mg/day in divided doses every 8 hours or as a continuous infusion for 48 hours; once patient is stable change to oral, 50 mg every 8 hours for 6 doses, then taper to 30-50 mg/day in divided doses

Anti-inflammatory or immunosuppressive:
Infants and Children:
Oral: 2.5-10 mg/kg/day or 75-300 mg/m^2/day divided every 6-8 hours
I.M., I.V.: 1-5 mg/kg/day or 30-150 mg/m^2/day divided every 12-24 hours
Adolescents and Adults: Oral, I.M., I.V., SubQ: 15-240 mg every 12 hours

Congenital adrenal hyperplasia: AAP Recommendations: Oral: Initial: 10-20 mg/m^2/day in 3 divided doses; usual requirement: Infants: 2.5-5 mg 3 times/day; Children: 5-10 mg 3 times/day; **Note:** Administer morning dose as early as possible; tablets may result in more reliable serum concentrations than oral liquid formulation (see Additional Information); individualize dose by monitoring growth, hormone levels, and bone age; mineralocorticoid (eg, fludrocortisone) and sodium supplement may be required in salt losers

Neonatal hypoglycemia (refractory to continuous glucose infusion of >12-15 mg/kg/minute): Neonates: I.V., oral: 5 mg/kg/day divided every 8-12 hours or 1-2 mg/kg/dose every 6 hours

Physiologic replacement: Children:
Oral: 0.5-0.75 mg/kg/day or 20-25 mg/m^2/day divided every 8 hours
I.M.: 0.25-0.35 mg/kg/day or 12-15 mg/m^2/day once daily

Shock: I.V.: **Sodium succinate:**
Children: Initial: 50 mg/kg as an I.V. bolus, followed by 50 mg/kg as a 24-hour infusion (see Carcillo, 2002 and Han, 2003). Some centers use: 50 mg/kg then repeated in 4 hours and/or every 24 hours if needed
Adolescents and Adults: 500 mg to 2 g every 2-6 hours

Status asthmaticus:
Children: I.V.: Optional loading dose: 4-8 mg/kg; maximum: 250 mg; then maintenance: 2 mg/kg/dose every 6 hours
Adults: 100-500 mg every 6 hours

Rectal: Adolescents and Adults: Insert 1 application 1-2 times/day for 2-3 weeks
Ulcerative colitis: One enema nightly for 21 days, or until remission occurs; clinical symptoms should subside within 3-5 days; discontinue use if no improvement within 2-3 weeks; some patients may require 2-3 months of therapy; if therapy lasts >21 days, discontinue slowly by decreasing use to every other night for 2-3 weeks

Topical: Children and Adults: Usual: Apply 2-3 times/day (depending on severity); may be applied up to 4 times/day

Administration
Oral: Administer with food or milk to decrease GI upset (see Additional Information)
Parenteral:
I.V. bolus: Dilute to 50 mg/mL and administer over 3-5 minutes
I.V. intermittent infusion: Dilute to 1 mg/mL and administer over 20-30 minutes; usual maximum concentration: 5 mg/mL
Note: In adult patients when administration of a small volume of fluid is needed, concentrations up to 60 mg/mL (100-3000 mg in 50 mL D_5W or NS) may be administered by direct I.V. or I.V. piggyback
Rectal: Patient should lie on left side during administration and for 30 minutes after; retain enema for at least 1 hour, preferably all night
Topical: Apply a thin film to clean, dry skin and rub in gently; avoid contact with eyes. Do not apply to face, underarms, or groin unless directed by physician. Do not wrap or bandage affected area unless directed by physician. Do not apply to diaper areas because diapers or plastic pants may be occlusive.

Monitoring Parameters Blood pressure, weight, serum glucose, electrolytes; growth in pediatric patients; assess HPA axis suppression in patients using topical steroids applied to a large surface area or to areas under occlusion (eg, ACTH stimulation test, morning plasma cortisol test, urinary free cortisol test). Monitor IOP with therapy >6 weeks.

Reference Range Hydrocortisone (normal endogenous morning levels) 4-30 mcg/mL

◀ **Test Interactions** Skin tests

Patient Information Limit caffeine; avoid alcohol; do not decrease dose or discontinue without physician's approval; avoid exposure to measles or chicken pox, advise physician immediately if exposed; notify physician if condition being treated persists or worsens. Topical: Avoid contact with eyes; do not use for longer than directed; contact physician if no improvement is seen in 2 weeks

Additional Information Cortef® oral suspension was reformulated in July 1998; the suspending agent was changed from tragacanth to xanthan gum; this suspension was found **not** to be bioequivalent to hydrocortisone tablets in the treatment of children with congenital adrenal hyperplasia; children required higher doses of the suspension (19.6 mg/m^2/day) compared to the tablets (15.2 mg/m^2/day); based on these findings, Cortef® suspension was voluntarily recalled from the market on July 18, 2000 (see Merke, 2001).

To facilitate retention of enema, prior antidiarrheal medication or sedation may be required (especially when beginning therapy)

Dosage Forms Excipient information presented when available (limited, particularly for generics); consult specific product labeling. [DSC] = Discontinued product

Aerosol, rectal, as acetate:
  Cortifoam®: 10% (15 g) [90 mg/applicator]
Cream, rectal, as acetate:
  Nupercainal® Hydrocortisone Cream: 1% (30 g) [strength expressed as base]
Cream, topical, as acetate: 0.5% (9 g, 30 g, 60 g) [available with aloe]; 1% (30 g, 454 g) [available with aloe]
  U-Cort™: 1% (28 g) [contains sodium bisulfite]
Cream, topical, as base: 0.5% (30 g); 1% (1.5 g, 30 g, 114 g, 454 g); 2.5% (20 g, 30 g, 454 g)
  Anusol-HC®: 2.5% (30 g) [contains benzyl alcohol]
  Caldecort®: 1% (30 g) [contains aloe vera gel]
  Cortaid® Intensive Therapy: 1% (60 g)
  Cortaid® Maximum Strength: 1% (15 g, 30 g, 40 g, 60 g) [contains aloe vera gel and benzyl alcohol]
  Cortaid® Sensitive Skin: 0.5% (15 g) [contains aloe vera gel]
  Cortizone-10® Maximum Strength: 1% (15 g, 30 g, 60 g) [contains aloe]
  Cortizone-10® Maximum Strength Intensive Healing Formula: 1% (28 g, 56 g) [contains aloe, benzyl alcohol]
  Cortizone-10® Plus Maximum Strength: 1% (30 g, 60 g) [contains vitamins A, D, E and aloe]
  Dermarest® Dricort®: 1% (15 g, 30 g)
  HydroZone Plus [DSC], Proctocort®, Procto-Pak™: 1% (30 g)
  Hytone®: 1% (30 g), 2.5% (30 g, 60 g) [DSC]
  IvySoothe®: 1% (30 g) [contains aloe]
  Post Peel Healing Balm: 1% (23 g)
  Preparation H® Hydrocortisone: 1% (27 g) [contains sodium benzoate]
  ProctoCream® HC: 2.5% (30 g) [contains benzyl alcohol]
  Procto-Kit™: 1% (30 g) [packaged with applicator tips and finger cots]; 2.5% (30 g) [packaged with applicator tips and finger cots]
  Proctosol-HC®, Proctozone-HC™: 2.5% (30 g)
  Summer's Eve® SpecialCare™ Medicated Anti-Itch Cream: 1% (30 g) [DSC]
Cream, topical, as butyrate: 0.1% (15 g, 45 g)
  Locoid®: 0.1% (15 g, 45 g)
  Locoid Lipocream®: 0.1% (15 g, 45 g)

Cream, topical, as probutate:
  Pandel®: 0.1% (15 g, 45 g, 80 g)
Cream, topical, as valerate: 0.2% (15 g, 45 g, 60 g)
  Westcort®: 0.2% (15 g, 45 g, 60 g)
Gel, topical, as base:
  Corticool®: 1% (45 g)
  Cortizone-10® Maximum Strength Cooling Relief: 1% (28 g) [contains aloe, ethanol 15%]
Injection, powder for reconstitution, as sodium succinate:
  A-Hydrocort®: 100 mg [contains monobasic sodium phosphate 0.8 mg, anhydrous dibasic sodium phosphate 8.73 mg; strength expressed as base]
  Solu-Cortef®: 100 mg, 250 mg, 500 mg, 1 g [diluent contains benzyl alcohol; strength expressed as base]
Lotion, topical, as base [spray]:
  Cortizone-10® Maximum Strength Easy Relief: 1% (36 mL) [contains aloe, ethanol 45%]
Lotion, topical, as base: 1% (120 mL); 2.5% (60 mL, 118 mL)
  Aquanil™ HC: 1% (120 mL)
  Beta-HC®
  Cetacort® [DSC]
  HydroZone Plus: 1% (120 mL) [DSC]
  Hytone®: 2.5% (60 mL) [DSC]
  Nutracort®: 1% (60 mL, 120 mL); 2.5% (60 mL, 120 mL)
  Sarnol®-HC: 1% (60 mL)
Lotion, topical, as butyrate:
  Locoid®: 0.1% (60 mL)
Ointment, topical, as acetate: 1% (30 g) [strength expressed as base; available with aloe]
  Anusol® HC-1: 1% (21 g) [strength expressed as base]
  Cortaid® Maximum Strength: 1% (15 g, 30 g) [strength expressed as base]
Ointment, topical, as base: 0.5% (30 g); 1% (30 g, 454 g); 2.5% (20 g, 30 g, 454 g)
  Cortizone-10® Maximum Strength: 1% (30 g, 60 g)
  Hytone®: 2.5% (30 g) [DSC]
Ointment, topical, as butyrate: 0.1% (15 g, 45 g)
  Locoid®: 0.1% (15 g, 45 g)
Ointment, topical, as valerate: 0.2% (15 g, 45 g, 60 g)
  Westcort®: 0.2% (15 g, 45 g, 60 g)
Powder, for prescription compounding [micronized]: USP: 100% (10 g, 25 g, 50 g, 100g)
  HYDRO-Rx: USP: 100% (10 g, 25 g, 50 g, 100 g)
Powder, for prescription compounding, as acetate [micronized]: USP (10 g, 25 g, 50 g)
Solution, topical, as base: 2.5% (30 mL)
  Texacort®: 2.5% (30 mL) [contains ethanol 48%]
Solution, topical, as butyrate: 0.1% (20 mL, 60 mL)
  Locoid®: 0.1% (20 mL, 60 mL) [contains alcohol 50%]
Solution, topical, as base [spray]:
  Cortaid® Intensive Therapy: 1% (60 mL) [contains alcohol]
  Cortizone-10® Quick Shot: 1% (44 mL) [contains benzyl alcohol] [DSC]
  Dermtex® HC: 1% (52 mL) [contains menthol 1%]
Suppository, rectal, as acetate: 25 mg (12s [DSC]; 24s, 100s)
  Anucort-HC®: 25 mg (12s, 24s, 100s)
  Anusol-HC®, Proctosol-HC®: 25 mg (12s, 24s)
  Encort™, Proctocort®: 30 mg (12s)
  Hemril®-30, Proctosert: 30 mg (12s, 24s)
Suspension, rectal, as base: 100 mg/60 mL (1s, 7s)
  Colocort®, Cortenema®: 100 mg/60 mL (1s, 7s)
Tablet, as base: 20 mg
  Cortef®: 5 mg, 10 mg, 20 mg
Extemporaneous Preparations A 2.5 mg/mL oral suspension prepared from tablets (with a vehicle containing sodium carboxymethylcellulose, syrup, hydroxybenzoate 0.1% preservatives, polysorbate 80, and citric acid) and stored in the dark in amber high density polyethylene bottles was stable for 90 days when stored at 5°C or 25°C and stable for 30 days when stored at 40°C; a 2.5 mg/mL

oral suspension prepared from powder and the same vehicle was stable for 90 days when stored in the dark in amber polyethylene bottles at 40°C (Fawcett, 1995).

Fawcett JP, Boulton DW, Jiang R, et al, "Stability of Hydrocortisone Oral Suspensions Prepared From Tablets and Powder," *Ann Pharmacother*, 1995, 29 (10):987-90.

References

American Academy of Pediatrics, Section on Endocrinology and Committee on Genetics, "Technical Report: Congenital Adrenal Hyperplasia," *Pediatrics*, 2000, 106(6):1511-8.

Carcillo JA and Fields AI, "Clinical Practice Parameters for Hemodynamic Support of Pediatric and Neonatal Patients in Septic Shock," *Crit Care Med*, 2002, 30(6):1365-78.

Cowett RM and Loughead JL, "Neonatal Glucose Metabolism: Differential Diagnoses, Evaluation, and Treatment of Hypoglycemia," *Neonatal Netw*, 2002, 21(4):9-19.

Halamek LP and Stevenson DK, "Neonatal Hypoglycemia, Part II: Pathophysiology and Therapy," *Clin Pediatr (Phila)*, 1998, 37(1):11-6.

Han YY, Carcillo JA, Dragotta MA, et al, "Early Reversal of Pediatric-Neonatal Septic Shock by Community Physicians is Associated With Improved Outcome," *Pediatrics*, 2003, 112(4):793-9.

Merke DP, Cho D, Calis KA, et al, "Hydrocortisone Suspension and Hydrocortisone Tablets are not Bioequivalent in the Treatment of Children With Congenital Adrenal Hyperplasia," *J Clin Endocrinol Metab*, 2001, 86(1):441-5.

♦ **Hydrocortisone Acetate** *see* Hydrocortisone *on page 685*

♦ **Hydrocortisone and Ciprofloxacin** *see* Ciprofloxacin and Hydrocortisone *on page 315*

♦ **Hydrocortisone Butyrate** *see* Hydrocortisone *on page 685*

♦ **Hydrocortisone, Neomycin, and Polymyxin B** *see* Neomycin, (Bacitracin) Polymyxin B, and Hydrocortisone *on page 980*

♦ **Hydrocortisone Probutate** *see* Hydrocortisone *on page 685*

♦ **Hydrocortisone Sodium Succinate** *see* Hydrocortisone *on page 685*

♦ **Hydrocortisone Valerate** *see* Hydrocortisone *on page 685*

♦ **Hydrodiuril** *see* Hydrochlorothiazide *on page 682*

♦ **Hydrogen Dioxide** *see* Hydrogen Peroxide *on page 689*

Hydrogen Peroxide (HYE droe jen per OKS ide)

Therapeutic Category Antibacterial, Otic; Antibacterial, Topical; Antibiotic, Oral Rinse

Use Cleanse wounds, suppurating ulcers, and local infections; used in the treatment of inflammatory conditions of the external auditory canal and as a mouthwash or gargle; hydrogen peroxide concentrate (30%) has been used as a hair bleach and as a tooth bleaching agent

Contraindications Should not be used in abscesses

Warnings Hydrogen peroxide concentrate (30%) is a caustic liquid; it should not be tasted since it is strongly irritating to skin or mucous membranes

Precautions Repeat use as a mouthwash or gargle may produce irritation of the buccal mucous membrane or "hairy tongue"; bandages should not be applied too quickly after its use

Adverse Reactions

Dermatologic: Bleaching effect on hair, irritating burn

Gastrointestinal: Rupture of the colon, proctitis, ulcerative colitis, gas embolism, hairy tongue

Local: Irritation of the buccal mucous membrane

Stability Protect from light and heat; decomposes upon standing, upon repeated agitation, or when in contact with oxidizing or reducing substances

Mechanism of Action Antiseptic oxidant that slowly releases oxygen and water upon contact with serum or tissue catalase

Pharmacodynamics Duration: Only while bubbling action occurs

Usual Dosage Children and Adults:

Mouthwash or gargle: Dilute the 3% solution with an equal volume of water; swish around in the mouth over the affected area for at least 1 minute and then expel; use up to 4 times/day (after meals and at bedtime)

Topical:

1.5% to 3% solution for cleansing wounds

1.5% gel for cleansing wounds or mouth/gum irritations: Apply a small amount to the affected area for at least 1 minute, then expectorate; use up to 4 times/day (after meals and at bedtime)

Administration Topical: Do not inject or instill into closed body cavities from which released oxygen cannot escape; strong solutions (30.5%) of hydrogen peroxide should not be applied undiluted to tissues

Dosage Forms

Gel, oral: 1.5% (15 g)

Solution:

Concentrate: 30.5% (480 mL)

Topical: 3% (120 mL, 480 mL)

♦ **Hydromorph Contin® (Can)** *see* HYDROmorphone *on page 689*

♦ **Hydromorph-IR® (Can)** *see* HYDROmorphone *on page 689*

HYDROmorphone (hye droe MOR fone)

Medication Safety Issues

Sound-alike/look-alike issues:

Dilaudid® may be confused with Demerol®, Dilantin®

HYDROmorphone may be confused with morphine; significant overdoses have occurred when hydromorphone products have been inadvertently administered instead of morphine sulfate. Commercially available prefilled syringes of both products looks similar and are often stored in close proximity to each other. **Note:** Hydromorphone 1 mg oral is approximately equal to morphine 4 mg oral; hydromorphone 1 mg I.V. is approximately equal to morphine 5 mg I.V.

High alert medication: The Institute for Safe Medication Practices (ISMP) includes this medication among its list of drug classes which have a heightened risk of causing significant patient harm when used in error.

Dilaudid®, Dilaudid-HP®: Extreme caution should be taken to avoid confusing the highly-concentrated (Dilaudid-HP®) injection with the less-concentrated (Dilaudid®) injectable product.

Exalgo™: Extreme caution should be taken to avoid confusing the extended release Exalgo™ 8 mg tablets with immediate release hydromorphone 8 mg tablets

Significant differences exist between oral and I.V. dosing. Use caution when converting from one route of administration to another.

Related Information

Laboratory Detection of Drugs in Urine *on page 1706*

Opioid Analgesics Comparison *on page 1510*

U.S. Brand Names Dilaudid-HP®; Dilaudid®; Exalgo™

Canadian Brand Names Dilaudid-HP-Plus®; Dilaudid-HP®; Dilaudid-XP®; Dilaudid®; Dilaudid® Sterile Powder; Hydromorph Contin®; Hydromorph-IR®; Hydromorphone HP; Hydromorphone HP® 10; Hydromorphone HP® 20; Hydromorphone HP® 50; Hydromorphone HP® Forte; Hydromorphone Hydrochloride Injection, USP; Jurnista™; PMS-Hydromorphone

Therapeutic Category Analgesic, Narcotic; Antitussive

Generic Available Yes: Excludes capsule, extended release tablet, liquid, powder for injection

Use Management of moderate to severe pain (FDA approved in adults); Dilaudid-HP® injection is indicated for use in opioid-tolerant patients who require larger than usual doses of opioids for pain relief (FDA approved in adults); has also been used as an antitussive at lower doses

Restrictions C-II

Medication Guide An FDA-approved patient medication guide for Exalgo™, which is available with the product information and at http://www.fda.gov/downloads/Drugs/DrugSafety/UCM204267.pdf, must be dispensed with this medication every time it is dispensed. Medication guides are also available at http://www.exalgorems.com.

Pregnancy Risk Factor C

Pregnancy Considerations Hydromorphone was teratogenic in some, but not all, animal studies; however, maternal toxicity was also reported. Hydromorphone crosses the placenta. Chronic opioid use during pregnancy may lead to a withdrawal syndrome in the neonate. Symptoms include irritability, hyperactivity, loss of sleep pattern, abnormal crying, tremor, vomiting, diarrhea, weight loss, or failure to gain weight.

Lactation Enters breast milk/not recommended

Breast-Feeding Considerations Low concentrations of hydromorphone can be found in breast milk. Withdrawal symptoms may be observed in breast-feeding infants when opioid analgesics are discontinued. Breast-feeding is not recommended.

Contraindications Hypersensitivity to hydromorphone or any component (see Warnings); significant respiratory depression (especially in settings without resuscitative equipment or without adequate respiratory monitoring); severe CNS depression; patients with severe or acute asthma, paralytic ileus (known or suspected); pregnancy (prolonged use or high doses at term); obstetrical analgesia

Warnings Respiratory depression may occur **[U.S. Boxed Warning]**; use with extreme caution in patients with pre-existing respiratory depression, decreased respiratory reserve, hypoxia, hypercapnia, significant COPD, or cor pulmonale. Hypotension may occur, especially in hypovolemic patients or those receiving medications that compromise vasomotor tone; use with extreme caution in patients with circulatory shock. Orthostatic hypotension may occur in ambulatory patients. Physical and psychological dependence may occur; abrupt discontinuation after prolonged use may result in withdrawal symptoms or seizures. Warn patient of possible impairment of alertness or physical coordination (see Patient Information). Interactions with other CNS drugs may occur (see Drug Interactions) **[U.S. Boxed Warning]**. Healthcare provider should be alert to problems of abuse, misuse, and diversion **[U.S. Boxed Warning]**. Infants born to women physically dependent on opioids will also be physically dependent and may experience respiratory difficulties or opioid withdrawal symptoms.

Do not confuse the highly-concentrated (Dilaudid-HP®) injection with the less-concentrated (Dilaudid®) injectable product **[U.S. Boxed Warning]**; significant overdose or death could result. Extended release capsules are not recommended for use in patients with severe hepatic impairment (studies have not been conducted). Injection (4 mg/mL, 10 mg/mL, and powder for reconstitution), oral liquid, and 8 mg tablets may contain sodium metabisulfite, which may cause allergic reactions in susceptible individuals. Rubber stopper of multiple dose vials contains latex which may cause allergic reactions in susceptible individuals; avoid use in patients with allergy to latex.

Precautions Use with caution in patients with hypersensitivity reactions to other phenanthrene derivative opioid agonists (morphine, hydrocodone, levorphanol, oxycodone, oxymorphone, codeine). Use with caution

and reduce the initial dose in patients with significant liver, respiratory, or renal disease; hypothyroidism or myxedema; head injury; increased intracranial pressure; CNS depression or coma; respiratory depression; adrenocortical insufficiency; toxic psychosis; seizures; acute abdominal conditions; post-GI surgery; biliary tract disease; pancreatitis; prostatic hypertrophy or urethral stricture; acute alcoholism; delirium tremens; kyphoscoliosis and in debilitated patients. Seizures and myoclonus have been reported in severely compromised patients receiving high doses of parenteral hydromorphone. Use with caution in patients undergoing biliary tract surgery (narcotics may cause spasm of the sphincter of Oddi).

Adverse Reactions
Cardiovascular: Bradycardia, hypotension, palpitations, peripheral vasodilation
Central nervous system: CNS depression, dizziness, drowsiness, intracranial pressure increased, sedation
Dermatologic: Pruritus
Endocrine & metabolic: Antidiuretic hormone release
Gastrointestinal: Biliary tract spasm, constipation, nausea, vomiting
Genitourinary: Urinary tract spasm
Ocular: Miosis
Respiratory: Respiratory depression
Miscellaneous: Histamine release, physical and psychological dependence with prolonged use

Drug Interactions

Avoid Concomitant Use
Avoid concomitant use of HYDROmorphone with any of the following: MAO Inhibitors

Increased Effect/Toxicity
HYDROmorphone may increase the levels/effects of: Alcohol (Ethyl); Alvimopan; CNS Depressants; Desmopressin; Selective Serotonin Reuptake Inhibitors; Thiazide Diuretics

The levels/effects of HYDROmorphone may be increased by: Amphetamines; Antipsychotic Agents (Phenothiazines); MAO Inhibitors; Succinylcholine

Decreased Effect
HYDROmorphone may decrease the levels/effects of: Pegvisomant

The levels/effects of HYDROmorphone may be decreased by: Ammonium Chloride; Mixed Agonist / Antagonist Opioids

Food Interactions Food does not significantly affect bioavailability of extended release capsules; food decreased the peak serum concentration by 25%, prolonged the time to peak by 0.8 hours, and increased the AUC of a single tablet dose by 35% (effects may not be clinically significant).

Stability Protect from light; store suppositories in refrigerator; store other dosage forms at room temperature; a slight yellow discoloration of injection has not been associated with a loss of potency; injection is stable for at least 24 hours when protected from light and stored at 25°C in most common large volume parenteral solutions

Mechanism of Action Binds to opiate receptors in the CNS, causing inhibition of ascending pain pathways, altering the perception of and response to pain; causes cough suppression by direct central action in the medulla; produces generalized CNS depression

Pharmacodynamics Analgesic effects:
Onset of action:
Oral: Immediate release formulations: Within 15-30 minutes
I.V.: Within 5 minutes
Maximum effect:
Oral: Immediate release formulations: Within 30-90 minutes
I.V.: 10-20 minutes

Duration: Oral: Immediate release formulations, I.V.: 4-5 hours; suppository may provide longer duration of effect

Pharmacokinetics (Adult data unless noted)

Absorption:

I.M.: Variable

Oral: Rapidly absorbed; extensive first-pass effect

Distribution: V_d: Adults: 4 L/kg; crosses the placenta; distributes into breast milk

Protein binding: ~8% to 19%

Metabolism: Primarily in the liver via glucuronidation to inactive metabolites; >95% is metabolized to hydro-morphone-3-glucuronide; minor amounts as 6-hydroxy reduction metabolites

Bioavailability: Oral: 62%

Half-life: 1-3 hours

Time to peak serum concentration: Oral: 30-60 minutes

Elimination: In urine, principally as glucuronide conjugates

Usual Dosage

Antitussive: Oral:

Children 6-12 years: 0.5 mg every 3-4 hours as needed

Children >12 years and Adults: 1 mg every 3-4 hours as needed

Pain: Doses should be titrated to appropriate analgesic effects, while minimizing adverse effects; when changing routes of administration, note that oral doses are less than one-half as effective as parenteral doses (may be only 1/5 as effective):

Infants >6 months who weigh >10 kg (see Friedrichsdorf, 2007 and Zernikow, 2009):

Oral: Usual initial: 0.03 mg/kg/dose every 4 hours as needed; usual range: 0.03-0.06 mg/kg/dose

I.V.: Usual initial: 0.01 mg/kg/dose every 3-6 hours as needed

I.V. continuous infusion: Usual initial: 0.003-0.005 mg/kg/hour

Children <50 kg:

Oral: 0.03-0.08 mg/kg/dose every 3-4 hours as needed

Note: The American Pain Society (2008) recommends an initial oral dose of 0.06 mg/kg for severe pain in children.

I.V.: 0.015 mg/kg/dose every 3-6 hours as needed

I.V. continuous infusion: Usual initial: 0.003-0.005 mg/kg/hour (maximum: 0.2 mg/hour) (see Friedrichsdorf, 2007 and Zernikow, 2009)

I.V.: Patient-controlled analgesia (PCA): Opiate-naïve:

Children ≥5 years and <50 kg: **Note:** PCA has been used in children as young as 5 years of age; however, clinicians need to assess children 5-8 years of age to determine if they are able to use the PCA device correctly. All patients should receive an initial loading dose of an analgesic (to attain adequate control of pain) before starting PCA for maintenance. Adjust doses, lockouts, and limits based on required loading dose, age, state of health, and presence of opioid tolerance. Use lower end of dosing range for opioid-naïve. Assess patient and pain control at regular intervals and adjust settings if needed (see American Pain Society, 2008):

Usual concentration: 0.2 mg/mL

Demand dose: Usual initial: 0.003-0.004 mg/kg/dose; usual range: 0.003-0.005 mg/kg/dose

Lockout: Usual initial: 5 doses/hour

Lockout interval: Range: 6-10 minutes

Usual basal rate: 0-0.004 mg/kg/hour

Children >50 kg and Adolescents >50 kg: See Adult PCA dose

Children >50 kg, Adolescents >50 kg, and Adults:

Oral: Initial: Opiate-naïve: 1-2 mg/dose every 3-4 hours as needed; patients with prior opiate exposure may tolerate higher initial doses; usual adult dose: 2-4 mg/dose; doses up to 8 mg have been used in adults

Note: The American Pain Society (2008) recommends an initial oral dose of 4-8 mg for severe pain in adults.

I.V.: Initial: Opiate-naïve: 0.2-0.6 mg/dose every 2-4 hours as needed; patients with prior opiate exposure may tolerate higher initial doses.

Patient-controlled analgesia (PCA): **Note:** All patients should receive an initial loading dose of an analgesic (to attain adequate control of pain) before starting PCA for maintenance. Adjust doses, lockouts, and limits based on required loading dose, age, state of health, and presence of opioid tolerance. Use lower end of dosing range for opioid-naïve. Assess patient and pain control at regular intervals and adjust settings if needed (see American Pain Society, 2008):

Usual concentration: 0.2 mg/mL

Demand dose: Usual initial: 0.1-0.2 mg; usual range: 0.05-0.4 mg

Lockout interval: Usual initial: 6 minutes; usual range: 5-10 minutes

I.M., SubQ: **Note:** I.M. use may result in variable absorption and a lag time to peak effect.

Initial: Opiate-naïve: 0.8-1 mg every 4-6 hours as needed; patients with prior opioid exposure may require higher initial doses; usual dosage range: 1-2 mg every 3-6 hours as needed

Rectal: 3 mg (1 suppository) every 4-8 hours as needed

Adult:

I.V.: Critically ill adult patients: 0.7-2 mg (based on 70 kg patient) every 1-2 hours as needed. **Note:** More frequent dosing may be needed (eg, mechanically ventilated patients).

I.V. continuous infusion: Usual dosage range: 0.5-1 mg/hour (based on 70 kg patient) or 7-15 mcg/kg/hour

Epidural:

Bolus dose: 0.8-1.5 mg

Infusion concentration: 0.05-0.075 mg/mL

Infusion rate: 0.04-0.4 mg/hour

Demand dose: 0.15 mg

Lockout interval: 30 minutes

Chronic pain: Adults: Oral: **Note:** Patients taking opioids chronically may become tolerant and require doses higher than the usual dosage range to maintain the desired effect. Tolerance can be managed by appropriate dose titration. There is no optimal or maximal dose for hydromorphone in chronic pain. The appropriate dose is one that relieves pain throughout its dosing interval without causing unmanageable side effects.

Administration

Oral: Administer with food or milk to decrease GI upset

Parenteral: I.V.: Administer via slow I.V. injection over at least 2-3 minutes

Rectal: Insert suppository rectally and retain

Monitoring Parameters Pain relief, respiratory rate, heart rate, blood pressure

Patient Information Avoid alcohol. Hydromorphone may cause drowsiness and impair ability to perform activities requiring mental alertness or physical coordination; may be habit-forming; avoid abrupt discontinuation after prolonged use; if oral liquid spills on skin, remove contaminated clothing and rinse area with cool water

Additional Information Equianalgesic doses: Morphine 10 mg I.M. = hydromorphone 1.5 mg I.M.

Dosage Forms Excipient information presented when available (limited, particularly for generics); consult specific product labeling. [DSC] = Discontinued product; [CAN] = Canadian brand name

Capsule, controlled release:

Hydromorph Contin® [CAN]: 3 mg, 6 mg, 12 mg, 18 mg, 24 mg, 30 mg [not available in U.S.]

Injection, powder for reconstitution, as hydrochloride:
  Dilaudid-HP®: 250 mg [contains sodium metabisulfite]
Injection, solution, as hydrochloride: 1 mg/mL (1 mL);
  2 mg/mL (1 mL, 20 mL); 4 mg/mL (1 mL)
  Dilaudid®: 1 mg/mL (1 mL); 2 mg/mL (1 mL; 20 mL
  [DSC]) [20 mL size contains edetate sodium; natural
  rubber/natural latex in packaging]; 4 mg/mL (1 mL)
  [contains sodium metabisulfite]
  Dilaudid-HP®: 10 mg/mL (1 mL, 5 mL) [contains sodium
  metabisulfite]
  Dilaudid-HP®: 10 mg/mL (50 mL) [contains sodium
  metabisulfite; natural rubber/natural latex in packaging]
Injection, solution, as hydrochloride [preservative free]:
  10 mg/mL (1 mL, 5 mL, 50 mL)
Liquid, oral, as hydrochloride:
  Dilaudid®: 1 mg/mL (480 mL) [contains sodium meta-
  bisulfite (may have trace amounts)]
Powder, for prescription compounding: USP: 100% (15
  grain)
Suppository, rectal, as hydrochloride: 3 mg
Tablet, as hydrochloride: 2 mg, 4 mg, 8 mg
  Dilaudid®: 2 mg, 4 mg, 8 mg [contains sodium meta-
  bisulfite (may have trace amounts)]
Tablet, extended release, as hydrochloride:
  Exalgo™: 8 mg, 12 mg, 16 mg

References

Berde CB and Sethna NF, "Analgesics for the Treatment of Pain in
  Children," N Engl J Med, 2002, 347(14):1094-103.
Carr D, Jacox A, Chapman CR, et al, "Clinical Practice Guideline
  Number 1: Acute Pain Management: Operative or Medical
  Procedures and Trauma," Rockville, Maryland: U.S. Department of
  Health and Human Services, Public Health Service, Agency for
  Health Care Policy and Research, AHCPR Publication No 92-0032,
  1992.
Friedrichsdorf SJ and Kang TI, "The Management of Pain in Children
  With Life-Limiting Illnesses," Pediatr Clin North Am, 2007, 54
  (5):645-72.
Jacox A, Carr D, Payne R, et al, "Clinical Practice Guideline Number 9:
  Management of Cancer Pain," Rockville, Maryland: U.S. Department
  of Health and Human Services, Public Health Service, Agency for
  Health Care Policy and Research, AHCPR Publication No. 94-0592,
  1994.
"Principles of Analgesic Use in the Treatment of Acute Pain and Cancer
  Pain," 6th ed, Glenview, IL: American Pain Society, 2008.
Zernikow B, Michel E, Craig F, et al, "Pediatric Palliative Care: Use of
  Opioids for the Management of Pain," Paediatr Drugs, 2009, 11
  (2):129-51.

◆ **Hydromorphone HP (Can)** see HYDROmorphone
  on page 689

◆ **Hydromorphone HP® 10 (Can)** see HYDROmorphone
  on page 689

◆ **Hydromorphone HP® 20 (Can)** see HYDROmorphone
  on page 689

◆ **Hydromorphone HP® 50 (Can)** see HYDROmorphone
  on page 689

◆ **Hydromorphone HP® Forte (Can)** see HYDROmorphone on page 689

◆ **Hydromorphone Hydrochloride** see HYDROmorphone
  on page 689

◆ **Hydromorphone Hydrochloride Injection, USP (Can)**
  see HYDROmorphone on page 689

◆ **HYDRO-Rx** see Hydrocortisone on page 685

◆ **Hydro-Tussin™-CBX [DSC]** see Carbinoxamine and
  Pseudoephedrine on page 249

◆ **Hydro-Tussin™ DM [DSC]** see Guaifenesin and Dextromethorphan on page 658

◆ **HydroVal® (Can)** see Hydrocortisone on page 685

Hydroxocobalamin (hye droks oh koe BAL a min)

U.S. Brand Names Cyanokit®

Therapeutic Category Antidote, Cyanide; Nutritional
Supplement; Vitamin, Water Soluble

Generic Available Yes: Excludes powder for injection

Use

I.M. injection: Treatment of pernicious anemia and other
vitamin B_{12} deficiency states; dietary supplement particularly in conditions of increased requirements (eg,
pregnancy, thyrotoxicosis, hemorrhage, malignancy, liver
or kidney disease)

I.V. infusion (Cyanokit®): Treatment of cyanide poisoning

Pregnancy Risk Factor C

Pregnancy Considerations Animal studies are insufficient to determine the effect, if any, on pregnancy or fetal
development. There are no adequate and well-controlled
studies in pregnant women. Data on the use of
hydroxocobalamin in pregnancy for the treatment of
cyanide poisoning and cobalamin defects are limited.

Lactation Excretion in breast milk unknown/use caution

Contraindications Hypersensitivity to hydroxocobalamin,
cyanocobalamin, cobalt, or any component

Warnings Anaphylactic shock has occurred after parenteral vitamin B_{12} administration; intradermal skin testing
may be used prior to administration in individuals sensitive
to cobalt

When using Cyanokit®: Increased blood pressure
(>180 mm Hg systolic or >110 mm Hg diastolic) is
associated with infusion; elevations usually noted at
beginning of infusion, peak toward the end of infusion,
and return to baseline within 4 hours of infusion. Collection
of pretreatment blood cyanide concentrations does not
preclude administration and should not delay administration in the emergency management of highly suspected
or confirmed cyanide toxicity. Pretreatment levels may be
useful as postinfusion levels may be inaccurate. Treatment
of cyanide poisoning should include decontamination and
supportive therapy. Photosensitivity is a potential concern;
avoid direct sunlight while skin remains discolored. Safety
and efficacy for use in children has not been established.
Will produce chromaturia which may last up to 5 weeks
after administration.

Precautions When using solution for I.M. injection as
treatment of severe vitamin B_{12} deficiency: Serum
potassium concentrations should be monitored early as
severe hypokalemia has occurred after the conversion of
megaloblastic anemia to normal erythropoiesis; the
increase in nucleic acid degradation produced by
administration of hydroxocobalamin to deficient patients
may result in gout in susceptible individuals; use of
hydroxocobalamin in folic acid deficient individuals may
improve folate-deficient megaloblastic anemia and
obscure the true diagnosis

Adverse Reactions

I.M. injection:
  Cardiovascular: Peripheral vascular thrombosis
  Dermatologic: Itching, exanthema, urticaria
  Endocrine & metabolic: Hypokalemia
  Gastrointestinal: Diarrhea
  Local: Pain at injection site
  Miscellaneous: Hypersensitivity reactions

I.M. infusion (Cyanokit®):
  Cardiovascular: Hypertension (18% to 28%; see Warn-
    ings), chest discomfort, tachycardia, bradycardia, hot
    flashes, peripheral edema, angioneurotic edema
  Central nervous system: Headache, dizziness, memory
    impairment, restlessness
  Dermatologic: Erythema (94% to 100%; may last up to 2
    weeks), rash (predominantly acneiform; 20% to 44%;
    can appear 7-28 days after administration and usually
    resolves within a few weeks), pruritus, urticaria;
    photosensitivity

Gastrointestinal: Nausea, abdominal discomfort, diarrhea, dyspepsia, dysphagia, hematochezia, vomiting

Genitourinary: Chromaturia (100%; may last up to 5 weeks after administration)

Hematologic: Lymphocytes decreased

Local: Infusion site reaction (6% to 39%)

Ocular: Irritation, redness, swelling

Respiratory: Dry throat, dyspnea, throat tightness

Miscellaneous: Hypersensitivity reactions including anaphylaxis

Drug Interactions

Avoid Concomitant Use There are no known interactions where it is recommended to avoid concomitant use.

Increased Effect/Toxicity There are no known significant interactions involving an increase in effect.

Decreased Effect There are no known significant interactions involving a decrease in effect.

Stability Stable at room temperature; protect from light. Cyanokit® may be exposed at short intervals to temperatures outside of room temperature:

Usual transport: <15 days at 41°F to 104°F (5°C to 40°C)

Desert transport: <4 days at 41°F to 104°F (5°C to 40°C)

Freezing/defrosting cycles: <15 days at -4°F to 104°F (-20°C to 40°C)

Reconstituted vials (Cyanokit®) are stable for 6 hours at temperatures not exceeding 104°F (40°C). Hydroxocobalamin infusion (Cyanokit®) is physically incompatible if mixed with diazepam, dobutamine, dopamine, fentanyl, nitroglycerin, pentobarbital, propofol, and thiopental. It is also chemically incompatible with sodium thiosulfate, sodium nitrate, and ascorbic acid. It should not be infused either in the same solution or into the same I.V. line with these medications.

Mechanism of Action Hydroxocobalamin (vitamin B_{12a}) is a precursor to cyanocobalamin (vitamin B_{12}). Cyanocobalamin acts as a coenzyme for various metabolic functions, including fat and carbohydrate metabolism and protein synthesis, used in cell replication and hematopoiesis. In the presence of cyanide, each hydroxocobalamin molecule can bind one cyanide ion by substituting it for the hydroxo ligand linked to the trivalent cobalt ion, forming cyanocobalamin.

Pharmacodynamics

Onset of action: I.M.:

Megaloblastic anemia:

Conversion of megaloblastic to normoblastic erythroid hyperplasia within bone marrow: 8 hours

Increased reticulocytes: 2-5 days

Complicated vitamin B_{12} deficiency:

Psychiatric sequelae: 24 hours

Thrombocytopenia: 10 days

Granulocytopenia: 2 weeks

Pharmacokinetics (Adult data unless noted)

Distribution: Principally stored in the liver; also stored in the kidneys and adrenals

Protein binding: I.M. solution: Bound to transcobalamin II; I.V.: Cyanokit®: Significant; forms various cobalamin-(III) complexes

Half-life: I.V.: 26-31 hours

Metabolism: Converted in the tissues to active coenzymes methylcobalamin and deoxyadenosylcobalamin

Time to peak serum concentration: 2 hours

Elimination: Urine (50% to 98%)

Usual Dosage

I.M.:

Schilling test (diagnostic for vitamin B_{12} deficiency): Children and Adults: 1000 mcg once

Congenital transcobalamin deficiency: Neonates: 1000 mcg twice weekly

Vitamin B_{12} deficiency or pernicious anemia: Varying regimens:

Uncomplicated disease:

Children: Initial: 100 mcg/day for 10-15 days (total dose: 1-5 mg); maintenance: 60 mcg/month

or as an alternative: 30-50 mcg/day for at least 2 weeks (total dose: 1-5 mg); maintenance: 100 mcg/month

Adults: Initial: 30 mcg/day for 5-10 days; maintenance: 100-200 mcg/monthly

or as an alternative: 1000 mcg/day for 5-10 days, followed by 100-200 mcg/month

or as an alternative: 100 mcg/day for 1 week, followed by 100 mcg every other day for 2 weeks; maintenance: 100 mcg/month

Complicated disease (eg, severe anemia with heart failure, thrombocytopenia with bleeding, granulocytopenia with infection, severe neurologic damage): Adults: 1000 mcg plus folic acid 15 mg once, followed by 100 mcg/day plus oral folic acid 5 mg/day for 1 week; maintenance dosing as above

I.V.: Cyanide toxicity (Cyanokit®):

Children (non-U.S. marketing experience per manufacturer): 70 mg/kg as a single infusion

Adults: Initial: 5 g as single infusion; may repeat a second 5 g dose depending on the severity of poisoning and clinical response: maximum cumulative dose: 10 g

Dosage interval in hepatic or renal impairment: A decrease in the interval between injections may be required

Administration Parenteral:

I.M.: Administer 1000 mcg/mL injection I.M. only; do not administer SubQ

I.V.: Cyanokit®: Reconstitute 2.5 g vial with 100 mL NS, LR, or 5% dextrose; after reconstitution, repeatedly invert or "rock" solution for at least 30 seconds; do not shake. Administer over 15 minutes; if repeat dose is needed, administer second dose over 15 minutes to 2 hours depending upon the patient's clinical state

Monitoring Parameters

Anemia and deficiency states: Vitamin B_{12}, serum potassium, erythrocyte and reticulocyte counts, hemoglobin, hematocrit

Cyanide toxicity: Blood pressure and heart rate during and after infusion, serum lactate levels, venous-arterial pO_2 gradient, blood cyanide concentrations (see Warnings)

Reference Range

Vitamin B_{12}: Normal: 200-900 pg/mL; vitamin B_{12} deficiency: <200 pg/mL; megaloblastic anemia: <100 pg/mL

Cyanide toxicity: Blood cyanide levels may be used for diagnosis confirmation; however, reliable levels require prompt testing and proper storage conditions

Cyanide levels related to clinical symptomatology:

Tachycardia/flushing: 0.5-1 mg/L

Obtundation: 1-2.5 mg/L

Coma: 2.5-3 mg/L

Death: >3 mg/L

Test Interactions The following values may be affected, *in vitro*, following hydroxocobalamin 5 g dose. Interference following hydroxocobalamin 10 g dose can be expected to last up to an additional 24 hours. **Note:** Extent and duration of interference dependant on analyzer used and patient variability.

Falsely elevated:

Basophils, hemoglobin, MCH, and MCHC [duration: 12-16 hours]

Albumin, alkaline phosphatase, cholesterol, creatinine, glucose, total protein, and triglycerides [duration: 24 hours]

Bilirubin [duration: up to 4 days]

Urinalysis: Glucose, protein, erythrocytes, leukocytes, ketones, bilirubin, urobilinogen, nitrite [duration: 2-8 days]

Falsely decreased: ALT and amylase [duration: 24 hours]

Unpredictable:

AST, CK, CKMB, LDH, phosphate, and uric acid [duration: 24 hours]

PT (quick or INR) and aPTT [duration: 24-48 hours]

Urine pH [duration: 2-8 days]

May also interfere with colorimetric tests

Patient Information Life-long therapy is required in patients with pernicious anemia or other absorption defects; do not discontinue therapy without consulting your physician; avoid alcohol; large doses (Cyanokit®) will result in red-colored urine for up to 5 weeks and skin and mucous membrane redness for up to 2 weeks after administration; may cause photosensitivity (eg, exposure to sunlight may cause severe sunburn, skin rash, redness, or itching) while skin is discolored; avoid exposure to sunlight and artificial light sources (sunlamps, tanning booth/bed); wear protective clothing, wide-brimmed hats, sunglasses, and lip sunscreen (SPF ≥15); use a sunscreen [broad-spectrum sunscreen or physical sunscreen (preferred) or sunblock with SPF ≥15]; contact physician if reaction occurs; an acne-like rash may occur 7-28 days after administration of Cyanokit®; this rash usually goes away without any treatment

Additional Information Cyanocobalamin is preferred over hydroxocobalamin as a treatment agent for anemia due to reports of antibody formation to the hydroxocobalamin-transcobalamin complex. Cyanide is a clear colorless gas or liquid with a faint bitter almond odor. Cyanide reacts with trivalent ions in cytochrome oxidase in the mitochondria leading to histotoxic hypoxia and lactic acidosis. Signs and symptoms of cyanide toxicity include headache, altered mental status, dyspnea, mydriasis, chest tightness, nausea, vomiting, tachycardia/hypertension (initially), bradycardia/hypotension (later), seizures, cardiovascular collapse, or coma. Expert advice from a regional poison control center for appropriate use may be obtained (1-800-222-1222).

Dosage Forms Excipient information presented when available (limited, particularly for generics); consult specific product labeling.

Injection, solution: 1000 mcg/mL (30 mL)

Injection, powder for reconstitution:

Cyanokit®: 2.5 g (2 vials) [provided in a kit which also contains one I.V. infusion set]

♦ **Hydroxy-1,4-naphthoquinone** see Atovaquone on page 153

♦ **Hydroxycarbamide** see Hydroxyurea on page 695

Hydroxychloroquine (hye droks ee KLOR oh kwin)

Medication Safety Issues

Sound-alike/look-alike issues:

Hydroxychloroquine may be confused with hydrocortisone

Plaquenil® may be confused with Platinol®

Related Information

Malaria on page 1652

Medications for Which A Single Dose May Be Fatal When Ingested By A Toddler on page 1709

U.S. Brand Names Plaquenil®

Canadian Brand Names Apo-Hydroxyquine®; Gen-Hydroxychloroquine; Mylan-Hydroxychloroquine; Plaquenil®; PRO-Hydroxyquine

Therapeutic Category Antimalarial Agent; Antirheumatic, Disease Modifying

Generic Available Yes

Use Suppression or treatment of malaria caused by susceptible *P. vivax*, *P. ovale*, *P. malariae*, and some strains of *P. falciparum* (not effective against chloroquine-resistant strains of *P. falciparum*; not active against pre-erythrocytic or exoerythrocytic tissue stages of *Plasmodium*); treatment of systemic lupus erythematosus (SLE) and acute or chronic rheumatoid arthritis

Pregnancy Considerations Malaria infection in pregnant women may be more severe than in nonpregnant women. Therefore, pregnant women and women who are likely to become pregnant are advised to avoid travel to malaria-risk areas. Hydroxychloroquine is recommended as an alternative treatment of pregnant women for uncomplicated malaria in chloroquine-sensitive regions. Women exposed to hydroxychloroquine for the treatment of rheumatoid arthritis or systemic lupus erythematosus during pregnancy may be enrolled in the Organization of Teratology Information Specialists (OTIS) Autoimmune Diseases Study pregnancy registry (877-311-8972).

Lactation Enters breast milk (AAP considers "compatible")

Contraindications Hypersensitivity to hydroxychloroquine, 4-aminoquinoline derivatives, or any component; retinal or visual field changes; patients with porphyria or psoriasis

Warnings Children are especially sensitive to 4-aminoquinoline compounds; long-term use in children is contraindicated; daily dose >6-6.5 mg/kg/day in patients with abnormal hepatic or renal function may be associated with an increased risk of retinal toxicity

Precautions Use with caution in patients with hepatic disease, G-6-PD deficiency, and patients on concurrent therapy with known hepatotoxic drugs

Adverse Reactions

Cardiovascular: Cardiomyopathy (rare)

Central nervous system: Insomnia, nervousness, nightmares, dizziness, psychosis, headache, confusion, agitation, ataxia

Dermatologic: Lichenoid dermatitis, bleaching of the hair, pruritus, alopecia, hyperpigmentation, photosensitivity, Stevens-Johnson syndrome, exfoliative dermatitis, urticaria, angioedema

Gastrointestinal: GI irritation, abdominal cramps, anorexia, nausea, vomiting, diarrhea

Hematologic: Bone marrow suppression, thrombocytopenia, aplastic anemia, agranulocytosis, anemia

Hepatic: Hepatic failure, abnormal liver function

Neuromuscular & skeletal: Muscle weakness, skeletal muscle palsies, neuromyopathy, depression of tendon reflexes, peripheral neuropathy, myopathy

Ocular: Visual field defects, blindness, retinitis, macular degeneration, night vision decreased, abnormal color vision, loss of visual acuity

Respiratory: Bronchospasm

Drug Interactions

Avoid Concomitant Use

Avoid concomitant use of Hydroxychloroquine with any of the following: Artemether; BCG; Lumefantrine; Mefloquine; Natalizumab; Pimecrolimus; Tacrolimus (Topical); Vaccines (Live)

Increased Effect/Toxicity

Hydroxychloroquine may increase the levels/effects of: Antipsychotic Agents (Phenothiazines); Beta-Blockers; Cardiac Glycosides; Dapsone; Dapsone (Systemic); Dapsone (Topical); Leflunomide; Lumefantrine; Mefloquine; Natalizumab; Vaccines (Live)

The levels/effects of Hydroxychloroquine may be increased by: Artemether; Dapsone; Dapsone (Systemic); Denosumab; Mefloquine; Pimecrolimus; Tacrolimus (Topical); Trastuzumab

Decreased Effect

Hydroxychloroquine may decrease the levels/effects of: Anthelmintics; BCG; Sipuleucel-T; Vaccines (Inactivated); Vaccines (Live)

The levels/effects of Hydroxychloroquine may be decreased by: Echinacea

Food Interactions Food increases bioavailability

Stability Store tablets at room temperature; protect from light

Mechanism of Action Interferes with digestive vacuole function within sensitive malarial parasites by increasing the pH and interfering with lysosomal degradation of hemoglobin; inhibits locomotion of neutrophils and chemotaxis of eosinophils; impairs complement-dependent antigen-antibody reactions

Pharmacodynamics Onset of action for JRA: 2-4 months, up to 6 months

Pharmacokinetics (Adult data unless noted)

Absorption: Highly variable (31% to 100%)

Distribution: Extensive distribution to most body fluids and tissues; excreted into breast milk; crosses the placenta

Metabolism: In the liver

Bioavailability: Increased when administered with food

Elimination: Metabolites and unchanged drug slowly excreted in the urine

Usual Dosage Oral:

Children:

Chemoprophylaxis of malaria: 5 mg/kg **(base)** once weekly; do not exceed the recommended adult dose; begin 2 weeks before exposure; continue for 4 weeks after leaving endemic area

Uncomplicated acute attack of malaria: 10 mg/kg **(base)** initial dose; followed by 5 mg/kg **(base)** in 6-8 hours on day 1; 5 mg/kg **(base)** as a single dose on day 2 and on day 3

JRA or SLE: 3-5 mg/kg/day **(as sulfate)** divided 1-2 times/day to a maximum of 400 mg/day **(as sulfate)**; not to exceed 7 mg/kg/day

Adults:

Chemoprophylaxis of malaria: 310 mg **(base)** once weekly on same day each week; begin 2 weeks before exposure; continue for 4 weeks after leaving endemic area

Uncomplicated acute attack of malaria: 620 mg **(base)** first dose day one; 310 mg **(base)** in 6-8 hours day one; 310 mg **(base)** as a single dose day 2; and 310 mg **(base)** as a single dose on day 3

Rheumatoid arthritis: 400-600 mg/day **(as sulfate)** once daily to start; increase dose until optimum response level is reached; usually after 4-12 weeks dose should be reduced by 50% and a maintenance dose given of 200-400 mg/day **(as sulfate)** divided 1-2 times/day

Lupus erythematosus: 400 mg **(as sulfate)** every day or twice daily for several weeks depending on response; 200-400 mg/day **(as sulfate)** for prolonged maintenance therapy

Administration Oral: Administer with food or milk to decrease GI distress

Monitoring Parameters Ophthalmologic examination at baseline and every 3 months with prolonged therapy (including visual acuity, slit-lamp, fundoscopic, and visual field exam), CBC with differential and platelet count; check for muscular weakness with prolonged therapy

Patient Information May cause photosensitivity reactions (eg, exposure to sunlight may cause severe sunburn, skin rash, redness, or itching); avoid exposure to sunlight and artificial light sources (sunlamps, tanning booth/bed); wear protective clothing, wide-brimmed hats, sunglasses, and lip sunscreen (SPF ≥15); use a sunscreen [broad-spectrum sunscreen or physical sunscreen (preferred) or sunblock with SPF ≥15]; contact physician if reaction occurs. Notify physician if blurring of vision, vision change, weakness, numbness, tremors, rash, persistent diarrhea, or emotional change occur. May cause dizziness and vision changes, so exercise caution when driving; avoid alcohol; contraindicated during breast-feeding.

Dosage Forms Excipient information presented when available (limited, particularly for generics); consult specific product labeling.

Tablet, as sulfate: 200 mg [equivalent to 155 mg base]

Extemporaneous Preparations A 25 mg/mL hydroxychloroquine sulfate suspension is made by removing the coating off of fifteen 200 mg hydroxychloroquine sulfate tablets with a towel moistened with alcohol; tablets are ground to a fine powder and levigated to a paste with 15 mL of Ora-Plus® suspending agent; add an additional 45 mL of suspending agent and levigate until a uniform mixture is obtained; qs ad to 120 mL with sterile water for irrigation; a 30 day expiration date is recommended, although stability testing has not been performed

Pesko LJ, "Compounding: Hydroxychloroquine," *Am Druggist*, 1993, 207:57.

References

Centers for Disease Control and Prevention, "Guidelines for the Treatment of Malaria in the United States," available at http://www.cdc.gov/malaria/diagnosis_treatment/tx_clinicians.htm and http://www.cdc.gov/malaria/pdf/treatmenttable.pdf; last accessed October 2, 2007.

Emery H, "Clinical Aspects of Systemic Lupus Erythematosus in Childhood," *Pediatr Clin North Am*, 1986, 33(5):1177-90.

Giannini EH and Cawkwell GD, "Drug Treatment in Children With Juvenile Rheumatoid Arthritis. Past, Present, and Future," *Pediatr Clin North Am*, 1995, 42(5):1099-125.

"Guidelines for the Management of Rheumatoid Arthritis. American College of Rheumatology Ad Hoc Committee on Clinical Guidelines," *Arthritis Rheum*, 1996, 39(5):713-22.

◆ **Hydroxychloroquine Sulfate** *see* Hydroxychloroquine *on page 694*

◆ **Hydroxydaunomycin Hydrochloride** *see* DOXOrubicin *on page 477*

◆ **Hydroxyethyl Starch** *see* Hetastarch *on page 677*

◆ **Hydroxyldaunorubicin Hydrochloride** *see* DOXOrubicin *on page 477*

Hydroxyurea (hye droks ee yoor EE a)

Medication Safety Issues

Sound-alike/look-alike issues:

Hydroxyurea may be confused with hydrOXYzine

High alert medication: The Institute for Safe Medication Practices (ISMP) includes this medication among its list of drugs which have a heightened risk of causing significant patient harm when used in error.

International issues:

Hydrea® may be confused with Hydra® which is a brand name for isoniazid in Japan

Related Information

Adult and Adolescent HIV *on page 1620*

Emetogenic Potential of Antineoplastic Agents *on page 1579*

U.S. Brand Names Droxia®; Hydrea®

Canadian Brand Names Apo-Hydroxyurea®; Gen-Hydroxyurea; Hydrea®; Mylan-Hydroxyurea

Therapeutic Category Antineoplastic Agent, Miscellaneous

Generic Available Yes

Use Treatment of refractory chronic myelocytic leukemia (CML), melanoma, and relapsed or refractory ovarian carcinoma (FDA approved in adults); used with radiation in treatment of primary squamous cell carcinomas of the head and neck (excluding lip cancer) (FDA approved in adults); adjunct in the management of sickle cell patients who have had at least three painful crises in the previous 12 months (to reduce frequency of these crises and the need for blood transfusions) (FDA approved in adults); has also been used in the treatment of HIV infection, psoriasis, hematologic conditions such as essential thrombocythemia, polycythemia vera, hypereosinophilia, and hyperleukocytosis due to acute leukemia; relapsed AML; treatment of uterine, cervix, and nonsmall cell lung cancers; radiosensitizing agent in the treatment of primary brain tumors

Pregnancy Risk Factor D

Pregnancy Considerations Animal studies have demonstrated teratogenicity and embryotoxicity. There are no adequate and well-controlled studies in pregnant women. Women of childbearing potential should be advised to avoid pregnancy.

Lactation Enters breast milk/contraindicated

Breast-Feeding Considerations Due to the potential for serious adverse reactions, breast-feeding is not recommended.

Contraindications Hypersensitivity to hydroxyurea or any component; severe anemia, severe bone marrow suppression; when hydroxyurea is used as an antineoplastic agent: WBC <2500/mm^3 or platelet count <100,000/mm^3, or severe anemia; when hydroxyurea is used in patients with sickle cell anemia: Neutrophil count <2000 cells/mm^3, platelet count <80,000/mm^3, hemoglobin <4.5 g/dL, reticulocyte count <80,000/mm^3 when hemoglobin <9 g/dL

Warnings Hazardous agent; use appropriate precautions for handling and disposal; hydroxyurea is mutagenic, clastogenic, and presumed to be a human carcinogen **[U.S. Boxed Warning]**. Secondary leukemia and skin cancer have been reported in patients receiving long-term hydroxyurea therapy. Hydroxyurea impairs fertility and is embryotoxic causing fetal malformations; women of childbearing potential should be advised to avoid becoming pregnant. Vasculitic ulcerations and gangrene have been reported in patients who received hydroxyurea for myeloproliferative disorders with a previous or concurrent history of interferon use; discontinue if cutaneous vasculitic ulcerations develop. Megaloblastic erythropoiesis may be seen early in treatment; plasma iron clearance may be delayed and the rate of utilization of iron by erythrocytes may be delayed. When treated with hydroxyurea and antiretroviral agents (including didanosine), HIV-infected patients are at higher risk for potentially fatal pancreatitis, hepatotoxicity, hepatic failure, and severe peripheral neuropathy; discontinue immediately if signs of these develop.

Precautions Hematologic status, renal function, and hepatic function should be determined prior to and monitored during treatment. Use with caution and modify dose in patients with renal impairment. Use with caution in patients who have received previous radiotherapy or chemotherapy. Severe anemia must be corrected prior to initiating therapy.

Adverse Reactions

Cardiovascular: Edema

Central nervous system: Chills, disorientation, dizziness, drowsiness, fever, hallucinations, headache, malaise, seizures

Dermatologic: Facial erythema, gangrene, hair loss, hyperpigmentation, maculopapular rash, nail changes, pruritus, thinning of the skin, vasculitic ulcerations

Endocrine & metabolic: Hyperuricemia, weight gain

Gastrointestinal: Anorexia, constipation, diarrhea, nausea, pancreatitis, stomatitis, vomiting

Genitourinary: Dysuria

Hematologic: Bleeding, megaloblastic anemia, myelosuppression (leukopenia, neutropenia, thrombocytopenia)

Hepatic: Hepatic enzymes increased, hepatotoxicity

Neuromuscular & skeletal: Peripheral neuropathy

Renal: BUN increased, renal tubular function impairment, serum creatinine increased

Respiratory: Dyspnea, pulmonary fibrosis (rare), pulmonary infiltrates

Miscellaneous: Dermatomyositis-like lesions, parvovirus B-19 infection, secondary leukemia, skin cancer

Drug Interactions

Avoid Concomitant Use

Avoid concomitant use of Hydroxyurea with any of the following: BCG; Didanosine; Natalizumab; Pimecrolimus; Stavudine; Tacrolimus (Topical); Vaccines (Live)

Increased Effect/Toxicity

Hydroxyurea may increase the levels/effects of: Didanosine; Leflunomide; Natalizumab; Stavudine; Vaccines (Live)

The levels/effects of Hydroxyurea may be increased by: Denosumab; Didanosine; Pimecrolimus; Stavudine; Tacrolimus (Topical); Trastuzumab

Decreased Effect

Hydroxyurea may decrease the levels/effects of: BCG; Sipuleucel-T; Vaccines (Inactivated); Vaccines (Live)

The levels/effects of Hydroxyurea may be decreased by: Echinacea

Food Interactions In sickle cell patients, supplemental administration of folic acid is recommended; hydroxyurea may mask development of folic acid deficiency

Stability Store in a tightly sealed container since the drug is degraded by moisture; store at 25°C (77°F); excursions permitted to 15°C to 30°C (59°F to 86°F)

Mechanism of Action Interferes with synthesis of DNA during the S-phase of cell division without interfering with RNA synthesis; inhibits ribonucleoside diphosphate reductase preventing conversion of ribonucleotides to deoxyribonucleotides; hydroxyurea also inhibits the incorporation of thymidine into DNA; in sickle cell patients, hydroxyurea increases the production of fetal hemoglobin and decreases neutrophils; increases water content of RBCs, increases deformability of sickled cells, and alters the adhesion of RBCs to endothelium.

Pharmacodynamics Maximum effect for sickle cell disease: 6-18 months

Pharmacokinetics (Adult data unless noted)

Absorption: Readily from the GI tract

Distribution: Readily crosses the blood-brain barrier and the placenta; distributes into ascitic fluid and peritoneal or pleural effusions with estimated volume of distribution approximating total body water; concentrates in leukocytes and erythrocytes; excreted in breast milk

Metabolism: 60% via hepatic metabolism and urease found in intestinal bacteria

Half-life: 3-4 hours

Time to peak serum concentration: Within 1-4 hours

Elimination: 50% of drug excreted unchanged in urine; renal excretion of urea (metabolite) and respiratory excretion of CO_2 (metabolic end product)

Usual Dosage Oral (refer to individual protocols): Base dosage on ideal body weight:

Children:

Treatment of pediatric astrocytoma, medulloblastoma, and primitive neuroectodermal tumors: No FDA approved dosage regimens have been established. Dosages of 1500-3000 mg/m^2 as a single dose in combination with other agents, followed by a second course 2 weeks later with subsequent courses every 4-6 weeks have been used (eight-in-one regimen).

CML: Initial: 10-20 mg/kg/day once daily; adjust dose according to hematologic response

Children and Adults: Sickle cell anemia: Initial dose: 15 mg/kg/day (range: 10-20 mg/kg/day) once daily; increase dose in increments of 5 mg/kg/day every 12 weeks to a maximum dose of 35 mg/kg/day; reduced dosage of hydroxyurea alternating with erythropoietin may decrease myelotoxicity and increase concentrations of fetal hemoglobin in patients who have not been helped by hydroxyurea alone.

If blood counts are toxic (neutrophil count <2000 cells/mm^3, platelet count <80,000/mm^3, hemoglobin <4.5 g/dL, and reticulocytes <80,000/mm^3 if the hemoglobin <9 g/dL), discontinue hydroxyurea until bone marrow recovers. Restart therapy after reducing the dose by 2.5 mg/kg/day less than the dose at which toxicity occurred. Dose may be titrated every 12 weeks in 2.5 mg/kg/day increments.

Adults:

Solid tumors:

Intermittent therapy: 80 mg/kg as a single dose every third day

Continuous therapy: 20-30 mg/kg/day given as a single dose/day

Concomitant therapy with irradiation: 80 mg/kg as a single dose every third day starting at least 7 days before initiation of irradiation

Resistant chronic myelocytic leukemia: 20-30 mg/kg/day once daily

HIV infection: 500 mg twice daily (15 mg/kg/day divided twice daily) in combination with didanosine 200 mg twice daily (**Note:** HIV Adult and Adolescent guidelines state that there is insufficient data to make a recommendation for or against its use; see February 4, 2002, http://www.aidsinfo.nih.gov)

Dosing adjustment in renal impairment: Adults:

Sickle cell anemia:

Cl$_{cr}$ ≥60 mL/minute: Initial dose: 15 mg/kg/day

Cl$_{cr}$ <60 mL/minute: Reduce initial dose to 7.5 mg/kg/day

Hemodialysis: Reduce initial dose to 7.5 mg/kg/dose and administer following hemodialysis (titrate dose to response and toxicity avoidance)

Other indications:

Cl$_{cr}$ 10-50 mL/minute: Administer 50% of normal dose

Cl$_{cr}$ <10 mL/minute: Administer 20% of normal dose

Hemodialysis: Administer dose following hemodialysis

Administration Oral: For patients unable to swallow capsules, contents of capsule may be emptied into a glass of water if administered immediately

Monitoring Parameters CBC with differential and platelet count, hemoglobin, renal function and liver function tests, serum uric acid

Sickle cell anemia: Monitor blood counts every 2 weeks throughout therapy

Test Interactions False-negative triglyceride measurement by a glycerol oxidase method

Patient Information Inform physician if fever, sore throat, bruising, or bleeding develops; advise women of child-bearing potential to avoid becoming pregnant while taking hydroxyurea and to use a contraceptive method. To minimize risk of exposure to hydroxyurea, wear disposable gloves when handling bottle or capsules. Wash hands before and after contact with the bottle or capsule. If the powder from the capsule is spilled, it should immediately be wiped up with a damp disposable towel and discarded in a closed container.

Nursing Implications When handling hydroxyurea, wear impervious gloves to minimize risk of dermal exposure.

Additional Information Myelosuppressive effects:

WBC: Moderate

Platelets: Moderate

Onset (days): 7

Nadir (days): 10

Recovery (days): 21

Dosage Forms Excipient information presented when available (limited, particularly for generics); consult specific product labeling.

Capsule: 500 mg

Droxia®: 200 mg, 300 mg, 400 mg

Hydrea®: 500 mg

Extemporaneous Preparations A 40 mg/mL oral suspension in a 1:1 mixture of Ora-Sweet® and Ora-Plus® was stable for 14 days at room temperature (25°C) and under refrigeration (4°C) in plastic prescription bottles (see Nahata, 2003); label "shake well." This study did not determine microbial growth; extended storage under refrigeration is recommended.

Nahata MC, "Stability of Hydroxyurea in Two Extemporaneously Prepared Oral Suspensions Stored at Two Temperatures," *ASHP Midyear Clinical Meeting*, 2003, 38; P-161(E).

References

Geyer JR, Finlay JL, Boyett JM, et al, "Survival of Infants With Malignant Astrocytomas. A Report From the Childrens Cancer Group," *Cancer*, 1995, 75(4):1045-50.

Geyer JR, Pendergrass TW, Milstein JM, et al, "Eight Drugs in One Day Chemotherapy in Children With Brain Tumors: A Critical Toxicity Appraisal," *J Clin Oncol*, 1988, 6(6):996-1000.

Maier-Redelsperger M, de Montalembert M, Flahault A, et al, "Fetal Hemoglobin and F-Cell Responses to Long-Term Hydroxyurea Treatment in Young Sickle Cell Patients. The French Study Group on Sickle Cell Disease," *Blood*, 1998, 91(12):4472-9.

Montaner JS, Zala C, Conway B, et al, "A Pilot Study of Hydroxyurea Among Patients With Advanced Human Immunodeficiency Virus (HIV) Disease Receiving Chronic Didanosine Therapy: Canadian HIV Trials Network Protocol 080," *J Infect Dis*, 1997, 175(4):801-6.

Panel on Clinical Practices for the Treatment of HIV Infection, "Guidelines for the Use of Antiretroviral Agents in HIV-Infected Adults and Adolescents," March 23, 2004, http://www.aidsinfo.nih.gov.

Rodgers GP, Dover GJ, Noguchi CT, et al, "Hematologic Responses of Patients With Sickle Cell Disease to Treatment With Hydroxyurea," *N Engl J Med*, 1990, 322(15):1037-45.

Rodgers GP, Dover GJ, Uyesaka N, et al, "Augmentation by Erythropoietin of the Fetal-Hemoglobin Response to Hydroxyurea in Sickle Cell Disease," *N Engl J Med*, 1993, 328(2):73-80.

Strouse JJ, Lanzkron S, Beach MC, et al, "Hydroxyurea for Sickle Cell Disease: A Systematic Review for Efficacy and Toxicity in Children," *Pediatrics*, 2008, 122(6):1332-42.

HydrOXYzine (hye DROKS i zeen)

Medication Safety Issues

Sound-alike/look-alike issues:

HydrOXYzine may be confused with hydrALAZINE, hydroxyurea

Atarax® may be confused with Ativan®

Vistaril® may be confused with Restoril™, Versed, Zestril®

Beers Criteria medication: This drug may be inappropriate for use in geriatric patients (high severity risk).

International issues:

Vistaril® may be confused with Vastarel® which is a brand name for trimetazidine in multiple international markets

Related Information

Acute Dystonic Reactions, Management *on page 1687*

Compatibility of Chemotherapy and Related Supportive Care Medications *on page 1580*

Compatibility of Medications Mixed in a Syringe *on page 1713*

U.S. Brand Names Vistaril®

Canadian Brand Names Apo-Hydroxyzine®; Atarax®; Hydroxyzine Hydrochloride Injection, USP; Novo-Hydroxyzin; PMS-Hydroxyzine; Vistaril®

Therapeutic Category Antianxiety Agent; Antiemetic; Antihistamine; Sedative

Generic Available Yes

Use Treatment of anxiety; preoperative sedative; antipruritic; antiemetic

Pregnancy Risk Factor C

Pregnancy Considerations Hydroxyzine-induced fetal abnormalities at high dosages in animal studies. Neonatal withdrawal symptoms have been reported following long-term maternal use or the use of large doses near term. Use in early pregnancy is contraindicated by the manufacturer.

Lactation Excretion in breast milk unknown/not recommended

Contraindications Hypersensitivity to hydroxyzine or any component (see Warnings); early pregnancy

Warnings Subcutaneous, intra-arterial and I.V. administration are **not** recommended since intravascular hemolysis, thrombosis, and digital gangrene can occur; extravasation can result in sterile abscess and marked tissue induration. Hydroxyzine causes sedation; caution must be used when performing tasks which require alertness (eg, operating machinery or driving). Sedative effects of CNS depressants or ethanol are potentiated (see Drug Interactions).

Injection may contain benzyl alcohol which may cause allergic reactions in susceptible individuals; syrup may contain sodium benzoate; benzoic acid (benzoate) is a metabolite of benzyl alcohol; large amounts of benzyl alcohol (≥99 mg/kg/day) have been associated with a potentially fatal toxicity ("gasping syndrome") in neonates; the "gasping syndrome" consists of metabolic acidosis, respiratory distress, gasping respirations, CNS dysfunction (including convulsions, intracranial hemorrhage), hypotension and cardiovascular collapse; avoid use of hydroxyzine products containing benzyl alcohol or sodium benzoate in neonates; *in vitro* and animal studies have shown that benzoate displaces bilirubin from protein binding sites

Precautions Use with caution in patients with narrow-angle glaucoma, prostatic hypertrophy, bladder neck obstruction, asthma, or COPD. Neonatal withdrawal symptoms, including seizures, have been reported following long-term maternal use or the use of large doses near term.

Adverse Reactions

Cardiovascular: Hypotension; supraventricular tachycardia (case report; see Wong, 2004)

Central nervous system: Drowsiness, dizziness, headache, ataxia, hallucination, seizure

Dermatologic: Pruritus, rash, urticaria

Gastrointestinal: Xerostomia

Genitourinary: Urinary retention

Local: Pain at injection site

Neuromuscular & skeletal: Weakness, involuntary movements, paresthesia, tremor

Ocular: Blurred vision

Respiratory: Thickening of bronchial secretions

Miscellaneous: Allergic reaction, anticholinergic effects

Drug Interactions

Metabolism/Transport Effects Inhibits CYP2D6 (weak)

Avoid Concomitant Use There are no known interactions where it is recommended to avoid concomitant use.

Increased Effect/Toxicity

HydrOXYzine may increase the levels/effects of: Alcohol (Ethyl); Anticholinergics; CNS Depressants

The levels/effects of HydrOXYzine may be increased by: Pramlintide

Decreased Effect

HydrOXYzine may decrease the levels/effects of: Acetylcholinesterase Inhibitors (Central); Betahistine

The levels/effects of HydrOXYzine may be decreased by: Acetylcholinesterase Inhibitors (Central); Amphetamines

Stability Injection: Store at 15°C to 30°C. Protect from light

Mechanism of Action Competes with histamine for H_1-receptor sites on effector cells in the GI tract, blood vessels, and respiratory tract

Pharmacodynamics

Onset of action: Within 15-30 minutes

Duration: 4-6 hours

Pharmacokinetics (Adult data unless noted)

Absorption: Oral: Well absorbed

Distribution: V_d, apparent:

Children 1-14 years: 18.5 ± 8.6 L/kg

Adults: 16 ± 3 L/kg

Metabolism: In the liver; forms metabolites

Half-life:

Children 1-14 years (mean age: 6.1 ± 4.6 years): 7.1 ± 2.3 hours; **Note:** Half-life increased with increasing age and was 4 hours in patients 1-year old and 11 hours in a 14-year old patient (see Simons, 1984)

Adults: 3 hours; one study reported a terminal half-life of 20 hours (see Simons, 1984a)

Time to peak serum concentration: Oral: 2 hours

Usual Dosage

Children:

Manufacturer's recommendation:

Preoperative sedation:

Oral: 0.6 mg/kg/dose

I.M.: 0.5-1 mg/kg/dose

Pruritus, anxiety: Oral:

<6 years: 50 mg/day in divided doses

≥6 years: 50-100 mg/day in divided doses

Alternative dosing: Pruritus, anxiety:

Oral: 2 mg/kg/day divided every 6-8 hours

I.M.: 0.5-1 mg/kg/dose every 4-6 hours as needed

Adults:

Antiemetic: I.M.: 25-100 mg/dose every 4-6 hours as needed

Anxiety: Oral: 25-100 mg 4 times/day; maximum dose: 600 mg/day

Preoperative sedation:

Oral: 50-100 mg

I.M.: 25-100 mg

Management of pruritus: Oral: 25 mg 3-4 times/day

Dosing interval in hepatic impairment: Change dosing interval to every 24 hours in patients with primary biliary cirrhosis

Administration

Oral: May be administered without regard to food; shake suspension well before use

Parenteral: **Not** recommended for subcutaneous, intra-arterial, or I.V. administration (see Warnings). Administer I.M. deep in large muscle. For I.M. administration in children, injections should be made into the midlateral muscles of the thigh. Hydroxyzine has been administered slow I.V. to oncology patients via central venous lines without problems

Monitoring Parameters Relief of symptoms, mental status, blood pressure

Patient Information May cause drowsiness and impair ability to perform activities requiring mental alertness or physical coordination. May cause dry mouth. Avoid alcohol. Do not use other prescription or OTC medications (especially sedatives, tranquilizers, antihistamines, or pain medications) without consulting prescriber. Report hallucinations, seizure activity, tremors or involuntary movements, or loss of sensation to physician.

Dosage Forms Excipient information presented when available (limited, particularly for generics); consult specific product labeling. [DSC] = Discontinued product

Capsule, as pamoate: 25 mg, 50 mg, 100 mg

Vistaril®: 25 mg, 50 mg

Injection, solution, as hydrochloride: 25 mg/mL (1 mL); 50 mg/mL (1 mL, 2 mL, 10 mL)

Solution, oral, as hydrochloride: 10 mg/5 mL (473 mL)

Syrup, as hydrochloride: 10 mg/5 mL (120 mL, 480 mL)

Tablet, as hydrochloride: 10 mg, 25 mg, 50 mg

References

Baumgartner TG, "Administration of Hydroxyzine Injection," *Am J Hosp Pharm*, 1979, 36(12):1660.

Berde C, Ablin A, Glazer J, et al, "American Academy of Pediatrics Report of the Subcommittee on Disease-Related Pain in Childhood Cancer," *Pediatrics*, 1990, 86(5 Pt 2):818-25.

Serreau R, Komiha M, Blanc F, et al, "Neonatal Seizures Associated With Maternal Hydroxyzine Hydrochloride in Late Pregnancy," *Reprod Toxicol*, 2005, 20(4):573-4.

Simons FE, Simons KJ, Becker AB, et al, "Pharmacokinetics and Antipruritic Effects of Hydroxyzine in Children With Atopic Dermatitis," *J Pediatr*, 1984, 104(1):123-7.

Simons FE, Simons KJ, and Frith EM, "The Pharmacokinetics and Antihistaminic of the H₁ Receptor Antagonist Hydroxyzine," *J Allergy Clin Immunol*, 1984, 73(1 Pt 1):69-75.

Wong AR and Rasool AH, "Hydroxyzine-Induced Supraventricular Tachycardia in a Nine-Year-Old Child," *Singapore Med J*, 2004, 45 (2):90-2.

◆ **Hydroxyzine Hydrochloride** *see* HydrOXYzine *on page 697*

◆ **Hydroxyzine Hydrochloride Injection, USP (Can)** *see* HydrOXYzine *on page 697*

◆ **Hydroxyzine Pamoate** *see* HydrOXYzine *on page 697*

◆ **HydroZone Plus [OTC] [DSC]** *see* Hydrocortisone *on page 685*

◆ **Hylenex™** *see* Hyaluronidase *on page 679*

◆ **HyoMax™-DT** *see* Hyoscyamine *on page 699*

◆ **HyoMax™-FT** *see* Hyoscyamine *on page 699*

◆ **HyoMax®-SR** *see* Hyoscyamine *on page 699*

◆ **Hyonatol** *see* Hyoscyamine, Atropine, Scopolamine, and Phenobarbital *on page 700*

◆ **Hyoscine Butylbromide** *see* Scopolamine *on page 1248*

◆ **Hyoscine Hydrobromide** *see* Scopolamine *on page 1248*

Hyoscyamine (hye oh SYE a meen)

Medication Safety Issues
Sound-alike/look-alike issues:
Anaspaz® may be confused with Anaprox®, Antispas®
Levbid® may be confused with Enbrel®, Lithobid®, Lopid®, Lorabid®
Levsinex® may be confused with Lanoxin®
Levsin/SL® maybe confused with Levaquin®

Beers Criteria medication: This drug may be inappropriate for use in geriatric patients (high severity risk).

U.S. Brand Names Anaspaz®; HyoMax®-SR; HyoMax™-DT; HyoMax™-FT; Hyosyne; Levbid®; Levsin®; Levsin®/SL; Symax® DuoTab; Symax® FasTab; Symax® SL; Symax® SR

Canadian Brand Names Levsin®

Therapeutic Category Anticholinergic Agent; Antispasmodic Agent, Gastrointestinal

Generic Available Yes: Elixir (oral), solution (oral), tablet (orally disintegrating)

Use Treatment of GI tract disorders caused by spasm; adjunctive therapy for peptic ulcers and hypermotility disorders of lower urinary tract; infant colic

Pregnancy Risk Factor C

Pregnancy Considerations Crosses the placenta, effects to the fetus not known; use during pregnancy only if clearly needed.

Lactation Enters breast milk/not recommended

Breast-Feeding Considerations Excreted in breast milk in trace amounts. May also suppress lactation. Breast-feeding is not recommended.

Contraindications Hypersensitivity to hyoscyamine or any component; narrow-angle glaucoma, GI and GU obstruction, paralytic ileus, severe ulcerative colitis, myasthenia gravis

Warnings Low doses may cause a paradoxical decrease in heart rate; heat prostration may occur in hot weather.

Some oral liquids contain sodium benzoate; benzoic acid (benzoate) is a metabolite of benzyl alcohol; large amounts of benzyl alcohol (≥99 mg/kg/day) have been associated with a potentially fatal toxicity ("gasping syndrome") in neonates; *in vitro* and animal studies have shown that benzoate displaces bilirubin from protein binding sites; avoid using products containing sodium benzoate in neonates

Precautions Use with caution in patients with hyperthyroidism, CHF, cardiac arrhythmias, prostatic hypertrophy, autonomic neuropathy, chronic lung disease, biliary tract disease, children with spastic paralysis. Disintegrating tablet (NuLev™) contains aspartame which is metabolized to phenylalanine and must be used with caution in patients with phenylketonuria.

Adverse Reactions
Cardiovascular: Tachycardia or palpitations, bradycardia (with very low doses), orthostatic hypotension

Central nervous system: Headache, lightheadedness, short-term memory loss, fatigue, delirium, restlessness, ataxia, dizziness, insomnia, psychosis, euphoria, nervousness, confusion, insomnia, fever

Dermatologic: Dry skin, photosensitivity, rash, urticaria

Gastrointestinal: Xerostomia, nausea, vomiting, constipation, dysphagia, dysgeusia, dry throat

Genitourinary: Difficult urination, urinary retention

Local: Irritation at injection site

Neuromuscular & skeletal: Weakness, tremor

Ocular: Blurred vision, photophobia, mydriasis, anisocoria, cycloplegia, intraocular pressure elevated

Respiratory: Dry nose

Miscellaneous: Diaphoresis decreased

Drug Interactions
Avoid Concomitant Use There are no known interactions where it is recommended to avoid concomitant use.

Increased Effect/Toxicity
Hyoscyamine may increase the levels/effects of: AbobotulinumtoxinA; Anticholinergics; Cannabinoids; OnabotulinumtoxinA; Potassium Chloride; RimabotulinumtoxinB

The levels/effects of Hyoscyamine may be increased by: Pramlintide

Decreased Effect
Hyoscyamine may decrease the levels/effects of: Acetylcholinesterase Inhibitors (Central); Secretin

The levels/effects of Hyoscyamine may be decreased by: Acetylcholinesterase Inhibitors (Central)

Mechanism of Action Blocks the action of acetylcholine at parasympathetic sites in smooth muscle, secretory glands, and the CNS; specific anticholinergic responses are dose-related; increases cardiac output, dries secretions, antagonizes histamine and serotonin

Pharmacodynamics
Onset of action:
Oral: 20-30 minutes
Sublingual: 5-20 minutes
I.V.: 2-3 minutes
Duration: 4-6 hours

Pharmacokinetics (Adult data unless noted)
Absorption: Well absorbed from the GI tract

Distribution: Crosses the placenta; small amounts appear in breast milk

Protein binding: 50%

Metabolism: In the liver

Half-life: 3.5 hours

Elimination: 30% to 50% eliminated unchanged in urine within 12 hours

Usual Dosage

GI tract disorders:

Infants <2 years: Oral: The following table lists the hyoscyamine dosage using the drop formulation; hyoscyamine drops are dosed every 4 hours as needed

Hyoscyamine Drops Dosage

Weight (kg)	Dose (drops)	Maximum Daily Dose (drops)
2.3	3	18
3.4	4	24
5	5	30
7	6	36
10	8	48
15	11	66

Oral, S.L.:

Children 2-12 years: 0.0625-0.125 mg every 4 hours as needed; maximum daily dosage 0.75 mg **or** timed release 0.375 mg every 12 hours; maximum daily dosage 0.75 mg

Children >12 years to Adults: 0.125-0.25 mg every 4 hours as needed; maximum daily dosage 1.5 mg **or** timed release 0.375-0.75 mg every 12 hours; maximum daily dosage 1.5 mg

I.V., I.M., SubQ: Children >12 years to Adults: 0.25-0.5 mg at 4-hour intervals for 1-4 doses

Adjunct to anesthesia: I.M., I.V., SubQ: Children >2 years to Adults: 5 mcg/kg given 30-60 minutes prior to induction of anesthesia

Hypermotility of lower urinary tract: Oral, S.L.: Adults: 0.15-0.3 mg four times daily; timed release: 0.375 mg every 12 hours

Reversal of neuromuscular blockage: I.V., I.M., SubQ: 0.2 mg for every 1 mg neostigmine

Administration

Oral: Administer before meals; timed release tablets are scored and may be cut for easier dosage titration; S.L.: Place under the tongue

Parenteral: May be administered I.M., I.V., and SubQ; no information is available for I.V. administration rate or dilution

Monitoring Parameters Pulse, anticholinergic effects, urine output, GI symptoms

Patient Information May cause dry mouth; maintain good oral hygiene habits, because lack of saliva may increase chance of cavities; notify physician if skin rash, flushing or eye pain occurs, or if difficulty in urinating, constipation, or sensitivity to light becomes severe or persists; may cause dizziness or blurred vision; may cause drowsiness and impair ability to perform activities requiring mental alertness or physical coordination. May rarely cause photosensitivity reactions (eg, exposure to sunlight may cause severe sunburn, skin rash, redness, or itching); avoid direct exposure to sunlight

Dosage Forms Excipient information presented when available (limited, particularly for generics); consult specific product labeling. [DSC] = Discontinued product

Capsule, extended release, oral, as sulfate: 0.375 mg [DSC]

Elixir, oral, as sulfate: 0.125 mg/5 mL (473 mL)

Hyosyne: 0.125 mg/5 mL (473 mL) [contains ethanol 20%; orange-lemon flavor]

Levsin®: 0.125 mg/5 mL (473 mL) [contains ethanol 20%; orange flavor] [DSC]

Injection, solution, as sulfate:

Levsin®: 0.5 mg/mL (1 mL)

Solution, oral, as sulfate [drops]: 0.125 mg/mL (15 mL)

Hyosyne: 0.125 mg/mL (15 mL) [contains ethanol 5%, sodium benzoate; orange-lemon flavor]

Levsin®: 0.125 mg/mL (15 mL) [contains ethanol 5%; orange flavor] [DSC]

Tablet, chewable/disintegrating, oral, as sulfate:

HyoMax™-FT: 0.125 mg

Symax® FasTab: 0.125 mg

Tablet, oral, as sulfate: 0.125 mg, 0.15 mg [DSC]

Levsin®: 0.125 mg

Tablet, sublingual, as sulfate: 0.125 mg

Levsin®/SL: 0.125 mg

Symax® SL: 0.125 mg

Tablet, extended release, oral, as sulfate: 0.375 mg

Levbid®: 0.375 mg

Tablet, orally disintegrating, oral, as sulfate: 0.125 mg

Anaspaz®: 0.125 mg [scored]

Tablet, sustained release, oral, as sulfate:

HydroMax®-SR: 0.375 mg

Symax® SR: 0.375 mg

Tablet, variable release, oral:

HyoMax™-DT: Hyoscyamine sulfate 0.125 mg [immediate release] and hyoscyamine sulfate 0.25 mg [sustained release]

Symax® DuoTab: Hyoscyamine sulfate 0.125 mg [immediate release] and hyoscyamine sulfate 0.25 mg [sustained release]

Hyoscyamine, Atropine, Scopolamine, and Phenobarbital

(hye oh SYE a meen, A troe peen, skoe POL a meen & fee noe BAR bi tal)

Medication Safety Issues

Sound-alike/look-alike issues:

Donnatal® may be confused with Donnagel®, Donnatal Extentabs®

Beers Criteria medication: This drug may be inappropriate for use in geriatric patients (high severity risk).

U.S. Brand Names Donnatal Extentabs®; Donnatal®; Hyonatol

Therapeutic Category Anticholinergic Agent; Antispasmodic Agent, Gastrointestinal

Generic Available Yes: Tablet

Use Adjunct in treatment of peptic ulcer disease, irritable bowel, spastic colitis, spastic bladder, and renal colic

Pregnancy Risk Factor C

Pregnancy Considerations Reproduction studies with this combination have not been done; refer to individual components.

Lactation Excretion in breast milk unknown/use caution

Contraindications Hypersensitivity to hyoscyamine, atropine, scopolamine, phenobarbital, or any component of the formulation; narrow-angle glaucoma; tachycardia; GI and GU obstruction; myasthenia gravis; paralytic ileus; intestinal atony; unstable cardiovascular status in acute hemorrhage; severe ulcerative colitis; hiatal hernia associated with reflux esophagitis; acute intermittent porphyria

Warnings Heat prostration can occur in the presence of high environmental temperature

Precautions Use with caution in patients with hepatic or renal disease, hyperthyroidism, CAD, CHF, cardiac arrhythmias, tachycardia, hypertension, autonomic neuropathy

Adverse Reactions

Cardiovascular: Tachycardia, palpitations, bradycardia (with very low doses of atropine)

Central nervous system: Headache, drowsiness, nervousness, confusion, insomnia, fever, dizziness

Gastrointestinal: Xerostomia, nausea, vomiting, constipation, dysphagia, paralytic ileus, dysgeusia

Genitourinary: Impotence, urinary retention

Neuromuscular & skeletal: Weakness, musculoskeletal pain

Ocular: Blurred vision, photophobia, mydriasis, cycloplegia, intraocular pressure elevated

Respiratory: Nasal congestion

Miscellaneous: Hypersensitivity reactions, diaphoresis decreased

Drug Interactions

Metabolism/Transport Effects Phenobarbital: **Substrate** of CYP2C9 (minor), 2C19 (major), 2E1 (minor); **Induces** CYP1A2 (strong), 2A6 (strong), 2B6 (strong), 2C8/9 (strong), 3A4 (strong)

Avoid Concomitant Use

Avoid concomitant use of Hyoscyamine, Atropine, Scopolamine, and Phenobarbital with any of the following: Darunavir; Dronedarone; Etravirine; Everolimus; Nilotinib; Pazopanib; Ranolazine; Romidepsin; Tolvaptan; Voriconazole

Increased Effect/Toxicity

Hyoscyamine, Atropine, Scopolamine, and Phenobarbital may increase the levels/effects of: AbobotulinumtoxinA; Alcohol (Ethyl); Anticholinergics; Cannabinoids; CNS Depressants; Meperidine; OnabotulinumtoxinA; Potassium Chloride; RimabotulinumtoxinB; Thiazide Diuretics

The levels/effects of Hyoscyamine, Atropine, Scopolamine, and Phenobarbital may be increased by: Carbonic Anhydrase Inhibitors; Chloramphenicol; CYP2C19 Inhibitors (Moderate); CYP2C19 Inhibitors (Strong); Divalproex; Felbamate; Pramlintide; Primidone; Rufinamide; Valproic Acid

Decreased Effect

Hyoscyamine, Atropine, Scopolamine, and Phenobarbital may decrease the levels/effects of: Acetaminophen; Acetylcholinesterase Inhibitors (Central); Bendamustine; Beta-Blockers; Calcium Channel Blockers; Chloramphenicol; Contraceptives (Estrogens); Contraceptives (Progestins); Corticosteroids (Systemic); CycloSPORINE; CycloSPORINE (Systemic); CYP1A2 Substrates; CYP2A6 Substrates; CYP2B6 Substrates; CYP2C8 Substrates (High risk); CYP2C9 Substrates (High risk); CYP3A4 Substrates; Darunavir; Deferasirox; Disopyramide; Divalproex; Doxycycline; Dronedarone; Etoposide; Etoposide Phosphate; Etravirine; Everolimus; Griseofulvin; GuanFACINE; Irinotecan; Lacosamide; LamoTRIgine; Maraviroc; Methadone; MetroNIDAZOLE; MetroNIDAZOLE (Systemic); Nilotinib; OXcarbazepine; Pazopanib; Propafenone; QuiNIDine; Ranolazine; Romidepsin; Rufinamide; Saxagliptin; Secretin; Sorafenib; Tadalafil; Teniposide; Theophylline Derivatives; Tipranavir; Tolvaptan; Treprostinil; Tricyclic Antidepressants; Valproic Acid; Vitamin K Antagonists; Voriconazole; Zonisamide

The levels/effects of Hyoscyamine, Atropine, Scopolamine, and Phenobarbital may be decreased by: Acetylcholinesterase Inhibitors (Central); Amphetamines; Cholestyramine Resin; CYP2C19 Inducers (Strong); Folic Acid; Ketorolac; Ketorolac (Systemic); Leucovorin Calcium-Levoleucovorin; Mefloquine; Methylfolate; Pyridoxine; Rifamycin Derivatives; Tipranavir

Mechanism of Action Anticholinergic agents (hyoscyamine, atropine, and scopolamine) inhibit the muscarinic actions of acetylcholine at the postganglionic parasympathetic neuroeffector sites including smooth muscle, secretory glands, and CNS sites; specific anticholinergic responses are dose-related

Pharmacokinetics (Adult data unless noted) Absorption: Well absorbed from the GI tract

Usual Dosage Oral:

Children: Donnatal®: 0.1 mL/kg/dose every 4 hours; maximum dose: 5 mL **or** see table for alternative.

Donnatal® Dosage

Weight (kg)	Dose (mL)	
	Every 4 Hours	Every 6 Hours
4.5	0.5	0.75
10	1	1.5
14	1.5	2
23	2.5	3.8
34	3.8	5
≥45	5	7.5

Adults: Donnatal®: 1-2 tablets or capsules 3-4 times/day **or** 5-10 mL 3-4 times/day or 1 extended release tablet every 12 hours (may increase to every 8 hours if needed)

Administration Oral: Administer 30-60 minutes before meals; do not crush or chew extended release tablets

Patient Information Maintain good oral hygiene habits because lack of saliva may increase chance of cavities; may cause dry mouth; notify physician if skin rash, flushing or eye pain occurs, or if difficulty in urinating, constipation, or sensitivity to light becomes severe or persists; observe caution while driving or performing other tasks requiring alertness, as may cause drowsiness, dizziness, or blurred vision

Dosage Forms Excipient information presented when available (limited, particularly for generics); consult specific product labeling. [DSC] = Discontinued product

Elixir: Hyoscyamine sulfate 0.1.37 mg, atropine sulfate 0.0194 mg, scopolamine hydrobromide 0.0065 mg, and phenobarbital 16.2 mg per 5 mL (480 mL) [DSC]

Donnatal®: Hyoscyamine sulfate 0.1037 mg, atropine sulfate 0.0194 mg, scopolamine hydrobromide 0.0065 mg, and phenobarbital 16.2 mg per 5 mL (120 mL, 480 mL) [contains ethanol 23.8%; citrus flavor] [DSC]

Donnatal®: Hyoscyamine sulfate 0.1037 mg, atropine sulfate 0.0194 mg, scopolamine hydrobromide 0.0065 mg, and phenobarbital 16.2 mg per 5 mL (120 mL, 480 mL) [contains ethanol 23.8%; grape flavor]

Tablet: Hyoscyamine sulfate 0.1037 mg, atropine sulfate 0.0194 mg, scopolamine hydrobromide 0.0065 mg, and phenobarbital 16.2 mg

Donnatal®: Hyoscyamine sulfate 0.1037 mg, atropine sulfate 0.0194 mg, scopolamine hydrobromide 0.0065 mg, and phenobarbital 16.2 mg

Hyonatol: Hyoscyamine sulfate 0.1037 mg, atropine sulfate 0.0194 mg, scopolamine hydrobromide 0.0065 mg, and phenobarbital 16.2 mg

Tablet, extended release:

Donnatal Extentabs®: Hyoscyamine sulfate 0.3111 mg, atropine sulfate 0.0582 mg, scopolamine hydrobromide 0.0195 mg, and phenobarbital 48.6 mg

◆ **Hyoscyamine Sulfate** *see* Hyoscyamine *on page 699*

◆ **Hyosyne** *see* Hyoscyamine *on page 699*

◆ **HyperHep B® (Can)** *see* Hepatitis B Immune Globulin *on page 673*

◆ **HyperHEP B™ S/D** *see* Hepatitis B Immune Globulin *on page 673*

◆ **HyperRAB™ S/D** *see* Rabies Immune Globulin (Human) *on page 1198*

◆ **HyperRHO™ S/D Full Dose** *see* Rh₀(D) Immune Globulin *on page 1207*

◆ **HyperRHO™ S/D Mini Dose** *see* Rh₀(D) Immune Globulin *on page 1207*

◆ **Hyper-Sal™** see Sodium Chloride on page 1270

◆ **HyperTET™ S/D** see Tetanus Immune Globulin (Human) on page 1328

◆ **Hypertonic Saline** see Sodium Chloride on page 1270

◆ **Hytone® [DSC]** see Hydrocortisone on page 685

◆ **Ibidomide Hydrochloride** see Labetalol on page 787

◆ **Ibu®** see Ibuprofen on page 702

◆ **Ibu-200 [OTC]** see Ibuprofen on page 702

Ibuprofen (eye byoo PROE fen)

Medication Safety Issues
Sound-alike/look-alike issues:
Haltran® may be confused with Halfprin®
Motrin® may be confused with Neurontin®

Injectable formulations: Both ibuprofen and ibuprofen lysine are available for parenteral use. Ibuprofen lysine is **only** indicated for closure of a clinically-significant patent ductus arteriosus.

U.S. Brand Names Addaprin [OTC]; Advil® Children's [OTC]; Advil® Infants' [OTC]; Advil® Migraine [OTC]; Advil® [OTC]; Caldolor™; Genpril® [OTC] [DSC]; I-Prin [OTC]; Ibu-200 [OTC]; Ibu®; Midol® Cramp and Body Aches [OTC]; Motrin® Children's [OTC]; Motrin® IB [OTC]; Motrin® Infants' [OTC]; Motrin® Junior [OTC]; Neo-Profen®; Proprinal [OTC]; Ultraprin [OTC]

Canadian Brand Names Advil®; Apo-Ibuprofen®; Motrin® (Children's); Motrin® IB; Novo-Profen; Nu-Ibuprofen

Therapeutic Category Analgesic, Non-narcotic; Anti-inflammatory Agent; Antipyretic; Nonsteroidal Anti-inflammatory Drug (NSAID), Oral; Nonsteroidal Anti-inflammatory Drug (NSAID), Parenteral

Generic Available Yes: Caplet, suspension, tablet

Use
Oral: Treatment of inflammatory diseases and rheumatoid disorders including juvenile rheumatoid arthritis (JRA) (FDA approved in pediatric patients (age not specified)], rheumatoid arthritis (FDA approved in adults), and osteoarthritis (FDA approved in adults); mild to moderate pain (FDA approved in ages ≥6 months and adults); reduction of fever (FDA approved in ages ≥6 months and adults); primary dysmenorrhea (FDA approved in adults); migraine pain; gout; cystic fibrosis

Ibuprofen injection (Caldolor™): Management of mild to moderate pain, management of moderate to severe pain when used concurrently with an opioid analgesic; reduction of fever (all indications FDA approved in ages ≥17 years)

Ibuprofen lysine injection (NeoProfen®): Treatment (ie, closure) of a clinically significant PDA when usual treatments are ineffective (FDA approved in premature neonates who weigh between 500-1500 g and who are ≤32 weeks gestational age). **Note:** The prophylactic use of ibuprofen is not currently indicated nor recommended (see Shah, 2006).

Medication Guide An FDA-approved patient medication guide, which is available with the product information and at http://www.fda.gov/downloads/Drugs/DrugSafety/ucm088647.pdf, must be dispensed with this medication for each new outpatient prescription and refill for oral administration.

Pregnancy Risk Factor C/D ≥30 weeks gestation

Pregnancy Considerations Adverse events were not observed in the initial animal reproduction studies; therefore, the manufacturer classifies ibuprofen as pregnancy category C (category D: ≥30 weeks gestation). NSAID exposure during the first trimester is not strongly associated with congenital malformations; however, cardiovascular anomalies and cleft palate have been observed following NSAID exposure in some studies. The use of a NSAID close to conception may be associated with an increased risk of miscarriage. Non-teratogenic effects have been observed following NSAID administration during the third trimester including: Myocardial degenerative changes, prenatal constriction of the ductus arteriosus, fetal tricuspid regurgitation, failure of the ductus arteriosus to close postnatally; renal dysfunction or failure, oligohydramnios; gastrointestinal bleeding or perforation, increased risk of necrotizing enterocolitis; intracranial bleeding (including intraventricular hemorrhage), platelet dysfunction with resultant bleeding; pulmonary hypertension. Because they may cause premature closure of the ductus arteriosus, use of NSAIDs late in pregnancy should be avoided (use after 31 or 32 weeks gestation is not recommended by some clinicians). Product labeling for Caldolor™ specifically notes that use at ≥30 weeks gestation should be avoided and therefore classifies ibuprofen as pregnancy category D at this time. The chronic use of NSAIDs in women of reproductive age may be associated with infertility that is reversible upon discontinuation of the medication. A registry is available for pregnant women exposed to autoimmune medications including ibuprofen. For additional information contact the Organization of Teratology Information Specialists, OTIS Autoimmune Diseases Study, at 877-311-8972.

Lactation Enters breast milk/not recommended (AAP rates "compatible")

Breast-Feeding Considerations Based on limited data, only very small amounts of ibuprofen are excreted into breast milk. Adverse events have not been reported in nursing infants. The AAP considers ibuprofen to be "usually compatible with breast-feeding." Because there is a potential for adverse events to occur in nursing infants, the manufacturer does not recommend the use of ibuprofen while breast-feeding. Use with caution in nursing women with hypertensive disorders of pregnancy or pre-existing renal disease.

Contraindications Hypersensitivity to ibuprofen or any component (see Warnings); history of asthma, urticaria, or allergic-type reaction to aspirin, or other NSAIDs; patients with the "aspirin triad" [asthma, rhinitis (with or without nasal polyps), and aspirin intolerance] (fatal asthmatic and anaphylactoid reactions may occur in these patients); perioperative pain in the setting of coronary artery bypass graft (CABG)

Ibuprofen lysine injection (NeoProfen®) is contraindicated in preterm neonates with untreated proven or suspected infection; congenital heart disease where patency of the PDA is necessary for pulmonary or systemic blood flow (eg, pulmonary atresia, severe tetralogy of Fallot, severe coarctation of aorta); bleeding (especially with active intracranial hemorrhage or GI bleed); thrombocytopenia; coagulation defects; proven or suspected necrotizing enterocolitis (NEC); significant renal dysfunction

Warnings NSAIDs are associated with an increased risk of adverse cardiovascular thrombotic events, including potentially fatal MI and stroke **[U.S. Boxed Warning]**; risk may be increased with duration of use or pre-existing cardiovascular risk factors or disease; carefully evaluate cardiovascular risk profile prior to prescribing; use the lowest effective dose for the shortest duration of time, taking into consideration individual patient treatment goals; alternate therapies should be considered for patients at high risk. Use is contraindicated for treatment of perioperative pain in the setting of CABG surgery **[U.S. Boxed Warning]**; an increased incidence of MI and stroke was found in patients receiving COX-2 selective NSAIDs for the treatment of pain within the first 10-14 days after CABG surgery (see Contraindications). NSAIDs may cause fluid retention, edema, and new onset or worsening of pre-existing hypertension; use with caution in patients with hypertension, CHF, or fluid retention. Response to ACE inhibitors, thiazides, or loop diuretics may be impaired with concurrent use of NSAIDs (see Drug Interactions). Concurrent administration of ibuprofen, and potentially other nonselective NSAIDs, may interfere with aspirin's cardioprotective effect (see Drug Interactions).

NSAIDs may increase the risk of gastrointestinal irritation, ulceration, bleeding, and perforation **[U.S. Boxed Warning]**. These events, which can be potentially fatal, may occur at any time during therapy, and without warning. Avoid the use of NSAIDs in patients with active GI bleeding or ulcer disease. Use NSAIDs with extreme caution in patients with a history of GI bleeding or ulcers (these patients have a 10-fold increased risk for developing a GI bleed). Use NSAIDs with caution in patients with other risk factors which may increase GI bleeding (eg, concurrent therapy with aspirin, anticoagulants, and/or corticosteroids, longer duration of NSAID use, smoking, use of alcohol, and poor general health). Use the lowest effective dose for the shortest duration of time, taking into consideration individual patient treatment goals; alternate therapies should be considered for patients at high risk.

NSAIDs may compromise existing renal function. Renal toxicity may occur in patients with impaired renal function, dehydration, heart failure, liver dysfunction, those taking diuretics and ACE inhibitors; use with caution in these patients; rehydrate patient before starting therapy; monitor renal function closely. NSAIDs are not recommended for use in patients with advanced renal disease. Long-term use of NSAIDs may cause renal papillary necrosis and other renal injury.

Fatal asthmatic and anaphylactoid reactions may occur in patients with the "aspirin triad" who receive NSAIDs (see Contraindications). NSAIDs may cause serious dermatologic adverse reactions including exfoliative dermatitis, Stevens-Johnson syndrome, and toxic epidermal necrolysis. Avoid use of NSAIDs in late pregnancy as they may cause premature closure of the ductus arteriosus.

Some products contain sodium benzoate (see Dosage Forms); benzoate is a metabolite of benzyl alcohol; large amounts of benzyl alcohol (≥99 mg/kg/day) have been associated with a potentially fatal toxicity ("gasping syndrome") in neonates; the "gasping syndrome" consists of metabolic acidosis, respiratory distress, gasping respirations, CNS dysfunction (including convulsions, intracranial hemorrhage), hypotension and cardiovascular collapse; avoid use of ibuprofen products containing benzyl alcohol or sodium benzoate in neonates; *in vitro* and animal studies have shown that benzoate displaces bilirubin from protein binding sites

Precautions Use with caution in patients with decreased hepatic function; closely monitor patients with abnormal LFTs; severe hepatic reactions (eg, fulminant hepatitis, liver failure) have occurred with NSAID use, rarely; discontinue if signs or symptoms of liver disease develop, or if systemic manifestations occur. Use with caution in patients with asthma; asthmatic patients may have aspirin-sensitive asthma which may be associated with severe and potentially fatal bronchospasm when aspirin or NSAIDs are administered (see Contraindications). Anemia (due to occult or gross blood loss from the GI tract, fluid retention, or other effect on erythropoiesis) may occur; monitor hemoglobin and hematocrit in patients receiving long-term therapy. Use with caution and monitor carefully in patients with coagulation disorders or those receiving anticoagulants; NSAIDs inhibit platelet aggregation and may prolong bleeding time. May increase the risk of aseptic meningitis, especially in patients with systemic lupus erythematosus (SLE) and related connective tissue disorders. May cause vision changes (blurred or diminished vision, changes in color vision, scotomata);

discontinue ibuprofen if such effects occur and obtain ophthalmologic examination with central visual fields and color vision testing.

Ibuprofen injection (Caldolor™): Additional precautions: Product must be diluted prior to administration; hemolysis can occur if not diluted. Patients must be well hydrated before administration (to reduce risk of adverse effects on the kidneys).

Ibuprofen lysine injection (NeoProfen®): Use with caution, avoid extravasation; I.V. solution may be irritating to tissues. Use with caution in neonates with controlled infection or those at risk for infection (ibuprofen may alter the usual signs of infection). May inhibit platelet aggregation; monitor for signs of bleeding. Use with caution in neonates when total bilirubin is elevated (ibuprofen may displace bilirubin from albumin-binding sites). Long-term evaluations of neurodevelopmental outcome, growth, or diseases associated with prematurity (eg, chronic lung disease, retinopathy of prematurity) following treatment have not been conducted (see Additional Information).

OTC labeling: Prior to self-medication, patients should contact healthcare provider if they have had recurring stomach pain or upset, ulcers, bleeding problems, high blood pressure, heart or kidney disease, other serious medical problems, or are currently taking a diuretic, aspirin, anticoagulant, or steroid drug. Recommended dosages should not be exceeded, due to an increased risk of GI bleeding. Consuming ≥3 alcoholic beverages/day or taking this medication longer than recommended may also increase the risk of GI bleeding. Stop use and consult a healthcare provider if symptoms do not improve within first 24 hours of use (children), symptoms get worse or newly appear (children and adults), fever lasts for >3 days (children and adults), or pain lasts >3 days (children) and >10 days (adults). Do not give for >10 days unless instructed by healthcare provider (children and adults). For children with severe or persistent sore throat or sore throat with symptoms such as high fever, headache, nausea, and vomiting, consult healthcare provider immediately; do not use for treatment of sore throat for >2 days or use in children <3 years of age with sore throat, unless directed by physician.

Chewable tablets contain phenylalanine which must be avoided (or used with caution) in patients with phenylketonuria. Safety and efficacy of oral dosage forms have not been established in infants <6 months of age.

Adverse Reactions

Oral:

Cardiovascular: Edema, hypertension, increased risk of cardiovascular thrombotic events (see Warnings)

Central nervous system: Aseptic meningitis, dizziness, headache, nervousness

Dermatologic: Exfoliative dermatitis, pruritus, rash, Stevens-Johnson syndrome, toxic epidermal necrolysis

Endocrine & metabolic: Fluid retention

Gastrointestinal: Abdominal pain or cramps, abdominal distress, appetite decreased, constipation, diarrhea, dyspepsia, epigastric pain, flatulence, GI bleed, GI perforation, GI ulceration (see Warnings), heartburn, nausea, vomiting

Hematologic: Anemia, bleeding time increased

Hepatic: Liver enzymes increased, hepatitis, liver failure

Ocular: Vision changes (blurred or diminished vision, changes in color vision, scotomata)

Otic: Tinnitus

Renal: Renal dysfunction, renal papillary necrosis and other renal injury with long term use (see Warnings)

Miscellaneous: Hypersensitivity reactions, anaphylactoid reactions

<1%, postmarketing, and/or case reports: Acute renal failure, agranulocytosis, allergic rhinitis, alopecia, amblyopia, anaphylaxis, anemia, aplastic anemia, arrhythmia, azotemia, blurred vision, bone marrow suppression, bronchospasm, CHF, confusion, conjunctivitis, creatinine clearance decreased, cystitis, depression, drowsiness, dry eyes, duodenal ulcer, edema, emotional lability, eosinophilia, epistaxis, erythema multiforme, gastritis, hallucinations, hearing decreased, hematuria, hematocrit decreased, hemoglobin decreased, hemolytic anemia, inhibition of platelet aggregation, insomnia, jaundice, liver function tests abnormal, leukopenia, melena, neutropenia, palpitation, pancreatitis, peptic ulcer, peripheral neuropathy, photosensitivity, polydipsia, polyuria, somnolence, tachycardia, thrombocytopenia, toxic amblyopia, urticaria, vesiculobullous eruptions, vision changes

Injection: Ibuprofen (Caldolor™):
Cardiovascular: Edema, hypertension, hypotension, increased risk of cardiovascular thrombotic events (see Warnings)
Central nervous system: Aseptic meningitis, dizziness, headache
Dermatologic: Exfoliative dermatitis, pruritus, Stevens-Johnson syndrome, toxic epidermal necrolysis
Endocrine & metabolic: Albumin decreased, hypernatremia, hypokalemia, hypoproteinemia
Gastrointestinal: Abdominal pain, diarrhea, dyspepsia, flatulence, nausea, vomiting; GI bleed, GI perforation, GI ulceration (see Warnings)
Hematologic: Anemia, eosinophilia, hemoglobin decreased, hemorrhage, neutropenia, thrombocytopenia
Hepatic: LDH increased, hepatitis, liver failure
Renal: BUN increased, renal failure
Respiratory: Cough
Urogenital: Urinary retention
Miscellaneous: Anaphylactoid reactions, hypersensitivity reactions

Injection: Ibuprofen lysine (NeoProfen®):
Cardiovascular: Cardiac failure, edema, hypotension, tachycardia
Central nervous system: Convulsions, intraventricular hemorrhage (29%; grade 3/4: 15%)
Dermatologic: Skin irritation (16%)
Endocrine & metabolic: Adrenal insufficiency (7%), hypocalcemia (12%), hypoglycemia (12%), hypernatremia (7%)
Gastrointestinal: GI disorders [non-NEC (22%)], GI perforation, necrotizing enterocolitis
Genitourinary: Urinary tract infection
Hematologic: Anemia (32%)
Hepatic: Cholestasis
Renal: BUN elevated (± hematuria), oliguria, renal failure, renal impairment, serum creatinine increased, urine output decreased (3%; small decrease reported on days 2-6 of life with compensatory increase in output on day 9)
Respiratory: Apnea (28%), atelectasis (4%), respiratory failure (10%), respiratory infection (19%); pulmonary hypertension [5 cases reported; 3 following early (prophylactic) administration of tromethamine ibuprofen and 2 cases following L-lysine ibuprofen for treatment of PDA (see Bellini, 2006; Gournay, 2002; Ohlsson, 2008)]
Miscellaneous: Infection, sepsis (43%)
<1%, postmarketing, and/or case reports: Abdominal distension, feeding problems, gastritis, gastroesophageal reflux, hyperglycemia, ileus, inguinal hernia, injection site reaction, jaundice, neutropenia, thrombocytopenia

Drug Interactions
Metabolism/Transport Effects Substrate (minor) of CYP2C9, 2C19; **Inhibits** CYP2C9 (strong)
Avoid Concomitant Use
Avoid concomitant use of Ibuprofen with any of the following: Ketorolac; Ketorolac (Systemic)
Increased Effect/Toxicity
Ibuprofen may increase the levels/effects of: Aminoglycosides; Anticoagulants; Antiplatelet Agents; Bisphosphonate Derivatives; Collagenase (Systemic); CycloSPORINE; CycloSPORINE (Systemic); Desmopressin; Digoxin; Drotrecogin Alfa; Eplerenone; Haloperidol; Ibrutumomab; Lithium; Methotrexate; Nonsteroidal Anti-Inflammatory Agents; Pemetrexed; Potassium-Sparing Diuretics; Pralatrexate; Quinolone Antibiotics; Salicylates; Thrombolytic Agents; Tositumomab and Iodine I 131 Tositumomab; Vancomycin; Vitamin K Antagonists

The levels/effects of Ibuprofen may be increased by: Antidepressants (Tricyclic, Tertiary Amine); Corticosteroids (Systemic); Dasatinib; Glucosamine; Herbs (Anticoagulant/Antiplatelet Properties); Ketorolac; Ketorolac (Systemic); Nonsteroidal Anti-Inflammatory Agents; Omega-3-Acid Ethyl Esters; Pentosan Polysulfate Sodium; Pentoxifylline; Probenecid; Prostacyclin Analogues; Selective Serotonin Reuptake Inhibitors; Serotonin/Norepinephrine Reuptake Inhibitors; Treprostinil
Decreased Effect
Ibuprofen may decrease the levels/effects of: ACE Inhibitors; Angiotensin II Receptor Blockers; Antiplatelet Agents; Beta-Blockers; Eplerenone; HydrALAZINE; Loop Diuretics; Potassium-Sparing Diuretics; Salicylates; Thiazide Diuretics

The levels/effects of Ibuprofen may be decreased by: Bile Acid Sequestrants; Nonsteroidal Anti-Inflammatory Agents; Salicylates
Food Interactions Food may decrease the rate but not the extent of oral absorption
Stability
Suspension: Store at controlled room temperature of 15°C to 30°C (59°F to 86°F).
Tablet: Store at controlled room temperature of 20°C to 25°C (68°F to 77°F).
Ibuprofen injection (Caldolor™): Store intact vials at room temperature of 20°C to 25°C (68°F to 77°F). Must be diluted prior to use. Dilute with D_5W, NS, or LR to a final concentration ≤4 mg/mL. Diluted solutions are stable for 24 hours at room temperature and room lighting.
Ibuprofen lysine injection (NeoProfen®): Store at controlled room temperature of 20°C to 25°C (68°F to 77°F). Protect from light; store injection vials in carton until ready to use. Stable in I.V. dextrose or saline solutions. Following dilution, administer within 30 minutes of preparation. Discard unused portion of vial (vial does not contain preservative). **Incompatible** with TPN solution.
Mechanism of Action Inhibits prostaglandin synthesis by decreasing the activity of the enzyme, cyclooxygenase, which results in decreased formation of prostaglandin precursors
Pharmacodynamics
Fever reduction:
Onset of action (single oral dose 8 mg/kg):
Infants ≤1 year: Mean ± SD: 69 ± 22 minutes
Children ≥6 years: 109 ± 64 minutes
Maximum effect: 2-4 hours
Duration: 6-8 hours (dose-related)
Pharmacokinetics (Adult data unless noted)
Absorption: Oral: Rapid (80%)
Distribution: Ibuprofen follows a 2-compartment open model

V_d, apparent: Preterm neonates, GA: 22-31 weeks and PNA: <1 day old (n=21): 62.1 ± 3.9 mL/kg (see Aranda, 1997)

V_d, central compartment: Preterm neonates, GA: 28.7 ± 1.3 weeks (n=13):

PNA 3 days old: 0.244 ± 0.084 L/kg (n=13); subset of 9 patients with ductal closure: 0.247 ± 0.102 L/kg

PNA 5 days old: 0.171 ± 0.077 L/kg (n=13); subset of 9 patients with ductal closure: 0.147 ± 0.075 L/kg

Note: The V_d of the central compartment was significantly decreased on day 5 of life versus day 3; the decrease was more pronounced in patients with ductal closure (see Van Overmeire, 2001).

V_d:

Febrile children <11 years: 0.2 L/kg

Adults: 0.12 L/kg

Protein binding: 90% to 99%

Metabolism: Oxidized in the liver; **Note:** Ibuprofen is a racemic mixture of R and S isomers; the R isomer (thought to be inactive) is slowly and incompletely (~60%) converted to the S isomer (active) in adults; the amount of conversion in children is not known, but it is thought to be similar to adults; a study in preterm neonates estimated the conversion to be 61% after prophylactic ibuprofen use and 86% after curative treatment (see Gregoire, 2004).

Half-life:

Alpha (distribution): I.V.: Preterm neonates: 1.04 ± 1.48 hours (see Van Overmeire, 2001)

Preterm newborn, GA: 22-31 weeks and PNA: <1 day old (n=21): Beta half-life: 30.5 ± 4.2 hours (see Aranda, 1997)

Preterm neonates, GA: 28.7 ± 1.3 weeks (n=13): Beta half-life: (see Van Overmeire, 2001):

PNA 3 days old: 43.1 ± 26.1 hours

PNA 5 days old: 26.8 ± 23.6 hours

Preterm neonates, GA 24-27.9 weeks (n=62): R-enantiomer: 10 hours; S-enantiomer: 25.5 hours (see Gregoire, 2004)

Children: 1-2 hours; children 3 months to 10 years: Mean: 1.6 hours

Adults: 2-4 hours

Time to peak serum concentration: Tablets: 1-2 hours; suspension: Mean: 1 hour

Children with cystic fibrosis:

Suspension (n=22): 0.74 ± 0.43 hours (median: 30 minutes)

Chewable tablet (n=4): 1.5 ± 0.58 hours (median: 1.5 hours)

Tablet (n=12): 1.33 ± 0.95 hours (median: 1 hour)

Elimination: ~1% excreted as unchanged drug and 14% as conjugated ibuprofen in urine; 45% to 80% eliminated in urine as metabolites; some biliary excretion

Usual Dosage

I.V.

Neonates: Treatment of PDA: Ibuprofen lysine (Neo-Profen®): Neonates between 500-1500 g and ≤32 weeks GA: Patent ductus arteriosus (treatment): Initial dose: Ibuprofen 10 mg/kg, followed by two doses of 5 mg/kg after 24 and 48 hours

Note: Use birth weight to calculate all doses. Hold second or third doses if urinary output is <0.6 mL/kg/hour; may give when laboratory studies indicate renal function is back to normal. A second course of treatment, alternative pharmacologic therapy, or surgery may be needed if the ductus arteriosus fails to close or reopens following the initial course of therapy.

Adolescents ≥17 years and adults: Ibuprofen injection (Caldolor™): **Note:** Patients should be well hydrated prior to administration.

Analgesic: 400-800 mg every 6 hours as needed (maximum: 3.2 g/day)

Antipyretic: Initial: 400 mg, then 400 mg every 4-6 hours or 100-200 mg every 4 hours as needed (maximum: 3.2 g/day)

Oral: **Note:** To reduce the risk of adverse cardiovascular and GI effects, use the lowest effective dose for the shortest period of time

Infants and Children:

Analgesic: 4-10 mg/kg/dose every 6-8 hours; maximum daily dose: 40 mg/kg/day

Antipyretic: 6 months to 12 years: Temperature <102.5°F (39°C): 5 mg/kg/dose; temperature ≥102.5°F: 10 mg/kg/dose; give every 6-8 hours; maximum daily dose: 40 mg/kg/day

Juvenile rheumatoid arthritis: 6 months to 12 years: Usual: 30-40 mg/kg/day in 3-4 divided doses; start at lower end of dosing range and titrate; patients with milder disease may be treated with 20 mg/kg/day; doses >40 mg/kg/day may increase risk of serious adverse effects; doses >50 mg/kg/day have not been studied and are not recommended; maximum dose: 2.4 g/day

OTC pediatric labeling (analgesic, antipyretic): 6 months to 11 years: 7.5 mg/kg/dose every 6-8 hours; maximum daily dose: 30 mg/kg

Manufacturer's recommendations: See table; use of weight to select dose is preferred; if weight is not available, then use age; doses may be repeated every 6-8 hours; maximum: 4 doses/day; treatment for >10 days is not recommended unless directed by healthcare provider; treatment of sore throat for >2 days or use in children <3 years of age with sore throat is not recommended, unless directed by healthcare provider (see Precautions)

Ibuprofen Dosing

Weight (lbs)	Age	Dosage (mg)
12-17	6-11 mo	50
18-23	12-23 mo	75
24-35	2-3 y	100
35-47	4-5 y	150
48-59	6-8 y	200
60-71	9-10 y	250
72-95	11 y	300

Cystic fibrosis: Ibuprofen when taken chronically (for 4 years) in doses to achieve peak plasma concentrations of 50-100 mcg/mL has been shown to slow the progression of lung disease in mild cystic fibrosis patients >5 years of age, and especially in patients who started therapy when <13 years of age. Doses administered twice daily ranged from 16.2-31.6 mg/kg/dose with 90% of patients requiring 20-30 mg/kg/dose (mean dose: ~25 mg/kg/dose), but individual patient's dose requirements were not predictable. Patients did not take pancreatic enzymes nor eat for 2 hours after the dose (see Konstan, 1995). In children with cystic fibrosis, an initial ibuprofen pharmacokinetic analyses is recommended using tablet doses of 20-30 mg/kg to optimize concentrations in the therapeutic range; blood sampling is recommended at 1, 2, and 3 hours postdose. A recent pharmacokinetic study in children with cystic fibrosis demonstrated that ibuprofen oral suspension also delivers therapeutic plasma concentrations; this study recommends using a 20 mg/kg dose of ibuprofen suspension for the initial pharmacokinetic analyses and obtaining blood samples at 30, 45, and 60 minutes postdose (see Scott, 1999); further studies are needed

◄

Adolescents and Adults:

Inflammatory disease: 400-800 mg/dose 3-4 times/day; maximum dose: 3.2 g/day

Pain/fever/dysmenorrhea: 200-400 mg/dose every 4-6 hours; maximum daily dose: 1.2 g

OTC labeling (analgesic, antipyretic): 200 mg every 4-6 hours as needed (maximum: 1200 mg/24 hours); treatment for >10 days is not recommended unless directed by healthcare provider

Dosing adjustment in hepatic impairment: Severe hepatic impairment: Avoid use

Dosing adjustment in renal impairment: Advanced renal disease: Use is not recommended

Administration

Oral: Administer with food or milk to decrease GI upset; shake suspension well before use

Ibuprofen lysine injection (NeoProfen®): I.V: For I.V. administration only; administration via umbilical arterial line has not been evaluated. Dilute with dextrose or saline to an appropriate volume. Infuse over 15 minutes through I.V. port closest to insertion site. Avoid extravasation. Do not administer simultaneously via same line with TPN. If needed, interrupt TPN for 15 minutes prior to and after ibuprofen administration, keeping line open with dextrose or saline.

Ibuprofen injection (Caldolor™) I.V.: For I.V. administration only; must be diluted to a final concentration of ≤4 mg/mL prior to administration; infuse over at least 30 minutes

Monitoring Parameters CBC, serum electrolytes, occult blood loss, liver enzymes; urine output, serum BUN, and creatinine in patients receiving I.V. ibuprofen, concurrent diuretics, those with decreased renal function, or in patients on chronic therapy. Monitor preterm neonates for signs of bleeding and infection; serum electrolytes, glucose, calcium and bilirubin; vital signs; monitor I.V. site for signs of extravasation. Patients receiving long-term therapy for JRA should receive periodic ophthalmological exams.

Reference Range Plasma concentrations >200 mcg/mL may be associated with severe toxicity; cystic fibrosis: therapeutic peak plasma concentration: 50-100 mcg/mL

Patient Information Ibuprofen is a nonsteroidal anti-inflammatory drug (NSAID); NSAIDs may cause serious adverse reactions, especially with overuse; use exactly as directed; do not increase dose or frequency; do not take longer than 3 days for fever (adults and children), 10 days for pain (adults), or 3 days for pain (children) without consulting healthcare professional. NSAIDs may increase the risk for heart attack, stroke, or ulcers and bleeding in stomach or intestines; GI bleeding, ulceration, or perforation can occur with or without pain. Notify physician before use if you have hypertension, heart failure, heart or kidney disease, history of stomach ulcers or bleeding in stomach or intestines, or other medical problems. Read the patient Medication Guide that you receive with each prescription and refill of ibuprofen.

While using this medication, do not use alcohol, excessive amounts of vitamin C, other prescription or OTC medications containing aspirin or salicylate, or other NSAIDs without consulting prescriber. Ibuprofen may cause dizziness or drowsiness and impair ability to perform activities requiring mental alertness or physical coordination. Notify physician if changes in vision occur, if pain worsens or lasts >10 days in adults or >3 days in children, if fever worsens or lasts >3 days, if stomach pain or upset occurs, if swelling or redness occurs in painful area, or if any new symptoms appear. Stop taking medication and report ringing in ears; persistent cramping or stomach pain; unresolved nausea or vomiting; respiratory difficulty or shortness of breath; unusual bruising or bleeding (mouth, urine, stool); skin rash; unusual swelling of extremities; chest pain; or palpitations.

OTC (pediatrics; also see above paragraphs): Notify physician if child's condition does not improve or if worsens within first 24 hours of use. Do not give for >10 days unless instructed by healthcare provider. For children with severe or persistent sore throat or sore throat with symptoms such as high fever, headache, nausea, and vomiting, consult healthcare provider immediately; do not use for treatment of sore throat for >2 days or use in children <3 years of age with sore throat, unless directed by physician.

Additional Information Nystagmus, dizziness, drowsiness, seizures, vomiting, hypotension, irregular heartbeat, breathing difficulties, apnea, kidney failure, and coma have been reported with overdose. Motrin® suspension contains sucrose 0.3 g/mL and 1.6 calories/mL. Due to its effects on platelet function, ibuprofen should be withheld for at least 4-6 half-lives prior to surgical or dental procedures.

Note: A study comparing the short-term use of acetaminophen and ibuprofen in 84,192 children (6 months to 12 years of age) found no significant difference in the rates of hospitalization for acute GI bleeding, acute renal failure, anaphylaxis or Reye's syndrome. (Four of 55,785 children in the ibuprofen group and zero of 28,130 children in the acetaminophen group were hospitalized with acute GI bleeding). A low WBC occurred more frequently in the ibuprofen group (8 vs 0) (see Lesko, 1995). A subanalysis of 27,065 children <2 years of age also found no significant difference in the rates of hospitalization. (Three of 17,938 children in the ibuprofen group and zero of 9,127 children in the acetaminophen group were hospitalized with GI bleeding) (see Lesko, 1999).

There is currently no scientific evidence to support alternating acetaminophen with ibuprofen in the treatment of fever (see Mayoral, 2000)

I.V. ibuprofen is as effective as I.V. indomethacin for the treatment of PDA in preterm neonates, but is less likely to cause adverse effects on renal function (eg, oliguria, increased serum creatinine) (see Aranda, 2006; Lago, 2002; Ohlsson, 2008; Van Overmeire, 2000). However, a trend towards an increase in the risk for the development of chronic lung disease has been noted for ibuprofen (see Ohlsson, 2008); in addition, five cases of pulmonary hypertension in neonates receiving ibuprofen have been reported (see Adverse Reactions; Bellini, 2006; Gournay 2002; Ohlsson, 2008). Further studies, especially long-term studies, are needed. **Note**: Although several studies have utilized oral ibuprofen for PDA closure, not enough data exists regarding safety and effectiveness to recommend the oral route at this time (see Amoozgar, 2009; Cherif, 2008; Erdeve, 2009; Ohlsson, 2008).

Dosage Forms Excipient information presented when available (limited, particularly for generics); consult specific product labeling. [DSC] = Discontinued product

Caplet: 200 mg [OTC]

Advil®: 200 mg [contains sodium benzoate]

Ibu-200: 200 mg

Motrin® IB: 200 mg

Motrin® Junior: 100 mg [scored]

Capsule, liquid-filled:

Advil®: 200 mg [solubilized ibuprofen; contains potassium 20 mg]

Advil® Migraine: 200 mg [solubilized ibuprofen; contains potassium 20 mg]

Gelcap:

Advil®: 200 mg [contains coconut oil]

Injection, solution:

Caldolor™: 100 mg/mL (4 mL, 8 mL)

Injection, solution, as lysine [preservative free]:

NeoProfen®: 17.1 mg/mL (2 mL) [equivalent to ibuprofen 10 mg/mL]

Suspension, oral: 100 mg/5 mL (5 mL, 10 mL, 120 mL, 240 mL, 480 mL)

Advil® Children's: 100 mg/5 mL (120 mL) [contains sodium benzoate, sodium, propylene glycol; blue raspberry, fruit, and grape flavors]

Motrin® Children's: 100 mg/5 mL (60 mL, 120 mL) [contains sodium benzoate; berry, dye free berry, bubble gum, and grape flavors]

Suspension, oral [concentrate, drops]: 40 mg/mL (15 mL)

Advil® Infants': 40 mg/mL (15 mL) [contains sodium benzoate; fruit, grape, and white grape flavors]

Motrin® Infants': 40 mg/mL (15 mL) [contains sodium benzoate; ethanol free; berry and dye-free berry flavors]

Tablet: 200 mg [OTC], 400 mg, 600 mg, 800 mg

Addaprin: 200 mg

Advil®: 200 mg [contains sodium benzoate]

Genpril®: 200 mg [DSC]

Ibu®: 400 mg, 600 mg, 800 mg

Ibu-200: 200 mg

I-Prin: 200 mg

Midol® Cramp and Body Aches: 200 mg

Motrin® IB: 200 mg

Proprinal: 200 mg [contains sodium benzoate]

Ultraprin: 200 mg [sugar free]

Tablet, chewable:

Advil® Children's: 50 mg [contains phenylalanine 2.1 mg; grape flavors]

Advil® Junior: 100 mg [contains phenylalanine 4.2 mg; grape flavors] [DSC]

Motrin® Junior: 100 mg [contains phenylalanine 2.1 mg; grape and orange flavors]

References

Amoozgar H, Ghodstehrani M, and Pishva N, "Oral Ibuprofen and Ductus Arteriosus Closure in Full-Term Neonates: A Prospective Case-Control Study," Pediatr Cardiol, 2009 [Epub ahead of print].

Aranda JV and Thomas R, "Systematic Review: Intravenous Ibuprofen in Preterm Newborns," Semin Perinatol, 2006, 30(3):114-20.

Aranda JV, Varvarigou A, Beharry K, et al, "Pharmacokinetics and Protein Binding of Intravenous Ibuprofen in the Premature Newborn Infant," Acta Paediatr, 1997, 86(3):289-93.

Bellini C, Campone F, and Serra G, "Pulmonary Hypertension Following L-lysine Ibuprofen Therapy in a Preterm Infant With Patent Ductus Arteriosus," CMAJ, 2006, 174(13):1843-4.

Berde C, Ablin A, Glazer J, et al, "American Academy of Pediatrics Report of the Subcommittee on Disease-Related Pain in Childhood Cancer," Pediatrics, 1990, 86(5 Pt 2):818-25.

Capone ML, Sciulli MG, Tacconelli S, et al. "Pharmacodynamic Interaction of Naproxen With Low-Dose Aspirin in Healthy Subjects," J Am Coll Cardiol, 2005, 45(8):1295-1301.

Catella-Lawson F, Reilly MP, Kapoor SC, et al. "Cyclooxygenase Inhibitors and the Antiplatelet Effects of Aspirin," N Engl J Med, 2001, 345(25):1809-17.

Cherif A, Khrouf N, Jabnoun S, et al, "Randomized Pilot Study Comparing Oral Ibuprofen With Intravenous Ibuprofen in Very Low Birth Weight Infants With Patent Ductus Arteriosus," Pediatrics, 2008, 122(6):e1256-61.

Cryer B, Berlin RG, Cooper SA, et al. "Double-Blind, Randomized, Parallel, Placebo-Controlled Study Of Ibuprofen Effects On Thromboxane B2 Concentrations In Aspirin-Treated Healthy Adult Volunteers," Clin Ther, 2005, 27(2):185-191.

Erdeve O, Gokmen T, Altug N, et al, "Oral Versus Intravenous Ibuprofen: Which Is Better in Closure of Patent Ductus Arteriosus?" Pediatrics, 2009, 123(4):e763.

Gal P, Ransom JL, and Davis SA, "Possible Ibuprofen-Induced Kernicterus in a Near-Term Infant With Moderate Hyperbilirubinemia," J Pediatr Pharmacol Ther, 2006, 11:245-50.

Gournay V, Savagner C, Thiriez G, et al, "Pulmonary Hypertension After Ibuprofen Prophylaxis in Very Preterm Infants," Lancet, 2002, 359 (9316):1486-8.

Gregoire N, Gualano V, Geneteau A, et al, "Population Pharmacokinetics of Ibuprofen Enantiomers in Very Premature Neonates," J Clin Pharmacol, 2004, 44(10):1114-24.

Kauffman RE and Nelson MV, "Effect of Age on Ibuprofen Pharmacokinetics and Antipyretic Response," J Pediatr, 1992, 121 (6):969-73.

Konstan MW, Byard PJ, Hoppel CL, et al, "Effect of High-Dose Ibuprofen in Patients With Cystic Fibrosis," N Engl J Med, 1995, 332 (13):848-54.

Lago P, Bettiol T, Salvadori S, et al, "Safety and Efficacy of Ibuprofen Versus Indomethacin in Preterm Infants Treated for Patent Ductus Arteriosus: A Randomised Controlled Trial," Eur J Pediatr, 2002, 161 (4):202-7.

Lesko SM and Mitchell AA, "An Assessment of the Safety of Pediatric Ibuprofen. A Practitioner-Based Randomized Clinical Trial," JAMA, 1995, 273(12):929-33.

Lesko SM and Mitchell A, "The Safety of Acetaminophen and Ibuprofen Among Children Younger Than Two Years Old," Pediatrics, 1999, 104 (4), http://www.pediatrics.org/cgi/content/full/104/4/e39.

Mayoral CE, Marino RV, Rosenfeld, W, et al, "Alternating Antipyretics: Is This an Alternative?" Pediatrics, 2000, 105(5):1009-12.

Ohlsson A, Walia R, and Shah S, "Ibuprofen for the Treatment of Patent Ductus Arteriosus in Preterm and/or Low Birth Weight Infants," Cochrane Database Syst Rev, 2008, Jan 23(1):CD003481.

Pai VB, Sakadjian A, and Puthoff TD, "Ibuprofen Lysine for the Prevention and Treatment of Patent Ductus Arteriosus," Pharmacotherapy, 2008, 28(9):1162-82.

Scott CS, Retsch-Bogart GZ, Kustra RP, et al, "The Pharmacokinetics of Ibuprofen Suspension, Chewable Tablets, and Tablets in Children With Cystic Fibrosis," J Pediatr, 1999, 134(1):58-63.

Shah SS and Ohlsson A, "Ibuprofen for the Prevention of Patent Ductus Arteriosus in Preterm and/or Low Birth Weight Infants," Cochrane Database Syst Rev, 2006, (1):CD004213.

Van Overmeire B, "Common Clinical and Practical Questions on the Use of Intravenous Ibuprofen Lysine for the Treatment of Patent Ductus Arteriosus," J Pediatr Pharmacol Ther, 2007, 12:194-206.

Van Overmeire B, Smets K, Lecoutere D, et al, "A Comparison of Ibuprofen and Indomethacin for Closure of Patent Ductus Arteriosus," N Engl J Med, 2000, 343(10):674-81.

Van Overmeire B, Touw D, Schepens PJ, et al, "Ibuprofen Pharmacokinetics in Preterm Infants With Patent Ductus Arteriosus," Clin Pharmacol Ther, 2001, 70(4):336-43.

◆ **Ibuprofen and Pseudoephedrine** see Pseudoephedrine and Ibuprofen on page 1184

◆ **Ibuprofen Lysine** see Ibuprofen on page 702

◆ **IC51** see Japanese Encephalitis Virus Vaccine (Inactivated) on page 776

◆ **ICI-204,219** see Zafirlukast on page 1439

◆ **ICL670** see Deferasirox on page 395

◆ **ICRF-187** see Dexrazoxane on page 413

◆ **Idamycin® (Can)** see IDArubicin on page 707

◆ **Idamycin PFS®** see IDArubicin on page 707

IDArubicin (eye da ROO bi sin)

Medication Safety Issues

Sound-alike/look-alike issues:

IDArubicin may be confused with DOXOrubicin, DAUNOrubicin, epirubicin

Idamycin PFS® may be confused with Adriamycin

High alert medication: The Institute for Safe Medication Practices (ISMP) includes this medication among its list of drugs which have a heightened risk of causing significant patient harm when used in error.

Related Information

Compatibility of Chemotherapy and Related Supportive Care Medications on page 1580

Emetogenic Potential of Antineoplastic Agents on page 1579

Extravasation Treatment on page 1522

U.S. Brand Names Idamycin PFS®

Canadian Brand Names Idamycin®

Therapeutic Category Antineoplastic Agent, Anthracycline; Antineoplastic Agent, Antibiotic

Generic Available Yes

Use Used in combination with other antineoplastic agents for treatment of acute myeloid leukemia (AML) (FDA approved in adults); has also been used for the treatment of acute lymphocytic leukemia (ALL)

Pregnancy Risk Factor D

Lactation Excretion in breast milk unknown

Contraindications Hypersensitivity to idarubicin or any component; patients with pre-existing bone marrow suppression unless the benefit warrants the risk; severe CHF, cardiomyopathy, or arrhythmias; pregnancy

Warnings Hazardous agent; use appropriate precautions for handling and disposal; I.V. use only, severe local tissue necrosis will result if extravasation occurs **[U.S. Boxed Warning]**. May cause myocardial toxicity (CHF, arrhythmias or cardiomyopathies) **[U.S. Boxed Warning]**; myocardial toxicity is more common in patients who have previously received anthracyclines or have pre-existing cardiac disease; the risk of myocardial toxicity is also increased in patients with concomitant or prior mediastinal/pericardial irradiation, patients with anemia, bone marrow depression, infections, leukemic pericarditis, or myocarditis. Monitor cardiac function during treatment; the maximum lifetime anthracycline dose for idarubicin is approximately 137.5 mg/m^2; may cause severe myelosuppression **[U.S. Boxed Warning]**; myelosuppression occurs in all patients given a therapeutic dose and is the dose-limiting adverse effect associated with idarubicin.

Precautions Use with caution and reduce dose in patients with impaired hepatic or renal function **[U.S. Boxed Warning]** and patients receiving concurrent radiation therapy

Adverse Reactions

Cardiovascular: Arrhythmias, cardiomyopathy, ECG changes, heart failure

Dermatologic: Alopecia, rash, urticaria

Gastrointestinal: Anorexia, diarrhea, mucositis, nausea, stomatitis, vomiting

Genitourinary: Discoloration of urine (pink or red)

Hematologic: Anemia, leukopenia (nadir: 8-29 days), thrombocytopenia (nadir: 10-15 days)

Hepatic: Liver enzymes or bilirubin increased

Local: Erythematous streaking, tissue necrosis upon extravasation

Miscellaneous: Anaphylaxis

<1%, postmarketing, and/or care reports: Hyperuricemia

Drug Interactions

Metabolism/Transport Effects Substrate of P-glycoprotein

Avoid Concomitant Use

Avoid concomitant use of IDArubicin with any of the following: BCG; Natalizumab; Pimecrolimus; Tacrolimus (Topical); Vaccines (Live)

Increased Effect/Toxicity

IDArubicin may increase the levels/effects of: Leflunomide; Natalizumab; Vaccines (Live)

The levels/effects of IDArubicin may be increased by: Bevacizumab; Denosumab; P-Glycoprotein Inhibitors; Pimecrolimus; Tacrolimus (Topical); Taxane Derivatives; Trastuzumab

Decreased Effect

IDArubicin may decrease the levels/effects of: BCG; Cardiac Glycosides; Sipuleucel-T; Vaccines (Inactivated); Vaccines (Live)

The levels/effects of IDArubicin may be decreased by: Cardiac Glycosides; Echinacea; P-Glycoprotein Inducers

Stability Store vials under refrigeration and protect from light; incompatible with acyclovir, ceftazidime, furosemide, hydrocortisone, sodium bicarbonate and heparin; inactivated by alkaline solutions

Mechanism of Action Intercalates with DNA causing strand breakage and affects topoisomerase II activity resulting in inhibition of chain elongation and inhibition of DNA and RNA synthesis

Pharmacokinetics (Adult data unless noted)

Distribution:

V_d: Large volume of distribution due to extensive tissue binding; distributes into CSF

V_{dss}: 1700 L/m^2

Protein binding:

Idarubicin: 97%

Idarubicinol: 94%

Metabolism: In the liver to idarubicinol (active metabolite)

Half-life:

Children: 18.7 hours (range: 2.5-22.4 hours)

Adults: 19 hours (range: 10.5-34.7 hours)

Idarubicinol: 45-56.8 hours

Elimination: Primarily by biliary excretion; 2.3% to 6.5% of a dose is eliminated renally

Usual Dosage AML: I.V. (refer to individual protocols):

Children: 10-12 mg/m^2 once daily for 3 days of treatment course

Adults:

Induction: 12 mg/m^2/day for 3 days

Consolidation: 10-12 mg/m^2/day for 2 days

Dosing adjustment in hepatic and/or renal impairment:

Serum creatinine ≥2 mg/dL: Reduce dose by 25%

Bilirubin >2.5 mg/dL: Reduce dose by 50%

Bilirubin >5 mg/dL: **Do not administer**

Administration Do not administer I.M. or SubQ

Parenteral: I.V.: Administer by I.V. intermittent infusion over 10-30 minutes into a free flowing I.V. solution of NS or D_5W; administer at a final concentration of 1 mg/mL

Monitoring Parameters CBC with differential, platelet count, ECHO, ECG, serum electrolytes, creatinine, uric acid, ALT, AST, bilirubin, signs of extravasation

Patient Information Notify physician if fever, sore throat, bleeding, bruising, or pain at infusion site occurs. Urine may turn pink or red. Contraceptive measures are recommended during therapy.

Nursing Implications Maintain adequate patient hydration; local erythematous streaking along the vein may indicate too rapid a rate of administration; care should be taken to avoid extravasation; if extravasation occurs, the manufacturer recommends that the affected extremity be elevated and that topical ice packs be placed over the affected area immediately for 30 minutes, then apply for 30 minutes 4 times/day for 3 days; alternative therapy includes topical application of dimethylsulfoxide

Dosage Forms Excipient information presented when available (limited, particularly for generics); consult specific product labeling.

Injection, solution, as hydrochloride [preservative free]:

1 mg/mL (5 mL, 10 mL, 20 mL)

Idamycin PFS®: 1 mg/mL (5 mL, 10 mL, 20 mL)

References

Dinndorf PA, Avramis VI, Wiersma S, et al, "Phase I/II Study of Idarubicin Given With Continuous Infusion Fludarabine Followed by Continuous Infusion Cytarabine in Children With Acute Leukemia: A Report From the Children's Cancer Group," *J Clin Oncol*, 1997, 15 (8):2780-5.

Leahey A, Kelly K, Rorke LB, et al, "A Phase I/II Study of Idarubicin (Ida) With Continuous Infusion Fludarabine (F-ara-A) and Cytarabine (ara-C) for Refractory or Recurrent Pediatric Acute Myeloid Leukemia (AML)," *J Pediatr Hematol Oncol*, 1997, 19(4):304-8.

Reid JM, Pendergrass TW, Krailo MD, et al, "Plasma Pharmacokinetics and Cerebrospinal Fluid Concentrations of Idarubicin and Idarubicinol in Pediatric Leukemia Patients: A Children's Cancer Study Group Report," *Cancer Res*, 1990, 50(20):6525-8.

◆ **Idarubicin Hydrochloride** *see* IDArubicin *on page* 707

◆ **IDEC-C2B8** *see* RiTUXimab *on page* 1227

◆ **IDR** *see* IDArubicin *on page* 707

◆ **Ifex** *see* Ifosfamide *on page* 709

Ifosfamide (eye FOSS fa mide)

Medication Safety Issues
Sound-alike/look-alike issues:
Ifosfamide may be confused with cyclophosphamide

High alert medication: The Institute for Safe Medication Practices (ISMP) includes this medication among its list of drugs which have a heightened risk of causing significant patient harm when used in error.

Related Information
Compatibility of Chemotherapy and Related Supportive Care Medications *on page 1580*
Emetogenic Potential of Antineoplastic Agents *on page 1579*

U.S. Brand Names Ifex
Canadian Brand Names Ifex
Therapeutic Category Antineoplastic Agent, Alkylating Agent
Generic Available Yes
Use In combination with other antineoplastics in treatment of testicular cancer (FDA approved in adults); has also been used in the treatment of bladder cancer, cervical cancer, ovarian cancer, nonsmall cell lung cancer, small cell lung cancer, Hodgkin's and non-Hodgkin's lymphoma; acute lymphocytic leukemia; brain tumors, germ cell tumors, Wilms' tumor, Ewing's sarcoma, osteosarcoma, and soft tissue sarcomas

Pregnancy Risk Factor D
Pregnancy Considerations Increased resorptions and embryotoxic effects have been observed in animal studies.
Lactation Enters breast milk/not recommended
Contraindications Hypersensitivity to ifosfamide or any component; patients with severely depressed bone marrow function; pregnancy
Warnings Hazardous agent; use appropriate precautions for handling and disposal. Severe bone marrow suppression may occur (dose-limiting toxicity); use with caution in patients with compromised bone marrow reserve; use is contraindicated in patients with severely depressed bone marrow function **[U.S. Boxed Warning]**; may cause CNS toxicity, including confusion and coma; may require therapy discontinuation, usually reversible upon discontinuation of treatment. Encephalopathy (ranging from mild somnolence to hallucinations and/or coma) may occur; risk factors may include hypoalbuminemia, renal dysfunction, and prior history of ifosfamide-induced encephalopathy **[U.S. Boxed Warning]**. Urotoxic side effects, primarily hemorrhagic cystitis, may occur (dose-limiting toxicity); hydration (at least 2 L/day) and/or mesna administration will protect against hemorrhagic cystitis **[U.S. Boxed Warning]**; risk factors for ifosfamide-induced nephrotoxicity include previous or concurrent cisplatin therapy, pre-existing renal impairment, prior nephrectomy, children ≤5 years, or patients who have received high cumulative ifosfamide doses of 50 g/m^2.
Precautions Use with caution in patients with impaired renal function or those with compromised bone marrow reserve

Adverse Reactions
Cardiovascular: Cardiotoxicity
Central nervous system: Ataxia, coma, confusion, depressive psychoses, dizziness, fever, hallucinations, lethargy, seizures, somnolence
Dermatologic: Alopecia, hyperpigmentation
Endocrine & metabolic: Metabolic acidosis
Gastrointestinal: Diarrhea, nausea, stomatitis, vomiting
Genitourinary: Dysuria, hemorrhagic cystitis
Hematologic: Myelosuppression (leukocyte nadir: 7-14 days), thrombocytopenia
Hepatic: Bilirubin and/or liver enzymes increased
Local: Phlebitis

Neuromuscular & skeletal: Polyneuropathy
Renal: BUN and serum creatinine increased, hematuria, renal tubular acidosis

Drug Interactions
Metabolism/Transport Effects Substrate of CYP2A6 (major), 2B6 (minor), 2C8 (minor), 2C9 (minor), 2C19 (major), 3A4 (major); **Inhibits** CYP3A4 (weak); **Induces** CYP2C8 (weak), 2C9 (weak)

Avoid Concomitant Use
Avoid concomitant use of Ifosfamide with any of the following: BCG; Natalizumab; Pimecrolimus; Tacrolimus (Topical); Vaccines (Live)

Increased Effect/Toxicity
Ifosfamide may increase the levels/effects of: Leflunomide; Natalizumab; Vaccines (Live); Vitamin K Antagonists

The levels/effects of Ifosfamide may be increased by: CYP2A6 Inhibitors (Moderate); CYP2A6 Inhibitors (Strong); CYP2C19 Inhibitors (Moderate); CYP2C19 Inhibitors (Strong); CYP3A4 Inhibitors (Moderate); CYP3A4 Inhibitors (Strong); Dasatinib; Denosumab; Pimecrolimus; Tacrolimus (Topical); Trastuzumab

Decreased Effect
Ifosfamide may decrease the levels/effects of: BCG; Sipuleucel-T; Vaccines (Inactivated); Vaccines (Live); Vitamin K Antagonists

The levels/effects of Ifosfamide may be decreased by: CYP2A6 Inducers (Strong); CYP2C19 Inducers (Strong); CYP3A4 Inducers (Strong); Deferasirox; Echinacea; Herbs (CYP3A4 Inducers)

Stability Store intact vials of powder for injection at room temperature. Store intact vials of solution under refrigeration. Reconstituted solutions may be stored under refrigeration for up to 21 days. Solutions diluted for administration are stable for 7 days at room temperature and for 6 weeks under refrigeration.

Mechanism of Action Causes cross-linking of DNA strands by binding with nucleic acids and other intracellular structures; inhibits protein synthesis and DNA synthesis

Pharmacokinetics (Adult data unless noted) Dose-dependent pharmacokinetics:
Distribution: Unchanged ifosfamide penetrates the blood-brain barrier; excreted into breast milk
Metabolism: Requires biotransformation by the cytochrome P450 enzyme system in the liver before it can act as an alkylating agent; following hydroxylation, the metabolite breaks down to acrolein (bladder irritant) and ifosfamide mustard (active drug)
Half-life: Terminal:
Low dose (1800 mg/m^2): 4-7 hours
High dose (3800-5000 mg/m^2): 11-15 hours
Elimination: 60% to 80% of a dose is excreted in urine as unchanged drug and metabolites

Usual Dosage I.V. (refer to individual protocols):
Children: 1200-1800 mg/m^2/day for 5 days every 21-28 days or 5000 mg/m^2 as a single 24-hour infusion or 3 g/m^2/day for 2 days
Adults: 700-2000 mg/m^2/day for 5 days or 1000-3000 mg/m^2/day for 3 days every 21-28 days; 5000 mg/m^2 as a single dose over 24 hours

Administration Parenteral: Administer as a slow I.V. intermittent infusion over at least 30 minutes at a final concentration for administration not to exceed 40 mg/mL (usual concentration for administration is between 0.6-20 mg/mL), or administer as a 24-hour infusion

Monitoring Parameters CBC with differential and platelet count, urine output, urinalysis, liver function and renal function tests, serum electrolytes, CNS changes

Patient Information Notify physician of pain or irritation in urination, CNS changes, fever, chills, bruising, or bleeding. Contraceptive measure are recommended during therapy.

◀ **Nursing Implications** Maintain adequate patient hydration

Additional Information Usually used in combination with mesna, an agent used to prevent hemorrhagic cystitis

Dosage Forms Excipient information presented when available (limited, particularly for generics); consult specific product labeling.

Injection, powder for reconstitution: 1 g
  Ifex: 1 g, 3 g
Injection, solution: 50 mg/mL (20 mL, 60 mL)

References
Ninane J, Baurain R, and de Kraker J, "Alkylating Activity in Serum, Urine, and CSF Following High-Dose Ifosfamide in Children," *Cancer Chemother Pharmacol*, 1989, 24(Suppl 1):S2-6.

Oberlin O, Fawaz O, Rey A, et al, "Long-Term Evaluation of Ifosfamide-Related Nephrotoxicity in Children," *J Clin Oncol*, 2009, 27 (32):5350-5.

Pinkerton CR, Rogers H, James C, et al, "A Phase II Study of Ifosfamide in Children With Recurrent Solid Tumors," *Cancer Chemother Pharmacol*, 1985, 15(3):258-62.

♦ **IG** *see* Immune Globulin (Intramuscular) *on page 718*

♦ **IGIM** *see* Immune Globulin (Intramuscular) *on page 718*

♦ **IGIV** *see* Immune Globulin (Intravenous) *on page 719*

♦ **IGIVnex® (Can)** *see* Immune Globulin (Intravenous) *on page 719*

♦ **IL-1Ra** *see* Anakinra *on page 108*

♦ **IL-2** *see* Aldesleukin *on page 60*

♦ **IL-11** *see* Oprelvekin *on page 1025*

Imatinib (eye MAT eh nib)

Medication Safety Issues

Sound-alike/look-alike issues:
Imatinib may be confused with dasatinib, erlotinib, nilotinib, sorafenib, sunitinib

High alert medication: The Institute for Safe Medication Practices (ISMP) includes this medication among its list of drug classes which have a heightened risk of causing significant patient harm when used in error.

Related Information

Emetogenic Potential of Antineoplastic Agents *on page 1579*

U.S. Brand Names Gleevec®

Canadian Brand Names Gleevec®

Therapeutic Category Antineoplastic Agent, Tyrosine Kinase Inhibitor

Generic Available No

Use Treatment of:

Newly-diagnosed Philadelphia chromosome-positive (Ph+) chronic myeloid leukemia (CML) in chronic phase (FDA approved in ages ≥2 years and adults)

Recurrent Ph+ CML in chronic phase following stem cell transplant or in patients resistant to interferon alpha therapy (FDA approved in ages ≥2 years)

Ph+ CML in blast crisis, accelerated phase, or chronic phase after failure of interferon therapy (FDA approved in adults)

Ph+ acute lymphoblastic leukemia (ALL) (relapsed or refractory), aggressive systemic mastocytosis (ASM) without D816V c-Kit mutation (or c-Kit mutation status unknown), dermatofibrosarcoma protuberans (DFSP) (unresectable, recurrent, and metastatic), hypereosinophilic syndrome (HES) and/or chronic eosinophilic leukemia (CEL), myelodysplastic/myeloproliferative disease (MDS/MPD) associated with platelet-derived growth factor receptor (PDGFR) gene rearrangements (FDA approved in adults)

Has also been used in the treatment of desmoid tumors (soft tissue sarcoma); poststem cell transplant (allogeneic) follow-up treatment in CML

Pregnancy Risk Factor D

Pregnancy Considerations There are no adequate and well-controlled studies in pregnant women. Animal studies have demonstrated teratogenic effects and fetal loss. Women of childbearing potential are advised not to become pregnant (female patients and female partners of male patients). Adequate contraception is recommended. Case reports of pregnancies while on therapy (both males and females) include reports of spontaneous abortion, minor abnormalities (hypospadias, pyloric stenosis, and small intestine rotation) at or shortly after birth, and other congenital abnormalities including skeletal malformations, hypoplastic lungs, exomphalos, kidney abnormalities, hydrocephalus, cerebellar hypoplasia, and cardiac defects.

Retrospective case reports of women with CML in complete hematologic response (CHR) with cytogenic response (partial or complete) who interrupted imatinib therapy due to pregnancy, demonstrated a loss of response in some patients while off treatment. At 18 months after treatment reinitiation following delivery, CHR was again achieved in all patients and cytogenic response was achieved in some patients. Cytogenetic response rates may not be as high as compared to patients with 18 months of uninterrupted therapy (Ault, 2006; Pye, 2008).

Lactation Enters breast milk/not recommended

Breast-Feeding Considerations Imatinib and its active metabolite are found in human breast milk; the milk/plasma ratio is 0.5 for imatinib and 0.9 for the active metabolite. Based on body weight, up to 10% of a therapeutic maternal dose could potentially be received by a breastfed infant. Due to the potential for serious adverse reactions in the nursing infant, breast-feeding is not recommended.

Contraindications Hypersensitivity to imatinib or any component

Warnings May cause fluid retention, weight gain, and edema which may lead to significant complications, including pleural effusion, pericardial effusion, pulmonary edema, and ascites. Use with caution in patients where fluid accumulation may be poorly tolerated, such as cardiovascular disease (HF or hypertension) and pulmonary disease. Severe HF and left ventricular dysfunction (LVD) have been reported (rare), usually in patients with comorbidities and/or risk factors. Carefully monitor patients with pre-existing cardiac disease or risk factors for heart failure. With initiation of imatinib treatment, cardiogenic shock and/or LVD have been reported in patients with hypereosinophilic syndrome and cardiac involvement (reversible with systemic steroids, circulatory support, and temporary cessation of imatinib). Patients with high eosinophil levels and an abnormal echocardiogram or abnormal serum troponin level may benefit from prophylactic systemic steroids with the initiation of imatinib.

Severe bullous dermatologic reactions (including erythema multiforme and Stevens-Johnson syndrome) have been reported. Successful resumption at a lower dose (with corticosteroids and/or antihistamine) has been described; however, some patients may experience recurrent reactions.

May cause hepatotoxicity (either as monotherapy or in combination with chemotherapy); may be severe; monitor; interruption of therapy or dose reductions may be necessary. Transaminase and bilirubin elevations and acute liver failure have been observed with imatinib in combination with chemotherapy.

May cause severe hemorrhage. Hematologic toxicity (anemia, neutropenia, and thrombocytopenia) may occur.

Precautions Use with caution in patients with pre-existing hepatic and/or renal impairment; may require dosage adjustment. Use caution in thyroidectomy patients (receiving levothyroxine thyroid replacement therapy); hypothyroidism has been reported; monitor TSH levels. May cause GI irritation. Opportunistic infections may be associated with use. Use with caution in patients receiving concurrent therapy with drugs which alter cytochrome P450 activity or require metabolism by these isoenzymes (avoid concomitant use of strong CYP3A4 inducers) (see Drug Interactions). Hazardous agent; use appropriate precautions for handling and disposal.

Adverse Reactions

Cardiovascular: Anasarca, ascites, chest pain, edema/fluid retention (includes aggravated edema, facial edema, flushing, pericardial effusion, peripheral edema, pleural effusion, pulmonary edema, and superficial edema) (see Warnings)

Central nervous system: Anxiety, chills, CNS/cerebral hemorrhage, depression, dizziness, fatigue, fever, headache, hyperesthesia, insomnia

Dermatologic: Alopecia, dry skin, erythema, erythema multiforme, photosensitivity reaction, pruritus, rash, Stevens-Johnson syndrome (see Warnings)

Endocrine & metabolic: Hyperglycemia, hypoalbuminemia, hypocalcemia, hypokalemia, weight gain

Gastrointestinal: Abdominal distention, abdominal pain, anorexia, constipation, diarrhea, dyspepsia, flatulence, gastritis, gastroesophageal reflux, gastrointestinal hemorrhage, mouth ulceration, nausea, stomatitis/mucositis, taste disturbance, vomiting, weight loss, xerostomia

Hematologic (see Warnings): Anemia, hemorrhage, leukopenia, lymphopenia, neutropenia, pancytopenia, thrombocytopenia

Hepatic: Alkaline phosphatase increased, ALT increased, ascites/pleural effusion, AST increased, hepatotoxicity, hyperbilirubinemia

Neuromuscular & skeletal: Arthralgia/joint pain, back pain, bone pain, joint swelling, limb pain, muscle cramps, musculoskeletal pain, myalgia, paresthesia, peripheral neuropathy, rigors weakness

Ocular: Blurred vision, conjunctival hemorrhage, conjunctivitis, dry eyes, eyelid edema, lacrimation increased, periorbital edema

Renal: Serum creatinine increased

Respiratory: Cough, dyspnea, epistaxis, nasopharyngitis, pharyngitis, pharyngolaryngeal pain, pneumonia, respiratory infection, rhinitis, sinusitis

Miscellaneous: Diaphoresis, infection without neutropenia, influenza, night sweats

<1%, postmarketing, and/or case reports (limited to important or life-threatening): Anaphylactic shock, angina, amylase increased, angioedema, aplastic anemia, arrhythmia, atrial fibrillation, avascular necrosis, blepharitis, bullous eruption, cardiac arrest, cardiac failure, cardiac tamponade, cardiogenic shock, cataract, cellulitis, cerebral edema, chelitis, CHF (severe), colitis, confusion, CPK increased, dehydration, diverticulitis, dysphagia, embolism, eosinophilia, esophagitis, exanthematous pustulosis (acute generalized), exfoliative dermatitis, gastric ulcer, gastroenteritis, gastrointestinal obstruction, gastrointestinal perforation, glaucoma, gout, hearing loss, hematemesis, hematoma, hematuria, hemolytic anemia, hemorrhagic corpus luteum, hemorrhagic ovarian cyst, hepatic failure, hepatic necrosis, hepatitis, herpes simplex, herpes zoster, hip osteonecrosis, hypercalcemia, hyperkalemia, hyperuricemia, hyper-/hypotension, hypomagnesemia, hyponatremia, hypophosphatemia, ileus, inflammatory bowel disease, interstitial lung disease, interstitial pneumonitis, intracranial pressure increased, jaundice, LDH increased, left ventricular dysfunction, leucocytoclastic vasculitis, lichen planus, lichenoid keratosis, lymphadenopathy, macular edema, melena, memory impairment, MI, migraine, myopathy, optic neuritis, palpitation, pancreatitis, papilledema, pericarditis, petechiae, pleuritic pain, pulmonary fibrosis, pulmonary hemorrhage, pulmonary hypertension, purpura, pustular rash, Raynaud's phenomenom, renal failure, respiratory failure, retinal hemorrhage, sciatica, scleral hemorrhage, seizure, sepsis, skin pigment changes, somnolence, syncope, tachycardia, thrombocythemia, thrombosis, tinnitus, toxic epidermal necrolysis, tremor, tumor hemorrhage, urinary tract infection, urticaria, vertigo, vesicular rash, vitreous hemorrhage

Drug Interactions

Metabolism/Transport Effects Substrate of CYP1A2 (minor), CYP2D6 (minor), CYP2C9 (minor), CYP2C19 (minor), CYP3A4 (major), P-glycoprotein; **Inhibits** CYP2C9 (weak), CYP2D6 (moderate), CYP3A4 (strong), ABCG2

Avoid Concomitant Use

Avoid concomitant use of Imatinib with any of the following: Alfuzosin; BCG; Dronedarone; Eplerenone; Everolimus; Halofantrine; Natalizumab; Nilotinib; Nisoldipine; Pimecrolimus; Ranolazine; Rivaroxaban; Romidepsin; Salmeterol; Silodosin; Tacrolimus (Topical); Tamsulosin; Thioridazine; Tolvaptan; Vaccines (Live)

Increased Effect/Toxicity

Imatinib may increase the levels/effects of: Acetaminophen; Alfuzosin; Almotriptan; Alosetron; Bortezomib; Brinzolamide; Ciclesonide; Colchicine; CycloSPORINE; CycloSPORINE (Systemic); CYP2D6 Substrates; CYP3A4 Substrates; Dienogest; Dronedarone; Dutasteride; Eplerenone; Everolimus; FentaNYL; Fesoterodine; GuanFACINE; Halofantrine; Ixabepilone; Leflunomide; Lumefantrine; Maraviroc; MethylPREDNISolone; Natalizumab; Nebivolol; Nilotinib; Nisoldipine; Paricalcitol; Pazopanib; Pimecrolimus; Ranolazine; Rivaroxaban; Romidepsin; Salmeterol; Saxagliptin; Silodosin; Simvastatin; Sorafenib; Tadalafil; Tamoxifen; Tamsulosin; Thioridazine; Tolvaptan; Topotecan; Vaccines (Live); Vitamin K Antagonists; Warfarin

The levels/effects of Imatinib may be increased by: Antifungal Agents (Azole Derivatives, Systemic); CYP3A4 Inhibitors (Moderate); CYP3A4 Inhibitors (Strong); Dasatinib; Denosumab; Lansoprazole; P-Glycoprotein Inhibitors; Pimecrolimus; Tacrolimus (Topical); Trastuzumab

Decreased Effect

Imatinib may decrease the levels/effects of: BCG; Cardiac Glycosides; Codeine; Fludarabine; Prasugrel; Sipuleucel-T; TraMADol; Vaccines (Inactivated); Vaccines (Live); Vitamin K Antagonists

The levels/effects of Imatinib may be decreased by: CYP3A4 Inducers (Strong); Deferasirox; Echinacea; Peginterferon Alfa-2b; P-Glycoprotein Inducers; Rifamycin Derivatives; St Johns Wort

Food Interactions Food may reduce gastrointestinal irritation. Avoid grapefruit juice (may increase imatinib plasma concentration).

Stability Store at controlled room temperature of 25°C (77°F); protect from moisture.

Mechanism of Action Inhibits Bcr-Abl tyrosine kinase, the constitutive abnormal gene product of the Philadelphia chromosome in chronic myeloid leukemia (CML). Inhibition of this enzyme blocks proliferation and induces apoptosis in Bcr-Abl positive cell lines as well as in fresh leukemic cells in Philadelphia chromosome positive CML. Also inhibits tyrosine kinase for platelet-derived growth factor (PDGF), stem cell factor (SCF), c-kit, and cellular events mediated by PDGF and SCF.

Pharmacokinetics (Adult data unless noted)
Absorption: Rapid

◀ Protein binding: ~95% to albumin and alpha$_1$-acid glycoprotein (parent drug and metabolite)

Metabolism: Hepatic via CYP3A4 (minor metabolism via CYP1A2, CYP2D6, CYP2C9, CYP2C19); primary metabolite (active): N-demethylated piperazine derivative (CGP74588); severe hepatic impairment (bilirubin >3-10 times ULN) increases AUC by 45% to 55% for imatinib and its active metabolite, respectively

Bioavailability: 98%

Half-life elimination:

Adults: Parent drug: ~18 hours; N-desmethyl metabolite: ~40 hours

Children: Parent drug: ~15 hours

Time to peak: 2-4 hours (adults and children)

Excretion: Feces (68% primarily as metabolites, 20% as unchanged drug); urine (≤13% primarily as metabolites, 5% as unchanged drug)

Usual Dosage Oral: **Note:** For concurrent use with a strong CYP3A4 enzyme-inducing agent (eg, rifampin, phenytoin), imatinib dosage should be increased by at least 50%. The optimal duration of therapy for CML is not yet determined; discontinuing treatment is not recommended after achieving remission due to the potential for relapse (NCCN CML guidelines v1.2010).

Children ≥2 years: **Note:** May be administered once daily or in 2 divided doses.

Ph+ CML (chronic phase, newly diagnosed): 340 mg/m^2/day; maximum: 600 mg/day

Ph+ CML (chronic phase and recurrent after stem cell transplant or resistant to interferon): 260 mg/m^2/day

Adults: **Note:** Doses ≤600 mg should be administered once daily; 800 mg doses should be administered as 400 mg/dose twice a day

Ph+ CML:

Chronic phase: 400 mg once daily; may be increased to 600 mg daily, if tolerated, for disease progression, lack of hematologic response after 3 months, lack of cytogenetic response after 6-12 months, or loss of previous hematologic or cytogenetic response; ranges up to 800 mg/day (400 mg twice daily) have also been used

Accelerated phase or blast crisis: 600 mg once daily; may be increased to 800 mg daily (400 mg/dose twice daily), if tolerated, for disease progression, lack of hematologic response after 3 months, lack of cytogenetic response after 6-12 months, or loss of previous hematologic or cytogenetic response

Ph+ ALL (relapsed or refractory): 600 mg once daily

GIST (adjuvant treatment following complete resection): 400 mg once daily

GIST (unresectable and/or metastatic malignant): 400 mg/day; may be increased up to 800 mg/day (400 mg/dose twice daily), if tolerated, for disease progression; **Note:** Significant improvement (progression-free survival, objective response rate) was demonstrated in patients with KIT exon 9 mutation with 800 mg (versus 400 mg), although overall survival (OS) was not impacted. The higher dose did not demonstrate a difference in time to progression or OS patients with Kit exon 11 mutation or wild-type status (Debiec-Rychter, 2006; Heinrich, 2008).

ASM with eosinophilia: Initiate at 100 mg once daily; titrate up to a maximum of 400 mg once daily (if tolerated) for insufficient response to lower dose

ASM without D816V c-Kit mutation or c-Kit mutation status unknown: 400 mg once daily

DFSP: 400 mg/dose twice daily

HES/CEL: 400 mg once daily

HES/CEL with FIP1L1-PDGFRα fusion kinase: Initiate at 100 mg once daily; titrate up to a maximum of 400 mg once daily (if tolerated) if insufficient response to lower dose

MDS/MPD: 400 mg once daily

Dosage adjustment with concomitant strong CYP3A4 inducers: Avoid concomitant use of strong CYP3A4 inducers (eg, dexamethasone, carbamazepine, phenobarbital, phenytoin, rifampin); if concomitant use cannot be avoided, increase imatinib dose by at least 50% with careful monitoring.

Dosage adjustment for renal impairment:

Mild impairment (Cl$_{cr}$ 40-59 mL/minute): Maximum recommended dose: 600 mg/day

Moderate impairment (Cl$_{cr}$ 20-39 mL/minute): Decrease recommended starting dose by 50%; dose may be increased as tolerated; maximum recommended dose: 400 mg/day

Severe impairment (Cl$_{cr}$ <20 mL/minute): Use caution; a dose of 100 mg/day has been tolerated in severe impairment (Gibbons, 2008)

Dosage adjustment for hepatic impairment:

Mild-to-moderate impairment: No adjustment necessary

Severe impairment: Manufacturer's FDA-approved labeling: Reduce dose by 25%

NCCN Soft tissue Sarcoma guidelines (v.1.2009): GIST: Reduce dose by 25% to 50%

Dosage adjustment for hepatotoxicity (during therapy) or other nonhematologic adverse reactions: Withhold treatment until toxicity resolves; may resume if appropriate (depending on initial severity of adverse event)

Hepatotoxicity (during therapy): If elevations of bilirubin >3 times upper limit of normal (ULN) or liver transaminases >5 times ULN occur, withhold treatment until bilirubin <1.5 times ULN or transaminases <2.5 times ULN. Resume treatment at a reduced dose as follows:

Children ≥2 years:

If initial dose 260 mg/m^2/day, reduce dose to 200 mg/m^2/day

If initial dose 340 mg/m^2/day, reduce dose to 260 mg/m^2/day

Adults:

If initial dose 400 mg, reduce dose to 300 mg

If initial dose 600 mg, reduce dose to 400 mg

If initial dose 800 mg, reduce dose to 600 mg

Dosage adjustment for hematologic adverse reactions:

Chronic phase CML (initial dose: 260-340 mg/m^2/day in children) or 400 mg/day in adults), ASM, MDS/MPD, and HES/CEL (initial dose: 400 mg/day), or GIST (initial dose: 400 mg): If ANC <1 x 10^9/L and/or platelets <50 x 10^9/L: Withhold until ANC ≥1.5 x 10^9/L and platelets ≥75 x 10^9/L; resume treatment at previous dose. For recurrent neutropenia or thrombocytopenia, withhold until recovery and reinstitute treatment at a reduced dose as follows:

Children ≥2 years:

If initial dose 260 mg/m^2/day, reduce dose to 200 mg/m^2/day

If initial dose 340 mg/m^2/day, reduce dose to 260 mg/m^2/day

Adults: If initial dose 400 mg, reduce dose to 300 mg

CML (accelerated phase or blast crisis) and PH+ ALL: Adults (initial dose: 600 mg): If ANC <0.5 x 10^9/L and/or platelets <10 x 10^9/L, establish whether cytopenia is related to leukemia (bone marrow aspirate or biopsy). If unrelated to leukemia, reduce dose to 400 mg. If cytopenia persists for an additional 2 weeks, further reduce dose to 300 mg. If cytopenia persists for 4 weeks and is still unrelated to leukemia, withhold treatment until ANC ≥1 x 10^9/L and platelets ≥20 x 10^9/L, then resume treatment at 300 mg.

ASM-associated with eosinophilia and HES/CEL with FIP1L1-PDGFRα fusion kinase (starting dose: 100 mg/day): If ANC <1 x 10^9/L and/or platelets <50 x 10^9/L: Withhold until ANC ≥1.5 x 10^9/L and platelets ≥75 x 10^9/L; resume treatment at previous dose.

DFSP (initial dose: 800 mg/day): If ANC <1 x 10^9/L and/or platelets <50 x 10^9/L, withhold until ANC ≥1.5 x 10^9/L and platelets ≥75 x 10^9/L; resume treatment at reduced dose of 600 mg/day. If depression in neutrophils or platelets recurs, withhold until recovery and reinstitute treatment with a further dose reduction to 400 mg/day.

Administration Should be administered orally with a meal and a large glass of water. Tablets may be dispersed in water or apple juice (using ~50 mL for 100 mg tablet, ~200 mL for 400 mg tablet); stir until tablet dissolves and use immediately. For daily dosing ≥800 mg, the 400 mg tablets should be used to reduce iron exposure (tablets are coated with ferric oxide). Avoid grapefruit juice.

Monitoring Parameters CBC (weekly for first month, biweekly for second month, then periodically thereafter), liver function tests [at baseline and monthly or as clinically indicated; more frequently (at least weekly) in patients with moderate-to-severe hepatic impairment (Ramanathan, 2008)], renal function, serum electrolytes, including calcium, phosphorus, potassium, and sodium levels; thyroid function tests (in thyroidectomy patients); fatigue, weight, and edema/fluid status; consider echocardiogram and serum troponin levels in patients with HES/CEL and in patients with MDS/MPD or ASM with high eosinophil levels.

Monitor for signs/symptoms of HF in patients at risk for cardiac failure or patients with pre-existing cardiac disease. Baseline evaluation of left ventricular ejection fraction may be considered prior to initiation of imatinib therapy in patients with known underlying heart disease or in elderly patients.

Patient Information Do not take any new prescriptions, OTC medications, or herbal products during therapy without consulting prescriber; avoid chronic use of acetaminophen or aspirin unless approved by prescriber. Take exactly as directed; do not alter or discontinue dose without consulting prescriber. Take with food or a large glass of water. If you have difficulty swallowing tablets, tablet may be dissolved in water or apple juice (using ~50 mL for 100 mg tablet or ~200 mL for 400 mg tablet), stir until dissolved and use immediately. Avoid grapefruit juice. Maintain adequate hydration unless instructed to restrict fluid intake. You will be required to have regularly scheduled laboratory tests while on this medication. You will be more susceptible to infection (avoid crowds or contagious people and do not receive any vaccination unless approved by prescriber). You may experience headache, dizziness, or fatigue (use caution when driving or engaging in tasks requiring alertness until response to drug is known); loss of appetite, nausea, vomiting, or mouth sores (small frequent meals, frequent mouth care, chewing gum, or sucking lozenges may help); constipation (increased exercise, fluids, fruit, or fiber may help); or diarrhea. Report immediately any chest pain, palpitations, or swelling of extremities; unusual cough, respiratory difficulty, or wheezing; weight gain >5 lb; skin rash; muscle or bone pain, tremors, or cramping; persistent fatigue or weakness; easy bruising or unusual bleeding (eg, tarry stools, blood in vomitus, stool, urine, or mouth); persistent GI problems or pain; or other adverse effects.

Nursing Implications Fluid accumulation may be poorly tolerated in certain patients, including those with CHF or hypertension. Use caution in patients with cardiac or pulmonary disease or renal or hepatic impairment. Assess closely any other pharmacological agents or herbal products patient may be taking for effectiveness and possible interactions prior to beginning therapy (especially

those drugs affected by cytochrome P450 actions). Assess results of laboratory tests on a regular basis (eg, CBC, LFTs, renal and thyroid function tests, calcium, phosphorus, potassium, and sodium levels). Monitor therapeutic effectiveness and adverse reactions at beginning of therapy and regularly during therapy (eg, weight and fluid status, hemorrhage, paresthesia, respiratory or CNS changes). Teach appropriate use, interventions to reduce side effects, and symptoms to report.

Dosage Forms Excipient information presented when available (limited, particularly for generics); consult specific product labeling.

Tablet:

Gleevec®: 100 mg; 400 mg

References

Carpenter PA, Snyder DS, Flowers ME, et al, "Prophylactic Administration of Imatinib After Hematopoietic Cell Transplantation for High-Risk Philadelphia Chromosome-Positive Leukemia," *Blood*, 2007, 109(7):2791-3.

Gibbons J, Egorin MJ, Ramanathan RK, et al, "Phase I and Pharmacokinetic Study of Imatinib Mesylate in Patients With Advanced Malignancies and Varying Degrees of Renal Dysfunction: A Study by the National Cancer Institute Organ Dysfunction Working Group," *J Clin Oncol*, 2008, 26(4):570-6.

National Comprehensive Cancer Network (NCCN)® "Practice Guidelines in Oncology™: Soft Tissue Sarcoma Version 1.2009." Available at http://www.nccn.org/professionals/physician_gls/PDF/sarcoma.pdf.

◆ **Imatinib Mesylate** *see* Imatinib *on page 710*

◆ **Imferon** *see* Iron Dextran Complex *on page 762*

◆ **IMI 30** *see* IDArubicin *on page 707*

◆ **Imidazole Carboxamide** *see* Dacarbazine *on page 380*

◆ **Imidazole Carboxamide Dimethyltriazene** *see* Dacarbazine *on page 380*

Imiglucerase (imi GLOO ser ase)

Medication Safety Issues

Sound-alike/look-alike issues:

Cerezyme® may be confused with Cerebyx®, Ceredase®

U.S. Brand Names Cerezyme®

Canadian Brand Names Cerezyme®

Therapeutic Category Enzyme, Glucocerebrosidase; Gaucher's Disease, Treatment Agent

Generic Available No

Use Long-term enzyme replacement therapy for patients with Type 1 Gaucher's disease

Pregnancy Risk Factor C

Pregnancy Considerations Reproduction studies have not been conducted.

Lactation Excretion in breast milk unknown/use caution

Contraindications Hypersensitivity to imiglucerase or any component

Warnings During clinical trials, 16% of patients developed IgG antibodies reactive with imiglucerase; <1% of patients experienced anaphylactoid reactions; most patients may continue therapy after a reduction in the infusion rate and pretreatment with an antihistamine and/or corticosteroid; close observation for hypersensitivity reactions is recommended

Precautions Patients experiencing respiratory symptoms during treatment should be evaluated for potential pulmonary hypertension

Adverse Reactions

Cardiovascular: Systemic hypertension (mild), pulmonary hypertension, tachycardia, flushing, peripheral edema (transient)

Central nervous system: Headache, dizziness, fatigue, fever

Dermatologic: Rash, pruritus

Gastrointestinal: Nausea, abdominal pain, diarrhea, vomiting

Genitourinary: Urinary frequency decreased

Local: Burning, swelling, pruritus, sterile abscess at injection site

Neuromuscular & skeletal: Back pain

Respiratory: Dyspnea, cough

Miscellaneous: Anaphylactoid reactions (see Warnings)

Drug Interactions

Avoid Concomitant Use There are no known interactions where it is recommended to avoid concomitant use.

Increased Effect/Toxicity There are no known significant interactions involving an increase in effect.

Decreased Effect There are no known significant interactions involving a decrease in effect.

Stability Store in refrigerator 2°C to 8°C (36°F to 46°F); after reconstitution, stable for 12 hours refrigerated or at room temperature; after dilution in NS, 40 units/mL solution is stable for 24 hours refrigerated; do not use if opaque particles or solution discoloration are seen

Mechanism of Action Imiglucerase, produced by recombinant DNA technology, is an analog of glucocerebrosidase; it acts by replacing the missing enzyme associated with Gaucher's disease; Gaucher's disease is an inherited metabolic disorder caused by the defective activity of beta-glucosidase and the resultant accumulation of glucosyl ceramide laden macrophages in the liver, bone, and spleen; this results in one or more of the following conditions: anemia, thrombocytopenia, bone disease, hepatomegaly, splenomegaly

Pharmacodynamics

Onset of significant improvement in symptoms:

Hepatosplenomegaly and hematologic abnormalities: Within 6 months

Improvement in bone mineralization: Noted at 80-104 weeks of therapy

Pharmacokinetics (Adult data unless noted)

Distribution: V_d: 0.09-0.15 L/kg

Half-life, elimination: 3.6-10.4 minutes

Clearance: 9.8-20.3 mL/minute/kg

Usual Dosage I.V.: Children and Adults: 30-60 units/kg every 2 weeks; range in dosage: 2.5 units/kg 3 times/week to 60 units/kg once weekly to every 4 weeks. Initial dose should be based on disease severity and rate of progression. Children at high risk for complications from Gaucher's disease (one or more of the following: symptomatic disease including manifestations of abdominal or bone pain, fatigue, exertional limitations, weakness, and cachexia; growth failure; evidence of skeletal involvement; platelet count ≤60,000 mm^3 and/or documented abnormal bleeding episode(s); Hgb ≥2.0 g/dL below lower limit for age and sex; impaired quality of life) should receive an initial dose of 60 units/kg; failure to respond to treatment within 6 months indicates the need for a higher dosage.

Maintenance: After patient response is well established a reduction in dosage may be attempted; progressive reductions may be made at intervals of 3-6 months; assess dosage frequently to maintain consistent dosage per kg body weight

Administration Parenteral: Visually inspect the powder in the vial for particulate matter prior to reconstitution. Reconstitute 200 unit vial with 5.1 mL SWI or 400 unit vial with 10.2 mL SWI resulting in a 40 units/mL concentration; visually inspect the solution following reconstitution for particulate matter; further dilute in 100-200 mL NS; infuse over 1-2 hours; may filter diluted solution through an in-line low protein-binding 0.2 micron filter during administration; do not administer products with visualized particulate matter.

Monitoring Parameters CBC, platelets, liver function tests, MRI or CT scan (spleen and liver volume), skeletal x-rays

Dosage Forms Excipient information presented when available (limited, particularly for generics); consult specific product labeling.

Injection, powder for reconstitution:

Cerezyme®: 200 units, 400 units [derived from Chinese hamster cells; contains mannitol and polysorbate 80]

References

Charrow J, Andersson HC, Kaplan P, et al, "Enzyme Replacement Therapy and Monitoring for Children With Type 1 Gaucher Disease: Consensus Recommendations," *J Pediatr*, 2004, 144(1):112-20.

◆ **Imipemide** *see* Imipenem and Cilastatin *on page 714*

Imipenem and Cilastatin

(i mi PEN em & sye la STAT in)

Medication Safety Issues

Sound-alike/look-alike issues:

Imipenem may be confused with ertapenem, meropenem

Primaxin® may be confused with Premarin®, Primacor®

U.S. Brand Names Primaxin®

Canadian Brand Names Primaxin®; Primaxin® I.V.

Therapeutic Category Antibiotic, Carbapenem

Generic Available No

Use Treatment of documented multidrug-resistant gram-negative infection of the lower respiratory tract, urinary tract, intra-abdominal, gynecologic, bone and joint, septicemias, endocarditis, and skin and skin structure due to organisms proven or suspected to be susceptible to imipenem/cilastatin (FDA approved in all ages); treatment of multiple organism infection in which other agents have an insufficient spectrum of activity or are contraindicated due to toxic potential; therapeutic alternative for treatment of gram-negative sepsis in immunocompromised patients

Pregnancy Risk Factor C

Pregnancy Considerations With the exception of slightly decreased fetal weights at the highest doses in rats and an increase in embryonic loss in cynomolgus monkeys, most animal studies have not shown an increased fetal risk or teratogenic effects. However, due to the adverse events observed in some animal studies, imipenem/cilastatin is classified as pregnancy category C. No adequate and well-controlled studies have been conducted in pregnant women and it is not known whether imipenem can cause fetal harm. Due to pregnancy induced physiologic changes, some pharmacokinetic parameters of imipenem/cilastatin may be altered. Pregnant women have a larger volume of distribution resulting in lower serum peak levels than for the same dose in nonpregnant women. Clearance is also increased.

Lactation Enters breast milk/use caution

Breast-Feeding Considerations Imipenem is excreted in human milk. The low concentrations and low oral bioavailability suggest minimal exposure risk to the infant. The manufacturer recommends that caution be exercised when administering imipenem/cilastatin to nursing women, however, most penicillins and carbapenems are safe for use in breast-feeding. Nondose-related effects could include modification of bowel flora.

Contraindications Hypersensitivity to imipenem/cilastatin or any component

Warnings Serious and occasionally fatal hypersensitivity reactions have been reported in patients receiving beta-lactam therapy; careful inquiry should be made concerning previous hypersensitivity reactions to penicillins, cephalosporins, or other beta-lactams before initiating imipenem. Valproic acid (VPA) serum concentrations may be significantly decreased by concurrent carbapenem use leading to breakthrough seizures (see Drug interactions); VPA dosage adjustment may not adequately compensate; concurrent use with valproic acid not recommended. Seizures have been reported with imipenem therapy in children with meningitis; imipenem is not recommended in pediatric patients with CNS infections. Pseudomembranous colitis has been reported in patients receiving imipenem; prolonged use may result in superinfection.

Precautions Use with caution in patients with history of seizures or who are predisposed and in patients with a history of hypersensitivity to penicillins; use with caution and adjust dose in patients with impaired renal function

Adverse Reactions

Cardiovascular: Hypotension, tachycardia

Central nervous system: Altered effect, seizures (see Warnings)

Gastrointestinal: Diarrhea, nausea, oral candidiasis, pseudomembranous colitis (see Warnings), vomiting

Genitourinary: Anuria, discoloration of urine, hematuria, oliguria

Hepatic: Transient increase in liver enzymes

Local: Irritation and pain at injection site, phlebitis

Miscellaneous: Hypersensitivity reaction (see Warnings)

<1%, postmarketing, and/or case reports: Abdominal pain, abnormal urinalysis, acute renal failure, alkaline phosphatase increased, anaphylaxis, anemia, angioneurotic edema, asthenia, bilirubin increased, bone marrow depression, BUN/creatinine increased, candidiasis, confusion, cyanosis, dizziness, drug fever, dyspnea, encephalopathy, eosinophilia, erythema multiforme, fever, flushing, gastroenteritis, glossitis, hallucinations, headache, hearing loss, hematocrit decreased, hemoglobin decreased, hemolytic anemia, hemorrhagic colitis, hepatitis (including fulminant onset), hepatic failure, hyperchloremia, hyperhidrosis, hyperkalemia, hyperventilation, hyponatremia, injection site erythema, jaundice, lactate dehydrogenase increased, leukocytosis, leukopenia, myoclonus, neutropenia (including agranulocytosis), palpitation, pancytopenia, paresthesia, pharyngeal pain, polyarthralgia, polyuria, positive Coombs' test, prothrombin time increased, pruritus, pruritus vulvae, psychic disturbances, rash, resistant *P. aeruginosa*, salivation increased, somnolence, staining of teeth, Stevens-Johnson syndrome, taste perversion, thoracic spine pain, thrombocythemia, thrombocytopenia, tinnitus, tongue/tooth discoloration, tongue papillar hypertrophy, toxic epidermal necrolysis, transaminases increased, tremor, urticaria, vertigo

Drug Interactions

Avoid Concomitant Use

Avoid concomitant use of Imipenem and Cilastatin with any of the following: BCG; Ganciclovir (Systemic); Ganciclovir-Valganciclovir

Increased Effect/Toxicity

Imipenem and Cilastatin may increase the levels/effects of: CycloSPORINE; CycloSPORINE (Systemic)

The levels/effects of Imipenem and Cilastatin may be increased by: CycloSPORINE; CycloSPORINE (Systemic); Ganciclovir (Systemic); Ganciclovir-Valganciclovir; Probenecid

Decreased Effect

Imipenem and Cilastatin may decrease the levels/effects of: BCG; CycloSPORINE; CycloSPORINE (Systemic); Divalproex; Typhoid Vaccine; Valproic Acid

Stability Powder for injection should be stored at a temperature below 25°C (77°F).

I.V.: When reconstituted suspension is further diluted with NS, it is stable for 10 hours at room temperature or 48 hours under refrigeration [Note: Final admixture concentration of 10 mg/mL shown to maintain solubility in NS for 4 hours at room temperature (Trissel, 1999)]; when reconstituted suspension is further diluted with D_5W, $D_{10}W$, D_5NS, or $D_5^1/_4NS$, it is stable for 4 hours at room temperature and 24 hours under refrigeration; compatible with TPN via Y-site injection; **incompatible** when mixed directly in TPN solution; inactivated at alkaline or acidic pH

I.M.: Reconstituted I.M. suspension in lidocaine HCl should be used within 1 hour after preparation

Mechanism of Action Inhibits cell wall synthesis by binding to all of the penicillin-binding proteins with greatest affinity for PBP 1 and PBP 2; cilastatin prevents renal metabolism of imipenem by competitive inhibition of dehydropeptidase along the brush border of the proximal renal tubules

Pharmacokinetics (Adult data unless noted)

Absorption: I.M.:

Imipenem: 75%

Cilastatin: 95%

Distribution: Imipenem appears in breast milk; crosses the placenta; only low concentrations penetrate into CSF

Protein binding:

Imipenem: 13% to 21%

Cilastatin: 40%

Metabolism: Imipenem is metabolized in the kidney by dehydropeptidase; cilastatin is partially metabolized in the kidneys

Half-life, both: Prolonged with renal insufficiency

Neonates: 1.5-3 hours

Infants and Children: 1-1.4 hours

Adults: 1 hour

Elimination: When imipenem is given with cilastatin, urinary excretion of unchanged imipenem increases to 70%; 70% to 80% of a cilastatin dose is excreted unchanged in the urine

Dialysis: Moderately dialyzable (20% to 50%)

Usual Dosage Dosage recommendation based on imipenem component for non-CNS infections: I.V. infusion: (I.M. is limited to mild-moderate infections):

Neonates:

0-4 weeks, <1200 g: 20 mg/kg/dose every 18-24 hours

Postnatal age ≤7 days, 1200-1500 g: 40 mg/kg/day divided every 12 hours

Postnatal age ≤7 days, >1500 g: 50 mg/kg/day divided every 12 hours

Postnatal age >7 days, 1200-1500 g: 40 mg/kg/day divided every 12 hours

Postnatal age >7 days, >1500 g: 75 mg/kg/day divided every 8 hours

Infants 4 weeks to 3 months: 100 mg/kg/day divided every 6 hours

Infants ≥3 months and Children: 60-100 mg/kg/day divided every 6 hours; maximum dose: 4 g/day

Adults:

Serious infections: 2-4 g/day divided every 6 hours

Mild to moderate infections: 1-2 g/day in 3-4 divided doses

Dosing adjustment in renal impairment: Imipenem doses should be reduced in patients with Cl_{cr} <41-70 mL/minute/1.73 m^2: See table.

Creatinine Clearance (mL/min/1.73 m^2)	Frequency	% Decrease in Daily Maximum Dose
41-70	Every 6 h	50
21-40	Every 8 h	63
6-20	Every 12 h	75

Patients with creatinine clearance ≤5 mL/minute/1.73 m^2 should not receive imipenem unless undergoing hemodialysis

Administration

I.M.: Administer suspension by deep I.M. injection into a large muscle mass such as the gluteal muscle or lateral part of the thigh; the I.M. powder for suspension should be reconstituted with lidocaine hydrochloride 1% injection (without epinephrine). **Note:** The I.M. formulation is not for I.V. use.

I.V.: Administer by I.V. intermittent infusion; final concentration should not exceed 5 mg/mL; in fluid-restricted patients, a final concentration of 7 mg/mL has been administered at some institutions (Taketomo, 2009); doses ≤500 mg may be infused over 15-30 minutes; doses >500 mg should be infused over 40-60 minutes

Monitoring Parameters Periodic renal, hepatic, and hematologic function tests

Test Interactions Interferes with urinary glucose determination using Clinitest®; Positive Coombs' [direct]

Nursing Implications If nausea and/or vomiting occur during administration, decrease the rate of I.V. infusion

Additional Information Sodium content of 1 g I.V. formulation: 3.2 mEq; sodium content of 500 mg I.M. formulation: 1.4 mEq

Dosage Forms Excipient information presented when available (limited, particularly for generics); consult specific product labeling.

Injection, powder for reconstitution [I.M.]:
Primaxin®: Imipenem 500 mg and cilastatin 500 mg [contains sodium 32 mg (1.4 mEq)]

Injection, powder for reconstitution [I.V.]:
Primaxin®: Imipenem 250 mg and cilastatin 250 mg [contains sodium 18.8 mg (0.8 mEq)]; imipenem 500 mg and cilastatin 500 mg [contains sodium 37.5 mg (1.6 mEq)]

References

Ahonkhai VI, Cyhan GM, Wilson SE, et al, "Imipenem-Cilastatin in Pediatric Patients: An Overview of Safety and Efficacy in Studies Conducted in the United States," *Pediatr Infect Dis J,* 1989, 8 (11):740-4.

Overturf GD, "Use of Imipenem-Cilastatin in Pediatrics," *Pediatr Infect Dis J,* 1989, 8(11):792-4.

Taketomo CK, personal communication, September 2009.

Trissel LA, Gilbert DL, and Wolkin AC, "Compatibility of Docetaxel With Selected Drugs During Simulated Y-Site Administration," *Int J Pharmaceut Compound,* 1999, 3(3):241-4.

Wong VK, Wright HT Jr, Ross LA, et al, "Imipenem/Cilastatin Treatment of Bacterial Meningitis in Children," *Pediatr Infect Dis J,* 1991, 10 (2):122-5.

Imipramine (im IP ra meen)

Medication Safety Issues
Sound-alike/look-alike issues:
Imipramine may be confused with amitriptyline, desipramine, Norpramin®

Related Information
Antidepressant Agents *on page 1484*
Medications for Which A Single Dose May Be Fatal When Ingested By A Toddler *on page 1709*

U.S. Brand Names Tofranil-PM®; Tofranil®

Canadian Brand Names Apo-Imipramine®; Novo-Pramine; Tofranil®

Therapeutic Category Antidepressant, Tricyclic (Tertiary Amine)

Generic Available Yes

Use Treatment of various forms of depression, often in conjunction with psychotherapy; enuresis in children; analgesic for certain chronic and neuropathic pain

Medication Guide An FDA-approved patient medication guide, which is available with the product information and at http://www.fda.gov/downloads/Drugs/DrugSafety/ucm089161.pdf, must be dispensed with this medication for each new outpatient prescription and refill.

Pregnancy Risk Factor D

Lactation Enters breast milk/not recommended (AAP rates "of concern")

Contraindications Hypersensitivity to imipramine (cross-sensitivity with other tricyclics may occur) or any component; use of MAO inhibitors within 14 days (potentially fatal reactions may occur, see Drug Interactions); narrow-angle glaucoma; use during acute recovery phase after MI

Warnings Imipramine is FDA approved for the treatment of nocturnal enuresis in children ≥6 years of age. Imipramine is not approved for the treatment of depression in pediatric patients. Clinical worsening of depression or suicidal ideation and behavior may occur in children and adults with major depressive disorder **[U.S. Boxed Warning]**. In clinical trials, antidepressants increased the risk of suicidal thinking and behavior (suicidality) in children, adolescents, and young adults (18-24 years of age) with major depressive disorder and other psychiatric disorders. This risk must be considered before prescribing antidepressants for any clinical use. Short-term studies did **not** show an increased risk of suicidality with antidepressant use in patients >24 years of age and showed a decreased risk in patients ≥65 years.

Patients of all ages who are treated with antidepressants for any indication require appropriate monitoring and close observation for clinical worsening of depression, suicidality, and unusual changes in behavior, especially during the first few months after antidepressant initiation or when the dose is adjusted. Family members and caregivers should be instructed to closely observe the patient (ie, daily) and communicate condition with healthcare provider. Patients should also be monitored for associated behaviors (eg, anxiety, agitation, panic attacks, insomnia, irritability, hostility, aggressiveness, impulsivity, akathisia, hypomania, mania) which may increase the risk for worsening depression or suicidality. Worsening depression or emergence of suicidality (or associated behaviors listed above) that is abrupt in onset, severe, or not part of the presenting symptoms, may require discontinuation or modification of drug therapy.

Do not discontinue abruptly in patients receiving high doses chronically (withdrawal symptoms may occur; see Adverse Reactions). To reduce risk of intentional overdose, write prescriptions for the smallest quantity consistent with good patient care. Screen individuals for bipolar disorder prior to treatment (using antidepressants alone may induce manic episodes in patients with this condition). May worsen psychosis in some patients. Do not exceed a dose of 2.5 mg/kg/day in children; ECG changes (of unknown significance) have been reported in pediatric patients who received twice this amount.

The American Heart Association recommends that all children diagnosed with ADHD who may be candidates for medication, such as imipramine, should have a thorough cardiovascular assessment prior to initiation of therapy. These recommendations are based upon reports of serious cardiovascular adverse events (including sudden death) in patients (both children and adults) taking usual doses of stimulant medications. Most of these patients were found to have underlying structural heart disease (eg, hypertrophic obstructive cardiomyopathy). This assessment should include a combination of thorough medical history, family history, and physical examination. An ECG is not mandatory but should be considered.

Precautions Use with caution in patients with cardiovascular disease, conduction disturbances, seizure disorders, urinary retention, anorexia, significant renal or hepatic dysfunction, hyperthyroidism or those receiving thyroid replacement. Use of capsules is generally **not** recommended in children due to high mg strength and increased potential for acute overdose. Safety of imipramine for long-term chronic use in the treatment of enuresis has not been established; long-term usefulness should be periodically re-evaluated for the individual patient; medication should be tapered off gradually to achieve drug-free period for reassessment; children who relapse with enuresis during drug-free period do not always respond to subsequent courses of therapy.

Adverse Reactions Less sedation and anticholinergic effects than amitriptyline

Cardiovascular: Arrhythmias, hypotension (especially orthostatic), CHF, ECG changes, heart block, hypertension, MI, palpitation, stroke, tachycardia

Central nervous system: Drowsiness, sedation, confusion, dizziness, fatigue, anxiety, nervousness, seizures, agitation, delusions, disorientation, hallucination, headache, hypomania, insomnia, nightmares, psychosis, restlessness, suicidal thinking and behavior (see Warnings)

Dermatologic: Rash, photosensitivity, alopecia, itching, petechiae, purpura, urticaria

Endocrine & metabolic: Hyperglycemia, hypoglycemia, breast enlargement, galactorrhea, gynecomastia, increase or decrease in libido, SIADH, weight gain or weight loss

Gastrointestinal: Nausea, vomiting, constipation, xerostomia, appetite decreased, abdominal cramps, black tongue, diarrhea, epigastric disorders, ileus, stomatitis, taste disturbance,

Genitourinary: Urinary retention, impotence, testicular swelling

Hematologic: Blood dyscrasias, agranulocytosis, eosinophilia, thrombocytopenia

Hepatic: Hepatitis, cholestatic jaundice, transaminases elevated

Neuromuscular & skeletal: Weakness, ataxia, extrapyramidal symptoms, incoordination, numbness, paresthesia, peripheral neuropathy, tingling, tremor

Ocular: Blurred vision, intraocular pressure elevated, disturbances of accommodation, mydriasis

Otic: Tinnitus

Miscellaneous: Hypersensitivity reactions, diaphoresis, proneness to falling; withdrawal symptoms following abrupt discontinuation (headache, nausea, malaise)

Drug Interactions

Metabolism/Transport Effects Substrate of CYP1A2 (minor), 2B6 (minor), 2C19 (major), 2D6 (major), 3A4 (minor); **Inhibits** CYP1A2 (weak), 2C19 (weak), 2D6 (moderate), 2E1 (weak)

Avoid Concomitant Use

Avoid concomitant use of Imipramine with any of the following: Artemether; Dronedarone; Iobenguane I 123; Lumefantrine; MAO Inhibitors; Metoclopramide; Nilotinib; Pimozide; QuiNINE; Sibutramine; Tetrabenazine; Thioridazine; Ziprasidone

Increased Effect/Toxicity

Imipramine may increase the levels/effects of: Alcohol (Ethyl); Alpha-/Beta-Agonists (Direct-Acting); Alpha1-Agonists; Amphetamines; Anticholinergics; Aspirin; Beta2-Agonists; CNS Depressants; Desmopressin; Dronedarone; Fesoterodine; Nebivolol; NSAID (COX-2 Inhibitor); NSAID (Nonselective); Pimozide; QTc-Prolonging Agents; QuiNIDine; QuiNINE; Serotonin Modulators; Sulfonylureas; Tamoxifen; Tetrabenazine; Thioridazine; TraMADol; Vitamin K Antagonists; Yohimbine; Ziprasidone

The levels/effects of Imipramine may be increased by: Alfuzosin; Altretamine; Artemether; BuPROPion; Chloroquine; Cimetidine; Cinacalcet; Ciprofloxacin; Ciprofloxacin (Systemic); CYP2C19 Inhibitors (Moderate); CYP2C19 Inhibitors (Strong); CYP2D6 Inhibitors (Moderate); CYP2D6 Inhibitors (Strong); Dexmethylphenidate; Divalproex; DULoxetine; Gadobutrol; Lithium; Lumefantrine; MAO Inhibitors; Methylphenidate; Metoclopramide; Nilotinib; Pramlintide; Propoxyphene; Protease Inhibitors; QuiNIDine; QuiNINE; Selective Serotonin Reuptake Inhibitors; Sibutramine; Terbinafine; Terbinafine (Systemic); Valproic Acid

Decreased Effect

Imipramine may decrease the levels/effects of: Acetylcholinesterase Inhibitors (Central); Alpha2-Agonists; Codeine; Iobenguane I 123

The levels/effects of Imipramine may be decreased by: Acetylcholinesterase Inhibitors (Central); Barbiturates; CarBAMazepine; CYP2C19 Inducers (Strong); Peginterferon Alfa-2b; St Johns Wort

Food Interactions Riboflavin dietary requirements may be increased; food does not alter bioavailability

Stability Store at controlled room temperature at 20°C to 25°C (68°F to 77°F); dispense in tightly closed container

Mechanism of Action Mechanism not fully defined. As an antidepressant, imipramine increases the synaptic concentration of serotonin and/or norepinephrine in the CNS by inhibition of their reuptake by the presynaptic neuronal membrane. Mechanism of action in controlling childhood enuresis is thought to be apart from the antidepressant effect.

Pharmacodynamics Maximum antidepressant effects usually occur after ≥2 weeks

Pharmacokinetics (Adult data unless noted)

Absorption: Oral: Well absorbed

Distribution: Crosses the placenta; distributes into breast milk

V_d: Children: 14.5 L/kg; Adults: ~17 L/kg

Protein binding: >90% (primarily to alpha$_1$ acid glycoprotein and lipoproteins; to a lesser extent albumin)

Metabolism: In the liver by microsomal enzymes to desipramine (active) and other metabolites; significant first-pass effect

Bioavailability: 20% to 80%

Half-life: Adults: Range: 6-18 hours

Mean: Children: 11 hours; Adults: 16-17 hours

Desipramine (active metabolite): Adults: 22-28 hours

Time to peak serum concentration: Within 1-2 hours

Elimination: In the urine

Usual Dosage Oral:

Children:

Depression: **Note:** Not FDA approved for the treatment of depression in pediatric patients; controlled clinical trials have not shown tricyclic antidepressants to be superior to placebo for the treatment of depression in children and adolescents (see Dopheide, 2006 and Wagner, 2005).

1.5 mg/kg/day with dosage increments of 1 mg/kg every 3-4 days to a maximum dose of 5 mg/kg/day in 1-4 divided doses; monitor carefully especially with doses ≥3.5 mg/kg/day

Enuresis: ≥6 years: Initial: 10-25 mg at bedtime, if inadequate response still seen after 1 week of therapy, increase by 25 mg/day; dose should not exceed 2.5 mg/kg/day or 50 mg at bedtime if 6-12 years of age or 75 mg at bedtime if ≥12 years of age

Adjunct in the treatment of cancer pain: Initial: 0.2-0.4 mg/kg at bedtime; dose may be increased by 50% every 2-3 days up to 1-3 mg/kg/dose at bedtime

Adolescents: Depression: Initial: 25-50 mg/day; increase gradually; maximum dose: 100 mg/day in single or divided doses

Adults: Depression:

Outpatients: Initial: 75 mg/day; may increase gradually to 150 mg/day. May be given in divided doses or as a single bedtime dose; maximum: 200 mg/day

Inpatients: Initial: 100-150 mg/day; may increase gradually to 200 mg/day; if no response after 2 weeks, may further increase to 250-300 mg/day. May be given in divided doses or as a single bedtime dose; maximum: 300 mg/day.

Note: Following remission, a maintenance dose may be required for a longer period of time; use lowest effective dose; adolescents can usually be maintained at a lower dose; usual adult maintenance dose: 75-150 mg/day

Administration Oral: May administer with food to decrease GI distress. For treatment of enuresis, administer dose 1 hour before bedtime; for early night bedwetters, drug has been shown to be more effective if given earlier and in divided amounts (eg, 25 mg in midafternoon and repeated at bedtime)

Monitoring Parameters Heart rate, ECG, supine and standing blood pressure (especially in children), liver enzymes, CBC, serum drug concentrations (see Reference Range). Obtain ECG before initiation of therapy and at appropriate intervals in patients with any evidence of cardiovascular disease and in all patients who will receive doses that are larger than usual. Monitor patient periodically for symptom resolution; monitor for worsening depression, suicidality, and associated behaviors (especially at the beginning of therapy or when doses are increased or decreased; see Warnings).

ADHD: Evaluate patients for cardiac disease prior to initiation of therapy for ADHD with thorough medical history, family history, and physical exam; consider ECG (see Warnings); perform ECG and echocardiogram if findings suggest cardiac disease; promptly conduct cardiac evaluation in patients who develop chest pain, unexplained syncope, or any other symptom of cardiac disease during treatment.

Reference Range

Therapeutic: Imipramine and desipramine 150-250 ng/mL (SI: 530-890 nmol/L); desipramine 150-300 ng/mL (SI: 560-1125 nmol/L)

Potentially toxic: >300 ng/mL (SI: >1070 nmol/L)

Toxic: >1000 ng/mL (SI: >3570 nmol/L)

Patient Information Read the patient Medication Guide that you receive with each prescription and refill of imipramine. An increased risk of suicidal thinking and behavior has been reported with the use of antidepressants in children, adolescents, and young adults (18-24 years of age). Notify physician if you feel more depressed, have thoughts of suicide, or become more agitated or irritable (see Warnings). Limit caffeine; avoid alcohol and the herbal medicine St. John's wort; may cause drowsiness and impair ability to perform activities requiring mental alertness or physical coordination; may cause dry mouth. May cause photosensitivity reactions (eg, exposure to sunlight may cause severe sunburn, skin rash, redness, or itching); avoid exposure to sunlight and artificial light sources (sunlamps, tanning booth/bed); wear protective clothing, wide-brimmed hats, sunglasses, and lip sunscreen (SPF ≥15); use a sunscreen [broad-spectrum sunscreen or physical sunscreen (preferred) or sunblock with SPF ≥15]; contact physician if reaction occurs.

Dosage Forms Excipient information presented when available (limited, particularly for generics); consult specific product labeling.

Capsule, as pamoate: 75 mg, 100 mg, 125 mg, 150 mg

Tofranil-PM®: 75 mg, 100 mg, 125 mg, 150 mg

Tablet, as hydrochloride: 10 mg, 25 mg, 50 mg

Tofranil®: 10 mg, 25 mg, 50 mg

References

American Academy of Pediatrics/American Heart Association Clarification of Statement on Cardiovascular Evaluation and Monitoring of Children and Adolescents With Heart Disease Receiving Medications for ADHD; available at: http://americanheart.mediaroon.com/index.php?s=43&item=422.

Berde C, Ablin A, Glazer J, et al, "American Academy of Pediatrics Report of the Subcommittee on Disease-Related Pain in Childhood Cancer," *Pediatrics*, 1990, 86(5 Pt 2):818-25.

Dopheide JA, "Recognizing and Treating Depression in Children and Adolescents," *Am J Health Syst Pharm*, 2006, 63(3):233-43.

Levy HB, Harper CR, and Weinberg WA, "A Practical Approach to Children Failing in School," *Pediatr Clin North Am*, 1992, 39 (4):895-928.

Vetter VL, Elia J, Erickson C, et al, "Cardiovascular Monitoring of Children and Adolescents With Heart Disease Receiving Stimulant Drugs: A Scientific Statement From the American Heart Association Council on Cardiovascular Disease in the Young Congenital Cardiac Defects Committee and the Council on Cardiovascular Nursing," *Circulation*, 2008, 117(18):2407-23.

Wagner KD, "Pharmacotherapy for Major Depression in Children and Adolescents," *Prog Neuropsychopharmacol Biol Psychiatry*, 2005, 29 (5):819-26.

◆ **Imipramine Hydrochloride** *see* Imipramine *on page 716*

◆ **Imipramine Pamoate** *see* Imipramine *on page 716*

◆ **Imitrex®** *see* SUMAtriptan *on page 1308*

◆ **Imitrex® DF (Can)** *see* SUMAtriptan *on page 1308*

◆ **Imitrex® Nasal Spray (Can)** *see* SUMAtriptan *on page 1308*

Immune Globulin (Intramuscular)
(i MYUN GLOB yoo lin, IN tra MUS kyoo ler)

U.S. Brand Names GamaSTAN™ S/D

Canadian Brand Names BayGam®

Therapeutic Category Immune Globulin

Generic Available No

Use Provide passive immunity in susceptible individuals (eg, household and sexual contacts; travelers to high-risk areas; staff, attendees, and parents of diapered attendees in daycare center outbreaks; illicit drug users; staff and residents of institutions for custodial care) if given within 14 days of exposure to hepatitis A and for whom immunization is contraindicated or there is insufficient time for active immunization to take effect; prophylaxis of measles in susceptible individuals if given within 6 days of exposure; replacement therapy in antibody deficiency disorders; postexposure prophylaxis of rubella if given within 72 hours of exposure in a susceptible pregnant woman who will not consider termination of pregnancy under any circumstances

Pregnancy Risk Factor C

Pregnancy Considerations Reproduction studies have not been conducted with this product. Immune globulins cross the placenta in increased amounts after 30 weeks gestation.

Contraindications Hypersensitivity to immune globulin or any component; IgA deficiency

Warnings As a product of human plasma, IGIM may potentially transmit disease; screening of donors, as well as testing and/or inactivation of certain viruses reduces this risk. Epidemiologic and laboratory data indicate current IGIM products do not have a discernible risk of transmitting HIV.

Precautions Use with caution in patients with thrombocytopenia or coagulation disorders since bleeding may occur following an I.M. injection. IGIM is **NOT** for I.V. administration.

Adverse Reactions

Cardiovascular: Flushing, chest pain

Central nervous system: Fever, chills, lethargy, headache

Dermatologic: Urticaria, erythema, angioedema

Gastrointestinal: Nausea, vomiting

Local: Pain, tenderness, discomfort, muscle stiffness at I.M. site

Neuromuscular & skeletal: Myalgia, arthralgia

Renal: Nephrotic syndrome

Respiratory: Dyspnea

Miscellaneous: Hypersensitivity reactions, anaphylaxis

Drug Interactions

Avoid Concomitant Use There are no known interactions where it is recommended to avoid concomitant use.

Increased Effect/Toxicity There are no known significant interactions involving an increase in effect.

Decreased Effect

Immune Globulin (Intramuscular) may decrease the *levels/effects of:* Vaccines (Live)

Stability Store in refrigerator; do not freeze

Mechanism of Action Provides passive immunity by increasing the antibody titer and antigen-antibody reaction potential

Pharmacodynamics Duration: Immune effect: Usually 3-4 weeks

Pharmacokinetics (Adult data unless noted)

Half-life: 23 days

Time to peak serum concentration: I.M.: Within 48 hours

Usual Dosage I.M.: Infants, Children, Adolescents, and Adults:

Hepatitis A:

Pre-exposure prophylaxis upon travel into endemic areas (hepatitis A vaccine preferred):

Anticipated risk of 1-3 months: 0.02 mL/kg single dose

Anticipated risk >3 months: 0.06 mL/kg once every 4-6 months if exposure continues

Postexposure prophylaxis: 0.02 mL/kg single dose given within 14 days of exposure

Measles:

Postexposure prophylaxis: 0.25 mL/kg (~40 mg/kg IgG) single dose given within 6 days of exposure; maximum dose: 15 mL

Postexposure prophylaxis, immunocompromised host: 0.5 mL/kg (~80 mg/kg IgG) single dose given within 6 days of exposure; maximum dose: 15 mL

Rubella: Postexposure prophylaxis: 0.55 mL/kg single dose within 72 hours of exposure

Replacement therapy in antibody deficiency disorders: Initial: 1.3 mL/kg (~200 mg/kg); maintenance dose: 0.66 mL/kg (~100 mg/kg IgG) every 2-4 weeks (infants and children maximum single dose: 20-30 mL; adult maximum single dose: 30-50 mL); determine frequency of administration on the basis of trough IgG concentrations and clinical response

Administration I.M.: **Do not give I.V. or SubQ.** Administer deep I.M. into a large muscle mass; infants and small children, administer I.M. into the anterolateral aspect of the thigh; larger children and adolescents, administer into the upper outer quadrant of the gluteal region.

Limit the volume at a single injection site: Infants and small children: 1-3 mL; large child and adolescent: 5 mL; use multiple injection sites if the dose volume exceeds the recommended limit at a single injection site

Dosage Forms Excipient information presented when available (limited, particularly for generics); consult specific product labeling.

Injection, solution [preservative free; solvent detergent-treated]:

GamaSTAN™ S/D: 15% to 18% (2 mL, 10 mL)

References

Advisory Committee on Immunization Practices (ACIP), "Prevention of Hepatitis A Through Active or Passive Immunization: Recommendations of the Advisory Committee on Immunization Practices (ACIP)," *MMWR Recomm Rep,* 2006, 55(RR-7):1-23.

American Academy of Pediatrics, *Red Book®, 2003 Report of the Committee on Infectious Diseases,* 26th ed, Pickering LK ed, Elk Grove Village, IL: American Academy of Pediatrics, 2003, 54-6,423.

Immune Globulin (Intravenous)

(i MYUN GLOB yoo lin, IN tra VEE nus)

Medication Safety Issues

Sound-alike/look-alike issues:

Gamimune® N may be confused with CytoGam®

Immune globulin (intravenous) may be confused with hepatitis B immune globulin

Related Information

Intravenous Immune Globulin *on page 1490*

U.S. Brand Names Carimune® NF; Flebogamma®; Gammagard Liquid; Gammagard S/D; Gamunex®; Octagam®; Privigen®

Canadian Brand Names Gamimune® N; Gammagard Liquid; Gammagard S/D; Gamunex®; IGIVnex®; Privigen®

Therapeutic Category Immune Globulin

Generic Available No

Use Treatment of immunodeficiency syndrome, idiopathic thrombocytopenic purpura (ITP) and B-cell chronic lymphocytic leukemia (CLL); used in conjunction with appropriate anti-infective therapy to prevent or modify acute bacterial or viral infections in patients with iatrogenically-induced or disease-associated immunodepression; autoimmune neutropenia, hematopoietic stem cell transplant patients, Kawasaki disease, pediatric HIV infection, HIV-associated thrombocytopenia, Guillain-Barré syndrome, dermatomyositis, polymyositis, demyelinating polyneuropathies

FDA (see FDA website for approval age groups) and NIH Recommendations for the use of IGIV:

Primary immunodeficiencies

Kawasaki disease

Pediatric HIV infection

Chronic B-cell lymphocytic leukemia

Recent stem cell transplantation

Immune-mediated thrombocytopenia

Chronic inflammatory demyelinating polyneuropathy

Pregnancy Risk Factor C

Pregnancy Considerations Reproduction studies have not been conducted. Immune globulins cross the placenta in increased amounts after 30 weeks gestation. Intravenous immune globulin has been recommended for use in fetal-neonatal alloimmune thrombocytopenia and pregnancy-associated ITP.

Lactation Excretion in breast milk unknown

Contraindications Hypersensitivity to immune globulin, blood products, or any component; IgA deficiency (except with the use of Gammagard® S/D or Polygam® S/D; these agents are contraindicated in selective IgA deficiency where IgA deficiency is the only abnormality of concern); Privigen® contains the stabilizer L-proline and is contraindicated in patients with hyperprolinemia.Patients may experience severe hypersensitivity reactions or anaphylaxis in the setting of detectable IgA levels following infusion of Polygam® S/D. The occurrence of severe hypersensitivity reactions or anaphylaxis under such conditions should prompt consideration of an alternative therapy. Polygam® S/D is contraindicated in patients with selective IgA deficiency where the IgA deficiency is the only abnormality of concern.

Warnings Acute renal dysfunction (increased serum creatinine, oliguria, acute renal failure, osmotic nephrosis) can rarely occur **[U.S. Boxed Warning]**; most cases usually occur within 7 days of use (more likely with products stabilized with sucrose). Due to risk of renal dysfunction, use caution in patients with renal disease, diabetes mellitus, volume depletion, sepsis, paraproteinemia, the elderly, and concomitant use of nephrotoxic medications; discontinue if renal function deteriorates. Reports of noncardiogenic pulmonary edema with severe respiratory distress, hypoxemia, and fever occurring within 1-6 hours after a dose have occurred. Thrombotic events have been reported; patients at risk include those with a history of atherosclerosis, multiple cardiovascular risk factors, impaired cardiac output, hyperviscosity/hypercoagulable disorders, and prolonged periods of immobilization. Hyperproteinemia, increased serum viscosity, and hyponatremia may occur; distinguishing true hyponatremia from a pseudohyponatremia as treatment aimed at decreasing free water in patients with pseudohyponatremia may lead to volume depletion, a further increase in serum viscosity, and a higher risk of thrombotic events. Hypersensitivity and anaphylactic reactions can occur; a severe fall in blood pressure may rarely occur with anaphylactic reaction; immediate treatment (including epinephrine 1:1000) should be available.

Aseptic meningitis syndrome has been reported which usually starts within several hours to 2 days following IVIG. Symptoms include severe headache, nuchal rigidity, drowsiness, fever, photophobia, painful eye movements, nausea, and vomiting. Aseptic meningitis syndrome may occur more frequently with high dose (2 g/kg) therapy. Intravenous immune globulin has been associated with antiglobulin hemolysis; monitor for signs of hemolytic anemia. High-dose regimens (1 g/kg for 1-2 days) are not recommended for individuals with fluid overload or where fluid volume may be of concern.

Precautions Use with caution in patients with a history of cardiovascular disease or thrombotic episodes. Rapid IVIG infusion may be a possible risk factor for vascular occlusive events associated with IVIG. Do not exceed manufacturer's recommended initial infusion rate, use a lower IVIG concentration, and advance slowly in patients at risk. Monitor for adverse events during and after the infusion. Discontinue administration with signs of infusion reaction (fever, chills, nausea, vomiting, and rarely shock). Risk of adverse events may be increased with initial treatment, when switching brands of immune globulin, and with treatment interruptions of >8 weeks. Assure that patients are not volume depleted prior to the initiation of an IVIG infusion. Product of human plasma; may potentially contain infectious agents which could transmit disease. Screening of donors, as well as testing and/or inactivation or removal of certain viruses, reduces the risk. Infections thought to be transmitted by this product should be reported to the manufacturer. Response to live vaccines may be reduced following immune globulin treatment, refer to package insert or current practice guidelines for recommendations on separation intervals. Products may contain maltose, sorbitol, sucrose, and some packaging may contain latex.

Adverse Reactions

Cardiovascular: Chest pain, flushing of the face, hypotension, pallor, pulmonary embolism, tachycardia, thromboembolism (see Warnings)

Central nervous system: Anxiety, aseptic meningitis syndrome, chills, dizziness, fever, headache, irritability, lightheadedness, malaise, seizures

Dermatologic: Contact dermatitis, eczema, erythema, pruritus, urticaria

Gastrointestinal: Abdominal pain, gastroenteritis, nausea, toothache, vomiting

Hematologic: Hemolytic anemia, transient neutropenia

Neuromuscular & skeletal: Arthralgia, back pain, myalgia, rigors

Ocular: Conjunctivitis

Renal: Acute renal failure

Respiratory: Acute respiratory distress syndrome, difficulty breathing, pulmonary edema (see Warnings), tightness in the chest, transfusion-related acute lung injury (see Warnings)

Miscellaneous: Aseptic meningitis, diaphoresis, hypersensitivity reactions, rigors

<1%, postmarketing, and/or case reports: Apnea, ARDS, autoimmune pure red cell aplasia (PRCA) exacerbation, bronchopneumonia, bronchospasm, bullous dermatitis, cardiac arrest, chest pain, coma, Coombs' test positive, cyanosis, epidermolysis, erythema multiforme, hepatic dysfunction, hypoxemia, leukopenia, loss of consciousness, pancytopenia, papular rash, pulmonary embolism, seizure, Stevens-Johnson syndrome, tremor, vascular collapse

Drug Interactions

Avoid Concomitant Use There are no known interactions where it is recommended to avoid concomitant use.

Increased Effect/Toxicity There are no known significant interactions involving an increase in effect.

Decreased Effect

Immune Globulin (Intravenous) may decrease the levels/effects of: Vaccines (Live)

Stability Do not mix with other drugs or I.V. infusion fluids. Stability is dependent upon the manufacturer and brand. Do not freeze. Dilution is dependent upon the manufacturer and brand. Gently swirl; do not shake; avoid foaming. Do not mix products from different manufacturers together. Discard unused portion of vials.

Carimune® NF: Prior to reconstitution, store ≤30°C (86°F). Reconstitute with NS, D$_5$W, or SWI. Following reconstitution, store under refrigeration. Begin infusion within 24 hours.

Flebogamma®: Store at 2°C to 25°C (36°F to 77°F). Dilution is not recommended.

Gammagard Liquid: May dilute in D$_5$W only. Prior to use, store at 2°C to 8°C (36°F to 46°F) for up to 36 months; do not freeze. May store at room temperature of 25°C (77°F) within the first 24 months of manufacturing. Storage time at room temperature varies with length of time previously refrigerated; refer to product labeling for details.

Gammagard S/D: Store at ≤25°C (≤77°F). Reconstitute with SWI; may store diluted solution under refrigeration for up to 24 hours.

Gamunex®: May be stored for up to 36 months at 2°C to 8°C (36°F to 46°F); may be stored at ≤25°C (≤77°F) for up to 6 months. Dilute in D$_5$W only.

Octagam®: Store at 2°C to 25°C (36°F to 77°F).

Privigen®: Store at ≤25°C (≤77°F); do not freeze (do not use if previously frozen). Protect from light. If necessary to further dilute, D$_5$W may be used.

Mechanism of Action Replacement therapy for primary and secondary immunodeficiencies; interference with F$_c$ receptors on the cells of the reticuloendothelial system for autoimmune cytopenias and ITP

Pharmacokinetics (Adult data unless noted) Half-life: 21-29 days

Usual Dosage Children and Adults: I.V.:

Primary immunodeficiency disorders: Adjust dose/frequency based on desired IgG concentration and clinical response: Manufacturers dosing recommendations vary based on individual product used.

General dosing range: 200-800 mg/kg every 3-4 weeks; maintain a trough IgG concentration of 500 mg/dL

Chronic lymphocytic leukemia (CLL): 400 mg/kg/dose every 3-4 weeks

Immune (idiopathic) thrombocytopenic purpura: 400-1000 mg/kg/day for 2-5 consecutive days (total dose: 2 g/kg); maintenance dose: 400-1000 mg/kg/dose every 3-6 weeks based on clinical response and platelet count

Pediatric HIV infection: 400 mg/kg/dose every 2-4 weeks in those patients with hypogammaglobulinemia (IgG <400 mg/dL). Consider IGIV for HIV-infected children who have recurrent, serious bacterial infections during a 1-year period.

HIV-associated thrombocytopenia: 500-1000 mg/kg/day for 3-5 days

Kawasaki disease (AHA guidelines): 2 g/kg as a single dose, given over 10-12 hours; if signs and symptoms persist, retreatment with a second 2 g/kg infusion should be considered. Must be used in combination with aspirin.

Hematopoietic stem cell transplantation with hypogamma-globulinemia (CDC guidelines):
Children: 400 mg/kg/month; increase dose or frequency to maintain IgG concentration >400 mg/dL
Adolescents and Adults: 500 mg/kg/week
Guillain-Barré syndrome: 400 mg/kg/day for 5 days **or** 1 g/kg/day for 2 days **or** 2 g/kg as a single dose
Refractory dermatomyositis: 2 g/kg per month administered over 2-5 days
Refractory polymyositis: 2 g/kg per month administered over 2-5 days
Chronic inflammatory demyelinating polyneuropathy: 400 mg/kg/day for 5 days once each month or 1 g/kg/day for 2 days once each month

Administration Do not administer I.M. or SubQ
I.V. infusion over 2-12 hours; for initial treatment, a lower concentration and/or a slower rate of infusion should be used. Administer in separate infusion line from other medications; if using primary line, flush with saline prior to administration. Refrigerated product should be warmed to room temperature prior to infusion. Some products require filtration; refer to individual product labeling. Antecubital veins should be used, especially with concentrations ≥10% to prevent injection site discomfort. Decrease dose, rate, and/or concentration of infusion in patients who may be at risk of renal impairment or thrombosis. Decreasing the rate or stopping the infusion may help relieve some adverse effects (flushing, changes in pulse rate, changes in blood pressure). Epinephrine should be available during administration. See Intravenous Immune Globulin Product Comparison on page 1490 for more information.

Monitoring Parameters Platelet count, blood pressure, vital signs, Quantitative Immunoglobulins (QUIGS), trough IgG concentration; periodic monitoring of renal function tests, including BUN, serum creatinine, and urine output in patients with an increased risk for developing acute renal failure; signs and symptoms of hemolysis; hemoglobin and hematocrit; signs of infusion reaction or anaphylaxis

Test Interactions IVIG products containing maltose (eg, Octagam®) may cause falsely elevated glucose readings when glucose dehydrogenase pyrroloquinolinequinone (GDH-PQQ) based methods are used.

Patient Information Notify physician of any sudden weight gain, fluid retention/edema, decreased urine output, and/or shortness of breath

Nursing Implications Appropriate agents for treatment of a hypersensitivity reaction (eg, epinephrine, diphenhydramine) should be readily available; patients may need to be pretreated with an antipyretic, antihistamine, and/or corticosteroid to prevent chills and fever; adverse reactions may also be alleviated by decreasing the rate or the concentration of infusion or utilizing a different IGIV preparation

Additional Information Octagam® contains sodium 30 mmol/L.

Dosage Forms Excipient information presented when available (limited, particularly for generics); consult specific product labeling.
Injection, powder for reconstitution [preservative free, nanofiltered]:
Carimune® NF: 3 g, 6 g, 12 g [contains sucrose]
Injection, powder for reconstitution [preservative free, solvent detergent-treated]:
Gammagard S/D: 2.5 g, 5 g, 10 g [stabilized with human albumin, glycine, glucose, and polyethylene glycol; packaging may contain natural latex/natural rubber]
Injection, solution [preservative free; solvent detergent-treated]:
Gammagard Liquid: 10% (10 mL, 25 mL, 50 mL, 100 mL, 200 mL) [latex free, sucrose free; stabilized with glycine]
Octagam®: 5% (20 mL, 50 mL, 100 mL, 200 mL) [sucrose free; contains sodium 30 mmol/L and maltose]

Injection, solution [preservative free]
Flebogamma®: 5% (10 mL, 50 mL, 100 mL, 200 mL) [contains polyethylene glycol and sorbitol]
Gamunex®: 10% (10 mL, 25 mL, 50 mL, 100 mL, 200 mL) [caprylate/chromatography purified]
Privigen®: 10% (50 mL, 100 mL, 200 mL) [sucrose free]

References
Anderson D, Ali K, Blanchette V, et al, "Guidelines on the Use of Intravenous Immune Globulin for Hematologic Conditions," *Transfus Med Rev*, 2007, 21(2 Suppl 1):S9-56.
ASHP Commission on Therapeutics, "ASHP Therapeutic Guidelines for Intravenous Immune Globulin," *Am J Hosp Pharm*, 1992, 49(3):652-4.
Blanchette VS, Luke B, Andrew M, et al, "A Prospective Randomized Trial of High-Dose Intravenous Immune Globulin G Therapy, Oral Prednisone Therapy, and No Therapy in Childhood Acute Immune Thrombocytopenic Purpura," *J Pediatr*, 1993, 123(6):989-95.
Centers for Disease Control and Prevention, Infectious Disease Society of America, and American Society of Blood and Marrow Transplantation, "Guidelines for Preventing Opportunistic Infections Among Hematopoietic Stem Cell Transplant Recipients," *MMWR Recomm Rep*, 2000, 49(RR-10):1-125, CE1-7.
Cherin P and Herson S, "Indications for Intravenous Gammaglobulin Therapy in Inflammatory Myopathies," *J Neurol Neurosurg Psychiatry*, 1994, 57 Suppl:50-4.
Dalakas MC and Hohlfeld R, "Polymyositis and Dermatomyositis," *Lancet*, 2003, 362(9388):971-82.
Dalakas MC, Illa I, Dambrosia JM, et al, "A Controlled Trial of High-Dose Intravenous Immune Globulin Infusions as Treatment for Dermatomyositis," *N Engl J Med*, 1993, 329(27):1993-2000.
Dalakas MC, "Intravenous Immunoglobulin in Autoimmune Neuromuscular Diseases," *JAMA*, 2004, 291(19):2367-75.
Eijkhout HW, van Der Meer JW, Kallenberg CG, et al, "The Effect of Two Different Dosages of Intravenous Immunoglobulin on the Incidence of Recurrent Infections in Patients With Primary Hypogammaglobulinemia. A Randomized, Double-Blind, Multicenter Crossover Trial," *Ann Intern Med*, 2001, 135(3):165-74.
Feasby T, Banwell B, Benstead T, et al, "Guidelines on the Use of Intravenous Immune Globulin for Neurologic Conditions," *Transfus Med Rev*, 2007, 21(2 Suppl 1):S57-107.
Gürcan HM and Ahmed AR, "Efficacy of Various Intravenous Immunoglobulin Therapy Protocols in Autoimmune and Chronic Inflammatory Disorders," *Ann Pharmacother*, 2007, 41(5):812-23.
Hughes RA, Raphael JC, Swan AV, et al, "Intravenous Immunoglobulin for Guillain-Barre Syndrome," *Cochrane Database of Systematic Reviews*, 2008, issue 2.
Hughes RA, Wijdicks EF, Barohn R, et al, "Practice Parameter: Immunotherapy for Guillain-Barré Syndrome: Report of the Quality Standards Subcommittee of the American Academy of Neurology," *Neurology*, 2003, 61(6):736-40.
Kaplan JE, Masur H, and Holmes KK, "Guidelines for Preventing Opportunistic Infections Among HIV-Infected Persons - 2002 Recommendations of the USPHS and IDSA," *MMWR*, 2002, 51 (RR-8):1-46.
Kaplan JE, Masur H, Holmes KK, et al, "Guidelines for Preventing Opportunistic Infections Among HIV-Infected Persons–2002. Recommendations of the U.S. Public Health Service and the Infectious Diseases Society of America," *MMWR Recomm Rep*, 2002, 51(RR-8):1-52.
Kuwabara S, "Guillain-Barré Syndrome: Epidemiology, Pathophysiology and Management," *Drugs*, 2004, 64(6):597-610.
Newburger JW, Takahashi M, Gerber MA, et al, "Diagnosis, Treatment, and Long-Term Management of Kawasaki Disease: A Statement for Health Professionals From the Committee on Rheumatic Fever, Endocarditis, and Kawasaki Disease, Council on Cardiovascular Disease in the Young, American Heart Association," *Pediatrics*, 2004, 114(6):1708-33.
NIH Consensus Conference, "Intravenous Immunoglobulin, Prevention and Treatment of Disease," *JAMA*, 1990, 264(24):3189-93.
Sansome A and Dubowitz V, "Intravenous Immunoglobulin in Juvenile Dermatomyositis - Four Year Review of Nine Cases," *Arch Dis Child*, 1995, 72(1):25-8.
Siegel J, "Intravenous Immune Globulins: Therapeutic, Pharmaceutical, & Cost Considerations," *Pharmacy Practice News*, 2006, Jan:33-7.
"University Hospital Consortium Expert Panel for Off-Label Use of Polyvalent Intravenously Administered Immunoglobulin Preparations Consensus Statement," *JAMA*, 1995, 273(23):1865-70.

♦ **Immune Serum Globulin** *see* Immune Globulin (Intramuscular) *on page 718*

♦ **Immunine® VH (Can)** *see* Factor IX *on page 557*

♦ **Imodium® (Can)** *see* Loperamide *on page 838*

♦ **Imodium® A-D [OTC]** *see* Loperamide *on page 838*

◆ **Imogam® Rabies-HT** *see* Rabies Immune Globulin (Human) *on page 1198*

◆ **Imogam® Rabies Pasteurized (Can)** *see* Rabies Immune Globulin (Human) *on page 1198*

◆ **Imovax® Rabies** *see* Rabies Virus Vaccine *on page 1199*

◆ **Imuran®** *see* AzaTHIOprine *on page 161*

Inamrinone (eye NAM ri none)

Medication Safety Issues
Sound-alike/look-alike issues:
Amrinone may be confused with aMILoride, amiodarone

High alert medication: The Institute for Safe Medication Practices (ISMP) includes this medication among its list of drug classes which have a heightened risk of causing significant patient harm when used in error.

Related Information
CPR Pediatric Drug Dosages *on page 1455*

Therapeutic Category Phosphodiesterase Enzyme Inhibitor

Generic Available Yes

Use Short-term treatment of CHF; **Note:** Due to potential serious adverse effects and limited experience, inamrinone should only be used in patients who have not responded to other therapies (ie, digoxin, diuretics, vasodilators); patients must be closely monitored. Use of inamrinone in controlled trials did not extend beyond 48 hours; inamrinone has not been shown to be safe or effective for long-term treatment of CHF; long-term oral use of inamrinone and similar agents for heart failure was associated with no improvement in symptoms, increased risk of hospitalization, and increased risk of sudden death; risk appears to be increased in patients with NYHA Class IV symptoms.

Pregnancy Risk Factor C

Contraindications Hypersensitivity to inamrinone lactate or any component (see Warnings)

Warnings Injection contains sodium metabisulfite which may cause allergic reactions in susceptible individuals

Precautions Avoid use in patients with severe obstructive aortic or pulmonic valvular disease; use in patients with hypertrophic subaortic stenosis may increase outflow tract obstruction. Use with caution and modify dosage in patients with impaired renal function. Hypotension may occur; monitor blood pressure and heart rate; infusion may require reduction in rate or temporary discontinuation if hypotension occurs; hypotension may be prolonged, especially in patients with renal dysfunction. Monitor also for arrhythmias, thrombocytopenia, hepatotoxicity, and GI effects; discontinue inamrinone if significant increase in liver enzymes with symptoms of idiosyncratic hypersensitivity reaction (ie, eosinophilia) occurs; monitor fluids and electrolytes. Diuresis may result from improvement in cardiac output and may require dosage reduction of diuretics. Inamrinone may exacerbate myocardial ischemia or worsen ventricular ectopy; not recommended for use in patients with acute MI.

Adverse Reactions
Cardiovascular: Hypotension (1.3% incidence), ventricular and supraventricular arrhythmias (3%) (may be related to infusion rate); chest pain (0.2%)

Central nervous system: Fever (0.9%)

Gastrointestinal: Nausea (1.7%), vomiting (0.9%), abdominal pain (0.4%), anorexia (0.4%); GI effects may be due to an increase in gastric acid secretion and intestinal motility, secondary to phosphodiesterase inhibition

Hematologic: Thrombocytopenia (2.4%), may be dose-related; in one study, 8 of 16 children (1.5 months to 11.2 years of age) developed thrombocytopenia (mean count 66 x 10^9 platelets/L). Inamrinone bolus doses ranged

from 1.2-3 mg/kg given in 4 divided doses over 1 hour and were followed by continuous infusions of 5-10 mcg/kg/minute. Thrombocytopenia developed 19-71 hours after starting inamrinone (mean ± SD = 51 ± 25 hours). Resolution of thrombocytopenia occurred 54 ± 15 hours after therapy was discontinued; thrombocytopenia developed in patients with a higher total dose, longer duration of infusion, higher plasma concentrations of N-acetylamrinone (major metabolite of inamrinone), and higher plasma ratios of N-acetylamrinone to inamrinone.

Hepatic: Hepatotoxicity (0.2%), liver enzymes elevated (rare), bilirubin elevated (rare), jaundice (rare)

Local: Burning at injection site (0.2%)

Miscellaneous: Hypersensitivity reactions

Drug Interactions
Avoid Concomitant Use There are no known interactions where it is recommended to avoid concomitant use.

Increased Effect/Toxicity There are no known significant interactions involving an increase in effect.

Decreased Effect There are no known significant interactions involving a decrease in effect.

Stability Store at controlled room temperature at 15°C to 30°C (59°F to 86°F). Protect from light; store in carton until ready for use. Dilute only with NS or ½NS; do not directly dilute with dextrose-containing solutions, chemical interaction occurs; may be administered I.V. (via Y-site) into running dextrose infusions. Furosemide forms a precipitate when injected in I.V. lines containing inamrinone; incompatible with sodium bicarbonate; use diluted solutions of inamrinone (1-3 mg/mL) within 24 hours.

Mechanism of Action Inhibits phosphodiesterase III (PDE III), the major PDE in cardiac and vascular tissues. Inhibition of PDE III increases cyclic adenosine monophosphate (cAMP) which potentiates the delivery of calcium to myocardial contractile systems and results in a positive inotropic effect. Inhibition of PDE III in vascular tissue results in relaxation of vascular muscle and vasodilatation.

Pharmacodynamics
Onset of action: I.V.: Within 2-5 minutes

Maximum effect: Within 10 minutes

Duration: Dose dependent with low doses lasting ~30 minutes and higher doses lasting ~2 hours

Pharmacokinetics (Adult data unless noted)
Distribution: V_d:
  Neonates: 1.8 L/kg
  Infants: 1.6 L/kg
  Adults: 1.2 L/kg

Protein binding: 10% to 49%

Metabolism: In the liver to several metabolites (N-acetate, N-glycolyl, N-glucuronide, and O-glucuronide)

Half-life:
  Neonates, 1-2 weeks of age: 22.2 hours
  Infants 6-38 weeks of age: 6.8 hours; negative correlation of age with half-life in infants 4-38 weeks of age
  Infants and Children (1 month to 15 years of age): 2.2-10.5 hours
  Adults, normal volunteers: 3.6 hours
  Adults with CHF: 5.8 hours

Elimination: Excreted in urine as metabolites and unchanged drug; 10% to 40% as unchanged drug in the urine within 24 hours

Usual Dosage I.V.: **Note:** Dose should not exceed 10 mg/kg/24 hours; doses of 18 mg/kg/day have been used in adults for a short duration; titrate infusion based on patient clinical response and adverse effects

Neonates: 0.75 mg/kg I.V. bolus over 2-3 minutes followed by maintenance infusion 3-5 mcg/kg/minute; I.V. bolus may need to be repeated in 30 minutes; see Additional Information

Infants and Children: 0.75 mg/kg I.V. bolus over 2-3 minutes followed by maintenance infusion 5-10 mcg/kg/minute; I.V. bolus may need to be repeated in 30 minutes; see Additional Information

Adults: 0.75 mg/kg I.V. bolus over 2-3 minutes followed by maintenance infusion of 5-10 mcg/kg/minute; I.V. bolus may need to be repeated in 30 minutes

PALS Guidelines 2005: I.V., I.O.: Loading dose: 0.75-1 mg/kg over 5 minutes; if tolerated, loading dose may be repeated up to 2 times; maximum total loading dose: 3 mg/kg; follow with maintenance infusion of 2-20 mcg/kg/minute; **Note:** If hypotension occurs during loading dose, administer 5-10 mL/kg of NS or other appropriate fluid and position patient flat or with head down (if patient can tolerate); if hypotension continues after fluid loading, administer a vasopressor agent and do not administer further inamrinone loading doses

ACLS Guidelines 2005: Adults: 0.75 mg/kg I.V. bolus over 2-3 minutes [give over 10-15 minutes in patients with LV dysfunction (eg, postresuscitation)] followed by maintenance infusion of 5-15 mcg/kg/minute; I.V. bolus may need to be repeated in 30 minutes

Dosing adjustment in renal impairment:
Infants and Children:
Cl_{cr} 30-50 mL/minute: Administer 100% of dose
Cl_{cr} 10-29 mL/minute: Administer 50% of dose
Cl_{cr} <10 mL/minute: Administer 25% of dose
Intermittent hemodialysis or peritoneal dialysis: Administer 25% of dose

Adults:
Cl_{cr} ≥10 mL/minute: Administer 100% of dose
Cl_{cr} <10 mL/minute: Administer 50% to 75% of dose

Administration Parenteral:
I.V. bolus: Infuse over 2-3 minutes; may be administered undiluted; **Note:** PALS Guidelines 2005 recommend infusing bolus dose over 5 minutes; ACLS Guidelines 2005 recommend infusing bolus over 2-3 minutes in adults **without** LV dysfunction and over 10-15 minutes in adults **with** LV dysfunction
Continuous infusion: Dilute with NS or 1/2NS to final concentration of 1-3 mg/mL; use controlled infusion device (eg, I.V. pump)

Monitoring Parameters Blood pressure, heart rate, ECG, CBC, platelet count, liver enzymes, renal function, fluid status, intake and output, body weight, serum electrolytes (especially potassium and magnesium), infusion site; if Swan-Ganz catheter is present, monitor cardiac index, stroke volume, systemic vascular resistance, pulmonary capillary wedge pressure, pulmonary vascular resistance

Reference Range Proposed: Adults: 3 mcg/mL; linear correlation with cardiac index observed from 0.5-7 mcg/mL

Nursing Implications Do **not** administer furosemide I.V. push via "Y" site into inamrinone solutions as precipitate will occur; monitor patients closely (see Monitoring Parameters)

Additional Information Preliminary pharmacokinetic studies estimate that total initial bolus doses of 3-4.5 mg/kg given in divided doses to neonates and infants are required to obtain serum concentrations similar to therapeutic adult levels. The use of these higher doses has been reported in a small number of infants and children. Some centers use a total loading dose of 3 mg/kg (administered as 4 doses of 0.75 mg/kg/dose given every 15 minutes; each of the 0.75 mg/kg doses is given over 5 minutes. Further pharmacodynamic studies are needed to define pediatric inamrinone dosing guidelines.

Effective July 1, 2000, the nonproprietary name of the drug (amrinone) was officially changed by the U.S. Pharmacopeia (USP) Nomenclature Committee and the U.S. Adopted Names (USAN) Council to inamrinone to prevent confusion with amiodarone; other countries will still use the name amrinone

Dosage Forms Excipient information presented when available (limited, particularly for generics); consult specific product labeling.
Injection, solution, as lactate: 5 mg/mL (20 mL) [contains sodium metabisulfite]

References
"ACC/AHA 2005 Guideline Update for the Diagnosis and Management of Chronic Heart Failure in the Adult: A Report of the American College of Cardiology/American Heart Association Task Force on Practice Guidelines (Writing Committee to Update the 2001 Guidelines for the Evaluation and Management of Heart Failure)," *J Am Coll Cardiol*, 2005, 46(6):e1-82.

Allen-Webb EM, Ross MP, Pappas JB, et al, "Age-Related Amrinone Pharmacokinetics in a Pediatric Population," *Crit Care Med*, 1994, 22 (6):1016-24.

"2005 American Heart Association (AHA) Guidelines for Cardiopulmonary Resuscitation (CPR) and Emergency Cardiovascular Care (ECC), Part 7.4: Monitoring and Medications and Part 12: Pediatric Advanced Life Support, The American Heart Association Emergency Cardiovascular Care Committee," *Circulation*, 2005, 112(24 Suppl): IV72-83, 167-87.

Drug Prescribing in Renal Failure: Dosing Guidelines for Adults and Children, 5th ed, Aronoff GR, et al, eds, Philadelphia, PA: American College of Physicians, 1993.

Heart Failure Society of America, "HFSA 2006 Comprehensive Heart Failure Practice Guideline," *J Card Fail*, 2006, 12(1):e1-122.

Lawless S, Burckart G, Diven W, et al, "Amrinone in Neonates and Infants After Cardiac Surgery," *Crit Care Med*, 1989, 17(8):751-4.

Lawless ST, Zaritsky A, and Miles MV, "The Acute Pharmacokinetics and Pharmacodynamics of Amrinone in Pediatric Patients," *J Clin Pharmacol*, 1991, 31(9):800-3.

Lynn AM, Sorensen GK, and Williams GD, "Hemodynamic Effects of Amrinone and Colloid Administration in Children Following Cardiac Surgery," *J Cardiothorac Vasc Anesth*, 1993, 7(5):560-5.

Ross MP, Allen-Webb EM, Pappas JB, et al, "Amrinone-Associated Thrombocytopenia: Pharmacokinetic Analysis," *Clin Pharmacol Ther*, 1993, 53(6):661-7.

◆ **Inapsine® [DSC]** *see* Droperidol *on page 483*

◆ **Inderal® [DSC]** *see* Propranolol *on page 1175*

◆ **Inderal® (Can)** *see* Propranolol *on page 1175*

◆ **Inderal® LA** *see* Propranolol *on page 1175*

Indinavir (in DIN a veer)

Medication Safety Issues
Sound-alike/look-alike issues:
Indinavir may be confused with Denavir™

Related Information
Adult and Adolescent HIV *on page 1620*
Management of Healthcare Worker Exposures to HBV, HCV, and HIV *on page 1661*
Pediatric HIV *on page 1613*
Perinatal HIV *on page 1628*

U.S. Brand Names Crixivan®

Canadian Brand Names Crixivan®

Therapeutic Category Antiretroviral Agent; HIV Agents (Anti-HIV Agents); Protease Inhibitor

Generic Available No

Use Treatment of HIV infection in combination with other antiretroviral agents; (**Note:** HIV regimens consisting of **three** antiretroviral agents are strongly recommended); postexposure chemoprophylaxis following occupational exposure to HIV

Pregnancy Risk Factor C

Pregnancy Considerations Adverse events were observed in some animal reproduction studies. No increased risk of overall birth defects has been observed according to data collected by the antiretroviral pregnancy registry. Plasma levels of indinavir were 74% lower at weeks 30-32 of gestation when compared to the same women at 14-28 weeks of gestation. Plasma levels were not measurable in some patients 8 hours post dose. It is not known if indinavir will exacerbate hyperbilirubinemia in neonates. Pregnancy and protease inhibitors are both associated with an increased risk of hyperglycemia.

Glucose levels should be closely monitored. Until optimal dosing during pregnancy has been established, the manufacturer does not recommend indinavir use in pregnant patients. The AIDSinfo guidelines consider indinavir an alternative agent if lopinavir/ritonavir cannot be used, however, indinavir should be used in combination with low-dose ritonavir during pregnancy (with ritonavir boosting, 82% of pregnant women reached target trough concentrations). Healthcare professionals are encouraged to contact the antiretroviral pregnancy registry to monitor outcomes of pregnant women exposed to antiretroviral medications (1-800-258-4263 or www.APRegistry.com).

Lactation Excretion in breast milk unknown/contraindicated

Breast-Feeding Considerations In infants born to mothers who are HIV positive, HAART while breast-feeding may decrease postnatal infection. However, maternal or infant antiretroviral therapy does not completely eliminate the risk of postnatal HIV transmission.

In the United States where formula is accessible, affordable, safe, and sustainable, complete avoidance of breast-feeding by HIV-infected women is recommended to decrease potential transmission of HIV.

Contraindications Hypersensitivity to indinavir or any component; concurrent therapy with amiodarone, cisapride, dihydroergotamine, ergonovine, ergotamine, methylergonovine, midazolam, pimozide, triazolam

Warnings Indinavir is a CYP3A4 isoenzyme inhibitor that interacts with numerous drugs. Due to potential serious and/or life-threatening drug interactions, some drugs are contraindicated (see Contraindications and Drug Interactions). Concurrent use with atazanavir, rifampin, St John's wort, or certain cholesterol-lowering agents (lovastatin, simvastatin) is **not** recommended. Alteration of dose or serum concentration monitoring may be required with other medications (see Drug Interactions).

Cases of nephrolithiasis and nephrolithiasis associated with renal insufficiency, acute renal failure, or pyelonephritis with or without bacteremia have been reported. Maintain adequate hydration in all patients to minimize risk. If signs and symptoms of nephrolithiasis occur (flank pain with or without hematuria or microscopic hematuria), temporarily interrupt or discontinue therapy. Tubulointerstitial nephritis with medullary calcification and cortical atrophy has been reported in patients with asymptomatic severe leukocyturia; consider discontinuation of indinavir in patients with severe leukocyturia. Immune reconstitution syndrome (an acute inflammatory response to residual or indolent opportunistic infections) may occur in HIV patients during initial treatment with combination antiretroviral agents, including indinavir; this syndrome may require further patient assessment and therapy. Hepatitis, including hepatic failure and death, has been reported (causal relationship not established). Spontaneous bleeding episodes have been reported in patients with hemophilia A and B. New onset diabetes mellitus, exacerbation of diabetes and hyperglycemia have been reported in HIV-infected patients receiving protease inhibitors. Acute hemolytic anemia has been reported. Indirect hyperbilirubinemia and elevated serum transaminases may occur.

Precautions Use with caution in patients with hepatic impairment; modify dose in patients with impaired liver function. Use of indinavir in HIV-infected pregnant patients is **not** recommended; significantly lower serum concentrations were observed in these patients receiving standard adult doses; optimal dose is not currently known. Fat redistribution and accumulation [ie, central obesity, peripheral wasting, facial wasting, breast enlargement, dorsocervical fat enlargement (buffalo hump), and cushingoid appearance] have been observed in patients receiving antiretroviral agents (causal relationship not established).

Adverse Reactions

Central nervous system: Insomnia, dizziness, headache, somnolence, asthenia, depression

Dermatologic: Rash, dry skin, urticaria, pruritus, paronychia

Endocrine & metabolic: Rare: Hyperglycemia, new onset diabetes, exacerbation of diabetes mellitus, ketoacidosis; serum cholesterol and triglycerides elevated; fat redistribution and accumulation (see Precautions)

Gastrointestinal: Nausea (10%), vomiting, diarrhea, abdominal pain, dyspepsia, metallic taste, pancreatitis

Genitourinary: Dysuria, pyelonephritis

Hematologic: Hemolytic anemia, spontaneous bleeding episodes in hemophiliacs (rare)

Hepatic: Hyperbilirubinemia (14%), liver function tests elevated, jaundice, liver cirrhosis, hepatitis (life-threatening in rare cases)

Neuromuscular & skeletal: Arthralgia

Renal: Nephrolithiasis, urolithiasis (pediatric patients: 29%; adult patients: 12.4%); hematuria, proteinuria, renal failure, interstitial nephritis; sterile leukocyturia (which may occur with elevations in serum creatinine) has been reported in pediatric patients without clinical symptoms of nephrolithiasis

Respiratory: Dry throat, pharyngitis

Miscellaneous: Immune reconstitution syndrome (see Warnings)

Drug Interactions

Metabolism/Transport Effects Substrate of CYP2D6 (minor), CYP3A4 (major), P-glycoprotein; **Inhibits** CYP2C9 (weak), 2C19 (weak), 2D6 (weak), 3A4 (strong)

Avoid Concomitant Use

Avoid concomitant use of Indinavir with any of the following: Alfuzosin; ALPRAZolam; Amiodarone; Atazanavir; Cisapride; Dronedarone; Eplerenone; Ergot Derivatives; Everolimus; Halofantrine; Lovastatin; Midazolam; Nilotinib; Nisoldipine; Pimozide; QuiNIDine; Ranolazine; Rivaroxaban; Romidepsin; Salmeterol; Silodosin; Simvastatin; St Johns Wort; Tamsulosin; Tolvaptan; Triazolam

Increased Effect/Toxicity

Indinavir may increase the levels/effects of: Alfuzosin; Almotriptan; Alosetron; ALPRAZolam; Amiodarone; Antifungal Agents (Azole Derivatives, Systemic); Atazanavir; Bortezomib; Brinzolamide; Calcium Channel Blockers (Dihydropyridine); Calcium Channel Blockers (Nondihydropyridine); CarBAMazepine; Ciclesonide; Cisapride; Clarithromycin; Colchicine; Corticosteroids (Orally Inhaled); CycloSPORINE; CycloSPORINE (Systemic); CYP3A4 Substrates; Dienogest; Digoxin; Dronedarone; Dutasteride; Enfuvirtide; Eplerenone; Ergot Derivatives; Etravirine; Everolimus; FentaNYL; Fesoterodine; Fusidic Acid; GuanFACINE; Halofantrine; HMG-CoA Reductase Inhibitors; Ixabepilone; Lovastatin; Lumefantrine; Maraviroc; Meperidine; MethylPREDNISolone; Midazolam; Nefazodone; Nilotinib; Nisoldipine; Paricalcitol; Pazopanib; Pimecrolimus; Pimozide; Protease Inhibitors; QuiNIDine; Ranolazine; Rifamycin Derivatives; Rivaroxaban; Romidepsin; Salmeterol; Saxagliptin; Sildenafil; Silodosin; Simvastatin; Sirolimus; Sorafenib; Tacrolimus; Tacrolimus (Systemic); Tacrolimus (Topical); Tadalafil; Tamsulosin; Temsirolimus; Tenofovir; Tolvaptan; TraZODone; Triazolam; Tricyclic Antidepressants; Vardenafil

The levels/effects of Indinavir may be increased by: Antifungal Agents (Azole Derivatives, Systemic); Atazanavir; Clarithromycin; CycloSPORINE; CycloSPORINE (Systemic); Delavirdine; Efavirenz; Enfuvirtide; Etravirine; Fusidic Acid; P-Glycoprotein Inhibitors

Decreased Effect

Indinavir may decrease the levels/effects of: Abacavir; Clarithromycin; Contraceptives (Estrogens); Delavirdine; Divalproex; Etravirine; Meperidine; Prasugrel; Theophylline Derivatives; Valproic Acid; Zidovudine

The levels/effects of Indinavir may be decreased by: Antacids; Atovaquone; CarBAMazepine; Contraceptives (Estrogens); CYP3A4 Inducers (Strong); Deferasirox; Didanosine; Efavirenz; Garlic; H2-Antagonists; Nevirapine; Peginterferon Alfa-2b; P-Glycoprotein Inducers; Proton Pump Inhibitors; Rifamycin Derivatives; St Johns Wort; Tenofovir; Venlafaxine

Food Interactions Decreased absorption when administered with food high in calories, protein, or fat; 27% decrease in AUC when administered with grapefruit juice

Stability Store capsules at room temperature in original container with desiccant (capsules are sensitive to moisture)

Mechanism of Action A protease inhibitor which acts on an enzyme late in the HIV replication process after the virus has entered into the cell's nucleus preventing cleavage of the gag-pol protein precursors resulting in the production of immature, noninfectious virions; cross-resistance with other protease inhibitors is possible

Pharmacokinetics (Adult data unless noted)

Absorption: Rapid (in the fasted state); presence of food high in calories, fat, and protein significantly decreases the extent of absorption

Protein binding: 60%

Metabolism: In the liver by CYP3A4 to inactive metabolites; 6 oxidative and 1 glucuronide conjugate metabolites have been identified

Bioavailability: Wide interpatient variability in children: 15% to 50%

Half-life:

Children 4-17 years (n=18): 1.1 hours

Adults: 1.8 ± 0.4 hours

Adults with mild to moderate hepatic dysfunction: 2.8 ± 0.5 hours

Time to peak serum concentration: 0.8 ± 0.3 hours

Elimination: 83% in feces as unabsorbed drug and metabolites; ~10% excreted in urine as unchanged drug

Usual Dosage Oral (use in combination with other antiretroviral agents):

Neonates and Infants: Not approved for use; should not be administered to neonates until further studies are performed due to side effect of hyperbilirubinemia and risk of kernicterus

Children: Not approved for use; optimal dose not established; clinical trials in children 4-15 years of age used doses of 500 mg/m^2/dose every 8 hours; maximum dose: 800 mg/dose every 8 hours; this dose produced AUCs and peak concentrations slightly higher than those seen in adults receiving the standard dose; however, in 50% of children studied, trough indinavir levels were lower than those observed in adults (see Additional Information).

Adolescents and Adults: 800 mg/dose every 8 hours

Adults:

Ritonavir-boosted regimens:

Indinavir 400 mg twice daily with ritonavir 400 mg twice daily

or

Indinavir 800 mg twice daily with ritonavir 100-200 mg twice daily

Concomitant therapy with delavirdine, itraconazole, or ketoconazole: Reduce dose of indinavir to 600 mg every 8 hours when used in combination with delavirdine 400 mg 3 times/day, itraconazole 200 mg twice daily or ketoconazole.

Concomitant therapy with efavirenz or nevirapine: Increase dose of indinavir to 1000 mg every 8 hours

Concomitant therapy with lopinavir and ritonavir (Kaletra®): Reduce dose of indinavir to 600 mg twice daily

Concomitant therapy with nelfinavir: Increase dose of indinavir to 1200 mg twice daily

Concomitant therapy with rifabutin: Increase dose of indinavir to 1000 mg every 8 hours and reduce dose of rifabutin to 1/2 the standard dose

Dosage adjustment in hepatic impairment:

Children: No dosing information is available

Adults:

Mild to moderate hepatic impairment: Decrease dose from 800 mg every 8 hours to 600 mg every 8 hours

Severe hepatic impairment: No dosing information is available

Administration Administer with water on an empty stomach or with a light snack 1 hour before or 2 hours after a meal; may administer with other liquids (ie, skim milk, coffee, tea, juice) or a light toast with jelly or cornflakes with skim milk); do not administer with grapefruit juice. May administer with food if taken in combination with ritonavir (ie, meal restrictions are not required). If coadministered with didanosine, give at least 1 hour apart on an empty stomach. Administer every 8 hours around-the-clock to avoid significant fluctuation in serum levels.

Monitoring Parameters Serum bilirubin, cholesterol, triglycerides, amylase, lipase, liver function tests, urinalysis, blood glucose levels, CD4 cell count, plasma levels of HIV RNA, CBC

Patient Information Indinavir is not a cure for HIV. Some medicines should not be taken with indinavir; report the use of other medications, nonprescription medications, and herbal or natural products to your healthcare provider. Avoid the herbal medicine St John's wort and grapefruit juice. Indinavir may cause kidney stones; drink plenty of fluids to decrease the risk of kidney stone formation; adults should drink at least 48 ounces of liquids per day. Take indinavir every day as prescribed; do not change dose or discontinue without physician's advice; if a dose is missed, take it as soon as possible, then return to normal dosing schedule; if a dose is skipped, do not double the next dose.

HIV medications may cause changes in body fat, including an increase in fat in the upper back and neck, breasts, and trunk; a loss of fat from the face, arms, and legs may also occur.

Nursing Implications Ensure adequate patient hydration to minimize the risk of nephrolithiasis; adults should drink at least 48 ounces of liquids per day.

Additional Information One study in children 4-17 years of age (n=18), adjusted the indinavir dose and dosing interval to maintain trough plasma concentrations. A mean daily dose of 2043 mg/m^2 was required with 9 of 18 children requiring doses every 6 hours (see Fletcher, 2000). Other pediatric studies have also suggested that every 6 hour dosing may be needed in some children (see Gatti, 2000) and that a wide range of doses (1250-2450 mg/m^2/day) may be required (see van Rossum, 2000a). However, it should be noted that the higher incidence of renal toxicity observed in children versus adults, may preclude studying higher doses of indinavir.

Two small studies assessed the use of indinavir in combination with ritonavir. One study used doses of indinavir 500 mg/m^2/dose **plus** ritonavir 100 mg/m^2/dose twice daily (n=4; 1-10 years of age); one patient attained high concentrations of both drugs and developed renal toxicity (see van Rossum, 2000). Another study used doses of indinavir 400 mg/m^2/dose **plus** ritonavir 125 mg/m^2/dose twice daily in children (n=14); AUC and trough concentrations were similar to adults receiving ritonavir boosted doses; however, peak concentrations were slightly decreased (see Bergshoeff, 2004). A pediatric clinical trial that used these same doses demonstrated good virologic efficacy; however, 4 of 21 patients developed nephrolithiasis; a high rate of overall side effects and intolerance to the dosing regimen was observed (see Fraaij, 2007). Further studies are needed.

Dosage Forms Excipient information presented when available (limited, particularly for generics); consult specific product labeling. [DSC] = Discontinued product

Capsule:

Crixivan®: 100 mg, 200 mg, 333 mg [DSC], 400 mg

Extemporaneous Preparations An indinavir 10 mg/mL oral solution is stable for 2 weeks stored at 4°C. The solution is made by first preparing an indinavir 100 mg/mL concentrate: Add contents of fifteen 400 mg capsules and 54 mL of purified distilled water into a 100 mL amber glass bottle. Place bottle in an ultrasonic water bath filled with water at 37°C for 60 minutes, stirring the solution every 10 minutes. Filter solution; wash bottle and filter with 6 mL purified distilled water; cool to room temperature. 50 mL of 100 mg/mL indinavir concentrate is added to 360 mL of viscous sweet base, 90 mL of simple syrup, 1.8 g citric acid, 45 mg azorubine, 0.1M sodium hydroxide solution to pH 3, and 12 drops of lemon oil to make a final volume of 500 mL. Mix solution until it is homogeneous.

Hugen PW, Burger DM, ter Hofstede HJ, et al, "Development of an Indinavir Oral Liquid for Children," *Am J Health Syst Pharm*, 2000, 57(14):1332-9.

References
Bergshoeff AS, Fraaij PL, van Rossum AM, et al, "Pharmacokinetics of Indinavir Combined With Low-Dose Ritonavir in Human Immunodeficiency Virus Type 1-Infected Children," *Antimicrob Agents Chemother*, 2004, 48(5):1904-7.

Briars LA, Hilao JJ, and Kraus DM, "A Review of Pediatric Human Immunodeficiency Virus Infection," *Journal of Pharmacy Practice*, 2004, 17(6):407-31.

Fletcher CV, Brundage RC, Remmel RP, et al, "Pharmacologic Characteristics of Indinavir, Didanosine, and Stavudine in Human Immunodeficiency Virus-Infected Children Receiving Combination Therapy," *Antimicrob Agents Chemother*, 2000, 44(4):1029-34.

Fraaij PL, Verweel G, van Rossum AM, et al, "Indinavir/Low-Dose Ritonavir Containing HAART in HIV-1 Infected Children has Potent Antiretroviral Activity, but Is Associated With Side Effects and Frequent Discontinuation of Treatment," *Infection*, 2007, 35(3):186-9.

Gatti G, Vigano' A, Sala N, et al, "Pharmacokinetics and Pharmacodynamics in Children With Human Immunodeficiency Virus Infection," *Antimicrob Agents Chemother*, 2000, 44(3):752-5.

Mueller BU, Smith S, Sleasman J, et al, "A Phase I/II Study of the Protease Inhibitor Indinavir (MK-0639) in Children With HIV Infection," *Eleventh International Conference on AIDS*, Vancouver, Canada, 1996.

Panel on Antiretroviral Guidelines for Adults and Adolescents, "Guidelines for the Use of Antiretroviral Agents in HIV-Infected Adults and Adolescents," December 1, 2009, http://www.aidsinfo.nih.gov.

Piscitelli SC, Burstein AH, Chaitt D, et al, "Indinavir Concentrations and St John's Wort," *Lancet*, 2000, 355(9203):547-8.

Stein DS, Fish DG, Bilello JA, et al, "A 24-Week Open-Label Phase I/II Evaluation of the HIV Protease Inhibitor MK-639 (Indinavir)," *AIDS*, 1996, 10(5):485-92.

U.S. Public Health Service, "Updated U.S. Public Health Service Guidelines for the Management of Occupational Exposures to HIV and Recommendations for Postexposure Prophylaxis," *MMWR Recomm Rep*, 2005, 54(RR-9):1-17.

van Rossum AM, de Groot R, Hartwig NG, et al, "Pharmacokinetics of Indinavir and Low-Dose Ritonavir in Children With HIV-1 Infection," *AIDS*, 2000, 14(14):2209-10.

van Rossum AM, Niesters HG, Geelen SP, et al, "Clinical and Virologic Response to Combination Treatment With Indinavir, Zidovudine, and Lamivudine in Children With Human Immunodeficiency Virus-1 Infection: A Multicenter Study in the Netherlands. On Behalf of the Dutch Study Group for Children with HIV-1 Infections," *J Pediatr*, 2000, 136(6):780-8.

Working Group on Antiretroviral Therapy and Medical Management of HIV-Infected Children, "Guidelines for the Use of Antiretroviral Agents in Pediatric HIV Infection," February 23, 2009. Available at http://www.aidsinfo.nih.gov.

◆ **Indinavir Sulfate** *see* Indinavir *on page 723*

◆ **Indocid® P.D.A. (Can)** *see* Indomethacin *on page 726*

◆ **Indocin®** *see* Indomethacin *on page 726*

◆ **Indocin® I.V.** *see* Indomethacin *on page 726*

◆ **Indometacin** *see* Indomethacin *on page 726*

Indomethacin (in doe METH a sin)

Medication Safety Issues
Sound-alike/look-alike issues:
Indocin® may be confused with Imodium®, Lincocin®, Minocin®, Vicodin®

Beers Criteria medication: This drug may be inappropriate for use in geriatric patients (high severity risk).

International issues:
Flexin® [Great Britain] may be confused with Floxin® which is a brand name for ofloxacin in the U.S.
Flexin® [Great Britain]: Brand name for orphenadrine in Israel

U.S. Brand Names Indocin®; Indocin® I.V.
Canadian Brand Names Apo-Indomethacin®; Indocid® P.D.A.; Novo-Methacin; Nu-Indo; Pro-Indo; ratio-Indomethacin; Sandoz-Indomethacin
Therapeutic Category Analgesic, Non-narcotic; Anti-inflammatory Agent; Antipyretic; Nonsteroidal Anti-inflammatory Drug (NSAID), Oral; Nonsteroidal Anti-inflammatory Drug (NSAID), Parenteral
Generic Available Yes: Excludes oral suspension
Use Management of inflammatory diseases and rheumatoid disorders; moderate pain; acute gouty arthritis; I.V. form used as alternative to surgery for closure of patent ductus arteriosus (PDA) in neonates
Medication Guide An FDA-approved patient medication guide, which is available with the product information and at http://www.fda.gov/downloads/Drugs/DrugSafety/ucm088612.pdf, must be dispensed with this medication for each new outpatient prescription and refill.
Pregnancy Risk Factor C
Pregnancy Considerations Adverse events have been observed in animal reproduction studies; therefore, the manufacturer classifies indomethacin as pregnancy category C. Indomethacin crosses the placenta and can be detected in fetal plasma and amniotic fluid. Indomethacin exposure during the first trimester is not strongly associated with congenital malformations; however, cardiovascular anomalies and cleft palate have been observed following NSAID exposure in some studies. The use of an NSAID close to conception may be associated with an increased risk of miscarriage. Non-teratogenic effects have been observed following NSAID administration during the third trimester, including myocardial degenerative changes, prenatal constriction of the ductus arteriosus, failure of the ductus arteriosus to close postnatally, and fetal tricuspid regurgitation; renal dysfunction or failure, oligohydramnios; gastrointestinal bleeding or perforation, increased risk of necrotizing enterocolitis; intracranial bleeding (including intraventricular hemorrhage), platelet dysfunction with resultant bleeding; and pulmonary hypertension. The risk of fetal ductal constriction following maternal use of indomethacin is increased with gestational age and duration of therapy. Because they may cause premature closure of the ductus arteriosus, use of NSAIDs late in pregnancy should be avoided (use after 31 or 32 weeks gestation is not recommended by some clinicians). Indomethacin has been used in the management of preterm labor. Indomethacin should be used with caution in pregnant women with hypertension. The chronic use of NSAIDs in women of reproductive age may be associated with infertility that is reversible upon discontinuation of the medication.
Lactation Enters breast milk/not recommended (AAP rates "compatible")

Breast-Feeding Considerations Indomethacin is excreted into breast milk and low amounts have been measured in the plasma of nursing infants. Seizures in a nursing infant were observed in one case report, although adverse events have not been noted in other cases. Breast-feeding is not recommended by the manufacturer. The AAP considers indomethacin to be "usually compatible with breast-feeding." (The therapeutic use of indomethacin is contraindicated in neonates with significant renal failure.) Hypertensive crisis and psychiatric side effects have been noted in case reports following use of indomethacin for analgesia in postpartum women. Use with caution in nursing women with hypertensive disorders of pregnancy or pre-existing renal disease.

Contraindications Hypersensitivity to indomethacin or any component; history of asthma, urticaria, or allergic-type reaction to aspirin, or other NSAIDs; patients with the "aspirin triad" [asthma, rhinitis (with or without nasal polyps), and aspirin intolerance] (fatal asthmatic and anaphylactoid reactions may occur in these patients); perioperative pain in the setting of coronary artery bypass graft (CABG)

Injection (ibuprofen lysine) is contraindicated in preterm infants with untreated proven or suspected infection; congenital heart disease where patency of the PDA is necessary for pulmonary or systemic blood flow (eg, pulmonary atresia, severe tetralogy of Fallot, severe coarctation of aorta); bleeding (especially with active intracranial hemorrhage or GI bleed); thrombocytopenia; coagulation defects; proven or suspected necrotizing enterocolitis (NEC); significant renal dysfunction

Suppositories are contraindicated for use in patients with a history of proctitis or recent rectal bleeding.

Warnings NSAIDs are associated with an increased risk of adverse cardiovascular thrombotic events, including potentially fatal MI and stroke **[U.S. Boxed Warning]**; risk may be increased with duration of use or pre-existing cardiovascular risk factors or disease; carefully evaluate cardiovascular risk profile prior to prescribing; use the lowest effective dose for the shortest duration of time, taking into consideration individual patient treatment goals; alternate therapies should be considered for patients at high risk. Use is contraindicated for treatment of perioperative pain in the setting of CABG surgery **[U.S. Boxed Warning]**; an increased incidence of MI and stroke was found in patients receiving COX-2 selective NSAIDs for the treatment of pain within the first 10-14 days after CABG surgery. NSAIDs may cause fluid retention, edema, and new-onset or worsening of pre-existing hypertension; use with caution in patients with hypertension, CHF, or fluid retention. Concurrent administration of ibuprofen, and potentially other nonselective NSAIDs, may interfere with aspirin's cardioprotective effect.

NSAIDs may increase the risk of gastrointestinal inflammation, ulceration, bleeding, and perforation **[U.S. Boxed Warning]**. These events, which can be potentially fatal, may occur at any time during therapy, and without warning. Avoid the use of NSAIDs in patients with active GI bleeding or ulcer disease. Use NSAIDs with extreme caution in patients with a history of GI bleeding or ulcers (these patients have a 10-fold increased risk for developing a GI bleed). Use NSAIDs with caution in patients with other risk factors which may increase GI bleeding (eg, concurrent therapy with aspirin, anticoagulants, and/or corticosteroids, longer duration of NSAID use, smoking, use of alcohol, and poor general health). Use the lowest effective dose for the shortest duration of time, taking into consideration individual patient treatment goals; alternate therapies should be considered for patients at high risk.

NSAIDs may compromise existing renal function. Renal toxicity may occur in patients with impaired renal function, dehydration, heart failure, liver dysfunction, and those taking diuretics and ACE inhibitors; use with caution in these patients; monitor renal function closely. NSAIDs are not recommended for use in patients with advanced renal disease. Long-term use of NSAIDs may cause renal papillary necrosis and other renal injury.

Fatal asthmatic and anaphylactoid reactions may occur in patients with the "aspirin triad" who receive NSAIDs (see Contraindications). NSAIDs may cause serious dermatologic adverse reactions including exfoliative dermatitis, Stevens-Johnson syndrome, and toxic epidermal necrolysis. Avoid use of NSAIDs in late pregnancy as they may cause premature closure of the ductus arteriosus.

Precautions Use with caution in patients with cardiac dysfunction, hypertension, renal or hepatic impairment, epilepsy, patients receiving anticoagulants and for treatment of JRA in children (fatal hepatitis has been reported; monitor children closely; assess liver function periodically)

Adverse Reactions

Cardiovascular: Hypertension, edema

Central nervous system: Somnolence, fatigue, depression, confusion, dizziness, headache

Dermatologic: Rash

Endocrine & metabolic: Hyperkalemia, dilutional hyponatremia (I.V.), hypoglycemia (I.V.)

Gastrointestinal: Nausea, vomiting, epigastric pain, abdominal pain, anorexia; GI bleeding, ulcers, perforation; necrotizing enterocolitis

Hematologic: Hemolytic anemia, bone marrow suppression, agranulocytosis, thrombocytopenia, inhibition of platelet aggregation

Hepatic: Hepatitis

Ocular: Corneal opacities

Otic: Tinnitus

Renal: Renal failure, oliguria

Miscellaneous: Hypersensitivity reactions

Drug Interactions

Metabolism/Transport Effects Substrate (minor) of CYP2C9, 2C19; **Inhibits** CYP2C9 (strong), 2C19 (weak)

Avoid Concomitant Use

Avoid concomitant use of Indomethacin with any of the following: Ketorolac; Ketorolac (Systemic)

Increased Effect/Toxicity

Indomethacin may increase the levels/effects of: Aminoglycosides; Anticoagulants; Antiplatelet Agents; Bisphosphonate Derivatives; Collagenase (Systemic); CycloSPORINE; CycloSPORINE (Systemic); Desmopressin; Digoxin; Drotrecogin Alfa; Eplerenone; Haloperidol; Ibritumomab; Lithium; Methotrexate; Nonsteroidal Anti-Inflammatory Agents; Pemetrexed; Potassium-Sparing Diuretics; Pralatrexate; Quinolone Antibiotics; Salicylates; Thrombolytic Agents; Tiludronate; Tositumomab and Iodine I 131 Tositumomab; Triamterene; Vancomycin; Vitamin K Antagonists

The levels/effects of Indomethacin may be increased by: Antidepressants (Tricyclic, Tertiary Amine); Corticosteroids (Systemic); Dasatinib; Glucosamine; Herbs (Anticoagulant/Antiplatelet Properties); Ketorolac; Ketorolac (Systemic); Nonsteroidal Anti-Inflammatory Agents; Omega-3-Acid Ethyl Esters; Pentosan Polysulfate Sodium; Pentoxifylline; Probenecid; Prostacyclin Analogues; Selective Serotonin Reuptake Inhibitors; Serotonin/Norepinephrine Reuptake Inhibitors; Treprostinil

Decreased Effect

Indomethacin may decrease the levels/effects of: ACE Inhibitors; Angiotensin II Receptor Blockers; Antiplatelet Agents; Beta-Blockers; Eplerenone; HydrALAZINE; Loop Diuretics; Potassium-Sparing Diuretics; Salicylates; Thiazide Diuretics

The levels/effects of Indomethacin may be decreased by: Bile Acid Sequestrants; Nonsteroidal Anti-Inflammatory Agents; Salicylates

Food Interactions Food may decrease the rate but not the extent of absorption

Stability

Oral suspension: Store below 86°F; do not freeze

I.V. product: Protect from light; not stable in alkaline solution; reconstitute just prior to administration; discard any unused portion; do not use preservative-containing diluents for reconstitution; will precipitate if reconstituted with solutions at pH <6 (product is not buffered)

Mechanism of Action Inhibits prostaglandin synthesis by decreasing the activity of the enzyme, cyclooxygenase, which results in decreased formation of prostaglandin precursors

Pharmacokinetics (Adult data unless noted)

Absorption: Oral:

Immediate Release:

Neonates: Incomplete, nonuniform

Adults: Rapid and well absorbed

Extended Release: Adults: 90% over 12 hours (**Note:** 75 mg product is designed to initially release 25 mg and then 50 mg over an extended period of time)

Distribution:

Neonates: PDA: 0.36 L/kg

Post-PDA closure: 0.26 L/kg

Adults: 0.34-1.57 L/kg

Protein binding: 99%

Metabolism: In the liver via glucuronide conjugation and other pathways

Bioavailability: Oral:

Neonates, premature: 13% to 20%

Adults: ~100%

Half-life:

Neonates:

Postnatal age (PNA) <2 weeks: ~20 hours

PNA >2 weeks: ~11 hours

Adults: 2.6-11.2 hours

Elimination: Significant enterohepatic recycling; 33% excreted in feces as demethylated metabolites with 1.5% as unchanged drug; 60% eliminated in urine as drug and metabolites

Usual Dosage

Patent ductus arteriosus:

Neonates: I.V.: Initial: 0.2 mg/kg, followed by 2 doses depending on postnatal age (PNA):

PNA **at time of first dose** <48 hours: 0.1 mg/kg at 12- to 24-hour intervals

PNA **at time of first dose** 2-7 days: 0.2 mg/kg at 12- to 24-hour intervals

PNA **at time of first dose** >7 days: 0.25 mg/kg at 12- to 24-hour intervals

In general, may use 12-hour dosing interval if urine output >1 mL/kg/hour after prior dose; use 24-hour dosing interval if urine output is <1 mL/kg/hour but >0.6 mL/kg/hour; doses should be withheld if patient has oliguria (urine output <0.6 mL/kg/hour) or anuria

Inflammatory/rheumatoid disorders: **Note:** Use lowest effective dose: Oral:

Children ≥2 years: 1-2 mg/kg/day in 2-4 divided doses; maximum dose: 4 mg/kg/day; do not exceed 150-200 mg/day

Adults: 25-50 mg/dose 2-3 times/day; maximum dose: 200 mg/day; extended release capsule should be given on a 1-2 times/day schedule

Administration

Oral: Administer with food, milk, or antacids to decrease GI adverse effects; extended release capsules must be swallowed whole, do not crush or chew

Parenteral: I.V.: Administer over 20-30 minutes at a concentration of 0.5-1 mg/mL in preservative free SWI or preservative free NS

Note: Do **not** administer via I.V. bolus or I.V. infusion via an umbilical catheter into vessels near the superior mesenteric artery, as these may cause vasoconstriction and can compromise blood flow to the intestines. Do not administer intra-arterially.

Monitoring Parameters BUN, serum creatinine, potassium, liver enzymes, CBC with differential; in addition, in neonates treated for PDA: heart rate, heart murmur, blood pressure, urine output, echocardiogram, serum sodium and glucose, platelet count, and serum concentrations of concomitantly administered drugs which are renally eliminated (eg, aminoglycosides, digoxin); periodic ophthalmic exams with chronic use

Patient Information Avoid alcohol; may cause dizziness

Additional Information Indomethacin may mask signs and symptoms of infections; fatalities in children have been reported, due to unrecognized overwhelming sepsis; drowsiness, lethargy, nausea, vomiting, seizures, paresthesia, headache, dizziness, tinnitus, GI bleeding, cerebral edema, and cardiac arrest have been reported with overdoses

Dosage Forms Excipient information presented when available (limited, particularly for generics); consult specific product labeling.

Capsule: 25 mg, 50 mg

Capsule, extended release, oral: 75 mg

Injection, powder for reconstitution: 1 mg

Indocin® I.V: 1 mg

Suppository, rectal: 50 mg (30s)

Suspension, oral:

Indocin®: 25 mg/5 mL (237 mL) [contains alcohol 1%; pineapple-coconut-mint flavor]

References
Coombs RC, Morgan ME, Durbin GM, et al, "Gut Blood Flow Velocities in the Newborn: Effects of Patent Ductus Arteriosus and Parenteral Indomethacin," *Arch Dis Child*, 1990, 65(10 Spec No):1067-71.

Gersony WM, Peckham GJ, Ellison RC, et al, "Effects of Indomethacin in Premature Infants With Patent Ductus Arteriosus: Results of a National Collaborative Study," *J Pediatr*, 1983, 102(6):895-906.

Kraus DM and Pham JT, "Neonatal Therapy," *Applied Therapeutics: The Clinical Use of Drugs*, 9th ed, Koda-Kimble MA, Young LY, Kradjan WA, et al, eds, Baltimore, MD: Lippincott Williams & Wilkins, 2009.

◆ **Indomethacin Sodium Trihydrate** *see* Indomethacin *on page 726*

◆ **INF-alpha 2** *see* Interferon Alfa-2b *on page 751*

◆ **Infanrix®** *see* Diphtheria, Tetanus Toxoids, and Acellular Pertussis Vaccine *on page 458*

◆ **Infantaire [OTC]** *see* Acetaminophen *on page 36*

◆ **Infantaire Gas Drops [OTC]** *see* Simethicone *on page 1262*

◆ **Infasurf®** *see* Calfactant *on page 240*

◆ **INFeD®** *see* Iron Dextran Complex *on page 762*

◆ **Inflamase® Mild (Can)** *see* PrednisoLONE *on page 1148*

InFLIXimab (in FLIKS e mab)

Medication Safety Issues

Sound-alike/look-alike issues:

Remicade® may be confused with Renacidin®, Rituxan® InFLIXimab may be confused with riTUXimab

U.S. Brand Names Remicade®

Canadian Brand Names Remicade®

Therapeutic Category Antirheumatic, Disease Modifying; Gastrointestinal Agent, Miscellaneous; Immunosuppressant Agent; Monoclonal Antibody; Tumor Necrosis Factor (TNF) Blocking Agent

Generic Available No

Use Reduction of signs and symptoms of Crohn's disease in patients with moderate to severely active disease who have had an inadequate response to conventional therapy (FDA approved in children ≥6 years and adults); reduction in the number of draining enterocutaneous fistulas in patients with fistulizing Crohn's disease (FDA approved in adults); treatment of refractory ulcerative colitis (FDA approved in adults); in combination with methotrexate for reducing signs and symptoms, inhibiting progression of structural damage, and improving physical function in patients with moderate to severe rheumatoid arthritis (FDA approved in adults); reduction of signs and symptoms of ankylosing spondylitis (FDA approved in adults); treatment of psoriatic arthritis (to reduce signs/symptoms of active arthritis and inhibit progression of structural damage and improve physical function); treatment of chronic severe plaque psoriasis (FDA approved in adults)

Medication Guide An FDA-approved patient medication guide, which is available with the product information and at http://www.remicade.com/remicade/assets/Med_Guide.pdf, must be dispensed with this medication for each new outpatient prescription and refill.

Pregnancy Risk Factor B

Pregnancy Considerations Reproduction studies have not been conducted. Use during pregnancy only if clearly needed. A Rheumatoid Arthritis and Pregnancy Registry has been established for women exposed to infliximab during pregnancy (Organization of Teratology Information Services, 877-311-8972).

Lactation Excretion in breast milk unknown/not recommended

Breast-Feeding Considerations It is not known whether infliximab is secreted in human milk. Because many immunoglobulins are secreted in milk and the potential for serious adverse reactions exists, a decision should be made whether to discontinue nursing or discontinue the drug, taking into account the importance of the drug to the mother.

Contraindications Hypersensitivity to infliximab, murine proteins, or any component; patients with any serious active infection or sepsis; patients with moderate or severe (NYHA class III/IV) congestive heart failure. Infliximab doses >5 mg/kg should not be administered to patients with moderate to severe heart failure; doses at 10 mg/kg have been associated with an increased incidence of death and worsening heart failure (see Warnings).

Warnings Patients receiving infliximab are at increased risk for serious infections which may result in hospitalization and/or fatality; infections usually developed in patients receiving concomitant immunosuppressive agents (eg, methotrexate or corticosteroids) and may present as disseminated (rather than local) disease. Active tuberculosis (or reactivation of latent tuberculosis), invasive fungal (including aspergillosis, blastomycosis, candidiasis, coccidioidomycosis, histoplasmosis, and pneumocystosis) and bacterial, viral, or other opportunistic infections have been reported in patients receiving TNF-blocking agents, including infliximab **[U.S. Boxed Warning]**. Monitor closely for signs/symptoms of infection; discontinue for serious infection or sepsis. Consider empiric antifungal therapy in patients who are at risk for invasive fungal infection and develop severe systemic illness. Other opportunistic infections (eg, invasive fungal infections, listeriosis, *Pneumocystis*) have occurred during therapy. Caution should be exercised when considering use in patients with conditions that predispose them to infections (eg, diabetes) or residence/travel from areas of endemic mycoses (blastomycosis, coccidioidomycosis, histoplasmosis), or with latent or localized infections. Do not give with clinically important active infection. Patients who develop a new infection while undergoing treatment should be monitored closely. Serious infections were reported when used in combination with anakinra or etanercept; combination of infliximab and anakinra is not recommended.

Reactivation of latent tuberculosis infections and active tuberculosis (may be disseminated or extrapulmonary) have been associated with infliximab therapy **[U.S. Boxed Warning]**. Tuberculosis (disseminated or extrapulmonary) has been reactivated in patients previously exposed to tuberculosis while on therapy. Most cases of reactivation have been reported within the first 3-6 months of treatment. Patients should be evaluated for tuberculosis risk factors and latent tuberculosis infection with a tuberculin skin test prior and during therapy; patients with initial negative tuberculin skin tests should receive continued monitoring for tuberculosis throughout treatment. Caution should be exercised when considering the use of infliximab in patients who have been exposed to tuberculosis. Treatment of latent tuberculosis should be initiated before therapy is used. The risk/benefit ratio should be weighed in patients who have resided in regions where histoplasmosis is endemic; infliximab has been associated with reactivation of hepatitis B in patients who are chronic carriers of this virus; patients who develop a new infection while receiving infliximab should be monitored closely; if a patient develops a serious infection while on treatment, infliximab therapy should be discontinued. Rare reactivation of hepatitis B virus (HBV) has occurred in chronic virus carriers; use with caution; evaluate prior to initiation and during treatment.

Hepatosplenic T-cell lymphoma has been reported in patients with Crohn's disease or ulcerative colitis treated with infliximab and concurrent or prior azathioprine or mercaptopurine use, usually reported in adolescent and young adult males **[U.S. Boxed Warning]**. Infliximab use has been associated with reports of leukopenia, neutropenia, thrombocytopenia, and pancytopenia (some fatal). Use with caution in patients with a history of significant hematologic abnormalities; discontinue therapy if significant hematologic abnormalities develop.

Infliximab administration has been associated with infusion-related hypersensitivity reactions which include urticaria, dyspnea, and/or hypotension that occurred during or within 2 hours of infusion; discontinue infliximab if severe reaction occurs; medications for treatment of hypersensitivity reactions must be readily available for use in case of a reaction. Pretreatment may be considered and may be warranted in all patients with prior infusion reactions. Serum sickness-like reactions have occurred; may be associated with a decreased response to treatment.

Rare cases of CNS demyelinating disorders, such as multiple sclerosis, optic neuritis, Guillain-Barre syndrome, and seizure disorders have been reported in patients undergoing infliximab therapy; consider discontinuing therapy in patients who develop significant CNS adverse reactions. Severe hepatic reactions (some fatal), including acute liver failure, hepatitis, and cholestasis have occurred between 2 weeks to more than a year after infliximab initiation. Severe hepatic reactions (including hepatitis, jaundice, acute hepatic failure, and cholestasis) have been reported during treatment; discontinue infliximab if jaundice and/or liver enzyme elevation (≥5 times the upper limit of normal) develops. Higher incidence of mortality and hospitalization for worsening heart failure have been reported in patients with CHF treated with infliximab, especially those patients treated at a higher dose of 10 mg/kg; do not initiate infliximab therapy in patients with moderate or severe CHF.

Precautions Use with caution in patients with a history of recurrent infections or illnesses which predispose the patient to infection. Positive antinuclear antibody titers have been detected in patients (with negative baselines). Rare cases of autoimmune disorder, including lupus-like syndrome, have been reported; monitor and discontinue if

◄ symptoms develop; if antibodies to double-stranded DNA are confirmed in a patient with lupus-like symptoms, infliximab should be discontinued. Patients should be brought up to date with all immunizations before initiating therapy. Live vaccines should not be given concurrently; there is no data available concerning secondary transmission of live vaccines in patients receiving therapy.

Adverse Reactions

Cardiovascular: Arrhythmia, bradycardia, cardiac arrest, chest pain, circulatory failure, edema, flushing, heart failure, hypertension, hypotension, MI, pericardial effusion, syncope, systemic vasculitis, tachycardia, thrombophlebitis (deep)

Central nervous system: Anxiety, chills, confusion, delirium, depression, dizziness, fatigue, fever, headache, multiple sclerosis, myelitis, seizures, somnolence, suicide attempt

Dermatologic: Abscess, angioedema, cellulitis, furunculosis, moniliasis, pruritus, rash, urticaria

Endocrine & metabolic: Dehydration, menstrual irregularity, weight decrease

Gastrointestinal: Abdominal pain, constipation, diarrhea, dyspepsia, GI hemorrhage, ileus, intestinal obstruction, intestinal perforation, intestinal stenosis, nausea, pancreatitis, peritonitis, stomatitis, vomiting

Genitourinary: Urinary tract infection

Hematologic: Agranulocytosis, anemia, hemolytic anemia, leukopenia, neutropenia, pancytopenia, thrombocytopenia

Hepatic: Acute liver failure, AST and ALT elevated, autoimmune hepatitis, biliary pain, cholecystitis, cholestatic jaundice, hepatitis, hepatitis B reactivation, hepatocellular damage, hepatosplenic T-cell lymphoma (HSTCL), jaundice

Neuromuscular & skeletal: Arthralgia, arthropathy, back pain, chronic osteomyelitis, myalgia, peripheral neuropathy, septic arthritis

Ophthalmologic: Endophthalmitis, optic neuritis

Renal: Renal calculus, renal failure

Respiratory: Adult respiratory distress syndrome, bronchitis, bronchospasm, cough, dyspnea, pleural effusion, pneumonia, pulmonary edema, pulmonary embolism, respiratory insufficiency, rhinitis, tuberculosis, upper respiratory tract infections

Miscellaneous: Allergic reaction; anaphylaxis; diaphoresis; hypersensitivity reactions; infection; laryngeal/pharyngeal edema; lupus-like syndrome; lymphadenopathy; lymphoma; malignancies; moniliasis; sepsis; serum sickness; serum-sickness-like reaction (antibodies to infliximab, dysphagia, fever, hand and facial edema, headache, loss of drug efficacy 3-12 days after reinstitution of infliximab following an extended period without treatment myalgias, polyarthralgias, rash, sore throat)

Drug Interactions

Avoid Concomitant Use

Avoid concomitant use of InFLIXimab with any of the following: Abatacept; Anakinra; BCG; Canakinumab; Certolizumab Pegol; Natalizumab; Pimecrolimus; Rilonacept; Tacrolimus (Topical); Vaccines (Live)

Increased Effect/Toxicity

InFLIXimab may increase the levels/effects of: Abatacept; Anakinra; Canakinumab; Certolizumab Pegol; Leflunomide; Natalizumab; Rilonacept; Vaccines (Live)

The levels/effects of InFLIXimab may be increased by: Abciximab; Denosumab; Pimecrolimus; Tacrolimus (Topical); Trastuzumab

Decreased Effect

InFLIXimab may decrease the levels/effects of: BCG; Sipuleucel-T; Vaccines (Inactivated); Vaccines (Live)

The levels/effects of InFLIXimab may be decreased by: Echinacea

Stability Store vial in refrigerator; do not freeze; infliximab solution should be used immediately after reconstitution since the vial contains no preservative; do not shake or agitate vigorously; do not use if discolored or cloudy; the reconstituted dose must be further diluted in NS and the infusion should begin within 3 hours of preparation

Mechanism of Action Chimeric monoclonal antibody which binds specifically to human tumor necrosis factor alpha (TNFα); inhibits binding of TNFα with its receptors

Pharmacodynamics

Onset:
  Crohn's disease: 1-2 weeks
  Rheumatoid arthritis: 3-7 days
Duration:
  Crohn's disease: 8-48 weeks
  Rheumatoid arthritis: 6-12 weeks

Pharmacokinetics (Adult data unless noted)

Distribution: Within the vascular compartment
  V_d: Adults: 3 L
Half-life, terminal: 8-9.5 days

Usual Dosage I.V. infusion: **Note:** Premedication with antihistamines (H_1-antagonist and/or H_2-antagonist), acetaminophen and/or corticosteroids may be considered to prevent and/or manage infusion-related reactions:

Children:
Crohn's disease: Initial: 5 mg/kg; repeat 5 mg/kg/dose at 2 and 6 weeks after the first infusion; maintenance: 5 mg/kg/dose every 8 weeks. **Note:** If the response is incomplete, dose has been increased up to 10 mg/kg (Stephens, 2003).

Juvenile idiopathic arthritis uncontrolled by conventional disease modifying drugs (in combination with methotrexate): Initial: 3 mg/kg; repeat 3 mg/kg/dose at 2 and 6 weeks after the first infusion, then 3-6 mg/kg/dose every 8 weeks thereafter (Ruperto, 2009). Alternatively, some studies used 6 mg/kg/dose starting at week 14 of methotrexate therapy; repeat 6 mg/kg/dose 2 and 6 weeks after the first infusion, then every 8 weeks thereafter (Ruperto, 2007).

Adults:
Crohn's disease or fistulizing disease: Initial: 5 mg/kg; repeat 5 mg/kg/dose at 2 and 6 weeks after the first infusion; maintenance: 5 mg/kg/dose every 8 weeks. If response is incomplete, may increase dose up to 10 mg/kg. Patients who do not respond by week 14 are unlikely to respond with continued infliximab dosing.

Rheumatoid arthritis (in combination with methotrexate): Initial: 3 mg/kg; repeat 3 mg/kg/dose at 2 and 6 weeks after the first infusion, then every 8 weeks thereafter. If the response is incomplete, may increase dose up to 10 mg/kg or treat as often as every 4 weeks.

Ankylosing spondylitis: Initial: 5 mg/kg; repeat 5 mg/kg/dose at 2 and 6 weeks after the first infusion, then every 6 weeks thereafter

Plaque psoriasis: 5 mg/kg at 0, 2, and 6 weeks, then every 8 weeks thereafter

Psoriatic arthritis: Initial: 5 mg/kg; repeat 5 mg/kg/dose at 2 and 6 weeks after the first infusion, then every 8 weeks thereafter

Ulcerative colitis: Initial: 5 mg/kg; repeat 5 mg/kg/dose at 2 and 6 weeks after the first infusion, then every 8 weeks thereafter

Administration Parenteral: Administer by I.V. infusion over 2-3 hours at a final concentration between 0.4-4 mg/mL in NS. A rate titration schedule may be used to prevent acute infusion reactions. For a total 250 mL volume to be infused, initiate at a rate of 10 mL/hour for first 15 minutes followed by 20 mL/hour for 15 minutes, 40 mL/hour for 15 minutes, 80 mL/hour for 15 minutes, 150 mL/hour for 30 minutes, and then 250 mL/hour until infusion is complete. Administer through an in-line, sterile, nonpyrogenic, low-protein-binding filter with pore size of

≤1.2 micrometers; do not infuse in the same I.V. line as other agents

Monitoring Parameters Urinalysis, blood chemistry, ESR, blood pressure, signs of infection, CBC; tuberculin skin test prior to initiation of therapy

Crohn's disease: C-reactive protein, frequency of stools, abdominal pain

Rheumatoid arthritis: C-reactive protein, rheumatoid factor, decrease in pain, swollen joints, stiffness

Patient Information Notify physician if persistent fever, bruising, cough, flu-like symptoms, severe fatigue, jaundice, abdominal pain, bleeding, pallor, shortness of breath, swelling of ankles or feet, vision change, weakness in arms and/or legs, numbness, or chest discomfort occurs.

Additional Information A retrospective study of 57 children receiving 361 infliximab infusions reported that the rate of infusion-related reactions in children was similar to that in adults (9.7% incidence shown). Female gender, immunosuppressive use for <4 months, and prior infusion reactions were risk factors for subsequent infusion reactions in children (see Crandall, 2003)

Dosage Forms Excipient information presented when available (limited, particularly for generics); consult specific product labeling.

Injection, powder for reconstitution [preservative free]:

Remicade®: 100 mg [contains sucrose 500 mg and polysorbate 80]

References

Crandall WV and Mackner LM, "Infusion Reactions to Infliximab in Children and Adolescents: Frequency, Outcome and a Predictive Model," *Aliment Pharmacol Ther*, 2003, 17(1):75-84.

Hyams JS, "Use of Infliximab in the Treatment of Crohn's Disease in Children and Adolescents," *J Pediatr Gastroenterol Nutr*, 2001, 33 (Suppl 1):S36-9.

Hyams JS, Markowitz J, and Wyllie R, "Use of Infliximab in the Treatment of Crohn's Disease in Children and Adolescents," *J Pediatr*, 2000, 137(2):192-6.

Ruperto N, Lovell DJ, Cuttica R, et al, "A Randomized, Placebo-Controlled Trial of Infliximab Plus Methotrexate for the Treatment of Polyarticular-Course Juvenile Rheumatoid Arthritis," *Arthritis Rheum*, 2007, 56(9):3096-106.

Ruperto N, Lovell DJ, Cuttica R, et al, "Long-Term Efficacy and Safety of Infliximab Plus Methotrexate for the Treatment of Polyarticular Course Juvenile Rheumatoid Arthritis: Findings From an Open-Label Treatment Extension," *Ann Rheum Dis*, 2009 [Epub ahead of print].

Serrano MS, Schmidt-Sommerfeld E, Kilbaugh TJ, et al, "Use of Infliximab in Pediatric Patients With Inflammatory Bowel Disease," *Ann Pharmacother*, 2001, 35(7-8):823-8.

Stephens MC, Shepanski MA, Mamula P, et al, "Safety and Steroid-Sparing Experience Using Infliximab for Crohn's Disease at a Pediatric Inflammatory Bowel Disease Center," *Am J Gastroenterol*, 2003, 98(1):104-11.

Wilkinson N, Jackson G, and Gardner-Medwin J, "Biologic Therapies for Juvenile Arthritis," *Arch Dis Child*, 2003, 88(3):186-91.

◆ **Influenza A (H1N1) 2009 Monovalent Vaccine** *see* Influenza Virus Vaccine (H1N1, Inactivated) *on page 731*

◆ **Influenza A (H1N1) 2009 Monovalent Vaccine** *see* Influenza Virus Vaccine (H1N1, Live/Attenuated) *on page 733*

Influenza Virus Vaccine (H1N1, Inactivated)

(in floo EN za VYE rus vak SEEN H1N1 in AK te VAT ed)

Medication Safety Issues

Sound-alike/look-alike issues:

Influenza virus vaccine may be confused with flumazenil

Influenza A (H1N1) 2009 vaccine may be confused with the avian strain (H5N1) of influenza virus vaccine or the seasonal influenza virus vaccine (human strain)

Canadian Brand Names Arepanrix™ H1N1

Therapeutic Category Vaccine, Inactivated Virus

Generic Available No

Use To provide active immunity to influenza disease caused by pandemic 2009 (H1N1) virus [previously referred to as novel swine-origin influenza A (H1N1) virus (S-OIV)] (FDA approved in ages >6 months and adults)

The Advisory Committee on Immunization Practices (ACIP) recommends initial vaccination for the following target groups as soon as vaccine is available:

• Pregnant women

• Persons who live with or care for infants <6 months of age

• Healthcare personnel (defined as persons working in healthcare settings who have the potential for exposure to patients with influenza or infectious materials)

• Children and young adults ages 6 months to 24 years

• Persons aged 25-64 years of age with medical conditions which put them at higher risk of complications from influenza infection and their close contacts. This includes chronic disorders of the pulmonary (including asthma) or cardiovascular systems (except hypertension), chronic metabolic diseases (including diabetes mellitus), hepatic disease, renal dysfunction, cognitive or neurologic/neuromuscular conditions, hematologic disorders, or immunosuppression (including immunosuppression caused by medications or HIV)

Pregnancy Risk Factor C

Pregnancy Considerations Animal reproduction studies have not been conducted; therefore, the manufacturer classifies influenza A (H1N1) 2009 vaccine as pregnancy category C. Pregnant women and women up to 2 weeks postpartum (including pregnancy loss) are at increased risk for influenza-related complications; therefore, the ACIP recommends vaccination of all pregnant women at any time during pregnancy. Pregnant women should observe the same precautions as nonpregnant persons to reduce the risk of exposure to influenza and other respiratory infections.

Lactation Excretion in breast milk unknown/use caution

Breast-Feeding Considerations It is not known if the vaccine is excreted into breast milk. The influenza A (H1N1) 2009 vaccine is made using the same processes as the seasonal influenza vaccine and breast-feeding has not been shown to decrease its immune response nor does the CDC consider breast-feeding a contraindication to vaccination. Vaccination with the influenza A (H1N1) 2009 vaccine is recommended for persons caring for infants and small children. The CDC recommends taking general precautions (eg, frequent hand washing) to decrease viral transmission to the child.

Contraindications Hypersensitivity to influenza virus vaccine or any component; allergy to eggs or egg products, chicken, chicken feathers, or chicken dander; presence of acute respiratory disease or other active infections or illnesses (delay immunization in a patient with an active neurological disorder); **Note:** Starting July 1, 2006, no vaccines containing greater than trace amounts of thimerosal may be administered to pregnant women or children <3 years of age in select states (check individual state statutes).

Warnings Severe allergic reactions including anaphylaxis may occur; immediate treatment for anaphylactic/anaphylactoid reaction should be available. Antigenic response may not be as great as expected in patients receiving immunosuppressive drugs. Inactivated influenza virus vaccine is preferred over live virus vaccine for household members, healthcare workers, and others coming in close contact with severely immunosuppressed persons requiring care in a protected environment.

◀

Precautions Use with caution in patients with history of febrile convulsions or Guillain-Barré syndrome (GBS) which has occurred within 6 weeks of receiving a prior influenza vaccine dose; patients with thrombocytopenia, any coagulation disorder, or receiving anticoagulants. Routine prophylactic administration of acetaminophen to prevent fever due to vaccines has been shown to decrease the immune response of some vaccines; the clinical significance of this reduction in immune response has not been established (see Prymula, 2009).

Administration of influenza A (H1N1) vaccine is not a substitute for seasonal influenza vaccine. Crossreactivity with seasonal influenza virus vaccine has not been observed. In order to maximize vaccination rates, the ACIP recommends simultaneous administration of all age-appropriate vaccines (live or inactivated) for which a person is eligible at a single clinic visit, unless contra-indications exist. Some products are manufactured using arginine, chicken egg protein, gelatin, gentamicin, neo-mycin, polymyxin, and/or thimerosal

Adverse Reactions All serious adverse reactions must be reported to the U.S. Department of Health and Human Services (DHHS) Vaccine Adverse Event Reporting System (VAERS) 1-800-822-7967 or online at https://secure.vaers.org. Note: The influenza A (H1N1) 2009 vaccine is manufactured by the same processes used for the seasonal influenza vaccine and similar adverse events may be expected. Refer to the Influenza Virus Vaccine (Inactivated) monograph for additional information.

The following data is presented from a preliminary study following 1 dose of a hemagglutinin antigen (HA) 15 mcg or HA 30 mcg product produced by CSL (n=240) (Greenberg, 2009):

Central nervous system: Chills, fever, headache, malaise

Gastrointestinal: Nausea

Local: Injection site reactions: Bruising, induration, pain, redness, tenderness

Neuromuscular & skeletal: Myalgia

<1%: Flu-like syndrome, vomiting

Drug Interactions

Avoid Concomitant Use There are no known inter-actions where it is recommended to avoid concomitant use.

Increased Effect/Toxicity There are no known signifi-cant interactions involving an increase in effect.

Decreased Effect

The levels/effects of Influenza Virus Vaccine (H1N1, Inactivated) may be decreased by: Immunosuppressants

Stability Store under refrigeration 2°C to 8°C (36°F to 46°F); do not freeze. Protect from light.

CSL and GSK product: Multidose vial: Store in refrigerator between uses. Discard within 28 days after piercing rubber stopper.

Novartis product, Sanofi Pasteur product: Multidose vial: Store in refrigerator between uses.

Mechanism of Action Promotes immunity to influenza H1N1 virus by inducing specific antibody production.

Pharmacokinetics (Adult data unless noted)

Onset: Protective antibody titers (1:40) were observed in 96.7% of healthy adults 21 days after vaccination following a single dose (preliminary data; Greenberg, 2009).

Usual Dosage Immunization: **Note:** Clinical studies are ongoing to determine the optimal dose and schedule of the influenza A (H1N1) 2009 vaccine.

CSL product and Sanofi Pasteur product: I.M.:

Children 6-35 months: 0.25 mL/dose; administer 2 doses, ~1 month apart

Children 36 months to 9 years: 0.5 mL/dose; administer 2 doses, ~1 month apart

Children ≥10 years and Adults: 0.5 mL as a single dose

Novartis product: I.M.:

Children 4-9 years: 0.5 mL/dose; administer 2 doses, ~1 month apart

Children 10-17 years and Adults: 0.5 mL as a single dose

GSK product: I.M.: Adults: 0.5 mL as a single dose

Elderly: Refer to adult dosing. **Note:** Intranasal: Not approved for use in individuals ≥50 years.

Administration I.M.: For I.M. administration only. Shake suspension well prior to use.

Infants: I.M. injection in the anterolateral aspect of the thigh

Children and Adults: I.M. injection in the deltoid muscle

Patients at risk of bleeding (eg, patient receiving antihemophilic factor): Schedule vaccination shortly after factor is administered. Use a fine needle (23-gauge or smaller) for vaccination and apply firm pressure to the site (without rubbing) for at least 2 minutes.

Monitoring Parameters Monitor for syncope for ≥15 minutes following vaccination.

Patient Information Notify physician if you experience a high fever, seizures, or allergic reaction (difficulty breath-ing, hives, weakness, dizziness, fast heart beat). Inacti-vated influenza virus vaccine is safe to administer to mothers who are breast-feeding.

Nursing Implications Federal law requires that the date of administration, the vaccine manufacturer, lot number of vaccine, and the administering person's name, title, and address be entered into the patient's permanent medical record.

Additional Information

When vaccine supply is limited: The ACIP recommends initial vaccination for the following target groups:

• Pregnant women

• Persons who live with or care for infants <6 months of age

• Healthcare personnel who have the potential for exposure to patients with influenza or infectious materials

• Children 6 months to 4 years of age

• Children and adolescents 5-18 years of age with medical conditions which put them at higher risk of complications from influenza infection

When vaccine supply is not limited: The ACIP recommends that decisions to expand vaccination out-side of the initial target population (refer to Use) should be made based on local availability and demand and should initially be expanded to include persons 25-64 years of age followed by vaccination of persons ≥65 years.

The influenza A (H1N1) vaccine approved in September 2009 contains an A/California/7/09-like virus, which is a subtype separate from that in the 2009 seasonal influenza vaccine. It will not protect against seasonal influenza and the seasonal influenza vaccine will not offer protection from the pandemic (H1N1) 2009 virus.

In order to maximize vaccination rates, the ACIP recommends simultaneous administration of all age-appropriate vaccines (live or inactivated) for which a person is eligible at a single visit, unless contraindications exist. The use of combination vaccines is generally preferred over separate infections, taking into consider-ation provider assessment, patient preference, and potential adverse events.

For additional information, please refer to the following website: http://www.cdc.gov/vaccines/vpd-vac/.

Dosage Forms Excipient information presented when available (limited, particularly for generics); consult specific product labeling. [CAN] = Canadian product

Injection, emulsion [inactivated]:

Arepanrix™ H1N1 [CAN]: Influenza A/California/7/2009 (H1N1) v-like strain HA 3.75 mcg/0.5 mL (5 mL) [contains chicken egg protein, sucrose (trace amounts), and thimerosal; AS03 adjuvant contains tocopherol, squalene and polysorbate 80] [not available in U.S.]

Injection, suspension [inactivated; preservative free]:

CSL product: Influenza A/California/7/2009 (H1N1) v-like virus HA 15 mcg/0.5 mL (0.25 mL, 0.5 mL) [contains chicken egg protein, neomycin, polymyxin B]

Novartis product: Influenza A/California/7/2009 (H1N1) v-like virus HA 15 mcg/0.5 mL (0.5 mL) [contains chicken egg protein, neomycin, polymyxin B, thimerosal (trace amounts)]

Sanofi Pasteur product: Influenza A/California/7/2009 (H1N1) v-like virus HA 15 mcg/0.5 mL (0.25 mL, 0.5 mL) [contains gelatin, sucrose ≤2%/0.5 mL]

Injection, suspension [inactivated]:

CSL product: Influenza A/California/7/2009 (H1N1) v-like virus HA 15 mcg/0.5 mL (5 mL) [contains chicken egg protein, neomycin, polymyxin B, thimerosal]

GSK product: Influenza A/California/7/2009 (H1N1) v-like virus HA 15 mcg/0.5 mL (10 mL) [contains chicken egg protein, thimerosal]

Novartis product: Influenza A/California/7/2009 (H1N1) v-like virus HA 15 mcg/0.5 mL (5 mL) [contains chicken egg protein, neomycin, polymyxin B, thimerosal]

Sanofi Pasteur product: Influenza A/California/7/2009 (H1N1) v-like virus HA 15 mcg/0.5 mL (5 mL) [contains gelatin, sucrose ≤2%/0.5 mL, thimerosal]

References

Centers for Disease Control and Prevention (CDC), "General Recommendations on Immunization. Recommendations of the Advisory Committee on Immunization Practices (ACIP)," *MMWR Recomm Rep*, 2006, 55(RR-15):1-48. Available at: http://www.cdc.gov/mmwr/preview/mmwrhtml/rr5515a1.htm.

Centers for Disease Control and Prevention (CDC), "Syncope After Vaccination – United States, January 2005-July 2007," *MMWR Morb Mortal Wkly Rep*, 2008, 57(17):457-60. Available at http://www.cdc.gov/mmwr/preview/mmwrhtml/mm5717a2.htm

Centers for Disease Control and Prevention, "Use of Influenza A (H1N1) 2009 Monovalent Vaccine," *MMWR Morb Mortal Wkly Rep*, 2009, 58(RR-10):1-8. Available at http://www.cdc.gov/mmwr/PDF/rr/rr5810.pdf

Greenberg ME, Lai MH, Hartel GF, et al, "Response After One Dose of a Monovalent Influenza A (H1N1) 2009 Vaccine – Preliminary Report," *N Engl J Med*, 2009. Available at: http://content.nejm.org/cgi/content/abstract/NEJMoa0907413v1

Novel Swine-Origin Influenza A (H1N1) Virus Investigation Team, Dawood FS, Jain S, Finelli L, et al, "Emergence of a Novel Swine-Origin Influenza A (H1N1) Virus in Humans," *N Engl J Med*, 2009, 360 (25):2605-15.

Prymula R, Siegrist CA, Chlibek R, et al, "Effect of Prophylactic Paracetamol Administration at Time of Vaccination on Febrile Reactions and Antibody Responses in Children: Two Open-Label, Randomised Controlled Trials," *Lancet*, 2009, 374(9698):1339-50.

Influenza Virus Vaccine (H1N1, Live/Attenuated) (in floo EN za VYE rus vak SEEN H1N1)

Medication Safety Issues

Sound-alike/look-alike issues:

Influenza virus vaccine may be confused with flumazenil

Influenza A (H1N1) 2009 vaccine may be confused with the avian strain (H5N1) of influenza virus vaccine or the seasonal influenza virus vaccine (human strain)

Therapeutic Category Vaccine, Live Virus; Vaccine, Live/Attenuated

Generic Available No

Use To provide active immunity against influenza disease caused by pandemic 2009 (H1N1) virus [previously referred to as novel swine-origin influenza A (H1N1) virus (S-OIV)] (FDA approved in ages 2-49 years)

Pregnancy Risk Factor C

Pregnancy Considerations Animal reproduction studies have not been conducted; therefore, the manufacturer classifies influenza A (H1N1) 2009 vaccine as pregnancy category C. Pregnant women and women up to 2 weeks postpartum (including pregnancy loss) are at increased risk for influenza related complications and should be vaccinated, however the nasal formulation of the influenza A (H1N1) 2009 vaccine should not be used in pregnant women. Pregnant women should observe the same precautions as nonpregnant persons to reduce the risk of exposure to influenza and other respiratory infections.

Lactation Excretion in breast milk unknown/use caution

Breast-Feeding Considerations It is not known if the vaccine is excreted into breast milk. The influenza A (H1N1) 2009 vaccine is made using the same processes as the seasonal influenza vaccine and breast-feeding has not been shown to decrease its immune response nor does the CDC consider breast-feeding a contraindication to vaccination. Vaccination with the influenza A (H1N1) 2009 vaccine is recommended for persons caring for infants and small children. The use of the nasal spray (live virus vaccine) should be used with caution in breast-feeding women (per manufacturer) due to the possibility of viral shedding from mother to infant; however, the CDC states that breast-feeding women may receive the nasal spray (live virus vaccine) after delivery. The CDC recommends taking general precautions (eg, frequent hand washing) to decrease viral transmission to the child.

Contraindications Hypersensitivity to influenza virus vaccine, egg or egg products, gentamicin, gelatin, arginine, or any component; children or adolescents receiving aspirin or aspirin-containing therapy due to the association of Reye syndrome with aspirin and wild-type influenza infection

Warnings Children <2 years of age who received the live, attenuated influenza virus vaccine intranasally had an increased risk of hospitalization and wheezing that was observed in clinical trials. Because safety and efficacy information is limited, the ACIP does not recommend the use of LAIV in patients with asthma or active wheezing or to children <5 years of age who have had wheezing in the past year; patients with chronic disorders of the cardiovascular and pulmonary systems; patients with cognitive or neurologic/neuromuscular disorders; pregnant women; patients requiring follow-up or hospitalization due to chronic metabolic diseases, such as diabetes, renal dysfunction, hepatic dysfunction, immunosuppression (including immunosuppression caused by medications or HIV), or hemoglobinopathies, such as sickle cell disease); residents of nursing homes and other chronic-care facilities; and to family members or close contacts of immunosuppressed persons requiring a protected environment (eg, hematopoietic stem cell transplant recipient).

Epinephrine injection must be readily available in the event of an acute anaphylactic reaction following vaccination.

Precautions Individuals receiving live, attenuated influenza virus vaccine intranasally should avoid close contact with immunocompromised individuals for at least 7 days. Avoid administering intranasal influenza virus vaccine during an acute phase of febrile and/or respiratory illness (postpone at least 72 hours until after the acute phase). If nasal congestion that might decrease delivery of the vaccine to the nasopharyngeal mucosa is present, postpone administration until illness resolves.

Use with caution in patients with history of Guillain-Barré syndrome (GBS); carefully consider risks and benefits to vaccination in patients known to have experienced GBS within 6 weeks following any previous influenza vaccination. Routine prophylactic administration of acetaminophen to prevent fever due to vaccines has been shown to decrease the immune response of some vaccines; the clinical significance of this reduction in immune response has not been established (see Prymula, 2009).

Administration of influenza A (H1N1) vaccine is not a substitute for seasonal influenza vaccine. Simultaneous administration of inactivated vaccines against seasonal and novel influenza A (H1N1) viruses is permissible if different anatomic sites are used; however, simultaneous administration of live, attenuated vaccines against seasonal and novel influenza A (H1N1) virus is not recommended.

Adverse Reactions All serious adverse reactions must be reported to the U.S. Department of Health and Human Services (DHHS) Vaccine Adverse Event Reporting System (VAERS) 1-800-822-7967 or online at https://secure.vaers.org. Note: The influenza A (H1N1) 2009 vaccine is manufactured by the same processes used for the seasonal influenza vaccine and similar adverse events may be expected. Refer to the Influenza Virus Vaccine (Inactivated) monograph for additional information.

Drug Interactions

Avoid Concomitant Use

Avoid concomitant use of Influenza Virus Vaccine (H1N1, Live/Attenuated) with any of the following: Immuno-suppressants

Increased Effect/Toxicity

The levels/effects of Influenza Virus Vaccine (H1N1, Live/Attenuated) may be increased by: Immunosuppressants

Decreased Effect

Influenza Virus Vaccine (H1N1, Live/Attenuated) may decrease the levels/effects of: Tuberculin Tests

The levels/effects of Influenza Virus Vaccine (H1N1, Live/Attenuated) may be decreased by: Antiviral Agents (Influenza A and B); Immune Globulins; Immunosuppressants; Influenza Virus Vaccine (Live/Attenuated)

Stability Refrigerate upon receipt and until use at 2°C to 8°C (35°F to 46°F); do not freeze.

Mechanism of Action Promotes immunity to influenza H1N1 virus by inducing specific antibody production.

Pharmacodynamics

Onset of action: Protective antibody levels achieved ~2 weeks after vaccination

Duration: Protective antibody levels persist approximately ≥6 months

Usual Dosage Immunization: **Note:** Clinical studies are ongoing to determine the optimal dose and schedule of the influenza A (H1N1) 2009 vaccine. Intranasal:

Children 2-9 years: 0.2 mL/dose; administer 2 doses, ~1 month apart

Children ≥10 years and Adults ≤49 years: 0.2 mL/dose as a single dose

Administration Intranasal: Administer 0.1 mL (half of the dose from a single sprayer) into each nostril while the recipient is in an upright position. Insert the tip of the sprayer just inside the nostril and depress the plunger to spray. Remove dose-divider clip from the sprayer to administer the second half of the dose into the other nostril. Do not administer by the I.M., SubQ, intradermal, or I.V. route.

Monitoring Parameters Monitor for syncope for ≥15 minutes following vaccination.

Patient Information If the patient sneezes after intranasal vaccine administration, the dose should not be repeated. Patients with an acute febrile illness should not receive the vaccine until symptoms improve. Report any suspected adverse effects to your physician.

Nursing Implications The used sprayer should be disposed of according to the standard procedures for biohazardous waste products. CDC has stated that the inactivated influenza virus vaccine injection is preferred over the live, intranasal influenza vaccine for physicians, nurses, family members, or individuals who will come in close contact with anyone with a severely weakened immune system (eg, people with hematopoietic stem cell transplants in a protective environment).

Federal law requires that the date of administration, the vaccine manufacturer, lot number of vaccine, and the administering person's name, title, and address be entered into the patient's permanent medical record.

Additional Information The influenza A (H1N1) vaccine approved in September 2009 contains an A/California/7/09-like virus, which is a subtype separate from that in the 2009 seasonal influenza vaccine. It will not protect against seasonal influenza and the seasonal influenza vaccine will not offer protection from the pandemic (H1N1) 2009 virus.

In order to maximize vaccination rates, the ACIP recommends simultaneous administration of all age-appropriate vaccines (live or inactivated) for which a person is eligible at a single visit, unless contraindications exist. The use of combination vaccines is generally preferred over separate infections, taking into consideration provider assessment, patient preference, and potential adverse events.

For additional information, please refer to the following website: http://www.cdc.gov/vaccines/vpd-vac/.

Dosage Forms Excipient information presented when available (limited, particularly for generics); consult specific product labeling.

Suspension, intranasal [live; preservative free; spray]:

MedImmune product: Influenza A/California/7/2009 (H1N1) v-like virus FFU 106.5-7.5 /0.2 mL (0.2 mL) [contains arginine, chicken egg protein, gelatin, and gentamicin]

References

Centers for Disease Control and Prevention (CDC), "General Recommendations on Immunization. Recommendations of the Advisory Committee on Immunization Practices (ACIP)," *MMWR Recomm Rep*, 2006, 55(RR-15):1-48. Available at: http://www.cdc.gov/mmwr/preview/mmwrhtml/rr5515a1.htm.

Centers for Disease Control and Prevention, "Use of Influenza A (H1N1) 2009 Monovalent Vaccine," *MMWR Morb Mortal Wkly Rep*, 2009, 58(RR-10):1-8. Available at http://www.cdc.gov/mmwr/PDF/rr/rr5810.pdf

Novel Swine-Origin Influenza A (H1N1) Virus Investigation Team, Dawood FS, Jain S, Finelli L, et al, "Emergence of a Novel Swine-Origin Influenza A (H1N1) Virus in Humans," *N Engl J Med*, 2009, 360 (25):2605-15.

Prymula R, Siegrist CA, Chlibek R, et al, "Effect of Prophylactic Paracetamol Administration at Time of Vaccination on Febrile Reactions and Antibody Responses in Children: Two Open-Label, Randomised Controlled Trials," *Lancet*, 2009, 374(9698):1339-50.

Influenza Virus Vaccine (Inactivated)

(in floo EN za VYE rus vak SEEN in AK te VAT ed)

Medication Safety Issues

Sound-alike/look-alike issues:

Fluarix® may be confused with Flarex®

Influenza virus vaccine may be confused with flumazenil

Influenza virus vaccine may be confused with tetanus toxoid and tuberculin products. Medication errors have occurred when tuberculin skin tests (PPD) have been inadvertently administered instead of tetanus toxoid products and influenza virus vaccine. These products are refrigerated and often stored in close proximity to each other.

Influenza virus vaccine (human strain) may be confused with the avian strain (H5N1) of influenza virus vaccine or the influenza A (H1N1) 2009 vaccine

U.S. Brand Names Afluria®; Agriflu®; Fluarix®; Flu-Laval®; Fluvirin®; Fluzone®

Canadian Brand Names Fluviral S/F®; Vaxigrip®

Therapeutic Category Vaccine; Vaccine, Inactivated Virus

Generic Available No

Use Provide active immunity to influenza A and B virus strains contained in the vaccine (Fluzone®, Afluria®: FDA approved in ages ≥6 months and adults; Fluvirin®: FDA approved in ages ≥4 years and adults; Agriflu®, FluLaval®, Fluarix®: FDA approved in ages ≥18 years)

Recommendations for annual seasonal influenza vaccination:
Persons at high risk for influenza-related complications and severe disease:
- All children 6-59 months of age
- Persons ≥50 years of age
- Residents of nursing homes and other chronic-care facilities that house persons of any age with chronic medical conditions
- Adults and children with chronic disorders of the pulmonary or cardiovascular systems, including children with asthma, bronchopulmonary dysplasia, cystic fibrosis, and congenital heart disease
- Adults and children who have required regular medical follow-up or hospitalization during the preceding year because of chronic metabolic diseases (including diabetes mellitus), renal dysfunction, sickle cell disease and other hemoglobinopathies, human immunodeficiency virus (HIV) infection, or immunosuppression (including immunosuppression caused by medications)
- Children and adolescents (6 months to 18 years of age) who are receiving long-term aspirin therapy and therefore, may be at risk for developing Reye's syndrome after influenza
- Women who will be pregnant during influenza season
- Adults and children with cognitive or neurologic/neuromuscular conditions including conditions such as spinal cord injuries or seizure disorders which may compromise respiratory function, the handling of respiratory secretions, or that can increase the risk of aspiration
- Persons who live with or care for persons at high risk for influenza-related complications
- Healthy household contacts and caregivers of children aged 0-59 months and persons at high risk for severe complications from influenza
- Healthcare workers

Pregnancy Risk Factor B/C (manufacturer specific)

Pregnancy Considerations Reproduction studies have not been conducted with all products; when conducted, adverse events were not observed in animal studies. Case reports and limited studies suggest pregnancy may increase the risk of serious medical complications from influenza infection. Vaccination is recommended regardless of stage of pregnancy. Vaccination with the injection during the third trimester of pregnancy has been shown to decrease the incidence of laboratory confirmed influenza and respiratory illness with fever in infants ≤6 months.

Lactation Excretion in breast milk unknown/use caution

Breast-Feeding Considerations Use of influenza vaccine has not been shown to affect the safety of breast-feeding mothers or their infants. The ACIP recommends use of either TIV or LAIV in breast-feeding women unless contraindicated due to other medical conditions.

Contraindications Hypersensitivity to influenza virus vaccine or any component; allergy to eggs or egg products, chicken, chicken feathers, or chicken dander

Warnings Severe allergic reactions including anaphylaxis may occur; immediate treatment for anaphylactic/anaphylactoid reaction should be available. Antigenic response may not be as great as expected in patients receiving immunosuppressive drugs. Inactivated influenza virus vaccine is preferred over live virus vaccine for household members, healthcare workers, and others coming in close contact with severely immunosuppressed persons requiring care in a protected environment. Influenza vaccines from previous seasons must not be used.

Precautions Use with caution in patients with history of febrile convulsions or Guillain-Barré syndrome (GBS) which has occurred within 6 weeks of receiving a prior influenza vaccine dose; patients with thrombocytopenia, any coagulation disorder, or receiving anticoagulants. ACIP recommends that persons with moderate to severe acute febrile illnesses should delay vaccination until symptoms have resolved. Products may contain gentamicin, kanamycin, neomycin, polymyxin, or polysorbate 80. Packaging may contain natural latex rubber; use caution in patients with known sensitivity. Routine prophylactic administration of acetaminophen to prevent fever due to vaccines has been shown to decrease the immune response of some vaccines; the clinical significance of this reduction in immune response has not been established (see Prymula, 2009).

Adverse Reactions All serious adverse reactions must be reported to the U.S. Department of Health and Human Services (DHHS) Vaccine Adverse Event Reporting System (VAERS) 1-800-822-7967.
Cardiovascular: Chest tightness, facial edema, migraine
Central nervous system: Chills, fatigue, fever, headache, malaise, shivering
Gastrointestinal: Diarrhea, nausea, sore throat, vomiting
Local: Injection site reactions including: Bruising, erythema, induration, inflammation, pain, soreness (10% to 64%; may last up to 2 days), swelling
Neuromuscular & skeletal: Arthralgia, back pain, myalgia (may start within 6-12 hours and last 1-2 days; incidence equal to placebo in adults; occurs more frequently than placebo in children)
Ocular: Red eyes
Respiratory: Cough, nasal congestion, nasopharyngitis, rhinitis, upper respiratory track infection, wheezing
Miscellaneous: Diaphoresis
<1% and/or postmarketing: Abdominal pain, allergic reactions, anaphylaxis, angioedema, autoimmune hemolytic anemia, bronchospasm, chest pain, conjunctivitis, convulsions, dizziness, dyspnea, erythema muliforme, eye pain, eye/eyelid swelling, facial palsy (Bell's palsy), flushing, Guillain-Barre syndrome (GBS), Henoch-Schonlein purpura, hypersensitivity reaction, hypoesthesia, lymphadenopathy, myasthenia, myelitis (including encephalomyelitis and transverse myelitis), neuralgia, oculorespiratory syndrome (ORS; acute, self-limited reaction with ocular and respiratory symptoms), optic neuritis/neuropathy, pain, paresthesia, pharyngitis, photophobia, pruritus, rash, serum sickness, Stevens-Johnson syndrome, syncope, tachycardia, thrombocytopenia, urticaria, vasculitis, vertigo, weakness

Drug Interactions

Avoid Concomitant Use There are no known interactions where it is recommended to avoid concomitant use.

Increased Effect/Toxicity There are no known significant interactions involving an increase in effect.

Decreased Effect
The levels/effects of Influenza Virus Vaccine (Inactivated) may be decreased by: Immunosuppressants

Stability Store between 2°C to 8°C (36°F to 46°F). Potency is destroyed by freezing; do not use if product has been frozen.
Afluria®, Agriflu®, Fluarix®: Protect from light.
Afluria®, FluLaval®: Discard 28 days after initial entry. Protect from light.

Fluzone®: Between uses, the multiple dose vial should be stored at 2°C to 8°C (36°F to 46°F).

Mechanism of Action Promotes immunity to influenza virus by inducing specific antibody production

Pharmacodynamics
Onset of action: Protective antibody levels achieved ~3 weeks after vaccination
Duration: Protective antibody levels persist approximately ≥6 months

Usual Dosage I.M.: It is important to note that influenza seasons vary in their timing and duration from year to year. In general, vaccination should begin soon after the vaccine becomes available and if possible, prior to October. However, vaccination should continue throughout the influenza season as long as vaccine is available.
Afluria®, Fluzone®:
Children 6-35 months: 0.25 mL (1 or 2 doses; see **Note**)
Children 3-8 years: 0.5 mL (1 or 2 doses; see **Note**)
Children ≥9 years and Adults: 0.5 mL (1 dose)
Fluarix®:
Children 3-8 years: 0.5 mL/dose (1 or 2 doses per season; see **Note**)
Children ≥9 years and Adults: 0.5 mL/dose (1 dose per season)
Fluvirin®:
Children 4-8 years: 0.5 mL (1 or 2 doses; see **Note**)
Children ≥9 years and Adults: 0.5 mL (1 dose)
Agriflu®, FluLaval®: Adults ≥18 years: 0.5 mL (1 dose)
Note: Previously unvaccinated children 6 months to <9 years of age should receive 2 doses, given >1 month apart in order to achieve a satisfactory antibody response. Second dose should preferably be administered before the onset of influenza season.

Administration I.M.: For I.M. administration only. Shake suspension well prior to use.
Infants: I.M. injection in the anterolateral aspect of the thigh
Children and Adults: I.M. injection in the deltoid muscle
Patients at risk of bleeding (eg, patient receiving antihemophilic factor): Schedule vaccination shortly after factor is administered. Use a fine needle (23 gauge or smaller) for vaccination and apply firm pressure to the site (without rubbing) for at least 2 minutes.
If a pediatric vaccine (0.25 mL) is inadvertently administered to an adult an additional 0.25 mL should be administered to provide the full adult dose (0.5 mL). If the error is discovered after the patient has left, an adult dose should be given as soon as the patient can return. If an adult vaccine (0.5 mL) is inadvertently given to a child, no action needs to be taken.

Patient Information Notify physician if you experience a high fever, seizures, or allergic reaction (difficulty breathing, hives, weakness, dizziness, fast heart beat). Inactivated influenza virus vaccine is safe to administer to mothers who are breast-feeding.

Nursing Implications Federal law requires that the date of administration, the vaccine manufacturer, lot number of vaccine, and the administering person's name, title, and address be entered into the patient's permanent medical record.

Additional Information Influenza is highly contagious. Incubation period is 1-3 days. Patients are most contagious during the 24 hours before the onset of symptoms and during their most symptomatic period.
Note: Starting July 1, 2006, no vaccines containing greater than trace amounts of thimerosal may be administered to pregnant women or children <3 years of age in select states (check individual state statutes).

In order to maximize vaccination rates, the ACIP recommends simultaneous administration of all age-appropriate vaccines (live or inactivated) for which a person is eligible at a single visit, unless contraindications exist. The use of combination vaccines is generally preferred over separate infections, taking into consideration provider assessment, patient preference, and potential adverse events.

For additional information, please refer to the following website: http://www.cdc.gov/vaccines/vpd-vac/.

Dosage Forms Excipient information presented when available (limited, particularly for generics); consult specific product labeling.
Injection, suspension [purified split-virus]:
Afluria®: 5 mL [TIV; contains chicken egg protein, thimerosal, neomycin (trace amounts), and polymyxin (trace amounts)]
FluLaval®: 5 mL [TIV; contains chicken egg protein and thimerosal]
Fluvirin®: 5 mL [TIV; contains chicken egg protein, thimerosal, neomycin (trace amounts), and polymyxin (trace amounts)]
Fluzone®: 5 mL [TIV; contains chicken egg protein and thimerosal]
Injection, suspension [purified split-virus; preservative free]:
Afluria®: 0.25 mL, 0.5 mL [TIV; contains chicken egg protein, neomycin (trace amounts), and polymyxin (trace amounts)]
Agriflu®: 0.5 mL [TIV; contains chicken egg protein, kanamycin (trace amounts), neomycin (trace amounts), polysorbate 80]
Fluarix®: 0.5 mL [TIV; contains chicken egg protein, gentamicin (trace amounts), polysorbate 80]
Fluvirin®: 0.5 mL [TIV; contains chicken egg protein, thimerosal (trace amounts), neomycin (trace amounts), and polymyxin (trace amounts)]
Fluzone®: 0.25 mL, 0.5 mL [TIV; contains chicken egg protein]

References
Centers for Disease Control and Prevention (CDC), "General Recommendations on Immunization. Recommendations of the Advisory Committee on Immunization Practices (ACIP)," *MMWR Recomm Rep*, 2006, 55(RR-15):1-48. Available at: http://www.cdc.gov/mmwr/preview/mmwrhtml/rr5515a1.htm.
Centers for Disease Control and Prevention, "Prevention and Control of Seasonal Influenza with Vaccines," *MMWR* Early Releas, July 24, 2009; Available at http://www.cdc.gov/mmwr/pdf/rr/rr58e0724.pdf.
Prymula R, Siegrist CA, Chlibek R, et al, "Effect of Prophylactic Paracetamol Administration at Time of Vaccination on Febrile Reactions and Antibody Responses in Children: Two Open-Label, Randomised Controlled Trials," *Lancet*, 2009, 374(9698):1339-50.

Influenza Virus Vaccine (Live/Attenuated) (in floo EN za VYE rus vak SEEN)

Medication Safety Issues
Sound-alike/look-alike issues:
Influenza virus vaccine may be confused with flumazenil
Influenza virus vaccine (human strain) may be confused with the avian strain (H5N1) of influenza virus vaccine or the influenza A (H1N1) 2009 vaccine

U.S. Brand Names FluMist®
Therapeutic Category Vaccine; Vaccine, Live/Attenuated
Generic Available No
Use Active immunization for the prevention of seasonal influenza A and B virus strains in healthy individuals (FDA approved in ages 2-49 years)
Pregnancy Risk Factor C
Pregnancy Considerations Reproduction studies have not been conducted. Case reports and limited studies suggest pregnancy may increase the risk of serious medical complications from influenza infection. The safety and efficacy of the nasal spray have not been studied in pregnant pregnant women; however, pregnant women do not need to avoid contact with persons recently vaccinated with LAIV.
Lactation Excretion in breast milk unknown/use caution

Breast-Feeding Considerations Use of influenza vaccine has not been shown to affect the safety of breast-feeding mothers or their infants. The use of the nasal spray (live virus vaccine) should be used with caution (per manufacturer) due to the possibility of viral shedding from mother to infant. The ACIP recommends use of either TIV or LAIV in breast-feeding women unless contraindicated due to other medical conditions.

Contraindications Hypersensitivity to influenza virus vaccine, egg or egg products, gentamicin, gelatin, arginine, or any component; children or adolescents receiving aspirin or aspirin-containing therapy due to the association of Reye syndrome with aspirin and wild-type influenza infection

Warnings Children <2 years of age who received the live, attenuated influenza virus vaccine intranasally had an increased risk of hospitalization and wheezing that was observed in clinical trials. Because safety and efficacy information is limited, the ACIP does not recommend the use of LAIV in patients with asthma or active wheezing or to children <5 years of age who have had wheezing in the past year; patients with chronic disorders of the cardiovascular and pulmonary systems; patients with cognitive or neurologic/neuromuscular disorders; pregnant women; patients requiring follow-up or hospitalization due to chronic metabolic diseases, such as diabetes, renal dysfunction, hepatic dysfunction, immunosuppression (including immunosuppression caused by medications or HIV), or hemoglobinopathies, such as sickle cell disease); residents of nursing homes and other chronic-care facilities; and to family members or close contacts of immunosuppressed persons requiring a protected environment (eg, hematopoietic stem cell transplant recipient.

Epinephrine injection must be readily available in the event of an acute anaphylactic reaction following vaccination.

Precautions Individuals receiving live, attenuated influenza virus vaccine intranasally should avoid close contact with immunocompromised individuals for at least 7 days. Avoid administering intranasal influenza virus vaccine during an acute phase of febrile and/or respiratory illness (postpone at least 72 hours until after the acute phase). If nasal congestion is present that might decrease delivery of the vaccine to the nasopharyngeal mucosa, postpone administration until illness resolves.

Use with caution in patients with history of Guillain-Barré syndrome (GBS); carefully consider risks and benefits to vaccination in patients known to have experienced GBS within 6 weeks following any previous influenza vaccination. Routine prophylactic administration of acetaminophen to prevent fever due to vaccines has been shown to decrease the immune response of some vaccines; the clinical significance of this reduction in immune response has not been established (see Prymula, 2009).

Simultaneous administration of inactivated vaccines against seasonal and novel influenza A (H1N1) viruses is permissible if different anatomic sites are used; however, simultaneous administration of live, attenuated vaccines against seasonal and novel influenza A (H1N1) virus is not recommended.

Adverse Reactions

Central nervous system: Chills, fever, headache, irritability, lethargy

Dermatologic: Urticaria

Gastrointestinal: Abdominal pain, anorexia, diarrhea, nausea, vomiting

Neuromuscular & skeletal: Myalgia, weakness

Otic: Otitis media

Respiratory: Cough, nasal congestion, runny nose, sinusitis, sneezing, sore throat, wheezing

Miscellaneous: Anaphylaxis, Guillain-Barré syndrome

<1% and/or postmarketing: Bell's palsy, epistaxis, exacerbation of mitochondrial encephalomyopathy, rash, syncope

Drug Interactions

Avoid Concomitant Use

Avoid concomitant use of Influenza Virus Vaccine (Live/Attenuated) with any of the following: Immunosuppressants

Increased Effect/Toxicity

The levels/effects of Influenza Virus Vaccine (Live/Attenuated) may be increased by: Immunosuppressants

Decreased Effect

Influenza Virus Vaccine (Live/Attenuated) may decrease the levels/effects of: Influenza Virus Vaccine (H1N1, Live/Attenuated); Tuberculin Tests

The levels/effects of Influenza Virus Vaccine (Live/Attenuated) may be decreased by: Antiviral Agents (Influenza A and B); Immune Globulins; Immunosuppressants

Stability Refrigerate upon receipt and until use at 2°C to 8°C (35°F to 46°F); do not freeze.

Mechanism of Action Promotes immunity to influenza virus by inducing influenza strain-specific serum antibodies

Pharmacodynamics

Onset of action: Protective antibody levels achieved ~2 weeks after vaccination

Duration: Protective antibody levels persist approximately ≥6 months

Usual Dosage Intranasal: Administer vaccine prior to exposure to influenza. It is important to note that influenza seasons vary in their timing and duration from year to year. In general, vaccination should begin soon after the vaccine becomes available and if possible, prior to October. However, vaccination should continue throughout the influenza season as long as vaccine is available. For children ages 2-8 years who have never received influenza vaccine, vaccinate in October or earlier since a second dose will need to be given one month after the initial dose.

Children 2-8 years:

Not previously vaccinated with influenza virus vaccine and those vaccinated for the first time during the previous influenza season but who only received one dose in the previous season: 2 doses (0.2 mL each); second dose one month after the initial dose

Previously vaccinated with influenza virus vaccine: 1 dose (0.2 mL) per season

Children and Adolescents 9-17 years: 1 dose (0.2 mL) per season

Adults 18-49 years: 1 dose (0.2 mL) per season

Administration Intranasal: Administer 0.1 mL (half of the dose from a single sprayer) into each nostril while the recipient is in an upright position. Insert the tip of the sprayer just inside the nostril and depress the plunger to spray. Remove dose-divider clip from the sprayer to administer the second half of the dose into the other nostril. Do not administer by the I.M., SubQ, intradermal, or I.V. route.

Monitoring Parameters Monitor for ≥15 minutes following vaccination

Patient Information If the patient sneezes after intranasal vaccine administration, the dose should not be repeated. Patients with an acute febrile illness should not receive the vaccine until symptoms improve. Report any suspected adverse effects to your physician.

Nursing Implications The used sprayer should be disposed of according to the standard procedures for biohazardous waste products. CDC has stated that the inactivated influenza virus vaccine injection is preferred over the live, intranasal influenza vaccine for physicians, nurses, family members, or individuals who will come in close contact with anyone with a severely weakened immune system (eg, people with hematopoietic stem cell transplants in a protective environment).

Federal law requires that the date of administration, the vaccine manufacturer, lot number of vaccine, and the administering person's name, title, and address be entered into the patient's permanent medical record.

Additional Information In order to maximize vaccination rates, the ACIP recommends simultaneous administration of all age-appropriate vaccines (live or inactivated) for which a person is eligible at a single visit, unless contraindications exist. The use of combination vaccines is generally preferred over separate infections, taking into consideration provider assessment, patient preference, and potential adverse events.

For additional information, please refer to the following website: http://www.cdc.gov/vaccines/vpd-vac/.

Dosage Forms Excipient information presented when available (limited, particularly for generics); consult specific product labeling.

Solution, intranasal [preservative free; spray]:
FluMist®: 0.2 mL [trivalent, LAIV; contains arginine, chicken egg protein, gelatin, and gentamicin]

References

Belshe RB, Mendelman PM, Treanor J, et al, "The Efficacy of Live Attenuated, Cold-Adapted, Trivalent, Intranasal Influenza Virus Vaccine in Children," *N Engl J Med*, 1998, 338(20):1405-12.

Centers for Disease Control and Prevention (CDC), "General Recommendations on Immunization. Recommendations of the Advisory Committee on Immunization Practices (ACIP)," *MMWR Recomm Rep*, 2006, 55(RR-15):1-48. Available at: http://www.cdc.gov/mmwr/preview/mmwrhtml/rr5515a1.htm.

Centers for Disease Control and Prevention, "Prevention and Control of Seasonal Influenza with Vaccines," *MMWR* Early Releas, July 24, 2009. Available at http://www.cdc.gov/mmwr/pdf/rr/rr58e0724.pdf.

Harper SA, Fukuda K, Cox NJ, et al, "Using Live, Attenuated Influenza Vaccine for Prevention and Control of Influenza: Supplemental Recommendations of the Advisory Committee on Immunization Practices (ACIP)," *MMWR Recomm Rep*, 2003, 52(RR-13):1-8.

Prymula R, Siegrist CA, Chlibek R, et al, "Effect of Prophylactic Paracetamol Administration at Time of Vaccination on Febrile Reactions and Antibody Responses in Children: Two Open-Label, Randomised Controlled Trials," *Lancet*, 2009, 374(9698):1339-50.

◆ **Influenza Virus Vaccine (Purified Surface Antigen)** *see* Influenza Virus Vaccine (Inactivated) *on page 734*

◆ **Influenza Virus Vaccine (Split-Virus)** *see* Influenza Virus Vaccine (Inactivated) *on page 734*

◆ **Influenza Virus Vaccine (Trivalent, Live)** *see* Influenza Virus Vaccine (Live/Attenuated) *on page 736*

◆ **Infufer® (Can)** *see* Iron Dextran Complex *on page 762*

◆ **Infumorph® 200** *see* Morphine Sulfate *on page 946*

◆ **Infumorph® 500** *see* Morphine Sulfate *on page 946*

◆ **INH** *see* Isoniazid *on page 767*

◆ **InnoPran XL®** *see* Propranolol *on page 1175*

◆ **Inova™** *see* Benzoyl Peroxide *on page 184*

◆ **Insta-Glucose® [OTC]** *see* Dextrose *on page 422*

Insulin Aspart (IN soo lin AS part)

Medication Safety Issues

Sound-alike/look-alike issues:
NovoLog® may be confused with Humalog®, Humulin® R, Novolin® N, Novolin® R, NovoLog® Mix 70/30

High alert medication: The Institute for Safe Medication Practices (ISMP) includes this medication among its list of drugs which have a heightened risk of causing significant patient harm when used in error. ***Due to the number of insulin preparations, it is essential to identify/clarify the type of insulin to be used.***

Cross-contamination may occur if insulin pens are shared among multiple patients. Steps should be taken to prohibit sharing of insulin pens.

U.S. Brand Names NovoLog®

Canadian Brand Names NovoRapid®

Therapeutic Category Antidiabetic Agent, Parenteral; Insulin, Rapid-Acting

Generic Available No

Use Treatment of type 1 diabetes mellitus (insulin dependent, IDDM); type 2 diabetes mellitus (noninsulin dependent, NIDDM) to control hyperglycemia

Pregnancy Risk Factor B

Pregnancy Considerations Adverse events have generally not been observed in animal reproduction studies; therefore, the manufacturer classifies insulin aspart as pregnancy category B. When compared to regular insulin, the use of insulin aspart during pregnancy has not been found to increase the risk of adverse events to the fetus. Maternal hyperglycemia can be associated with adverse effects in the fetus, including macrosomia, neonatal hyperglycemia, and hyperbilirubinemia; the risk of congenital malformations is increased when the Hb A_{1c} is above the normal range.

Insulin requirements tend to fall during the first trimester of pregnancy and increase in the later trimesters, peaking at 28-32 weeks of gestation. Following delivery, insulin requirements decrease rapidly. Diabetes can be associated with adverse effects in the mother. Poorly-treated diabetes may cause end-organ damage that may in turn negatively affect obstetric outcomes. Physiologic glucose levels should be maintained prior to and during pregnancy to decrease the risk of adverse events in the fetus and the mother. Insulin is the drug of choice for the control of diabetes mellitus during pregnancy. Insulin aspart has been demonstrated to be as safe and effective as regular human insulin when used during pregnancy and may have advantages over regular insulin during pregnancy.

Lactation Excretion in breast milk unknown/compatible

Breast-Feeding Considerations It is not known if insulin aspart is found in breast milk. Endogenous insulin can be found in breast milk. Plasma glucose concentrations in the mother affect glucose concentrations in breast milk. The gastrointestinal tract destroys insulin when administered orally; therefore, insulin is not expected to be absorbed intact by the breast-feeding infant. All types of insulin are safe for use while breast-feeding. Due to increased calorie expenditure, women with diabetes may require less insulin while nursing.

Contraindications Hypersensitivity insulin aspart or any component

Warnings Refer to information common to all insulin formulations found in Insulin Regular on page 748.

Precautions Refer to information common to all insulin formulations found in Insulin Regular on page 748.

Adverse Reactions Refer to information common to all insulin formulations found in Insulin Regular on page 748.

Drug Interactions

Metabolism/Transport Effects Refer to Insulin Regular on page 748.

Avoid Concomitant Use There are no known interactions where it is recommended to avoid concomitant use.

Increased Effect/Toxicity

Insulin Aspart may increase the levels/effects of: Antidiabetic Agents (Thiazolidinedione); Hypoglycemic Agents; Quinolone Antibiotics

The levels/effects of Insulin Aspart may be increased by: Beta-Blockers; Edetate CALCIUM Disodium; Edetate Disodium; Herbs (Hypoglycemic Properties); Pegvisomant

Decreased Effect

The levels/effects of Insulin Aspart may be decreased by: Corticosteroids (Orally Inhaled); Corticosteroids (Systemic); Luteinizing Hormone-Releasing Hormone Analogs; Somatropin; Thiazide Diuretics

Food Interactions Refer to information common to all insulin formulations found in Insulin Regular on page 748.

Stability Store unopened container in refrigerator; do not freeze; protect from heat and light. Once opened (in use) vials may be stored in refrigerator or at room temperature for up to 28 days. Cartridges that are in use should be stored at room temperature and used within 28 days; do not refrigerate. Insulin in reservoir should be replaced every 48 hours. Discard if exposed to temperatures ≥37°C (98.6°F). May be mixed in the same syringe with NPH insulin.

Mechanism of Action Refer to information common to all insulin formulations found in Insulin Regular on page 748. Insulin aspart is a rapid-acting insulin analog.

Pharmacodynamics Onset and duration of hypoglycemic effects depend upon the route of administration (adsorption and onset of action are more rapid after deeper I.M. injections than after SubQ), site of injection (onset and duration are progressively slower with SubQ injection into the abdomen, arm, buttock, or thigh respectively), volume and concentration of injection, and the preparation administered; local heat and massage also increase the rate of absorption.

Onset of action: 0.17-0.33 hours

Maximum effect: 1-3 hours

Duration: 3-5 hours

Pharmacokinetics (Adult data unless noted)

Protein binding: 0% to 9%

Half-life: Adults: 81 minutes

Time to peak serum concentration: 40-50 minutes

Elimination: Urine

Clearance: Adults: 1.22 L/hour/kg

Usual Dosage Refer to information common to all insulin formulations found in Insulin Regular on page 748. Insulin aspart is a rapid-acting insulin analog which is normally administered as a premeal component of the insulin regimen or as a continuous SubQ infusion.

Dosing adjustment in renal impairment: Insulin requirements are reduced with renal impairment; see Insulin Regular on page 748

Administration Parenteral:

SubQ: Administration is usually made into the subcutaneous fat of the thighs, arms, buttocks, or abdomen, with sites rotated; cold injections should be avoided. May be mixed in the same syringe with NPH insulin. When mixing insulin aspart with NPH insulin, aspart should be drawn into the syringe first. Administer immediately before meals (within 5-10 minutes of the start of a meal). Can be infused SubQ by external insulin pump; however, when used in an external pump, it is not recommended to be diluted with other insulin.

I.V.: Insulin aspart may be administered I.V. in selected clinical situations to control hyperglycemia. Appropriate medical supervision is required. May be diluted to a concentration between 0.05 and 1 unit/mL with NS, D$_5$W, or D$_{10}$W

Monitoring Parameters Urine sugar and acetone, serum glucose, electrolytes, Hb A$_{1c}$, lipid profile; when used intravenously, close monitoring of serum glucose and potassium are required to avoid hypoglycemia and/or hypokalemia

Reference Range Refer to information common to all insulin formulations found in Insulin Regular on page 748.

Patient Information Do not take any new medication during therapy unless approved by healthcare provider. This medication is used to control diabetes; it is not a cure. It is imperative to follow other components of prescribed treatment (eg, diet and exercise regimen). Take exactly as directed. Do not change dose or discontinue unless advised by healthcare provider. With insulin aspart (NovoLog®), you must start eating within 5-10 minutes after injection. If you experience hypoglycemic reaction, contact healthcare provider immediately. Always carry quick source of sugar with you. Monitor glucose levels as directed by healthcare provider. Report adverse side effects, including chest pain or palpitations; persistent fatigue, confusion, headache; skin rash or redness; numbness of mouth, lips, or tongue; muscle weakness or tremors; vision changes; respiratory difficulty; or nausea, vomiting, or flu-like symptoms.

Dosage Forms Excipient information presented when available (limited, particularly for generics); consult specific product labeling.

Injection, solution:

NovoLog®: 100 units/mL (3 mL) [FlexPen® prefilled syringe or PenFill® prefilled cartridge]; (10 mL) [vial]

♦ **Insulin Aspart and Insulin Aspart Protamine** *see Insulin Aspart Protamine and Insulin Aspart on page 739*

Insulin Aspart Protamine and Insulin Aspart (IN soo lin AS part PROE ta meen & IN soo lin AS part)

Medication Safety Issues

Sound-alike/look-alike issues:

NovoLog® Mix 70/30 may be confused with Humalog® Mix 75/25™, Humulin® 70/30, Novolin® 70/30, NovoLog®

High alert medication: The Institute for Safe Medication Practices (ISMP) includes this medication among its list of drugs which have a heightened risk of causing significant patient harm when used in error. *Due to the number of insulin preparations, it is essential to identify/clarify the type of insulin to be used.*

Cross-contamination may occur if insulin pens are shared among multiple patients. Steps should be taken to prohibit sharing of insulin pens.

U.S. Brand Names NovoLog® Mix 70/30

Canadian Brand Names NovoMix® 30

Therapeutic Category Antidiabetic Agent, Parenteral; Insulin, Combination

Generic Available No

Use Treatment of type 1 diabetes mellitus (insulin dependent, IDDM); type 2 diabetes mellitus (noninsulin dependent, NIDDM) to control hyperglycemia

Pregnancy Risk Factor C

Pregnancy Considerations Refer to Insulin Aspart on page 738.

Lactation Refer to Insulin Aspart on page 738.

Breast-Feeding Considerations Refer to Insulin Aspart on page 738.

Contraindications Hypersensitivity insulin aspart, insulin aspart protamine, or to any component; hypoglycemia

Warnings Refer to information common to all insulin formulations found in Insulin Regular; not for I.V. infusion or use in insulin infusion pumps

Precautions Refer to information common to all insulin formulations found in Insulin Regular.

Adverse Reactions Refer to information common to all insulin formulations found in Insulin Regular.

Drug Interactions

Metabolism/Transport Effects Refer to Insulin Regular on page 748.

Avoid Concomitant Use There are no known interactions where it is recommended to avoid concomitant use.

Increased Effect/Toxicity

Insulin Aspart Protamine and Insulin Aspart may increase the levels/effects of: Antidiabetic Agents (Thiazolidine-dione); Hypoglycemic Agents; Quinolone Antibiotics

The levels/effects of Insulin Aspart Protamine and Insulin Aspart may be increased by: Beta-Blockers; Edetate CALCIUM Disodium; Edetate Disodium; Herbs (Hypoglycemic Properties); Pegvisomant

Decreased Effect

The levels/effects of Insulin Aspart Protamine and Insulin Aspart may be decreased by: Corticosteroids (Orally Inhaled); Corticosteroids (Systemic); Luteinizing Hormone-Releasing Hormone Analogs; Somatropin; Thiazide Diuretics

Food Interactions Refer to information common to all insulin formulations found in Insulin Regular.

Stability Store unopened container in refrigerator; do not freeze; protect from light. If refrigeration is not possible, vial (in use) may be stored at room temperature for up to 28 days. The pen (in use) should not be refrigerated; store below 30°C (86°F) away from direct heat or light; discard after 14 days. Do not mix or dilute with other insulins.

Mechanism of Action Refer to information common to all insulin formulations found in Insulin Regular. Insulin aspart protamine and insulin aspart is a combination insulin product with intermediate-acting characteristics.

Pharmacodynamics

Onset of action: 10-20 minutes

Maximum effect: 1-4 hours

Duration: 18-24 hours

Pharmacokinetics (Adult data unless noted)

Half-life: 8-9 hours (mean)

Elimination: Urine

Usual Dosage Refer to information common to all insulin formulations found in Insulin Regular. Fixed ratio insulins (such as insulin aspart protamine and insulin aspart combination) are normally administered in 2 daily doses with each dose intended to cover two meals and a snack. Because of variability in the peak affect and individual patient variability in activities, meals, etc, it may be more difficult to achieve complete glycemic control using fixed combinations of insulins in all patients.

Dosing adjustment in renal impairment: Insulin requirements are reduced with renal impairment; see Insulin Regular

Administration

Parenteral: SubQ: Gently roll vial or pen in the palms of the hands to resuspend before use; administer into the subcutaneous fat of the thighs, arms, buttocks, or abdomen, with sites rotated. Cold injections should be avoided. Administer within 15 minutes before a meal (before breakfast and supper). Do not mix or dilute with other insulins. **Not for I.V. administration** or use in an insulin infusion pump.

Monitoring Parameters Refer to information common to all insulin formulations found in Insulin Regular.

Reference Range Refer to information common to all insulin formulations found in Insulin Regular.

Patient Information Refer to information common to all insulin formulations found in Insulin Regular.

Dosage Forms Excipient information presented when available (limited, particularly for generics); consult specific product labeling.

Injection, suspension:

NovoLog® Mix 70/30: Insulin aspart protamine suspension 70% [intermediate acting] and insulin aspart solution 30% [rapid acting]: 100 units/mL (3 mL) [FlexPen® prefilled syringe]; (10 mL) [vial]

Insulin Detemir (IN soo lin DE te mir)

Medication Safety Issues

High alert medication: The Institute for Safe Medication Practices (ISMP) includes this medication among its list of drugs which have a heightened risk of causing significant patient harm when used in error. *Due to the number of insulin preparations, it is essential to identify/clarify the type of insulin to be used.*

Note: Insulin detemir is a clear solution, but it is NOT intended for I.V. or I.M. administration.

Cross-contamination may occur if insulin pens are shared among multiple patients. Steps should be taken to prohibit sharing of insulin pens.

U.S. Brand Names Levemir®

Canadian Brand Names Levemir®

Therapeutic Category Antidiabetic Agent, Parenteral; Insulin, Intermediate-Acting

Generic Available No

Use Treatment of type 1 diabetes mellitus (insulin dependent, IDDM); type 2 diabetes mellitus (noninsulin dependent, NIDDM) to control hyperglycemia

Pregnancy Risk Factor C

Pregnancy Considerations Adverse events were observed in animal reproduction studies; therefore, the manufacturer classifies insulin detemir as pregnancy category C. Maternal hyperglycemia can be associated with adverse effects in the fetus, including macrosomia, neonatal hyperglycemia, and hyperbilirubinemia; the risk of congenital malformations is increased when the Hb A_{1c} is above the normal range. Insulin requirements tend to fall during the first trimester of pregnancy and increase in the later trimesters, peaking at 28-32 weeks of gestation. Following delivery, insulin requirements decrease rapidly. Diabetes can be associated with adverse effects in the mother. Poorly-treated diabetes may cause end-organ damage that may in turn negatively affect obstetric outcomes. Physiologic glucose levels should be maintained prior to and during pregnancy to decrease the risk of adverse events in the fetus and the mother. Insulin is the drug of choice for the control of diabetes mellitus during pregnancy. Pregnant women using insulin detemir should be switched to NPH insulin pending additional safety information with this agent.

Lactation Excretion in breast milk unknown/compatible

Breast-Feeding Considerations It is not known if insulin detemir is found in breast milk. Endogenous insulin can be found in breast milk. Plasma glucose concentrations in the mother affect glucose concentrations in breast milk. The gastrointestinal tract destroys insulin when administered orally; therefore, insulin is not expected to be absorbed intact by the breast-feeding infant. All types of insulin are safe for use while breast-feeding. Due to increased calorie expenditure, women with diabetes may require less insulin while nursing.

Contraindications Hypersensitivity to insulin detemir or any component; hypoglycemia

Warnings Refer to information common to all insulin formulations found in Insulin Regular on page 748. Safety and efficacy not established in children <6 years of age. **Not for I.V. administration** or use in insulin infusion pumps.

Precautions Refer to information common to all insulin formulations found in Insulin Regular on page 748.

Adverse Reactions Refer to information common to all insulin formulations found in Insulin Regular on page 748.

Drug Interactions

Metabolism/Transport Effects Refer to Insulin Regular on page 748.

Avoid Concomitant Use There are no known inter-actions where it is recommended to avoid concomitant use.

Increased Effect/Toxicity

Insulin Detemir may increase the levels/effects of: Antidiabetic Agents (Thiazolidinedione); Hypoglycemic Agents; Quinolone Antibiotics

The levels/effects of Insulin Detemir may be increased by: Beta-Blockers; Edetate CALCIUM Disodium; Edetate Disodium; Herbs (Hypoglycemic Properties); Peg-visomant

Decreased Effect

The levels/effects of Insulin Detemir may be decreased by: Corticosteroids (Orally Inhaled); Corticosteroids (Systemic); Luteinizing Hormone-Releasing Hormone Analogs; Somatropin; Thiazide Diuretics

Food Interactions Refer to information common to all insulin formulations found in Insulin Regular on page 748.

Stability Store unopened vial or cartridges in refrigerator; do not freeze. Unopened vials or cartridges are stable at room temperature for 42 days. Once opened (in use), vials may be stored in refrigerator or at room temperature (below 30°C) for up to 42 days. Cartridges and prefilled syringes that are in use should be stored at room temperature and used within 42 days; do not refrigerate. Do not store with needle in place. Do not dilute or mix with other insulins or solutions.

Mechanism of Action Refer to information common to all insulin formulations found in Insulin Regular on page 748. The product labeling identifies this product as a long-acting insulin analog; however, its pharmacodynamic character-istics and dosing are typical of intermediate insulin forms. In some patients, or at higher dosages, it may have a duration of action approaching long-acting insulins.

Pharmacodynamics

Onset of action: 3-4 hours

Duration: 6-23 hours (dose dependent)

Pharmacokinetics (Adult data unless noted)

Distribution: V_d: 0.1 L/kg

Bioavailability: 60%

Half-life: SubQ: 5-7 hours (dose dependent)

Time to peak serum concentration: 6-8 hours

Elimination: Urine

Usual Dosage Refer to information common to all insulin formulations found in Insulin Regular on page 748.

SubQ: Children and Adults: Type 1 or type 2 diabetes:

Previously receiving basal insulin alone (eg, insulin glargine) or basal insulin plus bolus insulin (eg, NPH + regular insulin): May be substituted on an equivalent unit-per-unit basis

Insulin-naive patients (adults with type 2 diabetes only): 0.1-0.2 units/kg once daily in the evening or 10 units once or twice daily. Adjust dose to achieve glycemic targets.

Dosage adjustment in renal impairment: Insulin require-ments are reduced due to changes in insulin clearance or metabolism. See Insulin Regular on page 748.

Administration Parenteral: SubQ: Administer into the thighs, arms, buttocks, or abdomen, with sites rotated. Cold injections should be avoided. **Not for I.V. infusion** or use in insulin infusion pumps. May not be diluted or mixed with other insulins or solutions. When treated once daily, administer with evening meal or at bedtime. When treated twice daily, administer evening dose with evening meal, at bedtime, or 12 hours following the morning dose.

Monitoring Parameters Urine sugar and acetone, serum glucose, electrolytes, Hb A_{1c}, lipid profile

Reference Range Refer to information common to all insulin formulations found in Insulin Regular on page 748.

Patient Information Refer to information common to all insulin formulations found in Insulin Regular on page 748.

Dosage Forms Excipient information presented when available (limited, particularly for generics); consult specific product labeling.

Injection, solution:

Levemir®: 100 units/mL (3 mL) [FlexPen® prefilled syringe]; (10 mL) [vial]

Insulin Glargine (IN soo lin GLAR jeen)

Medication Safety Issues

Sound-alike/look-alike issues:

Insulin glargine may be confused with insulin glulisine

Lantus® may be confused with latanoprost, Xalatan®

International issues:

Lantus® [U.S., Canada, and multiple international markets] may be confused with Lanvis® brand name for thioguanine [Canada and multiple international markets]

High alert medication: The Institute for Safe Medication Practices (ISMP) includes this medication among its list of drugs which have a heightened risk of causing significant patient harm when used in error. *Due to the number of insulin preparations, it is essential to identify/clarify the type of insulin to be used.*

Note: Insulin glargine is a clear solution, but it is NOT intended for I.V. or I.M. administration.

Cross-contamination may occur if insulin pens are shared among multiple patients. Steps should be taken to prohibit sharing of insulin pens.

U.S. Brand Names Lantus®

Canadian Brand Names Lantus®; Lantus® OptiSet®

Therapeutic Category Antidiabetic Agent, Parenteral; Insulin, Long-Acting

Generic Available No

Use Treatment of type 1 diabetes mellitus (insulin depend-ent, IDDM); type 2 diabetes mellitus (noninsulin depend-ent, NIDDM) requiring basal (long-acting) insulin to control hyperglycemia

Pregnancy Risk Factor C

Pregnancy Considerations Adverse events have been shown in some animal studies; therefore, the manufacturer classifies insulin glargine as pregnancy category C. Maternal hyperglycemia can be associated with adverse effects in the fetus, including macrosomia, neonatal hyperglycemia, and hyperbilirubinemia; the risk of con-genital malformations is increased when Hb A_{1c} is above the normal range.

Insulin requirements tend to fall during the first trimester of pregnancy and increase in the later trimesters, peaking at 28-32 weeks of gestation. Following delivery, insulin requirements decrease rapidly. Diabetes can be associ-ated with adverse effects in the mother. Poorly-treated diabetes may cause end-organ damage that may in turn negatively affect obstetric outcomes. Physiologic glucose levels should be maintained prior to and during pregnancy to decrease the risk of adverse events in the fetus and the mother. Insulin is the drug of choice for the control of diabetes mellitus during pregnancy. Pregnancy outcome information following the use of insulin glargine is available from case reports and small studies. Current reports indicate that insulin glargine is effective when used during pregnancy and may be an option for pregnant women with significantly uncontrolled diabetes; however, pregnant women using insulin glargine should be switched to NPH insulin pending additional safety information with this agent.

Lactation Excretion in breast milk unknown/compatible

Breast-Feeding Considerations It is not known if significant amounts of insulin glargine are found in breast milk. Endogenous insulin can be found in breast milk. Plasma glucose concentrations in the mother affect glucose concentrations in breast milk. The gastrointestinal tract destroys insulin when administered orally; therefore, insulin is not expected to be absorbed intact by the breast-feeding infant. All types of insulin are safe for use while breast-feeding. Due to increased calorie expenditure, women with diabetes may require less insulin while nursing.

Contraindications Hypersensitivity insulin glargine or any component

Warnings Refer to information common to all insulin formulations found in Insulin Regular on page 748. **Not for I.V. administration** or use in insulin infusion pumps

Precautions Refer to information common to all insulin formulations found in Insulin Regular on page 748.

Adverse Reactions Refer to information common to all insulin formulations found in Insulin Regular on page 748.

Drug Interactions

Metabolism/Transport Effects Refer to Insulin Regular on page 748.

Avoid Concomitant Use There are no known inter-actions where it is recommended to avoid concomitant use.

Increased Effect/Toxicity
Insulin Glargine may increase the levels/effects of: Antidiabetic Agents (Thiazolidinedione); Hypoglycemic Agents; Quinolone Antibiotics

The levels/effects of Insulin Glargine may be increased by: Beta-Blockers; Edetate CALCIUM Disodium; Edetate Disodium; Herbs (Hypoglycemic Properties); Peg-visomant

Decreased Effect
The levels/effects of Insulin Glargine may be decreased by: Corticosteroids (Orally Inhaled); Corticosteroids (Systemic); Luteinizing Hormone-Releasing Hormone Analogs; Somatropin; Thiazide Diuretics

Food Interactions Refer to information common to all insulin formulations found in Insulin Regular on page 748.

Stability Store unopened containers or cartridges in refrigerator at 2°C to 8°C (36°F to 46°F); do not freeze; protect from direct heat or light. Once opened (in use), vials may be stored in refrigerator or at room temperature for up to 28 days. Cartridges (in use; inserted into OptiClik™ delivery system) should not be refrigerated; store below 30°C (86°F) away from direct heat or light; discard after 28 days. May **not** be mixed with any other insulin or solution.

Mechanism of Action Refer to information common to all insulin formulations found in Insulin Regular on page 748. Insulin glargine is a long-acting insulin formulation.

Pharmacodynamics
Onset of action: 3-4 hours
Duration: 24 hours

Pharmacokinetics (Adult data unless noted)
Absorption: Slow; after injection it forms microprecipitates in the skin which allow small amounts to release over time
Metabolism: Partially metabolized in the skin to form two active metabolites
Time to peak serum concentration: No pronounced peak
Elimination: Urine

Usual Dosage SubQ: Refer to information common to all insulin formulations found in Insulin Regular on page 748.
Type 1 diabetes: Conversion from "conventional" insulin therapy to once daily insulin glargine:
Children <6 years: Limited data; thirty-five preschool-aged children (2.6-6.3 years) were converted to once-daily insulin glargine (with insulin lispro prior to each meal); 40% of the established total daily insulin dose

was administered as insulin glargine. Insulin glargine was well tolerated and this regimen resulted in a reduction in hypoglycemic episodes in the nonobese group (Alemzadeh, 2005).
Children ≥6 years and Adults: Current therapy: If once-daily NPH or Ultralente® insulin: Use the same total dose of insulin glargine as NPH or Ultralente®; if twice-daily NPH or Ultralente®: Use 80% of the total daily dose of NPH or Ultralente® (eg, 20% reduction); administer once daily; adjust dosage according to patient response
Type 2 diabetes: Adults:
Patient not already on insulin: 10 units once daily, adjusted according to patient response (range in clinical study: 2-100 units/day)
Patients already on insulin: See adult type 1 diabetes recommendation.
Dosage adjustment in renal impairment: Insulin require-ments are reduced with renal impairment; see Insulin Regular on page 748.

Administration Parenteral: SubQ: Administer into the subcutaneous fat of the thighs, arms, buttocks, or abdomen, with sites rotated. Cold injections should be avoided. Administer once daily, at any time of day, but at the same time each day. Do not mix with any other insulin or solution.

Monitoring Parameters Urine sugar and acetone, serum glucose, electrolytes, Hb A_{1c}, lipid profile

Reference Range Refer to information common to all insulin formulations found in Insulin Regular on page 748.

Patient Information Refer to information common to all insulin formulations found in Insulin Regular on page 748.

Dosage Forms Excipient information presented when available (limited, particularly for generics); consult specific product labeling.
Injection, solution:
Lantus®: 100 units/mL (3 mL) [OptiClik® prefilled cartridge or SoloStar® disposable insulin device]; (10 mL) [vial]

References
Alemzadeh R, Berhe T, and Wyatt DT, "Flexible Insulin Therapy With Glargine Insulin Improved Glycemic Control and Reduced Severe Hypoglycemia Among Preschool-Aged Children With Type 1 Diabetes Mellitus," *Pediatrics,* 2005, 115(5):1320-4.

Insulin Glulisine (IN soo lin gloo LIS een)

Medication Safety Issues
Sound-alike/look-alike issues:
Insulin glulisine may be confused with insulin glargine

High alert medication: The Institute for Safe Medication Practices (ISMP) includes this medication among its list of drugs which have a heightened risk of causing significant patient harm when used in error. *Due to the number of insulin preparations, it is essential to identify/clarify the type of insulin to be used.*

Cross-contamination may occur if insulin pens are shared among multiple patients. Steps should be taken to prohibit sharing of insulin pens.

U.S. Brand Names Apidra®
Canadian Brand Names Apidra®
Therapeutic Category Insulin, Rapid-Acting
Generic Available No

Use Treatment of type 1 diabetes mellitus (insulin depend-ent, IDDM); type 2 diabetes mellitus (noninsulin depend-ent, NIDDM) to control hyperglycemia

Pregnancy Risk Factor C

Pregnancy Considerations Adverse events were observed in some animal reproduction studies; therefore, the manufacturer classifies insulin glulisine as pregnancy category C. Maternal hyperglycemia can be associated with adverse effects in the fetus, including macrosomia, neonatal hyperglycemia, and hyperbilirubinemia; the risk of congenital malformations is increased when the Hb A_{1c} is above the normal range.

Insulin requirements tend to fall during the first trimester of pregnancy and increase in the later trimesters, peaking at 28-32 weeks of gestation. Following delivery, insulin requirements decrease rapidly. Diabetes can be associated with adverse effects in the mother. Poorly-treated diabetes may cause end-organ damage that may in turn negatively affect obstetric outcomes. Physiologic glucose levels should be maintained prior to and during pregnancy to decrease the risk of adverse events in the fetus and mother. Insulin is the drug of choice for the control of diabetes mellitus during pregnancy. Due to lack of clinical studies with insulin glulisine in pregnant women, the manufacturer recommends use during pregnancy only if the potential benefit to the mother justifies any potential risk to the fetus.

Lactation Excretion in breast milk unknown/compatible

Breast-Feeding Considerations It is not known if insulin glulisine is found in breast milk. Endogenous insulin can be found in breast milk. Plasma glucose concentrations in the mother affect glucose concentrations in breast milk. The gastrointestinal tract destroys insulin when administered orally; therefore, insulin is not expected to be absorbed intact by the breast-feeding infant. All types of insulin are safe for use while breast-feeding. Due to increased calorie expenditure, women with diabetes may require less insulin while nursing.

Contraindications Hypersensitivity to insulin glulisine or any component; do not use during episodes of hypoglycemia

Warnings Refer to information common to all insulin formulations found in Insulin Regular on page 748.

Precautions Refer to information common to all insulin formulations found in Insulin Regular on page 748. While regular insulin is the preferred formulation for I.V. use, insulin glulisine may be administered I.V. in carefully controlled clinical settings with medical supervision and close monitoring of blood glucose as well as serum potassium.

Adverse Reactions Refer to information common to all insulin formulations found in Insulin Regular on page 748.

Drug Interactions

Metabolism/Transport Effects Refer to Insulin Regular on page 748.

Avoid Concomitant Use There are no known interactions where it is recommended to avoid concomitant use.

Increased Effect/Toxicity

Insulin Glulisine may increase the levels/effects of: Antidiabetic Agents (Thiazolidinedione); Hypoglycemic Agents; Quinolone Antibiotics

The levels/effects of Insulin Glulisine may be increased by: Beta-Blockers; Edetate CALCIUM Disodium; Edetate Disodium; Herbs (Hypoglycemic Properties); Pegvisomant

Decreased Effect

The levels/effects of Insulin Glulisine may be decreased by: Corticosteroids (Orally Inhaled); Corticosteroids (Systemic); Luteinizing Hormone-Releasing Hormone Analogs; Somatropin; Thiazide Diuretics

Food Interactions Refer to information common to all insulin formulations found in Insulin Regular on page 748.

Stability Store unopened container in refrigerator; do not freeze; protect from heat and light. Once opened (in use) vials may be stored in refrigerator or at room temperature for up to 28 days. Cartridges that are in use should be stored at room temperature and used within 28 days; do not refrigerate. Insulin glulisine in reservoir should be replaced every 48 hours. Discard if exposed to temperatures $\geq 37°C$ (98.6°F). May be mixed in the same syringe with NPH insulin.

Mechanism of Action Refer to information common to all insulin formulations found in Insulin Regular on page 748. Insulin glulisine is a rapid-acting insulin analog.

Pharmacodynamics Onset and duration of hypoglycemic effects depend upon the route of administration (adsorption and onset of action are more rapid after deeper I.M. injections than after SubQ), site of injection (onset and duration are progressively slower with SubQ injection into the abdomen, arm, buttock, or thigh respectively), volume and concentration of injection, and the preparation administered; local heat and massage also increase the rate of absorption.

Onset of action: 5-15 minutes
Maximum effect: 45-75 minutes
Duration: 2-4 hours

Pharmacokinetics (Adult data unless noted)
Distribution: V_d: Adults: 13 L
Bioavailability: SubQ: ~70%
Half-life:
SubQ: 42 minutes
I.V.: 13 minutes
Time to peak serum concentration: SubQ: 60 minutes (range: 40-120 minutes)
Elimination: Urine

Usual Dosage Refer to information common to all insulin formulations found in Insulin Regular on page 748. Insulin glulisine is a rapid-acting insulin analog which is normally administered as a premeal component of the insulin regimen or as a continuous SubQ infusion. In carefully controlled clinical settings with medical supervision and close monitoring of blood glucose as well as serum potassium, insulin glulisine may also be administered I.V.

Dosing adjustment in renal impairment: Insulin requirements are reduced with renal impairment; see Insulin Regular on page 748.

Administration Parenteral:

SubQ: Administration is usually made into the subcutaneous fat of the thighs, arms, buttocks, or abdomen, with sites rotated; cold injections should be avoided. May be mixed in the same syringe with NPH insulin. When mixing insulin glulisine with NPH insulin, glulisine should be drawn into the syringe first. Administer 15 minutes before meals or within 20 minutes after starting a meal. Can be infused SubQ by external insulin pump; however, when used in an external pump, it is not recommended to be diluted with other insulins.

I.V.: Dilute with NS to a final concentration of 0.05-1 unit/mL and administer using polyvinyl chloride infusion bags into a dedicated infusion line (the use of other bags and tubing has not been studied).

Monitoring Parameters Urine sugar and acetone, serum glucose, electrolytes, Hb A_{1c}, lipid profile

Reference Range Refer to information common to all insulin formulations found in Insulin Regular on page 748.

Patient Information Do not take any new medication during therapy unless approved by healthcare provider. This medication is used to control diabetes; it is not a cure. It is imperative to follow other components of prescribed treatment (eg, diet and exercise regimen). Take exactly as directed. Do not change dose or discontinue unless advised by healthcare provider. With insulin glulisine (Apidra®), you must administer 15 minutes before or within 20 minutes after starting a meal. If you experience hypoglycemic reaction, contact healthcare provider immediately. Always carry quick source of sugar with you. Monitor glucose levels as directed by healthcare provider. Report adverse side effects, including chest pain or palpitations; persistent fatigue, confusion, headache; skin rash or redness; numbness of mouth, lips, or tongue; muscle weakness or tremors; vision changes; respiratory difficulty; or nausea, vomiting, or flu-like symptoms.

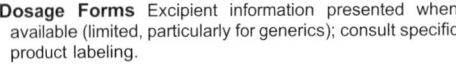

Dosage Forms Excipient information presented when available (limited, particularly for generics); consult specific product labeling.
Injection, solution:
Apidra®: 100 units/mL (3 mL [cartridge], 3 mL [SoloStar® prefilled pen], 10 mL [vial])

Insulin Lispro (IN su lin LIS pro)

Medication Safety Issues
Sound-alike/look-alike issues:
Humalog® may be confused with Humalog® Mix 50/50, Humira®, Humulin® N, Humulin® R, NovoLog®

High alert medication: The Institute for Safe Medication Practices (ISMP) includes this medication among its list of drugs which have a heightened risk of causing significant patient harm when used in error. *Due to the ·number of insulin preparations, it is essential to identify/clarify the type of insulin to be used.*

Cross-contamination may occur if insulin pens are shared among multiple patients. Steps should be taken to prohibit sharing of insulin pens.

U.S. Brand Names Humalog®
Canadian Brand Names Humalog®
Therapeutic Category Antidiabetic Agent, Parenteral; Insulin, Rapid-Acting
Generic Available No
Use Treatment of type 1 diabetes mellitus (insulin dependent, IDDM); type 2 diabetes mellitus (noninsulin dependent, NIDDM) to control hyperglycemia
Pregnancy Risk Factor B
Pregnancy Considerations Adverse events have not been observed in animal reproduction studies; therefore, the manufacturer classifies insulin lispro as pregnancy category B. Insulin lispro has not been shown to cross the placenta at standard clinical doses. Although congenital anomalies have been noted in case reports, when compared to regular insulin, insulin lispro has not been found to increase the risk of adverse events to the fetus in larger studies. Maternal hyperglycemia can be associated with adverse effects in the fetus, including macrosomia, neonatal hyperglycemia, and hyperbilirubinemia; the risk of congenital malformations is increased when Hb A$_{1c}$ is above the normal range.

Insulin requirements tend to fall during the first trimester of pregnancy and increase in the later trimesters, peaking at 28-32 weeks of gestation. Following delivery, insulin requirements decrease rapidly. Diabetes can be associated with adverse effects in the mother. Poorly-treated diabetes may cause end-organ damage that may in turn negatively affect obstetric outcomes. Physiologic glucose levels should be maintained prior to and during pregnancy to decrease the risk of adverse events in the fetus and mother. Insulin is the drug of choice for the control of diabetes mellitus during pregnancy. The use of insulin lispro has been shown to be as effective as regular insulin to treat diabetes in pregnancy and may have advantages over regular insulin during pregnancy.

Lactation Excretion in breast milk unknown/compatible
Breast-Feeding Considerations It is not known if significant amounts of insulin lispro are found in breast milk. Endogenous insulin can be found in breast milk. Plasma glucose concentrations in the mother affect glucose concentrations in breast milk. The gastrointestinal tract destroys insulin when administered orally; therefore, insulin is not expected to be absorbed intact by the breast-feeding infant. All types of insulin are safe for use while breast-feeding. Due to increased calorie expenditure, women with diabetes may require less insulin while nursing.

Contraindications Hypersensitivity lispro insulin or any component; hypoglycemia
Warnings Refer to information common to all insulin formulations found in Insulin Regular on page 748.
Precautions Refer to information common to all insulin formulations found in Insulin Regular on page 748.
Adverse Reactions Refer to information common to all insulin formulations found in Insulin Regular on page 748.
Drug Interactions
Metabolism/Transport Effects Refer to Insulin Regular on page 748.
Avoid Concomitant Use There are no known interactions where it is recommended to avoid concomitant use.
Increased Effect/Toxicity
Insulin Lispro may increase the levels/effects of: Antidiabetic Agents (Thiazolidinedione); Hypoglycemic Agents; Quinolone Antibiotics

The levels/effects of Insulin Lispro may be increased by: Beta-Blockers; Edetate CALCIUM Disodium; Edetate Disodium; Herbs (Hypoglycemic Properties); Pegvisomant
Decreased Effect
The levels/effects of Insulin Lispro may be decreased by: Corticosteroids (Orally Inhaled); Corticosteroids (Systemic); Luteinizing Hormone-Releasing Hormone Analogs; Somatropin; Thiazide Diuretics
Food Interactions Refer to information common to all insulin formulations found in Insulin Regular on page 748.
Stability Store unopened container in refrigerator; do not freeze; protect from heat and light. Once opened (in use) vials may be stored in refrigerator or at room temperature for up to 28 days. Cartridges that are in use should be stored at room temperature and used within 28 days; do not refrigerate. Insulin in reservoir should be replaced every 48 hours. Discard if exposed to temperatures ≥37°C (98.6°F). May be mixed in the same syringe with Humulin® N, Humulin® U and NPH insulins. A sterile diluent is available from the manufacturer for preparing dilutions of Humalog®.
Mechanism of Action Refer to information common to all insulin formulations found in Insulin Regular on page 748. Insulin lispro is a rapid-acting form of insulin.
Pharmacodynamics Onset and duration of hypoglycemic effects depend upon the route of administration (adsorption and onset of action are more rapid after deeper I.M. injections than after SubQ), site of injection (onset and duration are progressively slower with SubQ injection into the abdomen, arm, buttock, or thigh respectively), volume and concentration of injection, and the preparation administered; local heat, and massage also increase the rate of absorption.
Onset of action: 15-30 minutes
Maximum effect: 0.5-2.5 hours
Duration: 3-6.5 hours
Pharmacokinetics (Adult data unless noted)
Distribution: V$_d$: 0.26-0.36 L/kg
Bioavailability: 55% to 77%
Half-life: SubQ: 1 hour
Excretion: Urine
Usual Dosage Refer to information common to all insulin formulations found in Insulin Regular on page 748. Insulin lispro is a rapid-acting insulin analog which is normally administered as a premeal component of the insulin regimen or as a continuous SubQ infusion.
Dosing adjustment in renal impairment: Insulin requirements are reduced due to changes in insulin clearance or metabolism. Refer to Insulin Regular on page 748.
Administration Parenteral: SubQ: Administration is usually made into the subcutaneous fat of the thighs, arms, buttocks, or abdomen, with sites rotated; cold

injections should be avoided. May be mixed in the same syringe with Humulin® N, Humulin® U, or NPH insulin. When mixing insulin lispro with other insulins, lispro should be drawn into the syringe first. Administer 15 minutes before meals or immediately after. Can be infused SubQ by external insulin pump; however, when used in an external pump, it is not recommended to be diluted with other insulins.

Monitoring Parameters Urine sugar and acetone, serum glucose, electrolytes, Hb A$_{1c}$, lipid profile

Reference Range Refer to information common to all insulin formulations found in Insulin Regular on page 748.

Patient Information Do not take any new medication during therapy unless approved by healthcare provider. This medication is used to control diabetes; it is not a cure. It is imperative to follow other components of prescribed treatment (eg, diet and exercise regimen). Take exactly as directed. Do not change dose or discontinue unless advised by healthcare provider. With insulin lispro (Humalog®), you must administer 15 minutes before meals or immediately after. If you experience hypoglycemic reaction, contact healthcare provider immediately. Always carry quick source of sugar with you. Monitor glucose levels as directed by healthcare provider. Report adverse side effects, including chest pain or palpitations; persistent fatigue, confusion, headache; skin rash or redness; numbness of mouth, lips, or tongue; muscle weakness or tremors; vision changes; respiratory difficulty; or nausea, vomiting, or flu-like symptoms.

Dosage Forms Excipient information presented when available (limited, particularly for generics); consult specific product labeling.

Injection, solution:

Humalog®: 100 units/mL (3 mL) [prefilled cartridge or prefilled disposable pen]; (10 mL) [vial]

◆ Insulin Lispro and Insulin Lispro Protamine *see* Insulin Lispro Protamine and Insulin Lispro *on page 745*

Insulin Lispro Protamine and Insulin Lispro
(IN soo lin LYE sproe PROE ta meen & IN soo lin LYE sproe)

Medication Safety Issues

Sound-alike/look-alike issues:

Humalog® Mix 50/50™ may be confused with Humalog® and Humulin® 50/50

Humalog® Mix 75/25™ may be confused with Humulin® 70/30, Novolin® 70/30, and NovoLog® Mix 70/30

High alert medication: The Institute for Safe Medication Practices (ISMP) includes this medication among its list of drugs which have a heightened risk of causing significant patient harm when used in error. *Due to the number of insulin preparations, it is essential to identify/clarify the type of insulin to be used.*

Cross-contamination may occur if insulin pens are shared among multiple patients. Steps should be taken to prohibit sharing of insulin pens.

U.S. Brand Names Humalog® Mix 50/50™; Humalog® Mix 75/25™

Canadian Brand Names Humalog® Mix 25

Therapeutic Category Antidiabetic Agent, Parenteral; Insulin, Combination

Generic Available No

Use Treatment of type 1 diabetes mellitus (insulin dependent, IDDM); type 2 diabetes mellitus (noninsulin dependent, NIDDM) to control hyperglycemia

Pregnancy Risk Factor B

Pregnancy Considerations Refer to Insulin Lispro on page 744.

Lactation Refer to Insulin Lispro on page 744.

Breast-Feeding Considerations Refer to Insulin Lispro on page 744.

Contraindications Hypersensitivity to insulin lispro, insulin lispro protamine, or any component; hypoglycemia

Warnings Refer to information common to all insulin formulations found in Insulin Regular. Not for I.V. infusion or use in insulin infusion pumps

Precautions Refer to information common to all insulin formulations found in Insulin Regular.

Adverse Reactions Refer to information common to all insulin formulations found in Insulin Regular.

Drug Interactions

Metabolism/Transport Effects Refer to Insulin Regular on page 748.

Avoid Concomitant Use There are no known interactions where it is recommended to avoid concomitant use.

Increased Effect/Toxicity

Insulin Lispro Protamine and Insulin Lispro may increase the levels/effects of: Antidiabetic Agents (Thiazolidinedione); Hypoglycemic Agents; Quinolone Antibiotics

The levels/effects of Insulin Lispro Protamine and Insulin Lispro may be increased by: Beta-Blockers; Edetate CALCIUM Disodium; Edetate Disodium; Herbs (Hypoglycemic Properties); Pegvisomant

Decreased Effect

The levels/effects of Insulin Lispro Protamine and Insulin Lispro may be decreased by: Corticosteroids (Orally Inhaled); Corticosteroids (Systemic); Luteinizing Hormone-Releasing Hormone Analogs; Somatropin; Thiazide Diuretics

Food Interactions Refer to information common to all insulin formulations found in Insulin Regular.

Stability Store unopened container or pen in refrigerator; do not freeze; protect from light. If refrigeration is not possible, vial (in use) may be stored at room temperature for up to 28 days. The pen (in use) should **not** be refrigerated; store below 30°C (86°F) away from direct heat or light; discard after 10 days. Do not mix or dilute with other insulins.

Mechanism of Action Refer to information common to all insulin formulations found in Insulin Regular. Insulin lispro protamine and insulin lispro is a combination product with a rapid onset and a duration of action which is similar to intermediate-acting insulin products.

Pharmacodynamics

Onset of action: 0.25-0.5 hours

Maximum effect: 2 hours

Duration: 18-24 hours

Pharmacokinetics (Adult data unless noted)

Time to peak serum concentration: 1 hour (median; range: 0.5-4 hours)

Elimination: Urine

Usual Dosage Refer to information common to all insulin formulations found in Insulin Regular. Fixed ratio insulins (such as insulin lispro protamine and insulin lispro combination) are normally administered in 2 daily doses with each dose intended to cover two meals and a snack. Because of variability in the peak affect and individual patient variability in activities, meals, etc, it may be more difficult to achieve complete glycemic control with fixed combination formulations in all patients.

Dosage adjustment in renal impairment: Insulin requirements are reduced with renal impairment; see Insulin Regular.

Administration Parenteral: SubQ: Gently roll vial or pen in the palms of the hands to resuspend before use; administer into the subcutaneous fat of the thighs, arms, buttocks, or abdomen, with sites rotated. Cold injections should be avoided. Administer within 15 minutes before a meal (breakfast and supper). Do not mix or dilute with other insulins. **Not for I.V. administration** or use in an insulin infusion pump.

Monitoring Parameters Refer to information common to all insulin formulations found in Insulin Regular.

Reference Range Refer to information common to all insulin formulations found in Insulin Regular.

Patient Information Refer to information common to all insulin formulations found in Insulin Regular.

Dosage Forms Excipient information presented when available (limited, particularly for generics); consult specific product labeling.

Injection, suspension:

Humalog® Mix 50/50™: Insulin lispro protamine suspension 50% [intermediate acting] and insulin lispro solution 50% [rapid acting]: 100 units/mL (3 mL) [disposable pen]; (10 mL) [vial]

Humalog® Mix 75/25™: Insulin lispro protamine suspension 75% [intermediate acting] and insulin lispro solution 25% [rapid acting]: 100 units/mL (3 mL) [disposable pen]; (10 mL) [vial]

Insulin NPH (IN soo lin N P H)

Medication Safety Issues

Sound-alike/look-alike issues:

Humulin® N may be confused with Humulin® R, Humalog®, Humira®

Novolin® N may be confused with Novolin® R, NovoLog®

High alert medication: The Institute for Safe Medication Practices (ISMP) includes this medication among its list of drugs which have a heightened risk of causing significant patient harm when used in error. *Due to the number of insulin preparations, it is essential to identify/clarify the type of insulin to be used.*

Cross-contamination may occur if insulin pens are shared among multiple patients. Steps should be taken to prohibit sharing of insulin pens.

U.S. Brand Names Humulin® N; Novolin® N

Canadian Brand Names Humulin® N; Novolin® ge NPH

Therapeutic Category Antidiabetic Agent, Insulin; Insulin, Intermediate-Acting

Generic Available No

Use Treatment of type 1 diabetes mellitus (insulin dependent, IDDM); type 2 diabetes mellitus (noninsulin dependent, NIDDM) to control hyperglycemia

Pregnancy Considerations Maternal hyperglycemia can be associated with adverse effects in the fetus, including macrosomia, neonatal hyperglycemia, and hyperbilirubinemia; the risk of congenital malformations is increased when the Hb A_{1c} is above the normal range. Insulin requirements tend to fall during the first trimester of pregnancy and increase in the later trimesters, peaking at 28-32 weeks of gestation. Following delivery, insulin requirements decrease rapidly. Diabetes can be associated with adverse effects in the mother. Poorly-treated diabetes may cause end-organ damage that may in turn negatively affect obstetric outcomes. Physiologic glucose levels should be maintained prior to and during pregnancy to decrease the risk of adverse events in the fetus and the mother. Insulin is the drug of choice for the control of diabetes mellitus during pregnancy. NPH insulin is preferred over other intermediate-acting insulin products during pregnancy.

Lactation Excretion in breast milk unknown/compatible

Breast-Feeding Considerations Endogenous insulin can be found in breast milk. Plasma glucose concentrations in the mother affect glucose concentrations in breast milk. The gastrointestinal tract destroys insulin when administered orally; therefore, insulin is not expected to be absorbed intact by the breast-feeding infant. All types of insulin are safe for use while breast-feeding. Due to increased calorie expenditure, women with diabetes may require less insulin while nursing.

Contraindications Hypersensitivity to NPH insulin or any component

Warnings Refer to information common to all insulin formulations found in Insulin Regular on page 748.

Precautions Refer to information common to all insulin formulations found in Insulin Regular on page 748.

Adverse Reactions Refer to information common to all insulin formulations found in Insulin Regular on page 748.

Drug Interactions

Metabolism/Transport Effects Refer to Insulin Regular on page 748.

Avoid Concomitant Use There are no known interactions where it is recommended to avoid concomitant use.

Increased Effect/Toxicity

Insulin NPH may increase the levels/effects of: Antidiabetic Agents (Thiazolidinedione); Hypoglycemic Agents; Quinolone Antibiotics

The levels/effects of Insulin NPH may be increased by: Beta-Blockers; Edetate CALCIUM Disodium; Edetate Disodium; Herbs (Hypoglycemic Properties); Pegvisomant

Decreased Effect

The levels/effects of Insulin NPH may be decreased by: Corticosteroids (Orally Inhaled); Corticosteroids (Systemic); Luteinizing Hormone-Releasing Hormone Analogs; Somatropin; Thiazide Diuretics

Food Interactions Refer to information common to all insulin formulations found in Insulin Regular on page 748.

Stability Store unopened containers in refrigerator at 2°C to 8°C (36°F to 46°F); do not freeze; protect from direct heat or light. Once opened (in use), vials may be stored in refrigerator or at room temperature for up to 28 days. Cartridges should not be refrigerated; store below 30°C (86°F) away from direct heat or light; discard after 14 days. May be mixed with regular insulin, insulin lispro, insulin aspart, and insulin glulisine (always add the NPH insulin to the mixture last). A sterile diluent is available from the manufacturer for preparing dilutions of Humulin® N.

Mechanism of Action Refer to information common to all insulin formulations found in Insulin Regular on page 748. Insulin NPH is an intermediate-acting form of insulin.

Pharmacodynamics

Onset of action: 1-2 hours

Maximum effect: 6-14 hours

Duration: 18 to >24 hours

Pharmacokinetics (Adult data unless noted)

Elimination: Urine

Usual Dosage Refer to information common to all insulin formulations found in Insulin Regular on page 748. Insulin NPH is an intermediate-acting insulin formulation which is usually administered 1-2 times daily.

Dosing adjustment in renal impairment: Insulin requirements are reduced due to changes in insulin clearance or metabolism.

Administration Parenteral: SubQ: Gently roll vial or pen in the palms of the hands to resuspend before use; administer into the subcutaneous fat of the thighs, arms, buttocks, or abdomen, with sites rotated. Cold injections should be avoided. Administer within 15 minutes before a meal (before breakfast and supper). May be mixed with regular insulin, insulin aspart, insulin lispro, and insulin glulisine. **Not for I.V. administration** or use in insulin infusion pumps.

Monitoring Parameters Urine sugar and acetone, serum glucose, electrolytes, Hb A_{1c}, lipid profile

Reference Range Refer to information common to all insulin formulations found in Insulin Regular on page 748.

Patient Information Do not take any new medication during therapy unless approved by healthcare provider. This medication is used to control diabetes; it is not a cure. It is imperative to follow other components of prescribed treatment (eg, diet and exercise regimen). Take exactly as directed. Do not change dose or discontinue unless advised by healthcare provider. If you experience hypoglycemic reaction, contact healthcare provider immediately. Always carry quick source of sugar with you. Monitor glucose levels as directed by healthcare provider. Report adverse side effects, including chest pain or palpitations; persistent fatigue, confusion, headache; skin rash or redness; numbness of mouth, lips, or tongue; muscle weakness or tremors; vision changes; respiratory difficulty; or nausea, vomiting, or flu-like symptoms.

Dosage Forms Excipient information presented when available (limited, particularly for generics); consult specific product labeling. [CAN] = Canadian brand name; [DSC] = Discontinued product

Injection, suspension:
Humulin® N: 100 units/mL (3 mL) [disposable pen]; (10 mL) [vial]
Novolin® ge NPH [CAN]: 100 units/mL (3 mL) [NovolinSet® prefilled syringe or PenFill® prefilled cartridge]; 10 mL [vial]
Novolin® N: 100 units/mL (3 mL) [InnoLet® prefilled syringe or PenFill® prefilled cartridge] [DSC]; (10 mL) [vial]

Insulin NPH and Insulin Regular
(IN soo lin N P H & IN soo lin REG yoo ler)

Medication Safety Issues
Sound-alike/look-alike issues:
Humulin® 50/50 may be confused with Humalog® Mix 50/50
Humulin® 70/30 may be confused with Humalog® Mix 75/25, Humulin® R, Novolin® 70/30, NovoLog® Mix 70/30
Novolin® 70/30 may be confused with Humalog® Mix 75/25, Humulin® 70/30, Humulin® R, Novolin® R, and NovoLog® Mix 70/30

High alert medication: The Institute for Safe Medication Practices (ISMP) includes this medication among its list of drugs which have a heightened risk of causing significant patient harm when used in error. *Due to the number of insulin preparations, it is essential to identify/clarify the type of insulin to be used.*

Cross-contamination may occur if insulin pens are shared among multiple patients. Steps should be taken to prohibit sharing of insulin pens.

U.S. Brand Names Humulin® 50/50 [DSC]; Humulin® 70/30; Novolin® 70/30

Canadian Brand Names Humulin® 20/80; Humulin® 70/30; Novolin® ge 30/70; Novolin® ge 40/60; Novolin® ge 50/50

Therapeutic Category Antidiabetic Agent, Parenteral; Insulin, Combination

Generic Available No

Use Treatment of type 1 diabetes mellitus (insulin dependent, IDDM); type 2 diabetes mellitus (noninsulin dependent, NIDDM) to control hyperglycemia

Pregnancy Considerations See individual agents.

Breast-Feeding Considerations See individual agents.

Contraindications Hypersensitivity to regular insulin, NPH insulin, or any component; hypoglycemia

Warnings Refer to information common to all insulin formulations found in Insulin Regular. Not for I.V. infusion or use in insulin infusion pumps.

Precautions Refer to information common to all insulin formulations found in Insulin Regular.

Adverse Reactions Refer to information common to all insulin formulations found in Insulin Regular.

Drug Interactions
Metabolism/Transport Effects Refer to Insulin Regular on page 748.
Avoid Concomitant Use There are no known interactions where it is recommended to avoid concomitant use.
Increased Effect/Toxicity
Insulin NPH and Insulin Regular may increase the levels/ effects of: Antidiabetic Agents (Thiazolidinedione); Hypoglycemic Agents; Quinolone Antibiotics

The levels/effects of Insulin NPH and Insulin Regular may be increased by: Beta-Blockers; Edetate CALCIUM Disodium; Edetate Disodium; Herbs (Hypoglycemic Properties); Pegvisomant

Decreased Effect
The levels/effects of Insulin NPH and Insulin Regular may be decreased by: Corticosteroids (Orally Inhaled); Corticosteroids (Systemic); Luteinizing Hormone-Releasing Hormone Analogs; Somatropin; Thiazide Diuretics

Food Interactions Refer to information common to all insulin formulations found in Insulin Regular.

Stability Store unopened container in refrigerator; do not freeze; protect from light. If refrigeration is not possible, vial (in use) may be stored at room temperature for up to 28 days. The pen (in use) should **not** be refrigerated; store below 30°C (86°F) away from direct heat or light; discard after 10 days. Do not mix or dilute with other insulins.

Mechanism of Action Refer to information common to all insulin formulations found in Insulin Regular. Insulin NPH and insulin regular is a combination insulin product with intermediate-acting characteristics.

Pharmacodynamics
Onset of action:
Novolin® 70/30, Humulin® 70/30: 0.5 hours
Humulin® 50/50: 0.5-1 hour
Maximum effect:
Novolin® 70/30, Humulin® 70/30: 1.5-12 hours
Humulin® 50/50: 1.5-4.5 hours
Duration:
Novolin® 70/30, Humulin® 70/30: Up to 24 hours
Humulin® 50/50: 7.5-24 hours

Pharmacokinetics (Adult data unless noted)
Elimination: Urine

Usual Dosage Refer to information common to all insulin formulations found in Insulin Regular. Fixed ratio insulins (such as insulin aspart protamine and insulin aspart combination) are normally administered in 2 daily doses with each dose intended to cover two meals and a snack. Because of variability in the peak affect and individual patient variability in activities, meals, etc, it may be more difficult to achieve complete glycemic control using fixed combinations of insulins in all patients.
Dosing adjustment in renal impairment: Insulin requirements are reduced with renal impairment; see Insulin Regular

Administration Parenteral: SubQ: Gently roll vial or pen in the palms of the hands to resuspend before use; administer into the subcutaneous fat of the thighs, arms, buttocks, or abdomen, with sites rotated. Cold injections should be avoided. Administer within 15 minutes before a meal (before breakfast and supper). Do not mix or dilute with other insulins. **Not for I.V. administration** or use in an insulin infusion pump.

Monitoring Parameters Refer to information common to all insulin formulations found in Insulin Regular.

Reference Range Refer to information common to all insulin formulations found in Insulin Regular.

Patient Information Refer to information common to all insulin formulations found in Insulin Regular.

Dosage Forms Excipient information presented when available (limited, particularly for generics); consult specific product labeling. [DSC] = Discontinued product
Injection, suspension:
Humulin® 50/50: Insulin NPH suspension 50% [intermediate acting] and insulin regular solution 50% [short acting]: 100 units/mL (10 mL) [vial] [DSC]
Humulin® 70/30: Insulin NPH suspension 70% [intermediate acting] and insulin regular solution 30% [short acting]: 100 units/mL (3 mL) [disposable pen]; (10 mL) [vial]
Novolin® 70/30: Insulin NPH suspension 70% [intermediate acting] and insulin regular solution 30% [short acting]: 100 units/mL (3 mL) [InnoLet® prefilled syringe or PenFill® prefilled cartridge] [DSC]; (10 mL) [vial]

Additional formulations available in Canada: Injection, suspension:
Humulin® 20/80: Insulin regular solution 20% [short acting] and insulin NPH suspension 80% [intermediate acting]: 100 units/mL (3 mL) [PenFill® prefilled cartridge]
Novolin® ge 30/70: Insulin regular solution 30% [short acting] and insulin NPH suspension 70% [intermediate acting]: 100 units/mL (3 mL) [prefilled syringe or PenFill® prefilled cartridge]; (10 mL) [vial]
Novolin® ge 40/60: Insulin regular solution 40% [short acting] and insulin NPH suspension 60% [intermediate acting]: 100 units/mL (3 mL) [PenFill® prefilled cartridge]
Novolin® ge 50/50: Insulin regular solution 50% [short acting] and insulin NPH suspension 50% [intermediate acting]: 100 units/mL (3 mL) [PenFill® prefilled cartridge]

Insulin Regular (IN soo lin REG yoo ler)

Medication Safety Issues
Sound-alike/look-alike issues:
Humulin® R may be confused with Humalog®, Humira®, Humulin® 70/30, Humulin® N, Novolin® 70/30, Novolin® R, NovoLog®
Novolin® R may be confused with Humulin® R, Novolin® 70/30, Novolin® N, NovoLog®

High alert medication: The Institute for Safe Medication Practices (ISMP) includes this medication among its list of drugs which have a heightened risk of causing significant patient harm when used in error. *Due to the number of insulin preparations, it is essential to identify/clarify the type of insulin to be used.*

Concentrated solutions (eg, U-500) should not be available in patient care areas. U-500 regular insulin should be stored, dispensed, and administered separately from U-100 regular insulin. For patients who receive U-500 insulin in the hospital setting, highlighting the strength prominently on the patient's medical chart and medication record may help to reduce dispensing errors.

Cross-contamination may occur if insulin pens are shared among multiple patients. Steps should be taken to prohibit sharing of insulin pens.

U.S. Brand Names Humulin® R; Humulin® R U-500; Novolin® R

Canadian Brand Names Humulin® R; Novolin® ge Toronto

Therapeutic Category Antidiabetic Agent, Parenteral; Antidote; Hyperkalemia, Adjunctive Treatment Agent; Insulin, Short-Acting

Generic Available No

Use Treatment of insulin-dependent diabetes mellitus, also noninsulin-dependent diabetes mellitus unresponsive to treatment with diet and/or oral hypoglycemics; to assure proper utilization of glucose and reduce glucosuria in nondiabetic patients receiving parenteral nutrition (glucosuria cannot be adequately controlled with infusion rate adjustments or requires assistance in achieving optimal caloric intakes); treatment of hyperkalemia (use with glucose to shift potassium into cells to lower serum potassium levels)

Pregnancy Considerations Insulin has not been found to cross the placenta, but insulin bound to anti-insulin antibodies has been detected in cord blood. Maternal hyperglycemia can be associated with adverse effects in the fetus, including macrosomia, neonatal hyperglycemia, and hyperbilirubinemia; the risk of congenital malformations is increased when the Hb A_{1c} is above the normal range. Insulin requirements tend to fall during the first trimester of pregnancy and increase in the later trimesters, peaking at 28-32 weeks of gestation. Following delivery, insulin requirements decrease rapidly. Diabetes can be associated with adverse effects in the mother. Poorly-treated diabetes may cause end-organ damage that may in turn negatively affect obstetric outcomes. Physiologic glucose levels should be maintained prior to and during pregnancy to decrease the risk of adverse events in the fetus and the mother. Insulin is the drug of choice for the control of diabetes mellitus during pregnancy.

Lactation Excretion in breast milk unknown/compatible

Breast-Feeding Considerations Endogenous insulin can be found in breast milk. Plasma glucose concentrations in the mother affect glucose concentrations in breast milk. The gastrointestinal tract destroys insulin when administered orally; therefore, insulin is not expected to be absorbed intact by the breast-feeding infant. All types of insulin are safe for use while breast-feeding. Due to increased calorie expenditure, women with diabetes may require less insulin while nursing.

Contraindications Hypersensitivity to regular insulin or any component; hypoglycemia

Warnings Hypoglycemia is the most common adverse effect of insulin. The timing of hypoglycemia differs among various insulin formulations. Any change of insulin should be made cautiously; changing manufacturers, type, and/or method of manufacture may result in the need for a change of dosage. Human insulin differs from animal-source insulin. Hypoglycemia may result from increased work or exercise without eating; use of long-acting insulin preparations (insulin glargine, Ultralente®) with regular insulin may delay recovery from hypoglycemia.

Precautions Use with caution and adjust dosage in patients with renal impairment; use with caution and monitor closely in patient with hepatic impairment. While regular insulin is the preferred formulation for I.V. administration, both insulin aspart and insulin glulisine have been approved for I.V. use in selected clinical situations with close medical supervision and monitoring of serum potassium.

Adverse Reactions Primarily symptoms of hypoglycemia
Cardiovascular: Palpitation, pallor, tachycardia
Central nervous system: Fatigue, headache, hypothermia, loss of consciousness, mental confusion
Dermatologic: Urticaria, redness
Endocrine & metabolic: Hypoglycemia, hypokalemia
Gastrointestinal: Hunger, nausea, numbness of mouth
Local: Atrophy or hypertrophy of SubQ fat tissue; edema, itching, pain or warmth at injection site; stinging
Neuromuscular & skeletal: Muscle weakness, paresthesia, tremor
Ocular: Transient presbyopia or blurred vision
Miscellaneous: Anaphylaxis, diaphoresis, local and/or systemic hypersensitivity reactions

Drug Interactions
Metabolism/Transport Effects Induces CYP1A2 (weak)

Avoid Concomitant Use There are no known interactions where it is recommended to avoid concomitant use.

Increased Effect/Toxicity

Insulin Regular may increase the levels/effects of: Antidiabetic Agents (Thiazolidinedione); Hypoglycemic Agents; Quinolone Antibiotics

The levels/effects of Insulin Regular may be increased by: Beta-Blockers; Edetate CALCIUM Disodium; Edetate Disodium; Herbs (Hypoglycemic Properties); Pegvisomant

Decreased Effect

The levels/effects of Insulin Regular may be decreased by: Corticosteroids (Orally Inhaled); Corticosteroids (Systemic); Luteinizing Hormone-Releasing Hormone Analogs; Somatropin; Thiazide Diuretics

Food Interactions Use caution with chromium, garlic, gymnema (may increase hypoglycemia).

Stability Store unopened containers in refrigerator at 2°C to 8°C (36°F to 46°F); do not freeze; protect from direct heat or light. Once opened (in use) vials may be stored in refrigerator at room temperature for up to 28 days. Regular insulin should only be used if clear. May be mixed in the same syringe with NPH, Lente®, and Ultralente® insulins. For I.V. continuous infusion, may be diluted in NS, ¹/₂NS, D₅W, or D₁₀W.

Stability of parenteral admixture of regular insulin in NS or ¹/₂NS at room temperature (25°C) and at refrigeration temperature (4°C): 24 hours; all bags should be prepared fresh; tubing should be flushed 30 minutes prior to administration to allow adsorption as time permits. See Administration.

Mechanism of Action Insulin acts via specific membrane-bound receptors on target tissues to regulate metabolism of carbohydrate, protein, and fats. Insulin facilitates entry of glucose into muscle, adipose, and other tissues via hexose transporters, including GLUT4. Insulin stimulates the cellular uptake of amino acids and increases cellular permeability to several ions, including potassium, magnesium, and phosphate. By activating sodium-potassium ATPases, insulin promotes the intracellular movement of potassium.

Target organs for insulin include the liver, skeletal muscle, and adipose tissue. Within the liver, insulin stimulates hepatic glycogen synthesis through the activation of the enzymes hexokinase, phosphofructokinase, and glycogen synthase as well as the inhibition of glucose-6 phosphatase. Insulin promotes hepatic synthesis of fatty acids, which are released into the circulation as lipoproteins. Skeletal muscle effects of insulin include increased protein synthesis and increased glycogen synthesis. Within adipose tissue, insulin stimulates the processing of circulating lipoproteins to provide free fatty acids, facilitating triglyceride synthesis and storage by adipocytes. Insulin also directly inhibits the hydrolysis of triglycerides.

Normally secreted by the pancreas, insulin products are manufactured for pharmacologic use through recombinant DNA technology using either *E. coli* or *Saccharomyces cerevisiae*. Insulins are categorized based on promptness and duration of effect, including rapid-, short-, intermediate-, and long-acting insulins. Regular insulin is considered a "short-acting" insulin.

Pharmacodynamics Onset and duration of hypoglycemic effects depend upon the route of administration (adsorption and onset of action are more rapid after deeper I.M. injections than after SubQ), site of injection (onset and duration are progressively slower with SubQ injection into the abdomen, arm, buttock, or thigh respectively), volume and concentration of injection, and the preparation administered; local heat and massage also increase the rate of absorption.

Onset of action: Approximately 30-60 minutes
Maximum effect: 1-5 hours
Duration: 6-10 hours (may increase with dose)

Pharmacokinetics (Adult data unless noted)

Distribution: V$_d$: 0.26-0.36 L/kg
Half-life: SubQ: 1.5 hours
Excretion: Urine

Usual Dosage The general objective of insulin replacement therapy is to approximate the physiologic pattern of insulin secretion. This requires a basal level of insulin throughout the day, supplemented by additional insulin at mealtimes. Since combinations using different types of insulins are frequently used, dosage adjustment must address the individual component of the insulin regimen which most directly influences the blood glucose value in question, based on the known onset and duration of the insulin component. The frequency of doses and monitoring must be individualized in consideration of the patient's ability to manage therapy. Diabetic education and nutritional counseling are essential to maximize the effectiveness of therapy.

Type 1 diabetes mellitus: Children and Adults: **Note:** Multiple daily doses guided by blood glucose monitoring are the standard of diabetes care. The following daily doses are expressed as the total units/kg/day of all insulin formulations used.

Initial dose: SubQ: 0.2-0.6 units/kg/day in divided doses. Conservative initial doses of 0.2-0.4 units/kg/day are often recommended to avoid the potential for hypoglycemia. Regular insulin may be the only insulin formulation used initially.

Division of daily insulin requirement ("conventional therapy"): Generally, 50% to 75% of the daily insulin dose is given as an intermediate- or long-acting form of insulin (in 1-2 daily injections). The remaining portion of the 24-hour insulin requirement is divided and administered as either regular insulin or a rapid acting form of insulin at the same time before breakfast and dinner.

Division of daily insulin requirement ("intensive therapy"): Basal insulin delivery with one or two doses of intermediate- or long-acting insulin formulations superimposed with doses of rapid or very rapid-acting insulin formulations three or more times daily.

Adjustment of dose: Dosage must be titrated to achieve glucose control and avoid hypoglycemia. Adjust dose to maintain premeal and bedtime glucose in target range (see Reference Range). Since combinations of agents are frequently used, dosage adjustment must address the individual component of the insulin regimen which most directly influences the blood glucose value in question, based on the known onset and duration of the insulin component.

Usual maintenance range: 0.5-1 unit/kg/day in divided doses. An estimate of anticipated needs may be based on body weight and/or activity factors as follows:
Adolescents: May require ≤1.2 units/kg/day during growth spurts
Nonobese: 0.4-0.6 units/kg/day
Obese: 0.8-1.2 units/kg/day

Continuous SubQ insulin infusion (insulin pump): Regular insulin, insulin lispro, insulin aspart, and insulin glulisine: Combination of a "basal" continuous insulin infusion rate using one of these insulin formulations with preprogrammed, premeal bolus doses which are patient controlled. When converting from multiple daily SubQ doses of maintenance insulin, it is advisable to reduce the basal rate to less than the equivalent of the total daily units of longer acting insulin, eg NPH. Divide the total number of units by 24 to get the basal rate in units/hour. Do not include the total units of regular insulin or other rapid-acting insulin formulations in this calculation. The same premeal regular insulin dosage may be used.

Type 2 diabetes mellitus: Augmentation therapy (patients for which diet, exercise, weight reduction, and oral hypoglycemics have not been adequate): Adults: Initial dosage of 0.15-0.2 units/kg/day (10-12 units) of an intermediate- or long-acting insulin administered at bedtime has been recommended. As an alternative, regular insulin or rapid-acting insulin formulations administered before meals have also been used. Dosage must be carefully adjusted.

Diabetic ketoacidosis:
Children: I.V. continuous infusion: 0.05-0.1 units/kg/hour (range: 0.05-0.2 units/kg/hour) depending upon the rate of decrease of serum glucose (decreasing the serum glucose level too rapidly may lead to cerebral edema; optimum rate of decrease of serum glucose 80-100 mg/dL/hour). Continue infusion until acidosis clears (pH >7.3 and HCO_3 >25 mEq/L), not when the blood glucose normalizes. SubQ therapy may begin when the HCO_3 >16 mE/L, pH >7.3, and/or anion gap <16mEq/L. Continue I.V. insulin until the onset of the SubQ insulin dose (for regular insulin: 30-60 minutes).

Adults: I.V.: Regular insulin 0.15 units/kg (approximately 15-20 units) initially followed by an infusion of 0.1 units/kg/hour (approximately 7 units/hour); increase infusion rate achieve glucose serum reduction of 50-70 mg/dL/hour. Decrease dose to 0.05-0.1 units/kg/hour once serum glucose reaches 250 mg/dL and ketoacidosis/acid-base abnormalities have resolved.

Note: Newly-diagnosed patients with IDDM presenting in DKA and patients with blood sugars <800 mg/dL may be relatively "sensitive" to insulin and should receive loading and initial maintenance doses ~50% of those indicated.

Optimization of caloric intake while on parenteral nutrition: Neonates: Continuous I.V. infusion: 0.01-0.1 units/kg/hour; neonates are very sensitive to insulin; start at low end of infusion rate and monitor closely

Hyperkalemia (after treatment with calcium and sodium bicarbonate): I.V.
Children: Dextrose 0.5-1 g/kg (using $D_{25}W$ or $D_{50}W$) combined with regular insulin 1 unit for every 4-5 g dextrose; infuse over 2 hours **OR** as an alternative, dextrose 0.5-1 g/kg infused over 15-30 minutes followed by 0.1 unit/kg insulin SubQ or I.V.

Adults: 10 units regular insulin mixed with 25 g dextrose (50 mL $D_{50}W$) given over 15-30 minutes (see ACLS, 2005); alternatively, 50 mL $D_{50}W$ over 5 minutes followed by 10 units regular insulin I.V. push over seconds may be administered in the setting of imminent cardiac arrest. In patients with ongoing cardiac arrest (eg, PEA with presumed hyperkalemia), administration of $D_{50}W$ over <5 minutes is routine. Effects on potassium are temporary. As appropriate, consider methods of enhancing potassium removal/excretion.

Dosing adjustment in renal impairment (regular): Insulin requirements are reduced due to changes in insulin clearance or metabolism
Cl_{cr} 10-50 mL/minute: Administer at 75% of recommended dose
Cl_{cr} <10 mL/minute: Administer at 25% to 50% of recommended dose and monitor glucose closely
Hemodialysis: Because of a large molecular weight (6000 daltons), insulin is not significantly removed by either peritoneal or hemodialysis; supplemental dose is not necessary
Peritoneal dialysis: Supplemental dose is not necessary
Continuous arteriovenous or venovenous hemofiltration effects: Supplemental dose is not necessary

Administration Parenteral:
SubQ, I.M.: Administration is usually made into the subcutaneous fat of the thighs, arms, buttocks, or abdomen, with sites rotated; may be administered I.M.

however, SubQ is the preferred route. When mixing regular insulin with other insulin preparations, regular insulin should be drawn into the syringe first; administer 30-60 minutes before meals. May be infused SubQ by external insulin pump; however, when used in an external pump, it is not recommended to be diluted with other solutions.

I.V.: Regular insulin is the preferred insulin formulation approved for I.V. administration (insulin aspart and insulin glulisine have been approved for I.V. administration in carefully controlled clinical settings with medical supervision and close monitoring of blood glucose as well as serum potassium); to minimize absorption of insulin to I.V. solution bag or tubing:

If new tubing is **not** needed: Wait a minimum of 30 minutes between the preparation of the solution and the initiation of the infusion.

If new tubing is needed: After receiving the insulin continuous infusion solution, the administration set should be attached to the I.V. container and the line should be flushed with the insulin solution, wait 30 minutes, then flush the line again with the insulin solution prior to initiating the infusion.

Because of adsorption, the actual amount of insulin being administered could be substantially less than the apparent amount. Therefore, adjustment of the insulin drip rate should be based on the effect and not solely on the apparent insulin dose. Furthermore, the apparent I.V. infusion dose should not be used as the basis for determining the subsequent insulin dose upon discontinuing the insulin drip. Dosage adjustment requires continuous medical supervision.

Monitoring Parameters Urine sugar and acetone, serum glucose, electrolytes, Hb A_{1c}, lipid profile
DKA: Arterial blood gases (initial), venous pH, CBC with differential, urinalysis, serum glucose (baseline and every hour until reaches 250 mg/dL), BUN, creatinine, electrolytes, anion gap, I&O
Hyperkalemia: Serum potassium and glucose must be closely monitored to avoid hypoglycemia and/or hypokalemia.

Reference Range
Glucose, fasting:
Newborns: 30-90 mg/dL
Adults: 70-110 mg/dL
Recommendations for glycemic control with type 1 diabetes:
Hb A_{1c}:
<6 years: ≤8.5% and ≥7.5%
6-12 years: <8%
13-19 years: <7.5%
Adults: <7%
Plasma glucose*:
Preprandial:
<6 years: 90-130 mg/dL
6-12 years: 90-180 mg/dL
13 years to Adults: 90-130 mg/dL
Bedtime and overnight:
<6 years: 110-200 mg/dL
6-12 years: 100-180 mg/dL
13-19 years: 90-150 mg/dL
Peak postprandial**: Adults: <180 mg/dL
*Plasma glucose concentrations are generally 10% to 15% higher than those in whole blood
**Peak postprandial plasma glucose is measured 1-2 hours after a meal
Criteria for diagnosis of DKA:
Serum glucose:
Children: >200 mg/dL
Adults: >250 mg/dL
Arterial pH:
Children: <7.3
Adults: <7-7.24

Bicarbonate:
Children: <15 mEq/L
Adults: <10-15 mEq/L
Moderate ketonuria or ketonemia

Patient Information Do not take any new medication during therapy unless approved by healthcare provider. This medication is used to control diabetes; it is not a cure. It is imperative to follow other components of prescribed treatment (eg, diet and exercise regimen). Take exactly as directed. Do not change dose or discontinue unless advised by healthcare provider. If you experience hypoglycemic reaction, contact healthcare provider immediately. Always carry quick source of sugar with you. Monitor glucose levels as directed by healthcare provider. Report adverse side effects, including chest pain or palpitations; persistent fatigue, confusion, headache; skin rash or redness; numbness of mouth, lips, or tongue; muscle weakness or tremors; vision changes; respiratory difficulty; or nausea, vomiting, or flu-like symptoms.

Additional Information In mild diabetic ketoacidosis or unusual circumstances, for patients without I.V. access, SubQ or I.M. regular insulin has been used. Doses are similar to the doses recommended for bolus and the hourly infusion (total dose administered once per hour). If volume depletion and secondary sympathetic activation decrease local perfusion, insulin absorption may be inconsistent. For this reason, many clinicians do not recommend this approach.

Dosage Forms Excipient information presented when available (limited, particularly for generics); consult specific product labeling. [DSC] = Discontinued product

Injection, solution:
Humulin® R: 100 units/mL (10 mL)
Novolin® R: 100 units/mL (3 mL) [InnoLet® prefilled syringe or PenFill® prefilled cartridge] [DSC]; (10 mL) [vial]
Injection, solution [concentrate]:
Humulin® R U-500: 500 units/mL (20 mL vial)

References

"2005 American Heart Association Guidelines for Cardiopulmonary Resuscitation and Emergency Cardiovascular Care," *Circulation*, 2005, 112(24 Suppl): 1-211.
American Diabetes Association, "Standards of Medical Care in Diabetes," *Diabetes Care*, 2007, 30(Suppl 1):4-41.
Simeon PS, Geffner ME, Levin SR, et al, "Continuous Insulin Infusions in Neonates: Pharmacologic Availability of Insulin in Intravenous Solutions," *J Pediatr*, 1994, 124(5 Pt 1):818-20.

◆ **Insulin Regular and Insulin NPH** *see* Insulin NPH and Insulin Regular *on page* 747

◆ **Intal® [DSC]** *see* Cromolyn *on page* 363

◆ **Intal® (Can)** *see* Cromolyn *on page* 363

◆ **α-2-interferon** *see* Interferon Alfa-2b *on page* 751

◆ **Interferon Alfa-2b (PEG Conjugate)** *see* Peginterferon Alfa-2b *on page* 1071

Interferon Alfa-2b (in ter FEER on AL fa too bee)

Medication Safety Issues

Sound-alike/look-alike issues:
Interferon alfa-2b may be confused with interferon alfa-2a, interferon alfa-n3, pegylated interferon alfa-2b
Intron® A may be confused with PEG-Intron®

International issues:
Interferon alfa-2b may be confused with interferon alpha multi-subtype which is available in international markets

Related Information

Emetogenic Potential of Antineoplastic Agents *on page* 1579

U.S. Brand Names Intron® A
Canadian Brand Names Intron® A

Therapeutic Category Antineoplastic Agent, Miscellaneous; Biological Response Modulator; Interferon
Generic Available No
Use

Treatment of chronic hepatitis B (FDA approved in ages ≥1 year and adults); chronic hepatitis C (in combination with ribavirin) (FDA approved in ages ≥3 years and adults); chronic hepatitis C (without ribavirin) (FDA approved in adults); hairy cell leukemia (FDA approved in adults); treatment of AIDS-related Kaposi's sarcoma (FDA approved in adults); condylomata acuminata (FDA approved in adults); adjuvant therapy of malignant melanoma following surgical excision (FDA approved in adults); and follicular non-Hodgkin's lymphoma (FDA approved in adults)

Other uses include hemangiomas of infancy, AIDS-related thrombocytopenia, cutaneous ulcerations of Behçet's disease, neuroendocrine tumors (including carcinoid syndrome and islet cell tumor), cutaneous T-cell lymphoma, desmoid tumor, lymphomatoid granulomatosis, hepatitis D, chronic myelogenous leukemia (CML), non-Hodgkin's lymphomas (other than follicular lymphoma, see approved use), multiple myeloma, renal cell carcinoma, West Nile virus

Medication Guide An FDA-approved patient medication guide, which is available with the product information and at http://www.fda.gov/downloads/Drugs/DrugSafety/ucm111337.pdf, must be dispensed with this medication for each new outpatient prescription and refill.

Pregnancy Risk Factor C / X in combination with ribavirin

Pregnancy Considerations Animal studies have demonstrated abortifacient effects. Disruption of the normal menstrual cycle was also observed in animal studies; therefore, the manufacturer recommends that reliable contraception is used in women of childbearing potential. Alfa interferon is endogenous to normal amniotic fluid. *In vitro* administration studies have reported that when administered to the mother, it does not cross the placenta. Case reports of use in pregnant women are limited. The Perinatal HIV Guidelines Working Group does not recommend that interferon-alfa be used during pregnancy. Interferon alfa-2b monotherapy should only be used in pregnancy when the potential benefit to the mother justifies the possible risk to the fetus. Combination therapy with ribavirin is contraindicated in pregnancy (refer to Ribavirin monograph); two forms of contraception should be used during combination therapy and patients should have monthly pregnancy tests. A pregnancy registry has been established for women inadvertently exposed to ribavirin while pregnant (800-593-2214).

Lactation Enters breast milk/not recommended (AAP rates "compatible")

Breast-Feeding Considerations Breast milk samples obtained from a lactating mother prior to and after administration of interferon alfa-2b showed that interferon alfa is present in breast milk and administration of the medication did not significantly affect endogenous levels. The AAP considers interferon alfa to be "usually compatible with breast-feeding." Breast-feeding is not linked to the spread of hepatitis C virus; however, if nipples are cracked or bleeding, breast-feeding is not recommended. Mothers coinfected with HIV are discouraged from breast-feeding to decrease potential transmission of HIV.

Contraindications Hypersensitivity to interferon alfa or any component; autoimmune hepatitis, hepatic decompensation

Warnings Safety and efficacy in children <18 years of age have not been established. Hazardous agent; use appropriate precautions for handling and disposal. Alpha interferons suppress bone marrow function which may result in severe cytopenias or aplastic anemia. Alpha interferons may cause or aggravate fatal or life-threatening neuropsychiatric, autoimmune, ischemic, and infectious disorders **[U.S. Boxed Warning]**. Depression, suicidal ideation, suicidal attempts, and suicides in association with interferon alfa therapy in patients with and without previous psychiatric symptoms has been reported. Suicidal ideation or attempts may occur more frequently in pediatric patients as compared to adults. Patients should be monitored closely and those patients with severe or worsening signs or symptoms of these conditions should be withdrawn from therapy.

Ophthalmologic disorders including vision loss, retinopathy, optic neuritis, and papilledema have occurred; close monitoring is advised. Development of autoimmune diseases including vasculitis, ITP, rheumatoid arthritis, SLE, and hepatitis have been reported in patients on alfa interferon. Patients being treated for chronic hepatitis B or C with a history of autoimmune disease or who are immunosuppressed transplant recipients should not receive interferon alfa-2b. Do not treat patients with visceral AIDS-related Kaposi's sarcoma associated with rapidly-progressing or life-threatening disease.

May cause hepatotoxicity; monitor closely if abnormal liver function tests develop. A transient increase in ALT (≥2 times baseline) may occur in patients treated with interferon alfa-2b for chronic hepatitis B. Worsening and potentially fatal liver disease, including jaundice, hepatic encephalopathy, and hepatic failure have been reported in patients receiving interferon alfa for chronic hepatitis B and C with decompensated liver disease, autoimmune hepatitis, history of autoimmune disease, and immunosuppressed transplant recipients; avoid interferon treatment in these patients. Discontinue treatment in any patient developing signs or symptoms of liver failure.

Pulmonary infiltrates, pneumonitis, and pneumonia have been reported with interferon alfa therapy; occurs more frequently in patients being treated for chronic hepatitis C. Patients with fever, cough, dyspnea, or other respiratory symptoms should be evaluated with a chest x-ray; monitor closely and consider discontinuing treatment with evidence of impaired pulmonary function.

Diluent for interferon alfa-2b injection may contain benzyl alcohol which can cause allergic reactions in susceptible individuals; large amounts of benzyl alcohol (≥99 mg/kg/day) have been associated with a potentially fatal toxicity ("gasping syndrome") in neonates; the "gasping syndrome" consists of metabolic acidosis, respiratory distress, gasping respirations, CNS dysfunction (including convulsions, intracranial hemorrhage), hypotension and cardiovascular collapse; avoid use of interferon alfa-2b products containing benzyl alcohol in neonates; in vitro and animal studies have shown that benzoate, a metabolite of benzyl alcohol, displaces bilirubin from protein binding sites

Precautions Use with caution in patients with pulmonary function impairment, seizure disorders, brain metastases, compromised CNS, multiple sclerosis, arrhythmias, and patients with pre-existing cardiac disease, severe renal dysfunction (Cl_{cr} <50 mL/minute), hepatic impairment, or myelosuppression. Use caution in patients with diabetes, pre-existing thyroid disease, coagulopathy, hypertension, or in patients receiving drugs that may cause lactic acidosis. Product of human plasma; may potentially contain infectious agents which could transmit disease. Screening of donors, as well as testing and/or inactivation or removal of certain viruses, reduces the risk. Due to differences in dosage, patients should not change brands of interferons without the concurrence of their healthcare provider.

Adverse Reactions Flu-like symptoms (arthralgia, chills, fatigue/malaise, fever, headache, myalgia, rigors) begin about 2-6 hours after the dose is given and may persist as long as 24 hours; usually patient can build up a tolerance to side effects

Cardiovascular: Arrhythmias, cardiomyopathy, chest pain, edema, hypotension, MI, syncope, tachycardia, vasculitis

Central nervous system: Agitation, chills, confusion, depression, dizziness, EEG abnormalities, fatigue/malaise, fever, headache, impaired memory, psychiatric symptoms (depression, mania, psychosis, suicidal behavior), sensory neuropathy

Dermatologic: Angioedema, dry skin, partial alopecia, pruritus, rash, urticaria

Endocrine & metabolic: Growth retardation, hyperglycemia, hypertriglyceridemia, thyroid dysfunction, uric acid level elevated, weight loss

Gastrointestinal: Abdominal cramps, anorexia, diarrhea, dysgeusia, GI hemorrhage, nausea, pancreatitis, stomatitis, ulcerative colitis, vomiting, xerostomia

Hematologic: Anemia, leukopenia (mainly neutropenia), neutralizing antibodies, thrombocytopenia

Hepatic: ALT and AST elevated, ascites, hepatitis

Local: Burning, erythema, pain, rash at the site of injection

Neuromuscular & skeletal: Arthralgia, leg cramps, myalgia, rigors, spondylitis, tendonitis

Ocular: Blurred vision, optic neuritis, papilledema, retinal hemorrhage

Renal: BUN and serum creatinine elevated, interstitial nephritis, proteinuria

Respiratory: Coughing, dyspnea, interstitial pneumonitis, nasal congestion, pulmonary infiltrates

Miscellaneous: Anaphylaxis, diaphoresis, flu-like symptoms, SLE

Drug Interactions

Metabolism/Transport Effects Inhibits CYP1A2 (weak)

Avoid Concomitant Use

Avoid concomitant use of Interferon Alfa-2b with any of the following: Telbivudine

Increased Effect/Toxicity

Interferon Alfa-2b may increase the levels/effects of: Aldesleukin; Methadone; Ribavirin; Telbivudine; Theophylline Derivatives; Zidovudine

Decreased Effect There are no known significant interactions involving a decrease in effect.

Stability Refrigerate; do not freeze; do not shake; reconstituted solution from powder for injection is stable for 24 hours when refrigerated; after first use of prefilled pen, discard unused portion after 1 month

Mechanism of Action Inhibits cellular growth, alters the state of cellular differentiation, interferes with oncogene expression, alters cell surface antigen expression, increases phagocytic activity of macrophages, and augments cytotoxicity of lymphocytes for target cells

Pharmacokinetics (Adult data unless noted)

Metabolism: Majority of dose is thought to be metabolized in the kidney, filtered and absorbed at the renal tubule

Bioavailability:
I.M.: 83%
SubQ: 90%

Half-life, elimination:
I.M., I.V.: 2 hours
SubQ: 3 hours

Time to peak serum concentration: I.M., SubQ: ~3-8 hours

Usual Dosage Note: Withhold treatment for ANC <500/mm^3 or platelets <25,000/mm^3. Consider premedication with acetaminophen prior to administration to reduce the incidence of some adverse reactions. Not all dosage forms and strengths are appropriate for all indications; refer to product labeling for details.

Children: SubQ:
Chronic hepatitis B: 3 million units/m^2 3 times/week for 1 week; then 6 million units/m^2 3 times/week; maximum: 10 million units 3 times/week; total duration of therapy 16-24 weeks
Chronic hepatitis C: 3-5 million units/m^2 3 times/week
Hemangiomas: 3 million units/m^2 daily
Adults:
Hairy cell leukemia: I.M., SubQ: 2 million units/m^2 3 times/week for up to 6 months (may continue treatment with continued treatment response)
AIDS-related Kaposi's sarcoma: I.M., SubQ: 30 million units/m^2 3 times/week
Condylomata acuminata: Intralesionally: 1 million units/lesion 3 times/week (on alternate days) for 3 weeks; not to exceed 5 million units per treatment (maximum dose: 5 lesions at one time) (use only the 10 million units vial); may administer a second course at 12-16 weeks
Chronic hepatitis B: I.M., SubQ: 5 million units given once daily **or** 10 million units given 3 times/week for 4 months
Chronic hepatitis C: I.M., SubQ: 3 million units 3 times/week for 16 weeks. In patients with normalization of ALT at 16 weeks, continue treatment for 18-24 months; consider discontinuation if normalization does not occur at 16 weeks. **Note:** May be used in combination therapy with ribavirin in previously untreated patients or in patients who relapse following alpha interferon therapy.
Lymphoma (follicular): SubQ: 5 million units 3 times/week for ≤18 months
Malignant melanoma adjuvant therapy:
Induction: I.V.: 20 million units/m^2/dose 5 days/week for 4 weeks
Maintenance: SubQ: 10 million units/m^2/dose 3 days/week for 48 weeks
Administration Parenteral: SubQ (rather than I.M.) administration is suggested for those patients who are at risk for bleeding or are thrombocytopenic; rotate SubQ injection site to help minimize local reactions
Monitoring Parameters Baseline ECG, CBC with differential and platelet count, hemoglobin, hematocrit, blood glucose, liver function tests, renal function tests, TSH levels, triglyceride levels, electrolytes, weight, chest x-ray, neuropsychiatric monitoring (including depressive symptomatology), ophthalmologic examination
Patient Information Read the patient Medication Guide that you receive with each prescription and refill of interferon alfa-2b. Do not change brands of interferon as changes in dosage may result; do not operate heavy machinery while on therapy since changes in mental status may occur; may cause dry mouth. Report any signs of depression or suicidal ideation to your physician.
Nursing Implications Patient should be well hydrated; may pretreat with NSAID or acetaminophen to decrease fever and its severity and to alleviate headache
Additional Information Myelosuppressive effects:
WBC: Mild
Platelets: Mild
Onset (days): 7-10
Nadir (days): 14
Recovery (days): 21
Dosage Forms Excipient information presented when available (limited, particularly for generics); consult specific product labeling.
Injection, powder for reconstitution [preservative free]:
Intron® A: 10 million int. units; 18 million int. units; 50 million int. units [contains human albumin]
Injection, solution:
Intron® A: 6 million int. units/mL (3 mL); 10 million int. units/1 mL (2.5 mL) [contains edetate disodium, polysorbate 80]
Intron® A: 3 million int. units/0.2 mL (1.2 mL) [contains edetate disodium, polysorbate 80; delivers 6 doses of 0.2 mL each; 18 million int. units total per pen]
Intron® A: 5 million int. units/0.2 mL (1.2 mL) [contains edetate disodium, polysorbate 80; delivers 6 doses of 0.2 mL each; 30 million int. units total per pen]
Intron® A: 10 million int. units/0.2 mL (1.2 mL) [contains edetate disodium, polysorbate 80; delivers 6 doses of 0.2 mL each; 60 million int. units total per pen]

References
Davis GL, Balart LA, Schiff ER, et al, "Treatment of Chronic Hepatitis C With Recombinant Interferon Alfa. A Multicenter Randomized, Controlled Trial. Hepatitis Interventional Therapy Group," *N Engl J Med*, 1989, 321(22):1501-6.
Garmendia G, Miranda N, Borroso S, et al, "Regression of Infancy Hemangiomas With Recombinant IFN-Alpha 2b," *J Interferon Cytokine Res*, 2001, 21(1):31-8.
Gurakan F, Kocak N, Ozen H, et al, "Comparison of Standard and High Dosage Recombinant Interferon Alpha 2b for Treatment of Children With Chronic Hepatitis B Infection," *Pediatr Infect Dis J*, 2000, 19 (1):52-6.
Kirkwood JM, Ibrahim JG, Sondak VK, et al, "High- and Low-Dose Interferon Alfa-2b in High-Risk Melanoma: First Analysis of Intergroup Trial E1690/S9111/C9190," *J Clin Oncol*, 2000, 18(12):2444-58.
Zwiener RJ, Fielman BA, Cochran C, et al, "Interferon-Alpha-2b Treatment of Chronic Hepatitis C in Children With Hemophilia," *Pediatr Infect Dis J*, 1996, 15(10):906-8.

◆ **Interferon Alpha-2b** *see* Interferon Alfa-2b *on page 751*
◆ **Interleukin-1 Receptor Antagonist** *see* Anakinra *on page 108*
◆ **Interleukin 2** *see* Aldesleukin *on page 60*
◆ **Interleukin-11** *see* Oprelvekin *on page 1025*
◆ **Intralipid®** *see* Fat Emulsion *on page 563*
◆ **Intravenous Fat Emulsion** *see* Fat Emulsion *on page 563*
◆ **Intron® A** *see* Interferon Alfa-2b *on page 751*
◆ **Intropin** *see* DOPamine *on page 472*
◆ **Intuniv™** *see* GuanFACINE *on page 660*
◆ **Invanz®** *see* Ertapenem *on page 523*
◆ **Invirase®** *see* Saquinavir *on page 1245*
◆ **Iodex [OTC]** *see* Iodine *on page 753*

Iodine (EYE oh dyne)

Medication Safety Issues
Sound-alike/look-alike issues:
Iodine may be confused with codeine, Iopidine®, Lodine®
U.S. Brand Names Iodex [OTC]; Iodoflex™; Iodosorb®
Therapeutic Category Topical Skin Product
Generic Available Yes: Tincture
Use Used topically as an antiseptic in the management of minor, superficial skin wounds and has been used to disinfect the skin preoperatively
Pregnancy Considerations An adequate amount of iodine intake is essential for thyroid function. Iodine crosses the placenta and requirements are increased during pregnancy. Iodine deficiency in pregnancy can lead to neurologic damage in the newborn; an extreme form, cretinism, is characterized by gross mental retardation, short stature, deaf mutism, and spasticity. Large amounts of iodine during pregnancy can cause fetal goiter or hyperthyroidism. Transient hypothyroidism in the newborn has also been reported following topical or vaginal use prior to delivery.
Lactation Enters breast milk/use caution (AAP rates "compatible")
Breast-Feeding Considerations Iodine is excreted in breast milk and is a source of iodine for the nursing infant. Actual levels are variable, but have been reported as 113-270 mcg/L in American women. Application of topical iodine antiseptic solutions can be absorbed in amounts which may affect levels in breast milk. Exposure to excess iodine may cause thyrotoxicosis. Skin rash in the nursing

infant has been reported with maternal intake of potassium iodide.

Contraindications Hypersensitivity to iodine preparations or any component; neonates; Hashimoto thyroiditis, history of Grave's disease, or nontoxic nodular goiter

Warnings May be highly toxic if ingested; iodine may be absorbed systemically, especially when large wounds are treated or when used in neonates. Not for application to large areas of the body or for use with tight or air-excluding bandages. When used for self medication (OTC), do not use on deep wounds, puncture wounds, animal bites, or serious burns without consulting with healthcare provider. Notify healthcare provider if condition does not improve within 7 days. Iodosorb® is for use as topical application to wet wounds only.

Precautions Use with caution in patients with renal dysfunction; since iodine may be absorbed systemically, thyroid function may need to be monitored when used chronically or over a large area.

Adverse Reactions

Endocrine & metabolic: Increase TSH

Local: Skin irritation, discoloration, eczema, edema, pain, redness

Miscellaneous: Hypersensitivity, allergic reactions

Drug Interactions

Avoid Concomitant Use There are no known interactions where it is recommended to avoid concomitant use.

Increased Effect/Toxicity There are no known significant interactions involving an increase in effect.

Decreased Effect There are no known significant interactions involving a decrease in effect.

Stability Store at room temperature.

Mechanism of Action Free iodine oxidizes microbial protoplasm making it effective against bacteria, fungi, yeasts, protozoa, and viruses; complexes with amino groups in tissue compounds to form iodophors from which the iodine is slowly released causing a sustained action. Iodosorb® and Iodoflex™ contain iodine in hydrophilic beads of cadexomer which allows a slow release of iodine into the wound.

Pharmacokinetics (Adult data unless noted)

Absorption: Topical: Amount absorbed systemically depends upon the iodine concentration and skin characteristics

Metabolism: Degraded by amylases normally present in wound fluid

Excretion: Urine (>90%)

Usual Dosage Children and Adults:

Antiseptic for minor cuts, scrapes: Apply small amount to affected area 1-3 times/day

Cleaning wet ulcers and wounds (Iodosorb®, Iodoflex™): Apply to clean wound; maximum: 50 g/application and 150 g/week. Change dressing ~3 times/week; reduce applications as exudate decreases. Do not use for >3 months; discontinue when wound is free of exudate.

Administration Topical: Apply to affected areas; avoid tight bandages because iodine may cause burns on occluded skin.

Iodosorb®: Apply 1/8" to 1/4" thickness to dry sterile gauze, then place prepared gauze onto clean wound. Change dressing when gel changes color from brown to yellow/gray (~3 times/week). Remove with sterile water, saline, or wound cleanser; gently blot fluid from surface leaving wound slightly moist before reapplying gel.

Patient Information May stain skin and clothing; may experience transient pain within the first hour after application

Additional Information Sodium thiosulfate inactivates iodine and is an effective chemical antidote for iodine poisoning; solutions of sodium thiosulfate may be used to remove iodine stains from skin and clothing

Dosage Forms Excipient information presented when available (limited, particularly for generics); consult specific product labeling.

Dressing, topical [gel pad] (Iodoflex™): 0.9% (5 g, 10 g)

Gel, topical (Iodosorb®): 0.9% (40 g)

Ointment, topical (Iodex): 4.7% (30 g, 720 g)

Tincture, topical: 2% (30 mL, 480 mL); 7% (30 mL, 480 mL)

◆ **Iodine and Potassium Iodide** *see* Potassium Iodide and Iodine *on page 1140*

◆ **Iodine Sodium** *see* Trace Metals *on page 1366*

Iodixanol (EYE oh dix an ole)

Medication Safety Issues

Not for intrathecal use

High alert medication: The Institute for Safe Medication Practices (ISMP) includes this medication among its list of drugs which have a heightened risk of causing significant patient harm when used in error.

U.S. Brand Names Visipaque™

Canadian Brand Names Visipaque™

Therapeutic Category Radiological/Contrast Media, Nonionic

Generic Available No

Use Nonionic contrast media for radiological use intra-arterially: Digital subtraction angiography; angiocardiography (left ventriculography and selective coronary arteriography), peripheral arteriography, visceral arteriography, and cerebralarteriography. Intravenously: Contrast enhanced computed tomography (CECT) imaging of the head and body, excretory urography, and peripheral venography

Pregnancy Risk Factor B

Pregnancy Considerations Fetal harm was not observed in animal studies. There are no adequate and well-controlled studies in pregnant women. In general, iodinated contrast media agents are avoided during pregnancy unless essential for diagnosis.

Lactation Excretion in breast milk unknown/not recommended

Breast-Feeding Considerations Due to the potential for adverse reactions, temporary discontinuation of breast-feeding should be considered.

Contraindications Hypersensitivity to iodixanol or any component; intrathecal administration; administration to children who have experienced prolonged fasting or received recent laxative dose(s)

Warnings For I.V. or intra-arterial use only; **may be fatal if given intrathecally [U.S. Boxed Warning]**; intrathecal injection has also resulted in serious reactions (seizures, cerebral hemorrhage, coma, paralysis, arachnoiditis, ARF, cardiac arrest, rhabdomyolysis, hyperthermia, and brain edema). May cause rare but serious thromboembolic events including MI and stroke. Iodinated contrast media has been associated with severe hypersensitivity reactions including anaphylaxis; immediate treatment for anaphylactic reactions should be available during administration of iodixanol. Use with extreme caution in patients with or suspected of having pheochromocytoma; the amount of iodixanol used should be kept to an absolute minimum and blood pressure should be closely monitored throughout the procedure in these patients. Contrast media when administered intravascularly may promote sickling in patients who are homozygous for sickle cell disease. May worsen renal insufficiency in patients with multiple myeloma. Avoid use in patients with homocystinuria due to the risk of inducing thrombosis and embolism. Avoid extravasation.

Precautions Use with caution in children with asthma, hypersensitivity to other medication and/or allergens, cyanotic and acyanotic heart disease, CHF, serum creatinine >1.5 mg/dL, and neonates (immature renal function) due to an increased risk of adverse effects with iodixanol. Dehydration, particularly in children, may also increase the risk of adverse effects. Patients should be adequately hydrated both prior to and after iodixanol administration. Use caution in thyroid disease; thyroid storm has been reported in patients with history of hyperthyroidism.

Adverse Reactions

Cardiovascular: Cardiac arrest, chest pain, angina, syncope, arrhythmias, cardiac failure, hypotension, hypertension, MI, flushing, peripheral ischemia

Central nervous system: Agitation, anxiety, insomnia, nervousness, dizziness, headache, migraine, vertigo, fatigue, malaise, seizures, cerebral vascular disorder, stupor, confusion, amnesia

Dermatologic: Rash, pruritus, urticaria

Endocrine & metabolic: Hypoglycemia

Gastrointestinal: Diarrhea, nausea, vomiting, taste perversion, dyspepsia, pharyngeal edema

Genitourinary: Hematuria

Hematologic: DIC

Local: Injection site reactions (discomfort/pain/warmth)

Neuromuscular & skeletal: Back pain, dyskinesia, polymyalgia rheumatica

Ocular: Abnormal vision, cortical blindness (rare)

Otic: Tinnitus

Renal: Acute renal failure, abnormal renal function

Respiratory: Asthma, bronchitis, dyspnea, pulmonary edema, rhinitis, respiratory depression

Miscellaneous: Hypersensitivity reactions including anaphylaxis, diaphoresis

Drug Interactions

Avoid Concomitant Use There are no known interactions where it is recommended to avoid concomitant use.

Increased Effect/Toxicity

Iodixanol may increase the levels/effects of: Aldesleukin; MetFORMIN

Decreased Effect There are no known significant interactions involving a decrease in effect.

Stability Store at room temperature; do not mix with or inject in I.V. lines with other medications, solutions, or TPN solutions

Mechanism of Action Iodixanol is a nonionic, isosmolar, water soluble, iodinated x-ray contrast media for intravascular administration. It opacifies vessels in the path of flow permitting radiographic visualization of internal structures.

Pharmacodynamics Following administration, the increase in tissue density is related to blood flow, the concentration of the iodixanol solution used, and the extraction of iodixanol by various interstitial tissues. The degree of enhancement is directly related to the iodine content in an administered dose.

Kidney:

Visualization: Renal parenchyma: 30-60 seconds; calyces and pelves (normal renal function): 1-3 minutes

Optimum contrast: 5-15 minutes

Pharmacokinetics (Adult data unless noted)

Distribution: V_d: Adults: 0.26 L/kg

Metabolism: Metabolites have not been identified.

Time to peak level: I.V.: Children: 0.75-1.25 hours

Half-life:

Newborns to Infants <2 months: 4.1 ± 1.4 hours

Infants 2-6 months: 2.8 ± 0.6 hours

Infants 6-12 months: 2.4 ± 0.4 hours

Children 1 to <3 years: 2.2 ± 0.5 hours

Children 3 to <12 years: 2.3 ± 0.5 hours

Adults: 2.1 ± 0.1 hours

Elimination: 97% excreted unchanged in the urine within 24 hours; <2% excreted in feces

Clearance: Adults: 110 mL/minute

Dialysis: Dialyzable (36% to 49% depending upon the membrane)

Usual Dosage The concentration and volume of iodixanol to be used should be individualized depending upon age, weight, size of vessel, and rate of blood flow within the vessel.

Children >1 year:

Intra-arterial: Cerebral, cardiac chambers and related major arteries, and visceral studies: **320 mg iodine/mL**: 1-2 mL/kg; not to exceed 4 mL/kg

I.V.: Contrast-enhanced computerized tomography or excretory urography: **270 mg iodine/mL**: 1-2 mL/kg; not to exceed 2 mL/kg

Children >12 years and Adults: Maximum recommended total dose of iodine: 80 g

Intra-arterial: Iodixanol **320 mg iodine/mL**: Dose individualized based on injection site and study type; refer to product labeling

I.V.: Iodixanol **270 mg and 320 mg iodine/mL**: concentration and dose vary based on study type; refer to product labeling.

Dosage adjustment in renal impairment: Not studied; use caution

Administration I.V. or intra-arterial: Administer without further dilution. **Not for intrathecal administration** (see Warnings). Avoid extravasation.

Monitoring Parameters Monitor signs and symptoms of hypersensitivity reactions

Test Interactions False positive result for urine protein when using Multistix®; may affect urine specific gravity results immediately following administration (refractometry or urine osmolality may be used as an alternative); protein-bound iodine and radioactive iodine will not accurately reflect thyroid function for at least 16 days following iodixanol administration

Patient Information Inform healthcare provider if you are allergic to any drugs or food, or if you have had any reactions to previous injections of dyes used for x-ray procedures.

Dosage Forms Excipient information presented when available (limited, particularly for generics); consult specific product labeling.

Injection, solution [preservative free]:

Visipaque™ 270: 550 mg/mL (50 mL, 100 mL, 125 mL, 150 mL, 200 mL) [provides organically-bound iodine 270 mg/mL; contains tromethamine 1.2 mg/mL, edetate calcium disodium]

Visipaque™ 320: 652 mg/mL (50 mL, 100 mL, 125 mL, 150 mL, 200 mL) [provides organically-bound iodine 320 mg/mL; contains tromethamine 1.2 mg/mL, edetate calcium disodium]

References

Johnson WH, Lloyd TR, Victorica BE, et al, "Iodixanol Pharmacokinetics in Children," *Pediatr Cardiol*, 2001, 22(3):223-7.

◆ **Iodoflex™** *see* Iodine *on page 753*

Iodoquinol (eye oh doe KWIN ole)

U.S. Brand Names Yodoxin®

Canadian Brand Names Diodoquin®

Therapeutic Category Amebicide

Generic Available No

Use Treatment of acute and chronic intestinal amebiasis due to *Entamoeba histolytica*; asymptomatic cyst passers; *Blastocystis hominis* infections; iodoquinol alone is ineffective for amebic hepatitis or hepatic abscess

Pregnancy Considerations There is very limited data on the use of iodoquinol during pregnancy and safety has not been established. Adverse effects have occurred in children exposed to topical iodoquinol.

Lactation Excretion in breast milk unknown

Breast-Feeding Considerations It is unknown if iodoquinol is excreted in human milk and safety during lactation has not been established.

Contraindications Hypersensitivity to iodine, iodoquinol, or any component; hepatic or renal damage; pre-existing optic neuropathy

Precautions Use with caution in patients with thyroid disease or neurological disorders

Adverse Reactions

Central nervous system: Agitation, retrograde amnesia, fever, chills, headache, ataxia

Dermatologic: Anal pruritus, rash, acne

Endocrine & metabolic: Enlargement of the thyroid

Gastrointestinal: Nausea, vomiting, diarrhea, gastritis, anorexia, constipation

Neuromuscular & skeletal: Weakness, peripheral neuropathy, myalgia

Ocular: Optic neuritis, optic atrophy, visual impairment

Drug Interactions

Avoid Concomitant Use There are no known interactions where it is recommended to avoid concomitant use.

Increased Effect/Toxicity There are no known significant interactions involving an increase in effect.

Decreased Effect There are no known significant interactions involving a decrease in effect.

Mechanism of Action Contact amebicide that works in the lumen of the intestine by an unknown mechanism

Pharmacokinetics (Adult data unless noted)

Absorption: Oral: Poor and irregular

Metabolism: In the liver

Elimination: In feces; metabolites appear in urine

Usual Dosage Oral:

Children: 30-40 mg/kg/day in 3 divided doses for 20 days; not to exceed 1.95 g/day

Adults: 650 mg 3 times/day after meals for 20 days; not to exceed 2 g/day

Administration Oral: Administer medication after meals; tablets may be crushed and mixed with applesauce or chocolate syrup

Monitoring Parameters Ophthalmologic exam

Test Interactions May increase protein-bound serum iodine concentrations reflecting a decrease in iodine 131 uptake; false-positive ferric chloride test for phenylketonuria

Patient Information Notify physician if rash occurs

Dosage Forms Excipient information presented when available (limited, particularly for generics); consult specific product labeling.

Tablet: 210 mg, 650 mg

◆ **Iodosorb®** see Iodine on page 753

◆ **Ionil® [OTC]** see Salicylic Acid on page 1241

◆ **Ionil Plus® [OTC]** see Salicylic Acid on page 1241

◆ **Ionil T® Plus [OTC] [DSC]** see Coal Tar on page 349

◆ **Iosat™ [OTC]** see Potassium Iodide on page 1138

Ipecac Syrup (IP e kak SIR up)

Therapeutic Category Antidote, Emetic

Generic Available Yes

Use Treatment of acute oral drug overdosage and certain poisonings; use only in alert conscious patients who have ingested potentially toxic amounts of substance

Pregnancy Risk Factor C

Lactation Excretion in breast milk unknown/use caution

Contraindications Hypersensitivity to ipecac syrup or any component; do not use in unconscious patients, patients with absent gag reflex or seizures; ingestion of strong bases or acids, other corrosive substances, volatile oils, hydrocarbons with high potential for aspiration

Warnings Avoid use in patients with coagulopathy or bleeding problems (risk of gastroesophageal hemorrhage) and in patients receiving calcium channel blockers, beta-blockers, clonidine, or digitalis glycosides (risk of exaggerated vagal stimulation with gagging, resulting in severe bradycardia); do not confuse ipecac syrup with ipecac fluid extract; fluid extract is 14 times more potent than syrup

Precautions Use with caution in patients with cardiovascular disease and bulimics

Adverse Reactions

Cardiovascular: Cardiotoxicity

Central nervous system: Lethargy, drowsiness

Gastrointestinal: Protracted vomiting, diarrhea; Mallory-Weiss syndrome, gastric rupture

Neuromuscular & skeletal: Myopathy

Respiratory: Aspiration (can be fatal)

Drug Interactions

Avoid Concomitant Use There are no known interactions where it is recommended to avoid concomitant use.

Increased Effect/Toxicity There are no known significant interactions involving an increase in effect.

Decreased Effect There are no known significant interactions involving a decrease in effect.

Food Interactions Milk, carbonated beverages may decrease effectiveness

Mechanism of Action Irritates the gastric mucosa and stimulates the medullary chemoreceptor trigger zone to induce vomiting

Pharmacodynamics

Onset of vomiting after oral dose: Within 15-30 minutes; usual: 20 minutes

Duration: 20-25 minutes; can last longer, up to 1-2 hours

Usual Dosage Oral:

Children:

<6 months: Not recommended

6-12 months: 5-10 mL followed by 10-20 mL/kg or 120-240 mL of water; repeat dose one time if vomiting does not occur within 20-30 minutes

1-12 years: 15 mL followed by 10-20 mL/kg or 120-240 mL of water; repeat dose one time if vomiting does not occur within 20-30 minutes

Adolescents and Adults: 30 mL followed by 240 mL of water; repeat dose one time if vomiting does not occur within 20-30 minutes

Administration Oral: Administer within 60 minutes of ingestion; follow administration with water; do not administer with milk or carbonated beverages

Nursing Implications Do **not** administer to unconscious patients

Additional Information Patients should be kept active and moving following administration of ipecac; if vomiting does not occur after second dose, gastric lavage may be considered to remove ingested substance

The Position Statement of The American Academy of Clinical Toxicology and The European Association of Poisons Centres and Clinical Toxicologists does **not** recommend **routine** administration of ipecac syrup to poisoned patients; scientific literature does not support that ipecac improves patient outcome; this paper states that the **routine** administration of ipecac syrup in the emergency room should be abandoned. Also, scientific literature cannot support or exclude giving ipecac syrup soon after toxic ingestions; administration of ipecac syrup may delay the administration or decrease the effectiveness of activated charcoal, oral antidotes, or whole bowel irrigation; its use should be considered only if it can be given within 60 minutes after ingestion of poison.

A recent study suggests that the use of syrup of ipecac, selectively administered at home, does **not** improve patient outcome or reduce utilization of emergency services; thus, clear evidence of the benefit of at home use of ipecac syrup is lacking (see Bond, 2003). Furthermore, the American Academy of Pediatrics now recommends that ipecac syrup should no longer be used routinely as a home treatment strategy and that existing ipecac syrup in the home should be disposed of safely (see AAP, 2003).

Dosage Forms Excipient information presented when available (limited, particularly for generics); consult specific product labeling.

Syrup: USP: 7% (30 mL)

References

American Academy of Pediatrics Committee on Injury, Violence, and Poison Prevention, "Poison Treatment in the Home," *Pediatrics*, 2003, 112(5):1182-5.

Bond GR, "Home Syrup of Ipecac Use Does Not Reduce Emergency Department Use or Improve Outcome," *Pediatrics*, 2003, 112 (5):1061-4.

"Position Statement: Ipecac Syrup. American Academy of Clinical Toxicology; European Association of Poisons Centres and Clinical Toxicologists," *J Toxicol Clin Toxicol*, 1997, 35(7):699-709.

Quang LS and Woolf AD, "Past, Present, and Future Role of Ipecac Syrup," *Curr Opin Pediatr*, 2000, 12(2):153-62.

Shannon M, "Ingestion of Toxic Substances by Children," *N Engl J Med*, 2000, 342(3):186-91.

◆ **IPOL®** *see* Poliovirus Vaccine (Inactivated) *on page 1127*

Ipratropium (i pra TROE pee um)

Medication Safety Issues

Sound-alike/look-alike issues:

Atrovent® may be confused with Alupent®, Serevent®

Ipratropium may be confused with tiotropium

Related Information

Asthma *on page 1697*

U.S. Brand Names Atrovent®; Atrovent® HFA

Canadian Brand Names Alti-Ipratropium; Apo-Ipravent®; Atrovent®; Atrovent® HFA; Gen-Ipratropium; Mylan-Ipratropium Solution; Mylan-Ipratropium Sterinebs; Novo-Ipramide; Nu-Ipratropium; PMS-Ipratropium

Therapeutic Category Antiasthmatic; Anticholinergic Agent; Bronchodilator

Generic Available Yes: Solution for nebulization

Use Anticholinergic bronchodilator used in bronchospasm associated with asthma, COPD, bronchitis, and emphysema; symptomatic relief of rhinorrhea associated with allergic and nonallergic rhinitis (nasal spray)

Pregnancy Risk Factor B

Pregnancy Considerations Teratogenic effects were not observed in animal studies. Inhaled ipratropium is recommended for use as additional therapy for pregnant women with severe asthma exacerbations.

Lactation Excretion in breast milk unknown/use caution

Contraindications Hypersensitivity to ipratropium, atropine, or any component (see Additional Information)

Warnings Not indicated for first-line therapy; should be added to short-acting beta-agonists (SABA) therapy for severe exacerbations (NIH Guidelines, 2007)

Precautions Use with caution in patients with narrow-angle glaucoma, bladder neck obstruction, or prostatic hypertrophy

Adverse Reactions

Note: Ipratropium is poorly absorbed from the lung, so systemic effects are rare

Cardiovascular: Palpitations, tachycardia (including SVT), flushing, hypotension, hypertension, atrial fibrillation, angioedema

Central nervous system: Nervousness, dizziness, headache, fatigue, drowsiness, insomnia

Dermatologic: Rash, pruritus, alopecia, urticaria

Gastrointestinal: Nausea, xerostomia, constipation

Genitourinary: Dysuria, urinary retention

Ocular: Blurred vision, mydriasis

Respiratory: Cough, hoarseness, dry secretions, epistaxis (with nasal spray), laryngospasm, bronchospasm

Miscellaneous: Hypersensitivity reactions

Drug Interactions

Avoid Concomitant Use There are no known interactions where it is recommended to avoid concomitant use.

Increased Effect/Toxicity

Ipratropium may increase the levels/effects of: AbobotulinumtoxinA; Anticholinergics; Cannabinoids; OnabotulinumtoxinA; Potassium Chloride; RimabotulinumtoxinB

The levels/effects of Ipratropium may be increased by: Pramlintide

Decreased Effect

Ipratropium may decrease the levels/effects of: Acetylcholinesterase Inhibitors (Central); Secretin

The levels/effects of Ipratropium may be decreased by: Acetylcholinesterase Inhibitors (Central)

Stability Store at room temperature; compatible for 1 hour when mixed with albuterol or metaproterenol in a nebulizer

Mechanism of Action Blocks the action of acetylcholine at parasympathetic sites in bronchial smooth muscle causing bronchodilation; inhibits secretions from the serous and seromucous glands lining the nasal mucosa

Pharmacodynamics

Onset of bronchodilation: 1-3 minutes after administration

Maximum effect: Maximal effect within 1.5-2 hours

Duration: Bronchodilation persists for up to 4-6 hours

Pharmacokinetics (Adult data unless noted)

Absorption: Not readily absorbed into the systemic circulation from the surface of the lung or from the GI tract

Distribution: Following inhalation, 15% of dose reaches the lower airways

Half-life: 2 hours

Usual Dosage

Neonates: Nebulization: 25 mcg/kg/dose 3 times/day

Infants: Nebulization: 125-250 mcg 3 times/day

Acute exacerbation of asthma (has not been shown to provide further benefit once the patient is hospitalized, NIH guidelines, 2007):

Children: Nebulization: 250-500 mcg (0.25-0.5 mg) every 20 minutes for 3 doses then as needed

Metered inhaler: 4-8 puffs as needed

Children >12 years and Adults: Nebulization: 500 mcg (0.5 mg) every 30 minutes for 3 doses then as needed

Metered inhaler: 8 puffs as needed

Maintenance treatments (nonacute) (evidence is lacking for providing added benefit to beta$_2$-agonists in long-term control asthma therapy, NIH Guidelines, 2007):

Children:

Nebulization: 250-500 mcg every 6 hours

Metered inhaler: 1-2 inhalations every 6 hours; not to exceed 12 inhalations/day

Children ≥12 years and Adults:

Nebulization: 250 mcg every 6 hours

Metered inhaler: 2-3 inhalations every 6 hours; not to exceed 12 inhalations/day

Nasal spray:

Children >6 years and Adults: 0.03%: 2 sprays in each nostril 2-3 times/day

Children >5 years and Adults: 0.06%: 2 sprays in each nostril 3-4 times/day

Administration

Nasal spray: Pump must be primed before usage by 7 actuations into the air away from the face; if not used for >24 hours, pump must be reprimed with 2 actuations; if not used >7 days, reprime with 7 actuations

Nebulization: May be administered with or without dilution in NS; use of a nebulizer with a mouth piece rather than a face mask may be preferred to prevent contact with eyes

Oral Inhalation: Shake well before use (Atrovent® only; Atrovent® HFA does not require shaking); use spacer device in children <8 years

Patient Information May cause dry mouth; avoid spraying aerosol in eyes as this may cause blurred vision, eye pain or discomfort, and precipitate or worsen glaucoma in susceptible patients

Additional Information Atrovent® HFA does not contain soya lecithin or any soy ingredients like the previous formulation did. It is not contraindicated in patients with a history of peanut allergy. Generic ipratropium may still be available until supply runs out, it should not be used in patients allergic to soy related food products (soybeans, peanuts) as they may contain soya lecithin. No generic products for Atrovent® HFA will be available until after November 2009, when the patent is scheduled to expire.

Dosage Forms Excipient information presented when available (limited, particularly for generics); consult specific product labeling.

Aerosol for oral inhalation, as bromide:
Atrovent® HFA: 17 mcg/actuation (12.9 g)
Solution for nebulization, as bromide: 0.02% (2.5 mL)
Solution, intranasal, as bromide [spray]:
Atrovent®: 0.03% (30 mL); 0.06% (15 mL)

References

"Guidelines for the Diagnosis and Management of Asthma. NAEPP Expert Panel Report 3," August 2007, www.nhlbi.nih.gov/guidelines/asthma/asthgdln.pdf.

Henry RI, Hiller EG, Milner AD, et al, "Nebulised Ipratropium Bromide and Sodium Cromoglycate in the First 2 Years of Life," *Arch Dis Child*, 1984, 59(1):54-7.

Mann NP and Hiller RG, "Ipratropium Bromide in Children With Asthma," *Thorax*, 1982, 37(1):72-4.

"National Asthma Education and Prevention Program. Expert Panel Report: Guidelines for the Diagnosis and Management of Asthma Update on Selected Topics–2002," *J Allergy Clin Immunol*, 2002, 110 (5 Suppl):S141-219.

Schuh S, Johnson DW, Callahan S, et al, "Efficacy of Frequent Nebulized Ipratropium Added to Frequent High-Dose Albuterol Therapy in Severe Childhood Asthma," *J Pediatr*, 1995, 126 (4):639-45.

Schuh S, Johnson D, Canny G, et al, "Efficacy of Adding Nebulized Ipratropium Bromide to Nebulized Albuterol Therapy in Acute Bronchiolitis," *Pediatrics*, 1992, 90(6): 920-3.

Wang EE, Milner R, Allen U, et al, "Bronchodilators for Treatment of Mild Bronchiolitis: A Factorial Randomized Trial," *Arch Dis Child*, 1992, 67(3):289-93.

Wilkie RA and Bryan MH, "Effect of Bronchodilators on Airway Resistance in Ventilator-dependent Neonates With Chronic Lung Disease," *J Pediatr*, 1987, 111(2):278-82.

◆ **Ipratropium Bromide** see Ipratropium on page 757
◆ **I-Prin [OTC]** see Ibuprofen on page 702
◆ **Iproveratril Hydrochloride** see Verapamil on page 1416
◆ **IPV** see Poliovirus Vaccine (Inactivated) on page 1127
◆ **Iquix®** see Levofloxacin on page 813

Irbesartan (ir be SAR tan)

Medication Safety Issues

Sound-alike/look-alike issues:
Avapro® may be confused with Anaprox®

Related Information

Antihypertensive Agents by Class on page 1481

U.S. Brand Names Avapro®

Canadian Brand Names Avapro®

Therapeutic Category Angiotensin II Receptor Blocker; Antihypertensive Agent

Generic Available No

Use Treatment of hypertension alone or in combination with other antihypertensives (FDA approved in adults); treatment of diabetic nephropathy in patients with type 2 diabetes mellitus (noninsulin dependent, NIDDM) and hypertension (FDA approved in adults); has also been used to reduce proteinuria in children with chronic kidney disease either as monotherapy or in addition to ACE inhibitor therapy

Pregnancy Risk Factor C (1st trimester); D (2nd and 3rd trimesters)

Pregnancy Considerations Medications which act on the renin-angiotensin system are reported to have the following fetal/neonatal effects: Hypotension, neonatal skull hypoplasia, anuria, renal failure, and death; oligohydramnios is also reported. These effects are reported to occur with exposure during the second and third trimesters. There are no adequate and well-controlled studies in pregnant women. **[U.S. Boxed Warning]: Based on human data, drugs that act on the angiotensin system can cause injury and death to the developing fetus when used in the second and third trimesters. Angiotensin receptor blockers should be discontinued as soon as possible once pregnancy is detected.**

Lactation Excretion in breast milk unknown/contraindicated

Contraindications Hypersensitivity to irbesartan, any component, or other angiotensin II receptor blockers

Warnings When used in pregnancy during the second and third trimesters, drugs that act on the renin-angiotensin system can cause injury and death to the developing fetus. ARBs should be discontinued as soon as possible once pregnancy is detected **[U.S. Boxed Warning]**. Neonatal hypotension, skull hypoplasia, anuria, renal failure, oligohydramnios (associated with fetal limb contractures, craniofacial deformities, hypoplastic lung development), prematurity, intrauterine growth retardation, patent ductus arteriosus, and death have been reported with the use of ACE inhibitors, primarily in the second and third trimesters. Symptomatic hypotension may occur, especially in patients with an activated renin-angiotensin system (eg, volume- or salt-depleted patients receiving high doses of diuretic agents); use with caution in these patients; correct depletion before starting therapy or initiate therapy at a lower dose.

Precautions Use with caution in patients with impaired renal function; use is associated with deterioration of renal function and/or increases in serum creatinine, particularly in patients with low renal blood flow (eg, renal artery stenosis, heart failure); deterioration may result in oliguria, acute renal failure, or progressive azotemia. Small increases in serum creatinine may occur following initiation; consider discontinuation in patients with progressive and/or significant deterioration in renal function. Hyperkalemia may occur; risk factors include renal dysfunction, diabetes mellitus, concomitant use of potassium-sparing diuretics, potassium supplements, and/or potassium-containing salts; use with caution with these agents; monitor potassium closely.

Adverse Reactions

Cardiovascular: Hypotension, orthostatic hypotension, chest pain, edema, tachycardia

Central nervous system: Fatigue, anxiety, nervousness, dizziness, orthostatic dizziness, headache

Dermatology: Rash

Endocrine & metabolic: Hyperkalemia

Gastrointestinal: Diarrhea, dyspepsia, abdominal pain, nausea, vomiting, constipation

Hematologic: Anemia (case report; see Simonetti, 2007)

Hepatic: Rarely: Liver enzymes increased, jaundice, hepatitis

Neuromuscular & skeletal: Musculoskeletal pain, rhabdomyolysis (rare)

Renal: BUN and serum creatinine elevated, renal dysfunction

Respiratory: Pharyngitis, rhinitis, sinus abnormality

Miscellaneous: Influenza-type illness, UTI, angioedema (rare)

Drug Interactions

Metabolism/Transport Effects Substrate of CYP2C9 (minor); **Inhibits** CYP2C8 (moderate), 2C9 (moderate), 2D6 (weak), 3A4 (weak)

Avoid Concomitant Use There are no known interactions where it is recommended to avoid concomitant use.

Increased Effect/Toxicity

Irbesartan may increase the levels/effects of: ACE Inhibitors; Amifostine; Antihypertensives; Carvedilol; CYP2C8 Substrates (High risk); CYP2C9 Substrates (High risk); Hypotensive Agents; Lithium; Potassium-Sparing Diuretics; RiTUXimab

The levels/effects of Irbesartan may be increased by: Diazoxide; Eplerenone; Fluconazole; Herbs (Hypotensive Properties); MAO Inhibitors; Pentoxifylline; Phosphodiesterase 5 Inhibitors; Potassium Salts; Prostacyclin Analogues; Tolvaptan; Trimethoprim

Decreased Effect

The levels/effects of Irbesartan may be decreased by: Herbs (Hypertensive Properties); Methylphenidate; Nonsteroidal Anti-Inflammatory Agents; Rifamycin Derivatives; Yohimbine

Food Interactions Food does not significantly affect AUC. Limit salt substitutes or potassium-rich diet. Avoid natural licorice (causes sodium and water retention and increases potassium loss).

Stability Store at controlled room temperature of 25°C (77°F).

Mechanism of Action Irbesartan produces direct antagonism of the effects of angiotensin II. Unlike the ACE inhibitors, irbesartan blocks the binding of angiotensin II to the AT1 receptor subtype. It produces its blood pressure-lowering effects by antagonizing AT1-induced vasoconstriction, aldosterone release, catecholamine release, arginine vasopressin release, water intake, and hypertrophic responses. This action results in more efficient blockade of the cardiovascular effects of angiotensin II and fewer side effects than the ACE inhibitors. Irbesartan does not affect the ACE (kininase II) or the response to bradykinin.

Pharmacodynamics Antihypertensive effect:

Onset of action: 1-2 hours

Maximum effect: 3-6 hours postdose; with chronic dosing maximum effect: ~2 weeks

Duration: >24 hours

Pharmacokinetics (Adult data unless noted)

Absorption: Rapid and almost complete

Distribution: V_d: Adults: 53-93 L

Protein binding: 90%, primarily to albumin and alpha$_1$ acid gylcoprotein

Metabolism: Hepatic, via glucuronide conjugation and oxidation; oxidation occurs primarily by cytochrome P450 isoenzyme CYP2C9

Bioavailability: 60% to 80%

Half-life, elimination: Adults: 11-15 hours

Time to peak serum concentration: 1.5-2 hours

Elimination: Excreted via biliary and renal routes; feces (80%); urine (20%)

Dialysis: Not removed by hemodialysis

Usual Dosage Oral:

Children:

Hypertension: Not approved for use; limited information is available; dosing based on clinical trials (Sakarcan, 2001) and National High Blood Pressure Education Program Working Group on High Blood Pressure in Children and Adolescents, 2004 recommendations; **Note:** Use a starting dose of 50% of the recommended initial dose in volume- and salt-depleted patients.

6-12 years: Initial: 75 mg once daily; may be titrated to a maximum dose of 150 mg once daily

≥13 years: Initial: 150 mg once daily; may be titrated to a maximum dose of 300 mg once daily

Proteinuria reduction in children with chronic kidney disease: Not approved for use; limited information is available; dosing based on open-label clinical trials (see Franscini, 2002; Gartenmann, 2003; von Vigier, 2000):

4-18 years: Studies utilized a dosage based on weight categories (see below); initial doses were approximately 2 mg/kg once daily; doses were increased after 3-5 weeks and after 8-12 weeks if needed, according to specific blood pressure criteria; median final dose in the largest study (n=44; median age: 10 years): 4 mg/kg once daily

10-20 kg: Initial: 37.5 mg once daily

21-40 kg: Initial: 75 mg once daily

>40 kg: Initial: 150 mg once daily

Adults:

Hypertension: Initial: 150 mg once daily; may be titrated to a maximum dose of 300 mg once daily; **Note:** Use a starting dose of 75 mg once daily in volume- or salt-depleted patients.

Nephropathy with type 2 diabetes and hypertension: Target dose: 300 mg once daily

Dosage adjustment in renal impairment: No dosage adjustment necessary with mild-to-severe impairment unless the patient is also volume depleted.

Dosage adjustment in hepatic impairment: No dosage adjustment is needed.

Administration May be administered without regard to food. Capsules may be opened and mixed with small amount of applesauce prior to administration (see Sakaran, 2001).

Monitoring Parameters Blood pressure, BUN, serum creatinine, renal function, baseline and periodic serum electrolytes, urinalysis

Patient Information Do not take any new medication (prescription or OTC), herbal products, potassium supplements, or salt substitutes during therapy without consulting prescriber. Take exactly as directed and do not discontinue without consulting prescriber. Medication should be taken at the same time each day; may be taken without regard to meals. This drug does not eliminate need for diet or exercise regimen as recommended by prescriber. May cause dizziness or lightheadedness (use caution when driving or engaging in tasks that require alertness until response to drug is known); postural hypotension (use caution when rising from lying or sitting position or climbing stairs); or diarrhea. Report immediately swelling of face, lips, or mouth; difficulty swallowing; chest pain or palpitations, unrelenting headache; muscle weakness or pain; unusual cough; or other persistent adverse reactions. This medication may cause injury and death to the developing fetus when used during pregnancy; women of childbearing potential should be informed of potential risk; consult prescriber for appropriate contraceptive measures; this medication should be discontinued as soon as possible once pregnancy is detected (see Warnings).

Nursing Implications Assess effectiveness and interactions with other pharmacological agents and herbal products patient may be taking (eg, concurrent use of potassium supplements, ACE inhibitors, and potassium-sparing diuretics may increase risk of hyperkalemia).

Monitor laboratory tests at baseline and periodically during therapy. Monitor therapeutic effectiveness (reduced BP) and adverse response on a regular basis during therapy (eg, changes in renal function, dizziness, bradycardia, headache, nausea, hypotension, hyperkalemia). Teach patient proper use, possible side effects/appropriate interventions, and adverse symptoms to report.

Dosage Forms Excipient information presented when available (limited, particularly for generics); consult specific product labeling.

Tablet, oral:

Avapro®: 75 mg, 150 mg, 300 mg

References

Chobanian AV, Bakris GL, Black HR, et al, "The Seventh Report of the Joint National Committee on Prevention, Detection, Evaluation, and Treatment of High Blood Pressure: The JNC 7 Report," *JAMA*, 2003, 289(19):2560-72.

Franscini LM, Von Vigier RO, Pfister R, et al, "Effectiveness and Safety of the Angiotensin II Antagonist Irbesartan in Children With Chronic Kidney Diseases," *Am J Hypertens*, 2002, 15(12):1057-63.

Gartenmann AC, Fossali E, von Vigier RO, et al, "Better Renoprotective Effect of Angiotensin II Antagonist Compared to Dihydropyridine Calcium Channel Blocker in Childhood," *Kidney Int*, 2003, 64 (4):1450-4.

Hogg RJ, Portman RJ, Milliner D, et al, "Evaluation and Management of Proteinuria and Nephrotic Syndrome in Children: Recommendations From a Pediatric Nephrology Panel Established at the National Kidney Foundation Conference on Proteinuria, Albuminuria, Risk, Assessment, Detection, and Elimination (PARADE)," *Pediatrics*, 2000, 105(6):1242-9.

National High Blood Pressure Education Program Working Group on High Blood Pressure in Children and Adolescents, "The Fourth Report on the Diagnosis, Evaluation, and Treatment of High Blood Pressure in Children and Adolescents," *Pediatrics*, 2004, 114(2 Suppl):555-76.

Sakarcan A, Tenney F, Wilson JT, et al, "The Pharmacokinetics of Irbesartan in Hypertensive Children and Adolescents," *J Clin Pharmacol*, 2001, 41(7):742-9.

Simonetti GD, Bianchetti MG, Konrad M, et al, "Severe Anemia Caused by the Angiotensin Receptor Blocker Irbesartan After Renal Transplantation," *Pediatr Nephrol*, 2007, 22(5):756-7.

von Vigier RO, Zberg PM, Teuffel O, et al, "Preliminary Experience With the Angiotensin II Receptor Antagonist Irbesartan in Chronic Kidney Disease," *Eur J Pediatr*, 2000, 159(8):590-3.

Zaffanello M, Franchini M, and Fanos V, "New Therapeutic Strategies With Combined Renin-Angiotensin System Inhibitors for Pediatric Nephropathy," *Pharmacotherapy*, 2008, 28(1):125-30.

♦ **Ircon® [OTC]** *see* Ferrous Fumarate *on page 576*

Irinotecan (eye rye no TEE kan)

Medication Safety Issues

High alert medication: The Institute for Safe Medication Practices (ISMP) includes this medication among its list of drug classes which have a heightened risk of causing significant patient harm when used in error.

Related Information

Compatibility of Chemotherapy and Related Supportive Care Medications *on page 1580*
Emetogenic Potential of Antineoplastic Agents *on page 1579*

U.S. Brand Names Camptosar®

Canadian Brand Names Camptosar®; Irinotecan Hydrochloride Trihydrate

Therapeutic Category Antineoplastic Agent, Topoisomerase Inhibitor

Generic Available Yes

Use Treatment of metastatic carcinoma of the colon or rectum (FDA approved in adults); has also been used in the treatment of nonsmall cell lung cancer, small cell lung cancer, cervical cancer, gastric cancer, pancreatic cancer, brain tumors, hepatoblastoma, neuroblastoma, Ewing's sarcoma, and rhabdomyosarcoma

Pregnancy Risk Factor D

Pregnancy Considerations Teratogenic effects were noted in animal studies. There are no adequate and well-controlled studies in pregnant women. Women of child-bearing potential should avoid becoming pregnant while receiving treatment.

Lactation Excretion in breast milk unknown/not recommended

Breast-Feeding Considerations Due to the potential for serious adverse reactions in the nursing infant, breast-feeding is not recommended.

Contraindications Hypersensitivity to irinotecan or any component; concurrent use with St John's wort or ketoconazole (see Drug Interactions); patients with severe bone marrow failure

Warnings Hazardous agent; use appropriate precautions for handling and disposal. Irinotecan is potentially embryotoxic and teratogenic if administered to pregnant women. Do not use in patients with hereditary fructose intolerance (product contains sorbitol).

May cause severe, dose-limiting, and potentially fatal diarrhea **[U.S. Boxed Warning]**; early and late forms of severe diarrhea have been reported with irinotecan administration. Early diarrhea has occurred during or shortly after infusion and may be accompanied by symptoms of rhinitis, increased salivation, miosis, lacrimation, diaphoresis, flushing, and abdominal cramping. Atropine 0.01 mg/kg I.V. (maximum dose: 0.4 mg) may be used to prevent or treat symptoms of early diarrhea. Late diarrhea has occurred >24 hours after irinotecan administration and can be prolonged leading to life-threatening dehydration and electrolyte imbalance. Treat late diarrhea promptly with loperamide until a normal pattern of bowel movements returns (see Additional Information for loperamide dosing recommendation); fluid and electrolyte replacement may be needed for dehydration. Provide antibiotic support (cefixime has been used in children whose diarrhea persisted >24 hours despite loperamide) if patient develops persistent diarrhea, ileus, fever, or severe neutropenia. Interrupt or reduce subsequent irinotecan doses if National Cancer Institute (NCI) grade 3 (increase of 7-9 stools daily, or incontinence, or severe cramping) or grade 4 (increase ≥10 stools daily, grossly bloody stool, or need for parenteral support) late diarrhea occurs. Cases of colitis complicated by ulceration, bleeding, ileus, and infection have been reported. Renal impairment and acute renal failure have been reported, possibly due to dehydration secondary to diarrhea.

May cause severe myelosuppression **[U.S. Boxed Warning]**; deaths due to sepsis following severe myelosuppression have been reported with irinotecan administration. Therapy should be temporarily discontinued if neutropenic fever occurs or if the absolute neutrophil count is <1000/mm^3. The dose of irinotecan should be reduced if there is a clinically significant decrease in neutrophil count (<1500/mm^3) or platelet count (<100,000/mm^3). Patients homozygous for the UGT1A1*28 allele are at increased risk of neutropenia; initial one-level dose reduction should be considered for both single-agent and combination regimens. Heterozygous carriers of the UGT1A1*28 allele may also be at increased risk; however, most patients have tolerated normal starting doses. Patients with abnormal glucuronidation of bilirubin, such as Gilbert's syndrome, may also be at greater risk of myelosuppression when receiving irinotecan.

Precautions Use with caution and reduce initial irinotecan dose in patients with increased total serum bilirubin concentration (1-2 mg/dL) who previously received pelvic/abdominal radiation therapy or in patients with baseline total serum bilirubin concentration >2 mg/dL. Use with caution in patients with impaired renal function.

Adverse Reactions

Cardiovascular: Edema, facial flushing, hypotension, thromboembolic events

Central nervous system: Asthenia, chills, confusion, dizziness, fever, headache, insomnia, somnolence, tremor

Dermatologic: Alopecia, rash

Endocrine & metabolic: Dehydration, hypernatremia, hypokalemia, hyponatremia, metabolic acidosis, weight loss

Gastrointestinal: Abdominal pain, anorexia, colitis, constipation, diarrhea (see Warnings), dyspepsia, ileus, mucositis, nausea, vomiting

Genitourinary: Glucosuria, hematuria, proteinuria

Hematologic: Anemia, leukopenia, lymphocytopenia, neutropenia, thrombocytopenia

Hepatic: Alkaline phosphatase increased, bilirubin increased, transaminases increased

Local: Pain at infusion site

Neuromuscular & skeletal: Back pain, weakness

Renal: Acute renal failure (rare), serum creatinine increased

Respiratory: Cough, dyspnea, pneumonitis, pulmonary infiltrates

Miscellaneous: Anaphylaxis, cholinergic symptoms (diaphoresis, lacrimation, miosis, rhinitis, salivation increased)

<1%, postmarketing, and/or case reports: Amylase increased, anaphylactoid reaction, angina, arterial thrombosis, bleeding, bradycardia, cardiac arrest, cerebral infarct, cerebrovascular accident, circulatory failure, deep thrombophlebitis, dysrhythmia, gastrointestinal bleeding, gastrointestinal obstruction, hepatomegaly, hiccups, hyperglycemia, hypersensitivity, interstitial lung disease, intestinal perforation, lipase increased, megacolon, MI, muscle cramps, myocardial ischemia, pancreatitis, paresthesia, peripheral vascular disorder, pulmonary embolus; pulmonary toxicity (dyspnea, fever, reticulonodular infiltrates on chest x-ray); renal impairment, syncope, thrombophlebitis, typhlitis, ulceration, vertigo

Drug Interactions

Metabolism/Transport Effects Substrate (major) of CYP2B6, CYP3A4, P-glycoprotein, SLCO1B1, UGT1A1

Avoid Concomitant Use

Avoid concomitant use of Irinotecan with any of the following: Atazanavir; BCG; Natalizumab; Pimecrolimus; St Johns Wort; Tacrolimus (Topical); Vaccines (Live)

Increased Effect/Toxicity

Irinotecan may increase the levels/effects of: Leflunomide; Natalizumab; Vaccines (Live)

The levels/effects of Irinotecan may be increased by: Antifungal Agents (Azole Derivatives, Systemic); Atazanavir; Bevacizumab; CYP2B6 Inhibitors (Moderate); CYP2B6 Inhibitors (Strong); CYP3A4 Inhibitors (Moderate); CYP3A4 Inhibitors (Strong); Dasatinib; Denosumab; Eltrombopag; P-Glycoprotein Inhibitors; Pimecrolimus; Quazepam; Sorafenib; Tacrolimus (Topical); Trastuzumab

Decreased Effect

Irinotecan may decrease the levels/effects of: BCG; Sipuleucel-T; Vaccines (Inactivated); Vaccines (Live)

The levels/effects of Irinotecan may be decreased by: CarBAMazepine; CYP2B6 Inducers (Strong); CYP3A4 Inducers (Strong); Deferasirox; Echinacea; P-Glycoprotein Inducers; PHENobarbital; Phenytoin; St Johns Wort

Stability Store unopened Bedford irinotecan vials at 20°C to 25°C (68°F to 77°F); store unopened Camptosar® vials at 15°C to 30°C (59°F to 86°F). Protect from light. Once injectable solution is mixed with D$_5$W, solution is stable for 24 hours if stored at room temperature or 48 hours if stored refrigerated. Injectable solution mixed with NS is

stable for 24 hours if stored at room temperature. Do not refrigerate solutions mixed in NS since visible particulates may develop.

Mechanism of Action Prodrug undergoes de-esterification by cellular carboxylesterases to a potent active metabolite (SN-38) which is a topoisomerase I inhibitor. Binds to topoisomerase I-DNA complex preventing religation of single-strand DNA breaks, resulting in double-strand DNA breakage and cell death.

Pharmacokinetics (Adult data unless noted)

Distribution: Distributes to pleural fluid, sweat, and saliva

Protein binding:

Irinotecan: 30% to 68%

SN-38 (active metabolite): 95%

Half-life, terminal: Adults:

Irinotecan: 6-12 hours

SN-38 (active metabolite): 10-20 hours

Metabolism: Irinotecan is converted to its active metabolite SN-38 by carboxylesterase-mediated cleavage of the carbamate bond. SN-38 undergoes conjugation by the enzyme UDP-glucuronosyl transferase 1A1 (UGT1A1) to a glucuronide metabolite in the liver. Irinotecan also undergoes oxidation by cytochrome P450 3A4 to yield to 2 inactive metabolites.

Elimination: 11% to 20% of irinotecan and <1% SN-38 is excreted in the urine

Usual Dosage I.V. infusion (refer to individual protocols):

Children:

Refractory solid tumor (low-dose, protracted schedule): 20 mg/m^2/day for 5 days for 2 consecutive weeks followed by a week of rest; repeat cycle every 3 weeks

Refractory solid tumor or CNS tumor: 50 mg/m^2/day for 5 days; repeat cycle every 21 days; or for heavily pretreated patients: 125 mg/m^2/dose once weekly for 4 weeks, repeat cycle every 6 weeks; less heavily pretreated patients: 160 mg/m^2/dose once weekly for 4 weeks, repeat cycle every 6 weeks

Adults:

Colorectal cancer that has recurred or progressed following fluorouracil-containing chemotherapy: 300-350 mg/m^2/dose once every 3 weeks (maximum single dose: 700 mg) or 125 mg/m^2/dose once weekly (maximum dose: 150 mg/m^2) for 4 weeks followed by a 2-week rest period; repeat courses every 6 weeks (4 weeks of therapy followed by 2 weeks off)

Small cell lung cancer: 100-125 mg/m^2/dose once weekly (maximum dose: 150 mg/m^2) or 350 mg/m^2/dose once every 3 weeks; or 60-70 mg/m^2 once weekly for 3 weeks in combination with other agents

Note: A new cycle of irinotecan therapy should not begin until serious treatment-induced toxicity has fully resolved, granulocyte count recovers to ≥1500/mm^3, and platelet count recovers to ≥100,000/mm^3. Treatment should be delayed 1-2 weeks to allow for recovery from treatment-related toxicities. If the patient has not recovered after a 2-week delay, consider discontinuing irinotecan.

Administration Parenteral: I.V. infusion: Irinotecan can be further diluted in D$_5$W (preferred diluent) or NS to a final concentration of 0.12-2.8 mg/mL. Infuse over 30-90 minutes depending on protocol. Higher incidence of cholinergic symptoms have been reported with more rapid infusion rates.

Monitoring Parameters Signs of diarrhea and dehydration, serum electrolytes, serum BUN and creatinine; infusion site for signs of inflammation; CBC with differential and platelet count, hemoglobin, liver function tests, and serum bilirubin

Patient Information Advise women of childbearing potential to avoid becoming pregnant while receiving irinotecan. Avoid the use of laxatives. Notify physician if diarrhea, vomiting, fever, or symptoms of dehydration such as fainting, lightheadedness, or dizziness occur. Initiate ▶

loperamide therapy at the first episode of poorly formed or loose stools after irinotecan administration (see Additional Information).

Nursing Implications Avoid extravasation. If extravasation occurs, flush the site with sterile water and apply an ice pack. To prevent emesis, pretreat with a 5-HT$_3$ antagonist and dexamethasone 30 minutes prior to irinotecan therapy. Atropine may be used to prevent or treat symptoms of early diarrhea. Treat late diarrhea promptly with loperamide (see Additional Information).

Additional Information Loperamide dosing for treatment of late diarrhea: Oral:

8-10 kg: 1 mg after the first loose bowel movement followed by 0.5 mg every 3 hours until a normal pattern of bowel movement returns. Take 0.75 mg every 4 hours during the night rather than every 3 hours.

10.1-20 kg: 1 mg after the first loose bowel movement followed by 1 mg every 3 hours until a normal pattern of bowel movement returns. Take 1 mg every 4 hours during the night rather than every 3 hours.

20.1-30 kg: 2 mg after the first loose bowel movement followed by 1 mg every 3 hours until a normal pattern of bowel movement returns. Take 2 mg every 4 hours during the night rather than every 3 hours.

30.1-43 kg: 2 mg after the first loose bowel movement followed by 1 mg every 2 hours until a normal pattern of bowel movement returns. Take 2 mg every 4 hours during the night rather than every 2 hours.

>43 kg: 4 mg after the first loose bowel movement followed by 2 mg every 2 hours until the patient is diarrhea free for 12 hours. Take 4 mg every 4 hours during the night rather than every 2 hours.

Dosage Forms Excipient information presented when available (limited, particularly for generics); consult specific product labeling.

Injection, solution, as hydrochloride: 20 mg/mL (2 mL, 5 mL, 25 mL)

Camptosar®: 20 mg/mL (2 mL, 5 mL) [contains sorbitol 45 mg/mL]

References

Bomgaars L, Kerr J, Berg S, et al, "A Phase I Study of Irinotecan Administered on a Weekly Schedule in Pediatric Patients," *Pediatr Blood Cancer*, 2005, Mar 14.

Cosetti M, Wexler LH, Calleja E, et al, "Irinotecan for Pediatric Solid Tumors: The Memorial Sloan-Kettering Experience," *J Pediatr Hematol Oncol*, 2002, 24(2):101-5.

Furman WL, Crews K, Daw NC, et al, "Cefixime (CFX) Enables Further Dose-Escalation of Oral Irinotecan (IRN) in Pediatric Patients With Refractory Solid Tumors," American Society of Clinical Oncology Annual Meeting, 2003, abstract: 3210.

Gajjar A, Chintagumpala MM, Bowers DC, et al, "Effect of Intrapatient Dosage Escalation of Irinotecan on Its Pharmacokinetics in Pediatric Patients Who Have High-Grade Gliomas and Receive Enzyme-Inducing Anticonvulsant Therapy," *Cancer*, 2003, 97(9 Suppl):2374-80.

◆ **Irinotecan Hydrochloride Trihydrate (Can)** *see* Irinotecan *on page 760*

◆ **Iron Dextran** *see* Iron Dextran Complex *on page 762*

Iron Dextran Complex
(EYE ern DEKS tran KOM pleks)

Medication Safety Issues
Sound-alike/look-alike issues:
Dexferrum® may be confused with Desferal®
Iron dextran complex may be confused with ferumoxytol
U.S. Brand Names Dexferrum®; INFeD®
Canadian Brand Names Dexiron™; Infufer®
Therapeutic Category Iron Salt, Parenteral; Mineral, Parenteral
Generic Available No
Use Treatment of iron deficiency when oral iron administration is infeasible or ineffective (FDA approved in children ≥4 months and adults)

Pregnancy Risk Factor C

Pregnancy Considerations Adverse events have been observed in animal reproduction studies. It is not known if iron dextran (as iron dextran) crosses the placenta. It is recommended that pregnant women meet the dietary requirements of iron with diet and/or supplements in order to prevent adverse events associated with iron deficiency anemia in pregnancy. Treatment of iron deficiency anemia in pregnant women is the same as in nonpregnant women and in most cases, oral iron preparations may be used. Except in severe cases of maternal anemia, the fetus achieves normal iron stores regardless of maternal concentrations.

Lactation Enters breast milk/use caution

Breast-Feeding Considerations Trace amounts of iron dextran (as iron dextran) are found in human milk. Iron is normally found in breast milk. Breast milk or iron fortified formulas generally provide enough iron to meet the recommended dietary requirements of infants. The amount of iron in breast milk is generally not influenced by maternal iron status.

Contraindications Hypersensitivity to the iron formulation or any component (see Warnings); any anemia not associated with iron deficiency

Warnings Deaths associated with parenteral iron administration following anaphylactic-type reactions have been reported **[U.S. Boxed Warning]**; treatment agents for anaphylactic reactions (eg, epinephrine, steroids, diphenhydramine) should be immediately available; a test dose is recommended prior to initial therapy; however, anaphylactic and other hypersensitivity reactions have occurred after uneventful test doses. A history of drug allergy increases the risk for anaphylactic-type reactions. Rapid I.V. administration is associated with flushing, fatigue, weakness, hypotension, and chest, back, groin, or flank pain; use parenteral iron only in patients where the iron deficient state is not amenable to oral iron therapy; only iron dextran is approved for I.M. administration. Adverse events (including life-threatening) associated with iron dextran usually occur more with the high-molecular-weight formulation (DexFerrum®), compared to low-molecular-weight (INFeD®) (see Chertow, 2006). Delayed (1-2 days) infusion reaction, including arthralgia, back pain, chills, dizziness, and fever, may occur with large doses (eg, total dose infusion) of I.V. iron dextran; usually subsides within 3-4 days. May also occur (less commonly) with I.M. administration; subsiding within 3-7 days.

Precautions Use with caution in patients with histories of significant allergies, asthma, serious hepatic impairment, pre-existing cardiac disease (may exacerbate cardiovascular complications), and rheumatoid arthritis (may exacerbate joint pain and swelling); avoid use during acute kidney infection. Discontinue oral iron prior to initiating parenteral iron therapy. Exogenous hemosiderosis may result from excess iron stores; patients with refractory anemias and/or hemoglobinopathies may be prone to iron overload with unwarranted iron supplementation. Intramuscular injections of iron-carbohydrate complexes may have a risk of delayed injection site tumor development. Intramuscular iron dextran use in neonates may be associated with an increased incidence of gram negative sepsis.

In patients with chronic kidney disease (CKD) requiring iron supplementation, the I.V. route is preferred for hemodialysis patients; either oral iron or I.V. iron may be used for nondialysis and peritoneal dialysis CKD patients. In patients with cancer-related anemia (either due to cancer or chemotherapy-induced) requiring iron supplementation, the I.V. route is superior to oral therapy; I.M. administration is not recommended for parenteral iron supplementation.

Adverse Reactions Note: Adverse event risk is reported to be higher with the high-molecular-weight iron dextran formulation.

Anaphylactoid reactions: Respiratory difficulties and cardiovascular collapse have been reported and occur most frequently within the first several minutes of administration.

Cardiovascular: Arrhythmia, bradycardia, cardiac arrest, cardiovascular collapse, chest pain, chest tightness, flushing, hypovolemia, hyper-/hypotension, MI, shock, syncope, tachycardia, thrombosis

Central nervous system: Agitation, chills, convulsion, disorientation, dizziness, fever, headache, insomnia, malaise, seizure, shivering, somnolence, unconsciousness, unresponsiveness

Dermatologic: Angioedema, pruritus, purpura, rash, urticaria

Gastrointestinal: Abdominal pain, diarrhea, dyspepsia, eructation, flatulence, melena, metallic taste, nausea, taste alteration, vomiting

Genitourinary: Discoloration of urine, hematuria

Hematologic: Leukocytosis

Hepatic: Liver enzymes increased

Local: Injection site reactions (cellulitis, inflammation, soreness, swelling), muscle atrophy/fibrosis (with I.M. administration), pain, phlebitis, staining of skin/tissue at the site of I.M. injection, sterile abscess

Neuromuscular & skeletal: Arthralgia, arthritis/arthritis exacerbation, backache, leg cramps, myalgia, paresthesia, weakness

Ocular: Blurred vision, conjunctivitis

Renal: Hematuria

Respiratory: Bronchospasm, dyspnea, cough, rhinitis, upper respiratory infection, pulmonary edema, pharyngitis, pneumonia, respiratory arrest, wheezing

Miscellaneous: Anaphylactic reaction, diaphoresis, lymphadenopathy, tumor formation (at former injection site)

Note: Sweating, urticaria, arthralgia, fever, chills, dizziness, headache, and nausea may be delayed 24-48 hours after I.V. administration or 3-4 days after I.M. administration.

Drug Interactions

Avoid Concomitant Use

Avoid concomitant use of Iron Dextran Complex with any of the following: Dimercaprol

Increased Effect/Toxicity

The levels/effects of Iron Dextran Complex may be increased by: ACE Inhibitors; Dimercaprol

Decreased Effect There are no known significant interactions involving a decrease in effect.

Stability Store at room temperature. Product literature states parenteral iron formulations should not be mixed with other medications or in parenteral nutrition solutions.

Mechanism of Action Replaces iron found in hemoglobin, myoglobin, and specific enzymes; allows transportation of oxygen via hemoglobin

Pharmacodynamics

Onset of action: Hematologic response to either oral or parenteral iron salts is essentially the same; red blood cell form and color changes within 3-10 days

Maximum effect: Peak reticulocytosis occurs in 5-10 days, and hemoglobin values increase within 2-4 weeks; serum ferritin peak: 7-9 days after I.V. dose

Pharmacokinetics (Adult data unless noted)

Absorption: I.M.: 60% absorbed after 3 days; 90% after 1-3 weeks, the balance is slowly absorbed over months

Note: Following I.V. doses, the uptake of iron by the reticuloendothelial system appears to be constant at about 40-60 mg/hour

Half-life: 48 hours

Elimination: By the reticuloendothelial system and excreted in urine and feces (via bile)

Dialysis: Not dialyzable

Usual Dosage Multiple forms for parenteral iron exist; close attention must be paid to the specific product when ordering and administering; incorrect selection or substitution of one form for another without proper dosage adjustment may result in serious over- or under-dosing; test doses are recommended before starting therapy.

Iron deficiency anemia:

I.M. (INFeD®), I.V. (Dexferrum®, INFeD®): Test dose (given 1 hour prior to starting iron dextran therapy):

Infants <10 kg: 10 mg (0.2 mL)

Children 10-20 kg: 15 mg (0.3 mL)

Children >20 kg, Adolescents, and Adults: 25 mg (0.5 mL)

Total replacement dosage of iron dextran for iron deficiency anemia:

$(mL) = 0.0442 \times LBW\ (kg) \times (Hb_n - Hb_o) + [0.26 \times LBW\ (kg)]$

LBW = lean body weight

Hb_n = desired hemoglobin (g/dL) = 12 if <15 kg or 14.8 if >15 kg

Hb_o = measured hemoglobin (g/dL)

Total iron replacement dosage for acute blood loss: Assumes 1 mL of normocytic, normochromic red cells = 1 mg elemental iron

Iron dextran (mL) = 0.02 x blood loss (mL) x hematocrit (expressed as a decimal fraction)

Note: Total dose infusions have been used safely and are the preferred method of administration

I.M., I.V.: Maximum daily dose: Injected in daily or less frequent increments:

Infants <5 kg: 25 mg (0.5 mL)

Children 5-10 kg: 50 mg (1 mL)

Children >10 kg and Adults: 100 mg (2 mL)

Anemia of prematurity: I.V.: Neonates: 0.2-1 mg/kg/day or 20 mg/kg/week with epoetin alfa therapy

Anemia of chronic renal failure: I.V.: National Kidney Foundation DOQI Guidelines: **Note:** Initiation of iron therapy, determination of dose, and duration of therapy should be guided by results of iron status tests combined with the Hb level and the dose of the erythropoietin stimulating agent. See Reference Range for target levels. There is insufficient evidence to recommend I.V. iron if ferritin level >500 ng/mL.

Children: Predialysis or peritoneal dialysis: As a single dose repeated as often as necessary:

<10 kg: 125 mg

10-20 kg: 250 mg

>20 kg: 500 mg

Children: Hemodialysis: Given during each dialysis for 10 doses:

<10 kg: 25 mg

10-20 kg: 50 mg

>20 kg: 100 mg

Adults: Initial: 100 mg at every dialysis for 10 doses; maintenance: 25-100 mg once, twice, or three times/week for 10 weeks (should provide 250-1000 mg total dose within 12 weeks)

Cancer-associated anemia: Adults: I.V.: 25 mg slow I.V. push test dose, followed 1 hour later by 100 mg over 5 minutes; larger doses, up to total dose infusion (over several hours) may be administered

Administration

Parenteral: Avoid dilution in dextrose due to an increased incidence of local pain and phlebitis

I.M.: Use Z-track technique for I.M. administration (deep into the upper outer quadrant of buttock); alternate buttocks with subsequent injections; administer test dose at same recommended site using the same technique.

I.V.: Infuse test dose over at least 30 seconds (INFeD®) or 5 minutes (Dexferum®); may be injected undiluted at a rate not to exceed 50 mg/minute; dilute large or total replacement doses in NS (50-100 mL), maximum concentration 50 mg/mL and infuse over 1-6 hours at a maximum rate of 50 mg/minute

Monitoring Parameters Vital signs and other symptoms of anaphylactoid reactions (during I.V. infusion); reticulocyte count, serum ferritin, hemoglobin, serum iron concentrations, and transferrin saturation (TSAT). Ferritin and TSAT may be inaccurate if measured within 14 days of receiving a large single dose (1000 mg in adults).

Reference Range

Serum iron:
Newborns: 110-270 mcg/dL
Infants: 30-70 mcg/dL
Children: 55-120 mcg/dL
Adults: Male: 75-175 mcg/dL; female: 65-165 mcg/dL

Total iron binding capacity:
Newborns: 59-175 mcg/dL
Infants: 100-400 mcg/dL
Children and Adults: 230-430 mcg/dL

Transferrin: 204-360 mg/dL

Percent transferrin saturation (TSAT): 20% to 50%

Iron levels >300 mcg/dL may be considered toxic; should be treated as an overdosage

Ferritin: 13-300 ng/mL

Chronic kidney disease (CKD): Targets for iron therapy (KDOQI Guidelines, 2007) to maintain Hgb 11-12 g/dL:
Children: Nondialysis CKD, hemodialysis, or peritoneal dialysis: Ferritin: >100 ng/mL and TSAT >20%
Adults: Nondialysis (CKD) or peritoneal dialysis: Ferritin: >100 ng/mL and TSAT >20%
Hemodialysis: Ferritin >200 ng/mL and TSAT >20% or CHr (content of hemoglobin in reticulocytes) >29 pg/cell

Test Interactions May cause falsely elevated values of serum bilirubin and falsely decreased values of serum calcium. Residual iron dextran may remain in reticuloendothelial cells; may affect accuracy of examination of bone marrow iron stores. Bone scans with 99m Tc-labeled bone seeking agents may show reduced bony uptake, marked renal activity, and excess blood pooling and soft tissue accumulation following I.V. iron dextran infusion or with high serum ferritin levels. Following I.M. iron dextran, bones scans with 99m Tc-diphosphonate may show dense activity in the buttocks.

Nursing Implications Only iron dextran is approved for I.M. administration.

Additional Information Iron storage may lag behind the appearance of normal red blood cell morphology; use periodic hematologic determination to assess therapy

Dosage Forms Excipient information presented when available (limited, particularly for generics); consult specific product labeling.

Note: Strength expressed as elemental iron

Injection, solution:
Dexferrum®: 50 mg/mL (1 mL, 2 mL) [high-molecular-weight iron dextran]
INFeD®: 50 mg/mL (2 mL) [low-molecular-weight iron dextran]

References

Auerbach M, Ballard H, Trout JR, et al, "Intravenous Iron Optimizes the Response to Recombinant Human Erythropoietin in Cancer Patients With Chemotherapy-Related Anemia: A Multicenter, Open-Label, Randomized Trial," *J Clin Oncol*, 2004, 22(7):1301-7.

Auerbach M, Witt D, and Toler W, "Clinical Use of the Total Dose Intravenous Infusion of Iron Dextran," *J Lab Clin Med*, 1988, 111 (5):566-70.

Benito RP and Guerrero TC, "Response to a Single Intravenous Dose Versus Multiple Intramuscular Administration of Iron Dextran Complex: A Comparative Study," *Curr Ther Res Clin Exp*, 1973, 15 (7):373-82.

Chertow GM, Mason PD, Vaage-Nilsen O, et al, "Update on Adverse Drug Events Associated With Parenteral Iron," *Nephrol Dial Transplant*, 2006, 21(2):378-82.

"KDOQI Clinical Practice Guideline and Clinical Practice Recommendations for Anemia in Chronic Kidney Disease: 2007 Update of Hemoglobin Target," *Am J Kidney Dis*, 2007, 50(3):471-530.

National Comprehensive Cancer Network® (NCCN), "Practice Guidelines in Oncology™: Cancer- and Chemotherapy-Induced Anemia Version 3.2009." Available at http://www.nccn.org/professionals/physician_gls/PDF/anemia.pdf.

◆ **Iron Fumarate** *see* Ferrous Fumarate *on page 576*

◆ **Iron Gluconate** *see* Ferrous Gluconate *on page 577*

Iron Sucrose (EYE ern SOO krose)

Medication Safety Issues
Sound-alike/look-alike issues:
Iron sucrose may be confused with ferumoxytol

U.S. Brand Names Venofer®

Canadian Brand Names Venofer®

Therapeutic Category Iron Salt, Parenteral; Mineral, Parenteral

Generic Available No

Use Treatment of microcytic, hypochromic anemia resulting from iron deficiency in chronic kidney disease patients, either dialysis-dependent or nondialysis-dependent, who may or may not be receiving erythropoietin

Pregnancy Risk Factor B

Pregnancy Considerations Teratogenic effects were not observed in animal studies. There are no adequate and well-controlled studies in pregnant women. Based on limited data, iron sucrose may be effective for the treatment of iron-deficiency anemia in pregnancy. It is recommended that pregnant women meet the dietary requirements of iron with diet and/or supplements in order to prevent adverse events associated with iron deficiency anemia in pregnancy. Treatment of iron deficiency anemia in pregnant women is the same as in nonpregnant women and in most cases, oral iron preparations may be used. Except in severe cases of maternal anemia, the fetus achieves normal iron stores regardless of maternal concentrations.

Lactation Excretion in breast milk unknown/use caution

Breast-Feeding Considerations Iron is normally found in breast milk. Breast milk or iron fortified formulas generally provide enough iron to meet the recommended dietary requirements of infants. The amount of iron in breast milk is generally not influenced by maternal iron status.

Contraindications Hypersensitivity to the iron formulation or any component (see Warnings); anemias that are not associated with iron deficiency; hemochromatosis; hemolytic anemia; iron overload

Warnings Deaths associated with parenteral iron administration following anaphylactic-type reactions have been reported; treatment agents for anaphylactic reactions (eg, epinephrine, steroids, diphenhydramine) should be immediately available; a test dose is recommended prior to initial therapy; rapid I.V. administration is associated with flushing, fatigue, weakness, hypotension, and chest, back, groin, or flank pain; the incidence of hypotension in nondialysis patients is substantially lower. Hypotension may be related to total dose or rate of administration; use parenteral iron only in patients where the iron deficient state is not amenable to oral iron therapy; iron sucrose is not approved for I.M. administration.

Precautions Use with caution in patients with histories of significant allergies, asthma, hepatic impairment, rheumatoid arthritis

Adverse Reactions

Anaphylactoid reactions: Respiratory difficulties and cardiovascular collapse have been reported and occur most frequently within the first several minutes of administration.

Cardiovascular: Cardiovascular collapse, hypotension, flushing, chest pain, syncope, tachycardia, MI, hypovolemia, hypertension, thrombosis

Central nervous system: Dizziness, fever, headache, chills, shivering, malaise, insomnia, agitation, somnolence

Dermatologic: Urticaria, pruritus, rash

Gastrointestinal: Nausea, vomiting, diarrhea, metallic taste, abdominal pain, dyspepsia, flatulence, eructation, melena, pharyngitis

Genitourinary: Discoloration of urine

Hematologic: Leukocytosis

Hepatic: Liver enzymes elevated

Local: Pain, phlebitis

Neuromuscular & skeletal: Arthralgia, arthritic reactivation in patients with quiescent arthritis, backache, paresthesia, leg cramps, weakness

Ocular: Blurred vision, conjunctivitis

Renal: Hematuria

Respiratory: Dyspnea, cough, rhinitis, upper respiratory infection, pulmonary edema, pneumonia

Miscellaneous: Lymphadenopathy, diaphoresis

Note: Sweating, urticaria, arthralgia, fever, chills, dizziness, headache, and nausea may be delayed 24-48 hours after I.V. administration.

Drug Interactions

Avoid Concomitant Use

Avoid concomitant use of Iron Sucrose with any of the following: Dimercaprol

Increased Effect/Toxicity

The levels/effects of Iron Sucrose may be increased by: Dimercaprol

Decreased Effect There are no known significant interactions involving a decrease in effect.

Stability Store vials at room temperature; do not freeze; following dilution, solutions are stable for 48 hours at room temperature or under refrigeration. Product literature states parenteral iron formulations should not be mixed with other medications or in parenteral nutrition solutions.

Mechanism of Action Replaces iron found in hemoglobin, myoglobin, and specific enzymes; allows transportation of oxygen via hemoglobin

Pharmacodynamics

Onset of action: Hematologic response to either oral or parenteral iron salts is essentially the same; red blood cell form and color changes within 3-10 days

Maximum effect: Peak reticulocytosis occurs in 5-10 days, and hemoglobin values increase within 2-4 weeks

Pharmacokinetics (Adult data unless noted)

Following I.V. doses, the uptake of iron by the reticuloendothelial system appears to be constant at about 40-60 mg/hour

Distribution: V_{dss}: Healthy adults: 7.9 L

Metabolism: Dissociated into iron and sucrose by the reticuloendothelial system

Half-life: 6 hours

Excretion: Healthy adults: Urine (5%) within 24 hours

Dialysis: Not dialyzable

Usual Dosage Multiple forms for parenteral iron exist; close attention must be paid to the specific product when ordering and administering; incorrect selection or substitution of one form for another without proper dosage adjustment may result in serious over- or under-dosing; test doses are recommended before starting therapy.

Note: Per National Kidney Foundation DOQI Guidelines, initiation of iron therapy, determination of dose, and duration of therapy should be guided by results of iron status tests combined with the Hb level and the dose of the erythropoietin stimulating agent. See Reference Range for target levels. There is insufficient evidence to recommend I.V. iron if ferritin level >500 ng/mL.

Children: Limited data on 14 children (ages 2-14 years) with ESRD were treated with iron sucrose in 3 dosages: 3 mg/kg/dialysis (repletion treatment), 1 mg/kg/dialysis (repletion treatment), and 0.3 mg/kg/dialysis (maintenance treatment). Iron overload expressed by serum ferritin >400 occurred in all patients receiving 3 mg/kg dosage. The lower dosage (1 mg/kg) successfully increased ferritin therapeutic levels. The 0.3 mg/kg dose was successful in maintaining ferritin between 193-250 mcg/L (Leijn, 2004).

Adults **(doses expressed in mg of elemental iron):** Test dose: 50 mg (while product labeling does not indicate need for a test dose in product-naive patients, test doses were administered in some clinical trials)

Hemodialysis-dependent chronic renal failure: 100 mg (5 mL) administered 1-3 times/week during dialysis, for a total dose of 1000 mg (10 doses); administer no more than 3 times/week; may continue to administer at lowest dose necessary to maintain target hemoglobin, hematocrit, and iron storage parameters

Nonhemodialysis-dependent chronic renal failure: 200 mg (10 mL) administered on 5 different days over a 2-week period (total dose: 1000 mg). Single doses of 500 mg administered for 2 doses (day 1 and day 14) have been done in a limited number of patients, 6% (2 out of 30) experienced hypotension (manufacturer's information).

Administration Parenteral: Avoid dilution in dextrose due to an increased incidence of local pain and phlebitis

Slow I.V. injection: 100-200 mg (5-10 mL) over 2-5 minutes

Infusion: Dilute 1 vial (5 mL) in maximum of 100 mL NS; infuse over at least 15 minutes; dilute large doses (>200 mg) in a maximum of 250 mL NS; infuse 300 mg over at least 1.5 hours; infuse 400 mg over at least 2.5 hours; infuse 500 mg over at least 3.5 hours; **not for I.M. administration**

Monitoring Parameters Vital signs and other symptoms of anaphylactoid reactions (during I.V. infusion); reticulocyte count, serum ferritin, hemoglobin, serum iron concentrations, and transferrin saturation (TSAT). Ferritin and TSAT may be inaccurate if measured within 14 days of receiving a large single dose (1000 mg in adults).

Reference Range

Serum iron:

  Newborns: 110-270 mcg/dL

  Infants: 30-70 mcg/dL

  Children: 55-120 mcg/dL

  Adults: Male: 75-175 mcg/dL; female: 65-165 mcg/dL

Total iron binding capacity:

  Newborns: 59-175 mcg/dL

  Infants: 100-400 mcg/dL

  Children and Adults: 230-430 mcg/dL

Transferrin: 204-360 mg/dL

Percent transferrin saturation (TSAT): 20% to 50%

Iron levels >300 mcg/dL may be considered toxic; should be treated as an overdosage

Ferritin: 13-300 ng/mL

Chronic kidney disease (CKD): Targets for iron therapy (KDOQI Guidelines, 2007) to maintain Hgb 11-12 g/dL:

  Children: Nondialysis CKD, hemodialysis, or peritoneal dialysis: Ferritin: >100 ng/mL and TSAT >20%

  Adults: Nondialysis (CKD) or peritoneal dialysis: Ferritin: >100 ng/mL and TSAT >20%

    Hemodialysis: Ferritin >200 ng/mL and TSAT >20% or CHr (content of hemoglobin in reticulocytes) >29 pg/cell

Test Interactions May cause falsely elevated values of serum bilirubin and falsely decreased values of serum calcium.

Additional Information Iron storage may lag behind the appearance of normal red blood cell morphology; use periodic hematologic determination to assess therapy; VLBW infants receiving I.V. iron sucrose 2 mg/kg/day with erythropoietin showed improved erythropoiesis when compared with oral iron supplementation and erythropoietin (Pollak, 2001)

Dosage Forms Excipient information presented when available (limited, particularly for generics); consult specific product labeling.

Injection, solution [preservative free]:
Venofer®: 20 mg of elemental iron/mL (5 mL, 10 mL)

References

"KDOQI Clinical Practice Guideline and Clinical Practice Recommendations for Anemia in Chronic Kidney Disease: 2007 Update of Hemoglobin Target," *Am J Kidney Dis*, 2007, 50(3):471-530.

Leijn E, Monnens LA, and Cornelissen EA, "Intravenous Iron Supplementation in Children on Hemodialysis," *J Nephrol*, 2004, 17 (3):423-6.

Pollak A, Hayde M, Hayn M, et al, "Effect of Intravenous Iron Supplementation on Erythropoiesis in Erythropoietin-Treated Premature Infants," *Pediatrics*, 2001, 107(1):78-85.

◆ **Iron Sulfate** *see* Ferrous Sulfate *on page* 577

◆ **Iron Sulfate (Ferrous Sulfate)** *see* Iron Supplements (Oral/Enteral) *on page* 766

Iron Supplements (Oral/Enteral)
(EYE ern SUP la ments)

Therapeutic Category Iron Salt; Mineral, Oral

Generic Available Yes

Use Prevention and treatment of iron deficiency anemias; supplemental therapy for patients receiving epoetin alfa

Pregnancy Risk Factor A

Contraindications Hypersensitivity to iron salts or any component (see Warnings); hemochromatosis, hemolytic anemia

Warnings Avoid use in premature infants until the vitamin E stores, deficient at birth, are replenished; some products contain sulfites and/or tartrazine which may cause allergic reactions in susceptible individuals

Precautions Avoid using for longer than 6 months, except in patients with conditions that require prolonged therapy; avoid in patients with peptic ulcer, enteritis, or ulcerative colitis; avoid in patients receiving frequent blood transfusions

Adverse Reactions

Gastrointestinal: GI irritation, epigastric pain, nausea, diarrhea, dark stools, constipation

Genitourinary: Discoloration of urine (black or dark)

Miscellaneous: Liquid preparations may temporarily stain the teeth

Food Interactions Milk, cereals, dietary fiber, tea, coffee, or eggs decrease absorption of iron.

Mechanism of Action Iron is released from the plasma and eventually replenishes the depleted iron stores in the bone marrow where it is incorporated into hemoglobin

Pharmacodynamics

Onset of action: Hematologic response to either oral or parenteral iron salts is essentially the same; red blood cell form and color changes within 3-10 days

Maximum effect: Peak reticulocytosis occurs in 5-10 days, and hemoglobin values increase within 2-4 weeks

Pharmacokinetics (Adult data unless noted)

Absorption: Oral: Iron is absorbed in the duodenum and upper jejunum; in persons with normal iron stores 10% of an oral dose is absorbed, this is increased to 20% to 30% in persons with inadequate iron stores; food and achlorhydria will decrease absorption

Elimination: Iron is largely bound to serum transferrin and excreted in the urine, sweat, sloughing of intestinal mucosa, and by menses

Usual Dosage Note: Multiple salt forms of iron exist; close attention must be paid to the salt form when ordering and administering iron; incorrect selection or substitution of one salt for another without proper dosage adjustment may result in serious over- or underdosing.

Oral (dose expressed in terms of **elemental** iron):
Recommended Daily Allowance: See table.

Recommended Daily Allowance of Iron
(Dosage expressed as elemental iron)

Age	RDA (mg)
<5 mo	5
5 mo to 10 y	10
Male	
11-18 y	12
>18 y	10
Female	
11-50 y	15
>50 y	10

Premature neonates: 2-4 mg elemental iron/kg/day divided every 12-24 hours (maximum dose: 15 mg/day)

Infants and Children:

Severe iron deficiency anemia: 4-6 mg elemental iron/ kg/day in 3 divided doses

Mild to moderate iron deficiency anemia: 3 mg elemental iron/kg/day in 1-2 divided doses

Prophylaxis: 1-2 mg elemental iron/kg/day up to a maximum of 15 mg elemental iron/day

Adults:

Iron deficiency: 2-3 mg/kg/day or 60-100 mg elemental iron twice daily up to 60 mg elemental iron 4 times/ day, or 50 mg elemental iron (extended release) 1-2 times/day

Prophylaxis: 60-100 mg elemental iron/day

Elemental Iron Content of Iron Salts

Iron Salt	Elemental Iron Content (% of salt form)	Approximate Equivalent Doses (mg of iron salt)
Ferrous fumarate	33	197
Ferrous gluconate	11.6	560
Ferrous sulfate	20	324
Ferrous sulfate, exsiccated	30	217

Administration Oral: Do not chew or crush sustained release preparations; administer with water or juice between meals for maximum absorption; may administer with food if GI upset occurs; do not administer with milk or milk products

Monitoring Parameters Serum iron, total iron binding capacity, reticulocyte count, hemoglobin, ferritin

Reference Range

Serum iron:
Newborns: 110-270 mcg/dL
Infants: 30-70 mcg/dL
Children: 55-120 mcg/dL
Adults: Male: 75-175 mcg/dL; Female: 65-165 mcg/dL

Total iron binding capacity:
Newborns: 59-175 mcg/dL
Infants: 100-400 mcg/dL
Children and Adults: 230-430 mcg/dL

Transferrin: 204-360 mg/dL
Percent transferrin saturation: 20% to 50%

Iron levels >300 mcg/dL may be considered toxic; should be treated as an overdosage

Ferritin: 13-300 ng/mL

Test Interactions False-positive for blood in stool by the guaiac test

Patient Information May color the stools and urine black; do not take within 2 hours of tetracyclines or fluoroquinolones, do not take with milk or antacids; keep out of reach of children

Additional Information When treating iron deficiency anemias, treat for 3-4 months after hemoglobin/hematocrit return to normal in order to replenish total body stores; elemental iron dosages as high as 15 mg/kg/day have been used to supplement neonates receiving concomitant epoetin alpha in the treatment of anemia of prematurity

Dosage Forms See individual monographs.

◆ **Isagel® [OTC]** see Ethyl Alcohol on page 547
◆ **ISG** see Immune Globulin (Intramuscular) on page 718
◆ **Isoamyl Nitrite** see Amyl Nitrite on page 107

Isoniazid (eye soe NYE a zid)

Medication Safety Issues
International issues:
Hydra®, a brand name for isoniazid in Japan, may be confused with Hydrea®, a brand name for hydroxyurea in U.S.

Canadian Brand Names Isotamine®; PMS-Isoniazid

Therapeutic Category Antitubercular Agent

Generic Available Yes

Use Treatment of susceptible mycobacterial infection due to *M. tuberculosis* and prophylactically to those individuals exposed to tuberculosis

Pregnancy Risk Factor C

Pregnancy Considerations Isoniazid was found to be embryocidal in animal studies; teratogenic effects were not noted. Isoniazid crosses the human placenta. Due to the risk of tuberculosis to the fetus, treatment is recommended when the probability of maternal disease is moderate to high. The CDC recommends isoniazid as part of the initial treatment regimen (CDC, 2003). Pyridoxine supplementation is recommended (25 mg/day).

Lactation Enters breast milk/compatible

Breast-Feeding Considerations Small amounts of isoniazid are excreted in breast milk. However, women with tuberculosis should not be discouraged from breast-feeding. Pyridoxine supplementation is recommended for the mother and infant.

Contraindications Hypersensitivity to isoniazid or any component; acute liver disease; previous history of hepatic damage during isoniazid therapy

Warnings Severe and sometimes fatal hepatitis may occur **[U.S. Boxed Warning]**; usually occurs within the first 3 months of treatment, although may develop even after many months of treatment. The risk of developing hepatitis is age related; daily ethanol consumption may also increase the risk. Patients must report any prodromal symptoms of hepatitis, such as fatigue, weakness, malaise, anorexia, nausea, or vomiting.

Precautions Use with caution in patients with hepatic or renal impairment

Adverse Reactions
Central nervous system: Seizure, stupor, dizziness, agitation, euphoria, psychosis, fever, ataxia

Dermatologic: Skin eruptions, rash, acne

Endocrine & metabolic: Hyperglycemia, metabolic acidosis, pellagra

Gastrointestinal: Nausea, vomiting, epigastric distress; diarrhea (associated with administration of syrup formulation)

Hematologic: Agranulocytosis, hemolytic anemia, aplastic anemia, thrombocytopenia, eosinophilia, leukopenia

Hepatic: Hepatitis, 3% to 10% of children experience transient elevated liver transaminase levels

Local: Irritation at I.M. injection site

Neuromuscular & skeletal: Peripheral neuropathy

Ocular: Optic neuritis

Otic: Tinnitus

Miscellaneous: Hypersensitivity reaction

Drug Interactions
Metabolism/Transport Effects Substrate of CYP2E1 (major); **Inhibits** CYP1A2 (weak), 2A6 (moderate), 2C9 (weak), 2C19 (strong), 2D6 (moderate), 2E1 (moderate), 3A4 (strong); **Induces** CYP2E1 (after discontinuation) (weak)

Avoid Concomitant Use
Avoid concomitant use of Isoniazid with any of the following: Alfuzosin; Clopidogrel; Dronedarone; Eplerenone; Everolimus; Halofantrine; Nilotinib; Nisoldipine; Ranolazine; Rivaroxaban; Romidepsin; Salmeterol; Silodosin; Tamsulosin; Thioridazine; Tolvaptan

Increased Effect/Toxicity
Isoniazid may increase the levels/effects of: Acetaminophen; Alfuzosin; Almotriptan; Alosetron; Benzodiazepines (metabolized by oxidation); Bortezomib; Brinzolamide; CarBAMazepine; Chlorzoxazone; Ciclesonide; Colchicine; CycloSERINE; CYP2A6 Substrates; CYP2C19 Substrates; CYP2D6 Substrates; CYP2E1 Substrates; CYP3A4 Substrates; Dienogest; Dronedarone; Dutasteride; Eplerenone; Everolimus; FentaNYL; Fesoterodine; GuanFACINE; Halofantrine; Ixabepilone; Lumefantrine; Maraviroc; MethylPREDNISolone; Nebivolol; Nilotinib; Nisoldipine; Paricalcitol; Pazopanib; Phenytoin; Pimecrolimus; Ranolazine; Rivaroxaban; Romidepsin; Salmeterol; Saxagliptin; Silodosin; Sorafenib; Tadalafil; Tamoxifen; Tamsulosin; Theophylline Derivatives; Thioridazine; Tolvaptan

The levels/effects of Isoniazid may be increased by: Rifamycin Derivatives

Decreased Effect
Isoniazid may decrease the levels/effects of: Clopidogrel; Codeine; Prasugrel; TraMADol

The levels/effects of Isoniazid may be decreased by: Antacids; Corticosteroids (Systemic)

Food Interactions Rate and extent of isoniazid absorption may be reduced when administered with food; avoid foods with histamine or tyramine (cheese, broad beans, dry sausage, salami, nonfresh meat, liver pate, soya bean, liquid and powdered protein supplements, wine); increase dietary intake of folate, niacin, magnesium, and pyridoxine; the American Academy of Pediatrics recommends that pyridoxine supplementation (1-2 mg/kg/day) should be administered to patients with nutritional deficiencies including all symptomatic HIV-infected children, children or adolescents on meat or milk-deficient diets, breast-feeding infants and their mothers, pregnant adolescents and women, and those predisposed to neuritis to prevent peripheral neuropathy

Stability Protect from light and excessive heat; avoid freezing

Mechanism of Action Inhibits mycolic acid synthesis resulting in disruption of the bacterial cell wall

Pharmacokinetics (Adult data unless noted)
Absorption: Oral, I.M.: Rapid and complete

Distribution: Crosses the placenta; appears in breast milk; distributes into most body tissues and fluids including the CSF

Protein binding: 10% to 15%

Metabolism: By the liver to acetylisoniazid with decay rate determined genetically by acetylation phenotype; undergoes further hydrolysis to isonicotinic acid and acetylhydrazine

Half-life: May be prolonged in patients with impaired hepatic function or severe renal impairment

Fast acetylators: 30-100 minutes

Slow acetylators: 2-5 hours

Time to peak serum concentration: Oral: Within 1-2 hours

Elimination: 75% to 95% excreted in urine as unchanged drug and metabolites; small amounts excreted in feces and saliva

Dialysis: Dialyzable (50% to 100%)

Usual Dosage Oral, I.M.:

Infants and Children:

Treatment: 10-15 mg/kg/day in 1-2 divided doses; maximum dose: 300 mg/day

Prophylaxis: 10 mg/kg/day given once daily, not to exceed 300 mg/day

Adults:

Treatment: 5 mg/kg/day given daily (usual dose: 300 mg)

Prophylaxis: 300 mg/day given daily

American Thoracic Society and CDC currently recommend twice weekly therapy as part of a short-course regimen which follows 1-2 months of daily treatment for uncomplicated pulmonary tuberculosis in **compliant** patients

Children: 20-30 mg/kg/dose (up to 900 mg/dose) twice weekly

Adults: 15 mg/kg/dose (up to 900 mg/dose) twice weekly

Duration of therapy:

Asymptomatic infection (positive skin test):

Isoniazid susceptible: 9 months of isoniazid

Isoniazid resistant: 9 months of rifampin

Pulmonary, hilar adenopathy, and extrapulmonary infection other than meningitis, bone/joint, or disseminated infection:

6 months which includes 2-month therapy of isoniazid, rifampin, and pyrazinamide daily followed by 4 months of isoniazid and rifampin daily **or** 2 months of isoniazid, rifampin, and pyrazinamide daily, followed by 4 months of isoniazid and rifampin twice weekly under direct observation

alternatively

9 months of isoniazid and rifampin daily **or** 1 month of isoniazid and rifampin daily followed by 8 months of isoniazid and rifampin twice weekly under direct observation; if isoniazid resistance is identified, rifampin and ethambutol should be continued for a maximum of 12 months

Note: If drug resistance is possible, ethambutol or streptomycin should be added to the initial therapy regimen until susceptibility is determined.

Meningitis, bone/joint, and disseminated infection:

12 months which includes 2 months of isoniazid, rifampin, pyrazinamide, and streptomycin daily followed by 10 months of isoniazid and rifampin daily **or** 2 months of isoniazid, rifampin, pyrazinamide, and streptomycin daily followed by 10 months of isoniazid and rifampin twice weekly under direct observation

Administration

Oral: Administer 1 hour before or 2 hours after meals with water; administration of isoniazid syrup has been associated with diarrhea

Parenteral: I.M.: Administer I.M. when oral therapy is not possible

Monitoring Parameters Periodic liver function tests; monitor for prodromal signs of hepatitis; ophthalmologic exam; chest x-ray

Test Interactions False-positive urinary glucose with Clinitest®

Patient Information Report any prodromal symptoms of hepatitis (fatigue, weakness, nausea, vomiting, dark urine, or yellowing of eyes) or any burning, tingling, or numbness in the extremities; avoid alcohol

Dosage Forms Excipient information presented when available (limited, particularly for generics); consult specific product labeling.

Injection, solution: 100 mg/mL (10 mL)

Oral solution: 50 mg/5 mL (473 mL) [orange flavor]

Tablet: 100 mg, 300 mg

References

Ad Hoc Committee of the Scientific Assembly on Microbiology, Tuberculosis, and Pulmonary Infections, "Treatment of Tuberculosis and Tuberculosis Infection in Adults and Children," *Clin Infect Dis*, 1995, 21:9-27.

American Academy of Pediatrics, Committee on Infectious Diseases, "Chemotherapy for Tuberculosis in Infants and Children," *Pediatrics*, 1992, 89(1):161-5.

Starke JR, "Modern Approach to the Diagnosis and Treatment of Tuberculosis in Children," *Pediatr Clin North Am*, 1988, 35(3):441-64.

Starke JR, "Multidrug Therapy for Tuberculosis in Children," *Pediatr Infect Dis J*, 1990, 9(11):785-93.

Van Scoy RE and Wilkowske CJ, "Antituberculous Agents: Isoniazid, Rifampin, Streptomycin, Ethambutol, and Pyrazinamide," *Mayo Clin Proc*, 1983, 58(4):233-40.

◆ **Isonicotinic Acid Hydrazide** *see* Isoniazid *on page 767*

◆ **Isonipecaine Hydrochloride** *see* Meperidine *on page 880*

◆ **Isophane Insulin** *see* Insulin NPH *on page 746*

◆ **Isophane Insulin and Regular Insulin** *see* Insulin NPH and Insulin Regular *on page 747*

◆ **Isophosphamide** *see* Ifosfamide *on page 709*

Isoproterenol (eye soe proe TER e nole)

Medication Safety Issues

Sound-alike/look-alike issues:

Isuprel® may be confused with Disophrol®, Ismelin®, Isordil®

Related Information

Asthma *on page 1697*

Emergency Pediatric Drip Calculations *on page 1457*

U.S. Brand Names Isuprel®

Therapeutic Category Adrenergic Agonist Agent; Antiasthmatic; Beta$_1$ & Beta$_2$-Adrenergic Agonist Agent; Bronchodilator; Sympathomimetic

Generic Available No

Use Treatment of asthma or COPD (reversible airway obstruction); ventricular arrhythmias due to A-V nodal block; hemodynamically compromised bradyarrhythmias or atropine-resistant bradyarrhythmias, temporary use in third degree A-V block until pacemaker insertion; low cardiac output or vasoconstrictive shock states

Pregnancy Risk Factor C

Pregnancy Considerations Animal reproduction studies have not been conducted. Adequate studies have not been conducted in pregnant women; use during pregnancy when the potential benefit to the mother outweighs the possible risk to the fetus.

Lactation Excretion in breast milk unknown

Contraindications Hypersensitivity to isoproterenol, other sympathomimetic amines, or any component (see Warnings); angina, pre-existing cardiac arrhythmias (ventricular); tachycardia or A-V block caused by cardiac glycoside intoxication; narrow-angle glaucoma

Warnings Tolerance may occur with prolonged use; when discontinuing an isoproterenol continuous infusion used for bronchodilation, the infusion **must** be gradually tapered over a 24- to 48-hour period to prevent rebound bronchospasm; injection contains sulfites which may cause allergic reactions in susceptible individuals

Precautions Use with caution in diabetics, renal or cardiovascular disease, hyperthyroidism, prostatic hypertrophy

Adverse Reactions

Cardiovascular: Flushing of the face or skin, ventricular arrhythmias, tachycardia, hypotension, chest pain, palpitations, hypertension

Central nervous system: Nervousness, restlessness, anxiety, dizziness, headache, vertigo, insomnia

Endocrine & metabolic: Parotid glands swelling

Gastrointestinal: Heartburn, GI distress, nausea, vomiting, dry throat, xerostomia

Neuromuscular & skeletal: Tremor, weakness, trembling

Miscellaneous: Diaphoresis

Drug Interactions

Avoid Concomitant Use

Avoid concomitant use of Isoproterenol with any of the following: Inhalational Anesthetics

Increased Effect/Toxicity

The levels/effects of Isoproterenol may be increased by: COMT Inhibitors; Inhalational Anesthetics

Decreased Effect There are no known significant interactions involving a decrease in effect.

Mechanism of Action Stimulates beta$_1$- and beta$_2$-receptors resulting in relaxation of bronchial, GI, and uterine smooth muscle; increases heart rate and contractility; causes vasodilation of peripheral vasculature

Pharmacodynamics

Onset of action: I.V.: Immediately

Duration: I.V. (single dose): Few minutes

Pharmacokinetics (Adult data unless noted)

Metabolism: By conjugation in many tissues including the liver and lungs

Half-life: 2.5-5 minutes

Elimination: In urine principally as sulfate conjugates

Usual Dosage

Neonates, Infants, and Children: I.V. infusion: 0.05-2 mcg/kg/minute; rate (mL/hour) = dose (mcg/kg/minute) x weight (kg) x 60 minutes/hour divided by concentration (mcg/mL)

Adults: I.V. infusion: 2-20 mcg/minute

Administration Parenteral: For continuous infusions, dilute in dextrose or NS to a maximum concentration of 20 mcg/mL; concentrations as high as 64 mcg/mL have been used safely and with efficacy in situations of extreme fluid restriction

Monitoring Parameters Heart rate, blood pressure, respiratory rate, arterial blood gases, central venous pressure, ECG

Patient Information May cause dry mouth

Additional Information Hypotension is more common in hypovolemic patients

Dosage Forms Excipient information presented when available (limited, particularly for generics); consult specific product labeling.

Injection, solution, as hydrochloride:

Isuprel®: 0.2 mg/mL (1:5000) (1 mL, 5 mL) [contains sodium metabisulfite]

References

Rachelefsky GS and Siegel SC, "Asthma in Infants and Children - Treatment of Childhood Asthma: Part II," *J Allergy Clin Immunol*, 1985, 76(3):409-25.

◆ **Isoproterenol Hydrochloride** see Isoproterenol on page 768

◆ **Isoptin® SR** see Verapamil on page 1416

◆ **Isopto® Atropine** see Atropine on page 157

◆ **Isopto® Carpine** see Pilocarpine on page 1110

◆ **Isopto® Homatropine** see Homatropine on page 678

◆ **Isopto® Hyoscine** see Scopolamine on page 1248

◆ **Isotamine® (Can)** see Isoniazid on page 767

Isotretinoin (eye soe TRET i noyn)

Medication Safety Issues

Sound-alike/look-alike issues:

Accutane® may be confused with Accolate®, Accupril® Claravis™ may be confused with Cleviprex™

Isotretinoin may be confused with tretinoin

U.S. Brand Names Accutane® [DSC]; Amnesteem®; Claravis™; Sotret®

Canadian Brand Names Accutane®; Clarus™; Isotrex®

Therapeutic Category Acne Products; Retinoic Acid Derivative; Vitamin A Derivative

Generic Available No

Use Treatment of severe recalcitrant nodular acne unresponsive to conventional therapy, including systemic antibiotics (FDA approved in ages ≥12 years and adults); used investigationally for the treatment of children with high-risk neuroblastoma that does not respond to conventional therapy

Restrictions iPLEDGE is a risk minimization program designed by the FDA to decrease fetal exposures to isotretinoin. iPLEDGE requires that all wholesalers, prescribers, patients (male and female), and dispensing pharmacies register with a central clearinghouse. Registration is accessible through the internet at http://www.ipledgeprogram.com or by calling 866-495-0654. The Responsible Site Pharmacist must activate the iPLEDGE registration. Prescriptions for isotretinoin may not be dispensed unless authorized by the iPLEDGE system and Risk Management Authorization (RMA) number documented. Prescriptions may not be written for more than a 30-day supply. The iPLEDGE system will automatically calculate and provide the "Do Not Dispense To Patient After" date to the pharmacist. The pharmacist must not dispense the prescription after this date. Automatic refills are not allowed; a new prescription must be written and authorization from the iPLEDGE received.

Prescribers will be provided with qualification stickers after they have read the details of the program and have signed and mailed to the manufacturer their agreement to participate. Audits of pharmacies will be conducted to monitor program compliance.

Medication Guide An FDA-approved patient medication guide, which is available with the product information and as follows, must be dispensed with this medication for each new outpatient prescription and refill.

Accutane®: http://www.fda.gov/downloads/Drugs/DrugSafety/ucm085812.pdf

Sotret®: http://www.fda.gov/downloads/Drugs/DrugSafety/ucm089135.pdf

Pregnancy Risk Factor X

Pregnancy Considerations Major fetal abnormalities (both internal and external), spontaneous abortion, premature births and low IQ scores in surviving infants have been reported. [**U.S. Boxed Warning**]: **Because of the high likelihood of teratogenic effects, all patients (male and female), prescribers, wholesalers, and dispensing pharmacists must register and be active in the iPLEDGE™ risk management program; do not prescribe isotretinoin for women who are or who are likely to become pregnant while using the drug.** This medication is contraindicated in females of childbearing potential unless they are able to comply with the guidelines of the iPLEDGE™ pregnancy prevention program. Females of childbearing potential should not become pregnant during therapy or for 1 month following discontinuation of isotretinoin. Upon discontinuation of treatment, females of childbearing potential should have a pregnancy test after their last dose and again one month after their last dose. Two forms of contraception should be continued during this time. Any pregnancies should be reported to the iPLEDGE™ program (www.ipledge-pro-gram.com or 866-495-0654).

Lactation Excretion in breast milk unknown/contraindicated

Contraindications Hypersensitivity to isotretinoin, para-bens, soybeans, vitamin A or other retinoids; patients who are pregnant or intend to become pregnant during treatment; nursing mothers

Warnings Accutane® must not be used by female patients who are or may become pregnant **[U.S. Boxed Warning]**; major human fetal abnormalities to isotretinoin administration have been documented; during pregnancy, it can cause fetal defects in the CNS (cerebral abnormalities, hydrocephalus, microcephaly, cranial nerve deficit, cerebellar malformation), skull, ear, eye, and cardiovascular systems, cleft palate, and parathyroid hormone deficiency. Because of the high likelihood of teratogenic effects, all patients (male and female), prescribers, wholesalers, and dispensing pharmacists must register and be active in the iPLEDGE risk management program **[U.S. Boxed Warning]**; do not prescribe isotretinoin for women who are or who are likely to become pregnant while using the drug. Prescription for isotretinoin should not be issued until a female patient has had negative results from 2 urine or serum pregnancy tests, one performed in the prescriber's office when the patient is qualified for therapy, the second one performed on the second day of next normal menstrual period or 11 days after the last unprotected act of sexual intercourse, whichever is later. Pregnancy testing and counseling should be repeated monthly. Two forms of effective contraception must be used for at least 1 month before beginning therapy, during therapy, and for 1 month after discontinuation of therapy. Upon discontinuation of treatment, females of childbearing potential should have a pregnancy test after their last dose and again 1 month after their last dose. If pregnancy occurs during treatment, isotretinoin should be discontinued immediately and patient should be referred to a physician experienced in reproductive toxicity.

Isotretinoin may cause depression, psychosis, and suicidal ideations; all patients should be observed closely for symptoms of depression or suicidal thoughts. Discontinuation of treatment alone may not be sufficient; further evaluation may be necessary. Use with extreme caution in patients with a history of psychiatric disorder. Concomitant use with tetracyclines has been associated with cases of pseudotumor cerebri; avoid concomitant treatment with tetracyclines. Rare postmarketing cases of severe skin reactions (eg, erythema multiforme, Stevens-Johnson syndrome, toxic epidermal necrolysis), including fatalities, have been reported; monitor for severe skin reactions; discontinue use if severe skin reaction occurs. Dose-related elevations of serum triglycerides (in excess of 800 mg/dL) have been reported with use; acute pancreatitis and fatal hemorrhagic pancreatitis (rare) have been reported. Hearing impairment, which can continue after therapy is discontinued, may occur. Clinical hepatitis and elevated liver enzymes have been reported with use. May decrease bone mineral density; osteoporosis, osteopenia, and bone fractures have been reported with long-term, high-dose, or multiple courses of therapy. Use with caution in patients with a genetic predisposition to bone disorders (ie, osteoporosis, osteomalacia) and with disease states or concomitant medications that can induce bone disorders. Patients may be at risk when participating in activities with repetitive impact (such as sports). Skeletal hyperostosis, calcification of ligaments and tendons, and premature epiphyseal closure have also been reported with the use. Vision impairment, corneal opacities, and decreased night vision have also been reported with use.

Precautions Use with caution in patients with diabetes mellitus or hypertriglyceridemia; history of childhood osteoporosis, osteomalacia, or other disorders of bone metabolism including patients with anorexia nervosa or patients receiving drugs that cause osteoporosis/osteomalacia or affect vitamin D metabolism (ie, corticosteroids, anticonvulsants)

Adverse Reactions

Cardiovascular: Chest pain, edema, flushing, palpitations, syncope, tachycardia, vascular thrombotic stroke, vasculitis

Central nervous system: Aggressive behavior, dizziness, drowsiness, emotional instability, fatigue, headache, insomnia, lethargy, malaise, mental depression, nervousness, paresthesia, pseudotumor cerebri (see Warnings), psychosis, seizures, suicidal ideation/attempts (see Warnings), violent behavior

Dermatologic: Abnormal wound healing, acne fulminans, alopecia, bruising, cheilitis (dose-related), cutaneous allergic reactions, dry nose, dry skin, eczema, eruptive xanthomas, erythema multiforme, facial erythema, fragility of skin, hair abnormalities, hirsutism, hyper/hypopigmentation, nail dystrophy, paronychia, peeling of palms or soles, photosensitivity, pruritus, rash, Stevens-Johnson syndrome, toxic epidermal necrolysis (see Warnings)

Endocrine & metabolic: Abnormal menses, HDL decreased, hypercalcemia, hypercholesterolemia, hyperglycemia, hypertriglyceridemia (see Warnings), hyperuricemia, weight loss

Gastrointestinal: Acute pancreatitis, colitis, esophageal ulceration, esophagitis, gum inflammation or bleeding, ileitis, inflammatory bowel disease (see Warnings), nausea, vomiting, xerostomia

Hematologic: Agranulocytosis (rare), anemia, erythrocyte sedimentation rate increased, neutropenia, platelet count increased, pyogenic granuloma, thrombocytopenia

Hepatic: AST, ALT, GGTP, LDH, and alkaline phosphatase increased; hepatitis

Neuromuscular & skeletal: Arthralgia (22% in pediatric patients), arthritis, back pain (29% in pediatric patients), bone mineral density decreased, bone pain, CPK increased, myalgia, premature epiphyseal closure (see Warnings), rhabdomyolysis (rare), skeletal hyperostosis, tendonitis, weakness

Ocular: Blurred vision, cataracts, color vision disorder, conjunctivitis, corneal opacities, dry eyes, eyelid inflammation, keratitis, night vision decreased, optic neuritis, photophobia, visual disturbances

Otic: Hearing impairment, tinnitus

Renal: Glomerulonephritis, hematuria, proteinuria, pyuria, vasculitis

Respiratory: Bronchospasm, epistaxis, respiratory infection, Wegener's granulomatosis

Miscellaneous: Allergic reactions, anaphylactic reactions, diaphoresis, disseminated herpes simplex, infection, lymphadenopathy

Drug Interactions

Avoid Concomitant Use

Avoid concomitant use of Isotretinoin with any of the following: Tetracycline Derivatives; Vitamin A

Increased Effect/Toxicity

Isotretinoin may increase the levels/effects of: Vitamin A

The levels/effects of Isotretinoin may be increased by: Alcohol (Ethyl); Tetracycline Derivatives

Decreased Effect

Isotretinoin may decrease the levels/effects of: Contraceptives (Estrogens); Contraceptives (Progestins)

Food Interactions Food (high-fat meal) or milk increases isotretinoin bioavailability.

Stability Store at room temperature of 59°F to 86°F (15°C to 30°C). Protect from light.

Mechanism of Action Reduces sebaceous gland size and reduces sebum production; regulates cell proliferation and differentiation

Pharmacokinetics (Adult data unless noted) Note: Pharmacokinetic parameters in adolescents (12-15 years) are similar to adults.

Absorption: Oral: Demonstrates biphasic absorption

Distribution: Crosses the placenta; appears in breast milk, bile

Protein binding: 99% to 100%; primarily albumin

Metabolism: Hepatic via CYP2B6, 2C8, 2C9, 2D6, 3A4; forms metabolites; major metabolite: 4-oxo-isotretinoin (active)

Half-life, terminal: Parent drug: 21 hours; Metabolite: 21-24 hours

Time to peak serum concentration: Within 3 hours

Elimination: Excreted in feces as unchanged drug and in urine as metabolites

Usual Dosage Oral:

Children: Acne: 0.5-1 mg/kg/day in 2 divided doses; for severe cases (involving trunk, nuchal region, lower back, buttocks, thighs) may require higher doses up to 2 mg/kg/day in 2 divided doses. Duration of therapy is typically 15-20 weeks or until the total cyst count decreases by 70%, whichever is sooner; an alternate reported approach is continuation until a total cumulative dose of 120 mg/kg (eg, 1 mg/kg/day for 120 days). Lower dosages (0.3-0.5 mg/kg/day) continued for 6-12 months to cumulative dose 120 mg/kg have also been shown effective (see Brecher, 2003).

Children: Maintenance therapy for neuroblastoma: 160 mg/m^2/day in 2 divided doses for 14 consecutive days in a 28-day cycle (see Matthay, 1999)

Adults: Acne: 0.5-1 mg/kg/day in 2 divided doses (dosages as low as 0.05 mg/kg/day have been reported to be beneficial) for 15-20 weeks or until the total cyst count decreases by 70%, whichever is sooner. Adults with very severe disease/scarring or primarily involves the trunk may require dosage adjustment up to 2 mg/kg/day. A second course of therapy may be initiated after a period of ≥2 months of therapy.

Administration Oral: Capsules can be swallowed or chewed and swallowed; the capsule may be opened with a large needle and the contents placed on apple sauce or ice cream for patients unable to swallow the capsule; administer with meals

Monitoring Parameters CBC with differential, platelet count, baseline ESR, serum triglyceride, liver enzymes, CPK, ophthalmologic exam, blood glucose; pregnancy test in female patients of childbearing potential (see Warnings); bone density measurement; serious skin reactions

Patient Information Read the patient Medication Guide that you receive with each prescription and refill of isotretinoin. Do not take vitamin supplements containing vitamin A; use caution when driving at night since decreased night vision can develop suddenly; patients who wear contact lenses may experience decreased tolerance to the lenses; avoid alcohol; may cause dry mouth; notify physician of any headache, blurred vision, yellowing of skin or eyes, bone or muscle pain, vision changes, suicidal thoughts, dark urine, abdominal pain, rectal bleeding, severe diarrhea, or rashes. Female patients of childbearing potential must be counseled to use 2 effective forms of contraception simultaneously, unless absolute abstinence is the chosen method. Do not self-medicate with St John's wort due to a possible interaction with hormonal contraceptives; female patients should join the Accutane® survey and watch a videotape that provides information about contraceptive methods; inform prescriber if you are pregnant. This drug should not be used during pregnancy. Do not get pregnant 1 month before, during, or for 1 month following therapy. This drug may cause severe fetal defects. Two forms of

contraception and monthly tests to rule out pregnancy are required during therapy. It is important to note that any type of contraception may fail; it is the responsibility of the patient to be compliant with contraceptive therapy. Do not breast-feed. Inform patients not to donate blood during therapy and for 1 month following discontinuation of therapy.

May cause photosensitivity reactions (eg, exposure to sunlight may cause severe sunburn, skin rash, redness, or itching); avoid exposure to sunlight and artificial light sources (sunlamps, tanning booth/bed); wear protective clothing, wide-brimmed hats, sunglasses, and lip sunscreen (SPF ≥15); use a sunscreen [broad-spectrum sunscreen or physical sunscreen (preferred) or sunblock with SPF ≥15]; contact physician if reaction occurs.

Dosage Forms Excipient information presented when available (limited, particularly for generics); consult specific product labeling. [DSC] = Discontinued product

Capsule, oral:

Claravis™: 10 mg, 20 mg, 40 mg [contains soybean oil]

Capsule, softgel, oral:

Accutane®: 10 mg, 20 mg, 40 mg [contains soybean oil and parabens] [DSC]

Amnesteem®: 10 mg, 20 mg, 40 mg [contains soybean oil]

Sotret®: 10 mg, 20 mg, 30 mg, 40 mg [contains soybean oil and parabens]

References

American Academy of Pediatrics Committee on Drugs, "Retinoid Therapy for Severe Dermatological Disorders," *Pediatrics*, 1992, 90 (1 Pt 1):119-20.

Brecher AR and Orlow SJ, "Oral Retinoid Therapy for Dermatologic Conditions in Children and Adolescents," *J Am Acad Dermatol*, 2003, 49(2):171-82.

DiGiovanna JJ and Peck GL, "Oral Synthetic Retinoid Treatment in Children," *Pediatr Dermatol*, 1983, 1(1):77-88.

Matthay KK, Villablanca JG, Seeger RC, et al, "Treatment of High-Risk Neuroblastoma With Intensive Chemotherapy, Radiotherapy, Autologous Bone Marrow Transplantation, and 13-cis-Retinoic Acid. Children's Cancer Group," *N Engl J Med*, 1999, 341:1165-73.

Reynolds CP, Kane DJ, Einhorn PA, et al, "Response of Neuroblastoma to Retinoic Acid *In Vitro*, and *In Vivo*," *Prog Clin Biol Res*, 1991, 366:203-11.

◆ **Isotrex® (Can)** *see* Isotretinoin *on page 769*

Isradipine (iz RA di peen)

Medication Safety Issues

Sound-alike/look-alike issues:

DynaCirc® may be confused with Dynabac®, Dynacin®

Related Information

Antihypertensive Agents by Class *on page 1481*

U.S. Brand Names DynaCirc® CR

Canadian Brand Names DynaCirc®

Therapeutic Category Antihypertensive Agent; Calcium Channel Blocker; Calcium Channel Blocker, Nondihydropyridine

Generic Available Yes: Capsule

Use Treatment of hypertension

Pregnancy Risk Factor C

Pregnancy Considerations Teratogenic effects were not observed in animal studies. Israpidine crosses the human placenta. There are no adequate and well-controlled studies in pregnant women.

Lactation Excretion in breast milk unknown/not recommended

Contraindications Hypersensitivity to isradipine or any component

Warnings Symptomatic hypotension may occur; syncope and severe dizziness have been rarely reported, especially after initiation of recommended doses. May cause negative inotropic effects in some patients (use with caution in patients with CHF, especially when used in combination with beta-blockers). Dose-related peripheral edema may occur (use caution in differentiating this adverse effect from decreasing left ventricular function in patients with CHF).

Capsules may contain benzyl alcohol which may cause allergic reactions in susceptible individuals; large amounts of benzyl alcohol (≥99 mg/kg/day) have been associated with a potentially fatal toxicity ("gasping syndrome") in neonates; the "gasping syndrome" consists of metabolic acidosis, respiratory distress, gasping respirations, CNS dysfunction (including convulsions, intracranial hemor-rhage), hypotension and cardiovascular collapse; use isradipine capsules containing benzyl alcohol with caution in neonates; *in vitro* and animal studies have shown that benzoate, a metabolite of benzyl alcohol, displaces bilirubin from protein binding sites

Precautions Use with caution in patients with CHF or hepatic dysfunction. Use controlled release tablets with caution in patients with severe GI narrowing (obstructive symptoms have occurred in patients with GI strictures after ingestion of other nondeformable controlled release products). Safety and efficacy have not been established in pediatric patients.

Adverse Reactions

Cardiovascular: Edema (dose related, 1% to 9%), palpitation (dose related, 1% to 5%), flushing (dose related, 1% to 5%), tachycardia, chest pain; syncope (rare); slight prolongation of QT_c interval of 3% in one study

Central nervous system: Headache, dizziness, fatigue (dose related, 1% to 9%)

Dermatologic: Rash

Gastrointestinal: Nausea, abdominal discomfort, vomiting, diarrhea, constipation, abdominal distention

Genitourinary: Urinary frequency increased

Neuromuscular & skeletal: Weakness

Respiratory: Dyspnea

Drug Interactions

Metabolism/Transport Effects Substrate of CYP3A4 (major); **Inhibits** CYP3A4 (weak)

Avoid Concomitant Use

Avoid concomitant use of Isradipine with any of the following: Artemether; Dronedarone; Lumefantrine; Nilo-tinib; Pimozide; QuiNINE; Tetrabenazine; Thioridazine; Ziprasidone

Increased Effect/Toxicity

Isradipine may increase the levels/effects of: Amifostine; Antihypertensives; Calcium Channel Blockers (Nondihy-dropyridine); Dronedarone; Hypotensive Agents; Magne-sium Salts; Neuromuscular-Blocking Agents (Nondepolarizing); Nitroprusside; Phenytoin; Pimozide; QTc-Prolonging Agents; QuiNINE; RiTUXimab; Tacroli-mus; Tacrolimus (Systemic); Tetrabenazine; Thiorida-zine; Ziprasidone

The levels/effects of Isradipine may be increased by: Alfuzosin; Alpha1-Blockers; Antifungal Agents (Azole Derivatives, Systemic); Artemether; Calcium Channel Blockers (Nondihydropyridine); Chloroquine; Cimetidine; Ciprofloxacin; Ciprofloxacin (Systemic); CycloSPORINE; CycloSPORINE (Systemic); CYP3A4 Inhibitors (Moder-ate); CYP3A4 Inhibitors (Strong); Diazoxide; Flucona-zole; Gadobutrol; Herbs (Hypotensive Properties); Lumefantrine; Macrolide Antibiotics; Magnesium Salts; MAO Inhibitors; Nilotinib; Pentoxifylline; Phosphodiester-ase 5 Inhibitors; Prostacyclin Analogues; Protease Inhibitors; QuiNINE; Quinupristin

Decreased Effect

Isradipine may decrease the levels/effects of: Clopidog-rel; QuiNIDine

The levels/effects of Isradipine may be decreased by: Barbiturates; Calcium Salts; CarBAMazepine; CYP3A4

Inducers (Strong); Deferasirox; Herbs (CYP3A4 Indu-cers); Herbs (Hypertensive Properties); Methylphenidate; Nafcillin; Rifamycin Derivatives; Yohimbine

Food Interactions

Capsules: Food decreases the rate, but not the extent of absorption

Controlled release tablets: Food decreases bioavailability by up to 25%

Stability

Capsules: Store at controlled room temperature; dispense in a tight, light-resistant container

Controlled release tablets: Store below 30°C (86°F), in a tight container; protect from moisture and humidity

Mechanism of Action Inhibits calcium ions from entering the "slow channels" or select voltage-sensitive areas of vascular smooth muscle and myocardium during depola-rization; produces a relaxation of coronary vascular smooth muscle and coronary vasodilation; increases myocardial oxygen delivery in patients with vasospastic angina

Pharmacodynamics

Onset of action:

Immediate release capsule: ~1 hour

Controlled release tablet: 2 hours

Maximum effect: **Note:** Full hypotensive effect may not occur for 2-4 weeks

Immediate release capsule (single dose): 2-3 hours

Controlled release tablet (single dose): 8-10 hours

Duration:

Immediate release capsule: >12 hours

Controlled release tablet: 24 hours

Pharmacokinetics (Adult data unless noted)

Absorption: 90% to 95%, but large first-pass effect

Distribution: V_d (apparent): 3 L/kg; crosses the placenta

Protein binding: 95%

Metabolism: Extensive first-pass effect; hepatically metab-olized via cytochrome P450 isoenzyme CYP3A4; major metabolic pathways include oxidation and ester cleav-age; six inactive metabolites have been identified

Bioavailability: Oral: 15% to 24%

Patients with renal dysfunction (Cl_{cr} 30-80 mL/minute): Increased by 45%

Patients with severe renal failure (Cl_{cr} <10 mL/minute) who are on hemodialysis: Decreased by 20% to 50%

Patients with hepatic impairment: Increased by 52%

Half-life: Alpha half-life: 1.5-2 hours; terminal half-life: 8 hours

Time to peak serum concentration:

Immediate release capsule: 1.5 hours

Controlled release tablet: Plateaus between 7-18 hours

Elimination: 60% to 65% of the dose is eliminated in the urine (none as unchanged drug); 25% to 30% in the feces

Dialysis: Not significantly removed by hemodialysis (supplemental dose not required)

Usual Dosage

Children: Limited information exists; dose is not well established; only 3 retrospective pediatric studies have been published (see Flynn, 2002; Johnson, 1997; Strauser, 2000); further studies are needed. Some experts recommend the following:

Immediate release capsules (or extemporaneously prepared suspension): Initial: 0.05-0.15 mg/kg/dose given 3-4 times/day; titrate dose to response; usual dose: 0.3-0.4 mg/kg/day divided every 8 hours; max-imum dose 0.8 mg/kg/day up to 20 mg/day (see Flynn, 2000)

Controlled release tablet: Children who receive a total daily dose of 5 or 10 mg of an immediate release formulation may be switched to an equivalent daily dose of the controlled release tablets administered once or twice daily (Flynn, 2002).

Adults:

Immediate release capsules: Initial: 2.5 mg twice daily; titrate dose to response; may increase dose in increments of 5 mg/day at 2-4 week intervals; usual dosage range (JNC 7): 2.5-10 mg/day in 2 divided doses; maximum: 20 mg/day; **Note:** Most patients do not have any additional response to doses >10 mg/day, but may have increased adverse effects.

Controlled release tablet: Initial: 5 mg once daily; titrate dose to response; may increase dose in increments of 5 mg/day at 2-4 week intervals; maximum: 20 mg/day; **Note:** Doses >10 mg/day are associated with increased adverse effects.

Administration May be administered without regard to meals; swallow controlled release tablet whole, do not crush, break, chew, or divide.

Monitoring Parameters Blood pressure, heart rate, liver and renal function

Patient Information May cause dizziness and impair ability to perform activities requiring mental alertness or physical coordination. Do not discontinue abruptly. Report unrelieved headache, dizziness, shortness of breath, rapid heart beat, chest pain, swelling of extremities, or sudden weight gain. Some medicines may interact with isradipine; report the use of other medications, nonprescription medications, and herbal or natural products to your physician and pharmacist; avoid the herbal medicine St John's wort. Empty controlled release tablets may appear in stool after medication is absorbed (this is normal).

Nursing Implications Assess therapeutic effectiveness and adverse reactions on a regular basis during therapy. Monitor blood pressure. Instruct patient on appropriate use, side effects, appropriate interventions, and adverse symptoms to report.

Additional Information DynaCirc® CR is an osmotic controlled-release formulation; the tablet is nondeformable; drug is released from the tablet at a constant rate that is dependent on the osmotic gradient between the contents of the bilayer active drug core of the tablet and the fluid in the GI tract; drug release is independent of pH or GI motility.

Dosage Forms Excipient information presented when available (limited, particularly for generics); consult specific product labeling.

Capsule: 2.5 mg, 5 mg

Tablet, controlled release:

DynaCirc® CR: 5 mg, 10 mg

Extemporaneous Preparations A 1 mg/mL oral suspension made from isradipine capsules and simple syrup, NF was stable for 35 days when stored in amber glass prescription bottles in the dark at 4°C. Empty the contents of ten 5 mg isradipine capsules into a glass mortar; wet the powder with glycerin, USP and triturate to a fine paste; add 15 mL of simple syrup and triturate well; transfer contents to a 60 mL amber glass prescription bottle; use 10 mL of simple syrup to rinse the mortar and transfer to the prescription bottle; repeat and qsad to a final volume of 50 mL; label "refrigerate" and "shake well".

MacDonald JL, Johnson CE, and Jacobson P, "Stability of Isradipine in Extemporaneously Compounded Oral Liquids," *Am J Hosp Pharm*, 1994, 51(19):2409-11.

References

Ahmed K, Michael B, and Burke JF Jr, "Effects of Isradipine on Renal Hemodynamics in Renal Transplant Patients Treated With Cyclosporine," *Clin Nephrol*, 1997, 48(5):307-10.

Chobanian AV, Bakris GL, Black HR, et al, "The Seventh Report of the Joint National Committee on Prevention, Detection, Evaluation, and Treatment of High Blood Pressure: The JNC 7 Report," *JAMA*, 2003, 289(19):2560-72.

Flynn JT and Pasko DA, "Calcium Channel Blockers: Pharmacology and Place in Therapy of Pediatric Hypertension," *Pediatr Nephrol*, 2000, 15(3-4):302-16.

Flynn JT and Warnick SJ, "Isradipine Treatment of Hypertension in Children: A Single-Center Experience," *Pediatr Nephrol*, 2002, 17(9):748-53.

Johnson CE, Jacobson PA, and Song MH, "Isradipine Therapy in Hypertensive Pediatric Patients," *Ann Pharmacother*, 1997, 31 (6):704-7.

McCrea JB, Francos GF, and Burke JF, "The Beneficial Effects of Isradipine on Renal Hemodynamics in Cyclosporine-Treated Renal Transplant Recipients," *Transplantation*, 1993, 55(3):672-4.

Rodicio JL, "Calcium Antagonists and Renal Protection From Cyclosporine Nephrotoxicity: Long-Term Trial in Renal Transplantation Patients," *J Cardiovasc Pharmacol*, 2000, 35(3 Suppl 1):S7-11.

Steele RM, Schuna AA, and Schreiber RT, "Calcium Antagonist-Induced Gingival Hyperplasia," *Ann Intern Med*, 1994, 120(8):663-4.

Strauser LM, Groshong T, and Tobias JD, "Initial Experience With Isradipine for the Treatment of Hypertension in Children," *South Med J*, 2000, 93(3):287-93.

◆ **Istalol®** *see* Timolol *on page 1351*

◆ **Isuprel®** *see* Isoproterenol *on page 768*

Itraconazole (i tra KOE na zole)

Medication Safety Issues

Sound-alike/look-alike issues:

Itraconazole may be confused with fluconazole

Sporanox® may be confused with Suprax®, Topamax®

U.S. Brand Names Sporanox®

Canadian Brand Names Sporanox®

Therapeutic Category Antifungal Agent, Systemic

Generic Available Yes: Capsule

Use Treatment of susceptible systemic fungal infections in immunocompromised and nonimmunocompromised patients including blastomycosis, coccidioidomycosis, paracoccidioidomycosis, histoplasmosis, and aspergillosis in patients who do not respond to or cannot tolerate amphotericin B; treatment of oropharyngeal or esophageal candidiasis (oral solution only)

Pregnancy Risk Factor C

Pregnancy Considerations Should not be used to treat onychomycosis during pregnancy. Effective contraception should be used during treatment and for 2 months following treatment. Congenital abnormalities have been reported during postmarketing surveillance, but a causal relationship has not been established.

Lactation Enters breast milk/not recommended

Contraindications Hypersensitivity to itraconazole or any component; concurrent administration with cisapride, dofetilide, ergot derivatives, levomethadyl, lovastatin, midazolam (oral), nisoldipine, pimozide, quinidine, simvastatin, or triazolam; treatment of onychomycosis in patients with evidence of left ventricular dysfunction, CHF, a history of CHF, pregnant women, or women intending to become pregnant

Warnings Not recommended for treatment of onychomycosis in patients with left ventricular dysfunction or a history of CHF **[U.S. Boxed Warning]**. Negative inotropic effects have been observed following intravenous administration. Discontinue or reassess use if signs or symptoms of CHF occur during treatment **[U.S. Boxed Warning]**. Calcium channel blockers (CCBs) may cause additive negative inotropic effects when used concurrently with itraconazole. Itraconazole may also inhibit the metabolism of CCBs; therefore, use caution with concurrent use of itraconazole and CCBs due to an increased risk of heart failure. Coadministration of cisapride, pimozide, quinidine, dofetilide, or levacetylmethadol (levomethadyl) with itraconazole is contraindicated **[U.S. Boxed Warning]**. Rare cases of serious cardiovascular adverse events (including death), ventricular tachycardia, and torsade de pointes have been observed due to increased cisapride, pimozide, quinidine, dofetilide, or levomethadyl concentrations induced by itraconazole. Serious (and rarely fatal) hepatic toxicity (eg, hepatitis, cholestasis, fulminant failure) has been observed with azole therapy; monitor liver function closely and dosage adjustment may be warranted. Not recommended for use in patients with active liver disease, elevated liver enzymes, or prior hepatotoxic reactions to other drugs; **itraconazole solution and capsules should not be used interchangeably**.

Precautions Use with caution in patients with hypersensitivity to other azole antifungal agents, patients with left ventricular dysfunction or a history of CHF, and in patients with hepatic impairment; discontinue if signs and symptoms of liver disease or CHF develop. Large differences in itraconazole pharmacokinetic parameters have been observed in cystic fibrosis patients receiving the solution; if a patient with cystic fibrosis does not respond to therapy, alternate therapies should be considered. Transient or permanent hearing loss has been reported. Quinidine (a contraindicated drug) was used concurrently in several of these cases. Hearing loss usually resolves after discontinuation, but may persist in some patients.

Adverse Reactions

Cardiovascular: Hypertension, ventricular fibrillation, edema, CHF

Central nervous system: Headache, dizziness, somnolence, fever, fatigue

Dermatologic: Rash, pruritus, urticaria, angioedema, toxic epidermal necrolysis

Endocrine & metabolic: Hypokalemia, adrenal insufficiency, gynecomastia

Gastrointestinal: Nausea, vomiting, diarrhea, abdominal pain, anorexia

Hematologic: Thrombocytopenia, leukopenia

Hepatic: Liver enzymes elevated, hepatitis

Otic: Tinnitus

Renal: Albuminuria

Drug Interactions

Metabolism/Transport Effects Substrate of CYP3A4 (major); **Inhibits** CYP3A4 (strong), P-glycoprotein

Avoid Concomitant Use

Avoid concomitant use of Itraconazole with any of the following: Alfuzosin; Cisapride; Conivaptan; Dabigatran Etexilate; Dofetilide; Dronedarone; Eplerenone; Ergot Derivatives; Everolimus; Halofantrine; Nilotinib; Nisoldipine; Pimozide; QuiNIDine; Ranolazine; Rivaroxaban; Romidepsin; Salmeterol; Silodosin; Tamsulosin; Tolvaptan; Topotecan

Increased Effect/Toxicity

Itraconazole may increase the levels/effects of: Alfentanil; Alfuzosin; Almotriptan; Alosetron; Aprepitant; Benzodiazepines (metabolized by oxidation); Bortezomib; Bosentan; Brinzolamide; BusPIRone; Busulfan; Calcium Channel Blockers; CarBAMazepine; Cardiac Glycosides; Ciclesonide; Cilostazol; Cisapride; Colchicine; Conivaptan; Corticosteroids (Orally Inhaled); Corticosteroids (Systemic); CycloSPORINE; CycloSPORINE (Systemic); CYP3A4 Substrates; Dabigatran Etexilate; Dienogest; Docetaxel; Dofetilide; Dronedarone; Dutasteride; Eletriptan; Eplerenone; Ergot Derivatives; Erlotinib; Eszopiclone; Everolimus; FentaNYL; Fesoterodine; Fexofenadine; Fosaprepitant; Gefitinib; GuanFACINE; Halofantrine; HMG-CoA Reductase Inhibitors; Imatinib; Irinotecan; Ixabepilone; Losartan; Lumefantrine; Macrolide Antibiotics; Maraviroc; Methadone; MethylPREDNISolone; Nilotinib; Nisoldipine; Paliperidone; Paricalcitol; Pazopanib; P-Glycoprotein Substrates; Phenytoin; Phosphodiesterase 5 Inhibitors; Pimecrolimus; Pimozide; Protease Inhibitors; QuiNIDine; Ramelteon; Ranolazine; Repaglinide; Rifamycin Derivatives; Rivaroxaban; Romidepsin; Salmeterol; Saxagliptin; Silodosin; Sirolimus; Solifenacin; Sorafenib; Sunitinib; Tacrolimus; Tacrolimus (Systemic); Tacrolimus (Topical); Tadalafil; Tamsulosin; Temsirolimus; Tolterodine; Tolvaptan; Topotecan; VinBLAStine; VinCRIStine; Vitamin K Antagonists; Ziprasidone; Zolpidem

The levels/effects of Itraconazole may be increased by: Grapefruit Juice; Macrolide Antibiotics; Protease Inhibitors

Decreased Effect

Itraconazole may decrease the levels/effects of: Amphotericin B; Prasugrel; Saccharomyces boulardii

The levels/effects of Itraconazole may be decreased by: Antacids; CYP3A4 Inducers (Strong); Deferasirox; Didanosine; Efavirenz; H2-Antagonists; Herbs (CYP3A4 Inducers); Phenytoin; Proton Pump Inhibitors; Rifamycin Derivatives; Sucralfate

Food Interactions Grapefruit juice decreases itraconazole AUC by 30%; avoid drinking grapefruit juice while taking oral itraconazole; absorption of capsule and oral solution are increased when taken with a cola beverage

Capsule: Food increases bioavailability

Solution: 31% increase in AUC if taken without food

Stability Store at room temperature; protect from light. Avoid freezing.

Mechanism of Action Inhibits ergosterol synthesis in fungal cell membranes by inhibiting fungal cytochrome P450

Pharmacokinetics (Adult data unless noted)

Absorption:

Capsule: Rapid and complete when capsule is given immediately after a meal (bioavailability: 100%); decreased absorption reported when administered via nasogastric tube

Oral solution: Solution better absorbed on empty stomach

Distribution: High affinity for tissues (liver, lung, kidney, adipose tissue, brain, vagina, dermis, epidermis); poor penetration into CSF, eye fluid, saliva; distributes into breast milk, bronchial exudate, and sputum

Protein binding: 99%

Metabolism: Saturable hepatic metabolism to active and inactive metabolites

Bioavailability: Capsules:

Fasted state: 40%

Fed state: Dose administered immediately after a meal: 100%

Half-life: 17-30 hours

Elimination: Metabolites are excreted in urine (35%) and bile (55%)

Dialysis: Nondialyzable

Usual Dosage

Oral:

Children: Efficacy of itraconazole has not been established; a limited number of children have been treated with itraconazole using doses of 3-5 mg/kg/day once daily; doses as high as 5-10 mg/kg/day divided every 12-24 hours have been used in 32 patients with chronic granulomatous disease for prophylaxis against *Aspergillus* infection; doses of 6-8 mg/kg/day have been used in the treatment of disseminated histoplasmosis

Prophylaxis for first episode of *Cryptococcus neoformans* or *Histoplasma capsulatum* in HIV-infected infants and children: 2-5 mg/kg/dose every 12-24 hours

Prophylaxis for recurrence of opportunistic disease in HIV-infected infants and children:

Cryptococcus neoformans: 2-5 mg/kg/dose every 12-24 hours

Histoplasma capsulatum: 2-5 mg/kg/dose every 12-48 hours

Adults:

Blastomycosis and nonmeningeal histoplasmosis: Initial: 200 mg once daily; if poor response, increase dose in 100 mg increments to a maximum of 400 mg/day in 2 divided doses

Life-threatening infection and aspergillosis: Initial loading dose can be administered as follows: 600 mg/day in 3 divided doses for the first 3-4 days; maintenance dose: 200-400 mg/day in 2 divided doses; maximum dose: 600 mg/day in 3 divided doses

Esophageal candidiasis: Vigorously swish 100 mg (10 mL) in the mouth for several seconds and then swallow daily; maximum dose: 200 mg/day

Oropharyngeal candidiasis: Vigorously swish 200 mg (20 mL) in the mouth for several seconds at a time once daily or 100 mg (10 mL) twice daily in patients refractory to oral fluconazole

Dosing adjustment in renal impairment: Limited data, use with caution

Administration
Oral: Avoid grapefruit juice

Capsules: Administer with food

Solution: Administer on an empty stomach

Monitoring Parameters Periodic liver function tests, serum potassium; monitor for prodromal signs of hepatitis

Reference Range Therapeutic blood concentration: >1 mcg/mL (severe infection)

Patient Information Report any prodromal symptoms of hepatitis (fatigue, weakness, nausea, vomiting, dark urine, or yellowing of eyes); avoid grapefruit juice

Nursing Implications Do not administer with antacids or H_2 antagonists

Dosage Forms Excipient information presented when available (limited, particularly for generics); consult specific product labeling.

Capsule: 100 mg

Sporanox®: 100 mg

Solution, oral:

Sporanox®: 100 mg/10 mL (150 mL) [cherry flavor]

References
Cowie F, Meller ST, Cushing P, et al, "Chemoprophylaxis for Pulmonary Aspergillosis During Intensive Chemotherapy," *Arch Dis Child*, 1994, 70(2):136-8.

Mouy R, Veber F, Blanche S, et al, "Long-Term Itraconazole Prophylaxis Against *Aspergillus* Infections in Thirty-Two Patients With Chronic Granulomatous Disease," *J Pediatr*, 1994, 125(6 Pt 1):998-1003.

Tobon AM, Franco L, Espinal D, et al, "Disseminated Histoplasmosis in Children: The Role of Itraconazole Therapy," *Pediatr Infect Dis J*, 1996; 15:1002-8.

"1999 USPHS/IDSA Guidelines for the Prevention of Opportunistic Infections in Persons Infected With Human Immunodeficiency Virus. USPHS/IDSA Prevention of Opportunistic Infections Working Group," *MMWR Morb Mortal Wkly Rep*, 1999, 48 (RR-10):1-66.

Ivermectin (eye ver MEK tin)

U.S. Brand Names Stromectol®

Therapeutic Category Anthelmintic; Anti-ectoparasitic Agent

Generic Available No

Use Treatment of intestinal strongyloidiasis; treatment of onchocerciasis due to the immature form of *Onchocerca volvulus* (**Note:** Ivermectin does not kill the adult *Onchocerca* worm). Other uses includes treatment of ascariasis, Bancroftian filariasis, gnathostomiasis, cutaneous larva migrans, mansonella, pediculosis (used in patients who have failed first-line therapy), scabies (used alone or in combination with a topical scabicide for severe or crusted scabies in immunocompromised patients; used when infestation is refractory or patient cannot tolerate topical therapy), and trichuriasis

Pregnancy Risk Factor C

Pregnancy Considerations Teratogenic effects have been observed in animal studies. Safety has not been established in pregnant women. The manufacturer and the Centers for Disease Control and Prevention (CDC) do not recommend use in pregnant women.

Lactation Enters breast milk/not recommended

Breast-Feeding Considerations Safety and efficacy for use in children <15 kg have not been established in the U.S.; therefore, ivermectin use is not recommended during lactation.

Contraindications Hypersensitivity to ivermectin or any component

Warnings Microfilaricidal drugs like ivermectin may cause cutaneous and/or systemic reactions of varying severity (Mazzoti reaction) and ophthalmological reactions in patients with onchocerciasis. These reactions are probably due to allergic and inflammatory responses to the death of microfilariae. Supportive treatment of Mazzoti reaction includes oral hydration, recumbency, NS, and/or parenteral corticosteroids to treat postural hypotension; antihistamines, corticosteroids, and/or aspirin have been used to treat mild to moderate cases.

Serious and/or fatal encephalopathy has been reported rarely following treatment with ivermectin in patients with onchocerciasis and loiasis. In addition, back pain, conjunctival hemorrhage, dyspnea, urinary and/or fecal incontinence, difficulty standing/walking, mental status changes, confusion, lethargy, stupor, seizures, or coma has also been reported. Pretreatment assessment for *Loa loa* infection is recommended in any patient with significant exposure to endemic areas (West and Central Africa) prior to treatment with ivermectin. Safety and efficacy has not been established in children <15 kg. The American Academy of Pediatrics (AAP) cautions against using ivermectin in children weighing <15 kg or <2 years of age since their blood-brain barrier may be less developed than in older patients.

Precautions Use with caution in patients with hyperreactive onchodermatitis who are more likely than others to experience severe adverse reactions such as edema and aggravation of onchodermatitis after treatment with ivermectin. Repeated courses of treatment for intestinal strongyloidiasis may be required in immunocompromised patients (eg, HIV); control of extraintestinal strongyloidiasis may necessitate suppressive (once monthly) therapy.

Adverse Reactions
Cardiovascular: Peripheral and facial edema, orthostatic hypotension, tachycardia, chest discomfort

Central nervous system: Dizziness, somnolence, vertigo, headache, seizures, encephalopathy, coma, confusion, chills, fatigue, mental status change, lethargy, stupor

Dermatologic: Pruritus, rash, urticaria, toxic epidermal necrolysis, Stevens-Johnson syndrome

Gastrointestinal: Abdominal pain, anorexia, constipation, diarrhea, nausea, vomiting, fecal incontinence

Genitourinary: Urinary incontinence

Hematologic: Leukopenia, anemia, eosinophilia, hemoglobin elevated

Hepatic: ALT, AST, and bilirubin elevated

Neuromuscular & skeletal: Tremor, asthenia, myalgia, back pain, neck pain, difficulty standing/walking

Ocular: Abnormal sensation in eye, eyelid edema, anterior uveitis, conjunctivitis, limbitis, keratitis, chorioretinitis, choroiditis, conjunctival hemorrhage, punctuate opacity, red eye, transient vision loss

Respiratory: Bronchial asthma exacerbation, dyspnea

Miscellaneous: Mazzotti reaction (with onchocerciasis), usually reported during the first 4 days after treatment and includes reactions such as arthralgia, synovitis, lymph node enlargement and tenderness, pruritus, edema, urticarial rash, hypotension, and fever

Drug Interactions
Metabolism/Transport Effects Substrate of CYP3A4 (minor), P-glycoprotein

Avoid Concomitant Use

Avoid concomitant use of Ivermectin with any of the following: BCG

Increased Effect/Toxicity

Ivermectin may increase the levels/effects of: Vitamin K Antagonists

The levels/effects of Ivermectin may be increased by: P-Glycoprotein Inhibitors

Decreased Effect

Ivermectin may decrease the levels/effects of: BCG; Typhoid Vaccine

The levels/effects of Ivermectin may be decreased by: P-Glycoprotein Inducers

Food Interactions Bioavailability is increased 2.5-fold when administered following a high-fat meal.

Stability Store at room temperature.

Mechanism of Action Ivermectin binds selectively and with high affinity to glutamate-gated chloride ion channels which occur in invertebrate nerve and muscle cells. This leads to increased permeability of cell membranes to chloride ions then hyperpolarization of the nerve or muscle cell, resulting in paralysis and death of the parasite.

Pharmacokinetics (Adult data unless noted)

Absorption: Well absorbed

Distribution: High concentration in the liver and adipose tissue; excreted in breast milk in low concentrations; does not readily cross the blood-brain barrier

Protein binding: 93% primarily to albumin

Half-life: 18 hours (range: 16-35 hours)

Time to peak serum concentration: 4 hours

Metabolism: >97% in the liver by CYP3A4; substrate of the p-glycoprotein transport system

Elimination: <1% in urine; feces

Usual Dosage Oral: Children ≥15 kg and Adults:

Onchocerciasis: 150 mcg/kg as a single dose; may repeat every 3-12 months until asymptomatic

Strongyloidiasis: 200 mcg/kg/day once daily for 2 days. In immunocompromised patients or patients with disseminated disease, may need to repeat therapy at 2-week intervals.

Ascariasis: 150-200 mcg/kg as a single dose

Cutaneous larva migrans: 200 mcg/kg once daily for 1-2 days

Mansonella streptocerca: 150 mcg/kg as a single dose

Mansonella ozzardi: 200 mcg/kg as a single dose

Pediculosis: 200 mcg/kg as a single dose; repeat in 10 days; some clinicians recommend 200 mcg/kg for 3 doses (on days 1, 2, and 10). Ivermectin is effective against adult lice, but has no effect on nits.

Scabies: 200 mcg/kg as a single dose; may need to repeat in 10-14 days

Trichuriasis: 200 mcg/kg once daily for 3 days

Alternatively, the following weight-based dosing can be used: See tables.

Weight-Based Dosage to Provide ~150 mcg/kg

Patient Weight (kg)	Single Oral Dose
15-25	3 mg
26-44	6 mg
45-64	9 mg
65-84	12 mg
≥85	150 mcg/kg

Weight-Based Dosage to Provide ~200 mcg/kg

Patient Weight (kg)	Single Oral Dose
15-24	3 mg
25-35	6 mg
36-50	9 mg
51-65	12 mg
66-79	15 mg
≥80	200 mcg/kg

Administration Oral: Administer on an empty stomach with water

Monitoring Parameters Periodic ophthalmologic exams; stool exam to document clearance of worms; skin and eye microfilarial counts when treating onchocerciasis

Dosage Forms Excipient information presented when available (limited, particularly for generics); consult specific product labeling.

Tablet [scored]:
Stromectol®: 3 mg

References
Frankowski BL, Weiner LB, Committee on School Health The Committee on Infectious Diseases, American Academy of Pediatrics, "Head Lice," *Pediatrics,* 2002, 110(3):638-43.

◆ **IVIG** *see* Immune Globulin (Intravenous) *on page* 719

◆ **IV Immune Globulin** *see* Immune Globulin (Intravenous) *on page* 719

◆ **Ivy-Rid® [OTC]** *see* Benzocaine *on page* 182

◆ **IvySoothe® [OTC]** *see* Hydrocortisone *on page* 685

◆ **Ixiaro®** *see* Japanese Encephalitis Virus Vaccine (Inactivated) *on page* 776

◆ **JAMP-Amlodipine (Can)** *see* AmLODIPine *on page* 91

◆ **JAMP-Citalopram (Can)** *see* Citalopram *on page* 319

◆ **JAMP-Ondansetron (Can)** *see* Ondansetron *on page* 1022

◆ **JAMP-Simvastatin (Can)** *see* Simvastatin *on page* 1263

◆ **Jantoven®** *see* Warfarin *on page* 1432

Japanese Encephalitis Virus Vaccine (Inactivated)

(jap a NEESE en sef a LYE tis VYE rus vak SEEN, in ak ti VAY ted)

Related Information
Immunization Guidelines *on page* 1636

U.S. Brand Names Ixiaro®; JE-VAX®

Canadian Brand Names JE-VAX®

Therapeutic Category Vaccine, Inactivated Virus

Generic Available No

Use Provide active immunity to Japanese encephalitis virus (Je-Vax® FDA approved in children ≥1 year and adults, Ixiaro® FDA approved for use in patients ≥17 years).

Active immunization against Japanese encephalitis

Japanese encephalitis vaccine is not recommended for all persons traveling to or residing in Asia. The Advisory Committee on Immunization Practices (ACIP) recommends vaccination for:
• Persons spending ≥1 month in endemic areas during transmission season.
• Research laboratory workers who may be exposed to the Japanese encephalitis virus.

Vaccination may also be considered for persons spending <30 days in endemic areas, such as:
• Travel to areas with an ongoing outbreak

- Travelers planning to go outside of urban areas and have an increased risk of exposure. For example, high-risk activities include extensive outdoor activity in rural areas especially at night; extensive outdoor activities such as camping, hiking, etc; staying in accommodations without air conditioning, screens or bed nets
- Travelers to endemic areas who are unsure of specific destination, activities, or duration of travel

Pregnancy Risk Factor B (Ixiaro®) / C (Je-Vax®)

Pregnancy Considerations

Ixiaro®: Adverse events were not observed in animal reproduction studies.

Je-Vax®: Reproduction studies have not been conducted. Risks of vaccine administration should be carefully considered and in general, pregnant women should only be vaccinated if they are at high risk for exposure. Infection from Japanese encephalitis during the 1st or 2nd trimesters of pregnancy may increase risk of miscarriage. Intrauterine transmission of the Japanese encephalitis virus has been reported.

Lactation Excretion in breast milk unknown/use caution

Breast-Feeding Considerations It is not known if the vaccine is excreted into breast milk; however, the ACIP does not consider breast-feeding to be a contraindication to vaccination.

Contraindications

Ixiaro®: Severe allergic reaction to a previous dose of the vaccine

Je-Vax®: Hypersensitivity to the vaccine, any component, or to proteins of rodent or neural origin

Warnings Immediate treatment for severe hypersensitivity reactions should be available during vaccine use.

Je-Vax®: Severe adverse reactions manifesting as generalized urticaria or angioedema may occur within minutes following vaccination, or up to 17 days later; most reactions occur within 10 days, with the majority within 48 hours; observe vaccinees for 30 minutes after vaccination; warn them of the possibility of delayed generalized urticaria and to remain where medical care is readily available for 10 days following any dose of the vaccine. Due to the potential for severe adverse reactions, Japanese encephalitis (JE) vaccine is **not** recommended for all persons traveling to or residing in Asia; safety and efficacy in infants <1 year of age have not been established; therefore, immunization of infants should be deferred whenever possible; it is not known whether the vaccine is excreted in breast milk.

Precautions The CDC recommends that the following individuals should not generally receive JE vaccine unless the benefit to the individual clearly outweighs the risk: Individuals acutely ill or with active infections, heart, kidney, or liver disorders, generalized malignancies such as leukemia or lymphoma, a history of multiple allergies, urticaria after hymenoptera envenomation, and pregnant women (unless there is a very high risk of Japanese encephalitis during the woman's stay in Asia). Routine prophylactic administration of acetaminophen to prevent fever due to vaccines has been shown to decrease the immune response of some vaccines; the clinical significance of this reduction in immune response has not been established (see Prymula, 2009).

Ixiaro®: Contains protamine sulfate which may cause hypersensitivity reactions in certain individuals. Immunization should be completed ≥7 days prior to potential exposure. Safety and efficacy have not been established in children <17 years of age.

Je-Vax®: Unusual alcohol intake immediately after vaccination has been associated with an increased incidence of hypersensitivity reactions; avoid excessive alcohol intake during the 48 hours following vaccination. Individuals receiving other vaccinations within 7 days prior to this vaccine also had an increased incidence of hypersensitivity reactions; where possible, JE vaccine should be administered concurrently with other vaccines.

Adverse Reactions Report allergic or unusual adverse reactions to the Vaccine Adverse Event Reporting System (VAERS) 1-800-822-7967.

Cardiovascular: Hypotension, angioedema (rare)

Central nervous system: Fever, fatigue, headache, malaise, chills, dizziness, seizure (rare), encephalitis (rare), encephalopathy (rare)

Dermatologic: Rash, urticaria, itching with or without accompanying rash, facial swelling, erythema multiforme (rare), erythema nodosum (rare)

Gastrointestinal: Nausea, vomiting, abdominal pain, diarrhea

Local: Pain, induration, pruritus, tenderness, redness, and swelling at injection site

Neuromuscular & skeletal: Myalgia, peripheral neuropathy (rare), joint swelling (rare), back pain

Respiratory: Dyspnea, nasopharyngitis, pharyngolaryngeal pain, upper respiratory tract infection, cough, rhinitis

Miscellaneous: Severe hypersensitivity reactions including anaphylaxis (see Warnings), flu-like illness

Drug Interactions

Avoid Concomitant Use There are no known interactions where it is recommended to avoid concomitant use.

Increased Effect/Toxicity There are no known significant interactions involving an increase in effect.

Decreased Effect

The levels/effects of Japanese Encephalitis Virus Vaccine (Inactivated) may be decreased by: Immunosuppressants

Stability Ixiaro®: Refrigerate; do not freeze; store in original packaging to protect from light.

Je-Vax®: Refrigerate; do not freeze; discard 8 hours after reconstitution.

Mechanism of Action An inactivated vaccine which offers immunity to disease caused by the Japanese encephalitis virus. Je-Vax® is prepared from the homogenate of infected mice brains. Ixiaro® is a purified Japanese encephalitis vaccine made from the SA_{14}-14-2 strain grown in Vero cells.

Usual Dosage

Ixiaro®: I.M.:

Adults ≥17 years of age: 0.5 mL/dose; a total of 2 doses given on days 0 and 28. Immunization should be completed ≥7 days prior to potential exposure.

Je-Vax®: SubQ:

Children 1-3 years: Three 0.5 mL doses given on days 0, 7, and 30

Children >3 years and Adults: Three 1 mL doses given on days 0, 7, and 30

An abbreviated schedule with the third dose administered on day 14 should be used only when time does not permit waiting; 2 doses a week apart produce immunity in about 80% of recipients; the longest regimen yields highest titers after 6 months.

Booster dose: Give after 2 years, or according to current recommendation

Note: Travel should not commence for at least 10 days after the last dose of vaccine, to allow adequate antibody formation and recognition of any delayed adverse reaction

Administration Ixiaro®: I.M.: Shake well prior to use to form a homogeneous suspension. Do not use if discolored or if coarse particulate matter remains; inject I.M. into the deltoid muscle; **not for I.V., SubQ, or intradermal administration**

Je-Vax®: **SubQ:** Use entire contents of provided diluent to reconstitute vaccine; gently agitate to mix thoroughly; discard if powder does not dissolve; use within 8 hours following reconstitution; **not for I.V., I.M., or intradermal administration**

Patient Information Adverse reactions may occur shortly after vaccination or up to 17 days (usually within 10 days) after vaccination; advise concurrent use of other means to reduce the risk of mosquito exposure when possible, including bed nets, insect repellents, protective clothing, avoidance of travel in endemic areas, and avoidance of outdoor activity during twilight and evening periods

Nursing Implications Federal law requires that the date of administration, name of manufacturer, lot number, and administering person's name, title and address be entered into patient's permanent medical record.

Additional Information Ixiaro® is a purified Japanese encephalitis vaccine made from the SA$_{14}$-14-2 strain grown in Vero cells. It was developed due to neurologic side effects observed with Je-Vax®, a vaccine derived from mice-brain cells that contains additives which may contribute to the adverse effects. In studies comparing the two vaccines, seroconversion rates were similar following two doses of Ixiaro® as opposed to three doses of Je-Vax®. Safety profile of Ixiaro® was found to be similar to placebo. Based on antibody titers, protection following Ixiaro® remains for at least 1 year and studies are currently planned to determine the need for booster doses.

In order to maximize vaccination rates, the ACIP recommends simultaneous administration of all age-appropriate vaccines (live or inactivated) for which a person is eligible at a single visit, unless contraindications exist. The use of combination vaccines is generally preferred over separate infections, taking into consideration provider assessment, patient preference, and potential adverse events.

For additional information, please refer to the following website: http://www.cdc.gov/vaccines/vpd-vac/.

Dosage Forms Excipient information presented when available (limited, particularly for generics); consult specific product labeling.

Injection, powder for reconstitution:

JE-VAX®: [contains mouse serum protein, thimerosal, gelatin, polysorbate 80]

Injection, suspension:

Ixiaro®: Inactivated JEV proteins 6 mcg/0.5 mL (0.5 mL) [contains sodium metabisulphite, bovine serum, and protamine sulfate]

References

Centers for Disease Control and Prevention (CDC), "General Recommendations on Immunization. Recommendations of the Advisory Committee on Immunization Practices (ACIP)," *MMWR Recomm Rep*, 2006, 55(RR-15):1-48. Available at: http://www.cdc.gov/mmwr/preview/mmwrhtml/rr5515a1.htm.

Centers for Disease Control and Prevention (CDC), "Syncope After Vaccination-United States, January 2005-July 2007," *MMWR Morb Mortal Wkly Rep*, 2008, 57(17):457-60.

"Inactivated Japanese Encephalitis Virus Vaccine. Recommendations of the Advisory Committee on Immunization Practices (ACIP)," *MMWR Recomm Rep*, 1993, 42(RR-1):1-15.

Prymula R, Siegrist CA, Chlibek R, et al, "Effect of Prophylactic Paracetamol Administration at Time of Vaccination on Febrile Reactions and Antibody Responses in Children: Two Open-Label, Randomised Controlled Trials," *Lancet*, 2009, 374(9698):1339-50.

◆ **JE-VAX®** *see* Japanese Encephalitis Virus Vaccine (Inactivated) *on page 776*

◆ **Jolivette™** *see* Norethindrone *on page 1001*

◆ **Jurnista™ (Can)** *see* HYDROmorphone *on page 689*

◆ **Just for Kids™ [OTC]** *see* Fluoride *on page 595*

◆ **K-10® (Can)** *see* Potassium Chloride *on page 1136*

◆ **Kadian®** *see* Morphine Sulfate *on page 946*

◆ **Kala® [OTC]** *see* Lactobacillus *on page 790*

◆ **Kaletra®** *see* Lopinavir and Ritonavir *on page 839*

◆ **Kalexate** *see* Sodium Polystyrene Sulfonate *on page 1279*

◆ **Kank-A® Soft Brush™ [OTC]** *see* Benzocaine *on page 182*

◆ **Kaon-Cl-10®** *see* Potassium Chloride *on page 1136*

◆ **Kao-Paverin® [OTC] [DSC]** *see* Loperamide *on page 838*

◆ **Kaopectate® [OTC]** *see* Bismuth *on page 195*

◆ **Kaopectate® [OTC] (Can)** *see* Attapulgite *on page 159*

◆ **Kaopectate® Children's [OTC] (Can)** *see* Attapulgite *on page 159*

◆ **Kaopectate® Extra Strength [OTC]** *see* Bismuth *on page 195*

◆ **Kaopectate® Extra Strength [OTC] (Can)** *see* Attapulgite *on page 159*

◆ **Kao-Tin [OTC]** *see* Bismuth *on page 195*

◆ **Kapectolin [OTC] [DSC]** *see* Bismuth *on page 195*

◆ **Kayexalate®** *see* Sodium Polystyrene Sulfonate *on page 1279*

◆ **KCI** *see* Potassium Chloride *on page 1136*

◆ **K-Dur® (Can)** *see* Potassium Chloride *on page 1136*

◆ **Keflex®** *see* Cephalexin *on page 282*

◆ **Keftab® (Can)** *see* Cephalexin *on page 282*

◆ **Kenalog®** *see* Triamcinolone *on page 1376*

◆ **Kenalog®-10** *see* Triamcinolone *on page 1376*

◆ **Kenalog®-40** *see* Triamcinolone *on page 1376*

◆ **Keppra®** *see* Levetiracetam *on page 808*

◆ **Keppra XR™** *see* Levetiracetam *on page 808*

◆ **Keralyt® [OTC]** *see* Salicylic Acid *on page 1241*

◆ **Kerr Insta-Char® [OTC]** *see* Charcoal, Activated *on page 284*

◆ **Ketalar®** *see* Ketamine *on page 778*

Ketamine (KEET a meen)

Medication Safety Issues

Sound-alike/look-alike issues:

Ketalar® may be confused with Kenalog®, ketorolac

High alert medication: The Institute for Safe Medication Practices (ISMP) includes this medication among its list of drugs which have a heightened risk of causing significant patient harm when used in error.

Related Information

Adult ACLS Algorithms *on page 1463*

Preprocedure Sedatives in Children *on page 1688*

U.S. Brand Names Ketalar®

Canadian Brand Names Ketalar®; Ketamine Hydrochloride Injection, USP

Therapeutic Category General Anesthetic

Generic Available Yes

Use Anesthesia, short surgical procedures, dressing changes

Restrictions C-III

Pregnancy Considerations Adverse events have not been observed in animal reproduction studies. Ketamine crosses the placenta and can be detected in fetal tissue. Ketamine produces dose dependant increases in uterine contractions; effects may vary by trimester. The plasma clearance of ketamine is reduced during pregnancy. Dose related neonatal depression and decreased APGAR scores have been reported with large doses administered at delivery.

Contraindications Hypersensitivity to ketamine or any component; patients in whom a significant elevation in blood pressure would be hazardous (eg, patients with elevated intracranial pressure, hypertension, aneurysms, thyrotoxicosis, CHF, angina, or psychotic disorders)

Warnings Use only by or under the direct supervision of physicians experienced in administering general anesthetics. Resuscitative equipment should be available for use; respiratory depression may occur with rapid administration rates or with overdose. Postanesthetic emergence reactions which can manifest as vivid dreams, hallucinations and/or frank delirium occur in 12% of patients **[U.S. Boxed Warning]**; these reactions are less common in pediatric patients; emergence reactions may occur up to 24 hours postoperatively and may be reduced by minimization of verbal, tactile, and visual patient stimulation during recovery, or by pretreatment with a benzodiazepine (using lower recommended doses of ketamine). Severe emergent reactions may require treatment with a small hypnotic dose of a short or ultra-short acting barbiturate. Prolonged use may cause physical dependence (withdrawal symptoms on discontinuation) and tolerance. Cardiac function should be continuously monitored in patients with hypertension or cardiac decompensation.

Precautions Use with caution in patients with gastroesophageal reflux. Use with caution and decrease the dose in patients with hepatic dysfunction. Use with caution in patients with a full stomach, patients should fast (ie, be NPO) for an appropriate time before being sedated for elective procedures. Use with caution in patients with elevated CSF pressure, chronic alcoholics, and in acutely intoxicated patients. Do not use as sole anesthetic in surgery or diagnostic procedures of the pharynx, larynx, or bronchial tree or in surgical procedures involving visceral pain pathways

Adverse Reactions

Cardiovascular: Hypertension, tachycardia, cardiac output increased, paradoxical direct myocardial depression, hypotension, bradycardia, increases cerebral blood flow, arrhythmias

Central nervous system: Tonic-clonic movements, intracranial pressure elevated, hallucinations

Dermatologic: Transient erythema, morbilliform rash

Endocrine & metabolic: Metabolic rate increased

Gastrointestinal: Hypersalivation, vomiting, postoperative nausea, anorexia

Local: Pain and exanthema at injection site

Neuromuscular & skeletal: Skeletal muscle tone increased, tremor, purposeless movement, fasciculations

Ocular: Diplopia, nystagmus, intraocular pressure elevated

Respiratory: Airway resistance increased, cough reflex may be depressed, bronchospasm decreased; respiratory depression or apnea with large doses or rapid infusions, laryngospasm; bronchial mucous gland secretion increased

Miscellaneous: Emergence reactions; anaphylaxis; physical and psychological dependence with prolonged use

Drug Interactions

Metabolism/Transport Effects Substrate (major) of CYP2B6, 2C9, 3A4

Avoid Concomitant Use There are no known interactions where it is recommended to avoid concomitant use.

Increased Effect/Toxicity

The levels/effects of Ketamine may be increased by: CYP2B6 Inhibitors (Moderate); CYP2B6 Inhibitors (Strong); CYP2C9 Inhibitors (Moderate); CYP2C9 Inhibitors (Strong); CYP3A4 Inhibitors (Moderate); CYP3A4 Inhibitors (Strong); Dasatinib; Quazepam

Decreased Effect

The levels/effects of Ketamine may be decreased by: CYP2C9 Inducers (Highly Effective); Peginterferon Alfa-2b

Stability Protect from light; do not mix with barbiturates or diazepam as precipitation may occur

Mechanism of Action Produces dissociative anesthesia by direct action on the cortex and limbic system; does not usually impair pharyngeal or laryngeal reflexes

Pharmacodynamics

Onset of action:
Anesthesia:
I.M.: 3-4 minutes
I.V.: Within 30 seconds
Analgesia:
Oral: Within 30 minutes
I.M.: Within 10-15 minutes
Duration: Following single dose:
Anesthesia:
I.M.: 12-25 minutes
I.V.: 5-10 minutes
Analgesia: I.M.: 15-30 minutes
Recovery:
I.M.: 3-4 hours
I.V.: 1-2 hours

Pharmacokinetics (Adult data unless noted)

Metabolism: In the liver via N-dealkylation, hydroxylation of cyclohexone ring, glucuronide conjugation, and dehydration of hydroxylated metabolites
Half-life:
Alpha: 10-15 minutes
Terminal: 2.5 hours

Usual Dosage Titrate dose to effect
Children:
Oral: 6-10 mg/kg for 1 dose (mixed in cola or other beverage) given 30 minutes before the procedure
I.M.: 3-7 mg/kg
I.V.: Range: 0.5-2 mg/kg, use smaller doses (0.5-1 mg/kg) for sedation for minor procedures; usual induction dosage: 1-2 mg/kg
Continuous I.V. infusion: Sedation: 5-20 mcg/kg/minute; start at lower dosage listed and titrate to effect
Adults:
I.M.: 3-8 mg/kg
I.V.: Range: 1-4.5 mg/kg; usual induction dosage: 1-2 mg/kg
Children and Adults: Maintenance: Supplemental doses of $1/3$ to $1/2$ of initial dose

Administration

Oral: Use 100 mg/mL I.V. solution and mix the appropriate dose in 0.2-0.3 mL/kg of cola or other beverage
Parenteral: I.V.: Administer slowly, do not exceed 0.5 mg/kg/minute; do not administer faster than 60 seconds; maximum concentration for slow I.V. push: 50 mg/mL; **Note:** Do not inject 100 mg/mL concentration I.V. without proper dilution; dilute with an equal volume of SWI, NS, or D_5W to produce 50 mg/mL concentration for slow I.V. push. Maximum concentration for intermittent or continuous infusion: 2 mg/mL

Monitoring Parameters Cardiovascular effects, heart rate, blood pressure, respiratory rate, transcutaneous O_2 saturation

Patient Information May cause drowsiness and impair ability to perform activities requiring mental alertness or physical coordination; do not engage in such activities for at least 24 hours after ketamine anesthesia.

Nursing Implications Resuscitative equipment should be available for use. Ensure that outpatients have fully recovered from ketamine anesthesia before being released and that they are accompanied by a responsible adult.

◀ **Additional Information** Used in combination with anticholinergic agents to decrease hypersalivation; should not be used for sedation for procedures that require a total lack of movement (eg, MRI, radiation therapy) due to association with purposeless movements

Dosage Forms Excipient information presented when available (limited, particularly for generics); consult specific product labeling.

Injection, solution: 10 mg/mL (20 mL); 50 mg/mL (10 mL); 100 mg/mL (5 mL, 10 mL)

Ketalar®: 10 mg/mL (20 mL); 50 mg/mL (10 mL); 100 mg/mL (5 mL)

References

Cote CJ, "Sedation for the Pediatric Patient: A Review," *Pediatr Clin North Am*, 1994, 41(1):31-58.

Gutstein HB, Johnson KL, Heard MN, et al, "Oral Ketamine Premedication in Children," *Anesthesiology*, 1992, 76(1):28-33.

Tobias JD, Phipps S, Smith B, et al, "Oral Ketamine Premedication to Alleviate the Distress of Invasive Procedures in Pediatric Oncology Patients," *Pediatrics*, 1992, 90(4):537-41.

Tobias JD and Rasmussen GE, "Pain Management and Sedation in the Pediatric Intensive Care Unit," *Pediatr Clin North Am*, 1994, 41(6):1269-92.

◆ **Ketamine Hydrochloride** see Ketamine on page 778

◆ **Ketamine Hydrochloride Injection, USP (Can)** see Ketamine on page 778

Ketoconazole (kee toe KOE na zole)

Medication Safety Issues

Sound-alike/look-alike issues:

Kuric™ may be confused with Carac®

Nizoral® may be confused with Nasarel®, Neoral®, Nitrol®

U.S. Brand Names Extina®; Kuric™; Nizoral®; Nizoral® A-D [OTC]; Xolegel®

Canadian Brand Names Apo-Ketoconazole®; Ketoderm®; Novo-Ketoconazole; Xolegel®

Therapeutic Category Antifungal Agent, Systemic; Antifungal Agent, Topical

Generic Available Yes: Cream, shampoo, tablet

Use Treatment of susceptible fungal infections, including candidiasis, oral thrush, blastomycosis, coccidioidomycosis, histoplasmosis, paracoccidioidomycosis, chronic mucocutaneous candidiasis, as well as certain recalcitrant cutaneous dermatophytoses (FDA approved in ages ≥2 years of age and adults); used topically for treatment of tinea corporis, tinea cruris, tinea versicolor, cutaneous candidiasis, and seborrheic dermatitis (FDA approved in adults); shampoo is used for dandruff (1% shampoo: FDA approved in ages ≥12 years and adults), seborrheic dermatitis (foam: FDA approved in ages ≥12 years and adults), and tinea versicolor (shampoo: FDA approved in adults)

Pregnancy Risk Factor C

Pregnancy Considerations Adverse effects were noted in animal reproduction studies.

Lactation Enters breast milk/not recommended

Breast-Feeding Considerations In a case report, ketoconazole in concentrations of ≤0.22 mcg/mL were detected in the breast milk of a woman 1 month postpartum. She had been taking oral ketoconazole 200 mg/day for 5 days at the time of sampling. The maximum milk concentration occurred 3.25 hours after the dose and concentrations were undetectable 24 hours after the dose. Based on the highest milk concentration, the estimated dose to the nursing infant was 1.4% of the maternal dose. Breast-feeding is not recommended by the manufacturer.

Contraindications Hypersensitivity to ketoconazole or any component; single agent in the treatment of CNS fungal infections (due to poor CNS penetration); concomitant administration of astemizole, terfenadine, cisapride, or oral triazolam (see Drug Interactions)

Warnings Has been associated with hepatotoxicity, including some fatalities [U.S. Boxed Warning]; perform periodic liver function tests, use with caution in patients with impaired hepatic function; high doses of ketoconazole may depress adrenocortical function and decrease serum testosterone concentrations; concomitant use with cisapride is contraindicated due to the occurrence of ventricular arrhythmias [U.S. Boxed Warning]. Hypersensitivity reactions (including rare cases of anaphylaxis) have been reported.

Precautions Gastric acidity is necessary for the dissolution and absorption of ketoconazole; avoid concomitant (within 2 hours) administration of antacids, H_2 blockers, anticholinergics. Foam contains alcohol and propane/butane; do not expose to open flame or smoking during or immediately after application.

Adverse Reactions

Cardiovascular: Ventricular dysrhythmias

Central nervous system: Lethargy, nervousness

Dermatologic: Application site burning (foam), contact sensitization (foam), dry skin

Endocrine & metabolic: Adrenocortical insufficiency, libido decreased

Gastrointestinal: Abdominal discomfort, GI bleeding, nausea, vomiting

Hepatic: AST, ALT, and alkaline phosphatase increased; hepatotoxicity, jaundice

Local: Stinging

Miscellaneous: Anaphylaxis, hypersensitivity

<1% and/or postmarketing:

Topical: Alopecia, dryness, erythema, irritation, paresthesia, pruritus, rash, and warmth

Systemic: Bulging fontanelles, chills, diarrhea, dizziness, fever, gynecomastia, headache, hemolytic anemia, hypertriglyceridemia, impotence, leukopenia, neuropsychiatric disturbances, oligospermia, papilledema, photophobia, severe depression, somnolence, suicidal tendencies, thrombocytopenia

Drug Interactions

Metabolism/Transport Effects Substrate of CYP3A4 (major); Inhibits CYP1A2 (strong), CYP2A6 (moderate), CYP2B6 (weak), CYP2C8 (weak), CYP2C9 (strong), CYP2C19 (moderate), CYP2D6 (moderate), CYP3A4 (strong), P-glycoprotein

Avoid Concomitant Use

Avoid concomitant use of Ketoconazole with any of the following: Alfuzosin; Cisapride; Clopidogrel; Conivaptan; Dabigatran Etexilate; Dofetilide; Domperidone; Dronedarone; Eplerenone; Everolimus; Halofantrine; Nilotinib; Nisoldipine; Pimozide; QuiNIDine; Ranolazine; Rivaroxaban; Romidepsin; Salmeterol; Silodosin; Tamsulosin; Thioridazine; Tolvaptan; Topotecan

Increased Effect/Toxicity

Ketoconazole may increase the levels/effects of: Alfentanil; Alfuzosin; Aliskiren; Almotriptan; Alosetron; Aprepitant; Bendamustine; Benzodiazepines (metabolized by oxidation); Bortezomib; Bosentan; Brinzolamide; BusPIRone; Busulfan; Calcium Channel Blockers; CarBAMazepine; Carvedilol; Ciclesonide; Cilostazol; Cinacalcet; Cisapride; Colchicine; Conivaptan; Corticosteroids (Orally Inhaled); Corticosteroids (Systemic); CycloSPORINE; CycloSPORINE (Systemic); CYP1A2 Substrates; CYP2A6 Substrates; CYP2C19 Substrates; CYP2C9 Substrates (High risk); CYP2D6 Substrates; CYP3A4 Substrates; Dabigatran Etexilate; Dienogest; Docetaxel; Dofetilide; Domperidone; Dronedarone; Dutasteride; Eletriptan; Eplerenone; Erlotinib; Eszopiclone; Everolimus; FentaNYL; Fesoterodine; Fexofenadine; Fosaprepitant; Gefitinib; GuanFACINE; Halofantrine; HMG-CoA Reductase Inhibitors; Imatinib; Irinotecan; Ixabepilone; Losartan; Lumefantrine; Macrolide Antibiotics; Maraviroc; Methadone; MethylPREDNISolone; Nebivolol; Nilotinib; Nisoldipine; Paricalcitol;

Pazopanib; P-Glycoprotein Substrates; Phenytoin; Phosphodiesterase 5 Inhibitors; Pimecrolimus; Pimozide; Praziquantel; Protease Inhibitors; Proton Pump Inhibitors; QuiNIDine; Ramelteon; Ranolazine; Repaglinide; Rifamycin Derivatives; Rivaroxaban; Romidepsin; Salmeterol; Saxagliptin; Silodosin; Sirolimus; Solifenacin; Sorafenib; Sunitinib; Tacrolimus; Tacrolimus (Systemic); Tacrolimus (Topical); Tadalafil; Tamoxifen; Tamsulosin; Temsirolimus; Thioridazine; Tolterodine; Tolvaptan; Topotecan; Vitamin K Antagonists; Ziprasidone; Zolpidem

The levels/effects of Ketoconazole may be increased by: Grapefruit Juice; Macrolide Antibiotics; Protease Inhibitors

Decreased Effect

Ketoconazole may decrease the levels/effects of: Amphotericin B; Clopidogrel; Codeine; Prasugrel; Saccharomyces boulardii; TraMADol

The levels/effects of Ketoconazole may be decreased by: Antacids; CYP3A4 Inducers (Strong); Deferasirox; Didanosine; H2-Antagonists; Herbs (CYP3A4 Inducers); Phenytoin; Proton Pump Inhibitors; Rifamycin Derivatives; Sucralfate

Food Interactions Food may increase ketoconazole absorption; administration with an acidic beverage (eg, Coca-Cola, Pepsi, citrus juice) increases ketoconazole absorption

Mechanism of Action Alters the permeability of the cell wall; inhibits fungal biosynthesis of triglycerides and phospholipids; inhibits several fungal enzymes that results in a build-up of toxic concentrations of hydrogen peroxide

Pharmacokinetics (Adult data unless noted)

Absorption: Oral: Rapid (~75%)

Distribution: Minimal penetration into the CNS; distributes to bile, saliva, urine, sweat, synovial fluid, lungs, liver, kidney and bone marrow

Protein binding: 84% to 99%

Metabolism: Partially in the liver via CYP3A4 to inactive compounds

Bioavailability: Decreases as pH of the gastric contents increase

Half-life, biphasic:
Alpha: 2 hours
Terminal: 8 hours

Time to peak serum concentration: Oral: Within 1-2 hours

Elimination: Primarily in feces (57%) with smaller amounts excreted in urine (~13%)

Dialysis: Not dialyzable (0% to 5%)

Usual Dosage

Infants and Children: Oral: 3.3-6.6 mg/kg/day once daily
Prophylaxis for recurrence of mucocutaneous candidiasis with HIV infection: 5-10 mg/kg/day divided every 12-24 hours; maximum: 800 mg/day divided twice daily

Adults: Oral: 200-400 mg/day as a single daily dose; maximum: 800 mg/day divided twice daily

Shampoo (ketoconazole 2%): Apply to damp skin, lather, leave on 5 minutes, and rinse (one application should be sufficient)

Children and Adults:
Shampoo (ketoconazole 1%): Shampoo twice weekly (at least 3 days should elapse between each shampoo) for up to 8 weeks

Topical: Apply once daily to twice daily

Administration

Oral: May administer with or without food or with juice; administer with food to decrease nausea and vomiting; administer 2 hours prior to antacids, didanosine, proton pump inhibitors, or H2-receptor antagonists to prevent decreased ketoconazole absorption; shake suspension well before use

Shampoo:
1%: Apply to wet hair and massage over entire scalp for 1 minute; rinse hair thoroughly and reapply shampoo for 3 minutes; rinse

2%: Apply to damp skin covering affected area and a wide margin surrounding the area; lather, leave on 5 minutes, and rinse

Topical: Apply a sufficient amount and rub gently into the affected and surrounding area. For external use only. Avoid exposure to flame or smoking immediately following application of gel or foam.

Monitoring Parameters Liver function tests, signs of adrenal dysfunction

Patient Information Cream is for topical application to the skin only; avoid contact with the eye; notify physician of unusual fatigue, weakness, vomiting, dark urine, or yellowing of eyes; avoid alcohol

Dosage Forms Excipient information presented when available (limited, particularly for generics); consult specific product labeling.

Aerosol, topical [foam]:
Extina®: 2% (50 g, 100 g)
Cream, topical: 2% (15 g, 30 g, 60 g)
Kuric™: 2%: (75 g)
Gel, topical:
Xolegel®: 2% (15 g, 45 g) [contains dehydrated alcohol 34%]
Shampoo, topical: 1% (120 mL), 2% (120 mL)
Nizoral®: 2% (120 mL)
Nizoral® A-D: 1% (120 mL, 210 mL)
Tablet: 200 mg

Extemporaneous Preparations A 20 mg/mL suspension may be made by pulverizing twelve 200 mg ketoconazole tablets to a fine powder; add 40 mL Ora-Plus® in small portions with thorough mixing; incorporate Ora-Sweet® to make a final volume of 120 mL and mix thoroughly; shake well before using; protect from light; stable for 60 days when stored without light at 5°C and 25°C

Allen LV and Erickson MA, "Stability of Ketoconazole, Metolazone, Metronidazole, Procainamide, Hydrochloride, and Spironolactone in Extemporaneously Compounded Oral Liquids," *AM J Health-Syst Pharm*, 1996, 53:2073-8.

References

Como JA and Dismukes WE, "Oral Azole Drugs as Systemic Antifungal Therapy," *N Engl J Med*, 1994, 330(4):263-72.

Ginsburg AM, McCracken GH Jr, and Olsen K, "Pharmacology of Ketoconazole Suspension in Infants and Children," *Antimicrob Agents Chemother*, 1983, 23(5):787-9.

Herrod HG, "Chronic Mucocutaneous Candidiasis in Childhood and Complications of non-*Candida* Infection: A Report of the Pediatric Immunodeficiency Collaborative Study Group," *J Pediatr*, 1990, 116 (3):377-82.

◆ **Ketoderm® (Can)** *see Ketoconazole on page 780*

Ketorolac (KEE toe role ak)

Medication Safety Issues

Sound-alike/look-alike issues:
Acular® may be confused with Acthar®, Ocular®
Ketorolac may be confused with Ketalar®
Toradol® may be confused with Foradil®, Inderal®, Tegretol®, Torecan®, traMADol, tromethamine

Beers Criteria medication: This drug may be inappropriate for use in geriatric patients (high severity risk).

International issues:
Toradol® may be confused with Theradol® which is a brand name for tramadol in the Netherlands

U.S. Brand Names Acular LS®; Acular®; Acular® PF [DSC]; Acuvail™; Sprix™

Canadian Brand Names Acular LS®; Acular®; Apo-Ketorolac Injectable®; Apo-Ketorolac®; Ketorolac Tromethamine Injection, USP; Novo-Ketorolac; Nu-Ketorolac; ratio-Ketorolac; Toradol®; Toradol® IM

Therapeutic Category Analgesic, Non-narcotic; Anti-inflammatory Agent; Antipyretic; Nonsteroidal Anti-inflammatory Drug (NSAID), Ophthalmic; Nonsteroidal Anti-inflammatory Drug (NSAID), Oral; Nonsteroidal Anti-inflammatory Drug (NSAID), Parenteral

Generic Available Yes

Use

I.M., I.V.: Single-dose administration for moderately severe acute pain (FDA approved in ages ≥2 years and adults). Short-term (≤5 days) management of moderate to severe pain, usually postoperative pain (FDA approved in adults); has also been used to treat visceral pain associated with cancer, pain associated with trauma

Oral: Short-term (≤5 days) management of moderate to severe pain, usually postoperative pain, and only as continuation therapy of I.M. or I.V. ketorolac (FDA approved in adults); the combined duration of oral and parenteral ketorolac should not be >5 days due to the increased risk of serious adverse effects

Ophthalmic:

Acular®: Treatment of ocular itch associated with seasonal allergic conjunctivitis; postoperative inflammation following cataract extraction (FDA approved in ages ≥3 years and adults)

Acular LS™: Reduction of ocular pain, burning, and stinging after corneal refractive surgery (FDA approved in ages ≥3 years and adults)

Acular® P.F.: Reduction of ocular pain and photophobia after incisional refractive surgery (FDA approved in ages ≥3 years and adults)

Medication Guide An FDA-approved patient medication guide, which is available with the product information and at http://www.fda.gov/downloads/Drugs/DrugSafety/ucm089165.pdf, must be dispensed with this medication for each new outpatient prescription and refill.

Pregnancy Risk Factor C

Pregnancy Considerations Adverse events were not observed in the initial animal reproduction studies; therefore, the manufacturer classifies ketorolac as pregnancy category C. Ketorolac crosses the placenta. NSAID exposure during the first trimester is not strongly associated with congenital malformations; however, cardiovascular anomalies and cleft palate have been observed following NSAID exposure in some studies. The use of an NSAID close to conception may be associated with an increased risk of miscarriage. Non-teratogenic effects have been observed following NSAID administration during the third trimester including myocardial degenerative changes, prenatal constriction of the ductus arteriosus, fetal tricuspid regurgitation, failure of the ductus arteriosus to close postnatally; renal dysfunction or failure, oligohydramnios; gastrointestinal bleeding or perforation, increased risk of necrotizing enterocolitis; intracranial bleeding (including intraventricular hemorrhage), platelet dysfunction with resultant bleeding; pulmonary hypertension. Because they may cause premature closure of the ductus arteriosus, use of NSAIDs late in pregnancy should be avoided (use after 31 or 32 weeks gestation is not recommended by some clinicians). **[U.S. Boxed Warning]: Ketorolac is contraindicated during labor and delivery (may inhibit uterine contractions and adversely affect fetal circulation).** The chronic use of NSAIDs in women of reproductive age may be associated with infertility that is reversible upon discontinuation of the medication.

Lactation Enters breast milk/contraindicated (per manufacturer)

Breast-Feeding Considerations Low concentrations of ketorolac are found in breast milk. **[U.S. Boxed Warning]: Inhibition of prostaglandin synthesis may adversely affect neonates; use of systemic ketorolac is contraindicated in breast-feeding women.** The manufacturer of the ophthalmic product recommends that caution be used if administered to a breast-feeding woman. The AAP considers ketorolac to be "usually compatible with breast-feeding." The maternal pharmacokinetics of ketorolac were not found to change immediately postpartum.

Contraindications Hypersensitivity to ketorolac or any component; history of asthma, urticaria, or allergic-type reaction to aspirin, or other NSAIDs; patients with the "aspirin triad" [asthma, rhinitis (with or without nasal polyps), and aspirin intolerance] (fatal asthmatic and anaphylactoid reactions may occur in these patients); patients with active peptic ulcer disease (PUD), recent GI bleeding or perforation, or history of PUD or GI bleeding; advanced renal dysfunction; patients at risk for renal failure due to hypovolemia; women in late pregnancy; women in labor and delivery or breast-feeding; preoperative prophylactic analgesia; perioperative pain in the setting of coronary artery bypass graft (CABG); patients with cerebrovascular bleeding, incomplete hemostasis, hemorrhagic diathesis, or at high risk of bleeding; contraindicated for epidural or intrathecal use due to alcohol content; concomitant use of probenecid or pentoxifylline; do not administer with aspirin or other NSAIDs

Warnings NSAIDs are associated with an increased risk of adverse cardiovascular thrombotic events, including potentially fatal MI and stroke **[U.S. Boxed Warning]**; risk may be increased with duration of use or pre-existing cardiovascular risk factors or disease; carefully evaluate cardiovascular risk profile prior to prescribing; use the lowest effective dose for the shortest duration of time, taking into consideration individual patient treatment goals; alternate therapies should be considered for patients at high risk. NSAIDs may cause fluid retention, edema, and new onset or worsening of pre-existing hypertension; use with caution in patients with hypertension, CHF, or fluid retention. Concurrent administration of ibuprofen, and potentially other nonselective NSAIDs, may interfere with aspirin's cardioprotective effect. Due to the effects of platelets, use is contraindicated in patients with suspected or confirmed cerebrovascular bleeding, patients with hemorrhagic diathesis, incomplete hemostasis, those at high risk for bleeding, for use as prophylactic before any major surgery or intraoperatively when hemostats is critical due to increased risk of bleeding **[U.S. Boxed Warning]**.

NSAIDs may increase the risk of gastrointestinal inflammation, ulceration, bleeding, and perforation **[U.S. Boxed Warning]**. These events, which can be potentially fatal, may occur at any time during therapy, and without warning. Avoid the use of NSAIDs in patients with active GI bleeding or ulcer disease. Ketorolac is contraindicated in patients with active peptic ulcer disease, patients with recent or history of GI bleeding or perforation. Use NSAIDs with caution in patients with other risk factors which may increase GI bleeding (eg, concurrent therapy with aspirin, anticoagulants, and/or corticosteroids, longer duration of NSAID use, smoking, use of alcohol, and poor general health). Use the lowest effective dose for the shortest duration of time, taking into consideration individual patient treatment goals; alternate therapies should be considered for patients at high risk.

NSAIDs may compromise existing renal function. Renal toxicity may occur in patients with impaired renal function, dehydration, heart failure, liver dysfunction, and those taking diuretics and ACE inhibitors; use with caution in these patients; monitor renal function closely. Ketorolac is contraindicated in patients with advanced renal disease

[U.S. Boxed Warning]. Long-term use of NSAIDs may cause renal papillary necrosis and other renal injury.

Hypersensitivity reactions have been reported **[U.S. Boxed Warning]**; use is contraindicated in patients with a history of hypersensitivity to ketorolac or other NSAIDs; patients with the "aspirin triad" who receive NSAIDs may be at higher risk (see Contraindications). NSAIDs may cause serious dermatologic adverse reactions including exfoliative dermatitis, Stevens-Johnson syndrome, and toxic epidermal necrolysis.

Use is contraindicated for pregnant women during labor and delivery due to potential adverse effects on fetal circulation **[U.S. Boxed Warning]**; also avoid use in late pregnancy; contraindicated in nursing mothers due to potential adverse effects in neonates **[U.S. Boxed Warning]**.

Duration of ketorolac therapy should not exceed 5 days and should not exceed recommended dose due to adverse effects **[U.S. Boxed Warning]**; if multiple dosage forms are used, total duration of combined therapy should not exceed 5 days. Dosage adjustment is required for patients ≥65 years and those who weigh <50 kg **[U.S. Boxed Warning]**. Use is contraindicated in patients currently receiving aspirin or other NSAIDs due to risk of cumulative toxicity **[U.S. Boxed Warning]**.

Precautions Use with caution in patients with decreased hepatic function; closely monitor patients with abnormal LFTs; severe hepatic reactions (eg, fulminant hepatitis, liver failure) have occurred with NSAID use, rarely; discontinue if signs or symptoms of liver disease develop or if systemic manifestations occur. Use with caution in patients with asthma; asthmatic patients may have aspirin-sensitive asthma which may be associated with severe and potentially fatal bronchospasm when aspirin or NSAIDs are administered (see Contraindications). Anemia (due to occult or gross blood loss from the GI tract, fluid retention, or other effect on erythropoiesis) may occur; monitor hemoglobin and hematocrit in patients receiving long-term therapy. Use with caution and monitor carefully in patients with coagulation disorders or those receiving anticoagulants; NSAIDs inhibit platelet aggregation and may prolong bleeding time.

Use ocular product with caution in patients with complicated ocular surgeries, corneal denervation or epithelial defects, ocular surface diseases (eg, dry eye syndrome), repeated ocular surgeries within a short period of time, diabetes mellitus, rheumatoid arthritis; these patients may be at risk for corneal adverse events that may be sight threatening (see Adverse Reactions)

Adverse Reactions

Cardiovascular: Edema, hypertension, increased risk of cardiovascular thrombotic events (see Warnings)

Central nervous system: Dizziness, drowsiness, headache

Dermatologic: Exfoliative dermatitis, pruritus, purpura, rash, Stevens-Johnson syndrome, toxic epidermal necrolysis

Endocrine & metabolic: Fluid retention

Gastrointestinal: Abdominal pain, constipation, diarrhea, dyspepsia, flatulence, GI bleeding, GI fullness, GI perforation (see Warnings), GI ulceration, heartburn, nausea, peptic ulcer, stomatitis, vomiting

Hematologic: Anemia, bleeding time increased

Hepatic: Hepatitis, liver enzymes increased, liver failure

Local: Pain at injection site

Ocular: Blurred vision; ocular use: Allergic reactions, burning, conjunctival hyperemia, corneal edema or infiltrates, transient stinging; corneal erosion, perforation, thinning, or ulceration in susceptible patients (may be sight threatening; discontinue use; monitor closely), epithelial breakdown; delayed ocular healing; edema, inflammation, ocular irritation, or pain; keratitis; **Note:** Use >24 hours before surgery and >14 days after surgery may increase risk of corneal adverse events.

Otic: Tinnitus

Renal: Renal dysfunction, renal papillary necrosis and other renal injury with long-term use (see Warnings)

Miscellaneous: Anaphylaxis, hypersensitivity reactions (see Warnings), sweating

<1%, postmarketing, and/or case reports: Abnormal dreams, abnormal taste, abnormal thinking, abnormal vision, acute pancreatitis, alopecia, angioedema, anorexia, anxiety, appetite increased, aseptic meningitis, asthenia, asthma, blurred vision, bronchospasm, cholestatic jaundice, CHF, confusion, cough, depression, dry mouth, dyspnea, ecchymosis, eosinophilia, epistaxis, eructation, esophagitis, euphoria, excessive thirst, extrapyramidal symptoms, fever, flank pain with or without hematuria and/or azotemia, flushing, gastritis, glossitis, hallucinations, hearing loss, hematemesis, hematuria, hemolytic uremic syndrome, hyperkalemia, hyperkinesis, hyponatremia, hypotension, inability to concentrate, increased urinary frequency, infections, insomnia, interstitial nephritis, jaundice, leucopenia, Lyell's syndrome, maculopapular rash, malaise, melena, myalgia, nervousness, oliguria, pallor, palpitation, paresthesia, photosensitivity, polyuria, postoperative wound hemorrhage, proteinuria, psychosis, pulmonary edema, rectal bleeding, renal failure, rhinitis, seizures, sepsis, somnolence, stupor, syncope, tachycardia, thrombocytopenia, tremors, urinary retention, urticaria, vertigo, weight gain

Drug Interactions

Avoid Concomitant Use

Avoid concomitant use of Ketorolac with any of the following: Aspirin; Ketorolac (Systemic); Nonsteroidal Anti-Inflammatory Agents; Pentoxifylline; Probenecid

Increased Effect/Toxicity

Ketorolac may increase the levels/effects of: Aminoglycosides; Anticoagulants; Antiplatelet Agents; Aspirin; Bisphosphonate Derivatives; Collagenase (Systemic); CycloSPORINE; CycloSPORINE (Systemic); Desmopressin; Digoxin; Drotrecogin Alfa; Eplerenone; Haloperidol; Ibritumomab; Lithium; Methotrexate; Neuromuscular-Blocking Agents (Nondepolarizing); Nonsteroidal Anti-Inflammatory Agents; Pemetrexed; Pentoxifylline; Potassium-Sparing Diuretics; Pralatrexate; Quinolone Antibiotics; Salicylates; Thrombolytic Agents; Tositumomab and Iodine I 131 Tositumomab; Vancomycin; Vitamin K Antagonists

The levels/effects of Ketorolac may be increased by: Antidepressants (Tricyclic, Tertiary Amine); Corticosteroids (Systemic); Dasatinib; Glucosamine; Herbs (Anticoagulant/Antiplatelet Properties); Ketorolac (Systemic); Omega-3-Acid Ethyl Esters; Pentosan Polysulfate Sodium; Probenecid; Prostacyclin Analogues; Selective Serotonin Reuptake Inhibitors; Serotonin/Norepinephrine Reuptake Inhibitors; Treprostinil

Decreased Effect

Ketorolac may decrease the levels/effects of: ACE Inhibitors; Angiotensin II Receptor Blockers; Anticonvulsants; Antiplatelet Agents; Beta-Blockers; Eplerenone; HydrALAZINE; Latanoprost; Loop Diuretics; Potassium-Sparing Diuretics; Salicylates; Thiazide Diuretics

The levels/effects of Ketorolac may be decreased by: Bile Acid Sequestrants; Salicylates

◀ **Food Interactions** High-fat meals may delay time to peak (by ~1 hour) and decrease peak concentrations

Stability

Injection: Store at room temperature of 15°C to 30°C (59°F to 86°F). Protect from light; store in carton until use. Injection is clear and has a slight yellow color; additional color change indicates degradation; precipitation may occur at relatively low pH values; do not mix in same syringe with morphine, meperidine, promethazine, or hydroxyzine (precipitation will occur)

Ophthalmic solution: Store at room temperature of 15°C to 25°C (59°F to 77°F). Protect from light. Discard single-use Acular® P.F. vial immediately after administration (solution does not contain preservative).

Tablet: Store at room temperature of 15°C to 30°C (59°F to 86°F).

Mechanism of Action Inhibits prostaglandin synthesis by decreasing the activity of the enzyme, cyclooxygenase, which results in decreased formation of prostaglandin precursors

Pharmacodynamics Analgesia:

Onset of action:

Oral: 30-60 minutes

I.M., I.V.: ~30 minutes

Maximum effect:

Oral: 1.5-4 hours

I.M., I.V.: 2-3 hours

Duration: 4-6 hours

Pharmacokinetics (Adult data unless noted)

Absorption:

Oral: Well absorbed; 100%

I.M.: Rapid and complete

Distribution: Crosses placenta, crosses into breast milk, poor penetration into CSF; follows two-compartment model

V_d beta:

Children 4-8 years: 0.19-0.44 L/kg (mean: 0.26 L/kg)

Adults: 0.11-0.33 L/kg (mean: 0.18 L/kg)

Protein binding: 99%

Metabolism: In the liver; undergoes hydroxylation and glucuronide conjugation; in children 4-8 years, V_{dss} and plasma clearance were twice as high as adults

Bioavailability: Oral, I.M.: 100%

Half-life, terminal:

Infants 6-18 months of age (n=25): S-enantiomer: 0.83 ± 0.7 hours; R-enantiomer: 4 ± 0.8 hours (see Lynn, 2007)

Children:

1-16 years (n=36): Mean: 3 ± 1.1 hours (see Dsida, 2002)

3-18 years (n=24): Mean: 3.8 ± 2.6 hours

4-8 years (n=10): Mean: 6 hours; range: 3.5-10 hours

Adults: Mean: ~5 hours; range: 2-9 hours [S-enantiomer ~2.5 hours (biologically active); R-enantiomer ~5 hours]

With renal impairment: S_{cr} 1.9-5 mg/dL: Mean: ~11 hours; range: 4-19 hours

Renal dialysis patients: Mean: ~14 hours; range: 8-40 hours

Time to peak serum concentration:

Oral: ~45 minutes

I.M.: 30-45 minutes

I.V.: 1-3 minutes

Elimination: Renal excretion: 60% in urine as unchanged drug with 40% as metabolites; 6% of dose excreted in feces

Usual Dosage Note: To reduce the risk of adverse cardiovascular and GI effects, use the lowest effective dose for the shortest period of time.

Neonates: Note: Due to a lack of substantial evidence, NSAIDs are **not** recommended for use in neonates as an adjunct to postoperative analgesia, other than in a prospective clinical trial (see AAP, 2006). Full-term Neonates: Multiple-dose treatment: I.V.: Dose not established; limited data exists; one retrospective study

(n=10; mean PNA: 3 ± 4 weeks) recommends 0.5 mg/kg/ dose every 8 hours for up to 1-2 days postoperatively; do not exceed 48 hours of treatment (see Burd, 2002)

Infants ≥1 month and Children <2 years: Multiple-dose treatment: I.V.: 0.5 mg/kg every 6-8 hours, not to exceed 48-72 hours of treatment (see Burd, 2002; Dawkins, 2009; Gupta, 2004; Moffett, 2006)

Children 2-16 years and Children >16 years who are <50 kg: Do not exceed adult doses; see Additional Information

Single-dose treatment:

Manufacturer's recommendations:

I.M.: 1 mg/kg as a single dose; maximum dose: 30 mg

I.V.: 0.5 mg/kg as a single dose; maximum dose: 15 mg

Alternative dosing:

I.M., I.V.: 0.4-1 mg/kg as a single dose; **Note:** Limited information exists. Single I.V. doses of 0.5-1 mg/kg have been studied in children 2-16 years of age for postoperative analgesia. In one study (Maunuksela, 1992), the median required single I.V. dose was 0.4 mg/kg.

Oral: One study used 1 mg/kg as a single dose for analgesia in 30 children (mean ± SD age: 3 ± 2.5 years) undergoing bilateral myringotomy.

Multiple-dose treatment:

I.M., I.V.: 0.5 mg/kg every 6 hours, not to exceed 5 days of treatment (see Buck, 1994; Dsida, 2002; Gupta, 2004; Gupta, 2005)

Oral: No pediatric studies exist

Children >16 years and >50 kg and Adults <65 years:

Single-dose treatment:

I.M.: 60 mg as a single dose

I.V.: 30 mg as a single dose

Multiple-dose treatment:

I.M., I.V.: 30 mg every 6 hours; maximum dose: 120 mg/day

Oral: Initial: 20 mg, then 10 mg every 4-6 hours; maximum dose: 40 mg/day

Adults ≥65 years, renally impaired, or <50 kg:

Single-dose treatment:

I.M.: 30 mg as a single dose

I.V.: 15 mg as a single dose

Multiple-dose treatment:

I.M., I.V.: 15 mg every 6 hours; maximum dose: 60 mg/ day

Oral: 10 mg every 4-6 hours; maximum dose: 40 mg/ day

Children ≥3 years and Adults: Ophthalmic:

Seasonal allergic conjunctivitis (Acular®): Instill 1 drop in eye(s) 4 times/day

Postoperative inflammation (Acular®): Instill 1 drop in affected eye(s) 4 times/day starting 24 hours after cataract surgery and through 14 days after surgery

Postoperative pain, burning, and stinging (Acular LS™): Instill 1 drop in affected eye 4 times/day as needed for up to 4 days after corneal refractive surgery

Postoperative pain and photophobia (Acular® P.F.): Instill 1 drop in affected eye(s) 4 times/day as needed for up to 3 days after incisional refractive surgery

Administration

Ophthalmic: Instill drops into affected eye(s); avoid contact of container tip with skin or eyes; apply finger pressure to lacrimal sac during and for 1-2 minutes after instillation to decrease risk of absorption and systemic effects. Acular® P.F.: Administer to one or both eyes immediately after opening single-use vial; discard vial immediately after use

Oral: May administer with food or milk to decrease GI upset

Parenteral:

I.M.: Administer slowly and deeply into muscle; 60 mg/ 2 mL vial is for I.M. use only

I.V. bolus: Administer over at least 15 seconds; maximum concentration: 30 mg/mL; **Note:** I.V. ketorolac has been infused over 1-5 minutes in children.

Monitoring Parameters Signs of pain relief (eg, increased appetite and activity); BUN, serum creatinine, liver enzymes, CBC, serum electrolytes, occult blood loss, urinalysis, urine output; signs and symptoms of GI bleeding

Reference Range Serum concentration:

Therapeutic: 0.3-5 mcg/mL

Toxic: >5 mcg/mL

Patient Information Avoid alcohol; may cause dizziness or drowsiness and impair ability to perform activities requiring mental alertness or physical coordination; do not exceed 5 days total use (I.M., I.V., oral). Do not use ophthalmic solution while wearing contact lenses.

Additional Information 30 mg provides analgesia comparable to 12 mg of morphine or 100 mg of meperidine; ketorolac may possess an opioid-sparing effect; diarrhea, pallor, vomiting, and labored breathing may occur with overdose

Note: A single I.V. dose of ketorolac (0.75 mg/kg) in 21 children (2.5-9 years of age) undergoing outpatient strabismus surgery was associated with less postoperative emesis than morphine plus metoclopramide (Munro, 1994). However, a single dose of I.V. ketorolac (1 mg/kg) in 25 children (2-15 years of age) undergoing tonsillectomy was associated with an increase in surgical bleeding, more patients requiring extra hemostatic measures (eg, synthetic collagen, extra Neo-Synephrine® packing), and a higher estimated blood loss compared to rectal acetaminophen (Rusy, 1995); further studies are needed.

Product Availability

Sprix™: FDA approved May 2010; availability expected in early 2011

Sprix™ is a nasal spray indicated for short-term (≤5 days) management of moderate-to-moderately severe acute pain requiring analgesia at the opioid level.

Dosage Forms Excipient information presented when available (limited, particularly for generics); consult specific product labeling. [DSC] = Discontinued product

Injection, solution, as tromethamine: 15 mg/mL (1 mL); 30 mg/mL (1 mL, 2 mL, 10 mL) [contains ethanol]

Solution, ophthalmic, as tromethamine [drops]: 0.4% (5 mL); 0.5% (3 mL, 5 mL, 10 mL)

Acular®: 0.5% (3 mL, 5 mL, 10 mL) [contains benzalkonium chloride]

Acular LS®: 0.4% (5 mL) [contains benzalkonium chloride]

Solution, ophthalmic, as tromethamine [drops; preservative free]:

Acular® PF: 0.5% (0.4 mL) [DSC]

Acuvail™: 0.45% (0.4 mL)

Tablet, as tromethamine: 10 mg

References

American Academy of Pediatrics Committee on Fetus and Newborn, American Academy of Pediatrics Section on Surgery, Canadian Paediatric Society Fetus and Newborn Committee, et al, "Prevention and Management of Pain in the Neonate: An Update," *Pediatrics*, 2006, 118(5):2231-41.

Buck ML, "Clinical Experience With Ketorolac in Children," *Ann Pharmacother*, 1994, 28(9):1009-13.

Burd RS and Tobias JD, "Ketorolac for Pain Management After Abdominal Surgical Procedures in Infants," *South Med J*, 2002, 95 (3):331-3.

Dawkins TN, Barclay CA, Gardiner RL, et al, "Safety of Intravenous Use of Ketorolac in Infants Following Cardiothoracic Surgery," *Cardiol Young*, 2009, 19(1):105-8.

Dsida RM, Wheeler M, Birmingham PK, et al, "Age-Stratified Pharmacokinetics of Ketorolac Tromethamine in Pediatric Surgical Patients," *Anesth Analg*, 2002, 94(2):266-70.

Gupta A, Daggett C, Drant S, et al, "Prospective Randomized Trial of Ketorolac After Congenital Heart Surgery," *J Cardiothorac Vasc Anesth*, 2004, 18(4):454-7.

Gupta A, Daggett C, Ludwick J, et al, "Ketorolac After Congenital Heart Surgery: Does It Increase the Risk of Significant Bleeding Complications?" *Paediatr Anaesth*, 2005, 15(2):139-42.

Kumpulainen E, Kokki H, Laisalmi M, et al, "How Readily Does Ketorolac Penetrate Cerebrospinal Fluid in Children?" *J Clin Pharmacol*, 2008, 48(4):495-501.

Lynn AM, Bradford H, Kantor ED, et al, "Postoperative Ketorolac Tromethamine Use in Infants Aged 6-18 Months: The Effect on Morphine Usage, Safety Assessment, and Stereo-Specific Pharmacokinetics," *Anesth Analg*, 2007, 104(5):1040-51.

Maunuksela E, Kokki H, and Bullingham RES, "Comparison of Intravenous Ketorolac With Morphine for Postoperative Pain in Children," *Clin Pharmacol Ther*, 1992, 52(4):436-43.

Moffett BS, Wann TI, Carberry KE, et al, "Safety of Ketorolac in Neonates and Infants After Cardiac Surgery," *Paediatr Anaesth*, 2006, 16(4):424-8.

Munro HM, Reigger LQ, Reynolds PI, et al, "Comparison of the Analgesic and Emetic Properties of Ketorolac and Morphine for Paediatric Outpatient Strabismus Surgery," *Br J Anaesth*, 1994, 72 (6):624-8.

Rusy LM, Houck CS, Sullivan LJ, et al, "A Double-Blind Evaluation of Ketorolac Tromethamine Versus Acetaminophen in Pediatric Tonsillectomy: Analgesia and Bleeding," *Anesth Analg*, 1995, 80(2):226-9.

Watcha MF, Jones MB, Lagueruela RG, et al, "Comparison of Ketorolac and Morphine as Adjuvants During Pediatric Surgery," *Anesthesiology*, 1992, 76(3):368-72.

Zuppa AF, Mondick JT, Davis L, et al, "Population Pharmacokinetics of Ketorolac in Neonates and Young Infants," *Am J Ther*, 2009, 16 (2):143-6.

♦ **Ketorolac Tromethamine** see Ketorolac on page 781

♦ **Ketorolac Tromethamine Injection, USP (Can)** see Ketorolac on page 781

Ketotifen (kee toe TYE fen)

Medication Safety Issues

Sound-alike/look-alike issues:

Claritin™ Eye (ketotifen) may be confused with Claritin® (loratadine)

Ketotifen may be confused with ketoprofen

Zyrtec® Itchy Eye (ketotifen) may be confused with Zyrtec® (cetirizine)

U.S. Brand Names Alaway™ [OTC]; Claritin™ Eye [OTC]; Zaditor® [OTC]; Zyrtec® Itchy Eye [OTC]

Canadian Brand Names Novo-Ketotifen; Nu-Ketotifen®; Zaditen®; Zaditor®

Therapeutic Category Antiallergic, Ophthalmic; Histamine H_1 Antagonist, Ophthalmic

Generic Available Yes

Use Temporary relief of eye itching due to allergic conjunctivitis (FDA approved in children ≥3 years and adults)

Pregnancy Risk Factor C

Pregnancy Considerations Adverse fetal effects were found in some but not all animal studies. Topical ocular administration has not been studied.

Lactation Enters breast milk/not recommended

Contraindications Hypersensitivity to ketotifen or any component

Warnings Not indicated for use in eye irritation due to contact lenses; patients should be advised not to wear contact lens if their eye is red; solution contains benzalkonium chloride which may be absorbed by soft contact lenses; wait at least 10 minutes after administration before inserting contact lenses. When used for self-medication (OTC use), notify healthcare provider if symptoms worsen or do not improve within 3 days. Contact healthcare provider if change in vision, eye pain, or redness occur. Do not use if solution is cloudy or changes color.

Adverse Reactions

Dermatologic: Rash

Ocular: Allergic reactions, burning or stinging, conjunctivitis, discharge, dry eyes, eyelid disorder, itching, keratitis, lacrimation disorder, mydriasis, pain, photophobia, rash

Respiratory: Pharyngitis

Miscellaneous: Flu-like syndrome

Drug Interactions

Avoid Concomitant Use There are no known interactions where it is recommended to avoid concomitant use.

Increased Effect/Toxicity

Ketotifen may increase the levels/effects of: Anticholinergics; CNS Depressants; Methotrimeprazine

The levels/effects of Ketotifen may be increased by: Methotrimeprazine; Pramlintide

Decreased Effect

Ketotifen may decrease the levels/effects of: Acetylcholinesterase Inhibitors (Central)

The levels/effects of Ketotifen may be decreased by: Acetylcholinesterase Inhibitors (Central); Amphetamines

Stability Store at controlled room temperature (68°F to 77°F).

Mechanism of Action Ketotifen is an H_1 receptor antagonist and mast cell stabilizer which inhibits the release of mediators from cells involved in hypersensitivity reactions. Decreased chemotaxis and activation of eosinophils has also been demonstrated.

Pharmacodynamics

Onset of action: 5-15 minutes

Duration: 5-8 hours

Usual Dosage Ophthalmic: Children ≥3 years and Adults: Instill 1 drop into lower conjunctival sac of affected eye(s) twice daily, every 8-12 hours

Administration Ophthalmic: Instill into conjunctival sac avoiding contact of bottle tip with skin or eye; apply finger pressure to lacrimal sac during and for 1-2 minutes after instillation to decrease risk of absorption and systemic effects. Administer other topical ophthalmic medications at least 5 minutes apart.

Monitoring Parameters Improvement in symptomatology (eg, reduction in itching, tearing, and hyperaemia)

Patient Information Do not let tip of the applicator touch eye; do not contaminate tip of applicator (may cause eye infection, eye damage, or vision loss); wait at least 10 minutes before putting soft contact lenses in; do not wear contact lenses if eyes are red

Dosage Forms Excipient information presented when available (limited, particularly for generics); consult specific product labeling. [CAN] = Canadian brand name

Solution, ophthalmic [drops]: 0.025% (5 mL)

Alaway™: 0.025% (10 mL) [contains benzalkonium chloride]

Claritin™ Eye: 0.025% (5 mL) [contains benzalkonium chloride]

Zaditor®: 0.025% (5 mL) [contains benzalkonium chloride]

Zyrtec® Itchy Eye: 0.025% (5 mL) [contains benzalkonium chloride]

Syrup: 1 mg/5 mL (250 mL) [not available in U.S.]

Novo-Ketotifen® [CAN]: 1 mg/5 mL (250 mL) [not available in U.S.; contains alcohol, benzoate compounds; strawberry flavor]

Nu-Ketotifen® [CAN]: 1 mg/5 mL (250 mL) [not available in U.S.]

Zaditen® [CAN]: 1 mg/5 mL (250 mL) [not available in U.S.]

Tablet: 1 mg [not available in U.S.]

Novo-Ketotifen® [CAN]: 1 mg [not available in U.S.]

Zaditen® [CAN]: 1 mg [not available in U.S.]

References

Horak F, et al, "Onset and Duration of Action of Ketotifen 0.025% and Emedastine 0.05% in Seasonal Allergic Conjunctivitis," *Clin Drug Invest*, 2003, 23(5): 329-37.

◆ **Ketotifen Fumarate** *see* Ketotifen *on page 785*

◆ **Key-E® [OTC]** *see* Vitamin E *on page 1427*

◆ **Key-E® Kaps [OTC]** *see* Vitamin E *on page 1427*

◆ **KI** *see* Potassium Iodide *on page 1138*

◆ **Kidrolase® (Can)** *see* Asparaginase *on page 139*

◆ **Kineret®** *see* Anakinra *on page 108*

◆ **Kinrix™** *see* Diphtheria and Tetanus Toxoids, Acellular Pertussis, and Poliovirus Vaccine *on page 453*

◆ **Kionex®** *see* Sodium Polystyrene Sulfonate *on page 1279*

◆ **Kivexa™ (Can)** *see* Abacavir and Lamivudine *on page 29*

◆ **Klaron®** *see* Sulfacetamide *on page 1298*

◆ **Klean-Prep® (Can)** *see* Polyethylene Glycol-Electrolyte Solution *on page 1129*

◆ **Klonopin®** *see* ClonazePAM *on page 337*

◆ **Klonopin® Wafers [DSC]** *see* ClonazePAM *on page 337*

◆ **Klor-Con®** *see* Potassium Chloride *on page 1136*

◆ **Klor-Con® 8** *see* Potassium Chloride *on page 1136*

◆ **Klor-Con® 10** *see* Potassium Chloride *on page 1136*

◆ **Klor-Con®/25** *see* Potassium Chloride *on page 1136*

◆ **Klor-Con®/EF** *see* Potassium Bicarbonate and Potassium Citrate *on page 1135*

◆ **Klor-Con® M10** *see* Potassium Chloride *on page 1136*

◆ **Klor-Con® M15** *see* Potassium Chloride *on page 1136*

◆ **Klor-Con® M20** *see* Potassium Chloride *on page 1136*

◆ **K-Lyte®** *see* Potassium Bicarbonate and Potassium Citrate *on page 1135*

◆ **K-Lyte/Cl® [DSC]** *see* Potassium Bicarbonate and Potassium Chloride *on page 1135*

◆ **K-Lyte®/Cl (Can)** *see* Potassium Chloride *on page 1136*

◆ **K-Lyte® DS** *see* Potassium Bicarbonate and Potassium Citrate *on page 1135*

◆ **Koffex DM-Expectorant (Can)** *see* Guaifenesin and Dextromethorphan *on page 658*

◆ **Koffex Expectorant (Can)** *see* GuaiFENesin *on page 656*

◆ **Kogenate® (Can)** *see* Antihemophilic Factor (Recombinant) *on page 112*

◆ **Kogenate® FS** *see* Antihemophilic Factor (Recombinant) *on page 112*

◆ **Kolephrin® GG/DM [OTC]** *see* Guaifenesin and Dextromethorphan *on page 658*

◆ **Konakion (Can)** *see* Phytonadione *on page 1109*

◆ **Kondremul® [OTC]** *see* Mineral Oil *on page 933*

◆ **Konsyl® [OTC]** *see* Psyllium *on page 1185*

◆ **Konsyl-D™ [OTC]** *see* Psyllium *on page 1185*

◆ **Konsyl® Easy Mix™ [OTC]** *see* Psyllium *on page 1185*

◆ **Konsyl® Orange [OTC]** *see* Psyllium *on page 1185*

◆ **Konsyl® Original [OTC]** *see* Psyllium *on page 1185*

◆ **Koāte®-DVI** *see* Antihemophilic Factor (Human) *on page 109*

◆ **K-Pek II [OTC]** *see* Loperamide *on page 838*

◆ **K-Phos® MF** *see* Potassium Phosphate and Sodium Phosphate *on page 1143*

◆ **K-Phos® Neutral** *see* Potassium Phosphate and Sodium Phosphate *on page 1143*

- ◆ **K-Phos® No. 2** *see* Potassium Phosphate and Sodium Phosphate *on page 1143*
- ◆ **Kristalose®** *see* Lactulose *on page 791*
- ◆ **K-Tab®** *see* Potassium Chloride *on page 1136*
- ◆ **Kuric™** *see* Ketoconazole *on page 780*
- ◆ **kutrase® [DSC]** *see* Pancreatin *on page 1050*
- ◆ **ku-zyme® [DSC]** *see* Pancreatin *on page 1050*
- ◆ **Kwellada-P™ (Can)** *see* Permethrin *on page 1094*
- ◆ **Kytril®** *see* Granisetron *on page 653*
- ◆ **L-735,524** *see* Indinavir *on page 723*
- ◆ **L-749,345** *see* Ertapenem *on page 523*
- ◆ **L-M-X® 4 [OTC]** *see* Lidocaine *on page 818*
- ◆ **L-M-X® 5 [OTC]** *see* Lidocaine *on page 818*
- ◆ **L 754030** *see* Aprepitant/Fosaprepitant *on page 125*

Labetalol (la BET a lole)

Medication Safety Issues
Sound-alike/look-alike issues:
Labetalol may be confused with betaxolol, Hexadrol®, lamoTRIgine, Lipitor®
Normodyne® may be confused with Norpramin®
Trandate® may be confused with traMADol, Trendar®, Trental®, Tridrate®

High alert medication: The Institute for Safe Medication Practices (ISMP) includes this medication among its list of drugs which have a heightened risk of causing significant patient harm when used in error.

Significant differences exist between oral and I.V. dosing. Use caution when converting from one route of administration to another.

Related Information
Antihypertensive Agents by Class *on page 1481*

U.S. Brand Names Trandate®
Canadian Brand Names Apo-Labetalol®; Labetalol Hydrochloride Injection, USP; Normodyne®; Trandate®
Therapeutic Category Alpha-/Beta- Adrenergic Blocker; Antihypertensive Agent
Generic Available Yes
Use Treatment of mild to severe hypertension; I.V. for hypertensive emergencies
Pregnancy Risk Factor C
Pregnancy Considerations Because adverse events were observed in some animal reproduction studies, labetalol is classified as pregnancy category C. Labetalol crosses the placenta and can be detected in cord blood and infant serum after delivery. It has been shown to decrease maternal blood pressure without significantly effecting placental blood flow. In a cohort study, an increased risk of cardiovascular defects was observed following maternal use of beta-blockers during pregnancy. Nonteratogenic adverse events, including bradycardia, hypoglycemia, hypotension, and respiratory depression, have been observed in the infant following maternal use of labetalol during pregnancy; adequate facilities for monitoring infants at birth should be available. Untreated chronic maternal hypertension and pre-eclampsia are also associated with adverse events in the fetus/infant and mother. The pharmacokinetics of labetalol are not significantly changed during the third trimester of pregnancy. Labetalol is considered an appropriate agent for the treatment of hypertension in pregnancy; intravenous labetalol is also used for the management of pre-eclampsia.
Lactation Enters breast milk/use caution (AAP rates "compatible")
Breast-Feeding Considerations Low amounts of labetalol are found in breast milk and can be detected in the serum of nursing infants. The manufacturer recommends that caution be exercised when administering labetalol to nursing women. The AAP considers labetalol to be "usually compatible with breast-feeding."
Contraindications Hypersensitivity to labetalol or any component; asthma, obstructive airway disease, cardiogenic shock, uncompensated CHF, bradycardia, pulmonary edema, or heart block; history of asthma or obstructive airway disease
Warnings Orthostatic hypotension may occur with I.V. administration; patient should remain supine during and for up to 3 hours after I.V. administration; use with extreme caution when reducing severely elevated blood pressure; cerebral and cardiac adverse effects (infarction/ischemia) may occur if blood pressure is decreased too rapidly; blood pressure should be lowered over as long a period of time that is compatible with the status of the patient

Tablets may contain sodium benzoate; benzoic acid (benzoate) is a metabolite of benzyl alcohol; large amounts of benzyl alcohol (≥99 mg/kg/day) have been associated with a potentially fatal toxicity ("gasping syndrome") in neonates; the "gasping syndrome" consists of metabolic acidosis, respiratory distress, gasping respirations, CNS dysfunction (including convulsions, intracranial hemorrhage), hypotension and cardiovascular collapse; avoid use of labetalol products containing sodium benzoate in neonates; *in vitro* and animal studies have shown that benzoate displaces bilirubin from protein binding sites
Precautions Paradoxical increase in blood pressure has been reported with treatment of pheochromocytoma or clonidine withdrawal syndrome; use with extreme caution in patients with hyper-reactive airway disease, CHF, diabetes mellitus, hepatic dysfunction

Adverse Reactions
Cardiovascular: Orthostatic hypotension especially with I.V. administration, edema, CHF, A-V conduction disturbances (but less than with propranolol), bradycardia
Central nervous system: Drowsiness, fatigue, dizziness, behavior disorders, headache
Dermatologic: Rash, tingling in scalp or skin (transient with initiation of therapy)
Gastrointestinal: Nausea, xerostomia
Genitourinary: Sexual dysfunction, urinary problems
Neuromuscular & skeletal: Reversible myopathy has been reported in 2 children, paresthesia
Respiratory: Bronchospasm, nasal congestion

Drug Interactions
Avoid Concomitant Use
Avoid concomitant use of Labetalol with any of the following: Methacholine
Increased Effect/Toxicity
Labetalol may increase the levels/effects of: Alpha-/Beta-Agonists (Direct-Acting); Alpha1-Blockers; Alpha2-Agonists; Amifostine; Antihypertensives; Antipsychotic Agents (Phenothiazines); Bupivacaine; Cardiac Glycosides; Hypotensive Agents; Insulin; Lidocaine; Lidocaine (Systemic); Lidocaine (Topical); Mepivacaine; Methacholine; Midodrine; RiTUXimab; Sulfonylureas

The levels/effects of Labetalol may be increased by: Acetylcholinesterase Inhibitors; Aminoquinolines (Antimalarial); Amiodarone; Anilidopiperidine Opioids; Antipsychotic Agents (Phenothiazines); Calcium Channel Blockers (Nondihydropyridine); Diazoxide; Dipyridamole; Disopyramide; Dronedarone; Herbs (Hypotensive Properties); MAO Inhibitors; Pentoxifylline; Phosphodiesterase 5 Inhibitors; Propafenone; Propoxyphene; Prostacyclin Analogues; QuiNIDine; Reserpine; Selective Serotonin Reuptake Inhibitors
Decreased Effect
Labetalol may decrease the levels/effects of: Beta2-Agonists; Theophylline Derivatives

The levels/effects of Labetalol may be decreased by: Barbiturates; Herbs (Hypertensive Properties); Methylphenidate; Nonsteroidal Anti-Inflammatory Agents; Rifamycin Derivatives; Yohimbine

Food Interactions Avoid natural licorice (causes sodium and water retention and increases potassium loss); food may increase bioavailability

Stability

Injection: Store at room temperature; do not freeze; protect from light; stable in D_5W, NS, dextrose/saline combinations, D_5/LR, D_5/Ringer's, LR, and Ringer's injection for 24 hours; incompatible with sodium bicarbonate, furosemide; most stable in pH of 2-4

Tablets: Store at room temperature; protect unit dose boxes from excessive moisture

Mechanism of Action Blocks alpha-, beta$_1$- and beta$_2$-adrenergic receptor sites; elevated renins are reduced

Pharmacodynamics

Onset of action:
Oral: 20 minutes to 2 hours
I.V.: 2-5 minutes
Maximum effect:
Oral: 1-4 hours
I.V.: 5-15 minutes
Duration:
Oral: 8-24 hours (dose dependent)
I.V.: 2-4 hours

Pharmacokinetics (Adult data unless noted)

Distribution: Crosses the placenta; small amounts in breast milk
V_d: Adults: 3-16 L/kg; mean: 9.4 L/kg
Protein-binding: 50%
Metabolism: In the liver primarily via glucuronide conjugation; extensive first-pass effect
Bioavailability: Oral: 25%; increased bioavailability with liver disease, elderly
Half-life: 5-8 hours
Elimination: Possible decreased clearance in neonates/infants; <5% excreted in urine unchanged
Dialysis: Not removed by hemo- or peritoneal dialysis; supplemental dose is not necessary

Usual Dosage

Children: **Note:** Limited information regarding labetalol use in pediatric patients is currently available in the literature; labetalol should be initiated cautiously in pediatric patients (using the lower doses listed) with careful dosage adjustment and blood pressure monitoring

Oral: Some centers recommend initial oral doses of 4 mg/kg/day in 2 divided doses. (Reported oral doses have started at 3 mg/kg/day and 20 mg/kg/day and have increased up to 40 mg/kg/day.)

I.V., intermittent bolus doses: Initial doses of 0.2-0.5 mg/kg/dose with a range of 0.2-1 mg/kg/dose have been suggested; maximum dose: 20 mg/kg/dose

Treatment of pediatric hypertensive emergencies: Initial continuous infusions of 0.4-1 mg/kg/hour with a maximum of 3 mg/kg/hour have been used; one study used initial bolus dose of 0.2-1 mg/kg (maximum dose: 20 mg, mean: 0.5 mg/kg) followed by a continuous infusion of 0.25-1.5 mg/kg/hour (mean: 0.78 mg/kg/hour)

Adults:
Oral:
Outpatient: Initial: 100 mg twice daily, may increase as needed every 2-3 days by 100 mg until desired response is obtained; usual dose: 200-400 mg twice daily; not to exceed 2.4 g/day; usual dosage range (JNC 7): 200-800 mg/day in 2 divided doses

Inpatient (following acute loading with I.V. infusion): Initial: 200 mg; administer next dose as 200 mg or 400 mg after 6-12 hours, depending on blood pressure response; thereafter, for **inpatient** titration of dose, dose may be increased at 1-day intervals to obtain desired blood pressure control; increase dose as needed according to the following: 400 mg/day given in 2-3 divided doses; 800 mg/day given in 2-3 divided doses; 1600 mg/day given in 2-3 divided doses; up to a maximum of 2400 mg/day given in 2-3 divided doses (see Outpatient dosing).

I.V.: Initial: 20 mg; may give 40-80 mg at 10-minute intervals, up to 300 mg total dose

I.V. infusion (acute loading): Initial: 2 mg/minute; titrate to response; usual effective total dose: 50-200 mg total; maximum: 300 mg total dose; discontinue infusion and start oral tablets once satisfactory response in blood pressure is obtained

Note: Only acute loading dose infusions are described in the I.V. product labeling. Limited documentation of prolonged continuous infusions exists. In rare clinical situations, higher dosages (2-6 mg/**minute**) have been used in the critical care setting (eg, in patients with aortic dissection). Continuous infusions at relatively low doses (2-6 mg/**hour** - note difference in units) have been used in some settings (eg, following loading infusion in patients who are unable to be converted to oral regimens or as a continuation of outpatient oral regimens). These prolonged infusions should not be confused with loading infusions. Careful clarification of orders and specific infusion rates/units is required to avoid confusion.

Dosage adjustment in hepatic impairment: Dosage reduction may be necessary.

Administration

Oral: May administer with food but should be administered in a consistent manner with regards to meals

Parenteral:
I.V. bolus: Administer over 2-3 minutes; do not administer faster than 2 mg/minute; maximum concentration: 5 mg/mL

I.V. continuous infusion: Dilute to 1 mg/mL; undiluted labetalol injection (5 mg/mL) has been administered to a very small number of adult patients who were extremely fluid restricted

Monitoring Parameters Blood pressure, heart rate, pulse, ECG; **Note:** I.V. use: Monitor closely; due to the prolonged duration of action, careful monitoring should be extended for the duration of the infusion and for several hours after the infusion; excessive administration may result in prolonged hypotension and/or bradycardia

Test Interactions False-positive urine catecholamines, VMA if measured by fluorometric or photometric methods; use HPLC or specific catecholamine radioenzymatic technique

Patient Information Limit alcohol; may cause dizziness or drowsiness and impair ability to perform activities requiring mental alertness or physical coordination; do not stop medication abruptly; may cause dry mouth

Nursing Implications Instruct patient regarding compliance; do **not** abruptly withdraw medication in patients with ischemic heart disease; labetalol may mask other signs and symptoms of diabetes mellitus, but sweating can still occur

Dosage Forms Excipient information presented when available (limited, particularly for generics); consult specific product labeling.

Injection, solution, as hydrochloride: 5 mg/mL (4 mL, 8 mL, 20 mL, 40 mL)
Trandate®: 5 mg/mL (20 mL, 40 mL) [contains edetate disodium]

Tablet, as hydrochloride: 100 mg, 200 mg, 300 mg
Trandate®: 100 mg, 200 mg [contains sodium benzoate], 300 mg

Extemporaneous Preparations

A 40 mg/mL labetalol hydrochloride oral liquid preparation made from tablets and 3 different vehicles (cherry syrup, a 1:1 mixture of Ora-Sweet® and Ora-Plus®, or a

1:1 mixture of Ora-Sweet® SF and Ora-Plus®) was stable for 60 days when stored in amber plastic prescription bottles in the dark at room temperature (25°C) or under refrigeration (5°C); grind sixteen 300 mg tablets in a mortar into a fine powder; add 20 mL of the vehicle and mix well to form a uniform paste; mix while adding the vehicle in geometric proportions to **almost** 120 mL; transfer to a calibrated bottle and qsad with vehicle to make 120 mL; label "shake well" and "protect from light" (Allen, 1996).

Extemporaneously prepared solutions of labetalol hydrochloride (approximate concentrations 7-10 mg/mL) prepared in distilled water, simple syrup, apple juice, grape juice, and orange juice were stable for 4 weeks when stored in amber glass or plastic prescription bottles at 23°C and 4°C (Nahata, 1991).

Allen LV and Erickson MA, "Stability of Labetalol Hydrochloride, Metoprolol Tartrate, Verapamil Hydrochloride, and Spironolactone With Hydrochlorothiazide in Extemporaneously Compounded Oral Liquids," *Am J Health Syst Pharm*, 1996, 53(19):2304-9.

Nahata MC, "Stability of Labetolol Hydrochloride in Distilled Water, Simple Syrup, and Three Fruit Juices," *DICP*, 1991, 25(5):465-9.

References

Bunchman TE, Lynch RE, and Wood EG, "Intravenously Administered Labetalol for Treatment of Hypertension in Children," *J Pediatr*, 1992, 120(1):140-4.

Chobanian AV, Bakris GL, Black HR, et al, "The Seventh Report of the Joint National Committee on Prevention, Detection, Evaluation, and Treatment of High Blood Pressure: The JNC 7 report," *JAMA*, 2003, 289(19):2560-72.

Farine M, and Arbus GS, "Management of Hypertensive Emergencies in Children," *Pediatr Emerg Care*, 1989, 5(1):51-5.

Ishisaka DY, Yonan CD, Housel BF, "Labetalol for Treatment of Hypertension in a Child," *Clin Pharm*, 1991, 10(7):500-1 (case report).

Jones SE, "Coarctation in Children. Controlled Hypotension Using Labetalol and Halothane," *Anaesthesia*, 1979, 34(10):1052-5.

Jureidini KF, "Oral Labetalol in a Child With Phaeochromocytoma and Five Children With Renal Hypertension," *N Z Med J*, 1980, 10:479 (abstract).

Mueller JB and Solhaug MJ, "Labetalol in Pediatric Hypertensive Emergencies," *Pediatr Res*, 1988, 23(Pt 2):543A (abstract).

Wesley AG, Hariprasad D, Pather M, et al, "Labetalol in Tetanus. The Treatment of Sympathetic Nervous System Overactivity," *Anaesthesia*, 1983, 38(3):243-9.

♦ **Labetalol Hydrochloride** *see* Labetalol *on page 787*

♦ **Labetalol Hydrochloride Injection, USP (Can)** *see* Labetalol *on page 787*

♦ **Lac-Hydrin®** *see* Lactic Acid and Ammonium Hydroxide *on page 789*

♦ **Lac-Hydrin® Five [OTC]** *see* Lactic Acid and Ammonium Hydroxide *on page 789*

♦ **LAClotion™** *see* Lactic Acid and Ammonium Hydroxide *on page 789*

♦ **LaCrosse Complete [OTC]** *see* Sodium Phosphate *on page 1276*

Lactic Acid and Ammonium Hydroxide
(LAK tik AS id with a MOE nee um hye DROKS ide)

U.S. Brand Names AmLactin® [OTC]; Geri-Hydrolac™ [OTC]; Geri-Hydrolac™-12 [OTC]; Lac-Hydrin®; Lac-Hydrin® Five [OTC]; LAClotion™

Therapeutic Category Topical Skin Product

Generic Available Yes

Use Topical humectant used in the treatment of ichthyosis vulgaris, ichthyosis xerosis, and dry skin conditions

Pregnancy Risk Factor B

Pregnancy Considerations Lactic acid is a normal component in blood and tissues. Topical application in animals has not shown fetal harm.

Lactation Use caution

Breast-Feeding Considerations It is not known how this medication affects normal levels of lactic acid in human milk. Because studies have not been done in nursing women, use with caution when needed.

Contraindications Hypersensitivity to ammonium lactate, parabens, or any component

Warnings May cause photosensitivity reaction (see Patient Information)

Precautions Use with caution on face due to potential irritation, particularly in fair-skinned individuals

Adverse Reactions
Dermatologic: Rash, erythema, peeling, photosensitivity
Local: Burning, stinging

Drug Interactions
Avoid Concomitant Use There are no known interactions where it is recommended to avoid concomitant use.
Increased Effect/Toxicity There are no known significant interactions involving an increase in effect.
Decreased Effect There are no known significant interactions involving a decrease in effect.

Stability Store at room temperature

Mechanism of Action Ammonium lactate is a formulation of lactic acid neutralized with ammonium hydroxide. Lactic acid is an alpha-hydroxy acid which increases hydration of the skin, decreases corneocyte adhesion, reduces excessive epidermal keratinization in hyperkeratotic conditions, and induces synthesis of mucopolysaccharides and collagen in photodamaged skin.

Pharmacodynamics Onset of action: Ichthyosis xerosis: 3-7 days

Pharmacokinetics (Adult data unless noted) Bioavailability: 6%

Usual Dosage Infants, Children, and Adults: Topical: Apply twice daily

Administration Topical: Apply a small amount to the affected area(s) and rub in thoroughly; avoid contact with eyes, lips, or mucous membranes; shake lotion well before use

Monitoring Parameters Physical examination of skin condition

Patient Information Avoid contact with eyes, lips, or mucous membranes; may cause stinging or burning when applied to skin with fissures, erosions, or abrasions. May cause photosensitivity reactions (eg, exposure to sunlight may cause severe sunburn, skin rash, redness, or itching); avoid exposure to sunlight and artificial light sources (sunlamps, tanning booth/bed); wear protective clothing, wide-brimmed hats, sunglasses, and lip sunscreen (SPF ≥15); use a sunscreen [broad-spectrum sunscreen or physical sunscreen (preferred) or sunblock with SPF ≥15]; contact physician if reaction occurs. Do not use cosmetics or other skin care products on the treated skin area.

Dosage Forms Excipient information presented when available (limited, particularly for generics); consult specific product labeling.
Cream, topical: Lactic acid 12% with ammonium hydroxide (140 g, 280 g, 385 g)
  AmLactin®: Lactic acid 12% with ammonium hydroxide (140 g)
  Lac-Hydrin®: Lactic acid 12% with ammonium hydroxide (280 g, 385 g)
Lotion, topical:
  AmLactin®, Lac-Hydrin®, LAClotion™: Lactic acid 12% with ammonium hydroxide (225 g, 400 g)
  Geri-Hydrolac™, Lac-Hydrin® Five: Lactic acid 5% with ammonium hydroxide (120 mL, 240 mL)
  Geri-Hydrolac™-12: Lactic acid 12% with ammonium hydroxide (120 mL, 240 mL)

♦ **Lactinex™ [OTC]** *see* Lactobacillus *on page 790*

Lactobacillus (lak toe ba SIL us)

U.S. Brand Names Bacid® [OTC]; Culturelle® [OTC]; Dofus [OTC]; Flora-Q™ [OTC]; Floranex™ [OTC]; Kala® [OTC]; Lactinex™ [OTC]; Lacto-Bifidus [OTC]; Lacto-Key [OTC]; Lacto-Pectin [OTC]; Lacto-TriBlend [OTC]; Megadophilus® [OTC]; MoreDophilus® [OTC]; RisaQuad™ [OTC]; Superdophilus® [OTC]; VSL #3® [OTC]; VSL #3®-DS

Canadian Brand Names Bacid®; Fermalac

Therapeutic Category Antidiarrheal

Generic Available Yes

Use Treatment of uncomplicated diarrhea particularly that caused by antibiotic therapy; re-establish normal physiologic and bacterial flora of the intestinal tract

Contraindications Allergy to milk or lactose

Warnings Discontinue if high fever present

Adverse Reactions Gastrointestinal: Intestinal flatus

Drug Interactions

Avoid Concomitant Use There are no known interactions where it is recommended to avoid concomitant use.

Increased Effect/Toxicity There are no known significant interactions involving an increase in effect.

Decreased Effect There are no known significant interactions involving a decrease in effect.

Stability Store in the refrigerator

Mechanism of Action Creates an environment unfavorable to potentially pathogenic fungi or bacteria through the production of lactic acid, and favors establishment of an aciduric flora, thereby suppressing the growth of pathogenic microorganisms; helps re-establish normal intestinal flora

Pharmacokinetics (Adult data unless noted)

Absorption: Not orally absorbed

Distribution: Locally, primarily in the colon

Elimination: In feces

Usual Dosage Children and Adults: Oral:

Capsule: 1-2 capsules 2-4 times/day

Granules: 1 packet added to or taken with cereal, food, milk, fruit juice, or water, 3-4 times/day

Powder: ¼-1 teaspoon 1-3 times/day with liquid

Tablet, chewable: 4 tablets 3-4 times/day; may follow each dose with a small amount of milk, fruit juice, or water

Recontamination protocol for BMT unit: 1 packet 3 times/day for 6 doses for those patients who refuse yogurt

Administration Oral: Granules, powder, or contents of capsules may be added to or administered with cereal, food, milk, fruit juice, or water

Dosage Forms Excipient information presented when available (limited, particularly for generics); consult specific product labeling.

Capsule:

Culturelle®: *L. rhamnosus* GG 10 billion colony-forming units [contains casein and whey]

Dofus: *L. acidophilus* and *L. bifidus* 10:1 ratio [beet root powder base]

Flora-Q™: *L. acidophilus* and *L. paracasei* ≥8 billion colony-forming units [also contains *Bifidobacterium* and *S. thermophilus*]

Lacto-Key:

100: *L. acidophilus* 1 billion colony-forming units [milk, soy, and yeast free; rice derived]

600: *L. acidophilus* 6 billion colony-forming units [milk, soy, and yeast free; rice derived]

Lacto-Bifidus:

100: *L. bifidus* 1 billion colony-forming units [milk, soy, and yeast free; rice derived]

600: *L. bifidus* 6 billion colony-forming units [milk, soy, and yeast free; rice derived]

Lacto-Pectin: *L. acidophilus* and *L. casei* ≥5 billion colony-forming units [also contains *Bifidobacterium lactis* and citrus pectin cellulose complex]

Lacto-TriBlend:

100: *L. acidophilus, L. bifidus,* and *L. bulgaricus* 1 billion colony-forming units [milk, soy and yeast free; rice derived]

600: *L. acidophilus, L. bifidus,* and *L. bulgaricus* 6 billion colony-forming units [milk, soy and yeast free; rice derived]

Megadophilus®, Superdophilus®: *L. acidophilus* 2 billion units [available in dairy based or dairy free formulations]

RisaQuad™: *L. acidophilus* and *L. paracasei* 8 billion colony-forming units [also includes *Bifidobacterium* and *Streptococcus thermophilus*]

VSL #3®: *L. acidophilus, L. plantarum, L. paracasei, L. bulgaricus* 112 billion live cells [also contains *Bifidobacterium breve, B. longum, B. infantis,* and *Streptococcus thermophilus*]

Capsule, softgel: *L. acidophilus* 100 active units

Caplet:

Bacid®: *L. acidophilus* and *L. bulgaricus* [also contains *Bifidobacterium biffidum* and *Streptococcus thermophilus*]

Granules:

Lactinex™: *L. acidophilus* and *L. bulgaricus* 100 million live cells per 1 g packet (12s) [gluten free; contains calcium [5 mg/packet], lactose [380 mg/packet], potassium [20 mg/packet], sodium [5 mg/packet], sucrose [34 mg/packet], whey, evaporated milk, and soy peptone]

Powder:

Lacto-TriBlend: *L. acidophilus, L. bifidus,* and *L. bulgaricus*10 billion colony-forming units per ¼ teaspoon (60 g) [milk, soy, and yeast free; rice derived]

Megadophilus®, Superdophilus®: *L. acidophilus* 2 billion units per half-teaspoon (49 g, 70 g, 84 g, 126 g) [available in dairy based or dairy free (garbanzo bean) formulations]

MoreDophilus®: *L. acidophilus* 12.4 billion units per teaspoon (30 g, 120 g) [dairy free, yeast free; soy and carrot derived]

VSL #3®: *L. acidophilus, L. plantarum, L. paracasei, L. bulgaricus* 450 billion live cells per sachet (10s, 30s) [gluten free; also contains *Bifidobacterium breve, B. longum, B. infantis,* and *Streptococcus thermophilus*; lemon cream flavor and unflavored]

VSL #3®-DS: *L. acidophilus, L. plantarum, L. paracasei, L. bulgaricus* 900 billion live cells per packet (20s,) [gluten free; also contains *Bifidobacterium breve, B. longum, B. infantis,* and *Streptococcus thermophilus*]

Tablet:

Kala®: *L. acidophilus* 200 million units [dairy free, yeast free; soy based]

Tablet, chewable: *L. reuteri* 100 million organisms

Floranex™: *L. acidophilus* and *L. bulgaricus* 1 million colony-forming units [contains lactose, nonfat dried milk, whey]

Lactinex™: *L. acidophilus* and *L. bulgaricus* 1 million live cells [gluten free; contains calcium [5.2 mg/4 tablets, lactose [960 mg/4 tablets], potassium [20 mg/4 tablets], sodium [5.6 mg/4 tablets, and sucrose [500 sucrose/4 tablets]; contains whey, evaporated milk, and soy peptone]

Wafer: *L. acidophilus* 90 mg and *L. bifidus* 25 mg (100s) [provides 1 billion organisms/wafer at time of manufacture; milk free]

◆ **Lactobacillus acidophilus** *see Lactobacillus on page 790*

◆ **Lactobacillus bifidus** *see Lactobacillus on page 790*

◆ **Lactobacillus bulgaricus** *see Lactobacillus on page 790*

♦ **Lactobacillus casei** *see Lactobacillus on page 790*

♦ **Lactobacillus paracasei** *see Lactobacillus on page 790*

♦ **Lactobacillus plantarum** *see Lactobacillus on page 790*

♦ **Lactobacillus reuteri** *see Lactobacillus on page 790*

♦ **Lactobacillus rhamnosus GG** *see Lactobacillus on page 790*

♦ **Lacto-Bifidus [OTC]** *see Lactobacillus on page 790*

♦ **Lactoflavin** *see Riboflavin on page 1213*

♦ **Lacto-Key [OTC]** *see Lactobacillus on page 790*

♦ **Lacto-Pectin [OTC]** *see Lactobacillus on page 790*

♦ **Lacto-TriBlend [OTC]** *see Lactobacillus on page 790*

Lactulose (LAK tyoo lose)

Medication Safety Issues
Sound-alike/look-alike issues:
Lactulose may be confused with lactose
U.S. Brand Names Constulose; Enulose; Generlac; Kristalose®
Canadian Brand Names Acilac; Apo-Lactulose®; Laxilose; PMS-Lactulose
Therapeutic Category Ammonium Detoxicant; Hyperammonemia Agent; Laxative, Miscellaneous
Generic Available Yes
Use Adjunct in the prevention and treatment of portalsystemic encephalopathy (PSE); treatment of chronic constipation
Pregnancy Risk Factor B
Lactation Excretion in breast milk unknown
Contraindications Hypersensitivity to lactulose or any component; galactosemia or patients requiring low galactose diet
Warnings Accumulation of hydrogen gas in intestine could result in an explosion if the patient were to undergo electrocautery procedure
Precautions Use with caution in patients with diabetes mellitus; do not use with other laxatives especially when initiating PSE treatment as increased loose stools may falsely suggest adequate lactulose dosage
Adverse Reactions Gastrointestinal: Flatulence, abdominal discomfort, diarrhea, nausea, vomiting
Drug Interactions
Avoid Concomitant Use There are no known interactions where it is recommended to avoid concomitant use.
Increased Effect/Toxicity There are no known significant interactions involving an increase in effect.
Decreased Effect There are no known significant interactions involving a decrease in effect.
Food Interactions Contraindicated in patients on galactose-restricted diet
Stability Store at room temperature to reduce viscosity; discard solution if cloudy or very dark
Mechanism of Action The bacterial degradation of lactulose resulting in an acidic pH inhibits the diffusion of NH_3 into the blood by causing the conversion of NH_3 to NH_4+; also enhances the diffusion of NH_3 from the blood into the gut where conversion to NH_4+ occurs; produces an osmotic effect in the colon with resultant distention promoting peristalsis and elimination of NH_4+ from the body
Pharmacokinetics (Adult data unless noted)
Absorption: Oral: Not absorbed appreciably
Metabolism: By colonic flora to lactic acid and acetic acid
Elimination: Primarily in feces and urine (~3%)

Usual Dosage
Prevention and treatment of portal systemic encephalopathy (PSE): Oral:
Infants: 2.5-10 mL/day divided 3-4 times/day, adjust dosage to produce 2-3 soft stools per day
Children: 40-90 mL/day divided 3-4 times/day, adjust dosage to produce 2-3 soft stools per day
Adults:
Oral:
Acute episodes of PSE: 30-45 mL (20-30 g) at 1- to 2-hour intervals until laxative effect observed, then adjust dosage to produce 2-3 soft stools per day
Chronic therapy: 30-45 mL/dose (20-30 g/dose) 3-4 times/day; titrate dose every 1-2 days to produce 2-3 soft stools per day
Rectal: 300 mL diluted with 700 mL of water or NS, and given via a rectal balloon catheter and retained for 30-60 minutes; may give every 4-6 hours
Constipation: Oral:
Children: 7.5 mL/day (5 g/day) after breakfast
Adults: 15-30 mL/day (10-20 g/day); increase to a maximum of 60 mL/day (40 g/day) if needed
Administration
Oral: Administer with juice, milk, or water; dissolve crystals in 4 ounces of water or juice
Rectal: See Usual Dosage
Monitoring Parameters Serum ammonia, serum potassium, fluid status, stool output
Additional Information Upon discontinuation of therapy, allow 24-48 hours for resumption of normal bowel movements
Dosage Forms Excipient information presented when available (limited, particularly for generics); consult specific product labeling.
Crystals for solution, oral:
Kristalose®: 10 g/packet (30s), 20 g/packet (30s)
Solution, oral: 10 g/15 mL (15 mL, 30 mL, 237 mL, 473 mL, 946 mL, 1890 mL)
Constulose: 10 g/15 mL (240 mL, 960 mL)
Enulose: 10 g/15 mL (480 mL)
Generlac: 10 g/15 mL (480 mL, 1920 mL)
Solution, oral/rectal: 10 g/15 mL (237 mL, 473 mL, 946 mL)

♦ **L-AmB** *see Amphotericin B Liposome on page 103*

♦ **Lamictal®** *see LamoTRIgine on page 795*

♦ **Lamictal® ODT™** *see LamoTRIgine on page 795*

♦ **Lamictal® XR™** *see LamoTRIgine on page 795*

♦ **Lamisil®** *see Terbinafine on page 1322*

♦ **Lamisil AT® [OTC]** *see Terbinafine on page 1322*

LamiVUDine (la MI vyoo deen)

Medication Safety Issues
Sound-alike/look-alike issues:
LamiVUDine may be confused with lamoTRIgine
Epivir® may be confused with Combivir®
Related Information
Adult and Adolescent HIV *on page 1620*
Management of Healthcare Worker Exposures to HBV, HCV, and HIV *on page 1661*
Pediatric HIV *on page 1613*
Perinatal HIV *on page 1628*
U.S. Brand Names Epivir-HBV®; Epivir®
Canadian Brand Names 3TC®; Heptovir®
Therapeutic Category Antiretroviral Agent; HIV Agents (Anti-HIV Agents); Nucleoside Reverse Transcriptase Inhibitor (NRTI)
Generic Available No

Use

Epivir®: Treatment of HIV infection in combination with other antiretroviral agents. (**Note:** HIV regimens consisting of **three** antiretroviral agents are strongly recommended); chemoprophylaxis after occupational exposure to HIV

Epivir-HBV®: Management of chronic hepatitis B infection associated with evidence of hepatitis B viral replication and active liver inflammation

Pregnancy Risk Factor C

Pregnancy Considerations Adverse events were observed in some animal reproduction studies. Lamivudine crosses the human placenta. No increased risk of overall birth defects has been observed following 1st trimester exposure according to data collected by the antiretroviral pregnancy registry. The pharmacokinetics of lamivudine during pregnancy are not significantly altered and dosage adjustment is not required. The Perinatal HIV Guidelines Working Group recommends lamivudine for use during pregnancy; the combination of lamivudine with zidovudine is the recommended dual combination NRTI in pregnancy. It may also be used in combination with zidovudine in HIV-infected women who are in labor, but have had no prior antiretroviral therapy, in order to reduce the maternal-fetal transmission of HIV. Cases of lactic acidosis/hepatic steatosis syndrome have been reported in pregnant women receiving nucleoside analogues. It is not known if pregnancy itself potentiates this known side effect; however, pregnant women may be at increased risk of lactic acidosis and liver damage. Hepatic enzymes and electrolytes should be monitored frequently during the 3rd trimester of pregnancy in women receiving nucleoside analogues. Use caution with hepatitis B coinfection; hepatitis B flare may occur if lamivudine is discontinued postpartum. Health professionals are encouraged to contact the antiretroviral pregnancy registry to monitor outcomes of pregnant women exposed to antiretroviral medications (1-800-258-4263 or www.APRegistry.com).

Lactation Enters breast milk/contraindicated

Breast-Feeding Considerations In infants born to mothers who are HIV positive, HAART while breast-feeding may decrease postnatal infection. However, maternal or infant antiretroviral therapy does not completely eliminate the risk of postnatal HIV transmission.

In the United States where formula is accessible, affordable, safe, and sustainable, complete avoidance of breast-feeding by HIV-infected women is recommended to decrease potential transmission of HIV.

Contraindications Hypersensitivity to lamivudine or any component

Warnings The major clinical toxicity of lamivudine in pediatric patients is pancreatitis which has occurred in 14% of patients in one open-label, uncontrolled study; discontinue lamivudine therapy if clinical signs, symptoms, or laboratory abnormalities suggestive of pancreatitis occur. Cases of lactic acidosis, severe hepatomegaly with steatosis, and death have been reported in patients receiving nucleoside analogues **[U.S. Boxed Warning]**; most of these cases have been in women; prolonged nucleoside use, obesity, and prior liver disease may be risk factors; use with extreme caution in patients with other risk factors for liver disease; discontinue therapy in patients who develop laboratory or clinical evidence of lactic acidosis or pronounced hepatotoxicity.

HIV-infected patients should **not** receive lamivudine products intended for the treatment of hepatitis B (Epivir-HBV® tablets or oral solution); these products contain lower amounts of lamivudine compared to products intended to treat HIV (Epivir® tablets and oral solution) **[U.S. Boxed Warning]**. If treatment doses used for chronic hepatitis B are administered as monotherapy to a patient with unrecognized or untreated HIV infection, rapid emergence of HIV resistance will occur; this is due to the lower lamivudine doses used to treat hepatitis B compared to HIV; thus, all patients infected with hepatitis B should receive HIV counseling and testing prior to starting lamivudine for treatment of hepatitis B and periodically during treatment **[U.S. Boxed Warning]**.

HIV-infected patients who are coinfected with hepatitis B and patients infected only with hepatitis B may experience severe acute exacerbations and clinical symptoms or laboratory evidence of hepatitis when lamivudine is discontinued **[U.S. Boxed Warning]**; most cases are self-limited, but fatalities have been reported; monitor patients closely for at least several months after discontinuation of lamivudine; initiation of antihepatitis B therapy may be required. **Note:** HIV-infected patients should be screened for hepatitis B infection prior to starting lamivudine therapy. Concomitant use of combination antiretroviral therapy with interferon alfa (with or without ribavirin) has resulted in hepatic decompensation (with some fatalities) in patients coinfected with HIV and HCV; monitor patients closely, especially for hepatic decompensation; consider discontinuation of lamivudine if needed; consider dose reduction or discontinuation of interferon alfa, ribavirin, or both if clinical toxicities, including hepatic decompensation, worsen.

Precautions Use with extreme caution and only if there is no satisfactory alternative therapy in pediatric patients with a history of pancreatitis or other significant risk factors for the development of pancreatitis. Use with caution and reduce dosage in patients with impaired renal function. Fat redistribution and accumulation [ie, central obesity, peripheral wasting, facial wasting, breast enlargement, dorsocervical fat enlargement (buffalo hump), and cushingoid appearance] have been observed in patients receiving antiretroviral agents (causal relationship not established). Immune reconstitution syndrome (an acute inflammatory response to residual or indolent opportunistic infections) may occur in HIV patients during initial treatment with combination antiretroviral agents; this syndrome may require further patient assessment and therapy.

Adverse Reactions

Central nervous system: Headache, fatigue, insomnia, fever, psychomotor disorders, dizziness, depressive disorder

Dermatologic: Rash, pruritus, urticaria, alopecia

Endocrine & metabolic: Lactic acidosis, hyperglycemia; fat redistribution and accumulation (see Precautions)

Gastrointestinal: Nausea, feeding problem, abdominal discomfort, pancreatitis (children: 14%; primarily seen in children with advanced HIV receiving multiple medications), diarrhea, vomiting, anorexia, stomatitis

Hematologic: Neutropenia, anemia, thrombocytopenia

Hepatic: ALT, AST, bilirubin, and amylase elevated; hepatic steatosis, severe hepatomegaly

Neuromuscular & skeletal: Paresthesias, peripheral neuropathy, musculoskeletal pain, gait disorder, myalgia, muscle weakness, rhabdomyolysis, CPK elevated

Respiratory: Cough, wheezing

Miscellaneous: Immune reconstitution syndrome

Drug Interactions

Avoid Concomitant Use

Avoid concomitant use of LamiVUDine with any of the following: Emtricitabine

Increased Effect/Toxicity

LamiVUDine may increase the levels/effects of: Emtricitabine

The levels/effects of LamiVUDine may be increased by: Ganciclovir-Valganciclovir; Ribavirin; Trimethoprim

Decreased Effect There are no known significant interactions involving a decrease in effect.

Food Interactions Food delays the rate but not the extent of absorption (bioavailability is not significantly affected).

Stability Store tablets and oral solution at room temperature in tightly closed bottles

Mechanism of Action A synthetic nucleoside analogue that is converted intracellularly to the active triphosphate metabolite which inhibits reverse transcription via viral DNA chain termination after incorporation of the nucleoside analogue. Lamivudine triphosphate is a weak inhibitor of DNA polymerase alpha- and beta-mitochondrial DNA polymerase.

Pharmacokinetics (Adult data unless noted)

Absorption: Oral: Rapid

Distribution: Into extravascular spaces; distributes into breast milk

Children (n=38): CSF/plasma ratio: Median: 0.12; range: 0.04-0.47

V_d: Adults: 1.3 ± 0.4 L/kg

Protein binding: <36%

Metabolism: Converted intracellularly to the active triphosphate form

Bioavailability:

Children: Oral solution: 66% ± 26%

Adolescents and Adults:

150 mg tablet: 86% ± 16%

Oral solution: 87% ± 13%

Half-life:

Intracellular: 10-15 hours

Elimination:

Children 4 months to 14 years: 2 ± 0.6 hours

Adults with normal renal function: 5-7 hours

Time to peak serum concentration:

Fasting state: 0.9 hours

Fed state: 3.2 hours

Elimination: 70% of dose eliminated unchanged in urine via active organic secretion; 5.2% of dose is eliminated as a trans-sulfoxide metabolite

Usual Dosage Oral (use in combination with other antiretroviral agents):

HIV:

Neonates <30 days: 2 mg/kg/dose twice daily

Infants 1-3 months of age: 4 mg/kg/dose twice daily (see Tremoulet, 2007; Working Group, 2008)

Infants >3 months and Children <16 years: 4 mg/kg/dose twice daily; maximum dose: 150 mg every 12 hours

Alternate weight-based dosing using scored 150 mg tablets:

14-21 kg: 75 mg/dose twice daily (150 mg/day)

>21 kg to <30 kg: 75 mg in the morning, 150 mg in the evening (225 mg/day)

≥30 kg: 150 mg/dose twice daily (300 mg/day)

Adolescents ≥16 years and Adults, body weight <50 kg: 4 mg/kg/dose twice daily; maximum dose: 150 mg every 12 hours

Adolescents ≥16 years and Adults, body weight ≥50 kg: 150 mg twice daily or 300 mg once daily

HIV postexposure prophylaxis: Adolescents ≥16 years and Adults: 150 mg/dose twice daily or 300 mg/dose once daily (in combination with zidovudine, tenofovir, stavudine, or didanosine, with or without a protease inhibitor depending on risk)

Chronic hepatitis B infection: Note: Patients coinfected with HIV and hepatitis B should receive HIV doses of lamivudine (see above).

Children 2-17 years: 3 mg/kg/dose once daily; maximum dose: 100 mg/day

Adolescents ≥18 years and Adults: 100 mg/dose once daily

Dosing adjustment in renal impairment for HIV:

Neonates, Infants, Children, and Adolescents <30 kg: Insufficient data exists to recommend specific dosing adjustments for renal impairment; consider reducing the dose or increasing the dosing interval; use with caution; monitor closely

Adolescents ≥30 kg and Adults:

Cl_{cr} 30-49 mL/minute: 150 mg once daily

Cl_{cr} 15-29 mL/minute: 150 mg first dose, then 100 mg once daily

Cl_{cr} 5-14 mL/minute: 150 mg first dose, then 50 mg once daily

Cl_{cr} <5 mL/minute: 50 mg first dose, then 25 mg once daily

Note: Additional dose of lamivudine after routine (4 hour) peritoneal or hemodialysis is not required

Dosing adjustment in renal impairment for chronic hepatitis B:

Neonates, Infants, Children, and Adolescents: Insufficient data exists to recommend specific dosing adjustments for renal impairment; reduction in the dose should be considered; use with caution; monitor closely

Adults:

Cl_{cr} 30-49 mL/minute: 100 mg first dose, then 50 mg once daily

Cl_{cr} 15-29 mL/minute: 100 mg first dose, then 25 mg once daily

Cl_{cr} 5-14 mL/minute: 35 mg first dose, then 15 mg once daily

Cl_{cr} <5 mL/minute: 35 mg first dose, then 10 mg once daily

Note: Additional dose of lamivudine after routine (4 hour) peritoneal or hemodialysis is not required

Dosing adjustment in hepatic impairment: Dosage adjustment not required; use with caution in patients with decompensated liver disease (safety and efficacy not established with these patients)

Administration Oral: May be administered without regard to meals

Monitoring Parameters CBC with differential, hemoglobin, ALT, AST, serum amylase, bilirubin; signs and symptoms of pancreatitis, lactic acidosis, and pronounced hepatotoxicity; CD4 cell count, HIV RNA plasma levels in patients with HIV; HIV patients should be screened for hepatitis B infection before starting lamivudine (see Warnings)

Patient Information Lamivudine is not a cure for HIV; notify physician if persistent severe abdominal pain, nausea, vomiting, numbness, or tingling occur; avoid alcohol. Take lamivudine every day as prescribed; do not change dose or discontinue without physician's advice; if a dose is missed, take it as soon as possible, then return to normal dosing schedule; if a dose is skipped, do **not** double the next dose.

HIV medications may cause changes in body fat, including an increase in fat in the upper back and neck, breasts, and trunk; a loss of fat from the face, arms, and legs may also occur.

Additional Information Epivir® oral solution contains sucrose 1 g/5 mL.

A high rate of early virologic failure in therapy-naive adult HIV patients has been observed with the once-daily three-drug combination therapy of didanosine enteric-coated beadlets (Videx® EC), lamivudine, and tenofovir and the once-daily three-drug combination therapy of abacavir, lamivudine, and tenofovir. These combinations should not be used as a new treatment regimen for naive or pretreated patients. Any patient currently receiving either of these regimens should be closely monitored for virologic failure and considered for treatment modification.

Dosage Forms Excipient information presented when available (limited, particularly for generics); consult specific product labeling.

Solution, oral:
Epivir®: 10 mg/mL (240 mL) [strawberry-banana flavor]
Epivir-HBV®: 5 mg/mL (240 mL) [strawberry-banana flavor]
Tablet:
Epivir®: 150 mg [scored], 300 mg
Epivir-HBV®: 100 mg

References

Briars LA, Hilao JJ, and Kraus DM, "A Review of Pediatric Human Immunodeficiency Virus Infection," *Journal of Pharmacy Practice*, 2004, 17(6):407-31.

Eron JJ, Benoit SL, Jemsek J, et al, "Treatment With Lamivudine, Zidovudine, or Both in HIV-Positive Patients With 200 to 500 CD4$^+$ Cells Per Cubic Millimeter," *N Engl J Med*, 1995, 333(25):1662-9.

Lai CL, Chien RN, Leung NW, et al, "A One-Year Trial of Lamivudine for Chronic Hepatitis B," *N Engl J Med*, 1998, 339(2):61-8.

Lewis LL, Mueller B, Schock R, et al, "A Phase I/II Study to Evaluate the Safety, Toxicity, and Preliminary Efficacy of Combinations of Lamivudine (3TC), Zidovudine (AZT) and Didanosine (ddI) in Children With HIV Infection," Natl Conf Hum Retroviruses Relat Infect (2nd), 1995, Jan 29-Feb 2:103.

Lewis LL, Venzon D, Church J, et al, "Lamivudine in Children With Human Immunodeficiency Virus Infection: A Phase I/II Study," *J Infect Dis*, 1996, 174(1):16-25.

Panel on Antiretroviral Guidelines for Adults and Adolescents, "Guidelines for the Use of Antiretroviral Agents in HIV-Infected Adults and Adolescents," December 1, 2009, http://www.aidsinfo.nih.gov.

Tremoulet AH, Capparelli EV, Patel P, et al, "Population Pharmacokinetics of Lamivudine in Human Immunodeficiency Virus-Exposed and -Infected Infants," *Antimicrob Agents Chemother*, 2007, 51 (12):4297-302.

"Updated U.S. Public Health Service Guidelines for the Management of Occupational Exposures to HIV and Recommendations for Post-exposure Prophylaxis," *MMWR Recomm Rep*, 2005, 54(RR-9):1-17.

Working Group on Antiretroviral Therapy and Medical Management of HIV-Infected Children, "Guidelines for the Use of Antiretroviral Agents in Pediatric HIV Infection," February 23, 2009. Available at http://www.aidsinfo.nih.gov.

♦ **Lamivudine, Abacavir, and Zidovudine** *see* Abacavir, Lamivudine, and Zidovudine *on page 31*

♦ **Lamivudine and Abacavir** *see* Abacavir and Lamivudine *on page 29*

Lamivudine and Zidovudine
(la MI vyoo deen & zye DOE vyoo deen)

Medication Safety Issues
Sound-alike/look-alike issues:
Combivir® may be confused with Combivent®, Epivir®

AZT is an error-prone abbreviation (mistaken as azaTHIOprine, aztreonam)

Related Information
Management of Healthcare Worker Exposures to HBV, HCV, and HIV *on page 1661*

U.S. Brand Names Combivir®

Canadian Brand Names Combivir®

Therapeutic Category Antiretroviral Agent; HIV Agents (Anti-HIV Agents); Nucleoside Reverse Transcriptase Inhibitor (NRTI)

Generic Available No

Use Treatment of HIV-1 infection in combination with at least one other antiretroviral agent (FDA approved in children ≥30 kg, adolescents ≥30 kg, and adults). (**Note:** HIV regimens consisting of **three** antiretroviral agents are strongly recommended)

Pregnancy Risk Factor C

Pregnancy Considerations See individual agents.

Lactation See individual agents.

Breast-Feeding Considerations See individual agents.

Contraindications Hypersensitivity to lamivudine, zidovudine, or any component

Warnings This product contains lamivudine and zidovudine as a fixed-dose combination; concomitant use of Combivir® with drug products that contain lamivudine, zidovudine, or emtricitabine is not recommended. The major clinical toxicity of lamivudine in pediatric patients is pancreatitis; discontinue therapy if clinical signs, symptoms, or laboratory abnormalities suggestive of pancreatitis occur. HIV-infected patients who are coinfected with hepatitis B may experience severe acute exacerbations and clinical symptoms or laboratory evidence of hepatitis when a lamivudine-containing medication is discontinued **[U.S. Boxed Warning]**; most cases are self-limited, but fatalities have been reported; monitor patients closely for at least several months after discontinuation of lamivudine and zidovudine; initiation of antihepatitis B therapy may be required. **Note:** HIV-infected patients should be screened for hepatitis B infection prior to starting lamivudine therapy. Concomitant use of combination antiretroviral therapy with interferon alfa (with or without ribavirin) has resulted in hepatic decompensation (with some fatalities) in patients coinfected with HIV and HCV; monitor patients closely, especially for hepatic decompensation, neutropenia, and anemia; consider discontinuation of lamivudine and zidovudine if needed; consider dose reduction or discontinuation of interferon alfa, ribavirin, or both if clinical toxicities, including hepatic decompensation, worsen. Concomitant use of ribavirin and zidovudine may also result in exacerbation of anemia (concurrent use is **not** recommended).

Zidovudine is associated with hematologic toxicity including granulocytopenia and severe anemia requiring transfusions **[U.S. Boxed Warning]**; use with caution in patients with ANC <1000 cells/mm^3 or hemoglobin <9.5 g/dL; discontinue treatment in children with an ANC <500 cells/mm^3 until marrow recovery is observed; use of erythropoietin, filgrastim, or reduced zidovudine dosage may be necessary in some patients. Prolonged use of zidovudine may cause myositis and myopathy **[U.S. Boxed Warning]**. Zidovudine has been shown to be carcinogenic in rats and mice.

Cases of lactic acidosis, severe hepatomegaly with steatosis, and death have been reported with the use of lamivudine, zidovudine and other antiretroviral agents **[U.S. Boxed Warning]**; most of these cases have been in women; prolonged nucleoside use, obesity, and prior liver disease may be risk factors; use with extreme caution in patients with other risk factors for liver disease; discontinue therapy in patients who develop laboratory or clinical evidence of lactic acidosis or pronounced hepatotoxicity.

Precautions Always use Combivir® in combination with another antiretroviral agent. Use with extreme caution and only if there is no satisfactory alternative therapy in pediatric patients with a history of pancreatitis or other significant risk factors for pancreatitis. Use with caution in patients with bone marrow compromise or in patients with impaired renal or hepatic function. The dose of lamivudine should be reduced in patients with renal dysfunction; the dose of zidovudine should be reduced or therapy interrupted in patients with anemia, granulocytopenia, myopathy, renal or hepatic impairment, or liver cirrhosis. Use of the fixed-dose combination product (Combivir®) is **not** recommended for patients who need a dosage reduction, including children <30 kg, patients with renal or hepatic impairment, or those patients experiencing dose-limiting adverse effects (use individual antiretroviral agents to appropriately adjust dosages).

Fat redistribution and accumulation [ie, central obesity, peripheral wasting, facial wasting, breast enlargement, dorsocervical fat enlargement (buffalo hump), and cushingoid appearance] have been observed in patients receiving antiretroviral agents (causal relationship not established). Immune reconstitution syndrome (an acute inflammatory response to residual or indolent opportunistic infections) may occur in HIV patients during initial treatment with combination antiretroviral agents; this syndrome may require further patient assessment and therapy.

Adverse Reactions See individual agents.

Drug Interactions

Metabolism/Transport Effects Zidovudine: **Substrate** (minor) of CYP2A6, 2C9, 2C19, 3A4

Avoid Concomitant Use

Avoid concomitant use of Zidovudine and Lamivudine with any of the following: Emtricitabine; Stavudine

Increased Effect/Toxicity

Zidovudine and Lamivudine may increase the levels/ effects of: Emtricitabine; Ribavirin

The levels/effects of Zidovudine and Lamivudine may be increased by: Acyclovir-Valacyclovir; Clarithromycin; Divalproex; DOXOrubicin; DOXOrubicin (Liposomal); Fluconazole; Ganciclovir-Valganciclovir; Interferons; Methadone; Probenecid; Ribavirin; Trimethoprim; Valproic Acid

Decreased Effect

Zidovudine and Lamivudine may decrease the levels/ effects of: Stavudine

The levels/effects of Zidovudine and Lamivudine may be decreased by: Clarithromycin; DOXOrubicin; DOXOrubicin (Liposomal); Protease Inhibitors; Rifamycin Derivatives

Food Interactions Food does not affect the extent of absorption

Mechanism of Action See individual agents.

Pharmacokinetics (Adult data unless noted) One Combivir® tablet is bioequivalent to one lamivudine 150 mg tablet plus one zidovudine 300 mg tablet; see individual agents

Usual Dosage Oral (use in combination with at least one other antiretroviral agent): Children ≥30 kg, Adolescents ≥30 kg, and Adults: One tablet twice daily

Dosage adjustment in hepatic impairment: Not recommended (use individual antiretroviral agents to reduce dosage)

Dosage adjustment in renal impairment: Cl$_{cr}$ <50 mL/ minute: Not recommended (use individual antiretroviral agents to reduce dosage)

Administration Oral: May be administered without regard to meals

Monitoring Parameters CBC with differential, hemoglobin, MCV, reticulocyte count, liver enzymes, serum amylase, bilirubin, CD4 cell count, HIV RNA plasma levels, renal and hepatic function tests; signs and symptoms of pancreatitis, lactic acidosis, pronounced hepatotoxicity, anemia, and bone marrow suppression; HIV patients should be screened for hepatitis B infection before starting lamivudine (see Warnings)

Patient Information Avoid alcohol; Combivir® is not a cure; notify physician if persistent severe abdominal pain, nausea, or vomiting occurs; take Combivir® every day as prescribed; do not change dose or discontinue without physician's advice. If a dose is missed, take it as soon as possible, then return to normal dosing schedule; if a dose is skipped, do **not** double the next dose

HIV medications may cause changes in body fat, including an increase in fat in the upper back and neck, breasts, and trunk; a loss of fat from the face, arms, and legs may also occur.

Dosage Forms Excipient information presented when available (limited, particularly for generics); consult specific product labeling.

Tablet:

Combivir®: Zidovudine 300 mg and lamivudine 150 mg

References

Briars LA, Hilao JJ, and Kraus DM, "A Review of Pediatric Human Immunodeficiency Virus Infection," *Journal of Pharmacy Practice*, 2004, 17(6):407-31.

Panel on Antiretroviral Guidelines for Adults and Adolescents, "Guidelines for the Use of Antiretroviral Agents in HIV-Infected Adults and Adolescents," December 1, 2009, http://www.aidsinfo.nih.gov.

Working Group on Antiretroviral Therapy and Medical Management of HIV-Infected Children, "Guidelines for the Use of Antiretroviral Agents in Pediatric HIV Infection," February 23, 2009. Available at http://www.aidsinfo.nih.gov.

LamoTRIgine (la MOE tri jeen)

Medication Safety Issues

Sound-alike/look-alike issues:

LamoTRIgine may be confused with labetalol, Lamisil®, lamiVUDine, levothyroxine, Lomotil®, ludiomil

Lamictal® may be confused with Lamisil®, Lomotil®, ludiomil

Potential exists for medication errors to occur among different formulations of Lamictal® (tablets, extended release tablets, orally disintegrating tablets, and chewable/dispersible tablets). Patients should be instructed to visually inspect tablets dispensed to verify receiving the correct medication and formulation. The medication guide includes illustrations to aid in tablet verification.

Related Information

Antiepileptic Drugs *on page 1693*

U.S. Brand Names Lamictal®; Lamictal® ODT™; Lamictal® XR™

Canadian Brand Names Apo-Lamotrigine®; Lamictal®; Mylan-Lamotrigine; Novo-Lamotrigine; PMS-Lamotrigine; ratio-Lamotrigine

Therapeutic Category Anticonvulsant, Miscellaneous

Generic Available Yes; excludes extended release tablet, orally disintegrating tablet

Use

Tablets, chewable dispersible tablets, and orally disintegrating tablets: Adjunctive treatment of generalized seizures of Lennox-Gastaut syndrome, primary generalized tonic-clonic seizures, and partial seizures (FDA approved in ages ≥2 years and adults); monotherapy of partial seizures in patients who are converted from valproic acid or a single enzyme-inducing AED (specifically, carbamazepine, phenytoin, phenobarbital, or primidone) (FDA approved in ages ≥16 years and adults); maintenance treatment of bipolar disorder (FDA approved in ages ≥18 years and adults)

Extended-release tablets: Adjunctive treatment of primary generalized tonic-clonic seizures and partial onset seizures with or without secondary generalization (FDA approved in ages ≥13 years and adults)

Note: Preliminary investigations have shown potential efficacy as add-on therapy for absence, atypical absence, atonic, tonic, and myoclonic seizures; and as monotherapy in adults and adolescents for idiopathic generalized tonic-clonic seizures; additional studies are underway

Medication Guide An FDA-approved patient medication guide, which is available with the product information, must be dispensed with this medication for each new outpatient prescription and refill. Medication guides are available at:

Lamictal, Lamictal® ODT™: http://www.accessdata.fda.gov/drugsatfda_docs/label/2009/022251,020764s029,020241s036lbl.pdf

Lamictal® XR™: http://www.fda.gov/downloads/Drugs/DrugSafety/UCM166013.pdf

Pregnancy Risk Factor C

Pregnancy Considerations Lamotrigine has been found to decrease folate concentrations in animal studies. Teratogenic effects in animals were not observed. Lamotrigine crosses the human placenta and can be measured in the plasma of exposed newborns. Preliminary data from the North American Antiepileptic Drug Pregnancy Registry (NAAED) suggest an increased incidence of cleft lip and/or cleft palate following first trimester exposure. Healthcare providers may enroll patients in the Lamotrigine Pregnancy Registry by calling (800) 336-2176. Patients may enroll themselves in the NAAED registry by calling (888) 233-2334. Additional information is available at www.aedpregnancyregistry.org. Dose of lamotrigine may need adjustment during pregnancy to maintain clinical response; lamotrigine serum levels may decrease during pregnancy and return to prepartum levels following delivery. Monitor frequently during pregnancy, following delivery, and when adding or discontinuing combination hormonal contraceptives.

Lactation Enters breast milk/not recommended (AAP rates "of concern")

Breast-Feeding Considerations Lamotrigine is found in breast milk. In one study, the relative dose to the infant was 9% (range: 2% to 20%) of the weight-adjusted maternal dose. Lamotrigine was measurable in the plasma of nursing infants; adverse events were not observed.

Contraindications Hypersensitivity to lamotrigine or any component

Warnings Skin rash may occur (10% incidence in patients with epilepsy; 14% incidence in patients with bipolar disorder). Skin rash can be serious enough to require hospitalization or discontinuation of drug **[U.S. Boxed Warning]**; serious skin rashes (including Stevens-Johnson syndrome) occur in 0.8% of pediatric epilepsy patients (2-16 years of age) and 0.3% of adult epilepsy patients and in up to 0.13% of adult patients treated for bipolar and other mood disorders; rare cases of toxic epidermal necrolysis have been reported; rash-related deaths have occurred in pediatric and adult patients. In addition to pediatric age, the risk of rash may be increased in patients receiving valproic acid, high initial doses, or with rapid dosage increases; rash usually appears in the first 2-8 weeks of therapy, but may occur after prolonged treatment (eg, 6 months). Benign rashes may occur, but one cannot predict which rashes will become serious or life-threatening; the manufacturer recommends (ordinarily) discontinuation of lamotrigine at the first sign of rash (unless rash is clearly not drug related); discontinuation of lamotrigine may not prevent rash from becoming life-threatening or permanently disfiguring or disabling. Risk of nonserious rash may also be increased when the initial recommended dose or dose escalation rate is exceeded in patients with a history of rash or allergy to other AEDs.

Potentially fatal hypersensitivity reactions may occur; these may include multiorgan failure or dysfunction; early symptoms of hypersensitivity reaction (eg, lymphadenopathy, fever) may occur without rash; discontinue lamotrigine if another cause for symptoms cannot be established. Blood dyscrasias may occur.

Preliminary data from the North American Antiepileptic Drug Pregnancy Registry (NAAED) suggest a possible association of lamotrigine exposure in the first trimester of pregnancy with an increased chance of cleft lip and/or cleft palate. More research and data collection is needed to confirm this possible association. Pregnant women who are currently taking lamotrigine or who are thinking about taking lamotrigine should talk with their physician first, before stopping or starting this medication.

Antiepileptic drugs (AEDs) increase the risk of suicidal behavior and ideation in patients receiving these medications for any indication. Pooled analyses of placebo-controlled trials involving 11 different AEDs (regardless of indication) showed a twofold increased risk of suicidal thoughts or behavior (estimated incidence rate: 0.43% in AED treated patients compared to 0.24% of patients receiving placebo); increased risk was observed as early as 1 week after initiation of AED and continued through duration of trials (most trials ≤24 weeks); risk did not vary significantly by age (age range: 5-100 years). Consider risks and benefits of AEDs before prescribing. Monitor all patients receiving an AED for emergence of suicidal thoughts or behavior, thoughts of self-harm, any unusual changes in behavior or mood, or the emergence or worsening of depressive symptoms; notify heathcare provider immediately if symptoms or concerning behavior occur. **Note:** The FDA is requiring that a Medication Guide be developed for all antiepileptic drugs informing patients of this risk.

Precautions Use with caution and decrease the dose in patients with renal or moderate to severe hepatic dysfunction. Use with caution in patients with impaired cardiac function (clinical experience is limited). Use with caution and adjust the dose in patients receiving estrogen-containing oral contraceptives; estrogen-containing oral contraceptives may decrease the serum concentration of lamotrigine; dosage adjustment of lamotrigine will be necessary in most women when starting or stopping estrogen-containing oral contraceptives (see Drug Interactions and Usual Dosage fields). Valproic acid may cause an increase in lamotrigine serum concentrations requiring dose adjustment (see Drug Interactions). Patients treated for bipolar disorder should be monitored closely for clinical worsening of depressive symptoms or suicidality, especially with initiation of therapy or dosage changes; prescriptions should be written for the smallest quantity consistent with good patient care.

Do not abruptly discontinue; when discontinuing therapy, gradually reduce the dose by ~50% per week and taper over at least 2 weeks unless safety concerns require a more rapid withdrawal. Lamotrigine should **not** be restarted in patients who discontinued therapy due to lamotrigine-associated rash, unless benefits clearly outweigh risks; if restarting lamotrigine after withholding for >5 half-lives, use the initial dosing recommendations and titrate dosage accordingly (ie, do **not** restart at the previous maintenance dose). Lamotrigine binds to melanin and may possibly accumulate in the eye and other tissues rich in melanin; long-term ophthalmologic effects are unknown. A potential for the occurrence of medication errors exists with similar-sounding medications and among the different lamotrigine formulations.

Lamotrigine is **not** approved for acute treatment of mood episodes or for use in epilepsy as initial monotherapy, conversion to monotherapy from AEDs other than carbamazepine, phenytoin, phenobarbital, primidone, or valproic acid, or for conversion to monotherapy from 2 or more AEDs (safety and efficacy is not established). A small randomized, double-blind, placebo-controlled study in pediatric patients 1-24 months of age did **not** demonstrate safety and efficacy of immediate-release lamotrigine when used as adjunctive treatment for partial seizures; lamotrigine was associated with an increased risk for infectious and respiratory adverse reactions.

Adverse Reactions

Cardiovascular: Chest pain, edema, facial edema, hot flash

Central nervous system: Abnormal gait, agitation, anxiety, ataxia, depression, difficulty concentrating, dizziness, emotional lability, fatigue, fever, headache, incoordination, insomnia, irritability, nervousness, sedation, seizure exacerbation, somnolence, speech disorder; suicidal thinking and behavior (see Warnings), vertigo

Dermatologic: Angioedema, dry skin, photosensitivity; pruritus, rash (higher incidence in children and in patients receiving valproic acid, high initial lamotrigine doses, or rapid dosage increases), Stevens-Johnson syndrome, toxic epidermal necrolysis

Endocrine & metabolic: Amenorrhea, dysmenorrhea, vaginitis, weight gain, weight loss

Gastrointestinal: Abdominal pain, anorexia, constipation, diarrhea, dyspepsia, nausea, peptic ulcer, vomiting, xerostomia

Genitourinary: Urinary frequency (1% to 5%)

Neuromuscular & skeletal: Arthralgia, asthenia, back pain, myalgia, neck pain, tremor

Ocular: Abnormal vision, amblyopia, blurred vision, diplopia, nystagmus

Respiratory: Cough, dyspnea, epistaxis, pharyngitis, pharyngolaryngeal pain, rhinitis, sinusitis

Miscellaneous: Acute multiorgan failure (rare), diaphoresis, hypersensitivity reactions, lymphadenopathy

<1%, postmarketing, and/or case reports: Agranulocytosis, alopecia, anemia, aplastic anemia, apnea, arthritis, aseptic meningitis, bilirubinemia, bruising, chills, confusion, esophagitis, extrapyramidal syndrome, gastritis, gingivitis, hallucinations, hematuria, hemolytic anemia, hirsutism, hostility, hypertension, incontinence, kidney failure, leg cramps, leukopenia, liver function tests abnormal, lupus-like reaction, malaise, menorrhagia, mouth ulceration, myoclonus, neutropenia, palpitations, pancreatitis, pancytopenia, parethesia, parkinsonian symptom exacerbation, photophobia, progressive immunosuppression, psychosis, pure red cell aplasia, rhabdomyolysis (in association with hypersensitivity reaction), skin discoloration, syncope, tachycardia, thrombocytopenia, tics, tinnitus, urticaria, vasculitis, vasodilation

Drug Interactions

Avoid Concomitant Use There are no known interactions where it is recommended to avoid concomitant use.

Increased Effect/Toxicity

LamoTRIgine may increase the levels/effects of: Alcohol (Ethyl); CarBAMazepine; CNS Depressants; Desmopressin; Methotrimeprazine; OLANZapine

The levels/effects of LamoTRIgine may be increased by: Divalproex; Methotrimeprazine; Valproic Acid

Decreased Effect

LamoTRIgine may decrease the levels/effects of: Contraceptives (Progestins)

The levels/effects of LamoTRIgine may be decreased by: Barbiturates; CarBAMazepine; Contraceptives (Estrogens); Ketorolac; Ketorolac (Systemic); Mefloquine; Phenytoin; Primidone; Rifampin; Ritonavir

Food Interactions Absorption is not affected by food

Stability

Lamictal® tablets and chewable dispersible tablets: Store at controlled room temperature at 25°C (77°F); excursions permitted to 15°C to 30°C (59°F to 86°F); store in a dry place; protect 100 mg, 150 mg, and 200 mg tablets from light

Lamictal® orally disintegrating tablets: Store between 20°C to 25°C (68°F to 77°F); excursions permitted to 15°C to 30°C (59°F to 86°F)

Lamictal® XR™ tablets: Store at controlled room temperature at 25°C (77°F); excursions permitted to 15°C to 30°C (59°F to 86°F)

Mechanism of Action A triazine derivative which affects voltage-sensitive sodium channels and inhibits presynaptic release of glutamate and aspartate (excitatory amino acid CNS neurotransmitters); mechanism of action for treatment of bipolar disorder has not been established

Pharmacokinetics (Adult data unless noted)

Absorption: Oral: Immediate release: Rapid, 97.6% absorbed; **Note:** Orally disintegrating tablets (either swallowed whole with water or disintegrated in the mouth) are equivalent to regular tablets (swallowed whole with water) in terms of rate and extent of absorption.

Distribution: V_d: Adults: 1.1 L/kg; range: 0.9-1.3 L/kg; crosses into breast milk

Protein binding: 55% (primarily albumin)

Metabolism: >75% metabolized in the liver via glucuronidation; autoinduction may occur

Bioavailability: Immediate release: 98%; **Note:** AUCs were similar for immediate release and extended release preparations in patients receiving nonenzyme-inducing AEDs. In subjects receiving concomitant enzyme-inducing AEDs, bioavailability of extended release product was ~21% lower than immediate-release product; in some of these subjects, a decrease in AUC of up to 70% was observed when switching from immediate-release to extended-release tablets.

Half-life:

Infants and children:

With enzyme-inducing AEDs (ie, phenytoin, phenobarbital, carbamazepine, primidone):

Infants 10 months of age to children 5.3 years: 7.7 hours (range: 6-11 hours)

Children 5-11 years: 7 hours (range: 4-10 hours)

With enzyme-inducing AED and valproic acid (VPA): Children 5-11 years: 19 hours (range: 7-31 hours)

With VPA:

Infants 10 months of age to children 5.3 years: 45 hours (range: 30-52 hours)

Children 5-11 years: 66 hours (range 50-74 hours)

Adults:

Normal: Single dose: 33 hours; multiple dose: ~25 hours (range: 12-62 hours)

With enzyme-inducing AEDs: 13 hours (range: 8-23 hours)

With enzyme-inducing AED and VPA: ~27 hours (range: 11-52 hours)

With VPA: 59 hours (range: 30-89 hours)

Hepatic dysfunction: Child-Pugh classification:

Mild liver impairment: 46 ± 20 hours

Moderate liver impairment: 72 ± 44 hours

Severe liver impairment without ascites: 67± 11 hours

Severe liver impairment with ascites: 100 ± 48 hours

Renal dysfunction (Cl_{cr} 13 mL/minute): ~43 hours

Severe renal dysfunction (Cl_{cr} <10 mL/minute): 57.4 hours

During dialysis: 13 hours

Time to peak serum concentration: Oral: Immediate release: ~2 hours (range: 1.4-4.8 hours); select patients may have second peak at 4-6 hours due to enterohepatic recirculation. Extended release: 4-11 hours (dependent on adjunct therapy) (see Additional Information)

Elimination: 75% to 90% excreted as glucuronide metabolites and 10% as unchanged drug

Dialysis: ~20% is removed during 4-hour hemodialysis period

Usual Dosage Note: Dosage depends on patient's concomitant medications, ie, valproic acid; enzyme-inducing AEDs (specifically phenytoin, phenobarbital, carbamazepine, and primidone); or AEDS other than carbamazepine, phenytoin, phenobarbital, primidone, or valproic acid. Patients receiving concomitant rifampin or other drugs that induce lamotrigine glucuronidation and increase clearance should follow the same dosing regimen as that used with anticonvulsants that have this effect (eg, phenytoin, phenobarbital, carbamazepine, and primidone).

Anticonvulsant: Adjunctive (add-on) therapy:

Children 2-12 years: Immediate-release formulation: **Note: Only whole tablets should be used for dosing**; children 2-6 years will likely require maintenance doses at the higher end of recommended range; patients weighing <30 kg may need as much as a 50% increase in maintenance dose, compared with patients weighing >30 kg; titrate dose to clinical effect

◄ Patients receiving AEDs **other than carbamazepine, phenytoin, phenobarbital, primidone, or valproic acid:**

Weeks 1 and 2: 0.3 mg/kg/day in 1-2 divided doses; round dose down to the nearest whole tablet

Weeks 3 and 4: 0.6 mg/kg/day in 2 divided doses; round dose down to the nearest whole tablet

Maintenance dose: Titrate dose to effect; after week 4, increase dose every 1-2 weeks by a calculated increment; calculate increment as 0.6 mg/kg/day rounded down to the nearest whole tablet; add this amount to the previously administered daily dose; usual maintenance: 4.5-7.5 mg/kg/day in 2 divided doses; maximum: 300 mg/day

Patients receiving AED regimens **containing valproic acid**:

Weeks 1 and 2: 0.15 mg/kg/day in 1-2 divided doses; round dose down to the nearest whole tablet; use 2 mg every other day for patients weighing >6.7 kg and <14 kg

Weeks 3 and 4: 0.3 mg/kg/day in 1-2 divided doses; round dose down to the nearest whole tablet

Maintenance dose: Titrate dose to effect; after week 4, increase dose every 1-2 weeks by a calculated increment; calculate increment as 0.3 mg/kg/day rounded down to the nearest whole tablet; add this amount to the previously administered daily dose; usual maintenance: 1-5 mg/kg/day in 1-2 divided doses; maximum: 200 mg/day. **Note:** Usual maintenance dose in children adding lamotrigine to valproic acid **alone**: 1-3 mg/kg/day

Patients receiving **enzyme-inducing** AED regimens **without valproic acid**:

Weeks 1 and 2: 0.6 mg/kg/day in 2 divided doses; round dose down to the nearest whole tablet

Weeks 3 and 4: 1.2 mg/kg/day in 2 divided doses; round dose down to the nearest whole tablet

Maintenance dose: Titrate dose to effect; after week 4, increase dose every 1-2 weeks by a calculated increment; calculate increment as 1.2 mg/kg/day rounded down to the nearest whole tablet; add this amount to the previously administered daily dose; usual maintenance: 5-15 mg/kg/day in 2 divided doses; maximum: 400 mg/day

Children >12 years and Adults: Immediate-release formulations:

Patients receiving AEDs **other than carbamazepine, phenytoin, phenobarbital, primidone, or valproic acid:**

Weeks 1 and 2: 25 mg every day

Weeks 3 and 4: 50 mg every day

Maintenance dose: Titrate dose to effect; after week 4, increase dose every 1-2 weeks by 50 mg/day; usual maintenance: 225-375 mg/day in 2 divided doses

Patients receiving AED regimens **containing valproic acid**:

Weeks 1 and 2: 25 mg every other day

Weeks 3 and 4: 25 mg every day

Maintenance dose: Titrate dose to effect; after week 4, increase dose every 1-2 weeks by 25-50 mg/day; usual maintenance in patients receiving valproic acid and other drugs that induce glucuronidation: 100-400 mg/day in 1-2 divided doses; usual maintenance in patients adding lamotrigine to valproic acid **alone**: 100-200 mg/day

Patients receiving **enzyme-inducing** AED regimens **without valproic acid**:

Weeks 1 and 2: 50 mg/day

Weeks 3 and 4: 100 mg/day in 2 divided doses

Maintenance dose: Titrate dose to effect; after week 4, increase dose every 1-2 weeks by 100 mg/day; usual maintenance: 300-500 mg/day in 2 divided doses; doses as high as 700 mg/day in 2 divided doses have been used

Children ≥13 years and Adults: Extended-release formulation: **Note:** Dose increases after week 8 should not exceed 100 mg/day at weekly intervals

Regimens **containing** valproic acid: Initial: Week 1 and 2: 25 mg every other day; Week 3 and 4: 25 mg once daily; Week 5: 50 mg once daily; Week 6: 100 mg once daily; Week 7: 150 mg once daily; Maintenance: 200-250 mg once daily

Regimens **containing** carbamazepine, phenytoin, phenobarbital, or primidone and **without** valproic acid: Initial: Week 1 and 2: 50 mg once daily; Week 3 and 4: 100 mg once daily; Week 5: 200 mg once daily; Week 6: 300 mg once daily; Week 7: 400 mg once daily; Maintenance: 400-600 mg once daily

Regimens **not containing** carbamazepine, phenytoin, phenobarbital, primidone, or valproic acid: Initial: Week 1 and 2: 25 mg once daily; Week 3 and 4: 50 mg once daily; Week 5: 100 mg once daily; Week 6: 150 mg once daily; Week 7: 200 mg once daily; Maintenance: 300-400 mg once daily

Conversion from immediate release to extended release (Lamictal® XR™): Initial dose of the extended release tablet should match the total daily dose of the immediate-release formulation; monitor for seizure control, especially in patients on AED agents. Adjust dose as needed within the recommended dosing guidelines.

Anticonvulsant: Monotherapy: Children ≥16 years and Adults: Immediate-release formulations:

Conversion from adjunctive therapy with a **single enzyme-inducing** AED to lamotrigine monotherapy: **Note:** First add lamotrigine and titrate it (as outlined below) to the recommended maintenance monotherapy dose (500 mg/day in 2 divided doses), while maintaining the enzyme-inducing AED at a fixed level; then gradually taper the enzyme-inducing AED by 20% decrements each week to fully withdraw over a 4-week period.

Weeks 1 and 2: 50 mg/day

Weeks 3 and 4: 100 mg/day in 2 divided doses

Maintenance dose: After week 4, increase dose every 1-2 weeks by 100 mg/day; recommended maintenance monotherapy dose: 500 mg/day in 2 divided doses

Conversion from adjunctive therapy with **valproate** to lamotrigine monotherapy: **Note:** This is a 4 step conversion process to achieve the lamotrigine recommended monotherapy dose (500 mg/day in 2 divided doses).

First: Add lamotrigine and titrate it to a dose of 200 mg/day as follows (if not already receiving 200 mg/day), while maintaining the valproate dose at a fixed level:

Weeks 1 and 2: 25 mg every other day

Weeks 3 and 4: 25 mg every day

Then increase dose every 1-2 weeks by 25-50 mg/day

Second: Keep lamotrigine dose at 200 mg/day; slowly taper valproate dose in decrements of ≤500 mg/day per week, to a dose of 500 mg/day; maintain this dose for one week

Third: Increase lamotrigine to 300 mg/day and decrease valproate to 250 mg/day; maintain this dose for one week

Fourth: Discontinue valproate and increase lamotrigine by 100 mg/day at weekly intervals to achieve recommended maintenance monotherapy dose of 500 mg/day in 2 divided doses

Conversion from adjunctive therapy with AEDs other than enzyme-inducing AEDs or valproate to lamotrigine monotherapy: No specific guidelines available

Bipolar disorder: Adolescents ≥18 years and Adults: Immediate-release formulations:

Patients **not** receiving enzyme-inducing drugs (eg, carbamazepine, phenytoin, phenobarbital, primidone, rifampin) or valproate:

Weeks 1 and 2: 25 mg/day

Weeks 3 and 4: 50 mg/day

Week 5: 100 mg/day

Week 6 and thereafter: 200 mg/day

Patients receiving **valproate**:

Weeks 1 and 2: 25 mg every other day

Weeks 3 and 4: 25 mg/day

Week 5: 50 mg/day

Week 6 and thereafter: 100 mg/day

Note: If valproate is discontinued, increase daily lamotrigine dose in 50 mg increments at weekly intervals until dosage of 200 mg/day is attained.

Patients receiving **enzyme-inducing drugs** (eg, carbamazepine, phenytoin, phenobarbital, primidone, rifampin) **without valproate**:

Weeks 1 and 2: 50 mg/day

Weeks 3 and 4: 100 mg/day in divided doses

Week 5: 200 mg/day in divided doses

Week 6: 300 mg/day in divided doses

Week 7 and thereafter: May increase to 400 mg/day in divided doses

Note: If carbamazepine (or other enzyme-inducing drug) is discontinued, maintain current lamotrigine dose for 1 week, then decrease daily lamotrigine dose in 100 mg increments at weekly intervals until dosage of 200 mg/day is attained.

Dosage adjustment with concomitant estrogen-containing oral contraceptives: Follow initial lamotrigine dosing guidelines, maintenance dose should be adjusted as follows:

Patients **taking** concomitant carbamazepine, phenytoin, phenobarbital, primidone, or other drugs, such as rifampin, that induce lamotrigine glucuronidation: No dosing adjustment required

Patients **not taking** concomitant carbamazepine, phenytoin, phenobarbital, primidone, or other drugs, such as rifampin, that induce lamotrigine glucuronidation: If already taking estrogen-containing oral contraceptives, the maintenance dose of lamotrigine may need to be increased by as much as twofold over the target maintenance dose listed above. If already taking a stable dose of lamotrigine and starting an oral contraceptive agent, the lamotrigine maintenance dose may need to be increased by as much as twofold. Dose increases should start when contraceptive agent is started and titrated to clinical response increasing no more rapidly than 50-100 mg/day every week. Gradual increases of lamotrigine plasma levels may occur during the inactive "pill-free" week and will be greater when dose increases are made the week before. If increased adverse events consistently occur during "pill-free" week, overall dose adjustments may be required. Dose adjustments during "pill-free" week are not recommended. When discontinuing combination hormonal contraceptive, dose of lamotrigine may need decreased by as much as 50%; do not decrease by more than 25% of total daily dose over a 2-week period unless clinical response or plasma levels indicate otherwise.

Discontinuing therapy: Children and Adults: Do not abruptly discontinue; when discontinuing lamotrigine therapy, gradually decrease the dose by ~50% per week and taper over at least 2 weeks unless safety concerns require a more rapid withdrawal. **Note:** If

discontinuing other anticonvulsants and maintaining lamotrigine therapy, keep in mind that discontinuing carbamazepine, phenytoin, phenobarbital, primidone, or other drugs, such as rifampin, that induce lamotrigine glucuronidation should prolong the half-life of lamotrigine; discontinuing valproic acid should shorten the half-life of lamotrigine; monitor patient closely; dosage change may be needed

Dosage adjustment in renal impairment: Use with caution; has not been adequately studied; base initial dose on patient's AED regimen; decreased maintenance dosage may be effective in patients with significant renal impairment

Dosage adjustment in hepatic impairment:

Mild hepatic impairment: No dosage adjustment required

Moderate and severe hepatic impairment without ascites: Reduce initial, escalation, and maintenance doses by ~25%

Severe hepatic impairment with ascites: Reduce initial escalation, and maintenance doses by 50%

Note: Adjust escalation and maintenance doses by clinical response.

Administration Oral: May be administered without regard to food. If medication is received in blisterpack, examine blisterpack before use; do not use if blisters are broken, torn, or missing.

Regular tablet: Do not chew, as a bitter taste may result; swallow tablet whole

Chewable, dispersible tablet: Only whole tablets should be administered; may swallow whole, chew, or disperse in water or diluted fruit juice; if chewed, administer a small amount of water or diluted fruit juice to help in swallowing. To disperse, add tablets to a small amount of liquid (~1 teaspoon or enough to cover the medication); when the tablets are completely dispersed (in about 1 minute), swirl the solution and administer the entire amount immediately. Do not attempt to administer partial quantities of dispersed tablets.

Extended-release tablet (Lamictal® XR™): May be administered without regard to meals. Swallow tablet whole; do not chew, crush, or break.

Orally disintegrating tablet (Lamictal® ODT™): Place tablet on tongue and move around in the mouth. Tablet will dissolve rapidly and can be swallowed with or without food or water.

Monitoring Parameters All patients: Monitor for hypersensitivity reactions, especially rash; CBC with differential; liver and renal function

Epilepsy: Seizure frequency, duration, and severity; serum levels of concurrent anticonvulsants; signs and symptoms of suicidality (eg, anxiety, depression, behavior changes) (see Warnings)

Bipolar disorder: Clinical worsening of depressive symptoms or suicidality, especially with initiation of therapy or dosage changes

Reference Range The clinical value of monitoring lamotrigine plasma concentrations has not been established. Dosing should be based on therapeutic response. Proposed therapeutic range: 1-5 mcg/mL. Lamotrigine plasma concentrations of 0.25-29.1 mcg/mL have been reported in the literature.

Patient Information Read the patient Medication Guide that you receive with each prescription and refill of lamotrigine. Carefully look at your medication after each refill; contact the prescriber if the medication looks different or the label name has changed. Antiepileptic agents may increase the risk of suicidal thoughts and behavior; notify physician if you feel more depressed or have thoughts of suicide or self harm (see Warnings). Take exactly as directed; do not increase dose or frequency or discontinue without consulting prescriber. Do not abruptly discontinue therapy (an increase in seizure activity may result). Taking other medications may require a dosage change in lamotrigine; report the use of other medications, non-prescription medications, and herbal or natural products to your physician and pharmacist; do not use alcohol and other prescription or OTC medications (especially pain medications, sedatives, antihistamines, or hypnotics) without consulting prescriber. Notify physician if you will be starting or stopping oral contraceptives or other female hormonal products (a dosage adjustment of lamotrigine may be needed; efficacy of oral contraceptives may be decreased; report any changes in menstrual pattern such as breakthrough bleeding). Report any rash, fever, or swelling of glands to the physician immediately (skin rash may indicate a serious medical problem). Lamotrigine may cause dizziness, drowsiness, or blurred vision and impair ability to perform activities requiring mental alertness or physical coordination. May cause photosensitivity reactions (eg, exposure to sunlight may cause severe sunburn, skin rash, redness, or itching); avoid exposure to sunlight and artificial light sources (sunlamps, tanning booth/bed); wear protective clothing, wide-brimmed hats, sunglasses, and lip sunscreen (SPF ≥15); use a sunscreen [broad-spectrum sunscreen or physical sunscreen (preferred) or sunblock with SPF ≥15]; contact physician if reaction occurs. Report CNS changes, mentation changes, or changes in cognition; persistent GI symptoms (cramping, constipation, vomiting, anorexia); swelling of face, lips, or tongue; easy bruising or bleeding (mouth, urine, stool); vision changes; worsening of seizure activity, or loss of seizure control to prescriber.

Additional Information Low water solubility. Does **not** induce P450 microsomal enzymes. The clinical usefulness of lamotrigine should be periodically re-evaluated in patients with bipolar disorder who are receiving the drug for extended intervals (ie, >16 weeks).

The extended-release tablets contain a modified-release eroding formulation as the core of the tablet. The clear enteric coating has an aperture drilled through it on both sides of the tablet; this allows an extended release of the medication in the acidic environment within the stomach. The design of the table controls the dissolution rate of the medication over a 12-15 hour period.

Three different lamotrigine "Starter Kits" are available for adult patients for three different dosage forms (tablets, extended release tablets, and orally disintegrating tablets); each starter kit contains a blisterpack with a certain number and mg strength of tablets that are specific for initiating doses in different patient populations (see Dosage Forms).

Dosage Forms Excipient information presented when available (limited, particularly for generics); consult specific product labeling.
Tablet, oral: 25 mg, 100 mg, 150 mg, 200 mg
  Lamictal®: 25 mg, 100 mg, 150 mg, 200 mg
Tablet, oral [combination package; each unit-dose starter kit contains]:
  Lamictal® [blue kit; for patients taking valproic acid]:
    25 mg (35s)
  Lamictal® [green kit; for patients taking carbamazepine, phenytoin, phenobarbital, primidone, or rifampin and **not** taking valproic acid]:
    25 mg (84s)
    100 mg (14s)
  Lamictal® [orange kit; for patients **not** taking carbamazepine, phenytoin, phenobarbital, primidone, rifampin, or valproic acid]:
    25 mg (42s)
    100 mg (7s)
Tablet, dispersible/chewable, oral: 5 mg, 25 mg
  Lamictal®: 2 mg, 25 mg [black currant flavor]
  Lamictal®: 5 mg [scored; black currant flavor]
Tablet, extended release, oral:
  Lamictal® XR™: 25 mg, 50 mg, 100 mg, 200 mg

Tablet, extended release, oral [combination package; each patient titration kit contains]:
  Lamictal® XR™ [blue XR kit; for patients taking valproic acid]:
    25 mg (21s)
    50 mg (7s)
  Lamictal® XR™ [green XR kit; for patients taking carbamazepine, phenytoin, phenobarbital, or primidone and **not** taking valproic acid]:
    50 mg (14s)
    100 mg (14s)
    200 mg (7s)
  Lamictal® XR™ [orange XR kit; for patients **not** taking carbamazepine, phenytoin, phenobarbital, primidone, or valproic acid]:
    25 mg (14s)
    50 mg (14s)
    100 mg (7s)
Tablet, orally disintegrating, oral:
  Lamictal® ODT™: 25 mg, 50 mg, 100 mg, 200 mg [cherry flavor]
Tablet, orally disintegrating, oral [combination package; each patient titration kit contains]:
  Lamictal® ODT™ [blue ODT kit; for patients taking valproic acid; cherry flavor]:
    25 mg (21s)
    50 mg (7s)
  Lamictal® ODT™ [green ODT kit; for patients taking carbamazepine, phenytoin, phenobarbital, primidone, or rifampin and **not** taking valproic acid; cherry flavor]:
    50 mg (42s)
    100 mg (14s)
  Lamictal® ODT™ [orange ODT kit; for patients **not** taking carbamazepine, phenytoin, phenobarbital, primidone, rifampin, or valproic acid; cherry flavor]:
    25 mg (14s)
    50 mg (14s)
    100 mg (7s)

Extemporaneous Preparations A 1 mg/mL oral suspension made from tablets and 2 different vehicles (a 1:1 mixture of Ora-Sweet® and Ora-Plus®, or a 1:1 mixture of Ora-Sweet® SF and Ora-Plus®) was stable for 91 days when stored in amber plastic prescription bottles at room temperature (25°C) or under refrigeration (4°C); grind one 100 mg tablet in a mortar into a fine powder; add a small amount of the vehicle and mix well to form a uniform paste; mix while adding the vehicle in geometric proportions to **almost** 100 mL; transfer the mixture to a graduated cylinder and qsad with vehicle to make 100 mL; label "shake well" and "protect from light" (Nahata, 1999)

  Nahata MC, Morosco RS, and Hipple TF, "Stability of Lamotrigine in Two Extemporaneously Prepared Oral Suspensions at 4°C and 25°C," *Am J Health Syst Pharm*, 1999, 56(3):240-2.

References
Barr PA, Buettiker VE, and Antony JH, "Efficacy of Lamotrigine in Refractory Neonatal Seizures," *Pediatr Neurol*, 1999, 20(2):161-3.
Battino D, Estienne M, and Avanzini G, "Clinical Pharmacokinetics of Antiepileptic Drugs in Paediatric Patients: Part II. Phenytoin, Carbamazepine, Sulthiame, Lamotrigine, Vigabatrin, Oxcarbazepine, and Felbamate," *Clin Pharmacokinet*, 1995, 29(5):341-69.
Besag FM, Wallace SJ, Dulac O, et al, "Lamotrigine for the Treatment of Epilepsy in Childhood," *J Pediatr*, 1995, 127(6):991-7.
Burstein AH, "Lamotrigine," *Pharmacotherapy*, 1995, 15(2):129-43.
Dooley J, Camfield P, Gordon K, et al, "Lamotrigine-Induced Rash in Children," *Neurology*, 1996, 46(1):240-2.
Fitton A, and Goa KL, "Lamotrigine: An Update of its Pharmacology and Therapeutic Use in Epilepsy," *Drugs*, 1995, 50(4):691-713.
Messenheimer JA, "Lamotrigine," *Epilepsia*, 1995, 36(Suppl 2):S87-94.
Messenheimer JA, Giorgi L, and Risner ME, "The Tolerability of Lamotrigine in Children," *Drug Saf*, 2000, 22(4):303-12.
Mikati MA, Fayad M, Koleilat M, et al, "Efficacy, Tolerability, and Kinetics of Lamotrigine in Infants," *J Pediatr*, 2002, 141(1):31-5.

◆ **Lanacane® [OTC]** *see* Benzocaine *on page 182*

◆ **Lanacane® Maximum Strength [OTC]** *see* Benzocaine *on page 182*

◆ **Lanoxin®** *see* Digoxin *on page 437*

Lansoprazole (lan SOE pra zole)

Medication Safety Issues
Sound-alike/look-alike issues:
Lansoprazole may be confused with aripiprazole, dexlansoprazole
Prevacid® may be confused with Pravachol®, Prevpac®, Prilosec®, Prinivil®

U.S. Brand Names Prevacid®; Prevacid® 24 HR [OTC]; Prevacid® SoluTab™

Canadian Brand Names Apo-Lansoprazole®; Novo-Lansoprazole; Prevacid®; Prevacid® FasTab

Therapeutic Category Gastric Acid Secretion Inhibitor; Gastrointestinal Agent, Gastric or Duodenal Ulcer Treatment; Proton Pump Inhibitor

Generic Available Yes: Capsule

Use Short-term treatment of symptomatic gastroesophageal reflux disease (GERD) (FDA approved in ages ≥1 year and adults); short-term treatment (up to 8 weeks) for healing and symptomatic relief of all grades of erosive esophagitis (FDA approved in ages ≥1 year and adults); maintenance of healed erosive esophagitis (FDA approved in adults); short-term treatment (≤4 weeks) for healing and symptomatic relief of active duodenal ulcer (FDA approved in adults); treatment of pathological hypersecretory conditions, including Zollinger-Ellison syndrome (FDA approved in adults); adjuvant therapy in the treatment of *Helicobacter pylori*-associated antral gastritis (FDA approved in adults); prevention and treatment of NSAID-associated gastric ulcers (FDA approved in adults)

OTC labeling: Relief of frequent heartburn (≥2 days/week) (FDA approved in adults)

Pregnancy Risk Factor B

Pregnancy Considerations Animal studies have not shown teratogenic effects to the fetus. However, there are no adequate and well-controlled studies in pregnant women; use during pregnancy only if clearly needed.

Lactation Excretion in breast milk unknown/not recommended

Contraindications Hypersensitivity to lansoprazole, pantoprazole, esomeprazole, omeprazole, or any component

Warnings Long-term effects are not known; enterochromaffin (ECF)-like hyperplasia and subsequent carcinoids have developed in rats following lifetime exposure to high doses (150 mg/kg/day). Use of gastric acid inhibitors including proton pump inhibitors and H₂ blockers has been associated with an increased risk for development of acute gastroenteritis and community-acquired pneumonia (Canani, 2006).

Precautions Symptomatic response to therapy does not preclude the presence of gastric malignancy; use with caution in patients with liver disease, reduce dosage with severe impairment; Prevacid® SoluTabs™ contain aspartame which is metabolized to phenylalanine and must be used with caution in patients with phenylketonuria

Adverse Reactions
Central nervous system: Confusion, dizziness, fatigue, headache
Gastrointestinal: Abdominal pain, anorexia, appetite increased, constipation, diarrhea, nausea
Renal: Proteinuria
Miscellaneous: Hypersensitivity reactions
<1%, postmarketing, and/or case reports: Abnormal dreams, abnormal menses, acne, agitation, agranulocytosis, alopecia, amblyopia, amnesia, angina, anemia, aplastic anemia, arrhythmia, arthralgia, arthritis, asthenia, back pain, bezoar formation, bilirubinemia, blurred vision, bradycardia, breast enlargement, breast pain, candidiasis, cerebrovascular accident, chest pain, chills, cholelithiasis, colitis, creatinine increased, deafness, depression, diplopia, discoloration of feces, dry eyes, dysmenorrhea, dyspepsia, dysuria, edema, eructation, erythema multiforme, eye pain, fever, flatulence, flu-like syndrome, gastritis, glossitis, halitosis, hallucinations, hemolysis, hemolytic anemia, hepatotoxicity, hypergastrinemia, hyperglycemia, hypertension, hypertonia, hypoglycemia, hypotension, hypothyroidism, increased thirst, insomnia, interstitial nephritis, leg cramps, leukopenia, lymphadenopathy, malaise, melena, migraine, MI, myalgia, myositis, neck pain, nephrolithiasis, neutropenia, pain, palpitations, pancreatitis, pancytopenia, paresthesia, peripheral edema, photophobia, pruritus, rash, retinal degeneration, rhinitis, seizure, serum transaminases elevated, sinusitis, Stevens-Johnson syndrome, sweating, syncope, synovitis, tachycardia, taste perversion, tenesmus, thrombocytopenia, thrombotic thrombocytopenic purpura, tinnitus, toxic epidermal necrolysis, tremor, vasodilation, urinary frequency, urinary retention, vaginitis, vertigo, visual field defect, vomiting, weight changes, xerostomia

Drug Interactions
Metabolism/Transport Effects Substrate of CYP2C9 (minor), 2C19 (major), 3A4 (major); **Inhibits** CYP2C9 (weak), 2C19 (moderate), 2D6 (weak), 3A4 (weak); **Induces** CYP1A2 (weak)

Avoid Concomitant Use
Avoid concomitant use of Lansoprazole with any of the following: Delavirdine; Erlotinib; Nelfinavir; Posaconazole

Increased Effect/Toxicity
Lansoprazole may increase the levels/effects of: CYP2C19 Substrates; Imatinib; Methotrexate; Raltegravir; Saquinavir; Tacrolimus; Tacrolimus (Systemic); Vitamin K Antagonists; Voriconazole

The levels/effects of Lansoprazole may be increased by: Clopidogrel; Fluconazole; Ketoconazole; Ketoconazole (Systemic)

Decreased Effect
Lansoprazole may decrease the levels/effects of: Atazanavir; Cefditoren; Clopidogrel; Dabigatran Etexilate; Dasatinib; Delavirdine; Erlotinib; Indinavir; Iron Salts; Itraconazole; Ketoconazole; Ketoconazole (Systemic); Mesalamine; Mycophenolate; Nelfinavir; Posaconazole

The levels/effects of Lansoprazole may be decreased by: CYP2C19 Inducers (Strong); CYP3A4 Inducers (Strong); Deferasirox; Herbs (CYP3A4 Inducers); Tipranavir

Food Interactions Food decreases lansoprazole's bioavailability by 50%

Stability Store at room temperature; protect from light and moisture

Mechanism of Action Suppresses gastric acid secretion by selectively inhibiting the parietal cell membrane enzyme (H+, K+)-ATPase or proton pump; demonstrates antimicrobial activity against *Helicobacter pylori*

Pharmacodynamics
Duration of antisecretory activity: ≥24 hours
Relief of symptoms:
Gastric or duodenal ulcers: 1 week
Reflux esophagitis: 1-4 weeks
Ulcer healing:
Duodenal: 2 weeks
Gastric: 4 weeks

Pharmacokinetics (Adult data unless noted)
Absorption: Extremely acid labile and will degrade in acid pH of stomach; enteric coated granules improve bioavailability (80%)
Distribution: V_d:
Children: 0.61-0.9 L/kg
Adults: 15.7 ± 1.9 L

Protein binding: 97%

Metabolism: Extensive by the liver to inactive metabolites; in acid media of gastric parietal cell, lansoprazole is transformed to active sulfanilamide metabolite

Bioavailability: 80% (reduced by 50% if given 30 minutes after food)

Half-life:

Children: 1.2-1.5 hours

Adults: 1.3-1.7 hours

Time to peak serum concentration: 1.7 hours

Elimination: 14% to 25% in urine as metabolites; <1% as unchanged drug; biliary excretion is major route of elimination

Clearance:

Children: 0.57-0.71 L/hour/kg

Adults: 11.1 ± 3.8 L/hour

Adults: Hepatic impairment: 3.2-7.2 hours

Usual Dosage

Infants ≥3 months: One study of 68 patients suggests that 7.5 mg twice daily or 15 mg once daily provides better symptom relief compared to dietary management (Khoshoo, 2008). Pharmacokinetics studies have used a dosage range of 1-2 mg/kg/day (Springer, 2008; Zhang, 2008). **Note:** Treatment of GERD in children <12 months is controversial as a recent clinical trial did not demonstrate efficacy in this age group (Orenstein, 2009).

Children 1-11 years: GERD and erosive esophagitis:

≤30 kg: 15 mg once daily for up to 12 weeks

>30 kg: 30 mg once daily for up to 12 weeks

Children ≥12 years and Adults:

Duodenal ulcer: Oral: 15 mg once daily for 4 weeks; maintenance therapy: 15 mg once daily

Primary gastric ulcer (and also associated with NSAID use): Oral: 30 mg once daily for up to 8 weeks

Erosive esophagitis: Oral: 30 mg once daily for up to 8 weeks; additional 8 weeks may be tried in those patients who failed to respond or for a recurrence of esophagitis; maintenance: 15 mg once daily

GERD: Oral: 15 mg once daily for up to 8 weeks

Pathological hypersecretory conditions: Oral: Initial: 60 mg once daily; adjust dosage based upon patient response; doses of 90 mg twice daily have been used; administer doses >120 mg/day in divided doses

Reflux esophagitis: Oral: 30-60 mg once daily for 8 weeks

Helicobacter pylori-associated antral gastritis: Oral: 30 mg twice daily for 2 weeks (in combination with 1 g amoxicillin and 500 mg clarithromycin given twice daily for 14 days). Alternatively, in patients allergic to or intolerant of clarithromycin or in whom resistance to clarithromycin is known or suspected, lansoprazole 30 mg every 8 hours and amoxicillin 1 g every 8 hours may be given for 2 weeks

NSAID-associated gastric ulcer: Oral:

Healing: 30 mg once daily for up to 8 weeks

Prevention: 15 mg once daily for up to 12 weeks

Adults: Heartburn: OTC labeling: Oral: 15 mg once daily for 14 days; may repeat 14 days of therapy every 4 months. Do not take for >14 days or more often than every 4 months, unless instructed by healthcare provider.

Dosage adjustment in hepatic impairment: Reduce dosage for severe impairment

Administration Oral: Administer before eating

Capsules: Capsules may be opened and mixed with small amount of applesauce prior to administration without affecting the bioavailability; do not chew or crush granules; for nasogastric tube administration, the capsules can be opened, the granules mixed with 40 mL of apple, cranberry, grape, orange, pineapple, prune, tomato, and V-8® vegetable juice, and then administered through the NG tube; granules remain intact when mixed and stored for up to 30 minutes

Tablet, orally-disintegrating: Place the tablet on the tongue and allow to disintegrate with or without water until the particles can be swallowed; do not chew or crush

Monitoring Parameters Patients with Zollinger-Ellison syndrome should be monitored for gastric acid output, which should be maintained at 10 mEq/hour or less during the last hour before the next lansoprazole dose; lab monitoring should include CBC, liver function, renal function, and serum gastrin levels

Reference Range Plasma levels do not correlate with pharmacologic activity

Patient Information May cause dry mouth

Dosage Forms Excipient information presented when available (limited, particularly for generics); consult specific product labeling. [DSC] = Discontinued product

Capsule, delayed release: 15 mg, 30 mg

Prevacid®: 15 mg, 30 mg

Prevacid® 24 HR: 15 mg

Tablet, delayed release, orally disintegrating:

Prevacid® SoluTab™: 15 mg [contains phenylalanine 2.5 mg; strawberry flavor]; 30 mg [contains phenyl-alanine 5.1 mg; strawberry flavor]

Extemporaneous Preparations A 3 mg/mL suspension of lansoprazole is prepared by emptying the contents of ten 30 mg capsules and adding 100 mL 8.4% sodium bicarbonate solution; stir for 30 minutes; protect from light; stable for 8 hours at room temperature and for 14 days refrigerated (DiGiacinto, 2000). **Note:** The same formulation was studied by Phillips, et al. A 2-week stability at room temperature and 4-week stability under refrigeration were reported.

DiGiacinto JL, Olsen KM, Bergman KL, et al, "Stability of Suspension Formulations of Lansoprazole and Omeprazole Stored in Amber-Colored Plastic Oral Syringes," *Ann Pharmacother*, 2000, 34(5):600-4.

Phillips JO, Metzler MH, and Olsen K, "The Stability of SImplified Lansoprazole Suspension (SLS)," *Gastroen*, 1999, 116:A89.

References

Canani RB, Cirillo P, Roggero P, et al, "Therapy With Gastric Acidity Inhibitors Increases the Risk of Acute Gastroenteritis and Community-Acquired Pneumonia in Children," *Pediatrics*, 2006, 117(5):e817-20.

Chun AH, Eason CJ, Shi HH, et al, "Lansoprazole: An Alternative Method of Administration of a Capsule Dosage Formulation," *Clin Ther*, 1995, 17(3):441-7.

Gibbons TE and Gold BD, "The Use of Proton Pump Inhibitors in Children: A Comprehensive Review," *Paediatr Drugs*, 2003, 5 (1):25-40.

Khoshoo V and Dhume P, "Clinical Response to 2 Dosing Regimens of Lansoprazole in Infants With Gastroesophageal Reflux," *J Pediatr Gastroenterol Nutr*, 2008, 46(3):352-4.

Oderda G, Chiorboli E, Haitink AR, "Inhibition of Gastric Acidity in Children by Lansoprazole Granules," *Gastroent*, 1998, 114(4pt2): A295.

Orenstein SR, Hassall E, Furmaga-Jablonska W, et al, "Multicenter, Double-Blind, Randomized, Placebo-Controlled Trial Assessing the Efficacy and Safety of Proton Pump Inhibitor Lansoprazole in Infants With Symptoms of Gastroesophageal Reflux Disease," *J Pediatr*, 2009, 154(4):514-520.

Scott LJ, "Lansoprazole: In the Management of Gastroesophageal Reflux Disease in Children," *Paediatr Drugs*, 2003, 5(1):57-61.

Springer M, Atkinson S, North J, et al, "Safety and Pharmacodynamics of Lansoprazole in Patients With Gastroesophageal Reflux Disease Aged <1 Year," *Paediatr Drugs*, 2008, 10(4):255-63.

Tran A, et al, "Pharmacokinetics/Pharmacodynamics Study of Oral Lansoprazole in Children," *Fundam Clin Pharmacol*, 1996, 10:A221.

Zhang W, Kukulka M, Witt G, et al, "Age-Dependent Pharmacokinetics of Lansoprazole in Neonates and Infants," *Paediatr Drugs*, 2008, 10 (4):265-74.

◆ **Lantus®** *see* Insulin Glargine *on page 741*

◆ **Lantus® OptiSet® (Can)** *see* Insulin Glargine *on page 741*

◆ **Lanvis® (Can)** *see* Thioguanine *on page 1339*

◆ **Lapase [DSC]** *see* Pancreatin *on page 1050*

◆ **Largactil® (Can)** *see* ChlorproMAZINE *on page 298*

◆ **L-Arginine** *see* Arginine *on page 131*

◆ **L-Arginine Hydrochloride** *see* Arginine *on page 131*

◆ **Lariam® [DSC]** *see* Mefloquine *on page 872*

◆ **Lariam® (Can)** *see* Mefloquine *on page 872*

Laronidase (lair OH ni days)

U.S. Brand Names Aldurazyme®

Canadian Brand Names Aldurazyme®

Therapeutic Category Enzyme; Mucopolysaccharidosis I (MPS I) Disease, Treatment Agent

Generic Available No

Use Treatment of patients with mucopolysaccharidosis I (MPS I) lysosomal storage disease who have one of the following clinical syndromes: Hurler's syndrome (severe), Hurler-Scheie syndrome (intermediate), or patients with the Scheie form who have moderate to severe symptoms

Pregnancy Risk Factor B

Pregnancy Considerations Teratogenic effects were not observed in animal studies; however, there are no adequate and well-controlled studies in pregnant women. Use during pregnancy only if clearly needed. Patients are encouraged to enroll in the MPS I registry.

Lactation Excretion in breast milk unknown/use caution

Breast-Feeding Considerations Patients are encouraged to enroll in the MPS I registry.

Contraindications Hypersensitivity to laronidase or any component

Warnings Hypersensitivity reactions can occur at any time during laronidase therapy. Resuscitation equipment, oxygen, diphenhydramine, and a corticosteroid should be readily available to treat hypersensitivity or anaphylactic reactions. Use epinephrine with caution in patients with MPS I due to an increased prevalence of coronary artery disease in these patients.

Precautions The risks and benefits of administering laronidase following a severe anaphylactic or hypersensitivity reaction should be considered. If laronidase is to be readministered, use caution and have appropriate resuscitation measures available.

Adverse Reactions

Cardiovascular: Flushing, chest pain, edema, hypotension

Central nervous system: Chills, fever, headache

Dermatologic: Rash, urticaria, pruritus, angioedema

Hematologic: Thrombocytopenia

Local: Injection site reaction

Neuromuscular & skeletal: Hyper-reflexia, paresthesia

Respiratory: Dyspnea, cough, bronchospasm

Miscellaneous: Anaphylaxis, antibodies to laronidase

Drug Interactions

Avoid Concomitant Use There are no known interactions where it is recommended to avoid concomitant use.

Increased Effect/Toxicity There are no known significant interactions involving an increase in effect.

Decreased Effect There are no known significant interactions involving a decrease in effect.

Stability Store vials in refrigerator at 2°C to 8°C (36°F to 46°F). Do not freeze or shake. Diluted infusion solution is stable for up to 32 hours when stored at 2°C to 8°C (36°F to 46°F). Do not mix laronidase with any other drugs.

Mechanism of Action MPS I is a mucopolysaccharide storage disorder caused by a deficiency of the lysosomal enzyme, α-L-iduronidase which is required for the catabolism of glycosaminoglycans (GAG). Laronidase catalyses the hydrolysis of terminal α-L-iduronic acid residues of dermatan sulfate and heparan sulfate decreasing the accumulation of GAG substrates.

Pharmacokinetics (Adult data unless noted)

Distribution: V_d: 0.24 to 0.6 L/kg

Half-life: 1.5-3.6 hours

Clearance: Plasma: 1.7 to 2.7 mL/minute/kg

Usual Dosage Children, Adolescents, and Adults: I.V. infusion:

Patients ≤20 kg: 0.58 mg/kg/dose once weekly. Dose is delivered in a total volume of 100 mL.

Patients >20 kg: 0.58 mg/kg/dose once weekly. Dose is delivered in a total volume of 250 mL.

Administration I.V. infusion:

Determine the number of vials to be diluted. Remove vials from the refrigerator and allow them to reach room temperature. Do not use if the solution is discolored or contains particulate matter. Determine the total infusion volume based on the patient's weight (dose delivered in a total volume of 100 mL or 250 mL); prepare an infusion bag of 0.1% albumin in NS; gently rotate infusion bag after addition of albumin.

Remove and discard volume of 0.1% albumin in NS equal to volume of laronidase injection solution to be added to the infusion bag. Add laronidase; do not agitate solution as it denatures the enzyme. Administer with an in-line, low protein binding 0.2 micron filter.

An initial 10 mcg/kg/hour infusion rate may be incrementally increased every 15 minutes during the first hour if tolerated; increase to a maximum infusion rate of 200 mcg/kg/hour which is maintained for the remainder of the infusion (approximately 3 hours). See the following:

Initial infusion rate: 10 mcg/kg/hour for 15 minutes: If stable, increase rate to:

20 mcg/kg/hour for 15 minutes: If stable, increase rate to:

50 mcg/kg/hour for 15 minutes: If stable, increase rate to:

100 mcg/kg/hour for 15 minutes: If stable, increase rate to:

200 mcg/kg/hour for ~3 hours (remainder of the infusion)

Monitoring Parameters Vital signs, FVC, height, weight, range of motion, serum antibodies to α-L-iduronidase, urine levels of glycosaminoglycans (GAG), change in liver size

Nursing Implications Premedication with acetaminophen and/or diphenhydramine should be administered 30-60 minutes prior to starting infusion. If an infusion reaction occurs, decrease the infusion rate, temporarily stop the infusion, and/or administer antipyretics, antihistamines, and/or steroids

Dosage Forms Excipient information presented when available (limited, particularly for generics); consult specific product labeling.

Injection, solution [preservative free]:

Aldurazyme®: 2.9 mg/5 mL (5 mL) [contains polysorbate 80; derived from Chinese hamster cells]

References

Kakkis ED, Muenzer J, Tiller GE, et al, "Enzyme-Replacement Therapy in Mucopolysaccharidosis I," *N Engl J Med*, 2001, 344(3):182-8.

◆ **Lasix®** *see* Furosemide *on page 632*

◆ **Lasix® Special (Can)** *see* Furosemide *on page 632*

◆ **LASP** *see* Asparaginase *on page 139*

◆ **L-asparaginase** *see* Asparaginase *on page 139*

◆ **L-asparaginase with Polyethylene Glycol** *see* Pegaspargase *on page 1068*

◆ **Lassar's Zinc Paste** *see* Zinc Oxide *on page 1445*

◆ *Latrodectus* **Antivenin** *see* Antivenin (*Latrodectus mactans*) *on page 121*

◆ *Latrodectus mactans* **Antivenin** *see* Antivenin (*Latrodectus mactans*) *on page 121*

◆ **Lavacol® [OTC]** *see* Ethyl Alcohol *on page 547*

◆ **Laxilose (Can)** *see* Lactulose *on page 791*

◆ *l*-**Bunolol Hydrochloride** *see* Levobunolol *on page 811*

◆ **L-Carnitine** *see* Carnitine *on page 253*

◆ **L-Carnitine® [OTC]** *see* Carnitine *on page 253*

◆ **LCD** *see* Coal Tar *on page 349*

◆ **Lepargylic Acid** *see* Azelaic Acid *on page 162*

◆ **Lescol®** *see* Fluvastatin *on page 614*

◆ **Lescol® XL** *see* Fluvastatin *on page 614*

◆ **Leucovorin** *see* Leucovorin Calcium *on page 804*

Leucovorin Calcium (loo koe VOR in KAL see um)

Medication Safety Issues
Sound-alike/look-alike issues:

Leucovorin may be confused with Leukeran®, Leukine®, LEVOleucovorin

Folinic acid may be confused with folic acid

Folinic acid is an error prone synonym and should not be used

Related Information
Compatibility of Chemotherapy and Related Supportive Care Medications *on page 1580*

Therapeutic Category Antidote, Methotrexate; Folic Acid Derivative

Generic Available Yes

Use Reduction of toxic effects of high dose methotrexate ("leucovorin rescue"); to diminish the toxicity and counteract the effects of impaired methotrexate elimination or as an antidote for folic acid antagonist overdosage; treatment of folate deficient megaloblastic anemias of infancy, sprue, or pregnancy; nutritional deficiency when oral folate therapy is not possible; adjunctive treatment with sulfadiazine and pyrimethamine to prevent hematologic toxicity; combined with fluorouracil to prolong survival in the palliative treatment of patients with advanced colorectal cancer

Pregnancy Risk Factor C

Pregnancy Considerations Animal reproduction studies have not been conducted. Leucovorin is a biologically active form of folic acid. Adequate amounts of folic acid are recommended during pregnancy. Refer to Folic Acid monograph.

Lactation Excretion in breast milk unknown/use caution

Breast-Feeding Considerations Leucovorin is a biologically active form of folic acid. Adequate amounts of folic acid are recommended in breast-feeding women. Refer to Folic Acid monograph.

Contraindications Hypersensitivity to leucovorin or any component; pernicious anemia and other megaloblastic anemias secondary to the lack of vitamin B_{12}; not to be administered by intrathecal or intraventricular route (may be harmful or fatal)

Warnings Administer promptly; when the time interval between administration of folic acid antagonists and leucovorin rescue increases, its effectiveness in treatment of toxicity diminishes. In the treatment of accidental overdosages of intrathecally administered folic acid antagonists, do not administer leucovorin intrathecally as it **may be harmful or fatal if administered intrathecally**. Leucovorin enhances the toxicity of fluorouracil; when used in combination, the dosage of fluorouracil should be reduced. Combination therapy should not be initiated or continued in patients who have symptoms of GI toxicity of any severity until the symptoms have resolved; rapid clinical deterioration including death may occur; monitor combination use closely. Concomitant use with trimethoprim/sulfamethoxazole for the acute treatment of *Pneumocystis jiroveci* pneumonia in patients with HIV infection as been associated with increased rates of treatment failure and morbidity.

Precautions Parenteral therapy is recommended over oral therapy in cases where the patient is unable to tolerate oral treatment due to vomiting. Due to saturation of oral absorption with oral doses >25 mg, I.V. administration is recommended for doses >25 mg. Methotrexate serum levels should be monitored closely to determine the dose and duration of leucovorin rescue. Leucovorin doses may be increased, frequencies of administration altered, and duration of therapy increased depending upon the methotrexate clearance. Ascites, pleural effusion, renal insufficiency, and inadequate hydration may prolong methotrexate clearance. Refer to individual protocols or "Leucovorin Rescue Dose" graph on next page for leucovorin dosage adjustment recommendations.

Adverse Reactions
Dermatologic: Rash, pruritus, erythema, urticaria

Hematologic: Thrombocytosis

Respiratory: Wheezing

Miscellaneous: Hypersensitivity including anaphylactoid reactions

Drug Interactions
Avoid Concomitant Use
Avoid concomitant use of Leucovorin Calcium with any of the following: Raltitrexed

Increased Effect/Toxicity
Leucovorin Calcium may increase the levels/effects of: Capecitabine; Fluorouracil; Fluorouracil (Systemic); Fluorouracil (Topical)

Decreased Effect
Leucovorin Calcium may decrease the levels/effects of: PHENobarbital; Phenytoin; Primidone; Raltitrexed; Trimethoprim

Stability When powder for injection is reconstituted with bacteriostatic SWI, stability is 7 days at room temperature; protect from light; when doses >10 mg/m^2 are used, prepare leucovorin with preservative free SWI to decrease the amount of benzyl alcohol intake; do not mix in the same solution with 5-fluorouracil as precipitation occurs

Mechanism of Action A derivative of tetrahydrofolic acid, a reduced form of folic acid; does not require a reduction by dihydrofolate reductase for activation; allows for purine and thymidine synthesis, a necessity for normal erythropoiesis; leucovorin supplies the necessary cofactor blocked by methotrexate, enters the cells via the same active transport system as methotrexate

Pharmacodynamics Onset of action:

Oral: Within 30 minutes

I.V.: Within 5 minutes

Pharmacokinetics (Adult data unless noted)
Absorption: Oral, I.M.: Rapid

Metabolism: Rapidly converted to (5MTHF) 5-methyltetrahydrofolate (active) in the intestinal mucosa and by the liver

Bioavailability:

Oral absorption is saturable in doses >25 mg; apparent bioavailability:

Tablet, 25 mg: 97%

Tablet, 50 mg: 75%

Tablet, 100 mg: 37%

Tablet, 200 mg: 31%

Injection solution, when administered orally, provides equivalent bioavailability

Half-life: Adults: ~4-8 hours

Time to peak serum concentration:

Oral: ~2 hours

I.V. total folates: 10 minutes

5MTHF: ~1 hour

Elimination: Primarily in urine (80% to 90%) with small losses appearing in feces (5% to 8%)

Usual Dosage Children and Adults:

Treatment of folic acid antagonist overdosage (eg, pyrimethamine, trimethoprim): Oral: 5-15 mg/day for 3 days or until blood counts are normal or 5 mg every 3 days; doses of 6 mg/day are needed for patients with platelet counts <100,000/mm^3

Folate deficient megaloblastic anemia: I.M.: ≤1 mg/day

Megaloblastic anemia secondary to congenital deficiency of dihydrofolate reductase: I.M.: 3-6 mg/day

Leucovorin rescue (following methotrexate dosing of 12-15 g/m^2): I.V.: 10 mg/m^2 (15 mg in adults) to start, then 10 mg/m^2 (15 mg in adults) every 6 hours orally for 72 hours; if serum creatinine 24 hours after methotrexate administration is elevated ≥50% **or** the serum methotrexate concentration is >5 x 10^{-6} M, increase leucovorin dose to 100 mg/m^2/dose (150 mg in adults) every 3 hours until serum methotrexate level is less than 1 x 10^{-8} M (see graph for further dosing recommendations as a function of plasma methotrexate level vs time); if methotrexate clearance is delayed, continue leucovorin therapy until methotrexate level is 0.05 x 10^{-8} M

LEUCOVORIN RESCUE DOSE

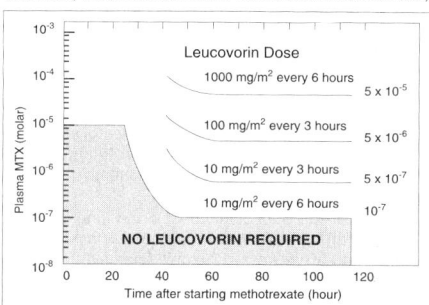

Adjunctive treatment with sulfadiazine to prevent hematologic toxicity (for toxoplasmosis): Infants, Children, and Adults: Oral, I.V.: 5-10 mg once daily; repeat every 3 days (see Sulfadiazine on page 1300)

Adjunctive treatment with pyrimethamine to prevent hematologic toxicity (*Pneumocystis jiroveci*): Adolescents and Adults: Oral, I.V.: 25 mg once weekly

Colorectal cancer: Adults: I.V.: 200 mg/m^2 in combination with fluorouracil 370 mg/m^2 or 20 mg/m^2 used in combination with fluorouracil 425 mg/m^2; treatment is daily for 5 days and repeated at 4-5 week intervals; refer to individual protocols

Investigational: Post I.T. methotrexate: Oral, I.V.: 12 mg/m^2 as a single dose; post high-dose methotrexate: 100-1000 mg/m^2/dose until the serum methotrexate level is less than 1 x 10^{-7} molar

Administration

Oral: **This drug should be given parenterally instead of orally in patients with GI toxicity, nausea, vomiting, and when individual doses are >25 mg.**

Parenteral: I.M., I.V.: Reconstitute 50 mg or 100 mg powder for injection vials with 5-10 mL SWI (350 mg vial requires 17 mL diluent resulting in 20 mg/mL final concentration); for I.V. administration, infuse at a maximum rate of 160 mg/minute; **not for intrathecal or intraventricular administration.**

Monitoring Parameters Leucovorin rescue: CBC with differential; plasma methotrexate levels, serum creatinine. Leucovorin is continued until the plasma methotrexate level is less than 1 x 10^{-7} molar or <0.5 x 10^{-7} molar in situations of delayed methotrexate clearance. Each dose

of leucovorin is increased if the plasma methotrexate concentration is excessively high. With 4- to 6-hour high-dose methotrexate infusions, plasma drug values in excess of 5 x 10^{-5} and 10^{-6} molar at 24 and 48 hours after starting the infusion, respectively, are often predictive of delayed methotrexate clearance; see leucovorin rescue dose graph.

When used with fluorouracil: CBC with differential, platelets, LFTs, electrolytes

Dosage Forms Excipient information presented when available (limited, particularly for generics); consult specific product labeling. **Note:** Strength expressed as base

Injection, powder for reconstitution: 50 mg, 100 mg, 200 mg, 350 mg

Injection, solution [preservative free]: 10 mg/mL (50 mL)

Tablet: 5 mg, 10 mg, 15 mg, 25 mg

◆ **Leukeran®** *see* Chlorambucil *on page* 287

◆ **Leukine®** *see* Sargramostim *on page* 1247

Leuprolide (loo PROE lide)

Medication Safety Issues
Sound-alike/look-alike issues:
Lupron® may be confused with Nuprin®
Lupron Depot®-3 Month may be confused with Lupron Depot-Ped®

U.S. Brand Names Eligard®; Lupron Depot-Ped®; Lupron Depot®; Lupron®

Canadian Brand Names Eligard®; Lupron®; Lupron® Depot®

Therapeutic Category Antineoplastic Agent, Hormone (Gonadotropin Hormone-Releasing Analog); Luteinizing Hormone-Releasing Hormone Analog

Generic Available Yes: Injection (solution)

Use Treatment of precocious puberty (FDA approved in females ages <8 years and males ages <9 years); palliative treatment of advanced prostate carcinoma (FDA approved in adults); treatment of anemia caused by uterine leiomyomata (fibroids) (FDA approved in adults); management of endometriosis (FDA approved in adults); has also been used in the treatment of breast cancer, infertility

Pregnancy Risk Factor X

Pregnancy Considerations Pregnancy must be excluded prior to the start of treatment. Although leuprolide usually inhibits ovulation and stops menstruation, contraception is not ensured and a nonhormonal contraceptive should be used. Fetal abnormalities and increased fetal mortality have been noted in animal studies.

Lactation Excretion in breast milk unknown/contraindicated

Contraindications Hypersensitivity to leuprolide, gonadotropin-releasing hormone (GnRH), GnRH agonist analogs, or any component (see Warnings); pernicious anemia; pregnancy, breast-feeding. Eligard® 45 mg is contraindicated in women and in pediatric patients.

Warnings Hazardous agent; use appropriate precautions for handling and disposal; gonadotropin-releasing hormone (GnRH) analog treatment of rodents has shown an increased incidence of pituitary tumors; urinary tract obstruction, bone pain, neuropathy, hematuria, or spinal cord compression may occur upon initiation of therapy. Decreased bone density has been reported and may not be reversible. Leuprolide may cause spontaneous abortion or fetal harm when administered to a pregnant woman.

Leuprolide injection for subcutaneous use contains benzyl alcohol which may cause allergic reactions in susceptible individuals; large amounts of benzyl alcohol (≥99 mg/kg/day) have been associated with a potentially fatal toxicity ("gasping syndrome") in neonates; avoid use of leuprolide products containing benzyl alcohol in neonates; *in vitro* and animal studies have shown that benzoate, a metabolite of benzyl alcohol, displaces bilirubin from protein binding sites

Precautions Use with caution in patients with risk factors for decreased bone mineral density (BMD) (ie, chronic alcohol or tobacco use, strong family history of osteoporosis, or chronic use of medications that can impact BMD, such as corticosteroids or anticonvulsants).

Adverse Reactions

Cardiovascular: Cardiac arrhythmias, edema, hypertension, hypotension

Central nervous system: Depression, dizziness, emotional lability, headache, insomnia, lethargy, memory disorders, pain

Dermatologic: Acne, pruritus, rash

Endocrine & metabolic: Estrogenic effects (breast tenderness, gynecomastia), hot flashes, hyperglycemia

Gastrointestinal: Anorexia, constipation, diarrhea, GI bleeding, nausea, vomiting

Genitourinary: Urinary frequency, vaginitis

Hematologic: Hemoglobin and hematocrit decreased

Neuromuscular & skeletal: Arthralgia, bone density decreased, bone pain, myalgia, neuropathy, paresthesia, weakness

Ocular: Blurred vision

Renal: BUN increased, hematuria

Miscellaneous: Anaphylaxis, diaphoresis

<1%, postmarketing and/or case reports: Asthmatic reactions; fibromyalgia-like symptoms (arthralgia/myalgia, headaches, GI distress); hemoptysis, hepatic dysfunction, hypokalemia, hypoproteinemia, injection site induration/abscess, MI, pelvic fibrosis, penile swelling, photosensitivity; pituitary apoplexy (cardiovascular collapse, mental status altered, ophthalmoplegia, sudden headache, visual changes, vomiting); prostate pain, pulmonary embolism, pulmonary infiltrate, spinal fracture/paralysis, stroke, tenosynovitis-like symptoms, thrombocytopenia, transient ischemia attack, uric acid increased, urticaria, WBC increased

Drug Interactions

Avoid Concomitant Use There are no known interactions where it is recommended to avoid concomitant use.

Increased Effect/Toxicity There are no known significant interactions involving an increase in effect.

Decreased Effect

Leuprolide may decrease the levels/effects of: Antidiabetic Agents

Stability Refrigerate leuprolide acetate injection; leuprolide (Depot®) powder for suspension and its diluent may be stored at room temperature; upon reconstitution, the suspension is stable for 24 hours; protect from light and heat; do not freeze vials; leuprolide implant may be stored at room temperature

Mechanism of Action Continuous daily administration results in suppression of ovarian and testicular steroidogenesis due to decreased levels of LH and FSH so that puberty and the pubertal growth spurt are arrested; produces a "medical castration" in prostate cancer patients; inhibits pituitary gonadotropin secretion

Pharmacodynamics Onset of action: Serum testosterone levels first increase within 3 days of therapy, then decrease after 2-4 weeks with continued therapy

Pharmacokinetics (Adult data unless noted)

Absorption: Requires parenteral administration since it is rapidly destroyed within the GI tract

Protein binding: 43% to 49%

Bioavailability:
  Oral: 0%
  SubQ: 94%
Half-life: 3 hours
Elimination: Not well defined

Usual Dosage Refer to individual protocol

Children: Precocious puberty:
  I.M. (Depot®) formulation: 0.15-0.3 mg/kg/dose given every 28 days; minimum dose: 7.5 mg; younger children generally require higher dosages on a mg/kg basis than older children. Consider discontinuing leuprolide therapy in girls by age 11 and boys by age 12.
  Initial dose for girls <8 years or boys <9 years (titrate dose in 3.75 mg increments every 4 weeks until clinical or laboratory tests indicate no disease progression):
    <25 kg: 7.5 mg every 4 weeks
    25-37.5 kg: 11.25 mg every 4 weeks
    >37.5 kg: 15 mg every 4 weeks
  SubQ: 35-50 mcg/kg once daily; may titrate dose upward by 10 mcg/kg/day if suppression of ovarian or testicular steroidogenesis is not achieved.

Adults: Advanced prostatic carcinoma:
  I.M. (Depot® formulation): 7.5 mg/dose given monthly, **or** 22.5 mg once every 3 months, **or** 30 mg once every 4 months
  Implant: Insert 65 mg implant subcutaneously every 12 months
  SubQ: 1 mg/day
  SubQ (Eligard™ Depot): 7.5 mg/dose given monthly, **or** 22.5 mg once every 3 months, **or** 30 mg once every 4 months, **or** 45 mg once every 6 months

Administration

Implant: Insert subcutaneously in the inner aspect of the upper arm. Keep site clean and dry for 24 hours after insertion. Remove at 12-month intervals.

Parenteral: Do not administer I.V.:
  Eligard®: Packaged in 2 syringes whose contents are mixed immediately prior to administration; one contains the Atrigel polymer system, and the second contains leuprolide acetate powder. Must be administered within 30 minutes of mixing. Injection site should be rotated periodically.
  Lupron Depot®: I.M.: Diluent is added to the vial to form a milky suspension; reconstitute only with diluent provided. Do not use needles smaller than 22 gauge.
  Lupron®: SubQ: 5 mg/mL solution is administered undiluted into areas on the arm, thigh, or abdomen

Monitoring Parameters Precocious puberty: Height, weight, bone age, Tanner staging test, GnRH testing (blood LH and FSH levels), testosterone in males and estradiol in females; closely monitor patients with prostatic carcinoma for plasma testosterone, acid phosphatase, and signs of weakness, paresthesias, and urinary tract obstruction during the first few weeks of therapy

Test Interactions Interferes with diagnostic tests of pituitary gonadotropic and gonadal function for up to 3 months after therapy

Patient Information Female patients should be informed that menstruation or spotting may occur for the first 2 months of therapy; notify physician if vaginal bleeding continues after 2 months of drug therapy

Nursing Implications Rotate SubQ and I.M. injection sites periodically

Dosage Forms Excipient information presented when available (limited, particularly for generics); consult specific product labeling. [DSC] = Discontinued product

Injection, solution, as acetate: 5 mg/mL (2.8 mL)
  Lupron®: 5 mg/mL (2.8 mL) [contains benzyl alcohol]
  Lupron®: 5 mg/mL (2.8 mL) [contains benzyl alcohol; packaged with syringes and alcohol swabs] [DSC]

Injection, powder for reconstitution, as acetate [depot formulation]:

Eligard®:

7.5 mg [released over 1 month; contains polylactide-co-glycolide]

22.5 mg [released over 3 months; contains polylactide-co-glycolide]

30 mg [released over 4 months; contains polylactide-co-glycolide]

45 mg [released over 6 months; contains polylactide-co-glycolide]

Lupron Depot®: 3.75 mg, 7.5 mg [released over 1 month; contains polysorbate 80, polylactide-co-glycolide]

Lupron Depot®-3 Month: 11.25 mg, 22.5 mg [released over 3 months; contains polysorbate 80, polylactide-co-glycolide]

Lupron Depot®-4 Month: 30 mg [released over 4 months; contains polysorbate 80, polylactide-co-glycolide]

Lupron Depot-Ped®: 7.5 mg, 11.25 mg, 15 mg [released over 1 month; contains polysorbate 80, polylactide-co-glycolide]

References

Kappy MS, Stuart T, and Perelman A, "Efficacy of Leuprolide Therapy in Children With Central Precocious Puberty," *Am J Dis Child*, 1988, 142 (10):1061-4.

Lee PA and Page JG, "Effects of Leuprolide in the Treatment of Central Precocious Puberty," *J Pediatr*, 1989, 114(2):321-4.

♦ **Leuprolide Acetate** *see* Leuprolide *on page* 805

♦ **Leuprorelin Acetate** *see* Leuprolide *on page* 805

♦ **Leurocristine Sulfate** *see* VinCRIStine *on page* 1425

♦ **Leustatin®** *see* Cladribine *on page* 323

Levalbuterol (leve al BYOO ter ole)

Medication Safety Issues

Sound-alike/look-alike issues:

Xopenex® may be confused with Xanax®

U.S. Brand Names Xopenex HFA™; Xopenex®

Canadian Brand Names Xopenex®

Therapeutic Category Adrenergic Agonist Agent; Anti-asthmatic; Beta$_2$-Adrenergic Agonist Agent; Bronchodilator; Sympathomimetic

Generic Available Yes: Excludes aerosol

Use Treatment and prevention of bronchospasm in patients with reversible obstructive airway disease

Pregnancy Risk Factor C

Pregnancy Considerations Teratogenic effects were not observed in animal studies; however, racemic albuterol was teratogenic in some species. There are no adequate and well-controlled studies in pregnant women. This drug should be used during pregnancy only if benefit exceeds risk. Use caution if needed for bronchospasm during labor and delivery; has potential to interfere with uterine contractions.

Lactation Excretion in breast milk unknown/use caution

Breast-Feeding Considerations It is not known whether levalbuterol is excreted in human milk. Plasma levels following oral inhalation are low. Racemic albuterol was shown to be tumorigenic in animal studies.

Contraindications Hypersensitivity to levalbuterol, any component, albuterol, or adrenergic amine

Warnings Paradoxical bronchospasm may occur, especially with the first use. Excessive use of inhaled sympathomimetics has been associated with death possibly due to cardiac arrest. Increasing use (>2 days/week) for symptom relief generally indicates inadequate control of asthma and the need for initiating or intensifying anti-inflammatory treatment. Regularly scheduled, daily, chronic use of short-acting beta agonists (eg, levalbuterol) is not recommended (NAEPP, 2007).

Precautions Use with caution in patients with hyperthyroidism, hypokalemia, diabetes mellitus, cardiovascular disorders including coronary insufficiency, hypertension, or history of cardiac arrhythmias; excessive or prolonged use can lead to tolerance

Adverse Reactions

Cardiovascular: Tachycardia, hypertension, hypotension, syncope, ECG abnormalities, chest pain, angioedema, arrhythmias

Central nervous system: Nervousness, dizziness, anxiety, headache, insomnia

Dermatologic: Rash, urticaria

Endocrine & metabolic: Hyperglycemia, hypokalemia, dysmenorrhea

Gastrointestinal: Dyspepsia, diarrhea, xerostomia, dry throat, gastroenteritis, nausea, pharyngitis, constipation

Genitourinary: Hematuria, vaginal moniliasis

Neuromuscular & skeletal: Leg cramps, pain, tremor

Ocular: Eye itching, conjunctivitis

Otic: Ear pain

Respiratory: Cough, rhinitis, sinusitis, turbinate edema, paradoxical bronchospasm, dyspnea

Miscellaneous: Hypersensitivity reactions, flu-like syndrome

Drug Interactions

Avoid Concomitant Use

Avoid concomitant use of Levalbuterol with any of the following: Iobenguane I 123

Increased Effect/Toxicity

Levalbuterol may increase the levels/effects of: Sympathomimetics

The levels/effects of Levalbuterol may be increased by: Atomoxetine; Cannabinoids; MAO Inhibitors; Tricyclic Antidepressants

Decreased Effect

Levalbuterol may decrease the levels/effects of: Iobenguane I 123

The levels/effects of Levalbuterol may be decreased by: Alpha-/Beta-Blockers; Beta-Blockers (Beta1 Selective); Beta-Blockers (Nonselective); Betahistine

Food Interactions Caffeinated beverages may increase side effects of levalbuterol

Stability Store all formulations at room temperature; protect from light; discard nebulized solution if it is not colorless; after the foil covering is opened, use within 2 weeks; if removed from the foil pouch, use within 1 week; vials of concentrated solution should be used immediately after removing from foil pouch; store aerosol with mouthpiece up; discard after 200 actuations

Mechanism of Action R-enantiomer of racemic albuterol; relaxes bronchial smooth muscle by action on beta$_2$-receptors with little effect on heart rate

Pharmacodynamics

Onset of action: Nebulized: 10-17 minutes; aerosol: 5.5-10 minutes

Maximum effect: Nebulized: 1.5 hours; aerosol: 77 minutes

Duration: Nebulized: 5-6 hours; aerosol: 3-6 hours

Pharmacokinetics (Adult data unless noted)

Nebulization:

Distribution: V_d: Adults: 1900 L

Metabolism: In the liver to an inactive sulfate

Half-life: 3.3-4.0 hours

Time to peak serum concentration: 0.2-1.8 hours

Elimination: 3% to 6% excreted unchanged in urine

Usual Dosage

Acute asthma exacerbation (NAEPP, 2007) **(dosage expressed in terms of mg levalbuterol):**

Nebulization:

Children: 0.075 mg/kg (minimum dose: 1.25 mg) every 20 minutes for 3 doses then 0.075-0.15 mg/kg (not to exceed 5 mg) every 1-4 hours as needed

Adults: 1.25-2.5 mg every 20 minutes for 3 doses then 1.25-5 mg every 1-4 hours as needed

Inhalation: MDI: 45 mcg/spray:

Children: 4-8 puffs every 20 minutes for 3 doses then every 1-4 hours

Adults: 4-8 puffs every 20 minutes for up to 4 hours then every 1-4 hours as needed

Maintenance therapy (nonacute) (NAEPP, 2007): Not recommended for long-term, daily maintenance treatment; regular use exceeding 2 days/week for symptom control indicates the need for additional long-term control therapy

Nebulization:

Children 0-4 years: 0.31-1.25 mg every 4-6 hours as needed

Children ≥5 years and Adults: 0.31-0.63 mg every 8 hours as needed

Inhalation: MDI: 45 mcg/spray:

Children <5 years: Not FDA approved

Children ≥5 years and Adults: 2 inhalations every 4-6 hours as needed

Administration

Inhalation: Nebulization: dilution required for concentrated solution

Oral inhalation: Prime the inhaler (before first use or if it has not been used for more than 2 weeks) by releasing 4 test sprays into the air away from the face; shake well before use; use spacer for children <8 years of age

Monitoring Parameters Serum potassium, oxygen saturation, heart rate, pulmonary function tests, respiratory rate, use of accessory muscles during respiration, suprasternal retractions; arterial or capillary blood gases (if patient's condition warrants)

Patient Information Do not exceed recommended dosage; may cause dry mouth; rinse mouth with water following each inhalation to help with dry throat and mouth; if more than one inhalation is necessary, wait at least 1 full minute between inhalations; notify physician if palpitations, tachycardia, chest pain, muscle tremors, dizziness, or headache occur, or if breathing difficulty persists; limit caffeinated beverages

Additional Information Levalbuterol administered in $1/2$ the mg dose of albuterol (eg, 0.63 mg levalbuterol to 1.25 mg albuterol) provides comparable efficacy and safety. Levalbuterol has not been evaluated by continuous nebulization (NIH Guidelines, 2007).

Dosage Forms Excipient information presented when available (limited, particularly for generics); consult specific product labeling.

Note: Strength expressed as base.

Aerosol, for oral inhalation, as tartrate:

Xopenex HFA™: 45 mcg/actuation (15 g) [200 actuations; chlorofluorocarbon free]

Solution for nebulization, as hydrochloride [preservative free]:

Xopenex®: 0.31 mg/3 mL (24s); 0.63 mg/3 mL (24s); 1.25 mg/3 mL (24s)

Solution for nebulization, as hydrochloride [concentrate; preservative free]: 1.25 mg/0.5 mL (30s)

Xopenex®: 1.25 mg/0.5 mL (30s)

References

Gawchik SM, Saccar CL, Noonan M, et al, "The Safety and Efficacy of Nebulized Levalbuterol Compared With Racemic Albuterol and Placebo in the Treatment of Asthma in Pediatric Patients," *J Allergy Clin Immunol*, 1999, 103(4):615-21.

Lotvall J, Palmqvist M, Arvidsson P, et al, "The Therapeutic Ratio of R-Albuterol Is Comparable With That of RS-Albuterol in Asthmatic Patients," *J Allergy Clin Immunol*, 2001, 108(5):726-31.

Milgrom H, Skoner DP, Bensch G, et al, "Low-Dose Levalbuterol in Children With Asthma: Safety and Efficacy in Comparison With Placebo and Racemic Albuterol," *J Allergy Clin Immunol*, 2001, 108(6):938-45.

"National Asthma Education and Prevention Program. Expert Panel Report: Guidelines for the Diagnosis and Management of Asthma Update on Selected Topics–2002," *J Allergy Clin Immunol*, 2002, 110 (5 Suppl):S141-219.

National Asthma Education and Prevention Program (NAEPP), "Expert Panel Report 3 (EPR-3): Guidelines for the Diagnosis and Management of Asthma," *Clinical Practice Guidelines*, National Institutes of Health, National Heart, Lung, and Blood Institute, NIH Publication No. 08-4051, prepublication 2007; available at http://www.nhlbi.nih.gov/guidelines/asthma/asthgdln.htm.

♦ **Levalbuterol Hydrochloride** *see* Levalbuterol *on page 807*

♦ **Levalbuterol Tartrate** *see* Levalbuterol *on page 807*

♦ **Levaquin®** *see* Levofloxacin *on page 813*

♦ **Levarterenol Bitartrate** *see* Norepinephrine *on page 1000*

♦ **Levate® (Can)** *see* Amitriptyline *on page 89*

♦ **Levbid®** *see* Hyoscyamine *on page 699*

♦ **Levemir®** *see* Insulin Detemir *on page 740*

Levetiracetam (lee va tye RA se tam)

Medication Safety Issues

Sound-alike/look-alike issues:

Keppra® may be confused with Keflex®, Keppra XR™

Levetiracetam may be confused with levocarnitine, levofloxacin

Potential for dispensing errors between Keppra® and Kaletra® (lopinavir/ritonavir)

U.S. Brand Names Keppra XR™; Keppra®

Canadian Brand Names Apo-Levetiracetam®; CO Levetiracetam; Dom-Levetiracetam; Keppra®; PHL-Levetiracetam; PMS-Levetiracetam; PRO-Levetiracetam

Therapeutic Category Anticonvulsant, Miscellaneous

Generic Available Yes: Oral solution, tablet

Use

Oral:

Oral solution and immediate release tablets: Adjunctive therapy in the treatment of partial onset seizures (FDA approved in ages ≥4 years and adults); adjunctive therapy in the treatment of juvenile myoclonic epilepsy (FDA approved in ages ≥12 years) and myoclonic seizures (FDA approved in adults); adjunctive therapy in the treatment of primary generalized tonic-clonic seizures (FDA approved in ages ≥6 years and adults)

Extended release tablets: Adjunctive therapy in the treatment of partial onset seizures (FDA approved in ages ≥16 years and adults)

I.V.: Adjunctive therapy in the treatment of partial onset seizures (FDA approved in ages ≥16 years and adults); adjunctive therapy in the treatment of myoclonic seizures in patients with juvenile myoclonic epilepsy (FDA approved in ages ≥16 years and adults); temporary use in patients in whom oral administration is not feasible (FDA approved in ages ≥16 years and adults)

Note: Studies have reported the use of oral levetiracetam as adjunctive therapy for the treatment of generalized epilepsy with photosensitivity and Lennox-Gastaut syndrome; has also been used investigationally as monotherapy for the treatment of various seizures types. Studies have also reported its use for treatment of tics in patients with Tourette syndrome; prophylaxis in pediatric migraine; and bipolar disorder.

Medication Guide An FDA-approved patient medication guide, which is available with the product information and at http://www.fda.gov/downloads/Drugs/DrugSafety/UCM152832.pdf, must be dispensed with this medication for each new outpatient prescription and refill.

Pregnancy Risk Factor C

Pregnancy Considerations Developmental toxicities were observed in animal studies. There are no adequate and well-controlled studies in pregnant women. Two registries are available for women exposed to levetiracetam during pregnancy:

Antiepileptic Drug Pregnancy Registry (888-233-2334 or http://www.mgh.harvard.edu/aed/)

Keppra® pregnancy registry (888-537-7734 or http://www.keppra.com)

Lactation Enters breast milk/not recommended

Contraindications Hypersensitivity to levetiracetam or any component

Warnings Neuropsychiatric adverse events including somnolence, fatigue, coordination difficulties, behavioral abnormalities (eg, aggression, agitation, anxiety, anger, hostility, irritability, depression) and psychotic symptoms (psychosis, hallucinations) may occur; incidence of behavioral abnormalities may be increased in children; dosage reductions may be required. Do not abruptly discontinue therapy; withdraw gradually to lessen chance for increased seizure frequency.

Antiepileptic drugs (AEDs) increase the risk of suicidal behavior and ideation in patients receiving these medications for any indication. Pooled analyses of placebo-controlled trials involving 11 different AEDs (regardless of indication) showed a twofold increased risk of suicidal thoughts or behavior (estimated incidence rate: 0.43% in AED treated patients compared to 0.24% of patients receiving placebo); increased risk was observed as early as 1 week after initiation of AED and continued through duration of trials (most trials ≤24 weeks); risk did not vary significantly by age (age range: 5–100 years). Consider risks and benefits of AEDs before prescribing. Monitor all patients receiving an AED for emergence of suicidal thoughts or behavior, thoughts of self-harm, any unusual changes in behavior or mood, or the emergence or worsening of depressive symptoms; notify heathcare provider immediately if symptoms or concerning behavior occur. **Note:** The FDA is requiring that a Medication Guide be developed for all antiepileptic drugs informing patients of this risk.

Precautions Use with caution and decrease dose in patients with renal dysfunction. Hematologic abnormalities (small but statistically significant decreases in RBC count, Hgb, Hct, WBC count, and neutrophils) may occur. Safety and efficacy of oral solution and immediate release tablets in children <4 years and I.V. formulation and extended release tablets in children <16 years have not been established.

Adverse Reactions Note: Adverse reactions are listed for oral levetiracetam when used to treat partial onset seizures; spectrum and frequency of adverse reactions is expected to be similar for treatment of myoclonic epilepsy, primary generalized tonic-clonic seizures and with I.V. use. The most frequently reported adverse reactions in pediatric clinical trials were somnolence, accidental injury, hostility, nervousness, and asthenia; unless otherwise noted, percent incidence is from pediatric studies; in adults, asthenia, somnolence, dizziness, and coordination difficulties occurred most frequently during the first 4 weeks of therapy (but may occur at anytime during treatment)

Cardiovascular: Facial edema (2%)

Central nervous system: Behavioral symptoms (agitation, aggression, anger, anxiety, apathy, depersonalization, depression, emotional lability, hostility, hyperkinesias, irritability, nervousness, neurosis, and personality disorder; incidence: adults 13%; children 38%); somnolence (adults 8% to 15%; children 23%); headache (adults 14%); hostility (adults 2%; children 12%); nervousness (adults 4%; children 10%); dizziness (adults 5% to 9%; children 7%); personality disorder (8%); pain (adults 7%;

children 6%); agitation (6%); emotional lability (adults 2%; children 6%); depression (adults 4%; children 3%); ataxia (adults 3%); vertigo (adults 3%); amnesia (adults 2%); anxiety (adults 2%); confusion (2%); psychotic symptoms (adults 0.7%); suicidal thinking and behavior (see Warnings)

Dermatologic: Bruising (4%), pruritus (2%), rash (2%), skin discoloration (2%)

Gastrointestinal: Vomiting (15%), anorexia (adults 3%; children 13%), diarrhea (8%), nausea (5%), gastroenteritis (4%), constipation (3%), dehydration (2%)

Hematologic: Leukocytes decreased (3%), hematocrit decreased, hemoglobin decreased, RBC decreased (see Precautions)

Neuromuscular & skeletal: Asthenia (adults 15%; children 9%), neck pain (2%), paresthesia (adults 2%), reflexes increased (2%)

Ocular: Conjunctivitis (3%), diplopia (adults 2%), amblyopia (2%)

Otic: Ear pain (2%)

Renal: Albuminuria (4%), urine abnormality (2%)

Respiratory: Rhinitis (adults 4%; children 13%), cough (adults 2%; children 11%), pharyngitis (adults 6%; children 10%), asthma (2%), sinusitis (adults 2%)

Miscellaneous: Accidental injury (children 17%); infection (adults 13%; children 2%); flu-like symptoms (3% to 8%)

Drug Interactions

Avoid Concomitant Use There are no known interactions where it is recommended to avoid concomitant use.

Increased Effect/Toxicity

Levetiracetam may increase the levels/effects of: Alcohol (Ethyl); CNS Depressants; Methotrimeprazine

The levels/effects of Levetiracetam may be increased by: Methotrimeprazine

Decreased Effect

The levels/effects of Levetiracetam may be decreased by: Ketorolac; Ketorolac (Systemic); Mefloquine

Food Interactions Oral: Immediate release: Food delays the rate, but not the extent of absorption (bioavailability is not affected); Extended release: Ingestion of a high fat, high caloric meal prior to administration results in a higher peak concentration and longer time to peak (median time to peak delayed by 2 hours)

Stability

Oral solution, tablets: Store at 25°C (77°F), away from heat and light

I.V. solution: Store at 25°C (77°F); dilute dose in 100 mL of D_5W, NS, or LR; admixed solution is stable for at least 24 hours in polyvinyl chloride bags stored at controlled room temperature. Stable when mixed with lorazepam, diazepam, or valproate sodium (concentrations not specified; see package insert)

Mechanism of Action The exact mechanism of the antiepileptic effects of levetiracetam is unknown. Several studies suggest one or more of the following central pharmacologic effects may be involved: Inhibition of voltage-dependent N-type calcium channels; blockade of GABA-ergic inhibitory transmission through displacement of negative modulators; reversal of the inhibition of glycine currents; reduction of delayed rectifier potassium current; and/or binding to synaptic proteins which modulate neurotransmitter release.

Pharmacokinetics (Adult data unless noted)

Absorption: Oral: Rapid and complete

Distribution: V_d approximates volume of intracellular and extracellular water; V_d Adults: 0.5-0.7 L/kg

Protein binding: <10%

Metabolism: Not extensive; 24% of dose is metabolized by enzymatic hydrolysis of acetamide group (major metabolic pathway; hydrolysis occurs primarily in the blood; not cytochrome P450 dependent); two minor metabolites ▶

(one via hydroxylation of 2-oxo-pyrrolidine ring and one via opening of the 2-oxo-pyrrolidine ring in position 5) are also formed; metabolites are inactive and renally excreted

Bioavailability: Oral: 100%; tablets, oral solution, and injection are bioequivalent; bioavailability of extended release tablets is similar to immediate release tablets

Half-life: Increased in patients with renal dysfunction
Children 4-12 years: 5 hours
Adults: 6-8 hours; extended release tablets: 7 hours

Time to peak serum concentration: Oral:
Immediate release: Fasting adults and children: 1 hour
Extended release: Adults: 4 hours (**Note:** Median time to peak is 2 hours longer in the fed state)

Excretion: 66% excreted in urine as unchanged drug and 27% as inactive metabolites; undergoes glomerular filtration and subsequent partial tubular reabsorption

Clearance: Correlated with creatinine clearance; clearance is decreased in patients with renal dysfunction
Children 6-12 years: 40% higher than adults on a per kg basis

Dialysis: Hemodialysis: Standard 4-hour treatment removes ~50% of the drug from the body; supplemental doses after dialysis are recommended

Usual Dosage Anticonvulsant:
Oral:
Infants 6 months of age to Children 4 years: Not approved for use; dose not established; limited information is available from prospective open-label clinical trials that involved a wider age range of children: Immediate release: Initial: 5-10 mg/kg/day given in 2-3 divided doses; may increase every week by 10 mg/kg/day, if tolerated, to a maximum of 60 mg/kg/day (see Grosso, 2005 and Lagae, 2005).

Myoclonic seizures: Children ≥12 years: Immediate release: Initial 500 mg twice daily; increase dosage every 2 weeks by 500 mg/dose given twice daily, to the recommended dose of 1500 mg twice daily. Efficacy of doses other than 3000 mg/day has not been established.

Partial onset seizures:
Children 4 to <16 years: Immediate release: Initial: 10 mg/kg/dose given twice daily; may increase every 2 weeks by 10 mg/kg/dose given twice daily, if tolerated, to a maximum of 30 mg/kg/dose twice daily (60 mg/kg/day); mean required dose: 52 mg/kg/day.

Adolescents ≥16 years and Adults:
Immediate release: Initial: 500 mg twice daily; may increase every 2 weeks by 500 mg/dose given twice daily, if tolerated, to a maximum of 1500 mg twice daily. Doses >3000 mg/day have been used in trials; however, there is no evidence of increased benefit.

Extended release: Initial: 1000 mg once daily; may increase every 2 weeks by 1000 mg/day to a maximum of 3000 mg once daily.

Primary generalized tonic-clonic seizures:
Children 6 to <16 years: Immediate release: Initial: 10 mg/kg/dose given twice daily; increase dosage every 2 weeks by 10 mg/kg/dose given twice daily, to the recommended dose of 30 mg/kg/dose twice daily (60 mg/kg/day). Efficacy of doses other than 60 mg/kg/day has not been established.

Adolescents ≥16 years and Adults: Immediate release: Initial: 500 mg twice daily; increase dosage every 2 weeks by 500 mg/dose given twice daily, to the recommended dose of 1500 mg twice daily. Efficacy of doses other than 3000 mg/day has not been established.

I.V.:
Infants and Children <16 years: Not approved for use; dose not established; very limited information is available. One small retrospective study (n=10) used I.V. levetiracetam in pediatric patients 3 weeks to 19

years of age. Dosing for patients taking oral levetiracetam was substituted on a mg per mg basis; for acute repetitive seizures or status epilepticus, 20-40 mg/kg/dose was given every 8 hours in infants and every 12 hours in older children; maintenance treatment and seizure prophylaxis dose was 10-20 mg/kg/dose every 12 hours (mean dose used: 50.4 mg/kg/day; mean duration of use: 4.9 days). Further studies are needed before these doses can be recommended for routine use (see Goraya, 2008).

Myoclonic seizures: Adolescents ≥16 years and Adults: Initial: 500 mg twice daily; increase dosage every 2 weeks by 500 mg/dose given twice daily, to the recommended dose of 1500 mg twice daily. Efficacy of doses <3000 mg/day has not been studied.

Partial onset seizures: Adolescents ≥16 years and Adults: Initial: 500 mg twice daily; may increase every 2 weeks by 500 mg/dose given twice daily, if tolerated, to a maximum of 1500 mg twice daily. Oral doses >3000 mg/day have been used in trials; however, there is no evidence of increased benefit.

Note: When switching from oral to I.V. formulation, the total daily dose should be the same.

Dosing adjustment in renal impairment:
Children (see Aronoff, 2007):
Cl_{cr} <50 mL/minute/1.73 m^2: Administer 50% of the dose
Hemodialysis: Administer 50% of normal dose every 24 hours; a supplemental dose after hemodialysis is recommended
CAPD: Administer 50% of normal dose
CRRT: Administer 50% of normal dose

Adults (manufacturer recommendations):
Immediate release formulations:
Cl_{cr} >80 mL/minute: 500-1500 mg every 12 hours
Cl_{cr} 50-80 mL/minute: 500-1000 mg every 12 hours
Cl_{cr} 30-50 mL/minute: 250-750 mg every 12 hours
Cl_{cr} <30 mL/minute: 250-500 mg every 12 hours
End-stage renal disease patients using dialysis: 500-1000 mg every 24 hours; a supplemental dose of 250-500 mg following dialysis is recommended

Extended release tablets:
Cl_{cr} >80 mL/minute: 1000-3000 mg every 24 hours
Cl_{cr} 50-80 mL/minute: 1000-2000 mg every 24 hours
Cl_{cr} 30-50 mL/minute: 500-1500 mg every 24 hours
Cl_{cr} <30 mL/minute: 500-1000 mg every 24 hours
End-stage renal disease patients using dialysis: Use immediate release product

Administration
Oral: May be administered without regard to meals; swallow immediate release and extended release tablets whole; do not break, crush, or chew. Manufacturer recommends use of calibrated measuring device to measure oral solution.

Parenteral: I.V.: **Injection is for I.V. use only and must be diluted prior to use.** In patients ≥16 years, dilute dose in 100 mL of D$_5$W, NS, or LR; infuse over 15 minutes. Do not use if solution contains particulate matter or is discolored. Discard unused portion of vial (does not contain preservative).

Monitoring Parameters Seizure frequency, duration, and severity; behavioral abnormalities and neuropsychiatric adverse events (see Warnings); renal function; CBC; signs and symptoms of suicidality (eg, anxiety, depression, behavior changes) (see Warnings)

Reference Range Therapeutic range and benefit of therapeutic drug monitoring have not been established; concentrations of 6-20 mg/L (35-120 micromol/L) were attained in adult study patients receiving doses of 1000-3000 mg/day

Patient Information Read the patient Medication Guide that you receive with each prescription and refill of levetiracetam. Antiepileptic agents may increase the risk of suicidal thoughts and behavior; notify physician if you feel more depressed or have thoughts of suicide or self harm (see Warnings). May cause dizziness or drowsiness and impair ability to perform activities requiring mental alertness or physical coordination. Avoid abrupt discontinuation after prolonged use (an increase in seizure activity may result). Inform healthcare provider immediately if any of the following symptoms occur: Extreme weakness, tiredness, or sleepiness; problems walking or moving; unusual thoughts or behavior; hallucinations or delusions; changes in behavior or mood (such as aggression, agitation, anger, anxiety, apathy, mood swings, hostility, and irritability); or depression or thoughts of suicide (**Note:** Suicide, attempted suicide, and thoughts of suicide have been reported in patients receiving levetiracetam). Avoid ethanol (may increase adverse effects). Inform healthcare provider if taking other prescription and nonprescription medications, especially pain medications, sedatives, antihistamines, or hypnotics, which may increase adverse effects. Report worsening of seizure activity or loss of seizure control.

Nursing Implications Doses should be titrated based on clinical response. Be aware of neuropsychiatric adverse events (see Warnings). Taper dosage slowly when discontinuing therapy. Injection must be diluted before I.V. use.

Additional Information A recent, small, retrospective study used a rapid dosage titration of levetiracetam in 8 children, 19 months to 17 years of age (mean age: 8.6 years). Full maintenance doses of levetiracetam were achieved over a titration period of 2-14 days (mean: 10 days). The drug was effective and well-tolerated; however, one patient developed adverse behavioral effects. Further studies are needed before rapid titration of levetiracetam can be routinely recommended (see Vaisleib, 2008).

In a preliminary report, levetiracetam-associated behavioral abnormalities were successfully treated with pyridoxine in 5 of 6 children, 2-10 years of age; further studies are needed before this treatment can be recommended (see Miller, 2002). Levetiracetam- induced psychosis (including visual and auditory hallucinations and persecutive delusions) has been reported in pediatric patients (see Kossoff, 2001).

Injection solution for I.V. administration is buffered to a pH of ~5.5

Dosage Forms Excipient information presented when available (limited, particularly for generics); consult specific product labeling.

Injection, solution:
Keppra®: 100 mg/mL (5 mL)
Solution, oral: 100 mg/mL (500 mL)
Keppra®: 100 mg/mL (480 mL) [dye free; grape flavor]
Tablet: 250 mg, 500 mg, 750 mg, 1000 mg
Keppra®: 250 mg, 500 mg, 750 mg, 1000 mg
Tablet, extended release:
Keppra XR™: 500 mg, 750 mg

References

Aronoff GR, Bennett WM, Berns JS, et al, *Drug Prescribing in Renal Failure: Dosing Guidelines for Adults and Children*, 5th ed. Philadelphia, PA: American College of Physicians, 2007, 89, 165.

Awaad Y, Michon AM, and Minarik S, "Use of Levetiracetam to Treat Tics in Children and Adolescents With Tourette Syndrome," *Mov Disord*, 2005, 20(6):714-8.

Glauser TA, Pellock JM, Bebin EM, et al, "Efficacy and Safety of Levetiracetam in Children with Partial Seizures: An Open-Label Trial," *Epilepsia*, 2002, 43(5):518-24.

Goraya JS, Khurana DS, Valencia I, et al, "Intravenous Levetiracetam in Children With Epilepsy," *Pediatr Neurol*, 2008, 38(3):177-80.

Grosso S, Franzoni E, Coppola G, et al, "Efficacy and Safety of Levetiracetam: An Add-On Trial in Children With Refractory Epilepsy," *Seizure*, 2005, 14(4):248-53.

Grunewald R, "Levetiracetam in the Treatment of Idiopathic Generalized Epilepsies," *Epilepsia*, 2005, 46(Suppl 9):154-60.

Kossoff EH, Bergey GK, Freeman JM, et al, "Levetiracetam Psychosis in Children With Epilepsy," *Epilepsia*, 2001, 42(12):1611-3.

Lagae L, Buyse G, and Ceulemans B, "Clinical Experience With Levetiracetam in Childhood Epilepsy: An Add-On and Monotherapy Trial," *Seizure*, 2005, 14(1):66-71.

Mandelbaum DE, Bunch M, Kugler SL, et al, "Efficacy of Levetiracetam at 12 Months in Children Classified By Seizure Type, Cognitive Status, and Previous Anticonvulsant Drug Use," *J Child Neurol*, 2005, 20(7):590-4.

Miller GS, "Pyridoxine Ameliorates Adverse Behavioral Effects of Levetiracetam in Children," *Epilepsia*, 2002, 43(Suppl 7):S62.

Miller GS, "Efficacy and Safety of Levetiracetam in Pediatric Migraine," *Headache*, 2004, 44(3):238-43.

Opp J, Tuxhorn I, May T, et al, "Levetiracetam in Children With Refractory Epilepsy: A Multicenter Open Label Study in Germany," *Seizure*, 2005, 14(7):476-84.

Patsalos PN, "Clinical Pharmacokinetics of Levetiracetam," *Clin Pharmacokinet*, 2004, 43(11):707-24.

Sankar R and Holmes GL, "Mechanisms of Action for the Commonly Used Antiepileptic Drugs: Relevance to Antiepileptic Drug-Associated Neurobehavioral Adverse Effects," *J Child Neurol*, 2004, 19(Suppl 1):6-14.

Vaisleib II and Neft RA, "Rapid Dosage Titration of Levetiracetam in Children," *Pharmacotherapy*, 2008, 28(3):393-6.

Vigevano F, "Levetiracetam in Pediatrics," *J Child Neurol*, 2005, 20(2):87-93.

Levobunolol (lee voe BYOO noe lole)

Medication Safety Issues
Sound-alike/look-alike issues:
Levobunolol may be confused with levocabastine
Betagan® may be confused with Betadine®, Betoptic® S

International issues:
Betagan® may be confused with Betagon® which is a brand name for mepindolol in Italy

U.S. Brand Names Betagan®

Canadian Brand Names Apo-Levobunolol®; Betagan®; Novo-Levobunolol; Optho-Bunolol®; PMS-Levobunolol; Sandoz-Levobunolol

Therapeutic Category Beta-Adrenergic Blocker, Ophthalmic

Generic Available Yes

Use To lower intraocular pressure in chronic open-angle glaucoma or ocular hypertension

Pregnancy Risk Factor C

Pregnancy Considerations Adverse events were observed in some animal reproduction studies.

Lactation Excretion in breast milk unknow/use caution

Contraindications Hypersensitivity to levobunolol or any component (see Warnings); asthma, severe COPD, sinus bradycardia, second or third degree A-V block, cardiogenic shock

Warnings Contains metabisulfite which may cause allergic reactions in susceptible individuals; use only in combination with miotic for patients with angle closure glaucoma; products contain sulfites which may cause allergic reactions in susceptible individuals

Precautions Use with caution in patients with CHF, diabetes mellitus, hyperthyroidism, myasthenia gravis

Adverse Reactions
Cardiovascular: Bradycardia, arrhythmias, hypotension, palpitations, cerebral ischemia, cerebral vascular accident, syncope, heart block, CHF
Central nervous system: Dizziness, headache, depression, ataxia, cerebral ischemia
Dermatologic: Rash, alopecia, itching
Endocrine & metabolic: Masked symptoms of hypoglycemia in diabetics
Gastrointestinal: Nausea, heartburn, diarrhea
Ocular: Stinging, burning, erythema, itching, blepharoconjunctivitis, keratitis, ptosis, visual acuity decreased, conjunctivitis, tearing
Respiratory: Bronchospasm

Drug Interactions

Avoid Concomitant Use
Avoid concomitant use of Levobunolol with any of the following: Methacholine

Increased Effect/Toxicity
Levobunolol may increase the levels/effects of: Alpha-/ Beta-Agonists (Direct-Acting); Bupivacaine; Hypotensive Agents; Lidocaine (Systemic); Lidocaine (Topical); Mepivacaine; Methacholine; Midodrine

The levels/effects of Levobunolol may be increased by: Anilidopiperidine Opioids; Dronedarone; MAO Inhibitors; QuiNIDine; Reserpine

Decreased Effect
Levobunolol may decrease the levels/effects of: Beta2-Agonists; Theophylline Derivatives

Mechanism of Action A nonselective beta-adrenergic blocking agent that lowers intraocular pressure by reducing aqueous humor production

Pharmacodynamics
Onset of action: Following ophthalmic instillation, decreases in intraocular pressure can be noted within 1 hour

Maximum effect: Within 2-6 hours

Maximal effectiveness: 2-3 weeks

Duration: 1-7 days

Pharmacokinetics (Adult data unless noted)
Absorption: May be absorbed systemically and produce systemic side effects

Metabolism: Extensively metabolized into several metabolites; primary metabolite (active) dihydrolevobunolol

Elimination: Not well defined

Usual Dosage Adults: 1-2 drops of 0.5% solution in eye(s) once daily or 1-2 drops of 0.25% solution twice daily; may increase to 1 drop of 0.5% solution twice daily

Administration Intraocular: Apply drops into conjunctival sac of affected eye(s); avoid contacting bottle tip with skin; apply gentle pressure to lacrimal sac during and immediately following instillation (1-2 minutes) to decrease systemic absorption; see manufacturer's information regarding proper usage of C Cap (compliance cap)

Monitoring Parameters Intraocular pressure

Dosage Forms Excipient information presented when available (limited, particularly for generics); consult specific product labeling.

Solution, ophthalmic, as hydrochloride: 0.25% (5 mL, 10 mL); 0.5% (5 mL, 10 mL, 15 mL) [contains benzalkonium chloride and sodium metabisulfite]

Betagan®: 0.25% (5 mL, 10 mL); 0.5% (2 mL, 5 mL, 10 mL, 15 mL) [contains benzalkonium chloride and sodium metabisulfite]

◆ **Levobunolol Hydrochloride** see Levobunolol on page 811

◆ **Levocarnitine** see Carnitine on page 253

Levocetirizine (LEE vo se TI ra zeen)

Medication Safety Issues
Sound-alike/look-alike issues:
Levocetirizine may be confused with cetirizine

U.S. Brand Names Xyzal®

Therapeutic Category Antihistamine

Generic Available No

Use Relief of symptoms associated with perennial allergic rhinitis (FDA approved in ages ≥6 months and adults), seasonal allergic rhinitis (FDA approved in ages ≥2 years and adults), and treatment of the uncomplicated skin manifestations of chronic idiopathic urticaria (FDA approved in ages ≥6 months and adults)

Pregnancy Risk Factor B

Pregnancy Considerations Levocetirizine was not shown to be teratogenic in animal studies. There are no adequate and well-controlled studies in pregnant women. Use during pregnancy only if clearly needed.

Lactation Excretion in breast milk unknown/not recommended

Breast-Feeding Considerations Cetirizine is excreted in breast milk; therefore, levocetirizine would be expected to enter breast milk. Use is not recommended while breast-feeding.

Contraindications Hypersensitivity to levocetirizine, cetirizine, hydroxyzine, or any component; end stage renal disease (Cl_{cr} <10 mL/minute); patients undergoing dialysis; children 6 months to 11 years with impaired renal function

Warnings Safety and efficacy for the use of cough and cold products in children <2 years of age is limited. Serious adverse effects including death have been reported. The FDA notes that there are no approved OTC uses for these products in children <2 years of age. Healthcare providers are reminded to ask caregivers about the use of OTC cough and cold products in order to avoid exposure to multiple medications containing the same ingredient. May cause drowsiness; avoid concurrent use with alcohol.

Precautions Use with caution in patients with mild to moderate renal dysfunction and adjust dosage.

Adverse Reactions
Central nervous system: Drowsiness, fatigue, pyrexia, somnolence

Gastrointestinal: Constipation (children 7%), diarrhea (children 4% to 13%), epistaxis pharyngitis, vomiting, xerostomia

Neuromuscular & skeletal: Weakness

Respiratory: Cough, nasopharyngitis

<1% and/or postmarketing: Aggressive reactions, agitation, anaphylaxis, angioneurotic edema, cholestasis, convulsions, dyspnea, glomerulonephritis, hallucinations, hepatitis, hypersensitivity, hypotension, myalgia, nausea, orofacial dyskinesia, palpitation, pruritus, rash, stillbirth, suicidal ideation, syncope, transient hepatic enzyme elevation, urticaria, visual disturbances, weight increased

Drug Interactions

Avoid Concomitant Use
There are no known interactions where it is recommended to avoid concomitant use.

Increased Effect/Toxicity
Levocetirizine may increase the levels/effects of: Alcohol (Ethyl); Anticholinergics; CNS Depressants

The levels/effects of Levocetirizine may be increased by: Pramlintide

Decreased Effect
Levocetirizine may decrease the levels/effects of: Acetylcholinesterase Inhibitors (Central); Betahistine

The levels/effects of Levocetirizine may be decreased by: Acetylcholinesterase Inhibitors (Central); Amphetamines

Stability Store at room temperature.

Mechanism of Action Levocetirizine is the R-enantiomer of cetirizine, a metabolite of hydroxyzine. It competes with histamine for H_1-receptor sites on effector cells in the GI tract, blood vessels, and respiratory tract.

Pharmacodynamics
Duration: 24 hours

Pharmacokinetics (Adult data unless noted)
Absorption: Well absorbed from the GI tract

Distribution: V_d:
Children: 0.4 L/kg
Adults: 0.4 L/kg

Protein binding: 91% to 92%

Metabolism: Limited hepatic metabolism (~14% of a dose); metabolic pathways include aromatic oxidation, N- and O-dealkylation, and taurine conjugation

Half-life:
Children 1-2 years: ~4 hours
Children 6-11 years: ~6 hours (24% less than adult half-life)
Adults: 8 hours
Time to peak serum concentration:
Children: 1.2 hours
Adults: Oral solution: 0.5 hours; Tablet: 0.9 hours
Elimination: 85.4% excreted unchanged in urine; 12.9% in feces
Clearance:
Children 1-2 years: 1 mL/kg/minute
Children 6-11 years: 0.82 mL/kg/minute
Adults: 0.63 mL/kg/minute
Dialysis: <10% removed during hemodialysis

Usual Dosage Oral:
Children 6 months to 5 years: 1.25 mg once daily
Children 6-11 years: 2.5 mg once daily
Children ≥12 years and Adults: 5 mg once daily

Dosage adjustments in renal impairment:
Children 6 months to 11 years: Avoid use
Children ≥12 years and Adults:
Cl_{cr} 50-80 mL/minute: 2.5 mg once daily
Cl_{cr} 30-50 mL/minute: 2.5 mg once every other day
Cl_{cr} 10-30 mL/minute: 2.5 mg twice weekly
Cl_{cr} <10 mL/minute or on hemodialysis: Contraindicated
Dosing adjustment in hepatic impairment: No dosage adjustment necessary.

Administration Administer without regard to food in the evening.

Patient Information May cause drowsiness and impair ability to perform activities requiring mental alertness or physical coordination; do not exceed daily dosage; may cause dry mouth. Although not reported with levocetirizine, cetirizine may cause photosensitivity reactions and avoiding exposure to sunlight may be appropriate.

Dosage Forms Excipient information presented when available (limited, particularly for generics); consult specific product labeling.
Solution, oral, as dihydrochloride:
Xyzal®: 0.5 mg/mL (150 mL)
Tablet, as dihydrochloride [scored]:
Xyzal®: 5 mg

References
Cranswick N, Turzíkova J, Fuchs M, et al, "Levocetirizine in 1-2 Year Old Children: Pharmacokinetic and Pharmacodynamic Profile," *Int J Clin Pharmacol Ther*, 2005, 43(4):172-7.
Simons FE and Simons KJ, "Levocetirizine: Pharmacokinetics and Pharmacodynamics in Children Age 6 to 11 Years," *J Allergy Clin Immunol*, 2005, 116(2):355-61.

◆ **Levocetirizine Dihydrochloride** *see* Levocetirizine *on page 812*

◆ **Levoclen™-4** *see* Benzoyl Peroxide *on page 184*

◆ **Levoclen™-8** *see* Benzoyl Peroxide *on page 184*

◆ **Levoclen™ Acne Wash** *see* Benzoyl Peroxide *on page 184*

Levofloxacin (lee voe FLOKS a sin)

Medication Safety Issues
Sound-alike/look-alike issues:
Levaquin® may be confused with Levoxyl®, Levsin/SL®, Lovenox®
Levofloxacin may be confused with levetiracetam, levodopa, Levophed®, levothyroxine
U.S. Brand Names Iquix®; Levaquin®; Quixin®
Canadian Brand Names Apo-Levofloxacin®; CO Levofloxacin; Levaquin®; Mylan-Levofloxacin; Novo-Levofloxacin; PMS-Levofloxacin; Sandoz-Levofloxacin
Therapeutic Category Antibiotic, Ophthalmic; Antibiotic, Quinolone

Generic Available No
Use Treatment of acute bacterial sinusitis, lower respiratory tract infections, skin and skin structure infections (uncomplicated or complicated), chronic bacterial prostatitis, complicated urinary tract infections and acute pyelonephritis due to multidrug-resistant organisms susceptible to levofloxacin including *Streptococcus pneumoniae* (including penicillin-resistant strains), *S. aureus, Haemophilus influenzae, H. parainfluenzae, Moraxella catarrhalis, Klebsiella pneumoniae, Legionella pneumophila, Chlamydia pneumoniae, Mycoplasma pneumoniae, E. coli, Enterococcus fecalis, S. pyogenes, Proteus mirabilis, Enterobacter cloacae,* (less active than ciprofloxacin against *Pseudomonas aeruginosa*; combination therapy with a beta-lactam antipseudomonal is recommended); treatment of community-acquired pneumonia; infectious diarrhea due to enterotoxigenic *E. coli, Shigella, Salmonella, Campylobacter* spp, *Vibrio parahaemolyticus*; post-exposure prevention of inhalational anthrax.

Used ophthalmically for treatment of bacterial conjunctivitis due to *S. aureus* (methicillin-susceptible strains), *S. epidermidis, S. pneumoniae, Streptococcus* (groups C/F), *Streptococcus* (group G), Viridans group *Streptococci, Corynebacterium* spp, *H. influenzae, Acinetobacter iwoffii,* or *Serratia marcescens*; treatment of bacterial corneal ulcer due to susceptible organisms

Medication Guide An FDA-approved patient medication guide, which is available with the product information and at http://www.fda.gov/downloads/Drugs/DrugSafety/ucm088619.pdf, must be dispensed with this medication for each new outpatient prescription and refill.

Pregnancy Risk Factor C

Pregnancy Considerations Adverse events have been observed in some animal studies; therefore, the manufacturer classifies levofloxacin as pregnancy category C. Levofloxacin crosses the placenta. Quinolone exposure during human pregnancy has been reported with other agents (see Ciprofloxacin and Ofloxacin monographs). To date, no specific teratogenic effect or increased pregnancy risk has been identified; however, because of concerns of cartilage damage in immature animals exposed to quinolones and the limited levofloxacin specific data, levofloxacin should only be used during pregnancy if a safer option is not available.

Lactation Enters breast milk/not recommended

Breast-Feeding Considerations Based on data from a case report, small amounts of levofloxacin are excreted in breast milk. Breast-feeding is not recommended by the manufacturer. Levofloxacin is the L-isomer of ofloxacin. Ofloxacin has also been shown to have minimal concentrations in human milk and is considered "usually compatible with breast-feeding" by the AAP. Nondose-related effects could include modification of bowel flora.

Contraindications Hypersensitivity to levofloxacin, any component, or other quinolones; not recommended for use in pregnant women or during breast-feeding

Warnings Oral and parenteral formulations are not recommended in children <18 years of age; levofloxacin increased osteochondrosis in immature rats and dogs. Fluoroquinolones have caused arthropathy with erosions of the cartilage in weight-bearing joints of immature animals; Achilles tendonitis and tendon rupture have been reported with fluoroquinolones in patients of all ages **[U.S. Boxed Warning]**; risk increased in patients taking concomitant corticosteroids, patients >60 years of age, and in patients with kidney, heart, or lung transplants. Prolonged use may result in superinfection, including *C. difficile*-associated diarrhea and pseudomembranous colitis; CNS stimulation and increased intracranial pressure may occur resulting in tremors, restlessness, confusion, and rarely hallucinations, depression, nightmares, suicidal ideation, or convulsive seizures; serious and occasionally fatal hypersensitivity and/or anaphylactic reactions have been reported often following the first dose. Hypersensitivity reactions have been accompanied by cardiovascular collapse, hypotension/shock, seizure, loss of consciousness, tingling, angioedema, airway obstruction, dyspnea, urticaria, itching, and skin reactions. If these reactions occur, discontinue levofloxacin. Resuscitation equipment, oxygen, epinephrine, antihistamine, and a corticosteroid should be readily available to treat hypersensitivity reactions.

Idiosyncratic reactions including toxic epidermal necrolysis, vasculitis, pneumonitis, nephritis, hepatic failure, and/or cytopenias have usually occurred after multiple doses. Discontinue drug if these reactions occur.

Oral solution contains benzyl alcohol and propylene glycol which may be toxic to newborns in high doses; benzyl alcohol may cause allergic reactions in susceptible individuals; large amounts of benzyl alcohol (≥99 mg/kg/day) have been associated with a potentially fatal toxicity ("gasping syndrome") in neonates; the "gasping syndrome" consists of metabolic acidosis, respiratory distress, gasping respirations, CNS dysfunction (including convulsions, intracranial hemorrhage), hypotension and cardiovascular collapse; *in vitro* and animal studies have shown that benzoate, a metabolite of benzyl alcohol, displaces bilirubin from protein binding sites

Precautions Use with caution in patients with known or suspected CNS disorders, myasthenia gravis, seizure disorders, severe cerebral arteriosclerosis, or renal impairment; modify dosage in patients with renal impairment. The use of quinolones has been linked to peripheral neuropathy (rare); discontinue if symptoms of sensory or sensorimotor neuropathy occur. Rare cases of torsade de pointes have been reported in patients taking levofloxacin so use with caution in patients on concurrent therapy with Class Ia or Class III antiarrhythmics or in patients with known prolongation of QT interval, bradycardia, cardiomyopathy, recent myocardial ischemia, hypokalemia, or hypomagnesemia. Use with caution in patients with diabetes (fluoroquinolones have been associated with serious and sometimes fatal hypoglycemia). Avoid excessive sunlight and take precautions to limit exposure (eg, loose-fitting clothing, sunscreen); may rarely cause moderate-to-severe phototoxicity reactions. Discontinue use if phototoxicity occurs.

Adverse Reactions

Cardiovascular: Cardiac failure, hypertension, hypotension, bradycardia, tachycardia, edema, torsade de pointes (rare), prolongation of QT interval, vasodilation, vasculitis

Central nervous system: Dizziness, fever, headache, insomnia, intracranial pressure increased, seizures, fatigue, nervousness, restlessness, confusion, hallucinations, anxiety, psychosis, lightheadedness, suicidal thoughts, depression, encephalopathy, abnormal EEG, nightmares

Dermatologic: Photosensitivity, pruritus, urticaria, rash, angioedema, Stevens-Johnson syndrome, toxic epidermal necrolysis, erythema multiforme

Endocrine & metabolic: Hypoglycemia, hyperglycemia, electrolyte abnormality

Gastrointestinal: Nausea, vomiting, diarrhea, constipation, anorexia, abdominal pain, pseudomembranous colitis, pancreatitis, dyspepsia

Genitourinary: Vaginitis

Hematologic: Granulocytopenia, leukopenia, thrombocytopenia, hemolytic anemia, eosinophilia, aplastic anemia, INR/prothrombin time elevated, agranulocytosis, pancytopenia

Hepatic: Liver enzymes elevated, hepatic failure (including fatal cases), jaundice, hepatitis

Local: With I.V.: Phlebitis, burning, pain, erythema, swelling

Neuromuscular & skeletal: Tremor, arthralgia, tendonitis, tendon rupture (usually involves the Achilles, hand, or shoulder tendons and can occur during therapy or up to a few months after therapy completion), myalgia, peripheral neuropathy, rhabdomyolysis, paresthesias

Ocular: Ophthalmic solution: Allergic reaction, foreign body sensation, transient decreased vision; ocular pain, burning, itching, dryness, discomfort, photophobia, corneal erosion, hyperemia, lid edema, lid erythema

Renal: Interstitial nephritis, acute renal insufficiency

Respiratory: Bronchospasm, respiratory distress, dyspnea, allergic pneumonitis, pharyngitis

Miscellaneous: Anaphylaxis, serum sickness, hypersensitivity reactions (see Warnings)

Drug Interactions

Avoid Concomitant Use

Avoid concomitant use of Levofloxacin with any of the following: Artemether; BCG; Dronedarone; Lumefantrine; Nilotinib; Pimozide; QuiNINE; Tetrabenazine; Thioridazine; Ziprasidone

Increased Effect/Toxicity

Levofloxacin may increase the levels/effects of: Corticosteroids (Systemic); Dronedarone; Pimozide; QTc-Prolonging Agents; QuiNINE; Sulfonylureas; Tetrabenazine; Thioridazine; Vitamin K Antagonists; Ziprasidone

The levels/effects of Levofloxacin may be increased by: Alfuzosin; Artemether; Chloroquine; Ciprofloxacin; Ciprofloxacin (Systemic); Gadobutrol; Insulin; Lumefantrine; Nilotinib; Nonsteroidal Anti-Inflammatory Agents; Probenecid; QuiNINE

Decreased Effect

Levofloxacin may decrease the levels/effects of: BCG; Mycophenolate; Sulfonylureas; Typhoid Vaccine

The levels/effects of Levofloxacin may be decreased by: Antacids; Calcium Salts; Didanosine; Iron Salts; Magnesium Salts; Quinapril; Sevelamer; Sucralfate; Zinc Salts

Food Interactions Iron and mineral supplements decrease levofloxacin concentrations

Stability Store ophthalmic solution, vial, premixed injection, tablet, and oral solution at room temperature; protect from light. Injection is stable for 72 hours when diluted to 5 mg/mL in a compatible I.V. fluid (ie, D₅W, NS, D₅W with NaCl and KCl, D₅LR) and stored at room temperature; stable for 14 days when stored under refrigeration; incompatible with mannitol, sodium bicarbonate, multivalent cations (eg, magnesium).

Mechanism of Action L-isomer of the racemate, ofloxacin, levofloxacin inhibits DNA gyrase (bacterial topoisomerase II) thereby inhibiting relaxation of supercoiled DNA and promoting breakage of DNA strands. DNA gyrase maintains the superhelical structure of DNA and is required for DNA replication, transcription, repair, recombination and transposition.

Pharmacokinetics (Adult data unless noted)

Absorption: Well absorbed; levofloxacin oral tablet and solution formulations are bioequivalent

Distribution: Widely distributed in the body including blister fluid, skin tissue, macrophages, prostate, lung tissue; excreted in breast milk

V_d: Adults: 1.25 L/kg

Protein binding: 24% to 38%

Bioavailability: Oral: 99%

Half-life: Adults: 6-8 hours

Time to peak serum concentration: Oral: Within 1-2 hours; food prolongs the time to peak by approximately 1 hour and decreases the peak concentration by 14% (tablet) or 25% (oral solution)

Elimination: 87% excreted unchanged in urine over 48 hours by tubular secretion and glomerular filtration; 4% in feces

Clearance: I.V.:

Children <5 years: 0.32 ± 0.08 L/hour/kg
Children 5-10 years: 0.25 ± 0.05 L/hour/kg
Children 10-12 years: 0.19 ± 0.05 L/hour/kg
Children 12-16 years: 0.18 ± 0.03 L/hour/kg
Adults: 0.15 ± 0.02 L/hour/kg

Dialysis: Not removed by hemodialysis or peritoneal dialysis; supplemental levofloxacin doses are not required

Usual Dosage

Oral, I.V.:

Children: **Note:** Limited information regarding levofloxacin use in pediatric patients is currently available in the literature; some centers recommend the following dose:

Children 6 months to 5 years: 10 mg/kg/dose every 12 hours

Children ≥5 years: 10 mg/kg/dose every 24 hours; maximum dose: 500 mg

Adults:

Chronic bacterial prostatitis: 500 mg every 24 hours for 28 days

Chronic bronchitis: 500 mg every 24 hours for 7 days

Community-acquired pneumonia: 500 mg every 24 hours for 7-14 days or 750 mg every 24 hours for 5 days

Nosocomial pneumonia: 750 mg every 24 hours for 7-14 days

Acute bacterial sinusitis: 500 mg every 24 hours for 10-14 days or 750 mg every 24 hours for 5 days

Complicated skin infection: 750 mg every 24 hours for 7-14 days

Uncomplicated skin infections: 500 mg every 24 hours for 7-10 days

Complicated UTI or acute pyelonephritis: 250 mg every 24 hours for 10 days or 750 mg every 24 hours for 5 days

Uncomplicated UTI: 250 mg every 24 hours for 3 days

Drug-resistant tuberculosis: 500-1000 mg every 24 hours (maximum dose: 1 g)

Travelers' diarrhea: 500 mg every 24 hours for up to 3 days

Inhalational anthrax (postexposure): 500 mg every 24 hours for 60 days beginning as soon as possible after exposure

Ophthalmic:

Children ≥1 year and Adults: Bacterial conjunctivitis: 0.5% solution:

Treatment day 1 and day 2: Instill 1-2 drops into affected eye(s) every 2 hours while awake, up to 8 times/day

Treatment day 3 through 7: Instill 1-2 drops into affected eye(s) every 4 hours while awake, up to 4 times/day

Children ≥6 years and Adults: Bacterial corneal ulcer: 1.5% solution

Treatment days 1-3: Instill 1-2 drops into affected eye(s) every 30 minutes to 2 hours while awake and ~4 and 6 hours after retiring

Treatment day 4 through treatment completion: Instill 1-2 drops into affected eye(s) every 1-4 hours while awake

Dosing interval in renal impairment: Adults:

Complicated UTI/pyelonephritis, chronic bronchitis, community-acquired pneumonia, acute maxillary sinusitis, uncomplicated skin infection, chronic bacterial prostatitis, or inhalational anthrax:

Cl$_{cr}$ 20-49 mL/minute: Administer 250 mg every 24 hours (initial dose: 500 mg)

Cl$_{cr}$ 10-19 mL/minute: Administer 250 mg every 48 hours (initial dose: 500 mg for most infections; 250 mg for UTI or pyelonephritis)

Uncomplicated UTI: No dosing adjustment required

Complicated skin infection, nosocomial pneumonia:

Cl$_{cr}$ 20-49 mL/minute: Administer 750 mg every 48 hours

Cl$_{cr}$ 10-19 mL/minute: Administer 500 mg every 48 hours (initial dose: 750 mg)

Administration

Oral: May administer levofloxacin tablets with or without food; administer levofloxacin oral solution 1 hour before or 2 hours after eating; avoid antacid use within 2 hours of administration; drink plenty of fluids to maintain proper hydration and urine output

Parenteral: I.V. infusion: Not for I.M., SubQ, or intrathecal administration; final concentration for administration should not exceed 5 mg/mL; administer by slow I.V. infusion over 60-90 minutes (250-500 mg over 60 minutes; 750 mg over 90 minutes); avoid rapid or bolus I.V. infusion due to risk of hypotension

Ophthalmic: Not for subconjunctival injection or for use into anterior chamber of the eye. Contact lenses should not be worn during treatment; instill drops into conjunctival sac of affected eye(s); apply finger pressure to lacrimal sac during and for 1-2 minutes after instillation to decrease risk of absorption and systemic effects; avoid contacting bottle tip with skin

Monitoring Parameters Patient receiving concurrent levofloxacin and theophylline should have serum levels of theophylline monitored; monitor INR in patients receiving warfarin; monitor blood glucose in patients receiving antidiabetic agents or patients with a history of diabetes; monitor renal, hepatic, and hematopoietic function periodically; number and type of stools/day for diarrhea

Test Interactions May produce false-positive urine screening results for opiates using commercially available immunoassay kits

Patient Information Drink plenty of fluids; may cause dizziness or lightheadedness and impair ability to perform activities requiring mental alertness or physical coordination. Notify physician if tendon pain or swelling occurs; palpitations, chest pain, loss of consciousness, signs of allergy, burning, tingling, numbness, or weakness develops; difficulty breathing, or if persistent diarrhea occurs. May cause photosensitivity reactions (eg, exposure to sunlight may cause severe sunburn, skin rash, redness, or itching); avoid exposure to sunlight and artificial light sources (sunlamps, tanning booth/bed); wear protective clothing, wide-brimmed hats, sunglasses, and lip sunscreen (SPF ≥15); use a sunscreen [broad-spectrum sunscreen or physical sunscreen (preferred) or sunblock with SPF ≥15]; contact physician if reaction occurs.

Nursing Implications Do not administer antacids containing calcium, aluminum, or magnesium, iron, sucralfate, multivitamin preparations with zinc, or didanosine chewable/buffered tablets or pediatric powder for oral solution with or within 2 hours before or 2 hours after a levofloxacin dose; ensure adequate patient hydration

Dosage Forms Excipient information presented when available (limited, particularly for generics); consult specific product labeling. [DSC] = Discontinued product

Infusion, premixed in D$_5$W [preservative free]:

Levaquin®: 250 mg (50 mL); 500 mg (100 mL); 750 mg (150 mL)

Injection, solution [preservative free]

Levaquin®: 25 mg/mL (20 mL, 30 mL)

Solution, ophthalmic [drops]:

Iquix®: 1.5% (5 mL)

Quixin®: 0.5% (5 mL) [contains benzalkonium chloride]

Solution, oral:

Levaquin®: 25 mg/mL (480 mL) [contains benzyl alcohol, propylene glycol]

Tablet, oral:
Levaquin®: 250 mg, 500 mg, 750 mg
Levaquin® Leva-Pak: 750 mg (5s) [DSC]
Extemporaneous Preparations A 50 mg/mL oral suspension made from tablets and two different vehicles (a 1:1 mixture of Ora-Plus® and strawberry syrup NF) was stable for 57 days when stored in amber plastic prescription bottles at room temperature (23°C to 25°C) or under refrigeration (3°C to 5°C); crush six 500 mg tablets in a mortar into a fine powder; add a small amount of the vehicle and mix well to form a uniform paste; mix while adding the vehicle in geometric proportions to **almost** 60 mL; transfer the mixture to a graduated cylinder and qsad with vehicle to make 60 mL; label "shake well."

VandenBussche HL, Johnson CE, Fontana EM, et al, "Stability of Levofloxacin in an Extemporaneously Compounded Oral Liquid," *Am J Health Syst Pharm*, 1999, 56(22):2316-8.

References
Chien S, Wells TG, Blumer JL, et al, "Levofloxacin Pharmacokinetics in Children," *J Clin Pharmacol*, 2005, 45(2):153-60.
Ernst ME, Ernst EJ, and Klepser ME, "Levofloxacin and Trovafloxacin: The Next Generation of Fluoroquinolones?" *Am J Health Syst Pharm*, 1997, 54(22):2569-84.
Schaad UB, "Role of the New Quinolones in Pediatric Practice," *Pediatr Infect Dis J*, 1992, 11(12):1043-6.

◆ **Levophed®** *see* Norepinephrine *on page 1000*
◆ **Levothroid®** *see* Levothyroxine *on page 816*

Levothyroxine (lee voe thye ROKS een)

Medication Safety Issues
Sound-alike/look-alike issues:
Levothyroxine may be confused with lamoTRIgine, Lanoxin®, levofloxacin, liothyronine
Levoxyl® may be confused with Lanoxin®, Levaquin®, Luvox®
Synthroid® may be confused with Symmetrel®

To avoid errors due to misinterpretation of a decimal point, always express dosage in mcg (**not** mg).

Significant differences exist between oral and I.V. dosing. Use caution when converting from one route of administration to another.
U.S. Brand Names Levothroid®; Levoxyl®; Synthroid®; Unithroid®
Canadian Brand Names Eltroxin®; Euthyrox; Levothyroxine Sodium; Synthroid®
Therapeutic Category Thyroid Product
Generic Available Yes
Use Replacement or supplemental therapy in congenital or acquired hypothyroidism; pituitary TSH suppression
Pregnancy Risk Factor A
Pregnancy Considerations Untreated maternal hypothyroidism may have adverse effects on fetal growth and development and is associated with higher rate of complications (spontaneous abortion, pre-eclampsia, stillbirth, premature delivery). Treatment should not be discontinued during pregnancy. TSH levels should be monitored during each trimester and 6-8 weeks postpartum. Increased doses may be needed during pregnancy.
Lactation Enters breast milk/compatible
Breast-Feeding Considerations Minimally excreted in human milk; adequate levels are needed to maintain normal lactation
Contraindications Hypersensitivity to levothyroxine sodium or any component; acute MI; thyrotoxicosis of any etiology; uncorrected adrenal insufficiency
Warnings Not for use in the treatment of obesity or for weight loss **[U.S. Boxed Warning]**; in euthyroid patients, doses within the range of daily hormonal requirements are ineffective for weight reduction; larger doses may produce serious or even life-threatening toxic effects particularly when used with some anorectic drugs (sympathomimetic amines). Overtreatment may result in craniosynostosis in infants and premature closure of epiphyses in children; monitor use closely.

Precautions Use with extreme caution in patients with cardiovascular disease, adrenal insufficiency, hypertension or coronary artery disease; patients with diabetes mellitus and insipidus may have their symptoms exaggerated or aggravated; routine use of T_4 for TSH suppression is not recommended in patients with benign thyroid nodules and should never be fully suppressive (TSH <0.1 mIU/mL) (Copper, 2006; Gharib, 2006); in the first 2 weeks of therapy, neonates and infants should be monitored for cardiac overload, arrhythmias, and aspiration from avid suckling

Adverse Reactions
Cardiovascular: Palpitations, tachycardia, cardiac arrhythmias, angina, CHF, hypertension
Central nervous system: Nervousness, insomnia, fever, headache, pseudotumor cerebri
Dermatologic: Alopecia
Endocrine & metabolic: Weight loss
Gastrointestinal: Diarrhea, abdominal cramps, appetite increased
Neuromuscular & skeletal: Tremor, slipped capital femoral epiphysis
Miscellaneous: Diaphoresis

Drug Interactions
Avoid Concomitant Use
Avoid concomitant use of Levothyroxine with any of the following: Sodium Iodide I131
Increased Effect/Toxicity
Levothyroxine may increase the levels/effects of: Vitamin K Antagonists
Decreased Effect
Levothyroxine may decrease the levels/effects of: Sodium Iodide I131; Theophylline Derivatives

The levels/effects of Levothyroxine may be decreased by: Bile Acid Sequestrants; Calcium Polystyrene Sulfonate; Calcium Salts; CarBAMazepine; Estrogen Derivatives; Iron Salts; Orlistat; Phenytoin; Raloxifene; Rifampin; Sevelamer; Sodium Polystyrene Sulfonate; Sucralfate

Food Interactions Limit intake of goitrogenic foods (asparagus, cabbage, peas, turnip greens, broccoli, spinach, brussel sprouts, lettuce, soybeans); soybean-based formulas, cottonseed meal, walnuts, and dietary fiber may decrease absorption

Stability Store at room temperature; protect from light and moisture; I.V. form must be administered immediately after preparation

Mechanism of Action Primary active compound is T_3 (triiodothyronine), which may be converted from T_4 (thyroxine) by deiodination in liver and peripheral tissues; exact mechanism of action is unknown; however, it is believed the thyroid hormone exerts its many metabolic effects through control of DNA transcription and protein synthesis; involved in normal metabolism, growth, and development; promotes gluconeogenesis, increases utilization and mobilization of glycogen stores, and stimulates protein synthesis, increases basal metabolic rate

Pharmacodynamics
Onset of action:
Oral: 3-5 days for therapeutic effects
I.V.: Within 6-8 hours
Maximum effect: 4-6 weeks

Pharmacokinetics (Adult data unless noted)
Absorption: Oral: Erratic (40% to 80%); decreases with age
Protein binding: >99%

Metabolism: In the liver and other peripheral sites by deiodination to triiodothyronine (active) T_3

Half-life: 6-7 days

Time to peak serum concentration: Within 2-4 hours

Elimination: Thyroid hormones are eliminated primarily in urine with 20% of T_4 excreted in feces

Usual Dosage

Neonates, Infants, and Children: Daily dosage:

Oral:

0-3 months: 10-15 mcg/kg; if the infant is at risk for development of cardiac failure use a lower starting dose ~25 mcg/day; if the initial serum T_4 is very low (<5 mcg/dL) begin treatment at a higher dosage ~50 mcg/day

3-6 months: 8-10 mcg/kg or 25-50 mcg

6-12 months: 6-8 mcg/kg or 50-75 mcg

1-5 years: 5-6 mcg/kg or 75-100 mcg

6-12 years: 4-5 mcg/kg or 100-125 mcg

12 years: 2-3 mcg/kg or ≥150 mcg

Growth and puberty complete: 1.7 mcg/kg

Note: Hyperactivity in older children may be minimized by starting at one-quarter of the recommended dose and increasing each week by that amount until the full dose is achieved (4 weeks).

Note: Children with severe or chronic hypothyroidism should be started at 25 mcg/day; adjust dose by 25 mcg every 2-4 weeks.

I.V., I.M.: 50% to 75% of the oral dose

Adults:

Hypothyroidism:

Oral: 1.7 mcg/kg/day or 100-200 mcg/day; if severe hypothyroidism, use 12.5-50 mcg/day to start, then increase by 25 mcg/day at intervals of 2-4 weeks

I.V., I.M.: 50% of the oral dose

Subclinical hypothyroidism (if treated): Oral: 1 mcg/kg

Myxedema coma or stupor: I.V.: 200-500 mcg one time, then 75-300 mcg daily; due to potential poor absorption of oral levothyroxine, avoid oral use in acute treatment

TSH suppression:

Well-differentiated thyroid cancer: Highly individualized; doses >2 mcg/kg/day may be needed to suppress TSH to <0.1 mIU/mL. High-risk tumors may need a target level of <0.01 mIU/mL for TSH suppression.

Benign nodules and nontoxic multinodular goiter: Routine use of T_4 for TSH suppression is not recommended in patients with benign thyroid nodules. In patients deemed appropriate candidates, treatment should never be fully suppressive (TSH <0.1 mIU/mL) (Cooper, 2006; Gharib, 2006); **Note:** Avoid use if TSH is already suppressed.

Administration

Oral: Administer on an empty stomach; 1-1.5 hours prior to breakfast

Parenteral: Dilute vial with 5 mL NS; use immediately after reconstitution; administer by direct I.V. infusion over 2- to 3-minute period; may administer I.M.

Monitoring Parameters T_4, TSH, heart rate, blood pressure, clinical signs of hypo- and hyperthyroidism; growth, bone development (children); TSH is the most reliable guide for evaluating adequacy of thyroid replacement dosage. TSH may be elevated during the first few months of thyroid replacement despite patients being clinically euthyroid. In cases where T_4 remains low and TSH is within normal limits, an evaluation of "free" (unbound) T_4 is needed to evaluate further increase in dosage.

In congenital hypothyroidism, adequacy of replacement should be determined using both TSH and total- or free-T_4. During the first 3 years of life, total- or free-T_4 should be maintained in the upper 1/2 of the normal range; this should result in normalization of the TSH. In some patients, TSH

may not normalize due to a resetting of the pituitary-thyroid feedback as a result of *in utero* hypothyroidism.

Suggested frequency for monitoring thyroid function tests in children: Every 1-2 months during the first year of life, every 2-3 months between ages 1-3 years, and every 3-12 months thereafter until growth is completed; repeat tests two weeks after any change in dosage.

Reference Range See normal values in Normal Laboratory Values for Children on page 1672

Test Interactions Many drugs may have effects on thyroid function tests: para-aminosalicylic acid, aminoglutethimide, amiodarone, barbiturates, carbamazepine, chloral hydrate, clofibrate, colestipol, corticosteroids, danazol, diazepam, estrogens, ethionamide, fluorouracil, I.V. heparin, insulin, lithium, methadone, methimazole, mitotane, nitroprusside, oxyphenbutazone, phenylbutazone, PTU, perphenazine, phenytoin, propranolol, salicylates, sulfonylureas, and thiazides

Patient Information Do not change brands without physician's knowledge; report immediately to physician any chest pain, increased pulse, palpitations, heat intolerances, excessive sweating; do not discontinue without notifying physician

Additional Information 15-37.5 mcg liothyronine = 50-60 mcg levothyroxine = 60 mg thyroid USP = 45 mg Thyroid Strong® = 60 mg thyroglobulin = 50-60 mcg liotrix

Dosage Forms Excipient information presented when available (limited, particularly for generics); consult specific product labeling.

Injection, powder for reconstitution, as sodium: 0.2 mg, 0.5 mg

Tablet, as sodium: 25 mcg, 50 mcg, 75 mcg, 88 mcg, 100 mcg, 112 mcg, 125 mcg, 137 mcg, 150 mcg, 175 mcg, 200 mcg, 300 mcg

Levothroid®: 25 mcg, 75 mcg, 88 mcg, 100 mcg, 112 mcg, 125 mcg, 137 mcg, 150 mcg, 175 mcg, 200 mcg, 300 mcg [scored]

Levothroid®: 50 mcg [scored; dye free]

Levoxyl®: 25 mcg, 75 mcg, 88 mcg, 100 mcg, 112 mcg, 125 mcg, 137 mcg, 150 mcg, 175 mcg, 200 mcg [scored]

Levoxyl®: 50 mcg [scored; dye free]

Synthroid®: 25 mcg, 75 mcg, 88 mcg, 100 mcg, 112 mcg, 125 mcg, 137 mcg, 150 mcg, 175 mcg, 200 mcg, 300 mcg [scored]

Synthroid®: 50 mcg [scored; dye free]

Unithroid®: 25 mcg, 75 mcg, 88 mcg, 100 mcg, 112 mcg, 125 mcg, 150 mcg, 175 mcg, 200 mcg, 300 mcg [scored]

Unithroid®: 50 mcg [scored; dye free]

Extemporaneous Preparations A 25 mcg/mL extemporaneous suspension may be compounded by crushing twenty-five 0.1 mg tablets; measure 40 mL glycerol; triturate powder into a pourable suspension with a small amount of glycerol and transfer to a calibrated 100 mL amber bottle; rinse the mortar with about 10 mL of the glycerol and pour into the bottle; repeat until the glycerol is used up; add water to bring the oral liquid to a total volume of 100 mL; label "shake well" and "refrigerate." The suspension is stable 8 days refrigerated.

Boulton DV, Fawcett JP, and Woods DJ, "Stability of an Extemporaneously Compounded Levothyroxine Sodium Oral Liquid," *Am J Health-Syst Pharm*, 1996; 53:1157-61.

References

Cooper DS, Doherty GM, Haugen BR, et al, "Management Guidelines for Patients With Thyroid Nodules and Differentiated Thyroid Cancer," *Thyroid*, 2006, 16(2):109-42.

de Groot JW, Zonnenberg BA, Plukker JT, et al, "Imatinib Induces Hypothyroidism in Patients Receiving Levothyroxine," *Clin Pharmacol Ther*, 2005, 78(4):433-8.

Gharib H, Papini E, Valcavi R, et al, "American Association of Clinical Endocrinologists and Associazione Medici Endocrinologi Medical Guidelines for Clinical Practice for the Diagnosis and Management of Thyroid Nodules," Endocr Pract, 2006, 12(1):63-102.

◆ **Levothyroxine Sodium** see Levothyroxine on page 816

◆ **Levoxyl®** see Levothyroxine on page 816

◆ **Levsin®** see Hyoscyamine on page 699

◆ **Levsin®/SL** see Hyoscyamine on page 699

◆ **Lexapro®** see Escitalopram on page 529

◆ **Lexiva®** see Fosamprenavir on page 623

◆ *l*-**Hyoscyamine Sulfate** see Hyoscyamine on page 699

◆ **Lialda™** see Mesalamine on page 887

◆ **LidaMantle®** see Lidocaine on page 818

◆ **Lidemol® (Can)** see Fluocinonide on page 595

◆ **Lidex** see Fluocinonide on page 595

◆ **Lidex® (Can)** see Fluocinonide on page 595

Lidocaine (LYE doe kane)

Medication Safety Issues

High alert medication: The Institute for Safe Medication Practices (ISMP) includes this medication (epidural administration; I.V. formulation) among its list of drugs which have a heightened risk of causing significant patient harm when used in error.

Transdermal patch may contain conducting metal (eg, aluminum); remove patch prior to MRI.

International issues:
  Lidpen® may be confused with Linoten® which is a brand name for pamidronate in Spain

Related Information

Adult ACLS Algorithms on page 1463
CPR Pediatric Drug Dosages on page 1455
Emergency Pediatric Drip Calculations on page 1457
Pediatric ALS Algorithms on page 1460

U.S. Brand Names Akten™; Anestacon® [DSC]; Anestafoam™ [OTC]; Band-Aid® Hurt-Free™ Antiseptic Wash [OTC]; Burn Jel® Plus [OTC]; Burn Jel® [OTC]; Burn-O-Jel [OTC]; L-M-X® 4 [OTC]; L-M-X® 5 [OTC]; LidaMantle®; Lidoderm®; LTA® 360; Premjact® [OTC]; Regenecare®; Regenecare® HA [OTC]; Solarcaine® Aloe Extra Burn Relief [OTC] [DSC]; Solarcaine® cool aloe Burn Relief [OTC]; Topicaine® [OTC]; Unburn®; Xylocaine®; Xylocaine® Dental; Xylocaine® MPF; Xylocaine® Viscous [DSC]

Canadian Brand Names Betacaine®; Lidodan™; Lidoderm®; Maxilene®; Xylocaine®; Xylocard®

Therapeutic Category Analgesic, Topical; Antiarrhythmic Agent, Class I-B; Local Anesthetic, Injectable; Local Anesthetic, Ophthalmic; Local Anesthetic, Topical; Local Anesthetic, Transdermal

Generic Available Yes: Infusion, injection, jelly, ointment, solution

Use

Injection: Treatment of ventricular arrhythmias (FDA approved in adults); local or regional anesthetic [FDA approved in pediatric patients (age not specified) and adults]

Topical: Local anesthetic for dermal, dental, and ophthalmic procedures [FDA approved in adults, refer to product specific information regarding FDA approval in pediatric patients]

Transdermal: Pain relief of postherpetic neuralgia (FDA approved in adults)

PALS guidelines recommend lidocaine as an alternative to amiodarone for cardiac arrest with pulseless VT or VF (unresponsive to defibrillation, CPR, and vasopressor administration); consider in patients with cocaine overdose to prevent arrhythmias secondary to MI

ACLS guidelines recommend lidocaine as an alternative to amiodarone for cardiac arrest with pulseless VT or VF (unresponsive to defibrillation, CPR, and vasopressor administration); it is not considered to be the drug of choice but may be considered for stable monomorphic VT (in patients with preserved ventricular function) and for polymorphic VT (with normal baseline or prolonged QT interval).

Pregnancy Risk Factor B

Pregnancy Considerations Animal studies with lidocaine have not shown teratogenic effects. Lidocaine and the MEGX metabolite cross the placenta. Use is not contraindicated during labor and delivery. Topical lidocaine is used locally to provide analgesia prior to episiotomy and during repair of obstetric lacerations. Administration by the perineal route may result in greater absorption than administration by the epidural route. Adverse events have been reported in the infant following maternal administration, however, when used in appropriate doses, the risk to the fetus is low. Cumulative exposure from all routes of administration should be considered.

Lactation Enters breast milk/use caution (AAP rates "compatible")

Breast-Feeding Considerations Small amounts of lidocaine and the MEGX metabolite are found in breast milk. The actual amount may depend on route and duration of administration. When administered topically at recommended doses, the amount of lidocaine available to the nursing infant would not be expected to cause adverse events. Cumulative exposure from all routes of administration should be considered.

Contraindications Hypersensitivity to lidocaine, amide-type local anesthetics, or any component (see Warnings); patients with Adams-Stokes syndrome, Wolff-Parkinson-White syndrome, or with severe degree of S-A, A-V, or intraventricular heart block (without a pacemaker)

Warnings Decrease dose in patients with decreased cardiac output or hepatic disease; do not use lidocaine solutions containing epinephrine for treatment of arrhythmias; do not use preservative-containing solution for epidural, spinal, or I.V. administration.

Topical anesthetic use prior to cosmetic or other medical procedures can result in high systemic levels and lead to toxic effects (eg, arrhythmias, methemoglobinemia, seizures, coma, respiratory depression, and death). Children may be at an increased risk for adverse effects. Toxic effects may occur, particularly when topical anesthetics are applied in large amounts or to large areas of the skin; left on for long periods of time; used with materials, wraps, or dressings to cover the skin after application; or applied to broken skin, rashes, or areas of skin irritation. These practices may increase the degree of systemic absorption and should be avoided. Consumers should consult their healthcare provider for instructions on safe use prior to applying topical anesthetics for medical or cosmetic purposes. Use a product with the lowest amount of anesthetic and apply the least amount possible to relieve pain. Some topical products are not recommended for use on otic or mucous membranes; specific product labeling should be consulted. Ophthalmic gel is for topical ophthalmic use only; not for injection; prolonged use may cause permanent corneal ulceration and/or opacification with loss of vision.

Safety and efficacy of transdermal patch have not been established in pediatric patients. Transdermal patches (both used and unused) may cause toxicities in children; used patches still contain large amounts of lidocaine; store and dispose patches out of the reach of children. Applying the transdermal patch to larger areas, for longer than recommended, or to broken or inflamed skin may result in increased absorption, high serum concentrations, and serious adverse effects; apply transdermal patch to intact skin only. Do not expose transdermal patch application site to external heat sources (eg, electric blankets, heating pads, heated water beds, heat lamps, tanning lamps, hot tubs, hot baths, saunas, sunbathing); although not evaluated, temperature-dependent increases in drug released from patch may occur. Transdermal patch may contain conducting metal (eg, aluminum) which may cause a burn to the skin during an MRI scan; remove patch prior to MRI; reapply patch after scan is completed. Due to the potential for altered electrical conductivity, remove transdermal patch before cardioversion or defibrillation.

Chondrolysis (necrosis and destruction of cartilage) has been reported following continuous intra-articular infusion of local anesthetics for extended periods of time (48-72 hours); patients presented as early as 2 months following the infusion with joint pain, stiffness, and loss of motion; more than 50% of patients required additional surgery, including arthroscopy or joint replacement; intra-articular administration of local anesthetics is not an FDA-approved route of administration.

Premixed infusions containing dextrose may cause hypersensitivity reactions in patients allergic to corn or corn products; some products contain tartrazine, benzyl alcohol, or bisulfites (consult specific product information) which may cause allergic reactions in susceptible individuals; large amounts of benzyl alcohol (≥99 mg/kg/day) have been associated with a potentially fatal toxicity ("gasping syndrome") in neonates; the "gasping syndrome" consists of metabolic acidosis, respiratory distress, gasping respirations, CNS dysfunction (including convulsions, intracranial hemorrhage), hypotension and cardiovascular collapse; avoid use of lidocaine products containing benzyl alcohol in neonates; *in vitro* and animal studies have shown that benzoate, a metabolite of benzyl alcohol, displaces bilirubin from protein-binding sites.

Precautions Use with caution in patients with hepatic disease, heart failure, marked hypoxia, severe respiratory depression, hypovolemia, or shock; incomplete heart block or bradycardia, atrial fibrillation; pseudocholinesterase deficiency

Adverse Reactions Adverse effects vary with route of administration and many are dose-related.

Cardiovascular: Arrhythmias, bradycardia, cardiovascular collapse, heart block, hypotension

Central nervous system: Agitation, anxiety, coma, confusion, euphoria, hallucinations, headache, lethargy, seizures, slurred speech

Dermatologic: Angioedema, bruising, contact dermatitis, edema, petechia, pruritus, rash

Transdermal patch: Depigmentation

Gastrointestinal: Nausea, vomiting

Local: Thrombophlebitis

Transdermal patch: Abnormal sensation, edema, erythema

Neuromuscular & skeletal: Chondrolysis (with continuous intra-articular administration; see Warnings), muscle twitching, paresthesia

Ocular: Blurred vision, diplopia

Ophthalmic gel: Burning upon instillation, conjunctival hyperemia, corneal epithelial changes; prolonged use may result in permanent corneal opacification, ulceration, and vision loss

Respiratory: Dyspnea, respiratory depression or arrest

Miscellaneous: Allergic and anaphylactoid reactions (rare)

Drug Interactions

Metabolism/Transport Effects Substrate of CYP1A2 (minor), CYP2A6 (minor), CYP2B6 (minor), CYP2C9 (minor), CYP2D6 (major), CYP3A4 (major), P-glycoprotein; **Inhibits** CYP1A2 (strong), 2D6 (moderate), 3A4 (moderate)

Avoid Concomitant Use

Avoid concomitant use of Lidocaine with any of the following: Thioridazine; Tolvaptan

Increased Effect/Toxicity

Lidocaine may increase the levels/effects of: Bendamustine; Colchicine; CYP1A2 Substrates; CYP2D6 Substrates; CYP3A4 Substrates; Eplerenone; Everolimus; Fesoterodine; Halofantrine; Pimecrolimus; Ranolazine; Salmeterol; Saxagliptin; Tamoxifen; Thioridazine; Tolvaptan

The levels/effects of Lidocaine may be increased by: Amiodarone; Beta-Blockers; CYP2D6 Inhibitors (Moderate); CYP2D6 Inhibitors (Strong); CYP3A4 Inhibitors (Moderate); CYP3A4 Inhibitors (Strong); Darunavir; Dasatinib; Disopyramide; P-Glycoprotein Inhibitors

Decreased Effect

Lidocaine may decrease the levels/effects of: TraMADol

The levels/effects of Lidocaine may be decreased by: CYP3A4 Inducers (Strong); Deferasirox; Herbs (CYP3A4 Inducers); Peginterferon Alfa-2b; P-Glycoprotein Inducers

Stability

Injection: Store at room temperature. Stability of parenteral admixture at room temperature (25°C): Use the expiration date on premixed bag; once out of overwrap, stability is 30 days.

Jelly: Store at controlled room temperature at 20°C to 25°C (68°F to 77°F)

Ophthalmic: Store at 15°C to 25°C (59°F to 77°F). Protect from light. Discard after use.

Transdermal System: Store at controlled room temperature of 25°C (77°F)

Mechanism of Action Class IB antiarrhythmic; suppresses automaticity of conduction tissue by increasing electrical stimulation threshold of ventricle, His-Purkinje system, and spontaneous depolarization of the ventricles during diastole by a direct action on the tissues; blocks both the initiation and conduction of nerve impulses by decreasing the neuronal membrane's permeability to sodium ions, which results in inhibition of depolarization with resultant blockade of conduction

Pharmacodynamics

Antiarrhythmic effect:

Onset of action (single I.V. bolus dose): 45-90 seconds

Duration: 10-20 minutes

Local anesthetic effect:

Onset of action:

Ophthalmic: 20 seconds to 5 minutes (median: 40 seconds)

Topical: (Jelly): 3-5 minutes

Duration: 1-2 hours; Ophthalmic: 5-30 minutes (mean: 15 minutes)

Pharmacokinetics (Adult data unless noted)

Absorption: Transdermal system: Adults: 3% ± 2% is expected to be absorbed with recommended doses

Distribution: Crosses blood-brain and placental barriers; distributes into breast milk; breast milk to plasma ratio: 0.4

V_d: Adults: 1.5 ± 0.6 L/kg; range: 0.7-2.7 L/kg; V_d alterable by many patient factors; decreased in CHF and liver disease

Protein binding: 60% to 80%; binds to alpha$_1$-acid glycoprotein

Metabolism: 90% in the liver; active metabolites monoethylglycinexylidide (MEGX) and glycinexylidide (GX) can accumulate and may cause CNS toxicity

819

Half-life, biphasic:
Alpha: 7-30 minutes
Beta, terminal: Infants, premature: 3.2 hours; Adults: 1.5-2 hours
CHF, liver disease, shock, severe renal disease: Prolonged half-life
Elimination: <10% excreted unchanged in urine; ~90% as metabolite
Dialysis: Dialyzable (0% to 5%)

Usual Dosage
Antiarrhythmic:
Children (PALS 2005 Guidelines):
I.V., I.O.: (**Note:** For use in pulseless VT or VF; give after defibrillation and epinephrine): Loading dose: 1 mg/kg/dose (maximum: 100 mg/dose); follow with continuous infusion; may administer second bolus of 0.5-1 mg/kg/dose if delay between bolus and start of infusion is >15 minutes; continuous infusion: 20-50 mcg/kg/minute. Use 20 mcg/kg/minute in patients with shock, hepatic disease, cardiac arrest, mild CHF; moderate-to-severe CHF may require 1/2 loading dose and lower infusion rates to avoid toxicity.
E.T.: 2-3 mg/kg/dose; flush with 5 mL of NS and follow with 5 assisted manual ventilations
Adults (decrease the dose in patients with CHF, acute MI with hypotension, shock, poor peripheral perfusion states, or hepatic disease; usual bolus dose, but 1/2 of normal maintenance infusion should be used in these patients):
I.V.:
Antiarrhythmic: Initial bolus: 1-1.5 mg/kg/dose; may repeat doses of 0.5-0.75 mg/kg/dose every 5-10 minutes if needed to a total of 3 mg/kg; continuous infusion: Initial: 1-4 mg/minute
Ventricular fibrillation or pulseless VT (after defibrillation and epinephrine or vasopressin) (ACLS 2005 guidelines): Initial dose: I.V./I.O.: 1-1.5 mg/kg/dose; may repeat 0.5-0.75 mg/kg/dose at 5-10 minute intervals; maximum total dose: 3 mg/kg; follow with continuous I.V. infusion after return of perfusion; continuous I.V. infusion: 1-4 mg/minute; **Note:** Use only bolus doses for cardiac arrest caused by VF or pulseless VT.
Patients with impaired cardiac function: Initial bolus: 0.5-0.75 mg/kg/dose IVP; may repeat every 5-10 minutes; follow with continuous infusion: Initial: 1-4 mg/minute; maximum total dose: 3 mg/kg (administered over 1 hour)
Prevention of ventricular fibrillation: I.V.: Initial bolus: 0.5 mg/kg/dose; repeat every 5-10 minutes to a total dose of 2 mg/kg
E.T.: (loading dose only): 2-2.5 times the I.V. bolus dose; dilute in 10 mL NS or distilled water
I.M.: Prehospital post-MI antiarrhythmic prophylaxis: 300 mg
Anesthesia, local injectable: Children and Adults: Dose varies with procedure, degree of anesthesia needed, vascularity of tissue, duration of anesthesia required, and physical condition of patient; maximum dose: 4.5 mg/kg; do not repeat within 2 hours.
Anesthesia, ocular: Ophthalmic gel (Akten™): Children and Adults: Apply 2 drops to ocular surface in area where procedure to occur; may reapply to maintain effect.
Anesthetic, topical: Note: Unless otherwise noted, the following traditional pediatric guideline for topical lidocaine dosage may be observed: Apply to affected area as needed; maximum dose: 3 mg/kg/dose; do not repeat within 2 hours (see Benitz, 1988).
Cream:
LidaMantle®: Skin irritation: Children and Adults: Apply a thin film to affected area 2-3 times/day as needed; reduce dose in pediatric patients according to age, body weight, and physical condition

L-M-X™ 4: Children ≥2 years and Adults: Apply 1/4 inch thick layer to intact skin. Leave on until adequate anesthetic effect is obtained. Remove cream and cleanse area before beginning procedure.
L-M-X™ 5: Children ≥12 years and Adults: Rectal: Apply topically to clean, dry area **or** using applicator, insert rectally, up to 6 times/day for anorectal pain and itching
Gel, ointment, solution: Adults: Apply to affected area ≤3 times/day as needed (maximum dose: 4.5 mg/kg, not to exceed 300 mg)
Jelly:
Children: Dose varies with age and weight; maximum dose: 4.5 mg/kg
Adults: Maximum dose: 30 mL (600 mg) in any 12-hour period
Anesthesia urethra: Male: 5-30 mL; Female: 3-5 mL
Lubrication of endotracheal tube: Apply a moderate amount to external surface only.
Transdermal (Lidoderm® patch): Adults: Postherpetic neuralgia: Apply patch to most painful areas; up to 3 patches may be applied per application; patch may remain in place for up to 12 hours in any 24-hour period

Administration
Endotracheal:
Children: Flush with 5 mL of NS after E.T. administration; follow with 5 assisted manual ventilations
Adults: Dilute in 10 mL NS or distilled water prior to E.T. administration (**Note:** Use of distilled water results in greater absorption, but a greater adverse effect on PaO_2)
Parenteral: I.V.: Solutions of 40-200 mg/mL must be diluted for I.V. use; final concentration not to exceed 20 mg/mL for I.V. push or 8 mg/mL for I.V. infusion; I.V. push rate of administration should not exceed 0.7 mg/minute or 50 mg/minute, whichever is less; I.V. continuous infusion must be administered with a calibrated infusion device
Transdermal: Apply patch to intact skin so most painful area is covered; do not apply to broken or inflamed skin. Patch may be cut to appropriate size prior to removal of release liner. Remove immediately if burning sensation occurs. Wash hands after applying patch; avoid eye contact. Avoid exposing application site to external heat sources (eg, electric blankets, heating pads, heated water beds, heat lamps, tanning lamps, hot tubs, hot baths, saunas, sunbathing). Keep used and unused patches out of the reach of children (see Warnings); fold used patch so adhesive side sticks to itself; dispose of used patch properly.
Monitoring Parameters Monitor ECG continuously; serum concentrations with continuous infusion; I.V. site (local thrombophlebitis may occur with prolonged infusions)

Reference Range
Therapeutic: 1.5-5 mcg/mL (SI: 6-21 micromoles/L)
Potentially toxic: >6 mcg/mL (SI: >26 micromoles/L)
Toxic: >9 mcg/mL (SI: >38 micromoles/L)

Patient Information
I.V. infusions: Report dizziness, numbness, double vision, nausea, pain or burning at infusion site, or respiratory difficulty immediately to your healthcare provider.
Dental/local anesthesia: Avoid eating or drinking for 1 hour after use because some numbness of the tongue and throat may occur. Begin with small sips of water to ensure swallowing without difficulty. Immediately report swelling of face, lips, or tongue.
Topical/cosmetic procedures: The FDA recommends checking with your healthcare provider prior to administration of product to ensure proper technique; may cause decreased sensation to pain, heat, or cold in the area and/or decreased muscle strength (depending on area of application) until effects wear off; use necessary

caution to reduce incidence of possible injury until full sensation returns. Report irritation, pain, persistent numbness, tingling, or swelling; restlessness, dizziness, or acute weakness; blurred vision; ringing in ears; or respiratory difficulty to your healthcare provider.

Transdermal patch: Patch may be cut to appropriate size. Remove immediately if burning sensation occurs. Wash hands after application. Keep used and unused patches out of the reach of children; used patches still contain large amounts of lidocaine; fold used patch so adhesive side sticks to itself; dispose of used patch properly and out of the reach of children.

Nursing Implications Multiple products and concentrations exist; use of an I.V. fluid filter is recommended where possible

Additional Information A needle-free powder lidocaine intradermal delivery system (Zingo®) was withdrawn from the market in November 2008 due to nonsafety issues; the company does not plan to market this product in the future.

Dosage Forms Excipient information presented when available (limited, particularly for generics); consult specific product labeling. [DSC] = Discontinued product

Aerosol, topical [foam]:
Anestafoam™: 4% (30 g) [contains benzalkonium chloride and benzyl alcohol]

Aerosol, topical [spray]:
Solarcaine® cool aloe Burn Relief: 0.5% (127 g) [contains aloe, vitamin E]

Cream, rectal:
L-M-X® 5: 5% (15 g, 30 g) [contains benzyl alcohol]

Cream, topical:
L-M-X® 4: 4% (5 g, 15 g, 30 g) [contains benzyl alcohol]

Cream, topical, as hydrochloride:
LidaMantle®: 3% (85 g)

Gel, ophthalmic, as hydrochloride [preservative free]:
Akten™: 3.5% (5 mL)

Gel, topical:
Burn-O-Jel: 0.5% (90 g)
Topicaine®: 4% (10 g, 30 g, 113 g); 5% (10 g, 30 g, 113 g) [contains aloe vera, benzyl alcohol, ethanol 35%, and jojoba]

Gel, topical, as hydrochloride:
Burn Jel®: 2% (3.5 g, 60 mL, 120 mL)
Burn Jel Plus: 2.5% (118 mL) [contains vitamin E]
Regenecare®: 2% (14 g, 85 g) [contains aloe, calcium alginate]
Regenecare® HA: 2% (85 g) [contains aloe, hyaluronic acid]
Solarcaine® Aloe Extra Burn Relief: 0.5% (113 g, 226 g) [contains aloe vera gel and tartrazine] [DSC]
Solarcaine® cool aloe Burn Relief: 0.5% (113 g, 226 g) [contains aloe, isopropyl alcohol, menthol, tartrazine]
Unburn®: 2.5% (59 mL) [contains vitamin E]

Infusion, premixed in D5, as hydrochloride: 0.4% [4 mg/mL] (250 mL, 500 mL); 0.8% [8 mg/mL] (250 mL, 500 mL)

Injection, solution, as hydrochloride: 0.5% [5 mg/mL] (50 mL); 1% [10 mg/mL] (2 mL, 10 mL, 20 mL, 30 mL, 50 mL); 2% [20 mg/mL] (2 mL, 5 mL, 20 mL, 50 mL)
Xylocaine®: 0.5% [5 mg/mL] (50 mL); 1% [10 mg/mL] (10 mL, 20 mL, 50 mL); 2% [20 mg/mL] (10 mL, 20 mL, 50 mL) [contains methylparaben]

Injection, solution, as hydrochloride [for dental use]:
Xylocaine® Dental: 2% [20 mg/mL] (1.8 mL)

Injection, solution, premixed in D7.5, as hydrochloride [preservative free]: 5% [50 mg/mL] (2 mL) [DSC]

Injection, solution, as hydrochloride [preservative free]: 0.5% [5 mg/mL] (50 mL); 1% [10 mg/mL] (2 mL, 5 mL, 30 mL); 1.5% [15 mg/mL] (20 mL); 2% [20 mg/mL] (2 mL, 5 mL, 10 mL); 4% [40 mg/mL] (5 mL)
Xylocaine®: 2% [20 mg/mL] (5 mL)

Xylocaine® MPF: 0.5% [5 mg/mL] (50 mL); 1% [10 mg/mL] (2 mL, 5 mL, 10 mL, 30 mL); 1.5% [15 mg/mL] (10 mL, 20 mL); 2% [20 mg/mL] (2 mL, 5 mL, 10 mL); 4% [40 mg/mL] (5 mL)

Jelly, topical, as hydrochloride: 2% (5 mL, 30 mL)
Anestacon®: 2% (15 mL) [contains benzalkonium chloride] [DSC]
Xylocaine®: 2% (5 mL, 30 mL)

Jelly, topical, as hydrochloride [preservative free]: 2% (5 mL, 10 mL, 20 mL)

Lotion, topical, as hydrochloride:
LidaMantle®: 3% (177 mL)

Ointment, topical: 5% (30 g [DSC], 35.4 g, 50 g [DSC])

Patch, transdermal:
Lidoderm®: 5% (30s)

Solution, topical, as hydrochloride: 4% [40 mg/mL] (50 mL)
Band-Aid® Hurt-Free™ Antiseptic Wash: 2% [20 mg/mL] (180 mL)
LTA® 360: 4% [40 mg/mL] (4 mL) [packaged with cannula for laryngotracheal administration]
Xylocaine®: 4% [40 mg/mL] (50 mL)

Solution, topical, as hydrochloride [preservative free]: 4% [40 mg/mL] (4 mL)

Solution, topical [spray]:
Premjact®: 9.6% (13 mL)
Solarcaine® Aloe Extra Burn Relief: 0.5% (127 g) [contains aloe vera] [DSC]

Solution, viscous, oral, as hydrochloride: 2% [20 mg/mL] (20 mL, 100 mL)
Xylocaine® Viscous: 2% [20 mg/mL] (100 mL) [DSC]

References

American Heart Association Emergency Cardiovascular Care Committee," 2005 American Heart Association (AHA) Guidelines for Cardiopulmonary Resuscitation (CPR) and Emergency Cardiovascular Care (ECC), Part 7.2: Management of Cardiac Arrest, Part 7.3: Management of Symptomatic Bradycardia and Tachycardia, and Part 12: Pediatric Advanced Life Support," *Circulation*, 2005, 112(24 Suppl):IV58-77,167-87.

Benitz WE and Tatro DS, "The Pediatric Drug Handbook," 2nd edition, Year Book Medical Publishers, Inc, 1988.

Busbee BG, Alam A, and Reichel E, "Lidocaine Hydrochloride Gel for Ocular Anesthesia: Results of a Prospective, Randomized Study," *Ophthalmic Surg Lasers Imaging*, 2008, 39(5):386-90.

Lidocaine and Epinephrine

(LYE doe kane & ep i NEF rin)

Medication Safety Issues
Transdermal patch may contain conducting metal (eg, aluminum); remove patch prior to MRI.

U.S. Brand Names LidoSite™ [DSC]; Lignospan® Forte; Lignospan® Standard; Xylocaine® MPF With Epinephrine; Xylocaine® With Epinephrine

Canadian Brand Names Xylocaine® With Epinephrine

Therapeutic Category Local Anesthetic, Injectable

Generic Available Yes: Excludes transdermal system

Use Local infiltration anesthesia [FDA approved in pediatric patients (age not specified) and adults]

Pregnancy Risk Factor B

Pregnancy Considerations See individual agents.

Lactation Lidocaine enters breast milk/use caution

Breast-Feeding Considerations Refer to Lidocaine monograph.

Contraindications Hypersensitivity to epinephrine, lidocaine, amide-type local anesthetics, or any component (see Warnings)

Warnings Topical anesthetic use prior to cosmetic or other medical procedures can result in high systemic levels and lead to toxic effects (eg, arrhythmias, methemoglobinemia, seizures, coma, respiratory depression, and death). Children may be at an increased risk for adverse effects. Toxic effects may occur, particularly when topical anesthetics are applied in large amounts or to large areas of the skin; left on for long periods of time; used with materials, wraps, or dressings to cover the skin after application; or applied to broken skin, rashes, or areas of skin irritation. These practices may increase the degree of systemic absorption and should be avoided. Consumers should consult their healthcare provider for instructions on safe use, prior to applying topical anesthetics for medical or cosmetic purposes. Use a product with the lowest amount of anesthetic and apply the least amount possible to relieve pain. Some topical products are not recommended for use on otic or mucous membranes; specific product labeling should be consulted.

Chondrolysis (necrosis and destruction of cartilage) has been reported following continuous intra-articular infusion of local anesthetics for extended periods of time (48-72 hours); patients presented as early as 2 months following the infusion with joint pain, stiffness, and loss of motion; more than 50% of patients required additional surgery, including arthroscopy or joint replacement; intra-articular administration of local anesthetics is not an FDA-approved route of administration.

Transdermal patch may contain conducting metal (eg, aluminum) which may cause a burn to the skin during an MRI scan; remove patch prior to MRI; reapply patch after scan is completed. Due to the potential for altered electrical conductivity, remove transdermal patch before cardioversion or defibrillation. Some products contain sodium or potassium metabisulfite which may cause allergic reactions in susceptible individuals.

Precautions Do not use solutions in distal portions of the body (digits, nose, ears, penis); do not use large doses in patients with conduction defects (ie, heart block)

Adverse Reactions

Cardiovascular: Bradycardia, hypotension

Central nervous system: Confusion, convulsions, dizziness, drowsiness, lightheadedness, nervousness

Dermatologic: Urticaria

Neuromuscular & skeletal: Chondrolysis (with continuous intra-articular administration; see Warnings), tremor

Ocular: Blurred vision

Otic: Tinnitus

Drug Interactions

Metabolism/Transport Effects Lidocaine: **Substrate** of CYP1A2 (minor), CYP2A6 (minor), CYP2B6 (minor), CYP2C9 (minor), CYP2D6 (major), CYP3A4 (major), P-glycoprotein; **Inhibits** CYP1A2 (strong), 2D6 (moderate), 3A4 (moderate)

Avoid Concomitant Use

Avoid concomitant use of Lidocaine and Epinephrine with any of the following: Iobenguane I 123

Increased Effect/Toxicity

Lidocaine and Epinephrine may increase the levels/ effects of: Bromocriptine; Sympathomimetics

The levels/effects of Lidocaine and Epinephrine may be increased by: Antacids; Atomoxetine; Beta-Blockers; Cannabinoids; Carbonic Anhydrase Inhibitors; COMT Inhibitors; Inhalational Anesthetics; MAO Inhibitors; Serotonin/Norepinephrine Reuptake Inhibitors; Tricyclic Antidepressants

Decreased Effect

Lidocaine and Epinephrine may decrease the levels/ effects of: Iobenguane I 123

The levels/effects of Lidocaine and Epinephrine may be decreased by: Spironolactone

Mechanism of Action Lidocaine blocks both the initiation and conduction of nerve impulses via decreased permeability of sodium ions; epinephrine increases the duration of action of lidocaine by causing vasoconstriction (via alpha effects) which slows the vascular absorption of lidocaine

Pharmacodynamics

Maximum effect: Within 5 minutes

Duration: 2-6 hours, dependent on dose and anesthetic procedure

Usual Dosage Dosage varies with the anesthetic procedure

Children: Use lidocaine concentrations of 0.5% or 1% (or even more dilute) to decrease possibility of toxicity; lidocaine dose (when using combination product of lidocaine and epinephrine) should not exceed 7 mg/kg/ dose; do not repeat within 2 hours

Administration Local injection: Before injecting, withdraw syringe plunger to make sure that injection is not into vein or artery; do not administer I.V. or intra-arterially

Additional Information Use preservative free solutions for epidural or caudal use

Dosage Forms Excipient information presented when available (limited, particularly for generics); consult specific product labeling. [DSC] = Discontinued product

Injection, solution:

0.5% / 1:200,000: Lidocaine hydrochloride 0.5% and epinephrine 1:200,000 (50 mL)

1% / 1:100,000: Lidocaine hydrochloride 1% and epinephrine 1:100,000 (20 mL, 30 mL, 50 mL)

2% / 1:100,000: Lidocaine hydrochloride 2% and epinephrine 1:100,000 (30 mL, 50 mL)

Xylocaine® with Epinephrine:

0.5% / 1:200,000: Lidocaine hydrochloride 0.5% and epinephrine 1:200,000 (50 mL) [contains methylparaben]

1% / 1:100,000: Lidocaine hydrochloride 1% and epinephrine 1:100,000 (10 mL, 20 mL, 50 mL) [contains methylparaben]

2% / 1:100,000: Lidocaine hydrochloride 2% and epinephrine 1:100,000 (10 mL, 20 mL, 50 mL) [contains methylparaben]

Injection, solution [preservative free]:

1% / 1:200,000: Lidocaine hydrochloride 1% and epinephrine 1:200,000 (30 mL)

1.5% / 1:200,000: Lidocaine hydrochloride 1.5% and epinephrine 1:200,000 (5 mL, 30 mL)

2% / 1:200,000: Lidocaine hydrochloride 2% and epinephrine 1:200,000 (20 mL)

Xylocaine®-MPF with Epinephrine:

1% / 1:200,000: Lidocaine hydrochloride 1% and epinephrine 1:200,000 (5 mL, 10 mL, 30 mL) [contains sodium metabisulfite]

1.5% / 1:200,000: Lidocaine hydrochloride 1.5% and epinephrine 1:200,000 (5 mL, 10 mL, 30 mL) [contains sodium metabisulfite]

2% / 1:200,000: Lidocaine hydrochloride 2% and epinephrine 1:200,000 (5 mL, 10 mL, 20 mL) [contains sodium metabisulfite]

Injection, solution [for dental use]:

2% / 1:50,000: Lidocaine hydrochloride 2% and epinephrine 1:50,000 (1.7 mL, 1.8 mL)

2% / 1:100,000: Lidocaine hydrochloride 2% and epinephrine 1:100,000 (1.7 mL, 1.8 mL)

Lignospan® Forte: 2% / 1:50,000: Lidocaine hydrochloride 2% and epinephrine 1:50,000 (1.7 mL) [contains edetate disodium, potassium metabisulfite]

Lignospan® Standard: 2% / 1:100,000: Lidocaine hydrochloride 2% and epinephrine 1:100,000 (1.7 mL) [contains edetate disodium, potassium metabisulfite]

Xylocaine® with Epinephrine:

2% / 1:50,000: Lidocaine hydrochloride 2% and epinephrine 1:50,000 (1.7 mL; 1.8 mL [DSC]) [contains sodium metabisulfite]

2% / 1:100,000: Lidocaine hydrochloride 2% and epinephrine 1:100,000 (1.7 mL; 1.8 mL [DSC]) [contains sodium metabisulfite]

Patch, transdermal:
LidoSite™: Lidocaine hydrochloride 10% and epinephrine 0.1% (25s) [contains sodium metabisulfite; for use only with LidoSite™ controller] [DSC]

Lidocaine and Prilocaine
(LYE doe kane & PRIL oh kane)

U.S. Brand Names EMLA®; Oraqix®
Canadian Brand Names EMLA®
Therapeutic Category Analgesic, Topical; Antipruritic, Topical; Local Anesthetic, Topical
Generic Available Yes: Cream
Use Topical anesthetic for use on normal intact skin to provide local analgesia for minor procedures such as I.V. cannulation or venipuncture; topical anesthetic for superficial minor surgery of genital mucous membranes and as an adjunct for local infiltration anesthesia in genital mucous membranes; has also been used for painful procedures such as lumbar puncture and skin graft harvesting
Pregnancy Risk Factor B
Pregnancy Considerations Refer to Lidocaine monograph.
Lactation Lidocaine enters breast milk/use caution
Breast-Feeding Considerations See individual agents.
Contraindications Hypersensitivity to lidocaine, prilocaine, amide-type local anesthetics, or any component; patients with congenital or idiopathic methemoglobinemia; neonates <37 weeks gestation, infants <12 months of age who are receiving concurrent treatment with methemoglobin-inducing agents (ie, sulfas, acetaminophen, benzocaine, chloroquine, dapsone, nitrofurantoin, nitroglycerin, nitroprusside, phenobarbital, phenytoin, primaquine, quinine)
Warnings Topical use prior to cosmetic procedures can result in high systemic levels and lead to toxic effects (eg, arrhythmias, seizures, coma, respiratory depression, and death). Toxic effects may occur particularly when topical anesthetics are applied in large amounts or to large areas of the skin; left on for long periods of time; used with materials, wraps, or dressings to cover the skin after application; or applied to broken skin, rashes, or areas of skin irritation. These practices may increase the degree of systemic absorption and should be avoided. The FDA recommends that consumers consult their healthcare provider for instructions on safe use, prior to applying topical anesthetics for medical or cosmetic purposes. Use of products with the lowest amount of anesthetic and applying the least amount possible to relieve pain is also recommended.
Precautions Use with caution in patients with severe hepatic disease, patients with G-6-PD deficiency, and patients taking drugs associated with drug-induced methemoglobinemia; adjust dosage by using smaller areas for application in small children (especially infants <3 months of age) or patients with impaired renal or hepatic function
Adverse Reactions
Cardiovascular: Bradycardia, hypotension, shock, angioedema
Central nervous system: Nervousness, euphoria, confusion, dizziness, drowsiness, convulsions, CNS excitation, alteration in temperature sensation
Dermatologic: Rash, urticaria
Hematologic: Methemoglobinemia
Local: Blanching, itching, erythema, edema
Neuromuscular & skeletal: Tremor
Ocular: Blurred vision
Otic: Tinnitus
Respiratory: Respiratory depression, bronchospasm

Drug Interactions
Metabolism/Transport Effects Lidocaine: **Substrate** of CYP1A2 (minor), CYP2A6 (minor), CYP2B6 (minor), CYP2C9 (minor), CYP2D6 (major), CYP3A4 (major), P-glycoprotein; **Inhibits** CYP1A2 (strong), 2D6 (moderate), 3A4 (moderate)
Avoid Concomitant Use There are no known interactions where it is recommended to avoid concomitant use.
Increased Effect/Toxicity There are no known significant interactions involving an increase in effect.
Decreased Effect There are no known significant interactions involving a decrease in effect.
Stability Store at room temperature
Mechanism of Action Local anesthetic action occurs by stabilization of neuronal membranes and inhibiting the ionic fluxes required for the initiation and conduction of impulses
Pharmacodynamics
Onset of action: 1 hour for sufficient dermal analgesia
Maximum effect: 2-3 hours
Duration: 1-2 hours after removal of the cream
Pharmacokinetics (Adult data unless noted)
Absorption: Topical: Related to the duration of application and to the area over which it is applied
3-hour application: 3.6% lidocaine and 6.1% prilocaine were absorbed
24-hour application: 16.2% lidocaine and 33.5% prilocaine were absorbed
Distribution: Both cross the blood-brain barrier; lidocaine and probably prilocaine are excreted in breast milk; V_d:
Lidocaine: 1.1-2.1 L/kg
Prilocaine: 0.7-4.4 L/kg
Protein binding:
Lidocaine: 70%
Prilocaine: 55%
Metabolism:
Lidocaine: Metabolized by the liver to inactive and active metabolites
Prilocaine: Metabolized in both the liver and kidneys
Half-life:
Lidocaine: 65-150 minutes, prolonged with cardiac or hepatic dysfunction
Prilocaine: 10-150 minutes, prolonged in hepatic or renal dysfunction
Usual Dosage Topical:
Newborns ≥37 weeks gestation, Infants, Children, and Adults: For minor procedures, apply 2.5 g/site for at least 60 minutes; for painful procedures, apply 2 g/10 cm² of skin and leave on for at least 2 hours; see table.
Note: Preliminary results in a study of 30 preterm neonates (n=30) using a single 0.5 g dose of EMLA® applied to the heel for 1 hour resulted in no measurable changes in methemoglobin levels

EMLA® Cream Maximum Recommended Dose and Application Area for Infants and Children Based on Application to Intact Skin

Age and Body Weight Requirements	Maximum Total Dose of EMLA®	Maximum Application Area	Maximum Application Time
Birth to 3 mo or <5 kg	1g	10 cm²	1 h
3-12 mo and >5 kg	2 g	20 cm²	4 h
1-6 y and >10 kg	10 g	100 cm²	4 h
7-12 y and >20 kg	20 g	200 cm²	4 h

Adult male genital skin as an adjunct prior to local anesthetic infiltration: Apply 1 g/10 cm² to skin surface for 15 minutes followed immediately by local anesthetic infiltration after removal of EMLA® cream

Administration Topical: Do not use on mucous membranes or the eyes; apply a thick layer of cream to intact skin and cover with an occlusive dressing

Patient Information Not for ophthalmic use; for external use only. EMLA® may block sensation in the treated skin.

Nursing Implications In small infants and children, an occlusive bandage should be placed over the EMLA® cream to prevent the child from placing the cream in his/her mouth or smearing the cream on the eyes

Dosage Forms Excipient information presented when available (limited, particularly for generics); consult specific product labeling. [CAN] = Canadian product

Cream, topical: Lidocaine 2.5% and prilocaine 2.5% (5 g, 30 g)

EMLA®: Lidocaine 2.5% and prilocaine 2.5% (5 g, 30 g)

Patch, transdermal:

EMLA® Patch [CAN]: Lidocaine 2.5% and prilocaine 2.5% per patch (2s, 20s) [active contact surface area of each 1 g patch: 10 cm^2; surface area of entire patch: 40 cm^2] [not available in U.S.]

Gel, periodontal:

Oraqix®: Lidocaine 2.5% and prilocaine 2.5% (1.7 g)

References

Broadman LM, Soliman IE, Hannallah RS, et al, "Analgesic Efficacy of Eutectic Mixture of Local Anesthetics (EMLA®) vs Intradermal Infiltration Prior to Venous Cannulation in Children," Am J Anaesth, 1987, 34:S56.

Halperin DL, Koren G, Attias D, et al, "Topical Skin Anesthesia for Venous Subcutaneous Drug Reservoir and Lumbar Puncture in Children," Pediatrics, 1989, 84(2):281-4.

Robieux I, Kumar R, Radhakrishnan S, et al, "Assessing Pain and Analgesia With a Lidocaine-Prilocaine Emulsion in Infants and Toddlers During Venipuncture," J Pediatr, 1991, 118(6):971-3.

Taddio A, Shennan AT, Stevens B, et al, "Safety of Lidocaine-Prilocaine Cream in the Treatment of Preterm Neonates," J Pediatr, 1995, 127 (6):1002-5.

Lidocaine and Tetracaine
(LYE doe kane & TET ra kane)

U.S. Brand Names Pliaglis™; Synera™

Therapeutic Category Analgesic, Topical; Local Anesthetic, Topical

Generic Available No

Use Topical anesthetic for use on intact skin to provide local analgesia for superficial venous access, including venipuncture, and for superficial dermatological procedures, including excision, electrodesiccation, and shave biopsy of skin lesions.

Pregnancy Risk Factor B

Pregnancy Considerations See individual agents.

Lactation Lidocaine enters breast milk/use caution

Breast-Feeding Considerations Refer to Lidocaine monograph.

Contraindications Hypersensitivity to lidocaine, tetracaine, local anesthetics of the amide or ester type, para-aminobenzoic acid, or any component

Warnings Since the heating element in the patch contains iron powder, **remove patch before** magnetic resonance imaging. Do not cut patch or remove the top cover since this could result in the patch heating to temperatures that can cause thermal injury. Keeping a patch on longer than recommended or applying multiple patches simultaneously or sequentially can result in systemic absorption sufficient to cause serious adverse effects due to the local anesthetic components.

Topical use prior to cosmetic procedures can result in high systemic levels and lead to toxic effects (eg, arrhythmias, seizures, coma, respiratory depression, and death). Toxic effects may occur particularly when topical anesthetics are applied in large amounts or to large areas of the skin; left on for long periods of time; used with materials, wraps, or dressings to cover the skin after application; or applied to broken skin, rashes, or areas of skin irritation. These practices may increase the degree of systemic absorption and should be avoided. The FDA recommends that consumers consult their healthcare provider for instructions on safe use, prior to applying topical anesthetics for medical or cosmetic purposes. Use of products with the lowest amount of anesthetic and applying the least amount possible to relieve pain is also recommended.

Precautions Use with caution in patients who are more sensitive to the systemic effects of lidocaine and tetracaine, including acutely ill, debilitated patients. Use with caution in patients with severe liver disease, pseudocholinesterase deficiency, and patients receiving class I antiarrhythmics and/or local anesthetics (systemic toxic effects may be additive or synergistic with lidocaine and tetracaine).

Adverse Reactions

Cardiovascular: Shock, bradycardia, hypotension

Central nervous system: Dizziness, headache, somnolence, nervousness, confusion, seizures, CNS excitation, insomnia

Dermatologic: Erythema (71%), blanching (12%), edema (12%), urticaria, angioedema, rash, contact dermatitis, skin discoloration at application site, pruritus, blister

Gastrointestinal: Nausea, vomiting

Neuromuscular & skeletal: Paresthesia, back pain

Respiratory: Bronchospasm

Miscellaneous: Anaphylactoid reactions

Drug Interactions

Metabolism/Transport Effects Lidocaine: **Substrate** of CYP1A2 (minor), CYP2A6 (minor), CYP2B6 (minor), CYP2C9 (minor), CYP2D6 (major), CYP3A4 (major), P-glycoprotein; **Inhibits** CYP1A2 (strong), 2D6 (moderate), 3A4 (moderate)

Avoid Concomitant Use There are no known interactions where it is recommended to avoid concomitant use.

Increased Effect/Toxicity There are no known significant interactions involving an increase in effect.

Decreased Effect There are no known significant interactions involving a decrease in effect.

Stability Store at room temperature.

Mechanism of Action Lidocaine (amide-type local anesthetic) and tetracaine (ester-type local anesthetic) block sodium ion channels required for the initiation and conduction of neuronal impulses. Heating element enhances delivery of the local anesthetics

Pharmacodynamics Onset of action: 20 minutes

Pharmacokinetics (Adult data unless noted)

Distribution: Lidocaine crosses the placental and blood-brain barriers; lidocaine is excreted in breast milk

V$_d$: Lidocaine:

Neonates: 2.75 L/kg

Adults: 1.1 L/kg

Protein binding: Lidocaine: 70%

Metabolism:

Lidocaine: Metabolized in the liver by cytochrome P450 CYP1A2 and partially by CYP3A4 to inactive and active metabolites monoethylglycinexylidide (MEGX) and glycinexylidide (GX)

Tetracaine: Hydrolysis by plasma esterases to primary metabolites para-aminobenzoic acid and diethyl-aminoethanol

Half-life: Lidocaine: Adults: 1.8 hours

Elimination: Lidocaine: Excreted in urine as metabolites and parent drug

Usual Dosage Topical: Children ≥3 years and Adults:

Venipuncture or I.V. cannulation: Apply to intact skin for 20-30 minutes before venous access

Superficial dermatologic procedures: Apply to intact skin for 30 minutes before procedure

Note: Maximum dose: Current patch removed and one additional patch applied at a new location to facilitate venous access is acceptable after a failed attempt. Otherwise, simultaneous or sequential application of multiple patches is **not recommended**.

Administration Topical: Do not use on mucous membranes or the eyes; apply to **intact skin** immediately after opening the pouch. Do **not** cut or remove the top cover of the patch as this could result in **thermal injury**. Do not cover the holes on the top of the patch as this could cause the patch to not heat up. Avoid contact with the eyes due to potential irritation or abrasion. If contact occurs, immediately wash out the eye with water or saline, and protect the eye until sensation returns.

Monitoring Parameters Pain assessment

Patient Information Chewing or ingesting a new or used patch may result in toxicity. Avoid inadvertent trauma (rubbing, scratching, or exposure to extreme heat or cold) since application of the patch may lead to diminished or blocked sensation in the treated skin.

Nursing Implications Not for home use by patient. Wash hands after handling patch; avoid eye contact with patch. The adhesive sides of a used patch should be folded together; used patch should be disposed immediately.

Additional Information Contains CHADD® self-warming heating element which facilitates drug delivery (when used appropriately, the patch is designed to increase skin temperature by <5°C); patch is latex free. A used patch will still contain large amounts of lidocaine and tetracaine (at least 90% of the initial amount).

Dosage Forms Excipient information presented when available (limited, particularly for generics); consult specific product labeling.

Cream, topical:
Pliaglis™: Lidocaine 7% and tetracaine 7% (30 g)
Patch, transdermal:
Synera™: Lidocaine 70 mg and tetracaine 70 mg (10s) [contains heating component; each patch is ~50 cm^2]

References

Sethna NF, Verghese ST, Hannallah RS, et al, "A Randomized Controlled Trial to Evaluate S-Caine Patch for Reducing Pain Associated With Vascular Access in Children," *Anesthesiology*, 2005, 102(2):403-8.

♦ **Lidocaine Hydrochloride** *see* Lidocaine *on page 818*

♦ **Lidodan™ (Can)** *see* Lidocaine *on page 818*

♦ **Lidoderm®** *see* Lidocaine *on page 818*

♦ **LidoSite™ [DSC]** *see* Lidocaine and Epinephrine *on page 821*

♦ **LID-Pack® (Can)** *see* Bacitracin and Polymyxin B *on page 170*

♦ **Lignocaine Hydrochloride** *see* Lidocaine *on page 818*

♦ **Lignospan® Forte** *see* Lidocaine and Epinephrine *on page 821*

♦ **Lignospan® Standard** *see* Lidocaine and Epinephrine *on page 821*

♦ **Lin-Amox (Can)** *see* Amoxicillin *on page 96*

♦ **Lin-Buspirone (Can)** *see* BusPIRone *on page 222*

Lindane (LIN dane)

Canadian Brand Names Hexit™; PMS-Lindane

Therapeutic Category Antiparasitic Agent, Topical; Pediculocide; Scabicidal Agent; Shampoos

Generic Available Yes

Use Alternative treatment of scabies (*Sarcoptes scabiei*), *Pediculus capitis* (head lice), and *Pediculus pubis* (crab lice); (the AAP and CDC consider permethrin 5% to be the scabicide of choice due to its safety and efficacy profile; many clinicians no longer recommend lindane as initial therapy for pediculosis due to reports of resistance and neurotoxicity)

Medication Guide An FDA-approved patient medication guide, which is available with the product information and as follows, must be dispensed with this medication for each new outpatient prescription and refill.

Lindane lotion: http://www.fda.gov/downloads/Drugs/DrugSafety/UCM133687.pdf
Lindane shampoo: http://www.fda.gov/downloads/Drugs/DrugSafety/UCM133688.pdf.

Pregnancy Risk Factor C

Pregnancy Considerations There are no well-controlled studies in pregnant women.

Lactation Enters breast milk/contraindicated

Breast-Feeding Considerations Nursing mothers should interrupt breast-feeding, express and discard milk for at least 24 hours following use.

Contraindications Hypersensitivity to lindane or any component; premature neonates; pregnant or lactating women; acutely inflamed skin or raw, weeping surfaces

Warnings May be associated with severe neurologic toxicities (contraindicated in premature infants and uncontrolled seizure disorders) **[U.S. Boxed Warning]**. Seizures and death have been reported with use; use with caution in infants, small children, patients <50 kg, or patients with a history of seizures; use caution with conditions which may increase risk of seizures or medications which decrease seizure threshold. Avoid contact with the face, eyes, mucous membranes, and urethral meatus.

Precautions Cover hands to prevent accidental lindane ingestion from thumbsucking; **consider alternative therapy for the treatment of scabies in infants and young children <2 years of age (ie, permethrin)**

Adverse Reactions

Cardiovascular: Cardiac arrhythmia

Central nervous system: Dizziness, restlessness, seizures, headache, ataxia

Dermatologic: Eczematous eruptions, contact dermatitis, rash

Gastrointestinal: Nausea, vomiting

Hematologic: Aplastic anemia

Hepatic: Hepatitis

Local: Burning and stinging

Ocular: Conjunctivitis

Renal: Hematuria

Respiratory: Pulmonary edema

Drug Interactions

Avoid Concomitant Use There are no known interactions where it is recommended to avoid concomitant use.

Increased Effect/Toxicity There are no known significant interactions involving an increase in effect.

Decreased Effect There are no known significant interactions involving a decrease in effect.

Mechanism of Action Directly absorbed by parasites and ova through the exoskeleton; stimulates the nervous system resulting in seizures and death of parasitic arthropods

Pharmacokinetics (Adult data unless noted)

Absorption: Topical: Up to 13% absorbed systemically (absorption is greater when applied to damaged skin, face, scalp, neck, or scrotum)

Distribution: Stored in body fat and accumulates in the brain; skin and adipose tissue may act as repositories

Metabolism: By the liver

Half-life, children: 17-22 hours

Time to peak serum concentration: Children: Topical: 6 hours

Elimination: In urine and feces

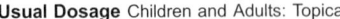

Usual Dosage Children and Adults: Topical:

Scabies: Apply a thin layer of lotion and massage it on skin from the neck to the toes (head to toe in infants).

Infants: Wash off 6 hours after application

Children: Wash off 6-8 hours after application

Adults: Bathe and remove drug 8-12 hours after application

Do not reapply sooner than 1 week later if live mites appear

Pediculosis: 15-30 mL of shampoo is applied and lathered for 4 minutes; rinse hair thoroughly and comb with a fine tooth comb to remove nits; repeat treatment in 7 days if lice or nits are still present

Pediculosis of the eyelashes: Do not treat with lindane; instead, apply an occlusive ophthalmic ointment like petrolatum to the eyelid margins twice daily for 10 days

Administration

For topical use only; do not apply to face; avoid getting in eyes; do **not** apply lotion immediately after a hot, soapy bath; lotion should be applied to dry, cool skin

Before applying lindane shampoo, wash hair with a plain shampoo, then dry

Patient Information Read the patient Medication Guide that you receive with each prescription and refill of lindane. Clothing and bedding should be washed in hot water or by dry cleaning to kill the scabies mite; combs and brushes may be washed with lindane shampoo then thoroughly rinsed with water

Nursing Implications

Children <6 years: ~30 mL lotion is sufficient volume for one application

Children ≥6 years and Adults: ~30-60 mL lotion is sufficient volume for one application

Pruritus associated with scabies or pediculosis may persist for longer than 1 week following treatment with drug. Oral antihistamine and/or topical corticosteroid may be used to help relieve pruritus.

Additional Information Excessive absorption may result in overdose with signs and symptoms which include nausea, vomiting, seizures, headaches, arrhythmias, apnea, pulmonary edema, hematuria, hepatitis, coma, and even death

Dosage Forms Excipient information presented when available (limited, particularly for generics); consult specific product labeling.

Lotion, topical: 1% (60 mL)

Shampoo, topical: 1% (60 mL) [contains alcohol 0.5%]

References

Eichenfield LF, Honig PJ, "Blistering Disorders in Childhood," *Pediatr Clin North Am*, 1991, 38(4):959-76.

Hogan DJ, Schachner L, Tanglertsampan C, "Diagnosis and Treatment of Childhood Scabies and Pediculosis," *Pediatr Clin North Am*, 1991, 38(4):941-57.

Pramanik AK and Hansen RC, "Transcutaneous Gamma Benzene Hexachloride Absorption and Toxicity in Infants and Children," *Arch Dermatol*, 1979, 115(10):1224-5.

Linezolid (li NE zoh lid)

Medication Safety Issues

Sound-alike/look-alike issues:

Zyvox® may be confused with Ziox™, Zosyn®, Zovirax®

U.S. Brand Names Zyvox®

Canadian Brand Names Zyvoxam®

Therapeutic Category Antibiotic, Oxazolidinone

Generic Available No

Use Treatment of community-acquired pneumonia, hospital-acquired pneumonia, complicated and uncomplicated skin and soft tissue infections (including diabetic foot infections without concomitant osteomyelitis), bacteremia caused by susceptible vancomycin-resistant *Enterococcus faecium* (VREF), *Enterococcus faecalis*, *Streptococcus pneumoniae* including multidrug resistant strains, *Staphylococcus aureus* including MRSA, *Streptococcus pyogenes*, or *Streptococcus agalactiae*. **Note:** There have been reports of vancomycin-resistant *E. faecium* and *S. aureus* (methicillin-resistant) developing resistance to linezolid during its clinical use.

Pregnancy Risk Factor C

Pregnancy Considerations Because adverse effects were observed in some animal studies, linezolid is classified pregnancy category C. There are no adequate and well-controlled studies in pregnant women.

Lactation Excretion in breast milk unknown/use caution

Breast-Feeding Considerations It is not known if linezolid is excreted in human milk. Linezolid has low protein binding and is 100% bioavailable orally which may increase the exposure to a nursing infant. The manufacturer advises caution if administering linezolid to a breast-feeding woman. Linezolid is used therapeutically in infants. Nondose-related effects could include modification of bowel flora.

Contraindications Hypersensitivity to linezolid or any component

Warnings Linezolid is a reversible, nonselective MAO inhibitor with the potential to have the same interactions as other MAO inhibitors. Avoid use with serotonergic agents such as tricyclic antidepressants, venlafaxine, trazodone, sibutramine, meperidine, dextromethorphan, and SSRIs due to risk of serotonin syndrome. Thrombocytopenia, anemia, leukopenia, and pancytopenia have been reported in patients receiving linezolid and may be dependent on duration of therapy (generally >2 weeks of treatment); monitor patients' CBC weekly during linezolid therapy; discontinuation of therapy may be required in patients who develop or have worsening myelosuppression. *C. difficile*-associated colitis has been reported; fluid and electrolyte management, protein supplementation, antibiotic treatment, and surgical evaluation may be indicated. Peripheral and optic neuropathy with vision loss have been reported primarily in patients treated for longer then 28 days with linezolid. Cases of lactic acidosis in which patients experienced repeated episodes of nausea and vomiting, acidosis, and low bicarbonate levels have been reported. The manufacturer does not recommend the use of linezolid for empiric treatment of pediatric CNS infections since therapeutic linezolid concentrations are not consistently achieved or maintained in the CSF of patients with ventriculoperitoneal shunts. However, limited data in the form of case reports in pediatric and adult patients suggest that linezolid may be useful in treating gram positive CNS infections that have failed to respond to other treatment options.

Oral suspension contains sodium benzoate; benzoic acid (benzoate) is a metabolite of benzyl alcohol; large amounts of benzyl alcohol (≥99 mg/kg/day) have been associated with a potentially fatal toxicity ("gasping syndrome") in neonates; use caution when administering oral suspension containing sodium benzoate to neonates; *in vitro* and animal studies have shown that benzoate displaces bilirubin from protein binding sites

Precautions Use with caution in patients with uncontrolled hypertension, history of seizures, pheochromocytoma, carcinoid syndrome, severe renal or hepatic impairment, pre-existing myelosuppression, patients receiving other drugs which may cause bone marrow suppression, or untreated hyperthyroidism; linezolid suspension contains aspartame which is metabolized to phenylalanine and must be used with caution in patients with phenylketonuria.

Adverse Reactions

Cardiovascular: Hypertension

Central nervous system: Headache, insomnia, dizziness, fever, vertigo, seizures

Dermatologic: Rash, pruritus

Endocrine & metabolic: Lactic acidosis

Gastrointestinal: Nausea, diarrhea, vomiting, constipation, pseudomembranous colitis, dyspepsia, taste alteration, tongue discoloration, pancreatitis, abdominal pain, *C. difficile*-associated diarrhea

Genitourinary: Vaginal moniliasis

Hematologic: Neutropenia, thrombocytopenia, anemia, leukopenia, pancytopenia, eosinophilia

Hepatic: ALT elevated

Neuromuscular & skeletal: Peripheral neuropathy

Ocular: Optic neuropathy, blurred vision, loss of vision

Renal: BUN and creatinine elevated

Respiratory: Dyspnea

Miscellaneous: Anaphylaxis

Drug Interactions

Avoid Concomitant Use

Avoid concomitant use of Linezolid with any of the following: Alpha-/Beta-Agonists (Indirect-Acting); Alpha1-Agonists; Alpha2-Agonists (Ophthalmic); Amphetamines; Anilidopiperidine Opioids; Atomoxetine; BuPROPion; BusPIRone; CarBAMazepine; Cyclobenzaprine; Dexmethylphenidate; Dextromethorphan; HYDROmorphone; MAO Inhibitors; Maprotiline; Meperidine; Methyldopa; Methylphenidate; Mirtazapine; Propoxyphene; Selective Serotonin Reuptake Inhibitors; Serotonin 5-HT1D Receptor Agonists; Serotonin/Norepinephrine Reuptake Inhibitors; Sibutramine; Tapentadol; Tetrabenazine; Tetrahydrozoline; Tetrahydrozoline (Nasal); Tricyclic Antidepressants

Increased Effect/Toxicity

Linezolid may increase the levels/effects of: Alpha-/Beta-Agonists (Direct-Acting); Alpha-/Beta-Agonists (Indirect-Acting); Alpha1-Agonists; Alpha2-Agonists (Ophthalmic); Amphetamines; Antihypertensives; Atomoxetine; Beta2-Agonists; BuPROPion; Dexmethylphenidate; Dextromethorphan; HYDROmorphone; Lithium; Meperidine; Methadone; Methyldopa; Methylphenidate; Mirtazapine; Orthostatic Hypotension Producing Agents; Rauwolfia Alkaloids; Selective Serotonin Reuptake Inhibitors; Serotonin 5-HT1D Receptor Agonists; Serotonin Modulators; Serotonin/Norepinephrine Reuptake Inhibitors; Tetrahydrozoline; Tetrahydrozoline (Nasal); Tricyclic Antidepressants

The levels/effects of Linezolid may be increased by: Altretamine; Anilidopiperidine Opioids; BusPIRone; CarBAMazepine; COMT Inhibitors; Cyclobenzaprine; Levodopa; MAO Inhibitors; Maprotiline; Propoxyphene; Sibutramine; Tapentadol; Tetrabenazine; TraMADol

Decreased Effect There are no known significant interactions involving a decrease in effect.

Food Interactions Ingestion of tyramine-containing foods and/or beverages may cause hypertensive crisis; limit intake of tyramine-containing foods and/or beverages to less than 100 mg/meal

Stability Store at room temperature; protect from light. Store infusion bags in overwrap until ready for use. The yellow color of the injectable solution may intensify over time without adversely affecting potency. Store reconstituted oral suspension at room temperature and use within 21 days. Linezolid injection is physically incompatible with amphotericin B, chlorpromazine, diazepam, erythromycin lactobionate, pentamidine, phenytoin, sulfamethoxazole and trimethoprim, and ceftriaxone. Linezolid injection is compatible with D_5W, NS, and LR.

Mechanism of Action Inhibits initiation of protein synthesis by binding to a site on the bacterial 23S ribosomal RNA of the 50S subunit preventing the formation of a functional 70S initiation complex which is an essential component of the bacterial translation process

Pharmacokinetics (Adult data unless noted)

Absorption: Well absorbed orally

Distribution: Well-perfused tissues

V_d:
Children: 0.73 ± 0.18 L/kg
Adults: 0.6 L/kg

Protein binding: 31%

Metabolism: Oxidation to 2 inactive metabolites

Bioavailability: 100%

Half-life:
Preterm neonate <1 week: 5.6 hours
Full term neonate <1 week: 3 hours
Full term neonate ≥1 week to ≤28 days: 1.5 hours
Infants >28 days to <3 months: 1.8 hours
Children 3 months to 11 years: 2.9 hours
Adolescents: 4.1 hours
Adults: 4-5 hours

Time to peak serum concentration: Oral: 1-2 hours

Elimination: 65% nonrenal; 30% renal; 2 metabolites of linezolid may accumulate in patients with severe renal impairment

Clearance: Children: 0.34 ± 0.15 L/hour/kg

Dialysis: 30% removed in a 3-hour hemodialysis session (linezolid dose should be given after hemodialysis)

Usual Dosage Note: No dosage adjustment needed when switching from I.V. to oral

Neonates 0-4 weeks and birthweight <1200 g: Oral, I.V.: 10 mg/kg/dose every 8-12 hours (**Note:** Use every 12 hours in patients <34 weeks gestation and <1 week of age.)

Neonates <7 days and birthweight ≥1200 g: Oral, I.V.: 10 mg/kg/dose every 8-12 hours (**Note:** Use every 12 hours in patients <34 weeks gestation and <1 week of age.)

Neonates ≥7 days and birthweight ≥1200 g, Infants, and Children:
Complicated skin and skin structure infections, nosocomial or community-acquired pneumonia including concurrent bacteremia: Oral, I.V.: 10 mg/kg/dose every 8 hours for 10-14 days
VREF: Oral, I.V.: 10 mg/kg/dose every 8 hours for 14-28 days
Uncomplicated skin and skin structure infections: Oral:
Children <5 years: 10 mg/kg/dose every 8 hours for 10-14 days
Children 5-11 years: 10 mg/kg/dose every 12 hours for 10-14 days
Sixty-six children 12 months to 17 years of age with community-acquired pneumonia were enrolled in a Phase II, open-label multicenter study of I.V. linezolid followed by oral linezolid with a mean total treatment duration of 12.2 ± 6.2 days (range: 6-41 days); 92.4% of patients were considered cured, one failed (methicillin-resistant *Staphylococcus aureus*) and 4 were considered indeterminate (Kaplan, 2001); pharmacokinetic data obtained in pediatric patients 0.3-16 years of age support an I.V. linezolid dose of 10 mg/kg/dose 2-3 times/day (Kearns, 2000)

Children ≥12 years and Adolescents:
Uncomplicated skin and skin structure infections: Oral: 600 mg every 12 hours for 10-14 days
Complicated skin and skin structure infections, nosocomial or community-acquired pneumonia including concurrent bacteremia: Oral, I.V.: 600 mg every 12 hours for 10-14 days
VREF infections: Oral, I.V.: 600 mg every 12 hours for 14-28 days

Adults:
Uncomplicated skin and skin structure infections: Oral: 400 mg every 12 hours for 10-14 days
Complicated skin and skin structure infection, nosocomial or community-acquired pneumonia including concurrent bacteremia: Oral, I.V.: 600 mg every 12 hours for 10-14 days
VREF infections: Oral, I.V.: 600 mg every 12 hours for 14-28 days

Dosage adjustment in renal impairment: No adjustment is recommended.

Hemodialysis: No dose adjustment is recommended; however, dose should be given after hemodialysis session.

Continuous venovenous hemofiltration, continuous venovenous hemodialysis, and continuous venovenous hemodiafiltration: No dosage adjustment is recommended.

Dosage adjustment in hepatic impairment: Mild to moderate impairment (Child Pugh class A or B): No adjustment is recommended.

Administration

Oral: Administer with or without food. Gently invert suspension bottle 3-5 times before use. Do not shake. Store at room temperature.

Parenteral: I.V.: Check infusion bag for minute leaks and solution for particulate matter prior to administration. Infuse over 30-120 minutes. 2 mg/mL solution should be administered without further dilution. Do not mix or infuse with other medications. Flush line before and after infusion with a linezolid-compatible I.V. solution like D₅W, NS, or LR.

Monitoring Parameters CBC; platelet counts and hemoglobin, particularly in patients at increased risk for bleeding, patients with pre-existing thrombocytopenia or myelosuppression, patients with chronic infection who have received or who are on concomitant antibiotics, or concomitant medications that decrease platelet count or function or produce bone marrow suppression, and inpatients requiring >2 weeks of therapy; number and type of stools/day for diarrhea; visual function in patients requiring ≥3 months of therapy or in patients reporting new visual symptoms

Patient Information Complete entire course of therapy even if symptoms improve.

Avoid alcohol and excessive amounts of tyramine-containing foods while taking linezolid: Red wine, aged cheese, smoked or pickled fish, beef or chicken liver, sauerkraut, soy sauce, dried sausage, fava or broad bean pods. Notify physician of changes in vision, persistent or worsening symptoms of infection, diarrhea, nausea, or vomiting; watery and bloody stools (with or without stomach cramps and fever) can develop as late as 2 or more months after the last dose of antibiotic.

Dosage Forms Excipient information presented when available (limited, particularly for generics); consult specific product labeling.

Infusion [premixed]:
Zyvox®: 200 mg (100 mL) [contains sodium 1.7 mEq]; 600 mg (300 mL) [contains sodium 5 mEq]

Powder for oral suspension:
Zyvox®: 20 mg/mL (150 mL) [contains phenylalanine 20 mg/5 mL, sodium benzoate, and sodium 0.4 mEq/ 5 mL; orange flavor]

Tablet:
Zyvox®: 600 mg [contains sodium 0.1 mEq/tablet]

References

Clemett D and Markham A, "Linezolid," *Drugs*, 2000, 59(4):815-27.

Cook AM, Ramsey CN, Martin CA, et al, "Linezolid for the Treatment of a Heteroresistant *Staphylococcus aureus* Shunt Infection," *Pediatr Neurosurg*, 2005, 41(2):102-4.

da Silva PS, Monteiro Neto H, and Sejas LM, "Successful Treatment of Vancomycin-Resistant Enterococcus Ventriculitis in a Child," *Braz J Infect Dis*, 2007, 11(2):297-9.

Kaplan SL, Patterson L, Edwards KM, et al, "Linezolid for the Treatment of Community-Acquired Pneumonia in Hospitalized Children. Linezolid Pediatric Pneumonia Study Group," *Pediatr Infect Dis J*, 2001, 20(5):488-94.

Kearns GL, Jungbluth GL, Abdel-Rahman SM, et al, "Impact of Ontogeny on Linezolid Disposition in Neonates and Infants," *Clin Pharmacol Ther*, 2003, 74(5):413-22.

Kearns GL, Abdel-Rahman SM, Blumer JL, et al, "Single Dose Pharmacokinetics of Linezolid in Infants and Children," *Pediatr Infect Dis J*, 2000, 19(12):1178-84.

Meyer B, Kornek GV, Nikfardjam M, et al, "Multiple-Dose Pharmacokinetics of Linezolid During Continuous Venovenous Haemofiltration," *J Antimicrob Chemother*, 2005, 56(1):172-9.

Milstone AM, Dick J, Carcon B, et al, "Cerebrospinal Fluid Penetration and Bacteriostatic Activity of Linezolid Against *Enterococcus faecalis* in a Child With a Ventriculoperitoneal Shunt Infection," *Pediatr Neurosurg*, 2007, 43(5):406-9.

Shaikh ZH, Peloquin CA, and Ericsson CD, "Successful Treatment of Vancomycin-Resistant *Enterococcus faecium* Meningitis With Linezolid: Case Report and Literature Review," *Scand J Infect Dis*, 2001, 33(5):375-9.

Tan TQ, "Update on the Use of Linezolid: A Pediatric Perspective," *Pediatr Infect Dis J*, 2004, 23(10):955-6.

Taylor JJ, Wilson JW, and Estes LL, "Linezolid and Serotonergic Drug Interactions: A Retrospective Survey," *Clin Infect Dis*, 2006, 43 (2):180-7.

Villani P, Regazzi MB, Marubbi F, et al, "Cerebrospinal Fluid Linezolid Concentrations in Postneurosurgical Central Nervous System Infections," *Antimicrob Agents Chemother*, 2002, 46(3):936-7.

◆ **Lioresal®** *see* Baclofen *on page 171*

◆ **Liotec (Can)** *see* Baclofen *on page 171*

Liothyronine (lye oh THYE roe neen)

Medication Safety Issues

Sound-alike/look-alike issues:
Liothyronine may be confused with levothyroxine

T3 is an error-prone abbreviation (mistaken as acetaminophen and codeine [ie, Tylenol® #3])

U.S. Brand Names Cytomel®; Triostat®

Canadian Brand Names Cytomel®

Therapeutic Category Thyroid Product

Generic Available Yes

Use Replacement or supplemental therapy in congenital or acquired hypothyroidism, treatment or prevention of euthyroid goiters including thyroid nodules and chronic lymphocytic thyroiditis; as a diagnostic aid in suppression tests to differentiate suspected mild hyperthyroidism or thyroid gland autonomy

Pregnancy Risk Factor A

Pregnancy Considerations Untreated hypothyroidism may have adverse effects on fetal growth and development, and is associated with higher rate of complications; treatment should not be discontinued during pregnancy.

Lactation Enters breast milk (small amounts)/compatible

Contraindications Hypersensitivity to liothyronine sodium or any component; recent MI or thyrotoxicosis; uncorrected adrenal insufficiency

Warnings Not for use in the treatment of obesity or for weight loss **[U.S. Boxed Warning]**; in euthyroid patients, doses within the range of daily hormonal requirements are ineffective for weight reduction; larger doses may produce serious or even life-threatening toxic effects particularly when used with some anorectic drugs (sympathomimetic amines). Short duration of action permits more rapid assessment of dosage changes and rapid diminution of adverse effects upon discontinuation; transient partial loss of hair in pediatrics may be seen in the first few months of therapy.

Precautions Use with extreme caution in patients with cardiovascular disease, adrenal insufficiency, or coronary artery disease; use with extreme caution in patients receiving digoxin or vasopressors (see Drug Interactions); use with caution in patients with diabetes mellitus and diabetes insipidus as symptoms of their disease may be exaggerated or aggravated; myxedematous patients are very sensitive to thyroid supplements; initiate therapy at very low doses and increase gradually

Adverse Reactions

Cardiovascular: Palpitations, tachycardia, cardiac arrhythmias, angina, CHF, hypertension

Central nervous system: Nervousness, insomnia, fever, headache, irritability

Dermatologic: Alopecia, dermatitis herpetiformis, hair loss (transient)

Endocrine & metabolic: Weight loss

Gastrointestinal: Diarrhea, abdominal cramps, appetite increased

Local: Phlebitis with parenteral form

Neuromuscular & skeletal: Tremor

Miscellaneous: Diaphoresis

Drug Interactions

Avoid Concomitant Use

Avoid concomitant use of Liothyronine with any of the following: Sodium Iodide I131

Increased Effect/Toxicity

Liothyronine may increase the levels/effects of: Vitamin K Antagonists

Decreased Effect

Liothyronine may decrease the levels/effects of: Sodium Iodide I131; Theophylline Derivatives

The levels/effects of Liothyronine may be decreased by: Bile Acid Sequestrants; Calcium Polystyrene Sulfonate; Calcium Salts; CarBAMazepine; Estrogen Derivatives; Phenytoin; Rifampin; Sodium Polystyrene Sulfonate

Food Interactions Limit intake of goitrogenic foods (asparagus, cabbage, peas, turnip greens, broccoli, spinach, brussel sprouts, lettuce, soybeans)

Stability Store tablets at controlled room temperature; refrigerate parenteral solution at temperatures between 2°C and 8°C (36°F to 46°F)

Mechanism of Action Primary active compound is T_3 (triiodothyronine), which may be converted from T_4 (thyroxine) by deiodination in liver and peripheral tissues; exact mechanism of action is unknown; however, it is believed the thyroid hormone exerts its many metabolic effects through control of DNA transcription and protein synthesis; involved in normal metabolism, growth, and development; promotes gluconeogenesis, increases utilization and mobilization of glycogen stores, and stimulates protein synthesis, increases basal metabolic rate

Pharmacodynamics I.V., Oral:

Onset of action: Within a few hours

Maximum effect: Within 48 hours

Duration: Up to 72 hours

Pharmacokinetics (Adult data unless noted)

Absorption: Oral: Well absorbed (~85% to 90%)

Metabolism: In the liver to inactive compounds

Half-life: 25 hours (range: 16-49 hours); hypothyroid 1.4 days; hyperthyroid 0.6 days

Elimination: 76% to 83% In urine

Usual Dosage

Congenital hypothyroidism (Cretinism): Neonates, Infants, and Children <3 years: Oral: 5 mcg/day; increase by 5 mcg every 3 days to a maximum dosage of 20 mcg/day for neonates and infants, 50 mcg/day for children 1-3 years of age

Hypothyroidism:

Children: Oral: 5 mcg/day increase in 5 mcg/day increments every 3-4 days;

Usual maintenance dose:

Infants: 20 mcg/day

Children 1-3 years: 50 mcg/day

Children >3 years: Full adult dosage may be necessary

Adults: Oral: 25 mcg/day increase in 12.5-25 mcg/day increments every 1-2 weeks to a maximum of 100 mcg/day

Goiter, nontoxic:

Children: Oral: 5 mcg/day increase in 5 mcg/day increments every 1-2 weeks; usual maintenance dose 15-20 mcg/day

Adults: Oral: 5 mcg/day; increase in 5-10 mcg/day increments every 1-2 weeks; when 25 mcg is reached, increase dosage in 12.5-25 mcg increments every 1-2 weeks; usual maintenance dosage: 75 mcg/day

T_3 suppression test: Adults: Oral: 75-100 mcg/day for 7 days

Myxedema coma: Adults:

I.V.: 25-50 mcg; reduce dosage in patients with known or suspected cardiovascular disease to 10-20 mcg

Note: Normally, at least 4 hours should be allowed between I.V. doses to adequately assess therapeutic response and no more than 12 hours should elapse between doses to avoid fluctuations in hormone levels.

Oral (**Note:** Due to potential poor oral absorption in the acute phase of myxedema, oral therapy should be avoided until the clinical situation has been stabilized): 5 mcg/day; increase in 5-10 mcg/day increments every 1-2 weeks; when 25 mcg/day is reached; increase by 5-25 mcg/day increments every 1-2 weeks; usual maintenance dose: 50-100 mcg/day

Administration

Oral: Administer on an empty stomach

Parenteral: I.V.: For I.V. use only; do not administer SubQ or I.M.; should not be admixed with other solutions

Monitoring Parameters T_3, TSH, heart rate, blood pressure, clinical signs of hypo- and hyperthyroidism; TSH is the most reliable guide for evaluating adequacy of thyroid replacement dosage. TSH may be elevated during the first few months of thyroid replacement despite patients being clinically euthyroid.

Suggested frequency for monitoring thyroid function tests in children: Every 1-2 months during the first year of life, every 2-3 months between ages 1-3 years, and every 3-12 months thereafter until growth is completed; repeat tests two weeks after any change in dosage.

Reference Range See normal values in Normal Laboratory Values for Children on page 1672

Test Interactions Many drugs may have effects on thyroid function tests (ie, para-aminosalicylic acid, aminoglutethimide, amiodarone, barbiturates, carbamazepine, chloral hydrate, clofibrate, colestipol, corticosteroids, danazol, diazepam, estrogens, ethionamide, fluorouracil, I.V. heparin, insulin, lithium, methadone, methimazole, mitotane, nitroprusside, oxyphenbutazone, phenylbutazone, PTU, perphenazine, phenytoin, propranolol, salicylates, sulfonylureas, and thiazides)

Patient Information Do not change brands without physician's knowledge; report immediately to physician any chest pain, increased pulse, palpitations, heat intolerance, excessive sweating; do not discontinue without notifying physician

Additional Information 15-37.5 mcg liothyronine = 50-60 mcg levothyroxine = 60 mg thyroid USP

Dosage Forms Excipient information presented when available (limited, particularly for generics); consult specific product labeling.

Injection, solution: 10 mcg/mL (1 mL)

Triostat®: 10 mcg/mL (1 mL) [contains ethanol 6.8%]

Tablet, oral: 5 mcg, 25 mcg, 50 mcg

Cytomel®: 5 mcg, 25 mcg, 50 mcg

◆ **Liothyronine Sodium** see Liothyronine on page 828

◆ **Lipancreatin** see Pancrelipase on page 1051

◆ **Lipase, Protease, and Amylase** see Pancrelipase on page 1051

◆ **Lipitor®** see Atorvastatin on page 151

◆ **Liposyn® II [DSC]** see Fat Emulsion on page 563

◆ **Liposyn® II (Can)** see Fat Emulsion on page 563

◆ **Liposyn® III** see Fat Emulsion on page 563

◆ **Liquadd™ [DSC]** see Dextroamphetamine on page 416

◆ **Liquid Antidote** *see* Charcoal, Activated *on page 284*
◆ **Liqui-Doss® [OTC] [DSC]** *see* Mineral Oil *on page 933*
◆ **Liquid Paraffin** *see* Mineral Oil *on page 933*

Lisdexamfetamine (lis dex am FET a meen)

Medication Safety Issues
Sound-alike/look-alike issues:
Vyvanse™ may be confused with Vytorin®, Glucovance®, Vivactil®

Beers Criteria medication: This drug may be inappropriate for use in geriatric patients (high severity risk).

Related Information
Laboratory Detection of Drugs in Urine *on page 1706*

U.S. Brand Names Vyvanse™
Canadian Brand Names Vyvanse™
Therapeutic Category Amphetamine; Central Nervous System Stimulant
Generic Available No
Use Treatment of attention-deficit/hyperactivity disorder (ADHD)
Restrictions C-II
Medication Guide An FDA-approved patient medication guide, which is available with the product information and at http://www.fda.gov/downloads/Drugs/DrugSafety/ucm089823.pdf, must be dispensed with this medication for each new outpatient prescription and refill.

Pregnancy Risk Factor C
Pregnancy Considerations Animal studies have shown that amphetamines may cause embryotoxic and teratogenic effects and that pre- or early postnatal exposure to amphetamines may lead to lasting changes in behavior, including impaired learning, memory, and motor skills, as well as changes to libido. There are no adequate and well-controlled studies in pregnant women. No reproductive studies have been performed with lisdexamfetamine. Infants born to mothers dependent on amphetamines are more likely to arrive prematurely with low birth weight and may experience withdrawal symptoms including irritation, restlessness, anxiousness, weakness, listlessness, or lethargy.

Lactation Enters breast milk/not recommended
Breast-Feeding Considerations Manufacturer advises nursing mothers taking amphetamines to refrain from breast-feeding.
Contraindications Hypersensitivity or idiosyncrasy to lisdexamfetamine, dextroamphetamine, other sympathomimetic amines, or any component; advanced arteriosclerosis, symptomatic cardiovascular disease, moderate to severe hypertension, hyperthyroidism, glaucoma, agitated states, history of drug abuse, concurrent use or use within 14 days of MAO inhibitors (hypertensive crisis may occur)

Warnings Serious cardiovascular events including sudden death may occur in patients with pre-existing structural cardiac abnormalities or other serious heart problems. Sudden death has been reported in children and adolescents; sudden death, stroke, and MI have been reported in adults. Avoid the use of amphetamines in patients with known serious structural cardiac abnormalities, cardiomyopathy, serious heart rhythm abnormalities, coronary artery disease, or other serious cardiac problems that could place patients at an increased risk to the sympathomimetic effects of amphetamines. Patients should be carefully evaluated for cardiac disease prior to initiation of therapy. **Note:** The American Heart Association recommends that all children diagnosed with ADHD who may be candidates for medication, such as lisdexamfetamine, should have a thorough cardiovascular assessment prior to initiation of therapy. This assessment should include a combination of medical history, family history, and physical examination focusing on cardiovascular disease risk factors. An ECG is not mandatory but should be considered.

Stimulant medications may increase blood pressure (average increase 2-4 mm Hg) and heart rate (average increase 3-6 bpm); some patients may experience greater increases; use stimulant medications with caution in patients with hypertension and other cardiovascular conditions that may be exacerbated by increases in blood pressure or heart rate; use is contraindicated in patients with moderate to severe hypertension. Psychiatric adverse events may occur. Stimulants may exacerbate symptoms of behavior disturbance and thought disorder in patients with pre-existing psychosis. New-onset psychosis or mania may occur with stimulant use. May induce mixed/manic episode in patients with bipolar disorder. May be associated with aggressive behavior or hostility (monitor for development or worsening of these behaviors).

Safety and efficacy of amphetamines have not been established in children <3 years of age (use in children <3 years is **not** recommended); lisdexamfetamine has not been studied in children <6 years of age or >12 years of age; long-term effects in pediatric patients have not been determined. Use of stimulants in children has been associated with growth suppression (monitor growth; treatment interruption may be needed). Appetite suppression may occur; monitor weight during therapy, particularly in children. Stimulants may lower seizure threshold leading to new-onset or breakthrough seizure activity (use with caution in patients with a history of seizure disorder). Visual disturbances (difficulty in accommodation and blurred vision) have been reported.

Amphetamines possess a high potential for abuse **[U.S. Boxed Warning]**; misuse may cause sudden death and serious cardiovascular adverse events **[U.S. Boxed Warning]**; prolonged administration may lead to drug dependence; abrupt discontinuation following high doses or for prolonged periods may result in symptoms of withdrawal; avoid abrupt discontinuation in patients who have received amphetamines for prolonged periods; use is contraindicated in patients with history of ethanol or drug abuse. Amphetamines may impair the ability to engage in potentially hazardous activities. May exacerbate motor and phonic tics and Tourette's syndrome.

Precautions Prescriptions should be written for the smallest quantity consistent with good patient care to minimize possibility of overdose.

Adverse Reactions
Cardiovascular: Hypertension, tachycardia, palpitations, MI, cardiac arrhythmias, ventricular hypertrophy (by ECG criteria); cardiomyopathy with chronic use (case reports); serious cardiovascular events including sudden death in patients with pre-existing structural cardiac abnormalities or other serious heart problems (see Warnings)

Central nervous system: Insomnia, headache, nervousness, dizziness, irritability, aggression, overstimulation, fever, somnolence, affect lability, anxiety, agitation, restlessness, psychomotor activity, euphoria, dyskinesia, dysphoria, depression, tic, exacerbation of phonic and motor tics, Tourette's syndrome, seizures, stroke, psychotic episodes (rare with recommended doses); psychiatric adverse effects (see Warnings)

Dermatologic: Rash, hyperhidrosis, urticaria; Stevens-Johnson syndrome, toxic epidermal necrolysis

Endocrine & metabolic: Growth suppression, weight loss, libido changes

Gastrointestinal: Anorexia, nausea, vomiting, diarrhea, abdominal cramps, unpleasant taste, xerostomia, constipation

Genitourinary: Impotence

Neuromuscular and Skeletal: Tremor

Ocular: Mydriasis, difficulty in accommodation, blurred vision

Respiratory: Dyspnea

Miscellaneous: Hypersensitivity reactions, angioedema, anaphylaxis; physical and psychologic dependence with long-term use

Drug Interactions

Avoid Concomitant Use

Avoid concomitant use of Lisdexamfetamine with any of the following: Iobenguane I 123; MAO Inhibitors

Increased Effect/Toxicity

Lisdexamfetamine may increase the levels/effects of: Analgesics (Opioid); Sympathomimetics

The levels/effects of Lisdexamfetamine may be increased by: Alkalinizing Agents; Antacids; Atomoxetine; Cannabinoids; Carbonic Anhydrase Inhibitors; MAO Inhibitors; Tricyclic Antidepressants

Decreased Effect

Lisdexamfetamine may decrease the levels/effects of: Antihistamines; Ethosuximide; Iobenguane I 123; PHENobarbital; Phenytoin

The levels/effects of Lisdexamfetamine may be decreased by: Ammonium Chloride; Antipsychotics; Gastrointestinal Acidifying Agents; Lithium; Methenamine

Food Interactions Acidic foods, juices, or vitamin C may decrease GI absorption. Food does not affect the extent of absorption (ie, AUC of dextroamphetamine); a high-fat meal delays the time to peak concentration of dextroamphetamine by 1 hour

Stability Store at controlled room temperature; protect from light; dispense in tightly-closed container.

Mechanism of Action Lisdexamfetamine dimesylate is a prodrug that is converted to the active component dextroamphetamine (an amphetamine). Amphetamines are noncatecholamine, sympathomimetic amines that promote the release of catecholamines (primarily dopamine and norepinephrine) from their storage sites in the presynaptic nerve terminals, thus increasing the amounts of circulating dopamine and norepinephrine in the cerebral cortex and reticular activating system. A less significant mechanism may include their ability to block the reuptake of catecholamines by competitive inhibition. Amphetamines also weakly inhibit the action of monoamine oxidase. They peripherally increase blood pressure and act as a respiratory stimulant and weak bronchodilator.

Pharmacokinetics (Adult data unless noted)

Absorption: Rapid

Distribution: Dextroamphetamine: V_d: Adults: 3.5-4.6 L/kg; distributes into CNS; mean CSF concentrations are 80% of plasma; enters breast milk

Metabolism: Converted to dextroamphetamine and l-lysine via first-pass intestinal and/or hepatic metabolism; not metabolized by CYP P450

Half-life elimination: Adults: Lisdexamfetamine: <1 hour; dextroamphetamine: 12 hours

Time to peak serum concentration: Children 6-12 years: T_{max}: Lisdexamfetamine: 1 hour; Dextroamphetamine: 3.5 hours

Elimination: 96% of the dose is eliminated in the urine (42% of dose as amphetamine, 2% lisdexamfetamine, 25% hippuric acid); feces (minimal)

Usual Dosage Oral: Individualize dosage based on patient need and response to therapy. Administer at the lowest effective dose.

Children: 6-12 years and Adults: Initial: 30 mg once daily in the morning; may increase in increments of 10-20 mg/day at weekly intervals until optimal response is obtained; maximum: 70 mg/day; doses >70 mg/day have not been studied.

Administration Oral: Administer in the morning with or without food; avoid afternoon doses to prevent insomnia. Swallow capsule whole, do not chew; capsule may be opened and the entire contents dissolved in glass of water; consume the resulting solution immediately; do not store solution; do not divide capsule; do not take less than one capsule/day.

Monitoring Parameters Evaluate patients for cardiac disease prior to initiation of therapy with thorough medical history, family history, and physical exam; consider ECG (see Warnings); perform ECG and echocardiogram if findings suggest cardiac disease; promptly conduct cardiac evaluation in patients who develop chest pain, unexplained syncope, or any other symptom of cardiac disease during treatment. Monitor CNS activity, blood pressure, heart rate, height, weight, sleep, appetite, abnormal movements, growth in children. Patients should be re-evaluated at appropriate intervals to assess continued need of the medication. Observe for signs/symptoms of aggression or hostility, or depression.

Test Interactions Amphetamines may interfere with urinary steroid measurements; may cause significant increase in plasma corticosteroid levels

Patient Information Read the patient Medication Guide that you receive with each prescription and refill of dextroamphetamine. Serious cardiac effects or psychiatric adverse effects may occur; notify your physician of any heart problems, high blood pressure, or psychiatric conditions before starting therapy. May reduce the growth rate in children and has been associated with worsening of aggressive behavior; notify your physician if your child displays aggression or hostility; make sure your physician monitors your child's weight and height. May impair ability to perform activities requiring mental alertness or physical coordination. May be habit-forming; avoid abrupt discontinuation after prolonged use. Limit caffeine; avoid alcohol and the herbal medicine St. John's wort. May cause dry mouth.

Additional Information Treatment for ADHD should include "drug holiday" or periodic discontinuation in order to assess the patient's requirements, decrease tolerance, and limit suppression of linear growth and weight. Medications used to treat ADHD should be part of a total treatment program that may include other components such as psychological, educational, and social measures.

Dosage Forms

Capsule, as dimesylate:

Vyvanse™: 20 mg, 30 mg, 40 mg, 50 mg, 60 mg, 70 mg

References

American Academy of Pediatrics/American Heart Association Clarification of Statement on Cardiovascular Evaluation and Monitoring of Children and Adolescents With Heart Disease Receiving Medications for ADHD; available at: http://americanheart.mediaroon.com/index.-php?s=43&item=422.

Biederman J, Krishnan S, Zhang Y, et al, "Efficacy and Tolerability of Lisdexamfetamine Dimesylate (NRP-104) in Children With Attention-Deficit/Hyperactivity Disorder: A Phase III, Multicenter, Randomized, Double-Blind, Forced-Dose, Parallel-Group Study," *Clin Ther*, 2007, 29(3):450-63.

Chiang WK, "Amphetamines," *Goldfrank's Toxicologic Emergencies*, 8th ed, Flomenbaum NE, Goldfrank LR, Hoffman RS, eds, New York, NY: The McGraw-Hill Companies, 2006, 1119.

Nissen SE, "ADHD and Cardiovascular Risk," *N Engl J Med*, 2006, 354:1445-8.

Pliszka S and AACAP Work Group on Quality Issues, "Practice Parameter for the Assessment and Treatment of Children and Adolescents With Attention-Deficit/Hyperactivity Disorder," *J Am Acad Child Adolesc Psychiatry*, 2007, 46(7):894-921.

Vetter VL, Elia J, Erickson CH, et al, "Cardiovascular Monitoring of Children and Adolescents With Heart Disease Receiving Stimulant Drugs. A Scientific Statement from the American Heart Association Council on Cardiovascular Disease in the Young Congenital Cardiac Defects Committee and the Council on Cardiovascular Nursing," *Circulation*, 2008, 117:2407-23.

Westfall TC and Westfall DP, "Adrenergic Agonists and Antagonists," *Goodman and Gilman's The Pharmacological Basis of Therapeutics*, 11th ed, Brunton LL, ed, New York, NY: McGraw-Hill, 2006, 257-8.

♦ **Lisdexamfetamine Dimesylate** *see* Lisdexamfetamine *on page 830*

Lisinopril (lyse IN oh pril)

Medication Safety Issues
Sound-alike/look-alike issues:
Lisinopril may be confused with fosinopril, Lioresal®, Lipitor®, Risperdal®
Prinivil® may be confused with Plendil®, Pravachol®, Prevacid®, Prilosec®, Proventil®
Zestril® may be confused with Desyrel®, Restoril™, Vistaril®, Zegerid®, Zerit®, Zetia®, Zostrix®, Zyprexa®

International issues:
Acepril [Malaysia] may be confused with Accupril® which is a brand name for quinapril [U.S.]
Acepril: Brand name for lisinopril [Malaysia], but also the brand name for captopril [Great Britain]; enalapril [Hungary, Switzerland]
Carace [Ireland] may be confused with Carac™ which is a brand name for fluorouracil [U.S.]

Related Information
Antihypertensive Agents by Class *on page 1481*

U.S. Brand Names Prinivil®; Zestril®
Canadian Brand Names Apo-Lisinopril®; CO Lisinopril; Dom-Lisinopril; Mint-Lisinopril; Mylan-Lisinopril; Novo-Lisinopril; PHL-Lisinopril; PMS-Lisinopril; Prinivil®; PRO-Lisinopril; RAN™-Lisinopril; ratio-Lisinopril; Riva-Lisinopril; Sandoz-Lisinopril; Zestril®; ZYM-Lisinopril
Therapeutic Category Angiotensin-Converting Enzyme (ACE) Inhibitor; Antihypertensive Agent
Generic Available Yes

Use Treatment of hypertension, either alone or in combination with other antihypertensive agents (FDA approved in ages 6-16 years and adults); adjunctive therapy in treatment of heart failure (HF) (FDA approved in adults); treatment of acute myocardial infarction (MI) within 24 hours in hemodynamically-stable patients to improve survival (FDA approved in adults)

Pregnancy Risk Factor C (1st trimester); D (2nd and 3rd trimesters)

Pregnancy Considerations Due to adverse events observed in some animal studies, lisinopril is considered pregnancy category C during the first trimester. Based on human data, lisinopril is considered pregnancy category D if used during the second and third trimesters (per the manufacturer; however, one study suggests that fetal injury may occur at anytime during pregnancy). Lisinopril crosses the placenta. First trimester exposure to ACE inhibitors may cause major congenital malformations. An increased risk of cardiovascular and/or central nervous system malformations was observed in one study; however, an increased risk of teratogenic events was not observed in other studies. Second and third trimester use of an ACE inhibitor is associated with oligohydramnios. Oligohydramnios due to decreased fetal renal function may lead to fetal limb contractures, craniofacial deformation, and hypoplastic lung development. The use of ACE inhibitors during the second and third trimesters is also associated with anuria, hypotension, renal failure (reversible or irreversible), skull hypoplasia, and death in the fetus/neonate. Chronic maternal hypertension itself is also associated with adverse events in the fetus/infant. ACE inhibitors are not recommended during pregnancy to treat maternal hypertension or heart failure. Those who are planning a pregnancy should be considered for other medication options if an ACE inhibitor is currently prescribed or the ACE inhibitor should be discontinued as soon as possible once pregnancy is detected. The exposed fetus should be monitored for fetal growth, amniotic fluid volume, and organ formation. Infants exposed to an ACE inhibitor *in utero*, especially during the second and third trimester, should be monitored for hyperkalemia, hypotension, and oliguria.

[U.S. Boxed Warning]: Based on human data, ACE inhibitors can cause injury and death to the developing fetus when used in the second and third trimesters. ACE inhibitors should be discontinued as soon as possible once pregnancy is detected.

Lactation Excretion in breast milk unknown/not recommended

Breast-Feeding Considerations It is not known if lisinopril is excreted in breast milk. Breast-feeding is not recommended by the manufacturer.

Contraindications Hypersensitivity to lisinopril, any component, or other ACE inhibitors; patients with idiopathic or hereditary angioedema or a history of angioedema with previous ACE inhibitor use

Warnings Serious adverse effects including angioedema, anaphylactoid reactions, neutropenia, agranulocytosis, hypotension, and hepatic failure may occur (see also Adverse Reactions). Angioedema can occur at any time during treatment (especially following first dose) and may occur in the head, neck, extremities, or intestines. Angioedema of the larynx, glottis, or tongue may cause airway obstruction, especially in patients with a history of airway surgery; prolonged monitoring may be required, even in patients with swelling of only the tongue (ie, without respiratory distress) because treatment with corticosteroids and antihistamines may not be sufficient; very rare fatalities have occurred with angioedema of the larynx or tongue; aggressive early and appropriate management (eg, establishing patent airway and/or SubQ epinephrine) is critical in patients with angioedema of larynx, glottis, or tongue, in whom airway obstruction is likely to occur. Use in patients with idiopathic or hereditary angioedema or previous angioedema associated with ACE inhibitor therapy is contraindicated. Life-threatening anaphylactoid reactions have been reported in patients dialyzed with high-flux membranes receiving concomitant ACE inhibitor therapy; if this occurs, stop dialysis immediately and initiate treatment for anaphylactoid reactions; symptoms have not been relieved with antihistamines; anaphylactoid reactions may also occur in patients who undergo low-density lipoprotein apheresis with dextran sulfate absorption.

Neutropenia and agranulocytosis have been reported (rarely); risk may be increased in patients with renal dysfunction especially if the patients have collagen vascular diseases; periodic monitoring of WBC should be considered. Hepatic failure has been rarely reported in patients receiving ACE inhibitors; the reported syndrome starts with hepatitis or cholestatic jaundice and progresses to fulminant hepatic necrosis; discontinue ACE inhibitor if marked elevation of hepatic transaminases or jaundice occurs and initiate appropriate medical treatment

ACE inhibitors can cause injury and death to the developing fetus when used during pregnancy. ACE inhibitors should be discontinued as soon as possible once pregnancy is detected **[U.S. Boxed Warning]**. Neonatal hypotension, skull hypoplasia, anuria, renal failure, oligohydramnios (associated with fetal limb contractures, craniofacial deformities, hypoplastic lung development), prematurity, intrauterine growth retardation, patent ductus arteriosus, and death have been reported with the use of ACE inhibitors, primarily in the second and third trimesters. The risk of neonatal toxicity has been considered less when ACE inhibitors are used in the first trimester; however, major congenital malformations have been reported. The cardiovascular and/or central nervous systems are most commonly affected.

Precautions Use with caution and modify dosage in patients with renal impairment, especially renal artery stenosis; elevated BUN and serum creatinine may occur in these patients; discontinuation of concomitant diuretic or lisinopril may be needed. Severe hypotension may occur, usually with initiation of therapy; effect most often seen in patients who are sodium- and/or volume-depleted; initiate lower doses and monitor closely when starting therapy in these patients. Use with caution and modify dosage in patients with hyponatremia, hypovolemia, severe CHF, left ventricular outflow tract obstruction, or with concomitant diuretic therapy. Safety and efficacy in pediatric patients <6 years of age or in pediatric patients with GFR <30 mL/minute/1.73 m^2 has not been established.

Adverse Reactions Note: No relevant differences in adverse reactions between pediatric and adult patients have been identified.

Cardiovascular: Hypotension, chest discomfort, orthostatic effects, syncope

Central nervous system: Dizziness, headache, fatigue

Dermatologic: Rash, angioedema (see Warnings); **Note:** The relative risk of angioedema with ACE inhibitors is higher within the first 30 days of use (compared to >1 year of use), for Black Americans (compared to Whites), for lisinopril or enalapril (compared to captopril), and for patients previously hospitalized within 30 days (Brown, 1996).

Endocrine & metabolic: Hyperkalemia

Gastrointestinal: Diarrhea, nausea, vomiting, ageusia, intestinal angioedema (rare)

Hematologic: Neutropenia, agranulocytosis

Hepatic: Cholestatic jaundice, hepatitis, fulminant hepatic necrosis (rare, but potentially fatal)

Renal: BUN elevated, serum creatinine elevated

Respiratory: Cough, dyspnea, eosinophilic pneumonitis; **Note:** An isolated dry cough lasting >3 weeks was reported in 7 of 42 pediatric patients (17%) receiving ACE inhibitors (see von Vigier, 2000)

Neuromuscular & skeletal: Weakness, pain

Miscellaneous: Anaphylactoid reactions

Drug Interactions

Avoid Concomitant Use There are no known interactions where it is recommended to avoid concomitant use.

Increased Effect/Toxicity

Lisinopril may increase the levels/effects of: Allopurinol; Amifostine; Antihypertensives; AzaTHIOprine; CycloSPORINE; CycloSPORINE (Systemic); Ferric Gluconate; Gold Sodium Thiomalate; Hypotensive Agents; Iron Dextran Complex; Lithium; RiTUXimab

The levels/effects of Lisinopril may be increased by: Angiotensin II Receptor Blockers; Diazoxide; DPP-IV Inhibitors; Eplerenone; Everolimus; Herbs (Hypotensive Properties); Loop Diuretics; MAO Inhibitors; Pentoxifylline; Phosphodiesterase 5 Inhibitors; Potassium Salts; Potassium-Sparing Diuretics; Prostacyclin Analogues; Sirolimus; Temsirolimus; Thiazide Diuretics; Tolvaptan; Trimethoprim

Decreased Effect

The levels/effects of Lisinopril may be decreased by: Antacids; Aprotinin; Herbs (Hypertensive Properties); Methylphenidate; Nonsteroidal Anti-Inflammatory Agents; Salicylates; Yohimbine

Food Interactions Food does not affect oral absorption. Limit salt substitutes or potassium-rich diet. Avoid natural licorice (causes sodium and water retention and increases potassium loss).

Mechanism of Action Competitive inhibitor of angiotensin-converting enzyme (ACE); prevents conversion of angiotensin I to angiotensin II, a potent vasoconstrictor; results in lower levels of angiotensin II which causes an increase in plasma renin activity and a reduction in

aldosterone secretion; a CNS mechanism may also be involved in hypotensive effect as angiotensin II increases adrenergic outflow from CNS; vasoactive kallikreins may be decreased in conversion to active hormones by ACE inhibitors, thus reducing blood pressure

Pharmacodynamics

Onset of action (decrease in blood pressure): 1 hour

Maximum effect: 6-8 hours

Duration: 24 hours

Pharmacokinetics (Adult data unless noted)

Absorption: Oral:

Children:

2-15 years: Range: 20% to 36% (Hogg, 2007)

6-16 years: 28%

Adults: 25% (range: 6% to 60%)

Protein binding: 25%

Half-life: 11-13 hours; half-life increases with renal dysfunction

Time to peak serum concentration:

Infants and Children 6 months to 15 years: Median (range): 5-6 hours (Hogg, 2007)

Children 6-16 years: Within 6 hours

Adults: Within 7 hours

Elimination: Excreted in urine as unchanged drug

Dialysis: Removable by hemodialysis

Usual Dosage Oral: Dosage must be titrated according to patient's response; **reduce dose by 50% in patients with hyponatremia, hypovolemia, severe CHF, decreased renal function, or receiving diuretics:**

Hypertension (**Note:** If possible, discontinue diuretics 2-3 days prior to initiating lisinopril; restart diuretic, if needed, after blood pressure is stable):

Infants and Children <6 years: Not approved for use; limited information exists in the literature. One retrospective study (n=123; 59 with hypertension; age range: 2 months to 18 years; mean age: 10 years) used initial doses of 0.1 mg/kg once daily; treatment was initiated in the hospital with patients under close observation; doses were adjusted at subsequent clinic visits based on clinical response; maximum dose: 0.5 mg/kg/day; median maximum dose used in the study: 0.135 mg/kg/day (25th to 75th percentiles: 0.092-0.192 mg/kg/day) (see Raes, 2007). Further studies are needed before these doses can be routinely recommended.

Children ≥6 years: Initial: 0.07 mg/kg once daily; maximum initial dose: 5 mg once daily; increase dose at 1- to 2-week intervals; doses >0.61 mg/kg or >40 mg have not been evaluated

Adults: Initial: 10 mg/day given once daily; increase dose by 5-10 mg/day at 1- to 2-week intervals; usual dose: 20-40 mg/day given once daily; doses up to 80 mg/day have been used, but do not appear to have a greater effect; usual dosage range (JNC 7): 10-40 mg once daily

Note: Antihypertensive effect may diminish toward the end of the dosing interval especially with doses of 10 mg/day. An increased dose may aid in extending the duration of antihypertensive effect.

Heart failure: Adults: Initial: 2.5-5 mg once daily (with diuretics and usually digitalis); increase dose by ≤10 mg/day increments at ≥2 week intervals based on clinical response; usual maintenance dose: 5-40 mg/day given once daily; maximum dose: 40 mg/day. Target dose: 20-40 mg once daily (ACC/AHA 2005 Heart Failure Guidelines)

Note: If patient has hyponatremia (serum sodium <130 mEq/L) or renal impairment (Cl$_{cr}$ <30 mL/minute or serum creatinine >3 mg/dL), then initial dose should be 2.5 mg/day

Dosing adjustment in renal impairment:

Children: Cl$_{cr}$ <30 mL/minute/1.73 m^2: Use is not recommended

Adults:
Hypertension: Modify initial dose and cautiously titrate dose based on clinical response; maximum dose: 40 mg once daily
Cl$_{cr}$ >30 mL/minute: Initial: 10 mg once daily
Cl$_{cr}$ 10-30 mL/minute: Initial: 5 mg once daily
Cl$_{cr}$ <10 mL/minute (usually on hemodialysis): Initial: 2.5 mg once daily
CHF: Cl$_{cr}$ <30 mL/minute or serum creatinine >3 mg/dL: Initial: 2.5 mg/day

Administration Oral: May be administered without regard to food

Monitoring Parameters Blood pressure, BUN, serum creatinine, renal function, WBC, and serum potassium; monitor for angioedema and anaphylactoid reactions (see Warnings)

Patient Information Limit alcohol. Notify physician immediately if swelling of face, lips, tongue, or difficulty in breathing occurs; if these occur, do not take any more doses until a physician can be consulted. Notify physician if vomiting, diarrhea, excessive perspiration, dehydration, or persistent cough occurs. Do not use a salt substitute (potassium-containing) without physician advice. May cause dizziness, fainting, and lightheadedness, especially in first week of therapy; sit and stand up slowly. May cause rash. Report sore throat, fever, other signs of infection, or other side effects. This medication may cause injury and death to the developing fetus when used during pregnancy; women of childbearing potential should be informed of potential risk; consult prescriber for appropriate contraceptive measures; this medication should be discontinued as soon as possible once pregnancy is detected (see Warnings).

Nursing Implications Discontinue if angioedema occurs; observe closely for hypotension after the first dose or initiation of a new higher dose (keep in mind that maximum effect on blood pressure occurs at 6-8 hours)

Dosage Forms Excipient information presented when available (limited, particularly for generics); consult specific product labeling.
Tablet: 2.5 mg, 5 mg, 10 mg, 20 mg, 30 mg, 40 mg
Prinivil®: 5 mg, 10 mg, 20 mg [scored]
Zestril®: 2.5 mg, 10 mg, 20 mg, 30 mg, 40 mg
Zestril®: 5 mg [scored]

Extemporaneous Preparations
A 1 mg/mL lisinopril suspension made from tablets, Bicitra®, and Ora-Sweet SF® is stable for up to 4 weeks when stored at ≤25°C (77°F) in a polyethylene terephthalate bottle; add 10 mL of purified water (USP) to a bottle containing ten 20 mg lisinopril tablets; shake for ≥1 minute; add 30 mL of Bicitra® and 160 mL of Ora-Sweet SF® to the mixture in the bottle; shake gently to suspend the contents; label "shake well" [Thompson, 2003; Prinivil® (package insert), 2008; Zestril® (package insert), 2007].

A 1 mg/mL lisinopril suspension made from tablets and a 1:1 mixture of Ora-Plus® and Ora-Sweet® is stable for 13 weeks when stored at 4°C or 25°C in amber, plastic, prescription bottles; crush ten 10 mg tablets and triturate to a fine powder in a mortar. Levigate the powder with small amount of the vehicle into a uniform paste. Add the vehicle in geometric proportions with constant mixing and transfer to graduate. Rinse the mortar with vehicle, transfer to the graduate, and qs to 100 mL; label "shake well" (Nahata, 2004).

A 1 mg/mL lisinopril suspension made from tablets, methylcellulose 1% with parabens and simple syrup NF is stable for 13 weeks at 4°C or 8 weeks at 25°C in amber, plastic, prescription bottles; crush ten 10 mg tablets and triturate to a fine powder in a mortar. Levigate the powder with 7.7 mL of methylcellulose gel into a uniform paste. Add simple syrup in geometric proportions

with constant mixing and transfer to a graduate. Rinse the mortar with syrup, transfer to the graduate, and qs to 100 mL; label "shake well" (Nahata, 2004).

A 2 mg/mL lisinopril syrup made from powder (Sigma Chemical Company, St. Louis, MO) and simple syrup was stable for 30 days when stored in amber plastic prescription bottles at room temperature (23°C) or under refrigeration (5°C); dissolve 1 gram of lisinopril powder in 30 mL of distilled water; incorporate resultant solution into syrup using geometric dilution and qsad to 500 mL; label "shake well" and "refrigerate"; **Note:** Although no visual evidence of microbial growth was observed, the authors recommend storage at 5°C to inhibit microbial growth (Webster, 1997).

Nahata MC and Morosco RS, "Stability of Lisinopril in Two Liquid Dosage Forms," *Ann Pharmacother*, 2004, 38(3):396-9.
Prinivil® (package insert), Whitehouse Station, NJ: Merck & Co, Inc, 2008.
Thompson KC, Zhao Z, Mazakas JM, et al, "Characterization of an Extemporaneous Liquid Formulation of Lisinopril," *Am J Health Syst Pharm*, 2003, 60(1):69-74.
Webster AA, English BA, and Rose DJ, "The Stability of Lisinopril as an Extemporaneous Syrup," *Intr J Pharmaceut Compound*, 1997, 1:352-3.
Zestril® (package insert), Wilmington, DE: AstraZeneca Pharmaceuticals, 2007.

References
Brown NJ, Ray WA, Snowden M, et al, "Black Americans Have an Increased Rate of Angiotensin-Converting Enzyme Inhibitor-Associated Angioedema," *Clin Pharmacol Ther*, 1996, 60(1):8-13.
Chase SL and Sutton JD, "Lisinopril: A New Angiotensin-Converting Enzyme Inhibitor," *Pharmacotherapy*, 1989, 9(3):120-30.
Chobanian AV, Bakris GL, Black HR, et al, "The Seventh Report of the Joint National Committee on Prevention, Detection, Evaluation, and Treatment of High Blood Pressure: The JNC 7 Report," *JAMA*, 2003, 289(19):2560-72.
Hogg RJ, Delucchi A, Sakihara G, et al, "A Multicenter Study of the Pharmacokinetics of Lisinopril in Pediatric Patients With Hypertension," *Pediatr Nephrol*, 2007, 22(5):695-701.
National High Blood Pressure Education Program Working Group on High Blood Pressure in Children and Adolescents, "The Fourth Report on the Diagnosis, Evaluation, and Treatment of High Blood Pressure in Children and Adolescents," *Pediatrics*, 2004, 114(2 Suppl):555-76.
Raes A, Malfait F, Van Aken S, et al, "Lisinopril in Paediatric Medicine: A Retrospective Chart Review of Long-Term Treatment in Children," *J Renin Angiotensin Aldosterone Syst*, 2007, 8(1):3-12.
Raia JJ Jr, Barone JA, Byerly WG, et al, "Angiotensin-Converting Enzymes Inhibitors: A Comparative Review," *DICP*, 1990, 24 (5):506-25.
Soffer B, Zhang Z, Miller K, et al, "A Double-Blind, Placebo-Controlled, Dose-Response Study of the Effectiveness and Safety of Lisinopril for Children With Hypertension," *Am J Hypertens*, 2003, 16(10):795-800.
von Vigier RO, Mozzettini S, Truttmann AC, et al, "Cough is Common in Children Prescribed Converting Enzyme Inhibitors," *Nephron*, 2000, 84(1):98.

♦ **Lispro Insulin** *see* Insulin Lispro *on page 744*

♦ **Lithane™ (Can)** *see* Lithium *on page 834*

Lithium (LITH ee um)

Medication Safety Issues
Sound-alike/look-alike issues:
Eskalith® may be confused with Estratest®
Lithium may be confused with lanthanum
Lithobid® may be confused with Levbid®, Lithostat®

Do not confuse **mEq** (milliequivalent) with **mg** (milligram). **Note:** 300 mg lithium carbonate or citrate contain 8 mEq lithium. Dosage should be written in **mg** (milligrams) to avoid confusion.
Check prescriptions for unusually high volumes of the syrup for dosing errors.

Related Information
Serotonin Syndrome *on page 1695*

U.S. Brand Names Lithobid®

Canadian Brand Names Apo-Lithium® Carbonate; Apo-Lithium® Carbonate SR; Carbolith™; Duralith®; Euro-Lithium; Lithane™; PMS-Lithium Carbonate; PMS-Lithium Citrate

Therapeutic Category Antidepressant, Miscellaneous; Antimanic Agent

Generic Available Yes

Use Management of acute manic episodes (FDA approved in ages ≥12 years and adults); maintenance treatment of mania in individuals with bipolar disorder (maintenance treatment decreases frequency and diminishes intensity of subsequent manic episodes) (FDA approved in ages ≥12 years and adults); has also been used as adjunct treatment for depression; used investigationally to treat severe aggression in children and adolescents with conduct disorder (see Additional Information)

Pregnancy Risk Factor D

Pregnancy Considerations Cardiac malformations in the infant, including Ebstein's anomaly, are associated with use of lithium during the first trimester of pregnancy. Nontoxic effects to the newborn include shallow respiration, hypotonia, lethargy, cyanosis, diabetes insipidus, thyroid depression, and nontoxic goiter when lithium is used near term. Efforts should be made to avoid lithium use during the first trimester; if an alternative therapy is not appropriate, the lowest possible dose of lithium should be used throughout the pregnancy. Fetal echocardiography and ultrasound to screen for anomalies should be conducted between 16-20 weeks of gestation. Lithium levels should be monitored in the mother and may need to be adjusted following delivery.

Lactation Enters breast milk/contraindicated

Contraindications Hypersensitivity to lithium or any component (see Warnings)

Warnings Lithium toxicity is closely related to serum concentrations and can occur at therapeutic doses **[U.S. Boxed Warning]**; serum lithium determinations are required to monitor therapy. Lithium should generally be avoided in patients with severe cardiovascular or renal disease, severe dehydration or debilitation, sodium depletion, and in patients receiving ACE inhibitors or diuretics (these patients are at very high risk of lithium toxicity). Chronic lithium therapy may result in diminished renal concentrating ability (eg, nephrogenic diabetes insipidus) and has been associated with morphologic changes with glomerular and interstitial fibrosis and atrophy of nephrons. Renal function (including assessment of tubular and glomerular function) should be assessed before initiation of and during lithium therapy; treatment should be re-evaluated if progressive or sudden changes in renal function occur during therapy. An encephalopathic syndrome (resembling neuroleptic malignant syndrome) may occur in patients receiving lithium with haloperidol or other antipsychotic agents (see Drug Interactions). Patients and caregivers should be informed of the symptoms of lithium toxicity (see Patient Information).

Capsule may contain benzyl alcohol which may cause allergic reactions in susceptible individuals; solution may contain sodium benzoate; benzoic acid (benzoate) is a metabolite of benzyl alcohol; large amounts of benzyl alcohol (≥99 mg/kg/day) have been associated with a potentially fatal toxicity ("gasping syndrome") in neonates; avoid use of lithium products containing benzyl alcohol in neonates; in vitro and animal studies have shown that benzoate, a metabolite of benzyl alcohol, displaces bilirubin from protein binding sites

Precautions Use with extreme caution in patients with cardiovascular or renal disease, patients receiving medications that alter sodium excretion (eg, diuretics, ACE inhibitors, or NSAIDs), and in patients with significant fluid loss (protracted sweating, diarrhea, or prolonged fever); monitor lithium concentrations closely, lithium

dosage reduction or temporary cessation may be required. Use with caution and modify dose in patients with renal dysfunction.

Adverse Reactions

Cardiovascular: Arrhythmias, hypotension, severe bradycardia, sinus node dysfunction, syncope

Central nervous system: Ataxia, blackout spells, confusion, dizziness, dystonia, fatigue, headache, restlessness, sedation, seizures, slurred speech, somnolence, vertigo

Dermatologic: Alopecia, anesthesia of skin, chronic folliculitis, drying and thinning of hair, exacerbation of psoriasis, rash

Endocrine & metabolic: Goiter, hyperthyroidism (rare), hypothyroidism, nephrogenic diabetes insipidus (thirst, polyuria, polydipsia)

Gastrointestinal: Anorexia, diarrhea, excessive salivation, gastritis, nausea, salivary gland swelling, vomiting, xerostomia

Genitourinary: Albuminuria, glycosuria, oliguria, polyuria

Hematologic: Leukocytosis

Neuromuscular & skeletal: Choreoathetoid movements, muscle hyperirritability, muscle weakness, tremor

Ocular: Blurred vision, nystagmus

Miscellaneous: Coldness and painful discoloration of fingers and toes

Drug Interactions

Avoid Concomitant Use

Avoid concomitant use of Lithium with any of the following: Sibutramine

Increased Effect/Toxicity

Lithium may increase the levels/effects of: Antipsychotics; Neuromuscular-Blocking Agents; Serotonin Modulators; Tricyclic Antidepressants

The levels/effects of Lithium may be increased by: ACE Inhibitors; Angiotensin II Receptor Blockers; Calcium Channel Blockers (Nondihydropyridine); CarBAMazepine; Desmopressin; Loop Diuretics; MAO Inhibitors; Methyldopa; Nonsteroidal Anti-Inflammatory Agents; Phenytoin; Potassium Iodide; Selective Serotonin Reuptake Inhibitors; Sibutramine; Thiazide Diuretics; Topiramate

Decreased Effect

Lithium may decrease the levels/effects of: Amphetamines; Antipsychotics; Desmopressin

The levels/effects of Lithium may be decreased by: Calcitonin; Calcium Polystyrene Sulfonate; Carbonic Anhydrase Inhibitors; Loop Diuretics; Sodium Bicarbonate; Sodium Chloride; Sodium Polystyrene Sulfonate; Theophylline Derivatives

Food Interactions Avoid changes in sodium content of diet (reduction in sodium intake can increase lithium toxicity); syrup may precipitate in tube feedings

Stability

Extended release tablets: Store between 15°C and 30°C (59°F to 86°F). Protect from moisture; dispense in tightly closed container.

Immediate release tablets and capsules: Store at 25°C (77°F); excursions permitted to 15°C to 30°C (59°F to 86°F). Protect from moisture; dispense in tightly closed container.

Oral solution: Store at 25°C (77°F); excursions permitted to 15°C to 30°C (59°F to 86°F). Dispense in tightly closed container.

Mechanism of Action Alters cation transport across cell membrane in nerve and muscle cells and influences reuptake of serotonin and/or norepinephrine

Pharmacokinetics (Adult data unless noted)

Distribution: Crosses the placenta; appears in breast milk at 35% to 50% of the concentrations in serum

Adults:

V_d: Initial: 0.3-0.4 L/kg

V_{dss}: 0.7-1 L/kg

Half-life, terminal: Adults: 18-24 hours, can increase to more than 36 hours in patients with renal impairment

Time to peak serum concentration (immediate release product): Within 0.5-2 hours

Elimination: 90% to 98% of a dose is excreted in the urine as unchanged drug; other excretory routes include feces (1%) and sweat (4% to 5%)

Dialysis: Dialyzable (50% to 100%)

Usual Dosage Oral: Monitor serum concentrations and clinical response (efficacy and toxicity) to determine proper dose:

Bipolar Disorder:

Children 6-12 years: 15-60 mg/kg/day in 3-4 divided doses (immediate release); dose not to exceed usual adult dosage; initiate at lower dose and adjust dose weekly based on serum concentrations

Adolescents: 600-1800 mg/day in 3-4 divided doses (immediate release) or 2 divided doses for extended release tablets

Adults: 300 mg 3-4 times/day (immediate release) or 450-900 mg of extended release tablets twice daily; usual maximum maintenance dose: 2.4 g/day

Dosing adjustment in renal impairment:

Cl_{cr} 10-50 mL/minute: Administer 50% to 75% of normal dose

Cl_{cr} <10 mL/minute: Administer 25% to 50% of normal dose

Administration Oral: Administer with meals to decrease GI upset. Do not crush or chew extended release dosage form; swallow whole

Monitoring Parameters Serum lithium concentration every 3-4 days during initial therapy; once patient is clinically stable and serum concentrations are stable, serum lithium may be obtained every 1-2 months; obtain lithium serum concentrations 8-12 hours postdose (ie, just before next dose). Monitor renal, hepatic, thyroid and cardiovascular function; CBC with differential, urinalysis, serum sodium, calcium, potassium

Reference Range

Therapeutic: Acute mania: 0.6-1.2 mEq/L (SI: 0.6-1.2 mmol/L); protection against future episodes in most patients with bipolar disorder: 0.8-1 mEq/L (SI: 0.8-1 mmol/L). A higher rate of relapse is described in subjects who are maintained <0.4 mEq/L (SI: <0.4 mmol/L)

Toxic: >2 mEq/L (SI: >2 mmol/L)

Concentration-related adverse effects:

GI complaints/tremor: 1.5-2 mEq/L

Confusion/somnolence: 2-2.5 mEq/L

Seizures/death: >2.5 mEq/L

Patient Information Limit caffeine; limit alcohol; avoid tasks requiring psychomotor coordination until CNS effects are known; may cause dry mouth; blood concentration monitoring is required to determine the proper dose; maintain a steady salt and fluid intake especially during the summer months; avoid dehydration; notify physician if vomiting, diarrhea, muscle weakness, tremor, drowsiness, or ataxia occur (these may be signs of lithium toxicity)

Nursing Implications Avoid dehydration

Additional Information In terms of efficacy, the results of studies using lithium to treat severe aggression in children and adolescents with conduct disorders, are mixed. A double-blind, placebo-controlled trial in patients 10-17 years of age (n=40) demonstrated efficacy for lithium in reducing aggressive behavior in psychiatrically hospitalized patients with conduct disorder and severe aggression. Lithium was initiated at 600 mg/day and titrated upwards by 300 mg/day. Final lithium carbonate doses ranged from 900-2100 mg/day divided into 3 doses/day (mean ± SD: 1425 ± 321 mg/day); serum lithium concentrations ranged from 0.78-1.55 mmol/L (mean ± SD: 1.07 ± 0.19 mmol/L)

(see Malone, 2000). In an earlier double-blind, placebo-controlled study in 50 children 5-12 years of age (mean ± SD: 9.4 ± 1.8 years), lithium was also initiated at 600 mg/day in 3 divided doses. Doses were titrated upwards in 300 mg/day increments. The mean optimal lithium dose was 1248 mg/day (range: 600-1800 mg/day); serum lithium concentrations ranged from 0.53-1.79 mmol/L (mean: 1.12 mmol/L). Doses >1500 mg/day and serum concentrations >1.13 mmol/L did not provide additional benefit (see Campbell, 1995). Several other studies have not demonstrated efficacy; further studies are needed.

Dosage Forms Excipient information presented when available (limited, particularly for generics); consult specific product labeling.

Capsule, as carbonate: 150 mg, 300 mg, 600 mg

Solution, as citrate: 300 mg/5 mL (5 mL, 500 mL) [equivalent to amount of lithium in lithium carbonate]

Syrup, as citrate: 300 mg/5 mL (480 mL) [equivalent to amount of lithium in lithium carbonate]

Tablet, as carbonate: 300 mg

Tablet, extended release, as carbonate: 300, 450 mg

Lithobid®: 300 mg

References

Campbell M, Adams PB, Small AM, et al, "Lithium in Hospitalized Aggressive Children With Conduct Disorder: A Double-Blind and Placebo-Controlled Study," *J Am Acad Child Adolesc Psychiatry*, 1995, 34(4):445-53.

Campbell M, Kafantaris V, and Cueva JE, "An Update on the Use of Lithium Carbonate in Aggressive Children and Adolescents With Conduct Disorder," *Psychopharmacol Bull*, 1995a, 31(1):93-102.

Levy HB, Harper CR, and Weinberg WA, "A Practical Approach to Children Failing in School," *Pediatr Clin North Am*, 1992, 39 (4):895-928.

Malone RP, Delaney MA, Luebbert JF, et al, "A Double-Blind Placebo-Controlled Study of Lithium in Hospitalized Aggressive Children and Adolescents With Conduct Disorder," *Arch Gen Psychiatry*, 2000, 57 (7):649-54.

Weller EB, Weller RA, and Fristad MA, "Lithium Dosage Guide for Prepubertal Children: A Preliminary Report," *J Am Acad Child Psychiatry*, 1986, 25(1):92-5.

◆ **Lithium Carbonate** see Lithium on page 834

◆ **Lithium Citrate** see Lithium on page 834

◆ **Lithobid®** see Lithium on page 834

◆ **Little Fevers™ [OTC]** see Acetaminophen on page 36

◆ **Little Noses® Decongestant [OTC]** see Phenylephrine on page 1102

◆ **Little Noses® Saline [OTC]** see Sodium Chloride on page 1270

◆ **Little Noses® Stuffy Nose Kit [OTC]** see Sodium Chloride on page 1270

◆ **Little Teethers® [OTC]** see Benzocaine on page 182

◆ **Little Tummys® Gas Relief [OTC]** see Simethicone on page 1262

◆ **Little Tummys® Laxative [OTC]** see Senna on page 1253

◆ **Live Attenuated Influenza Vaccine (LAIV)** see Influenza Virus Vaccine (H1N1, Live/Attenuated) on page 733

◆ **Live Attenuated Influenza Vaccine (LAIV)** see Influenza Virus Vaccine (Live/Attenuated) on page 736

◆ **LMD®** see Dextran on page 415

◆ **Locoid®** see Hydrocortisone on page 685

◆ **Locoid Lipocream®** see Hydrocortisone on page 685

◆ **Lodrane® [DSC]** see Brompheniramine and Pseudoephedrine on page 205

◆ **Lodrane® 12D** see Brompheniramine and Pseudoephedrine on page 205

◆ **Lodrane® 24D** see Brompheniramine and Pseudoephedrine on page 205

◆ **Lodrane® D [DSC]** see Brompheniramine and Pseudoephedrine on page 205

♦ **LoHist 12D** *see* Brompheniramine and Pseudoephedrine *on page 205*

♦ **LoHist LQ** *see* Brompheniramine and Pseudoephedrine *on page 205*

♦ **LoHist PD [DSC]** *see* Brompheniramine and Pseudoephedrine *on page 205*

♦ **L-OHP** *see* Oxaliplatin *on page 1030*

♦ **Lomine (Can)** *see* Dicyclomine *on page 433*

♦ **Lomotil®** *see* Diphenoxylate and Atropine *on page 450*

Lomustine (loe MUS teen)

Medication Safety Issues

Sound-alike/look-alike issues:
Lomustine may be confused with bendamustine, carmustine

High alert medication: The Institute for Safe Medication Practices (ISMP) includes this medication among its list of drug classes which have a heightened risk of causing significant patient harm when used in error.

Lomustine should only be administered as a single dose once every 6 weeks; serious errors have occurred when lomustine was inadvertently administered daily.

Related Information

Emetogenic Potential of Antineoplastic Agents *on page 1579*

U.S. Brand Names CeeNU®

Canadian Brand Names CeeNU®

Therapeutic Category Antineoplastic Agent, Alkylating Agent (Nitrosourea)

Generic Available No

Use Treatment of primary or metastatic brain tumors; combination therapy of Hodgkin's disease in patients who relapsed while being treated with primary therapy or who failed to respond to primary therapy [FDA approved in pediatric patients (age not specified) and adults]; has also been used in the treatment of colon cancer, medulloblastoma, and melanoma

Pregnancy Risk Factor D

Pregnancy Considerations Teratogenic effects and embryotoxicity have been observed in animal studies. There are no adequate and well-controlled studies in pregnant women. May cause fetal harm when administered to a pregnant woman. Women of childbearing potential should be advised to avoid pregnancy and should be advised of the potential harm to the fetus.

Lactation Enters breast milk/not recommended

Breast-Feeding Considerations Due to the potential for serious adverse reactions in the nursing infant, breast-feeding is not recommended.

Contraindications Hypersensitivity to lomustine or any component

Warnings Hazardous agent; use appropriate precautions for handling and disposal. Lomustine should be administered under the supervision of a physician experienced in the use of cancer chemotherapy agents **[U.S. Boxed Warning]**. Since major toxicity is bone marrow suppression, monitor blood counts weekly for at least 6 weeks after a dose **[U.S. Boxed Warning]**; nadir: ~6 weeks; do not give courses more frequently than every 6 weeks because the toxicity is delayed and cumulative. May cause delayed pulmonary toxicity (infiltrates and/or fibrosis); usually related to cumulative doses >1100 mg/m^2; onset of toxicity of 6 months or longer (has been reported up to 17 years after childhood administration in combination with radiation therapy); patients with baseline forced vital capacity (FVC) or carbon monoxide diffusing capacity (DL$_{co}$) <70% of predicted levels are at particular risk. Lomustine has been found to be clastogenic, teratogenic, embryotoxic, and carcinogenic in animals. Long-term use may be associated with the development of secondary malignancies.

Precautions Use with caution in patients with depressed platelet, leukocyte, or erythrocyte counts; reduced dosages are recommended. Use with caution in patients with hepatic impairment; reversible hepatotoxicity (transaminase, alkaline phosphatase, and bilirubin elevations) has been reported; monitor liver function tests periodically. Kidney damage has been observed; azotemia, decreased kidney size, and renal failure have been reported with long-term use; use with caution in patients with renal impairment; monitor renal function tests periodically; dosage adjustment may be required

Adverse Reactions

Central nervous system: Ataxia, disorientation, lethargy
Dermatologic: Alopecia, rash
Gastrointestinal: Anorexia, diarrhea, nausea and vomiting (usually within 3-6 hours after oral administration), stomatitis
Genitourinary: Azoospermia
Hematologic: Anemia, bone marrow dysplasia, leukopenia, myelosuppression (occurs 4-6 weeks after a dose and may persist 1-2 weeks; dose-related), thrombocytopenia
Hepatic: ALT, AST, alkaline phosphatase, and bilirubin increased; hepatotoxicity
Neuromuscular & skeletal: Dysarthria
Ocular: Blindness, optic atrophy, visual disturbances
Renal: Azotemia, interstitial nephritis, kidney size decreased, renal damage, renal failure
Respiratory: Pulmonary fibrosis/infiltrate with total cumulative dose >1 g/m^2 with onset occurring after 6 months or longer from the start of therapy; delayed-onset fibrosis may occur up to 17 years after treatment
Miscellaneous: Secondary malignancies

Drug Interactions

Metabolism/Transport Effects Substrate of CYP2D6; Inhibits CYP2D6 (weak), 3A4 (weak)

Avoid Concomitant Use

Avoid concomitant use of Lomustine with any of the following: BCG; Natalizumab; Pimecrolimus; Tacrolimus (Topical); Vaccines (Live)

Increased Effect/Toxicity

Lomustine may increase the levels/effects of: Leflunomide; Natalizumab; Vaccines (Live)

The levels/effects of Lomustine may be increased by: Denosumab; Pimecrolimus; Tacrolimus (Topical); Trastuzumab

Decreased Effect

Lomustine may decrease the levels/effects of: BCG; Sipuleucel-T; Vaccines (Inactivated); Vaccines (Live)

The levels/effects of Lomustine may be decreased by: Echinacea; Peginterferon Alfa-2b

Food Interactions Avoid concurrent administration of food/drugs that cause vomiting

Stability Store at 25°C (77°F); excursions permitted to15°C to 30°C (59°F to 86°F). Avoid exposure to excessive heat (>40°C; 104°F) and prolonged exposure to moisture; protect from light

Mechanism of Action Inhibits DNA and RNA synthesis through DNA alkylation and DNA cross-linking; carbamoylates amine groups on proteins; inhibits DNA polymerase activity, RNA and protein synthesis

Pharmacokinetics (Adult data unless noted)

Absorption: Rapid and complete absorption from the GI tract (30-60 minutes)
Distribution: Widely distributed; lomustine and/or its metabolites penetrate into the CNS; CSF level is ≥50% of concurrent plasma concentration; metabolites are present in breast milk

Metabolism: Rapid conversion to 4-hydroxy metabolites (active) partially by liver microsomal enzymes during first pass through the liver

Half-life (metabolites): 16-48 hours

Time to peak serum concentration (of active metabolite): Within 3 hours

Elimination: Excreted primarily in urine as metabolites; <5% fecal excretion

Usual Dosage Note: Repeat courses should only be administered after adequate recovery of leukocytes to >4000/mm^3 and platelets to >100,000/mm^3. Details concerning dosage in combination regimens should also be consulted.

Oral (refer to individual protocol):

Children: 75-130 mg/m^2 as a single dose every 6 weeks; subsequent doses are readjusted after initial treatment according to platelet and leukocyte counts

Adults: 100-130 mg/m^2 as a single dose every 6 weeks

With compromised marrow function: Initial dose: 100 mg/m^2 as a single dose every 6 weeks

Dosage adjustment based on hematologic response (nadir) for subsequent cycles:

Leukocytes >3000/mm^3, platelets >75,000/mm^3: No adjustment required

Leukocytes 2000-2999/mm^3, platelets 25,000-74,999/mm^3: Administer 70% of prior dose

Leukocytes <2000/mm^3, platelets <25,000/mm^3: Administer 50% of prior dose

Dosage adjustment in renal impairment: The FDA-approved labeling does not contain renal dosing adjustment guidelines. The following guidelines have been used by some clinicians:

Aronoff, 2007: Adults:

Cl$_{cr}$ 10-50 mL/minute: Administer 75% of dose

Cl$_{cr}$ <10 mL/minute: Administer 25% to 50% of dose

Hemodialysis: Supplemental dose is not necessary

Continuous ambulatory peritoneal dialysis (CAPD): Administer 25% to 50% of dose

Dosage adjustment in hepatic impairment: The FDA-approved labeling does not contain hepatic adjustment guidelines; lomustine is hepatically metabolized and caution should be used in patients with hepatic dysfunction.

Administration Oral: Administer with fluids on an empty stomach and at bedtime; do not administer food or drink for 2 hours after lomustine administration to decrease incidence of nausea and vomiting. Standard antiemetics may be administered prior to lomustine if needed. Varying strengths of capsules may be required to obtain necessary dose. Do not break capsules; use appropriate precautions (eg, gloves) when handling; avoid exposure to broken capsules.

Monitoring Parameters CBC with differential and platelet count, hepatic and renal function tests, pulmonary function tests (forced vital capacity, carbon monoxide diffusing capacity)

Patient Information Wear gloves when handling lomustine capsules. Notify physician if fever, chills, sore throat, bleeding, bruising, dry cough, swelling of feet or lower legs, shortness of breath, mental confusion, or yellowing of the eyes or skin occur; avoid alcohol and aspirin (GI irritants) for short periods after taking lomustine. Women of childbearing potential should be advised to avoid becoming pregnant while taking lomustine.

Dosage Forms Excipient information presented when available (limited, particularly for generics); consult specific product labeling.

Capsule:

CeeNU®: 10 mg, 40 mg, 100 mg

References

Aronoff GR, Bennett WM, Berns JS, et al, *Drug Prescribing in Renal Failure: Dosing Guidelines for Adults and Children,* 5th ed, Philadelphia, PA: American College of Physicians, 2007, 97, 177.

Berg SL, Grisell DL, DeLaney TF, et al, "Principles of Treatment of Pediatric Solid Tumors," *Pediatr Clin North Am,* 1991, 38(2):249-67.

Jakacki RI, Yates A, Blaney SM, et al, "A Phase I Trial of Temozolomide and Lomustine in Newly Diagnosed High-Grade Gliomas of Childhood," *Neuro Oncol,* 2008, 10(4):569-76.

Medical Research Council Brain Tumor Working Party, "Randomized Trial of Procarbazine, Lomustine, and Vincristine in the Adjuvant Treatment of High-Grade Astrocytoma: A Medical Research Council Trial," *J Clin Oncol,* 2001, 19(2):509-18.

Packer RJ, Gajjar A, Vezina G, et al, "Phase III Study of Craniospinal Radiation Therapy Followed by Adjuvant Chemotherapy for Newly Diagnosed Average-Risk Medulloblastoma," *J Clin Oncol,* 2006, 24 (25):4202-8.

◆ **Lomustinum** *see* Lomustine *on page* 837

◆ **Longastatin** *see* Octreotide Acetate *on page* 1008

◆ **Loniten® (Can)** *see* Minoxidil *on page* 935

◆ **Loperacap (Can)** *see* Loperamide *on page* 838

Loperamide (loe PER a mide)

Medication Safety Issues

Sound-alike/look-alike issues:

Imodium® A-D may be confused with Indocin®

Loperamide may be confused with furosemide

U.S. Brand Names Diamode [OTC]; Imodium® A-D [OTC]; K-Pek II [OTC]; Kao-Paverin® [OTC] [DSC]

Canadian Brand Names Apo-Loperamide®; Diarr-Eze; Dom-Loperamide; Imodium®; Loperacap; Novo-Loperamide; PMS-Loperamine; Rhoxal-loperamide; Rho®-Loperamine; Riva-Loperamide; Sandoz-Loperamide

Therapeutic Category Antidiarrheal

Generic Available Yes

Use Treatment of acute diarrhea and chronic diarrhea associated with inflammatory bowel disease; chronic functional diarrhea (idiopathic), chronic diarrhea caused by bowel resection or organic lesions; to decrease the volume of ileostomy discharge

Pregnancy Risk Factor C

Pregnancy Considerations Teratogenic effects were not observed in animal studies.

Lactation Enters breast milk/not recommended.

Contraindications Hypersensitivity to loperamide or any component; abdominal pain in the absence of diarrhea; children <24 months of age; acute ulcerative colitis; patients who must avoid constipation; infectious diarrhea resulting from organisms that penetrate the intestinal mucosa (eg, *Shigella, Salmonella*); patients with pseudomembranous colitis; bloody diarrhea

Warnings Discontinue therapy if constipation, abdominal distension, or ileus develop. HIV-positive patients should have therapy discontinued with early signs of abdominal distension due to reports of toxic megacolon in these patients who, while receiving loperamide, developed infectious colitis from both viral and bacterial pathogens.

Imodium® A-D contains benzoic acid and sodium benzoate; benzoic acid (benzoate) is a metabolite of benzyl alcohol; large amounts of benzyl alcohol (≥99 mg/kg/day) have been associated with a potentially fatal toxicity ("gasping syndrome") in neonates; *in vitro* and animal studies have shown that benzoate displaces bilirubin from protein binding sites; avoid use in neonates

Precautions If clinical improvement in acute diarrhea is not observed in 48 hours, discontinue use; use with caution and monitor patients with hepatic dysfunction closely for CNS toxicity

Adverse Reactions

Central nervous system: Sedation, fatigue, dizziness

Dermatologic: Rash, pruritus, urticaria, angioedema, erythema multiforme (rare), Stevens-Johnson syndrome (rare), toxic epidermal necrolysis (rare)

Gastrointestinal: Nausea, vomiting, constipation, abdominal cramping, xerostomia, toxic megacolon, paralytic ileus

Genitourinary: Urinary retention

Miscellaneous: Hypersensitivity reactions

Drug Interactions

Metabolism/Transport Effects Substrate of CYP2B6 (minor), P-glycoprotein

Avoid Concomitant Use There are no known interactions where it is recommended to avoid concomitant use.

Increased Effect/Toxicity

The levels/effects of Loperamide may be increased by: P-Glycoprotein Inhibitors

Decreased Effect

The levels/effects of Loperamide may be decreased by: P-Glycoprotein Inducers

Mechanism of Action Acts directly on intestinal muscles to inhibit peristalsis and prolong transit time

Pharmacodynamics Onset of action: Within 30-60 minutes

Pharmacokinetics (Adult data unless noted)

Absorption: Oral: 40%

Protein binding: 97%

Metabolism: Hepatic (>50%) to inactive compounds

Half-life: Adults: 10.8 hours (range 9.1-14.4 hours)

Time to peak serum concentration:

Capsules: 5 hours

Liquid: 2.5 hours

Elimination: Fecal and urinary (1%) excretion of metabolites and unchanged drug (30% to 40%)

Usual Dosage Oral:

Acute diarrhea:

Children: Initial doses (in first 24 hours):

2-5 years (13-20 kg): 1 mg 3 times/day

6-8 years (21-30): 2 mg twice daily

9-12 years (>30 kg): 2 mg 3 times/day

After initial dosing, 0.1 mg/kg doses after each loose stool but not exceeding initial dosage

Children >12 years and Adults: 4 mg initially, followed by 2 mg after each loose stool, up to 16 mg/day

Chronic diarrhea:

Children: 0.08-0.24 mg/kg/day divided 2-3 times/day, maximum: 2 mg/dose

Adults: 4 mg initially followed by 2 mg after each unformed stool until diarrhea is controlled; reduce dosage to meet individual requirements. When optimal dosage is determined, may administer total dosage once daily or in divided doses. Average daily maintenance dosage: 4-8 mg; if improvement is not seen with 16 mg/day for at least 10 days, symptoms are unlikely to be controlled by further therapy

Administration Oral: Drink plenty of fluids to help prevent dehydration

Patient Information Do not exceed maximum daily dosage; may cause drowsiness and impair ability to perform activities requiring mental alertness or physical coordination; if acute diarrhea lasts longer than 48 hours, consult physician; may cause dry mouth; avoid alcohol

Dosage Forms Excipient information presented when available (limited, particularly for generics); consult specific product labeling. [DSC] = Discontinued product

Caplet, as hydrochloride: 2 mg

Diamode, Imodium® A-D, Kao-Paverin® [DSC]: 2 mg

Capsule, as hydrochloride: 2 mg

Liquid, oral, as hydrochloride: 1 mg/5 mL (5 mL, 10 mL, 120 mL)

Imodium® A-D: 1 mg/5 mL (60 mL, 120 mL) [contains alcohol, sodium benzoate, benzoic acid; cherry mint flavor]

Imodium® A-D [new formulation]: 1 mg/7.5 mL (60 mL, 120 mL, 360 mL) [contains sodium 10 mg/30 mL, sodium benzoate; creamy mint flavor]

Tablet, as hydrochloride: 2 mg

K-Pek II: 2 mg

◆ **Loperamide Hydrochloride** *see* Loperamide *on page 838*

Lopinavir and Ritonavir
(lop IN uh veer & rit ON uh veer)

Medication Safety Issues

Sound-alike/look-alike issues:

Potential for dispensing errors between Kaletra® and Keppra® (levetiracetam)

Administration issues:

Children's doses are based on weight and calculated by milligrams of lopinavir. Care should be taken to accurately calculate the dose. The oral solution contains lopinavir 80 mg and ritonavir 20 mg per one mL. Children <12 years of age (and ≤40 kg) who are not taking certain concomitant antiretroviral medications will receive <5 mL of solution per dose.

Related Information

Adult and Adolescent HIV *on page 1620*

Body Surface Area of Children and Adults *on page 1576*

Management of Healthcare Worker Exposures to HBV, HCV, and HIV *on page 1661*

Pediatric HIV *on page 1613*

Perinatal HIV *on page 1628*

U.S. Brand Names Kaletra®

Canadian Brand Names Kaletra®

Therapeutic Category Antiretroviral Agent; HIV Agents (Anti-HIV Agents); Protease Inhibitor

Generic Available No

Use Treatment of HIV infection in combination with other antiretroviral agents (**Note:** HIV regimens consisting of three antiretroviral agents are strongly recommended)

Medication Guide An FDA-approved patient medication guide, which is available with the product information and at http://www.fda.gov/downloads/Drugs/DrugSafety/UCM143461.pdf, must be dispensed with this medication for each new outpatient prescription and refill.

Pregnancy Risk Factor C

Pregnancy Considerations Adverse events were not seen in animal studies, except at doses which were also maternally toxic. Safety and pharmacokinetic studies of the tablet in pregnant women are not completed. Preliminary information suggests increased dosage may be needed during pregnancy, although specific recommendations with the tablet formulation are not yet available. Once-daily dosing is not recommended during pregnancy. Lopinavir/ritonavir crosses the placenta, however, teratogenic effects have not been observed in humans. The Perinatal HIV Guidelines Working Group considers this a recommended combination for use during pregnancy. Pregnancy and protease inhibitors are both associated with an increased risk of hyperglycemia. Glucose levels should be closely monitored. Health professionals are encouraged to contact the antiretroviral pregnancy registry to monitor outcomes of pregnant women exposed to antiretroviral medications (1-800-258-4263 or www.APRegistry.com).

Lactation Excretion in breast milk unknown/contraindicated

Breast-Feeding Considerations In infants born to mothers who are HIV positive, HAART while breast-feeding may decrease postnatal infection. However, maternal or infant antiretroviral therapy does not completely eliminate the risk of postnatal HIV transmission.

In the United States where formula is accessible, affordable, safe, and sustainable, complete avoidance of breast-feeding by HIV-infected women is recommended to decrease potential transmission of HIV.

Contraindications Hypersensitivity (eg, Stevens-Johnson syndrome, erythema multiforme) to lopinavir, ritonavir, or any component; concurrent therapy with medications that largely rely on cytochrome P450 isoenzymes CYP3A for clearance and that have an association between increased plasma concentrations and serious or life-threatening effects [eg, cisapride, dihydroergotamine, ergonovine, ergotamine, lovastatin, methylergonovine, midazolam (oral), pimozide, simvastatin, triazolam]; concurrent therapy with strong CYP3A4 inducers that significantly decrease lopinavir serum concentrations which may lead to treatment failure or development of resistance [eg, rifampin or the herbal medicine St John's wort (*Hypericum perforatum*)] (see Drug Interactions).

Warnings Lopinavir and ritonavir are potent CYP3A isoenzyme inhibitors that interact with numerous drugs. Due to potential serious and/or life-threatening drug interactions, some drugs are contraindicated (see Contraindications and Drug Interactions) and other medications may require concentration monitoring or dosage adjustment if coadministered with lopinavir and ritonavir (see Drug Interactions). Concomitant use with certain medications may require dosage adjustment of lopinavir and ritonavir (see Drug Interactions).

Potentially fatal pancreatitis may occur; markedly elevated serum triglycerides is a risk factor for developing pancreatitis; advanced HIV disease or a history of pancreatitis may also place patients at increased risk; discontinue lopinavir and ritonavir therapy if clinical signs, symptoms, or laboratory abnormalities suggestive of pancreatitis occur. New onset diabetes mellitus, exacerbations of diabetes, and hyperglycemia have been reported in HIV-infected patients receiving protease inhibitors. Immune reconstitution syndrome (an acute inflammatory response to residual or indolent opportunistic infections) may occur in HIV patients during initial treatment with combination antiretroviral agents, including lopinavir/ritonavir; this syndrome may require further patient assessment and therapy.

A fatal accidental overdose occurred in a 2.1 kg, 44-day old infant (born at 30 weeks gestational age) with HIV who received a single dose of 6.5 mL of lopinavir/ritonavir oral solution. The infant died of cardiogenic shock 9 days later. Healthcare providers are reminded that lopinavir/ritonavir oral solution is highly concentrated. To minimize the risk for medication errors, healthcare providers should pay special attention to accurate calculation of the dose, transcription of the medication order, dispensing information, dosing instructions, and proper measurement of the dose. This is especially important for infants and young children. New pediatric tablets containing lopinavir 100 mg and ritonavir 25 mg (ie, $\frac{1}{2}$ the amount in regular tablets) are now available; caution should be taken so that dosing and dispensing errors do not occur.

Precautions Use with caution in patients with hepatic impairment (lopinavir and ritonavir are primarily metabolized by the liver); hepatitis or markedly elevated transaminases prior to therapy may increase risk for developing or worsening elevations in liver enzymes or for hepatic decompensation; hepatic dysfunction (including fatalities) have been reported; in general, these occurred in patients with advanced HIV disease who were taking multiple concomitant medications and who had underlying chronic hepatitis or cirrhosis; a causal relationship with lopinavir/ritonavir has not been established; monitor liver enzymes prior to therapy and periodically during treatment; consider more frequent monitoring of liver enzymes in patients with concurrent chronic hepatitis or cirrhosis, especially during the first few months of lopinavir/ritonavir therapy. Spontaneous bleeding episodes have been reported in patients with hemophilia type A and B receiving protease inhibitors. Large increases in total cholesterol and triglycerides have been reported; patients should be monitored prior to therapy and periodically during treatment. Fat redistribution and accumulation [ie, central obesity, peripheral wasting, facial wasting, breast enlargement, dorsocervical fat enlargement (buffalo hump), and cushingoid appearance] have been observed in patients receiving antiretroviral agents (causal relationship not established). Safety, efficacy, and pharmacokinetic profiles of lopinavir and ritonavir have not been established in infants <14 days of age.

Adverse Reactions

Cardiovascular: Hypertension (up to 2%), vein distension (up to 3%)

Central nervous system: Headache (2% to 6%), insomnia (up to 3%), pain, depression (up to 2%), chills (up to 2%), fever (2%)

Dermatologic: Rash (1% to 5%; children 3%)

Endocrine & metabolic: Hyperglycemia (1% to 5%), hypertriglyceridemia (4% to 36%), hypercholesterolemia (3% to 39%; children 3%), hyperuricemia (up to 5%); new onset diabetes, exacerbation of diabetes mellitus; serum phosphorus decreased (1% to 2%); fat redistribution and accumulation (see Precautions); weight loss (up to 3%), libido decreased (up to 2%), hypogonadism (males: up to 2%), amenorrhea (up to 4.5%), hypernatremia (children 3%), hyponatremia (children 3%)

Gastrointestinal: Nausea (5% to 16%), vomiting (2% to 6%; children 21%), diarrhea (5% to 28%; **Note:** In one adult study, incidence of diarrhea was higher in patients receiving once-daily dosing compared to twice daily dosing; children 12%), taste aversion (children: 22%), abdominal pain (2% to 11%), amylase elevated (3% to 8%; children 7%), dyspepsia (up to 6%), flatulence (1% to 4%), anorexia (up to 2%), dysphagia (up to 2%)

Hematologic: Platelets decreased (grade 3/4: children 4%), neutropenia (grade 3/4: 1% to 5%), hemolytic anemia, spontaneous bleeding in hemophiliacs

Hepatic: ALT elevated (grade 3/4: 3% to 11%; children 7%), AST elevated (grade 3/4: 2% to 10%; children 8%), GGT elevated (10% to 29%), bilirubin elevated (1%; children 3%), hepatitis (may be life-threatening in rare cases)

Neuromuscular & skeletal: Asthenia (up to 9%), myalgia (up to 2%), paresthesia (up to 2%)

Miscellaneous: Immune reconstitution syndrome (see Warnings); rare: Allergic reaction (fever, rash, jaundice)

Drug Interactions

Metabolism/Transport Effects

Lopinavir: **Substrate** of CYP3A4 (major); **Inhibits** CYP2D6 (strong), CYP3A4 (strong), P-glycoprotein; **Induces** CYP1A2 (weak-moderate), CYP2C9 (weak-moderate), CYP2C19 (strong)

Ritonavir: **Substrate** of CYP1A2 (minor), CYP2B6 (minor), CYP2D6 (major), CYP3A4 (major), P-glycoprotein; **Inhibits** CYP2C8 (strong), CYP2C9 (weak), CYP2C19 (weak), CYP2D6 (strong), CYP2E1 (weak), CYP3A4 (strong), P-glycoprotein; **Induces** CYP1A2 (weak), 2C8 (weak), 2C9 (weak), 3A4 (weak)

Avoid Concomitant Use

Avoid concomitant use of Lopinavir and Ritonavir with any of the following: Alfuzosin; Amiodarone; Cisapride; Dabigatran Etexilate; Darunavir; Disulfiram; Dronedarone; Eplerenone; Ergot Derivatives; Etravirine; Everolimus; Flecainide; Fluticasone (Nasal); Halofantrine; Lovastatin; Midazolam; Nilotinib; Nisoldipine; Pimozide; Pitavastatin; Propafenone; QuiNIDine; Ranolazine; Rivaroxaban; Romidepsin; Salmeterol; Silodosin; Simvastatin; St Johns Wort; Tamoxifen; Tamsulosin; Thioridazine; Tolvaptan; Topotecan; Triazolam; Voriconazole

Increased Effect/Toxicity

Lopinavir and Ritonavir may increase the levels/effects of: Alfuzosin; Almotriptan; Alosetron; ALPRAZolam; Amiodarone; Antifungal Agents (Azole Derivatives, Systemic); Atomoxetine; Bortezomib; Bosentan; Brinzolamide; Calcium Channel Blockers (Dihydropyridine); Calcium Channel Blockers (Nondihydropyridine); CarBAMazepine; Ciclesonide; Cisapride; Clarithromycin; Clorazepate; Colchicine; Corticosteroids (Orally Inhaled); CycloSPORINE; CycloSPORINE (Systemic); CYP2C8 Substrates (High risk); CYP2D6 Substrates; CYP3A4 Substrates; Dabigatran Etexilate; Diazepam; Dienogest; Digoxin; Dronabinol; Dronedarone; Dutasteride; Enfuvirtide; Eplerenone; Ergot Derivatives; Estazolam; Etravirine; Everolimus; FentaNYL; Fesoterodine; Flecainide; Flurazepam; Fluticasone (Nasal); Fusidic Acid; GuanFACINE; Halofantrine; HMG-CoA Reductase Inhibitors; Ixabepilone; Lovastatin; Lumefantrine; Maraviroc; Meperidine; MethylPREDNISolone; Midazolam; Nebivolol; Nefazodone; Nilotinib; Nisoldipine; Paricalcitol; Pazopanib; P-Glycoprotein Substrates; Pimecrolimus; Pimozide; Pitavastatin; PrednisoLONE; PredniSONE; Propafenone; Protease Inhibitors; QuiNIDine; Ranolazine; Rifamycin Derivatives; Rivaroxaban; Romidepsin; Salmeterol; Saxagliptin; Sildenafil; Silodosin; Simvastatin; Sirolimus; Sorafenib; Tacrolimus; Tacrolimus (Systemic); Tacrolimus (Topical); Tadalafil; Tamoxifen; Tamsulosin; Temsirolimus; Tenofovir; Tetrabenazine; Thioridazine; Tolvaptan; Topotecan; TraZODone; Treprostinil; Triazolam; Tricyclic Antidepressants; Vardenafil; VinBLAStine; VinCRIStine

The levels/effects of Lopinavir and Ritonavir may be increased by: Antifungal Agents (Azole Derivatives, Systemic); Clarithromycin; CycloSPORINE; CycloSPORINE (Systemic); Delavirdine; Disulfiram; Efavirenz; Enfuvirtide; Etravirine; Fusidic Acid; MetroNIDAZOLE (Topical); P-Glycoprotein Inhibitors

Decreased Effect

Lopinavir and Ritonavir may decrease the levels/effects of: Abacavir; Atovaquone; BuPROPion; Clarithromycin; Codeine; Contraceptives (Estrogens); CYP2C19 Substrates; Darunavir; Deferasirox; Delavirdine; Didanosine; Divalproex; Etravirine; LamoTRIgine; Meperidine; Methadone; Phenytoin; Prasugrel; Theophylline Derivatives; TraMADol; Valproic Acid; Voriconazole; Warfarin; Zidovudine

The levels/effects of Lopinavir and Ritonavir may be decreased by: Antacids; CarBAMazepine; Contraceptives (Estrogens); CYP3A4 Inducers (Strong); Efavirenz; Garlic; Nevirapine; Peginterferon Alfa-2b; P-Glycoprotein Inducers; Phenytoin; Rifamycin Derivatives; St Johns Wort; Tenofovir

Food Interactions Compared to fasting, a moderate fat meal increased lopinavir AUC by 80% (oral solution), but by only 26.9% for the tablets; a high fat meal increased lopinavir AUC by 130% (oral solution), but by only 18.9% for the tablets

Stability

Oral solution: Store at 2°C to 8°C (36°F to 46°F) until dispensed; refrigerated products are stable until labeled expiration date; stability at room temperature: 2 months; avoid exposure to excessive heat.

Tablets: Store at controlled room temperature 20°C to 25°C (68°F to 77°F). Dispense in original container or USP equivalent tight container. Do not expose to high humidity outside original container or USP equivalent tight container for >2 weeks.

Mechanism of Action This product is a fixed-dose combination of lopinavir and ritonavir; antiretroviral effects are due to lopinavir, a protease inhibitor; lopinavir acts on an enzyme (protease) late in the HIV replication process after the virus has entered into the cell's nucleus. Lopinavir binds to the protease activity site and inhibits the activity of the enzyme, thus preventing cleavage of viral polyprotein precursors (gag-pol protein precursors) into individual functional proteins found in infectious HIV. This results in the formation of immature, noninfectious viral particles. Ritonavir inhibits the metabolism of lopinavir via the cytochrome P450 CYP3A isoenzyme pathway and significantly increases plasma concentrations of lopinavir.

Pharmacokinetics (Adult data unless noted) Information below refers to Lopinavir; see Ritonavir for additional information.

Protein binding: 98% to 99%; binds to both alpha$_1$ - acid glycoprotein and albumin; higher affinity for alpha$_1$-acid glycoprotein; decreased protein binding in patients with mild to moderate hepatic impairment

Metabolism: Primarily oxidative, via cytochrome P450 CYP3A isoenzyme; 13 oxidative metabolites identified; may induce its own metabolism

Bioavailability: Absolute bioavailability not established; AUC for oral solution was 22% lower than capsule when given under fasting conditions; concentrations were similar under nonfasting conditions

Half-life: Adults: Mean: 5-6 hours

Elimination: 2.2% of dose eliminated unchanged in urine; 83% of dose eliminated in feces

Clearance: (Apparent oral): Adults: 6-7 L/hour

Dialysis: Unlikely to remove significant amounts of drug (due to high protein binding)

Usual Dosage Oral (use in combination with other antiretroviral agents): **Note:** Pediatric dosage is based on patient body weight or surface area and is presented here based on lopinavir component. **Do not exceed recommended adult dose.** Use of tablets in patients <15 kg or <0.6 m^2 is **not** recommended (use oral solution). Once-daily dosing has not been studied in pediatric patients, and therefore, is **not** recommended.

Neonates <14 days: Not approved for use; dose is not established.

Neonates and Infants 14 days to 6 months:

Patients receiving concomitant antiretroviral therapy <u>without</u> amprenavir, efavirenz, fosamprenavir, nelfinavir, or nevirapine: Lopinavir 16 mg/kg or 300 mg/m^2 twice daily. **Note:** Infants <6 months of age, especially those <6 weeks of age, who receive this dose may have lower trough concentrations compared to adults; evaluate infants and adjust dose for incremental growth at frequent intervals (Working Group, 2008).

Patients receiving concomitant antiretroviral therapy **with amprenavir, efavirenz, fosamprenavir, nelfinavir, or nevirapine**: Dosage information does not exist; lopinavir/ritonavir is not recommended in patients <6 months of age who are receiving these agents.

Children 6 months to 18 years: (see also Additional Information)

Patients receiving concomitant antiretroviral therapy **without amprenavir, efavirenz, fosamprenavir, nelfinavir, or nevirapine:**

Body surface area dosing: Lopinavir 230 mg/m^2 twice daily

Weight-based dosing:

<15 kg: Lopinavir 12 mg/kg twice daily

≥15-40 kg: Lopinavir 10 mg/kg twice daily

>40 kg: See Adult dosing

Patients receiving concomitant antiretroviral therapy **with amprenavir, efavirenz, fosamprenavir, nelfinavir, or nevirapine:** (or treatment-experienced patients not receiving these agents in whom decreased susceptibility to lopinavir is suspected; Working Group, 2008):

Body surface area dosing: Lopinavir 300 mg/m^2 twice daily

Weight-based dosing:

<15 kg: Lopinavir 13 mg/kg twice daily

≥15-45 kg: Lopinavir 11 mg/kg twice daily

>45 kg: See Adult dosing

Adults:

Patients receiving concomitant antiretroviral therapy **without amprenavir, efavirenz, fosamprenavir, nelfinavir, or nevirapine:** Lopinavir 400 mg/ritonavir 100 mg twice daily

Once-daily dosing: Adults: **Antiretroviral-naive patients only**: Lopinavir 800 mg/ritonavir 200 mg once daily; **Note:** Once-daily dosing is **not** recommended for pediatric or antiretroviral-experienced patients, or for patients receiving amprenavir, efavirenz, fosamprenavir, nelfinavir, nevirapine, carbamazepine, phenobarbital, or phenytoin; once-daily dosing has not been evaluated with concurrent use of indinavir or saquinavir

Patients receiving concomitant antiretroviral therapy **with amprenavir, efavirenz, fosamprenavir, nelfinavir, or nevirapine: Note:** Once-daily dosing is **not** recommended:

Oral solution: Lopinavir 533 mg/ritonavir 133 mg (6.5 mL) twice daily

Tablets: Lopinavir 500 mg/ritonavir 125 mg twice daily

Dosing adjustment in renal impairment: Has not been studied in patients with renal impairment; however, a decrease in clearance is not expected

Dosing adjustment in hepatic impairment: Lopinavir AUC may be increased ~30% in patients with mild-to-moderate hepatic impairment; use with caution. No data available in patients with severe impairment.

Administration Oral:

Oral solution: Administer with food to enhance bioavailability and decrease kinetic variability; use a calibrated oral dosing syringe to measure and administer the oral solution; **Note:** Dose must be accurately measured and administered to pediatric patients as oral solution is very concentrated and a fatal accidental overdose has been reported (see Warnings)

Tablets: May be administered without regard to meals; swallow tablets whole, do not crush, break, or chew

Monitoring Parameters Signs and symptoms of pancreatitis; serum electrolytes, glucose, triglycerides, cholesterol, liver enzymes, bilirubin, amylase, CBC with differential, platelets, CD4 cell count, HIV RNA plasma level

Patient Information Lopinavir and ritonavir is not a cure for HIV. Notify physician if symptoms of pancreatitis occur (nausea, vomiting, abdominal pain). Report the use of other medications, nonprescription medications and herbal or natural products to your physician and pharmacist; avoid the herbal medicine St John's wort. Lopinavir and ritonavir may interfere with certain oral contraceptives and contraceptive patch; alternate contraceptive measures may be needed (consult with physician). Special care should be taken to accurately measure and administer oral solution to pediatric patients to decrease the risk of accidental overdose or underdose. Take lopinavir and ritonavir everyday as prescribed; do not change dose or discontinue without physician's advice; if a dose is missed, take it as soon as possible, then return to normal dosing schedule; if a dose is skipped, do not double the next dose

HIV medications may cause changes in body fat, including an increase in fat in the upper back and neck, breasts, and trunk; a loss of fat from the face, arms, and legs may also occur.

Additional Information Oral solution contains 42.4% alcohol (v/v); overdose in a child may cause potentially lethal alcohol toxicity; treatment should be supportive and include general poisoning management; activated charcoal may help remove unabsorbed medication; dialysis unlikely to be of benefit

Preliminary studies have reported response rates (defined as viral loads <400 copies/mL) of 91%, 81%, and 33% for patients with 0-5, 6-7, and 8-10 protease mutations at baseline, respectively (see Hurst, 2000).

The FDA-approved dose for pediatric patients 6 months to 18 years of age who are not receiving concomitant antiretroviral therapy with amprenavir, efavirenz, fosamprenavir, nelfinavir, or nevirapine is 230 mg/m² of lopinavir and 57.5 mg/m² of ritonavir per dose. The FDA-approved dose for pediatric patients who are receiving concomitant antiretroviral therapy with amprenavir, efavirenz, fosamprenavir, nelfinavir, or nevirapine is 300 mg/m² of lopinavir and 75 mg/m² of ritonavir per dose. The use of these doses twice daily in children 6 months to 12 years of age has resulted in lopinavir AUCs that are similar to those attained in adults receiving standard doses; however, trough levels in children were lower that those observed in adults. Therefore, some clinicians may elect to initiate lopinavir/ritonavir in higher doses (eg, 300 mg/m²/dose twice daily) in pediatric patients 6 months to 12 years of age, who are **not** receiving concomitant antiviral therapy with amprenavir, efavirenz, fosamprenavir, nelfinavir, or nevirapine, especially when used in PI-experienced patients suspected of having reduced susceptibility to protease inhibitors (see Working Group 2008, Supplement 1: Pediatric Antiretroviral Drug Information for details).

Dosage Forms Excipient information presented when available (limited, particularly for generics); consult specific product labeling.

Solution, oral:

Kaletra®: Lopinavir 80 mg and ritonavir 20 mg per mL (160 mL) [contains alcohol 42.4%]

Tablet:

Kaletra®:

Lopinavir 100 mg and ritonavir 25 mg

Lopinavir 200 mg and ritonavir 50 mg

References

Briars LA, Hilao JJ, and Kraus DM, "A Review of Pediatric Human Immunodeficiency Virus Infection," *Journal of Pharmacy Practice*, 2004, 17(6):407-31.

Hurst M and Faulds D, "Lopinavir," *Drugs*, 2000, 60(6):1371-9.

Mangum EM and Graham KK, "Lopinavir-Ritonavir: A New Protease Inhibitor," *Pharmacotherapy*, 2001, 21(11):1352-63.

Morris JL and Kraus DM, "New Antiretroviral Therapies for Pediatric HIV Infection," *J Pediatr Pharmacol Ther*, 2005, 10:215-47.

Panel on Antiretroviral Guidelines for Adults and Adolescents, "Guidelines for the Use of Antiretroviral Agents in HIV-Infected Adults and Adolescents," December 1, 2009, http://www.aidsinfo.nih.gov.

Piscitelli SC, Burstein AH, Chaitt D, et al, "Indinavir Concentrations and St John's Wort," *Lancet*, 2000, 355(9203):547-8.

Working Group on Antiretroviral Therapy and Medical Management of HIV-Infected Children, "Guidelines for the Use of Antiretroviral Agents in Pediatric HIV Infection," February 23, 2009. Available at http://www.aidsinfo.nih.gov.

◆ **Lopressor®** see Metoprolol *on page 918*

◆ **Loprox®** see Ciclopirox *on page 306*

◆ **Loradamed [OTC]** see Loratadine *on page 842*

Loratadine (lor AT a deen)

Medication Safety Issues

Sound-alike/look-alike issues:

Claritin® may be confused with clarithromycin

Claritin® (loratadine) may be confused with Claritin™ Eye (ketotifen)

U.S. Brand Names Alavert® Allergy 24 Hour [OTC]; Alavert® Children's Allergy [OTC]; Claritin® 24 Hour Allergy [OTC]; Claritin® Children's Allergy [OTC]; Claritin® Hives Relief [OTC] [DSC]; Claritin® Liqui-Gels® 24 Hour Allergy [OTC]; Claritin® RediTabs® 24 Hour Allergy [OTC]; Dimetapp® ND Children's [OTC] [DSC]; Loradamed [OTC]; Tavist® ND Allergy [OTC]

Canadian Brand Names Apo-Loratadine®; Claritin®; Claritin® Kids

Therapeutic Category Antihistamine

Generic Available Yes

Use Symptomatic relief of nasal and non-nasal symptoms of allergic rhinitis; treatment of chronic idiopathic urticaria

Pregnancy Risk Factor B

Pregnancy Considerations Loratadine was not found to be teratogenic in animal studies. There are no adequate and well-controlled studies in pregnant woman; use during pregnancy only if clearly needed.

Lactation Enters breast milk/not recommended (AAP rates "compatible")

Contraindications Hypersensitivity to loratadine or any component

Warnings Use with caution and adjust dosage in patients with severe liver impairment or renal impairment; Claritin® syrup contains sodium benzoate; benzoic acid (benzoate) is a metabolite of benzyl alcohol; large amounts of benzyl alcohol (≥99 mg/kg/day) have been associated with a potentially fatal toxicity ("gasping syndrome") in neonates; in vitro and animal studies have shown that benzoate displaces bilirubin from protein binding sites; avoid use in neonates

Precautions Use cautiously in patients who are also taking ketoconazole, itraconazole, fluconazole, erythromycin, clarithromycin, or other drugs which may impair loratadine's hepatic metabolism; although increased plasma levels of loratadine have been observed, no adverse effects with concomitant administration have been reported including QT interval prolongation which has occurred when similar antihistamines, terfenadine and astemizole, were combined with these agents; while less sedating than other antihistamines, loratadine may cause drowsiness and impair ability to perform hazardous activities requiring mental alertness. Use cautiously in breast-feeding women as breast milk levels of loratadine are equivalent to serum levels. Some tablets contain phenylalanine which must be avoided (or used with caution) in patients with phenylketonuria.

Adverse Reactions

Cardiovascular: Hypotension, hypertension, palpitations, tachycardia, chest pain, syncope

Central nervous system: Headache, somnolence, fatigue, anxiety, depression, dizziness, fever, migraine, agitation, nervousness, hyperactivity

Dermatologic: Alopecia, dermatitis, dry skin, rash, pruritus, photosensitivity

Gastrointestinal: Xerostomia, nausea, vomiting, gastritis, abdominal pain, diarrhea

Endocrine & metabolic: Breast pain and enlargement (rare), menorrhagia, dysmenorrhea

Neuromuscular & skeletal: Hyperkinesia, arthralgias, myalgias, leg cramps

Ocular: Blurred vision, altered lacrimation, eye pain, conjunctivitis

Genitourinary: Discoloration of urine

Respiratory: Nasal dryness, pharyngitis, dyspnea, nasal congestion, wheezing, nose bleed

Miscellaneous: Diaphoresis

Drug Interactions

Metabolism/Transport Effects Substrate of CYP2D6 (minor), CYP3A4 (minor), P-glycoprotein; **Inhibits** CYP2C8 (weak), 2C19 (moderate), 2D6 (weak)

Avoid Concomitant Use There are no known interactions where it is recommended to avoid concomitant use.

Increased Effect/Toxicity

Loratadine may increase the levels/effects of: Alcohol (Ethyl); Anticholinergics; CNS Depressants

The levels/effects of Loratadine may be increased by: Amiodarone; P-Glycoprotein Inhibitors; Pramlintide

Decreased Effect

Loratadine may decrease the levels/effects of: Acetylcholinesterase Inhibitors (Central); Betahistine

The levels/effects of Loratadine may be decreased by: Acetylcholinesterase Inhibitors (Central); Amphetamines; Peginterferon Alfa-2b; P-Glycoprotein Inducers

Food Interactions Administration with food increases loratadine's bioavailability by 40%

Mechanism of Action Long-acting tricyclic antihistamine with selective peripheral histamine H_1 receptor antagonistic properties

Pharmacodynamics

Onset of action: Within 1-3 hours

Maximum effect: 8-12 hours

Duration: >24 hours

Pharmacokinetics (Adult data unless noted)

Absorption: Rapid; food increases total bioavailability (AUC) by 40%

Distribution: Binds preferentially to peripheral nervous system H_1 receptors; no appreciable entry into CNS; loratadine and metabolite pass easily into breast milk and achieve concentrations equivalent to plasma levels; breast milk to plasma ratio: 1.17

Protein binding: 97% (loratadine), 73% to 77% (metabolite)

Metabolism: Extensive first-pass metabolism by cytochrome P450 system to an active metabolite (descarboethoxyloratadine)

Half-life: 8.4 hours (loratadine), 28 hours (metabolite)

Time to peak serum concentration: 1-2 hours

Elimination: 80% eliminated via urine & feces as metabolic products

Usual Dosage Oral:

Children 2-5 years: 5 mg once daily

Children ≥6 years and Adults: 10 mg once daily

Dosing interval in renal (GFR <30 mL/minute) or hepatic impairment: Administer dosage every other day

Administration Oral: Administer on an empty stomach or before meals; place Claritin® RediTab® (rapidly disintegrating tablet) on the tongue; tablet disintegration occurs rapidly; may administer with or without water

Monitoring Parameters Improvement in signs and symptoms of allergic rhinitis or chronic idiopathic urticaria

Reference Range Therapeutic serum levels (not used clinically): Loratadine: 2.5-100 ng/mL; active metabolite: 0.5-100 ng/mL

Test Interactions Antigen skin testing

Patient Information Drink plenty of water; may cause dry mouth; may color urine; may cause drowsiness and impair ability to perform activities requiring mental alertness or physical coordination; notify physician if fainting episode occurs; avoid alcohol. May rarely cause photosensitivity reactions (eg, exposure to sunlight may cause severe sunburn, skin rash, redness, or itching); avoid direct exposure to sunlight

Dosage Forms Excipient information presented when available (limited, particularly for generics); consult specific product labeling. [DSC] = Discontinued product

Capsule, liquid gel, oral:

Claritin® Liqui-Gels® 24 Hour Allergy: 10 mg

Solution, oral: 5 mg/5 mL (120 mL)

Syrup, oral: 5 mg/5 mL (120 mL)

Claritin® Children's Allergy: 5 mg/5 mL (60 mL, 120 mL) [dye free, ethanol free; contains propylene glycol, sodium benzoate; fruit flavor]

Claritin® Children's Allergy: 5 mg/5 mL (60 mL, 120 mL) [dye free, ethanol free, sugar free; contains propylene glycol, sodium 6 mg/5 mL, sodium benzoate; grape flavor]

Tablet, oral: 10 mg

Alavert® Allergy 24 Hour: 10 mg [dye free, gluten free, sucrose free]

Claritin® 24 Hour Allergy: 10 mg

Claritin® Hives Relief: 10 mg [DSC]

Loradamed: 10 mg

Tavist® ND Allergy: 10 mg

Tablet, chewable, oral:

Claritin® Children's Allergy: 5 mg [contains phenyl-alanine 1.4 mg/tablet; grape flavor]

Tablet, orally disintegrating, oral:

Alavert® Allergy 24 Hour: 10 mg [dye free, gluten free, sucrose free; contains phenylalanine 8.4 mg/tablet; Citrus Burst™ and mint flavors]

Alavert® Children's Allergy: 10 mg [dye free, gluten free, sucrose free; contains phenylalanine 8.4 mg/tablet; bubblegum and Citrus Burst™ flavors]

Claritin® RediTabs® 24 Hour Allergy: 10 mg [mint flavor]

Dimetapp® ND Children's: 10 mg [contains phenyl-alanine 8.4 mg/tablet] [DSC]

References

Lin CC, Radwanski E, Affrime M, et al, "Pharmacokinetics of Loratadine in Pediatric Subjects," *Am J Therapeut*, 1995, 2:504-8.

Luck JC and Evrard HM, "Atrial Fibrillation Associated With Loratadine Use," *J Allergy Clin Immunol*, 1995, 95(2):282.

Lutsky BN, Klose P, Melon J, et al, "A Comparative Study of the Efficacy and Safety of Loratadine Syrup and Terfenadine Suspension in the Treatment of 3 to 6 Year Old Children With Seasonal Allergic Rhinitis," *Clin Ther*, 1993, 15(5):855-65.

Salmun LM, Herron JM, Banfield C, et al, "The Pharmacokinetics, Electrocardiographic Effects, and Tolerability of Loratadine Syrup in Children Aged 2 to 5 Years," *Clin Ther*, 2000, 22(5):613-21.

Loratadine and Pseudoephedrine

(lor AT a deen & soo doe e FED rin)

Medication Safety Issues

Sound-alike/look-alike issues:

Claritin-D® may be confused with Claritin-D® 24

Claritin-D® 24 may be confused with Claritin-D®

U.S. Brand Names Alavert™ Allergy and Sinus [OTC]; Claritin-D® 12 Hour Allergy & Congestion [OTC]; Claritin-D® 24 Hour Allergy & Congestion [OTC]

Canadian Brand Names Chlor-Tripolon ND®; Claritin® Extra; Claritin® Liberator

Therapeutic Category Antihistamine/Decongestant Combination

Generic Available Yes

Use Symptomatic relief of symptoms of seasonal allergic rhinitis and nasal congestion

Pregnancy Risk Factor B

Pregnancy Considerations See individual agents.

Lactation Enters breast milk/not recommended

Contraindications Hypersensitivity to loratadine, pseudoephedrine, or any component; MAO inhibitor therapy; severe hypertension; severe coronary artery disease; narrow-angle glaucoma

Precautions Use with caution and adjust dosage in patients with renal impairment; use with caution in patients with hyperthyroidism, diabetes mellitus, prostatic hypertrophy, mild to moderate hypertension, arrhythmias; use cautiously in patients who are also taking ketoconazole, itraconazole, fluconazole, erythromycin, clarithromycin, or other drugs which may impair loratadine's hepatic metabolism; although increased plasma levels of loratadine have been observed, no adverse effects with concomitant administration have been reported including QT interval prolongation which has occurred when similar antihistamines, terfenadine and astemizole, were combined with these agents; while less sedating than other antihistamines, loratadine may cause drowsiness and impair ability to perform hazardous activities requiring mental alertness, the CNS stimulant properties of pseudoephedrine may counteract this effect. Use cautiously in breast-feeding women as breast milk levels of loratadine are equivalent to serum levels.

Adverse Reactions See individual agents.

Drug Interactions

Metabolism/Transport Effects Loratadine: **Substrate** of CYP2D6 (minor), CYP3A4 (minor), P-glycoprotein; **Inhibits** CYP2C8 (weak), 2C19 (moderate), 2D6 (weak)

Avoid Concomitant Use

Avoid concomitant use of Loratadine and Pseudoephedrine with any of the following: Iobenguane I 123; MAO Inhibitors

Increased Effect/Toxicity

Loratadine and Pseudoephedrine may increase the levels/effects of: Alcohol (Ethyl); Anticholinergics; Bromocriptine; CNS Depressants; Sympathomimetics

The levels/effects of Loratadine and Pseudoephedrine may be increased by: Amiodarone; Antacids; Atomoxetine; Cannabinoids; Carbonic Anhydrase Inhibitors; MAO Inhibitors; P-Glycoprotein Inhibitors; Pramlintide; Serotonin/Norepinephrine Reuptake Inhibitors

Decreased Effect

Loratadine and Pseudoephedrine may decrease the levels/effects of: Acetylcholinesterase Inhibitors (Central); Betahistine; Iobenguane I 123

The levels/effects of Loratadine and Pseudoephedrine may be decreased by: Acetylcholinesterase Inhibitors (Central); Amphetamines; Peginterferon Alfa-2b; P-Glycoprotein Inducers; Spironolactone

Food Interactions Administration with food increases loratadine's bioavailability by 40%

Mechanism of Action Loratadine is a long-acting tricyclic antihistamine with selective peripheral histamine H_1-receptor antagonistic properties. Pseudoephedrine directly stimulates alpha-adrenergic receptors of respiratory mucosa causing vasoconstriction and directly stimulates beta-adrenergic receptors causing bronchial relaxation, increased heart rate and contractility

Pharmacokinetics (Adult data unless noted) See individual agents.

Usual Dosage Oral: Children ≥12 years and Adults:

Claritin-D® 12-Hour: 1 tablet every 12 hours

Claritin-D® 24-Hour: 1 tablet every 24 hours

Dosage adjustment in renal impairment: Cl_{cr} <30 mL/minute:

Claritin-D® 12-Hour: 1 tablet every 24 hours

Claritin-D® 24-Hour: 1 tablet every other day

Administration Oral: Administer on an empty stomach or before meals; swallow extended release tablets whole, do not chew or crush

Monitoring Parameters Improvement in signs and symptoms of allergic rhinitis or nasal congestion

Reference Range Therapeutic serum levels (not used clinically): Loratadine: 2.5-100 ng/mL; active metabolite: 0.5-100 ng/mL

Test Interactions Antigen skin testing; false-positive test for amphetamines by EMIT assay

Patient Information Drink plenty of water; may cause dry mouth; may color urine; notify physician if fainting episode occurs; avoid alcohol. May rarely cause photosensitivity reactions (eg, exposure to sunlight may cause severe sunburn, skin rash, redness, or itching); avoid direct exposure to sunlight

Dosage Forms Excipient information presented when available (limited, particularly for generics); consult specific product labeling.

Tablet, extended release: Loratadine 10 mg and pseudoephedrine sulfate 240 mg

Alavert™ Allergy and Sinus: Loratadine 5 mg and pseudoephedrine sulfate 120 mg

Claritin-D® 12 Hour Allergy & Congestion: Loratadine 5 mg and pseudoephedrine sulfate 120 mg [contains calcium 30 mg/tablet]

Claritin-D® 24 Hour Allergy & Congestion: Loratadine 10 mg and pseudoephedrine sulfate 240 mg [contains calcium 25 mg/tablet]

LORazepam (lor A ze pam)

Medication Safety Issues

Sound-alike/look-alike issues:

LORazepam may be confused with ALPRAZolam, clonazePAM, diazepam, Lovaza®, temazepam, zolpidem

Ativan® may be confused with Ambien®, Atarax®, Atgam®, Avitene®

Injection dosage form contains propylene glycol. Monitor for toxicity when administering continuous lorazepam infusions.

Beers Criteria medication: This drug may be inappropriate for use in geriatric patients (high severity risk).

Related Information

Compatibility of Chemotherapy and Related Supportive Care Medications *on page 1580*

Preprocedure Sedatives in Children *on page 1688*

U.S. Brand Names Ativan®; Lorazepam Intensol™

Canadian Brand Names Apo-Lorazepam®; Ativan®; Dom-Lorazepam; Lorazepam Injection, USP; Novo-Lorazem; Nu-Loraz; PHL-Lorazepam; PMS-Lorazepam; PRO-Lorazepam

Therapeutic Category Antianxiety Agent; Anticonvulsant; Benzodiazepine; Antiemetic; Benzodiazepine; Hypnotic; Sedative

Generic Available Yes

Use Management of anxiety; status epilepticus; preoperative sedation and amnesia; adjunct to antiemetic therapy

Restrictions C-IV

Pregnancy Risk Factor D

Pregnancy Considerations Teratogenic effects have been observed in some animal studies. Lorazepam crosses the human placenta. Respiratory depression, withdrawal symptoms, or hypotonia may occur if administered late in pregnancy or near the time of delivery.

Lactation Enters breast milk/not recommended (AAP rates "of concern")

Breast-Feeding Considerations Sedation and impaired nursing may occur in infants exposed to lorazepam from breast milk.

Contraindications Hypersensitivity to lorazepam or any component (see Warnings); there may be a cross-sensitivity with other benzodiazepines; do not use in a comatose patient, those with pre-existing CNS depression, narrow-angle glaucoma, severe uncontrolled pain, severe hypotension

Warnings Benzodiazepines may cause significant and potentially fatal respiratory depression, both if used alone and if used in combination with other CNS depressants. May cause CNS depression, which may impair physical or mental abilities; patients must be cautioned about performing tasks which require mental alertness (eg, operating machinery or driving). May cause emergent or worsening of pre-existing depression; not recommended for use in patients with a primary depressive disorder or psychosis, particularly if suicidal risk may be present; do not use without adequate antidepressant therapy.

May cause physical and psychological dependence with prolonged use; do not abruptly discontinue; rebound or withdrawal symptoms (including seizures) may occur following abrupt discontinuation or large decreases in dose. Use caution when reducing dose or withdrawing therapy; decrease slowly and monitor for withdrawal symptoms. Flumazenil may cause acute withdrawal in patients receiving long-term benzodiazepine therapy. Potential for drug dependency exists; use benzodiazepines with caution in patients with a history of drug abuse, alcoholism, or significant personality disorders; risk of dependence increases with higher dosage and longer duration of therapy.

Dilute injection prior to I.V. use with equal volume of compatible diluent (D_5W, NS, SWI); do not inject intra-arterially, arteriospasm and gangrene may occur. Injection contains 2% benzyl alcohol, polyethylene glycol, and propylene glycol, which may be toxic to newborns in high doses; benzyl alcohol may cause allergic reactions in susceptible individuals; large amounts of benzyl alcohol (≥99 mg/kg/day) have been associated with a potentially fatal toxicity ("gasping syndrome") in neonates; the "gasping syndrome" consists of metabolic acidosis, respiratory distress, gasping respirations, CNS dysfunction (including convulsions, intracranial hemorrhage), hypotension and cardiovascular collapse; use lorazepam products containing benzyl alcohol with caution in neonates; *in vitro* and animal studies have shown that benzoate, a metabolite of benzyl alcohol, displaces bilirubin from protein binding sites.

Concentrated oral solution contains polyethylene glycol and propylene glycol which may have adverse effects (see Additional Information).

Precautions Use with caution in neonates, especially in preterm infants (several cases of neurotoxicity and myoclonus have been reported). Use with caution in patients with renal or hepatic impairment (benzodiazepines may worsen hepatic encephalopathy; decrease dosage in patients with severe hepatic insufficiency), compromised pulmonary function (including those with COPD or sleep apnea), CNS depression, or those receiving other CNS depressants. Debilitated patients may be more susceptible to the sedative effects of benzodiazepines; monitor closely; titrate dosage carefully according to patient response.

Benzodiazepines have been associated with anterograde amnesia; they do not have analgesic, antidepressant, or antipsychotic properties. Paradoxical reactions, including hyperactive or aggressive behavior, have been reported with benzodiazepines, particularly in pediatric/adolescent or psychiatric patients; discontinue drug if this occurs. As a hypnotic, should be used only after evaluation of potential causes of sleep disturbance. Failure of sleep disturbance to resolve after 7-10 days may indicate psychiatric or medical illness. A worsening of insomnia or the emergence of new abnormalities of thought or behavior may represent unrecognized psychiatric or medical illness and require immediate and careful evaluation.

Safety and efficacy of long-term use (>4 months) have not been established; long-term usefulness should be periodically re-evaluated for the individual patient. Safety and efficacy of oral lorazepam in children <12 years and safety of injectable lorazepam in children <18 years have not been established.

Adverse Reactions

Cardiovascular: Bradycardia, circulatory collapse, hypertension, or hypotension

Central nervous system: Confusion, CNS depression, sedation, drowsiness, lethargy, hangover effect, dizziness, transitory hallucinations, ataxia, rhythmic myoclonic jerking in preterm infants

Gastrointestinal: Constipation, xerostomia, nausea, vomiting

Genitourinary: Urinary incontinence or retention

Hematologic: Leukopenia

Hepatic: LDH elevated

Local: Pain with injection

Ocular: Diplopia, nystagmus

Respiratory: Respiratory depression, apnea

Miscellaneous: Physical and psychological dependence with prolonged use

Drug Interactions

Avoid Concomitant Use There are no known interactions where it is recommended to avoid concomitant use.

Increased Effect/Toxicity

LORazepam may increase the levels/effects of: Alcohol (Ethyl); Clozapine; CNS Depressants; Methotrimeprazine; Phenytoin

The levels/effects of LORazepam may be increased by: Divalproex; Loxapine; Methotrimeprazine; Probenecid; Valproic Acid

Decreased Effect

The levels/effects of LORazepam may be decreased by: Theophylline Derivatives; Yohimbine

Stability Do not use if injection is discolored or contains precipitate; protect from light; refrigerate injectable form and oral solution; injection is stable at room temperature for 8 weeks. Store tablets at controlled room temperature; dispense in tightly closed container.

Mechanism of Action Depresses all levels of the CNS, including the limbic and reticular formation, by binding to the benzodiazepine site on the gamma-aminobutyric acid (GABA) receptor complex and modulating GABA, which is a major inhibitory neurotransmitter in the brain

Pharmacodynamics Sedation:

Onset of action:
Oral: Within 60 minutes
I.M.: 30-60 minutes
I.V.: 15-30 minutes
Duration: 8-12 hours

Pharmacokinetics (Adult data unless noted)

Absorption: Oral, I.M.: Rapid, complete

Distribution: Crosses into placenta; crosses into breast milk

V_d:
Neonates: 0.76 L/kg
Adults: 1.3 L/kg

Protein binding: ~85%

Metabolism: Primarily by glucuronide conjugation in the liver to an inactive metabolite (lorazepam glucuronide)

Bioavailability: Oral: 90% to 93%

Half-life:
Full-term neonates: 40.2 hours; range: 18-73 hours
Older Children: 10.5 hours; range: 6-17 hours
Adults: 12.9 hours; range: 10-16 hours

Time to peak serum concentration: Oral: 2 hours

Elimination: In urine primarily as the glucuronide conjugate

Dialysis: Lorazepam: Poorly dialyzable; lorazepam glucuronide: May be highly dialyzable

Usual Dosage

Adjunct to antiemetic therapy:
Children: I.V.: Limited information exists in the literature, especially for multiple doses:
Single dose: 0.04-0.08 mg/kg/dose prior to chemotherapy (maximum dose: 4 mg)
Multiple doses: Some centers use 0.02-0.05 mg/kg/dose (maximum dose: 2 mg) every 6 hours as needed
Adults: Oral, I.V.: 0.5-2 mg every 4-6 hours as needed

Anxiety/sedation:
Infants and Children: Oral, I.V.: Usual: 0.05 mg/kg/dose (maximum dose: 2 mg/dose) every 4-8 hours; range: 0.02-0.1 mg/kg
Adults: Oral: 1-10 mg/day in 2-3 divided doses; usual dose: 2-6 mg/day in divided doses

Insomnia: Adults: Oral: 2-4 mg at bedtime

Operative amnesia: Adults: I.V.: Up to 0.05 mg/kg; maximum dose: 4 mg/dose

Preoperative: Adults: I.M.: 0.05 mg/kg administered 2 hours before surgery; maximum dose: 4 mg/dose; I.V.: 0.044 mg/kg 15-20 minutes before surgery; usual maximum dose: 2 mg/dose

Sedation (preprocedure): Infants and Children:
Oral, I.M., I.V.: Usual: 0.05 mg/kg; range: 0.02-0.09 mg/kg
I.V.: May use smaller doses (eg, 0.01-0.03 mg/kg) and repeat every 20 minutes, as needed to titrate to effect

Status epilepticus: I.V.:
Neonates: 0.05 mg/kg slow I.V. over 2-5 minutes; may repeat in 10-15 minutes (see Warnings regarding benzyl alcohol)
Infants and Children: 0.05-0.1 mg/kg (maximum: 4 mg/dose) slow I.V. over 2-5 minutes (maximum rate: 2 mg/minute); may repeat every 10-15 minutes if needed (see Hegenbarth, 2008; Sabo-Graham, 1998)
Adolescents: 0.07 mg/kg (maximum: 4 mg/dose) slow I.V. over 2-5 minutes (maximum rate: 2 mg/minute); may repeat in 10-15 minutes if needed; usual total maximum dose: 8 mg (see Crawford, 1987)
Adults: 4 mg/dose slow I.V. over 2-5 minutes (maximum rate: 2 mg/minute); may repeat in 10-15 minutes; usual total maximum dose: 8 mg

Dosage adjustment in renal impairment: I.V.: Risk of propylene glycol toxicity. Monitor closely if using for prolonged periods of time or at high doses.

Dosage adjustment in hepatic impairment: Use with caution; benzodiazepines may worsen hepatic encephalopathy; decrease dosage in patients with severe hepatic insufficiency.

Administration

Oral: May administer with food to decrease GI distress; dilute oral solution in water, juice, soda, or semisolid food (eg, applesauce, pudding)

Parenteral:
I.V.: Do not exceed 2 mg/minute or 0.05 mg/kg over 2-5 minutes; dilute I.V. dose with equal volume of compatible diluent (D_5W, NS, SWI); administer I.V. using repeated aspiration with slow I.V. injection, to make sure the injection is not intra-arterial and that perivascular extravasation has not occurred
I.M.: Administer undiluted by deep injection into muscle mass

Monitoring Parameters Respiratory rate, blood pressure, heart rate; CBC with differential and liver function with long-term use

Patient Information Avoid alcohol; limit caffeine; may be habit-forming; avoid abrupt discontinuation after prolonged use; may cause drowsiness and impair ability to perform activities requiring mental alertness or physical coordination; may cause dry mouth

Additional Information Single oral doses >0.09 mg/kg produced increased ataxia without increasing sedative benefit vs lower doses. Since both strengths of injection contain 2% benzyl alcohol, Neofax® recommends using the 4 mg/mL strength for dilution with **preservative free** SWI to make a 0.4 mg/mL dilution for I.V. use in neonates (in order to decrease the amount of benzyl alcohol delivered to the neonate); however, the stability of this dilution has not been studied.

Diarrhea in a 9-month old infant receiving high-dose oral lorazepam was attributed to the lorazepam oral solution that contains polyethylene glycol and propylene glycol (both are osmotically active); diarrhea resolved when crushed tablets were substituted for the oral solution (see Marshall, 1995). To avoid the adverse effects of polyethylene glycol and propylene glycol that are found in the commercially available oral solution, a 1 mg/mL oral suspension can also be made from tablets (see Extemporaneous Preparations).

Lorazepam crosses the placenta. Neonatal withdrawal symptoms (or symptoms of toxicity) may occur in infants of mothers who receive benzodiazepines during the late phase of pregnancy or at delivery. Reported symptoms include: Hypoactivity, hypotonia, feeding problems, respiratory depression, apnea, hypothermia, and impaired metabolic response to cold stress. Lorazepam enters breast milk. Sedation, irritability, and inability to suckle may occur in infants exposed to lorazepam from breast milk.

Dosage Forms Excipient information presented when available (limited, particularly for generics); consult specific product labeling. [DSC] = Discontinued product

Injection, solution: 2 mg/mL (1 mL, 10 mL); 4 mg/mL (1 mL, 10 mL)

Ativan®: 2 mg/mL (1 mL; 10 mL [DSC]); 4 mg/mL (1 mL, 10 mL) [contains benzyl alcohol, polyethylene glycol 400, and propylene glycol]

Injection, solution [preservative free]: 2 mg/mL (1 mL); 4 mg/mL (1 mL)

Solution, oral [concentrate]: 2 mg/mL (30 mL)

Lorazepam Intensol™: 2 mg/mL (30 mL) [ethanol free, sugar free, dye free; contains propylene glycol]

Tablet: 0.5 mg, 1 mg, 2 mg

Ativan®: 0.5 mg

Ativan®: 1 mg, 2 mg [scored]

Extemporaneous Preparations Two different 1 mg/mL oral suspensions made from different generic lorazepam tablets (Mylan Pharmaceuticals and Watson Laboratories), sterile water, Ora-Sweet®, and Ora-Plus® were both stable for 63 days when stored in amber glass prescription bottles at room temperature (22°C) or under refrigeration (4°C); both suspensions were stable for 91 days when stored under refrigeration; the Mylan suspension was also stable for 91 days when stored at room temperature, while the Watson suspension was not. Place one hundred eighty 2 mg tablets in a 12-ounce amber glass bottle; add sterile water to disperse the tablets (Mylan tablets: Add 144 mL sterile water; Watson tablets: Add 48 mL sterile water); shake until slurry is formed; add Ora-Plus® by geometric dilution (Mylan tablets: Add 108 mL Ora-Plus®; Watson tablets: Add 156 mL Ora-Plus®); qsad with Ora-Sweet® to a final volume of 360 mL (Mylan tablets: Add 83 mL Ora-Sweet®; Watson tablets: Add 146 mL Ora-Sweet®); label "shake well" and "store under refrigeration."

Lee ME, Lugo RA, Rusho WJ, et al, "Chemical Stability of Extemporaneously Prepared Lorazepam Suspension at Two Temperatures," *J Pediatr Pharmacol Ther*, 2004, 9 (4):254-58.

References

Crawford TO, Mitchell WG, and Snodgrass SR, "Lorazepam in Childhood Status Epilepticus and Serial Seizures: Effectiveness and Tachyphylaxis," *Neurology*, 1987, 37(2):190-5.

Deshmukh A, Wittert W, Schnitzler E, et al, "Lorazepam in the Treatment of Refractory Neonatal Seizures: A Pilot Study," *Am J Dis Child*, 1986, 140(10):1042-4.

Hegenbarth MA and American Academy of Pediatrics Committee on Drugs, "Preparing for Pediatric Emergencies: Drugs to Consider," *Pediatrics*, 2008, 121(2):433-43.

Henry DW, Burwinkle JW, and Klutman NE, "Determination of Sedative and Amnestic Doses of Lorazepam in Children," *Clin Pharm*, 1991, 10 (8):625-9.

Lee DS, Wong HA, and Knoppert DC, "Myoclonus Associated With Lorazepam Therapy in Very-Low-Birth-Weight Infants," *Biol Neonate*, 1994, 66(6):311-5.

Marshall JD, Farrar HC, and Kearns GL, "Diarrhea Associated With Enteral Benzodiazepine Solutions," *J Pediatr*, 1995, 126(4):657-9.

McDermott CA, Kowalczyk AL, Schnitzler ER, et al, "Pharmacokinetics of Lorazepam in Critically Ill Neonates With Seizures," *J Pediatr*, 1992, 120(3):479-83.

Sabo-Graham T and Seay AR, "Management of Status Epilepticus in Children," *Pediatr Rev*, 1998, 19(9):306-9.

◆ **Lorazepam Injection, USP (Can)** see LORazepam on page 845

◆ **Lorazepam Intensol™** see LORazepam on page 845

◆ **Lorcet® 10/650** see Hydrocodone and Acetaminophen on page 684

◆ **Lorcet® Plus** see Hydrocodone and Acetaminophen on page 684

◆ **Lortab®** see Hydrocodone and Acetaminophen on page 684

Losartan (loe SAR tan)

Medication Safety Issues

Sound-alike/look-alike issues:

Cozaar® may be confused with Colace®, Coreg®, Hyzaar®, Zocor®

Losartan may be confused with valsartan

Related Information

Antihypertensive Agents by Class on page 1481

U.S. Brand Names Cozaar®

Canadian Brand Names Cozaar®

Therapeutic Category Angiotensin II Receptor Blocker; Antihypertensive Agent

Generic Available Yes

Use Treatment of hypertension alone or in combination with other antihypertensive agents (FDA approved in ages 6-16 years and adults); treatment of diabetic nephropathy in patients with type 2 diabetes mellitus (noninsulin dependent, NIDDM) and hypertension (FDA approved in adults); reduction of the risk of stroke in patients with hypertension and left ventricular hypertrophy (FDA approved in adults; see Additional Information); has also been used to reduce proteinuria in children with chronic kidney disease, either as monotherapy or in addition to ACE inhibitor therapy, and in Marfan's Syndrome to slow the rate of progression of aortic-root dilation

Pregnancy Risk Factor C (1st trimester); D (2nd and 3rd trimesters)

Pregnancy Considerations Medications which act on the renin-angiotensin system are reported to have the following fetal/neonatal effects: Hypotension, neonatal skull hypoplasia, anuria, renal failure, and death; oligohydramnios is also reported. These effects are reported to occur with exposure during the second and third trimesters. There are no adequate and well-controlled studies in pregnant women. **[U.S. Boxed Warning]: Based on human data, drugs that act on the angiotensin system can cause injury and death to the developing fetus when used in the second and third trimesters. Angiotensin receptor blockers should be discontinued as soon as possible once pregnancy is detected.**

Lactation Excretion in breast milk unknown/not recommended

Breast-Feeding Considerations It is not known if losartan is found in breast milk; the manufacturer recommends discontinuing the drug or discontinuing nursing based on the importance of the drug to the mother.

Contraindications Hypersensitivity to losartan, any component, or other angiotensin II receptor blockers

Warnings When used in pregnancy during the second and third trimesters, drugs that act on the renin-angiotensin system can cause injury and death to the developing fetus. ARBs should be discontinued as soon as possible once pregnancy is detected **[U.S. Boxed Warning]**. Neonatal hypotension, skull hypoplasia, anuria, renal failure, oligohydramnios (associated with fetal limb contractures, craniofacial deformities, hypoplastic lung development), prematurity, intrauterine growth retardation, patent ductus arteriosus, and death have been reported with the use of ACE inhibitors, primarily in the second and third trimesters. Use with caution in volume-depleted patients (eg, those on thiazide diuretics); correct depletion first or use a lower starting dose. Symptomatic hypotension may occur, especially in patients with an activated renin-angiotensin system (eg, volume- or salt-depleted patients receiving high doses of diuretic agents); use with caution in these patients; correct depletion before starting therapy or initiate therapy at a lower dose.

Precautions Use with caution and reduce dosage in patients with hepatic impairment (clearance of losartan is reduced in these patients). Use with caution in patients with impaired renal function; use is associated with deterioration of renal function and/or increases in serum creatinine, particularly in patients with low renal blood flow (eg, renal artery stenosis, heart failure); deterioration may result in oliguria, acute renal failure, or progressive azotemia. Small increases in serum creatinine may occur following initiation; consider discontinuation in patients with progressive and/or significant deterioration in renal function. Hyperkalemia may occur; risk factors include renal dysfunction, diabetes mellitus, concomitant use of potassium-sparing diuretics, potassium supplements, and/or potassium-containing salts; use with caution in these patients and with these agents; monitor potassium closely. Not recommended for use in children <6 years of age or in children with GFR <30 mL/minute/1.73m^2 (no data exists).

Angioedema (although reported rarely) can occur at any time during treatment (especially following first dose) and may include swelling of the face, lips, pharynx, and tongue. Angioedema of the larynx, glottis, or tongue may cause airway obstruction. Some patients who experienced angioedema with losartan previously experienced angioedema with other medications, including ACI inhibitors.

Adverse Reactions Note: No significant differences in adverse reactions have been identified between children and adults.

Cardiovascular: Chest pain, hypotension, postural hypotension

Central nervous system: Headache, fatigue, dizziness, hypesthesia, fever, insomnia, syncope

Dermatology: Cellulitis

Endocrine & metabolic: Hypoglycemia, hyperkalemia, weight gain

Gastrointestinal: Diarrhea, gastritis, dyspepsia, abdominal pain, nausea

Hematologic: Anemia

Neuromuscular & skeletal: Weakness, back pain, lower limb pain, muscle cramps, myalgia

Renal: BUN and serum creatinine elevated, renal dysfunction

Respiratory: Cough, bronchitis, URI, nasal congestion, sinusitis

Miscellaneous: Infection, flu-like syndrome, angioedema (rare)

Drug Interactions

Metabolism/Transport Effects Substrate (major) of CYP2C9, 3A4; **Inhibits** CYP1A2 (weak), 2C8 (moderate), 2C9 (moderate), 2C19 (weak), 3A4 (weak)

Avoid Concomitant Use There are no known interactions where it is recommended to avoid concomitant use.

Increased Effect/Toxicity

Losartan may increase the levels/effects of: ACE Inhibitors; Amifostine; Antihypertensives; Carvedilol; CYP2C8 Substrates (High risk); CYP2C9 Substrates (High risk); Hypoglycemic Agents; Hypotensive Agents; Lithium; Potassium-Sparing Diuretics; RiTUXimab

The levels/effects of Losartan may be increased by: Antifungal Agents (Azole Derivatives, Systemic); CYP2C9 Inhibitors (Moderate); CYP2C9 Inhibitors (Strong); Diazoxide; Eplerenone; Fluconazole; Herbs (Hypoglycemic Properties); Herbs (Hypotensive Properties); MAO Inhibitors; Pentoxifylline; Phosphodiesterase 5 Inhibitors; Potassium Salts; Prostacyclin Analogues; Tolvaptan; Trimethoprim

Decreased Effect

The levels/effects of Losartan may be decreased by: CYP2C9 Inducers (Highly Effective); CYP3A4 Inducers (Strong); Deferasirox; Herbs (CYP3A4 Inducers); Herbs (Hypertensive Properties); Methylphenidate; Nonsteroidal Anti-Inflammatory Agents; Peginterferon Alfa-2b; Rifamycin Derivatives; Yohimbine

Food Interactions Food does not significantly affect the AUC of losartan or its active metabolite. Limit salt substitutes or potassium-rich diet. Avoid natural licorice (causes sodium and water retention and increases potassium loss).

Stability Store at controlled room temperature at 25°C (77°F) in tightly closed container. Protect from light.

Mechanism of Action Losartan produces direct antagonism of the effects of angiotensin II. Unlike the ACE inhibitors, losartan blocks the binding of angiotensin II to the AT1 receptor subtype. It produces its blood pressure-lowering effects by antagonizing AT1-induced vasoconstriction, aldosterone release, catecholamine release, arginine vasopressin release, water intake, and hypertrophic responses. This action results in more efficient blockade of the cardiovascular effects of angiotensin II and fewer side effects than the ACE inhibitors. Losartan does not affect the ACE (kininase II) or the response to bradykinin.

Pharmacodynamics Antihypertensive effect:

Maximum effect: 6 hours postdose; with chronic dosing, substantial hypotensive effects are seen within 1 week; maximum effect: 3-6 weeks

Duration: 24 hours

Pharmacokinetics (Adult data unless noted) Note: No significant differences in pharmacokinetic parameters have been identified across studied pediatric age groups (6-16 years) and adult population.

Absorption: Oral: Well-absorbed

Distribution: V_d: Adults:

Losartan: ~34 L

E-3174: ~12 L

Protein binding: Highly bound, >98%; primarily to albumin

Metabolism: Extensive first-pass effect; metabolized in the liver via CYP2C9 and 3A4 to active carboxylic metabolite, E-3174 (14% of dose; 40 times more potent than losartan) and several inactive metabolites

Bioavailability: Oral: 33%; AUC of E-3174 is four times greater than that of losartan; extemporaneously prepared suspension and tablet have similar bioavailability of losartan and E-3174

Half-life elimination:

Losartan:

Children 6-16 years: 2.3 ± 0.8 hours

Adults: 2.1 ± 0.7 hours

E-3174:

Children 6-16 years: 5.6 ± 1.2 hours

Adults: 7.4 ± 2.4 hours

Time to peak serum concentration:

Losartan:

Children: 2 hours

Adults: 1 hour

E-3174:

Children: 4 hours

Adults: 3.5 hours

Excretion: Biliary excretion plays a role in the elimination of parent drug and metabolites; 35% of an oral dose is eliminated in the urine and 60% in the feces; 4% of dose is eliminated as unchanged drug in the urine; 6% as E-3174

Clearance: Adults:

Plasma:

Losartan: 600 mL/minute

E-3174: 50 mL/minute

Renal:

Losartan: 75 mL/minute

E-3174: 25 mL/minute

Dialysis: Losartan and E-3174: Not removed by hemodialysis

Usual Dosage Oral:

Children:

Hypertension: Manufacturer's recommendations:

Infants and Children <6 years: Not recommended; dose not established

Children 6-16 years: Initial: 0.7 mg/kg once daily (maximum: 50 mg/day); dose may be increased to achieve desired effect; maximum: 100 mg/day; **Note:** Doses >1.4 mg/kg/day (or >100 mg/day) have not been studied (see also Shahinfar, 2005).

Proteinuria reduction in children with chronic kidney disease: Not approved for use; limited information is available; dosing based on 3 retrospective clinical trials (Chandar, 2007; Ellis, 2003; Ellis, 2004): Children 4-18 years: Initial: 0.4-0.8 mg/kg/day; increase dose if no adverse effects occur and blood pressure remains >90th percentile or proteinuria does not fall <50% of baseline excretion; doses can be increased slowly up to 1 mg/kg/day (maximum: 50 mg/day)

Marfan's syndrome aortic-root dilation: Not approved for use; limited information is available; dosing based on preliminary results of a small (n=18), nonrandomized, retrospective, clinical study (Brooke, 2008); further studies are needed: Children 14 months to 16 years: Initial: 0.6 mg/kg/day for 3 weeks (while assessing for adverse events); then gradually increase dose to 1.4 mg/kg/day (maximum: 100 mg/day)

Adults:

Hypertension: Initial: 50 mg once daily; can be administered once or twice daily; increase dose to achieve desired effect; total daily dosage range: 25-100 mg/day; **Note:** Patients receiving diuretics or with intravascular volume depletion: Initial dose: 25 mg once daily

Nephropathy in patients with type 2 diabetes and hypertension: Initial: 50 mg once daily; can be increased to 100 mg once daily based on blood pressure response

Stroke reduction (HTN with LVH): Initial: 50 mg once daily (maximum daily dose: 100 mg); may be used in combination with a thiazide diuretic

Dosing adjustment in renal impairment:

Children: Use is not recommended if Cl$_{cr}$ <30 mL/minute/1.73 m^2

Adults: No initial dosage adjustment necessary

Dosing adjustment in hepatic impairment:

Children: No specific dosing recommendations provided by manufacturer; however, it is advisable to initiate at a reduced dosage.

Adults: Reduce initial dose to 25 mg/day

Administration May be administered with or without food.

Monitoring Parameters Blood pressure, BUN, serum creatinine, renal function, baseline and periodic serum electrolytes, urinalysis

Patient Information Do not take any new medication (prescription or OTC), herbal products, potassium supplements, or salt substitutes during therapy without consulting prescriber. Take exactly as directed and do not discontinue without consulting prescriber. Medication should be taken at same time each day; may be taken without regard to meals. This drug does not eliminate need for diet or exercise regimen as recommended by prescriber. If you have diabetes, you may be cautioned to monitor glucose levels closely; may alter glucose control. May cause dizziness or lightheadedness (use caution when driving or engaging in tasks that require alertness until response to drug is known); postural hypotension (use caution when rising from lying or sitting position or climbing stairs); or diarrhea. Report immediately swelling of face, lips, or mouth; difficulty swallowing; chest pain or palpitations, unrelenting headache; muscle weakness or pain; unusual cough; or other persistent adverse reactions. This medication may cause injury and death to the developing fetus when used during pregnancy; women of childbearing potential should be informed of potential risk; consult prescriber for appropriate contraceptive measures; this medication should be discontinued as soon as possible once pregnancy is detected (see Warnings).

Nursing Implications Assess effectiveness and interactions with other pharmacological agents and herbal products patient may be taking (eg, concurrent use of potassium supplements, ACE inhibitors, and potassium-sparing diuretics may increase risk of hyperkalemia). Monitor laboratory tests at baseline and periodically during therapy. Monitor therapeutic effectiveness (reduced BP) and adverse response on a regular basis during therapy (eg, changes in renal function, dizziness, bradycardia, headache, nausea, hypotension, hyperkalemia). Caution patients with diabetes to monitor glucose levels closely; may alter glucose control. Teach patient proper use, possible side effects/appropriate interventions, and adverse symptoms to report.

Additional Information Potassium content: 25 mg tablets: 2.12 mg (0.054 mEq); 50 mg tablets: 4.24 mg (0.108 mEq; 100 mg tablets: 8.48 mg (0.216 mEq)

Evidence from the LIFE study (Dahlöf, 2002) suggests that when used to reduce the risk of stroke in patients with HTN and LVH, losartan may not be effective in the African-American population.

Dosage Forms Excipient information presented when available (limited, particularly for generics); consult specific product labeling.

Tablet, oral, as potassium: 25 mg, 50 mg, 100 mg

Cozaar®: 25 mg [contains potassium 2.12 mg (0.054 mEq)]

Cozaar®: 50 mg [contains potassium 4.24 mg (0.108 mEq)]

Cozaar®: 100 mg [contains potassium 8.48 mg (0.216 mEq)]

Extemporaneous Preparations A 2.5 mg/mL losartan suspension made from tablets, Ora-Plus® and Ora-Sweet® is stable for 4 weeks under refrigeration (2°C to 8°C [35°F to 46°F]) when stored in amber polyethylene terephthalate prescription bottles. Combine 10 mL of purified water and ten losartan 50 mg tablets in an 8-ounce amber polyethylene terephthalate bottle. Shake well for ≥2 minutes. Allow concentrate to stand for 1 hour, then shake for 1 minute. Separately, prepare 190 mL of a 50:50 mixture of Ora-Plus® and Ora-Sweet SF®. Add to tablet and water mixture in the bottle; shake for 1 minute. Resulting 200 mL suspension will contain losartan 2.5 mg/mL. Label "Shake well before use." Return promptly to refrigerator after each use. [Cozaar® (package insert), 2008].

Cozaar® (package insert), Whitehouse Station, NJ: Merck & Co, Inc., 2008.

References

Brooke BS, Habashi JP, Judge DP, et al, "Angiotensin II Blockade and Aortic-Root Dilation in Marfan's Syndrome," N Engl J Med, 2008, 358 (26):2787-95.

Butani L, "Angiotensin Blockade in Children With Chronic Glomerulonephritis and Heavy Proteinuria," Pediatr Nephrol, 2005, 20 (11):1651-4.

Chandar J, Abitbol C, Montané B, et al, "Angiotensin Blockade as Sole Treatment for Proteinuric Kidney Disease in Children," Nephrol Dial Transplant, 2007, 22(5):1332-7.

Dahlöf B, Devereux RB, Kjeldsen SE, et al, "Cardiovascular Morbidity and Mortality in the Losartan Intervention For Endpoint Reduction in Hypertension Study (LIFE): A Randomised Trial Against Atenolol," Lancet, 2002, 359(9311):995-1003.

Ellis D, Moritz ML, Vats A, et al, "Antihypertensive and Renoprotective Efficacy and Safety of Losartan. A Long-Term Study in Children With Renal Disorders," Am J Hypertens, 2004, 17(10):928-35.

Ellis D, Vats A, Moritz ML, et al, "Long-Term Antiproteinuric and Renoprotective Efficacy and Safety of Losartan in Children With Proteinuria," J Pediatr, 2003, 143(1):89-97.

Hogg RJ, Portman RJ, Milliner D, et al, "Evaluation and Management of Proteinuria and Nephrotic Syndrome in Children: Recommendations From a Pediatric Nephrology Panel Established at the National Kidney Foundation Conference on Proteinuria, Albuminuria, Risk, Assessment, Detection, and Elimination (PARADE)," *Pediatrics*, 2000, 105(6):1242-9.

Litwin M, Grenda R, Sladowska J, et al, "Add-On Therapy With Angiotensin II Receptor 1 Blocker in Children With Chronic Kidney Disease Already Treated With Angiotensin-Converting Enzyme Inhibitors," *Pediatr Nephrol*, 2006, 21(11):1716-22.

National High Blood Pressure Education Program Working Group on High Blood Pressure in Children and Adolescents, "The Fourth Report on the Diagnosis, Evaluation, and Treatment of High Blood Pressure in Children and Adolescents," *Pediatrics*, 2004, 114(2 Suppl):555-76.

Shahinfar S, Cano F, Soffer BA, et al, "A Double-Blind, Dose-Response Study of Losartan in Hypertensive Children," *Am J Hypertens*, 2005, 18(2 Pt 1):183-90.

White CT, Macpherson CF, Hurley RM, et al, "Antiproteinuric Effects of Enalapril and Losartan: A Pilot Study," *Pediatr Nephrol*, 2003, 18 (10):1038-43.

Zaffanello M, Franchini M, and Fanos V, "New Therapeutic Strategies With Combined Renin-Angiotensin System Inhibitors for Pediatric Nephropathy," *Pharmacotherapy*, 2008, 28(1):125-30.

- ◆ **Losartan** *see Losartan on page 847*
- ◆ **Losec® (Can)** *see Omeprazole on page 1016*
- ◆ **Losec MUPS® (Can)** *see Omeprazole on page 1016*
- ◆ **Lotensin®** *see Benazepril on page 179*
- ◆ **Lotio Calaminae** *see Calamine Lotion on page 227*
- ◆ **Lotrimin AF® [OTC]** *see Miconazole on page 927*
- ◆ **Lotrimin® AF Athlete's Foot Cream [OTC]** *see Clotrimazole on page 344*
- ◆ **Lotrimin® AF for Her [OTC]** *see Clotrimazole on page 344*
- ◆ **Lotrimin® AF Jock Itch Cream [OTC]** *see Clotrimazole on page 344*

Lovastatin (LOE va sta tin)

Medication Safety Issues

Sound-alike/look-alike issues:

Lovastatin may be confused with atorvastatin, Leustatin®, Livostin®, Lotensin®, nystatin, pitavastatin

Mevacor® may be confused with Benicar®, Lipitor®, Mivacron®

International issues:

Lovacol® [Chile and Finland] may be confused with Levatol® which is a brand name for penbutolol in the U.S.

Lovastin® [Poland] may be confused with Livostin® which is a brand name for levocabastine in the U.S.

Related Information

Normal Laboratory Values for Children *on page 1672*

U.S. Brand Names Altoprev®; Mevacor®

Canadian Brand Names Apo-Lovastatin®; CO Lovastatin; Dom-Lovastatin; Gen-Lovastatin; Mevacor®; Mylan-Lovastatin; Novo-Lovastatin; Nu-Lovastatin; PHL-Lovastatin; PMS-Lovastatin; PRO-Lovastatin; RAN™-Lovastatin; ratio-Lovastatin; Riva-Lovastatin; Sandoz-Lovastatin

Therapeutic Category Antilipemic Agent; HMG-CoA Reductase Inhibitor

Generic Available Yes: Immediate release tablet

Use Hyperlipidemia: Adjunct to dietary therapy to decrease elevated serum total and low density lipoprotein cholesterol (LDL-C), apolipoprotein B (apo-B), and triglyceride levels, and to increase high density lipoprotein cholesterol (HDL-C) in patients with primary hypercholesterolemia (heterozygous, familial and nonfamilial) and mixed dyslipidemia (Fredrickson types IIa and IIb) (see Additional Information for recommendations on initiating hypercholesterolemia pharmacologic treatment in children ≥8 years); treatment of isolated hypertriglyceridemia (Fredrickson type IV) and type III hyperlipoproteinemia; treatment of primary dysbetalipoproteinemia (Fredrickson Type III)

Primary prevention of cardiovascular disease in high risk patients; risk factors include: Age ≥55 years, smoking, hypertension, low HDL-C or family history of early coronary heart disease

Pregnancy Risk Factor X

Pregnancy Considerations Cholesterol biosynthesis may be important in fetal development. Contraindicated in pregnancy. Administer to women of childbearing potential only when conception is highly unlikely and patients have been informed of potential hazards.

Lactation Excretion in breast milk unknown/contraindicated

Contraindications Hypersensitivity to lovastatin or any component; active liver disease; unexplained persistent elevations of serum transaminases; pregnancy; breast-feeding

Warnings Rhabdomyolysis with or without acute renal failure secondary to myoglobinuria has occurred rarely and is dose-related. Risk is increased with concurrent use of clarithromycin, danazol, diltiazem, fluvoxamine, indinavir, nefazodone, nelfinavir, ritonavir, verapamil, troleandomycin, cyclosporine, fibric acid derivatives, erythromycin, niacin, azole antifungals and large quantities of grapefruit juice (>1 quart/day). Assess the risk versus benefit before combining any of these drugs with lovastatin. Temporarily discontinue lovastatin in any patient experiencing an acute or serious condition predisposing to renal failure secondary to rhabdomyolysis.

Precautions Persistent increases in serum transaminases have occurred; liver function must be monitored by laboratory assessment at the initiation of therapy in patients with a history of liver disease, prior to use of doses ≥40 mg daily or as clinically indicated. Use with caution in patients with history of heavy alcohol use or have a previous history of liver disease; use with caution and modify dose in patients with renal impairment or receiving concomitant amiodarone, cyclosporine, danazol, fibrates, lipid-lowering doses of niacin, or verapamil. Lovastatin is less effective in patients with rare **homozygous** familial hypercholesterolemia and may be more likely to elevate serum transaminases.

Adverse Reactions

Cardiovascular: Chest pain

Central nervous system: Headache, dizziness, insomnia, tremor, vertigo, memory loss, psychic disturbances, anxiety, depression

Dermatologic: Rash, alopecia, pruritus, dermatomyositis

Endocrine & metabolic: Gynecomastia, abnormal thyroid function tests

Gastrointestinal: Abdominal pain, constipation, diarrhea, dyspepsia, flatulence, nausea, acid regurgitation, xerostomia, vomiting, anorexia

Hepatic: Hepatitis, cholestatic jaundice, cirrhosis, hepatic necrosis, hepatoma, hepatic enzymes elevated

Neuromuscular & skeletal: CPK increased, myalgia, weakness, muscle cramps, leg pain, arthralgia, paresthesia, rhabdomyolysis

Ocular: Blurred vision, eye irritation, cataracts, ophthalmoplegia

Miscellaneous: Hypersensitivity syndrome (including one or more of the following features: Anaphylaxis, angioedema, lupus erythematous-like syndrome, polymyalgia rheumatica, dermatomyositis, vasculitis, purpura, leukopenia, hemolytic anemia, erythema multiforme)

Drug Interactions

Metabolism/Transport Effects Substrate of CYP3A4 (major), P-glycoprotein; **Inhibits** CYP2C9 (weak), 2D6 (weak), 3A4 (weak)

Avoid Concomitant Use

Avoid concomitant use of Lovastatin with any of the following: Protease Inhibitors

Increased Effect/Toxicity

Lovastatin may increase the levels/effects of: DAPTO-mycin; Diltiazem; Vitamin K Antagonists

The levels/effects of Lovastatin may be increased by: Amiodarone; Antifungal Agents (Azole Derivatives, Systemic); Colchicine; CycloSPORINE; CycloSPORINE (Systemic); CYP3A4 Inhibitors (Moderate); CYP3A4 Inhibitors (Strong); Danazol; Dasatinib; Diltiazem; Dronedarone; Fenofibrate; Fenofibric Acid; Fluconazole; Gemfibrozil; Grapefruit Juice; Macrolide Antibiotics; Nefazodone; Niacin; Niacinamide; P-Glycoprotein Inhibitors; Protease Inhibitors; QuiNINE; Rifamycin Derivatives; Sildenafil; Verapamil

Decreased Effect

The levels/effects of Lovastatin may be decreased by: Antacids; Bosentan; CYP3A4 Inducers (Strong); Deferasirox; Etravirine; P-Glycoprotein Inducers; Phenytoin; Rifamycin Derivatives; St Johns Wort

Food Interactions Food **increases** the absorption of lovastatin immediate release tablets (serum concentrations of active drug under fasting conditions are approximately two-thirds of that when administered with food). Food **decreases** the absorption of lovastatin extended release tablets. Lovastatin serum concentrations may be increased if taken with grapefruit juice; the risk of myopathy/rhabdomyolysis is increased with daily intake of large quantities of grapefruit juice (>1 quart/day); avoid concurrent use.

Stability Immediate release tablets should be stored at temperatures between 5°C to 30°C (41°F to 86°F); extended release tablets should be stored at temperatures between 20°C to 25°C (68°F to 77°F); avoid excessive heat and humidity

Mechanism of Action Lovastatin acts by competitively inhibiting 3-hydroxyl-3-methylglutaryl-coenzyme A (HMG-CoA) reductase, the enzyme that catalyzes the rate-limiting step in cholesterol biosynthesis

Pharmacodynamics

Onset of action: 3 days

Maximum effect: 4-6 weeks

LDL-C reduction: 40 mg/day: 31% (for each doubling of this dose, LDL-C is lowered by ~6%)

Average HDL-C increase: 5% to 15%

Average triglyceride reduction: 7% to 30%

Pharmacokinetics (Adult data unless noted)

Absorption: Oral: 30% absorbed but less than 5% reaches the systemic circulation due to an extensive first-pass effect; absorption increased with extended release tablets

Protein binding: 95%

Half-life: 1.1-1.7 hours

Time to peak serum concentration: 2-4 hours

Elimination: ~80% to 85% of dose excreted in feces and 10% in urine

Usual Dosage Oral:

Treatment of heterozygous familial hypercholesterolemia: Children and Adolescents 10-17 years: Begin treatment if after adequate trial of diet the following are present: LDL-C >189 mg/dL or LDL-C remains >160 mg/dL and positive family history of premature cardiovascular disease or meets NCEP classification:

Initial (using immediate release formulation): 10 mg once daily, increase to 20 mg once daily after 8 weeks and 40 mg once daily after 16 weeks as needed. (**Note:** Girls must be at least 1 year post-menarche)

Adults: Initial:

Immediate release tablet: 20 mg once daily; adjust dosage at 4-week intervals; range: 10-80 mg/day in single or 2 divided doses; maximum dose: 80 mg/day; for patients requiring LDL-C reductions <20%, a lower initial dose of 10 mg once daily may be used.

Extended release tablet: 20 mg once daily; adjust dosage at 4-week intervals; maximum dose: 60 mg/day

Dosing adjustment in patients who are concomitantly receiving amiodarone or verapamil: Dose should not exceed 40 mg/day

Dosage adjustment in patients who are concomitantly receiving cyclosporine or danazol: Initial: 10 mg once daily, not to exceed 20 mg/day

Dosage adjustment in patients who are concomitantly receiving fibrates or lipid-lowering doses of niacin (≥1 g/day): Dose should not exceed 20 mg/day

Dosing adjustment in renal impairment: Cl_{cr} <30 mL/minute: Doses exceeding 20 mg/day should be carefully considered and implemented cautiously

Administration Oral: Administer immediate release tablets with the evening meal. Administer extended release tablet at bedtime; do not crush or chew; avoid administration with grapefruit juice

Monitoring Parameters Serum cholesterol (total and fractionated), creatine phosphokinase levels (CPK); liver function tests (see Precautions)

Reference Range See Related Information for age- and gender-specific serum cholesterol, LDL-C, TG, and HDL concentrations.

Patient Information Avoid grapefruit juice and the herbal medicine, St John's wort. Report severe and unresolved gastric upset, any vision changes, unexplained muscle pain or weakness, changes in color of urine or stool, yellowing of skin or eyes, and any unusual bruising. Female patients of childbearing age must be counseled to use 2 effective forms of contraception simultaneously, unless absolute abstinence is the chosen method; this drug may cause severe fetal defects.

Additional Information The current recommendation for pharmacologic treatment of hypercholesterolemia in children is limited to children ≥8 years of age and is based on LDL-C concentrations and the presence of coronary vascular disease (CVD) risk factors (see table and Daniels, 2008). In adults, for each 1% lowering in LDL-C, the relative risk for major cardiovascular events is reduced by ~1%. For more specific risk assessment and treatment recommendations for adults, see NCEP ATPIII, 2001.

Recommendations for Initiating Pharmacologic Treatment in Children ≥8 Years[1]

No risk factors for CVD	LDL ≥190 mg/dL despite 6-month to 1-year diet therapy
Family history of premature CVD or ≥2 CVD risk factors present, including obesity, hypertension, or cigarette smoking	LDL ≥160 mg/dL despite 6-month to 1-year diet therapy
Diabetes mellitus present	LDL ≥130 mg/dL

[1]Adapted from Daniels SR, Greer FR, and Committee on Nutrition, "Lipid Screening and Cardiovascular Health in Childhood," *Pediatrics*, 2008, 122(1):198-208.

Dosage Forms Excipient information presented when available (limited, particularly for generics); consult specific product labeling.

Tablet: 10 mg, 20 mg, 40 mg

Mevacor®: 20 mg, 40 mg

Tablet, extended release:

Altoprev®: 20 mg, 40 mg, 60 mg

References

American Academy of Pediatrics Committee on Nutrition, "Cholesterol in Childhood," *Pediatrics*, 1998, 101(1 Pt 1):141-7.

American Academy of Pediatrics, "National Cholesterol Education Program: Report of the Expert Panel on Blood Cholesterol Levels in Children and Adolescents," *Pediatrics*, 1992, 89(3 Pt 2):525-84.

Daniels SR, Greer FR, and Committee on Nutrition, "Lipid Screening and Cardiovascular Health in Childhood," *Pediatrics*, 2008, 122(1):198-208.

Duplaga BA, "Treatment of Childhood Hypercholesterolemia With HMG-CoA Reductase Inhibitors," *Ann Pharmacother*, 1999, 33 (11):1224-7.

Grundy SM, Cleeman JI, Merz CN, et al, "Implications of Recent Clinical Trials for the National Cholesterol Education Program Adult Treatment Panel III Guidelines," *Circulation*, 2004, 110(2):227-39.

Lambert M, Lupien PJ, Gagne C, et al, "Treatment of Familial Hypercholesterolemia in Children and Adolescents: Effect of Lovastatin. Canadian Lovastatin in Children Study Group," *Pediatrics*, 1996, 97(5):619-28.

McCrindle BW, Urbina EM, Dennison BA, et al, "Drug Therapy of High-Risk Lipid Abnormalities in Children and Adolescents: A Scientific Statement from the American Heart Association Atherosclerosis, Hypertension, and Obesity in Youth Committee, Council of Cardiovascular Disease in the Young, With the Council on Cardiovascular Nursing," *Circulation*, 2007, 115(14):1948-67.

Stein EA, Illingworth DR, Kwiterovich PO Jr, et al, "Efficacy and Safety of Lovastatin in Adolescent Males With Heterozygous Familial Hypercholesterolemia: A Randomized Controlled Trial," *JAMA*, 1999, 281(2):137-44.

"Third Report of the National Cholesterol Education Program Expert Panel on Detection, Evaluation, and Treatment of High Blood Cholesterol in Adults (Adult Treatment Panel III)," May 2001, www.nhlbi.nih.gov/guidelines/cholesterol.

◆ **Lovenox®** *see* Enoxaparin *on page* 505

◆ **Lovenox® HP (Can)** *see* Enoxaparin *on page* 505

◆ **Low-molecular-weight iron dextran (INFeD®)** *see* Iron Dextran Complex *on page* 762

◆ **Lozi-Flur™** *see* Fluoride *on page* 595

◆ **L-PAM** *see* Melphalan *on page* 875

◆ **L-Phenylalanine Mustard** *see* Melphalan *on page* 875

◆ **L-Sarcolysin** *see* Melphalan *on page* 875

◆ **LTA® 360** *see* Lidocaine *on page* 818

◆ **LTG** *see* LamoTRIgine *on page* 795

◆ ***L*-Thyroxine Sodium** *see* Levothyroxine *on page* 816

◆ **Lu-26-054** *see* Escitalopram *on page* 529

◆ **Lugol's Solution** *see* Potassium Iodide and Iodine *on page* 1140

◆ **Lumefantrine and Artemether** *see* Artemether and Lumefantrine *on page* 136

◆ **Luminal® Sodium** *see* PHENobarbital *on page* 1097

◆ **Lumizyme™** *see* Alglucosidase Alfa *on page* 64

◆ **LupiCare® Dandruff [OTC]** *see* Salicylic Acid *on page* 1241

◆ **LupiCare® Psoriasis [OTC]** *see* Salicylic Acid *on page* 1241

◆ **LupiCare® Psoriasis Scalp [OTC] [DSC]** *see* Salicylic Acid *on page* 1241

◆ **Lupron®** *see* Leuprolide *on page* 805

◆ **Lupron Depot®** *see* Leuprolide *on page* 805

◆ **Lupron® Depot® (Can)** *see* Leuprolide *on page* 805

◆ **Lupron Depot-Ped®** *see* Leuprolide *on page* 805

◆ **Luride® [DSC]** *see* Fluoride *on page* 595

◆ **Luride® Lozi-Tab®** *see* Fluoride *on page* 595

◆ **LuSonal™** *see* Phenylephrine *on page* 1102

◆ **Luvox** *see* Fluvoxamine *on page* 615

◆ **Luvox® (Can)** *see* Fluvoxamine *on page* 615

◆ **Luvox® CR** *see* Fluvoxamine *on page* 615

◆ **Luxiq®** *see* Betamethasone *on page* 189

◆ **LY139603** *see* Atomoxetine *on page* 149

◆ **LY146032** *see* DAPTOmycin *on page* 389

◆ **Lyderm® (Can)** *see* Fluocinonide *on page* 595

◆ **Lymphocyte Immune Globulin** *see* Antithymocyte Globulin (Equine) *on page* 118

◆ **Lymphocyte Mitogenic Factor** *see* Aldesleukin *on page* 60

◆ **Lysteda™** *see* Tranexamic Acid *on page* 1369

◆ **Maalox® Children's [OTC]** *see* Calcium Carbonate *on page* 232

◆ **Maalox® Quick Dissolve [OTC]** *see* Calcium Supplements *on page* 239

◆ **Maalox® Regular Chewable [OTC] [DSC]** *see* Calcium Carbonate *on page* 232

◆ **Maalox® Total Relief® [OTC]** *see* Bismuth *on page* 195

◆ **Macrobid®** *see* Nitrofurantoin *on page* 995

◆ **Macrodantin®** *see* Nitrofurantoin *on page* 995

Mafenide (MA fe nide)

U.S. Brand Names Sulfamylon®
Therapeutic Category Antibiotic, Topical
Generic Available No
Use Adjunct in the treatment of second and third degree burns to prevent septicemia caused by susceptible organisms such as *Pseudomonas aeruginosa*
Pregnancy Risk Factor C
Pregnancy Considerations Teratogenic effects were not observed in animal studies using an oral preparation. Safety and efficacy have not been established in pregnant women. The manufacturer does not recommended use in women of childbearing potential unless the burn area covers >20% of the total body surface or when benefits of treatment outweigh possible risks to the fetus.
Lactation Excretion in breast milk unknown/not recommended
Contraindications Hypersensitivity to mafenide or any component (see Warnings)
Warnings Superinfection with nonsusceptible organisms has occurred in burn wounds treated with mafenide; some products contain sulfites which may cause allergic reactions in susceptible individuals
Precautions Use with caution in patients with renal impairment and in patients with G-6-PD deficiency
Adverse Reactions
Dermatologic: Erythema, rash, pruritus, urticaria
Endocrine & metabolic: Hyperchloremia, metabolic acidosis
Hematologic: Bone marrow suppression, hemolytic anemia, bleeding, porphyria, eosinophilia
Local: Burning sensation, excoriation, pain, swelling
Respiratory: Hyperventilation, tachypnea
Miscellaneous: Hypersensitivity reactions, facial edema
Drug Interactions
Avoid Concomitant Use
Avoid concomitant use of Mafenide with any of the following: BCG
Increased Effect/Toxicity There are no known significant interactions involving an increase in effect.
Decreased Effect
Mafenide may decrease the levels/effects of: BCG
Stability Prepared topical solution is stable for 48 hours at room temperature
Mechanism of Action Interferes with bacterial cellular metabolism and bacterial folic acid synthesis through competitive inhibition of para-aminobenzoic acid
Pharmacokinetics (Adult data unless noted)
Absorption: Diffuses through devascularized areas and is rapidly absorbed from burned surface
Metabolism: To para-carboxybenzene sulfonamide which is a carbonic anhydrase inhibitor
Time to peak serum concentration: Topical: 2-4 hours
Elimination: In urine as metabolites
Usual Dosage Children ≥3 months and Adults: Topical
Cream: Apply once or twice daily; apply to a thickness of approximately 16 mm; the burned area should be covered with cream at all times

Solution: Irrigate dressing every 4 hours or as needed to keep gauze moistened

Administration Topical:

Cream: Apply to cleansed, debrided, burned area with a sterile-gloved hand

Solution: Reconstitute 50 g powder by adding to 1 liter sterile water or 1 liter NS for irrigation; mix until completely dissolved; filter solution through a 0.22 micron filter before use; cover area with gauze and the dressing wetted with mafenide solution; wound dressing may be left undisturbed for up to 5 days

Monitoring Parameters Acid base balance, improvement of wound healing

Patient Information Inform physician if rash, blisters, or swelling appear

Nursing Implications For external use only

Dosage Forms Excipient information presented when available (limited, particularly for generics); consult specific product labeling.

Cream, topical:

Sulfamylon®: 85 mg/g (60 g, 120 g, 454 g) [contains sodium metabisulfite]

Powder, for topical solution, as acetate:

Sulfamylon®: 50 g/packet (5s)

◆ **Mafenide Acetate** see Mafenide on page 852

◆ **Mag 64™ [OTC]** see Magnesium Chloride on page 853

◆ **Mag Delay® [OTC]** see Magnesium Chloride on page 853

◆ **Mag Delay® [OTC]** see Magnesium Supplements on page 859

◆ **Mag G® [OTC]** see Magnesium Gluconate on page 855

◆ **Mag G® [OTC]** see Magnesium Supplements on page 859

◆ **MagGel™ [OTC]** see Magnesium Supplements on page 859

◆ **MagGel™ 600 [OTC]** see Magnesium Oxide on page 857

◆ **Maginex™ [OTC]** see Magnesium L-aspartate Hydrochloride on page 856

◆ **Maginex™ [OTC]** see Magnesium Supplements on page 859

◆ **Maginex™ DS [OTC]** see Magnesium L-aspartate Hydrochloride on page 856

◆ **Maginex™ DS [OTC]** see Magnesium Supplements on page 859

◆ **Magnacet™ [DSC]** see Oxycodone and Acetaminophen on page 1041

◆ **Magnesia Magma** see Magnesium Hydroxide on page 855

◆ **Magnesia Magma (Magnesium Hydroxide)** see Magnesium Supplements on page 859

Magnesium Chloride (mag NEE zhum KLOR ide)

U.S. Brand Names Chloromag®; Mag 64™ [OTC]; Mag Delay® [OTC]; Mag-SR with Calcium [DSC]; Mag-SR [DSC]; Slow-Mag® [OTC]

Therapeutic Category Electrolyte Supplement, Oral; Electrolyte Supplement, Parenteral; Magnesium Salt

Generic Available Yes

Use Treatment and prevention of hypomagnesemia; dietary supplement

Pregnancy Risk Factor C

Pregnancy Considerations Reproduction studies have not been conducted. Magnesium crosses the placenta; serum levels in the fetus correlate with those in the mother.

Lactation Enters breast milk/compatible

Breast-Feeding Considerations Magnesium is found in breast milk. The amount is not influenced by dietary intake under normal conditions.

Contraindications Hypersensitivity to magnesium salt(s) or any component (see Warnings); serious renal impairment, myocardial damage, heart block; patients with colostomy or ileostomy, intestinal obstruction, impaction, or perforation, appendicitis, abdominal pain

Warnings Multiple salt forms of magnesium exist; close attention must be paid to the salt form when ordering and administering magnesium; **incorrect selection or substitution of one salt for another without proper dosage adjustment may result in serious over- or underdosing**

Magnesium chloride injection contains benzyl alcohol which may cause allergic reactions in susceptible individuals; large amounts of benzyl alcohol (≥99 mg/kg/day) have been associated with a potentially fatal toxicity ("gasping syndrome") in neonates; the "gasping syndrome" consists of metabolic acidosis, respiratory distress, gasping respirations, CNS dysfunction (including convulsions, intracranial hemorrhage), hypotension and cardiovascular collapse; avoid or use magnesium chloride injection with caution in neonates

Precautions See Magnesium Supplements on page 859.

Adverse Reactions See Magnesium Supplements on page 859.

Drug Interactions

Avoid Concomitant Use There are no known interactions where it is recommended to avoid concomitant use.

Increased Effect/Toxicity

Magnesium Chloride may increase the levels/effects of: Calcium Channel Blockers; Neuromuscular-Blocking Agents

The levels/effects of Magnesium Chloride may be increased by: Calcitriol; Calcium Channel Blockers

Decreased Effect

Magnesium Chloride may decrease the levels/effects of: Bisphosphonate Derivatives; Eltrombopag; Mycophenolate; Phosphate Supplements; Quinolone Antibiotics; Tetracycline Derivatives; Trientine

The levels/effects of Magnesium Chloride may be decreased by: Trientine

Mechanism of Action Magnesium is important as a cofactor in many enzymatic reactions in the body. There are at least 300 enzymes which are dependent upon magnesium for normal functioning. Actions on lipoprotein lipase have been found to be important in reducing serum cholesterol. Magnesium is necessary for the maintaining of serum potassium and calcium levels due to its effect on the renal tubule. In the heart, magnesium acts as a calcium channel blocker. It also activates sodium potassium ATPase in the cell membrane to promote resting polarization and produce arrhythmias.

Pharmacodynamics See Magnesium Supplements on page 859.

Pharmacokinetics (Adult data unless noted) See Magnesium Supplements on page 859.

Usual Dosage

Hypomagnesemia:

Neonates: I.V.: **Magnesium chloride:** 0.2-0.4 mEq/kg/dose every 8-12 hours for 2-3 doses

Children:

I.M., I.V.: **Magnesium chloride:** 0.2-0.4 mEq/kg/dose every 4-6 hours for 3-4 doses; maximum single dose: 16 mEq

Oral: **Note:** Achieving optimal magnesium levels using oral therapy may be difficult due to the propensity for magnesium to cause diarrhea; I.V. replacement may be more appropriate particularly in situations of severe deficit: **Magnesium chloride:** 10-20 mg/kg elemental magnesium per dose up to 4 times/day

Dietary supplement: Adults: Oral: (Mag 64™, Mag Delay®, Slow-Mag®): 2 tablets once daily

Daily maintenance magnesium: I.V.: **Magnesium chloride:**

Neonates, Infants, and Children ≤45 kg: 0.25-0.5 mEq/kg/day

Adolescents >45 kg and Adults: 0.2-0.5 mEq/kg/day or 3-10 mEq/1000 kcal/day (maximum: 8-20 mEq/day)

Dosing adjustment in renal impairment: Patients in severe renal failure should not receive magnesium due to toxicity from accumulation. Patients with a Cl_{cr} <25 mL/minute receiving magnesium should have serum magnesium levels monitored.

Administration

Oral: Tablet: Take with full glass of water; do not chew or crush sustained release formulations

Parenteral: Intermittent infusion: Dilute to a concentration of 0.5 mEq/mL (maximum concentration: 1.6 mEq/mL, and infuse over 2-4 hours; do not exceed 1 mEq/kg/hour; in severe circumstances, half of the dosage to be administered may be infused over the first 15-20 minutes

Monitoring Parameters See Magnesium Supplements on page 859.

Reference Range See Magnesium Supplements on page 859.

Additional Information Magnesium chloride 500 mg = 59 mg **elemental** magnesium= 4.9 mEq magnesium

Dosage Forms Excipient information presented when available (limited, particularly for generics); consult specific product labeling. [DSC] = Discontinued product

Injection, solution, as hexahydrate: 200 mg/mL (50 mL) [equivalent to elemental magnesium 1.97 mEq/mL]

Chloromag®: 200 mg/mL (50 mL) [contains benzyl alcohol; equivalent to elemental magnesium 1.97 mEq/mL]

Tablet, delayed release, enteric coated, oral:

Mag 64™, Mag Delay®: Elemental magnesium 64 mg [contains elemental calcium 110 mg]

Tablet, enteric coated, oral:

Slow-Mag®: Elemental magnesium 64 mg [contains elemental calcium 113 mg]

Tablet, oral:

Mag-SR: Elemental magnesium 64 mg [DSC]

Mag-SR with Calcium: Elemental magnesium 64 mg [contains elemental calcium 106 mg] [DSC]

Magnesium Citrate (mag NEE zhum SIT rate)

U.S. Brand Names Citroma® [OTC]

Canadian Brand Names Citro-Mag®

Therapeutic Category Laxative, Osmotic; Magnesium Salt

Generic Available Yes

Use Short-term treatment of constipation

Pregnancy Risk Factor B

Contraindications Hypersensitivity to magnesium salt(s) or any component (see Warnings); serious renal impairment, myocardial damage, heart block; patients with colostomy or ileostomy, intestinal obstruction, impaction, or perforation, appendicitis, abdominal pain

Warnings Multiple salt forms of magnesium exist; close attention must be paid to the salt form when ordering and administering magnesium; **incorrect selection or substitution of one salt for another without proper dosage adjustment may result in serious over- or underdosing**.

Precautions See Magnesium Supplements on page 859.

Adverse Reactions See Magnesium Supplements on page 859.

Drug Interactions

Avoid Concomitant Use

Avoid concomitant use of Magnesium Citrate with any of the following: Calcium Polystyrene Sulfonate; Sodium Polystyrene Sulfonate

Increased Effect/Toxicity

Magnesium Citrate may increase the levels/effects of: Aluminum Hydroxide; Calcium Channel Blockers; Neuromuscular-Blocking Agents

The levels/effects of Magnesium Citrate may be increased by: Calcitriol; Calcium Channel Blockers; Calcium Polystyrene Sulfonate; Sodium Polystyrene Sulfonate

Decreased Effect

Magnesium Citrate may decrease the levels/effects of: Bisphosphonate Derivatives; Eltrombopag; Mycophenolate; Phosphate Supplements; Quinolone Antibiotics; Tetracycline Derivatives; Trientine

The levels/effects of Magnesium Citrate may be decreased by: Trientine

Mechanism of Action Promotes bowel evacuation by causing osmotic retention of fluid which distends the colon and produces increased peristaltic activity when taken orally.

Pharmacodynamics See Magnesium Supplements on page 859.

Pharmacokinetics (Adult data unless noted) See Magnesium Supplements on page 859.

Usual Dosage Cathartic: Oral:

Children <6 years: 2-4 mL/kg/dose given once or in divided doses

Children 6-12 years: 100-150 mL/dose given once or in divided doses

Children >12 years and Adults: 150-300 mL/dose given once or in divided doses

Dosing adjustment in renal impairment: Patients in severe renal failure should not receive magnesium due to toxicity from accumulation. Patients with a Cl_{cr} <25 mL/minute receiving magnesium should have serum magnesium levels monitored.

Administration Oral:

Solution: Mix with water and administer on an empty stomach.

Tablet: Take with full glass of water.

Monitoring Parameters See Magnesium Supplements on page 859.

Reference Range See Magnesium Supplements on page 859.

Dosage Forms Excipient information presented when available (limited, particularly for generics); consult specific product labeling.

Solution, oral: 290 mg/5 mL (300 mL) [cherry and lemon flavors]

Citroma®: 290 mg/5 mL (300 mL) [contains magnesium 48 mg/5 mL, potassium 13 mg/5 mL; cherry and lemon flavors]

Citroma®: 290 mg/5 mL (300 mL) [contains magnesium 48 mg/5 mL, sodium 7.5 mg/5 mL; grape and lemony flavors]

Citroma®: 290 mg/5 mL (340 mL) [contains benzoic acid, magnesium 48 mg/5 mL, sodium 0.5 mg/5 mL; grape flavor]

Tablet: Elemental magnesium 100 mg

Magnesium Gluconate
(mag NEE zhum GLOO koe nate)

U.S. Brand Names Mag G® [OTC]; Magonate® [OTC]; Magtrate® [OTC]

Therapeutic Category Electrolyte Supplement, Oral; Magnesium Salt

Generic Available Yes: Tablet

Use Treatment and prevention of hypomagnesemia; dietary supplement

Pregnancy Considerations Magnesium crosses the placenta; serum levels in the fetus correlate with those in the mother.

Lactation Enters breast milk/compatible

Breast-Feeding Considerations Magnesium is found in breast milk. The amount is not influenced by dietary intake under normal conditions.

Contraindications Hypersensitivity to magnesium salt(s) or any component (see Warnings); serious renal impairment, myocardial damage, heart block; patients with colostomy or ileostomy, intestinal obstruction, impaction, or perforation, appendicitis, abdominal pain

Warnings Multiple salt forms of magnesium exist; close attention must be paid to the salt form when ordering and administering magnesium; **incorrect selection or substitution of one salt for another without proper dosage adjustment may result in serious over- or under-dosing**

Magonate® solution contains sodium benzoate; benzoic acid (benzoate) is a metabolite of benzyl alcohol; large amounts of benzyl alcohol (≥99 mg/kg/day) have been associated with a potentially fatal toxicity ("gasping syndrome") in neonates; in vitro and animal studies have shown that benzoate displaces bilirubin from protein binding sites; avoid use of Magonate® solution in neonates

Precautions See Magnesium Supplements on page 859.

Adverse Reactions See Magnesium Supplements on page 859.

Drug Interactions

Avoid Concomitant Use There are no known interactions where it is recommended to avoid concomitant use.

Increased Effect/Toxicity

Magnesium Gluconate may increase the levels/effects of: Calcium Channel Blockers; Neuromuscular-Blocking Agents

The levels/effects of Magnesium Gluconate may be increased by: Calcitriol; Calcium Channel Blockers

Decreased Effect

Magnesium Gluconate may decrease the levels/effects of: Bisphosphonate Derivatives; Eltrombopag; Mycophenolate; Phosphate Supplements; Quinolone Antibiotics; Tetracycline Derivatives; Trientine

The levels/effects of Magnesium Gluconate may be decreased by: Trientine

Mechanism of Action Magnesium is important as a cofactor in many enzymatic reactions in the body. There are at least 300 enzymes which are dependent upon magnesium for normal functioning. Actions on lipoprotein lipase have been found to be important in reducing serum cholesterol. Magnesium is necessary for the maintaining of serum potassium and calcium levels due to its effect on the renal tubule. In the heart, magnesium acts as a calcium channel blocker. It also activates sodium potassium ATPase in the cell membrane to promote resting polarization and produce arrhythmias.

Pharmacodynamics See Magnesium Supplements on page 859.

Pharmacokinetics (Adult data unless noted) See Magnesium Supplements on page 859.

Usual Dosage Oral: **Note:** Achieving optimal magnesium levels using oral therapy may be difficult due to the propensity for magnesium to cause diarrhea; I.V. replacement may be more appropriate particularly in situations of severe deficit.

Prevention and treatment of hypomagnesemia:

Children: 10-20 mg/kg **elemental** magnesium per dose up to 4 times/day

Adults: 500-1000 mg 3 times/day

Dosing adjustment in renal impairment: Patients in severe renal failure should not receive magnesium due to toxicity from accumulation. Patients with a Cl_{cr} <25 mL/minute receiving magnesium should have serum magnesium levels monitored.

Administration Oral:

Solution: Mix with water and administer on an empty stomach.

Tablet: Take with full glass of water.

Monitoring Parameters See Magnesium Supplements on page 859.

Reference Range See Magnesium Supplements on page 859.

Additional Information Magnesium gluconate 500 mg = 27 mg **elemental** magnesium = 2.4 mEq magnesium

Dosage Forms Excipient information presented when available (limited, particularly for generics); consult specific product labeling.

Liquid, oral:

Magonate®: 1000 mg/5 mL (355 mL) [contains sodium benzoate; melon flavor; equivalent to elemental magnesium 54 mg (4.8 mEq) per 5 mL]

Tablet, oral: 500 mg [equivalent to elemental magnesium 27 mg (2.4 mEq)]; 550 mg [equivalent to elemental magnesium 30 mg)]

Mag G®: 500 mg [equivalent to elemental magnesium 27 mg (2.4 mEq)]

Magonate®: 500 mg [scored; equivalent to elemental magnesium 27 mg (2.4 mEq)]

Magtrate®: 500 mg [equivalent to elemental magnesium 27 mg (2.4 mEq)]

Magnesium Hydroxide
(mag NEE zhum hye DROKS ide)

U.S. Brand Names Dulcolax® Milk of Magnesia [OTC]; Phillips'® M-O [OTC]; Phillips'® Milk of Magnesia [OTC]

Therapeutic Category Antacid; Laxative, Osmotic

Generic Available Yes: Liquid

Use Short-term treatment of constipation; treatment of hyperacidity symptoms

Contraindications Hypersensitivity to magnesium salt(s) or any component (see Warnings); serious renal impairment, myocardial damage, heart block; patients with colostomy or ileostomy, intestinal obstruction, impaction, or perforation, appendicitis, abdominal pain

Warnings Multiple salt forms of magnesium exist; close attention must be paid to the salt form when ordering and administering magnesium; **incorrect selection or substitution of one salt for another without proper dosage adjustment may result in serious over- or under-dosing**

Precautions See Magnesium Supplements on page 859.

Adverse Reactions See Magnesium Supplements on page 859.

Drug Interactions

Avoid Concomitant Use

Avoid concomitant use of Magnesium Hydroxide with any of the following: Calcium Polystyrene Sulfonate; QuiNINE; Sodium Polystyrene Sulfonate

Increased Effect/Toxicity

Magnesium Hydroxide may increase the levels/effects of: Alpha-/Beta-Agonists; Amphetamines; Calcium Channel Blockers; Misoprostol; Neuromuscular-Blocking Agents; QuiNIDine

The levels/effects of Magnesium Hydroxide may be increased by: Calcitriol; Calcium Channel Blockers; Calcium Polystyrene Sulfonate; Sodium Polystyrene Sulfonate

Decreased Effect

Magnesium Hydroxide may decrease the levels/effects of: ACE Inhibitors; Allopurinol; Anticonvulsants (Hydantoin); Antifungal Agents (Azole Derivatives, Systemic); Antipsychotic Agents (Phenothiazines); Atazanavir; Bisacodyl; Bisphosphonate Derivatives; Cefditoren; Cefpodoxime; Cefuroxime; Chloroquine; Corticosteroids (Oral); Dabigatran Etexilate; Dasatinib; Delavirdine; Eltrombopag; Erlotinib; Fexofenadine; HMG-CoA Reductase Inhibitors; Iron Salts; Isoniazid; Mesalamine; Methenamine; Mycophenolate; Penicillamine; Phosphate Supplements; Protease Inhibitors; QuiNINE; Quinolone Antibiotics; Tetracycline Derivatives; Trientine; Ursodiol

The levels/effects of Magnesium Hydroxide may be decreased by: Trientine

Mechanism of Action Promotes bowel evacuation by causing osmotic retention of fluid which distends the colon and produces increased peristaltic activity when taken orally. To reduce stomach acidity, it reacts with hydrochloric acid in stomach to form magnesium chloride.

Pharmacodynamics See Magnesium Supplements on page 859.

Pharmacokinetics (Adult data unless noted) See Magnesium Supplements on page 859.

Usual Dosage Oral:

Liquid: Dosage based upon regular strength liquid (400 mg/5 mL); when using concentrated magnesium hydroxide solution, reduce recommended dose by $1/2$:

Children <2 years: 0.5 mL/kg/dose

Children 2-5 years: 5-15 mL/day once before bedtime or in divided doses

Children 6-11 years: 15-30 mL/day once before bedtime or in divided doses

Children ≥12 years and Adults: 30-60 mL/day once before bedtime or in divided doses

Tablet:

Children 2-5 years: 311-622 mg (1-2 tablets) once before bedtime or in divided doses

Children 6-11 years: 933-1244 mg (3-4 tablets) once before bedtime or in divided doses

Children ≥12 years and Adults: 1866-2488 mg (6-8 tablets) once before bedtime or in divided doses

Magnesium hydroxide and mineral oil (Phillips'® M-O) (infant dosage to provide equivalent dosage of magnesium hydroxide listed above):

Children <2 years: 0.6 mL/kg/dose

Children 2-5 years: 5-15 mL/day once or in divided doses

Children 6-11 years: 15-30 mL/day once or in divided doses

Children ≥12 years and Adults: 30-60 mL once or in divided doses

Antacid: Oral:

Children:

Liquid: 2.5-5 mL/dose, up to 4 times/day

Tablet: 311 mg (1 tablet) up to 4 times/day

Adults:

Liquid: 5-15 mL/dose, up to 4 times/day

Liquid concentrate: 2.5-7.5 mL/dose, up to 4 times/day

Tablet: 622-1244 mg/dose (2-4 tablets) up to 4 times/day

Dosing adjustment in renal impairment: Patients in severe renal failure should not receive magnesium due to toxicity from accumulation. Patients with a Cl_{cr} <25 mL/minute receiving magnesium should have serum magnesium levels monitored.

Administration Oral:

Solution: Mix with water and administer on an empty stomach.

Tablet: Take with full glass of water.

Monitoring Parameters See Magnesium Supplements on page 859.

Reference Range See Magnesium Supplements on page 859.

Dosage Forms Excipient information presented when available (limited, particularly for generics); consult specific product labeling.

Magnesium hydroxide:

Liquid, oral: 400 mg/5 mL (360 mL, 480 mL, 960 mL, 3780 mL)

Dulcolax® Milk of Magnesia: 400 mg/5 mL (360 mL, 780 mL) [regular and mint flavors]

Phillips'® Milk of Magnesia: 400 mg/5 mL (120 mL, 360 mL, 780 mL) [original, French vanilla, cherry, and mint flavors]

Liquid, oral concentrate: 800 mg/5 mL (100 mL, 400 mL)

Phillips'® Milk of Magnesia [concentrate]: 800 mg/5 mL (240 mL) [strawberry créme flavor]

Tablet, chewable (Phillips'® Milk of Magnesia): 311 mg [mint flavor]

Magnesium hydroxide and mineral oil:

Suspension, oral (Phillips'® M-O): Magnesium hydroxide 300 mg and mineral oil 1.25 mL per 5 mL (360 mL, 780 mL) [original and mint flavors]

Magnesium L-aspartate Hydrochloride

(mag NEE zhum el as PAR tate hye droe KLOR ide)

U.S. Brand Names Maginex™ DS [OTC]; Maginex™ [OTC]

Therapeutic Category Electrolyte Supplement, Oral; Magnesium Salt

Generic Available No

Use Magnesium supplement

Pregnancy Considerations Magnesium crosses the placenta; serum levels in the fetus correlate with those in the mother.

Lactation Enters breast milk/compatible

Breast-Feeding Considerations Magnesium is found in breast milk. The amount is not influenced by dietary intake under normal conditions.

Contraindications Hypersensitivity to magnesium salt(s) or any component (see Warnings); serious renal impairment, myocardial damage, heart block; patients with colostomy or ileostomy, intestinal obstruction, impaction, or perforation, appendicitis, abdominal pain

Warnings Multiple salt forms of magnesium exist; close attention must be paid to the salt form when ordering and administering magnesium; **incorrect selection or substitution of one salt for another without proper dosage adjustment may result in serious over- or underdosing**

Precautions See Magnesium Supplements on page 859.

Adverse Reactions See Magnesium Supplements on page 859.

Drug Interactions

Avoid Concomitant Use There are no known interactions where it is recommended to avoid concomitant use.

Increased Effect/Toxicity

Magnesium L-aspartate Hydrochloride may increase the levels/effects of: Calcium Channel Blockers; Neuromuscular-Blocking Agents

The levels/effects of Magnesium L-aspartate Hydrochloride may be increased by: Calcitriol; Calcium Channel Blockers

Decreased Effect

Magnesium L-aspartate Hydrochloride may decrease the levels/effects of: Bisphosphonate Derivatives; Eltrombopag; Mycophenolate; Phosphate Supplements; Quinolone Antibiotics; Tetracycline Derivatives; Trientine

The levels/effects of Magnesium L-aspartate Hydrochloride may be decreased by: Trientine

Mechanism of Action Magnesium is important as a cofactor in many enzymatic reactions in the body. There are at least 300 enzymes which are dependent upon magnesium for normal functioning. Actions on lipoprotein lipase have been found to be important in reducing serum cholesterol. Magnesium is necessary for the maintaining of serum potassium and calcium levels due to its effect on the renal tubule. In the heart, magnesium acts as a calcium channel blocker. It also activates sodium potassium ATPase in the cell membrane to promote resting polarization and produce arrhythmias.

Pharmacodynamics See Magnesium Supplements on page 859.

Pharmacokinetics (Adult data unless noted) See Magnesium Supplements on page 859.

Usual Dosage Oral:

Hypomagnesemia: **Note:** Achieving optimal magnesium levels using oral therapy may be difficult due to the propensity for magnesium to cause diarrhea: I.V. replacement may be more appropriate particularly in situations of severe deficit:

Children: 10-20 mg/kg elemental magnesium per dose up to 4 times/day

Dietary supplement: Adults: 1230 mg up to 3 times/day

Dosing adjustment in renal impairment: Patients in severe renal failure should not receive magnesium due to toxicity from accumulation. Patients with a Cl_{cr} <25 mL/minute receiving magnesium should have serum magnesium levels monitored.

Administration Oral:

Granules: Mix each packet in 4 ounces water or juice prior to administration

Tablet: Take with full glass of water

Monitoring Parameters See Magnesium Supplements on page 859.

Reference Range See Magnesium Supplements on page 859.

Additional Information Magnesium L-aspartate 500 mg = 49.6 mg **elemental** magnesium = 4.1 mEq magnesium

Dosage Forms Excipient information presented when available (limited, particularly for generics); consult specific product labeling.

Granules, for solution, oral [preservative free]:

Maginex™ DS: 1230 mg/packet (30s) [equivalent to magnesium 122 mg (10 mEq); sugar free; lemon flavor]

Tablet, enteric coated, oral [preservative free]:

Maginex™: 615 mg [equivalent to magnesium 61 mg (5 mEq)]

Magnesium Oxide (mag NEE zhum OKS ide)

U.S. Brand Names Mag-Ox® 400 [OTC]; MagGel™ 600 [OTC]; MAGnesium-Oxide™ [OTC]; Phillips'® Laxative Dietary Supplement Cramp-Free [OTC]; Uro-Mag® [OTC]

Therapeutic Category Electrolyte Supplement, Oral; Laxative, Osmotic; Magnesium Salt

Generic Available Yes

Use Magnesium supplement; short-term treatment of constipation; treatment of hyperacidity symptoms

Pregnancy Considerations Magnesium crosses the placenta; serum levels in the fetus correlate with those in the mother.

Lactation Enters breast milk/compatible

Breast-Feeding Considerations Magnesium is found in breast milk. The amount is not influenced by dietary intake under normal conditions.

Contraindications Hypersensitivity to magnesium salt(s) or any component (see Warnings); serious renal impairment, myocardial damage, heart block; patients with colostomy or ileostomy, intestinal obstruction, impaction, or perforation, appendicitis, abdominal pain

Warnings Multiple salt forms of magnesium exist; close attention must be paid to the salt form when ordering and administering magnesium; **incorrect selection or substitution of one salt for another without proper dosage adjustment may result in serious over- or under-dosing**

Precautions See Magnesium Supplements on page 859.

Adverse Reactions See Magnesium Supplements on page 859.

Drug Interactions

Avoid Concomitant Use

Avoid concomitant use of Magnesium Oxide with any of the following: Calcium Polystyrene Sulfonate; Sodium Polystyrene Sulfonate

Increased Effect/Toxicity

Magnesium Oxide may increase the levels/effects of: Calcium Channel Blockers; Neuromuscular-Blocking Agents

The levels/effects of Magnesium Oxide may be increased by: Calcitriol; Calcium Channel Blockers; Calcium Polystyrene Sulfonate; Sodium Polystyrene Sulfonate

Decreased Effect

Magnesium Oxide may decrease the levels/effects of: Bisphosphonate Derivatives; Eltrombopag; Mycophenolate; Phosphate Supplements; Quinolone Antibiotics; Tetracycline Derivatives; Trientine

The levels/effects of Magnesium Oxide may be decreased by: Trientine

Mechanism of Action Magnesium is important as a cofactor in many enzymatic reactions in the body. There are at least 300 enzymes which are dependent upon magnesium for normal functioning. Actions on lipoprotein lipase have been found to be important in reducing serum cholesterol. Magnesium is necessary for the maintaining of serum potassium and calcium levels due to its effect on the renal tubule. In the heart, magnesium acts as a calcium channel blocker. It also activates sodium potassium ATPase in the cell membrane to promote resting polarization and produce arrhythmias. Promotes bowel evacuation by causing osmotic retention of fluid which distends the colon and produces increased peristaltic activity when taken orally. To reduce stomach acidity, it reacts with hydrochloric acid in the stomach to form magnesium chloride

Pharmacodynamics See Magnesium Supplements on page 859.

Pharmacokinetics (Adult data unless noted) See Magnesium Supplements on page 859.

Usual Dosage Oral:

Antacid: Adults: 140 mg 3-4 times/day or 400-840 mg/day

Cathartic: Adults: 2-4 g at bedtime

Hypomagnesemia: **Note:** Achieving optimal magnesium levels using oral therapy may be difficult due to the propensity for magnesium to cause diarrhea: I.V. replacement may be more appropriate particularly in situations of severe deficit.

Children: 10-20 mg/kg elemental magnesium per dose up to 4 times/day

Dosing adjustment in renal impairment: Patients in severe renal failure should not receive magnesium due to toxicity from accumulation. Patients with a Cl_{cr} <25 mL/minute receiving magnesium should have serum magnesium levels monitored.

Administration Oral: Tablet: Take with full glass of water.

Monitoring Parameters See Magnesium Supplements on page 859.

Reference Range See Magnesium Supplements on page 859.

Additional Information Magnesium oxide 500 mg = 302 mg **elemental** magnesium = 25 mEq magnesium

Dosage Forms Excipient information presented when available (limited, particularly for generics); consult specific product labeling.

Caplet, oral: Elemental magnesium 250 mg
   Phillips'® Laxative Dietary Supplement Cramp-Free: Elemental magnesium 500 mg

Capsule, oral:
   Uro-Mag®: 140 mg [equivalent to elemental magnesium 84.5 mg (6.93 mEq)]

Capsule, softgel, oral:
   MagGel™ 600: 600 mg [equivalent to elemental magnesium 348 mg (28.64 mEq)]

Tablet, oral: 400 mg, 500 mg
   Mag-Ox® 400: 400 mg [scored; equivalent to elemental magnesium 240 mg (20 mEq)]
   MAGnesium-Oxide™: 400 mg [equivalent to elemental magnesium 240 mg (20 mEq)]

◆ **MAGnesium-Oxide™ [OTC]** *see* Magnesium Oxide *on page 857*

Magnesium Sulfate (mag NEE zhum SUL fate)

Medication Safety Issues

Sound-alike/look-alike issues:
   Magnesium sulfate may be confused with manganese sulfate, morphine sulfate
   $MgSO_4$ is an error-prone abbreviation (mistaken as morphine sulfate)

High alert medication: The Institute for Safe Medication Practices (ISMP) includes this medication (I.V. formulation) among its list of drugs which have a heightened risk of causing significant patient harm when used in error.

Related Information

Adult ACLS Algorithms *on page 1463*
CPR Pediatric Drug Dosages *on page 1455*
Pediatric ALS Algorithms *on page 1460*

Therapeutic Category Anticonvulsant; Electrolyte Supplement, Oral; Electrolyte Supplement, Parenteral; Magnesium Salt

Generic Available Yes

Use Treatment and prevention of hypomagnesemia, treatment of hypertension, torsade de pointes, and encephalopathy and seizures associated with acute nephritis; prevention and treatment of seizures in severe pre-eclampsia or eclampsia; prevention of premature labor; adjunctive treatment for bronchodilation in moderate to severe acute asthma

Pregnancy Risk Factor A/C (manufacturer dependent)

Pregnancy Considerations Magnesium crosses the placenta; serum levels in the fetus correlate with those in the mother. Magnesium sulfate is used during pregnancy for the treatment of eclampsia and severe pre-eclampsia.

Lactation Enters breast milk/compatible

Breast-Feeding Considerations Magnesium is found in breast milk. The amount is not influenced by dietary intake under normal conditions. In women receiving parenteral magnesium sulfate for the treatment of eclampsia, magnesium levels in breast milk returned to normal 24 hours following discontinuation of treatment.

Contraindications Hypersensitivity to magnesium salt(s) or any component (see Warnings); serious renal impairment, myocardial damage, heart block; patients with colostomy or ileostomy, intestinal obstruction, impaction, or perforation, appendicitis, abdominal pain

Warnings Multiple salt forms of magnesium exist; close attention must be paid to the salt form when ordering and administering magnesium; **incorrect selection or substitution of one salt for another without proper dosage adjustment may result in serious over- or underdosing**

Precautions See Magnesium Supplements on page 859.

Adverse Reactions See Magnesium Supplements on page 859.

Drug Interactions

Avoid Concomitant Use
Avoid concomitant use of Magnesium Sulfate with any of the following: Calcium Polystyrene Sulfonate; Sodium Polystyrene Sulfonate

Increased Effect/Toxicity
Magnesium Sulfate may increase the levels/effects of: Alcohol (Ethyl); Calcium Channel Blockers; CNS Depressants; Methotrimeprazine; Neuromuscular-Blocking Agents

The levels/effects of Magnesium Sulfate may be increased by: Calcitriol; Calcium Channel Blockers; Calcium Polystyrene Sulfonate; Methotrimeprazine; Sodium Polystyrene Sulfonate

Decreased Effect
Magnesium Sulfate may decrease the levels/effects of: Bisphosphonate Derivatives; Eltrombopag; Mycophenolate; Phosphate Supplements; Quinolone Antibiotics; Tetracycline Derivatives; Trientine

The levels/effects of Magnesium Sulfate may be decreased by: Ketorolac; Ketorolac (Systemic); Mefloquine; Trientine

Mechanism of Action Magnesium is important as a cofactor in many enzymatic reactions in the body. There are at least 300 enzymes which are dependent upon magnesium for normal functioning. Actions on lipoprotein lipase have been found to be important in reducing serum cholesterol. Magnesium is necessary for the maintaining of serum potassium and calcium levels due to its effect on the renal tubule. In the heart, magnesium acts as a calcium channel blocker. It also activates sodium potassium ATPase in the cell membrane to promote resting polarization and produce arrhythmias. Magnesium prevents premature labor by inhibiting myometrial contractions. In the CNS, magnesium prevents or controls seizures by blocking neuromuscular transmission and decreasing the amount of acetylcholine liberated at the end-plate by the motor nerve impulse. It also has a depressant effect on the CNS.

Pharmacodynamics See Magnesium Supplements on page 859.

Pharmacokinetics (Adult data unless noted) See Magnesium Supplements on page 859.

Usual Dosage Note: 1 g of magnesium sulfate = 98.6 mg **elemental** magnesium = 8.12 mEq magnesium

Hypomagnesemia:
   Neonates: I.V.: 25-50 mg magnesium sulfate/kg/dose (equal to 0.2-0.4 mEq magnesium/kg/dose) every 8-12 hours for 2-3 doses
   Children: I.M., I.V.: 25-50 mg magnesium sulfate/kg/dose (equal to 0.2-0.4 mEq magnesium/kg/dose) every 4-6 hours for 3-4 doses; maximum single dose: 2000 mg magnesium sulfate (equal to 16 mEq magnesium)
   Adults: I.M., I.V.: 1 g magnesium sulfate every 6 hours for 4 doses, or 250 mg magnesium sulfate/kg over a 4-hour period; for severe hypomagnesemia: 8-12 g magnesium sulfate/day in divided doses has been used

Daily maintenance magnesium: I.V.: **Note:** mEq denotes amount of magnesium ion only not the total salt form

Neonates, Infants, and Children ≤45 kg: 0.25-0.5 mEq magnesium/kg/day

Adolescents >45 kg and Adults: 0.2-0.5 mEq magnesium/kg/day or 3-10 mEq magnesium/1000 kcal/day (maximum: 8-24 mEq magnesium/day)

Management of seizures and hypertension: I.M., I.V.:

Children: 20-100 mg magnesium sulfate/kg/dose every 4-6 hours as needed; in severe cases, doses as high as 200 mg magnesium sulfate/kg/dose have been used

Adults: 1 g magnesium sulfate every 6 hours for 4 doses as needed

Prevention of premature labor: I.V.: Adolescents and Adults: Initial loading dose: 4-6 g magnesium sulfate followed by a continuous infusion of 2-3 g/hour

Treatment and prevention of seizures in severe pre-eclampsia or eclampsia: I.V.: Adolescents and Adults: 4-6 g magnesium sulfate over 15-20 minutes; followed by a 1-2 g magnesium sulfate/hour continuous infusion; or may follow with I.M. doses of 4-5 g magnesium sulfate in each buttock every 4 hours. **Note:** Initial infusion may be given over 3-4 minutes if eclampsia is severe, maximum: 40 g magnesium/24 hours

Treatment of torsade de pointes VT: I.V.:

Infants and Children: 25-50 mg magnesium sulfate/kg/dose; not to exceed 2 g magnesium sulfate/dose

Adults: 1-2 g magnesium sulfate/dose

Bronchodilation (adjunctive treatment in severe acute asthma for patients who have life-threatening exacerbations and in those whose exacerbations remain in the severe category after 1 hour of intensive conventional therapy, NIH Guidelines, 2007): I.V.:

Children: 25-75 mg magnesium sulfate/kg/dose (maximum dose: 2 g) as a single dose

Adults: 2 g magnesium sulfate as a single dose

Note: Literature evaluating magnesium sulfate's efficacy in the relief of bronchospasm has utilized single dosages in patients with acute symptomatology who have received aerosol β-agonist therapy (see References) with inconsistent results. A recent study (Ciarallo, 2000) showed significant improvement in pulmonary function in children who received a single dose of 40 mg/kg magnesium sulfate vs. placebo; pulmonary index scores after magnesium sulfate 75 mg/kg (maximum: 2.5 g) vs. placebo were not statistically different in 54 children between 1-18 years of age (Scarfone, 2000). See Additional Information.

Dosing adjustment in renal impairment: Patients in severe renal failure should not receive magnesium due to toxicity from accumulation. Patients with a Cl_{cr} <25 mL/minute receiving magnesium should have serum magnesium levels monitored.

Administration Parenteral:

Intermittent infusion: Dilute to a concentration of 0.5 mEq/mL (60 mg/mL of **magnesium sulfate**) (maximum concentration: 1.6 mEq/mL, 200 mg/mL of magnesium sulfate) and infuse over 2-4 hours; do not exceed 1 mEq/kg/hour (125 mg/kg/hour of magnesium sulfate); in severe circumstances, half of the dosage to be administered may be infused over the first 15-20 minutes; in medical emergencies (eg, prevention of seizures in pre-eclampsia), the loading dose (4-6 g) may be infused over 15-20 minutes (smaller doses, eg, treatment of torsade de pointes, may be infused over 5-20 minutes).

For I.M. administration, dilute magnesium sulfate to a maximum concentration of 200 mg/mL prior to injection

Monitoring Parameters See Magnesium Supplements on page 859.

Reference Range See Magnesium Supplements on page 859.

Additional Information Magnesium sulfate 500 mg = 49.3 mg **elemental** magnesium = 4.1 mEq magnesium. Nebulized magnesium sulfate in varying concentrations/dosages has been used successfully with and without $beta_2$-adrenergic agonists in the treatment of acute asthma (Blitz, 2006).

Dosage Forms Excipient information presented when available (limited, particularly for generics); consult specific product labeling.

Infusion [premixed in D_5W]: 10 mg/mL (100 mL); 20 mg/mL (500 mL)

Infusion [premixed in water for injection]: 40 mg/mL (100 mL, 500 mL, 1000 mL); 80 mg/mL (50 mL)

Injection, solution: 500 mg/mL (2 mL, 10 mL, 20 mL, 50 mL)

Powder, oral/topical: USP: 100% (227 g, 454 g, 480 g, 1810 g, 1920 g, 2720 g)

References

"2005 American Heart Association (AHA) Guidelines for Cardiopulmonary Resuscitation (CPR) and Emergency Cardiovascular Care (ECC) of Pediatric and Neonatal Patients: Pediatric Advanced Life Support," *Pediatrics*, 2006, 117(5):1005-28.

Blitz M, Blitz S, Beasely R, et al, "Inhaled Magnesium Sulfate in the Treatment of Acute Asthma," *Cochrane Database Syst Rev*, 2005, 19 (4):CD003898.

Briggs GG and Wan SR, "Drug Therapy During Labor and Delivery, Part 2," *Am J Health Syst Pharm*, 2006, 63(12):1131-9.

Bloch H, Silverman R, Mancherje N, et al, "Intravenous Magnesium Sulfate as an Adjunct in the Treatment of Acute Asthma," *Chest*, 1995, 107(6):1576-81.

Chernow B, Smith J, Rainey TG, et al, "Hypomagnesemia: Implications for the Critical Care Specialist," *Crit Care Med*, 1982, 10(3):193-6.

Cheuk DK, Chau TC, and Lee SL, "A Meta-analysis on Intravenous Magnesium Sulphate for Treating Acute Asthma," *Arch Dis Child*, 2005, 90(1):74-7.

Ciarallo L, Brousseau D, and Reinert S, "Higher-Dose Intravenous Magnesium Therapy for Children With Moderate to Severe Acute Asthma," *Arch Pediatr Adolesc Med*, 2000, 154(10):979-83.

Ciarallo L, Sauer AH, and Shannon MW, "Intravenous Magnesium Therapy for Moderate to Severe Pediatric Asthma: Results of a Randomized, Placebo-Controlled Trial," *J Pediatr*, 1996, 129 (6):809-14.

"Dietary Reference Intakes for Calcium, Phosphorus, Magnesium, Vitamin D, and Fluoride. Standing Committee on the Scientific Evaluation of Dietary Reference Intakes, Food and Nutrition Board, Institute of Medicine," National Academy of Sciences, Washington, DC: National Academy Press, 1997.

"Guidelines for the Diagnosis and Management of Asthma. NAEPP Expert Panel Report 3," August 2007, www.nhlbi.nih.gov/guidelines/asthma/asthgdln.pdf.

Scarfone RJ, Loiselle JM, Joffe MD, et al, "A Randomized Trial of Magnesium in the Emergency Department Treatment of Children With Asthma," *Ann Emerg Med*, 2000, 36(6):572-8.

Magnesium Supplements
(mag NEE zee um SUP la ments)

Related Information

U.S. Brand Names Almora® [OTC]; Chloromag®; Dulcolax® Milk of Magnesia [OTC]; Mag Delay® [OTC]; Mag G® [OTC]; Mag-Ox 400® [OTC]; MagGel™ [OTC]; Maginex™ DS [OTC]; Maginex™ [OTC]; Magonate® Sport [OTC] [DSC]; Magonate® [OTC]; Magtrate® [OTC]; May-SR® [OTC]; Phillips'® M-O [OTC]; Phillips'® Milk of Magnesia [OTC]; Slow-Mag® [OTC]; Uro-Mag® [OTC]

Therapeutic Category Antacid; Anticonvulsant, Miscellaneous; Electrolyte Supplement, Oral; Electrolyte Supplement, Parenteral; Laxative, Osmotic; Magnesium Salt

Generic Available Yes

Use

Treatment and prevention of hypomagnesemia (see individual monographs for magnesium chloride, magnesium sulfate, magnesium gluconate, magnesium l-aspartate hydrochloride, and magnesium oxide)

Treatment of hypertension (see individual monograph for magnesium sulfate)

Treatment of torsade de pointes (see individual monograph for magnesium sulfate)

Treatment of encephalopathy and seizures associated with acute nephritis (see individual monograph for magnesium sulfate)

Short-term treatment of constipation (see individual monographs for magnesium citrate, magnesium hydroxide, and magnesium oxide)

Treatment of hyperacidity symptoms (see individual monographs for magnesium hydroxide and magnesium oxide)

Adjunctive treatment for bronchodilation in moderate to severe acute asthma (see individual monograph for magnesium sulfate)

Contraindications Hypersensitivity to magnesium salt(s) or any component (see Warnings); serious renal impairment, myocardial damage, heart block; patients with colostomy or ileostomy, intestinal obstruction, impaction, or perforation, appendicitis, abdominal pain

Warnings Multiple salt forms of magnesium exist; close attention must be paid to the salt form when ordering and administering magnesium; **incorrect selection or substitution of one salt for another without proper dosage adjustment may result in serious over- or underdosing.**

Precautions Use with caution in patients with impaired renal function (accumulation of magnesium may lead to magnesium intoxication); use with caution in digitalized patients (may alter cardiac conduction leading to heart block)

Adverse Reactions Adverse effects with magnesium therapy are primarily related to the magnesium serum level

>3 mg/dL: Depressed CNS, blocked peripheral neuromuscular transmission leading to anticonvulsant effects

>5 mg/dL: Depressed deep tendon reflexes, flushing, somnolence

>12 mg/dL: Respiratory paralysis, complete heart block

Other effects:

Cardiovascular: Hypotension

Endocrine & metabolic: Hypermagnesemia

Gastrointestinal: Diarrhea, abdominal cramps, gas formation

Neuromuscular & skeletal: Muscle weakness

Pharmacodynamics

Onset of action:

Anticonvulsant:

I.M.: 60 minutes

I.V.: Immediately

Laxative: Oral: 4-8 hours

Duration: Anticonvulsant:

I.M.: 3-4 hours

I.V.: 30 minutes

Pharmacokinetics (Adult data unless noted)

Absorption: Oral: Up to 30%

Elimination: Renal with unabsorbed drug excreted in feces

Usual Dosage

Recommended daily allowance of magnesium: Oral: See table.

Magnesium – Recommended Daily Allowance (RDA) and Estimated Average Requirement (EAR) (in terms of elemental magnesium)

Age	RDA (mg/day)	EAR (mg/day)
<6 mo	40	30
6-12 mo	60	75
1-3 y	80	65
4-8 y	130	110
Male		
9-13 y	240	200
14-18 y	410	340
19-30 y	400	330
Female		
9-13 y	240	200
14-18 y	360	300
19-30 y	310	255

Elemental Magnesium Content of Magnesium Salts

Magnesium Salt	Elemental Magnesium (mg/500 mg salt)	Magnesium (mEq/500 mg salt)
Magnesium chloride	59	4.9
Magnesium gluconate	27	2.4
Magnesium L-aspartate	49.6	4.1
Magnesium oxide	302	25
Magnesium sulfate	49.3	4.1

Treatment and prevention of hypomagnesemia:

I.V.: See magnesium chloride on page 853 and magnesium sulfate on page 858

Oral: See magnesium chloride on page 853, magnesium gluconate on page 855, magnesium L-aspartate on page 856, and magnesium oxide on page 857.

Management of hypertension & seizures: I.V.: See magnesium sulfate on page 858

Treatment of torsade de pointes VT: I.V.: See magnesium sulfate on page 858

Bronchodilation: I.V: See magnesium sulfate on page 858

Cathartic: Oral: See magnesium citrate on page 854, magnesium hydroxide on page 855, and magnesium oxide on page 857

Antacid: Oral: See magnesium hydroxide on page 855 and magnesium oxide on page 857

Administration See individual monographs.

Monitoring Parameters Serum magnesium, deep tendon reflexes, respiratory rate, renal function, blood pressure, stool output (laxative use)

Reference Range

Neonates and Infants: 1.5-2.3 mEq/L

Children: 1.5-2.0 mEq/L

Adults: 1.4-2.0 mEq/L

Additional Information 1 g elemental magnesium = 83.3 mEq = 41.1 mmol

Dosage Forms See individual monographs.

References

"2005 American Heart Association (AHA) Guidelines for Cardiopulmonary Resuscitation (CPR) and Emergency Cardiovascular Care (ECC) of Pediatric and Neonatal Patients: Pediatric Advanced Life Support," *Pediatrics*, 2006, 117(5):1005-28.

Bloch H, Silverman R, Mancherje N, et al, "Intravenous Magnesium Sulfate as an Adjunct in the Treatment of Acute Asthma," *Chest*, 1995, 107(6):1576-81.

Chernow B, Smith J, Rainey TG, et al, "Hypomagnesemia: Implications for the Critical Care Specialist," *Crit Care Med*, 1982, 10(3):193-6.

Ciarallo L, Brousseau D, and Reinert S, "Higher-Dose Intravenous Magnesium Therapy for Children With Moderate to Severe Acute Asthma," *Arch Pediatr Adolesc Med*, 2000, 154(10):979-83.

Ciarallo L, Sauer AH, and Shannon MW, "Intravenous Magnesium Therapy for Moderate to Severe Pediatric Asthma: Results of a Randomized, Placebo-Controlled Trial," *J Pediatr*, 1996, 129 (6):809-14.

"Dietary Reference Intakes for Calcium, Phosphorus, Magnesium, Vitamin D, and Fluoride. Standing Committee on the Scientific Evaluation of Dietary Reference Intakes, Food and Nutrition Board, Institute of Medicine," National Academy of Sciences, Washington, DC: National Academy Press, 1997.

Engel J, "Normal Laboratory Values," *Pocket Guide to Pediatric Assessment*, St Louis, MO: CV Mosby, 1989, 259.

Scarfone RJ, Loiselle JM, Joffe MD, et al, "A Randomized Trial of Magnesium in the Emergency Department Treatment of Children With Asthma," *Ann Emerg Med*, 2000, 36(6):572-8.

◆ **Magonate® [OTC]** *see* Magnesium Gluconate *on page 855*

◆ **Magonate® [OTC]** *see* Magnesium Supplements *on page 859*

◆ **Magonate® Sport [OTC] [DSC]** *see* Magnesium Supplements *on page 859*

◆ **Mag-Ox® 400 [OTC]** *see* Magnesium Oxide *on page 857*

◆ **Mag-Ox 400® [OTC]** *see* Magnesium Supplements *on page 859*

◆ **Mag-SR [DSC]** *see* Magnesium Chloride *on page 853*

◆ **Mag-SR with Calcium [DSC]** *see* Magnesium Chloride *on page 853*

◆ **Magtrate® [OTC]** *see* Magnesium Gluconate *on page 855*

◆ **Magtrate® [OTC]** *see* Magnesium Supplements *on page 859*

◆ **MAH** *see* Magnesium L-aspartate Hydrochloride *on page 856*

◆ **Malarone®** *see* Atovaquone and Proguanil *on page 154*

◆ **Malarone® Pediatric (Can)** *see* Atovaquone and Proguanil *on page 154*

◆ **Mandelamine® (Can)** *see* Methenamine *on page 896*

◆ **Mandrake** *see* Podophyllum Resin *on page 1126*

◆ **Manganese Chloride** *see* Trace Metals *on page 1366*

◆ **Manganese Sulfate** *see* Trace Metals *on page 1366*

Mannitol (MAN i tole)

Medication Safety Issues
Sound-alike/look-alike issues:
Osmitrol® may be confused with esmolol

Related Information
Antihypertensive Agents by Class *on page 1481*

U.S. Brand Names Osmitrol®; Resectisol®

Canadian Brand Names Osmitrol®

Therapeutic Category Diuretic, Osmotic

Generic Available Yes

Use Reduction of increased intracranial pressure (ICP) associated with cerebral edema; promotion of diuresis in the prevention and/or treatment of oliguria or anuria due to acute renal failure; reduction of increased intraocular pressure; promotion of urinary excretion of toxic substances. Resectisol® is used for urologic irrigation for transurethral prostatic resection (see package insert for further information on this use).

Pregnancy Risk Factor C

Pregnancy Considerations
Reproduction studies have not been conducted.

Lactation Excretion in breast milk unknown/use caution

Contraindications Hypersensitivity to mannitol or any component; severe renal disease, dehydration, active intracranial bleeding, severe pulmonary edema or congestion

Adverse Reactions
Cardiovascular: Circulatory overload, CHF (due to inadequate urine output and overexpansion of extracellular fluid)
Central nervous system: Convulsions, headache
Endocrine & metabolic: Fluid and electrolyte imbalance, hyponatremia or hypernatremia, hypokalemia or hyperkalemia, water intoxication, dehydration and hypovolemia secondary to rapid diuresis
Gastrointestinal: Xerostomia
Local: Tissue necrosis
Respiratory: Pulmonary edema
Miscellaneous: Allergic reactions

Drug Interactions
Avoid Concomitant Use There are no known interactions where it is recommended to avoid concomitant use.
Increased Effect/Toxicity
Mannitol may increase the levels/effects of: Amifostine; Antihypertensives; Hypotensive Agents; RiTUXimab

The levels/effects of Mannitol may be increased by: Diazoxide; Herbs (Hypotensive Properties); MAO Inhibitors; Pentoxifylline; Phosphodiesterase 5 Inhibitors; Prostacyclin Analogues
Decreased Effect
The levels/effects of Mannitol may be decreased by: Herbs (Hypertensive Properties); Methylphenidate; Yohimbine

Stability Store at room temperature (15°C to 30°C); protect from freezing; crystallization may occur at low temperatures; do not use solutions that contain crystals; heating in a hot water bath and vigorous shaking may be utilized for resolubilization of crystals; cool solutions to body temperature before using; incompatible with strongly acidic or alkaline solutions; potassium chloride or sodium chloride may cause precipitation of mannitol 20% or 25% solution

Mechanism of Action Increases the osmotic pressure of glomerular filtrate, which inhibits tubular reabsorption of water and electrolytes and increases urinary output

Pharmacodynamics After I.V. injection:
Diuresis: Onset of action: Within 1-3 hours
Reduction in ICP:
Onset of action: Within 15 minutes
Duration: 3-6 hours

Pharmacokinetics (Adult data unless noted)
Distribution: Remains confined to extracellular space; does not penetrate blood-brain barrier (except in very high concentrations or with acidosis)
Metabolism: Minimal amounts in the liver to glycogen
Half-life: 1.1-1.6 hours
Elimination: Primarily unchanged in urine by glomerular filtration

Usual Dosage I.V.:
Children:
Test dose (to assess adequate renal function): 200 mg/kg (maximum dose: 12.5 g) over 3-5 minutes to produce a urine flow of at least 1 mL/kg/hour for 1-3 hours
Initial: 0.5-1 g/kg
Maintenance: 0.25-0.5 g/kg every 4-6 hours
Adults:
Test dose: 12.5 g (200 mg/kg) over 3-5 minutes to produce a urine flow of at least 30-50 mL of urine per hour over the next 2-3 hours
Initial: 0.5-1 g/kg
Maintenance: 0.25-0.5 g/kg every 4-6 hours

Administration Parenteral: In-line filter set (≤5 micron) should always be used for mannitol infusion with concentrations ≥20%; administer test dose (for oliguria) I.V. push over 3-5 minutes; for cerebral edema or elevated ICP, administer over 20-30 minutes; maximum concentration for administration: 25%

◀ **Monitoring Parameters** Renal function, daily fluid intake and output, serum electrolytes, serum and urine osmolality; for treatment of elevated intracranial pressure, maintain serum osmolality 310-320 mOsm/kg

Patient Information May cause dry mouth

Nursing Implications Avoid extravasation; crenation and agglutination of red blood cells may occur if administered with whole blood

Additional Information Approximate osmolarity: Mannitol 20%: 1100 mOsm/L; mannitol 25%: 1375 mOsm/L

Dosage Forms Excipient information presented when available (limited, particularly for generics); consult specific product labeling.

Injection, solution: 5% [50 mg/mL] (1000 mL); 10% [100 mg/mL] (500 mL, 1000 mL); 15% [150 mg/mL] (500 mL); 20% [200 mg/mL] (150 mL, 250 mL, 500 mL); 25% [250 mg/mL] (50 mL)

Osmitrol®: 5% [50 mg/mL] (1000 mL); 10% [100 mg/mL] (500 mL, 1000 mL); 15% [150 mg/mL] (500 mL); 20% [200 mg/mL] (250 mL, 500 mL)

Solution, urogenital (Resectisol®): 5% [50 mg/mL] (2000 mL, 4000 mL)

◆ **Mapap® [OTC] [DSC]** *see* Acetaminophen *on page 36*

◆ **Mapap® Arthritis Pain [OTC]** *see* Acetaminophen *on page 36*

◆ **Mapap® Children's [OTC]** *see* Acetaminophen *on page 36*

◆ **Mapap® Children's Rapid Tabs [OTC]** *see* Acetaminophen *on page 36*

◆ **Mapap® Extra Strength [OTC]** *see* Acetaminophen *on page 36*

◆ **Mapap® Infants [OTC]** *see* Acetaminophen *on page 36*

◆ **Mapap® Junior Rapid Tabs [OTC]** *see* Acetaminophen *on page 36*

◆ **Mapezine® (Can)** *see* CarBAMazepine *on page 244*

◆ **Marcaine®** *see* Bupivacaine *on page 213*

◆ **Marcaine® Spinal** *see* Bupivacaine *on page 213*

◆ **Mar-Cof® CG** *see* Guaifenesin and Codeine *on page 657*

◆ **Margesic® H** *see* Hydrocodone and Acetaminophen *on page 684*

◆ **Marinol®** *see* Dronabinol *on page 482*

◆ **Matulane®** *see* Procarbazine *on page 1159*

◆ **3M™ Avagard™ [OTC]** *see* Chlorhexidine Gluconate *on page 291*

◆ **Maxair® Autohaler®** *see* Pirbuterol *on page 1117*

◆ **Maxidex®** *see* Dexamethasone *on page 406*

◆ **Maxidone®** *see* Hydrocodone and Acetaminophen *on page 684*

◆ **Maxilene® (Can)** *see* Lidocaine *on page 818*

◆ **Maximum D3® [OTC]** *see* Cholecalciferol *on page 300*

◆ **Maxipime®** *see* Cefepime *on page 264*

◆ **Maxitrol®** *see* Dexamethasone, Neomycin, and Polymyxin B *on page 408*

◆ **May Apple** *see* Podophyllum Resin *on page 1126*

◆ **May-SR® [OTC]** *see* Magnesium Supplements *on page 859*

◆ **MCT** *see* Medium Chain Triglycerides *on page 870*

◆ **MCT Oil® [OTC]** *see* Medium Chain Triglycerides *on page 870*

◆ **MCT Oil® (Can)** *see* Medium Chain Triglycerides *on page 870*

◆ **MCV** *see* Meningococcal (Groups A / C / Y and W-135) Diphtheria Conjugate Vaccine *on page 877*

◆ **MCV4** *see* Meningococcal (Groups A / C / Y and W-135) Diphtheria Conjugate Vaccine *on page 877*

◆ **MDL 73,147EF** *see* Dolasetron *on page 469*

Measles, Mumps, and Rubella Vaccines (Combined)
(MEE zels, mumpz & roo BEL a vak SEENS, kom BINED)

Medication Safety Issues
Sound-alike/look-alike issues:
MMR (measles, mumps and rubella virus vaccine) may be confused with MMRV (measles, mumps, rubella, and varicella) vaccine

Related Information
Immunization Guidelines *on page 1636*

U.S. Brand Names M-M-R® II

Canadian Brand Names M-M-R® II; Priorix™

Therapeutic Category Vaccine, Live Virus

Generic Available No

Use Provide active immunity to measles, mumps, and rubella viruses (FDA approved in ages ≥12 months and adults)

Pregnancy Risk Factor C

Pregnancy Considerations Animal reproduction studies have not been conducted. It is not known whether the drug can cause fetal harm or affect reproduction capacity (contracting natural measles during pregnancy can increase fetal risk). Do not administer to pregnant females. The Advisory Committee on Immunization Practices (ACIP) recommends that pregnancy should be avoided for 1 month following vaccination. Also refer to individual monographs.

Lactation
Measles/mumps: Excretion in breast milk unknown/use caution
Rubella: Enters breast milk/use caution

Breast-Feeding Considerations Evidence of rubella infection has occurred in breast-fed infants following maternal immunization, most without severe disease.

Contraindications Hypersensitivity to measles, mumps, and rubella vaccine, gelatin or any component of the formulation; history of anaphylactic reactions to neomycin; individuals with blood dyscrasias, leukemia, lymphomas, or other malignant neoplasms affecting the bone marrow or lymphatic systems; concurrent immunosuppressive therapy; primary and acquired immunodeficiency states; family history of congenital or hereditary immunodeficiency; active/untreated tuberculosis; current febrile illness or active febrile infection; pregnancy; known anaphylactoid reaction to eggs

Warnings Avoid pregnancy for at least 1 month following vaccination (ACIP, 2001); manufacturer recommends waiting 3 months following vaccination; women who are pregnant when vaccinated or who become pregnant within 28 days of vaccination should be counseled on the theoretical risks to the fetus. Use in patients with existing thrombocytopenia may result in more severe reduction in platelets; avoid use in patients with previous history of postvaccination thrombocytopenia, as rechallenge has resulted in recurrence of thrombocytopenia; severe allergic reactions including anaphylaxis have been reported rarely. Immediate treatment for anaphylactic/anaphylactoid reaction should be available during vaccine use. Use with extreme caution in patients with immediate-type hypersensitivity reactions to eggs.

MMR vaccine should not be administered to severely immunocompromised persons with the exception of asymptomatic children with HIV. Severely immunocompromised patients and symptomatic HIV-infected patients who are exposed to measles should receive immune globulin, regardless of prior vaccination status. Patients with minor illnesses (diarrhea, mild upper respiratory tract infection with or without low grade fever or other illnesses with low-grade fever) may receive vaccine. Leukemia patients who are in remission and who have not received chemotherapy for at least 3 months may be vaccinated.

Precautions Use with caution in patients with history of cerebral injury, convulsions, or other conditions where stress due to fever should be avoided; defer vaccination for at least 3 months after receiving blood and plasma transfusions or immune globulin (See Appendix Immuniza-tion Guidelines, "Suggested Intervals Between Adminis-tration of Antibody-Containing Products for Different Indications and Measles-Containing Vaccine and Vari-cella-Containing Vaccine"). Routine prophylactic admin-istration of acetaminophen to prevent fever due to vaccines has been shown to decrease the immune response of some vaccines; the clinical significance of this reduction in immune response has not been established (see Prymula, 2009).

Adverse Reactions All serious adverse reactions must be reported to the U.S. Department of Health and Human Services (DHHS) Vaccine Adverse Event Reporting System (VAERS) 1-800-822-7967.

Cardiovascular: Syncope, vasculitis

Central nervous system: Ataxia, dizziness, febrile con-vulsions, fever, encephalitis (rare), encephalopathy (rare), Guillain-Barré syndrome (rare), headache, irrita-bility, malaise, measles inclusion body encephalitis, polyneuritis, polyneuropathy, seizures, subacute scleros-ing panencephalitis

Dermatologic: Angioneurotic edema, erythema multiforme, purpura, rash, Stevens-Johnson syndrome, urticaria

Endocrine & metabolic: Diabetes mellitus, parotitis

Gastrointestinal: Diarrhea, nausea, pancreatitis, sore throat, vomiting

Genitourinary: Orchitis

Hematologic: Leukocytosis, thrombocytopenia

Local: Injection site reactions which include burning, induration, redness, stinging, swelling, tenderness, wheal and flare, vesiculation

Neuromuscular & skeletal: Arthralgia/arthritis (variable; highest rates in women, 12% to 26% versus children, up to 3%), myalgia, paresthesia

Ocular: Ocular palsies, conjunctivitis, retinitis, optic neuritis, papillitis, retrobulbar neuritis

Otic: Otitis media

Respiratory: Bronchospasm, cough, pneumonitis, rhinitis

Miscellaneous: Anaphylactoid reactions, anaphylaxis, atypical measles, panniculitis, regional lymphadenop-athy, aseptic meningitis (associated with Urabe strain of mumps vaccine)

Drug Interactions

Avoid Concomitant Use

Avoid concomitant use of Measles, Mumps, and Rubella Virus Vaccine with any of the following: Immuno-suppressants

Increased Effect/Toxicity

The levels/effects of Measles, Mumps, and Rubella Virus Vaccine may be increased by: Immunosuppressants

Decreased Effect

Measles, Mumps, and Rubella Virus Vaccine may decrease the levels/effects of: Tuberculin Tests

The levels/effects of Measles, Mumps, and Rubella Virus Vaccine may be decreased by: Immune Globulins; Immunosuppressants

Stability Prior to reconstitution, store the powder at 2°C to 8°C (36°F to 46°F) or colder (freezing does not affect potency). Protect from light. Diluent may be stored with powder or at room temperature. Discard if not used within 8 hours of reconstitution.

Mechanism of Action As a live, attenuated vaccine, MMR vaccine offers active immunity to disease caused by the measles, mumps, and rubella viruses.

Usual Dosage SubQ: 0.5 mL per dose

Infants <12 months: If there is risk of exposure to measles, single-antigen measles vaccine should be administered at 6-11 months of age with a second dose (of MMR) at ≥12 months of age.

Children ≥12 months: 2 doses, the first at 12 months of age, then repeated at 4-6 years of age. If the second dose was not received, the schedule should be completed by the 11- to 12-year old visit. (The second dose may be administered at any time provided at least 4 weeks have elapsed since the first dose.)

Adults: Adults born in or after 1957 (adults born before 1957 are generally considered to be immune to measles and mumps) without documentation of live vaccine on or after first birthday, or without physician-diagnosed measles or mumps, or without laboratory evidence of immunity, should be vaccinated with at least one dose; a second dose, separated by no less than 1 month, is indicated for those previously vaccinated with one dose of measles vaccine, students entering institutions of higher learning, recently exposed in an outbreak setting, healthcare workers at time of employment, and for travelers to endemic areas.

Administration Use entire contents of the provided diluent to reconstitute vaccine. Gently agitate to mix thoroughly. Discard if powder does not dissolve. Use as soon as possible following reconstitution; administer by SubQ injection into the anterolateral aspect of the thigh or arm; **not for I.V. administration**

Test Interactions Temporary suppression of TB skin test reactivity with onset approximately 3 days after administration

Patient Information Soreness or swelling may occur at the site of injection; fever, mild rash, swelling in the glands of the cheeks or neck, and temporary pain or stiffness in the joints may occur. Some effects may not occur until 1-2 weeks after the injection. Notify your healthcare provider immediately if these effects continue or are severe, or for a high fever, seizures or allergic reaction (respiratory difficulty, hives, weakness, dizziness, fast heartbeat). Not to be used during pregnancy; do not get pregnant for 28 days after getting the vaccine. Pregnant women should wait until after giving birth to get the vaccine.

Nursing Implications Federal law requires that the date of administration, the vaccine manufacturer, lot number of vaccine, and the administering person's name, title, and address be entered into the patient's permanent medical record.

Additional Information Using separate sites and syringes, MMR may be administered concurrently with DTaP or *Haemophilus* b conjugate vaccine (PedvaxHIB®). Varicella vaccine may be administered with MMR using separate sites and syringes; however, if not administered simultaneously, doses should be separated by at least 30 days. Unless otherwise specified, MMR should be given 1 month before or 1 month after live viral vaccines.

In order to maximize vaccination rates, the ACIP recommends simultaneous administration of all age-appropriate vaccines (live or inactivated) for which a person is eligible at a single visit, unless contraindications exist. The use of combination vaccines is generally preferred over separate infections, taking into consider-ation provider assessment, patient preference, and potential adverse events.

For additional information, please refer to the following website: http://www.cdc.gov/vaccines/vpd-vac/.

Dosage Forms Excipient information presented when available (limited, particularly for generics); consult specific product labeling.

Injection, powder for reconstitution [preservative free]:
M-M-R® II: Measles virus ≥1000 $TCID_{50}$, mumps virus ≥20,000 $TCID_{50}$, and rubella virus ≥1000 $TCID_{50}$ [contains albumin (human), bovine serum, chicken egg protein, gelatin, neomycin, sorbitol, and sucrose 1.9 mg/vial]

References

Centers for Disease Control and Prevention (CDC), "General Recommendations on Immunization. Recommendations of the Advisory Committee on Immunization Practices (ACIP)," *MMWR Recomm Rep*, 2006, 55(RR-15):1-48. Available at: http://www.cdc.gov/mmwr/preview/mmwrhtml/rr5515a1.htm.

Centers for Disease Control and Prevention (CDC), "Recommended Adult Immunization Schedule – United States, 2009" *MMWR Morb Mortal Wkly Rep*, 2009, 57(53):Q1-4.

Centers for Disease Control and Prevention (CDC), "Recommended Immunization Schedules for Persons Aged 0 Through 18 Years – United States, 2009," *MMWR Morb Mortal Wkly Rep*, 2009, 57 (51 and 52):Q1-4.

Centers for Disease Control and Prevention (CDC), "Revised ACIP Recommendation for Avoiding Pregnancy After Receiving a Rubella-Containing Vaccine," *MMWR Morb Mortal Wkly Rep*, 2001, 50 (49):1117.

Centers for Disease Control and Prevention (CDC), "Syncope After Vaccination – United States, January 2005-July 2007," *MMWR Morb Mortal Wkly Rep*, 2008, 57(17):457-60.

"General Recommendations on Immunization. Recommendations of the Advisory Committee on Immunization Practices (ACIP)," *MMWR Recomm Rep*, 1994, 43(RR-1):1-38.

Prymula R, Siegrist CA, Chlibek R, et al, "Effect of Prophylactic Paracetamol Administration at Time of Vaccination on Febrile Reactions and Antibody Responses in Children: Two Open-Label, Randomised Controlled Trials," *Lancet*, 2009, 374(9698):1339-50.

Watson JC, Hadler SC, Dykewicz CA, et al, "Measles, Mumps, and Rubella–Vaccine Use and Strategies for Elimination of Measles, Rubella, and Congenital Rubella Syndrome and Control of Mumps: Recommendations of the Advisory Committee on Immunization Practices (ACIP)," *MMWR Recomm Rep*, 1998, 47(RR-8):1-57.

Measles, Mumps, Rubella, and Varicella Virus Vaccine

(MEE zels, mumpz, roo BEL a, & var i SEL a VYE rus vak SEEN)

Related Information

Immunization Guidelines *on page 1636*

U.S. Brand Names ProQuad®

Therapeutic Category Vaccine, Live Virus

Generic Available No

Use To provide active immunity to measles, mumps, rubella, and varicella viruses (FDA approved in ages 12 months to 12 years)

The Advisory Committee on Immunization Practices (ACIP) recommends routine vaccination against measles, mumps, rubella, and varicella in healthy children 12 months to 12 years of age. For children receiving their first dose at 12-47 months of age, either the MMRV combination vaccine or separate MMR and varicella vaccines can be used. The ACIP prefers administration of separate MMR and varicella vaccines as the first dose in this age group unless the parent or caregiver expresses preference for the MMRV combination. For children receiving the first dose at ≥48 months or their second dose at any age, use of MMRV is preferred.

Pregnancy Risk Factor C

Pregnancy Considerations Animal reproduction studies have not been conducted. Do not administer to pregnant females and pregnancy should be avoided for 3 months (per manufacturer labeling) following vaccination. The ACIP recommends that pregnancy should be avoided for 1 month following vaccination with any of the individual components of this vaccine. Refer to individual monographs. A pregnancy registry has been established for pregnant women exposed to varicella virus vaccine (800-986-8999).

Lactation

Measles, mumps, varicella: Excretion in breast milk unknown/use caution

Rubella: Enters breast milk/use caution

Breast-Feeding Considerations
Following vaccination of the mother, rubella virus may be transmitted to the nursing infant via breast milk.

Contraindications Hypersensitivity to any component of the vaccine including gelatin; known anaphylactic reaction to neomycin or eggs; individuals with blood dyscrasias, leukemia, lymphomas, or other malignant neoplasms affecting the bone marrow or lymphatic systems; concurrent immunosuppressive therapy; primary and acquired immunodeficiency states including HIV or a family history of congenital or hereditary immunodeficiency; cellular immune deficiencies; hypogammaglobulinemic and dysgammaglobulinemic states; active untreated tuberculosis; current febrile illness (>38.5°C); pregnancy

Warnings Individuals of childbearing age should avoid pregnancy for at least 1 month following vaccination (see ACIP, 2001); manufacturer recommendation is 3 months; individuals who are pregnant when vaccinated or who become pregnant within 28 days of vaccination should be counseled on the theoretical risks to the fetus. Immediate treatment for anaphylactic/anaphylactoid reaction should be available during vaccine use. Use extreme caution in patients with immediate-type hypersensitivity reactions to eggs. Varicella virus transmission may occur; vaccinated individuals should not have close association with susceptible high risk individuals (newborns, pregnant women, immunocompromised persons) for 6 weeks following vaccination. While safety and efficacy of this combination vaccine has not been established in patients with HIV infection, MMR and varicella individual vaccines have been recommended in children with HIV infection who are asymptomatic and not immunosuppressed (CDC immunologic category 1). Avoid use of salicylates for 6 weeks following vaccination; varicella may increase the risk of Reye's syndrome.

Precautions Use caution with history of cerebral injury, seizures, or other conditions where stress due to fever should be avoided. Children 12-23 months of age have been reported to have a twofold higher risk of developing febrile seizures with the use of the combination product MMRV compared to administration of MMR and varicella separately. Because it is uncommon for a child to have their first febrile seizure after 4 years of age, the ACIP recommends the use of the combination MMRV vaccine for children receiving their first dose at ≥48 months or their second dose at any age. The ACIP recommends that children with a personal or family history of seizures be vaccinated with separate MMR and varicella vaccines, as opposed to the MMRV combination vaccine. Routine prophylactic administration of acetaminophen to prevent fever due to vaccines has been shown to decrease the immune response of some vaccines; the clinical significance of this reduction in immune response has not been established (see Prymula, 2009).

Use caution in patients with thrombocytopenia and in patients who develop thrombocytopenia after first dose; thrombocytopenia may worsen. Defer vaccination at least 3 months after receiving blood and plasma transfusions or immune globulin (see Appendix Immunization Guidelines "Suggested Intervals Between Administration of Antibody-Containing Products for Different Indications and Measles-Containing Vaccine and Varicella-Containing Vaccine").

Adverse Reactions All serious adverse reactions must be reported to the U.S. Department of Health and Human Services (DHHS) Vaccine Adverse Event Reporting System (VAERS) 1-800-822-7967.

With the exception of fever and measles-like rash, the incidence of adverse events was similar to that reported in patients receiving M-M-R® II and Varivax®. Also refer to M-M-R® II and Varivax® monographs for additional adverse reactions reported with those agents. Local injection site reactions appear to be slightly less than reported with individual vaccine formulations.

Central nervous system: Febrile seizures, fever ≥38.9°C (≥102°F) (20%), irritability

Dermatologic: Measles-like rash, rash, varicella-like rash, viral exanthema

Gastrointestinal: Diarrhea

Local: Bruising, erythema (11% to 24%); injection site reaction including pain, pruritus, soreness (21% to 41%), tenderness; swelling (8% to 16%)

Respiratory: Rhinorrhea, upper respiratory tract infection

Miscellaneous: Hypersensitivity reactions (see Warnings)

<1%, postmarketing, and/or case reports: Anorexia, cough, crying, dermatitis, headache, injection site hemorrhage, injection site rash, insomnia, malaise, miliaria ruba, nasal congestion, otitis, otitis media, pharyngitis, respiratory congestion, rhinorrhea, rubella-like rash, sleep disorder, somnolence, viral infection, vomiting

Drug Interactions

Avoid Concomitant Use

Avoid concomitant use of Measles, Mumps, Rubella, and Varicella Virus Vaccine with any of the following: Immunosuppressants

Increased Effect/Toxicity

The levels/effects of Measles, Mumps, Rubella, and Varicella Virus Vaccine may be increased by: 5-ASA Derivatives; Immunosuppressants; Salicylates

Decreased Effect

Measles, Mumps, Rubella, and Varicella Virus Vaccine may decrease the levels/effects of: Tuberculin Tests

The levels/effects of Measles, Mumps, Rubella, and Varicella Virus Vaccine may be decreased by: Immune Globulins; Immunosuppressants

Stability Vaccine: Stable in a freezer for up to 18 months at temperatures at or below -15°C (-5°F). During shipment, powder should be stored at or below -20°C (-4°F). May store under refrigeration at 2°C to 8°C (36°F to 46°F) for up to 72 hours prior to reconstitution. Protect from light; use within 30 minutes following reconstitution.

Diluent: Store at under refrigeration at 2°C to 8°C (36°F to 46°F) or at room temperature of 20°C to 25°C (68°F to 77°F).

Mechanism of Action A live, attenuated virus; offers active immunity to disease caused by the measles, mumps, rubella, and varicella-zoster virus.

Usual Dosage SubQ: Children 12 months to 12 years: One dose (0.5 mL). The first dose is usually administered at 12-15 months of age. If a second dose is needed, ProQuad® can be used and is usually administered at 4-6 years of age; second dose may be administered before age 4 if needed, as long as ≥3 months have elapsed since the first dose

ACIP recommendations: For children receiving their first dose at 12-47 months of age, either the MMRV combination vaccine or separate MMR and varicella vaccines can be used; however, the ACIP prefers administration of separate MMR and varicella vaccines as the first dose in this age group unless the parent or caregiver expresses preference for the MMRV combination. For children receiving the first dose at ≥48 months or their second dose at any age, use of MMRV is preferred. The ACIP recommends that children with a personal or family history of seizures be vaccinated with separate MMR and varicella vaccines, as opposed to the MMRV combination vaccine.

Allow at least 1 month between administering a dose of a measles-containing vaccine (eg, M-M-R® II) and ProQuad®.

Allow at least 3 months between administering a varicella-containing vaccine (eg, Varivax®) and ProQuad®.

Administration Parenteral: Use entire contents of provided diluent to reconstitute vaccine. Gently agitate to mix thoroughly. Discard if powder does not dissolve. Use as soon as possible following reconstitution; administer by SubQ injection into the anterolateral aspect of the thigh or deltoid region of arm; **not for I.V. administration**

Monitoring Parameters Monitor for syncope for ≥15 minutes following vaccination.

Test Interactions Temporary suppression of TB skin test reactivity with onset approximately 3 days after administration.

Patient Information Soreness or swelling may occur at the site of injection; fever, mild rash, swelling in the glands of the cheeks or neck, and temporary pain or stiffness in the joints may occur. Some effects may not occur until 1-2 weeks after the injection. Notify your healthcare provider immediately if these effects continue or are severe, or for a high fever, seizures, or allergic reaction (respiratory difficulty, hives, weakness, dizziness, fast heartbeat) occurs. Not to be given during pregnancy; do not get pregnant for 28 days after getting the vaccine. Do not use aspirin or aspirin-containing products for 6 weeks following vaccination.

Nursing Implications Federal law requires that the date of administration, name of manufacturer, lot number, and administering person's name, title, and address be entered into patient's permanent medical record.

Additional Information In order to maximize vaccination rates, the ACIP recommends simultaneous administration of all age-appropriate vaccines (live or inactivated) for which a person is eligible at a single visit, unless contraindications exist. The use of combination vaccines is generally preferred over separate infections, taking into consideration provider assessment, patient preference, and potential adverse events.

For additional information, please refer to the following website: http://www.cdc.gov/vaccines/vpd-vac/.

Dosage Forms Excipient information presented when available (limited, particularly for generics); consult specific product labeling.

Injection, powder for reconstitution [preservative free]:

ProQuad®: Measles virus ≥3.00 log_{10} TCID$_{50}$, mumps virus ≥4.3 log_{10} TCID$_{50}$, rubella virus ≥3.00 log_{10} TCID$_{50}$, and varicella virus ≥3.99 log_{10} PFU [contains albumin (human), bovine serum, chicken egg protein, gelatin, neomycin, sorbitol, and sucrose (≤21 mg/vial)]

References

ACIP Provisional Recommendations for Use of Measles, Mumps, Rubella and Varicella (MMRV) Vaccine October 20, 2009. Available at: http://www.cdc.gov/vaccines/recs/provisional/downloads/mmrv-oct2009-508.pdf.

Centers for Disease Control and Prevention (CDC), "General Recommendations on Immunization. Recommendations of the Advisory Committee on Immunization Practices (ACIP)," *MMWR Recomm Rep*, 2006, 55(RR-15):1-48. Available at: http://www.cdc.gov/mmwr/preview/mmwrhtml/rr5515a1.htm.

Centers for Disease Control and Prevention (CDC), "Recommended Adult Immunization Schedule – United States, 2010," *MMWR Morb Mortal Wkly Rep*, 2010, 57(59):Q1-4.

Centers for Disease Control and Prevention (CDC), "Recommended Immunization Schedules for Persons Aged 0 Through 18 Years – United States, 2010," *MMWR Morb Mortal Wkly Rep*, 2010, 58 (51 and 52):Q1-4.

Centers for Disease Control and Prevention (CDC), "Revised ACIP Recommendation for Avoiding Pregnancy After Receiving a Rubella-Containing Vaccine," *MMWR Morb Mortal Wkly Rep*, 2001, 50 (49):1117.

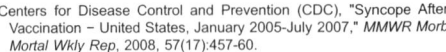

Centers for Disease Control and Prevention (CDC), "Syncope After Vaccination – United States, January 2005-July 2007," *MMWR Morb Mortal Wkly Rep*, 2008, 57(17):457-60.

Nolan T, Bernstein DI, Block SL, et al, "Safety and Immunogenicity of Concurrent Administration of Live Attenuated Influenza Vaccine With Measles-Mumps-Rubella and Varicella Vaccines to Infants 12 to 15 Months of Age," *Pediatrics*, 2008, 121(3):508-16.

Prymula R, Siegrist CA, Chlibek R, et al, "Effect of Prophylactic Paracetamol Administration at Time of Vaccination on Febrile Reactions and Antibody Responses in Children: Two Open-Label, Randomised Controlled Trials," *Lancet*, 2009, 374(9698):1339-50.

Watson JC, Hadler SC, Dykewicz CA, et al, "Measles, Mumps, and Rubella–Vaccine Use and Strategies for Elimination of Measles, Rubella, and Congenital Rubella Syndrome and Control of Mumps: Recommendations of the Advisory Committee on Immunization Practices (ACIP)," *MMWR Recomm Rep*, 1998, 47(RR-8):1-57.

Measles Virus Vaccine (Live)
(MEE zels VYE rus vak SEEN, live)

Medication Safety Issues
Sound-alike/look-alike issues:
Attenuvax® may be confused with Meruvax®

Related Information
Immunization Guidelines *on page 1636*

U.S. Brand Names Attenuvax® [DSC]

Therapeutic Category Vaccine, Live Virus

Generic Available No

Use Provide active immunity to measles virus (FDA approved in ages ≥12 months and adults); immunization is also recommended for infants 6-12 months of age in outbreak situations; revaccination is recommended for students entering colleges and other institutions of higher education, for healthcare workers at the time of employment, and for international travelers who visit endemic areas. Adults born before 1957 are generally considered to be immune.

MMR is the vaccine of choice if recipients are likely to be susceptible to rubella and/or mumps as well as to measles. Persons vaccinated between 1963 and 1967 with a killed measles vaccine, followed by live vaccine within 3 months, or with a vaccine of unknown type, should be revaccinated with live measles virus vaccine.

Pregnancy Risk Factor C

Pregnancy Considerations Reproduction studies have not been conducted. Vaccine should not be administered to pregnant women and the ACIP recommends that pregnancy be avoided for 1 month following vaccination. Infection with natural measles during pregnancy may increase the risk of spontaneous abortion, stillbirth, congenital defects and prematurity.

Lactation Excretion in breast milk unknown/use caution

Breast-Feeding Considerations Breast-feeding is not a contraindication to vaccination.

Contraindications Hypersensitivity to neomycin, gelatin, or any component of the formulation; acute respiratory infections, active, untreated tuberculosis, immunosuppressed patients; pregnancy; patients with blood dyscrasias, leukemia, lymphomas, or other malignant neoplasms affecting the bone marrow or lymphatic systems, primary and acquired immunodeficiency states, including HIV, cellular immune deficiencies, hypogammaglobulinemic and dysgammaglobulinemic states; known anaphylactoid reaction to eggs

Warnings Use in patients with existing thrombocytopenia may result in more severe reduction in platelets; avoid use in patients with previous history of postvaccination thrombocytopenia as rechallenge has resulted in recurrence of thrombocytopenia; avoid pregnancy for at least 1 month following vaccination (ACIP, 2001); manufacturer recommends waiting 3 months following vaccination; severe allergic reactions including anaphylaxis have been reported rarely; use with extreme caution in patients with immediate-type hypersensitivity reactions to eggs

Precautions Use with caution in patients with history of cerebral injury or seizures. Routine prophylactic administration of acetaminophen to prevent fever due to vaccines has been shown to decrease the immune response of some vaccines; the clinical significance of this reduction in immune response has not been established (see Prymula, 2009). Defer vaccination for at least 3 months after receiving blood and plasma transfusions or immune globulin (See Appendix Immunization Guidelines, "Suggested Intervals Between Administration of Antibody-Containing Products for Different Indications and Measles-Containing Vaccine and Varicella-Containing Vaccine")

Adverse Reactions All serious adverse reactions must be reported to the U.S. Department of Health and Human Services (DHHS) Vaccine Adverse Event Reporting System (VAERS) 1-800-822-7967.

Cardiovascular: Edema, vasculitis, angioneurotic edema

Central nervous system: Fever between 100°F and 103°F usually between 5th and 12th days postvaccination, fatigue, convulsions, encephalitis, confusion, severe headache, ataxia, syncope, dizziness, malaise, irritability, Guillain-Barré syndrome, subacute sclerosing panencephalitis

Dermatologic: Rash (rarely generalized), pruritus, reddening of skin (especially around ears and eyes), erythema multiforme, urticaria, thrombocytopenic purpura, Stevens-Johnson syndrome

Gastrointestinal: Diarrhea

Hematologic: Thrombocytopenia

Local: Burning or stinging, induration, vesiculation at injection site

Neuromuscular & skeletal: Palsies, stiff neck

Ocular: Diplopia, coryza, ocular palsies, retinitis, optic neuritis, papillitis, retrobulbar neuritis, conjunctivitis

Respiratory: Cough, rhinitis, bronchospasm

Miscellaneous: Anaphylaxis and anaphylactoid reactions, lymphadenopathy

Drug Interactions

Avoid Concomitant Use
Avoid concomitant use of Measles Virus Vaccine (Live) with any of the following: Immunosuppressants

Increased Effect/Toxicity
The levels/effects of Measles Virus Vaccine (Live) may be increased by: Immunosuppressants

Decreased Effect
Measles Virus Vaccine (Live) may decrease the levels/ effects of: Tuberculin Tests

The levels/effects of Measles Virus Vaccine (Live) may be decreased by: Immune Globulins; Immunosuppressants

Stability Refrigerate at 2°C to 8°C (36°F to 46°F); discard if left at room temperature for over 8 hours; protect from light

Mechanism of Action Promotes active immunity to measles virus by inducing specific measles IgG and IgM antibodies.

Usual Dosage Children ≥15 months and Adults: SubQ: 0.5 mL

Administration Reconstitute with provided diluent only; agitate to mix thoroughly until completely dissolved; administer by SubQ injection into the anterolateral aspect of the thigh or arm; **not for I.V. administration**

Monitoring Parameters Monitor for syncope for ≥15 minutes following vaccination.

Test Interactions May temporarily depress tuberculin skin test sensitivity

Patient Information Parents should monitor children closely for fever for 5-11 days after vaccination; females should not become pregnant for at least 1 month after vaccination

Nursing Implications Federal law requires that the date of administration, the vaccine manufacturer, lot number of vaccine, and the administering person's name, title, and address be entered into the patient's permanent medical record

Additional Information Contains 25 mcg neomycin per dose. Measles vaccine given immediately after exposure to natural measles may provide some protection if the vaccine is administered within 72 hours of exposure; vaccination even a few days prior to natural exposure may provide significant protection; DTP, IPV, Hib, and hepatitis B vaccines may be given concurrently.

In order to maximize vaccination rates, the ACIP recommends simultaneous administration of all age-appropriate vaccines (live or inactivated) for which a person is eligible at a single visit, unless contraindications exist. The use of combination vaccines is generally preferred over separate infections, taking into consideration provider assessment, patient preference, and potential adverse events.

For additional information, please refer to the following website: http://www.cdc.gov/vaccines/vpd-vac/.

Dosage Forms Excipient information presented when available (limited, particularly for generics); consult specific product labeling. [DSC] = Discontinued product

Injection, powder for reconstitution [preservative free]:

Attenuvax®: ≥1000 $TCID_{50}$ [contains albumin (human), bovine serum, chicken egg protein, gelatin, neomycin, sorbitol, and sucrose (1.9 mg/vial)] [DSC]

References

Centers for Disease Control and Prevention (CDC), "General Recommendations on Immunization. Recommendations of the Advisory Committee on Immunization Practices (ACIP)," *MMWR Recomm Rep*, 2006, 55(RR-15):1-48. Available at: http://www.cdc.gov/mmwr/preview/mmwrhtml/rr5515a1.htm.

Centers for Disease Control and Prevention (CDC), "Recommended Adult Immunization Schedule – United States, 2009," *MMWR Morb Mortal Wkly Rep*, 2009, 57(53):Q1-4.

Centers for Disease Control and Prevention (CDC), "Recommended Immunization Schedules for Persons Aged 0 Through 18 Years – United States, 2009," *MMWR Morb Mortal Wkly Rep*, 2009, 57 (51 and 52):Q1-4.

Centers for Disease Control and Prevention (CDC), "Revised ACIP Recommendation for Avoiding Pregnancy After Receiving a Rubella-Containing Vaccine," *MMWR Morb Mortal Wkly Rep*, 2001, 50 (49):1117.

Centers for Disease Control and Prevention (CDC), "Syncope After Vaccination – United States, January 2005-July 2007," *MMWR Morb Mortal Wkly Rep*, 2008, 57(17):457-60.

Gardner P and Schaffner W, "Immunization of Adults," *N Engl J Med*, 1993, 328(17):1252-8.

Prymula R, Siegrist CA, Chlibek R, et al, "Effect of Prophylactic Paracetamol Administration at Time of Vaccination on Febrile Reactions and Antibody Responses in Children: Two Open-Label, Randomised Controlled Trials," *Lancet*, 2009, 374(9698):1339-50.

Watson JC, Hadler SC, Dykewicz CA, et al, "Measles, Mumps, and Rubella–Vaccine Use and Strategies for Elimination of Measles, Rubella, and Congenital Rubella Syndrome and Control of Mumps: Recommendations of the Advisory Committee on Immunization Practices (ACIP)," *MMWR Recomm Rep*, 1998, 47(RR-8):1-57.

◆ **Mebaral®** *see* Mephobarbital *on page 882*

Mebendazole (me BEN da zole)

Medication Safety Issues
Sound-alike/look-alike issues:
Mebendazole may be confused with metroNIDAZOLE

Canadian Brand Names Vermox®

Therapeutic Category Anthelmintic

Generic Available Yes

Use Treatment of enterobiasis (pinworm infection), trichuriasis (whipworm infection), ascariasis (roundworm infection), and hookworm infections caused by *Necator americanus* or *Ancylostoma duodenale*; drug of choice in the treatment of capillariasis

Pregnancy Risk Factor C

Lactation Excretion in breast milk unknown/use caution

Breast-Feeding Considerations Since only 2% to 10% of mebendazole is absorbed, it is unlikely that it is excreted in breast milk in significant quantities.

Contraindications Hypersensitivity to mebendazole or any component

Warnings Pregnancy and children <2 years of age are relative contraindications since safety has not been established

Adverse Reactions

Central nervous system: Dizziness, fever, headache

Dermatologic: Rash, pruritus, alopecia

Gastrointestinal: Diarrhea, abdominal pain, nausea, vomiting

Hematologic: Neutropenia, anemia, leukopenia

Hepatic: Transient abnormalities in liver function tests

Otic: Tinnitus

Renal: Hematuria

Drug Interactions

Avoid Concomitant Use There are no known interactions where it is recommended to avoid concomitant use.

Increased Effect/Toxicity
Mebendazole may increase the levels/effects of: MetroNIDAZOLE; MetroNIDAZOLE (Systemic); MetroNIDAZOLE (Topical)

Decreased Effect
The levels/effects of Mebendazole may be decreased by: Aminoquinolines (Antimalarial); CarBAMazepine; Phenytoin

Food Interactions Food increases mebendazole absorption

Mechanism of Action Selectively and irreversibly blocks uptake of glucose and other nutrients in susceptible intestine-dwelling helminths

Pharmacokinetics (Adult data unless noted)

Absorption: Oral: 2% to 10%

Distribution: To liver, fat, muscle, plasma, and hepatic cysts

Protein binding: 95%

Metabolism: Extensive in the liver

Half-life: 2.8-9 hours

Time to peak serum concentration: Variable (0.5-7 hours)

Elimination: Primarily in feces as inactive metabolites with 5% to 10% eliminated in urine

Dialysis: Not dialyzable

Usual Dosage Children and Adults: Oral:

Pinworms: Single chewable tablet (100 mg); may need to repeat after 2 weeks

Whipworms, roundworms, hookworms: 100 mg twice daily, morning and evening on 3 consecutive days; if patient is not cured within 3-4 weeks, a second course of treatment may be administered

Capillariasis: 200 mg twice daily for 20 days

Administration Oral: Administer with food; tablet can be crushed and mixed with food, swallowed whole, or chewed

Monitoring Parameters For treatment of trichuriasis, ascariasis, hookworm, or mixed infections, check for helminth ova in the feces within 3-4 weeks following the initial therapy

Dosage Forms Excipient information presented when available (limited, particularly for generics); consult specific product labeling.

Tablet, chewable: 100 mg

References

Hotez PJ, "Hookworm Disease in Children," *Pediatr Infect Dis J*, 1989, 8(8):516-20.

Mechlorethamine (me klor ETH a meen)

Medication Safety Issues
High alert medication: The Institute for Safe Medication Practices (ISMP) includes this medication among its list of drugs which have a heightened risk of causing significant patient harm when used in error.

Related Information
Compatibility of Chemotherapy and Related Supportive Care Medications *on page 1580*
Emetogenic Potential of Antineoplastic Agents *on page 1579*
Extravasation Treatment *on page 1522*

U.S. Brand Names Mustargen®
Canadian Brand Names Mustargen®
Therapeutic Category Antineoplastic Agent, Alkylating Agent (Nitrogen Mustard)
Generic Available No
Use Combination therapy of Hodgkin's disease, brain tumors, non-Hodgkin's lymphoma, and malignant lymphomas; palliative treatment of lung, breast, and ovarian carcinoma; sclerosing agent in intracavitary therapy of pleural, pericardial, and other malignant effusions

Pregnancy Risk Factor D
Pregnancy Considerations Animal studies have demonstrated teratogenic effects. There are no adequate and well-controlled studies in pregnant women. Women of childbearing potential are advised not to become pregnant. Use only when potential benefit justifies potential risk to the fetus. **[U.S. Boxed Warning]: Avoid exposure during pregnancy.**

Lactation Excretion in breast milk unknown/not recommended
Breast-Feeding Considerations It is not known if mechlorethamine is excreted in human breast milk. Due to the potential for serious adverse reactions in the nursing infant, breast-feeding is not recommended.

Contraindications Hypersensitivity to mechlorethamine or any component; pre-existing profound myelosuppression; pregnancy

Warnings Hazardous agent; use appropriate precautions for handling and disposal; disposal of mechlorethamine powder and solution must be followed **[U.S. Boxed Warning]**; avoid inhalation of dust or vapors and contact with skin or mucous membranes. Avoid contact during pregnancy **[U.S. Boxed Warning]**; mechlorethamine is potentially carcinogenic, teratogenic, and mutagenic. It may cause permanent sterility and birth defects. Mechlorethamine is a potent vesicant **[U.S. Boxed Warning]**; extravasation of the drug into subcutaneous tissues results in painful inflammation, erythema, and induration; severe tissue damage (leading to ulceration and necrosis) and pain may occur; promptly infiltrate the area with sterile isotonic sodium thiosulfate ($^1/_6$ molar) and apply a cold compress for 6-12 hours. See Extravasation Treatment on page 1522.

Precautions Use with caution in patients with myelosuppression; patients with lymphoma should receive adequate hydration, alkalinization of the urine and/or prophylactic allopurinol to prevent complications such as uric acid nephropathy and hyperuricemia

Adverse Reactions
Cardiovascular: Thrombosis
Central nervous system: Vertigo, fever, headache, drowsiness, lethargy, encephalopathy (high dose)
Dermatologic: Rash, alopecia
Endocrine & metabolic: Amenorrhea, impaired spermatogenesis, hyperuricemia
Gastrointestinal: Nausea, vomiting, anorexia, diarrhea, metallic taste, mucositis
Hematologic: Myelosuppression (leukopenia, thrombocytopenia), hemolytic anemia
Local: Thrombophlebitis, tissue necrosis upon extravasation
Neuromuscular & skeletal: Weakness
Ocular: Lacrimation
Otic: Tinnitus, deafness
Miscellaneous: Hypersensitivity reactions, diaphoresis, anaphylaxis

Drug Interactions
Avoid Concomitant Use
Avoid concomitant use of Mechlorethamine with any of the following: BCG; Natalizumab; Pimecrolimus; Tacrolimus (Topical); Vaccines (Live)

Increased Effect/Toxicity
Mechlorethamine may increase the levels/effects of: Leflunomide; Natalizumab; Vaccines (Live)

The levels/effects of Mechlorethamine may be increased by: Denosumab; Pimecrolimus; Tacrolimus (Topical); Trastuzumab

Decreased Effect
Mechlorethamine may decrease the levels/effects of: BCG; Sipuleucel-T; Vaccines (Inactivated); Vaccines (Live)

The levels/effects of Mechlorethamine may be decreased by: Echinacea

Stability Highly unstable in neutral or alkaline solutions; use immediately after reconstitution; discard any unused drug after 60 minutes (although manufacturer reports only 15 minutes of stability after reconstitution, other studies indicate it is stable longer)

Mechanism of Action Alkylating agent that inhibits DNA and RNA synthesis via formation of carbonium ions which can attach to nucleic acids at the N^7 position of guanine; cross-links strands of DNA causing miscoding, breakage, and failure of replication

Pharmacokinetics (Adult data unless noted)
Absorption: Incomplete after intracavitary administration secondary to rapid deactivation by body fluids
Distribution: Following I.V. administration, drug undergoes rapid hydrolysis to a highly reactive alkylating intermediate; unchanged drug is undetectable in the blood within a few minutes
Half-life: <1 minute
Elimination: <0.01% of unchanged drug is recovered in urine

Usual Dosage Refer to individual protocols
Children:
Lymphoma: MOPP regimen: Mustargen® (mechlorethamine), Oncovin® (vincristine), procarbazine, and prednisone: I.V.: 6 mg/m^2 on days 1 and 8 of a 28-day cycle
Brain tumors: MOPP regimen: I.V.: 3 mg/m^2 on days 1 and 8 of a 28-day cycle
Adults:
I.V.: 0.4 mg/kg or 12-16 mg/m^2 as a single monthly dose or divided into 0.1 mg/kg/day once daily for 4 days, repeated at 4- to 6-week intervals
Intracavitary: 10-30 mg or 0.2-0.4 mg/kg

Administration
Intracavitary: Dilute dose in up to 100 mL NS; paracentesis is performed to remove most of the fluid from the cavity prior to administration; inject drug slowly with frequent aspiration to ensure that a free flow of fluid is present; change patient's position every 5-10 minutes for 1 hour following injection to distribute drug uniformly throughout the cavity
Parenteral: **DO NOT ADMINISTER I.M. or SubQ** Administer I.V. push through a side port of an established I.V. line over 1-5 minutes at a concentration not to exceed 1 mg/mL

Monitoring Parameters CBC with differential and platelet count, hemoglobin; serum uric acid in lymphoma patients

Patient Information Report to physician any pain or irritation at the site of injection, fever, sore throat, bruising, bleeding, shortness of breath, itching, or wheezing

Nursing Implications Avoid extravasation, inhalation of vapors, or contact with skin, mucous membranes, and eyes since mechlorethamine is a potent vesicant. If accidental eye contact occurs, copious irrigation for at least 15 minutes with NS or a balanced salt ophthalmic irrigating solution should be instituted immediately followed by prompt ophthalmologic consultation. If accidental skin contact occurs, irrigate the affected area with copious amounts of water for at least 15 minutes while removing contaminated clothing, followed by application of a 2% sodium thiosulfate solution; contaminated clothing should be destroyed. Medical attention should be sought immediately. For mechlorethamine extravasations, infiltrate area with a $1/6$ molar sodium thiosulfate solution and apply cold compresses for 6-12 hours; $1/6$ molar sodium thiosulfate solution can be prepared by diluting 4 mL of 10% sodium thiosulfate injection with 6 mL of SWI; Dorr recommends to inject 2 mL of the $1/6$ molar solution into site for each milligram of mechlorethamine extravasated

Additional Information Myelosuppressive effects:

WBC: Severe
Platelets: Severe
Onset (days): 4-7
Nadir (days): 14
Recovery (days): 21

Dosage Forms Excipient information presented when available (limited, particularly for generics); consult specific product labeling.

Injection, powder for reconstitution, as hydrochloride:
Mustargen®: 10 mg

References

Ater JL, van Eys J, Woo SY, et al, "MOPP Chemotherapy Without Irradiation as Primary Postsurgical Therapy for Brain Tumors in Infants and Young Children," *J Neurooncol*, 1997, 32(3):243-52.

Berg SL, Grisell DL, DeLaney TF, et al, "Principles of Treatment of Pediatric Solid Tumors," *Pediatr Clin North Am*, 1991, 38(2):249-67.

Dorr RT, Soble M, and Alberts DS, "Efficacy of Sodium Thiosulfate as a Local Antidote to Mechlorethamine Skin Toxicity in the Mouse," *Cancer Chemother Pharmacol*, 1988, 22(4):299-302.

Krischer JP, Ragab AH, Kun L, et al, "Nitrogen Mustard, Vincristine, Procarbazine, and Prednisone as Adjuvant Chemotherapy in the Treatment of Medulloblastoma. A Pediatric Oncology Group Study," *J Neurosurg*, 1991, 74(6):905-9.

♦ **Mechlorethamine Hydrochloride** *see* Mechlorethamine *on page 868*

Meclizine (MEK li zeen)

Medication Safety Issues

Sound-alike/look-alike issues:
Antivert® may be confused with Anzemet®, Axert®

U.S. Brand Names Antivert®; Bonine® [OTC]; Dramamine® Less Drowsy Formula [OTC]; Medi-Meclizine [OTC]; Trav-L-Tabs® [OTC]

Canadian Brand Names Bonamine™; Bonine®

Therapeutic Category Antiemetic; Antihistamine

Generic Available Yes

Use Prevention and treatment of motion sickness; management of vertigo

Pregnancy Risk Factor B

Pregnancy Considerations No data available on crossing the placenta. Probably no effect on the fetus (insufficient data). Available evidence suggests safe use during pregnancy.

Lactation Excretion in breast milk unknown/not recommended

Contraindications Hypersensitivity to meclizine or any component

Precautions Use with caution in patients with angle-closure glaucoma or obstructive diseases of the GI or GU tract

Adverse Reactions

Cardiovascular: Hypotension, palpitations, tachycardia

Central nervous system: Drowsiness, fatigue, auditory and visual hallucinations, restlessness, excitation, insomnia, nervousness

Dermatologic: Urticaria, rash

Endocrine & metabolic: Weight gain

Gastrointestinal: Xerostomia, anorexia, nausea, vomiting, diarrhea, constipation, appetite increase

Hepatic: Cholestatic jaundice, hepatitis

Neuromuscular & skeletal: Myalgia, tremor, paresthesia

Ocular: Blurred vision, diplopia

Otic: Tinnitus

Respiratory: Bronchospasm, epistaxis

Drug Interactions

Avoid Concomitant Use There are no known interactions where it is recommended to avoid concomitant use.

Increased Effect/Toxicity

Meclizine may increase the levels/effects of: Alcohol (Ethyl); Anticholinergics; CNS Depressants

The levels/effects of Meclizine may be increased by: Pramlintide

Decreased Effect

Meclizine may decrease the levels/effects of: Acetylcholinesterase Inhibitors (Central); Betahistine

The levels/effects of Meclizine may be decreased by: Acetylcholinesterase Inhibitors (Central); Amphetamines

Mechanism of Action Has central anticholinergic action and CNS depressant activity; decreases excitability of the middle ear labyrinth and blocks conduction in the middle ear vestibular-cerebellar pathways

Pharmacodynamics

Onset of action: Oral: 30-60 minutes

Duration: 12-24 hours

Pharmacokinetics (Adult data unless noted)

Metabolism: In the liver

Half-life: 6 hours

Elimination: As metabolites in urine and as unchanged drug in feces

Usual Dosage Children >12 years and Adults: Oral:

Motion sickness: 25-50 mg 1 hour before travel, repeat dose every 24 hours if needed

Vertigo: 25-100 mg/day in divided doses

Administration Oral: Administer with food to decrease GI distress

Patient Information May cause drowsiness and impair ability to perform activities requiring mental alertness or physical coordination; may cause dry mouth; avoid alcohol

Dosage Forms Excipient information presented when available (limited, particularly for generics); consult specific product labeling.

Caplet, as hydrochloride: 12.5 mg

Tablet, as hydrochloride: 12.5 mg, 25 mg
Antivert®: 12.5 mg, 25 mg, 50 mg
Dramamine® Less Drowsy Formula: 25 mg
Medi-Meclizine: 25 mg
Trav-L-Tabs®: 25 mg

Tablet, chewable, as hydrochloride: 25 mg
Bonine®: 25 mg [raspberry flavor]

♦ **Meclizine Hydrochloride** *see* Meclizine *on page 869*

♦ **Meclozine Hydrochloride** *see* Meclizine *on page 869*

♦ **Med-Atenolol (Can)** *see* Atenolol *on page 147*

♦ **Med-Baclofen (Can)** *see* Baclofen *on page 171*

♦ **Med-Diltiazem (Can)** *see* Diltiazem *on page 443*

♦ **Med-Glybe (Can)** *see* GlyBURIDE *on page 648*

◆ **Medicinal Carbon** see Charcoal, Activated *on page 284*

◆ **Medicinal Charcoal** see Charcoal, Activated *on page 284*

◆ **Medicone® Hemorrhoidal [OTC]** see Benzocaine *on page 182*

◆ **Medicone® Suppositories [OTC]** see Phenylephrine *on page 1102*

◆ **Medi-First™ Sinus Decongestant [OTC]** see Phenylephrine *on page 1102*

◆ **Medi-Meclizine [OTC]** see Meclizine *on page 869*

◆ **Medi-Phenyl [OTC]** see Phenylephrine *on page 1102*

◆ **Mediproxen [OTC]** see Naproxen *on page 967*

Medium Chain Triglycerides
(mee DEE um chane trye GLIS er ides)

U.S. Brand Names MCT Oil® [OTC]
Canadian Brand Names MCT Oil®
Therapeutic Category Caloric Agent; Nutritional Supplement
Generic Available No
Use Nutritional supplement for those who cannot digest long chain fats; malabsorption associated with disorders such as pancreatic insufficiency, bile salt deficiency, and bacterial overgrowth of the small bowel; induce ketosis as a prevention for seizures (akinetic, clonic, and petit mal)
Contraindications Hypersensitivity to medium chain triglycerides or any component; should not be used in patients with hepatic encephalopathy due to earlier observations which report that short chain fatty acids may have a narcotic effect on the CNS and inhibit oxidative phosphorylation
Warnings Patients with cirrhosis demonstrate higher concentrations of medium chain fatty acids in the serum and CSF than normal individuals; impaired hepatic clearance of medium chain fatty acids due to parenchymal dysfunction of medium chain fatty acid oxidation, portal systemic shunt, and impaired protein binding of fatty acid enhance the passive diffusion of medium chain fatty acids into the CSF
Precautions Use with caution in patients with hepatic cirrhosis and complications such as portacaval shunts or encephalopathy
Adverse Reactions
Central nervous system: Sedation, narcosis, coma (cirrhotics)
Endocrine & metabolic: Ketosis
Gastrointestinal: Nausea, vomiting, abdominal pain, diarrhea, borborygmi
Mechanism of Action A semisynthetic class of lipids; medium chain triglycerides (MCT) are composed of fatty acids with chain length varying from 6-12 carbon atoms; preparations contain approximately 75% octanoic (caprylic), 20% to 25% decanoic (capric), 1% hexanoic (caproic), and 1% dodecanoic (lauric) acids

MCT are hydrolyzed in the stomach and in the small intestine by pancreatic lipase to form medium chain fatty acids; the medium chain fatty acids are incorporated into bile salts for more rapid solubilization and entrance into the mucosal cell and into the portal venous blood; MCT can also be absorbed unchanged as a triglycerides into the mucosal cell; medium chain fatty acids presented to the liver are minimally converted to hepatic lipid and are rapidly oxidized to carbon dioxide, ketones, and acetate; the medium chain fatty acids are also esterified to long chain triglycerides
Pharmacodynamics Onset of action: Octanoic acid appeared in each subject by 30 minutes following ingestion; effect on seizures in children: Within 6 weeks

Pharmacokinetics (Adult data unless noted)
Absorption: Up to 30% of dose can be absorbed unchanged as a triglyceride in the mucosal cell
Metabolism: Almost entirely oxidized by the liver to acetyl CoA fragments and to carbon dioxide; little deposited in adipose tissue or elsewhere
Elimination: As much as 20% of oral dose of MCT, recovered in expired CO_2 in 50 minutes; <10% elimination of medium chain fatty acids in feces
Usual Dosage Oral:
Infants: Nutritional supplement: Initial: 0.5 mL every other feeding, then advance to every feeding, then increase in increments of 0.25-0.5 mL/feeding at intervals of 2-3 days as tolerated
Children: Seizures: About 40 mL with each meal or 50% to 70% (800-1120 kcal) of total calories (1600 kcal) as the oil will induce the ketosis necessary for seizure control
Children and Adults: Cystic fibrosis: 3 tablespoons/day in divided doses
Adults: Malabsorption syndromes: 15 mL 3-4 times/day
Administration Oral:
Dilute with at least an equal volume of water or mix with some other vehicle such as fruit juice (should not be cold; flavoring may be added); mixture should be sipped slowly; administer no more than 15-20 mL at any one time (up to 100 mL may be administered in divided doses in a 24-hour period)
Possible GI side effects from medication can be prevented if therapy is initiated with small supplements at meals and gradually increased according to patient's tolerance
Monitoring Parameters
Nutritional supplement and malabsorption: Weight gain, height, stool output
Seizure treatment: Reduction in seizures, urine ketones
Patient Information GI symptoms may occur during the first few days of administration and then disappear; it is important to continue therapy with at least the smallest dose
Additional Information Does not provide any essential fatty acids; contains only saturated fats; supplementation with safflower, corn oil, or other polyunsaturated vegetable oil must be given to provide the patient with the essential fatty acids; caloric content: 8.3 calories/g; 115 calories/15 mL
Dosage Forms Excipient information presented when available (limited, particularly for generics); consult specific product labeling.
Oil: 14 g/15 mL (960 mL) [115 calories/15 mL; derived from coconut oil]

◆ **Med-Metformin (Can)** see MetFORMIN *on page 891*

◆ **Med-Ranitidine (Can)** see Ranitidine *on page 1200*

◆ **Medrol®** see MethylPREDNISolone *on page 912*

◆ **Medrol Dose Pack** see MethylPREDNISolone *on page 912*

MedroxyPROGESTERone
(me DROKS ee proe JES te rone)

Medication Safety Issues
Sound-alike/look-alike issues:
Depo-Provera® may be confused with depo-subQ provera 104™
depo-subQ provera 104™ may be confused with Depo-Provera®
MedroxyPROGESTERone may be confused with hydroxyprogesterone, methylPREDNISolone, methylTESTOSTERone
Provera® may be confused with Covera®, Femara®, Parlodel®, Premarin®, Proscar®, Prozac®

The injection dosage form is available in different formulations. Carefully review prescriptions to assure the correct formulation and route of administration.

U.S. Brand Names Depo-Provera®; Depo-Provera® Contraceptive; depo-subQ provera 104™; Provera®

Canadian Brand Names Alti-MPA; Apo-Medroxy®; Depo-Prevera®; Depo-Provera®; Gen-Medroxy; Novo-Medrone; Provera-Pak; Provera®

Therapeutic Category Contraceptive, Progestin Only; Progestin

Generic Available Yes

Use Secondary amenorrhea or abnormal uterine bleeding due to hormonal imbalance; prevention of pregnancy; reduction of endometrial hyperplasia in nonhysterectomized postmenopausal women receiving conjugated estrogens; endometrial or renal carcinoma; management of endometriosis-associated pain (FDA approved in adults)

Pregnancy Risk Factor X

Pregnancy Considerations There is an increased risk of minor birth defects in children whose mothers take progesterones during the first 4 months of pregnancy. Hypospadias has been reported in male and mild masculinization of the external genitalia has been reported in female babies exposed during the first trimester. High doses are used to impair fertility. Low birth weight has been reported in neonates from unexpected pregnancies which occurred 1-2 months following injection of medroxyprogesterone (MPA) contraceptive. Ectopic pregnancies have been reported with use of the MPA contraceptive injection. When therapy is discontinued, fertility returns sooner in women of lower body weight. Median time to conception/return to ovulation following discontinuation of MPA contraceptive injection is 10 months following the last injection.

Lactation Enters breast milk/compatible

Breast-Feeding Considerations Composition, quality, and quantity of breast milk are not affected; adverse developmental and behavioral effects have not been noted following exposure of infant to MPA while breast-feeding.

Contraindications Hypersensitivity to medroxyprogesterone or any component; thrombophlebitis; cerebral vascular disease, undiagnosed vaginal bleeding, liver dysfunction, thromboembolic disorders, breast cancer, pregnancy (known or suspected)

Warnings Discontinue if there is a sudden partial or complete loss of vision, proptosis, diplopia, migraine, if papilledema or retinal vascular lesions are present, or any other symptom of a thromboembolic event. Prolonged use of medroxyprogesterone as a contraceptive reduces estrogen levels and has been associated with increased bone mineral density (BMD) losses **[U.S. Boxed Warning]**. Use as a long-term contraceptive agent (≥2 years) should be reserved for situations when other contraceptives are not effective or contraindicated **[U.S. Boxed Warning]**. Monitor BMD if prolonged use is necessary.

Precautions Use with caution in patients with mental depression, diabetes, epilepsy, asthma, migraines, renal or cardiac dysfunction

Adverse Reactions

Cardiovascular: Edema, thromboembolic disorders

Central nervous system: Depression, dizziness, insomnia, nervousness

Dermatologic: Acne, alopecia, urticaria

Endocrine & metabolic: Amenorrhea, bone mineral density loss (contraceptive use), breakthrough bleeding, breast tenderness, ectopic pregnancy, galactorrhea, libido increased, menstrual irregularities, oligomenorrhea, weight gain or weight loss

Gastrointestinal: Anorexia, rectal bleeding

Hepatic: Cholestatic jaundice

Local: Pain at injection site

Neuromuscular & skeletal: Osteoporotic fractures (contraceptive use), paresthesia, weakness

Miscellaneous: Anaphylaxis

<1%, postmarketing, and/or case reports: Allergic reaction, anemia, angioedema, appetite changes, asthma, axillary swelling, blood dyscrasia, body odor, breast cancer, breast changes, cervical cancer, chest pain, chills, chloasma, convulsions, deep vein thrombosis, diaphoresis, drowsiness, dry skin, dysmenorrhea, dyspareunia, dyspnea, facial palsy, fever, galactorrhea, genitourinary infections, glucose tolerance decreased, hirsutism, hoarseness, jaundice, lack of return to fertility, lactation decreased, libido increased, melasma, nipple bleeding, osteoporosis, osteoporotic fractures, paralysis, paresthesia, pruritus, pulmonary embolus, rectal bleeding, scleroderma, sensation of pregnancy, somnolence, syncope, tachycardia, thirst, thrombophlebitis, uterine hyperplasia, vaginal cysts, varicose veins; residual lump, sterile abscess, or skin discoloration at the injection site

Drug Interactions

Metabolism/Transport Effects Substrate of CYP3A4 (major); **Induces** CYP3A4 (weak)

Avoid Concomitant Use

Avoid concomitant use of MedroxyPROGESTERone with any of the following: Griseofulvin

Increased Effect/Toxicity

MedroxyPROGESTERone may increase the levels/effects of: Benzodiazepines (metabolized by oxidation); Selegiline; Tranexamic Acid; Voriconazole

The levels/effects of MedroxyPROGESTERone may be increased by: Herbs (Progestogenic Properties); Voriconazole

Decreased Effect

MedroxyPROGESTERone may decrease the levels/effects of: Saxagliptin; Vitamin K Antagonists

The levels/effects of MedroxyPROGESTERone may be decreased by: Acitretin; Aminoglutethimide; Aprepitant; Artemether; Barbiturates; Bile Acid Sequestrants; Bosentan; CarBAMazepine; CYP3A4 Inducers (Strong); Deferasirox; Felbamate; Fosaprepitant; Griseofulvin; LamoTRIgine; Mycophenolate; OXcarbazepine; Phenytoin; Retinoic Acid Derivatives; Rifamycin Derivatives; St Johns Wort; Topiramate

Mechanism of Action Inhibits secretion of pituitary gonadotropins, which prevents follicular maturation and ovulation, transforms a proliferative endometrium into a secretory one

Pharmacodynamics Time to ovulation (after last injection): 10 months (range: 6-12 months)

Pharmacokinetics (Adult data unless noted)

Absorption: I.M.: Slow

Protein binding: 86% to 90%

Metabolism: In the liver

Bioavailability: 0.6% to 10%

Half-life: 30 days

Time to peak serum concentration: SubQ (depo-subQ provera 104™): 1 week

Elimination: Oral: In urine and feces

Usual Dosage

Adolescents and Adults:

Amenorrhea: Oral: 5-10 mg/day for 5-10 days or 2.5 mg/day

Abnormal uterine bleeding: Oral: 5-10 mg for 5-10 days starting on day 16 or day 21 of menstrual cycle

Contraception: **Note:** First dose to be given only during first 5 days of normal menstrual period; only within 5 days postpartum if not breast-feeding, or only at sixth postpartum week if exclusively breast-feeding. When switching from other contraceptive methods, depo-subQ provera 104™ should be administered within 7 days after the last day of using the last method (pill, ring, patch).

I.M. (Depo-Provera®): 150 mg every 3 months

SubQ (depo-subQ provera 104™): 104 mg every 3 months (every 12-14 weeks)

Endometriosis-associated pain: SubQ (depo-subQ provera 104™): 104 mg every 3 months; treatment longer than 2 years is not recommended due to impact of long-term use on bone mineral density

Adults: Accompanying cyclic estrogen therapy (postmenopausal): Oral: 5-10 mg for 12-14 consecutive days each month, starting on day 1 or day 16 of cycle; lower doses may be used if given with estrogen continuously throughout the cycle

Administration

Oral: Administer with food

Parenteral: I.M. injection, suspension only: In upper arm or buttock; SubQ (depo-subQ provera 104™ only): Into anterior thigh or abdomen; not for I.V. use; shake well before drawing into syringe

Monitoring Parameters BMD (see Warnings), menstrual bleeding patterns

Test Interactions Altered thyroid and liver function tests, prothrombin time, factors VII, VIII, IX, X, metyrapone test

Patient Information Notify physician if sudden loss of vision, severe headache, sharp chest pain, coughing up blood, weakness or numbness in an arm or leg, severe pain or swelling in calf, unusual heavy vaginal bleeding or severe pain or tenderness in lower abdominal area

Additional Information I.M. dosing is recommended only for contraceptive purposes or in the treatment of endometrial or renal carcinoma

Dosage Forms Excipient information presented when available (limited, particularly for generics); consult specific product labeling.

Injection, suspension, as acetate: 150 mg/mL (1 mL)
Depo-Provera®: 400 mg/mL (2.5 mL)
Depo-Provera® Contraceptive: 150 mg/mL (1 mL) [prefilled syringe or vial]
depo-subQ provera 104™: 104 mg/0.65 mL (0.65 mL) [prefilled syringe]
Tablet, as acetate: 2.5 mg, 5 mg, 10 mg
Provera®: 2.5 mg, 5 mg, 10 mg

♦ **Medroxyprogesterone Acetate** see MedroxyPROGESTERone on page 870

♦ **Med-Sotalol (Can)** see Sotalol on page 1284

♦ **Med-Verapamil (Can)** see Verapamil on page 1416

Mefloquine (ME floe kwin)

Related Information
Malaria on page 1652
U.S. Brand Names Lariam® [DSC]
Canadian Brand Names Apo-Mefloquine®; Lariam®
Therapeutic Category Antimalarial Agent
Generic Available Yes
Use Treatment of acute malarial infections and prevention of malaria due to Plasmodium vivax and Plasmodium flaciparum (including chloroquine-resistant strains) (FDA approved in ages ≥6 months and adults)
Medication Guide An FDA-approved patient medication guide, which is available with the product information and at http://www.fda.gov/downloads/Drugs/DrugSafety/ucm088616.pdf, must be dispensed with this medication for each new outpatient prescription and refill.

Pregnancy Risk Factor C
Pregnancy Considerations Mefloquine crosses the placenta and is teratogenic in animals. There are no adequate and well-controlled studies in pregnant women, however, clinical experience has not shown teratogenic or embryotoxic effects; use with caution during pregnancy if travel to endemic areas cannot be postponed. Non-pregnant women of childbearing potential are advised to use contraception and avoid pregnancy during malaria prophylaxis and for 3 months thereafter. In case of an unplanned pregnancy, treatment with mefloquine is not considered a reason for pregnancy termination. CDC treatment guidelines are available for the treatment of malaria during pregnancy (CDC, 2007).

Lactation Enters breast milk/not recommended

Breast-Feeding Considerations Excreted in small quantities; effect to nursing infant is unknown. Breast-feeding is not recommended during therapy and the long half-life of mefloquine should also be considered once therapy is complete.

Contraindications Hypersensitivity to mefloquine, related compounds such as quinine and quinidine, or any component; history of convulsions or psychiatric disorder (including active or recent history of depression, generalized anxiety disorder, psychosis, or schizophrenia)

Warnings Mefloquine may cause a range of psychiatric symptoms (anxiety, paranoia, depression, hallucinations and psychosis). Rare cases of suicidal ideation and suicide have been reported (no causal relationship established). The appearance of psychiatric symptoms such as acute anxiety, depression, restlessness, or confusion may be considered a prodrome to more serious events. When used as prophylaxis, substitute an alternative medication. Discontinue if unexplained neuropsychiatric disturbances occur. Dizziness, loss of balance, and other CNS disorders have been reported; due to long half-life, effects may persist long after mefloquine has been discontinued.

In cases of life-threatening, serious, or overwhelming malaria infections due to Plasmodium falciparum, patients should be treated with an intravenous malarial drug. Mefloquine may be given orally to complete the course.

Precautions Use with caution in patients with a previous history of depression (see Contraindications regarding psychiatric illness, including active/recent depression). Use with caution in patients with significant cardiac disease; EKG changes have been reported. If mefloquine is to be used for a prolonged period, periodic evaluations including liver function tests and ophthalmic examinations should be performed. Use caution in activities requiring mental alertness and fine motor coordination such as driving or operating machinery. Hypersensitivity reactions ranging from mild skin reactions to anaphylaxis have occurred.

Adverse Reactions
Cardiovascular: Extrasystoles, syncope
Central nervous system: Anxiety, chills, depression, dizziness, fatigue, fever, hallucinations, headache, mood changes, panic attacks, paranoia, seizure, suicidal ideation (rare)
Dermatologic: Rash
Gastrointestinal: Abdominal pain, appetite decreased, diarrhea, nausea, vomiting
Hematologic: Leukocytosis, leucopenia, thrombocytopenia
Neuromuscular & skeletal: Myalgia
Miscellaneous: Anaphylaxis
<1% and/or postmarketing: Agitation, aggression, alopecia, arthralgia, ataxia, AV block, bradycardia, cardiopulmonary arrest, chest pain, confusion, diaphoresis, dyspepsia, dyspnea, edema, emotional lability, encephalopathy, erythema multiforme, extrasystoles, flushing, hearing impairment, hypertension, hypotension, liver

function tests elevated, memory impairment, muscle cramps, palpitations, paresthesia, pruritus, somnolence, Stevens-Johnson syndrome, syncope, tachycardia, tinnitus, tremor, urticaria, vertigo, vestibular disorders, visual disturbances, weakness

Drug Interactions

Metabolism/Transport Effects Substrate of CYP3A4 (major); **Inhibits** CYP2D6 (weak), CYP3A4 (weak), P-glycoprotein

Avoid Concomitant Use

Avoid concomitant use of Mefloquine with any of the following: Aminoquinolines (Antimalarial); Artemether; Dabigatran Etexilate; Dronedarone; Halofantrine; Lumefantrine; Nilotinib; Pimozide; QuiNIDine; QuiNINE; Silodosin; Tetrabenazine; Thioridazine; Topotecan; Ziprasidone

Increased Effect/Toxicity

Mefloquine may increase the levels/effects of: Aminoquinolines (Antimalarial); Antipsychotic Agents (Phenothiazines); Colchicine; Dabigatran Etexilate; Dapsone; Dapsone (Systemic); Dapsone (Topical); Dronedarone; Halofantrine; Lumefantrine; P-Glycoprotein Substrates; Pimozide; QTc-Prolonging Agents; QuiNINE; Rivaroxaban; Silodosin; Tetrabenazine; Thioridazine; Topotecan; Typhoid Vaccine; Ziprasidone

The levels/effects of Mefloquine may be increased by: Alfuzosin; Aminoquinolines (Antimalarial); Artemether; Chloroquine; Ciprofloxacin; Ciprofloxacin (Systemic); CYP3A4 Inhibitors (Moderate); CYP3A4 Inhibitors (Strong); Dapsone; Dapsone (Systemic); Gadobutrol; Lumefantrine; Nilotinib; QuiNIDine; QuiNINE

Decreased Effect

Mefloquine may decrease the levels/effects of: Anticonvulsants; Lumefantrine

The levels/effects of Mefloquine may be decreased by: CYP3A4 Inducers (Strong); Deferasirox; Herbs (CYP3A4 Inducers)

Food Interactions Food increases bioavailability of mefloquine by ~40%.

Stability Store at room temperature.

Mechanism of Action Mefloquine which is structurally similar to quinine, destroys the asexual blood forms of *Plasmodium falciparum, P. vivax, P. malariae, P. ovale*; interferes with the malaria parasite's ability to metabolize and utilize erythrocyte hemoglobin; produces swelling of the parasitic food vacuoles

Pharmacokinetics (Adult data unless noted)

Absorption: Slowly absorbed; more complete absorption when administered as a suspension compared with tablets

Distribution: Distributes into tissues, erythrocytes, urine, CSF

V_d:

Children 6-24 months of age: 11.95 L/kg

Children 5-12 years: 8.84 L/kg

Adults: 19 L/kg

Protein binding: ~98%

Metabolism: Hepatic; main metabolite is inactive

Half-life:

Children: 9.8-10.7 days

Adults: 21-22 days (range: 13-33 days)

Time to peak serum concentration: ~17 hours (range: 6-24 hours)

Elimination: Primarily bile and feces; urine (9% of total dose as unchanged drug, 4% of total dose as primary metabolite)

Dialysis: Not removed by hemodialysis

Usual Dosage Oral (dose is expressed in terms of mefloquine hydrochloride):

Children: ≥6 months and >5 kg: **Note:** Experience with dosing patients <20 kg is limited.

Malaria treatment: (mild-to-moderate infection):

Manufacturer's labeling: 20-25 mg/kg/day in 2 divided doses, taken 6-8 hours apart (maximum dose: 1250 mg)

Unlabeled dosing (CDC): 15 mg/kg followed 12 hours later by 10 mg/kg/dose. If clinical improvement is not seen within 48-72 hours, an alternative therapy should be used for retreatment.

Malaria prophylaxis: 5 mg/kg/dose once weekly (maximum dose: 250 mg) starting 1-2 weeks before arrival in the area with endemic infection, continuing weekly during travel, and for 4 weeks after leaving endemic area. **Note:** Prophylaxis may begin 2-3 weeks prior to travel to ensure tolerance if patient is on multiple medications.

Labeled dosing for prophylaxis:

20-30 kg: 1/2 of 250 mg tablet (125 mg) once weekly

30-45 kg: 3/4 of 250 mg tablet (187.5 mg) once weekly

>45 kg: 1 tablet (250 mg) once weekly

Unlabeled dosing (CDC) for prophylaxis:

≤9 kg: 5 mg/kg/dose once weekly

10-19 kg: 1/4 of 250 mg tablet (62.5 mg) once weekly

20-30 kg: 1/2 of 250 mg tablet (125 mg) once weekly

31-45 kg: 3/4 of a 250 mg tablet (187.5 mg) once weekly

≥46 kg: 1 tablet (250 mg) once weekly

Adults:

Malaria treatment (mild to moderate infection): 5 tablets (1250 mg) as a single dose **or** 750 mg followed 6-12 hours later by 500 mg. If clinical improvement is not seen within 48-72 hours, an alternative therapy should be used for retreatment.

Malaria prophylaxis: 250 mg once weekly on the same day each week, starting 1-2 weeks before arrival in endemic area, continuing weekly during travel, and for 4 weeks after leaving endemic area. **Note:** Prophylaxis may begin 2-3 weeks prior to travel to ensure tolerance in patients on multiple medications.

Dosage adjustment in renal impairment: No dosage adjustment needed in patients with renal impairment or on dialysis.

Dosage adjustment in hepatic impairment: Half-life may be prolonged and plasma levels may be higher. Specific dosing adjustments are not available.

Administration Oral: Administer with food and an ample amount of water, at least 8 oz of water for adults. If vomiting occurs within 30 minutes after a dose, repeat dose. If vomiting occurs within 30-60 minutes after a dose, an additional half-dose should be administered. If vomiting recurs, monitor closely and consider alternative treatment. Administering mefloquine on a full stomach may minimize nausea and vomiting. For patients unable to swallow tablets or unable to tolerate its bitter taste, crush tablets and mix with a small amount of water, milk, applesauce, chocolate syrup, jelly, or food immediately before administration. Pulverized dose of mefloquine can be enclosed in a gelatin capsule to mask bitter taste.

Monitoring Parameters Sequential blood smears for percent parasitemia; periodic hepatic function tests, ophthalmologic exam

Patient Information Do not take mefloquine on an empty stomach. May cause dizziness or drowsiness and impair ability to perform activities requiring mental alertness or physical coordination. Advise women of childbearing potential to use effective contraceptive measures during malaria prophylaxis and for 3 months after the last dose. Report any symptoms of anxiety, confusion, depression, or restlessness.

Additional Information Information on recommendations for travelers can be obtained by contacting the Centers for Disease Control and Prevention (CDC) Malaria Hotline (770-488-7788) or visit the CDC website: http://www.cdc.gov/travel/diseases.htm#malaria.

Dosage Forms Excipient information presented when available (limited, particularly for generics); consult specific product labeling. [DSC] = Discontinued product

Tablet, as hydrochloride: 250 mg [equivalent to 228 mg base]

Lariam®: 250 mg [equivalent to 228 mg base] [DSC]

References

American Academy of Pediatrics, "Drugs for Parasitic Infections," In: Pickering LK, ed. Red Book: 2009 Report of the Committee on Infectious Diseases. 28th ed. Elk Grove Village, IL: American Academy of Pediatrics; 2009:783-816. Available at: http://aapredbook.aappublications.org/cgi/content/full/2009/1/4.10. Accessed October 8, 2009

Centers for Disease Control and Prevention, "Treatment of Malaria (Guidelines for Clinicians)." Available at http://www.cdc.gov/malaria/pdf/clinicalguidance.pdf.

Dubos F, Delattre P, Demer M, et al, "Safety of Mefloquine in Infants With Acute Falciparum Malaria," *Pediatr Infect Dis J*, 2004, 23 (7):679-81.

Fryauff DJ, Owusu-agyei S, Utz G, et al, "Mefloquine Treatment for Uncomplicated Falciparum Malaria in Young Children 6-24 months of Age in Northern Ghana," *Am J Trop Med Hyg*, 2007, 76 (2):224-31.

◆ **Mefloquine Hydrochloride** see Mefloquine on page 872

◆ **Megace®** see Megestrol on page 874

◆ **Megace® ES** see Megestrol on page 874

◆ **Megace® OS (Can)** see Megestrol on page 874

◆ **Megadophilus® [OTC]** see Lactobacillus on page 790

Megestrol (me JES trole)

Medication Safety Issues
Sound-alike/look-alike issues:
Megace® may be confused with Reglan®
Megestrol may be confused with mesalamine

U.S. Brand Names Megace®; Megace® ES

Canadian Brand Names Apo-Megestrol®; Megace®; Megace® OS; Nu-Megestrol

Therapeutic Category Antineoplastic Agent, Miscellaneous; Progestin

Generic Available Yes: Excludes Megace® ES

Use Appetite stimulation and promotion of weight gain in cachexia (particularly in HIV patients) which is unresponsive to nutritional supplementation; palliative treatment of breast and endometrial carcinomas

Pregnancy Risk Factor D (tablet) / X (suspension)

Pregnancy Considerations Adverse effects were demonstrated in animal studies. Use during pregnancy is contraindicated (suspension).

Lactation Enters breast milk/not recommended

Breast-Feeding Considerations Due to the potential for adverse reaction in the newborn, the manufacturer recommends discontinuing breast-feeding while receiving megestrol. In addition, HIV-infected mothers are discouraged from breast-feeding to decrease the potential transmission of HIV.

Contraindications Hypersensitivity to megestrol or any component; pregnancy (known or suspected); concomitant use with dofetilide

Warnings Hazardous agent; use appropriate precautions for handling and disposal. May cause fetal harm when administered during pregnancy; women of childbearing age should use appropriate contraceptive measures. May suppress HPA axis during chronic administration; acute adrenal insufficiency may occur with abrupt withdrawal after long-term use or with stress; withdrawal or discontinuation of megestrol should be done carefully. Consider providing exogenous glucocorticoids during periods of stress or severe infection.

Oral suspensions contain sodium benzoate; benzoic acid (benzoate) is a metabolite of benzyl alcohol; large amounts of benzyl alcohol (≥99 mg/kg/day) have been associated with a potentially fatal toxicity ("gasping syndrome") in neonates; *in vitro* and animal studies have shown that benzoate, a metabolite of benzyl alcohol, displaces bilirubin from protein-binding sites; avoid use of products containing sodium benzoate in neonates. Megestrol may inhibit the elimination of dofetilide resulting in increased dofetilide plasma concentrations and potential serious ventricular arrhythmias associated with QT interval prolongation; concomitant use with dofetilide is not recommended. Megestrol may reduce indinavir serum levels resulting in a need for increase in indinavir dose.

Precautions Use with caution in patients with history of thromboembolic disease; use caution in patients with diabetes mellitus as increased insulin requirements have been reported in association with megestrol use

Adverse Reactions

Cardiovascular: Cardiomyopathy, palpitations, edema, hypertension, chest pain, thromboembolic disorders

Central nervous system: Insomnia, depression, fever, headache, confusion, mood changes, lethargy, malaise, asthenia, seizures

Dermatologic: Rash, alopecia, pruritus, vesiculobullous rash

Endocrine & metabolic: Breakthrough bleeding and amenorrhea, spotting, changes in menstrual flow or vaginal bleeding pattern, changes in cervical erosion and secretions, breast tenderness increased, glucose intolerance, HPA axis suppression, adrenal insufficiency, Cushing's syndrome, hypercalcemia, weight gain

Gastrointestinal: Constipation, xerostomia, nausea, vomiting, diarrhea, flatulence, abdominal pain, dyspepsia

Genitourinary: Impotence, gynecomastia, urinary incontinence

Hematologic: Leukopenia, anemia

Hepatic: Hepatomegaly, cholestatic jaundice, hepatotoxicity

Local: Thrombophlebitis

Neuromuscular & skeletal: Weakness, paresthesia, carpal tunnel syndrome, neuropathy

Ocular: Amblyopia

Renal: Albuminuria

Respiratory: Hyperpnea, dyspnea, pulmonary embolism, hyperventilation

Miscellaneous: Diaphoresis, moniliasis, herpes

Drug Interactions

Avoid Concomitant Use
Avoid concomitant use of Megestrol with any of the following: Dofetilide

Increased Effect/Toxicity
Megestrol may increase the levels/effects of: Dofetilide

The levels/effects of Megestrol may be increased by: Herbs (Progestogenic Properties)

Decreased Effect
The levels/effects of Megestrol may be decreased by: Aminoglutethimide

Food Interactions A high fat meal significantly increases plasma levels; avoid herbs with progestogenic properties (eg, bloodroot, chasteberry, damiana, oregano, and yucca) as they may enhance the adverse/toxic effects of megestrol

Stability Store tablets and oral suspension at room temperature; protect from heat

Mechanism of Action A synthetic progestin with antiestrogenic properties which disrupt the estrogen receptor cycle. Megestrol interferes with the normal estrogen cycle and results in a lower LH titer. It may also have a direct effect on the endometrium. As an antineoplastic progestin, it is thought to act through an antileutenizing effect mediated via the pituitary. The exact mechanism for appetite stimulation has not been determined but is postulated to be due in part to a direct effect on the hypothalamus.

Pharmacodynamics Onset of action:

Antineoplastic: 2 months of continuous therapy

Weight gain: 2-4 weeks

Pharmacokinetics (Adult data unless noted)

Absorption: Well absorbed

Metabolism: In the liver

Half-life: Adults: 10-120 hours

Time to peak serum concentration:

Tablet: 2-3 hours

Suspension: 3-5 hours

Elimination: In urine (57% to 78%) and feces (8% to 30%) within 10 days

Usual Dosage Oral: **Note:** Megace® ES is not equivalent mg per mg with other megestrol formulations (625 mg Megace® ES is equivalent to 800 mg megestrol tablets or suspension).

Appetite stimulant in cachexia: Titrate dosage to response; decrease dose if weight gain is excessive:

Children: Limited data has been reported in cachectic children with cystic fibrosis, HIV, and solid tumors: Megestrol (tablets or 40 mg/mL suspension): 7.5-10 mg/kg/day in 1-4 divided doses; not to exceed 800 mg/day or 15 mg/kg/day

Adolescents and Adults:

Megestrol (tablets or 40 mg/mL suspension): 800 mg/day in 1-4 divided doses; titrate dose to response; doses between 400-800 mg/day have been clinically effective

Megace® ES: 625 mg once daily

Breast carcinoma: Female Adults: Megestrol (tablets or 40 mg/mL suspension): 40 mg 4 times/day

Endometrial carcinoma: Female Adults: Megestrol (tablets or 40 mg/mL suspension): 40-320 mg/day in divided doses; not to exceed 800 mg/day

Uterine bleeding: Female Adults: Megestrol (tablets or 40 mg/mL suspension): 40 mg 2-4 times/day

Administration Oral: Shake oral suspension well before administering; administer without regard to food

Monitoring Parameters Monitor for signs of thromboembolic phenomena and adrenal axis suppression

Appetite stimulation: Weight, caloric intake, basal cortisol level

Antineoplastic: Tumor response

Patient Information Follow dosage schedule and do not take more than prescribed. May cause photosensitivity reactions (eg, exposure to sunlight may cause severe sunburn, skin rash, redness, or itching); avoid exposure to sunlight and artificial light sources (sunlamps, tanning booth/bed); wear protective clothing, wide-brimmed hats, sunglasses, and lip sunscreen (SPF ≥15); use a sunscreen [broad-spectrum sunscreen or physical sunscreen (preferred) or sunblock with SPF ≥15]; contact physician if reaction occurs. May cause dry mouth. Report absent or altered menses, abdominal pain, vaginal itching, irritation, or discharge; report warmth, redness, or swelling of extremities, sudden onset of difficulty breathing, severe headache, or change in vision. May cause fetal harm particularly in the first 4 months of pregnancy; use appropriate contraception.

Dosage Forms Excipient information presented when available (limited, particularly for generics); consult specific product labeling.

Suspension, oral, as acetate: 40 mg/mL (10 mL, 20 mL, 240 mL, 480 mL)

Megace®: 40 mg/mL (240 mL) [contains ethanol 0.06% and sodium benzoate; lemon-lime flavor]

Megace® ES: 125 mg/mL (150 mL) [contains ethanol 0.06% and sodium benzoate; lemon-lime flavor]

Tablet, as acetate: 20 mg, 40 mg

References

Eubanks V, Koppersmith N, Wooldridge N, et al, "Effects of Megestrol Acetate on Weight Gain, Body Composition, and Pulmonary Function in Patients With Cystic Fibrosis," *J Pediatr*, 2002, 140(4):439-44.

Nasr SZ, Hurwitz ME, Brown RW, et al, "Treatment of Anorexia and Weight Loss With Megestrol Acetate in Patients With Cystic Fibrosis," *Pediatr Pulmonol*, 1999, 28(5):380-2.

Stockheim JA, Daaboul JJ, Yogev R, et al, "Adrenal Suppression in Children With the Human Immunodeficiency Virus Treated With Megestrol Acetate," *J Pediatr*, 1999, 134(3):368-70.

Tchekmedyian NS, Hickman M, and Heber D, "Treatment of Anorexia and Weight Loss With Megestrol Acetate in Patients With Cancer or Acquired Immunodeficiency Syndrome," *Semin Oncol*, 1991, 18(1 Suppl 2):35-42.

◆ **Megestrol Acetate** see Megestrol on page 874

◆ **Mellaril® (Can)** see Thioridazine on page 1341

Melphalan (MEL fa lan)

Medication Safety Issues

Sound-alike/look-alike issues:

Melphalan may be confused with Mephyton®, Myleran® Alkeran® may be confused with Alferon®, Leukeran®, Myleran®

High alert medication: This medication is in a class of medications the Institute for Safe Medication Practices (ISMP) includes among its list of drug classes which have a heightened risk of causing significant patient harm when used in error.

Related Information

Compatibility of Chemotherapy and Related Supportive Care Medications on page 1580

Emetogenic Potential of Antineoplastic Agents on page 1579

U.S. Brand Names Alkeran®

Canadian Brand Names Alkeran®

Therapeutic Category Antineoplastic Agent, Alkylating Agent (Nitrogen Mustard)

Generic Available Yes: Excludes tablet

Use Palliative treatment of multiple myeloma and non-resectable epithelial ovarian carcinoma (FDA approved in adults); has also been used for the treatment of neuroblastoma, rhabdomyosarcoma, breast cancer, brain tumor, AML, Ewing's sarcoma, medulloblastoma, Hodgkin's disease; part of a conditioning regimen for bone marrow and stem cell transplantation

Pregnancy Risk Factor D

Pregnancy Considerations Animal studies have demonstrated embryotoxicity and teratogenicity. Therapy may suppress ovarian function leading to amenorrhea. There are no adequate and well-controlled studies in pregnant women. Women of childbearing potential should be advised to avoid pregnancy while on melphalan therapy.

Lactation Excretion in breast milk unknown/not recommended

Contraindications Hypersensitivity to melphalan or any component; patients whose disease was resistant to prior therapy

Warnings The FDA currently recommends that procedures for proper handling and disposal of antineoplastic agents be considered; potentially mutagenic, carcinogenic, and teratogenic **[U.S. Boxed Warning]**; bone marrow suppression resulting in infection or bleeding may occur **[U.S. Boxed Warning]**; hypersensitivity has been reported with I.V. and oral administration **[U.S. Boxed Warning]**; long-term oral therapy and cumulative dose >600 mg can increase the chance of developing secondary leukemia; produces amenorrhea

Precautions Use with extreme caution in patients with bone marrow suppression due to prior irradiation or chemotherapy. Use with caution and consider dose reduction in patients with renal impairment. Avoid administration of live vaccines to immunocompromised patients. Cross-sensitivity may exist between melphalan and chlorambucil.

Adverse Reactions

Cardiovascular: Cardiac arrest, diaphoresis, and hypotension and have been reported following I.V. administration; chest pain

Dermatologic: Alopecia, urticaria

Endocrine & metabolic: Amenorrhea

Gastrointestinal: Anorexia, mucositis, nausea, stomatitis, vomiting

Hematologic: Anemia, leukopenia, neutropenia, thrombocytopenia

Local: Burning, discomfort, skin ulceration at injection site, tissue necrosis

Renal: BUN and serum creatinine increased

Respiratory: Bronchospasm, dyspnea, pulmonary fibrosis

Miscellaneous: Anaphylaxis, hypersensitivity reaction, secondary malignancies

<1%, frequency undefined, postmarketing, and/or case reports: Agranulocytosis, allergic reactions, bladder irritation, bone marrow failure (irreversible), diarrhea, hemolytic anemia, hemorrhagic cystitis, hemorrhagic necrotic enterocolitis, hepatic veno-occlusive disease (I.V. melphalan), hepatitis, interstitial pneumonitis, jaundice, ovarian suppression, pruritus, radiation myelopathy, rash, secondary carcinoma, secondary myeloproliferative syndrome, SIADH, skin hypersensitivity, skin vesiculation, sterility, testicular suppression, transaminases increased, vasculitis

Drug Interactions

Avoid Concomitant Use

Avoid concomitant use of Melphalan with any of the following: BCG; Nalidixic Acid; Natalizumab; Pimecrolimus; Tacrolimus (Topical); Vaccines (Live)

Increased Effect/Toxicity

Melphalan may increase the levels/effects of: Carmustine; CycloSPORINE; CycloSPORINE (Systemic); Leflunomide; Natalizumab; Vaccines (Live); Vitamin K Antagonists

The levels/effects of Melphalan may be increased by: Denosumab; Nalidixic Acid; Pimecrolimus; Tacrolimus (Topical); Trastuzumab

Decreased Effect

Melphalan may decrease the levels/effects of: BCG; Cardiac Glycosides; Sipuleucel-T; Vaccines (Inactivated); Vaccines (Live); Vitamin K Antagonists

The levels/effects of Melphalan may be decreased by: Echinacea

Food Interactions Food interferes with oral absorption

Stability

Tablet: Store in refrigerator at 2°C to 8°C (36°F to 46°F); protect from light

Injection: Store at controlled room temperature 15°C to 30°C (59°F to 86°F); protect from light. Dose from reconstituted 5 mg/mL solution should be immediately diluted in NS to a concentration no greater than 0.45 mg/mL and administered completely within 60 minutes of reconstitution; do not refrigerate since it may precipitate

Mechanism of Action Alkylating agent that inhibits DNA and RNA synthesis via interstrand cross-linking with DNA, probably binding at the N^7 position of guanine.

Pharmacokinetics (Adult data unless noted)

Absorption: Oral: Variable and incomplete

Distribution: Distributes throughout total body water; low penetration into CSF; V_{dss}: 0.5 L/kg

Protein binding: 60% to 90%

Metabolism: Nonenzymatic hydrolysis to mono- or dihydroxy products; some conjugation to glutathione

Bioavailability: Ranges from 49% to 95% depending on the presence of food; average: 60%

Half-life: 75-120 minutes

Time to peak serum concentration: Oral: Within 2 hours

Elimination: 10% to 15% of dose excreted unchanged in urine; after oral administration, 20% to 50% excreted in stool

Usual Dosage Refer to individual protocols

Children:

I.V.:

Pediatric rhabdomyosarcoma: 10-35 mg/m²/dose every 21-28 days

High-dose melphalan with bone marrow transplantation for neuroblastoma: 70-100 mg/m²/day on day 7 and 6 before BMT; or 140-220 mg/m² single dose before BMT; or 50 mg/m²/day for 4 days; or 70 mg/m²/day for 3 days

Oral: 4-20 mg/m²/day for 1-21 days

Adults:

Multiple myeloma:

Oral: 6 mg/day once daily initially adjusted as indicated or 0.15 mg/kg/day for 7 days; or 0.25 mg/kg/day for 4 days or 8-10 mg/m² for 4 days, repeat at 4- to 6-week intervals

I.V.: 16 mg/m²/dose every 2 weeks for 4 doses, then repeat monthly as per protocol for multiple myeloma

Ovarian carcinoma: Oral: 0.2 mg/kg/day for 5 days, repeat in 4-5 weeks

Dosing adjustment in renal impairment: BUN ≥30 mg/dL: Reduce dose by 50%

The following guidelines have been used by some clinicians (see Aronoff, 2007): Adults:

Cl_{cr} 10-50 mL/minute: Administer 75% of dose

Cl_{cr} <10 mL/minute: Administer 50% of dose

Administration

Oral: Administer on an empty stomach

Parenteral: I.V.: Reconstitute 50 mg vial for injection with special diluent to yield a 5 mg/mL solution; dilute the reconstituted solution with NS to a final concentration not to exceed 2 mg/mL for I.V. central line administration or 0.45 mg/mL for peripheral I.V. administration; administer by I.V. infusion over 15-30 minutes at a rate not to exceed 10 mg/minute but total infusion should be administered within 1 hour

Monitoring Parameters CBC with differential and platelet count, serum electrolytes, hemoglobin; monitor infusion site for redness and irritation

Test Interactions Positive Coombs' [direct]

Patient Information Notify physician if fever, shortness of breath, skin rash, unusual lumps/masses, nausea, vomiting, weight loss, amenorrhea, persistent cough, sore throat, bleeding, or bruising occurs. Women of childbearing potential should be advised to avoid becoming pregnant.

Nursing Implications Ensure adequate patient hydration; care should be taken to avoid extravasation. If accidental skin contact occurs, immediately wash the affected area with soap and water.

Additional Information Myelosuppressive effects:

WBC: Moderate

Platelets: Moderate

Onset (days): 7

Nadir (days): 14-21

Recovery (days): 42-50

Dosage Forms Excipient information presented when available (limited, particularly for generics); consult specific product labeling.

Injection, powder for reconstitution: 50 mg

Alkeran®: 50 mg [diluent contains ethanol and propylene glycol]

Tablet:

Alkeran®: 2 mg

References

Aronoff GR, Bennett WM, Berns JS, et al, Drug Prescribing in Renal Failure: Dosing Guidelines for Adults and Children, 5th ed. Philadelphia, PA: American College of Physicians, 2007, 97, 177.

Berg SL, Grisell DL, DeLaney TF, et al, "Principles of Treatment of Pediatric Solid Tumors," Pediatr Clin North Am, 1991, 38(2):249-67.

Lazarus HM, Phillips GL, Herzig RH, et al, "High-Dose Melphalan and the Development of Hematopoietic Stem-Cell Transplantation: 25 Years Later," *J Clin Oncol*, 2008, 26(14):2240-3.

Ozkaynak MF, Sahdev I, Gross TG, et al, "A Pilot Study of Addition of Amifostine to Melphalan, Carboplatin, Etoposide, and Cyclophosphamide With Autologous Hematopoietic Stem Cell Transplantation in Pediatric Solid Tumors - A Pediatric Blood and Marrow Transplant Consortium Study," *J Pediatr Hematol Oncol*, 2008, 30(3):204-9.

Pole JG, Casper J, Elfenbein G, et al, "High-Dose Chemoradiotherapy Supported by Marrow Infusions for Advanced Neuroblastoma: A Pediatric Oncology Group Study," *J Clin Oncol*, 1991, 9(1):152-8.

Schroeder H, Pinkerton CR, Powles RL, et al, "High-Dose Melphalan and Total Body Irradiation With Autologous Marrow Rescue in Childhood Acute Lymphoblastic Leukemia After Relapse," *Bone Marrow Transplant*, 1991, 7(1):11-15.

◆ **Menactra®** see Meningococcal (Groups A / C / Y and W-135) Diphtheria Conjugate Vaccine *on page 877*

◆ **MenACWY-D (Menactra®)** see Meningococcal (Groups A / C / Y and W-135) Diphtheria Conjugate Vaccine *on page 877*

◆ **MenACWY-CRM (Menveo®)** *see* Meningococcal (Groups A / C / Y and W-135) Diphtheria Conjugate Vaccine *on page 877*

◆ **Meningococcal Conjugate Vaccine** see Meningococcal (Groups A / C / Y and W-135) Diphtheria Conjugate Vaccine *on page 877*

Meningococcal (Groups A / C / Y and W-135) Diphtheria Conjugate Vaccine

(me NIN joe kok al groops aye, see, why & dubl yoo won thur tee fyve dif THEER ee a KON joo gate vak SEEN)

Medication Safety Issues

Administration issue:

Menactra® (MCV4) should be administered by intramuscular (I.M.) injection only. Inadvertent subcutaneous (SubQ) administration has been reported; possibly due to confusion of this product with Menomume® (MPSV4), also a meningococcal polysaccharide vaccine, which is administered by the SubQ route.

Related Information

Immunization Guidelines *on page 1636*

U.S. Brand Names Menactra®; Menveo®

Therapeutic Category Vaccine, Inactivated Bacteria

Generic Available No

Use Prevention of invasive meningococcal disease in children and adults at risk (Menactra®: FDA approved in ages ≥2 years and adults ≤55 years; Menveo®: FDA approved in ages ≥11 years and adults ≤55 years); individuals with anatomic or functional asplenia, those with terminal complement component deficiencies, military recruits, and residents of or travelers to epidemic or highly endemic areas. The American College Health Association recommends immunization of college students who will be living in dormitories for the first time.

Vaccinations should be considered for household or institutional contacts of persons with meningococcal disease as an adjunct to appropriate antibiotic chemoprophylaxis as well as medical and laboratory personnel at risk of exposure to meningococcal disease.

Meningococcal conjugate vaccine [MCV4 (Menactra®) should be used in children 2-10 years of age; MenACWY-CRM (Menveo®) or MCV4; Menactra®] is preferred for persons aged 11-55 years; meningococcal polysaccharide vaccine [MPSV4; Menomune®] may be used if the conjugate vaccine is not available. MPSV4 is preferred in adults ≥56 years of age.

Pregnancy Risk Factor B/C (manufacturer dependent)

Pregnancy Considerations Animal reproduction studies have not been conducted with Menactra® (therefore classified as pregnancy category C). An isolated teratogenic effect was observed in an animal developmental toxicity study; not necessarily vaccine related. Carcinogenic or mutagenic studies have not been performed. Patients should contact the Sanofi Pasteur Inc vaccine registry at 1-800-822-2463 if they are pregnant or become aware they were pregnant at the time of Menactra® vaccination.

Adverse events were not observed in animal reproduction studies conducted with Menveo® (therefore classified as pregnancy category B). Patients should contact the Novartis Vaccines and Diagnostics Inc. pregnancy registry at 1-877-311-8972 if they are pregnant or become aware they were pregnant at the time of Menveo® vaccination.

Limited information is available following inadvertent use of meningococcal diphtheria conjugate vaccine during pregnancy; safety and effectiveness have not been established.

Lactation Excretion in breast milk unknown/use caution

Contraindications Hypersensitivity to any component of the formulation, including diphtheria toxoid or CRM₁₉₇ (a diphtheria toxin carrier protein) or other meningococcal containing vaccines; Menactra®: History of Guillain-Barré Syndrome (GBS)

Warnings Immediate treatment for anaphylactoid or acute hypersensitivity reactions should be available during vaccine use; patients receiving immunosuppressive therapy may have diminished response; GBS has been reported in a temporal relationship following Menactra® administration. Individuals with a previous history of GBS should not receive Menactra®; data not currently available to assess possible risk of GBS following use of MenACWY-CRM (Menveo®).

Safety and efficacy in children <2 years of age (Menactra®) or <11 years of age (Menveo®) have not been established. Latex is used in stopper of the vial; patients with known hypersensitivity should avoid doses from vial formulation and use prefilled syringe for dose.

Precautions Use with caution in patients with coagulation disorders including thrombocytopenia, due to an increased risk for bleeding following I.M. administration; if the patient receives antihemophilia or other similar therapy, I.M. injection can be scheduled shortly after such therapy is administered; defer vaccination for persons with moderate or severe acute febrile illness until recovery; may administer to patient with mild acute illness (with or without fever). Routine prophylactic administration of acetaminophen to prevent fever due to vaccines has been shown to decrease the immune response of some vaccines; the clinical significance of this reduction in immune response has not been established (see Prymula, 2009).

Adverse Reactions All serious adverse reactions must be reported to the U.S. Department of Health and Human Services (DHHS) Vaccine Adverse Event Reporting System (VAERS) 1-800-822-7967. Incidence of erythema, swelling, or tenderness may be higher in children

Central nervous system: Chills, drowsiness, fatigue, fever, GBS (see Warnings), headache, irritability, malaise, pain

Dermatologic: Rash

Gastrointestinal: Anorexia, diarrhea, nausea, vomiting

Local: Erythema, induration, pain at injection site, swelling

Neuromuscular & skeletal: Arthralgia

<1%, postmarketing, and/or case reports: Acute disseminated encephalomyelitis, anaphylactic/anaphylactoid reactions, breathing difficulties, facial palsy, hypotension, myalgia, pruritus, transverse myelitis, upper airway swelling, urticaria, vasovagal syncope, wheezing

Drug Interactions

Avoid Concomitant Use There are no known interactions where it is recommended to avoid concomitant use.

Increased Effect/Toxicity There are no known significant interactions involving an increase in effect.

Decreased Effect

The levels/effects of Meningococcal (Groups A / C / Y and W-135) Diphtheria Conjugate Vaccine may be decreased by: Immunosuppressants

Stability

Menactra®: Store at 2°C to 8°C (35°F to 46°F); do not freeze; protect from light

Menveo®: Prior to reconstitution, store between 2°C to 8°C (36°F to 46°F); protect from light and do not freeze. Discard product exposed to freezing.

Mechanism of Action Induces the formation of bactericidal antibodies to meningococcal antigens; the presence of these antibodies is strongly correlated with immunity to meningococcal disease caused by *Neisseria meningitides* groups A, C, Y and W-135.

Usual Dosage I.M.:

Menactra®: Children >2 years and Adults ≤55 years of age: 0.5 mL

Menveo®: Children ≥11 years and Adults ≤55 years: 0.5 mL

Note: Revaccination with MCV4 (Menactra®) is indicated in patients who were previously vaccinated with MPSV4 (Menomune®) or MCV4 (Menactra®) and remain at an increased risk for meningococcal infection. Persons at high risk for infection (those with prolonged increased risk for meningococcal disease) have increased susceptibility, such as persistent complement component deficiencies; persons with anatomic or functional asplenia; and persons with prolonged exposure, including lab workers or travelers to hyperendemic or epidemic areas. If previously vaccinated at ages 2-6 years, revaccinate 3 years after the last dose. If previously vaccinated at ≥7 years of age, revaccinate 5 years after the last dose. Persons who remain at high risk should then be revaccinated every 5 years. Revaccination with MCV4 (Menactra®) is not indicated for persons living in dormitories if on-campus housing is their only risk factor; however, revaccination is indicated for college freshmen living in dormitories if they received MPSV4 (Menomune®) ≥5 years previously.

Administration Administer by I.M. injection; **not for intradermal, subcutaneous, or I.V. administration**

Menveo®: Prior to use, remove liquid contents from vial of MenCYW-135 and inject into vial containing MenA powder. Gently invert or swirl until dissolved. The resulting solution should be clear and colorless. A small amount of liquid will remain in the vial after withdrawing the 0.5 mL dose. Use immediately after reconstitution but may be stored at ≤25°C (77°F) for up to 8 hours. Do not mix with other vaccines in the same syringe.

Patient Information Inform patients about common side effects; patients should report serious and unusual effects to physician

Nursing Implications Federal law requires that the date of administration, the vaccine manufacturer, lot number of vaccine, and the administering person's name, title, and address be entered into the patient's permanent medical record.

Additional Information In order to maximize vaccination rates, the ACIP recommends simultaneous administration of all age-appropriate vaccines (live or inactivated) for which a person is eligible at a single visit, unless contraindications exist. The use of combination vaccines is generally preferred over separate injections, taking into consideration provider assessment, patient preference, and potential adverse events.

For additional information, please refer to the following website: http://www.cdc.gov/vaccines/vpd-vac/.

Dosage Forms Excipient information presented when available (limited, particularly for generics); consult specific product labeling.

Injection, solution [preservative free]:

Menactra®: 4 mcg each of polysaccharide antigen groups A, C, Y, and W-135 [bound to diphtheria toxoid 48 mcg] per 0.5 mL [MCV4 or MenACWY-D; contains natural rubber/natural latex in packaging of vials]

Menveo®: MenA oligosaccharide 10 mcg, MenC oligosaccharide 5 mcg, MenY oligosaccharide 5 mcg, and MenW-135 oligosaccharide 5 mcg [bound to CRM$_{197}$ protein 32.7-64.1 mcg] per 0.5 mL (0.5 mL) [MenACWY-CRM; supplied in two vials, one containing MenA powder and one containing MenCYW-135 liquid]

References

Centers for Disease Control and Prevention (CDC), "General Recommendations on Immunization. Recommendations of the Advisory Committee on Immunization Practices (ACIP)," *MMWR Recomm Rep*, 2006, 55(RR-15):1-48. Available at: http://www.cdc.gov/mmwr/preview/mmwrhtml/rr5515a1.htm.

Centers for Disease Control and Prevention (CDC), "Licensure of a Meningococcal Conjugate Vaccine (Menveo) and Guidance for Use – Advisory Committee on Immunization Practices (ACIP), 2010," *MMWR Morb Mortal Wkly Rep*, 2010, 59(9):273.

Centers for Disease Control and Prevention (CDC), "Recommended Adult Immunization Schedule – United States, 2010" *MMWR Morb Mortal Wkly Rep*, 2010, 59(01):Q1-4.

Centers for Disease Control and Prevention (CDC), "Recommended Immunization Schedules for Persons Aged 0 Through 18 Years – United States, 2010," *MMWR Morb Mortal Wkly Rep*, 2009, 58 (51-2):1-4.

Centers for Disease Control and Prevention (CDC), "Updated Recommendation From the Advisory Committee on Immunization Practices (ACIP) for Revaccination of Persons at Prolonged Increased Risk for Meningococcal Disease," *MMWR Morb Mortal Wkly Rep*, 2009, 58(37):1042-3. Available at: http://www.cdc.gov/mmwr/preview/mmwrhtml/mm5837a4.htm?s_cid=mm5837a4_e.

Prymula R, Siegrist CA, Chlibek R, et al, "Effect of Prophylactic Paracetamol Administration at Time of Vaccination on Febrile Reactions and Antibody Responses in Children: Two Open-Label, Randomised Controlled Trials," *Lancet*, 2009, 374(9698):1339-50.

◆ **Meningococcal Polysaccharide Vaccine** *see* Meningococcal Polysaccharide Vaccine (Groups A / C / Y and W-135) *on page 878*

Meningococcal Polysaccharide Vaccine (Groups A / C / Y and W-135)

(me NIN joe kok al pol i SAK a ride vak SEEN groops aye, see, why & dubl yoo won thur tee fyve)

Medication Safety Issues

Administration issue:

Menomume® (MPSV4) should be administered by subcutaneous (SubQ) injection. Menactra® (MCV4), also a meningococcal polysaccharide vaccine, is to be administered by intramuscular (I.M.) injection only.

Related Information

Immunization Guidelines *on page 1636*

U.S. Brand Names Menomune®-A/C/Y/W-135

Therapeutic Category Vaccine

Generic Available No

Use Provide active immunity to meningococcal serogroups contained in the vaccine (FDA approved in ages ≥2 years and adults); prevention and control of outbreaks of serogroup C meningococcal disease; recommended for use in children ≥2 years and adults at risk (anatomic or functional asplenia, those with terminal complement component or properdin deficiencies), and residents of or travelers to epidemic or highly endemic areas. The American College Health Association recommends immunization of college students who will be living in dormitories for the first time.

Vaccinations should be considered for household or institutional contacts of persons with meningococcal disease as an adjunct to appropriate antibiotic chemoprophylaxis as well as medical and laboratory personnel at risk of exposure to meningococcal disease.

Meningococcal conjugate vaccine (MCV4; Menactra®) is preferred for persons aged 2-55 years; MPSV4 may be used if MCV4 is not available

Pregnancy Risk Factor C

Pregnancy Considerations Animal studies have not been conducted. Based on limited data, teratogenic effects have not been reported when used during pregnancy. Pregnancy should not preclude vaccination with MPSV4 if indicated. Patients may contact the Sanofi Pasteur Inc vaccine registry at 1-800-822-2463 if they are pregnant or become aware they were pregnant at the time of vaccination.

Lactation Excretion in breast milk unknown/use caution

Contraindications Hypersensitivity to any component of the formulation; defer vaccination for persons with acute febrile illness until recovery

Warnings Avoid administration at the same time as whole-cell pertussis or whole-cell typhoid vaccines due to the combined endotoxin content; patients receiving immuno-suppressive therapy may have diminished response. Safety and efficacy in pediatric patients <2 years of age have not been established. Some dosage forms contain thimerosal.

Precautions Immediate treatment for anaphylactoid or acute hypersensitivity reactions should be available during vaccine use. Routine prophylactic administration of acetaminophen to prevent fever due to vaccines has been shown to decrease the immune response of some vaccines; the clinical significance of this reduction in immune response has not been established (see Prymula, 2009).

Adverse Reactions All serious adverse reactions must be reported to the U.S. Department of Health and Human Services (DHHS) Vaccine Adverse Event Reporting System (VAERS) 1-800-822-7967. Incidence of erythema, swelling, or tenderness may be higher in children.

Central nervous system: Chills, fever, headache, malaise
Local: Erythema, induration, pain at injection site, tenderness

Drug Interactions

Avoid Concomitant Use There are no known inter-actions where it is recommended to avoid concomitant use.

Increased Effect/Toxicity There are no known signifi-cant interactions involving an increase in effect.

Decreased Effect

The levels/effects of Meningococcal Polysaccharide Vaccine (Groups A / C / Y and W-135) may be decreased by: Immunosuppressants

Stability Prior to and following reconstitution, store at 2°C to 8°C (35°F to 46°F); single use vial stable for 30 minutes after reconstitution; use multidose vial within 35 days of reconstitution

Mechanism of Action Induces the formation of bacter-icidal antibodies to meningococcal antigens; the presence of these antibodies is strongly correlated with immunity to meningococcal disease caused by *Neisseria meningitidis* groups A, C, Y and W-135.

Pharmacodynamics

Onset of action: Antibody levels: 7-10 days

Duration: Antibodies against group A and C polysacchar-ides decline markedly (to prevaccination levels) over the first 3 years following a single dose of vaccine, especially in children <4 years of age

Usual Dosage SubQ: Children ≥2 years and Adults: 0.5 mL

Note: Revaccination with MCV4 (Menactra®) is indicated in patients who were previously vaccinated with MPSV4 (Menomune®) or MCV4 (Menactra®) and remain at an increased risk for meningococcal infection. Persons at high risk for infection (those with prolonged increased risk for meningococcal disease) have increased suscepti-bility, such as persistent complement component defi-ciencies; persons with anatomic or functional asplenia; and persons with prolonged exposure, including lab workers or travelers to hyperendemic or epidemic areas. If previously vaccinated at ages 2-6 years, revaccinate 3 years after the last dose. If previously vaccinated at ≥7 years of age, revaccinate 5 years after the last dose. Persons who remain at high risk should then be revaccinated every 5 years. Revaccination with MCV4 (Menactra®) is not indicated for persons living in dormitories if on-campus housing is their only risk factor; however, revaccination is indicated for college freshmen living in dormitories if they received MPSV4 (Meno-mune®) ≥5 years previously.

Administration Reconstitute using provided diluent; shake well; administer by SubQ injection; **not for intra-dermal, I.M., or I.V. administration**

Patient Information Inform patients about common side effects; patients should report serious and unusual effects to physician

Nursing Implications Federal law requires that the date of administration, the vaccine manufacturer, lot number of vaccine, and the administering person's name, title and address be entered into the patient's permanent medical record.

Additional Information In order to maximize vaccination rates, the ACIP recommends simultaneous administration of all age-appropriate vaccines (live or inactivated) for which a person is eligible at a single visit, unless contraindications exist. The use of combination vaccines is generally preferred over separate infections, taking into consideration provider assessment, patient preference, and potential adverse events.

For additional information, please refer to the following website: http://www.cdc.gov/vaccines/vpd-vac/.

Dosage Forms Excipient information presented when available (limited, particularly for generics); consult specific product labeling.

Injection, powder for reconstitution [MPSV4]:

Menomune®-A/C/Y/W-135: 50 mcg each of polysacchar-ide antigen groups A, C, Y, and W-135 per 0.5 mL dose [contains lactose 2.5-5 mg/0.5 mL, natural rubber/natural latex in packaging, thimerosal in diluent for multidose vial]

References

Centers for Disease Control and Prevention (CDC), "General Recommendations on Immunization. Recommendations of the Advisory Committee on Immunization Practices (ACIP)," *MMWR Recomm Rep*, 2006, 55(RR-15):1-48. Available at: http://www.cdc.gov/mmwr/preview/mmwrhtml/rr5515a1.htm.

Centers for Disease Control and Prevention (CDC), "Recommended Adult Immunization Schedule – United States, 2009" *MMWR Morb Mortal Wkly Rep*, 2009, 57(53):Q1-4.

Centers for Disease Control and Prevention (CDC), "Recommended Immunization Schedules for Persons Aged 0 Through 18 years – United States, 2009," *MMWR Morb Mortal Wkly Rep*, 2009, 57(51): Q1-4.

Centers for Disease Control and Prevention (CDC), "Updated Recommendation From the Advisory Committee on Immunization Practices (ACIP) for Revaccination of Persons at Prolonged Increased Risk for Meningococcal Disease," *MMWR Morb Mortal Wkly Rep*, 2009, 58(37):1042-3. Available at http://www.cdc.gov/mmwr/preview/mmwrhtml/mm5837a4.htm?s_cid=mm5837a4_e.

Prymula R, Siegrist CA, Chlibek R, et al, "Effect of Prophylactic Paracetamol Administration at Time of Vaccination on Febrile Reactions and Antibody Responses in Children: Two Open-Label, Randomised Controlled Trials," *Lancet*, 2009, 374(9698):1339-50.

◆ **Menomune®-A/C/Y/W-135** *see* Meningococcal Polysac-charide Vaccine (Groups A / C / Y and W-135) *on page 878*

◆ **Menostar®** *see* Estradiol *on page 536*

◆ **Menveo®** *see* Meningococcal (Groups A / C / Y and W-135) Diphtheria Conjugate Vaccine *on page 877*

Meperidine (me PER i deen)

Medication Safety Issues

Avoid the use of meperidine for pain control, especially in elderly and renally-compromised patients because of the risk of neurotoxicity (American Pain Society, 2008; Institute for Safe Medication Practices [ISMP], 2007)

Sound-alike/look-alike issues:

Meperidine may be confused with meprobamate

Demerol® may be confused with Demulen®, Desyrel®, dicumarol, Dilaudid®, Dymelor®, Pamelor®

High alert medication: The Institute for Safe Medication Practices (ISMP) includes this medication among its list of drug classes which have a heightened risk of causing significant patient harm when used in error.

Beers Criteria medication: This drug may be inappropriate for use in geriatric patients (high severity risk).

Related Information

Adult ACLS Algorithms *on page 1463*

Compatibility of Medications Mixed in a Syringe *on page 1713*

Opioid Analgesics Comparison *on page 1510*

Preprocedure Sedatives in Children *on page 1688*

Serotonin Syndrome *on page 1695*

U.S. Brand Names Demerol®

Canadian Brand Names Demerol®

Therapeutic Category Analgesic, Narcotic

Generic Available Yes

Use Management of moderate to severe pain; adjunct to anesthesia and preoperative sedation

Restrictions C-II

Pregnancy Risk Factor C

Pregnancy Considerations Meperidine is known to cross the placenta, which may result in respiratory or CNS depression in the newborn.

Lactation Enters breast milk/contraindicated (AAP rates "compatible")

Breast-Feeding Considerations Meperidine is excreted in breast milk and may cause CNS and/or respiratory depression in the nursing infant.

Contraindications Hypersensitivity to meperidine or any component (see Warnings); use of MAO inhibitors within 14 days (potentially fatal reactions may occur, see Drug Interactions)

Warnings CNS and respiratory depression may occur. Neonates and young infants may be at higher risk for adverse effects, especially respiratory depression (due to decreased elimination); use with caution and in reduced doses in this age group. Use with great caution (and only if essential) in patients with head injury, increased ICP, or other intercranial lesions (potential to depress respiration and increase ICP may be greatly exaggerated in these patients). Use with extreme caution in patients with COPD, cor pulmonale, acute asthmatic attacks, hypoxia, hypercapnia, pre-existing respiratory depression, significantly decreased respiratory reserve. Severe hypotension may occur; use with caution in postoperative patients, in patients with hypovolemia, or in those receiving drugs which may exaggerate hypotensive effects (including phenothiazines or general anesthetics). Meperidine may be given I.V., but should be administered very slowly and as a diluted solution; rapid I.V. administration may result in increased adverse effects including severe respiratory depression, apnea, hypotension, peripheral circulatory collapse, or cardiac arrest; do not administer I.V. unless a narcotic antagonist and respiratory support are immediately available.

Physical and psychological dependence may occur; abrupt discontinuation after prolonged use may result in withdrawal symptoms or seizures. Warn patient of possible impairment of alertness or physical coordination and orthostatic hypotension (see Patient Information). Interactions with other CNS drugs may occur (see Drug Interactions). Healthcare provider should be alert to problems of abuse, misuse, and diversion. Infants born to women physically dependent on opioids will also be physically dependent and may experience respiratory difficulties or opioid withdrawal symptoms.

Multiple dose vial may contain sulfites which may cause allergic reactions in susceptible individuals; oral liquid may contain benzoic acid or sodium benzoate; benzoic acid (benzoate) is a metabolite of benzyl alcohol; large amounts of benzyl alcohol (≥99 mg/kg/day) have been associated with a potentially fatal toxicity ("gasping syndrome") in neonates; the "gasping syndrome" consists of metabolic acidosis, respiratory distress, gasping respirations, CNS dysfunction (including convulsions, intracranial hemorrhage), hypotension, and cardiovascular collapse; use meperidine products containing benzoic acid or sodium benzoate with caution in neonates; *in vitro* and animal studies have shown that benzoate displaces bilirubin from protein binding sites

Precautions Use with caution in patients with pulmonary, hepatic, or renal disorders; use with caution in patients with tachycardias, biliary colic, seizure disorders, or those receiving prolonged use or high-dose meperidine [normeperidine (an active metabolite and CNS stimulant) may accumulate and precipitate twitches, tremors, or seizures]; decrease the dose in patients with renal or hepatic impairment (normeperidine metabolite may accumulate in these patients; **Note:** Due to the accumulation of normeperidine and its adverse effects, meperidine is not considered to be an opioid of choice for the treatment of pain. The Institute for Safe Medication Practices (ISMP) recommends avoiding its use for pain control, especially in the elderly and in patients with renal impairment (ISMP, 2007). The American Pain Society (2003) recommends that meperidine should not be used for chronic pain control; if used for treatment of acute pain it should only be used in patients without renal or CNS disease, treatment should be limited to ≤48 hours, and (adult) doses should not exceed 600 mg/24 hours.

Use with caution and decrease initial dose in patients with sickle cell anemia, Addison's disease, hypothyroidism, urethral stricture, prostatic hypertrophy, or pheochromocytoma (meperidine may precipitate hypertension in patients with pheochromocytoma). Meperidine may obscure diagnosis or clinical course of patients with acute abdominal conditions. Safe use in pregnancy prior to labor has not been established; when administered to a pregnant woman, meperidine passes into the fetal circulation and may result in respiratory and CNS depression in the newborn; resuscitative equipment and naloxone should be available for the neonate.

Adverse Reactions

Cardiovascular: Palpitations, hypotension, bradycardia, peripheral vasodilation, tachycardia, syncope, orthostatic hypotension

Central nervous system: CNS depression, dizziness, drowsiness, lightheadedness, sedation, intracranial pressure elevated, headache, euphoria, dysphoria, agitation, transient hallucinations, disorientation; active metabolite (normeperidine) may precipitate twitches, tremors, or seizures

Dermatologic: Pruritus, rash, urticaria

Endocrine & metabolic: Antidiuretic hormone release

Gastrointestinal: Nausea, vomiting, constipation, biliary tract spasm, xerostomia

Genitourinary: Urinary tract spasm, urinary retention

Local: Pain at injection site; phlebitis, wheal, and flare over the vein (with I.V. use); induration, irritation (repeated SubQ use)

Neuromuscular and skeletal: Tremor, weakness, uncoordinated muscle movements

Ocular: Miosis, visual disturbances

Respiratory: Respiratory depression, respiratory arrest

Miscellaneous: Physical and psychological dependence, histamine release, anaphylaxis, hypersensitivity reactions, diaphoresis

Drug Interactions

Metabolism/Transport Effects Substrate (minor) of CYP2B6, 2C19, 3A4

Avoid Concomitant Use

Avoid concomitant use of Meperidine with any of the following: MAO Inhibitors; Sibutramine

Increased Effect/Toxicity

Meperidine may increase the levels/effects of: Alcohol (Ethyl); Alvimopan; CNS Depressants; Desmopressin; Selective Serotonin Reuptake Inhibitors; Serotonin Modulators; Thiazide Diuretics

The levels/effects of Meperidine may be increased by: Amphetamines; Antipsychotic Agents (Phenothiazines); Barbiturates; MAO Inhibitors; Protease Inhibitors; Sibutramine; Succinylcholine

Decreased Effect

Meperidine may decrease the levels/effects of: Pegvisomant

The levels/effects of Meperidine may be decreased by: Ammonium Chloride; Mixed Agonist / Antagonist Opioids; Phenytoin; Protease Inhibitors

Stability Incompatible with aminophylline, heparin, phenobarbital, phenytoin, and sodium bicarbonate

Mechanism of Action Binds to opiate receptors in the CNS, causing inhibition of ascending pain pathways, altering the perception of and response to pain; produces generalized CNS depression

Pharmacodynamics Analgesia:

Onset of action:
Oral, I.M., SubQ: Within 10-15 minutes
I.V.: Within 5 minutes
Maximum effect:
Oral, I.M., SubQ: Within 1 hour
I.V.: 5-7 minutes
Duration:
Oral, I.M., SubQ: 2-4 hours
I.V.: 2-3 hours

Pharmacokinetics (Adult data unless noted)

Distribution: Crosses the placenta; appears in breast milk
V_{dss}:
Neonates: Preterm 1-7 days: 8.8 L/kg; term 1-7 days: 5.6 L/kg
Infants: 1 week to 2 months: 8 L/kg; 3-18 months: 5 L/kg; 5-8 years: 2.8 L/kg
Adults: 3-4 L/kg

Protein binding: (to alpha$_1$-acid glycoprotein)
Neonates: 52%
Infants: 3-18 months: 85%
Adults: ~60% to 80%

Metabolism: In the liver via hydrolysis and N-demethylation

Bioavailability: ~50% to 60%, increased bioavailability with liver disease

Half-life, terminal:
Preterm infants 3.6-65 days of age: 11.9 hours (range: 3.3-59.4 hours)
Term infants:
0.3-4 days of age: 10.7 hours (range: 4.9-16.8 hours)
26-73 days of age: 8.2 hours (range: 5.7-31.7 hours)
Neonates: 23 hours (range: 12-39 hours)
Infants 3-18 months: 2.3 hours
Children 5-8 years: 3 hours

Adults: 2.5-4 hours
Adults with liver disease: 7-11 hours
Normeperidine (active metabolite): Neonates: 30-85 hours; Adults: 8-16 hours; normeperidine half-life is dependent on renal function and can accumulate with high doses or in patients with decreased renal function; normeperidine may precipitate tremors or seizures

Elimination: ~5% meperidine eliminated unchanged in urine

Usual Dosage Doses should be titrated to appropriate analgesic effect; **when changing route of administration, note that oral doses are about half as effective as parenteral dose**

Children:
Oral, I.M., I.V., SubQ: Usual: 1-1.5 mg/kg/dose every 3-4 hours as needed; 1-2 mg/kg as a single dose preoperative medication may be used; maximum dose: 100 mg/dose
I.V. continuous infusion: Loading dose: 0.5-1 mg/kg followed by initial rate: 0.3 mg/kg/hour; titrate dose to effect; may require 0.5-0.7 mg/kg/hour

Adults: Oral, I.M., I.V.: SubQ: 50-150 mg/dose every 3-4 hours as needed

AHCPR dosing guidelines: Opioid naive patients: **Note:** Oral route not recommended (see Carr, 1992 and Jacox, 1994):
Children and Adults <50 kg: Moderate to severe pain: I.M., I.V., SubQ: Usual initial dose: 0.75 mg/kg every 2-3 hours
Children and Adults ≥50 kg: Moderate to severe pain: I.M., I.V., SubQ: Usual initial dose: 100 mg every 3 hours

Dosing adjustment in renal impairment: Use with caution and reduce dose; accumulation of meperidine and its active metabolite (normeperidine) may occur (see Precautions)
Cl$_{cr}$ 10-50 mL/minute: Administer 75% of normal dose
Cl$_{cr}$ <10 mL/minute: Administer 50% of normal dose

Dosing adjustment in hepatic impairment: Use with caution and reduce dose; accumulation of meperidine and its active metabolite (normeperidine) may occur (see Precautions)

Administration

Oral: Administer with water; dilute oral liquid in water prior to use (use 4 oz water for adults)
Parenteral:
SubQ: Suitable for occasional use; when repeated doses are required, the I.M. route of administration is preferred
Slow I.V. push: Do not administer rapid I.V., administer over at least 5 minutes and dilute to ≤10 mg/mL (see Warnings)
Intermittent infusion: Dilute to 1 mg/mL and administer over 15-30 minutes

Monitoring Parameters Respiratory and cardiovascular status; relief of pain, level of sedation

Patient Information Avoid alcohol and the herbal medicine St John's wort. May cause dry mouth. May be habit-forming; avoid abrupt discontinuation after prolonged use. May cause drowsiness and impair ability to perform activities requiring mental alertness or physical coordination. May cause postural hypotension (use caution when changing position from lying or sitting to standing).

Additional Information Equianalgesic doses: morphine 10 mg I.M. = meperidine 75-100 mg I.M.. **Note:** Although meperidine has been used in combination with chlorpromazine and promethazine as a premedication ("Lytic Cocktail"), this combination may have a higher rate of adverse effects compared to alternative sedatives and analgesics (See American Academy of Pediatrics Committee on Drugs, 1995)

◄ **Dosage Forms** Excipient information presented when available (limited, particularly for generics); consult specific product labeling. [DSC] = Discontinued product

Injection, solution, as hydrochloride [ampul]: 25 mg/0.5 mL (0.5 mL); 25 mg/mL (1 mL); 50 mg/mL (1 mL, 1.5 mL, 2 mL); 75 mg/mL (1 mL); 100 mg/mL (1 mL)

Injection, solution, as hydrochloride [prefilled syringe]: 25 mg/mL (1 mL); 50 mg/mL (1 mL); 75 mg/mL (1 mL); 100 mg/mL (1 mL)

Injection, solution, as hydrochloride [for PCA pump]: 10 mg/mL (30 mL, 50 mL [DSC], 60 mL)

Injection, solution, as hydrochloride [vial]: 25 mg/mL (1 mL); 50 mg/mL (1 mL, 30 mL); 75 mg/mL (1 mL) [DSC]; 100 mg/mL (1 mL, 20 mL) [may contain sodium metabisulfite]

Solution, oral, as hydrochloride: 50 mg/5 mL (500 mL)

Tablet, as hydrochloride: 50 mg, 100 mg

Demerol®: 50 mg, 100 mg

References

American Academy of Pediatrics Committee on Drugs, "Reappraisal of Lytic Cocktail/Demerol®, Phenergan®, and Thorazine® (DPT) for the Sedation of Children," *Pediatrics*, 1995, 95(4):598-602.

Carr D, Jacox A, Chapman CR, et al, "Clinical Practice Guideline Number 1: Acute Pain Management: Operative or Medical Procedures and Trauma," Rockville, Maryland: U.S. Department of Health and Human Services, Public Health Service, Agency for Health Care Policy and Research, AHCPR Publication No 92-0032, 1992.

Cole TB, Sprinkle RH, Smith SJ, et al, "Intravenous Narcotic Therapy for Children With Severe Sickle Cell Pain Crisis," *Am J Dis Child*, 1986, 140(12):1255-9.

Institute for Safe Medication Practice, "High Alert Medication Feature: Reducing Patient Harm From Opiates," ISMP Medication Safety Alert, February 22, 2007. Available at http://www.ismp.org/Newsletters/acutecare/articles/20070222.asp.

Jacox A, Carr D, Payne R, et al, "Clinical Practice Guideline Number 9: Management of Cancer Pain," Rockville, Maryland: U.S. Department of Health and Human Services, Public Health Service, Agency for Health Care Policy and Research, AHCPR Publication No. 94-0592, 1994.

Olkkola KT, Hamunen K, and Maunuksela EL, "Clinical Pharmacokinetics and Pharmacodynamics of Opioid Analgesics in Infants and Children," *Clin Pharmacokinet*, 1995, 28(5):385-404.

Pokela ML, Olkkola KT, Koivisto ME, et al, "Pharmacokinetics and Pharmacodynamics of Intravenous Meperidine in Neonates and Infants," *Clin Pharmacol Ther*, 1992, 52(4):342-9.

"Principles of Analgesic Use in the Treatment of Acute Pain and Chronic Cancer Pain," 5th ed, Glenview, IL: American Pain Society, 2003.

♦ **Meperidine Hydrochloride** *see* Meperidine *on page 880*

Mephobarbital (me foe BAR bi tal)

Medication Safety Issues

Sound-alike/look-alike issues:

Mephobarbital may be confused with methocarbamol

Mebaral® may be confused with Medrol®, Mellaril®, Tegretol®

Beers Criteria medication: This drug may be inappropriate for use in geriatric patients (high severity risk).

U.S. Brand Names Mebaral®

Canadian Brand Names Mebaral®

Therapeutic Category Anticonvulsant, Barbiturate; Barbiturate; Sedative

Generic Available No

Use Treatment of generalized tonic-clonic and simple partial seizures

Restrictions C-IV

Pregnancy Risk Factor D

Contraindications Hypersensitivity to mephobarbital or any component; pre-existing CNS depression; respiratory depression; severe uncontrolled pain; history of porphyria

Precautions Use with caution in patients with hepatic or renal impairment or respiratory diseases

Adverse Reactions

Central nervous system: Drowsiness, lethargy, paradoxical excitement (especially in children)

Dermatologic: Rash, including Stevens-Johnson syndrome or erythema multiforme

Gastrointestinal: Nausea, vomiting

Hematologic: Agranulocytosis, thrombocytopenic purpura

Miscellaneous: Psychological and physical dependence

Drug Interactions

Metabolism/Transport Effects Substrate of CYP2B6 (minor), 2C9 (minor), 2C19 (major); **Inhibits** CYP2C19 (weak); **Induces** CYP2A6 (weak)

Avoid Concomitant Use

Avoid concomitant use of Mephobarbital with any of the following: Voriconazole

Increased Effect/Toxicity

Mephobarbital may increase the levels/effects of: Alcohol (Ethyl); CNS Depressants; Meperidine; Thiazide Diuretics

The levels/effects of Mephobarbital may be increased by: Chloramphenicol; CYP2C19 Inhibitors (Moderate); CYP2C19 Inhibitors (Strong); Divalproex; Felbamate; Primidone; Valproic Acid

Decreased Effect

Mephobarbital may decrease the levels/effects of: Acetaminophen; Beta-Blockers; Calcium Channel Blockers; Chloramphenicol; Contraceptives (Estrogens); Contraceptives (Progestins); Corticosteroids (Systemic); CycloSPORINE; CycloSPORINE (Systemic); Disopyramide; Divalproex; Doxycycline; Etoposide; Etoposide Phosphate; Griseofulvin; LamoTRIgine; Methadone; Propafenone; QuiNIDine; Teniposide; Theophylline Derivatives; Tricyclic Antidepressants; Valproic Acid; Vitamin K Antagonists; Voriconazole

The levels/effects of Mephobarbital may be decreased by: CYP2C19 Inducers (Strong); Pyridoxine; Rifamycin Derivatives

Food Interactions High doses of pyridoxine may decrease drug effect; barbiturates may increase the metabolism of vitamin D & K; dietary requirements of vitamin D, K, C, B_{12}, folate and calcium may be increased with long-term use

Mechanism of Action Increases seizure threshold in the motor cortex; depresses monosynaptic and polysynaptic transmission in the CNS; depresses CNS activity by binding to barbiturate site at GABA-receptor complex enhancing GABA activity; depresses reticular activating system; higher doses may be gabamimetic

Pharmacokinetics (Adult data unless noted) Values listed are for mephobarbital; see also Phenobarbital on page 1097

Absorption: Oral: ~50%

Metabolism: In the liver via N-demethylation to phenobarbital

Usual Dosage Epilepsy: Oral:

Children: 4-10 mg/kg/day in 2-4 divided doses

Adults: 200-600 mg/day in 2-4 divided doses

Administration Oral: Administer with water, milk, or juice

Monitoring Parameters Phenobarbital serum concentrations; CBC with differential, platelet count, hepatic and renal function

Reference Range Phenobarbital level should be in the range of 15-40 mcg/mL (SI: 65-172 micromoles/L)

Patient Information May cause drowsiness and impair ability to perform activities requiring mental alertness or physical coordination; avoid alcohol; limit caffeine; may be habit-forming; avoid abrupt discontinuation after prolonged use

Additional Information Sometimes used in specific patients who have excessive sedation or hyperexcitability from phenobarbital

Dosage Forms Excipient information presented when available (limited, particularly for generics); consult specific product labeling.
Tablet: 32 mg, 50 mg, 100 mg

◆ **Mephyton®** see Phytonadione on page 1109

Mepivacaine (me PIV a kane)

Medication Safety Issues
Sound-alike/look-alike issues:
Mepivacaine may be confused with bupivacaine
Polocaine® may be confused with prilocaine

High alert medication: The Institute for Safe Medication Practices (ISMP) includes this medication (epidural administration) among its list of drug classes which have a heightened risk of causing significant patient harm when used in error.

U.S. Brand Names Carbocaine®; Polocaine®; Polocaine® Dental; Polocaine® MPF; Scandonest® 3% Plain

Canadian Brand Names Carbocaine®; Polocaine®

Therapeutic Category Local Anesthetic, Injectable

Generic Available No

Use Local or regional analgesia; anesthesia by local infiltration, peripheral and central neural techniques including epidural and caudal blocks; **not** for use in spinal anesthesia

Pregnancy Risk Factor C

Pregnancy Considerations Animal reproduction studies have not been conducted. Mepivacaine has been used in obstetrical analgesia.

Lactation Excretion in breast milk unknown/use caution

Contraindications Hypersensitivity to mepivacaine, other amide-type local anesthetics, or any component

Warnings Local anesthetics have been associated with rare occurrences of sudden respiratory arrest; convulsions due to systemic toxicity leading to cardiac arrest have been reported presumably due to intravascular injection. A test dose is recommended prior to epidural administration and all reinforcing doses with continuous catheter technique. Do not use solutions containing preservatives for caudal or epidural block. Chondrolysis has been reported following continuous intra-articular infusion; intra-articular administration of local anesthetics is not an FDA-approved route of administration.

Precautions Use with extreme caution as lumbar or caudal anesthesia in patients with existing neurologic disease, spinal deformities, or severe hypertension. Use with caution in patients with cardiac disease, hepatic or renal disease. Use caution in debilitated, elderly, or acutely-ill patients; dose reduction may be required.

Adverse Reactions Degree of adverse effects in the CNS and cardiovascular system is directly related to the blood levels of mepivacaine, route of administration, and physical status of the patient. The effects below are more likely to occur after systemic administration rather than infiltration.

Cardiovascular: Bradycardia, cardiac arrest, cardiac output decreased, heart block, hypertension, hypotension, myocardial depression, syncope, tachycardia, ventricular arrhythmias
Central nervous system: Anxiety, chills, depression, dizziness, excitation, fever, headache, restlessness, seizures, tremors
Dermatologic: Angioneurotic edema, erythema, pruritus, urticaria
Gastrointestinal: Fecal incontinence, nausea, vomiting
Genitourinary: Incontinence, urinary retention
Neuromuscular & skeletal: Chondrolysis (continuous intra-articular administration), paralysis, paresthesia, tremors, weakness

Ocular: Blurred vision, pupil constriction
Otic: Tinnitus
Respiratory: Apnea, hypoventilation, sneezing
Miscellaneous: Allergic reaction, anaphylactoid reaction, diaphoresis

Drug Interactions
Avoid Concomitant Use There are no known interactions where it is recommended to avoid concomitant use.

Increased Effect/Toxicity
The levels/effects of Mepivacaine may be increased by: Beta-Blockers

Decreased Effect There are no known significant interactions involving a decrease in effect.

Stability Store at controlled room temperature of 15°C to 30°C (59°F to 86°F). Brief exposure up to 40°C (104°F) does not adversely affect the product. Solutions may be sterilized.

Mechanism of Action Blocks both the initiation and conduction of nerve impulses by decreasing the neuronal membrane's permeability to sodium ions, which results in inhibition of depolarization with resultant blockade of conduction

Pharmacodynamics Route and dose dependent:
Onset of action: Range: 3-20 minutes
Duration: 2-2.5 hours

Pharmacokinetics (Adult data unless noted)
Protein binding: ~75%
Metabolism: Primarily hepatic via N-demethylation, hydroxylation, and glucuronidation
Half-life:
Neonates: 8.7-9 hours
Adults: 1.9-3 hours
Elimination: Urine (95% as metabolites)

Usual Dosage Injectable local anesthetic: Dose varies with procedure, degree of anesthesia needed, vascularity of tissue, duration of anesthesia required, and physical condition of patient. The smaller dose/concentration (0.5%) will produce more superficial blockade, a higher dose (1%) will block sensory and sympathetic conduction without loss of motor function, a higher dose (1.5%) will provide extensive and often complete motor blockade, and 2% will produce complete sensory and motor blockade. The smallest dose and concentration required to produce the desired effect should be used.

Children: Maximum dose: 5-6 mg/kg; only concentrations <2% should be used in children <3 years or <14 kg (30 lbs)
Adults: Maximum dose: 400 mg; do not exceed 1000 mg/24 hours
Cervical, brachial, intercostal, pudendal nerve block: 5-40 mL of a 1% solution (maximum: 400 mg) **or** 5-20 mL of a 2% solution (maximum: 400 mg). For pudendal block: Inject ¹/₂ the total dose each side.
Transvaginal block (paracervical plus pudendal): Up to 30 mL (both sides) of a 1% solution (maximum: 300 mg). Inject ¹/₂ the total dose into each side.
Paracervical block: Up to 20 mL (both sides) of a 1% solution (maximum: 200 mg). Inject ¹/₂ the total dose into each side. This is the maximum recommended dose per 90-minute procedure; inject slowly with 5 minutes between sides.
Caudal and epidural block (**preservative free solutions only**): 15-30 mL of a 1% solution (maximum: 300 mg) **or** 10-25 mL of a 1.5% solution (maximum: 375 mg) **or** 10-20 mL of a 2% solution (maximum: 400 mg)
Infiltration: Up to 40 mL of a 1% solution (maximum: 400 mg)
Therapeutic block (pain management): 1-5 mL of a 1% solution (maximum: 50 mg) **or** 1-5 mL of a 2% solution (maximum: 100 mg)

◀ **Administration** Parenteral: Administer in small incremental doses; when using continuous intermittent catheter techniques, use frequent aspirations before and during the injection to avoid intravascular injection

Monitoring Parameters
Blood pressure, heart rate, respiration, signs of CNS toxicity (lightheadedness, dizziness, tinnitus, restlessness, tremors, twitching, drowsiness, circumoral paresthesia)

Patient Information You will experience decreased sensation to pain, heat, or cold in the area and/or decreased muscle strength (depending on area of application) until effects wear off; use necessary caution to reduce incidence of possible injury until full sensation returns. Report irritation, pain, burning at injection site; chest pain or palpitations; or respiratory difficulty.

Oral injection: This will cause numbness of your mouth. Do not eat or drink for 1 hour after use. Take small sips of water at first to ensure that you can swallow without difficulty. Your tongue and/or mouth may be numb, use caution to avoid biting yourself. Report irritation, pain, burning at injection site; chest pain or palpitations; or respiratory difficulty.

Dosage Forms Excipient information presented when available (limited, particularly for generics); consult specific product labeling. [DSC] = Discontinued product

Injection, solution, as hydrochloride:
 Carbocaine®: 1% (50 mL); 2% (50 mL) [contains methylparaben]
 Polocaine®: 1% (50 mL); 2% (50 mL) [contains methylparaben]
Injection, solution, as hydrochloride [for dental use]: 3% (1.8 mL)
 Carbocaine®: 3% (1.7 mL)
 Polocaine® Dental: 3% (1.7 mL, 1.8 mL [DSC])
 Scandonest® 3% Plain: 3% (1.7 mL)
Injection, solution, as hydrochloride [preservative free]:
 Carbocaine®: 1% (30 mL); 1.5% (30 mL); 2% (20 mL)
 Polocaine® MPF: 1% (30 mL); 1.5% (30 mL); 2% (20 mL)

References
Dodson WE, Hillman RE, and Hillman LS, "Brain Tissue Levels in a Fatal Case of Neonatal Mepivacaine (Carbocaine®) Poisoning," *J Pediatr*, 1975, 86(4):624-7.
Torres MJ, Garcia JJ, del Cano Moratinos AM, et al, "Fixed Drug Eruption Induced by Mepivacaine," *J Allergy Clin Immunol*, 1995, 96 (1):130-1.

◆ **Mepivacaine Hydrochloride** *see* Mepivacaine *on page 883*

◆ **Mepron®** *see* Atovaquone *on page 153*

◆ **Mercaptoethane Sulfonate** *see* Mesna *on page 888*

Mercaptopurine (mer kap toe PYOOR een)

Medication Safety Issues
Sound-alike/look-alike issues:
Mercaptopurine may be confused with methotrexate
Purinethol® may be confused with propylthiouracil

High alert medication: The Institute for Safe Medication Practices (ISMP) includes this medication among its list of drugs which have a heightened risk of causing significant patient harm when used in error.

To avoid potentially serious dosage errors, the terms "6-mercaptopurine" or "6-MP" should be avoided; use of these terms has been associated with sixfold overdosages.

Azathioprine is metabolized to mercaptopurine; concurrent use of these commercially-available products has resulted in profound myelosuppression.

Related Information
Emetogenic Potential of Antineoplastic Agents *on page 1579*

U.S. Brand Names Purinethol®
Canadian Brand Names Purinethol®
Therapeutic Category Antineoplastic Agent, Antimetabolite; Antineoplastic Agent, Purine
Generic Available Yes
Use Use in conjunction with methotrexate for maintenance therapy in childhood ALL; use in combination regimens for the treatment of AML, CML; non-Hodgkin's lymphoma
Pregnancy Risk Factor D
Lactation Enters breast milk/contraindicated
Contraindications Hypersensitivity to mercaptopurine or any component; severe liver disease; severe bone marrow suppression; patients whose disease showed prior resistance to mercaptopurine or thioguanine
Warnings Hazardous agent; use appropriate precautions for handling and disposal; mercaptopurine may cause birth defects; potentially carcinogenic

Avoid using the terms "6-mercaptopurine" or "6-MP" which have been associated with medication errors resulting in sixfold overdosages.

Precautions Use with caution and adjust dosage in patients with renal impairment or hepatic failure; patients who receive allopurinol concurrently should have the mercaptopurine dose reduced by 66% to 75%
Adverse Reactions
Central nervous system: Drug fever
Dermatologic: Rash, hyperpigmentation, alopecia
Endocrine & metabolic: Hyperuricemia
Gastrointestinal: Mild nausea or vomiting, diarrhea, stomatitis, anorexia
Genitourinary: Oligospermia
Hematologic: Myelosuppression (leukopenia, thrombocytopenia, anemia), eosinophilia
Hepatic: Hepatotoxicity, hyperbilirubinemia, jaundice, elevation of liver enzymes
Renal: Renal toxicity (oliguria, hematuria)
Drug Interactions
Avoid Concomitant Use
Avoid concomitant use of Mercaptopurine with any of the following: BCG; Febuxostat; Natalizumab; Pimecrolimus; Tacrolimus (Topical); Vaccines (Live)
Increased Effect/Toxicity
Mercaptopurine may increase the levels/effects of: Leflunomide; Natalizumab; Vaccines (Live); Vitamin K Antagonists

The levels/effects of Mercaptopurine may be increased by: 5-ASA Derivatives; Allopurinol; AzaTHIOprine; Denosumab; Febuxostat; Pimecrolimus; Tacrolimus (Topical); Trastuzumab
Decreased Effect
Mercaptopurine may decrease the levels/effects of: BCG; Sipuleucel-T; Vaccines (Inactivated); Vaccines (Live); Vitamin K Antagonists

The levels/effects of Mercaptopurine may be decreased by: Echinacea
Food Interactions Food decreases bioavailability
Stability Intact vials and tablets should be stored at room temperature and protected from light; reconstitute 500 mg vial with 49.8 mL SWI; the 10 mg/mL solution is stable for 24 hours
Mechanism of Action Prodrug incorporated into DNA and RNA; blocks purine synthesis and inhibits DNA and RNA synthesis
Pharmacokinetics (Adult data unless noted)
Absorption: Oral: Variable and incomplete (16% to 50%)
Distribution: Distributed throughout total body water; penetrates into CSF at low concentrations

Protein binding: 19%

Metabolism: Undergoes first-pass metabolism in the GI mucosa and liver; metabolized in the liver to sulfate conjugates, 6-thiouric acid, and other inactive compounds

Bioavailability: Oral: <20% (variable)

Half-life: Age dependent

Children: <60 minutes

Adults: 36-90 minutes

Time to peak serum concentration: Oral: Within 2 hours

Elimination: 20% excreted unchanged in urine

Usual Dosage Refer to individual protocols

Children:

Oral:

Induction: 2.5-5 mg/kg/day given once daily, or 70-100 mg/m^2/day once daily

Maintenance: 1.5-2.5 mg/kg/day given once daily or 50-75 mg/m^2/day once daily

I.V. continuous infusion (investigational; distributed under the auspices of the NCI for authorized studies): 50 mg/m^2/hour for 24-48 hours, or 1000 mg/m^2/day for 24 hours

Adults: Oral:

Induction: 2.5-5 mg/kg/day given once daily, or 80-100 mg/m^2/day given once daily

Maintenance: 1.5-2.5 mg/kg/day given once daily

Dosing adjustment in renal impairment: Children and Adults: Cl$_{cr}$ <50 mL/minute: Administer every 48 hours

Administration

Oral: Do not administer with meals. For pediatric patients with ALL, studies suggest that evening administration may lower the risk of relapse compared to morning administration.

Parenteral: Administer by slow I.V. push over several minutes or by slow I.V. continuous infusion to reduce the incidence of vein irritation; further dilute the 10 mg/mL reconstituted solution in NS or D$_5$W to a final concentration for administration of 1-2 mg/mL

Monitoring Parameters CBC with differential and platelet count, liver function tests, uric acid, urinalysis

Patient Information Report to physician if fever, sore throat, bleeding, bruising, shortness of breath, or painful urination occurs; avoid alcohol

Nursing Implications Avoid extravasation

Additional Information Myelosuppressive effects:

WBC: Moderate

Platelets: Moderate

Onset (days): 7-10

Nadir (days): 14

Recovery (days): 21

Dosage Forms Excipient information presented when available (limited, particularly for generics); consult specific product labeling.

Tablet, oral [scored]: 50 mg

Purinethol®: 50 mg

Extemporaneous Preparations A 50 mg/mL oral suspension can be prepared in a vertical flow hood using a 1:1 mixture of methylcellulose 1% and simple syrup; crush thirty 50 mg tablets into a fine powder in a mortar; add a small amount of methylcellulose and simple syrup mixture to make a uniform paste; mix while adding 1:1 mixture of methylcellulose 1% and simple syrup to a final volume of 30 mL. **Note:** May use ultrasonication dispersal. Preparation is stable for 14 days when stored at room temperature; label "shake well" and "caution chemotherapy"

Nahata MC and Hipple TF, *Pediatric Drug Formulations*, 4th ed, Cincinnati, OH: Harvey Whitney Books, 2000.

References

Zimm S, Ettinger LJ, Holcenberg JS, et al, "Phase I and Clinical Pharmacological Study of Mercaptopurine Administered as a Prolonged Intravenous Infusion," *Cancer Res*, 1985, 45(4):1869-73.

♦ **6-Mercaptopurine (error-prone abbreviation)** *see* Mercaptopurine *on page 884*

♦ **Mercapturic Acid** *see* Acetylcysteine *on page 43*

Meropenem (mer oh PEN em)

Medication Safety Issues

Sound-alike/look-alike issues:

Meropenem may be confused with ertapenem, imipenem, metronidazole.

U.S. Brand Names Merrem® I.V.

Canadian Brand Names Merrem®

Therapeutic Category Antibiotic, Carbapenem

Generic Available No

Use Treatment of multidrug-resistant infection caused by gram-negative and gram-positive aerobic and anaerobic pathogens documented or suspected to be susceptible to meropenem; used in treatment of meningitis (FDA approved in pediatric patients ages ≥3 months), intra-abdominal infections and complicated skin and skin structure infections caused by susceptible *S. aureus, S. pyogenes, S. agalactiae, S. pneumoniae, H. influenzae, N. meningitidis, M. catarrhalis, E. coli, Klebsiella, Enterobacter, Serratia, P. aeruginosa, B. cepacia,* and *B. fragilis* (FDA approved in ages ≥3 months and adults); has been used for treatment of lower respiratory tract infections, acute pulmonary exacerbations in cystic fibrosis, urinary tract infections, empiric treatment of febrile neutropenia, and sepsis

Pregnancy Risk Factor B

Pregnancy Considerations Meropenem is classified as pregnancy category B because no evidence of impaired fertility or fetal harm has been found in animals. Adequate and well-controlled studies have not been conducted in pregnant women and it is not known whether meropenem can cause fetal harm.

Lactation Excretion in breast milk unknown/use caution

Breast-Feeding Considerations It is not known if meropenem is excreted in breast milk. The manufacturer recommends that caution be exercised when administering meropenem to breast-feeding women. Most penicillins and carbapenems are safe for use in breast-feeding. Nondose-related effects could include modification of bowel flora.

Contraindications Hypersensitivity to meropenem, any component, other carbapenems, or in patients who have experienced anaphylactic reactions to beta-lactams

Warnings Serious and occasionally fatal hypersensitivity reactions have been reported in patients receiving beta-lactam therapy; careful inquiry should be made concerning previous hypersensitivity reactions to penicillins, cephalosporins, or other beta-lactams before initiating meropenem. Pseudomembranous colitis has been reported with the use of meropenem; prolonged use may result in superinfection. Seizures and other CNS adverse events have been reported, most commonly in patients with renal impairment and/or underlying neurologic disorders. Valproic acid (VPA) serum concentrations may be significantly decreased by concurrent carbapenem use leading to breakthrough seizures (see Drug Interactions); serum VPA concentrations should be closely monitored after initiation of meropenem. VPA dosage adjustment may not adequately compensate for this interaction. Thrombocytopenia has been reported in patients with renal dysfunction who are receiving meropenem.

Precautions Use with caution in patients with a history of seizures, CNS disease, CNS infection, and/or compromised renal function; dosage adjustment required in patients with renal impairment

Adverse Reactions

Cardiovascular: Hypotension, syncope

Central nervous system: Hallucinations, headache, pain, seizures (<0.38%; see Warnings)

Dermatologic: Pruritus, rash (1.4%)

Gastrointestinal: Constipation, diarrhea (4.3%), GI hemorrhage, leukopenia, melena, nausea, neutropenia, oral moniliasis, pseudomembranous colitis (see Warnings), vomiting (1%)

Hematologic: Anemia, thrombocytopenia (see Warnings)

Local: Pain, edema, and inflammation at the injection site; phlebitis (1.2%)

Respiratory: Apnea

Miscellaneous: Hypersensitivity (see Warnings)

<1%, postmarketing, and/or case reports: Abdominal enlargement, abdominal pain, agitation/delirium, agranulocytosis, alkaline phosphatase increased, ALT increased, angioedema, anemia (hypochromic), anorexia, anxiety, aPTT decreased, asthma, AST increased, back pain, bilirubin increased, bradycardia, BUN increased, cardiac arrest, chest pain, chills, cholestatic jaundice/jaundice, confusion, cough, creatinine increased, depression, diaphoresis, dizziness, dyspepsia, dyspnea, dysuria, eosinophilia, epistaxis, erythema multiforme, fever, flatulence, heart failure, hematuria, hemoglobin/hematocrit decreased, hemolytic anemia, hemoperitoneum, hepatic failure, hypertension, hypervolemia, hypokalemia, hypoxia, ileus, injection pain, injection site edema, insomnia, intestinal obstruction, LDH increased, leukocytosis, leukopenia, MI, nervousness, neutropenia, paresthesia, pelvic pain, peripheral edema, platelets increased, pleural effusion, positive Coomb's test, prothrombin time decreased, pulmonary edema, pulmonary embolism, renal failure, respiratory disorder, skin ulcer, somnolence, Stevens-Johnson syndrome, tachycardia, toxic epidermal necrolysis, urinary incontinence, urticaria, vaginal moniliasis, weakness, WBC decreased, whole body pain

Drug Interactions

Avoid Concomitant Use

Avoid concomitant use of Meropenem with any of the following: BCG; Probenecid

Increased Effect/Toxicity

The levels/effects of Meropenem may be increased by: Probenecid

Decreased Effect

Meropenem may decrease the levels/effects of: BCG; Divalproex; Typhoid Vaccine; Valproic Acid

Stability Store intact vials at 20°C to 25°C (68°F to 77°F); meropenem reconstituted with SWI is stable for up to 2 hours at room temperature or for up to 12 hours when refrigerated; when reconstituted with NS to a final concentration between 2.5-50 mg/mL, the solution is stable for up to 2 hours at room temperature or 18 hours when refrigerated; when reconstituted with D5W to a final concentration between 2.5-50 mg/mL, the solution is stable for up to 1 hour at room temperature or 8 hours when refrigerated; solutions prepared for infusion in plastic I.V. bags with NS at concentrations ranging from 2.5-20 mg/mL are stable for 4 hours at room temperature or 24 hours when refrigerated

Mechanism of Action Inhibits cell wall synthesis by binding to penicillin-binding proteins (PBPs) with its strongest affinities for PBPs 2, 3 and 4 of *E. coli* and *P. aeruginosa* and PBPs 1, 2 and 4 of *S. aureus*

Pharmacokinetics (Adult data unless noted)

Distribution: Penetrates into most tissues and body fluids including CSF, urinary tract, peritoneal fluid, bone, bile, lung, bronchial mucosa, muscle tissue, and heart valves

Protein binding: 2%

Metabolism: 20% is hydrolyzed in plasma to an inactive metabolite

Half-life:

Premature newborns: 3 hours

Full-term newborns: 2 hours

Infants 3 months to 2 years: 1.5 hours

Children 2-12 years and Adults: 1 hour

Time to peak tissue and fluid concentrations: 1 hour after the start of infusion except in bile, lung, muscle, and CSF which peak at 2-3 hours

Elimination: Cleared by the kidney with 70% excreted unchanged in urine

Usual Dosage I.V.:

Neonates:

Postnatal age 0-7 days: 20 mg/kg/dose every 12 hours

Postnatal age >7 days:

Weight 1200-2000 g: 20 mg/kg/dose every 12 hours

Weight ≥2000 g: 20 mg/kg/dose every 8 hours

Children ≥3 months:

Complicated skin and skin structure infection: 10 mg/kg/dose every 8 hours; maximum dose: 500 mg

Intra-abdominal infection: 20 mg/kg/dose every 8 hours; maximum dose: 1000 mg

Meningitis: 40 mg/kg/dose every 8 hours; maximum dose: 2000 mg

Fever/Neutropenia empiric treatment: 20 mg/kg/dose every 8 hours; maximum dose: 1000 mg

Pulmonary exacerbation in patients with cystic fibrosis: 40 mg/kg/dose every 8 hours; maximum dose: 2000 mg

Adults:

Complicated skin and skin structure infection: 500 mg every 8 hours

Intra-abdominal infection: 1000 mg every 8 hours

Fever/Neutropenia empiric treatment: 1000 mg every 8 hours

Meningitis: 2000 mg every 8 hours

Dosage adjustment in renal impairment: Adults:

Cl$_{cr}$ 26-50 mL/minute: Standard dose every 12 hours

Cl$_{cr}$ 10-25 mL/minute: One-half dose every 12 hours

Cl$_{cr}$ <10 mL/minute: One-half dose every 24 hours

Intermittent hemodialysis: Meropenem and its metabolites are dialyzable: Administer standard dose after dialysis

Continuous arteriovenous or venous hemofiltration: Dose as Cl$_{cr}$ 10-50 mL/minute

Administration Administer by I.V. push or I.V. intermittent infusion; infuse I.V. push injection over 3-5 minutes at a final concentration not to exceed 50 mg/mL; intermittent infusion dose should be administered over 15-30 minutes at a final concentration ranging from 1-20 mg/mL in D5W or NS

Monitoring Parameters Periodic renal, hepatic, and hematologic function tests. Observe for changes in bowel frequency.

Test Interactions Positive Coombs' [direct]

Patient Information Inform physician if taking valproic acid or divalproex sodium since an alternative treatment may be needed; inform physician of prolonged diarrhea.

Additional Information Sodium content 1 g: 3.92 mEq

Dosage Forms Excipient information presented when available (limited, particularly for generics); consult specific product labeling.

Injection, powder for reconstitution:

Merrem® I.V: 500 mg [contains sodium 45.1 mg as sodium carbonate (1.96 mEq)]; 1 g [contains sodium 90.2 mg as sodium carbonate (3.92 mEq)]

References

Aronoff GR, Bennett WM, Berns JS, et al, *Drug Prescribing in Renal Failure: Dosing Guidelines for Adults and Children*, 5th ed, Philadelphia, PA: American College of Physicians, 2007, 97, 177.

Blumer JL, Saiman L, Konstan MW, et al, "The Efficacy and Safety of Meropenem and Tobramycin Vs Ceftazidime and Tobramycin in the Treatment of Acute Pulmonary Exacerbations in Patients With Cystic Fibrosis," *Chest*, 2005, 128(4):2336-46.

Blummer JL, "Pharmacokinetic Determinants of Carbapenem Therapy in Neonates and Children," *Pediatr Infect Dis J*, 1996, 15(8):733-7.

Blummer JL, Reed MD, Kearns GL, et al, "Sequential, Single-Dose Pharmacokinetic Evaluation of Meropenem in Hospitalized Infants and Children," *Antimicrob Agents Chemother*, 1995, 39(8):1721-5.

Bradley, JS, "Meropenem: A New, Extremely Broad Spectrum Beta-lactam Antibiotic for Serious Infections in Pediatrics," *Pediatr Infect Dis J*, 1997, 16:263-8.

Latzin P, Fehling M, Bauernfeind A, et al, "Efficacy and Safety of Intravenous Meropenem and Tobramycin Versus Ceftazidime and Tobramycin in Cystic Fibrosis," *J Cyst Fibros*, 2008, 7(2):142-6.

Odio CM, Puig JR, Feris JM, et al, "Prospective, Randomized, Investigator-Blinded Study of the Efficacy and Safety of Meropenem vs. Cefotaxime Therapy in Bacterial Meningitis in Children. Meropenem Meningitis Study Group," *Pediatr Infect Dis J*, 1999, 18(7):581-90.

Ververs TF, van Dijk A, Vinks SA, et al, "Pharmacokinetics and Dosing Regimen of Meropenem in Critically Ill Patients Receiving Continuous Venovenous Hemofiltration," *Crit Care Med*, 2000, 28(10):3412-6.

Wiseman LR, Wagstaff AJ, Brogden RN, et al, "Meropenem. A Review of its Antibacterial Activity, Pharmacokinetic Properties and Clinical Efficacy," *Drugs*, 1995, 50(1):73-101.

Yildirim I, Aytac S, Ceyhan M, et al, "Piperacillin/Tazobactam Plus Amikacin Versus Carbapenem Monotherapy as Empirical Treatment of Febrile Neutropenia in Childhood Hematological Malignancies," *Pediatr Hematol Oncol*, 2008, 25(4):291-9.

♦ **Merrem® (Can)** *see* Meropenem *on page 885*

♦ **Merrem® I.V.** *see* Meropenem *on page 885*

♦ **Meruvax® II [DSC]** *see* Rubella Virus Vaccine (Live) *on page 1238*

Mesalamine (me SAL a meen)

Medication Safety Issues
Sound-alike/look-alike issues:
Mesalamine may be confused with mecamylamine, megestrol, memantine, metaxalone, methenamine
Apriso™ may be confused with Apri®
Asacol® may be confused with Ansaid®, Os-Cal®, Visicol®
Lialda™ may be confused with Aldara®
Pentasa® may be confused with Pancrease®, Pangestyme™

U.S. Brand Names Apriso™; Asacol®; Asacol® HD; Canasa®; Lialda™; Pentasa®; Rowasa®; sfRowasa™

Canadian Brand Names Asacol®; Asacol® 800; Mesasal®; Mezavant®; Novo-5 ASA; Pentasa®; Salofalk®

Therapeutic Category 5-Aminosalicylic Acid Derivative; Anti-inflammatory Agent; Anti-inflammatory Agent, Rectal

Generic Available Yes: Rectal suspension

Use Treatment of ulcerative colitis (UC), proctosigmoiditis, and proctitis

Pregnancy Risk Factor B

Pregnancy Considerations Animal studies have not demonstrated teratogenicity or fertility impairment. There are no adequate and well-controlled studies in pregnant women. Mesalamine is known to cross the placenta.

Lactation Enters breast milk/use caution

Breast-Feeding Considerations Adverse effects (diarrhea) in a nursing infant have been reported while the mother received rectal administration of mesalamine within 12 hours after the first dose. The AAP recommends to monitor the infant stool for consistency and to use with caution. Low concentrations of the parent drug and higher concentrations of the N-acetyl metabolite of the parent drug have been detected in human breast milk.

Contraindications Hypersensitivity to mesalamine, aminosalicylates, salicylates, or any component (see Warnings); Canasa™ suppositories contain saturated vegetable fatty acid esters (contraindicated in patients with allergy to these components)

Warnings Myocarditis and pericarditis should be considered in patients with chest pain; this cardiac hypersensitivity reaction has occurred rarely with mesalamine-containing products; pancreatitis should be considered in any patient with new abdominal complaints; has been implicated in the production of an acute intolerance

syndrome or exacerbation of colitis (<3%), prompt discontinuation is required if this develops.

Some products may contain sulfites which may cause allergic reactions in susceptible individuals. Apriso™ contains phenylalanine. Rowasa® suspension contains sodium benzoate; benzoic acid (benzoate) is a metabolite of benzyl alcohol; large amounts of benzyl alcohol (≥99 mg/kg/day) have been associated with a potentially fatal toxicity ("gasping syndrome") in neonates; *in vitro* and animal studies have shown that benzoate displaces bilirubin from protein binding sites; avoid use of Rowasa® suspension in neonates.

Precautions Some capsules contain phenylalanine which must be avoided in patients with phenylketonuria. Use with caution in patients with hypersensitivity to sulfasalazines or patients with renal or hepatic impairment and patients with conditions predisposing to the development of myocarditis or pericarditis; use delayed release formulations with caution in patients with pyloric stenosis due to prolonged gastric retention; Asacol® HD 800 mg tablet has not been shown to be bioequivalent to two Asacol® 400 mg tablets.

Adverse Reactions
Cardiovascular: Chest pain, edema, myocarditis, pericarditis, T-wave abnormalities

Central nervous system: Anxiety, chills, depression, dizziness, fatigue, fever, headache, insomnia, malaise, somnolence, vertigo

Dermatologic: Acne, alopecia, dry skin, erythema nodosum, lichen planus, photosensitivity, prurigo, psoriasis, pyoderma gangrenosum, rash, urticaria

Endocrine & metabolic: Amenorrhea, breast pain, menorrhagia, triglycerides increased

Gastrointestinal: Abdominal pain, anal irritation, anorexia, bloody diarrhea, constipation, cramps, discoloration of urine (yellow-brown), dysgeusia, dyspepsia, eructation, exacerbation of colitis (see Warnings), flatulence, gastritis, hemorrhoids, nausea, pancreatitis, pharyngolaryngeal pain, vomiting

Genitourinary: Dysuria, epididymitis

Hematologic: Rare: Agranulocytosis, thrombocytopenia, eosinophilia, aplastic anemia, hemoglobin/hematocrit decreased

Hepatic: Cholestatic jaundice, jaundice, liver enzymes elevated liver necrosis/failure

Neuromuscular & skeletal: Arthralgia, arthritis, myalgia, tremor, weakness

Ocular: Conjunctivitis

Otic: Ear pain, tinnitus

Renal: Creatinine clearance decreased, hematuria, interstitial nephritis, nephrotic syndrome, renal papillary necrosis

Respiratory: Asthma exacerbation, dyspnea, fibrosing alveolitis, interstitial pneumonitis, pharyngitis, pleuritis, pulmonary infiltrates, sinusitis

Miscellaneous: Intolerance syndrome, Kawasaki-like syndrome, lupus-like syndrome

Drug Interactions
Avoid Concomitant Use There are no known interactions where it is recommended to avoid concomitant use.

Increased Effect/Toxicity
Mesalamine may increase the levels/effects of: Heparin; Heparin (Low Molecular Weight); Thiopurine Analogs; Varicella Virus-Containing Vaccines

Decreased Effect
Mesalamine may decrease the levels/effects of: Cardiac Glycosides

The levels/effects of Mesalamine may be decreased by: Antacids; H2-Antagonists; Proton Pump Inhibitors

Stability Store tablets and capsules at room temperature; unstable in presence of water or light; once foil has been removed, unopened bottles have an expiration of 1 year following the date of manufacture; store suppositories at room temperature; do not refrigerate

Mechanism of Action Mesalamine (5-aminosalicylic acid) is the active component of sulfasalazine; the specific mechanism of action of mesalamine is unknown; however, it is thought that it modulates local chemical mediators of the inflammatory response, especially leukotrienes; action appears topical rather than systemic

Pharmacokinetics (Adult data unless noted)

Absorption:
Capsule: 20% to 30%
Rectal: ~15%; variable and dependent upon retention time, underlying GI disease, and colonic pH
Tablet: 20% to 28%

Distribution: Breast milk to plasma ratio:
5-ASA: 0.27
Acetyl 5-ASA: 5.1

Protein binding: 43%

Metabolism: In the liver by acetylation to acetyl-5-amino-salicylic acid (acetyl-5-ASA, an active metabolite) and to glucuronide conjugates; intestinal metabolism may also occur

Half-life:
5-ASA: 0.5-15 hours
Acetyl 5-ASA: 5-10 hours

Time to peak serum concentration: Capsule: Apriso™: ~4 hours; Pentasa®: 3 hours; rectal: Within 4-7 hours; delayed release tablet: Asacol®: 4-12 hours; Asacol® HD: 10-16 hours; Lialda™: 9-12 hours (average)

Elimination: Most metabolites are excreted in urine with <2% appearing in feces

Usual Dosage Oral (usual course of therapy is 3-6 weeks):
(Oral products are formulated to slowly release therapeutic quantities of drug throughout the GI tract):
Capsule (ethylcellulose-coated, controlled release):
Children: 50 mg/kg/day divided every 6-12 hours
Adults: 1 g 4 times/day for up to 8 weeks
Capsule (enteric coating in polymer matrix, extended release): Adults: 1.5 g once daily in the morning
Tablet (coated with acrylic-based resin; drug released after reaches terminal ileum):
Children: 50 mg/kg/day divided every 8-12 hours
Adults: Treatment:
Asacol®: 800 mg 3 times/day for 6 weeks; maintenance for remission of UC: 1.6 g daily in divided doses up to 6 months
Asacol® HD: 1.6 g 3 times/day for 6 weeks
Lialda™: 2.4-4.8 g once daily for up to 8 weeks
Retention enema: Adults: 60 mL (4 g) at bedtime, retained overnight, approximately 8 hours for 3-6 weeks
Rectal suppository: Adults: Insert 1 suppository (500 mg) in rectum twice daily or 1 suppository (1000 mg) in rectum once daily at bedtime, for 3-6 weeks; may increase to 3 times daily (500 mg only) if ineffective response noted after 2 weeks of therapy

Administration

Oral: Administer with food; swallow tablets or capsules whole, do not chew or crush; do not break outer coating of Asacol®, Asacol® HD, or Lialda™ tablets; Apriso™: Do not administer concurrently with antacids

Rectal: Retain enema for 8 hours or as long as practical; shake rectal suspension well before use; retain suppository for 1-3 hours

Patient Information May discolor urine yellow-brown. May rarely cause photosensitivity reactions (eg, exposure to sunlight may cause severe sunburn, skin rash, redness, or itching); avoid direct exposure to sunlight. Suppositories will cause staining of direct contact surfaces including fabrics.

Dosage Forms Excipient information presented when available (limited, particularly for generics); consult specific product labeling. [CAN] = Canadian brand name

Capsule, controlled release:
Pentasa®: 250 mg, 500 mg
Capsule, delayed and extended release:
Apriso™: 0.375 g [contains phenylalanine 0.56 mg/capsule]
Suppository, rectal:
Canasa®: 1000 mg [contains saturated vegetable fatty acid esters]
Suspension, rectal: 4 g/60 mL (7s, 28s) [contains potassium metabisulfite and sodium benzoate]
Rowasa®: 4 g/60 mL (7s, 28s) [contains potassium metabisulfite and sodium benzoate; packaged as kit with wipes]
sfRowasa™: 4 g/60 mL (7s, 28s) [contains sodium benzoate]
Tablet, delayed release [enteric coated]:
Asacol®: 400 mg
Asacol® HD: 800 mg
Lialda™: 1.2 g
Tablet, delayed and extended release:
Mezavant® [CAN]: 1.2 g [not available in U.S.]

References

Grand RJ, Ramakrishna J, and Calenda KA, "Inflammatory Bowel Disease in the Pediatric Patient," *Gastroenterol Clin North Am,* 1995, 24(3):613-32.

♦ **Mesalazine** *see* Mesalamine *on page 887*

♦ **Mesasal® (Can)** *see* Mesalamine *on page 887*

♦ **M-Eslon® (Can)** *see* Morphine Sulfate *on page 946*

Mesna (MES na)

Related Information
Compatibility of Chemotherapy and Related Supportive Care Medications *on page 1580*

U.S. Brand Names Mesnex®

Canadian Brand Names Mesnex®; Uromitexan

Therapeutic Category Antidote, Cyclophosphamide-induced Hemorrhagic Cystitis; Antidote, Ifosfamide-induced Hemorrhagic Cystitis

Generic Available Yes: Solution for injection

Use Detoxifying agent used as a protectant against hemorrhagic cystitis induced by ifosfamide and cyclophosphamide [FDA approved in pediatrics (age not specified) and adults]

Pregnancy Risk Factor B

Pregnancy Considerations Teratogenic effects were not observed in animal studies. There are no adequate and well-controlled studies in pregnant women. Use during pregnancy only if clearly needed.

Lactation Excretion in breast milk unknown/not recommended

Breast-Feeding Considerations Due to the potential for adverse reactions in the nursing infant, breast-feeding is not recommended.

Contraindications Hypersensitivity to mesna, other thiol compounds, or any component (see Warnings)

Warnings Mesna injection contains benzyl alcohol which may cause allergic reactions in susceptible individuals; large amounts of benzyl alcohol (≥99 mg/kg/day) have been associated with a potentially fatal toxicity ("gasping syndrome") in neonates; the "gasping syndrome" consists of metabolic acidosis, respiratory distress, gasping respirations, CNS dysfunction (including convulsions, intracranial hemorrhage), hypotension and cardiovascular collapse; avoid use of mesna products containing benzyl alcohol in children <2 years of age; *in vitro* and animal studies have shown that benzoate, a metabolite of benzyl alcohol, displaces bilirubin from protein binding sites.

Allergic reactions have been reported; symptoms ranged from mild hypersensitivity to systemic anaphylactic reactions and may include fever, hypotension, and/or tachycardia; patients with autoimmune disorders receiving cyclophosphamide and mesna may be at increased risk.

Precautions Examine morning urine specimen for hematuria prior to ifosfamide or cyclophosphamide treatment; if hematuria develops, reduce the ifosfamide/cyclophosphamide dose or discontinue the drug and consider increasing the mesna dosage. Mesna will not prevent or alleviate other toxicities associated with ifosfamide or cyclophosphamide and will not prevent hemorrhagic cystitis in all patients. Mesna will not reduce the risk of thrombocytopenia-related hematuria. Patients should receive adequate hydration during treatment.

Adverse Reactions

Cardiovascular: Flushing, hypotension, tachycardia (see Warnings)

Central nervous system: Dizziness, fever, headache, hyperesthesia, somnolence

Dermatologic: Skin rash

Gastrointestinal: Anorexia, constipation, diarrhea, dysgeusia (with oral administration), flatulence, nausea, vomiting

Neuromuscular & skeletal: Arthralgia, back pain, rigors

Ocular: Conjunctivitis

Respiratory: Cough, pharyngitis, rhinitis

Miscellaneous: Allergic reaction, anaphylactic reaction, or hypersensitivity (see Warnings); flu-like symptoms

<1%, postmarketing, and/or case reports: Hypertension, injection site erythema, injection site pain, limb pain, malaise, myalgia, platelets decreased, ST-segment increased, tachypnea, transaminases increased

Drug Interactions

Avoid Concomitant Use There are no known interactions where it is recommended to avoid concomitant use.

Increased Effect/Toxicity There are no known significant interactions involving an increase in effect.

Decreased Effect There are no known significant interactions involving a decrease in effect.

Stability Store intact vials and tablets at room temperature of 20°C to 25°C (68°F to 77°F). Opened multidose vials may be stored and used for up to 8 days after opening. Diluted solutions in D_5W, D_5/NS, NS, or LR are chemically and physically stable for 48 hours at room temperature (the manufacturer recommends a final concentration of 20 mg/mL); compatible with solutions containing ifosfamide or cyclophosphamide (variable based on concentration, pH, and storage temperature); incompatible with cisplatin. Solutions of mesna (0.5-3.2 mg/mL) and cyclophosphamide (1.8-10.8 mg/mL) in D_5W are stable for 48 hours refrigerated or 6 hours at room temperature (Menard, 2003).

Mechanism of Action In the urinary bladder, mesna binds with and detoxifies acrolein and other urotoxic metabolites of ifosfamide and cyclophosphamide via an active sulfhydryl group on mesna

Pharmacokinetics (Adult data unless noted)

Distribution: No tissue penetration; following glomerular filtration, mesna disulfide is reduced in the renal tubules back to mesna and delivered to the bladder in the active form

Protein binding: 69% to 75%

Bioavailability: Oral: 50%

Half-life: 22 minutes (mesna); after I.V. administration, mesna is rapidly oxidized intravascularly to mesna disulfide (half-life: 70 minutes). I.V. followed by oral therapy has a half-life of 1-8 hours.

Elimination: Unchanged drug and metabolite are excreted primarily in the urine; time for maximum urinary mesna excretion: 1 hour after I.V. and 2-3 hours after an oral mesna dose

Usual Dosage Note: Mesna dosing schedule should be repeated each day ifosfamide is received. If ifosfamide dose is adjusted, the mesna dose should also be modified to maintain the mesna-to-ifosfamide ratio. Children and Adults (refer to individual protocols): **Mesna dose depends on dose of antineoplastic agent used:**

Short infusion standard-dose ifosfamide (<2.5 g/m^2/day): Mesna dose is equal to 60% of the ifosfamide dose given in 3 divided doses (0, 4, and 8 hours after the start of ifosfamide)

Continuous infusion standard-dose ifosfamide (<2.5 g/m^2/day): ASCO Guidelines: Mesna dose (as an I.V. bolus) is equal to 20% of the ifosfamide dose, followed by a continuous infusion of mesna at 40% of the ifosfamide dose; continue mesna infusion for 12-24 hours after completion of ifosfamide infusion (Hensley, 2009)

High-dose ifosfamide (>2.5 g/m^2/day): ASCO Guidelines: Evidence for use is inadequate; more frequent and prolonged mesna administration regimens may be required

I.V. followed by Oral (for ifosfamide doses ≤2 g/m^2/day): Mesna dose is equal to 100% of the ifosfamide dose, given as 20% of the ifosfamide dose I.V. at hour 0, followed by 40% of the ifosfamide dose given orally 2 and 6 hours after start of ifosfamide

When used with ifosfamide: I.V.: Mesna dose is 20% w/w of ifosfamide dose 15 minutes before and 4 and 8 hours later or combined with ifosfamide administration; for high-dose ifosfamide, mesna has been administered at a dose of 20% w/w 15 minutes before and every 3 hours for 3-6 doses or combined with ifosfamide administration; (**Note:** In clinical protocols, total daily mesna dose ranged between 60% to 160% w/w of the daily ifosfamide dose)

When used with cyclophosphamide: I.V.: Mesna dose is 20% w/w of cyclophosphamide dose 15 minutes before and every 3 hours for 3-4 doses or combined with cyclophosphamide administration; (**Note:** In clinical protocols, total daily mesna dose ranged between 60% to 160% w/w of the daily cyclophosphamide dose)

I.V. continuous infusion: Mesna doses equivalent to 60% to 100% of the ifosfamide or cyclophosphamide dose have been used

Oral: Mesna dose is 40% w/w of the antineoplastic agent dose in 3 doses at 4-hour intervals or 20 mg/kg/dose every 4 hours x 3 (oral mesna is not recommended for the first dose before ifosfamide or cyclophosphamide)

Administration

Oral: Administer orally in tablet form or dilute mesna injection solution for oral use before oral administration to decrease sulfur odor; mesna can be diluted 1:1 to 1:10 in carbonated cola drinks, fruit juices (grape, apple, tomato, and orange juice), or in plain or chocolate milk (most palatable in chilled grape juice). Patients who vomit within 2 hours after taking oral mesna should repeat the dose or receive I.V. mesna.

Parenteral: Administer by I.V. infusion over 15-30 minutes, or by continuous I.V. infusion (maintain continuous infusion for 12-24 after completion of ifosfamide infusion), or per protocol; mesna may be diluted in D_5W or NS to a final concentration of 1-20 mg/mL; may be added to solutions containing ifosfamide or cyclophosphamide

Monitoring Parameters Urinalysis

Test Interactions False-positive urinary ketones with Chemstrip®, Multistix®, or Labstix®

Nursing Implications Used concurrently with and/or following high-dose ifosfamide or cyclophosphamide; ensure adequate patient hydration; report vomiting within 1 hour of an oral mesna dose to physician so that I.V. mesna can be administered

Additional Information pH of the commercial 100 mg/mL solution: 6.5-8.5. A preservative free formulation of Mesnex® injection may be obtained directly from the manufacturer. It is restricted for use in children <2 years and others who are sensitive to benzyl alcohol. Contact Bristol-Myers Squibb Company at 800-437-0994 for additional information.

Dosage Forms Excipient information presented when available (limited, particularly for generics); consult specific product labeling.

Injection, solution: 100 mg/mL (10 mL) [contains benzyl alcohol]

Mesnex®: 100 mg/mL (10 mL) [contains benzyl alcohol]

Tablet:

Mesnex®: 400 mg

References

Ben Yehuda A, Heyman A and Steiner Salz D, "False Positive Reaction for Urinary Ketones With Mesna," *Drug Intell Clin Pharm*, 1987, 21(6): 547-8.

Brock N and Pohl J, "The Development of Mesna for Regional Detoxification," *Cancer Treat Rev*, 1983, 10(Suppl A):33-43.

"Cancer Chemotherapy," *Med Lett Drugs Ther*, 1989, 31(793):49-56.

Hensley ML, Hagerty KL, Kewalramani T, et al, "American Society of Clinical Oncology 2008 Clinical Practice Guideline Update: Use of Chemotherapy and Radiation Therapy Protectants," *J Clin Oncol*, 2009, 27(1):127-45.

Khaw SL, Downie PA, Waters KD, et al, "Adverse Hypersensitivity Reactions to Mesna as Adjunctive Therapy for Cyclophosphamide," *Pediatr Blood Cancer*, 2007, 49(3):341-3.

Menard C, Bourguignon C, Schlatter J, et al, "Stability of Cyclophosphamide and Mesna Admixtures in Polyethylene Infusion Bags," *Ann Pharmacother*, 2003, 37(12):1789-92.

Schoenike SE and Dana WJ, "Ifosfamide and Mesna," *Clin Pharm*, 1990, 9(3):179-91.

Schuchter LM, Hensley ML, Meropol NJ, et al, "2002 Update of Recommendations for the Use of Chemotherapy and Radiotherapy Protectants: Clinical Practice Guidelines of the American Society of Clinical Oncology," *J Clin Oncol*, 2002, 20(12):2895-903.

♦ **Mesnex®** *see* Mesna *on page 888*

♦ **Mestinon®** *see* Pyridostigmine *on page 1189*

♦ **Mestinon®-SR (Can)** *see* Pyridostigmine *on page 1189*

♦ **Mestinon® Timespan®** *see* Pyridostigmine *on page 1189*

♦ **Metacortandralone** *see* PrednisoLONE *on page 1148*

♦ **Metadate CD®** *see* Methylphenidate *on page 908*

♦ **Metadate® ER** *see* Methylphenidate *on page 908*

♦ **Metadol™ (Can)** *see* Methadone *on page 893*

♦ **Metadol-D™ (Can)** *see* Methadone *on page 893*

♦ **Metamucil® [OTC]** *see* Psyllium *on page 1185*

♦ **Metamucil® (Can)** *see* Psyllium *on page 1185*

♦ **Metamucil® Plus Calcium [OTC]** *see* Psyllium *on page 1185*

♦ **Metamucil® Smooth Texture [OTC]** *see* Psyllium *on page 1185*

Metaproterenol (met a proe TER e nol)

Medication Safety Issues

Sound-alike/look-alike issues:

Metaproterenol may be confused with metipranolol, metoprolol

Alupent® may be confused with Atrovent®

Related Information

Asthma *on page 1697*

U.S. Brand Names Alupent® [DSC]

Canadian Brand Names Apo-Orciprenaline®; ratio-Orciprenaline®; Tanta-Orciprenaline®

Therapeutic Category Adrenergic Agonist Agent; Antiasthmatic; Beta$_2$-Adrenergic Agonist Agent; Bronchodilator; Sympathomimetic

Generic Available Yes: Excludes inhaler

Use Bronchodilator in reversible airway obstruction due to asthma or COPD

Pregnancy Risk Factor C

Pregnancy Considerations No data on crossing the placenta. Reported association with polydactyly in 1 study; may be secondary to severe maternal disease or chance.

Lactation Excretion in breast milk unknown

Breast-Feeding Considerations No data on crossing into breast milk or clinical effects on the infant.

Contraindications Hypersensitivity to metaproterenol or any component; pre-existing cardiac arrhythmias associated with tachycardia; narrow-angle glaucoma

Warnings Excessive use may result in cardiac arrest and death; do not use concurrently with other sympathomimetic bronchodilators. Some products contain sodium benzoate; benzoic acid (benzoate) is a metabolite of benzyl alcohol; large amounts of benzyl alcohol (≥99 mg/kg/day) have been associated with a potentially fatal toxicity ("gasping syndrome") in neonates; *in vitro* and animal studies have shown that benzoate displaces bilirubin from protein binding sites; avoid use of sodium benzoate containing products in neonates.

Precautions Use with caution in patients with ischemic heart disease, hypertension, hyperthyroidism, seizure disorders, CHF, cardiac arrhythmias, and diabetes mellitus

Adverse Reactions

Cardiovascular: Tachycardia, palpitations, hypertension

Central nervous system: Nervousness, dizziness, headache, fatigue, vertigo

Gastrointestinal: Nausea, vomiting, diarrhea, GI distress, xerostomia, dysgeusia, throat irritation

Neuromuscular & skeletal: Tremor, weakness, muscle cramps

Respiratory: Exacerbation of asthma, hoarseness, cough, nasal congestion

Drug Interactions

Avoid Concomitant Use

Avoid concomitant use of Metaproterenol with any of the following: Iobenguane I 123

Increased Effect/Toxicity

Metaproterenol may increase the levels/effects of: Sympathomimetics

The levels/effects of Metaproterenol may be increased by: Atomoxetine; Cannabinoids; MAO Inhibitors; Tricyclic Antidepressants

Decreased Effect

Metaproterenol may decrease the levels/effects of: Iobenguane I 123

The levels/effects of Metaproterenol may be decreased by: Alpha-/Beta-Blockers; Beta-Blockers (Beta1 Selective); Beta-Blockers (Nonselective); Betahistine

Stability Protect from light

Mechanism of Action Relaxes bronchial smooth muscle and peripheral vasculature by action on beta$_2$-receptors

Pharmacodynamics

Onset of bronchodilation:

Oral: Within 30 minutes

Inhalation: Within 60 seconds

Maximum effect: Oral: Within 1 hour

Duration: (approximately 1-5 hours) regardless of route administered

Pharmacokinetics (Adult data unless noted)

Absorption: Oral: Well absorbed

Metabolism: Extensive first-pass in the liver (~40% of oral dose is available)

Elimination: Mainly as glucuronic acid conjugates

Usual Dosage

Oral:

Children:

<2 years: 0.4 mg/kg/dose given 3-4 times/day; in infants, the dose can be given every 8-12 hours

2-6 years: 1.3-2.6 mg/kg/day divided every 6-8 hours

6-9 years: 10 mg/dose given 3-4 times/day

Children >9 years and Adults: 20 mg/dose given 3-4 times/day

Inhalation: Children >12 years and Adults: 2-3 inhalations every 3-4 hours, up to 12 inhalations in 24 hours

Nebulizer:

Infants and Children: 0.01-0.02 mL/kg (0.5-1 mg/kg) of 5% solution; minimum dose: 0.1 mL (5 mg); maximum dose: 0.3 mL (15 mg) every 4-6 hours (may be given more frequently according to need); equivalent doses using more dilute solutions may be administered at the same frequency

Adolescents and Adults: 0.2 to 0.3 mL (10-15 mg) of 5% metaproterenol every 4-6 hours (can be given more frequently according to need); equivalent doses using more dilute solutions may be administered at the same frequency

Administration

Nebulization: Dilute 5% solution in 2-3 mL NS; more dilute solutions may be used without dilution

Oral: Administer with food to decrease GI distress

Monitoring Parameters Heart rate, respiratory rate, blood pressure, arterial or capillary blood gases if applicable, pulmonary function tests

Patient Information May cause dry mouth

Dosage Forms Excipient information presented when available (limited, particularly for generics); consult specific product labeling. [DSC] = Discontinued product

Aerosol for oral inhalation, as sulfate:

Alupent®: 0.65 mg/inhalation (14 g) [contains chlorofluorocarbon; 200 doses] [DSC]

Solution for nebulization, as sulfate [preservative free]: 0.4% [4 mg/mL] (2.5 mL); 0.6% [6 mg/mL] (2.5 mL)

Syrup, as sulfate: 10 mg/5 mL (480 mL)

Tablet, as sulfate: 10 mg, 20 mg

References

"National Asthma Education and Prevention Program. Expert Panel Report: Guidelines for the Diagnosis and Management of Asthma Update on Selected Topics–2002," *J Allergy Clin Immunol*, 2002, 110 (5 Suppl):S141-219.

◆ **Metaproterenol Sulfate** *see* Metaproterenol *on page 890*

MetFORMIN (met FOR min)

Medication Safety Issues

Sound-alike/look-alike issues:

MetFORMIN may be confused with metroNIDAZOLE

Glucophage® may be confused with Glucotrol®, Glutofac®

International issues:

Dianben [Spain] may be confused with Diovan® brand name for valsartan [U.S., Canada, and multiple international markets]

U.S. Brand Names Fortamet®; Glucophage®; Glucophage® XR; Glumetza®; Riomet®

Canadian Brand Names Apo-Metformin®; CO Metformin; Dom-Metformin; Glucophage®; Glumetza®; Glycon; Med-Metformin; Mylan-Metformin; Novo-Metformin; Nu-Metformin; PHL-Metformin; PMS-Metformin; PRO-Metformin; RAN™-Metformin; ratio-Metformin; Riva-Metformin; Sandoz-Metformin FC

Therapeutic Category Antidiabetic Agent, Biguanide; Antidiabetic Agent, Oral; Hypoglycemic Agent, Oral

Generic Available Yes: Excludes solution

Use Management of type II diabetes mellitus (noninsulindependent, NIDDM) as monotherapy when hyperglycemia cannot be managed with diet and exercise alone; may be used concomitantly with a sulfonylurea or insulin to improve glycemic control

Pregnancy Risk Factor B

Pregnancy Considerations Adverse events have not been observed in animal studies; therefore, metformin is classified as pregnancy category B. Metformin has been found to cross the placenta in levels which may be comparable to those found in the maternal plasma. Pharmacokinetic studies suggest that clearance of metformin may be increased during pregnancy and dosing may need adjusted in some women when used during the third trimester.

Fetal, neonatal, and maternal outcomes have been evaluated following maternal use of metformin for the treatment of GDM and type 2 diabetes. Available information suggests that metformin use during pregnancy may be safe as long as good glycemic control is maintained; however, many studies used metformin during the second or third trimester only. Maternal hyperglycemia can be associated with adverse effects in the fetus, including macrosomia, neonatal hyperglycemia, and hyperbilirubinemia; the risk of congenital malformations is increased when the Hb A_{1c} is above the normal range. Diabetes can also be associated with adverse effects in the mother. Poorly-treated diabetes may cause end-organ damage that may negatively affect obstetric outcomes. Physiologic glucose levels should be maintained prior to and during pregnancy to decrease the risk of adverse events in the mother and the fetus. Until additional safety and efficacy data are obtained, the use of oral agents is generally not recommended as routine management of GDM or type 2 diabetes mellitus during pregnancy. Insulin is the drug of choice for the control of diabetes mellitus during pregnancy.

Metformin has also been evaluated for the treatment of PCOS, a syndrome which may exhibit oligomenorrhea and in some women, hyperinsulinemia. When used to treat infertility related to PCOS, current guidelines restrict the use of metformin to women with glucose intolerance.

Lactation Enters breast milk/not recommended

Breast-Feeding Considerations Low amounts of metformin (generally ≤1% of the weight-adjusted maternal dose) are excreted into breast milk. Breast-feeding is not recommended by the manufacturer. Because breast milk levels of metformin stay relatively constant, avoiding nursing around peak plasma concentrations in the mother would not be helpful in reducing metformin exposure to the infant. Growth and development were not found to be affected in infants born to mothers with PCOS and who took metformin while breast-feeding.

Contraindications Hypersensitivity to metformin or any component; renal disease or renal dysfunction (S_{cr} ≥1.5 mg/dL in males or ≥1.4 mg/dL in females) or abnormal creatinine clearance which may result from clinical conditions such as cardiovascular collapse, respiratory failure, acute MI, acute CHF, and septicemia (see Warnings); acute or chronic metabolic acidosis with or without coma (including diabetic ketoacidosis)

Warnings Lactic acidosis is a rare, but potentially severe consequence of therapy with metformin **[U.S. Boxed Warning]**; withhold therapy in clinical conditions which may predispose to the development of lactic acidosis (eg, hypoxemia, dehydration, hypoperfusion, sepsis) or in any patient with CHF requiring pharmacologic management; the risk of accumulation and lactic acidosis increases with the degree of impairment of renal function and age; avoid use in patients with renal function below the limit of normal for their age; measure baseline renal function and monitor annually; more frequent monitoring may be necessary depending upon the patient's clinical condition; therapy should be suspended for any surgical procedures (resume only after normal intake resumed and normal renal function is verified); temporarily discontinue therapy for 48 hours in patients undergoing radiologic studies involving the intravascular administration of iodinated contrast materials

◄ (potential for acute alteration in renal function); avoid use in patients with impaired liver function; avoid excessive acute or chronic alcohol use (alcohol potentiates the effect of metformin on lactate metabolism); lactic acidosis should be suspected in any diabetic patient receiving metformin who has evidence of acidosis when evidence of ketoacidosis is lacking

Precautions Use with caution in patients receiving medications that may affect renal function, particularly tubular secretion, as they may also affect metformin disposition; hypoglycemia (rare with metformin) may occur with inadequate caloric intake, strenuous exercise, or concurrent use with other hypoglycemic drugs

Adverse Reactions

Cardiovascular: Chest discomfort, flushing, palpitation

Central nervous system: Headache, chills, dizziness, lightheadedness

Dermatologic: Rash, urticaria

Endocrine & metabolic: Hypoglycemia (rare), lactic acidosis

Gastrointestinal: Anorexia, nausea, vomiting, diarrhea, flatulence, indigestion, abdominal discomfort, abdominal distention, abnormal stools, constipation, dyspepsia, heartburn, metallic taste

Hematologic: Megaloblastic anemia (rare)

Neuromuscular & skeletal: Weakness, myalgia

Respiratory: Dyspnea, upper respiratory tract infection

Miscellaneous: Vitamin B_{12} levels decreased, sweating increased, flu-like syndrome, nail disorder

Drug Interactions

Avoid Concomitant Use There are no known interactions where it is recommended to avoid concomitant use.

Increased Effect/Toxicity

The levels/effects of MetFORMIN may be increased by: Cephalexin; Cimetidine; Iodinated Contrast Agents; Pegvisomant

Decreased Effect

The levels/effects of MetFORMIN may be decreased by: Corticosteroids (Orally Inhaled); Corticosteroids (Systemic); Luteinizing Hormone-Releasing Hormone Analogs; Somatropin; Thiazide Diuretics

Food Interactions Food decreases the extent and slightly delays the absorption (clinical significance unknown); may decrease absorption of vitamin B_{12} and folic acid

Stability Tablets and oral solution: Store at 20°C to 25°C (68°F to 77°F); protect from light

Mechanism of Action Decreases hepatic glucose production, decreases intestinal absorption of glucose, and improves insulin sensitivity (increases peripheral glucose uptake and utilization)

Pharmacodynamics

Onset of action: Within days, maximum effects up to 2 weeks

Average decrease in fasting blood glucose: Children >10 years and Adults: 60-70 mg/dL

Pharmacokinetics (Adult data unless noted)

Absorption: Oral: Slowly and incompletely absorbed

Distribution: Adults: V_d: 654 ± 358 L

Protein binding, plasma: Negligible

Bioavailability: Oral: 50% to 60% (under fasting conditions)

Half-life, plasma elimination: 3-6 hours

Time to peak serum concentration: Immediate release formulation: 2-4 hours; extended release formulation: 4-8 hours (median: 7 hours)

Elimination: Renal; tubular secretion is major route; excretion: 90% in urine as unchanged drug

Dialysis: Removed by hemodialysis; clearance up to 170 mL/minute

Usual Dosage Oral: **Note:** While significant responses may not be seen at doses <1500 mg daily, a lower recommended starting dose and gradual increase in dosage is recommended to minimize GI symptoms

Treatment of type 2 diabetes mellitus (noninsulin-dependent) in previously untreated patients or patients currently receiving sulfonylurea oral antidiabetic agents:

Children 10-16 years: Initial: 500 mg twice daily; dosage increases should be made weekly, in increments of 500 mg/day in divided doses, up to a maximum of 2000 mg/day.

Children ≥17 years and Adults:

Initial: 500 mg twice daily; dosage increases should be made weekly, in increments of 500 mg/day in 2 divided doses, up to a maximum of 2500 mg/day; doses >2000 mg/day may be better tolerated divided 3 times/day

Alternative dose: Initial: 850 mg once daily; dosage increases should be made in increments of 850 mg every 2 weeks, given in divided doses, up to a maximum of 2550 mg/day

Glucophage® XR (extended release tablets): Initial: 500 mg once daily; dosage may be increased by 500 mg weekly; maximum dose: 2000 mg once daily. If glycemic control is not achieved at maximum dose, may divide dose to 1000 mg twice daily; if doses >2000 mg/day are needed, switch to regular release tablets and titrate to maximum dose of 2550 mg/day

Glumetza™ (extended release tablet): Initial: 1000 mg once daily; may increase weekly as needed in 500 mg increments; not to exceed 2000 mg/day; if 2000 mg/day is ineffective, may consider using 1000 mg twice daily

Adjunctive agent to diabetic patient receiving insulin: Children ≥17 years and Adults: Initial: 500 mg metformin or metformin extended release once daily, continue current insulin dose; increase by 500 mg every week; maximum dose: 2500 mg metformin or 2000 mg metformin extended release; decrease insulin dose by 10% to 25% when fasting blood glucose <120 mg/dL

Dosing adjustment in renal impairment: Metformin is contraindicated in the presence of renal dysfunction (see Contraindications)

Dosing adjustment in hepatic impairment: Avoid metformin; liver disease is a risk factor for the development of lactic acidosis during metformin therapy.

Administration Oral:

Glucophage®, Riomet™: Administer in divided doses with meals

Glucophage® XR, Glumetza™: Administer with evening meal; extended release tablets should be swallowed whole; do not cut, crush, or chew

Monitoring Parameters Fasting blood glucose, hemoglobin A_{1c}, initial and periodic monitoring of hemoglobin, hematocrit, and red blood cell indices; renal function (baseline and annually)

Reference Range Target range:

Blood glucose: Fasting and preprandial: 80-120 mg/dL; bedtime: 100-140 mg/dL

Glycosylated hemoglobin (hemoglobin A_{1c}): <7%

Patient Information Do not change dose or discontinue without consulting prescriber; avoid alcohol while taking this medication, could cause severe reaction; maintain regular dietary intake and exercise routine; always carry quick source of sugar with you; during the first weeks of therapy, side effects such as headache, nausea, vomiting, or diarrhea may occur; consult prescriber if these persist; report severe or persistent side effects, extended vomiting or flu-like symptoms, skin rash, easy bruising or bleeding, or change in color of urine or stool; contact your healthcare provider immediately if you feel very weak, tired, or uncomfortable, have unusual muscle pain, trouble breathing, unusual stomach discomfort, are dizzy or lightheaded, or suddenly develop a slow or irregular heartbeat; parts of the extended release tablet (which do not contain active ingredient) may be found excreted in the stool

Additional Information When transferring therapy from chlorpropamide to metformin, monitor the patient closely during the first 2 weeks due to the prolonged retention of chlorpropamide in the body, leading to overlapping drug effects and possible hypoglycemia; if the patient has not responded to 4 weeks at the maximum metformin dosage, consider a gradual addition of a sulfonylurea antidiabetic agent, even if prior primary or secondary failure to a sulfonylurea has occurred; continue metformin at the maximum dose

Dosage Forms Excipient information presented when available (limited, particularly for generics); consult specific product labeling.

Solution, oral, as hydrochloride:
Riomet®: 100 mg/mL (118 mL, 473 mL) [dye free, ethanol free, sugar free; contains saccharin; cherry flavor]
Tablet, as hydrochloride: 500 mg, 850 mg, 1000 mg
Glucophage®: 500 mg, 850 mg
Glucophage®: 1000 mg [scored]
Tablet, extended release, as hydrochloride: 500 mg, 750 mg
Fortamet®: 500 mg, 1000 mg
Glucophage® XR: 500 mg, 750 mg
Glumetza®: 500 mg, 1000 mg

References

DeFronzo RA, "Pharmacologic Therapy for Type 2 Diabetes Mellitus," *Ann Intern Med*, 1999, 131(4):281-303.

Jones K, Arlanian S, McVie R, et al, "Metformin Improves Glycemic Control in Children With Type 2 Diabetes," *Diabetes*, 2000, 49(Suppl 1):A75.

"Type 2 Diabetes in Children and Adolescents. American Diabetes Association," *Diabetes Care*, 2000, 23(3):381-9.

◆ **Metformin Hydrochloride** *see* MetFORMIN *on page 891*

Methadone (METH a done)

Medication Safety Issues
Sound-alike/look-alike issues:
Methadone may be confused with dexmethylphenidate, Mephyton®, methylphenidate, Metadate® CD, Metadate® ER, morphine

High alert medication: The Institute for Safe Medication Practices (ISMP) includes this medication among its list of drug classes which have a heightened risk of causing significant patient harm when used in error.

Related Information
Compatibility of Chemotherapy and Related Supportive Care Medications *on page 1580*
Medications for Which A Single Dose May Be Fatal When Ingested By A Toddler *on page 1709*
Opioid Analgesics Comparison *on page 1510*

U.S. Brand Names Dolophine®; Methadone Diskets®; Methadone Intensol™; Methadose®
Canadian Brand Names Metadol-D™; Metadol™
Therapeutic Category Analgesic, Narcotic
Generic Available Yes
Use Management of moderate to severe pain unresponsive to non-narcotics; used in narcotic detoxification maintenance programs and for the treatment of iatrogenic narcotic dependency
Restrictions C-II

Treatment of narcotic addiction (detoxification or maintenance programs): Methadone may only be dispensed by pharmacies or maintenance programs certified by the Federal Substance Abuse and Mental Health Service Administration, registered by the Drug Enforcement Agency, and approved by the designated state authority. Exceptions include: During inpatient care, when patients are admitted for conditions other than concurrent opioid addiction (parenteral methadone may be used for those patients unable to take oral methadone) and during an emergency period ≤3 days while opioid addiction treatment is being sought in an appropriately licensed facility.

Pregnancy Risk Factor C
Pregnancy Considerations Teratogenic effects have been observed in some, but not all, animal studies. Data collected by the Teratogen Information System are complicated by maternal use of illicit drugs, nutrition, infection, and psychosocial circumstances. However, pregnant women in methadone treatment programs are reported to have improved fetal outcomes compared to pregnant women using illicit drugs. Methadone can be detected in the amniotic fluid, cord plasma, and newborn urine. Fetal growth, birth weight, length, and/or head circumference may be decreased in infants born to narcotic-addicted mothers treated with methadone during pregnancy. Growth deficits do not appear to persist; however, decreased performance on psychometric and behavioral tests has been found to continue into childhood. Abnormal fetal nonstress tests have also been reported. Withdrawal symptoms in the neonate may be observed up to 2-4 weeks after delivery. The manufacturer states that methadone should be used during pregnancy only if clearly needed. Because methadone clearance in pregnant women is increased and half-life is decreased during the 2nd and 3rd trimesters of pregnancy, withdrawal symptoms may be observed in the mother; dosage of methadone may need increased or dosing interval decreased during pregnancy.

Lactation Enters breast milk/not recommended (AAP rates "compatible")
Breast-Feeding Considerations Peak methadone levels appear in breast milk 4-5 hours after an oral dose. Methadone has been detected in the plasma of some breast-fed infants whose mothers are taking methadone. Use during breast-feeding is not recommended, and the manufacturer recommends that women on high dose methadone maintenance who already are breast-feeding be instructed to wean breast-feeding gradually to avoid neonatal abstinence syndrome. Sedation and respiratory depression have been reported in nursing infants. Unless otherwise contraindicated (concurrent medical conditions, other medications of abuse), the AAP rates methadone "compatible" with breast-feeding.

Contraindications Hypersensitivity to methadone or any component; severe respiratory depression (in absence of resuscitative equipment or ventilatory support); acute or severe asthma; hypercarbia; known or suspected ileus

Warnings Death and life-threatening adverse events (eg, respiratory depression, cardiac arrhythmias) in patients receiving methadone for pain control have been reported **[U.S. Boxed Warning].** These events may be the result of unintentional overdoses, drug interactions, and cardiac toxicities associated with methadone (QT prolongation, torsade de pointes). Particular vigilance and patient monitoring is necessary during treatment initiation (including conversion from another opioid) and dose titration. Incomplete cross-tolerance between methadone and other opioids may occur; fatalities have been reported when converting patients from chronic, high dose treatment with other opioids to methadone; knowledge of the pharmacokinetics of methadone is essential for appropriate conversion from other opioids (see package insert for conversion tables). Methadone's elimination half-life is significantly longer than its duration of analgesic action. The respiratory depressant effects of methadone occur later and persist longer than its peak analgesic effects. Carefully select initial methadone dose for pain control and slowly titrate to analgesic effect in all patients, including those who are opioid-tolerant. Instruct patients to take methadone as prescribed; do not take more methadone than prescribed without first talking with physician.

Methadone may cause prolongation of the QT interval or torsade de pointes (especially at higher doses, eg, in adults with doses >200 mg/day) **[U.S. Boxed Warning]**; use with caution in patients at risk for QT prolongation (eg, patients with cardiac hypertrophy, hypokalemia, hypomagnesemia, concomitant diuretic use), with medications known to prolong the QT interval, or with history of conduction abnormalities. Monitoring of the QT_c interval prior to and during therapy has been recommended by the Center for Substance Abuse and Treatment (CSAT) (see Additional Information).

May cause respiratory depression **[U.S. Boxed Warning]**; use with extreme caution in patients with respiratory disease or pre-existing respiratory depression; methadone's effect on respiration lasts longer than analgesic effects. Use with extreme caution (and only if essential) in patients with head injury, increased ICP, or other intracranial lesions. May cause severe hypotension; use with caution in patients with severe volume depletion or circulatory shock. Tablets are to be used only for oral administration and **must not** be used for injection. Abrupt discontinuation after prolonged use may result in withdrawal symptoms or seizures.

Concentrated oral solution may contain propylene glycol or sodium benzoate; benzoic acid (benzoate) is a metabolite of benzyl alcohol; large amounts of benzyl alcohol (≥99 mg/kg/day) have been associated with a potentially fatal toxicity ("gasping syndrome") in neonates; the "gasping syndrome" consists of metabolic acidosis, respiratory distress, gasping respirations, CNS dysfunction (including convulsions, intracranial hemorrhage), hypotension, and cardiovascular collapse; avoid use of methadone products containing sodium benzoate in neonates; *in vitro* and animal studies have shown that benzoate displaces bilirubin from protein binding sites

Precautions Due to the cumulative effects of methadone, the dose and frequency of administration need to be reduced with repeated use; use with caution in patients with hepatic, renal, pulmonary, or cardiovascular disease; use with caution and decrease dose in patients who are debilitated and those with severe renal or hepatic dysfunction, hypothyroidism, Addison's disease, urethral stricture, or prostatic hypertrophy.

Adverse Reactions

Cardiovascular: Hypotension, bradycardia, peripheral vasodilation; prolongation of QT interval, torsade de pointes (see Warnings)

Central nervous system: CNS depression, intracranial pressure elevated, drowsiness, dizziness, sedation (marked sedation seen after repeated administration)

Endocrine & metabolic: Antidiuretic hormone release

Gastrointestinal: Nausea, vomiting, constipation, xerostomia, biliary tract spasm

Genitourinary: Urinary tract spasm

Ocular: Miosis

Respiratory: Respiratory depression

Miscellaneous: Histamine release, physical and psychological dependence with prolonged use

Drug Interactions

Metabolism/Transport Effects Substrate of CYP2B6 (major), 2C9 (minor), 2C19 (minor), 2D6 (minor), 3A4 (major); **Inhibits** CYP2D6 (moderate), 3A4 (weak)

Avoid Concomitant Use

Avoid concomitant use of Methadone with any of the following: Artemether; Dronedarone; Lumefantrine; Nilotinib; Pimozide; QuiNINE; Tetrabenazine; Thioridazine; Ziprasidone

Increased Effect/Toxicity

Methadone may increase the levels/effects of: Alcohol (Ethyl); Alvimopan; CNS Depressants; CYP2D6

Substrates; Desmopressin; Dronedarone; Fesoterodine; Nebivolol; Pimozide; QTc-Prolonging Agents; QuiNINE; Selective Serotonin Reuptake Inhibitors; Tamoxifen; Tetrabenazine; Thiazide Diuretics; Thioridazine; Zidovudine; Ziprasidone

The levels/effects of Methadone may be increased by: Alfuzosin; Amphetamines; Antifungal Agents (Azole Derivatives, Systemic); Antipsychotic Agents (Phenothiazines); Artemether; Chloroquine; Ciprofloxacin; Ciprofloxacin (Systemic); CYP2B6 Inhibitors (Moderate); CYP2B6 Inhibitors (Strong); CYP3A4 Inhibitors (Moderate); CYP3A4 Inhibitors (Strong); Gadobutrol; Interferons (Alfa); Lumefantrine; MAO Inhibitors; Nilotinib; Quazepam; QuiNINE; Selective Serotonin Reuptake Inhibitors; Succinylcholine

Decreased Effect

Methadone may decrease the levels/effects of: Codeine; Didanosine; Pegvisomant; TraMADol

The levels/effects of Methadone may be decreased by: Ammonium Chloride; Barbiturates; CarBAMazepine; CYP2B6 Inducers (Strong); CYP3A4 Inducers (Strong); Deferasirox; Etravirine; Herbs (CYP3A4 Inducers); Mixed Agonist / Antagonist Opioids; Phenytoin; Protease Inhibitors; Reverse Transcriptase Inhibitors (Non-Nucleoside); Rifamycin Derivatives

Stability Store at controlled room temperature; protect from light

Tablets: Protect from moisture

Mechanism of Action Binds to opiate receptors in the CNS, causing inhibition of ascending pain pathways, altering the perception of and response to pain; produces generalized CNS depression

Pharmacodynamics Analgesia:

Onset of action:

Oral: Within 30-60 minutes

Parenteral: Within 10-20 minutes

Maximum effect: Parenteral: 1-2 hours

Duration: Oral: 6-8 hours; after repeated doses, duration increases to 22-48 hours

Pharmacokinetics (Adult data unless noted)

Distribution: Crosses the placenta; appears in breast milk

V_d: (Mean ± SD):

Children: 7.1 ± 2.5 L/kg

Adults: 6.1 ± 2.4 L/kg

V_{dss}: Adults: 2-6 L/kg

Protein binding: 85% to 90% (primarily to alpha$_1$-acid glycoprotein)

Metabolism: N-demethylated in the liver to an inactive metabolite

Half-life: May be prolonged with alkaline pH

Children: 19 ± 14 hours (range: 4-62 hours)

Adults: 35 ± 22 hours (range: 9-87 hours)

Elimination: In urine (<10% as unchanged drug); increased renal excretion with urine pH <6; **Note:** Methadone may persist in the liver and other tissues; slow release from tissues may prolong the pharmacologic effect despite low serum concentrations

Dialysis: Hemodialysis, peritoneal dialysis: Not established as effective for increasing the elimination of methadone (or metabolite)

Usual Dosage Doses should be titrated to appropriate effects:

Neonatal abstinence syndrome: Oral, I.V.: Initial: 0.05-0.2 mg/kg/dose given every 12-24 hours or 0.5 mg/kg/day divided every 8 hours; individualize dose and tapering schedule to control symptoms of withdrawal; usually taper dose by 10% to 20% per week over 1 to 1½ months. **Note**: Due to long elimination half-life, tapering is difficult; consider alternate agent.

Children:

Analgesia: **Note:** Dosing interval may range from 4-12 hours during initial therapy; decrease in dose or frequency may be required (~2-5 days after initiation of therapy or dosage increase) due to accumulation with repeated doses.

I.V.: Initial: 0.1 mg/kg/dose every 4 hours for 2-3 doses, then every 6-12 hours as needed; maximum dose: 10 mg/dose

Oral, I.M., SubQ: Initial: 0.1 mg/kg/dose every 4 hours for 2-3 doses, then every 6-12 hours as needed or 0.7 mg/kg/24 hours divided every 4-6 hours as needed; maximum dose: 10 mg/dose

Iatrogenic narcotic dependency: Oral: Controlled studies have not been conducted; several clinically used dosing regimens have been reported. Methadone dose **must be individualized** and will depend upon patient's previous narcotic dose and severity of opioid withdrawal; patients who have received higher doses of narcotics will require higher methadone doses.

General guidelines: Initial: 0.05-0.1 mg/kg/dose every 6 hours; increase by 0.05 mg/kg/dose until withdrawal symptoms are controlled; after 24-48 hours, the dosing interval can be lengthened to every 12-24 hours; to taper dose, wean by 0.05 mg/kg/day; if withdrawal symptoms recur, taper at a slower rate

Adults:

Analgesia:

Oral: Initial 5-10 mg; dosing interval may range from 4-12 hours during initial therapy; decrease in dose or frequency may be required (~2-5 days after initiation of therapy or dosage increase) due to accumulation with repeated doses

Manufacturer's recommendations: 2.5-10 mg every 3-4 hours as needed

I.V.: Manufacturer's recommendations: Opioid-naive patients: Initial: 2.5-10 mg every 8-12 hours; titrate slowly to effect; may also be administered by SubQ or I.M. injection

Detoxification: Oral: 15-40 mg/day

Maintenance of opiate dependence: Oral: 20-120 mg/day

Dosing adjustment in renal impairment: Children and Adults: Cl_{cr} <10 mL/minute: Administer 50% to 75% of normal dose

Administration Oral: Administer with juice or water; dispersible tablet should be completely dissolved before administration; oral dose for detoxification and maintenance may be administered in Tang®, Kool-Aid®, apple juice, grape Crystal Light®

Monitoring Parameters Respiratory, cardiovascular, and mental status, pain relief (if used for analgesia), abstinence scoring system (if used for neonatal abstinence syndrome); ECG for monitoring QT_c interval prior to and during therapy (see Additional Information).

Patient Information Avoid alcohol; may be habit-forming; avoid abrupt discontinuation after prolonged use; may cause drowsiness and impair ability to perform activities requiring mental alertness or physical coordination; may cause dry mouth; may cause postural hypotension (use with caution when changing positions from lying or sitting to standing); seek medical attention immediately if you experience heart palpitations, dizziness, lightheadedness, or fainting (these may be symptoms of an arrhythmia)

Additional Information Methadone accumulates with repeated doses and dosage may need to be adjusted downward after 3-5 days to prevent toxic effects. Some patients may benefit from every 8- to 12-hour dosing interval (pain control).

Methadone 10 mg I.M. = morphine 10 mg I.M.

The Center for Substance Abuse and Treatment (CSAT) of the Substance Abuse and Mental Health Services Administration has developed a consensus guideline statement outlining recommendations regarding ECG monitoring in patients being considered for and being treated with methadone regardless of indication. Of note, these recommendations should not supersede clinical judgment or patient preferences and may not apply to patients with terminal, intractable cancer pain. Five recommendations have been developed:

Recommendation 1: Disclosure: Clinicians should inform patients of arrhythmia risk when methadone is prescribed.

Recommendation 2: Clinical History: Clinicians should inquire about any history of structural heart disease, arrhythmia, and syncope.

Recommendation 3: Screening: Clinicians should obtain pretreatment ECG for all patients to measure QT_c interval, follow up ECG within 30 days, then annually (monitor more frequently if patient receiving >100 mg/day or if unexplained syncope or seizure occurs while on methadone).

Recommendation 4: Risk Stratification: If before or at anytime during therapy the QT_c *>450-499 msecs*: Discuss potential risks and benefits; monitor QT_c more frequently. If before or anytime during therapy the QT_c ≥*500 msecs*: Consider discontinuation or reducing methadone dose or eliminate factors promoting QT_c prolongation (eg, potassium-wasting drugs) or use alternative therapy (eg, buprenorphine).

Recommendation 5: Drug Interactions: Clinicians should be aware of interactions between methadone and other drugs that either prolong the QT interval or reduce methadone elimination.

The panel also concluded that the arrhythmia risk is directly associated with methadone's ability to block the delayed rectifier potassium channel (Ikr) and prolong repolarization. The guideline further states that the use of the Bazett formula is adequate even though it is likely to overcorrect with high heart rates. The patient should remain supine for at least 5 minutes prior to obtaining ECG. In addition, screening for QT_c prolongation using automated readings does not require a specialist (eg, cardiologist) and may be performed in a primary care setting. However, in cases when uncertainty exists about whether or not clinically significant QT_c prolongation is present, the ECG should be repeated or interpreted by a cardiologist. For more information, see Krantz, 2009.

Dosage Forms Excipient information presented when available (limited, particularly for generics); consult specific product labeling.

Injection, solution, as hydrochloride: 10 mg/mL (20 mL)

Solution, oral, as hydrochloride: 5 mg/5 mL (500 mL); 10 mg/5 mL (500 mL)

Solution, oral, as hydrochloride [concentrate]: 10 mg/mL (946 mL)

Methadone Intensol™: 10 mg/mL (30 mL) [dye free; sugar free; contains sodium benzoate; unflavored]

Methadose®: 10 mg/mL (1000 mL) [contains propylene glycol; cherry flavor]

Methadose®: 10 mg/mL (1000 mL) [dye free, sugar free; contains sodium benzoate; unflavored]

Tablet, as hydrochloride: 5 mg, 10 mg

Dolophine®: 5 mg, 10 mg

Tablet, dispersible, as hydrochloride: 40 mg

Methadose®: 40 mg [scored]

Methadone Diskets®: 40 mg [scored] [orange-pineapple flavor]

References

Anand KJ and Arnold JH, "Opioid Tolerance and Dependence in Infants and Children," *Crit Care Med*, 1994, 22(2):334-42.

Berde C, Ablin A, Glazer J, et al, "American Academy of Pediatrics Report of the Subcommittee on Disease-Related Pain in Childhood Cancer," *Pediatrics*, 1990, 86(5 Pt 2):818-25.

Krantz MJ, Lewkowiez L, Hays H, et al, "Torsade de Pointes Associated With Very-High-Dose Methadone," *Ann Intern Med*, 2002, 137 (6):501-4.

Krantz MJ, Martin J, Stimmel B, et al, "QT$_c$ Interval Screening in Methadone Treatment," *Ann Intern Med*, 2009, 150(6):387-95.

Lauriault G, LeBelle MJ, Lodge BA, et al, "Stability of Methadone in Four Vehicles for Oral Administration," *Am J Hosp Pharm*, 1991, 48 (6):1252-6.

Olkkola KT, Hamunen K, and Maunuksela EL, "Clinical Pharmacokinetics and Pharmacodynamics of Opioid Analgesics in Infants and Children," *Clin Pharmacokinet*, 1995, 28(5):385-404.

◆ **Methadone Diskets®** *see* Methadone *on page* 893

◆ **Methadone Hydrochloride** *see* Methadone *on page* 893

◆ **Methadone Intensol™** *see* Methadone *on page* 893

◆ **Methadose®** *see* Methadone *on page* 893

Methenamine (meth EN a meen)

Medication Safety Issues
Sound-alike/look-alike issues:
Hiprex® may be confused with Mirapex®
Methenamine may be confused with mesalamine, methazolamide, methionine
Urex® may be confused with Eurax®, Serax®

International issues:
Urex®: Brand name for methenamine [U.S., Canada], but also the brand name for furosemide [Australia, China, Turkey]

U.S. Brand Names Hiprex®; Urex™

Canadian Brand Names Dehydral®; Hiprex®; Mandelamine®; Urasal®; Urex™

Therapeutic Category Antibiotic, Miscellaneous

Generic Available Yes

Use Prophylaxis or suppression of recurrent urinary tract infections

Pregnancy Risk Factor C (methenamine mandelate)

Pregnancy Considerations Because animal reproduction studies were not conducted, methenamine mandelate is classified pregnancy category C. Methenamine hippurate did not cause adverse fetal effects in animals. Methenamine crosses the placenta and distributes to amniotic fluid. Adverse fetal effects were not observed in two human trials. Methenamine use has been shown to interfere with urine estriol concentrations if measured via acid hydrolysis. Use of enzyme hydrolysis prevents this lab interference.

Lactation Enters breast milk

Breast-Feeding Considerations Small amounts of methenamine are secreted in human milk.

Contraindications Hypersensitivity to methenamine or any component (see Warnings); severe dehydration, renal insufficiency (methenamine is ineffective in patients with renal impairment), hepatic insufficiency in patients receiving hippurate salt; concurrent therapy with sulfonamides

Warnings Dosage of 8 g/day for 3-4 weeks has been associated with bladder irritation, albuminuria, and hematuria; Hiprex® tablets contain tartrazine which may cause allergic reactions in susceptible individuals

Precautions Use with caution in patients with hepatic impairment. Use care to maintain an acidic pH of the urine when treating infections due to urea-splitting organisms such as *Proteus* and *Pseudomonas*.

Adverse Reactions
Central nervous system: Headache
Dermatologic: Rash, pruritus, urticaria
Gastrointestinal: Nausea, vomiting, diarrhea, abdominal cramping, anorexia, stomatitis
Genitourinary: Bladder irritation, painful and frequent micturition, dysuria, crystalluria

Hepatic: AST and ALT elevated (with hippurate formulation)
Otic: Tinnitus
Renal: Hematuria
Respiratory: Lipoid pneumonitis (with mandelate suspension), dyspnea

Drug Interactions
Avoid Concomitant Use
Avoid concomitant use of Methenamine with any of the following: BCG; Sulfonamide Derivatives

Increased Effect/Toxicity
Methenamine may increase the levels/effects of: Sulfonamide Derivatives

Decreased Effect
Methenamine may decrease the levels/effects of: Amphetamines; BCG; Typhoid Vaccine

The levels/effects of Methenamine may be decreased by: Antacids; Carbonic Anhydrase Inhibitors

Food Interactions Foods/diets which alkalinize urine pH >5.5 decrease activity of methenamine; cranberry juice can be used to acidify urine and increase activity of methenamine

Stability Protect from excessive heat

Mechanism of Action Methenamine is hydrolyzed to formaldehyde and ammonia in acidic urine; formaldehyde has nonspecific bactericidal action

Pharmacokinetics (Adult data unless noted)
Absorption: Readily from the GI tract; 10% to 30% of the drug will be hydrolyzed by gastric juices unless it is protected by an enteric coating

Distribution: Distributes into breast milk; crosses the placenta

Metabolism: ~10% to 25% in the liver

Half-life: 3-6 hours

Elimination: Excretion occurs via glomerular filtration and tubular secretion with ~70% to 90% of dose excreted unchanged in urine within 24 hours

Usual Dosage Oral:
Children >2 years to 12 years: Mandelate: 50-75 mg/kg/day divided every 6-8 hours; maximum dose: 4 g/day
Children 6-12 years: Hippurate: 0.5-1 g twice daily
Children >12 years and Adults:
Hippurate: 1 g twice daily
Mandelate: 1 g 4 times/day after meals and at bedtime

Administration Oral: Administer with food to minimize GI upset; shake suspension well before use; patient should drink plenty of fluids to ensure adequate urine flow; administer with cranberry juice, ascorbic acid, or ammonium chloride to acidify urine; avoid intake of alkalinizing agents (sodium bicarbonate, antacids)

Monitoring Parameters Urinary pH, urinalysis, urine cultures, periodic liver function tests in patients receiving hippurate salt

Test Interactions Formaldehyde interferes with fluorometric procedures causing falsely increased results for catecholamines and VMA (U); falsely decreased urine estriol concentration with tests using acid hydrolysis

Nursing Implications Urine should be acidic, pH <5.5 for maximum effect

Additional Information Should not be used to treat infections outside of the lower urinary tract (ie, pyelonephritis)

Dosage Forms Excipient information presented when available (limited, particularly for generics); consult specific product labeling. [DSC] = Discontinued product
Tablet, as hippurate: 1 g
Hiprex®, Urex™: 1 g [Hiprex® contains tartrazine dye]
Tablet, as mandelate: 500 mg, 1000 mg

References

"Practice Parameter: The Diagnosis, Treatment, and Evaluation of the Initial Urinary Tract Infection in Febrile Infants and Young Children. American Academy of Pediatrics. Committee on Quality Improvement. Subcommittee on Urinary Tract Infection," *Pediatrics*, 1999, 103 (4 Pt 1):843-52.

◆ **Methenamine Hippurate** *see* Methenamine *on page 896*

◆ **Methenamine Mandelate** *see* Methenamine *on page 896*

Methimazole (meth IM a zole)

Medication Safety Issues
Sound-alike/look-alike issues:
 Methimazole may be confused with metolazone
U.S. Brand Names Northyx™ [DSC]; Tapazole®
Canadian Brand Names Dom-Methimazole; PHL-Methimazole; Tapazole®
Therapeutic Category Antithyroid Agent
Generic Available Yes
Use Palliative treatment of hyperthyroidism, to return the hyperthyroid patient to a normal metabolic state prior to thyroidectomy, and to control thyrotoxic crisis that may accompany thyroidectomy
Pregnancy Risk Factor D
Pregnancy Considerations Methimazole crosses the placenta. Rare cases of aplasia cutis congenital have been reported in the neonate, as well as a syndrome which includes choanal atresia, facial abnormalities, growth restriction and developmental abnormalities. Additional data is needed to determine any association of these adverse events with maternal methimazole use. To avoid these potential congenital defects, propylthiouracil treatment should be considered for use during the first trimester; however, methimazole may be used during the second and third trimesters. Fetal thyroid function may also be transiently suppressed. Untreated hyperthyroidism may also cause adverse events in the mother (eg, heart failure, miscarriage, preeclampsia, thyroid storm); fetus (eg, goiter, growth restriction, hypo/hyperthyroidism, still birth); and neonate (eg, hyper-/hypothyroidism, neuropsychologic damage). The thioamides are treatment of choice for hyperthyroidism during pregnancy. In order to prevent adverse events to the fetus, the lowest effective dose should be used in order to achieve maternal levels of T_4 in the high euthyroid or low hyperthyroid range. Since thyroid dysfunction may diminish as pregnancy advances, the dose may be decreased or use may be discontinued 2-3 weeks prior to delivery. Thyroid function should be monitored closely.
Lactation Enters breast milk/contraindicated (per manufacturer) (AAP rates "compatible")
Breast-Feeding Considerations Methimazole is found in breast milk at levels ~0.14% of the weight adjusted maternal dose. Although breast-feeding is contraindicated by the manufacturer, the AAP and other expert analysis have concluded that breast-feeding is generally considered safe. Reviews of thioamide use in breast-feeding have not shown that thyroid function of the breast-fed infant is significantly affected.
Contraindications Hypersensitivity to methimazole or any component, nursing mothers per manufacturer, however, expert analysis and the American Academy of Pediatrics state this drug may be used with caution in nursing mothers (see Breast-Feeding and Drugs on page 1710)
Warnings May cause significant bone marrow depression; the most severe manifestation is agranulocytosis. Aplastic anemia, thrombocytopenia, and leukopenia may also occur; use with extreme caution in patients receiving other drugs known to cause myelosuppression, particularly agranulocytosis. Avoid doses >40 mg/day. Discontinue if significant bone marrow suppression occurs, particularly

agranulocytosis or aplastic anemia. May cause fetal harm when administered to a pregnant woman; readily crosses the placenta and can induce goiter and cretinism in the developing fetus; however, thioamides are the treatment of choice for hyperthyroidism in pregnancy. The lowest effective dose should be used; monitor thyroid function tests closely. Rare, severe hepatic reactions (hepatic necrosis, hepatitis) may occur; discontinue use in the presence of hepatitis. May cause hypoprothrombinemia; monitor PT.

Adverse Reactions
Cardiovascular: Edema, ANCA-positive vasculitis, leukocytoclastic vasculitis, periarteritis
Central nervous system: Drowsiness, vertigo, headache, CNS stimulation, neuropathies, CNS depression, fever, dizziness
Dermatologic: Rash, urticaria, pruritus, alopecia, skin pigmentation, exfoliative dermatitis, acneiform eruptions
Endocrine & metabolic: Weight gain, goiter
Gastrointestinal: Ageusia, nausea, vomiting, epigastric distress, splenomegaly, constipation, salivary gland swelling
Hematologic: Agranulocytosis, aplastic anemia, granulocytopenia, leukopenia, hypoprothrombinemia
Hepatic: Cholestatic jaundice, hepatitis
Neuromuscular & skeletal: Arthralgia, myalgia, paresthesia, neuritis
Renal: Nephritis
Respiratory: Interstitial pneumonitis
Miscellaneous: Lupus-like syndrome, lymphadenopathy, insulin autoimmune syndrome

Drug Interactions
Metabolism/Transport Effects Inhibits CYP1A2 (weak), 2A6 (weak), 2B6 (weak), 2C9 (weak), 2C19 (weak), 2D6 (moderate), 2E1 (weak), 3A4 (weak)
Avoid Concomitant Use
Avoid concomitant use of Methimazole with any of the following: Sodium Iodide I131
Increased Effect/Toxicity There are no known significant interactions involving an increase in effect.
Decreased Effect
Methimazole may decrease the levels/effects of: Sodium Iodide I131; Vitamin K Antagonists
Stability Store at room temperature; protect from light
Mechanism of Action Inhibits the synthesis of thyroid hormones by blocking the oxidation of iodine in the thyroid gland, blocking iodine's ability to combine with tyrosine to form thyroxine (T_4) and triiodothyronine (T_3)
Pharmacodynamics Antithyroid effect:
Onset of action: 12-18 hours
Duration: 36-72 hours
Pharmacokinetics (Adult data unless noted)
Distribution: Concentrated in thyroid gland; crosses placenta; found in high concentrations in breast milk; breast milk to plasma ratio: 1:1
Bioavailability: 80% to 95%
Metabolism: Hepatic
Half-life: 5-13 hours
Time to peak serum concentration: 1 hour
Elimination: Excreted in urine
Usual Dosage Oral:
Children:
 Initial: 0.4 mg/kg/day in 3 divided doses; maintenance: 0.2 mg/kg/day in 3 divided doses
 or
 Initial: 0.5-0.7 mg/kg/day or 15-20 mg/m^2/day in 3 divided doses
 Maintenance: $1/3$ to $2/3$ of initial dose; maximum dose: 30 mg/day

Adults: Initial: 5 mg every 8 hours for mild hyperthyroidism; 10 mg every 8 hours for moderately severe disease and up to 20 mg every 8 hours for severe hyperthyroidism; maintenance: 5-15 mg/day

Thyrotoxic crisis: Adults: **Note:** Recommendations vary widely and have not been evaluated in comparative trials: 20-30 mg every 6-12 hours for short-term initial therapy; followed by gradual reduction to maintenance dosage: 5-15 mg/day

Dosage adjustment in renal impairment: No adjustment necessary

Administration Oral: Administer with meals

Monitoring Parameters Signs of hyper- or hypothyroidism, CBC with differential, liver function (baseline and as needed); serum thyroxine, free thyroxine index, prothrombin time

Patient Information Notify physician of fever, sore throat, unusual bleeding or bruising, headache, rash, or yellowing of skin

Dosage Forms Excipient information presented when available (limited, particularly for generics); consult specific product labeling. [DSC] = Discontinued product

Tablet: 5 mg, 10 mg, 20 mg
Northyx™: 5 mg, 10 mg, 15 mg, 20 mg [DSC]
Tapazole®: 5 mg, 10 mg

References

Raby C, Lagorce JF, Jambut-Absil AC, et al, "The Mechanism of Action of Synthetic Antithyroid Drugs: Iodine Complexation During Oxidation of Iodide," *Endocrinology*, 1990, 126(3):1683-91.

Methocarbamol (meth oh KAR ba mole)

Medication Safety Issues
Sound-alike/look-alike issues:
Methocarbamol may be confused with mephobarbital
Robaxin® may be confused with ribavirin, Rubex®, Skelaxin®

Beers Criteria medication: This drug may be inappropriate for use in geriatric patients (high severity risk).

U.S. Brand Names Robaxin®; Robaxin®-750

Canadian Brand Names Robaxin®

Therapeutic Category Skeletal Muscle Relaxant, Nonparalytic

Generic Available Yes: Tablet

Use Treatment of muscle spasm associated with acute painful musculoskeletal conditions; supportive therapy in tetanus

Pregnancy Risk Factor C

Pregnancy Considerations Animal reproduction studies have not been conducted. The manufacturer notes that fetal and congenital abnormalities have been rarely reported following *in utero* exposure. Use during pregnancy only if clearly needed.

Lactation Excretion in breast milk unknown/use caution

Contraindications Hypersensitivity to methocarbamol or any component; injectable formulation in patients with renal impairment

Warnings Solution is hypertonic, avoid extravasation; avoid using injection in patients with impaired renal function because the polyethylene glycol vehicle may be irritating to the kidneys

Precautions Use injectable form cautiously in patients with suspected or known seizure disorders; use with caution in myasthenia gravis patients receiving pyridostigmine (see Drug Interactions); use oral formulation with caution in patients with renal or hepatic impairment; monitor these patients closely

Adverse Reactions
Cardiovascular: Syncope, bradycardia, hypotension
Central nervous system: Drowsiness, dizziness, light-headedness, headache, fever, vertigo, seizures, amnesia, confusion

Dermatologic: Urticaria, pruritus, rash
Gastrointestinal: Nausea, metallic taste, GI upset, vomiting, dyspepsia
Genitourinary: Discoloration of urine (brown, black, or green)
Hematologic: Leukopenia
Hepatic: Cholestatic jaundice
Local: Pain and phlebitis at injection site, thrombophlebitis
Ocular: Blurred vision, conjunctivitis, nystagmus, diplopia
Respiratory: Nasal congestion
Miscellaneous: Hypersensitivity reactions including anaphylaxis and angioneurotic edema

Drug Interactions

Avoid Concomitant Use There are no known interactions where it is recommended to avoid concomitant use.

Increased Effect/Toxicity
Methocarbamol may increase the levels/effects of: Alcohol (Ethyl); CNS Depressants; Methotrimeprazine

The levels/effects of Methocarbamol may be increased by: Methotrimeprazine

Decreased Effect
Methocarbamol may decrease the levels/effects of: Pyridostigmine

Stability Injection when diluted to 4 mg/mL in SWI, D$_5$W, or NS is stable for 6 days at room temperature; do **not** refrigerate after dilution

Mechanism of Action CNS depressant with sedative and skeletal muscle relaxant effects; exact mechanism of action is unknown

Pharmacodynamics Onset of action: 30 minutes

Pharmacokinetics (Adult data unless noted) Oral:
Protein binding: 46% to 50%
Metabolism: Extensive in the liver via dealkylation and hydroxylation
Half-life: 1-2 hours
Time to peak serum concentration: Within ~1-2 hours
Elimination: Clearance: Adults: 0.2-0.8 L/hour/kg

Usual Dosage
Tetanus: I.V.:
Children (recommended **only** for use in tetanus): 15 mg/kg/dose or 500 mg/m^2/dose, may repeat every 6 hours if needed; maximum dose: 1.8 g/m^2/day for 3 days only
Adults: 1-2 g by direct I.V. injection followed by additional 1-2 g (maximum dose: 3 g total); repeat with 1-2 g every 6 hours until NG tube or oral therapy possible; total daily dose of up to 24 g may be needed

Muscle spasm: Adults:
Oral: 1.5 g 4 times/day for 2-3 days (up to 8 g/day may be used for severe conditions); decrease dose to 4-4.5 g/day as 1 g 4 times/day or 750 mg every 4 hours or 1.5 g 3 times/day
I.M., I.V.: 1 g every 8 hours if oral not possible; maximum dose: 3 g/day for 3 consecutive days (except when treating tetanus); may be reinstituted after 2 drug-free days

Dosing adjustment in renal impairment: Clearance is reduced by as much as 40% in patients with renal failure on hemodialysis; avoid use or reduce dosage and monitor closely; do not administer parenteral formulation to patients with renal dysfunction

Dosing adjustment in hepatic impairment: Clearance may be reduced by as much as 70% in cirrhotic patients; avoid use or reduce dosage and monitor patient closely

Administration
Parenteral: I.V.: May be injected directly I.V. without dilution at a maximum rate of 180 mg/m^2/minute but not >3 mL/minute; may also be diluted in NS or D$_5$W to a concentration of 4 mg/mL and infused more slowly; patient should be in the recumbent position during and for 10-15 minutes after I.V. administration

I.M.: Do not inject more than 3 mL per site; not recommended for SubQ administration

Test Interactions May cause color interference in certain screening tests for 5-hydroxyindoleacetic acid (5-HIAA) using nitrosonaphthol reagent and in screening tests for vanillylmandelic acid (VMA) using the Gitlow method

Patient Information May cause drowsiness and impair ability to perform activities requiring mental alertness or physical coordination; urine may darken to brown, black, or green

Nursing Implications Avoid infiltration, extremely irritating to tissues

Dosage Forms Excipient information presented when available (limited, particularly for generics); consult specific product labeling.

Injection, solution:
Robaxin®: 100 mg/mL (10 mL) [contains natural rubber/natural latex in packaging, polyethylene glycol 300]
Tablet, oral: 500 mg, 750 mg
Robaxin®: 500 mg [scored]
Robaxin®-750: 750 mg

Methohexital (meth oh HEKS i tal)

Medication Safety Issues
Sound-alike/look-alike issues:
Brevital® may be confused with Brevibloc®

High alert medication: The Institute for Safe Medication Practices (ISMP) includes this medication among its list of drugs which have a heightened risk of causing significant patient harm when used in error.

Related Information
Adult ACLS Algorithms *on page 1463*
Preprocedure Sedatives in Children *on page 1688*

U.S. Brand Names Brevital® Sodium

Canadian Brand Names Brevital®

Therapeutic Category Barbiturate; General Anesthetic; Sedative

Generic Available No

Use Induction of anesthesia prior to the use of other general anesthetic agents (I.M., rectal: FDA approved in ages >1 month; I.V.: FDA approved in adults); adjunct to subpotent inhalational anesthetic agents for short surgical procedures (I.M., rectal: FDA approved in ages >1 month; I.V.: FDA approved in adults); anesthesia for short surgical, diagnostic, or therapeutic procedures associated with minimal painful stimuli (I.M., rectal: FDA approved in ages >1 month; I.V.: FDA approved in adults); anesthesia for use with other parenteral agents, usually narcotic analgesics, to supplement subpotent inhalational anesthetic agents for longer surgical procedures (FDA approved in adults); induction of hypnotic state (FDA approved in adults)

Restrictions C-IV

Pregnancy Risk Factor B

Pregnancy Considerations Animal studies have not shown fetal or maternal harm. There are no adequate and well-controlled studies in pregnant women. Methohexital crosses the placenta. Use only if potential benefit outweighs risk to fetus.

Lactation Enters breast milk/use caution

Breast-Feeding Considerations Methohexital is minimally excreted in breast milk and levels decline rapidly after administration. Interruption of breast-feeding is unnecessary.

Contraindications Hypersensitivity to methohexital, barbiturates, or any component; porphyria; patients in whom general anesthesia is contraindicated

Warnings Continuously monitor respiratory function, pulse oximetry, and cardiac function. Resuscitative drugs, ventilation and intubation equipment, and trained personnel should be immediately available **[U.S. Boxed Warning]**. For deep sedation, a designated individual (other than the person performing the procedure) should be present to continuously monitor the patient.

Precautions Use with extreme caution in patients with liver impairment, asthma, cardiovascular instability; may precipitate seizures in patients with history of convulsions, especially partial seizure disorders; prolonged administration may result in increased CNS, respiratory, and cardiovascular effects; use with caution in patients with obstructive pulmonary disease, severe hypertension or hypotension, myocardial disease, CHF, severe anemia, extreme obesity, renal impairment, or endocrine disorders. Safety and efficacy of I.V. administration in pediatric patients have not been established.

Adverse Reactions
Cardiovascular: Hypotension, circulatory depression, peripheral vascular collapse, tachycardia (following induction), cardiorespiratory arrest
Central nervous system: Seizures, headache, somnolence, unconsciousness; anxiety, emergence delirium, restlessness (especially if postoperative pain is present)
Dermatologic: Erythema, pruritus, urticaria
Gastrointestinal: Nausea, vomiting, abdominal pain, salivation
Hepatic: Liver enzymes elevated
Local: Pain on I.M. injection, thrombophlebitis, nerve injury adjacent to injection site
Neuromuscular & skeletal: Twitching, rigidity, tremor, involuntary muscle movement
Respiratory: Apnea, respiratory depression, laryngospasm, coughing, bronchospasm, dyspnea, rhinitis
Miscellaneous: Hiccups, anaphylaxis (rare)

Drug Interactions
Avoid Concomitant Use There are no known interactions where it is recommended to avoid concomitant use.

Increased Effect/Toxicity
Methohexital may increase the levels/effects of: Alcohol (Ethyl); CNS Depressants; Meperidine; Thiazide Diuretics

The levels/effects of Methohexital may be increased by: Chloramphenicol; Divalproex; Felbamate; Primidone; Valproic Acid

Decreased Effect
Methohexital may decrease the levels/effects of: Acetaminophen; Beta-Blockers; Calcium Channel Blockers; Chloramphenicol; Contraceptives (Estrogens); Contraceptives (Progestins); Corticosteroids (Systemic); CycloSPORINE; CycloSPORINE (Systemic); Disopyramide; Divalproex; Doxycycline; Etoposide; Etoposide Phosphate; LamoTRIgine; Methadone; Propafenone; QuiNIDine; Teniposide; Theophylline Derivatives; Tricyclic Antidepressants; Valproic Acid; Vitamin K Antagonists

The levels/effects of Methohexital may be decreased by: Pyridoxine; Rifamycin Derivatives

Stability Store vials at controlled room temperature of 20°C to 25°C (68°F to 77°F). Solutions should be freshly prepared and used promptly. Reconstituted solutions are chemically stable at room temperature for 24 hours; 0.2% (2 mg/mL) solutions in D_5W or NS are stable at room temperature for 24 hours.

Do not dilute with solutions containing bacteriostatic agents; acceptable diluents: D_5W, NS, SWI, or accompanying diluent (for 500 mg vial to make a 1% solution); SWI is the preferred diluent except for making the 0.2% solution for I.V. continuous infusion (use of SWI to make the 0.2% solution will result in extreme hypotonicity; D_5W

or NS should be used); dilute with D_5W for I.V. or rectal administration only (not for I.M. use). Do not use I.V./I.M. solutions if not clear and colorless. Solutions are alkaline (pH 9.5-11) and incompatible with acids (eg, atropine sulfate, succinylcholine chloride); incompatible with phenol-containing solutions, silicone, and LR

Mechanism of Action Ultra short-acting I.V. barbiturate anesthetic; depresses CNS activity by binding to barbiturate site at GABA-receptor complex enhancing GABA activity; depresses reticular activating system; higher doses may be gabamimetic

Pharmacodynamics

Onset of action:

I.M. (pediatric patients): 2-10 minutes

I.V.: 1 minute

Rectal (pediatric patients): 5-15 minutes

Duration:

I.M.: 1-1.5 hours

I.V.: 7-10 minutes

Rectal: 1-1.5 hours

Pharmacokinetics (Adult data unless noted)

Metabolism: In the liver via demethylation and oxidation

Bioavailability: Rectal: 17%

Elimination: Through the kidney via glomerular filtration

Usual Dosage Doses must be titrated to effect

Manufacturer's recommendations:

Infants <1 month: Safety and efficacy not established

Infants ≥1 month and Children:

I.M.: Induction: 6.6-10 mg/kg of a 5% solution

Rectal: Induction: Usual: 25 mg/kg of a 1% solution

Alternative pediatric dosing:

Children:

I.M.: Preoperative: 5-10 mg/kg/dose of a 5% solution

I.V.:

Induction: 1-2 mg/kg/dose of a 1% solution (see Björkman, 1987)

Procedural sedation: Initial: 0.5 mg/kg of a 1% solution given immediately prior to procedure; titrate dose to achieve level of sedation as needed, in increments of 0.5 mg/kg to a maximum dose of 2 mg/kg; **Note:** In the prospective phase of a study, 20 children (mean age: 26 months) undergoing emergency CT scans required a mean dose of 1 ± 0.5 mg/kg/dose with a mean total dose of 14 ± 7.5 mg/kg (see Sedik, 2001).

Rectal: Preoperative, anesthesia induction, or preprocedural: Usual: 25 mg/kg/dose; range: 20-35 mg/kg/dose; maximum dose: 500 mg/dose; give as 10% (100 mg/mL) aqueous solution 5-15 minutes prior to procedure (see Bjorkman, 1987; Pomeranz, 2000)

Adults: I.V.:

Induction: Range: 1-1.5 mg/kg or 50-120 mg/dose

Maintenance: Intermittent I.V. bolus injection: 20-40 mg (2-4 mL of a 1% solution) every 4-7 minutes

Administration

Parenteral:

I.M.: Reconstitute with NS to a maximum concentration of 50 mg/mL (5% solution)

I.V.: Adults:

Bolus: Dilute with SWI (preferred), NS, or D_5W to a maximum concentration of 10 mg/mL (1% solution); for induction, infuse a 1% solution at a rate of 1 mL/5 seconds

Continuous infusion: Dilute with D_5W or NS to prepare a 0.2% solution (see Usual Dosage)

Rectal: Dilute with acceptable diluent (see Stability) to a recommended concentration of 10 mg/mL (1% solution); **Note:** 10% solution has been given rectally (see Bjorkman, 1987; Pomeranz, 2000).

Monitoring Parameters Blood pressure, heart rate, respiratory rate, oxygen saturation, pulse oximetry

Patient Information May cause drowsiness and impair ability to perform activities requiring mental alertness or physical coordination; do not drive a motor vehicle or operate machinery until 8-12 hours after medication was administered, or until normal functions return (whichever is longer)

Nursing Implications Check catheter placement prior to I.V. injection; avoid extravasation; avoid intra-arterial administration (thrombosis, necrosis, and gangrene may occur)

Additional Information Does not possess analgesic properties; Brevital® has FDA-approved labeling for I.V. use in adults, and for rectal and I.M. use only in pediatric patients >1 month of age; 100 pediatric patients (3 months to 5 years of age) received rectal methohexital (25 mg/kg) for sedation prior to computed tomography (CT) scan; sedation was adequate in 95% of patients; mean time for full sedation = 8.2 ± 3.9 minutes; mean duration of action = 79.3 ± 30.9 minutes; 10% of patients had transient side effects (see Pomeranz, 2000)

Dosage Forms Excipient information presented when available (limited, particularly for generics); consult specific product labeling.

Injection, powder for reconstitution, as sodium:

Brevital® Sodium: 500 mg, 2.5 g

References

Björkman S, Gabrielsson J, Quaynor H, et al, "Pharmacokinetics of I.V. and Rectal Methohexitone in Children," Br J Anaesth, 1987, 59 (12):1541-7.

Coté CJ, "Sedation for the Pediatric Patient," Pediatr Clin North Am, 1994, 41(1):31-58.

Elman DS and Denson JS, "Preanesthetic Sedation of Children With Intramuscular Methohexital Sodium," Anesth Analg, 1965, 44 (5):494-8.

Miller JR, Grayson M, and Stoelting VK, "Sedation With Intramuscular Methohexital Sodium for Office and Clinic Ophthalmic Procedures in Children," Am J Ophthalmol, 1966, 62(1):38-43.

Pomeranz ES, Chudnofsky CR, Deegan TJ, et al, "Rectal Methohexital Sedation for Computed Tomography Imaging of Stable Pediatric Emergency Department Patients," Pediatrics, 2000, 105(5):1110-4.

Sedik H, "Use of Intravenous Methohexital as a Sedative in Pediatric Emergency Departments," Arch Pediatr Adolesc Med, 2001, 155 (6):665-8.

◆ **Methohexital Sodium** see Methohexital on page 899

Methotrexate (meth oh TREKS ate)

Medication Safety Issues

Sound-alike/look-alike issues:

Methotrexate may be confused with mercaptopurine, methylPREDNISolone sodium succinate, metolazone, metroNIDAZOLE, mitoxantrone, pralatrexate

MTX is an error-prone abbreviation (mistaken as mitoxantrone)

High alert medication: The Institute for Safe Medication Practices (ISMP) includes this medication among its list of drugs which have a heightened risk of causing significant patient harm when used in error.

Intrathecal medication safety: The American Society of Clinical Oncology (ASCO)/Oncology Nursing Society (ONS) chemotherapy administration safety standards (Jacobson, 2009) encourage the following safety measures for intrathecal chemotherapy:

• Intrathecal medication should not be prepared during the preparation of any other agents

• After preparation, store in an isolated location or container clearly marked with a label identifying as "intrathecal" use only

• Delivery to the patient should only be with other medications intended for administration into the central nervous system

Errors have occurred (resulting in death) when methotrexate was administered as "daily" dose instead of the recommended "weekly" dose.

International issues:

Trexall™ may be confused with Truxal® which is a brand name for chlorprothixene in Belgium

Trexall™ may be confused with Trexol® which is a brand name for tramadol in Mexico

Related Information
Compatibility of Chemotherapy and Related Supportive Care Medications *on page 1580*
Emetogenic Potential of Antineoplastic Agents *on page 1579*

U.S. Brand Names Rheumatrex®; Trexall™

Canadian Brand Names Apo-Methotrexate®; ratio-Methotrexate

Therapeutic Category Antineoplastic Agent, Antimetabolite; Antirheumatic, Disease Modifying

Generic Available Yes

Use Treatment of trophoblastic neoplasms (gestational choriocarcinoma, choriadenoma destruens, and hydatidiform mole), acute lymphocytic leukemias, meningeal leukemia, osteosarcoma, breast cancer, head and neck cancer (epidermoid), cutaneous T-Cell lymphoma (advanced mycosis fungoides), lung cancer (squamous cell and small cell), advanced non-Hodgkin's lymphoma [FDA approved in pediatrics (age not specified) and adults]; children with severe polyarticular juvenile rheumatoid arthritis who have failed to respond to other agents (FDA approved in ages 2-16 years); psoriasis (severe, recalcitrant, disabling), severe rheumatoid arthritis (FDA approved in adults)

Has also been used for the treatment and maintenance of remission in Crohn's disease; ectopic pregnancy; dermatomyositis; bladder cancer, central nervous system tumors (including nonleukemic meningeal cancers), acute promyelocytic leukemia (maintenance treatment), soft tissue sarcoma (desmoid tumors)

Pregnancy Risk Factor X (psoriasis, rheumatoid arthritis)

Pregnancy Considerations [U.S. Boxed Warning]: Methotrexate may cause fetal death and/or congenital abnormalities. Studies in animals and pregnant women have shown evidence of fetal abnormalities; therefore, the manufacturer classifies methotrexate as pregnancy category X (for psoriasis or RA). A pattern of congenital malformations associated with maternal methotrexate use is referred to as the aminopterin/methotrexate syndrome. Features of the syndrome include CNS, skeletal, and cardiac abnormalities. Low birth weight and developmental delay have also been reported. The use of methotrexate may impair fertility and cause menstrual irregularities or oligospermia during treatment and following therapy. Methotrexate is approved for the treatment of trophoblastic neoplasms (gestational choriocarcinoma, chorioadenoma destruens, and hydatidiform mole) and has been used for the medical management of ectopic pregnancy and the medical management of abortion. **[U.S. Boxed Warning]: Use is contraindicated for the treatment of psoriasis or RA in pregnant women.** Pregnancy should be excluded prior to therapy in women of childbearing potential. Use for the treatment of neoplastic diseases only when the potential benefit to the mother outweighs the possible risk to the fetus. Pregnancy should be avoided for ≥3 months following treatment in male patients and ≥1 ovulatory cycle in female patients. A registry is available for pregnant women exposed to autoimmune medications including methotrexate. For additional information contact the Organization of Teratology Information Specialists, OTIS Autoimmune Diseases Study, at 877-311-8972.

Lactation Enters breast milk/contraindicated

Breast-Feeding Considerations Low amounts of methotrexate are excreted into breast milk. Due to the potential for serious adverse reactions in a breast-feeding infant, use is contraindicated in nursing mothers. The AAP considers methotrexate to be a "cytotoxic drug that may interfere with cellular metabolism of the nursing infant."

Contraindications Hypersensitivity to methotrexate or any component (see Warnings); nursing mothers

Additional contraindications for patients with psoriasis or rheumatoid arthritis: Pregnancy, alcoholism, alcoholic liver disease or other chronic liver disease, immunodeficiency syndrome (overt or laboratory evidence); pre-existing blood dyscrasias (eg, bone marrow hypoplasia, leukopenia, thrombocytopenia, significant anemia)

Warnings Hazardous agent; use appropriate precautions for handling and disposal. Due to the possibility of severe toxic reactions, fully inform patient of the risks involved; do not use in women of childbearing age unless benefit outweighs risks; methotrexate has been reported to cause fetal death and/or congenital anomalies **[U.S. Boxed Warning]**; women of childbearing potential should not be started on methotrexate until pregnancy is excluded; do not use in pregnant women for treatment of RA or psoriasis. Bone marrow suppression may occur **[U.S. Boxed Warning]**; may result in anemia, aplastic anemia, pancytopenia, leukopenia, neutropenia, and/or thrombocytopenia. Use caution in patients with pre-existing bone marrow suppression. Discontinue therapy in RA or psoriasis if a significant decrease in hematologic components is noted; immune suppression may lead to potentially fatal opportunistic infections **[U.S. Boxed Warning]**. Use of low-dose methotrexate has been associated with the development of malignant lymphomas **[U.S. Boxed Warning]**; may regress upon discontinuation of therapy; treat lymphoma appropriately if regression is not induced by cessation of methotrexate.

Methotrexate has been associated with acute (elevated transaminases) and potentially fatal chronic (fibrosis, cirrhosis) hepatotoxicity **[U.S. Boxed Warning]**. Risk is related to cumulative dose (total dose: ≥1.5 g) and prolonged exposure (duration: ≥2 years). Monitor closely (with liver function tests, including serum albumin) for liver toxicities. Liver enzyme elevations may be noted, but may not be predictive of hepatic disease in long-term treatment for psoriasis [but generally is predictive in rheumatoid arthritis (RA) treatment]. With long-term use, liver biopsy may show histologic changes, fibrosis, or cirrhosis; periodic liver biopsy is recommended with long-term use for psoriasis in patients with risk factors for hepatotoxicity, in patients with persistent abnormal liver function tests, and in RA patients; discontinue methotrexate with moderate-to-severe change in liver biopsy. Risk factors for hepatotoxicity include history of above moderate alcohol consumption, persistant abnormal liver chemistries, history of chronic liver disease (including hepatitis B or C), family history of inheritable liver disease, diabetes, obesity, hyperlipidemia, lack of folate supplementation during methotrexate therapy, and history of significant exposure to heptatotoxic drugs. Use caution with pre-existing liver impairment; may require dosage reduction. Use caution when used with other hepatotoxic agents (azathioprine, retinoids, sulfasalazine). May cause renal damage leading to acute renal failure, especially with high-dose methotrexate; monitor renal function and methotrexate concentrations closely, maintain adequate hydration and urinary alkalinization. Use caution in osteosarcoma patients treated with high-dose methotrexate in combination with nephrotoxic chemotherapy (eg, cisplatin). Methotrexate elimination is reduced in patients with renal impairment **[U.S. Boxed Warning]**. Elimination is reduced in patients with ascites and/or pleural fluid **[U.S. Boxed**

Warning]; may require dose reduction or discontinuation. Monitor closely for toxicity.

May cause potentially life-threatening pneumonitis (may occur at any time during therapy and at any dosage) **[U.S. Boxed Warning]**; monitor closely for pulmonary symptoms, particularly dry, nonproductive cough. Other potential symptoms include fever, dyspnea, hypoxemia, or pulmonary infiltrate. Neurotoxicity manifested as generalized or focal seizures has been reported in pediatric patients with acute lymphoblastic leukemia treated with I.V. methotrexate (1 g/m^2). Symptomatic patients were commonly noted to have leukoencephalopathy and/or microangiopathic calcifications. An acute, neurologic syndrome (confusion, hemiparesis, transient blindness, seizures, coma) has been reported in patients receiving high-dose methotrexate. Any dose level or route of administration may cause severe and potentially fatal dermatologic reactions, including toxic epidermal necrolysis, Stevens-Johnson syndrome, exfoliative dermatitis, skin necrosis, and erythema multiforme **[U.S. Boxed Warning]**. Radiation dermatitis and sunburn may be precipitated by methotrexate administration. Psoriatic lesions may be worsened by concomitant exposure to ultraviolet radiation. Tumor lysis syndrome may occur in patients with high tumor burden **[U.S. Boxed Warning]**; use appropriate prevention and treatment.

Concurrent administration with NSAIDs may cause severe bone marrow suppression, aplastic anemia, and GI toxicity **[U.S. Boxed Warning]**. Do not administer NSAIDs prior to or during high-dose methotrexate therapy; may increase and prolong serum methotrexate concentrations. Doses used for psoriasis may still lead to unexpected toxicities; use caution when administering NSAIDs or salicylates with lower doses of methotrexate for RA. Methotrexate may increase the concentrations and effects of mercaptopurine; may require dosage adjustments. Vitamins containing folate may decrease response to systemic methotrexate; folate deficiency may increase methotrexate toxicity. Concomitant methotrexate administration with radiotherapy may increase the risk of soft tissue necrosis and osteonecrosis **[U.S. Boxed Warning]**. Diarrhea and ulcerative stomatitis may require interruption of therapy **[U.S. Boxed Warning]**; death from hemorrhagic enteritis or intestinal perforation has been reported. Use with caution in patients with peptic ulcer disease, ulcerative colitis.

When used for intrathecal administration, should not be prepared during the preparation of any other agents; after preparation, store intrathecal medications in an isolated location or container clearly marked with a label identifying as "intrathecal" use only; delivery of intrathecal medications to the patient should only be with other medications intended for administration into the central nervous system (see Jacobson, 2009).

Some injections contain benzyl alcohol which may cause allergic reactions in susceptible individuals; large amounts of benzyl alcohol (≥99 mg/kg/day) have been associated with a potentially fatal toxicity ("gasping syndrome") in neonates; the "gasping syndrome" consists of metabolic acidosis, respiratory distress, gasping respirations, CNS dysfunction (including convulsions, intracranial hemorrhage), hypotension and cardiovascular collapse; avoid use of methotrexate products containing benzyl alcohol in neonates; *in vitro* and animal studies have shown that benzoate, a metabolite of benzyl alcohol, displaces bilirubin from protein binding sites. Methotrexate formulations and/or diluents containing preservatives should not be used for intrathecal or high-dose therapy **[U.S. Boxed Warning]**.

Adverse Reactions

Cardiovascular: Chest pain, hypotension, pericarditis, vasculitis

Central nervous system: Chills, confusion, dizziness, encephalopathy, fatigue, fever, malaise, seizures (see Warnings)

  I.T.: Acute chemical arachnoiditis (back pain, headache, nuchal rigidity); leukoencephalopathy (ataxia, coma, confusion, dementia, irritability, seizures, somnolence)

Dermatitis: Alopecia, depigmentation or hyperpigmentation of skin, erythema multiforme (see Warnings), exfoliative dermatitis, photosensitivity, pruritus, rash, Stevens-Johnson syndrome, toxic epidermal necrolysis, urticaria

Endocrine & metabolic: Hyperuricemia

Gastrointestinal: Anorexia, diarrhea, enteritis, nausea, pancreatitis, stomatitis, vomiting

Genitourinary: Cystitis

Hematologic: Anemia, aplastic anemia, hemorrhage, leukopenia, myelosuppression (see Warnings), neutropenia, thrombocytopenia

Hepatic: Hepatotoxicity (see Warnings), hyperbilirubinemia, liver enzymes increased; hepatic fibrosis or cirrhosis (in psoriatic patients, hepatotoxicity has occurred after ≥2 years and after a total dose of at least 1.5 g)

Neuromuscular & skeletal: I.T.: Subacute myelopathy (paraparesis/paraplegia)

Ocular: Blurred vision, conjunctivitis

Renal: Nephropathy (azotemia, hematuria, renal failure)

Respiratory: Dyspnea, hypoxemia, interstitial pneumonitis

Miscellaneous: Anaphylaxis

<1%, postmarketing, and/or case reports: Arthralgias, coughing, dysuria, epistaxis, eye discomfort, hematocrit decreased, infection, sweating, tinnitus, upper respiratory infection, vaginal discharge

Drug Interactions

Metabolism/Transport Effects Substrate of P-glycoprotein, SLCO1B1

Avoid Concomitant Use

Avoid concomitant use of Methotrexate with any of the following: Acitretin; BCG; Natalizumab; Pimecrolimus; Tacrolimus (Topical); Vaccines (Live)

Increased Effect/Toxicity

Methotrexate may increase the levels/effects of: CycloSPORINE; CycloSPORINE (Systemic); Leflunomide; Natalizumab; Vaccines (Live); Vitamin K Antagonists

The levels/effects of Methotrexate may be increased by: Acitretin; Ciprofloxacin; Ciprofloxacin (Systemic); CycloSPORINE; CycloSPORINE (Systemic); Denosumab; Eltrombopag; Nonsteroidal Anti-Inflammatory Agents; Penicillins; P-Glycoprotein Inhibitors; Pimecrolimus; Probenecid; Proton Pump Inhibitors; Salicylates; Sulfonamide Derivatives; Tacrolimus (Topical); Trastuzumab; Trimethoprim

Decreased Effect

Methotrexate may decrease the levels/effects of: BCG; Cardiac Glycosides; Sapropterin; Sipuleucel-T; Vaccines (Inactivated); Vaccines (Live); Vitamin K Antagonists

The levels/effects of Methotrexate may be decreased by: Bile Acid Sequestrants; Echinacea; P-Glycoprotein Inducers

Food Interactions Milk-rich foods may decrease methotrexate absorption; folate may decrease drug response; folate deficiency states may increase methotrexate toxicity

Stability Store tablets and intact vials at room temperature (15°C to 25°C). Protect from light. Solution diluted in D$_5$W or NS is stable for 24 hours at room temperature (21°C to 25°C). Reconstituted solutions with a preservative may be stored under refrigeration for up to 3 months, and up to 4 weeks at room temperature. Intrathecal dilutions are stable at room temperature for 7 days, but it is generally recommended that they be used within 4-8 hours. Injection is incompatible with chlorpromazine, gemcitabine, ifosfamide, midazolam, promethazine, and propofol

Intrathecal mediations should not be prepared during the preparation of any other agents. After preparation, store intrathecal medications in an isolated location or container clearly marked with a label identifying as "intrathecal" use only.

Mechanism of Action An antimetabolite that binds to dihydrofolate reductase blocking the reduction of dihydrofolate to tetrahydrofolic acid; depletion of tetrahydrofolic acid leads to depletion of DNA precursors and inhibition of DNA and purine synthesis

Pharmacodynamics Approximate time to benefit in treatment of rheumatoid arthritis: 3-6 weeks

Pharmacokinetics (Adult data unless noted)

Absorption:

Oral: Average: 30%; variable absorption at low doses (<30 mg/m^2); incomplete absorption after large doses

I.M.: Completely absorbed

Distribution: Small amounts excreted into breast milk; crosses the placenta; does not achieve therapeutic concentrations in the CSF; distributes to gallbladder, spleen, and skin; sustained concentrations are retained in the kidney and liver; V_{dss}: 0.4-0.8 L/kg

Metabolism: In the liver to 7-hydroxymethotrexate; polyglutamates are produced intracellularly (active metabolites)

Protein binding: 50% to 60%

Time to peak serum concentration:

Oral: 0.5-4 hours

Parenteral: 0.5-2 hours

Half-life (terminal): Low dose <30 mg/m^2: 3-10 hours; high dose: 8-15 hours

Elimination: Small amounts in feces; primarily excreted unchanged in urine (90%) via glomerular filtration and active secretion by the renal tubule; 1% to 11% of a dose is excreted as the 7-hydroxy metabolite

Usual Dosage Refer to individual protocols:

Children:

Dermatomyositis: Oral: 15-20 mg/m^2/week as a single dose once weekly or 0.3-1 mg/kg/dose once weekly

Juvenile rheumatoid arthritis: Oral, I.M., SubQ: Initial: 10 mg/m^2 once weekly; dosing may be increased to 15-20 mg/m^2/week as a single dose or in 3 divided doses given 12 hours apart; **Note:** Subcutaneous administration is recommended with doses >10 mg/m^2 since oral absorption decreases with higher doses; folic acid 1 mg daily or leucovorin calcium ≤5 mg weekly are often used to prevent folate depletion from methotrexate

Antineoplastic dosage range: **Note:** Doses between 100-500 mg/m^2 **may require** leucovorin calcium rescue. Doses >500 mg/m^2 **require** leucovorin calcium rescue

Oral, I.M.: 7.5-30 mg/m^2/week or every 2 weeks

I.V.: 10 mg to 33,000 mg/m^2 bolus dosing or continuous infusion over 6-42 hours

Antineoplastic dosing schedules (adapted from Dorr RT and Von Hoff DD, *Cancer Chemotherapy Handbook*, 2nd ed, 1994): See table

Pediatric solid tumors:

<12 years: 12 g/m^2 (dosage range: 12-18 g)

≥12 years: 8 g/m^2 (maximum dose: 18 g)

Meningeal leukemia: I.T.: 6-12 mg/dose (maximum: 15 mg) based on age:

<1 year: 6 mg dose

1 year: 8 mg dose

2 years: 10 mg dose

≥3 years: 12 mg dose

I.T. doses are administered at 2- to 5-day intervals until CSF counts return to normal followed by a dose once weekly for 2 weeks then monthly thereafter

Methotrexate Dosing Schedules

	Dose	Route	Frequency
Conventional dose	15-20 mg/m^2	Oral	Twice weekly
	30-50 mg/m^2	Oral, I.V.	Weekly
	15 mg/day for 5 days	Oral, I.M.	Every 2-3 weeks
Intermediate dose	50-150 mg/m^2	I.V. push	Every 2-3 weeks
	240 mg/m^{2*}	I.V. infusion	Every 4-7 days
	0.5-1 g/m^{2*}	I.V. infusion	Every 2-3 weeks
High dose	1-12 g/m^{2*}	I.V. infusion	Every 1-3 weeks

*Followed with leucovorin rescue.

ALL (high-dose): I.V.: Loading dose: 200 mg/m^2 followed by a 24-hour infusion of 1200 mg/m^2/day

ANLL: I.V.: 7.5 mg/m^2/day on days 1-5 of treatment course

Resistant ANLL: I.V.: 100 mg/m^2/dose on day 1 of treatment course

Non-Hodgkin's lymphoma: I.V.: 200-500 mg/m^2; repeat every 28 days

Induction of remission in acute lymphoblastic leukemias: Oral: 3.3 mg/m^2/day for 4-6 weeks

Remission maintenance: Oral, I.M.: 20-30 mg/m^2 2 times/week

Adults:

Trophoblastic neoplasms: Oral, I.M.: 15-30 mg/day for 5 days, repeat in 7 days for 3-5 courses

Head and neck cancer: Oral, I.M., I.V.: 25-50 mg/m^2 once weekly

Meningeal leukemia: I.T.: Usual dose: 12 mg/dose (maximum dose: 15 mg)

Rheumatoid arthritis: **Note:** Some experts recommend concomitant folic acid at a dose of at least 5 mg/week (except the day of methotrexate) to reduce hematologic, gastrointestinal, and hepatic adverse events related to methotrexate.

Oral: 7.5 mg once weekly **or** 2.5 mg every 12 hours for 3 doses/week; dosage exceeding 20 mg/week may cause a higher incidence and severity of adverse events; alternative dose: 10-15 mg once weekly; increase by 5 mg every 4 weeks to highest tolerated dose (maximum: 30 mg/week) (see Visser, 2009)

I.M., SubQ: 15 mg once weekly (dosage varies, similar to oral) (see Braun, 2008)

Psoriasis: **Note:** Some experts recommend concomitant folic acid 1-5 mg/day (except the day of methotrexate) to reduce hematologic, gastrointestinal, and hepatic adverse events related to methotrexate.

Oral: 2.5-5 mg/dose every 12 hours for 3 doses given weekly

or

Oral, I.M., SubQ: 10-25 mg given once weekly; titrate to lowest effective dose

Note: An initial test dose of 2.5-5 mg is recommended in patients with risk factors for hematologic toxicity or renal impairment (see Kalb, 2009).

Dosing adjustment in renal impairment:

Cl$_{cr}$ 61-80 mL/minute: Decrease dose by 25%

Cl$_{cr}$ 51-60 mL/minute: Decrease dose by 33%

Cl$_{cr}$ 10-50 mL/minute: Decrease dose by 50% to 70%

Administration

Oral: Administer on an empty stomach.

Parenteral:

Methotrexate may be administered I.V. push, I.V. intermittent infusion, or I.V. continuous infusion at a concentration <25 mg/mL; doses >100-300 mg/m^2 are usually administered by I.V. continuous infusion and are followed by a course of leucovorin calcium rescue

For intrathecal use, mix methotrexate without preservatives with NS, Elliotts B solution, or LR to a concentration not greater than 2 mg/mL

Monitoring Parameters CBC with differential and platelet count, creatinine clearance, serum creatinine, BUN, hepatic function tests, serum electrolytes, urinalysis, plasma methotrexate concentrations (see Leucovorin calcium rescue graph to evaluate plasma methotrexate concentration versus leucovorin calcium rescue dose); periodic liver biopsy for psoriatic patients with risk factors for hepatotoxicity receiving long-term treatment; patients with persistent abnormal liver function tests and RA patients; chest x-ray; pulmonary function tests if methotrexate-induced lung disease is suspected

Reference Range Serum concentrations >1 x 10^{-7} mol/L for more than 40 hours are toxic

Patient Information Report to physician any fever, sore throat, black or tarry stools, yellowing of skin or eyes, bleeding or bruising, shortness of breath, painful urination; avoid alcohol. May cause photosensitivity reactions (eg, exposure to sunlight may cause severe sunburn, skin rash, redness, or itching); avoid exposure to sunlight and artificial light sources (sunlamps, tanning booth/bed); wear protective clothing, wide-brimmed hats, sunglasses, and lip sunscreen (SPF ≥15); use a sunscreen [broad-spectrum sunscreen or physical sunscreen (preferred) or sunblock with SPF ≥15]; contact physician if reaction occurs. Pregnancy should be avoided if either partner is receiving methotrexate; effective contraceptive measures must be used; avoid pregnancy for a minimum of 3 months after completion of therapy in male patients and for at least one ovulatory cycle in female patients.

Nursing Implications Intensive hydration should be administered and urine should be alkalinized prior to high doses to enhance methotrexate solubility

Additional Information Myelosuppressive effects:
WBC: Mild
Platelets: Moderate
Onset (days): 7
Nadir (days): 10
Recovery (days): 21
Methotrexate overexposure: The investigational rescue agent, glucarpidase, is an enzyme which rapidly hydrolyzes extracellular methotrexate into inactive metabolites, resulting in a rapid reduction of methotrexate concentrations. Glucarpidase is available for intrathecal (I.T.) use through an Emergency Use IND and for I.V. use under an Open-Label Treatment protocol.

Dosage Forms Excipient information presented when available (limited, particularly for generics); consult specific product labeling.
Injection, powder for reconstitution: 1 g
Injection, solution: 25 mg/mL (2 mL, 10 mL) [contains benzyl alcohol]
Injection, solution [preservative free]: 25 mg/mL (2 mL, 4 mL, 8 mL, 10 mL, 40 mL)
Tablet: 2.5 mg
Trexall™: 5 mg, 7.5 mg, 10 mg, 15 mg
Tablet [dose pack]: 2.5 mg (4 cards with 2, 3, 4, 5, or 6 tablets each)
Rheumatrex®: 2.5 mg (4 cards with 2, 3, 4, 5, or 6 tablets each)

References
American Academy of Pediatrics Committee on Drugs, "Transfer of Drugs and Other Chemicals Into Human Milk," *Pediatrics*, 2001, 108 (3):776-89.
Barnhart KT, "Clinical Practice. Ectopic Pregnancy," *N Engl J Med*, 2009, 361(4):379-87.
Bell EA, "Pharmacotherapy of Juvenile Idiopathic Arthritis," *J Pharmacy Practice*, 2009, 22(1):17-28.
Benz C, Tillis T, Tattelman E, et al, "Optimal Schedule of Methotrexate and 5-Fluorouracil in Human Breast Cancer," *Cancer Res*, 1982, 42 (5):2081-6.
Berg SL, Grisell DL, DeLaney TF, et al, "Principles of Treatment of Pediatric Solid Tumors," *Pediatr Clin North Am*, 1991, 38(2):249-67.
Bleyer AW, "Clinical Pharmacology of Intrathecal Methotrexate II. An Approved Dosage Regimen Derived From Age-Related Pharmacokinetics," *Cancer Treat Rep*, 1977, 61(8):1419-25.

Braun J, Kästner P, Flaxenberg P, et al, "Comparison of the Clinical Efficacy and Safety of Subcutaneous Versus Oral Administration of Methotrexate in Patients With Active Rheumatoid Arthritis: Results of a Six-Month, Multicenter, Randomized, Double-Blind, Controlled, Phase IV Trial," *Arthritis Rheum*, 2008, 58(1):73-81.
Crom WR, Glynn-Barnhart AM, Rodman JH, et al, "Pharmacokinetics of Anticancer Drugs in Children," *Clin Pharmacokinet*, 1987, 12 (3):168-213.
Giannini EH, Brewer EJ, Kuzmina N, et al, "Methotrexate in Resistant Juvenile Rheumatoid Arthritis. Results of the USA-USSR Double-Blind, Placebo-Controlled Trial," *N Engl J Med*, 1992, 326(16):1043-9.
Glantz MJ, Cole BF, Recht L, et al, "High-Dose Intravenous Methotrexate for Patients With Nonleukemic Leptomeningeal Cancer: Is Intrathecal Chemotherapy Necessary?" *J Clin Oncol*, 1998, 16 (4):1561-7.
Glantz MJ, Jaeckle KA, Chamberlain MC, et al, "A Randomized Controlled Trial Comparing Intrathecal Sustained-Release Cytarabine (DepoCyt) to Intrathecal Methotrexate in Patients With Neoplastic Meningitis From Solid Tumors," *Clin Cancer Res*, 1999, 5 (11):3394-402.
Greaves MW and Weinstein GD, "Treatment of Psoriasis," *N Engl J Med*, 1995, 332(9):581-8.
Jacobson JO, Polovich M, McNiff KK, et al, "American Society of Clinical Oncology/Oncology Nursing Society Chemotherapy Administration Safety Atandards," *J Clin Oncol*, 2009, 27(32):5469-75.
Kalb RE, Strober B, Weinstein G, et al, "Methotrexate and Psoriasis: 2009 National Psoriasis Foundation Consensus Conference," *J Am Acad Dermatol*, 2009, 60(5):824-37.
National Comprehensive Cancer Network (NCCN)®, "Clinical Practice Guidelines in Oncology™: Central Nervous System Cancers," Version 2.2009. Available at: http://www.nccn.org/professionals/physician_gls/PDF/cns.pdf.
Schwartz S, Borner K, Müller K, et al, "Glucarpidase (Carboxypeptidase G2) Intervention in Adult and Elderly Cancer Patients With Renal Dysfunction and Delayed Methotrexate Elimination After High-Dose Methotrexate Therapy," *Oncologist*, 2007, 12(11):1299-308.
Rose CD, Singsen BH, and Eichenfield AH, "Safety and Efficacy of Methotrexate Therapy for Juvenile Rheumatoid Arthritis," *J Pediatr*, 1990, 117(4):653-9.
Visser K, Katchamart W, Loza E, et al, "Multinational Evidence-Based Recommendations for the Use of Methotrexate in Rheumatic Disorders With a Focus on Rheumatoid Arthritis: Integrating Systematic Literature Research and Expert Opinion of a Broad International Panel of Rheumatologists in the 3E Initiative," *Ann Rheum Dis*, 2009, 68(7):1086-93.
Widemann BC, Balis FM, Murphy RF, et al, "Carboxypeptidase-G2, Thymidine, and Leucovorin Rescue in Cancer Patients With Methotrexate-Induced Renal Dysfunction," *J Clin Oncol*, 1997, 15 (5):2125-34.
Widemann BC, Balis FM, Shalabi A, et al, "Treatment of Accidental Intrathecal Methotrexate Overdose With Intrathecal Carboxypeptidase G2," *J Natl Cancer Inst*, 2004, 96(20):1557-9.

◆ **Methotrexate Sodium** *see* Methotrexate *on page 900*

◆ **Methotrexatum** *see* Methotrexate *on page 900*

Methsuximide (meth SUKS i mide)

Medication Safety Issues
Sound-alike/look-alike issues:
Methsuximide may be confused with ethosuximide
Related Information
Antiepileptic Drugs *on page 1693*
U.S. Brand Names Celontin®
Canadian Brand Names Celontin®
Therapeutic Category Anticonvulsant, Succinimide
Generic Available No
Use Control of refractory absence (petit mal) seizures (FDA approved in children and adults); useful adjunct in refractory, partial complex (psychomotor) seizures
Pregnancy Considerations Patients exposed to methsuximide during pregnancy are encouraged to enroll themselves into the NAAED Pregnancy Registry by calling 1-888-233-2334. Additional information is available at www.aedpregnancyregistry.org.
Contraindications Hypersensitivity to methsuximide, other succinimides, or any component

Warnings Blood dyscrasias (sometimes fatal) have been reported (monitor hematologic function periodically or if signs/symptoms of infection develop); SLE has been reported with the use of succinimides

Antiepileptic drugs (AEDs) increase the risk of suicidal behavior and ideation in patients receiving these medications for any indication. Pooled analyses of placebo-controlled trials involving 11 different AEDs (regardless of indication) showed a twofold increased risk of suicidal thoughts or behavior (estimated incidence rate: 0.43% in AED-treated patients compared to 0.24% in patients receiving placebo); increased risk was observed as early as one week after initiation of AED and continued through duration of trials (most trials ≤24 weeks); risk did not vary significantly by age (age range: 5–100 years). Consider risks and benefits of AEDs before prescribing. Monitor all patients receiving an AED for emergence of suicidal thoughts or behavior, thoughts of self-harm, any unusual changes in behavior or mood, or the emergence or worsening of depressive symptoms; notify heathcare provider immediately if symptoms or concerning behavior occur. **Note:** The FDA is requiring that a Medication Guide be developed for all antiepileptic drugs, informing patients of this risk.

Precautions Use with caution in patients with hepatic or renal disease. Avoid abrupt withdrawal (may precipitate absence status). When used alone, methsuximide may increase tonic-clonic seizures in patients with mixed seizure disorders; methsuximide must be used in combination with other anticonvulsants in patients with both absence and tonic-clonic seizures. May cause CNS depression, which may impair physical or mental abilities; patients must be cautioned about performing tasks which require mental alertness.

Adverse Reactions

Cardiovascular: Hyperemia

Central nervous system: Aggressiveness, ataxia, auditory hallucinations (rare), confusion, dizziness, depression, drowsiness, euphoria, headache, hypochondriacal behavior, insomnia, irritability, lethargy, mental instability, mental slowness, nervousness, psychosis (rare), suicidal thinking and behavior (see Warnings)

Dermatologic: Pruritus, rash, Stevens-Johnson syndrome, urticaria

Endocrine & metabolic: Weight loss

Gastrointestinal: Abdominal pain, anorexia, constipation, diarrhea, epigastric pain, nausea, vomiting

Genitourinary: Microscopic hematuria, proteinuria

Hematologic: Eosinophilia, leukopenia, monocytosis, pancytopenia (with and without bone marrow suppression) (see Warnings)

Neuromuscular & skeletal: Systemic lupus erythematosus (case reports)

Ocular: Blurred vision, periorbital edema, photophobia

Miscellaneous: Hiccups

Drug Interactions

Metabolism/Transport Effects Substrate of CYP2C19 (major); **Inhibits** CYP2C19 (weak)

Avoid Concomitant Use There are no known interactions where it is recommended to avoid concomitant use.

Increased Effect/Toxicity

Methsuximide may increase the levels/effects of: Alcohol (Ethyl); CNS Depressants; Methotrimeprazine

The levels/effects of Methsuximide may be increased by: CYP2C19 Inhibitors (Moderate); CYP2C19 Inhibitors (Strong); Methotrimeprazine

Decreased Effect

The levels/effects of Methsuximide may be decreased by: CYP2C19 Inducers (Strong); Ketorolac; Ketorolac (Systemic); Mefloquine

Stability Store at 25°C (77°F); protect from light, moisture, and excessive heat 40°C (104°F); **Note:** Methsuximide has a relatively low melting temperature (124°F); do not store in conditions that promote high temperatures (eg, in a closed vehicle)

Mechanism of Action Increases the seizure threshold and suppresses paroxysmal spike-and-wave pattern in absence seizures; depresses nerve transmission in the motor cortex

Pharmacokinetics (Adult data unless noted)

Metabolism: Rapidly demethylated in the liver to N-desmethylmethsuximide (active metabolite)

Half-life: 2-4 hours

N-desmethylmethsuximide:

Children: 26 hours

Adults: 28-80 hours

Time to peak serum concentration: Within 1-3 hours

Elimination: <1% in urine as unchanged drug

Usual Dosage Oral:

Children: Initial: 10-15 mg/kg/day in 3-4 divided doses; increase weekly up to maximum of 30 mg/kg/day; mean dose required:

<30 kg: 20 mg/kg/day

>30 kg: 14 mg/kg/day

Adults: 300 mg/day for the first week; may increase by 300 mg/day at weekly intervals up to 1.2 g in 2-4 divided doses/day

Administration Oral: Administer with food

Monitoring Parameters CBC with differential, liver enzymes, urinalysis; measure trough serum levels for efficacy and 3-hour postdose concentrations for toxicity; signs and symptoms of suicidality (eg, anxiety, depression, behavior changes) (see Warnings)

Reference Range Measure N-desmethylmethsuximide concentrations:

Therapeutic: 10-40 mcg/mL (SI: 53-212 micromoles/L)

Toxic: >40 mcg/mL (SI: >212 micromoles/L)

Patient Information May cause drowsiness and impair ability to perform activities requiring mental alertness or physical coordination. Do not discontinue abruptly (seizures may occur). Antiepileptic agents may increase the risk of suicidal thoughts and behavior; notify physician if you feel more depressed or have thoughts of suicide or self-harm (see Warnings). Notify physician if sore throat or fever develop. Report worsening of seizure activity or loss of seizure control. Do not store capsules in conditions that promote high temperatures (eg, in closed cars or other vehicles), as medication may melt.

Dosage Forms Excipient information presented when available (limited, particularly for generics); consult specific product labeling.

Capsule:

Celontin®: 150 mg, 300 mg

References

Miles MV, Tennison MB, and Greenwood RS, "Pharmacokinetics of N-desmethylmethsuximide in Pediatric Patients," *J Pediatr,* 1989, 114(4 Pt 1):647-50.

Tennison MB, Greenwood RS, Miles MV, "Methsuximide for Intractable Childhood Seizures," *Pediatrics,* 1991, 87(2):186-9.

◆ **Methylacetoxyprogesterone** *see* MedroxyPROGES-TERone *on page 870*

Methyldopa (meth il DOE pa)

Medication Safety Issues

Sound-alike/look-alike issues:

Methyldopa may be confused with L-dopa, levodopa

Beers Criteria medication: This drug may be inappropriate for use in geriatric patients (high severity risk).

Related Information

Antihypertensive Agents by Class *on page 1481*

Canadian Brand Names Apo-Methyldopa®; Nu-Medopa ▶

Therapeutic Category Alpha-Adrenergic Inhibitors, Central; Antihypertensive Agent

Generic Available Yes

Use Management of moderate to severe hypertension

Pregnancy Risk Factor B

Pregnancy Considerations Crosses the placenta. Hypotension reported. A large amount of clinical experience with the use of these drugs for the management of hypertension during pregnancy is available. Available evidence suggests safe use during pregnancy.

Lactation Enters breast milk/compatible

Breast-Feeding Considerations Crosses into breast milk at extremely low levels. AAP considers **compatible** with breast-feeding.

Contraindications Hypersensitivity to methyldopa or any component (see Warnings); liver disease, pheochromocytoma

Warnings Injection contains sodium bisulfite which may cause allergic reactions in susceptible individuals

Precautions Use with caution and adjust dose in patients with renal dysfunction; active metabolite may accumulate in uremia

Adverse Reactions

Cardiovascular: Orthostatic hypotension, bradycardia, edema

Central nervous system: Drowsiness, sedation, vertigo, headache, depression, memory lapse, fever

Dermatologic: Rash

Endocrine & metabolic: Gynecomastia, sexual dysfunction, sodium retention

Gastrointestinal: Nausea, vomiting, diarrhea, xerostomia, "black" tongue

Genitourinary: Discoloration of urine (red or brown)

Hematologic: Hemolytic anemia, positive Coombs' test, leukopenia

Hepatic: Hepatitis, liver enzymes elevated, jaundice, cirrhosis

Neuromuscular & skeletal: Weakness

Respiratory: Nasal congestion

Drug Interactions

Avoid Concomitant Use

Avoid concomitant use of Methyldopa with any of the following: Iobenguane I 123; MAO Inhibitors

Increased Effect/Toxicity

Methyldopa may increase the levels/effects of: Lithium

The levels/effects of Methyldopa may be increased by: COMT Inhibitors; MAO Inhibitors

Decreased Effect

Methyldopa may decrease the levels/effects of: Iobenguane I 123

The levels/effects of Methyldopa may be decreased by: Iron Salts

Food Interactions Avoid natural licorice (causes sodium and water retention and increases potassium loss); dietary requirements for vitamin B_{12} and folate may be increased with high doses of methyldopa

Mechanism of Action Stimulates inhibitory alpha-adrenergic receptors via alpha-methylnorepinephrine (false transmitter); this results in a decreased sympathetic outflow to the heart, kidneys, and peripheral vasculature; may decrease plasma renin activity

Pharmacodynamics Hypotensive effects:

Maximum effect: Oral, I.V.: Single-dose: Within 3-6 hours; multiple-dose: 2-3 days

Duration:

Oral: Single-dose: 12-24 hours; multiple-dose: 1-2 days

I.V.: 10-16 hours

Pharmacokinetics (Adult data unless noted)

Absorption: Oral: ~50%

Distribution: Crosses placenta; appears in breast milk

Protein binding: <15%

Metabolism: In the intestine and the liver

Half-life: Elimination:

Neonates: 10-20 hours

Adults: 1-3 hours

Elimination: ~70% of systemic dose eliminated in urine as drug and metabolites

Dialysis: Slightly dialyzable (5% to 20%)

Usual Dosage

Children:

Oral: Initial: 10 mg/kg/day in 2-4 divided doses; increase every 2 days as needed to maximum dose of 65 mg/kg/day; do not exceed 3 g/day

I.V.: Initial: 2-4 mg/kg/dose; if response is not seen within 4-6 hours, may increase to 5-10 mg/kg/dose; administer doses every 6-8 hours; maximum daily dose: 65 mg/kg or 3 g, whichever is less

Adults:

Oral: Initial: 250 mg 2-3 times/day; increase every 2 days as needed; usual dose 500 mg to 2 g daily in 2-4 divided doses; maximum dose: 3 g/day; usual dosage range (JNC 7): 250-1000 mg/day in 2 divided doses

I.V.: 250-1000 mg every 6-8 hours; maximum dose: 4 g/day

Dosing interval in renal impairment: Children and Adults:

Cl_{cr} >50 mL/minute: Administer normal dose every 8 hours

Cl_{cr} 10-50 mL/minute: Administer normal dose every 8-12 hours

Cl_{cr} <10 mL/minute: Administer normal dose every 12-24 hours

Administration

Oral: May be administered without regard to food; administer new dosage increases in the evening to minimize sedation

Parenteral: I.V.: Infuse I.V. dose slowly over 30-60 minutes at a concentration ≤10 mg/mL

Monitoring Parameters Blood pressure, CBC with differential, hemoglobin, hematocrit, Coombs' test [direct], liver enzymes

Test Interactions Urinary uric acid, serum creatinine (alkaline picrate method), AST (colorimetric method), and urinary catecholamines (falsely high levels)

Patient Information Avoid alcohol; may cause drowsiness and impair ability to perform activities requiring mental alertness or physical coordination; may cause dry mouth; rise slowly from prolonged sitting or lying position; may cause urine to turn red or brown; notify physician of unexplained prolonged general tiredness, fever, or jaundice

Nursing Implications Transient sedation or depression may occur for first 72 hours of therapy, or when doses are increased

Additional Information Most effective if used with diuretic; titrate dose to optimal blood pressure control with minimal side effects

Dosage Forms Excipient information presented when available (limited, particularly for generics); consult specific product labeling.

Injection, solution, as methyldopate hydrochloride: 50 mg/mL (5 mL) [contains sodium bisulfite]

Tablet: 250 mg, 500 mg

Extemporaneous Preparations A 50 mg/mL oral liquid preparation made from tablets and 2 different vehicles [unpreserved simple syrup (Syrup, USP) and a 1:1 mixture of simple syrup (containing 0.5% citric acid) and hydrochloric acid 0.2 N] was stable for 14 days when stored in glass prescription bottles in the dark, at room temperature (25°C) or under refrigeration (5°C); grind ten 250 mg tablets in a glass mortar into a fine powder. To make formulation with unpreserved simple syrup (Syrup, USP), levigate with Syrup, USP to form a uniform paste; add a small amount of Syrup, USP; mix well; transfer to a calibrated bottle; rinse the mortar and pestle several times with vehicle; transfer to calibrated bottle and qsad to 50 mL. To make formulation with second vehicle, levigate powdered tablets with 25 mL of hydrochloric acid 0.2 N (0.73% w/v); dilute this mixture to 50 mL with simple syrup containing 0.5% citric acid by the method described above. Label "shake well" and "protect from light."

Newton DW, Rogers AG, Becker CH, et al, "Extemporaneous Preparation of Methyldopa in Two Syrup Vehicles," *Am J Hosp Pharm*, 1975, 32(8):817-21.

References

Chobanian AV, Bakris GL, Black HR, et al, "The Seventh Report of the Joint National Committee on Prevention, Detection, Evaluation, and Treatment of High Blood Pressure: The JNC 7 report," *JAMA*, 2003, 289(19):2560-72.

◆ **Methyldopate Hydrochloride** *see* Methyldopa *on page 905*

Methylene Blue (METH i leen bloo)

Medication Safety Issues Due to potential toxicity (hemolytic anemia), do not use methylene blue to color enteral feedings to detect aspiration.

Therapeutic Category Antidote, Cyanide; Antidote, Drug-induced Methemoglobinemia

Generic Available Yes

Use Antidote for cyanide poisoning and drug-induced methemoglobinemia (FDA approved use), indicator dye, bacteriostatic genitourinary antiseptic; other uses include treatment/prevention of ifosfamide-induced encephalopathy; topically, in conjunction with polychromatic light to photoinactivate viruses such as herpes simplex; alone or in combination with vitamin C for the management of chronic urolithiasis

Pregnancy Risk Factor C

Contraindications Hypersensitivity to methylene blue or any component; renal insufficiency; intraspinal injection

Warnings Do not inject subcutaneously or intrathecally as necrotic abscesses (SubQ) and neural damage (I.T.) including paraplegia have occurred. Methylène blue should not be added to enteral feeding products (Wessel, 2005); safety and efficacy has not been established.

Precautions Use with caution in patients with severe renal insufficiency or G-6-PD deficiency; continued use can cause profound anemia; inject slowly to avoid high local concentrations and the production of methemoglobin

Adverse Reactions

Cardiovascular: Cyanosis, hypertension, large I.V. doses have been associated with precordial pain and hypotension

Central nervous system: Dizziness, fever, headache, mental confusion

Dermatologic: Phototoxicity, skin staining

Gastrointestinal: Abdominal pain, diarrhea, discoloration of feces (blue-green), nausea, vomiting

Genitourinary: Bladder irritation, discoloration of urine (blue-green)

Hematologic: Formation of methemoglobin, hemolytic anemia

Miscellaneous: Diaphoresis

Drug Interactions

Avoid Concomitant Use There are no known interactions where it is recommended to avoid concomitant use.

Increased Effect/Toxicity There are no known significant interactions involving an increase in effect.

Decreased Effect There are no known significant interactions involving a decrease in effect.

Stability Store at 20°C to 25°C (68°F to 77°F); excursions permitted to 15°C to 30°C (59°F to 86°F)

Mechanism of Action Weak germicide; in low concentrations hastens the conversion of methemoglobin to hemoglobin; has opposite effect at high concentrations by converting ferrous iron of reduced hemoglobin to ferric iron to form methemoglobin; in cyanide toxicity, it combines with cyanide to form cyanmethemoglobin preventing the interference of cyanide with the cytochrome system

Pharmacokinetics (Adult data unless noted)

Absorption: Well-absorbed from GI tract

Bioavailability, oral: 50% to 100%

Time to peak effect: 30 minutes

Metabolism: Peripheral reduction to leukomethylene blue

Elimination: In bile, feces, and urine as leukomethylene blue

Usual Dosage

Methemoglobinemia: Children and Adults: I.V.: 1-2 mg/kg or 25-50 mg/m^2; may be repeated after 1 hour if necessary

Chronic methemoglobinemia: Adults: Oral: 100-300 mg/day

NADPH-methemoglobin reductase deficiency: Children: Oral: 1-1.5 mg/kg/day (maximum dose: 300 mg/day) given with 5-8 mg/kg/day ascorbic acid

Genitourinary antiseptic: Adults: Oral: 65-130 mg 3 times/day; maximum dose: 390 mg/day

Chronic urolithiasis: Adults: Oral: 65 mg 3 times/day

Ifosfamide-induced encephalopathy: Adults: Oral, I.V.:

Note: Treatment may not be necessary; encephalopathy may improve spontaneously

Prevention: 50 mg every 6-8 hours

Treatment: 50 mg as a single dose or every 4-8 hours until symptoms resolve

Administration

Parenteral: Administer undiluted by direct I.V. injection over several minutes; when administered for the treatment of ifosfamide-induced encephalopathy, may be administered either undiluted as a slow I.V. push over at least 5 minutes or diluted in 50 mL NS or D$_5$W and infused over at least 5 minutes; may be administered intraosseously

Oral: Administer after meals with a full glass of water; may be mixed with fruit juice to mask unpleasant taste

Monitoring Parameters CBC; of note, pulse oximetry is not reliable as methylene blue interferes with light emission, resulting in falsely depressed readings

Patient Information May discolor urine and feces blue-green; may discolor skin on contact

Additional Information Has been used topically (0.1% solutions) in conjunction with polychromatic light to photoinactivate viruses such as herpes simplex; has been used alone or in combination with vitamin C for the management of chronic urolithiasis; skin stains may be removed using a hypochlorite solution

Dosage Forms Excipient information presented when available (limited, particularly for generics); consult specific product labeling.

Injection, solution: 10 mg/mL (1 mL, 10 mL)

References

Albert M, Lessin MS, and Gilchrist BF, "Methylene Blue: Dangerous Dye for Neonates," *J Pediatr Surg*, 2003, 38(8):1244-5.

Clifton J 2nd and Leikin JB, "Methylene Blue," *Am J Ther*, 2003, 10 (4):289-91.

David KA and Picus J, "Evaluating Risk Factors for the Development of Ifosfamide Encephalopathy," *Am J Clin Oncol*, 2005, 28(3):277-80.

Maloney JP, Ryan TA, Brasel KJ, et al, "Food Dye Use in Enteral Feedings: A Review and a Call for a Moratorium," *Nutr Clin Pract*, 2002, 17(3):169-81.

Patel PN, "Methylene Blue for Management of Ifosfamide-Induced Encephalopathy," *Ann Pharmacother*, 2006, 40(2):299-303.

Pelgrims J, DeVos F, Van den Brande J, et al, "Methylene Blue in the Treatment and Prevention of Ifosfamide-Induced Encephalopathy: Report of 12 Cases and a Review of the Literature," *Br J Cancer*, 2000, 82(2) 291-4.

Sills MR and Zinkham WH, "Methylene Blue-Induced Heinz Body Hemolytic Anemia," *Arch Pediatr Adolesc Med*, 1994, 148(3):306-10.

Wessel J, Balint J, Crill C, et al, "Standards for Specialized Nutrition Support: Hospitalized Pediatric Patients," *Nutr Clin Pract*, 2005, 20 (1):103-16.

◆ **Methylin®** *see* Methylphenidate *on page 908*

◆ **Methylin® ER** *see* Methylphenidate *on page 908*

◆ **Methylmorphine** *see* Codeine *on page 351*

Methylphenidate (meth il FEN i date)

Medication Safety Issues
Sound-alike/look-alike issues:
Metadate CD® may be confused with Metadate® ER
Metadate® ER may be confused with Metadate CD®, methadone
Methylphenidate may be confused with methadone
Ritalin® may be confused with Ismelin®, Rifadin®, ritodrine
Ritalin LA® may be confused with Ritalin-SR®
Ritalin-SR® may be confused with Ritalin LA®
U.S. Brand Names Concerta®; Daytrana™; Metadate CD®; Metadate® ER; Methylin®; Methylin® ER; Ritalin LA®; Ritalin-SR®; Ritalin®
Canadian Brand Names Apo-Methylphenidate®; Apo-Methylphenidate® SR; Biphentin®; Concerta®; Novo-Methylphenidate ER-C; PHL-Methylphenidate; PMS-Methylphenidate; ratio-Methylphenidate; Ritalin®; Ritalin® SR; Sandoz-Methylphenidate SR
Therapeutic Category Central Nervous System Stimulant
Generic Available Yes: Immediate release tablet, extended release tablet, sustained release tablet
Use Treatment of attention-deficit/hyperactivity disorder (ADHD); narcolepsy
Restrictions C-II
Medication Guide An FDA-approved patient medication guide, which is available with the product information and as follows, must be dispensed with this medication for each new prescription prescription and refill.
Concerta®: http://www.fda.gov/downloads/Drugs/DrugSafety/ucm088575.pdf
Daytrana™: http://www.fda.gov/downloads/Drugs/DrugSafety/ucm088581.pdf
Metadate CD®: http://www.fda.gov/downloads/Drugs/DrugSafety/ucm088635.pdf
Methylin® chewable tablet: http://www.fda.gov/downloads/Drugs/DrugSafety/ucm088639.pdf
Methylin® oral solution: http://www.fda.gov/downloads/Drugs/DrugSafety/ucm088640.pdf
Ritalin®: http://www.fda.gov/downloads/Drugs/DrugSafety/ucm089090.pdf
Ritalin LA®: http://www.fda.gov/downloads/Drugs/DrugSafety/ucm089092.pdf
Ritalin-SR®: http://www.fda.gov/downloads/Drugs/DrugSafety/ucm089826.pdf
Pregnancy Risk Factor C
Pregnancy Considerations Animal studies have shown teratogenic effects to the fetus. There are no adequate and well-controlled studies in pregnant women. Do not use in women of childbearing age unless the potential benefit outweighs the possible risk.
Lactation Enters breast milk/use caution
Breast-Feeding Considerations Methylphenidate excretion into breast milk has been noted in case reports. In both cases, the authors calculated the relative infant dose to be ≤0.2% of the weight adjusted maternal dose. Adverse events were not noted in either infant, however, both were older (6 months of age and 11 months of age) and exposure was limited.
Contraindications Hypersensitivity to methylphenidate or any component; glaucoma; motor tics; Tourette's syndrome (diagnosis or family history); patients with marked agitation, tension, and anxiety; use with or within 14 days

following MAO inhibitor therapy (hypertensive crisis may occur)

Metadate CD® is also contraindicated in patients with severe hypertension, heart failure, arrhythmia, hyperthyroidism, recent MI, or angina.

Warnings Serious cardiovascular events including sudden death may occur in patients with pre-existing structural cardiac abnormalities or other serious heart problems. Sudden death has been reported in children and adolescents; sudden death, stroke, and MI have been reported in adults. Avoid the use of CNS stimulants in patients with known serious structural cardiac abnormalities, cardiomyopathy, serious heart rhythm abnormalities, coronary artery disease, or other serious cardiac problems that could place patients at an increased risk to the sympathomimetic effects of CNS stimulants. Patients should be carefully evaluated for cardiac disease prior to initiation of therapy (see Monitoring Parameters). **Note:** The American Heart Association recommends that all children diagnosed with ADHD who may be candidates for medication, such as methylphenidate, should have a thorough cardiovascular assessment prior to initiation of therapy. This assessment should include a combination of medical history, family history, and physical examination focusing on cardiovascular disease risk factors. An ECG is not mandatory but should be considered. **Note:** ECG abnormalities and 4 cases of sudden cardiac death have been reported in children receiving clonidine with methylphenidate; reduce dose of methylphenidate by 40% when used concurrently with clonidine; consider ECG monitoring.

Stimulant medications may increase blood pressure (average increase 2-4 mm Hg) and heart rate (average increase 3-6 bpm); some patients may experience greater increases; use stimulant medications with caution in patients with hypertension and other cardiovascular conditions that may be exacerbated by increases in blood pressure or heart rate. Psychiatric adverse events may occur. Stimulants may exacerbate symptoms of behavior disturbance and thought disorder in patients with pre-existing psychosis. New-onset psychosis or mania may occur with stimulant use. May induce mixed/manic episode in patients with bipolar disorder. May be associated with aggressive behavior or hostility (monitor for development or worsening of these behaviors).

Safety and efficacy have not been established in children <6 years of age (use is **not** recommended in children <6 years of age). Long-term effects in pediatric patients have not been determined. Use of stimulants in children has been associated with growth suppression (monitor growth; treatment interruption may be needed). Appetite suppression may occur; monitor weight during therapy, particularly in children. Stimulants may lower seizure threshold leading to new onset or breakthrough seizure activity (use with caution in patients with a history of seizure disorder). Visual disturbances (difficulty in accommodation and blurred vision) have been reported.

CNS stimulants possess a high potential for abuse; misuse may cause sudden death and serious cardiovascular adverse events; prolonged administration may lead to drug dependence; abrupt discontinuation following high doses or for prolonged periods may result in symptoms of withdrawal; avoid abrupt discontinuation in patients who have received methylphenidate for prolonged periods; use with caution in patients with history of ethanol or drug abuse. Do not use for severe depression or normal fatigue states.

A potential for GI obstruction exists with Concerta® (tablet is nondeformable); do not ordinarily use in patients with severe GI narrowing (eg, esophageal motility disorders, small bowel inflammatory disease, short gut syndrome, history of cystic fibrosis, peritonitis, chronic intestinal pseudo-obstruction, or Meckel's diverticulum). Transdermal system may cause allergic contact sensitization, characterized by intense local reactions (edema, vesicles, papules); remove patch and monitor application site if reaction occurs; seek further evaluation if erythema, edema, and/or papules do not significantly decrease or resolve within 24 hours of patch removal. Allergic sensitization may subsequently manifest systemically when methylphenidate is administered orally or via other routes; systemic sensitization reactions may include dermatitis, generalized skin eruptions, headache, fever, vomiting, diarrhea, arthralgia, or malaise; initiate oral methylphenidate under close medical supervision in patients who have experienced a contact sensitization to the transdermal system; some of these patients may **not** be able to take methylphenidate in any dosage form. Do not expose transdermal application site to direct external heat sources (eg, electric blankets, heating pads, heated water beds), a >2-fold increase in drug release may occur.

Precautions Use with caution in patients with heart failure, recent MI, hyperthyroidism, seizures, acute stress reactions, emotional instability. Hematological monitoring is advised with long term use (see Monitoring Parameters). Stimulants like methylphenidate have a demonstrated value as part of a comprehensive treatment program for ADHD.

Chewable tablets contain aspartame which is metabolized to phenylalanine and must be avoided (or used with caution) in patients with phenylketonuria. Chewable tablets must be taken with adequate amount of liquid, otherwise tablet may swell and block the throat or esophagus and cause choking; do not use chewable tablets in patients who have difficulty swallowing; instruct patients to seek immediate medical attention if chest pain, vomiting, difficulty in breathing or swallowing occur after taking chewable tablet.

Adverse Reactions

Cardiovascular: Tachycardia, hypertension, hypotension, palpitations, angina, cardiac arrhythmias; cerebral arteritis, cerebral occlusion (case reports); serious cardiovascular events including sudden death in patients with preexisting structural cardiac abnormalities or other serious heart problems (see Warnings)

Central nervous system: Nervousness, insomnia, irritability, aggression, emotional lability, dizziness, drowsiness, movement disorders, motor tics, precipitation of Tourette's syndrome; fever, headache, toxic psychosis (rare); neuroleptic malignant syndrome (very rare and usually in patients receiving medications associated with the syndrome; one case with concurrent first dose of venlafaxine has been reported); transient depression

Dermatologic: Rash, urticaria, exfoliative dermatitis, erythema multiforme, necrotizing vasculitis, scalp hair loss

Endocrine & metabolic: Growth suppression, weight loss

Gastrointestinal: Anorexia, nausea, vomiting, abdominal pain, diarrhea, potential for GI obstruction with Concerta® (see Warnings)

Hematologic: Thrombocytopenia, anemia, leukopenia, thrombocytopenic purpura

Hepatic: Abnormal liver function, transaminases elevated, hepatic coma

Local: Transdermal system: Application site reactions, erythema, itching; papules, edema, vesicles (allergic contact dermatitis)

Neuromuscular & skeletal: Arthralgia, dyskinesia

Ocular: Visual disturbances, blurred vision, problems with accommodation

Miscellaneous: Hypersensitivity reactions; physical and psychological dependence

Drug Interactions

Metabolism/Transport Effects Inhibits CYP2D6 (weak)

Avoid Concomitant Use

Avoid concomitant use of Methylphenidate with any of the following: Inhalational Anesthetics; Iobenguane I 123; MAO Inhibitors

Increased Effect/Toxicity

Methylphenidate may increase the levels/effects of: CloNIDine; Inhalational Anesthetics; Phenytoin; Sympathomimetics; Tricyclic Antidepressants

The levels/effects of Methylphenidate may be increased by: Atomoxetine; Cannabinoids; MAO Inhibitors

Decreased Effect

Methylphenidate may decrease the levels/effects of: Antihypertensives; Iobenguane I 123

Food Interactions Food may increase oral absorption

Concerta®: A high fat meal does not alter pharmacokinetics or pharmacodynamics; no evidence of dose dumping occurs when administered with or without food

Metadate CD®: Food delays the early peak by ~1 hour; a high fat meal increases peak concentrations by 30% and AUC by 17%; one adult study showed no difference in bioavailability when Metadate CD® capsules were opened and contents sprinkled onto 1 tablespoon of applesauce (compared to fasting conditions; see Pentikin, 2002).

Methylin®:

Chewable tablets: A high fat meal delays peak concentrations by ~1 hour, but increases AUC by ~20% (**Note:** Magnitude of food effect is similar to immediate release tablets).

Oral solution: A high fat meal delays peak concentrations by ~1 hour, but increases peak by ~13% and AUC by ~25% (**Note:** Increase in peak concentration and AUC are similar to immediate release tablets).

Ritalin LA®: Compared to fasting, food does not affect the first peak concentration, extent of absorption, or time to second peak concentration; however, the second peak was 25% lower. A high fat meal delays absorption. Compared to fasting, no differences in pharmacokinetics occurred when Ritalin LA® capsules were administered with applesauce. No evidence of dose dumping occurs when administered with or without food.

Stability Store at room temperature; dispense oral formulations in tight, light-resistant container; **Note:** Metadate CD® should be dispensed in the original dose pack of 30 capsules

Methylin® chewable tablets, Methylin® ER, Ritalin-SR®: Protect from moisture

Concerta®: Protect from humidity

Transdermal system: Keep patches stored in protective pouch; use patches within 2 months after tray is opened

Mechanism of Action Produces stimulant effect by activating the brain stem arousal system and cerebral cortex; blocks the reuptake of norepinephrine and dopamine into presynaptic neurons, thus increasing the concentrations of these neurotransmitters in the extraneuronal space.

Pharmacodynamics Cerebral stimulation:

Maximum effect:

Immediate release tablet: Within 2 hours

Sustained release tablet: Within 4-7 hours

Duration (AAP, 2001):

Immediate release tablet (short-acting): Methylin®, Ritalin®: 3-5 hours

Sustained release, extended release (intermediate-acting): Metadate® ER, Methylin® ER, Ritalin-SR®: 3-8 hours

Extended release (long-acting): Concerta®, Metadate CD®, Ritalin LA®: 8-12 hours

Pharmacokinetics (Adult data unless noted)

Absorption: Oral:

Immediate release products: Readily absorbed

Transdermal: Absorption is increased when applied to inflamed skin or exposed to heat; transdermal absorption may increase with chronic therapy

Protein binding: 15%

Metabolism: In the liver via hydroxylation (de-esterification) to ritalinic acid (alpha-phenyl-2-piperidine acetic acid), which has little or no pharmacologic activity

Bioavailability: Chewable tablets and oral solution are bioequivalent to immediate release tablets. **Note:** A much lower first pass effect occurs with transdermal (vs oral) administration; thus, much lower doses (on a mg/kg basis) given via the transdermal route may still produce higher AUCs, compared to the oral route.

Half-life: 2-4 hours

Time to peak serum concentration:

Chewable tablets, oral solution: 1-2 hours

Extended release tablet (Concerta®): 6-10 hours

Elimination: 90% of dose is eliminated in the urine as metabolites and unchanged drug; main urinary metabolite (ritalinic acid) accounts for 80% of the dose; drug is also excreted in feces via bile

Usual Dosage Note: Discontinue medication if no improvement is seen after appropriate dosage adjustment over a one-month period of time:

Oral:

Immediate release product (Methylin®, Ritalin®):

Children ≥6 years: ADHD: Initial: 0.3 mg/kg/dose or 2.5-5 mg/dose given before breakfast and lunch; increase by 0.1 mg/kg/dose or by 5-10 mg/day at weekly intervals; usual dose: 0.3-1 mg/kg/day; maximum dose: 2 mg/kg/day or 60 mg/day; specific patients may require 3 doses/day (ie, additional dose at 4 PM)

Adults: Narcolepsy: 10 mg 2-3 times/day; maximum dose: 60 mg/day

Metadate® ER, Methylin® ER, Ritalin-SR®: Children ≥6 years and Adults: Sustained release and extended release tablets (duration of action ~8 hours) may be given in place of regular tablets, once the daily dose is titrated using the regular tablets and the titrated 8-hour dosage corresponds to sustained release tablet size

Concerta®: Children ≥6 years and Adults:

Initial: Methylphenidate naive patients: 18 mg once daily

Switching from methylphenidate immediate release 5 mg 2-3 times/day: Concerta® 18 mg once daily

Switching from methylphenidate immediate release 10 mg 2-3 times/day: Concerta® 36 mg once daily

Switching from methylphenidate immediate release 15 mg 2-3 times/day: Concerta® 54 mg once daily

Dosage adjustment: May increase by 18 mg/day increments at weekly intervals

Maximum dose:

Children 6-12 years: 54 mg/day

Adolescent and Adults: 72 mg/day; do not exceed 2 mg/kg/day

Metadate CD®: Children ≥6 years and Adults: Initial: 20 mg once daily; may increase by 20 mg/day increments at weekly intervals; maximum dose: 60 mg once daily

Ritalin LA®: Children ≥6 years and Adults:

Methylphenidate naive patients: Initial: 20 mg once daily; may increase by 10 mg/day increments at weekly intervals; maximum dose: 60 mg once daily; **Note:** If a lower initial dose is desired, patients may begin with Ritalin LA® 10 mg once daily. Alternatively, patients may begin therapy with an immediate release product, and switch to Ritalin LA® once immediate release dosage is titrated to 5 mg twice daily

Patients currently receiving methylphenidate: Initial dose: See table; may increase by 10 mg/day increments at weekly intervals; maximum dose: 60 mg once daily

Recommended Ritalin LA® Dose for Patients Receiving Methylphenidate

Previous Methylphenidate Dose	Recommended Ritalin LA® Dose
5 mg methylphenidate twice daily	10 mg once daily
10 mg methylphenidate twice daily or 20 mg methylphenidate sustained release	20 mg once daily
15 mg methylphenidate twice daily	30 mg once daily
20 mg methylphenidate twice daily or 40 mg methylphenidate sustained release	40 mg once daily
30 mg methylphenidate twice daily or 60 mg methylphenidate sustained release	60 mg once daily

Transdermal (Daytrana™): Children 6-12 years: Initial: 10 mg patch once daily; apply to hip 2 hours before effect is needed and remove 9 hours after application (see Administration); titrate dose based on response and tolerability; may increase to next transdermal patch dosage size no more frequently than every week. **Note:** Doses >20 mg/9 hours do not appear to provide additional benefit. Patch may be removed before 9 hours if a shorter duration of action is required or if late day adverse effects appear. Plasma concentrations usually start to decline when the patch is removed but drug absorption may continue for several hours after patch removal.

Administration

Oral: Immediate and sustained release tablets: Administer on an empty stomach ~30-45 minutes before meals; do not crush, chew, or break sustained or extended release dosage form, swallow whole; to avoid insomnia, last daily dose should be administered several hours before retiring.

Concerta®: May be administered without regard to food, but must be taken with water, milk, or juice; administer dose once daily in the morning; do not crush, chew, or divide tablets

Metadate CD®: Administer dose once daily in the morning, before breakfast, with water, milk, or juice; capsule may be swallowed whole or opened and contents sprinkled on a small amount (one tablespoonful) of applesauce; immediately consume drug/applesauce mixture; do not store for future use; drink fluids after consuming drug/applesauce mixture to ensure complete swallowing of beads; do not crush, chew, or divide capsules or its contents

Methylin® chewable tablet: Children and Adults: Administer with at least 8 ounces of water or other fluid (choking may occur if not enough fluids are taken; see Precautions)

Ritalin LA®: Administer dose once daily in the morning; may be administered with or without food (but some food may delay absorption); capsule may be swallowed whole or may be opened and contents sprinkled on a small amount (one spoonful) of applesauce (**Note:** Applesauce should not be warm); immediately consume drug/applesauce mixture; do not store for future use; do not crush, chew, or divide capsule or its contents

Topical: Transdermal (Daytrana™): Apply patch immediately after opening pouch and removing protective liner; do not use patch if pouch seal is broken; do not use patches that are cut or damaged. Apply to clean, dry, healthy skin on the hip; do not apply to oily, damaged, or irritated skin; do not apply to the waistline. Apply at the same time each day, 2 hours before effect is needed. Alternate site of application daily (ie, use alternate hip). Press patch firmly for 30 seconds to ensure proper adherence. Remove patch 9 hours after application. Patch may be removed earlier if a shorter duration of action is required or if late day adverse effects occur.

Avoid exposure of application site to external heat source (eg, electric blankets, heating pads, heated water beds), which may significantly increase the amount of drug absorbed. If patch should become dislodged, may replace with new patch (to different site) but total wear time should not exceed 9 hours. If adhesive residue remains on child's skin after patch removal, use oil or lotion and gently rub area to remove adhesive. Avoid touching the sticky side of the patch. Wash hands with soap and water after handling.

Dispose of used patch by folding adhesive side onto itself, and discard in toilet or appropriate lidded container; discard unused patches that are no longer needed in the same manner; protective pouch and liner should be discarded in an appropriate lidded container. **Note:** Used patches contain residual drug; keep all transdermal patches out of the reach of children.

Monitoring Parameters Evaluate patients for cardiac disease prior to initiation of therapy with thorough medical history, family history, and physical exam; consider ECG (see Warnings); perform ECG and echocardiogram if findings suggest cardiac disease; promptly conduct cardiac evaluation in patients who develop chest pain, unexplained syncope, or any other symptom of cardiac disease during treatment. Monitor CBC with differential, platelet count, blood pressure, heart rate, height, weight, appetite, abnormal movements, growth in children. Patients should be re-evaluated at appropriate intervals to assess continued need of the medication. Observe for signs/symptoms of aggression or hostility, or depression. Transdermal system: Also monitor the application site for local adverse reactions and allergic contact sensitization (see Warnings).

Patient Information Read the patient Medication Guide that you receive with each prescription and refill of methylphenidate. Serious cardiac effects or psychiatric adverse effects may occur; notify your physician of any heart problems, high blood pressure, or psychiatric conditions before starting therapy. May reduce the growth rate in children and has been associated with worsening of aggressive behavior; notify your physician if your child displays aggression or hostility; make sure your physician monitors your child's weight and height. Avoid caffeine and the herbal medicine St John's wort. May be habit-forming; avoid abrupt discontinuation after prolonged use. May cause dizziness or drowsiness and impair ability to perform activities requiring mental alertness or physical coordination. Notify physician if blurred vision occurs. Intact Concerta® tablet shell may appear in stool (this is normal). Report the use of other medications and herbal or natural products to your physician and pharmacist. Seek immediate medical attention if chest pain, vomiting, or difficulty in breathing or swallowing occur after taking chewable tablet. When using transdermal patches, avoid exposing application site to external heat sources (eg, electric blankets, heating pads, heated water bed); patches may be irritating to the skin; inform physician if skin rash or irritation occurs; do not use patch if swelling or blistering occurs; see Administration for details of patch application

Additional Information Methylphenidate is a racemic mixture of d- and l-enantiomers; the d-enantiomer is more active than the l-enantiomer. Treatment with methylphenidate should include "drug holidays" or periodic discontinuation in order to assess the patient's requirements, decrease tolerance and limit suppression of linear growth and weight. Medications used to treat ADHD should be part of a total treatment program that may include other components such as psychological, educational, and social measures. Concerta®, Metadate CD®, and Ritalin LA® are formulated to deliver methylphenidate in a biphasic release profile; Concerta® is an osmotic controlled release formulation, with an immediate release (within 1 hour) outer coating; once daily Concerta® has been shown to be as effective as immediate release methylphenidate tablets administered 3 times/day (see Pelham, 2001). Metadate CD® capsules contain both immediate release beads (30% of the dose) and extended release beads (70% of the dose). Ritalin LA® capsules contain both immediate release beads (50% of the dose) and enteric coated, delayed release beads (50% of the dose). Methylin®, Methylin® ER, and Ritalin-SR® tablets are color and additive free; Methylin® oral solution is colorless. Concerta® tablets may be seen on abdominal x-ray under certain conditions (eg, when digital enhancing techniques are used).

Daytrana™ Transdermal System consists of an adhesive-based matrix containing active drug which is dispersed in acrylic adhesive that is dispersed in a silicone adhesive. The patch consists of 3 layers: A polyester/ethylene vinyl acetate laminate (outside) film backing, the adhesive layer containing methylphenidate, and a flouropolymer-coated polyester protective liner (which must be removed before application). Long-term use of the transdermal system (ie, >7 weeks) has not been studied; long-term usefulness should be periodically re-evaluated for the individual patient.

Dosage Forms Excipient information presented when available (limited, particularly for generics); consult specific product labeling. [DSC] = Discontinued product

Capsule, extended release, oral, as hydrochloride [bimodal release]:

Metadate CD®: 10 mg [contains sucrose; 3 mg immediate release, 7 mg extended release]

Metadate CD®: 20 mg [contains sucrose; 6 mg immediate release, 14 mg extended release]

Metadate CD®: 30 mg [contains sucrose; 9 mg immediate release, 21 mg extended release]

Metadate CD®: 40 mg [contains sucrose; 12 mg immediate release, 28 mg extended release]

Metadate CD®: 50 mg [contains sucrose; 15 mg immediate release, 35 mg extended release]

Metadate CD®: 60 mg [contains sucrose; 18 mg immediate release, 42 mg extended release]

Ritalin LA®: 10 mg [5 mg immediate release, 5 mg extended release]

Ritalin LA®: 20 mg [10 mg immediate release, 10 mg extended release]

Ritalin LA®: 30 mg [15 mg immediate release, 15 mg extended release]

Ritalin LA®: 40 mg [20 mg immediate release, 20 mg extended release]

Patch, transdermal [once-daily patch]:

Daytrana™: 10 mg/9 hours (10s [DSC], 30s) [12.5 cm^2, total methylphenidate 27.5 mg]

Daytrana™: 15 mg/9 hours (10s [DSC], 30s) [18.75 cm^2, total methylphenidate 41.3 mg]

Daytrana™: 20 mg/9 hours (10s [DSC], 30s) [25 cm^2, total methylphenidate 55 mg]

Daytrana™: 30 mg/9 hours (10s [DSC], 30s) [37.5 cm^2, total methylphenidate 82.5 mg]

Solution, oral, as hydrochloride:

Methylin®: 5 mg/5 mL (500 mL) [grape flavor]; 10 mg/5 mL (500 mL) [grape flavor]

Tablet, as hydrochloride: 5 mg, 10 mg, 20 mg

Methylin®, Ritalin®: 5 mg, 10 mg, 20 mg

Tablet, chewable, as hydrochloride:

Methylin®: 2.5 mg [contains phenylalanine 0.42 mg/tablet; grape flavor]; 5 mg [contains phenylalanine 0.84 mg/tablet; grape flavor]; 10 mg [scored; contains phenylalanine 1.68 mg/tablet; grape flavor]

Tablet, extended release, as hydrochloride: 20 mg [DSC]

Metadate® ER: 10 mg [contains lactose] [DSC]; 20 mg [contains lactose]

Methylin® ER: 10 mg, 20 mg

Tablet, extended release, as hydrochloride [bi-modal release]:

Concerta®: 18 mg [4 mg immediate release, 14 mg extended release]

Concerta®: 27 mg [6 mg immediate release, 21 mg extended release]

Concerta®: 36 mg [8 mg immediate release, 28 mg extended release]

Concerta®: 54 mg [12 mg immediate release, 42 mg extended release]

Tablet, sustained release, as hydrochloride: 20 mg

Ritalin-SR®: 20 mg [dye free]

References

American Academy of Pediatrics/American Heart Association Clarification of Statement on Cardiovascular Evaluation and Monitoring of Children and Adolescents With Heart Disease Receiving Medications for ADHD; available at: http://americanheart.mediaroon.com/index.php?s=43&item=422.

American Academy of Pediatrics. Subcommittee on Attention-Deficit/Hyperactivity Disorder, "Clinical Practice Guideline: Treatment of the School-Aged Child With Attention-Deficit/Hyperactivity Disorder," *Pediatrics*, 2001, 108(4):1033-44.

Greenhill LL, "Pharmacologic Treatment of Attention Deficit Hyperactivity Disorder," *Psychiatr Clin North Am*, 1992, 15(1):1-27.

Greenhill LL, Pliszka S, Dulcan MK, et al, "Practice Parameter for the Use of Stimulant Medications in the Treatment of Children, Adolescents, and Adults," *J Am Acad Child Adolesc Psychiatry*, 2002, 41(2 Suppl):26S-49S.

Kelly DP and Aylward GP, "Attention Deficits in School-Aged Children and Adolescents," *Pediatr Clin North Am*, 1992, 39(3):487-512.

Pelham WE, Gnagy EM, Burrows-Maclean L, et al, "Once-a-Day Concerta Methylphenidate Versus Three-Times-Daily Methylphenidate in Laboratory and Natural Settings," *Pediatrics*, 2001, 107(6), http://www.pediatrics.org/cgi/content/full/107/6/e105.

Pentikis HS, Simmons RD, Benedict MF, et al, "Methylphenidate Bioavailability in Adults When an Extended-Release Multiparticulate Formulation is Administered Sprinkled on Food or as an Intact Capsule," *J Am Acad Child Adolesc Psychiatry*, 2002, 41(4):443-9.

Vetter VL, Elia J, Erickson C, et al, "Cardiovascular Monitoring of Children and Adolescents With Heart Disease Receiving Stimulant Drugs: A Scientific Statement From the American Heart Association Council on Cardiovascular Disease in the Young Congenital Cardiac Defects Committee and the Council on Cardiovascular Nursing," *Circulation*, 2008, 117(18):2407-23.

Wilens TE and Biederman J, "The Stimulants," *Psychiatr Clin North Am*, 1992, 15(1):191-222.

◆ **Methylphenidate Hydrochloride** see Methylphenidate on page 908

◆ **Methylphenobarbital** see Mephobarbital on page 882

◆ **Methylphenoxy-Benzene Propanamine** see Atomoxetine on page 149

◆ **Methylphenyl Isoxazolyl Penicillin** see Oxacillin on page 1029

◆ **Methylphytyl Napthoquinone** see Phytonadione on page 1109

MethylPREDNISolone (meth il pred NIS oh lone)

Medication Safety Issues

Sound-alike/look-alike issues:

MethylPREDNISolone may be confused with medroxyPROGESTERone, methotrexate, predniSONE

Depo-Medrol® may be confused with Solu-Medrol®

Medrol® may be confused with Mebaral®

Solu-Medrol® may be confused with Depo-Medrol®, salmeterol, Solu-Cortef®

International issues:

Medor® may be confused with Medral® which is a brand name for omeprazole in Mexico

Related Information

Asthma on page 1697

Corticosteroids on page 1487

U.S. Brand Names A-Methapred®; Depo-Medrol®; Medrol®; Solu-Medrol®

Canadian Brand Names Depo-Medrol®; Medrol®; Methylprednisolone Acetate; Solu-Medrol®

Therapeutic Category Adrenal Corticosteroid; Anti-inflammatory Agent; Antiasthmatic; Corticosteroid, Systemic; Glucocorticoid

Generic Available Yes

Use

Systemic: Anti-inflammatory or immunosuppressant agent in the treatment of a variety of diseases including those of hematologic, allergic, inflammatory, neoplastic, and autoimmune origin (FDA approved in ages >1 month and adults)

Intra-articular (or soft tissue): Acute gouty arthritis, acute/subacute bursitis, acute nonspecific tenosynovitis, epicondylitis, rheumatoid arthritis, synovitis of osteoarthritis

Intralesional (injectable suspension): Alopecia areata; discoid lupus erythematosus; infiltrated, inflammatory lesions associated with granuloma annulare, lichen planus, neurodermatitis, and psoriatic plaques; keloids; necrobiosis lipoidica diabeticorum; possibly helpful in cystic tumors of an aponeurosis or tendon (ganglia)

Pregnancy Considerations Adverse events have been observed with corticosteroids in animal reproduction studies. Methylprednisolone crosses the placenta. Some studies have shown an association between first trimester systemic corticosteroid use and oral clefts; adverse events in the fetus/neonate have been noted in case reports following large doses of systemic corticosteroids during pregnancy. Pregnant women exposed to methylprednisolone for antirejection therapy following a transplant may contact the National Transplantation Pregnancy Registry (NTPR) at 215-955-4820. Women exposed to methylprednisolone during pregnancy for the treatment of an autoimmune disease may contact the OTIS Autoimmune Diseases Study at 877-311-8972.

Lactation Enters breast milk/use caution

Breast-Feeding Considerations Low levels of methylprednisolone are excreted in breast milk

Contraindications Hypersensitivity to methylprednisolone or any component (see Warnings); systemic fungal infections (except intra-articular injection in localized joint conditions); varicella infections; intrathecal administration of methylprednisolone acetate suspension.

Formulations containing benzyl alcohol preservative: Contraindicated in premature infants (see Warnings).

Immunosuppressive doses: Contraindicated with immunization with live or live-attenuated vaccines.

I.M.: Contraindicated with idiopathic thrombocytopenic purpura

Warnings Hypothalamic pituitary adrenal (HPA) suppression may occur; acute adrenal insufficiency (adrenal crisis) may occur with abrupt withdrawal after long-term therapy or with stress; withdrawal or discontinuation of corticosteroids should be done carefully; patients with HPA axis suppression may require increased doses of systemic glucocorticosteroids prior to, during, and after unusual stress (eg, surgery). Immunosuppression may occur; patients may be more susceptible to infections; avoid exposure to chickenpox and measles. Corticosteroids may mask signs of infection. Corticosteroids may activate latent opportunistic infections or exacerbate systemic fungal infections. Amebiasis should be ruled out in any patient with recent travel to tropical climates or unexplained diarrhea prior to initiation of corticosteroids. Use with great caution in patients with known or suspected *Strongyloides* infection. Corticosteroids should not be used for cerebral malaria. May cause osteoporosis (at any age) or inhibition of bone growth in pediatric patients. Acute myopathy may occur with high doses, CNS effects (ranging from euphoria to psychosis) may occur. Rare cases of anaphylactoid reactions have been reported with corticosteroids.

High-dose corticosteroids should not be used for the management of traumatic brain injury (an increase in mortality was observed in patients with cranial trauma who received high-dose I.V. methylprednisolone hemisuccinate). Depressions in the skin, due to dermal and/or subdermal atrophy, may occur at the site of methylprednisolone acetate injection; do not exceed recommended dose per injection; avoid injection or leakage into the dermis; avoid injection into deltoid muscle (high incidence of subcutaneous atrophy).

Methylprednisolone **acetate** I.M. injection (multiple-dose vial) and the diluent for methylprednisolone **sodium succinate** injection contain benzyl alcohol which may cause allergic reactions in susceptible individuals; large amounts of benzyl alcohol (≥99 mg/kg/day) have been associated with a potentially fatal toxicity ("gasping syndrome") in neonates; the "gasping syndrome" consists of metabolic acidosis, respiratory distress, gasping respirations, CNS dysfunction (including convulsions, intracranial hemorrhage), hypotension and cardiovascular collapse; avoid use of methylprednisolone products containing benzyl alcohol in neonates; *in vitro* and animal studies have shown that benzoate, a metabolite of benzyl alcohol, displaces bilirubin from protein binding sites. Benzyl alcohol is also potentially toxic to neural tissue when administered locally.

Precautions Avoid using higher than recommended doses; suppression of HPA axis function, suppression of linear growth (ie, reduction of growth velocity), reduced bone mineral density, hypercorticism (Cushing's syndrome), hyperglycemia, or glucosuria, may occur; titrate to lowest effective dose. Reduction in growth velocity may occur when corticosteroids are administered to pediatric patients by any route; monitor growth. Use with extreme caution in patients with respiratory tuberculosis or untreated systemic infections. Use with caution in patients with thyroid dysfunction, cirrhosis, nonspecific ulcerative colitis, fresh intestinal anastomoses, diverticulitis, hypertension, renal impairment, osteoporosis, thromboembolic disorders, CHF, recent MI (left ventricular free wall rupture has been reported), convulsive disorders, myasthenia gravis, thrombophlebitis, peptic ulcer disease, diabetes, or hepatic impairment. Avoid injection into an infected site. Response to killed or inactivated vaccines cannot be predicted in patients receiving immunosuppressive doses of corticosteroids.

Use with caution in patients with cataracts and/or glaucoma; increased intraocular pressure, open-angle glaucoma, and cataracts have occurred with prolonged use. Corticosteroids should not be used in active ocular herpes simplex. Systemic use is not recommended in the treatment of optic neuritis (an increased risk of new episodes may occur).

Adverse Reactions

Cardiovascular: Arrhythmias, bradycardia, cardiac arrest, cardiomegaly, circulatory collapse, CHF, edema, fat embolism, hypertension, hypertrophic cardiomyopathy in premature infants, myocardial rupture (post MI), syncope, tachycardia, thromboembolism, vasculitis

Central nervous system: Depression, emotional instability, euphoria, headache, insomnia, intracranial hypertension, malaise, mood swings, nervousness, neuritis, personality changes, pseudotumor cerebri, psychoses, seizures, vertigo

Dermatologic: Acne, allergic dermatitis, bruising, dermal thinning, dry scaly skin, erythema, hirsutism, hyperpigmentation, hypopigmentation, hypertrichosis, impaired wound healing, petechiae, rash, skin atrophy, skin test reaction impaired, sterile abscess, striae, urticaria

Endocrine & metabolic: Adrenal suppression, alkalosis, amenorrhea, appetite increased, calcium absorption decreased, calcium excretion increased, Cushing's syndrome, diabetes mellitus, glucose intolerance, growth suppression, HPA axis suppression, hyperglycemia, hypokalemia, menstrual irregularities, negative nitrogen balance, protein catabolism, sodium and water retention, weight gain

Gastrointestinal: Abdominal distention, GI hemorrhage, GI perforation, nausea, pancreatitis, peptic ulcer, perforation of the small and large intestine, ulcerative esophagitis, vomiting

Hematologic: Transient leukocytosis

Hepatic: Hepatomegaly, liver enzymes increased

Local: Postinjection flare (intra-articular use), sterile abscess

Neuromuscular & skeletal: Arthralgia, arthropathy, aseptic necrosis (femoral and humeral heads; rare), bone mineral density decreased, fractures, muscle mass loss, muscle weakness, myopathy, neuropathy, osteoporosis, parasthesia, tendon rupture, vertebral compression fractures, weakness

Ocular: Cataracts, exophthalmoses, glaucoma, IOP elevated

Renal: Glycosuria

Miscellaneous: Abnormal fat disposition, anaphylactoid reactions (rare), anaphylaxis, angioedema, diaphoresis, fungal infection exacerbation, hiccups, hypersensitivity reactions, immunosuppression, infection symptoms masked, Kaposi's sarcoma (with prolonged systemic use), susceptibility to infection increased, tuberculosis reactivation, secondary malignancy

Drug Interactions

Metabolism/Transport Effects Substrate of CYP3A4 (major); **Inhibits** CYP2C8 (weak), 3A4 (weak)

Avoid Concomitant Use

Avoid concomitant use of MethylPREDNISolone with any of the following: Aldesleukin; BCG; Natalizumab; Pimecrolimus; Tacrolimus (Topical); Vaccines (Live)

Increased Effect/Toxicity

MethylPREDNISolone may increase the levels/effects of: Acetylcholinesterase Inhibitors; Amphotericin B; CycloSPORINE; CycloSPORINE (Systemic); Leflunomide; Loop Diuretics; Natalizumab; NSAID (COX-2 Inhibitor); NSAID (Nonselective); Thiazide Diuretics; Vaccines (Live); Warfarin

The levels/effects of MethylPREDNISolone may be increased by: Antifungal Agents (Azole Derivatives, Systemic); Aprepitant; Calcium Channel Blockers (Nondihydropyridine); CYP3A4 Inhibitors (Strong); Denosumab; Estrogen Derivatives; Fluconazole; Fosaprepitant; Macrolide Antibiotics; Neuromuscular-Blocking Agents (Nondepolarizing); Pimecrolimus; Quinolone Antibiotics; Salicylates; Tacrolimus (Topical); Trastuzumab

Decreased Effect

MethylPREDNISolone may decrease the levels/effects of: Aldesleukin; Antidiabetic Agents; BCG; Calcitriol; Corticorelin; Isoniazid; Salicylates; Sipuleucel-T; Vaccines (Inactivated); Vaccines (Live)

The levels/effects of MethylPREDNISolone may be decreased by: Aminoglutethimide; Antacids; Barbiturates; Bile Acid Sequestrants; Echinacea; Mitotane; Primidone; Rifamycin Derivatives

Food Interactions Systemic use of corticosteroids may require a diet with increased potassium, vitamins A, B_6, C, D, folate, calcium, zinc and phosphorus and decreased sodium; grapefruit juice may significantly increase the bioavailability of oral methylprednisolone

Stability

Methylprednisolone sodium succinate: Store intact vials at controlled room temperature of 20°C to 25°C (68°F to 77°F). Protect from light. Store reconstituted solutions at room temperature of 20°C to 25°C (68°F to 77°F); use within 48 hours. Reconstitute with accompanying diluent or bacteriostatic water for injection with benzyl alcohol. May further dilute in D_5W. Stability of parenteral admixture at room temperature (25°C) and at refrigeration temperature (4°C) is 48 hours.

Methylprednisolone acetate: Store at controlled room temperature of 20°C to 25°C (68°F to 77°F). Do **not** dilute or mix with other solutions.

Mechanism of Action Decreases inflammation by suppression of migration of polymorphonuclear leukocytes and reversal of increased capillary permeability

Pharmacodynamics The time of maximum effects and the duration of these effects is dependent upon the route of administration. See table.

Route	Maximum Effect	Duration
Oral	1-2 h	30-36 h
I.M. (acetate)	4-8 d	1-4 wk
Intra-articular	1 wk	1-5 wk

Pharmacokinetics (Adult data unless noted)

Half-life:

Adolescents: 1.9 + 0.7 hours (n=6; patients 12-20 years of age; see Rouster-Stevens, 2008)

Adults: 2.4-3.3 hours (see Rohatagi, 1997)

Usual Dosage Note: Adjust dose depending upon condition being treated and response of patient. The lowest possible dose should be used to control the condition; when dose reduction is possible, the dose should be reduced gradually. In life-threatening situations, parenteral doses larger than the oral dose may be needed. **Only sodium succinate salt may be given I.V.**

NIH Asthma Guidelines (NAEPP, 2007):

Children <12 years:

Asthma exacerbations (emergency medical care or hospital doses): Oral, I.V.: 1-2 mg/kg/day in 2 divided doses (maximum: 60 mg/day) until peak expiratory flow is 70% of predicted or personal best

Short-course "burst" (acute asthma):

Oral: 1-2 mg/kg/day in divided doses 1-2 times/day for 3-10 days; maximum dose: 60 mg/day; **Note:** Burst should be continued until symptoms resolve or patient achieves peak expiratory flow 80% of personal best; usually requires 3-10 days of treatment (~5 days on average); longer treatment may be required

I.M. (acetate): **Note:** This may be given in place of short-course "burst" of oral steroids in patients who are vomiting or if compliance is a problem

Children ≤4 years: 7.5 mg/kg as a one-time dose; maximum dose: 240 mg

Children 5-11 years: 240 mg as a one-time dose

Long-term treatment: Oral: 0.25-2 mg/kg/day given as a single dose in the morning or every other day as needed for asthma control; maximum dose: 60 mg/day

Children ≥12 years and Adults:

Asthma exacerbations (emergency medical care or hospital doses): Oral, I.V.: 40-80 mg/day in divided doses 1-2 times/day until peak expiratory flow is 70% of predicted or personal best

Short-course "burst" (acute asthma):

Oral: 40-60 mg/day in divided doses 1-2 times/day for 3-10 days; **Note:** Burst should be continued until symptoms resolve and peak expiratory flow is at least 80% of personal best; usually requires 3-10 days of treatment (~5 days on average); longer treatment may be required

I.M. **(acetate)**: 240 mg as a one-time dose (**Note:** This may be given in place of short-course "burst" of oral steroids in patients who are vomiting or if compliance is a problem)

Long-term treatment: Oral: 7.5-60 mg daily given as a single dose in the morning or every other day as needed for asthma control

Children:

Anti-inflammatory or immunosuppressive: Oral, I.M., I.V.: 0.5-1.7 mg/kg/day or 5-25 mg/m^2/day in divided doses every 6-12 hours

"Pulse" therapy: 15-30 mg/kg/dose over ≥30 minutes given once daily for 3 days

Status asthmaticus (previous NAEPP guidelines still used by some clinicians): I.V.: Loading dose: 2 mg/kg/dose, then 0.5-1 mg/kg/dose every 6 hours; **Note:** See new NAEPP guidelines for asthma exacerbations (emergency medical care or hospital doses) listed above.

Lupus nephritis: I.V.: 30 mg/kg over ≥30 minutes every other day for 6 doses

Acute spinal cord injury: I.V.: 30 mg/kg over 15 minutes followed in 45 minutes by a continuous infusion of 5.4 mg/kg/hour for 23 hours

Adults:

Oral: Initial: 2-60 mg/day in 1-4 divided doses; gradually reduce dose to lowest effective dose

High-dose therapy: I.V. **(sodium succinate)**: 30 mg/kg over ≥30 minutes; repeat as needed every 4-6 hours for 48-72 hours

I.M. **(sodium succinate)**: 10-80 mg/day once daily

I.M. **(acetate)**: 10-80 mg every 1-2 weeks (once daily dosing, in an amount equal to the total daily oral dose of the tablets, may be used as a temporary or short-term substitute for oral therapy)

I.V. **(sodium succinate)**: 40-250 mg every 4-6 hours

Lupus nephritis: High-dose "pulse" therapy: I.V. **(sodium succinate)**: 1 g/day for 3 days

Intra-articular, intralesional **(acetate)**: 4-40 mg, up to 80 mg for large joints every 1-5 weeks

Administration

Oral: Administer after meals or with food or milk; do not administer with grapefruit juice

Parenteral: I.V.: **Succinate:** Low dose (eg, ≤1.8 mg/kg or ≤125 mg/dose): I.V. push over 3-15 minutes; moderate dose (eg, ≥2 mg/kg or 250 mg/dose): administer over 15-30 minutes; high dose (eg, 15 mg/kg or ≥500 mg/dose): administer over ≥30 minutes; doses >15 mg/kg or ≥1 g: administer over 1 hour. Do **not** administer high-dose I.V. push; hypotension, cardiac arrhythmia, and sudden death have been reported in patients given high-dose methylprednisolone I.V. push over <20 minutes; administer intermittent infusion over 15-60 minutes; maximum concentration: I.V. push: 125 mg/mL; I.V. infusion: 2.5 mg/mL. **Do not give acetate form I.V.**

I.M.: Acetate: Avoid injection into the deltoid muscle due to a high incidence of subcutaneous atrophy. Do not inject into areas that have evidence of acute local infection. Discard contents of single-dose vial after use.

Monitoring Parameters Blood pressure, serum glucose, potassium, and calcium and clinical presence of adverse effects. Monitor intraocular pressure (if therapy >6 weeks), linear growth of pediatric patients (with chronic use), assess HPA suppression

Test Interactions Interferes with skin tests

Patient Information Avoid alcohol; avoid grapefruit juice if taking oral methylprednisolone; limit caffeine. Notify physician if condition being treated persists or worsens; do not decrease or discontinue dose without physician's approval. Avoid exposure to chicken pox or measles, if exposed seek medical advice without delay

Additional Information Sodium content of 1 g sodium succinate injection: 2.01 mEq; methylprednisolone sodium succinate 53 mg = methylprednisolone base 40 mg

Dosage Forms Excipient information presented when available (limited, particularly for generics); consult specific product labeling. [DSC] = Discontinued product

Injection, powder for reconstitution, as sodium succinate: 40 mg, 125 mg, 500 mg, 1 g [strength expressed as base]

A-Methapred®: 40 mg, 125 mg [strength expressed as base]

Solu-Medrol®: 40 mg [DSC], 125 mg [DSC], 500 mg [DSC], 1 g [DSC], 2 g [contains benzyl alcohol (in diluent); strength expressed as base]

Solu-Medrol®: 500 mg, 1 g [strength expressed as base]

Injection, powder for reconstitution, as sodium succinate [preservative free]:

Solu-Medrol®: 40 mg, 125 mg, 500 mg, 1 g [strength expressed as base]

Injection, suspension, as acetate: 40 mg/mL (1 mL, 5 mL, 10 mL); 80 mg/mL (1 mL, 5 mL)

Depo-Medrol®: 20 mg/mL (5 mL); 40 mg/mL (5 mL, 10 mL); 80 mg/mL (5 mL) [contains benzyl alcohol, polysorbate 80]

Depo-Medrol®: 40 mg/mL (1 mL); 80 mg/mL (1 mL)

Tablet, oral: 4 mg

Medrol®: 2 mg, 4 mg, 8 mg, 16 mg, 32 mg

Tablet, oral [dose-pack]: 4 mg (21s) [scored]

Medrol® Dosepak™: 4 mg (21s) [scored]

References

National Asthma Education and Prevention Program (NAEPP), "Expert Panel Report 3 (EPR-3): Guidelines for the Diagnosis and Management of Asthma," *Clinical Practice Guidelines*, National Institutes of Health, National Heart, Lung, and Blood Institute, NIH Publication No. 08-4051, prepublication 2007; available at http://www.nhlbi.nih.gov/guidelines/asthma/asthgdln.htm.

Rohatagi S, Barth J, Möllmann H, et al, "Pharmacokinetics of Methylprednisolone and Prednisolone After Single and Multiple Oral Administration," *J Clin Pharmacol*, 1997, 37(10):916-25.

Rouster-Stevens KA, Gursahaney A, Ngai KL, et al, "Pharmacokinetic Study of Oral Prednisolone Compared With Intravenous Methylprednisolone in Patients With Juvenile Dermatomyositis," *Arthritis Rheum*, 2008, 59(2):222-6.

◆ **6-α-Methylprednisolone** see MethylPREDNISolone on page 912

◆ **Methylprednisolone Acetate** see MethylPREDNISolone on page 912

◆ **Methylprednisolone Sodium Succinate** see MethylPREDNISolone on page 912

◆ **4-Methylpyrazole** see Fomepizole on page 620

◆ **Methylrosaniline Chloride** see Gentian Violet on page 645

◆ **Methylthionine Chloride** see Methylene Blue on page 907

Metoclopramide (met oh kloe PRA mide)

Medication Safety Issues

Sound-alike/look-alike issues:

Metoclopramide may be confused with metolazone, metoprolol, metroNIDAZOLE

Reglan® may be confused with Megace®, Regonol®, Renagel®

Related Information

Compatibility of Chemotherapy and Related Supportive Care Medications on page 1580

Compatibility of Medications Mixed in a Syringe on page 1713

U.S. Brand Names Metozolv™ ODT; Reglan®

Canadian Brand Names Apo-Metoclop®; Metoclopramide Hydrochloride Injection; Metoclopramide Omega; Nu-Metoclopramide; PMS-Metoclopramide

Therapeutic Category Antiemetic; Gastrointestinal Agent, Prokinetic

Generic Available Yes: Excludes oral-disintegrating tablet

Use Treatment of gastroesophageal reflux; prevention of nausea and vomiting associated with chemotherapy; prevention of postoperative nausea and vomiting; facilitates intubation of the small intestine and symptomatic treatment of diabetic gastroparesis (FDA approved in adults)

Medication Guide An FDA-approved patient medication guide, which is available with the product information and as follows, must be dispensed with this medication for each new outpatient prescription and refill for oral administration.

Metozolv™ ODT: http://www.accessdata.fda.gov/drugsatfda_docs/label/2009/022246s000lbl.pdf

Reglan® injection: http://www.fda.gov/downloads/Drugs/DrugSafety/UCM176362.pdf

Reglan® tablet: http://www.alavenpharm.com/downloads/ReglanTablets_MedicationGuide.pdf

Pregnancy Risk Factor B

Pregnancy Considerations Teratogenic effects were not observed in animal studies; however, there are no adequate and well-controlled studies in pregnant women. Crosses the placenta; available evidence suggests safe use during pregnancy.

Lactation Enters breast milk/use caution

Breast-Feeding Considerations Enters breast milk; may increase milk production

Contraindications Hypersensitivity to metoclopramide or any component; GI obstruction, pheochromocytoma, history of seizure disorder or patients receiving drugs likely to cause extrapyramidal reactions

Warnings May cause tardive dyskinesia, which is often irreversible; duration of treatment and total cumulative dose are associated with an increased risk. Therapy durations >12 weeks should be avoided (except in rare cases following risk:benefit assessment). Risk appears to be increased in the elderly, women, and diabetics; however, it is not possible to predict which patients will develop tardive dyskinesia. Therapy should be discontinued in any patient if signs or symptoms appear.

Extrapyramidal symptoms (EPS) may occur, generally manifested as acute dystonic reactions within the initial 24-48 hours of use. Risk of these reactions is increased at higher doses, in pediatric patients, and in adults <30 years of age.

Pseudoparkinsonism (eg, bradykinesia, tremor, rigidity) may also occur (usually within first 6 months of therapy) and is generally reversible following discontinuation. Rare reports of neuroleptic malignant syndrome; patients with NADH-cytochrome b5 reductase deficiency are at increased risk for developing methemoglobinemia and/or sulfhemoglobinemia. Neonates have prolonged clearance of metoclopramide which may lead to increased serum concentrations. In addition, neonates may have decreased NADH-cytochrome b5 reductase activity. Both conditions increase the risk of developing methemoglobinemia.

Some products contain sodium benzoate; benzoic acid (benzoate) is a metabolite of benzyl alcohol; large amounts of benzyl alcohol (≥99 mg/kg/day) have been associated with a potentially fatal toxicity ("gasping syndrome") in neonates; in vitro and animal studies have shown that benzoate displaces bilirubin from protein binding sites; avoid use of sodium benzoate containing products in neonates.

Precautions Use with caution and reduce dosage in patients with renal impairment, hypertension, or depression; transient increases in plasma aldosterone may occur which could result in fluid retention or volume overload. Patients with CHF or cirrhosis of the liver may be at increased risk for development of fluid retention and volume overload. Use with caution in these patients and discontinue therapy if symptoms of excessive body fluids occurs. Abrupt discontinuation may (rarely) result in withdrawal symptoms (dizziness, headache, nervousness).

Adverse Reactions Extrapyramidal reactions occur most frequently in children and young adults and following I.V. administration of high doses, usually within 24-48 hours after starting therapy

Cardiovascular: A-V block, bradycardia, CHF, hypertension, hypotension, SVT

Central nervous system: Agitation, anxiety, depression, drowsiness, dystonia, fatigue, hallucinations, lassitude, neuroleptic malignant syndrome (rare), restlessness, seizures, tardive dyskinesia (see Warnings)

Endocrine & metabolic: Amenorrhea, galactorrhea, gynecomastia, hyperprolactinemia

Gastrointestinal: Constipation, diarrhea

Genitourinary: Impotence, urinary frequency

Hematologic: Agranulocytosis, leukopenia, methemoglobinemia (see Warnings), neutropenia, sulfhemoglobinemia (see Warnings)

Hepatic: Jaundice, porphyria

Ocular: Visual disturbances

Miscellaneous: Hypersensitivity reactions

Drug Interactions

Metabolism/Transport Effects Substrate (minor) of CYP1A2, 2D6; **Inhibits** CYP2D6 (weak)

Avoid Concomitant Use

Avoid concomitant use of Metoclopramide with any of the following: Antipsychotics; Droperidol; Promethazine; Selective Serotonin Reuptake Inhibitors; Tetrabenazine; Tricyclic Antidepressants

Increased Effect/Toxicity

Metoclopramide may increase the levels/effects of: Antipsychotics; CycloSPORINE; CycloSPORINE (Systemic); Promethazine; Selective Serotonin Reuptake Inhibitors; Tetrabenazine; Tricyclic Antidepressants; Venlafaxine

The levels/effects of Metoclopramide may be increased by: Droperidol

Decreased Effect

Metoclopramide may decrease the levels/effects of: Anti-Parkinson's Agents (Dopamine Agonist); Posaconazole; Quinagolide

The levels/effects of Metoclopramide may be decreased by: Peginterferon Alfa-2b

Stability Protect from light; stable for 48 hours at room temperature when admixed with ascorbic acid, cimetidine (in NS only), cytarabine, dexamethasone sodium phosphate, diphenhydramine, doxorubicin, heparin, benztropine, dexamethasone hydrochloride, hydrocortisone sodium phosphate, lidocaine, magnesium sulfate, mannitol, potassium acetate, potassium chloride, and potassium phosphate; stable for 24 hours at room temperature when admixed with clindamycin (in NS only) and cyclophosphamide; incompatible with cephalothin, chloramphenicol, and sodium bicarbonate

. **Mechanism of Action** Potent dopamine receptor antagonist; blocks dopamine receptors in chemoreceptor trigger zone of the CNS, preventing emesis; accelerates gastric emptying and intestinal transit time without stimulating gastric, biliary, or pancreatic secretions

Pharmacodynamics

Onset of action:
Oral: Within 30-60 minutes
I.M.: Within 10-15 minutes
I.V.: Within 1-3 minutes

Duration: Therapeutic effects persist for 1-2 hours, regardless of route administered

Pharmacokinetics (Adult data unless noted)

Absorption: Oral: Rapid

Distribution: V_d: 3.5 L/kg; crosses the placenta; appears in breast milk; breast milk to plasma ratio: 0.5-4.06

Protein binding: ~30%

Bioavailability: Oral: 80 ± 15.5%

Half-life: Normal renal function:
Adults: 5-6 hours
Children: ~4 hours (half-life and clearance may be dose-dependent)

Elimination: Primarily in the urine (~85%) and feces

Usual Dosage

Intubation of small intestine to facilitate radiographic examination of upper GI tract: I.V.:
Children:
<6 years: 0.1 mg/kg as a single dose
6-14 years: 2.5-5 mg as a single dose
Children >14 years and Adults: 10 mg as a single dose

Gastroesophageal reflux: Oral, I.M., I.V.:
Neonates, Infants and Children: 0.4-0.8 mg/kg/day in 4 divided doses
Adults: 10-15 mg 4 times/day; single doses of 20 mg are occasionally needed prior to provoking situations. Treatment >12 weeks has not been evaluated and is not recommended.

Postoperative nausea and vomiting: I.V.:
Children: 0.1-0.2 mg/kg/dose; repeat every 6-8 hours as needed
Children >14 years and Adults: 10 mg; repeat every 6-8 hours as needed

Antiemetic **(chemotherapy-induced emesis)**: Oral, I.V.:
Children and Adults: 1-2 mg/kg/dose every 2-4 hours (maximum: 5 doses/day); pretreatment with diphenhydramine will decrease risk of extrapyramidal reactions to this dosage

Diabetic gastroparesis: Adults: Oral, I.V.: 10 mg before each meal and at bedtime for 2-8 weeks

Dosing adjustment in renal impairment: Children and Adults:
Cl_{cr} 40-50 mL/minute: Administer 75% of recommended dose
Cl_{cr} 10-40 mL/minute: Administer 50% of recommended dose
Cl_{cr} <10 mL/minute: Administer 25% to 50% of recommended dose

Administration

Oral: Administer 30 minutes before meals and at bedtime

Parenteral: Dilute to 0.2 mg/mL (maximum concentration: 5 mg/mL) and infuse over 15-30 minutes (maximum rate of infusion: 5 mg/minute); higher doses (>10 mg) to be diluted in 50 mL of compatible solution (preferably NS) and administered over at least 15 minutes; rapid I.V. administration is associated with a transient but intense feeling of anxiety and restlessness, followed by drowsiness

Monitoring Parameters Renal function; blood pressure and heart rate (when rapid I.V. administration is used)

Patient Information May cause drowsiness and impair ability to perform activities requiring mental alertness or physical coordination

Additional Information In February 2009, the U.S. Food and Drug Administration (FDA) notified healthcare professionals of the requirement for manufacturers to add a boxed warning to the metoclopramide prescribing information related to a link between chronic use and the development of tardive dyskinesia (involuntary and repetitive movements of the body). Current labeling warns of the risk, but the warning will now become a boxed warning. The labeling change was prompted by study data analysis and continued spontaneous reports of tardive dyskinesia to the FDA. The majority of reports are associated with higher doses, long-term use (>3 months), and use in the elderly, particularly older women.

Metoclopramide-induced tardive dyskinesia symptoms include impaired movement of the fingers, lip smacking, rapid eye movements or blinking, and tongue protrusion. These symptoms are rarely reversible following discontinuation of metoclopramide and treatment is not available at this time. The FDA is also requiring manufacturers to provide a medication guide to patients discussing the risk of tardive dyskinesia. Additional information can be found at http://www.fda.gov/Safety/MedWatch/SafetyInformation/SafetyAlertsforHumanMedicalProducts/ucm106942.htm.

Dosage Forms Excipient information presented when available (limited, particularly for generics); consult specific product labeling.

Injection, solution [preservative free]: 5 mg/mL (2 mL)
  Reglan®: 5 mg/mL (2 mL, 10 mL, 30 mL)
Solution, oral: 5 mg/5 mL (10 mL, 480 mL)
Tablet: 5 mg, 10 mg
  Reglan®: 5 mg, 10 mg
Tablet, orally disintegrating:
  Metozolv™ ODT: 5 mg, 10 mg [mint flavor]

◆ **Metoclopramide Hydrochloride Injection (Can)** *see* Metoclopramide *on page 915*

◆ **Metoclopramide Omega (Can)** *see* Metoclopramide *on page 915*

Metolazone (me TOLE a zone)

Medication Safety Issues
Sound-alike/look-alike issues:
  Metolazone may be confused with metaxalone, methazolamide, methimazole, methotrexate, metoclopramide, metoprolol, minoxidil
  Zaroxolyn® may be confused with Zarontin®

Related Information
Antihypertensive Agents by Class *on page 1481*

U.S. Brand Names Zaroxolyn®

Canadian Brand Names Zaroxolyn®

Therapeutic Category Antihypertensive Agent; Diuretic, Miscellaneous

Generic Available Yes

Use Management of mild to moderate hypertension (Zaroxolyn® only); treatment of edema in CHF, nephrotic syndrome, and impaired renal function

Pregnancy Risk Factor B

Pregnancy Considerations Teratogenic effects were not observed in animal studies. Metolazone crosses the placenta and appears in cord blood. Hypoglycemia, hypokalemia, hyponatremia, jaundice, and thrombocytopenia are reported as complications to the fetus or newborn following maternal use of thiazide diuretics.

Lactation Enters breast milk/not recommended

Contraindications Hypersensitivity to metolazone, any component, other thiazide diuretics, or sulfonamide-derived drugs; anuria; patients with hepatic coma

Warnings Chemical similarities are present among sulfonamides, sulfonylureas, carbonic anhydrase inhibitors, thiazides, and loop diuretics (except ethacrynic acid). Use in patients with thiazide or sulfonamide allergy is specifically contraindicated in product labeling, however, there is potential for cross-reaction with any of these compounds; avoid use in patients allergic to these compounds particularly if the reaction was severe. Large or prolonged fluid and electrolyte losses may occur with concomitant furosemide administration.

Precautions Use with caution in patients with severe renal disease, impaired hepatic function, gout, lupus erythematosus, diabetes mellitus, moderate-high cholesterol concentrations, and/or high triglycerides

Adverse Reactions
Cardiovascular: Palpitations, chest pain, orthostatic hypotension, precordial pain, syncope, venous thrombosis, necrotizing angiitis
Central nervous system: Vertigo, headache, chills, drowsiness, fatigue, restlessness, depression, dizziness
Dermatologic: Rash, dry skin, photosensitivity, toxic epidermal necrolysis, Stevens-Johnson syndrome, cutaneous vasculitis, urticaria
Endocrine & metabolic: Hypokalemia, hyponatremia, hypochloremia, metabolic alkalosis, hyperglycemia, hyperuricemia, hypomagnesemia, gout, hypercalcemia
Gastrointestinal: Abdominal bloating, GI irritation, bitter taste, nausea, vomiting, anorexia, xerostomia, abdominal pain, epigastric distress
Hematologic: Blood dyscrasias, aplastic anemia, hemolytic anemia, leukopenia, agranulocytosis, thrombocytopenia
Hepatic: Hepatitis, cholestatic jaundice
Neuromuscular & skeletal: Arthralgia, back pain, paresthesias, joint pain, muscle cramps/spasm, weakness
Ocular: Eye itching, transient blurred vision
Otic: Tinnitus
Renal: Polyuria, prerenal azotemia, uremia
Respiratory: Cough, sinus congestion, epistaxis

Drug Interactions
Avoid Concomitant Use
Avoid concomitant use of Metolazone with any of the following: Dofetilide

Increased Effect/Toxicity
Metolazone may increase the levels/effects of: ACE Inhibitors; Allopurinol; Amifostine; Antihypertensives; Calcitriol; Calcium Salts; CarBAMazepine; Dofetilide; Hypotensive Agents; Lithium; OXcarbazepine; RiTUXimab

The levels/effects of Metolazone may be increased by: Alcohol (Ethyl); Analgesics (Opioid); Barbiturates; Corticosteroids (Orally Inhaled); Corticosteroids (Systemic); Herbs (Hypotensive Properties); MAO Inhibitors; Pentoxifylline; Phosphodiesterase 5 Inhibitors; Prostacyclin Analogues

Decreased Effect
Metolazone may decrease the levels/effects of: Antidiabetic Agents

The levels/effects of Metolazone may be decreased by: Bile Acid Sequestrants; Herbs (Hypertensive Properties); Methylphenidate; Nonsteroidal Anti-Inflammatory Agents; Yohimbine

Food Interactions Avoid natural licorice (causes sodium and water retention and increases potassium loss); avoid garlic (may have increased antihypertensive effect); avoid ephedra, yohimbe, ginseng (may worsen hypertension)

Mechanism of Action Inhibits sodium reabsorption in the cortical diluting site and proximal convoluted tubules causing increased excretion of sodium and water as well as potassium and hydrogen ions

Pharmacodynamics
Onset of action: 1 hour
Duration: 12-24 hours

Pharmacokinetics (Adult data unless noted)
Absorption: Oral: Rate and extent vary with the preparation
Protein binding: 95%
Half-life: 6-20 hours
Elimination: Enterohepatic recycling; 70% to 95% excreted unchanged in urine

Usual Dosage Oral:
Children: 0.2-0.4 mg/kg/day divided every 12-24 hours
Adults:
  Edema: 5-10 mg/dose every 24 hours
  Edema associated with renal disease or cardiac failure (ACC/AHA 2005 Heart Failure Guidelines): 2.5-20 mg/dose every 24 hours
  Hypertension: 2.5-5 mg/dose every 24 hours

Administration Oral: Administer with food to decrease GI distress; administer early in day to avoid nocturia

Monitoring Parameters Serum electrolytes, renal function, blood pressure, body weight, fluid balance

Patient Information May cause dry mouth; may cause drowsiness and impair ability to perform activities requiring mental alertness or physical coordination. May cause photosensitivity reactions (eg, exposure to sunlight may cause severe sunburn, skin rash, redness, or itching); avoid exposure to sunlight and artificial light sources (sunlamps, tanning booth/bed); wear protective clothing, wide-brimmed hats, sunglasses, and lip sunscreen (SPF ≥15); use a sunscreen [broad-spectrum sunscreen or physical sunscreen (preferred) or sunblock with SPF ≥15]; contact physician if reaction occurs.

Additional Information Metolazone 5 mg is approximately equivalent to hydrochlorothiazide 50 mg

Dosage Forms Excipient information presented when available (limited, particularly for generics); consult specific product labeling. [DSC] = Discontinued product
Tablet: 2.5 mg, 5 mg, 10 mg
Zaroxolyn®: 2.5 mg, 5 mg; 10 mg [DSC]

Extemporaneous Preparations

A 1 mg/mL suspension may be made by crushing twelve 10 mg Zaroxolyn® tablets; add Ora-Sweet®, Ora-Sweet® SF, Ora-Plus®, or cherry syrup diluted 1:4 with simple syrup to total volume of 120 mL. Label "shake well"; stable 60 days refrigerated.

A 0.25 mg/mL suspension may be made by crushing one 2.5 mg tablet; add 1:1 mixture 1% methylcellulose:simple syrup mixture to a total volume of 10 mL; label "shake well"; refrigerate; stable 91 days refrigerated; 28 days at room temperature in plastic and 14 days at room temperature in glass.

Nahata, MC, Pai VB, and Hipple TF, *Pediatric Drug Formulations*, 5th ed, Cincinnati, OH: Harvey Whitney Books Co, 2004.

References
Arnold WC, "Efficacy of Metolazone and Furosemide in Children With Furosemide-Resistant Edema," *Pediatrics*, 1984, 74(5):872-5.
Chobanian AV, Bakris GL, Black HR, et al, "The Seventh Report of the Joint National Committee on Prevention, Detection, Evaluation, and Treatment of High Blood Pressure: The JNC 7 Report," *JAMA*, 2003, 289(19):2560-72.
Wells TG, "The Pharmacology and Therapeutics of Diuretics in the Pediatric Patient," *Pediatr Clin North Am*, 1990, 37(2):463-504.

◆ **Metopirone®** *see* Metyrapone *on page 923*

Metoprolol (me toe PROE lole)

Medication Safety Issues
Sound-alike/look-alike issues:
Lopressor® may be confused with Lyrica®
Metoprolol may be confused with metaproterenol, metoclopramide, metolazone, misoprostol
Metoprolol succinate may be confused with metoprolol tartrate
Toprol-XL® may be confused with Tegretol®, Tegretol®-XR, Topamax®

High alert medication: The Institute for Safe Medication Practices (ISMP) includes this medication among its list of drugs which have a heightened risk of causing significant patient harm when used in error.

Significant differences exist between oral and I.V. dosing. Use caution when converting from one route of administration to another.

Related Information
Antihypertensive Agents by Class *on page 1481*

U.S. Brand Names Lopressor®; Toprol-XL®

Canadian Brand Names Apo-Metoprolol SR®; Apo-Metoprolol®; Betaloc®; Dom-Metoprolol; Gen-Metoprolol; Lopressor®; Metoprolol Tartrate Injection, USP; Metoprolol-25; Metoprolol-L; Mylan-Metoprolol (Type L); Novo-Metoprol; Nu-Metop; PHL-Metoprolol; PMS-Metoprolol; Riva-Metoprolol; Sandoz-Metoprolol

Therapeutic Category Antianginal Agent; Antiarrhythmic Agent, Class II; Antihypertensive Agent; Antimigraine Agent; Beta-Adrenergic Blocker

Generic Available Yes

Use
Immediate release tablets and injection: Treatment of hypertension, alone or in combination with other agents (FDA approved in adults), angina pectoris (FDA approved in adults), and hemodynamically-stable acute myocardial infarction (to reduce cardiovascular mortality) (FDA approved in adults)

Extended release tablets: Treatment of hypertension, alone or in combination with other agents (FDA approved in ages ≥6 years and adults); angina pectoris (FDA approved in adults); and patients with heart failure (stable NYHA Class II or III) already receiving ACE inhibitors, diuretics, and/or digoxin (to reduce mortality/hospitalization) (FDA approved in adults)

Metoprolol has also been used for the treatment of ventricular arrhythmias, atrial ectopy; prevention and treatment of atrial fibrillation and atrial flutter; multifocal atrial tachycardia; symptomatic treatment of hypertrophic obstructive cardiomyopathy; essential tremor; and migraine headache prophylaxis

Pregnancy Risk Factor C (manufacturer); D (2nd and 3rd trimesters - expert analysis)

Pregnancy Considerations Teratogenic effects were not observed in animal studies. Metoprolol crosses the placenta. Maternal use of beta-blockers has been associated with fetal bradycardia, hypotension, and IUGR; IUGR is probably related to maternal hypertension. Available evidence suggests beta-blockers are generally safe during pregnancy (JNC 7). Cases of neonatal hypoglycemia have been reported following maternal use of beta-blockers at parturition. Information specific to metoprolol is limited.

Lactation Enters breast milk/use caution (AAP rates "compatible")

Breast-Feeding Considerations Metoprolol is considered compatible by the AAP. However, monitor the infant for signs of beta-blockade (hypotension, bradycardia, etc) with long-term use.

Contraindications Hypersensitivity to metoprolol, any component of the formulation, or other beta-blockers; **Note:** Additional contraindications are formulation and/or indication specific.

Immediate release tablets and injection:
Hypertension and angina: Sinus bradycardia; second- and third-degree heart block; cardiogenic shock; overt cardiac failure; sick sinus syndrome (except in patients with a functioning artificial pacemaker); severe peripheral arterial disease; pheochromocytoma (without alpha blockade)

Myocardial infarction: Severe sinus bradycardia (heart rate <45 beats/minute); significant first-degree heart block (P-R interval ≥0.24 seconds); second- and third-degree heart block; systolic blood pressure <100 mm Hg; moderate-to-severe cardiac failure

Extended release tablet: Severe bradycardia; second- and third-degree heart block; cardiogenic shock; decompensated heart failure; sick sinus syndrome (except in patients with a functioning artificial pacemaker)

Warnings May depress myocardial activity and precipitate or worsen heart failure; use with caution and monitor closely, especially in patients with compensated heart failure and during upwards titration of dose; if heart failure worsens, may need to increase diuretics and not advance the dose of metoprolol; a reduction in dose or discontinuation of metoprolol may be needed. Beta-blocker therapy should not be withdrawn abruptly (particularly in patients with CAD), but gradually tapered over 1-2 weeks to avoid acute tachycardia, hypertension, and/or ischemia **[U.S. Boxed Warning]**. Beta-blockers should generally be avoided in patients with bronchospastic disease; metoprolol, with relative beta$_1$ selectivity, should be used with caution and closely monitored in patients with bronchospastic disease; beta$_2$ stimulants and the lowest possible dose of metoprolol should be used in these patients. Metoprolol may block hypoglycemia-induced tachycardia and blood pressure changes; use with caution in patients with diabetes mellitus. Metoprolol decreases the ability of the heart to respond to reflex adrenergic stimuli and may increase the risk of general anesthesia and surgical procedures. May mask clinical signs of hyperthyroidism (exacerbation of symptoms of hyperthyroidism, including thyroid storm, may occur following abrupt discontinuation). Use with caution with potent inhibitors of cytochrome P450 CYP2D6 isoenzyme (see Drug Interactions). Use with caution with verapamil, diltiazem, or anesthetic agents that decrease myocardial function (bradycardia or heart block may occur). Beta-blocker use has been associated with induction or exacerbation of psoriasis, but cause and effect have not been firmly established.

Precautions Use with caution in patients with hepatic dysfunction and in patients with peripheral vascular disease (beta-blockers may aggravate arterial insufficiency). Patients who have a history of severe anaphylactic hypersensitivity reactions to various substances may be more reactive while receiving beta-blockers; these patients may not be responsive to the normal doses of epinephrine used to treat hypersensitivity reactions. Contraindicated in patients with pheochromocytoma; if required, these patients should receive an alpha-blocking agent before receipt of any beta-blocking agent.

Adverse Reactions

Cardiovascular: Bradycardia, CHF, heart block (second- and third-degree), hypotension, palpitations, peripheral circulation reduced, peripheral edema, worsening of AV conduction disturbances

Central nervous system: Depression, dizziness, insomnia, mental confusion, tiredness

Dermatologic: Pruritus, rash, worsening of psoriasis

Gastrointestinal: Abdominal pain, constipation, diarrhea, nausea, vomiting, xerostomia

Hematologic (potential): Agranulocytosis, thrombocytopenia

Hepatic: Hepatic dysfunction, hepatitis, jaundice; rare: alkaline phosphatase, LDH, transaminase elevated

Respiratory: Bronchospasm, dyspnea, wheezing

Drug Interactions

Metabolism/Transport Effects Substrate of CYP2C19 (minor), 2D6 (major); **Inhibits** CYP2D6 (weak)

Avoid Concomitant Use

Avoid concomitant use of Metoprolol with any of the following: Methacholine

Increased Effect/Toxicity

Metoprolol may increase the levels/effects of: Alpha-/Beta-Agonists (Direct-Acting); Alpha1-Blockers; Alpha2-Agonists; Amifostine; Antihypertensives; Antipsychotic Agents (Phenothiazines); Bupivacaine; Cardiac Glycosides; Hypotensive Agents; Insulin; Lidocaine; Lidocaine (Systemic); Lidocaine (Topical); Mepivacaine; Methacholine; Midodrine; RiTUXimab; Sulfonylureas

The levels/effects of Metoprolol may be increased by: Acetylcholinesterase Inhibitors; Aminoquinolines (Antimalarial); Amiodarone; Anilidopiperidine Opioids; Antipsychotic Agents (Phenothiazines); Calcium Channel

Blockers (Nondihydropyridine); CYP2D6 Inhibitors (Moderate); CYP2D6 Inhibitors (Strong); Darunavir; Diazoxide; Dipyridamole; Disopyramide; Dronedarone; Herbs (Hypotensive Properties); MAO Inhibitors; Pentoxifylline; Phosphodiesterase 5 Inhibitors; Propafenone; Propoxyphene; Prostacyclin Analogues; QuiNIDine; Reserpine; Selective Serotonin Reuptake Inhibitors

Decreased Effect

Metoprolol may decrease the levels/effects of: Beta2-Agonists; Theophylline Derivatives

The levels/effects of Metoprolol may be decreased by: Barbiturates; Herbs (Hypertensive Properties); Methylphenidate; Nonsteroidal Anti-Inflammatory Agents; Peginterferon Alfa-2b; Rifamycin Derivatives; Yohimbine

Food Interactions

Metoprolol tartrate: Food may enhance the extent of oral absorption

Metoprolol succinate (extended release tablets): Food does not significantly affect bioavailability

Stability

All formulations: Store at controlled room temperature of 25°C (77°F); excursions permitted to 15°C to 30°C (59°F to 86°F)

Tablets: Protect from moisture and dispense in tight, light-resistant container

Injection: Protect from light

Mechanism of Action Selective inhibitor of beta$_1$-adrenergic receptors at lower doses; competitively blocks beta$_1$ adrenergic receptors with little or no effect on beta$_2$-receptors at doses in adults <100 mg/day; inhibits beta$_2$-receptors at higher doses; does not exhibit membrane stabilizing or intrinsic sympathomimetic activity

Pharmacodynamics

Beta blockade:

Onset of action: Oral: Metoprolol tartrate tablets: Within 1 hour

Maximum effect: I.V.: 20 minutes

Duration: Dose dependent

Antihypertensive effect:

Onset of action: Oral: Metoprolol tartrate tablets: Within 15 minutes

Maximum effect: Oral (multiple dosing): After 1 week

Duration: Oral: Metoprolol tartrate tablets (single dose): 6 hours; metoprolol succinate (extended release tablets): Up to 24 hours

Pharmacokinetics (Adult data unless noted) Note: The pharmacokinetics of metoprolol in hypertensive children 6-17 years of age were found to be similar to adults.

Absorption: Rapid and complete, with large first-pass effect

Distribution: Crosses the blood brain barrier; CSF concentrations are 78% of plasma concentrations

Protein binding: 12% bound to albumin

Metabolism: Significant first-pass metabolism; extensive metabolism in the liver via isoenzyme CYP2D6

Bioavailability: Oral: 50%

Half-Life:

Neonates: 5-10 hours

Adults: CYP2D6 poor metabolizers: 7.5 hours; CYP2D6 extensive metabolizers: 2.8 hours

Adults with chronic renal failure: Similar to normal adults

Elimination: 10% of an I.V. dose and <5% of an oral dose is excreted unchanged in the urine

Usual Dosage (See Additional Information)

Oral: Hypertension:

Immediate release tablets: Children and Adolescents 1-17 years: Initial: 1-2 mg/kg/day, administered in 2 divided doses; adjust dose based on patient response; maximum: 6 mg/kg/day (≤200 mg/day) (National High Blood Pressure Education Program Working Group on High Blood Pressure in Children and Adolescents, 2004)

Extended release tablets: Manufacturer's recommendation: Children ≥6 years: Initial: 1 mg/kg once daily (maximum initial dose: 50 mg/day); adjust dose based on patient response (maximum: 2 mg/kg/day or 200 mg/day; higher doses have not been studied)

Adults:

Immediate release tablets: Initial: 100 mg/day in single or divided doses, increase at weekly intervals to desired effect; usual dosage range: 100-450 mg/day; doses >450 mg/day have not been studied; usual dosage range (JNC 7): 50-100 mg/day in 1-2 divided doses

Note: Lower once-daily dosing (especially 100 mg/day) may not control blood pressure for 24 hours; larger or more frequent dosing may be needed. Patients with bronchospastic diseases should receive the lowest possible daily dose; dose should initially be divided into 3 doses per day (to avoid high plasma concentrations).

Extended release tablets: Initial: 25-100 mg/day as a single dose; increase at weekly intervals to desired effect; doses >400 mg/day have not been studied; usual dosage range (JNC 7): 50-100 mg once daily

Oral: Congestive heart failure: Adults: Extended release tablets: Initial: NYHA Class II heart failure: 25 mg once daily; more severe heart failure: 12.5 mg once daily; may double the dose every 2 weeks as tolerated; maximum: 200 mg/day

Administration Oral:

Metoprolol tartrate tablets: Administer with food or immediately after meals

Metoprolol succinate extended release tablets: May be administered without regard to meals; Toprol-XL® tablets are scored and may be divided; do not chew or crush the half or whole tablets; swallow whole. Do not chew, crush, or break generic nonscored extended release tablets; swallow whole.

Monitoring Parameters Blood pressure, heart rate, respirations, circulation in extremities

Additional Information Do not abruptly discontinue therapy, taper dosage gradually over 1-2 weeks. Beta-blockers without intrinsic sympathomimetic activity (such as metoprolol) have been shown to decrease morbidity and mortality when initiated in the acute treatment of MI and continued long term; metoprolol injection is used for early treatment of definitive or suspected MI; consult adult reference for further information.

A limited number of studies assessing the use of metoprolol in hypertensive pediatric patients are available. A recent article examined the use of metoprolol extended release tablets in children 6-16 years of age (mean age: 12.5 ± 2.8 years). In part one (a 4-week double-blind dose ranging study), patients were randomized to receive placebo (n=23) or metoprolol 0.2 mg/kg/day (n=45), 1 mg/kg/day (n=23), or 2 mg/kg/day (n=49) given as once daily dosing. For patients in the higher dosing groups, doses were initiated at 0.5 mg/kg/day, and increased after 1 week to 1 mg/kg/day if tolerated. Doses were increased again after 1 week to 2 mg/kg/day if tolerated in the 2 mg/kg/day dosing group. At the end of 4 weeks, metoprolol significantly decreased systolic blood pressure in the 1 mg/kg/day and 2 mg/kg/day groups compared to placebo. Diastolic blood pressure was significantly reduced only in the 2 mg/kg/day group. In part two (a 52-week open-label trial), 100 patients received initial doses of 25 mg or 12.5 mg once daily; doses were increased every 2 weeks in 25 mg or 50 mg increments based on blood pressure and tolerability, to a maximum dose of 200 mg once daily. The mean doses were 37 ± 33 mg at study entry, 97 ± 64 mg at week 16, and 112 ± 69 mg at study end (see Batisky, 2007). In an older study using nonsustained release tablets, 16 hypertensive adolescents

(≥13 years of age) were treated with an initial metoprolol dose of 50 mg twice daily; patients were seen every 4-6 weeks and doses were increased to 100 mg twice daily if blood pressure was not controlled (see Falkner, 1982).

Pediatric dosing information for metoprolol, for use in indications other than hypertension, is also limited; in one case report, oral metoprolol (2 mg/kg/day in 3 divided doses) helped control paroxysmal supraventricular tachycardia in a 6-month old infant receiving digoxin (see Hepner, 1983). Low dose oral metoprolol (initial: 0.1 mg/kg/dose given twice daily, then increased slowly as needed to a maximum of 0.9 ± 0.7 mg/kg/day) was used to treat severe CHF that failed conventional therapy in four children (mean age: 7.8 years) with cardiomyopathy who were under consideration for heart transplantation (see Shaddy, 1998). A follow-up report in 15 children, 2.5-15 years of age (mean: 8.6 ± 1.3 years) used low dose oral metoprolol [Initial: 0.1-0.2 mg/kg/dose given twice daily, then increased slowly as needed to a maximum of 1.1 ± 0.1 mg/kg/day (range: 0.5-2.3 mg/kg/day)] to treat dilated cardiomyopathy and CHF; all patients received ACE inhibitors, digoxin, and diuretics before starting metoprolol (see Shaddy, 1999). Two studies (Muller, 1993; O'Marcaigh, 1994) assessed metoprolol for unexplained syncope in children at I.V. doses of 0.1-0.2 mg/kg for tilt table testing; in both studies, oral metoprolol was given after tilt table testing to select patients; initial oral doses of 0.8-2.8 mg/kg/day were used in 15 patients (8-20 years of age), but treatment was discontinued in three patients receiving 1.8-2.8 mg/kg/day due to adverse effects (Muller, 1993); oral doses of 1-2 mg/kg/day, rounded to the nearest 25 mg/day and divided into 2 doses daily were used in 19 patients (7-18 years of age) with unexplained syncope; the mean effective dose was 1.5 mg/kg/day (O'Marcaigh, 1994). High-dose beta-blocker therapy has been recommended to treat childhood hypertrophic cardiomyopathy (see Ostman-Smith, 1999). Further pediatric studies are required before these doses can be recommended.

Dosage Forms Excipient information presented when available (limited, particularly for generics); consult specific product labeling.

Injection, solution, as tartrate: 1 mg/mL (5 mL)

Lopressor®: 1 mg/mL (5 mL)

Tablet, as tartrate: 25 mg, 50 mg, 100 mg

Lopressor®: 50 mg, 100 mg

Tablet, extended release, as succinate: 25 mg, 50 mg, 100 mg, 200 mg [expressed as mg equivalent to tartrate]

Toprol-XL®: 25 mg, 50 mg, 100 mg, 200 mg [expressed as mg equivalent to tartrate]

Extemporaneous Preparations A 10 mg/mL metoprolol tartrate oral liquid preparation made with twelve 100 mg tablets and qsad to 120 mL with 3 different vehicles (a 1:1 mixture of Ora-Sweet® and Ora-Plus®, a 1:1 mixture of Ora-Sweet® SF and Ora-Plus®, or cherry syrup) was found to be stable for 60 days when stored in amber plastic bottles in the dark at 5°C and 25°C. Microbial growth was not determined. Label "shake well" and "protect from light".

Allen LV and Erickson MA, "Stability of Labetalol Hydrochloride, Metoprolol Tartrate, Verapamil Hydrochloride, and Spironolactone With Hydrochlorothiazide in Extemporaneously Compounded Oral Liquids," *Am J Health Syst Pharm*, 1996, 53(19):2304-9.

References

Batisky DL, Sorof JM, Sugg J, et al, "Efficacy and Safety of Extended Release Metoprolol Succinate in Hypertensive Children 6 to 16 Years of Age: A Clinical Trial Experience," *J Pediatr*, 2007, 150(2):134-9.

Brauchli YB, Jick SS, Curtin F, et al, "Association Between Beta-Blockers, Other Antihypertensive Drugs and Psoriasis: Population-Based Case-Control Study," *Br J Dermatol*, 2008, 158(6):1299-307.

Chobanian AV, Bakris GL, Black HR, et al, "The Seventh Report of the Joint National Committee on Prevention, Detection, Evaluation, and Treatment of High Blood Pressure: The JNC 7 report," *JAMA*, 2003, 289(19):2560-72.

Falkner B, Lowenthal DT, and Affrime MB, "The Pharmacodynamic Effectiveness of Metoprolol in Adolescent Hypertension," *Pediatr Pharmacol (New York)*, 1982, 2(1):49-55.

Gold MH, Holy AK, and Roenigk HH Jr, "Beta-Blocking Drugs and Psoriasis. A Review of Cutaneous Side Effects and Retrospective Analysis of Their Effects on Psoriasis," *J Am Acad Dermatol*, 1988, 19 (5 Pt 1):837-41.

Hepner SI, and Davoli E, "Successful Treatment of Supraventricular Tachycardia With Metoprolol, a Cardioselective Beta Blocker," *Clin Pediatr (Phila)*, 1983, 22(7):522-3.

Morselli PL, Boutroy MJ, Bianchetti G, et al, "Pharmacokinetics of Antihypertensive Drugs in the Neonatal Period," *Dev Pharmacol Ther*, 1989, 13(2-4):190-8.

Muller G, Deal BJ, Strasburger JF, et al, "Usefulness of Metoprolol for Unexplained Syncope and Positive Response to Tilt Testing in Young Persons," *Am J Cardiol*, 1993, 71(7):592-5.

National High Blood Pressure Education Program Working Group on High Blood Pressure in Children and Adolescents, "The Fourth Report on the Diagnosis, Evaluation, and Treatment of High Blood Pressure in Children and Adolescents," *Pediatrics*, 2004, 114(2 Suppl 4th Report):555-76.

O'Marcaigh AS, MacLellan-Tobert SG, and Porter CJ, "Tilt-Table Testing and Oral Metoprolol Therapy in Young Patients With Unexplained Syncope," *Pediatrics*, 1994, 93(2):278-83.

Ostman-Smith I, Wettrell G, and Riesenfield T, "A Cohort Study of Childhood Hypertrophic Cardiomyopathy: Improved Survival Following High-Dose Beta-Adrenoceptor Antagonist Treatment," *J Am Coll Cardiol*, 1999, 34(6):1813-22.

Schön MP and Boehncke WH, "Psoriasis," *N Engl J Med*, 2005, 352 (18):1899-912.

Shaddy RE, "Beta-Blocker Therapy in Young Children With Congestive Heart Failure Under Consideration for Heart Transplantation," *Am Heart J*, 1998, 136(1):19-21.

Shaddy RE, Tani LY, Gidding SS, et al, "Beta-Blocker Treatment of Dilated Cardiomyopathy With Congestive Heart Failure in Children: A Multi-Institutional Experience," *J Heart Lung Transplant*, 1999, 18 (3):269-74.

◆ **Metoprolol-25 (Can)** *see* Metoprolol *on page 918*

◆ **Metoprolol-L (Can)** *see* Metoprolol *on page 918*

◆ **Metoprolol Succinate** *see* Metoprolol *on page 918*

◆ **Metoprolol Tartrate** *see* Metoprolol *on page 918*

◆ **Metoprolol Tartrate Injection, USP (Can)** *see* Metoprolol *on page 918*

◆ **Metozolv™ ODT** *see* Metoclopramide *on page 915*

◆ **MetroCream®** *see* MetroNIDAZOLE *on page 921*

◆ **MetroGel®** *see* MetroNIDAZOLE *on page 921*

◆ **Metrogel® (Can)** *see* MetroNIDAZOLE *on page 921*

◆ **MetroGel-Vaginal®** *see* MetroNIDAZOLE *on page 921*

◆ **MetroLotion®** *see* MetroNIDAZOLE *on page 921*

MetroNIDAZOLE (me troe NI da zole)

Medication Safety Issues
Sound-alike/look-alike issues:
MetroNIDAZOLE may be confused with mebendazole, meropenem, metFORMIN, methotrexate, metoclopramide, miconazole

Related Information
Compatibility of Chemotherapy and Related Supportive Care Medications *on page 1580*

U.S. Brand Names Flagyl®; Flagyl® 375; Flagyl® ER; MetroCream®; MetroGel-Vaginal®; MetroGel®; MetroLotion®; Noritate®; Vandazole®

Canadian Brand Names Apo-Metronidazole®; Flagyl®; Florazole® ER; MetroCream®; Metrogel®; Nidagel™; Noritate®; Trikacide

Therapeutic Category Amebicide; Antibiotic, Anaerobic; Antibiotic, Topical; Antiprotozoal

Generic Available Yes: Capsule, cream, gel, infusion, lotion, tablet

Use Treatment of susceptible anaerobic bacterial and protozoal infections in the following conditions: Amebiasis (liver abscess, dysentery), giardiasis, symptomatic and asymptomatic trichomoniasis; skin and skin structure infections, bone and joint infections, CNS infections, endocarditis, gynecological infections, intra-abdominal infections, respiratory tract (lower) infections and systemic anaerobic bacterial infections; surgical prophylaxis (colorectal); topically for the treatment of acne rosacea; treatment of antibiotic-associated pseudomembranous colitis (AAPC) caused by *C. difficile*; bacterial vaginosis (FDA approved in adults)

Pregnancy Risk Factor B

Pregnancy Considerations Teratogenic effects have not been observed in animal reproduction studies; therefore, the manufacturer classifies metronidazole as pregnancy category B. Metronidazole crosses the placenta and rapidly distributes into the fetal circulation. Although there have been a few reports of facial anomalies after *in utero* exposure, most studies have not found an increased risk of congenital abnormalities following maternal use of metronidazole during the first trimester of pregnancy. In studies that included women taking metronidazole during all trimesters of pregnancy, an increased risk of adverse fetal and neonatal outcomes has not been observed. Because metronidazole has been carcinogenic in some animal species, concern has been raised whether metronidazole should be used during pregnancy; however, a strong carcinogenic potential in humans has not been observed, including one study of prenatal exposure.

Metronidazole pharmacokinetics are similar between pregnant and nonpregnant patients. Bacterial vaginosis has been associated with adverse pregnancy outcomes (including preterm labor); metronidazole is recommended for the treatment of symptomatic bacterial vaginosis in pregnant patients. Vaginal trichomoniasis has been also associated with adverse pregnancy outcomes (including preterm labor). Treatment may relieve symptoms and prevent further sexual transmission; however, metronidazole has not resulted in reduced perinatal morbidity and should not be used solely to prevent preterm delivery. Some clinicians consider deferring therapy in asymptomatic women until >37 weeks gestation. Use of oral metronidazole is contraindicated during the first trimester (per the FDA approved labeling). Consult current CDC guidelines for appropriate use in pregnant women.

Lactation Enters breast milk/not recommended (AAP rates "of concern")

Breast-Feeding Considerations Metronidazole and its active metabolite are measurable in the breast milk and infant plasma. Milk concentrations are similar to those in the maternal plasma and are highly variable. Peak concentrations of metronidazole in breast milk occur ~2-4 hours after the oral dose. In studies, the calculated relative infant doses have ranged from 0.13% to 36% of the weight-adjusted maternal dose. Use of metronidazole in a lactating patient is not recommended by the manufacturer. The AAP considers metronidazole to be a "drug for which the effect on the nursing infant is unknown, but may be of concern." If metronidazole is given, breast-feeding should be withheld for 12-24 hours after the dose.

Contraindications Hypersensitivity to metronidazole, nitroimidazole derivatives, or any component; 1st trimester of pregnancy

Warnings Has been shown to be carcinogenic in rodents **[U.S. Boxed Warning]**; aseptic meningitis, encephalopathy, seizures, and neuropathies (peripheral and optic) have been reported especially with increased doses and chronic treatment; if this occurs, discontinue therapy. Use with caution in patients with a history of seizure disorder; consider reduced doses in patients who have non-infectious CNS disease

Precautions Use with caution in patients with liver impairment, blood dyscrasias, CNS disease; metronidazole injection should be used with caution in patients receiving corticosteroids or patients predisposed to edema (injection contains 28 mEq of sodium/g metronidazole);

reduce dosage in patients with severe liver impairment; dosage adjustment is not necessary in patients with moderate to severe renal insufficiency. Prolonged use may result in fungal or bacterial superinfection, including *C. difficile*-associated diarrhea (CDAD) and pseudomembranous colitis; CDAD has been observed >2 months postantibiotic treatment.

Adverse Reactions

Cardiovascular: Flattening of the T-wave, flushing, syncope

Central nervous system: Aseptic meningitis, ataxia, confusion, coordination impaired, depression, dizziness, encephalopathy, fever, seizures, headache, insomnia, irritability, seizures, vertigo

Dermatologic: Erythematous rash, pruritus, Stevens-Johnson syndrome, urticaria

Endocrine & metabolic: Disulfiram-type reaction with alcohol, dysmenorrhea

Gastrointestinal: Anorexia, abdominal cramping, constipation, diarrhea, epigastric distress, furry tongue, glossitis, metallic taste, nausea (~12%), pancreatitis (rare), proctitis, stomatitis, vomiting, xerostomia

Genitourinary: Cystitis, discoloration of urine (dark or reddish brown), dyspareunia, dysuria, incontinence, libido decreased, pelvic pressure, polyuria, vaginal dryness, vaginitis

Hematologic: Neutropenia (reversible), thrombocytopenia (reversible, rare)

Local: Thrombophlebitis

Neuromuscular & skeletal: Dysarthria, peripheral neuropathy, weakness

Ocular: Optic neuropathy

Respiratory: Nasal congestion, pharyngitis, rhinitis, sinusitis

Miscellaneous: Flu-like syndrome, joint pains resembling serum sickness, moniliasis

Drug Interactions

Metabolism/Transport Effects Inhibits CYP2C9 (weak), 3A4 (moderate)

Avoid Concomitant Use

Avoid concomitant use of MetroNIDAZOLE with any of the following: BCG; Disulfiram; Tolvaptan

Increased Effect/Toxicity

MetroNIDAZOLE may increase the levels/effects of: Alcohol (Ethyl); Busulfan; Calcineurin Inhibitors; Colchicine; CYP3A4 Substrates; Disulfiram; Eplerenone; Everolimus; FentaNYL; Halofantrine; Phenytoin; Pimecrolimus; Ranolazine; Salmeterol; Saxagliptin; Tipranavir; Tolvaptan; Vitamin K Antagonists

The levels/effects of MetroNIDAZOLE may be increased by: Mebendazole

Decreased Effect

MetroNIDAZOLE may decrease the levels/effects of: BCG; Mycophenolate; Typhoid Vaccine

The levels/effects of MetroNIDAZOLE may be decreased by: PHENobarbital; Phenytoin

Food Interactions Peak concentration is decreased and delayed when administered with food

Stability

Injection: Store at controlled room temperature; protect from light. Keep in overwrap until ready to use. Product may be refrigerated but crystals may form. Crystals redissolve on warming to room temperature. Prolonged exposure to light will cause a darkening of the product; however, short-term exposure to normal room light does not adversely affect metronidazole stability. Direct sunlight should be avoided. Stability of parenteral admixture at room temperature (25°C): Out of overwrap stability: 30 days.

Tablets: Store at room temperature; protect from light and moisture.

Mechanism of Action Reduced to a product which interacts with DNA to cause a loss of helical DNA structure and strand breakage resulting in inhibition of protein synthesis and cell death in susceptible organisms

Pharmacokinetics (Adult data unless noted)

Absorption: Oral: Well absorbed

Distribution: Excreted in breast milk; widely distributed into body tissues, fluids including bile, liver, bone, pleural fluid, vaginal secretions, CSF, erythrocytes, and hepatic abscesses

Protein binding: <20%

Metabolism: 30% to 60% in the liver to hydroxylated metabolite (60% to 80% bioactive), acetic acid metabolites, glucuronide, and sulfated conjugates

Half-life (increases with hepatic impairment):
Neonates: 25-75 hours
Children and Adults:
Metronidazole: 6-12 hours
Hydroxymetronidazole: 9.5-20 hours

Time to peak serum concentration: Within 1-2 hours

Elimination: Excreted via the urine (20% as unchanged drug) and feces (6% to 15%)

Dialysis: Extensively removed by hemodialysis and peritoneal dialysis

Usual Dosage

Neonates: Anaerobic infections: Oral, I.V.:
0-4 weeks, <1200 g: 7.5 mg/kg every 48 hours
Postnatal age ≤7 days:
1200-2000 g: 7.5 mg/kg/day given every 24 hours
>2000 g: 15 mg/kg/day in divided doses every 12 hours
Postnatal age >7 days:
1200-2000 g: 15 mg/kg/day in divided doses every 12 hours
>2000 g: 30 mg/kg/day in divided doses every 12 hours

Infants and Children:
Amebiasis: Oral: 35-50 mg/kg/day in divided doses every 8 hours
Other parasitic infections: Oral: 15-30 mg/kg/day in divided doses every 8 hours
Anaerobic infections: Oral, I.V.: 30 mg/kg/day in divided doses every 6 hours; maximum dose: 4 g/day
AAPC: Oral: 30 mg/kg/day divided every 6 hours for 7-10 days
Helicobacter pylori infection (has been used in combination with amoxicillin and bismuth subsalicylate): Oral: 15-20 mg/kg/day in 2 divided doses for 4 weeks

Adults:
Amebiasis: Oral: 500-750 mg every 8 hours
Anaerobic infections: Oral, I.V.: 30 mg/kg/day in divided doses every 6 hours; not to exceed 4 g/day; **Note:** Initial: 1 g I.V. loading dose may be administered
AAPC: Oral: 250-500 mg 3-4 times/day for 10-14 days
Bacterial vaginosis or vaginitis due to *Gardnerella*, *Mobiluncus*: Oral:
Regular release: 500 mg twice daily
Extended release: 750 mg once daily for 7 days
Helicobacter pylori infection: Oral: 250-500 mg 3 times/day in combination with at least one other agent active against *H. pylori*
Trichomoniasis: Oral: 500 mg every 12 hours for 7 days or 2 g as a single dose
Surgical prophylaxis (colorectal): I.V. 15 mg/kg 1 hour prior to surgery; followed by 7.5 mg/kg 6 and 12 hours after initial dose
Topical: Apply a thin film twice daily to affected areas
Vaginal: One applicatorful (5 g) intravaginally 1-2 times/day for 5 days

Dosing adjustment in hepatic impairment: 50% to 67% decrease in dosage

Administration

Intravaginal: Use only **vaginal gel** intravaginally; do not apply to the eye

Oral: Administer on an empty stomach; may administer with food if GI upset occurs

Parenteral: Administer I.V. by slow intermittent infusion over 30-60 minutes at a final concentration for administration of 5-8 mg/mL

Topical: Wash affected areas with a mild cleanser; wait 15-20 minutes, then apply a thin film of drug to the affected area and rub in. Do not apply to the eye.

Monitoring Parameters WBC count

Test Interactions May cause falsely decreased AST and ALT levels

Patient Information May discolor urine dark or reddish brown; avoid alcohol; do not take alcohol for at least 48 hours after the last dose; may cause dry mouth

Nursing Implications Avoid contact between the drug and aluminum in the infusion set

Additional Information Sodium content of 500 mg ready-to-use vial: 14 mEq

Dosage Forms Excipient information presented when available (limited, particularly for generics); consult specific product labeling.

Capsule, oral: 375 mg
Flagyl® 375: 375 mg
Cream, topical: 0.75% (45 g)
MetroCream®: 0.75% (45 g) [contains benzyl alcohol]
Noritate®: 1% (60 g)
Gel, topical: 1% (45 g)
MetroGel®: 1% (60 g) [60 g tube also packaged in a kit with Cetaphil® skin cleanser]
Gel, vaginal: 0.75% (70 g)
MetroGel-Vaginal®, Vandazole®: 0.75% (70 g)
Infusion [premixed iso-osmotic sodium chloride solution]: 500 mg (100 mL)
Lotion, topical: 0.75% (60 mL)
MetroLotion®: 0.75% (60 mL) [contains benzyl alcohol]
Tablet, oral: 250 mg, 500 mg
Flagyl®: 250 mg, 500 mg
Tablet, extended release, oral:
Flagyl® ER: 750 mg

Extemporaneous Preparations A 50 mg/mL oral suspension can be made using a 1:1 mixture of Ora-Sweet® and Ora-Plus®; crush twenty-four 250 mg tablets into a fine powder in a mortar; add a small amount of vehicle and mix to make a uniform paste; mix while adding the vehicle in geometric portions to almost 120 mL; transfer to a calibrated bottle and qsad with vehicle to 120 mL; preparation is stable for 60 days when stored at room temperature or under refrigeration; label "shake well"

Allen LV Jr and Erickson MA III, "Stability of Ketoconazole, Metolazone, Metronidazole, Procainamide Hydrochloride, and Spironolactone in Extemporaneously Compounded Oral Liquids," *Am J Health Syst Pharm*, 1996, 53(17):2073-8.

References

Centers for Disease Control and Prevention, "Sexually Transmitted Diseases Treatment Guidelines - 2006," *MMWR Recomm Rep*, 2006, 55(RR-11):1-100. Available at http://www.cdc.gov/std/treatment/2006/rr5511.pdf.

Committee on Adolescence, American Academy of Pediatrics, "Sexual Assault and the Adolescent," *Pediatrics*, 1994, 94(5):761-5.

Israel DM and Hassall E, "Treatment and Long-Term Follow-up of *Helicobacter pylori*-Associated Duodenal Ulcer Disease in Children," *J Pediatr*, 1993, 123(1):53-8.

Kelly CP, Pothoulakis C, and LaMont JT, "*Clostridium difficile* Colitis," *N Engl J Med*, 1994, 330(4):257-62.

Oldenburg B and Speck WT, "Metronidazole," *Pediatr Clin North Am*, 1983, 30(1):71-5.

◆ **Metronidazole Hydrochloride** *see* MetroNIDAZOLE *on page 921*

Metyrapone (me TEER a pone)

Medication Safety Issues
Sound-alike/look-alike issues:
Metyrapone may be confused with metyrosine

U.S. Brand Names Metopirone®

Therapeutic Category Diagnostic Agent, Hypothalamic-Pituitary ACTH Function

Generic Available No

Use Diagnostic drug for testing hypothalamic-pituitary ACTH function

Pregnancy Risk Factor C

Pregnancy Considerations Use during pregnancy only if clearly needed. Subnormal response may occur in pregnant women and the fetal pituitary may be affected.

Lactation Excretion in breast milk unknown/use caution

Contraindications Hypersensitivity to metyrapone or any component; adrenal cortical insufficiency

Warnings All corticosteroid therapy should be discontinued prior to and during the metyrapone test; administration of metyrapone may induce acute adrenal insufficiency in patients with reduced adrenal secretory capacity; patients with suspected adrenocortical insufficiency should be observed closely over 24 hours

Precautions The test may be abnormal in the presence of thyroid dysfunction; demonstrate the ability of the adrenals to respond to exogenous ACTH before using metyrapone

Adverse Reactions
Cardiovascular: Hypotension, tachycardia
Central nervous system: Dizziness, headache, sedation
Dermatologic: Rash
Gastrointestinal: Abdominal discomfort, nausea, vomiting
Hematologic: Bone marrow suppression (rare)

Drug Interactions
Metabolism/Transport Effects Inhibits CYP2A6 (weak); **Induces** CYP3A4 (weak)
Avoid Concomitant Use There are no known interactions where it is recommended to avoid concomitant use.
Increased Effect/Toxicity There are no known significant interactions involving an increase in effect.
Decreased Effect
Metyrapone may decrease the levels/effects of: Saxagliptin

The levels/effects of Metyrapone may be decreased by: Phenytoin

Stability Protect from light

Mechanism of Action Reduces cortisol and corticosterone production by inhibition of 11-beta-hydroxylation of precursors in the adrenal cortex. Continued inhibition stimulates increased ACTH production by the pituitary; increased precursor levels have a weak suppressive activity on ACTH release. Elevated levels of precursor metabolites (17-hydroxycorticosteroids [17-OHCS] or 17-ketogenic steroids [17-KGS]) appear in the urine which can easily serve as an index of pituitary ACTH responsiveness. Production of aldosterone may also be suppressed by metyrapone. The adrenal cortex must have the ability to respond to ACTH before metyrapone is employed to test the capacity of the pituitary to respond to a decreased concentration of plasma cortisol.

Pharmacodynamics Maximum effect: Peak excretion of steroid during the first 24 hours after administration

Pharmacokinetics (Adult data unless noted)
Absorption: Oral: Well absorbed
Half-life, elimination: 1.9 ± 0.7 hours
Time to peak serum concentration: 1 hour
Elimination: 5.3% of dose excreted in urine unchanged

Usual Dosage Oral:

Children: 15 mg/kg/dose or 300 mg/m^2/dose every 4 hours for 6 doses; minimum: 250 mg/dose **or as an alternative** 30 mg/kg as a single dose (maximum: 3 g) given at midnight the night before the test

Adults: 750 mg every 4 hours for 6 doses **or as an alternative** 3 g as a single dose given at midnight the night before the test

Administration Oral: May administer with food or milk to reduce GI irritation

Reference Range

Normal response to metyrapone:

Plasma ACTH: 44 pmol/L (200 ng/L)

Plasma II desoxycortisol: 0.2 micromoles/L (70 mcg/L)

24 hour urinary excretion of 17-OHCS: 2-4 time increase

24 hour urinary excretion of 17-KGS: 2 time increase

A subnormal response may be indicative of panhypopituitarism or partial hypopituitarism. An excessive response is suggestive of Cushing's syndrome associated with adrenal hyperplasia.

Patient Information Arise slowly from prolonged sitting or lying position; may cause drowsiness and impair ability to perform activities requiring mental alertness or physical coordination

Dosage Forms Excipient information presented when available (limited, particularly for generics); consult specific product labeling.

Capsule: 250 mg

◆ **Mevacor®** see Lovastatin *on page 850*

◆ **Mevinolin** see Lovastatin *on page 850*

Mexiletine (MEKS i le teen)

Canadian Brand Names Novo-Mexiletine

Therapeutic Category Antiarrhythmic Agent, Class I-B

Generic Available Yes

Use Management of serious ventricular arrhythmias; suppression of premature ventricular contractions; diabetic neuropathy

Pregnancy Risk Factor C

Lactation Enters breast milk/compatible

Contraindications Hypersensitivity to mexiletine or any component; cardiogenic shock; second or third degree heart block (except in patients with a functioning artificial pacemaker)

Warnings Antiarrhythmic agents should be reserved for patients with life-threatening ventricular arrhythmias **[U.S. Boxed Warning]**. In the Cardiac Arrhythmia Suppression Trial (CAST), recent (>6 days but <2 years ago) myocardial infarction patients with asymptomatic, nonlife-threatening ventricular arrhythmias did not benefit and may have been harmed by attempts to suppress the arrhythmia with flecainide or encainide. An increased mortality or nonfatal cardiac arrest rate (7.7%) was seen in the active treatment group compared with patients in the placebo group (3%). The applicability of the CAST results to other populations is unknown. Worsening of arrhythmia (including ventricular tachycardia or ventricular fibrillation) may occur.

Blood dyscrasias (including leukopenia, agranulocytosis, and thrombocytopenia) have been reported.

Precautions Use with caution in patients with seizure disorders, severe heart failure, hypotension, hepatic impairment; avoid dietary regimens or concomitant drug therapy that markedly change urine pH (see Drug and Food Interactions)

Adverse Reactions

Cardiovascular: Palpitations, bradycardia, chest pain, syncope, hypotension, atrial or ventricular arrhythmias

Central nervous system: Dizziness, confusion, ataxia

Dermatologic: Rash

Gastrointestinal: Nausea, vomiting, diarrhea

Hematologic: Rarely thrombocytopenia, leukopenia, agranulocytosis

Hepatic: Liver enzymes elevated, hepatitis

Neuromuscular & skeletal: Paresthesia, tremor

Ocular: Diplopia

Otic: Tinnitus

Respiratory: Dyspnea

Miscellaneous: Positive antinuclear antibody

Drug Interactions

Metabolism/Transport Effects Substrate (major) of CYP1A2, 2D6; **Inhibits** CYP1A2 (strong)

Avoid Concomitant Use There are no known interactions where it is recommended to avoid concomitant use.

Increased Effect/Toxicity

Mexiletine may increase the levels/effects of: Bendamustine; CYP1A2 Substrates; Theophylline Derivatives

The levels/effects of Mexiletine may be increased by: CYP1A2 Inhibitors (Moderate); CYP1A2 Inhibitors (Strong); CYP2D6 Inhibitors (Moderate); CYP2D6 Inhibitors (Strong); Darunavir; Selective Serotonin Reuptake Inhibitors

Decreased Effect

The levels/effects of Mexiletine may be decreased by: CYP1A2 Inducers (Strong); Peginterferon Alfa-2b; Phenytoin

Food Interactions Food may decrease the rate, but not the extent of oral absorption; diets which affect urine pH can increase or decrease excretion of mexiletine; avoid dietary changes that alter urine pH

Mechanism of Action Class IB antiarrhythmic; structurally related to lidocaine; may cause increase in systemic vascular resistance and decrease in cardiac output; no significant negative inotropic effect

Pharmacodynamics Onset of action: Oral: 30-120 minutes

Pharmacokinetics (Adult data unless noted)

Distribution: V_d: 5-7 L/kg; found in breast milk in similar concentrations as plasma

Protein-binding: 50% to 70%

Metabolism: Extensive in the liver (some minor active metabolites)

Bioavailability: Oral: 88%

Half-life, adults: 10-14 hours; increase in half-life with hepatic or heart failure

Elimination: 10% to 15% excreted unchanged in urine; urinary acidification increases excretion

Usual Dosage Oral:

Children: Range: 1.4-5 mg/kg/dose (mean: 3.3 mg/kg/dose) given every 8 hours; start with lower initial dose and increase according to effects and serum concentrations

Adults: Initial: 200 mg every 8 hours (may load with 400 mg if necessary); adjust dose every 2-3 days; usual dose: 200-300 mg every 8 hours; some patients may respond to the same daily dose divided every 12 hours; maximum dose: 1.2 g/day

Dosing adjustment in renal impairment: Children and Adults: Cl$_{cr}$ <10 mL/minute: Administer 50% to 75% of normal dose

Dosing adjustment in hepatic disease: Children and Adults: Administer 25% to 30% of normal dose; patients with severe liver disease may require even lower doses, monitor closely

Administration Oral: Administer with food, milk, or antacids to decrease GI upset

Monitoring Parameters Liver enzymes, CBC, ECG, heart rate, serum concentrations

Reference Range
Therapeutic range: 0.5-2 mcg/mL
Potentially toxic: >2 mcg/mL

Patient Information Limit caffeine; may cause dizziness; notify physician if persistent abdominal pain, nausea, vomiting, yellowing of the eyes or skin, pale stools, dark urine, fever, sore throat, bleeding, or bruising occurs

Additional Information I.V. form under investigation

Dosage Forms Excipient information presented when available (limited, particularly for generics); consult specific product labeling.

Capsule, as hydrochloride: 150 mg, 200 mg, 250 mg

Extemporaneous Preparations A 10 mg/mL oral suspension can be made using capsules and distilled water or sorbitol USP; grind the contents of eight 150 mg capsules to a powder in a mortar and pestle; then add a small amount of distilled water or sorbitol; mix to make a uniform paste; add distilled water or sorbitol in geometric amounts (while mixing) to **almost** 120 mL; transfer to a graduated cylinder and qsad 120 mL while mixing; suspension made with sorbitol is stable in plastic prescription bottles for 2 weeks at room temperature (25°C) and 4 weeks if refrigerated (4°C); suspension made with distilled water is stable in plastic prescription bottles for 7 weeks at room temperature (25°C) and 13 weeks if refrigerated (4°C); extended storage at 4°C is recommended to minimize microbial contamination; shake well before use

Nahata MC, Morosco RS, and Hipple TF, "Stability of Mexiletine in Two Extemporaneous Liquid Formulations Stored Under Refrigeration and at Room Temperature," *J Am Pharm Assoc*, 2000, 40(2):257-9.

References
Moak JP, Smith RT, and Garson A Jr, "Mexiletine: An Effective Antiarrhythmic Drug for Treatment of Ventricular Arrhythmias in Congenital Heart Disease," *J Am Coll Cardiol*, 1987, 10(4):824-9.

◆ **Mezavant® (Can)** see Mesalamine on page 887

◆ **MG 217® [OTC]** see Coal Tar on page 349

◆ **MG 217® Medicated Tar [OTC]** see Coal Tar on page 349

◆ **MgSO₄ (error-prone abbreviation)** see Magnesium Sulfate on page 858

◆ **Miacalcin®** see Calcitonin on page 227

◆ **Miacalcin® NS (Can)** see Calcitonin on page 227

◆ **Micaderm® [OTC]** see Miconazole on page 927

Micafungin (mi ka FUN gin)

U.S. Brand Names Mycamine®
Canadian Brand Names Mycamine®
Therapeutic Category Antifungal Agent, Echinocandin; Antifungal Agent, Systemic
Generic Available No
Use Treatment of patients with esophageal candidiasis (FDA approved in adults); treatment of candidemia, acute disseminated candidiasis, *Candida* peritonitis and abscess (FDA approved in adults); prophylaxis of *Candida* infections in patients undergoing hematopoietic stem cell transplant (FDA approved in adults); has been used for treatment of invasive *Aspergillosis*; micafungin is ineffective against cryptococcosis, fusariosis, and zygomycosis
Pregnancy Risk Factor C
Pregnancy Considerations Visceral teratogenic and abortifacient effects were noted in animal studies. There are no adequate and well-controlled studies in pregnant women. Use only if benefit outweighs risk.
Lactation Excretion in breast milk unknown/use caution
Contraindications Hypersensitivity to micafungin, other echinocandins, or any component
Warnings Cases of hypersensitivity reactions including anaphylactoid reactions and anaphylaxis with shock have

been reported in patients who received micafungin; if reaction occurs, discontinue infusion and provide appropriate treatment. Rare cases of acute intravascular hemolysis, hemoglobinuria, and hemolytic anemia have been reported. Isolated cases of hepatitis, hepatic failure, and acute renal failure have also been reported; monitor for evidence of worsening of these conditions.

Precautions Use with caution in patients with renal impairment, hepatic impairment, and in patients receiving concomitant hepatotoxic drugs; monitor for evidence of worsening function.

Adverse Reactions
Cardiovascular: Atrial fibrillation, bradycardia, edema, facial swelling, hypertension, hypotension, shock, tachycardia, vasodilation

Central nervous system: Delirium, dizziness, fever, headache, insomnia, rigors, somnolence

Dermatologic: Erythema multiforme, pruritus, rash, urticaria

Endocrine & metabolic: Hypernatremia, hypoglycemia, hypokalemia, hypomagnesemia

Gastrointestinal: Abdominal pain, anorexia, diarrhea, nausea, vomiting

Hematologic: Anemia, hemolysis, hemolytic anemia, leukopenia, lymphopenia, neutropenia, thrombocytopenia

Hepatic: Alkaline phosphatase, AST, ALT, and blood LDH increased; hepatic failure; hepatitis

Local: Infusion site inflammation, phlebitis, thrombophlebitis (local reactions occur more frequently when micafungin is administered via peripheral line)

Renal: Acute renal failure, BUN and serum creatinine increased

Respiratory: Cough, dyspnea, epistaxis, pneumonia

Miscellaneous: Anaphylactoid reactions, anaphylaxis, histamine-mediated reactions, sepsis

<1%, postmarketing, and/or case reports: Acidosis, anuria, apnea, arrhythmia, arthralgia, cardiac arrest, coagulopathy, cyanosis, deep vein thrombosis, encephalopathy, facial edema, hemoglobinuria, hepatic dysfunction, hepatocellular damage, hepatomegaly, hyperbilirubinemia, hyponatremia, hypoxia, intracranial hemorrhage, jaundice, MI, mucosal inflammation, oliguria, pancytopenia, pulmonary embolism, renal impairment, renal tubular necrosis, seizure, site thrombosis, skin necrosis, thrombotic thrombocytopenia purpura

Drug Interactions
Metabolism/Transport Effects Substrate of CYP3A4 (minor); **Inhibits** CYP3A4 (weak)

Avoid Concomitant Use There are no known interactions where it is recommended to avoid concomitant use.

Increased Effect/Toxicity There are no known significant interactions involving an increase in effect.

Decreased Effect
Micafungin may decrease the levels/effects of: Saccharomyces boulardii

Stability Store unopened vials at 25°C (77°F); excursions permitted to 15°C to 30°C (59°F to 86°F); reconstituted solution may be stored in the original vial for up to 24 hours at 25°C (77°F); diluted infusion may be stored for up to 24 hours at 25°C (77°F); protect from light.

Mechanism of Action Inhibits synthesis of beta (1,3)-D-glucan, an essential cell wall component of susceptible fungi, disrupting the cell wall structure and leading to osmotic stress and lysis of the fungal cell.

Pharmacokinetics (Adult data unless noted)
Distribution: Distributes into lung, liver, spleen, and kidney
Neonates: V_d: 0.34-0.76 L/kg
Children 2-8 years: V_{dss}: 0.35 ± 0.18 L/kg
Children 9-17 years: V_{dss}: 0.28 ± 0.09 L/kg
Adults: V_d: 0.39 ± 0.11 L/kg

Protein binding: >99% to albumin

Metabolism: In the liver to M-1, catechol form by arylsulfatase; further metabolized to M-2, methoxy form by catechol-O-methyltransferase; hydroxylation to M-5 by CYP3A

Half-life:

Neonates: 6.7 ± 2.2 hours

Children 2-8 years: 11.6 ± 2.8 hours

Children 9-17 years: 13.3 ± 4.3 hours

Healthy Adults: 14-15 hours

Adults receiving bone marrow or peripheral stem-cell transplantation: 10.7-13.5 hours

Elimination: <1% of dose is eliminated unchanged renally; 71% is eliminated in the feces

Clearance:

Neonates: 0.45-57 mL/minute/kg

Children 2-8 years: 0.385 ± 0.15 mL/minute/kg

Children 9-17 years: 0.285 ± 0.12 mL/minute/kg

Dialysis: Not dialyzable

Usual Dosage I.V.: **Note:** Not currently FDA approved for use in children; studies in children are limited to pharmacokinetic modeling studies, short-duration trials, and case reports.

Prophylaxis of *Candida* infections in hematopoietic stem cell transplant recipients:

Infants, Children, and Adolescents: 1.5-2 mg/kg/day once daily

Adults: 50 mg once daily

Disseminated candidiasis:

Neonates:

<1000 g: 10 mg/kg/day once daily; doses as high as 10-15 mg/kg/day have been used in extremely low birth weight neonates

≥1000 g: 7 mg/kg/day once daily

Infants, Children, and Adolescents: 2-4 mg/kg/day once daily (maximum dose: 200 mg)

Adults: 100 mg once daily

Aspergillosis, esophageal candidiasis:

Neonates: 8-12 mg/kg/day once daily

Infants, Children, and Adolescents: 4-8.6 mg/kg/day once daily (maximum dose: 325 mg)

Adults: 150 mg once daily

Dosing adjustment in renal impairment: No adjustment needed

Dosing adjustment in hepatic impairment: No adjustment needed in mild-to-moderate hepatic impairment; the effect of severe hepatic impairment on micafungin pharmacokinetics has not been studied

Administration Parenteral: I.V.: Flush line with NS prior to administration. Infuse over one hour at a final concentration of 0.5-1.5 mg/mL in NS or D_5W; more rapid infusions may result in a higher incidence of histamine-mediated reactions. Do not coinfuse with other medications since precipitation may occur.

Reconstitute vial with NS or D_5W by gently dissolving powder by swirling the vial. Do **not** vigorously shake the vial. Further dilute the reconstituted dose in 100 mL of NS or D_5W or to a final concentration between 0.5-1.5 mg/mL.

Monitoring Parameters Periodic liver function tests, renal function tests, CBC with differential

Nursing Implications
Infuse slowly over 1 hour; possible histamine-mediated reactions have been reported to occur with more rapid infusions.

Dosage Forms Excipient information presented when available (limited, particularly for generics); consult specific product labeling.

Injection, powder for reconstitution, as sodium [preservative-free]:

Mycamine®: 50 mg, 100 mg [contains lactose]

References

Arrieta AC, Seibel N, Kovanda L, et al, "Safety, Efficacy and Pharmacokinetics of Micafungin in Pediatric Patients," Program and Abstracts of the 46th Interscience Conference on Antimicrobial Agents and Chemotherapy, San Francisco, 2006, September 27-30, (abstract M-876).

Antachopoulos C and Walsh TJ, "New Agents for Invasive Mycoses in Children," *Curr Opin Pediatr*, 2005, 17(1):78-87.

Benjamin DK Jr, Driscoll T, Seibel NL, et al, "Safety and Pharmacokinetics of Intravenous Anidulafungin in Children With Neutropenia at High Risk for Invasive Fungal Infections," *Antimicrob Agents Chemother*, 2006, 50(2):632-8.

Benjamin DK Jr, Smith PB, Arrieta A, et al, "Safety and Pharmacokinetics of Repeat-Dose Micafungin in Young Infants," *Clin Pharmacol Ther*, 2010, 87(1):93-9.

Carver PL, "Micafungin," *Ann Pharmacother*, 2004, 38(10):1707-21.

Denning DW, Marr KA, Lau WM, et al, "Micafungin (FK463), Alone or in Combination With Other Systemic Antifungal Agents, for the Treatment of Acute Invasive Aspergillosis," *J Infect*, 2006, 53(5):337-49.

Flynn PM, Seibel N, Arrieta A, et al, "Treatment of Invasive Aspergillosis in Pediatric Patients With Micafungin Alone or in Combination with Other Systemic Antifungal Agents," Program and abstracts of the 46th Interscience Conference on Antimicrobial Agents and Chemotherapy, San Francisco, 2006, September 27-30 (abstract M-891).

Heresi GP, Gerstmann DR, Reed MD, et al, "The Pharmacokinetics and Safety of Micafungin, a Novel Echinocandin, in Premature Infants," *Pediatr Infect Dis J*, 2006, 25(12):1110-5.

Hope WW, Mickiene D, Petraitis V, et al, "The Pharmacokinetics and Pharmacodynamics of Micafungin in Experimental Hematogenous Candida Meningoencephalitis: Implications for Echinocandin Therapy in Neonates," *J Infect Dis*, 2008, 197(1):163-71.

Hope WW, Seibel NL, Schwartz CL, et al, "Population Pharmacokinetics of Micafungin in Pediatric Patients and Implications for Antifungal Dosing," *Antimicrob Agents Chemother*, 2007, 51 (10):3714-9.

Kawada M, Fukuoka N, Kondo M, et al, "Pharmacokinetics of Prophylactic Micafungin in Very-Low-Birth-Weight Infants," *Pediatr Infect Dis J*, 2009, 28(9):840-2.

Kobayashi S, Murayama S, Tatsuzawa O, et al, "X-Linked Severe Combined Immunodeficiency (X-SCID) With High Blood Levels of Immunoglobulins and *Aspergillus* Pneumonia Successfully Treated With Micafungin Followed by Unrelated Cord Blood Stem Cell Transplantation," *Eur J Pediatr*, 2007, 166(3):207-10.

Kontoyiannis DP, Ratanatharathorn V, Young JA, et al, "Micafungin Alone or in Combination With Other Systemic Antifungal Therapies in Hematopoietic Stem Cell Transplant Recipients With Invasive Aspergillosis," *Transpl Infect Dis*, 2009, 11(1):89-93.

Kusuki S, Hashii Y, Yoshida H, et al, "Antifungal Prophylaxis With Micafungin in Patients Treated for Childhood Cancer," *Pediatr Blood Cancer*, 2009, 53(4):605-9.

Ostrosky-Zeichner L, Kontoyiannis D, Raffalli J, et al, "International, Open-Label, Noncomparative, Clinical Trial of Micafungin Alone and in Combination for Treatment of Newly Diagnosed and Refractory Candidemia," *Eur J Clin Microbiol Infect Dis*, 2005, 24(10):654-61.

Pappas PG, Kauffman CA, Andes D, et al, "Clinical Practice Guidelines for the Management of Candidiasis: 2009 Update by the Infectious Diseases Society of America," *Clin Infect Dis*, 2009, 48(5):503-35.

Queiroz-Telles F, Berezin E, Leverger G, et al, "Micafungin Versus Liposomal Amphotericin B for Pediatric Patients With Invasive Candidiasis: Substudy of a Randomized Double-Blind Trial," *Pediatr Infect Dis J*, 2008, 27(9):820-6.

Santos RP, Sánchez PJ, Mejias A, et al, "Successful Medical Treatment of Cutaneous *Aspergillosis* in a Premature Infant Using Liposomal Amphotericin B, Voriconazole and Micafungin," *Pediatr Infect Dis J*, 2007, 26(4):364-6.

Seibel NL, Schwartz C, Arrieta A, et al, "Safety, Tolerability, and Pharmacokinetics of Micafungin (FK463) in Febrile Neutropenic Pediatric Patients," *Antimicrob Agents Chemother*, 2005, 49 (8):3317-24.

Singer MS, Seibel NL, Vezina G, et al, "Successful Treatment of Invasive *Aspergillosis* in Two Patients With Acute Myelogenous Leukemia," *J Pediatr Hematol Oncol*, 2003, 25(3):252-6.

Smith PB, Walsh TJ, Hope W, et al, "Pharmacokinetics of an Elevated Dosage of Micafungin in Premature Neonates," *Pediatr Infect Dis J*, 2009, 28(5):412-5.

van Burik JA, Ratanatharathorn V, Stepan DE, et al, "Micafungin Versus Fluconazole for Prophylaxis Against Invasive Fungal Infections During Neutropenia in Patients Undergoing Hematopoietic Stem Cell Transplantation," *Clin Infect Dis*, 2004, 39(10):1407-16.

◆ **Micafungin Sodium** *see* Micafungin *on page 925*

◆ **Micatin® [OTC]** *see* Miconazole *on page 927*

◆ **Micatin® (Can)** *see* Miconazole *on page 927*

Miconazole (mi KON a zole)

Medication Safety Issues
Sound-alike/look-alike issues:
Miconazole may be confused with metroNIDAZOLE, Micronase®, Micronor®
Lotrimin® may be confused with Lotrisone®, Otrivin®
Micatin® may be confused with Miacalcin®

U.S. Brand Names Aloe Vesta® Antifungal [OTC]; Baza® Antifungal [OTC]; Carrington Antifungal [OTC]; Critic-Aid® Clear AF [OTC]; DermaFungal [OTC]; Dermagran® AF [OTC]; DiabetAid™ Antifungal Foot Bath [OTC]; Fungoid® [OTC]; Lotrimin AF® [OTC]; Micaderm® [OTC]; Micatin® [OTC]; Micro-Guard® [OTC]; Miranel AF™ [OTC]; Mitrazol™ [OTC]; Monistat® 1 [OTC]; Monistat® 3 [OTC]; Monistat® 7 [OTC]; Neosporin® AF [OTC]; Oravig™; Podactin Cream [OTC]; Secura® Antifungal Extra Thick [OTC]; Secura® Antifungal Greaseless [OTC]; Zeasorb®-AF [OTC]

Canadian Brand Names Dermazole; Micatin®; Micozole; Monistat®; Monistat® 3

Therapeutic Category Antifungal Agent, Topical; Antifungal Agent, Vaginal

Generic Available Yes

Use Treatment of vulvovaginal candidiasis; topical treatment of superficial fungal infections

Pregnancy Risk Factor C

Lactation Excretion in breast milk unknown/use caution

Contraindications Hypersensitivity to miconazole or any component; vaginal preparation should not be used in the first trimester of pregnancy unless the drug is essential to patient's welfare

Warnings The safety of miconazole in infants <1 year of age has not been established

Precautions Use with caution in patients allergic to other imidazole-derivative antifungals (eg, clotrimazole, econazole, ketoconazole)

Adverse Reactions
Central nervous system: Headache
Dermatologic: Maceration, urticaria, rash, pruritus, allergic contact dermatitis
Genitourinary: Pelvic cramps
Local: Irritation, burning, itching, phlebitis

Drug Interactions
Metabolism/Transport Effects Substrate of CYP3A4 (major); **Inhibits** CYP1A2 (moderate), 2A6 (strong), 2B6 (strong), 2C9 (strong), 2C19 (strong), 2D6 (strong), 2E1 (moderate), 3A4 (strong)

Avoid Concomitant Use There are no known interactions where it is recommended to avoid concomitant use.

Increased Effect/Toxicity
Miconazole may increase the levels/effects of: Vitamin K Antagonists

Decreased Effect There are no known significant interactions involving a decrease in effect.

Stability Store at room temperature

Mechanism of Action Inhibits biosynthesis of ergosterol, damaging the fungal cell wall membrane which increases permeability and causes leaking of nutrients

Pharmacokinetics (Adult data unless noted)
Absorption: Vaginal: Small amount absorbed systemically
Distribution: Into body tissues, joints, and fluids; poor penetration into sputum, saliva, urine, and CSF
Protein binding: 91% to 93%
Metabolism: In the liver
Half-life: Multiphasic degradation:
Alpha: 40 minutes
Beta: 126 minutes
Terminal: 24 hours

Elimination: ~50% excreted in feces and <1% in urine as unchanged drug

Usual Dosage
Infants, Children, Adolescents, and Adults: Topical:
Tinea pedis and tinea corporis: Apply twice daily for 4 weeks
Tinea cruris: Apply twice daily for 2 weeks
Adolescents and Adults:
Vaginal: Insert contents of 1 applicator of 2% vaginal cream or 100 mg vaginal suppository at bedtime for 7 days; or 1 applicator of 4% vaginal cream or 200 mg vaginal suppository at bedtime for 3 days; or 1200 mg vaginal suppository one-time dose at bedtime or during the day
Note: Many products are available as a combination pack (contains a suppository for vaginal instillation and external cream which is applied twice daily for up to 7 days to relieve external symptoms)

Administration For external use only.
Topical: Apply sparingly to the cleansed, dry affected area; if intertriginous areas are involved, rub cream gently into the skin
Vaginal: Wash hands before using; gently insert tablet or full applicator of cream high into vagina at bedtime. Wash applicator with soap and water following use. Remain lying down for 30 minutes following administration.

Monitoring Parameters Hematocrit, hemoglobin, serum electrolytes and lipids

Patient Information Avoid contact with the eyes; do not use vaginal cream or suppositories for self-medication if patient has abdominal pain, fever, or malodorous vaginal discharge; inform physician if abdominal pain, hives, skin rash, vaginal pruritus or discomfort occurs; avoid intercourse during therapy if using vaginal product. Condoms and diaphragms may not be effective if using vaginal product. Do not use tampons, douches, spermicides, or other vaginal products during treatment. Use deodorant-free sanitary napkins or pads instead.

Product Availability
Oravig™: FDA approved April 2010; availability expected in the third quarter of 2010
Oravig™ is a buccal tablet indicated for the local treatment of oropharyngeal candidiasis in adults.

Dosage Forms Excipient information presented when available (limited, particularly for generics); consult specific product labeling. [DSC] = Discontinued product
Aerosol, topical, as nitrate:
Micatin®: 2% (90 g)
Micatin®: 2% (105 mL) [contains benzyl alcohol]
Neosporin® AF: 2% (105 mL)
Aerosol, topical, as nitrate [powder]:
Micatin®: 2% (90 g)
Neosporin® AF: 2% (85 g)
Combination package, topical/vaginal, as nitrate: Cream, topical 2% (9 g); cream, vaginal 4% (3 x 5 g); cream, topical 2% (9 g); suppository, vaginal 200 mg (3s)
Monistat® 1: Cream, topical 2% (9 g); insert, vaginal 1200 mg (1) [contains benzoic acid (in cream), soya lecithin (in insert)]
Monistat® 1 Day or Night: Cream, topical 2% (9 g); insert, vaginal 1200 mg (1) [contains benzoic acid (in cream), mineral oil (in insert), soya lecithin (in insert)]
Monistat® 3: Cream, topical 2% (9 g); insert, vaginal 200 mg (3)
Monistat® 3: Cream, topical 2% (9 g); cream, vaginal 4% (25 g); cream, topical 2% (9 g); cream, vaginal 4% (3 x 5 g) [contains benzoic acid; vaginal cream 200 mg/applicator]
Monistat® 7: Cream, topical 2% (9 g); cream, vaginal 2% (45 g); cream, topical 2% (9 g); cream, vaginal 2% (7 x 5 g) [contains benzoic acid]
Monistat® 7: Cream, topical 2% (9 g); suppository, vaginal 100 mg (7s) [contains benzoic acid (in cream)]

Cream, topical, as nitrate: 2% (15 g, 30 g, 45 g)
  Baza® Antifungal: 2% (4 g, 57 g, 142 g) [zinc oxide-based formula]
Carrington Antifungal: 2% (150 g)
Micaderm®, Podactin Cream: 2% (30 g)
Micatin®: 2% (14 g) [contains benzoic acid]
Micro-Guard®, Mitrazol™: 2% (60 g)
Miranel AF™: 2% (14 g) [contains benzoic acid]
Neosporin® AF: 2% (14 g) [contains benzoic acid]
Secura® Antifungal Extra Thick: 2% (97.5 g) [contains zinc oxide]
Secura® Antifungal Greaseless: 2% (60 g)
Cream, vaginal, as nitrate [prefilled or refillable applicator]: 2% (45 g), 4% (25 g)
Monistat® 3: 4% (15 g, 25 g) [contains benzoic acid; 200 mg/applicator]
Monistat® 7: 2% (45 g) [contains benzoic acid; 100 mg/applicator]
Gel, topical, as nitrate:
  Zeasorb®-AF: 2% (24 g)
Lotion, powder, as nitrate:
  Zeasorb®-AF: 2% (56 g) [contains alcohol 36%] [DSC]
Ointment, topical, as nitrate:
  Aloe Vesta® Antifungal: 2% (60 g, 150 g) [contains aloe]
  Critic-Aid® Clear AF: 2% (4 g, 57 g, 142 g)
  DermaFungal: 2% (120 g)
  Dermagran® AF: (120 g) [zinc oxide-based formula]
Powder, topical, as nitrate:
  Lotrimin AF®: 2% (90 g)
  Micro-Guard®: 2% (90 g)
  Mitrazol™: 2% (30 g)
  Zeasorb®-AF: 2% (70 g)
Suppository, vaginal, as nitrate: 100 mg (7s); 200 mg (3s)
Tablet, for solution, topical, as nitrate [effervescent]:
  DiabetAid™ Antifungal Foot Bath: 2% (10s)
Tincture, topical, as nitrate: 2% (30 mL, 473 mL)
  Fungoid®: 2% (30 mL, 473 mL) [contains isopropyl alcohol 30%; 30 mL size also available in a treatment kit which contains nail scrub and nail brush]

- ◆ **Miconazole Nitrate** see Miconazole on page 927
- ◆ **Micozole (Can)** see Miconazole on page 927
- ◆ **MICRhoGAM®** see Rh$_o$(D) Immune Globulin on page 1207
- ◆ **Micro-Guard® [OTC]** see Miconazole on page 927
- ◆ **microK®** see Potassium Chloride on page 1136
- ◆ **microK® 10** see Potassium Chloride on page 1136
- ◆ **Micro-K Extencaps® (Can)** see Potassium Chloride on page 1136
- ◆ **Micronase® [DSC]** see GlyBURIDE on page 648
- ◆ **Micronor® (Can)** see Norethindrone on page 1001
- ◆ **Microzide®** see Hydrochlorothiazide on page 682

Midazolam (MID aye zoe lam)

Medication Safety Issues
Sound-alike/look-alike issues:
  Versed may be confused with VePesid®, Vistaril®

High alert medication: The Institute for Safe Medication Practices (ISMP) includes this medication among its list of drugs which have a heightened risk of causing significant patient harm when used in error.

Related Information
Adult ACLS Algorithms on page 1463
Compatibility of Medications Mixed in a Syringe on page 1713
Preprocedure Sedatives in Children on page 1688

Canadian Brand Names Apo-Midazolam®; Midazolam Injection

Therapeutic Category Anticonvulsant, Benzodiazepine; Benzodiazepine; Hypnotic; Sedative

Generic Available Yes

Use Sedation, anxiolysis, amnesia prior to procedure or before induction of anesthesia; conscious sedation prior to diagnostic or radiographic procedures; continuous I.V. sedation of intubated and mechanically ventilated patients; status epilepticus

Restrictions C-IV

Pregnancy Risk Factor D

Pregnancy Considerations Midazolam has been found to cross the placenta; not recommended for use during pregnancy.

Lactation Enters breast milk/not recommended (AAP rates "of concern")

Contraindications Hypersensitivity to midazolam, any component (see Warnings), or cherries (syrup); cross-sensitivity with other benzodiazepines may occur; uncontrolled pain; existing CNS depression; shock; narrow-angle glaucoma

Warnings Midazolam may cause respiratory depression/arrest **[U.S. Boxed Warning]**; deaths and hypoxic encephalopathy have resulted when these were not promptly recognized and treated appropriately; dose must be individualized and patients must be appropriately monitored; serious respiratory adverse events occur most often when midazolam is used in combination with other CNS depressants; personnel and equipment needed for standard respiratory resuscitation should be immediately available during midazolam use; a dedicated individual (other than the one performing the procedure) should monitor the deeply sedated pediatric patient throughout the procedure; use with extreme caution, particularly in noncritical care settings. Initial I.V. dose in adults should not exceed 2.5 mg. Pediatric dosing is age, weight, procedure, and route dependant. Use lower doses in elderly or debilitated patients **[U.S. Boxed Warning]**. Do not administer by rapid I.V. injection in neonates **[U.S. Boxed Warning]**; severe hypotension and seizures have been reported; risk may be increased with concomitant fentanyl use. Paradoxical reactions, including hyperactive or aggressive behavior, have been reported in both adult and pediatric patients.

Syrup contains sodium benzoate and injection may contain benzyl alcohol which may cause allergic reactions in susceptible individuals; large amounts of benzyl alcohol (≥99 mg/kg/day) have been associated with a potentially fatal toxicity ("gasping syndrome") in neonates; the "gasping syndrome" consists of metabolic acidosis, respiratory distress, gasping respirations, CNS dysfunction (including convulsions, intracranial hemorrhage), hypotension and cardiovascular collapse; avoid use of midazolam products containing benzyl alcohol or sodium benzoate in neonates; a benzyl alcohol free (preservative free) injection is available; in vitro and animal studies have shown that benzoate, a metabolite of benzyl alcohol, displaces bilirubin from protein binding sites

Precautions Use with caution in patients with heart failure, renal impairment, pulmonary disease, hepatic dysfunction and in neonates (especially premature neonates); several cases of myoclonus have been reported in premature infants; benzodiazepine withdrawal may occur if abruptly discontinued in patients receiving prolonged I.V. continuous infusions; doses should be tapered slowly with prolonged use; does not have analgesic, antidepressant, or antipsychotic properties. Does not protect against increases in heart rate or blood pressure during intubation. Should not be used in shock, coma, or acute alcohol intoxication. Avoid intra-arterial administration or extravasation of parenteral formulation. Use during upper airway procedures may increase risk of hypoventilation. Prolonged responses have been noted following extended administration by continuous infusion (possibly due to metabolite accumulation) or in the presence of drugs which inhibit midazolam metabolism.

Adverse Reactions

Cardiovascular: Cardiac arrest, hypotension, bradycardia

Central nervous system: Drowsiness, sedation, amnesia, dizziness, paradoxical excitement, hyperactivity, combativeness, headache, ataxia, rhythmic myoclonic jerking in preterm infants (~8% incidence), nystagmus

Gastrointestinal: Nausea, vomiting

Local:

I.M., I.V.: Pain and local reactions at injection site (severity less than diazepam)

Nasal: Burning, irritation, discomfort

Neuromuscular & skeletal: Tonic/clonic movements, muscle tremor

Ocular: Blurred vision, diplopia, lacrimation

Respiratory: Respiratory depression, oxygen desaturation, apnea, laryngospasm, bronchospasm, cough

Miscellaneous: Physical and psychological dependence with prolonged use, hiccups

Drug Interactions

Metabolism/Transport Effects Substrate of CYP2B6 (minor), 3A4 (major); **Inhibits** CYP2C8 (weak), 2C9 (weak), 3A4 (weak)

Avoid Concomitant Use

Avoid concomitant use of Midazolam with any of the following: Efavirenz; Protease Inhibitors

Increased Effect/Toxicity

Midazolam may increase the levels/effects of: Alcohol (Ethyl); Clozapine; CNS Depressants; Methotrimeprazine; Phenytoin; Propofol

The levels/effects of Midazolam may be increased by: Antifungal Agents (Azole Derivatives, Systemic); Aprepitant; Atorvastatin; Calcium Channel Blockers (Nondihydropyridine); Cimetidine; Contraceptives (Estrogens); Contraceptives (Progestins); CYP3A4 Inhibitors (Moderate); CYP3A4 Inhibitors (Strong); Dasatinib; Efavirenz; Fluconazole; Fosaprepitant; Grapefruit Juice; Isoniazid; Macrolide Antibiotics; Methotrimeprazine; Nefazodone; Propofol; Protease Inhibitors; Proton Pump Inhibitors; Selective Serotonin Reuptake Inhibitors

Decreased Effect

The levels/effects of Midazolam may be decreased by: CarBAMazepine; CYP3A4 Inducers (Strong); Deferasirox; Ginkgo Biloba; Rifamycin Derivatives; St Johns Wort; Theophylline Derivatives; Yohimbine

Food Interactions Grapefruit juice delays the absorption and significantly increases bioavailability of oral midazolam

Stability Stable at a concentration of 0.5 mg/mL for 24 hours in D_5W or NS and for 4 hours in LR

Mechanism of Action Depresses all levels of the CNS, including the limbic and reticular formation, by binding to the benzodiazepine site on the gamma-aminobutyric acid (GABA) receptor complex and modulating GABA, which is a major inhibitory neurotransmitter in the brain

Pharmacodynamics Sedation:

Onset of action:

Oral: Children: Within 10-20 minutes

I.M.:

Children: Within 5 minutes

Adults: Within 15 minutes

I.V.: Within 1-5 minutes

Intranasal: Within 5 minutes

Maximum effect:

I.M.:

Children: 15-30 minutes

Adults: 30-60 minutes

I.V.: 5-7 minutes

Intranasal: 10 minutes

Duration:

I.M.: Mean: 2 hours, up to 6 hours

I.V.: 20-30 minutes

Intranasal: 30-60 minutes

Note: Full recovery may take more than 24 hours

Pharmacokinetics (Adult data unless noted)

Absorption: Oral, nasal: Rapid

Distribution: V_d:

Preterm infants (n=24; GA: 26-34 weeks; PNA: 3-11 days): Median: 1.1 L/kg (range: 0.4-4.2 L/kg)

Infants and Children 6 months to 16 years: 1.24-2.02 L/kg

Adults: 1-3.1 L/kg

Increased V_d with CHF and chronic renal failure; widely distributed in body including CSF and brain; crosses placenta; enters fetal circulation; crosses into breast milk

Protein binding: Children >1 year and Adults: 97%; primarily to albumin

Metabolism: Extensive in the liver via cytochrome P450 CYP3A4 enzyme; undergoes hydroxylation and then glucuronide conjugation; primary metabolite (alpha-hydroxy-midazolam) is active and equipotent to midazolam

Bioavailability: Oral: 15% to 45% (syrup: 36%); I.M.: >90%; intranasal: ~60%; rectal: ~40% to 50%

Half-life, elimination: Increased half-life with cirrhosis, CHF, obesity, elderly, and acute renal failure

Preterm infants (n=24; GA: 26-34 weeks; PNA: 3-11 days): Median: 6.3 hours (range: 2.6-17.7 hours)

Neonates: 4-12 hours; seriously ill neonates: 6.5-12 hours

Children: I.V.: 2.9-4.5 hours; syrup: 2.2-6.8 hours

Adults: 3 hours (range: 1.8-6.4 hours)

Elimination: 63% to 80% excreted as alpha-hydroxy-midazolam glucuronide in urine; ~2% to 10% in feces, <1% eliminated as unchanged drug in the urine

Clearance:

Preterm infants (n=24; GA: 26-34 weeks; PNA: 3-11 days): Median: 1.8 mL/minute/kg (range: 0.7-6.7 mL/minute/kg)

Neonates <39 weeks GA: 1.17 mL/minute/kg

Neonates >39 weeks GA: 1.84 mL/minute/kg

Seriously ill neonates: 1.2-2 mL/minute/kg

Infants >3 months: 9.1 mL/minute/kg

Children >1 year: 3.2-13.3 mL/minute/kg

Healthy adults: 4.2-9 mL/minute/kg

Adults with acute renal failure: 1.9 mL/minute/kg

Usual Dosage Dosage must be individualized and based on patient's age, underlying diseases, concurrent medications, and desired effect; decrease dose (by ~30%) if narcotics or other CNS depressants are administered concomitantly; use multiple small doses and titrate to desired sedative effect; allow 3-5 minutes between doses to decrease the chance of oversedation

Neonates:

Conscious sedation during mechanical ventilation:

I.V. continuous infusion:

<32 weeks: Initial: 0.03 mg/kg/hour (0.5 mcg/kg/minute)

>32 weeks: Initial: 0.06 mg/kg/hour (1 mcg/kg/minute)

Note: Do not use I.V. loading doses in neonates; for faster achievement of sedation, infuse the continuous infusion at a faster rate for the first several hours; use the smallest dose possible.

Infants >2 months and Children:

Status epilepticus refractory to standard therapy: I.V.: Loading dose: 0.15 mg/kg followed by a continuous infusion of 1 mcg/kg/minute; titrate dose upward every 5 minutes until clinical seizure activity is controlled; mean infusion rate required in 24 children was 2.3 mcg/kg/minute with a range of 1-18 mcg/kg/minute (Rivera, 1993)

◄ **Infants ≥6 months and Children:**
Sedation, anxiolysis, and amnesia prior to procedure or before induction of anesthesia: Oral: Single dose; 0.25-0.5 mg/kg, depending on patient status and desired effect, usual: 0.5 mg/kg; maximum dose: 20 mg;
Patient-specific dosing:
Infants 6 months to <6 years, and less cooperative patients: Higher doses (up to 1 mg/kg) may be required
Children 6 to <16 years, or cooperative patients (especially if intensity and duration of sedation is less critical): 0.25 mg/kg may suffice
High risk pediatric patients (respiratory or cardiac compromised, concomitant CNS depressants, higher risk surgical patients): 0.25 mg/kg should be considered

Children:
Preoperative sedation or conscious sedation for procedures:
I.M.: Usual: 0.1-0.15 mg/kg 30-60 minutes before surgery or procedure; range: 0.05-0.15 mg/kg; doses up to 0.5 mg/kg have been used in more anxious patients; maximum total dose: 10 mg
I.V.:
Infants <6 months: Limited information is available in nonintubated infants; dosing recommendations are unclear; infants <6 months are at higher risk for airway obstruction and hypoventilation; titrate dose with small increments to desired clinical effect; monitor carefully
Infants 6 months to Children 5 years: Initial: 0.05-0.1 mg/kg; titrate dose carefully; total dose of 0.6 mg/kg may be required; usual total dose maximum dose: 6 mg
Children 6-12 years: Initial: 0.025-0.05 mg/kg; titrate dose carefully; total doses of 0.4 mg/kg may be required; usual total dose maximum: 10 mg
Children 12-16 years: Dose as adults; usual total dose maximum: 10 mg
Intranasal: Usual: 0.2 mg/kg; may repeat in 5-15 minutes; range: 0.2-0.3 mg/kg/dose
Conscious sedation during mechanical ventilation:
I.V.: Continuous infusion: Loading dose: 0.05-0.2 mg/kg given slow I.V. over 2-3 minutes, then follow with initial continuous infusion: 0.06-0.12 mg/kg/hour (1-2 mcg/kg/minute); titrate to the desired effect; range: 0.024-0.36 mg/kg/hour (0.4-6 mcg/kg/minute)

Adults:
Preoperative sedation: I.M.: 0.07-0.08 mg/kg 30-60 minutes presurgery; usual dose: 5 mg
Conscious sedation: I.V.: Titrate dose slowly to desired effect; administer slowly over at least 2 minutes and wait another 2 or more minutes to evaluate effect. Some adults may respond to doses as low as 1 mg; do not give more than 2.5 mg over a period of 2 minutes. Titrate as needed, using small increments every 2-3 minutes. Usual total dose: 2.5-5 mg; total dose >5 mg is generally not needed; maintenance doses may be given by slow titration, if needed, in increments of 25% of the original dose used to reach sedative endpoint.
Conscious sedation during mechanical ventilation:
I.V.: Optional loading dose: 0.01-0.05 mg/kg (~0.5-4 mg/dose); may repeat at 10- to 15-minute intervals until patient is adequately sedated, then begin continuous infusion
Continuous infusion: Initial: 0.02-0.1 mg/kg/hour (1-7 mg/hour); use lowest doses listed for patients receiving other sedatives, or opioids, or having residual anesthetic effects; titrate the infusion to achieve adequate level of sedation; use lowest effective dose

Administration
Intranasal: Administer using a 1 mL needleless syringe into the nares over 15 seconds; use the 5 mg/mL injection; 1/2 of the dose may be administered to each nare; **Note:** The 5 mg/mL injection has also been administered as a nasal spray using a graded pump device (see Ljungman, 2000),
Oral: Administer on empty stomach (feeding is usually contraindicated prior to sedation for procedures); do not administer with grapefruit juice
Parenteral:
I.V.: Administer by slow I.V. injection over at least 2-5 minutes at a concentration of 1-5 mg/mL (maximum concentration: 5 mg/mL) or by I.V. infusion; avoid extravasation; do not administer intra-arterially
I.M.: Maximum concentration: 1 mg/mL

Monitoring Parameters Level of sedation, respiratory rate, heart rate, blood pressure, oxygen saturation (ie, pulse oximetry)

Patient Information Report the use of other medications, nonprescription medications, and herbal or natural products to your physician and pharmacist; avoid alcohol; avoid grapefruit juice if taking oral midazolam

Nursing Implications Abrupt discontinuation after prolonged use may result in withdrawal symptoms

Additional Information Sodium content of injection: 0.14 mEq/mL. For Neonates: Since both concentrations of Versed® injection contain 1% benzyl alcohol, use the 5 mg/mL injection and dilute to 0.5 mg/mL with SWI without preservatives to decrease the amount of benzyl alcohol delivered to the neonate, or use preservative free injection. With continuous infusion, midazolam may accumulate in peripheral tissues; use lowest effective infusion rate to reduce accumulation effects. Midazolam is 3-4 times as potent as diazepam. Paradoxical reactions associated with midazolam use in children (eg, agitation, restlessness, combativeness) have been successfully treated with flumazenil (see Massanari, 1997)

Dosage Forms Excipient information presented when available (limited, particularly for generics); consult specific product labeling.
Injection, solution: 1 mg/mL (2 mL, 5 mL, 10 mL); 5 mg/mL (1 mL, 2 mL, 5 mL, 10 mL) [contains benzyl alcohol 1%]
Injection, solution [preservative free]: 1 mg/mL (2 mL, 5 mL); 5 mg/mL (1 mL, 2 mL)
Syrup: 2 mg/mL (118 mL) [contains sodium benzoate; cherry flavor]

References
Adrian ER, "Intranasal Versed®: The Future of Pediatric Conscious Sedation," *Pediatr Nurs*, 1994, 20(3):287-92.
Booker PD, Beechey A, and Lloyd-Thomas AR, "Sedation of Children Requiring Artificial Ventilation Using an Infusion of Midazolam," *Br J Anaesth*, 1986, 58(10):1104-8.
Burtin P, Jacqz-Aigrain E, Girard P, et al, "Population Pharmacokinetics of Midazolam in Neonates," *Clin Pharmacol Ther*, 1994, 56(6 Pt 1):615-25.
de Wildt SN, Kearns GL, Hop WC, et al, "Pharmacokinetics and Metabolism of Intravenous Midazolam in Preterm Infants," *Clin Pharmacol Ther*, 2001, 70(6):525-31.
Jacqz-Aigrain E, Daoud P, Burtin P, et al, "Placebo-Controlled Trial of Midazolam Sedation in Mechanically Ventilated Newborn Babies," *Lancet*, 1994, 344(8923):646-50.
Kupietzky A and Houpt MI, "Midazolam: A Review of Its Use for Conscious Sedation of Children," *Pediatr Dent*, 1993, 15(4):237-41.
Ljungman G, Kreuger A, Andreasson S, et al, "Midazolam Nasal Spray Reduces Procedural Anxiety in Children," *Pediatrics*, 2000, 105(1 Pt 1):73-8.
Lugo RA, Fishbein M, Nahata MC, et al, "Complication of Intranasal Midazolam," *Pediatrics*, 1993, 92(4):638.
Magny JF, Zupan V, Dehan M, et al, "Midazolam and Myoclonus in Neonate," *Eur J Pediatr*, 1994, 153(5):389-90.
Malinovsky JM, Populaire C, Cozian A, et al, "Premedication With Midazolam in Children, Effect of Intranasal, Rectal and Oral Routes on Plasma Midazolam Concentrations," *Anaesthesia*, 1995, 50 (4):351-4.

Massanari M, Novitsky J, and Reinstein LJ, "Paradoxical Reactions in Children Associated With Midazolam Use During Endoscopy," *Clin Pediatr*, 1997, 36(12):681-4.

Riva J, Lejbusiewicz G, Papa M, et al, "Oral Premedication With Midazolam in Paediatric Anaesthesia. Effects on Sedation and Gastric Contents," *Paediatr Anaesth*, 1997, 7(3):191-6.

Rivera R, Segnini M, Baltodano A, et al, "Midazolam in the Treatment of Status Epilepticus in Children," *Crit Care Med*, 1993, 21(7):991-4.

Silvasi DL, Rosen DA, and Rosen KR, "Continuous Intravenous Midazolam Infusion for Sedation in the Pediatric Intensive Care Unit," *Anesth Analg*, 1988, 67(3):286-8.

Wang Z, Gorski JC, Hamman MA, et al, "The Effects of St John's Wort (*Hypericum perforatum*) on Human Cytochrome P450 Activity," *Clin Pharmacol Ther*, 2001, 70(4):317-26.

◆ **Midazolam Hydrochloride** *see* Midazolam *on page 928*

◆ **Midazolam Injection (Can)** *see* Midazolam *on page 928*

◆ **Midol® Cramp and Body Aches [OTC]** *see* Ibuprofen *on page 702*

◆ **Midol® Extended Relief [OTC]** *see* Naproxen *on page 967*

◆ **Migergot** *see* Ergotamine and Caffeine *on page 522*

◆ **Migranal®** *see* Dihydroergotamine *on page 442*

◆ **Mild-C® [OTC]** *see* Ascorbic Acid *on page 138*

◆ **Milk of Magnesia** *see* Magnesium Hydroxide *on page 855*

◆ **Milk of Magnesia (Magnesium Hydroxide)** *see* Magnesium Supplements *on page 859*

◆ **Millipred™** *see* PrednisoLONE *on page 1148*

Milrinone (MIL ri none)

Medication Safety Issues
Sound-alike/look-alike issues:
Primacor® may be confused with Primaxin®

High alert medication: The Institute for Safe Medication Practices (ISMP) includes this medication among its list of drugs which have a heightened risk of causing significant patient harm when used in error.

Related Information
CPR Pediatric Drug Dosages *on page 1455*

U.S. Brand Names Primacor® [DSC]

Canadian Brand Names Milrinone Lactate Injection; Primacor®

Therapeutic Category Phosphodiesterase Enzyme Inhibitor

Generic Available Yes

Use Short-term treatment of acute decompensated heart failure

Pregnancy Risk Factor C

Lactation Excretion in breast milk unknown/use caution

Contraindications Hypersensitivity to milrinone, any component, or inamrinone (amrinone)

Warnings Longer treatment of heart failure (>48 hours) has not been shown to be safe and effective (there are no controlled trials using milrinone infusions for >48 hours); long-term oral use for heart failure was associated with no improvement in symptoms, increased risk of hospitalization, and increased risk of sudden death; monitor ECG continuously to promptly detect and manage ventricular arrhythmias. Long-term, regularly scheduled intermittent infusions are strongly discouraged (see ACC/AHA 2005 Guidelines).

Precautions Avoid use in patients with severe obstructive aortic or pulmonic valvular disease; use in patients with hypertrophic subaortic stenosis may increase outflow tract obstruction. Use with caution in patients with a history of ventricular arrhythmias, atrial fibrillation, or atrial flutter. Use with caution and modify dosage in patients with impaired renal function. Hypotension may occur; monitor blood pressure and heart rate; infusion may require reduction in rate or temporary discontinuation if hypotension occurs; hypotension may be prolonged, especially in patients with renal dysfunction. Infusion site reactions may occur; monitor infusion site carefully. Milrinone is not recommended for use in patients with acute MI.

Adverse Reactions
Central nervous system: Headaches (mild to moderate, 2.9%)

Cardiovascular: Ventricular arrhythmias (12.1%) including ventricular ectopic activity (8.5%), nonsustained ventricular tachycardia (2.8%), sustained ventricular tachycardia (1%), and ventricular fibrillation (0.2%); supraventricular arrhythmias (3.8%); hypotension (2.9%); angina/chest pain (1.2%); torsade de pointes (rare)

Dermatological: Rash

Endocrine & metabolic: Hypokalemia (0.6%)

Hematologic: Thrombocytopenia (0.4%)

Hepatic: Abnormal liver function tests

Local: Infusion site reaction

Neuromuscular & skeletal: Tremor (0.4%)

Respiratory: Bronchospasm (rare)

Miscellaneous: Anaphylactic shock (rare)

Drug Interactions
Avoid Concomitant Use There are no known interactions where it is recommended to avoid concomitant use.

Increased Effect/Toxicity There are no known significant interactions involving an increase in effect.

Decreased Effect There are no known significant interactions involving a decrease in effect.

Stability
Storage:
Injection: Store at controlled room temperature 15°C to 30°C (59°F to 86°F); avoid freezing

Premixed infusion: Store at room temperature at 25°C (77°F); brief exposure up to 40°C (104°F) will not adversely affect drug; minimize exposure to heat; avoid excessive heat; protect from freezing

Compatibility: Stable in D5W, LR, 1/2NS, NS

Y-site administration: Compatible: Atracurium, bumetanide, calcium gluconate, cimetidine, digoxin, diltiazem, dobutamine, dopamine, epinephrine, fentanyl, heparin, hydromorphone, insulin (regular), isoproterenol, labetalol, lorazepam, magnesium sulfate, midazolam, morphine, nicardipine, nitroglycerin, norepinephrine, pancuronium, potassium chloride, propofol, propranolol, quinidine gluconate, ranitidine, rocuronium, sodium bicarbonate, sodium nitroprusside, theophylline, thiopental, torsemide, vecuronium. **Incompatible:** Furosemide, imipenem-cilastin, procainamide.

Compatibility in syringe: Compatible: Atropine, calcium chloride, digoxin, epinephrine, lidocaine, morphine, propranolol, sodium bicarbonate, verapamil. **Incompatible:** Furosemide.

Compatibility when admixed: Compatible: Quinidine gluconate. **Incompatible:** Bumetanide, furosemide, procainamide.

Mechanism of Action Inhibits phosphodiesterase III (PDE III), the major PDE in cardiac and vascular tissues. Inhibition of PDE III increases cyclic adenosine monophosphate (cAMP) which potentiates the delivery of calcium to myocardial contractile systems and results in a positive inotropic effect. Inhibition of PDE III in vascular tissue results in relaxation of vascular muscle and vasodilatation.

Pharmacodynamics Onset of action (improved hemodynamic function): Within 5-15 minutes

Pharmacokinetics (Adult data unless noted)
Distribution: V_d beta:
Infants (after cardiac surgery): 0.9 ± 0.4 L/kg
Children (after cardiac surgery): 0.7 ± 0.2 L/kg

Adults:
After cardiac surgery: 0.3 ± 0.1 L/kg
CHF (with single injection): 0.38 L/kg
CHF (with infusion): 0.45 L/kg
Protein binding: 70%
Half-life:
Infants (after cardiac surgery): 3.15 ± 2 hours
Children (after cardiac surgery): 1.86 ± 2 hours
Adults:
After cardiac surgery: 1.69 ± 0.18 hours
CHF: 2.3-2.4 hours
Renal impairment: Prolonged half-life
Elimination: Excreted in the urine as unchanged drug (83%) and glucuronide metabolite (12%)
Clearance:
Infants (after cardiac surgery): 3.8 ± 1 mL/kg/minute
Children (after cardiac surgery): 5.9 ± 2 mL/kg/minute
Children (with septic shock): 10.6 ± 5.3 mL/kg/minute
Adults:
After cardiac surgery: 2 ± 0.7 mL/kg/minute
CHF: 2.2-2.3 mL/kg/minute
Renal impairment: Decreased clearance

Usual Dosage

Neonates, Infants, and Children: I.V.: A limited number of studies have used different dosing schemes (see Additional Information). Two pharmacokinetic studies propose per kg doses for pediatric patients with septic shock that are greater than those recommended for adults (Lindsay, 1998) and in infants and children after cardiac surgery (Ramamoorthy, 1998). Further pharmacodynamic studies are needed to define pediatric milrinone guidelines. Several centers are using the following guidelines:
Loading dose: 50 mcg/kg administered over 15 minutes followed by a continuous infusion of 0.5 mcg/kg/minute; range: 0.25-0.75 mcg/kg/minute; titrate dose to effect
PALS Guidelines 2005: I.V., I.O.: Loading dose: 50-75 mcg/kg administered over 10-60 minutes followed by a continuous infusion of 0.5-0.75 mcg/kg/minute
Adults: I.V.: Loading dose: 50 mcg/kg slow I.V. over 10 minutes, followed by a continuous infusion of 0.5 mcg/kg/minute; range: 0.375-0.75 mcg/kg/minute; titrate dose to effect; maximum daily dose: 1.13 mg/kg/day
Dosing adjustment in renal impairment: For continuous infusion:
Cl_{cr} 50 mL/minute/1.73 m^2: Administer 0.43 mcg/kg/minute
Cl_{cr} 40 mL/minute/1.73 m^2: Administer 0.38 mcg/kg/minute
Cl_{cr} 30 mL/minute/1.73 m^2: Administer 0.33 mcg/kg/minute
Cl_{cr} 20 mL/minute/1.73 m^2: Administer 0.28 mcg/kg/minute
Cl_{cr} 10 mL/minute/1.73 m^2: Administer 0.23 mcg/kg/minute
Cl_{cr} 5 mL/minute/1.73 m^2: Administer 0.2 mcg/kg/minute

Administration

Loading dose: Administer slow I.V. push over 15 minutes for pediatric patients and over 10 minutes in adults; loading dose may be given as undiluted solution, but may dilute to 10-20 mL (in adults) for ease of administration.
I.V. continuous infusion: Dilute with ½NS, NS, or D$_5$W and administer via infusion pump or syringe pump; usual concentration: ≤200 mcg/mL; 250 mcg/mL in NS has been used (see Barton, 1996). **Note:** Some pediatric centers use a concentration of 500 mcg/mL but only if infused via a central line.
Monitoring Parameters Blood pressure, heart rate, cardiac output, CI, SVR, PVR, CVP, ECG, CBC, platelet count, serum electrolytes (especially potassium and magnesium), liver enzymes, renal function; clinical signs and symptoms of CHF; monitor infusion site carefully (avoid extravasation)

Nursing Implications Do not administer furosemide I.V. push via "Y" site into milrinone solutions as precipitate will occur; decrease the infusion rate if significant hypotension occurs

Additional Information Dosing schemes and proposed dosing based on pharmacokinetic data:

Neonates: A loading dose of 50 mcg/kg administered over 15 minutes, followed by a continuous infusion of 0.5 mcg/kg/minute for 30 minutes in 10 neonates (3-27 days old, median age 5 days) improved hemodynamic parameters and was well tolerated (see Chang, 1995). Further neonatal studies of longer duration are needed.

Infants and children with septic shock: Twelve patients (9 months to 15 years of age) were administered a loading dose of 50 mcg/kg, followed by a continuous infusion of 0.5 mcg/kg/minute. At 1 hour after the loading dose, if patients did not respond (defined as a ≥20% increase in CI or an improvement in peripheral perfusion), an additional loading dose of 25 mcg/kg was given and the infusion rate was increased to 0.75 mcg/kg/minute. Nine of 12 patients required the additional loading dose and increased rate of infusion (see Barton, 1996). A subsequent pharmacokinetic analysis of these patients recommended larger loading doses of 75 mcg/kg and infusion rates of 0.75-1 mcg/kg/minute. However, these doses were based on a one-compartment pharmacokinetic model and are higher then the mean infusion rate of 0.69 mcg/kg/minute used in the study (see Lindsay, 1998). Further studies are needed.

Infants and Children after open heart surgery: A prospective, open-label trial compared a lower dose of milrinone (Group A) to a higher dose (Group B). Group A: Eleven patients received a loading dose of 25 mcg/kg given over 5 minutes followed by an infusion of 0.25 mcg/kg/minute; 30 minutes later, a second 25 mcg/kg loading dose was given and the infusion was increased to 0.5 mcg/kg/minute. Group B: 8 patients received a loading dose of 50 mcg/kg given over 10 minutes followed by an infusion of 0.5 mcg/kg/minute; 30 minutes later, a second loading dose of 25 mcg/kg was given and the infusion was increased to 0.75 mcg/kg/minute. Patients in both groups received a third loading dose of 25 mcg/kg if needed. A two-compartment model and NONMEM pharmacokinetic analyses were performed. Based on the NONMEM analysis, the authors propose the following doses: Infants: Loading dose: 104 mcg/kg and continuous infusion of 0.49 mcg/kg/minute; children: loading dose: 67 mcg/kg and continuous infusion of 0.61 mcg/kg/minute (see Ramamoorthy, 1998). Further studies are needed before these proposed doses can routinely be used in the pediatric population.

A double-blind placebo-controlled trial, compared low dose (loading dose: 25 mcg/kg given over 60 minutes followed by an infusion of 0.25 mcg/kg/minute for 35 hours) with high-dose (loading dose: 75 mcg/kg given over 60 minutes followed by an infusion of 0.75 mcg/kg/minute for 35 hours) milrinone for the prevention of low cardiac output syndrome in 227 pediatric patients, ranging in age from 2 days to 6.9 years (median age: 3 months). High-dose milrinone decreased the risk of low cardiac output syndrome by 48% (see Hoffman, 2003). Further studies are needed.

Dosage Forms Excipient information presented when available (limited, particularly for generics); consult specific product labeling. [DSC] = Discontinued product

Infusion [premixed in D$_5$W]: 200 mcg/mL (100 mL, 200 mL)

Primacor®: 200 mcg/mL (200 mL) [DSC]

Injection, solution: 1 mg/mL (10 mL, 20 mL, 50 mL)

References

"2005 American Heart Association (AHA) Guidelines for Cardiopulmonary Resuscitation (CPR) and Emergency Cardiovascular Care (ECC), Part 12: Pediatric Advanced Life Support, The American Heart Association Emergency Cardiovascular Care Committee," *Circulation*, 2005, 112(24 Suppl):IV58-77, 167-87.

"ACC/AHA 2005 Guideline Update for the Diagnosis and Management of Chronic Heart Failure in the Adult: A Report of the American College of Cardiology/American Heart Association Task Force on Practice Guidelines (Writing Committee to Update the 2001 Guidelines for the Evaluation and Management of Heart Failure)," *J Am Coll Cardiol*, 2005, 46(6):e1-82.

Barton P, Garcia J, Kouatli A, et al, "Hemodynamic Effects of I.V. Milrinone Lactate in Pediatric Patients With Septic Shock. A Prospective Double-Blinded, Randomized, Placebo-Controlled, Interventional Study," *Chest*, 1996, 109(5):1302-12.

Chang AC, Atz AM, Wernovsky G, et al, "Milrinone: Systemic and Pulmonary Hemodynamic Effects in Neonates After Cardiac Surgery," *Crit Care Med*, 1995, 23(11):1907-14.

Cuffe MS, Califf RM, Adams KF Jr, et al, "Short-Term Intravenous Milrinone for Acute Exacerbation of Chronic Heart Failure: A Randomized Controlled Trial," *JAMA*, 2002, 287(12):1541-7.

Heart Failure Society of America, "HFSA 2006 Comprehensive Heart Failure Practice Guideline," *J Card Fail*, 2006, 12(1):e1-122.

Hoffman TM, Wernovsky G, Atz AM, et al, "Efficacy and Safety of Milrinone in Preventing Low Cardiac Output Syndrome in Infants and Children After Corrective Surgery for Congenital Heart Disease," *Circulation*, 2003, 107(7):996-1002.

Hoffman TM, Wernovsky G, Atz AM, et al, "Prophylactic Intravenous Use of Milrinone After Cardiac Operation in Pediatrics (PRIMACORP) Study," *Am Heart J*, 2002, 143(1):15-21.

Lindsay CA, Barton P, Lawless S, et al, "Pharmacokinetics and Pharmacodynamics of Milrinone Lactate in Pediatric Patients With Septic Shock," *J Pediatr*, 1998, 132(2):329-34.

Ramamoorthy C, Anderson GD, Williams GD, et al, "Pharmacokinetics and Side Effects of Milrinone in Infants and Children After Open Heart Surgery," *Anesth Analg*, 1998, 86(2):283-9.

◆ **Milrinone Lactate** *see* Milrinone *on page 931*

◆ **Milrinone Lactate Injection (Can)** *see* Milrinone *on page 931*

Mineral Oil (MIN er al oyl)

Medication Safety Issues
Beers Criteria medication: This drug may be inappropriate for use in geriatric patients (high severity risk).

U.S. Brand Names Fleet® Mineral Oil Enema [OTC]; Kondremul® [OTC]; Liqui-Doss® [OTC] [DSC]

Therapeutic Category Laxative, Lubricant

Generic Available Yes: Oral oil

Use Temporary relief of constipation, to relieve fecal impaction, preparation for bowel studies or surgery

Contraindications Patients with a colostomy or an ileostomy, appendicitis, ulcerative colitis, diverticulitis, dysphagia or hiatal hernia

Warnings Oral form should be avoided in children <4 years of age because of the risk of aspiration

Adverse Reactions
Gastrointestinal: Nausea, vomiting, diarrhea, abdominal cramps, anal itching, anal seepage

Respiratory: Lipid pneumonitis with aspiration

Drug Interactions
Avoid Concomitant Use There are no known interactions where it is recommended to avoid concomitant use.

Increased Effect/Toxicity There are no known significant interactions involving an increase in effect.

Decreased Effect
Mineral Oil may decrease the levels/effects of: Phytonadione

Food Interactions May decrease absorption of fat-soluble vitamins, carotene, calcium, and phosphorus

Mechanism of Action Eases passage of stool by decreasing water absorption, softens stool, and lubricates the intestine

Pharmacodynamics Onset of action: ~6-8 hours

Pharmacokinetics (Adult data unless noted)
Absorption: Minimal following oral or rectal administration

Distribution: Into intestinal mucosa, liver, spleen, and mesenteric lymph nodes

Elimination: In feces

Usual Dosage
Children:
Oral: 5-11 years: 5-15 mL once daily or in divided doses; should not be used for longer than 1 week

Rectal: 2-11 years: 30-60 mL as a single dose

Children ≥12 years and Adults:
Oral: 15-45 mL/day once daily or in divided doses; should not be used for longer than 1 week

Rectal: Contents of one retention enema (range 60-150 mL)/day as a single dose

Administration
Oral: Nonemulsified mineral oil may be administered at bedtime on an empty stomach; emulsified mineral oil should be shaken before using; may be administered with meals (more palatable than nonemulsified mineral oil)

Rectal: Gently insert enema tip into rectum with a slight side-to-side movement with tip pointing toward the navel; have patient bear down

Monitoring Parameters Evacuation of stool; anal leakage indicates dose too high or need for disimpaction

Patient Information Do not take if experiencing abdominal pain, nausea, or vomiting. Rectal enema: Do not take if experiencing rectal bleeding

Dosage Forms Excipient information presented when available (limited, particularly for generics); consult specific product labeling.

Liquid, oral:
Liqui-Doss®: 13.5 mL/15 mL (480 mL) [self-emulsifying oily liquid; alcohol free, sugar free] [DSC]

Microemulsion, oral:
Kondremul®: 2.5 mL/5 mL (480 mL) [sugar free; mint flavor]

Oil, rectal [enema]:
Fleet® Mineral Oil: 100% (118 mL)

Oil, oral: 100% (30 mL, 480 mL, 3840 mL)

Oil, topical: 100% (480 mL) [light]

References
Baker SS, Liptak GS, Colletti RB, et al, "A Medical Position Statement of the North American Society for Pediatric Gastroenterology and Nutrition; Constipation in Infants and Children: Evaluation and treatment," www.naspgn.org/constipation, 2000, 1-34.

◆ **Minipress®** *see* Prazosin *on page 1147*

◆ **Minirin® (Can)** *see* Desmopressin *on page 404*

◆ **Minitran™** *see* Nitroglycerin *on page 996*

◆ **Minocin®** *see* Minocycline *on page 933*

◆ **Minocin® PAC** *see* Minocycline *on page 933*

Minocycline (mi noe SYE kleen)

Medication Safety Issues
Sound-alike/look-alike issues:
Dynacin® may be confused with Dyazide®, Dynabac®, DynaCirc®, Dynapen®

Minocin® may be confused with Indocin®, Lincocin®, Minizide®, Mithracin®, niacin

U.S. Brand Names Dynacin®; Minocin®; Minocin® PAC; Myrac™ [DSC]; Solodyn®

Canadian Brand Names Apo-Minocycline®; Arestin Microspheres; Dom-Minocycline; Minocin®; Mylan-Minocycline; Novo-Minocycline; PHL-Minocycline; PMS-Minocycline; ratio-Minocycline; Riva-Minocycline; Sandoz-Minocycline

Therapeutic Category Antibiotic, Tetracycline Derivative

Generic Available Yes: Excludes extended release tablet, injection, pellet-filled capsule

Use Treatment of susceptible gram-negative and gram-positive infections involving the respiratory tract, urinary tract, and skin/soft tissue; treatment of anthrax (inhalational, cutaneous, and gastrointestinal); brucellosis; asymptomatic meningococcal carrier state; rickettsial diseases (including Rocky Mountain spotted fever, typhus fever, Q fever); nongonococcal urethritis caused by *Ureaplasma urealyticum* or *C. trachomatis*, and gonorrhea; chlamydial infections (FDA approved in ages >8 years and adults); inflammatory acne vulgaris (FDA approved in ages ≥12 years); has been used to treat *Nocardia*, cutaneous (non-CNS) infections; *Mycobacterium marinum* cutaneous infections

Pregnancy Risk Factor D

Pregnancy Considerations Tetracyclines, including minocycline, cross the placenta, enter fetal circulation, and may cause permanent discoloration of teeth if used during the second or third trimester. Congenital anomalies after minocycline use have been reported postmarketing. Because use during pregnancy may cause fetal harm, minocycline is classified as pregnancy category D.

Lactation Enters breast milk/not recommended

Breast-Feeding Considerations Small amounts of minocycline are excreted in breast milk and therefore, breast-feeding is not recommended by the manufacturer. Minocycline absorption is not affected by dairy products. This may lead to increased absorption from maternal milk when compared to other tetracyclines which are bound by the calcium in the maternal milk. Nondose-related effects could include modification of bowel flora. There have been case reports of black discoloration of breast milk in women taking minocycline.

Contraindications Hypersensitivity to minocycline, other tetracyclines, or any component

Warnings Use of tetracyclines during tooth development may cause permanent discoloration of the teeth (yellow-gray to brown) and enamel hypoplasia; adult-onset tooth discoloration following long-term minocycline administration has also been reported. Do not administer to children ≤8 years of age due to permanent discoloration of teeth and retardation of skeletal development and bone growth (risk being greatest for children <4 years and in those receiving high doses). Minocycline has been associated with increases in BUN secondary to antianabolic effects. Pseudotumor cerebri has been reported rarely in infants and adolescents; use with isotretinoin has been associated with cases of pseudotumor cerebri; avoid concomitant treatment with isotretinoin. CNS effects (dizziness, lightheadedness, vertigo) may occur; patients must be cautioned about performing tasks which require mental alertness. Photosensitivity reaction may occur; avoid prolonged exposure to sunlight or tanning equipment; discontinue if skin erythema occurs. Azotemia, hyperphosphatemia, and acidosis have been reported in patients with significant renal dysfunction. Prolonged use may result in superinfection including *C. difficile*-associated diarrhea and pseudomembranous colitis. Minocycline can cause fetal harm if used during pregnancy; avoid use during pregnancy. Severe, sometimes fatal, hepatic injury has been associated with minocycline use; discontinue therapy if liver injury is suspected.

Precautions Use with caution in patients with renal or hepatic impairment; consider dosage modification in patients with renal impairment

Adverse Reactions

Cardiovascular: Myocarditis, pericarditis, vasculitis

Central nervous system: Ataxia, bulging fontanels, dizziness, fatigue, fever, headache, malaise, mood alteration, pseudotumor cerebri (see Warnings), sedation, seizure, somnolence, vertigo

Dermatologic: Alopecia, angioedema, erythema multiforme, erythema nodosum, exfoliative dermatitis, hyperpigmentation of nails, photosensitivity, pruritus, rash, skin hyperpigmentation (blue-black), Stevens-Johnson syndrome, toxic epidermal necrolysis, urticaria

Endocrine & metabolic: Acidosis, hyperphosphatemia, thyroid dysfunction, thyroid gland discoloration (brown-black)

Gastrointestinal: Anorexia, diarrhea, dyspepsia, dysphagia, enterocolitis, esophagitis, glossitis, moniliasis, nausea, oral cavity discoloration, pancreatitis, pseudomembranous colitis (see Warnings), stomatitis, vomiting, xerostomia

Genitourinary: Balanitis, vulvovaginitis

Hematologic: Agranulocytosis, eosinophilia, hemolytic anemia, leukopenia, neutropenia, pancytopenia, thrombocytopenia

Hepatic: Autoimmune hepatitis, hepatic cholestasis, hepatic failure (see Warnings), hepatitis, hyperbilirubinemia, jaundice, liver enzymes increased

Local: Injection site reaction, thrombophlebitis (I.V. administration)

Neuromuscular & skeletal: Arthralgia, arthritis, bone discoloration, hypoesthesia, injury to growing bones and teeth (see Warnings), joint stiffness, myalgia, paresthesia

Ophthalmic: Blurred vision

Otic: Hearing loss, tinnitus

Renal: Acute renal failure, BUN increased, interstitial nephritis

Respiratory: Asthma, bronchospasm, cough, dyspnea, pneumonitis, pulmonary infiltrates with eosinophilia

Miscellaneous: Anaphylaxis, enamel hypoplasia (see Warnings), serum sickness, systemic lupus erythematosus, tooth discoloration (yellow-gray-brown) (see Warnings)

Drug Interactions

Avoid Concomitant Use

Avoid concomitant use of Minocycline with any of the following: BCG; Retinoic Acid Derivatives

Increased Effect/Toxicity

Minocycline may increase the levels/effects of: Neuromuscular-Blocking Agents; Retinoic Acid Derivatives; Vitamin K Antagonists

Decreased Effect

Minocycline may decrease the levels/effects of: Atazanavir; BCG; Penicillins; Typhoid Vaccine

The levels/effects of Minocycline may be decreased by: Antacids; Bile Acid Sequestrants; Bismuth; Bismuth Subsalicylate; Iron Salts; Magnesium Salts; Quinapril; Sucralfate; Zinc Salts

Food Interactions Administration with iron, calcium, milk, or dairy products may decrease minocycline absorption; minocycline may decrease absorption of calcium, iron, magnesium, and zinc.

Stability

Oral formulations: Store at room temperature; protect from light, moisture, and excessive heat

Injection: Store vials at 20°C to 25°C (68°F to 77°F) prior to reconstitution. Reconstituted solution should be further diluted immediately. Final dilution should be administered immediately; stable at room temperature for 24 hours. Incompatible with adrenocorticotropic hormone, aminophylline, amobarbital, amphotericin B, bicarbonate infusion mixtures, calcium, cefazolin, heparin, hydrocortisone, penicillin, pentobarbital, phenytoin, whole blood.

Mechanism of Action Inhibits bacterial protein synthesis by binding with the 30S and possibly the 50S ribosomal subunit(s) of susceptible bacteria

934

Pharmacokinetics (Adult data unless noted)

Absorption: Oral: Well absorbed

Distribution: Widely distributed to most body fluids, bile, and tissues; poor CNS penetration; deposits in fat for extended periods; crosses placenta; appears in breast milk

V_d: Adults: 0.14-0.7 L/kg

Protein binding: 55% to 96%

Bioavailability: 90% to 100%

Half-life: Adults: I.V.: 15-23 hours; Oral: 16 hours (range: 11-26 hours)

Time to peak serum concentration:

Capsules and pellet filled capsules: 1-4 hours

Tablet: 1-3 hours

Extended release tablet: 3.5-4 hours

Elimination: 5% to 12% excreted unchanged in urine

Usual Dosage

I.V.:

Children >8 years: Initial: 4 mg/kg, followed by 2 mg/kg/ dose every 12 hours (maximum: 400 mg/day)

Adults: Initial: 200 mg, followed by 100 mg every 12 hours (maximum: 400 mg/day)

Oral:

Children >8 years: Initial: 4 mg/kg followed by 2 mg/kg/ dose every 12 hours

Children ≥12 years and Adolescents: Inflammatory, non-nodular, moderate-to-severe acne: Extended release tablet (Solodyn™):

45-54 kg: 45 mg once daily

55-77 kg: 65 mg once daily

78-102 kg: 90 mg once daily

103-125 kg: 115 mg once daily

126-136 kg: 135 mg once daily

Note: Therapy should be continued for 12 weeks. Higher doses do not confer greater efficacy and may be associated with more acute vestibular side effects.

Adults: Infections: Initial: 200 mg, followed by 100 mg every 12 hours; more frequent dosing intervals may be used (100-200 mg initially, followed by 50 mg 4 times daily)

Acne: Oral: 50-100 mg once or twice daily

Asymptomatic meningococcal carrier state: Oral: 100 mg every 12 hours for 5 days; **Note:** CDC recommendations do not mention use of minocycline for eradicating nasopharyngeal carriage of meningococcus.

Chlamydial or *Ureaplasma urealyticum* infection, uncomplicated (urethral, endocervical, or rectal): Oral, I.V.: 100 mg every 12 hours for at least 7 days

Gonococcal infection, uncomplicated (males): Oral, I.V.: Without urethritis or anorectal infection: Initial: 200 mg, followed by 100 mg every 12 hours for at least 4 days

Gonococcal infection, uncomplicated urethritis: Oral, I.V.: 100 mg every 12 hours for 5 days

Mycobacterium marinum cutaneous infection: Oral: 100 mg every 12 hours for 6-8 weeks (**Note:** Optimal dosing has not been established)

Nocardiosis, cutaneous (non-CNS): Oral: 100-200 mg every 12 hours

Syphilis: Oral, I.V.: Initial: 200 mg, followed by 100 mg every 12 hours for 10-15 days

Dosage adjustment in renal impairment: Consider decreasing dose or extending interval between doses; Cl_{cr} <80 mL/minute; maximum dose: 200 mg/day (minocycline serum level may need to be monitored)

Administration

I.V.: Reconstitute vial with 5 mL of SWI and further dilute in NS, D_5W, D_5NS, Ringer's injection, or LR to a final concentration not to exceed 0.4 mg/mL; infuse slowly; avoid rapid administration; the manufacturer's labeling does not provide a recommended administration rate; other tetracyclines are typically infused over 1-2 hours; the injectable route should be used only if the oral route is not feasible or adequate; prolonged intravenous therapy may be associated with thrombophlebitis

Oral: Administer with adequate fluid to decrease the risk of esophageal irritation and ulceration. Administer tablets 1 hour before or 2 hours after meals; capsule, pellet-filled capsule, and extended release tablet may be taken with or without food or milk. Swallow pellet-filled capsule and extended release tablet whole; do not chew, crush, or split. Administer antacids, calcium supplements, iron supplements, magnesium-containing laxatives, and cholestyramine 2 hours before or after minocycline.

Monitoring Parameters CBC, serum BUN, creatinine, liver function tests. Observe for changes in bowel frequency.

Test Interactions May cause interference with fluorescence test for urinary catecholamines (false elevation)

Patient Information Contact physician if watery or bloody stools develop. May discolor nails, skin, and teeth. May cause photosensitivity reactions (eg, exposure to sunlight may cause severe sunburn, skin rash, redness, or itching); avoid exposure to sunlight and artificial light sources (sunlamps, tanning booth/bed); wear protective clothing, wide-brimmed hats, sunglasses, and lip sunscreen (SPF ≥15); use a sunscreen [broad-spectrum sunscreen or physical sunscreen (preferred) or sunblock with SPF ≥15]; contact physician if reaction occurs. May cause light-headedness/dizziness and impair ability to perform activities requiring mental alertness or physical coordination. Women of childbearing potential should be advised to avoid becoming pregnant.

Dosage Forms Excipient information presented when available (limited, particularly for generics); consult specific product labeling. [DSC] = Discontinued product

Capsule: 50 mg, 75 mg, 100 mg

Dynacin®: 75 mg [DSC], 100 mg [DSC]

Capsule, pellet filled:

Minocin®: 50 mg, 100 mg

Minocin® PAC: 50 mg, 100 mg [packaged with wipes, serum, and masque]

Injection, powder for reconstitution:

Minocin®: 100 mg

Tablet: 50 mg, 75 mg, 100 mg

Dynacin®: 50 mg, 75 mg, 100 mg

Myrac™ [DSC]: 50 mg, 75 mg

Myrac™ [DSC]: 100 mg [scored]

Tablet, extended release:

Solodyn®: 45 mg, 65 mg, 90 mg, 115 mg, 135 mg

References

Garner SE, Eady EA, Popescu C, et al, "Minocycline for Acne Vulgaris: Efficacy and Safety," *Cochrane Database Syst Rev*, 2003, (1): CD002086.

Sanchez AR, Rogers RS 3rd, and Sheridan PJ, "Tetracycline and Other Tetracycline-Derivative Staining of the Teeth and Oral Cavity," *Int J Dermatol*, 2004, 43(10):709-15.

Zhanel GG, Homeniuk K, Nichol K, et al, "The Glycylcyclines: A Comparative Review With the Tetracyclines," *Drugs*, 2004, 64 (1):63-88.

Zouboulis CC and Piquero-Martin J, "Update and Future of Systemic Acne Treatment," *Dermatology*, 2003, 206(1):37-53.

◆ **Minocycline Hydrochloride** *see* Minocycline *on page 933*

◆ **Minox (Can)** *see* Minoxidil *on page 935*

Minoxidil (mi NOKS i dil)

Medication Safety Issues

Sound-alike/look-alike issues:

Loniten® may be confused with Lipitor®

Minoxidil may be confused with metolazone, midodrine, Minipress®, Minocin®, Monopril®, Noxafil®

International issues:
Noxidil® [Thailand] may be confused with Noxafil® which is a brand name for posaconazole in the U.S.

Related Information
Antihypertensive Agents by Class *on page 1481*

U.S. Brand Names Rogaine® Extra Strength for Men [OTC]; Rogaine® for Men [OTC]; Rogaine® for Women [OTC]

Canadian Brand Names Apo-Gain®; Loniten®; Minox; Rogaine®

Therapeutic Category Antihypertensive Agent; Vasodilator

Generic Available Yes: Excludes aerosol, topical solution

Use Management of severe hypertension; topically for management of alopecia or male pattern alopecia

Pregnancy Risk Factor C

Pregnancy Considerations Adverse events were observed in some animal studies.

Lactation Enters breast milk/not recommended

Breast-Feeding Considerations Excretion in breast milk has been reported in one case report of a woman receiving 10 mg/day orally.

Contraindications Hypersensitivity to minoxidil or any component; pheochromocytoma

Warnings May cause pericardial effusion progressing to tamponade **[U.S. Boxed Warning]**; pericarditis, angina, and sodium and water retention may also occur; use of minoxidil should be reserved for treatment of hypertension in patients who have not adequately responded to maximum doses of a diuretic and two other antihypertensive agents **[U.S. Boxed Warning]**; minoxidil is usually used with a beta-blocker (to treat minoxidil-induced tachycardia) and a diuretic (for treatment of water retention/edema); avoid concomitant use of minoxidil with guanethidine (see Drug Interactions); minoxidil may rapidly control blood pressure; too rapid control of blood pressure may lead to syncope, CVA, MI, or ischemia. Myocardial lesions and other adverse cardiac effects have been shown in experimental animals **[U.S. Boxed Warning]**; significance of these findings in humans is unclear.

Precautions Use with caution in patients with coronary artery disease or with recent MI, pulmonary hypertension, significant renal dysfunction, heart failure; renal failure or dialysis patients may require dosage reduction. Elongations, thickening, and enhanced pigmentation of fine body hair between eyebrows and hairline, sideburns, cheek, and eventually back, arms, legs, and scalp is seen in ~80% of patients within the first 3-6 weeks; may take 1-6 months for hypertrichosis to reverse itself after discontinuation of the drug.

Adverse Reactions
Cardiovascular: Edema, CHF, tachycardia, angina, pericardial effusion and tamponade, ECG changes
Central nervous system: Dizziness, fatigue, headache
Dermatologic: Hypertrichosis (commonly occurs within 1-2 months of therapy), coarsening facial features, dermatologic reactions, rash, Stevens-Johnson syndrome, photosensitivity
Endocrine & metabolic: Sodium and water retention, weight gain
Respiratory: Pulmonary hypertension, pulmonary edema

Drug Interactions
Avoid Concomitant Use There are no known interactions where it is recommended to avoid concomitant use.

Increased Effect/Toxicity
Minoxidil may increase the levels/effects of: Amifostine; Antihypertensives; Hypotensive Agents; RiTUXimab

The levels/effects of Minoxidil may be increased by: CycloSPORINE; CycloSPORINE (Systemic); Diazoxide; Herbs (Hypotensive Properties); MAO Inhibitors;

Pentoxifylline; Phosphodiesterase 5 Inhibitors; Prostacyclin Analogues

Decreased Effect
The levels/effects of Minoxidil may be decreased by: Herbs (Hypertensive Properties); Methylphenidate; Yohimbine

Food Interactions Avoid natural licorice (causes sodium and water retention and increases potassium loss)

Stability Store at controlled room temperature 20°C to 25°C (68°F to 77°F); topical 5% solution is flammable, keep away from fire or flame

Mechanism of Action Produces vasodilation by directly relaxing arteriolar smooth muscle, with little effect on veins; effects may be mediated by cyclic AMP; stimulation of hair growth is secondary to vasodilation, increased cutaneous blood flow and stimulation of resting hair follicles

Pharmacodynamics Hypotensive effects:
Onset of action: Oral: Within 30 minutes
Maximum effect: Within 2-8 hours
Duration: Up to 2-5 days

Pharmacokinetics (Adult data unless noted)
Metabolism: 88% primarily via glucuronidation
Protein-binding: None
Bioavailability: Oral: 90%
Half-life, adults: 3.5-4.2 hours
Elimination: 12% excreted unchanged in urine
Dialysis: Dialyzable (50% to 100%)

Usual Dosage
Hypertension: Oral:
Children <12 years: Initial: 0.1-0.2 mg/kg once daily; maximum dose: 5 mg/day; increase gradually every 3 days; usual dosage: 0.25-1 mg/kg/day in 1-2 divided doses; maximum dose: 50 mg/day
Children >12 years and Adults: Initial: 5 mg once daily, increase gradually every 3 days; usual dose: 10-40 mg/day in 1-2 divided doses; maximum dose: 100 mg/day; **Note:** Usual dosage range for Adolescents ≥18 years and Adults (JNC 7): 2.5-80 mg/day in 1-2 divided doses
Alopecia: Adults: Topical: Apply twice daily

Administration Oral: May be administered without regard to food

Monitoring Parameters Fluids and electrolytes, body weight, blood pressure

Patient Information May cause dizziness; rise slowly from prolonged lying or sitting position. May cause photosensitivity reactions (eg, exposure to sunlight may cause severe sunburn, skin rash, redness, or itching); avoid exposure to sunlight and artificial light sources (sunlamps, tanning booth/bed); wear protective clothing, wide-brimmed hats, sunglasses, and lip sunscreen (SPF ≥15); use a sunscreen [broad-spectrum sunscreen or physical sunscreen (preferred) or sunblock with SPF ≥15]; contact physician if reaction occurs.

Additional Information May take 1-6 months for hypertrichosis to totally reverse after oral minoxidil therapy is discontinued

Dosage Forms Excipient information presented when available (limited, particularly for generics); consult specific product labeling. [DSC] = Discontinued product
Aerosol, topical [foam]:
Rogaine for Men®: 5% (60 g)
Solution, topical: 2% (60 mL); 5% (60 mL)
Rogaine® for Men: 2% (60 mL) [DSC] [supplied with dropper applicator]
Rogaine® for Women: 2% (60 mL) [supplied with dropper applicator]
Rogaine® Extra Strength for Men: 5% (60 mL) [supplied with dropper applicator]
Tablet: 2.5 mg, 10 mg

References

Chobanian AV, Bakris GL, Black HR, et al, "The Seventh Report of the Joint National Committee on Prevention, Detection, Evaluation, and Treatment of High Blood Pressure: The JNC 7 report," *JAMA*, 2003, 289(19):2560-72.

Misoprostol (mye soe PROST ole)

Medication Safety Issues

Sound-alike/look-alike issues:

Cytotec® may be confused with Cytoxan, Sytobex®

Misoprostol may be confused with metoprolol, mifepristone

U.S. Brand Names Cytotec®

Canadian Brand Names Apo-Misoprostol®; Novo-Misoprostol; PMS-Misoprostol

Therapeutic Category Gastrointestinal Agent, Gastric Ulcer Treatment; Prostaglandin

Generic Available Yes

Use Prevention of NSAID-induced gastric ulcers (FDA approved in adults)

Pregnancy Risk Factor X

Pregnancy Considerations Teratogenic effects were not observed in animal reproduction studies; however, congenital anomalies following first trimester exposure, fetal death, uterine perforation, and abortion have been reported after the use of misoprostol in human pregnancy. **[U.S. Boxed Warning]: Not to be used to reduce NSAID-induced ulcers in women of childbearing potential unless woman is capable of complying with effective contraceptive measures.** Do not use in women of childbearing potential without a negative serum pregnancy test within 2 weeks prior to therapy; therapy is normally begun on the second or third day of next normal menstrual period. Use to prevent NSAID-induced ulcers is contraindicated in pregnant women. Written and verbal warnings concerning the hazards of misoprostol should be provided. During pregnancy, misoprostol may induce or augment uterine contractions; the manufacturer states that misoprostol should not be used as a cervical-ripening agent for induction of labor. However, The American College of Obstetricians and Gynecologists (ACOG) supports this off-label use in women who have not had a prior cesarean delivery or major uterine surgery. Hyperstimulation of the uterus, uterine rupture, or adverse events in the fetus or mother may occur with this use. Misoprostol is FDA approved for the medical termination of pregnancy of ≤49 days in conjunction with mifepristone.

Lactation Enters breast milk/use caution

Breast-Feeding Considerations Misoprostol acid (the active metabolite of misoprostol) has been detected in breast milk. Concentrations following a single oral dose were 7.6-20.9 pg/mL after 1 hour and decreased to <1 pg/mL by 5 hours. Adverse events have not been reported in nursing infants.

Contraindications Hypersensitivity to prostaglandins; pregnancy (when used to prevent NSAID-induced ulcers)

Warnings May cause abortion, premature labor, or birth defects if given to pregnant women **[U.S. Boxed Warning]**; not to be used for reducing the risk of NSAID-induced ulcers in pregnant women or women of child-bearing potential unless the woman is capable of complying with effective contraceptive measures; women should have a negative serum pregnancy test within 2 weeks prior to initiating therapy with therapy begun on the second or third day of next menstrual period. **Due to the abortifacient property of this medication, patients must be warned not to give this drug to others [U.S. Boxed Warning].**

Precautions Use with caution in patients with inflammatory bowel disease (due to potential for development of diarrhea with misoprostol), cardiovascular disease, and renal impairment

Adverse Reactions

Central nervous system: Headache

Gastrointestinal: Abdominal pain, constipation, diarrhea, flatulence, nausea, vomiting

Genitourinary: Uterine rupture (when taken after the eighth week of pregnancy)

<1%, postmarketing, and case reports: Abnormal taste, abnormal vision, alkaline phosphatase increased, alopecia, amylase increase, anaphylaxis, anemia, anxiety, appetite changes, arrhythmia, arterial thrombosis, arthralgia, back pain, breast pain, bronchitis, bronchospasm, cardiac enzymes increased, chest pain, chills, confusion, conjunctivitis, CVA, deafness, depression, dermatitis, diaphoresis, dizziness, drowsiness, dysphagia, dyspnea, dysuria, earache, edema, epistaxis, ESR increased, fatigue, fetal or infant death (when used during pregnancy), fever, GI bleeding, GI inflammation, gingivitis, glycosuria, gout, gynecological disorders (cramps, dysmenorrhea, hypermenorrhea, postmenopausal vaginal bleeding, spotting, and other menstrual disorders) hematuria, hepatobiliary function abnormal, hyper-/hypotension, impotence, loss of libido, MI, muscle cramps, myalgia, neuropathy, neurosis, nitrogen increased, pallor, phlebitis, pneumonia, polyuria, pulmonary embolism, purpura, rash, reflux, rigors, stiffness, syncope, thirst, thrombocytopenia, tinnitus, upper respiratory tract infection, urinary tract infection, uterine rupture, weakness, weight changes

Drug Interactions

Avoid Concomitant Use

Avoid concomitant use of Misoprostol with any of the following: Carbetocin

Increased Effect/Toxicity

Misoprostol may increase the levels/effects of: Carbetocin; Oxytocin

The levels/effects of Misoprostol may be increased by: Antacids

Decreased Effect There are no known significant interactions involving a decrease in effect.

Food Interactions Misoprostol peak serum concentrations may be decreased if taken with food (not clinically significant)

Mechanism of Action Misoprostol, a gastric antisecretory agent, is a synthetic prostaglandin E_1 analog that replaces the protective prostaglandins consumed with prostaglandin-inhibiting therapies (eg, NSAIDs) resulting in reduction of acid secretion from the gastric parietal cell and stimulation of bicarbonate production from the gastric and duodenal mucosa

Pharmacodynamics Inhibition of gastric acid secretion:

Onset of action: 30 minutes

Maximum effect: 60-90 minutes

Duration: 3 hours

Pharmacokinetics (Adult data unless noted)

Absorption: Rapid and extensive

Protein binding (misoprostol acid): 80% to 90%

Metabolism: Extensive "first pass" de-esterification to misoprostol acid (active metabolite)

Bioavailability: 88%

Half-life (metabolite): Terminal: 20-40 minutes

Time to peak serum concentration (active metabolite): Fasting: 14 ± 8 minutes

Elimination: In urine (~80%)

Usual Dosage Oral: Prevention of NSAID-induced ulcers: Adults: 200 mcg 4 times/day; if not tolerated, may decrease dose to 100 mcg 4 times/day; take for the duration of NSAID therapy

Dosage adjustment in renal impairment: Half-life, maximum plasma concentration, and bioavailability may be increased; however, a correlation has not been observed with degree of dysfunction. Decrease dose if recommended dose is not tolerated

Administration Oral: Administer after meals and at bedtime

Patient Information May initially cause diarrhea which usually resolves after 8 days of therapy; avoid taking with magnesium-containing antacids; do not take if you are pregnant. An effective form of birth control should be used during treatment. Do not share this medication with others.

Nursing Implications Incidence of diarrhea may be lessened by having patient take dose right after meals

Additional Information Has also been used to improve absorption in cystic fibrosis patients 8-16 years of age at doses of 100 mcg 4 times daily, in conjunction with pancreatic enzyme supplements (limited data available)

Dosage Forms Excipient information presented when available (limited, particularly for generics); consult specific product labeling.

Tablet: 100 mcg, 200 mcg

Cytotec®: 100 mcg, 200 mcg

References

Cleghorn GJ, Shepherd RW, and Holt TL, "The Use of a Synthetic Prostaglandin E1 Analogue (Misoprostol) as an Adjunct to Pancreatic Enzyme Replacement in Cystic Fibrosis," Scand J Gastroenterol Suppl, 1988, 143:142-7.

Robinson PJ, Smith AL, and Sly PD, "Duodenal pH in Cystic Fibrosis and Its Relationship to Fat Malabsorption," Dig Dis Sci, 1990, 35 (10):1299-304.

Mitoxantrone (mye toe ZAN trone)

Medication Safety Issues

Sound-alike/look-alike issues:

Mitoxantrone may be confused with methotrexate, mitomycin, mitotane, Mutamycin®

High alert medication: The Institute for Safe Medication Practices (ISMP) includes this medication among its list of drug classes which have a heightened risk of causing significant patient harm when used in error.

Related Information

Compatibility of Chemotherapy and Related Supportive Care Medications on page 1580

Emetogenic Potential of Antineoplastic Agents on page 1579

Extravasation Treatment on page 1522

U.S. Brand Names Novantrone®

Canadian Brand Names Mitoxantrone Injection®; Novantrone®

Therapeutic Category Antineoplastic Agent, Anthracenedione; Antineoplastic Agent, Antibiotic

Generic Available Yes

Use Treatment of acute nonlymphocytic leukemias (ANLL; includes myelogenous, promyelocytic, monocytic, and erythroid leukemias); advanced hormone-refractory prostate cancer, secondary progressive, or relapsing-remitting multiple sclerosis (MS); mitoxantrone is also active in pediatric sarcoma, Hodgkin's lymphoma, non-Hodgkin's lymphomas (NHL), acute lymphocytic leukemia (ALL), myelodysplastic syndrome, breast cancer; has been used as part of a conditioning regimen in adults for autologous hematopoietic stem-cell transplantation (HSCT) (FDA approved in adults)

Pregnancy Risk Factor D

Pregnancy Considerations Adverse effects were noted in animal studies. May cause fetal harm if administered to a pregnant woman. There are no adequate and well-controlled studies in pregnant women. Pregnancy should be avoided while on treatment. Women with multiple sclerosis and who are biologically capable of becoming pregnant should have a pregnancy test prior to each dose.

Lactation Enters breast milk/not recommended

Breast-Feeding Considerations Mitoxantrone is excreted in human milk and significant concentrations (180 mg/mL) have been reported for 28 days after the last administration. Because of the potential for serious adverse reactions in infants from mitoxantrone, breast-feeding should be discontinued before starting treatment.

Contraindications Hypersensitivity to mitoxantrone or any component

Warnings Mitoxantrone can cause severe myelosuppression; use with caution in patients with pre-existing myelosuppression; do not use if baseline neutrophil count is <1500 cells/mm^3 (except for in the treatment of ANLL); monitor blood counts and monitor for infection due to neutropenia **[U.S. Boxed Warning]**. May cause myocardial toxicity and potentially-fatal heart failure (HF); increases with cumulative dosing. Effects may occur during therapy or may be delayed (months or years after completion of therapy). Predisposing factors for mitoxantrone-induced cardiotoxicity are prior anthracycline or anthracenedione therapy, prior cardiovascular disease, concomitant use of cardiotoxic drugs, and mediastinal/pericardial irradiation, although may also occur in patients without risk factors. Prior to therapy initiation, evaluate all patients for cardiac-related signs/symptoms, including history, physical exam, and ECG; and evaluate baseline left ventricular ejection fraction (LVEF) with echocardiogram or multigated radionuclide angiography (MUGA) or MRI. Not recommended for use in MS patients when LVEF <50%, or baseline LVEF below the lower limit of normal (LLN). Evaluate for cardiac signs/symptoms (by history, physical exam, and ECG) and evaluate LVEF (using same method as baseline LVEF) in MS patients prior to each dose and if signs/symptoms of HF develop. Use in MS should be limited to a cumulative dose ≤140 mg/m^2, and discontinued if LVEF falls below LLN or a significant decrease in LVEF is observed; decreases in LVEF and HF have been observed in patients with MS who have received cumulative doses <100 mg/m^2. Patients with MS should undergo annual LVEF evaluation following discontinuation of therapy to monitor for delayed cardiotoxicity **[U.S. Boxed Warning]**. For I.V. administration only, into a free-flowing I.V.; may cause severe local tissue damage if extravasation occurs **[U.S. Boxed Warning]**; extravasation resulting in burning, erythema, pain, swelling, and skin discoloration (blue) has been reported; extravasation may result in tissue necrosis and requires debridement for skin graft. Do not administer SubQ, I.M., or intra-arterial injections (have resulted in local/regional neuropathy); do not administer intrathecally (may cause serious and permanent neurologic damage) **[U.S. Boxed Warning]**, including local nerve demyelination, seizures, coma, and paraplegia. Hazardous agent; use appropriate precautions for handling and disposal. Secondary acute myelogenous leukemia has been reported in patients treated with mitoxantrone (in both patients with cancer and with MS) **[U.S. Boxed Warning]**; monitor CBC, platelet count; signs and symptoms of infection prior to each course and after discontinuation of mitoxantrone; occurrence of secondary leukemia is more common when anthracyclines are given in combination with DNA-damaging agents, when patients have been heavily pretreated with cytotoxic drugs, or when anthracycline doses have been escalated. Rapid lysis of tumor cells may lead to hyperuricemia.

Precautions Dosage should be reduced in patients with pre-existing bone marrow suppression, previous treatment with cardiotoxic agents, and patients with impaired hepatobiliary function. May cause urine, saliva, tears, and sweat to turn blue-green for 24 hours postinfusion; whites of eyes may have blue-green tinge. Mitoxantrone is excreted in breast milk; breast-feeding should be discontinued prior to initiating therapy due to risk of adverse effects on infant.

Adverse Reactions

Cardiovascular: Cardiomyopathy, cardiotoxicity [arrhythmias, CHF, ECG changes, ischemia, LVEF decreased (see Warnings), chest pain, edema, hypertension, hypotension, tachycardia

Central nervous system: Anxiety, chills, depression, fatigue, fever, headache, pain, seizures

Dermatologic: Alopecia, cutaneous mycosis, discoloration of skin (blue-green), nail bed changes, petechiae/bruising, pruritus, rash, skin desquamation, skin infection, urticaria

Endocrine & metabolic: Amenorrhea, dehydration, hyperglycemia, hyperuricemia, hypocalcemia, hypokalemia, hyponatremia, menorrhagia, menstrual disorder, weight gain/loss

Gastrointestinal: Abdominal pain, anorexia, aphthosis, constipation, diarrhea, dyspepsia, GI bleeding, mucositis, nausea, stomatitis (occurs more frequently with "daily times 3 day" regimens than once every 3 week schedules), vomiting

Genitourinary: Abnormal urine, discoloration of urine (blue-green), impotence, sterility, urinary tract infection

Hematologic: Hemorrhage, lymphopenia, mild anemia, myelosuppression [granulocytopenia, leukopenia, neutropenia, pancytopenia (see Warnings)], neutropenic fever, thrombocytopenia

Hepatic: Alkaline phosphatase increased, GGT increased, jaundice, transient elevation of liver enzymes

Local: Phlebitis, tissue necrosis (or burning, erythema, pain, skin discoloration, swelling) with extravasation

Neuromuscular & skeletal: Arthralgia, back pain, myalgia, weakness

Ocular: Blurred vision, conjunctivitis, sclera discoloration (blue)

Renal: BUN increased, creatinine increased, hematuria, proteinuria, renal failure

Respiratory: Cough, dyspnea, interstitial pneumonitis, pharyngitis, pneumonia, rhinitis, sinusitis, upper respiratory tract infection

Miscellaneous: Allergic reaction, anaphylaxis, development of secondary leukemia (see Warnings), diaphoresis, fungal infection, infection, sepsis, systemic infection

Drug Interactions

Metabolism/Transport Effects Inhibits CYP3A4 (weak)

Avoid Concomitant Use

Avoid concomitant use of Mitoxantrone with any of the following: BCG; Natalizumab; Pimecrolimus; Tacrolimus (Topical); Vaccines (Live)

Increased Effect/Toxicity

Mitoxantrone may increase the levels/effects of: Leflunomide; Natalizumab; Vaccines (Live)

The levels/effects of Mitoxantrone may be increased by: Denosumab; Pimecrolimus; Tacrolimus (Topical); Trastuzumab

Decreased Effect

Mitoxantrone may decrease the levels/effects of: BCG; Sipuleucel-T; Vaccines (Inactivated); Vaccines (Live)

The levels/effects of Mitoxantrone may be decreased by: Echinacea

Stability After penetration of the stopper, undiluted mitoxantrone solution is stable for 7 days at room temperature or 14 days when refrigerated; solutions diluted for administration are stable for 7 days at room temperature or under refrigeration, although the manufacturer recommends immediate use; incompatible with heparin; physically compatible with ondansetron for at least 4 hours

Mechanism of Action Inhibits DNA and RNA synthesis by intercalating with DNA and causing template disordering and steric obstruction; replication is decreased by binding to DNA topoisomerase II (enzyme responsible for DNA helix supercoiling); active throughout entire cell cycle. Mitoxantrone inhibits B-cell, T-cell, and macrophage proliferation; impairs antigen presentation and secretion of interferon gamma, TNF$_\alpha$, IL-2.

Pharmacokinetics (Adult data unless noted)

Distribution: Distributes into thyroid, liver, pancreas, spleen, heart, bone marrow, and red blood cells; prolonged retention in tissues; excreted in breast milk
V_{dss}: >1000 L/m^2

Protein binding: 78%

Half-life, terminal: 23-215 hours (median: 75 hours); may be prolonged with liver impairment

Elimination: 11% of dose excreted in urine (65% as unchanged drug) and 25% in bile as unchanged drug and metabolites

Usual Dosage I.V. (details concerning dosing in combination regimens should also be consulted):

Leukemias:

Children ≤2 years: 0.4 mg/kg/day once daily for 3-5 days

Children >2 years and Adults: 12 mg/m^2/day once daily for 2-3 days; acute leukemia in relapse: 8-12 mg/m^2/day once daily for 5 days; ANLL: 10 mg/m^2/day once daily for 3-5 days

Solid tumors:

Children: 18-20 mg/m^2 once every 3-4 weeks **or** 5-8 mg/m^2 every week

Adults: 12-14 mg/m^2 once every 3-4 weeks (maximum total: 80-120 mg/m^2)

Multiple sclerosis: Adults: 12 mg/m^2/dose every 3 months; maximum cumulative dose: 140 mg/m^2 (discontinue use with LVEF <50% or clinically significant reduction in LVEF)

Prostate cancer (advanced hormone-refractory): Adults: 12-14 mg/m^2 every 3 weeks (in combination with corticosteroids)

Non-Hodgkin's lymphoma (unlabeled use): Adults: 8-10 mg/m^2 every 21-28 days (as part of a combination chemotherapy regimen)

Dosing adjustment in hepatic impairment: Although official dosage adjustment recommendations have not been established, dosage reduction of 50% in patients with serum bilirubin of 1.5-3 mg/dL and dosage reduction of 75% in patients with serum bilirubin >3 mg/dL have been recommended; **Note:** MS patients with hepatic impairment should not receive mitoxantrone.

Dosing adjustment for toxicity:

ANLL patients: Severe or life-threatening nonhematologic toxicity: Withhold treatment until toxicity resolves

MS Patients:

Neutrophils <1500/mm^3: Use is not recommended

Signs/symptoms of HF: Evaluate for cardiac signs/symptoms and LVEF

LVEF <50% or baseline LVEF below the lower limit of normal (LLN): Use is not recommended

Administration Do not administer by SubQ, I.M., intrathecal, or intra-arterial injection (intra-arterial injection has resulted in local/regional neuropathy; seizures, coma, paralysis with bowel and bladder dysfunction, and neurotoxicity have been reported following intrathecal injection of mitoxantrone).

Parenteral: I.V.: Do **not** administer I.V. push over <3 minutes; may administer by I.V. bolus over 5-15 minutes **or** I.V. intermittent infusion over 15-60 minutes. Must be diluted prior to use.

Monitoring Parameters CBC with differential, platelet count, serum uric acid (for leukemia treatment), liver function tests, women with multiple sclerosis of childbearing potential must have a pregnancy test prior to each dose; injection site for signs of extravasation

Cardiac monitoring: Prior to initiation, evaluate all patients for cardiac-related signs/symptoms, including history, physical exam, and ECG; evaluate baseline and periodic left ventricular ejection fraction (LVEF) with ECG or multigated radionuclide angiography (MUGA) or MRI. In patients with MS, evaluate for cardiac signs/symptoms (by history, physical exam, and ECG) and evaluate LVEF (using same method as baseline LVEF) prior to each dose and if signs/symptoms of HF develop. Patients with MS should undergo annual LVEF evaluation following discontinuation of therapy to monitor for delayed cardiotoxicity.

Patient Information May discolor skin, sclera, tears, sweat, and urine to a blue-green color; women of childbearing potential should be advised to avoid becoming pregnant; contraceptive measures are recommended during therapy; do not breast-feed. Notify physician if fever, chills, sore throat, cough, pain with urinating, trouble breathing, swelling of legs or ankles, uneven or fast heartbeat, or unusual bleeding or bruising occurs.

Nursing Implications Mitoxantrone is an irritant (is considered a vesicant by some institutions). If extravasation occurs, the drug should be discontinued and restarted in another vein; extravasation may result in erythema, swelling, pain, burning, and/or a blue discoloration of the skin. If extravasation occurs, place ice pack over the affected area and elevate extremity.

Additional Information Myelosuppression (leukocyte nadir: 10-14 days; recovery: 21 days); injection contains 0.14 mEq of sodium/mL

Dosage Forms Excipient information presented when available (limited, particularly for generics); consult specific product labeling. [DSC] = Discontinued product

Injection, solution [concentrate; preservative free]: 2 mg/mL (10 mL, 12.5 mL, 15 mL, 20 mL)

Novantrone®: 2 mg/mL (10 mL, 15 mL [DSC])

References

Koeller J and Eble M, "Mitoxantrone: A Novel Anthracyline Derivative," *Clin Pharm*, 1988, 7(8):574-81.

National Comprehensive Cancer Network® (NCCN), "Clinical Practice Guidelines in Oncology™: Non-Hodgkin's Lymphomas," Version 1, 2009. Available at http://www.nccn.org/professionals/physician_gls/PDF/nhl.pdf.

Pratt CB, Vietti TJ, Etcubanas E, et al, "Novantrone® for Childhood Malignant Solid Tumors. A Pediatric Oncology Group Phase II Study," *Invest New Drugs*, 1986, 4(1):43-8.

Stevens RF, Hann IM, Wheatley K, et al, "Marked Improvements in Outcome With Chemotherapy Alone in Paediatric Acute Myeloid Leukemia: Results of the United Kingdom Medical Research Council's 10th AML Trial. MRC Childhood Leukaemia Working Party," *Br J Haematol*, 1998, 101(1):130-40.

Wells RJ, Adams MT, Alonzo TA, et al, "Mitoxantrone and Cytarabine Induction, High-Dose Cytarabine, and Etoposide Intensification for Pediatric Patients With Relapsed or Refractory Acute Myeloid Leukemia: Children's Cancer Group Study 2951," *J Clin Oncol*, 2003, 21(15):2940-7.

♦ **Mitoxantrone Dihydrochloride** *see* Mitoxantrone on page 938

♦ **Mitoxantrone HCl** *see* Mitoxantrone on page 938

♦ **Mitoxantrone Hydrochloride** *see* Mitoxantrone on page 938

♦ **Mitoxantrone Injection® (Can)** *see* Mitoxantrone on page 938

♦ **Mitozantrone** *see* Mitoxantrone on page 938

♦ **Mitrazol™ [OTC]** *see* Miconazole on page 927

♦ **MK-639** *see* Indinavir on page 723

♦ **MK0826** *see* Ertapenem on page 523

♦ **MK 869** *see* Aprepitant/Fosaprepitant on page 125

♦ **MMF** *see* Mycophenolate on page 956

♦ **MMR** *see* Measles, Mumps, and Rubella Vaccines (Combined) on page 862

♦ **M-M-R® II** *see* Measles, Mumps, and Rubella Vaccines (Combined) on page 862

♦ **MMR-V** *see* Measles, Mumps, Rubella, and Varicella Virus Vaccine on page 864

♦ **MMRV** *see* Measles, Mumps, Rubella, and Varicella Virus Vaccine on page 864

♦ **MOAB anti-Tac** *see* Daclizumab on page 382

Modafinil (moe DAF i nil)

U.S. Brand Names Provigil®

Canadian Brand Names Alertec®; Apo-Modafinil®

Therapeutic Category Central Nervous System Stimulant

Generic Available No

Use Improve wakefulness in patients with excessive daytime sleepiness associated with narcolepsy and shift work sleep disorder (SWSD); adjunctive therapy for obstructive sleep apnea/hypopnea syndrome (OSAHS); attention-deficit/hyperactivity disorder (ADHD); treatment of fatigue in multiple sclerosis (MS) and other disorders

Restrictions C-IV

Pregnancy Risk Factor C

Pregnancy Considerations Embryotoxic effects have been observed in some, but not all animal studies. There are no adequate and well-controlled studies in pregnant women; use only when the potential risk of drug therapy is outweighed by the drug's benefits. Efficacy of steroidal contraceptives may be decreased; alternate means of contraception should be considered during therapy and for 1 month after modafinil is discontinued.

Lactation Excretion in breast milk unknown/use caution

Contraindications Hypersensitivity to modafinil, armodafinil, or any component

Warnings Serious and life-threatening rashes, including Stevens-Johnson syndrome and toxic epidermal necrolysis, have been reported with modafinil. Although initially reported in children during clinical trials, postmarketing cases have occurred in both children and adults. Most cases have occurred within the first 5 weeks of therapy; however, rare cases have occurred after long-term use. No risk factors have been identified to predict occurrence or severity. Patients should be advised to discontinue at first sign of rash.

May impair the ability to engage in potentially hazardous activities. The degree of sleepiness should be reassessed frequently; some patients may not return to a normal level of wakefulness. Produces psychoactive and euphoric effects, alterations of mood, perception, thinking, and feelings typical of other CNS stimulants. No clinical symptoms of withdrawal have been reported; patients should be monitored closely for abuse potential, particularly those with a prior history of drug and/or stimulant abuse.

Rare cases of multiorgan hypersensitivity reactions in association with modafinil use and lone cases of angioedema and anaphylactoid reactions with armodafinil have been reported. Signs and symptoms are diverse, reflecting the involvement of specific organs. Patients typically present with fever and rash associated with organ-system dysfunction. Patients should be advised to report any signs and symptoms related to these effects; discontinuation of therapy is recommended.

The American Heart Association recommends that all children diagnosed with ADHD who may be candidates for stimulant medication, such as modafinil, should have a thorough cardiovascular assessment prior to initiation of therapy. These recommendations are based upon reports of serious cardiovascular adverse events (including sudden death) in patients (both children and adults) taking usual doses of stimulant medications. Most of these patients were found to have underlying structural heart disease (eg, hypertrophic obstructive cardiomyopathy). This assessment should include a combination of thorough medical history, family history, and physical examination. An ECG is not mandatory but should be considered. Modafinil use is not recommended in patients with a history of angina, cardiac ischemia, recent history of MI, left ventricular hypertrophy, or patients with mitral valve prolapse who have developed mitral valve prolapse syndrome with previous CNS stimulant use. Increase monitoring in patients with hypertension; additional antihypertensive therapy may be necessary.

Effectiveness of steroidal contraceptives may be reduced when administered concomitantly with modafinil; alternative or concomitant methods of contraception are recommended for patients receiving modafinil and for 1 month following discontinuation. Cyclosporine serum levels may be reduced with modafinil use; monitor cyclosporine levels.

Precautions Use with caution in patients with hepatic impairment; dosage reduction is recommended. Use with caution in patients with pre-existing psychosis or bipolar disorder (may induce mixed/manic episode). May exacerbate symptoms of behavior and thought disorder in psychotic patients; new-onset psychosis or mania may occur with stimulant use; observe for symptoms of aggression, hostility, or suicidal ideation. Use with caution in patients with renal impairment. Use with caution in patients with Tourette syndrome; stimulants may unmask tics.

Adverse Reactions

Cardiovascular: Chest pain, hypertension, palpitation, tachycardia, vasodilation, edema, angioedema

Central nervous system: Insomnia (children: 29%; adults: 5%), headache (children: 20%; adults: 34%; dose related), nervousness, dizziness, depression, anxiety, somnolence, chills, agitation, confusion, emotional lability, vertigo, mania, psychosis, fever. Tourette syndrome, hostility, cataplexy increased, hypnagogic hallucinations increased, and suicidal ideation were reported in controlled, open label clinical studies in children.

Dermatologic: Rash (includes some severe cases requiring hospitalization), Stevens-Johnson syndrome (see Warnings), toxic epidermal necrolysis

Endocrine & metabolic: Weight loss (children: 5%), dysmenorrhea

Gastrointestinal: Appetite decreased (children: 16%; adults: 4%), nausea, diarrhea, dyspepsia, xerostomia, constipation, flatulence, mouth ulceration, taste perversion, abdominal pain (children: 12%), vomiting

Genitourinary: Abnormal urine, hematuria, pyuria

Hematologic: Eosinophilia, agranulocytosis, transient leukopenia

Hepatic: Abnormal LFTs

Neuromuscular & skeletal: Back pain, paresthesia, dyskinesia, hyperkinesia, hypertonia, neck rigidity, tremor

Ocular: Amblyopia, eye pain, vision abnormal

Respiratory: Pharyngitis, rhinitis, lung disorder, asthma, epistaxis, cough

Miscellaneous: Diaphoresis, drug rash with eosinophilia and systemic symptoms (DRESS syndrome), hypersensitivity syndrome (multiorgan), infection

Drug Interactions

Metabolism/Transport Effects Substrate of CYP3A4 (major); **Inhibits** CYP1A2 (weak), 2A6 (weak), 2C9 (weak), 2C19 (strong), 2E1 (weak), 3A4 (weak); **Induces** CYP1A2 (weak), 2B6 (weak), 3A4 (weak)

Avoid Concomitant Use

Avoid concomitant use of Modafinil with any of the following: Clopidogrel; Iobenguane I 123

Increased Effect/Toxicity

Modafinil may increase the levels/effects of: CYP2C19 Substrates; Sympathomimetics

The levels/effects of Modafinil may be increased by: Atomoxetine; Cannabinoids; CYP3A4 Inhibitors (Moderate); CYP3A4 Inhibitors (Strong); Dasatinib

Decreased Effect

Modafinil may decrease the levels/effects of: Clopidogrel; Contraceptives (Estrogens); Iobenguane I 123; Saxagliptin

The levels/effects of Modafinil may be decreased by: CYP3A4 Inducers (Strong); Deferasirox; Herbs (CYP3A4 Inducers)

Food Interactions Delays absorption (by ~1 hour), but does not affect bioavailability.

Stability Store at controlled room temperature.

Mechanism of Action The exact mechanism of action is unclear. It does not appear to alter the release of dopamine or norepinephrine and it may exert its stimulant effects by decreasing GABA-mediated neurotransmission, although this theory has not yet been fully evaluated. Several studies also suggest that an intact central alpha-adrenergic system is required for modafinil's activity; the drug increases high-frequency alpha waves while decreasing both delta and theta wave activity, and these effects are consistent with generalized increases in mental alertness.

Pharmacokinetics (Adult data unless noted) Modafinil is a racemic compound (at steady state total exposure to the l-isomer is ~3 times that for the d-isomer) whose enantiomers have different pharmacokinetics and do not interconvert.

Distribution: V_d: Adults: 0.9 L/kg

Protein binding: 60%, primarily to albumin

Metabolism: Hepatic; multiple pathways including CYP3A4

Half-life: Adults: Effective half-life: 15 hours; steady-state: 2-4 days

Time to peak serum concentration: 2-4 hours

Elimination: Urine (as metabolites; <10% as unchanged drug)

Usual Dosage Oral:

ADHD:

Children <30 kg: 200-340* mg once daily

Children >30 kg: 300-425* mg

Adults: 100-300 mg once daily

*Randomized, double-blind, placebo-controlled pediatric studies have utilized an 85 mg film-coated tablet (currently not commercially available) to provide these dosages. All studies utilized a titration method but varied the length of titration (3 weeks vs 7-9 days); clinical improvement was noted earlier in the shorter titration period.

Narcolepsy, obstructive sleep apnea/hypopnea syndrome (OSAHS), and shift work sleep disorder (SWSD): Adults: Initial: 200 mg as a single daily dose. **Note:** Doses of up to 400 mg/day, given as a single dose, have been well tolerated, but there is no consistent evidence that this dose confers additional benefit.

Dosing adjustment in renal impairment: Safety and efficacy have not been established in severe renal impairment.

Dosing adjustment in hepatic impairment: Dose should be reduced to one-half of that recommended for patients with normal liver function.

Administration Oral: May be administer without regard to food, as a single dose in the morning; administer 1 hour prior to the start of work shift in those patients with SWSD

Monitoring Parameters Monitor CNS activity, blood pressure (if hypertensive patient), heart rate, appetite

Patient Information Take exactly as prescribed; do not exceed recommended dosage without consulting health-care provider. Avoid alcohol; may cause drowsiness and impair ability to perform activities requiring mental alertness or physical coordination; may cause dry mouth.

Dosage Forms Excipient information presented when available (limited, particularly for generics); consult specific product labeling.

Tablet:
  Provigil®: 100 mg, 200 mg

References

Amiri S, Mohammadi MR, Mohammadi M, et al, "Modafinil as a Treatment for Attention-Deficit/Hyperactivity Disorder in Children and Adolescents: A Double-Blind, Randomized Clinical Trial," *Prog Neuropsychopharmacol Biol Psychiatry*, 2007, August 8 [Epub ahead of print].

Biederman J, Swanson JM, Wigal SB, et al, "Efficacy and Safety of Modafinil Film-Coated Tablets in Children and Adolescents With Attention-Deficit/Hyperactivity Disorder: Results of a Randomized, Double-Blind, Placebo-Controlled, Flexible-Dose Study," *Pediatrics*, 2005, 116(6):e777-84.

Broughton RJ, Fleming JA, George, CF, et al, "Randomized, Double-Blind, Placebo-Controlled Crossover Trial of Modafinil in the Treatment of Excessive Daytime Sleepiness in Narcolepsy," *Neurology*, 1997, 49(2):444-51.

Greenhill LL, Biederman J, Boellner SW, etal, "A Randomized, Double-Blind, Placebo-Controlled Study of Modafinil Film-Coated Tablets in Children and Adolescents With Attention-Deficit/Hyperactivity Disorder," *J AM Acad Child Adolesc Psychiatry*, 2006, 45(5):503-11.

Grozinger M, "Interaction of Modafinil and Clomipramine as Comedication in a Narcoleptic Patient," *Clin Neuropharmacol*, 1998, 21(2):127-9.

Rugino TA and Copley TC, "Effects of Modafinil in Children With Attention-Deficit/Hyperactivity Disorder: An Open-Label Study," *J Am Acad Child Adolesc Psychiatry*, 2001, 40(2):230-5.

Swanson JM, Greenhill LL, Lopez FA, et al, "Modafinil Film-Coated Tablets in Children and Adolescents With Attention-Deficit/Hyperactivity Disorder: Results of a Randomized, Double-Blind, Placebo-Controlled, Fixed-Dose Study Followed by Abrupt Discontinuation," *J Clin Psychiatry*, 2006, 67(1):137-47.

U.S. Modafinil in Narcolepsy Multicenter Study Group, "Randomized Trial of Modafinil for the Treatment of Pathological Somnolence in Narcolepsy," *Ann Neurol*, 1998, 43(1):88-97.

Wigal SB, Biederman J, Swanson JM, et al, "Efficacy and Safety of Modafinil Film-Coated Tablets in Children and Adolescents With or Without Prior Stimulant Treatment for Attention-Deficit/Hyperactivity Disorder: Pooled Analysis of 3 Randomized, Double-Blind, Placebo-Controlled Studies," *Prim Care Companion J Clin Psychiatry*, 2006, 8(6):352-60.

◆ **MOM** *see* Magnesium Hydroxide *on page 855*

Mometasone Furoate
(moe MET a sone FYOOR oh ate)

Medication Safety Issues
Sound-alike/look-alike issues:
Elocon® lotion may be confused with ophthalmic solutions. Manufacturer's labeling emphasizes the product is **NOT** for use in the eyes.

Related Information
Corticosteroids *on page 1487*

U.S. Brand Names Asmanex® Twisthaler®; Elocon®; Nasonex®

Canadian Brand Names Elocom®; Nasonex®; PMS-Mometasone; ratio-Mometasone; Taro-Mometasone

Therapeutic Category Adrenal Corticosteroid; Anti-inflammatory Agent; Antiasthmatic; Corticosteroid, Inhalant (Oral); Corticosteroid, Intranasal; Corticosteroid, Topical; Glucocorticoid

Generic Available Yes: Cream, lotion, ointment

Use
Oral inhalation: Maintenance treatment of asthma as prophylactic therapy (FDA approved in ages ≥4 years and adults); **NOT** indicated for the relief of acute bronchospasm. Also used to help reduce or discontinue oral corticosteroid therapy for asthma (see Additional Information)

Intranasal: Treatment of seasonal and perennial allergic rhinitis (FDA approved in ages ≥2 years and adults); prevention of seasonal allergic rhinitis (FDA approved in ages ≥12 years and adults); treatment of nasal polyps (FDA approved in adults)

Topical: Relief of the inflammation and pruritus associated with corticosteroid-responsive dermatoses [medium potency topical corticosteroid]; **Note:** Due to lack of established safety and efficacy in specific age groups, the cream and ointment are not recommended for use in children <2 years of age and the lotion is not recommended for use in children <12 years of age (see also Additional Information)

Pregnancy Risk Factor C

Pregnancy Considerations Adverse events were observed in animal studies following topical and SubQ administration. Hypoadrenalism may occur in infants born to women receiving corticosteroids during pregnancy. Monitor these infants closely after birth. A decrease in fetal growth has not been observed with inhaled corticosteroid use during pregnancy. Inhaled corticosteroids are recommended for the treatment of asthma (most information available using budesonide) and allergic rhinitis during pregnancy. In general, the use of topical corticosteroids during pregnancy is not considered to have significant risk; however, intrauterine growth retardation in the infant has been reported (rare). The use of large amounts or for prolonged periods of time should be avoided.

Lactation Excretion in breast milk unknown/use caution

Breast-Feeding Considerations Systemic corticosteroids are excreted in human milk; however, information for mometasone is not available. The use of inhaled corticosteroids is not considered a contraindication to breast-feeding. Hypertension in the nursing infant has been reported following corticosteroid ointment applied to the nipples. Use with caution.

Contraindications Hypersensitivity to mometasone or any component (see Warnings); primary treatment of status asthmaticus

Warnings
Oral inhalation: Fatalities have occurred due to adrenal insufficiency in asthmatic patients during and after switching from systemic corticosteroids to aerosol steroids (see Additional Information); several months may be required for full recovery of hypothalamic-pituitary-adrenal (HPA) function; patients receiving higher doses of systemic corticosteroids (eg, adults receiving ≥20 mg of prednisone per day) may be at greater risk; during this period of HPA suppression, aerosol steroids do **not** provide the systemic glucocorticoid or mineralocorticoid activity needed to treat patients requiring stress doses (ie, patients with major stress such as trauma, surgery, infections, or other conditions associated with severe electrolyte loss). When used at high doses or for a prolonged time, hypercorticism and HPA suppression (including adrenal crisis) may occur; use with inhaled or systemic corticosteroids (even alternate-day dosing) may increase risk of HPA suppression. Acute adrenal insufficiency may occur with abrupt withdrawal after long-term use or with stress; withdrawal and

discontinuation of corticosteroids should be done carefully; patients with HPA axis suppression may require doses of systemic glucocorticosteroids prior to, during, and after unusual stress (eg, surgery). Immunosuppression may occur; patients may be more susceptible to infections; avoid exposure to chickenpox and measles. Switching patients from systemic corticosteroids to aerosol steroids may unmask allergic conditions previously treated by the systemic steroid. Bronchospasm may occur after use of inhaled asthma medications (see Additional Information).

Powder for oral inhalation (Asmanex® Twisthaler®) contains lactose (milk proteins) which may cause allergic reactions in patients with severe milk protein allergy.

Nasal: Acute adrenal insufficiency or corticosteroid withdrawal may occur when replacing a systemic corticosteroid with a nasal corticosteroid; hypothalamic-pituitary-adrenal (HPA) axis suppression or hypercorticism may occur, especially in younger children or in patients receiving high doses for a prolonged period of time. Immunosuppression may occur; avoid exposure to chickenpox and measles.

Topical: Adverse systemic effects may occur when topical steroids are used on large areas of the body, denuded areas, for prolonged periods of time, with an occlusive dressing, and/or in infants or small children; infants and small children may be more susceptible to HPA axis suppression or other systemic toxicities due to a larger skin surface area to body mass ratio; use with caution in pediatric patients and for no longer than 3 weeks

Precautions Avoid using higher than recommended doses; suppression of HPA axis function, suppression of linear growth (ie, reduction of growth velocity), reduced bone mineral density, hypercorticism (Cushing's syndrome), hyperglycemia, or glucosuria may occur; titrate to lowest effective dose; these adverse effects (as well as intracranial hypertension) may also occur with topical use and have been reported in pediatric patients (see also Additional Information). Do not use topical mometasone furoate products for the treatment of diaper dermatitis. Use with extreme caution in patients with respiratory tuberculosis, untreated systemic infections, ocular herpes simplex. Nasal corticosteroids are not recommended for patients with recent nasal trauma, nasal surgery, or nasal septum ulcers, due to inhibition of wound healing. Rarely, local fungal infections, immediate hypersensitivity reactions, nasal septum perforation, or increased intraocular pressure may occur with intranasal corticosteroid use; glaucoma and/or cataracts have also been reported.

Adverse Reactions

Nasal/oral inhalation:

Cardiovascular: Chest pain

Central nervous system: Headache; fatigue (oral inhalation), depression (oral inhalation), insomnia (oral inhalation), fever (oral inhalation)

Endocrine & metabolic: Dysmenorrhea; HPA suppression, Cushing's syndrome, growth suppression (oral inhalation)

Gastrointestinal: Vomiting, nausea, diarrhea, dyspepsia, abdominal pain, oral candidiasis; taste disturbance (rare)

Hematologic: Bruising

Neuromuscular & skeletal: Musculoskeletal pain, arthralgia, myalgia; bone mineral density decreased (oral inhalation)

Ocular: Conjunctivitis, rarely: IOP increased, glaucoma, cataracts (oral inhalation)

Otic: Earache, otitis media

Respiratory: Pharyngitis, cough, dysphonia, epistaxis, upper respiratory tract infection, sinusitis, asthma, bronchitis, nasal irritation, rhinitis, wheezing; nasal burning and irritation; nasal ulcers (rare), nasal

candidiasis (rare), nasal septum perforation (rare), smell disturbance (rare)

Miscellaneous: Viral infection, flu-like symptoms; cases of hypersensitivity reactions, anaphylaxis, and angioedema have been reported

Topical use: Dermatologic: Bacterial skin infection, burning, tingling, stinging, furunculosis, pruritus, skin atrophy, folliculitis, moniliasis, paresthesia, skin depigmentation, acneform reaction, itching, rosacea

Drug Interactions

Metabolism/Transport Effects Substrate of CYP3A4 (minor)

Avoid Concomitant Use

Avoid concomitant use of Mometasone with any of the following: Aldesleukin; BCG; Natalizumab; Pimecrolimus; Tacrolimus (Topical); Vaccines (Live)

Increased Effect/Toxicity

Mometasone may increase the levels/effects of: Leflunomide; Natalizumab; Vaccines (Live)

The levels/effects of Mometasone may be increased by: Denosumab; Pimecrolimus; Tacrolimus (Topical); Trastuzumab

Decreased Effect

Mometasone may decrease the levels/effects of: Aldesleukin; BCG; Corticorelin; Sipuleucel-T; Vaccines (Inactivated); Vaccines (Live)

The levels/effects of Mometasone may be decreased by: Echinacea

Stability

Cream: Store between 2°C to 25°C (36°F to 77°F)

Lotion: Store between 2°C to 30°C (36°F to 86°F)

Nasal spray: Store between 2°C to 25°C (36°F to 77°F); protect from light

Ointment: Store at 25°C (77°F); excursions permitted to 15°C to 30°C (59°F to 86°F)

Oral inhaler: Store at 25°C (77°F) in a dry place; excursions permitted to 15°C to 30°C (59°F to 86°F); discard inhaler 45 days after opening foil pouch (or when dose counter reads "00")

Mechanism of Action Controls the rate of protein synthesis, depresses the migration of polymorphonuclear leukocytes and fibroblasts, reverses capillary permeability, and stabilizes lysosomal membranes at the cellular level to prevent or control inflammation

Pharmacodynamics Clinical effects are due to direct local effect rather than systemic absorption

Onset of action: Intranasal: Improvement in allergic rhinitis symptoms may be seen within 11 hours

Maximum effect: Intranasal: Within 1-2 weeks after starting therapy; oral inhalation: 1-2 weeks or more

Duration after discontinuation: Oral inhalation: Several days or more

Pharmacokinetics (Adult data unless noted)

Absorption:

Intranasal: Undetectable in plasma

Oral inhalation: Systemic absorption: Adults (single dose): <1%

Topical: 0.4% of the applied dose of the cream and 0.7% of the applied dose of the ointment enter the circulation after 8 hours of contact with normal skin (without occlusion); absorption is increased by occlusive dressings or with decreased integrity of skin (eg, inflammation or skin disease)

Distribution: V_{dss}: Adults: 152 L

Protein binding: 98% to 99%

Metabolism: Extensive in the liver to multiple metabolites; no major metabolites are detectable in the plasma; *in vitro* incubation studies identified one minor metabolite, 6 Beta-hydroxymometasone furoate, formed via cytochrome P450 CYP3A4 pathway

Bioavailability: Oral inhalation: Single dose: <1%

◀ Half-life: Adults: Mean: 5 hours

Elimination: Metabolites are excreted primarily via the bile with a limited amount via urine; after oral inhalation 74% of the dose was excreted in the feces and 8% in the urine (none as unchanged drug)

Usual Dosage

Nasal spray: Titrate to lowest effective dose

Allergic rhinitis:

Children 2-11 years: 1 spray (50 mcg) in each nostril once daily

Children ≥12 years and Adults: 2 sprays (100 mcg) in each nostril once daily; when used for the prevention of allergic rhinitis, treatment should begin 2-4 weeks prior to pollen season

Nasal polyps: Adults ≥18 years: 2 sprays (100 mcg) in each nostril twice daily; 2 sprays (100 mcg) in each nostril once daily may be effective in some patients

Oral inhalation: **Note:** Maximum effects may not be seen until 1-2 weeks or longer; doses should be titrated to the lowest effective dose once asthma is controlled

Children 4-11 years (regardless of prior therapy): **Note:** Use 110 mcg inhaler: Initial: 1 inhalation (110 mcg) once daily, administered in the evening. Maximum dose: 1 inhalation/day (110 mcg/day)

Children ≥12 years and Adults:

Patients previously treated with bronchodilators only or with inhaled corticosteroids: Initial: 1 inhalation (220 mcg) once daily, administered in the evening; may increase dose after 2 weeks if adequate response not obtained. Maximum dose: 2 inhalations/day (440 mcg/day); may be administered as 1 inhalation twice daily or 2 inhalations once daily in the evening

Patients previously treated with oral corticosteroids: Initial: 2 inhalations (440 mcg) twice daily. Maximum dose: 4 inhalations/day (880 mcg/day)

NIH Asthma Guidelines (NAEPP, 2007) [give in divided doses]: **Note:** 220 mcg inhaler delivers 200 mcg mometasone furoate per actuation; NAEPP uses doses based on delivery, while manufacturer recommended doses are based on inhaler amount

Children ≥12 years and Adults:

"Low" dose: 200 mcg/day (200 mcg/puff: 1 puff/day)

"Medium" dose: 400 mcg/day (200 mcg/puff: 2 puffs/day)

"High" dose: >400 mcg/day (200 mcg/puff: >2 puffs/day)

Topical: Apply sparingly, do not use occlusive dressings. Discontinue therapy when control is achieved; reassess diagnosis if no improvement is seen in 2 weeks.

Cream, ointment: Children ≥2 years and Adults: Apply a thin film to affected area once daily; do not use in pediatric patients for >3 weeks

Lotion: Children ≥12 years and Adults: Apply a few drops to affected area once daily; massage lightly into skin

Administration

Oral inhalation: Remove inhaler from foil pouch; write date on cap label. Keep inhaler upright while removing cap, twisting in a counterclockwise direction; lifting the cap loads the device with the medication. Exhale fully prior to bringing the inhaler up to the mouth. Place inhaler in mouth, while holding it in a horizontal position. Close lips around the mouthpiece and inhale quickly and deeply. Remove the inhaler from your mouth and hold your breath for about 10 seconds, if possible. Do not exhale into inhaler. Wipe the mouthpiece dry and replace the cap immediately after each inhalation; rotate fully until click is heard. Rinse mouth with water (without swallowing) after inhalation to decrease chance of oral candidiasis. Avoid contact of the inhaler with any liquids; do not wash; wipe with dry cloth or tissue if needed. Discard the inhaler 45 days after opening foil pouch or when dose counter reads "00".

Intranasal spray: Shake well prior to each use; clear nasal passages by blowing nose prior to use; occlude one nostril while administering to the other. Nasal spray must be primed before first use (10 actuations or until a fine spray appears) or after >1 week of nonuse (2 actuations or until a fine spray appears); discard unit after 120 metered sprays are used. Spray should be administered once or twice daily, at a regular interval. Do not spray into eyes or directly onto nasal septum. After removing nasal spray from container, avoid prolonged exposure of product to direct light; brief exposure to light (with normal use) is acceptable.

Topical: Apply sparingly; avoid contact with eyes. Do not apply to face, underarms, or groin unless directed by physician. Do not wrap or bandage affected area unless directed by physician. Do not use for treatment of diaper dermatitis or in diaper area.

Lotion: Hold nozzle of bottle close to affected area and gently squeeze bottle

Monitoring Parameters Monitor growth in pediatric patients; assess HPA axis suppression in patients using topical steroids applied to a large surface area or to areas under occlusion. Intranasal and oral inhalation: Check mucous membranes for signs of fungal infection. Oral inhalation: Monitor pulmonary function tests (eg, FEV_1, peak flow); monitor for decreased bone density in patients at higher risk (eg, family history of osteoporosis; prolonged immobilization; chronic use of anticonvulsants, cortico-steroids or other medications that can reduce bone mass).

Patient Information Notify physician if condition being treated persists or worsens. Do not decrease dose or discontinue without physician approval. Avoid exposure to chickenpox or measles; if exposed, seek medical advice without delay

Oral inhalation: Not a bronchodilator and not indicated for relief of bronchospasm or acute episodes of asthma. May take 1-2 weeks before effects of medication are seen. May cause systemic effects including hypercorticism, adrenal suppression, reduced growth velocity in children, or reduction in bone mineral density. Report sore mouth or mouth lesions to physician; carefully read and follow the Patient's Instructions for Use leaflet that accompanies the product

Topical: Avoid contact with eyes; do not use occlusive dressings or other corticosteroid-containing products unless directed by physician; do not use for longer than directed; contact physician if no improvement is seen in 2 weeks

Additional Information When using mometasone oral inhalation to help reduce or discontinue oral corticosteroid therapy, begin prednisone taper after at least 1 week of mometasone inhalation therapy; do not decrease predni-sone faster than 2.5 mg/day on a weekly basis; monitor patients for signs of asthma instability and adrenal insufficiency (see Warnings); decrease mometasone to lowest effective dose **after** prednisone reduction is complete. If bronchospasm with wheezing occurs after oral inhalation use, a fast-acting bronchodilator may be used; discontinue orally inhaled corticosteroid and initiate alternative chronic therapy.

Several studies conducted in children 6-23 months of age with atopic dermatitis demonstrated a high incidence of adrenal suppression when topical mometasone furoate products were applied once daily for approximately 3 weeks over an average body surface area of about 40%. Of the patients with normal baseline adrenal function, adrenal suppression occurred in 16% of patients using the cream, 27% of patients using the ointment, and 29% of patients using the lotion. Follow-up testing 2-4 weeks after discontinuation of therapy demonstrated suppressed HPA axis function in 1 of 5 patients who used the cream, 3 of 8 patients who used the ointment, and 1 of 8 patients who used the lotion.

Dosage Forms Excipient information presented when available (limited, particularly for generics); consult specific product labeling.

Cream, topical, as furoate: 0.1% (15 g, 45 g)
Elocon®: 0.1% (15 g, 45 g)
Lotion, topical, as furoate: 0.1% (30 mL, 60 mL)
Elocon®: 0.1% (30 mL, 60 mL) [contains isopropyl alcohol 40%]
Ointment, topical, as furoate: 0.1% (15 g, 45 g)
Elocon®: 0.1% (15 g, 45 g)
Powder for oral inhalation, as furoate:
Asmanex® Twisthaler®: 110 mcg (30 units) [contains lactose; delivers 100 mcg/actuation]; 220 mcg (14 units, 30 units, 60 units, 120 units) [contains lactose; delivers 200 mcg/actuation]
Suspension, intranasal, as furoate [spray]:
Nasonex®: 50 mcg/spray (17 g) [delivers 120 sprays; contains benzalkonium chloride]

References

National Asthma Education and Prevention Program (NAEPP), "Expert Panel Report 3 (EPR-3): Guidelines for the Diagnosis and Management of Asthma," *Clinical Practice Guidelines*, National Institutes of Health, National Heart, Lung, and Blood Institute, NIH Publication No. 08-4051, prepublication 2007; available at http://www.nhlbi.nih.gov/guidelines/asthma/asthgdln.htm.

◆ **Mometasone Furoate** *see* Mometasone Furoate *on page 942*

◆ **MOM (Magnesium Hydroxide)** *see* Magnesium Supplements *on page 859*

◆ **Monacolin K** *see* Lovastatin *on page 850*

◆ **Monarc-M™** *see* Antihemophilic Factor (Human) *on page 109*

◆ **Monistat® (Can)** *see* Miconazole *on page 927*

◆ **Monistat® 1 [OTC]** *see* Miconazole *on page 927*

◆ **Monistat® 3 [OTC]** *see* Miconazole *on page 927*

◆ **Monistat® 3 (Can)** *see* Miconazole *on page 927*

◆ **Monistat® 7 [OTC]** *see* Miconazole *on page 927*

◆ **Monoclate-P®** *see* Antihemophilic Factor (Human) *on page 109*

◆ **Monoclonal Antibody** *see* Muromonab-CD3 *on page 955*

◆ **Monodox®** *see* Doxycycline *on page 479*

◆ **Mononine®** *see* Factor IX *on page 557*

◆ **Monopril® [DSC]** *see* Fosinopril *on page 627*

◆ **Monopril® (Can)** *see* Fosinopril *on page 627*

Montelukast (mon te LOO kast)

Medication Safety Issues
Sound-alike/look-alike issues:
Singulair® may be confused with Sinequan®
Related Information
Asthma *on page 1697*
U.S. Brand Names Singulair®
Canadian Brand Names Singulair®
Therapeutic Category Antiasthmatic; Leukotriene Receptor Antagonist
Generic Available No
Use Prophylaxis and chronic treatment of asthma (FDA approved in ages ≥12 months and adults); relief of symptoms of seasonal allergic rhinitis (FDA approved in ages ≥2 years and adults) and perennial allergic rhinitis (FDA approved in ages ≥6 months and adults); prevention of exercise-induced bronchospasm (FDA approved in ages ≥15 years and adults)
Pregnancy Risk Factor B

Pregnancy Considerations Montelukast was not teratogenic in animal studies, however, there are no adequate and well-controlled studies in pregnant women. Based on limited data, structural defects have been reported in neonates exposed to montelukast *in utero*; however, a specific pattern and relationship to montelukast has not been established. Healthcare providers should report any prenatal exposures to the montelukast pregnancy registry at (800) 986-8999.

Lactation Excretion in breast milk unknown/use caution

Contraindications Hypersensitivity to montelukast or any component

Warnings Montelukast is not indicated for use in the reversal of bronchospasm in acute asthma attacks, including status asthmaticus; therapy with montelukast can be continued during acute exacerbations of asthma; rare cases of systemic eosinophilia, sometimes presenting with clinical features of vasculitis (consistent with Churg-Strauss syndrome) have been reported; these reactions may also be associated with a reduction in oral corticosteroid dosage; a causal association with montelukast has not been established. Postmarketing reports of behavioral changes (eg, agitation, aggression, depression, insomnia, tremor) have been noted in pediatric and adult patients. In a retrospective analysis performed by Merck, serious behavior-related events were rare (Philip, 2009); monitor.

Precautions Phenobarbital reduces the AUC of montelukast ~40% following a single 10 mg dosage; no dosage adjustment of montelukast is indicated, however, appropriate clinical monitoring is indicated when potent cytochrome P450 enzyme inducers, such as phenobarbital or rifampin, are coadministered with montelukast. Chewable tablets contain phenylalanine which must be avoided (or used with caution) in patients with phenylketonuria.

Adverse Reactions
Cardiovascular: Vasculitis (rare)

Central nervous system: Agitation, aggression, anxiety, asthenia, behavior mood changes, depression, dizziness, dream abnormalities, drowsiness, fatigue, fever, hallucinations, headache, hostility, irritability, restlessness, somnambulism, suicidality

Dermatologic: Dermatitis, eczema, rash, urticaria

Gastrointestinal: Abdominal pain, diarrhea, dyspepsia, gastroenteritis, nausea

Hematologic: Eosinophilia

Hepatic: Liver enzymes elevated

Ocular: Conjunctivitis

Otic: Ear pain, otitis

Respiratory: Cough, laryngitis, nasal congestion, pharyngitis, pneumonia, rhinorrhea, sinusitis, tonsillitis, upper respiratory infection, wheezing

Miscellaneous: Hypersensitivity reactions, influenza, viral infection

<1% and/or post-marketing: Angioedema, arthralgia, bruising, cholestatic hepatitis, cramps, edema, epistaxis, eosinophilia, erythema nodosum, hepatic eosinophilic infiltration, hepatic injury, mylagia, palpitations, pancreatitis, seizure, tremor, vomiting

Drug Interactions
Metabolism/Transport Effects **Substrate** (major) of CYP2C9, 3A4; **Inhibits** CYP2C8 (weak), 2C9 (weak)

Avoid Concomitant Use There are no known interactions where it is recommended to avoid concomitant use.

Increased Effect/Toxicity
The levels/effects of Montelukast may be increased by: CYP2C9 Inhibitors (Moderate); CYP2C9 Inhibitors (Strong)

Decreased Effect

The levels/effects of Montelukast may be decreased by:
CYP2C9 Inducers (Highly Effective); CYP3A4 Inducers (Strong); Deferasirox; Herbs (CYP3A4 Inducers); Peginterferon Alfa-2b

Stability Store at room temperature; protect from moisture and light; granules must be administered within 15 minutes of opening the packet

Mechanism of Action Montelukast is a selective leukotriene receptor antagonist that inhibits the cysteinyl leukotriene CysLT$_1$ receptor. This activity produces inhibition of the effects of this leukotriene on bronchial smooth muscle resulting in the attenuation of bronchoconstriction and decreased vascular permeability, mucosal edema, and mucus production.

Pharmacokinetics (Adult data unless noted)

Absorption: Rapid

Distribution: V$_d$: Adults: 8-11 L

Protein binding: >99%

Metabolism: Extensive by cytochrome P450 3A4 and 2C9

Bioavailability: Tablet:
5 mg: 63% to 73%
10 mg: 64%

Time to peak serum concentration: Tablet:
4 mg: 2 hours
5 mg: 2-2.5 hours
10 mg: 3-4 hours

Elimination: Exclusively via bile; <0.2% excreted in urine

Usual Dosage Oral:

Treatment of asthma and allergic rhinitis (safety and efficacy for treatment of asthma in children <12 months or perennial allergic rhinitis in infants <6 months has not been established):

Children
6 months to 5 years: 4 mg/day
6-14 years: 5 mg/day

Adolescents >14 years and Adults: 10 mg/day

Prevention of exercise-induced bronchospasm: Adolescents ≥15 years and Adults: 10 mg at least 2 hours prior to exercise; additional doses should not be administered within 24 hours. Daily administration to prevent exercise-induced bronchospasm has not been evaluated.

Note: None of the clinical trials evaluated the safety and efficacy of therapy with morning dosing; the pharmacokinetics of montelukast are similar whether dosed in the morning or evening.

Administration Oral: Administer in the evening without regard to meals. Granules may be administered directly into the mouth or mixed in cold or room temperature soft foods; based on stability studies, only applesauce, mashed carrots, rice, and ice cream should be used; granules are not intended to be dissolved in liquid and must be administered within 15 minutes of opening the packet; liquids may be taken subsequent to administration

Monitoring Parameters Pulmonary function tests (FEV-1), improvement in asthma symptoms, behavioral effects

Patient Information Take regularly as prescribed, even during symptom-free periods. Do not use to treat acute episodes of asthma. Do not decrease the dose or stop taking any other asthma medications unless instructed by a physician.

Additional Information Recent studies of montelukast use in acute asthma and RSV bronchiolitis have shown promising results. Pulmonary function tests improved significantly in adult patients receiving a single dose (10 mg) montelukast along with I.V. prednisolone at the onset of an acute asthma exacerbation (Cylly, 2003). Pediatric patients with RSV positive bronchiolitis receiving daily montelukast demonstrated fewer symptoms when compared with placebo treated controls (Bisgaard, 2003).

Dosage Forms Excipient information presented when available (limited, particularly for generics); consult specific product labeling.

Granules:
Singulair®: 4 mg/packet (30s)
Tablet:
Singulair®: 10 mg
Tablet, chewable:
Singulair®: 4 mg [contains phenylalanine 0.674 mg; cherry flavor]; 5 mg [contains phenylalanine 0.842 mg; cherry flavor]

References

Bisgaard H, "A Randomized Trial of Montelukast in Respiratory Syncytial Virus Postbronchiolitis," *Am J Respir Crit Care Med*, 2003, 167(3):379-83.

Cylly A, Kara A, Ozdemir T, et al, "Effects of Oral Montelukast on Airway Function in Acute Asthma," *Respir Med*, 2003, 97(5):533-6.

"Guidelines for the Diagnosis and Management of Asthma. NAEPP Expert Panel Report 3," August 2007, www.nhlbi.nih.gov/guidelines/asthma/asthgdln.pdf.

"National Asthma Education and Prevention Program. Expert Panel Report: Guidelines for the Diagnosis and Management of Asthma Update on Selected Topics–2002," *J Allergy Clin Immunol*, 2002, 110 (5 Suppl):S141-219.

Philip G, Hustad CM, Malice MP, et al, "Analysis of Behavior-Related Adverse Experiences in Clinical Trials of Montelukast," *J Allergy Clin Immunol*, 2009, 124(4):699-706.

Philip G, Hustad C, Noonan G, et al, "Reports of Suicidality in Clinical Trials of Montelukast," *J Allergy Clin Immunol*, 2009, 124(4):691-6.

◆ **Montelukast Sodium** *see* Montelukast *on page* 945

◆ **More Attenuated Enders Strain** *see* Measles Virus Vaccine (Live) *on page* 866

◆ **MoreDophilus® [OTC]** *see* Lactobacillus *on page* 790

◆ **Morphine HP® (Can)** *see* Morphine Sulfate *on page* 946

◆ **Morphine LP® Epidural (Can)** *see* Morphine Sulfate *on page* 946

Morphine Sulfate (MOR feen SUL fate)

Medication Safety Issues

Sound-alike/look-alike issues:
Morphine may be confused with HYDROmorphone, methadone
Morphine sulfate may be confused with magnesium sulfate
Kadian® may be confused with Kapidex™ [DSC]
MS Contin® may be confused with Oxycontin®
MSO$_4$ and MS are error-prone abbreviations (mistaken as magnesium sulfate)
Avinza® may be confused with Evista®, Invanz®
Roxanol™ may be confused with OxyFast®, Roxicet™, Roxicodone®

High alert medication: The Institute for Safe Medication Practices (ISMP) includes this medication (I.V. formulation) among its list of drug classes which have a heightened risk of causing significant patient harm when used in error.

Use care when prescribing and/or administering morphine solutions. These products are available in different concentrations. Always prescribe dosage in mg; **not** by volume (mL).

Use caution when selecting a morphine formulation for use in neurologic infusion pumps (eg, Medtronic delivery systems). The product should be appropriately labeled as "preservative-free" and suitable for intraspinal use via continuous infusion. In addition, the product should be formulated in a pH range that is compatible with the device operation specifications.

Significant differences exist between oral and I.V. dosing. Use caution when converting from one route of administration to another.

Related Information

Adult ACLS Algorithms *on page 1463*
Compatibility of Medications Mixed in a Syringe *on page 1713*
Laboratory Detection of Drugs in Urine *on page 1706*
Medications for Which A Single Dose May Be Fatal When Ingested By A Toddler *on page 1709*
Opioid Analgesics Comparison *on page 1510*
Preprocedure Sedatives in Children *on page 1688*

U.S. Brand Names Astramorph/PF™; Avinza®; Depo-Dur®; Duramorph®; Infumorph® 200; Infumorph® 500; Kadian®; MS Contin®; Oramorph® SR; Roxanol™ [DSC]

Canadian Brand Names Doloral; Kadian®; M-Eslon®; M.O.S.-SR®; M.O.S.-Sulfate®; M.O.S.® 10; M.O.S.® 20; M.O.S.® 30; Morphine HP®; Morphine LP® Epidural; MS Contin®; MS-IR®; Novo-Morphine SR; PMS-Morphine Sulfate SR; ratio-Morphine; ratio-Morphine SR; Statex®

Therapeutic Category Analgesic, Narcotic

Generic Available Yes: Excludes capsule, controlled release tablet, sustained release tablet, extended release liposomal suspension for injection

Use Relief of moderate to severe acute and chronic pain (FDA approved in adults); has also been used for pain of MI; relief from dyspnea of acute left ventricular failure and pulmonary edema; preanesthetic medication

Astramorph/PF™, Duramorph®: I.V., epidural, or intrathecal (both at the lumbar level) management of pain unresponsive to non-narcotic analgesics (FDA approved in adults)

Controlled, extended, and sustained release products (eg, Avinza®, Kadian®, MS Contin®, Oramorph® SR): Management of moderate to severe **chronic** pain when continuous, around-the-clock opioid analgesia is required for an extended amount of time (FDA approved in adults) (**not** for PRN use; **Note:** Kadian® is **not** indicated for relief of pain for the first 12-24 hour after surgery)

DepoDur®: Epidural (at the lumbar level) single-dose management of surgical pain in adults; may be used in women undergoing cesarean section following clamping of the umbilical cord (FDA approved in adults) (not for use in vaginal labor and delivery)

Infumorph®: Intrathecal (at the lumbar level) or epidural infusion via microinfusion device for the treatment of intractable chronic pain (FDA approved in adults)

Restrictions C-II

Medication Guide An FDA-approved patient medication guide, which is available with the product information and as follows, must be dispensed with this medication for each new outpatient prescription and refill.

Oral solution: http://www.fda.gov/downloads/Drugs/Drug-Safety/UCM199333.pdf

Pregnancy Risk Factor C

Pregnancy Considerations Teratogenic effects were not observed in animal studies; however reduced growth and behavioral abnormalities in offspring have been observed. Morphine crosses the human placenta. The frequency of congenital malformations has not been reported to be greater than expected in children from mothers treated with morphine during pregnancy. However, following *in utero* exposure infants may exhibit withdrawal, decreased brain volume (reversible), small size, decreased ventilatory response to CO2, and increased risk of sudden infant death syndrome. In patients with chronic, noncancer pain, minimal (if any) opioids should be used during pregnancy. Neonates born to mothers receiving chronic opioids during pregnancy should be monitored for neonatal withdrawal syndrome.

DepoDur® may be used in women undergoing cesarean section following clamping of the umbilical cord; not for use in vaginal labor and delivery.

Lactation Enters breast milk/use caution (AAP rates "compatible")

Breast-Feeding Considerations Morphine concentrates in breast milk, with a milk to plasma AUC ratio of 2.5:1. Detectable serum levels of morphine can be found in infants following morphine administration to nursing mothers. Treatment of the mother with single doses of morphine is not expected to cause detrimental effects in nursing infants. Breast-feeding following chronic use or in neonates with hepatic or renal dysfunction may lead to higher levels of morphine in the infant and a risk of adverse effects. Breast-feeding should be delayed for 48 hours after DepoDur® administration.

Contraindications Hypersensitivity to morphine sulfate or any component (see Warnings); severe respiratory depression or respiratory depression in a setting without resuscitative equipment or appropriate monitoring; acute or severe asthma; hypercarbia; upper airway obstruction; severe liver or renal insufficiency; GI obstruction especially known or suspected paralytic ileus; pregnancy (prolonged use or high doses at term). DepoDur® is also contra-indicated in patients with suspected or known CNS injury, increased ICP, circulatory shock, or conditions that preclude an epidural injection. Duramorph® is also labeled as being contraindicated in patients with depleted blood volume or concurrent administration of phenothiazines or general anesthetics (severe hypotension may occur).

Warnings CNS and respiratory depression may occur; neonates and infants <3 months of age are more susceptible to respiratory depression, use with caution and in reduced doses in this age group. Use only preservative free injections for epidural or intrathecal administration and in neonates. Use with extreme caution in patients with COPD, cor pulmonale, hypoxia, hypercapnia, pre-existing respiratory depression, significantly decreased respiratory reserve, head injury, increased ICP, other intracranial lesions. Severe hypotension may occur; use with caution in patients with circulatory shock, hypovolemia, impaired myocardial function or those receiving drugs which may exaggerate hypotensive effects (including phenothiazines or general anesthetics). Morphine may obscure diagnosis or clinical course of patients with acute abdominal conditions.

Physical and psychological dependence may occur; abrupt discontinuation after prolonged use may result in withdrawal symptoms or seizures. Warn patient of possible impairment of alertness or physical coordination (see Patient Information). Interactions with other CNS drugs may occur (see Drug Interactions). Healthcare provider should be alert to problems of abuse, misuse, and diversion. Infants born to women physically dependent on opioids will also be physically dependent and may experience respiratory difficulties or opioid withdrawal symptoms.

A toxic or potentially fatal dose of morphine may be rapidly released if extended, sustained, or controlled release products are chewed, crushed, broken or dissolved (see Administration) or if these products are abused by crushing, chewing, snorting, or injecting the dissolved product (see Additional Information). Consumption of alcoholic beverages or ethanol-containing products (prescription or nonprescription) while receiving Avinza® therapy may disrupt the extended-release formulation, causing a rapid release of morphine and potentially fatal overdose. Kadian® capsules are indicated for the treatment of moderate to severe chronic pain and are not intended for PRN use (see Use). Kadian® 100 mg and 200 mg capsules are for use in opioid-tolerant patients only; fatal respiratory depression may occur if these capsules or their contents are administered to patients who are not tolerant to high-dose opioids. MS Contin® 100 mg and 200 mg tablets are for use only in opioid-tolerant patients requiring >400 mg/day of morphine. Patients should be warned not to let others use these products, since severe adverse effects, including death, may result.

Prior to administration via epidural or intrathecal route, evaluate benefits versus risks in patients with infection at injection site, bleeding diatheses, or anticoagulation therapy. Only physicians experienced in the techniques and familiar with the clinical management of the adverse effects of epidural and intrathecal drug administration should administer drugs via the intraspinal route. When morphine is used via the epidural or intrathecal routes, severe adverse effects may occur, including significant respiratory depression; facilities must be properly equipped to resuscitate patients; monitor patients for delayed sedation. When DepoDur® is used, patients must be closely monitored for a minimum of 48 hours (due to prolonged effects of extended release epidural preparation). Monitor patients closely for a minimum of 24 hours after the initial epidural or intrathecal dose of Duramorph®. When Infumorph® is used, patients must be closely monitored for a minimum of 24 hours after the initial (single) test dose and as appropriate for the first several days after catheter implantation. Due to fewer potential adverse effects, the epidural route is preferred over the intrathecal route (intrathecal route is associated with a higher incidence of respiratory depression). Tolerance to morphine and increased epidural or intrathecal dosage requirements may occur (patients may require hospitalization and detoxification). Seizures may occur with high doses of intraspinal morphine. Myoclonic spasm of the lower extremities has been reported in adults receiving high doses of intrathecal morphine. Safety and efficacy of spinal morphine products have not been established in pediatric patients. Freezing may adversely affect modified-release mechanism of DepoDur®; check freeze indicator within carton prior to administration (see Stability).

Parenteral products are designed for administration by specific routes (I.V., intrathecal, epidural). Use caution when prescribing, dispensing, or administering so as to use formulations only by intended route(s). Injection may contain sodium metabisulfite which may cause allergic reactions in susceptible individuals; oral solution may contain sodium benzoate; benzoic acid (benzoate) is a metabolite of benzyl alcohol; large amounts of benzyl alcohol (≥99 mg/kg/day) have been associated with a potentially fatal toxicity ("gasping syndrome") in neonates; the "gasping syndrome" consists of metabolic acidosis, respiratory distress, gasping respirations, CNS dysfunction (including convulsions, intracranial hemorrhage), hypotension and cardiovascular collapse; avoid use of morphine sulfate products containing sodium benzoate in neonates; in vitro and animal studies have shown that benzoate displaces bilirubin from protein binding sites

Precautions Use with caution in patients with hypersensitivity reactions to other phenanthrene derivative opioid agonists (codeine, hydrocodone, hydromorphone, levorphanol, oxycodone, oxymorphone). Use with caution in patients with biliary tract disease or acute pancreatitis (morphine may cause spasm of the sphincter of Oddi); use with caution and decrease the dose in patients with Addison's disease, hypothyroidism, renal impairment, hepatic dysfunction (eg, cirrhosis), urethral stricture, prostatic hypertrophy, or in debilitated patients; use with caution in patients with CNS depression, toxic psychosis, seizure disorders, acute alcoholism, and delirium tremens.

Kadian® should be discontinued 24 hours prior to cordotomy or other interruption of pain transmission pathways (use parenteral short-acting opioids to control pain). Use Kadian® with great caution and decrease the dose in patients who are receiving other CNS depressants (respiratory depression, hypotension, profound sedation, or coma may result). The pharmacokinetics of Avinza® and Kadian® have not been studied in patients <18 years of age; the available capsule mg strength may not be appropriate for pediatric patients who are very young; sprinkling capsule contents on applesauce is **not** a suitable alternative for these patients; other oral products should be used.

When administered to a pregnant woman, I.V., epidural, and intrathecal morphine readily pass into the fetal circulation and may result in respiratory depression in the newborn; resuscitative equipment and naloxone should be available for the neonate

Adverse Reactions

Cardiovascular: Atrial fibrillation, bradycardia, chest pain, edema, hypotension, orthostatic hypotension, palpitations, peripheral vasodilation, syncope, tachycardia

Central nervous system: Amnesia, anxiety, apathy, ataxia, chills, CNS depression, depression, dizziness, drowsiness, euphoria, fever, headache (especially following epidural or intrathecal use), hypoesthesia, insomnia, intracranial pressure increased, lethargy, malaise, restlessness, sedation, seizure, vertigo; dysphoric reactions and toxic psychoses have been reported

Dermatologic: Pruritus (more common with epidural or intrathecal administration; may be due to histamine release; may be dose-related), urticaria

Endocrine & metabolic: Antidiuretic hormone release, gynecomastia, hyponatremia

Gastrointestinal: Anorexia, biliary tract spasm, constipation, dyspepsia, dysphagia, GERD, GI irritation, intestinal obstruction, nausea, paralytic ileus, vomiting, xerostomia

Genitourinary: Urinary retention (may be prolonged, up to 20 hours, following epidural or intrathecal use), urinary tract spasm (may be more common with epidural or intrathecal administration), urination decreased

Hematologic: Anemia, leukopenia, thrombocytopenia

Hepatic: Liver enzymes increased

Local: Pain at injection site

Neuromuscular & skeletal: Arthralgia, back pain, bone pain, paresthesia, trembling, weakness

Ocular: Miosis, vision problems

Respiratory: Asthma, atelectasis, dyspnea, hiccups, hypoxia, noncardiogenic pulmonary edema, respiratory depression, rhinitis

Miscellaneous: Anaphylaxis (extremely rare), diaphoresis, flu-like syndrome, histamine release, physical and psychological dependence

Drug Interactions

Metabolism/Transport Effects Substrate of CYP2D6 (minor)

Avoid Concomitant Use There are no known interactions where it is recommended to avoid concomitant use.

Increased Effect/Toxicity

Morphine Sulfate may increase the levels/effects of: Alcohol (Ethyl); Alvimopan; CNS Depressants; Desmopressin; Selective Serotonin Reuptake Inhibitors; Thiazide Diuretics

The levels/effects of Morphine Sulfate may be increased by: Amphetamines; Antipsychotic Agents (Phenothiazines); Succinylcholine

Decreased Effect

Morphine Sulfate may decrease the levels/effects of: Pegvisomant

The levels/effects of Morphine Sulfate may be decreased by: Ammonium Chloride; Mixed Agonist / Antagonist Opioids; Peginterferon Alfa-2b; Rifamycin Derivatives

Food Interactions

Avinza®: A high fat meal may delay absorption

Kadian®: Food may decrease the rate, but not the extent of absorption

MS Contin®: A fatty meal may slightly decrease peak plasma concentrations

Oral solution: Food may increase bioavailability

Oramorph® SR: Food has little to no effect on bioavailability

Stability

Suppositories: Refrigerate; do not freeze

Injection: Store at controlled room temperature. Protect from light. Degradation depends on pH and presence of oxygen; relatively stable in pH ≤4; darkening of solutions indicates degradation. Morphine solutions for injection are stable in $D_5^1/4NS$, $D_5^1/2NS$, D_5NS, D_5W, $D_{10}W$, LR, D_5LR, $^1/2NS$, NS, dextran 6% in dextrose, dextran 6% in NS.

Avinza® and Kadian®: Store at controlled room temperature. Protect from light and moisture

Duramorph®: Store in carton at controlled room temperature of 20°C to 25°C (65°F to 77°F); excursions permitted to 15°C to 30°C (59°F to 86°F). Protect from light; do not freeze. Discard unused portion of vial (vial does not contain preservative). Do not heat sterilize.

DepoDur®: Store in carton under refrigeration, 2°C to 8°C (36°F to 46°F). Do not freeze; do not use if product has been frozen or is suspected of having been frozen. Check freeze indicator (located on carton) before administration; do not administer if indicator bulb is pink or purple (this indicates drug may have been frozen). May store unopened vials at room temperature for up to 7 days. After withdrawal from vial, drug may be held at room temperature for ≤4 hours before use. Do not heat or gas sterilize. Discard unused portion of vial (vial does not contain preservatives). Do not mix with other medications.

Mechanism of Action Binds to opiate receptors in the CNS, causing inhibition of ascending pain pathways, altering the perception of and response to pain; produces generalized CNS depression

Pharmacodynamics See table.

Dosage Form / Route	Analgesia	
	Peak	Duration
Tablets	1 h	3-5 h
Oral solution	1 h	3-5 h
Epidural	1 h	12-20 h
Extended release tablets	3-4 h	8-12 h
Suppository	20-60 min	3-7 h
Subcutaneous injection	50-90 min	3-5 h
I.M. injection	30-60 min	3-5 h
I.V. injection	20 min	3-5 h

Pharmacokinetics (Adult data unless noted)

Absorption: Oral: Variable

Distribution: Distributes to skeletal muscle, liver, kidneys, lungs, intestinal tract, spleen, brain, and into breast milk; crosses placenta

V_d, apparent: Children 1.7-18.7 years with cancer: Median: 5.2 L/kg; a significantly higher V_d was observed in children <11 years (median: 7.1 L/kg) versus >11 years (median: 4.7 L/kg) (see Hunt, 1999)

V_d, apparent: Adults: 1-4.7 L/kg

Protein binding:

Premature Infants: <20%

Adults: 20% to 35%

Metabolism: In the liver via glucuronide conjugation to morphine-6-glucuronide (active) and morphine-3-glucuronide (inactive)

Half-life:

Preterm: 10-20 hours

Neonates: 7.6 hours (range: 4.5-13.3 hours)

Infants 1-3 months: 6.2 hours (range: 5-10 hours)

Infants 6 months to Children 2.5 years: 2.9 hours (range: 1.4-7.8 hours)

Preschool Children: 1-2 hours

Children 6-19 years with sickle cell disease: Mean ~1.3 hours

Adults: 2-4 hours

Elimination: Excreted unchanged in urine:

Neonates: 3% to 15%

Adults: 2% to 12%

Clearance: **Note:** Adult values are reached by 6 months to 2.5 years of age

Preterm: 0.5-3 mL/minute/kg

Neonates 1-7 days: Median: 5.5 mL/minute/kg (range: 3.2-8.4 mL/minute/kg)

Neonates 8-30 days: Median: 7.4 mL/minute/kg (range: 3.4-13.8 mL/minute/kg)

Infants 1-3 months: Median: 10.5 mL/minute/kg (range: 9.8-20.1 mL/minute/kg)

Infants 3-6 months: Median: 13.9 mL/minute/kg (range: 8.3-24.1 mL/minute/kg)

Infants 6 months to Children 2.5 years: Median: 21.7 mL/minute/kg (range: 5.8-28.6 mL/minute/kg)

Preschool Children: 20-40 mL/minute/kg

Children 1.7-18.7 years with cancer: Median: 23.1 mL/minute/kg; a significantly higher clearance was observed in children <11 years (median: 37.4 mL/minute/kg) versus >11 years (median: 21.9 mL/minute/kg) (see Hunt, 1999)

Children 6-19 years with sickle cell disease: Mean ~36 mL/minute/kg (range: 6-59 mL/minute/kg)

Adults: 10-20 mL/minute/kg

Usual Dosage Doses should be titrated to appropriate effect; when changing routes of administration in chronically treated patients, please note that oral doses are approximately one-half as effective as parenteral dose

Neonates (see Warnings; **Note: Use preservative free formulation**):

I.M., I.V., SubQ: Initial: 0.05 mg/kg every 4-8 hours; titrate carefully to effect; maximum dose: 0.1 mg/kg/dose

I.V. continuous infusion: Initial: 0.01 mg/kg/hour (10 mcg/kg/hour); do **not** exceed infusion rates of 0.015-0.02 mg/kg/hour due to decreased elimination, increased CNS sensitivity, and adverse effects; **Note:** Some centers may use slightly higher doses, especially in neonates who develop tolerance.

International Evidence-Based Group for Neonatal Pain recommendations (Anand, 2001): I.V.:

Intermittent dose: 0.05-0.1 mg/kg/dose

Continuous infusion: Range: 0.01-0.03 mg/kg/hour

Infants and Children:

Oral: Tablet and solution (prompt release): 0.2-0.5 mg/kg/dose every 4-6 hours as needed

Note: The American Pain Society (2008) recommends an initial oral dose of 0.3 mg/kg for children with severe pain.

I.M., I.V., SubQ: 0.1-0.2 mg/kg/dose every 2-4 hours as needed; may initiate at 0.05 mg/kg/dose; usual maximum dose: Infants: 2 mg/dose; Children 1-6 years: 4 mg/dose; Children 7-12 years: 8 mg/dose; Adolescents: 15 mg/dose; **Note:** Infants <3 months of age are more susceptible to respiratory depression; use with caution and in reduced doses in this age group (see Warnings)

I.V., SubQ continuous infusion:

Sickle cell or cancer pain: Initial: Infants: 0.02 mg/kg/hour (20 mcg/kg/hour); Children: 0.03 mg/kg/hour (30 mcg/kg/hour); conversion from intermittent I.V. morphine: Administer the patient's total daily I.V. morphine dose over 24 hours as a continuous infusion; titrate dose to appropriate effect; in one study (Miser, 1980), children with severe pain from terminal cancer required a median dose of 0.04-0.07 mg/kg/hour (40-70 mcg/kg/hour); range: 0.025-2.6 mg/kg/hour

Postoperative pain: 0.01-0.04 mg/kg/hour

I.V.: Patient-controlled analgesia (PCA): Opioid-naïve:

Children ≥5 years and <50 kg: **Note:** PCA has been used in children as young as 5 years of age; however, clinicians need to assess children 5-8 years of age to determine if they are able to use the PCA device correctly. All patients should receive an initial loading dose of an analgesic (to attain adequate control of pain) before starting PCA for maintenance. Adjust doses, lockouts, and limits based on required loading dose, age, state of health, and presence of opioid tolerance. Use lower end of dosing range for opioid-naïve. Assess patient and pain control at regular intervals and adjust settings if needed (see American Pain Society, 2008).

Usual concentration: 1 mg/mL

Demand dose: Usual initial: 0.02 mg/kg/dose; usual range: 0.01-0.03 mg/kg/dose

Lockout: Usual initial: 5 doses/hour

Lockout interval: Range: 6-8 minutes

Usual basal rate: 0-0.03 mg/kg/hour

Children and Adolescents >50 kg: See Adult PCA dose

Sedation/analgesia for procedures: I.V.: 0.05-0.1 mg/kg 5 minutes before the procedure

Epidural (**Note: Must use preservative free**): 0.03-0.05 mg/kg (30-50 mcg/kg); maximum dose: 0.1 mg/kg (100 mcg/kg) or 5 mg/24 hours

Children: Oral: Controlled release tablet: 0.3-0.6 mg/kg/dose every 12 hours

Conversion from prompt release tablets and solution: Administer 1/2 of the patient's total daily oral morphine dose every 12 hours or 1/3 of the patient's total daily oral morphine dose every 8 hours

Adolescents >12 years: Sedation/analgesia for procedures: I.V.: 3-4 mg; may repeat in 5 minutes if necessary

Adults:

Oral:

Prompt release: 10-30 mg every 4 hours as needed

Controlled release: 15-30 mg every 8-12 hours

Avinza® extended release capsules (chronic pain): Conversion from other oral morphine products: Administer the patient's total daily oral morphine dose as Avinza® capsules once daily; do not administer more often than every 24 hours; supplemental pain medication may be needed (up to 4 days) until response to daily Avinza® dosage has been stabilized; see package insert for more details; maximum dose: 1600 mg/day; higher doses contain quantity of fumaric acid that may result in nephrotoxicity

Kadian® extended release capsules (chronic pain): Conversion from other oral morphine products: Administer 1/2 of the patient's total daily oral morphine dose as Kadian® capsules every 12 hours or administer the total daily oral morphine dose as Kadian® capsules every 24 hours; do not administer more often than every 12 hours; see package insert for more details

I.M., I.V., SubQ: 2.5-20 mg/dose every 2-6 hours as needed; usual: 10 mg/dose every 4 hours as needed

I.V., SubQ continuous infusion: 0.8-10 mg/hour; may increase depending on pain relief/adverse effects; usual range up to 80 mg/hour

I.V.: Patient-controlled analgesia (PCA): Opioid-naïve: >50 kg:

Note: All patients should receive an initial loading dose of an analgesic (to attain adequate control of pain) before starting PCA for maintenance. Adjust doses, lockouts, and limits based on required loading dose, age, state of health, and presence of opioid tolerance. Use lower end of dosing range for opioid-naïve. Assess patient and pain control at regular intervals and adjust settings if needed (see American Pain Society, 2008):

Usual concentration: 1 mg/mL

Demand dose: Usual initial: 1 mg; usual range: 0.5-2.5 mg

Lockout interval: Usual initial: 6 minutes; usual range: 5-10 minutes

Epidural (**Note: Use preservative free**; use lower doses and with extreme caution in debilitated patients):

Astramorph/PF™, Duramorph®:

Single dose: Initial: 5 mg in lumbar region; if inadequate pain relief within 1 hour, give 1-2 mg; maximum dose: 10 mg/24 hours (single doses may provide adequate relief for up to 24 hours)

Continuous infusion: Initial: 2 mg/24 hours to 4 mg/24 hours; may give further doses of 1-2 mg if pain relief is not achieved initially; maximum total dose: 10 mg/24 hours

Note: The American Pain Society (2008) recommends 1-6 mg/dose as a single epidural dose or an epidural infusion of 0.1-1 mg/hour; adjust dose for age, injection site, and patient's medical condition and degree of opioid tolerance.

DepoDur® (extended release liposome injection): Surgical pain: Single-dose:

Cesarean section: 10 mg

Lower abdominal or pelvic surgery: 10-15 mg; **Note:** Some patients may benefit from a 20 mg dose; however, the incidence of adverse respiratory effects may be increased.

Major orthopedic surgery of the lower extremity: 15 mg

Intrathecal (1/10 of epidural dose; **Note: Must use preservative free**; use lower doses and with extreme caution in debilitated patients):

Single dose: Opioid-naive: 0.2-1 mg/dose (single doses may provide adequate relief for up to 24 hours); repeat doses **not** recommended; **Note:** The American Pain Society (2008) recommends 0.1-0.3 mg/dose as a single intrathecal dose for acute pain; adjust dose for age, injection site, and patient's medical condition and degree of opioid tolerance. Doses of 1-10 mg/day have been used in opioid-tolerant patients.

Note: Consider use of low-dose continuous I.V. naloxone infusion (0.6 mg/hour) for 24 hours after intrathecal injection to help reduce potential side effects (eg, nausea, vomiting, pruritus, urinary retention); weigh risk of using narcotic antagonist in patients receiving opioids chronically.

Continuous microinfusion (Infumorph®):

Opioid-naive: Initial: 0.2-1 mg/day

Opioid-tolerant: Initial: 1-10 mg/day, titrate to effect; usual maximum: ~20 mg/day; doses >20 mg/day may be associated with higher risk of serious adverse effects

Note: Consider use of low-dose naloxone (0.2 mg) to help reduce side effects (eg, nausea, vomiting, pruritus, urinary retention); weigh risk of using narcotic antagonist in patients receiving opioids chronically.

Dosing adjustment in renal impairment: Children and Adults:

Cl_{cr} 10-50 mL/minute: Administer 75% of normal dose

Cl_{cr} <10 mL/minute: Administer 50% of normal dose

Dosing adjustment in hepatic impairment: Use with caution; specific guidelines are not available; clearance is decreased in patients with cirrhosis; accumulation of morphine is not expected with single-dose use, but may occur with multiple doses; lower doses may be needed with multiple dose regimens

Administration

Oral: Administer with food; swallow extended, sustained, and controlled release products whole; do not chew, crush, break, or dissolve (this would result in rapid release and absorption of a potentially toxic dose of drug) Avinza® and Kadian® capsules may be administered without regard to meals. Do not administer Avinza® with alcohol (see Patient Information). Avinza® and Kadian® (extended release capsules) may be opened and contents sprinkled on a small amount of applesauce immediately prior to ingestion; swallow mixture; rinse mouth with water and swallow to ensure all beads have been ingested; do not chew, crush, or dissolve beads or pellets from capsule (this would result in rapid release and absorption of a potentially toxic dose of drug). Kadian® capsules may be opened and contents sprinkled into ~10 mL of water, then flushed while swirling through a pre-wetted 16-French gastrostomy tube fitted with a funnel at the port end; flush with water to transfer all pellets and flush the tube; do not attempt to administer via NG tube.

Parenteral: **Note:** Solutions for injection should be visually inspected for particulate matter and discoloration prior to administration. Do not use if it contains a precipitate or is darker in color than pale yellow or discolored in any other way.

I.V. push: Administer over at least 5 minutes at a final concentration of 0.5-5 mg/mL (rapid I.V. administration may increase adverse effects)

Intermittent infusion: Administer over 15-30 minutes at a final concentration of 0.5-5 mg/mL

Continuous I.V. infusion: 0.1-1 mg/mL in D_5W, $D_{10}W$, or NS

Epidural and intrathecal: Use only preservative free injections. Adults: Infumorph® was developed for use in continuous microinfusion devices only; it may require dilution before use, as determined by the individual patient's dosage requirements and the characteristics of the continuous microinfusion device; not recommended for single dose I.V., I.M., or SubQ administration; filter through ≤5 micron microfilter before injecting into microinfusion device

Epidural, extended release liposome suspension (Depo-Dur®): Adults: For epidural use only (at the lumbar level); do not administer I.V., I.M., or by the intrathecal route; not recommended for administration into thoracic epidural space or higher (has not been studied); do not use if suspect vial has been frozen (see Stability). Gently invert vial to resuspend particles immediately before use (avoid aggressive agitation). May administer undiluted or may dilute up to 5 mL total volume in preservative free NS. Product does not contain preservative; drug must be administered within 4 hours after withdrawal from vial. Do not use in-line filter during administration. Do not administer within 15 minutes of epidural lidocaine and epinephrine (see Drug Interactions); do not administer any other medication into the epidural space for at least 48 hours after DepoDur®

Monitoring Parameters

Respiratory and cardiovascular status, oxygen saturation, pain relief (if used for analgesia), level of sedation. **Note:** Resedation may occur following epidural administration; when DepoDur® is used, monitor patients closely for ≥48 hours due to prolonged effects of extended release epidural preparation. Monitor patients receiving Infumorph® closely for ≥24 hours after initiation and as appropriate for the first several days after catheter implantation.

Patient Information

Use exactly as directed; do not increase dose or frequency. Do not crush, chew, break, or dissolve any extended, sustained, or controlled release product. Avoid alcohol. Do not drink any alcohol (including beer, wine, distilled spirits) or take over-the-counter or other prescription medications which may contain alcohol, when taking Avinza® (alcohol may cause a sudden and dangerous release of medication from this product which may cause decreased breathing, coma, or death). Morphine may cause drowsiness and impair ability to perform activities requiring mental alertness or physical coordination. May be habit-forming; avoid abrupt discontinuation after prolonged use. Do not let others use your morphine products; severe adverse effects, including death, may occur (see Warnings).

Morphine may cause itching, low blood pressure, or blurred vision (use caution when climbing stairs or changing position from sitting or lying to standing), loss of appetite, dry mouth, nausea, vomiting, or constipation (consult prescriber about use of stool softeners and/or laxatives). Report chest pain, slow or rapid heartbeat, acute dizziness, or persistent headache; changes in mental status; swelling of extremities or unusual weight gain; changes in urinary elimination or pain on urination; acute headache; back or flank pain; muscle spasms; blurred vision; skin rash; or shortness of breath.

Nursing Implications

Do not administer rapidly I.V. Accidental dermal exposure to Duramorph® should be treated by removing contaminated clothing and rinsing the affected area with water. See also Monitoring Parameters.

Additional Information

Less adverse effects are associated with epidural compared to intrathecal route of administration; equianalgesic doses: Codeine: 120 mg I.M. = morphine 10 mg I.M. = single dose oral morphine 60 mg **or** chronic dosing oral morphine 15-25 mg

DepoDur® is an extended release sterile suspension of multivesicular liposomes in NS; liposomes range in size from 17-23 micrometers (median diameter); the pharmacokinetics, safety, and efficacy of DepoDur® have not been studied in patients <18 years of age and use in these patients is **not** recommended

Avinza® capsules contain both immediate release and extended release beads; also contains fumaric acid (as an osmotic agent and local pH modifier); this product is intended for once daily oral administration only; not for PRN or postoperative use. Kadian® capsules contain extended release pellets that are polymer-coated; this product is intended for every 12 hour or every 24 hour dosing. Kadian® capsules also contain talc; parenteral abuse may result in local tissue necrosis, infection, pulmonary granulomas, endocarditis, and valvular heart injury.

Dosage Forms

Excipient information presented when available (limited, particularly for generics); consult specific product labeling. [DSC] = Discontinued product; [CAN] = Canadian brand name

Capsule, extended release, oral:

Avinza®: 30 mg, 45 mg, 60 mg, 75 mg, 90 mg, 120 mg

Kadian®: 10 mg, 20 mg, 30 mg, 50 mg, 60 mg, 80 mg, 100 mg, 200 mg

Infusion [premixed in D_5W]: 1 mg/mL (100 mL, 250 mL)

Injection, extended release liposomal suspension [lumbar epidural injection, preservative free]:

DepoDur®: 10 mg/mL (1 mL, 1.5 mL)

Injection, solution: 1 mg/mL (10 mL); 2 mg/mL (1 mL); 4 mg/mL (1 mL); 5 mg/mL (1 mL); 8 mg/mL (1 mL); 10 mg/0.7 mL (0.7 mL); 10 mg/mL (1 mL, 10 mL); 15 mg/mL (1 mL, 20 mL); 25 mg/mL (4 mL, 10 mL); 20 mL, 40 mL, 50 mL, 100 mL, 250 mL); 50 mg/mL (20 mL, 40 mL, 50 mL) [some preparations contain sodium metabisulfite]

Injection, solution [epidural, intrathecal, or I.V. infusion; preservative free]:
Astramorph/PF™: 0.5 mg/mL (2 mL, 10 mL); 1 mg/mL (2 mL, 10 mL)
Duramorph®: 0.5 mg/mL (10 mL); 1 mg/mL (10 mL)

Injection, solution [epidural or intrathecal infusion via microinfusion device; preservative free]:
Infumorph® 200: 10 mg/mL (20 mL)
Infumorph® 500: 25 mg/mL (20 mL)

Injection, solution [for PCA pump]: 1 mg/mL (30 mL; 50 mL [DSC]); 5 mg/mL (30 mL; 50 mL [DSC])

Injection, solution [for PCA pump, preservative free]: 0.5 mg/mL (30 mL); 1 mg/mL (30 mL); 5 mg/mL (30 mL)

Injection, solution [preservative free]: 0.5 mg/mL (10 mL); 1 mg/mL (10 mL); 25 mg/mL (10 mL)

Solution, oral: 10 mg/5 mL (5 mL, 100 mL, 500 mL); 20 mg/5 mL (100 mL, 500 mL)
Doloral [CAN]: 1 mg/mL (10 mL, 250 mL, 500 mL); 5 mg/mL (10 mL, 250 mL, 500 mL) [not available in U.S.]

Solution, oral, as sulfate [concentrate]: 100 mg/5 mL (15 mL [DSC], 30 mL, 120 mL, 240 mL)
Roxanol™: 100 mg/5 mL (30 mL, 120 mL, 240 mL) [DSC]

Suppository, rectal: 5 mg (12s), 10 mg (12s), 20 mg (12s), 30 mg (12s)

Tablet, oral: 10 mg [DSC], 15 mg, 30 mg

Tablet, controlled release, oral: 15 mg, 30 mg, 60 mg, 100 mg, 200 mg
MS Contin®: 15 mg, 30 mg, 60 mg, 100 mg, 200 mg

Tablet, extended release, oral: 15 mg, 30 mg, 60 mg, 100 mg, 200 mg

Tablet, sustained release, oral:
Oramorph® SR: 15 mg, 30 mg, 60 mg, 100 mg

References

Berde C, Ablin A, Glazer J, et al, "American Academy of Pediatrics Report of the Subcommittee on Disease-Related Pain in Childhood Cancer," *Pediatrics*, 1990, 86(5 Pt 2):818-25.

Dampier CD, Setty BN, Logan J, et al, "Intravenous Morphine Pharmacokinetics in Pediatric Patients With Sickle Cell Disease," *J Pediatr*, 1995, 126(3):461-7.

Henneberg SW, Hole P, Madsen de Haas I, et al, "Epidural Morphine for Postoperative Pain Relief in Children," *Acta Anaesthesiol Scand*, 1993, 37(7):664-7.

Hunt A, Joel S, Dick G, et al, "Population Pharmacokinetics of Oral Morphine and Its Glucuronides in Children Receiving Morphine as Immediate-Release Liquid or Sustained-Release Tablets for Cancer Pain," *J Pediatr*, 1999, 135(1):47-55.

McRorie TI, Lynn AM, Nespeca MK, et al, "The Maturation of Morphine Clearance and Metabolism," *Am J Dis Child*, 1992, 147(8):972-6.

Miser AW, Davis DM, Hughes CS, et al, "Continuous Subcutaneous Infusion of Morphine in Children With Cancer," *Am J Dis Child*, 1983, 137(4):383-5.

Miser AW, Miser JS, and Clark BS, "Continuous Intravenous Infusion of Morphine Sulfate for Control of Severe Pain in Children With Terminal Malignancy," *J Pediatr*, 1980, 96(5):930-2.

Olkkola KT, Hamunen K, and Maunuksela EL, "Clinical Pharmacokinetics and Pharmacodynamics of Opioid Analgesics in Infants and Children," *Clin Pharmacokinet*, 1995, 28(5):385-404.

"Principles of Analgesic Use in the Treatment of Acute Pain and Cancer Pain," 6th ed, Glenview, IL: American Pain Society, 2008.

◆ **M.O.S.® 10 (Can)** *see* Morphine Sulfate *on page 946*

◆ **M.O.S.® 20 (Can)** *see* Morphine Sulfate *on page 946*

◆ **M.O.S.® 30 (Can)** *see* Morphine Sulfate *on page 946*

◆ **Mosco® Callus & Corn Remover [OTC]** *see* Salicylic Acid *on page 1241*

◆ **M.O.S.-SR® (Can)** *see* Morphine Sulfate *on page 946*

◆ **M.O.S.-Sulfate® (Can)** *see* Morphine Sulfate *on page 946*

◆ **Motrin® Children's [OTC]** *see* Ibuprofen *on page 702*

◆ **Motrin® (Children's) (Can)** *see* Ibuprofen *on page 702*

◆ **Motrin® IB [OTC]** *see* Ibuprofen *on page 702*

◆ **Motrin® IB (Can)** *see* Ibuprofen *on page 702*

◆ **Motrin® Infants' [OTC]** *see* Ibuprofen *on page 702*

◆ **Motrin® Junior [OTC]** *see* Ibuprofen *on page 702*

◆ **MoviPrep®** *see* Polyethylene Glycol-Electrolyte Solution *on page 1129*

◆ **Moxatag™** *see* Amoxicillin *on page 96*

◆ **4-MP** *see* Fomepizole *on page 620*

◆ **MPA** *see* MedroxyPROGESTERone *on page 870*

◆ **MPA** *see* Mycophenolate *on page 956*

◆ **6-MP (error-prone abbreviation)** *see* Mercaptopurine *on page 884*

◆ **MPSV** *see* Meningococcal Polysaccharide Vaccine (Groups A / C / Y and W-135) *on page 878*

◆ **MPSV4** *see* Meningococcal Polysaccharide Vaccine (Groups A / C / Y and W-135) *on page 878*

◆ **MS Contin®** *see* Morphine Sulfate *on page 946*

◆ **MS (error-prone abbreviation and should not be used)** *see* Morphine Sulfate *on page 946*

◆ **MS-IR® (Can)** *see* Morphine Sulfate *on page 946*

◆ **MSO$_4$ (error-prone abbreviation and should not be used)** *see* Morphine Sulfate *on page 946*

◆ **MTX (error-prone abbreviation)** *see* Methotrexate *on page 900*

◆ **Mucinex® [OTC]** *see* GuaiFENesin *on page 656*

◆ **Mucinex® Children's [OTC] [DSC]** *see* GuaiFENesin *on page 656*

◆ **Mucinex® Children's Cough [OTC] [DSC]** *see* Guaifenesin and Dextromethorphan *on page 658*

◆ **Mucinex® DM [OTC]** *see* Guaifenesin and Dextromethorphan *on page 658*

◆ **Mucinex® DM Maximum Strength [OTC]** *see* Guaifenesin and Dextromethorphan *on page 658*

◆ **Mucinex® Full force™ [OTC] [DSC]** *see* Oxymetazoline *on page 1043*

◆ **Mucinex® Kid's Mini-Melts™ [OTC]** *see* GuaiFENesin *on page 656*

◆ **Mucinex® Kid's [OTC]** *see* GuaiFENesin *on page 656*

◆ **Mucinex® Kid's Cough [OTC]** *see* Guaifenesin and Dextromethorphan *on page 658*

◆ **Mucinex® Kid's Cough Mini-Melts™ [OTC]** *see* Guaifenesin and Dextromethorphan *on page 658*

◆ **Mucinex® Maximum Strength [OTC]** *see* GuaiFENesin *on page 656*

◆ **Mucinex® Mini-Melts™ [OTC] [DSC]** *see* GuaiFENesin *on page 656*

◆ **Mucinex® Mini-Melts™ Junior Strength [OTC] [DSC]** *see* GuaiFENesin *on page 656*

◆ **Mucinex® moisture smart™ [OTC] [DSC]** *see* Oxymetazoline *on page 1043*

◆ **Muco-Fen® [DSC]** *see* GuaiFENesin *on page 656*

◆ **Muco-Fen® 1200 [DSC]** *see* GuaiFENesin *on page 656*

◆ **Mucomyst** *see* Acetylcysteine *on page 43*

◆ **Mucomyst® (Can)** *see* Acetylcysteine *on page 43*

◆ **Multiple Trace Metals** *see* Trace Metals *on page 1366*

◆ **Multitrace®-4** *see* Trace Metals *on page 1366*

◆ **Multitrace®-4 Concentrate** *see* Trace Metals *on page 1366*

◆ **Multitrace®-4 Neonatal** *see* Trace Metals *on page 1366*

◆ **Multitrace®-4 Pediatric** *see* Trace Metals *on page 1366*

◆ **Multitrace®-5** *see* Trace Metals *on page 1366*

◆ **Multitrace®-5 Concentrate** *see* Trace Metals *on page 1366*

◆ **Mumps, Measles and Rubella Vaccines** *see* Measles, Mumps, and Rubella Vaccines (Combined) *on page 862*

◆ **Mumps, Rubella, Varicella, and Measles Vaccine** *see* Measles, Mumps, Rubella, and Varicella Virus Vaccine *on page 864*

◆ **Mumpsvax® [DSC]** *see* Mumps Virus Vaccine (Live/Attenuated) *on page 953*

Mumps Virus Vaccine (Live/Attenuated)
(mumpz VYE rus vak SEEN, live, a ten YOO ate ed)

Related Information
Immunization Guidelines *on page 1636*

U.S. Brand Names Mumpsvax® [DSC]

Therapeutic Category Vaccine, Live Virus

Generic Available No

Use Provide active immunity against mumps virus (FDA approved in ages ≥12 months and adults)

Note: Trivalent measles-mumps-rubella (MMR) vaccine is the preferred agent for most children and many adults; persons born prior to 1957 are generally considered immune and need not be vaccinated

Pregnancy Risk Factor C

Pregnancy Considerations Reproduction studies have not been conducted. Rates of spontaneous abortion may be increased if mumps infection occurs during the first trimester. Although mumps vaccine virus can infect the placenta and fetus, there is not good evidence that it causes congenital malformations. Vaccine should not be administered to pregnant women and the ACIP recommends that pregnancy be avoided for 1 month following vaccination.

Lactation
Excretion in breast milk unknown/use caution

Contraindications Hypersensitivity to mumps vaccine, gelatin, or any component of the formulation; history of anaphylactic reactions to neomycin; individuals with blood dyscrasias, leukemia, lymphomas, or other malignant neoplasms affecting the bone marrow or lymphatic systems; concurrent immunosuppressive therapy; primary and acquired immunodeficiency states; family history of congenital or hereditary immunodeficiency; active/ untreated tuberculosis; current febrile illness or active febrile infection

Warnings Avoid pregnancy for at least 1 month following vaccination (ACIP, 2001); manufacturer recommends waiting 3 months following vaccination; use in patients with existing thrombocytopenia may result in more severe reduction in platelets; avoid use in patients with previous history of post vaccination thrombocytopenia, as rechallenge has resulted in recurrence of thrombocytopenia; severe allergic reactions including anaphylaxis have been reported rarely. Immediate treatment for anaphylactic/ anaphylactoid reaction should be available during vaccine use. Use extreme caution in patients with immediate-type hypersensitivity reactions to eggs.

Mumps vaccine should not be administered to severely immunocompromised persons with the exception of asymptomatic children with HIV. Patients with minor illnesses (diarrhea, mild upper respiratory tract infection with or without low grade fever or other illnesses with low-grade fever) may receive vaccine. Leukemia patients who are in remission and who have not received chemotherapy for at least 3 months may be vaccinated.

Precautions Immediate treatment for anaphylactic reactions should be available during vaccine use; defer vaccination for persons with acute febrile illness until recovery. Routine prophylactic administration of acetaminophen to prevent fever due to vaccines has been shown to decrease the immune response of some vaccines; the clinical significance of this reduction in immune response has not been established (see Prymula, 2009).

Adverse Reactions All serious adverse reactions must be reported to the U.S. Department of Health and Human Services (DHHS) Vaccine Adverse Event Reporting System (VAERS) 1-800-822-7967.
Cardiovascular: Vasculitis

Central nervous system: Fever, seizures, syncope, irritability, confusion, headache, encephalitis, Guillain-Barré syndrome

Dermatologic: Rash, Stevens-Johnson syndrome, erythema multiforme, urticaria

Endocrine & metabolic: Parotitis

Genitourinary: Orchitis in postpubescent and adult males

Gastrointestinal: Pancreatitis, diarrhea, parotitis

Hematologic: Thrombocytopenia, purpura, leukocytosis

Local: Burning or stinging at injection site

Ocular: Ocular palsies, optic neuritis, papillitis, retrobulbar neuritis, conjunctivitis

Otic: Nerve deafness, otitis media

Respiratory: Cough, rhinitis

Miscellaneous: Hypersensitivity reactions, lymphadenopathy

Drug Interactions
Avoid Concomitant Use
Avoid concomitant use of Mumps Virus Vaccine with any of the following: Immunosuppressants

Increased Effect/Toxicity
The levels/effects of Mumps Virus Vaccine may be increased by: Immunosuppressants

Decreased Effect
Mumps Virus Vaccine may decrease the levels/effects of: Tuberculin Tests

The levels/effects of Mumps Virus Vaccine may be decreased by: Immune Globulins; Immunosuppressants

Stability Prior to reconstitution, store the powder at 2°C to 8°C (36°F to 46°F) or colder (freezing does not affect potency). Protect from light. Diluent may be stored with powder or at room temperature. Discard if not used within 8 hours of reconstitution.

Mechanism of Action Promotes active immunity to mumps virus by inducing specific antibodies.

Usual Dosage Children ≥12 months and Adults: SubQ: 0.5 mL as a single dose

Administration Use entire contents of the provided diluent to reconstitute vaccine. Gently agitate to mix thoroughly. Discard if powder does not dissolve. Use as soon as possible following reconstitution; discard if not used within 8 hours; administer by SubQ injection into the anterolateral aspect of the thigh or arm; **not for I.M. or I.V. administration**

Monitoring Parameters Monitor for syncope for ≥15 minutes following vaccination.

Test Interactions Temporary suppression of tuberculosis skin test

Patient Information Pregnancy should be avoided for at least 1 month following vaccination. A little swelling of the glands in the cheeks and under the jaw may occur that lasts for a few days; this could happen from 1-2 weeks after getting the mumps vaccine; this happens rarely.

Nursing Implications Federal law requires that the date of administration, the vaccine manufacturer, lot number of vaccine, and the administering person's name, title, and address be entered into the patient's permanent medical record.

◀ **Additional Information** All adults without documentation of live vaccine on or after the first birthday or physician-diagnosed mumps, or laboratory evidence or immunity (particularly males and young adults who work in or congregate in hospitals, colleges, and on military bases) should be vaccinated. It is reasonable to consider persons born before 1957 immune, but there is no contraindication to vaccination of older persons. Susceptible travelers should be vaccinated.

In order to maximize vaccination rates, the ACIP recommends simultaneous administration of all age-appropriate vaccines (live or inactivated) for which a person is eligible at a single visit, unless contraindications exist. The use of combination vaccines is generally preferred over separate infections, taking into consideration provider assessment, patient preference, and potential adverse events.

For additional information, please refer to the following website: http://www.cdc.gov/vaccines/vpd-vac/.

Dosage Forms Excipient information presented when available (limited, particularly for generics); consult specific product labeling. [DSC] = Discontinued product

Injection, powder for reconstitution [preservative free]:

Mumpsvax®: ≥20,000 $TCID_{50}$ [contains albumin (human), bovine serum, chicken egg protein, gelatin, sorbitol, and sucrose (1.9 mg/vial)] [DSC]

References

Centers for Disease Control and Prevention (CDC), "General Recommendations on Immunization. Recommendations of the Advisory Committee on Immunization Practices (ACIP)," *MMWR Recomm Rep*, 2006, 55(RR-15):1-48. Available at: http://www.cdc.gov/mmwr/preview/mmwrhtml/rr5515a1.htm.

Centers for Disease Control and Prevention (CDC), "Recommended Adult Immunization Schedule – United States, 2009" *MMWR Morb Mortal Wkly Rep*, 2009, 57(53):Q1-4.

Centers for Disease Control and Prevention (CDC), "Recommended Immunization Schedules for Persons Aged 0 Through 18 Years – United States, 2009," *MMWR Morb Mortal Wkly Rep*, 2009, 57 (51 and 52):Q1-4.

Centers for Disease Control and Prevention (CDC), "Revised ACIP Recommendation for Avoiding Pregnancy After Receiving a Rubella-Containing Vaccine," *MMWR Morb Mortal Wkly Rep*, 2001, 50 (49):1117.

Centers for Disease Control and Prevention (CDC), "Syncope After Vaccination – United States, January 2005-July 2007," *MMWR Morb Mortal Wkly Rep*, 2008, 57(17):457-60.

Prymula R, Siegrist CA, Chlibek R, et al, "Effect of Prophylactic Paracetamol Administration at Time of Vaccination on Febrile Reactions and Antibody Responses in Children: Two Open-Label, Randomised Controlled Trials," *Lancet*, 2009, 374(9698):1339-50.

Watson JC, Hadler SC, Dykewicz CA, et al, "Measles, Mumps, and Rubella–Vaccine Use and Strategies for Elimination of Measles, Rubella, and Congenital Rubella Syndrome and Control of Mumps: Recommendations of the Advisory Committee on Immunization Practices (ACIP)," *MMWR Recomm Rep*, 1998, 47(RR-8):1-57.

Mupirocin (myoo PEER oh sin)

Medication Safety Issues

Sound-alike/look-alike issues:

Bactroban® may be confused with bacitracin, baclofen, Bactrim™

U.S. Brand Names Bactroban Cream®; Bactroban Nasal®; Bactroban®

Canadian Brand Names Bactroban®

Therapeutic Category Antibiotic, Topical

Generic Available Yes: Topical ointment

Use Ointment: Topical treatment of impetigo caused by *Staphylococcus aureus* and *Streptococcus pyogenes*; topical treatment of folliculitis, furunculosis, minor wounds, burns, and ulcers caused by susceptible organisms; Cream: Treatment of secondarily-infected traumatic skin lesions due to susceptible strains of *S. aureus* and *S. pyogenes*; prophylactic agent applied to intravenous catheter exit sites; Intranasal ointment: Eradication of *S. aureus* from nasal and perineal carriage sites

Pregnancy Risk Factor B

Pregnancy Considerations Teratogenic effects were not observed in animal studies. There are no adequate and well-controlled studies in pregnant women; use during pregnancy only if clearly needed.

Lactation Excretion in breast milk unknown/use caution

Contraindications Hypersensitivity to mupirocin, poly-ethylene glycol, or any component

Warnings Potentially toxic amounts of polyethylene glycol (PEG) contained in the vehicle may be absorbed percutaneously in patients with extensive burns or open wounds; the PEG vehicle may irritate mucous membranes and increase nasal secretions if applied intranasally; prolonged use may result in overgrowth of nonsusceptible organisms

Precautions Use with caution in patients with impaired renal function and in burn patients

Adverse Reactions

Dermatologic: Pruritus, rash, erythema, dry skin

Local: Burning, stinging, pain, tenderness, local edema

Drug Interactions

Avoid Concomitant Use

Avoid concomitant use of Mupirocin with any of the following: BCG

Increased Effect/Toxicity There are no known significant interactions involving an increase in effect.

Decreased Effect

Mupirocin may decrease the levels/effects of: BCG; Typhoid Vaccine

Stability Do not mix with Aquaphor®, coal tar solution, or salicylic acid

Mechanism of Action Binds to bacterial isoleucyl trans-fer-RNA synthetase preventing isoleucine incorporation resulting in the inhibition of protein and RNA synthesis

Pharmacokinetics (Adult data unless noted)

Absorption: Following topical administration, penetrates the outer layers of the skin; systemic absorption is minimal through intact skin

Protein binding: 95%

Metabolism: Extensive in the liver and skin to monic acid

Half-life: 17-36 minutes

Elimination: Metabolite is excreted in urine

Usual Dosage

Intranasal: Children and Adults: Apply small amount 2-4 times/day for 5-14 days

Topical:

Cream: Infants ≥3 months, Children, and Adults: Apply small amount 3 times/day for 10 days

Ointment: Infants ≥2 months, Children, and Adults: Apply a small amount 3-5 times/day for 5-14 days

Administration Cream and ointment: For topical use only; do not apply into the eye; may cover with gauze dressing; Intranasal: Avoid contact with eyes; apply one-half of the ointment from the single-use tube into each nostril

Additional Information Contains polyethylene glycol vehicle

Dosage Forms Excipient information presented when available (limited, particularly for generics); consult specific product labeling.

Note: Strength expressed as base

Cream, topical, as calcium:

Bactroban Cream®: 2% (15 g, 30 g) [contains benzyl alcohol]

Ointment, intranasal, as calcium:

Bactroban Nasal®: 2% (1 g) [single-use tube]

Ointment, topical: 2% (0.9 g, 22 g)

Bactroban®: 2% (22 g) [contains polyethylene glycol]

References

Britton JW, Fajardo JE, and Krafte-Jacobs B, "Comparison of Mupirocin and Erythromycin in the Treatment of Impetigo," *J Pediatr*, 1990, 117 (5):827-9.

Hayakawa T, Hayashidera T, Katsura S, et al, "Nasal Mupirocin Treatment of Pharynx-Colonized Methicillin Resistant *Staphylococcus aureus*: Preliminary Study With 10 Carrier Infants," *Pediatr Int*, 2000, 42(1):67-70.

Hitomi S, Kubota M, Mori N, et al, "Control of a Methicillin-Resistant *Staphylococcus aureus* Outbreak in a Neonatal Intensive Care Unit by Unselective Use of Nasal Mupirocin Ointment," *J Hosp Infect*, 2000, 46(2):123-9.

Oh J, von Baum H, Klaus G, et al, "Nasal Carriage of *Staphylococcus aureus* in Families of Children on Peritoneal Dialysis. European Pediatric Peritoneal Dialysis Study Group (EPPS)," *Adv Perit Dial*, 2000, 16:324-7.

♦ **Mupirocin Calcium** *see* Mupirocin *on page 954*

♦ **Murine® Ear Wax Removal System [OTC]** *see* Carbamide Peroxide *on page 248*

♦ **Muro 128® [OTC]** *see* Sodium Chloride *on page 1270*

Muromonab-CD3 (myoo roe MOE nab see dee three)

U.S. Brand Names Orthoclone OKT® 3 [DSC]

Therapeutic Category Immunosuppressant Agent

Generic Available No

Use Treatment of acute allograft rejection in renal transplant patients; effective in reversing acute hepatic, cardiac, and bone marrow transplant rejection episodes resistant to conventional treatment

Pregnancy Risk Factor C

Lactation Excretion in breast milk unknown/contraindicated

Contraindications Hypersensitivity to OKT3 or any Murine® product; patients in fluid overload or those with >3% weight gain within 1 week prior to start of OKT3

Warnings It is imperative, especially prior to the first few doses, that there be no clinical evidence of volume overload, uncontrolled hypertension, or uncompensated heart failure, including a clear chest x-ray and weight restriction of ≤3% above the patient's minimum weight during the week prior to injection.

Risk of development of lymphoproliferative disorders (particularly of the skin) is increased. May result in an increased susceptibility to infection; dosage of concomitant immunosuppressants should be reduced during OKT3 therapy (see Additional Information); cyclosporine should be decreased to 50% of the usual maintenance dose and maintenance therapy should be resumed about 4 days before stopping OKT3.

Severe pulmonary edema has occurred in patients with fluid overload. Seizures, encephalopathy, cerebral edema, aseptic meningitis, and headache have been reported following muromonab-CD3. Contraindicated for use in patients with a history of seizures or those who are predisposed to seizures. Arterial, venous, and capillary thrombosis of allografts and other vascular beds have been reported with use; use with caution in patients with history of thrombosis or underlying vascular disease.

Anaphylactic and anaphylactoid reactions may occur after administration of any dose of muromonab-CD3 **[U.S. Boxed Warning]**; acute hypersensitivity reactions may be characterized by cardiovascular collapse, cardiorespiratory arrest, loss of consciousness, shock, tachycardia, tingling, angioedema, airway obstruction, bronchospasm, dyspnea, urticaria, and pruritus. These reactions may be difficult to differentiate from the cytokine release syndrome associated with use; however, hypersensitivity reactions are more likely to occur within the first 10 minutes after administration. Cytokine release syndrome may occur in a significant proportion of patients following the first couple of doses of muromonab-CD3; symptoms usually begin 30-60 minutes after administration of dose and may persist for several hours; symptoms range from a mild, self-limiting

"flu-like reaction" to severe, life-threatening shock-like reaction.

Patients at higher risk for serious complications include those with unstable angina, recent MI or ischemic heart disease, heart failure, pulmonary edema, COPD, intravascular volume overload or depletion, cerebrovascular disease, patients with advanced symptomatic vascular disease or neuropathy, history of seizures, and septic shock. Pretreatment with corticosteroids may decrease serum levels of cytokines and manifestations of the syndrome, but it is not known if this decreases organ damage and sequelae associated with it.

Precautions Cardiopulmonary resuscitation may be needed. If the patient's temperature is >37.8°C, reduce before administering OKT3. Should be administered under the supervision of a physician experienced in immunosuppressive therapy in a facility appropriate for monitoring and resuscitation **[U.S. Boxed Warning]**.

Adverse Reactions

Cardiovascular: Tachycardia, hypertension, hypotension, perioral and peripheral cyanosis

Central nervous system: Aseptic meningitis, seizures, headache, pyrexia, confusion

Dermatologic: Pruritus, rash

Gastrointestinal: Diarrhea, nausea, vomiting

Neuromuscular & skeletal: Arthralgia, tremor, myalgia

Ocular: Photophobia

Renal: BUN elevated, serum creatinine elevated

Respiratory: Dyspnea, chest pain, tightness, wheezing, pulmonary edema

Miscellaneous: Flu-like symptoms (ie, fever, chills), anaphylactic-type reactions

Drug Interactions

Avoid Concomitant Use

Avoid concomitant use of Muromonab-CD3 with any of the following: BCG; Natalizumab; Pimecrolimus; Tacrolimus (Topical); Vaccines (Live)

Increased Effect/Toxicity

Muromonab-CD3 may increase the levels/effects of: Leflunomide; Natalizumab; Vaccines (Live)

The levels/effects of Muromonab-CD3 may be increased by: Denosumab; Pimecrolimus; Tacrolimus (Topical); Trastuzumab

Decreased Effect

Muromonab-CD3 may decrease the levels/effects of: BCG; Sipuleucel-T; Vaccines (Inactivated); Vaccines (Live)

The levels/effects of Muromonab-CD3 may be decreased by: Echinacea

Stability Store in refrigerator; do not freeze or shake; OKT3 left out of the refrigerator for more than 4 hours must not be used

Mechanism of Action Coats the circulating T lymphocytes subjecting these cells to opsonization by the reticuloendothelial system; modulates the T lymphocyte antigen receptor CD3 complex which results in the removal of all CD3 molecules from the cell surface so that the cell lacks the ability to function as a T lymphocyte

Pharmacokinetics (Adult data unless noted)

Distribution: V_d is closely related to the apparent volume of distribution for albumin

Half-life: 18 hours

Elimination: Binds to T lymphocytes with resultant opsonization and removal by the reticuloendothelial system

Usual Dosage I.V. (refer to individual protocols):

Note: Children and Adults: Methylprednisolone sodium succinate 1 mg/kg I.V. given 2-6 hours prior to first OKT3 administration and I.V. hydrocortisone sodium succinate 50-100 mg given 30 minutes after administration are strongly recommended to decrease the incidence of reactions to the first dose; patient temperature should not exceed 37.8°C (100°F) at time of administration

Children <12 years: 0.1 mg/kg/day once daily for 10-14 days **or** patients ≤30 kg: 2.5 mg once daily for 10-14 days; patients >30 kg: 5 mg once daily for 10-14 days

Children ≥12 years and Adults: 5 mg/day once daily for 10-14 days

Administration Parenteral: Filter each dose through a low protein-binding 0.22 micron filter (Millex GV) before administration; administer I.V. push over 1 minute at a final concentration of 1 mg/mL

Monitoring Parameters Chest x-ray, weight gain, CBC with differential, BUN and S_{cr}, vital signs (blood pressure, temperature, pulse, respiration) and immunologic monitoring of T cells, serum levels of OKT3, CD3+ cell count

Reference Range Mean serum trough levels rise during the first 3 days, then average 0.9 mcg/mL on days 3-14; if serum trough OKT3 concentrations are maintained at 1 mcg/mL, then CD3 counts remain low

Nursing Implications Inform patient of expected first dose effects which may include fever, chills, chest tightness, wheezing, nausea, vomiting, and diarrhea; first-dose reaction usually starts 40-60 minutes after the injection and lasts for several hours; first-dose effects are markedly reduced with subsequent doses; monitor patient closely for 48 hours after the first dose; corticosteroids are recommended; acetaminophen and antihistamines can be given concomitantly with OKT3 to reduce early reactions

Additional Information Recommend decreasing dose of prednisone to 0.5 mg/kg, azathioprine to 0.5 mg/kg (approximate 50% decrease in dose), and discontinuing cyclosporine or decreasing cyclosporine dose by 50% while patient is receiving OKT3

Product Availability Orthoclone OKT® 3: Due to diminishing use, the manufacturer of muromonab is discontinuing production; supplies are expected to be available through the end of 2010.

Dosage Forms Excipient information presented when available (limited, particularly for generics); consult specific product labeling. [DSC] = Discontinued product

Injection, solution:
  Orthoclone OKT® 3: 1 mg/mL (5 mL) [contains polysorbate 80] [DSC]

References
Ettenger RB, Marik JL, Rosenthal JT, et al, "OKT₃ for Rejection Reversal in Pediatric Renal Transplantation," *Clin Transpl*, 1988, 2:180-4.

Hooks MA, Wade CS, and Millikan WJ Jr, "Muromonab CD-3: A Review of Its Pharmacology, Pharmacokinetics, and Clinical Use in Transplantation," *Pharmacotherapy*, 1991, 11(1):26-37.

Niaudet P, Murcia I, Jean G, et al, "A Comparative Trial of OKT₃ and Antilymphocyte Serum in the Preventive Treatment of Rejection After Kidney Transplantation in Children," *Ann Pediatr Paris*, 1990, 37 (2):83-5.

Todd PA and Brogden RN, "Muromonab CD3 A Review of Its Pharmacology and Therapeutic Potential," *Drugs*, 1989, 37 (6):871-99.

Mycophenolate (mye koe FEN oh late)

U.S. Brand Names CellCept®; Myfortic®
Canadian Brand Names CellCept®; Myfortic®
Therapeutic Category Immunosuppressant Agent
Generic Available Yes: Capsule, tablet

Use Immunosuppressant agent used in conjunction with other immunosuppressive therapies (eg, cyclosporine and corticosteroids with or without antithymocyte induction) for the prophylaxis of organ rejection in patients receiving allogeneic renal, hepatic, or cardiac transplants; add-on immunosuppressant agent that is typically used in place of azathioprine in combination regimens for the treatment of refractory acute kidney graft rejection. Use of mycophenolate is also being studied in intestine, small bowel, and bone marrow transplant patients; moderate-to-severe psoriasis; chronic graft-versus-host disease; myasthenia gravis; proliferative lupus nephritis; and frequently relapsing nephrotic syndrome

Medication Guide An FDA-approved medication guide must be distributed when dispensing an outpatient prescription (new or refill) if this medication is to be used without direct supervision of a healthcare provider. Medication guides are available:
  Myfortic®: http://www.fda.gov/downloads/Drugs/DrugSafety/UCM172735.pdf
  CellCept®: http://www.fda.gov/downloads/Drugs/DrugSafety/UCM170919.pdf

Pregnancy Risk Factor D
Pregnancy Considerations [U.S. Boxed Warning]: Mycophenolate is associated with an increased risk of congenital malformations and spontaneous abortions when used during pregnancy. Adverse events have been reported in animal studies at doses less than the equivalent recommended human dose. Data from the National Transplantation Pregnancy Registry (NTPR) have observed an increase in structural malformations (including ear malformations) in infants born to mothers taking mycophenolate during pregnancy. Spontaneous abortions have also been noted. Females of childbearing potential should have a negative pregnancy test within 1 week prior to beginning therapy. Two reliable forms of contraception should be used beginning 4 weeks prior to, during, and for 6 weeks after therapy. The effectiveness of hormonal contraceptive agents may be affected by mycophenolate.

The National Transplantation Pregnancy Registry (NTPR, Temple University) is a registry for pregnant women taking immunosuppressants following any solid organ transplant. The NTPR encourages reporting of all immunosuppressant exposures during pregnancy in transplant recipients at 877-955-6877.

Lactation Excretion in breast milk unknown/not recommended

Breast-Feeding Considerations It is unknown if mycophenolate is excreted in human milk. Due to potentially serious adverse reactions, the decision to discontinue the drug or discontinue breast-feeding should be considered. Breast-feeding is not recommended during therapy or for 6 weeks after treatment is complete.

Contraindications Hypersensitivity to mycophenolate mofetil, mycophenolate sodium, mycophenolic acid, polysorbate 80 (I.V. formulation), or any component

Warnings Hazardous agent: Use appropriate precautions for handling and disposal. Immunosuppression with mycophenolate may result in an increased susceptibility to infection and an increased risk of developing lymphomas and other malignancies, particularly of the skin **[U.S. Boxed Warning]**; risk appears to be associated with the intensity and duration of immunosuppression; patients should be instructed to limit exposure to sunlight and ultraviolet light. Lymphoproliferative disorder has been reported in pediatric patients. Mycophenolate is associated with an increased risk of first trimester pregnancy loss, teratogenic effects, and congenital malformations, including external ear, facial abnormalities, cleft lip and palate, and anomalies of the distal limbs, heart, esophagus, and kidney **[U.S. Boxed Warning]**; women using mycophenolate during pregnancy should be encouraged to enroll in the National Transplantation Pregnancy Registry. In women of childbearing potential, two reliable forms of contraception must be initiated 4 weeks before starting mycophenolate therapy, maintained during therapy, and continued for 6 weeks after it has been discontinued.

Cases of progressive multifocal leukoencephalopathy (PML) have been associated with mycophenolate use; consider PML in the differential diagnosis in patients reporting neurological symptoms.

Note: CellCept® and Myfortic® dosage forms should not be used interchangeably due to differences in absorption.

Precautions Use with caution in patients with active serious digestive disease and in patients with renal impairment; modify dosage in patients with severe chronic renal impairment (GFR <25 mL/minute/1.73 m^2 outside of the immediate post-transplant period) and in patients with neutropenia. Avoid use in patients with rare hereditary deficiency of hypoxanthineguanine phosphoribosyl-transferase (HGPRT) such as Lesch-Nyhan and Kelley-Seegmiller syndrome. The oral suspension contains aspartame which is metabolized to phenylalanine and must be used with caution in patients with phenylketonuria.

Adverse Reactions

Cardiovascular: Chest pain, hypertension, hypotension, peripheral edema, tachycardia

Central nervous system: Anxiety, dizziness, fever, headache, insomnia

Dermatologic: Acne, rash

Endocrine & metabolic: Hypercholesterolemia, hyperglycemia, hyperkalemia, hypocalcemia, hypokalemia, hypophosphatemia

Gastrointestinal: Abdominal pain, anorexia, colitis, constipation, diarrhea, dyspepsia, gastric and duodenal ulcers, GI tract hemorrhage, intestinal perforation, nausea, oral moniliasis, pancreatitis, vomiting

Genitourinary: Hematuria, urinary tract infection

Hematologic: Anemia, leukocytosis, leukopenia, neutropenia, pure red cell aplasia, thrombocytopenia

Local: Phlebitis, thrombosis

Neuromuscular & skeletal: Back pain, myalgia, paresthesia, tremor, weakness

Renal: BUN elevated, creatinine elevated, renal tubular necrosis

Respiratory: Cough, dyspnea, pharyngitis, pulmonary fibrosis, respiratory tract infection

Miscellaneous: 1% incidence of infection, lymphoproliferative disease, malignancy, progressive multifocal leukoencephalopathy, sepsis

Drug Interactions

Avoid Concomitant Use

Avoid concomitant use of Mycophenolate with any of the following: BCG; Cholestyramine Resin; Natalizumab; Pimecrolimus; Rifamycin Derivatives; Tacrolimus (Topical); Vaccines (Live)

Increased Effect/Toxicity

Mycophenolate may increase the levels/effects of: Acyclovir-Valacyclovir; Ganciclovir-Valganciclovir; Leflunomide; Natalizumab; Vaccines (Live)

The levels/effects of Mycophenolate may be increased by: Acyclovir-Valacyclovir; Denosumab; Ganciclovir-Valganciclovir; Pimecrolimus; Probenecid; Tacrolimus (Topical); Trastuzumab

Decreased Effect

Mycophenolate may decrease the levels/effects of: BCG; Contraceptives (Estrogens); Contraceptives (Progestins); Sipuleucel-T; Vaccines (Inactivated); Vaccines (Live)

The levels/effects of Mycophenolate may be decreased by: Antacids; Cholestyramine Resin; CycloSPORINE; CycloSPORINE (Systemic); Echinacea; Magnesium Salts; MetroNIDAZOLE; MetroNIDAZOLE (Systemic); Penicillins; Proton Pump Inhibitors; Quinolone Antibiotics; Rifamycin Derivatives; Sevelamer

Food Interactions Presence of food decreases mycophenolate peak concentration by 40% following mycophenolate mofetil and 33% following mycophenolate delayed release oral tablet, but has no effect on the extent of absorption; avoid echinacea (has immunostimulant property)

Stability Store capsules, tablets, delayed release tablets, dry powder for oral suspension, and intact I.V. vials at room temperature of 15°C to 30°C (59°F to 86°F); protect from light

Suspension: Store reconstituted suspension in refrigerator or at room temperature; stable for 60 days after reconstitution. Do not freeze.

Injection: Mycophenolate I.V. infusion solution is stable for 12 hours at room temperature after preparation; administration of the infusion solution should begin within 4 hours from reconstitution and dilution of the drug. Do not mix mycophenolate with any other drugs.

Mechanism of Action Hydrolyzed to form mycophenolic acid (MPA), the active metabolite, which is a potent, uncompetitive reversible inhibitor of inosine monophosphate dehydrogenase (IMPDH) in the purine biosynthesis pathway; inhibition of IMPDH results in a depletion of guanosine triphosphate and deoxyguanosine triphosphate, thereby inhibiting T- and B-cell proliferation, cytotoxic T-cell generation and antibody secretion.

Pharmacokinetics (Adult data unless noted)

Absorption: Rapid and extensive; early post-transplant period MPA AUC values are approximately 45% to 53% lower than later post-transplant period (>3 months) MPA AUC values in pediatric patients 1-18 years.

Distribution: Mean V_d (adults):

Mycophenolate mofetil: MPA: Oral: 4 L/kg; I.V. 3.6 L/kg

Mycophenolate delayed release tablet: MPA: Oral: 54 L (at steady state)

Protein binding:

Mycophenolate: 97%

Mycophenolate glucuronide: 82%

Metabolism: Mycophenolate mofetil and enteric-coated mycophenolate sodium undergo hydrolysis by esterases to mycophenolic acid (MPA is the active metabolite); MPA is metabolized by glucuronyl transferase to mycophenolic acid glucuronide (MPAG is inactive). MPAG is converted to MPA via enterohepatic recirculation.

Bioavailability:

Mycophenolate mofetil: 80.7% to 94%; enterohepatic recirculation contributes to MPA concentration; two 500 mg tablets have been shown to be bioequivalent to four 250 mg capsules or 1000 mg of oral suspension

Enteric-coated mycophenolate sodium: 72%

Half-life:

Mycophenolate mofetil: MPA: Oral: 18 hours; I.V.: 17 hours

Mycophenolate delayed release: MPA: Oral: 8-16 hours; MPAG: 13-17 hours

Time to peak serum concentration: Oral:

Mycophenolate mofetil: 0.5-1 hour

Mycophenolate sodium: 1.5-2.75 hours

Elimination:

Mycophenolate mofetil: 6% in feces; 87% of mycophenolic acid dose recovered as MPAG in urine; <1% of dose excreted as MPA in urine

Mycophenolate delayed release: 3% excreted as MPA in urine and in feces; >60% recovered as MPAG in urine

Dialysis: Not dialyzable

Usual Dosage

Oral: Mycophenolate mofetil tablets, capsules, and suspension should **not** be used interchangeably with the delayed-release tablet formulation due to differences in the rate of absorption.

Children:

Mycophenolate mofetil: 600 mg/m^2/dose twice daily; maximum dose: 2 g/day; **Note:** Limited information regarding mycophenolate use in pediatric patients is currently available in the literature: 32 pediatric patients (14 underwent living donor and 18 receiving cadaveric donor renal transplants) received mycophenolate 8-30 mg/kg/dose orally twice daily with cyclosporine, prednisone, and Atgam® induction. However, pharmacokinetic studies suggest that doses of mycophenolate adjusted to body surface area resulted in AUCs which better approximated those of adults versus doses adjusted for body weight which resulted in lower AUCs in pediatric patients.

or

BSA 1.25 m^2 to 1.5 m^2: 750 mg twice daily

BSA >1.5 m^2: 1 g twice daily

Mycophenolate delayed-release tablet: 400-450 mg/m^2/dose twice daily; maximum dose: 720 mg

BSA <1.19 m^2: Use of this formulation is not recommended.

or

BSA 1.19-1.58 m^2: 540 mg twice daily

BSA >1.58 m^2: 720 mg twice daily; **Note:** Mycophenolate delayed release 720 mg twice daily was shown to be bioequivalent to mycophenolate mofetil 1000 mg twice daily

Adults:

Mycophenolate mofetil:

Renal transplant: 1 g twice daily in combination with corticosteroids and cyclosporine; dosages as high as 3-3.5 g/day were used in clinical trials, but no efficacy advantage was established

Cardiac transplant: 1.5 g twice daily

Hepatic transplant: 1.5 g twice daily

Mycophenolate delayed-release tablet:

Renal transplant: 720 mg twice daily

Cardiac transplant: 1080 mg twice daily has been shown to be therapeutically similar to mycophenolate mofetil 1.5 g twice daily in a study of 154 *de novo* heart transplant recipients and has a comparable safety profile (Kobashigawa, 2006).

I.V. infusion (administer within 24 hours following transplantation; can be given for up to 14 days; patients should be switched to oral formulation as soon as oral medication is tolerated):

Adults:

Renal transplant: 1 g twice daily

Cardiac transplant: 1.5 g twice daily

Hepatic transplant: 1 g twice daily

Dosing adjustment in renal impairment: Renal transplant: GFR <25 mL/minute/1.73 m^2 outside the immediate post-transplant period:

Mycophenolate mofetil: Avoid doses >1 g twice daily

Mycophenolate delayed release tablet: Monitor carefully

Dosing adjustment for toxicity (neutropenia): ANC <1.3 x 10^3/µL; dosing should be interrupted or the dose reduced

Administration

Oral: Administer on an empty stomach one hour before or two hours after food; one center has mixed the contents of the capsule in chocolate syrup; mycophenolate suspension can be administered orally or via a nasogastric tube with a minimum size of 8 French; shake suspension well before use. Swallow delayed-release tablet whole; do not crush, chew, or cut.

I.V.: **Do not administer I.V. push** or by rapid I.V. bolus injection; reconstitute vial with D$_5$W and further dilute to a final concentration of 6 mg/mL using D$_5$W. Administer by slow I.V. infusion over a period of no less than 2 hours.

Monitoring Parameters CBC with differential, platelet count, serum electrolytes, glucose, phosphate, cholesterol, and renal function tests; blood pressure. Pregnancy test in female patients of childbearing potential within 1 week prior to beginning therapy.

Patient Information Do not take within 1 hour before or 2 hours after antacids or cholestyramine; maintain adequate hydration. You will be susceptible to infection (avoid crowds and people with infections). Report to physician any diarrhea, vomiting, stomach pain, leg swelling, chest pain, acute headache or dizziness, respiratory infection symptoms, difficulty breathing, fatigue, lethargy, abnormal skin paleness, or unusual bleeding or bruising. You may be at increased risk for skin cancer (wear protective clothing and use sunscreen). Women of childbearing age should use two effective forms of contraception simultaneously for 4 weeks before starting mycophenolate therapy, during therapy, and for 6 weeks after discontinuing mycophenolate, unless abstinence is the chosen method of contraception.

Nursing Implications Mycophenolate capsules should not be opened or crushed; avoid inhalation or direct contact of the capsule contents with skin or mucous membranes; mycophenolate tablets should not be crushed. Avoid direct contact of I.V. mycophenolate solution with skin or mucous membranes. If contact occurs, wash thoroughly with soap and water; rinse eyes with plain water.

Dosage Forms Excipient information presented when available (limited, particularly for generics); consult specific product labeling.

Capsule, oral, as mofetil: 250 mg

CellCept®: 250 mg

Injection, powder for reconstitution, as mofetil hydrochloride:

CellCept®: 500 mg [contains polysorbate 80]

Powder for suspension, oral, as mofetil:

CellCept®: 200 mg/mL (175 mL) [contains phenylalanine 0.56 mg/mL; mixed fruit flavor]

Tablet, oral, as mofetil: 500 mg

CellCept®: 500 mg [may contain ethyl alcohol]

Tablet, delayed release, as mycophenolic acid:

Myfortic®: 180 mg, 360 mg [formulated as a sodium salt]

Extemporaneous Preparations A 50 mg/mL suspension can be prepared in a vertical flow hood by emptying six 250 mg mycophenolate mofetil capsules into a mortar wetted and triturated with 7.5 mL Ora-Plus® to a smooth paste. Add 15 mL of cherry syrup and triturate to make a final volume of 30 mL. The suspension is stable for 210 days when stored at 5°C, stable for 28 days when stored at 37°C or 25°C, and stable for 11 days when stored at 45°C.

Venkataramanan R, McCombs JR, Zudarnan S, et al, "Stability of Mycophenolate Mofetil as an Extemporaneous Suspension," *Ann Pharmacother*, 1998, 32:755-7.

References
Ettenger R, Warshaw B, Menster M, et al, "Mycophenolate Mofetil in Pediatric Renal Transplantation: A Report of the Ped MMF Study Group." Abstract: 1996, Annual Meeting, ASTP.

Hogg RJ, Fitzgibbons L, Bruick J, et al, "Mycophenolate Mofetil in Children With Frequently Relapsing Nephrotic Syndrome: A Report From the Southwest Pediatric Nephrology Study Group," *Clin J Am Soc Nephrol*, 2006, 1(6):1173-8.

Kobashigawa JA, Renlund DG, Gerosa G, et al, "Similar Efficacy and Safety of Enteric-Coated Mycophenolate Sodium (EC-MPS, Myfortic) Compared With Mycophenolate Mofetil (MMF) in *de novo* Heart Transplant Recipients: Results of a 12-Month, Single-Blind, Randomized, Parallel-Group, Multicenter Study," *J Heart Lung Transplant*, 2006, 25(8):935-41.

Sollinger HW, "Mycophenolate Mofetil for the Prevention of Acute Rejection in Primary Cadaveric Renal Allograft Recipients. U.S. Renal Transplant Mycophenolate Mofetil Study Group," *Transplantation*, 1995, 60:225-32.

Staatz CE and Tett SE, "Clinical Pharmacokinetics and Pharmacodynamics of Mycophenolate in Solid Organ Transplant Recipients," *Clin Pharmacokinet*, 2007, 46(1):13-58.

◆ **Mylanta® Children's [OTC]** *see* Calcium Supplements *on page 239*

◆ **Mylanta® Gas Maximum Strength [OTC]** *see* Simethicone *on page 1262*

◆ **Mylan-Terbinafine (Can)** *see* Terbinafine *on page 1322*

◆ **Mylan-Timolol (Can)** *see* Timolol *on page 1351*

◆ **Mylan-Topiramate (Can)** *see* Topiramate *on page 1360*

◆ **Mylan-Trazodone (Can)** *see* TraZODone *on page 1371*

◆ **Mylan-Triazolam (Can)** *see* Triazolam *on page 1381*

◆ **Mylan-Valacyclovir (Can)** *see* Valacyclovir *on page 1394*

◆ **Mylan-Valproic (Can)** *see* Valproic Acid and Derivatives *on page 1398*

◆ **Mylan-Venlafaxine XR (Can)** *see* Venlafaxine *on page 1412*

◆ **Mylan-Verapamil (Can)** *see* Verapamil *on page 1416*

◆ **Mylan-Verapamil SR (Can)** *see* Verapamil *on page 1416*

◆ **Mylan-Warfarin (Can)** *see* Warfarin *on page 1432*

◆ **Myleran®** *see* Busulfan *on page 223*

◆ **Mylicon® Infants [OTC]** *see* Simethicone *on page 1262*

◆ **Mylotarg®** *see* Gemtuzumab Ozogamicin *on page 640*

◆ **Myobloc®** *see* RimabotulinumtoxinB *on page 1216*

◆ **Myochrysine®** *see* Gold Sodium Thiomalate *on page 652*

◆ **Myozyme®** *see* Alglucosidase Alfa *on page 64*

◆ **Myrac™ [DSC]** *see* Minocycline *on page 933*

◆ **Mysoline®** *see* Primidone *on page 1154*

◆ **Na₂EDTA** *see* Edetate Disodium *on page 489*

◆ **Nabi-HB®** *see* Hepatitis B Immune Globulin *on page 673*

Nabilone (NA bi lone)

U.S. Brand Names Cesamet®
Canadian Brand Names Cesamet®
Therapeutic Category Antiemetic
Generic Available No
Use Treatment of refractory nausea and vomiting associated with cancer chemotherapy
Restrictions C-II
Pregnancy Risk Factor C
Pregnancy Considerations Animal studies did not demonstrate teratogenic effects; however, dose-related decreased fetal weights and increased fetal resorptions were observed. There are no adequate and well-controlled studies in pregnant women. Use during pregnancy only if clearly needed.
Lactation Excretion in breast milk unknown/not recommended
Breast-Feeding Considerations Because some cannabinoids are excreted in breast milk, use in breast-feeding is not recommended.
Contraindications Hypersensitivity to nabilone, cannabinoids, tetrahydrocannabinol, or any component
Warnings Nabilone has potential for abuse and/or dependence; use caution in patients with substance abuse history; limit antiemetic therapy availability to current cycle of chemotherapy. Safety and efficacy in children have not been established.
Precautions Use with caution in patients with cardiovascular disease (may cause tachycardia and orthostatic hypotension), history of substance abuse, and those with pre-existing CNS depression; use caution with current or previous history of mental illness; cannabinoid use may reveal symptoms of psychiatric disorders. Psychiatric adverse reactions may persist for up to 3 days after discontinuing treatment.

Adverse Reactions
Cardiovascular: Orthostatic hypotension, arrhythmia, chest pain, hypertension, syncope, tachycardia
Central nervous system: Dizziness (59%), drowsiness (52% to 66%), vertigo (52% to 59%), euphoria (11% to 38%), ataxia, depression, concentration decreased, sleep disturbance, dysphoria, headache, sedation, depersonalization, disorientation, abnormal dreams, anxiety, apathy, cerebral vascular accident, chills, fatigue, fever, emotional disorder, emotional lability, hallucinations, insomnia, mood swings, memory disturbance, nervousness, neurosis (phobic), panic disorder, paranoia, psychosis (toxic)
Dermatologic: Photosensitivity, rash, pruritus
Gastrointestinal: Xerostomia (22% to 36%), anorexia, nausea, appetite increased, abdominal pain, aphthous ulcer, constipation, diarrhea, dyspepsia, gastritis, epistaxis, mouth irritation, taste perversion, vomiting
Genitourinary: Urinary retention, polyuria
Hematologic: Anemia, leukopenia
Neuromuscular & skeletal: Weakness, akathisia, back pain, dystonia, joint pain, muscle pain, neck pain, numbness, paresthesia, tremor
Ocular: Visual disturbance (13%), amblyopia, eye irritation, xerophthalmia, photophobia, pupil dilation
Otic: Tinnitus
Respiratory: Cough, dyspnea, nasal congestion, wheezing
Miscellaneous: Hypersensitivity reactions, diaphoresis, anhydrosis

Drug Interactions
Avoid Concomitant Use There are no known interactions where it is recommended to avoid concomitant use.

Increased Effect/Toxicity
Nabilone may increase the levels/effects of: Alcohol (Ethyl); CNS Depressants; Methotrimeprazine; Sympathomimetics

The levels/effects of Nabilone may be increased by: Anticholinergic Agents; Cocaine; Methotrimeprazine
Decreased Effect There are no known significant interactions involving a decrease in effect.
Stability Store at room temperature between 15°C and 30°C (59°F and 86°F).
Mechanism of Action Not fully characterized; antiemetic activity may be due to effect on cannabinoid receptors (CB1) within the central nervous system
Pharmacokinetics (Adult data unless noted)
Absorption: Rapid and complete
Distribution: ~12.5 L/kg
Metabolism: To several active metabolites by oxidation and stereospecific enzyme reduction; CYP450 enzymes may also be involved
Half-life: Parent compound: 2 hours; Metabolites: 35 hours
Time to peak serum concentration: Within 2 hours
Elimination: Feces (~60%); renal (~24%)
Usual Dosage
Oral:
Children >4 years:
 <18 kg: 0.5 mg twice daily
 18-30 kg: 1 mg twice daily
 >30 kg: 1 mg 3 times/day
Adults: 1-2 mg twice daily (maximum: 6 mg divided in 3 doses daily)
Dosage adjustment in renal impairment: No adjustment required.
Administration Oral: Initial dose should be given 1-3 hours before chemotherapy; may be given 2-3 times/day during the entire chemotherapy course and for up to 48 hours after the last dose of chemotherapy; a dose the night before chemotherapy may be useful
Monitoring Parameters Blood pressure, heart rate; signs and symptoms of excessive use, abuse, or misuse

Patient Information May cause drowsiness and impair ability to perform activities requiring mental alertness or physical coordination; may cause dry mouth; avoid alcohol. May cause photosensitivity reactions; avoid exposure to sunlight and artificial light sources. Report excessive or persistent CNS changes (euphoria, anxiety, depression, memory lapse, bizarre thought patterns, excitability, inability to control thoughts or behavior, fainting); respiratory difficulties; rapid heartbeat; or other adverse reactions.

Dosage Forms Excipient information presented when available (limited, particularly for generics); consult specific product labeling.

Capsule:
Cesamet®: 1 mg

References
Chan HS, Correia JA, and MacLeod SM, "Nabilone Versus Prochlorperazine for Control of Cancer Chemotherapy-Induced Emesis in Children: A Double-Blind, Crossover Trial," *Pediatrics*, 1987, 79(6):946-52.

Dupuis LL and Nathan PC, "Options for the Prevention and Management of Acute Chemotherapy-Induced Nausea and Vomiting in Children," *Pediatr Drug*, 2003, 5(9):597-613.

Tramer MR, Carroll D, Campbell FA, et al, "Cannabinoids for Control of Chemotherapy Induced Nausea and Vomiting: Quantitative Systematic Review," *BMJ*, 2001, 323(7303):16-21.

Ward A and Holmes B, "Nabilone: A Preliminary Review of Its Pharmacological Properties and Therapeutic Use," *Drugs*, 1985, 30(2):127-44.

◆ *NAC* see Acetylcysteine *on page 43*

◆ *N-Acetyl-L-cysteine* see Acetylcysteine *on page 43*

◆ *N-Acetylcysteine* see Acetylcysteine *on page 43*

◆ *N-Acetyl-P-Aminophenol* see Acetaminophen *on page 36*

◆ *NaCl* see Sodium Chloride *on page 1270*

Nadolol (nay DOE lole)

Medication Safety Issues
Sound-alike/look-alike issues:
Nadolol may be confused with Mandol®
Corgard® may be confused with Cognex®, Coreg®

Related Information
Antihypertensive Agents by Class *on page 1481*

U.S. Brand Names Corgard®

Canadian Brand Names Alti-Nadolol; Apo-Nadol®; Corgard®; Novo-Nadolol

Therapeutic Category Antianginal Agent; Antiarrhythmic Agent, Class II; Antihypertensive Agent; Antimigraine Agent; Beta-Adrenergic Blocker

Generic Available Yes

Use Treatment of hypertension, alone or in combination with other agents (FDA approved in adults); treatment of angina pectoris (FDA approved in adults); prophylaxis of migraine headaches

Pregnancy Risk Factor C

Pregnancy Considerations Adverse events were observed in some animal reproduction studies; therefore, the manufacturer classifies nadolol as pregnancy category C. Nadolol crosses the placenta and is measurable in infant serum after birth. In a cohort study, an increased risk of cardiovascular defects was observed following maternal use of beta-blockers during pregnancy. Bradycardia, respiratory depression, and hypoglycemia have been observed in neonates following maternal use of nadolol during pregnancy. In addition, intrauterine growth restriction (IUGR) and small placentas have been observed in neonates following *in utero* exposure to other nonselective beta-blockers; adequate facilities for monitoring infants at birth should be available. Severe, untreated chronic hypertension during pregnancy may be associated with maternal and fetal adverse events; however, nadolol is currently not recommended for the initial treatment of hypertension in pregnancy. Refer to the Propranolol monograph for additional information on a nonselective beta-blocking agent.

Lactation Enters breast milk/use caution consider risk: benefit (AAP rates "compatible")

Breast-Feeding Considerations Nadolol is excreted into breast milk in concentrations higher than the maternal serum. According to the manufacturer, the decision to continue or discontinue breast-feeding during therapy should take into account the risk of exposure to the infant and the benefits of treatment to the mother. The AAP considers nadolol to be "usually compatible with breast-feeding." The time to peak milk concentration is 6 hours after the oral dose, the half-life of nadolol in breast milk is similar to that in the maternal serum, and nadolol can still be detected in breast milk for several days after the last maternal dose.

Contraindications Hypersensitivity to nadolol or any component; overt cardiac failure, cardiogenic shock, sinus bradycardia, greater than first degree conduction block, bronchial asthma

Warnings May depress myocardial activity and precipitate or worsen heart failure; use with caution and monitor closely, especially in patients with compensated heart failure and during upwards titration of dose; if heart failure worsens, may need to increase diuretics and not advance the dose of nadolol; a reduction in dose or discontinuation of nadolol may be needed. Beta-blocker therapy should not be withdrawn abruptly (particularly in patients with CAD), but gradually tapered over 1-2 weeks to avoid acute tachycardia, hypertension, and/or ischemia **[U.S. Boxed Warning]**. Beta-blockers should generally be avoided in patients with bronchospastic disease; nadolol is contra-indicated for patients with asthma. Nadolol may block hypoglycemia-induced tachycardia and blood pressure changes; use with caution in patients with diabetes mellitus. Nadolol decreases the ability of the heart to respond to reflex adrenergic stimuli and may increase the risk of general anesthesia and surgical procedures. May mask clinical signs of hyperthyroidism (exacerbation of symptoms of hyperthyroidism, including thyroid storm, may occur following abrupt discontinuation). Beta-blocker use has been associated with induction or exacerbation of psoriasis, but cause and effect have not been firmly established.

Precautions Increase dosing interval in patients with renal dysfunction; use with caution in patients with diabetes mellitus

Adverse Reactions
Cardiovascular: CHF, edema, orthostatic hypotension, persistent bradycardia, Raynaud's syndrome
Central nervous system: Dizziness, fatigue
Dermatological: Psoriasis exacerbation, rash
Gastrointestinal: GI discomfort
Respiratory: Bronchospasm

Drug Interactions
Metabolism/Transport Effects Substrate of P-glycoprotein

Avoid Concomitant Use
Avoid concomitant use of Nadolol with any of the following: Methacholine

Increased Effect/Toxicity
Nadolol may increase the levels/effects of: Alpha-/Beta-Agonists (Direct-Acting); Alpha1-Blockers; Alpha2-Agonists; Amifostine; Antihypertensives; Bupivacaine; Cardiac Glycosides; Hypotensive Agents; Insulin; Lidocaine; Lidocaine (Systemic); Lidocaine (Topical); Mepivacaine; Methacholine; Midodrine; RiTUXimab; Sulfonylureas

The levels/effects of Nadolol may be increased by: Acetylcholinesterase Inhibitors; Amiodarone; Anilidopiperidine Opioids; Calcium Channel Blockers ▷

(Nondihydropyridine); Diazoxide; Dipyridamole; Disopyramide; Dronedarone; Herbs (Hypotensive Properties); MAO Inhibitors; Pentoxifylline; P-Glycoprotein Inhibitors; Phosphodiesterase 5 Inhibitors; Prostacyclin Analogues; Reserpine

Decreased Effect

Nadolol may decrease the levels/effects of: Beta2-Agonists; Theophylline Derivatives

The levels/effects of Nadolol may be decreased by: Herbs (Hypertensive Properties); Methylphenidate; Nonsteroidal Anti-Inflammatory Agents; P-Glycoprotein Inducers; Yohimbine

Food Interactions Avoid natural licorice (causes sodium and water retention and increases potassium loss)

Stability Store at room temperature in tightly closed bottle; avoid excessive heat; protect from light

Mechanism of Action Competitively blocks response to beta-adrenergic stimulation; nonselective beta-blocker

Pharmacodynamics Duration: 24 hours

Pharmacokinetics (Adult data unless noted)

Absorption: Oral: 30% to 40%

Distribution: Concentration in human breast milk is 4.6 times higher than serum

Protein-binding: 28%

Half-life, elimination:

Increased half-life with decreased renal function

Infants 3-22 months (n=3): 3.2-4.3 hours

Children 10 years (n=1): 15.7 hours

Children ~15 years (n=1): 7.3 hours

Adults: 10-24 hours

Dialysis: Moderately dialyzable (20% to 50%)

Usual Dosage Oral:

Children: Very limited information (ie, one study) regarding pediatric dosage currently available in literature: The study used oral nadolol to control supraventricular tachycardia (SVT) in 26 children 3 months to 15 years of age. SVT was well controlled in 23 out of 26 children; recommended initial dose: 0.5-1 mg/kg once daily; monitor carefully, gradually increase dose; median dose required: 1 mg/kg/day; maximum dose: 2.5 mg/kg/day.

Adults: Initial: 40 mg once daily; increase gradually; usual dosage: 40-80 mg/day; may need up to 240-320 mg/day; doses as high as 640 mg/day have been used; usual dosage range for hypertension (JNC 7): 40-120 mg once daily

Dosage adjustment in adults with renal impairment:

Cl$_{cr}$ 10-50 mL/minute: Administer 50% of normal dose

Cl$_{cr}$ <10 mL/minute: Administer 25% of normal dose

Administration Oral: May administer without regard to meals

Monitoring Parameters Blood pressure, heart rate, fluid intake and output, weight

Patient Information Limit alcohol; do not abruptly discontinue; may mask symptoms of hypoglycemia, but sweating may still occur

Dosage Forms Excipient information presented when available (limited, particularly for generics); consult specific product labeling. [DSC] = Discontinued product

Tablet: 20 mg, 40 mg, 80 mg

Corgard®: 20 mg, 40 mg, 80 mg, 120 mg [DSC], 160 mg [DSC]

References

Brauchli YB, Jick SS, Curtin F, et al, "Association Between Beta-Blockers, Other Antihypertensive Drugs and Psoriasis: Population-Based Case-Control Study," *Br J Dermatol*, 2008, 158(6):1299-307.

Chobanian AV, Bakris GL, Black HR, et al, "The Seventh Report of the Joint National Committee on Prevention, Detection, Evaluation, and Treatment of High Blood Pressure: The JNC 7 report," *JAMA*, 2003, 289(19):2560-72.

Devlin RG and Duchin KL, "Nadolol in Human Serum and Breast Milk," *Br J Clin Pharmacol*, 1981, 12(3):393-6.

Gold MH, Holy AK, and Roenigk HH Jr, "Beta-Blocking Drugs and Psoriasis. A Review of Cutaneous Side Effects and Retrospective Analysis of Their Effects on Psoriasis," *J Am Acad Dermatol*, 1988, 19 (5 Pt 1):837-41.

Mehta AV and Chidambaram B, "Efficacy and Safety of Intravenous and Oral Nadolol for Supraventricular Tachycardia in Children," *J Am Coll Cardiol*, 1992, 19(3):630-5.

Mehta AV and Chidambaram B, and Rice PJ, "Pharmacokinetics of Nadolol in Children With Supraventricular Tachycardia," *J Clin Pharmacol*, 1992, 32(1):1023-7.

Schön MP and Boehncke WH, "Psoriasis," *N Engl J Med*, 2005, 352 (18):1899-912.

Nafcillin (naf SIL in)

Related Information

Extravasation Treatment *on page 1522*

Canadian Brand Names Nallpen®; Unipen®

Therapeutic Category Antibiotic, Penicillin (Antistaphylococcal)

Generic Available Yes

Use Treatment of bacterial infections such as osteomyelitis, septicemia, endocarditis, and CNS infections due to susceptible penicillinase-producing strains of *Staphylococcus*

Pregnancy Risk Factor B

Pregnancy Considerations Adverse events have not been observed in animal studies; therefore, nafcillin is classified as pregnancy category B. There is no available data on the placental transfer of nafcillin. Human experience with the penicillins during pregnancy has not shown any positive evidence of adverse effects on the fetus.

Lactation Enters breast milk/use caution

Breast-Feeding Considerations It is not known if nafcillin crosses into human milk. The manufacturer recommends that caution be exercised when administering nafcillin to nursing women. Other penicillins distribute into human milk and are considered safe for use during breast-feeding. Nondose-related effects could include modification of bowel flora.

Contraindications Hypersensitivity to nafcillin, any component, or penicillins. Premixed nafcillin solutions containing dextrose may be contraindicated in patients with allergies to corn or corn products.

Warnings Elimination rate will be decreased in neonates; avoid using in neonates during the first 2 weeks of life. Serious hypersensitivity reactions including anaphylaxis have been reported; immediate treatment for anaphylactic reaction should be available during administration. Pseudomembranous colitis has been reported in patients receiving nafcillin.

Precautions Extravasation of I.V. infusions should be avoided; modification of dosage is necessary in patients with both severe renal and hepatic impairment; use with caution in patients with cephalosporin hypersensitivity

Adverse Reactions

Central nervous system: Fever, seizures

Dermatologic: Skin rash

Endocrine & metabolic: Hypokalemia

Gastrointestinal: Nausea, diarrhea, pseudomembranous colitis

Hematologic: Neutropenia, anemia, eosinophilia

Hepatic: AST elevated

Local: Pain, thrombophlebitis

Neuromuscular & skeletal: Arthralgia, myalgia

Renal: Acute interstitial nephritis (rare), hematuria

Miscellaneous: Hypersensitivity reactions

Drug Interactions

Metabolism/Transport Effects Induces CYP3A4 (strong)

Avoid Concomitant Use

Avoid concomitant use of Nafcillin with any of the following: BCG; Dienogest; Dronedarone; Everolimus; Nilotinib; Pazopanib; Ranolazine; Romidepsin; Tolvaptan

Increased Effect/Toxicity

Nafcillin may increase the levels/effects of: Methotrexate

The levels/effects of Nafcillin may be increased by: Probenecid

Decreased Effect

Nafcillin may decrease the levels/effects of: BCG; Calcium Channel Blockers; Contraceptives (Estrogens); CycloSPORINE; CycloSPORINE (Systemic); CYP3A4 Substrates; Dienogest; Dronedarone; Everolimus; GuanFACINE; Maraviroc; Mycophenolate; Nilotinib; Pazopanib; Ranolazine; Romidepsin; Saxagliptin; Sorafenib; Tadalafil; Tolvaptan; Typhoid Vaccine; Vitamin K Antagonists

The levels/effects of Nafcillin may be decreased by: Fusidic Acid; Tetracycline Derivatives

Food Interactions Food decreases GI absorption

Stability Reconstituted nafcillin 250 mg/mL solution for injection is stable for 3 days at room temperature and 7 days when refrigerated; when diluted for I.V. intermittent infusion in D_5W or NS, solution is stable for 24 hours at room temperature and 96 hours when refrigerated. Thawed premixed frozen solution is stable for 21 days under refrigeration or 72 hours at room temperature. Incompatible with aminoglycosides.

Mechanism of Action Interferes with bacterial cell wall synthesis during active multiplication by binding to one or more of the penicillin-binding proteins; inhibits the final transpeptidation step of peptidoglycan synthesis causing cell wall death and resultant bactericidal activity against susceptible bacteria

Pharmacokinetics (Adult data unless noted)

Distribution: Distributes into bile, synovial, pleural, ascitic, and pericardial fluids and into bone and liver; CSF penetration is poor unless meninges are inflamed; crosses the placenta; excreted into breast milk

V_d:

Neonates: 0.24-0.53 L/kg
Children: 0.85-0.91 L/kg
Adults: 0.57-1.55 L/kg

Protein binding: 90%
Metabolism: 70% to 90%
Half-life:

Neonates:

<3 weeks: 2.2-5.5 hours
4-9 weeks: 1.2-2.3 hours

Children 1 month to 14 years: 0.75-1.9 hours
Adults with normal renal and hepatic function: 0.5-1.5 hours

Time to peak serum concentration: I.M.: Within 30-60 minutes

Elimination: Primarily in bile and 10% to 30% in urine as unchanged drug; undergoes enterohepatic recycling

Dialysis: Not dialyzable (0% to 5%)

Usual Dosage

Neonates: I.M., I.V.:

0-4 weeks, <1200 g: 50 mg/kg/day in divided doses every 12 hours

≤7 days:

1200-2000 g: 50 mg/kg/day in divided doses every 12 hours
>2000 g: 75 mg/kg/day in divided doses every 8 hours

>7 days:

1200-2000 g: 75 mg/kg/day in divided doses every 8 hours
>2000 g: 100-140 mg/kg/day in divided doses every 6 hours

Children:

I.M., I.V.:

Mild to moderate infections: 50-100 mg/kg/day in divided doses every 6 hours
Severe infections: 100-200 mg/kg/day in divided doses every 4-6 hours
Maximum dose: 12 g/day

Staphylococcal endocarditis:

Native valve: 200 mg/kg/day in divided doses every 4-6 hours for 6 weeks
Prosthetic valve: 200 mg/kg/day in divided doses every 4-6 hours for 6 weeks or longer with rifampin and with gentamicin for the first 2 weeks of therapy

Adults:

I.M.: 500 mg every 4-6 hours
I.V.: 500-2000 mg every 4-6 hours

Dosing adjustment in patients with both severe renal/ hepatic impairment: Use lower range of usual dose or reduce dose 33% to 50%

Administration Parenteral:

I.M.: Administer deep I.M. into a large muscle (ie, gluteus maximus) using a solution containing 250 mg/mL

I.V.: Nafcillin may be administered by I.V. push over 5-10 minutes or by I.V. intermittent infusion over 15-60 minutes at a final concentration not to exceed 40 mg/mL; in fluid-restricted patients, a maximum concentration of 100 mg/ mL may be administered

Monitoring Parameters Periodic CBC with differential, urinalysis, BUN, serum creatinine, AST, and ALT; initial culture and susceptibility test

Test Interactions False-positive urinary and serum proteins

Patient Information Report any redness, swelling, burning, or pain at injection site; report any difficulty in swallowing or respiration.

Nursing Implications Extravasation may cause tissue sloughing and necrosis; hyaluronidase infiltration may help avoid injury

Additional Information Sodium content of 1 g injection: 3.33 mEq

Dosage Forms Excipient information presented when available (limited, particularly for generics); consult specific product labeling.

Infusion [premixed iso-osmotic dextrose solution]: 1 g (50 mL); 2 g (100 mL)

Injection, powder for reconstitution, as sodium: 1 g, 2 g, 10 g

References

Banner W Jr, Gooch WM 3d, Burckart G, et al, "Pharmacokinetics of Nafcillin in Infants With Low Birth Weights," *Antimicrob Agents Chemother*, 1980, 17(4):691-4.

Zenk KE, Dungy CL, and Greene CR, "Nafcillin Extravasation Injury: Use of Hyaluronidase as an Antidote," *Am J Dis Child*, 1981, 135 (12):1113-4.

◆ **Nafcillin Sodium** *see* Nafcillin *on page 962*

◆ **NaHCO₃** *see* Sodium Bicarbonate *on page 1269*

Nalbuphine (NAL byoo feen)

Medication Safety Issues

Sound-alike/look-alike issues:

Nubain® may be confused with Navane®, Nebcin®

High alert medication: The Institute for Safe Medication Practices (ISMP) includes this medication among its list of drug classes which have a heightened risk of causing significant patient harm when used in error.

U.S. Brand Names Nubain®

Therapeutic Category Analgesic, Narcotic; Opioid Partial Agonist

Generic Available Yes

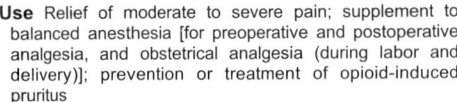

Use Relief of moderate to severe pain; supplement to balanced anesthesia [for preoperative and postoperative analgesia, and obstetrical analgesia (during labor and delivery)]; prevention or treatment of opioid-induced pruritus

Pregnancy Risk Factor C

Pregnancy Considerations Severe fetal bradycardia has been reported following use in labor/delivery. Fetal bradycardia may occur when administered earlier in pregnancy (not documented). Use only if clearly needed, with monitoring to detect and manage possible adverse fetal effects. Naloxone has been reported to reverse bradycardia. Newborn should be monitored for respiratory depression or bradycardia following nalbuphine use in labor.

Lactation Enters breast milk/use caution

Contraindications Hypersensitivity to nalbuphine or any component

Warnings Abrupt discontinuation after prolonged use may result in narcotic withdrawal; administration to patients receiving chronic opiates may precipitate narcotic withdrawal

Neonatal and fetal adverse reactions have occurred after administration of nalbuphine to pregnant women during labor; these adverse reactions, which may be life-threatening, include: Bradycardia, respiratory depression, apnea, cyanosis, and hypotonia; use with caution in pregnancy; monitor neonates closely with maternal use in labor and delivery.

Precautions Reduce dose in patients with hepatic impairment; use with caution in patients with CNS depression, impaired respiration, recent MI, or biliary tract surgery; may produce respiratory depression or bradycardia; use with caution in patients with a history of drug dependence, head trauma or increased intracranial pressure, decreased hepatic or renal function, or patients suspected to be opioid dependent

Adverse Reactions

Cardiovascular: Hypotension, tachycardia, bradycardia, peripheral vasodilation

Central nervous system: CNS depression, drowsiness, headache, dizziness, sedation, ICP elevated

Dermatologic: Urticaria, pruritus, rash

Gastrointestinal: Anorexia, nausea, vomiting, xerostomia, biliary tract spasm

Genitourinary: Urinary tract spasm, urinary retention

Ocular: Blurred vision, miosis

Respiratory: Respiratory depression

Miscellaneous: Histamine release, physical and psychological dependence, narcotic withdrawal in patients receiving opiate agonists chronically, sweating; anaphylaxis, anaphylactoid reactions (may be life-threatening)

Drug Interactions

Avoid Concomitant Use There are no known interactions where it is recommended to avoid concomitant use.

Increased Effect/Toxicity

Nalbuphine may increase the levels/effects of: Alcohol (Ethyl); Alvimopan; CNS Depressants; Desmopressin; Selective Serotonin Reuptake Inhibitors; Thiazide Diuretics

The levels/effects of Nalbuphine may be increased by: Amphetamines; Antipsychotic Agents (Phenothiazines); Succinylcholine

Decreased Effect

Nalbuphine may decrease the levels/effects of: Analgesics (Opioid); Pegvisomant

The levels/effects of Nalbuphine may be decreased by: Ammonium Chloride; Mixed Agonist / Antagonist Opioids

Stability Store at controlled room temperature at 25°C (77°F); protect from excessive light; store product in carton until used; not physically compatible with nafcillin and ketorolac

Mechanism of Action Binds to opiate receptors in the CNS, causing inhibition of ascending pain pathways, altering the perception of and response to pain; produces generalized CNS depression; opiate antagonistic effect may result from competitive inhibition at the opiate mu receptor

Pharmacodynamics

Onset of action:

I.M., SubQ: Within 15 minutes

I.V.: 2-3 minutes

Maximum effect:

I.M.: 30 minutes

I.V.: 1-3 minutes

Duration: 3-6 hours

Pharmacokinetics (Adult data unless noted)

Distribution: Crosses placenta; distributes into breast milk in small amounts (<1% of dose)

Metabolism: In the liver; extensive first-pass metabolism

Protein binding: ~50%

Half-life, terminal:

Children 1-8 years: 0.9 hours

Adults 23-32 years: ~2 hours; range: 3.5-5 hours

Adults 65-90 years: 2.3 hours

Time to peak serum concentration:

I.M.: 30 minutes

I.V.: 1-3 minutes

Elimination: Metabolites primarily in feces (via bile) and in urine; 4% to 7% eliminated unchanged in the urine

Usual Dosage

Children 1-14 years: Premedication: I.M., I.V., SubQ: 0.2 mg/kg; maximum dose: 20 mg/dose

Children: Analgesia: I.M., I.V., SubQ: 0.1-0.15 mg/kg every 3-6 hours as needed; maximum single-dose: 20 mg/dose; maximum daily dose: 160 mg/day

Adults:

Analgesia: I.M., I.V., SubQ: 10 mg/70 kg every 3-6 hours as needed; maximum single-dose: 20 mg/dose; maximum daily dose: 160 mg/day

Surgical anesthesia supplement: I.V.: Induction: 0.3-3 mg/kg administered over 10-15 minutes; maintenance doses of 0.25-0.5 mg/kg may be given as required

Opioid-induced pruritus: I.V.: 2.5-5 mg; may repeat dose (see Cohen, 1992)

Administration Parenteral: I.V.: Administer over 5-10 minutes; larger doses should be administered over 10-15 minutes

Monitoring Parameters Relief of pain, respiratory and mental status, blood pressure

Test Interactions May interfere with certain enzymatic methods used to detect opioids, depending on sensitivity and specificity of the test (refer to test manufacturer for details)

Patient Information Avoid alcohol; may cause drowsiness and impair ability to perform activities requiring mental alertness or physical coordination; may impair judgment; may be habit-forming; avoid abrupt discontinuation after prolonged use; will cause withdrawal in patients currently dependent on narcotics; may cause dry mouth

Nursing Implications Observe patient for excessive sedation, respiratory depression, implement safety measures, assist with ambulation; observe for narcotic withdrawal (nausea, vomiting, abdominal cramps, lacrimation, rhinorrhea, piloerection, anxiety, restlessness, increased temperature)

Additional Information Analgesic potency: 1 mg nalbuphine ~1 mg morphine

Dosage Forms Excipient information presented when available (limited, particularly for generics); consult specific product labeling. [DSC] = Discontinued product

Injection, solution, as hydrochloride: 10 mg/mL (10 mL); 20 mg/mL (10 mL)

Nubain®: 10 mg/mL (10 mL) [DSC]; 20 mg/mL (10 mL)

Injection, solution, as hydrochloride [preservative free]: 10 mg/mL (1 mL); 20 mg/mL (1 mL)

Nubain®: 10 mg/mL (1 mL); 20 mg/mL (1 mL)

References
Cohen SE, Ratner EF, Kreitzman TR, et al, "Nalbuphine is Better Than Naloxone for Treatment of Side Effects After Epidural Morphine," *Anesth Analg*, 1992, 75(5):747-52.

Jaillon P, Gardin ME, Lecocq B, et al, "Pharmacokinetics of Nalbuphine in Infants, Young Healthy Volunteers, and Elderly Patients," *Clin Pharmacol Ther*, 1989, 46(2):226-33.

Kendrick WD, Woods AM, Daly MY, et al, "Naloxone Versus Nalbuphine Infusion for Prophylaxis of Epidural Morphine-Induced Pruritus," *Anesth Analg*, 1996, 82:641-7.

Kjellberg F and Tramer MR, "Pharmacological Control of Opioid-Induced Pruritus: A Quantitative Systematic Review of Randomized Trials," *Eur J Anaesthesiol*, 2001, 18(6):346-57.

Nakatsuka N, Minogue SC, Lim J, et al, "Intravenous Nalbuphine 50 Microg x kg(-1) is Ineffective for Opioid-Induced Pruritus in Pediatrics," *Can J Anaesth*, 2006, 53(11):1103-10.

◆ **Nalbuphine Hydrochloride** see Nalbuphine on page 963

◆ **Nalcrom® (Can)** see Cromolyn on page 363

◆ **Nallpen** see Nafcillin on page 962

◆ **Nallpen® (Can)** see Nafcillin on page 962

◆ ***N*-allylnoroxymorphine Hydrochloride** see Naloxone on page 965

Naloxone (nal OKS one)

Medication Safety Issues
Sound-alike/look-alike issues:
Naloxone may be confused with Lanoxin®, naltrexone
Narcan® may be confused with Marcaine®, Norcuron®

International issues:
Narcan® may be confused with Marcen® which is a brand name for ketazolam in Spain

Related Information
CPR Pediatric Drug Dosages on page 1455

Canadian Brand Names Naloxone Hydrochloride Injection®

Therapeutic Category Antidote for Narcotic Agonists

Generic Available Yes

Use Reverses CNS and respiratory depression in suspected narcotic overdose; neonatal opiate depression; coma of unknown etiology; used as low dose I.V. continuous infusion for the prevention and treatment of narcotic-induced pruritus; adjunct in the treatment of septic shock (see Additional Information); used investigationally for phencyclidine and alcohol ingestion

Pregnancy Risk Factor C

Pregnancy Considerations Consider benefit to the mother and the risk to the fetus before administering to a pregnant woman who is known or suspected to be opioid dependent. May precipitate withdrawal in both the mother and fetus.

Lactation Excretion in breast milk unknown/not recommended

Breast-Feeding Considerations No data reported. Since naloxone is used for opiate reversal the concern should be on opiate drug levels in a breast-feeding mother and transfer to the infant rather than naloxone exposure. The safest approach would be **not** to breast-feed.

Contraindications Hypersensitivity to naloxone or any component

Warnings May precipitate withdrawal symptoms (hypertension, sweating, agitation, irritability, shrill cry, failure to feed) in patients with physical dependence to opiates (including newborns of narcotic dependent mothers)

Precautions Use with caution in patients with chronic cardiac or pulmonary disease or coronary artery disease. Following the use of narcotics during surgery, naloxone may reverse analgesia and increase blood pressure; use with caution and administer in smaller increments to patients suspected to be opioid dependent and in postoperative patients (to avoid large cardiovascular changes)

Adverse Reactions
Cardiovascular: Hypertension, hypotension, tachycardia, ventricular arrhythmias, cardiac arrest
Gastrointestinal: Nausea, vomiting
Miscellaneous: Diaphoresis increased

Drug Interactions
Avoid Concomitant Use There are no known interactions where it is recommended to avoid concomitant use.

Increased Effect/Toxicity There are no known significant interactions involving an increase in effect.

Decreased Effect There are no known significant interactions involving a decrease in effect.

Stability Protect from light; stable in NS and D_5W at 4 mcg/mL for 24 hours; do not mix with alkaline solutions

Mechanism of Action Competes and displaces narcotics at narcotic receptor sites

Pharmacodynamics
Onset of action:
E.T., I.M., SubQ: Within 2-5 minutes
I.V.: Within 2 minutes
Duration: (20-60 minutes) is shorter than that of most opioids; therefore, repeated doses are usually needed

Pharmacokinetics (Adult data unless noted)
Distribution: Crosses the placenta
Metabolism: Primarily by glucuronidation in the liver
Half-life:
Neonates: 1.2-3 hours
Adults: 0.5-1.5 hours (mean: ~1 hour)
Elimination: In urine as metabolites

Usual Dosage
PALS 2000 Guidelines: I.V. (**Note:** May be administered I.M., SubQ, or E.T., but onset of action may be delayed, especially if patient has poor perfusion; recommended PALS E.T. doses are 2-10 times the I.V. dose; see also Administration):
For total reversal of narcotic effect: **Note:** Doses may need to be repeated:
Infants and Children ≤ 5 years or ≤20 kg: 0.1 mg/kg
Children >5 years or >20 kg: 2 mg/dose
Alternative dosing to avoid sudden hemodynamic effects from opioid reversal: Use repeated doses of 0.01-0.03 mg/kg

Neonatal opioid-induced depression: I.V., I.M., SubQ: Manufacturer's recommendations: Initial: Usual: 0.01 mg/kg; may repeat every 2-3 minutes as needed based on response; may need to repeat every 1-2 hours

I.M., I.V. (preferred), E.T. (preferred if I.V. route not available), SubQ: **Note:** The dose for pediatric postoperative narcotic reversal is **one-tenth** of the dose used for opiate intoxication:

Opiate intoxication:
Birth (including premature infants) to 5 years or <20 kg: 0.1 mg/kg; repeat every 2-3 minutes if needed; may need to repeat doses every 20-60 minutes
>5 years or ≥20 kg: 2 mg/dose; if no response, repeat every 2-3 minutes; may need to repeat doses every 20-60 minutes

Children and Adults: I.V. continuous infusion: If continuous infusion is required, calculate the initial dosage/hour based on the effective intermittent dose used and duration of adequate response seen; titrate dose; a range of: 2.5-160 mcg/kg/hour has been reported; taper continuous infusion gradually to avoid relapse

Adults: 0.4-2 mg every 2-3 minutes as needed; may need to repeat doses every 20-60 minutes; **Note:** Use 0.1-0.2 mg increments in patients who are opioid dependent and in postoperative patients to avoid large cardiovascular changes.

Postanesthesia opioid reversal: Infants and Children: **0.01 mg/kg;** may repeat every 2-3 minutes as needed based on response

Manufacturer's recommendations (postoperative opioid depression): I.V.: Initial: 0.005-0.01 mg/dose every 2-3 minutes as needed based on response; may need to repeat every 1-2 hours

Opioid-induced pruritus:

Children and Adolescents: Limited pediatric information is available

Prevention: One double-blind, prospective, randomized, placebo-controlled study used the following dose: Children and adolescents 6-17 years (n=20): I.V.: Continuous infusion: 0.25 mcg/kg/hour; **Note:** Patients who received this dose experienced a lower incidence and severity of opioid-induced side effects (ie, pruritus, nausea) without a loss of pain control (see Maxwell, 2005).

Treatment: One retrospective study reported the following doses: Children and Adolescents 3-20 years (n=30): I.V.: Continuous infusion: Initial: 2 mcg/kg/hour; **Note:** Most initial nonresponders received antihistamines; may increase by 0.5 mcg/kg/hour every few hours if pruritus continues; mean (± SD) dose: 2.3 ± 0.68 mcg/kg/hour; monitor closely; doses ≥3 mcg/kg/hour may increase risk for loss of pain control and patients may require an increase in opioid dose (see Vrchoticky, 2000).

Adults: I.V.: Continuous infusion: Initial 0.25 mcg/kg/hour; **Note:** Doses ranging from 0.25-2.4 mcg/kg/hour have been used in randomized clinical trials; monitor closely; doses ≥2 mcg/kg/hour may increase risk for loss of pain control and patients may require an increase in opioid dose (see Kjellberg, 2001).

Administration

Endotracheal: Dilute to 1-2 mL with NS; PALS Guidelines 2000 recommendations: Dilute to 3-5 mL with NS; follow with several positive-pressure ventilations

Parenteral:

I.V. continuous infusion: Dilute to 4 mcg/mL in D_5W or NS

I.V. push: Administer over 30 seconds as undiluted preparation

Note: I.M. or SubQ administration in hypotensive patients or patients with peripheral vasoconstriction or hypoperfusion may result in erratic or delayed absorption

Monitoring Parameters Respiratory rate, heart rate, blood pressure

Nursing Implications Use of neonatal naloxone (0.02 mg/mL) is no longer recommended because unacceptably high fluid volumes will result, especially in small neonates; the 0.4 mg/mL preparation is available and can be accurately dosed with appropriately sized syringes (1 mL)

Additional Information Some products contain methyl and propylparabens. Naloxone has been used to increase blood pressure in patients with septic shock; increases in blood pressure may last several hours; however, an increase in patient survival has not been demonstrated and in some studies serious adverse effects (eg, agitation, pulmonary edema, hypotension, cardiac arrhythmias, seizures) have been reported; naloxone should be used with caution for septic shock, especially in patients with

underlying pain or opioid tolerance; optimal dosage for this indication has not been established; one neonatal study (n=2) reported a positive blood pressure response, but one neonate developed intractable seizures and died.

Dosage Forms Excipient information presented when available (limited, particularly for generics); consult specific product labeling.

Injection, solution, as hydrochloride: 0.4 mg/mL (1 mL, 10 mL)

Injection, solution, as hydrochloride [preservative free]: 0.4 mg/mL (1 mL); 1 mg/mL (2 mL)

References

American Academy of Pediatrics Committee on Drugs, "Naloxone Dosage and Route of Administration for Infants and Children: Addendum to Emergency Drug Doses for Infants and Children," *Pediatrics*, 1990, 86(3):484-5.

Chamberlain JM and Klein BL, "A Comprehensive Review of Naloxone for the Emergency Physician," *Am J Emerg Med*, 1994, 12(6):650-60.

"Guidelines 2000 for Cardiopulmonary Resuscitation and Emergency Cardiovascular Care, Part 10: Pediatric Advanced Life Support, The American Heart Association in Collaboration With the International Liaison Committee on Resuscitation," *Circulation*, 2000, 102(8 Suppl): I291-342.

"Guidelines 2000 for Cardiopulmonary Resuscitation and Emergency Cardiovascular Care, Part 11: Neonatal Resuscitation, The American Heart Association in Collaboration With the International Liason Committee on Resuscitation," *Circulation*, 2000, 102(8 Suppl): I343-357.

Kjellberg F and Tramer MR, "Pharmacological Control of Opioid-Induced Pruritus: A Quantitative Systematic Review of Randomized Trials," *Eur J Anaesthesiol*, 2001, 18(6):346-57.

Maxwell LG, Kaufmann SC, and Bitzer S, "The Effects of a Small-Dose Naloxone Infusion on Opioid-Induced Side Effects and Analgesia in Children and Adolescents Treated With Intravenous Patient-controlled Analgesia: A Double-Blind, Prospective, Randomized, Controlled Study," *Anesth Analg*, 2005, 100(4):953-8.

Vrchoticky T, "Naloxone for the Treatment of Narcotic Indiced Pruritus," *Journal of Pediatric Pharmacy Practice*, 2000, 5(2):92-7.

♦ **Naloxone and Buprenorphine** *see* Buprenorphine and Naloxone *on page 216*

♦ **Naloxone Hydrochloride** *see* Naloxone *on page 965*

♦ **Naloxone Hydrochloride Dihydrate and Buprenorphine Hydrochloride** *see* Buprenorphine and Naloxone *on page 216*

♦ **Naloxone Hydrochloride Injection® (Can)** *see* Naloxone *on page 965*

♦ **NAPA and NABZ** *see* Sodium Phenylacetate and Sodium Benzoate *on page 1274*

Naphazoline (naf AZ oh leen)

U.S. Brand Names AK-Con™; Clear eyes® for Dry Eyes and ACR Relief [OTC]; Clear eyes® for Dry Eyes and Redness Relief [OTC]; Clear eyes® Redness Relief [OTC]; Clear eyes® Seasonal Relief [OTC]; Privine® [OTC]

Canadian Brand Names Naphcon Forte®; Vasocon®

Therapeutic Category Adrenergic Agonist Agent, Ophthalmic; Decongestant, Nasal; Nasal Agent, Vasoconstrictor; Ophthalmic Agent, Vasoconstrictor

Generic Available No

Use Topical ocular vasoconstrictor (to soothe, refresh, moisturize, and relieve redness due to minor eye irritation); temporarily relieves nasal congestion associated with rhinitis, sinusitis, hay fever, or the common cold

Pregnancy Risk Factor C

Pregnancy Considerations Animal reproduction studies have not been conducted.

Lactation Excretion in breast milk unknown/use caution

Contraindications Hypersensitivity to naphazoline or any component; narrow-angle glaucoma; prior to peripheral iridectomy (in patients susceptible to angle block)

Warnings Excessive dosage may cause marked sedation in children, particularly infants

Precautions Rebound congestion may occur with extended use (use no longer than 3-5 days); use with caution in the presence of hypertension, diabetes mellitus, hyperthyroidism, heart disease, coronary artery disease, cerebral arteriosclerosis, or long-standing asthma

Adverse Reactions

Cardiovascular: Systemic cardiovascular stimulation (rare), pallor

Central nervous system: Dizziness, headache, nervousness, anxiety, tenseness, drowsiness, hallucinations, convulsions, CNS depression, prolonged psychosis

Gastrointestinal: Nausea, vomiting

Local: Transient stinging, nasal mucosa irritation, dryness

Ocular: Mydriasis, intraocular pressure elevated, blurring of vision, blepharospasm (ophthalmic formulations)

Respiratory: Respiratory difficulty, sneezing, rebound nasal congestion (nasal formulations)

Miscellaneous: Diaphoresis

Drug Interactions

Avoid Concomitant Use

Avoid concomitant use of Naphazoline with any of the following: Iobenguane I 123; MAO Inhibitors

Increased Effect/Toxicity

Naphazoline may increase the levels/effects of: Sympathomimetics

The levels/effects of Naphazoline may be increased by: Atomoxetine; Cannabinoids; MAO Inhibitors; Tricyclic Antidepressants

Decreased Effect

Naphazoline may decrease the levels/effects of: Iobenguane I 123

Mechanism of Action Stimulates alpha-adrenergic receptors in the arterioles of the conjunctiva and the nasal mucosa to produce vasoconstriction

Pharmacodynamics

Onset of action: Following topical administration, decongestion occurs within 10 minutes

Duration: 2-6 hours

Pharmacokinetics (Adult data unless noted) Elimination: Not well defined

Usual Dosage

Nasal: Intranasal not recommended for use in children <6 years of age (especially in infants) due to CNS depression; therapy should not exceed 3-5 days

Children 6-12 years: 0.05%, 1 drop or spray every 6 hours if needed

Children >12 years to Adults: 0.05%, 1-2 drops or sprays every 3-6 hours if needed

Ophthalmic: Therapy should generally not exceed 3-4 days; not recommended for use in children <6 years of age due to CNS depression (especially in infants)

Children >6 years and Adults (0.01% to 0.1%): Instill 1-2 drops every 3-4 hours

Administration

Ophthalmic: Instill drops into conjunctival sac of affected eye; finger pressure should be applied to lacrimal sac during and for 1-2 minutes after instillation to decrease risk of absorption and systemic reactions; avoid contact of bottle tip with skin or eye

Nasal: Spray or drop medication into one nostril while gently occluding the other; then reverse procedure

Patient Information Discontinue eye drops if visual changes or ocular pain occur

Dosage Forms Excipient information presented when available (limited, particularly for generics); consult specific product labeling.

Solution, intranasal, as hydrochloride [drops]:

Privine®: 0.05% (25 mL)

Solution, intranasal, as hydrochloride [spray]:

Privine®: 0.05% (20 mL)

Solution, ophthalmic, as hydrochloride:

AK-Con™: 0.1% (15 mL) [contains benzalkonium chloride]

Clear eyes® for Dry Eyes and ACR Relief: 0.025% (15 mL) [contains hypromellose, and zinc sulfate]

Clear eyes® for Dry Eyes and Redness Relief: 0.012% (15 mL) [contains hypromellose, glycerin and benzalkonium chloride]

Clear eyes® Redness Relief: 0.012% (6 mL, 15 mL, 30 mL) [contains glycerin and benzalkonium chloride]

Clear eyes® Seasonal Relief: 0.012% (15 mL, 30 mL) [contains glycerin, zinc sulfate and benzalkonium chloride]

◆ **Naphazoline Hydrochloride** *see* Naphazoline *on page 966*

◆ **Naphcon Forte® (Can)** *see* Naphazoline *on page 966*

◆ **Naprelan®** *see* Naproxen *on page 967*

◆ **Naprelan™ (Can)** *see* Naproxen *on page 967*

◆ **Naprosyn®** *see* Naproxen *on page 967*

Naproxen (na PROKS en)

Medication Safety Issues

Sound-alike/look-alike issues:

Naproxen may be confused with Natacyn®, Nebcin®

Aleve® may be confused with Alesse®

Anaprox® may be confused with Anaspaz®, Avapro®

Naprelan® may be confused with Naprosyn®

Naprosyn® may be confused with Naprelan®, Natacyn®, Nebcin®

Beers Criteria medication: This drug may be inappropriate for use in geriatric patients (high severity risk).

International issues:

Flogen® [Mexico] may be confused with Flovent® which is a brand name for fluticasone in the U.S.

Flogen® [Mexico] may be confused with Floxin® which is a brand name for ofloxacin in the U.S.

U.S. Brand Names Aleve® [OTC]; Anaprox®; Anaprox® DS; EC-Naprosyn®; Mediproxen [OTC]; Midol® Extended Relief [OTC]; Naprelan®; Naprosyn®; Pamprin® Maximum Strength All Day Relief [OTC]

Canadian Brand Names Anaprox®; Anaprox® DS; Apo-Napro-Na DS®; Apo-Napro-Na®; Apo-Naproxen EC®; Apo-Naproxen SR®; Apo-Naproxen®; Mylan-Naproxen EC; Naprelan™; Naprosyn®; Novo-Naproc EC; Novo-Naprox; Novo-Naprox Sodium; Novo-Naprox Sodium DS; Novo-Naprox SR; Nu-Naprox; PMS-Naproxen EC; PRO-Naproxen EC; Riva-Naproxen

Therapeutic Category Analgesic, Non-narcotic; Anti-inflammatory Agent; Antipyretic; Nonsteroidal Anti-inflammatory Drug (NSAID), Oral

Generic Available Yes

Use Management of inflammatory disease and rheumatoid disorders (including rheumatoid arthritis, juvenile rheumatoid arthritis, osteoarthritis, ankylosing spondylitis); acute gout; mild to moderate pain; primary dysmenorrhea; fever; tendonitis, bursitis. **Note:** Due to delayed absorption, the delayed-release tablets are **not** recommended for initial treatment of pain

Medication Guide An FDA-approved patient medication guide, which is available with the product information and at http://www.fda.gov/downloads/Drugs/DrugSafety/ucm088657.pdf, must be dispensed with this medication for each new outpatient prescription and refill.

Pregnancy Risk Factor C

Pregnancy Considerations Adverse events were not observed in the initial animal reproduction studies; therefore, the manufacturer classifies naproxen as pregnancy category C. Naproxen crosses the placenta and can be detected in fetal tissue and the serum of newborn infants following *in utero* exposure. NSAID exposure during the first trimester is not strongly associated with congenital malformations; however, cardiovascular anomalies and cleft palate have been observed following NSAID exposure in some studies. The use of a NSAID close to conception may be associated with an increased risk of miscarriage. Nonteratogenic effects have been observed following NSAID administration during the third trimester including: Myocardial degenerative changes, prenatal constriction of the ductus arteriosus, fetal tricuspid regurgitation, failure of the ductus arteriosus to close postnatally; renal dysfunction or failure, oligohydramnios; gastrointestinal bleeding or perforation, increased risk of necrotizing enterocolitis; intracranial bleeding (including intraventricular hemorrhage), platelet dysfunction with resultant bleeding; pulmonary hypertension. Because they may cause premature closure of the ductus arteriosus, use of NSAIDs late in pregnancy should be avoided (use after 31 or 32 weeks gestation is not recommended by some clinicians). The chronic use of NSAIDs in women of reproductive age may be associated with infertility that is reversible upon discontinuation of the medication. A registry is available for pregnant women exposed to autoimmune medications including naproxen. For additional information contact the Organization of Teratology Information Specialists, OTIS Autoimmune Diseases Study, at (877) 311-8972.

Lactation Enters breast milk/not recommended (AAP rates "compatible")

Breast-Feeding Considerations Small amounts of naproxen are excreted into breast milk. Naproxen has been detected in the urine of a breast-feeding infant. Breast-feeding is not recommended by the manufacturer. The AAP considers naproxen to be "usually compatible with breast-feeding." In a study which included 20 mother-infant pairs, there were two cases of drowsiness and one case of vomiting in the breast-fed infants. Maternal naproxen dose, duration, and relationship to breast-feeding were not provided.

Contraindications Hypersensitivity to naproxen or any component; history of asthma, urticaria, or allergic-type reaction to aspirin, or other NSAIDs; patients with the "aspirin triad" [asthma, rhinitis (with or without nasal polyps), and aspirin intolerance] (fatal asthmatic and anaphylactoid reactions may occur in these patients); perioperative pain in the setting of coronary artery bypass graft (CABG)

Warnings NSAIDs are associated with an increased risk of adverse cardiovascular thrombotic events, including potentially fatal MI and stroke **[U.S. Boxed Warning]**; risk may be increased with duration of use or pre-existing cardiovascular risk factors or disease; carefully evaluate cardiovascular risk profile prior to prescribing; use the lowest effective dose for the shortest duration of time, taking into consideration individual patient treatment goals; alternate therapies should be considered for patients at high risk. Use is contraindicated for treatment of perioperative pain in the setting of CABG surgery **[U.S. Boxed Warning]**; an increased incidence of MI and stroke was found in patients receiving COX-2 selective NSAIDs for the treatment of pain within the first 10-14 days after CABG surgery (see Contraindications). NSAIDs may cause fluid retention, edema, and new onset or worsening of pre-existing hypertension; use with caution in patients with hypertension, heart failure, or fluid retention; be aware of sodium content of sodium naproxen products in patients with sodium restriction. Concurrent administration of ibuprofen, and potentially other nonselective NSAIDs, may interfere with aspirin's cardioprotective effect.

NSAIDs may increase the risk of gastrointestinal irritation, ulceration, bleeding, and perforation **[U.S. Boxed Warning]**. These events, which can be potentially fatal, may occur at any time during therapy and without warning. Avoid the use of NSAIDs in patients with active GI bleeding or ulcer disease. Use NSAIDs with extreme caution in patients with a history of GI bleeding or ulcers (these patients have a 10-fold increased risk for developing a GI bleed). Use NSAIDs with caution in patients with other risk factors which may increase GI bleeding (eg, concurrent therapy with aspirin, anticoagulants and/or corticosteroids, longer duration of NSAID use, smoking, use of alcohol, and poor general health). Use the lowest effective dose for the shortest duration of time, taking into consideration individual patient treatment goals; alternate therapies should be considered for patients at high risk.

NSAIDs may compromise existing renal function. Renal toxicity may occur in patients with impaired renal function, dehydration, salt depletion, heart failure, liver dysfunction, those taking diuretics and ACE inhibitors; use with caution in these patients; monitor renal function closely. Naproxen is not recommended for use in patients with moderate to severe or severe renal impairment (Cl_{cr} <30 mL/minute). Long-term use of NSAIDs may cause renal papillary necrosis and other renal injury.

Fatal asthmatic and anaphylactoid reactions may occur in patients with the "aspirin triad" who receive NSAIDs (see Contraindications). Avoid use of NSAIDs in late pregnancy as they may cause premature closure of the ductus arteriosus. NSAIDs can cause serious skin reactions including exfoliative dermatitis, Stevens-Johnson Syndrome, and toxic epidermal necrolysis; these events may occur without warning; discontinue use at risk appearance of rash or other sign of hypersensitivity.

Precautions Use with caution in patients with decreased hepatic function; closely monitor patients with abnormal LFTs; severe hepatic reactions (eg, fulminant hepatitis, liver failure) have occurred with NSAID use, rarely; discontinue if signs or symptoms of liver disease develop, or if systemic manifestations occur. Use with caution in patients with asthma. Safety and efficacy have not been established in children <2 years of age.

OTC labeling: Prior to self-medication, patients should contact healthcare provider if they have had recurring stomach pain or upset, heartburn, ulcers, bleeding problems, asthma, allergy to aspirin or any other pain reliever or fever reducer, high blood pressure, heart or kidney disease, other serious medical problems, or are currently taking a diuretic, steroid, anticoagulant, aspirin, other NSAID, or any other drug. Recommended dosages and duration should not be exceeded, due to an increased risk of GI bleeding, MI, and stroke. Stop use and consult a healthcare provider if symptoms get worse, newly appear, or continue; if an allergic reaction occurs; if the patient feels faint, vomits blood, or has bloody or black stools; if the patient has difficulty swallowing or heartburn; if fever worsens or lasts >3 days; or if pain worsens or lasts >10 days in adults or >3 days in children. Consuming ≥3 alcoholic beverages/day or taking this medication longer than recommended may increase the risk of GI bleeding. Not for OTC use in children <12 years of age without consulting with physician. See also Patient Information.

Adverse Reactions

Cardiovascular: Edema, hypertension, palpitations

Central nervous system: Drowsiness, fatigue, headache, vertigo; aseptic meningitis (<1%)

Dermatologic: Pruritus, rash; pseudoporphyria (ie, skin fragility increased and blistering with scarring in sun-exposed skin), incidence: 12% in naproxen-treated children with JRA (discontinue therapy if this occurs);

exfoliative dermatitis, Stevens-Johnson syndrome, toxic epidermal necrolysis

Endocrine & metabolic: Fluid retention

Gastrointestinal: Abdominal pain, constipation, diarrhea, dyspepsia, GI bleed, heartburn, nausea, perforation, stomatitis, ulcers, vomiting

Hematologic: Agranulocytosis, anemia, inhibition of platelet aggregation, prolongation of bleeding time, thrombocytopenia

Hepatic: Liver enzymes elevated; rarely: hepatic necrosis, hepatitis, jaundice, liver failure

Ocular: Visual disturbances

Otic: Tinnitus

Renal: Renal dysfunction

Miscellaneous: Anaphylactoid reactions, hypersensitivity reactions

Drug Interactions

Metabolism/Transport Effects Substrate (minor) of CYP1A2, 2C9

Avoid Concomitant Use

Avoid concomitant use of Naproxen with any of the following: Ketorolac; Ketorolac (Systemic)

Increased Effect/Toxicity

Naproxen may increase the levels/effects of: Aminoglycosides; Anticoagulants; Antiplatelet Agents; Bisphosphonate Derivatives; Collagenase (Systemic); CycloSPORINE; CycloSPORINE (Systemic); Desmopressin; Digoxin; Drotrecogin Alfa; Eplerenone; Haloperidol; Ibritumomab; Lithium; Methotrexate; Nonsteroidal Anti-Inflammatory Agents; Pemetrexed; Potassium-Sparing Diuretics; Pralatrexate; Quinolone Antibiotics; Salicylates; Thrombolytic Agents; Tositumomab and Iodine I 131 Tositumomab; Vancomycin; Vitamin K Antagonists

The levels/effects of Naproxen may be increased by: Antidepressants (Tricyclic, Tertiary Amine); Corticosteroids (Systemic); Dasatinib; Glucosamine; Herbs (Anticoagulant/Antiplatelet Properties); Ketorolac; Ketorolac (Systemic); Nonsteroidal Anti-Inflammatory Agents; Omega-3-Acid Ethyl Esters; Pentosan Polysulfate Sodium; Pentoxifylline; Probenecid; Prostacyclin Analogues; Selective Serotonin Reuptake Inhibitors; Serotonin/Norepinephrine Reuptake Inhibitors; Treprostinil

Decreased Effect

Naproxen may decrease the levels/effects of: ACE Inhibitors; Angiotensin II Receptor Blockers; Antiplatelet Agents; Beta-Blockers; Eplerenone; HydrALAZINE; Loop Diuretics; Potassium-Sparing Diuretics; Salicylates; Thiazide Diuretics

The levels/effects of Naproxen may be decreased by: Bile Acid Sequestrants; Nonsteroidal Anti-Inflammatory Agents; Salicylates

Food Interactions Delayed-release tablets: Food delays the time to peak concentrations.

Stability Store tablets and suspension at room temperature [15°C to 30°C (59°F to 86°F)]; avoid exposure of suspension to excessive heat >40°C (104°F); dispense naproxen tablets and suspension in light-resistant, well-closed containers

Mechanism of Action Inhibits prostaglandin synthesis by decreasing the activity of the enzyme, cyclooxygenase, which results in decreased formation of prostaglandin precursors

Pharmacokinetics (Adult data unless noted)

Absorption: Oral: Almost 100%

Distribution: Crosses the placenta; ~1% distributed into breast milk

V_d: Adults: 0.16 L/kg

Protein binding: >99%

Metabolism: Extensively metabolized in the liver to 6-0-desmethyl naproxen; parent drug and desmethyl metabolite undergo further metabolism to their respective acylglucuronide conjugated metabolites

Bioavailability: 95%

Half-life, elimination: Children: Range: 8-17 hours

Children 8-14 years: 8-10 hours

Adults: 12-17 hours

Time to peak serum concentration:

Tablets, naproxen: 2-4 hours

Tablets, naproxen sodium: 1-2 hours

Tablets, delayed-release (empty stomach): 4-6 hours; range 2-12 hours

Tablets, delayed-release (with food): 12 hours; range: 4-24 hours

Suspension: 1-4 hours

Elimination: 95% excreted in urine (<1% as unchanged drug; <1% as 6-0-desmethyl naproxen; 66% to 92% as their conjugates); ≤3% excreted in feces

Usual Dosage Note: Dosage expressed as naproxen base; 200 mg naproxen base is equivalent to 220 mg naproxen sodium

Oral:

Children >2 years:

Analgesia: 5-7 mg/kg/dose every 8-12 hours

Inflammatory disease, including JRA: Usual: 10-15 mg/kg/day in 2 divided doses; range: 7-20 mg/kg/day; maximum dose: 1000 mg/day. Manufacturer's recommendation for JRA: 10 mg/kg/day in 2 divided doses

Children >12 and Adults ≤65 years: OTC labeling for pain and fever: 200 mg every 8-12 hours; if needed may take 400 mg for the initial dose; maximum dose: 600 mg/day

Adults:

Rheumatoid arthritis, osteoarthritis, and ankylosing spondylitis: 500-1000 mg/day in 2 divided doses

Acute gout: Initial: 750 mg, followed by 250 mg every 8 hours until attack subsides. **Note:** Delayed release tablet is not recommended due to delayed absorption.

Mild to moderate pain, dysmenorrhea, acute tendonitis, or bursitis: Initial: 500 mg, then 500 mg every 12 hours or 250 mg every 6-8 hours as needed; maximum dose: 1250 mg/day initially, then 1000 mg/day thereafter. **Note:** Delayed release tablet is not recommended for treatment of acute pain, due to delayed absorption.

Dosage adjustment in renal impairment: Moderate to severe and severe renal impairment (Cl$_{cr}$ <30 mL/minute): Not recommended for use

Administration Oral: Administer with food, milk, or antacids to decrease GI adverse effects. Shake suspension well before use. Do not chew, crush, or break delayed or controlled release tablet, swallow whole. Separate administration of naproxen and antacids, sucralfate, or cholestyramine by 2 hours.

Monitoring Parameters CBC with differential, platelets, BUN, serum creatinine, liver enzymes, occult blood loss, periodic ophthalmologic exams, hemoglobin, hematocrit, blood pressure

Test Interactions Naproxen may interfere with urinary tests for 17-ketogenic steroids, due to an interaction with m-di-nitrobenzene; interaction with the measurement of 17-hydroxy-corticosteroids does not appear to occur; however, naproxen should be discontinued 72 hours before adrenal function testing if the Porter-Silber test is used. Naproxen may interfere with urinary assays of 5-hydroxy indoleacetic acid (5HIAA).

Patient Information Naproxen is a nonsteroidal anti-inflammatory drug (NSAID); NSAIDs may cause serious adverse reactions, especially with overuse; use exactly as directed; do not increase dose or frequency; do not take longer than 3 days for fever (adults and children), 10 days for pain (adults), or 3 days for pain (children) without consulting healthcare professional. NSAIDs may increase the risk for heart attack, stroke, or ulcers and bleeding in stomach or intestines; GI bleeding, ulceration, or perforation can occur with or without pain. Notify physician before use if you have hypertension, heart failure, heart or kidney disease, history of stomach ulcers or bleeding in stomach or intestines, or other medical problems. Read the patient Medication Guide that you receive with each prescription and refill of naproxen.

While using this medication, do not use alcohol, excessive amounts of vitamin C, other prescription or OTC medications containing aspirin or salicylate, or other NSAIDs without consulting prescriber. Naproxen may cause dizziness or drowsiness and impair ability to perform activities requiring mental alertness or physical coordination. Children with JRA: Protect skin from sun; use sunscreen, wide-brimmed hats, etc.

Notify physician if changes in vision occur, if pain worsens or lasts >10 days in adults or >3 days in children, if fever worsens or lasts >3 days, if stomach pain or upset occurs, if swelling or redness occurs in painful area, or if any new symptoms appear. Stop taking medication and report ringing in ears; persistent cramping or stomach pain; unresolved nausea or vomiting; respiratory difficulty or shortness of breath; unusual bruising or bleeding (mouth, urine, stool); skin rash; unusual swelling of extremities; chest pain; or palpitations. Report weight gain or edema to physician.

OTC (pediatrics): Do not administer to children for >3 days unless recommended by physician or other healthcare professional; notify physician if child's condition does not improve or if worsens within 24 hours

Additional Information In a multicenter, retrospective chart review, 19 children, 4-14 years of age (mean: 9.1 ± 2.9) with rheumatic fever (but without carditis, chorea, or rashes), were treated solely with naproxen (10-20 mg/kg/day divided in 2 doses) until ESR normalized (between 4-8 weeks); fever and arthritis resolved within a median of 1 day of starting therapy; no patient had side effects, or developed carditis over the following 6 months; comparative studies with aspirin that include patients with mild carditis are needed to confirm these findings (see Uziel, 2000)

Due to its effects on platelet function, naproxen should be withheld for at least 4-6 half-lives prior to surgical or dental procedures.

Dosage Forms Excipient information presented when available (limited, particularly for generics); consult specific product labeling. [DSC] = Discontinued product
  Caplet, as sodium: 220 mg [equivalent to naproxen 200 mg and sodium 20 mg]
    Aleve®, Midol® Extended Relief, Pamprin® Maximum Strength All Day Relief: 220 mg [equivalent to naproxen 200 mg and sodium 20 mg]
  Capsule, liquid gel, as sodium:
    Aleve®: 220 mg [equivalent to naproxen 200 mg and sodium 20 mg]
  Combination package, oral [dose-pack]:
  Naprelan® [each package contains]:
    Day 1-3: Tablet, controlled release, oral, as sodium: 825 mg (6s) [equivalent to naproxen base 750 mg and sodium 75 mg]
    Day 4-10: Tablet, controlled release, oral, as sodium: 550 mg (14s) [equivalent to naproxen base 500 mg and sodium 50 mg]
  Gelcap, as sodium:
    Aleve®: 220 mg [equivalent to naproxen 200 mg and sodium 20 mg]
  Suspension, oral: 125 mg/5 mL (500 mL)
    Naprosyn®: 125 mg/5 mL (473 mL) [contains sodium 39 mg (1.5 mEq)/5 mL; orange-pineapple flavor]
  Tablet: 250 mg, 375 mg, 500 mg
    Naprosyn®: 250 mg, 375 mg, 500 mg

Tablet, as sodium: 220 mg [equivalent to naproxen 200 mg and sodium 20 mg]; 275 mg [equivalent to naproxen 250 mg and sodium 25 mg]; 550 mg [equivalent to naproxen 500 mg and sodium 50 mg]
    Aleve®: 220 mg [equivalent to naproxen 200 mg and sodium 20 mg]
    Anaprox®: 275 mg [equivalent to naproxen 250 mg and sodium 25 mg]
    Anaprox® DS: 550 mg [equivalent to naproxen 500 mg and sodium 50 mg]
    Mediproxen: 220 mg [equivalent to naproxen 200 mg and sodium 20 mg]
  Tablet, controlled release, as sodium:
    Naprelan®: 412.5 mg [equivalent to naproxen 375 mg and sodium 37.5 mg]
    Naprelan®: 550 mg [equivalent to naproxen 500 mg and sodium 50 mg]
    Naprelan®: 825 mg [equivalent to naproxen 750 mg and sodium 75 mg]
  Tablet, delayed release, enteric coated: 375 mg, 500 mg
    EC-Naprosyn®: 375 mg, 500 mg
  Tablet, extended release, as sodium: 550 mg [equivalent to naproxen 500 mg and sodium 50 mg] [DSC]

References
Berde C, Ablin A, Glazer J, et al, "American Academy of Pediatrics Report of the Subcommittee on Disease-Related Pain in Childhood Cancer," *Pediatrics*, 1990, 86(5 Pt 2):818-25.
Lang BA and Finlayson LA, "Naproxen-Induced Pseudoporphyria in Patients With Juvenile Rheumatoid Arthritis," *J Pediatr*, 1994, 124 (4):639-42.
Uziel Y, Hashkes PJ, Kassem E, et al, "The Use of Naproxen in the Treatment of Children With Rheumatic Fever," *J Pediatr*, 2000, 137 (2):269-71.
Wells TG, Mortensen ME, Dietrich A, et al, "Comparison of the Pharmacokinetics of Naproxen Tablets and Suspension in Children," *J Clin Pharmacol*, 1994, 34(1):30-3.

Nedocromil (ne doe KROE mil)

Related Information
  Asthma *on page 1697*
U.S. Brand Names Alocril®; Tilade® [DSC]
Canadian Brand Names Alocril®; Tilade®
Therapeutic Category Antiallergic, Ophthalmic; Antiasthmatic; Inhalation, Miscellaneous
Generic Available No

Use

Aerosol: Maintenance therapy in patients with mild to moderate asthma

Ophthalmic: Treatment of itching associated with allergic conjunctivitis

Pregnancy Risk Factor B

Pregnancy Considerations There are no well-controlled studies in pregnant women. Animal studies show no evidence of teratogenicity or harm to fetus. Additionally, nedocromil has minimal systemic absorption.

Lactation Excretion in breast milk unknown/use caution

Contraindications Hypersensitivity to nedocromil or any component

Warnings If systemic or inhaled steroid therapy is at all reduced, monitor patients carefully; nedocromil is **not** a bronchodilator and, therefore, should not be used for reversal of acute bronchospasm

Precautions Refrain from wearing contact lenses while exhibiting the signs and symptoms of allergic conjunctivitis

Adverse Reactions

Cardiovascular: Chest pain

Central nervous system: Dizziness, dysphonia, headache, fatigue

Dermatologic: Rash

Gastrointestinal: Nausea, vomiting, dyspepsia, diarrhea, abdominal pain, xerostomia, dysgeusia, unpleasant taste

Hepatic: ALT elevated

Neuromuscular and skeletal: Arthritis, tremor

Ocular: Burning, irritation, stinging, conjunctivitis, eye redness, photophobia (ophthalmic formulation)

Respiratory: Cough, pharyngitis, rhinitis, bronchitis, upper respiratory infection, bronchospasm, sputum production increased, pneumonitis with eosinophilia (PIE syndrome) (inhalation formulation)

Drug Interactions

Avoid Concomitant Use There are no known interactions where it is recommended to avoid concomitant use.

Increased Effect/Toxicity There are no known significant interactions involving an increase in effect.

Decreased Effect There are no known significant interactions involving a decrease in effect.

Stability Store at room temperature; do not freeze; the remaining contents of Alocril® unit dose solution should be discarded immediately after use

Mechanism of Action Inhibits the activation of and mediator release from a variety of inflammatory cell types associated with asthma including eosinophils, neutrophils, macrophages, mast cells, monocytes, and platelets; it inhibits the release of histamine, leukotrienes, and slow-reacting substance of anaphylaxis; it inhibits the development of early and late bronchoconstriction responses to inhaled antigen

Pharmacodynamics Inhalation: Duration: 2 hours; maximum therapeutic benefit is seen after at least 1 week of therapy

Pharmacokinetics (Adult data unless noted)

Absorption: Systemic: Inhalation: 7% to 9%; ophthalmic: <4%

Protein binding, plasma: 89%

Elimination: Excreted unchanged in urine 70%; feces 30%

Usual Dosage

Inhalation: Children ≥6 years and Adults: 2 inhalations 4 times/day; may reduce dosage to 2-3 times/day once desired clinical response to initial dose is observed

Ophthalmic: Children ≥3 years and Adults: 1-2 drops in each eye twice daily throughout the period of exposure to allergen

Administration

Oral inhalation: Shake well before use; must be primed by 3 actuations prior to first use; if canister remains unused for >7 days, reprime with 3 actuations; discard canister after 104 actuations

Ophthalmic: Instill drops into conjunctival sac; avoid contact of bottle tip with skin or eye

Patient Information May cause dry mouth

Additional Information Has no known therapeutic systemic activity when delivered by inhalation

Dosage Forms Excipient information presented when available (limited, particularly for generics); consult specific product labeling. [DSC] = Discontinued product

Aerosol for oral inhalation, as sodium:

Tilade®: 1.75 mg/activation (16.2 g; at least 104 inhalations) [DSC]

Solution, ophthalmic, as sodium:

Alocril®: 2% (5 mL) [contains benzalkonium chloride]

◆ **Nedocromil Sodium** see Nedocromil on page 970

Nefazodone (nef AY zoe done)

Medication Safety Issues

Sound-alike/look-alike issues:

Serzone® may be confused with selegiline, Serentil®, Seroquel®, sertraline

Related Information

Antidepressant Agents on page 1484

Serotonin Syndrome on page 1695

Therapeutic Category Antidepressant, Serotonin Reuptake Inhibitor/Antagonist

Generic Available Yes

Use Treatment of depression (FDA approved in adults)

Note: Due to the risk of hepatic failure, other antidepressant agents are generally tried first (see Warnings)

Medication Guide An FDA-approved patient medication guide, which is available with the product information and at http://dailymed.nlm.nih.gov/dailymed/drugInfo.cfm?id=4522, must be dispensed with this medication for each new outpatient prescription and refill.

Pregnancy Risk Factor C

Pregnancy Considerations Nefazodone is classified as pregnancy category C due to adverse effects observed in animal studies. When nefazodone is taken during pregnancy, an increased risk of major malformations has not been observed in the small number of pregnancies studied. The long-term effects on neurobehavior have not been evaluated.

Women treated for major depression and who are euthymic prior to pregnancy are more likely to experience a relapse when medication is discontinued as compared to pregnant women who continue taking antidepressant medications. Therapy during pregnancy should be individualized; treatment of depression during pregnancy should incorporate the clinical expertise of the mental health clinician, obstetrician, primary healthcare provider, and pediatrician. If treatment during pregnancy is required, consider tapering therapy during the third trimester to prevent potential withdrawal symptoms in the infant. If this is done and the woman is considered to be at risk of relapse from her major depressive disorder, the medication can be restarted following delivery. Treatment algorithms have been developed by the ACOG and the APA for the management of depression in women prior to conception and during pregnancy (Yonkers, 2009).

Lactation Enters breast milk/use caution

Breast-Feeding Considerations Nefazodone and its metabolites are excreted in breast milk. Drowsiness, lethargy, poor feeding, and failure to maintain body temperature have been reported in a premature nursing infant. Adverse events were not observed in two case reports of older infants. The long-term effects on neuro-behavior have not been studied. The manufacturer recommends that caution be exercised when administering nefazodone to nursing women.

Contraindications Hypersensitivity to nefazodone, related compounds (phenylpiperazine antidepressants), or any component; liver injury due to previous nefazodone treatment (see Warnings); concurrent use with astemizole, carbamazepine, cisapride, pimozide, or terfenadine; concurrent therapy with triazolam (see Warnings)

Warnings Nefazodone is not approved for use in pediatric patients. Clinical worsening of depression or suicidal ideation and behavior may occur in children and adults with major depressive disorder **[U.S. Boxed Warning]**. In clinical trials, antidepressants increased the risk of suicidal thinking and behavior (suicidality) in children, adolescents, and young adults (18-24 years of age) with major depressive disorder and other psychiatric disorders. This risk must be considered before prescribing antidepressants for any clinical use. Short-term studies did not show an increased risk of suicidality with antidepressant use in patients >24 years of age and showed a decreased risk in patients ≥65 years.

Patients of all ages who are treated with antidepressants for any indication require appropriate monitoring and close observation for clinical worsening of depression, suicidality, and unusual changes in behavior, especially during the first few months after antidepressant initiation or when the dose is adjusted. Family members and caregivers should be instructed to closely observe the patient (ie, daily) and communicate condition with healthcare provider. Patients should also be monitored for associated behaviors (eg, anxiety, agitation, panic attacks, insomnia, irritability, hostility, aggressiveness, impulsivity, akathisia, hypomania, mania) which may increase the risk for worsening depression or suicidality. Worsening depression or emergence of suicidality (or associated behaviors listed above) that is abrupt in onset, severe, or not part of the presenting symptoms, may require discontinuation or modification of drug therapy. If intolerable symptoms occur following a decrease in dosage or upon discontinuation of therapy, consider resuming the previous dose with a more gradual taper. Therapy should not be abruptly discontinued in patients receiving high doses for prolonged periods. To reduce risk of intentional overdose, write prescriptions for the smallest quantity consistent with good patient care.

Life-threatening hepatic failure has been reported in patients treated with nefazodone **[U.S. Boxed Warning]**. The estimated rate is 1 case of liver failure (resulting in liver transplant or death) per 250,000-300,000 patient-years of nefazodone treatment (3-4 times the background rate of liver failure); actual incidence may be higher due to under-reporting. Onset of liver injury has generally occurred between 2 weeks to 6 months of nefazodone therapy. Nefazodone should not routinely be started in patients with active liver disease or elevated baseline serum transaminases (baseline abnormalities may complicate patient monitoring). Nefazodone should be discontinued if clinical signs or symptoms suggestive of liver failure occur or if serum AST or ALT levels increase to ≥3 times the upper limit of normal. Do not reinitiate nefazodone in these patients.

Concurrent use with triazolam is contraindicated; nefazodone significantly increases triazolam serum concentrations; initial triazolam dosage must be reduced by 75% if drugs are used concomitantly; such reductions may not be possible with available dosage forms; thus, use with triazolam is contraindicated. Nefazodone significantly increases alprazolam serum concentrations; initial alprazolam dosage should be reduced by 50% if drugs are used concomitantly. Concurrent use of MAO inhibitors, use of MAO inhibitors within previous 14 days, and use of MAO inhibitors within 1 week of stopping nefazodone is not recommended; serious, potentially fatal reactions may occur. Nefazodone may potentially significantly increase plasma concentrations of astemizole, cisapride, pimozide, and terfenadine, resulting in QT prolongation and serious cardiovascular adverse events; concurrent use with any of these drugs is contraindicated. Carbamazepine will significantly decrease nefazodone serum concentrations; concurrent use is contraindicated.

May precipitate a shift to mania or hypomania in patients with bipolar disorder. Monotherapy in patients with bipolar disorder should be avoided. Patients presenting with depressive symptoms should be screened for bipolar disorder. Use with caution in patients with a history of mania. Nefazodone is not FDA approved for the treatment of bipolar depression.

Precautions Use with caution in patients with a history of seizures; seizures have been reported with nefazodone use. May cause orthostatic or postural hypotension; use with caution in patients with known cardiovascular or cerebrovascular disease or predisposing hypotensive conditions like dehydration, hypovolemia, or concurrent antihypertensive therapy. Priapism has been reported (rarely) during postmarketing surveillance; if condition occurs, therapy should be discontinued and physician contacted. Use with caution in patients with recent history of MI or unstable heart disease; nefazodone has not been studied in these patients; sinus bradycardia may occur with nefazodone use. Use with caution and decrease the dose in debilitated patients. May impair physical or mental abilities; patients must be cautioned about performing tasks which require mental alertness (eg, operating machinery or driving) until certain nefazodone does not adversely affect abilities. Visual disturbances, including blurred vision, scotoma, and visual trials have been reported. No clinical studies have assessed the combined use of nefazodone and electroconvulsive therapy; however, similar drugs may increase the risks associated with electroconvulsive therapy; consider discontinuing, when possible, prior to ECT treatment. Discontinue use prior to elective surgery (unknown interactions with general anesthetics may exist).

Adverse Reactions

Cardiovascular: Postural hypotension, peripheral edema, hypotension, bradycardia, vasodilation

Central nervous system: Headache, drowsiness, dizziness, insomnia, lightheadedness, confusion, memory impairment, abnormal dreams, concentration decreased, chills, fever, ataxia, incoordination, psychomotor retardation, agitation; suicidal thinking and behavior (see Warnings)

Dermatologic: Pruritus, rash

Endocrine & metabolic: Breast pain, libido decreased

Gastrointestinal: Xerostomia, nausea, constipation, dyspepsia, diarrhea, appetite increased, vomiting, thirst, taste perversion

Genitourinary: Urinary frequency, UTI, urinary retention, vaginitis

Hematologic: Hematocrit decreased

Hepatic: Liver enzymes elevated, hepatic failure (see Warnings)

Neuromuscular & skeletal: Weakness, parasthesia, tremor, hypertonia, arthralgia, neck rigidity

Ocular: Blurred vision, abnormal vision (scotoma, visual trails), visual field defect

Otic: Tinnitus

Respiratory: Pharyngitis, cough increased

Miscellaneous: Infection, flu syndrome

Drug Interactions

Metabolism/Transport Effects Substrate (major) of CYP2D6, 3A4; **Inhibits** CYP1A2 (weak), 2B6 (weak), 2C8 (weak), 2D6 (weak), 3A4 (strong); **Induces** P-glycoprotein

Avoid Concomitant Use

Avoid concomitant use of Nefazodone with any of the following: Alfuzosin; CarBAMazepine; Cisapride; Dronedarone; Eplerenone; Everolimus; Halofantrine; Nilotinib; Nisoldipine; Pimozide; Ranolazine; Rivaroxaban; Romidepsin; Salmeterol; Sibutramine; Silodosin; Tamsulosin; Tolvaptan

Increased Effect/Toxicity

Nefazodone may increase the levels/effects of: Alcohol (Ethyl); Alfuzosin; Almotriptan; Alosetron; Benzodiazepines (metabolized by oxidation); Bortezomib; Brinzolamide; CarBAMazepine; Cardiac Glycosides; Ciclesonide; Cisapride; Clozapine; CNS Depressants; Colchicine; CYP3A4 Substrates; Dienogest; Dronedarone; Dutasteride; Eplerenone; Everolimus; FentaNYL; Fesoterodine; GuanFACINE; Halofantrine; HMG-CoA Reductase Inhibitors; Ixabepilone; Lumefantrine; Maraviroc; Methyl-PREDNISolone; Nilotinib; Nisoldipine; Paricalcitol; Pazopanib; Pimecrolimus; Pimozide; Ranolazine; Rivaroxaban; Romidepsin; Salmeterol; Saxagliptin; Serotonin Modulators; Silodosin; Sorafenib; Tacrolimus; Tacrolimus (Systemic); Tacrolimus (Topical); Tadalafil; Tamsulosin; Tolvaptan

The levels/effects of Nefazodone may be increased by: BusPIRone; CYP2D6 Inhibitors (Moderate); CYP2D6 Inhibitors (Strong); CYP3A4 Inhibitors (Moderate); CYP3A4 Inhibitors (Strong); Dasatinib; MAO Inhibitors; Protease Inhibitors; Selective Serotonin Reuptake Inhibitors; Sibutramine

Decreased Effect

Nefazodone may decrease the levels/effects of: Dabigatran Etexilate; P-Glycoprotein Substrates; Prasugrel

The levels/effects of Nefazodone may be decreased by: CarBAMazepine; CYP3A4 Inducers (Strong); Deferasirox; Peginterferon Alfa-2b

Food Interactions Food delays absorption and decreases bioavailability by ~20%

Stability Store at controlled room temperature at 20°C to 25°C (68°F to 77°F); dispense in a tightly-closed, light-resistant container.

Mechanism of Action Inhibits neuronal reuptake of serotonin and norepinephrine; also blocks 5-HT_2 and alpha$_1$ receptors; has no significant affinity for alpha$_2$, beta-adrenergic, 5-HT_{1A}, cholinergic, dopaminergic, or benzodiazepine receptors

Pharmacodynamics

Maximum antidepressant effect: Adults: 4-6 weeks

Pharmacokinetics (Adult data unless noted)

Absorption: Oral: Rapid and complete

Distribution: Distributes into CNS; V_d: 0.22-0.87 L/kg

Protein binding: >99%

Metabolism: Hepatic, via N-dealkylation and aliphatic and aromatic hydroxylation, to three active metabolites: A triazoledione metabolite, hydroxynefazodone, and m-chlorophenylpiperazine (mCPP); other metabolites have also been identified but not tested for activity

Bioavailability: Oral: Absolute: 20% (variable); AUC increased by 25% in patients with cirrhosis of the liver

Half-life elimination: **Note:** Active metabolites persist longer in all populations.

Children: 4.1 hours

Adolescents: 3.9 hours

Adults: 2-4 hours

Time to peak serum concentration: **Note:** Prolonged in presence of food

Children and Adolescents: 0.5 -1 hour

Adults: 1 hour

Elimination: Primarily urine, as metabolites (<1% is eliminated as unchanged drug in urine); feces

Dialysis: Not likely to be of benefit

Usual Dosage Oral: Depression:

Children and Adolescents: **Note:** Not FDA approved; see Warnings. Limited information is available: Based on primary outcome measures, no randomized, placebo-controlled trial has shown nefazodone to be effective for the treatment of depression in pediatric patients (Findling, 2006; Laughren, 2004; Wagner, 2005); one study showed a positive trend toward efficacy (Emslie, 2000); two open-label trials [(n=28; age range: 7-17 years) and (n=10; adolescents)] showed nefazodone improved depressive symptom severity scores in children and adolescents (Findling, 2000; Goodnick, 2000); a small case series (n=7; age range: 9-17 years) showed improvement in depression severity scores in treatment refractory children and adolescents with multiple comorbid conditions (Wilens, 1997). Because efficacy has not been established in controlled clinical trials and due to the risk of hepatotoxicity, nefazodone is seldom prescribed in children and adolescents (Dopheide, 2006). If use is indicated, some experts recommend the following doses: Initial: 50 mg twice daily (100 mg/day) for at least 7 days; then increase to 100 mg twice daily (200 mg/day) for at least 7 days; then titrate at weekly intervals using 50 mg/day increments in children and 100 mg/day increments in adolescents; usual target range: 300-400 mg/day

Adults: Initial: 200 mg/day given in 2 divided doses; titrate in 100-200 mg/day increments at ≥1 week intervals; effective dosage: 300-600 mg/day in 2 divided doses

Administration May be administered with or without food

Monitoring Parameters Blood pressure, mental status, liver enzymes, clinical signs and symptoms of liver failure (discontinue nefazodone if clinical signs or symptoms suggestive of liver failure occur or if serum AST or ALT levels increase to ≥3 times the upper limit of normal; do not reinitiate nefazodone in these patients). Monitor patient periodically for symptom resolution; monitor for worsening depression, suicidality, and associated behaviors (especially at the beginning of therapy or when doses are increased or decreased; see Warnings).

Patient Information Read the patient Medication Guide that you receive with each prescription and refill of citalopram. An increased risk of suicidal thinking and behavior has been reported with the use of antidepressants in children, adolescents, and young adults (18-24 years of age). Notify physician if you feel more depressed, have thoughts of suicide, or become more agitated or irritable (see Warnings). Avoid alcohol, caffeine, CNS stimulants, tryptophan supplements, and the herbal medicine St John's wort. May cause dizziness or drowsiness and impair ability to perform activities requiring mental alertness or physical coordination; may cause dry mouth. Nefazodone may cause liver abnormalities ranging from increased liver enzymes to cases of liver failure resulting in death or liver transplantation; notify physician if you have yellowing of skin or the whites of eyes, lack of appetite for several days or longer, unusually dark urine, severe nausea, abdominal pain, or general weakness. Notify physician if you have any changes in vision or eye pain; hives, rash, or other allergic reactions. Discontinue use and consult physician immediately if prolonged or inappropriate erections occur. Some medicines should not be taken with nefazodone or should not be taken for a while after nefazodone has been discontinued; report the use of other medications, nonprescription medications, and herbal or natural products to your physician and pharmacist. It may take up to 4-6 weeks to see the full therapeutic effects from this medication. Take as directed; do not alter dose or frequency without consulting prescriber; avoid abrupt discontinuation.

Nursing Implications Assess other medications patient may be taking for possible interaction (especially MAO inhibitors, P450 inhibitors, and other CNS active agents). Assess mental status for depression, suicidal ideation, anxiety, social functioning, mania, or panic attack. Monitor liver enzymes and for clinical signs and symptoms of liver failure (see Monitoring Parameters and Warnings).

Dosage Forms Excipient information presented when available (limited, particularly for generics); consult specific product labeling.

Tablet, as hydrochloride: 50 mg, 100 mg, 150 mg, 200 mg, 250 mg

References

Dopheide JA, "Recognizing and Treating Depression in Children and Adolescents," *Am J Health Syst Pharm*, 2006, 63(3):233-43.

Dubitsky GM, "Review and Evaluation of Clinical Data: Placebo-Controlled Antidepressant Studies in Pediatric Patients. Available at www.fda.gov/ohrms/dockets/ac/04/briefing/20044065b1-08-TAB06-Dubitsky-Review.pdf. Accessed on April 21, 2009.

Emslie GJ, Findling RL, Rynn MA, et al, "Efficacy and Safety of Nefazodone in the Treatment of Adolescents with Major Depressive Disorder," *J Child Adolesc Psychopharmacol*, 2000, 12(4):299.

Findling RL, McNamara NK, Stansbrey RJ, et al, "The Relevance of Pharmacokinetic Studies in Designing Efficacy Trials in Juvenile Major Depression," *J Child Adolesc Psychopharmacol*, 2006, 16 (1-2):131-45.

Findling RL, Preskorn SH, Marcus RN, et al, "Nefazodone Pharmacokinetics in Depressed Children and Adolescents," *J Am Acad Child Adolesc Psychiatry*, 2000, 39(8):1008-16.

Goodnick PJ, Jorge CA, Hunter T, et al, "Nefazodone Treatment of Adolescent Depression: An Open-Label Study of Response and Biochemistry," *Ann Clin Psychiatry*, 2000, 12(2):97-100.

Laughren TP, "Memorandum to Members of PDAC and Peds AC: Background Comments for February 2, 2004 Meeting of Psychopharmacological Advisory Committee (PDAC) and Pediatric Subcommittee of the Anti-Infective Drugs Advisory Committee (Peds AC)." Available at www.fda.gov/ohrms/dockets/ac/04/briefing/2004–4065b1–04-Tab02-Laughren-Jan5.pdf. Accessed on April 21, 2009.

Wagner KD, "Pharmacotherapy for Major Depression in Children and Adolescents," *Prog Neuropsychopharmacol Biol Psychiatry*, 2005, 29 (5):819-26.

Wilens TE, Spencer TJ, Biederman J, et al, "Case Study: Nefazodone for Juvenile Mood Disorders," *J Am Acad Child Adolesc Psychiatry*, 1997, 36(4):481-5.

◆ **Nefazodone Hydrochloride** *see* Nefazodone *on page 971*

Nelarabine (nel AY re been)

Medication Safety Issues

High alert medication: The Institute for Safe Medication Practices (ISMP) includes this medication among its list of drug classes which have a heightened risk of causing significant patient harm when used in error.

Related Information

Emetogenic Potential of Antineoplastic Agents *on page 1579*

U.S. Brand Names Arranon®

Canadian Brand Names Atriance™

Therapeutic Category Antineoplastic Agent, Antimetabolite

Generic Available No

Use Treatment of relapsed or refractory T-cell acute lymphoblastic leukemia (ALL) and T-cell lymphoblastic lymphoma [FDA approved in pediatrics (age not specified) and adults]

Pregnancy Risk Factor D

Pregnancy Considerations Teratogenic effects were observed in animal studies. There are no adequate and well-controlled studies in pregnant women. May cause fetal harm if administered during pregnancy. Women of childbearing potential should be advised to use effective contraception and avoid becoming pregnant during therapy.

Lactation Excretion in breast milk unknown/not recommended

Breast-Feeding Considerations Due to the potential for serious adverse reactions in the nursing infant, breast-feeding is not recommended.

Contraindications Hypersensitivity to nelarabine or any component

Warnings Hazardous agent; use appropriate precautions for handling and disposal. Severe neurotoxicity, including severe somnolence, seizure, and peripheral neuropathy, has been reported **[U.S. Boxed Warning]**. Observe closely for signs and symptoms of neurotoxicity; discontinue if ≥grade 2. Adverse effects associated with demyelination or similar to Guillain-Barré syndrome (ascending peripheral neuropathies) have also been reported. Neurologic toxicities may not fully resolve and neurologic function return to baseline after treatment cessation. Neurologic toxicity is dose-limiting. Risk of neurotoxicity may increase in patients with concurrent or previous intrathecal chemotherapy or history of craniospinal irradiation.

Precautions Bone marrow suppression, including leukopenia, thrombocytopenia, anemia, neutropenia, and febrile neutropenia are associated with treatment; monitor blood counts regularly. Use extreme caution in patients with elevated uric acid, gout, and history of uric acid stones (monitor for hyperuricemia, consider allopurinol, and hydrate accordingly). Use caution in patients with renal impairment and severe hepatic impairment. Avoid administration of live vaccines in immunocompromised patients on nelarabine therapy.

Adverse Reactions

Cardiovascular: Chest pain, edema, hypotension, peripheral edema, tachycardia

Central nervous system: Amnesia, aphasia, ataxia (2%), attention disturbance, cerebral hemorrhage, coma, confusion, depression, dizziness, fatigue, fever, headache (17%), hemiparesis, hydrocephalus, insomnia, intracranial hemorrhage, lethargy, nerve palsy, nerve paralysis, progressive multifocal leukoencephalopathy, seizures (6%; see Warnings), somnolence (7%; see Warnings)

Dermatologic: Petechiae

Endocrine & metabolic: Anorexia, dehydration, hyperglycemia, hypocalcemia (8%), hypoglycemia (6%), hypokalemia (11%), hypomagnesemia (6%)

Gastrointestinal: Abdominal distention, abdominal pain, constipation, diarrhea, nausea, stomatitis, taste perversion, vomiting (10%)

Hematologic: Anemia (95%), leukopenia (38%), neutropenia (94%), thrombocytopenia (88%)

Hepatic: AST and ALT increased (12%), hyperbilirubinemia (10%), hypoalbuminemia (10%)

Neuromuscular & skeletal: Abnormal gait (6%), arthralgia, ascending peripheral neuropathy (similar to Guillain-Barré syndrome; see Warnings), back pain, demyelination, dysarthria, hypertonia, hypoesthesia (6%), hyporeflexia, incoordination, limb pain, motor dysfunction (4%), myalgia, neuropathic pain, paresthesia (4%), rigors, sciatica, tremor (4%), weakness

Ocular: Blurred vision, nystagmus

Renal: Serum creatinine increased (6%)

Respiratory: Cough, dyspnea, epistaxis, pleural effusion, pneumonia, sinusitis, wheezing

Miscellaneous: Infection

<1%, postmarketing, and/or case reports: Effusion, opportunistic infection, pneumothorax, progressive multifocal leukoencephalopathy, respiratory arrest, tumor lysis syndrome

Drug Interactions

Avoid Concomitant Use

Avoid concomitant use of Nelarabine with any of the following: BCG; Natalizumab; Pentostatin; Pimecrolimus; Tacrolimus (Topical); Vaccines (Live)

Increased Effect/Toxicity

Nelarabine may increase the levels/effects of: Leflunomide; Natalizumab; Vaccines (Live)

The levels/effects of Nelarabine may be increased by: Denosumab; Pimecrolimus; Tacrolimus (Topical); Trastuzumab

Decreased Effect

Nelarabine may decrease the levels/effects of: BCG; Sipuleucel-T; Vaccines (Inactivated); Vaccines (Live)

The levels/effects of Nelarabine may be decreased by: Echinacea; Pentostatin

Stability Store unopened vials at room temperature. Undiluted injection solution is stable in a PVC infusion bag or glass container for up to 8 hours at room temperature.

Mechanism of Action Nelarabine is a prodrug that is demethylated by adenosine deaminase to ara-G. Ara-G is phosphorylated by deoxyguanosine kinase and deoxycytidine kinase to ara-GTP (active). Ara-GTP is incorporated into the DNA of leukemic blasts leading to inhibition of DNA synthesis and cell death. Ara-GTP appears to accumulate at higher levels in T-cells compared with B-cells correlating to its differential activity.

Pharmacokinetics (Adult data unless noted)

Distribution: V_{ss}:

Nelarabine: Adults: 197 ± 216 L/m²; Children: 213 ± 358 L/m²

Ara-G: Adults: 50 ± 24 L/m²; Children: 33 ± 9.3 L/m²

Protein binding: Nelarabine and ara-G: <25%

Metabolism: Nelarabine is O-demethylated to ara-G by adenosine deaminase; ara-G undergoes hydrolysis to guanine; guanine is N-deaminated to xanthine which is further oxidized to form uric acid and then oxidized to form allantoin

Half-life:

Children:

Nelarabine: 13 minutes

Ara-G: 2 hours

Adults:

Nelarabine: 18 minutes

Ara-G: 3 hours

Elimination: Nelarabine 6.6% and ara-G 27% are excreted in urine within 24 hours of infusion on day 1

Clearance: Nelarabine clearance is ~30% higher in children (259 ± 409 L/hour/m²) than in adults (197 ± 189 L/hour/m²); ara-G clearance in children (11.3 ± 4.2 L/hour/m²) is similar to adults (10.5 ± 4.5 L/hour/m²)

Usual Dosage Refer to individual protocols: I.V.:

T-cell ALL, T-cell lymphoblastic lymphoma:

Children: 650 mg/m²/dose on days 1 through 5; repeat cycle every 21 days

Adults: 1500 mg/m²/dose on days 1, 3, and 5; repeat cycle every 21 days

Dosage adjustment for toxicity:

For neurologic toxicity ≥ grade 2 of NCI Common Toxicity Criteria: Discontinue treatment

For hematologic or other non-neurologic toxicity: Consider treatment delay

Dosage adjustment in renal impairment:

Cl_{cr} ≥50 mL/minute: No adjustment recommended

Cl_{cr} <50 mL/minute: Data are insufficient for a dosing recommendation; monitor closely

Dosage adjustment in hepatic impairment: Safety has not been established

Bilirubin >3 times ULN: Monitor closely

Administration I.V.: The appropriate nelarabine dose is transferred into an empty PVC infusion bag or glass container and administered undiluted.

Children: Infuse over 1 hour daily for 5 consecutive days

Adults: Infuse over 2 hours on days 1, 3, and 5

Monitoring Parameters Monitor for neurologic toxicity (severe somnolence, seizure, peripheral neuropathy, confusion, ataxia, paresthesia, hypoesthesia, coma, or craniospinal demyelination); signs and symptoms of tumor lysis syndrome; hydration status; CBC with platelet counts, renal and liver function tests

Patient Information May cause drowsiness and impair ability to perform activities requiring mental alertness or physical coordination. Notify physician if unusual bleeding, bruising, breathing difficulty, somnolence, confusion, seizures, coma, peripheral neuropathy (numbness and tingling in the hands, fingers, feet, or toes), problems with fine motor skills, unsteady gait, weakness, or paralysis occurs. Women of childbearing potential should be advised to avoid becoming pregnant while receiving nelarabine treatment.

Nursing Implications Appropriate measures must be taken to prevent hyperuricemia in patients at risk for tumor lysis syndrome (eg, hydration, urine alkalinization, and prophylaxis with allopurinol).

Dosage Forms Excipient information presented when available (limited, particularly for generics); consult specific product labeling. [CAN] = Canadian brand name

Injection, solution:

Arranon®: 5 mg/mL (50 mL)

Atriance™ [CAN]: 5 mg/mL (50 mL)

References

Berg SL, Blaney SM, Devidas M, et al, "Phase II Study of Nelarabine (Compound 506U78) in Children and Young Adults With Refractory T-Cell Malignancies: A Report From the Children's Oncology Group," *J Clin Oncol*, 2005, 23(15):3376-82.

Gandhi V, Plunkett W, Weller S, et al, "Evaluation of the Combination of Nelarabine and Fludarabine in Leukemias: Clinical Response, Pharmacokinetics, and Pharmacodynamics in Leukemia Cells," *J Clin Oncol*, 2001, 19(8):2142-52.

Kurtzberg J, Ernst TJ, Keating MJ, et al, "Phase I Study of 506U78 Administered on a Consecutive 5-Day Schedule in Children and Adults With Refractory Hematologic Malignancies," *J Clin Oncol*, 2005, 23(15):3396-403.

Nelfinavir (nel FIN a veer)

Medication Safety Issues

Sound-alike/look-alike issues:

Nelfinavir may be confused with nevirapine

Viracept® may be confused with Viramune®

Related Information

Adult and Adolescent HIV *on page 1620*

Management of Healthcare Worker Exposures to HBV, HCV, and HIV *on page 1661*

Pediatric HIV *on page 1613*

Perinatal HIV *on page 1628*

U.S. Brand Names Viracept®

Canadian Brand Names Viracept®

Therapeutic Category Antiretroviral Agent; HIV Agents (Anti-HIV Agents); Protease Inhibitor

Generic Available No

Use Treatment of HIV infection in combination with other antiretroviral agents. (**Note:** HIV regimens consisting of **three** antiretroviral agents are strongly recommended)

Pregnancy Risk Factor B

Pregnancy Considerations Adverse events were not observed in animal studies and no increased risk of overall birth defects has been observed following 1st trimester exposure in humans according to data collected by the antiretroviral pregnancy registry. Nelfinavir crosses the placenta. The Perinatal HIV Guidelines Working Group recommends nelfinavir as an alternative PI in combination regimens during pregnancy with HAART for perinatal prophylaxis. A dose of 1250 mg twice daily has been shown to provide adequate plasma concentrations although lower and variable levels may occur late in pregnancy. Pregnancy and protease inhibitors are both associated with an increased risk of hyperglycemia. Glucose levels should be closely monitored. Health professionals are encouraged to contact the antiretroviral pregnancy registry to monitor outcomes of pregnant women exposed to antiretroviral medications (1-800-258-4263 or www.APRegistry.com).

Lactation Excretion in breast milk unknown/contraindicated

Breast-Feeding Considerations In infants born to mothers who are HIV positive, HAART while breast-feeding may decrease postnatal infection. However, maternal or infant antiretroviral therapy does not completely eliminate the risk of postnatal HIV transmission.

In the United States where formula is accessible, affordable, safe, and sustainable, complete avoidance of breast-feeding by HIV-infected women is recommended to decrease potential transmission of HIV.

Contraindications Hypersensitivity to nelfinavir or any component; concurrent therapy with amiodarone, dihydroergotamine, ergonovine, ergotamine, midazolam, methylergonovine, pimozide, quinidine, or triazolam

Warnings Nelfinavir inhibits cytochrome P450 isoenzyme CYP3A and interacts with numerous drugs. Due to potential serious and/or life-threatening drug interactions, some drugs are contraindicated (see Contraindications and Drug Interactions) and the following drugs should **not** be coadministered with nelfinavir: Astemizole, cisapride, terfenadine, rifampin, St John's wort, lovastatin, simvastatin, or proton pump inhibitors; concurrent use with some anticonvulsants may significantly limit nelfinavir's effectiveness. Spontaneous bleeding episodes have been reported in patients with hemophilia type A and B receiving protease inhibitors. New onset diabetes mellitus, exacerbations of diabetes, and hyperglycemia have been reported in HIV-infected patients receiving protease inhibitors.

Precautions Use with caution in patients with mild hepatic impairment; use is **not** recommended in patients with moderate or severe hepatic impairment; nelfinavir is metabolized in the liver and may also cause hepatitis and/or exacerbate pre-existing hepatic dysfunction. Fat redistribution and accumulation [ie, central obesity, peripheral wasting, facial wasting, breast enlargement, dorsocervical fat enlargement (buffalo hump), and cushingoid appearance] have been observed in patients receiving antiretroviral agents (causal relationship not established). Immune reconstitution syndrome (an acute inflammatory response to residual or indolent opportunistic infections) may occur in HIV patients during initial treatment with combination antiretroviral agents, including nelfinavir; this syndrome may require further patient assessment and therapy. Powder formulation contains aspartame which is metabolized to phenylalanine and should be avoided or used with caution in patients with phenylketonuria. For information concerning a manufacturing process-related impurity (ethyl methanesulfonate; EMS), see Additional Information.

Adverse Reactions Note: Adverse effects are similar in children and adults, with diarrhea being the most common adverse effect in both age groups

Cardiovascular: Hypertension

Central nervous system: Concentration decreased, anxiety, depression, dizziness, emotional lability, hyperkinesia, insomnia, migraine, seizures, sleep disorder, somnolence, suicide ideation, fever, headache, asthenia, malaise

Dermatologic: Rash, pruritus, urticaria, diaphoresis

Endocrine & metabolic: Hyperlipemia, hyperuricemia; rare: hyperglycemia, diabetes, ketoacidosis; fat redistribution and accumulation (see Precautions); **Note:** Lipodystrophy was observed in 28% of children after a median of 49 months of receiving a nelfinavir-containing antiretroviral regimen (see Scherpbier, 2006)

Gastrointestinal: Diarrhea (adults: 14% to 20%; children: 39% to 47%; **Note:** A secretory diarrhea, mediated via a calcium-dependent process, may occur; calcium carbonate, administered at the same time as nelfinavir, has been used to treat this adverse effect in adults without affecting plasma concentrations of nelfinavir or its major metabolite), nausea, flatulence, abdominal pain, anorexia, dyspepsia, epigastric pain, mouth ulceration, GI bleeding, pancreatitis, vomiting

Genitourinary: Kidney calculus, sexual dysfunction

Hematologic: Anemia, leukopenia, thrombocytopenia; rare: spontaneous bleeding episodes in hemophiliacs

Hepatic: Hepatitis, liver function tests elevated, worsening of chronic liver disease

Neuromuscular & skeletal: Weakness, arthralgia, arthritis, cramps, myalgia, myasthenia, myopathy, paresthesia, back pain

Ocular: Acute iritis

Respiratory: Dyspnea, pharyngitis, rhinitis, sinusitis

Drug Interactions

Metabolism/Transport Effects **Substrate** of CYP2C9 (minor), CYP2C19 (major), CYP2D6 (minor), CYP3A4 (major), P-glycoprotein; **Inhibits** CYP1A2 (weak), CYP2B6 (weak), CYP2C9 (weak), CYP2C19 (weak), CYP2D6 (weak), CYP3A4 (strong), P-glycoprotein

Avoid Concomitant Use

Avoid concomitant use of Nelfinavir with any of the following: Alfuzosin; Amiodarone; Cisapride; Dabigatran Etexilate; Dronedarone; Eplerenone; Ergot Derivatives; Everolimus; Halofantrine; Lovastatin; Midazolam; Nilotinib; Nisoldipine; Pimozide; Proton Pump Inhibitors; QuiNIDine; Ranolazine; Rivaroxaban; Romidepsin; Salmeterol; Silodosin; Simvastatin; St Johns Wort; Tamsulosin; Tolvaptan; Topotecan; Triazolam

Increased Effect/Toxicity

Nelfinavir may increase the levels/effects of: Alfuzosin; Almotriptan; Alosetron; ALPRAZolam; Amiodarone; Antifungal Agents (Azole Derivatives, Systemic); Azithromycin; Bortezomib; Brinzolamide; Calcium Channel Blockers (Dihydropyridine); Calcium Channel Blockers (Nondihydropyridine); CarBAMazepine; Ciclesonide; Cisapride; Clarithromycin; Colchicine; Corticosteroids (Orally Inhaled); CycloSPORINE; CycloSPORINE (Systemic); CYP3A4 Substrates; Dabigatran Etexilate; Dienogest; Digoxin; Dronedarone; Dutasteride; Enfuvirtide; Eplerenone; Ergot Derivatives; Etravirine; Everolimus; FentaNYL; Fesoterodine; Fusidic Acid; GuanFACINE; Halofantrine; HMG-CoA Reductase Inhibitors; Ixabepilone; Lovastatin; Lumefantrine; Maraviroc; Meperidine; MethylPREDNISolone; Midazolam; Nefazodone; Nilotinib; Nisoldipine; Paricalcitol; Pazopanib; P-Glycoprotein Substrates; Pimecrolimus; Pimozide; Protease Inhibitors; QuiNIDine; Ranolazine; Rifamycin Derivatives; Rivaroxaban; Romidepsin; Salmeterol; Saxagliptin; Sildenafil; Silodosin; Simvastatin; Sirolimus; Sorafenib; Tacrolimus; Tacrolimus (Systemic); Tacrolimus (Topical); Tadalafil; Tamsulosin; Temsirolimus; Tenofovir; Tolvaptan; Topotecan; TraZODone; Triazolam; Tricyclic Antidepressants; Vardenafil

The levels/effects of Nelfinavir may be increased by: Antifungal Agents (Azole Derivatives, Systemic); Clarithromycin; CycloSPORINE; CycloSPORINE (Systemic); Delavirdine; Efavirenz; Enfuvirtide; Etravirine; Fusidic Acid; P-Glycoprotein Inhibitors

Decreased Effect
Nelfinavir may decrease the levels/effects of: Abacavir; Clarithromycin; Contraceptives (Estrogens); Delavirdine; Divalproex; Etravirine; Meperidine; Methadone; Prasugrel; Theophylline Derivatives; Valproic Acid; Zidovudine

The levels/effects of Nelfinavir may be decreased by: Antacids; CarBAMazepine; Contraceptives (Estrogens); CYP2C19 Inducers (Strong); CYP3A4 Inducers (Strong); Deferasirox; Efavirenz; Garlic; H2-Antagonists; Nevirapine; Peginterferon Alfa-2b; P-Glycoprotein Inducers; Proton Pump Inhibitors; Rifamycin Derivatives; St Johns Wort; Tenofovir

Food Interactions Food enhances bioavailability and decreases pharmacokinetic variability. A bitter taste will result if the oral powder formulation is mixed with acidic food or juice (see Administration)

Stability Store at room temperature of 15°C to 30°C (59°F to 86°F). Dispense in original container; keep container tightly closed.

Mechanism of Action A protease inhibitor which acts on an enzyme (protease) late in the HIV replication process after the virus has entered into the cell's nucleus; nelfinavir binds to the protease activity site and inhibits the activity of the enzyme, thus preventing cleavage of viral polyprotein precursors (gag-pol protein precursors) into individual functional proteins found in infectious HIV; this results in the formation of immature, noninfectious viral particles

Pharmacokinetics (Adult data unless noted)
Absorption: AUC is two- to threefold higher under fed conditions versus fasting; AUC is highly variable in pediatric patients due to increased clearance, problems with compliance, and inconsistent food intake with dosing

Distribution: V_d: Adults: 2-7 L/kg

Protein binding: >98%

Metabolism: Via multiple cytochrome P450 isoforms including CYP3A4 and CYP2C19; one active oxidative metabolite with comparable activity to the parent drug and several minor oxidative metabolites are formed

Bioavailability: Adults: 20% to 80%; **Note:** The 625 mg and 250 mg tablet formulations were shown to be bioequivalent in HIV-infected patients receiving multiple doses of 1250 mg twice daily (under fed conditions). In healthy volunteers, the 250 mg and 625 mg tablets were **not** bioequivalent; the AUC for the 625 mg tablets was 34% higher than the 250 mg tablets in fasted adults and 24% higher than the 250 mg tablets under fed conditions. Nelfinavir concentrations following a single 750 mg dose using the 250 mg tablets were similar to those after administration of the oral powder, under fed conditions in healthy volunteers.

Half-life: Adults: 3.5-5 hours

Time to peak serum concentration: 2-4 hours

Elimination: 98% to 99% excreted in feces (78% as metabolites and 22% as unchanged nelfinavir); 1% to 2% excreted in urine (primarily as unchanged drug)

Usual Dosage Oral (use in combination with other antiretroviral agents):
Neonates and Infants: Not approved for use; a reliable, effective dose has not been established. **Note:** 40 mg/kg/dose twice daily given to neonates and infants (age: birth to 6 weeks) resulted in high interpatient variability in serum drug concentrations; nelfinavir dosing is problematic in young infants, since the drug is best absorbed when taken with a high fat meal; higher doses are currently being studied. **Note:** Three times daily dosing may be required in infants <2 months of age; further studies are needed (see Hirt, 2006; Working Group, 2008).

Infants and Children <2 years: Not approved for use; a reliable, effective dose has not been established. **Note:** Current guidelines recommend nelfinavir (as an alternative PI) for initial therapy only in children >2 years of age; this is due to a lower virologic response observed in children <2 years and the lack of appropriate dosing recommendations (see Working Group, 2008).

Children 2-13 years (oral powder or 250 mg tablets): 45-55 mg/kg/dose (maximum: 1250 mg) twice daily or 25-35 mg/kg/dose (maximum: 750 mg) 3 times/day; **Note:** Doses >2500 mg/day have not been studied in children

Adolescents ≥14 years and Adults: 1250 mg/dose twice daily or 750 mg 3 times/day

Dosing adjustment in hepatic impairment:
Mild hepatic impairment (Child-Pugh Class A): Use with caution; no dosage adjustment is necessary. In adults, nelfinavir AUC and C_{max} were not significantly different compared to subjects with normal hepatic function.

Moderate hepatic impairment (Child-Pugh Class B): Not recommended for use. In adults, nelfinavir AUC was increased by 62% and C_{max} was increased by 22% compared to subjects with normal hepatic function.

Severe hepatic impairment (Child-Pugh Class C): Has not been studied; not recommended for use.

Dosing adjustment in renal impairment: Has not been studied; however, since <2% of the drug is eliminated in the urine, renal impairment should have minimal effect on nelfinavir elimination

Administration Administer with food to enhance bioavailability and decrease kinetic variability. **Note:** Due to problems with administration of the oral powder to infants, use of the tablets may be preferred. Tablets can be readily dissolved in water and consumed or mixed with milk or chocolate milk; consume immediately; rinse glass with water and swallow to make sure total dose is consumed; tablets can also be crushed and administered with pudding. Oral powder can be mixed with a small amount of water, milk, formula, dietary supplements, ice cream, or pudding; mixture must be stored under refrigeration if not used immediately; do not store mixture for more than 6 hours; do not mix oral powder with any acidic food or juice (eg, grapefruit, orange, or apple juice or applesauce) because of resulting bitter taste. If coadministered with didanosine, nelfinavir should be administered 2 hours before or 1 hour after didanosine.

Monitoring Parameters Liver function tests, blood glucose levels, CBC with differential, CD4 cell count, plasma levels of HIV RNA

Patient Information Nelfinavir is not a cure for HIV. Some medications should not be taken with nelfinavir; report the use of other medications, nonprescription medications, and herbal or natural products to your physician and pharmacist; avoid the herbal medicine St John's wort. Use an alternative method of contraception to birth control pills during nelfinavir therapy. If a nelfinavir dose is missed, take the dose as soon as possible and then return to the normal schedule. However, if a dose is skipped, do not double the next dose.

HIV medications may cause changes in body fat, including an increase in fat in the upper back and neck, breasts, and trunk; a loss of fat from the face, arms, and legs may also occur.

Nursing Implications Do not add water to bottles of oral powder; a special scoop is provided with powder for measuring purposes. If diarrhea occurs, it may be treated with an antimotility agent like loperamide

Additional Information Due to the higher variability of nelfinavir plasma concentrations in infants and children, dosage adjustment utilizing measurement of plasma concentrations and pharmacokinetics may be beneficial (see Crommentuyn, 2006; Fletcher, 2008). Further studies are needed.

In September 2007, a notice was mailed to healthcare providers concerning a possible manufacturing process-related impurity (ethyl methanesulfonate; EMS) in

◀ Viracept® (nelfinavir). EMS has been shown to be teratogenic, mutagenic, and carcinogenic in animal studies. No human data is available. Nelfinavir had been recalled in Europe because of unacceptably high levels of EMS. Testing revealed that levels of EMS in Viracept® manufactured by Pfizer in the U.S. were lower than those in Viracept® manufactured by Roche in Europe. At the time, Pfizer was working to refine the manufacturing process in order to ensure that the product met specifications for the amount of EMS that is acceptable. Until that issue was resolved, as a precaution, the "Dear Health Care Professional" letter of September 2007 recommended that pediatric and pregnant patients should not be started on nelfinavir; pediatric patients who were stable on nelfinavir-containing regimens could continue to receive nelfinavir; pregnant women receiving nelfinavir should be switched to an alternative agent (unless other treatment options were not available). An acceptable limit of EMS in nelfinavir has now been agreed upon by the FDA and Pfizer. As of March 31, 2008, all Viracept® manufactured by Pfizer meets the acceptable limit. Pfizer notified healthcare providers in May 2008 that nelfinavir may once again be prescribed as indicated to all patient populations (including children and pregnant women). For additional information concerning the May 2008 notice, refer to the following AIDsinfo website: http://aidsinfo.nih.gov/contentfiles/NFV_prescribing_info.pdf. For additional information concerning the September 2007 notices, refer to the following FDA website: http://www.fda.gov/Safety/MedWatch/SafetyInformation/SafetyAlertsforHumanMedicalProducts/ucm152969.htm

Dosage Forms Excipient information presented when available (limited, particularly for generics); consult specific product labeling.

Powder, oral:
  Viracept®: 50 mg/g (144 g) [contains phenylalanine 11.2 mg/g]
Tablet:
  Viracept®: 250 mg, 625 mg

References
Briars LA, Hilao JJ, and Kraus DM, "A Review of Pediatric Human Immunodeficiency Virus Infection," *Journal of Pharmacy Practice*, 2004, 17(6):407-31.

Crommentuyn KM, Scherpbier HJ, Kuijpers TW, et al, "Population Pharmacokinetics and Pharmacodynamics of Nelfinavir and Its Active Metabolite M8 in HIV-1-Infected Children," *Pediatr Infect Dis J*, 2006, 25(6):538-43.

Fletcher CV, Brundage RC, Fenton T, et al, "Pharmacokinetics and Pharmacodynamics of Efavirenz and Nelfinavir in HIV-Infected Children Participating in an Area-Under-the-Curve Controlled Trial," *Clin Pharmacol Ther*, 2008, 83(2):300-6.

Hirt D, Urien S, Jullien V, et al, "Age-Related Effects on Nelfinavir and M8 Pharmacokinetics: A Population Study With 182 Children," *Antimicrob Agents Chemother*, 2006, 50(3):910-6.

McDonald CK and Kuritzkes DR, "Human Immunodeficiency Virus Type I Protease Inhibitors," *Arch Intern Med*, 1997, 157(9):951-9.

Panel on Antiretroviral Guidelines for Adults and Adolescents, "Guidelines for the Use of Antiretroviral Agents in HIV-Infected Adults and Adolescents," December 1, 20098, http://www.aidsinfo.nih.gov.

Scherpbier HJ, Bekker V, van Leth F, et al, "Long-Term Experience With Combination Antiretroviral Therapy That Contains Nelfinavir for Up to 7 Years in a Pediatric Cohort," *Pediatrics*, 2006, 117(3):e528-36.

Working Group on Antiretroviral Therapy and Medical Management of HIV-Infected Children, "Guidelines for the Use of Antiretroviral Agents in Pediatric HIV Infection," February 23, 2009. Available at http://www.aidsinfo.nih.gov.

◆ **Nembutal®** *see* PENTobarbital *on page* 1087

◆ **Nembutal® Sodium (Can)** *see* PENTobarbital *on page* 1087

◆ **NeoBenz® Micro [DSC]** *see* Benzoyl Peroxide *on page* 184

◆ **NeoBenz® Micro SD [DSC]** *see* Benzoyl Peroxide *on page* 184

◆ **NeoBenz® Micro Wash [DSC]** *see* Benzoyl Peroxide *on page* 184

◆ **Neo-Fradin™** *see* Neomycin *on page* 978

◆ **Neofrin™** *see* Phenylephrine *on page* 1102

Neomycin (nee oh MYE sin)

U.S. Brand Names Neo-Fradin™; Neo-Rx

Therapeutic Category Ammonium Detoxicant; Antibiotic, Aminoglycoside; Antibiotic, Topical; Hyperammonemia Agent

Generic Available Yes

Use Administered orally to prepare GI tract for surgery; treat minor skin infections; treat diarrhea caused by *E. coli*; adjunct in the treatment of hepatic encephalopathy

Pregnancy Risk Factor D

Pregnancy Considerations Aminoglycosides cross the placenta; however, neomycin has limited maternal absorption. Therefore the portion of an orally administered maternal dose available to cross the placenta is very low. Teratogenic effects have not been observed following maternal use of neomycin. Because of several reports of total irreversible bilateral congenital deafness in children whose mothers received another aminoglycoside (streptomycin) during pregnancy, the manufacturer classifies neomycin as pregnancy category D.

Lactation Excretion in breast milk unknown/not recommended

Breast-Feeding Considerations It is not known if neomycin is excreted into breast milk; however, limited oral absorption by both the mother and infant would minimize exposure to the nursing infant. Nondose-related effects could include modification of bowel flora. Breast-feeding is not recommended by the manufacturer.

Contraindications Hypersensitivity to neomycin or any component, or other aminoglycosides; patients with intestinal obstruction, inflammatory or ulcerative gastrointestinal disease

Warnings Neomycin is more toxic than other aminoglycosides when given parenterally; **do not administer parenterally**; topical neomycin is a contact sensitizer with sensitivity occurring in 5% to 15% of patients treated with the drug; systemic absorption can occur when neomycin is utilized for irrigation of wounds or surgical sites. Systemic absorption occurs following oral administration; toxic reactions may occur **[U.S. Boxed Warning]**. Concurrent and/or sequential use of any form of other aminoglycosides should be avoided because toxicity may be additive **[U.S. Boxed Warning]**. May cause nephrotoxicity **[U.S. Boxed Warning]**; usual risk factors include pre-existing renal impairment, concomitant nephrotoxic medications, advanced age, and dehydration. Discontinue treatment if signs of nephrotoxicity occur; renal damage is usually reversible. May cause neurotoxicity **[U.S. Boxed Warning]**; usual risk factors include pre-existing renal impairment, concomitant neuro-/nephrotoxic medications, advanced age, and dehydration. Ototoxicity is proportional to the amount of drug given and the duration of treatment. Tinnitus or vertigo may be indications of vestibular injury and impending bilateral irreversible damage. Discontinue treatment if signs of ototoxicity occur; risk of hearing loss continues after drug withdrawal. Avoid concurrent use of potent diuretics due to risk of ototoxicity **[U.S. Boxed Warning]**; intravenous use of diuretics may enhance neomycin toxicity by altering concentration in serum and tissue. May cause neuromuscular blockade and respiratory paralysis **[U.S. Boxed Warning]**, especially when given soon after anesthesia or muscle relaxants.

Precautions Use with caution in patients with renal impairment, pre-existing hearing impairment, neuromuscular disorders; modify dosage in patients with renal impairment. Oral doses of 12 g/day may produce a malabsorption syndrome for a variety of substances (fat, nitrogen, cholesterol, carotene, glucose, xylose, lactose, sodium, calcium, cyanocobalamin, and iron).

Adverse Reactions

Dermatologic: Contact dermatitis, erythema, rash, urticaria

Gastrointestinal: Nausea, vomiting, diarrhea, colitis, malabsorption

Local: Burning

Neuromuscular & skeletal: Neuromuscular blockade

Ocular: Contact conjunctivitis

Otic: Ototoxicity

Renal: Nephrotoxicity

Miscellaneous: Candidiasis

Drug Interactions

Avoid Concomitant Use

Avoid concomitant use of Neomycin with any of the following: BCG; Gallium Nitrate

Increased Effect/Toxicity

Neomycin may increase the levels/effects of: AbobotulinumtoxinA; Bisphosphonate Derivatives; CARBOplatin; Colistimethate; CycloSPORINE; CycloSPORINE (Systemic); Gallium Nitrate; Neuromuscular-Blocking Agents; OnabotulinumtoxinA; RimabotulinumtoxinB

The levels/effects of Neomycin may be increased by: Amphotericin B; Capreomycin; CISplatin; Loop Diuretics; Nonsteroidal Anti-Inflammatory Agents; Vancomycin

Decreased Effect

Neomycin may decrease the levels/effects of: BCG; Cardiac Glycosides

The levels/effects of Neomycin may be decreased by: Penicillins

Stability Reconstituted neomycin solution is stable for 7 days when refrigerated

Mechanism of Action Interferes with bacterial protein synthesis by binding to 30S ribosomal subunits

Pharmacokinetics (Adult data unless noted)

Absorption: Poor orally (3%) or percutaneously; readily absorbed through denuded or abraded skin and body cavities

Distribution: V_d: 0.36 L/kg

Half-life: 2-3 hours (age and renal function dependent)

Time to peak serum concentration:

I.M.: Within 2 hours

Oral: 1-4 hours

Elimination: In urine (30% to 50% as unchanged drug); 97% of an oral dose eliminated unchanged in feces

Dialysis: Dialyzable (50% to 100%)

Usual Dosage

Neonates: Oral: Diarrhea: 50 mg/kg/day divided every 6 hours

Children: Oral: 50-100 mg/kg/day in divided doses every 6-8 hours

Preoperative bowel antisepsis: 90 mg/kg/day divided every 4 hours for 2 days; or 25 mg/kg at 1, 2, and 11 PM on the day preceding surgery as an adjunct to mechanical cleansing of the intestine and in combination with erythromycin base

Hepatic coma: 2.5-7 g/m²/day divided every 4-6 hours for 5-6 days not to exceed 12 g/day

Diarrhea caused by enteropathogenic *E. coli*: 50 mg/kg/day divided every 6 hours for 2-3 days

Children and Adults: Topical: Apply ointment 1-3 times/day; topical solutions containing 0.1% to 1% neomycin have been used for irrigation

Adults: Oral: 500-2000 mg every 6-8 hours

Preoperative bowel antisepsis: 1 g each hour for 4 doses then 1 g every 4 hours for 5 doses; or 1 g at 1 PM, 2 PM, and 11 PM with oral erythromycin on day preceding surgery as an adjunct to mechanical cleansing of the bowel; or 6 g/day divided every 4 hours for 2-3 days

Hepatic coma: 4-12 g/day divided every 4-6 hours

Diarrhea caused by enteropathogenic *E. coli*: 3 g/day divided every 6 hours

Monitoring Parameters Renal function tests

Patient Information Notify physician if ringing in the ears, hearing impairment, or dizziness occurs

Dosage Forms Excipient information presented when available (limited, particularly for generics); consult specific product labeling.

Powder, for prescription compounding, as sulfate [micronized]:

Neo-Rx: USP: 100% (10 g, 100 g) [neomycin base ≥600 mcg/mg neomycin sulfate]

Solution, oral, as sulfate (Neo-Fradin™): 125 mg/5 mL (60 mL, 480 mL) [contains benzoic acid; cherry flavor]

Tablet, oral, as sulfate: 500 mg

References

Feigin RD and Cherry JD, *Textbook of Pediatric Infectious Diseases*, 4th ed, Philadelphia, PA: WB Saunders Co, 1997.

Neomycin and Polymyxin B
(nee oh MYE sin & pol i MIKS in bee)

U.S. Brand Names Neosporin® G.U. Irrigant

Canadian Brand Names Neosporin® Irrigating Solution

Therapeutic Category Antibiotic, Topical; Antibiotic, Urinary Irrigation; Genitourinary Irrigant

Generic Available Yes

Use Short-term use as a continuous irrigant or rinse in the urinary bladder to prevent bacteriuria and gram-negative rod septicemia associated with the use of indwelling catheters

Pregnancy Risk Factor D

Pregnancy Considerations Because of several reports of total irreversible bilateral congenital deafness in children whose mothers received streptomycin during pregnancy, the manufacturer classifies neomycin and polymyxin B as pregnancy risk factor D. See individual agents.

Lactation Excretion in breast milk unknown

Breast-Feeding Considerations It is not known if neomycin or polymyxin B are excreted into breast milk. See individual agents.

Contraindications Hypersensitivity to neomycin, polymyxin B, or any component; ophthalmic use; irrigation should be avoided in patients with defects in the bladder mucosa or wall

Warnings Topical neomycin is a contact sensitizer

Precautions Use with caution in patients with impaired renal function, dehydrated patients, burn patients, and patients receiving a high dose for prolonged treatment

Adverse Reactions

Dermatologic: Contact dermatitis, erythema, rash, urticaria

Genitourinary: Bladder irritation

Local: Burning

Neuromuscular & skeletal: Neuromuscular blockade

Otic: Ototoxicity

Renal: Nephrotoxicity

Drug Interactions

Avoid Concomitant Use

Avoid concomitant use of Neomycin and Polymyxin B with any of the following: BCG; Gallium Nitrate

Increased Effect/Toxicity

Neomycin and Polymyxin B may increase the levels/effects of: AbobotulinumtoxinA; Bisphosphonate Derivatives; CARBOplatin; Colistimethate; CycloSPORINE; CycloSPORINE (Systemic); Gallium Nitrate;

Neuromuscular-Blocking Agents; OnabotulinumtoxinA; RimabotulinumtoxinB

The levels/effects of Neomycin and Polymyxin B may be increased by: Amphotericin B; Capreomycin; CISplatin; Loop Diuretics; Nonsteroidal Anti-Inflammatory Agents; Vancomycin

Decreased Effect

Neomycin and Polymyxin B may decrease the levels/ effects of: BCG; Cardiac Glycosides

The levels/effects of Neomycin and Polymyxin B may be decreased by: Penicillins

Stability Store irrigant solution in the refrigerator

Mechanism of Action Neomycin inhibits bacterial protein synthesis by binding to the 30S ribosomal subunits; polymyxin B interacts with phospholipid components in the cytoplasmic membranes of susceptible bacteria disrupting the osmotic integrity of the cell membrane

Pharmacokinetics (Adult data unless noted) Absorption: Not absorbed following topical application to intact skin; absorbed through denuded or abraded skin, peritoneum, wounds, or ulcers

Usual Dosage Children and Adults: Bladder irrigation: 1 mL is added to 1 L of NS with administration rate adjusted to patient's urine output; usually administered via a 3-way catheter (approximately 40 mL/hour); continuous irrigation or rinse of the urinary bladder should not exceed 10 days

Administration Bladder irrigant: Do not inject irrigant solution; concentrated irrigant solution must be diluted in 1 liter NS before administration; connect irrigation container to the inflow lumen of a 3-way catheter to permit continuous irrigation of the urinary bladder

Monitoring Parameters Urinalysis, renal function

Patient Information Notify physician if condition worsens or if rash/irritation develops

Additional Information GU irrigant contains methylparaben

Dosage Forms Excipient information presented when available (limited, particularly for generics); consult specific product labeling.

Solution, irrigation: Neomycin 40 mg and polymyxin B 200,000 units per mL (1 mL, 20 mL)

Neosporin® G.U. Irrigant: Neomycin 40 mg and polymyxin B 200,000 units per mL (1 mL, 20 mL)

◆ **Neomycin, Bacitracin, and Polymyxin B** *see* Bacitracin, Neomycin, and Polymyxin B *on page 170*

Neomycin, (Bacitracin) Polymyxin B, and Hydrocortisone

(nee oh MYE sin, bas i TRAY sin, pol i MIKS in bee, & hye droe KOR ti sone)

U.S. Brand Names Cortisporin® Cream; Cortisporin® Ophthalmic [DSC]; Cortisporin® Otic; PediOtic® [DSC]

Canadian Brand Names Cortimyxin®; Cortisporin® Otic

Therapeutic Category Antibacterial, Otic; Antibiotic, Ophthalmic; Antibiotic, Otic; Antibiotic, Topical; Corticosteroid, Ophthalmic; Corticosteroid, Otic; Corticosteroid, Topical

Generic Available Yes

Use Steroid-responsive inflammatory condition for which a corticosteroid is indicated and where bacterial infection or a risk of bacterial infection exists

Pregnancy Risk Factor C

Contraindications Hypersensitivity to hydrocortisone, polymyxin B sulfate, bacitracin, neomycin sulfate, or any component (see Warnings); herpes simplex, vaccinia and varicella; otic use: perforated tympanic membrane

Warnings Neomycin may cause cutaneous and conjunctival sensitization; children are more susceptible to topical corticosteroid-induced hypothalamic pituitary-adrenal axis suppression and Cushing's syndrome; otic solution contains potassium metabisulfate which may cause allergic reactions in susceptible individuals

Precautions Use with caution in patients with chronic otitis media and when the integrity of the tympanic membrane is in question

Adverse Reactions

Dermatologic: Contact dermatitis

Local: Itching, pain, stinging, burning, local edema

Ocular: Intraocular pressure elevated, glaucoma, cataracts, conjunctival erythema; blurring of vision (ophthalmic formulation)

Otic: Ototoxicity

Miscellaneous: Sensitization to neomycin, secondary infections

Drug Interactions

Metabolism/Transport Effects Hydrocortisone: **Substrate** of CYP3A4 (minor), P-glycoprotein; **Induces** CYP3A4 (weak)

Avoid Concomitant Use

Avoid concomitant use of Neomycin, Polymyxin B, and Hydrocortisone with any of the following: Aldesleukin; BCG; Gallium Nitrate; Natalizumab; Pimecrolimus; Tacrolimus (Topical); Vaccines (Live)

Increased Effect/Toxicity

Neomycin, Polymyxin B, and Hydrocortisone may increase the levels/effects of: AbobotulinumtoxinA; Acetylcholinesterase Inhibitors; Amphotericin B; Bisphosphonate Derivatives; CARBOplatin; Colistimethate; CycloSPORINE; CycloSPORINE (Systemic); Gallium Nitrate; Leflunomide; Loop Diuretics; Natalizumab; Neuromuscular-Blocking Agents; NSAID (COX-2 Inhibitor); NSAID (Nonselective); OnabotulinumtoxinA; RimabotulinumtoxinB; Thiazide Diuretics; Vaccines (Live); Warfarin

The levels/effects of Neomycin, Polymyxin B, and Hydrocortisone may be increased by: Amphotericin B; Antifungal Agents (Azole Derivatives, Systemic); Aprepitant; Calcium Channel Blockers (Nondihydropyridine); Capreomycin; CISplatin; Denosumab; Estrogen Derivatives; Fluconazole; Fosaprepitant; Loop Diuretics; Macrolide Antibiotics; Neuromuscular-Blocking Agents (Nondepolarizing); P-Glycoprotein Inhibitors; Pimecrolimus; Quinolone Antibiotics; Salicylates; Tacrolimus (Topical); Trastuzumab; Vancomycin

Decreased Effect

Neomycin, Polymyxin B, and Hydrocortisone may decrease the levels/effects of: Aldesleukin; Antidiabetic Agents; BCG; Calcitriol; Cardiac Glycosides; Corticorelin; Isoniazid; Salicylates; Sipuleucel-T; Vaccines (Inactivated); Vaccines (Live)

The levels/effects of Neomycin, Polymyxin B, and Hydrocortisone may be decreased by: Aminoglutethimide; Antacids; Barbiturates; Bile Acid Sequestrants; Echinacea; Mitotane; Penicillins; P-Glycoprotein Inducers; Primidone; Rifamycin Derivatives

Usual Dosage

Children: Otic: Solution and suspension: 3 drops into affected ear 3-4 times/day

Adults: Otic: Solution and suspension: 4 drops into affected ear 3-4 times/day

Children and Adults:

Topical ointment: Apply thin layer to affected area 2-4 times/day

Ophthalmic:

Ointment: Apply 1/2" ribbon to inside of lower lid every 3-4 hours until improvement occurs then 1-3 times/day

Suspension: Instill 1-2 drops in the affected eye every 3-4 hours

Administration Shake ophthalmic and otic suspension well before use

Ophthalmic: Avoid contamination of the tip of the eye dropper or ointment tube; solution and suspension: Apply finger pressure to lacrimal sac during and for 1-2 minutes after instillation to decrease risk of absorption and systemic effects

Otic: Drops can be instilled directly into the affected ear, or a cotton wick may be saturated with suspension and inserted in ear canal. Keep wick moist with suspension every 4 hours; wick should be replaced every 24 hours.

Topical: Apply a thin layer to the cleansed, dry affected area; may cover with a sterile bandage

Patient Information Ophthalmic: May cause sensitivity to bright light; may cause temporary blurring of vision or stinging following administration

Additional Information Otic **suspension** is the preferred otic preparation; otic **suspension** can be used for the treatment of infections of mastoidectomy and fenestration cavities caused by susceptible organisms; otic **solution** is used **only** for superficial infections of the external auditory canal (ie, swimmer's ear)

Dosage Forms Excipient information presented when available (limited, particularly for generics); consult specific product labeling. [DSC] = Discontinued product

Cream, topical (Cortisporin®): Neomycin 3.5 mg, polymyxin B 10,000 units, and hydrocortisone acetate 5 mg per g (7.5 g)

Solution, otic (Cortisporin®): Neomycin 3.5 mg, polymyxin B 10,000 units, and hydrocortisone 10 mg per mL (10 mL) [contains potassium metabisulfite]

Suspension, ophthalmic (Cortisporin® [DSC]): Neomycin 3.5 mg, polymyxin B 10,000 units, and hydrocortisone 10 mg per mL (7.5 mL) [contains thimerosal]

Suspension, otic: Neomycin 3.5 mg, polymyxin B 10,000 units, and hydrocortisone 10 mg per mL (10 mL)

Cortisporin®: Neomycin 3.5 mg, polymyxin B 10,000 units, and hydrocortisone 10 mg per mL (10 mL) [contains thimerosal]

PediOtic®: Neomycin 3.5 mg, polymyxin B 10,000 units, and hydrocortisone 10 mg per mL (7.5 mL) [contains thimerosal] [DSC]

Neomycin, Polymyxin B, and Prednisolone

(nee oh MYE sin, pol i MIKS in bee, & pred NIS oh lone)

U.S. Brand Names Poly-Pred®

Therapeutic Category Antibiotic, Ophthalmic; Corticosteroid, Ophthalmic

Generic Available No

Use Used for steroid-responsive inflammatory ocular condition in which bacterial infection or a risk of bacterial ocular infection exists

Pregnancy Risk Factor C

Contraindications Hypersensitivity to neomycin, polymyxin B, prednisolone, or any component; dendritic keratitis, viral disease of the cornea and conjunctiva, mycobacterial infection of the eye, fungal disease of the ocular structure, or after uncomplicated removal of a corneal foreign body

Warnings Symptoms of neomycin sensitization include itching, reddening, edema, or failure to heal

Precautions Prolonged use may result in overgrowth of nonsusceptible organisms, glaucoma, damage to the optic nerve, defects in visual acuity, and cataract formation

Adverse Reactions

Dermatologic: Cutaneous sensitization, skin rash, delayed wound healing

Ocular: Intraocular pressure elevated, glaucoma, optic nerve damage, cataracts, conjunctival sensitization

Drug Interactions

Metabolism/Transport Effects Prednisolone: **Substrate** of CYP3A4 (minor); **Inhibits** CYP3A4 (weak)

Avoid Concomitant Use

Avoid concomitant use of Neomycin, Polymyxin B, and Prednisolone with any of the following: Aldesleukin; BCG; Gallium Nitrate; Natalizumab; Pimecrolimus; Tacrolimus (Topical); Vaccines (Live)

Increased Effect/Toxicity

Neomycin, Polymyxin B, and Prednisolone may increase the levels/effects of: AbobotulinumtoxinA; Acetylcholinesterase Inhibitors; Amphotericin B; Bisphosphonate Derivatives; CARBOplatin; Colistimethate; CycloSPORINE; CycloSPORINE (Systemic); Gallium Nitrate; Leflunomide; Loop Diuretics; Natalizumab; Neuromuscular-Blocking Agents; NSAID (COX-2 Inhibitor); NSAID (Nonselective); OnabotulinumtoxinA; RimabotulinumtoxinB; Thiazide Diuretics; Vaccines (Live); Warfarin

The levels/effects of Neomycin, Polymyxin B, and Prednisolone may be increased by: Amphotericin B; Antifungal Agents (Azole Derivatives, Systemic); Aprepitant; Calcium Channel Blockers (Nondihydropyridine); Capreomycin; CISplatin; CycloSPORINE; CycloSPORINE (Systemic); Denosumab; Estrogen Derivatives; Fluconazole; Fosaprepitant; Loop Diuretics; Macrolide Antibiotics; Neuromuscular-Blocking Agents (Nondepolarizing); Pimecrolimus; Quinolone Antibiotics; Ritonavir; Salicylates; Tacrolimus (Topical); Trastuzumab; Vancomycin

Decreased Effect

Neomycin, Polymyxin B, and Prednisolone may decrease the levels/effects of: Aldesleukin; Antidiabetic Agents; BCG; Calcitriol; Cardiac Glycosides; Corticorelin; Isoniazid; Salicylates; Sipuleucel-T; Vaccines (Inactivated); Vaccines (Live)

The levels/effects of Neomycin, Polymyxin B, and Prednisolone may be decreased by: Aminoglutethimide; Antacids; Barbiturates; Bile Acid Sequestrants; Echinacea; Mitotane; Penicillins; Primidone; Rifamycin Derivatives

Usual Dosage Children and Adults:

Ophthalmic: Instill 1-2 drops every 3-4 hours; acute infections may require every 30-minute instillation initially with frequency of administration reduced as the infection is brought under control

To treat the eye lids: Instill 1-2 drops every 3-4 hours, close the eye and rub the excess on the lids and lid margins.

Administration Ophthalmic: Avoid contamination of the dropper tip; shake suspension well before using; apply finger pressure to lacrimal sac during and for 1-2 minutes after instillation to decrease risk of absorption and systemic effects

Patient Information Ophthalmic: May cause sensitivity to bright light; may cause temporary blurring of vision or stinging following administration

Dosage Forms Excipient information presented when available (limited, particularly for generics); consult specific product labeling.

Suspension, ophthalmic: Neomycin 0.35%, polymyxin B 10,000 units per mL, and prednisolone acetate 0.5% (5 mL; 10 mL [DSC]) [contains thimerosal]

- **Neosporin® AF [OTC]** *see* Miconazole *on page* 927
- **Neosporin® G.U. Irrigant** *see* Neomycin and Polymyxin B *on page* 979
- **Neosporin® Irrigating Solution (Can)** *see* Neomycin and Polymyxin B *on page* 979
- **Neosporin® Neo To Go® [OTC]** *see* Bacitracin, Neomycin, and Polymyxin B *on page* 170
- **Neosporin® Topical [OTC]** *see* Bacitracin, Neomycin, and Polymyxin B *on page* 170

Neostigmine (nee oh STIG meen)

Medication Safety Issues
Sound-alike/look-alike issues:
Prostigmin® may be confused with physostigmine

U.S. Brand Names Prostigmin®

Canadian Brand Names Prostigmin®

Therapeutic Category Antidote; Neuromuscular Blocking Agent; Cholinergic Agent; Diagnostic Agent; Myasthenia Gravis

Generic Available Yes: Injection

Use Treatment of myasthenia gravis; prevention and treatment of postoperative bladder distention and urinary retention; reversal of the effects of nondepolarizing neuromuscular blocking agents after surgery

Pregnancy Risk Factor C

Lactation Excretion in breast milk unknown/not recommended

Contraindications Hypersensitivity to neostigmine, bromides, or any component; GI or GU obstruction, peritonitis

Warnings Does **not** antagonize, and may prolong the phase I block of depolarizing muscle relaxants (eg, succinylcholine); adequate facilities should be available for cardiopulmonary resuscitation when testing and adjusting dose for myasthenia gravis; have atropine and epinephrine ready to treat hypersensitivity reactions; anticholinesterase insensitivity can develop for brief or prolonged periods

Precautions Use with caution in patients with epilepsy, asthma, bradycardia, hyperthyroidism, cardiac arrhythmias, peptic ulcer, vagotonia, or recent coronary occlusion

Adverse Reactions
Cardiovascular: Bradycardia, hypotension, asystole, A-V block, nodal rhythms, flushing, syncope
Central nervous system: Restlessness, agitation, seizures, dysphonia, dizziness, drowsiness, headache
Dermatologic: Rash, urticaria
Gastrointestinal: Hyperperistalsis, nausea, vomiting, diarrhea, dysphagia, flatulence, abdominal cramps; salivary, gastric, and intestinal secretions increased
Genitourinary: Urinary frequency and incontinence
Local: Thrombophlebitis
Neuromuscular & skeletal: Weakness, muscle cramps, arthralgia, tremor, dysarthria
Ocular: Miosis, lacrimation, diplopia, conjunctival hyperemia
Respiratory: Bronchoconstriction, secretions increased, laryngospasm, dyspnea, respiratory arrest, bronchospasm, respiratory paralysis
Miscellaneous: Allergic reactions, diaphoresis

Drug Interactions
Avoid Concomitant Use There are no known interactions where it is recommended to avoid concomitant use.

Increased Effect/Toxicity
Neostigmine may increase the levels/effects of: Beta-Blockers; Cholinergic Agonists; Succinylcholine

The levels/effects of Neostigmine may be increased by: Corticosteroids (Systemic)

Decreased Effect
Neostigmine may decrease the levels/effects of: Neuromuscular-Blocking Agents (Nondepolarizing)

Mechanism of Action Competitively inhibits the hydrolysis of acetylcholine by acetylcholinesterase facilitating transmission of impulses across the myoneural junction and producing cholinergic activity

Pharmacodynamics
Onset of action:
Oral: 45-75 minutes
I.M.: Within 20-30 minutes
I.V.: Within 1-20 minutes
Duration:
Oral: 2-4 hours
I.M.: 2-4 hours
I.V.: 1-2 hours

Pharmacokinetics (Adult data unless noted)
Absorption: Oral: Poor (~1% to 2%)
Metabolism: In the liver
Half-life: 0.5-2.1 hours
Elimination: 50% excreted renally as unchanged drug

Usual Dosage
Myasthenia gravis:
Diagnosis: I.M. (all cholinesterase medications should be discontinued at least 8 hours before; atropine should be administered I.V. immediately prior to or I.M. 30 minutes before neostigmine):
Children: 0.025-0.04 mg/kg as a single dose
Adults: 0.02 mg/kg as a single dose
Treatment (dosage requirements are variable; adjust dosage so patient takes larger doses at times of greatest fatigue):
Children:
Oral: 2 mg/kg/day or 60 mg/m^2/day every 3-4 hours; not to exceed 375 mg/day
I.M., I.V., SubQ: 0.01-0.04 mg/kg every 2-4 hours
Adults:
Oral: Initial: 15 mg/dose every 3-4 hours, gradually increase every 1-2 days; usual daily range: 15-375 mg
I.M., I.V., SubQ: 0.5-2.5 mg every 1-3 hours up to 10 mg/24 hours maximum
Reversal of nondepolarizing neuromuscular blockade after surgery in conjunction with atropine or glycopyrrolate: I.V.:
Infants: 0.025-0.1 mg/kg/dose
Children: 0.025-0.08 mg/kg/dose
Adults: 0.5-2.5 mg; total dose not to exceed 5 mg
Bladder atony: Adults: I.M., SubQ:
Prevention: 0.25 mg every 4-6 hours for 2-3 days
Treatment: 0.5-1 mg every 3 hours for 5 doses after bladder has emptied

Dosing adjustment in renal impairment:
Cl_{cr} 10-50 mL/minute: Administer 50% of normal dose
Cl_{cr} <10 mL/minute: Administer 25% of normal dose

Administration
Parenteral: May be administered undiluted by slow I.V. injection over several minutes; may be administered I.M. or SubQ
Oral: Divide dosages so patient receives larger doses at times of greatest fatigue; may be administered with or without food

Monitoring Parameters Muscle strength, heart rate, respiratory rate

Patient Information The side effects are generally due to exaggerated pharmacologic effects; the most common side effects are salivation and muscle fasciculations; notify physician if nausea, vomiting, muscle weakness, severe abdominal pain, or difficulty breathing occurs

Dosage Forms Excipient information presented when available (limited, particularly for generics); consult specific product labeling.

Injection, solution, as methylsulfate: 0.5 mg/mL (1 mL, 10 mL); 1 mg/mL (10 mL)

Tablet, as bromide: 15 mg

♦ **Neostigmine Bromide** see Neostigmine on page 982

♦ **Neostigmine Methylsulfate** see Neostigmine on page 982

♦ **Neo-Synephrine® (Can)** see Phenylephrine on page 1102

♦ **Neo-Synephrine® 12 Hour [OTC]** see Oxymetazoline on page 1043

♦ **Neo-Synephrine® 12 Hour Extra Moisturizing [OTC]** see Oxymetazoline on page 1043

♦ **Neo-Synephrine® Extra Strength [OTC]** see Phenylephrine on page 1102

♦ **Neo-Synephrine® Injection [DSC]** see Phenylephrine on page 1102

♦ **Neo-Synephrine® Mild [OTC]** see Phenylephrine on page 1102

♦ **Neo-Synephrine® Regular Strength [OTC]** see Phenylephrine on page 1102

♦ **Nephro-Calci® [OTC]** see Calcium Carbonate on page 232

♦ **Nephro-Calci® [OTC]** see Calcium Supplements on page 239

♦ **Nephro-Fer® [OTC] [DSC]** see Ferrous Fumarate on page 576

♦ **Nesacaine®** see Chloroprocaine on page 292

♦ **Nesacaine®-CE (Can)** see Chloroprocaine on page 292

♦ **Nesacaine®-MPF** see Chloroprocaine on page 292

♦ **NESP** see Darbepoetin Alfa on page 390

♦ **Neulasta®** see Pegfilgrastim on page 1070

♦ **Neumega®** see Oprelvekin on page 1025

♦ **Neupogen®** see Filgrastim on page 580

♦ **Neurontin®** see Gabapentin on page 634

♦ **Neut®** see Sodium Bicarbonate on page 1269

♦ **NeutraCare®** see Fluoride on page 595

♦ **NeutraGard® [OTC]** see Fluoride on page 595

♦ **NeutraGard® Advanced** see Fluoride on page 595

♦ **NeutraGard® Plus** see Fluoride on page 595

♦ **Neutra-Phos® [OTC] [DSC]** see Potassium Phosphate and Sodium Phosphate on page 1143

♦ **Neutra-Phos®-K [OTC] [DSC]** see Potassium Phosphate on page 1140

♦ **Neutrogena® Advanced Solutions™ [OTC]** see Salicylic Acid on page 1241

♦ **Neutrogena® Blackhead Eliminating™ 2-in-1 Foaming Pads [OTC]** see Salicylic Acid on page 1241

♦ **Neutrogena® Blackhead Eliminating™ Astringent [OTC] [DSC]** see Salicylic Acid on page 1241

♦ **Neutrogena® Blackhead Eliminating™ Daily Scrub [OTC]** see Salicylic Acid on page 1241

♦ **Neutrogena® Blackhead Eliminating™ Treatment Mask [OTC] [DSC]** see Salicylic Acid on page 1241

♦ **Neutrogena® Body Clear® [OTC]** see Benzoyl Peroxide on page 184

♦ **Neutrogena® Body Clear® [OTC]** see Salicylic Acid on page 1241

♦ **Neutrogena® Clear Pore™ [OTC]** see Benzoyl Peroxide on page 184

♦ **Neutrogena® Clear Pore™ Oil-Controlling Astringent [OTC]** see Salicylic Acid on page 1241

♦ **Neutrogena® Oil-Free Acne Wash [OTC]** see Benzoyl Peroxide on page 184

♦ **Neutrogena® Oil-Free Acne Wash [OTC]** see Salicylic Acid on page 1241

♦ **Neutrogena® Oil-Free Acne Wash 60 Second Mask Scrub [OTC]** see Salicylic Acid on page 1241

♦ **Neutrogena® Oil-Free Acne Wash Cream Cleanser [OTC]** see Salicylic Acid on page 1241

♦ **Neutrogena® Oil-Free Acne Wash Foam Cleanser [OTC]** see Salicylic Acid on page 1241

♦ **Neutrogena® On The Spot® Acne Treatment [OTC]** see Benzoyl Peroxide on page 184

♦ **Neutrogena® Rapid Clear® Acne Defense [OTC]** see Salicylic Acid on page 1241

♦ **Neutrogena® Rapid Clear® Acne Eliminating [OTC]** see Salicylic Acid on page 1241

♦ **Neutrogena® T/Gel [OTC]** see Coal Tar on page 349

♦ **Neutrogena® T/Gel Extra Strength [OTC]** see Coal Tar on page 349

♦ **Neutrogena® T/Gel Stubborn Itch Control [OTC]** see Coal Tar on page 349

Nevirapine (ne VYE ra peen)

Medication Safety Issues

Sound-alike/look-alike issues:

Nevirapine may be confused with nelfinavir

Viramune® may be confused with Viracept®

Related Information

Adult and Adolescent HIV on page 1620

Pediatric HIV on page 1613

Perinatal HIV on page 1628

U.S. Brand Names Viramune®

Canadian Brand Names Viramune®

Therapeutic Category Antiretroviral Agent; HIV Agents (Anti-HIV Agents); Non-nucleoside Reverse Transcriptase Inhibitor (NNRTI)

Generic Available No

Use Treatment of HIV infection in combination with other antiretroviral agents. (**Note:** HIV regimens consisting of **three** antiretroviral agents are strongly recommended). Do not start nevirapine therapy in women with CD4$^+$ counts >250 cells/mm^3 or in men with CD4$^+$ counts >400 cells/mm^3 unless benefit of therapy outweighs the risk (see Warnings). Nevirapine is also used as chemoprophylaxis to prevent maternal-fetal HIV transmission (see Related Information, Perinatal HIV).

Medication Guide An FDA-approved patient medication guide, which is available with the product information and at http://www.fda.gov/downloads/Drugs/DrugSafety/ucm089818.pdf, must be dispensed with this medication for each new outpatient prescription and refill.

Pregnancy Risk Factor B

Pregnancy Considerations Nevirapine crosses the placenta. No increased risk of overall birth defects has been observed following 1st trimester exposure according to data collected by the antiretroviral pregnancy registry. Pharmacokinetics are not altered during pregnancy and dose adjustment is not needed. The Perinatal HIV Guidelines Working Group recommends nevirapine as the NNRTI for use during pregnancy. When used to prevent perinatal transmission in women who do not need therapy for their own health, use is not recommended if CD4$^+$ lymphocyte counts >250/mm^3 (monitor for liver toxicity during first 18 weeks of therapy). It may also be used in combination with zidovudine in HIV-infected women who are in labor, but have had no prior antiretroviral therapy, in order to reduce the maternal-fetal transmission of HIV; consider adding intrapartum and postpartum zidovudine and lamivudine to reduce nevir-apine resistance. Health professionals are encouraged to contact the antiretroviral pregnancy registry to monitor outcomes of pregnant women exposed to antiretroviral medications (1-800-258-4263 or www.APRegistry.com).

Lactation Enters breast milk/contraindicated

Breast-Feeding Considerations In infants born to mothers who are HIV positive, HAART while breast-feeding may decrease postnatal infection. Infant prophy-laxis with zidovudine in combination with nevirapine or nevirapine alone may also decrease the risk of HIV transmission to the infant. However, maternal or infant antiretroviral therapy does not completely eliminate the risk of postnatal HIV transmission.

In the United States where formula is accessible, affordable, safe, and sustainable, complete avoidance of breast-feeding by HIV-infected women is recommended to decrease potential transmission of HIV.

Contraindications Hypersensitivity to nevirapine or any component; moderate or severe hepatic impairment (Child Pugh Class B or C)

Warnings Severe, life-threatening, and fatal cases of skin reactions (eg, Stevens-Johnson syndrome, toxic epider-mal necrolysis, and hypersensitivity reactions accompa-nied by rash, constitutional symptoms, and organ dysfunction) have occurred in patients receiving nevirapine **[U.S. Boxed Warning]**. Discontinue nevirapine in patients who develop a severe rash or rash accompanied by fever, blistering, oral lesions, conjunctivitis, facial edema, muscle or joint aches, general malaise, fatigue, hepatitis, renal dysfunction, granulocytopenia, eosinophilia, or lympha-denopathy; do not restart nevirapine in these patients. Initiating therapy at a lower dose for the first 14 days of therapy (lead-in dose) has been shown to reduce the frequency of rash. If nonsevere rash (in the absence of transaminase elevations) occurs, do not increase dose until rash has resolved. If rash continues beyond 28 days, use an alternative regimen. Concomitant use of predni-sone during the first 6 weeks of therapy was associated with an increase in incidence and severity of rash. Use of prednisone to prevent nevirapine-associated rash is not recommended. Obtain liver function tests immediately in all patients who develop a rash within the first 18 weeks of therapy.

Severe, life-threatening, and fatal cases of hepatotoxicity have been reported with the use of nevirapine **[U.S. Boxed Warning]**. Hepatitis or hepatic failure may be associated with hypersensitivity reactions and may include severe rash, rash with fever, malaise, fatigue, blisters, oral lesions, conjunctivitis, facial edema, muscle or joint aches, eosinophilia, granulocytopenia, lymphadenopathy, and renal dysfunction. Rhabdomyolysis has occurred in some patients in conjunction with skin and/or hepatic reactions associated with nevirapine therapy.

Intensive monitoring is required during the initial 18 weeks of therapy to detect potentially life-threatening hepatotox-icity or skin reactions **[U.S. Boxed Warning]** (see Monitoring Parameters). The greatest risk for these reactions occurs in the first 6 weeks of therapy. Patients with elevated AST or ALT levels, coinfection with hepatitis B or C, women with CD4+ counts >250 cells/mm^3, and men with CD4+ counts >400 cells/mm^3 may be at higher risk for rash-associated hepatic adverse events. Women with high CD4+ counts are at the greatest risk of hepatotoxicity including potentially fatal hepatic events. Serious hepatotoxicity has been reported in patients receiving multiple-dose regimens of nevirapine for post-exposure prophylaxis. Symptomatic liver toxicity has **not** been reported after single doses of nevirapine (when used for chemoprophylaxis) and may be less common in HIV-infected children. Permanently discontinue nevirapine

therapy if clinical hepatotoxicity, severe skin reactions, hypersensitivity reactions or elevated transaminases with rash or other systemic symptoms occur; do not restart after recovery.

Nevirapine induces hepatic cytochrome P450 3A and has the potential for interacting with numerous drugs; drugs having suspected interactions and that should only be used with careful monitoring include rifampin, rifabutin, triazolam, midazolam, oral contraceptives, oral antico-agulants, digoxin, phenytoin, and theophylline.

Precautions Use with caution in patients with either renal or hepatic dysfunction; not recommended for use in patients with severe hepatic impairment; elevated AST or ALT levels and/or a history of chronic hepatitis (B or C) infection are associated with a greater risk of hepatic adverse events; nevirapine may accumulate in patients with worsening hepatic function and ascites. Fat redis-tribution and accumulation [ie, central obesity, peripheral wasting, facial wasting, breast enlargement, dorsocervical fat enlargement (buffalo hump), and cushingoid appear-ance] have been observed in patients receiving antire-troviral agents (causal relationship not established). Immune reconstitution syndrome (an acute inflammatory response to residual or indolent opportunistic infections) may occur in HIV patients during initial treatment with combination antiretroviral agents, including nevirapine; this syndrome may require further patient assessment and therapy.

Adverse Reactions

Central nervous system: Headache, fever, sedation, malaise

Dermatologic: Rash (usually maculopapular erythematous cutaneous eruptions with or without pruritus, located on the trunk, face, and extremities; women may be at a higher risk for development of rash; 21% of pediatric patients developed rash), toxic epidermal necrolysis, angioedema, Stevens-Johnson syndrome (see Warnings)

Endocrine & metabolic: Fat redistribution and accumu-lation (see Precautions)

Gastrointestinal: Nausea, diarrhea, vomiting, abdominal pain

Hematologic: Eosinophilia, neutropenia (children: 8.9%), granulocytopenia [more common in younger pediatric patients (2 weeks to < 3 months of age) compared to older children and adults; also more common in pediatric patients receiving concomitant zidovudine], thrombocy-topenia; anemia (7.3%; reported more commonly in children in postmarketing reports; however, effects of concomitant medications cannot be separated out)

Hepatic: Liver enzymes elevated, hepatotoxicity (children 2.4%), liver failure, cholestatic hepatitis, hepatic necrosis, jaundice (see Warnings)

Neuromuscular & skeletal: Myalgia, arthralgia, paresthesia

Miscellaneous: Anaphylaxis, hypersensitivity reactions

Drug Interactions

Metabolism/Transport Effects Substrate of CYP2B6 (minor), 2D6 (minor), 3A4 (major); **Inhibits** CYP1A2 (weak), 2D6 (weak), 3A4 (weak); **Induces** CYP2B6 (strong), 3A4 (strong)

Avoid Concomitant Use

Avoid concomitant use of Nevirapine with any of the following: Atazanavir; Dienogest; Dronedarone; Etravir-ine; Everolimus; Nilotinib; Nisoldipine; Pazopanib; Rano-lazine; Romidepsin; St Johns Wort; Tolvaptan

Increased Effect/Toxicity

Nevirapine may increase the levels/effects of: Etravirine; Paclitaxel; Rifabutin

The levels/effects of Nevirapine may be increased by: Atazanavir; Voriconazole

Decreased Effect

Nevirapine may decrease the levels/effects of: Atazanavir; Caspofungin; CYP2B6 Substrates; CYP3A4 Substrates; Dienogest; Dronedarone; Etravirine; Everolimus; GuanFACINE; Maraviroc; Methadone; NIFEdipine; Nilotinib; Nisoldipine; Pazopanib; Protease Inhibitors; Ranolazine; Rifabutin; Romidepsin; Saxagliptin; Sorafenib; Tadalafil; Tolvaptan; Voriconazole

The levels/effects of Nevirapine may be decreased by: CYP3A4 Inducers (Strong); Deferasirox; Peginterferon Alfa-2b; Rifabutin; Rifampin; St Johns Wort

Stability Store at controlled room temperature at 25°C (77°F); excursions permitted to 15°C to 30°C (59°F to 86°F)

Mechanism of Action A non-nucleoside reverse transcriptase inhibitor which specifically binds to HIV-1 reverse transcriptase blocking the RNA-dependent and DNA-dependent DNA polymerase activity and disrupting the virus' life cycle. Nevirapine does not inhibit HIV-2 reverse transcriptase or human DNA polymerase.

Pharmacokinetics (Adult data unless noted)

Absorption: Rapid and readily absorbed

Distribution: V_d: 1.21 L/kg; widely distributed; crosses the placenta; excreted in breast milk; 45% of the plasma concentration in CSF

Metabolism: Metabolized by cytochrome P450 isozymes from the CYP3A family to hydroxylated metabolites; autoinduction of metabolism occurs in 2-4 weeks with a 1.5-2 times increase in clearance; nevirapine is more rapidly metabolized in pediatric patients than in adults

Protein binding, plasma: 60%

Bioavailability: 91% to 93%

Half-life: Adults: Single dose (45 hours); multiple dosing (25-30 hours)

Time to peak serum concentration: 4 hours

Elimination: 81.3% in urine as metabolites, 10.1% in feces; <3% of the total dose is eliminated in urine as parent drug

Clearance: Women have a 13.8% lower clearance compared to men; body size does not totally explain the gender difference

Usual Dosage Oral:

HIV Infection (treatment) (use in combination with other antiretroviral agents):

Note: If patient experiences a nonsevere rash (in the absence of transaminase elevations) during the first 14 days of therapy, do not increase dose until rash has resolved. If rash continues beyond 28 days, use an alternative regimen. Discontinue nevirapine if severe rash, rash with constitutional symptoms, or rash with elevated hepatic transaminases occurs (see Warnings). If nevirapine therapy is interrupted for >7 days, restart at the initial recommended dose (ie, once daily for the first 14 days) before increasing to twice daily dosing.

Neonates <14 days of age: Treatment dose is not defined

Neonates ≥15 days, Infants, and Children: Initial: 150 mg/m²/dose (maximum: 200 mg/dose) once daily for the first 14 days of therapy; increase to 150 mg/m²/dose every 12 hours if no rash or other adverse effects occur (maximum: 200 mg/dose every 12 hours). Children ≤8 years of age may require 200 mg/m²/dose every 12 hours (see Working Group, 2008).

Adolescents and Adults: Initial: 200 mg/dose once daily for the first 14 days; increase to 200 mg every 12 hours if no rash or other adverse effects occur

Prevention of maternal-fetal HIV transmission: (Perinatal HIV Guidelines Working Group, 2008); see also Related Information, Perinatal HIV; **Note:** Nevirapine is used in combination with zidovudine (and possibly lamivudine) in select situations (eg, infants born to mothers with no antiretroviral therapy prior to labor or during labor; infants born to mothers with only intrapartum antiretroviral therapy; infants born to mothers with suboptimal viral suppression at delivery; or infants born to mothers with known antiretroviral drug-resistant virus):

Mother: 200 mg as a single dose at onset of labor; **Note:** This dose is recommended for use in combination with I.V. zidovudine infusion during labor. Single-dose nevirapine is not recommended for women in the U.S. who are receiving standard antiretroviral prophylaxis regimens. If single-dose nevirapine is given to the mother, alone or in combination with zidovudine, consideration should be given to adding maternal zidovudine/lamivudine starting as soon as possible (during labor or immediately postpartum) and continuing for 7 days, in an effort to reduce development of nevirapine resistance.

Neonates ≤14 days: 2 mg/kg as a single dose between birth and 72 hours of age if mother received intrapartum single-dose nevirapine. If maternal dose was given ≤2 hours prior to delivery (or **not** given), administer infant dose as soon as possible following birth. Recommended for use with 6 weeks of zidovudine prophylaxis to the infant; consideration should be given to adding 7 days of neonatal lamivudine in an effort to reduce development of nevirapine resistance (see Related Information, Perinatal HIV).

Dosage adjustment in renal impairment: Adults:

Cl_{cr} ≥20 mL/minute: No dosage adjustment required

Hemodialysis: An additional 200 mg dose is recommended following dialysis. **Note:** Nevirapine metabolites may accumulate in patients on dialysis (clinical significance is unknown)

Dosage adjustment in hepatic impairment: Use is contraindicated in patients with moderate or severe hepatic impairment (Child Pugh Class B or C). Permanently discontinue if symptomatic hepatic events occur (see Warnings and Precautions). Monitor patients with hepatic impairment carefully for symptoms of drug induced toxicity (increased trough concentrations have been observed in some patients with hepatic fibrosis or cirrhosis).

Administration Oral: May be administered with water, milk, or soda, with or without meals; may be administered with an antacid or didanosine; shake suspension gently prior to administration

Monitoring Parameters Clinical chemistry tests, CBC with differential, CD4 cell count, plasma levels of HIV RNA; liver function tests at baseline, closely during first 18 weeks of treatment, prior to dose escalation, 2 weeks postdose escalation, and at frequent intervals thereafter; obtain liver function tests immediately if patient develops signs or symptoms consistent with hepatitis or hypersensitivity reactions; obtain liver function tests immediately in all patients who develop a rash within the first 18 weeks of therapy

Patient Information Nevirapine is not a cure for HIV; take nevirapine as prescribed; read the patient Medication Guide that you receive with each prescription and refill of nevirapine; avoid the herbal medicine St John's wort; inform physician immediately of any rash or symptoms of fatigue, malaise, jaundice, liver tenderness, anorexia, or nausea; use an alternative method of contraception from birth control pills during nevirapine therapy; if a dose is missed, take the next dose as soon as possible, however, if a dose is skipped, do not double the next dose

HIV medications may cause changes in body fat, including an increase in fat in the upper back and neck, breasts, and trunk; a loss of fat from the face, arms, and legs may also occur.

Additional Information Early virologic failure and rapid emergence of resistant mutations have been observed in therapy-naive adult HIV patients treated with tenofovir, didanosine enteric-coated beadlets (Videx® EC) and either efavirenz or nevirapine; the combination of tenofovir, didanosine, and any non-nucleoside reverse transcriptase inhibitor is **not** recommended as initial antiretroviral therapy.

Dosage Forms Excipient information presented when available (limited, particularly for generics); consult specific product labeling.

Suspension, oral:
Viramune®: 50 mg/5 mL (240 mL)
Tablet:
Viramune®: 200 mg

References
Briars LA, Hilao JJ, and Kraus DM, "A Review of Pediatric Human Immunodeficiency Virus Infection," *Journal of Pharmacy Practice*, 2004, 17(6):407-31.

D'Aquila RT, Hughes MD, Johnson VA, et al, "Nevirapine, Zidovudine, and Didanosine Compared With Zidovudine and Didanosine in Patients With HIV-1 Infection. A Randomized, Double-Blind, Placebo-Controlled Trial. National Institute of Allergy and Infectious Diseases AIDS Clinical Trials Group Protocol 241 Investigators," *Ann Intern Med*, 1996, 124(12):1019-30.

Mueller BU, Sei S, Anderson B, et al, "Comparison of Virus Burden in Blood and Sequential Lymph Node Biopsy Specimens From Children Infected With Human Immunodeficiency Virus," *J Pediatr*, 1996, 129 (3):410-8.

Panel on Antiretroviral Guidelines for Adults and Adolescents, "Guidelines for the Use of Antiretroviral Agents in HIV-Infected Adults and Adolescents," December 1, 2009, http://www.aidsinfo.nih.gov.

Perinatal HIV Guidelines Working Group, "Recommendations for the Use of Antiretroviral Drugs in Pregnant HIV-1-Infected Women for Maternal Health and Interventions to Reduce Perinatal HIV-1 Transmission in the United States," July 8, 2008, http://www.aidsinfo.nih.gov.

Working Group on Antiretroviral Therapy and Medical Management of HIV-Infected Children, "Guidelines for the Use of Antiretroviral Agents in Pediatric HIV Infection," February 23, 2009. Available at http://www.aidsinfo.nih.gov.

◆ **Nexium®** *see* Esomeprazole *on page 534*
◆ **NFV** *see* Nelfinavir *on page 975*
◆ **NG-Citalopram (Can)** *see* Citalopram *on page 319*
◆ **NH₄Cl** *see* Ammonium Chloride *on page 94*

Niacin (NYE a sin)

Medication Safety Issues
Sound-alike/look-alike issues:
Niacin may be confused with Minocin®, Niaspan®, Nispan®
Niaspan® may be confused with niacin
Nicobid® may be confused with Nitro-Bid®

International issues:
Niacor® may be confused with Nacor® which is a brand name for enalapril in Spain

Related Information
Normal Laboratory Values for Children *on page 1672*

U.S. Brand Names Niacin-Time®; Niacor®; Niaspan®; Slo-Niacin® [OTC]

Canadian Brand Names Niaspan®

Therapeutic Category Antilipemic Agent; Nutritional Supplement; Vitamin, Water Soluble

Generic Available Yes

Use Adjunctive treatment of hyperlipidemias (FDA approved in adults) (see Additional Information for recommendations on initiating hypercholesterolemia pharmacologic treatment in children ≥8 years); adjunctive treatment of hypertriglyceridemia in patients at risk of pancreatitis (FDA approved in adults); to lower the risk of recurrent MI in patients with hyperlipidemia (FDA approved in adults); in combination with a bile acid sequestrant to slow progression (or promote regression) of atherosclerotic disease in patients with CAD and hyperlipidemia (FDA approved in adults); peripheral vascular disease and circulatory disorders; treatment of pellagra; dietary supplement; **Note:** Niacin may be used in combination with lovastatin, simvastatin, or bile acid sequestrants for treatment of hyperlipidemias in patients who fail monotherapy; combination therapy is not indicated as initial therapy

Pregnancy Risk Factor A/C (dose exceeding RDA recommendation)

Pregnancy Considerations Animal reproduction studies have not been conducted. It is unknown whether or not niacin at lipid-lowering doses is harmful to the developing fetus. If a woman becomes pregnant while receiving niacin for primary hypercholesterolemia, niacin should be discontinued. If a woman becomes pregnant while receiving niacin for hypertriglyceridemia, the benefits and risks of continuing niacin should be assessed on an individual basis.

Lactation Enters breast milk/consider risk:benefit

Breast-Feeding Considerations Niacin is excreted in human breast milk. Because lipid-lowering doses of niacin may cause serious adverse reactions in nursing infants, a decision should be made whether to discontinue nursing or discontinue the drug, taking into account the importance of the drug to the mother.

Contraindications Hypersensitivity to niacin or any component; active liver disease, unexplained persistent increases in liver enzymes, significant or unexplained hepatic dysfunction, active peptic ulcer disease, arterial hemorrhaging; GERD (relative contraindication)

Warnings Hepatotoxicity may occur and may be more common if extended release product is substituted for immediate release product at same dosage; do not interchange extended or sustained release products for immediate release at same dosage. Cases of myopathy and rhabdomyolysis have occurred during concomitant use of niacin with HMG-CoA reductase inhibitors; risk may be increased in patients with diabetes, renal failure, or uncontrolled hypothyroidism; monitor all patients receiving both medications for clinical signs of rhabdomyolysis (muscle pain, tenderness, or weakness) and serum CPK and potassium.

Precautions Use with caution in patients with diabetes mellitus; niacin may increase fasting blood glucose (monitor glucose; adjustment of hypoglycemic therapy may be needed). May elevate uric acid levels, use with caution in patients predisposed to gout; large doses should be administered with caution to patients with gallbladder disease, jaundice, history of liver disease, diabetes, unstable angina, MI, renal dysfunction or heavy alcohol use; niacin may cause small increases in prothrombin time (use with caution in patients receiving anticoagulants; monitor closely)

Adverse Reactions
Cardiovascular: Arrhythmias, edema, flushing, hypotension, orthostasis, palpitations, syncope, tachycardia, vasovagal attacks
Central nervous system: Chills, dizziness, headache, insomnia, nervousness
Dermatologic: Acanthosis nigricans (reversible), burning, dry skin, hyperpigmentation, pruritus, rash, sebaceous gland activity increased, tingling skin, urticaria
Endocrine & metabolic: Hyperglycemia, hyperuricemia, hypophosphatemia transient
Gastrointestinal: Anorexia, diarrhea, eructation, flatulence, GI upset, heartburn, nausea, peptic ulcers, vomiting
Hematologic: Slight reduction in platelet counts, small increases in prothrombin time

Hepatic: Abnormal liver function tests, chronic liver damage, hepatitis, jaundice

Neuromuscular & skeletal: Asthenia, leg cramps, myalgia, myasthenia, myopathy, paresthesia

Ocular: Blurred vision

Respiratory: Cough increased, dyspnea

Miscellaneous: Hypersensitivity reactions (rare), sweating

Drug Interactions

Avoid Concomitant Use There are no known interactions where it is recommended to avoid concomitant use.

Increased Effect/Toxicity
Niacin may increase the levels/effects of: HMG-CoA Reductase Inhibitors

Decreased Effect
The levels/effects of Niacin may be decreased by: Bile Acid Sequestrants

Food Interactions Concurrent intake of hot drinks, alcohol, or spicy food may increase flushing and pruritus (avoid around the time of niacin administration)

Mechanism of Action Component of two coenzymes necessary for tissue respiration, lipid metabolism, and glycogenolysis; inhibits the synthesis of very low density lipoproteins

Pharmacodynamics Vasodilation:
Onset of action: Within 20 minutes
Extended release: Within 1 hour
Duration: 20-60 minutes
Extended release: 8-10 hours

Pharmacokinetics (Adult data unless noted)
Absorption: Oral: Rapid and extensive; ≥60% to 76% of dose is absorbed

Distribution: Crosses into breast milk

Metabolism: Extensive first-pass effect; niacin in smaller doses is converted to niacinamide which is metabolized in the liver; niacin undergoes conjugation with glycine to form nicotinuric acid; nicotinamide, nicotinamide adenine dinucleotide (NAD), and other niacin metabolites are formed via saturable pathways; **Note:** It is not clear whether nicotinamide is formed before or after the synthesis of NAD

Bioavailability: Single dose studies indicate that only certain Niaspan® tablet strengths are interchangeable (ie, two 500 mg tablets are equivalent to one 1000 mg tablet; however, three 500 mg tablets are **not** equivalent to two 750 mg tablets)

Half-life: 45 minutes

Time to peak serum concentration: Immediate release: ~45 minutes; extended release: 4-5 hours

Elimination: In urine, with ~33% as unchanged drug; with larger doses, a greater percentage is excreted unchanged in urine

Usual Dosage Oral:
Children:
Recommended daily allowances (RDA):
0-0.5 years: 5 mg/day
0.5-1 year: 6 mg/day
1-3 years: 9 mg/day
4-6 years: 12 mg/day
7-10 years: 13 mg/day
Male:
11-14 years: 17 mg/day
15-18 years: 20 mg/day
19-24 years: 19 mg/day
Female: 11-24 years: 15 mg/day
Hyperlipidemia: Initial: 100-250 mg/day (maximum dose: 10 mg/kg/day) in 3 divided doses with meals; increase weekly by 100 mg/day or increase every 2-3 weeks by 250 mg/day as tolerated; evaluate efficacy and adverse effects with laboratory tests at 20 mg/kg/day or 1000 mg/day (whichever is less); continue to increase if needed and as tolerated; re-evaluate at each 500 mg

increment; doses up to 2250 mg/day have been used; **Note:** Routine use in children and adolescents is not recommended due to limited safety and efficacy information

Pellagra: 50-100 mg/dose 3 times/day

Adults:
Recommended daily allowances (RDA):
Male:
25-50 years: 19 mg/day
>51 years: 15 mg/day
Female:
25-50 years: 15 mg/day
>51 years: 13 mg/day
Hyperlipidemia:
Immediate release products: Initial: 50-100 mg twice daily for 1 week; increase slowly over 1 month (by doubling daily dose every week) to 1-1.5 g/day divided in 2-3 doses; assess therapy at 4 and 8 weeks of therapy; if needed, dose may be increased slowly to 3 g/day or until desired result is attained; maximum dose: 3 g/day in 3 divided doses; **Note:** Some patients may require a slower dose titration

Extended release products: Initial: 500 mg/day divided in 2 doses for 1 week; increase to 500 mg twice daily for 3 weeks; if needed, dose may be increased to 2 g/day or until desired result is attained; maximum dose: 2 g/day

Niaspan®: Initial: 500 mg daily at bedtime for 4 weeks; increase to 1 g daily at bedtime for 4 weeks; adjust dose to patient response and tolerance; may increase by 500 mg/day at 4-week intervals; maximum dose: 2 g/day; **Note:** Women may respond at lower doses than men.

Niacin deficiency: 10-20 mg/day, maximum dose: 100 mg/day

Pellagra: 50-100 mg 3-4 times/day, maximum dose: 500 mg/day

Dosage adjustment in renal impairment: Use with caution

Dosage adjustment in hepatic impairment: Contraindicated in patients with active liver disease, unexplained liver enzyme elevations, significant or unexplained hepatic dysfunction. Use with caution in patients with history of liver disease or those with suspected liver disease (eg, those who consume large quantities of alcohol)

Administration Oral: Administer with food or milk to decrease GI upset; administer Niaspan® with a low-fat snack (do not administer on an empty stomach). Swallow timed release tablet and capsule whole; do not break, chew, or crush. To minimize flushing, administer dose at bedtime, take aspirin (adults: 325 mg) 30 minutes before niacin, and avoid alcohol, hot drinks, or spicy food around the time of administration. Separate administration of bile acid sequestrants by at least 4-6 hours (bile acid sequestrants may decrease the absorption of niacin).

Monitoring Parameters Blood glucose, serum uric acid, periodic liver function tests, platelet count and prothrombin time (if on concurrent anticoagulant), serum phosphorus (if predisposed to hypophosphatemia). Treatment of hyperlipidemias: Baseline: Liver enzymes, uric acid, fasting glucose, and minimum of two fasting lipid profiles; repeat 4-6 weeks after dose is stabilized; once LDL-C goal is reached, repeat every 2-3 months for first year and then every 6-12 months if no sign of toxicity develops and dose remains stable. Monitor CPK and serum potassium (if on concurrent HMG-CoA reductase inhibitor).

Reference Range See Related Information for age- and gender-specific serum cholesterol, LDL-C, TG, and HDL concentrations.

Test Interactions False elevations in some fluorometric determinations of urinary catecholamines; false-positive urine glucose (Benedict's reagent)

Patient Information Transient flushing of the skin and a sensation of warmth (especially of face and upper body), itching, tingling or headache may occur; if dizziness occurs, avoid sudden changes in posture and notify physician; notify physician if taking vitamins or other products that contain niacin or nicotinamide; do not change brands once dosage is stabilized; report signs and symptoms of hepatotoxicity (nausea, vomiting, loss of appetite, yellow skin, dark urine, general feeling of weakness) to physician

Additional Information The current recommendation for pharmacologic treatment of hypercholesterolemia in children is limited to children ≥8 years of age and is based on LDL-C concentrations and the presence of coronary vascular disease (CVD) risk factors (see table and Daniels, 2008). In adults, for each 1% lowering in LDL-C, the relative risk for major cardiovascular events is reduced by ~1%. For more specific risk assessment and treatment recommendations for adults, see NCEP ATPIII, 2001.

Recommendations for Initiating Pharmacologic Treatment in Children ≥8 Years[1]

No risk factors for CVD	LDL ≥190 mg/dL despite 6-month to 1-year diet therapy
Family history of premature CVD or ≥2 CVD risk factors present, including obesity, hypertension, or cigarette smoking	LDL ≥160 mg/dL despite 6-month to 1-year diet therapy
Diabetes mellitus present	LDL ≥130 mg/dL

[1]Adapted from Daniels SR, Greer FR, and Committee on Nutrition, "Lipid Screening and Cardiovascular Health in Childhood," *Pediatrics*, 2008, 122(1):198-208.

Dosage Forms Excipient information presented when available (limited, particularly for generics); consult specific product labeling. [DSC] = Discontinued product

Caplet, timed release, oral: 500 mg

Capsule, oral: 50 mg, 250 mg

Capsule, extended release, oral: 250 mg; 400 mg [DSC]; 500 mg

Capsule, timed release, oral: 250 mg, 400 mg, 500 mg

Tablet, oral: 50 mg, 100 mg, 250 mg, 500 mg

Niacor®: 500 mg [scored]

Tablet, controlled release, oral:

Slo-Niacin®: 250 mg, 500 mg, 750 mg [scored]

Tablet, extended release, oral:

Niaspan®: 500 mg, 750 mg, 1000 mg

Tablet, timed release, oral: 250 mg, 500 mg, 750 mg, 1000 mg

Niacin-Time®: 500 mg

References

American Academy of Pediatrics Committee on Nutrition, "Cholesterol in Childhood," *Pediatrics*, 1998, 101(1 Pt 1):141-7.

"ASHP Therapeutic Position Statement on the Safe Use of Niacin in the Management of Dyslipidemias. American Society of Health-System Pharmacists," *Am J Health Syst Pharm*, 1997, 54(24):2815-9.

Colletti RB, Neufeld EJ, Roff NK, et al, "Niacin Treatment of Hypercholesterolemia in Children," *Pediatrics*, 1993, 92(1):78-82.

Daniels SR, Greer FR, and Committee on Nutrition, "Lipid Screening and Cardiovascular Health in Childhood," *Pediatrics*, 2008, 122(1):198-208.

McCrindle BW, Urbina EM, Dennison BA, et al, "Drug Therapy of High-Risk Lipid Abnormalities in Children and Adolescents: A Scientific Statement from the American Heart Association Atherosclerosis, Hypertension, and Obesity in Youth Committee, Council of Cardiovascular Disease in the Young, With the Council on Cardiovascular Nursing," *Circulation*, 2007, 115(14):1948-67.

Schuna AA, "Safe Use of Niacin," *Am J Health Syst Pharm*, 1997, 54 (24):2803.

"Third Report of the National Cholesterol Education Program Expert Panel on Detection, Evaluation, and Treatment of High Blood Cholesterol in Adults (Adult Treatment Panel III)," May 2001, www.nhlbi.nih.gov/guidelines/cholesterol.

◆ **Niacin-Time®** *see* Niacin *on page 986*

◆ **Niacor®** *see* Niacin *on page 986*
◆ **Niaspan®** *see* Niacin *on page 986*
◆ **Niastase® (Can)** *see* Factor VIIa (Recombinant) *on page 556*

NiCARdipine (nye KAR de peen)

Medication Safety Issues
Sound-alike/look-alike issues:
NiCARdipine may be confused with niacinamide, NIFEdipine, niMODipine
Cardene® may be confused with Cardizem®, Cardura®, codeine

International issues:
Cardene® may be confused with Cardem® which is a brand name for celiprolol in Spain
Cardene® may be confused with Cardin® which is a brand name for methyldopa in Brazil and a brand name for simvastatin in Poland

Significant differences exist between oral and I.V. dosing. Use caution when converting from one route of administration to another.

Related Information
Antihypertensive Agents by Class *on page 1481*

U.S. Brand Names Cardene®; Cardene® I.V.; Cardene® SR

Therapeutic Category Antianginal Agent; Antihypertensive Agent; Calcium Channel Blocker; Calcium Channel Blocker, Nondihydropyridine

Generic Available Yes: Capsule, injection

Use
Immediate release product: Treatment of chronic stable angina; hypertension
Sustained release product: Treatment of hypertension
Parenteral: Short-term treatment of hypertension when oral treatment is not possible

Pregnancy Risk Factor C

Pregnancy Considerations Adverse events were observed in some animal reproduction studies. Nicardipine crosses the placenta; changes in fetal heart rate have been observed following maternal use.

Lactation Enters breast milk

Breast-Feeding Considerations Nicardipine is minimally excreted into breast milk. In one study, peak milk concentrations ranged from 1.9-18.8 mcg/mL following oral maternal doses of 40-150 mg/day. The estimated exposure to the breast-feeding infant was calculated to be 0.073% of the weight-adjusted maternal oral dose or 0.14% of the weight-adjusted maternal I.V. dose.

Contraindications Hypersensitivity to nicardipine or any component; advanced aortic stenosis

Warnings Symptomatic hypotension may occur; monitor blood pressure carefully (see Monitoring Parameters); lowering of blood pressure should be done at a rate appropriate for the patient's condition; rapid drops in blood pressure may lead to arterial insufficiency; avoid systemic hypotension in patients following an acute cerebral infarct or hemorrhage.

Nicardipine may increase frequency, duration, or severity of angina with initiation of therapy or dosage increase (use with caution in patients with CAD). May cause negative inotropic effects in some patients (use with caution in patients with CHF or significant left ventricular dysfunction, especially when used in combination with beta-blockers).

Precautions Use with caution and carefully titrate the dose in patients with cardiac, renal, or hepatic dysfunction or reduced liver blood flow; decrease the starting dose for patients with severe hepatic dysfunction. Use I.V. formulation with caution in patients with pheochromocytoma (limited clinical experience) and portal hypertension (may cause increase hepatic venous pressure gradient). Peripheral infusion sites (for I.V. therapy) should be changed every 12 hours to minimize venous irritation. Abrupt withdrawal may cause rebound angina in patients with CAD. Use of immediate release product for treatment of hypertension may result in relatively large differences in peak and trough blood pressures (compared to sustained release product). Safety and efficacy have not been demonstrated in pediatric patients.

Adverse Reactions

Cardiovascular: Flushing, vasodilation, palpitation, tachycardia, peripheral edema (dose related), angina increased (dose related), hypotension (I.V.: 6%), orthostasis, syncope, abnormal ECG, facial edema, MI

Central nervous system: Headache, dizziness, somnolence, paresthesia, nervousness, insomnia, abnormal dreams; intracranial hemorrhage (I.V.: 0.7%)

Dermatologic: Rash

Endocrine & metabolic: Hypokalemia (I.V.: 0.7%)

Gastrointestinal: Nausea, vomiting, dyspepsia, xerostomia, constipation, diarrhea, abdominal pain; gingival hyperplasia (1 case report)

Genitourinary: Polyuria, nocturia; hematuria (I.V.: 0.7%)

Local: Injection site reaction (I.V.: 1.4%); injection site pain (0.7%)

Neuromuscular & skeletal: Asthenia, myalgia, malaise, tremor, hypesthesia

Ocular: Blurred vision

Respiratory: Dyspnea

Miscellaneous: Diaphoresis

Drug Interactions

Metabolism/Transport Effects Substrate of CYP1A2 (minor), CYP2C9 (minor), CYP2D6 (minor), CYP2E1 (minor), CYP3A4 (major), P-glycoprotein; **Inhibits** CYP2C9 (strong), CYP2C19 (moderate), CYP2D6 (moderate), CYP3A4 (strong), P-glycoprotein

Avoid Concomitant Use

Avoid concomitant use of NiCARdipine with any of the following: Alfuzosin; Dabigatran Etexilate; Dronedarone; Eplerenone; Everolimus; Halofantrine; Nilotinib; Nisoldipine; Ranolazine; Rivaroxaban; Romidepsin; Salmeterol; Silodosin; Tamsulosin; Thioridazine; Tolvaptan; Topotecan

Increased Effect/Toxicity

NiCARdipine may increase the levels/effects of: Alfuzosin; Almotriptan; Alosetron; Amifostine; Antihypertensives; Bortezomib; Brinzolamide; Calcium Channel Blockers (Nondihydropyridine); Ciclesonide; Colchicine; CYP2C19 Substrates; CYP2C9 Substrates (High risk); CYP2D6 Substrates; CYP3A4 Substrates; Dabigatran Etexilate; Dienogest; Dronedarone; Dutasteride; Eplerenone; Everolimus; FentaNYL; Fesoterodine; GuanFACINE; Halofantrine; Hypotensive Agents; Ixabepilone; Lumefantrine; Magnesium Salts; Maraviroc; MethylPREDNISolone; Neuromuscular-Blocking Agents (Nondepolarizing); Nilotinib; Nisoldipine; Nitroprusside; Paricalcitol; Pazopanib; P-Glycoprotein Substrates; Phenytoin; Pimecrolimus; Ranolazine; RiTUXimab; Rivaroxaban; Romidepsin; Salmeterol; Saxagliptin; Silodosin; Sorafenib; Tacrolimus; Tacrolimus (Systemic); Tadalafil; Tamoxifen; Tamsulosin; Thioridazine; Tolvaptan; Topotecan

The levels/effects of NiCARdipine may be increased by: Alpha1-Blockers; Antifungal Agents (Azole Derivatives, Systemic); Calcium Channel Blockers (Nondihydropyridine); CycloSPORINE; CycloSPORINE (Systemic); CYP3A4 Inhibitors (Moderate); CYP3A4 Inhibitors (Strong); Dasatinib; Diazoxide; Fluconazole; Grapefruit

Juice; Herbs (Hypotensive Properties); Macrolide Antibiotics; Magnesium Salts; MAO Inhibitors; Pentoxifylline; P-Glycoprotein Inhibitors; Phosphodiesterase 5 Inhibitors; Prostacyclin Analogues; Protease Inhibitors; Quinupristin

Decreased Effect

NiCARdipine may decrease the levels/effects of: Clopidogrel; Codeine; Prasugrel; QuiNIDine; TraMADol

The levels/effects of NiCARdipine may be decreased by: Barbiturates; Calcium Salts; CarBAMazepine; CYP3A4 Inducers (Strong); Deferasirox; Herbs (CYP3A4 Inducers); Herbs (Hypertensive Properties); Methylphenidate; Nafcillin; Peginterferon Alfa-2b; P-Glycoprotein Inducers; Rifamycin Derivatives; Yohimbine

Food Interactions A high-fat meal may decrease nicardipine peak concentrations and the extent of absorption; however, in the clinical trials that established safety and efficacy, the immediate and sustained release capsules were administered without regard to meals. Administration of sustained release capsule with a high-fat meal reduces fluctuations in serum concentrations.

Grapefruit juice may increase nicardipine serum concentrations (avoid concurrent use); avoid natural licorice (causes sodium and water retention and increases potassium loss)

Stability

Capsules (immediate and sustained-release): Store at 15°C to 30°C (59°F to 86°F); dispense in light-resistant container

Injection: Store at room temperature; protect from light (store ampuls in carton before use); avoid exposure to elevated temperatures; freezing does not affect stability; diluted solution (0.1 mg/mL) is stable for 24 hours at room temperature

Compatible in D_5W, D_5W with KCl 40 mEq, D_5NS, $D_51/2NS$, NS, $1/2NS$ for 24 hours when stored at controlled room temperature in glass or polyvinyl chloride containers; **not** compatible with sodium bicarbonate 5% or LR

Y-site administration: Compatible: Diltiazem, dobutamine, dopamine, epinephrine, fentanyl, gatifloxacin, hydromorphone, labetalol, linezolid, lorazepam, midazolam, milrinone, morphine, nitroglycerin, norepinephrine, ranitidine, vecuronium. **Incompatible:** Furosemide, heparin, thiopental

Mechanism of Action Inhibits calcium ions from entering the "slow channels" or select voltage-sensitive areas of vascular smooth muscle and myocardium during depolarization; produces a relaxation of coronary vascular smooth muscle and coronary vasodilation; increases myocardial oxygen delivery in patients with vasospastic angina

Pharmacodynamics Antihypertensive effects:

Onset of action:

I.V.: Within minutes

Oral: 0.5-2 hours

Maximum effect:

Immediate capsules: 1-2 hours

Sustained release capsules (at steady state): Sustained from 2-6 hours postdose

I.V. continuous infusion: 50% of the maximum effect is seen by 45 minutes; final effect of a continuously infused dose is seen by 50 hours

Duration:

Immediate release capsules: <8 hours

Sustained release capsules: 12 hours

I.V.: Single dose: 3 hours

I.V. continuous infusion: Upon discontinuation, a 50% decrease in effect is seen in ~30 minutes with gradual discontinuing antihypertensive effects for ~50 hours.

Pharmacokinetics (Adult data unless noted) Absorption: Oral: ~100%, but large first-pass effect

Distribution: V_d: Adults: 8.3 L/kg

Protein binding: >95%

◄ Metabolism: Extensive, saturable, first-pass effect; dose-dependent (nonlinear) pharmacokinetics; extensive hepatic metabolism; major pathway is via cytochrome P450 isoenzyme CYP3A4

Bioavailability: Oral: 35%

Half-life: Follows dose-dependent (nonlinear) pharmacokinetics; "apparent" or calculated half-life is dependant upon serum concentrations. Half-life over the first 8 hours after oral dosing is 2-4 hours; terminal half-life (oral): 8.6 hours. After I.V. infusion, serum concentrations decrease tri-exponentially; alpha half-life: 2.7 minutes; beta half-life: 44.8 minutes; terminal half-life: 14.4 hours (**Note:** Terminal half-life can only be seen after long-term infusions)

Time to peak serum concentration: Oral:

Immediate release capsule: 30-120 minutes (mean: 1 hour)

Sustained release capsule: 1-4 hours

Elimination: 60% of an oral dose is excreted in the urine (<1% as unchanged drug); 35% excreted in feces.

Clearance: Decreased in patients with hepatic dysfunction; may be decreased in patients with renal impairment

Usual Dosage Note: Oral and I.V. doses are **not** equivalent on a mg per mg basis.

Neonates: **Note:** Very limited information exists.

I.V. continuous infusion: One prospective open-label study of 20 hypertensive neonates (15 preterm; median PNA 15 days) used initial nicardipine doses of 0.5 mcg/kg/minute (n=17). Doses were titrated according to blood pressure; the mean maximal required dose was 0.74 ± 0.41 mcg/kg/minute (range: 0.5-2 mcg/kg/minute) and occurred at 12 ± 19 hours of nicardipine infusion. The median duration of treatment was 11 days (range: 2-43 days) (see Milou, 2000). Similar doses were required in a smaller study of 8 preterm infants and in one case report of a neonate who received ECMO therapy (see Gouyon, 1997 and McBride, 2003). Further studies are needed.

Oral: No information is available.

Children: Note: Limited information exists; dose is not well established. Further studies are needed.

I.V. continuous infusion: Some experts recommend the following: Initial: 0.5-1 mcg/kg/minute; titrate dose according to blood pressure; rate of infusion may be increased every 15-30 minutes; maximum dose: 4-5 mcg/kg/minute (see Flynn, 2000 and Flynn, 2001; see also Additional Information).

Note: Other smaller studies support the use of an initial pediatric nicardipine dose of 1 mcg/kg/minute (see Nakagawa, 2004 and Treluyer, 1993). However, several studies used a higher initial dose of 5 mcg/kg/minute; once blood pressure was controlled, the dose was decreased to a lower maintenance dose. Mean maintenance doses have been reported to be 2.4 mcg/kg/minute (range: 1-5 mcg/kg/minute in 10 PICU patients) and 3 mcg/kg/minute (range: 2.1-5.5 mcg/kg/minute in 9 post-op cardiac surgery patients) (see Tobias, 2001).

Oral: One case report used 20 mg every 8 hours in a 14-year old boy following cardiac transplant (see Larsen, 1994). Another case used 30 mg every 8 hours in a 14-year old girl with renal disease (see Michael, 1998).

Adults:

Oral:

Immediate release: Initial: 20 mg 3 times/day; titrate to response; usual: 20-40 mg 3 times/day; allow at least 3 days between increases in dose

Sustained release: Initial: 30 mg twice daily; titrate to response; usual: 30-60 mg twice daily; **Note:** Usual dosage range (JNC 7): 30-60 mg twice daily.

Note: Use caution and re-examine blood pressure control when converting patients from the immediate release to the sustained release product; the total daily dose of immediate release product may not be equivalent to the daily sustained-release dose.

I.V. continuous infusion:

Hypertension in patients **not** receiving oral nicardipine: Initial: 5 mg/hour; titrate dose according to blood pressure; increase infusion by 2.5 mg/hour every 15 minutes to a maximum of 15 mg/hour; may increase infusion rate every 5 minutes if a more rapid blood pressure reduction is required; once desired blood pressure is achieved, decrease infusion rate to 3 mg/hour. Monitor and titrate to lowest dose necessary to maintain stable blood pressure.

Substitution for oral nicardipine therapy (approximate equivalents):

Oral dose of 20 mg every 8 hours = 0.5 mg/hour I.V. infusion

Oral dose of 30 mg every 8 hours = 1.2 mg/hour I.V. infusion

Oral dose of 40 mg every 8 hours = 2.2 mg/hour I.V. infusion

Dosing adjustment in renal impairment: Specific guidelines are not available; careful monitoring and dosage adjustment is warranted. Adult: Oral: Titrate dose carefully beginning with usual initial dose.

Dosing adjustment in hepatic impairment: Specific guidelines are not available; use with caution in patients with severe hepatic impairment; careful monitoring and dosage adjustment is warranted. Adult: Oral: Initial:

Immediate release: Titrate dose carefully beginning with 20 mg twice daily

Sustained release: Has not been studied

Administration

Oral: May be administered without regard to meals; avoid concurrent administration with high-fat meals or grapefruit juice. Swallow sustained release capsule whole; do not crush, break, or chew.

I.V.: Administer by slow I.V. continuous infusion; I.V. product must be diluted prior to administration; may dilute with D_5W, D_5W with KCl 40 mEq, D_5NS, $D_5^1/2NS$, NS, $^1/2NS$; manufacturer recommended concentration for infusion: 0.1 mg/mL; **Note:** One pediatric study used infusions of 0.5 mg/mL in D_5W, NS, or other compatible solution (see Flynn, 2001). Avoid extravasation.

Monitoring Parameters Blood pressure, heart rate, liver and renal function; **Note:** Monitor blood pressure carefully during initiation of therapy and with dosage adjustments.

Immediate release product: Measure blood pressure at peak effects (1-2 hours after the dose) especially during initiation of therapy, and just prior to the next dose (to ensure control of blood pressure throughout dosing interval).

Sustained release product: Measure blood pressure 2-4 hours after the first dose or dosage increase and just prior to the next dose

I.V.: Monitor infusion site for extravasation; monitor blood pressure continuously during I.V. administration

Patient Information May cause dizziness or drowsiness and impair ability to perform activities requiring mental alertness or physical coordination; may cause dry mouth. May cause low blood pressure upon standing; rise slowly from prolonged sitting or lying position. Avoid alcohol and grapefruit juice.

Do not discontinue abruptly; report any dizziness, shortness of breath, palpitations, chest pain, rapid heart beat, swelling of extremities, muscle weakness or pain, or nervousness. Some medicines may interact with nicardipine; report the use of other medications, nonprescription medications, and herbal or natural products to your physician and pharmacist; avoid the herbal medicine St John's wort.

Nursing Implications Do not crush or break sustained release capsules.

I.V.: Avoid extravasation; closely monitor I.V. site for swelling, redness, burning, or pain; change peripheral infusion sites every 12 hours

Assess therapeutic effectiveness, and adverse reactions on a regular basis during therapy. Monitor blood pressure (see Monitoring Parameters). Instruct patient on appropriate use, side effects, appropriate interventions, and adverse symptoms to report.

Additional Information A retrospective study in 29 hypertensive children (mean age: 7.8 years; range: 2 days to 18 years) used initial nicardipine doses of 0.5-1 mcg/kg/minute; doses were titrated according to blood pressure and the rate of infusion was increased every 15-30 minutes; the mean effective dose was 1.8 ± 0.3 mcg/kg/minute (range: 0.3-4 mcg/kg/minute); blood pressure was controlled within 2.7 ± 2.1 hours (range: 0.5-9 hours) after starting nicardipine continuous infusion (see Flynn, 2001). Nicardipine has also been used in children for controlled hypotension to limit intraoperative blood loss (see Tobias, 2002).

The sustained release capsule contains a powder component (containing 25% of the dose) and a spherical granule component (containing 75% of the dose). The I.V. product is buffered to a pH of 3.5.

Dosage Forms Excipient information presented when available (limited, particularly for generics); consult specific product labeling.

Capsule, oral, as hydrochloride: 20 mg, 30 mg
Cardene®: 20 mg, 30 mg
Capsule, sustained release, oral, as hydrochloride:
Cardene® SR: 30 mg, 45 mg, 60 mg
Infusion, premixed in iso-osmotic dextrose, as hydrochloride:
Cardene® I.V.: 20 mg (200 mL); 40 mg (200 mL)
Infusion, premixed in iso-osmotic sodium chloride, as hydrochloride:
Cardene® I.V.: 20 mg (200 mL); 40 mg (200 mL)
Injection, solution, as hydrochloride: 2.5 mg/mL (10 mL)
Cardene® I.V.: 2.5 mg/mL (10 mL)

References

Chobanian AV, Bakris GL, Black HR, et al, "The Seventh Report of the Joint National Committee on Prevention, Detection, Evaluation, and Treatment of High Blood Pressure: The JNC 7 Report," *JAMA*, 2003, 289(19):2560-72.

Flynn JT and Pasko DA, "Calcium Channel Blockers: Pharmacology and Place in Therapy of Pediatric Hypertension," *Pediatr Nephrol*, 2000, 15(3-4):302-16.

Flynn JT, Mottes TA, Brophy PD, et al, "Intravenous Nicardipine for Treatment of Severe Hypertension in Children," *J Pediatr*, 2001, 139(1):38-43.

Gouyon JB, Geneste B, Semama DS, et al, "Intravenous Nicardipine in Hypertensive Preterm Infants," *Arch Dis Child Fetal Neonatal Ed*, 1997, 76(2):F126-7.

Larsen A and Tobias J, "Nicardipine for the Treatment of Hypertension Following Cardiac Transplantation in a 14-Year-Old Boy," *Clin Pediatr (Phila)*, 1994, 33(5):309-11.

McBride BF, White CM, Campbell M, et al, "Nicardipine to Control Neonatal Hypertension During Extracorporeal Membrane Oxygen Support," *Ann Pharmacother*, 2003, 37(5):667-70.

Michael J, Groshong T, and Tobias JD, "Nicardipine for Hypertensive Emergencies in Children With Renal Disease," *Pediatr Nephrol*, 1998, 12(1):40-2.

Milou C, Debuche-Benouachkou V, Semama DS, et al, "Intravenous Nicardipine as a First-Line Antihypertensive Drug in Neonates," *Intensive Care Med*, 2000, 26(7):956-8.

Nakagawa TA, Sartori SC, Morris A, et al, "Intravenous Nicardipine for Treatment of Postcoarctectomy Hypertension in Children," *Pediatr Cardiol*, 2004, 25(1):26-30.

Steele RM, Schuna AA, and Schreiber RT, "Calcium Antagonist-Induced Gingival Hyperplasia," *Ann Intern Med*, 1994, 120(8):663-4.

Tobias JD, "Nicardipine to Control Mean Arterial Pressure After Cardiothoracic Surgery in Infants and Children," *Am J Ther*, 2001, 8(1):3-6.

Treluyer JM, Hubert P, Jouvet P, et al, "Intravenous Nicardipine in Hypertensive Children," *Eur J Pediatr*, 1993, 152(9):712-4.

◆ **Nicardipine Hydrochloride** see NiCARdipine on page 988
◆ **Nicotinic Acid** see Niacin on page 986
◆ **Nidagel™ (Can)** see MetroNIDAZOLE on page 921
◆ **Nifediac CC®** see NIFEdipine on page 991
◆ **Nifedical XL®** see NIFEdipine on page 991

NIFEdipine (nye FED i peen)

Medication Safety Issues
Sound-alike/look-alike issues:
NIFEdipine may be confused with niCARdipine, niMODipine, nisoldipine
Procardia XL® may be confused with Cartia XT®

Beers Criteria medication: This drug may be inappropriate for use in geriatric patients (high severity risk).

International issues:
Nipin® [Italy and Singapore] may be confused with Nipent® which is a brand name for pentostatin in the U.S.

Related Information
Antihypertensive Agents by Class on page 1481
Medications for Which A Single Dose May Be Fatal When Ingested By A Toddler on page 1709

U.S. Brand Names Adalat® CC; Afeditab® CR; Nifediac CC®; Nifedical XL®; Procardia XL®; Procardia®

Canadian Brand Names Adalat® XL®; Apo-Nifed PA®; Apo-Nifed®; Gen-Nifedipine XL; Mylan-Nifedipine Extended Release; Nifedipine PA; Nu-Nifed; Nu-Nifedipine-PA; PMS-Nifedipine

Therapeutic Category Antianginal Agent; Antihypertensive Agent; Calcium Channel Blocker; Calcium Channel Blocker, Nondihydropyridine

Generic Available Yes

Use Treatment of chronic stable or vasospastic angina; treatment of hypertension (extended release products only)

Pregnancy Risk Factor C

Pregnancy Considerations Adverse events were observed in animal reproduction studies. Nifedipine crosses the placenta. Use in pregnancy only when clearly needed and when the benefits outweigh the potential hazard to the fetus. Hypotension, IUGR reported. IUGR probably related to maternal hypertension. May be used for the treatment of preterm labor.

Lactation Enters breast milk/not recommended (AAP considers "compatible")

Contraindications Hypersensitivity to nifedipine or any component (see Warnings); recent MI

Warnings Excessive hypotension may occur, especially during initiation of therapy or dosage increase (more common with concurrent beta-blocker therapy; monitor blood pressure closely; profound hypotension, MI, and death have been reported in adults when immediate release nifedipine has been used (orally or sublingually) for acute reduction of blood pressure (manufacturer does **not** recommended use of capsules for acute reduction of blood pressure); immediate release nifedipine is not FDA approved for long-term control of essential hypertension (appropriate studies to determine optimal dose or dosing interval have not been conducted); 90 mg tablet may contain tartrazine which may cause allergic reactions in susceptible individuals (see Dosage Forms)

Precautions May increase frequency, duration, and severity of angina or precipitate acute MI during initiation of therapy; use with caution in patients with CHF or aortic stenosis (especially with concomitant beta-blocker)

Adverse Reactions
Cardiovascular: Flushing, hypotension, tachycardia, palpitations, syncope, peripheral edema

◀

Central nervous system: Dizziness, fever, headache, chills, fatigue

Dermatologic: Dermatitis, urticaria, purpura; photosensitivity (rare)

Gastrointestinal: Nausea, diarrhea, constipation, gingival hyperplasia

Hematologic: Thrombocytopenia, leukopenia, anemia

Hepatic: Liver enzymes elevated, cholestasis, jaundice; allergic hepatitis (rare)

Neuromuscular & skeletal: Joint stiffness, arthritis with ANA elevated

Ocular: Blurred vision, transient blindness

Respiratory: Shortness of breath

Miscellaneous: Diaphoresis

Drug Interactions

Metabolism/Transport Effects Substrate of CYP2D6 (minor), 3A4 (major); **Inhibits** CYP1A2 (moderate), 2C9 (weak), 2D6 (weak), 3A4 (weak)

Avoid Concomitant Use

Avoid concomitant use of NIFEdipine with any of the following: Grapefruit Juice

Increased Effect/Toxicity

NIFEdipine may increase the levels/effects of: Amifostine; Antihypertensives; Calcium Channel Blockers (Nondihydropyridine); CYP1A2 Substrates; Hypotensive Agents; Magnesium Salts; Neuromuscular-Blocking Agents (Nondepolarizing); Nitroprusside; Phenytoin; RiTUXimab; Tacrolimus; Tacrolimus (Systemic); VinCRIStine

The levels/effects of NIFEdipine may be increased by: Alcohol (Ethyl); Alpha1-Blockers; Antifungal Agents (Azole Derivatives, Systemic); Calcium Channel Blockers (Nondihydropyridine); Cimetidine; Cisapride; CycloSPORINE; CycloSPORINE (Systemic); CYP3A4 Inhibitors (Moderate); CYP3A4 Inhibitors (Strong); Dasatinib; Diazoxide; Fluconazole; Grapefruit Juice; Herbs (Hypotensive Properties); Macrolide Antibiotics; Magnesium Salts; MAO Inhibitors; Pentoxifylline; Phosphodiesterase 5 Inhibitors; Prostacyclin Analogues; Protease Inhibitors; Quinupristin

Decreased Effect

NIFEdipine may decrease the levels/effects of: Clopidogrel; QuiNIDine

The levels/effects of NIFEdipine may be decreased by: Barbiturates; Calcium Salts; CarBAMazepine; CYP3A4 Inducers (Strong); Deferasirox; Herbs (CYP3A4 Inducers); Herbs (Hypertensive Properties); Methylphenidate; Nafcillin; Peginterferon Alfa-2b; Rifamycin Derivatives; Yohimbine

Food Interactions Capsule is rapidly absorbed orally if it is administered without food but may result in vasodilator side effects; administration with low-fat meals may decrease flushing; grapefruit juice may significantly increase the oral bioavailability of nifedipine (avoid concurrent use); food may decrease the rate but not the extent of absorption of Procardia XL®; a high fat meal does not effect the extent of absorption of Adalat® CC, but delays the time to peak and increases the peak concentration

Stability Store at room temperature; protect from light and moisture

Mechanism of Action Inhibits calcium ions from entering the "slow channels" or select voltage-sensitive areas of vascular smooth muscle and myocardium during depolarization; produces a relaxation of coronary vascular smooth muscle and coronary vasodilation; increases myocardial oxygen delivery in patients with vasospastic angina

Pharmacodynamics

Onset of action:

S.L. or "bite and swallow": Within 1-5 minutes

Oral:

Immediate release: Within 20-30 minutes

Extended release: 2-2.5 hours

Duration:

Immediate release: 4-8 hours

Extended release: 24 hours

Pharmacokinetics (Adult data unless noted)

Protein-binding: 92% to 98% (concentration-dependent); **Note:** Protein-binding may be significantly decreased in patients with renal or hepatic impairment

Metabolism: In the liver to inactive metabolites

Bioavailability:

Capsules: 45% to 75%

Extended release: 84% to 89% relative to immediate release capsules

Half-life:

Normal adults: 2-5 hours

Cirrhosis: 7 hours

Elimination: In the urine with >90% of the dose excreted as inactive metabolites

Usual Dosage Oral, S.L. or "bite and swallow" (eg, patient bites capsule to release liquid contents and then swallows) (see Warnings):

Note: Doses are usually titrated upward over 7 to 14 days; may increase over 3 days if clinically necessary:

Children:

Hypertensive emergencies: Immediate release: 0.25-0.5 mg/kg/dose; maximum dose: 10 mg/dose; may repeat if needed every 4-6 hours; monitor carefully; maximum dose: 1-2 mg/kg/day; **Note:** Initial doses ≤0.25 mg/kg/dose may result in a less dramatic decrease in blood pressure and be safer than larger initial doses (see Blaszak, 2001); some centers use initial doses of 0.1 mg/kg/dose (see Egger, 2002).

Hypertension (chronic treatment): Extended release: Initial: 0.25-0.5 mg/kg/day given once daily or divided in 2 doses per day; titrate dose to effect; maximum dose: 3 mg/kg/day up to 120 mg/day (National High Blood Pressure Education Program Working Group on High Blood Pressure in Children and Adolescents, 2004); some centers use maximum dose: 3 mg/kg/day up to 180 mg/day (see Flynn, 2000)

Adolescents and Adults:

Angina: Immediate release: Initial: 10 mg 3 times/day; usual dose: 10-20 mg 3 times/day; some patients may require 20-30 mg 3-4 times/day; doses >120 mg/day are rarely needed; maximum dose: 180 mg/24 hours; **Note:** Do not use for acute anginal episodes; may precipitate myocardial infarction

Hypertension: Extended release tablet: Initial: 30 mg once daily; usual dosage range (JNC 7): Adolescents ≥18 years and Adults: 30-60 mg once daily; maximum dose: 120 mg/day

Administration Oral: Administer with food; Adalat® CC: Administer on an empty stomach; do not administer nifedipine with grapefruit juice; swallow sustained release tablets whole, do not crush, break, or chew; liquid-filled capsule may be punctured and drug solution administered sublingually or orally; when measuring smaller doses from the liquid-filled capsules, consider the following concentrations (for Procardia®) 10 mg capsule = 10 mg/0.34 mL; 20 mg capsule = 20 mg/0.45 mL

Note: When nifedipine is administered sublingually, only a small amount is absorbed sublingually; the observed effects are actually due to swallowing of the drug with subsequent rapid oral absorption

Monitoring Parameters Blood pressure, CBC, platelets, periodic liver enzymes

Patient Information Avoid alcohol and grapefruit juice; rise slowly from prolonged sitting or lying position; insoluble shell of extended release tablet may appear in the stool (this is normal). May rarely cause photosensitivity reactions; avoid exposure to sunlight and artificial light sources (sunlamps, tanning booth/bed); use a sunscreen; contact physician if reaction occurs

Dosage Forms Excipient information presented when available (limited, particularly for generics); consult specific product labeling.

Capsule, softgel: 10 mg, 20 mg

Procardia®: 10 mg

Tablet, extended release: 30 mg, 60 mg, 90 mg

Adalat® CC, Procardia XL®: 30 mg, 60 mg, 90 mg

Afeditab® CR, Nifedical XL®: 30 mg, 60 mg

Nifediac CC®: 30 mg, 60 mg, 90 mg [90 mg tablet contains tartrazine]

References

Adcock KG and Wilson JT, "Nifedipine Labeling Illustrates the Pediatric Dilemma for Off-Patent Drugs," *Pediatrics*, 2002, 109(2):319-21.

Blaszak RT, Savage JA, and Ellis EN, "The Use of Short-Acting Nifedipine in Pediatric Patients With Hypertension," *J Pediatr*, 2001, 139(1):34-7.

Chobanian AV, Bakris GL, Black HR, et al, "The Seventh Report of the Joint National Committee on Prevention, Detection, Evaluation, and Treatment of High Blood Pressure: The JNC 7 report," *JAMA*, 2003, 289(19):2560-72.

Dilmen U, Cagfülar MK, Senses A, et al, "Nifedipine in Hypertensive Emergencies of Children," *Am J Dis Child*, 1983, 137(12):1162-5.

Egger DW, Deming DD, Hamada N, et al, "Evaluation of the Safety of Short-Acting Nifedipine in Children With Hypertension," *Pediatr Nephrol*, 2002, 17(1):35-40.

Flynn JT and Pasko DA, "Calcium Channel Blockers: Pharmacology and Place in Therapy of Pediatric Hypertension," *Pediatr Nephrol*, 2000, 15(3-4):302-16.

Lopez-Herce J, Albajara L, Cagigas P, et al, "Treatment of Hypertensive Crisis in Children With Nifedipine," *Intensive Care Med*, 1988, 14 (5):519-21.

National High Blood Pressure Education Program Working Group on High Blood Pressure in Children and Adolescents, "The Fourth Report on the Diagnosis, Evaluation, and Treatment of High Blood Pressure in Children and Adolescents," *Pediatrics*, 2004, 114(2 Suppl):555-76.

Rosen WJ and Johnson CE, "Evaluation of Five Procedures for Measuring Nonstandard Doses of Nifedipine Liquid," *Am J Hosp Pharm*, 1989, 46(11):2313-7.

Yiu V, Orrbine E, Rosychuk RJ, et al, "The Safety and Use of Short-Acting Nifedipine in Hospitalized Hypertensive Children," *Pediatr Nephrol*, 2004, 19(6):644-50.

◆ **Nifedipine PA (Can)** see NIFEdipine on page 991

◆ **Nimbex®** see Cisatracurium on page 317

◆ **Nipent®** see Pentostatin on page 1088

◆ **Niravam™** see ALPRAZolam on page 68

◆ **Nitalapram** see Citalopram on page 319

Nitazoxanide (nye ta ZOX a nide)

U.S. Brand Names Alinia®

Therapeutic Category Antiprotozoal

Generic Available No

Use Treatment of diarrhea caused by *Cryptosporidium parvum* or *Giardia lamblia* in immunocompetent patients; manufacturer is pursuing approval for treatment of *Cryptosporidium*-induced diarrhea in HIV-infected patients and patients with immunodeficiency; treatment of intestinal amebiasis; treatment of refractory or recurrent *Clostridium difficile*-associated diarrhea

Pregnancy Risk Factor B

Pregnancy Considerations Teratogenic effects were not observed in animal studies. There are no adequate and well-controlled studies in pregnant women.

Lactation Excretion in breast milk unknown/use caution

Contraindications Hypersensitivity to nitazoxanide or any component

Warnings Suspension contains sodium benzoate; benzoic acid (benzoate) is a metabolite of benzyl alcohol; large amounts of benzyl alcohol (≥99 mg/kg/day) have been associated with a potentially fatal toxicity ("gasping syndrome") in neonates; avoid use of sodium benzoate containing products in neonates; *in vitro* and animal studies have shown that benzoate displaces bilirubin from protein binding sites

Precautions Use with caution in patients with renal, hepatic, or biliary disease since pharmacokinetics of nitazoxanide have not been studied in these patients. Use suspension dosage form with caution in diabetic patients due to sucrose content.

Adverse Reactions

Cardiovascular: Tachycardia, syncope, hypertension

Central nervous system: Headache (1.1%), fever, malaise, dizziness, chills, somnolence, insomnia

Dermatologic: Pruritus, rash

Endocrine and metabolic: Amenorrhea

Gastrointestinal: Abdominal pain (7.8%), diarrhea (2.1%), vomiting (1.1%), nausea, anorexia, flatulence, constipation

Genitourinary: Discoloration of urine (bright yellow); dysuria

Hepatic: ALT elevated

Neuromuscular and skeletal: Myalgia, leg cramps

Ophthalmologic: Discoloration of eye (yellow sclerae)

Renal: Serum creatinine elevated

Miscellaneous: Diaphoresis

Drug Interactions

Avoid Concomitant Use There are no known interactions where it is recommended to avoid concomitant use.

Increased Effect/Toxicity There are no known significant interactions involving an increase in effect.

Decreased Effect There are no known significant interactions involving a decrease in effect.

Food Interactions

Suspension: Administration with food increases AUC two-fold and peak concentrations by 50%

Tablet: Administration with food increases AUC by 45% to 50% and peak concentrations by ≤10%

Stability Store tablets and powder for oral suspension at room temperature. Reconstituted oral suspension is stable for 7 days at room temperature.

Mechanism of Action Appears to interfere with the pyruvate:ferredoxin oxidoreductase (PFOR) enzyme-dependent electron transfer reaction which is essential for anaerobic energy metabolism

Pharmacokinetics (Adult data unless noted)

Protein binding: Tizoxanide: >99%

Metabolism: Hydrolyzed in plasma to tizoxanide (active); conjugated to tizoxanide glucuronide in the liver

Bioavailability: Relative bioavailability of the suspension to the tablet is 70%

Half-life: Tizoxanide: 1-1.6 hours

Time to peak serum concentration: Tizoxanide: 1-4 hours

Elimination: Tizoxanide is excreted in urine (<10%), bile, and feces (60%); tizoxanide glucuronide is excreted in urine and bile

Usual Dosage Oral:

Diarrhea caused by *Cryptosporidium parvum* or *Giardia lamblia*:

Children 12-47 months: 100 mg every 12 hours for 3 days

Children 4-11 years: 200 mg every 12 hours for 3 days

Children ≥12 years, Adolescents, and Adults: 500 mg every 12 hours for 3 days

C. difficile-associated diarrhea: Adults: 500 mg every 12 hours for 7-10 days

Dosage adjustment in renal and/or hepatic impairment: Specific recommendations are not available; use with caution

Administration Minimize gastric irritation by administering with food; shake suspension well prior to use

Monitoring Parameters Periodic liver function tests, stool frequency

▶

Patient Information May discolor eyes or urine to a yellow tint

Additional Information The oral suspension contains sucrose 1.48 g/5 mL.

A randomized, placebo-controlled study of 89 adults and adolescents receiving a 3-day course of nitazoxanide 500 mg twice daily for 3 days to treat enteric protozoa found a cure rate of 81% versus a cure rate of 40% for placebo (Rossignol, 2001).

Dosage Forms Excipient information presented when available (limited, particularly for generics); consult specific product labeling.

Powder for suspension, oral: 100 mg/5 mL (60 mL) [contains sucrose 1.48 g/5 mL, sodium benzoate; strawberry flavor]

Tablet: 500 mg

Alinia® 3-Day Therapy Packs™ [unit-dose pack]: 500 mg (6s)

References

Bobak DA, "Use of Nitazoxanide for Gastrointestinal Tract Infections: Treatment of Protozoan Parasitic Infection and Beyond," *Curr Infect Dis Rep*, 2006, 8(2):91-5.

Rossignol JF, Ayoub A, and Ayers MS, "Treatment of Diarrhea Caused by *Giardia intestinalis* and *Entamoeba histolytica* or *E. dispar*: A Randomized, Double-Blind, Placebo-Controlled Study of Nitazoxanide," *J Infect Dis*, 2001, 184(3):381-4.

Nitisinone (ni TIS i known)

U.S. Brand Names Orfadin®

Therapeutic Category Tyrosinemia Type 1, Treatment Agent

Generic Available No

Use Adjunct to dietary restriction of tyrosine and phenylalanine in the treatment of hereditary tyrosinemia type 1 (HT-1)

Pregnancy Risk Factor C

Pregnancy Considerations Adverse events were observed in some animal reproduction studies.

Lactation Excretion in breast milk unknown/use caution

Contraindications Hypersensitivity to nitisinone or any component

Warnings Nitisinone therapy should be initiated by individuals experienced in the treatment of HT-1. Dietary restriction of tyrosine and phenylalanine must be used in conjunction with nitisinone; inadequate dietary restriction can result in elevations in plasma tyrosine leading to toxic ophthalmic effects (corneal ulcers, corneal opacities, keratitis, conjunctivitis, eye pain, and photophobia), skin effects (painful hyperkeratotic plaques on the soles and palms), and variable degrees of mental retardation and developmental delay. Nitisinone dosage should not be adjusted in order to lower the plasma tyrosine level. Transient thrombocytopenia has been reported; platelet and WBC counts should be monitored regularly during nitisinone therapy.

Precautions Slit-lamp examination of the eyes should be done prior to initiation of nitisinone therapy; patients who develop photophobia, eye pain or signs of inflammation such as redness, swelling, or burning of the eyes during treatment should be re-examined and a plasma tyrosine level measured; if the plasma tyrosine level is >500 micromoles/L a more restrictive diet is indicated. Patients with HT-1 are at risk for developing porphyric crises, liver failure, or hepatic neoplasm; regular liver monitoring by imaging (ultrasound, CT scan, MRI), liver function tests, and measurement of serum alpha-fetoprotein concentration is recommended; an increase in serum alpha-fetoprotein or signs of nodules in the liver during treatment may be a sign of inadequate therapy or hepatic malignancy.

Adverse Reactions Many adverse reactions noted in clinical trials are consistent with symptomatology of HT-1

Cardiovascular: Cyanosis

Central nervous system: Headache, seizures, encephalopathy, brain tumor, nervousness, somnolence

Endocrine & metabolic: Dehydration, hypoglycemia, amenorrhea

Dermatologic: Pruritus, exfoliative dermatitis, dry skin, maculopapular rash, alopecia

Gastrointestinal: Abdominal pain, diarrhea, gastritis, gastroenteritis, GI hemorrhage, melena, tooth discoloration

Hematologic: Thrombocytopenia, leukopenia, porphyria

Hepatic: Liver failure, hepatic neoplasm, hepatomegaly, liver enzymes elevated

Ocular: Conjunctivitis, corneal opacity, keratitis, photophobia, blepharitis, eye pain, cataracts

Respiratory: Bronchitis, respiratory insufficiency, epistaxis

Miscellaneous: Infection, septicemia

Drug Interactions

Avoid Concomitant Use There are no known interactions where it is recommended to avoid concomitant use.

Increased Effect/Toxicity There are no known significant interactions involving an increase in effect.

Decreased Effect There are no known significant interactions involving a decrease in effect.

Stability Store in refrigerator 2°C to 8°C (36°F to 46°F)

Mechanism of Action Nitisinone is a competitive inhibitor of 4-hydroxyphenyl-pyruvate dioxygenase, an enzyme of the tyrosine metabolic pathway. Hereditary tyrosinemia type 1 occurs due to a deficiency in fumarylacetoacetase (FAH) the final enzyme in the tyrosine metabolic pathway. This deficiency results in an accumulation of maleylacetoacetate and fumarylacetoacetate. These catabolic intermediates are converted to the toxic metabolites succinylacetone and succinylacetoacetate which are responsible for progressive liver failure, increased risk of hepatocellular carcinoma, coagulopathy, painful neurologic crises, and renal tubular dysfunction with rickets. Nitisinone prevents the formation of these toxic metabolites.

Pharmacokinetics (Adult data unless noted)

Half-life: Adults: 54 hours

Time to peak serum concentration: 3 hours

Usual Dosage Oral: Infants, Children, and Adults: 1 mg/kg/day twice daily; may increase after 1 month of treatment to 1.5 mg/kg/day if needed; not to exceed 2 mg/kg/day

Administration Oral: Administer on an empty stomach, at least one hour before a meal. Capsules may be opened and mixed with a small amount of water, formula, or applesauce immediately before use.

Monitoring Parameters Urine succinylacetone level, alpha-fetoprotein, plasma tyrosine level, liver function, CBC, platelets, ophthalmic exams (see Warnings and Precautions)

Reference Range Plasma tyrosine level <500 micromoles/L

Patient Information Advise patients and caregivers of the need to maintain a diet low in tyrosine and phenylalanine; report eye symptoms (see Precautions), rash, jaundice, or excessive bleeding to a physician promptly

Dosage Forms Excipient information presented when available (limited, particularly for generics); consult specific product labeling.

Capsule:

Orfadin®: 2 mg, 5 mg, 10 mg

References

Holme E and Lindstedt S, "Diagnosis and Management of Tyrosinemia Type I," *Curr Opin Pediatr*, 1995, 7(6):726-32.

◆ **Nitro-Bid®** *see* Nitroglycerin *on page 996*

◆ **Nitro-Dur®** *see* Nitroglycerin *on page 996*

Nitrofurantoin (nye troe fyoor AN toyn)

Medication Safety Issues

Sound alike/look alike issues:
Macrobid® may be confused with microK®, Nitro-Bid®
Nitrofurantoin may be confused with Neurontin®, nitroglycerin

Beers Criteria medication: This drug may be inappropriate for use in geriatric patients (high severity risk).

International issues:
Macrobid® may be confused with Mikrozid® which is a brand name for ethanol/propanol combination in Great Britain

U.S. Brand Names Furadantin®; Macrobid®; Macrodantin®

Canadian Brand Names Apo-Nitrofurantoin®; Macrobid®; Macrodantin®; Novo-Furantoin

Therapeutic Category Antibiotic, Miscellaneous

Generic Available Yes: Excludes suspension

Use Prevention and treatment of urinary tract infections caused by susceptible gram-negative and some gram-positive organisms including *E. coli*, *Klebsiella*, *Enterobacter*, enterococci, *S. saprophyticus*, and *S. aureus*; *Pseudomonas*, *Serratia*, and most species of *Proteus* are generally resistant to nitrofurantoin.
Macrodantin® and Furadantin® (FDA approved in ages ≥1 month)
Macrobid® (FDA approved in ages ≥12 years)

Pregnancy Risk Factor B (contraindicated at term)

Pregnancy Considerations Because adverse effects have not been observed in animals, nitrofurantoin is classified pregnancy category B. Nitrofurantoin crosses the placenta, but very little reaches the amniotic fluid. Most published experiences with nitrofurantoin use during pregnancy have failed to identify any increased obstetric or teratogenic risks. Isolated reports of a potential increased risk for cardiovascular defects and a case report of upper limb paralysis have not been replicated in other studies. Use of nitrofurantoin during pregnancy has been generally well tolerated with rare reports of maternal toxicity including severe pulmonary reactions or hematologic adverse effects. Nitrofurantoin is contraindicated in pregnant patients at term (38-42 weeks gestation), during labor and delivery, or when the onset of labor is imminent due to the possibility of hemolytic anemia in the neonate.

Lactation Enters breast milk/not recommended (infants <1 month); AAP rates "compatible"

Breast-Feeding Considerations Minimal, if any, nitrofurantoin distributes to human milk. Although use of nitrofurantoin during breast-feeding is not recommended by the manufacturer, the AAP considers nitrofurantoin to be "usually compatible with breast-feeding." Use with caution in patients at risk for G6PD deficiency or in newborns at risk for hyperbilirubinemia. Nondose-related effects could include modification of bowel flora.

Contraindications Hypersensitivity to nitrofurantoin or any component; anuria, oliguria, or significant renal impairment (Cl_{cr} <60 mL/minute or significant serum creatinine elevation); infants <1 month of age, pregnant patients at term (38-42 weeks gestation), during labor and delivery (due to the possibility of hemolytic anemia); in patients with a history of cholestatic jaundice or hepatic impairment with previous nitrofurantoin therapy

Warnings Nitrofurantoin should not be used to treat UTIs in febrile infants and young children in whom renal involvement is likely; not indicated for the treatment of pyelonephritis or perinephric abscesses; therapeutic concentrations of nitrofurantoin are not attained in the urine of patients with renal insufficiency (Cl_{cr} <60 mL/minute, anuria, or oliguria). Acute, subacute, or chronic (usually after 6 months of therapy) pulmonary reactions, including fatalities have been reported; monitor for dyspnea, cough, fever, malaise, radiologic evidence of diffuse interstitial pneumonitis or fibrosis; if these reactions occur, discontinue nitrofurantoin immediately. Hepatitis, cholestatic jaundice, chronic active hepatitis (onset may be insidious) and hepatic necrosis resulting in death may occur; monitor patients for changes in liver function; if hepatitis occurs, discontinue nitrofurantoin immediately. Peripheral neuropathy may occur; risk is increased by renal impairment, anemia, diabetes mellitus, electrolyte imbalance, vitamin B deficiency, and debilitating disease. Optic neuritis has been reported. Prolonged use may result in fungal or bacterial superinfection, including *C. difficile*-associated diarrhea (CDAD) and pseudomembranous colitis; CDAD has been observed >2 months postantibiotic treatment.

Precautions Use with caution in patients with G-6-PD deficiency (hemolytic anemia-induced by nitrofurantoin appears to be linked to G-6-PD deficiency in the red blood cells of affected patients), patients with anemia, vitamin B deficiency, diabetes mellitus, or electrolyte abnormalities

Adverse Reactions

Cardiovascular: Chest pain, cyanosis, ECG changes (associated with pulmonary toxicity)

Central nervous system: Dizziness, headache, chills, fever, vertigo, drowsiness, malaise, pseudotumor cerebri, confusion, depression, psychotic changes

Dermatologic: Rash, exfoliative dermatitis, urticaria, pruritus, alopecia, Stevens-Johnson syndrome, angioedema, erythema multiforme

Endocrine & metabolic: Hyperphosphatemia

Gastrointestinal: Nausea, vomiting, anorexia, pancreatitis, pseudomembranous colitis (rare), diarrhea, abdominal pain, flatulence, dyspepsia, constipation

Genitourinary: Discoloration of urine (dark yellow or brown), crystalluria

Hematologic: Hemolytic anemia, eosinophilia, leukopenia, granulocytopenia, thrombocytopenia, megaloblastic anemia, methemoglobinemia; G-6-PD deficiency anemia, aplastic anemia, hemoglobin decreased

Hepatic: Hepatotoxicity, cholestatic jaundice, hepatitis; AST, ALT, and alkaline phosphatase elevated

Neuromuscular & skeletal: Arthralgia, peripheral neuropathy, muscle weakness, asthenia, paresthesia, myalgia

Ocular: Optic neuritis (rare), amblyopia, nystagmus

Respiratory: Interstitial pneumonitis and/or fibrosis, dyspnea, cough

Miscellaneous: Hypersensitivity reactions, lupus-like syndrome, anaphylaxis

Drug Interactions

Avoid Concomitant Use

Avoid concomitant use of Nitrofurantoin with any of the following: BCG; Magnesium Trisilicate; Norfloxacin

Increased Effect/Toxicity

The levels/effects of Nitrofurantoin may be increased by: Probenecid

Decreased Effect

Nitrofurantoin may decrease the levels/effects of: BCG; Norfloxacin; Typhoid Vaccine

The levels/effects of Nitrofurantoin may be decreased by: Magnesium Trisilicate

Food Interactions Food increases the total amount absorbed; cranberry juice and other urinary acidifiers may enhance the action of nitrofurantoin; ensure diet is adequate in protein and vitamin B complex

Stability Protect oral suspension from light; store capsules and suspension at room temperature (59°F to 86°F or 15°C to 30°C)

Mechanism of Action Inhibits several bacterial enzyme systems including acetyl coenzyme A; reduced by bacterial enzymes to active intermediates that may alter ribosomal proteins resulting in inhibition of protein, DNA, RNA, and cell wall synthesis

Pharmacokinetics (Adult data unless noted)

Absorption: Well absorbed from the GI tract; macrocrystalline form is absorbed more slowly due to slower dissolution, but causes less GI distress than formulations containing microcrystals of the drug

Distribution: V_d: 0.8 L/kg; crosses the placenta; appears in breast milk and bile

Protein binding: ~40% to 60%

Metabolism: Partially in the liver

Bioavailability: Presence of food increases bioavailability

Half-life: 20-60 minutes and is prolonged with renal impairment

Elimination: As metabolites and unchanged drug (40%) in the urine and small amounts in the bile; renal excretion is via glomerular filtration and tubular secretion

Dialysis: Dialyzable

Usual Dosage Oral:

Infants >1 month and Children: 5-7 mg/kg/day divided every 6 hours; maximum dose: 400 mg/day

Macrocrystal/monohydrate: Children >12 years: 100 mg every 12 hours for 7 days

Prophylaxis of UTI: 1-2 mg/kg/day as a single daily dose; maximum dose: 100 mg/day

Adults: 50-100 mg/dose every 6 hours; macrocrystal/monohydrate: 100 mg twice daily for 7 days

Prophylaxis of UTI: 50-100 mg/dose at bedtime

Dosing adjustment in renal impairment: Cl_{cr} <60 mL/minute: Avoid use

Administration Oral: Administer with food or milk; do not administer with antacid preparations containing magnesium trisilicate; suspension may be mixed with water, milk, fruit juice, or infant formula. Shake suspension well before use.

Monitoring Parameters Signs of pulmonary reaction; signs of numbness or tingling of the extremities; periodic liver and renal function tests; CBC; urine culture and *in vitro* susceptibility tests. Observe for change in bowel frequency.

Test Interactions Causes false-positive urine glucose with Clinitest®

Patient Information May discolor urine to a dark yellow or brown color; avoid alcohol. Inform physician if diarrhea, chest pain, dyspnea, or cough occur.

Dosage Forms Excipient information presented when available (limited, particularly for generics); consult specific product labeling. [DSC] = Discontinued product

Capsule [macrocrystal]: 50 mg, 100 mg

Macrodantin®: 25 mg, 50 mg, 100 mg

Capsule [macrocrystal/monohydrate]: 100 mg [nitrofurantoin macrocrystal 25% and nitrofurantoin monohydrate 75%]

Macrobid®: 100 mg [nitrofurantoin macrocrystal 25% and nitrofurantoin monohydrate 75%]

Suspension, oral:

Furadantin®: 25 mg/5 mL (230 mL; 470 mL [DSC])

References

Brendstrup L, Hjelt K, Petersen KE, et al, "Nitrofurantoin Versus Trimethoprim Prophylaxis in Recurrent Urinary Tract Infections in Children," *Acta Paediatr Scand,* 1990. 79(12):1225-34.

Coraggio MJ, Gross TP, and Roscelli JD, "Nitrofurantoin Toxicity in Children," *Pediatr Infect Dis J,* 1989, 8(3):163-6.

"Practice Parameter: The Diagnosis, Treatment, and Evaluation of the Initial Urinary Tract Infection in Febrile Infants and Young Children. American Academy of Pediatrics. Committee on Quality Improvement. Subcommittee on Urinary Tract Infection," *Pediatrics,* 1999, 103 (4 Pt 1):843-52.

♦ **Nitrogen Mustard** *see* Mechlorethamine *on page 868*

Nitroglycerin (nye troe GLI ser in)

Medication Safety Issues

Sound-alike/look-alike issues:

Nitroglycerin may be confused with nitrofurantoin, nitroprusside

Nitro-Bid® may be confused with Macrobid®, Nicobid®

Nitroderm may be confused with NicoDerm®

Nitrol® may be confused with Nizoral®

Nitrostat® may be confused with Nilstat®, nystatin

Nitroglycerin transdermal patches should be removed prior to defibrillation or MRI study.

International issues:

Nitrocor® [Chile and Italy] may be confused with Natrecor® which is a brand name for nesiritide in the U.S.

Nitrocor® [Chile and Italy] may be confused with Nutracort® which is a brand name for hydrocortisone in the U.S.

Nitro-Dur® may be confused with Nitrocor® [Chile and Italy]

Related Information

Antihypertensive Agents by Class *on page 1481*

U.S. Brand Names Minitran™; Nitro-Bid®; Nitro-Dur®; Nitro-Time®; Nitrolingual®; NitroQuick® [DSC]; Nitrostat®

Canadian Brand Names Gen-Nitro; Minitran™; Mylan-Nitro Sublingual Spray; Nitro-Dur®; Nitroglycerin Injection, USP; Nitrol®; Nitrostat™; Rho®-Nitro; Transderm-Nitro®; Trinipatch® 0.2; Trinipatch® 0.4; Trinipatch® 0.6

Therapeutic Category Antianginal Agent; Antihypertensive Agent; Nitrate; Vasodilator; Vasodilator, Coronary

Generic Available Yes: Capsule, injection, patch, tablet

Use Acute treatment and prophylaxis of angina pectoris; I.V. for treatment of CHF (especially when associated with acute MI); pulmonary hypertension; hypertensive emergencies occurring perioperatively (especially during cardiovascular surgery)

Pregnancy Risk Factor C

Lactation Excretion in breast milk unknown/use caution

Contraindications Hypersensitivity to nitroglycerin, organic nitrates, or any component (including adhesives in transdermal patches); glaucoma; severe anemia; increased ICP; concurrent use with sildenafil or other phosphodiesterase-5 (PDE-5) inhibitors (see Drug Interactions); I.V. product is also contraindicated in hypotension, uncontrolled hypokalemia, pericardial tamponade, or constrictive pericarditis

Warnings May cause severe hypotension; use with caution in hypovolemia, hypotension, and right ventricular infarctions. Transdermal patch may contain conducting metal (eg, aluminum) which may cause a burn to the skin during an MRI scan; remove patch prior to MRI; reapply patch after scan is completed. Due to the potential for altered electrical conductivity, remove transdermal patch before cardioversion or defibrillation.

Adverse Reactions

Cardiovascular: Flushing, hypotension, pallor, reflex tachycardia, cardiovascular collapse; severe hypotension, bradycardia, and acute coronary vascular insufficiency with abrupt withdrawal

Central nervous system: Dizziness, restlessness, headache

Dermatologic: Allergic contact dermatitis, exfoliative dermatitis

Endocrine & metabolic: Alcohol intoxication from one I.V. formulation

Gastrointestinal: Nausea, vomiting

Miscellaneous: Perspiration

Drug Interactions

Avoid Concomitant Use
Avoid concomitant use of Nitroglycerin with any of the following: Phosphodiesterase 5 Inhibitors

Increased Effect/Toxicity
Nitroglycerin may increase the levels/effects of: Hypotensive Agents; Rosiglitazone

The levels/effects of Nitroglycerin may be increased by: Phosphodiesterase 5 Inhibitors

Decreased Effect
Nitroglycerin may decrease the levels/effects of: Alteplase; Heparin

Stability Nitroglycerin adsorbs to plastics; I.V. must be prepared in glass bottles and special administration sets intended for nitroglycerin (nonpolyvinyl chloride) must be used; do not mix with other drugs; store sublingual tablets and ointment in tightly closed container; store at 15°C to 30°C

Mechanism of Action Reduces cardiac oxygen demand by decreasing left ventricular end diastolic pressure and systemic vascular resistance; dilates coronary arteries and improves collateral flow to ischemic regions; vasodilates veins more than arteries

Pharmacodynamics Onset and duration of action is dependent upon dosage form administered; see table.

Nitroglycerin[1]

Dosage Form	Onset (min)	Duration
I.V.	1-2	3-5 min
Sublingual	1-3	30-60 min
Translingual spray	2	30-60 min
Buccal, extended release	2-3	3-5 h
Oral, sustained release	40	4-8 h
Topical ointment	20-60	2-12 h
Transdermal	40-60	18-24 h

[1]Hemodynamic and antianginal tolerance often develops within 24-48 h of continuous nitrate administration.

Adapted from Corwin S and Reiffel, JA, "Nitrate Therapy for Angina Pectoris," *Arch Intern Med*, 1985, 145:538-43 and Franciosa JA, "Nitroglycerin and Nitrates in Congestive Heart Failure," *Heart and Lung*, 1980, 9(5):873-82.

Pharmacokinetics (Adult data unless noted)
Protein binding: 60%
Metabolism: Extensive first-pass
Half-life: 1-4 minutes
Elimination: Excretion of inactive metabolites in urine

Usual Dosage Tolerance to the hemodynamic and antianginal effects can develop within 24-48 hours of continuous use

Children: I.V. continuous infusion: Initial: 0.25-0.5 mcg/kg/minute; titrate by 0.5-1 mcg/kg/minute every 3-5 minutes as needed; usual dose: 1-3 mcg/kg/minute; usual maximum dose: 5 mcg/kg/minute; doses up to 20 mcg/kg/minute may be used

Adults:
Oral: 2.5-9 mg every 8-12 hours
I.V. continuous infusion: **Note:** Do **not** dose per kg; adult dose is in units of mcg/minute; Initial: 5 mcg/minute, increase by 5 mcg/minute every 3-5 minutes to 20 mcg/minute, then increase as needed by 10 mcg/minute every 3-5 minutes, up to 200 mcg/minute
Sublingual: 0.2-0.6 mg every 5 minutes for maximum of 3 doses in 15 minutes
Ointment: 1" to 2" every 8 hours
Patch, transdermal: Initial: 0.2-0.4 mg/hour, titrate to 0.4-0.8 mg/hour; use a "patch-on" period of 12-14 hours per day and a "patch-off" period of 10-12 hours per day to minimize tolerance

Lingual: 1-2 sprays into mouth onto or under tongue every 3-5 minutes for maximum of 3 sprays in 15 minutes; may administer 5-10 minutes before activities that may precipitate angina
Buccal: Initial: 1 mg every 5 hours while awake (3 times/day); titrate dosage upward if angina occurs with tablet in place

Administration
Oral:
Buccal tablet: Place in buccal pouch and allow to dissolve; do not swallow, chew, or crush
Lingual spray: Do not shake container. Pump spray must be primed prior to first use with 5 sprays; direct priming sprays into the air, away from patient and others; if unused for 6 weeks, a single priming spray is needed; storage >6 weeks without use may require up to 5 repriming sprays. Monitor amount of medication in container; the end of the pump should be covered by the fluid in the bottle; replace container when fluid falls below the level of the center tub. To administer dose, spray onto or under tongue with container as close to mouth as possible; do not inhale spray; avoid swallowing immediately after spray; do not expectorate or rinse mouth for 5-10 minutes after use
Sublingual tablet: Place under tongue and allow to dissolve, do not swallow, chew, or crush; do not eat or drink while tablet dissolves
Regular or sustained release capsule/tablet: Administer with a full glass of water on an empty stomach; swallow sustained release capsules/tablets whole, do not crush or chew
Parenteral: I.V. continuous infusion: Dilute in D$_5$W or NS to 50-100 mcg/mL; maximum concentration not to exceed 400 mcg/mL; rate of infusion (mL/hour) = dose (mcg/kg/minute) x weight (kg) x 60 minutes/hour divided by the concentration (mcg/mL); administer via controlled infusion device
Transdermal: Place on hair-free area of skin; rotate patch sites; **Note:** Some products are a membrane-controlled system (eg, Transderm-Nitro®); do **not** cut these patches to deliver partial doses; rate of drug delivery, reservoir contents, and adhesion may be affected; if partial dose is needed, surface area of patch can be blocked proportionally using adhesive bandage (see Lee, 1997 and see specific product labeling)

Monitoring Parameters Blood pressure, heart rate (continuously with I.V. use)

Patient Information Avoid alcohol; may cause dizziness, headache; if no relief of chest pains after 3 sublingual doses, seek emergency care immediately

Nursing Implications Transdermal patches are now labeled as mg/hour (rates of release used to be described as mg/24 hours)

Additional Information I.V. preparations contain alcohol and/or propylene glycol; may need to use nitrate-free interval (10-12 hours/day) to avoid tolerance development; tolerance may possibly be reversed with acetylcysteine; gradually decrease dose in patients receiving NTG for prolonged period to avoid withdrawal reaction; lingual spray contains 20% alcohol, do not spray toward flames

Dosage Forms Excipient information presented when available (limited, particularly for generics); consult specific product labeling. [DSC] = Discontinued product
Capsule, extended release: 2.5 mg, 6.5 mg, 9 mg
Nitro-Time®: 2.5 mg, 6.5 mg, 9 mg
Infusion [premixed in D$_5$W]: 25 mg (250 mL) [0.1 mg/mL]; 50 mg (250 mL) [0.2 mg/mL]; 50 mg (500 mL) [0.1 mg/mL]; 100 mg (250 mL) [0.4 mg/mL]; 200 mg (500 mL) [0.4 mg/mL]
Injection, solution: 5 mg/mL (5 mL, 10 mL) [contains ethanol and propylene glycol]
Ointment, topical:
Nitro-Bid®: 2% [20 mg/g] (1 g, 30 g, 60 g)

Patch, transdermal [once-daily patch]: 0.1 mg/hour (30s); 0.2 mg/hour (30s); 0.4 mg/hour (30s); 0.6 mg/hour (30s)

Minitran™: 0.1 mg/hour (30s); 0.2 mg/hour (30s); 0.4 mg/hour (30s); 0.6 mg/hour (30s)

Nitro-Dur®: 0.1 mg/hour (30s); 0.2 mg/hour (30s); 0.3 mg/hour (30s); 0.4 mg/hour (30s); 0.6 mg/hour (30s); 0.8 mg/hour (30s)

Solution, translingual [spray]:

Nitrolingual®: 0.4 mg/spray (4.9 g) [contains ethanol 20%; 60 metered sprays]; (12 g) [contains ethanol 20%; 200 metered sprays]; (16.9 g) [DSC] [contains ethanol 20%; 260 metered sprays]

Tablet, sublingual: 0.3 mg, 0.4 mg, 0.6 mg

NitroQuick® [DSC], Nitrostat®: 0.3 mg, 0.4 mg, 0.6 mg

References

Elkayam U, "Tolerance to Organic Nitrates: Evidence, Mechanisms, Clinical Relevance, and Strategies for Prevention," *Ann Intern Med,* 1991, 114(8):667-77.

Lee HA and Anderson PO, "Giving Partial Doses of Transdermal Patches," *Am J Health Syst Pharm,* 1997, 54(15):1759-60.

◆ **Nitroglycerin Injection, USP (Can)** *see* Nitroglycerin *on page 996*

◆ **Nitroglycerol** *see* Nitroglycerin *on page 996*

◆ **Nitrol® (Can)** *see* Nitroglycerin *on page 996*

◆ **Nitrolingual®** *see* Nitroglycerin *on page 996*

◆ **Nitropress®** *see* Nitroprusside *on page 998*

Nitroprusside (nye troe PRUS ide)

Medication Safety Issues

Sound-alike/look-alike issues:

Nitroprusside may be confused with nitroglycerin

High alert medication: The Institute for Safe Medication Practices (ISMP) includes this medication among its list of drugs which have a heightened risk of causing significant patient harm when used in error.

Related Information

Antihypertensive Agents by Class *on page 1481*

CPR Pediatric Drug Dosages *on page 1455*

U.S. Brand Names Nitropress®

Therapeutic Category Antihypertensive Agent; Vasodilator

Generic Available Yes

Use Management of hypertensive crises; CHF; used for controlled hypotension during anesthesia

Pregnancy Risk Factor C

Lactation Excretion in breast milk unknown

Contraindications Hypersensitivity to nitroprusside or any component of the formulation; treatment of compensatory hypertension (aortic coarctation, arteriovenous shunting); high output failure; congenital optic atrophy or tobacco amblyopia

Warnings Use only as an infusion with D₅W **[U.S. Boxed Warning]**; continuously monitor patient's blood pressure **[U.S. Boxed Warning]**; may cause precipitous decreases in blood pressure. Except when used briefly or at low (<2 mcg/kg/minute) infusion rates, nitroprusside gives rise to large cyanide quantities **[U.S. Boxed Warning]**; cyanide or thiocyanate toxicity may occur; risk increased in patients with decreased renal or liver function or when using excessive doses. Do not use the maximum dose for more than 10 minutes; if blood pressure is not controlled, then discontinue infusion. Monitor for cyanide toxicity via acid-base balance and venous oxygen concentration.

Precautions Use with caution in patients with severe renal impairment, hepatic failure, hypothyroidism, hyponatremia, increased intracranial pressure

Adverse Reactions

Cardiovascular: Excessive hypotensive response, palpitations, substernal distress

Central nervous system: Restlessness, disorientation, psychosis, headache, intracranial pressure elevated

Endocrine & metabolic: Thyroid suppression

Gastrointestinal: Nausea, vomiting

Hematologic: Thiocyanate toxicity

Neuromuscular & skeletal: Weakness

Miscellaneous: Diaphoresis, cyanide toxicity

Drug Interactions

Avoid Concomitant Use There are no known interactions where it is recommended to avoid concomitant use.

Increased Effect/Toxicity

Nitroprusside may increase the levels/effects of: Amifostine; Antihypertensives; Hypotensive Agents; RiTUXimab

The levels/effects of Nitroprusside may be increased by: Calcium Channel Blockers; Diazoxide; Herbs (Hypotensive Properties); MAO Inhibitors; Pentoxifylline; Phosphodiesterase 5 Inhibitors; Prostacyclin Analogues

Decreased Effect

The levels/effects of Nitroprusside may be decreased by: Herbs (Hypertensive Properties); Methylphenidate; Yohimbine

Stability Discard solution 24 hours after reconstitution and dilution; discard highly colored solutions

Mechanism of Action Causes peripheral vasodilation by direct action on venous and arteriolar smooth muscle, thus reducing peripheral resistance; will increase cardiac output by decreasing afterload; reduces aortal and left ventricular impedance

Pharmacodynamics Hypotensive effects:

Onset of action: Within 2 minutes

Duration: 1-10 minutes

Pharmacokinetics (Adult data unless noted)

Metabolism: Converted to cyanide by erythrocyte and tissue sulfhydryl group interactions; cyanide is converted in the liver by the enzyme rhodanase to thiocyanate

Half-life: <10 minutes

Thiocyanate: 2.7-7 days

Elimination: Thiocyanate is excreted in the urine

Usual Dosage Children and Adults: I.V. continuous infusion: Start 0.3-0.5 mcg/kg/minute, titrate to effect; usual dose: 3 mcg/kg/minute; rarely need >4 mcg/kg/minute; maximum dose: 8-10 mcg/kg/minute

Rate (mL/hour) = dose (mcg/kg/minute) x weight (kg) x 60 minutes/hour divided by concentration (mcg/mL)

Administration Parenteral: I.V. continuous infusion only via controlled infusion device; not for direct injection; dilute in plain dextrose solutions only (eg, D₅W); solution should be protected from light, but not necessary to wrap administration set or I.V. tubing. Final concentration for administration: Usual maximum: 200 mcg/mL; in fluid restricted patients a final maximum concentration of 1000 mcg/mL in D₅W has been used. Do not add other medications to nitroprusside solutions.

Monitoring Parameters Blood pressure, heart rate; monitor for cyanide and thiocyanate toxicity; monitor acid-base status as acidosis can be the earliest sign of cyanide toxicity; monitor thiocyanate levels if requiring prolonged infusion (>3 days) or dose ≥4 mcg/kg/minute or patient has renal dysfunction; monitor cyanide blood levels in patients with decreased hepatic function

Reference Range

Thiocyanate:

Toxic: 35-100 mcg/mL

Fatal: >200 mcg/mL

Cyanide:

Normal <0.2 mcg/mL

Normal (smoker): <0.4 mcg/mL

Toxic: >2 mcg/mL

Potentially lethal: >3 mcg/mL

Additional Information Thiocyanate toxicity includes psychoses, blurred vision, confusion, weakness, tinnitus, seizures; cyanide toxicity includes metabolic acidosis, tachycardia, pink skin, decreased pulse, decreased reflexes, altered consciousness, coma, almond smell on breath, methemoglobinemia, dilated pupils

Dosage Forms Excipient information presented when available (limited, particularly for generics); consult specific product labeling.

Injection, solution, as sodium: 25 mg/mL (2 mL)

◆ **Nitroprusside Sodium** *see* Nitroprusside *on page 998*

◆ **NitroQuick® [DSC]** *see* Nitroglycerin *on page 996*

◆ **Nitrostat®** *see* Nitroglycerin *on page 996*

◆ **Nitrostat™ (Can)** *see* Nitroglycerin *on page 996*

◆ **Nitro-Time®** *see* Nitroglycerin *on page 996*

◆ **Nix® [OTC]** *see* Permethrin *on page 1094*

◆ **Nix® (Can)** *see* Permethrin *on page 1094*

Nizatidine (ni ZA ti deen)

Medication Safety Issues

Sound-alike/look-alike issues:

Axid® may be confused with Ansaid®

International issues:

Tazac® [Australia] may be confused with Tiazac® which is a brand name for diltiazem in the U.S.

U.S. Brand Names Axid®; Axid® AR [OTC]

Canadian Brand Names Apo-Nizatidine®; Axid®; Gen-Nizatidine; Novo-Nizatidine; Nu-Nizatidine; PMS-Nizatidine

Therapeutic Category Gastrointestinal Agent, Gastric or Duodenal Ulcer Treatment; Histamine H_2 Antagonist

Generic Available Yes: Capsule

Use Treatment and maintenance therapy of duodenal ulcer; treatment of active benign gastric ulcer; esophagitis; gastroesophageal reflux disease (GERD); over-the-counter (OTC) formulation for use in the relief of heartburn, acid indigestion, and sour stomach; adjunctive therapy in the treatment of *Helicobacter pylori*-associated duodenal ulcer

Pregnancy Risk Factor B

Pregnancy Considerations Teratogenic effects were not observed in animal studies.

Lactation Enters breast milk/may be compatible

Breast-Feeding Considerations The amount of nizatidine excreted in breast milk is 0.1%.

Contraindications Hypersensitivity to nizatidine, H_2 antagonists, or any component

Warnings Use of gastric acid inhibitors including proton pump inhibitors and H_2 blockers has been associated with an increased risk for development of acute gastroenteritis and community-acquired pneumonia (Canani, 2006). A large epidemiological study has suggested an increased risk for developing pneumonia in patients receiving H_2 receptor antagonists; however, a causal relationship with nizatidine has not been demonstrated.

Precautions Use with caution and modify dosage in patients with impaired renal function

Adverse Reactions

Cardiovascular: Chest pain, ventricular tachycardia (short, asymptomatic episodes)

Central nervous system: Headache, fever, dizziness, insomnia, somnolence, anxiety, nervousness, irritability

Dermatologic: Rash, pruritus

Endocrine & metabolic: Hyperuricemia

Gastrointestinal: Nausea, vomiting, diarrhea, flatulence, dyspepsia, constipation, dry mouth, anorexia, abdominal pain

Genitourinary: Impotence

Hematologic: Anemia, thrombocytopenia, eosinophilia, leukopenia

Hepatic: Liver enzymes elevated, jaundice, hepatitis

Neuromuscular & skeletal: Back pain, asthenia, myalgia

Ocular: Amblyopia

Respiratory: Rhinitis, pharyngitis, sinusitis, cough, nasal congestion, pneumonia (causal relationship has not been established; see Warnings)

Miscellaneous: Hypersensitivity reactions, serum sickness

Drug Interactions

Metabolism/Transport Effects Inhibits 3A4 (weak)

Avoid Concomitant Use

Avoid concomitant use of Nizatidine with any of the following: Delavirdine; Erlotinib

Increased Effect/Toxicity

Nizatidine may increase the levels/effects of: Saquinavir

Decreased Effect

Nizatidine may decrease the levels/effects of: Antifungal Agents (Azole Derivatives, Systemic); Atazanavir; Cefditoren; Cefpodoxime; Cefuroxime; Dasatinib; Delavirdine; Erlotinib; Fosamprenavir; Indinavir; Iron Salts; Mesalamine; Nelfinavir

Food Interactions Limit xanthine-containing foods and beverages; administration with apple juice decreases absorption by 27%

Stability Nizatidine is stable for 48 hours at room temperature when the contents of a capsule are mixed in Gatorade® lemon-lime, Cran-Grape® grape-cranberry drink, V8®, or aluminum- and magnesium hydroxide suspension (approximate concentration 2.5 mg/mL)

Mechanism of Action Competitive inhibition of histamine at H_2-receptors of the gastric parietal cells, which inhibits gastric acid secretion

Pharmacodynamics Maximum effect: Duodenal ulcer: 4 weeks

Pharmacokinetics (Adult data unless noted)

Distribution: V_d: Adults: 0.8-1.5 L/kg; breast milk: 0.1% excreted into breast milk

Protein binding: 35%

Bioavailability: Oral: 70%

Half-life, elimination: Adults: 1-2 hours; anuric: 3.5-11 hours

Time to peak serum concentration: 0.5-3 hours

Elimination: 60% excreted unchanged in urine

Usual Dosage Oral:

Infants 6 months to Children 11 years: Limited information available: 5-10 mg/kg/day divided twice daily (see References)

GERD, esophagitis: Children ≥12 years and Adults: 150 mg twice daily

Active duodenal and gastric ulcers: Adults: 300 mg once daily at bedtime or 150 mg twice daily

Maintenance of healed duodenal ulcer: Adults: 150 mg once daily

Relief of heartburn, acid indigestion, sour stomach (OTC use): Adults: 75 mg 30-60 minutes before meals; no more than 2 tablets/day

Helicobacter pylori-associated duodenal ulcer (limited information): Adults: 150 mg twice daily for 4 weeks (combined with clarithromycin and bismuth formulation; followed by 300 mg/day)

Dosing adjustment in renal impairment: Adults:

Active treatment:

Cl_{cr} 20-50 mL/minute: 150 mg once daily

Cl_{cr} <20 mL/minute: 150 mg every other day

Maintenance treatment:

Cl_{cr} 20-50 mL/minute: 150 every other day

Cl_{cr} <20 mL/minute: 150 mg every 3 days

Administration Oral: May administer with or without food; do not administer or mix with apple juice (see Food Interactions and Stability)

Test Interactions False-positive urobilinogen with Multistix®

Patient Information Avoid excessive amounts of caffeinated beverages and aspirin; do not take with apple juice; with self medication, if the symptoms of heartburn, acid indigestion, or sour stomach persist after 2 weeks of continuous use of the drug, consult clinician

Dosage Forms Excipient information presented when available (limited, particularly for generics); consult specific product labeling.

Capsule:
Axid®: 150 mg, 300 mg [DSC]
Solution, oral:
Axid®: 15 mg/mL (120 mL, 480 mL) [bubble gum flavor]
Tablet:
Axid® AR: 75 mg

Extemporaneous Preparations A 2.5 mg/mL solution may be made by opening a 300 mg capsule into a mortar and grinding to a fine powder. Add incremental amounts of Gatorade® lemon-lime, Ocean Spray® cran-grape, apple juice, or V8® 100% vegetable juice to a total volume of 120 mL; shake well; stable for 2 days refrigerated.

Nahata, MC, Pai VB, and Hipple TF, *Pediatric Drug Formulations*, 5th ed, Cincinnati, OH: Harvey Whitney Books Co, 2004.

References
Canani RB, Cirillo P, Roggero P, et al, "Therapy With Gastric Acidity Inhibitors Increases the Risk of Acute Gastroenteritis and Community-Acquired Pneumonia in Children," *Pediatrics*, 2006, 117(5):e817-20.
Mikawa K, Nishina K, Maekawa N, et al, "Effects of Oral Nizatidine on Preoperative Gastric Fluid pH and Volume in Children," *Br J Anaesth*, 1994, 73(5):600-4.
Simeone D, Caria MC, Miele E, et al, "Treatment of Childhood Peptic Esophagitis: A Double-Blind Placebo-Controlled Trial of Nizatidine," *J Pediatr Gastroenterol Nur*, 1997, 25(1):51-5.

◆ **Nizoral®** *see* Ketoconazole *on page 780*

◆ **Nizoral® A-D [OTC]** *see* Ketoconazole *on page 780*

◆ **N-Methylhydrazine** *see* Procarbazine *on page 1159*

◆ **No Doz® Maximum Strength [OTC]** *see* Caffeine *on page 225*

◆ **Nora-BE™** *see* Norethindrone *on page 1001*

◆ **Noradrenaline** *see* Norepinephrine *on page 1000*

◆ **Noradrenaline Acid Tartrate** *see* Norepinephrine *on page 1000*

◆ **Norco®** *see* Hydrocodone and Acetaminophen *on page 684*

◆ **Norcuron** *see* Vecuronium *on page 1411*

◆ **Norcuron® (Can)** *see* Vecuronium *on page 1411*

◆ **Nordeoxyguanosine** *see* Ganciclovir *on page 636*

◆ **Norditropin®** *see* Somatropin *on page 1281*

◆ **Norditropin® FlexPro®** *see* Somatropin *on page 1281*

◆ **Norditropin NordiFlex®** *see* Somatropin *on page 1281*

Norepinephrine (nor ep i NEF rin)

Medication Safety Issues
Sound-alike/look-alike issues:
Levophed® may be confused with levofloxacin

High alert medication: The Institute for Safe Medication Practices (ISMP) includes this medication among its list of drugs which have a heightened risk of causing significant patient harm when used in error.

Related Information
CPR Pediatric Drug Dosages *on page 1455*
Emergency Pediatric Drip Calculations *on page 1457*
Extravasation Treatment *on page 1522*

U.S. Brand Names Levophed®
Canadian Brand Names Levophed®

Therapeutic Category Adrenergic Agonist Agent; Alpha-Adrenergic Agonist; Sympathomimetic

Generic Available Yes

Use Treatment of shock which persists after adequate fluid volume replacement; severe hypotension; cardiogenic shock

Pregnancy Risk Factor C

Lactation Excretion in breast milk unknown

Contraindications Hypersensitivity to norepinephrine, bisulfites (contains metabisulfite), or any component of the formulation; hypotension from hypovolemia except as an emergency measure to maintain coronary and cerebral perfusion until volume could be replaced; mesenteric or peripheral vascular thrombosis unless it is a lifesaving procedure; during anesthesia with cyclopropane or halothane anesthesia (risk of ventricular arrhythmias)

Warnings Potent drug; must be diluted prior to use; monitor hemodynamic status; injection contains sodium metabisulfite which may cause allergic reactions in susceptible individuals. Extravasation may cause tissue necrosis (treat extravasation with phentolamine; see Extravasation Treatment on page 1522) **[U.S. Boxed Warning]**

Precautions Blood/volume depletion should be corrected, if possible, before norepinephrine therapy; extravasation may cause severe tissue necrosis; do **not** give to patients with peripheral or mesenteric vascular thrombosis because ischemia may be increased and the area of infarct extended; use with caution during cyclopropane or halothane anesthesia and in patients with occlusive vascular disease

Adverse Reactions
Cardiovascular: Cardiac arrhythmias, palpitations, bradycardia, tachycardia, hypertension, chest pain, pallor
Central nervous system: Anxiety, headache
Endocrine & metabolic: Uterine contractions
Gastrointestinal: Vomiting
Local: Organ ischemia (due to vasoconstriction of renal and mesenteric arteries), ischemic necrosis and sloughing of superficial tissue after extravasation
Ocular: Photophobia
Respiratory: Respiratory distress
Miscellaneous: Diaphoresis

Drug Interactions
Avoid Concomitant Use
Avoid concomitant use of Norepinephrine with any of the following: Inhalational Anesthetics; Iobenguane I 123

Increased Effect/Toxicity
Norepinephrine may increase the levels/effects of: Bromocriptine; Sympathomimetics

The levels/effects of Norepinephrine may be increased by: Antacids; Atomoxetine; Beta-Blockers; Cannabinoids; Carbonic Anhydrase Inhibitors; COMT Inhibitors; Inhalational Anesthetics; MAO Inhibitors; Serotonin/Norepinephrine Reuptake Inhibitors; Tricyclic Antidepressants

Decreased Effect
Norepinephrine may decrease the levels/effects of: Iobenguane I 123

The levels/effects of Norepinephrine may be decreased by: Spironolactone

Stability Readily oxidized, do not use if brown coloration; dilute with D_5W, D_5W/NS, or NS (dilution in NS is not recommended by the manufacturer; however, stability in NS has been proven by others; see Tremblay, 2008); not stable with alkaline solutions

Mechanism of Action Stimulates beta$_1$-adrenergic receptors and alpha-adrenergic receptors causing increased contractility and heart rate as well as vasoconstriction, thereby increasing systemic blood pressure and coronary blood flow; clinically, alpha effects (vasoconstriction) are greater than beta effects (inotropic and chronotropic effects)

Pharmacodynamics

Onset of action: Very rapid

Duration: Limited duration following I.V. injection

Pharmacokinetics (Adult data unless noted)

Metabolism: By catechol-o-methyltransferase (COMT) and monoamine oxidase (MAO)

Elimination: In urine (84% to 96% as inactive metabolites)

Usual Dosage I.V. (dose stated in terms of **norepinephrine base**):

Children: Initial: 0.05-0.1 mcg/kg/minute, titrate to desired effect; maximum dose: 1-2 mcg/kg/minute

Rate (mL/hour) = dose (mcg/kg/minute) x weight (kg) x 60 minutes/hour divided by concentration (mcg/mL)

Adults: Initial: 0.5-1 mcg/minute; titrate to desired response

Usual range: 8-30 mcg/minute as an infusion

ACLS dosage range: 0.5-30 mcg/minute

Administration Parenteral: Administer into large vein to avoid potential extravasation; standard concentration: 4 mcg/mL but 16 mcg/mL has been used safely and with efficacy in situations of extreme fluid restriction

Monitoring Parameters Blood pressure, heart rate, urine output, peripheral perfusion

Additional Information Treat extravasations with local injections of phentolamine (see Extravasation Treatment on page 1522)

Dosage Forms Excipient information presented when available (limited, particularly for generics); consult specific product labeling. Strength expressed as base:

Injection, solution: 1 mg/mL (4 mL) [contains sodium metabisulfite]

References

Tremblay M, Lessard MR, Trépanier CA, et al, "Stability of Norepinephrine Infusions Prepared in Dextrose and Normal Saline Solutions," *Can J Anaesth*, 2008, 55(3):163-7.

◆ **Norepinephrine Bitartrate** *see* Norepinephrine on page 1000

Norethindrone (nor eth IN drone)

Medication Safety Issues

Sound-alike/look-alike issues:

Micronor® may be confused with miconazole, Micronase®

U.S. Brand Names Aygestin®; Camila™; Errin™; Jolivette™; Nor-QD®; Nora-BE™; Ortho Micronor®

Canadian Brand Names Micronor®; Norlutate®

Therapeutic Category Contraceptive, Oral; Contraceptive, Progestin Only; Progestin

Generic Available Yes

Use Treatment of amenorrhea, abnormal uterine bleeding, endometriosis, oral contraceptive

Pregnancy Risk Factor X

Pregnancy Considerations First trimester exposure may cause genital abnormalities including hypospadias in male infants and mild virilization of external female genitalia. Significant adverse events related to growth and development have not been observed (limited studies). Use is contraindicated during pregnancy. May be started immediately postpartum if not breast-feeding.

Lactation Enters breast milk/use caution

Breast-Feeding Considerations Small amounts of progestins are found in breast milk (1% to 6% of maternal serum concentration). Norethindrone can cause changes in milk production in the mother. When used for contraception, may start 3 weeks after delivery in women who are partially breast-feeding, or 6 weeks after delivery in women who are fully breast-feeding.

Contraindications Hypersensitivity to norethindrone or any component; thromboembolic disorders, severe hepatic disease, breast cancer, cerebral hemorrhage, undiagnosed vaginal bleeding; known or suspected pregnancy; as a diagnostic test for pregnancy

Warnings Discontinue if sudden partial or complete loss of vision, proptosis, diplopia, or migraine occur; **there is a higher rate of failure with progestin only contraceptives**; progestin-induced withdrawal bleeding occurs within 3-7 days after discontinuation of drug

Precautions Use with caution in patients with asthma, diabetes mellitus, seizure disorder, migraine, cardiac or renal dysfunction, psychic depression; may affect lipid and carbohydrate metabolism; women with diabetes mellitus or hyperlipidemias should be monitored closely

Adverse Reactions

Cardiovascular: Edema, thromboembolic disorders, hypertension

Central nervous system: Mental depression, nervousness, dizziness, fatigue, headache, migraine, insomnia, mood swings

Dermatologic: Hirsutism, rash, melasma or chloasma, acne

Endocrine & metabolic: Breakthrough bleeding, spotting, changes in menstrual flow, amenorrhea, changes in cervical erosion and cervical secretions, weight gain or weight loss, breast enlargement and tenderness

Gastrointestinal: Nausea

Hepatic: Cholestatic jaundice, abnormal liver function tests

Ophthalmic: Optic neuritis

Miscellaneous: Hypersensitivity reactions including anaphylactic reactions

Drug Interactions

Metabolism/Transport Effects Substrate of CYP3A4 (major); **Induces** CYP2C19 (weak)

Avoid Concomitant Use

Avoid concomitant use of Norethindrone with any of the following: Griseofulvin

Increased Effect/Toxicity

Norethindrone may increase the levels/effects of: Benzodiazepines (metabolized by oxidation); Selegiline; Tranexamic Acid; Voriconazole

The levels/effects of Norethindrone may be increased by: Herbs (Progestogenic Properties); Voriconazole

Decreased Effect

Norethindrone may decrease the levels/effects of: Vitamin K Antagonists

The levels/effects of Norethindrone may be decreased by: Acitretin; Aminoglutethimide; Aprepitant; Artemether; Barbiturates; Bile Acid Sequestrants; Bosentan; CarBAMazepine; Colesevelam; CYP3A4 Inducers (Strong); Darunavir; Deferasirox; Felbamate; Fosaprepitant; Griseofulvin; LamoTRIgine; Mycophenolate; OXcarbazepine; Phenytoin; Retinoic Acid Derivatives; Rifamycin Derivatives; Rufinamide; St Johns Wort; Topiramate

Food Interactions Avoid bloodroot, chasteberry, damiana, oregano, and yucca; may enhance the adverse/toxic effect of progestins. Avoid St John's wort; may diminish the therapeutic effect of progestin contraceptives; contraceptive failure is possible.

Mechanism of Action Inhibits secretion of pituitary gonadotropin (LH) which prevents follicular maturation and ovulation; in the presence of adequate endogenous estrogen, transforms a proliferative endometrium to a secretory one

Pharmacokinetics (Adult data unless noted)

Absorption: Oral: Rapidly absorbed

Distribution: V_d: 4 L/kg

Protein binding: 61% to albumin and 36% to sex hormone-binding globulin (SHBG)

Metabolism: Hepatic via reduction and conjugation; first-pass effect

Bioavailability: ~65%

Half-life: ~8 hours

Time to peak serum concentration: 1 hour (range: 0.5-2 hours)

Elimination: Urine (>50% as metabolites); feces (20% to 40% as metabolites)

Usual Dosage Adolescents and Adults: Female: Oral: Not indicated for use before menarche

Amenorrhea and abnormal uterine bleeding: Norethindrone acetate 2.5-10 mg/day for 5-10 days beginning during the latter half of the menstrual cycle

Endometriosis: Norethindrone acetate 5 mg/day for 14 days; increase at increments of 2.5 mg/day every 2 weeks up to 15 mg/day

Contraception: Progesterone only: Norethindrone 0.35 mg every day of the year starting on first day of menstrual period or the day after a miscarriage or abortion. If switching from a combined oral contraceptive, begin the day after finishing the last active combined tablet. If dose is missed, take as soon as remembered. An additional method of contraception should be used for 48 hours if dose is taken >3 hours late.

Administration Oral: Administer at the same time each day; may administer with food

Test Interactions Thyroid function test, metyrapone test, liver function tests, coagulation tests (prothrombin time, factors VII, VIII, IX, X)

Patient Information Progestin-induced withdrawal bleeding occurs within 3-7 days after discontinuation of the drug; for contraception, take at the same time every day; use an additional method of contraception for the next 48 hours if dose is taken >3 hours late

Dosage Forms Excipient information presented when available (limited, particularly for generics); consult specific product labeling.

Tablet:

Camila™, Errin™, Jolivette™, Ortho Micronor®, Nora-BE™, Nor-QD®: 0.35 mg

Tablet, as acetate:

Aygestin®: 5 mg

References

American College of Obstetricians and Gynecologists, "ACOG Committee Opinion. Number 310, April 2005. Endometriosis in Adolescents," *Obstet Gynecol*, 2005, 105(4):921-7.

ACOG Committee on Practice Bulletins-Gynecology, "ACOG Practice Bulletin. No. 73: Use of Hormonal Contraception in Women With Coexisting Medical Conditions," *Obstet Gynecol*, 2006, 107 (6):1453-72.

Nortriptyline (nor TRIP ti leen)

Medication Safety Issues

Sound-alike/look-alike issues:

Aventyl® HCl may be confused with Bentyl®

Nortriptyline may be confused with amitriptyline, desipramine, Norpramin®

Pamelor® may be confused with Demerol®, Dymelor®, Panlor® DC, Tambocor™

Related Information

Antidepressant Agents *on page 1484*

U.S. Brand Names Pamelor®

Canadian Brand Names Alti-Nortriptyline; Apo-Nortriptyline®; Aventyl®; Gen-Nortriptyline; Norventyl; Novo-Nortriptyline; Nu-Nortriptyline; PMS-Nortriptyline

Therapeutic Category Antidepressant, Tricyclic (Secondary Amine)

Generic Available Yes: Excludes solution

Use Treatment of various forms of depression, often in conjunction with psychotherapy; nocturnal enuresis

Medication Guide An FDA-approved patient medication guide, which is available with the product information and at http://www.fda.gov/downloads/Drugs/DrugSafety/ucm088671.pdf, must be dispensed with this medication for each new outpatient prescription and refill.

Pregnancy Considerations Animal reproduction studies are inconclusive. Nortriptyline and its metabolites cross the human placenta and can be detected in cord blood. According to the manufacturer, the decision to use nortriptyline during pregnancy or in women of childbearing potential should take into account the potential benefits and possible risks. Treatment algorithms have been developed by the ACOG and the APA for the management of depression in women prior to conception and during pregnancy.

Lactation Enters breast milk/not recommended (AAP rates "of concern")

Breast-Feeding Considerations Nortriptyline is excreted into breast milk and the M/P ratio ranged from 0.87 to 3.71 in one study. Based on available information, nortriptyline has not been detected in the serum of nursing infants, however low levels of the active metabolite E-10-hydroxynortriptyline have been detected in the serum of newborns following breast-feeding. The AAP considers nortriptyline to be a "drug for which the effect on the nursing infant is unknown, but may be of concern."

Contraindications Hypersensitivity to nortriptyline or amitriptyline (cross-sensitivity with other tricyclics may occur) or any component (see Warnings); use of MAO inhibitors within 14 days (potentially fatal reactions may occur, see Drug Interactions); use during acute recovery period after MI

Warnings Nortriptyline is not approved for use in pediatric patients. Clinical worsening of depression or suicidal ideation and behavior may occur in children and adults with major depressive disorder **[U.S. Boxed Warning]**. In clinical trials, antidepressants increased the risk of suicidal thinking and behavior (suicidality) in children, adolescents, and young adults (18-24 years of age) with major depressive disorder and other psychiatric disorders. This risk must be considered before prescribing antidepressants for any clinical use. Short-term studies did **not** show an increased risk of suicidality with antidepressant use in patients >24 years of age and showed a decreased risk in patients ≥65 years.

Patients of all ages who are treated with antidepressants for any indication require appropriate monitoring and close observation for clinical worsening of depression, suicidality, and unusual changes in behavior, especially during the first few months after antidepressant initiation or when the dose is adjusted. Family members and caregivers should be instructed to closely observe the patient (ie, daily) and communicate condition with healthcare provider. Patients should also be monitored for associated behaviors (eg, anxiety, agitation, panic attacks, insomnia, irritability, hostility, aggressiveness, impulsivity, akathisia, hypomania, mania) which may increase the risk for worsening depression or suicidality. Worsening depression or emergence of suicidality (or associated behaviors listed above) that is abrupt in onset, severe, or not part of the presenting symptoms, may require discontinuation or modification of drug therapy.

Do not discontinue abruptly in patients receiving high doses chronically (withdrawal symptoms may occur). To reduce risk of intentional overdose, write prescriptions for the smallest quantity consistent with good patient care. Screen individuals for bipolar disorder prior to treatment (using antidepressants alone may induce manic episodes in patients with this condition). May worsen psychosis in some patients.

Use with extreme caution with renal or hepatic impairment. Capsule may contain sodium bisulfite and/or benzyl alcohol, both of which may cause allergic reactions in susceptible individuals; solution contains benzoic acid; benzoic acid (benzoate) is a metabolite of benzyl alcohol; large amounts of benzyl alcohol (≥99 mg/kg/day) have been associated with a potentially fatal toxicity ("gasping syndrome") in neonates; avoid use of nortriptyline products containing benzoic acid or benzyl alcohol in neonates; *in vitro* and animal studies have shown that benzoate displaces bilirubin from protein binding sites

Precautions Use with caution in patients with cardiac conduction disturbances, cardiovascular disease, seizure disorder, history of urinary retention, hyperthyroidism, or those receiving thyroid hormone replacement

Adverse Reactions Nortriptyline has lower anticholinergic and sedative effects compared to amitriptyline

Cardiovascular: Postural hypotension, arrhythmias, tachycardia, sudden death

Central nervous system: Sedation, fatigue, anxiety, impaired cognitive function, seizures; suicidal thinking and behavior (see Warnings)

Dermatologic: Photosensitivity

Endocrine & metabolic: SIADH (rare), weight gain

Gastrointestinal: Xerostomia, constipation, appetite increased

Genitourinary: Urinary retention

Hematologic: Rarely agranulocytosis, leukopenia, eosinophilia

Hepatic: Cholestatic jaundice, liver enzymes elevated

Neuromuscular & skeletal: Tremor, weakness

Ocular: Blurred vision, intraocular pressure elevated

Miscellaneous: Allergic reactions

Drug Interactions

Metabolism/Transport Effects Substrate of CYP1A2 (minor), 2C19 (minor), 2D6 (major), 3A4 (minor); **Inhibits** CYP2D6 (weak), 2E1 (weak)

Avoid Concomitant Use

Avoid concomitant use of Nortriptyline with any of the following: Artemether; Dronedarone; Iobenguane I 123; Lumefantrine; MAO Inhibitors; Metoclopramide; Nilotinib; Pimozide; QuiNINE; Sibutramine; Tetrabenazine; Thioridazine; Ziprasidone

Increased Effect/Toxicity

Nortriptyline may increase the levels/effects of: Alcohol (Ethyl); Alpha-/Beta-Agonists (Direct-Acting); Alpha1-Agonists; Amphetamines; Anticholinergics; Beta2-Agonists; CNS Depressants; Desmopressin; Dronedarone; Pimozide; QTc-Prolonging Agents; QuiNIDine; QuiNINE; Serotonin Modulators; Sulfonylureas; Tetrabenazine; Thioridazine; TraMADol; Vitamin K Antagonists; Yohimbine; Ziprasidone

The levels/effects of Nortriptyline may be increased by: Alfuzosin; Altretamine; Artemether; BuPROPion; Chloroquine; Cimetidine; Cinacalcet; Ciprofloxacin; Ciprofloxacin (Systemic); CYP2D6 Inhibitors (Moderate); CYP2D6 Inhibitors (Strong); Dexmethylphenidate; Divalproex; DULoxetine; Gadobutrol; Lithium; Lumefantrine; MAO Inhibitors; Methylphenidate; Metoclopramide; Nilotinib; Pramlintide; Propoxyphene; Protease Inhibitors; QuiNIDine; QuiNINE; Selective Serotonin Reuptake Inhibitors; Sibutramine; Terbinafine; Terbinafine (Systemic); Valproic Acid

Decreased Effect

Nortriptyline may decrease the levels/effects of: Acetylcholinesterase Inhibitors (Central); Alpha2-Agonists; Iobenguane I 123

The levels/effects of Nortriptyline may be decreased by: Acetylcholinesterase Inhibitors (Central); Barbiturates; CarBAMazepine; Peginterferon Alfa-2b; St Johns Wort

Food Interactions Riboflavin dietary requirements may be increased

Stability Protect from light

Mechanism of Action Increases the synaptic concentration of serotonin and/or norepinephrine in the CNS by inhibition of their reuptake by the presynaptic neuronal membrane

Pharmacodynamics Onset of action: Therapeutic antidepressant effects begin in 7-21 days; maximum effects may not occur for ≥2-3 weeks

Pharmacokinetics (Adult data unless noted)

Absorption: Oral: Rapid; well absorbed

Distribution: V_d: 14-22 L/kg; crosses placenta; enters breast milk

Protein binding: 93% to 95%

Metabolism: Undergoes significant first-pass metabolism; primarily detoxified in the liver via hydroxylation followed by glucuronide conjugation

Half-life:

Children (mean ± SD): 18 ± 4 hours

Adults (mean ± SD): 46 ± 24 hours

Time to peak serum concentration: Oral: Within 7-8.5 hours

Elimination: Metabolites and small amounts of unchanged drug excreted in urine; small amounts of biliary elimination occur

Dialysis: Not Dialyzable

Usual Dosage Oral:

Nocturnal enuresis: Children (give dose 30 minutes before bedtime):

6-7 years (20-25 kg): 10 mg/day

8-11 years (25-35 kg): 10-20 mg/day

>11 years (35-54 kg): 25-35 mg/day

Depression: **Note:** Not FDA approved for use in pediatric patients; controlled clinical trials have not shown tricyclic antidepressants to be superior to placebo for the treatment of depression in children and adolescents (see Dopheide, 2006 and Wagner, 2005).

Children 6-12 years: 1-3 mg/kg/day or 10-20 mg/day in 3-4 divided doses

Adolescents: 1-3 mg/kg/day or 30-50 mg/day in 3-4 divided doses; usual maximum dose: 150 mg/day

Adults: 25 mg 3-4 times/day up to 150 mg/day

Dosing adjustment in hepatic impairment: Use lower doses and slower titration; individualization of dosage is recommended

Administration Oral: May administer with food to decrease GI upset; dilute oral solution in water, milk, or fruit juice immediately before use; do not dilute in grape juice or carbonated beverages

Monitoring Parameters Heart rate, blood pressure, mental status, weight, plasma concentrations. Monitor patient periodically for symptom resolution; monitor for worsening depression, suicidality, and associated ▶

behaviors (especially at the beginning of therapy or when doses are increased or decreased; see Warnings).

Reference Range Therapeutic: 50-150 ng/mL (SI: 190-570 nmol/L)

Patient Information Read the patient Medication Guide that you receive with each prescription and refill of nortriptyline. An increased risk of suicidal thinking and behavior has been reported with the use of antidepressants in children, adolescents, and young adults (18-24 years of age). Notify physician if you feel more depressed, have thoughts of suicide, or become more agitated or irritable (see Warnings). Avoid alcohol and the herbal medicine St John's wort; limit caffeine; do not discontinue medication abruptly; may cause drowsiness and impair ability to perform activities requiring mental alertness or physical coordination; may cause dry mouth. May cause photosensitivity reactions (eg, exposure to sunlight may cause severe sunburn, skin rash, redness, or itching); avoid exposure to sunlight and artificial light sources (sunlamps, tanning booth/bed); wear protective clothing, wide-brimmed hats, sunglasses, and lip sunscreen (SPF ≥15); use a sunscreen [broad-spectrum sunscreen or physical sunscreen (preferred) or sunblock with SPF ≥15]; contact physician if reaction occurs.

Nursing Implications Treatment duration of nocturnal enuresis is usually ≤3 months

Dosage Forms Excipient information presented when available (limited, particularly for generics); consult specific product labeling.

Capsule: 10 mg, 25 mg, 50 mg, 75 mg

Pamelor®: 10 mg, 25 mg, 50 mg, 75 mg [may contain benzyl alcohol; 50 mg may also contain sodium bisulfite]

Solution:

Pamelor®: 10 mg/5 mL (473 mL) [contains ethanol 4% and benzoic acid]

References

Dopheide JA, "Recognizing and Treating Depression in Children and Adolescents," *Am J Health Syst Pharm,* 2006, 63(3):233-43.

Levy HB, Harper CR, and Weinberg WA, "A Practical Approach to Children Failing in School," *Pediatr Clin North Am,* 1992, 39 (4):895-928

Wagner KD, "Pharmacotherapy for Major Depression in Children and Adolescents," *Prog Neuropsychopharmacol Biol Psychiatry,* 2005, 29 (5):819-26.

- **Novo-Ferrogluc (Can)** *see* Ferrous Gluconate *on page 577*
- **Novo-Fluconazole (Can)** *see* Fluconazole *on page 584*
- **Novo-Fluoxetine (Can)** *see* FLUoxetine *on page 600*
- **Novo-Flurprofen (Can)** *see* Flurbiprofen *on page 605*
- **Novo-Fluvoxamine (Can)** *see* Fluvoxamine *on page 615*
- **Novo-Furantoin (Can)** *see* Nitrofurantoin *on page 995*
- **Novo-Gesic (Can)** *see* Acetaminophen *on page 36*
- **Novo-Glyburide (Can)** *see* GlyBURIDE *on page 648*
- **Novo-Hydrazide (Can)** *see* Hydrochlorothiazide *on page 682*
- **Novo-Hydroxyzin (Can)** *see* HydrOXYzine *on page 697*
- **Novo-Hylazin (Can)** *see* HydrALAZINE *on page 680*
- **Novo-Ipramide (Can)** *see* Ipratropium *on page 757*
- **Novo-Ketoconazole (Can)** *see* Ketoconazole *on page 780*
- **Novo-Ketorolac (Can)** *see* Ketorolac *on page 781*
- **Novo-Ketotifen (Can)** *see* Ketotifen *on page 785*
- **Novo-Lamotrigine (Can)** *see* LamoTRIgine *on page 795*
- **Novo-Lansoprazole (Can)** *see* Lansoprazole *on page 801*
- **Novo-Levobunolol (Can)** *see* Levobunolol *on page 811*
- **Novo-Levofloxacin (Can)** *see* Levofloxacin *on page 813*
- **Novo-Lexin (Can)** *see* Cephalexin *on page 282*
- **Novolin® 70/30** *see* Insulin NPH and Insulin Regular *on page 747*
- **Novolin® ge 30/70 (Can)** *see* Insulin NPH and Insulin Regular *on page 747*
- **Novolin® ge 40/60 (Can)** *see* Insulin NPH and Insulin Regular *on page 747*
- **Novolin® ge 50/50 (Can)** *see* Insulin NPH and Insulin Regular *on page 747*
- **Novolin® ge NPH (Can)** *see* Insulin NPH *on page 746*
- **Novolin® ge Toronto (Can)** *see* Insulin Regular *on page 748*
- **Novolin® N** *see* Insulin NPH *on page 746*
- **Novolin® R** *see* Insulin Regular *on page 748*
- **Novo-Lisinopril (Can)** *see* Lisinopril *on page 832*
- **NovoLog®** *see* Insulin Aspart *on page 738*
- **NovoLog 70/30** *see* Insulin Aspart Protamine and Insulin Aspart *on page 739*
- **NovoLog® Mix 70/30** *see* Insulin Aspart Protamine and Insulin Aspart *on page 739*
- **Novo-Loperamide (Can)** *see* Loperamide *on page 838*
- **Novo-Lorazem (Can)** *see* LORazepam *on page 845*
- **Novo-Lovastatin (Can)** *see* Lovastatin *on page 850*
- **Novo-Medrone (Can)** *see* MedroxyPROGESTERone *on page 870*
- **Novo-Metformin (Can)** *see* MetFORMIN *on page 891*
- **Novo-Methacin (Can)** *see* Indomethacin *on page 726*
- **Novo-Methylphenidate ER-C (Can)** *see* Methylphenidate *on page 908*
- **Novo-Metoprol (Can)** *see* Metoprolol *on page 918*
- **Novo-Mexiletine (Can)** *see* Mexiletine *on page 924*
- **Novo-Minocycline (Can)** *see* Minocycline *on page 933*
- **Novo-Misoprostol (Can)** *see* Misoprostol *on page 937*
- **NovoMix® 30 (Can)** *see* Insulin Aspart Protamine and Insulin Aspart *on page 739*
- **Novo-Morphine SR (Can)** *see* Morphine Sulfate *on page 946*
- **Novo-Nadolol (Can)** *see* Nadolol *on page 961*

- **Novo-Naproc EC (Can)** *see* Naproxen *on page 967*
- **Novo-Naprox (Can)** *see* Naproxen *on page 967*
- **Novo-Naprox Sodium (Can)** *see* Naproxen *on page 967*
- **Novo-Naprox Sodium DS (Can)** *see* Naproxen *on page 967*
- **Novo-Naprox SR (Can)** *see* Naproxen *on page 967*
- **Novo-Nizatidine (Can)** *see* Nizatidine *on page 999*
- **Novo-Nortriptyline (Can)** *see* Nortriptyline *on page 1002*
- **Novo-Ofloxacin (Can)** *see* Ofloxacin *on page 1011*
- **Novo-Ondansetron (Can)** *see* Ondansetron *on page 1022*
- **Novo-Oxybutynin (Can)** *see* Oxybutynin *on page 1037*
- **Novo-Oxycodone Acet (Can)** *see* Oxycodone and Acetaminophen *on page 1041*
- **Novo-Pantoprazole (Can)** *see* Pantoprazole *on page 1054*
- **Novo-Paroxetine (Can)** *see* PARoxetine *on page 1064*
- **Novo-Pen-VK (Can)** *see* Penicillin V Potassium *on page 1082*
- **Novo-Peridol (Can)** *see* Haloperidol *on page 666*
- **Novo-Pheniram (Can)** *see* Chlorpheniramine *on page 296*
- **Novo-Pirocam (Can)** *see* Piroxicam *on page 1118*
- **Novo-Pramine (Can)** *see* Imipramine *on page 716*
- **Novo-Pranol (Can)** *see* Propranolol *on page 1175*
- **Novo-Pravastatin (Can)** *see* Pravastatin *on page 1145*
- **Novo-Prazin (Can)** *see* Prazosin *on page 1147*
- **Novo-Prednisolone (Can)** *see* PrednisoLONE *on page 1148*
- **Novo-Prednisone (Can)** *see* PredniSONE *on page 1151*
- **Novo-Profen (Can)** *see* Ibuprofen *on page 702*
- **Novo-Purol (Can)** *see* Allopurinol *on page 66*
- **Novo-Quinidin (Can)** *see* QuiNIDine *on page 1192*
- **Novo-Quinine (Can)** *see* QuiNINE *on page 1194*
- **Novo-Rabeprazole EC (Can)** *see* Rabeprazole *on page 1197*
- **Novo-Ranidine (Can)** *see* Ranitidine *on page 1200*
- **NovoRapid® (Can)** *see* Insulin Aspart *on page 738*
- **Novo-Risperidone (Can)** *see* Risperidone *on page 1218*
- **Novo-Rythro Estolate (Can)** *see* Erythromycin *on page 525*
- **Novo-Rythro Ethylsuccinate (Can)** *see* Erythromycin *on page 525*
- **Novo-Semide (Can)** *see* Furosemide *on page 632*
- **Novo-Sertraline (Can)** *see* Sertraline *on page 1254*
- **NovoSeven® RT** *see* Factor VIIa (Recombinant) *on page 556*
- **Novo-Sotalol (Can)** *see* Sotalol *on page 1284*
- **Novo-Soxazole (Can)** *see* SulfiSOXAZOLE *on page 1305*
- **Novo-Spiroton (Can)** *see* Spironolactone *on page 1289*
- **Novo-Spirozine (Can)** *see* Hydrochlorothiazide and Spironolactone *on page 683*
- **Novo-Sucralate (Can)** *see* Sucralfate *on page 1296*
- **Novo-Sumatriptan (Can)** *see* SUMAtriptan *on page 1308*
- **Novo-Sundac (Can)** *see* Sulindac *on page 1307*
- **Novo-Terbinafine (Can)** *see* Terbinafine *on page 1322*
- **Novo-Theophyl SR (Can)** *see* Theophylline *on page 1335*
- **Novo-Topiramate (Can)** *see* Topiramate *on page 1360*

◆ **Novo-Trazodone (Can)** see TraZODone on page 1371
◆ **Novo-Trifluzine (Can)** see Trifluoperazine on page 1382
◆ **Novo-Trimel (Can)** see Sulfamethoxazole and Trimethoprim on page 1302
◆ **Novo-Trimel D.S. (Can)** see Sulfamethoxazole and Trimethoprim on page 1302
◆ **Novo-Triptyn (Can)** see Amitriptyline on page 89
◆ **Novo-Veramil (Can)** see Verapamil on page 1416
◆ **Novo-Veramil SR (Can)** see Verapamil on page 1416
◆ **Novo-Warfarin (Can)** see Warfarin on page 1432
◆ **Noxafil®** see Posaconazole on page 1132
◆ **NPH Insulin** see Insulin NPH on page 746
◆ **NPH Insulin and Regular Insulin** see Insulin NPH and Insulin Regular on page 747
◆ **NRP104** see Lisdexamfetamine on page 830
◆ **NRS® [OTC]** see Oxymetazoline on page 1043
◆ **NSC-750** see Busulfan on page 223
◆ **NSC-755** see Mercaptopurine on page 884
◆ **NSC-71423** see Megestrol on page 874
◆ **NSC-105014** see Cladribine on page 323
◆ **NSC-109229 (E. coli)** see Asparaginase on page 139
◆ **NSC-218321** see Pentostatin on page 1088
◆ **NSC-241240** see CARBOplatin on page 250
◆ **NSC-312887** see Fludarabine on page 587
◆ **NSC606869** see Clofarabine on page 332
◆ **NSC-613795** see Sargramostim on page 1247
◆ **NSC-614629** see Filgrastim on page 580
◆ **NSC-628503** see Docetaxel on page 465
◆ **NSC-644468** see Deferoxamine on page 397
◆ **NSC-720568** see Gemtuzumab Ozogamicin on page 640
◆ **NSC-725961** see Pegfilgrastim on page 1070
◆ **NTBC** see Nitisinone on page 994
◆ **NTG** see Nitroglycerin on page 996
◆ **NTZ** see Nitazoxanide on page 993
◆ **Nu-Acyclovir (Can)** see Acyclovir on page 46
◆ **Nu-Alpraz (Can)** see ALPRAZolam on page 68
◆ **Nu-Amoxi (Can)** see Amoxicillin on page 96
◆ **Nu-Ampi (Can)** see Ampicillin on page 104
◆ **Nu-Atenol (Can)** see Atenolol on page 147
◆ **Nu-Baclo (Can)** see Baclofen on page 171
◆ **Nubain®** see Nalbuphine on page 963
◆ **Nu-Beclomethasone (Can)** see Beclomethasone on page 176
◆ **Nu-Buspirone (Can)** see BusPIRone on page 222
◆ **Nu-Capto (Can)** see Captopril on page 242
◆ **Nu-Carbamazepine (Can)** see CarBAMazepine on page 244
◆ **Nu-Cefaclor (Can)** see Cefaclor on page 260
◆ **Nu-Cephalex (Can)** see Cephalexin on page 282
◆ **Nu-Cimet (Can)** see Cimetidine on page 309
◆ **Nu-Clonazepam (Can)** see ClonazePAM on page 337
◆ **Nu-Clonidine (Can)** see CloNIDine on page 338
◆ **Nu-Cotrimox (Can)** see Sulfamethoxazole and Trimethoprim on page 1302
◆ **Nu-Cromolyn (Can)** see Cromolyn on page 363
◆ **Nu-Cyclobenzaprine (Can)** see Cyclobenzaprine on page 367
◆ **Nu-Desipramine (Can)** see Desipramine on page 401
◆ **Nu-Diclo (Can)** see Diclofenac on page 429

◆ **Nu-Diclo-SR (Can)** see Diclofenac on page 429
◆ **Nu-Diltiaz (Can)** see Diltiazem on page 443
◆ **Nu-Diltiaz-CD (Can)** see Diltiazem on page 443
◆ **Nu-Divalproex (Can)** see Valproic Acid and Derivatives on page 1398
◆ **Nu-Doxycycline (Can)** see Doxycycline on page 479
◆ **Nu-Erythromycin-S (Can)** see Erythromycin on page 525
◆ **Nu-Famotidine (Can)** see Famotidine on page 561
◆ **Nu-Fluoxetine (Can)** see FLUoxetine on page 600
◆ **Nu-Flurprofen (Can)** see Flurbiprofen on page 605
◆ **Nu-Fluvoxamine (Can)** see Fluvoxamine on page 615
◆ **Nu-Furosemide (Can)** see Furosemide on page 632
◆ **Nu-Glyburide (Can)** see GlyBURIDE on page 648
◆ **Nu-Hydral (Can)** see HydrALAZINE on page 680
◆ **Nu-Hydro (Can)** see Hydrochlorothiazide on page 682
◆ **Nu-Ibuprofen (Can)** see Ibuprofen on page 702
◆ **Nu-Indo (Can)** see Indomethacin on page 726
◆ **Nu-Ipratropium (Can)** see Ipratropium on page 757
◆ **Nu-Ketorolac (Can)** see Ketorolac on page 781
◆ **Nu-Ketotifen® (Can)** see Ketotifen on page 785
◆ **Nu-Loraz (Can)** see LORazepam on page 845
◆ **Nu-Lovastatin (Can)** see Lovastatin on page 850
◆ **NuLYTELY®** see Polyethylene Glycol-Electrolyte Solution on page 1129
◆ **Nu-Medopa (Can)** see Methyldopa on page 905
◆ **Nu-Megestrol (Can)** see Megestrol on page 874
◆ **Nu-Metformin (Can)** see MetFORMIN on page 891
◆ **Nu-Metoclopramide (Can)** see Metoclopramide on page 915
◆ **Nu-Metop (Can)** see Metoprolol on page 918
◆ **Nu-Naprox (Can)** see Naproxen on page 967
◆ **Nu-Nifed (Can)** see NIFEdipine on page 991
◆ **Nu-Nifedipine-PA (Can)** see NIFEdipine on page 991
◆ **Nu-Nizatidine (Can)** see Nizatidine on page 999
◆ **Nu-Nortriptyline (Can)** see Nortriptyline on page 1002
◆ **Nu-Oxybutyn (Can)** see Oxybutynin on page 1037
◆ **Nu-Pentoxifylline SR (Can)** see Pentoxifylline on page 1090
◆ **Nu-Pen-VK (Can)** see Penicillin V Potassium on page 1082
◆ **Nupercainal® [OTC]** see Dibucaine on page 428
◆ **Nupercainal® Hydrocortisone Cream [OTC]** see Hydrocortisone on page 685
◆ **Nu-Pirox (Can)** see Piroxicam on page 1118
◆ **Nu-Pravastatin (Can)** see Pravastatin on page 1145
◆ **Nu-Prazo (Can)** see Prazosin on page 1147
◆ **Nu-Prochlor (Can)** see Prochlorperazine on page 1161
◆ **Nu-Propranolol (Can)** see Propranolol on page 1175
◆ **Nu-Ranit (Can)** see Ranitidine on page 1200
◆ **Nu-Salbutamol (Can)** see Albuterol on page 57
◆ **Nu-Sertraline (Can)** see Sertraline on page 1254
◆ **Nu-Simvastatin (Can)** see Simvastatin on page 1263
◆ **Nu-Sotalol (Can)** see Sotalol on page 1284
◆ **Nu-Sucralate (Can)** see Sucralfate on page 1296
◆ **Nu-Sundac (Can)** see Sulindac on page 1307
◆ **Nu-Tetra (Can)** see Tetracycline on page 1331
◆ **Nu-Timolol (Can)** see Timolol on page 1351
◆ **Nutracort®** see Hydrocortisone on page 685

◆ **Nutralox® [OTC]** *see* Calcium Carbonate *on page 232*
◆ **Nutralox® [OTC]** *see* Calcium Supplements *on page 239*
◆ **Nu-Trazodone (Can)** *see* TraZODone *on page 1371*
◆ **Nutropin®** *see* Somatropin *on page 1281*
◆ **Nutropin AQ®** *see* Somatropin *on page 1281*
◆ **Nutropin® AQ (Can)** *see* Somatropin *on page 1281*
◆ **Nu-Verap (Can)** *see* Verapamil *on page 1416*
◆ **Nu-Verap SR (Can)** *see* Verapamil *on page 1416*
◆ **NVP** *see* Nevirapine *on page 983*
◆ **Nyaderm (Can)** *see* Nystatin *on page 1007*
◆ **Nyamyc™** *see* Nystatin *on page 1007*
◆ **Nycoff [OTC]** *see* Dextromethorphan *on page 421*

Nystatin (nye STAT in)

Medication Safety Issues
Sound-alike/look-alike issues:
Nystatin may be confused with HMG-CoA reductase inhibitors (also known as "statins"; eg, atorvastatin, fluvastatin, lovastatin, pitavastatin, pravastatin, rosuvastatin, simvastatin), Nitrostat®

U.S. Brand Names Nyamyc™; Nystat-Rx®; Nystop®; Pedi-Dri®

Canadian Brand Names Candistatin®; Nyaderm; PMS-Nystatin

Therapeutic Category Antifungal Agent, Oral Nonabsorbed; Antifungal Agent, Topical; Antifungal Agent, Vaginal

Generic Available Yes: Cream, ointment, powder, suspension, tablet

Use Treatment of susceptible cutaneous, mucocutaneous, oral cavity and vaginal fungal infections normally caused by the *Candida* species

Pregnancy Risk Factor A (vaginal)/C (oral, topical)

Pregnancy Considerations Animal reproduction studies have not been conducted. Adverse events in the fetus or newborn have not been reported following maternal use of vaginal nystatin during pregnancy. Absorption following oral use is poor and nystatin is not absorbed following application to mucous membranes or intact skin.

Lactation Excretion in breast milk unknown/use caution

Breast-Feeding Considerations Excretion into breast milk is not known; however, absorption following oral use is poor and nystatin is not absorbed following application to mucous membranes or intact skin.

Contraindications Hypersensitivity to nystatin or any component

Adverse Reactions
Dermatologic: Contact dermatitis, Stevens-Johnson syndrome, pruritus, rash
Gastrointestinal: Nausea, vomiting, diarrhea
Local: Irritation, burning, pain

Drug Interactions
Avoid Concomitant Use There are no known interactions where it is recommended to avoid concomitant use.

Increased Effect/Toxicity There are no known significant interactions involving an increase in effect.

Decreased Effect
Nystatin may decrease the levels/effects of: Saccharomyces boulardii

Stability Store vaginal inserts in refrigerator; protect from moisture and light

Mechanism of Action Binds to sterols in fungal cell membrane, changing the cell wall permeability allowing for leakage of cellular contents

Pharmacodynamics Onset of action: Symptomatic relief from candidiasis: Within 24-72 hours

Pharmacokinetics (Adult data unless noted)
Absorption: Not absorbed through mucous membranes or intact skin; poorly absorbed from the GI tract
Elimination: In feces as unchanged drug

Usual Dosage
Oral candidiasis:
Neonates: 100,000 units 4 times/day or 50,000 units to each side of mouth 4 times/day
Infants: 200,000 units 4 times/day or 100,000 units to each side of mouth 4 times/day
Children and Adults: 400,000-600,000 units 4 times/day
Cutaneous candidal infections: Children and Adults: Topical: Apply 2-4 times/day
Intestinal infections: Adults: Oral: 500,000-1,000,000 units every 8 hours
Vaginal infections: Adolescents and Adults: Vaginal tablets: Insert 1 tablet/day at bedtime for 2 weeks

Administration
Oral: Shake suspension well before use; suspension should be swished about the mouth and retained in the mouth for as long as possible (several minutes) before swallowing. For neonates and infants, paint nystatin suspension into recesses of the mouth.
Topical:
Cream or ointment: Gently massage formulation into the skin
Intravaginal: Insert vaginal tablet high in the vagina
Powder: Dust in shoes, in stockings, and on feet for treatment of candidal infection of the feet; also used on very moist lesions

Monitoring Parameters KOH smears or cultures should be used to confirm diagnosis of cutaneous or mucocutaneous candidiasis

Patient Information Inform physician if irritation or sensitization occur during therapy

Dosage Forms Excipient information presented when available (limited, particularly for generics); consult specific product labeling.
Cream, topical: 100,000 units/g (15 g, 30 g)
Ointment, topical: 100,000 units/g (15 g, 30 g)
Powder, for prescription compounding: 50 million units (10 g); 150 million units (30 g); 500 million units (100 g)
Nystat-Rx®: 50 million units (10 g); 150 million units (30 g); 500 million units (100 g); 1 billion units (190 g); 2 billion units (350 g)
Powder, topical: 100,000 units/g (15 g, 30 g, 60 g)
Nyamyc™: 100,000 units/g (15 g, 30 g, 60 g) [contains talc]
Nystop®: 100,000 units/g (15 g, 30 g, 60 g) [contains talc]
Pedi-Dri®: 100,000 units/g (56.7 g) [contains talc]
Suspension, oral: 100,000 units/mL (5 mL, 60 mL, 480 mL)
Tablet, oral: 500,000 units
Tablet, vaginal: 100,000 units (15s) [packaged with applicator]

References
Dismukes WE, Wade JS, Lee JY, et al, "A Randomized, Double-Blind Trial of Nystatin Therapy for the Candidiasis Hypersensitivity Syndrome," *N Engl J Med*, 1990, 323(25):1717-23.

◆ **Nystat-Rx®** *see* Nystatin *on page 1007*
◆ **Nystop®** *see* Nystatin *on page 1007*
◆ **Nytol® (Can)** *see* DiphenhydrAMINE *on page 448*
◆ **Nytol® Extra Strength (Can)** *see* DiphenhydrAMINE *on page 448*
◆ **Nytol® Quick Caps [OTC]** *see* DiphenhydrAMINE *on page 448*
◆ **Nytol® Quick Gels [OTC]** *see* DiphenhydrAMINE *on page 448*
◆ **NāSal™ [OTC]** *see* Sodium Chloride *on page 1270*
◆ **Nōstrilla® [OTC]** *see* Oxymetazoline *on page 1043*
◆ **OCBZ** *see* OXcarbazepine *on page 1035*

◆ **Occlusal®-HP [OTC] [DSC]** *see* Salicylic Acid *on page 1241*

◆ **Occlusal™-HP (Can)** *see* Salicylic Acid *on page 1241*

◆ **Ocean® [OTC]** *see* Sodium Chloride *on page 1270*

◆ **Ocean® for Kids [OTC]** *see* Sodium Chloride *on page 1270*

◆ **Octagam®** *see* Immune Globulin (Intravenous) *on page 719*

◆ **Octostim® (Can)** *see* Desmopressin *on page 404*

Octreotide Acetate (ok TREE oh tide AS e tate)

Medication Safety Issues

Sound-alike/look-alike issues:
Sandostatin® may be confused with Sandimmune®, Sandostatin LAR®, sargramostim, simvastatin

U.S. Brand Names Sandostatin LAR®; Sandostatin®

Canadian Brand Names Octreotide Acetate Injection; Octreotide Acetate Omega; Sandostatin LAR®; Sandostatin®

Therapeutic Category Antidiarrheal; Antidote; Antihemorrhagics; Antisecretory Agent; Somatostatin Analog

Generic Available Yes: Injection solution (excludes depot formulation)

Use Control of symptoms, including secretory diarrhea in patients with metastatic carcinoid or vasoactive intestinal peptide-secreting tumors (VIPomas) (FDA approved in adults); treatment of acromegaly (FDA approved in adults). Other uses include control of bleeding of esophageal varices, Cushing's syndrome, insulinomas, glucagonoma, small bowel fistulas, postgastrectomy dumping syndrome, chemotherapy-induced diarrhea, graft-versus-host disease (GVHD)-associated diarrhea, Zollinger-Ellison syndrome, persistent hyperinsulinemic hypoglycemia of infancy (nesidioblastosis), postoperative chylothorax, second-line treatment for thymic malignancies; islet cell tumors; treatment of malignant bowel obstruction; treatment of sulfonylurea overdosage (nondepot formulation); hypothalamic obesity

Pregnancy Risk Factor B

Pregnancy Considerations Teratogenic effects were not observed in animal studies. Octreotide crosses the human placenta; data concerning use in pregnancy is limited. Women of childbearing potential should use adequate contraception during treatment with octreotide; normalization of IGF-1 and GH may restore fertility in women with acromegaly. In case reports of acromegalic women who received normal doses of octreotide during pregnancy, no congenital malformations were reported.

Lactation Excretion in breast milk unknown/use caution

Contraindications Hypersensitivity to octreotide or any component

Warnings Dosage adjustment may be required to maintain symptomatic control; octreotide may affect glucose regulation; insulin requirements may be reduced in type I diabetic patients; symptomatic hypoglycemia which may be severe, has been reported; in nondiabetics and type II diabetics with partially intact insulin reserves, octreotide may decrease insulin levels and hyperglycemia may occur; monitor glucose tolerance and antidiabetic treatment closely; may worsen hypoglycemia in patients with insulinomas; patients must be monitored closely for biliary tract abnormalities (including biliary obstruction, cholecystitis, and cholelithiasis). The incidence of gallbladder stone or sludge increases with a duration of therapy ≥12 months. In patients with neuroendocrine tumors, the NCCN guidelines (v.2.2009) recommend considering prophylactic cholecystectomy in patients undergoing abdominal surgery if octreotide treatment is planned. Postmarketing cases of serious and fatal events, including hypoxia and necrotizing enterocolitis, have been reported with octreotide use in children (usually with serious underlying conditions), particularly in children <2 years of age. In studies with octreotide depot, the incidence of cholelithiasis in children is higher than the reported incidences for adults.

Precautions Hypothyroidism, with or without goiter, has been reported in acromegalic patients; use with caution in patients with renal impairment and consider dosage modification in patients with severe renal failure requiring dialysis; use with caution in patients with hepatic impairment; dosage adjustment required in patients with established cirrhosis; use caution in diabetic patients with gastroparesis; chronic usage is associated with abnormal Schillings test and depressed vitamin B$_{12}$ levels; monitor vitamin B$_{12}$ levels in patients receiving long-term therapy; suppression of growth hormone (animal data) is of concern when used as long-term therapy in children. Use with caution in patients with heart failure or concomitant medications that alter heart rate or rhythm; bradycardia, conduction abnormalities, and arrhythmia have been observed in acromegalic and carcinoid syndrome patients; cardiovascular medication requirements may change; may enhance the adverse/toxic effects of other QT$_c$-prolonging agents. Vehicle used in depot injectable (polylactide-co-glycolide microspheres) has rarely been associated with retinal artery occlusion in patients with abnormal arteriovenous anastomosis.

Adverse Reactions

Cardiovascular: Angina, arrhythmia, bradycardia, chest pain, conduction abnormalities, edema, flushing, palpitation, peripheral edema

Central nervous system: Abnormal gait, amnesia, dizziness, dysphonia, fatigue, fever, hallucinations, headache, malaise, nervousness, neuralgia, neuropathy, somnolence, vertigo

Dermatologic: Acne, alopecia, bruising, cellulitis, pruritus

Endocrine & metabolic: Anorexia, cachexia, goiter, hyperglycemia, hypoglycemia (see Warnings), hypokalemia, hypothyroidism

Gastrointestinal: Abdominal pain, biliary duct dilatation, biliary sludge (see Warnings), cholelithiasis (children: 33% reported), constipation, cramping, dehydration, diarrhea, dyspepsia, fat malabsorption, feces discoloration, flatulence, nausea, steatorrhea, tenesmus, vomiting, xerostomia

Genitourinary: Incontinence, polyuria, urinary tract infection

Hematologic: Anemia, epistaxis hematoma

Local: Injection site pain, phlebitis

Neuromuscular & skeletal: Arthralgia, arthropathy, back pain, muscle cramps, muscle spasm, myalgia, paresthesia, rigors, tremors, weakness

Ocular: Blurred vision, visual disturbance

Otic: Earache, tinnitus

Renal: Oliguria, urinary hyperosmolarity

Respiratory: Cold symptoms, pulmonary hypertension, shortness of breath, upper respiratory tract infection

Miscellaneous: Allergic reaction, anaphylactoid reaction, antibody formation, flu-like symptoms,

<1%, postmarketing, and/or case reports (limited to important or life-threatening): Anaphylactic shock, aneurysm, aphasia, appendicitis, arthritis, ascending cholangitis, ascites, atrial fibrillation, basal cell carcinoma, Bell's palsy, biliary obstruction, breast carcinoma, cardiac arrest, cerebral vascular disorder, CHF, cholecystitis, cholestatic hepatitis, CK increased, creatinine increased, deafness, diabetes insipidus, diabetes mellitus, facial edema, fatty liver, galactorrhea, gallbladder polyp, GI bleeding, GI hemorrhage, GI ulcer, glaucoma, gynecomastia, hearing loss, hematuria, hemiparesis, hemorrhoids, hepatitis, hyperesthesia, hypertensive reaction, hypoadrenalism, hypoxia, intestinal obstruction, intracranial hemorrhage, intraocular pressure increased,

ischemia, jaundice, joint effusion, lactation, LFTs increased, libido decreased, malignant hyperpyrexia, menstrual irregularities, MI, migraine, necrotizing enterocolitis, nephrolithiasis, neuritis, orthostatic hypotension, pancreatitis, pancytopenia, paresis, petechiae, pituitary apoplexy, pleural effusion, pneumonia, pneumothorax, pulmonary embolism, pulmonary nodule, Raynaud's syndrome, rectal bleeding, renal failure, renal insufficiency, retinal vein thrombosis, scotoma, seizure, status asthmaticus, suicide attempt, syncope, tachycardia, thrombocytopenia, thrombophlebitis, thrombosis, urticaria, visual field defect, wheal/erythema

Drug Interactions

Avoid Concomitant Use

Avoid concomitant use of Octreotide with any of the following: Artemether; Dronedarone; Lumefantrine; Nilotinib; Pimozide; QuiNINE; Tetrabenazine; Thioridazine; Ziprasidone

Increased Effect/Toxicity

Octreotide may increase the levels/effects of: Codeine; Dronedarone; Hypoglycemic Agents; Pegvisomant; Pimozide; QTc-Prolonging Agents; QuiNINE; Tetrabenazine; Thioridazine; Ziprasidone

The levels/effects of Octreotide may be increased by: Alfuzosin; Artemether; Chloroquine; Ciprofloxacin; Ciprofloxacin (Systemic); Gadobutrol; Herbs (Hypoglycemic Properties); Lumefantrine; Nilotinib; QuiNINE

Decreased Effect

Octreotide may decrease the levels/effects of: CycloSPORINE; CycloSPORINE (Systemic)

Food Interactions Schedule injections between meals to decrease GI effects; may decrease vitamin B_{12} levels and decrease absorption of dietary fats. Avoid hypoglycemic herbs that may enhance the hypoglycemic effect of octreotide, including alfalfa, aloe, bilberry, bitter melon, burdock, celery, damiana, fenugreek, garcinia, garlic, ginger, ginseng, gymnema, marshmallow, and stinging nettle.

Stability Store in refrigerator between 2°C and 8°C (36°F and 46°F); protect from light; Sandostatin® injection at room temperature at 20°C to 30°C (70°F and 86°F) and protected from light is stable for 14 days; parenteral admixtures are stable in NS for 4 days and D_5W for 24 hours at room temperature; stable for up to 7 days in a polypropylene syringe; not compatible in TPN solutions due to glycosyl octreotide conjugate which may have decreased activity. Sandostatin LAR® Depot must be used immediately after reconstitution

Mechanism of Action A synthetic polypeptide which mimics natural somatostatin by inhibiting serotonin release, and the secretion of gastrin, vasoactive intestinal peptide (VIP), insulin, glucagon, secretin, motilin, thyrotropin, cholecystokinin, serotonin, and pancreatic polypeptide; in animals, also a potent inhibitor of growth hormone; decreases GI motility and inhibits intestinal secretion of water and electrolytes, and decreases splanchnic blood flow

Pharmacodynamics Duration (immediate release formulation): SubQ: 6-12 hours

Pharmacokinetics (Adult data unless noted)

Absorption: SubQ: Rapid; I.M. (depot formulation): Released slowly (via microsphere degradation in the muscle)

Bioavailability: SubQ: 100%; I.M.: 60% to 63% of SubQ dose

Distribution: V_d:

Adults: 13.6 L

Adults with acromegaly: 21.6 ± 8.5 L

Protein binding: 65% primarily to lipoprotein (41% in acromegaly)

Metabolism: Extensive by the liver

Half-life: 1.7-1.9 hours; up to 3.7 hours with cirrhosis; up to 3.4 hours with fatty liver disease; up to 3.1 hours in renal impairment

Time to peak serum concentration: SubQ: 0.4 hours (0.7 hours acromegaly); I.M.: 1 hour

Elimination: 32% excreted unchanged in urine

Clearance:

Adults: 10 L/hour

Adults with acromegaly: 18 L/hour

Note: When using Sandostatin LAR® Depot formulation, steady-state levels are achieved after 3 injections (3 months of therapy)

Usual Dosage Dosage should be individualized according to the patient's response

Sandostatin®:

Infants and Children (data limited to small studies and case reports): **Note:** The following are effective dosing ranges for specific therapies: I.V., SubQ:

Diarrhea:

I.V., SubQ: Doses of 1-10 mcg/kg every 12 hours have been used in children beginning at the low end of the range and increasing based upon the clinical response

I.V. continuous infusion: Initial 1 mcg/kg bolus dose, followed by a continuous infusion of 1 mcg/kg/hour has been used successfully in several cases of severe diarrhea secondary to graft-vs-host disease

Chylothorax (see Chan, 2006; Roehr, 2006):

SubQ: 40 mcg/kg/day; case reports of effective dosage range from 2-68 mcg/kg/day

I.V. continuous infusion: 0.5-4 mcg/kg/hour continuous infusion; titrate dose to response; case reports of effective dosage range from 0.3-10 mcg/kg/hour (median 2.8 mcg/kg/hour); treatment duration is usually 1-2 weeks but may vary with the clinical response

Esophageal varices/GI bleed: 1-2 mcg/kg initial I.V. bolus followed by 1-2 mcg/kg/hour continuous infusion; titrate infusion rate to response; taper dose by 50% every 12 hours when no active bleeding occurs for 24 hours; may discontinue when dose is 25% of initial dose (see Eroglu, 2004)

Hypothalamic obesity (from cranial insult): SubQ: 5 mcg/kg/day divided into 3 daily doses; dose may be increased bimonthly at 5 mcg/kg/day increments to a maximum of 15 mcg/kg/day divided into 3 daily doses (see Lustig, 2003)

Persistent hyperinsulinemic hypoglycemia of infancy (nesidioblastosis): 2-10 mcg/kg/day initially divided every 12 hours; increase dosage depending upon patient response by either using a more frequent interval (every 6-8 hours) or larger dose; doses of 40 mcg/kg/day have been used

Treatment of sulfonylurea overdose: **Note:** SubQ is the preferred route of administration; repeat dosing, dose escalation, or initiation of a continuous infusion may be required in patients who experience recurrent hypoglycemia. Duration of treatment may exceed 24 hours. Optimal care decisions should be made based upon patient-specific details; SubQ: 1-1.5 mcg/kg/dose; repeat in 6-12 hours as needed based upon blood glucose concentrations

Adults:

Acromegaly:

SubQ, I.V.: Initial: 50 mcg 3 times/day; titrate to achieve growth hormone levels <5 ng/mL or IGF-I (somatomedin C) levels <1.9 units/mL in males and <2.2 units/mL in females. Usual effective dose is 100-200 mcg 3 times/day; range: 300-1500 mcg/day. **Note:** Should be withdrawn yearly for a 4-week interval (8 weeks for depot injection) in patients who have received irradiation. Resume if levels increase and signs/symptoms recur.

I.M. depot injection: Patients must be stabilized on subcutaneous octreotide for at least 2 weeks before switching to the long-acting depot. Upon switch: 20 mg I.M. intragluteally every 4 weeks for 3 months, then the dose may be modified based upon response.

Dosage adjustment: After 3 months of depot injections, the dosage may be continued or modified as follows:

GH ≤1 ng/mL, IGF-1 normal, and symptoms controlled: Reduce octreotide LAR® to 10 mg I.M. every 4 weeks

GH ≤2.5 ng/mL, IGF-1 normal, and symptoms controlled: Maintain octreotide LAR® at 20 mg I.M. every 4 weeks

GH >2.5 ng/mL, IGF-1 elevated, and/or symptoms uncontrolled: Increase octreotide LAR® to 30 mg I.M. every 4 weeks

Note: Patients not adequately controlled at a dose of 30 mg may increase dose to 40 mg every 4 weeks. Dosages >40 mg are not recommended.

Carcinoid tumors:

SubQ, I.V.: Initial 2 weeks: 100-600 mcg/day in 2-4 divided doses; usual range: 50-750 mcg/day (some patients may require up to 1500 mcg/day)

I.M. depot injection: Patients must be stabilized on subcutaneous octreotide for at least 2 weeks before switching to the long-acting depot. Upon switch: 20 mg I.M. intragluteally every 4 weeks for 2 months, then the dose may be modified based upon response

Note: Patients should continue to receive their SubQ injections for the first 2 weeks at the same dose in order to maintain therapeutic levels (some patients may require 3-4 weeks of continued SubQ injections). Patients who experience periodic exacerbations of symptoms may require temporary SubQ injections in addition to depot injections (at their previous SubQ dosing regimen) until symptoms have resolved.

Dosage adjustment: See dosing adjustment for VIPomas.

VIPomas:

SubQ, I.V.: Initial 2 weeks: 200-300 mcg/day in 2-4 divided doses; titrate dose based on response/tolerance; range: 150-750 mcg/day (doses >450 mcg/day are rarely required)

I.M. depot injection: Patients must be stabilized on subcutaneous octreotide for at least 2 weeks before switching to the long-acting depot. Upon switch: 20 mg I.M. intragluteally every 4 weeks for 2 months, then the dose may be modified based upon response.

Note: Patients receiving depot injection should continue to receive their SubQ injections for the first 2 weeks at the same dose in order to maintain therapeutic levels (some patients may require 3-4 weeks of continued SubQ injections). Patients who experience periodic exacerbations of symptoms may require temporary SubQ injections in addition to depot injections (at their previous SubQ dosing regimen) until symptoms have resolved.

Dosage adjustment: After 2 months of depot injections, the dosage may be continued or modified as follows:

Increase to 30 mg I.M. every 4 weeks if symptoms are inadequately controlled

Decrease to 10 mg I.M. every 4 weeks, for a trial period, if initially responsive to 20 mg dose

Dosage >30 mg is not recommended

Dosage adjustment in renal impairment: Clearance is decreased by 50% in patients with severe renal failure requiring dialysis; consider dosage modification in these patients as follows:

- Nondialysis-dependent renal impairment: No dosage adjustment required
- Dialysis-dependent renal impairment: Depot injection: Initial dose: I.M.: 10 mg every 4 weeks; titrate based upon response (clearance is reduced by ~50%

Dosage adjustment in hepatic impairment: Patients with established cirrhosis of the liver: Depot injection: Initial dose: I.M.: 10 mg every 4 weeks; titrate based upon response

Administration Parenteral: Only Sandostatin® injection may be administered I.V. and SubQ; Sandostatin LAR® Depot may only be administered I.M.

SubQ: Use the concentration with smallest volume to deliver dose to reduce injection site pain; rotate injection site; may bring to room temperature prior to injection

I.V. infusion: Dilute Sandostatin® injection in 50-200 mL NS or D_5W and infuse over 15-30 minutes or over 24 hours as a continuous infusion; in emergency situations, may be administered by direct I.V. push over 3 minutes; see Stability for compatibility information; allow solution to come to room temperature before administration

I.M. administration: Reconstitute with provided diluent; see detailed instruction booklet for complete instructions; use immediately after reconstitution; administer into gluteal area only (avoid deltoid injections due to significant pain and discomfort at injection site)

Monitoring Parameters Baseline and periodic ultrasound evaluations for cholelithiasis, blood sugar, baseline and periodic thyroid function tests, fluid and electrolyte balance, fecal fat, and serum carotene determinations; for carcinoid, monitor urinary 5-hydroxyindole acetic acid (5-HIAA), plasma serotonin, plasma substance P; for VIPoma, monitor VIP; vitamin B_{12} levels (chronic therapy); for acromegaly: growth hormone levels, IGF-I (somatomedin C), glycemic control, and antidiabetic regimen (patients with diabetes mellitus)

Reference Range Vasoactive intestinal peptide (VIP): <75 ng/L; levels vary considerably between laboratories; growth hormone level: <5 ng/mL; IGF-I (somatomedin C): males: <1.9 units/mL, females: <2.2 units/mL

Patient Information May cause dry mouth

Dosage Forms Excipient information presented when available (limited, particularly for generics); consult specific product labeling.

Injection, microspheres for suspension, as acetate [depot formulation]:

Sandostatin LAR®: 10 mg, 20 mg, 30 mg [contains polylactide-co-glycolide; packaged with diluent and syringe]

Injection, solution, as acetate: 0.2 mg/mL (5 mL); 1 mg/mL (5 mL)

Sandostatin®: 0.2 mg/mL (5 mL); 1 mg/mL (5 mL)

Injection, solution, as acetate [preservative free]: 0.05 mg/mL (1 mL); 0.1 mg/mL (1 mL); 0.5 mg/mL (1 mL)

Sandostatin®: 0.05 mg/mL (1 mL); 0.1 mg/mL (1 mL); 0.5 mg/mL (1 mL)

References

Beckman RA, Siden R, Yanik GA, et al, "Continuous Octreotide Infusion for the Treatment of Secretory Diarrhea Caused by Acute Intestinal Graft-Versus-Host Disease in a Child," *J Pediatr Hematol Oncol*, 2000, 22(4):344-50.

Calello DP, Osterhoudt KC, Henretig FM, et al, "Octreotide for Pediatric Sulfonylurea Overdose: Review of 5 Cases," *Clin Toxicol*, 2005, 43:671.

Chan SY, Lau W, Wong WH, et al, "Chylothorax in Children After Congenital Heart Surgery," *Ann Thorac Surg*, 2006, 82(5):1650-6.

Cheung Y, Leung MP, and Yip M, "Octreotide for Treatment of Postoperative Chylothorax," *J Pediatr*, 2001, 139(1):157-9.

Couper RT, Berzen A, Berall G, et al, "Clinical Response to the Long-Acting Somatostatin Analogue SMS 201-995 in a Child With Congenital Microvillus Atrophy," *Gut*, 1989, 30(7):1020-4.

Eroglu Y, Emerick KM, Whitingon PF, et al, "Octreotide Therapy for Control of Acute Gastrointestinal Bleeding in Children," *J Pediatr Gastroenterol Nutr*, 2004, 38(1):41-7.

Fasano CJ, O'Malley G, Dominici P, et al, "Comparison of Octreotide and Standard Therapy Versus Standard Therapy Alone for the Treatment of Sulfonylurea-Induced Hypoglycemia," *Ann Emerg Med*, 2008, 51(4):400-6.

Jaros W, Biller J, Greer S, et al, "Successful Treatment of Idiopathic Secretory Diarrhea of Infancy With the Somatostatin Analogue SMS 201-995," *Gastroenterology*, 1988, 94(1):189-93.

Katz MD and Erstad BL, "Octreotide, A New Somatostatin Analogue," *Clin Pharm*, 1989, 8(4):255-73.

Kalomenidis I, "Octreotide and chylothorax," *Curr Opin Pulm Med*, 2006, 12(4):264-7.

Lugassy DM, Nelson LS, Hoffman RS, et al, "Failure of Standard Octreotide Dosing to Prevent Recurrent Hypoglycemia Following Sulfonylurea Exposure in a Child," *J Toxicol Clin Toxicol*, 2009, 47 (7):760.

Lustig RH, Hinds PS, Ringwald-Smith K, et al, "Octreotide Therapy of Pediatric Hypothalamic Obesity: A Double-Blind, Placebo-Controlled Trial," *J Clin Endocrinol Metab*, 2003, 88(6):2586-92.

McLaughlin SA, Crandall CS, and McKinney PE, "Octreotide: An Antidote for Sulfonylurea-Induced Hypoglycemia," *Ann Emerg Med*, 2000, 36(2):133-8.

Mordel A, Sivilotti ML, Old AC, et al, "Octreotide for Pediatric Sulfonylurea Poisoning," *J Toxicol Clin Toxicol*, 1998, 36(5):437.

Pratap U, Slavik Z, Ofoe VD, et al, "Octreotide to Treat Postoperative Chylothorax After Cardiac Operations in Children," *Ann Thorac Surg*, 2001, 72(5):1740-2.

Roehr CC, Jung A, Proquitté H, et al, "Somatostatin or Octreotide as Treatment Options for Chylothorax in Young Children: A Systematic Review," *Intensive Care Med*, 2006, 32(5):650-7.

Siafakas C, Fox VL, and Nurko S, "Use of Octreotide for the Treatment of Severe Gastrointestinal Bleeding in Children," *J Pediatr Gastroenterol Nutr*, 1998, 26(3):356-9.

Stanley CA, "Hyperinsulinism in Infants and Children," *Pediatr Clin North Am*, 1997, 44(2):363-74.

Tang J and Weiter JJ, "Branch Retinal Artery Occlusion After Injection of a Long-Acting Risperidone Preparation," *Ann Intern Med*, 2007, 147(4):283-4.

◆ **Octreotide Acetate** *see* Octreotide Acetate *on page 1008*

◆ **Octreotide Acetate Injection (Can)** *see* Octreotide Acetate *on page 1008*

◆ **Octreotide Acetate Omega (Can)** *see* Octreotide Acetate *on page 1008*

◆ **Ocufen®** *see* Flurbiprofen *on page 605*

◆ **Ocuflox®** *see* Ofloxacin *on page 1011*

Ocular Lubricant (OK yoo lar LOO bri kant)

Therapeutic Category Lubricant, Ocular; Ophthalmic Agent, Miscellaneous

Use Ocular lubricant

Contraindications Hypersensitivity to any component

Warnings Discontinue if eye pain, vision change, redness or eye irritation occurs or if condition worsens or persists >72 hours

Adverse Reactions Ocular: Temporary blurring of vision, irritation

Stability Store away from heat

Mechanism of Action Forms an occlusive film on the surface of the eye to lubricate and protect the eye from drying

Usual Dosage Children and Adults: Ophthalmic: Apply 1/4" of ointment to the inside of the lower lid as needed

Administration Ophthalmic: Do not use with contact lenses; to avoid contamination, do not touch tip of container to any surface

Additional Information Contains petrolatum, mineral oil, chlorobutanol and lanolin alcohols

---

Dosage Forms Excipient information presented when available (limited, particularly for generics); consult specific product labeling.

Ointment, ophthalmic: 3.5 g

◆ **OcuNefrin™ [OTC]** *see* Phenylephrine *on page 1102*

◆ **Oesclim® (Can)** *see* Estradiol *on page 536*

◆ **Off-Ezy® Wart Remover [OTC] [DSC]** *see* Salicylic Acid *on page 1241*

Ofloxacin (oh FLOKS a sin)

Medication Safety Issues

Sound-alike/look-alike issues:

Floxin® may be confused with Flexeril®

Ocuflox® may be confused with Occlusal®-HP, Ocufen®

International issues:

Floxin® may be confused with Flogen® which is a brand name for naproxen in Mexico

Floxin® may be confused with Fluoxin® which is a brand name for fluoxetine in the Czech Republic and Romania

Floxin® may be confused with Flexin® which is a brand name for orphenadrine in Israel and indomethacin in Great Britain

U.S. Brand Names Floxin®; Ocuflox®

Canadian Brand Names Apo-Ofloxacin®; Apo-Oflox®; Floxin®; Novo-Ofloxacin; Ocuflox®; PMS-Ofloxacin

Therapeutic Category Antibiotic, Ophthalmic; Antibiotic, Otic; Antibiotic, Quinolone

Generic Available Yes

Use Treatment of acute bacterial exacerbations of chronic bronchitis, community-acquired pneumonia, uncomplicated skin and skin structure infections, urethral and cervical gonorrhea (acute, uncomplicated), urethritis and cervicitis (nongonococcal), pelvic inflammatory disease, uncomplicated cystitis, complicated urinary tract infections, and prostatitis caused by susceptible organisms including *S. pneumoniae, S. aureus, S. pyogenes, C. koseri, E. aerogenes, E. coli, H. influenzae, K. pneumoniae, N. gonorrhoeae, P. mirabilis, C. trachomatis,* and *P. aeruginosa*

Ophthalmic: Treatment of bacterial keratitis due to susceptible organisms including *P. aeruginosa, Propionibacterium acnes, S. marcescens, S. aureus, S. epidermidis,* and *S. pneumoniae;* treatment of severe bacterial conjunctivitis due to susceptible organisms including *Enterobacter cloacae, H. influenzae, P. mirabilis, P. aeruginosa, S. aureus, S. epidermidis,* or *S. pneumoniae*

Otic: Treatment of chronic suppurative otitis media with or without perforation of the tympanic membrane; instillation into the ear canal of patients with tympanostomy tubes for treatment of acute otitis media caused by susceptible *S. aureus, S. pneumoniae, H. influenzae, M. catarrhalis,* or *P. aeruginosa;* otitis externa caused by susceptible *S. aureus* or *P. aeruginosa*

Medication Guide An FDA-approved patient medication guide, which is available with the product information and at http://www.fda.gov/downloads/Drugs/DrugSafety/ucm088599.pdf, must be dispensed with this medication for each new outpatient prescription and refill.

Pregnancy Risk Factor C

Pregnancy Considerations Adverse events have been observed in some animal studies; therefore, the manufacturer classifies ofloxacin as pregnancy category C. Ofloxacin crosses the placenta and produces measurable concentrations in the amniotic fluid. An increased risk of teratogenic effects has not been observed in animals or humans following ofloxacin use during pregnancy; however, because of concerns of cartilage damage in immature animals, ofloxacin should only be used during pregnancy if a safer option is not available. Serum concentrations of ofloxacin may be lower during pregnancy than in nonpregnant patients.

Lactation Enters breast milk/not recommended (AAP rates "compatible")

Breast-Feeding Considerations Ofloxacin is excreted in breast milk. Breast-feeding is not recommended by the manufacturer. The AAP considers ofloxacin to be "usually compatible with breast-feeding." Due to the low concentrations in human milk, minimal toxicity would be expected in the nursing infant. Nondose-related effects could include modification of bowel flora.

Contraindications Hypersensitivity to ofloxacin, any component, or other quinolones; not recommended for use in pregnant women or during breast-feeding

Otic formulation: Patients with viral infections of the external ear canal

Warnings Oral formulation not recommended for use in children <18 years of age; ofloxacin has caused osteochondrosis in immature rats and dogs. Fluoroquinolones have caused arthropathy with erosions of the cartilage in weight-bearing joints of immature animals; Achilles tendonitis and tendon rupture have been reported with fluoroquinolones in patients of all ages **[U.S. Boxed Warning]**; risk increased in patients taking concomitant corticosteroids, patients >60 years of age, and in patients with kidney, heart, or lung transplants. Prolonged use may result in superinfection, including *C. difficile*-associated diarrhea and pseudomembranous colitis; CNS stimulation and increased intracranial pressure may occur resulting in tremors, restlessness, confusion, and rarely hallucinations, depression, nightmares, suicidal ideation, or convulsive seizures; serious and occasionally fatal hypersensitivity and/or anaphylactic reactions have been reported often following the first dose. Hypersensitivity reactions have been accompanied by cardiovascular collapse, hypotension/shock, seizure, loss of consciousness, tingling, angioedema, airway obstruction, dyspnea, urticaria, itching, and skin reactions. If these reactions occur, discontinue ofloxacin.

Precautions Use with caution in patients with known or suspected CNS disorders, seizure disorders, severe cerebral arteriosclerosis or renal impairment; modify dosage in patients with renal impairment. The use of quinolones has been linked to peripheral neuropathy (rare); discontinue if symptoms of sensory or sensorimotor neuropathy occur. Rare cases of torsade de pointes have been reported in patients taking ofloxacin so use with caution in patients on concurrent therapy with Class Ia or Class III antiarrhythmics or in patients with known prolongation of QT interval, bradycardia, cardiomyopathy, hypokalemia, or hypomagnesemia. Avoid excessive sunlight and take precautions to limit exposure (eg, loose-fitting clothing, sunscreen); may rarely cause moderate-to-severe phototoxicity reactions. Discontinue use if phototoxicity occurs.

Adverse Reactions

Cardiovascular: Cardiac failure, hypertension, hypotension, bradycardia, tachycardia, edema, torsade de pointes (rare), prolongation of QT interval, chest pain

Central nervous system: Dizziness, lightheadedness, vertigo, insomnia (more common with ofloxacin than other quinolones), fever, headache, intracranial pressure increased, seizures, fatigue, nervousness, restlessness, confusion, hallucinations, anxiety, suicidal thoughts, depression, encephalopathy, abnormal EEG

Dermatologic: Rash, pruritus, Stevens-Johnson syndrome, photosensitivity, urticaria, angioedema, toxic epidermal necrolysis, erythema multiforme

Endocrine & metabolic: Hypoglycemia, hyperglycemia, electrolyte abnormality

Gastrointestinal: Bitter taste, nausea, vomiting, diarrhea, constipation, anorexia, abdominal pain, pseudomembranous colitis, pancreatitis

Genitourinary: Vaginitis

Hematologic: Granulocytopenia, leukopenia, thrombocytopenia, hemolytic anemia

Hepatic: Liver enzymes elevated, hepatic failure, jaundice

Neuromuscular & skeletal: Tremor, arthralgia, tendonitis, tendon rupture, myalgia, peripheral neuropathy

Ocular: Ophthalmic solution: Burning, stinging, itching, foreign body sensation, conjunctival hyperemia, ocular edema, redness, photophobia, blurred vision

Otic: Otic solution: Earache, tinnitus, otorrhagia

Renal: Interstitial nephritis, acute renal insufficiency, hematuria

Respiratory: Bronchospasm, respiratory distress, dyspnea

Miscellaneous: Anaphylaxis, serum sickness syndrome

Drug Interactions

Metabolism/Transport Effects Inhibits CYP1A2 (strong)

Avoid Concomitant Use

Avoid concomitant use of Ofloxacin with any of the following: BCG

Increased Effect/Toxicity

Ofloxacin may increase the levels/effects of: Bendamustine; Corticosteroids (Systemic); CYP1A2 Substrates; Sulfonylureas; Theophylline Derivatives; Vitamin K Antagonists

The levels/effects of Ofloxacin may be increased by: Insulin; Nonsteroidal Anti-Inflammatory Agents; Probenecid

Decreased Effect

Ofloxacin may decrease the levels/effects of: BCG; Mycophenolate; Sulfonylureas; Typhoid Vaccine

The levels/effects of Ofloxacin may be decreased by: Antacids; Calcium Salts; Didanosine; Iron Salts; Magnesium Salts; Quinapril; Sevelamer; Sucralfate; Zinc Salts

Food Interactions Calcium, dairy products, iron, mineral supplements, and enteral products may decrease ofloxacin concentrations.

Stability Store tablets, ophthalmic solution, and otic solution at room temperature.

Mechanism of Action Ofloxacin inhibits DNA gyrase (bacterial topoisomerase II) thereby inhibiting relaxation of supercoiled DNA and promoting breakage of DNA strands. DNA gyrase maintains the superhelical structure of DNA and is required for DNA replication, transcription, repair, recombination, and transposition.

Pharmacokinetics (Adult data unless noted)

Absorption:

Oral: Well absorbed

Ocular: Minimal absorption unless inflammation or epithelial defect is present

Otic: Minimal absorption unless tympanic membrane is perforated

Distribution: Widely distributed into body tissues and fluids including blister fluid, cervix, lung, ovary, prostatic tissue, skin, and sputum; crosses the placenta; excreted into breast milk

V_d: 2.4-3.5 L/kg

Protein binding: 20% to 32%

Bioavailability: Oral: 98%

Half-life, biphasic: 4-7.4 hours and 20-25 hours; prolonged with renal impairment

Time to peak serum concentration: Oral 1-2 hours

Elimination: 68% to 90% is excreted unchanged in urine; 4% to 8% excreted in feces; <10% is metabolized

Usual Dosage

Oral:

Children: **Note:** Limited information regarding ofloxacin use in pediatric patients is currently available in the literature; some centers recommend doses of 15 mg/kg/day divided every 12 hours.

Adults:

Chronic bronchitis (acute exacerbation), community-acquired pneumonia, skin and skin structure infections (uncomplicated): 400 mg every 12 hours for 10 days

Urethral and cervical gonorrhea (acute, uncomplicated): 400 mg as a single dose

Cervicitis/urethritis (nongonococcal) due to *C. trachomatis* or mixed infections due to *C. trachomatis* and *N. gonorrhoeae*: 300 mg every 12 hours for 7 days

Pelvic inflammatory disease: 400 mg every 12 hours for 10-14 days

Cystitis (uncomplicated): 200 mg every 12 hours for 3-7 days

UTI (complicated): 200 mg every 12 hours for 10 days

Prostatitis: 300 mg every 12 hours for 6 weeks

Ophthalmic: Children >1 year and Adults:

Conjunctivitis: Instill 1-2 drops in affected eye(s) every 2-4 hours while awake for the first 2 days, then 4 times/day for an additional 5 days

Corneal ulcer: Instill 1-2 drops in affected eye(s) every 30 minutes while awake and every 4-6 hours at night for the first 2 days; then starting day 3, instill 1-2 drops every hour while awake for 4-6 additional days; thereafter, 1-2 drops 4 times/day until clinical cure is achieved.

Otic:

Acute otitis media with tympanostomy tubes: Children >1 year to 12 years: Instill 5 drops (0.25 mL) into the affected ear(s) twice daily for 10 days

Chronic suppurative otitis media with perforated tympanic membranes: Adolescents ≥12 years and Adults: Instill 10 drops (0.5 mL) into the affected ear(s) twice daily for 10-14 days

Otitis externa:

Children 6 months to 13 years: Instill 5 drops into the affected ear(s) once daily for 7 days

Adolescents ≥13 years and Adults: Instill 10 drops into the affected ear(s) once daily for 7 days

Dosage adjustment in renal impairment: Adults: Oral:

Cl_{cr} 20-50 mL/minute: Administer usual dose every 24 hours

Cl_{cr} <20 mL/minute: Administer half the usual dose every 24 hours

Dosage adjustment in hepatic impairment: Severe impairment: Maximum dose: 400 mg/day

Administration

Oral: May administer ofloxacin tablets with or without food; avoid antacids, vitamins with iron or minerals, sucralfate, or didanosine; use within 2 hours of administration; drink plenty of fluids to maintain proper hydration and urine output

Ophthalmic: Not for subconjunctival or direct injection into the anterior chamber of the eye. Apply gentle pressure to lacrimal sac during and immediately following instillation (1 minute) or instruct patient to gently close eyelid after administration, to decrease systemic absorption of ophthalmic drops; avoid contact of bottle tip with skin or eye. Remove contact lenses prior to administration (ophthalmic solution contains benzalkonium chloride which may adsorb to soft contact lenses); lenses may be inserted 15 minutes after administration.

Otic: Not for ophthalmic use or injection. Gently clean any discharge that can be easily removed from the outer ear. Warm otic solution by holding bottle in hand for 1-2 minutes prior to instillation. The tip of the bottle should not touch the fingers, ear, or any surface. Patient should lie on side with affected ear upward. For middle ear infections, gently press the tragus 4 times in a pumping motion to allow the drops to pass through the hole or tube in the eardrum and into the middle ear. For otitis externa infection, pull the outer ear upward and backward to allow the ear drops to flow down into the ear canal. Patient should remain on his/her side for at least 5 minutes. If necessary, repeat procedure for the other ear.

Monitoring Parameters Patients receiving concurrent ofloxacin and theophylline should have serum levels of theophylline monitored; monitor INR in patients receiving warfarin; monitor blood glucose in patients receiving antidiabetic agents; monitor renal, hepatic, hematopoietic function, and electrolytes periodically; number and type of stools/day for diarrhea

Ophthalmic: Slit-lamp biomicroscopy and fluorescein staining may be necessary

Otic: Presence of otorrhea, cultures

Patient Information Avoid contaminating otic and ophthalmic solution containers. Drink plenty of fluids; may cause dizziness or lightheadedness and impair ability to perform activities requiring mental alertness or physical coordination; notify physician if tendon pain or swelling, burning, tingling, numbness, or weakness develops, or if palpitations, chest pains, signs of allergy occurs; burning, tingling, numbness, or weakness develop; difficulty breathing, or persistent diarrhea occurs. May cause photosensitivity reactions (eg, exposure to sunlight may cause severe sunburn, skin rash, redness, or itching); avoid exposure to sunlight and artificial light sources (sunlamps, tanning booth/bed); wear protective clothing, wide-brimmed hats, sunglasses, and lip sunscreen (SPF ≥15); use a sunscreen [broad-spectrum sunscreen or physical sunscreen (preferred) or sunblock with SPF ≥15]; contact physician if reaction occurs.

Nursing Implications Do not administer antacids containing calcium, aluminum, or magnesium, iron, sucralfate, multivitamin preparations with zinc, didanosine chewable/buffered tablets or pediatric powder for oral solution with or within 2 hours before or 2 hours after a ofloxacin dose; ensure adequate patient hydration

Dosage Forms Excipient information presented when available (limited, particularly for generics); consult specific product labeling. [DSC] = Discontinued product

Solution, ophthalmic [drops]: 0.3% (5 mL, 10 mL)

Ocuflox®: 0.3% (5 mL) [contains benzalkonium chloride]

Solution, otic [drops]: 0.3% (5 mL, 10 mL)

Floxin®: 0.3% (5 mL, 10 mL) [contains benzalkonium chloride] [DSC]

Floxin® Otic Singles™: 0.3% (0.25 mL) [contains benzalkonium chloride; packaged as 2 single-dose containers per pouch, 10 pouches per carton, total net volume 5 mL] [DSC]

Tablet: 200 mg, 300 mg, 400 mg

References

Alghasham AA and Nahata MC, "Clinical Use of Fluoroquinolones in Children," *Ann Pharmacother*, 2000, 34(3):347-59.

♦ **Oforta™** *see* Fludarabine *on page 587*

♦ **OKT3** *see* Muromonab-CD3 *on page 955*

♦ **Oleovitamin A** *see* Vitamin A *on page 1426*

♦ **Oleptro™** *see* TraZODone *on page 1371*

♦ **Oleum Ricini** *see* Castor Oil *on page 259*

Olsalazine (ole SAL a zeen)

Medication Safety Issues

Sound-alike/look-alike issues:

Olsalazine may be confused with OLANZapine

Dipentum® may be confused with Dilantin®

U.S. Brand Names Dipentum®

Canadian Brand Names Dipentum®

◀ **Therapeutic Category** 5-Aminosalicylic Acid Derivative; Anti-inflammatory Agent

Generic Available No

Use Maintenance of remission of ulcerative colitis in patients intolerant to sulfasalazine (FDA approved in adults)

Pregnancy Risk Factor C

Pregnancy Considerations Animal studies have demonstrated fetal developmental toxicities. There are no well-controlled studies in pregnant women. Use during pregnancy only if clearly necessary.

Lactation Enters breast milk/not recommended

Breast-Feeding Considerations The active metabolite, 5-aminosalicylic acid may pass into breast milk. Diarrhea has been reported in breast-fed infants whose mothers took olsalazine.

Contraindications Hypersensitivity to olsalazine, salicylates, or any component

Warnings Diarrhea is a common adverse effect of olsalazine. May exacerbate symptoms of colitis.

Precautions Use with caution in patients with hypersensitivity to sulfasalazine or mesalamine. Use with caution in patients with asthma, severe allergies, hepatic impairment, or renal impairment.

Adverse Reactions

Cardiovascular: Chest pain, edema, heart block (second degree), hypertension, myocarditis, orthostatic hypotension, pericarditis, tachycardia

Central nervous system: Depression, dizziness, fever, insomnia, vertigo

Dermatologic: Erythema nodosum, photosensitivity, pruritus, rash

Gastrointestinal: Bloating, cramps, diarrhea, nausea, pancreatitis, rectal bleeding, vomiting, xerostomia

Genitourinary: Dysuria, urinary frequency

Hematologic: Anemia, eosinophilia, leukopenia, lymphopenia, neutropenia, pancytopenia, reticulocytosis, thrombocytopenia

Hepatic: AST and ALT increased, hepatic failure, hepatic necrosis, mild cholestatic hepatitis,

Neuromuscular & skeletal: Arthralgia, myalgia, paresthesia, peripheral neuropathy, tremor

Ocular: Blurred vision, dry eyes

Otic: Tinnitus

Renal: Hematuria, interstitial nephritis, proteinuria

Respiratory: Bronchospasm, respiratory infection

<1% and postmarketing: Angioneurotic edema, aplastic anemia, bilirubin increased, cirrhosis, dyspnea, hepatitis, interstitial lung disease, jaundice, Kawasaki-like syndrome, pancytopenia, paraesthesia, peripheral neuropathy, pyrexia

Drug Interactions

Avoid Concomitant Use There are no known interactions where it is recommended to avoid concomitant use.

Increased Effect/Toxicity

Olsalazine may increase the levels/effects of: Heparin; Heparin (Low Molecular Weight); Thiopurine Analogs; Varicella Virus-Containing Vaccines

Decreased Effect

Olsalazine may decrease the levels/effects of: Cardiac Glycosides

Mechanism of Action Olsalazine is a sodium salt of a salicylate compound that is effectively bioconverted by colonic bacteria to 5-aminosalicylic acid (5-ASA). The exact mechanism of action appears to be topical rather than systemic. It may diminish colonic inflammation by blocking cyclooxygenase and inhibiting colon prostaglandin production in the bowel mucosa.

Pharmacokinetics (Adult data unless noted)

Absorption: <3%; very little intact olsalazine is systemically absorbed

Protein binding: >99%

Metabolism: Mostly by colonic bacteria to the active drug, 5-aminosalicylic acid

Bioavailability: 2.4%

Half-life, elimination: 54 minutes (in serum)

Elimination: Primarily in feces; <1% eliminated in urine

Usual Dosage Adults: Oral: 1 g/day in 2 divided doses

Administration Oral: Administer with food in evenly divided doses

Patient Information Contact physician if diarrhea occurs. May cause dry mouth. May rarely cause photosensitivity reactions (eg, exposure to sunlight may cause severe sunburn, skin rash, redness, or itching); avoid direct exposure to sunlight.

Dosage Forms Excipient information presented when available (limited, particularly for generics); consult specific product labeling.

Capsule, as sodium:
  Dipentum®: 250 mg

◆ **Olsalazine Sodium** *see* Olsalazine *on page 1013*

◆ **Olux®** *see* Clobetasol *on page 331*

◆ **Olux-E™** *see* Clobetasol *on page 331*

◆ **Olux®/Olux-E™ CP** *see* Clobetasol *on page 331*

Omalizumab (oh mah lye ZOO mab)

Medication Safety Issues

Sound-alike/look-alike issues:
  Omalizumab may be confused with ofatumumab

U.S. Brand Names Xolair®

Canadian Brand Names Xolair®

Therapeutic Category Monoclonal Antibody, Anti-Asthmatic

Generic Available No

Use Treatment of moderate to severe, persistent allergic asthma not adequately controlled with inhaled corticosteroids

Medication Guide An FDA-approved patient medication guide, which is available with the product information and at http://www.fda.gov/downloads/Drugs/DrugSafety/ucm089829.pdf, must be dispensed with this medication for each new outpatient prescription and refill.

Pregnancy Risk Factor B

Pregnancy Considerations Teratogenic effects were not observed in animal studies. There are no adequate and well-controlled studies in pregnant women. IgG molecules are known to cross the placenta; use during pregnancy only if clearly needed. A registry has been established to monitor outcomes of women exposed to omalizumab during pregnancy or within 8 weeks prior to pregnancy (866-496-5247).

Lactation Excretion in breast milk unknown/use caution

Breast-Feeding Considerations IgG is excreted in human milk and excretion of omalizumab is expected. Effects to nursing infant are not known; use with caution.

Contraindications Hypersensitivity to omalizumab or any component

Warnings Not indicated for use in the control of acute asthma symptoms. Anaphylaxis, including delayed-onset anaphylaxis, has been reported following administration **[U.S. Boxed Warning]**; reactions usually occur within 2 hours of administration, but may occur up to 24 hours and in some cases >24 hours after treatment. Patients should receive treatment only under direct medical supervision and be observed for a minimum of 2 hours following administration; providers and patients should have appropriate treatment for anaphylaxis available. Hypersensitivity reactions may occur following any dose, even during chronic therapy; discontinue therapy following any severe reaction. Injection site reactions typically occur within 1 hour postinjection, last <8 days, and generally decrease in frequency after subsequent doses. Due to the risk of delayed anaphylaxis, patients should be fully prepared and trained on the appropriate emergency self-treatment of an anaphylactic reaction. Safety and efficacy in children <12 years of age has not been established.

Malignant neoplasms of varying types (breast, non-melanoma skin, prostate, and parotid) were observed in 0.5% of patients during clinical trials (compared with 0.2% in controls); the majority of these patients received omalizumab for <1 year; risk of long-term exposure to omalizumab is not known. Systemic or inhaled cortico-steroid use should not be abruptly discontinued upon initiation of omalizumab therapy; gradual tapering under medical supervision is recommended. In a one year clinical trial in Brazil, patients with increased risk of geohelminthic infections (roundworm, hookworm, whipworm, thread-worm) experienced an increase in geohelminthic infections when compared with the control group (42% vs 53%).

Preliminary findings of an ongoing safety review suggest an increased risk of cardiovascular (eg, arrhythmias, cardiomyopathy, ischemic heart disease, heart failure, pulmonary hypertension), cerebrovascular, and throm-boembolic adverse events in patients treated with omalizumab.

Precautions Dosage and frequency of administration are dependent upon the serum total IgE level and body weight. Total IgE level must be measured prior to beginning treatment. Total IgE levels are elevated during treatment and remain elevated for up to one year after the discontinuation of treatment. Remeasurement of IgE levels during omalizumab treatment should not be used as a guide to dosage. Remeasurement of IgE levels may be used after treatment has been discontinued for at least one year.

Adverse Reactions

Cardiovascular: Hot flushes

Central nervous system: Headache, dizziness, fatigue

Dermatologic: Urticaria, dermatitis, pruritus, alopecia

Hematologic: Thrombocytopenia

Local: Injection site reactions (bruising, redness, warmth, burning, stinging, pain, induration, and inflammation occurring within 1 hour of injection and persisting up to 8 days decreasing in frequency with repeated administration)

Neuromuscular & skeletal: Arthralgia, leg pain, arm pain

Respiratory: Upper respiratory infections, sinusitis, phar-yngitis, wheezing

Miscellaneous: Anaphylaxis (see Warnings), hypersensi-tivity reactions, rate of infections increased including viral infections

Drug Interactions

Avoid Concomitant Use

Avoid concomitant use of Omalizumab with any of the following: BCG; Natalizumab; Pimecrolimus; Tacrolimus (Topical); Vaccines (Live)

Increased Effect/Toxicity

Omalizumab may increase the levels/effects of: Lefluno-mide; Natalizumab; Vaccines (Live)

The levels/effects of Omalizumab may be increased by: Denosumab; Pimecrolimus; Tacrolimus (Topical); Trastuzumab

Decreased Effect

Omalizumab may decrease the levels/effects of: BCG; Sipuleucel-T; Vaccines (Inactivated); Vaccines (Live)

The levels/effects of Omalizumab may be decreased by: Echinacea

Stability Store in refrigerator at 2°C to 8°C (36°F to 46°F); omalizumab is provided in a single use vial with no preservatives; the reconstituted solution is stable for 4 hours at room temperature and 8 hours refrigerated

Mechanism of Action Omalizumab is an IgG monoclonal antibody which binds to free (unbound) IgE and prevents the binding of IgE to the high-affinity IgE receptor on the surface of mast cells and basophils. By decreasing bound IgE, the activation and release of mediators in the allergic response (early and late phase) is limited. Both the free (unbound) IgE serum level and the number of high-affinity IgE receptors are decreased. Long-term treatment in patients with allergic asthma showed a decrease in asthma exacerbations and corticosteroid usage.

Pharmacodynamics Response to therapy: ~12-16 weeks (87% of patients had measurable response in 12 weeks)

Pharmacokinetics (Adult data unless noted)

Absorption: Slow after SubQ administration

Distribution: V_d: 78 ± 32 mL/kg

Metabolism: Hepatic: IgG degradation by reticuloendothe-lial system and endothelial cells

Bioavailability: Absolute: 62%

Half-life: Adults: 1-4 weeks

Time to peak serum concentration: 7-8 days

Excretion: Primarily via hepatic degradation; intact IgG may be secreted in bile

Clearance: 2.4 ± 1.1 mL/kg/day

Usual Dosage Dosage and frequency of administration are dependent upon the serum total IgE level and body weight. Measure total IgE level prior to beginning treat-ment. Total IgE levels are elevated during treatment and remain elevated for up to one year after the discontinuation of treatment. Remeasurement of IgE levels during omalizumab treatment should not be used as a guide to dosage.

Asthma: Children ≥12 years and Adults: SubQ: 0.016 mg/ kg/international unit of IgE every 4 weeks.

The following is the manufacturer's recommendation:

IgE ≥30-100 international units/mL:
  30-90 kg: 150 mg every 4 weeks
  >90-150 kg: 300 mg every 4 weeks

IgE >100-200 international units/mL:
  30-90 kg: 300 mg every 4 weeks
  >90-150 kg: 225 mg every 2 weeks

IgE >200-300 international units/mL:
  30-60 kg: 300 mg every 4 weeks
  >60-90 kg: 225 mg every 2 weeks
  >90-150 kg: 300 mg every 2 weeks

IgE >300-400 international units/mL:
  30-70 kg: 225 mg every 2 weeks
  >70-90 kg: 300 mg every 2 weeks
  >90 kg: Do not use*

IgE >400-500 international units/mL:
  30-70 kg: 300 mg every 2 weeks
  >70-90 kg: 375 mg every 2 weeks
  >90 kg: Do not use*

IgE >500-600 international units/mL:
  30-60 kg: 300 mg every 2 weeks
  >60-70 kg: 375 mg every 2 weeks
  >70 kg: Do not use*

IgE >600-700 international units/mL:
  30-60 kg: 375 mg every 2 weeks
  >60 kg: Do not use*

*Dosage has not been studied and approved for this weight and IgE level

Administration SubQ: Reconstitute 150 mg vial with 1.4 mL SWI; swirl vial for approximately 1 minute to evenly wet powder; repeat swirling for 5-10 seconds every 5 minutes in order to dissolve remaining solids; dissolution time is at least 20 minutes. Reconstituted solution will be viscous with no visible gel-like particles present in solution. Do not use if contents of vial do not dissolve within 40 minutes. Resulting concentration is 150 mg/1.2 mL (125 mg/mL). Due to viscosity, injection may take 5-10 seconds to administer. Doses >150 mg should be divided into more than one injection site.

Monitoring Parameters Baseline total serum IgE, pulmonary function tests, anaphylactic/hypersensitivity reactions

Reference Range See Usual Dosage

Patient Information Do not alter asthma medications without consulting physician. Patient should read the accompanying Medication Guide before starting treatment and before each subsequent treatment. Report any signs and symptoms of allergic reactions including difficulty breathing, difficulty swallowing, swelling of the throat or tongue, cough, chest tightness, and generalized itching to your healthcare provider immediately.

Additional Information Omalizumab was used successfully in a double-blind, randomized, placebo-controlled study of 334 children between the ages of 6-12 years; omalizumab dosage was based on body weight and serum total IgE. Patients received omalizumab at either 2- or 4-week intervals with a dosage equal to 0.016 mg/kg/IgE (international units/mL) per 4 weeks. 55% of patients were able to discontinue corticosteroid use (Milgrom, 2003). A registry has been established to monitor outcomes of women exposed to omalizumab during pregnancy or within 8 weeks prior to pregnancy (866-496-5247).

Dosage Forms Excipient information presented when available (limited, particularly for generics); consult specific product labeling.
Injection, powder for reconstitution [preservative free]:
Xolair®: 150 mg [contains sucrose 145.5 g]

References
Berger W, Gupta N, McAlary M, et al, "Evaluation of Long-Term Safety of the Anti-IgE Antibody, Omalizumab, in Children with Allergic Asthma," *Ann Allergy Asthma Immunol*, 2003, 91(2):182-8.
Casale TB, Condemi J, LaForce C, et al, "Effect of Omalizumab on Symptoms of Seasonal Allergic Rhinitis: A Randomized Controlled Trial," *JAMA*, 2001, 286(23):2956-67.
Milgrom H, Berger W, Nayak A, et al, "Treatment of Childhood Asthma With Anti-Immunoglobulin E Antibody (Omalizumab)," *Pediatrics*, 2001, 108(2):E36.
Milgrom H, Fick RB Jr, Su JQ, et al, "Treatment of Allergic Asthma With Monoclonal Anti-IgE Antibody. rhuMAb-E25 Study Group," *Engl J Med*, 1999, 341(26):1966-73.
Strunk RC and Bloomberg GR, "Omalizumab for Asthma," *N Engl J Med*, 2006, 354(25):2689-95.

Omeprazole (oh ME pray zol)

Medication Safety Issues
Sound-alike/look-alike issues:
Omeprazole may be confused with aripiprazole, fomepizole
Prilosec® may be confused with Plendil®, Prevacid®, predniSONE, prilocaine, Prinivil®, Proventil®, Prozac®

International issues:
Losec [multiple international markets] may be confused with Lasix®, a brand name for furosemide [U.S., Canada, and multiple international markets]
Norpramin: Brand name for omeprazole [Spain], but also the brand name for desipramine [U.S., Canada] and enalapril/hydrochlorothiazide [Portugal]

U.S. Brand Names Prilosec OTC™ [OTC]; Prilosec®

Canadian Brand Names Apo-Omeprazole®; Losec MUPS®; Losec®; Mylan-Omeprazole; PMS-Omeprazole; PMS-Omeprazole DR; ratio-Omeprazole; Sandoz-Omeprazole

Therapeutic Category Gastric Acid Secretion Inhibitor; Gastrointestinal Agent, Gastric or Duodenal Ulcer Treatment; Proton Pump Inhibitor

Generic Available Yes: Excludes granules for suspension

Use Treatment and maintenance of healing of severe erosive esophagitis (grade 2 or above) (FDA approved for children ≥1 year and adults); treatment of active duodenal ulcer; treatment of active benign gastric ulcers; treatment of symptomatic gastroesophageal reflux disease (GERD) (FDA approved for children ≥1 year and adults); treatment of pathological hypersecretory conditions; treatment of peptic ulcer disease; adjunctive treatment of duodenal ulcers associated with *Helicobacter pylori*; relief of frequent heartburn (OTC products)

Pregnancy Risk Factor C

Pregnancy Considerations Adverse events were observed in some animal reproduction studies. Based on data collected by the Teratogen Information System (TERIS), it was concluded that therapeutic doses used during pregnancy would be unlikely to pose a substantial teratogenic risk (quantity/quality of data: fair). Because the possibility of harm still exists, the manufacturer recommends use during pregnancy only if the potential benefit to the mother outweighs the possible risk to the fetus.

Lactation Enters breast milk/not recommended

Contraindications Hypersensitivity to omeprazole, substituted benzimidazole proton pump inhibitors (eg, esomeprazole, lansoprazole), or any component

Warnings In long-term (2-year) studies in rats, omeprazole produced a dose-related increase in gastric carcinoid tumors. While available endoscopic evaluations and histologic examinations of biopsy specimens from human stomachs have not detected a risk from short-term exposure to omeprazole, further human data on the effect of sustained hypochlorhydria and hypergastrinemia are needed to rule out the possibility of an increased risk for the development of tumors in humans receiving long-term therapy. Atrophic gastritis has been reported occasionally in gastric corpus biopsies from patients treated long-term with omeprazole. Symptomatic response to therapy does not prelude the presence of GI malignancy. Use of gastric acid inhibitors, including proton pump inhibitors and H_2 blockers, has been associated with an increased risk for development of acute gastroenteritis and community-acquired pneumonia (Canani, 2006).

Precautions Bioavailability may be increased in patients with hepatic dysfunction or patients of Asian descent; consider dosage reductions, especially for maintenance healing of erosive esophagitis

Adverse Reactions
Cardiovascular: Chest pain, tachycardia, bradycardia, palpitations, hypertension
Central nervous system: Headache, dizziness, vertigo, insomnia, confusion, anxiety, hemifacial dysesthesia, nervousness, fever, fatigue, malaise, depression, aggression, hallucinations
Dermatologic: Rash, dry skin, urticaria, pruritus, alopecia, toxic epidermal necrolysis (rare), Stevens-Johnson syndrome (rare), erythema multiforme, hyperhydrosis
Endocrine & metabolic: Hypoglycemia, hyponatremia, weight gain, gynecomastia
Gastrointestinal: Diarrhea, nausea, abdominal pain, vomiting, constipation, flatulence, discoloration of feces, irritable colon, xerostomia, anorexia, dysgeusia, abdominal pain, atrophic gastritis, pancreatitis (some fatal), anorexia, fecal discoloration, gastric fundic polyps, mucosal atrophy of tongue, taste perversion
Genitourinary: Urinary frequency
Hematologic: Agranulocytosis, pancytopenia, thrombocytopenia, anemia, leukocytosis, hemolytic anemia
Hepatic: Hepatitis, liver function tests elevated, jaundice, liver necrosis
Neuromuscular & skeletal: Muscle cramps, myalgia, arthralgia, leg pain, paresthesia, back pain, joint pain

Ocular: Blurred vision, ocular irritation, optic atrophy, dry eyes, anterior ischemic optic neuropathy, optic neuritis, double vision

Otic: Tinnitus, otitis media

Renal: Hematuria, pyuria, proteinuria, glycosuria, interstitial nephritis, UTI, serum creatinine elevated

Respiratory: Pharyngeal pain, cough, epistaxis, URI, bronchospasm

Miscellaneous: Hypersensitivity reactions

Drug Interactions

Metabolism/Transport Effects Substrate of CYP2A6 (minor), 2C9 (minor), 2C19 (major), 2D6 (minor), 3A4 (major); **Inhibits** CYP1A2 (weak), 2C9 (moderate), 2C19 (strong), 2D6 (weak), 3A4 (weak); **Induces** CYP1A2 (weak)

Avoid Concomitant Use

Avoid concomitant use of Omeprazole with any of the following: Delavirdine; Erlotinib; Nelfinavir; Posaconazole

Increased Effect/Toxicity

Omeprazole may increase the levels/effects of: Benzodiazepines (metabolized by oxidation); Carvedilol; Cilostazol; Clozapine; CycloSPORINE; CycloSPORINE (Systemic); CYP2C19 Substrates; CYP2C9 Substrates (High risk); Methotrexate; Phenytoin; Raltegravir; Saquinavir; Tacrolimus; Tacrolimus (Systemic); Vitamin K Antagonists; Voriconazole

The levels/effects of Omeprazole may be increased by: Clopidogrel; Fluconazole; Ketoconazole; Ketoconazole (Systemic)

Decreased Effect

Omeprazole may decrease the levels/effects of: Atazanavir; Cefditoren; Clopidogrel; Clozapine; Dabigatran Etexilate; Dasatinib; Delavirdine; Erlotinib; Indinavir; Iron Salts; Itraconazole; Ketoconazole; Ketoconazole (Systemic); Mesalamine; Mycophenolate; Nelfinavir; Posaconazole

The levels/effects of Omeprazole may be decreased by: CYP2C19 Inducers (Strong); Peginterferon Alfa-2b; Tipranavir

Food Interactions A 25% reduction in peak plasma concentration was measured when the 20 mg capsule was mixed with applesauce; there was no change in AUC; the clinical significance is unknown. There was no change in peak plasma level or AUC when the 40 mg capsule was mixed with applesauce.

Stability Omeprazole stability is a function of pH; it is rapidly degraded in acidic media but has acceptable stability under alkaline conditions. Each capsule of omeprazole contains enteric-coated granules to prevent omeprazole degradation by gastric acidity.

Delayed release capsules and oral suspension: Store at 25°C (77°F); excursions permitted to 15°C to 30°C (59°F to 86°F)

Mechanism of Action Suppresses gastric acid secretion by inhibiting the parietal cell membrane enzyme (H^+/K^+)-ATPase or proton pump; demonstrates antimicrobial activity against *Helicobacter pylori*

Pharmacodynamics

Onset of action: 1 hour

Maximum effect: 2 hours

Duration: 72 hours; 50% of maximum effect at 24 hours; after stopping treatment, secretory activity gradually returns over 3-5 days

Maximum secretory inhibition: 4 days

Pharmacokinetics (Adult data unless noted)

Absorption: Rapid

Protein binding: 95%

Metabolism: Extensively hepatic by cytochrome P450 system; saturable first pass effect

Bioavailability: 30% to 40%; improves slightly with repeated administration; increased in Asians and those with hepatic disease; excreted into breast milk (peak concentration in breast milk <7% of corresponding peak plasma concentration)

Half-life: Adults: 0.5-1 hour; chronic hepatic disease: 3 hours

Time to peak serum concentration: 0.5-3.5 hours

Elimination:

Clearance: Adults: 500-600 mL/minute; chronic hepatic disease: 70 mL/minute

Note: Half-life and AUC were significantly reduced for omeprazole suspension when compared with an equivalent dose via the commercially available capsule in 7 adults (Song, 2001).

Usual Dosage Oral:

Children:

GERD, ulcers, esophagitis: Manufacturer's recommendations: Children 1-16 years:

5 kg to <10 kg: 5 mg once daily

10 kg to ≤20 kg: 10 mg once daily

>20 kg: 20 mg once daily

Alternate dosing: 1 mg/kg/dose once or twice daily; range of effective dosages in the literature: 0.2-3.5 mg/kg/day (Hassall, 2000; Zimmermann, 2001). Higher doses may be necessary in children between 1-6 years of age due to increased metabolic clearance (Andersson, 2000). In critically ill children to maintain gastric pH >5, administration every 6-8 hours may be necessary (1.5-2 mg/kg/day) (Kaufman, 2002)

Adjunctive therapy of duodenal ulcers associated with *Helicobacter pylori* (in combination with antibiotic therapy either clarithromycin or clarithromycin and amoxicillin) in children (Gottrand, 2001):

15-30 kg: 10 mg twice daily

>30 kg: 20 mg twice daily

Adolescents and Adults:

Active duodenal ulcer: 20 mg/day for 4-8 weeks

Gastric ulcers: 40 mg/day for 4-8 weeks

GERD or severe erosive esophagitis: 20 mg/day for 4-8 weeks

Maintenance of healing of erosive esophagitis: 20 mg/day

Pathological hypersecretory conditions: 60 mg/day to start; doses up to 120 mg 3 times/day have been administered; administer daily doses >80 mg in divided doses

Frequent heartburn (≥2 times/week): 20 mg/day for 14 days

Adjunctive therapy of duodenal ulcers associated with *Helicobacter pylori* (in combination with antibiotic therapy either clarithromycin or clarithromycin and amoxicillin): 20 mg twice daily for 10 days (in combination with two antibiotics) or 40 mg once daily for 14 days

Note: If an ulcer is present at the time of initial therapy, the recommended duration of treatment should be extended an additional 18 days (dual therapy) or 14 days (triple therapy).

Dosage adjustment in hepatic impairment: Bioavailability is increased with chronic liver disease. Consider dosage adjustment, especially for maintenance healing of erosive esophagitis. Specific guidelines are not available.

Administration

Oral:

Capsule: Should be swallowed whole; do not chew or crush. Delayed release capsule may be opened and contents added to 1 tablespoon of applesauce and pellets swallowed whole (use immediately after adding to applesauce).

Oral suspension: Empty the contents of the 2.5 mg packet or 10 mg packet into 5 mL or 15 mL of water, respectively; stir, the suspension should be left to thicken for 2-3 minutes and administered within 30 minutes. If any material remains after administration, add more water, stir, and administer immediately.

Tablet: Should be swallowed whole; do not crush or chew.

Nasogastric tube administration:

Capsule: When using capsules to extemporaneously prepare a solution for NG administration, the manufacturers of Prilosec® recommend the use of an acidic juice for preparation and administration.

Oral suspension: Add 5 mL of water to a catheter-tipped syringe and then add the contents of a 2.5 mg packet (or 15 mL of water for the 10 mg packet), shake the suspension well and leave to thicken for 2-3 minutes. Administer within 30 minutes of reconstitution. Use an NG or gastric tube that is a French size 6 or larger; flush the syringe and tube with water.

Patient Information May cause dry mouth; do not chew or crush granules

Dosage Forms Excipient information presented when available (limited, particularly for generics); consult specific product labeling.

Capsule, delayed release: 10 mg, 20 mg, 40 mg

Prilosec®: 10 mg, 20 mg, 40 mg

Granules for suspension, delayed release, enteric coated, oral:

Prilosec®: 2.5 mg/packet (30s); 10 mg/packet (30s)

Tablet, delayed release: 20 mg

Prilosec OTC™: 20 mg

Extemporaneous Preparations

Omeprazole 2 mg/mL suspension may be made by adding 100 mL 8.4% sodium bicarbonate solution to the contents of ten 20 mg omeprazole capsules; stir for 30 minutes; protect from light; stable 14 days at room temperature and 45 days refrigerated

DiGiacinto JL, Olsen KM, Bergman KL, et al, "Stability of Suspension Formulations of Lansoprazole and Omeprazole Stored in Amber-Colored Plastic Oral Syringes," *Ann Pharmacother*, 2000, 34(5):600-4.

References

Andersson T, Hassall E, Lundborg P, et al, "Pharmacokinetics of Orally Administered Omeprazole in Children. International Pediatric Omeprazole Pharmacokinetic Group," *Am J Gastroenterol*, 2000, 95 (11):3101-6.

Canani RB, Cirillo P, Roggero P, et al, "Therapy With Gastric Acidity Inhibitors Increases the Risk of Acute Gastroenteritis and Community-Acquired Pneumonia in Children," *Pediatrics*, 2006, 117(5):e817-20.

Gibbons TE and Gold BD, "The Use of Proton Pump Inhibitors in Children: A Comprehensive Review," *Paediatr Drugs*, 2003, 5 (1):25-40.

Gottrand F, Kalach N, Spyckerelle C, et al, "Omeprazole Combined With Amoxicillin and Clarithromycin in the Eradication of *Helicobacter pylori* in Children With Gastritis: A Prospective Randomized Double-Blind Trial," *J Pediatr*, 2001, 139(5):664-8.

Gunasekaran TS and Hassall EG, "Efficacy and Safety of Omeprazole for Severe Gastroesophageal Reflux in Children," *J Pediatr*, 1993, 123(1):148-54.

Hassall E, Israel D, Shepherd R, "Omeprazole for Treatment of Chronic Erosive Esophagitis in Children: A Multicenter Study of Efficacy, Safety, Tolerability and Dose Requirements. International Pediatric Omeprazole Study Group," *J Pediatr*, 2000, 137(6):800-7.

Kane DL, "Administration of Omeprazole (Prilosec™) in the Atypical Patient," *Int J Pharm Compounding*, 1997, 1(1):13.

Kato S, Ebina K, Fujii K, et al, "Effect of Omeprazole in the Treatment of Refractory Acid-Related Diseases in Childhood: Endoscopic Healing and Twenty-Four Hour Intragastric Acidity," *J Pediatr*, 1996, 128 (3):415-21.

Kaufman SS, Lyden ER, Brown CR, et al, "Omeprazole Therapy in Pediatric Patients After Liver and Intestinal Transplantation," *J Pediatr Gastroenterol Nutr*, 2002, 34(2):194-8.

Song JC, Quercia RA, Fan C, et al, "Pharmacokinetic Comparison of Omeprazole Capsules and a Simplified Omeprazole Suspension," *Am J Health Syst Pharm*, 2001, 58(8):689-94.

Zimmermann AE, Walters JK, Katona BG, et al, "A Review of Omeprazole Use in the Treatment of Acid-Related Disorders in Children," *Clin Ther*, 2001, 23(5):660-79.

Omeprazole and Sodium Bicarbonate

(oh MEP ra zole & SOW dee um bye KAR bun ate)

Medication Safety Issues

Sound-alike/look-alike issues:

Zegerid® may be confused with Zestril®

Related Information

Sodium Content of Selected Medicinals *on page 1724*

U.S. Brand Names Zegerid OTC™ [OTC]; Zegerid®

Therapeutic Category Proton Pump Inhibitor; Substituted Benzimidazole

Generic Available No

Use Short-term (4-8 weeks) treatment of active duodenal ulcer disease or active benign gastric ulcer; treatment of symptomatic gastroesophageal reflux disease (GERD) (FDA approved in adults); treatment and maintenance healing of erosive esophagitis; reduction of risk of upper gastrointestinal bleeding in critically ill patients (FDA approved in adults)

OTC labeling: Relief of frequent (≥2 days/week), uncomplicated heartburn (FDA approved in adults)

Pregnancy Risk Factor C

Pregnancy Considerations Adverse events were observed in some animal reproduction studies. Based on data collected by the Teratogen Information System (TERIS), it was concluded that therapeutic doses used during pregnancy would be unlikely to pose a substantial teratogenic risk (quantity/quality of data: fair). Because the possibility of harm still exists, the manufacturer recommends use during pregnancy only if the potential benefit to the mother outweighs the possible risk to the fetus. Chronic use of sodium bicarbonate-containing products may lead to systemic alkalosis, edema, and weight gain; metabolic alkalosis and fluid overload may occur in mother and fetus.

Lactation Enters breast milk/not recommended

Contraindications Hypersensitivity to omeprazole, substituted benzimidazole proton pump inhibitors (eg, esomeprazole, lansoprazole), or any component.

Warnings

Use of proton pump inhibitors may increase the risk of gastrointestinal infections (eg, *Salmonella, Campylobacter*). Relief of symptoms does not preclude the presence of a gastric malignancy. Atrophic gastritis (by biopsy) has been noted with long-term omeprazole therapy. In long-term (2-year) studies in rats, omeprazole produced a dose-related increase in gastric carcinoid tumors. While available endoscopic evaluations and histologic examinations of biopsy specimens from human stomachs have not detected a risk from short-term exposure to omeprazole, further human data on the effect of sustained hypochlorhydria and hypergastrinemia are needed to rule out the possibility of an increased risk for the development of tumors in humans receiving long-term therapy. Bioavailability may be increased in the elderly, Asian population, and those with hepatic dysfunction.

Precautions Use with caution in patients with Bartter's syndrome, hypokalemia, and respiratory alkalosis due to high content of sodium bicarbonate; avoid use in patients on sodium-restrictive diets; chronic use may lead to systemic alkalosis, edema, and weight gain

Adverse Reactions

Cardiovascular: Atrial fibrillation, bradycardia, edema (see Warnings), hyper/hypotension, tachycardia

Central nervous system: Agitation, dizziness, fever, headache

Dermatologic: Rash

Endocrine & metabolic: Hyper/hypoglycemia, hyper/hypo-kalemia, hyper/hyponatremia, hypocalcemia, hypomagnesemia, hypophosphatemia

Gastrointestinal: Abdominal pain, constipation, diarrhea, flatulence, hypomotility, nausea, oral candidiasis, vomiting

Hematologic: Anemia, thrombocytopenia

Neuromuscular & skeletal: Back pain

Respiratory: Cough

Miscellaneous: Infections

<1%, postmarketing, and/or case reports: Abdominal swelling, abnormal dreams, aggression, agranulocytosis, alkaline phosphatase increased, allergic reactions, alopecia, anaphylaxis, angina, angioedema, anorexia, anxiety, apathy, atrophic gastritis, benign gastric polyps, blurred vision, confusion, creatinine increased, depression, diaphoresis, double vision, dry mouth, dry skin, epistaxis, erythema multiforme, esophageal candidiasis, fatigue, fecal discoloration, glycosuria, gynecomastia, hallucinations, hematuria, hemifacial dysesthesia, hemolytic anemia, hepatic encephalopathy, hepatic failure, hepatic necrosis, hyperhidrosis, interstitial nephritis, irritable colon, jaundice, joint pain, leg pain, leukocytosis, leukopenia, liver disease (hepatocellular, cholestatic, mixed), malaise, microscopic pyuria, mucosal atrophy (tongue), muscle cramps, muscle weakness, myalgia, nervousness, neutropenia, ocular irritation, optic neuropathy, pain, palpitation, pancreatitis, pancytopenia, paresthesia, peripheral edema, petechiae, pharyngeal pain, photosensitivity, pneumothorax, proteinuria, pruritus, psychic disturbance, purpura, skin inflammation, somnolence, Stevens-Johnson syndrome, stomatitis, taste perversion, testicular pain, tinnitus, toxic epidermal necrolysis, tremor, urinary frequency, urinary tract infection, urticaria, vertigo, weight gain

Drug Interactions

Metabolism/Transport Effects **Substrate** of CYP2A6 (minor), 2C9 (minor), 2C19 (major), 2D6 (minor), 3A4 (minor); **Inhibits** CYP1A2 (weak), 2C9 (moderate), 2C19 (strong), 2D6 (weak), 3A4 (weak); **Induces** CYP1A2 (weak)

Avoid Concomitant Use

Avoid concomitant use of Omeprazole and Sodium Bicarbonate with any of the following: Delavirdine; Erlotinib; Nelfinavir; Posaconazole

Increased Effect/Toxicity

Omeprazole and Sodium Bicarbonate may increase the levels/effects of: Alpha-/Beta-Agonists; Amphetamines; Benzodiazepines (metabolized by oxidation); Cilostazol; Clozapine; CycloSPORINE; CycloSPORINE (Systemic); CYP2C19 Substrates; CYP2C9 Substrates (High risk); Flecainide; Memantine; Methotrexate; Phenytoin; QuiNIDine; QuiNINE; Raltegravir; Saquinavir; Tacrolimus; Tacrolimus (Systemic); Vitamin K Antagonists; Voriconazole

The levels/effects of Omeprazole and Sodium Bicarbonate may be increased by: Calcium Polystyrene Sulfonate; Clopidogrel; Fluconazole; Ketoconazole; Ketoconazole (Systemic)

Decreased Effect

Omeprazole and Sodium Bicarbonate may decrease the levels/effects of: ACE Inhibitors; Anticonvulsants (Hydantoin); Antifungal Agents (Azole Derivatives, Systemic); Antipsychotic Agents (Phenothiazines); Atazanavir; Bisacodyl; Cefditoren; Cefpodoxime; Cefuroxime; Chloroquine; Clopidogrel; Clozapine; Corticosteroids (Oral); Dabigatran Etexilate; Dasatinib; Delavirdine; Erlotinib; Flecainide; HMG-CoA Reductase Inhibitors; Indinavir; Iron Salts; Isoniazid; Itraconazole; Ketoconazole; Ketoconazole (Systemic); Lithium; Mesalamine; Methenamine; Mycophenolate; Nelfinavir; Penicillamine;

Phosphate Supplements; Posaconazole; Protease Inhibitors; Tetracycline Derivatives; Trientine; Ursodiol

The levels/effects of Omeprazole and Sodium Bicarbonate may be decreased by: CYP2C19 Inducers (Strong); Peginterferon Alfa-2b; Tipranavir

Food Interactions Administration of omeprazole powder for suspension 1 hour after a meal reduced the AUC by 24% and peak plasma level by 63%.

Stability Omeprazole stability is a function of pH; it is rapidly degraded in acidic media but has acceptable stability under alkaline conditions. Each capsule of omeprazole contains enteric-coated granules to prevent omeprazole degradation by gastric acidity. Store at 25°C (77°F); excursions permitted to 15°C to 30°C (59°F to 86°F).

Mechanism of Action Suppresses gastric acid secretion by inhibiting the parietal cell membrane enzyme (H$^+$/K$^+$)-ATPase or proton pump; demonstrates antimicrobial activity against *Helicobacter pylori*

Pharmacodynamics

Onset of action: 1 hour

Maximum effect: 2 hours

Duration: 72 hours; 50% of maximum effect at 24 hours

Maximum secretory inhibition: 4 days

Pharmacokinetics (Adult data unless noted)

Absorption: Rapid

Protein binding: 95%

Metabolism: Extensively hepatic by cytochrome P450 system; saturable first pass effect

Bioavailability: 30% to 40%; improves slightly with repeated administration; increased in Asian patients and patients with hepatic dysfunction; excreted into breast milk (peak concentration in breast milk <7% of corresponding peak plasma concentration)

Half-life: Adults: ~1 hour (range: 0.4-3.2 hours); chronic hepatic disease: 3 hours

Time to peak serum concentration: ~30 minutes

Elimination:

Clearance: Adults: 500-600 mL/minute; chronic hepatic disease: 70 mL/minute

Usual Dosage Oral: Dosage listed that of omeprazole component

Children: GERD, ulcers, esophagitis; **Note:** Recognizing that this formulation has not received FDA approval for use in children despite an approved dosage for omeprazole in children and considering that omeprazole has been used safely in children as an extemporaneous formulation with sodium bicarbonate, the following dosage is recommended:

5 kg to <10 kg: 5 mg once daily

10 kg to ≤20 kg: 10 mg once daily

>20 kg: 20 mg once daily

Alternate dosing: 1 mg/kg/day once or twice daily; range of effective dosages in the literature: 0.2-3.5 mg/kg/day (see Hassall, 2000; Zimmermann, 2001). Higher doses may be necessary in children between 1-6 years of age due to increased metabolic clearance (see Andersson, 2000). To maintain gastric pH >5 in critically-ill children, administration every 6-8 hours may be necessary (1.5-2 mg/kg/day) (see Kaufman, 2002).

Adults:

Active duodenal ulcer: 20 mg/day for 4-8 weeks

Gastric ulcers: 40 mg/day for 4-8 weeks

GERD or severe erosive esophagitis: 20 mg/day for 4-8 weeks

Heartburn: OTC labeling: 20 mg once daily for 14 days. Do not take for >14 days or more often than every 4 months, unless instructed by healthcare provider.

Maintenance of healing of erosive esophagitis: 20 mg/day

Administration

Capsule: Should be swallowed whole; do not chew or crush. Capsules should **not** be opened, sprinkled on food, or administered via NG.

Powder for oral suspension:

Oral: Administer 1 hour before a meal. Mix with 2 tablespoons of water; stir well and drink immediately. Rinse cup with water and drink.

Nasogastric/orogastric tube: Mix well with 20 mL of water and administer immediately; flush tube with an additional 20 mL of water. Suspend enteral feeding for 3 hours before and 1 hour after administering.

Patient Information See individual agents.

Additional Information Each capsule of omeprazole-sodium bicarbonate contains 1100 mg (13 mEq) of sodium bicarbonate; total Na content is 304 mg and 303 mg for the prescription and OTC product, respectively. Each packet of omeprazole-sodium bicarbonate powder for oral suspension contains 1680 mg (20 mEq) of sodium bicarbonate; total Na content is 460 mg.

Dosage Forms Excipient information presented when available (limited, particularly for generics); consult specific product labeling.

Capsule, immediate release:

Zegerid®: Omeprazole 20 mg and sodium bicarbonate 1100 mg [contains sodium 304 mg (13 mEq) per capsule]

Zegerid®: Omeprazole 40 mg and sodium bicarbonate 1100 mg [contains sodium 304 mg (13 mEq) per capsule]

Zegerid OTC™: Omeprazole 20 mg and sodium bicarbonate 1100 mg [contains sodium 303 mg (13 mEq) per capsule]

Powder for oral suspension:

Zegerid®: Omeprazole 20 mg and sodium bicarbonate 1680 mg per packet (30s) [contains sodium 460 mg (20 mEq) per packet]

Zegerid®: Omeprazole 40 mg and sodium bicarbonate 1680 mg per packet (30s) [contains sodium 460 mg (20 mEq) per packet]

Extemporaneous Preparations Omeprazole-sodium bicarbonate 2 mg/mL may be made by adding six 20 mg omeprazole-sodium bicarbonate packets to a glass mortar, add 30 mL of water to the packets, mix well, and transfer to 60 mL bottle. Rinse mortar with additional water to reach a final volume of 60 mL. Solution is stable for 45 days refrigerated.

Johnson CE, Cober MP, and Ludwig JL, "Stability of Partial Doses of Omeprazole-Sodium Bicarbonate Oral Suspension," *Ann Pharmacother*, 2007, 41:1954-61.

References

Andersson T, Hassall E, Lundborg P, et al, "Pharmacokinetics of Orally Administered Omeprazole in Children. International Pediatric Omeprazole Pharmacokinetic Group," *Am J Gastroenterol*, 2000, 95 (11):3101-6.

Canani RB, Cirillo P, Roggero P, et al, "Therapy With Gastric Acidity Inhibitors Increases the Risk of Acute Gastroenteritis and Community-Acquired Pneumonia in Children," *Pediatrics*, 2006, 117(5):e817-20.

Gibbons TE and Gold BD, "The Use of Proton Pump Inhibitors in Children: A Comprehensive Review," *Paediatr Drugs*, 2003, 5 (1):25-40.

Gottrand F, Kalach N, Spyckerelle C, et al, "Omeprazole Combined With Amoxicillin and Clarithromycin in the Eradication of Helicobacter pylori in Children With Gastritis: A Prospective Randomized Double-Blind Trial," *J Pediatr*, 2001, 139(5):664-8.

Gunasekaran TS and Hassall EG, "Efficacy and Safety of Omeprazole for Severe Gastroesophageal Reflux in Children," *J Pediatr*, 1993, 123(1):148-54.

Hassall E, Israel D, Shepherd R, "Omeprazole for Treatment of Chronic Erosive Esophagitis in Children: A Multicenter Study of Efficacy, Safety, Tolerability and Dose Requirements. International Pediatric Omeprazole Study Group," *J Pediatr*, 2000, 137(6):800-7.

Johnson CE, Cober MP, and Ludwig JL, "Stability of Partial Doses of Omeprazole-Sodium Bicarbonate Oral Suspension," *Ann Pharmacother*, 2007, 41(12):1954-61.

Kane DL, "Administration of Omeprazole (Prilosec™) in the Atypical Patient," *Int J Pharm Compounding*, 1997, 1(1):13.

Kato S, Ebina K, Fujii K, et al, "Effect of Omeprazole in the Treatment of Refractory Acid-Related Diseases in Childhood: Endoscopic Healing and Twenty-Four Hour Intragastric Acidity," *J Pediatr*, 1996, 128 (3):415-21.

Kaufman SS, Lyden ER, Brown CR, et al, "Omeprazole Therapy in Pediatric Patients After Liver and Intestinal Transplantation," *J Pediatr Gastroenterol Nutr*, 2002, 34(2):194-8.

Song JC, Quercia RA, Fan C, et al, "Pharmacokinetic Comparison of Omeprazole Capsules and a Simplified Omeprazole Suspension," *Am J Health Syst Pharm*, 2001, 58(8):689-94.

Zimmermann AE, Walters JK, Katona BG, et al, "A Review of Omeprazole Use in the Treatment of Acid-Related Disorders in Children," *Clin Ther*, 2001, 23(5):660-79.

◆ **Omeprazole Magnesium** see Omeprazole on page 1016

◆ **Omnicef®** see Cefdinir on page 263

◆ **Omnii Gel™ [OTC]** see Fluoride on page 595

◆ **Omnipred™** see PrednisoLONE on page 1148

◆ **Omnitrope®** see Somatropin on page 1281

OnabotulinumtoxinA
(oh nuh BOT yoo lin num TOKS in aye)

Medication Safety Issues

Botulinum products are not interchangeable; potency differences may exist between the products.

U.S. Brand Names Botox®; Botox® Cosmetic

Canadian Brand Names Botox®; Botox® Cosmetic; Xeomin®

Therapeutic Category Muscle Contracture, Treatment; Ophthalmic Agent, Toxin

Generic Available No

Use Treatment of strabismus and blepharospasm associated with dystonia (including benign essential blepharospasm or VII nerve disorders) (FDA approved in ages >12 years and adults); treatment of dynamic muscle contracture in pediatric cerebral palsy patients (orphan drug); treatment of cervical dystonia dystonia (FDA approved in ages >16 and adults); treatment of severe primary axillary hyperhidrosis (not adequately controlled with topical treatments) (FDA approved in adults); temporary improvement in the appearance of lines and wrinkles of the face (moderate to severe glabellar lines associated with corrugator and/or procerus muscle activity) in adult patients ≤65 years of age. Other uses include treatment of sialorrhea; palmar hyperhidrosis, esophageal achalasia, chronic anal fissure; migraine headache.

Medication Guide An FDA-approved patient medication guide, which is available with the product information and at http://www.fda.gov/downloads/Drugs/DrugSafety/UCM176360.pdf, must be dispensed with this medication for each new outpatient prescription and refill.

Pregnancy Risk Factor C

Pregnancy Considerations Decreased fetal body weight, delayed ossification, maternal toxicity, abortions, and fetal malformations were observed in animal studies. Human reproduction studies have not been conducted. Avoid use in pregnancy. Based on limited case reports, adverse fetal effects have not been observed with inadvertent administration during pregnancy. It is currently recommended to ensure adequate contraception in women of childbearing potential.

Lactation Excretion in breast milk unknown/use caution

Contraindications Hypersensitivity to botulinum toxin or any component of the formulation; infection at the site of injection

Warnings The U.S. Food and Drug Administration (FDA) and Health Canada have issued respective early communications to healthcare professionals alerting them of serious adverse events in association with the use of onabotulinumtoxinA (Botox®, Botox® Cosmetic) and rimabotulinumtoxinB (Myobloc®). Events reported are suggestive of botulism, indicating systemic spread of the botulinum toxin beyond the site of injection. Reactions were observed in both adult and pediatric patients treated for a variety of conditions with varying doses. However, the most serious outcomes, including respiratory failure and death, were associated with the use in children for cerebral palsy limb spasticity. The FDA has evaluated postmarketing cases and now reports that systemic and potentially fatal toxicity may result from local injection of the botulinum toxins in the treatment of other underlying conditions such as cerebral palsy associated with limb spasticity. Monitor patients closely for signs/ symptoms of systemic toxic effects (possibly occurring 1 day to several weeks after treatment) and instruct patients to seek immediate medical attention with worsening symptoms or dysphagia, dyspnea, muscle weakness, or difficulty speaking.

AbobotulinumtoxinA (Dysport®) is not equivalent in potency to Botox®; the Dysport®:Botox® equivalency ratio is ~3:1 or 4:1, respectively; patients treated for cervical dystonia may experience dysphagia which rarely may result in dyspnea, aspiration, and pneumonia; weakness of hand muscles and blepharoptosis may occur in patients who also receive treatment for palmar and facial hyperhidrosis respectively

Precautions Presence of antibodies to onabotulinumtoxinA may reduce the effectiveness of therapy; to minimize the development of antibodies, keep the dose of onabotulinumtoxinA as low as possible. Reduced blinking from onabotulinumtoxinA injection of the orbicularis muscle can lead to corneal exposure, persistent epithelial defect, and corneal ulceration, especially in patients with VII nerve disorders; carefully test corneal sensation in eyes previously operated upon. Avoid injection into the lower lid area to avoid ectropion, and vigorously treat any epithelial defect (this may require protective drops, ointment, therapeutic soft contact lenses, or closure of the eye by patching). Retrobulbar hemorrhages sufficient to compromise retinal circulation have occurred from needle penetrations into the orbit; have appropriate instruments to decompress the orbit accessible; ocular (globe) penetrations by needles have also occurred (an ophthalmoscope to diagnose this condition should be available).

Use with caution in patients with peripheral motor neuropathic diseases (eg, amyotrophic lateral sclerosis or motor neuropathy) or neuromuscular junction disorders (eg, myasthenia gravis or Lambert-Eaton syndrome) as these patients may be at increased risk for development of significant systemic side effects including severe dysphagia and respiratory compromise; use cautiously if there is inflammation present at the proposed injection site or when excessive weakness or atrophy is present in the target muscles

Adverse Reactions

Cardiovascular: Arrhythmia, MI (rare)

Central nervous system: Anxiety, dizziness, drowsiness, fever, speech disorder

Dermatologic: Erythema multiforme, keratitis, nonaxillary sweating (after primary hyperhidrosis treatment), pruritus, psoriasiform eruption, rash

Gastrointestinal: Dyspepsia, dysphagia (particularly after treatment of cervical dystonia), pharyngitis, xerostomia

Local: Erythema and bruising at injection site, pain, tenderness

Neuromuscular & skeletal: Muscle weakness, temporary loss of function around injection site

Ocular: Blepharospasm, diplopia, dry eyes, ectropion, entropion, eyelid edema, lagophthalmos, photophobia, ptosis, retrobulbar hemorrhage, spatial disorientation, tearing, vertical deviation

Respiratory: Cough, respiratory failure, rhinitis

Miscellaneous: Flu-like syndrome, hypersensitivity reactions, infection

Drug Interactions

Avoid Concomitant Use There are no known interactions where it is recommended to avoid concomitant use.

Increased Effect/Toxicity
OnabotulinumtoxinA may increase the levels/effects of: AbobotulinumtoxinA; RimabotulinumtoxinB

The levels/effects of OnabotulinumtoxinA may be increased by: Aminoglycosides; Anticholinergic Agents; Neuromuscular-Blocking Agents

Decreased Effect There are no known significant interactions involving a decrease in effect.

Stability Store lyophilized product in refrigerator at 2°C to 8°C (36°F to 46°F); administer within 4 hours after reconstitution; reconstituted solution may be stored in the refrigerator (2°C to 8°C/36°F to 46°F) until administered; do not freeze reconstituted solution

Mechanism of Action OnabotulinumtoxinA (formerly botulinum A toxin) is a neurotoxin produced by *Clostridium botulinum*, a spore-forming anaerobic bacillus; it blocks neuromuscular conduction by binding to receptor sites on motor nerve terminals, entering the nerve terminals and inhibiting the release of acetylcholine. When injected intramuscularly at therapeutic doses, it produces a localized chemical denervation muscle paralysis. When the muscle is chemically denervated, it atrophies and may develop extrajunctional acetylcholine receptors. There is evidence that the nerve can sprout and reinnervate the muscle, with the weakness being reversible. Following several weeks of paralysis, alignment of the eye is measurably changed, despite return of innervation to the injected muscle. When injected intradermally, a temporary chemical denervation of the sweat gland reduces local sweating.

Pharmacodynamics

Strabismus:
Onset of action: 1-2 days after injection
Duration of paralysis: 2-6 weeks
Blepharospasm:
Onset of action: 3 days after injection
Maximum effect: 1-2 weeks
Duration of paralysis: 3 months
Spasticity associated with cerebral palsy
Onset of action: Several days
Duration of paralysis: 3-8 months
Reduction in axillary sweat production:
Duration of effect: 201 days (mean)

Usual Dosage I.M.:

Strabismus:
Children 2 months to 12 years:
Horizontal or vertical deviations <20 prism diopters: 1.25 units into any one muscle
Horizontal or vertical deviations 20-25 prism diopters: 1-2.5 units into any one muscle
Persistent VI nerve palsy of ≥1 month duration: 1-1.25 units into the medial rectus muscle
Children ≥12 years and Adults:
Horizontal or vertical deviations <20 prism diopters: 1.25-2.5 units into any one muscle
Horizontal or vertical deviations 20-50 prism diopters: 2.5-5 units into any one muscle
Persistent VI nerve palsy of ≥1 month duration: 1.25-2.5 units into the medial rectus muscle

Note: Re-examine patient 7-14 days after each injection to assess effects; dosage may be increased up to twofold of the previously administered dose; do not exceed 25 units as a single injection for any one muscle

Blepharospasm: Adults: Initial: 1.25-2.5 units injected into the medial and lateral pretarsal orbicularis oculi of the upper lid and into the lateral pretarsal orbicularis oculi of the lower lid; dose may be increased up to 2.5-5 units at repeat treatment sessions; do not exceed 5 units per injection or cumulative dose of 200 units in a 30-day period

Spasticity associated with cerebral palsy: Children >18 months to Adolescents: Small muscle: 1-2 units/kg; large muscle: 3-6 units/kg; maximum dose per injection site: 50 units; maximum dose for any one visit: 12 units/kg, up to 400 units; no more than 400 units should be administered during a 3-month period

Cervical dystonia: Adults: Initial and sequential doses should be individualized related to the patient's head and neck position, localization of pain, muscle hypertrophy, and patient response; mean dosage used in research trials: 236 units (range: 198-300 units) divided among affected muscles; limit total dose into sternocleidomastoid muscles to ≤100 units

Severe primary axillary hyperhidrosis: Adults: Intradermal: 50 units per axilla injected in 0.1-0.2 mL aliquots

Reduction of glabellar lines: Adults ≤65 years: I.M.: An effective dose is determined by gross observation of the patient's ability to activate the superficial muscles injected. The location, size and use of muscles may vary markedly among individuals. Inject 0.1 mL dose into each of five sites, two in each corrugator muscle and one in the procerus muscle (total dose 0.5 mL).

Administration Parenteral: For I.M. or intradermal administration only by individuals understanding the relevant neuromuscular and orbital anatomy and any alterations to the anatomy due to prior surgical procedures and standard electromyographic techniques; reconstitute vial with preservative-free NS to obtain an optimal injection volume of 0.1 mL; suggested diluent volumes and resulting concentrations: 1 mL (10 units/0.1 mL); 2 mL (5 units/0.1 mL), 4 mL (2.5 units/0.1 mL) or 8 mL (1.25 units/0.1 mL); gently swirl as onabotulinumtoxinA is denatured by violent agitation. Local site reactions may be minimized by careful injection into the target muscle, using a minimal volume, and slowing the rate of injection. Application of ice and topical anesthetics to the injection site may also be used.

Monitoring Parameters Monitor patients closely for signs/symptoms of systemic toxic effects (possibly occurring 1 day to several weeks after treatment; see Warnings)

Cervical dystonia: Toronto Western Spasmodic Torticollis Rating Scale (TWSTRS) which evaluates severity, disability, and pain

Cerebral palsy: Modified Ashworth Scale, Tardieu Scale, Gross Motor Function Measure; treatment goals include: Improved gait and balance, facilitation of patient care, increased comfort with therapy, improved tolerance of bracing, and prevention of musculoskeletal complications

Patient Information Patients with blepharospasm may have been extremely sedentary for a long time; sedentary patients should be cautioned to resume activity slowly and carefully following injection; may cause dry mouth

Dosage Forms Excipient information presented when available (limited, particularly for generics); consult specific product labeling. [CAN] = Canadian product; not available in U.S.

Injection, powder for reconstitution [preservative free]:

Botox®: *Clostridium botulinum* type A neurotoxin complex 100 units [contains albumin (human)]; *Clostridium botulinum* type A neurotoxin complex 200 units [contains albumin (human)]

Botox® Cosmetic: *Clostridium botulinum* type A neurotoxin complex 50 units [contains albumin (human)]; *Clostridium botulinum* type A neurotoxin complex 100 units [contains albumin (human)]

Botox® [CAN]: Botulinum toxin A 50 units [contains albumin (human)], 100 units [contains albumin (human)], 200 units [contains albumin (human)]

Botox Cosmetic® [CAN]: Botulinum toxin A 50 units [contains albumin (human)], 100 units [contains albumin (human)], 200 units [contains albumin (human)]

Xeomin® [CAN]: Botulinum toxin A 100 units [contains albumin (human) and sucrose]

References

"Botulinum Toxin," *NIH Consens Statement*, 1990, 12-14, 8(8):1-20.

Benson J and Daugherty KK, "Botulinum Toxin A in the Treatment of Sialorrhea," *Ann Pharmacother*, 2007, 41(1):79-85.

Charles PD, "Botulinum Neurotoxin Serotype A: A Clinical Update on Non-cosmetic Uses," *Am J Health Syst Pharm*, 2004, 61(22 Suppl 6): S11-23.

Cheng CM, Chen JS, and Patel RP, "Unlabeled Uses of Botulinum Toxins: A Review, Part 1," *Am J Health Syst Pharm*, 2006, 63 (2):145-52.

Cheng CM, Chen JS, and Patel RP, "Unlabeled Uses of Botulinum Toxins: A Review, Part 2," *Am J Health Syst Pharm*, 2006, 63 (3):225-32.

Criswell SR, Crowner BE, and Racette BA, "The Use of Botulinum Toxin Therapy for Lower-Extremity Spasticity in Children With Cerebral Palsy," *Neurosurg Focus*, 2006, 21(2):e1.

Russman BS, Tilton A, and Gormley ME Jr, "Cerebral Palsy: A Rational Approach to a Treatment Protocol, and the Role of Botulinum Toxin in Treatment," *Muscle Nerve Suppl*, 1997, 6:S181-S193.

Scott AB, Magoon EH, McNeer KW, et al, "Botulinum Treatment of Childhood Strabismus," *Ophthalmology*, 1990, 97(11):1434-8.

♦ **Oncaspar®** *see* Pegaspargase *on page 1068*

♦ **Oncovin** *see* VinCRIStine *on page 1425*

Ondansetron (on DAN se tron)

Medication Safety Issues

Sound-alike/look-alike issues:

Ondansetron may be confused with dolasetron, granisetron, palonosetron

Zofran® may be confused with Zantac®, Zosyn®

Related Information

Compatibility of Chemotherapy and Related Supportive Care Medications *on page 1580*

U.S. Brand Names Zofran®; Zofran® ODT

Canadian Brand Names Apo-Ondansetron®; CO Ondansetron; Dom-Ondansetron; JAMP-Ondansetron; Mint-Ondansetron; Mylan-Ondansetron; Novo-Ondansetron; Ondansetron Injection; Ondansetron-Omega; PHL-Ondansetron; PMS-Ondansetron; RAN™-Ondansetron; ratio-Ondansetron; Sandoz-Ondansetron; Zofran®; Zofran® ODT; ZYM-Ondansetron

Therapeutic Category 5-HT$_3$ Receptor Antagonist; Antiemetic

Generic Available Yes

Use Prevention of nausea and vomiting associated with highly emetogenic cancer chemotherapy or radiotherapy (Injection: FDA approved in ages ≥6 months and adults; oral formulations: FDA approved in ages ≥4 years and adults); prevention of postoperative nausea and vomiting (Injection: FDA approved in ages 1 month to 12 years and adults; oral formulations: FDA approved in adults); has also been used in the treatment of hyperemesis gravidarum

Pregnancy Risk Factor B

Pregnancy Considerations Teratogenic effects were not observed in animal studies; however, there are no adequate and well-controlled studies in pregnant women. Use of ondansetron for the treatment of nausea and vomiting of pregnancy (NVP) has been evaluated. Additional studies are needed to determine safety to the fetus, particularly during the first trimester. Based on preliminary data, use is generally reserved for severe NVP (hyperemesis gravidarum) or when conventional treatments are not effective.

Lactation Excretion in breast milk unknown/use caution

Contraindications Hypersensitivity to ondansetron, other 5-HT$_3$ receptor antagonists, or any component

Warnings Selective 5-HT$_3$ antagonists, including ondansetron, have been associated with a number of dose-dependent increases in ECG intervals (eg, PR, QRS duration, QT/QT$_c$, JT), usually occurring 1-2 hours after I.V. administration. In general, these changes are not clinically relevant; however, when used in conjunction with other agents that prolong these intervals, arrhythmia may occur. When used with agents that prolong the QT interval (eg, Class I and III antiarrhythmics), clinically relevant QT interval prolongation may occur resulting in torsade de pointes. A number of trials have shown that 5-HT$_3$ antagonists produce QT interval prolongation to variable degrees. Reduction in heart rate may also occur with the 5-HT$_3$ antagonists. I.V. formulations of 5-HT$_3$ antagonists have more association with ECG interval changes compared to oral formulations.

Zofran® solution contains sodium benzoate; benzoic acid (benzoate) is a metabolite of benzyl alcohol; large amounts of benzyl alcohol (≥99 mg/kg/day) have been associated with a potentially fatal toxicity ("gasping syndrome") in neonates; *in vitro* and animal studies have shown that benzoate displaces bilirubin from protein binding sites; avoid use of Zofran® solution in neonates.

Precautions Use with caution in patients at risk of QT prolongation and/or ventricular arrhythmia, including patients with congenital long QT syndrome or other risk factors for QT prolongation [eg, medications known to prolong QT interval, electrolyte abnormalities (hypokalemia or hypomagnesemia), and cumulative high-dose anthracycline therapy].

Adverse Reactions

Cardiovascular: ECG changes, flushing, QT interval increased

Central nervous system: Dizziness, drowsiness, fatigue, fever, headache, lightheadedness, sedation, seizures, shivers

Dermatologic: Local injection site reaction, rash

Gastrointestinal: Abdominal pain, constipation, diarrhea, hiccups, xerostomia

Hepatic: Transient increase in liver enzymes

Neuromuscular & skeletal: Ataxia, musculoskeletal pain, tremor, twitching, weakness

Miscellaneous: Anaphylaxis

<1%, postmarketing, and/or case reports: Angina, anaphylactoid reactions, angioedema, arrhythmia, blindness (transient/following infusion; lasting ≤48 hours), blurred vision (transient/following infusion), bradycardia, bronchospasm, cardiopulmonary arrest, dyspnea, dystonic reaction, electrocardiographic alterations (second-degree heart block and ST-segment depression), extrapyramidal symptoms, flushing, hypersensitivity reaction, hypokalemia, hypotension, laryngeal edema, laryngospasm, oculogyric crisis, palpitations, premature ventricular contractions (PVC), shock, stridor, supraventricular tachycardia, syncope, tachycardia, tonic clonic seizures, urticaria, vascular occlusive events, ventricular arrhythmia

Drug Interactions

Metabolism/Transport Effects Substrate of CYP1A2 (minor), CYP2C9 (minor), CYP2D6 (minor), CYP2E1 (minor), CYP3A4 (major), P-glycoprotein; **Inhibits** CYP1A2 (weak), 2C9 (weak), 2D6 (weak)

Avoid Concomitant Use

Avoid concomitant use of Ondansetron with any of the following: Apomorphine

Increased Effect/Toxicity

Ondansetron may increase the levels/effects of: Apomorphine

The levels/effects of Ondansetron may be increased by: P-Glycoprotein Inhibitors

Decreased Effect

The levels/effects of Ondansetron may be decreased by: CYP3A4 Inducers (Strong); Deferasirox; Herbs (CYP3A4 Inducers); Peginterferon Alfa-2b; P-Glycoprotein Inducers; Rifamycin Derivatives

Stability

Compatible for 7 days at room temperature when diluted in saline or dextrose solutions; Y-site injection compatibility with bleomycin, carboplatin, carmustine, chlorpromazine, cisplatin, cyclophosphamide, cytarabine, dacarbazine, dactinomycin, daunorubicin, dexamethasone, diphenhydramine, doxorubicin, droperidol, etoposide, fludarabine, ifosfamide, mechlorethamine, methotrexate, mesna, metoclopramide, mitoxantrone, prochlorperazine, promethazine, teniposide, vinblastine, and vincristine

Incompatible with acyclovir, ampicillin, aminophylline, furosemide, ganciclovir, lorazepam, methylprednisolone, and piperacillin

Mechanism of Action Selective 5-HT$_3$ receptor antagonist, blocking serotonin, both peripherally on vagal nerve terminals and centrally in the chemoreceptor trigger zone

Pharmacokinetics (Adult data unless noted)

Absorption: Oral: 100%; nonlinear absorption occurs with increasing oral doses; Zofran® ODT tablets are bio-equivalent to Zofran® tablets; absorption does not occur via oral mucosa

Distribution: V$_d$:

Children: Surgical patients:

1-4 months: 3.5 L/kg

5-24 months: 2.3 L/kg

3-12 years: 1.65 L/kg

Children: Cancer patients: 4-18 years: 1.9 L/kg

Adults: 1.9 L/kg

Protein binding, plasma: 70% to 76%

Metabolism: Extensive first-pass metabolism; primarily by hydroxylation, followed by glucuronidation and sulfate conjugation

Bioavailability: Oral: 50% to 70% due to significant first-pass metabolism; in cancer patients (adult) 85% to 87% bioavailability possibly related to changes in metabolism

Half-life:

Children: 1-4 months: 6.7 hours; 5 months to 12 years: 2.9 hours

Adults: 3.5-5.5 hours

Elimination: In urine and feces; <5% of the parent drug is recovered unchanged in urine

Clearance:

Children: Surgical patients:

1-4 months: 0.401 L/kg/hour

5-24 months: 0.581 L/kg/hour

3-12 years: 0.439 L/kg/hour

Children: Cancer patients: 4-18 years: 0.599 L/kg/hour

Adults (normal):

19-40 years: 0.381 L/kg/hour

61-74 years: 0.319 L/kg/hour

>75 years: 0.262 L/kg/hour

Usual Dosage

Prevention of chemotherapy- or radiotherapy-induced nausea and vomiting:

Oral (all doses given 30 minutes before chemotherapy or 1-2 hours prior to radiotherapy and repeated at 8-hour intervals):

Children <4 years: No FDA-approved oral dosage; however, the following dosages based upon body surface area have been used:

<0.3 m^2: 1 mg 3 times/day

0.3-0.6 m^2: 2 mg 3 times/day

0.6-1 m^2: 3 mg 3 times/day
>1 m^2: 4 mg 3 times/day
or
Children 4-11 years: 4 mg 3 times/day
Children >11 years and Adults: 8 mg 3 times/day or 24 mg once daily
Adults: Total body irradiation: 8 mg 1-2 hours before each fraction of radiotherapy administered each day
Single high-dose fraction radiotherapy to abdomen: 8 mg 1-2 hours before irradiation, then 8 mg every 8 hours after first dose for 1-2 days after completion of radiotherapy
Daily fractionated radiotherapy to abdomen: 8 mg 1-2 hours before irradiation, then 8 mg every 8 hours after first dose for each day of radiotherapy
I.V.:
Children 6 months to 18 years: 0.15 mg/kg/dose infused 30 minutes before the start of emetogenic chemotherapy, with subsequent doses administered 4 and 8 hours after the first dose
Adults: A single 32 mg dose/day or 0.15 mg/kg/dose or 45-80 kg: 8 mg, >80 kg: 12 mg infused 30 minutes before the start of emetogenic chemotherapy with subsequent doses administered 4 and 8 hours after the first dose; a few studies have evaluated a single 8 mg loading dose followed by a continuous 1 mg/hour infusion
Prevention of postoperative nausea and vomiting: I.V., I.M. (this route has only been recommended in adults): Give immediately before induction of anesthesia, or postoperatively if the patient is symptomatic:
Children ≥2 years <40 kg: 0.1 mg/kg
Children >40 kg and Adults: 4 mg
Note: Repeating a second ondansetron dose in patients who did not achieve adequate control of postoperative nausea and vomiting after a single dose will not provide additional control.
Treatment of hyperemesis gravidarum: I.V.: 8 mg every 12 hours or 1 mg/hour infused continuously for up to 24 hours
Dosing adjustment in severe hepatic impairment (Child-Pugh score ≥10): Adults: Once daily dosage; maximum 8 mg per dose
Administration
Oral: May administer without regard to meals; Zofran® ODT tablet: Place tablet on tongue, it will disintegrate immediately; may also swallow with fluids as whole tablet
Parenteral:
I.V.: Dilute in 50 mL I.V. fluid (maximum concentration: 1 mg/mL) and infuse over 15 minutes; single doses for prevention of postoperative nausea/vomiting may be administered I.V. undiluted over 2-5 minutes
I.M.: Administer as undiluted injection
Patient Information May cause dry mouth
Dosage Forms Excipient information presented when available (limited, particularly for generics); consult specific product labeling. [DSC] = Discontinued product
Infusion, premixed in D$_5$ [preservative free]: 32 mg (50 mL)
Zofran®: 32 mg (50 mL) [DSC]
Infusion, premixed in sodium chloride [preservative free]: 32 mg (50 mL)
Injection, solution: 2 mg/mL (2 mL, 20 mL)
Zofran®: 2 mg/mL (2 mL, 20 mL)
Injection, solution [preservative free]: 2 mg/mL (2 mL)
Solution, oral: 4 mg/5 mL (50 mL)
Zofran®: 4 mg/5 mL (50 mL) [contains sodium benzoate; strawberry flavor]
Tablet: 4 mg; 8 mg
Zofran®: 4 mg; 8 mg
Tablet, orally disintegrating: 4 mg; 8 mg
Zofran® ODT: 4 mg, 8 mg [each strength contains phenylalanine <0.03 mg/tablet; strawberry flavor]

References
"ASHP Therapeutic Guidelines on the Pharmacologic Management of Nausea and Vomiting in Adult and Pediatric Patients Receiving Chemotherapy or Radiation Therapy or Undergoing Surgery," *Am J Health Syst Pharm*, 1999, 56(8):729-64.
Carden PA, Mitchell SL, Waters KD, et al, "Prevention of Cyclophosphamide/Cytarabine-Induced Emesis With Ondansetron in Children With Leukemia," *J Clin Oncol*, 1990, 8(9):1531-5.
Marty M, Pouillart P, Scholl S, et al, "Comparison of the 5-hydroxytryptamine 3 (Serotonin) Antagonist Ondansetron (GR 38032F) With High-Dose Metoclopramide in the Control of Cisplatin-Induced Emesis," *N Engl J Med*, 1990, 322(12):816-21.
Pinkerton CR, Williams D, Wootton C, et al, "5-HT$_3$ Antagonist Ondansetron - An Effective Outpatient Antiemetic in Cancer Treatment," *Arch Dis Child*, 1990, 65(8):822-5.
Roila F and Del Favero A, "Ondansetron Clinical Pharmacokinetics," *Clin Pharmacokinet*, 1995, 29(2):95-109.
Seynaeve C, Schuller J, Buser K, et al, "Comparison of the Anti-emetic Efficacy of Different Doses of Ondansetron, Given as Either a Continuous Infusion or a Single Intravenous Dose, in Acute Cisplatin-Induced Emesis," *Br J Cancer* 1992, 66(1):192-7.
Spahr-Schopfer IA, Lerman J, Sikich N, et al, "Pharmacokinetics of Intravenous Ondansetron in Healthy Children Undergoing Ear, Nose, and Throat Surgery," *Clin Pharmacol Ther*, 1995, 58(3):316-21.
Spector JI, Lester EP, Chevlen EM, et al, "A Comparison of Oral Ondansetron and Intravenous Granisetron for the Prevention of Nausea and Emesis Associated With Cisplatin-Based Chemotherapy," *Oncologist*, 1998, 3(6):432-438.

◆ **Ondansetron Hydrochloride** *see* Ondansetron *on page 1022*

◆ **Ondansetron Injection (Can)** *see* Ondansetron *on page 1022*

◆ **Ondansetron-Omega (Can)** *see* Ondansetron *on page 1022*

◆ **One Gram C [OTC]** *see* Ascorbic Acid *on page 138*

◆ **Onsolis™** *see* FentaNYL *on page 567*

◆ **Onxol® [DSC]** *see* Paclitaxel *on page 1044*

◆ **OPC-14597** *see* Aripiprazole *on page 132*

◆ **Operand® Chlorhexidine Gluconate [OTC]** *see* Chlorhexidine Gluconate *on page 291*

◆ **Ophthetic® [DSC]** *see* Proparacaine *on page 1168*

◆ **Ophtho-Dipivefrin™ (Can)** *see* Dipivefrin *on page 461*

◆ **Ophtho-Tate® (Can)** *see* PrednisoLONE *on page 1148*

◆ **Opium and Belladonna** *see* Belladonna and Opium *on page 178*

Opium Tincture (OH pee um TING chur)

Medication Safety Issues
Sound-alike/look-alike issues:
Opium tincture may be confused with camphorated tincture of opium (paregoric)

High alert medication: The Institute for Safe Medication Practices (ISMP) includes this medication among its list of drugs which have a heightened risk of causing significant patient harm when used in error.

Use care when prescribing opium tincture; each mL contains the equivalent of morphine 10 mg; paregoric contains the equivalent of morphine 0.4 mg/mL

DTO is an error-prone abbreviation (mistaken as Diluted Tincture of Opium; dose equivalency of paregoric)
Therapeutic Category Analgesic, Narcotic; Antidiarrheal
Generic Available Yes
Use Treatment of diarrhea or relief of pain; **a 25-fold dilution with water** (final concentration 0.4 mg/mL morphine) can be used to treat neonatal abstinence syndrome (opiate withdrawal)
Restrictions C-II
Pregnancy Risk Factor B/D (prolonged use or high doses at term)
Lactation Enters breast milk/use caution

Contraindications Hypersensitivity to opium, morphine, or any component; diarrhea caused by poisoning until the toxic material has been removed; increased intracranial pressure, severe respiratory depression, severe liver or renal insufficiency

Warnings Do not confuse opium tincture with pare-goric; opium tincture is 25 times as potent as paregoric; opium shares the toxic potential of opiate agonists, usual precautions of opiate agonist therapy should be observed; opium may mask dehydration by producing fluid retention in the bowel; monitor patients with prolonged or severe diarrhea carefully; abrupt discontinuation after prolonged use may result in withdrawal symptoms

Precautions Use with caution in patients with respiratory, hepatic, or renal dysfunction, severe prostatic hypertrophy, or history of narcotic abuse; infants <3 months of age are more susceptible to respiratory depression, use with caution and in reduced doses in this age group

Adverse Reactions

Cardiovascular: Hypotension, bradycardia, peripheral vasodilation

Central nervous system: CNS depression, intracranial pressure elevated, drowsiness, dizziness, sedation

Dermatologic: Pruritus

Endocrine & metabolic: Antidiuretic hormone release

Gastrointestinal: Nausea, vomiting, constipation

Genitourinary: Urinary tract spasm, urinary retention

Hepatic: Biliary tract spasm

Ocular: Miosis

Respiratory: Respiratory depression

Miscellaneous: Physical and psychological dependence, histamine release

Drug Interactions

Avoid Concomitant Use There are no known inter-actions where it is recommended to avoid concomitant use.

Increased Effect/Toxicity

Opium Tincture may increase the levels/effects of: Alcohol (Ethyl); Alvimopan; CNS Depressants; Desmo-pressin; Selective Serotonin Reuptake Inhibitors; Thia-zide Diuretics

The levels/effects of Opium Tincture may be increased by: Amphetamines; Antipsychotic Agents (Phenothia-zines); Succinylcholine

Decreased Effect

Opium Tincture may decrease the levels/effects of: Pegvisomant

The levels/effects of Opium Tincture may be decreased by: Ammonium Chloride; Mixed Agonist / Antagonist Opioids

Stability Protect from light and excessive heat; do not refrigerate, decreased solubility and precipitation may occur

Mechanism of Action Contains many narcotic alkaloids including morphine; gastric motility inhibition is primarily due to morphine content; decreases digestive secretions, increases GI muscle tone, and reduces GI propulsion

Pharmacodynamics Duration: 4-5 hours

Pharmacokinetics (Adult data unless noted)

Absorption: Variable from GI tract

Metabolism: In the liver

Elimination: In urine and bile

Usual Dosage Oral:

Neonates (full-term): Neonatal abstinence syndrome (opiate withdrawal): **Use a 25-fold dilution of opium tincture** (final concentration: 0.4 mg/mL morphine): Initial: Give 0.1 mL/kg or 2 drops/kg of the 25-fold dilution per dose with feedings every 3-4 hours; increase as needed by 0.1 mL/kg or 2 drops/kg of the 25-fold dilution every 3-4 hours until withdrawal symptoms are con-trolled; usual dose: 0.2-0.5 mL of the 25-fold dilution per

dose given every 3-4 hours; it is rare to exceed 0.7 mL of the 25-fold dilution per dose; stabilize withdrawal symptoms for 3-5 days, then gradually decrease the dosage (keeping the same dosage interval) over a 2- to 4-week period

Children:

Diarrhea: 0.005-0.01 mL/kg/dose every 3-4 hours for a maximum of 6 doses/24 hours

Analgesia: 0.01-0.02 mL/kg/dose every 3-4 hours

Adults:

Diarrhea: Usual: 0.6 mL/dose; range: 0.3-1 mL/dose every 3-6 hours to maximum of 6 mL/24 hours

Analgesia: 0.6-1.5 mL/dose every 3-4 hours; usual maximum dose: 6 mL/24 hours

Administration Oral: May administer with food to decrease GI upset; for neonatal abstinence syndrome (opiate withdrawal), use a 25-fold dilution of opium tincture

Monitoring Parameters Respiratory rate, blood pressure, heart rate, resolution of diarrhea or pain, mental status; if using a 25-fold dilution to treat neonatal abstinence syndrome, monitor for resolution of withdrawal symptoms (such as irritability, high-pitched cry, stuffy nose, rhinor-rhea, vomiting, poor feeding, diarrhea, sneezing, yawning etc), and signs of overtreatment (such as bradycardia, lethargy, hypotonia, irregular respirations, respiratory depression etc). An abstinence scoring system (eg, Finnegan abstinence scoring system) can be used to more objectively assess neonatal opiate withdrawal symptoms and the need for dosage adjustment. Monitor fluid and electrolyte balance in young children being treated for prolonged or severe diarrhea.

Patient Information Avoid alcohol; may cause drowsi-ness and impair ability to perform activities requiring mental alertness or physical coordination; may be habit-forming; avoid abrupt discontinuation after prolonged use

Nursing Implications Observe patient for excessive sedation, respiratory depression; implement safety meas-ures; assist with ambulation; do not abruptly discontinue after prolonged use

Additional Information Opium tincture contains 10 mg/mL morphine and 17% to 21% alcohol; for treatment of neonatal abstinence syndrome, a 25-fold dilution of opium tincture (final concentration: 0.4 mg/mL morphine) is preferred over paregoric; the 25-fold dilution of opium tincture contains the same morphine concentration as paregoric, but without the high amount of alcohol or additives of paregoric

Dosage Forms Excipient information presented when available (limited, particularly for generics); consult specific product labeling.

Tincture: Anhydrous morphine 10 mg/mL (120 mL, 480 mL) [0.6 mL equivalent to morphine 6 mg; contains alcohol 19%]

References

Kraus DM and Pham JT, "Neonatal Therapy," *Applied Therapeutics: The Clinical Use of Drugs,* 9th ed, Koda-Kimble MA, Young LY, Kradjan WA, et al, eds, Baltimore, MD: Lippincott Williams & Wilkins, 2009.

Levy M and Spino M, "Neonatal Withdrawal Syndrome: Associated Drugs and Pharmacologic Management," *Pharmacotherapy,* 1993, 13 (3):202-11.

"Neonatal Drug Withdrawal. American Academy of Pediatrics Commit-tee on Drugs," *Pediatrics,* 1998, 101(6):1079-88.

♦ **Opium Tincture, Deodorized** *see* Opium Tincture *on page 1024*

Oprelvekin (oh PREL ve kin)

Medication Safety Issues

Sound-alike/look-alike issues:

Oprelvekin may be confused with aldesleukin, Proleukin®

Neumega® may be confused with Neulasta®, Neupogen®

U.S. Brand Names Neumega®

Therapeutic Category Biological Response Modulator; Thrombopoietic Growth Factor

Generic Available No

Use Prevention of severe thrombocytopenia and the reduction of the need for platelet transfusions following myelosuppressive chemotherapy in adult patients with nonmyeloid malignancies who are at high risk of severe thrombocytopenia (FDA approved in adults)

Pregnancy Risk Factor C

Pregnancy Considerations Animal studies have demonstrated adverse fetal effects. There are no adequate and well-controlled studies in pregnant women. Use during pregnancy only if the potential benefits outweigh the potential risk to the fetus.

Lactation Excretion in breast milk unknown/not recommended

Breast-Feeding Considerations Due to the potential for serious adverse reactions in the nursing infant, breast-feeding is not recommended.

Contraindications Hypersensitivity to oprelvekin or any component

Warnings Treatment has been associated with severe hypersensitivity reactions including anaphylaxis [U.S. Boxed Warning]; may occur with the first or with subsequent doses; permanently discontinue oprelvekin in any patient developing an allergic reaction. Not indicated following myeloablative chemotherapy as effectiveness was not significant vs placebo and toxicity (edema, conjunctival bleeding, hypotension, and tachycardia) was increased vs placebo in these patients. Severe hypokalemia and/or sudden death have been reported in patients receiving chronic diuretic therapy, ifosfamide, and oprelvekin. Moderate decreases in hemoglobin, hematocrit, and RBC without a decrease in red cell mass have been observed; this is predominately related to an increase in plasma volume (dilutional anemia) from renal sodium and water retention. Onset of dilutional anemia is within 3-5 days of oprelvekin therapy and is reversible over approximately 7 days following discontinuation of oprelvekin. Stroke has been reported in patients who develop atrial fibrillation/flutter while receiving oprelvekin. Animal studies were predictive of an effect of oprelvekin on developing bone in children; thickening of femoral and tibial growth plates was noted. Papilledema has been reported in 2% of adult patients and 16% of pediatric patients receiving oprelvekin; use with caution in patients with pre-existing papilledema, as this may worsen with oprelvekin therapy. Per the manufacturer, oprelvekin should not be used in children, particularly those <12 years of age, except as part of a controlled clinical trial.

Precautions Oprelvekin may cause serious fluid retention resulting in peripheral edema, facial edema, dyspnea on exertion, pulmonary edema, capillary leak syndrome, atrial arrhythmias, and exacerbation of pre-existing pleural effusions. Use cautiously in patients with conditions where expansion of plasma volume should be avoided (eg, left ventricular dysfunction, CHF, hypertension). Use caution in patients with cardiac arrhythmias or conduction defects (ventricular arrhythmias generally occurring within 2-7 days of initiation of treatment have been reported postmarketing); use with caution in patients with respiratory disease; history of thromboembolic problems or stroke, and hepatic or renal dysfunction; modify dosage in patients with severe renal dysfunction

Adverse Reactions

Cardiovascular: Atrial arrhythmias, cardiomegaly (children: 21%), edema, palpitations, syncope, tachycardia (children: 84%), vasodilation

Central nervous system: Dizziness, fever, headache, insomnia, neutropenic fever

Dermatologic: Rash

Endocrine & metabolic: Fluid retention

Gastrointestinal: Diarrhea, mucositis, nausea, oral moniliasis, vomiting, weight gain

Hematologic: Anemia (dilutional; see Warnings)

Neuromuscular & skeletal: Arthralgia, periosteal changes (children: 11%), weakness

Ocular: Conjunctival injection (children: 57%), papilledema (frequency estimated to be up to 16% in children, 2% in adults)

Respiratory: Cough, dyspnea, pharyngitis, pleural effusion, pneumonia, rhinitis

<1%, postmarketing, and/or case reports: Allergic reaction, amblyopia, anaphylaxis/anaphylactoid reactions, blindness, blurred vision, capillary leak syndrome, cardiac arrest, chest pain, dehydration, dysarthria, exfoliative dermatitis, eye hemorrhage, facial edema, fibrinogen increased, fluid overload, HF, hypoalbuminemia, hypocalcemia, hypokalemia, hypotension, injection site reactions (dermatitis, pain, discoloration), loss of consciousness, mental status changes, optic neuropathy, paresthesia, pericardial effusion, peripheral edema, pneumonia, pulmonary edema, renal failure, shock, skin discoloration, stroke, urticaria, ventricular arrhythmia, visual acuity changes, visual field defect, von Willebrand factor concentration increased, wheezing

Drug Interactions

Avoid Concomitant Use There are no known interactions where it is recommended to avoid concomitant use.

Increased Effect/Toxicity There are no known significant interactions involving an increase in effect.

Decreased Effect There are no known significant interactions involving a decrease in effect.

Stability Store vials under refrigeration between 2°C to 8°C (36°F to 46°F); protect from light; do not freeze. Use reconstituted oprelvekin within 3 hours of reconstitution; store reconstituted solution at either 2°C to 8°C (36°F to 46°F) or room temperature (≤25°C/70°F). Do not freeze reconstituted solution.

Mechanism of Action Oprelvekin stimulates multiple stages of megakaryocytopoiesis and thrombopoiesis, resulting in proliferation of megakaryocyte progenitors and megakaryocyte maturation

Pharmacodynamics

Onset of action: 5-9 days

Maximum effect: 14-19 days

Duration: Up to 7 days after discontinuation

Pharmacokinetics (Adult data unless noted)

Distribution: V_d: Adults: 112-152 mL/kg

Bioavailability: >80%

Metabolism: Uncertain

Half-life: Terminal: 6.9-8.1 hours

Time to peak serum concentration: 3.2 ± 2.4 hours

Elimination: Urine (primarily as metabolites)

Clearance: Adults: 2.2-2.7 mL/min/kg; clearance decreases with age and is about 1.2-1.6 times faster in children than in adults

Usual Dosage SubQ: **Note:** First dose should not be administered until 6-24 hours after the end of chemotherapy. Discontinue the drug at least 48 hours before beginning the next cycle of chemotherapy.

Children: 25-50 mcg/kg once daily for 27 days was shown to be efficacious with decreased toxicities as compared to higher doses in one study with 47 pediatric patients (see Cairo, 2005); dosing should continue until postnadir platelet count ≥50,000/mm³

Note: The manufacturer states that, until efficacy/toxicity parameters are established, the use of oprelvekin in pediatric patients (particularly those <12 years of age) should be restricted to use in controlled clinical trials.

Adults: 50 mcg/kg once daily for 10-21 days (until postnadir platelet count ≥50,000/mm³)

Dosage adjustment in renal failure: Adults: Cl_{cr} <30 mL/minute: 25 mcg/kg once daily for 10-21 days (until postnadir platelet count ≥50,000/mm³)

Administration SubQ: Reconstitute to a final concentration of 5 mg/mL with SWI; direct diluent down side of vial, gently swirl, do not shake. Administer subcutaneously in either the abdomen, thigh, hip, or upper arm (if not self-injected).

Monitoring Parameters Monitor electrolytes and fluid balance during therapy; obtain a CBC at regular intervals during therapy; monitor platelet counts until adequate recovery has occurred; renal function (at baseline)

Patient Information Report any swelling in the arms or legs (peripheral edema), shortness of breath (congestive failure, anemia), irregular heartbeat, headaches, or hypersensitivity reactions.

Dosage Forms Excipient information presented when available (limited, particularly for generics); consult specific product labeling.

Injection, powder for reconstitution:
Neumega®: 5 mg [packaged with diluent]

References

Adams VR and Brenner TL, "Oprelvekin (Neumega®)," *J Oncol Pharm Pract*, 1999, 5(3):117-24.

Cairo MS, Davenport V, Bessmertny O, et al, "Phase I/II Dose Escalation Study of Recombinant Human Interleukin-11 Following Ifosfamide, Carboplatin and Etoposide in Children, Adolescents and Young Adults With Solid Tumours or Lymphoma: A Clinical, Haematological and Biological Study," *Br J Haematol*, 2005, 128 (1):49-58.

Du X and Williams DA, "Interleukin-11: Review of Molecular, Cell Biology, and Clinical Use," *Blood*, 1997, 89(11):3897-908.

Gordon MS, "Thrombopoietic Activity of Recombinant Human Interleukin 11 in Cancer Patients Receiving Chemotherapy," *Cancer Chemother Pharmacol*, 1996, 38 (Suppl):96-8.

Milman E, Berdon WE, Garvin JH, et al, "Periostitis Secondary to Interleukin-11 (Oprelvekin, Neumega®). Treatment for Thrombocytopenia in Pediatric Patients," *Pediatr Radiol*, 2003, 33(7):450-2.

Tepler I, Elias L, Smith JW 2d, et al, "A Randomized Placebo-Controlled Trial of Recombinant Human Interleukin-11 in Cancer Patients With Severe Thrombocytopenia Due to Chemotherapy," *Blood*, 1996, 87 (9):3607-14.

Teramura M, Kobayashi S, Yoshinaga K, et al, "Effect of Interleukin 11 on Normal and Pathological Thrombopoiesis," *Cancer Chemother Pharmacol*, 1996, 38 (Suppl):99-102.

◆ **Optho-Bunolol® (Can)** see Levobunolol on page 811

◆ **Opticrom® (Can)** see Cromolyn on page 363

◆ **Optimyxin® (Can)** see Bacitracin and Polymyxin B on page 170

◆ **Optivar®** see Azelastine on page 163

◆ **Orabase® with Benzocaine [OTC]** see Benzocaine on page 182

◆ **Oracea™** see Doxycycline on page 479

◆ **Oracort (Can)** see Triamcinolone on page 1376

◆ **Orajel® Baby Daytime and Nighttime [OTC]** see Benzocaine on page 182

◆ **Orajel® Baby Teething [OTC]** see Benzocaine on page 182

◆ **Orajel® Baby Teething Nighttime [OTC]** see Benzocaine on page 182

◆ **Orajel® Denture Plus [OTC]** see Benzocaine on page 182

◆ **Orajel® Dry Mouth [OTC]** see Glycerin on page 650

◆ **Orajel® Maximum Strength [OTC]** see Benzocaine on page 182

◆ **Orajel® Maximum Strength Overnight Cold Sore [OTC]** see Dyclonine on page 486

◆ **Orajel® Medicated Toothache [OTC]** see Benzocaine on page 182

◆ **Orajel® Mouth Sore [OTC]** see Benzocaine on page 182

◆ **Orajel® Multi-Action Cold Sore [OTC]** see Benzocaine on page 182

◆ **Orajel PM® Maximum Strength [OTC]** see Benzocaine on page 182

◆ **Orajel® Ultra Mouth Sore [OTC]** see Benzocaine on page 182

◆ **Oralone®** see Triamcinolone on page 1376

◆ **Oramorph® SR** see Morphine Sulfate on page 946

◆ **Oranyl [OTC]** see Pseudoephedrine on page 1183

◆ **Orap®** see Pimozide on page 1112

◆ **Orapred®** see PrednisoLONE on page 1148

◆ **Orapred ODT®** see PrednisoLONE on page 1148

◆ **Oraqix®** see Lidocaine and Prilocaine on page 823

◆ **OraVerse™** see Phentolamine on page 1101

◆ **Oravig™** see Miconazole on page 927

◆ **Oraxyl™** see Doxycycline on page 479

◆ **Orazinc® [OTC]** see Zinc Supplements on page 1445

◆ **Orciprenaline Sulfate** see Metaproterenol on page 890

◆ **Orencia®** see Abatacept on page 34

◆ **Orfadin®** see Nitisinone on page 994

◆ **ORG 946** see Rocuronium on page 1230

◆ **Organidin® NR [OTC]** see GuaiFENesin on page 656

◆ **ORG NC 45** see Vecuronium on page 1411

◆ **ORO-Clense (Can)** see Chlorhexidine Gluconate on page 291

◆ **Orthoclone OKT® 3 [DSC]** see Muromonab-CD3 on page 955

◆ **Ortho Micronor®** see Norethindrone on page 1001

◆ **Oscal** see Calcium Carbonate on page 232

◆ **Os-Cal® (Can)** see Calcium Carbonate on page 232

◆ **Os-Cal® 500 [OTC]** see Calcium Supplements on page 239

Oseltamivir (o sel TAM e veer)

Medication Safety Issues

Sound-alike/look-alike issues:
Tamiflu® may be confused with Thera-Flu®
Tamiflu® may be confused with Tambocor™

Dispensing issues:
Oseltamivir (Tamiflu®) oral suspension is packaged with an oral syringe. Healthcare providers dispensing this medication should be aware that the syringe is calibrated in 30 mg, 45 mg, and 60 mg graduations. **When the oral syringe is dispensed, instructions to the patient should be provided based on these units of measure (not mL or teaspoon). When dispensing the oral suspension for children <1 year of age, the oral syringe provided from the manufacturer should be removed and NOT provided to the caregiver.** Pharmacists and healthcare providers should instead supply an oral syringe capable of measuring mL doses. Patients should always be provided with a measuring device calibrated the same way as their labeled instructions.

Oseltamivir (Tamiflu®) 75 mg capsules can be compounded into a suspension when oseltamivir oral suspension is not commercially available. The commercially-available oral suspension concentration is 12 mg/mL; however, the extemporaneously prepared suspension concentration is 15 mg/mL. Prescriptions written in mL or teaspoons should specify the oral suspension concentration to be dispensed.

◄ **U.S. Brand Names** Tamiflu®
Canadian Brand Names Tamiflu®
Therapeutic Category Antiviral Agent, Oral; Neuraminidase Inhibitor
Generic Available No
Use Treatment of uncomplicated acute illness due to influenza A and B infection in patients who have been symptomatic for **no more than 2 days** (FDA approved in ages ≥1 year and adults); prophylaxis of influenza A and B exposures that occur before (or less than 2 weeks after) vaccination with inactivated vaccine, or in years when circulating strains differ from those included in the vaccine (oseltamivir is not a substitute for annual flu vaccination); or preventing influenza (FDA approved in ages ≥1 year and adults)

Treatment and prevention of influenza (FDA emergency use authorization in ages <1 year); treatment of influenza in patients symptomatic for >2 days and/or in patients with severe illness (ie, sick enough to require hospitalization) (Emergency Use Authorization).

Pregnancy Risk Factor C
Pregnancy Considerations In animal reproduction studies, a dose-dependent increase in the rates of minor skeleton abnormalities was found in exposed offspring; therefore, the manufacturer classifies oseltamivir as pregnancy category C. The rate of each abnormality remained within the background rate of occurrence in the species studied. In an *in vitro* study using human placentas, placental transfer of oseltamivir carboxylate, the active metabolite of oseltamivir phosphate, was found to be incomplete, resulting in minimal accumulation in the fetus. Adverse events have not been reported in the infants of mothers who have taken oseltamivir during pregnancy. Influenza infection may be more severe in pregnant women. Oseltamivir and zanamivir are currently recommended for the treatment or prophylaxis of 2009 H1N1 influenza (previously known as novel influenza A [H1N1]) in pregnant women and women up to 2 weeks postpartum (including following pregnancy loss). For seasonal influenza, oseltamivir and zanamivir are currently recommended as an adjunct to vaccination and should not be used as a substitute for vaccination in pregnant women (consult current CDC guidelines).

Lactation Enters breast milk/not recommended
Breast-Feeding Considerations Oseltamivir and its carboxylate metabolite have been detected in breast milk. Breast milk samples were obtained from a single patient (~9 months postpartum) over the course of 5 days of treatment. The maximum total concentration of oseltamivir (expressed as parent drug and metabolite) was 81.6 ng/mL. Using a milk concentration of 81.6 ng/mL, the estimated exposure to the breastfeeding infant would be ~0.5% of the weight adjusted maternal dose (in a 60 kg woman).

Contraindications Hypersensitivity to oseltamivir, any component, or other sialic acid-based neuraminidase inhibitors

Warnings There have been postmarketing reports of neuropsychiatric events in children (including self-injury with fatalities, hallucination, confusion, and delirium). Closely monitor patients for signs of any unusual behavior. Oral suspension contains sodium benzoate; benzoic acid (benzoate) is a metabolite of benzyl alcohol; large amounts of benzyl alcohol (≥99 mg/kg/day) have been associated with a potentially fatal toxicity ("gasping syndrome") in neonates; use oral suspension containing sodium benzoate with caution in neonates; *in vitro* and animal studies have shown that benzoate displaces bilirubin from protein binding sites.

Precautions Use with caution and modify dosage in patients with renal impairment; oseltamivir does not prevent complication of serious bacterial infection which may begin with or coexist with influenza. Use suspension with caution in patients with hereditary fructose intolerance since 75 mg oral suspension delivers 2 g sorbitol which is greater than the maximum daily limit; may cause diarrhea and dyspepsia.

Adverse Reactions
Cardiovascular: Arrhythmia, unstable angina
Central nervous system: Abnormal behavior, confusion, delirium, dizziness, fatigue, hallucinations, headache, insomnia, nightmares, self-injury, seizure, vertigo
Dermatologic: Erythema multiforme, rash, Stevens-Johnson syndrome, toxic epidermal necrolysis,
Endocrine & metabolic: Aggravation of diabetes mellitus
Gastrointestinal: Abdominal pain, diarrhea, nausea, pseudomembranous colitis, vomiting
Hematologic: Anemia
Hepatic: Hepatitis
Ocular: Conjunctivitis
Respiratory: Bronchitis, epistaxis
Miscellaneous: Anaphylaxis, swelling of face or tongue

Drug Interactions
Avoid Concomitant Use There are no known interactions where it is recommended to avoid concomitant use.
Increased Effect/Toxicity
The levels/effects of Oseltamivir may be increased by: Probenecid
Decreased Effect
Oseltamivir may decrease the levels/effects of: Influenza Virus Vaccine (H1N1, Live/Attenuated); Influenza Virus Vaccine (Live/Attenuated)
Food Interactions Food has no significant effect on peak oseltamivir plasma concentration or AUC
Stability Store capsule and powder for oral suspension at room temperature. Reconstituted, commercially-available oral suspension is stable for 10 days if refrigerated; do not freeze.
Mechanism of Action Inhibits influenza virus neuraminidase which is responsible for detachment of virions from the infected cell's membrane and for viral penetration through respiratory secretions resulting in the inability of the virus to spread within the respiratory tract
Pharmacodynamics Reduction in the median time to improvement: 1.3 days
Pharmacokinetics (Adult data unless noted)
Absorption: Well absorbed from the GI tract
Distribution: Adults: V_{dss}: 23-26 L
Protein binding: 3% (oseltamivir carboxylate); 42% (oseltamivir phosphate)
Metabolism: Prodrug oseltamivir phosphate is metabolized by hepatic esterases to oseltamivir carboxylate (active); neither oseltamivir phosphate or oseltamivir carboxylate are a substrate, inducer, or inhibitor of cytochrome P450 isoenzymes
Half-life:
Oseltamivir phosphate: 1-3 hours
Oseltamivir carboxylate: 6-10 hours
Elimination: >99% of oseltamivir carboxylate is eliminated by renal excretion via glomerular filtration and tubular secretion
Usual Dosage Oral:
Treatment of influenza: **Note:** Hospitalized patients with severe 2009 H1N1 influenza infection may require longer (eg, ≥10 days) treatment courses. Some experts also recommend empirically doubling the treatment dose. Doubling the dose in adult outpatients was not associated with increased adverse events. As no double dose studies have been published in children, use caution. Initiate as early as possible in any hospitalized patient with suspected/confirmed influenza [interim recommendations (CDC, 2009)]; may be administered via naso- or orogastric tube in mechanically-ventilated

patients (see Taylor, 2008). Treatment should ideally begin within 48 hours; however, if initiated after 48 hours it may decrease mortality or duration of illness.

Infants <1 year [interim recommendations for treatment of H1N1 influenza A (CDC, 2009)]: **Note:** Weight-based dosing recommendations are not intended for premature neonates.

<12 months: 3 mg/kg/dose twice daily for 5 days

Alternate dosing based on age (use if weight not available):

<3 months: 12 mg twice daily for 5 days

3-5 months: 20 mg twice daily for 5 days

6-11 months: 25 mg twice daily for 5 days

Children ≥1-12 years:

≤15 kg: 30 mg twice daily for 5 days; 2 mg/kg/dose (maximum dose: 30 mg) twice daily has been used in the original influenza work done in children (Whitley, 2001).

>15 kg to 23 kg: 45 mg/dose twice daily for 5 days

>23 kg to 40 kg: 60 mg/dose twice daily for 5 days

>40 kg: 75 mg/dose twice daily for 5 days

Children >12 years and Adults: 75 mg/dose twice daily for 5 days

Prophylaxis of influenza (Initiate treatment within 2 days of contact with an infected individual; duration of treatment: 10 days):

Infants <1 year [interim recommendations for chemoprophylaxis of H1N1 influenza A (CDC, 2009)]: **Note:** Weight-based dosing recommendations are not intended for premature neonates.

<3 months: Not recommended unless clinically critical

3-11 months: 3 mg/kg/dose once daily

Alternate dosing based on age (use only if weight not available):

<3 months: Not recommended unless clinically critical

3-5 months: 20 mg once daily

6-11 months: 25 mg once daily

Children: 1-12 years (Harper, 2009):

≤15 kg: 30 mg once daily

>15 kg to ≤23 kg: 45 mg once daily

>23 kg to ≤40 kg: 60 mg once daily

>40 kg: 75 mg once daily

Children ≥13 years and Adults: 75 mg once daily

Dosing adjustment in renal impairment: Adults:

Cl_{cr} 10-30 mL/minute:

Treatment of influenza: Decrease dose to 75 mg once daily

High-dose treatment (ie, critically-ill H1N1 patients): Currently no data are available; consider 150 mg once daily

Prophylaxis of influenza: Decrease dose to 75 mg every other day

Cl_{cr} <10 mL/minute: No recommended dosage regimens are available for patients with end-stage renal disease

Administration May administer with or without food; may decrease stomach upset if administered with food; shake suspension well before use. Capsules may be opened and mixed with sweetened liquid (eg, chocolate syrup).

Monitoring Parameters Renal function, serum glucose in patients with diabetes mellitus; signs of unusual behavior

Patient Information Oseltamivir is not a substitute for the annual flu vaccination. Report any unusual behavior to physician.

Additional Information Tamiflu® oral suspension: 75 mg dose delivers 2 g sorbitol

Dosage Forms Excipient information presented when available (limited, particularly for generics); consult specific product labeling.

Capsule, as phosphate:

Tamiflu®: 30 mg, 45 mg, 75 mg

Powder for oral suspension:

Tamiflu®: 12 mg/mL (25 mL) [contains sodium benzoate; tutti-frutti flavor]

Extemporaneous Preparations Emergency Compounding of an oral suspension when commercially-manufactured suspension is not available: A 15 mg/mL suspension is made by transferring the contents of ten 75 mg capsules into a clean mortar; triturate to a fine powder. Add one-third of the 48 mL volume of vehicle [cherry syrup (HUMCO) or Ora-Sweet SF (Paddock)] and triturate until a uniform suspension is achieved. Transfer suspension to an amber glass bottle; add another one-third of the vehicle to the mortar, rinse mortar and pestle, and transfer the vehicle into the bottle. Repeat the rinsing step with the remainder of the vehicle. Stable for 35 days when stored in a refrigerator; stable for 5 days when stored at room temperature. Label "shake gently before using." **Note:** This compounding procedure results in 15 mg/mL suspension which differs from the commercially-available Tamiflu® oral suspension with a 12 mg/mL concentration.

References

Centers for Disease Control, "Intensive-Care Patients with Severe Novel Influenza A (H1N1) Virus Infection," July, 17, 2009. Available at: http://www.cdc.gov/mmwr/preview/mmwrhtml/mm5827a4.htm.

Centers for Disease Control, "Updated Interim Recommendations for the Use of Antiviral Medications in the Treatment and Prevention of Influenza for the 2009-2010 Season," October 16, 2009. Available at http://www.cdc.gov/H1N1flu/recommendations.htm.

Centers for Disease Control, "Updated Recommendations for Health Care Providers of Children and Adolescents on the Use of Antiviral Medications for the Management of 2009 H1N1 and Seasonal Influenza for the 2009-2010 Season," December 2, 2009. Available at: http://www.cdc.gov/h1n1flu/recommendations_pediatric_supplement.htm.

Harper SA, Bradley JS, Englund JA, et al, "Seasonal Influenza in Adults and Children - Diagnosis, Treatment, Chemoprophylaxis, and Institutional Outbreak Management: Clinical Practice Guidelines of the Infectious Diseases Society of America," *Clin Infect Dis*, 2009, 48 (8):1003-32.

Hayden FG, Atmar RL, Schilling M, et al, "Use of the Selective Oral Neuraminidase Inhibitor Oseltamivir to Prevent Influenza," *N Engl J Med*, 1999, 341(18):1336-43.

Kimberlin DW, Shalabi M, Abzug MJ, et al, "Safety of Oseltamivir Compared With the Adamantanes in Children Less Than 12 Months of Age," *Pediatr Infect Dis J*, 2009, Nov 25.

Taylor WRJ, Thinh BN, Anh GT, et al, "Oseltamivir is Adequately Absorbed Following Nasogastric Administration to Adult Patients With Severe H5N1 Influenza," *PLoS One*, 2008, 3(10):e3410.

Treanor JJ, Hayden FG, Vrooman PS, et al, "Efficacy and Safety of the Oral Neuraminidase Inhibitor Oseltamivir in Treating Acute Influenza: A Randomized Controlled Trial. US Oral Neuraminidase Study Group," *JAMA*, 2000, 283(8):1016-24.

Whitley RJ, Hayden FG, Reisinger KS, et al, "Oral Oseltamivir Treatment of Influenza in Children," *Pediatr Infect Dis J*, 2001, 20 (2):127-33.

◆ **Osmitrol®** *see* Mannitol *on page 861*

◆ **OsmoPrep®** *see* Sodium Phosphate *on page 1276*

◆ **Osteocit® (Can)** *see* Calcium Citrate *on page 234*

◆ **Ostoforte® (Can)** *see* Ergocalciferol *on page 519*

◆ **OTFC (Oral Transmucosal Fentanyl Citrate)** *see* FentaNYL *on page 567*

◆ **Otix® [OTC]** *see* Carbamide Peroxide *on page 248*

◆ **Outgro® [OTC]** *see* Benzocaine *on page 182*

◆ **Ovace®** *see* Sulfacetamide *on page 1298*

◆ **Ovace® Plus** *see* Sulfacetamide *on page 1298*

◆ **Ovol® (Can)** *see* Simethicone *on page 1262*

Oxacillin (oks a SIL in)

Therapeutic Category Antibiotic, Penicillin (Antistaphylococcal)

Generic Available Yes

Use Treatment of bacterial infections such as osteomyelitis, septicemia, endocarditis, and CNS infections due to susceptible penicillinase-producing strains of *Staphylococcus*

Pregnancy Risk Factor B

Pregnancy Considerations Adverse events have not been observed in animal studies; therefore, oxacillin is classified as pregnancy category B. Oxacillin is distributed into the amniotic fluid and is detected in cord blood. There was not an increased risk of teratogenic effects with oxacillin observed in an epidemiologic study.

Lactation Enters breast milk/use caution

Breast-Feeding Considerations Low levels of oxacillin are found in breast milk. The manufacturer recommends that caution be exercised when administering oxacillin to nursing women. Other penicillins distribute into human milk and are considered safe for use during breast-feeding. Nondose-related effects could include modification of bowel flora.

Contraindications Hypersensitivity to oxacillin, other penicillins, or any component

Warnings Prolonged use may result in superinfection. Elimination rate will be decreased in neonates; monitor patients closely.

Precautions Use with caution in patients with hypersensitivity to cephalosporins, severe renal impairment; dosage modification required in patients with renal impairment

Adverse Reactions

Central nervous system: Fever

Dermatologic: Rash, urticaria, pruritus

Gastrointestinal: Diarrhea, nausea, vomiting, *C. difficile* colitis

Hematologic: Mild leukopenia, agranulocytosis, thrombocytopenia, neutropenia, eosinophilia

Hepatic: AST elevated, hepatotoxicity

Local: Thrombophlebitis

Renal: Acute interstitial nephritis; hematuria and azotemia have occurred in neonates and infants receiving high-dose oxacillin; albuminuria

Miscellaneous: Hypersensitivity reactions, serum sickness-like reactions, anaphylaxis

Drug Interactions

Avoid Concomitant Use

Avoid concomitant use of Oxacillin with any of the following: BCG

Increased Effect/Toxicity

Oxacillin may increase the levels/effects of: Methotrexate

The levels/effects of Oxacillin may be increased by: Probenecid

Decreased Effect

Oxacillin may decrease the levels/effects of: BCG; Mycophenolate; Typhoid Vaccine

The levels/effects of Oxacillin may be decreased by: Fusidic Acid; Tetracycline Derivatives

Stability Reconstituted oxacillin 250 mg/1.5 mL solution for injection is stable for 3 days at room temperature or 7 days when refrigerated; injection is incompatible with aminoglycosides and tetracyclines

Mechanism of Action Interferes with bacterial cell wall synthesis during active multiplication by binding to one or more of the penicillin-binding proteins; inhibits the final transpeptidation step of peptidoglycan synthesis causing cell wall death and resultant bactericidal activity against susceptible bacteria

Pharmacokinetics (Adult data unless noted)

Distribution: Distributes into bile, pleural, synovial, and pericardial fluids and into lungs and bone; penetrates the blood-brain barrier only when meninges are inflamed; crosses the placenta; appears in breast milk

Protein binding: 90% to 95%

Metabolism: In the liver to active and inactive metabolites

Half-life (prolonged with reduced renal function):

Neonates 8-15 days: 1.6 hours

Children 1 week to 2 years: 0.9-1.8 hours

Adults: 0.3-0.8 hours

Time to peak serum concentration: I.M.: Within 30-60 minutes

Elimination: By the kidneys and to small degree via bile as parent drug and metabolites

Dialysis: Not dialyzable (0% to 5%)

Usual Dosage

Neonates: I.M., I.V.:

0-4 weeks, <1200 g: 50 mg/kg/day in divided doses every 12 hours

Postnatal age <7 days:

1200-2000 g: 50-100 mg/kg/day in divided doses every 12 hours

>2000 g: 75-150 mg/kg/day in divided doses every 8 hours

Postnatal age ≥7 days:

1200-2000 g: 75-150 mg/kg/day in divided doses every 8 hours

>2000 g: 100-200 mg/kg/day in divided doses every 6 hours

Infants and Children: I.M., I.V.:

Mild to moderate infections: 100-150 mg/kg/day in divided doses every 6 hours; maximum dose: 4 g/day

Severe infections: 150-200 mg/kg/day in divided doses every 4-6 hours; maximum dose: 12 g/day

Adults: I.M., I.V.:

Mild to moderate infections: 500 mg to 1 g/dose every 6 hours

Severe infections: 1-2 g/dose every 4-6 hours

Dosing interval in renal impairment: Cl_{cr} <10 mL/minute: Use lower range of the usual dosage

Administration Parenteral:

I.M. injection: Reconstitute each gram of oxacillin with 5.7 mL of SWI to make a 167 mg/mL solution; shake well until a clear solution is obtained. Administer by deep I.M. injection into a large muscle mass (eg, gluteus maximus).

I.V. push: Administer over 10 minutes at a maximum concentration of 100 mg/mL

I.V. intermittent infusion: Administer over 15-30 minutes at a final concentration ≤40 mg/mL

I.M. injection: May dilute with SWI to a final concentration of 167 mg/mL; administer I.M. injections deep into a large muscle mass

Monitoring Parameters Periodic CBC with differential, urinalysis, BUN, serum creatinine, AST and ALT; number and type of stools/day for diarrhea

Test Interactions False-positive urinary and serum proteins

Additional Information Sodium content: 1 g injection: 2.5 mEq

Dosage Forms Excipient information presented when available (limited, particularly for generics); consult specific product labeling.

Infusion [premixed iso-osmotic dextrose solution]: 1 g (50 mL); 2 g (50 mL)

Injection, powder for reconstitution: 1 g, 2 g, 10 g

References

Olans RN and Weiner LB, "Reversible Oxacillin Hepatotoxicity," *J Pediatr*, 1976, 89(5):835-8.

Prober CG, Stevenson DK, and Benitz WE, "The Use of Antibiotics in Neonates Weighing Less Than 1200 Grams," *Pediatr Infect Dis J*, 1990, 9(2):111-21.

◆ **Oxacillin Sodium** *see* Oxacillin *on page 1029*

◆ **Oxalatoplatin** *see* Oxaliplatin *on page 1030*

◆ **Oxalatoplatinum** *see* Oxaliplatin *on page 1030*

Oxaliplatin (ox AL i pla tin)

Medication Safety Issues

Sound-alike/look-alike issues:

Oxaliplatin may be confused with Aloxi®, carboplatin, cisplatin

High alert medication: The Institute for Safe Medication Practices (ISMP) includes this medication among its list of drug classes which have a heightened risk of causing significant patient harm when used in error.

Related Information

Emetogenic Potential of Antineoplastic Agents *on page 1579*

U.S. Brand Names Eloxatin®

Canadian Brand Names Eloxatin®

Therapeutic Category Antineoplastic Agent, Alkylating Agent

Generic Available Yes

Use Treatment of stage III colon cancer (adjuvant) and advanced colorectal carcinoma (FDA approved in adults); has also been used in the treatment of esophageal cancer, gastric cancer, hepatobiliary cancer, nonsmall cell lung cancer, non-Hodgkin's lymphoma, ovarian cancer, pancreatic cancer, testicular cancer, relapsed/refractory childhood solid tumors including CNS and non-CNS tumors

Pregnancy Risk Factor D

Pregnancy Considerations Decreased fetal weight, decreased ossification, and increased fetal deaths were observed in animal studies at one-tenth the equivalent human dose. There are no adequate and well-controlled studies in pregnant women. Women of childbearing potential should be advised to avoid pregnancy and use effective contraception during treatment.

Canadian labeling: Use in pregnant women is contraindicated in the Canadian labeling. Males should be advised not to father children during and for up to 6 months following therapy. May cause permanent infertility in males. Prior to initiating therapy, advise males desiring to father children, to seek counseling on sperm storage.

Lactation Excretion in breast milk unknown/not recommended

Breast-Feeding Considerations Due to the potential for serious adverse reactions in the nursing infant, breast-feeding is not recommended.

Contraindications Hypersensitivity to oxaliplatin, other platinum-containing compounds, or any component; pregnancy; grade 3 to 4 neuropathy usually due to prior exposure

Warnings Hazardous agent; use appropriate precautions for handling and disposal. Oxaliplatin should be administered under the supervision of a physician experienced in the use of cancer chemotherapy agents **[U.S. Boxed Warning]**. Anaphylactic-like reactions may occur within minutes of oxaliplatin administration **[U.S. Boxed Warning]**; manage reactions with supportive therapy, epinephrine, corticosteroids, and antihistamines. Two different types of neuropathy may occur: 1) an acute (within first 2 days), reversible (resolves within 14 days) sensory neuropathy with peripheral symptoms that are often exacerbated by cold (may include pharyngolaryngeal dysesthesia); 2) persistent (>14 days) sensory neuropathy which presents with paresthesias, dysesthesias, hypoesthesias, and impaired proprioception that often interferes with daily activities (eg, writing, buttoning, swallowing); these symptoms may improve in some patients upon discontinuing treatment. May cause pulmonary fibrosis or hepatotoxicity (including rare cases of hepatitis and hepatic failure). The presence of hepatic vascular disorders, including veno-occlusive disease, should be considered, especially in individuals developing portal hypertension or who present with elevated liver function tests. When administered as sequential infusions, taxane derivatives (docetaxel, paclitaxel) should be administered before platinum derivatives to limit myelosuppression and enhance efficacy. Oxaliplatin may cause fetal harm (pregnancy should be avoided during therapy).

Precautions Use caution in patients with renal impairment since increased toxicity may occur.

Adverse Reactions

Cardiovascular: Chest pain, edema, flushing, hypotension, peripheral edema, thromboembolism

Central nervous system: Fatigue, fever, headache, insomnia, dizziness, pain

Dermatologic: Alopecia, angioedema, erythema, hand-foot syndrome, pruritus, rash, urticaria

Endocrine & metabolic: Dehydration, hypokalemia, metabolic acidosis

Gastrointestinal: Abdominal pain, anorexia, colitis, constipation, diarrhea, dyspepsia, dysphagia, gastroesophageal reflux, GI bleed, ileus, mucositis, nausea, pancreatitis, rectal hemorrhagestomatitis, taste perversion, vomiting

Genitourinary: Dysuria, hematuria

Hematologic: Anemia, hemolytic anemia, hemorrhage, leukopenia, neutropenia, neutropenic fever, neutropenic sepsis, thrombocytopenia

Hepatic: Alkaline phosphatase, ALT, AST and bilirubin elevated; hepatotoxicity, nodular regenerative hyperplasia peliosis, veno-occlusive liver disease

Local: Erythema, injection site reaction, pain, swelling

Neuromuscular & skeletal: Arthralgia, back pain, dysesthesia, hypoesthesia, jaw spasm paresthesia, peripheral neuropathy, rigors

Ocular: Abnormal lacrimation, ocular pain, optic neuritis, transient vision loss, visual acuity decreased, visual field disturbance

Renal: Serum creatinine elevated

Respiratory: Bronchospasm, cough, dyspnea, epistaxis, hypoxia, interstitial lung disease, pharyngitis, pharyngolaryngeal dysesthesia, pulmonary fibrosis, rhinitis, shortness of breath, URI

Miscellaneous: Anaphylaxis, hiccup, hypersensitivity

Drug Interactions

Avoid Concomitant Use

Avoid concomitant use of Oxaliplatin with any of the following: BCG; Natalizumab; Pimecrolimus; Tacrolimus (Topical); Vaccines (Live)

Increased Effect/Toxicity

Oxaliplatin may increase the levels/effects of: Leflunomide; Natalizumab; Taxane Derivatives; Topotecan; Vaccines (Live); Vitamin K Antagonists

The levels/effects of Oxaliplatin may be increased by: Denosumab; Pimecrolimus; Tacrolimus (Topical); Trastuzumab

Decreased Effect

Oxaliplatin may decrease the levels/effects of: BCG; Cardiac Glycosides; Sipuleucel-T; Vaccines (Inactivated); Vaccines (Live); Vitamin K Antagonists

The levels/effects of Oxaliplatin may be decreased by: Echinacea

Stability Store at room temperature; protect from light; do not freeze. Diluted solution is stable up to 6 hours at room temperature or up to 24 hours under refrigeration. Do not dilute using chloride-containing solutions (eg, NaCl) due to rapid conversion to monochloroplatinum, dichloroplatinum, and diaquoplatinum; all highly reactive in sodium chloride (Takimoto, 2007). Diluted infusion solutions do not require protection from light. Do not reconstitute or dilute oxaliplatin using needles containing aluminum. Incompatible with alkaline solutions (eg, fluorouracil), chloride-containing solutions, and diazepam.

Mechanism of Action Oxaliplatin, a platinum derivative alkylating agent, binds to DNA forming cross-links which inhibit DNA replication and transcription, resulting in cell death; cytotoxicity is cell-cycle nonspecific

Pharmacokinetics (Adult data unless noted)

Distribution: V_d: Adults: 440 L

Protein binding: >90%

Metabolism: Nonenzymatic biotransformation (rapid and extensive), forms active and inactive derivatives

Half-life:

Adults: Oxaliplatin ultrafilterable platinum:

Distribution:

Alpha phase: 0.4 hours

Beta phase: 16.8 hours

Terminal: 391 hours

Children:

Oxaliplatin: Beta: 200.6 hours (median range: 162.5-299 hours)

Oxaliplatin ultrafilterable platinum: Beta: 217.6 hours (median range: 79.7-936.6 hours)

Elimination: Urine (~54%); feces (~2%)

Usual Dosage I.V.: Details concerning dosing in combination regimens should also be consulted. Delay dosage in subsequent cycles until recovery of neutrophils ≥1.5 x 10^9/L and platelets ≥75 x 10^9/L.

Children: Protocol ADVL0421 for relapsed/recurrent childhood solid tumors:

≤12 months: 4.3 mg/kg over 2 hours every 3 weeks

>12 months: 130 mg/m^2 over 2 hours every 3 weeks

Adults:

Advanced colorectal cancer: 85 mg/m^2 every 2 weeks until disease progression or unacceptable toxicity (in combination with fluorouracil/leucovorin calcium)

Stage III colon cancer (adjuvant): 85 mg/m^2 every 2 weeks for 12 cycles (in combination with fluorouracil/leucovorin calcium)

Colon/colorectal cancer (unlabeled doses or combinations): 85 mg/m^2/dose on days 1, 15, and 29 of an 8-week treatment cycle in combination with fluorouracil/leucovorin calcium (Kuebler, 2007) **or** 85 mg/m^2 every 2 weeks in combination with fluorouracil/leucovorin calcium/irinotecan (Falcone, 2007) **or** 130 mg/m^2 every 3 weeks in combination with capecitabine (Cassidy, 2008)

Dosage adjustments for toxicity: Adults:

Acute toxicities: Longer infusion times (up to 6 hours) may mitigate acute toxicities

Persistent grade 2 neurosensory event: Reduce dose to 75 mg/m^2 for Stage III colon cancer adjuvant treatment or 65 mg/m^2 for advanced colorectal cancer

Grade 3 neurosensory event: Consider discontinuing therapy

Recovery from grade 3/4 GI or grade 4 neutropenia or grade 3/4 thrombocytopenia: Reduce dose to 75 mg/m^2 for Stage III colon cancer adjuvant treatment

Recovery from grade 3/4 GI or grade 4 neutropenia or grade 3/4 thrombocytopenia: Reduce dose to 65 mg/m^2 for advanced colorectal cancer; next dose should be delayed until neutrophils >1.5 x10^9/L and platelets >75 x10^9/L

Dosage adjustment in renal impairment: Adults: The FDA-approved labeling does not contain renal dosing adjustment guidelines. Oxaliplatin is primarily eliminated renally; in patients with Cl$_{cr}$ <30 mL/minute, the AUC is increased ~190%. Oxaliplatin use has been studied in 25 patients with renal dysfunction; treatment was well tolerated in patients with mild-to-moderate impairment (Cl$_{cr}$ 20-59 mL/minute), suggesting that dose reduction is not necessary in this patient population (Takimoto, 2003). Patients with severe renal impairment (Cl$_{cr}$ <20 mL/minute) have not been adequately studied; consider omitting dose or changing chemotherapy regimen if Cl$_{cr}$ <20 mL/minute.

Dosage adjustment in hepatic impairment: Mild, moderate, or severe hepatic impairment: Dosage adjustment not necessary (Doroshow, 2003; Synold, 2007)

Administration I.V.: Administer as I.V. infusion over 2-6 hours. The final concentration should not be less than 0.2 mg/mL. For patients in which volume may be of concern, a final concentration of 0.3-0.6 mg/mL is acceptable. Flush infusion line with D$_5$W prior to administration of any concomitant medication. Do **not** use I.V. administration sets containing aluminum.

Monitoring Parameters CBC with differential, hemoglobin, platelet count, blood chemistries including serum creatinine and liver function tests; signs of neuropathy, hypersensitivity reaction, and respiratory effects.

Patient Information Maintain adequate hydration. Inform physician of sore throat, fever, chills, unusual fatigue or unusual bruising/bleeding, persistent diarrhea, rash, cough, swelling of throat, difficulty breathing, muscle cramps or twitching, tingling/numbness in arms, fingers, legs, or toes (avoid exposure to cold temperature, cold drinks, or cold objects since symptoms of acute sensory neuropathy may be exacerbated by cold temperature). Avoid becoming pregnant during or for 1 month following therapy; effective contraceptive measures must be used. Do not breast-feed.

Nursing Implications Patients should receive an antiemetic premedication regimen. Longer infusion times (up to 6 hours) may mitigate acute toxicities. Observe closely for anaphylactic-like reactions which can occur within minutes of administration. Extravasation may result in tissue necrosis; care should be taken to avoid extravasation. If skin or mucous membranes come in contact with oxaliplatin, thoroughly wash skin immediately with soap and water; flush mucous membranes with water. Do not use ice for mucositis prophylaxis.

Dosage Forms Excipient information presented when available (limited, particularly for generics); consult specific product labeling. [CAN] = Canadian brand name

Injection, solution [preservative free; concentrate]: 5 mg/mL (10 mL, 20 mL)

Eloxatin®: 5 mg/mL (10 mL, 20 mL, 40 mL)

Injection, powder for reconstitution: 50 mg, 100 mg

Eloxatin® [CAN]: 50 mg [contains lactose], 100 mg [contains lactose] [not available in U.S.]

References

Cassidy J, Clarke S, Díaz-Rubio E, et al, "Randomized Phase III Study of Capecitabine Plus Oxaliplatin Compared With Fluorouracil/Folinic Acid Plus Oxaliplatin as First-Line Therapy for Metastatic Colorectal Cancer," *J Clin Oncol*, 2008, 26(12):2006-12.

Doroshow JH, Synold TW, Gandara D, et al, "Pharmacology of Oxaliplatin in Solid Tumor Patients With Chronic Dysfunction: A Preliminary Report of the National Cancer Institute Organ Dysfunction Working Group," *Semin Oncol*, 2003, 30(4 Suppl 15):14-9.

Falcone A, Ricci S, Brunetti I, et al, "Phase III Trial of Infusional Fluorouracil, Leucovorin, Oxaliplatin, and Irinotecan (FOLFOXIRI) Compared With Infusional Fluorouracil, Leucovorin, and Irinotecan (FOLFIRI) as First-Line Treatment for Metastatic Colorectal Cancer: The Gruppo Oncologico Nord Ovest," *J Clin Oncol*, 2007, 25 (13):1670-6.

Khushalani NI, Leichman CG, Proulx G, et al, "Oxaliplatin in Combination With Protracted-Infusion Fluorouracil and Radiation: Report of a Clinical Trial for Patients With Esophageal Cancer," *J Clin Oncol*, 2002, 20(12):2844-50.

Kuebler JP, Wieand HS, O'Connell MJ, et al, "Oxaliplatin Combined With Weekly Bolus Fluorouracil and Leucovorin as Surgical Adjuvant Chemotherapy for Stage II and III Colon Cancer: Results From NSABP C-07," *J Clin Oncol*, 2007, 25(16):2198-204.

Synold TW, Takimoto CH, Doroshow JH, et al, "Dose-Escalating and Pharmacologic Study of Oxaliplatin in Adult Cancer Patients With Impaired Hepatic Function: A National Cancer Institute Organ Dysfunction Working Group Study," *Clin Cancer Res*, 2007, 13 (12):3660-6.

Takimoto CH, Graham MA, Lockwood G, et al, "Oxaliplatin Pharmacokinetics and Pharmacodynamics in Adult Cancer Patients With Impaired Renal Function," *Clin Cancer Res*, 2007, 13 (16):4832-9.

Takimoto CH, Remick SC, Sharma S, et al, "Dose-Escalating and Pharmacological Study of Oxaliplatin in Adult Cancer Patients With Impaired Renal Function: A National Cancer Institute Organ Dysfunction Working Group Study," *J Clin Oncol*, 2003, 21 (14):2664-72.

Oxaprozin (oks a PROE zin)

Medication Safety Issues
Sound-alike/look-alike issues:
Daypro® may be confused with Diupres®
Oxaprozin may be confused with oxazepam

Beers Criteria medication: This drug may be inappropriate for use in geriatric patients (high severity risk).

U.S. Brand Names Daypro®

Canadian Brand Names Apo-Oxaprozin®; Daypro®

Therapeutic Category Analgesic, Non-narcotic; Anti-inflammatory Agent; Nonsteroidal Anti-inflammatory Drug (NSAID), Oral

Generic Available Yes

Use Symptomatic relief of the signs and symptoms of osteoarthritis; adult and juvenile rheumatoid arthritis

Medication Guide An FDA-approved patient medication guide, which is available with the product information and at http://www.fda.gov/downloads/Drugs/DrugSafety/ucm088580.pdf, must be dispensed with this medication for each new outpatient prescription and refill.

Pregnancy Risk Factor C

Pregnancy Considerations Adverse events were not observed in the initial animal reproduction studies; therefore, the manufacturer classifies oxaprozin as pregnancy category C. NSAID exposure during the first trimester is not strongly associated with congenital malformations; however, cardiovascular anomalies and cleft palate have been observed following NSAID exposure in some studies. The use of an NSAID close to conception may be associated with an increased risk of miscarriage. Non-teratogenic effects have been observed following NSAID administration during the third trimester including myocardial degenerative changes, prenatal constriction of the ductus arteriosus, fetal tricuspid regurgitation, failure of the ductus arteriosus to close postnatally; renal dysfunction or failure, oligohydramnios; gastrointestinal bleeding or perforation, increased risk of necrotizing enterocolitis; intracranial bleeding (including intraventricular hemorrhage), platelet dysfunction with resultant bleeding; pulmonary hypertension. Because they may cause premature closure of the ductus arteriosus, use of NSAIDs late in pregnancy should be avoided (use after 31 or 32 weeks gestation is not recommended by some clinicians). The chronic use of NSAIDs in women of reproductive age may be associated with infertility that is reversible upon discontinuation of the medication. A registry is available for pregnant women exposed to autoimmune medications including oxaprozin. For additional information contact the Organization of Teratology Information Specialists, OTIS Autoimmune Diseases Study, at 877-311-8972.

Lactation Excretion in breast milk unknown/not recommended

Breast-Feeding Considerations The amount of oxaprozin found in breast milk is not known; however, distribution into breast milk would be expected. Breast-feeding is not recommended by the manufacturer.

Contraindications Hypersensitivity to oxaprozin or any component; history of asthma, urticaria, or allergic-type reaction to aspirin, or other NSAIDs; patients with the "aspirin triad" [asthma, rhinitis (with or without nasal polyps), and aspirin intolerance] (fatal asthmatic and anaphylactoid reactions may occur in these patients); perioperative pain in the setting of coronary artery bypass graft (CABG)

Warnings NSAIDs are associated with an increased risk of adverse cardiovascular thrombotic events, including potentially fatal MI and stroke **[U.S. Boxed Warning]**; risk may be increased with duration of use or pre-existing cardiovascular risk factors or disease; carefully evaluate cardiovascular risk profile prior to prescribing; use the lowest effective dose for the shortest duration of time, taking into consideration individual patient treatment goals; alternate therapies should be considered for patients at high risk. Use is contraindicated for treatment of perioperative pain in the setting of CABG surgery **[U.S. Boxed Warning]**; an increased incidence of MI and stroke was found in patients receiving COX-2 selective NSAIDs for the treatment of pain within the first 10-14 days after CABG surgery. NSAIDs may cause fluid retention, edema, and new onset or worsening of pre-existing hypertension; use with caution in patients with hypertension, CHF, or fluid retention. Concurrent administration of ibuprofen, and potentially other nonselective NSAIDs, may interfere with aspirin's cardioprotective effect.

NSAIDs may increase the risk of gastrointestinal inflammation, ulceration, bleeding, and perforation **[U.S. Boxed Warning]**. These events, which can be potentially fatal, may occur at any time during therapy, and without warning. Avoid the use of NSAIDs in patients with active GI bleeding or ulcer disease. Use NSAIDs with extreme caution in patients with a history of GI bleeding or ulcers (these patients have a 10-fold increased risk for developing a GI bleed). Use NSAIDs with caution in patients with other risk factors which may increase GI bleeding (eg, concurrent therapy with aspirin, anticoagulants, and/or corticosteroids, longer duration of NSAID use, smoking, use of alcohol, and poor general health). Use the lowest effective dose for the shortest duration of time, taking into consideration individual patient treatment goals; alternate therapies should be considered for patients at high risk.

NSAIDs may compromise existing renal function. Renal toxicity may occur in patients with impaired renal function, dehydration, heart failure, liver dysfunction, and those taking diuretics and ACE inhibitors; use with caution in these patients; monitor renal function closely. NSAIDs are not recommended for use in patients with advanced renal disease. Long-term use of NSAIDs may cause renal papillary necrosis and other renal injury.

Fatal asthmatic and anaphylactoid reactions may occur in patients with the "aspirin triad" who receive NSAIDs (see Contraindications). NSAIDs may cause serious dermatologic adverse reactions including exfoliative dermatitis, Stevens-Johnson syndrome, and toxic epidermal necrolysis. Avoid use of NSAIDs in late pregnancy as they may cause premature closure of the ductus arteriosus.

Precautions Severe hepatic reactions (rare) may occur. Use with caution in patients with, asthma, dehydration (rehydrate patient before starting therapy), mild-to-moderate renal dysfunction, hepatic dysfunction, coagulation disorders, or those receiving anticoagulants. Safety and efficacy in pediatric patients <6 years of age have not been established. May cause photosensitivity reactions.

Adverse Reactions Note: Adverse reactions occurred in 45% of JRA patients, compared to ~30% of adult rheumatoid arthritis patients (see also Additional Information)

Cardiovascular: Fluid retention, edema, hypertension

Central nervous system: Confusion, depression, dizziness, headache, sedation, sleep disturbance, somnolence

Dermatologic: Pruritus, rash; mild photosensitivity reactions (reported in 30% of JRA patients; see Additional Information)

Gastrointestinal: Abdominal distress, abdominal pain, anorexia, constipation, diarrhea, flatulence, dyspepsia, nausea, vomiting; GI ulcer, bleeding or perforation

Hematologic: Anemia, bleeding time increased, inhibition of platelet aggregation; agranulocytosis, aplastic anemia (rare)

Hepatic: Liver enzymes elevated; Rarely: Severe hepatic reactions (jaundice, fatal fulminant hepatitis, liver necrosis, hepatic failure)

Ocular: Blurred vision, conjunctivitis

Otic: Tinnitus

Renal: Dysuria, renal dysfunction, urinary frequency, acute renal failure; renal injury, renal papillary necrosis (long-term use)

Miscellaneous: Anaphylaxis, anaphylactoid reactions

Drug Interactions

Avoid Concomitant Use

Avoid concomitant use of Oxaprozin with any of the following: Ketorolac; Ketorolac (Systemic)

Increased Effect/Toxicity

Oxaprozin may increase the levels/effects of: Amino-glycosides; Anticoagulants; Antiplatelet Agents; Bisphosphonate Derivatives; Collagenase (Systemic); CycloSPORINE; CycloSPORINE (Systemic); Desmo-pressin; Digoxin; Drotrecogin Alfa; Eplerenone; Haloperidol; Ibritumomab; Lithium; Methotrexate; Nonsteroidal Anti-Inflammatory Agents; Pemetrexed; Potassium-Sparing Diuretics; Pralatrexate; Quinolone Antibiotics; Salicylates; Thrombolytic Agents; Tositumomab and Iodine I 131 Tositumomab; Vancomycin; Vitamin K Antagonists

The levels/effects of Oxaprozin may be increased by: Antidepressants (Tricyclic, Tertiary Amine); Corticosteroids (Systemic); Dasatinib; Glucosamine; Herbs (Anticoagulant/Antiplatelet Properties); Ketorolac; Ketorolac (Systemic); Nonsteroidal Anti-Inflammatory Agents; Omega-3-Acid Ethyl Esters; Pentosan Polysulfate Sodium; Pentoxifylline; Probenecid; Prostacyclin Analogues; Selective Serotonin Reuptake Inhibitors; Serotonin/Norepinephrine Reuptake Inhibitors; Treprostinil

Decreased Effect

Oxaprozin may decrease the levels/effects of: ACE Inhibitors; Angiotensin II Receptor Blockers; Antiplatelet Agents; Beta-Blockers; Eplerenone; HydrALAZINE; Loop Diuretics; Potassium-Sparing Diuretics; Salicylates; Thiazide Diuretics

The levels/effects of Oxaprozin may be decreased by: Bile Acid Sequestrants; Nonsteroidal Anti-Inflammatory Agents; Salicylates

Food Interactions Food may decrease the rate, but not the extent of oral absorption

Stability Store at 25°C (77°F); protect from light; keep bottle tightly closed

Mechanism of Action Inhibits prostaglandin synthesis by decreasing the activity of the enzyme, cyclooxygenase, which results in decreased formation of prostaglandin precursors

Pharmacodynamics Maximum effect: Due to its long half-life, several days of treatment are required for oxaprozin to reach its full effect

Pharmacokinetics (Adult data unless noted)

Absorption: Oral: 95%

Distribution: Distributes into synovial tissues at twice the concentration of plasma and 3 times the concentration of synovial fluid; expected to distribute into breast milk (exact amount not known)

V_d (apparent): Adults: 11-17 L per 70 kg

Protein binding: 99%, primarily to albumin; protein binding is saturable (nonlinear protein binding)

Metabolism: Hepatic via microsomal oxidation (65%) and conjugation with glucuronic acid (35%); major conjugated metabolites are ester and ether glucuronide (inactive); small amounts of an active phenolic metabolite is produced (<5%) but has limited contribution to overall activity

Half-life: Adults: 41-55 hours

Time to peak serum concentration: 2.4-3.1 hours

Elimination: Excreted in the urine (5% as unchanged drug, 65% as metabolites) and feces (35% as metabolites)

Clearance: After adjusting for body weight, no clinically important age-related differences in apparent clearance of unbound drug were identified between adult and pediatric patients ≥6 years of age

Dialysis: Not significantly removed by hemodialysis or CAPD due to high protein binding

Usual Dosage Note: Use lowest effective dose; dose may be divided if patient does not tolerate once daily dosing; Oral:

Children 6-16 years: JRA: Dose according to body weight. **Note:** Doses greater than 1200 mg have not been evaluated:

22-31 kg: 600 mg once daily

32-54 kg: 900 mg once daily

≥55 kg: 1200 mg once daily

Adults: Osteoarthritis or Rheumatoid arthritis: Usual: 1200 mg once daily; titrate to lowest effective dose; patients with low body weight should start with 600 mg daily; a one-time loading dose of 1200 mg to 1800 mg or 26 mg/kg (whichever is lower) may be given if needed; maximum daily dose: 1800 mg or 26 mg/kg (whichever is lower) in divided doses

Note: Chronic administration of doses >1200 mg/day should be reserved for adult patients >50 kg with severe disease, low risk for peptic ulcer disease, and normal hepatic and renal function; ensure that patient tolerates lower doses before advancing to larger dose

Dosing adjustment in renal impairment: Severe renal impairment or patients on dialysis: Initial: 600 mg once daily; may increase dose if needed to 1200 mg once daily with close monitoring

Dosing adjustment in hepatic impairment: Use with caution in patients with severe hepatic dysfunction (dosage reduction is not required in patients with well compensated cirrhosis)

Administration May be administered without regard to food; administer with food or milk to decrease GI distress

Monitoring Parameters CBC, occult blood loss, liver enzymes, renal function tests; blood pressure, signs and symptoms of GI bleeding

Test Interactions False-positive urine immunoassay screening test for benzodiazepines may occur; test may remain positive for several days after discontinuing oxaprozin

Patient Information May cause dizziness and impair ability to perform activities requiring mental alertness or physical coordination; avoid alcohol; report any signs of blood in stool, GI bleeding, weight gain, edema, skin rash, unusual fatigue, persistent abdominal pain/tenderness or yellow skin to physician. May cause photosensitivity reactions (eg, exposure to sunlight may cause severe sunburn, skin rash, redness, or itching); avoid exposure to sunlight and artificial light sources (sunlamps, tanning booth/bed); wear protective clothing, wide-brimmed hats, sunglasses, and lip sunscreen (SPF ≥15); use a sunscreen [broad-spectrum sunscreen or physical sunscreen (preferred) or sunblock with SPF ≥15]; contact physician if reaction occurs.

Additional Information An open-label study of oxaprozin (10-20 mg/kg/dose once daily) in 59 JRA patients [3-16 years of age (mean age: 9 years)], reported adverse events in 58% of patients; GI symptoms occurred at a higher incidence than historically reported in adults; 9 of 30 patients (30%) who continued therapy for a total of 19-48 weeks, developed a vesicular rash on sun-exposed areas of skin; 5 of these 9 patients with rash discontinued the drug (see Bass, 1985).

Dosage Forms Excipient information presented when available (limited, particularly for generics); consult specific product labeling.
Tablet, oral: 600 mg
Daypro®: 600 mg
References
Bass JC, Athreya BH, Brewer EJ, et al, "A Once-Daily Anti-Inflammatory Drug, Oxaprozin, in the Treatment of Juvenile Rheumatoid Arthritis," *J Rheumatol*, 1985, 12(2):384-6.

OXcarbazepine (ox car BAZ e peen)

Medication Safety Issues
Sound-alike/look-alike issues:
OXcarbazepine may be confused with carBAMazepine
Trileptal® may be confused with TriLipix™
U.S. Brand Names Trileptal®
Canadian Brand Names Apo-Oxcarbazepine®; Trileptal®
Therapeutic Category Anticonvulsant, Miscellaneous
Generic Available Yes
Use Treatment of partial seizures in patients with epilepsy (FDA approved as monotherapy in ages ≥4 years and adults; FDA approved as adjunctive therapy in ages ≥2 years and adults)
Pregnancy Risk Factor C
Pregnancy Considerations Oxcarbazepine crosses the human placenta. Teratogenic effects have been observed in animal studies. There are no adequate and well-controlled studies in pregnant women; however, oxcarbazepine is structurally related to carbamazepine (teratogenic in humans); use during pregnancy only if the benefit to the mother outweighs the potential risk to the fetus. Nonhormonal forms of contraception should be used during therapy.

Patients exposed to oxcarbazepine during pregnancy are encouraged to enroll themselves into the AED Pregnancy Registry by calling 1-888-233-2334. Additional information is available at www.aedpregnancyregistry.org.
Lactation Enters breast milk/not recommended
Breast-Feeding Considerations Oxcarbazepine and its active metabolite (MHD) are excreted in human breast milk. A milk-to-plasma concentration ratio of 0.5 was found for both. Because of the potential for serious adverse reactions to oxcarbazepine in nursing infants, a decision should be made whether to discontinue nursing or to discontinue the drug in nursing women.
Contraindications Hypersensitivity to oxcarbazepine or any component
Warnings Significant hyponatremia may occur; a serum sodium <125 mEq/L has been reported in 2.5% of patients; consider monitoring serum sodium especially in patients who receive other drugs that may cause hyponatremia and in patients with symptoms of hyponatremia (eg, nausea, headache, malaise, confusion, lethargy, obtundation, or an increase in seizure frequency or severity). Do not abruptly discontinue therapy, withdraw gradually to lessen chance for increased seizure frequency (unless a more rapid withdrawal is required due to safety concerns). Serious dermatologic reactions (including potentially fatal Stevens-Johnson syndrome and toxic epidermal necrolysis) have been reported (median onset 19 days); consider discontinuation of oxcarbazepine and alternative therapy in patients who develop skin reactions. Rare cases of anaphylaxis and angioedema have been reported after the first or subsequent doses of oxcarbazepine; angioedema has occurred in the lips, eyelids, glottis, and larynx; angioedema of the larynx (laryngeal edema) can be fatal; permanently discontinue oxcarbazepine if any of these reactions occur; do not rechallenge or restart oxcarbazepine in these patients. Cross-hypersensitivity reactions with carbamazepine may occur (incidence: 25% to 30%);

serious and potentially fatal multiorgan hypersensitivity reactions have also been reported (see Adverse Reactions); discontinue oxcarbazepine immediately if signs or symptoms of hypersensitivity develop.

Antiepileptic drugs (AEDs) increase the risk of suicidal behavior and ideation in patients receiving these medications for any indication. Pooled analyses of placebo-controlled trials involving 11 different AEDs (regardless of indication) showed a twofold increased risk of suicidal thoughts or behavior (estimated incidence rate: 0.43% in AED treated patients compared to 0.24% of patients receiving placebo); increased risk was observed as early as 1 week after initiation of AED and continued through duration of trials (most trials ≤24 weeks); risk did not vary significantly by age (age range: 5–100 years). Consider risks and benefits of AEDs before prescribing. Monitor all patients receiving an AED for emergence of suicidal thoughts or behavior, thoughts of self-harm, any unusual changes in behavior or mood, or the emergence or worsening of depressive symptoms; notify healthcare provider immediately if symptoms or concerning behavior occur. **Note:** The FDA is requiring that a Medication Guide be developed for all antiepileptic drugs informing patients of this risk.
Precautions CNS adverse effects may occur including somnolence, fatigue, coordination abnormalities (ataxia and gait disturbances), and cognitive symptoms (difficulty concentrating, speech or language problems, and psychomotor slowing); these effects may be more common when oxcarbazepine is used as add-on therapy versus monotherapy. Use with caution and modify dose in patients with renal impairment. Multiple drug interactions may occur (see Drug Interactions).
Adverse Reactions
Central nervous system: Headache, dizziness, somnolence (incidence in children: Up to 34.8%), fatigue, ataxia or gait disturbances (children: Up to 23.2%), tremor, insomnia, cognitive symptoms (children: Up to 5.8%; psychomotor slowing, difficulty concentrating, speech or language problems), vertigo, anxiety, nervousness, emotional lability; suicidal thinking and behavior (see Warnings)
Dermatologic: Rash, maculopapular rash; rare: Stevens-Johnson syndrome, erythema multiforme, toxic epidermal necrolysis
Endocrine & metabolic: Hyponatremia (incidence: 2.5%; usually occurs within the first 3 months of therapy, but has been reported in patients more than 1 year after starting medication; serum sodium returns towards normal after discontinuation, reduction of dose, or with conservative treatment such as fluid restriction); reduction in T_4 levels
Gastrointestinal: Nausea, vomiting, abdominal pain, dyspepsia; rare: Pancreatitis, lipase elevated, amylase elevated
Neuromuscular & skeletal: Abnormal gait
Ocular: Diplopia, abnormal vision, nystagmus
Miscellaneous: Hypersensitivity reactions; anaphylaxis and angioedema (see Warnings); a rare, multiorgan hypersensitivity reaction with rash, lymphadenopathy, fever, abnormal liver function tests, hepatitis, nephritis, oliguria, hepatorenal syndrome, hematological abnormalities, pruritus, asthenia, and/or arthralgia has also been reported (median time to detection: 13 days post-therapy initiation)
Drug Interactions
Metabolism/Transport Effects **Inhibits** CYP2C19 (weak); **Induces** CYP3A4 (strong)
Avoid Concomitant Use
Avoid concomitant use of OXcarbazepine with any of the following: Dronedarone; Everolimus; Nilotinib; Nisoldipine; Pazopanib; Ranolazine; Romidepsin; Tolvaptan

Increased Effect/Toxicity

OXcarbazepine may increase the levels/effects of: Phenytoin

The levels/effects of OXcarbazepine may be increased by: Thiazide Diuretics

Decreased Effect

OXcarbazepine may decrease the levels/effects of: Contraceptives (Estrogens); Contraceptives (Progestins); CYP3A4 Substrates; Dronedarone; Everolimus; GuanFACINE; Maraviroc; NIFEdipine; Nilotinib; Nisoldipine; Pazopanib; Ranolazine; Romidepsin; Saxagliptin; Sorafenib; Tadalafil; Tolvaptan

The levels/effects of OXcarbazepine may be decreased by: Divalproex; PHENobarbital; Phenytoin; Valproic Acid

Food Interactions

Tablets: Food does not affect rate or extent of absorption
Suspension: Effect of food has not been studied, but bioavailability is not likely to be affected

Stability Store at controlled room temperature (25°C); dispense in tight container; suspension is stable for 7 weeks after first opening the bottle

Mechanism of Action Active 10-monohydroxy metabolite (MHD) is primarily responsible for anticonvulsant activity; exact mechanism unknown; both MHD and oxcarbazepine are thought to decrease the spread of seizure activity by blockade of sodium channels; also increases conductance of potassium and modulates activity of high-voltage activated calcium channels

Pharmacokinetics (Adult data unless noted)

Absorption: Oral: Complete

Distribution: MHD: V_d (apparent): Adults: 49 L

Protein binding: Oxcarbazepine: 67%; MHD: 40%, primarily to albumin; parent drug and metabolite do not bind to alpha-1 acid glycoprotein

Metabolism: Oxcarbazepine is extensively metabolized in the liver to its active 10-monohydroxy metabolite (MHD); MHD undergoes further metabolism via glucuronide conjugation; 4% of dose is oxidized to the 10,11-dihydroxy metabolite (DHD) (inactive); 70% of serum concentration appears as MHD, 2% as unchanged oxcarbazepine, and the rest as minor metabolites; **Note:** Unlike carbamazepine, autoinduction of metabolism has not been observed and biotransformation of oxcarbazepine does not result in an epoxide metabolite

Bioavailability: Tablets and suspension have similar bioavailability (based on MDH serum concentrations)

Half-life:
Adults:
Oxcarbazepine: 2 hours
MHD: 9 hours
Adults with renal impairment (Cl_{cr} <30 mL/minute): MHD: 19 hours

Time to peak serum concentration: Adults:
Tablets: 3-13 hours (median: 4.5 hours)
Suspension: Median: 6 hours

Elimination: >95% of dose is excreted in the urine with <1% as unchanged parent drug, 27% as unchanged MHD, 49% as MHD glucuronides, 3% as DHD (inactive), and 13% as conjugate of oxcarbazepine and MHD; <4% excreted in feces

Clearance (per body weight):
Children 2 to <4 years: Increased by ~80% compared to adults
Children 4-12 years: Increased by ~40% compared to adults
Children ≥13 years: Values approach adult clearance

Hepatic impairment: Mild to moderate: No effect on pharmacokinetics; Severe: Not studied

Usual Dosage Oral: **Note:** Oral suspension and tablets are interchangeable on a mg per mg basis:

Neonates, Infants, and Children <2 years: Not approved for use; limited information is available

Children 2-16 years:
Adjunctive therapy:
Children 2 to <4 years: Initial dose: 8-10 mg/kg/day given in 2 divided doses (usual maximum: 600 mg/ day); for children <20 kg, consider initial dose of 16-20 mg/kg/day given in 2 divided doses; increase dose slowly over 2-4 weeks; do not exceed 60 mg/kg/ day in 2 divided doses

Children 4-16 years: Initial dose: 8-10 mg/kg/day given in 2 divided doses (usual maximum: 600 mg/day); increase dose slowly over 2 weeks to the following weight-dependent target maintenance dose:
20-29 kg: 900 mg/day in 2 divided doses
29.1-39 kg: 1200 mg/day in 2 divided doses
>39 kg: 1800 mg/day in 2 divided doses

Note: Use of these pediatric target maintenance doses in one clinical trial resulted in doses ranging from 6-51 mg/ kg/day (median dose: 31 mg/kg/day) in children 4-16 years of age (see Glauser, 2000). In children 2-4 years of age, 50% of patients were titrated to a final dose of at least 55 mg/kg/day with target dose of 60 mg/kg/day. Due to a higher drug clearance, children 2 to <4 years of age may require up to twice the dose per body weight compared to adults; children 4 to ≤12 years of age may require a 50% higher dose per body weight compared to adults (see product information).

Children 4-16 years:
Conversion to monotherapy: Initial: 8-10 mg/kg/day given in 2 divided doses, with a simultaneous initial reduction of the dose of concomitant antiepileptic drugs (AEDs); withdraw concomitant AEDs completely over 3-6 weeks, while increasing oxcarbazepine dose as needed by no more than 10 mg/kg/day at approximately weekly intervals; increase oxcarbazepine dose to achieve the recommended monotherapy maintenance dose by weight listed below.

Initiation of monotherapy: Initial: 8-10 mg/kg/day given in 2 divided doses; increase dose every third day by 5 mg/ kg/day to achieve the recommended monotherapy maintenance dose by weight, as follows:
20 kg: 600-900 mg/day in 2 divided doses
25-30 kg: 900-1200 mg/day in 2 divided doses
35-40 kg: 900-1500 mg/day in 2 divided doses
45 kg: 1200-1500 mg/day in 2 divided doses
50-55 kg: 1200-1800 mg/day in 2 divided doses
60-65 kg: 1200-2100 mg/day in 2 divided doses
70 kg: 1500-2100 mg/day in 2 divided doses

Adults:
Adjunctive therapy: Initial: 300 mg twice daily; increase if needed by no more than 600 mg/day at approximately weekly intervals; recommended maintenance dose: 600 mg twice daily; **Note:** Doses >1200 mg/day may have greater efficacy, but most patients are not able to tolerate 2400 mg/day (mostly due to CNS effects); monitor patient closely and measure concentrations of concomitant antiepileptic agents during dosage titration and especially with oxcarbazepine doses >1200 mg/ day.

Conversion to monotherapy: Initial: 300 mg twice daily with a simultaneous initial reduction of the dose of concomitant antiepileptic drugs (AEDs); withdraw concomitant AEDs completely over 3-6 weeks, while increasing oxcarbazepine dose as needed by no more than 600 mg/day at approximately weekly intervals; recommended oxcarbazepine dose (1200 mg twice daily) should be reached in about 2-4 weeks; **Note:** A lower dose (1200 mg/day) was effective in one study in patients who initiated oxcarbazepine monotherapy.

Initiation of monotherapy: Initial: 300 mg twice daily; increase by 300 mg/day every third day to 1200 mg/ day; a higher dose (2400 mg/day) was effective in patients who were converted from other AEDs to oxcarbazepine monotherapy.

Dosing adjustment in renal impairment: Cl$_{cr}$ <30 mL/minute: Initial dose: Administer 50% of the normal starting dose; slowly increase the dose if needed, using a slower dosage titration than normal

Dosing adjustment in hepatic impairment:

Mild to moderate hepatic impairment: No dosage adjustment recommended

Severe hepatic impairment: Not evaluated

Administration Oral: May be taken without regard to meals

Suspension: Prior to using for the first time, firmly insert the manufacturer supplied plastic adapter into the neck of the bottle; cover the adapter with child-resistant cap when not in use; shake suspension well (for at least 10 seconds) before use; remove child-resistant cap and insert manufacturer supplied oral syringe to withdraw appropriate dose; dose may be administered directly from syringe or mixed in a small amount of water immediately prior to use; after use, rinse oral syringe with warm water and allow to dry thoroughly; discard any unused portion 7 weeks after first opening bottle

Monitoring Parameters Seizure frequency, duration and severity; symptoms of CNS depression (dizziness, headache, somnolence) and allergic reaction; consider monitoring serum sodium (particularly during first three months of therapy) especially in patients who receive other drugs that may cause hyponatremia and in patients with symptoms of hyponatremia (see Warnings); signs and symptoms of suicidality (eg, anxiety, depression, behavior changes) (see Warnings)

Patient Information Inform prescriber if allergic to carbamazepine. Severe allergic reactions (anaphylaxis) or swelling of the face, lips, eyes, tongue, or difficulty in swallowing or breathing may occur rarely after taking oxcarbazepine; report these reactions to physician immediately; stop taking oxcarbazepine until physician can be consulted. Report excessive somnolence or allergic reactions to physician immediately; report unusual symptoms such as nausea, headache, malaise, confusion, lethargy, obtundation, worsening of seizure activity, or loss of seizure control to physician immediately (blood test for serum sodium may be needed); report skin rash, fever, itching, joint pain, abdominal pain, lack of urination, and swollen glands to physician immediately (these may be signs of a serious or potentially fatal multiorgan hypersensitivity reaction). Antiepileptic agents may increase the risk of suicidal thoughts and behavior; notify physician if you feel more depressed or have thoughts of suicide or self-harm (see Warnings).

May cause drowsiness and impair ability to perform activities requiring mental alertness or physical coordination. Avoid alcohol. Oxcarbazepine may decrease the effectiveness of oral contraceptives (use an alternative, nonhormonal, form of contraception). Do not abruptly discontinue (an increase in seizure activity may result).

Additional Information Symptoms of overdose may include CNS depression (somnolence, ataxia, obtundation); treatment is symptomatic and supportive; consider general poisoning management (eg, gastric lavage, activated charcoal); largest reported overdose is 24 g; oxcarbazepine is a keto analogue of carbamazepine

Dosage Forms Excipient information presented when available (limited, particularly for generics); consult specific product labeling.

Suspension, oral: 300 mg/5 mL (250 mL)

Trileptal®: 300 mg/5 mL (250 mL) [contains ethanol, propylene glycol]

Tablet, oral: 150 mg, 300 mg, 600 mg

Trileptal®: 150 mg, 300 mg, 600 mg

References

Glauser TA, Nigro M, Sachdeo R, et al, "Adjunctive Therapy With Oxcarbazepine in Children With Partial Seizures. The Oxcarbazepine Pediatric Study Group," Neurology, 2000, 54(12):2237-44.

Tecoma ES, "Oxcarbazepine," Epilepsia, 1999, 40(Suppl 5): S37-46.

◆ **Oxeze® Turbuhaler® (Can)** see Formoterol on page 621

◆ **Oxipor® VHC [OTC]** see Coal Tar on page 349

◆ **Oxpentifylline** see Pentoxifylline on page 1090

◆ **Oxybutyn (Can)** see Oxybutynin on page 1037

Oxybutynin (oks i BYOO ti nin)

Medication Safety Issues

Sound-alike/look-alike issues:

Oxybutynin may be confused with OxyContin®

Ditropan® may be confused with Detrol®, diazepam, Diprivan®, dithranol

Beers Criteria medication: This drug may be inappropriate for use in geriatric patients (high severity risk).

Transdermal patch may contain conducting metal (eg, aluminum); remove patch prior to MRI.

U.S. Brand Names Ditropan XL®; Ditropan®; Gelnique™; Oxytrol®

Canadian Brand Names Apo-Oxybutynin®; Ditropan XL®; Ditropan®; Dom-Oxybutynin; Mylan-Oxybutynin; Novo-Oxybutynin; Nu-Oxybutyn; Oxybutyn; Oxybutynine; Oxytrol®; PHL-Oxybutynin; PMS-Oxybutynin; Riva-Oxybutynin; Uromax®

Therapeutic Category Antispasmodic Agent, Urinary

Generic Available Yes: Excludes gel, transdermal patch

Use Relief of bladder spasms associated with voiding in patients with uninhibited and reflex neurogenic bladder; treatment of overactive bladder with symptoms of urge urinary incontinence, urgency, and frequency (FDA approved in ages >5 and adults); symptoms of detrus or overactivity associated with a neurological condition (XL product FDA approved in ages >6 years)

Pregnancy Risk Factor B

Pregnancy Considerations Teratogenic effects were not observed in animal studies. There are no adequate and well-controlled studies in pregnant women; use during pregnancy only if clearly needed.

Lactation Excretion in breast milk unknown/use caution

Breast-Feeding Considerations Suppression of lactation has been reported.

Contraindications Hypersensitivity to oxybutynin or any component; glaucoma (angle-closure), partial or complete GI obstruction, GU obstruction; toxic megacolon

Warnings Transdermal patch may contain conducting metal (eg, aluminum); remove patch prior to MRI. The extended release formulation consists of drug within a nondeformable matrix; following drug release/absorption, the matrix/shell is expelled in the stool.

Precautions Use with caution in patients with hepatic or renal disease, myasthenia gravis, heart disease, hyperthyroidism, reflux esophagitis, hypertension, prostatic hypertrophy, autonomic neuropathy, ulcerative colitis, intestinal atony. After application of the alcohol-based gel product, avoid open fire or smoking until gel has dried. Once topical gel has dried, application site should be covered with clothing to avoid transfer of medicine to others.

Adverse Reactions

Cardiovascular: Arrhythmias, myocarditis, palpitations, peripheral edema, tachycardia, vasodilation

Central nervous system: Confusion, dizziness, drowsiness, fever, hallucinations, headache, insomnia, seizures, somnolence

Dermatologic: Rash

Endocrine & metabolic: Hot flashes, suppressed lactation

Gastrointestinal: Abdominal pain, constipation, diarrhea, dyspepsia, flatulence, GI motility decreased, nausea, vomiting, xerostomia

Genitourinary: Impotence, urinary hesitancy or retention, urinary tract infections

Local: Application site reactions, such as burning (transdermal formulation), erythema, macular rash, pruritus, and rash

Neuromuscular & skeletal: Weakness

Ocular: Amblyopia, blurred vision, cycloplegia, lacrimation decreased, mydriasis

Respiratory: Dry nasal and sinus mucous membranes

Miscellaneous: Diaphoresis decreased, hypersensitivity reactions

Drug Interactions
Metabolism/Transport Effects Substrate of CYP3A4 (minor); **Inhibits** CYP2C8 (weak), 2D6 (weak), 3A4 (weak)

Avoid Concomitant Use There are no known interactions where it is recommended to avoid concomitant use.

Increased Effect/Toxicity

Oxybutynin may increase the levels/effects of: AbobotulinumtoxinA; Anticholinergics; Cannabinoids; OnabotulinumtoxinA; Potassium Chloride; RimabotulinumtoxinB

The levels/effects of Oxybutynin may be increased by: Pramlintide

Decreased Effect

Oxybutynin may decrease the levels/effects of: Acetylcholinesterase Inhibitors (Central); Secretin

The levels/effects of Oxybutynin may be decreased by: Acetylcholinesterase Inhibitors (Central)

Food Interactions Food may slightly delay absorption and increase bioavailability of immediate release formulation by 25%. Absorption of extended release formulation is not affected by food.

Stability Store at controlled room temperature; protect syrup from light; keep transdermal patch in sealed pouch; protect from moisture or humidity; keep gel in sachet; protect from heat.

Mechanism of Action Direct antispasmodic effect on smooth muscle, also inhibits the action of acetylcholine on smooth muscle; does not block effects at skeletal muscle or at autonomic ganglia; increases bladder capacity, decreases uninhibited contractions, and delays desire to void resulting in decreased urgency and frequency

Pharmacodynamics
Immediate release formulation:
  Onset of action: Oral: Within 30-60 minutes
  Maximum effect: 3-6 hours
  Duration: 6-10 hours
Extended release formulation: Maximum effects: 3 days
Transdermal formulation: Duration: 96 hours

Pharmacokinetics (Adult data unless noted)
Absorption: Oral: Rapid and well absorbed

Distribution: V_d: Adults: 193 L

Metabolism: Hepatic via cytochrome isozyme CYP3A4 found mostly in liver and gut wall; extensive first pass effect (not with I.V. or transdermal use); metabolized in the liver to active and inactive metabolites

Bioavailability: Oral: Immediate release: 6% (range: 1.6% to 10.9%)

Half-life: Adults: 2-3 hours

Time to peak serum concentration:
  Immediate release: Within 60 minutes
  Extended release: 4-6 hours
  Transdermal: 24-48 hours

Elimination: <0.1% excreted unchanged in urine

Usual Dosage
Children: Oral:
  Immediate release:
    1-5 years: 0.2 mg/kg/dose 2-3 times/day
    >5 years: 5 mg twice daily, up to 5 mg 3 times/day
  Extended release: ≥6 years: 5 mg once daily; increase as tolerated in 5 mg increments to a maximum of 20 mg/day
Adults:
  Oral: 5 mg 2-3 times/day up to 5 mg 4 times/day maximum **or** extended release tablet (Ditropan® XL) 5-10 mg once daily; increase in 5 mg increments to a maximum of 30 mg/day
  Topical gel: Apply contents of one sachet (100 mg/g) once daily
  Transdermal: 3.9 mg/day system applied twice weekly (every 3-4 days)
Note: Should be discontinued periodically to determine whether the patient can manage without the drug and to minimize tolerance to the drug

Administration
Oral: May be administered with or without food; swallow extended release tablets whole; do not chew or crush.

Topical gel: For topical use only. Apply to clean, dry, intact skin on abdomen, thighs, or upper arms/shoulders. Rotate site; do not apply to same site on consecutive days. Wash hands after use. Cover treated area with clothing after gel has dried to prevent transfer of medication to others. Do not bathe, shower, or swim until 1 hour after gel applied.

Transdermal: Apply to dry intact skin on the abdomen, hip, or buttock. Rotate site of application with each administration and avoid application to the same site within 7 days

Patient Information May cause drowsiness and impair ability to perform activities requiring mental alertness or physical coordination; may cause heat prostration (fever and heat stroke due to decreased sweating) when used in hot climates; avoid alcohol; may cause dry mouth; nonabsorbable tablet shell may be seen in stool, but active drug has been released

Dosage Forms Excipient information presented when available (limited, particularly for generics); consult specific product labeling.
Gel, topical, as chloride:
  Gelnique™: 10% (1 g) [contains ethanol]
Patch, transdermal:
  Oxytrol®: 3.9 mg/day (8s) [39 cm²; total oxybutynin 36 mg]
Syrup, as chloride: 5 mg/5 mL (473 mL)
Tablet, as chloride: 5 mg
  Ditropan®: 5 mg
Tablet, extended release, as chloride: 5 mg, 10 mg, 15 mg
  Ditropan XL®: 5 mg, 10 mg, 15 mg

References
Humphreys MR and Reinberg YE, "Contemporary and Emerging Drug Treatments for Urinary Incontinence in Children," *Paediatr Drugs*, 2005, 7(3):151-62.

◆ **Oxybutynin Chloride** *see* Oxybutynin *on page 1037*

◆ **Oxybutynine (Can)** *see* Oxybutynin *on page 1037*

◆ **Oxycocet® (Can)** *see* Oxycodone and Acetaminophen *on page 1041*

◆ **Oxycodan® (Can)** *see* Oxycodone and Aspirin *on page 1042*

OxyCODONE (oks i KOE done)

Medication Safety Issues
Sound-alike/look-alike issues:
  OxyCODONE may be confused with HYDROcodone, OxyContin®, oxymorphone

OxyContin® may be confused with MS Contin®, oxybutynin, oxycodone

OxyFast® may be confused with Roxanol™

Roxicodone® may be confused with Roxanol™

High alert medication: The Institute for Safe Medication Practices (ISMP) includes this medication among its list of drug classes which have a heightened risk of causing significant patient harm when used in error.

International issues:

Supeudol® [Canada] may be confused with Supadol Mono which is a brand name for acetaminophen in Luxembourg

U.S. Brand Names OxyContin®; OxyIR® [DSC]; Roxicodone®

Canadian Brand Names Oxy.IR®; OxyContin®; PMS-Oxycodone; Supeudol®

Therapeutic Category Analgesic, Narcotic

Generic Available Yes

Use Relief of moderate to severe pain (FDA approved in adults)

Controlled release tablets (OxyContin®) are indicated for around-the-clock management of moderate to severe pain when an analgesic is needed for an extended period of time; **Note:** OxyContin® is not intended for use as a PRN analgesic or for treatment of mild pain, pain that is not expected to persist for an extended period of time, or for immediate postoperative pain (within 12-24 hours after surgery); OxyContin® may be used for postoperative pain only if the patient received it prior to surgery or if moderate to severe persistent pain is anticipated.

Restrictions C-II

Medication Guide An FDA-approved patient medication guide, which is available with the product information and as follows, must be dispensed with this medication for each new outpatient prescription and refill.

OxyContin®: http://www.fda.gov/downloads/Drugs/DrugSafety/UCM208530.pdf

Pregnancy Risk Factor C

Pregnancy Considerations Should be used in pregnancy only if clearly needed. Use of narcotics during pregnancy may produce physical dependence in the neonate; respiratory depression may occur in the newborn if narcotics are used prior to delivery (especially high doses).

Lactation Enters breast milk/use caution

Contraindications Hypersensitivity to oxycodone or any component (see Warnings); significant respiratory depression (in settings without resuscitative equipment or without adequate respiratory monitoring); patients with hypercarbia, severe or acute asthma, paralytic ileus (known or suspected)

Warnings Respiratory depression may occur; use with extreme caution in patients with pre-existing respiratory depression, decreased respiratory reserve, hypoxia, hypercapnia, significant COPD, or cor pulmonale. Hypotension may occur, especially in hypovolemic patients or those receiving medications that compromise vasomotor tone; use with extreme caution in patients with circulatory shock; orthostatic hypotension may occur in ambulatory patients. Physical and psychological dependence may occur; abrupt discontinuation after prolonged use may result in withdrawal symptoms; use of agonist/antagonist analgesics may precipitate withdrawal symptoms and/or reduce the analgesic efficacy in patients who have received or who are receiving a pure opioid agonist such as oxycodone. Warn patient of possible impairment of alertness or physical coordination (see Patient Information); interactions with other CNS drugs may occur (see Drug Interactions). OxyContin® is a controlled-release oral formulation indicated for the management of moderate-to-

severe pain when continuous analgesia is needed for an extended period of time; OxyContin® is not intended for use as an "as needed" analgesic or for immediately-postoperative pain management **[U.S. Boxed Warning]**. Controlled release 60 mg, 80 mg, and 160 mg tablets should only be used in patients who are opioid tolerant **[U.S. Boxed Warning]**; administration of these tablet strengths to opioid-naive patients may cause fatal respiratory depression. Do not crush, break, or chew controlled-release tablets **[U.S. Boxed Warning]**; taking broken, chewed, or crushed tablets may lead to rapid release and absorption of a potentially fatal dose. Healthcare provider should be alert to problems of abuse, misuse, and diversion **[U.S. Boxed Warning]**.

Oral concentrate contains sodium benzoate; benzoic acid (benzoate) is a metabolite of benzyl alcohol; large amounts of benzyl alcohol (≥99 mg/kg/day) have been associated with a potentially fatal toxicity ("gasping syndrome") in neonates; the "gasping syndrome" consists of metabolic acidosis, respiratory distress, gasping respirations, CNS dysfunction (including convulsions, intracranial hemorrhage), hypotension and cardiovascular collapse; avoid use of oxycodone products containing sodium benzoate in neonates; in vitro and animal studies have shown that benzoate displaces bilirubin from protein binding sites.

Precautions Use with caution in patients with hypersensitivity to other phenanthrene derivative opioid agonists (morphine, codeine, hydrocodone, hydromorphone, oxymorphone, levorphanol). Use with caution in patients with head injury; increased intracranial pressure; CNS depression; respiratory depression; coma; toxic psychosis; seizures; acute abdominal conditions; biliary tract disease, pancreatitis; severe renal, respiratory, or hepatic insufficiency; hypothyroidism; Addison's disease; urethral stricture and in debilitated patients. Use care in prescribing, dispensing, and administering the oral concentrated solution, inappropriate use may cause overdose.

Adverse Reactions

Cardiovascular system: Bradycardia, hypotension, orthostatic hypotension, peripheral vasodilation

Central nervous system: Abnormal dreams, abnormal thoughts, anxiety, chills, confusion, CNS depression, dizziness, drowsiness, dysphoria, fatigue, fever, headache, insomnia, intracranial pressure elevated, lightheadedness, nervousness, sedation, somnolence

Dermatologic: Pruritus, skin rash

Endocrine & metabolic: Antidiuretic hormone release

Gastrointestinal: Abdominal pain, anorexia, biliary tract spasm, constipation, dyspepsia, gastritis, nausea, vomiting, xerostomia

Genitourinary: Urinary retention, urinary tract spasm

Neuromuscular & skeletal: Asthenia

Ocular: Miosis

Respiratory: Dyspnea, hiccups, respiratory depression

Miscellaneous: Anaphylactoid reactions, anaphylaxis, diaphoresis, histamine release, physical and psychological dependence

Drug Interactions

Metabolism/Transport Effects Substrate of CYP2D6 (minor), 3A4 (major)

Avoid Concomitant Use There are no known interactions where it is recommended to avoid concomitant use.

Increased Effect/Toxicity

OxyCODONE may increase the levels/effects of: Alcohol (Ethyl); Alvimopan; CNS Depressants; Desmopressin; Selective Serotonin Reuptake Inhibitors; Thiazide Diuretics

The levels/effects of OxyCODONE may be increased by: Amphetamines; Antipsychotic Agents (Phenothiazines); CYP3A4 Inhibitors (Moderate); CYP3A4 Inhibitors (Strong); Dasatinib; Succinylcholine

Decreased Effect
OxyCODONE may decrease the levels/effects of: Pegvisomant

The levels/effects of OxyCODONE may be decreased by: Ammonium Chloride; CYP3A4 Inducers (Strong); Deferasirox; Mixed Agonist / Antagonist Opioids; Rifampin; St Johns Wort

Food Interactions Food does not significantly affect absorption of controlled release tablets; high fat meal may increase peak concentrations of OxyContin® 160 mg tablet by 25%

Stability Store at room temperature; protect from light and moisture
OxyFast® oral concentrate: Stable for 90 days after opening

Mechanism of Action Binds to opiate receptors in the CNS, causing inhibition of ascending pain pathways, altering the perception of and response to pain; produces generalized CNS depression

Pharmacodynamics Duration of pain relief: Oral:
Immediate release: 4-5 hours
Controlled release: 12 hours

Pharmacokinetics (Adult data unless noted)
Distribution: Distributes into skeletal muscle, liver, intestinal tract, lungs, spleen, brain, and breast milk; V_{dss}:
Children 2-10 years: Mean: 2.1 L/kg; range: 1.2-3.7 L/kg
Adults: 2.6 L/kg
Protein binding: 38% to 45%
Metabolism: In the liver primarily to noroxycodone (via demethylation) and oxymorphone (via CYP2D6); noroxycodone is the major circulating metabolite, but has much weaker activity than oxycodone; oxymorphone is active, but present in low concentrations; <15% of the dose is metabolized to oxymorphone via CYP2D6; drug and metabolites undergo glucuronide conjugation
Bioavailability: Adults: 60% to 87%
Half-life, apparent: Adults:
Immediate release: 3.2 hours
Controlled release (OxyContin®): 4.5 hours
Half-life, elimination:
Children 2-10 years: 1.8 hours; range: 1.2-3 hours
Adults: 3.7 hours
Adults with renal dysfunction (Cl_{cr} <60 mL/minute): Half-life increases by 1 hour, but peak oxycodone concentrations increase by 50% and AUC increases by 60%
Adults with mild to moderate hepatic dysfunction: Half-life increases by 2.3 hours, peak oxycodone concentrations increase by 50%, and AUC increases by 95%
Elimination: In the urine as unchanged drug (≤19%) and metabolites: Conjugated oxycodone (≤50%), conjugated oxymorphone (≤14%), noroxycodone, and conjugated noroxycodone

Usual Dosage Oral: Doses should be titrated to appropriate effect:
Immediate release products:
Children: 0.05-0.15 mg/kg/dose every 4-6 hours as needed
Adults: Initial: 5 mg every 6 hours as needed; usual: 10-30 mg every 4 hours as needed; more severe pain: ≥30 mg every 4 hours
AHCPR dosing guidelines: Opioid naive patients: (See Carr, 1992 and Jacox, 1994)
Children and Adults <50 kg: Moderate to severe pain: Usual initial dose: 0.2 mg/kg every 3-4 hours
Children and Adults ≥50 kg: Moderate to severe pain: Usual initial dose: 10 mg every 3-4 hours
Controlled release product: Adolescents ≥18 years and Adults: Initial: 10 mg every 12 hours; use immediate-release analgesics as needed for rescue from breakthrough pain or prior to predictable pain from procedures or activities; rescue analgesic should be 1/4 to 1/3 of the 12-hour controlled release oxycodone dose; increase the dose of controlled release oxycodone if >2 doses of rescue analgesic are required within 24 hours; dose of controlled release oxycodone may be adjusted every 1-2 days by 25% to 50% (initial increase may be from 10 mg to 20 mg every 12 hours). Mean doses used in open-label trials: Opioid naive patients: 40 mg/day; cancer patients: 105 mg/day (range: 20-720 mg/day)

Note: To convert patients from other opioid or nonopioid analgesics to oxycodone controlled release tablets: See OxyContin® package insert

Dosing adjustment in renal impairment: Cl_{cr} <60 mL/minute: Initiate doses conservatively and carefully titrate dose to appropriate effect

Dosing adjustment in hepatic impairment: Initial: 1/3 to 1/2 of the usual dose; carefully titrate dose to appropriate effect

Administration May administer with food to decrease GI upset; swallow controlled (sustained) release tablets whole; do not crush, chew, or break (this would result in rapid release and absorption of a potentially fatal dose of drug); avoid high fat meals when initiating controlled release 160 mg tablets

Monitoring Parameters Pain relief, respiratory rate, mental status, blood pressure

Patient Information May cause dry mouth; may cause drowsiness and impair ability to perform activities requiring mental alertness or physical coordination; may cause postural hypotension (use caution when changing positions from lying or sitting to standing); avoid alcohol; report the use of other prescription and nonprescription medications to your physician and pharmacist. May be habit-forming; do not discontinue abruptly if therapy lasts more than a few weeks; dose should be tapered to prevent withdrawal. Do not crush, chew, or break controlled release tablets (OxyContin®), as risk of overdose (and possibly death) may occur. Empty controlled release tablets may appear in stool after medication is absorbed (this is normal). Do not share OxyContin® with others (sharing is illegal and may cause severe medical adverse effects, including death).

Additional Information OxyContin® tablets deliver medication over 12 hours; release is pH independent. Equianalgesic doses: oral oxycodone 30 mg = morphine 10 mg I.M. = single oral dose morphine 60 mg **or** chronic dosing oral morphine 30 mg

Dosage Forms Excipient information presented when available (limited, particularly for generics); consult specific product labeling. [DSC] = Discontinued product
Capsule, immediate release, as hydrochloride: 5 mg
OxyIR®: 5 mg [DSC]
Liquid, oral, as hydrochloride [concentrate]:
Roxicodone®: 20 mg/mL (30 mL) [contains sodium benzoate]
Solution, oral, as hydrochloride: 5 mg/5 mL (100 mL, 500 mL)
Roxicodone®: 5 mg/5 mL (5 mL, 500 mL) [contains ethanol]
Solution, oral, as hydrochloride [concentrate]: 20 mg/mL (30 mL)
Tablet, as hydrochloride: 5 mg, 10 mg, 15 mg, 20 mg, 30 mg
Roxicodone®: 5 mg, 15 mg, 30 mg
Tablet, controlled release, as hydrochloride:
OxyContin®: 10 mg, 15 mg, 20 mg, 30 mg, 40 mg, 60 mg, 80 mg

References
Carr D, Jacox A, Chapman CR, et al, "Clinical Practice Guideline Number 1: Acute Pain Management: Operative or Medical Procedures and Trauma," Rockville, Maryland: U.S. Department of Health and Human Services, Public Health Service, Agency for Health Care Policy and Research, AHCPR Publication No 92-0032, 1992.

Jacox A, Carr D, Payne R, et al, "Clinical Practice Guideline Number 9: Management of Cancer Pain," Rockville, Maryland: U.S. Department of Health and Human Services, Public Health Service, Agency for Health Care Policy and Research, AHCPR Publication No. 94-0592, 1994.

Olkkola KT, Hamunen K, and Maunuksela EL, "Clinical Pharmacokinetics and Pharmacodynamics of Opioid Analgesics in Infants and Children," *Clin Pharmacokinet*, 1995, 28(5):385-404.

Olkkola KT, Hamunen K, Seppala T, et al, "Pharmacokinetics and Ventilatory Effects of Intravenous Oxycodone in Postoperative Children," *Br J Clin Pharmacol*, 1994, 38(1):71-6.

Oxycodone and Acetaminophen

(oks i KOE done & a seet a MIN oh fen)

Medication Safety Issues

Sound-alike/look-alike issues:

Endocet® may be confused with Indocid®

Percocet® may be confused with Darvocet®, Fioricet®, Percodan®

Roxicet™ may be confused with Roxanol™

Tylox® may be confused with Trimox®, Tylenol®, Wymox®, Xanax®

High alert medication: The Institute for Safe Medication Practices (ISMP) includes this medication among its list of drug classes which have a heightened risk of causing significant patient harm when used in error.

Duplicate therapy issues: This product contains acetaminophen, which may be a component of other combination products. Do not exceed the maximum recommended daily dose of acetaminophen.

Related Information

Opioid Analgesics Comparison *on page 1510*

U.S. Brand Names Endocet®; Magnacet™ [DSC]; Percocet®; Primalev™ [DSC]; Primlev™; Roxicet™; Roxicet™ 5/500; Tylox®

Canadian Brand Names Endocet®; Novo-Oxycodone Acet; Oxycocet®; Percocet®; Percocet®-Demi; PMS-Oxycodone-Acetaminophen

Therapeutic Category Analgesic, Narcotic

Generic Available Yes: Excludes caplet and solution

Use Relief of moderate to severe pain

Restrictions C-II

Pregnancy Risk Factor C

Pregnancy Considerations Use of opioids during pregnancy may produce physical dependence in the neonate; respiratory depression may occur in the newborn if opioids are used prior to delivery (especially high doses).

Lactation Enters breast milk/use caution

Breast-Feeding Considerations

Oxycodone: Excreted in breast milk. If occasional doses are used during breast-feeding, monitor infant for sedation, GI effects, and changes in feeding pattern.

Acetaminophen: May be taken while breast-feeding.

Contraindications Hypersensitivity to oxycodone, acetaminophen, or any component (see Warnings); severe respiratory depression, severe liver or renal insufficiency

Warnings Abrupt discontinuation after prolonged use may result in withdrawal symptoms; some preparations contain sodium metabisulfite which may cause allergic reactions in susceptible individuals; capsule may contain sodium benzoate; benzoic acid (benzoate) is a metabolite of benzyl alcohol; large amounts of benzyl alcohol (≥99 mg/kg/day) have been associated with a potentially fatal toxicity ("gasping syndrome") in neonates; the "gasping syndrome" consists of metabolic acidosis, respiratory distress, gasping respirations, CNS dysfunction (including convulsions, intracranial hemorrhage), hypotension and cardiovascular collapse; avoid use of oxycodone and acetaminophen products containing sodium benzoate in neonates; *in vitro* and animal studies have shown that benzoate displaces bilirubin from protein binding sites

Precautions Use with caution in patients with hypersensitivity to other phenanthrene derivative opioid agonists (morphine, codeine, hydrocodone, hydromorphone, oxymorphone, levorphanol)

Adverse Reactions

Cardiovascular: Hypotension, bradycardia, peripheral vasodilation

Central nervous system: CNS depression, intracranial pressure elevated, drowsiness, sedation

Dermatologic: Pruritus

Endocrine & metabolic: Antidiuretic hormone release

Gastrointestinal: Nausea, vomiting, constipation, biliary tract spasm

Genitourinary: Urinary tract spasm

Ocular: Miosis

Respiratory: Respiratory depression

Miscellaneous: Physical and psychological dependence, histamine release

Drug Interactions

Metabolism/Transport Effects

Oxycodone: **Substrate** of CYP2D6 (minor), 3A4 (major)

Acetaminophen: **Substrate** (minor) of CYP1A2, 2A6, 2C9, 2D6, 2E1, 3A4

Avoid Concomitant Use There are no known interactions where it is recommended to avoid concomitant use.

Increased Effect/Toxicity

Oxycodone and Acetaminophen may increase the levels/effects of: Alcohol (Ethyl); Alvimopan; CNS Depressants; Desmopressin; Selective Serotonin Reuptake Inhibitors; Thiazide Diuretics; Vitamin K Antagonists

The levels/effects of Oxycodone and Acetaminophen may be increased by: Amphetamines; Antipsychotic Agents (Phenothiazines); CYP3A4 Inhibitors (Moderate); CYP3A4 Inhibitors (Strong); Dasatinib; Imatinib; Isoniazid; Succinylcholine

Decreased Effect

Oxycodone and Acetaminophen may decrease the levels/effects of: Pegvisomant

The levels/effects of Oxycodone and Acetaminophen may be decreased by: Ammonium Chloride; Anticonvulsants (Hydantoin); Barbiturates; CarBAMazepine; Cholestyramine Resin; CYP3A4 Inducers (Strong); Deferasirox; Mixed Agonist / Antagonist Opioids; Peginterferon Alfa-2b; Rifampin; St Johns Wort

Food Interactions Rate of absorption of acetaminophen may be decreased when given with food high in carbohydrates

Mechanism of Action See individual agents.

Pharmacodynamics

Onset of action: Within 10-15 minutes

Maximum effect: Within 1 hour

Duration: 3-6 hours

Pharmacokinetics (Adult data unless noted) See individual agents.

Usual Dosage Oral (titrate dose to appropriate analgesic effects):

Children: Based on **oxycodone component**: 0.05-0.15 mg/kg/dose up to 5 mg/dose every 4-6 hours as needed

Adults: 1-2 tablets every 4-6 hours as needed for pain; maximum daily dose of acetaminophen: 4 g/day

Administration Oral: May administer with food or milk to decrease GI upset

Monitoring Parameters Pain relief, respiratory rate, mental status, blood pressure

◄ **Patient Information** Avoid alcohol; may cause drowsiness and impair ability to perform activities requiring mental alertness or physical coordination. May be habit-forming; do not discontinue abruptly if therapy lasts more than a few weeks; dose should be tapered to prevent narcotic withdrawal.

Dosage Forms Excipient information presented when available (limited, particularly for generics); consult specific product labeling. [DSC] = Discontinued product

Caplet:
Roxicet™ 5/500: Oxycodone hydrochloride 5 mg and acetaminophen 500 mg

Capsule: 5/500: Oxycodone hydrochloride 5 mg and acetaminophen 500 mg

Tylox®: 5/500: Oxycodone hydrochloride 5 mg and acetaminophen 500 mg [contains sodium benzoate and sodium metabisulfite]

Solution, oral:
Roxicet™: Oxycodone hydrochloride 5 mg and acetaminophen 325 mg per 5 mL (5 mL, 500 mL) [contains ethanol <0.5%; mint flavor]

Tablet: 2.5/325: Oxycodone hydrochloride 2.5 mg and acetaminophen 325 mg; 5/325: Oxycodone hydrochloride 5 mg and acetaminophen 325 mg; 7.5/325: Oxycodone hydrochloride 7.5 mg and acetaminophen 325 mg; 7.5/500: Oxycodone hydrochloride 7.5 mg and acetaminophen 500 mg; 10/325: Oxycodone hydrochloride 10 mg and acetaminophen 325 mg; 10/650: Oxycodone hydrochloride 10 mg and acetaminophen 650 mg

Endocet® 5/325 [scored]: Oxycodone hydrochloride 5 mg and acetaminophen 325 mg

Endocet® 7.5/325: Oxycodone hydrochloride 7.5 mg and acetaminophen 325 mg

Endocet® 7.5/500: Oxycodone hydrochloride 7.5 mg and acetaminophen 500 mg

Endocet® 10/325: Oxycodone hydrochloride 10 mg and acetaminophen 325 mg

Endocet® 10/650: Oxycodone hydrochloride 10 mg and acetaminophen 650 mg

Magnacet™ 2.5/400: Oxycodone hydrochloride 2.5 mg and acetaminophen 400 mg [DSC]

Magnacet™ 5/400: Oxycodone hydrochloride 5 mg and acetaminophen 400 mg [DSC]

Magnacet™ 7.5/400: Oxycodone hydrochloride 7.5 mg and acetaminophen 400 mg [DSC]

Magnacet™ 10/400: Oxycodone hydrochloride 10 mg and acetaminophen 400 mg [DSC]

Percocet® 2.5/325: Oxycodone hydrochloride 2.5 mg and acetaminophen 325 mg

Percocet® 5/325 [scored]: Oxycodone hydrochloride 5 mg and acetaminophen 325 mg

Percocet® 7.5/325: Oxycodone hydrochloride 7.5 mg and acetaminophen 325 mg

Percocet® 7.5/500: Oxycodone hydrochloride 7.5 mg and acetaminophen 500 mg

Percocet® 10/325: Oxycodone hydrochloride 10 mg and acetaminophen 325 mg

Percocet® 10/650: Oxycodone hydrochloride 10 mg and acetaminophen 650 mg

Primalev™ 2.5/300: Oxycodone hydrochloride 2.5 mg and acetaminophen 300 mg [DSC]

Primlev™ 5/300: Oxycodone hydrochloride 5 mg and acetaminophen 300 mg

Primlev™ 7.5/300: Oxycodone hydrochloride 7.5 mg and acetaminophen 300 mg

Primlev™ 10/300: Oxycodone hydrochloride 10 mg and acetaminophen 300 mg

Roxicet™ [scored]: Oxycodone hydrochloride 5 mg and acetaminophen 325 mg

References
Olkkola KT, Hamunen K, and Maunuksela EL, "Clinical Pharmacokinetics and Pharmacodynamics of Opioid Analgesics in Infants and Children," *Clin Pharmacokinet*, 1995, 28(5):385-404.

Oxycodone and Aspirin (oks i KOE done & AS pir in)

Medication Safety Issues
Sound-alike/look-alike issues:
Percodan® may be confused with Decadron®, Percocet®, Percogesic®, Periactin®

High alert medication: The Institute for Safe Medication Practices (ISMP) includes this medication among its list of drug classes which have a heightened risk of causing significant patient harm when used in error.

U.S. Brand Names Endodan®; Percodan®

Canadian Brand Names Endodan®; Oxycodan®; Percodan®

Therapeutic Category Analgesic, Narcotic

Generic Available Yes

Use Relief of moderate to moderately severe pain

Restrictions C-II

Pregnancy Risk Factor B (oxycodone); D (aspirin)

Pregnancy Considerations Use of opioids during pregnancy may produce physical dependence in the neonate; respiratory depression may occur in the newborn if opioids are used prior to delivery (especially high doses).

Lactation Enters breast milk/use caution

Breast-Feeding Considerations
Aspirin: Caution is suggested due to potential adverse effects in nursing infants.
Oxycodone: No data reported.

Contraindications Hypersensitivity to oxycodone, salicylates, other NSAIDs, or any component; patients with the aspirin "triad" [asthma, rhinitis (with or without nasal polyps), and aspirin intolerance] (fatal asthmatic and anaphylactoid reactions may occur in these patients); severe respiratory depression; hypercarbia; severe or acute asthma; paralytic ileus (known or suspected); severe liver or renal insufficiency; bleeding disorders

Warnings Contains aspirin, do not use aspirin-containing products in children <16 years of age for chickenpox or flu symptoms due to the association with Reye's syndrome. Contains oxycodone; respiratory depression may occur; use with extreme caution in patients with pre-existing respiratory depression, decreased resiratory reserve, hypoxia, hypercapnia, significant COPD, or cor pulmonale. Hypotension may occur, especially in hypovolemic patients or those receiving medications that compromise vasomotor tone; use with extreme caution in patients with circulatory shock. Orthostatic hypotension may occur in ambulatory patients; physical and psychological dependence may occur; abrupt discontinuation after prolonged use may result in withdrawal symptoms; warn patients of possible impairment of alertness or physical coordination (see Patient Information); interactions with other CNS drugs may occur (see Drug Interactions). Healthcare provider should be alert to problems of abuse, misuse, and diversion.

Precautions Contains aspirin, use with caution in patients with impaired hepatic or renal function, erosive gastritis, peptic ulcer, gout. Contains oxycodone. Use with caution in patients with hypersensitivity to other phenanthrene derivative opioid agonists (morphine, codeine, hydrocodone, hydromorphone, oxymorphone, levorphanol). Use with caution in patients with head injury; increased intracranial pressure; CNS depression; respiratory depression; coma; toxic psychosis; seizures; acute abdominal conditions; biliary tract disease, pancreatitis; severe renal, respiratory, or hepatic insufficiency; hypothyroidism; Addison's disease; urethral stricture and in debilitated patients.

Adverse Reactions

Cardiovascular: Hypotension, bradycardia, peripheral vasodilation

Central nervous system: CNS depression, intracranial pressure elevated, drowsiness, sedation

Dermatologic: Pruritus, rash

Endocrine & metabolic: Antidiuretic hormone release

Gastrointestinal: Nausea, vomiting, constipation, biliary tract spasm, GI distress, GI bleeding, ulcers

Genitourinary: Urinary tract spasm

Hematologic: Inhibition of platelet aggregation (due to aspirin)

Hepatic: Hepatotoxicity (due to aspirin)

Ocular: Miosis

Respiratory: Respiratory depression, bronchospasm

Miscellaneous: Histamine release, physical and psychological dependence

Drug Interactions

Metabolism/Transport Effects

Oxycodone: **Substrate** of CYP2D6 (minor), 3A4 (major)

Aspirin: **Substrate** of CYP2C9 (minor)

Avoid Concomitant Use

Avoid concomitant use of Oxycodone and Aspirin with any of the following: Ketorolac; Ketorolac (Systemic)

Increased Effect/Toxicity

Oxycodone and Aspirin may increase the levels/effects of: Alcohol (Ethyl); Alendronate; Alvimopan; Anticoagulants; Carbonic Anhydrase Inhibitors; CNS Depressants; Collagenase (Systemic); Corticosteroids (Systemic); Desmopressin; Divalproex; Drotrecogin Alfa; Heparin; Ibritumomab; Methotrexate; Pralatrexate; Salicylates; Selective Serotonin Reuptake Inhibitors; Sulfonylureas; Thiazide Diuretics; Thrombolytic Agents; Tositumomab and Iodine I 131 Tositumomab; Valproic Acid; Varicella Virus-Containing Vaccines; Vitamin K Antagonists

The levels/effects of Oxycodone and Aspirin may be increased by: Amphetamines; Antidepressants (Tricyclic, Tertiary Amine); Antiplatelet Agents; Antipsychotic Agents (Phenothiazines); Calcium Channel Blockers (Nondihydropyridine); CYP3A4 Inhibitors (Moderate); CYP3A4 Inhibitors (Strong); Dasatinib; Ginkgo Biloba; Glucosamine; Herbs (Anticoagulant/Antiplatelet Properties); Ketorolac; Ketorolac (Systemic); Loop Diuretics; Nonsteroidal Anti-Inflammatory Agents; NSAID (Nonselective); Omega-3-Acid Ethyl Esters; Pentosan Polysulfate Sodium; Pentoxifylline; Prostacyclin Analogues; Selective Serotonin Reuptake Inhibitors; Serotonin/Norepinephrine Reuptake Inhibitors; Succinylcholine; Treprostinil

Decreased Effect

Oxycodone and Aspirin may decrease the levels/effects of: ACE Inhibitors; Loop Diuretics; NSAID (Nonselective); Pegvisomant; Probenecid; Tiludronate

The levels/effects of Oxycodone and Aspirin may be decreased by: Ammonium Chloride; Corticosteroids (Systemic); CYP3A4 Inducers (Strong); Deferasirox; Mixed Agonist / Antagonist Opioids; Nonsteroidal Anti-Inflammatory Agents; NSAID (Nonselective); Rifampin; St Johns Wort

Food Interactions Aspirin may increase renal excretion of vitamin C and may decrease serum folate levels

Mechanism of Action See individual agents.

Pharmacokinetics (Adult data unless noted) See individual agents.

Usual Dosage Oral: Based on **oxycodone-combined salt component**:

Children: 0.05-0.15 mg/kg/dose every 4-6 hours as needed; maximum dose: 5 mg/dose (1 tablet Percodan®)

Adults: Percodan®: 1 tablet every 6 hours as needed for pain; **Note:** Maximum aspirin dose should not exceed 4 g/day

Dosing adjustment in renal impairment: Cl_{cr} <60 mL/minute: Initiate doses conservatively and carefully titrate dose to appropriate effect

Dosing adjustment in hepatic impairment: Initial: $1/3$ to $1/2$ of the usual dose; carefully titrate dose to appropriate effect

Administration Oral: May administer with food or milk to decrease GI upset

Monitoring Parameters Pain relief, respiratory rate, mental status, blood pressure

Patient Information Avoid alcohol; may cause drowsiness and impair ability to perform activities requiring mental alertness or physical coordination. May be habit-forming; do not discontinue abruptly if therapy lasts more than a few weeks; dose should be tapered to prevent narcotic withdrawal.

Additional Information One generic tablet contains ~5 mg oxycodone as combined salt

Dosage Forms Excipient information presented when available (limited, particularly for generics); consult specific product labeling.

Tablet: Oxycodone hydrochloride 4.5 mg, oxycodone terephthalate 0.38 mg, and aspirin 325 mg

Endodan®, Percodan®: Oxycodone hydrochloride 4.8355 mg and aspirin 325 mg

◆ **Oxycodone Hydrochloride** *see* OxyCODONE *on page 1038*

◆ **OxyContin®** *see* OxyCODONE *on page 1038*

◆ **Oxyderm™ (Can)** *see* Benzoyl Peroxide *on page 184*

◆ **OxyIR® [DSC]** *see* OxyCODONE *on page 1038*

◆ **Oxy.IR® (Can)** *see* OxyCODONE *on page 1038*

Oxymetazoline (oks i met AZ oh leen)

Medication Safety Issues

Sound-alike/look-alike issues:

Oxymetazoline may be confused with oxymetholone

Afrin® may be confused with aspirin

Afrin® (oxymetazoline) may be confused with Afrin® (saline)

Neo-Synephrine® (oxymetazoline) may be confused with Neo-Synephrine® (phenylephrine)

Visine® may be confused with Visken®

U.S. Brand Names 4-Way® 12 Hour [OTC]; Afrin® Extra Moisturizing [OTC]; Afrin® Original [OTC]; Afrin® Severe Congestion [OTC]; Afrin® Sinus [OTC]; Dristan™ 12-Hour [OTC]; Duramist® Plus [OTC]; Genasal [OTC]; Mucinex® Full force™ [OTC] [DSC]; Mucinex® moisture smart™ [OTC] [DSC]; Neo-Synephrine® 12 Hour Extra Moisturizing [OTC]; Neo-Synephrine® 12 Hour [OTC]; NRS® [OTC]; Nõstrilla® [OTC]; Sudafed OM® Sinus Congestion [OTC]; Vicks Sinex® 12 Hour Ultrafine Mist [OTC]; Vicks Sinex® 12 Hour [OTC]; Vicks® Early Defense™ [OTC]; Visine® L.R. [OTC]

Canadian Brand Names Claritin® Allergic Decongestant; Dristan® Long Lasting Nasal; Drixoral® Nasal

Therapeutic Category Adrenergic Agonist Agent; Decongestant, Nasal; Nasal Agent, Vasoconstrictor; Vasoconstrictor, Nasal; Vasoconstrictor, Ophthalmic

Generic Available Yes: Nasal spray

Use Symptomatic relief of nasal mucosal congestion associated with acute or chronic rhinitis, the common cold, sinusitis, hay fever, or other allergies

Contraindications Hypersensitivity to oxymetazoline or any component (see Warnings); patients on MAO inhibitor therapy

Warnings Use for periods exceeding 3 days may result in severe rebound nasal congestion; excessive dosage in children may cause profound CNS depression. Some products contain benzyl alcohol which may cause allergic reactions in susceptible individuals; large amounts of benzyl alcohol (≥99 mg/kg/day) have been associated with a potentially fatal toxicity ("gasping syndrome") in neonates; the "gasping syndrome" consists of metabolic acidosis, respiratory distress, gasping respirations, CNS dysfunction (including convulsions, intracranial hemorrhage), hypotension and cardiovascular collapse; *in vitro* and animal studies have shown that benzoate, a metabolite of benzyl alcohol, displaces bilirubin from protein binding sites; avoid use of these products in neonates

Precautions Use with caution in patients with hyperthyroidism, heart disease, hypertension, diabetes mellitus, increased intraocular pressure, or prostatic hypertrophy

Adverse Reactions

Cardiovascular: Hypertension, palpitations, reflex bradycardia, pallor

Central nervous system: Nervousness, dizziness, insomnia, headache, anxiety, tenseness, drowsiness, CNS depression, convulsions, hallucinations

Gastrointestinal: Nausea, vomiting

Ocular: Stinging to eye, mydriasis, intraocular pressure elevated, blurred vision

Respiratory: Sneezing, respiratory difficulty, rebound congestion with prolonged use, dryness of nasal mucosa

Miscellaneous: Diaphoresis

Drug Interactions

Avoid Concomitant Use

Avoid concomitant use of Oxymetazoline with any of the following: Iobenguane I 123; MAO Inhibitors

Increased Effect/Toxicity

Oxymetazoline may increase the levels/effects of: Sympathomimetics

The levels/effects of Oxymetazoline may be increased by: Atomoxetine; Cannabinoids; MAO Inhibitors; Tricyclic Antidepressants

Decreased Effect

Oxymetazoline may decrease the levels/effects of: Iobenguane I 123

Mechanism of Action Stimulates alpha-adrenergic receptors in the arterioles of the nasal mucosa and arterioles of the conjunctiva to produce vasoconstriction

Pharmacodynamics

Onset of action: Intranasal: Within 5-10 minutes

Duration: 5-6 hours

Pharmacokinetics (Adult data unless noted) Metabolic fate is unknown

Usual Dosage

Nasal: Therapy should not exceed 3-5 days; avoid use in children <6 years of age

Children ≥6 years and Adults: 2-3 drops or 2-3 sprays or 1-2 metered sprays (Nōstrilla®) into each nostril twice daily

Ophthalmic: Children ≥6 years and Adults: Instill 1-2 drops into the affected eye(s) 2-4 times/day (≥6 hours apart)

Administration

Nasal: Spray or apply drops into each nostril while gently occluding the other

Ophthalmic: Instill drops into conjunctival sac of affected eye(s); avoid contact of bottle tip with skin or eye; finger pressure should be applied to lacrimal sac during and for 1-2 minutes after instillation to decrease the risk of absorption and systemic reactions

Dosage Forms Excipient information presented when available (limited, particularly for generics); consult specific product labeling. [DSC] = Discontinued product

Gel, intranasal, as hydrochloride [spray]:

Vicks® Early Defense™: 0.05% (14.7 mL) [microgel; contains benzyl alcohol and menthol]

Solution, intranasal, as hydrochloride [spray]: 0.05% (15 mL, 30 mL)

Afrin® Extra Moisturizing: 0.05% (15 mL) [contains benzyl alcohol and glycerin; regular or no drip formula]

Afrin® Original: 0.05% (15 mL, 30 mL) [contains benzalkonium chloride]

Afrin® Original: 0.05% (15 mL) [contains benzyl alcohol and benzalkonium chloride; no drip formula]

Afrin® Severe Congestion: 0.05% (15 mL) [contains benzyl alcohol and menthol; regular or no drip formula]

Afrin® Sinus: 0.05% (15 mL) [contains benzyl alcohol, benzalkonium chloride, camphor, phenol; regular or no drip formula]

Dristan™ 12-Hour: 0.05% (15 mL) [contains benzyl alcohol and benzalkonium chloride]

Duramist® Plus, Neo-Synephrine® 12 Hour, Nōstrilla®, Vicks Sinex® 12 Hour Ultrafine Mist, Vicks Sinex® 12 Hour, 4-Way® 12 Hour: 0.05% (15 mL) [contains benzalkonium chloride]

Genasal, NRS®: 0.05% (15 mL, 30 mL) [contains benzalkonium chloride]

Mucinex® Full force™: 0.05% (22 mL) [contains benzalkonium chloride, camphor, and menthol] [DSC]

Mucinex® moisture smart™: 0.05% (22 mL) [contains benzalkonium chloride and glycerin] [DSC]

Neo-Synephrine® 12 Hour Extra Moisturizing: 0.05% (15 mL) [contains glycerin]

Sudafed OM® Sinus Congestion: 0.05% (15 mL) [contains benzalkonium chloride and glycerin]

Solution, ophthalmic, as hydrochloride:

Visine® L.R.: 0.025% (15 mL, 30 mL) [contains benzalkonium chloride]

◆ **Oxymetazoline Hydrochloride** see Oxymetazoline on page 1043

◆ **Oxytrol®** see Oxybutynin on page 1037

◆ **Oysco 500 [OTC]** see Calcium Carbonate on page 232

◆ **Oysco® 500 [OTC]** see Calcium Supplements on page 239

◆ **Oyst-Cal 500 [OTC]** see Calcium Carbonate on page 232

◆ **Oyst-Cal 500 [OTC]** see Calcium Supplements on page 239

◆ **Ozurdex™** see Dexamethasone on page 406

◆ **P-071** see Cetirizine on page 283

◆ **Pacerone®** see Amiodarone on page 84

Paclitaxel (PAK li taks el)

Medication Safety Issues

Sound-alike/look-alike issues:

Paclitaxel may be confused with paroxetine, Paxil®

Paclitaxel (conventional) may be confused with paclitaxel (protein-bound)

Taxol® may be confused with Abraxane®, Paxil®, Taxotere®

High alert medication: The Institute for Safe Medication Practices (ISMP) includes this medication among its list of drugs which have a heightened risk of causing significant patient harm when used in error.

Related Information

Compatibility of Chemotherapy and Related Supportive Care Medications on page 1580

Emetogenic Potential of Antineoplastic Agents on page 1579

Extravasation Treatment on page 1522

U.S. Brand Names Onxol® [DSC]; Taxol® [DSC]

Canadian Brand Names Abraxane® For Injectable Suspension; Apo-Paclitaxel®; Taxol®

Therapeutic Category Antineoplastic Agent, Anti-microtubular

Generic Available Yes

Use Treatment of breast cancer, advanced ovarian cancer, nonsmall cell lung cancer, and second-line treatment of AIDS-related Kaposi's sarcoma (FDA approved in adults); has also been used in head and neck cancer, bladder cancer, cervical cancer, small cell lung cancer, and unknown primary adenocarcinomas

Pregnancy Risk Factor D

Pregnancy Considerations Animal studies have demonstrated embryotoxicity, fetal toxicity, and maternal toxicity. There are no adequate and well-controlled studies in pregnant women. Women of childbearing potential should be advised to avoid becoming pregnant.

Lactation Excretion in breast milk unknown/contra-indicated

Breast-Feeding Considerations Due to the potential for serious adverse reactions, breast-feeding is contra-indicated.

Contraindications Hypersensitivity to paclitaxel, Cremophor® EL (polyoxyethylated castor oil) or any component

Warnings Hazardous agent; use appropriate precautions for handling and disposal. Anaphylaxis and severe hypersensitivity reactions have occurred in 2% to 4% of patients receiving paclitaxel in clinical trials during first or subsequent infusions **[U.S. Boxed Warning]**. All patients should be premedicated with a corticosteroid, diphenhydramine, and an H_2-receptor antagonist to prevent hypersensitivity reactions; fatal reactions have occurred despite premedication. Patients who experience severe hypersensitivity reactions to paclitaxel should not be rechallenged with the drug. Be prepared to treat a severe hypersensitivity reaction with epinephrine, I.V. fluids, diphenhydramine, and a corticosteroid.

CNS toxicity has been reported in pediatric patients receiving high doses of paclitaxel (350-420 mg/m^2 as a 3-hour infusion) which may have resulted from the ethanol contained in the formulation. With use, peripheral neuropathy may occur; patients with pre-existing neuropathies from chemotherapy or coexisting conditions (eg, diabetes mellitus) may be at a higher risk; reduce dose by 20% for severe neuropathy. Severe bone marrow suppression (primarily neutropenia) with resulting infection may occur **[U.S. Boxed Warning]**. In general, do not administer paclitaxel to patients with baseline neutrophil counts <1500/mm^3 (<1000 cells/mm^3 for patients with AIDS-related KS). Infusion-related hypotension, bradycardia, and/or hypertension may occur; frequent monitoring of vital signs is recommended, especially during the first hour of the infusion. Rare but severe conduction abnormalities have been reported; conduct cardiac monitoring during subsequent infusions for these patients.

Precautions Use with caution in patients with moderate or severe hepatic impairment; dosage adjustment may be necessary in patients with hepatic impairment, severe neutropenia, or peripheral neuropathy. Formulations contain dehydrated alcohol; may cause adverse CNS effects

Adverse Reactions

Cardiovascular: Arrhythmias, bradycardia, edema, flushing, hyper-/hypotension, syncope

Central nervous system: Confusion, fatigue, fever, headache

Dermatologic: Alopecia, changes in nail pigmentation, rash

Endocrine & metabolic: Serum triglyceride concentrations increased

Gastrointestinal: Diarrhea, mild to moderate nausea/vomiting, mucositis

Hematologic: Leukopenia, severe neutropenia [dose-limiting toxicity (see Warnings)], thrombocytopenia anemia

Hepatic: Alkaline phosphatase, AST increased, bilirubin increased

Local: Erythema, swelling at the injection site, tenderness

Neuromuscular & skeletal: Arthralgia, motor dysfunction, muscle weakness, myalgia, peripheral neuropathy (dose-dependent, characterized by paresthesia with numbness and tingling in a stocking-and-glove distribution)

Ocular: Diplopia, loss of visual acuity

Renal: Serum creatinine increased

Respiratory: Dyspnea

Miscellaneous: Anaphylactoid reactions (bronchospasm, dyspnea, generalized urticaria, hypotension), anaphylaxis, ethanol intoxication (see Warnings)

<1%, postmarketing, and/or case reports: Ataxia, atrial fibrillation, AV block, back pain, cardiac conduction abnormalities, cellulitis, heart failure, chills, conjunctivitis, dehydration, enterocolitis, extravasation recall, hepatic encephalopathy, hepatic necrosis, induration, intestinal obstruction, intestinal perforation, interstitial pneumonia, ischemic colitis, lacrimation increased, maculopapular rash, malaise, MI, necrotic changes and ulceration following extravasation, neuroencephalopathy, neutropenic enterocolitis, ototoxicity (tinnitus and hearing loss), pancreatitis, paralytic ileus, phlebitis, pulmonary embolism, pulmonary fibrosis, radiation recall, radiation pneumonitis, pruritus, renal insufficiency, seizure, skin exfoliation, skin fibrosis, skin necrosis, Stevens-Johnson syndrome, supraventricular tachycardia, toxic epidermal necrolysis, ventricular tachycardia (asymptomatic), visual disturbances (scintillating scotomata)

Drug Interactions

Metabolism/Transport Effects Substrate of CYP2C8 (major), CYP3A4 (major), P-glycoprotein; **Induces** CYP3A4 (weak)

Avoid Concomitant Use

Avoid concomitant use of Paclitaxel with any of the following: BCG; Natalizumab; Pimecrolimus; Tacrolimus (Topical); Vaccines (Live)

Increased Effect/Toxicity

Paclitaxel may increase the levels/effects of: Antineoplastic Agents (Anthracycline); DOXOrubicin; Leflunomide; Natalizumab; Trastuzumab; Vaccines (Live); Vinorelbine

The levels/effects of Paclitaxel may be increased by: CYP2C8 Inhibitors (Moderate); CYP2C8 Inhibitors (Strong); CYP2C9 Inhibitors (Moderate); CYP2C9 Inhibitors (Strong); CYP3A4 Inhibitors (Moderate); CYP3A4 Inhibitors (Strong); Dasatinib; Deferasirox; Denosumab; P-Glycoprotein Inhibitors; Pimecrolimus; Platinum Derivatives; Reverse Transcriptase Inhibitors (Non-Nucleoside); Tacrolimus (Topical); Trastuzumab

Decreased Effect

Paclitaxel may decrease the levels/effects of: BCG; Saxagliptin; Sipuleucel-T; Vaccines (Inactivated); Vaccines (Live)

The levels/effects of Paclitaxel may be decreased by: CYP2C8 Inducers (Highly Effective); CYP2C9 Inducers (Highly Effective); CYP3A4 Inducers (Strong); Deferasirox; Echinacea; Herbs (CYP3A4 Inducers); Peginterferon Alfa-2b; P-Glycoprotein Inducers; Trastuzumab

Stability Refrigerate intact vials or store at room temperature; undiluted vials of paclitaxel may precipitate upon refrigeration, but will redissolve at room temperature with no loss in potency; dilution of paclitaxel from 0.3 mg/mL to 1.2 mg/mL in NS or D$_5$W is stable for up to 48 hours at room temperature; incompatible with amphotericin B, chlorpromazine, hydroxyzine, methylprednisolone, and mitoxantrone

Mechanism of Action An antimicrotubule agent that promotes the assembly of microtubules from tubulin dimers and stabilizes microtubules by preventing depolymerization; results in the inhibition of mitotic cellular functions and cell replication by blocking cells in the late G2 phase and M phase of the cell cycle

Pharmacokinetics (Adult data unless noted)

Distribution: Biphasic with initial rapid distribution to the peripheral compartment; later phase is a slow efflux of paclitaxel from the peripheral compartment

V_d: 227-688 L/m^2

Protein binding: 89% to 98%

Metabolism: Cytochrome P450 hepatic isoenzymes metabolize paclitaxel to 6 alpha-hydroxypaclitaxel

Half-life (varies with dose and infusion duration):
Children: 4.6-17 hours
Adults: 1.5-8.4 hours

Elimination: Urinary recovery of unchanged drug: 1.3% to 12.6%

Dialysis: No significant drug removal by hemodialysis

Usual Dosage I.V. infusion (refer to individual protocols):

Children:
Treatment for refractory leukemia is still undergoing investigation: 250-360 mg/m^2/dose infused over 24 hours every 14 days
Recurrent Wilms' tumor: 250-350 mg/m^2/dose infused over 24 hours every 3 weeks

Adults:
Ovarian carcinoma: 135-175 mg/m^2/dose infused over 1-24 hours every 3 weeks
Metastatic breast cancer: 175 mg/m^2/dose infused over 3 hours every 3 weeks (protocols have used dosages ranging between 135-250 mg/m^2/dose over 1-24 hours every 3 weeks)
Kaposi's sarcoma: 135 mg/m^2/dose infused over 3 hours every 3 weeks, or 100 mg/m^2/dose infused over 3 hours every 2 weeks

Dosage adjustment in renal impairment: None

Dosage adjustment in hepatic impairment:
Total bilirubin ≤1.5 mg/dL and AST >2x normal limits: Total dose <135 mg/m^2
Total bilirubin 1.6-3.0 mg/dL: Total dose ≤75 mg/m^2
Total bilirubin ≥3.1 mg/dL: Total dose ≤50 mg/m^2

Administration Parenteral: I.V.: Patients should be premedicated with a corticosteroid, diphenhydramine and an H$_2$-receptor antagonist 30-60 minutes prior to paclitaxel administration. To minimize patient exposure to the plasticizer diethylhexylphthalate (DEHP) from polyoxyl 35 castor oil-induced leaching of polyvinyl chloride-containing I.V. infusion bags and administration sets, prepare paclitaxel infusions in glass or in polypropylene or polyolefin bags and administer through polyethylene lined administration sets with a 0.22 micron in-line filter. Paclitaxel can be further diluted in D$_5$W, NS, D$_5$/NS or D$_5$ in Ringer's injection to a final concentration of 0.3-1.2 mg/mL. Paclitaxel has been infused over short (1-3 hours) and long periods (24, 72, and 96 hours to 14 days continuous infusion)

Monitoring Parameters CBC with differential, platelet count, vital signs, ECG, liver function test; observe I.V. injection site for extravasation

Patient Information Avoid alcohol; may cause drowsiness and impair ability to perform activities requiring mental alertness or physical coordination

Dosage Forms Excipient information presented when available (limited, particularly for generics); consult specific product labeling. [DSC] = Discontinued product

Injection, solution: 6 mg/mL (5 mL, 16.7 mL, 25 mL, 50 mL) [contains ethanol and purified Cremophor® EL (polyoxyethylated castor oil)]

Onxol: 6 mg/mL (5 mL, 25 mL, 50 mL) [contains ethanol and purified Cremophor® EL (polyoxyethylated castor oil)] [DSC]

Taxol®: 6 mg/mL (5 mL, 16.7 mL, 50 mL) [contains ethanol and purified Cremophor® EL (polyoxyethylated castor oil)] [DSC]

References
Woo MH, Gregornik D, Shearer PD, et al, "Pharmacokinetics of Paclitaxel in an Anephric Patient," *Cancer Chemother Pharmacol*, 1999, 43(1):92-6.

◆ **Pacnex™** see Benzoyl Peroxide on page 184

◆ **Pain Eze [OTC]** see Acetaminophen on page 36

◆ **Palafer® (Can)** see Ferrous Fumarate on page 576

◆ **Palgic®** see Carbinoxamine on page 248

◆ **Palgic®-D [DSC]** see Carbinoxamine and Pseudoephedrine on page 249

◆ **Palgic®-DS [DSC]** see Carbinoxamine and Pseudoephedrine on page 249

Palivizumab (pah li VIZ u mab)

Medication Safety Issues
Sound-alike/look-alike issues:
Synagis® may be confused with Synalgos®-DC, Synvisc®

U.S. Brand Names Synagis®

Canadian Brand Names Synagis®

Therapeutic Category Monoclonal Antibody

Generic Available No

Use Prevention of serious lower respiratory tract disease caused by respiratory syncytial virus (RSV) in infants and children at high risk for RSV disease (FDA approved ≤24 months of age).

The American Academy of Pediatrics recommends RSV prophylaxis with palivizumab during RSV season for:

• Infants <3 months of age who were born between 32 and 34 6/7 weeks gestational age and have one of the following:
o Daycare attendance
o >1 sibling who is <5 years of age living in the same household

• Infants <6 months of age who were born between 29 and 31 6/7 weeks gestational age

• Infants <12 months of age who were born <28 weeks gestational age

• Infants <12 months of age with congenital airway abnormality or neuromuscular disorder that decreases the ability to manage airway secretions

• Infants and children <24 months of age with chronic lung disease (CLD) necessitating medical therapy within 6 months of age prior to the beginning of RSV season

• Infants and children <24 months with congenital heart disease and one of the following:
o Receiving medication to treat congestive heart failure
o Moderate to severe pulmonary hypertension
o Cyanotic heart disease

Pregnancy Risk Factor C

Pregnancy Considerations Not for adult use; reproduction studies have not been conducted

Contraindications Hypersensitivity to palivizumab or any component

Warnings Rare cases of anaphylaxis have been reported following re-exposure to palivizumab. Severe acute hypersensitivity reactions have also been reported following administration of palivizumab. Palivizumab should be permanently discontinued if a severe hypersensitivity reaction occurs. If anaphylaxis or severe allergic reaction occurs, administer epinephrine (1:1000) and provide supportive care as required.

Precautions Use with caution in patients with thrombocytopenia or any coagulation disorder. Safety and efficacy have not been demonstrated for treatment of established RSV disease.

Adverse Reactions

Cardiovascular: Arrhythmia, cyanosis

Central nervous system: Fever

Dermatologic: Rash

Gastrointestinal: Diarrhea, gastroenteritis, vomiting

Hepatic: AST increased

Respiratory: Cough, otitis media, pharyngitis, rhinitis, upper respiratory infection, wheezing

Miscellaneous: Anaphylaxis and hypersensitivity reactions (includes angioedema, dyspnea, hypotonia, pruritus, respiratory failure, unresponsiveness, and urticaria), hernia

<1%, postmarketing, and/or case reports: Injection site reaction, thrombocytopenia

Drug Interactions

Avoid Concomitant Use There are no known interactions where it is recommended to avoid concomitant use.

Increased Effect/Toxicity

The levels/effects of Palivizumab may be increased by: Abciximab

Decreased Effect There are no known significant interactions involving a decrease in effect.

Stability Store in refrigerator at a temperature between 2°C to 8°C (35.6°F to 46.4°F) in original container; do not freeze; do not shake, vigorously agitate, or dilute the solution. The single-use vial does not contain a preservative; solution should be administered within 6 hours of reconstitution

Mechanism of Action Humanized monoclonal antibody directed to an epitope in the A antigenic site of the respiratory syncytial virus F protein resulting in neutralizing and fusion-inhibitory activity against RSV

Pharmacodynamics Protective trough concentrations (>40 mcg/mL) are achieved following the second dose.

Pharmacokinetics (Adult data unless noted)

Half-life:

Children <24 months: 20 days

Adults: 18 days

Time to achieve adequate serum antibody titers: 48 hours

Usual Dosage Children:

I.M.: 15 mg/kg once monthly throughout RSV season; **Note:** For cardiopulmonary bypass patients, administer a dose as soon as possible after cardiopulmonary bypass procedure, even if <1 month from previous dose. AAP recommends a maximum of three doses for patients born 32-34 6/7 weeks without significant congenital heart disease or chronic lung disease and maximum of five doses for all others (AAP, 2009).

I.V. (I.V. route is investigational): 15 mg/kg has been administered to patients who could not receive I.M. injections; use has been investigated in hematopoietic stem cell transplant patients with active RSV upper respiratory tract infection.

Administration Parenteral:

I.M.: Administer undiluted solution I.M., preferably in the anterolateral aspect of the thigh; gluteal muscle should not be used routinely as an injection site because of the risk of damage to the sciatic nerve; injection volume over 1 mL should be given as a divided dose. Do **not** dilute product; do not shake or vigorously agitate the vial.

I.V. (I.V. route is investigational): Administer IVP or I.V. intermittent infusion at a rate not to exceed 1-2 mL/minute at a final concentration of 20 mg/mL in SWI. Filter through a 0.22 micron low protein binding filter (Millex-GV) prior to administration.

Monitoring Parameters Observe for anaphylactic or severe allergic reactions

Additional Information RSV prophylaxis should be initiated no earlier than July 1st in Southeast Florida, September 15th in Northcentral and Southwest Florida, and November 1st in most other areas of the United States.

Antipalivizumab antibodies may develop after the fourth injection in some patients (~1%). This has not been associated with any risk of adverse events or altered serum concentrations.

Dosage Forms Excipient information presented when available (limited, particularly for generics); consult specific product labeling.

Injection, solution [preservative free]:

Synagis®: 100 mg/mL (0.5 mL, 1 mL)

References

American Academy of Pediatrics Committee on Infectious Diseases, "Policy Statement - Modified Recommendations for Use of Palivizumab for Prevention of Respiratory Syncytial Virus Infections," *Pediatrics*, 2009, Sep 7 [epub ahead of print].

Boeckh M, Berrey MM, Bowden RA, et al, "Phase 1 Evaluation of the Respiratory Syncytial Virus-Specific Monoclonal Antibody Palivizumab in Recipients of Hematopoietic Stem Cell Transplants," *J Infect Dis*, 2001, 184(3):350-4.

Feltes TF, Cabalka AK, Meissner HC, et al, "Palivizumab Prophylaxis Reduces Hospitalization Due to Respiratory Syncytial Virus in Young Children With Hemodynamically Significant Congenital Heart Disease," *J Pediatr*, 2003, 143(4):532-40.

Giebels K, Marcotte JE, Podoba J, et al, "Prophylaxis Against Respiratory Syncytial Virus in Young Children With Cystic Fibrosis," *Pediatr Pulmonol*, 2008, 43(2):169-74.

"Palivizumab, a Humanized Respiratory Syncytial Virus Monoclonal Antibody, Reduces Hospitalization From Respiratory Syncytial Virus Infection in High-Risk Infants. The Impact-RSV Study Group," *Pediatrics*, 1998, 102(3 Pt 1):531-7.

◆ **Palmer's® Skin Success Acne Cleanser [OTC]** *see* Salicylic Acid *on page 1241*

◆ **Palmer's® Skin Success Invisible Acne [OTC]** *see* Benzoyl Peroxide *on page 184*

◆ **Palmitate-A® [OTC]** *see* Vitamin A *on page 1426*

Palonosetron (pal oh NOE se tron)

Medication Safety Issues

Sound-alike/look-alike issues:

Aloxi® may be confused with Eloxatin®, oxaliplatin

Palonosetron may be confused with dolasetron, granisetron, ondansetron

U.S. Brand Names Aloxi®

Therapeutic Category 5-HT$_3$ Receptor Antagonist; Antiemetic

Generic Available No

Use Prevention of acute and delayed chemotherapy-induced nausea and vomiting; prevention of postoperative nausea and vomiting (PONV) (FDA approved in adults)

Pregnancy Risk Factor B

Pregnancy Considerations Teratogenic effects were not observed in animal studies. There are no adequate and well-controlled studies in pregnant women; use during pregnancy only if clearly needed.

Lactation Excretion in breast milk unknown/not recommended

Breast-Feeding Considerations The extent to which palonosetron is excreted in breast milk, if at all, is unknown. Due to the potential for adverse effects in the nursing infant, breast-feeding is not recommended.

Contraindications Hypersensitivity to palonosetron or any component

Warnings Palonosetron may cause ECG interval changes (PR, QT_c, JT prolongation and QRS widening); interval prolongation could lead to cardiovascular consequences such as heart block or cardiac arrhythmias; hypersensitivity reactions may occur in patients who have exhibited hypersensitivity to other 5-HT$_3$ antagonists (eg, ondansetron, dolasetron)

Precautions Use with caution in patients with, or who may develop, prolongation of cardiac conduction intervals, particularly QT_c; conditions include hypokalemia, hypomagnesemia, or congenital QT syndrome; use with caution in patients receiving antiarrhythmic or other medications known to prolong the QT interval (eg, class I or III antiarrhythmic agents) or medications known to reduce potassium or magnesium levels (eg, diuretics)

Adverse Reactions
Cardiovascular: Arrhythmia, bradycardia, edema, extrasystoles, hypertension, hypotension, myocardial ischemia, prolonged QT interval and other ECG changes (see Warnings), tachycardia
Central nervous system: Anxiety, dizziness, euphoria, fatigue, fever, headache, insomnia
Dermatologic: Allergic dermatitis, erythema, pruritus, rash
Endocrine & metabolic: Hyperglycemia, hyperkalemia, metabolic acidosis
Gastrointestinal: Abdominal pain, anorexia, constipation, diarrhea, dyspepsia, flatulence, hiccups, taste disturbance, xerostomia
Genitourinary: Urinary retention
Hepatic: Bilirubin increased, transient elevations in liver enzymes
Local: Injection site reactions, vein discoloration
Neuromuscular & skeletal: Limb pain, weakness
Ocular: Amblyopia, eye irritation
Otic: Tinnitus
Respiratory: Epistaxis
Miscellaneous: Flu-like syndrome, hypersensitivity reactions

Drug Interactions
Metabolism/Transport Effects Substrate (minor) of CYP1A2, 2D6, 3A4
Avoid Concomitant Use
Avoid concomitant use of Palonosetron with any of the following: Apomorphine
Increased Effect/Toxicity
Palonosetron may increase the levels/effects of: Apomorphine
Decreased Effect
The levels/effects of Palonosetron may be decreased by: Peginterferon Alfa-2b

Stability Store at room temperature; protect from light. Do not freeze; do not mix with other drugs.
Mechanism of Action Palonosetron is a selective 5-HT$_3$ receptor antagonist, blocking serotonin, both peripherally on vagal nerve terminals and centrally in the chemoreceptor trigger zone
Pharmacokinetics (Adult data unless noted)
Distribution: Adults: 8.3 ± 2.5 L/kg
Protein binding: 62%
Metabolism: Metabolized to 2 minimally active metabolites (<1% activity of palonosetron)
Half-life:
Children: 21-37 hours
Adults: 40 hours
Elimination: Urine 80% to 93% (40% as unchanged drug); feces (5% to 8%)
Clearance: Adults: Total body: 160 mL/h/kg
Usual Dosage
Children and Adolescents: Information based on small clinical trials: I.V.: Prevention of acute chemotherapy-induced nausea and vomiting

Kadota (2007): A multicenter, stratified, double-blind randomized trial of 60 pediatric patients >2 years [12 patients (1 month to 2 years) treated in an open-label fashion] showed 3 mcg/kg (maximum dose: 0.25 mg) and 10 mcg/kg (maximum dose: 0.75 mg) were well-tolerated and effective (no emesis, no rescue first 0-24 hours)

Sepúlveda-Vildósola (2008): A randomized comparison of palonosetron (0.25 mg single dose 30 minutes before chemotherapy) and ondansetron (8 mg/m^2 every 8 hours beginning 30 minutes before chemotherapy) in children 2-15 years, evaluated 100 chemotherapy courses in each arm and showed a statistically significant reduction in emetic events on days 0-3 in the palonosetron group and clinically significant reduction in emetic events on days 4-7 (up to 6 emetic events in the ondansetron group vs none with palonosetron)

Adults: I.V.:
Prevention of acute and delayed chemotherapy-induced nausea and vomiting: 0.25 mg as a single dose administered 30 minutes before chemotherapy
PONV: 0.075 mg immediately prior to anesthesia induction
Dosage adjustment in hepatic or renal impairment: No dosage adjustment is indicated
Administration Infuse I.V. undiluted over 30 seconds; do not mix with other medications. Solutions of 5 mcg/mL and 30 mcg/mL in NS, D_5W, $D_5\frac{1}{2}NS$, and D_5LR injection are stable for 48 hours at room temperature and 14 days under refrigeration
Monitoring Parameters Baseline ECG in high-risk patients (see Warnings and Precautions), emesis episodes
Patient Information May cause dry mouth
Dosage Forms Excipient information presented when available (limited, particularly for generics); consult specific product labeling.
Injection, solution:
Aloxi®: 0.05 mg/mL (1.5 mL, 5 mL) [contains edetate disodium]

References
Eisenberg P, Figueroa-Vadillo J, Zamora R, et al, "Improved Prevention of Moderately Emetogenic Chemotherapy-Induced Nausea and Vomiting With Palonosetron, a Pharmacologically Novel 5-HT$_3$ Receptor Antagonist: Results of a Phase III, Single-Dose Trial Versus Dolasetron," *Cancer*, 2003, 98(11):2473-82.
Gralla R, Lichinitser M, Van Der Vegt S, et al, "Palonosetron Improves Prevention of Chemotherapy-Induced Nausea and Vomiting Following Moderately Emetogenic Chemotherapy: Results of a Double-Blind Randomized Phase III Trial Comparing Single Doses of Palonosetron With Ondansetron," *Ann Oncol*, 2003, 14(10):1570-7.
Kadota R, Shen V, and Messinger Y, "Safety, Pharmacokinetics, and Efficacy of Palonosetron in Pediatric Patients: A Multicenter, Stratified, Double-Blind, Phase 3, Randomized Study," *J Clin Oncol*, 2007, 25 (18S June 20 Suppl):9570.
Sepúlveda-Vildósola AC, Betanzos-Cabrera Y, Lastiri GG, et al, "Palonosetron Hydrochloride Is an Effective and Safe Option to Prevent Chemotherapy-Induced Nausea and Vomiting in Children," *Arch Med Res*, 2008, 39(6):601-6.
Siddiqui MA and Scott LJ, "Palonosetron," *Drugs*, 2004, 64 (10):1125-32.
Trissel LA and Xu QA, "Physical and Chemical Stability of Palonosetron HCl in 4 Infusion Solutions," *Ann Pharmacother*, 2004, 38 (10):1608-11.

◆ **Palonosetron Hydrochloride** *see* Palonosetron *on page 1047*

◆ **2-PAM** *see* Pralidoxime *on page 1144*

◆ **Pamelor®** *see* Nortriptyline *on page 1002*

Pamidronate (pa mi DROE nate)

Medication Safety Issues
Sound-alike/look-alike issues:
Aredia® may be confused with Adriamycin, Meridia®
Pamidronate may be confused with papaverine

International issues:

Linoten® [Spain] may be confused with Lidopen® which is a brand name for lidocaine in the U.S.

U.S. Brand Names Aredia®

Canadian Brand Names Aredia®; Pamidronate Disodium Omega; Pamidronate Disodium®; PMS-Pamidronate; Rhoxal-pamidronate

Therapeutic Category Antidote, Hypercalcemia; Bisphosphonate Derivative

Generic Available Yes

Use Symptomatic treatment of moderate to severe Paget's disease; hypercalcemia associated with malignancy; treatment of osteolytic bone lesions associated with multiple myeloma or metastatic breast cancer

Investigation use: Inhibit bone resorption in severe osteogenesis imperfecta

Pregnancy Risk Factor D

Pregnancy Considerations Pamidronate has been shown to cross the placenta and cause nonteratogenic embryo/fetal effects in animals. There are no adequate and well-controlled studies in pregnant women; manufacturer states pamidronate should not be used in pregnancy. Based on limited case reports, serum calcium levels in the newborn may be altered if pamidronate is administered during pregnancy. Bisphosphonates are incorporated into the bone matrix and gradually released over time. Theoretically, there may be a risk of fetal harm when pregnancy follows the completion of therapy. Women of childbearing potential should be advised to use effective contraception and avoid becoming pregnant during therapy.

Lactation Excretion in breast milk unknown/use caution

Contraindications Hypersensitivity to pamidronate or any component; pregnancy; severe renal impairment

Warnings Leukopenia has been observed with oral pamidronate; monitoring of white blood cell counts is suggested; vein irritation and thrombophlebitis may occur with I.V. infusions

Osteonecrosis of the jaw has been reported in cancer patients receiving biphosphonates; many of these patients were also receiving corticosteroids and chemotherapy, the majority of cases were associated with dental procedures; a dental exam should be considered prior to treatment in cancer patients, especially those with risk factors (chemotherapy, corticosteroids, poor oral hygiene); while on treatment, avoid invasive dental procedures

The Food and Drug Administration (FDA) is informing healthcare practitioners of the possible association between bisphosphonate use and the development of severe (possibly incapacitating) bone, muscle, and/or joint pain. The severe musculoskeletal pain may develop days, months, or years after initiating a bisphosphonate. This is a distinct event from the acute phase response (eg, fever, chills, bone pain, myalgia, arthralgia) that may occur following initial bisphosphonate administration which generally resolves within several days of continued use.

Single pamidronate doses should not exceed 90 mg. Initial or single doses have been associated with renal deterioration, progressing to renal failure and dialysis. Glomerulosclerosis (focal segmental) with or without nephrotic syndrome, has also been reported, particularly in patients with multiple myeloma and breast cancer. Longer infusion times (>2 hours) may reduce the risk for renal toxicity, especially in patients with pre-existing renal insufficiency. Withhold pamidronate treatment (until renal function returns to baseline) in patients with evidence of renal deterioration. Monitor serum creatinine prior to each dose.

Precautions Use with caution in patients with renal impairment; maintain adequate hydration and urinary output during treatment; use with caution with other potentially nephrotoxic drugs. Use has been associated with asymptomatic electrolyte abnormalities (including hypophosphatemia, hypokalemia, hypomagnesemia, and hypocalcemia). Rare cases of symptomatic hypocalcemia, including tetany have been reported. Use with caution in patients with a history of thyroid surgery; patients may have relative hypoparathyroidism, predisposing them to pamidronate-related hypocalcemia.

Adverse Reactions

Cardiovascular: Tachycardia, hypertension, syncope

Central nervous system: Malaise, fever, fatigue, somnolence, insomnia, seizures

Dermatologic: Rash

Endocrine & metabolic: Hypocalcemia, hypophosphatemia, hypothyroidism, hypokalemia, hypomagnesemia, fluid overload

Gastrointestinal: Nausea, anorexia, constipation, GI hemorrhage, abdominal pain, occult blood in stools, abnormal taste

Hematologic: Leukopenia, anemia

Local: Vein irritation, thrombophlebitis

Neuromuscular & skeletal: Bone pain, myalgia, osteonecrosis of the jaw

Ocular: Scleritis, uveitis, conjunctivitis

Renal: Uremia, renal failure, glomerulosclerosis (with or without nephrotic syndrome)

Respiratory: Rales, rhinitis

Miscellaneous: Moniliasis (associated with 90 mg dosage)

Drug Interactions

Avoid Concomitant Use There are no known interactions where it is recommended to avoid concomitant use.

Increased Effect/Toxicity

Pamidronate may increase the levels/effects of: Phosphate Supplements

The levels/effects of Pamidronate may be increased by: Aminoglycosides; Nonsteroidal Anti-Inflammatory Agents; Thalidomide

Decreased Effect There are no known significant interactions involving a decrease in effect.

Stability Reconstituted solution stable for 24 hours at room temperature or refrigerated; incompatible with calcium-containing I.V. fluids (ie, Ringer's solution)

Mechanism of Action Pamidronate, a biphosphonate, lowers serum calcium concentrations by binding to bone and inhibiting osteoclast-mediated calcium resorption; this agent does not appear to produce any significant effect on renal tubular calcium handling

Pharmacodynamics

Onset of hypocalcemic action: 24-48 hours

Maximum effect: 5-7 days

Pharmacokinetics (Adult data unless noted)

Absorption: Poorly from the GI tract; pharmacokinetic studies are lacking

Bone half-life: 300 days

Half-life, elimination: Adults with cancer: 28 ± 7 hours

Elimination:

Biphasic: ~50% excreted unchanged in urine within 72 hours

Clearance: Adults with cancer: Total: 107 ± 50 mL/minute; renal: 49 ± 28 mL/minute

Usual Dosage

Hypercalcemia: I.V.: **Note:** Due to increased risk of nephrotoxicity, single doses should not exceed 90 mg

Children (limited experience): 0.5-1 mg/kg

Adults: Dosage based upon serum calcium measurement:

Serum calcium 12-13.5 mg/dL: 60-90 mg

Serum calcium >13.5 mg/dL: 90 mg

Consider retreatment if the serum calcium becomes elevated again; allow a minimum of 7 days between each treatment to allow for a full response to the initial treatment

Osteogenesis imperfecta:

Children (limited experience): 0.5-3 mg/kg/day for 3 days; may repeat in 4- to 6-month intervals; or as an alternative 10-30 mg/m^2 monthly

Osteopenia in nonambulatory children with cerebral palsy: Limited experience (Henderson, 2002); 1 mg/kg/day for 3 days; each dose not <15 mg/day or >30 mg/day; repeat at 3-month intervals

Osteolytic bone lesions of breast cancer or multiple myeloma: Adults: 90 mg/month; treatment should be withheld for renal deterioration (as defined per manufacturer: Patients with normal baseline creatinine: An increase of 0.5 mg/dL; patients with abnormal baseline creatinine: An increase of 1 mg/dL)

Paget's disease: Adults: 30 mg for 3 consecutive days

Dosing adjustment in renal impairment: Not recommended for use in patients with severe renal impairment; safety and efficacy have not been established in patients with serum creatinine >5 mg/dL; limited studies have reported successful use in multiple myeloma patients with serum creatinine ≥3 mg/dL

The manufacturer recommends the following guidelines:

Treatment of bone metastases: Use is not recommended in patients with severe renal impairment.

Renal impairment in indications other than bone metastases: Use clinical judgement to determine if benefit outweighs risks.

Administration Reconstitute each vial with 10 mL SWI; dilute further in 250-1000 mL D$_5$W, 1/2NS, or NS (refer to manufacturer's information regarding dilution for specific treatments); do not mix with calcium-containing solutions (eg, LR); infuse over 2-24 hours; longer infusions (>2 hours) may reduce the risk for renal toxicity, particularly in patients with pre-existing renal insufficiency

Monitoring Parameters Monitor serum creatinine prior to each dose; monitor serum calcium, phosphate, potassium, and magnesium; patients with pre-existing anemia, leukopenia, or thrombocytopenia should have hemoglobin, hematocrit, and CBC with differential monitored closely, particularly in the first 2 weeks following treatment; in Paget's disease, monitor serum alkaline phosphatase and urinary hydroxyproline excretion; dental exam and preventative dentistry for patients at risk for osteonecrosis

Test Interactions Bisphosphonates may interfere with diagnostic imaging agents such as technetium-99m-diphosphonate in bone scans.

Dosage Forms Excipient information presented when available (limited, particularly for generics); consult specific product labeling.

Injection, powder for reconstitution, as disodium: 30 mg, 90 mg

Aredia®: 30 mg, 90 mg

Injection, solution, as disodium: 3 mg/mL (10 mL); 6 mg/mL (10 mL); 9 mg/mL (10 mL)

Injection, solution, as disodium [preservative free]: 3 mg/mL (10 mL)

References

Falk MJ, Heeger S, Lynch KA, et al, "Intravenous Bisphosphonate Therapy in Children With Osteogenesis Imperfecta," *Pediatrics*, 2003, 111(3):573-8.

Glorieux FH, Bishop NH, Plotkin H, et al, "Cyclic Administration of Pamidronate in Children With Severe Osteogenesis Imperfecta," *N Engl J Med*, 1998, 339(14):947-52.

Henderson RC, Lark RK, Kecskemethy HH, et al, "Bisphosphonates to Treat Osteopenia in Children With Quadriplegic Cerebral Palsy: A Randomized, Placebo-Controlled Clinical Trial," *J Pediatr*, 2002, 141 (5):644-51.

Lteif AN and Zimmerman D, "Bisphosphonates for Treatment of Childhood Hypercalcemia," *Pediatrics*, 1998, 102(4 Pt 1):990-3.

◆ **Pamidronate Disodium** see Pamidronate on page 1048

◆ **Pamidronate Disodium® (Can)** see Pamidronate on page 1048

◆ **Pamidronate Disodium Omega (Can)** see Pamidronate on page 1048

◆ **Pamprin® Maximum Strength All Day Relief [OTC]** see Naproxen on page 967

◆ **Pan-2400™ [OTC]** see Pancreatin on page 1050

◆ **Pancrease® (Can)** see Pancrelipase on page 1051

◆ **Pancrease® MT** see Pancrelipase on page 1051

◆ **Pancreatic Enzymes** see Pancrelipase on page 1051

Pancreatin (PAN kree a tin)

Medication Safety Issues

Sound-alike/look-alike issues:

Pancreatin may be confused with Panretin®

U.S. Brand Names Dygase [DSC]; Hi-Vegi-Lip [OTC]; kuzyme® [DSC]; kutrase® [DSC]; Lapase [DSC]; Pan-2400™ [OTC]

Therapeutic Category Enzyme, Pancreatic; Pancreatic Enzyme

Generic Available Yes

Use Replacement therapy in symptomatic treatment of malabsorption syndrome caused by pancreatic enzyme insufficiency

Pregnancy Risk Factor C

Lactation Excretion in breast milk unknown/use caution

Breast-Feeding Considerations Systemic absorption and concentration in the breast milk is unlikely, but unknown.

Contraindications Hypersensitivity to pancreatin, any component, or to bovine or pork protein; acute pancreatitis; acute exacerbations of chronic pancreatic diseases

Warnings Pancreatin is inactivated by acids; use microencapsulated products whenever possible, since these products permit better dissolution of enzymes in the duodenum and protect the enzyme preparations from acid degradation in the stomach; these products are not bioequivalent, do not substitute without consulting a physician or pharmacist; do not substitute generic pancreatic enzymes for brand name products

Colonic strictures have been reported in several pediatric patients. There is a possible association between the development of strictures and a high lipase intake (mean >16,000 units/kg/meal). Patients receiving doses >2500 lipase units/kg/meal or 4000 lipase units/g fat/day should be re-evaluated or titrated downward to lowest effective dose.

Precautions Do not spill powder on hands as is a skin irritant; inhalation of powder may produce an asthmatic attack

Adverse Reactions

Dermatologic: Rash

Endocrine & metabolic: Hyperuricemia

Gastrointestinal: Nausea, abdominal cramps, constipation, diarrhea, colonic strictures, mouth irritation, greasy stools, perianal irritation/inflammation, flatulence

Ocular: Lacrimation

Renal: Hyperuricosuria

Respiratory: Sneezing, bronchospasm

Miscellaneous: Hypersensitivity reactions

Food Interactions Avoid placing contents of opened capsules on alkaline foods (pH >5.5), such as dairy products (milk, custard, or ice cream); see Administration

Mechanism of Action Replaces endogenous pancreatic enzymes to assist in digestion of protein, starch and fats

Pharmacokinetics (Adult data unless noted)
Absorption: Not absorbed, acts locally in the GI tract
Elimination: In feces

Usual Dosage Oral: The following dosage recommendations are only an approximation for initial dosages. The actual dosage will depend on the digestive requirements of the individual patient. Adjust dose based upon body weight and stool fat content. Oral: Total daily dose in children and adults is divided into 3 meals/day plus 2-3 snacks/day with half the meal-time dose given with the snack:
Infants: 2000-4000 lipase units/120 mL (4 ounce) formula
Children ≤4 years: 1000 lipase units/kg/meal (maximum: 2500 lipase units/kg), with 1/2 dose with each snack
Children >4 years and Adults: 400-500 lipase units/kg/meal (maximum: 2500 lipase units/kg), with 1/2 dose with each snack

Administration Oral: Swallow capsules/tablets whole; retention in the mouth before swallowing may cause mucosal irritation and stomatitis; administer before or with meals; when administering to infants, may open capsule and spread over acidic foods (applesauce, mashed fruits, rice cereal) in a rubber-tipped teaspoon (use mixture immediately, do not make ahead of time). Place mixture onto the middle of the infant's tongue and then give bottle or breast. As an alternative, the parent may dip a clean finger into the food/enzyme mixture and then place finger into the infant's mouth and allow infant to suck on. Check infant's mouth after eating for lodged enzyme beads and remove.

Monitoring Parameters Stool fat content

Additional Information Concomitant administration of conventional pancreatin enzymes with an H_2-receptor antagonist has been used to decrease acid inactivation of enzyme activity.

Dosage Forms Excipient information presented when available (limited, particularly for generics); consult specific product labeling. [DSC] = Discontinued product
Capsule: Lipase 8500 units, protease 50,000 units, amylase 50,000 units [pancreatin 500 mg]
Dygase, kutrase®: Lipase 2400 units, protease 30,000 units, amylase 30,000 units [DSC]
ku-zyme®: Lipase 1200 units, protease 15,000 units, amylase 15,000 units [DSC]
Lapase: Lipase 1200 units, protease 15,000 units, and amylase 15,000 units [contains tartrazine] [DSC]
Pan-2400™: Lipase 9816 units, protease 60,214 units, amylase 75,900 units [pancreatin 2400 mg]
Tablet: Lipase 565 units, protease 8200 units, amylase 8200 units [pancreatin 325 mg]; lipase 2400 units, protease 30,000 units, amylase 30,000 units [pancreatin 1200 mg]
Hi-Vegi-Lip: Lipase 4800 units, protease 60,000 units, amylase 60,000 units [pancreatin 2400 mg; vegetable source]

References
Pettei MJ, Leonidas JC, Levinne JJ, et al, "Pancolonic Disease in Cystic Fibrosis and High-Dose Pancreatic Enzyme Therapy," *J Pediatr*, 1994, 125(4):587-9.
Taylor CJ, "Colonic Strictures in Cystic Fibrosis," *Lancet*, 1994, 343 (8898):615-6.

◆ **Pancrecarb MS® [DSC]** see Pancrelipase on page 1051

Pancrelipase (pan kre LI pase)

Medication Safety Issues
Sound-alike/look-alike issues:
Pancrease® may be confused with Pentasa®
Pangestyme™ may be confused with Pentasa®
Viokase® may be confused with Viokase® 8
Viokase® 8 may be confused with Viokase®

Related Information
Pancreatin on page 1050

U.S. Brand Names Creon®; Pancrease® MT; Pancrecarb MS® [DSC]; Pancrelipase™; Pangestyme™ CN [DSC]; Pangestyme™ EC [DSC]; Pangestyme™ [DSC]; Pangestyme™ UL [DSC]; Plaretase® 8000 [DSC]; Ultrase® MT [DSC]; Ultrase® [DSC]; Viokase® [DSC]; Zenpep™

Canadian Brand Names Cotazym®; Creon®; Pancrease®; Pancrease® MT; Ultrase®; Ultrase® MT; Viokase®

Therapeutic Category Enzyme, Pancreatic; Pancreatic Enzyme

Generic Available No

Use Treatment of exocrince pancreatic insufficiency caused by cystic fibrosis, chronic pancreatitis, pancreatectomy, or obstructed pancreatic ducts (FDA approved in children and adults); open occluded feeding tubes

Medication Guide An FDA-approved patient medication guide, which is available with the product information and as follows, must be dispensed with this medication for each new outpatient prescription and refill.
Creon®: http://www.fda.gov/downloads/Drugs/DrugSafety/UCM152847.pdf
Zenpep™: http://www.fda.gov/downloads/Drugs/Drug-Safety/UCM180714.pdf

Pregnancy Risk Factor B/C (product specific)

Pregnancy Considerations Reproduction studies have not been conducted with all products currently marketed (category C). When conducted, adverse events were not observed in animal reproduction studies at doses close to the maximum recommended human dose (category B). Nutrition should be optimized in pregnancy; in cystic fibrosis patients with malabsorption, pancreatic enzyme replacement is not considered to cause a risk to the pregnancy.

Lactation Excretion in breast milk unknown/use caution

Breast-Feeding Considerations Systemic absorption and concentration into the breast milk is unlikely, but unknown.

Contraindications Hypersensitivity to pancrelipase, any component, or to pork protein; acute pancreatitis; acute exacerbations of chronic pancreatic diseases

Warnings Pancrelipase is inactivated by acids; use microencapsulated products whenever possible, since these products permit better dissolution of enzymes in the duodenum and protect the enzyme preparations from acid degradation in the stomach; products are not bioequivalent, do not substitute without consulting a physician or pharmacist; do not substitute generic enzymes for brand name products

Fibrosing colonopathy and colonic strictures have been reported in several pediatric patients. Development of the strictures has been associated with high lipase intake (mean: >6,000 units/kg/meal) over a prolonged period of time in children <12 years. Patients receiving doses >2500 lipase units/kg/meal or 4000 lipase units/g fat/day should be re-evaluated or titrated downward to lowest effective dose.

Precautions Pancrealipase is an oral mucosa and skin irritant; care should be taken to ensure product is not retained in mouth nor powder on hands or area around mouth; inhalation of powder may produce an asthmatic attack. Use caution in patients with gout, hyperuricemia, or renal impairment; products contain purines which may increase uric acid levels.

Adverse Reactions
Central nervous system: Dizziness, headache
Endocrine & metabolic: Hyperuricemia, weight decreased

Gastrointestinal: Abdominal pain, abnormal feces, early satiety, fibrosing colonopathy, flatulence

Respiratory: Cough

Miscellaneous: Hypersensitivity reactions

Case reports: Allergic reactions (severe), anaphylaxis, asthma, carcinoma recurrence, distal intestinal obstruction syndrome (DIOS), hives, nausea, pruritus, rash, urticaria

Drug Interactions

Avoid Concomitant Use There are no known interactions where it is recommended to avoid concomitant use.

Increased Effect/Toxicity There are no known significant interactions involving an increase in effect.

Decreased Effect

Pancrelipase may decrease the levels/effects of: Iron Salts

Food Interactions Avoid placing contents of opened capsules on alkaline foods, such as dairy products (milk, custard, or ice cream); see Administration

Stability

Creon® [new formulation]: Store at room temperature of 25°C (77°F); protect from moisture and discard if moisture conditions are >70%. Keep bottle tightly closed.

Pancrease® MT: Store in a tightly-closed container and in a dry place at ≤25°C (77°F); do not refrigerate.

Ultrase®, Ultrase® MT: Store at room temperature of 15°C to 25°C (59°F to 77°F) in a dry place; do not refrigerate.

Viokase®: Store in a tightly-closed container and in a dry place at ≤25°C (77°F).

Zenpep™: Store at room temperature of 20°C to 25°C (68°F to 77°F); protect from moisture; keep bottle tightly-closed after opening.

Mechanism of Action Replaces endogenous pancreatic enzymes to assist in digestion of protein, starch and fats

Pharmacokinetics (Adult data unless noted)

Absorption: Not absorbed, acts locally in the GI tract

Elimination: In feces

Usual Dosage Oral: Adjust dose based on body weight, clinical symptoms, and stool fat content. Allow several days between dose adjustments. Total daily dose reflects ~3 meals/day and 2-3 snacks/day, with half the mealtime dose given with a snack. Doses of lipase >2500 units/kg/meal should be used with caution and only with documentation of 3-day fecal fat measures. Doses of lipase >6000 units/kg/meal are associated with colonic stricture and should be decreased.

Infants and Children:

≤1 year: Lipase 2000-4000 units per 120 mL of formula, breast milk, or per breast-feeding (see Administration)

>1 to <4 years: Initial dose: Lipase 1000 units/kg/meal. Dosage range: Lipase 1000-2500 units/kg/meal. Maximum dose: Lipase 10,000 units/kg/day or lipase 4000 units/g of fat/day

≥4 years: Refer to adult dosing

Adults: Initial: Lipase 500 units/kg/meal. Dosage range: Lipase 500-2500 units/kg/meal. Maximum dose: Lipase 10,000 units/kg/day or lipase 4000 units/g of fat/day

Occluded feeding tubes: Children and Adults: One tablet of Viokase® crushed with one 325 mg tablet of sodium bicarbonate (to activate the Viokase®) in 5 mL of water can be instilled into the nasogastric tube and clamped for 5 minutes; then flushed with 50 mL of water

Administration Administer with meals or snacks and swallow capsules whole with a generous amount of liquid, water, or juice. Do not crush or chew; retention in the mouth before swallowing may cause mucosal irritation and stomatitis. If necessary, capsules may also be opened and contents added to a small amount of an acidic food (pH ≤4), such as applesauce. The food should be at room temperature and swallowed immediately after mixing. The contents of the capsule should not be crushed or chewed.

Follow with water or juice to ensure complete ingestion and that no medication remains in the mouth. Creon® capsules contain enteric coated spheres which are 0.71-1.6 mm in diameter. Zenpep™ capsules contain enteric coated beads which are 1.8-2.5 mm in diameter.

When administering to infants <1 year, do not mix with breast milk or infant formula. Open capsule and place the contents directly into the mouth or mix with a small amount of applesauce, commercially prepared pears, or bananas baby food. Follow with water or infant formula to ensure complete ingestion.

Monitoring Parameters Stool fat content, abdominal symptoms, nutritional intake, weight, growth, stool character

Additional Information Concomitant administration with an H$_2$-receptor antagonist has been used to decrease acid inactivation of enzyme activity; concomitant antacid administration may decrease effectiveness of enzymes.

Dosage Forms Excipient information presented when available (limited, particularly for generics); consult specific product labeling. [DSC] = Discontinued product

Capsule, delayed release, enteric coated beads [porcine derived]:

Pancrelipase™: Lipase 5000 units, protease 17,000 units, amylase 27,000 units

Zenpep™: Lipase 5000 units, protease 17,000 units, amylase 27,000 units

Zenpep™: Lipase 10,000 units, protease 34,000 units, amylase 55,000 units

Zenpep™: Lipase 15,000 units, protease 51,000 units, amylase 82,000 units

Zenpep™: Lipase 20,000 units, protease 68,000 units, amylase 109,000 units

Capsule, delayed release, enteric coated granules [porcine derived]:

Pangestyme™ CN-10: Lipase 10,000 units, protease 37,500 units, amylase 33,200 units [DSC]

Pangestyme™ CN-20: Lipase 20,000 units, protease 75,000 units, amylase 66,400 units [DSC]

Pangestyme™ EC: Lipase 4500 units, protease 25,000 units, and amylase 20,000 units [DSC]

Pangestyme™ MT16: Lipase 16,000 units, protease 48,000 units, and amylase 48,000 units [DSC]

Pangestyme™ UL 12: Lipase 12,000 units, protease 39,000 units, and amylase 39,000 units [DSC]

Pangestyme™ UL 18: Lipase 18,000 units, protease 58,500 units, and amylase 58,500 units [DSC]

Pangestyme™ UL 20: Lipase 20,000 units, protease 65,000 units, and amylase 65,000 units [DSC]

Capsule, delayed release, enteric coated microspheres [porcine derived]: Lipase 4500 units, protease 25,000 units, and amylase 20,000 units [DSC]; Lipase 10,000 units, protease 30,000 units, and amylase 30,000 units [DSC]; Lipase 16,000 units, protease 48,000 units, and amylase 48,000 units [DSC]; Lipase 20,000 units, protease 44,000 units, and amylase 56,000 units [DSC]

Creon® 5: Lipase 5000 units, protease 18,750 units, and amylase 16,600 units [DSC]

Creon® 10: Lipase 10,000 units, protease 37,500 units, and amylase 33,200 units [DSC]

Creon® 20: Lipase 20,000 units, protease 75,000 units, and amylase 66,400 units [DSC]

Pancrecarb MS-4®: Lipase 4000 units, protease 25,000 units, and amylase 25,000 units [buffered] [DSC]

Pancrecarb MS-8®: Lipase 8000 units, protease 45,000 units, and amylase 40,000 units [buffered] [DSC]

Pancrecarb MS-16® Lipase 16,000 units, protease 52,000 units, and amylase 52,000 units [buffered] [DSC]

Capsule, delayed release, enteric coated microspheres [new formulation; porcine derived]:

Creon®: Lipase 6000 units, protease 19,000 units, and amylase 30,000 units

Creon®: Lipase 12000 units, protease 38,000 units, and amylase 60,000 units

Creon®: Lipase 24,000 units, protease 76,000 units, and amylase 120,000 units

Capsule, enteric coated microspheres [porcine derived]:

Ultrase®: Lipase 4500 units, protease 25,000 units, and amylase 20,000 units

Capsule, enteric coated microtablets [porcine derived]:

Pancrease® MT 4: Lipase 4000 units, protease 12,000 units, and amylase 12,000 units

Pancrease® MT 10: Lipase 10,000 units, protease 30,000 units, and amylase 30,000 units

Pancrease® MT 16: Lipase 16,000 units, protease 48,000 units, and amylase 48,000 units

Pancrease® MT 20: Lipase 20,000 units, protease 44,000 units, and amylase 56,000 units

Capsule, enteric coated minitablets [porcine derived]:

Ultrase® MT12: Lipase 12,000 units, protease 39,000 units, and amylase 39,000 units [DSC]

Ultrase® MT18: Lipase 18,000 units, protease 58,500 units, and amylase 58,500 units [DSC]

Ultrase® MT20: Lipase 20,000 units, protease 65,000 units, and amylase 65,000 units [DSC]

Powder [porcine derived]:

Viokase®: Lipase 16,800 units, protease 70,000 units, and amylase 70,000 units per 0.7 g (227 g) [DSC]

Tablet [porcine derived]:

Plaretase™ 8000: Lipase 8000 units, protease 30,000 units, and amylase 30,000 units [DSC]

Viokase® 8: Lipase 8000 units, protease 30,000 units, and amylase 30,000 units [DSC]

Viokase® 16: Lipase 16,000 units, protease 60,000 units, and amylase 60,000 units [DSC]

References

Borowitz DS, Grand RJ, and Durie PR, "Use of Pancreatic Enzyme Supplements for Patients With Cystic Fibrosis in the Context of Fibrosing Colonopathy. Consensus Committee," *J Pediatr*, 1995, 127 (5):681-4.

FitzSimmons SC, Burkhart GA, Borowitz D, et al, "High-Dose Pancreatic-Enzyme Supplements and Fibrosing Colonopathy in Children With Cystic Fibrosis," *N Engl J Med*, 1997, 336(18):1283-9.

Marcuard SP and Stegall KS, "Unclogging Feeding Tubes With Pancreatic Enzyme," *JPEN J Parenter Enteral Nutr*, 1990, 14 (2):198-200.

Marcuard SP, Stegall KL, and Trogdon S, "Clearing Obstructed Feeding Tubes," *JPEN J Parenter Enteral Nutr*, 1989, 13(1):81-3.

Pettei MJ, Leonidas JC, Levinne JJ, et al, "Pancolonic Disease in Cystic Fibrosis and High-Dose Pancreatic Enzyme Therapy," *J Pediatr*, 1994, 125(4):587-9.

Stallings VA, Stark LJ, Robinson KA, et al, "Evidence-Based Practice Recommendations for Nutrition-Related Management of Children and Adults With Cystic Fibrosis and Pancreatic Insufficiency: Results of a Systematic Review," *J Am Diet Assoc*, 2008, 108(5):832-9.

Taylor CG, "Colonic Strictures in Cystic Fibrosis," *Lancet*, 1994, 343 (8898):615-6.

◆ **Pancrelipase™** *see Pancrelipase on page 1051*

Pancuronium (pan kyoo ROE nee um)

Medication Safety Issues

Sound-alike/look-alike issues:

Pancuronium may be confused with pipecuronium

High alert medication: The Institute for Safe Medication Practices (ISMP) includes this medication among its list of drugs which have a heightened risk of causing significant patient harm when used in error.

United States Pharmacopeia (USP) 2006: The Interdisciplinary Safe Medication Use Expert Committee of the USP has recommended the following:

- Hospitals, clinics, and other practice sites should institute special safeguards in the storage, labeling, and use of these agents and should include these safeguards in staff orientation and competency training.

- Healthcare professionals should be on high alert (especially vigilant) whenever a neuromuscular-blocking agent (NMBA) is stocked, ordered, prepared, or administered.

Canadian Brand Names Pancuronium Bromide®

Therapeutic Category Neuromuscular Blocker Agent, Nondepolarizing; Skeletal Muscle Relaxant, Paralytic

Generic Available Yes

Use Produces skeletal muscle relaxation during surgery after induction of general anesthesia, increases pulmonary compliance during assisted mechanical respiration, facilitates endotracheal intubation

Pregnancy Risk Factor C

Lactation Excretion in breast milk unknown/not recommended

Contraindications Hypersensitivity to pancuronium, bromide, or any component (see Warnings)

Warnings Ventilation must be supported during neuromuscular blockade; electrolyte imbalance alters blockade; contains benzyl alcohol which may cause allergic reactions in susceptible individuals; large amounts of benzyl alcohol (≥99 mg/kg/day) have been associated with a potentially fatal toxicity ("gasping syndrome") in neonates; the "gasping syndrome" consists of metabolic acidosis, respiratory distress, gasping respirations, CNS dysfunction (including convulsions, intracranial hemorrhage), hypotension and cardiovascular collapse; *in vitro* and animal studies have shown that benzoate, a metabolite of benzyl alcohol, displaces bilirubin from protein binding sites; avoid use of benzyl alcohol containing products in neonates

Precautions Use with caution and decrease dose in patients with decreased renal function; many clinical conditions may affect the response to neuromuscular blockade, see table.

Clinical Conditions Affecting Neuromuscular Blockade

Potentiation	Antagonism
Electrolyte abnormalities	Alkalosis
Severe hyponatremia	Hypercalcemia
Severe hypocalcemia	Demyelinating lesions
Severe hypokalemia	Peripheral neuropathies
Hypermagnesemia	Diabetes mellitus
Neuromuscular diseases	
Acidosis	
Acute intermittent porphyria	
Renal failure	
Hepatic failure	

Adverse Reactions Most frequent adverse reactions are related to prolongation of pharmacologic actions

Cardiovascular: Tachycardia, hypertension

Dermatologic: Rash, erythema

Gastrointestinal: Excessive salivation

Local: Burning sensation along the vein

Neuromuscular & skeletal: Muscle weakness

Respiratory: Wheezes, bronchospasm

Miscellaneous: Hypersensitivity reactions

Drug Interactions

Avoid Concomitant Use

Avoid concomitant use of Pancuronium with any of the following: QuiNINE

Increased Effect/Toxicity

Pancuronium may increase the levels/effects of: Cardiac Glycosides; Corticosteroids (Systemic); Onabotulinumtoxin A; Rimabotulinumtoxin B

The levels/effects of Pancuronium may be increased by: Abobotulinumtoxin A; Aminoglycosides; Calcium Channel Blockers; Capreomycin; Colistimethate; Inhalational Anesthetics; Ketorolac; Ketorolac (Systemic); Lincosamide Antibiotics; Lithium; Loop Diuretics; Magnesium Salts; Polymyxin B; Procainamide; QuiNIDine; QuiNINE; Spironolactone; Tetracycline Derivatives; Vancomycin

Decreased Effect

The levels/effects of Pancuronium may be decreased by: Acetylcholinesterase Inhibitors; Loop Diuretics

Stability Refrigerate; however, stable for up to 6 months at room temperature; compatible with D_5W, NS, D_5NS, and LR injections

Mechanism of Action Nondepolarizing neuromuscular blocker which blocks acetylcholine from binding to receptors on motor endplate thus inhibiting depolarization

Pharmacodynamics

Maximum effect: I.V. injection: Within 2-3 minutes
Duration: 40-60 minutes (dose dependent)

Pharmacokinetics (Adult data unless noted)

Distribution: V_d: Adults: 0.23 L/kg
Protein binding: 87%
Metabolism: 30% to 40% metabolized in liver
Half-life: 110 minutes
Elimination: Primarily in urine (60%) as unchanged drug and bile (40%)
Clearance: Adults: 1.9 mL/kg/minute

Usual Dosage I.V.:

Neonates and Infants: 0.1 mg/kg every 30-60 minutes as needed or as continuous infusion of 0.02-0.04 mg/kg/hour or 0.4-0.6 mcg/kg/minute

Children: 0.15 mg/kg every 30-60 minutes as needed or as continuous infusion 0.03-0.1 mg/kg/hour or 0.5-1.7 mcg/kg/minute

Adolescents and Adults: 0.15 mg/kg every 30-60 minutes as needed or as a continuous infusion 0.02-0.04 mg/kg/hour or 0.4-0.6 mcg/kg/minute

Dosing adjustment in renal impairment:
Cl_{cr} 10-50 mL/minute: Administer 50% of normal dose
Cl_{cr} <10 mL/minute: Do not use

Administration Parenteral: May be administered undiluted by rapid I.V. injection; for continuous infusion, dilute to 0.01-0.8 mg/mL in D_5NS, D_5W, LR, or NS.

Monitoring Parameters Heart rate, blood pressure, assisted ventilation status, peripheral nerve stimulator measuring twitch response

Nursing Implications Does not alter the patient's state of consciousness; addition of sedation and analgesia are recommended

Additional Information Patients with hepatic and biliary disease have a larger V_d which may result in a higher total initial dose and possibly a slower onset of effect; the duration of neuromuscular blocking effects may be prolonged in patients with hepatic, biliary, or renal dysfunction

Dosage Forms Excipient information presented when available (limited, particularly for generics); consult specific product labeling.

Injection, solution, as bromide: 1 mg/mL (10 mL); 2 mg/mL (2 mL, 5 mL) [may contain benzyl alcohol]

References

Martin LD, Bratton SL, and O'Rourke PP, "Clinical Uses and Controversies of Neuromuscular Blocking Agents in Infants and Children," *Crit Care Med*, 1999, 27(7):1358-68.

♦ **Pancuronium Bromide** *see* Pancuronium *on page 1053*
♦ **Pancuronium Bromide® (Can)** *see* Pancuronium *on page 1053*

♦ **Pandel®** *see* Hydrocortisone *on page 685*
♦ **Pangestyme™ CN [DSC]** *see* Pancrelipase *on page 1051*
♦ **Pangestyme™ EC [DSC]** *see* Pancrelipase *on page 1051*
♦ **Pangestyme™ MT [DSC]** *see* Pancrelipase *on page 1051*
♦ **Pangestyme™ UL [DSC]** *see* Pancrelipase *on page 1051*
♦ **Panglobulin** *see* Immune Globulin (Intravenous) *on page 719*
♦ **PanOxyl® (Can)** *see* Benzoyl Peroxide *on page 184*
♦ **PanOxyl® Aqua Gel** *see* Benzoyl Peroxide *on page 184*
♦ **PanOxyl® Bar [OTC]** *see* Benzoyl Peroxide *on page 184*
♦ **Panto™ I.V. (Can)** *see* Pantoprazole *on page 1054*
♦ **Pantoloc® (Can)** *see* Pantoprazole *on page 1054*

Pantoprazole (pan TOE pra zole)

Medication Safety Issues

Sound-alike/look-alike issues:
Pantoprazole may be confused with aripiprazole
Protonix® may be confused with Lotronex®, Lovenox®, protamine

Vials containing Protonix® I.V. for injection are not recommended for use with spiked I.V. system adaptors. Nurses and pharmacists have reported breakage of the glass vials during attempts to connect spiked I.V. system adaptors, which may potentially result in injury to healthcare professionals.

International issues:
Protonix® may be confused with Pretanix® which is a brand name for indapamide in Hungary

U.S. Brand Names Protonix®

Canadian Brand Names Apo-Pantoprazole®; CO Pantoprazole; Mylan-Pantoprazole; Novo-Pantoprazole; Pantoloc®; Panto™ I.V.; PHL-Pantoprazole; PMS-Pantoprazole; Protonix®; RAN™-Pantoprazole; ratio-Pantoprazole; Riva-Pantoprazole; Sandoz-Pantoprazole; Tecta™; ZYM-Pantoprazole

Therapeutic Category Gastric Acid Secretion Inhibitor; Gastrointestinal Agent, Gastric or Duodenal Ulcer Treatment; Proton Pump Inhibitor

Generic Available Yes: Delayed release tablet

Use

Oral: Treatment and maintenance of healing of erosive esophagitis associated with gastroesophageal reflux disease (GERD); treatment of pathological hypersecretory conditions including Zollinger-Ellison syndrome; adjunctive therapy of duodenal ulcers associated with *Helicobacter pylori*

I.V.: Short-term treatment (7-10 days) of patients with GERD with a history of erosive esophagitis; an alternative to oral therapy in patients who are unable to continue taking oral pantoprazole; treatment of pathological hypersecretory conditions associated with Zollinger-Ellison syndrome or other GI hypersecretory disorders

Pregnancy Risk Factor B

Pregnancy Considerations Teratogenic effects were not observed in animal studies. There are no adequate and well-controlled studies in pregnant women. Use in pregnancy only if clearly needed.

Lactation Enters breast milk/not recommended

Breast-Feeding Considerations Not recommended due to carcinogenicity in animal studies.

Contraindications Hypersensitivity to pantoprazole, substituted benzimidazole proton pump inhibitors (eg, esomeprazole, omeprazole, lansoprazole), or any component

Warnings In long-term (2-year) studies in rodents, pantoprazole was carcinogenic and caused rare types of gastrointestinal tumors. While available endoscopic evaluations and histologic examinations of biopsy specimens from human stomachs have not detected a risk from short-term exposure to pantoprazole, further human data on the effect of sustained hypochlorhydria and hypergastrinemia are needed to rule out the possibility of an increased risk for the development of tumors in humans receiving long-term therapy. Symptomatic response to therapy does not preclude the presence of gastric malignancy. Use of gastric acid inhibitors including proton pump inhibitors and H_2 blockers has been associated with an increased risk for development of acute gastroenteritis and community-acquired pneumonia (Canani, 2006). Atrophic gastritis has been reported in gastric biopsies from patients treated long-term with pantoprazole, particularly in patients who were *H. pylori* positive.

Precautions Long-term treatment (>3 years) may lead to malabsorption of cyanocobalamin (vitamin B_{12}) caused by hypo or achlorhydria. Injection contains edetate sodium (EDTA); EDTA is a potent chelator of metal ions, particularly zinc; use with caution in patients prone to zinc deficiency or receiving other EDTA-containing products. Zinc supplementation may be necessary.

Adverse Reactions

Cardiovascular: Chest pain, tachycardia, angina, palpitations, hypertension, hypotension, syncope, angioedema (Quincke's edema)

Central nervous system: Headache, dizziness, vertigo, insomnia, anxiety, fever, nervousness, confusion, depression, emotional lability, hallucinations, migraine, speech disorder

Dermatologic: Urticaria, pruritus, acne, alopecia, dry skin, maculopapular rash; rare severe dermatologic conditions such as Stevens-Johnson syndrome, erythema multiforme, toxic epidural necrolysis

Endocrine & metabolic: Hyperglycemia, hyperlipemia, goiter, gout

Gastrointestinal: Diarrhea, nausea, abdominal pain, vomiting, constipation, flatulence, dyspepsia, eructation, xerostomia, anorexia, dysgeusia, duodenitis, dysphagia, glossitis, halitosis, abnormal stools, tongue discoloration, ulcerative colitis, taste perversion, pancreatitis (rare), salivation increased

Genitourinary: Urinary frequency, UTI, interstitial nephritis (rare)

Hematologic: Thrombocytopenia, leukopenia, leukocytosis, anemia, pancytopenia (rare), pernicious anemia (see Precautions)

Hepatic: Hepatitis, liver function tests elevated, cholestatic jaundice, biliary pain, hyperbilirubinemia, hepatic failure (rare)

Local: I.V.: Thrombophlebitis, abscess

Neuromuscular & skeletal: Muscle cramps, myalgia, arthralgia, neck pain, hypertonia, back pain, paresthesias, reflexes decreased, leg cramps, bone pain, bursitis, CPK elevated, rhabdomyolysis (rare)

Ocular: Amblyopia, diplopia, extraocular palsy, glaucoma, anterior ischemic optic neuropathy (rare), blurred vision

Otic: Ear pain, tinnitus

Renal: Hematuria, pyuria, proteinuria, glycosuria, interstitial nephritis (rare)

Respiratory: Rhinitis, bronchitis, cough, dyspnea, pharyngitis, sinusitis, URI

Miscellaneous: Anaphylaxis (I.V. formulation), flu-like syndrome, infection

Drug Interactions

Metabolism/Transport Effects Substrate of CYP2C19 (major), 2C9 (minor), 2D6 (minor), 3A4 (minor); **Inhibits** 2C9 (weak), ABCG2; **Induces** CYP1A2 (weak), 3A4 (weak)

Avoid Concomitant Use

Avoid concomitant use of Pantoprazole with any of the following: Delavirdine; Erlotinib; Nelfinavir; Posaconazole

Increased Effect/Toxicity

Pantoprazole may increase the levels/effects of: Methotrexate; Raltegravir; Saquinavir; Topotecan; Voriconazole

The levels/effects of Pantoprazole may be increased by: Clopidogrel; Fluconazole; Ketoconazole; Ketoconazole (Systemic)

Decreased Effect

Pantoprazole may decrease the levels/effects of: Atazanavir; Cefditoren; Clopidogrel; Dabigatran Etexilate; Dasatinib; Delavirdine; Erlotinib; Indinavir; Iron Salts; Itraconazole; Ketoconazole; Ketoconazole (Systemic); Mesalamine; Mycophenolate; Nelfinavir; Posaconazole

The levels/effects of Pantoprazole may be decreased by: CYP2C19 Inducers (Strong); Peginterferon Alfa-2b; Tipranavir

Stability Protect from light; store tablets at room temperature; refrigerate powder for injection (36°F to 46°F). Reconstituted injection is stable at room temperature for 24 hours; do not freeze; after further dilution with I.V. fluid, the solution is stable at room temperature for 24 hours. Neither the reconstituted solution or diluted solution need be protected from light. Pantoprazole stability is a function of pH; it is rapidly degraded in acidic media, but has acceptable stability under alkaline conditions. Each tablet of pantoprazole is enteric coated to prevent degradation by gastric acidity.

Mechanism of Action Suppresses gastric acid secretion by inhibiting the parietal cell membrane enzyme (H^+/K^+)-ATPase or proton pump; demonstrates antimicrobial activity against *Helicobacter pylori*

Pharmacodynamics Acid secretion:

Onset of action:

Oral: 2.5 hours

I.V.: 15-30 minutes

Maximum effect: I.V.: 2 hours

Duration: Oral, I.V.: 24 hours

Pharmacokinetics (Adult data unless noted)

Distribution: V_d: Adults: 11-23.6 L

Protein binding: 98%

Metabolism: Extensive liver metabolism; no evidence of active metabolites

Bioavailability: ~77%

Half-life: Adults: 1 hour; prolonged half-life (3.5-10 hours) in slow metabolizers

Time to peak serum concentration: Oral: 2.5 hours

Elimination: Renal: 71% (as metabolites); biliary/fecal: 18%

Clearance: Adults: 7.6-14 L/hour

Dialysis: Not appreciably removed by hemodialysis

Usual Dosage I.V. therapy should be discontinued as soon as the patient tolerates oral therapy

Erosive esophagitis associated with GERD:

Children: Oral: Limited data; 20 mg once daily (0.5-1 mg/kg/day) was used in 15 children, 6-13 years of age (20-40 kg) for 28 days (Madrazo-De La Garza, 2003)

Adults: Treatment and maintenance:

Oral: 40 mg/day for up to 8 weeks; in mild GERD, 20 mg/day has been effective

I.V.: 40 mg/day for 7-10 days

Hypersecretory conditions (including Zollinger-Ellison syndrome): Adults:

Oral: Initial: 40 mg twice daily; adjust dose based on patient response; doses up to 240 mg/day have been used

I.V.: Initial: 80 mg twice daily; adjust dosage to maintain acid output below 10 mEq/hour; doses up to 80 mg every 8 hours have been used; doses >240 mg/day or treatment duration >6 days have not been studied

Adjunctive therapy of duodenal ulcers associated with *Helicobacter pylori* (in combination with antibiotic therapy): Adults: Oral: 40 mg once or twice daily

Dosage adjustment in renal or hepatic Impairment: No dosage adjustment needed.

Administration

I.V.: Reconstitute powder for injection with 10 mL NS; further dilute in NS, D_5W, or LR to a final concentration 0.4-0.8 mg/mL; infuse over 15 minutes at a rate not to exceed 7 mL/minute; for more rapid infusion, dilute reconstituted solution to a final concentration of 4 mg/mL and infuse over 2 minutes; not for I.M. or SubQ use

Oral: Administer tablets without regard to food; tablet should be swallowed whole, do not chew or crush; may be administered with antacids. Protonix® delayed-release suspension should not be crushed or chewed and should be administered 30 minutes before a meal. Administer in 5 mL apple juice, stir for 5 seconds and swallow immediately. May administer in 1 teaspoonful of applesauce, swallow within 10 minutes of preparation. Do not adminster in water, other liquids, or foods. For nasogastric administration, empty granules into barrel of syringe, add 10 mL apple juice; may rinse syringe with additional apple juice to prevent granules from remaining in syringe.

Test Interactions Reports of false-positive urine screening tests for tetrahydrocannabinol in patients receiving pantoprazole

Patient Information May cause dry mouth; do not chew or crush tablets

Dosage Forms Excipient information presented when available (limited, particularly for generics); consult specific product labeling. [CAN] = Canadian brand name

Note: Strength expressed as base

Granules for suspension, delayed release, enteric coated, as sodium, oral:

Protonix®: 40 mg/packet (30s)

Injection, powder for reconstitution, as sodium:

Protonix®: 40 mg [contains edetate sodium 1 mg]

Tablet, delayed release, as sodium: 20 mg, 40 mg

Protonix®: 20 mg, 40 mg

Tablet, enteric coated, as magnesium:

Pantoloc® [CAN]: 40 mg [not available in the U.S.]

Extemporaneous Preparations A 2 mg/mL oral liquid may be prepared by first removing the Protonix® imprint from twenty 40 mg tablets by gently rubbing the tablets on a paper towel dampened with alcohol; allow to air dry; (this eliminates dark flecks in final product). Crush the tablets; place coarse powder in 600 mL beaker and add 340 mL SWI. Place beaker on a magnetic stirrer. While stirring, add 16.8 g sodium bicarbonate powder and stir for about 20 minutes until the tablet remnants have disintegrated and the coating has dissolved. While continuing to stir, add another 16.8 g sodium bicarbonate powder and stir for an additional 5 minutes until the powder dissolves. Add enough SWI to bring the final volume to 400 mL. Mix well. Stable 62 days refrigerated and protected from light. Label "shake well."

Dentinger PJ, Swenson CF, and Anaizi NH, "Stability of Pantoprazole in an Extemporaneously Compounded Oral Liquid," *Am J Health Syst Pharm*, 2002, 59 (10):953-6.

References
Canani RB, Cirillo P, Roggero P, et al, "Therapy With Gastric Acidity Inhibitors Increases the Risk of Acute Gastroenteritis and Community-Acquired Pneumonia in Children," *Pediatrics*, 2006, 117(5):e817-20.
Madrazo-De La Garza A, Dibildox M, Vargas A, et al, "Efficacy and Safety of Oral Pantoprazole 20 mg Given Once Daily for Reflux Esophagitis in Children," *J Pediatr Gastroenterol Nutr*, 2003, 36 (2):261-5.

Papaverine (pa PAV er een)

Medication Safety Issues
Sound-alike/look-alike issues:
Papaverine may be confused with pamidronate

U.S. Brand Names Para-Time SR® [DSC]

Therapeutic Category Antimigraine Agent; Vasodilator

Generic Available Yes

Use Relief of peripheral and cerebral ischemia associated with arterial spasm; investigationally for prophylaxis of migraine headache; intracavernosal injection for impotence

Pregnancy Risk Factor C

Lactation Excretion in breast milk unknown/not recommended

Contraindications Hypersensitivity to papaverine or any component; complete atrioventricular block; Parkinson's disease

Precautions Use with caution in patients with glaucoma; administer I.V. slowly and with caution since arrhythmias and apnea may occur with rapid I.V. use; should **not** be used in neonates due to the increased risk of drug-induced cerebral vasodilation and possibility of an intracranial bleed

Adverse Reactions
Cardiovascular: Flushing of the face, tachycardia, hypotension, arrhythmias with rapid I.V. use
Central nervous system: Depression, dizziness, vertigo, drowsiness, sedation, lethargy, headache
Dermatologic: Pruritus
Gastrointestinal: Xerostomia, nausea, constipation
Hepatic: Hepatic hypersensitivity
Local: Thrombosis at the I.V. administration site
Respiratory: Apnea with rapid I.V. use
Miscellaneous: Diaphoresis

Drug Interactions
Avoid Concomitant Use There are no known interactions where it is recommended to avoid concomitant use.

Increased Effect/Toxicity
Papaverine may increase the levels/effects of: Hypotensive Agents

Decreased Effect There are no known significant interactions involving a decrease in effect.

Stability Protect from heat or freezing; do not refrigerate injection; solutions should be clear to pale yellow; precipitates with LR

Mechanism of Action Smooth muscle spasmolytic producing a generalized smooth muscle relaxation including vasodilatation, GI sphincter relaxation, bronchiolar muscle relaxation, and potentially a depressed myocardium

Pharmacodynamics Onset of action: Oral: Rapid

Pharmacokinetics (Adult data unless noted)
Protein binding: 90%
Metabolism: Rapid in the liver
Bioavailability: Oral: ~54%
Half-life: 30-120 minutes
Elimination: Primarily as metabolites in urine

Usual Dosage
Children: I.M., I.V.: 1.5 mg/kg 4 times/day
Migraine prophylaxis: 6-15 years: Oral: Initial: 5 mg/kg/day given once daily; range: 5-10 mg/kg/day divided into 2-3 doses/day

Adults:
Oral: 75-300 mg 3-5 times/day
Oral, sustained release: 150-300 mg every 12 hours
I.M., I.V.: 30-120 mg every 3 hours as needed

Administration
Oral: Administer after or with meals, milk or antacids to decrease nausea; swallow sustained release capsule whole, do not crush or chew
Parenteral: Rapid I.V. administration may result in arrhythmias and fatal apnea; administer slow I.V. over 1-2 minutes

Monitoring Parameters Liver enzymes; intraocular pressure in glaucoma patients

Patient Information May cause dizziness, flushing, headache; may cause drowsiness and impair ability to perform activities requiring mental alertness or physical coordination; may cause dry mouth

Additional Information Evidence of therapeutic value of systemic use for relief of peripheral and cerebral ischemia related to arterial spasm is lacking

Further studies are needed to determine the benefit of adding papaverine (60 mg/500 mL) to arterial catheter infusions containing NS or 1/2NS and heparin 1 unit/mL. One investigation showed a lower risk of arterial catheter failure and longer duration of arterial catheter function in patients 7 months to 5.5 years of age who received papaverine in their arterial catheter solutions; these results should be verified by additional studies before the addition of papaverine to arterial catheter solutions can be recommended.

Dosage Forms Excipient information presented when available (limited, particularly for generics); consult specific product labeling. [DSC] = Discontinued product
Capsule, sustained release, as hydrochloride: 150 mg
Para-Time SR®: 150 mg [DSC]
Injection, solution, as hydrochloride: 30 mg/mL (2 mL, 10 mL)

References
Heulitt MJ, Farrington EA, O'Shea TM, et al, "Double-Blind, Randomized, Controlled Trial of Papaverine-Containing Infusions to Prevent Failure of Arterial Catheters in Pediatric Patients," *Crit Care Med*, 1993, 21(6):825-9.
Sillanpää M and Koponen M, "Papaverine in the Prophylaxis of Migraine and Other Vascular Headache in Children," *Acta Paediatr Scand*, 1978, 67(2):209-12.

◆ **Papaverine Hydrochloride** *see* Papaverine *on page 1056*

Papillomavirus (Types 6, 11, 16, 18) Recombinant Vaccine
(pap ih LO ma VYE rus typs six e LEV en SIX teen aye teen ree KOM be nant vak SEEN)

Medication Safety Issues
Sound-alike/look-alike issues:
Papillomavirus vaccine types 6, 11, 16, 18 (Gardasil®) may be confused with Papillomavirus vaccine types 16, 18 (Cervarix®)

Related Information
Immunization Guidelines *on page 1636*

U.S. Brand Names Gardasil®
Canadian Brand Names Gardasil®
Therapeutic Category Vaccine
Generic Available No

Use Prevention of cervical, vulvar, and vaginal cancer caused by Human Papillomavirus (HPV) types 16 and 18 and prevention of cervical adenocarcinoma *in situ*, and vulvar, vaginal, or cervical intraepithelial neoplasia caused by HPV types 6, 11, 16, 18 (FDA approved in girls ≥9 years and women through 26 years of age); prevention of genital warts caused by HPV types 6 and 11 (FDA approved in males and females ≥9 years through 26 years of age

Pregnancy Risk Factor B
Pregnancy Considerations Teratogenic effects were not observed in animal studies. In clinical trials, women who were found to be pregnant before the completion of the 3-dose regimen were instructed to defer any remaining dose until pregnancy resolution. Pregnancies detected within 30 days of vaccination had a higher rate of congenital anomalies (pyloric stenosis, congenital megacolon, congenital hydronephrosis, hip dysplasia, club foot) than the placebo group. Pregnancies with onset beyond 30 days of vaccination had a rate of congenital anomalies consistent with the general population. Overall, the type of teratogenic events were the same as those generally observed for this age group. A registry has been established for women exposed to the HPV vaccine during pregnancy (1-800-986-8999). Administration of the vaccine in pregnancy is not recommended; until additional information is available, the vaccine series (or completion of the series) should be delayed until pregnancy is completed.

Lactation Excretion in breast milk unknown/use caution.
Breast-Feeding Considerations Infants had a higher incidence of acute respiratory illness when breast-fed by mothers within 30 days postvaccination. Lactating women may receive vaccine.

Contraindications Hypersensitivity to human papillomavirus vaccine, yeast, or any component

Warnings Administration of HPV vaccine during pregnancy is not recommended. Pregnancies detected within 30 days of vaccination had a higher rate of congenital anomalies (pyloric stenosis, congenital megacolon, congenital hydronephrosis, hip dysplasia, club foot) than the placebo group. Pregnancies with onset beyond 30 days of vaccination had a rate of congenital anomalies consistent with the general population. A registry has been established for women exposed to the HPV vaccine during pregnancy (1-800-986-8999).

Immediate treatment for anaphylactic reactions should be available during vaccine use. There is no evidence that individuals already infected with HPV will be protected against disease by the same HPV types after vaccination. Consider deferring vaccination for patients with serious illness. May vaccinate patients with mild concurrent febrile illness. Syncope may occur following vaccination and is sometimes associated with tonic-clonic movements or other seizure-like activity; observe patients for 15 minutes after administration

Precautions Use with caution in patients with bleeding disorders such as hemophilia or thrombocytopenia or patients on anticoagulant therapy, due to an increased risk for bleeding following I.M. administration. Routine prophylactic administration of acetaminophen to prevent fever due to vaccines has been shown to decrease the immune response of some vaccines; the clinical significance of this reduction in immune response has not been established (see Prymula, 2009).

Adverse Reactions All serious adverse reactions must be reported to the U.S. Department of Health and Human Services (DHHS) Vaccine Adverse Event Reporting System (VAERS) 1-800-822-7967.
Cardiovascular: Hypertension, syncope
Central nervous system: Dizziness, fever, headache, insomnia, malaise, seizure, syncope (may result in falls with injury or be associated with tonic-clonic movements)
Gastrointestinal: Appendicitis, diarrhea, gastroenteritis, nausea, toothache, vomiting
Genitourinary: Pelvic inflammatory disease
Local: Bruising, erythema, injection site pain, pruritus, swelling
Neuromuscular & skeletal: Arthralgia, myalgia
Respiratory: Asthma, bronchospasm, cough, nasal congestion
Miscellaneous: Anaphylaxis

◄ <1%, postmarketing, and/or case reports: Acute disseminated encephalomyelitis, arrhythmia, arthritis, autoimmune hemolytic anemia and other autoimmune diseases, chills, DVT, fatigue, gastroenteritis, Guillain-Barré syndrome, hypersensitivity reaction, hyper/hypothyroidism, ITP, JRA, lymphadenopathy, motor neuron disease, pancreatitis, paralysis, pulmonary embolus, RA, renal failure (acute), sepsis, transverse myelitis, urticaria, weakness

Drug Interactions

Avoid Concomitant Use There are no known interactions where it is recommended to avoid concomitant use.

Increased Effect/Toxicity There are no known significant interactions involving an increase in effect.

Decreased Effect

The levels/effects of Papillomavirus (Types 6, 11, 16, 18) Vaccine (Human, Recombinant) may be decreased by: Immunosuppressants

Stability Store in the refrigerator; do not freeze. Protect from light. May be stored at temperatures ≤25°C (≤77°F) for a total time of ≤72 hours.

Mechanism of Action Promotes immunity to human HPV types 6, 11, 16, and 18 by inducing the production of neutralizing antibodies to the virus types

Usual Dosage I.M.: 0.5 mL

Preadolescents ≥9 years, Adolescents, and Adults ≤26 years: Initial dose: 0.5 mL followed by a second dose 2 months after first dose; third dose 6 months after first dose (immunization with HPV vaccine is usually initiated at 11-12 years; optimally, vaccination should be completed prior to onset of sexual activity)

Note: Minimum interval between the first and second dose of vaccine is 4 weeks; minimum interval between the second and third dose of vaccine is 12 weeks, minimum interval between first and third dose of the vaccine is 24 weeks. If the vaccine series is interrupted and only one dose was given, administer the second dose as soon as possible and give the third dose ≥12 weeks later. If the vaccine series is interrupted and the first two doses were given, administer the third dose as soon as possible. Inadequate doses or doses received following a shorter than recommended dosing interval should be repeated. The HPV vaccine series should be completed with the same product whenever possible.

Administration I.M.: Shake suspension well prior to use; do not use suspension if it is discolored or contains particulate matter; do not dilute or mix with other vaccines. Administer I.M. into the deltoid region of the upper arm or in the higher anterolateral area of the thigh; **not for I.V., intradermal, or SubQ administration**

Monitoring Parameters Observe patient for 15 minutes after they receive HPV vaccine for syncope.

Patient Information This vaccine does not substitute for regular, routine cervical cancer screening; the vaccine is not intended for the treatment of active genital warts or cervical cancer. This vaccine may be given during a minor illness, such as a cold or low-grade fever. Three doses will be required for effective immunity. Inform prescriber immediately if difficulty breathing, chest pain, acute headache, rash, difficulty swallowing, or excessive pain/swelling at injection site occurs.

Nursing Implications Federal law requires that the date of administration, the vaccine manufacturer, lot number of vaccine, and the administering person's name, title and address be entered into the patient's permanent medical record. Patients who develop syncope associated with tonic-clonic movements usually respond when maintained in a supine or Trendelenburg position.

Additional Information In order to maximize vaccination rates, the ACIP recommends simultaneous administration of all age-appropriate vaccines (live or inactivated) for which a person is eligible at a single visit, unless contraindications exist. The use of combination vaccines is generally preferred over separate infections, taking into consideration provider assessment, patient preference, and potential adverse events.

For additional information, please refer to the following website: http://www.cdc.gov/vaccines/vpd-vac/.

Dosage Forms Excipient information presented when available (limited, particularly for generics); consult specific product labeling.

Injection, suspension [preservative free]:

Gardasil®: HPV 6 L1 protein 20 mcg, HPV 11 L1 protein 40 mcg, HPV 16 L1 protein 40 mcg, and HPV 18 L1 protein 20 mcg per 0.5 mL (0.5 mL) [contains aluminum, polysorbate 80; manufactured using S. cerevisiae (baker's yeast)]

References

Advisory Committee on Immunization Practices, "Vaccines for Children Program, Vaccines to Prevent Human Papillomavirus (HPV) Infection," October 2009. Available at http://www.cdc.gov/vaccines/programs/vfc/downloads/resolutions/1009hpv-508.pdf.

American Academy of Pediatrics Committee on Infectious Diseases, "Recommended Childhood and Adolescent Immunization Schedules - United States, 2009," Pediatrics, 2009, 123(1):189-90.

Block SL, Nolan T, Sattler C, et al, "Comparison of the Immunogenicity and Reactogenicity of a Prophylactic Quadrivalent Human Papillomavirus (Types 6, 11, 16, and 18) L1 Virus-Like Particle Vaccine in Male and Female Adolescents and Young Adult Women," Pediatrics, 2006, 118(5):2135-45.

Centers for Disease Control and Prevention (CDC), "General Recommendations on Immunization. Recommendations of the Advisory Committee on Immunization Practices (ACIP)," MMWR Recomm Rep, 2006, 55(RR-15):1-48. Available at: http://www.cdc.gov/mmwr/preview/mmwrhtml/rr5515a1.htm.

Centers for Disease Control and Prevention (CDC), "Quadrivalent Human Papillomavirus Vaccine. Recommendations of the Advisory Committee on Immunization Practices (ACIP)," MMWR Recomm Rep, 2007, 56(RR-2):1-24.

Centers for Disease Control and Prevention (CDC), "Recommended Immunization Schedules for Persons Aged 0-18 Years – United States, 2009," MMWR, 2009, 57(51): Q1-4.

Prymula R, Siegrist CA, Chlibek R, et al, "Effect of Prophylactic Paracetamol Administration at Time of Vaccination on Febrile Reactions and Antibody Responses in Children: Two Open-Label, Randomised Controlled Trials," Lancet, 2009, 374(9698):1339-50.

Papillomavirus (Types 16, 18) Vaccine (Human, Recombinant)

(pap ih LO ma VYE rus typs SIX teen AYE teen vak SEEN YU man ree KOM be nant)

Medication Safety Issues

Sound-alike/look-alike issues:

Papillomavirus vaccine types 16, 18 (Cervarix®) may be confused with Papillomavirus vaccine types 6, 11, 16, 18 (Gardasil®)

Cervarix® may be confused with Cerebyx®, Celebrex®

Related Information

Immunization Guidelines on page 1636

U.S. Brand Names Cervarix®

Canadian Brand Names Cervarix®

Therapeutic Category Vaccine, Inactivated (Viral)

Generic Available No

Use

Prevention of cervical cancer and cervical intraepithelial neoplasia with or without cervical adenocarcinoma in situ caused by Human Papillomavirus (HPV) types 16 and 18 (FDA approved in girls ≥10 years and women ≤25 years of age)

The Advisory Committee on Immunization Practices (ACIP) recommends routine vaccination for females 11-12 years of age; catch-up vaccination is recommended for females 13-25 years of age

Pregnancy Risk Factor B

Pregnancy Considerations Adverse events were not observed in animal reproduction studies. In clinical trials, pregnancy testing was conducted prior to each vaccine administration and vaccination was discontinued if the woman was found to be pregnant; women were also instructed to avoid pregnancy for 2 months after receiving the vaccine. Pregnancies detected within 30 days prior or 45 days after vaccination had a higher rate of spontaneous abortions. A registry has been established for women exposed to the HPV vaccine during pregnancy (888-452-9622).

Lactation Excretion in breast milk unknown/use caution

Contraindications Hypersensitivity to human papillomavirus vaccine or any component

Warnings Administration of HPV vaccine during pregnancy is not recommended. Pregnancies detected within 30 days prior or 45 days after vaccination had a higher rate of spontaneous abortions and abnormal infant (other than congenital anomaly) births; causality with HPV vaccine has not been established. A registry has been established for women exposed to the HPV vaccine during pregnancy (1-888-452-9622).

Avoid use of prefilled syringes in latex hypersensitive patients; tip cap and plunger contain latex and may cause an allergic reaction to occur. The single dose vial stopper does not contain latex.

Immediate treatment for anaphylactic reactions should be available during vaccine use. There is no evidence that individuals already infected with HPV will be protected; those already infected with one or more HPV types were protected from disease in the remaining HPV types. Not for the treatment of active disease; does not protect against diseases caused by nonvaccine HPV types. Consider deferring vaccination for patients with serious illness. May vaccinate patients with mild concurrent febrile illness. Syncope may occur following vaccination and is sometimes associated with tonic-clonic movements or other seizure-like activity; observe patients for 15 minutes after administration.

Precautions Use with caution in patients with bleeding disorders such as hemophilia or thrombocytopenia or patients on anticoagulant therapy, due to an increased risk for bleeding following I.M. administration. Use with caution in immunocompromised patients including those receiving chemotherapy, radiation, or high dose steroids, as they may have decreased response to the vaccine. Routine prophylactic administration of acetaminophen to prevent fever due to vaccines has been shown to decrease the immune response of some vaccines; the clinical significance of this reduction in immune response has not been established (see Prymula, 2009).

Adverse Reactions All serious adverse reactions must be reported to the U.S. Department of Health and Human Services (DHHS) Vaccine Adverse Event Reporting System (VAERS) 1-800-822-7967.

Cardiovascular: Syncope (see Warnings)

Central nervous system: Fatigue, syncope (may be associated with tonic-clonic movements)

Dermatologic: Urticaria

Local: Injection site pain, pruritus, redness, swelling

Neuromuscular & skeletal: Arthralgia, myalgia

Respiratory: Nasopharyngitis, pharyngitis, pharyngolaryngeal pain, upper respiratory tract infection

Miscellaneous: Chlamydia infection, influenza, vaginal infection

<1%, postmarketing, and/or case reports: Allergic reactions, anaphylactic/anaphylactoid reactions, angioedema, erythema multiforme

Drug Interactions

Avoid Concomitant Use There are no known interactions where it is recommended to avoid concomitant use.

Increased Effect/Toxicity There are no known significant interactions involving an increase in effect.

Decreased Effect

The levels/effects of Papillomavirus (Types 16, 18) Vaccine (Human, Recombinant) may be decreased by: Immunosuppressants

Stability Store under refrigeration at 2°C to 8°C (36°F to 46°F); do not freeze; discard if frozen. May develop a fine, white deposit with a clear, colorless supernatant during storage (not a sign of deterioration).

Mechanism of Action Promotes immunity to human HPV types 16 and 18 by inducing the production of IgG neutralizing antibodies to the virus types

Pharmacodynamics

Onset of action: Peak seroconversion was observed 1 month following the last dose of vaccine

Duration: Not well defined; >5 years

Usual Dosage I.M.: 0.5 mL

Female: Preadolescents ≥10 years, Adolescents, and Adults ≤25 years: Initial dose: 0.5 mL followed by a second dose 1 month after first dose; third dose 6 months after first dose (immunization with HPV vaccine is usually initiated at 11-12 years; optimally, vaccination should be completed prior to onset of sexual activity)

Note: Minimum interval between the first and second dose of vaccine is 4 weeks; minimum interval between the second and third dose of vaccine is 12 weeks; minimum interval between first and third dose of the vaccine is 24 weeks. If the vaccine series is interrupted and only one dose was given, administer the second dose as soon as possible and give the third dose ≥12 weeks later. If the vaccine series is interrupted and the first two doses were given, administer the third dose as soon as possible. If the dose is given in an interval shorter than recommended, the dose should be repeated. The HPV vaccine series should be completed with the same product whenever possible.

Papillomavirus (Types 16, 18) Recombinant vaccine with other inactivated vaccines: May be given simultaneously or at any interval between doses

Papillomavirus (Types 16, 18) Recombinant vaccine with live vaccines: May be given simultaneously or at any interval between doses

Vaccine administration with antibody-containing products: Papillomavirus (Types 16, 18) Recombinant vaccine may be given simultaneously at different sites or at any interval between doses. Examples of antibody-containing products include I.M. and I.V. immune globulin, hepatitis B immune globulin, tetanus immune globulin, varicella zoster immune globulin, rabies immune globulin, whole blood, packed red cells, plasma, and platelet products.

Administration I.M.: Shake suspension well prior to use; do not use suspension if it is discolored or contains particulate matter; should be a homogenous, turbid, white suspension. Do not dilute or mix with other vaccines. Administer I.M. into the deltoid region of the upper arm; **not for I.V., intradermal, or SubQ administration**

Monitoring Parameters Observe patient for 15 minutes after they receive HPV vaccine for syncope. Patient should continue to be screened for cervical cancer per current guidelines after vaccination series is completed.

Patient Information This vaccine does not substitute for regular, routine cervical cancer screening; the vaccine is not intended for the treatment of active genital warts or cervical cancer. This vaccine should not be used in pregnant women. This vaccine may be given during a minor illness, such as a cold or low-grade fever. Three

◀

doses will be required for effective immunity. Inform prescriber immediately if difficulty breathing, chest pain, acute headache, rash, difficulty swallowing, or excessive pain/swelling at injection site occurs.

Nursing Implications Federal law requires that the date of administration, the vaccine manufacturer, lot number of vaccine, and the administering person's name, title and address be entered into the patient's permanent medical record. Patients who develop syncope associated with tonic-clonic movements usually respond when maintained in a supine or Trendelenburg position.

Additional Information In order to maximize vaccination rates, the ACIP recommends simultaneous administration of all age-appropriate vaccines (live or inactivated) for which a person is eligible at a single clinic visit, unless contraindications exist.

Comparison of HPV vaccines: Cervarix® and Gardasil® are both vaccines formulated to protect against infection with the human papillomavirus. Both are inactive vaccines which contain proteins HPV16 L1 and HPV 18 L1, the cause of >70% of invasive cervical cancer. The vaccines differ in that Gardasil® also contains HPV 6 L1 and HPV 11 L1 proteins which protect against 75% to 90% of genital warts. The vaccines also differ in their preparation and adjuvants used. The viral proteins in Cervarix® are prepared using *Trichoplusia ni* (insect cells) which are adsorbed onto an aluminum salt which is also combined with a monophosphoryl lipid. The viral proteins in Gardasil® are prepared using *S. cerevisiae* (baker's yeast) which are then adsorbed onto an aluminum salt. Results from a short-term study (measurements obtained 1 month following the third vaccination in the series) have shown that the immune response to HPV 16 and HPV 18 may be greater with Cervarix®; although the clinical significance of these differences is not known, local adverse events may also occur more frequently with this preparation. Both vaccines are effective and results from long-term studies are pending.

In order to maximize vaccination rates, the ACIP recommends simultaneous administration of all age-appropriate vaccines (live or inactivated) for which a person is eligible at a single visit, unless contraindications exist. The use of combination vaccines is generally preferred over separate infections, taking into consideration provider assessment, patient preference, and potential adverse events.

For additional information, please refer to the following website: http://www.cdc.gov/vaccines/vpd-vac/.

Dosage Forms Excipient information presented when available (limited, particularly for generics); consult specific product labeling.

Injection, suspension [preservative free]:
Cervarix®: HPV 16 L1 protein 20 mcg, and HPV 18 L1 protein 20 mcg per 0.5 mL (0.5 mL) [contains aluminum; packaging may contain natural latex rubber; manufactured using *Trichoplusia ni* (insect cells)]

References

Advisory Committee On Immunization Practices, "Vaccines for Children Program, Vaccines to Prevent Human Papillomavirus (HPV) Infection," October 2009. Available at http://www.cdc.gov/vaccines/programs/vfc/downloads/resolutions/1009hpv-508.pdf.

American Academy of Pediatrics Committee on Infectious Diseases, "Recommended Childhood and Adolescent Immunization Schedules – United States, 2009," *Pediatrics*, 2009, 123(1):189-90.

Centers for Disease Control and Prevention (CDC), "General Recommendations on Immunization. Recommendations of the Advisory Committee on Immunization Practices (ACIP)," *MMWR Recomm Rep*, 2006, 55(RR-15):1-48. Available at: http://www.cdc.gov/mmwr/preview/mmwrhtml/rr5515a1.htm.

◆ **Papillomavirus Vaccine, Recombinant** *see* Papillomavirus (Types 6, 11, 16, 18) Recombinant Vaccine *on page 1057*

◆ **Papillomavirus Vaccine, Recombinant** *see* Papillomavirus (Types 16, 18) Vaccine (Human, Recombinant) *on page 1058*

◆ **Paracetamol** *see* Acetaminophen *on page 36*

◆ **Parafon Forte® (Can)** *see* Chlorzoxazone *on page 300*

◆ **Parafon Forte® DSC** *see* Chlorzoxazone *on page 300*

◆ **Paraplatin-AQ (Can)** *see* CARBOplatin *on page 250*

◆ **Para-Time SR® [DSC]** *see* Papaverine *on page 1056*

◆ **Parcaine™** *see* Proparacaine *on page 1168*

Paregoric (par e GOR ik)

Medication Safety Issues
Sound-alike/look-alike issues:
Camphorated tincture of opium is an error-prone synonym (mistaken as opium tincture)
Paregoric may be confused with Percogesic®

High alert medication: The Institute for Safe Medication Practices (ISMP) includes this medication among its list of drug classes which have a heightened risk of causing significant patient harm when used in error.

Use care when prescribing opium tincture; each mL contains the equivalent of morphine 10 mg; paregoric contains the equivalent of morphine 0.4 mg/mL.

Therapeutic Category Analgesic, Narcotic; Antidiarrheal

Generic Available Yes

Use Treatment of diarrhea or relief of pain; neonatal abstinence syndrome (neonatal opiate withdrawal)

Restrictions C-III

Pregnancy Risk Factor B/D (prolonged use or high doses)

Lactation Enters breast milk/use caution

Breast-Feeding Considerations Information regarding use while breast-feeding is based on experience with morphine. Probably safe with low doses and by administering dose after breast-feeding to further minimize exposure to the drug. Monitor the infant for possible side effects related to opiates.

Contraindications Hypersensitivity to opium or any component (see Warnings and Additional Information); diarrhea caused by poisoning until the toxic material has been removed

Warnings Abrupt discontinuation after prolonged use may result in symptoms of withdrawal. Do **not** confuse this product (paregoric) with opium tincture which is 25 times **more** potent. Each 5 mL of paregoric contains 2 mg morphine equivalent, 0.02 mL anise oil, 20 mg benzoic acid, 20 mg camphor, 0.2 mL glycerin and alcohol; final alcohol content 45%; paregoric also contains papaverine and noscapine; because all of these additives may be harmful to neonates, **a 25-fold dilution of opium tincture** is often preferred for treatment of neonatal abstinence syndrome (opiate withdrawal); see Opium Tincture on page 1024. Some centers prefer to use morphine oral solution.

Paregoric contains benzoic acid; benzoic acid (benzoate) is a metabolite of benzyl alcohol; large amounts of benzyl alcohol (≥99 mg/kg/day) have been associated with a potentially fatal toxicity ("gasping syndrome") in neonates; the "gasping syndrome" consists of metabolic acidosis, respiratory distress, gasping respirations, CNS dysfunction (including convulsions, intracranial hemorrhage), hypotension and cardiovascular collapse; use paregoric products containing benzoic acid with caution in neonates; *in vitro* and animal studies have shown that benzoate displaces bilirubin from protein binding sites

Precautions Use with caution in patients with respiratory, hepatic or renal dysfunction, severe prostatic hypertrophy, or history of narcotic abuse; opium shares the toxic potential of opiate agonists, usual precautions of opiate agonist therapy should be observed; infants <3 months of age are more susceptible to respiratory depression, use with caution and in reduced doses in this age group

Adverse Reactions

Cardiovascular: Hypotension, bradycardia, vasodilation

Central nervous system: CNS depression, intracranial pressure elevated, drowsiness, dizziness, sedation

Endocrine & metabolic: Antidiuretic hormone release

Gastrointestinal: Nausea, vomiting, constipation, biliary tract spasm

Genitourinary: Urinary tract spasm, urinary retention

Ocular: Miosis

Respiratory: Respiratory depression

Miscellaneous: Physical and psychological dependence, histamine release

Drug Interactions

Avoid Concomitant Use There are no known interactions where it is recommended to avoid concomitant use.

Increased Effect/Toxicity

Paregoric may increase the levels/effects of: Alcohol (Ethyl); Alvimopan; CNS Depressants; Desmopressin; Selective Serotonin Reuptake Inhibitors; Thiazide Diuretics

The levels/effects of Paregoric may be increased by: Amphetamines; Antipsychotic Agents (Phenothiazines); Succinylcholine

Decreased Effect

Paregoric may decrease the levels/effects of: Pegvisomant

The levels/effects of Paregoric may be decreased by: Ammonium Chloride; Mixed Agonist / Antagonist Opioids

Stability Store in light-resistant, tightly closed container; protect from freezing

Mechanism of Action Increases smooth muscle tone in GI tract, decreases motility and peristalsis, diminishes digestive secretions

Pharmacokinetics (Adult data unless noted)

Metabolism: Opium is metabolized in the liver

Elimination: In urine, primarily as morphine glucuronide conjugates and as parent compound (morphine, codeine, papaverine, etc)

Usual Dosage Oral:

Neonates (full term): **Note:** Due to potential adverse effects from the additives in paregoric, other agents are preferred for treatment of neonatal abstinence syndrome (see Warnings): Neonatal abstinence syndrome (opiate withdrawal): Initial: 0.1 mL/kg or 2 drops/kg with feedings every 3-4 hours; increase dosage by 0.1 mL/kg or 2 drops/kg every 3-4 hours until withdrawal symptoms are controlled; it is rare to exceed 0.7 mL/dose. Stabilize withdrawal symptoms for 3-5 days, then gradually decrease the dosage (keeping the same dosing interval) over a 2- to 4-week period.

Children: 0.25-0.5 mL/kg 1-4 times/day

Adults: 5-10 mL 1-4 times/day

Administration Oral: May administer with food to decrease GI upset; shake well before use

Monitoring Parameters Respiratory rate, blood pressure, heart rate, level of sedation; neonatal abstinence syndrome (opiate withdrawal): Monitor for resolution of withdrawal symptoms (such as irritability, high-pitched cry, stuffy nose, rhinorrhea, vomiting, poor feeding, diarrhea, sneezing, yawning, etc) and signs of over treatment (such as bradycardia, lethargy, hypotonia, irregular respiration, respiratory depression, etc); an abstinence scoring system (eg, Finnegan abstinence scoring system) can be used to more objectively assess neonatal opiate withdrawal symptoms and the need for dosage adjustment

Patient Information Avoid alcohol; may cause drowsiness and impair ability to perform activities requiring mental alertness or physical coordination; may be habit-forming; avoid abrupt discontinuation after prolonged use

Dosage Forms Excipient information presented when available (limited, particularly for generics); consult specific product labeling.

Liquid, oral: Morphine equivalent 2 mg/5 mL (473 mL) [equivalent to opium 20 mg powder; contains ethanol ≤47.7% and benzoic acid]

References

Kraus DM and Pham JT, "Neonatal Therapy," *Applied Therapeutics: The Clinical Use of Drugs*, 9th ed, Koda-Kimble MA, Young LY, Kradjan WA, et al, eds, Baltimore, MD: Lippincott Williams & Wilkins, 2009.

Levy M and Spino M, "Neonatal Withdrawal Syndrome: Associated Drugs and Pharmacologic Management," *Pharmacotherapy*, 1993, 13 (3):202-11.

"Neonatal Drug Withdrawal. American Academy of Pediatrics Committee on Drugs," *Pediatrics*, 1998, 101(6):1079-88.

Paricalcitol (pah ri KAL si tole)

Medication Safety Issues

Sound alike/look alike issues:

Paricalcitol may be confused with calcitriol

U.S. Brand Names Zemplar®

Canadian Brand Names Zemplar®

Therapeutic Category Vitamin D Analog; Vitamin, Fat Soluble

Generic Available No

Use

I.V.: Prevention and treatment of secondary hyperparathyroidism associated with stage 5 chronic kidney disease (CKD) (FDA approved in children ≥5 years and adults)

Oral: Prevention and treatment of secondary hyperparathyroidism associated with stages 3 and 4 chronic kidney disease (CKD) and stage 5 CKD patients on hemodialysis or peritoneal dialysis (FDA approved in adults)

Pregnancy Risk Factor C

Pregnancy Considerations There are no adequate and well-controlled studies in pregnant women; use during pregnancy only if potential benefit to mother outweighs possible risk to fetus.

Lactation Excretion in breast milk unknown/not recommended

Contraindications Hypersensitivity to paricalcitol or any component; vitamin D toxicity; hypercalcemia

Warnings Excessive administration may lead to over suppression of PTH, hypercalcemia, hypercalciuria, hyperphosphatemia, and adynamic bone disease. Acute hypercalcemia may increase risk of cardiac arrhythmias and seizures. Chronic hypercalcemia may lead to generalized vascular and other soft-tissue calcification. Phosphate and vitamin D (and its derivatives) should be withheld during therapy to avoid hypercalcemia. Not indicated for use in patients with rapidly worsening kidney function or those who are noncompliant with medications or follow-up (K/DOQI Guidelines, 2003).

Precautions Hypercalcemia potentiates digoxin toxicity; use concomitantly with caution

Adverse Reactions

Cardiovascular: Arrhythmias, cardiomyopathy, chest pain, CHF, edema, hypertension, hypotension, palpitation, MI, postural hypotension, syncope

Central nervous system: Anxiety, chills, depression, dizziness, fever, headache, insomnia, lightheadedness, vertigo

Dermatologic: Bruising, facial edema, pruritus, rash, skin hypertrophy, skin ulcer, urticaria

Endocrine & metabolic: Acidosis, dehydration, hypoglycemia, hypokalemia

Gastrointestinal: Abdominal pain, constipation, diarrhea, dyspepsia, gastritis, gastroenteritis, GI bleeding, nausea (6% to 13%), peritonitis, vomiting, xerostomia

Genitourinary: Urinary tract infection

Neuromuscular & skeletal: Arthritis, back pain, leg cramps, neuropathy, weakness

Ocular: Amblyopia, retinal disorder

Respiratory: Bronchitis, cough, epistaxis, pneumonia, rhinitis, sinusitis

Miscellaneous: Allergic reaction, flu-like syndrome, infection (bacterial, fungal, viral); sepsis

<1% and/or postmarketing: Anorexia, arrhythmias, AST/ALT elevation, BUN elevation, conjunctivitis (calcific), ectopic calcification, hypercholesterolemia, hyperthermia, pancreatitis, photophobia, psychosis (rare), rhinorrhea, somnolence, taste perversion (metallic), weight loss

Drug Interactions

Metabolism/Transport Effects

Substrate of CYP3A4 (major)

Avoid Concomitant Use There are no known interactions where it is recommended to avoid concomitant use.

Increased Effect/Toxicity

The levels/effects of Paricalcitol may be increased by: CYP3A4 Inhibitors (Strong)

Decreased Effect There are no known significant interactions involving a decrease in effect.

Stability Store at room temperature.

Mechanism of Action Paricalcitol is a synthetic analog of cacitriol (1,25-hydroxy vitamin D_3) which binds to and activates the vitamin D receptor in kidney, parathyroid gland, intestine, and bone, thus reducing PTH levels and improving calcium and phosphate homeostasis. Decreased renal conversion of vitamin D to its primary active metabolite (1,25-hydroxyvitamin D) in chronic renal failure leads to reduced activation of vitamin D receptor, which subsequently removes inhibitory suppression of parathyroid hormone (PTH) release; increased serum PTH (secondary hyperparathyroidism) reduces calcium excretion and enhances bone resorption. Paricalcitol appears to have less effects on serum calcium and/or phosphorus levels than calcitriol.

Pharmacokinetics (Adult data unless noted)

Distribution: V_d:

Healthy subjects: Oral: 34 L; I.V.: 24 L

Stage 3 and 4 CKD: Oral: 44-46 L

Stage 5 CKD: I.V.: 31-35 L

Protein binding: >99%

Metabolism: Hydroxylation and glucuronidation via hepatic and nonhepatic enzymes, including CYP24, CYP3A4, UGT1A4; forms metabolites (at least one active)

Bioavailability: Oral: ~72% in healthy subjects

Time to peak serum concentration: Oral: 3 hours

Half-life: Adults:

Healthy subjects: Oral: 4-6 hours; I.V.: 5-7 hours

Stage 3 and 4 CKD: Oral: 17-20 hours

Stage 5 CKD: I.V.: 14-15 hours

Elimination: Healthy subjects: Feces (Oral: 70%; I.V.: 63%); urine (Oral: 18%, I.V.: 19%); 51% to 59% as metabolites

Usual Dosage In stage 3-5 CKD maintain Ca x P <55 mg²/dL² (adults and children >12 years) or <65 mg²/dL² (children <12 years), reduce or interrupt dosing if recommended Ca x P is exceeded or hypercalcemia is observed (K/DOQI Clinical Practice Guidelines, 2005).

Secondary hyperparathyroidism associated with chronic renal failure (stage 5 CKD): Children ≥5 years (limited small studies) and Adults: I.V.: 0.04-0.1 mcg/kg no more frequently than every other day; dose may be increased by 2-4 mcg every 2-4 weeks (0.04-0.1 mcg/kg for children); doses as high as 0.24 mcg/kg (16.8 mcg) have been administered safely; children may require higher weight-based doses; 0.2 ± 0.7 mcg/kg/dose (Seeherunvong, 2006); the dose of paricalcitol should be adjusted based on serum intact parathyroid hormone (iPTH) levels, as follows:

Same or increasing iPTH level: Increase paricalcitol dose

iPTH level decreased by <30%: Increase paricalcitol dose

iPTH level decreased by >30% and <60%: Maintain paricalcitol dose

iPTH level decrease by >60%: Decrease paricalcitol dose

iPTH level 1.5-3 times upper limit of normal: Maintain paricalcitol dose

Adults: Oral: Initial dose, in mcg, based on baseline iPTH level divided by 80. Administer 3 times weekly; no more frequently than every other day. **Note:** To reduce the risk of hypercalcemia initiate only after baseline serum calcium has been adjusted to ≤9.5 mg/dL.

Dose titration: Titration dose (mcg) = most recent iPTH level (pg/ml) divided by 80

Dosage adjustment for hypercalcemia or elevated Ca x P: Decrease calculated dose by 2-4 mcg. If further adjustment is required, dose should be reduced or interrupted until these parameters are normalized. If applicable, phosphate binder dosing may also be adjusted or withheld, or switch to a noncalcium-based phosphate binder

Secondary hyperparathyroidism associated with stage 3 and 4 CKD: Adults: Oral: Initial dose based on baseline serum iPTH:

iPTH ≤500 pg/mL: 1 mcg/day or 2 mcg 3 times/week*

iPTH >500 pg/mL: 2 mcg/day or 4 mcg 3 times/week*

*Do not administer 3 times/week regimen more frequently than every other day

Dosage adjustment based on iPTH level relative to baseline, adjust dose at 2-4 week intervals:

iPTH same or increased: Increase paricalcitol dose by 1 mcg/day or 2 mcg 3 times/week

iPTH decreased by <30%: Increase paricalcitol dose by 1 mcg/day or 2 mcg 3 times/week

iPTH decreased by ≥30% or ≤60%: Maintain paricalcitol dose

iPTH decreased by >60%: Decrease paricalcitol dose by 1 mcg/day* or 2 mcg 3 times/week

iPTH <60 pg/mL: Decrease paricalcitol dose by 1 mcg/day* or 2 mcg 3 times/week

*If patient is taking the lowest dose on an every other day regimen, but further dose reduction is needed, decrease dose to 1 mcg 3 times/week. If further dose reduction is required, withhold drug as needed and restart at a lower dose. If applicable, calcium-phosphate binder dosing may also be adjusted or withheld, or switch to noncalcium-based binder.

Dosage adjustment in hepatic impairment: Adjustment not needed for mild-to-moderate impairment. Paricalcitol has not been evaluated in severe hepatic impairment.

Administration Oral: May be administered with or without food. With the 3 times/week dosing schedule, doses should not be given more frequently than every other day.

Parenteral: Administer undiluted as an I.V. bolus dose at anytime during dialysis. Doses should not be administered more often than every other day.

Monitoring Parameters Signs and symptoms of vitamin D intoxication

Serum calcium and phosphorus (closely monitor levels during dosage titration and after initiation of a strong CYP3A4 inhibitor):

I.V.: Twice weekly during initial phase, then at least monthly once dose established

Oral: At least every 2 weeks for 3 months or following dose adjustment, then monthly for 3 months, then every 3 months

Calcium phosphorus product (Ca x P): Maintain Ca x P <55 mg^2/dL^2 (adults and children >12 years) or <65 mg^2/dL^2 (children <12 years) in stage 3-5 CKD

Serum or plasma intact parathyroid hormone (iPTH): At least every 2 weeks for 3 months or following dose adjustment, then monthly for 3 months, then as per K/DOQI Guidelines below

Per Kidney Disease Outcome Quality Initiative Practice Guidelines - Children (K/DOQI, 2005):

Stage 3 CKD: iPTH every 6 months

Stage 4 CKD: iPTH every 3 months

Stage 5 CKD: iPTH every 3 months

Per Kidney Disease Outcome Quality Initiative Practice Guidelines - Adults (K/DOQI, 2003):

Stage 3 CKD: iPTH every 12 months

Stage 4 CKD: iPTH every 3 months

Stage 5 CKD: iPTH every 3 months

Reference Range Chronic kidney disease (CKD) is defined either as kidney damage or GFR <60 mL/minute/1.73 m^2 for ≥3 months); stages of CKD are described below:

CKD Stage 1: Kidney damage with normal or increased GFR; GFR ≥90 mL/minute/1.73 m^2

CKD Stage 2: Kidney damage with mild decrease in GFR; GFR 60-89 mL/minute/1.73 m^2

CKD Stage 3: Moderate decrease in GFR; GFR 30-59 mL/minute/1.73 m^2

CKD Stage 4: Severe decrease in GFR; GFR 15-29 mL/minute/1.73 m^2

CKD Stage 5: Kidney failure; GFR <15 mL/minute/1.73 m^2 or dialysis

Target range for iPTH:

Stage 2 CKD: Children: 35-70 pg/mL (3.85-7.7 pmol/L)

Children and Adults:

Stage 3 CKD: Children and Adults: 35-70 pg/mL (3.85-7.7 pmol/L)

Stage 4 CKD: Children and Adults: 70-110 pg/mL (7.7-12.1 pmol/L)

Stage 5 CKD:

Children: 200-300 pg/mL (22-33 pmol/L)

Adults: 150-300 pg/mL (16.5-33 pmol/L)

Serum phosphorous:

Stages 1-4 CKD: Children: At or above the age-appropriate lower limits and no higher than age-appropriate upper limits

Stage 3 and 4 CKD: Adults: ≥2.7 to <4.6 mg/dL (≥0.87 to <1.49 mmol/L)

Stage 5 CKD:

Children 1-12 years: 4-6 mg/dL (1.29-1.94 mmol/L)

Children >12 years and Adults: 3.5-5.5 mg/dL (1.13-1.78 mmol/L)

Patient Information Take as directed; do not increase dosage without consulting prescriber. Adhere to diet as recommended (do not take any other phosphate or vitamin D related compounds while taking paricalcitol). You may experience nausea, vomiting, dry mouth (small frequent meals, frequent mouth care, chewing gums, or sucking lozenges may help); swelling of extremities (elevate feet when sitting); or lightheadedness or dizziness (use caution when driving or engaging in tasks requiring alertness until response to drug is known). Report persistent fever, gastric disturbances, abdominal pain or blood in stool, chest pain or palpitations, bone pain, irritability, muscular twitching, weakness, or signs of respiratory infection or flu.

Dosage Forms Excipient information presented when available (limited, particularly for generics); consult specific product labeling.

Capsule, gelatin: 1 mcg, 2 mcg, 4 mcg [contains alcohol and coconut or palm kernel oil]

Injection, solution: 2 mcg/mL (1 mL); 5 mcg/mL (1 mL, 2 mL) [contains alcohol 20% v/v and propylene glycol 30% v/v]

References

Greenbaum LA, Benador N, Goldstein SL, et al, "Intravenous Paricalcitol for Treatment of Secondary Hyperparathyroidism in Children on Hemodialysis," *Am J Kidney Dis*, 2007, 49(6):814-23.

"K/DOQI Clinical Practice Guidelines for Bone Metabolism and Disease in Children With Chronic Kidney Disease," *Am J Kidney Dis*, 2005, 46 (4 Suppl 1):S1-121.

"K/DOQI Clinical Practice Guidelines for Bone Metabolism and Disease in Chronic Kidney Disease. Guideline 1. Evaluation of Calcium and Phosphorus Metabolism," *Am J Kidney Dis*, 2003, 42(4 Suppl 3):52-7.

"K/DOQI Clinical Practice Guidelines for Bone Metabolism and Disease in Chronic Kidney Disease. Guideline 3. Evaluation of Serum Phosphorus Levels," *Am J Kidney Dis* , 2003, 42(4 Suppl 3):62-3.

"K/DOQI Clinical Practice Guidelines for Chronic Kidney Disease: Evaluation, Classification, and Stratification, Part 4. Definition and Classification of Stages of Chronic Kidney Disease," *Am J Kidney Dis*, 2002, 39(2 Suppl 1):46-75.

Sanchez CP, "Secondary Hyperparathyroidism in Children With Chronic Renal Failure: Pathogenesis and Treatment," *Paediatr Drugs*, 2003, 5 (11): 763-76.

Seeherunvong W, Nwobi, O, Abitbol CL, et al, "Paricalcitol Versus Calcitriol Treatment for Hyperparathyroidism in Pediatric Hemodialysis Patients," *Pediatr Nephrol*, 2006, 21(10):1434-9.

Ziolkowska H, "Minimizing Bone Abnormalities in Children With Renal Failure," *Paediatr Drugs*, 2006, 8(4):205-22.

♦ **Pariet® (Can)** see Rabeprazole *on page 1197*

♦ **Pariprazole** see Rabeprazole *on page 1197*

♦ **Parlodel®** see Bromocriptine *on page 203*

♦ **Parlodel® SnapTabs®** see Bromocriptine *on page 203*

Paromomycin (par oh moe MYE sin)

U.S. Brand Names Humatin® [DSC]

Canadian Brand Names Humatin®

Therapeutic Category Amebicide

Generic Available Yes

Use Treatment of acute and chronic intestinal amebiasis due to susceptible *Entamoeba histolytica* (not effective in the treatment of extraintestinal amebiasis); tapeworm infestations; adjunctive management of hepatic coma; treatment of cryptosporidial diarrhea

Pregnancy Considerations Paromomycin is poorly absorbed when given orally. Because it does not reach the maternal serum, it would not be expected to adversely affect the fetus. No adverse effects were observed in two infants whose mothers took paromomycin during pregnancy.

Breast-Feeding Considerations Paromomycin is poorly absorbed when given orally. Because it does not reach the maternal serum, it would not be expected to distribute into human milk.

Contraindications Hypersensitivity to paromomycin or any component; intestinal obstruction

Warnings May result in overgrowth of nonsusceptible organisms

Precautions Use with caution in patients with impaired GI motility or possible or proven ulcerative bowel lesions; use with caution in patients with impaired renal function

Adverse Reactions

Central nervous system: Headache, vertigo

Dermatologic: Exanthema, rash, pruritus

Endocrine & metabolic: Hypocholesterolemia

Gastrointestinal: Diarrhea, abdominal cramps, nausea, vomiting, anorexia, steatorrhea, secondary enterocolitis, pancreatitis

Hematologic: Eosinophilia

Otic: Ototoxicity

Renal: Hematuria

Drug Interactions

Avoid Concomitant Use There are no known interactions where it is recommended to avoid concomitant use.

Increased Effect/Toxicity There are no known significant interactions involving an increase in effect.

Decreased Effect There are no known significant interactions involving a decrease in effect.

Food Interactions Paromomycin may cause malabsorption of xylose, sucrose, and fats

Mechanism of Action Acts directly on ameba in the intestinal lumen; interferes with bacterial protein synthesis by binding to 30S ribosomal subunit of susceptible bacteria

Pharmacokinetics (Adult data unless noted)

Absorption: Poor from the GI tract

Elimination: Excreted unchanged in feces; portion of oral dose that may be absorbed is excreted in urine

Usual Dosage Oral:

Children:

Intestinal amebiasis (*Entamoeba histolytica*): 25-35 mg/kg/day divided every 8 hours for 7 days

Dientamoeba fragilis infection: 25-30 mg/kg/day divided every 8 hours for 7 days

Tapeworm:

T. saginata, T. solium, D. latum: 11 mg/kg/dose every 15 minutes for 4 doses

H. nana: 45 mg/kg/day once daily for 5-7 days

Adults:

Intestinal amebiasis (*Entamoeba histolytica*): 25-35 mg/kg/day divided every 8 hours for 7 days

Dientamoeba fragilis infection: 25-30 mg/kg/day divided every 8 hours for 7 days

Tapeworm:

T. saginata, T. solium, D. latum: 1 g every 15 minutes for 4 doses

H. nana: 45 mg/kg/day once daily for 5-7 days

Hepatic coma: 4 g/day in 2-4 divided doses for 5-6 days

Cryptosporidial diarrhea: 1.5-2 g/day in 3-4 divided doses for 10-14 days

Administration Oral: Administer with or after meals

Monitoring Parameters Periodic urinalysis and renal function tests; be alert to ototoxicity

Patient Information Notify physician if ringing in ears, hearing loss, or dizziness occurs

Additional Information With the treatment of cestodiasis caused by *T. solium*, paromomycin may cause disintegration of worm segments and release of viable eggs resulting in an increased risk for the development of cysticercosis

Dosage Forms Excipient information presented when available (limited, particularly for generics); consult specific product labeling. [DSC] = Discontinued product

Capsule: 250 mg

Humatin®: 250 mg [DSC]

References

Danziger LH, Kanyok TP, and Novak RM, "Treatment of Cryptosporidial Diarrhea in an AIDS Patient With Paromomycin," *Ann Pharmacother*, 1993, 27(12):1460-2.

Liu LX and Weller PF, "Antiparasitic Drugs," *N Engl J Med*, 1996, 334 (18):1178-84.

◆ **Paromomycin Sulfate** *see* Paromomycin *on page 1063*

PARoxetine (pa ROKS e teen)

Medication Safety Issues

Sound-alike/look-alike issues:

PARoxetine may be confused with FLUoxetine, paclitaxel, pyridoxine

Paxil® may be confused with Doxil®, paclitaxel, Plavix®, Prozac®, Taxol®

Related Information

Antidepressant Agents *on page 1484*

Serotonin Syndrome *on page 1695*

U.S. Brand Names Paxil CR®; Paxil®; Pexeva®

Canadian Brand Names Apo-Paroxetine®; CO Paroxetine; Dom-Paroxetine; Mylan-Paroxetine; Novo-Paroxetine; Paxil CR®; Paxil®; PHL-Paroxetine; PMS-Paroxetine; ratio-Paroxetine; Riva-paroxetine; Sandoz-Paroxetine; ZYM-Paroxetine

Therapeutic Category Antidepressant, Selective Serotonin Reuptake Inhibitor (SSRI)

Generic Available Yes: Excludes tablet (mesylate)

Use Treatment of depression, obsessive compulsive disorder, panic disorder, social anxiety disorder, generalized anxiety disorder, and post-traumatic stress disorder

Paxil CR®: Treatment of depression, panic disorder, social anxiety disorder, premenstrual dysphoric disorder

Pexeva®: Treatment of depression, obsessive compulsive disorder, panic disorder, generalized anxiety disorder

Medication Guide An FDA-approved patient medication guide, which is available with the product information and as follows, must be dispensed with this medication for each new outpatient prescription and refill.

Paxil CR®: http://www.fda.gov/downloads/Drugs/DrugSafety/ucm088676.pdf

Pexeva®: http://www.fda.gov/downloads/Drugs/DrugSafety/ucm088684.pdf

Pregnancy Risk Factor D

Pregnancy Considerations Due to adverse events observed in human studies, paroxetine is classified as pregnancy category D. Paroxetine crosses the placenta. The risk of cardiovascular and other congenital malformations may be higher with paroxetine than with other antidepressants. Nonteratogenic effects in the newborn following SSRI exposure late in the third trimester include respiratory distress, cyanosis, apnea, seizures, temperature instability, feeding difficulty, vomiting, hypoglycemia, hypo- or hypertonia, hyper-reflexia, jitteriness, irritability, constant crying, and tremor. An increased risk of low birth weight, lower Apgar scores, and blunted behavioral response to pain for a prolonged period after delivery has also been reported. Exposure to SSRIs after the twentieth week of gestation has been associated with persistent pulmonary hypertension of the newborn (PPHN). Adverse effects may be due to toxic effects of the SSRI or drug withdrawal due to discontinuation. The long-term effects of *in utero* SSRI exposure on infant development and behavior are not known.

Due to pregnancy-induced physiologic changes, women who are pregnant may require increased doses of paroxetine to achieve euthymia. Women treated for major depression and who are euthymic prior to pregnancy are more likely to experience a relapse when medication is discontinued as compared to pregnant women who continue taking antidepressant medications. The ACOG recommends that therapy with SSRIs or SNRIs during pregnancy be individualized; treatment of depression during pregnancy should incorporate the clinical expertise of the mental health clinician, obstetrician, primary healthcare provider, and pediatrician. The ACOG also recommends that therapy with paroxetine be avoided during pregnancy if possible and that fetuses exposed in early pregnancy be assessed with a fetal echocardiography. If treatment during pregnancy is required, consider tapering therapy during the third trimester in order to prevent withdrawal symptoms in the infant. If this is done and the woman is considered to be at risk of relapse from her major depressive disorder, the medication can be restarted following delivery, although the dose should be readjusted to that required before pregnancy. Treatment algorithms have been developed by the ACOG and the APA for the management of depression in women prior to conception and during pregnancy (Yonkers, 2009).

Lactation Enters breast milk/use caution (AAP rates "of concern")

Breast-Feeding Considerations Paroxetine is excreted in breast milk and concentrations in the hindmilk are higher than in foremilk. Paroxetine has not been detected in the serum of nursing infants and adverse events have not been reported. The AAP considers paroxetine to be a "drug for which the effect on the nursing infant is unknown but may be of concern." The manufacturer recommends that caution be exercised when administering paroxetine to nursing women.

The long-term effects on development and behavior have not been studied; therefore, one should prescribe paroxetine to a mother who is breast-feeding only when the benefits outweigh the potential risks.

Contraindications Hypersensitivity to paroxetine or any component; use of MAO inhibitors within 14 days (potentially fatal reactions may occur, see Drug Interactions); concurrent use of thioridazine or pimozide (see Drug Interactions)

Warnings Paroxetine is not approved for use in pediatric patients. Clinical worsening of depression or suicidal ideation and behavior may occur in children and adults with major depressive disorder **[U.S. Boxed Warning]**. In clinical trials, antidepressants increased the risk of suicidal thinking and behavior (suicidality) in children, adolescents, and young adults (18-24 years of age) with major depressive disorder and other psychiatric disorders. This risk must be considered before prescribing antidepressants for any clinical use. Short-term studies did **not** show an increased risk of suicidality with antidepressant use in patients >24 years of age and showed a decreased risk in patients ≥65 years of age.

Patients of all ages who are treated with antidepressants for any indication require appropriate monitoring and close observation for clinical worsening of depression, suicidality, and unusual changes in behavior, especially during the first few months after antidepressant initiation or when the dose is adjusted. Family members and caregivers should be instructed to closely observe the patient (ie, daily) and communicate condition with healthcare provider. All patients should also be monitored for associated behaviors (eg, anxiety, agitation, panic attacks, insomnia, irritability, hostility, aggressiveness, impulsivity, akathisia, hypomania, mania) which may increase the risk for worsening depression or suicidality. Worsening depression or emergence of suicidality (or associated behaviors listed above) that is abrupt in onset, severe, or not part of the presenting symptoms, may require discontinuation or modification of drug therapy.

Avoid abrupt discontinuation; discontinuation symptoms (including agitation, dysphoria, anxiety, confusion, dizziness, hypomania, nightmares, and other symptoms) may occur if therapy is abruptly discontinued or dose reduced; taper dosage gradually in patients receiving >20 mg/day to minimize risks of discontinuation symptoms; if intolerable symptoms occur following a decrease in dosage or upon discontinuation of therapy, consider resuming the previous dose with a more gradual taper. To reduce risk of intentional overdose, write prescriptions for the smallest quantity consistent with good patient care.

Screen individuals for bipolar disorder prior to treatment (using antidepressants alone may induce manic episodes in patients with this condition). Potentially fatal serotonin syndrome may occur when SSRIs are used in combination with serotonergic drugs (eg, triptans) or drugs that impair the metabolism of serotonin (eg, MAO inhibitors); see Drug Interactions.

An increased risk of birth defects (specifically cardiovascular malformations) has been reported when paroxetine was taken during the first trimester of pregnancy. The majority of heart defects were ventricular and atrial septal defects (VSD and ASD), some of which required surgical correction. Use paroxetine during pregnancy only if the potential benefits to the mother outweigh the possible risks to the fetus. Administration of paroxetine during late third trimester may result in adverse effects or paroxetine withdrawal syndrome in the newborn (consider risks and benefits; use with caution during late third trimester; see Additional Information). Exposure to SSRIs late in pregnancy may also be associated with an increased risk for persistent pulmonary hypertension of the newborn (see Chambers, 2006). Postmarketing reports of premature births in pregnant women receiving paroxetine or other SSRIs have been noted.

Precautions Use with caution in patients with a history of seizures, mania, renal disease, cardiac disease, or hepatic disease and in suicidal patients, children, or during breast-feeding in lactating women. Modify dosage in patients with renal or hepatic impairment. May cause hyponatremia, use with caution in patients with volume depletion or diuretic use. May cause abnormal bleeding (eg, ecchymosis, purpura, upper GI bleeding); use with caution in patients with impaired platelet aggregation and with concurrent use of aspirin, NSAIDs, or other drugs that affect coagulation. May cause akathisia (psychomotor restlessness), usually within the first few weeks of initiation of therapy. No clinical studies have assessed the combined use of paroxetine and electroconvulsive therapy

Adverse Reactions

Cardiovascular: Palpitations, tachycardia, vasodilation, postural hypotension, bradycardia, hypotension

Central nervous system: Headache, somnolence, dizziness, insomnia, nervousness, agitation, anxiety, migraine, impaired concentration, yawning, emotional lability, hostility, hyperkinesias, akathisia (psychomotor restlessness), hallucinations; suicidal thinking and behavior (see Warnings)

Note: SSRI-associated behavioral activation (ie, restlessness, hyperkinesis, hyperactivity, agitation) is 2- to 3-fold more prevalent in children compared to adolescents; it is more prevalent in adolescents compared to adults. Somnolence (including sedation and drowsiness) is more common in adults compared to children and adolescents (see Safer, 2006).

Dermatologic: Alopecia, purpura, ecchymosis, photosensitivity

Endocrine & metabolic: Hyponatremia (volume-depleted patients), SIADH, sexual dysfunction

Gastrointestinal: Nausea, xerostomia, constipation, vomiting, diarrhea, anorexia, flatulence, gastritis, abdominal pain

Note: SSRI-associated vomiting is 2- to 3-fold more prevalent in children compared to adolescents; it is more prevalent in adolescents compared to adults.

Hematologic: Anemia, leukopenia

Neuromuscular & skeletal: Weakness, tremor, arthritis, paresthesia, asthenia

Ocular: Eye pain, blurred vision

Otic: Ear pain

Respiratory: Asthma, rhinitis

Miscellaneous: Diaphoresis, thirst, bruxism, akinesia; withdrawal symptoms following abrupt discontinuation (see Warnings)

Drug Interactions

Metabolism/Transport Effects Substrate of CYP2D6 (major); **Inhibits** CYP1A2 (weak), 2B6 (moderate), 2C9 (weak), 2C19 (weak), 2D6 (strong), 3A4 (weak)

Avoid Concomitant Use

Avoid concomitant use of PARoxetine with any of the following: Iobenguane I 123; MAO Inhibitors; Metoclopramide; Pimozide; Sibutramine; Tamoxifen; Thioridazine

Increased Effect/Toxicity

PARoxetine may increase the levels/effects of: Alcohol (Ethyl); Alpha-/Beta-Blockers; Anticoagulants; Antidepressants (Serotonin Reuptake Inhibitor/Antagonist); Antiplatelet Agents; Aspirin; Atomoxetine; Beta-Blockers; BusPIRone; CarBAMazepine; Clozapine; CNS Depressants; Collagenase (Systemic); CYP2B6 Substrates; CYP2D6 Substrates; Desmopressin; Dextromethorphan; Drotrecogin Alfa; DULoxetine; Fesoterodine; Galantamine; Haloperidol; Ibritumomab; Lithium; Methadone; Methotrimeprazine; Mexiletine; NSAID (COX-2 Inhibitor); NSAID (Nonselective); Pimozide; Propafenone; Risperidone; Salicylates; Serotonin Modulators; Tamoxifen; Tetrabenazine; Thioridazine; Thrombolytic Agents; Tositumomab and Iodine I 131 Tositumomab; TraMADol; Tricyclic Antidepressants; Vitamin K Antagonists

The levels/effects of PARoxetine may be increased by: Analgesics (Opioid); Asenapine; BusPIRone; Cimetidine; CYP2D6 Inhibitors (Moderate); CYP2D6 Inhibitors (Strong); Dasatinib; Glucosamine; Herbs (Anticoagulant/Antiplatelet Properties); MAO Inhibitors; Methotrimeprazine; Metoclopramide; Omega-3-Acid Ethyl Esters; Pentosan Polysulfate Sodium; Pentoxifylline; Prostacyclin Analogues; Sibutramine; TraMADol; Tryptophan

Decreased Effect

PARoxetine may decrease the levels/effects of: Iobenguane I 123

The levels/effects of PARoxetine may be decreased by: CarBAMazepine; Cyproheptadine; Darunavir; Fosamprenavir; Peginterferon Alfa-2b

Food Interactions Tryptophan supplements may increase serious side effects; its use is **not recommended.**

Immediate release: Food or milk does not significantly affect extent of absorption; food may slightly increase AUC (by 6%), increase peak concentration by 29%, and decrease time to peak from 6.4 hours to 4.9 hours postdose

Controlled release: Bioavailability is not affected by food

Stability

Immediate release tablet: Hydrochloride: Store between 15°C to 30°C (59°F to 86°F); mesylate: Store at 25°C (77°F); excursions permitted to 15°C to 30°C (59°F to 86°F); protect from humidity

Oral suspension and controlled release tablet: Store ≤25°C (77°F)

Mechanism of Action Paroxetine is a selective serotonin reuptake inhibitor (SSRI), chemically unrelated to tricyclic, tetracyclic, or other antidepressants; the inhibition of serotonin reuptake from CNS neuronal synapses potentiates serotonin activity in the brain

Pharmacodynamics

Onset of action: Antidepressant effects: Within 1-4 weeks
Antiobsessional and antipanic effects: Up to several weeks

Pharmacokinetics (Adult data unless noted)

Absorption: Oral: Well absorbed

Distribution: V_d (adults): Mean: 8.7 L/kg; range: 3-28 L/kg
Protein binding: 95%

Metabolism: Extensive by cytochrome P450 enzymes via oxidation and methylation followed by glucuronide and sulfate conjugation; nonlinear kinetics may be seen with higher doses and longer duration of therapy due to saturation of P450 2D6 (CYP2D6), an enzyme partially responsible for metabolism. **Note:** Paroxetine pharmacokinetics have not been studied in patients deficient in CYP2D6 (ie, poor metabolizers)

Bioavailability: Immediate release tablet and oral suspension have equal bioavailability

Half-life: Adults: Mean: 21 hours; range: 3-65 hours
Time to peak serum concentration:
Immediate release tablet:
As hydrochloride: Mean: 5.2 hours
As mesylate: Mean: 8.1 hours
Controlled release tablet: 6-10 hours
Elimination: Metabolites are excreted in urine and bile; 2% of drug excreted unchanged in urine

Usual Dosage Oral: **Note:** For maintenance therapy, use lowest effective dose and periodically reassess need for continued treatment

Children and Adolescents: **Note:** Not FDA approved; see Warnings. Limited information is available.

Depression: The FDA recommends that paroxetine not be used in pediatric patients for the treatment of depression. Three well-controlled trials in pediatric patients with depression have failed to show therapeutic superiority over placebo; in addition, an increased risk for suicidal behavior was observed in patients receiving paroxetine when compared to other SSRIs (see Dopheide, 2006).

Obsessive-compulsive disorder (OCD): A 12-week open-label trial of paroxetine in 20 outpatients 8-17 years of age demonstrated the potential clinical usefulness in pediatric OCD; doses were initiated at 10 mg/day and could be increased every 2 weeks by no more than 10 mg/day increments, to a maximum of 60 mg/day (see Rosenberg, 1999). Efficacy of paroxetine was demonstrated in a 10-week, randomized, double-blind, placebo-controlled trial conducted in 207 pediatric patients (aged 7-17 years) with OCD; paroxetine doses were initiated at 10 mg/day and could be increased no more often than every 7 days by 10 mg/day increments, to a maximum dose of 50 mg/day; the overall mean dose was 20.3 mg/day for children and 26.8 mg/day for adolescents (see Geller, 2004). Further studies are needed.

Self-injurious behavior: A 15-year old autistic male with self-injurious behavior was successfully treated with paroxetine 20 mg/day (Snead, 1994). Further studies are needed.

Social phobia: A small case series reported the effective use of paroxetine in 5 pediatric patients with social phobia [2 children (7 and 11 years of age) and 3 adolescents (16, 17, and 18 years of age)]; comorbid diagnoses (obsessive compulsive disorder and/or dysthymia) existed in 3 patients; doses were adjusted on an individual basis; the 7-year old was started on 2.5 mg/day and increased to 5 mg/day after 4 weeks; the 11-year old was started on 5 mg/day and the dose was titrated upwards by 5 mg/day increments every 3-4 weeks to 15 mg/day; adolescents were started on ≤20 mg/day (see Mancini, 1999). A 16-week multicenter, randomized, double-blind, placebo-controlled trial reported the efficacy of paroxetine in pediatric patients (aged 8-17 years) with social anxiety disorder; 163 patients were randomized to receive paroxetine; doses were initiated at 10 mg/day and could be increased every 7 days by 10 mg/day increments, to a maximum dose of 50 mg/day; the overall mean dose was 21.7 mg/day for children and 26.1 mg/day for adolescents (see Wagner, 2004). Further studies are needed.

Adults:
Depression:
Paxil®, Pexeva®: Initial: 20 mg/day given once daily preferably in the morning; increase if needed by 10 mg/day increments at intervals of at least 1 week; maximum dose: 50 mg/day
Paxil CR®: Initial: 25 mg/day given once daily preferably in the morning; increase if needed by 12.5 mg/day increments at intervals of at least 1 week; maximum dose: 62.5 mg/day

Generalized anxiety disorder: Paxil®, Pexeva®: Initial: 20 mg/day given once daily preferably in the morning; recommended dose: 20 mg/day; range: 20-50 mg/day; doses >20 mg may not have additional benefit; if dose is increased, adjust in increments of 10 mg/day at intervals of at least 1 week

Obsessive compulsive disorder: Paxil®, Pexeva®: Initial: 20 mg/day given once daily preferably in the morning; increase by 10 mg/day increments at intervals of at least 1 week; recommended dose: 40 mg/day; range: 20-60 mg/day; maximum dose: 60 mg/day

Panic disorder:

Paxil®, Pexeva®: Initial: 10 mg/day given once daily preferably in the morning; increase by 10 mg/day increments at intervals of at least 1 week; recommended dose: 40 mg/day; range: 10-60 mg/day; maximum dose: 60 mg/day

Paxil CR®: Initial: 12.5 mg/day given once daily preferably in the morning; increase if needed by 12.5 mg/day increments at intervals of at least 1 week; maximum dose: 75 mg/day

Post-traumatic stress disorder: Paxil®: Initial: 20 mg/day given once daily preferably in the morning; recommended dose: 20 mg/day; range: 20-50 mg/day; doses of 40 mg/day have not been shown to be of greater benefit than 20 mg/day; if indicated, increase dose by 10 mg/day increments at intervals of at least 1 week

Premenstrual dysphoric disorder: Paxil CR®: Initial: 12.5 mg/day given once daily preferably in the morning; increase if needed to 25 mg/day after at least 1 week; may be given daily throughout the menstrual cycle **or** limited to the luteal phase

Social anxiety disorder:

Paxil®: Initial: 20 mg/day given once daily preferably in the morning; recommended dose: 20 mg/day; range: 20-60 mg/day; doses >20 mg may not have additional benefit

Paxil CR®: Initial: 12.5 mg/day given once daily preferably in the morning; increase if needed by 12.5 mg/day increments at intervals of at least 1 week; maximum dose: 37.5 mg/day

Dosing adjustment in severe hepatic or renal impairment: Adults:

Paxil®, Pexeva®: Initial: 10 mg/day; increase if needed by 10 mg/day increments at intervals of at least 1 week; maximum dose: 40 mg/day

Paxil CR®: Initial: 12.5 mg/day; increase if needed by 12.5 mg/day increments at intervals of at least 1 week; maximum dose: 50 mg/day

Administration May be administered without regard to meals; administration with food may decrease GI side effects; shake suspension well before use. Do not chew or crush immediate or controlled release tablet, swallow whole

Monitoring Parameters Blood pressure, heart rate, liver and renal function. Monitor patient periodically for symptom resolution; monitor for worsening depression, suicidality, and associated behaviors (especially at the beginning of therapy or when doses are increased or decreased; see Warnings)

Patient Information Read the patient Medication Guide that you receive with each prescription and refill of paroxetine. An increased risk of suicidal thinking and behavior has been reported with the use of antidepressants in children, adolescents, and young adults (18-24 years of age). Notify physician if you feel more depressed, have thoughts of suicide, or become more agitated or irritable (see Warnings). Avoid alcohol, tryptophan supplements, and the herbal medicine St John's wort; avoid aspirin, NSAIDs, or other drugs that affect coagulation (may increase risks of bleeding); may cause dizziness or drowsiness and impair ability to perform activities requiring mental alertness or physical coordination; may cause photosensitivity reactions; avoid exposure to sunlight and artificial light sources (sunlamps, tanning booth/bed); use a sunscreen; contact physician if reaction occurs; may cause dry mouth. Some medicines should not be taken with paroxetine or should not be taken for a while after paroxetine has been discontinued; report the use of other medications, nonprescription medications, and herbal or natural products to your physician and pharmacist. Take as directed; do not alter dose or frequency without consulting prescriber; avoid abrupt discontinuation.

Nursing Implications Assess other medications patient may be taking for possible interaction (especially MAO inhibitors, P450 inhibitors, and other CNS active agents). Assess mental status for depression, suicidal ideation, anxiety, social functioning, mania, or panic attack.

Additional Information Paroxetine is more potent and more selective than other SSRIs (eg, fluoxetine, fluvoxamine, sertraline, and clomipramine) in the inhibition of serotonin reuptake. If used for an extended period of time, long-term usefulness of paroxetine should be periodically re-evaluated for an individual patient. Paxil CR® tablets contain a degradable polymeric matrix (that controls the dissolution rate over ~4-5 hours) and an entering coating (that delays drug release until tablets leave the stomach). A recent report describes 5 children (age: 8-15 years) who developed epistaxis (n=4) or bruising (n=1) while receiving SSRI therapy (sertraline) (Lake, 2000). Another recent report describes the SSRI discontinuation syndrome in 6 children; the syndrome was similar to that reported in adults (see Diler, 2002).

Neonates born to women receiving SSRIs late during the third trimester may experience respiratory distress, apnea, cyanosis, temperature instability, vomiting, feeding difficulty, hypoglycemia, constant crying, irritability, hypotonia, hypertonia, hyper-reflexia, tremor, jitteriness, and seizures; these symptoms may be due to a direct toxic effect, withdrawal syndrome, or (in some cases) serotonin syndrome. Withdrawal symptoms occur in 30% of neonates exposed to SSRIs in *utero*; monitor newborns for at least 48 hours after birth; long-term effects of *in utero* exposure to SSRIs are unknown (see Levinson-Castiel, 2006).

Dosage Forms Excipient information presented when available (limited, particularly for generics); consult specific product labeling. [DSC] = Discontinued product

Note: Strength expressed as base:

Suspension, oral, as hydrochloride: 10 mg/5 mL (250 mL) [DSC]

Paxil®: 10 mg/5 mL (250 mL) [contains propylene glycol; orange flavor]

Tablet, as hydrochloride: 10 mg, 20 mg, 30 mg, 40 mg

Paxil®: 10 mg, 20 mg, 30 mg, 40 mg

Tablet, as mesylate:

Pexeva®: 10 mg, 20 mg, 30 mg, 40 mg

Tablet, controlled release, enteric coated, as hydrochloride: 37.5 mg

Paxil CR®: 12.5 mg, 25 mg, 37.5 mg

Tablet, extended release, enteric coated, as hydrochloride: 12.5 mg, 25 mg

References

Chambers CD, Hernandez-Diaz S, Van Marter LJ, et al, "Selective Serotonin-Reuptake Inhibitors and Risk of Persistent Pulmonary Hypertension of the Newborn," *N Engl J Med*, 2006, 354(6):579-87.

Diler RS and Avci A, "Selective Serotonin Reuptake Inhibitor Discontinuation Syndrome in Children: Six Case Reports," *Current Therapeutic Reseach*, 2002, 63(3):188-97.

Dopheide JA, "Recognizing and Treating Depression in Children and Adolescents," *Am J Health Syst Pharm*, 2006, 63(3):233-43.

Findling RL, Reed MD, and Blumer JL, "Pharmacological Treatment of Depression in Children and Adolescents," *Paediatr Drugs*, 1999, 1 (3):161-82.

Geller DA, Wagner KD, Emslie G, et al, "Paroxetine Treatment in Children and Adolescents With Obsessive-Compulsive Disorder: A Randomized, Multicenter, Double-Blind, Placebo-Controlled Trial," *J Am Acad Child Adolesc Psychiatry*, 2004, 43(11):1387-96.

Horrigan JP and Barnhill LJ, "Paroxetine-Pimozide Drug Interactions," *J Am Acad Child Adolesc Psychiatry*, 1994, 33(7):1060-1.

Keller MB, Ryan ND, Strober M, et al, "Efficacy of Paroxetine in the Treatment of Adolescent Major Depression: A Randomized, Controlled Trial," *J Am Acad Child Adolesc Psychiatry*, 2001, 40 (7):762-72.

Lake MB, Birmaher B, Wassick S, et al, "Bleeding and Selective Serotonin Reuptake Inhibitors in Childhood and Adolescence," *J Child Adolesc Psychopharmacol*, 2000, 10(1):35-8.

Levinson-Castiel R, Merlob P, Linder N, et al, "Neonatal Abstinence Syndrome After *in utero* Exposure to Selective Serotonin Reuptake Inhibitors in Term Infants," *Arch Pediatr Adolesc Med*, 2006, 160 (2):173-6.

Mancini C, Van Ameringen M, Oakman JM, et al, "Serotonergic Agents in the Treatment of Social Phobia in Children and Adolescents: A Case Series," *Depress Anxiety*, 1999, 10(1):33-9.

Markel H, Lee A, Holmes RD, et al, "LSD Flashback Syndrome Exacerbated by Selective Serotonin Reuptake Inhibitor Antidepressants in Adolescents," *J Pediatr*, 1994, 125(5 Pt 1):817-9.

Rey-Sanchez F and Guitierrez-Cassares JR, "Paroxetine in Children With Major Depressive Disorder: An Open Trial," *J Am Acad Child Adolesc Psychiatry*, 1997, 36(10):1443-7.

Rosenberg DR, Stewart CM, Fitzgerald KD, et al, "Paroxetine Open-Label Treatment of Pediatric Outpatients With Obsessive-Compulsive Disorder," *J Am Acad Child Adolesc Psychiatry*, 1999, 38(9):1180-5.

Safer DJ and Zito JM, "Treatment Emergent Adverse Effects of Selective Serotonin Reuptake Inhibitors by Age Group: Children vs. Adolescents," *J Child Adolesc Psychopharmacol*, 2006, 16(1/2):159-69.

Sharp SC and Hellings JA, "Efficacy and Safety of Selective Serotonin Reuptake Inhibitors in the Treatment of Depression in Children and Adolescents: Practitioner Review," *Clin Drug Investig*, 2006, 26 (5):247-55.

Snead RW, Boon F, and Presberg J, "Paroxetine for Self-Injurious Behavior," *J Am Acad Child Adolesc Psychiatry*, 1994, 33(6):909-10.

Stiskal JA, Kulin N, Koren G, et al, "Neonatal Paroxetine Withdrawal Syndrome," *Arch Dis Child Fetal Neonatal Ed*, 2001, 84(2):F134-5.

Wagner KD, Berard R, Stein MB, et al, "A Multicenter, Randomized, Double-Blind, Placebo-Controlled Trial of Paroxetine in Children and Adolescents With Social Anxiety Disorder," *Arch Gen Psychiatry*, 2004, 41(11):1153-62.

Wagner KD, "Pharmacotherapy for Major Depression in Children and Adolescents," *Prog Neuropsychopharmacol Biol Psychiatry*, 2005, 29 (5):819-26.

◆ **Paroxetine Hydrochloride** *see* PARoxetine *on page 1064*

◆ **Paroxetine Mesylate** *see* PARoxetine *on page 1064*

◆ **Parvolex® (Can)** *see* Acetylcysteine *on page 43*

◆ **Pathocil® (Can)** *see* Dicloxacillin *on page 432*

◆ **Pavabid [DSC]** *see* Papaverine *on page 1056*

◆ **Pavulon [DSC]** *see* Pancuronium *on page 1053*

◆ **Paxil®** *see* PARoxetine *on page 1064*

◆ **Paxil CR®** *see* PARoxetine *on page 1064*

◆ **PCA (error-prone abbreviation)** *see* Procainamide *on page 1156*

◆ **PCC** *see* Factor IX Complex (Human) *on page 558*

◆ **PCE®** *see* Erythromycin *on page 525*

◆ **PCEC** *see* Rabies Virus Vaccine *on page 1199*

◆ **PCV** *see* Penciclovir *on page 1076*

◆ **PCV** *see* Pneumococcal Conjugate Vaccine (7-Valent) *on page 1121*

◆ **PCV-7** *see* Pneumococcal Conjugate Vaccine (7-Valent) *on page 1121*

◆ **PCV-13** *see* Pneumococcal Conjugate Vaccine (13-Valent) *on page 1123*

◆ **PCV13-CRM(197)** *see* Pneumococcal Conjugate Vaccine (13-Valent) *on page 1123*

◆ **PediaCare® Children's Decongestant [OTC]** *see* Phenylephrine *on page 1102*

◆ **PediaCare® Children's Long-Acting Cough [OTC]** *see* Dextromethorphan *on page 421*

◆ **PediaCare® Children's Allergy [OTC]** *see* Diphenhydr-AMINE *on page 448*

◆ **PediaCare® Children's NightTime Cough [OTC]** *see* DiphenhydrAMINE *on page 448*

◆ **Pediacel® (Can)** *see* Diphtheria and Tetanus Toxoids, Acellular Pertussis, Poliovirus and *Haemophilus* b Conjugate Vaccine *on page 455*

◆ **Pediapred®** *see* PrednisoLONE *on page 1148*

◆ **Pediarix®** *see* Diphtheria, Tetanus Toxoids, Acellular Pertussis, Hepatitis B (Recombinant), and Poliovirus (Inactivated) Vaccine *on page 457*

◆ **PediaTan™** *see* Chlorpheniramine *on page 296*

◆ **Pediatex™-D [DSC]** *see* Carbinoxamine and Pseudoephedrine *on page 249*

◆ **Pediatex® TD** *see* Triprolidine and Pseudoephedrine *on page 1388*

◆ **Pediatric Digoxin CSD (Can)** *see* Digoxin *on page 437*

◆ **Pediatrix (Can)** *see* Acetaminophen *on page 36*

◆ **Pediazole® (Can)** *see* Erythromycin and Sulfisoxazole *on page 528*

◆ **Pedi-Dri®** *see* Nystatin *on page 1007*

◆ **PediOtic® [DSC]** *see* Neomycin, (Bacitracin) Polymyxin B, and Hydrocortisone *on page 980*

◆ **PedvaxHIB®** *see Haemophilus* b Conjugate Vaccine *on page 664*

◆ **PEG** *see* Polyethylene Glycol 3350 *on page 1128*

◆ **PEG-L-asparaginase** *see* Pegaspargase *on page 1068*

◆ **PEG-ASP** *see* Pegaspargase *on page 1068*

◆ **PEG-asparaginase** *see* Pegaspargase *on page 1068*

Pegaspargase (peg AS par jase)

Medication Safety Issues

Sound-alike/look-alike issues:

Oncaspar® may be confused with Elspar®

Pegaspargase may be confused with asparaginase

High alert medication: The Institute for Safe Medication Practices (ISMP) includes this medication among its list of drugs which have a heightened risk of causing significant patient harm when used in error.

Related Information

Emetogenic Potential of Antineoplastic Agents *on page 1579*

U.S. Brand Names Oncaspar®

Therapeutic Category Antineoplastic Agent, Miscellaneous

Generic Available No

Use First-line treatment of newly diagnosed acute lymphoblastic leukemia (ALL) as part of a multiple chemotherapeutic drug regimen (FDA approved in ages ≥1 year and adults); induction treatment of acute lymphoblastic leukemia in combination with other chemotherapeutic agents in patients who have developed hypersensitivity to native forms of L-asparaginase derived from *E. coli* and/or *Erwinia chrysanthemia* (FDA approved in ages ≥1 year and adults); has been used for the treatment of lymphoma and acute myelogenous leukemia (AML)

Pregnancy Risk Factor C

Pregnancy Considerations Reproduction studies have not been conducted with pegaspargase.

Lactation Excretion in breast milk unknown; since potential for serious adverse reaction in nursing infant exists, breast-feeding is not recommended

Breast-Feeding Considerations Due to the potential for serious adverse reactions in the nursing infant, breast-feeding is not recommended.

Contraindications Hypersensitivity to pegaspargase or any component; history of any of the following with prior L-asparaginase treatment: Pancreatitis, serious hemorrhagic events, serious thrombosis

Warnings Hazardous agent; use appropriate precautions for handling and disposal; inhalation of vapors and contact with skin, eyes, or mucous membranes must be avoided; be prepared to treat anaphylaxis at each administration. Risk of serious allergic reactions is higher in patients with hypersensitivity to other forms of L-asparaginase. Serious thrombotic events can occur in patients receiving pegaspargase. Pancreatitis can occur in patients receiving pegaspargase (promptly evaluate patients with abdominal pain). Discontinue pegaspargase if anaphylaxis or serious allergic reaction, thrombosis, or pancreatitis occur.

Glucose intolerance can occur in patients receiving pegaspargase. Coagulopathy with elevated prothrombin time, partial thromboplastin time, and hypofibrinogenemia can occur in patients receiving pegaspargase (monitor coagulation parameters at baseline and periodically during and after treatment). In patients with severe or symptomatic coagulopathy, treat with fresh-frozen plasma. Reversible hepatotoxicity (hyperbilirubinemia and liver enzyme elevation) may occur.

Precautions Use with caution in patients with an underlying coagulopathy or previous hematologic complication from asparaginase; patients receiving anticoagulation therapy, aspirin, or NSAIDs; use with caution in patients with hyperglycemia, diabetes, hepatic dysfunction, or in patients receiving hepatotoxic agents

Adverse Reactions

Cardiovascular: Chest pain, edema, hypotension, stroke, tachycardia

Central nervous system: CNS thrombosis, chills, coma, confusion, dizziness, fever, headache, malaise, mental status changes; seizures, somnolence

Dermatologic: Erythema, lip edema, pruritus, rash, urticaria

Endocrine & metabolic: Hyperammonemia, hyperglycemia, hyperuricemia, hypoglycemia, hypoproteinemia, thirst, transient diabetes mellitus

Gastrointestinal: Abdominal pain, amylase increased; anorexia, constipation, diarrhea, lipase increased; protracted nausea and vomiting

Genitourinary: Hematuria, hemorrhagic cystitis

Hematologic: Anemia, antithrombin III decreased; DIC, fibrinogen decreased; hemolytic anemia, hemorrhage, leukopenia, pancytopenia, prolonged prothrombin, thrombin and partial thromboplastin times; thrombocytopenia; thrombosis

Hepatic: ALT and AST elevated, ascites, hepatomegaly, hepatotoxicity, hyperbilirubinemia, jaundice

Local: Erythema, inflammation, pain, pruritus

Neuromuscular & skeletal: Arthralgia, limb pain, myalgia, paresthesia, weakness

Renal: BUN and serum creatinine elevated, renal failure

Respiratory: Bronchospasm, cough, dyspnea, epistaxis, laryngeal edema

Miscellaneous: Allergic reaction, anaphylaxis, sepsis, septic shock

<1% and/or postmarketing reports: alopecia, bacteremia, bone pain, bruising, coagulation time increased, colitis, DVT, emotional lability, endocarditis, face edema, fatigue, fatty liver deposits, hypertension, hypoalbuminemia, hyponatremia, liver failure, metabolic acidosis, mucositis, petechial rash, proteinuria, prothrombin time increased, purpura, sagittal sinus thrombosis, subacute bacterial endocarditis, superficial venous thrombosis, uric acid nephropathy

Drug Interactions
Avoid Concomitant Use

Avoid concomitant use of Pegaspargase with any of the following: BCG; Natalizumab; Pimecrolimus; Tacrolimus (Topical); Vaccines (Live)

Increased Effect/Toxicity

Pegaspargase may increase the levels/effects of: Leflunomide; Natalizumab; Vaccines (Live)

The levels/effects of Pegaspargase may be increased by: Denosumab; Pimecrolimus; Tacrolimus (Topical); Trastuzumab

Decreased Effect

Pegaspargase may decrease the levels/effects of: BCG; Sipuleucel-T; Vaccines (Inactivated); Vaccines (Live)

The levels/effects of Pegaspargase may be decreased by: Echinacea

Stability Store vials in refrigerator [2°C to 8°C (36°F to 46°F)]; do not freeze; do not administer if there is any indication that the drug has been frozen or that vial has been stored at room temperature [15°C to 25°C (59°F to 77°F)] for >48 hours. Solutions for infusion should be refrigerated immediately after aseptic preparation and administered within 24 hours of preparation. Avoid excessive agitation, do not shake; do not use if cloudy or discolored or if precipitate is present; use of a 0.2 micron filter may result in some loss of potency.

Mechanism of Action Hydrolyzes asparagine to aspartic acid and ammonia depleting the exogenous asparagine supply needed by leukemic cells for protein synthesis

Pharmacodynamics

Onset of action: Asparagine depletion: I.M.: Within 4 days

Duration: Asparagine depletion:

I.M.: ~21 days

I.V.: 2-4 weeks (in asparaginase-naïve adults)

Pharmacokinetics (Adult data unless noted)

Absorption: Not absorbed from the GI tract; therefore, requires parenteral administration; I.M.: Slow

Distribution:

Apparent V_d: Plasma volume:

I.M.: Children: 1.5 L/m^2

I.V.: Adults (asparaginase-naïve): 2.4 L/m^2

Half-life:

I.M.: Children: 5.8 days; Adults: 5.5-6 days; 3.2 ± 1.8 days in patients who previously had a hypersensitivity reaction to native L-asparaginase

I.V.: Adults (asparaginase-naïve): 7 days

Time to peak serum concentration: I.M.: 3-4 days

Elimination: Clearance is unaffected by age, renal function, or hepatic function; not detected in urine

Usual Dosage (Refer to individual protocols): I.M., I.V.: Children (>1 year) and Adults: 2500 international units/m^2/ dose ≥every 14 days (as part of a combination chemotherapy regimen)

Administration

I.M.: Limit the volume at a single injection site to 2 mL; for I.M. administration, if the volume to be administered is >2 mL, use multiple injection sites

I.V.: Administer dose as an I.V. infusion in 100 mL of D$_5$W or NS over a period of 1-2 hours through a running I.V. infusion line

Monitoring Parameters Vital signs during administration, CBC with differential, platelet count, urinalysis, serum amylase, liver enzymes, bilirubin, prothrombin time, renal function tests, urine glucose, blood glucose, uric acid, fibrinogen levels. Observe patients for 1 hour after administration for signs of anaphylaxis and serious allergic reactions.

◄ **Patient Information** Notify physician if fever, sore throat, severe abdominal pain, excessive thirst, painful/burning urination, increase in frequency of urination, severe headache, bruising, bleeding, chest tightness, rash, swelling, difficulty breathing, or shortness of breath occurs

Nursing Implications Patients should be observed for 1 hour following injection; appropriate agents for maintenance of an adequate airway and treatment of a hypersensitivity reaction (antihistamine, epinephrine, oxygen, I.V. corticosteroids) should be readily available

Dosage Forms Excipient information presented when available (limited, particularly for generics); consult specific product labeling.

Injection, solution [preservative free]:
Oncaspar®: 750 int. units/mL (5 mL)

References

Asselin BL, Whitin JC, Cappola DJ, et al, "Comparative Pharmacokinetic Studies of Three Asparaginase Preparations," *J Clin Oncol*, 1993, 11(9):1780-6.

Avramis VI and Panosyan EH, "Pharmacokinetic/Pharmacodynamic Relationships of Asparaginase Formulations: The Past, the Present and Recommendations for the Future," *Clin Pharmacokinet*, 2005, 44 (4):367-93.

Avramis VI and Spence SA, "Clinical Pharmacology of Asparaginases in the United States: Asparaginase Population Pharmacokinetic and Pharmacodynamic (PK-PD) Models (NONMEM) in Adult and Pediatric ALL Patients," *J Pediatr Hematol Oncol*, 2007, 29(4):239-47.

Avramis VI, Sencer S, Periclou AP, et al, "A Randomized Comparison of Native *Escherichia coli* Asparaginase and Polyethylene Glycol Conjugated Asparaginase for Treatment of Children With Newly Diagnosed Standard-Risk Acute Lymphoblastic Leukemia: A Children's Cancer Group Study," *Blood*, 2002, 99(6):1986-94.

Capizzi RL, "Asparaginase Revisited," *Leuk Lymphoma*, 1993, 10 (Suppl):147-50.

Douer D, Yampolsky H, Cohen LJ, et al, "Pharmacodynamics and Safety of Intravenous Pegaspargase During Remission Induction in Adults Aged 55 Years or Younger With Newly Diagnosed Acute Lymphoblastic Leukemia," *Blood*, 2007, 109(7):2744-50.

Jarrar M, Gaynon PS, Periclou AP, et al, "Asparagine Depletion After Pegylated *E. coli* Asparaginase Treatment and Induction Outcome in Children With Acute Lymphoblastic Leukemia in First Bone Marrow Relapse: A Children's Oncology Group Study (CCG-1941)," *Pediatr Blood Cancer*, 2006, 47(2):141-6.

Pegfilgrastim (peg fil GRA stim)

Medication Safety Issues

Sound-alike/look-alike issues:
Neulasta® may be confused with Neumega®, Neupogen®, and Lunesta®

U.S. Brand Names Neulasta®

Canadian Brand Names Neulasta®

Therapeutic Category Colony Stimulating Factor

Generic Available No

Use Reduction of the duration of neutropenia and the associated risk of infection in patients with nonmyeloid malignancies receiving myelosuppressive chemotherapeutic regimens associated with a significant incidence of febrile neutropenia

Pregnancy Risk Factor C

Pregnancy Considerations Animal studies have demonstrated adverse effects and fetal loss. There are no adequate and well-controlled studies in pregnant women; use only if potential benefit to mother justifies the potential risk to the fetus.

Lactation Excretion in breast milk unknown/use caution

Contraindications Hypersensitivity to filgrastim, pegfilgrastim, or any component; use in the period between 14 days before and 24 hours after administration of cytotoxic chemotherapy

Warnings Splenic rupture, including fatal cases, has been reported following the administration of pegfilgrastim. Patients experiencing left upper abdominal and/or shoulder tip pain should be evaluated for an enlarged spleen or splenic rupture. ARDS has been reported with use; evaluate patients with pulmonary symptoms such as fever, lung infiltrates, or respiratory distress; withhold or discontinue pegfilgrastim if ARDS occurs. Allergic reactions including anaphylaxis, angioedema, skin rash, erythema, and urticaria have occurred primarily with the initial dose and may recur after discontinuation (reaction may be delayed); close follow-up for several days and permanent discontinuation are recommended for severe reactions.

Do not administer 14 days prior to or within 24 hours following the administration of chemotherapy due to the potential sensitivity of rapidly dividing myeloid cells to cytotoxic chemotherapy. Benefit has not been demonstrated with regimens under a 2-week duration. Administration on the same day as chemotherapy is not recommended (NCCN Myeloid Growth Factor Guidelines, v.1, 2009). Safety and efficacy have not been evaluated for use in peripheral blood progenitor cell (PBPC) mobilization or in patients receiving radiation therapy. May precipitate sickle cell crises in patients with sickle cell disease; carefully evaluate potential risks vs benefits when considering use in this patient population. Use has not been evaluated in patients receiving chemotherapy associated with delayed myelosuppression (eg, nitrosoureas, mitomycin C).

Precautions Use with caution in any malignancy with myeloid characteristics due to pegfilgrastim's potential to act as a growth factor; use with caution in patients with gout; psoriasis; monitor patients with pre-existing cardiac conditions as cardiac events (MIs, arrhythmias) have been reported in premarketing clinical studies with the parent drug filgrastim. The 6 mg fixed dose should not be used in infants, children, and adolescents weighing <45 kg.

Adverse Reactions

Cardiovascular: Peripheral edema, flushing

Central nervous system: Fever, headache, insomnia, dizziness

Dermatologic: Erythema, rash, urticaria, Sweet's syndrome (acute febrile dermatosis), alopecia

Gastrointestinal: Splenomegaly, splenic rupture, nausea, vomiting, constipation, diarrhea, dyspepsia, abdominal pain, mucositis

Hematologic: Leukocytosis, sickle cell crisis, cytopenias (resulting from an antibody response to exogenous growth factors; have been reported on rare occasions in patients treated with other recombinant growth factors)

Local: Pain, erythema, and induration at injection site

Neuromuscular & skeletal: Bone pain (31% to 57%), myalgia, arthralgia, weakness

Respiratory: ARDS, hypoxia

Miscellaneous: Hypersensitivity reactions including anaphylaxis and allergic reaction, antibody formation

Drug Interactions

Avoid Concomitant Use There are no known interactions where it is recommended to avoid concomitant use.

Increased Effect/Toxicity There are no known significant interactions involving an increase in effect.

Decreased Effect There are no known significant interactions involving a decrease in effect.

Stability Store in refrigerator; do not freeze; if inadvertently frozen, allow to thaw in refrigerator; discard if frozen more than one time. Allow to reach room temperature prior to injection. May be kept at room temperature for up to 48 hours. Protect from light.

Mechanism of Action Pegfilgrastim is a covalent conjugate of filgrastim and monomethoxypolyethylene glycol. It stimulates the production, maturation, and activation of neutrophils to increase both their migration and cytotoxicity. Pegfilgrastim has reduced renal clearance and prolonged persistence *in vivo* when compared with filgrastim.

Pharmacokinetics (Adult data unless noted)

Half-life: Adults: 15-80 hours; Children (100 mcg/kg dose): ~20-30 hours (range: Up to 68 hours)

Elimination: Primarily through binding to neutrophils

Usual Dosage SubQ: **Note:** Do not administer in the period between 14 days before and 24 hours after administration of cytotoxic chemotherapy. According to the NCCN guidelines, efficacy has been demonstrated with every 2-week chemotherapy regimens; however, benefit has not been demonstrated with regimens under a 2-week duration (Myeloid Growth Factor Guidelines, v.1, 2009)

Children (limited studies in children): 100 mcg/kg (maximum dose: 6 mg) once per chemotherapy cycle, beginning 24-72 hours after completion of chemotherapy

Adolescents >45 kg and Adults: 6 mg once per chemotherapy cycle, beginning 24-72 hours after completion of chemotherapy

Dosage adjustment in renal impairment: No adjustment necessary

Administration Parenteral: SubQ: Administer undiluted solution; do not shake

Monitoring Parameters Temperature, CBC with differential and platelet count

Evaluate for left upper abdominal pain, shoulder tip pain, or splenomegaly. Monitor for sickle cell crisis (in patients with sickle cell anemia).

Test Interactions May interfere with bone imaging studies; increased hematopoietic activity of the bone marrow may appear as transient positive bone imaging changes

Patient Information Possible bone pain; notify physician of unusual fever or chills, severe bone pain, or chest pain and palpitations

Nursing Implications Bone pain management is usually successful with non-narcotic analgesic therapy.

Dosage Forms Excipient information presented when available (limited, particularly for generics); consult specific product labeling.

Injection, solution [preservative free]:

Neulasta®: 10 mg/mL (0.6 mL) [prefilled syringe; needle cover contains latex]

References

André N, Kababri ME, Bertrand P, et al, "Safety and Efficacy of Pegfilgrastim in Children With Cancer Receiving Myelosuppressive Chemotherapy," *Anticancer Drugs*, 2007, 18(3):277-81.

André N, Milano E, Rome A, et al, "Safety of Pegfilgrastim in Children," *Ann Pharmacother*, 2008, 42(2):290.

Fox E, Jayaprakash N, Widemann BC, et al, "Randomized Trial and Pharmacokinetic Study of Pegfilgrastim vs. Filgrastim in Children and Young Adults With Newly Diagnosed Sarcoma Treated With Dose Intensive Chemotherapy," *J Clin Oncol*, 2006, 24(18S):9020 [abstract from 2006 ASCO Annual Meeting Proceedings, Part I].

Koontz SE, Mohassel LR, Jaffe N, et al, "Safety and Efficacy of Pegfilgrastim in Pediatric Oncology Patients: The M.D. Anderson Cancer Center Experience," *J Clin Oncol*, 2004, 22(14S):8272.

National Comprehensive Cancer Network (NCCN), "Clinical Practice Guidelines in Oncology™: Myeloid Growth Factors," Version 1, 2009. Available at http://www.nccn.org/professionals/physician_gls/PDF/myeloid_growth.pdf.

Smith TJ, Khatcheressian J, Lyman GH, et al, "2006 Update of Recommendations for the Use of White Blood Cell Growth Factors: An Evidence-Based Clinical Practice Guideline," *J Clin Oncol*, 2006, 24(19):3187-205.

Snyder RL and Stringham DJ, "Pegfilgrastim-Induced Hyperleukocytosis," *Ann of Pharmacother*, 2007, 41(9):1524-30.

te Poele EM, Kamps WA, Tamminga, RY, et al, "Pegfilgrastim in Pediatric Cancer Patients," *J Pediat Hematol Oncol*, 2005, 27 (11):627-9.

Wendelin G, Lackner H, Schwinger W, et al, "Once-Per-Cycle Pegfilgrastim Versus Daily Filgrastim in Pediatric Patients With Ewing Sarcoma," *J Pediatr Hematol Oncol*, 2005, 27(8):449-51.

Peginterferon Alfa-2b

(peg in ter FEER on AL fa too bee)

Medication Safety Issues

Sound-alike/look-alike issues:

Peginterferon alfa-2b may be confused with interferon alfa-2a, interferon alfa-2b, interferon alfa-n3, peginterferon alfa-2a

PegIntron® may be confused with Intron® A

International issues:

Peginterferon alfa-2b may be confused with interferon alpha multi-subtype which is available in international markets

U.S. Brand Names PegIntron®; PegIntron® Redipen®

Canadian Brand Names PegIntron®

Therapeutic Category Biological Response Modulator; Interferon

Generic Available No

Use Treatment of chronic hepatitis C (in combination with ribavirin) in patients who have compensated liver disease (FDA approved in ages ≥3 years and adults); treatment of chronic hepatitis C (as monotherapy) in patients with compensated liver disease who have never received alfa interferons (FDA approved in adults)

Medication Guide An FDA-approved patient medication guide, which is available with the product information and as follows, must be dispensed with this medication for each new outpatient prescription and refill.

PegIntron®: http://www.fda.gov/downloads/Drugs/DrugSafety/UCM133677.pdf

PegIntron® Redipen®: http://www.fda.gov/downloads/Drugs/DrugSafety/UCM133675.pdf

Pregnancy Risk Factor C / X in combination with ribavirin

Pregnancy Considerations Reproduction studies with pegylated interferon alfa have not been conducted. Animal studies with nonpegylated interferon alfa-2b have demonstrated abortifacient effects. Disruption of the normal menstrual cycle was also observed in animal studies; therefore, the manufacturer recommends that reliable contraception is used in women of childbearing potential. Alfa interferon is endogenous to normal amniotic fluid. *In vitro* administration studies have reported that when administered to the mother, it does not cross the placenta. Case reports of use in pregnant women are limited. The Perinatal HIV Guidelines Working Group does not recommend that peginterferon alfa be used during pregnancy. Peginterferon alfa-2b monotherapy should only be used in pregnancy when the potential benefit to the mother justifies the possible risk to the fetus. **[U.S. Boxed Warning]: Combination therapy with ribavirin may cause birth defects and/or fetal mortality; avoid pregnancy in females and female partners of male patients;** combination therapy with ribavirin is contraindicated in pregnancy. Two forms of contraception should be used during combination therapy; patients should have monthly pregnancy tests. A pregnancy registry has been established for women inadvertently exposed to ribavirin while pregnant (800-593-2214).

Lactation Excretion in breast milk unknown/not recommended

Breast-Feeding Considerations Breast milk samples obtained from a lactating mother prior to and after administration of interferon alfa-2b showed that interferon alfa is present in breast milk and administration of the medication did not significantly affect endogenous levels. The AAP considers interferon alfa to be "usually compatible with breast-feeding." Breast-feeding is not linked to the spread of hepatitis C virus; however, if nipples are cracked or bleeding, breast-feeding is not recommended. Mothers coinfected with HIV are discouraged from breast-feeding to decrease potential transmission of HIV.

Contraindications Hypersensitivity to interferon alfa or any component; autoimmune hepatitis; decompensated liver disease. Combination therapy with ribavirin is contra-indicated in pregnancy, women who may become pregnant; males with pregnant partners; hemoglobinopa-thies (eg, thalassemia major, sickle-cell anemia); renal dysfunction (Cl_{cr} <50 mL/minute).

Warnings May cause or aggravate fatal or life-threatening autoimmune disorders, neuropsychiatric symptoms (including depression and/or suicidal thoughts/behaviors), infectious disorders, ischemic disorders **[U.S. Boxed Warning]**.

Neuropsychiatric effects (some life-threatening or fatal) including depression, suicidal/homicidal ideation, suicidal attempts, suicides, addiction relapse, and aggression in association with interferon alfa therapy in patients with and without previous psychiatric symptoms have been reported. Suicidal ideation or attempts may occur more frequently in pediatric patients as compared to adults (2.4% vs 1% respectively). Also observed are psychoses, hallucinations, bipolar disorders and mania. Use with extreme caution in patients with a history of psychiatric disorders, including depression. Patients should be monitored for signs and symptoms; if occurs, continued monitoring throughout therapy and for 6 months post-treatment recommended. If symptoms persist, worsen, or if suicidal behavior or aggression towards others develops, peginterferon should be discontinued and the patient should be followed with psychiatric care given when appropriate. In severe cases, discontinue immediately and complete a psychiatric intervention. Higher doses may be associated with the development of encephalopathy (higher risk in elderly patients).

Exacerbation or development of autoimmune disorders has been reported, including thyroiditis, thrombotic thrombocytopenic purpura, idiopathic thrombocytopenic purpura, rheumatoid arthritis, interstitial nephritis, systemic lupus erythematosus, and psoriasis; use with caution in patients with autoimmune disorders.

Cerebrovascular events (ischemic and hemorrhagic) have been reported in patients with no or few stroke risk factors (including age <45 years) receiving interferon alfa therapy.

Alpha interferons suppress bone marrow function which may result in severe cytopenias or aplastic anemia (rarely). Use with caution in patients who are chronically immunosuppressed (including those on myelosuppressive therapy) or at increased risk for severe anemia (eg, spherocytosis, history of GI bleeding). Combination therapy with ribavirin may also potentiate the neutropenic effects of alfa interferons. Hemolytic anemia has been reported in 10% of patients receiving combination therapy. An increased incidence of anemia was observed when using ribavirin weight-based dosing, as compared to flat-dose ribavirin. Dosage adjustment may be necessary for hematologic toxicity.

Patients with chronic hepatitis C (CHC) with cirrhosis receiving alpha interferons may be at risk for hepatic decompensation and death; immediately discontinue therapy if it occurs (Child-Pugh score >6). CHC patients coinfected with HIV are at increased risk for hepatic decompensation when receiving highly active antiretroviral therapy (HAART); monitor closely. A transient increase in ALT (2-5 times above baseline) not associated with deterioration of liver function may occur with peginterferon alfa-2b use; therapy generally may continue with monitoring.

Ophthalmologic disorders (including decreased/loss of vision, retinopathy, optic neuritis, papilledema) have occurred with peginterferon alfa-2b and/or with other alfa interferons. Discontinue treatment with new or worsening ophthalmic disorder.

May cause or aggravate dyspnea, pulmonary infiltrates, pneumonia, bronchiolitis obliterans, interstitial pneumo-nitis, pulmonary hypertension, and sarcoidosis which can result in respiratory failure (in some cases death reported); may recur upon rechallenge with treatment. Monitor closely; discontinue combination therapy with ribavirin if pulmonary infiltrate or pulmonary function impairment develops.

Pancreatitis has been observed with alfa interferon therapy; withhold treatment for suspected pancreatitis; discontinue therapy for known pancreatitis. Ulcerative or hemorrhagic/ischemic colitis has been observed with alfa interferons; discontinue therapy if signs of colitis (abdomi-nal pain, bloody diarrhea, fever) develop.

Acute hypersensitivity reactions (urticaria, angioedema, bronchoconstriction, anaphylaxis) and cutaneous reac-tions (Stevens-Johnson syndrome, toxic epidermal necrol-ysis) have been reported (rarely) with alfa interferons; prompt discontinuation is recommended; transient rashes do not require interruption of therapy.

Combination treatment with ribavirin may cause birth defects and/or fetal mortality (avoid pregnancy in females and female partners of male patients); hemolytic anemia (which may worsen cardiac disease), genotoxicity, muta-genicity, and may possibly be carcinogenic. Combination therapy with ribavirin is contraindicated in pregnancy **[U.S. Boxed Warning]**.

The FDA currently recommends that procedures for proper handling and disposal of antineoplastic agents be considered.

Precautions Use with caution in patients with renal impairment (Cl_{cr} <50 mL/minute); increases in serum creatinine have been reported. Dosage adjustment may be required; discontinue if serum creatinine >2 mg/dL in children. Do not use combination therapy with ribavirin in adults with Cl_{cr} <50 mL/minute.

Use with caution in patients with cardiovascular disease; hypotension, arrhythmia, tachycardia, cardiomyopathy, angina pectoris, and MI have been observed with treatment. Patients with pre-existing cardiac abnormalities should have baseline ECGs prior to combination treatment with ribavirin; closely monitor patients with a history of arrhythmia. Patients with a history of significant or unstable cardiac disease should not receive combination treatment with ribavirin.

Use caution in patients with a history of diabetes mellitus (particularly if prone to DKA) or with thyroid disorders. Diabetes mellitus, hyperglycemia, and thyroid disorders (aggravation of hyper- or hypothyroidism) have been reported; discontinue peginterferon alfa-2b if condition cannot be effectively managed with medication.

Severe inhibition of growth velocity, < 3rd percentile and affecting height and weight, was reported in 70% of pediatric patients during clinical trials on combination therapy; monitor closely; dosage adjustment may be required. After therapy, 20% continued to have severely inhibited growth; however, in majority of patients, growth velocity rates increased such that by 6 months post-treatment, weight gain stabilized to 53rd percentile (similar to predicted based on average baseline weight: 57th percentile) and height gain stabilized to 44th percentile (less than predicted based on average baseline height: 51st percentile).

Hypertriglyceridemia has been reported with use; discontinue if persistent and severe (triglycerides >1000 mg/dL), particularly if combined with symptoms of pancreatitis.

Dental/periodontal disorders have been reported with combination therapy; dry mouth may affect teeth and mucous membranes; instruct patients to brush teeth twice daily; encourage regular dental exams.

Combination therapy with ribavirin is preferred over monotherapy for the treatment of chronic hepatitis C (combination therapy provides a better response).

Use with caution with concurrent telbivudine therapy; peripheral neuropathy has been reported.

Safety and efficacy have not been established in patients who have received organ transplants, are coinfected with HIV or hepatitis B, or received treatment for >1 year. Patients with significant bridging fibrosis or cirrhosis, genotype 1 infection, or who have not responded to prior therapy, including previous pegylated interferon treatment, are less likely to benefit from combination therapy with peginterferon alfa-2b and ribavirin. Some formulations contain polysorbate 80.

Adverse Reactions Note: Includes adverse reaction reported during monotherapy trials

Cardiovascular: Chest pain, flushing

Central nervous system: Addiction relapse, aggression, agitation, anxiety/emotional liability/irritability, chills, concentration impaired, depression (see Warnings), dizziness, fatigue, fever (children: 80%; adults: 46%), headache, insomnia, irritability, malaise, nervousness, stroke, suicidal behavior (see Warnings)

Dermatologic: Alopecia, dry skin, pruritus, rash

Endocrine & metabolic: Anorexia, hyper-/hypothyroidism, hypertriglyceridemia, hyperuricemia, menstrual disorder, weight loss

Gastrointestinal: Abdominal pain (including upper right quadrant), constipation, diarrhea, dyspepsia, nausea, vomiting (children: 27%; adults: 14%), weight loss, xerostomia

Hematologic: Anemia (in combination with ribavirin), leukopenia, neutropenia, thrombocytopenia (see Warnings)

Hepatic: Hepatomegaly, hyperbilirubinemia, serum transaminases increased (transient)

Local: Inflammation, injection site erythema, pain, reaction

Neuromuscular & skeletal: Arthralgia, musculoskeletal pain, myalgia, rigors, weakness

Ocular: Blurred vision, conjunctivitis, optic neuritis, papilledema, vision loss/decreased (see Warnings)

Respiratory: Bronchiolitis obliterans, cough, dyspnea, interstitial pneumonitis, pharyngitis, pneumonia, pulmonary hypertension (see Warnings), pulmonary infiltrates, rhinitis, sarcoidosis, sinusitis

Miscellaneous: Acute hypersensitivity reactions (see Warnings), autoimmune disorders (see Warnings), diaphoresis, influenza-like illness, neutralizing antibodies, taste perversion, viral or fungal infection

≤1%, postmarketing, and/or case reports (limited to important or life-threatening): Abscess, angina, angioedema, aphthous stomatitis, aplastic anemia, arrhythmia, autoimmune thrombocytopenia (with or without purpura), bacterial infection, bronchoconstriction, cardiac arrest, cardiomyopathy, cellulitis, cotton wool spots, cytopenia, diabetes mellitus, drug overdose, emphysema, encephalopathy, erythema multiforme, fungal infection, gastroenteritis, gout, hallucinations, hearing impairment/loss, hemorrhagic colitis, hyperglycemia, hyper-/hypotension, injection site necrosis, interstitial nephritis, ischemic colitis, loss of consciousness, lupus-like syndrome, macular edema, memory loss, MI, migraine, myositis, nerve palsy (facial/oculomotor), palpitation, pancreatitis,

paresthesia, pericardial effusion, peripheral neuropathy, phototoxicity, pleural effusion, polyneuropathy, psoriasis, psychosis, pulmonary hypertension, pulmonary infiltrates, pure red cell aplasia, renal failure, renal insufficiency, retinal artery or vein thrombosis, retinal detachment (serous), retinal hemorrhage, retinal ischemia, rhabdomyolysis, rheumatoid arthritis, sarcoidosis, seizure, sepsis, serum creatinine increased, Stevens-Johnson syndrome, supraventricular arrhythmia, systemic lupus erythematosus, tachycardia, thrombotic thrombocytopenic purpura, thyroiditis, toxic epidermal necrolysis, transient ischemic attack, ulcerative colitis, urticaria, vasculitis, vertigo, visual acuity decreased, Vogt-Koyanagi-Harada syndrome

Drug Interactions

Metabolism/Transport Effects Inhibits CYP1A2 (weak)

Avoid Concomitant Use

Avoid concomitant use of Peginterferon Alfa-2b with any of the following: Telbivudine

Increased Effect/Toxicity ACE inhibitors, clozapine, erythropoietin may increase risk of bone marrow suppression. Fluorouracil, theophylline, zidovudine concentrations may increase. Warfarin's anticoagulant effect may increase.

Decreased Effect Melphalan concentrations may decrease. Prednisone may decrease effects of interferon alfa.

Stability Store vials at 25°C (77°F); excursions permitted to 15°C to 30°C (59°F to 86°F). Store Redipen® at 2°C to 8°C (36°F to 46°F). Once reconstituted, each product should be used immediately or may be stored for ≤24 hours at 2°C to 8°C (36°F to 46°F); do not freeze. Products do not contain preservative; do not reuse.

Mechanism of Action Inducer of the innate antiviral immune response; binds to the human type 1 interferon receptor which activates multiple intracellular signal transduction pathways, resulting in suppression of cell proliferation, immunomodulating activities (such as enhancement of the phagocytic activity of macrophages and augmentation of the specific cytotoxicity of lymphocytes for target cells), and inhibition of virus replication in virus-infected cells

Pharmacokinetics (Adult data unless noted)

Note: Peginterferon alfa-2b has a prolonged duration of effect relative to interferon alfa-2b and a reduced renal clearance (sevenfold lower). Data in children similar to adult values.

Bioavailability: Increases with chronic dosing

Half-life elimination: ~40 hours (range: 22-60 hours)

Time to peak serum concentration: 15-44 hours

Elimination: Urine (30%); clearance reduced in renal impairment by 17% in moderate dysfunction, 44% in severe dysfunction

Usual Dosage Note: Due to differences in dosage, patients should not change brands of interferon alfa therapy. SubQ:

Children:

Manufacturer recommendation: Children ≥3 years: 60 mcg/m^2 once weekly (in combination with ribavirin). Treatment duration: 48 weeks (genotype 1); 24 weeks (genotypes 2 and 3). Consider discontinuation of combination therapy in patients with HCV (genotype 1) at 12 weeks if a 2 log decrease in HCV-RNA has not been achieved or if HCV-RNA is still detectable at 24 weeks.

Note: Children who reach their 18th birthday during treatment should remain on the pediatric regimen.

Alternate dosing: American Association for the Study of Liver Diseases (AASLD) guideline recommendations: (age: 2-17 years): 60 mcg/m^2 once weekly (in combination with oral ribavirin) for 48 weeks (all genotypes) (see Ghany, 2009)

1073

Adults: Administer dose once weekly. Treatment duration: 48 weeks for genotype 1 and patients who previously failed therapy (regardless of genotype); 24 weeks (genotypes 2 and 3). Consider discontinuation in patients with HCV (genotype 1) at 12 weeks if a 2 log decrease in HCV-RNA has not been achieved or if HCV-RNA is still detectable at 24 weeks.

Monotherapy: Initial: 1 mcg/kg/week
≤45 kg: 40 mcg once weekly
46-56 kg: 50 mcg once weekly
57-72 kg: 64 mcg once weekly
73-88 kg: 80 mcg once weekly
89-106 kg: 96 mcg once weekly
107-136 kg: 120 mcg once weekly
137-160 kg: 150 mcg once weekly

Combination therapy with ribavirin: Initial: 1.5 mcg/kg/week
<40 kg: 50 mcg once weekly
40-50 kg: 64 mcg once weekly
51-60 kg: 80 mcg once weekly
61-75 kg: 96 mcg once weekly
76-85 kg: 120 mcg once weekly
86-105 kg: 150 mcg once weekly
>105 kg: 1.5 mcg/kg once weekly

Dosage adjustment for toxicity: For serious adverse reaction during treatment, modify dosage or discontinue; discontinue for persistent serious adverse reaction:

Children: Reduce to 40 mcg/m^2/week; may further reduce to 20 mcg/m^2/week if needed.

Adults:
Monotherapy dose reductions: Reduce to 0.5 mcg/kg/week as follows:
≤45 kg: 20 mcg once weekly
46-56 kg: 25 mcg once weekly
57-72 kg: 30 mcg once weekly
73-88 kg: 40 mcg once weekly
89-106 kg: 50 mcg once weekly
107-136 kg: 64 mcg once weekly
≥137 kg: 80 mcg once weekly

Combination therapy adult dosage reductions: Reduce to 1 mcg/kg/week; may further reduce to 0.5 mcg/kg/week if needed as follows:
<40 kg: 35 mcg once weekly; may further reduce to 20 mcg once weekly if needed
40-50 kg: 45 mcg once weekly; may further reduce to 25 mcg once weekly if needed
51-60 kg: 50 mcg once weekly; may further reduce to 30 mcg once weekly if needed
61-75 kg: 64 mcg once weekly; may further reduce to 35 mcg once weekly if needed
76-85 kg: 80 mcg once weekly; may further reduce to 45 mcg once weekly if needed
86-104 kg: 96 mcg once weekly; may further reduce to 50 mcg once weekly if needed
105-125 kg: 108 mcg once weekly; may further reduce to 64 mcg once weekly if needed
>125 kg: 135 mcg once weekly; may further reduce to 72 mcg once weekly if needed

Dosage adjustment for depression (severity based upon DSM-IV criteria)

Mild depression: No dosage adjustment required; evaluate once weekly by visit/phone call. If depression remains stable, continue weekly visits. If depression improves, resume normal visit schedule. For worsening depression, see "Moderate depression" below.

Moderate depression:
Children: Decrease to 40 mcg/m^2/week, may further decrease to 20 mcg/m^2/week if needed

Adults:
Monotherapy: Decrease to 0.5 mcg/kg once weekly
Combination therapy: Decrease peginterferon alfa-2b dose to 1 mcg/kg once weekly; may further reduce to 0.5 mcg/kg once weekly if needed
Note: Evaluate once weekly with an office visit at least every other week. If depression remains stable, consider psychiatric evaluation and continue with reduced dosing. If symptoms improve and remain stable for 4 weeks, resume normal visit schedule; continue reduced dosing or return to normal dose. For worsening depression or development of severe depression, discontinue therapy permanently and obtain immediate psychiatric consultation.

Dosage adjustment in hematologic toxicity: Refer to ribavirin monograph for additional adjustments information if combination therapy.

Children:
Hemoglobin decrease ≥2 g/dL in any 4-week period in patients with pre-existing cardiac disease: Monitor and evaluate weekly
Hemoglobin <10 g/dL: Decrease ribavirin dose to 12 mg/kg/day; may further reduce to 8 mg/kg/day
WBC <1.5 x 10^9/L, neutrophils <0.75 x 10^9/L, or platelets <70 x 10^9/L: Reduce peginterferon alfa-2b dose to 40 mcg/m^2/week; may further reduce to 20 mcg/m^2/week
Hemoglobin <8.5 g/dL, WBC <1.0 x 10^9/L, neutrophils <0.5 x 10^9/L, or platelets <50 x 10^9/L: Permanently discontinue peginterferon alfa-2b

Adults:
Hemoglobin decrease >2 g/dL in any 4-week period and stable cardiac disease: Decrease peginterferon alfa-2b dose by 50%; decrease ribavirin dose by 200 mg/day.
Hemoglobin <12 g/dL after dose reductions: Permanently discontinue both peginterferon alfa-2b and ribavirin.
Hemoglobin <10 g/dL in patients with cardiac disease: Reduce peginterferon alfa-2b dose by 50%; decrease ribavirin dose by 200 mg/day (patients receiving 1400 mg/day should decrease dose by 400 mg/day); may further reduce ribavirin dose by additional 200 mg/day if needed
WBC <1.5 x 10^9/L, neutrophils <0.75 x 10^9/L, or platelets <50 x 10^9/L:
Peginterferon alfa-2b combination therapy: Reduce peginterferon alfa-2b dose to 1 mcg/kg once weekly; may further reduce dose to 0.5 mcg/kg once weekly if needed
Peginterferon alfa-2b monotherapy: Reduce peginterferon alfa-2b dose to 0.5 mcg/kg once weekly
Hemoglobin <8.5 g/dL, WBC <1.0 x 10^9/L, neutrophils <0.5 x 10^9/L, or platelets <25 x 10^9/L: Permanently discontinue peginterferon alfa-2b and ribavirin.

Dosage adjustment in renal impairment: Combination with ribavirin: Children: Serum creatinine >2 mg/dL: Discontinue treatment

Administration
Redipen®: Hold cartridge upright and press the two halves together until there is a "click." Gently invert to mix; do not shake.
Vial: Add 0.7 mL of SWI (supplied diluent) to the vial. Gently swirl. Do not re-enter vial after dose removed. Discard unused reconstituted portion; do not reuse.
For SubQ administration. Rotate injection site; thigh, outer surface of upper arm, and abdomen are preferred injection sites; do not inject near navel or waistline; patients who are thin should only use thigh or upper arm. Do not inject into bruised, infected, irritated, red, or scarred skin.

Monitoring Parameters Baseline and periodic TSH, hematology (including hemoglobin, CBC with differential, platelets), chemistry (including LFTs) testing, renal function, triglycerides. Clinical studies for combination therapy tested as follows: CBC (including hemoglobin, WBC, and platelets) and chemistries (including liver function tests and uric acid) measured at weeks 2, 4, 8, and 12, and then every 6 weeks; TSH measured every 12 weeks during treatment.

Serum HCV RNA levels (pretreatment, 12 and 24 weeks after therapy initiation, 24 weeks after completion of therapy). **Note:** Discontinuation of therapy may be considered after 12 weeks in patients with HCV (genotype 1) who fail to achieve an early virologic response (EVR) (defined as ≥2-log decrease in HCV RNA compared to pretreatment) or after 24 weeks with detectable HCV RNA. Treat patients with HCV (genotypes 2,3) for 24 weeks (if tolerated) and then evaluate HCV RNA levels (see Ghany, 2009).

Evaluate for depression and other psychiatric symptoms before and after initiation of therapy; baseline ophthalmic eye examination; periodic ophthalmic exam in patients with diabetic or hypertensive retinopathy; baseline ECG in patients with cardiac disease; serum glucose or Hb A_{1c} (for patients with diabetes mellitus). In combination therapy with ribavirin, pregnancy tests (for women of childbearing age who are receiving treatment or who have male partners who are receiving treatment), continue monthly up to 6 months after discontinuation of therapy.

Reference Range

Early viral response (EVR): ≥2 log decrease in HCV RNA after 12 weeks of treatment

End of treatment response (ETR): Absence of detectable HCV RNA at end of the recommended treatment period

Sustained treatment response (STR): Absence of HCV RNA in the serum 6 months following completion of full treatment course

Patient Information Read the patient Medication Guide that you receive with each prescription and refill of peginterferon alfa-2b. Do not operate heavy machinery while on therapy since changes in mental status may occur; may cause dry mouth. Report any signs of depression or suicidal ideation, breathing problems, bleeding or easy bruising, or vision changes to your physician. If also taking ribavirin, avoid pregnancy (female patients or female partners of male patients).

Nursing Implications Patient should be well-hydrated; may pretreat with NSAID or acetaminophen to decrease fever and its severity and to alleviate headache. Assess results of laboratory tests on a regular basis, therapeutic effectiveness, and adverse reactions. Patients with pre-existing cardiac abnormalities, or in advanced stages of cancer should have ECGs taken before and during treatment. Monitor for neuropsychiatric changes. Assess knowledge/instruct patient/caregiver on appropriate reconstitution, injection and needle disposal, possible side effects, and symptoms to report.

Dosage Forms Excipient information presented when available (limited, particularly for generics); consult specific product labeling.

Injection, powder for reconstitution [preservative free]:

PegIntron®: 50 mcg, 80 mcg, 120 mcg, 150 mcg [contains polysorbate 80 and sucrose]

PegIntron® Redipen®: 50 mcg, 80 mcg, 120 mcg, 150 mcg [contains polysorbate 80 and sucrose]

References

American College of Obstetricians and Gynecologists, "ACOG Practice Bulletin No. 86: Viral Hepatitis in Pregnancy," *Obstet Gynecol*, 2007, 110(4):941-56.

American Academy of Pediatrics Committee on Drugs, "Transfer of Drugs and Other Chemicals Into Human Milk," *Pediatrics*, 2001, 108(3):776-89.

Dienstag JL and McHutchison JG, "American Gastroenterological Association Medical Position Statement on the Management of Hepatitis C," *Gastroenterology*, 2006, 130(1):225-30.

Ghany MG, Strader DB, Thomas DL, et al, "Diagnosis, Management, and Treatment of Hepatitis C: An Update," *Hepatology*, 2009, 49 (4):1335-74.

Kumar AR, Hale TW, and Moke RE, "Transfer of Interferon Alfa Into Human Breast Milk," *J Hum Lact*, 2000, 16:226-8.

Lebon P, Girard S, Thépot F, et al, "The Presence of Alpha-Interferon in Human Amniotic Fluid," *J Gen Virol*, 1982, 59(Pt 2):393-6.

"Perinatal HIV Guidelines Working Group. Public Health Service Task Force Recommendations for Use of Antiretroviral Drugs in Pregnant HIV-Infected Women for Maternal Health and Interventions to Reduce Perinatal HIV Transmission in the United States," April 29, 2009, 1-90. Available at: http://aidsinfo.nih.gov/ContentFiles/PerinatalGL.pdf.

Waysbort A, Giroux M, Mansat V, et al, "Experimental Study of Transplacental Passage of Alpha Interferon by Two Assay Techniques," *Antimicrob Agents Chemother*, 1993, 37(6):1232-7.

◆ **PegIntron®** *see* Peginterferon Alfa-2b *on page 1071*

◆ **PegIntron® Redipen®** *see* Peginterferon Alfa-2b *on page 1071*

◆ **PEGLA** *see* Pegaspargase *on page 1068*

◆ **PegLyte® (Can)** *see* Polyethylene Glycol-Electrolyte Solution *on page 1129*

◆ **Pegylated G-CSF** *see* Pegfilgrastim *on page 1070*

◆ **Pegylated Interferon Alfa-2b** *see* Peginterferon Alfa-2b *on page 1071*

Pemirolast (pe MIR oh last)

U.S. Brand Names Alamast®

Canadian Brand Names Alamast®

Therapeutic Category Antiallergic, Ophthalmic; Ophthalmic Agent, Miscellaneous

Generic Available No

Use Prevention of itching of the eye due to allergic conjunctivitis

Pregnancy Risk Factor C

Pregnancy Considerations There are no adequate and well-controlled studies in pregnant women. Should only be used during pregnancy if the benefit outweighs the risk to the fetus.

Lactation Excretion in breast milk unknown/use caution

Contraindications Hypersensitivity to pemirolast or any component

Warnings Not for treatment of contact lens related irritation; the preservative in pemirolast, lauralkonium chloride, may be absorbed by soft contact lenses; wait at least 10 minutes after administration before inserting soft contact lenses.

Adverse Reactions

Central nervous system: Headache, fever

Ocular: Burning, dry eyes, ocular discomfort, foreign body sensation

Respiratory: Rhinitis, bronchitis, cough, sinusitis, nasal congestion

Miscellaneous: Hypersensitivity reactions; cold/flu-like symptoms

Drug Interactions

Avoid Concomitant Use There are no known interactions where it is recommended to avoid concomitant use.

Increased Effect/Toxicity There are no known significant interactions involving an increase in effect.

Decreased Effect There are no known significant interactions involving a decrease in effect.

Stability Store at controlled room temperature

Mechanism of Action Pemirolast is a mast cell stabilizer that inhibits immediate hypersensitivity reactions by preventing the release of antigen-induced inflammatory mediators (eg, histamine, leukotriene C_4, D_4, E_4). It also inhibits the chemotaxis of eosinophils into ocular tissue and blocks the release of mediators from eosinophils.

Pharmacodynamics
Onset of action: A few days
Maximum effect: Up to 4 weeks
Pharmacokinetics (Adult data unless noted)
Half-life: Adults: 4.5 ± 0.2 hours
Excretion: 10% to 15% excreted unchanged in the urine
Usual Dosage Ophthalmic: Children >3 years and Adults: 1-2 drops into affected eye(s) four times daily
Administration Ophthalmic: Apply finger pressure to lacrimal duct during and for 1-2 minutes after instillation to decrease risk of systemic effects; avoid contact of bottle tip with skin or eye; the preservative in pemirolast, lauralkonium chloride, may be absorbed by soft contact lenses; wait at least 10 minutes after administration before inserting soft contact lenses.
Monitoring Parameters Local symptomatology
Patient Information May cause.dry eyes
Dosage Forms Excipient information presented when available (limited, particularly for generics); consult specific product labeling.
Solution, ophthalmic, as potassium: 0.1% (10 mL) [contains lauralkonium chloride]

Penciclovir (pen SYE kloe veer)

Medication Safety Issues
Sound-alike/look-alike issues:
Denavir® may be confused with indinavir
U.S. Brand Names Denavir®
Therapeutic Category Antiviral Agent, Topical
Generic Available No
Use Topical treatment of recurrent herpes labialis (cold sores, fever blisters)
Pregnancy Risk Factor B
Lactation Excretion in breast milk unknown
Contraindications Hypersensitivity to penciclovir or any component; previous or significant adverse reactions to famciclovir
Precautions No data available on safety and efficacy of penciclovir application to mucous membranes. Efficacy has not been established in immunocompromised patients or children <18 years of age.
Adverse Reactions
Central nervous system: Headache
Dermatologic: Erythematous rash
Local: Local anesthesia, application site reaction
Drug Interactions
Avoid Concomitant Use There are no known interactions where it is recommended to avoid concomitant use.
Increased Effect/Toxicity There are no known significant interactions involving an increase in effect.
Decreased Effect There are no known significant interactions involving a decrease in effect.
Stability Store at room temperature; do not freeze
Mechanism of Action In cells infected with HSV-1 or HSV-2, viral thymidine kinase phosphorylates penciclovir to a monophosphate form which is converted to penciclovir triphosphate by cellular kinases. Penciclovir triphosphate inhibits HSV polymerase by competing with deoxyguanosine triphosphate inhibiting viral DNA synthesis and replication.
Pharmacodynamics Resolution of pain and cutaneous healing: 3.5-4.8 days
Pharmacokinetics (Adult data unless noted) Absorption: Topical: Negligible
Usual Dosage Topical: Adolescents and Adults: Apply every 2 hours during waking hours for 4 days

Administration Topical: Apply only to herpes labialis on the lips and face. Apply sufficient amount to cover lesions and gently rub into the affected area. Avoid application in or near eyes since it may cause irritation.
Monitoring Parameters Resolution of pain and healing of cold sore lesion
Patient Information Start treatment at the first sign or symptom of cold sore; report if you experience significant burning, itching, stinging, or redness when applying this medication
Additional Information Penciclovir is the active metabolite of the prodrug famciclovir.
Dosage Forms Excipient information presented when available (limited, particularly for generics); consult specific product labeling.
Cream: 1% (1.5 g)
References
Dekker CL and Prober CG, "Pediatric Uses of Valacyclovir, Penciclovir and Famciclovir," *Pediatr Infect Dis J*, 2001, 20(11):1079-81.

Penicillamine (pen i SIL a meen)

Medication Safety Issues
Sound-alike/look-alike issues:
Penicillamine may be confused with penicillin

International issues:
Depen® may be confused with Depon® which is a brand name for acetaminophen in Greece
Depen® may be confused with Dipen® which is a brand name for diltiazem in Greece
Pemine® [Italy] may be confused with Pamine® which is a brand name for methscopolamine in the U.S.
U.S. Brand Names Cuprimine®; Depen®
Canadian Brand Names Cuprimine®; Depen®
Therapeutic Category Antidote, Copper Toxicity; Antidote, Lead Toxicity; Chelating Agent, Oral
Generic Available No
Use Treatment of Wilson's disease, cystinuria, adjunct in the treatment of severe rheumatoid arthritis (FDA approved in adults); has also been used for lead poisoning, primary biliary cirrhosis (as adjunctive therapy following initial treatment with calcium EDTA or BAL); has also been used in lead poisoning
Pregnancy Risk Factor D
Pregnancy Considerations Birth defects, including congenital cutix laxa and associated defects, have been reported in infants following penicillamine exposure during pregnancy. Use for the treatment of rheumatoid arthritis during pregnancy is contraindicated. Use for the treatment of cystinuria only if the possible benefits to the mother outweigh the potential risks to the fetus. Continued treatment of Wilson's disease during pregnancy protects the mother against relapse. Discontinuation has detrimental maternal and fetal effects. Daily dosage should be limited to 750 mg. For planned cesarean section, reduce dose to 250 mg/day for the last 6 weeks of pregnancy, and continue at this dosage until wound healing is complete.
Lactation Excretion in breast milk unknown/contraindicated
Contraindications Rheumatoid arthritic patients with renal insufficiency; patients with previous penicillamine-related aplastic anemia or agranulocytosis; concomitant administration with other hematopoietic-depressant drugs (eg, gold, immunosuppressants, antimalarials, phenylbutazone), pregnancy (except for the treatment of Wilson's disease or certain cases of cystinuria), breast-feeding
Warnings Penicillamine has been associated with fatalities due to agranulocytosis, aplastic anemia, thrombocytopenia, Goodpasture's syndrome, and myasthenia gravis; discontinue therapy if WBC <3500/mm^3; temporarily discontinue treatment if the platelet count is <100,000/mm^3; patients should be warned to promptly

report any symptoms suggesting toxicity **[U.S. Boxed Warning]**; due to the potential severity of these effects, patients should be monitored closely (see Monitoring Parameters). Proteinuria and/or hematuria may develop and are early warning signs of membraneous glomerulopathy which can progress to nephrotic syndrome; these symptoms may disappear with continued therapy; close observation is warranted; follow 24-hour urine protein excretion rates; excretion >1 g protein in urine per 24 hours or proteinuria which is progressively increasing requires decreasing the dosage or discontinuation in patients treated for rheumatoid arthritis; in Wilson's disease and cystinuria, the risks versus benefits of continuing must be considered.

Drug fever, sometimes accompanied with a skin eruption, necessitates temporary discontinuation of penicillamine in Wilson's disease and cystinuria patients and discontinuation in rheumatoid arthritic patients. Treatment may be resumed with a small dose and gradually increased to the desired dose once the symptoms have subsided. Early rashes (first few months) associated with penicillamine usually disappear within days after discontinuation of therapy and seldom return when treatment is restarted at a lower dose; late rashes (>6 months of treatment) require discontinuation of therapy.

Interruption of continuous therapy for Wilson's disease or cystinuria even for a few days has been associated with sensitivity reactions upon reinstitution of therapy; approximately 33% of patients will experience an allergic reaction. When used for cystinuria, renal stones may develop; an annual x-ray for renal stones is recommended

Precautions Patients on penicillamine for Wilson's disease or cystinuria should receive pyridoxine supplementation 25-50 mg/day; when treating rheumatoid arthritis, daily pyridoxine supplementation is also recommended. A positive ANA for lupus erythematosus may occur possibly progressing to a lupus-like syndrome. Patients who are allergic to penicillin may theoretically have cross-sensitivity to penicillamine. This possibility has been eliminated now that penicillamine is synthetically produced and no longer contains trace amounts of penicillin.

Adverse Reactions

Cardiovascular: Edema of the face, feet, or lower legs; vasculitis

Central nervous system: Agitation, anxiety, chills, dystonia, fatigue, fever, hyperpyrexia, myasthenic syndrome, psychiatric disturbances, worsening neurologic symptoms

Dermatologic: Alopecia, angioedema dermatomyositis, exfoliative dermatitis (dose-related) (see Warnings), friability of the skin increased, lichen planus, pemphigus, pruritus, rash (early and late 5%), skin friability increased, toxic epidermal necrolysis, urticaria, wrinkling (excessive), yellow nail syndrome

Endocrine & metabolic: Hypoglycemia, iron deficiency, thyroiditis, weight gain

Gastrointestinal: Ageusia, anorexia, cheilosis (rare), colitis, diarrhea, dysgeusia, epigastric pain, gingivostomatitis, glossitis, nausea (dose-related), oral ulcerations, pancreatitis, peptic ulcer reactivation, sore throat, taste alteration, vomiting (in children with doses >60 mg/kg/day)

Genitourinary: Bloody or cloudy urine, urinary incontinence

Hematologic: Agranulocytosis (see Warnings), aplastic anemia, eosinophilia, hemolytic anemia, leukocytosis, leukopenia, monocytosis, red cell aplasia, thrombocytopenia, thrombocytosis, thrombotic thrombocytopenia purpura

Hepatic: Alkaline phosphatase increased, hepatic cholestasis, hepatic failure, hepatitis, toxic hepatitis

Neuromuscular & skeletal: Arthralgia, dermatomyositis, muscle weakness, peripheral neuropathy, polyarthralgia (migratory, often with objective synovitis), polymyositis

Ocular: Diplopia, extraocular muscle weakness, optic neuritis, ptosis, visual disturbances

Otic: Tinnitus

Renal: Goodpasture's syndrome (see Warnings), hematuria, nephrotic syndrome, proteinuria, renal vasculitis

Respiratory: Asthma, coughing, interstitial pneumonitis, obliterative bronchiolitis, pulmonary fibrosis, wheezing

Miscellaneous: Allergic alveolitis, allergic reactions (see Warnings), anetoderma, elastosis perforans serpiginosa, lactic dehydrogenase increased, lymphadenopathy, mammary hyperplasia, positive ANA test, SLE-like syndrome, white spots on lips or mouth

Drug Interactions

Avoid Concomitant Use There are no known interactions where it is recommended to avoid concomitant use.

Increased Effect/Toxicity There are no known significant interactions involving an increase in effect.

Decreased Effect

Penicillamine may decrease the levels/effects of: Digoxin

The levels/effects of Penicillamine may be decreased by: Antacids; Iron Salts

Food Interactions Do not administer with milk or food (food decreases absorption by 50%); iron and zinc may decrease drug action; increase dietary intake or supplement with pyridoxine; for Wilson's disease, decrease copper in diet and omit chocolate, nuts, shellfish, mushrooms, liver, raisins, broccoli, and molasses; for lead poisoning, decrease calcium in diet

Mechanism of Action Chelates with lead, copper, mercury, iron, and other heavy metals to form stable, soluble complexes that are excreted in the urine; depresses circulating IgM rheumatoid factor levels and *in vitro*, depresses T-cell but not B-cell activity; combines with cystine to form a more soluble compound which prevents the formation of cystine calculi

Pharmacodynamics Onset of action:

Rheumatoid arthritis: 2-3 months

Wilson's disease: 1-3 months

Pharmacokinetics (Adult data unless noted)

Absorption: 40% to 70%

Protein binding: 80%

Metabolism: In the liver

Half-life: 1.7-7 hours

Time to peak serum concentration: Within 1-3 hours

Elimination: Primarily (30% to 60%) in urine as unchanged drug

Usual Dosage Oral:

Rheumatoid arthritis: **Note:** The optimal duration of therapy has not been determined; in patients experiencing a remission for ≥6 months, the daily dosage may be decreased in a stepwise fashion in 3-month intervals:

Children: Initial: 3 mg/kg/day (≤250 mg/day) for 3 months, then 6 mg/kg/day (≤500 mg/day) in 2 divided doses for 3 months to a maximum of 10 mg/kg/day (≤1-1.5 g/day) in 3-4 divided doses

Adults: 125-250 mg/day, may increase dose by 125-250 mg/day; if therapy still ineffective after 2-3 months of treatment and no signs of adverse effects, increases of 250 mg/day at 2-3 month intervals up to a maximum daily dose of 1.5 g may be done; doses >500 mg/day should be given in divided doses

Wilson's disease: **Note:** Dose that results in an initial 24-hour urinary copper excretion >2 mg/day should be continued for ~3 months; maintenance dose defined by amount resulting in <10 mcg serum free copper/dL.

Children: AASLD guidelines: 20 mg/kg/day in 2-3 divided doses, round off to the nearest 250 mg dose; reduce dose by 25% when clinically stable; administer with a pyridoxine supplement (25-50 mg/day)

Adults: 750-1500 mg/day in divided doses; maximum dose: 2000 mg/day; administer with a pyridoxine supplement (25-50 mg/day)

Note: In pregnant patients, limit daily dose to 1 g; if a cesarean section is planned, limit daily dose to 250 mg during the last 6 weeks before delivery and post-operatively until the wound has healed.

AASLD guidelines recommend to increase tolerability, therapy may be initiated at 250-500 mg/day and then titrated upward by 250 mg every 4-7 days; usual maintenance dose: 750-1000 mg/day in 2 divided doses; maximum: 1000-1500 mg/day in 2-4 divided doses; reduce dose by 25% when clinically stable (see Roberts, 2008)

Cystinuria (doses titrated to maintain urinary cystine excretion at <100-200 mg/day in patients without a history of stones and <100 mg/day in patients who have had stone formation and/or pain):

Children: 30 mg/kg/day in 4 divided doses; maximum dose: 4 g/day

Adults: Initial: 2 g/day divided every 6 hours (range: 1-4 g/day)

Lead poisoning (treatment duration varies from 4-12 weeks depending upon the pretreatment blood lead level; goal of therapy is to reduce the total body content so that the blood lead level does not rebound to unacceptable levels post-treatment):

Children: 20-30 mg/kg/day in 3-4 divided doses; initiating treatment at 25% of this dose and gradually increasing to the full dose over 2-3 weeks may minimize adverse reactions; maximum dose: 1.5 g/day; a reduced dosage of 15 mg/kg/day in 2 divided doses has been shown to be effective in the treatment of mild to moderate lead poisoning (blood lead concentration 20-40 mcg/dL) with a reduction in adverse effects (see Shannon, 2000)

Adults: 1-1.5 g/day in 3-4 divided doses; initiating treatment at 25% of this dose and gradually increasing to the full dose over 2-3 weeks may minimize adverse reactions

Primary biliary cirrhosis: Adults: 250 mg/day to start, increase by 250 mg every 2 weeks up to a maintenance dose of 1 g/day, as 250 mg 4 times/day

Dosing adjustment in renal impairment: Cl_{cr} <50 mL/minute: Avoid use

Administration Oral: Administer on an empty stomach 1 hour before or 2 hours after meals, milk, or other medications; patients unable to swallow capsules may mix contents of capsule with fruit juice or chilled pureed fruit; patients with cystinuria should drink copious amounts of water

Monitoring Parameters Urinalysis, CBC with differential, hemoglobin, and platelet count are recommended twice weekly for the first month then every 2 weeks for 6 months and monthly thereafter; in addition, monitor the patient's skin, lymph nodes, and body temperature; liver function tests are recommended every 6 months; weekly measurements of urinary and blood concentrations of the intoxicating metal are indicated; quantitative 24-hour urine protein at 1- to 2-week intervals initially (first 2-3 months); annual x-ray for renal stones (when used for cystinuria)

Wilson's disease: Periodic ophthalmic exam; 24-hour urinary copper excretion; copper excretion is highest initially after treatment and may exceed 1000 mcg/day; chronic treatment should produce urinary copper excretion

of 200-500 mcg/day on treatment; values <200 mcg/day may be due to either noncompliance or overtreatment which may be differentiated by measuring nonceruloplasmin bound copper (high in noncompliance and low in overtreatment)

Reference Range Wilson's disease: Adequate treatment: "Free" (unbound) serum copper <10 mcg/dL (Free serum copper = Total copper - ceruloplasmin copper); 24-hour urinary copper excretion 200-500 mcg (3-8 micromoles)/day

Patient Information Possible severe allergic reaction if patient allergic to penicillin; notify physician if unusual bleeding or bruising, or persistent fever, sore throat, or fatigue occur. Report any unexplained cough, shortness of breath, or rash; loss of taste may occur; do not skip or miss doses or discontinue without notifying physician; cystinuric patients should drink copious amounts of fluid particularly before bed and once during the night

Additional Information The racemic mixture interferes with pyridoxine action and is no longer used; however, supplemental pyridoxine is still recommended.

Dosage Forms Excipient information presented when available (limited, particularly for generics); consult specific product labeling.

Capsule:
Cuprimine®: 250 mg

Tablet:
Depen®: 250 mg

Extemporaneous Preparations A 50 mg/mL suspension may be made by mixing sixty 250 mg capsules with 3 g carboxymethylcellulose, 150 g sucrose, 300 mg citric acid, parabens (methylparaben 120 mg, propylparaben 12 mg, propylene glycol qsad to 100 mL), and purified water to a total volume of 300 mL; cherry flavor may be added. Stability is 30 days refrigerated.

DeCastro FJ, Jaeger RQ, and Rolfe UT, "An Extemporaneously Prepared Penicillamine Suspension Used to Treat Lead Intoxication," *Hosp Pharm*, 1977, 2:446-8.

References

Piomelli S, "Childhood Lead Poisoning," *Pediatr Clin North Am*, 2002, 49(6):1285-304.

Roberts EA, Schilsky ML, and American Association for Study of Liver Diseases (AASLD)," Diagnosis and Treatment of Wilson Disease: An Update," *Hepatology*, 2008, 47(6):2089-111.

Shannon MW and Townsend MK, "Adverse Effects of Reduced-Dose d-Penicillamine in Children With Mild-to-Moderate Lead Poisoning," *Ann Pharmacother*, 2000, 34(1):15-8.

"Treatment Guidelines for Lead Exposure in Children. American Academy of Pediatrics Committee on Drugs," *Pediatrics*, 1995, 96(1 Pt 1):155-60.

Penicillin G Benzathine
(pen i SIL in jee BENZ a theen)

Medication Safety Issues

Sound-alike/look-alike issues:

Penicillin may be confused with penicillamine

Bicillin® may be confused with Wycillin®

Bicillin® C-R (penicillin G benzathine and penicillin G procaine) may be confused with Bicillin® L-A (penicillin G benzathine). Penicillin G benzathine is the only product currently approved for the treatment of syphilis. Administration of penicillin G benzathine and penicillin G procaine combination instead of Bicillin® L-A may result in inadequate treatment response.

Penicillin G benzathine may only be administered by deep intramuscular injection; intravenous administration of penicillin G benzathine has been associated with cardiopulmonary arrest and death.

U.S. Brand Names Bicillin® L-A

Canadian Brand Names Bicillin® L-A

Therapeutic Category Antibiotic, Penicillin

Generic Available No

Use Active against many gram-positive organisms and some spirochetes; treatment of syphilis; used only for the treatment of mild-to-moderate infections (ie, *Streptococcus* pharyngitis) caused by organisms susceptible to low concentrations of penicillin G, or for prophylaxis of infections caused by these organisms, such as rheumatic fever disease and acute glomerulonephritis [FDA approved in children (age not specified) and adults]

Pregnancy Risk Factor B

Pregnancy Considerations Adverse events have not been observed in animal studies; therefore, penicillin G is classified as pregnancy category B. Penicillin crosses the placenta and distributes into amniotic fluid. There is no evidence of adverse fetal effects after penicillin use during pregnancy in humans. Penicillin G is the drug of choice for treatment of syphilis during pregnancy.

Lactation Enters breast milk/use caution

Breast-Feeding Considerations Penicillins are excreted in breast milk. The manufacturer recommends that caution be exercised when administering penicillin to nursing women. Nondose-related effects could include modification of bowel flora and allergic sensitization.

Contraindications Hypersensitivity to penicillin or any component

Warnings Do not administer I.V.; do not admix with other I.V. solutions; inadvertent I.V. administration has resulted in cardiac arrest and death **[U.S. Boxed Warning]**. Injection into or near a nerve may result in permanent neurovascular and neurological damage, gangrene requiring amputation of proximal portions of extremities, necrosis, and sloughing at the injection site; effects have most often occurred in infants and small children. Serious hypersensitivity reactions, including anaphylaxis, have been reported; supportive therapy and medication for the management of anaphylactic reactions should be available for immediate use. Superinfection and *C. difficile*-associated diarrhea have been reported with use of penicillin G benzathine.

Precautions Use with caution in patients with impaired renal function, impaired cardiac function, pre-existing seizure disorder, history of significant allergies and/or asthma, or hypersensitivity to cephalosporins. Repeated I.M. injections into anterolateral thigh may result in quadriceps femoris fibrosis or atrophy.

Adverse Reactions

Cardiovascular: Cardiac arrest, hypotension, palpitations, syncope, tachycardia

Central nervous system: Coma, confusion, convulsions, dizziness, fever, lethargy, nervousness

Dermatologic: Pruritus, rash, urticaria

Gastrointestinal: Nausea, pseudomembranous colitis, vomiting

Genitourinary: Hematuria, neurogenic bladder, proteinuria

Hematologic: Eosinophilia, hemolytic anemia, leukopenia, thrombocytopenia

Hepatic: AST increased

Local: Abscess, ecchymosis, gangrene, inflammation, neurovascular damage, pain at injection site, swelling

Neuromuscular & skeletal: Myoclonus, neuropathy, tremor

Ophthalmic: Blurred vision

Renal: BUN and creatinine increased, interstitial nephritis, renal failure

Respiratory: Apnea, dyspnea, hypoxia

Miscellaneous: Anaphylaxis, hypersensitivity reactions, Jarisch-Herxheimer reaction, serum sickness-like reaction

Drug Interactions

Avoid Concomitant Use

Avoid concomitant use of Penicillin G Benzathine with any of the following: BCG

Increased Effect/Toxicity

Penicillin G Benzathine may increase the levels/effects of: Methotrexate

The levels/effects of Penicillin G Benzathine may be increased by: Probenecid

Decreased Effect

Penicillin G Benzathine may decrease the levels/effects of: BCG; Mycophenolate; Typhoid Vaccine

The levels/effects of Penicillin G Benzathine may be decreased by: Fusidic Acid; Tetracycline Derivatives

Stability Store in the refrigerator at 2°C to 8°C (36°F to 46°F); avoid freezing

Mechanism of Action Inhibits bacterial cell wall synthesis by binding to one or more of the penicillin-binding proteins; inhibits the final transpeptidation step of peptidoglycan synthesis in bacterial cell wall

Pharmacokinetics (Adult data unless noted)

Absorption: I.M.: Slow

Distribution: Minimal concentrations attained in CSF with inflamed or uninflamed meninges; highest levels in the kidneys; lesser amounts in liver, skin, intestine; excreted in breast milk

Protein binding: ~60%

Time to peak serum concentration: Within 12-24 hours; serum levels are usually detectable for 1-4 weeks depending on the dose; larger doses result in more sustained levels rather than higher levels

Elimination: Excreted by renal tubular excretion; penicillin G is detected in urine for up to 12 weeks after a single I.M. injection; renal clearance is delayed in neonates, young infants, and patients with impaired renal function

Usual Dosage I.M. (dosage frequency depends on infection being treated):

Neonates >1200 g: Asymptomatic congenital syphilis: 50,000 units/kg for 1 dose

Infants and Children:

Group A streptococcal upper respiratory infection (see Gerber, 2009):

Rheumatic fever, primary prevention:

≤27 kg: 600,000 units as a single dose

>27 kg: 1.2 million units as a single dose

Rheumatic fever, secondary prevention; **Note:** Duration of secondary rheumatic fever prophylaxis varies: Rheumatic fever with carditis and residual heart disease: 10 years or until 40 years of age (whichever is longer), sometimes lifelong prophylaxis; rheumatic fever with carditis but no residual heart disease: 10 years or until 21 years of age (whichever is longer); rheumatic fever without carditis: 5 years or until 21 years of age (whichever is longer)

≤27 kg: 600,000 units every 3-4 weeks

>27 kg: 1.2 million units every 3-4 weeks

Early syphilis: 50,000 units/kg as a single dose; maximum dose: 2.4 million units/dose (divided in 2 injection sites)

Syphilis of more than 1-year duration: 50,000 units/kg every week for 3 successive weeks; maximum dose: 2.4 million units/dose (divided in 2 injection sites)

Adults:

Group A streptococcal upper respiratory infection: 1.2 million units as a single dose

Rheumatic fever, secondary prevention: 600,000 units twice monthly or 1.2 million units every 4 weeks

Early syphilis: 2.4 million units as a single dose in 2 injection sites

Syphilis of more than 1-year duration: 2.4 million units/dose (divided in 2 injection sites) once weekly for 3 doses

Administration Administer undiluted as deep I.M. injection in the upper outer quadrant of the buttock (adolescents and adults) or into the midlateral aspect of the thigh (neonates, infants, and children); do **not** give I.V., intra-arterially or SubQ; **inadvertent I.V. administration has resulted in thrombosis, severe neurovascular damage, cardiac arrest, and death** (see Warnings)

Monitoring Parameters CBC, urinalysis, culture, renal function tests, stool frequency

Test Interactions Positive Coombs' [direct], false-positive urinary and/or serum proteins

Nursing Implications SubQ administration may cause pain and induration; avoid repeated I.M. injections into the anterolateral thigh in neonates and infants since quadriceps femoris fibrosis and atrophy may occur. Warm medication to room temperature before administration to decrease discomfort associated with I.M. injection.

Additional Information Use a penicillin G benzathine/penicillin G procaine combination (ie, Bicillin® C-R) to achieve early peak levels in acute infections. Do not administer Bicillin® C-R to treat patients infected with syphilis since this may result in inadequate treatment.

Dosage Forms Excipient information presented when available (limited, particularly for generics); consult specific product labeling.

Injection, suspension [prefilled syringe]:

Bicillin® L-A: 600,000 units/mL (1 mL, 2 mL, 4 mL)

References

Centers for Disease Control and Prevention, "Sexually Transmitted Diseases Treatment Guidelines - 2006," *MMWR Recomm Rep*, 2006, 55(RR-11):1-100. Available at http://www.cdc.gov/std/treatment/2006/rr5511.pdf. Accessed September 18, 2008.

Gerber MA, Baltimore RS, Eaton CB, et al, "Prevention of Rheumatic Fever and Diagnosis and Treatment of Acute *Streptococcal pharyngitis*: A Scientific Statement from the American Heart Association Rheumatic Fever, Endocarditis, and Kawasaki Disease Committee of the Council on Cardiovascular Disease in the Young, the Interdisciplinary Council on Functional Genomics and Translational Biology, and the Interdisciplinary Council on Quality of Care and Outcomes Research: Endorsed by the American Academy of Pediatrics," *Circulation*, 2009, 119(11):1541-51.

Kaplan EL, Berrios X, Speth J, et al, "Pharmacokinetics of Benzathine Penicillin G: Serum Levels During the 28 Days After Intramuscular Injection of 1,200,000 Units," *J Pediatr*, 1989, 115(1):146-50.

Paryani SG, Vaughn AJ, Crosby M, et al, "Treatment of Asymptomatic Congenital Syphilis: Benzathine Versus Procaine Penicillin G Therapy," *J Pediatr*, 1994, 125(3):471-5.

Penicillin G (Parenteral/Aqueous)

(pen i SIL in jee, pa REN ter al, AYE kwee us)

Medication Safety Issues

Sound-alike/look-alike issues:

Penicillin may be confused with penicillamine

U.S. Brand Names Pfizerpen®

Canadian Brand Names Crystapen®

Therapeutic Category Antibiotic, Penicillin

Generic Available Yes

Use Treatment of sepsis, meningitis, pericarditis, endocarditis, pneumonia, and other infections due to susceptible gram-positive organisms (except *Staphylococcus aureus*), some gram-negative organisms such as *Neisseria gonorrhoeae*, or *N. meningitidis* and some anaerobes and spirochetes

Pregnancy Risk Factor B

Pregnancy Considerations Adverse events have not been observed in animal studies; therefore, penicillin G is classified as pregnancy category B. Penicillin crosses the placenta and distributes into amniotic fluid. There is no evidence of adverse fetal effects after penicillin use during pregnancy in humans. Penicillin G is the drug of choice for treatment of syphilis during pregnancy and penicillin G (parenteral/aqueous) is the drug of choice for the prevention of early-onset Group B Streptococcal (GBS) disease in newborns.

Lactation Enters breast milk/compatible

Breast-Feeding Considerations Very small amounts of penicillin G transfer into breast milk. Peak milk concentrations occur at approximately 1 hour after an IM dose and are higher if multiple doses are given. The manufacturer recommends that caution be exercised when administering penicillin to nursing women. Nondose-related effects could include modification of bowel flora and allergic sensitization.

Contraindications Hypersensitivity to penicillin or any component

Precautions Use with caution in patients with renal impairment, hypersensitivity to cephalosporins, or pre-existing seizure disorder; dosage modification required in patients with renal impairment; further dosage reduction recommended in patients with impaired hepatic and renal function

Adverse Reactions

Central nervous system: Convulsions, confusion, lethargy, fever, dizziness

Dermatologic: Rash, urticaria

Endocrine & metabolic: Electrolyte imbalance

Gastrointestinal: Diarrhea

Hematologic: Hemolytic anemia, neutropenia

Local: Thrombophlebitis

Neuromuscular & skeletal: Myoclonus

Renal: Acute interstitial nephritis

Miscellaneous: Jarisch-Herxheimer reaction, hypersensitivity reactions, anaphylaxis

Drug Interactions

Avoid Concomitant Use

Avoid concomitant use of Penicillin G (Parenteral/Aqueous) with any of the following: BCG

Increased Effect/Toxicity

Penicillin G (Parenteral/Aqueous) may increase the levels/effects of: Methotrexate

The levels/effects of Penicillin G (Parenteral/Aqueous) may be increased by: Probenecid

Decreased Effect

Penicillin G (Parenteral/Aqueous) may decrease the levels/effects of: BCG; Mycophenolate; Typhoid Vaccine

The levels/effects of Penicillin G (Parenteral/Aqueous) may be decreased by: Fusidic Acid; Tetracycline Derivatives

Food Interactions Food or milk decreases absorption

Stability Reconstituted parenteral solution is stable for 7 days when refrigerated; incompatible with aminoglycosides; inactivated in acidic or alkaline solutions

Mechanism of Action Inhibits bacterial cell wall synthesis by binding to one or more of the penicillin-binding proteins; inhibits the final transpeptidation step of peptidoglycan synthesis in bacterial cell wall

Pharmacokinetics (Adult data unless noted)

Absorption: Oral: <30%

Distribution: Penetration across the blood-brain barrier is poor with uninflamed meninges; crosses the placenta; appears in breast milk

Protein binding: 65%

Metabolism: In the liver (10% to 30%) to penicilloic acid

Half-life:

Neonates:

<6 days: 3.2-3.4 hours

7-13 days: 1.2-2.2 hours

>14 days: 0.9-1.9 hours

Infants and Children: 0.5-1.2 hours

Adults: 0.5-0.75 hours with normal renal function

Time to peak serum concentration:

Oral: Within 30-60 minutes

I.M.: Within 30 minutes

Elimination: Penicillin G and its metabolites are excreted in urine mainly by tubular secretion

Dialysis: Moderately dialyzable (20% to 50%)

Usual Dosage

Neonates: I.M., I.V.:

Postnatal age ≤7 days:

≤2000 g: 50,000 units/kg/day in divided doses every 12 hours

Meningitis: 100,000 units/kg/day in divided doses every 12 hours

>2000 g: 75,000 units/kg/day in divided doses every 8 hours

Meningitis: 150,000 units/kg/day in divided doses every 8 hours

Congenital syphilis: 100,000 units/kg/day in divided doses every 12 hours

Group B streptococcal meningitis: 250,000-450,000 units/kg/day in divided doses every 8 hours

Postnatal age >7 days:

<1200 g: 50,000 units/kg/day in divided doses every 12 hours

Meningitis: 100,000 units/kg/day in divided doses every 12 hours

1200-2000 g: 75,000 units/kg/day in divided doses every 8 hours

Meningitis: 150,000 units/kg/day in divided doses every 8 hours

>2000 g: 100,000 units/kg/day in divided doses every 6 hours

Meningitis: 200,000 units/kg/day in divided doses every 6 hours

Congenital syphilis: 150,000 units/kg/day in divided doses every 8 hours

Group B streptococcal meningitis: I.V.: 450,000 units/kg/day in divided doses every 6 hours

Infants and Children:

I.M., I.V.: 100,000 to 250,000 units/kg/day in divided doses every 4-6 hours

Severe infections: 250,000-400,000 units/kg/day in divided doses every 4-6 hours; maximum dose: 24 million units/day

Adults: I.M., I.V.: 2-24 million units/day in divided doses every 4-6 hours

Dosing interval in renal impairment:

Cl$_{cr}$ 10-30 mL/minute: Administer normal dose every 8-12 hours

Cl$_{cr}$ <10 mL/minute: Administer normal dose every 12-18 hours

Administration Parenteral: Administer by I.V. intermittent infusion over 15-60 minutes at a final concentration for administration of 100,000-500,000 units/mL. A final concentration of 50,000 units/mL infused over 15-30 minutes is recommended for neonates and infants. The potassium or sodium content of the dose should be considered when determining the infusion rate.

Monitoring Parameters Periodic serum electrolytes, renal and hematologic function tests

Test Interactions False-positive or negative urinary glucose determination using Clinitest®; positive Coombs' [direct]; false-positive urinary and/or serum proteins

Additional Information

Penicillin G potassium: 1.7 mEq of potassium and 0.3 mEq of sodium per 1 million units of penicillin G

Penicillin G sodium: 2 mEq of sodium per 1 million units of penicillin G

Dosage Forms Excipient information presented when available (limited, particularly for generics); consult specific product labeling.

Infusion, as potassium [premixed iso-osmotic dextrose solution, frozen]: 1 million units (50 mL), 2 million units (50 mL), 3 million units (50 mL) [contains sodium 1.02 mEq and potassium 1.7 mEq per 1 million units]

Injection, powder for reconstitution, as potassium (Pfizerpen®): 5 million units, 20 million units [contains sodium 6.8 mg (0.3 mEq) and potassium 65.6 mg (1.68 mEq) per 1 million units]

Injection, powder for reconstitution, as sodium: 5 million units [contains sodium 1.68 mEq per 1 million units]

References

American Academy of Pediatrics Committee on Infectious Diseases, "Treatment of Bacterial Meningitis," *Pediatrics*, 1988, 81(6):904-7.

Prober CG, Stevenson DK, and Benitz WE, "The Use of Antibiotics in Neonates Weighing Less Than 1200 Grams," *Pediatr Infect Dis J*, 1990, 9(2):111-21.

◆ **Penicillin G Potassium** *see* Penicillin G (Parenteral/Aqueous) *on page 1080*

Penicillin G Procaine (pen i SIL in jee PROE kane)

Medication Safety Issues

Sound-alike/look-alike issues:

Penicillin G procaine may be confused with penicillin V potassium

Wycillin® may be confused with Bicillin®

Canadian Brand Names Pfizerpen-AS®; Wycillin®

Therapeutic Category Antibiotic, Penicillin

Generic Available Yes

Use Moderately severe infections due to *Treponema pallidum* and other penicillin G-sensitive microorganisms that are susceptible to low but prolonged serum penicillin concentrations

Pregnancy Risk Factor B

Pregnancy Considerations Adverse events have not been observed in animal studies; therefore, penicillin G is classified as pregnancy category B. Penicillin crosses the placenta and distributes into amniotic fluid. There is no evidence of adverse fetal effects after penicillin use during pregnancy in humans.

Lactation Enters breast milk/compatible

Breast-Feeding Considerations Penicillins are excreted in breast milk. The manufacturer recommends that caution be exercised when administering penicillin to nursing women. Nondose-related effects could include modification of bowel flora and allergic sensitization.

Contraindications Hypersensitivity to penicillin, procaine, or any component (see Warnings)

Warnings Some formulations contain sulfites which may cause allergic reactions in susceptible individuals

Precautions Use with caution in patients with renal impairment, hypersensitivity to cephalosporins, or history of seizures; modify dosage in patients with severe renal impairment

Adverse Reactions

Cardiovascular: Myocardial depression, vasodilation, conduction disturbances

Central nervous system: Seizures, confusion, lethargy, dizziness, disorientation, agitation, hallucinations

Hematologic: Hemolytic anemia

Local: Sterile abscess and pain at injection site

Neuromuscular & skeletal: Myoclonus

Renal: Interstitial nephritis

Miscellaneous: Pseudoanaphylactic reactions, Jarisch-Herxheimer reaction, hypersensitivity reactions

Drug Interactions

Avoid Concomitant Use

Avoid concomitant use of Penicillin G Procaine with any of the following: BCG

Increased Effect/Toxicity

Penicillin G Procaine may increase the levels/effects of: Methotrexate

The levels/effects of Penicillin G Procaine may be increased by: Probenecid

◄ **Decreased Effect**
Penicillin G Procaine may decrease the levels/effects of:
BCG; Mycophenolate; Typhoid Vaccine

The levels/effects of Penicillin G Procaine may be decreased by: Fusidic Acid; Tetracycline Derivatives
Stability Store in refrigerator
Mechanism of Action Inhibits bacterial cell wall synthesis by binding to one or more of the penicillin-binding proteins; inhibits the final transpeptidation step of peptidoglycan synthesis in bacterial cell wall
Pharmacokinetics (Adult data unless noted)
Absorption: I.M.: Slow
Distribution: Penetration across the blood-brain barrier is poor, despite inflamed meninges; appears in breast milk
Time to peak serum concentration: Within 1-4 hours and can persist within the therapeutic range for 15-24 hours
Elimination: Renal clearance is delayed in neonates, young infants, and patients with impaired renal function
Dialysis: Moderately dialyzable (20% to 50%)
Usual Dosage I.M.:
Neonates ≥1200 g: Avoid using in this age group since sterile abscesses and procaine toxicity occur more frequently with neonates than older patients
Congenital syphilis: 50,000 units/kg/day once daily for 10 days; if more than 1 day of therapy is missed, the entire course should be restarted
Infants and Children: 25,000-50,000 units/kg/day in divided doses every 12-24 hours; not to exceed 4.8 million units/24 hours
Congenital syphilis: 50,000 units/kg/day once daily for 10 days; if more than 1 day of therapy is missed, the entire course should be restarted
Adults: 0.6-4.8 million units/day in divided doses every 12-24 hours
When used in conjunction with an aminoglycoside for the treatment of endocarditis caused by susceptible *S. viridans*: 1.2 million units every 6 hours for 2-4 weeks
Neurosyphilis: 2.4 million units once daily for 10 days with probenecid 500 mg every 6 hours
Administration Parenteral: **Do not give I.V., intra-arterially, or SubQ**; procaine suspension for deep I.M. injection only; inadvertent I.V. administration has resulted in neurovascular damage; in infants and children it is preferable to administer I.M. into the midlateral muscles of the thigh; in adults, administer into the gluteus maximus or into the midlateral muscles of the thigh
Monitoring Parameters Periodic renal and hematologic function tests with prolonged therapy
Test Interactions Positive Coombs' [direct], false-positive urinary and/or serum proteins
Nursing Implications Avoid repeated I.M. injections into the anterolateral thigh in neonates and infants since quadriceps femoris fibrosis and atrophy may occur
Dosage Forms Excipient information presented when available (limited, particularly for generics); consult specific product labeling.
Injection, suspension: 600,000 units/mL (1 mL, 2 mL)
References
Paryani SG, Vaughn AJ, Crosby M, et al, "Treatment of Asymptomatic Congenital Syphilis: Benzathine Versus Procaine Penicillin G Therapy," *J Pediatr*, 1994, 125(3):471-5.

◆ **Penicillin G Sodium** *see* Penicillin G (Parenteral/Aqueous) *on page 1080*

Penicillin V Potassium
(pen i SIL in vee poe TASS ee um)

Medication Safety Issues
Sound-alike/look-alike issues:
Penicillin V procaine may be confused with penicillin G potassium

Canadian Brand Names Apo-Pen VK®; Novo-Pen-VK; Nu-Pen-VK
Therapeutic Category Antibiotic, Penicillin
Generic Available Yes
Use Treatment of mild to moderately severe susceptible bacterial infections involving the upper respiratory tract, skin, and urinary tract; prophylaxis of pneumococcal infections and rheumatic fever (FDA approved in ages ≥12 years and adults)
Pregnancy Risk Factor B
Pregnancy Considerations Adverse events have not been observed in animal studies; therefore, penicillin V is classified as pregnancy category B. Penicillin crosses the placenta and distributes into amniotic fluid. There is no evidence of adverse fetal effects after penicillin use during pregnancy in humans. Due to pregnancy-induced physiologic changes, some pharmacokinetic parameters of penicillin V may be altered in the second and third trimester. Higher doses or increased dosing frequency may be required.
Lactation Enters breast milk/compatible
Breast-Feeding Considerations Penicillins are excreted in breast milk. The manufacturer recommends that caution be exercised when administering penicillin to nursing women. Nondose-related effects could include modification of bowel flora and allergic sensitization.
Contraindications Hypersensitivity to penicillin or any component
Warnings Oral solution contains sodium benzoate; benzoic acid (benzoate) is a metabolite of benzyl alcohol; large amounts of benzyl alcohol (≥99 mg/kg/day) have been associated with a potentially fatal toxicity ("gasping syndrome") in neonates; the "gasping syndrome" consists of metabolic acidosis, respiratory distress, gasping respirations, CNS dysfunction (including convulsions, intracranial hemorrhage), hypotension and cardiovascular collapse; use oral solution containing sodium benzoate with caution in neonates; *in vitro* and animal studies have shown that benzoate displaces bilirubin from protein binding sites
Precautions Use with caution in patients with renal impairment, hypersensitivity to cephalosporins, or history of seizures; dosage adjustment may be necessary in patients with renal impairment; oral solution may contain aspartame which is metabolized to phenylalanine and must be avoided (or used with caution) in patients with phenylketonuria
Adverse Reactions
Central nervous system: Convulsions, fever
Dermatologic: Rash
Gastrointestinal: Black hairy tongue, diarrhea, nausea, pseudomembranous colitis, vomiting
Hematologic: Hemolytic anemia
Renal: Acute interstitial nephritis
Miscellaneous: Anaphylaxis, hypersensitivity reactions
Drug Interactions
Avoid Concomitant Use
Avoid concomitant use of Penicillin V Potassium with any of the following: BCG
Increased Effect/Toxicity
Penicillin V Potassium may increase the levels/effects of: Methotrexate

The levels/effects of Penicillin V Potassium may be increased by: Probenecid
Decreased Effect
Penicillin V Potassium may decrease the levels/effects of: BCG; Mycophenolate; Typhoid Vaccine

The levels/effects of Penicillin V Potassium may be decreased by: Fusidic Acid; Tetracycline Derivatives
Food Interactions Food or milk may decrease absorption

Stability Refrigerate suspension after reconstitution; discard after 14 days

Mechanism of Action Interferes with bacterial cell wall synthesis during active multiplication by binding to one or more of the penicillin-binding proteins; inhibits the final transpeptidation step of peptidoglycan synthesis causing cell wall death and resultant bactericidal activity against susceptible bacteria

Pharmacokinetics (Adult data unless noted)

Absorption: Oral: 60% to 73% from the GI tract

Distribution: Widely distributed to kidneys, liver, skin, tonsils, and into synovial, pleural, and pericardial fluids; appears in breast milk

Protein binding: 80%

Metabolism: 10% to 30%

Half-life: 30 minutes and is prolonged in patients with renal impairment

Time to peak serum concentration: Within 30-60 minutes

Elimination: Penicillin V and its metabolites are excreted in urine mainly by tubular secretion

Usual Dosage Oral:

Systemic infections:

Children <12 years: 25-50 mg/kg/day in divided doses every 6-8 hours; maximum dose: 3 g/day

Children ≥12 years and Adults: 125-500 mg every 6-8 hours

Primary prevention of rheumatic fever (treatment of streptococcal tonsillopharyngitis):

Children ≤27 kg: 250 mg 2-3 times/day for 10 days

Children >27 kg, Adolescents, and Adults: 500 mg 2-3 times/day for 10 days

Prophylaxis of pneumococcal infections in children with sickle cell disease (SCD) and functional or anatomic asplenia: Children:

Before 2 months of age or as soon as SCD or asplenia occurs up to 3 years of age: 125 mg twice daily

>3 years: 250 mg twice daily; the decision to discontinue penicillin prophylaxis after 5 years of age in children who have not experienced invasive pneumococcal infection and have received recommended pneumococcal immunizations is patient and clinician dependent

Recurrent rheumatic fever, prophylaxis: Children and Adults: 250 mg twice daily

Administration Oral: Administer with water on an empty stomach 1 hour before or 2 hours after meals; may be administered with food to decrease GI upset

Monitoring Parameters Periodic renal and hematologic function tests during prolonged therapy

Test Interactions False-positive or negative urinary glucose determination using Clinitest®; positive Coombs' [direct]; false-positive urinary and/or serum proteins

Additional Information 0.7 mEq of potassium/250 mg penicillin V; 250 mg = 400,000 units of penicillin

Dosage Forms Excipient information presented when available (limited, particularly for generics); consult specific product labeling.

Note: 250 mg = 400,000 units

Powder for oral solution: 125 mg/5 mL (100 mL, 200 mL); 250 mg/5 mL (100 mL, 200 mL)

Tablet: 250 mg, 500 mg

References

"American Academy of Pediatrics. Committee on Infectious Diseases. Policy Statement: Recommendations for the Prevention of Pneumococcal Infections, Including the Use of Pneumococcal Conjugate Vaccine (Prevnar™), Pneumococcal Polysaccharide Vaccine, and Antibiotic Prophylaxis," *Pediatrics*, 2000, 106(2 Pt 1):362-6.

Dajani A, Taubert K, Ferrieri P, et al, "Treatment of Acute Streptococcal Pharyngitis and Prevention of Rheumatic Fever: A Statement for Health Professionals. Committee on Rheumatic Fever, Endocarditis, and Kawasaki Disease of the Council on Cardiovascular Disease in the Young, the American Heart Association," *Pediatrics*, 1995, 96(4 Pt 1):758-64.

Gerber MA, Baltimore RS, Eaton CB, et al, "Prevention of Rheumatic Fever and Diagnosis and Treatment of Acute *Streptococcal pharyngitis*: A Scientific Statement from the American Heart Association Rheumatic Fever, Endocarditis, and Kawasaki Disease Committee of the Council on Cardiovascular Disease in the Young, the Interdisciplinary Council on Functional Genomics and Translational Biology, and the Interdisciplinary Council on Quality of Care and Outcomes Research: Endorsed by the American Academy of Pediatrics," *Circulation*, 2009, 119(11):1541-51.

◆ **Penlac®** see Ciclopirox on page 306

◆ **Pennsaid®** see Diclofenac on page 429

◆ **Pentacel®** see Diphtheria and Tetanus Toxoids, Acellular Pertussis, Poliovirus and *Haemophilus* b Conjugate Vaccine on page 455

◆ **Pentahydrate** see Sodium Thiosulfate on page 1280

◆ **Pentam®-300** see Pentamidine on page 1083

Pentamidine (pen TAM i deen)

U.S. Brand Names NebuPent®; Pentam®-300

Therapeutic Category Antibiotic, Miscellaneous; Antiprotozoal

Generic Available No

Use Treatment and prevention of pneumonia caused by *Pneumocystis jiroveci* (formerly *carinii*) (PCP) (I.V., I.M.: FDA approved in ages ≥5 months and adults; aerosol: FDA approved in ages ≥17 years and adults); Note: The CDC recommends pentamidine for patients who cannot tolerate or who fail to respond to sulfamethoxazole and trimethoprim. Has also been used in the treatment of African trypanosomiasis, cutaneous leishmaniasis, and amebic meningoencephalitis

Pregnancy Risk Factor C

Pregnancy Considerations Animal reproductive studies were not conducted by the manufacturer; therefore, pentamidine is classified pregnancy category C. In postmarketing studies, pentamidine was embryocidal but not teratogenic when administered to animals. Pentamidine crosses the human placenta. Administration via the aerosolized route may minimize maternal serum concentrations. Concern regarding occupational exposure of pregnant healthcare workers has been discussed in the literature. Healthcare workers should avoid aerolized exposure if possible. If avoidance is not possible, they should wear a mask and gloves and ensure proper ventilation. Pentamidine may be used in pregnancy for prophylaxis or treatment of PCP if the patient is unable to take first line medications.

Lactation Excretion in breast milk unknown/not recommended

Breast-Feeding Considerations It is not known if pentamidine is excreted in human milk and use of pentamidine during breast-feeding is not recommended by the manufacturer. In the United States where formula is accessible, affordable, safe, and sustainable, complete avoidance of breast-feeding by HIV-infected women is recommended by the AAP and the CDC to decrease potential transmission of HIV.

Contraindications Hypersensitivity to pentamidine isethionate or any component

Warnings Sudden, severe hypotension (including some fatalities) has been observed, even after a single dose; may occur with either I.V. or I.M. administration, although more common with rapid I.V. administration; monitor blood pressure. Aerosolized pentamidine may induce bronchospasm or cough, especially in patients with asthma (inhaled bronchodilator therapy prior to pentamidine may control symptoms); acute pancreatitis has been reported in patients receiving aerosolized pentamidine; acute PCP may develop despite aerosolized pentamidine prophylaxis; although rare, extrapulmonary *Pneumocystis jiroveci* disease may occur and has been associated with

▶

aerosolized pentamidine. Healthcare personnel who administer aerosolized pentamidine inhalation therapy should be aware of the possibility of secondary exposure to tuberculosis or other infections from patients with undiagnosed pulmonary disease; use appropriate precautions to minimize exposure to healthcare personnel. Extravasations which have proceeded to ulceration, tissue necrosis, and/or sloughing at the injection site have been reported; closely monitor I.V. site. Stevens-Johnson syndrome has been reported with use.

Precautions Use with caution in patients with diabetes mellitus, renal or hepatic dysfunction, pancreatitis, leukopenia, thrombocytopenia, anemia, cardiovascular disease, hypertension, hypotension, or hypocalcemia; adjust dose in renal impairment. Concurrent use with other bone marrow suppressants may increase the risk for myelotoxicity; use with other nephrotoxic drugs (ie, aminoglycosides, amphotericin B, cisplatin, foscarnet, vancomycin) may increase the risk for nephrotoxicity

Adverse Reactions

Aerosol:
Cardiovascular: Chest pain
Central nervous system: Dizziness/light-headedness, fatigue, fever, headache
Dermatologic: Stevens-Johnson syndrome
Gastrointestinal: Appetite decreased, diarrhea, nausea, oral candida, taste alteration
Hematologic: Anemia
Respiratory: Bronchitis, bronchospasm, chest pain, cough, dyspnea, pharyngitis, sinusitis, upper respiratory tract infection, wheezing
Miscellaneous: Extrapulmonary *Pneumocystis jiroveci* disease, herpes infection, infection, influenza, night sweats

Injection:
Cardiovascular: Hypotension, ST segment abnormal, ventricular tachycardia
Central nervous system: Confusion/hallucinations
Dermatologic: Rash, Stevens-Johnson syndrome
Endocrine & metabolic: Hyperglycemia, hyperkalemia, hypocalcemia, hypoglycemia
Gastrointestinal: Nausea/anorexia, pancreatitis, taste alteration
Hematologic: Anemia, leukopenia, thrombocytopenia
Hepatic: Hepatic dysfunction, liver function tests increased
Local: Extravasation (tissue ulceration, necrosis, and/or sloughing), local reactions at I.M. injection site (includes induration, necrosis, pain, sterile abscess)
Renal: Azotemia, BUN increased, creatinine increased, renal function impaired

Aerosol or injection: <1%, postmarketing, and/or case reports: Allergic reaction, anaphylaxis, asthma, blepharitis, blurred vision, cardiac arrhythmia, central venous line related sepsis, cerebrovascular accident, chills, clotting time prolonged, CMV infection, colitis, congestion (chest, nasal), conjunctivitis, cryptococcal meningitis, cyanosis, defibrination, dermatitis, desquamation, diabetes mellitus/ketoacidosis, eosinophilia, erythema, esophagitis, extrapulmonary pneumocystosis, facial edema, flank pain, gait unsteady, gagging, gingivitis, hearing loss, hematochezia, hematuria, hemoptysis, hepatitis, hepatomegaly, histoplasmosis, hypersalivation, hypertension, hyperventilation, hypesthesia, hypomagnesemia, incontinence, insomnia, Jarisch-Herxheimer-like reaction, laryngitis, laryngospasm, leg edema, megaloblastic anemia, melena, memory loss, nephritis, nervousness, neuralgia, neuropathy, neutropenia, palpitation, pancytopenia, paronoia, paresthesia, peripheral neuropathy, phlebitis, pleuritis, pneumonitis (eosinophilic or interstitial), pneumothorax, pruritus, rales, renal failure, rhinitis, seizure, splenomagaly, syncope, syndrome of inappropriate antidiuretic hormone (SIADH), tachypnea, temperature abnormal, torsades de pointes, transient arterial desaturation, tremor, vasodilation, vasculitis, vertigo, vomiting, urticaria, xerostomia

Drug Interactions

Metabolism/Transport Effects Substrate of CYP2C19 (major); **Inhibits** CYP2C8/9 (weak), 2C19 (weak), 2D6 (weak), 3A4 (weak)

Avoid Concomitant Use

Avoid concomitant use of Pentamidine with any of the following: Artemether; BCG; Dronedarone; Lumefantrine; Nilotinib; Pimozide; QuiNINE; Tetrabenazine; Thioridazine; Ziprasidone

Increased Effect/Toxicity

Pentamidine may increase the levels/effects of: Dronedarone; Pimozide; QTc-Prolonging Agents; QuiNINE; Tetrabenazine; Thioridazine; Ziprasidone

The levels/effects of Pentamidine may be increased by: Alfuzosin; Artemether; Chloroquine; Ciprofloxacin; Ciprofloxacin (Systemic); CYP2C19 Inhibitors (Moderate); CYP2C19 Inhibitors (Strong); Gadobutrol; Lumefantrine; Nilotinib; QuiNINE

Decreased Effect

Pentamidine may decrease the levels/effects of: BCG; Typhoid Vaccine

The levels/effects of Pentamidine may be decreased by: CYP2C19 Inducers (Strong)

Stability Store intact vials at 20°C to 25°C (68°F to 77°F); protect from light; do not reconstitute with NS because precipitation will occur.
Aerosol: The manufacturer recommends the use of freshly prepared solutions for inhalation; once reconstituted, the solution is stable for up to 48 hours in the vial at room temperature; protect from light. Do **not** mix with other nebulizer solutions.
Injection: After reconstitution with SWI, solution is stable for 48 hours in the vial at room temperature if protected from light. Store at 22°C to 30°C (72°F to 86°F) to avoid crystallization. Solutions for infusion (1-2.5 mg/mL) in D_5W are stable for at least 24 hours at room temperature.

Mechanism of Action Interferes with RNA/DNA, phospholipids and protein synthesis through inhibition of oxidative phosphorylation and/or interference with incorporation of nucleotides and nucleic acids into RNA and DNA in protozoa

Pharmacokinetics (Adult data unless noted)

Absorption: I.M.: Well absorbed; Aerosol: Limited systemic absorption
Distribution: Binds to tissues and plasma protein; high concentrations are found in the liver, kidney, adrenals, spleen, lungs and pancreas; poor penetration into CNS; following oral inhalation, high concentrations are found in bronchoalveolar fluid; V_{dss}: I.V.: 821 ± 535 L; I.M.: 2724 ± 1066 L
Half-life: 5-8 hours; I.M.: 7-11 hours; half-life may be prolonged in patients with severe renal impairment
Elimination: I.V.: ≤12% in urine as unchanged drug
Dialysis: Not appreciably removed by hemodialysis or peritoneal dialysis

Usual Dosage

Children:
PCP:
Treatment: (Infants ≥5 months, Children, and Adolescents): I.M., I.V. (I.V. preferred): 4 mg/kg/dose once daily for 14-21 days
CDC recommendation:
Prevention (Children ≥5 years and Adolescents): Inhalation: 300 mg/dose monthly via Respirgard® II nebulizer
Treatment: I.V.: 3-4 mg/kg/dose once daily for 21 days

AIDS Info guidelines (2009):

Prevention (Children ≥5 years and Adolescents): Inhalation: 300 mg/dose monthly via Respirgard® II nebulizer

Treatment: I.V.: 4 mg/kg/dose once daily, if clinical improvement may change to atovaquone after 7-10 days

Prevention in pediatric oncology patients ≥2 years (intolerant to trimethoprim-sulfamethoxazole): 4 mg/kg/dose I.V. once a month (see Kim, 2008; Prasad, 2007)

Trypanosomiasis: Treatment: I.M.: 4 mg/kg/dose once daily for 7 days

Cutaneous leishmaniasis: Treatment: I.M., I.V.: 2-3 mg/kg/dose once daily or every 2 days for 4-7 doses

Adults: PCP:

FDA approved labeling:

Treatment: I.M., I.V. (I.V. preferred): 4 mg/kg/dose once daily for 14-21 days

Prevention: Inhalation: 300 mg/dose every 4 weeks via Respirgard® II nebulizer

CDC recommendation:

Prevention: Inhalation: 300 mg/dose monthly via Respirgard® II nebulizer

Treatment: I.V.: 3-4 mg/kg/dose once daily for 21 days

AIDS Info guidelines (2009):

Prevention: Inhalation: 300 mg/dose monthly via Respirgard® II nebulizer

Treatment: I.V.: 4 mg/kg/dose once daily; 3 mg/kg/dose may be used by some clinicians due to toxicities

Dosing adjustment in renal impairment: The FDA-approved labeling recommends that caution should be used in patients with renal impairment; however, no specific dosage adjustment guidelines are available. The following guidelines have been used by some clinicians (Aronoff, 2007):

Children: I.V.:

Cl_{cr} >30 mL/minute: No adjustment required

Cl_{cr} 10-30 mL/minute: Administer 4 mg/kg/dose every 36 hours

Cl_{cr} <10 mL/minute and peritoneal dialysis: Administer 4 mg/kg/dose every 48 hours

Hemodialysis: Administer 4 mg/kg/dose every 48 hours, after dialysis on dialysis days

Adults: I.V.:

Cl_{cr} >10 mL/minute: No adjustment required

Cl_{cr} <10 mL/minute: Administer 4 mg/kg/dose every 24-36 hours

Administration

Oral inhalation: Safe and effective administration via nebulization in children is dependent on patients wearing an appropriately sized pediatric face mask. Deliver via Respirgard® II nebulizer until nebulizer is emptied (30-45 minutes). Use appropriate precautions to minimize exposure to healthcare personnel; refer to individual institutional policy. Reconstitute with 6 mL SWI. The manufacturer recommends the use of freshly prepared solutions for inhalation. Do not mix with other nebulizer solutions.

Parenteral:

I.M.: Reconstitute vial with 3 mL SWI to a final concentration of 100 mg/mL; administer deep I.M.

I.V.: Reconstitute with 3-5 mL SWI or D_5W; the manufacturer recommends further dilution in D_5W; however, stability with further dilution in NS has also been documented. Administer by slow I.V. infusion over a period of at least 60-120 minutes at a final concentration for administration not to exceed 6 mg/mL; rapid I.V. administration can cause severe hypotension. Avoid extravasation; assess catheter position before and during infusion

Monitoring Parameters Liver function tests, renal function tests, blood glucose, serum potassium and calcium, CBC with differential and platelet count, ECG, blood pressure

Patient Information Maintain adequate fluid intake; notify physician if fever, cough, or shortness of breath occurs; avoid alcohol

Nursing Implications Patients should receive parenteral pentamidine while lying down and blood pressure should be monitored closely during administration and after completion of the infusion until blood pressure is stabilized; if hypotension occurs due to rapid I.V. administration, slow infusion rate to administer dose over 1-2 hours

Additional Information 1 mg pentamidine: 1.74 mg pentamidine isethionate

Dosage Forms Excipient information presented when available (limited, particularly for generics); consult specific product labeling.

Injection, powder for reconstitution, as isethionate [preservative free]:

Pentam®-300: 300 mg

Powder for solution, for nebulization, as isethionate [preservative free]:

NebuPent®: 300 mg

References

Aronoff GR, Bennett WM, Berns JS, et al, *Drug Prescribing in Renal Failure: Dosing Guidelines for Adults and Children*, 5th ed, Philadelphia, PA: American College of Physicians, 2007, 97, 177.

Centers for Disease Control and Prevention, "Amebic Meningoence-phalitis, Primary and Granulomatous." Available at: http://www.dpd.cdc.gov/dpdx/HTML/PDF_Files/MedLetter/AmebicMeningo-encephalitis.pdf.

Centers for Disease Control, "Guidelines for Prevention and Treatment of Opportunistic Infections Among HIV-Exposed and HIV-Infected Children," *MMWR Recomm Rep*, 2009, 58(RR-11):1-176. Available at: http://aidsinfo.nih.gov/contentfiles/Pediatric_OI.pdf .

Centers for Disease Control, "Guidelines for Prevention and Treatment of Opportunistic Infections in HIV-Infected Adults and Adolescents," *MMWR Recomm Rep*, 2009, 58(RR-4):1-194. Available at: http://www.cdc.gov/mmwr/pdf/rr/rr5804.pdf.

Centers for Disease Control and Prevention, "Leishmania." Available at: http://www.dpd.cdc.gov/dpdx/HTML/PDF_Files/MedLetter/Leishmania.pdf.

Centers for Disease Control and Prevention, "*Pneumocystis jiroveci* (formerly *carinii*) Pneumonia (PCP)." Available at: http://www.dpd.cdc.gov/dpdx/HTML/PDF_Files/MedLetter/Pneumo-cystis_jiroveci.pdf.

Centers for Disease Control and Prevention, "Trypanosomiasis." Available at: http://www.dpd.cdc.gov/dpdx/HTML/PDF_Files/MedLet-ter/Trypanosomiasis.pdf.

Kim SY, Dabb AA, Glenn DJ, et al, "Intravenous Pentamidine Is Effective as Second Line Pneumocystis Pneumonia Prophylaxis in Pediatric Oncology Patients," *Pediatr Blood Cancer*, 2008, 50 (4):779-83.

Prasad P, Nania JJ, and Shankar SM, "Pneumocystis Pneumonia in Children Receiving Chemotherapy," *Pediatr Blood Cancer*, 2008, 50 (4):896-8.

◆ **Pentamidine Isethionate** *see* Pentamidine *on page 1083*

◆ **Pentamycetin® (Can)** *see* Chloramphenicol *on page 289*

◆ **Pentasa®** *see* Mesalamine *on page 887*

◆ **Pentasodium Colistin Methanesulfonate** *see* Colistimethate *on page 357*

◆ **Pentavalent Human-Bovine Reassortant Rotavirus Vaccine (PRV)** *see* Rotavirus Vaccine *on page 1237*

Pentazocine (pen TAZ oh seen)

Medication Safety Issues

High alert medication: The Institute for Safe Medication Practices (ISMP) includes this medication among its list of drug classes which have a heightened risk of causing significant patient harm when used in error.

Beers Criteria medication: This drug may be inappropriate for use in geriatric patients (high severity risk).

Related Information

Compatibility of Medications Mixed in a Syringe *on page 1713*

Opioid Analgesics Comparison *on page 1510*

U.S. Brand Names Talwin®

Canadian Brand Names Talwin®

Therapeutic Category Analgesic, Narcotic; Opioid Partial Agonist; Sedative

Generic Available No

Use Relief of moderate to severe pain (FDA approved in adults); a sedative prior to surgery (FDA approved in ages ≥1 year and adults); supplement to surgical anesthesia (FDA approved in adults)

Restrictions C-IV

Pregnancy Risk Factor C

Pregnancy Considerations Pentazocine was not found to be teratogenic in animal studies. Pentazocine has been shown to cross the human placenta. Use should be avoided during labor and delivery of premature infants. Abstinence syndromes in the newborn have been reported after long-term use of pentazocine during pregnancy. Other adverse effects in the newborn have been reported following abuse of pentazocine during pregnancy; these effects may be due to pentazocine, other drugs abused, the mother's lifestyle, or a combination of all factors.

Lactation Enters breast milk/use caution

Breast-Feeding Considerations Pentazocine is excreted in human breast milk. Treatment of the mother with single doses of pentazocine is not expected to cause detrimental effects in nursing infants.

Contraindications Hypersensitivity to pentazocine or any component (see Warnings)

Warnings Pentazocine is a potent opioid analgesic which may cause physical and psychological dependence; abrupt discontinuation after prolonged use may result in withdrawal symptoms or seizures; use with caution in patients with a history of prior opioid dependence or abuse. Pentazocine is also a mild opioid antagonist and may precipitate opiate withdrawal symptoms in patients who have been receiving opiates regularly. Use with extreme caution in patients with head injury, intracranial lesions, or elevated intracranial pressure; exaggerated elevation of ICP may occur. Respiratory depression has been reported (rarely); use with caution in patients with respiratory depression, limited respiratory reserve, severe asthma, other obstructive respiratory conditions, or cyanosis; do not use if appropriate rescue respiratory therapy equipment is unavailable. May cause acute CNS manifestations such as hallucinations, disorientation, and confusion; most cases resolve within a few hours without intervention; monitor closely; use caution if drug is reintroduced after these effects subside; CNS effects may recur.

Severe sclerosis of skin, subcutaneous tissue, and underlying muscle have occurred at injection site; avoid SubQ use unless absolutely necessary; rotate injection site to minimize risk. Injection may contain sodium bisulfite which may cause allergic reactions in susceptible individuals.

Precautions Use with caution in seizure-prone patients, acute MI, patients undergoing biliary tract surgery, and patients with renal, hepatic, or respiratory dysfunction; decrease dosage in patients with decreased hepatic or renal function. Use with caution in ambulatory patients; pentazocine may cause CNS depression and dizziness, which may impair physical or mental abilities; patients must be cautioned against performing tasks which require mental alertness (eg, operating machinery or driving). Use with alcohol or other CNS depressants may increase CNS depressant effects; use with caution.

Adverse Reactions

Cardiovascular: Circulatory depression, hypertension, hypotension, palpitations, peripheral vasodilation, shock, systemic vascular resistance increased

Central nervous system: CNS depression, confusion, disorientation, disturbed dreams, dizziness, drowsiness, euphoria, hallucinations, headache, insomnia, intracranial pressure elevated, lightheadedness (more frequently than morphine), sedation, syncope; seizures may occur in seizure-prone patients especially with large I.V. doses

Dermatologic: Pruritus, rash; serious skin reactions (eg, erythema multiforme, Stevens-Johnson syndrome)

Endocrine & metabolic: Antidiuretic hormone release

Gastrointestinal: Biliary tract spasm, constipation, nausea (more frequently than morphine), vomiting, xerostomia

Genitourinary: Urinary retention, urinary tract spasm

Local: Dermatitis, flushed skin, injection site reaction (tissue damage and irritation; see Warnings), pain on injection, pruritus

Neuromuscular & skeletal: Paresthesia, weakness

Otic: Tinnitus

Respiratory: Dyspnea, laryngospasm, respiratory depression

Miscellaneous: Diaphoresis, histamine release, physical and psychological dependence

<1%, postmarketing, and/or case reports: Allergic reactions, chills, diarrhea, diplopia, eosinophilia, excitement, facial edema, granulocytopenia, irritability, leukopenia, miosis, muscle tremor, nystagmus, tachycardia, taste alteration, toxic epidermal necrolysis, vision blurred

Drug Interactions

Avoid Concomitant Use There are no known interactions where it is recommended to avoid concomitant use.

Increased Effect/Toxicity

Pentazocine may increase the levels/effects of: Alcohol (Ethyl); Alvimopan; CNS Depressants; Desmopressin; Selective Serotonin Reuptake Inhibitors; Thiazide Diuretics

The levels/effects of Pentazocine may be increased by: Amphetamines; Antipsychotic Agents (Phenothiazines); Succinylcholine

Decreased Effect

Pentazocine may decrease the levels/effects of: Analgesics (Opioid); Pegvisomant

The levels/effects of Pentazocine may be decreased by: Ammonium Chloride

Stability Store injection at controlled room temperature at 20°C to 25°C (68°F to 77°F); do not mix injection with barbiturates, precipitation will occur

Mechanism of Action Binds to opiate receptors in the CNS, causing inhibition of ascending pain pathways, altering the perception of and response to pain; produces generalized CNS depression; partial agonist antagonist

Pharmacodynamics

Onset of action:

I.M., SubQ: Within 15-30 minutes

I.V.: Within 2-3 minutes

Duration: Parenteral: 2-3 hours

Pharmacokinetics (Adult data unless noted)

Distribution: Children 4-8 years (mean ± SD): V_{dss}: 4 ± 1.2 L/kg (see Hanunen, 1993)

Protein binding: 60%

Metabolism: In the liver via oxidative and glucuronide conjugation pathways

Half-life: Increased half-life with decreased hepatic function

Neonates: 8-12 hours (estimated; see Osifo, 2008)

Children 4-8 years (mean ± SD): 3 ± 1.5 hours (see Hanunen, 1993)

Adults: 2-3 hours

Elimination: Small amounts excreted unchanged in urine

Usual Dosage

Neonates: Not recommended for use; safety, efficacy, and dose are not established (see Additional Information)

Children: Limited information available

Preoperative sedation: Manufacturer recommendations:

Infants <1 year: Safety, efficacy, and dose not established

Children 1-16 years: I.M.: 0.5 mg/kg as a single dose

Note: In 300 children (1-14 years) I.M. doses ranging from approximately 0.45-1.5 mg/kg in children <27 kg to 0.65-1.9 mg/kg in children >27 kg were used preoperatively (Rita, 1970)

Postoperative pain: I.M.: Doses of 15 mg for children 5-8 years of age and 30 mg for children 9-14 years of age have been used (n=30) (Waterworth, 1974)

Intraoperative analgesia: I.V.: Titrating doses of 0.5 mg/kg every 30-45 minutes as needed have been given in 50 children 5-9 years of age; total dose required: 1-1.5 mg/kg (Ray, 1994)

Adults:

Analgesia (excluding labor pain):

I.M., SubQ: 30-60 mg every 3-4 hours; do **not** exceed 60 mg/dose; maximum: 360 mg/day

I.V.: 30 mg every 3-4 hours; do **not** exceed 30 mg/dose; maximum: 360 mg/day

Labor pain:

I.M.: 30 mg once

I.V.: 20 mg every 2-3 hours as needed; maximum total dose: 60 mg

Dosing adjustment in renal impairment: Children and Adults:

Cl_{cr} 10-50 mL/minute: Administer 75% of normal dose

Cl_{cr} <10 mL/minute: Administer 50% of normal dose

Administration SubQ route not advised due to tissue damage; rotate injection site for I.M., SubQ use; avoid intra-arterial injection

Monitoring Parameters Respiratory and cardiovascular status; level of pain relief and sedation; blood pressure

Patient Information Avoid alcohol; may cause drowsiness and impair ability to perform activities requiring mental alertness or physical coordination; may be habit-forming; avoid abrupt discontinuation after prolonged use; will cause narcotic withdrawal symptoms in patients currently dependent on narcotics; may cause dry mouth

Additional Information Use only in patients who are not tolerant to or physically dependent upon narcotics

A retrospective study assessed the use of pentazocine 0.5 mg/kg every 8 hours in neonates undergoing surgery; pentazocine use was associated with life-threatening morbidity and unacceptable high mortality due to persistent respiratory depression; the authors of the study recommend the use of alternative neonatal analgesics (see Osifo, 2008).

Dosage Forms Excipient information presented when available (limited, particularly for generics); consult specific product labeling.

Injection, solution:

Talwin®: 30 mg/mL (1 mL, 10 mL) [10 mL size contains sodium bisulfite]

References

Hanunen K, Olkkola KT, Seppala T, et al, "Pharmacokinetics and Pharmacodynamics of Pentazocine in Children," *Pharmacol Toxicol*, 1993, 73(2):120-3.

Osifo OD and Aghahowa SE, "Hazards of Pentazocine for Neonatal Analgesia: A Single-Centre Experience Over 10 Years," *Ann Trop Paediatr*, 2008, 28(3):205-10.

Ray AD and Gupta M, "Clinical Trial of Pentazocine as Analgesic in Pediatric Cases," *J Indian Med Assoc*, 1994, 92(3):77-9.

Rita L, Seleny FL, and Levin RM, "A Comparison of Pentazocine and Morphine for Pediatric Premedication," *Anesth Analg*, 1970, 49 (3):377-82.

Waterworth TA, "Pentazocine (Fortal) as Postoperative Analgesic in Children," *Arch Dis Child*, 1974, 49(6):488-90.

♦ **Pentazocine Lactate** see Pentazocine on page 1085

PENTobarbital (pen toe BAR bi tal)

Medication Safety Issues

Sound-alike/look-alike issues:

PENTobarbital may be confused with PHENobarbital

Nembutal® may be confused with Myambutol®

Related Information

Compatibility of Medications Mixed in a Syringe on page 1713

Laboratory Detection of Drugs in Urine on page 1706

Preprocedure Sedatives in Children on page 1688

U.S. Brand Names Nembutal®

Canadian Brand Names Nembutal® Sodium

Therapeutic Category Anticonvulsant, Barbiturate; Barbiturate; General Anesthetic; Hypnotic; Sedative

Generic Available No

Use Preoperative sedation; high-dose barbiturate coma for treatment of increased intracranial pressure or status epilepticus unresponsive to other therapy

Restrictions C-II

Pregnancy Risk Factor D

Lactation Enters breast milk/contraindicated

Contraindications Hypersensitivity to barbiturates or any component; marked liver function impairment or latent porphyria; chronic or acute pain

Warnings Abrupt discontinuation after prolonged use may result in withdrawal symptoms or seizures; commercially available injection contains 40% propylene glycol

Precautions Use with caution in patients with hypovolemic shock, CHF, or hepatic impairment

Adverse Reactions

Cardiovascular: Arrhythmias, bradycardia, hypotension

Central nervous system: Drowsiness, lethargy, CNS excitation or depression, impaired judgment, hypothermia

Dermatologic: Rash

Gastrointestinal: Nausea, vomiting

Local: Arterial spasm, gangrene with inadvertent intra-arterial injection, thrombophlebitis

Renal: Oliguria

Respiratory: Laryngospasm, respiratory depression, apnea (especially with rapid I.V. use)

Miscellaneous: Physical and psychological dependency with chronic use

Drug Interactions

Metabolism/Transport Effects Induces CYP2A6 (strong), 3A4 (strong)

Avoid Concomitant Use

Avoid concomitant use of PENTobarbital with any of the following: Dronedarone; Everolimus; Nilotinib; Pazopanib; Ranolazine; Romidepsin; Tolvaptan

Increased Effect/Toxicity

PENTobarbital may increase the levels/effects of: Alcohol (Ethyl); CNS Depressants; Meperidine; Thiazide Diuretics

The levels/effects of PENTobarbital may be increased by: Carbonic Anhydrase Inhibitors; Chloramphenicol; Divalproex; Felbamate; Primidone; Valproic Acid

Decreased Effect

PENTobarbital may decrease the levels/effects of: Acetaminophen; Beta-Blockers; Calcium Channel Blockers; Chloramphenicol; Contraceptives (Estrogens); Contraceptives (Progestins); Corticosteroids (Systemic);

CycloSPORINE; CycloSPORINE (Systemic); CYP2A6 Substrates; CYP3A4 Substrates; Disopyramide; Divalproex; Doxycycline; Dronedarone; Etoposide; Etoposide Phosphate; Everolimus; Griseofulvin; GuanFACINE; LamoTRIgine; Maraviroc; Methadone; Nilotinib; Pazopanib; Propafenone; QuiNIDine; Ranolazine; Romidepsin; Saxagliptin; Sorafenib; Tadalafil; Teniposide; Theophylline Derivatives; Tolvaptan; Tricyclic Antidepressants; Valproic Acid; Vitamin K Antagonists

The levels/effects of PENTobarbital may be decreased by: Ketorolac; Ketorolac (Systemic); Mefloquine; Pyridoxine; Rifamycin Derivatives

Food Interactions High doses of pyridoxine may decrease drug effect; barbiturates may increase the metabolism of vitamins D and K; dietary requirements of vitamins D, K, C, B_{12}, folate, and calcium may be increased with long-term use

Stability Protect from light; aqueous solutions are not stable; low pH may cause precipitate; use only clear solution

Mechanism of Action Short-acting barbiturate with sedative, hypnotic, and anticonvulsant properties; depresses CNS activity by binding to barbiturate site at GABA-receptor complex enhancing GABA activity; depresses reticular activating system; higher doses may be gabamimetic

Pharmacodynamics

Onset of action:
I.M.: Within 10-15 minutes
I.V.: Within 1 minute
Duration: I.V.: 15 minutes

Pharmacokinetics (Adult data unless noted)

Distribution: V_d:
Children: 0.8 L/kg
Adults: 1 L/kg
Protein binding: 35% to 55%
Metabolism: Extensive in the liver via hydroxylation and oxidation pathways
Half-life, terminal:
Children: 25 hours
Normal adults: 22 hours; range: 35-50 hours
Elimination: <1% excreted unchanged renally

Usual Dosage

Infants ≥6 months and Children: (**Note:** Limited information is available for infants <6 months of age):
Preoperative/preprocedure sedation:
I.M.: 2-6 mg/kg; maximum dose: 100 mg/dose
I.V.: 1-3 mg/kg to a maximum of 100 mg until asleep
Children:
Hypnotic: I.M.: 2-6 mg/kg; maximum dose: 100 mg/dose
Conscious sedation prior to a procedure: Children >18 months: I.V.: Initial: 2 mg/kg, additional doses of 1-2 mg/kg may be given every 5-10 minutes until adequate sedation is achieved; maximum total dose: 6 mg/kg or 150-200 mg; mean total dose required (for CT scan sedation): 3.3-4.5 mg/kg
Adolescents: Conscious sedation: I.V.: 100 mg prior to a procedure
Children and Adults: Pentobarbital coma: I.V. (see Additional Information):
Loading dose: 10-15 mg/kg given slowly over 1-2 hours; monitor blood pressure and respiratory rate
Maintenance infusion: Initial: 1 mg/kg/hour; may increase to 2-3 mg/kg/hour; maintain burst suppression on EEG
Adults:
Hypnotic:
I.M.: 150-200 mg
I.V.: Initial: 100 mg, may repeat every 1-3 minutes up to 200-500 mg total
Preoperative sedation: I.M.: 150-200 mg

Administration Parenteral: I.V.: Do not inject >50 mg/minute; rapid I.V. injection may cause respiratory depression, apnea, laryngospasm, bronchospasm, and hypotension; administer over 10-30 minutes; maximum concentration: 50 mg/mL for slow I.V. push; may dilute in D_5W, $D_{10}W$, NS, ½NS, LR, Ringer's injection, D_5LR, and dextrose/saline combinations for continuous infusion

Monitoring Parameters Vital signs, respiratory status (includes pulse oximetry for conscious sedation), cardiovascular status, CNS status; monitor ICP and cerebral perfusion pressure (CPP) (CPP = MAP - ICP) when using pentobarbital coma to reduce ICP

Reference Range Therapeutic:
Sedation: 1-5 mcg/mL (SI: 4-22 micromoles/L)
Sleep: 5-15 mcg/mL (SI: 22-66 micromoles/L)
Coma: 20-40 mcg/mL (SI: 88-177 micromoles/L)

Patient Information Avoid alcohol; limit caffeine; may be habit-forming; avoid abrupt discontinuation after prolonged use; may cause drowsiness and impair ability to perform activities requiring mental alertness or physical coordination

Nursing Implications Parenteral solutions are very alkaline; avoid extravasation; avoid intra-arterial injection

Additional Information Tolerance to hypnotic effect can occur; taper dose to prevent withdrawal; **Note:** Loading doses of 15-35 mg/kg (given over 1-2 hours) have been utilized in pediatric patients for pentobarbital coma but these higher loading doses often cause hypotension requiring vasopressor therapy

I.V. continuous infusions of pentobarbital using initial bolus doses of 1-2 mg/kg followed by initial continuous infusions of 1-2 mg/kg/hour have been used for PICU sedation in six intubated, mechanically ventilated infants (age: 2-17 months) who "failed" sedation with fentanyl and midazolam infusions; doses were titrated to effect and supplemental boluses were administered as needed; further studies are needed (see Tobias, 1995)

Dosage Forms Excipient information presented when available (limited, particularly for generics); consult specific product labeling.
Injection, solution, as sodium: 50 mg/mL (20 mL, 50 mL) [contains alcohol 10% and propylene glycol 40%]

References

Fischer JH and Raineri DL, "Pentobarbital Anesthesia for Status Epilepticus," Clin Pharm, 1987, 6(8):601-2.
Hubbard AM, Markowitz RI, Kimmel B, et al, "Sedation for Pediatric Patients Undergoing CT and MRI," J Comput Assist Tomogr, 1992, 16 (1):3-6.
Pereira JK, Burrows PE, Richards HM, et al, "Comparison of Sedation Regimens for Pediatric Outpatient CT," Pediatr Radiol, 1993, 23 (5):341-4.
Schaible DH, Cupit GC, Swedlow DB, et al, "High-Dose Pentobarbital Pharmacokinetics in Hypothermic Brain-Injured Children," J Pediatr, 1982, 100(4):655-60.
Tobias JD, Deshpande JK, Pietsch JB, et al, "Pentobarbital Sedation for Patients in the Pediatric Intensive Care Unit," South Med J, 1995, 88 (3):290-4.

◆ **Pentobarbital Sodium** see PENTobarbital on page 1087

Pentostatin (PEN toe stat in)

Medication Safety Issues

Sound-alike/look-alike issues:
Pentostatin may be confused with pentamidine, pentosan

High alert medication: The Institute for Safe Medication Practices (ISMP) includes this medication among its list of drug classes which have a heightened risk of causing significant patient harm when used in error.

International issues:
Nipent® may be confused with Nipin® which is a brand name for nifedipine in Italy and Singapore

Related Information

Emetogenic Potential of Antineoplastic Agents *on page 1579*

U.S. Brand Names Nipent®

Canadian Brand Names Nipent®

Therapeutic Category Antineoplastic Agent, Antibiotic; Antineoplastic Agent, Antimetabolite (Purine Antagonist)

Generic Available Yes

Use Treatment of hairy cell leukemia; other uses include treatment of cutaneous T-cell lymphoma, chronic lymphocytic leukemia (CLL), and acute and chronic graft-versus-host disease (GVHD)

Pregnancy Risk Factor D

Pregnancy Considerations Animal studies have demonstrated teratogenicity, maternal toxicity, and fetal loss. There are no adequate and well-controlled studies in pregnant women. Women of childbearing potential should be advised to avoid becoming pregnant.

Lactation Excretion in breast milk unknown/not recommended

Breast-Feeding Considerations Due to the potential for serious adverse reactions in nursing the infant, breast-feeding is not recommended.

Contraindications Hypersensitivity to pentostatin or any component

Warnings Hazardous agent; use appropriate precautions for handling and disposal; should be administered under the supervision of an experienced cancer chemotherapy physician **[U.S. Boxed Warning]**. Severe CNS, renal, and liver toxicity have occurred with doses higher than recommended; do not exceed the recommended dose **[U.S. Boxed Warning]**; may cause elevations (reversible) in liver function tests. Severe pulmonary toxicities have occurred with doses higher than recommended; do not exceed the recommended dose. Do not administer concurrently with fludarabine; concomitant use has resulted in serious or fatal pulmonary toxicity **[U.S. Boxed Warning]**. Fatal pulmonary edema and hypotension have also been reported in patients treated with pentostatin in combination with carmustine, etoposide, or high-dose cyclophosphamide as part of a myeloablative regimen for bone marrow transplant. Bone marrow suppression may occur, primarily early in treatment and frequent monitoring of CBC during this time is necessary; if neutropenia persists beyond early cycles, evaluate for disease status. Safety and efficacy have not been established in children.

Precautions Use with caution in patients with renal dysfunction (Cl_{cr} <60 mL/minute); the terminal half-life is prolonged; appropriate dosing guidelines in renal insufficiency have not been determined. Severe rashes may occur and worsen with therapy continuation; may require withholding of treatment or discontinuation. Treatment should be temporarily withheld for active infections during therapy.

Adverse Reactions

Central nervous system: Fever (42% to 46%), fatigue (29% to 42%), pain (8% to 20%), chills (11% to 19%), headache (13% to 17%), CNS toxicity (1% to 11%), anxiety (3% to 10%), confusion (3% to 10%), depression (3% to 10%), dizziness (3% to 10%), insomnia (3% to 10%), nervousness (3% to 10%), somnolence (3% to 10%), abnormal dreams/thinking, amnesia, ataxia, emotional lability, encephalitis, hallucination, hostility, meningism, neurosis, seizure, vertigo, lethargy

Cardiovascular: Chest pain (3% to 10%), hypotension (3% to 10%), peripheral edema, angina, arrhythmias, AV block, bradycardia, cardiac arrest, deep thrombophlebitis, CHF, hypertension, pericardial effusion, sinus arrest, syncope, tachycardia, vasculitis

Dermatologic: Rash (26% to 43%), pruritus (10% to 21%), skin disorder (4% to 17%), cellulitis (6%), furunculosis (4%), dry skin (3% to 10%), urticaria (3% to 10%), acne, alopecia, eczema, petechial rash, photosensitivity, abscess, fungal infection (skin)

Endocrine & metabolic: Amenorrhea, hypercalcemia, hyponatremia, gout, decrease or loss of libido

Gastrointestinal: Nausea/vomiting (22% to 63%), diarrhea (15% to 17%), anorexia (13% to 16%), abdominal pain (4% to 16%), stomatitis (5% to 12%), dyspepsia (3% to 10%), flatulence (3% to 10%), gingivitis (3% to 10%), constipation, dysphagia, glossitis, ileus, taste perversion, oral moniliasis

Genitourinary: Urinary tract infection (3%), impotence, dysuria, hematuria

Hematologic: Myelosuppression (nadir: 7 days; recovery: 10-14 days), leukopenia (22% to 60%), anemia (8% to 35%), thrombocytopenia (6% to 32%), agranulocytosis (3% to 10%), hemorrhage (3% to 10%), acute leukemia, aplastic anemia, hemolytic anemia

Hepatic: Transaminases elevated (2% to 19%)

Local: Phlebitis (<3%)

Neuromuscular & skeletal: Myalgia (11% to 19%), weakness (10% to 12%), neuritis, arthralgia (3% to 10%), paresthesia (3% to 10%), arthritis, dysarthria, hyperkinesia, neuralgia, neuropathy, paralysis, twitching, osteomyelitis

Ocular: Conjunctivitis, amblyopia, eyes nonreactive, lacrimation disorder, photophobia, retinopathy, vision abnormal, watery eyes, xerophthalmia, uveitis/vision loss

Otic: Deafness, earache, labyrinthitis, tinnitus

Renal: Creatinine elevated (3% to 10%), nephropathy, renal failure, renal insufficiency, renal function abnormal, renal stone

Respiratory: Cough (17% to 20%), upper respiratory infection (13% to 16%), rhinitis (10% to 11%), dyspnea (8% to 11%), pharyngitis (8% to 10%), sinusitis (6%), pneumonia (5%), asthma (3% to 10%), bronchitis (3%), bronchospasm, laryngeal edema, pulmonary embolus, pulmonary toxicity (fatal; in combination with fludarabine), pulmonary edema

Miscellaneous: Infection (7% to 36%), hypersensitivity reactions (2% to 11%), diaphoresis (8% to 10%), herpes zoster (8%), viral infection (≤8%), bacterial infection (5%), herpes simplex (4%), sepsis (3%), flu-like syndrome (<3%)

Drug Interactions

Avoid Concomitant Use

Avoid concomitant use of Pentostatin with any of the following: BCG; Fludarabine; Natalizumab; Nelarabine; Pegademase Bovine; Pimecrolimus; Tacrolimus (Topical); Vaccines (Live)

Increased Effect/Toxicity

Pentostatin may increase the levels/effects of: Cyclophosphamide; Fludarabine; Leflunomide; Natalizumab; Vaccines (Live)

The levels/effects of Pentostatin may be increased by: Denosumab; Fludarabine; Pimecrolimus; Tacrolimus (Topical); Trastuzumab

Decreased Effect

Pentostatin may decrease the levels/effects of: BCG; Nelarabine; Pegademase Bovine; Sipuleucel-T; Vaccines (Inactivated); Vaccines (Live)

The levels/effects of Pentostatin may be decreased by: Echinacea; Pegademase Bovine

Stability Store intact vials under refrigeration at 2°C to 8°C (36°F to 46°F); reconstituted vials and further dilutions are stable at room temperature for 8 hours

Stable in LR, NS; **variable stability (consult detailed reference)** in D_5W

Y-site administration: Compatible: Fludarabine, melphalan, ondansetron, paclitaxel, sargramostim

Mechanism of Action Pentostatin is a purine antimetabolite that inhibits adenosine deaminase (ADA), preventing the deamination of adenosine to inosine. The resulting accumulation of deoxyadenosine (dAdo) and deoxyadenosine 5'-triphosphate (dATP) reduces purine metabolism and DNA and RNA synthesis. The greatest activity of ADA is in the cells of the lymphoid system, with T-cells having higher activity than B-cells.

Pharmacokinetics (Adult data unless noted)
Distribution: I.V.: V_d: Adults: 36.1 L (20.1 L/m^2); rapidly to body tissues
Protein binding: ~4%
Half-life elimination: Adults:
    Distribution half-life: 11-85 minutes
    Terminal half-life: 3-7 hours; renal impairment (Cl_{cr} <50 mL/minute): 4-18 hours
Elimination: Urine (~50% to 96%) within 24 hours (30% to 90% as unchanged drug)
Clearance: Adults: 68 mL/minute/m^2 (mean)

Usual Dosage I.V.: Adults (refer to individual protocols): Hydration with 500-1000 mL fluid prior to infusion and 500 mL after infusion is recommended:
Hairy cell leukemia: 4 mg/m^2 every 2 weeks
CLL: 4 mg/m^2 weekly for 3 weeks, then every 2 weeks
Cutaneous T-cell lymphoma: 3.75-5 mg/m^2 daily for 3 days every 3 weeks
Acute GVHD: 1.5 mg/m^2 daily for 3 days; may repeat after 2 weeks if needed
Chronic GVHD: 4 mg/m^2 every 2 weeks for 12 doses; then 4 mg/m^2 every 3-4 weeks (if still improving)

Dosage adjustment in renal impairment: The FDA-approved labeling does not contain renal dosage adjustment guidelines; use with caution in patients with Cl_{cr} <60 mL/minute. Two patients with Cl_{cr} 50-60 mL/minute achieved responses when treated with 2 mg/m^2/dose. The following guidelines have been used by some clinicians:
Kintzel, 1995:
    Cl_{cr} 46-60 mL/minute: Administer 70% of dose
    Cl_{cr} 31-45 mL/minute: Administer 60% of dose
    Cl_{cr} <30 mL/minute: Consider use of alternative drug
Lathia, 2002:
    Cl_{cr} 40-59 mL/minute: Administer 3 mg/m^2/dose
    Cl_{cr} 20-39 mL/minute: Administer 2 mg/m^2/dose

Administration I.V.: Reconstitute with 5 mL SWI to a concentration of 2 mg/mL. The solution may be further diluted in 25-50 mL NS or D$_5$W for infusion. Administer I.V. as a 20- to 30-minute infusion or as an I.V. bolus over 5 minutes.

Monitoring Parameters CBC with differential, platelet count, liver function, serum uric acid, renal function (creatinine clearance), bone marrow evaluation

Patient Information Do not take any new medication during therapy unless approved by prescriber. This drug can only be given by infusion on a specific schedule. Report immediately any redness, swelling, burning, or pain at infusion site; or signs of hypersensitivity (eg, respiratory difficulty or swallowing, chest tightness, rash, hives, swelling of lips or mouth). Maintain adequate hydration unless instructed to restrict fluid intake. You may be more susceptible to infection (avoid crowds and exposure to infection and do not have any vaccinations without consulting prescriber. May cause nausea and vomiting, or loss of appetite (small, frequent meals or frequent mouth care may help - or request medication from prescriber); headache (consult prescriber for approved analgesic); dizziness, confusion or lethargy (use caution when driving); or mouth sores (use frequent oral care with soft toothbrush or cotton swabs). Report signs of infection (eg, fever, chills, sore throat, mouth sores, burning urination, perianal itching, or vaginal discharge); unusual bruising or bleeding (eg, tarry stools, blood in urine, stool, or vomitus); vision changes or hearing; muscle tremors, weakness, or pain; CNS changes (eg, hallucinations, confusion, insomnia, seizures); or respiratory difficulty.

Dosage Forms Excipient information presented when available (limited, particularly for generics); consult specific product labeling.
Injection, powder for reconstitution: 10 mg [contains mannitol]
Nipent®: 10 mg [contains mannitol]

References
al-Razzak LA, Benedetti AE, Waugh WN, et al, "Chemical Stability of Pentostatin (NSC-218321), a Cytotoxic and Immunosuppressant Agent," *Pharm Res*, 1990, 7(5):452-60.
Bolanos-Meade J, Jacobsohn DA, Margolis J, et al, "Pentostatin in Steroid-Refractory Acute Graft-Versus-Host Disease," *J Clin Oncol*, 2005, 23(12):2661-8.
Brogden RN and Sorkin EM, "Pentostatin. A Review of Its Pharmacodynamic and Pharmacokinetic Properties, and Therapeutic Potential in Lymphoproliferative Disorders," *Drugs*, 1993, 46 (4):652-77.
Catovsky D, "Clinical Experience With 2'-Deoxycoformycin," *Hematol Cell Ther*, 1996, 38(Suppl 2):103-7.
Dillman RO, "A New Chemotherapeutic Agent: Deoxycoformycin (Pentostatin)," *Semin Hematol*, 1994, 31(1):16-27.
Dillman RO, Mick R, and McIntyre OR, "Pentostatin in Chronic Lymphocytic Leukemia: A Phase II Trial of Cancer and Leukemia Group B," *J Clin Oncol*, 1989, 7(4):433-8.
Grever MR, Siaw MFE, Jacob WF, et al, "The Biochemical and Clinical Consequences of 2'-Deoxycoformycin in Refractory Lymphoproliferative Malignancy," *Blood*, 1981, 57(3):406-17.
Jacobsohn DA, Chen AR, Zahurak M, et al, "Phase II Study of Pentostatin in Patients With Corticosteroid-Refractory Chronic Graft-Versus-Host Disease," *J Clin Oncol*, 2007, 25(27):4255-61.
Kane BJ, Kuhn JG, and Roush MK, "Pentostatin: An Adenosine Deaminase Inhibitor For the Treatment of Hairy Cell Leukemia," *Ann Pharmacother*, 1992, 26(7-8):939-47.
Kintzel PE and Dorr RT, "Anticancer Drug Renal Toxicity and Elimination: Dosing Guidelines for Altered Renal Function," *Cancer Treat Rev*, 1995, 21(1):33-64.
Kurzrock R, Pilat S, and Duvic M, "Pentostatin Therapy of T-Cell Lymphomas With Cutaneous Manifestations," *J Clin Oncol*, 1999, 17 (10):3117-21.
Lathia C, Fleming GF, Meyer M, et al, "Pentostatin Pharmacokinetics and Dosing Recommendations in Patients With Mild Renal Impairment," *Cancer Chemother Pharmacol*, 2002, 50(2):121-6.
Margolis J and Grever MR, "Pentostatin (Nipent): A Review of Potential Toxicity and Its Management," *Semin Oncol*, 2000, 27(2 Suppl 5):9-14.
Tsimberidou AM, Giles F, Duvic M, et al, "Phase II Study of Pentostatin in Advanced T-Cell Lymphoid Malignancies: Update of an M.D. Anderson Cancer Center Series," *Cancer*, 2004, 100(2):342-9.

◆ **Pentothal®** *see* Thiopental *on page 1340*

Pentoxifylline (pen toks I fi leen)

Medication Safety Issues
Sound-alike/look-alike issues:
    Pentoxifylline may be confused with tamoxifen
    Trental® may be confused with Bentyl®, Tegretol®, Trandate®

U.S. Brand Names Pentoxil® [DSC]; Trental®
Canadian Brand Names Albert® Pentoxifylline; Apo-Pentoxifylline SR®; Nu-Pentoxifylline SR; ratio-Pentoxifylline; Trental®
Therapeutic Category Blood Viscosity Reducer Agent
Generic Available Yes
Use Symptomatic management of peripheral vascular disease, mainly intermittent claudication (FDA approved in adults)

Has also been studied for use in AIDS patients with increased tumor necrosis factor, cerebrovascular accidents, cerebrovascular diseases, new onset type I diabetes mellitus, diabetic atherosclerosis, diabetic neuropathy, diabetic nephropathy, gangrene, cutaneous polyarteritis nodosa, hemodialysis shunt thrombosis, cerebral malaria, septic shock, sepsis in premature neonates, sickle cell syndromes, vasculitis, Kawasaki disease, Raynaud's syndrome, cystic fibrosis, bone marrow transplant-related toxicities (ie, graft-versus-host disease, veno-occlusive disease, and interstitial pneumonitis), and persistent pulmonary hypertension of the newborn

Pregnancy Risk Factor C

Pregnancy Considerations Teratogenic effects were not observed in animal studies. There are no adequate and well-controlled studies in pregnant women.

Lactation Enters breast milk/not recommended

Contraindications Hypersensitivity to pentoxifylline, any component, or other xanthine derivatives (eg, caffeine, theophylline, theobromine); recent cerebral or retinal hemorrhage

Warnings Use with caution in patients with renal or hepatic impairment, insulin-treated diabetics, chronic occlusive arterial disease of the limbs, recent surgery, or peptic ulcerations

Adverse Reactions
Cardiovascular: Mild hypotension, angina
Central nervous system: Headache, dizziness, agitation
Gastrointestinal: Dyspepsia, nausea, vomiting
Ocular: Blurred vision

Drug Interactions
Metabolism/Transport Effects Inhibits CYP1A2 (weak)

Avoid Concomitant Use
Avoid concomitant use of Pentoxifylline with any of the following: Ketorolac; Ketorolac (Systemic)

Increased Effect/Toxicity
Pentoxifylline may increase the levels/effects of: Anti-hypertensives; Antiplatelet Agents; Heparin; Heparin (Low Molecular Weight); Theophylline Derivatives; Vitamin K Antagonists

The levels/effects of Pentoxifylline may be increased by: Cimetidine; Ciprofloxacin; Ciprofloxacin (Systemic); Ketorolac; Ketorolac (Systemic)

Decreased Effect There are no known significant interactions involving a decrease in effect.

Food Interactions Food may decrease rate but not extent of absorption

Mechanism of Action Mechanism of action remains unclear; is thought to reduce blood viscosity and improve blood flow by altering the rheology of red blood cells; inhibits production of tumor necrosis factor-alpha; inhibits neutrophil activation and adhesion; increases tissue oxygen levels in patients with peripheral arterial disease; inhibits platelet aggregation

Pharmacodynamics Onset of action: 2-4 weeks with multiple doses

Pharmacokinetics (Adult data unless noted)
Absorption: Oral: Well absorbed
Distribution: Pentoxifylline and metabolites distribute into breast milk
Metabolism: Undergoes first-pass in the liver, dose-related (nonlinear) pharmacokinetics; 2 active metabolites (M-I and M-V); **Note:** Plasma concentrations of M-1 and M-V are 5 and 8 times greater, respectively, than pentoxifylline
Half-life, apparent:
Parent drug: 24-48 minutes
Metabolites: 60-96 minutes
Time to peak serum concentration: Within 2-4 hours
Elimination: Metabolites excreted in urine; 0% eliminated unchanged in the urine: 50% to 80% eliminated as M-V metabolite in the urine; 20% as other metabolites

Usual Dosage Oral:
Children: Minimal information available; one investigation (Furukawa, 1994) found a lower incidence of coronary artery lesions in 22 children (mean age: 2 years) treated for acute Kawasaki disease with versus without pentox-ifylline 20 mg/kg/day (given in 3 divided doses); all patients received aspirin and I.V. gamma globulin therapy; a lower dose (10 mg/kg/day) was not effective; higher doses have been used investigationally for the treatment of cystic fibrosis (Aronoff, 1994)

Adults: 400 mg 3 times/day with meals; decrease to 400 mg twice daily if CNS or GI side effects occur. **Note:** Although clinical benefit may be seen within 2-4 weeks, treatment should be continued for at least 8 weeks.

Dosing adjustment in renal impairment: Use with caution; monitor for enhanced therapeutic and toxic effects; **Note:** Pentoxifylline is not eliminated unchanged in the urine; however, the pharmacologically active metabolite (M-V) is; M-V may accumulate in patients with renal impairment and add to pharmacologic and toxic effects.

Adults: Dosage adjustments not listed by manufacturer; adjust dose based on degree of renal impairment (see Aronoff, 2007)
Cl_{cr} >50 mL/minute: 400 mg every 8-12 hours
Cl_{cr} 10-50 mL/minute: 400 mg every 12-24 hours
Cl_{cr} <10 mL/minute: 400 mg every 24 hours; **Note:** Further dosage reduction may be required; Paap (1996) suggests a further reduction to 200 mg once daily but current products (extended or controlled release; unscored) may require adaptation to 400 mg once every other day

Administration Oral: Administer with food or antacids to decrease GI upset. Do not crush, break, or chew extended or controlled release tablet, swallow whole.

Test Interactions False-positive theophylline level

Patient Information Limit caffeine; if GI or CNS side effects continue, contact physician; while beneficial effects may be seen in 2-4 weeks, continue treatment for at least 8 weeks

Dosage Forms Excipient information presented when available (limited, particularly for generics); consult specific product labeling. [DSC] = Discontinued product
Tablet, controlled release:
Trental®: 400 mg
Tablet, extended release: 400 mg
Pentoxil®: 400 mg [DSC]

References

Aronoff GR, Bennett WM, Berns JS, et al, *Drug Prescribing in Renal Failure: Dosing Guidelines for Adults and Children*, 5th ed, Philadelphia, PA: American College of Physicians, 2007, 117.

Aronoff SC, Quinn FJ, Carpenter LS, et al, "Effects of Pentoxifylline on Sputum Neutrophil Elastase and Pulmonary Function in Patients With Cystic Fibrosis: Preliminary Observations," *J Pediatr*, 1994, 125(6 Pt 1):992-7.

Berman W Jr, Berman N, Pathak D, et al, "Effects of Pentoxifylline (Trental®) on Blood Flow, Viscosity, and Oxygen Transport in Young Adults With Inoperable Cyanotic Congenital Heart Disease," *Pediatr Cardiol*, 1994, 15(2):66-70.

Furukawa S, Matsubara T, Umezawa Y, et al, "Pentoxifylline and Intravenous Gamma Globulin Combination Therapy for Acute Kawasaki Disease," *Eur J Pediatr*, 1994, 153(9):663-7.

Lauterbach R, "Pentoxifylline Treatment of Persistent Pulmonary Hypertension of Newborn," *Eur J Pediatr*, 1993, 152(5):460. (I.V. use)

Lauterbach R, Pawlik D, Tomaszczyk B, et al, "Pentoxifylline Treatment of Sepsis of Premature Infants; Preliminary Clinical Observations," *Eur J Pediatr*, 1994, 153(9):672-4. (I.V. use)

MacDonald MJ, Shahidi NT, Allen DB, et al, "Pentoxifylline in the Treatment of Children With New-Onset Type I Diabetes Mellitus," *JAMA*, 1994, 271(1):27-8.

Paap CM, Simpson KS, Horton MW, et al, "Multiple-Dose Pharmaco-kinetics of Pentoxifylline and Its Metabolites During Renal Insufficiency," *Ann Pharmacother*, 1996, 30(7-8):724-9.

◆ **Pepto-Bismol® Maximum Strength [OTC]** *see* Bismuth *on page 195*

◆ **Pepto Relief [OTC]** *see* Bismuth *on page 195*

Peramivir (pe RA mi veer)

Therapeutic Category Antiviral Agent; Neuraminidase Inhibitor

Generic Available No

Use Treatment of certain **hospitalized** patients with suspected or laboratory-confirmed 2009 H1N1 infection or infection due to nonsubtypable influenza A virus suspected to be 2009 H1N1 (Not FDA approved, Emergency Use Authorization only). Eligible patients include:

• Adult or pediatric patients not responding to appropriate oral or inhaled antiviral therapy

• Adult or pediatric patients for whom drug delivery by a route other than I.V. (eg, enteral oseltamivir or inhaled zanamivir) is not feasible or not expected to be dependable

• Adult patients that the clinician judges I.V. therapy is appropriate due to other circumstances

Restrictions Investigational agent (not FDA approved); only available in the U.S. under an Emergency Use Authorization (EUA). For information on eligibility or to request the emergency use, refer to http://www.cdc.gov/h1n1flu/eua/.

Peramivir is **not** for the treatment of seasonal influenza A or B virus infections, for outpatients with acute uncomplicated 2009 H1N1 virus infection, patients with documented or highly suspected oseltamivir resistant H1N1 virus infection, or for pre- or postexposure chemoprophylaxis (prevention) of influenza.

Under the terms of the EUA, reporting of all medication errors and selected adverse events occurring during treatment is mandatory (within 7 days from event onset) using the FDA MedWatch Form 3500 (available online at http://www.fda.gov/medwatch/safety/FDA-3500_fillable.-pdf). The patient's healthcare provider is also required to provide any follow-up request by the FDA or CDC. Adverse events which require reporting to the FDA include death, neuropsychiatric events, renal events, serious skin reactions (eg, Stevens-Johnson syndrome, toxic epidermal necrolysis), hypersensitivity reactions (eg, anaphylaxis, urticaria, angioedema), severe I.V. administration adverse events (eg, infiltrated I.V.), and other serious events (eg, congenital anomaly, birth defect, permanent disability).

Pregnancy Considerations Adverse events were not observed in animal reproduction studies. Pregnant women have not been included in clinical trials; pharmacokinetic and safety information is not available.

Lactation
Excretion unknown

Breast-Feeding Considerations Breast-feeding women have not been included in clinical trials; pharmacokinetic and safety information is not available.

Contraindications Hypersensitivity to peramivir, other neuraminidase inhibitors, or any component

Warnings Diarrhea, nausea, and vomiting have commonly occurred during clinical trials. Rare occurrences of neuropsychiatric events, including confusion, delirium, hallucinations, and/or self-injury have been reported with the use of other neuraminidase inhibitors from postmarketing surveillance; direct causality is difficult to establish since influenza infection may also be associated with behavioral and neurologic changes. Serious hypersensitivity reactions (eg, anaphylaxis, urticaria, angioedema) have been reported with other neuraminidase inhibitors. Although these reactions have not yet been observed with peramivir,

discontinue infusion immediately and treat reaction if hypersensitivity is suspected. Recommended pediatric doses are based on modeling from adult use; peramivir has not been administered to pediatric patients in clinical trials.

Precautions Use with caution in patients with documented or highly suspected zanamivir resistance. Neutropenia has occurred during clinical trials; monitor CBC during therapy. Elimination is primarily renal; dosage adjustment is required in renal impairment. Patients with known or suspected renal impairment must have creatinine clearance determined prior to dose calculation and first dose administration. Prior to use, patients must be informed and understand that peramivir is an investigational agent whose safety and efficacy have not been established.

Adverse Reactions Note: Investigational agent: Due to limited patient exposure, frequency of adverse events is unknown and risk of additional, undocumented, serious, or unexpected adverse events exists.

Cardiovascular: Blood pressure increased, ECG abnormalities (prolonged QT_c interval)

Central nervous system: Dizziness, headache, nervousness, neuropsychiatric events (including anxiety, confusion, delirium, depression, insomnia, mood alterations, nightmares, and restlessness), somnolence

Endocrine & metabolic: Hyperglycemia

Gastrointestinal: Anorexia, diarrhea, nausea, vomiting

Genitourinary: Cystitis, hematuria, proteinuria

Hematologic: Neutropenia

Hepatic: Hyperbilirubinemia

Drug Interactions

Avoid Concomitant Use There are no known interactions where it is recommended to avoid concomitant use.

Increased Effect/Toxicity

The levels/effects of Peramivir may be increased by: Probenecid

Decreased Effect

Peramivir may decrease the levels/effects of: Influenza Virus Vaccine (H1N1, Live/Attenuated); Influenza Virus Vaccine (Live/Attenuated)

Stability Store vials at 15°C to 30°C (59°F to 86°F). Once diluted, use immediately or refrigerate. If refrigerated, use within 24 hours following preparation (allow to reach room temperature prior to administration). Any unused portion of the single use vial must be discarded. Maintain adequate records of all vials of peramivir showing receipt, use, and disposition of product, including unused, intact vials.

Mechanism of Action Peramivir, a cyclopentane analogue, selectively inhibits the neuraminidase enzyme, thus preventing the release of particles from infected cells.

Pharmacokinetics (Adult data unless noted)

Bioavailability: Oral: ≤3% (agent investigated only as a parenteral formulation due to low oral bioavailability)

Protein binding: <30%

Half-life elimination: Range: 8-21 hours (normal renal function)

Elimination: Urine: 90% (primarily unchanged); peramivir is removed by dialysis

Usual Dosage I.V.:

Children: **Note:** Treatment duration >10 days may be permitted in certain situations, such as critical illness (eg, respiratory failure or intensive care unit admission), continued viral shedding, or unresolved clinical influenza illness.

≤30 days of life: 6 mg/kg once daily for 5 to 10 days

31-90 days of life: 8 mg/kg once daily for 5 to 10 days

91-180 days of life: 10 mg/kg once daily for 5 to 10 days

181 days of life through 5 years: 12 mg/kg once daily for 5 to 10 days (maximum dose: 600 mg)

6-17 years: 10 mg/kg once daily for 5 to 10 days (maximum dose: 600 mg)

Adults: 600 mg once daily for 5 to 10 days

Dosing adjustment in renal impairment: Dosage must be adjusted in patients with a Cl_{cr} <50 mL/minute. **Note:** Dosage adjustments based on Schwartz formula (children) and Cockroft and Gault equation (adults).

Children:

Cl_{cr} 31-49 mL/minute/1.73 m^2:
- ≤30 days of life: 1.5 mg/kg once daily for 5 to 10 days
- 31-90 days of life: 2 mg/kg once daily for 5 to 10 days
- 91-180 days of life: 2.5 mg/kg once daily for 5 to 10 days
- 181 days of life through 5 years: 3 mg/kg once daily for 5 to 10 days (maximum dose: 150 mg)
- 6-17 years: 2.5 mg/kg once daily for 5 to 10 days (maximum dose: 150 mg)

Cl_{cr} 10-30 mL/minute/1.73 m^2:
- ≤30 days of life: 1 mg/kg once daily for 5 to 10 days
- 31-90 days of life: 1.3 mg/kg once daily for 5 to 10 days
- 91-180 days of life: 1.6 mg/kg once daily for 5 to 10 days
- 181 days of life through 5 years: 1.9 mg/kg once daily for 5 to 10 days (maximum dose: 100 mg)
- 6-17 years: 1.6 mg/kg once daily for 5 to 10 days (maximum dose: 100 mg)

Cl_{cr} <10 mL/minute/1.73 m^2 (**not** on intermittent HD or CRRT):
- ≤30 days of life: 1 mg/kg on day 1, followed by 0.15 mg/kg once daily for 5 to 10 days
- 31-90 days of life: 1.3 mg/kg on day 1, followed by 0.2 mg/kg once daily for 5 to 10 days
- 91-180 days of life: 1.6 mg/kg on day 1, followed by 0.25 mg/kg once daily for 5 to 10 days
- 181 days of life through 5 years: 1.9 mg/kg on day 1, followed by 0.3 mg/kg once daily for 5 to 10 days (maximum dose: 15 mg)
- 6-17 years: 1.6 mg/kg on day 1 (maximum dose day 1: 100 mg), followed by 0.25 mg/kg once daily for 5 to 10 days (maximum dose: 15 mg)

Cl_{cr} <10 mL/minute/1.73 m^2 (**on** intermittent HD):
- ≤30 days of life: 1 mg/kg on day 1, followed by 1 mg/kg given 2 hours after each HD session **on dialysis days only**
- 31-90 days of life: 1.3 mg/kg on day 1, followed by 1.3 mg/kg given 2 hours after each HD session **on dialysis days only**
- 91-180 days of life: 1.6 mg/kg on day 1, followed by 1.6 mg/kg given 2 hours after each HD session **on dialysis days only**
- 181 days of life through 5 years: 1.9 mg/kg on day 1, followed by 1.9 mg/kg given 2 hours after each HD session **on dialysis days only** (maximum dose: 100 mg)
- 6-17 years: 1.6 mg/kg on day 1, followed by 1.6 mg/kg given 2 hours after each HD session **on dialysis days only** (maximum dose: 100 mg)

Continuous renal replacement therapy (CRRT): Limited data exist. Estimate total clearance by calculating CLCRRT depending on CRRT modality used (eg, CVVHD, SCUF), plus any residual renal function, and adjust dosage according to Cl_{cr} recommendation.

Adults:

Cl_{cr} 31-49 mL/minute: 150 mg once daily

Cl_{cr} 10-30 mL/minute: 100 mg once daily

Cl_{cr} <10 mL/minute (**not** on intermittent HD or CRRT): 100 mg on day 1, followed by 15 mg once daily

Cl_{cr} <10 mL/minute (**on** intermittent HD): 100 mg on day 1, followed by 100 mg given 2 hours after each HD session **on dialysis days only**

Continuous renal replacement therapy (CRRT): Limited data exist. Estimate total clearance by calculating CLCRRT depending on CRRT modality used (eg, CVVHD, SCUF), plus any residual renal function, and adjust dosage according to Cl_{cr} recommendation.

Peritoneal dialysis: No information available

Administration Parenteral: **Do not administer intramuscularly.** Administer diluted dose intravenously over 60 minutes (children) or 30 minutes (adults), not to exceed an infusion rate of 40 mg/minute. Add calculated dose to an empty sterile I.V. container and dilute with either NS or 0.45% sodium chloride solution not containing other electrolytes. Do not dilute with dextrose-containing solutions. Dilute calculated dose to make a final concentration ≤6 mg/mL. Alternatively, in children, may administer undiluted dose using an infusion device (eg, piggy back system, timed syringe system, or pump) to allow infusion into an open I.V. line with NS. Administer peramivir through a separate I.V. line or separate I.V. lumen in a multilumen catheter; flush I.V. line with NS between any other medication and peramivir. When administering via heparin lock, flush port with NS; after infusion, the port should be flushed again with NS and then heparin may be added to maintain catheter patency.

Monitoring Parameters CBC with differential and a basic metabolic profile (BMP) (initiation, day 3, and end of therapy); liver function tests, including AST, ALT, alkaline phosphatase, and total and direct bilirubin (initiation, end of therapy, and as needed); urinalysis (initiation, end of therapy, and as needed); renal function (prior to initiation and during therapy); vital signs (daily at minimum); development of diarrhea; signs or symptoms of unusual behavior (including attempts at self-injury, confusion, and/or delirium)

Dosage Forms Excipient information presented when available (limited, particularly for generics); consult specific product labeling.

Injection, solution: 10 mg/mL (20 mL)

References

Birnkrant D and Cox E, "The Emergency Use Authorization of Peramivir for Treatment of 2009 H1N1 Influenza," N Engl J Med, 2009, 361 (23):2204-7.

Hayden F, "Developing New Antiviral Agents for Influenza Treatment: What Does the Future Hold?" Clin Infect Dis, 2009, 48(Suppl 1):3-13.

Kohono S, MY Yen, HJ Cheong, et al, "Single-Intravenous Peramivir vs Oral Oseltamivir to Treat Acute, Uncomplicated Influenza in the Outpatient Setting: A Phase III Randomized, Double-Blind Trial," ICAAC , 2009, Abstract V-537a.

Ong AK and Hayden FG, "John F. Enders Lecture 2006: Antivirals for Influenza," J Infect Dis, 2007, 196(2):181-90.

◆ **Percocet®** *see* Oxycodone and Acetaminophen *on page 1041*

◆ **Percocet®-Demi (Can)** *see* Oxycodone and Acetaminophen *on page 1041*

◆ **Percodan®** *see* Oxycodone and Aspirin *on page 1042*

◆ **Perdiem® Overnight Relief [OTC]** *see* Senna *on page 1253*

◆ **Perforomist™** *see* Formoterol *on page 621*

◆ **Periactin** *see* Cyproheptadine *on page 375*

◆ **Peri-Colace® [OTC]** *see* Docusate and Senna *on page 469*

◆ **Peridex®** *see* Chlorhexidine Gluconate *on page 291*

◆ **Peridex® Oral Rinse (Can)** *see* Chlorhexidine Gluconate *on page 291*

◆ **Peridol (Can)** *see* Haloperidol *on page 666*

◆ **PerioChip®** *see* Chlorhexidine Gluconate *on page 291*

◆ **PerioGard®** *see* Chlorhexidine Gluconate *on page 291*

◆ **PerioMed™** *see* Fluoride *on page 595*

◆ **Periostat®** *see* Doxycycline *on page 479*

Permethrin (per METH rin)

U.S. Brand Names A200® Lice [OTC]; Acticin®; Elimite®; Nix® [OTC]; Rid® Spray [OTC]

Canadian Brand Names Kwellada-P™; Nix®

Therapeutic Category Antiparasitic Agent, Topical; Pediculocide; Scabicidal Agent

Generic Available Yes: Excludes spray

Use Single application treatment of infestation with *Pediculus humanus capitis* (head louse) and its nits; treatment of *Sarcoptes scabiei* (scabies)

Pregnancy Risk Factor B

Lactation Effect on infant unknown

Contraindications Hypersensitivity to pyrethroid, pyrethrin, any component, or to chrysanthemums

Precautions For external use only; do not use near the eyes or on mucous membranes such as inside the nose, mouth, or vagina

Adverse Reactions

Dermatologic: Pruritus, erythema, rash of the scalp

Local: Burning, stinging, pain, edema, tingling, numbness, scalp discomfort

Drug Interactions

Avoid Concomitant Use There are no known interactions where it is recommended to avoid concomitant use.

Increased Effect/Toxicity There are no known significant interactions involving an increase in effect.

Decreased Effect There are no known significant interactions involving a decrease in effect.

Mechanism of Action Inhibits sodium ion influx through nerve cell membrane channels in parasites resulting in delayed repolarization, paralysis, and death of organism

Pharmacokinetics (Adult data unless noted)

Absorption: Topical: Minimal (<2%)

Metabolism: By ester hydrolysis to inactive metabolites

Usual Dosage Topical: Children >2 months and Adults:

Head lice: After hair has been washed with shampoo, rinsed with water and towel dried, apply a sufficient volume of creme rinse to saturate the hair and scalp; also apply behind the ears and at the base of the neck; leave on hair for 10 minutes before rinsing off with water; remove remaining nits. May repeat in 1 week if lice or nits still present; in areas of head lice resistance to 1% permethrin, 5% permethrin has been applied to clean, dry hair and left on overnight (8-14 hours) under a shower cap.

Scabies: Apply cream from head to toe; leave on for 8-14 hours before washing off with water; for infants, also apply on the hairline, neck, scalp, temple, and forehead; may reapply in 1 week if live mites appear. Permethrin 5% cream was shown to be safe and effective when applied to an infant <1 month of age with neonatal scabies; time of application was limited to 6 hours before rinsing with soap and water.

Administration Topical: Avoid contact with eyes during application; shake creme rinse well before using

Patient Information Clothing and bedding should be washed in hot water or by dry cleaning to kill the scabies mite

Nursing Implications

To remove nits: Comb hair with a fine-toothed nit comb and apply a damp towel to the scalp for 30-60 minutes

For infestation of eyelashes: Apply petroleum ointment to eyelashes 3-4 times/day for 8-10 days; remove nits mechanically from the eyelashes

For scabies: Itching may continue for several weeks despite successful treatment; oral antihistamines and/or topical corticosteroids may be helpful in relieving symptoms

Additional Information Topical cream formulation contains formaldehyde which is a contact allergen

Dosage Forms Excipient information presented when available (limited, particularly for generics); consult specific product labeling.

Cream, topical (Acticin®, Elimite®): 5% (60 g) [contains coconut oil]

Lotion, topical: 1% (59 mL)

Liquid, topical [creme rinse formulation] (Nix®): 1% (60 mL) [contains isopropyl alcohol 20%]

Solution, spray [for bedding and furniture]:

A200® Lice: 0.5% (180 mL)

Nix®: 0.25% (148 mL)

Rid®: 0.5% (150 mL)

References

"Drugs for Head Lice," *Med Lett Drugs Ther*, 1997, 39(992):6-7.

Hogan DJ, Schachner L, Tanglertsampan C, "Diagnosis and Treatment of Childhood Scabies and Pediculosis," *Pediatr Clin North Am*, 1991, 38(4):941-57.

Krowchuk DP, Tunnessen WW Jr, and Hurwitz S, "Pediatric Dermatology Update," *Pediatrics*, 1992, 90(2 Pt 1):259-64.

Quarterman MJ and Lesher JL, "Neonatal Scabies Treated With Permethrin 5% Cream," *Pediatr Dermatol*, 1994, 11(3):264-6.

◆ **Peroxide** *see* Hydrogen Peroxide *on page 689*

Perphenazine (per FEN a zeen)

Medication Safety Issues

Sound-alike/look-alike issues:

Trilafon® may be confused with Tri-Levlen®

Canadian Brand Names Apo-Perphenazine®

Therapeutic Category Antiemetic; Antipsychotic Agent, Typical, Phenothiazine; Phenothiazine Derivative

Generic Available Yes

Use Treatment of schizophrenia (FDA approved in ages ≥12 years and adults); severe nausea and vomiting (FDA approved in adults); other psychotic disorders (eg, schizoaffective disorder), psychotic depression

Pregnancy Risk Factor C

Lactation Enters breast milk/not recommended (AAP rates "of concern")

Contraindications Hypersensitivity to perphenazine or any component; cross-sensitivity with other phenothiazines may exist; severe CNS depression; subcortical brain damage; bone marrow suppression; blood dyscrasias; coma

Warnings May cause extrapyramidal symptoms, including pseudoparkinsonism, acute dystonic reactions, akathisia, and tardive dyskinesia (risk of these reactions is moderate-high relative to other neuroleptics, and is dose-dependent; to decrease risk of tardive dyskinesia: Use smallest dose and shortest duration possible; evaluate continued need periodically; risk of dystonia is increased with the use of high potency and higher doses of conventional antipsychotics and in males and younger patients). May be associated with neuroleptic malignant syndrome (NMS); monitor for mental status changes, fever, muscle rigidity, and/or autonomic instability; risk may be increased in patients with Parkinson's disease or Lewy body dementia. Safety for use during pregnancy and lactation has not been established; prolonged jaundice, hyper-reflexia, hyporeflexia, or extrapyramidal signs may occur in newborn infants of mothers who received phenothiazines; clinical benefits should clearly outweigh risks before initiating use during pregnancy. May cause pigmentary retinopathy; discontinue drug if ophthalmoscopic or visual field exam demonstrated retinal changes.

Leukopenia, neutropenia, and agranulocytosis (sometimes fatal) have been reported in clinical trials and postmarketing reports with antipsychotic use; presence of risk factors (eg, pre-existing low WBC or history of drug-induced leuko/neutropenia) should prompt periodic blood count assessment. Discontinue therapy at first signs of blood dyscrasias or if absolute neutrophil count <1000/mm^3. Use is contraindicated in patients with existing blood dyscrasias or bone marrow suppression.

An increased risk of death has been reported with the use of antipsychotics in elderly patients with dementia-related psychosis **[U.S. Boxed Warning]**; most deaths seemed to be cardiovascular (eg, sudden death, heart failure) or infectious (eg, pneumonia) in nature; perphenazine is not approved for this indication.

Precautions Use with caution in patients with hemodynamic instability; may cause hypotension; predisposition to seizures; cardiac, hepatic, renal, or respiratory disease; psychic depression. May cause sedation, which may impair physical or mental abilities; patients must be cautioned about performing tasks which require mental alertness (eg, operating machinery or driving); use with caution in disorders where CNS depression is a feature. Use with caution in Parkinson's disease. Esophageal dysmotility and aspiration have been associated with antipsychotic use; use with caution in patients at risk of pneumonia. Use with caution in breast cancer or other prolactin-dependent tumors; may elevate prolactin levels. May alter temperature regulation; use with caution with strenuous exercise, heat exposure, dehydration, and concomitant medication possessing anticholinergic effects. May mask toxicity of other drugs due to antiemetic effects. May alter cardiac conduction; life-threatening arrhythmias have occurred with therapeutic doses of phenothiazines. May cause orthostatic hypotension; use with caution in patients at risk of this effect or those who would not tolerate transient hypotensive episodes (cerebrovascular disease, cardiovascular disease, or other medications which may predispose). May cause photosensitization; avoid prolonged exposure to sunlight (see Patient Information). Perphenazine has not been shown to be effective for the treatment of behavioral complications in patients with mental retardation. Safety and efficacy in children <12 years of age has not been established.

Cholestatic jaundice, liver damage, and hepatitis may occur; obtain appropriate liver tests; discontinue treatment if liver tests are abnormal. Monitor renal function in patients with long-term therapy; discontinue treatment if BUN becomes abnormal. Phenothiazines may cause anticholinergic effects (confusion, agitation, constipation, xerostomia, blurred vision, urinary retention); therefore, they should be used with caution in patients with decreased GI motility, urinary retention, benign prostatic hypertrophy, xerostomia, or visual problems. Conditions which also may be exacerbated by cholinergic blockade include narrow-angle glaucoma (screening is recommended) and worsening of myasthenia gravis. Relative to other neuroleptics, perphenazine has a low potency of cholinergic blockade.

Adverse Reactions

Cardiovascular: Bradycardia, cardiac arrest, dizziness, hypertension, hypotension, orthostatic hypotension, tachycardia

Central nervous system: Cerebral edema, dizziness, drowsiness, extrapyramidal symptoms (akathisia, dystonias, pseudoparkinsonism, tardive dyskinesia), headache, hyperactivity, impairment of temperature regulation, insomnia, neuroleptic malignant syndrome (NMS), paradoxical excitement, restlessness, seizure

Dermatologic: Discoloration of skin (blue-gray), photosensitivity, rash

Endocrine & metabolic: Amenorrhea, breast enlargement, galactorrhea, gynecomastia, hyperglycemia, hypoglycemia, lactation, libido (changes in), menstrual irregularity, SIADH, weight gain

Gastrointestinal: Anorexia, constipation, diarrhea, ileus, nausea, salivation, stomach pain, vomiting, xerostomia

Genitourinary: Difficult urination, ejaculatory disturbances, ejaculating dysfunction, incontinence, polyuria, priapism

Hematologic: Agranulocytosis, eosinophilia, hemolytic anemia, leukopenia, neutropenia, pancytopenia, thrombocytopenic purpura

Hepatic: Cholestatic jaundice, hepatotoxicity

Neuromuscular & skeletal: Tremor

Ocular: Blurred vision, cornea and lens changes, pigmentary retinopathy

Respiratory: Nasal congestion

Miscellaneous: Diaphoresis, hypersensitivity reactions

Drug Interactions

Metabolism/Transport Effects Substrate of CYP1A2 (minor), 2C9 (minor), 2C19 (minor), 2D6 (major), 3A4 (minor); **Inhibits** CYP1A2 (weak), 2D6 (weak)

Avoid Concomitant Use

Avoid concomitant use of Perphenazine with any of the following: Metoclopramide

Increased Effect/Toxicity

Perphenazine may increase the levels/effects of: Alcohol (Ethyl); Analgesics (Opioid); Anticholinergics; Anti-Parkinson's Agents (Dopamine Agonist); Beta-Blockers; CNS Depressants; Methotrimeprazine

The levels/effects of Perphenazine may be increased by: Acetylcholinesterase Inhibitors (Central); Antimalarial Agents; Beta-Blockers; CYP2D6 Inhibitors (Moderate); CYP2D6 Inhibitors (Strong); Darunavir; Lithium formulations; Methotrimeprazine; Metoclopramide; Pramlintide; Tetrabenazine

Decreased Effect

Perphenazine may decrease the levels/effects of: Amphetamines; Quinagolide

The levels/effects of Perphenazine may be decreased by: Antacids; Anti-Parkinson's Agents (Dopamine Agonist); Lithium formulations; Peginterferon Alfa-2b

Food Interactions May cause increase in dietary riboflavin requirements

Stability Store at controlled room temperature at 20°C to 25°C (68°F to 77°F); dispense in tight, light-resistant container

Mechanism of Action Perphenazine is a piperazine phenothiazine antipsychotic which blocks postsynaptic mesolimbic dopaminergic receptors in the brain; exhibits alpha-adrenergic blocking effect and depresses the release of hypothalamic and hypophyseal hormones

Pharmacodynamics

Onset of action: 2-4 weeks for control of psychotic symptoms (hallucinations, disorganized thinking or behavior, delusions)

Adequate trial: 6 weeks at moderate to high dose based on tolerability

Duration: Variable

Pharmacokinetics (Adult data unless noted)

Absorption: Well absorbed

Distribution: Crosses placenta

Metabolism: Extensively hepatic to metabolites via sulfoxidation, hydroxylation, dealkylation, and glucuronidation; **Note:** Metabolism is subject to genetic polymorphism; CYP2D6 poor metabolizers will have higher plasma concentrations of perphenazine compared with normal or extensive metabolizers.

Half-life: Perphenazine: 9-12 hours; 7-hydroxyperphenazine: 9.9-18.8 hours

Time to peak serum concentration: Perphenazine: 1-3 hours; 7-hydroxyperphenazine: 2-4 hours

Elimination: Urine and feces, primarily as metabolites

Dialysis: Not dialyzable (0% to 5%)

Usual Dosage Oral: **Note:** Dosage should be individualized; use lowest effective dose and shortest effective duration; periodically reassess the need for continued treatment

Children: **Note:** Safety and efficacy have not been established in children <12 years of age; use in this age group is not recommended by manufacturer. Some centers use the following doses:

Schizophrenia/psychoses:

<1 year: Dosage not established

1-6 years: 4-6 mg/day in divided doses

6-12 years: 6 mg/day in divided doses

>12 years: 4-16 mg 2-4 times/day

Postoperative vomiting: Dosage not established; use not recommended. Previous studies used an I.V. dose of 70 mcg/kg (maximum: 5 mg/dose) in children 2-12 years of age to decrease postoperative vomiting; perphenazine was shown to be more effective than placebo (Splinter, 1997), more effective than dexamethasone (Splinter, 1997a), and similar in efficacy to ondansetron (Splinter, 1998). However, I.V. granisetron was shown to be more effective than I.V. perphenazine (Fujii, 1999). Only one study has assessed oral perphenazine; doses of 70 mcg/kg were administered 1 hour prior to surgery to 100 children, 4-10 years of age, to reduce postoperative vomiting; oral granisetron was more effective than oral perphenazine (Fujii, 1999a).

Adults:

Schizophrenia/psychoses: 4-16 mg 2-4 times/day; maximum: 64 mg/day (exceptions occur; indication specific)

Nausea/vomiting: 8-16 mg/day in divided doses; maximum: 24 mg/day

Dosing adjustment in hepatic impairment: Specific guidelines are not available; consider dosage reduction in patients with liver disease

Administration May be administered without regard to meals; do not administer within 2 hours of antacids

Monitoring Parameters Vital signs; periodic eye exam, CBC with differential, liver enzyme tests; renal function in patients with long-term use; fasting blood glucose/Hgb A$_{1c}$; BMI; therapeutic response (mental status, mood, affect, gait), and adverse reactions at beginning of therapy and periodically with long-term use [eg, excess sedation, extrapyramidal symptoms, tardive dyskinesia, CNS changes, abnormal involuntary movement scale (AIMS)]

Reference Range 2-6 nmol/L

Patient Information Use exactly as directed; do not increase dose or frequency. It may take 2-3 weeks to achieve desired results; do not discontinue without consulting prescriber. Do not take within 2 hours of any antacid. Avoid alcohol, caffeine, and other prescription or nonprescription medications not approved by prescriber. May cause drowsiness, dizziness, lightheadedness, or blurred vision and impair ability to perform activities requiring mental alertness or physical coordination; use caution driving or when engaging in tasks requiring alertness until response to drug is known. May cause dry mouth. May cause photosensitivity reactions (eg, exposure to sunlight may cause severe sunburn, skin rash, redness, or itching); avoid exposure to sunlight and artificial light sources (sunlamps, tanning booth/bed); wear protective clothing, wide-brimmed hats, sunglasses, and lip sunscreen (SPF ≥15); use a sunscreen [broad-spectrum sunscreen or physical sunscreen (preferred) or sunblock with SPF ≥15]; contact physician if reaction occurs.

Maintain adequate hydration unless instructed to restrict fluid intake. Avoid skin contact with medication; may cause contact dermatitis (wash immediately with warm, soapy water). May cause nausea, vomiting (small frequent meals, frequent mouth care, chewing gum, or sucking lozenges may help); constipation; postural hypotension (use caution climbing stairs or when changing position from lying or sitting to standing); urinary retention (void before taking medication); or decreased perspiration (avoid strenuous exercise in hot environments). Report persistent CNS effects (eg, trembling fingers, altered gait

or balance, excessive sedation, seizures, unusual movements, anxiety, abnormal thoughts, confusion, personality changes); chest pain, palpitations, rapid heartbeat, severe dizziness; unresolved urinary retention or changes in urinary pattern; menstrual pattern, change in libido, swelling or pain in breasts (male or female); vision changes; skin rash or yellowing of skin; respiratory difficulty; or worsening of condition.

Nursing Implications Review ophthalmic exam and monitor laboratory results, therapeutic effectiveness (according to rationale for therapy), and adverse reactions at beginning of therapy and periodically with long-term use. Monitor blood pressure; can cause orthostatic hypotension. Initiate at lower doses and taper dosage slowly when discontinuing.

Additional Information Long-term usefulness of perphenazine should be periodically re-evaluated in patients receiving the drug for extended periods; consideration should be given whether to decrease the maintenance dose or discontinue drug therapy

Dosage Forms Excipient information presented when available (limited, particularly for generics); consult specific product labeling.

Tablet: 2 mg, 4 mg, 8 mg, 16 mg

References

Azaz-Livshits TL, Symmer LI, and Fraenkel YM, "Atypical Neuroleptic Malignant Syndrome Presenting as Rhabdomyolysis, Altered Consciousness, and Leukocytosis," *J Pharm Technol*, 1995, 11:173-5.

Fujii Y, Saitoh Y, Tanaka H, et al, "Anti-Emetic Efficacy of Prophylactic Granisetron Compared With Perphenazine for the Prevention of Postoperative Vomiting in Children," *Eur J Anaesthesiol*, 1999, 16 (5):304-7.

Fujii Y, Saitoh Y, Tanaka H, et al, "Preoperative Oral Antiemetics for Reducing Postoperative Vomiting After Tonsillectomy in Children: Granisetron Versus Perphenazine," *Anesth Analg*, 1999a, 88 (6):1298-301.

Hansen LB and Larsen NE, "Metabolic Interaction Between Perphenazine and Disulfiram," *Lancet*, 1982, 2(8313):1472.

Harper G, Dawes M, Azlin C, et al, "Small Bowel Obstruction in a Child on an Antipsychotic," *J Child Adolesc Psychopharmacol*, 1995, 5:81-4.

Lieberman JA, Stroup TS, McEvoy JP, et al, "Effectiveness of Antipsychotic Drugs in Patients With Chronic Schizophrenia," *N Engl J Med*, 2005, 353(12):1209-23.

Miyamoto S, Duncan GE, Marx CE, et al, "Treatments for Schizophrenia: A Critical Review of Pharmacology and Mechanisms of Action of Antipsychotic Drugs," *Mol Psychiatry*, 2005, 10(1):79-104.

Remington G, "Tardive Dyskinesia: Eliminated, Forgotten, or Overshadowed?" *Curr Opin Psychiatry*, 2007, 20(2):131-7.

Splinter WM and Roberts DJ, "Perphenazine Decreases Vomiting by Children After Tonsillectomy," *Can J Anaesth*, 1997, 44(12):1308-10.

Splinter WM and Roberts DJ, "Prophylaxis for Vomiting by Children After Tonsillectomy: Dexamethasone Versus Perphenazine," *Anesth Analg*, 1997a, 85(3):534-7.

Splinter WM and Rhine EJ, "Prophylaxis for Vomiting by Children After Tonsillectomy: Ondansetron Compared With Perphenazine," *Br J Anaesth*, 1998, 80(2):155-8.

◆ **Persantine®** *see* Dipyridamole *on page 461*

◆ **Pertussis, Acellular (Adsorbed)** *see* Diphtheria and Tetanus Toxoids, Acellular Pertussis, Poliovirus and *Haemophilus* b Conjugate Vaccine *on page 455*

◆ **Pethidine Hydrochloride** *see* Meperidine *on page 880*

◆ **Petrolatum White and Mineral Oil Ophthalmic Ointment** *see* Ocular Lubricant *on page 1011*

◆ **Pexeva®** *see* PARoxetine *on page 1064*

◆ **PFA** *see* Foscarnet *on page 626*

◆ **Pfizerpen®** *see* Penicillin G (Parenteral/Aqueous) *on page 1080*

◆ **Pfizerpen-AS® (Can)** *see* Penicillin G Procaine *on page 1081*

◆ **PGE$_1$** *see* Alprostadil *on page 69*

◆ **PGI$_2$** *see* Epoprostenol *on page 517*

◆ **PGX** *see* Epoprostenol *on page 517*

◆ **Phanasin® [OTC] [DSC]** *see* GuaiFENesin *on page 656*

◆ **Phanasin® Diabetic Choice® [OTC] [DSC]** *see* Guai-FENesin *on page 656*

◆ **Phanatuss® DM [OTC] [DSC]** *see* Guaifenesin and Dextromethorphan *on page 658*

◆ **Pharmaflur® [DSC]** *see* Fluoride *on page 595*

◆ **Pharmaflur® 1.1 [DSC]** *see* Fluoride *on page 595*

◆ **Phazyme™ (Can)** *see* Simethicone *on page 1262*

◆ **Phazyme® Ultra Strength [OTC]** *see* Simethicone *on page 1262*

◆ **Phenadoz™** *see* Promethazine *on page 1163*

◆ **Phenazo™ (Can)** *see* Phenazopyridine *on page 1097*

Phenazopyridine (fen az oh PEER i deen)

Medication Safety Issues
Sound-alike/look-alike issues:
Phenazopyridine may be confused with phenoxy-•benzamine
Pyridium® may be confused with Dyrenium®, Perdiem®, pyridoxine, pyrithione

U.S. Brand Names AZO-Gesic® [OTC]; AZO-Standard® Maximum Strength [OTC]; AZO-Standard® [OTC]; Baridium® [OTC]; Prodium® [OTC]; Pyridium®; ReAzo [OTC]; UTI Relief® [OTC]

Canadian Brand Names Phenazo™

Therapeutic Category Analgesic, Urinary; Local Anesthetic, Urinary

Generic Available Yes

Use Symptomatic relief of urinary burning, itching, frequency and urgency in association with urinary tract infection, or following urologic procedures

Pregnancy Risk Factor B

Lactation Excretion in breast milk unknown

Contraindications Hypersensitivity to phenazopyridine or any component; liver or kidney disease (do not use in patients with Cl_{cr} <50 mL/minute)

Warnings Does not treat infection, acts only as an analgesic; drug should be discontinued if skin or sclera develop a yellow color.

Precautions Use with caution in patients with renal impairment (Cl_{cr} 50-80 mL/minute)

Adverse Reactions
Central nervous system: Vertigo, headache
Dermatologic: Skin pigmentation, rash, pruritus
Gastrointestinal: Stomach cramps
Genitourinary: Discoloration of urine (orange or red)
Hematologic: Methemoglobinemia, hemolytic anemia
Hepatic: Hepatitis
Renal: Transient acute renal failure

Drug Interactions
Avoid Concomitant Use There are no known interactions where it is recommended to avoid concomitant use.
Increased Effect/Toxicity There are no known significant interactions involving an increase in effect.
Decreased Effect There are no known significant interactions involving a decrease in effect.

Mechanism of Action Exerts local topical anesthetic or analgesic action on urinary tract mucosa through an unknown mechanism

Pharmacokinetics (Adult data unless noted)
Metabolism: In the liver and other tissues
Elimination: In urine (where it exerts its action); renal excretion (as unchanged drug) is rapid and accounts for 65% of the drug's elimination

Usual Dosage Oral:
Children: 12 mg/kg/day in 3 divided doses for 2 days if used concomitantly with an antibacterial agent for UTI
Adults: 95-200 mg 3-4 times/day for 2 days if used concomitantly with an antibacterial agent for UTI

Dosing interval in renal impairment:
Cl_{cr} 50-80 mL/minute: Administer every 8-16 hours
Cl_{cr} <50 mL/minute: Avoid use

Administration Oral: Administer with food to decrease GI distress

Test Interactions False-negative Clinistix®, Tes-Tape®, Ictotest®, Acetest®, Ketostix®, urinalysis based upon spectrometry or color reactions

Patient Information May discolor urine orange or red; may stain contact lenses and fabric; not an antibiotic and does not treat infection; contact physician for antibiotic therapy

Dosage Forms Excipient information presented when available (limited, particularly for generics); consult specific product labeling. [DSC] = Discontinued product
Tablet, as hydrochloride: 100 mg, 200 mg
AZO-Gesic®, Prodium®, ReAzo: 95 mg
AZO-Standard®: 95 mg [gluten free]
AZO Standard® Maximum Strength: 97.5 mg [gluten free]
Baridium®, UTI Relief®: 97.2 mg
Pyridium®: 100 mg, 200 mg

Extemporaneous Preparations A 10 mg/mL suspension may be made by crushing three 200 mg tablets. Mix with a small amount of distilled water or glycerin. Add 20 mL Cologel® [DSC] and levigate until a uniform mixture is obtained. Add sufficient 2:1 simple syrup/cherry syrup mixture to make a final volume of 60 mL. Store in an amber container. Label "shake well". Stability is 60 days refrigerated.
Handbook on Extemporaneous Formulations, Bethesda MD: American Society of Hospital Pharmacists, 1987.

◆ **Phenazopyridine Hydrochloride** *see* Phenazopyridine *on page 1097*

◆ **Phenergan®** *see* Promethazine *on page 1163*

PHENobarbital (fee noe BAR bi tal)

Medication Safety Issues
Sound-alike/look-alike issues:
PHENobarbital may be confused with PENTobarbital, Phenergan®, phenytoin
Luminal® may be confused with Tuinal®

Related Information
Antiepileptic Drugs *on page 1693*
Febrile Seizures *on page 1690*
Laboratory Detection of Drugs in Urine *on page 1706*
Therapeutic Drug Monitoring: Blood Sampling Time Guidelines *on page 1704*

U.S. Brand Names Luminal® Sodium

Canadian Brand Names PMS-Phenobarbital

Therapeutic Category Anticonvulsant, Barbiturate; Barbiturate; Hypnotic; Sedative

Generic Available Yes

Use Management of generalized tonic-clonic (grand mal) and partial seizures; neonatal seizures; febrile seizures in children; sedation; may also be used for prevention and treatment of neonatal hyperbilirubinemia and lowering of bilirubin in chronic cholestasis; management of sedative/hypnotic withdrawal

Restrictions C-IV

Pregnancy Risk Factor D

Pregnancy Considerations Crosses the placenta. Cardiac defect reported; hemorrhagic disease of newborn due to fetal vitamin K depletion may occur; may induce maternal folic acid deficiency; withdrawal symptoms observed in infant following delivery. Epilepsy itself, number of medications, genetic factors, or a combination of these probably influence the teratogenicity of anticonvulsant therapy. Benefit:risk ratio usually favors continued use during pregnancy and breast-feeding.

◀ **Lactation** Enters breast milk/not recommended (AAP recommends use "with caution")

Breast-Feeding Considerations Sedation has been reported in nursing infants; infantile spasms may occur after weaning from breast milk. AAP recommends USE WITH CAUTION.

Contraindications Hypersensitivity to phenobarbital or any component; pre-existing CNS depression, severe uncontrolled pain, porphyria (manifest and latent), severe respiratory disease with dyspnea or obstruction; intra-arterial administration; use in nephritic patients (large doses)

Warnings Tolerance and/or psychological and physical dependence may occur; abrupt discontinuation after prolonged use may result in withdrawal symptoms, seizures, or status epilepticus; withdraw gradually if used over extended periods of time. Rapid I.V. administration may cause respiratory depression, apnea, laryngospasm, or hypotension. Phenobarbital may cause CNS depression, which may impair physical or mental abilities; patients must be cautioned about performing tasks which require mental alertness (eg, operating machinery or driving). Effects with other sedative drugs or ethanol may be potentiated. Commercially available injection contains 10% alcohol and 67.8% propylene glycol.

Antiepileptic drugs (AEDs) increase the risk of suicidal behavior and ideation in patients receiving these medications for any indication. Pooled analyses of placebo-controlled trials involving 11 different AEDs (regardless of indication) showed a two fold increased risk of suicidal thoughts or behavior (estimated incidence rate: 0.43% in AED treated patients compared to 0.24% of patients receiving placebo); increased risk was observed as early as 1 week after initiation of AED and continued through duration of trials (most trials ≤24 weeks); risk did not vary significantly by age (age range: 5–100 years). Consider risks and benefits of AEDs before prescribing. Monitor all patients receiving an AED for emergence of suicidal thoughts or behavior, thoughts of self-harm, any unusual changes in behavior or mood, or the emergence or worsening of depressive symptoms; notify heathcare provider immediately if symptoms or concerning behavior occur. **Note:** The FDA is requiring that a Medication Guide be developed for all antiepileptic drugs informing patients of this risk.

Precautions Use with caution in patients with renal or hepatic impairment or respiratory diseases. Use with caution in patients with acute or chronic pain (paradoxical excitement may occur or important symptoms may be masked), hepatic dysfunction (decreased dosage may be needed; avoid use in patients with premonitory signs of hepatic coma), pregnancy (fetal abnormalities may occur; infants may experience withdrawal symptoms with chronic maternal use), or debilitated patients (paradoxical excitement, depression, or confusion may occur). Use with caution (if at all) in patients with depression or suicidal tendencies or in patients with a history of drug abuse (use in patients with a history of sedative/hypnotic addiction is not recommended).

Solution for injection is highly alkaline and extravasation may cause local tissue damage leading to necrosis; ensure patient has adequate intravenous access with I.V. use. Intra-arterial administration may cause reactions ranging from transient pain to gangrene and is contra-indicated. Subcutaneous administration may cause tissue irritation (eg, redness, tenderness, necrosis) and is not recommended.

Adverse Reactions

Cardiovascular: Hypotension, circulatory collapse, brady-cardia, syncope

Central nervous system: Drowsiness, somnolence, CNS depression, paradoxical excitement, hyperkinetic activity, cognitive impairment, defects in general comprehension, short-term memory deficits, attention span decreased, ataxia, fever; suicidal thinking and behavior (see Warnings)

Dermatologic: Skin eruptions, skin rash, exfoliative dermatitis

Gastrointestinal: Nausea, vomiting, constipation

Hematologic: Megaloblastic anemia (chronic use)

Hepatic: Hepatitis

Local: Injection site reactions

Respiratory: Respiratory depression, apnea (especially with rapid I.V. use)

Miscellaneous: Psychological and physical dependence, hypersensitivity reactions

Drug Interactions

Metabolism/Transport Effects Substrate of CYP2C9 (minor), 2C19 (major), 2E1 (minor); **Induces** CYP1A2 (strong), 2A6 (strong), 2B6 (strong), 2C8 (strong), 2C9 (strong), 3A4 (strong)

Avoid Concomitant Use

Avoid concomitant use of PHENobarbital with any of the following: Darunavir; Dronedarone; Etravirine; Everolimus; Nilotinib; Pazopanib; Ranolazine; Romidepsin; Tolvaptan; Voriconazole

Increased Effect/Toxicity

PHENobarbital may increase the levels/effects of: Alcohol (Ethyl); CNS Depressants; Meperidine; Thiazide Diuretics

The levels/effects of PHENobarbital may be increased by: Carbonic Anhydrase Inhibitors; Chloramphenicol; CYP2C19 Inhibitors (Moderate); CYP2C19 Inhibitors (Strong); Divalproex; Felbamate; Primidone; Rufinamide; Valproic Acid

Decreased Effect

PHENobarbital may decrease the levels/effects of: Acetaminophen; Bendamustine; Beta-Blockers; Calcium Channel Blockers; Chloramphenicol; Contraceptives (Estrogens); Contraceptives (Progestins); Corticosteroids (Systemic); CycloSPORINE; CycloSPORINE (Systemic); CYP1A2 Substrates; CYP2A6 Substrates; CYP2B6 Substrates; CYP2C8 Substrates (High risk); CYP2C9 Substrates (High risk); CYP3A4 Substrates; Darunavir; Deferasirox; Disopyramide; Divalproex; Doxycycline; Dronedarone; Etoposide; Etoposide Phosphate; Etravir-ine; Everolimus; Griseofulvin; GuanFACINE; Irinotecan; Lacosamide; LamoTRIgine; Maraviroc; Methadone; Met-roNIDAZOLE; MetroNIDAZOLE (Systemic); Nilotinib; OXcarbazepine; Pazopanib; Propafenone; QuiNIDine; Ranolazine; Romidepsin; Rufinamide; Saxagliptin; Sor-afenib; Tadalafil; Teniposide; Theophylline Derivatives; Tipranavir; Tolvaptan; Treprostinil; Tricyclic Antidepres-sants; Valproic Acid; Vitamin K Antagonists; Voricona-zole; Zonisamide

The levels/effects of PHENobarbital may be decreased by: Amphetamines; Cholestyramine Resin; CYP2C19 Inducers (Strong); Folic Acid; Ketorolac; Ketorolac (Systemic); Leucovorin Calcium-Levoleucovorin; Meflo-quine; Methylfolate; Pyridoxine; Rifamycin Derivatives; Tipranavir

Food Interactions High doses of pyridoxine may decrease drug effect; barbiturates may increase the metabolism of vitamins D and K; dietary requirements of vitamins D, K, C, B$_{12}$, folate, and calcium may be increased with long-term use

Stability

Elixir: Protect from light

Injection: Protect from light; not stable in aqueous solutions; use only clear solutions; do not add to acidic solutions, precipitation may occur

Mechanism of Action Depresses CNS activity by binding to barbiturate site at GABA-receptor complex enhancing GABA activity; depresses reticular activating system; higher doses may be gabamimetic

Pharmacodynamics Hypnosis:

Onset of action:

Oral: Within 20-60 minutes

I.V.: Within 5 minutes

Maximum effect: I.V.: Within 30 minutes

Duration:

Oral: 6-10 hours

I.V.: 4-10 hours

Pharmacokinetics (Adult data unless noted)

Absorption: Oral: 70% to 90%

Distribution: V_d:

Neonates: 0.8-1 L/kg

Infants: 0.7-0.8 L/kg

Children: 0.6-0.7 L/kg

Protein binding: 35% to 50%, decreased protein binding in neonates

Metabolism: In the liver via hydroxylation and glucuronide conjugation

Half-life:

Neonates: 45-500 hours

Infants: 20-133 hours

Children: 37-73 hours

Adults: 53-140 hours

Time to peak serum concentration: Oral: Within 1-6 hours

Elimination: 20% to 50% excreted unchanged in urine; clearance can be increased with alkalinization of urine or with oral multiple-dose activated charcoal

Dialysis: Moderately dialyzable (20% to 50%)

Usual Dosage

Anticonvulsant: Status epilepticus: **Loading dose:** I.V.: **Note:** Be prepared to support respiration, especially when maximizing loading dose (see also Additional Information)

Neonates: Initial: 15-20 mg/kg in a single or divided dose; may repeat doses of 5-10 mg/kg every 15-20 minutes as needed (maximum total dose: 40 mg/kg)

Infants and Children: Initial: 15-20 mg/kg (maximum: 1000 mg/dose); may repeat dose after 15 minutes as needed (maximum total dose: 40 mg/kg)

Adults: Initial: 10-20 mg/kg; may repeat dose in 20-minute intervals as needed (maximum total dose: 30 mg/kg)

Anticonvulsant **maintenance dose**: Oral, I.V. (**Note:** Maintenance dose usually starts 12 hours after loading dose):

Neonates: 3-4 mg/kg/day given once daily; assess serum concentrations; increase to 5 mg/kg/day if needed (usually by second week of therapy)

Infants: 5-6 mg/kg/day in 1-2 divided doses

Children:

1-5 years: 6-8 mg/kg/day in 1-2 divided doses

5-12 years: 4-6 mg/kg/day in 1-2 divided doses

>12 years and adults: 1-3 mg/kg/day in 1-2 divided doses

Children:

Sedation: Oral: 2 mg/kg/dose 3 times/day

Hypnotic: I.M., I.V.: 3-5 mg/kg at bedtime

Hyperbilirubinemia: <12 years: Oral: 3-8 mg/kg/day in 2-3 divided doses; doses up to 12 mg/kg/day have been used

Preoperative sedation: Oral, I.M., I.V.: 1-3 mg/kg 1-1.5 hours before procedure

Adults:

Sedation: Oral, I.M.: 30-120 mg/day in 2-3 divided doses

Hypnotic: Oral, I.M., I.V.: 100-320 mg at bedtime

Hyperbilirubinemia: Oral: 90-180 mg/day in 2-3 divided doses

Preoperative sedation: I.M.: 100-200 mg 1-1.5 hours before procedure

Administration

Oral: Administer elixir with water, milk, or juice

Parenteral: Do not inject I.V. faster than 1 mg/kg/minute with a maximum of 30 mg/minute for infants and children and 60 mg/minute for adults >60 kg. Do not administer intra-arterially (contraindicated); avoid extravasation; SubQ administration is not recommended. For I.M. administration, inject deep into muscle; do not exceed 5 mL per injection site (adults) due to potential for tissue irritation

Monitoring Parameters CNS status, seizure activity, liver enzymes, CBC with differential, renal function, serum concentrations; signs and symptoms of suicidality (eg, anxiety, depression, behavior changes) (see Warnings). With I.V. use: Respiratory rate, heart rate, blood pressure, I.V. site (stop injection if patient complains of pain in the limb; see Precautions). For treatment of hyperbilirubinemia: Monitor bilirubin (total and direct)

Reference Range

Therapeutic: 15-40 mcg/mL (SI: 65-172 micromoles/L)

Potentially toxic: >40 mcg/mL (SI: >172 micromoles/L)

Coma: >50 mcg/mL (SI: >215 micromoles/L)

Potentially lethal: >80 mcg/mL (SI: >344 micromoles/L)

Patient Information Avoid alcohol; limit caffeine. May be habit-forming; avoid abrupt discontinuation after prolonged use (withdrawal symptoms or an increase in seizure activity may occur). May cause dizziness or drowsiness and impair ability to perform activities requiring mental alertness or physical coordination. Antiepileptic agents may increase the risk of suicidal thoughts and behavior; notify physician if you feel more depressed or have thoughts of suicide or self-harm (see Warnings). Report worsening of seizure activity or loss of seizure control.

Nursing Implications Parenteral solutions are very alkaline; avoid extravasation (see Precautions and Administration)

Additional Information Allow adequate time to elapse between I.V. doses when treating active seizures; peak concentrations in the brain may require ≥15 minutes to occur; repeating I.V. doses of phenobarbital until convulsions stop may cause the concentration in the brain to exceed the amount required to control seizure activity and result in severe barbiturate-induced CNS depression

A retrospective study (Relling, 2000) demonstrated that enzyme-inducing antiepileptic drugs (AEDs) (carbamazepine, phenobarbital, and phenytoin) increased systemic clearance of antileukemic drugs (teniposide and methotrexate) and were associated with a worse event-free survival, CNS relapse, and hematologic relapse (ie, lower efficacy), in B-lineage ALL children receiving chemotherapy; the authors recommend using nonenzyme-inducing AEDs in patients receiving chemotherapy for ALL.

Dosage Forms Excipient information presented when available (limited, particularly for generics); consult specific product labeling.

Elixir: 20 mg/5 mL (5 mL, 7.5 mL, 15 mL, 480 mL) [contains ethanol]

Injection, solution, as sodium: 65 mg/mL (1 mL); 130 mg/mL (1 mL) [contains ethanol and propylene glycol]

Luminal® Sodium: 60 mg/mL (1 mL); 130 mg/mL (1 mL) [contains ethanol 10% and propylene glycol 67.8%]

Tablet: 15 mg, 30 mg, 60 mg, 100 mg

Extemporaneous Preparations An alcohol-free 10 mg/mL phenobarbital suspension made from tablets and 2 different vehicles (a 1:1 mixture of Ora-Plus® and Ora-Sweet® and a 1:1 mixture of Ora-Plus® and Ora-Sweet® SF) was stable for 115 days when stored in amber plastic prescription bottles at room temperature (23°C to 25°C). Grind ten phenobarbital 60 mg tablets in a glass mortar into a fine powder. Mix 30 mL of Ora-Plus® and 30 mL of either Ora-Sweet® or Ora-Sweet® SF; stir vigorously. Add 15 mL of the vehicle to the powder; triturate well. Transfer the mixture to a 2 ounce amber plastic prescription bottle. Add 15 mL aliquots of the vehicle to the mortar and triturate to rinse mortar and pestle; transfer to bottle. Repeat to qsad to a final volume of 60 mL. Label "shake well prior to use." May mix dose with chocolate syrup (1:1 volume) immediately before administration to mask the bitter aftertaste (Cober, 2007).

Cober MP and Johnson CE, "Stability of an Extemporaneously Prepared Alcohol-Free Phenobarbital Suspension," *Am J Health Syst Pharm*, 2007, 64(6):644-6.

References
Hegenbarth MA and American Academy of Pediatrics Committee on Drugs, "Preparing for Pediatric Emergencies: Drugs to Consider," *Pediatrics*, 2008, 121(2):433-43.

Kraus DM and Pham JT, "Neonatal Therapy," *Applied Therapeutics: The Clinical Use of Drugs*, 9th ed, Koda-Kimble MA, Young LY, Kradjan WA, et al, eds, Baltimore, MD: Lippincott Williams & Wilkins, 2009.

Relling MV, Pui CH, Sandlund JT, et al, "Adverse Effect of Anticonvulsants on Efficacy of Chemotherapy for Acute Lymphoblastic Leukaemia," *Lancet*, 2000, 356(9226):285-90.

Sabo-Graham T and Seay AR, "Management of Status Epilepticus in Children," *Pediatr Rev*, 1998, 19(9):306-9.

♦ **Phenobarbital, Hyoscyamine, Atropine, and Scopolamine** see Hyoscyamine, Atropine, Scopolamine, and Phenobarbital on page 700

♦ **Phenobarbital Sodium** see PHENobarbital on page 1097

♦ **Phenobarbitone** see PHENobarbital on page 1097

Phenoxybenzamine (fen oks ee BEN za meen)

Medication Safety Issues
Sound-alike/look-alike issues:
Phenoxybenzamine may be confused with phenazopyridine

Related Information
Antihypertensive Agents by Class on page 1481

U.S. Brand Names Dibenzyline®

Canadian Brand Names Dibenzyline®

Therapeutic Category Alpha-Adrenergic Blocking Agent, Oral; Antihypertensive Agent; Vasodilator

Generic Available No

Use Symptomatic management of hypertension and sweating in patients with pheochromocytoma

Pregnancy Risk Factor C

Pregnancy Considerations Adequate animal reproduction studies have not been conducted. It is not known whether phenoxybenzamine can cause fetal harm when administered to a pregnant woman or can affect reproduction capacity.

Lactation Excretion in breast milk unknown/not recommended

Contraindications Hypersensitivity to phenoxybenzamine or any component (see Warnings); shock

Warnings Capsule contains benzyl alcohol which may cause allergic reactions in susceptible individuals; large amounts of benzyl alcohol (≥99 mg/kg/day) have been associated with a potentially fatal toxicity ("gasping syndrome") in neonates; avoid use of phenoxybenzamine products containing benzyl alcohol in neonates; *in vitro* and animal studies have shown that benzoate, a metabolite of benzyl alcohol, displaces bilirubin from protein binding sites

Precautions Use with caution in patients with renal dysfunction, cerebral or coronary arteriosclerosis

Adverse Reactions
Cardiovascular: Postural hypotension, tachycardia, syncope, shock

Central nervous system: Lethargy, headache, dizziness

Gastrointestinal: Vomiting, nausea, diarrhea

Neuromuscular & skeletal: Weakness

Ocular: Miosis

Respiratory: Nasal congestion

Drug Interactions
Avoid Concomitant Use
Avoid concomitant use of Phenoxybenzamine with any of the following: Alfuzosin; Silodosin; Tamsulosin

Increased Effect/Toxicity
Phenoxybenzamine may increase the levels/effects of: Alfuzosin; Amifostine; Antihypertensives; Calcium Channel Blockers; RiTUXimab; Silodosin; Tamsulosin

The levels/effects of Phenoxybenzamine may be increased by: Alfuzosin; Beta-Blockers; Diazoxide; Herbs (Hypotensive Properties); MAO Inhibitors; Pentoxifylline; Phosphodiesterase 5 Inhibitors; Prostacyclin Analogues; Silodosin; Tamsulosin

Decreased Effect
The levels/effects of Phenoxybenzamine may be decreased by: Herbs (Hypertensive Properties); Methylphenidate; Yohimbine

Mechanism of Action Produces long-lasting noncompetitive alpha-adrenergic blockade of postganglionic synapses in exocrine glands and smooth muscle

Pharmacodynamics Oral:
Onset of action: Within 2 hours
Maximum effect: Within 4-6 hours
Duration: Effects can continue for up to 4 days

Pharmacokinetics (Adult data unless noted)
Absorption: Oral: ~20% to 30%
Distribution: Distributes to and may accumulate in adipose tissues
Half-life: Adults: 24 hours
Elimination: Primarily in urine and bile

Usual Dosage Oral:
Children: Initial: 0.2 mg/kg once daily; maximum dose: 10 mg/dose; increase every 4 days by 0.2 mg/kg/day increments; usual maintenance dose: 0.4-1.2 mg/kg/day every 6-8 hours; maximum doses of up to 2-4 mg/kg/day have been recommended

Adults: Initial: 10 mg twice daily; increase dose every other day to usual dose of 10-40 mg every 8-12 hours; higher doses may be needed

Administration Oral: May administer with milk to decrease GI upset

Monitoring Parameters Blood pressure, orthostasis, heart rate

Patient Information Avoid alcohol; may cause dizziness; avoid sudden changes in posture; may cause nasal congestion and constricted pupils; avoid cough, cold, or allergy medications containing sympathomimetics

Dosage Forms Excipient information presented when available (limited, particularly for generics); consult specific product labeling.

Capsule, as hydrochloride:
Dibenzyline®: 10 mg [contains benzyl alcohol]

Extemporaneous Preparations
A 2 mg/mL oral liquid preparation made from capsules and with 1% propylene glycol and 0.15% citric acid in distilled water was stable for 7 days when stored in amber glass prescription bottles under refrigeration (4°C). The vehicle is made by dissolving 150 mg of citric acid in a minimal amount of distilled water; then 1 mL of propylene glycol is added and the solution is mixed well; qsad to 100 mL with distilled water. Grind the contents of two 10 mg capsules in a mortar into a fine powder; add a small amount of the vehicle and mix well; transfer to a graduated cylinder and qsad with vehicle to 10 mL; transfer to an amber glass prescription bottle with tight-fitting cap; label "shake well" and "refrigerate" (Lim, 1997).

A stock solution of 10 mg/mL in propylene glycol was stable for 30 days when stored under refrigeration (4°C); when this stock solution was diluted 1:4 (v/v) with syrup (66.7% sucrose) to 2 mg/mL, the preparation was stable for 1 hour at 4°C (see Lim, 1997). **Note**: Although the stock solution is stable for 30 days, it **must be diluted** before administration to decrease the amount of propylene glycol delivered to the patient.

Lim LY, Tan LL, Chan EW, et al "Stability of Phenoxybenzamine Hydrochloride in Various Vehicles," *Am J Health Syst Pharm*, 1997, 54(18):2073-8.

◆ **Phenoxybenzamine Hydrochloride** *see* Phenoxybenzamine *on page 1100*

◆ **Phenoxymethyl Penicillin** *see* Penicillin V Potassium *on page 1082*

Phentolamine (fen TOLE a meen)

Medication Safety Issues
Sound-alike/look-alike issues:
Phentolamine may be confused with phentermine, Ventolin®

Related Information
Antihypertensive Agents by Class *on page 1481*
Extravasation Treatment *on page 1522*

U.S. Brand Names OraVerse™

Canadian Brand Names Regitine®; Rogitine®

Therapeutic Category Alpha-Adrenergic Blocking Agent, Parenteral; Antidote; Extravasation; Antihypertensive Agent; Diagnostic Agent, Pheochromocytoma; Vasodilator

Generic Available Yes

Use Diagnosis of pheochromocytoma; treatment of hypertension associated with pheochromocytoma or other causes of excess sympathomimetic amines; local treatment and prevention of dermal necrosis after extravasation of drugs with alpha-adrenergic effects (dobutamine, dopamine, epinephrine, metaraminol, norepinephrine, phenylephrine) (see Additional Information)

Pregnancy Risk Factor C

Lactation Excretion in breast milk unknown

Contraindications Hypersensitivity to phentolamine or any component; renal impairment; coronary or cerebral arteriosclerosis; MI

Precautions Use with caution in patients with gastritis, peptic ulcer; history of cardiac arrhythmias; MI, cerebrovascular spasm, and cerebrovascular occlusion may occur

Adverse Reactions
Cardiovascular: Hypotension, tachycardia, angina, arrhythmias
Central nervous system: Dizziness, headache
Gastrointestinal: Nausea, vomiting, diarrhea, exacerbation of peptic ulcer
Neuromuscular & skeletal: Weakness
Respiratory: Nasal congestion

Drug Interactions
Avoid Concomitant Use
Avoid concomitant use of Phentolamine with any of the following: Alfuzosin; Silodosin; Tamsulosin

Increased Effect/Toxicity
Phentolamine may increase the levels/effects of: Alfuzosin; Amifostine; Antihypertensives; Calcium Channel Blockers; RiTUXimab; Silodosin; Tamsulosin

The levels/effects of Phentolamine may be increased by: Alfuzosin; Beta-Blockers; Diazoxide; Herbs (Hypotensive Properties); MAO Inhibitors; Pentoxifylline; Phosphodiesterase 5 Inhibitors; Prostacyclin Analogues; Silodosin; Tamsulosin

Decreased Effect
The levels/effects of Phentolamine may be decreased by: Herbs (Hypertensive Properties); Methylphenidate; Yohimbine

Stability Reconstituted solution is stable for 48 hours at room temperature and 1 week when refrigerated

Mechanism of Action
Systemic: Competitively blocks alpha-adrenergic receptors to produce brief antagonism of circulating epinephrine and norepinephrine; reduces hypertension caused by alpha effects of catecholamines; also has positive inotropic and chronotropic effects on the heart
SubQ: Blocks alpha-adrenergic receptors and reverses vasoconstriction caused by extravasation of medications with alpha-adrenergic effects

Pharmacodynamics
Onset of action:
I.M.: Within 15-20 minutes
I.V.: Immediate
Maximum effect:
I.M.: Within 20 minutes
I.V.: Within 2 minutes
Duration:
I.M.: 30-45 minutes
I.V.: Within 15-30 minutes

Pharmacokinetics (Adult data unless noted)
Metabolism: In the liver
Half-life: Adults: 19 minutes
Elimination: 10% to 13% excreted in urine as unchanged drug

Usual Dosage
Treatment of alpha-adrenergic agonist drug extravasation: SubQ (see Administration) (**Note**: Total dose required depends on the size of extravasation; dose may be repeated if required):
Neonates: Infiltrate area of extravasation with a small amount (eg, 1 mL given in 0.1-0.2 mL aliquots) of a 0.25-0.5 mg/mL solution (made by diluting 2.5-5 mg in 10 mL of preservative free NS) within 12 hours of extravasation; in general, do not exceed 2.5 mg total; monitor blood pressure, especially when dose exceeds the recommended I.M./I.V. pediatric dose of 0.1 mg/kg.
Infants, Children, and Adults: Infiltrate area of extravasation with a small amount (eg, 1 mL given in 0.2 mL aliquots) of a 0.5-1 mg/mL solution (made by diluting 5-10 mg in 10 mL of NS) within 12 hours of extravasation; in general, do not exceed 0.1-0.2 mg/kg or 5 mg total; **Note**: Doses of <5 mg total are usually effective; one **adult** case using a total dose of 50 mg (given over 1 hour in 0.5 ml aliquots of a 1 mg/mL solution) for a large extravasation has been reported (Cooper, 1989).

Diagnosis of pheochromocytoma: I.M., I.V.:
Children: 0.05-0.1 mg/kg/dose, maximum single dose: 5 mg
Adults: 5 mg

Hypertension (prior to surgery for pheochromocytoma): I.M., I.V.:
Children: 0.05-0.1 mg/kg/dose given 1-2 hours before pheochromocytomectomy; repeat as needed to control blood pressure; maximum single dose: 5 mg
Adults: 5 mg given 1-2 hours before pheochromocytomectomy; repeat as needed to control blood pressure

Hypertensive crisis due to MAO inhibitor/sympathomimetic amine interaction: I.M., I.V.: Adults: 5-20 mg

Administration Parenteral: Treatment of extravasation: Infiltrate area of extravasation with multiple small injections of a diluted solution (see Usual Dosage); use 27- or 30-gauge needles and change needle between each skin entry to prevent bacterial contamination and minimize pain; do not inject a volume such that swelling of the extremity or digit with resultant compartment syndrome occurs

Monitoring Parameters Blood pressure, heart rate, orthostasis; treatment of extravasation: site of extravasation, skin color, local perfusion

Nursing Implications Monitor the site of extravasation closely, as repeat doses of SubQ phentolamine may be needed

Additional Information When drugs with alpha-adrenergic effects extravasate, they cause local vasoconstriction which causes blanching of the skin and a pale, cold, hard appearance; SubQ phentolamine blocks the alpha-adrenergic receptors and reverses the vasoconstriction; the extravasation area should "pink up" and return to normal skin color following SubQ administration of phentolamine. Dobutamine primarily stimulates beta$_1$-adrenergic receptors, but does possess alpha (and beta$_2$) adrenergic effects; the alpha-adrenergic effects (vasoconstriction) may be seen when dobutamine extravasates (since high concentrations of dobutamine would be present locally); although infrequent, cases of dermal necrosis from dobutamine extravasation have been reported; thus, phentolamine may help prevent dermal necrosis following dobutamine extravasations (see Hoff, 1979; MacCara, 1983). Injection contains mannitol 25 mg/vial

Dosage Forms Excipient information presented when available (limited, particularly for generics); consult specific product labeling.

Injection, powder for reconstitution, as mesylate: 5 mg
Injection, solution, as mesylate [preservative free]:
OraVerse™: 0.4 mg/1.7 mL (1.7 mL) [contains edetate disodium; dental cartridge]

References

Cooper BE, "High-Dose Phentolamine for Extravasation of Pressors," *Clin Pharm*, 1989, 8(10):689.

Flemmer L and Chan JS, "A Pediatric Protocol for Management of Extravasation Injuries," *Pediatr Nurs*, 1993, 19(4):355-8, 424.

Hoff JV, Peatty PA, and Wade JL, "Dermal Necrosis From Dobutamine," *N Engl J Med*, 1979, 300(22):1280.

MacCara ME, "Extravasation: A Hazard of Intravenous Therapy," *Drug Intell Clin Pharm*, 1983, 17(10):713-7.

Siwy BK and Sadove AM, "Acute Management of Dopamine Infiltration Injury With Regitine," *Plast Reconstr Surg*, 1987, 80(4):610-2.

Subhani M, Sridhar S, and DeCristofaro JD, "Phentolamine Use in a Neonate for the Prevention of Dermal Necrosis Caused by Dopamine: A Case Report," *J Perinatol*, 2001, 21(5):324-6.

Thigpen JL, "Peripheral Intravenous Extravasation: Nursing Procedure for Initial Treatment," *Neonatal Netw*, 2007, 26(6):379-84.

Zenk KE, "Management of Intravenous Extravasations," *Infusion*, 1981, 5:77-9.

♦ **Phentolamine Mesylate** *see* Phentolamine *on page 1101*

♦ **Phenylalanine Mustard** *see* Melphalan *on page 875*

♦ **Phenylazo Diamino Pyridine Hydrochloride** *see* Phenazopyridine *on page 1097*

Phenylephrine (fen il EF rin)

Medication Safety Issues

Sound-alike/look-alike issues:
Mydfrin® may be confused with Midrin®
Neo-Synephrine® (phenylephrine) may be confused with Neo-Synephrine® (oxymetazoline)
Sudafed PE™ may be confused with Sudafed®

High alert medication: The Institute for Safe Medication Practices (ISMP) includes this medication among its list of drugs which have a heightened risk of causing significant patient harm when used in error.

Related Information

Extravasation Treatment *on page 1522*

U.S. Brand Names 4 Way® Fast Acting [OTC]; 4 Way® Menthol [OTC]; AK-Dilate®; Altafrin; Anu-Med [OTC]; Little Noses® Decongestant [OTC]; LusonaI™; Medi-First™ Sinus Decongestant [OTC]; Medi-Phenyl [OTC]; Medicone® Suppositories [OTC]; Mydfrin®; Nasop12™ [DSC]; Neo-Synephrine® Extra Strength [OTC]; Neo-Synephrine® Injection [DSC]; Neo-Synephrine® Mild [OTC]; Neo-Synephrine® Regular Strength [OTC]; Neofrin™; OcuNefrin™ [OTC]; PediaCare® Children's Decongestant [OTC]; Preparation H® [OTC]; Rectacaine [OTC]; Rhinall [OTC];

Sudafed PE® Children's [OTC]; Sudafed PE® Congestion [OTC]; Sudafed PE® Nasal Decongestant [OTC]; Sudogest™ PE [OTC]; Triaminic Thin Strips® Children's Cold with Stuffy Nose [OTC]; Triaminic Thin Strips® Cold [OTC] [DSC]; Tronolane® Suppository [OTC]; Vicks® Sinex® Nasal Spray [OTC] [DSC]; Vicks® Sinex® UltraFine Mist [OTC] [DSC]; Vicks® Sinex® VapoSpray 4-Hour™ Decongestant [OTC]

Canadian Brand Names Dionephrine®; Mydfrin®; Neo-Synephrine®

Therapeutic Category Adrenergic Agonist Agent; Adrenergic Agonist Agent, Ophthalmic; Alpha-Adrenergic Agonist; Hemorrhoidal Treatment Agent; Nasal Agent; Vasoconstrictor; Ophthalmic Agent, Mydriatic; Sympathomimetic

Generic Available Yes: Excludes chewable tablet, cream, filmstrip, liquid, suspension

Use Treatment of hypotension and vascular failure in shock; supraventricular tachycardia; as a vasoconstrictor in regional analgesia; symptomatic relief of nasal and nasopharyngeal mucosal congestion; as a mydriatic in ophthalmic procedures and treatment of wide-angle glaucoma; symptomatic relief of hemorrhoidal symptoms (rectal cream and ointment)

Pregnancy Risk Factor C

Pregnancy Considerations Animal reproduction studies have not been conducted.

Lactation Excretion in breast milk unknown/use caution

Contraindications Hypersensitivity to phenylephrine or any component (see Warnings); pheochromocytoma, severe hypertension, ventricular tachycardia; acute pancreatitis, hepatitis; peripheral or mesenteric vascular thrombosis, myocardial disease, severe coronary disease, asthma, narrow-angle glaucoma (ophthalmic preparation); MAO inhibitor therapy or within 2 weeks of discontinuation of MAO inhibitor

Warnings Safety and efficacy for the use of cough and cold products in children <2 years of age is limited. Serious adverse effects including death have been reported. The FDA notes that there are no approved OTC uses for these products in children <2 years of age. Healthcare providers are reminded to ask caregivers about the use of OTC cough and cold products in order to avoid exposure to multiple medications containing the same ingredient.

Do not use if solution turns brown or contains a precipitate. Injection and ophthalmic agents may contain sulfites which may cause allergic reactions in susceptible individuals. Some formulations contain sodium benzoate; benzoic acid (benzoate) is a metabolite of benzyl alcohol; large amounts of benzyl alcohol (≥99 mg/kg/day) have been associated with a potentially fatal toxicity ("gasping syndrome") in neonates; *in vitro* and animal studies have shown that benzoate displaces bilirubin from protein binding sites; avoid use of benzyl alcohol containing products in neonates. Rebound nasal congestion may occur if abruptly discontinued after prolonged use.

Precautions Use as pressor therapy for treatment of hypotension and vascular failure is **not** a substitute for replacement of blood, plasma, and body fluids; use with caution in patients with hyperthyroidism, bradycardia, partial heart block, myocardial disease, or severe arteriosclerosis; infuse into large veins to prevent extravasation which may cause severe necrosis

Adverse Reactions

Cardiovascular: Hypertension, angina, reflex severe bradycardia, arrhythmias, peripheral vasoconstriction, precordial pain

Central nervous system: Restlessness, excitability, headache, anxiety, nervousness, dizziness

Dermatologic: Pilomotor response, skin blanching

Local: Necrosis if extravasation occurs

Neuromuscular & skeletal: Tremor

Ocular: (Ophthalmic preparation): Transient stinging, brow-ache, blurred vision, photophobia, lacrimation

Respiratory: Respiratory distress, rebound nasal congestion, sneezing, burning, stinging, dryness

Drug Interactions

Avoid Concomitant Use

Avoid concomitant use of Phenylephrine with any of the following: Iobenguane I 123; MAO Inhibitors

Increased Effect/Toxicity

Phenylephrine may increase the levels/effects of: Sympathomimetics

The levels/effects of Phenylephrine may be increased by: Atomoxetine; Cannabinoids; MAO Inhibitors; Tricyclic Antidepressants

Decreased Effect

Phenylephrine may decrease the levels/effects of: Iobenguane I 123

Stability Store at room temperature; protect from light; compatible when admixed with dextrose, dextrose-saline, Ringer's, LR, NS, and 1/6 M sodium lactate injection; do not use if solution turns brown or contains a precipitate

Mechanism of Action Potent, direct-acting alpha-adre-nergic stimulator with weak beta-adrenergic activity; causes vasoconstriction of the arterioles of the nasal mucosa and conjunctiva; activates the dilator muscle of the pupil to cause contraction; produces systemic arterial vasoconstriction

Pharmacodynamics

Onset of action:

I.M.: Within 10-15 minutes

I.V.: Following parenteral injection, effects occur immediately

Oral: 15-20 minutes

SubQ: 10-15 minutes

Duration:

I.M.: 30 minutes to 2 hours

I.V.: 15-20 minutes

Oral: 2-4 hours

SubQ: 1 hour

Pharmacokinetics (Adult data unless noted)

Metabolism: In the liver and intestine by the enzyme monoamine oxidase

Half-life: 2.5 hours

Elimination: Metabolites, routes, and rates of excretion have not been identified

Usual Dosage

Ophthalmic procedures:

Infants <1 year: Instill 1 drop of 2.5% 15-30 minutes before procedures

Children and Adults: Instill 1 drop of 2.5% or 10% solution, may repeat in 10-60 minutes as needed

Ophthalmic irritation (OTC formulation for relief of eye redness): Adults: Instill 1-2 drops 0.12% solution into affected eye, up to 4 times/day; do not use for >72 hours

Nasal decongestant: Intranasal (therapy should not exceed 3-5 days):

Infants >6 months: 1-2 drops of 0.16% every 3 hours

Children:

1-6 years: 2-3 drops every 4 hours of 0.125% solution as needed

6-12 years: 2-3 drops every 4 hours of 0.25% solution as needed

Children >12 years and Adults: 2-3 drops or 1-2 sprays every 4 hours of 0.25% to 0.5% solution as needed; 1% solution may be used in adults in cases of extreme nasal congestion

Nasal decongestant: Oral: Manufacturer's recommendations:

Phenylephrine hydrochloride salt:

Children's Sudafed PE®: Children 4-5 years: 5 mL (2.5 mg) every 4 hours; not to exceed 6 doses/24 hours

Triaminic® Thin Strips® Cold with Stuffy Nose:

Children 4-6 years: 1 strip (2.5 mg/strip) every 4 hours; not to exceed 6 doses/24 hours

Children >6 to 12 years: 2 strips (2.5 mg/strip) every 4 hours; not to exceed 6 doses/24 hours

Phenylephrine tannate salt: Ah-Chew D®:

Children 6-12 years: 5-10 mg (2.5-5 mL) every 12 hours

Children >12 years and Adults: 10-20 mg (5-10 mL) every 12 hours

Hypotension/shock:

Children:

I.M., SubQ: 0.1 mg/kg/dose or 3 mg/m^2/dose every 1-2 hours as needed; (maximum dose: 5 mg)

I.V. bolus: 5-20 mcg/kg/dose every 10-15 minutes as needed

I.V. infusion: 0.1-0.5 mcg/kg/minute, titrate to desired effect

Adults:

I.M., SubQ: 2-5 mg/dose every 1-2 hours as needed; reported effective dosage range: 1-10 mg; (initial dose should not exceed 5 mg)

I.V. bolus: 0.2 mg/dose (range: 0.1-0.5 mg/dose) every 10-15 minutes as needed (initial dose should not exceed 0.5 mg)

I.V. infusion: 100-180 mcg/minute, **or alternatively,** 0.5 mcg/kg/minute; titrate to desired response. Dosing ranges between 0.4-9.1 mcg/kg/minute have been reported (Gregory, 1991)

Paroxysmal supraventricular tachycardia: I.V.:

Children: 5-10 mcg/kg over 20-30 seconds

Adults: Initial: 0.25-0.5 mg over 20-30 seconds; subsequent doses may be increased in 0.1-0.2 mg increments; not to exceed 1 mg/dose (maximum dose of 2 mg is recommended by some clinicians)

Treatment of hemorrhoidal symptoms: Children ≥12 years and Adults: Apply to rectal area or by applicator into rectum up to 4 times/day

Administration

Intranasal: Spray or apply drops into each nostril while gently occluding the other

Ophthalmic: Instill drops into conjunctival sac of affected eye(s); avoid contact of bottle tip with skin or eye; finger pressure should be applied to the lacrimal sac during and for 1-2 minutes after instillation to decrease risk of absorption and systemic reactions

Oral: Administer without regard to food; place orally dissolving tablet (NāSop™) or Triaminic® Thin Strips® on tongue and allow to dissolve

Parenteral: For direct I.V. administration, dilute to 1 mg/mL by adding 1 mL to 9 mL of SWI, then administer dose over 20-30 seconds; continuous infusion concentrations are usually 20-60 mcg/mL by adding 5 mg to 250 mL I.V. solution (20 mcg/mL) or 15 mg to 250 mL (60 mcg/mL); rate of infusion (mL/hour) = dose (mcg/kg/minute) x weight (kg) x 60 minutes/hour divided by concentration (mcg/mL); administer into a large vein to prevent the possibility of extravasation; use infusion device to control rate of flow; administration into an umbilical arterial catheter is **not** recommended

Rectal: Apply to clean and dry rectal area at night, in the morning, or after each bowel movement; when using applicator, remove protective cover from applicator and attach to tube. Lubricate applicator well, then gently insert into rectum. Thoroughly cleanse applicator after each use and replace protective cover.

Monitoring Parameters Heart rate, blood pressure, central venous pressure, arterial blood gases (hypotension/shock treatment)

Nursing Implications Extravasant; avoid I.V. infiltration; extravasation may be treated with local infiltration of phentolamine 5-10 mg diluted in 10-15 mL NS solution

◀ **Dosage Forms** Excipient information presented when available (limited, particularly for generics); consult specific product labeling. [DSC] = Discontinued product
Injection, solution, as hydrochloride: 1% [10 mg/mL] (1 mL, 5 mL, 10 mL)
 Neo-Synephrine®: 1% (1 mL) [contains sodium metabisulfite] [DSC]
Liquid, oral, as hydrochloride:
 LuSonal™: 7.5 mg/5 mL (480 mL) [contains phenylalanine; strawberry flavor]
 PediaCare® Children's Decongestant: 2.5 mg/5 mL (118 mL) [contains sodium 14 mg/5 mL, sodium benzoate; raspberry flavor]
 Sudafed PE® Children's: 2.5 mg/5 mL (118 mL) [ethanol free, sugar free; contains sodium 14 mg/5 mL, sodium benzoate; raspberry flavor]
Ointment, rectal, as hydrochloride:
 Formulation R™, Preparation H®: 0.25% (30 g, 60 g) [contains benzoic acid]
 Rectacaine: 0.25% (60 g)
Solution, intranasal, as hydrochloride [drops]:
 Little Noses® Decongestant: 0.125% (15 mL) [contains benzalkonium chloride]
 Rhinall: 0.25% (30 mL) [contains benzalkonium chloride and sodium bisulfite]
Solution, intranasal, as hydrochloride [spray]:
 4 Way® Fast Acting: 1% (15 mL, 30 mL, 37 mL) [contains benzalkonium chloride]
 4 Way® Menthol: 1% (15 mL) [contains benzalkonium chloride, menthol]
 Neo-Synephrine® Extra Strength: 1% (15 mL) [contains benzalkonium chloride]
 Neo-Synephrine® Mild: 0.25% (15 mL) [contains benzalkonium chloride]
 Neo-Synephrine® Regular Strength: 0.5% (15 mL) [contains benzalkonium chloride]
 Rhinall: 0.25% (40 mL) [contains benzalkonium chloride, sodium bisulfite]
 Vicks® Sinex® [DSC], Vicks® Sinex® UltraFine Mist [DSC]: 0.5% (15 mL) [contains benzalkonium chloride]
 Vicks® Sinex® VapoSpray™ 4 Hour Decongestant: 0.5% (15 mL) [contains benzalkonium chloride, menthol]
Solution, ophthalmic, as hydrochloride: 2.5% (2 mL, 3 mL, 5 mL, 15 mL)
 AK-Dilate®: 2.5% (2 mL, 15 mL); 10% (5 mL) [contains benzalkonium chloride]
 Altrafrin: 2.5% (15 mL) [contains benzalkonium chloride]; 10% (5 mL) [contains benzalkonium chloride]
 Mydfrin®: 2.5% (3 mL, 5 mL) [contains sodium bisulfite]
 Neofrin™: 2.5% (15 mL); 10% (15 mL)
 OcuNefrin™: 0.12% (15 mL)
 Relief®: 0.12% (15 mL) [contains benzalkonium chloride] [DSC]
Strip, orally disintegrating, as hydrochloride:
 Triaminic Thin Strips® Cold: 2.5 mg [raspberry flavor] [DSC]
 Triaminic Thin Strips® Children's Cold with Stuffy Nose: 2.5 mg [raspberry flavor]
Suppository, rectal, as hydrochloride: 0.25% (12s)
 Anu-Med: 0.25% (12s)
 Preparation H®: 0.25% (12s, 24s, 48s)
 Medicone®, Tronolane®: 0.25% (12s, 24s)
 Rectacaine: 0.25% (12s)
Tablet, chewable, as tannate:
 Nasop12™: 10 mg [grape flavor] [DSC]
Tablet, as hydrochloride: 10 mg
 Medi-First™ Sinus Decongestant: 10 mg
 Medi-Phenyl: 5 mg
 Sudafed PE® Congestion: 10 mg
 Sudafed PE® Nasal Decongestant: 10 mg
 Sudogest™ PE: 10 mg

References
Gregory JS, Bonfiglio MF, Dasta JF, et al, "Experience With Phenylephrine as a Component of the Pharmacologic Support of Septic Shock," *Crit Care Med*, 1991, 19(11):1395-400.

◆ **Phenylephrine and Cyclopentolate** *see* Cyclopentolate and Phenylephrine *on page 369*
◆ **Phenylephrine and Promethazine** *see* Promethazine and Phenylephrine *on page 1166*
◆ **Phenylephrine Hydrochloride** *see* Phenylephrine *on page 1102*
◆ **Phenylephrine, Promethazine, and Codeine** *see* Promethazine, Phenylephrine, and Codeine *on page 1167*
◆ **Phenylephrine Tannate** *see* Phenylephrine *on page 1102*
◆ **Phenylethylmalonylurea** *see* PHENobarbital *on page 1097*
◆ **Phenytek®** *see* Phenytoin *on page 1104*

Phenytoin (FEN i toyn)

Medication Safety Issues
Sound-alike/look-alike issues:
 Phenytoin may be confused with phenelzine, phentermine, PHENobarbital
 Dilantin® may be confused with Dilaudid®, diltiazem, Dipentum®

High alert medication: The Institute for Safe Medication Practices (ISMP) includes this medication (I.V. formulation) among its list of drug classes which have a heightened risk of causing significant patient harm when used in error.

International issues:
 Dilantin® may be confused with Dolantine® which is a brand name for pethidine in Belgium and Switzerland
Related Information
 Adult ACLS Algorithms *on page 1463*
 Antiepileptic Drugs *on page 1693*
 Therapeutic Drug Monitoring: Blood Sampling Time Guidelines *on page 1704*
U.S. Brand Names Dilantin®; Phenytek®
Canadian Brand Names Dilantin®
Therapeutic Category Antiarrhythmic Agent, Class I-B; Anticonvulsant, Hydantoin
Generic Available Yes: Excludes chewable tablet
Use Management of generalized tonic-clonic (grand mal), simple partial and complex partial seizures; prevention of seizures following head trauma/neurosurgery; ventricular arrhythmias, including those associated with digitalis intoxication, prolonged QT interval and surgical repair of congenital heart diseases in children; epidermolysis bullosa
Pregnancy Risk Factor D
Pregnancy Considerations Phenytoin crosses the placenta. Congenital malformations (including a pattern of malformations termed the "fetal hydantoin syndrome" or "fetal anticonvulsant syndrome") have been reported in infants. Isolated cases of malignancies (including neuroblastoma) and coagulation defects in the neonate following delivery have also been reported. Epilepsy itself, the number of medications, genetic factors, or a combination of these probably influence the teratogenicity of anticonvulsant therapy.

Total plasma concentrations of phenytoin are decreased by 56% in the mother during pregnancy; unbound plasma (free) concentrations are decreased by 31%. Because protein binding is decreased, monitoring of unbound plasma concentrations is recommended. Concentrations should be monitored through the 8th week postpartum.

The use of folic acid throughout pregnancy and vitamin K during the last month of pregnancy is recommended.

Patients exposed to phenytoin during pregnancy are encouraged to enroll themselves into the AED Pregnancy Registry by calling 1-888-233-2334. Additional information is available at www.aedpregnancyregistry.org.

Lactation Enters breast milk/not recommended (AAP rates "compatible")

Breast-Feeding Considerations Phenytoin is excreted in breast milk; however, the amount to which the infant is exposed is considered small. The manufacturers of phenytoin do not recommend breast-feeding during therapy, however, the AAP considers it to be usually compatible. Women should be counseled of the possible risks and benefits associated with breast-feeding while on phenytoin.

Contraindications Hypersensitivity to phenytoin or any component; heart block, sinus bradycardia

Warnings Abrupt withdrawal of phenytoin may precipitate status epilepticus in epileptic patients; do not discontinue abruptly; phenytoin should be withdrawn gradually, unless safety concerns (eg, allergic or hypersensitivity reaction) require a more rapid withdrawal. Serious skin reactions, including toxic epidermal necrolysis (TEN) and Stevens-Johnson syndrome (SJS), although rarely reported, have resulted in fatalities; phenytoin should be discontinued if there are any signs of rash. Preliminary data suggests that patients testing positive for the human leukocyte antigen (HLA) allele HLA-B*1502 have an increased risk of developing SJS and/or TEN. The risk appears to be highest in the early months of therapy initiation. The presence of this genetic variant exists in up to 15% of people of Asian descent in China, Thailand, Malaysia, Indonesia, Taiwan, and the Philippines, and may vary from <1% in Japanese and Koreans, to 2% to 4% of South Asians and Indians. This variant is virtually absent in those of Caucasian, African-American, Hispanic, or European ancestry. Of note, carbamazepine, another antiepileptic with a chemical structure similar to phenytoin, updated its prescribing information (December, 2007) to include a warning of an increased risk of SJS and TEN in patients carrying the HLA-B*1502 allele and a recommendation to screen patients of Asian descent for the allele prior to initiating therapy. In contrast to carbamazepine, the FDA is not recommending testing for the presence of HLA-B*1502 prior to initiating phenytoin therapy until more information is available. In the interim, the FDA is advising that prescribers avoid phenytoin or fosphenytoin as alternatives to carbamazepine therapy in patients positive for HLA-B*1502.

Antiepileptic drugs (AEDs) increase the risk of suicidal behavior and ideation in patients receiving these medications for any indication. Pooled analyses of placebo-controlled trials involving 11 different AEDs (regardless of indication) showed a twofold increased risk of suicidal thoughts or behavior (estimated incidence: 0.43% in AED treated patients compared to 0.24% of patients receiving placebo); increased risk was observed as early as 1 week after initiation of AED and continued through duration of trials (most trials ≤24 weeks); risk did not vary significantly by age (age range: 5–100 years). Consider risks and benefits of AEDs before prescribing. Monitor all patients receiving an AED for emergence of suicidal thoughts or behavior, thoughts of self-harm, any unusual changes in behavior or mood, or the emergence or worsening of depressive symptoms; notify heathcare provider immediately if symptoms or concerning behavior occur. **Note:** The FDA is requiring that a Medication Guide be developed for all antiepileptic drugs informing patients of this risk.

Dilantin® 30 mg capsule and oral suspension contain sodium benzoate; benzoic acid (benzoate) is a metabolite of benzyl alcohol; large amounts of benzyl alcohol (≥99 mg/kg/day) have been associated with a potentially fatal toxicity ("gasping syndrome") in neonates; the "gasping syndrome" consists of metabolic acidosis, respiratory distress, gasping respirations, CNS dysfunction (including convulsions, intracranial hemorrhage), hypotension and cardiovascular collapse; use phenytoin products containing sodium benzoate with caution in neonates; *in vitro* and animal studies have shown that benzoate displaces bilirubin from protein binding sites. Injection contains 40% propylene glycol and 10% alcohol.

Precautions Use with caution in patients with porphyria; discontinue if rash or lymphadenopathy occurs; modify dosage in patients with hepatic or renal dysfunction

Adverse Reactions
Dose-related:
Central nervous system: Slurred speech, dizziness, drowsiness, lethargy, coma, ataxia, dyskinesias
Ocular: Nystagmus, blurred vision, diplopia

Cardiovascular: I.V.: Hypotension, bradycardia, arrhythmias, cardiovascular collapse (especially with rapid I.V. use)
Central nervous system: Fever, mood changes; suicidal thinking and behavior (see Warnings)
Dermatologic: Hirsutism, coarsening of facial features, Stevens-Johnson syndrome, rash, exfoliative dermatitis
Endocrine & metabolic: Folic acid depletion, hyperglycemia
Gastrointestinal: Nausea, vomiting, gingival hyperplasia, gum tenderness
Hematologic: Blood dyscrasias, pseudolymphoma, lymphoma
Hepatic: Hepatitis
Local: Venous irritation and pain, thrombophlebitis
Neuromuscular & skeletal: Peripheral neuropathy, osteomalacia
Miscellaneous: Lymphadenopathy, SLE-like syndrome

Drug Interactions
Metabolism/Transport Effects Substrate of CYP2C9 (major), 2C19 (major), 3A4 (minor); **Induces** CYP2B6 (strong), 2C8 (strong), 2C9 (strong), 2C19 (strong), 3A4 (strong)

Avoid Concomitant Use
Avoid concomitant use of Phenytoin with any of the following: Darunavir; Dronedarone; Etravirine; Everolimus; Nilotinib; Pazopanib; Ranolazine; Romidepsin; Tolvaptan

Increased Effect/Toxicity
Phenytoin may increase the levels/effects of: Alcohol (Ethyl); CNS Depressants; Fosamprenavir; Lithium; Methotrimeprazine; Vitamin K Antagonists

The levels/effects of Phenytoin may be increased by: Allopurinol; Amiodarone; Antifungal Agents (Azole Derivatives, Systemic); Benzodiazepines; Calcium Channel Blockers; Capecitabine; CarBAMazepine; Carbonic Anhydrase Inhibitors; Chloramphenicol; Cimetidine; CYP2C19 Inhibitors (Moderate); CYP2C19 Inhibitors (Strong); CYP2C9 Inhibitors (Moderate); CYP2C9 Inhibitors (Strong); Dexmethylphenidate; Disulfiram; Efavirenz; Felbamate; Floxuridine; Fluconazole; Fluorouracil; Fluorouracil (Systemic); Fluorouracil (Topical); Isoniazid; Methotrimeprazine; Methylphenidate; MetroNIDAZOLE; MetroNIDAZOLE (Systemic); OXcarbazepine; Proton Pump Inhibitors; Rufinamide; Selective Serotonin Reuptake Inhibitors; Sulfonamide Derivatives; Tacrolimus; Tacrolimus (Systemic); Ticlopidine; Topiramate; Trimethoprim; Vitamin K Antagonists

Decreased Effect

Phenytoin may decrease the levels/effects of: Acetaminophen; Amiodarone; Antifungal Agents (Azole Derivatives, Systemic); CarBAMazepine; Caspofungin; Chloramphenicol; Clozapine; Contraceptives (Estrogens); Contraceptives (Progestins); CycloSPORINE; CycloSPORINE (Systemic); CYP2B6 Substrates; CYP2C19 Substrates; CYP2C8 Substrates (High risk); CYP2C9 Substrates (High risk); CYP3A4 Substrates; Darunavir; Deferasirox; Disopyramide; Divalproex; Doxycycline; Dronedarone; Efavirenz; Etoposide; Etoposide Phosphate; Etravirine; Everolimus; Felbamate; Flunarizine; GuanFACINE; HMG-CoA Reductase Inhibitors; Irinotecan; Lacosamide; LamoTRIgine; Levodopa; Loop Diuretics; Lopinavir; Maraviroc; Mebendazole; Meperidine; Methadone; MetroNIDAZOLE; MetroNIDAZOLE (Systemic); Metyrapone; Mexiletine; Nilotinib; OXcarbazepine; Pazopanib; Primidone; QUEtiapine; QuiNIDine; Ranolazine; Ritonavir; Romidepsin; Rufinamide; Saxagliptin; Sirolimus; Sorafenib; Tacrolimus; Tacrolimus (Systemic); Tadalafil; Temsirolimus; Teniposide; Theophylline Derivatives; Thyroid Products; Tipranavir; Tolvaptan; Topiramate; Treprostinil; Valproic Acid; Vecuronium; Zonisamide

The levels/effects of Phenytoin may be decreased by: Amphetamines; Antacids; CarBAMazepine; Ciprofloxacin; Ciprofloxacin (Systemic); CISplatin; Colesevelam; CYP2C19 Inducers (Strong); CYP2C9 Inducers (Highly Effective); Diazoxide; Divalproex; Folic Acid; Fosamprenavir; Ketorolac; Ketorolac (Systemic); Leucovorin Calcium-Levoleucovorin; Lopinavir; Mefloquine; Methylfolate; Peginterferon Alfa-2b; Pyridoxine; Rifamycin Derivatives; Ritonavir; Theophylline Derivatives; Tipranavir; Valproic Acid; Vigabatrin

Food Interactions Food may effect absorption of phenytoin, depending on product formulation; a high fat meal decreases the rate, but not the extent of absorption of 100 mg Dilantin® Kapseals (Cook, 2001); a high fat meal decreased the bioavailability of a generic extended phenytoin sodium capsule (Mylan) by 13% compared to Dilantin® Kapseals; when taken with a high fat meal, substituting the generic product for Dilantin® could result in a 37% decrease in serum phenytoin concentrations; substituting Dilantin® for the generic could result in 102% increase in plasma phenytoin concentrations; thus, when taking phenytoin sodium with food, switching products may result in decreased efficacy or increased toxicity (see Wilder, 2001)

Tube feedings decrease phenytoin bioavailability; to avoid decreased serum levels with continuous NG feeds, hold feedings for 2 hours prior to and 2 hours after phenytoin administration, if possible; phenytoin may increase the metabolism of vitamins D and K; dietary requirements of vitamins D, K, B_{12}, folate, and calcium may be increased with long-term use; high doses of folate may decrease bioavailability of phenytoin; avoid giving calcium or magnesium supplements at the same time as phenytoin, space administration by ≥2 hours

Stability Parenteral solution may be used as long as there is no precipitate and it is not hazy; slightly yellowed solution may be used; refrigeration may cause precipitate, sometimes the precipitate is resolved by allowing the solution to reach room temperature again; drug may precipitate with pH ≤11.5; do not mix with other medications. I.V. intermittent infusion: No consensus exists in the literature regarding phenytoin stability in I.V. solutions; due to a low solubility, phenytoin may precipitate in aqueous solutions; some centers have successfully used dilutions of 1-10 mg/mL in NS or LR; infusions should begin as soon as possible after preparation (eg, within 1 hour); diluted solutions should **not** be refrigerated; inspect for particulate matter; discard 4 hours after preparation (see Gannaway, 1983).

Mechanism of Action Stabilizes neuronal membranes and decreases seizure activity by increasing efflux or decreasing influx of sodium ions across cell membranes in the motor cortex during generation of nerve impulses; prolongs effective refractory period and suppresses ventricular pacemaker automaticity, shortens action potential in the heart

Pharmacokinetics (Adult data unless noted)

Absorption: Oral: Slow, variable; dependent on product formulation (see Food Interactions); decreased in neonates

Distribution: V_d:

Neonates:

Premature: 1-1.2 L/kg

Full-term: 0.8-0.9 L/kg

Infants: 0.7-0.8 L/kg

Children: 0.7 L/kg

Adults: 0.6-0.7 L/kg

Protein binding: Adults: 90% to 95%; increased free fraction (decreased protein binding) in neonates (up to 20% free), infants (up to 15% free), and patients with hyperbilirubinemia, hypoalbuminemia, renal dysfunction, or uremia

Metabolism: Follows dose-dependent (Michaelis-Menten) pharmacokinetics; "apparent" or calculated half-life is dependent upon serum concentration, therefore, metabolism is best described in terms of K_m and V_{max}; V_{max} is increased in infants >6 months and children compared to adults; major metabolite (via oxidation) HPPA undergoes enterohepatic recycling and elimination in urine as glucuronides

Bioavailability: Formulation dependent

Time to peak serum concentration: Oral: Dependent upon formulation

Extended release capsule: Within 4-12 hours

Immediate release preparation: Within 2-3 hours

Elimination: <5% excreted unchanged in urine; increased clearance and decreased serum concentrations with febrile illness; highly variable clearance, dependent upon intrinsic hepatic function and dose administered

Usual Dosage

Status epilepticus: I.V.:

Loading dose:

Neonates: 15-20 mg/kg in a single or divided dose;

Infants, Children, and Adults: 15-18 mg/kg in a single or divided dose

Maintenance dose, anticonvulsant (**Note:** Maintenance dose usually starts 12 hours after the loading dose):

Neonates: Initial: 5 mg/kg/day in 2 divided doses; usual: 5-8 mg/kg/day in 2 divided doses; some patients may require dosing every 8 hours

Infants and Children: Initial: 5 mg/kg/day in 2-3 divided doses; usual doses:

0.5-3 years: 8-10 mg/kg/day

4-6 years: 7.5-9 mg/kg/day

7-9 years: 7-8 mg/kg/day

10-16 years: 6-7 mg/kg/day

Some patients require every 8 hours dosing due to fast apparent half-life

Adults: Usual: 300 mg/day or 4-6 mg/kg/day in 2-3 divided doses

Anticonvulsant: Infants, Children and Adults: Oral:

Loading dose: 15-20 mg/kg; based on phenytoin serum concentrations and recent dosing history; administer oral loading dose in 3 divided doses given every 2-4 hours to decrease GI adverse effects and to ensure complete oral absorption

Maintenance dose: Same as I.V. maintenance dose/day listed above. Divide daily dose into 3 doses/day when using suspension, chewable tablets or nonextended release preparations. Extended release preparations may be dosed in adults every 12 or 24 hours if patient is not receiving concomitant enzyme-inducing drugs and apparent half-life is sufficiently long.

Administration

Oral: To ensure consistent absorption, phenytoin should be administered at the same time with regards to meals; may administer with food or milk to decrease GI upset; 100 mg Dilantin® Kapseals may be administered without regard to meals; shake oral suspension well prior to each dose; separate administration of antacids or tube feedings and oral phenytoin by 2 hours

Parenteral: I.V.: Neonates: Do not exceed I.V. infusion rate of 0.5 mg/kg/minute; Infants, Children, Adults: Do not exceed I.V. infusion rate of 1-3 mg/kg/minute, maximum rate: 50 mg/minute; I.V. injections should be followed by NS flushes through the same needle or I.V. catheter to avoid local irritation of the vein; I.V. intermittent infusion: Dilute with NS to a concentration of 1-10 mg/mL (see Stability), use an in-line 0.22 micron filter; avoid extravasation; avoid I.M. use due to erratic absorption, pain on injection, and precipitation of drug at injection site

Monitoring Parameters Serum concentrations, CBC with differential, liver enzymes; blood pressure with I.V. use; free and total serum concentrations in patients with hyperbilirubinemia, hypoalbuminemia, renal dysfunction, or uremia; signs and symptoms of suicidality (eg, anxiety, depression, behavior changes) (see Warnings)

Reference Range

Neonates: Therapeutic: 8-15 mcg/mL

Children and Adults:

Therapeutic: 10-20 mcg/mL (SI: 40-79 micromoles/L); toxicity is measured clinically, some patients require levels outside the suggested therapeutic range

Toxic: >20 mcg/mL (SI: >79 micromoles/L)

Lethal: >100 mcg/mL (SI: >400 micromoles/L)

Commonly accepted therapeutic free (unbound) concentration: 1-2 mcg/mL

Patient Information Avoid alcohol. May cause drowsiness and impair ability to perform activities requiring mental alertness or physical coordination. Do not change brand or dosage without consulting physician. Do not abruptly discontinue (an increase in seizure activity may result). Maintain good oral hygiene. Antiepileptic agents may increase the risk of suicidal thoughts and behavior; notify physician if you feel more depressed or have thoughts of suicide or self harm (see Warnings). Report chest pain, irregular heartbeat, or palpitations; slurred speech, unsteady gait, coordination difficulties, or change in mentation; skin rash; unresolved nausea, vomiting, or constipation; swollen glands; swollen, sore, or bleeding gums; unusual bruising or bleeding; acute persistent fatigue; vision changes; or other persistent adverse effects. Report worsening of seizure activity or loss of seizure control.

Additional Information The 30 mg/5 mL oral suspension is no longer made; possible permanent cerebellum damage may occur with chronic toxic serum concentrations

A recent study (Relling, 2000) demonstrated that enzyme-inducing antiepileptic drugs (AEDs) (carbamazepine, phenobarbital, and phenytoin) increased systemic clearance of antileukemic drugs (teniposide and methotrexate) and were associated with a worse event-free survival, CNS relapse, and hematologic relapse, (ie, lower efficacy), in B-lineage ALL children receiving chemotherapy; the authors recommend using nonenzyme-inducing AEDs in patients receiving chemotherapy for ALL.

Dosage Forms Excipient information presented when available (limited, particularly for generics); consult specific product labeling.

Capsule, extended release, as sodium: 100 mg

Dilantin®: 30 mg [contains sodium benzoate], 100 mg

Phenytek®: 200 mg, 300 mg

Capsule, prompt release, as sodium: 100 mg

Injection, solution, as sodium: 50 mg/mL (2 mL, 5 mL) [contains alcohol and propylene glycol]

Suspension, oral: 100 mg/4 mL (4 mL); 125 mg/5 mL (240 mL)

Dilantin®: 125 mg/5 mL (240 mL) [contains alcohol <0.6%, sodium benzoate; orange vanilla flavor]

Tablet, chewable:

Dilantin®: 50 mg

References

Bauer LA and Blouin RA, "Phenytoin Michaelis-Menten Pharmacokinetics in Caucasian Pediatric Patients," *Clin Pharmacokinet*, 1983, 8 (6):545-9.

Chiba K, Ishizaki T, Miura H, et al, "Michaelis-Menten Pharmacokinetics of Diphenylhydantoin and Application in the Pediatric Age Patient," *J Pediatr*, 1980, 96(3 Pt 1):479-84.

Cook J, Randinitis E, and Wilder BJ, "Effect of Food on the Bioavailability of 100-mg Dilantin® Kapseals," *Neurology*, 2001, 57 (4):698-700.

Gannaway WL, Wilding DC, Siepler JK, et al, "Clinical Use of Intravenous Phenytoin Sodium Infusions," *Clin Pharm*, 1983, 2 (2):135-8.

Relling MV, Pui CH, Sandlund JT, et al, "Adverse Effect of Anticonvulsants on Efficacy of Chemotherapy for Acute Lymphoblastic Leukaemia," *Lancet*, 2000, 356(9226):285-90.

Suzuki Y, Mimaki T, Cox S, et al, "Phenytoin Age-Dose-Concentration Relationship in Children," *Ther Drug Monit*, 1994, 16(2):145-50.

Wilder BJ, Leppik I, Hietpas TJ, et al, "Effect of Food on Absorption of Dilantin® Kapseals and Mylan Extended Phenytoin Sodium Capsules," *Neurology*, 2001, 57(4):582-9.

◆ **Phenytoin Sodium** *see* Phenytoin *on page 1104*

◆ **Phenytoin Sodium, Extended** *see* Phenytoin *on page 1104*

◆ **Phenytoin Sodium, Prompt** *see* Phenytoin *on page 1104*

◆ **Phillips'® M-O [OTC]** *see* Magnesium Hydroxide *on page 855*

◆ **Phillips'® M-O [OTC]** *see* Magnesium Supplements *on page 859*

◆ **Phillips'® Laxative Dietary Supplement Cramp-Free [OTC]** *see* Magnesium Oxide *on page 857*

◆ **Phillips'® Milk of Magnesia [OTC]** *see* Magnesium Hydroxide *on page 855*

◆ **Phillips'® Milk of Magnesia [OTC]** *see* Magnesium Supplements *on page 859*

◆ **Phillips'® Stool Softener Laxative [OTC]** *see* Docusate *on page 468*

◆ **pHisoHex®** *see* Hexachlorophene *on page 677*

◆ **PHL-Amiodarone (Can)** *see* Amiodarone *on page 84*

◆ **PHL-Amlodipine (Can)** *see* AmLODIPine *on page 91*

◆ **PHL-Amoxicillin (Can)** *see* Amoxicillin *on page 96*

◆ **PHL-Atenolol (Can)** *see* Atenolol *on page 147*

◆ **PHL-Azithromycin (Can)** *see* Azithromycin *on page 164*

◆ **PHL-Baclofen (Can)** *see* Baclofen *on page 171*

◆ **PHL-Carbamazepine (Can)** *see* CarBAMazepine *on page 244*

◆ **PHL-Carvedilol (Can)** *see* Carvedilol *on page 254*

◆ **PHL-Ciprofloxacin (Can)** *see* Ciprofloxacin *on page 310*

◆ **PHL-Citalopram (Can)** *see* Citalopram *on page 319*

◆ **PHL-Cyclobenzaprine (Can)** *see* Cyclobenzaprine *on page 367*

◆ **PHL-Divalproex (Can)** *see* Valproic Acid and Derivatives *on page 1398*

◆ **PHL-Doxycycline (Can)** *see* Doxycycline *on page 479*

◆ **Phlemex** *see* Guaifenesin and Dextromethorphan *on page 658*

◆ **PHL-Fluconazole (Can)** *see* Fluconazole *on page 584*

◆ **PHL-Fluoxetine (Can)** *see* FLUoxetine *on page 600*

Physostigmine (fye zoe STIG meen)

Medication Safety Issues
Sound-alike/look-alike issues:
Physostigmine may be confused with Prostigmin®, pyridostigmine

Therapeutic Category Antidote, Anticholinergic Agent; Cholinergic Agent; Cholinergic Agent, Ophthalmic

Generic Available Yes

Use Reverse toxic, life-threatening delirium caused by atropine, diphenhydramine, dimenhydrinate, *Atropa belladonna* (deadly nightshade), or jimson weed (*Datura* spp)

Pregnancy Risk Factor C

Lactation Excretion in breast milk unknown

Contraindications Hypersensitivity to physostigmine or any component (see Warnings); GI or GU obstruction, asthma, diabetes mellitus, gangrene, severe cardiovascular disease; patients receiving depolarizing neuromuscular blockers (eg, succinylcholine)

Warnings Because physostigmine has the potential for producing severe adverse effects, (ie, seizures, bradycardia), routine use as an antidote is controversial. Patients must have a normal QRS interval, as measured by ECG, in order to receive; use caution in poisoning with agents known to prolong intraventricular conduction. Atropine should be readily available to treat severe adverse effects. Injection contains benzyl alcohol and bisulfite which may cause allergic reactions in susceptible individuals; large amounts of benzyl alcohol (≥99 mg/kg/day) have been associated with a potentially fatal toxicity ("gasping syndrome") in neonates; the "gasping syndrome" consists of metabolic acidosis, respiratory distress, gasping respirations, CNS dysfunction (including convulsions, intracranial hemorrhage), hypotension and cardiovascular collapse; *in vitro* and animal studies have shown that benzoate, a metabolite of benzyl alcohol, displaces bilirubin from protein-binding sites; use injection with caution in neonates.

Precautions Use with caution in patients with epilepsy, narrow-angle glaucoma, marked vagotonia, parkinsonism, bradycardia

Adverse Reactions
Cardiovascular: Asystole, bradycardia, palpitations
Central nervous system: Hallucinations, nervousness, restlessness, seizures
Dermatologic: Burning, redness
Gastrointestinal: Diarrhea, epigastric pain, nausea, salivation, vomiting
Genitourinary: Urinary frequency
Neuromuscular & skeletal: Twitching, weakness
Ocular: Lacrimation, miosis
Respiratory: Bronchospasm, dyspnea, pulmonary edema, respiratory paralysis
Miscellaneous: Diaphoresis

Drug Interactions
Avoid Concomitant Use There are no known interactions where it is recommended to avoid concomitant use.

Increased Effect/Toxicity
Physostigmine may increase the levels/effects of: Beta-Blockers; Cholinergic Agonists; Succinylcholine

The levels/effects of Physostigmine may be increased by: Corticosteroids (Systemic)

Decreased Effect
Physostigmine may decrease the levels/effects of: Neuromuscular-Blocking Agents (Nondepolarizing)

Mechanism of Action Inhibits destruction of acetylcholine by acetylcholinesterase which prolongs the central and peripheral effects of acetylcholine

Pharmacodynamics Parenteral:
Onset of action: Within 3-8 minutes
Duration: 30 minutes to 1 hour
Pharmacokinetics (Adult data unless noted)
Distribution: Widely distributed throughout the body; crosses into the CNS
Half-life: 1-2 hours
Elimination: Via hydrolysis by cholinesterases
Usual Dosage
Reversal of toxic anticholinergic effects: **Note:** Administer slowly over 5 minutes to prevent respiratory distress and seizures. Continuous infusions of physostigmine should never be used.
Children: Reserve for life-threatening situations only: I.V.: 0.01-0.03 mg/kg/dose; may repeat after 15-20 minutes to a maximum total dose of 2 mg
Adults: I.M., I.V., SubQ: 0.5-2 mg initially, repeat every 20 minutes until response or adverse effect occurs; repeat 1-4 mg every 30-60 minutes as life-threatening symptoms recur
Preanesthetic reversal: Children and Adults:
I.M., I.V.: Give twice the dose, on a weight basis, of the anticholinergic drug (atropine, scopolamine)
Administration Parenteral: Infuse slowly I.V. without additional dilution over 5 minutes. Too rapid administration can cause bradycardia and hypersalivation leading to respiratory distress and seizures.
Monitoring Parameters Heart rate, respiratory rate, ECG
Dosage Forms Excipient information presented when available (limited, particularly for generics); consult specific product labeling.
Injection, solution, as salicylate: 1 mg/mL (2 mL) [contains benzyl alcohol and sodium metabisulfite]

♦ **Physostigmine Salicylate** see Physostigmine on page 1108
♦ **Physostigmine Sulfate** see Physostigmine on page 1108
♦ **Phytomenadione** see Phytonadione on page 1109

Phytonadione (fye toe na DYE one)

Medication Safety Issues
Sound-alike/look-alike issues:
Mephyton® may be confused with melphalan, methadone
Related Information
Compatibility of Chemotherapy and Related Supportive Care Medications on page 1580
U.S. Brand Names Mephyton®
Canadian Brand Names AquaMEPHYTON®; Konakion; Mephyton®
Therapeutic Category Nutritional Supplement; Vitamin, Fat Soluble
Generic Available Yes
Use Prevention and treatment of hypoprothrombinemia caused by vitamin K deficiency or anticoagulant-induced hypoprothrombinemia; hemorrhagic disease of the newborn
Pregnancy Risk Factor C
Lactation Enters breast milk/use caution (AAP rates "compatible")
Contraindications Hypersensitivity to phytonadione or any component (see Warnings)
Warnings Ineffective in hereditary hypoprothrombinemia and hypoprothrombinemia caused by severe liver disease; severe hemolytic anemia and hyperbilirubinemia has been reported rarely in neonates following large doses (10-20 mg) of phytonadione. Injection contains 0.9% benzyl alcohol which may cause allergic reactions in susceptible individuals; large amounts of benzyl alcohol (≥99 mg/kg/day) have been associated with a potentially

fatal toxicity ("gasping syndrome") in neonates; the "gasping syndrome" consists of metabolic acidosis, respiratory distress, gasping respirations, CNS dysfunction (including convulsions, intracranial hemorrhage), hypotension and cardiovascular collapse; in vitro and animal studies have shown that benzoate, a metabolite of benzyl alcohol, displaces bilirubin from protein-binding sites; injection is safe in neonates when used in appropriate doses.
Precautions Severe reactions resembling anaphylaxis or hypersensitivity have occurred rarely during or immediately after I.V. administration (even with proper dilution and rate of administration) **[U.S. Boxed Warning]** and with I.M. administration; restrict I.V. and I.M. administration for situations where the subcutaneous route is not feasible
Adverse Reactions See Warnings and Precautions
Cardiovascular: Flushing, hypotension, cyanosis
Central nervous system: Dizziness
Endocrine & metabolic: Hyperbilirubinemia (neonates; greater than recommended dose)
Gastrointestinal: GI upset, dysgeusia, hyperbilirubinemia (neonates)
Hematologic: Hemolysis, hemolytic anemia (neonates; greater than recommended dose)
Local: Pain, edema, tenderness at injection site
Respiratory: Dyspnea
Miscellaneous: Anaphylactoid reactions, diaphoresis
Drug Interactions
Avoid Concomitant Use There are no known interactions where it is recommended to avoid concomitant use.
Increased Effect/Toxicity There are no known significant interactions involving an increase in effect.
Decreased Effect
Phytonadione may decrease the levels/effects of: Vitamin K Antagonists

The levels/effects of Phytonadione may be decreased by: Mineral Oil; Orlistat
Stability Stable at room temperature; protect from light
Mechanism of Action Cofactor in the liver synthesis of clotting factors (II, VII, IX, X)
Pharmacodynamics Onset of action: Blood coagulation factors increase within 6-12 hours after oral doses and within 1-2 hours following parenteral administration; after parenteral administration prothrombin time may become normal after 12-14 hours
Pharmacokinetics (Adult data unless noted)
Absorption: Oral: From the intestines in the presence of bile
Metabolism: Rapidly in the liver
Elimination: In bile and urine
Usual Dosage SubQ route is preferred; I.V. and I.M. routes should be restricted for situations when the SubQ route is not feasible
Hemorrhagic disease of the newborn: Neonates: SubQ, I.M.:
Prophylaxis: 0.5-1 mg within 1 hour of birth; may repeat if necessary 6-8 hours later
Treatment: 1-2 mg/day
Oral anticoagulant overdose:
Infants and Children:
No bleeding, rapid reversal needed, patient will require further oral anticoagulant therapy: SubQ, I.V.: 0.5-2 mg
No bleeding, rapid reversal needed, patient will **not** require further oral anticoagulant therapy: SubQ, I.V.: 2-5 mg
Significant bleeding, not life-threatening: SubQ, I.V.: 0.5-2 mg
Significant bleeding, life-threatening: I.V.: 5 mg

Adolescents and Adults: SubQ, I.V.: 2.5-10 mg/dose (rarely up to 25-50 mg has been used in adults); may repeat in 6-8 hours if given by SubQ, I.V. route; may repeat 12-48 hours after oral route

Vitamin K deficiency due to drugs, malabsorption, or decreased synthesis of vitamin K:

Infants and Children:

Oral: 2.5-5 mg/24 hours

SubQ, I.M., I.V.: 1-2 mg/dose as a single dose

Adolescents and Adults:

Oral: 2.5-25 mg/24 hours

SubQ, I.M., I.V.: 10 mg

Minimum daily requirement: Oral: Not well established

Infants: 1-5 mcg/kg/day

Adults: 0.03 mcg/kg/day

Adequate intake:

0-6 months: 2 mcg/day

7-12 months: 2.5 mcg/day

1-3 years: 30 mcg/day

4-8 years: 55 mcg/day

9-13 years: 60 mcg/day

14-18 years: 75 mcg/day

Adults, male: 120 mcg/day

Adults, female: 90 mcg/day

Pregnant, <18 years of age: 75 mcg/day

Pregnant, >19 years of age: 90 mcg/day

Breast-feeding, <18 years of age: 75 mcg/day

Breast-feeding, >19 years of age: 90 mcg/day

Administration

Oral: May be administered with or without food

Parenteral: SubQ administration is the preferred method (see Precautions); for I.V. administration, dilute in 5-10 mL I.V. fluid (D_5W or NS) (maximum concentration: 10 mg/mL); infuse over 15-30 minutes; maximum rate of infusion: 1 mg/minute

Monitoring Parameters PT, INR (if applicable)

Additional Information Phytonadione is more effective and is preferred to other vitamin K preparations in the presence of impending hemorrhage; oral absorption depends on the presence of bile salts

Dosage Forms Excipient information presented when available (limited, particularly for generics); consult specific product labeling.

Injection, aqueous colloidal: 2 mg/mL (0.5 mL); 10 mg/mL (1 mL) [contains benzyl alcohol]

Injection, aqueous colloidal [preservative free]: 2 mg/mL (0.5 mL) [contains polysorbate 80, propylene glycol 10.4 mg/0.5 mL]

Tablet: 100 mcg [OTC]

Mephyton®: 5 mg

Extemporaneous Preparations A 1 mg/mL suspension may be made by crushing six 5 mg tablets, add 5 mL purified water and 5 mL 1% methylcellulose, mix well, add 70% sorbitol to a total volume of 30 mL; shake well, refrigerate, expected stability: 3 days.

Nahata, MC, Pai VB, and Hipple TF, *Pediatric Drug Formulations*, 5th ed, Cincinnati, OH: Harvey Whitney Books Co, 2004.

References

Michelson AD, Bovill E, Monagle P, et al, "Antithrombic Therapy in Children," *Chest*, 1998, 114(5 Suppl):748S-69S.

Pilocarpine (pye loe KAR peen)

Medication Safety Issues

Sound-alike/look-alike issues:

Isopto® Carpine may be confused with Isopto® Carbachol

Salagen® may be confused with Salacid®, selegiline

International issues:

Salagen® may be confused with Poagen® which is a brand name for grass pollen extract in Portugal

U.S. Brand Names Isopto® Carpine; Pilopine HS®; Salagen®

Canadian Brand Names Diocarpine; Isopto® Carpine; Pilopine HS®; Salagen®

Therapeutic Category Cholinergic Agent; Cholinergic Agent, Ophthalmic; Ophthalmic Agent, Miotic

Generic Available Yes: Hydrochloride solution, tablet

Use

Ophthalmic: Management of chronic simple glaucoma; chronic and acute angle-closure glaucoma; counter effects of cycloplegics

Oral: Symptomatic treatment of xerostomia caused by salivary gland hypofunction resulting from radiotherapy for cancer of the head and neck; and in Sjögren's syndrome

Pregnancy Risk Factor C

Pregnancy Considerations Adverse events were observed in some animal studies following oral administration.

Lactation Excretion in breast milk unknown/not recommended

Contraindications Hypersensitivity to pilocarpine or any component; when cholinergic effects such as constriction are undesirable, eg, acute inflammatory disease of anterior chamber, acute iritis; severe hepatic impairment (oral use)

Warnings Reduce dosage in hepatic impairment

Precautions Use with caution in patients with pre-existing retinal disease, CHF, asthma, peptic ulcer, urinary tract obstruction, Parkinson's disease, corneal abrasion, or those predisposed to retinal tears; may occasionally precipitate angle closure by increased resistance to aqueous flow from the posterior to anterior eye chamber

Adverse Reactions

Cardiovascular: Rare hypertension, tachycardia, flushing

Central nervous system: Headache, chills, dizziness

Gastrointestinal (rare): Nausea, vomiting, diarrhea, salivation

Genitourinary: Polyuria

Local: Stinging, burning

Neuromuscular & skeletal: Weakness

Ocular: Ophthalmic formulation: Miosis, ciliary spasm, blurred vision, retinal detachment, photophobia, acute iritis, keratitis, corneal opacities, lacrimation, browache, conjunctival and ciliary congestion early in therapy

Otic: Tinnitus

Respiratory: Rhinitis

Miscellaneous: Hypersensitivity reactions, diaphoresis

Drug Interactions

Metabolism/Transport Effects Inhibits CYP2A6 (weak), 2E1 (weak), 3A4 (weak)

Avoid Concomitant Use There are no known interactions where it is recommended to avoid concomitant use.

Increased Effect/Toxicity

The levels/effects of Pilocarpine may be increased by: Acetylcholinesterase Inhibitors

Decreased Effect There are no known significant interactions involving a decrease in effect.

Food Interactions High fat meals decrease the rate of oral absorption and maximum serum concentration; the time to reach maximum concentrations is also increased

Mechanism of Action Directly stimulates cholinergic receptors in the eye causing miosis (by contraction of the iris sphincter), loss of accommodation (by constriction of ciliary muscle), and lowering of intraocular pressure (with decreased resistance to aqueous humor outflow)

Pharmacodynamics

Ophthalmic solution instillation: Miosis:

Onset of action: Within 10-30 minutes

Duration: 4-8 hours

Intraocular pressure reduction:
Onset of action: 1 hour
Duration: 4-12 hours
Oral: Increased salivary flow
Onset of action: 20 minutes
Maximum effect: 1 hour
Duration: 3-5 hours

Pharmacokinetics (Adult data unless noted) Adults:
Half-life, elimination: Oral: 0.76-1.35 hours
Mild to moderate hepatic impairment: 2.1 hours
Elimination: Urine

Usual Dosage
Ophthalmic: Children and Adults:
Gel: 0.5" (1.3 cm) ribbon applied to lower conjunctival sac once daily at bedtime; adjust dosage as required to control elevated intraocular pressure
Solution: Instill 1-2 drops up to 6 times/day; adjust the concentration and frequency as required to control elevated intraocular pressure
To counteract the mydriatic effects of sympathomimetic agents: Instill 1 drop of a 1% solution in the affected eye
Xerostomia: Adults: Oral:
Following head and neck cancer: 5 mg 3 times/day, titration up to 10 mg 3 times/day may be considered for patients who have not responded adequately; not to exceed 10 mg/dose
Sjögren's syndrome: 5 mg 4 times/day

Dosage adjustment in hepatic impairment: Adults: Oral: Patients with moderate impairment 5 mg 2 times/day regardless of indication; avoid use in severe hepatic impairment

Administration
Ophthalmic gel: Instill gel into affected eye(s); close the eye for 1-2 minutes and instruct patient to roll the eyeball in all directions; avoid contact of bottle tip with eye or skin
Ophthalmic solution: Shake well before use; instill into affected eye(s); apply finger pressure to lacrimal sac during and for 1-2 minutes after instillation to decrease drainage into the nose and throat and minimize possible systemic absorption
Oral: May be administered with or without food; avoid administration with high fat meal

Monitoring Parameters Intraocular pressure, funduscopic exam, visual field testing; salivation (xerostomia treatment)

Patient Information May sting on instillation; notify physician of sweating, urinary retention; usually causes difficulty in dark adaptation; use caution when driving at night or doing hazardous activities in poor light

Dosage Forms Excipient information presented when available (limited, particularly for generics); consult specific product labeling. [DSC] = Discontinued product
Gel, ophthalmic, as hydrochloride:
Pilopine HS®: 4% (4 g) [contains benzalkonium chloride]
Solution, ophthalmic, as hydrochloride: 0.5% (15 mL) [DSC]; 1% (2 mL, 15 mL); 2% (2 mL, 15 mL); 3% (15 mL) [DSC]; 4% (2 mL, 15 mL); 6% (15 mL) [may contain benzalkonium chloride]
Isopto® Carpine: 1% (15 mL); 2% (15 mL); 4% (15 mL) [contains benzalkonium chloride]
Tablet, as hydrochloride: 5 mg, 7.5 mg
Salagen®: 5 mg, 7.5 mg

◆ **Pilocarpine Hydrochloride** see Pilocarpine on page 1110

◆ **Pilopine HS®** see Pilocarpine on page 1110

Pimecrolimus (pim e KROE li mus)

Medication Safety Issues
Sound-alike/look-alike issues:
Pimecrolimus may be confused with tacrolimus

U.S. Brand Names Elidel®
Canadian Brand Names Elidel®
Therapeutic Category Immunomodulating Agent, Topical
Generic Available No
Use Second-line agent for short-term and intermittent treatment of mild to moderate atopic dermatitis in non-immunocompromised patients unresponsive to, or intolerant of other treatments
Medication Guide An FDA-approved patient medication guide, which is available with the product information and at http://www.fda.gov/downloads/Drugs/DrugSafety/ucm088587.pdf, must be dispensed with this medication for each new outpatient prescription and refill.
Pregnancy Risk Factor C
Pregnancy Considerations There are no adequate and well-controlled studies in pregnant women; use only if clearly needed.
Lactation Excretion in breast milk unknown/not recommended
Breast-Feeding Considerations Due to the potential for serious adverse reactions in the nursing infant, breast-feeding is not recommended.
Contraindications Hypersensitivity to pimecrolimus or any component; Netherton's syndrome due to potential for increased systemic absorption; application to site with active cutaneous viral infection (treat and clear infection prior to the start of therapy); application on malignant or premalignant skin conditions
Warnings Pimecrolimus therapy may be associated with an increased risk for eczema herpeticum, varicella zoster, or herpes simplex virus infection; consider discontinuing therapy in patients who develop lymphadenopathy or in patients who have skin papillomas which worsen. Cream contains benzyl alcohol which may cause allergic reactions in susceptible individuals; large amounts of benzyl alcohol (≥99 mg/kg/day) have been associated with a potentially fatal toxicity ("gasping syndrome") in neonates; the "gasping syndrome" consists of metabolic acidosis, respiratory distress, gasping respirations, CNS dysfunction (including convulsions, intracranial hemorrhage), hypotension and cardiovascular collapse.
Precautions Use with caution in immunocompromised patients and in patients who have experienced adverse effects to topical cyclosporine or tacrolimus.
Adverse Reactions
Cardiovascular: Facial edema
Central nervous system: Headache, fever
Dermatologic: Pruritus, acne, infected hair follicles, skin cancer, skin discoloration, skin papilloma, impetigo
Gastrointestinal: Nausea
Local: Burning sensation, stinging
Respiratory: Nasopharyngitis, cough, wheezing
Miscellaneous: Lymphoma, lymphadenopathy, anaphylactic reaction
Drug Interactions
Metabolism/Transport Effects Substrate of CYP3A4 (minor)
Avoid Concomitant Use
Avoid concomitant use of Pimecrolimus with any of the following: Immunosuppressants
Increased Effect/Toxicity
Pimecrolimus may increase the levels/effects of: Immunosuppressants

The levels/effects of Pimecrolimus may be increased by: CYP3A4 Inhibitors (Moderate); CYP3A4 Inhibitors (Strong)
Decreased Effect There are no known significant interactions involving a decrease in effect.
Stability Store at room temperature; do not freeze

Mechanism of Action Binds with high affinity to macrophilin-12 (FKBP-12) inhibiting the calcium-dependent phosphatase activity of calcineurin. Inhibits T-cell activation by blocking the transcription and synthesis in human T-cells of early cytokines interleukin-2, interferon gamma (T_h1-type), interleukin-4, and interleukin-10 (T_h2-type). Prevents the release of inflammatory cytokines and mediators from mast cells after stimulation by antigen/IgE.

Pharmacodynamics Onset of action: Time to significant improvement: 8 days

Pharmacokinetics (Adult data unless noted)

Absorption: Topical: Low systemic absorption; blood concentration of pimecrolimus was routinely <2 ng/mL with treatment of atopic dermatitis in adult patients (13% to 62% BSA involvement); blood concentration of pimecrolimus was <3 ng/mL in 26 pediatric patients 2-14 years of age with atopic dermatitis (20% to 69% BSA involvement). Detectable blood levels were observed in a higher proportion of children as compared to adults and may be due to the larger surface area to body mass ratio seen in pediatric patients.

Protein binding: 99.5%, primarily to various lipoproteins

Metabolism: In the liver by the cytochrome P450 3A4 system

Half-life: Terminal: 30-40 hours

Time to peak serum concentration: Topical: 2-6 hours

Elimination: 80% in the feces as metabolites

Usual Dosage Children ≥2 years of age and Adults: Topical: Apply twice daily; use smallest amount of cream needed to control symptoms; continue therapy for as long as symptoms persist; re-evaluate patient at 6 weeks. **Note:** Pimecrolimus is not approved for use in children <2 years of age since the drug's long-term effect on the developing immune system is unknown. Detectable blood levels were observed in a higher proportion of children as compared to adults and may be due to the larger surface area to body mass ratio seen in pediatric patients. Children <2 years of age treated with pimecrolimus had a higher rate of upper respiratory infections than those treated with placebo.

Administration Topical: Avoid contact with eyes, nose, mouth, and cut, scraped, or infected skin areas. Wash hands with soap and water prior to and after cream application. If applying cream after a bath or shower, make sure skin is dry. Apply thin layer of cream by gently rubbing it in over affected skin surfaces which may include head and neck areas. The use of occlusive dressings is not recommended.

Monitoring Parameters Check skin for signs of worsening condition (increase in pruritus, erythema, excoriation, and lichenification)

Patient Information Avoid exposure to sunlight and artificial light sources (sunlamps, tanning booth/bed); wear protective clothing, wide-brimmed hats, and lip sunscreen (SPF ≥15); use a sunscreen [broad-spectrum sunscreen or physical sunscreen (preferred) or sunblock with SPF ≥15]; contact physician if any signs of serious infection occurs or if symptoms of atopic dermatitis do not improve within 6 weeks

Dosage Forms Excipient information presented when available (limited, particularly for generics); consult specific product labeling.

Cream, topical:

Elidel®: 1% (30 g, 60 g, 100 g)

References

Eichenfield LF, Lucky AW, Boguniewicz M, et al, "Safety and Efficacy of Pimecrolimus (ASM 981) Cream 1% in the Treatment of Mild and Moderate Atopic Dermatitis in Children and Adolescents," *J Am Acad Dermatol*, 2002, 46(4):495-504.

Wahn U, Bos JD, Goodfield M, et al, "Efficacy and Safety of Pimecrolimus Cream in the Long-Term Management of Atopic Dermatitis in Children," *Pediatrics*, 2002, 110(1 Pt 1):e2.

Wellington K and Jarvis B, "Topical Pimecrolimus: A Review of Its Clinical Potential in the Management of Atopic Dermatitis," *Drugs*, 2002, 62(5):817-40.

Pimozide (PI moe zide)

U.S. Brand Names Orap®

Canadian Brand Names Apo-Pimozide®; Orap®; PMS-Pimozide

Therapeutic Category Antipsychotic Agent, Typical

Generic Available No

Use Suppression of severe motor and phonic (vocal) tics in patients with Tourette's disorder who have failed to respond satisfactorily to standard treatment and whose daily life function and/or development is severely compromised by the presence of motor and phonic tics (FDA approved in ages ≥2 years and adults)

Note: A trial of standard treatment is currently recommended before a trial of pimozide because of pimozide's potential cardiac toxicity (see Warnings). See also Scahill, 2006 for the Tourette Syndrome Association Medical Advisory Board: Practice Committee's treatment guidelines.

Pregnancy Risk Factor C

Pregnancy Considerations No evidence of teratogenicity reported in animal studies. However, developmental toxicity and decreased pregnancies have been observed. There are no adequate and well-controlled studies in pregnant women. Use only if potential benefit justifies risk to the fetus.

Lactation Excretion in breast milk unknown/not recommended

Contraindications Hypersensitivity to pimozide or any component; simple tics or tics other than Tourette's disorder; patients receiving medications that can cause motor and phonic tics (eg, amphetamines, methylphenidate, pemoline) until these medications can be withdrawn to determine whether or not the drug (rather than Tourette's Disorder) is causing the tics; severe toxic CNS depression; coma; history of cardiac arrhythmias; congential long QT syndrome; concurrent use with QT_c-prolonging agents; hypokalemia or hypomagnesemia; concurrent use of drugs that are inhibitors of cytochrome P450 CYP3A4, including azole antifungals (itraconazole, ketoconazole), macrolide antibiotics [ie, clarithromycin, erythromycin (**Note:** The manufacturer lists azithromycin and dirithromycin in its list of contraindicated macrolides; however, these drugs do not inhibit CYP3A4 and are not expected to interact with pimozide)], citalopram, escitalopram, nefazodone, sertraline, protease inhibitors (eg, atazanavir, indinavir, nelfinavir, ritonavir, saquinavir), and other less potent inhibitors of CYP3A4 (eg, fluvoxamine, zileuton)

Warnings May alter cardiac conduction; sudden unexplained deaths have occurred in patients taking high doses (~1 mg/kg); deaths may be due to prolongation of the QT interval predisposing patients to ventricular arrhythmias; monitor ECG at baseline and periodically during dosage titration; correct any hypokalemia prior to initiation of therapy and maintain normal serum potassium during therapy. May cause hypotension at high doses (minimal hypotension at adult doses <5 mg/day) or orthostatic hypotension. Use with caution in patients with autonomic instability, hypovolemia, cerebrovascular or cardiovascular disease, or concurrent medications which may predispose to hypotension/bradycardia). Do not use in Parkinson's disease. Use with caution in patients with hemodynamic instability; bone marrow suppression (use of antipsychotic agents has been associated with neutropenia, leukopenia, and agranulocytosis; monitor patients with history of low WBC or drug-induced leukopenia or neutropenia); predisposition to seizures (antipsychotics may lower the seizure threshold); predisposition to seizures; subcortical brain damage; severe cardiac, hepatic, renal, or respiratory disease; patients with hypersensitivity to other antipsychotic drugs.

Esophageal dysmotility and aspiration have been associated with antipsychotic use; use with caution in patients at risk of pneumonia (ie, Alzheimer's disease). Use with caution in breast cancer or other prolactin-dependent tumors (may elevate prolactin levels). May alter temperature regulation. May mask other conditions or toxicity of other drugs due to antiemetic effects. May cause extrapyramidal symptoms, including pseudoparkinsonism, acute dystonic reactions, akathisia, and tardive dyskinesia (risk of these reactions is high relative to other neuroleptics, and is dose-dependent; to decrease risk of tardive dyskinesia: Use smallest dose and shortest duration possible; evaluate continued need periodically; risk of dystonia is increased with the use of high potency and higher doses of conventional antipsychotics and in males and younger patients. Use may be associated with neuroleptic malignant syndrome (NMS); monitor for mental status changes, fever, muscle rigidity, and/or autonomic instability; may also be associated with increased CPK, myogloburia, and acute renal failure; discontinue use if these symptoms occur; NMS may recur upon rechallenge.

Leukopenia, neutropenia, and agranulocytosis (sometimes fatal) have been reported in clinical trials and postmarketing reports with antipsychotic use; presence of risk factors (eg, pre-existing low WBC or history of drug-induced leuko/neutropenia) should prompt periodic blood count assessment. Discontinue therapy at first signs of blood dyscrasias or if absolute neutrophil count <1000/mm^3.

An increased risk of death has been reported with the use of antipsychotics in elderly patients with dementia-related psychosis **[U.S. Boxed Warning]**; most deaths seemed to be cardiovascular (eg, sudden death, heart failure) or infectious (eg, pneumonia) in nature; pimozide is not approved for this indication.

Precautions May cause anticholinergic effects (confusion, agitation, constipation, xerostomia, blurred vision, urinary retention); use with caution in patients with decreased GI motility, urinary retention, BPH, xerostomia, or visual problems. Use with caution in patients with narrow-angle glaucoma; condition may be exacerbated by cholinergic blockade; screening is recommended. Use with caution in patients with myasthenia gravis; condition may be exacerbated by cholinergic blockade. Relative to neuroleptics, pimozide has a moderate potency of cholinergic blockade.

May be moderately sedating, use with caution in disorders where CNS depression is a feature; patients must be cautioned about performing tasks which require mental alertness (eg, operating machinery or driving). Pimozide may have a tumorigenic potential; a dose-related increase in pituitary tumors was observed in studies of mice; full significance in humans is unknown; however, this finding should be considered when deciding to use pimozide chronically in a young patient. Limited information about the use of pimozide in children <12 years of age exists.

Avoid abrupt discontinuation after prolonged use; abrupt discontinuation in patients receiving maintenance treatment may result in transient dyskinetic signs in some patients; these dyskinetic movements may not be distinguishable from tardive dyskinesia (except for duration).

Adverse Reactions

Cardiovascular: Abnormal ECG

Central nervous system: Abnormal dreams, akathisia, akinesia, behavior changes, depression, drowsiness, headache, hyperkinesias, insomnia, nervousness, neuroleptic malignant syndrome, sedation, somnolence, speech disorder

Dermatologic: Rash

Endocrine & metabolic: Prolactin levels elevated

Gastrointestinal: Appetite increased, constipation, diarrhea, dysphagia, salivation increased, taste disturbance, thirst, xerostomia

Genitourinary: Impotence

Hematologic: Agranulocytosis, leukopenia, neutropenia

Neuromuscular & skeletal: Handwriting changes, muscle tightness, myalgia, rigidity, stooped posture, torticollis, tremor, weakness

Ocular: Accommodation decreased, photophobia, visual disturbance

Frequency not defined, postmarketing and/or case reports (some reported for disorders other than Tourette's disorder): Anorexia, blurred vision, cataracts, chest pain, diaphoresis, dizziness, excitement; extrapyramidal symptoms (dystonia, pseudoparkinsonism, tardive dyskinesia); GI distress, gingival hyperplasia (case report), hemolytic anemia, hyper-/hypotension, hyponatremia, libido decreased, nausea, nocturia, palpitation, periorbital edema, polyuria, postural hypotension, QT$_c$ prolongation, seizure, skin irritation, syncope, tachycardia, ventricular arrhythmia, vomiting, weight gain/loss

Drug Interactions

Metabolism/Transport Effects Substrate (major) of CYP1A2, 3A4; **Inhibits** CYP2C19 (weak), 2D6 (weak), 2E1 (weak), 3A4 (weak)

Avoid Concomitant Use

Avoid concomitant use of Pimozide with any of the following: Antifungal Agents (Azole Derivatives, Systemic); Aprepitant; Artemether; Dronedarone; Efavirenz; Fosaprepitant; Lumefantrine; Macrolide Antibiotics; Metoclopramide; Nefazodone; Nilotinib; Protease Inhibitors; QTc-Prolonging Agents; QuiNINE; Selective Serotonin Reuptake Inhibitors; Tetrabenazine; Thioridazine; Ziprasidone

Increased Effect/Toxicity

Pimozide may increase the levels/effects of: Alcohol (Ethyl); Anticholinergics; Anti-Parkinson's Agents (Dopamine Agonist); CNS Depressants; Dronedarone; QTc-Prolonging Agents; QuiNINE; Tetrabenazine; Thioridazine; Ziprasidone

The levels/effects of Pimozide may be increased by: Acetylcholinesterase Inhibitors (Central); Alfuzosin; Antifungal Agents (Azole Derivatives, Systemic); Aprepitant; Artemether; Chloroquine; Ciprofloxacin; Ciprofloxacin (Systemic); CYP1A2 Inhibitors (Moderate); CYP1A2 Inhibitors (Strong); CYP3A4 Inhibitors (Moderate); CYP3A4 Inhibitors (Strong); Efavirenz; Fosaprepitant; Gadobutrol; Lithium formulations; Lumefantrine; Macrolide Antibiotics; Metoclopramide; Nefazodone; Nilotinib; Pramlintide; Protease Inhibitors; QTc-Prolonging Agents; QuiNINE; Selective Serotonin Reuptake Inhibitors; Tetrabenazine

Decreased Effect

Pimozide may decrease the levels/effects of: Amphetamines; Quinagolide

The levels/effects of Pimozide may be decreased by: Anti-Parkinson's Agents (Dopamine Agonist); CYP1A2 Inducers (Strong); CYP3A4 Inducers (Strong); Deferasirox; Herbs (CYP3A4 Inducers); Lithium formulations

Food Interactions Grapefruit juice may increase pimozide serum concentrations; avoid use.

Stability Store at controlled room temperature at 25°C (77°F); excursions permitted to 15°C to 30°C (59°F to 86°F). Dispense in a tight, light-resistant container.

Mechanism of Action Pimozide, a diphenylbutylperidine conventional antipsychotic, is a potent centrally-acting dopamine receptor antagonist; effects which result in its characteristic neuroleptic effects

Pharmacodynamics Onset of action: Within one week
Maximum effect: 4-6 weeks
Duration: Variable

◄ **Pharmacokinetics (Adult data unless noted)**
Absorption: Oral: >50%
Protein binding: 99%
Metabolism: Hepatic; significant first-pass effect; metabolized primarily via N-dealkylation
Half-life:
  Tourette's disorder (see Sallee, 1987):
    Children 6-13 years (n=4): Mean ± SD: 66 ± 49 hours
    Adults 23-39 years (n=7): Mean ± SD: 111 ± 57 hours
  Schizophrenia: Adults: Mean: 55 hours
Time to peak serum concentration: 6-8 hours; range: 4-12 hours
Elimination: Urine

Usual Dosage Oral: **Note:** Slow titration is recommended to improve tolerability; use lowest effective dose (see Additional Information).
Children ≤12 years: Initial: 0.05 mg/kg (maximum: 1 mg/dose) once daily (preferably at bedtime); gradually titrate dose every 1-2 weeks as tolerated; may increase dose every third day if needed; maintenance: 2-4 mg once daily; maximum: 10 mg/day or 0.2 mg/kg/day (whichever is less)
Children >12 years and Adults: Initial: 1-2 mg/day in divided doses; gradually titrate dose every 1-2 weeks as tolerated; may increase dose every other day if needed; maintenance: 7-10 mg/day in divided doses; maximum: 10 mg/day or 0.2 mg/kg/day (whichever is less)

Dosing adjustment in hepatic impairment: Reduction of dose is necessary in patients with liver disease

Administration May be administered without regard to meals

Monitoring Parameters ECG should be performed at baseline and periodically thereafter, especially during dosage adjustment; vital signs; serum potassium; magnesium, sodium; renal and hepatic function; height, weight, BMI; mental status, abnormal involuntary movement scale (AIMS), extrapyramidal symptoms (EPS) screening; CBC with differential (patients with a history of low WBC or drug-induced leukopenia or neutropenia)

Patient Information Use exactly as directed; do not increase dose or frequency. It may take 2-3 weeks to achieve desired results; do not discontinue without consulting prescriber. Avoid alcohol, caffeine, other prescription and nonprescription medications not approved by prescriber. Avoid grapefruit juice. Maintain adequate hydration unless instructed to restrict fluid intake. This medication may cause changes in the rhythm of the heart; deaths have been reported in patients taking high doses; an ECG prior to starting treatment and periodically thereafter is required. This medication may cause excess drowsiness, restlessness, dizziness, or blurred vision (use caution driving or when engaging in tasks requiring alertness until response to drug is known); constipation, dry mouth, anorexia. Report persistent CNS effects (eg, trembling fingers, altered gait or balance, excessive sedation, seizures, unusual muscle or facial movements, anxiety, abnormal thoughts, confusion, personality changes); unresolved constipation or GI effects; breast swelling (male and female); decreased sexual ability; vision changes; respiratory difficulty; palpitations, unusual cough or flu-like symptoms; or worsening of condition.

Nursing Implications Assess results of ophthalmic exam and laboratory tests, blood pressure, therapeutic effectiveness, and adverse reactions at beginning of therapy and periodically with long-term use. Conduct baseline ECG and periodically during therapy (especially during dosage adjustment). Initiate at lower doses (see Usual Dosage) and decrease dosage slowly when discontinuing. Refer to Contraindications for medicines which may predispose patients to potentially fatal cardiac arrhythmias.

Additional Information Twenty-two children 7-16 years of age (mean age: 10.2 years) with Tourette's disorder were enrolled in a randomized, double-blind, crossover study of pimozide versus haloperidol; both medications were initiated at 1 mg/day and increased on a flexible dosage schedule of 2 mg/week within a 4-week time period; the mean effective pimozide dose was 3.4 mg/day (range: 1-6 mg/day); pimozide was found to be more effective than placebo while haloperidol was not; more adverse effects, including extrapyramidal reactions were observed with haloperidol (Sallee, 1997).

In a multicenter, double-blind, parallel-group comparative study, 50 patients 11-50 years of age were treated for Tourette's disorder with pimozide (n=24; median age: 23.5 years) versus risperidone (n=26); a fixed-dose titration of pimozide from 1 mg/day to 2 mg/day was used for the first week of therapy; this was followed by a flexible dosing period of 7 weeks; doses were increased by ≤1 mg/week up to a maximum of 6 mg/day and were given once daily; final pimozide dose: 1-6 mg/day (mean: 2.9 mg/day); both drugs significantly improved tics; although there was no difference in efficacy between drugs, risperidone was better tolerated (Bruggeman, 2001).

In a randomized, double-blind, crossover pediatric trial of patients with Tourette's disorder and chronic motor tic disorder (n=19; age: 7-17 years), risperidone was shown to be superior to pimozide in decreasing tic severity scores, but was associated with greater weight gain; pimozide was initiated at 1 mg/day, administered at bedtime; the dose was titrated weekly if needed to a maximum of 4 mg/day; final dosage of pimozide ranged from 1-4 mg/day (mean: 2.4 mg/day); initial risperidone dosage was 0.5 mg twice daily; doses were titrated to a maximum of 4 mg/day (2 mg/dose twice daily); final dosage of risperidone ranged from 1-4 mg/day (mean: 2.5 mg/day) (Gilbert, 2004).

Dosage Forms Excipient information presented when available (limited, particularly for generics); consult specific product labeling.
Tablet:
  Orap®: 1 mg, 2 mg

References
Bruggeman R, van der Linden C, Buitelaar JK, et al, "Risperidone Versus Pimozide in Tourette's Disorder: A Comparative Double-Blind Parallel-Group Study," *J Clin Psychiatry*, 2001, 62(1):50-6.

Bruun RD, "Subtle and Under-Recognized Side Effects of Neuroleptic Treatment in Children With Tourette's Disorder," *Am J Psychiatry*, 1988, 145(5):621-4.

Gilbert DL, Batterson JR, Sethuraman G, et al, "Tic Reduction With Risperidone Versus Pimozide in a Randomized, Double-Blind, Crossover Trial," *J Am Acad Child Adolesc Psychiatry*, 2004, 43 (2):206-14.

Jankovic J, "Tourette's Syndrome," *NEJM*, 2001, 345(16):1184-92.

Jimenez-Jimenez FJ and Garcia-Ruiz PJ, "Pharmacological Options for the Treatment of Tourette's Disorder," *Drugs*, 2001, 61(15):2207-20.

Krähenbühl S, Sauter B, Kupferschmidt H, et al, "Case Report: Reversible QT Prolongation With Torsade de Pointes in a Patient With Pimozide Intoxication," *Am J Med Sci*, 1995, 309(6):315-6.

Larkin S, "Epileptogenic Effect of Pimozide," *Am J Psychiatry*, 1983, 140(3):372-3.

Muller-Vahl JT, "The Treatment of Tourette's Syndrome: Current Opinions," *Expert Opin Pharmacother*, 2002, 3(7):899-914.

"Pimozide (Orap) Contraindicated With Clarithromycin (Biaxin™) and Other Macrolide Antibiotics," *FDA Medical Bulletin*, October 1996, 3.

Sallee FR, Dougherty D, Sethuraman G, et al, "Prolactin Monitoring of Haloperidol and Pimozide Treatment in Children With Tourette's Syndrome," *Biol Psychiatry*, 1996, 40(10):1044-50.

Sallee FR, Nesbitt L, Jackson C, et al, "Relative Efficacy of Haloperidol and Pimozide in Children and Adolescents With Tourette's Disorder," *Am J Psychiatry*, 1997, 154(8):1057-62.

Sallee FR, Pollock BG, Stiller RL, et al, "Pharmacokinetics of Pimozide in Adults and Children With Tourette's Syndrome," *J Clin Pharmacol*, 1987, 27(10):776-81.

Scahill L, Erenberg G, Berlin CM Jr, et al, "Contemporary Assessment and Pharmacotherapy of Tourette Syndrome," *NeuroRx*, 2006, 3 (2):192-206.

◆ **Pin-X® [OTC]** *see* Pyrantel Pamoate *on page 1187*

◆ **Pink Bismuth** *see* Bismuth *on page 195*

Piperacillin (pi PER a sil in)

Canadian Brand Names Piperacillin for Injection, USP
Therapeutic Category Antibiotic, Penicillin (Antipseudomonal)
Generic Available Yes
Use Treatment of serious infections caused by susceptible strains of gram-positive, gram-negative, and anaerobic bacilli; mixed aerobic-anaerobic bacterial infections or empiric antibiotic therapy in granulocytopenic patients. Primary use is in the treatment of serious carbenicillin-resistant or ticarcillin-resistant *Pseudomonas aeruginosa* infections susceptible to piperacillin.
Pregnancy Risk Factor B
Pregnancy Considerations Adverse events have not been observed in animal studies; therefore, piperacillin is classified as pregnancy category B. Piperacillin crosses the placenta and distributes into the amniotic fluid. Due to pregnancy induced physiologic changes, some pharmacokinetic parameters of piperacillin may be altered. At term, the apparent volume of distribution of piperacillin is increased and peak concentrations are significantly lower. Total clearance is normal to increased at term. These changes continue into the early postpartum period.
Lactation Enters breast milk/compatible
Breast-Feeding Considerations Small amounts of piperacillin are excreted in breast milk. The manufacturer recommends that caution be exercised when administering piperacillin to nursing women. Other penicillins are considered safe for use during breast-feeding. Nondose-related effects could include modification of bowel flora.
Contraindications Hypersensitivity to piperacillin, penicillins, or any component
Warnings Superinfection has been reported in up to 6% to 8% of patients receiving an extended spectrum penicillin; piperacillin therapy has been associated with an increased incidence of fever and rash in cystic fibrosis patients
Precautions Use with caution in patients with hypersensitivity to cephalosporins; dosage modification required in patients with impaired renal function
Adverse Reactions
Central nervous system: Seizures, fever, headache, dizziness, confusion, drowsiness
Dermatologic: Rash, exfoliative dermatitis
Endocrine & metabolic: Hypokalemia
Gastrointestinal: Diarrhea, vomiting
Hematologic: Hemolytic anemia, eosinophilia, neutropenia, prolonged bleeding time, thrombocytopenia
Hepatic: Liver enzymes elevated, cholestatic hepatitis
Local: Thrombophlebitis
Neuromuscular & skeletal: Myoclonus
Renal: Acute interstitial nephritis
Miscellaneous: Hypersensitivity reactions, anaphylaxis, serum sickness-like reaction
Drug Interactions
Avoid Concomitant Use
Avoid concomitant use of Piperacillin with any of the following: BCG
Increased Effect/Toxicity
Piperacillin may increase the levels/effects of: Methotrexate

The levels/effects of Piperacillin may be increased by: Probenecid
Decreased Effect
Piperacillin may decrease the levels/effects of: Aminoglycosides; BCG; Mycophenolate; Typhoid Vaccine

The levels/effects of Piperacillin may be decreased by: Fusidic Acid; Tetracycline Derivatives

Stability Reconstituted piperacillin solution is stable for 24 hours at room temperature and 7 days when refrigerated; incompatible with aminoglycosides
Mechanism of Action Inhibits bacterial cell wall synthesis by binding to one or more of the penicillin-binding proteins; inhibits the final transpeptidation step of peptidoglycan synthesis in bacterial cell walls
Pharmacokinetics (Adult data unless noted)
Absorption: I.M.: 70% to 80%
Distribution: Crosses the placenta; distributes into breast milk at low concentrations; penetration across the blood-brain barrier is poor when meninges are uninflamed; good biliary concentration (30-60 times higher than serum concentration)
Protein binding: 22%
Metabolism: 5% to 10%
Half-life: Prolonged with moderately severe renal or hepatic impairment
Neonates:
1-5 days: 3.6 hours
>6 days: 2.1-2.7 hours
Children:
1-6 months: 0.5-1 hours
6 months to 12 years: 0.39-0.5 hours
Adults: 36-80 minutes (dose-dependent)
Time to peak serum concentration: I.M.: Within 30-50 minutes
Elimination: Principally in urine and partially in feces (via bile)
Dialysis: Dialyzable (20% to 50%)
Usual Dosage
I.M., I.V.:
Neonates:
≤7 days: 150 mg/kg/day divided every 8 hours
>7 days: 200 mg/kg/day divided every 6 hours
Infants and Children: 200-300 mg/kg/day in divided doses every 4-6 hours; maximum dose: 24 g/day
Higher doses have been used in cystic fibrosis: 350-500 mg/kg/day in divided doses every 4 hours
Adults: 2-4 g/dose every 4-8 hours; maximum dose: 24 g/day
Dosing interval in renal impairment:
Cl$_{cr}$ 20-40 mL/minute: Administer every 8 hours
Cl$_{cr}$ <20 mL/minute: Administer every 12 hours
Administration Parenteral:
I.M.: Reconstitute each gram of piperacillin with at least 2 mL of SWI, NS, or 0.5% or 1% lidocaine hydrochloride (without epinephrine) to make a 400 mg/mL solution; administer by deep I.M. injection into the gluteus maximus
I.V. push: Administer over 3-5 minutes at a maximum concentration of 200 mg/mL
I.V. intermittent infusion: Administer over 30-60 minutes at a final concentration ≤20 mg/mL
Monitoring Parameters Serum electrolytes, bleeding time especially in patients with renal impairment; periodic tests of renal, hepatic and hematologic function
Test Interactions False-positive urinary and serum proteins, positive Coombs' [direct]
Nursing Implications If the patient is on concurrent aminoglycoside therapy, separate piperacillin administration from the aminoglycoside by at least 30-60 minutes
Additional Information Sodium content of 1 g: 1.85 mEq
Dosage Forms Excipient information presented when available (limited, particularly for generics); consult specific product labeling.
Injection, powder for reconstitution: 2 g, 3 g, 4 g, 40 g
References
Placzek M, Whitelaw A, Want S, et al, "Piperacillin in Early Neonatal Infection," *Arch Dis Child*, 1983, 58(12):1006-9.
Prince AS and Neu HC, "Use of Piperacillin, A Semisynthetic Penicillin, in the Therapy of Acute Exacerbations of Pulmonary Disease in Patients With Cystic Fibrosis," *J Pediatr*, 1980, 97(1):148-51.

Thirumoorthi MC, Asmar BI, Buckley JA, et al, "Pharmacokinetics of Intravenously Administered Piperacillin in Preadolescent Children," *J Pediatr*, 1983, 102(6):941-6.

Piperacillin and Tazobactam
(pi PER a sil in & ta zoe BAK tam)

Medication Safety Issues
Sound-alike/look-alike issues:
Zosyn® may be confused with Zofran®, Zyvox®

U.S. Brand Names Zosyn®

Canadian Brand Names Tazocin®

Therapeutic Category Antibiotic, Beta-lactam and Beta-lactamase Inhibitor Combination; Antibiotic, Penicillin (Antipseudomonal)

Generic Available Yes: Excludes infusion

Use Treatment of sepsis, postpartum endometritis or pelvic inflammatory disease, intra-abdominal infections, including appendicitis (complicated by rupture or abscess) and peritonitis; uncomplicated or complicated infections involving skin and skin structures, the lower respiratory tract, and urinary tract caused by piperacillin-resistant, beta-lactamase-producing strains that are piperacillin/tazobactam susceptible. Tazobactam expands activity of piperacillin to include beta-lactamase producing strains of *S. aureus, H. influenzae, B. fragilis, Klebsiella, E. coli*, and *Acinetobacter*. When piperacillin and tazobactam is used to treat nosocomial pneumonia caused by *P. aeruginosa*, combination therapy with an aminoglycoside is recommended.

Pregnancy Risk Factor B

Pregnancy Considerations Adverse events have not been observed in animal studies; therefore, piperacillin/tazobactam is classified as pregnancy category B. Piperacillin and tazobactam both cross the placenta and are found in the fetal serum, placenta, amniotic fluid, and fetal urine. When used during pregnancy, the clearance and volume of distribution of piperacillin/tazobactam are increased; half-life and AUC are decreased.

Lactation Enters breast milk/use caution

Breast-Feeding Considerations Low concentrations of piperacillin are excreted in breast milk; information for tazobactam is not available. The manufacturer recommends that caution be exercised when administering piperacillin/tazobactam to nursing women. Other penicillins are considered safe for use during breast-feeding. Non-dose-related effects could include modification of bowel flora. When given alone in the early postpartum period, some pharmacokinetic parameters of piperacillin may be altered (refer to Piperacillin monograph for details).

Contraindications Hypersensitivity to piperacillin, tazobactam, penicillins, cephalosporins, beta-lactamase inhibitors, or any component

Warnings Prolonged use may result in superinfection, including pseudomembranous colitis; abnormal platelet aggregation and prolonged bleeding have been reported in patients with renal failure; piperacillin therapy has been associated with an increased incidence of fever and rash in cystic fibrosis patients. Severe anaphylactic reactions, including shock, have been reported in patients receiving piperacillin and tazobactam; be prepared to treat anaphylaxis when administering Zosyn®

Precautions Use with caution in patients requiring restricted salt intake, and in patients with renal impairment or pre-existing seizure disorder; dosage modification required in patients with impaired renal function

Adverse Reactions
Cardiovascular: Hypertension, hypotension, edema, chest pain, arrhythmia, tachycardia, cardiac arrest

Central nervous system: Insomnia, headache, dizziness, agitation, confusion, fever, anxiety, convulsions, confusion

Dermatologic: Rash, pruritus, erythema multiforme, Stevens-Johnson syndrome, urticaria

Endocrine & metabolism: Hypokalemia

Gastrointestinal: Diarrhea, constipation, nausea, vomiting, dyspepsia, melena, abdominal pain, pseudomembranous colitis

Hematologic: Leukopenia, thrombocytopenia, neutropenia, decrease in hemoglobin/hematocrit, eosinophilia, prolonged prothrombin time, hemolytic anemia, agranulocytosis

Hepatic: AST elevated, ALT, bilirubin; hepatitis, cholestatic jaundice

Local: Phlebitis, pain, injection site reaction

Otic: Tinnitus

Renal: BUN and serum creatinine elevated, interstitial nephritis, renal failure

Respiratory: Dyspnea, rhinitis, pharyngitis

Miscellaneous: Hypersensitivity reactions, anaphylaxis

Drug Interactions
Avoid Concomitant Use
Avoid concomitant use of Piperacillin and Tazobactam Sodium with any of the following: BCG

Increased Effect/Toxicity
Piperacillin and Tazobactam Sodium may increase the levels/effects of: Methotrexate

The levels/effects of Piperacillin and Tazobactam Sodium may be increased by: Probenecid

Decreased Effect
Piperacillin and Tazobactam Sodium may decrease the levels/effects of: Aminoglycosides; BCG; Mycophenolate; Typhoid Vaccine

The levels/effects of Piperacillin and Tazobactam Sodium may be decreased by: Fusidic Acid; Tetracycline Derivatives

Stability Reconstituted piperacillin/tazobactam solution is stable for 24 hours at room temperature and 2 days when refrigerated; incompatible with LR solution and aminoglycosides (especially tobramycin)

Note: Reformulated Zosyn® containing EDTA has been shown to be compatible *in vitro* for Y-site infusion with amikacin and gentamicin, but not compatible with tobramycin.

Premixed solution: Store frozen; thawed solution is stable for 24 hours at room temperature or 14 days refrigerated; do not refreeze

Mechanism of Action Inhibits bacterial cell wall synthesis by binding to one or more of the penicillin-binding proteins; inhibits the final transpeptidation step of peptidoglycan synthesis in bacterial cell walls; tazobactam prevents degradation of piperacillin by binding to beta-lactamases

Pharmacokinetics (Adult data unless noted) Both AUC and peak concentrations are dose proportional

Distribution: Widely distributed into tissues and body fluids including lungs, intestinal mucosa, female reproductive tissues, interstitial fluid, gallbladder, and bile; penetration into CSF is poor when meninges are uninflamed; piperacillin and tazobactam cross the placenta; piperacillin is excreted into breast milk

V_d: Children and Adults: 0.243 L/kg

Protein binding:
Piperacillin: ~26% to 33%
Tazobactam: 31% to 32%

Metabolism:
Piperacillin: 6% to 9% to desethyl metabolite (weak activity)
Tazobactam: ~22% to inactive metabolite

Bioavailability: I.M.:
Piperacillin: 71%
Tazobactam: 84%

Half-life:
Piperacillin:
Infants 2-5 months: 1.4 hours
Children 6-23 months: 0.9 hour
Children 2-12 years: 0.7 hour
Adults: 0.7-1.2 hours
Metabolite: 1-1.5 hours
Tazobactam:
Infants 2-5 months: 1.6 hours
Children 6-23 months: 1 hour
Children 2-12 years: 0.8-0.9 hour
Adults: 0.7-0.9 hour
Elimination: Piperacillin and tazobactam are both elimi-nated by renal tubular secretion and glomerular filtration. Piperacillin, tazobactam, and desethylpiperacillin are also secreted into bile.
Piperacillin: 50% to 70% eliminated unchanged in urine
Tazobactam: Found in urine at 24 hours, with 20% as the inactive metabolite and 80% as unchanged drug
Clearance: Children 9 months to 12 years: 5.64 mL/minute/kg
Dialysis: Hemodialysis removes 30% to 40% of a piperacillin/tazobactam dose; peritoneal dialysis removes 21% of tazobactam and 6% of piperacillin

Usual Dosage Zosyn® (piperacillin and tazobactam) is a combination product; each 3.375 g vial contains 3 g piperacillin sodium and 0.375 g tazobactam sodium in a 8:1 ratio. Dosage recommendations are based on the **piperacillin** component.
Infants <6 months of age: I.V.: 150-300 mg of piperacillin component/kg/day in divided doses every 6-8 hours
Infants and Children ≥6 months: I.V.: 240 mg of piperacillin component/kg/day in divided doses every 8 hours; higher doses have been used for serious pseudomonal infections: 300-400 mg of piperacillin component/kg/day in divided doses every 6 hours; maximum dose: 16 g of piperacillin component/day
Appendicitis and/or peritonitis:
Infants 2-9 months: 240 mg of piperacillin component/kg/day in divided doses every 8 hours
Children ≥9 months and ≤40 kg: 300 mg piperacillin component/kg/day in divided doses every 8 hours
Children >40 kg and Adults: I.V.: 3.375 g (3 g piperacillin/0.375 g tazobactam) every 6 hours; maximum dose: 16 g of piperacillin component/day
Adults: Nosocomial pneumonia: I.V.: 4.5 g (4 g piperacillin/0.5 g tazobactam) every 6 hours for 7-14 days
Dosage adjustment in renal impairment: Adults:
Cl_{cr} 20-40 mL/minute: Decrease dose by 30% and administer every 6 hours
Cl_{cr} <20 mL/minute: Decrease dose by 30% and administer every 8 hours
Hemodialysis: Adults: Administer 2.25 g every 8-12 hours with an additional dose of 0.75 g after each dialysis
CAPD: Adults: Administer 2.25 g every 8-12 hours
Dosage adjustment in patients with hepatic cirrhosis: No dosing adjustment required

Administration Parenteral: I.V. intermittent infusion: May administer over 30 minutes at a maximum concentration of 200 mg/mL (piperacillin component); however, concentrations ≤20 mg/mL are preferred. Piperacillin has been shown to inactivate aminoglycosides *in vitro*. Concurrent aminoglycoside administration with piperacillin may pose a risk of reduced antibacterial efficacy *in vivo*, particularly in patients with end-stage renal disease requiring hemodialysis. If the patient is on concurrent aminoglycoside therapy, separate piperacillin and tazobactam administration from the aminoglycoside by at least 30-60 minutes.

Monitoring Parameters Serum electrolytes, bleeding time especially in patients with renal impairment; periodic tests of renal, hepatic, and hematologic function; observe for changes in bowel frequency

Test Interactions Positive Coombs' [direct], false-positive urinary and serum proteins; false-positive urine glucose using Clinitest®; false positive test results using the Platelia® *Aspergillus* enzyme immunoassay (EIA)

Additional Information Sodium content of 1 g piperacillin component in the combination product: 2.79 mEq

Dosage Forms Excipient information presented when available (limited, particularly for generics); consult specific product labeling.
Note: 8:1 ratio of piperacillin sodium/tazobactam sodium
Infusion [premixed iso-osmotic solution, frozen]:
Zosyn®: 2.25 g: Piperacillin 2 g and tazobactam 0.25 g (50 mL) [contains sodium 5.58 mEq (128 mg) and EDTA]
Zosyn®: 3.375 g: Piperacillin 3 g and tazobactam 0.375 g (50 mL) [contains sodium 8.38 mEq (192 mg) and EDTA]
Zosyn®: 4.5 g: Piperacillin 4 g and tazobactam 0.5 g (100 mL) [contains sodium 11.17 mEq (256 mg) and EDTA]
Injection, powder for reconstitution: 2.25 g: Piperacillin 2 g and tazobactam 0.25 g; 3.375 g: Piperacillin 3 g and tazobactam 0.375 g; 4.5 g: Piperacillin 4 g and tazobactam 0.5 g; 40.5 g: Piperacillin 36 g and tazobactam 4.5 g
Zosyn®: 2.25 g: Piperacillin 2 g and tazobactam 0.25 g [contains sodium 5.58 mEq (128 mg) and EDTA]
Zosyn®: 3.375 g: Piperacillin 3 g and tazobactam 0.375 g [contains sodium 8.38 mEq (192 mg) and EDTA]
Zosyn®: 4.5 g: Piperacillin 4 g and tazobactam 0.5 g [contains sodium 11.17 mEq (256 mg) and EDTA]
Zosyn®: 40.5 g: Piperacillin 36 g and tazobactam 4.5 g [contains sodium 100.4 mEq (2304 mg) and EDTA; bulk pharmacy vial]

References
Bryson HM and Brogden RN, "Piperacillin/Tazobactam. A Review of its Antibacterial Activity, Pharmacokinetic Properties, and Therapeutic Potential," *Drugs*, 1994, 47(3):506-35.
Reed MD, Goldfarb J, Yamashita T, et al, "Single-Dose Pharmacokinetics of Piperacillin and Tazobactam in Infants and Children," *Antimicrob Agents Chemother*, 1994, 38(12):2817-26.

◆ **Piperacillin for Injection, USP (Can)** *see* Piperacillin *on page 1115*

◆ **Piperacillin Sodium** *see* Piperacillin *on page 1115*

◆ **Piperacillin Sodium and Tazobactam Sodium** *see* Piperacillin and Tazobactam *on page 1116*

Pirbuterol (peer BYOO ter ole)

U.S. Brand Names Maxair® Autohaler®
Therapeutic Category Adrenergic Agonist Agent; Antiasthmatic; Beta$_2$-Adrenergic Agonist Agent; Bronchodilator; Sympathomimetic
Generic Available No
Use Prevention and treatment of bronchospasm in patients with reversible airway obstruction due to asthma or COPD
Pregnancy Risk Factor C
Lactation Excretion in breast milk unknown
Contraindications Hypersensitivity to pirbuterol or or any component
Warnings Paradoxical bronchospasm may occur, especially with the first use of a new cannister
Precautions Use with caution in patients with hyperthyroidism, diabetes mellitus, cardiovascular disorders (including coronary insufficiency or hypertension); excessive or prolonged use can lead to tolerance
Adverse Reactions
Cardiovascular: Tachycardia, palpitations, hypertension, chest pain
Central nervous system: Nervousness, CNS stimulation, anxiety, syncope, hyperactivity, insomnia, dizziness, depression, lightheadedness, drowsiness, headache

Dermatologic: Rash, pruritus, alopecia

Endocrine & metabolic: Hypokalemia

Gastrointestinal: GI upset, xerostomia, glossitis, abdominal pain, vomiting, nausea, unusual taste, hoarseness

Neuromuscular & skeletal: Tremor, weakness, muscle cramping

Respiratory: Irritation of oropharynx, cough, paradoxical bronchospasm

Miscellaneous: Diaphoresis

Drug Interactions

Avoid Concomitant Use

Avoid concomitant use of Pirbuterol with any of the following: Iobenguane I 123

Increased Effect/Toxicity

Pirbuterol may increase the levels/effects of: Sympathomimetics

The levels/effects of Pirbuterol may be increased by: Atomoxetine; Cannabinoids; MAO Inhibitors; Tricyclic Antidepressants

Decreased Effect

Pirbuterol may decrease the levels/effects of: Iobenguane I 123

The levels/effects of Pirbuterol may be decreased by: Alpha-/Beta-Blockers; Beta-Blockers (Beta1 Selective); Beta-Blockers (Nonselective); Betahistine

Stability Store at room temperature

Mechanism of Action Relaxes bronchial smooth muscle by action on beta$_2$-adrenergic receptors with little effect on heart rate

Pharmacodynamics

Onset of action: 5 minutes

Maximum effect: 30-60 minutes

Duration: 5 hours

Pharmacokinetics (Adult data unless noted)

Metabolism: Liver (by sulfate conjugation)

Half-life: 2 hours

Elimination: 51% excreted in the urine as pirbuterol plus its sulfate conjugate

Usual Dosage Oral inhalation:

Acute asthma exacerbation (NIH guidelines):

Children: 4-8 inhalations every 20 minutes for 3 doses then every 1-4 hours

Children >12 years and Adults: 4-8 inhalations every 20 minutes for up to 4 hours then every 1-4 hours

Maintenance therapy (nonacute) (NIH guidelines): Children and Adults: 2 inhalations 3-4 times/day

Administration Oral inhalation: Shake well before administration; "prime" (test spray) inhaler prior to first use and if it has not been used for 48 hours; use spacer for children <8 years of age (Maxair™ Inhaler only); Maxair™ Autohaler™ is breath activated; after sealing lips around mouthpiece, inhale deeply with steady, moderate force; inhalation triggers the release "puff" of medication; do not stop inhalation when puff occurs, but continue to take a deep, full breath; hold breath for 10 seconds, then exhale slowly

Monitoring Parameters Serum potassium, heart rate, pulmonary function tests, respiratory rate; arterial or capillary blood gases (if patient's condition warrants)

Patient Information Do not exceed recommended dosage; may cause dry mouth; rinse mouth with water following each inhalation to help with dry throat and mouth; if more than one inhalation is necessary, wait at least 1 full minute between inhalations; notify physician if palpitations, tachycardia, chest pain, muscle tremors, dizziness, headache, flushing occur, or if breathing difficulty persists

Dosage Forms Excipient information presented when available (limited, particularly for generics); consult specific product labeling.

Aerosol for oral inhalation, as acetate:

Maxair™ Autohaler™: 200 mcg/actuation (14 g) [400 actuations; contains chlorofluorocarbons]

References

"Guidelines for the Diagnosis and Management of Asthma. NAEPP Expert Panel Report 3," August 2007, www.nhlbi.nih.gov/guidelines/asthma/asthgdln.pdf.

"National Asthma Education and Prevention Program. Expert Panel Report: Guidelines for the Diagnosis and Management of Asthma Update on Selected Topics–2002," *J Allergy Clin Immunol*, 2002, 110 (5 Suppl):S141-219.

◆ **Pirbuterol Acetate** *see* Pirbuterol *on page 1117*

Piroxicam (peer OKS i kam)

Medication Safety Issues

Sound-alike/look-alike issues:

Feldene® may be confused with FLUoxetine

Beers Criteria medication: This drug may be inappropriate for use in geriatric patients (high severity risk).

U.S. Brand Names Feldene®

Canadian Brand Names Apo-Piroxicam®; Dom-Piroxicam; Gen-Piroxicam; Novo-Pirocam; Nu-Pirox; PMS-Piroxicam; PRO-Piroxicam

Therapeutic Category Analgesic, Non-narcotic; Anti-inflammatory Agent; Nonsteroidal Anti-inflammatory Drug (NSAID), Oral

Generic Available Yes

Use Management of inflammatory diseases and rheumatoid disorders; dysmenorrhea

Medication Guide An FDA-approved patient medication guide, which is available with the product information and at http://www.fda.gov/downloads/Drugs/DrugSafety/ucm088596.pdf, must be dispensed with this medication for each new outpatient prescription and refill.

Pregnancy Risk Factor C

Pregnancy Considerations Adverse events were not observed in the initial animal reproduction studies; therefore, the manufacturer classifies piroxicam as pregnancy category C. NSAID exposure during the first trimester is not strongly associated with congenital malformations; however, cardiovascular anomalies and cleft palate have been observed following NSAID exposure in some studies. The use of a NSAID close to conception may be associated with an increased risk of miscarriage. Nonteratogenic effects have been observed following NSAID administration during the third trimester including: Myocardial degenerative changes, prenatal constriction of the ductus arteriosus, fetal tricuspid regurgitation, failure of the ductus arteriosus to close postnatally; renal dysfunction or failure, oligohydramnios; gastrointestinal bleeding or perforation, increased risk of necrotizing enterocolitis; intracranial bleeding (including intraventricular hemorrhage), platelet dysfunction with resultant bleeding; pulmonary hypertension. Because they may cause premature closure of the ductus arteriosus, use of NSAIDs late in pregnancy should be avoided (use after 31 or 32 weeks gestation is not recommended by some clinicians). The chronic use of NSAIDs in women of reproductive age may be associated with infertility that is reversible upon discontinuation of the medication.

Lactation Enters breast milk/not recommended (AAP rates "compatible")

Breast-Feeding Considerations Piroxicam is excreted into breast milk. Breast-feeding is not recommended by the manufacturer. The AAP considers piroxicam to be "usually compatible with breast-feeding."

Contraindications Hypersensitivity to piroxicam or any component; history of asthma, urticaria, or allergic-type reaction to aspirin, or other NSAIDs; patients with the "aspirin triad" [asthma, rhinitis (with or without nasal polyps), and aspirin intolerance] (fatal asthmatic and anaphylactoid reactions may occur in these patients); perioperative pain in the setting of coronary artery bypass graft (CABG)

Warnings NSAIDs are associated with an increased risk of adverse cardiovascular thrombotic events, including potentially fatal MI and stroke **[U.S. Boxed Warning]**; risk may be increased with duration of use or pre-existing cardiovascular risk factors or disease; carefully evaluate cardiovascular risk profile prior to prescribing; use the lowest effective dose for the shortest duration of time, taking into consideration individual patient treatment goals; alternate therapies should be considered for patients at high risk. Use is contraindicated for treatment of perioperative pain in the setting of CABG surgery **[U.S. Boxed Warning]**; an increased incidence of MI and stroke was found in patients receiving COX-2 selective NSAIDs for the treatment of pain within the first 10-14 days after CABG surgery. NSAIDs may cause fluid retention, edema, and new onset or worsening of pre-existing hypertension; use with caution in patients with hypertension, CHF, or fluid retention. Concurrent administration of ibuprofen, and potentially other nonselective NSAIDs, may interfere with aspirin's cardioprotective effect.

Oral use: NSAIDs may increase the risk of gastrointestinal inflammation, ulceration, bleeding, and perforation **[U.S. Boxed Warning]**. These events, which can be potentially fatal, may occur at any time during therapy, and without warning. Avoid the use of NSAIDs in patients with active GI bleeding or ulcer disease. Use NSAIDs with extreme caution in patients with a history of GI bleeding or ulcers (these patients have a 10-fold increased risk for developing a GI bleed). Use NSAIDs with caution in patients with other risk factors which may increase GI bleeding (eg, concurrent therapy with aspirin, anticoagulants, and/or corticosteroids, longer duration of NSAID use; smoking; use of alcohol; and poor general health). Use the lowest effective dose for the shortest duration of time, taking into consideration individual patient treatment goals; alternate therapies should be considered for patients at high risk.

NSAIDs may compromise existing renal function. Renal toxicity may occur in patients with impaired renal function, dehydration, heart failure, liver dysfunction, those taking diuretics and ACE inhibitors; use with caution in these patients; monitor renal function closely. NSAIDs are not recommended for use in patients with advanced renal disease. Long-term use of NSAIDs may cause renal papillary necrosis and other renal injury.

Fatal asthmatic and anaphylactoid reactions may occur in patients with the "aspirin triad" who receive NSAIDs (see Contraindications). NSAIDs may cause serious dermatologic adverse reactions including exfoliative dermatitis, Stevens-Johnson syndrome, and toxic epidermal necrolysis. A serum sickness-like reaction can rarely occur; watch for arthralgias, pruritus, fever, fatigue, and rash. Avoid use of NSAIDs in late pregnancy as they may cause premature closure of the ductus arteriosus.

Precautions Use with caution in patients with decreased hepatic function; closely monitor patients with abnormal LFTs; severe hepatic reactions (eg, fulminant hepatitis, liver failure) have occurred with NSAID use, rarely; discontinue if signs or symptoms of liver disease develop, or if systemic manifestations occur. Use with caution in patients with asthma; asthmatic patients may have aspirin-sensitive asthma which may be associated with severe and potentially fatal bronchospasm when aspirin or NSAIDs are administered (see also Contraindications). Anemia (due to occult or gross blood loss from the GI tract, fluid retention, or other effect on erythropoiesis) may occur; monitor hemoglobin and hematocrit in patients receiving long-term therapy. Use with caution and monitor carefully in patients with coagulation disorders or those receiving anticoagulants, as NSAIDs inhibit platelet aggregation and may prolong bleeding time.

Adverse Reactions

Cardiovascular: Edema

Central nervous system: Dizziness, headache

Dermatologic: Rash, phototoxic skin eruptions, photosensitivity

Gastrointestinal: Nausea, epigastric distress, anorexia, abdominal discomfort, vomiting, GI bleeding, ulcers, perforation

Hematologic: Reduction in hemoglobin and hematocrit, inhibition of platelet aggregation

Hepatic: Liver enzymes elevated, hepatitis

Renal: Acute renal failure, BUN elevated, serum creatinine elevated

Miscellaneous: Anaphylactoid reactions

Drug Interactions

Metabolism/Transport Effects Substrate of CYP2C9 (minor); **Inhibits** CYP2C9 (strong)

Avoid Concomitant Use

Avoid concomitant use of Piroxicam with any of the following: Ketorolac; Ketorolac (Systemic)

Increased Effect/Toxicity

Piroxicam may increase the levels/effects of: Aminoglycosides; Anticoagulants; Antiplatelet Agents; Bisphosphonate Derivatives; Collagenase (Systemic); CycloSPORINE; CycloSPORINE (Systemic); Desmopressin; Digoxin; Drotrecogin Alfa; Eplerenone; Haloperidol; Ibritumomab; Lithium; Methotrexate; Nonsteroidal Anti-Inflammatory Agents; Pemetrexed; Potassium-Sparing Diuretics; Pralatrexate; Quinolone Antibiotics; Salicylates; Thrombolytic Agents; Tositumomab and Iodine I 131 Tositumomab; Vancomycin; Vitamin K Antagonists

The levels/effects of Piroxicam may be increased by: Antidepressants (Tricyclic, Tertiary Amine); Corticosteroids (Systemic); Dasatinib; Glucosamine; Herbs (Anticoagulant/Antiplatelet Properties); Ketorolac; Ketorolac (Systemic); Nonsteroidal Anti-Inflammatory Agents; Omega-3-Acid Ethyl Esters; Pentosan Polysulfate Sodium; Pentoxifylline; Probenecid; Prostacyclin Analogues; Selective Serotonin Reuptake Inhibitors; Serotonin/Norepinephrine Reuptake Inhibitors; Treprostinil

Decreased Effect

Piroxicam may decrease the levels/effects of: ACE Inhibitors; Angiotensin II Receptor Blockers; Antiplatelet Agents; Beta-Blockers; Eplerenone; HydrALAZINE; Loop Diuretics; Potassium-Sparing Diuretics; Salicylates; Thiazide Diuretics

The levels/effects of Piroxicam may be decreased by: Bile Acid Sequestrants; Nonsteroidal Anti-Inflammatory Agents; Salicylates

Food Interactions Food may decrease the rate but not the extent of absorption

Mechanism of Action Inhibits prostaglandin synthesis by decreasing the activity of the enzyme, cyclooxygenase, which results in decreased formation of prostaglandin precursors

Pharmacodynamics Analgesia:

Onset of action: Oral: Within 1 hour

Maximum effect: 3-5 hours

Pharmacokinetics (Adult data unless noted)

Distribution: Distributes into breast milk at a concentration of about 1% to 3% of maternal plasma

V_d: Adults: 0.14 L/kg

Protein binding: 99%

Metabolism: In the liver

Half-life: Adults: 50 hours

Elimination: Excreted as metabolites and unchanged drug (~5% to 10%) in the urine; small amount excreted in feces

Usual Dosage Oral:
Children: 0.2-0.3 mg/kg/day once daily; maximum dose: 15 mg/day
Adults: 10-20 mg/day once daily; although associated with increase in GI adverse effects, doses >20 mg/day have been used (ie, 30-40 mg/day)
Administration Oral: May administer with food or milk to decrease GI upset
Monitoring Parameters CBC, BUN, serum creatinine, liver enzymes; periodic ophthalmologic exams with chronic use
Patient Information Avoid alcohol. May cause photosensitivity reactions (eg, exposure to sunlight may cause severe sunburn, skin rash, redness, or itching); avoid exposure to sunlight and artificial light sources (sunlamps, tanning booth/bed); wear protective clothing, wide-brimmed hats, sunglasses, and lip sunscreen (SPF ≥15); use a sunscreen [broad-spectrum sunscreen or physical sunscreen (preferred) or sunblock with SPF ≥15]; contact physician if reaction occurs.
Dosage Forms Excipient information presented when available (limited, particularly for generics); consult specific product labeling.
Capsule, oral: 10 mg, 20 mg
Feldene®: 10 mg, 20 mg

- ◆ *p*-Isobutylhydratropic Acid *see* Ibuprofen *on page 702*
- ◆ **Pitressin®** *see* Vasopressin *on page 1410*
- ◆ **Pitrex (Can)** *see* Tolnaftate *on page 1358*
- ◆ **Pix Carbonis** *see* Coal Tar *on page 349*
- ◆ **Plantago Seed** *see* Psyllium *on page 1185*
- ◆ **Plantain Seed** *see* Psyllium *on page 1185*
- ◆ **Plaquenil®** *see* Hydroxychloroquine *on page 694*
- ◆ **Plaretase® 8000 [DSC]** *see* Pancrelipase *on page 1051*
- ◆ **Plasbumin®** *see* Albumin *on page 55*
- ◆ **Plasbumin®-5 (Can)** *see* Albumin *on page 55*
- ◆ **Plasbumin®-25 (Can)** *see* Albumin *on page 55*
- ◆ **Platinol** *see* CISplatin *on page 318*
- ◆ **Platinol-AQ** *see* CISplatin *on page 318*
- ◆ **Plavix®** *see* Clopidogrel *on page 341*
- ◆ **Pliaglis™** *see* Lidocaine and Tetracaine *on page 824*
- ◆ **PMPA** *see* Tenofovir *on page 1319*
- ◆ **PMS-Amantadine (Can)** *see* Amantadine *on page 77*
- ◆ **PMS-Amiodarone (Can)** *see* Amiodarone *on page 84*
- ◆ **PMS-Amitriptyline (Can)** *see* Amitriptyline *on page 89*
- ◆ **PMS-Amlodipine (Can)** *see* AmLODIPine *on page 91*
- ◆ **PMS-Amoxicillin (Can)** *see* Amoxicillin *on page 96*
- ◆ **PMS-Atenolol (Can)** *see* Atenolol *on page 147*
- ◆ **PMS-Atorvastatin (Can)** *see* Atorvastatin *on page 151*
- ◆ **PMS-Azithromycin (Can)** *see* Azithromycin *on page 164*
- ◆ **PMS-Baclofen (Can)** *see* Baclofen *on page 171*
- ◆ **PMS-Bethanechol (Can)** *see* Bethanechol *on page 191*
- ◆ **PMS-Brimonidine Tartrate (Can)** *see* Brimonidine *on page 202*
- ◆ **PMS-Bromocriptine (Can)** *see* Bromocriptine *on page 203*
- ◆ **PMS-Bupropion SR (Can)** *see* BuPROPion *on page 217*
- ◆ **PMS-Buspirone (Can)** *see* BusPIRone *on page 222*
- ◆ **PMS-Captopril (Can)** *see* Captopril *on page 242*
- ◆ **PMS-Carbamazepine (Can)** *see* CarBAMazepine *on page 244*
- ◆ **PMS-Carvedilol (Can)** *see* Carvedilol *on page 254*
- ◆ **PMS-Cefaclor (Can)** *see* Cefaclor *on page 260*
- ◆ **PMS-Cephalexin (Can)** *see* Cephalexin *on page 282*

- ◆ **PMS-Cetirizine (Can)** *see* Cetirizine *on page 283*
- ◆ **PMS-Chloral Hydrate (Can)** *see* Chloral Hydrate *on page 286*
- ◆ **PMS-Cholestyramine (Can)** *see* Cholestyramine Resin *on page 302*
- ◆ **PMS-Cimetidine (Can)** *see* Cimetidine *on page 309*
- ◆ **PMS-Ciprofloxacin (Can)** *see* Ciprofloxacin *on page 310*
- ◆ **PMS-Citalopram (Can)** *see* Citalopram *on page 319*
- ◆ **PMS-Clarithromycin (Can)** *see* Clarithromycin *on page 324*
- ◆ **PMS-Clindamycin (Can)** *see* Clindamycin *on page 327*
- ◆ **PMS-Clobetasol (Can)** *see* Clobetasol *on page 331*
- ◆ **PMS-Clonazepam (Can)** *see* ClonazePAM *on page 337*
- ◆ **PMS-Clozapine (Can)** *see* Clozapine *on page 345*
- ◆ **PMS-Cyclobenzaprine (Can)** *see* Cyclobenzaprine *on page 367*
- ◆ **PMS-Deferoxamine (Can)** *see* Deferoxamine *on page 397*
- ◆ **PMS-Desipramine (Can)** *see* Desipramine *on page 401*
- ◆ **PMS-Desmopressin (Can)** *see* Desmopressin *on page 404*
- ◆ **PMS-Dexamethasone (Can)** *see* Dexamethasone *on page 406*
- ◆ **PMS-Diclofenac (Can)** *see* Diclofenac *on page 429*
- ◆ **PMS-Diclofenac-K (Can)** *see* Diclofenac *on page 429*
- ◆ **PMS-Diclofenac SR (Can)** *see* Diclofenac *on page 429*
- ◆ **PMS-Digoxin (Can)** *see* Digoxin *on page 437*
- ◆ **PMS-Dimenhydrinate (Can)** *see* DimenhyDRINATE *on page 446*
- ◆ **PMS-Diphenhydramine (Can)** *see* DiphenhydrAMINE *on page 448*
- ◆ **PMS-Dipivefrin (Can)** *see* Dipivefrin *on page 461*
- ◆ **PMS-Docusate Calcium (Can)** *see* Docusate *on page 468*
- ◆ **PMS-Docusate Sodium (Can)** *see* Docusate *on page 468*
- ◆ **PMS-Doxycycline (Can)** *see* Doxycycline *on page 479*
- ◆ **PMS-Enalapril (Can)** *see* Enalapril/Enalaprilat *on page 499*
- ◆ **PMS-Erythromycin (Can)** *see* Erythromycin *on page 525*
- ◆ **PMS-Famciclovir (Can)** *see* Famciclovir *on page 560*
- ◆ **PMS-Fentanyl MTX (Can)** *see* FentaNYL *on page 567*
- ◆ **PMS-Fluconazole (Can)** *see* Fluconazole *on page 584*
- ◆ **PMS-Flunisolide (Can)** *see* Flunisolide *on page 592*
- ◆ **PMS-Fluorometholone (Can)** *see* Fluorometholone *on page 597*
- ◆ **PMS-Fluoxetine (Can)** *see* FLUoxetine *on page 600*
- ◆ **PMS-Fluvoxamine (Can)** *see* Fluvoxamine *on page 615*
- ◆ **PMS-Fosinopril (Can)** *see* Fosinopril *on page 627*
- ◆ **PMS-Furosemide (Can)** *see* Furosemide *on page 632*
- ◆ **PMS-Gabapentin (Can)** *see* Gabapentin *on page 634*
- ◆ **PMS-Glyburide (Can)** *see* GlyBURIDE *on page 648*
- ◆ **PMS-Haloperidol LA (Can)** *see* Haloperidol *on page 666*
- ◆ **PMS-Hydrochlorothiazide (Can)** *see* Hydrochlorothiazide *on page 682*
- ◆ **PMS-Hydromorphone (Can)** *see* HYDROmorphone *on page 689*
- ◆ **PMS-Hydroxyzine (Can)** *see* HydrOXYzine *on page 697*
- ◆ **PMS-Ipratropium (Can)** *see* Ipratropium *on page 757*

Pneumococcal Conjugate Vaccine (7-Valent)
(noo moe KOK al KON ju gate vak SEEN, seven vay lent)

Medication Safety Issues
Sound-alike/look-alike issues:
Pneumococcal 7-Valent Conjugate Vaccine (Prevnar®) may be confused with Pneumococcal 13-Valent Conjugate Vaccine (Prevnar 13™) or with Pneumococcal 23-Valent Polysaccharide Vaccine (Pneumovax® 23)

Related Information
Immunization Guidelines *on page 1636*

U.S. Brand Names Prevnar®
Canadian Brand Names Prevnar®
Therapeutic Category Vaccine
Generic Available No
Use
Immunization of infants and toddlers against *Streptococcus pneumoniae* infection caused by serotypes included in the vaccine

Advisory Committee on Immunization Practices (ACIP) guidelines recommend PCV7 for use in:

All infants and children 2-23 months

Children ≥2-59 months with cochlear implants

Children ages 24-59 months with: Sickle cell disease (including other sickle cell hemoglobinopathies, asplenia, splenic dysfunction), HIV infection, immunocompromising conditions (congenital immunodeficiencies, renal failure, nephrotic syndrome, diseases associated with immunosuppressive or radiation therapy, solid organ transplant), chronic illnesses (cardiac disease, cerebrospinal fluid leaks, diabetes mellitus, pulmonary disease excluding asthma unless on high dose corticosteroids)

Consider use in all children 24-59 months with priority given to:

Children 24-35 months

Children 24-59 months who are of Alaska native, American Indian, or African-American descent

Children 24-59 months who attend group day care centers

Pregnancy Risk Factor C

Pregnancy Considerations Reproduction studies have not been conducted. This product is indicated for use in infants and toddlers.

Lactation

Excretion in breast milk unknown/not recommended

Contraindications Hypersensitivity to pneumococcal vaccine or any component of the formulation, including diphtheria toxoid; defer vaccination for persons with acute febrile illness until recovery

Warnings Immediate treatment for anaphylactoid or acute hypersensitivity reactions should be available during vaccine use; children with impaired immune responsiveness may have a reduced response to active immunization; use of this vaccine does not replace the use of 23-valent pneumococcal polysaccharide vaccine in children >24 months of age with sickle cell disease, asplenia, HIV infection, chronic illness, or who are immunocompromised

Precautions Administer with caution to patients with thrombocytopenia or any coagulation disorder that would be compromised by I.M. injection; if the patient receives antihemophilia or other similar therapy, I.M. injection can be scheduled shortly after such therapy is administered. Routine prophylactic administration of acetaminophen to prevent fever due to vaccines has been shown to decrease the immune response of some vaccines; the clinical significance of this reduction in immune response has not been established (see Prymula, 2009).

Adverse Reactions All serious adverse reactions must be reported to the U.S. Department of Health and Human Services (DHHS) Vaccine Adverse Event Reporting System (VAERS) 1-800-822-7967.

Central nervous system: Fever, irritability, drowsiness, restlessness

Dermatologic: Erythema, rash

Gastrointestinal: Appetite decreased, vomiting, diarrhea

Local: Induration, tenderness, nodules

Drug Interactions

Avoid Concomitant Use There are no known interactions where it is recommended to avoid concomitant use.

Increased Effect/Toxicity There are no known significant interactions involving an increase in effect.

Decreased Effect

The levels/effects of Pneumococcal Conjugate Vaccine (7-Valent) may be decreased by: Immunosuppressants

Stability Store refrigerated at 2°C to 8°C (36°F to 46°F).

Mechanism of Action Contains saccharides of capsular antigens of serotypes 4, 6B, 9V, 18C, 19F, and 23F, individually conjugated to CRM197 protein

Usual Dosage I.M.: 0.5 mL; **Note:** Preterm infants should be vaccinated according to their chronological age from birth

Recommended schedule: Age at initiation of immunization: (**Note:** For "catch up" schedule recommendations see Appendix, Immunization Guidelines)

Infants 2-6 months: 4 total doses with the first three doses at least 6-8 weeks apart and the last dose at 12-15 months of age (eg, at ages 2, 4, 6, and 12-15 months); the first dose may be given as young as 6 weeks of age, but is typically given at 2 months of age. In case of a moderate shortage of vaccine, defer the fourth dose until shortage is resolved; in case of a severe shortage of vaccine, defer third and fourth doses until shortage is resolved.

7-11 months: 3 total doses; 2 doses at least 6-8 weeks apart, followed by a third dose at 12-15 months; in case of a severe shortage of vaccine, defer the third dose until shortage is resolved.

12-23 months: 2 total doses, at least 6-8 weeks apart. In case of a severe shortage of vaccine, defer the second dose until shortage is resolved.

24-59 months:

Healthy Children: 1 dose. In case of a severe shortage of vaccine, defer dosing until shortage is resolved.

Children with sickle cell disease, asplenia, HIV infection, chronic illness, or immunocompromising conditions: 2 total doses at least 6-8 weeks apart

Children 24-59 months of age at high risk for pneumococcal disease but have already received the 23-valent pneumococcal polysaccharide vaccine (PS23) may benefit from the immunologic response induced by PCV7. Suggested dosing: Starting ≥2 months after last PPV23 dose: One dose of PCV7, followed by a second dose ≥2 months later.

Children ≥5 years: Children at high risk for pneumococcal disease due to chronic underlying disease may benefit from PCV7 and the 23-valent pneumococcal polysaccharide vaccine (PS23): One dose PCV7; followed with one dose PS23 6-8 weeks later

Administration I.M.: Shake vial well before withdrawing the dose; administer I.M. in either the anterolateral aspect of the thigh or arm; **not for I.V. or SubQ administration**

Patient Information This vaccine is used to prevent bacterial meningitis and ear infections in infants and toddlers. This vaccine will help prevent the disease and stop its spread from person to person. It may be given with other childhood vaccines. Children who are moderately to severely ill should not get this vaccine until they have recovered. This vaccine may be given during a minor illness, such as a cold. Side effects from this vaccine include redness, tenderness, or swelling at the injection site and mild fever. Contact your healthcare provider immediately for high fever, unusual behavior, or signs of allergic reaction (respiratory difficulty, hoarseness or wheezing, hives, paleness, weakness, fast heartbeat, dizziness, or swelling of the throat).

Nursing Implications Federal law requires that the date of administration, the vaccine manufacturer, lot number of vaccine, and the administering person's name, title and address be entered into the patient's permanent medical record

Additional Information In order to maximize vaccination rates, the ACIP recommends simultaneous administration of all age-appropriate vaccines (live or inactivated) for which a person is eligible at a single visit, unless contraindications exist. The use of combination vaccines is generally preferred over separate infections, taking into consideration provider assessment, patient preference, and potential adverse events.

For additional information, please refer to the following website: http://www.cdc.gov/vaccines/vpd-vac/.

Dosage Forms Excipient information presented when available (limited, particularly for generics); consult specific product labeling.

Injection, suspension:

Prevnar®: 2 mcg of each capsular saccharide for serotypes 4, 9V, 14, 18C, 19F, and 23F, and 4 mcg of serotype 6B [bound to diphtheria CRM$_{197}$ protein ~20 mcg] per 0.5 mL (0.5 mL) [contains aluminum, natural rubber/natural latex in packaging, soy, and yeast]

References

Advisory Committee on Immunization Practices, "Preventing Pneumococcal Disease Among Infants and Young Children. Recommendations of the Advisory Committee on Immunization Practices (ACIP)," *MMWR Recomm Rep*, 2000, 49(RR-9):1-35.

American Academy of Pediatrics Committee on Infectious Diseases, "Recommended Immunization Schedules for Children and Adolescents – United States, 2007," *Pediatrics*, 2007, 119(1):207-8.

Centers for Disease Control and Prevention (CDC), Advisory Committee on Immunization Practices, "Pneumococcal Vaccination for Cochlear Implant Candidates and Recipients: Updated Recommendations of the Advisory Committee on Immunization Practices," *MMWR Morb Mortal Wkly Rep*, 2003, 52(31):739-40.

Centers for Disease Control and Prevention (CDC), "General Recommendations on Immunization. Recommendations of the Advisory Committee on Immunization Practices (ACIP)," *MMWR Recomm Rep*, 2006, 55(RR-15):1-48. Available at: http://www.cdc.gov/mmwr/preview/mmwrhtml/rr5515a1.htm.

Centers for Disease Control and Prevention (CDC), "Updated Recommendations on the Use of Pneumococcal Conjugate Vaccine: Suspension of Recommendation for Third and Fourth Dose," *MMWR Dispatch*, 53(Dispatch):1-2. Available at: http://www.cdc.gov/mmwr/preview/mmwrhtml/mm53d302a1.htm.

Centers for Disease Control and Prevention, "Recommended Childhood and Adolescent Immunization Schedule – United States, July-December 2004," *MMWR Morb Mortal Wkly Rep*, 2004, 53(16):Q1-4.

"Pneumococcal Vaccination for Cochlear Implant Recipients," *MMWR Morb Mortal Wkly Rep*, 2002, 51(41):931.

Prymula R, Siegrist CA, Chlibek R, et al, "Effect of Prophylactic Paracetamol Administration at Time of Vaccination on Febrile Reactions and Antibody Responses in Children: Two Open-Label, Randomised Controlled Trials," *Lancet*, 2009, 374(9698):1339-50.

Reefhuis J, Honein MA, Whitney CG, et al, "Risk of Bacterial Meningitis in Children With Cochlear Implants," *N Engl J Med*, 2003, 349 (5):435-45.

Pneumococcal Conjugate Vaccine (13-Valent)

(noo moe KOK al KON ju gate vak SEEN, thur TEEN vay lent)

Medication Safety Issues

Sound-alike/look-alike issues:

Pneumococcal 13-Valent Conjugate Vaccine (Prevnar 13™) may be confused with Pneumococcal 7-Valent Conjugate Vaccine (Prevnar®) or with Pneumococcal 23-Valent Polysaccharide Vaccine (Pneumovax® 23)

Related Information

Immunization Guidelines *on page 1636*

U.S. Brand Names Prevnar 13™

Therapeutic Category Vaccine, Inactivated (Bacterial)

Generic Available No

Use

Immunization of infants and children against *Streptococcus pneumoniae* infection caused by serotypes 1, 3, 4, 5, 6A, 6B, 7F, 9V, 14, 18C, 19A, 19F, and 23F (FDA approved in ages 6 weeks to 5 years). Prevention of otitis media in infants and children caused by *Streptococcus pneumoniae* serotypes 4, 6B, 9V, 14, 18C, 19F, and 23F (FDA approved in ages 6 weeks to 5 years)

The Advisory Committee on Immunization Practices (ACIP) recommends routine vaccination for the following:

All children age 2-59 months; ACIP recommends using 13-valent pneumococcal conjugate vaccine (PCV13; Prevnar 13™) as a replacement for the previously recommended 7-valent pneumococcal conjugate vaccine (PCV7; Prevnar®) for the immunization schedule

Children 24-71 months who have underlying medical conditions increasing their risk of pneumococcal disease or complications including: Cochlear implants, sickle cell disease (including other sickle cell hemoglobinopathies, asplenia, splenic dysfunction); HIV infection, chronic illnesses [including chronic heart disease, cerebrospinal fluid leaks, diabetes mellitus, chronic lung disease (includes asthma if on high-dose corticosteroids)]; immunocompromising conditions (diseases associated with immunosuppressive or radiation therapy, solid organ transplant, renal failure, nephrotic syndrome, congenital immunodeficiencies excluding chronic granulomatous disease)

Children 6-18 years old at increased risk for invasive pneumococcal disease due to sickle cell disease, HIV infection, or other immunocompromising condition, cochlear implant, or cerebrospinal fluid leaks (regardless of previous receipt of PCV7) in addition to PPSV23 vaccination

Pregnancy Risk Factor C

Pregnancy Considerations Reproduction studies have not been conducted. This product is indicated for use in infants and children.

Contraindications Hypersensitivity to pneumococcal vaccine or any component, including diphtheria toxoid

Warnings Immediate treatment for anaphylactoid or acute hypersensitivity reactions should be available during vaccine administration.

Precautions Defer vaccination for persons with acute febrile illness until recovery. Children with impaired immune responsiveness may have a reduced response to active immunization. Administer with caution to patients with thrombocytopenia or any coagulation disorder that would be compromised by I.M. injection; if the patient receives antihemophilia or other similar therapy, I.M. injection can be scheduled shortly after such therapy is administered. Febrile seizures have been reported. Routine prophylactic administration of acetaminophen to prevent fever due to vaccines has been shown to decrease the immune response of some vaccines; the clinical significance of this reduction in immune response has not been established (see Prymula, 2009). Apnea has occurred following intramuscular vaccine administration in premature infants; consider clinical status implications.

Adverse Reactions All serious adverse reactions must be reported to the U.S. Department of Health and Human Services (DHHS) Vaccine Adverse Event Reporting System (VAERS) 1-800-822-7967. **Note:** Due to similar vaccine components, adverse reactions reported with 7-valent pneumococcal conjugate vaccine may also occur with 13-valent pneumococcal conjugate vaccine.

Central nervous system: Drowsiness, febrile seizure (see Precautions), fever, insomnia, irritability

Dermatologic: Rash

Gastrointestinal: Appetite decreased, diarrhea, vomiting

Local: Erythema, swelling, tenderness

Miscellaneous: Anaphylactic reaction (see Warnings), hypersensitivity reaction (bronchospasm, dyspnea, facial edema)

<1%, postmarketing, and/or case reports: Angioneurotic edema, apnea (premature infants), breath holding, crying abnormal edema, erythema multiforme, hypotonic hyporesponsive episode, injection site reaction (dermatitis, pruritus), lymphadenopathy, seizure, shock, urticaria, urticaria-like rash

Drug Interactions

Avoid Concomitant Use There are no known interactions where it is recommended to avoid concomitant use.

Increased Effect/Toxicity There are no known significant interactions involving an increase in effect.

Decreased Effect
The levels/effects of Pneumococcal Conjugate Vaccine (13-Valent) may be decreased by: Immunosuppressants

Stability Store refrigerated at 2°C to 8°C (36°F to 46°F); do not freeze.

Mechanism of Action Contains saccharides of capsular antigens of serotypes 1, 3, 4, 5, 6A, 6B, 7F, 9V, 14, 18C, 19F, and 23F, individually conjugated to CRM197 protein

Usual Dosage I.M.: 0.5 mL per dose; **Note:** Preterm infants should be vaccinated according to their chronological age from birth.

Recommended schedule:
Infants (6 weeks and ≤6 months): 0.5 mL/dose for 4 total doses; the first dose may be given as young as 6 weeks of age, but is typically given at 8 weeks (2 months of age); the 3 remaining doses are usually given at 4, 6, and 12-15 months of age. The recommended dosing interval is 4-8 weeks. The minimum interval between doses in children <1 year of age is 4 weeks. The minimum interval between the third and fourth dose is 8 weeks.

Infants 7-11 months: 0.5 mL for 3 total doses; 2 doses at least 4 weeks apart, followed by a third dose at 12-15 months, separated from second dose by at least 8 weeks

Children 12-23 months: 0.5 mL for 2 total doses, at least 8 weeks apart

Children 24-59 months: Healthy children: 0.5 mL as a single dose

Children 24-71 months with underlying medical conditions: ACIP recommendations: 0.5 mL for a total of 2 doses, separated by 8 weeks

Previously vaccinated with PCV7 and/or PCV13 with a lapse in administration (ACIP recommendations):
Infants 7-11 months and previously received 1 or 2 doses: 0.5 mL dose at 7-11 months of age, followed by a second dose ≥8 weeks later at 12-15 months of age

Children 12-23 months:
Previously received 1 dose at ≤12 months of age: 0.5 mL dose, followed by a second dose ≥8 weeks later
Previously received 1 dose at ≥12 months of age: 0.5 mL dose ≥8 weeks after the most recent dose
Previously received 2 or 3 doses before age 12 months: 0.5 mL dose ≥8 weeks after the most recent dose

Children 24-59 months (healthy children with any incomplete schedule): 0.5 mL dose ≥8 weeks after the most recent dose

Children 24-71 months with an underlying medical condition:
Previously received <3 doses: 0.5 mL dose ≥8 weeks after the most recent dose, followed by a second dose ≥8 weeks later
Previously received 3 doses: 0.5 mL as a single dose ≥8 weeks after the most recent dose

Previously completed vaccination series with PCV7 (4 doses) (ACIP recommendations):
Children 14-59 months: 0.5 mL as a single supplemental dose ≥8 weeks after the most recent dose
Children 24-71 months with an underlying medical condition: 0.5 mL as a single supplemental dose ≥8 weeks after the most recent dose of PCV7 or PPSV23

High risk for invasive pneumococcal disease (ACIP recommendations): Children 6-18 years: 0.5 mL as a single dose ≥8 weeks after the most recent dose of PCV7 or PPSV23 (if applicable)

In order to maximize vaccination rates, the ACIP recommends simultaneous administration of all age-appropriate vaccines (live or inactivated) for which a person is eligible at a single clinic visit, unless contraindications exist.

Administration I.M.: Shake vial well before withdrawing the dose; administer I.M. in either the anterolateral aspect of the thigh or arm; **not for I.V. or SubQ administration**

Monitoring Parameters Monitor for syncope for ≥15 minutes following vaccination

Patient Information This vaccine is used to prevent bacterial meningitis and ear infections in infants and children. This vaccine will help prevent the disease and stop its spread from person to person. It may be given with other childhood vaccines. If you are moderately to severely ill, you should not get this vaccine until you have recovered. This vaccine may be given during a minor illness, such as a cold. Side effects from this vaccine include redness, tenderness, or swelling at the injection site and mild fever. Contact your healthcare provider immediately for high fever, unusual behavior, or signs of allergic reaction (respiratory difficulty, hoarseness or wheezing, hives, paleness, weakness, fast heartbeat, dizziness, or swelling of the throat).

Nursing Implications Federal law requires that the date of administration, the vaccine manufacturer, lot number of vaccine, and the administering person's name, title, and address be entered into the patient's permanent medical record.

Additional Information Pneumococcal 13-valent conjugate vaccine (PCV13; Prevnar 13™) is the successor to the previously-marketed pneumococcal 7-valent conjugate vaccine (PCV7; Prevnar®). Prevnar 13™ contains an additional six serotypes of Streptococcus pneumoniae, compared to the seven serotypes provided in the original Prevnar® formulation.

In the event of a severe vaccine shortage, the last dose of a series may be deferred until shortage is resolved. **Note:** Exception: Infants ≥6 months with two previous doses: May defer third and/or fourth dose during a severe shortage until resolution; if moderate shortage, may defer fourth dose.

In order to maximize vaccination rates, the ACIP recommends simultaneous administration of all age-appropriate vaccines (live or inactivated) for which a person is eligible at a single visit, unless contraindications exist. The use of combination vaccines is generally preferred over separate infections, taking into consideration provider assessment, patient preference, and potential adverse events.

For additional information, please refer to the following website: http://www.cdc.gov/vaccines/vpd-vac/.

Dosage Forms Excipient information presented when available (limited, particularly for generics); consult specific product labeling.

Injection, suspension:
Prevnar 13™: 2 mcg of each capsular saccharide for serotypes 1, 3, 4, 5, 6A, 7F, 9V, 14, 18C, 19A, 19F, and 23F, and 4 mcg of serotype 6B [bound to diphtheria CRM_{197} protein ~34 mcg] per 0.5 mL (0.5 mL) [contains aluminum, polysorbate 80, soy, and yeast]

References

Advisory Committee on Immunization Practices (ACIP), "Pneumococcal Vaccination for Cochlear Implant Recipients," MMWR, 2002, 51(41):931.

Centers for Disease Control and Prevention (CDC), "General Recommendations on Immunization. Recommendations of the Advisory Committee on Immunization Practices (ACIP)," MMWR Recomm Rep, 2006, 55(RR-15):1-48. Available at: http://www.cdc.gov/mmwr/preview/mmwrhtml/rr5515a1.htm.

Centers for Disease Control and Prevention, "Recommended Immunization Schedules for Persons Aged 0 Through 18 Years – United States, 2010," MMWR Morb Mortal Wkly Rep, 2010, 58(51&52):Q1-4.

Centers for Disease Control and Prevention (CDC), "Licensure of a 13-Valent Pneumococcal Conjugate Vaccine (PCV13) and Recommendations for Use Among Children – Advisory Committee on Immunization Practices (ACIP), 2010," MMWR Morb Mortal Wkly Rep, 2010, 59(9):258. Available at: http://www.cdc.gov/mmwr/preview/mmwrhtml/mm5909a2.htm?s_cid=mm5909a2_e.

Prymula R, Siegrist CA, Chlibek R, et al, "Effect of Prophylactic Paracetamol Administration at Time of Vaccination on Febrile Reactions and Antibody Responses in Children: Two Open-Label, Randomised Controlled Trials," *Lancet*, 2009, 374(9698):1339-50.

Reefhuis J, Honein MA, Whitney CG, et al, "Risk of Bacterial Meningitis in Children With Cochlear Implants," *N Engl J Med*, 2003, 349 (5):435-45.

Pneumococcal Polysaccharide Vaccine (Polyvalent)

(noo moe KOK al pol i SAK a ride vak SEEN, pol i VAY lent)

Medication Safety Issues

Sound-alike/look-alike issues:

Pneumococcal 23-Valent Polysaccharide Vaccine (Pneumovax® 23) may be confused with Pneumococcal 7-Valent Conjugate Vaccine (Prevnar®) or with Pneumococcal 13-Valent Conjugate Vaccine (Prevnar 13™)

Related Information

Immunization Guidelines *on page 1636*

U.S. Brand Names Pneumovax® 23

Canadian Brand Names Pneumo 23™; Pneumovax® 23

Therapeutic Category Vaccine

Generic Available No

Use

Children >2 years of age and adults who are at increased risk of pneumococcal disease and its complications due to underlying health conditions (including patients with sickle cell disease, splenectomy, HIV infection, leukemia, lymphoma, Hodgkin's disease, multiple myeloma, generalized immunosuppression, and those receiving immunosuppressive chemotherapy, and patients with cochlear implants)

Current Advisory Committee on Immunization Practices (ACIP) guidelines recommend **pneumococcal 7-valent conjugate vaccine (PCV7)** be used for children 2-23 months of age and, in certain situations, children up to 59 months of age

Pregnancy Risk Factor C

Pregnancy Considerations Animal reproduction studies have not been conducted. Vaccination should be considered in pregnant women at high risk for infection.

Lactation Excretion in breast milk unknown/use caution

Contraindications Hypersensitivity to pneumococcal vaccine or any component of the formulation; defer vaccination for persons with acute febrile illness until recovery

Warnings Immediate treatment for anaphylactoid or acute hypersensitivity reactions should be available during vaccine use; intradermal administration may cause severe local reactions

Precautions Use caution in patients with severe cardiovascular or pulmonary disease where a systemic reaction may pose a significant risk. Patients who will be receiving immunosuppressive therapy (including Hodgkin's disease, cancer chemotherapy, or transplantation) should be vaccinated at least 2 weeks prior to the initiation of immunosuppressive therapy. Immune responses may be impaired for several months following intensive immunosuppressive therapy (up to 2 years in Hodgkin's disease patients). Patients who will undergo splenectomy should also be vaccinated at least 2 weeks prior to surgery, if possible. Patients with HIV should be vaccinated as soon as possible (following confirmation of the diagnosis). Not recommended in children ≤2 years of age.

Administer with caution to patients with thrombocytopenia or any coagulation disorder that would be compromised by I.M. injection; if the patient receives antihemophilia or other similar therapy, I.M. injection can be scheduled shortly after such therapy is administered. Routine prophylactic administration of acetaminophen to prevent fever due to vaccines has been shown to decrease the immune response of some vaccines; the clinical significance of this reduction in immune response has not been established (see Prymula, 2009).

Adverse Reactions All serious adverse reactions must be reported to the U.S. Department of Health and Human Services (DHHS) Vaccine Adverse Event Reporting System (VAERS) 1-800-822-7967.

Central nervous system: Fever, malaise, headache, Guillain-Barré syndrome

Dermatologic: Rash, cellulitis, urticaria

Gastrointestinal: Nausea, vomiting

Hematologic: Thrombocytopenia (stabilized ITP patients); hemolytic anemia (patients with previous history of hematologic disorders)

Local: Erythema, induration and soreness at the injection site (~72%) (2-3 days)

Neuromuscular & skeletal: Arthralgia, myalgia, arthritis, paresthesia, radiculoneuropathy

Miscellaneous: Anaphylaxis, serum sickness, angioneurotic edema

Drug Interactions

Avoid Concomitant Use There are no known interactions where it is recommended to avoid concomitant use.

Increased Effect/Toxicity There are no known significant interactions involving an increase in effect.

Decreased Effect

Pneumococcal Polysaccharide Vaccine (Polyvalent) may decrease the levels/effects of: Zoster Vaccine

The levels/effects of Pneumococcal Polysaccharide Vaccine (Polyvalent) may be decreased by: Immunosuppressants

Stability Refrigerate

Mechanism of Action Although there are more than 80 known pneumococcal capsular types, pneumococcal disease is mainly caused by only a few types of pneumococci. Pneumococcal vaccine contains capsular polysaccharides of 23 pneumococcal types which represent at least 98% of pneumococcal disease isolates in the United States and Europe. The pneumococcal vaccine with 23 pneumococcal capsular polysaccharide types became available in 1983. The 23 capsular pneumococcal vaccine contains purified capsular polysaccharides of pneumococcal types 1, 2, 3, 4, 5, 8, 9, 12, 14, 17, 19, 20, 22, 23, 26, 34, 43, 51, 56, 57, 67, 70 (American Classification). These are the main pneumococcal types associated with serious infections in the United States.

Usual Dosage I.M., SubQ: 0.5 mL

Children ≥2 years at high risk for pneumococcal disease:

One dose PS23 6-8 weeks after last of 1-4 doses of PCV7; revaccinate with PPV23 3-5 years later

One dose PS23 followed by 2 doses PCV7 6-8 weeks apart; revaccinate with PS23 3-5 years later

Following bone marrow transplant: Administer one dose PPV23 at 12- and 24-months following BMT

Adults <65 years at high risk for pneumococcal disease: One dose; revaccinate 5 years later

Administration Administer SubQ or I.M. either the anterolateral aspect of the thigh or arm; **not for I.V. or intradermal administration**

Patient Information This vaccine is used to prevent pneumococcal disease which causes bacterial meningitis and pneumonia. Side effects from this vaccine include redness, tenderness, or swelling at the injection site and mild fever. Contact your healthcare provider immediately for high fever or signs of allergic reaction (respiratory difficulty, hoarseness or wheezing, hives, paleness, weakness, fast heartbeat, dizziness, swelling of the throat).

Nursing Implications Federal law requires that the date of administration, the vaccine manufacturer, lot number of vaccine, and the administering person's name, title, and address be entered into the patient's permanent medical record.

Additional Information In order to maximize vaccination rates, the ACIP recommends simultaneous administration of all age-appropriate vaccines (live or inactivated) for which a person is eligible at a single visit, unless contraindications exist. The use of combination vaccines is generally preferred over separate infections, taking into consideration provider assessment, patient preference, and potential adverse events.

For additional information, please refer to the following website: http://www.cdc.gov/vaccines/vpd-vac/.

Dosage Forms Excipient information presented when available (limited, particularly for generics); consult specific product labeling.

Injection, solution:

Pneumovax® 23: 25 mcg each of 23 capsular polysaccharide isolates/0.5 mL (0.5 mL, 2.5 mL)

References

Advisory Committee on Immunization Practices, "Preventing Pneumococcal Disease Among Infants and Young Children. Recommendations of the Advisory Committee on Immunization Practices (ACIP)," *MMWR Recomm Rep*, 2000, 49(RR-9):1-35.

American Academy of Pediatrics Committee on Infectious Diseases, "Recommended Immunization Schedules for Children and Adolescents – United States, 2007," *Pediatrics*, 2007, 119(1):207-8.

Centers for Disease Control and Prevention (CDC), "General Recommendations on Immunization. Recommendations of the Advisory Committee on Immunization Practices (ACIP)," *MMWR Recomm Rep*, 2006, 55(RR-15):1-48. Available at: http://www.cdc.gov/mmwr/preview/mmwrhtml/rr5515a1.htm.

Davidson M, Bulkow LR, Grabman J, et al, "Immunogenicity of Pneumococcal Revaccination in Patients With Chronic Disease," *Arch Intern Med*, 1994, 154(19):2209-14.

Gardner P and Schaffner W, "Immunization of Adults," *N Engl J Med*, 1993, 328(17):1252-8.

"Pneumococcal Vaccination for Cochlear Implant Recipients," *MMWR Morb Mortal Wkly Rep*, 2002, 51(41):931.

"Prevention of Pneumococcal Disease: Recommendations of the Advisory Committee on Immunization Practices (ACIP)," *MMWR Recomm Rep*, 1997, 46(RR-8):1-24.

Prymula R, Siegrist CA, Chlibek R, et al, "Effect of Prophylactic Paracetamol Administration at Time of Vaccination on Febrile Reactions and Antibody Responses in Children: Two Open-Label, Randomised Controlled Trials," *Lancet*, 2009, 374(9698):1339-50.

◆ **Pneumovax® 23** *see* Pneumococcal Polysaccharide Vaccine (Polyvalent) *on page 1125*

◆ **PNU-100766** *see* Linezolid *on page 826*

◆ **Podactin Cream [OTC]** *see* Miconazole *on page 927*

◆ **Podactin Powder [OTC]** *see* Tolnaftate *on page 1358*

◆ **Podocon-25®** *see* Podophyllum Resin *on page 1126*

◆ **Podofilm® (Can)** *see* Podophyllum Resin *on page 1126*

◆ **Podophyllin** *see* Podophyllum Resin *on page 1126*

Podophyllum Resin (po DOF fil um REZ in)

U.S. Brand Names Podocon-25®
Canadian Brand Names Podofilm®
Therapeutic Category Keratolytic Agent
Generic Available No
Use Topical treatment of benign growths including external genital and perianal warts (condylomata acuminata), papillomas, fibroids
Pregnancy Risk Factor X
Lactation Enters breast milk/contraindicated
Contraindications Not to be used on birthmarks, moles, or warts with hair growth; cervical, urethral, oral warts; not to be used by diabetic patients or patients with poor circulation; pregnant women; do not apply to normal tissue

Warnings Avoid contact with the eyes as it can cause severe corneal damage; 25% solution should not be applied to or near mucous membranes; podophyllum resin has caused teratogenic effects (skin tags, polyneuritis, limb malformations, septal heart defects) and fetal death when used during pregnancy

Precautions Topical application to large areas or in excessive amounts for prolonged periods should be avoided

Adverse Reactions
Central nervous system: Confusion, lethargy, hallucinations, ataxia, apnea, agitation, seizures
Dermatologic: Pruritus, erythema, scarring
Gastrointestinal: Nausea, vomiting, abdominal pain, diarrhea
Hematologic: Leukopenia, thrombocytopenia
Hepatic: Hepatotoxicity
Local: Pain, local edema
Neuromuscular & skeletal: Peripheral neuropathy, weakness
Renal: Renal failure

Drug Interactions
Avoid Concomitant Use There are no known interactions where it is recommended to avoid concomitant use.
Increased Effect/Toxicity There are no known significant interactions involving an increase in effect.
Decreased Effect There are no known significant interactions involving a decrease in effect.

Stability Protect from light; avoid exposure to excessive heat

Mechanism of Action Directly affects epithelial cell metabolism by arresting mitosis through binding to a protein subunit of spindle microtubules (tubulin)

Usual Dosage Children and Adults: Topical: 10% to 25% solution in compound benzoin tincture; use 1 drop at a time allowing drying between drops until area is covered; total volume should be limited to <0.5 mL to an area <10 cm^2 for genital or perianal warts or <2 cm^2 for vaginal warts per treatment session; therapy may be repeated once weekly for up to 4 applications for the treatment of genital or perianal warts; use 10% solution when applied to or near mucous membranes

Verrucae: 25% solution is applied directly to the wart; remove drug from area of application within 6 hours

Administration Topical: Shake well before using; use protective occlusive dressing around warts to prevent contact with unaffected skin; apply drug to dry surface of affected area

Patient Information Notify physician if undue skin irritation develops

Nursing Implications Solution should be washed off within 1-4 hours for genital and perianal warts and within 1-2 hours for accessible meatal warts

Dosage Forms Excipient information presented when available (limited, particularly for generics); consult specific product labeling.

Liquid, topical: 25% (15 mL) [in benzoin tincture]

References
"1993 Sexually Transmitted Diseases Treatment Guidelines," *MMWR Morb Mortal Wkly Rep*, 1993, 42(RR-14):1-102.

Goldfarb MT, Gupta AK, Gupta MA, et al, "Office Therapy for Human Papillomavirus Infection in Nongenital Sites," *Dermatol Clin*, 1991, 9 (2):287-96.

◆ **Poliovirus, Inactivated (IPV)** *see* Diphtheria and Tetanus Toxoids, Acellular Pertussis, and Poliovirus Vaccine *on page 453*

◆ **Poliovirus, Inactivated (IPV)** *see* Diphtheria and Tetanus Toxoids, Acellular Pertussis, Poliovirus and *Haemophilus* b Conjugate Vaccine *on page 455*

Poliovirus Vaccine (Inactivated)
(POE lee oh VYE rus vak SEEN, in ak ti VAY ted)

Related Information
Immunization Guidelines *on page 1636*
U.S. Brand Names IPOL®
Canadian Brand Names IPOL®
Therapeutic Category Vaccine, Inactivated Bacteria
Generic Available No
Use Provide active immunity to poliovirus (FDA approved in ages ≥6 weeks and adults)
Pregnancy Risk Factor C
Pregnancy Considerations Animal reproduction studies have not been conducted. Although adverse effects of IPV have not been documented in pregnant women or their fetuses, vaccination of pregnant women should be avoided on theoretical grounds. Pregnant women at increased risk for infection and requiring immediate protection against polio may be administered the vaccine.
Lactation Excretion into breast milk unknown/use caution
Contraindications Hypersensitivity to any component including neomycin, streptomycin, or polymyxin B; defer vaccination for persons with acute febrile illness until recovery
Warnings Immediate treatment for anaphylactoid or acute hypersensitivity reactions should be available during vaccine use. Although there is no convincing evidence documenting adverse effects of polio vaccine to the pregnant woman or developing fetus, it is prudent on theoretical grounds to avoid vaccinating pregnant women unless the woman is at increased risk of infection and requires immediate protection.
Precautions Routine prophylactic administration of acetaminophen to prevent fever due to vaccines has been shown to decrease the immune response of some vaccines; the clinical significance of this reduction in immune response has not been established (see Prymula, 2009).
Adverse Reactions All serious adverse reactions must be reported to the U.S. Department of Health and Human Services (DHHS) Vaccine Adverse Event Reporting System (VAERS) 1-800-822-7967.
Central nervous system: Fever (>101.3°F), crying, fatigue, fussiness, sleepiness, Guillain-Barré
Dermatologic: Rash, erythema
Gastrointestinal: Appetite decreased, vomiting
Local: Tenderness or pain at injection site, reddening of skin
Respiratory: Dyspnea
Drug Interactions
Avoid Concomitant Use There are no known interactions where it is recommended to avoid concomitant use.
Increased Effect/Toxicity There are no known significant interactions involving an increase in effect.
Decreased Effect
The levels/effects of Poliovirus Vaccine (Inactivated) may be decreased by: Immunosuppressants
Stability Refrigerate; do not freeze
Usual Dosage I.M., SubQ: 0.5 mL per dose
Infants and Children: Recommended schedule: A total of 4 doses administered at 2 months, 4 months, between 6-18 months, and between 4-6 years of age
Catch-up schedule: **Note:** Age at initiation of vaccination series:
4 months-17 years: A total of 3 injections 4 weeks apart
Adolescents ≥18 years and Adults: Not routinely recommended unless at increased risk of exposure; a total of 3 doses with second and third doses administered 1-2 months and 6-12 months later; if sufficient time is not available, alternative schedules with three doses given

1 month apart, or two doses given 1 month apart, or a single dose have been used depending upon the expediency desired
Administration Administer I.M. or SubQ into midlateral aspect of the thigh in infants and small children; administer in the deltoid area to older children and adults; **not for I.V. administration**
Test Interactions May temporarily suppress tuberculin skin test sensitivity (4-6 weeks)
Nursing Implications Federal law requires that the date of administration, the vaccine manufacturer, lot number of vaccine, and the administering person's name, title, and address be entered into the patient's permanent medical record.
Additional Information DTP, MMR, HIB, and hepatitis B vaccines may be given concurrently if at different sites; oral polio vaccine (OPV) is no longer distributed in the United States; OPV is the vaccine of choice for global eradication in areas with continued or recent circulation of wild-type poliovirus, most developing countries where the higher cost of IPV prohibits its use or where inadequate sanitation necessitates an optimal barrier to wild-type virus circulation (American Academy of Pediatrics, *Red Book*, 27th ed)

In order to maximize vaccination rates, the ACIP recommends simultaneous administration of all age-appropriate vaccines (live or inactivated) for which a person is eligible at a single visit, unless contraindications exist. The use of combination vaccines is generally preferred over separate infections, taking into consideration provider assessment, patient preference, and potential adverse events.

For additional information, please refer to the following website: http://www.cdc.gov/vaccines/vpd-vac/.
Dosage Forms Excipient information presented when available (limited, particularly for generics); consult specific product labeling.
Injection, suspension:
IPOL®: Type 1 poliovirus 40 D-antigen units, type 2 poliovirus 8 D-antigen units, and type 3 poliovirus 32 D-antigen units per 0.5 mL (0.5 mL, 5 mL) [contains 2-phenoxyethanol, formaldehyde, calf serum protein, neomycin (may have trace amounts), streptomycin (may have trace amounts), and polymyxin B (may have trace amounts)]

References
Centers for Disease Control and Prevention (CDC), "General Recommendations on Immunization. Recommendations of the Advisory Committee on Immunization Practices (ACIP)," *MMWR Recomm Rep*, 2006, 55(RR-15):1-48. Available at: http://www.cdc.gov/mmwr/preview/mmwrhtml/rr5515a1.htm.
Centers for Disease Control and Prevention, "Recommended Immunization Schedules for Persons Aged 0 Through 18 Years – United States, 2009," *MMWR Morb Mortal Wkly Rep*, 2009, 57(51-52):Q1-4.
Committee on Infectious Diseases, American Academy of Pediatrics, *Red Book: 2006 Report of the Committee on Infectious Diseases*, 27th ed, Pickering L, ed, Elk Grove Village, IL: American Academy of Pediatrics, 2006, 545.
Gardner P and Schaffner W, "Immunization of Adults," *N Engl J Med*, 1993, 328(17):1252-8.
Prevots DR, Burr RK, and Sutter RW, "Poliomyelitis Prevention in the United States: Updated Recommendations of the Advisory Committee on Immunization Practices (ACIP)," *MMWR Recomm Rep*, 2000, 49(RR-5):1-22.
Prymula R, Siegrist CA, Chlibek R, et al, "Effect of Prophylactic Paracetamol Administration at Time of Vaccination on Febrile Reactions and Antibody Responses in Children: Two Open-Label, Randomised Controlled Trials," *Lancet*, 2009, 374(9698):1339-50.

♦ **Polocaine®** *see* Mepivacaine *on page 883*

♦ **Polocaine® Dental** *see* Mepivacaine *on page 883*

♦ **Polocaine® MPF** *see* Mepivacaine *on page 883*

♦ **Poly-Dex™** *see* Dexamethasone, Neomycin, and Polymyxin B *on page 408*

◆ **Polyethylene Glycol-L-asparaginase** *see* Pegaspargase *on page 1068*

Polyethylene Glycol 3350
(pol i ETH i leen GLY kol 3350)

Medication Safety Issues
Sound-alike/look-alike issues:
MiraLax™ may be confused with Mirapex®
Polyethylene glycol 3350 may be confused with polyethylene glycol electrolyte solution

International issues:
MiraLax™ may be confused with Murelax® which is a brand name for oxazepam in Australia

U.S. Brand Names Dulcolax Balance® [OTC]; MiraLax® [OTC]

Therapeutic Category Laxative, Osmotic

Generic Available Yes

Use Treatment of occasional constipation (FDA approved in ages ≥17 years)

Pregnancy Risk Factor C

Pregnancy Considerations Reproduction studies have not been conducted in animals or in humans.

Lactation Excretion in breast milk unknown/use caution

Contraindications Hypersensitivity to polyethylene glycol or any component; GI obstruction, ileus, gastric retention, bowel perforation, toxic colitis, megacolon

Warnings Evaluate patients with symptoms of bowel obstruction (nausea, vomiting, abdominal pain, or distension) prior to use. 1-3 days may be required to produce bowel movement. Prolonged, frequent, or excessive use may lead to electrolyte imbalance.

Precautions Use with caution in patients with renal dysfunction.

Adverse Reactions
Dermatologic: Urticaria
Gastrointestinal: Abdominal bloating, cramping, diarrhea, flatulence, nausea
Miscellaneous: Anaphylactic shock

Drug Interactions
Avoid Concomitant Use There are no known interactions where it is recommended to avoid concomitant use.

Increased Effect/Toxicity There are no known significant interactions involving an increase in effect.

Decreased Effect There are no known significant interactions involving a decrease in effect.

Stability Store at room temperature before reconstitution.

Mechanism of Action An osmotic agent, polyethylene glycol 3350 causes water retention in the stool; increases stool frequency

Pharmacodynamics
Onset of action: Produces bowel movement in 1-3 days

Usual Dosage
Occasional constipation: Dulcolax Balance®, MiraLax™:
Children >6 months: 0.5-1.5 g/kg daily (initial dose: 0.5 g/kg; titrate to effect); not to exceed 17 g/day
Adults: Oral: 17 g (~1 heaping tablespoon) daily
Fecal impaction: >3 years: 1-1.5 g/kg daily (maximum daily dose: 100 g) for 3 days
Bowel preparation:
Children >2 years: 1.5 g/kg/day (maximum daily dose: 100 g) for 4 days
Adults: Mix 17 g in 8 oz of clear liquid and administer the entire mixture every 10 minutes until 2 liters are consumed (start within 6 hours after administering 20 mg bisacodyl delayed-release tablets) (see Wexner, 2006)

Administration Oral: Dulcolax Balance®, MiraLax™: 17 g (dose may be measured using bottle cap) added to 4-8 ounces of beverage (cold, hot, or room temperature)

Monitoring Parameters Stool frequency

Patient Information Consult healthcare provider prior to use if you have nausea, vomiting, abdominal pain, irritable bowel syndrome, kidney disease, or a sudden change in bowel habits for >2 weeks. Discontinue use and consult healthcare provider if you have diarrhea or rectal bleeding. Discontinue use if abdominal pain, bloating, cramping, or nausea gets worse, or if need to use for >1 week.

Dosage Forms Excipient information presented when available (limited, particularly for generics); consult specific product labeling.
Powder, for solution, oral: 17 g/packet (14s); 17 g/dose (119 g, 238 g, 255 g, 510 g, 527 g)
Dulcolax Balance®: 17 g/dose (119 g, 238 g, 510 g)
MiraLax®: 17 g/packet (10s, 12s); 17 g/dose (119 g, 238 g, 510 g)

References
Bell EA and Wall GC, "Pediatric Constipation Therapy Using Guidelines and Polyethylene Glycol 3350," *Ann Pharmacother*, 2004, 38 (4):686-93.

Candy D and Belsey J, "Macrogol (Polyethylene Glycol) Laxatives in Children With Functional Constipation and Faecal Impaction: A Systematic Review," *Arch Dis Child*, 2009, 94(2):156-60.

Co-Minh HB, Demoly P, Guillot B, et al, "Anaphylactic Shock After Oral Intake and Contact Urticaria Due to Polyethylene Glycols," *Allergy*, 2007, 62(1):92-3.

Loening-Baucke V, "Prevalence, Symptoms and Outcome of Constipation in Infants and Toddlers," *J Pediatr*, 2005, 146(3):359-63.

Loening-Baucke V, Krishna R, and Pashankar DS, "Polyethylene Glycol 3350 Without Electrolytes for the Treatment of Functional Constipation in Infants and Toddlers," *J Pediatr Gastroenterol Nutr*, 2004, 39(5):536-9.

Michail S, Gendy E, Preud'Homme D, et al, "Polyethylene Glycol for Constipation in Children Younger Than Eighteen Months Old," *J Pediatr Gastroenterol Nutr*, 2004, 39(2):197-9.

North American Society for Pediatric Gastroenterology, Hepatology and Nutrition, "Evaluation and Treatment of Constipation in Children: Summary of Updated Recommendations of the North American Society for Pediatric Gastroenterology, Hepatology and Nutrition," *J Pediatr Gastroenterol Nutr*, 2006, 43(3):405-7.

Nurko S, Youssef NN, Sabri M, et al, "PEG3350 in the Treatment of Childhood Constipation: A Multicenter, Double-Blinded, Placebo-Controlled Trial," *J Pediatr*, 2008, 153(2):254-61, 261.e1.

Pashankar DS, Bishop WP, and Loening-Baucke V, "Long-Term Efficacy of Polyethylene Glycol 3350 for the Treatment of Chronic Constipation in Children With and Without Encopresis," *Clin Pediatr (Phila)*, 2003, 42(9):815-9.

Pashankar DS, Loening-Baucke V, and Bishop WP, "Safety of Polyethylene Glycol 3350 for the Treatment of Chronic Constipation in Children," *Arch Pediatr Adolesc Med*, 2003, 157(7):661-4.

Pashankar DS, Uc A, and Bishop WP, "Polyethylene Glycol 3350 Without Electrolytes: A New Safe, Effective, and Palatable Bowel Preparation for Colonoscopy in Children," *J Pediatr*, 2004, 144 (3):358-62.

Pelham RW, Nix LC, Chavira RE, et al, "Clinical Trial: Single- and Multiple-Dose Pharmacokinetics of Polyethylene Glycol (PEG-3350) in Healthy Young and Elderly Subjects," *Aliment Pharmacol Ther*, 2008, 28(2):256-65.

Safder S, Demintieva Y, Rewalt M, et al, "Stool Consistency and Stool Frequency are Excellent Clinical Markers for Adequate Colon Preparation After Polyethylene Glycol 3350 Cleansing Protocol: A Prospective Clinical Study in Children," *Gastrointest Endosc*, 2008, 68(6):1131-5.

van den Berg MM, van Rossum CH, de Lorijn F, et al, "Functional Constipation in Infants: A Follow-Up Study," *J Pediatr*, 2005, 147 (5):700-4.

Voskuijl W, de Lorijn F, Verwijs W, et al, "PEG 3350 (Transipeg) Versus Lactulose in the Treatment of Childhood Functional Constipation: A Double Blind, Randomised, Controlled, Multicentre Trial," *Gut*, 2004, 53(11):1590-4.

Wexner SD, Beck DE, Baron TH, et al, "A Consensus Document on Bowel Preparation Before Colonoscopy: Prepared by a Task Force From the American Society of Colon and Rectal Surgeons (ASCRS), the American Society for Gastrointestinal Endoscopy (ASGE), and the Society of American Gastrointestinal and Endoscopic Surgeons (SAGES)," *Surg Endosc*, 2006, 20(7):1161.

Youssef NN, Peters JM, Henderson W, et al, "Dose Response of PEG 3350 for the Treatment of Childhood Fecal Impaction," *J Pediatr*, 2002, 141(3):410-4.

Polyethylene Glycol-Electrolyte Solution
(pol i ETH i leen GLY kol ee LEK troe lite soe LOO shun)

Medication Safety Issues

Sound-alike/look-alike issues:

GoLYTELY® may be confused with NuLYTELY®

NuLYTELY® may be confused with GoLYTELY®

TriLyte® may be confused with TriLipix™

U.S. Brand Names Colyte®; GoLYTELY®; MoviPrep®; NuLYTELY®; TriLyte®

Canadian Brand Names Colyte™; Klean-Prep®; PegLyte®

Therapeutic Category Laxative, Bowel Evacuant; Laxative, Osmotic

Generic Available Yes

Use Bowel cleansing prior to GI examination

Pregnancy Risk Factor C

Pregnancy Considerations Reproduction studies have not been conducted in animals or in humans.

Lactation Excretion in breast milk unknown/use caution

Breast-Feeding Considerations Significant changes in the mother's fluid or electrolyte balance would not be expected.

Contraindications Hypersensitivity to polyethylene glycol or any component; GI obstruction, illeus, gastric retention, bowel perforation, toxic colitis, megacolon

Warnings Seizures associated with electrolyte abnormalities (eg, hyponatremia, hypokalemia) have been reported. Do not add flavorings as additional ingredients before use

Precautions May interfere with barium coating of intestinal wall using the double contrast technique; use with caution in patients with ulcerative colitis; use with caution and observe in patients with impaired gag reflex or those who are otherwise prone to regurgitation or aspiration during administration; treatment duration for occasional constipation should not exceed 2 weeks. Use MoviPrep® with caution in patients with G6PD deficiency; contains ascorbic acid. MoviPrep® contains phenylalanine which must be avoided (or used with caution) in patients with phenylketonuria.

Adverse Reactions

Central nervous system: Malaise, dizziness, headache

Dermatologic: Irritative perineal rashes

Endocrine & metabolic: Mild metabolic acidosis with prolonged irrigation periods, electrolyte disturbances

Gastrointestinal: Nausea, cramps, vomiting, abdominal distention, bloating, dyspepsia

Neuromuscular & skeletal: Rigors

Drug Interactions

Avoid Concomitant Use There are no known interactions where it is recommended to avoid concomitant use.

Increased Effect/Toxicity There are no known significant interactions involving an increase in effect.

Decreased Effect There are no known significant interactions involving a decrease in effect.

Stability

Store at room temperature before reconstitution; use Colyte®, GoLYTELY®, NuLYTELY®, and TriLyte™ within 48 hours of reconstitution; use MoviPrep® within 24 hours of preparation; refrigerate reconstituted solution

Mechanism of Action Induces catharsis by strong electrolyte and osmotic effects

Pharmacodynamics Onset of action: Bowel cleansing: Within 1-2 hours; constipation: 2-4 days

Usual Dosage

Bowel cleansing (to prevent excessive fluid and electrolyte changes, use only products containing supplemental electrolytes for bowel cleansing): Patient should fast at least 2 hours (preferably 3-4 hours) prior to ingestion:

Children: Oral, nasogastric: Colyte®, GoLYTELY®, NuLYTELY®, and TriLyte™: 25-40 mL/kg/hour until rectal effluent is clear (usually in 4-10 hours)

Adults:

Oral: Drink 240 mL (8 oz) every 10 minutes until 4 liters are consumed or the rectal effluent is clear

Nasogastric: 20-30 mL/minute (1.2-1.8 L/hour) until 4 liters are administered

MoviPrep®: Split-dose regimen: The evening prior to colonoscopy: 1 L over 1 hour (one 8 oz glass every 15 minutes) followed by 0.5 L (16 oz) clear fluid; repeat the morning of the study and complete at least 1 hour prior to the start of the study

MoviPrep® Full-dose regimen: Beginning at 6 pm the night before the study and completed before bed: 1 L over 1 hour (one 8 oz glass every 15 minutes) followed 1.5 hours later with a second 1 L over 1 hour; administer an additional 1 L (approximately 32 oz) clear fluid

Administration Oral: Colyte®, GoLYTELY®, NuLYTELY®, and TriLyte™: Add tap water to "fill-line" for reconstitution of powder for solution; MoviPrep®: Add 1 L lukewarm water to the contents of 1 pouch A and 1 pouch B and mix together. No solid foods for 2 hours prior to initiation of therapy; rapid drinking is preferred to drinking small amounts continuously; chilled solution often more palatable; do not add flavorings as additional ingredients before use

Monitoring Parameters Electrolytes, BUN, serum glucose, urine osmolality

Patient Information Chilled solution is often more palatable

Nursing Implications First bowel movement should occur in 1 hour

Dosage Forms Excipient information presented when available (limited, particularly for generics); consult specific product labeling.

Powder, for oral solution, oral: PEG 3350 240 g, sodium sulfate 22.72 g, sodium bicarbonate 6.72 g, sodium chloride 5.84 g, and potassium chloride 2.98 g (4000 mL); PEG 3350 236 g, sodium sulfate 22.74 g, sodium bicarbonate 6.74 g, sodium chloride 5.86 g, and potassium chloride 2.97 g (4000 mL)

Colyte®: PEG 3350 240 g, sodium sulfate 22.72 g, sodium bicarbonate 6.72 g, sodium chloride 5.84 g, and potassium chloride 2.98 g (4000 mL) [available with citrus berry, lemon lime, cherry, orange, and pineapple flavor packets]

GoLYTELY®:

PEG 3350 236 g, sodium sulfate 22.74 g, sodium bicarbonate 6.74 g, sodium chloride 5.86 g, and potassium chloride 2.97 g (4000 mL) [regular and pineapple flavor]

PEG 3350 227.1 g, sodium sulfate 21.5 g, sodium bicarbonate 6.36 g, sodium chloride 5.53 g, and potassium chloride 2.82 g per packet (1s) [regular flavor; makes 1 gallon of solution after mixing]

MoviPrep®: Pouch A: PEG 3350 100g, sodium sulfate 7.5 g, sodium chloride 2.69 g, potassium chloride 1.015 g; Pouch B: Ascorbic acid 4.7 g, sodium ascorbate 5.9 g (1000 mL) [contains phenylalanine 2.33 mg/treatment; lemon flavor; packaged with 2 of Pouch A and 2 of Pouch B in carton and a disposable reconstitution container]

NuLYTELY®: PEG 3350 420 g, sodium bicarbonate 5.72 g, sodium chloride 11.2 g, and potassium chloride 1.48 g (4000 mL) [cherry, lemon-lime, orange, and pineapple flavors]

TriLyte®: PEG 3350 420 g, sodium bicarbonate 5.72 g, sodium chloride 11.2 g, and potassium chloride 1.48 g (4000 mL) [supplied with flavor packets]

References

Sondheimer JM, Sokol RJ, Taylor SF, et al, "Safety, Efficacy and Tolerance of Intestinal Lavage in Pediatric Patients Undergoing Diagnostic Colonoscopy," *J Pediatr*, 1991, 119(1):148-52.

Tuggle DW, Hoelzer DJ, Tunell WP, et al, "The Safety and Cost-Effectiveness of Polyethylene Glycol Electrolyte Solution Bowel Preparation in Infants and Children," *J Pediatr Surg*, 1987, 22 (6):513-5.

Polymyxin B (pol i MIKS in bee)

Medication Safety Issues

High alert medication: The Institute for Safe Medication Practices (ISMP) includes this medication (intrathecal administration) among its list of drug classes which have a heightened risk of causing significant patient harm when used in error.

U.S. Brand Names Poly-Rx

Therapeutic Category Antibiotic, Miscellaneous; Antibiotic, Ophthalmic; Antibiotic, Urinary Irrigation

Generic Available Yes

Use
Topically for wound irrigation and bladder irrigation against *Pseudomonas aeruginosa*; used occasionally for gut decontamination. Parenteral use of polymyxin B has mainly been replaced by less toxic antibiotics. Reserved for life-threatening infections caused by organisms resistant to the preferred drugs; used as inhalation therapy for gram-negative respiratory infections resistant to preferred drugs; used intrathecally for meningeal infections due to susceptible organisms which are resistant to less toxic antibiotics

Pregnancy Risk Factor B

Pregnancy Considerations [U.S. Boxed Warning]:
Safety in pregnant women has not been established. A teratogenic potential has not been identified for polymyxin B, but very limited data is available. Based on the relative toxicity compared to other antibiotics, systemic use in pregnancy cannot be recommended. Due to limited absorption through the maternal skin, limited fetal exposure would be expected after topical polymyxin use.

Lactation Excretion in breast milk unknown/use caution

Breast-Feeding Considerations
It is not known if polymyxin B is excreted in human milk. Due to the limited oral bioavailability, toxicity in a breastfed infant may be unlikely. Infant exposure would be even less after topical use due to the limited maternal skin absorption. Nondose-related effects could include modification of the bowel flora.

Contraindications
Hypersensitivity to polymyxin or any component

Warnings
May cause nephrotoxicity; renal function should be evaluated prior to initiation; patients with renal damage and nitrogen retention should receive reduced dosage **[U.S. Boxed Warning]**; polymyxin B-induced nephrotoxicity may be manifested by albuminuria, cellular casts, and azotemia; discontinue therapy with decreasing urinary output and increasing BUN. May cause neurotoxicity **[U.S. Boxed Warning]**; neurotoxic reactions may be manifested by irritability, weakness, drowsiness, ataxia, perioral paresthesia, numbness of the extremities, and blurring of vision. These reactions are usually associated with high serum levels found in patients with impaired renal function or nephrotoxicity. Avoid concurrent or sequential use of other nephrotoxic and neurotoxic drugs, particularly bacitracin, kanamycin, streptomycin, paromomycin, colistin, tobramycin, neomycin, gentamicin, and amikacin **[U.S. Boxed Warning]**. The drug's neurotoxicity can result in respiratory paralysis from neuromuscular blockade, especially when the drug is given soon after anesthesia or muscle relaxants. Polymyxin B sulfate is toxic when

given parenterally; **avoid parenteral use whenever possible**.

Precautions
Use with caution in patients with myasthenia gravis, patients receiving neuromuscular blocking agents or anesthetics, and in patients with impaired renal function; modify dosage in patients with renal impairment; **I.M. use is not recommended in infants and children due to severe pain at injection site**. Safety in pregnant women has not been established.

Adverse Reactions

Cardiovascular: Facial flushing

Central nervous system: Drowsiness, ataxia, fever, dizziness

Dermatologic: Rash, urticaria

Endocrine & metabolic: Hypocalcemia, hyponatremia, hypokalemia, hypochloremia

Local: Pain at injection site, thrombophlebitis

Neuromuscular & skeletal: Neuromuscular blockade, paresthesia

Ocular: Diplopia

Renal: Nephrotoxicity (hematuria, proteinuria, azotemia)

Respiratory: Respiratory arrest

Miscellaneous: Hypersensitivity reactions

Drug Interactions

Avoid Concomitant Use

Avoid concomitant use of Polymyxin B with any of the following: BCG

Increased Effect/Toxicity

Polymyxin B may increase the levels/effects of: Colistimethate; Neuromuscular-Blocking Agents

The levels/effects of Polymyxin B may be increased by: Capreomycin

Decreased Effect

Polymyxin B may decrease the levels/effects of: BCG

Stability
Protect from light; incompatible with calcium, magnesium, cephalothin, chloramphenicol, heparin, penicillins; inactivated by acidic or alkaline solutions

Mechanism of Action
Binds to phospholipids, alters permeability and damages the bacterial cytoplasmic membrane permitting leakage of intracellular constituents

Pharmacokinetics (Adult data unless noted)

Absorption: Well absorbed from the peritoneum; minimal absorption (<10%) from the GI tract (except in neonates), from mucous membranes or intact skin

Distribution: Widely distributed to body tissues in the liver, kidneys, heart, muscle; does not penetrate into CSF or synovial fluid; does not cross the placenta

Half-life: 4.5-6 hours, increased with reduced renal function

Time to peak serum concentration: I.M.: Within 2 hours

Elimination: Primarily as unchanged drug (>60%) in urine via glomerular filtration

Dialysis: Not removed by hemodialysis

Usual Dosage Note: Avoid parenteral use when possible

Infants <2 years:

I.M.: 25,000-40,000 units/kg/day divided every 6 hours

I.V.: 15,000-45,000 units/kg/day by continuous I.V. infusion or divided every 12 hours

Intrathecal: 20,000 units once daily for 3-4 days or 25,000 units once every other day; continue 25,000 units once every other day for at least 2 weeks after cultures of the CSF are negative

Children ≥2 years and Adults:

I.M.: 25,000-30,000 units/kg/day divided every 6 hours

I.V.: 15,000-25,000 units/kg/day divided every 12 hours or by continuous infusion; total daily dose should not exceed 2,000,000 units/day

Bladder irrigation: Continuous irrigation of the urinary bladder for up to 10 days using 20 mg (equal to 200,000 units) added to 1 L of NS; usually no more than 1 L of irrigant is used per day unless urine flow rate is high; administration rate is adjusted to patient's urine output

Topical irrigation or topical solution: 0.1% to 0.3% solution used to irrigate infected wounds; should not exceed 2 million units/day in adults

Gut sterilization: Oral: 100,000-200,000 units/kg/day divided every 6-8 hours

Inhalation: 2-2.5 mg/kg/day divided every 6 hours; final concentration for administration should not exceed 10 mg/mL

Intrathecal: 50,000 units once daily for 3-4 days, then reduce to once every other day for at least 2 weeks after cultures of the CSF are negative

Dosing adjustment in renal impairment:

Cl_{cr} 5-20 mL/minute: Administer 50% of usual daily dose divided every 12 hours

Cl_{cr} <5 mL/minute: Administer 15% of the usual daily dose divided every 12 hours

Administration Parenteral (avoid parenteral use whenever possible):

I.M.: Not recommended for routine use in infants and children because of the severe pain which occurs with I.M. injection; administer I.M. injections deep into the upper outer quadrant of the gluteal muscles at a final concentration of 250,000 units/mL

I.V.: Infuse drug slowly over 60-90 minutes or by continuous infusion at a concentration of 1000-1667 units/mL in D_5W

Intrathecal: Reconstitute vial with 10 mL NS without preservatives to provide a final concentration of 50,000 units/mL

Monitoring Parameters WBC, serum electrolytes, renal function tests, serum drug concentration, urine output

Reference Range Serum concentration >5 mcg/mL are toxic in adults

Additional Information 1 mg = 10,000 units; neuromuscular blockade may be reversed with calcium chloride

Dosage Forms Excipient information presented when available (limited, particularly for generics); consult specific product labeling.

Injection, powder for reconstitution: 500,000 units

Powder [for prescription compounding]:

Poly-Rx: 100 million units (13 g)

◆ **Polymyxin B and Bacitracin** see Bacitracin and Polymyxin B on page 170

◆ **Polymyxin B and Neomycin** see Neomycin and Polymyxin B on page 979

◆ **Polymyxin B, Bacitracin, and Neomycin** see Bacitracin, Neomycin, and Polymyxin B on page 170

◆ **Polymyxin B, Neomycin, and Dexamethasone** see Dexamethasone, Neomycin, and Polymyxin B on page 408

◆ **Polymyxin B, Neomycin, and Hydrocortisone** see Neomycin, (Bacitracin) Polymyxin B, and Hydrocortisone on page 980

◆ **Polymyxin B, Neomycin, and Prednisolone** see Neomycin, Polymyxin B, and Prednisolone on page 981

◆ **Polymyxin B Sulfate** see Polymyxin B on page 1130

◆ **Poly-Pred®** see Neomycin, Polymyxin B, and Prednisolone on page 981

◆ **Poly-Rx** see Polymyxin B on page 1130

◆ **Polysporin® [OTC]** see Bacitracin and Polymyxin B on page 170

◆ **Polytar® [OTC] [DSC]** see Coal Tar on page 349

◆ **Pontocaine® [DSC]** see Tetracaine on page 1330

◆ **Pontocaine® (Can)** see Tetracaine on page 1330

◆ **Pontocaine® Niphanoid®** see Tetracaine on page 1330

Poractant Alfa (por AKT ant AL fa)

U.S. Brand Names Curosurf® [DSC]
Canadian Brand Names Curosurf®
Therapeutic Category Lung Surfactant
Generic Available No
Use Treatment of respiratory distress syndrome (RDS) in premature infants
Warnings Rapidly affects oxygenation and lung compliance and should be restricted to a highly supervised use in a clinical setting with immediate availability of clinicians experienced with intubation and ventilatory management of premature infants; if transient episodes of bradycardia and decreased oxygen saturation occur, discontinue the dosing procedure and initiate measures to alleviate the condition; produces rapid improvements in lung oxygenation and compliance that may require immediate reductions in ventilator settings and FiO_2.

Pulmonary hemorrhage is a known complication of premature birth and very low birth weight. It has been reported in both clinical trials and postmarketing reports in infants who have received poractant.

Precautions Correction of acidosis, hypotension, anemia, hypoglycemia, and hypothermia is recommended prior to administration

Adverse Reactions

Cardiovascular: Transient bradycardia, hypotension

Local: Endotracheal tube blockage

Respiratory: Oxygen desaturation

Postmarketing reports: Pulmonary hemorrhage

Drug Interactions

Avoid Concomitant Use There are no known interactions where it is recommended to avoid concomitant use.

Increased Effect/Toxicity There are no known significant interactions involving an increase in effect.

Decreased Effect There are no known significant interactions involving a decrease in effect.

Stability Store in refrigerator; protect from light; prior to administration, allow to slowly warm to room temperature; artificial warming methods should **not** be used; unused, unopened vials warmed to room temperature may be returned to the refrigerator within 24 hours of warming only once; vials are for single use only

Mechanism of Action Poractant alfa, an extract of natural porcine lung surfactant, replaces deficient or ineffective endogenous lung surfactant in neonates with respiratory distress syndrome (RDS); surfactant prevents the alveoli from collapsing during expiration by lowering surface tension between air and alveolar surfaces

Usual Dosage Neonates: Intratracheal: Initial: 2.5 mL/kg/dose (200 mg/kg/dose); may repeat 1.25 mL/kg/dose (100 mg/kg/dose) at 12-hour intervals for up to 2 additional doses; maximum total dose: 5 mL/kg

Administration Intratracheal: For intratracheal administration only; suction infant prior to administration; inspect solution to verify complete mixing of the suspension; do not shake; gently turn vial upside-down to obtain uniform suspension; administer intratracheally by instillation through a 5-French end-hole catheter inserted into the infant's endotracheal tube; each dose should be administered as two aliquots, with each aliquot administered into one of the two main bronchi by positioning the infant with either the right or left side dependent; alternatively, it may be administered through a secondary lumen of a dual lumen endotracheal tube as a single dose administered over 1 minute without interrupting mechanical ventilation

Monitoring Parameters Continuous heart rate and transcutaneous O_2 saturation should be monitored during administration; frequent ABG sampling is necessary to prevent postdosing hyperoxia and hypocarbia

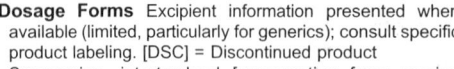

Dosage Forms Excipient information presented when available (limited, particularly for generics); consult specific product labeling. [DSC] = Discontinued product
Suspension, intratracheal [preservative free; porcine derived]:
Curosurf®: 80 mg/mL (1.5 mL, 3 mL) [DSC]

◆ **Porcine Lung Surfactant** *see* Poractant Alfa *on page 1131*

Posaconazole (poe sa KON a zole)

Medication Safety Issues
Sound-alike/look-alike issues:
Noxafil® may be confused with minoxidil

International issues:
Noxafil® may be confused with Noxidil® which is a brand name for minoxidil in Thailand
U.S. Brand Names Noxafil®
Canadian Brand Names Posanol™
Therapeutic Category Antifungal Agent, Systemic; Antifungal Agent, Triazole
Generic Available No
Use Prophylaxis of invasive *Aspergillus* and *Candida* infections in high-risk, severely immunocompromised patients such as hematopoietic stem cell transplant recipients with graft-versus-host disease or those with hematologic malignancies with prolonged neutropenia secondary to chemotherapy; treatment of oropharyngeal candidiasis (including patients refractory to itraconazole and/or fluconazole); treatment of serious invasive fungal infections, including zygomycosis and coccidioidomycosis in patients intolerant of, or refractory to, conventional antifungal therapy
Pregnancy Risk Factor C
Pregnancy Considerations Posaconazole has been shown to be teratogenic in animal studies. There are no adequate and well-controlled studies in pregnant women. Use only if the benefit to the mother justifies potential risk to the fetus.
Lactation Excretion in breast milk unknown/not recommended
Breast-Feeding Considerations Excretion in breast milk has not been investigated; use only if the benefit to the mother justifies potential risk to the fetus.
Contraindications Hypersensitivity to posaconazole or any component; concurrent therapy with ergot alkaloids (see Drug Interactions); coadministration with terfenadine, astemizole, cisapride, pimozide, halofantrine, or quinidine (posaconazole may increase plasma concentrations of these agents resulting in QT$_c$ prolongation and rarely, torsade de pointes)
Warnings Hepatotoxicity including hepatitis, cholestasis, hepatic failure and elevations in ALT, AST, alkaline phosphatase, and total bilirubin have been reported. Liver function tests and bilirubin should be monitored at the start and during posaconazole therapy.

Elevated cyclosporine levels resulting in nephrotoxicity, leukoencephalopathy, and death have been reported in patients on concurrent therapy with posaconazole. Dose adjustment and more frequent clinical monitoring of cyclosporine, tacrolimus, and sirolimus should be performed when posaconazole therapy is initiated in patients on these medications.

Oral suspension contains sodium benzoate; benzoic acid (benzoate) is a metabolite of benzyl alcohol; large amounts of benzyl alcohol (≥99 mg/kg/day) have been associated with a potentially fatal toxicity ("gasping syndrome") in neonates; use oral suspension containing sodium benzoate with caution in neonates; *in vitro* and animal studies

have shown that benzoate displaces bilirubin from protein-binding sites
Precautions Use caution in patients with hypersensitivity to other azole antifungal agents since cross-reaction may occur but has not yet been established. Use with caution in patients with proarrhythmic conditions since posaconazole has been associated with QT interval prolongation and torsade de pointes; do not administer with medications known to prolong the QT$_c$ interval and are metabolized through the CYP3A4 system. Use with caution in patients with hepatic impairment or severe renal impairment (CL$_{cr}$ <20 mL/minute/1.73m^2); monitor for breakthrough fungal infection in patients with severe renal impairment.
Adverse Reactions
Cardiovascular: Edema, hypertension, tachycardia, QT/QT$_c$ prolongation
Central nervous system: Headache, fever, dizziness, fatigue, insomnia, anxiety
Dermatologic: Rash, pruritus
Endocrine & metabolic: Hypokalemia, hypomagnesemia, hyperglycemia, hypocalcemia
Gastrointestinal: Nausea, vomiting, abdominal pain, diarrhea, dry mouth, anorexia, mucositis, dyspepsia, taste perversion, constipation
Hematologic: Anemia, neutropenia, thrombocytopenia
Hepatic: Bilirubin elevated, ALT, AST, and alkaline phosphatase; hepatitis
Neuromuscular & skeletal: Weakness, myalgia, tremor, arthralgia
Ocular: Blurred vision
Renal: Serum creatinine elevated
Respiratory: Coughing, dyspnea
Drug Interactions
Metabolism/Transport Effects Inhibits CYP3A4 (strong)
Avoid Concomitant Use
Avoid concomitant use of Posaconazole with any of the following: Alfuzosin; Cisapride; Conivaptan; Dofetilide; Dronedarone; Efavirenz; Eplerenone; Ergot Derivatives; Everolimus; Halofantrine; Nilotinib; Nisoldipine; Pimozide; Proton Pump Inhibitors; QuiNIDine; Ranolazine; Rivaroxaban; Romidepsin; Salmeterol; Silodosin; Sirolimus; Tamsulosin; Tolvaptan
Increased Effect/Toxicity
Posaconazole may increase the levels/effects of: Alfentanil; Alfuzosin; Almotriptan; Alosetron; Antineoplastic Agents (Vinca Alkaloids); Aprepitant; Benzodiazepines (metabolized by oxidation); Bortezomib; Bosentan; Brinzolamide; BusPIRone; Busulfan; Calcium Channel Blockers; CarBAMazepine; Cardiac Glycosides; Ciclesonide; Cilostazol; Cinacalcet; Cisapride; Colchicine; Conivaptan; Corticosteroids (Orally Inhaled); Corticosteroids (Systemic); CycloSPORINE; CycloSPORINE (Systemic); CYP3A4 Substrates; Dienogest; Docetaxel; Dofetilide; Dronedarone; Dutasteride; Eletriptan; Eplerenone; Ergot Derivatives; Erlotinib; Eszopiclone; Everolimus; FentaNYL; Fesoterodine; Fosaprepitant; Gefitinib; GuanFACINE; Halofantrine; HMG-CoA Reductase Inhibitors; Imatinib; Irinotecan; Ixabepilone; Losartan; Lumefantrine; Macrolide Antibiotics; Maraviroc; Methadone; MethylPREDNISolone; Nilotinib; Nisoldipine; Paricalcitol; Pazopanib; Phenytoin; Phosphodiesterase 5 Inhibitors; Pimecrolimus; Pimozide; Protease Inhibitors; QuiNIDine; Ramelteon; Ranolazine; Repaglinide; Rifamycin Derivatives; Rivaroxaban; Romidepsin; Salmeterol; Saxagliptin; Silodosin; Sirolimus; Solifenacin; Sorafenib; Sunitinib; Tacrolimus; Tacrolimus (Systemic); Tacrolimus (Topical); Tadalafil; Tamsulosin; Temsirolimus; Tolterodine; Tolvaptan; Vitamin K Antagonists; Ziprasidone; Zolpidem

The levels/effects of Posaconazole may be increased by: Grapefruit Juice; Macrolide Antibiotics; Protease Inhibitors

Decreased Effect

Posaconazole may decrease the levels/effects of: Amphotericin B; Prasugrel; Saccharomyces boulardii

The levels/effects of Posaconazole may be decreased by: Antacids; Didanosine; Efavirenz; H2-Antagonists; Metoclopramide; Phenytoin; Proton Pump Inhibitors; Rifamycin Derivatives; Sucralfate

Food Interactions Posaconazole AUC and C_{max} are 3 times higher when administered with a nonfat meal and 4 times higher if administered with a high fat meal relative to a fasted state

Stability Store at room temperature; do not freeze.

Mechanism of Action Inhibits the enzyme 14 α-sterol demethylase, an essential enzyme in ergosterol biosynthesis resulting in the inhibition of fungal cell membrane formation.

Pharmacokinetics (Adult data unless noted)

Absorption: Food and/or liquid nutritional supplements increase absorption

Distribution: V_d: Adults: 1774 L; extensive extravascular distribution and penetration into body tissues

Protein binding: >98%

Metabolism: Undergoes hepatic glucuronidation to form glucuronide conjugates; substrate for p-glycoprotein efflux

Half-life: 35 hours (range: 20-66 hours)

Time to peak serum concentration: 3-5 hours

Elimination: 71% (66% as unchanged drug) eliminated in feces; <0.2% as unchanged drug excreted in urine

Dialysis: Not removed by hemodialysis

Usual Dosage Oral: Children ≥13 years and Adults:

Prophylaxis of invasive Aspergillus and Candida infections: 200 mg 3 times/day

Treatment of refractory invasive fungal infections: 800 mg/day in divided doses (ie, 400 mg 2 times/day or 200 mg 4 times/day)

Treatment of oropharyngeal candidiasis: Initial: 100 mg 2 times/day on day 1; maintenance: 100 mg once daily for 13 days

Treatment of refractory oropharyngeal candidiasis: 400 mg 2 times/day

Dosage adjustment in renal impairment: No adjustment is necessary; monitor for breakthrough fungal infection in patients with Cl_{cr} <20 mL/minute/1.73 m^2

Dosage adjustment in hepatic impairment: No adjustment necessary

Administration Oral: Shake suspension before use. Administer with a full meal or with a liquid nutritional supplement. For patients who cannot tolerate a full meal or an oral liquid nutritional supplement, alternative antifungal therapy should be considered.

Monitoring Parameters Hepatic function tests and bilirubin, serum electrolytes, serum creatinine, ECG

Patient Information Inform physician if severe diarrhea or vomiting, chest pain or palpitations, yellowing of eyes or skin, changes in color of urine or stool, weakness or tremor, or changes in vision occur.

Additional Information Dextrose content (oral suspension): 350 mg/mL

Dosage Forms Excipient information presented when available (limited, particularly for generics); consult specific product labeling.

Suspension, oral:

Noxafil®: 40 mg/mL (123 mL) [contains sodium benzoate; delivers 105 mL of suspension; cherry flavor; packaged with calibrated dosing spoon]

References

Greenberg RN, Mullane K, vanBurik JA, et al, "Posaconazole As Salvage Therapy for Zygomycosis," Antimicrob Agents Chemother, 2006, 50(1):126-33.

Gubbins PO, Krishna G, Sansone-Parsons A, et al, "Pharmacokinetics and Safety of Oral Posaconazole in Neutropenic Stem Cell Transplant Recipients," Antimicrob Agents Chemother, 2006, 50(6):1993-9.

Walsh TJ, Raad I, Patterson TF, et al, "Treatment of Invasive Aspergillosis With Posaconazole in Patients Who Are Refractory to or Intolerant of Conventional Therapy: An Externally Controlled Trial," Clin Infect Dis, 2007, 44(1):2-12.

◆ **Posanol™ (Can)** see Posaconazole on page 1132

◆ **Post Peel Healing Balm [OTC]** see Hydrocortisone on page 685

◆ **Posture® [OTC]** see Calcium Phosphate (Tribasic) on page 238

◆ **Posture®** see Calcium Supplements on page 239

Potassium Acetate (poe TASS ee um AS e tate)

Medication Safety Issues

Consider special storage requirements for intravenous potassium salts; I.V. potassium salts have been administered IVP in error, leading to fatal outcomes.

Therapeutic Category Electrolyte Supplement, Parenteral

Generic Available Yes

Use Treatment and prevention of hypokalemia when it is necessary to avoid chloride or acid/base status requires an additional source of bicarbonate

Pregnancy Risk Factor C

Contraindications Hypersensitivity to any component of the potassium supplement; severe renal impairment, untreated Addison's disease, heat cramps, hyperkalemia, severe tissue trauma

Warnings Potassium acetate should be administered only in patients with adequate urine flow; must be diluted before I.V. use and infused slowly (see Administration)

Precautions Use with caution in patients with cardiac disease, patients receiving potassium-sparing drugs; patients should be on a cardiac monitor during intermittent infusions for doses >0.5 mEq/kg/hour or 5 mEq/hour (adults); solution for injection contains aluminum; use caution with impaired renal function and in premature infants

Adverse Reactions

Cardiovascular (with rapid I.V. administration): Arrhythmias and cardiac arrest, heart block, hypotension

Central nervous system: Mental confusion

Endocrine & metabolic: Hyperkalemia, metabolic alkalosis

Local: Pain at the site of injection, phlebitis

Neuromuscular & skeletal: Muscle weakness, paresthesia, flaccid paralysis

Respiratory: Dyspnea

Drug Interactions

Avoid Concomitant Use There are no known interactions where it is recommended to avoid concomitant use.

Increased Effect/Toxicity

Potassium Acetate may increase the levels/effects of: ACE Inhibitors; Angiotensin II Receptor Blockers; Potassium-Sparing Diuretics

The levels/effects of Potassium Acetate may be increased by: Eplerenone

Decreased Effect There are no known significant interactions involving a decrease in effect.

Stability Store at room temperature; do not freeze

Mechanism of Action Potassium is the major cation of intracellular fluid and is essential for the conduction of nerve impulses in heart, brain, and skeletal muscle; contraction of cardiac, skeletal, and smooth muscles;

maintenance of normal renal function, acid-base balance, carbohydrate metabolism, and gastric secretion

Pharmacokinetics (Adult data unless noted)

Distribution: Enters cells via active transport from extracellular fluid

Elimination: Primarily urine; skin and feces (small amounts); most intestinal potassium reabsorbed

Usual Dosage I.V. doses should be incorporated into the patient's maintenance I.V. fluids; intermittent I.V. potassium administration should be reserved for severe depletion situations; continuous ECG monitoring should be used for intermittent doses >0.5 mEq/kg/hour. **Note:** Doses listed as mEq of **potassium**.

Normal daily requirement: I.V.:
Neonates >24 hours of age and Infants: 2-6 mEq/kg/day
Children: 2-3 mEq/kg/day
Adults: 40-80 mEq/day
Treatment of hypokalemia:
Neonates, Infants, and Children:
I.V. intermittent infusion (must be diluted prior to administration): 0.5-1 mEq/kg/dose (maximum dose: 40 mEq) to infuse at 0.3-0.5 mEq/kg/hour (maximum dose/rate: 1 mEq/kg/hour); then repeated as needed based on frequently obtained lab values; severe depletion or ongoing losses may require >200% of normal daily limit needs
Adults:
I.V. intermittent infusion: 5-10 mEq/hour (continuous cardiac monitor recommended for rates >5 mEq/hour), not to exceed 40 mEq/hour; usual adult maximum per 24 hours: 400 mEq
Potassium dosage/rate of infusion guidelines:
Serum potassium ≥2.5 mEq/L (and <desired): 10 mEq with additional doses if needed; maximum infusion rate: 10 mEq/hour; maximum 24-hour dose: 200 mEq
Serum potassium <2.5 mEq/L: Up to 40 mEq with additional doses based upon frequent lab monitoring; maximum infusion rate: 40 mEq/hour; maximum 24-hour dose: 400 mEq; deficits at a plasma level of 2 mEq/L may be as high as 400-800 mEq of potassium

Administration Parenteral: Potassium must be diluted prior to parenteral administration; maximum recommended concentration (peripheral line): 80 mEq/L; maximum recommended concentration (central line): 150 mEq/L or 15 mEq/100 mL; in severely fluid-restricted patients (with central lines): 200 mEq/L or 20 mEq/100 mL has been used; maximum rate of infusion, see Usual Dosage, I.V. intermittent infusion

Monitoring Parameters Serum potassium, glucose, chloride, pH, urine output (if indicated), cardiac monitor [if intermittent I.V. infusion or potassium I.V. infusion rates >0.5 mEq/kg/hour or 5 mEq/hour (adults)]

Additional Information 1 mEq of acetate is equivalent to the alkalinizing effect of 1 mEq of bicarbonate. Hypokalemia is highly arrhythmogenic, particularly in the setting of ischemia or digitalis toxicity. ECG evidence of hypokalemia includes flattening of the T wave. As the T wave shrinks, U waves may appear. There is no prolongation of the QT interval. Hyperkalemia may present as tall peaked symmetrical T waves. S-T elevation may present in severe hyperkalemia. QRS complex progressively widens with eventual apparent sine waves on the ECG. Hyperkalemia will also induce cardiac slowing and AV conduction abnormalities.

Dosage Forms Excipient information presented when available (limited, particularly for generics); consult specific product labeling.

Injection, solution: 2 mEq/mL (20 mL, 50 mL, 100 mL) [contains aluminum]

Injection, solution [concentrate]: 4 mEq/mL (50 mL) [contains aluminum]

References
Hamill RJ, Robinson LM, Wexler HR, et al, "Efficacy and Safety of Potassium Infusion Therapy in Hypokalemic Critically Ill Patients," *Crit Care Med*, 1991, 19(5):694-9.
Khilnani P, "Electrolyte Abnormalities in Critically Ill Children," *Crit Care Med*, 1992, 20(2):241-50.

Potassium Bicarbonate
(poe TASS ee um bye KAR bun ate)

Therapeutic Category Electrolyte Supplement, Oral

Generic Available Yes

Use Treatment and prevention of hypokalemia when it is necessary to avoid chloride or acid/base status requires bicarbonate

Pregnancy Risk Factor C

Contraindications Hypersensitivity to any component of the potassium supplement; severe renal impairment, untreated Addison's disease, heat cramps, hyperkalemia, severe tissue trauma; solid oral dosage forms are contraindicated in patients in whom there is a structural, pathological, and/or pharmacologic cause for delay or arrest in passage through the GI tract

Precautions Use with caution in patients with cardiac and/or renal disease, patients receiving potassium-sparing drugs

Adverse Reactions
Central nervous system: Mental confusion
Endocrine & metabolic: Hyperkalemia, metabolic alkalosis
Gastrointestinal: Nausea, vomiting, diarrhea, abdominal pain, GI lesions, flatulence
Neuromuscular & skeletal: Muscle weakness, paresthesia, flaccid paralysis

Drug Interactions
Avoid Concomitant Use There are no known interactions where it is recommended to avoid concomitant use.
Increased Effect/Toxicity
Potassium Bicarbonate may increase the levels/effects of: ACE Inhibitors; Angiotensin II Receptor Blockers; Potassium-Sparing Diuretics

The levels/effects of Potassium Bicarbonate may be increased by: Eplerenone
Decreased Effect There are no known significant interactions involving a decrease in effect.

Stability Store at room temperature.

Mechanism of Action Potassium is the major cation of intracellular fluid and is essential for the conduction of nerve impulses in heart, brain, and skeletal muscle; contraction of cardiac, skeletal, and smooth muscles; maintenance of normal renal function, acid-base balance, carbohydrate metabolism, and gastric secretion. Bicarbonate neutralizes hydrogen ion concentration and raises blood and urinary pH.

Pharmacokinetics (Adult data unless noted)
Absorption: Well absorbed from upper GI tract
Distribution: Enters cells via active transport from extracellular fluid
Elimination: Primarily urine; skin and feces (small amounts); most intestinal potassium reabsorbed

Usual Dosage Oral (doses listed as mEq of **potassium**):
Normal daily requirement:
Children: 2-3 mEq/kg/day
Adults: 40-80 mEq/day
Prevention of hypokalemia during diuretic therapy:
Children: 1-2 mEq/kg/day in 1-2 divided doses
Adults: 25-100 mEq/day in 2-4 divided doses

Administration Oral: Dissolve completely in 3-8 oz cold water, juice, or other suitable beverage and drink slowly

Monitoring Parameters Serum potassium, chloride, glucose, pH, urine output (if indicated)

Additional Information Hypokalemia is highly arrhythmogenic, particularly in the setting of ischemia or digitalis toxicity. ECG evidence of hypokalemia includes flattening of the T wave. As the T wave shrinks, U waves may appear. There is no prolongation of the QT interval. Hyperkalemia may present as tall peaked symmetrical T waves. S-T elevation may present in severe hyperkalemia. QRS complex progressively widens with eventual apparent sine waves on the ECG. Hyperkalemia will also induce cardiac slowing and AV conduction abnormalities.

Dosage Forms Excipient information presented when available (limited, particularly for generics); consult specific product labeling.

Tablet for oral solution, effervescent: Potassium 25 mEq

Potassium Bicarbonate and Potassium Chloride

(poe TASS ee um bye KAR bun ate & poe TASS ee um KLOR ide)

Related Information
Potassium Bicarbonate on page 1134
Potassium Chloride on page 1136

U.S. Brand Names K-Lyte/Cl® [DSC]

Therapeutic Category Electrolyte Supplement, Oral

Generic Available Yes

Use Treatment or prevention of hypokalemia

Pregnancy Risk Factor C

Lactation Enters breast milk/compatible

Contraindications Hypersensitivity to any component of the potassium supplement; severe renal impairment, untreated Addison's disease, heat cramps, hyperkalemia, severe tissue trauma

Precautions Use with caution in patients with cardiac and/or renal disease, patients receiving potassium-sparing drugs

Adverse Reactions
Central nervous system: Mental confusion
Endocrine & metabolic: Hyperkalemia, metabolic alkalosis
Gastrointestinal: Nausea, vomiting, diarrhea, abdominal pain, GI lesions, flatulence
Neuromuscular & skeletal: Muscle weakness, paresthesia, flaccid paralysis

Drug Interactions
Avoid Concomitant Use There are no known interactions where it is recommended to avoid concomitant use.

Increased Effect/Toxicity
Potassium Bicarbonate and Potassium Chloride may increase the levels/effects of: ACE Inhibitors; Angiotensin II Receptor Blockers; Potassium-Sparing Diuretics

The levels/effects of Potassium Bicarbonate and Potassium Chloride may be increased by: Anticholinergic Agents; Eplerenone

Decreased Effect There are no known significant interactions involving a decrease in effect.

Stability Store at room temperature.

Usual Dosage Oral (doses listed as mEq of **potassium**):
Normal daily requirement:
Children: 2-3 mEq/kg/day
Adults: 40-80 mEq/day
Prevention of hypokalemia during diuretic therapy:
Children: 1-2 mEq/kg/day in 1-2 divided doses
Adults: 25-100 mEq/day in 2-4 divided doses

Administration Dissolve tablets in 3-4 ounces cold water or juice; solution should be sipped slowly, over 5-10 minutes; administer with meals

Monitoring Parameters Serum potassium, glucose, chloride, pH, urine output (if indicated)

Additional Information Hypokalemia is highly arrhythmogenic, particularly in the setting of ischemia or digitalis toxicity. ECG evidence of hypokalemia includes flattening of the T wave. As the T wave shrinks, U waves may appear. There is no prolongation of the QT interval. Hyperkalemia may present as tall peaked symmetrical T waves. S-T elevation may present in severe hyperkalemia. QRS complex progressively widens with eventual apparent sine waves on the ECG. Hyperkalemia will also induce cardiac slowing and AV conduction abnormalities.

Dosage Forms Excipient information presented when available (limited, particularly for generics); consult specific product labeling. [DSC] = Discontinued product

Tablet for solution, oral [effervescent]: Potassium chloride 25 mEq [potassium bicarbonate 0.5 g and potassium chloride 1.5 g]

K-Lyte/Cl®: Potassium chloride 25 mEq [potassium bicarbonate 0.5 g and potassium chloride 1.5 g; citrus or fruit punch flavor] [DSC]

◆ **Potassium Bicarbonate and Potassium Chloride (Effervescent)** *see* Potassium Bicarbonate and Potassium Chloride *on page 1135*

Potassium Bicarbonate and Potassium Citrate

(poe TASS ee um bye KAR bun ate & poe TASS ee um SIT rate)

Medication Safety Issues
Sound-alike/look-alike issues:
Klor-Con® may be confused with Klaron®

Related Information
Potassium Bicarbonate on page 1134

U.S. Brand Names K-Lyte/Cl®; K-Lyte® DS; Klor-Con®/EF

Therapeutic Category Electrolyte Supplement, Oral

Generic Available Yes

Use Treatment or prevention of hypokalemia, particularly when it is necessary to avoid chloride or the acid/base status requires bicarbonate

Pregnancy Risk Factor C

Contraindications Hypersensitivity to any component of the potassium supplement; severe renal impairment, untreated Addison's disease, heat cramps, hyperkalemia, severe tissue trauma

Precautions Use with caution in patients with cardiac and/or renal disease, patients receiving potassium-sparing drugs

Adverse Reactions
Central nervous system: Mental confusion
Endocrine & metabolic: Hyperkalemia, metabolic alkalosis
Gastrointestinal: Nausea, vomiting, diarrhea, abdominal pain, GI lesions, flatulence
Neuromuscular & skeletal: Muscle weakness, paresthesia, flaccid paralysis

Drug Interactions
Avoid Concomitant Use There are no known interactions where it is recommended to avoid concomitant use.

Increased Effect/Toxicity
Potassium Bicarbonate and Potassium Citrate may increase the levels/effects of: ACE Inhibitors; Aluminum Hydroxide; Angiotensin II Receptor Blockers; Potassium-Sparing Diuretics

The levels/effects of Potassium Bicarbonate and Potassium Citrate may be increased by: Eplerenone

Decreased Effect There are no known significant interactions involving a decrease in effect.

Stability Store at room temperature.

Mechanism of Action Potassium is the major cation of intracellular fluid and is essential for the conduction of nerve impulses in heart, brain, and skeletal muscle;

contraction of cardiac, skeletal, and smooth muscles; maintenance of normal renal function, acid-base balance, carbohydrate metabolism, and gastric secretion. Bicarbonate neutralizes hydrogen ion concentration and raises blood and urinary pH

Pharmacokinetics (Adult data unless noted)
Absorption: Well absorbed from upper GI tract
Distribution: Enters cells via active transport from extracellular fluid
Elimination: Primarily urine; skin and feces (small amounts); most intestinal potassium reabsorbed

Usual Dosage Oral (doses listed as mEq of **potassium**):
Normal daily requirement:
Children: 2-3 mEq/kg/day
Adults: 40-80 mEq/day
Prevention of hypokalemia during diuretic therapy:
Children: 1-2 mEq/kg/day in 1-2 divided doses
Adults: 25-100 mEq/day in 2-4 divided doses

Administration Oral: Dissolve completely in 3-8 oz cold water, juice, or other suitable beverage and drink slowly.

Monitoring Parameters Serum potassium, chloride, glucose, pH, urine output (if indicated)

Additional Information Hypokalemia is highly arrhythmogenic, particularly in the setting of ischemia or digitalis toxicity. ECG evidence of hypokalemia includes flattening of the T wave. As the T wave shrinks, U waves may appear. There is no prolongation of the QT interval. Hyperkalemia may present as tall peaked symmetrical T waves. S-T elevation may present in severe hyperkalemia. QRS complex progressively widens with eventual apparent sine waves on the ECG. Hyperkalemia will also induce cardiac slowing and AV conduction abnormalities.

Dosage Forms Excipient information presented when available (limited, particularly for generics); consult specific product labeling.
Tablet, effervescent:
Klor-Con®/EF: Potassium 25 mEq [sugar free; orange flavor]
K-Lyte®: Potassium 25 mEq [orange flavor]
K-Lyte® DS: Potassium 50 mEq [orange flavor]

♦ **Potassium Bicarbonate and Potassium Citrate (Effervescent)** *see* Potassium Bicarbonate and Potassium Citrate *on page 1135*

Potassium Chloride (poe TASS ee um KLOR ide)

Medication Safety Issues
Sound-alike/look-alike issues:
Kaon-Cl-10® may be confused with kaolin
KCl may be confused with HCl
Klor-Con® may be confused with Klaron®
microK® may be confused with Macrobid®, Micronase®

High alert medication: The Institute for Safe Medication Practices (ISMP) includes this medication (I.V. formulation) among its list of drugs which have a heightened risk of causing significant patient harm when used in error.
Per JCAHO recommendations, concentrated electrolyte solutions should not be available in patient care areas.
Consider special storage requirements for intravenous potassium salts; I.V. potassium salts have been administered IVP in error, leading to fatal outcomes.

U.S. Brand Names Epiklor™; Epiklor™/25; K-Tab®; Kaon-Cl-10®; Klor-Con®; Klor-Con® 10; Klor-Con® 8; Klor-Con® M10; Klor-Con® M15; Klor-Con® M20; Klor-Con®/25; microK®; microK® 10

Canadian Brand Names Apo-K®; K-10®; K-Dur®; K-Lyte®/Cl; Micro-K Extencaps®; Roychlor®; Slo-Pot; Slow-K®

Therapeutic Category Electrolyte Supplement, Oral; Electrolyte Supplement, Parenteral

Generic Available Yes

Use Treatment or prevention of hypokalemia

Pregnancy Risk Factor C

Pregnancy Considerations Reproduction studies have not been conducted. Potassium supplementation (that does not cause maternal hyperkalemia) would not be expected to cause adverse fetal events.

Lactation Enters breast milk/compatible

Breast-Feeding Considerations The normal content of potassium in human milk is ~13 mEq/L. Supplementation (that does not cause maternal hyperkalemia) would not be expected to affect normal levels.

Contraindications Hypersensitivity to any component of the potassium supplement; severe renal impairment, untreated Addison's disease, heat cramps, hyperkalemia, severe tissue trauma; solid oral dosage forms are contraindicated in patients in whom there is a structural, pathological, and/or pharmacologic cause for delay or arrest in passage through the GI tract; an oral liquid potassium preparation should be used in patients with esophageal compression or delayed gastric emptying time

Warnings Potassium chloride injection should be administered only in patients with adequate urine flow; injection must be diluted before I.V. use and infused slowly (see Administration)

Precautions Use with caution in patients with cardiac disease and/or renal disease, patients receiving potassium-sparing drugs; patients should be on a cardiac monitor during intermittent infusions for doses >0.5 mEq/kg/hour

Adverse Reactions
Cardiovascular (with rapid I.V. administration): Arrhythmias and cardiac arrest, heart block, hypotension
Central nervous system: Mental confusion
Endocrine & metabolic: Hyperkalemia
Gastrointestinal (with oral administration): Nausea, vomiting, diarrhea, abdominal pain, GI lesions, flatulence
Local: Pain at the site of injection, phlebitis
Neuromuscular & skeletal: Muscle weakness, paresthesia, flaccid paralysis

Drug Interactions
Avoid Concomitant Use There are no known interactions where it is recommended to avoid concomitant use.

Increased Effect/Toxicity
Potassium Chloride may increase the levels/effects of: ACE Inhibitors; Angiotensin II Receptor Blockers; Potassium-Sparing Diuretics

The levels/effects of Potassium Chloride may be increased by: Anticholinergic Agents; Eplerenone

Decreased Effect There are no known significant interactions involving a decrease in effect.

Stability Store at room temperature; do not freeze

Mechanism of Action Potassium is the major cation of intracellular fluid and is essential for the conduction of nerve impulses in heart, brain, and skeletal muscle; contraction of cardiac, skeletal, and smooth muscles; maintenance of normal renal function, acid-base balance, carbohydrate metabolism, and gastric secretion

Pharmacokinetics (Adult data unless noted)
Absorption: Well absorbed from upper GI tract; enters cells via active transport from extracellular fluid
Distribution: Enters cells via active transport from extracellular fluid
Elimination: Primarily urine; skin and feces (small amounts); most intestinal potassium reabsorbed

Usual Dosage I.V. doses should be incorporated into the patient's maintenance I.V. fluids; intermittent I.V. potassium administration should be reserved for severe depletion situations; continuous ECG monitoring should be used for intermittent doses >0.5 mEq/kg/hour. Doses listed as mEq of **potassium**. When using microencapsulated or wax matrix formulations, use no more than 20 mEq as a single dose.

Normal daily requirements: Oral, I.V.:
Neonates >24 hours of age and Infants: 2-6 mEq/kg/day
Children: 2-3 mEq/kg/day
Adults: 40-80 mEq/day
Prevention of hypokalemia during diuretic therapy: Oral:
Neonates, Infants, and Children: 1-2 mEq/kg/day in 1-2
divided doses
Adults: 20-40 mEq/day in 1-2 divided doses
Treatment of hypokalemia: **Note:** High variability exists in
dosing/infusion rate recommendations; therapy should
be guided by patient condition and specific institutional
guidelines.
Neonates, Infants, and Children:
Oral: 2-5 mEq/kg/day in divided doses; not to exceed
1-2 mEq/kg as a single dose; if deficits are severe or
ongoing losses are great, I.V. route should be
considered preferred route of administration
I.V. intermittent infusion (must be diluted prior to
administration): 0.5-1 mEq/kg/dose (maximum dose:
40 mEq) to infuse at 0.3-0.5 mEq/kg/hour (maximum
dose/rate: 1 mEq/kg/hour); then repeated as needed
based on frequently obtained lab values; severe
depletion or ongoing losses may require >200% of
normal daily limit needs
Adults:
I.V. intermittent infusion: 5-10 mEq/hour (continuous
cardiac monitor recommended for rates >5 mEq/hour),
not to exceed 40 mEq/hour; usual adult maximum per
24 hours: 400 mEq
Potassium dosage/rate of infusion guidelines:
Serum potassium ≥2.5 mEq/L (and <desired): 10
mEq with additional doses if needed; maximum
infusion rate: 10 mEq/hour; maximum 24-hour
dose: 200 mEq
Serum potassium <2.5 mEq/L: Up to 40 mEq, with
additional doses based upon frequent lab monitoring; maximum infusion rate: 40 mEq/hour; maximum 24-hour dose: 400 mEq; deficits at a plasma
level of 2 mEq/L may be as high as 400-800 mEq of
potassium
Oral:
Asymptomatic, mild hypokalemia: Usual dosage
range: 40-100 mEq/day divided in 2-5 doses;
generally recommended to limit doses to 20-25
mEq/dose to avoid GI discomfort
Mild to moderate hypokalemia: Some clinicians may
administer up to 120-240 mEq/day divided in 3-4
doses; limit doses to 40-60 mEq/dose. If deficits are
severe or ongoing losses are great, I.V. route should
be considered.

Administration

Oral: Sustained release and wax matrix tablets (K-Tab®,
Kaon-Cl-10®, Klor-Con®) should be swallowed whole,
do not crush or chew; administer with food; powder (Klor-
Con®) should be dissolved in 4-5 ounces of water or
juice; capsule (microK®) should be swallowed whole, do
not chew; may also be opened and contents sprinkled on
a spoonful of applesauce or pudding and swallowed
immediately without chewing; do not administer liquid
formulations full strength, must be diluted in 2-6 parts of
water or juice. Klor-Con® M tablet may be broken in half
and each half swallowed separately; the whole tablet
may be dissolved in approximately 4 ounces of water
(allow approximately 2 minutes to dissolve, stir well, and
drink immediately).
Parenteral: Potassium must be diluted prior to parenteral
administration; maximum recommended concentration
(peripheral line): 80 mEq/L; maximum recommended
concentration (central line): 150 mEq/L or 15 mEq/
100 mL; in severely fluid-restricted patients (with central
lines): 200 mEq/L or 20 mEq/100 mL has been used;

maximum rate of infusion, see Usual Dosage, I.V.
intermittent infusion
Monitoring Parameters Serum potassium, glucose,
chloride, pH, urine output (if indicated), cardiac monitor [if
intermittent I.V. infusion or potassium I.V. infusion rates
>0.5 mEq/kg/hour or >10 mEq/hour (adults)]
Additional Information Hypokalemia is highly arrhythmogenic, particularly in the setting of ischemia or digitalis
toxicity. ECG evidence of hypokalemia includes flattening
of the T wave. As the T wave shrinks, U waves may
appear. There is no prolongation of the QT interval.
Hyperkalemia may present as tall peaked symmetrical T
waves. S-T elevation may present in severe hyperkalemia.
QRS complex progressively widens with eventual apparent sine waves on the ECG. Hyperkalemia will also induce
cardiac slowing and AV conduction abnormalities.
Dosage Forms Excipient information presented when
available (limited, particularly for generics); consult specific
product labeling.
Capsule, extended release, microencapsulated: 8 mEq
[600 mg]; 10 mEq [750 mg]
microK®: 8 mEq [600 mg]
microK® 10: 10 mEq [750 mg]
Infusion [premixed in D_5W]: 20 mEq (1000 mL); 40 mEq
(1000 mL)
Infusion [premixed in D_5W and LR]: 20 mEq (1000 mL); 30
mEq (1000 mL); 40 mEq (1000 mL)
Infusion [premixed in D_5W and sodium chloride 0.2%]: 5
mEq (250 mL); 10 mEq (500 mL, 1000 mL); 20 mEq
(1000 mL); 30 mEq (1000 mL); 40 mEq (1000 mL)
Infusion [premixed in D_5W and sodium chloride 0.3%]: 10
mEq (500 mL); 20 mEq (1000 mL)
Infusion [premixed in D_5W and sodium chloride 0.45%]: 10
mEq (500 mL, 1000 mL); 20 mEq (1000 mL); 30 mEq
(1000 mL); 40 mEq (1000 mL)
Infusion [premixed in D_5W and NS]: 20 mEq (1000 mL); 40
mEq (1000 mL)
Infusion [premixed in $D_{10}W$ and sodium chloride 0.2%]: 5
mEq (250 mL)
Infusion [premixed in sodium chloride 0.45%]: 20 mEq
(1000 mL)
Infusion [premixed in NS]: 20 mEq (1000 mL); 40 mEq
(1000 mL)
Infusion [premixed in SWFI; highly concentrated]: 10 mEq
(50 mL, 100 mL); 20 mEq (50 mL, 100 mL); 30 mEq
(100 mL); 40 mEq (100 mL)
Injection, solution [concentrate]: 2 mEq/mL (5 mL, 10 mL,
15 mL, 20 mL, 30 mL, 250 mL, 500 mL)
Injection, solution [concentrate, preservative free]: 2
mEq/mL (5 mL, 10 mL, 15 mL, 20 mL)
Powder, for oral solution: 20 mEq/packet (30s, 100s,
1000s)
Epiklor™: 20 mEq/packet (30s, 100s) [sugar free; orange
flavor]
Epiklor™/25: 25 mEq/packet (30s, 100s) [sugar free;
orange flavor]
Klor-Con®: 20 mEq/packet (30s, 100s) [sugar free; fruit
flavor]
Klor-Con®/25: 25 mEq/packet (30s, 100s) [sugar free;
fruit flavor]
Solution, oral: 20 mEq/15 mL (15 mL, 30 mL, 480 mL); 40
mEq/15 mL (15 mL, 480 mL)
Tablet, extended release, microencapsulated: 10 mEq,
20 mEq
Klor-Con® M10: 10 mEq [750 mg]
Klor-Con® M15: 15 mEq [1125 mg; scored]
Klor-Con® M20: 20 mEq [1500 mg; scored]
Tablet, extended release, wax matrix: 8 mEq, 10 mEq
K-Tab®: 10 mEq [750 mg]
Kaon-Cl-10®: 10 mEq [750 mg]
Klor-Con® 8: 8 mEq [600 mg]
Klor-Con® 10: 10 mEq [750 mg]

References

Hamill RJ, Robinson LM, Wexler HR, et al, "Efficacy and Safety of Potassium Infusion Therapy in Hypokalemic Critically Ill Patients," *Crit Care Med*, 1991, 19(5):694-9.

Khilnani P, "Electrolyte Abnormalities in Critically Ill Children," *Crit Care Med*, 1992, 20(2):241-50.

Potassium Gluconate
(poe TASS ee um GLOO coe nate)

Therapeutic Category Electrolyte Supplement, Oral

Generic Available Yes

Use Treatment or prevention of hypokalemia

Pregnancy Risk Factor A

Contraindications Hypersensitivity to any component of the potassium supplement; severe renal impairment, untreated Addison's disease, heat cramps, hyperkalemia, severe tissue trauma; solid oral dosage forms are contraindicated in patients in whom there is a structural, pathological, and/or pharmacologic cause for delay or arrest in passage through the GI tract

Precautions Use with caution in patients with cardiac and/or renal disease, patients receiving potassium-sparing drugs

Adverse Reactions
Central nervous system: Mental confusion
Endocrine & metabolic: Hyperkalemia
Gastrointestinal: Abdominal pain, diarrhea, flatulence, GI lesions, nausea, vomiting
Neuromuscular & skeletal: Flaccid paralysis, muscle weakness, paresthesia

Drug Interactions
Avoid Concomitant Use There are no known interactions where it is recommended to avoid concomitant use.
Increased Effect/Toxicity
Potassium Gluconate may increase the levels/effects of: ACE Inhibitors; Angiotensin II Receptor Blockers; Potassium-Sparing Diuretics

The levels/effects of Potassium Gluconate may be increased by: Eplerenone
Decreased Effect There are no known significant interactions involving a decrease in effect.

Stability Store at room temperature.

Mechanism of Action Potassium is the major cation of intracellular fluid and is essential for the conduction of nerve impulses in heart, brain, and skeletal muscle; contraction of cardiac, skeletal, and smooth muscles; maintenance of normal renal function, acid-base balance, carbohydrate metabolism, and gastric secretion

Pharmacokinetics (Adult data unless noted)
Absorption: Well absorbed from upper GI tract
Distribution: Enters cells via active transport from extracellular fluid
Elimination: Primarily urine; skin and feces (small amounts); most intestinal potassium reabsorbed

Usual Dosage Oral: **Note:** Doses listed as mEq of potassium (approximately 4.3 mEq potassium/g potassium gluconate; 1 mEq potassium is equivalent to 39 mg elemental potassium)
Normal daily requirement:
Children: 2-3 mEq/kg/day
Adults: 40-80 mEq/day
Prevention of hypokalemia during diuretic therapy:
Children: 1-2 mEq/kg/day in 1-2 divided doses
Adults: 20-40 mEq/day in 1-2 divided doses
Treatment of hypokalemia:
Children: 2-5 mEq/kg/day in divided doses; not to exceed 1-2 mEq/kg as a single dose; if deficits are severe or ongoing losses are great, I.V. route should be considered preferred route of administration
Adults: 40-100 mEq/day in 2-4 divided doses

Administration Oral: Sustained release and wax matrix tablets should be swallowed whole, do not crush or chew; administer with food

Monitoring Parameters Serum potassium, chloride, glucose, pH, urine output (if indicated)

Additional Information 9.4 g potassium gluconate is approximately equal to 40 mEq potassium (4.3 mEq potassium/g potassium gluconate). Hypokalemia is highly arrhythmogenic, particularly in the setting of ischemia or digitalis toxicity. ECG evidence of hypokalemia includes flattening of the T wave. As the T wave shrinks, U waves may appear. There is no prolongation of the QT interval. Hyperkalemia may present as tall peaked symmetrical T waves. S-T elevation may present in severe hyperkalemia. QRS complex progressively widens with eventual apparent sine waves on the ECG. Hyperkalemia will also induce cardiac slowing and AV conduction abnormalities.

Dosage Forms Excipient information presented when available (limited, particularly for generics); consult specific product labeling.
Caplet: 595 mg [equivalent to potassium 99 mg]
Capsule: 99 mg [strength expressed as base]
Tablet: 99 mg [strength expressed as base]; 550 mg [equivalent to potassium 90 mg]; 595 mg [equivalent to potassium 99 mg]
Tablet, timed release: 95 mg [strength expressed as base]

Potassium Iodide (poe TASS ee um EYE oh dide)

Medication Safety Issues
Sound-alike/look-alike issues:
Potassium iodide products, including saturated solution of potassium iodide (SSKI®) may be confused with potassium iodide and iodine (Strong Iodide Solution or Lugol's solution)

U.S. Brand Names Iosat™ [OTC]; SSKI®; ThyroSafe™ [OTC]; ThyroShield™ [OTC]

Therapeutic Category Antithyroid Agent; Expectorant

Use Expectorant for the symptomatic treatment of chronic pulmonary diseases complicated by mucous; reduce thyroid vascularity prior to thyroidectomy and management of thyrotoxic crisis; block thyroidal uptake of radioactive isotopes of iodine in a radiation emergency or other exposure to radioactive iodine; treat cutaneous sporotrichosis

Pregnancy Risk Factor D

Pregnancy Considerations Iodide crosses the placenta (may cause hypothyroidism and goiter in fetus/newborn). Use as an expectorant during pregnancy is contraindicated by the AAP. Use for protection against thyroid cancer secondary to radioactive iodine exposure is considered acceptable based upon risk/benefit, keeping in mind the dose and duration. Repeat dosing should be avoided if possible. Refer to Iodine on page 753 for additional information.

Lactation Enters breast milk/use caution (AAP rates "compatible")

Breast-Feeding Considerations AAP considers this drug compatible, but recommends avoiding breast-feeding following radioactive iodine exposure unless no alternative is available. May cause skin rash in nursing infant. Refer to Iodine on page 753 for additional information.

Contraindications Hypersensitivity to iodides or any component; hyperkalemia, pulmonary edema, hyperthyroidism, impaired renal function, iodine-induced goiter, dermatitis herpetiformis, hypocomplementemic vasculitis

Warnings Prolonged use can lead to hypothyroidism.

Precautions Use with caution in patients with cystic fibrosis (may have exaggerated susceptibility to goitrogenic effects); use caution in patients with myotonia congenital, patients with a history of thyroid disease, and in patients with cardiac disease, Addison's disease, tuberculosis, or acute bronchitits; treatment may cause flare-up of acne

Adverse Reactions

Cardiovascular: Arrhythmia

Central nervous system: Fever, headache, confusion

Dermatologic: Urticaria, acne, angioedema, cutaneous hemorrhage

Endocrine & metabolic: Goiter with hypothyroidism, thyroid adenoma, acute parotitis

Gastrointestinal: Metallic taste, GI upset, GI bleeding, soreness of teeth and gums, cutaneous and mucosal hemorrhage, nausea, vomiting, diarrhea

Hematologic: Eosinophilia

Neuromuscular & skeletal: Arthralgia, numbness, paresthesia

Respiratory: Rhinitis, wheezing

Miscellaneous: Lymph node enlargement, swelling of face, lips, tongue, throat, hands, and feet

Drug Interactions

Avoid Concomitant Use

Avoid concomitant use of Potassium Iodide with any of the following: Sodium Iodide I131

Increased Effect/Toxicity

Potassium Iodide may increase the levels/effects of: ACE Inhibitors; Angiotensin II Receptor Blockers; Lithium; Potassium-Sparing Diuretics

The levels/effects of Potassium Iodide may be increased by: Eplerenone

Decreased Effect

Potassium Iodide may decrease the levels/effects of: Sodium Iodide I131; Vitamin K Antagonists

Stability Store at room temperature; SSKI® if exposed to cold temperatures may develop crystallization; warming with shaking will redissolve crystals; if solution becomes brown/yellow in color, it should be discarded

Mechanism of Action Reduces viscosity of mucus by increasing respiratory tract secretions; inhibits the release of thyroid hormone; following radioactive iodine exposure, potassium iodide blocks the uptake of radioiodine by the thyroid, reducing the risk of thyroid cancer

Pharmacodynamics Antithyroid effects:

Onset of action: 24-48 hours

Maximum effect: 10-15 days after continuous therapy

Duration: May persist up to 6 weeks

Usual Dosage Oral:

Expectorant:

Children:

SSKI®: 60-250 mg 4 times/day; maximum single dose: 500 mg

Pima®:

<3 years: 162 mg 3 times/day

>3 years: 325 mg 3 times/day

Adults:

SSKI®: 300-600 mg 3-4 times/day

Pima®: 325-650 mg 3 times/day

Preoperative thyroidectomy: Children and Adults: Given 10-14 days before surgery: 50-250 mg (1-5 drops, 1 g/mL SSKI®) 3 times/day

Thyrotoxic crisis:

Infants <1 year: 150-250 mg (3-5 drops, 1 g/mL SSKI®) 3 times/day

Children and Adults: 300-500 mg (6-10 drops 1 g/mL SSKI®) 3 times/day

Cutaneous Sporotrichosis:

Children: 250-500 mg (5-10 drops, 1 g/mL SSKI®) 3 times/day; increase gradually to a maximum of 1.25-2 g (25-40 drops SSKI®)

Adults: 250-500 mg (5-10 drops, 1 g/mL SSKI®) 3 times/day; increase gradually to a maximum of 2-2.5 g (40-50 drops SSKI®)

Note: Therapy is continued at the maximum tolerated dosage until the cutaneous lesions have resolved, usually 6-12 weeks

Radiation protectant to radioactive isotopes of iodine (Pima®):

Infants and children <1 year: 65 mg once daily for 10 days; start 24 hours prior to exposure

Children >1 year: 130 mg once daily for 10 days; start 24 hours prior to exposure

Adults: 195 mg once daily for 10 days; start 24 hours prior to exposure

Prevention of thyroidal uptake of radioactive isotopes of iodine to reduce risk of thyroid cancer following nuclear accident (Iosat™, ThyroSafe™, ThyroShield™):

Infants <1 month: 16.25 mg once daily

Infants ≥1 month and Children <3 years: 32.5 mg once daily

Children 3-18 years (≤150 lbs): 65 mg once daily

Children >18 years (>150 lbs) and Adults (including pregnant and lactating women): 130 mg once daily

Note: Treatment should continue until the risk of exposure has passed and/or until other measures (evacuation, sheltering, control of the food and milk supply) have been successfully implemented.

Administration Oral: Administer after meals with food or milk or dilute with a large quantity of water, fruit juice, milk, or broth

Monitoring Parameters Thyroid function tests; sign/symptoms of hyperthyroidism; thyroid function should be monitored in pregnant women, neonates, and young infants if repeat doses are required following radioactive iodine exposure

Additional Information 10 drops SSKI® = potassium iodide 500 mg

Dosage Forms Excipient information presented when available (limited, particularly for generics); consult specific product labeling.

Solution, oral:

SSKI®: 1 g/mL (30 mL, 240 mL) [contains sodium thiosulfate]

ThyroShield™: 65 mg/mL (30 mL) [black raspberry flavor]

Tablet:

Iosat™: 130 mg

ThyroSafe™: 65 mg [equivalent to iodine 50 mg]

Extemporaneous Preparations Preparation of oral solution:

Concentration of 16.25 mg/5 mL oral solution: Crush one 130 mg tablet into a fine powder. Add 20 mL of water and mix until powder is dissolved. Add an additional 20 mL of low-fat milk (white or chocolate), orange juice, flat soda, raspberry syrup, or infant formula. Final concentration will be 16.25 mg/5 mL.

Concentration of 8.125 mg/5 mL oral solution: Crush one 65 mg tablet into a fine powder. Add 20 mL of water and mix until powder is dissolved. Add an additional 20 mL of low-fat milk (white or chocolate), orange juice, flat soda, raspberry syrup, or infant formula. Final concentration will be 8.125 mg/5 mL.

References

"American Academy of Pediatrics Committee on Environmental Health. Radiation Disasters and Children," *Pediatrics*, 2003, 111(6 Pt 1):1455-66.

Kauffman CA, Hajjeh R, and Chapman SW, "Practice Guidelines for the Management of Patients With Sporotrichosis. For the Mycoses Study Group. Infectious Diseases Society of America," *Clin Infect Dis*, 2000, 30(4):684-7.

"Potassium Iodide as a Thyroid Blocking Agent in a Radiation Emergency: Final Recommendations on Use," Washington DC, Bureau of Radiological Health and Bureau of Drugs, Food and Drug Administration, 1982.

U.S. Food and Drug Administration, "FDA's Guidance on Protection of Children and Adults Against Thyroid Cancer in Case of Nuclear Accident," FDA Talk Paper. Available at: http://www.fda.gov/bbs/topics/answers/2001/ans01126.html. Accessed January 11, 2002.

Potassium Iodide and Iodine
(poe TASS ee um EYE oh dide & EYE oh dine)

Medication Safety Issues
Sound-alike/look-alike issues:
Potassium iodide and iodine (Strong Iodide Solution or Lugol's solution) may be confused with potassium iodide products, including saturated solution of potassium iodide (SSKI®)

Therapeutic Category Antithyroid Agent

Generic Available Yes

Use Reduce thyroid vascularity prior to thyroidectomy and management of thyrotoxic crisis

Pregnancy Risk Factor D (potassium iodide)

Pregnancy Considerations Iodide crosses the placenta (may cause hypothyroidism and goiter in fetus/newborn). Use for protection against thyroid cancer secondary to radioactive iodine exposure is considered acceptable based upon risk/benefit, keeping in mind the dose and duration. Repeat dosing should be avoided if possible. Refer to Iodine on page 753 for additional information.

Lactation Enters breast milk/use caution (AAP rates "compatible")

Breast-Feeding Considerations AAP considers this drug "compatible," but recommends avoiding breast-feeding following radioactive iodine exposure unless no alternative is available. Skin rash in the nursing infant has been reported with maternal intake of potassium iodide. Refer to Iodine monograph for additional information.

Contraindications Hypersensitivity to iodine or any component; hyperkalemia, pulmonary edema, hyperthyroidism, impaired renal function, iodine-induced goiter, dermatitis herpetiformis, hypocomplementemic vasculitis

Warnings Prolonged use can lead to hypothyroidism.

Precautions Use with caution in patients with cystic fibrosis (may have exaggerated susceptibility to goitrogenic effects); use caution in patients with myotonia congenital, patients with a history of thyroid disease, and in patients with cardiac disease, Addison's diseases, tuberculosis, or acute bronchitis; treatment may cause flare-up of acne

Adverse Reactions
Cardiovascular: Arrhythmia

Central nervous system: Fever, headache, confusion

Dermatologic: Urticaria, acne, angioedema, cutaneous hemorrhage, skin rash

Endocrine & metabolic: Goiter with hypothyroidism, thyroid adenoma, acute parotitis

Gastrointestinal: Metallic taste, GI upset, GI bleeding, soreness of teeth and gums, cutaneous and mucosal hemorrhage, nausea, vomiting, diarrhea

Hematologic: Eosinophilia

Neuromuscular & skeletal: Arthralgia, numbness, paresthesia

Respiratory: Rhinitis, wheezing

Miscellaneous: Lymph node enlargement, swelling of face, lips, tongue, throat, hands, and feet

Drug Interactions
Avoid Concomitant Use
Avoid concomitant use of Potassium Iodide and Iodine with any of the following: Sodium Iodide I131

Increased Effect/Toxicity
Potassium Iodide and Iodine may increase the levels/effects of: ACE Inhibitors; Angiotensin II Receptor Blockers; Lithium; Potassium-Sparing Diuretics

The levels/effects of Potassium Iodide and Iodine may be increased by: Eplerenone

Decreased Effect
Potassium Iodide and Iodine may decrease the levels/effects of: Sodium Iodide I131; Vitamin K Antagonists

Stability Store at room temperature; excursions permitted to 15°C to 30°C (59°F to 86°F); protect from light and keep container tightly closed

Mechanism of Action Inhibits the release of thyroid hormone; following radioactive iodine exposure, potassium iodide blocks the uptake of radioiodine by the thyroid, reducing the risk of thyroid cancer

Pharmacodynamics Antithyroid effects:
Onset of action: 24-48 hours
Maximum effect: 10-15 days after continuous therapy
Duration: May persist up to 6 weeks

Usual Dosage Oral:
Preoperative thyroidectomy: Children and Adults: Given 10-14 days before surgery: 0.1-0.3 mL (3-5 drops) strong iodine (Lugol's solution) 3 times/day

Graves' disease in neonates: 1 drop strong iodine (Lugol's solution) 3 times/day

Thyrotoxic crisis: Children and Adults: 1 mL strong iodine (Lugol's solution) 3 times/day

Administration Oral: Administer after meals with food or milk or dilute with a large quantity of water, fruit juice, milk, or broth

Monitoring Parameters
Thyroid function tests, signs/symptoms of hyperthyroidism; thyroid function should be monitored in pregnant women, neonates, and young infants if repeat doses are required following radioactive iodine exposure

Dosage Forms Excipient information presented when available (limited, particularly for generics); consult specific product labeling.
Solution, oral: Potassium iodide 100 mg/mL and iodine 50 mg/mL (480 mL)
Solution, topical: Potassium iodide 100 mg/mL and iodine 50 mg/mL (8 mL)

References
"American Academy of Pediatrics Committee on Environmental Health. Radiation Disasters and Children," *Pediatrics*, 2003, 111(6 Pt 1):1455-66.

Kauffman CA, Hajjeh R, and Chapman SW, "Practice Guidelines for the Management of Patients With Sporotrichosis. For the Mycoses Study Group. Infectious Diseases Society of America," *Clin Infect Dis*, 2000, 30(4):684-7.

"Potassium Iodide as a Thyroid Blocking Agent in a Radiation Emergency: Final Recommendations on Use," Washington DC, Bureau of Radiological Health and Bureau of Drugs, Food and Drug Administration, 1982.

U.S. Food and Drug Administration, "FDA's Guidance on Protection of Children and Adults Against Thyroid Cancer in Case of Nuclear Accident," FDA Talk Paper. Available at: http://www.fda.gov/bbs/topics/answers/2001/ans01126.html. Accessed January 11, 2002.

Potassium Phosphate (poe TASS ee um FOS fate)

Medication Safety Issues
Sound-alike/look-alike issues:
Neutra-Phos®-K may be confused with K-Phos Neutral®

High alert medication: The Institute for Safe Medication Practices (ISMP) includes this medication (I.V. formulation) among its list of drugs which have a heightened risk of causing significant patient harm when used in error.

Per JCAHO recommendations, concentrated electrolyte solutions should not be available in patient care areas.

Consider special storage requirements for intravenous potassium salts; I.V. potassium salts have been administered IVP in error, leading to fatal outcomes.

Safe Prescribing: Because inorganic phosphate exists as monobasic and dibasic anions, with the mixture of valences dependent on pH, ordering by mEq amounts is unreliable and may lead to large dosing errors. In addition, I.V. phosphate is available in the sodium and potassium salt; therefore, the content of these cations must be considered when ordering phosphate. The most reliable method of ordering I.V. phosphate is by millimoles, then specifying the potassium or sodium salt. For example, an order for 15 mmol of phosphate as potassium phosphate in one liter of normal saline.

U.S. Brand Names Neutra-Phos®-K [OTC] [DSC]

Therapeutic Category Electrolyte Supplement, Oral; Electrolyte Supplement, Parenteral; Phosphate Salt; Potassium Salt

Generic Available Yes: Injection

Use Treatment and prevention of hypophosphatemia; source of phosphate in large volume I.V. fluids

Pregnancy Risk Factor C

Pregnancy Considerations Reproduction studies have not been conducted with this product.

Breast-Feeding Considerations Phosphorus, sodium, and potassium are normal constituents of human milk.

Contraindications Hypersensitivity to phosphate (salts) or any component; hyperphosphatemia, hyperkalemia, hypocalcemia, hypomagnesemia, severe renal impairment, severe tissue trauma, heat cramps, CHF, patients with phosphate kidney stones

Warnings Parenteral **potassium** salt forms should be administered only in patients with adequate urine flow; must be diluted before I.V. use and infused slowly (see Administration), and patients must be on a cardiac monitor during intermittent infusions

Precautions Use with caution in patients with renal impairment, patients receiving potassium-sparing drugs (potassium salt forms), patients with adrenal insufficiency, cirrhosis

Adverse Reactions

Cardiovascular: Hypotension, edema, arrhythmias, heart block, cardiac arrest

Central nervous system: Tetany, mental confusion, seizures, dizziness, headache

Endocrine & metabolic: Hyperphosphatemia, hyperkalemia, hypocalcemia

Gastrointestinal: Nausea, vomiting, diarrhea, flatulence (oral use)

Local: Phlebitis (parenteral forms)

Neuromuscular & skeletal: Paresthesia, bone and joint pain, arthralgia, weakness, muscle cramps

Renal: Acute renal failure

Clinical manifestations of hypophosphatemia by systems:

Neuromuscular: Muscle weakness, anorexia, tremor, paresthesia, convulsions, coma, hyporeflexia, irritability, numbness, abnormal EEG, cardiomyopathy, respiratory failure, inability to wean from ventilator

Hematologic: Rhabdomyolysis, hemolytic anemia, oxygen release decreased, chemotaxis decreased, phagocytosis decreased, platelet survival decreased, myoglobinuria, thrombocytopenia

Skeletal: Osteomalacia, joint arthralgias, pathologic fractures

Drug Interactions

Avoid Concomitant Use There are no known interactions where it is recommended to avoid concomitant use.

Increased Effect/Toxicity

Potassium Phosphate may increase the levels/effects of: ACE Inhibitors; Angiotensin II Receptor Blockers; Potassium-Sparing Diuretics

The levels/effects of Potassium Phosphate may be increased by: Bisphosphonate Derivatives; Eplerenone

Decreased Effect

The levels/effects of Potassium Phosphate may be decreased by: Antacids; Calcium Salts; Iron Salts; Magnesium Salts; Sucralfate

Food Interactions Avoid giving with oxalate (ie, berries, nuts, chocolate, beans, celery, tomatoes) or phytate-containing foods (ie, bran, whole wheat)

Stability Phosphate salts may precipitate when mixed with calcium salts; solubility is improved in parenteral nutrition solutions which contain amino acids; check with a pharmacist to determine compatibility

Mechanism of Action Phosphorus is an essential mineral that is usually found in nature combined with oxygen as phosphate. It participates in bone deposition, calcium metabolism, as part of molecules that regulate many coenzymes, steps in the clotting cascade, and functions of the immune system. It is a component of the lipid bilayer of cell membranes in the form of phospholipids and of other intracellular compounds like nucleic acids and nucleoproteins. It acts as a buffer for the maintenance of plasma and urinary pH.

Pharmacokinetics (Adult data unless noted)

Absorption: Oral: 1% to 20%

Elimination: Oral forms excreted in feces; I.V. forms are excreted in the urine with over 80% to 90% of dose reabsorbed by the kidney

Usual Dosage Note: Consider the contribution of potassium when determining the appropriate phosphate replacement.

Phosphorus - Recommended Daily Allowance (RDA) and Estimated Average Requirement (EAR):

0-6 months:
  EAR: 3.2 mmol/day (adequate intake)
7-12 months:
  EAR: 8.9 mmol/day (adequate intake)
1-3 years:
  RDA: 14.8 mmol/day
  EAR: 12.3 mmol/day
4-8 years:
  RDA: 16.1 mmol/day
  EAR: 13.1 mmol/day
9-18 years:
  RDA: 40.3 mmol/day
  EAR: 34 mmol/day
19-30 years:
  RDA: 22.6 mmol/day
  EAR: 18.7 mmol/day

Hypophosphatemia: Hypophosphatemia does not necessarily equate with phosphate depletion. Hypophosphatemia may occur in the presence of low, normal, or high total body phosphate and conversely, phosphate depletion may exist with normal, low, or elevated levels of serum phosphate (Gaasbeek, 2005). It is difficult to provide concrete guidelines for the treatment of severe hypophosphatemia because the extent of total body deficits and response to therapy are difficult to predict. Aggressive doses of phosphate may result in a transient serum elevation followed by redistribution into intracellular compartments or bone tissue. Various regimens for replacement of phosphate in adults have been studied. The regimens below have only been studied in adult patients, however, many institutions have used them in children safely and successfully.

I.V. doses may be incorporated into the patient's maintenance I.V. fluids; intermittent I.V. infusion should be reserved for severe depletion situations. **Note:** Doses listed as mmol of **phosphate** (see also Additional Information).

Intermittent I.V. infusion: It is recommended that repletion of severe hypophosphatemia be done I.V. because large doses of oral phosphate may cause diarrhea and intestinal absorption may be unreliable.

Children and Adults: **Note:** There are no prospective studies of parenteral phosphate replacement in children. The following weight-based guidelines for adult dosing may be cautiously employed in pediatric patients. Guidelines differ based on degree of illness, use of TPN, and severity of hypophosphatemia.

General replacement guidelines (Lentz, 1978): **Note:** The initial dose may be increased by 25% to 50% if the patient is symptomatic secondary to hypophosphatemia and lowered by 25% to 50% if the patient is hypercalcemic.

Low dose: 0.08 mmol/kg over 6 hours; use if losses are recent and uncomplicated

Intermediate dose: 0.16-0.24 mmol/kg over 4-6 hours; use if serum phosphorus level 0.5-1 mg/dL (0.16-0.32 mmol/L)

High dose: 0.36 mmol/kg over 6 hours; use if serum phosphorus <0.5 mg/dL (<0.16 mmol/L)

Patients receiving TPN (Clark, 1995):

Low dose: 0.16 mmol/kg over 4-6 hours; use if serum phosphorus level 2.3-3 mg/dL (0.73- 0.96 mmol/L)

Intermediate dose: 0.32 mmol/kg over 4-6 hours; use if serum phosphorus level 1.6-2.2 mg/dL (0.51-0.72 mmol/L)

High dose: 0.64 mmol/kg over 8-12 hours; use if serum phosphorus <1.5 mg/dL (< 0.5 mmol/L)

Critically ill adult trauma patients receiving TPN (Brown, 2006):

Low dose: 0.32 mmol/kg over 4-6 hours; use if serum phosphorus level 2.3-3 mg/dL (0.73-0.96 mmol/L)

Intermediate dose: 0.64 mmol/kg over 4-6 hours; use if serum phosphorus level 1.6-2.2 mg/dL (0.51-0.72 mmol/L)

High dose: 1 mmol/kg over 8-12 hours; use if serum phosphorus <1.5 mg/dL (<0.5 mmol/L)

Alternative method in critically ill patients (Kingston, 1985):

Low dose: 0.25 mmol/kg over 4 hours; use if serum phosphorus level 0.5-1 mg/dL (0.16-0.32 mmol/L)

Moderate dose: 0.5 mmol/kg over 4 hours; use if serum phosphorus level <0.5 mg/dL (<0.16 mmol/L)

Adults: 15 mmol/dose over 2 hours; use if serum phosphorus <2 mg/dL (0.65 mmol/L); may repeat in 6- to 8-hour intervals if repeat serum phosphorus (at least 6 hours postdose) <2 mg/dL (0.65 mmol/L); not to exceed 45 mmol/24 hours (Rosen, 1995)

Maintenance:

Children:

I.V.:

Neonates: 0.8-1.5 mmol/kg/day

Infants and Children < 25 kg: 0.5-1.5 mmol/kg/day

Children 25-45 kg: 0.5-1 mmol/kg/day

Oral: 2-3 mmol/kg/day in divided doses (including dietary intake; see Additional Information)

Adults:

I.V.: 50-70 mmol/day

Oral: 50-150 mmol/day in divided doses (including dietary intake; see Additional Information)

Administration

Oral: Administer with food to reduce the risk of diarrhea; contents of 1 packet should be diluted in 75 mL water before administration; administer tablets with a full glass of water; maintain adequate fluid intake

Parenteral: For intermittent I.V. infusion: Peripheral line: Dilute to a maximum concentration of 0.05 mmol/mL; Central line: Dilute to a maximum concentration of 0.12 mmol/mL (maximum concentrations were determined with consideration for maximum potassium concentrations); maximum rate of infusion: 0.06 mmol/kg/hour; do **not** infuse with calcium-containing I.V. fluids

Monitoring Parameters Serum potassium, calcium, phosphorus, renal function, reflexes; cardiac monitor (when intermittent infusion or high-dose I.V. replacement of potassium salts needed)

Reference Range Note: There is a diurnal variation with the nadir at 1100, plateau at 1600, and peak in the early evening (Gaasbeek, 2005); 1 mmol/L phosphate = 3.1 mg/dL phosphorus

Newborns: 4.2-9 mg/dL phosphorus (1.36-2.91 mmol/L phosphate)

6 weeks to 18 months: 3.8-6.7 mg/dL phosphorus (1.23-2.16 mmol/L phosphate)

18 months to 3 years: 2.9-5.9 mg/dL phosphorus (0.94-1.91 mmol/L phosphate)

3-15 years: 3.6-5.6 mg/dL phosphorus (1.16-1.81 mmol/L phosphate)

>15 years: 2.5-5 mg/dL phosphorus (0.81-1.62 mmol/L phosphate)

Hypophosphatemia:

Moderate: 1-2 mg/dL phosphorus (0.32-0.65 mmol/L phosphate)

Severe: <1 mg/dL phosphorus (<0.32 mmol/L phosphate)

Additional Information Each mmol of phosphate contains 31 mg elemental phosphorus; 1 mmol/L phosphate = 3.1 mg/dL phosphorus; cow's milk is a good source of phosphate with 1 mg elemental (0.032 mmol) elemental phosphate per mL

With orders for I.V. phosphate, there is considerable confusion associated with the use of millimoles (mmol) versus milliequivalents (mEq) to express the phosphate requirement. Because inorganic phosphate exists as monobasic and dibasic anions, with the mixture of valences dependent on pH, ordering by mEq amounts is unreliable and may lead to large dosing errors. In addition, I.V. phosphate is available in the sodium and potassium salt; therefore, the content of these cations must be considered when ordering phosphate. The most reliable method of ordering I.V. phosphate is by millimoles, then specifying the potassium or sodium salt.

Dosage Forms Excipient information presented when available (limited, particularly for generics); consult specific product labeling. [DSC] = Discontinued product

Injection, solution: Potassium 4.4 mEq and phosphorus 3 mmol per mL (5 mL, 15 mL, 50 mL) [equivalent to potassium 170 mg and elemental phosphorus 93 mg per mL]

Powder for oral solution:

Neutra-Phos®-K: Monobasic potassium phosphate and dibasic potassium phosphate per packet (100s) [equivalent to elemental potassium 556 mg (14.25 mEq) and phosphorus 250 mg (14.25 mEq) per packet; sodium and sugar free; fruit flavor] [DSC]

References

Brown KA, Dickerson, RN, Morgan, RN, et al, "A New Graduated Dosing Regimen for Phosphorus Replacement in Patients Receiving Nutrition Support," *JPEN*, 2006, 30(3):209-14.

Clark CL, Sacks GS, Dickerson RN, et al, "Treatment of Hypophosphatemia in Patients Receiving Specialized Nutrition Support Using a Graduated Dosing Scheme: Results From a Prospective Clinical Trial," *Crit Care Med*, 1995, 23(9):1504-11.

"Dietary Reference Intakes for Calcium, Phosphorus, Magnesium, Vitamin D, and Fluoride. Standing Committee on the Scientific Evaluation of Dietary Reference Intakes, Food and Nutrition Board, Institute of Medicine," National Academy of Sciences, Washington, DC: National Academy Press, 1997.

Gaasbeek A and Meinders AE, "Hypophosphatemia: An Update on Its Etiology and Treatment," *Am J Med*, 2005, 118(10):1094-101.

Kingston M and Al-Siba'i MB, "Treatment of Severe Hypophosphatemia," *Crit Care Med*, 1985, 13(1):16-8

Lentz RD, Brown DM, and Kjellstrand CM, "Treatment of Severe Hypophosphatemia," *Ann Intern Med*, 1978, 89(6):941-4.

Lloyd CW and Johnson CE, "Management of Hypophosphatemia," *Clin Pharm*, 1988, 7(2):123-8.

Rosen GH, Boullata JI, O'Rangers EA, et al, "Intravenous Phosphate Repletion Regimen for Critically III Patients With Moderate Hypophosphatemia," *Crit Care Med*, 1995, 23(7):1204-10.

Potassium Phosphate and Sodium Phosphate

(poe TASS ee um FOS fate & SOW dee um FOS fate)

Medication Safety Issues

Sound-alike/look-alike issues:

K-Phos® Neutral may be confused with Neutra-Phos-K®

U.S. Brand Names K-Phos® MF; K-Phos® Neutral; K-Phos® No. 2; Neutra-Phos® [OTC] [DSC]; Phos-Nak; Phospha 250™ Neutral; Uro-KP-Neutral®

Therapeutic Category Electrolyte Supplement, Oral; Phosphate Salt; Potassium Salt; Sodium Salt

Generic Available Yes

Use Treatment and prevention of hypophosphatemia; short-term treatment of constipation

Pregnancy Risk Factor C

Contraindications Hypersensitivity to phosphate (salts) or any component; hyperphosphatemia, hyperkalemia, hypocalcemia, hypomagnesemia, hypernatremia, severe renal impairment, severe tissue trauma, heat cramps, CHF, patients with phosphate kidney stones

Precautions Use with caution in patients with renal impairment, patients receiving potassium-sparing drugs (potassium salt forms), patients with adrenal insufficiency, cirrhosis

Adverse Reactions

Cardiovascular: Hypotension, edema, arrhythmias, heart block, cardiac arrest

Central nervous system: Tetany, mental confusion, seizures, dizziness, headache

Endocrine & metabolic: Hyperphosphatemia, hyperkalemia, hypocalcemia, hypernatremia

Gastrointestinal: Nausea, vomiting, diarrhea, flatulence (oral use)

Neuromuscular & skeletal: Paresthesia, bone and joint pain, arthralgia, weakness, muscle cramps

Renal: Acute renal failure

Drug Interactions

Avoid Concomitant Use There are no known interactions where it is recommended to avoid concomitant use.

Increased Effect/Toxicity

Potassium Phosphate and Sodium Phosphate may increase the levels/effects of: ACE Inhibitors; Angiotensin II Receptor Blockers; Potassium-Sparing Diuretics

The levels/effects of Potassium Phosphate and Sodium Phosphate may be increased by: Bisphosphonate Derivatives; Eplerenone

Decreased Effect

The levels/effects of Potassium Phosphate and Sodium Phosphate may be decreased by: Antacids; Calcium Salts; Iron Salts; Magnesium Salts; Sucralfate

Food Interactions Avoid giving with oxalate (ie, berries, nuts, chocolate, beans, celery, tomatoes) or phytate-containing foods (ie, bran, whole wheat)

Stability Store at room temperature.

Mechanism of Action Phosphorus is an essential mineral that is usually found in nature combined with oxygen as phosphate. It participates in bone deposition, calcium metabolism, as part of molecules that regulate many coenzymes, steps in the clotting cascade, and functions of the immune system. It is a component of the lipid bilayer of cell membranes in the form of phospholipids and of other intracellular compounds like nucleic acids and nucleoproteins. It acts as a buffer for the maintenance of plasma and urinary pH. When administered orally or rectally as a laxative, it exerts osmotic effect in the small intestine by drawing water into the lumen of the gut, producing distension, promoting peristalsis, and evacuation of the bowel.

Pharmacodynamics Onset of action (catharsis):

Oral: 3-6 hours

Pharmacokinetics (Adult data unless noted)

Absorption: Oral: 1% to 20%

Elimination: Oral forms excreted in feces

Usual Dosage Note: Consider the contribution of sodium and potassium cations when determining appropriate phosphate replacement.

Phosphorus-Recommended Daily Allowance (RDA) and Estimated Average Requirement (EAR)

0-6 months:

EAR: 3.2 mmol/day (adequate intake)

7-12 months:

EAR: 8.9 mmol/day (adequate intake)

1-3 years:

RDA: 14.8 mmol/day

EAR: 12.3 mmol/day

4-8 years:

RDA: 16.1 mmol/day

EAR: 13.1 mmol/day

9-18 years:

RDA: 40.3 mmol/day

EAR: 34 mmol/day

19-30 years:

RDA: 22.6 mmol/day

EAR: 18.7 mmol/day

Maintenance: Oral:

Children: 2-3 mmol/kg/day in divided doses

Adults: 50-150 mmol/day in divided doses

Laxative: Oral: Uro-KP-Neutral®:

Children ≤4 years: 1 capsule or packet (250 mg phosphorus/8 mmol) 4 times/day; dilute as instructed

Children >4 years and Adults: 1-2 capsules or packets (250-500 mg phosphorus/8-16 mmol) 4 times/day; dilute as instructed

Administration Oral: Administer with food to reduce the risk of diarrhea; contents of 1 packet should be diluted in 75 mL water before administration; administer tablets/caplets with a full glass of water; maintain adequate fluid intake; dilute oral solution with an equal volume of cool water

Monitoring Parameters Serum potassium, sodium, calcium, phosphorus, renal function, reflexes; stool output (laxative use)

Reference Range Note: There is a diurnal variation with the nadir at 1100, plateau at 1600, and peak in the early evening (Gaasbeek, 2005); 1 mmol/L phosphate = 3.1 mg/dL phosphorus

Newborns: 4.2-9 mg/dL phosphorus (1.36-2.91 mmol/L phosphate)

6 weeks to 18 months: 3.8-6.7 mg/dL phosphorus (1.23-2.16 mmol/L phosphate)

18 months to 3 years: 2.9-5.9 mg/dL phosphorus (0.94-1.91 mmol/L phosphate)

3-15 years: 3.6-5.6 mg/dL phosphorus (1.16-1.81 mmol/L phosphate)

>15 years: 2.5-5 mg/dL phosphorus (0.81-1.62 mmol/L phosphate)

Hypophosphatemia:

Moderate: 1-2 mg/dL phosphorus (0.32-0.65 mmol/L phosphate)

Severe: <1 mg/dL phosphorus (<0.32 mmol/L phosphate)

Additional Information Each mmol of phosphate contains 31 mg elemental phosphorus; 1 mmol/L phosphate = 3.1 mg/dL phosphorus; cow's milk is a good source of phosphate with 1 mg elemental (0.032 mmol) elemental phosphate per mL

Dosage Forms Excipient information presented when available (limited, particularly for generics); consult specific product labeling. [DSC] = Discontinued product

Caplet:

Uro-KP-Neutral®: Dipotassium phosphate, disodium phosphate, and monobasic sodium phosphate [equivalent to elemental phosphorus 258 mg, sodium 262.4 mg (10.8 mEq), and potassium 49.4 mg (1.3 smEq)]

Powder, for oral solution:

Neutra-Phos®: Dibasic potassium phosphate, monobasic potassium phosphate, dibasic sodium phosphate, and monosodium phosphate per packet (100s) [equivalent to elemental phosphorus 250 mg (14.25 mEq), sodium 164 mg (7.1 mEq), and potassium 278 mg (7.1 mEq) per packet] [DSC]

Phos-NaK: Dibasic potassium phosphate, monobasic potassium phosphate, dibasic sodium phosphate, and monosodium phosphate per packet (100s) [sugar free; equivalent to elemental phosphorus 250 mg, sodium 160 mg (6.9 mEq), and potassium 280 mg (7.1 mEq) per packet; fruit flavor]

Tablet:

K-Phos® MF: Potassium acid phosphate 155 mg and sodium acid phosphate 350 mg [equivalent to elemental phosphorus 125.6 mg, sodium 67 mg (2.9 mEq), and potassium 44.5 mg (1.1 mEq)]

K-Phos® Neutral: Monobasic potassium phosphate 155 mg, dibasic sodium phosphate 852 mg, and monobasic sodium phosphate 130 mg [equivalent to elemental phosphorus 250 mg, sodium 298 mg (13 mEq), and potassium 45 mg (1.1 mEq)]

K-Phos® No. 2: Potassium acid phosphate 305 mg and sodium acid phosphate 700 mg [equivalent to elemental phosphorus 250 mg, sodium 134 mg (5.8 mEq), and potassium 88 mg (2.3 mEq)]

Phospha 250™ Neutral: Monobasic potassium phosphate 155 mg, dibasic sodium phosphate 852 mg, and monobasic sodium phosphate 130 mg [equivalent to elemental phosphorus 250 mg, sodium 298 mg (13 mEq), and potassium 45 mg (1.1 mEq)]

References

Gaasbeek A and Meinders AE, "Hypophosphatemia: An Update on Its Etiology and Treatment," *Am J Med*, 2005, 118(10):1094-101.

◆ **PPSV** *see* Pneumococcal Polysaccharide Vaccine (Polyvalent) *on page 1125*

◆ **PPSV23** *see* Pneumococcal Polysaccharide Vaccine (Polyvalent) *on page 1125*

◆ **PPV23** *see* Pneumococcal Polysaccharide Vaccine (Polyvalent) *on page 1125*

Pralidoxime (pra li DOKS eem)

Medication Safety Issues

Sound-alike/look-alike issues:

Pralidoxime may be confused with pramoxine, pyridoxine

Protopam® may be confused with protamine, Protropin®

U.S. Brand Names Protopam®

Canadian Brand Names Protopam®

Therapeutic Category Antidote, Anticholinesterase; Antidote, Organophosphate Poisoning

Generic Available No

Use Reverse muscle paralysis associated with toxic exposure to organophosphate anticholinesterase pesticides and chemicals; control of overdosage by anticholinesterase drugs used to treat myasthenia gravis (neostigmine, pyridostigmine)

Pregnancy Risk Factor C

Lactation Excretion in breast milk unknown/not recommended

Contraindications Hypersensitivity to pralidoxime or any component; poisonings due to phosphorus, inorganic phosphates, or organic phosphates without anticholinesterase activity

Warnings Not indicated as an antidote for carbamate classes of pesticides and may increase toxicity of carbaryl

Precautions Use with caution in patients with myasthenia gravis; dosage modification required in patients with impaired renal function; use with caution in patients receiving theophylline, succinylcholine, phenothiazines, respiratory depressants (eg, narcotic, barbiturates); rapid I.V. infusion has been associated with tachycardia, laryngospasm, and muscle rigidity

Adverse Reactions

Cardiovascular: Tachycardia (after rapid I.V. infusion), hypertension

Central nervous system: Dizziness, headache, drowsiness

Dermatologic: Rash

Gastrointestinal: Nausea

Local: Pain at injection site after I.M. use

Neuromuscular & skeletal: Muscular weakness, muscle rigidity (after rapid I.V. infusion), CPK elevated (transient)

Ocular: Blurred vision, diplopia

Respiratory: Hyperventilation, laryngospasm (after rapid I.V. administration)

Drug Interactions

Avoid Concomitant Use There are no known interactions where it is recommended to avoid concomitant use.

Increased Effect/Toxicity There are no known significant interactions involving an increase in effect.

Decreased Effect There are no known significant interactions involving a decrease in effect.

Mechanism of Action Reactivates cholinesterase that had been inactivated by phosphorylation as a result of exposure to organophosphate pesticides; removes the phosphoryl group from the active site of the inactivated enzyme

Pharmacokinetics (Adult data unless noted)

Half-life: 74-77 minutes

Time to peak serum concentration: I.V.: Within 5-15 minutes

Elimination: 80% to 90% excreted unchanged in urine 12 hours after administration

Usual Dosage

Organophosphate poisoning:

Children: I.M., I.V. (use in conjunction with atropine): 20-50 mg/kg/dose; repeat in 1-2 hours if muscle weakness has not been relieved, then at 10- to 12-hour intervals if cholinergic signs recur

Adults: I.M., I.V. (use in conjunction with atropine): 1-2 g; repeat in 1-2 hours if muscle weakness has not been relieved, then at 10- to 12-hour intervals if cholinergic signs recur

Treatment of toxicity from medications used to treat myasthenia gravis: Adults: I.V.: 1-2 g followed by increments of 250 mg every 5 minutes

Administration Parenteral: Reconstitute with 20 mL SWI (preservative free) resulting in 50 mg/mL solution; dilute in NS to 20 mg/mL and infuse over 15-30 minutes; if a more rapid onset of effect is desired or in a fluid-restricted situation, the maximum concentration is 50 mg/mL; the maximum rate of infusion is over 5 minutes and not exceeding 200 mg/minute

Monitoring Parameters Heart rate, respiratory rate, blood pressure, continuous ECG, muscle strength

Dosage Forms Excipient information presented when available (limited, particularly for generics); consult specific product labeling.

Injection, powder for reconstitution, as chloride:

Protopam®: 1 g

Injection, solution: 300 mg/mL (2 mL) [contains benzyl alcohol; prefilled auto injector]

◆ **Pralidoxime Chloride** *see* Pralidoxime *on page 1144*

◆ **Pravachol®** *see* Pravastatin *on page 1145*

Pravastatin (PRA va stat in)

Medication Safety Issues
Sound-alike/look-alike issues:
Pravachol® may be confused with atorvastatin, Prevacid®, Prinivil®, propranolol
Pravastatin may be confused with nystatin, pitavastatin, prasugrel

Related Information
Normal Laboratory Values for Children on page 1672

U.S. Brand Names Pravachol®

Canadian Brand Names Apo-Pravastatin®; CO Pravastatin; Dom-Pravastatin; Mylan-Pravastatin; Novo-Pravastatin; Nu-Pravastatin; PHL-Pravastatin; PMS-Pravastatin; Pravachol®; RAN™-Pravastatin; ratio-Pravastatin; Riva-Pravastatin; Sandoz-Pravastatin; ZYM-Pravastatin

Therapeutic Category Antilipemic Agent; HMG-CoA Reductase Inhibitor

Generic Available Yes

Use Hyperlipidemia: Adjunct to dietary therapy to decrease elevated serum total and low density lipoprotein cholesterol (LDL-C), apolipoprotein B (apo-B), and triglyceride levels, and to increase high density lipoprotein cholesterol (HDL-C) in patients with primary hypercholesterolemia (heterozygous, familial and nonfamilial) and mixed dyslipidemia (Fredrickson types IIa and IIb); treatment of homozygous familial hypercholesterolemia (see Additional Information for recommendations on initiating hypercholesterolemia pharmacologic treatment in children ≥8 years); treatment of isolated hypertriglyceridemia (Fredrickson type IV) and type III hyperlipoproteinemia; treatment of primary dysbetalipoproteinemia (Fredrickson Type III)

Primary prevention of cardiovascular disease in high risk patients; risk factors include: Age ≥55 years, smoking, hypertension, low HDL-C or family history of early coronary heart disease

Pregnancy Risk Factor X

Pregnancy Considerations Cholesterol biosynthesis may be important in fetal development. Contraindicated in pregnancy. Administer to women of childbearing potential only when conception is highly unlikely and patients have been informed of potential hazards.

Lactation Enters breast milk/contraindicated

Contraindications Hypersensitivity to pravastatin or any component; active liver disease; unexplained persistent elevations of serum transaminases; pregnancy; breast-feeding

Warnings Rhabdomyolysis with or without acute renal failure secondary to myoglobinuria has occurred rarely. Risk is increased with concurrent use of HMG-CoA reductase inhibitors and amiodarone, clarithromycin, danazol, diltiazem, fluvoxamine, amprenavir, delavirdine, indinavir, nefazodone, nelfinavir, ritonavir, verapamil, troleandomycin, cyclosporine, fibric acid derivatives, erythromycin, niacin, or azole antifungals. Assess the risk versus benefit before combining any of these medications with pravastatin. Temporarily discontinue pravastatin in any patient experiencing an acute or serious condition predisposing to renal failure secondary to rhabdomyolysis (eg, sepsis, hypotension, major surgery, trauma, severe metabolic, endocrine or electrolyte disorders, or uncontrolled seizures).

Precautions Persistent increases in serum transaminases have occurred (incidence in clinical trials ≤1.2%); liver function tests must be monitored at the initiation of therapy, prior to an increase in dosage, and then periodically (eg, semiannually), thereafter. Use with caution in patients with a recent history of liver disease, clinical signs of liver disease, or heavy users of alcohol.

Adverse Reactions
Cardiovascular: Angina, chest pain

Central nervous system: Dizziness, headache, somnolence, fatigue, sleep disturbances, depression, anxiety, nervousness, libido change, fever, vertigo

Dermatologic: Rash, pruritus, urticaria, dry skin, alopecia, dermatitis; rare: Photosensitivity, toxic epidermal necrolysis, erythema multiforme including Stevens-Johnson syndrome

Endocrine & metabolic: Gynecomastia

Gastrointestinal: Constipation, heartburn, flatulence, abdominal pain, diarrhea, nausea, pancreatitis, gastroenteritis, vomiting, appetite decreased, taste perversion

Genitourinary: Urinary frequency, dysuria, nocturia

Hematologic: Hemolytic anemia (rare)

Hepatic: Serum transaminases elevated, hepatitis, cholestatic jaundice; rare: Cirrhosis, fulminant hepatic necrosis, hepatoma

Neuromuscular & skeletal: CPK elevated, myalgia, muscle cramps, myopathy, peripheral nerve palsy, rhabdomyolysis, arthralgias, muscle weakness, dermatomyositis

Ocular: Blurred vision, diplopia

Respiratory: Rhinitis, cough, dyspnea, URI

Miscellaneous: Hypersensitivity reactions, influenza, lupus erythematosus-like syndrome

Drug Interactions
Metabolism/Transport Effects Substrate of CYP3A4 (minor), P-glycoprotein, SLCO1B1; **Inhibits** CYP2C9 (weak), 2D6 (weak), 3A4 (weak)

Avoid Concomitant Use There are no known interactions where it is recommended to avoid concomitant use.

Increased Effect/Toxicity
Pravastatin may increase the levels/effects of: DAPTOmycin; Vitamin K Antagonists

The levels/effects of Pravastatin may be increased by: Antifungal Agents (Azole Derivatives, Systemic); Colchicine; CycloSPORINE; CycloSPORINE (Systemic); Eltrombopag; Fenofibrate; Fenofibric Acid; Gemfibrozil; Niacin; Niacinamide; P-Glycoprotein Inhibitors; Protease Inhibitors; Rifamycin Derivatives

Decreased Effect
The levels/effects of Pravastatin may be decreased by: Antacids; Bile Acid Sequestrants; P-Glycoprotein Inducers; Phenytoin; Rifamycin Derivatives

Stability Tablets should be stored in well closed containers at controlled room temperature between 20°C to 25°C (68°F to 77°F); protect from light

Mechanism of Action Pravastatin is a selective, competitive inhibitor of 3-hydroxy-3-methylglutaryl-coenzyme A (HMG-CoA) reductase, the enzyme that catalyzes the rate-limiting step in cholesterol biosynthesis

Pharmacodynamics
Onset of action: 2 weeks
Maximum effect: After 4 weeks
LDL-reduction: 40 mg/day: 34% (for each doubling of this dose, LDL-C is lowered by ~6%)

Pharmacokinetics (Adult data unless noted)
Absorption: Oral: Rapidly absorbed
Distribution: V_d: Adults: 0.46 L/kg
Protein binding: 43% to 55%
Metabolism: Extensive first-pass metabolism to metabolites with minimal activity
Bioavailability: Absolute: 17%
Half-life:
Children: 1.6 hours (range: 0.85-4.2 hours)
Adults: 2.6-3.2 hours
Time to peak serum concentration: 1-1.5 hours
Elimination: ~20% excreted in urine unchanged and 70% in feces

Usual Dosage Oral: Dosage should be individualized according to the baseline LDL-C level, the recommended goal of therapy, and patient response; adjustments should be made at intervals of 4 weeks

Hyperlipidemia:

Children 8-13 years: 20 mg once daily; doses >20 mg have not been studied

Adolescents 14-18 years: 40 mg once daily; doses >40 mg have not been studied

Adolescents >18 years and Adults: 40 mg once daily; may increase dosage up to 80 mg once daily as indicated

Dosing adjustment in renal impairment: Adults: Initiate dosage at 10 mg once daily

Dosing adjustment in hepatic impairment: Adults: Initiate dosage at 10 mg once daily; avoid use in active liver disease

Dosing adjustment in patient's receiving concomitant cyclosporine: 20 mg once daily

Administration Oral: May be taken without regard to meals or time of day

Monitoring Parameters Serum cholesterol (total and fractionated), CPK; liver function tests (see Precautions)

Reference Range See Related Information for age- and gender-specific serum cholesterol, LDL-C, TG, and HDL concentrations.

Patient Information May rarely cause photosensitivity reactions (eg, exposure to sunlight may cause severe sunburn, skin rash, redness, or itching); avoid direct exposure to sunlight. Report severe and unresolved gastric upset, any vision changes, muscle pain and weakness, changes in color of urine or stool, yellowing of skin or eyes, and any unusual bruising. Female patients of childbearing age must be counseled to use 2 effective forms of contraception simultaneously, unless absolute abstinence is the chosen method; this drug may cause severe fetal defects. Avoid the herbal medicine St John's wort.

Additional Information The current recommendation for pharmacologic treatment of hypercholesterolemia in children is limited to children ≥8 years of age and is based on LDL-C concentrations and the presence of coronary vascular disease (CVD) risk factors (see table and Daniels, 2008). In adults, for each 1% lowering in LDL-C, the relative risk for major cardiovascular events is reduced by ~1%. For more specific risk assessment and treatment recommendations for adults, see NCEP ATPIII, 2001.

Recommendations for Initiating Pharmacologic Treatment in Children ≥8 Years[1]

No risk factors for CVD	LDL ≥190 mg/dL despite 6-month to 1-year diet therapy
Family history of premature CVD or ≥2 CVD risk factors present, including obesity, hypertension, or cigarette smoking	LDL ≥160 mg/dL despite 6-month to 1-year diet therapy
Diabetes mellitus present	LDL ≥130 mg/dL

[1]Adapted from Daniels SR, Greer FR, and Committee on Nutrition, "Lipid Screening and Cardiovascular Health in Childhood," *Pediatrics*, 2008, 122(1):198-208.

Dosage Forms Excipient information presented when available (limited, particularly for generics); consult specific product labeling.

Tablet, as sodium: 10 mg, 20 mg, 40 mg, 80 mg

Pravachol®: 10 mg, 20 mg, 40 mg, 80 mg

References

American Academy of Pediatrics. Committee on Nutrition, "Cholesterol in Childhood," *Pediatrics*, 1998, 101(1 Pt 1):141-7.

American Academy of Pediatrics, "National Cholesterol Education Program: Report of the Expert Panel on Blood Cholesterol Levels in Children and Adolescents," *Pediatrics*, 1992, 89(3 Pt 2):525-84.

Daniels SR, Greer FR, and Committee on Nutrition, "Lipid Screening and Cardiovascular Health in Childhood," *Pediatrics*, 2008, 122(1):198-208.

Duplaga BA, "Treatment of Childhood Hypercholesterolemia With HMG-CoA Reductase Inhibitors," *Ann Pharmacother*, 1999, 33(11):1224-7.

Grundy SM, Cleeman JI, Merz CN, et al, "Implications of Recent Clinical Trials for the National Cholesterol Education Program Adult Treatment Panel III Guidelines," *Circulation*, 2004, 110(2):227-39.

Hedman M, Neuvonen PJ, Neuvonen M, et al, "Pharmacokinetics and Pharmacodynamics of Pravastatin in Children With Familial Hypercholesterolemia," *Clin Pharmacol Ther*, 2003, 74(2):178-85.

McCrindle BW, Urbina EM, Dennison BA, et al, "Drug Therapy of High-Risk Lipid Abnormalities in Children and Adolescents: A Scientific Statement from the American Heart Association Atherosclerosis, Hypertension, and Obesity in Youth Committee, Council of Cardiovascular Disease in the Young, With the Council on Cardiovascular Nursing," *Circulation*, 2007, 115(14):1948-67.

"Third Report of the National Cholesterol Education Program Expert Panel on Detection, Evaluation, and Treatment of High Blood Cholesterol in Adults (Adult Treatment Panel III)," May 2001, www.nhlbi.nih.gov/guidelines/cholesterol.

Wiegman A, Hutten BA, de Groot E, et al, "Efficacy and Safety of Statin Therapy in Children With Familial Hypercholesterolemia: A Randomized Controlled Trial," *JAMA*, 2004, 292(3):331-7.

◆ **Pravastatin Sodium** see Pravastatin *on page 1145*

◆ **Praxis ASA EC 81 Mg Daily Dose (Can)** see Aspirin *on page 141*

Praziquantel (pray zi KWON tel)

U.S. Brand Names Biltricide®

Canadian Brand Names Biltricide®

Therapeutic Category Anthelmintic

Generic Available No

Use Treatment of all stages of schistosomiasis caused by *Schistosoma* species pathogenic to humans; also active in the treatment of clonorchiasis, opisthorchiasis, cysticercosis, and many intestinal tapeworm and trematode infections

Pregnancy Risk Factor B

Lactation Enters breast milk

Contraindications Hypersensitivity to praziquantel or any component; ocular cysticercosis, spinal cysticercosis

Precautions Use with caution in patients with severe hepatic disease and in patients with a history of seizures

Adverse Reactions

Central nervous system: Dizziness, drowsiness, fever, headache, vertigo, malaise, CSF reaction syndrome in patients being treated for neurocysticercosis (syndrome includes headache, seizures, intracranial hypertension, CSF protein concentrations elevated, hyperthermia)

Dermatologic: Urticarial rash, itching

Gastrointestinal: Abdominal pain, nausea, vomiting, anorexia, diarrhea

Hematologic: Eosinophilia

Miscellaneous: Diaphoresis

Drug Interactions

Metabolism/Transport Effects Substrate of CYP3A4 (major); **Inhibits** CYP2D6 (weak)

Avoid Concomitant Use

Avoid concomitant use of Praziquantel with any of the following: Rifampin

Increased Effect/Toxicity

The levels/effects of Praziquantel may be increased by: Cimetidine; CYP3A4 Inhibitors (Moderate); CYP3A4 Inhibitors (Strong); Dasatinib; Ketoconazole; Ketoconazole (Systemic)

Decreased Effect

The levels/effects of Praziquantel may be decreased by: Aminoquinolines (Antimalarial); CYP3A4 Inducers (Strong); Deferasirox; Herbs (CYP3A4 Inducers); Rifampin

Mechanism of Action Increases the cell permeability to calcium in schistosomes; causes strong contractions and paralysis of worm musculature leading to detachment of suckers from the blood vessel walls and to dislodgment

Pharmacokinetics (Adult data unless noted)
Absorption: Oral: ~80%
Distribution: CSF concentration is 14% to 20% of plasma concentration; excreted in breast milk
Protein binding: ~80%
Metabolism: Extensive first-pass effect; metabolized by the liver to hydroxylated and conjugated metabolites
Half-life: 0.8-1.5 hours
Metabolites: 4.5 hours
Time to peak serum concentration: Within 1-3 hours
Elimination: Praziquantel and metabolites excreted mainly in urine (99% as metabolites)

Usual Dosage Children and Adults: Oral:
Schistosomiasis:
S. mansoni, S. haematobium: 20 mg/kg/dose twice daily for 1 day
S. japonicum, S. mekongi: 20 mg/kg/dose 3 times/day for 1 day at 4- to 6-hour intervals
Flukes:
Liver, intestine: 75 mg/kg/day divided every 8 hours for 1 day
Lung: 75 mg/kg/day divided every 8 hours for 2 days
Nanophyetus salmincola: 60 mg/kg/day divided every 8 hours for 1 day
Cysticercosis: 50 mg/kg/day divided every 8 hours for 15 days (adjunctive therapy with dexamethasone is recommended for patients with numerous cysts and for those in whom neurologic symptoms or intracranial hypertension develops); for neurocysticercosis, steroids should be administered **prior** to starting praziquantel
Tapeworms: 5-10 mg/kg as a single dose (25 mg/kg for *H. nana*)

Administration Oral: Administer with food; tablets can be halved or quartered; do not chew tablets due to bitter taste

Patient Information Avoid alcohol (increased CNS depression); may cause drowsiness and impair ability to perform activities requiring mental alertness or physical coordination

Dosage Forms Excipient information presented when available (limited, particularly for generics); consult specific product labeling.
Tablet [tri-scored]: 600 mg

References
King CH and Mahmoud AA, "Drug Five Years Later: Praziquantel," *Ann Intern Med*, 1989, 110(4):290-6.
Liu LX and Weller PF, "Antiparasitic Drug," *N Engl J Med*, 1996, 334 (18):1178-84.

Prazosin (PRA zoe sin)

Medication Safety Issues
Sound-alike/look-alike issues:
Prazosin may be confused with predniSONE

International issues:
Prazac® [Denmark] may be confused with Prozac® which is a brand name for fluoxetine in the U.S.
Prazepam [multiple international markets] may be confused with prazosin.

Related Information
Antihypertensive Agents by Class *on page 1481*

U.S. Brand Names Minipress®

Canadian Brand Names Apo-Prazo®; Minipress®; Novo-Prazin; Nu-Prazo

Therapeutic Category Alpha-Adrenergic Blocking Agent, Oral; Antihypertensive Agent; Vasodilator

Generic Available Yes

Use Management of hypertension; severe CHF (in conjunction with diuretics and cardiac glycosides)

Pregnancy Risk Factor C

Lactation Excretion in breast milk unknown/use caution

Contraindications Hypersensitivity to prazosin, quinazolines, or any component

Precautions Marked orthostatic hypotension, syncope, and loss of consciousness may occur with first dose ("first dose phenomenon"). This reaction is more likely to occur in patients receiving beta-blockers, diuretics, low sodium diets or larger first doses (ie, >1 mg/dose in adults); avoid rapid increase in dose; use with caution in patients with renal impairment.

Adverse Reactions
Cardiovascular: Orthostatic hypotension, syncope, palpitations, tachycardia, edema
Central nervous system: Dizziness, lightheadedness, nightmares, drowsiness, headache, hypothermia
Dermatologic: Rash
Endocrine & metabolic: Fluid retention, sexual dysfunction
Gastrointestinal: Nausea, xerostomia
Genitourinary: Urinary frequency
Neuromuscular & skeletal: Weakness
Respiratory: Nasal congestion

Drug Interactions
Metabolism/Transport Effects Induces P-glycoprotein
Avoid Concomitant Use
Avoid concomitant use of Prazosin with any of the following: Alfuzosin; Silodosin; Tamsulosin
Increased Effect/Toxicity
Prazosin may increase the levels/effects of: Alfuzosin; Amifostine; Antihypertensives; Calcium Channel Blockers; Hypotensive Agents; RiTUXimab; Silodosin; Tamsulosin

The levels/effects of Prazosin may be increased by: Alfuzosin; Beta-Blockers; Diazoxide; Herbs (Hypotensive Properties); MAO Inhibitors; Pentoxifylline; Phosphodiesterase 5 Inhibitors; Prostacyclin Analogues; Silodosin; Tamsulosin
Decreased Effect
Prazosin may decrease the levels/effects of: Dabigatran Etexilate; P-Glycoprotein Substrates

The levels/effects of Prazosin may be decreased by: Herbs (Hypertensive Properties); Methylphenidate; Yohimbine

Food Interactions Avoid natural licorice (causes sodium and water retention and increases potassium loss); food has variable effects on absorption

Mechanism of Action Competitively inhibits postsynaptic alpha-adrenergic receptors which results in vasodilation of veins and arterioles and a decrease in total peripheral resistance and blood pressure

Pharmacodynamics Hypotensive effect:
Onset of action: Within 2 hours
Maximum decrease: 2-4 hours
Duration: 10-24 hours

Pharmacokinetics (Adult data unless noted)
Distribution: V_d: 0.5 L/kg (hypertensive adults)
Protein-binding: 92% to 97%
Metabolism: Extensive in the liver, metabolites may be active
Bioavailability, oral: 43% to 82%
Half-life, adults: 2-4 hours, increased half-life with CHF
Elimination: 6% to 10% excreted renally as unchanged drug

Usual Dosage Oral:
Children: Initial: 5 mcg/kg/dose (to assess hypotensive effects); usual dosing interval every 6 hours; increase dosage gradually up to 25 mcg/kg/dose every 6 hours; maximum daily dose: 15 mg or 0.4 mg/kg/day (400 mcg/kg/day); may be divided in 2 or 3 doses/day for treatment of hypertension

Adults: Initial: 1 mg/dose 2-3 times/day; usual maintenance dose: 3-15 mg/day in divided doses 2-4 times/day; maximum daily dose: 20 mg; usual dosage range for hypertension (JNC 7): 2-20 mg/day in 2-3 divided doses

Administration Oral: Administer in a consistent manner with respect to meals

Monitoring Parameters Blood pressure (standing and sitting or supine)

Test Interactions False positive screening tests for pheochromocytoma (increases urinary VMA by 17%; increases norepinephrine metabolite by 42%)

Patient Information Avoid alcohol; rise slowly from sitting or lying position; may cause dizziness or drowsiness and impair ability to perform activities requiring mental alertness or physical coordination; may cause dry mouth

Nursing Implications Be aware of "first-dose phenomenon" (see Precautions); syncope may occur usually within 90 minutes of initial dose

Dosage Forms Excipient information presented when available (limited, particularly for generics); consult specific product labeling.
Capsule, as hydrochloride: 1 mg, 2 mg, 5 mg

References
Chobanian AV, Bakris GL, Black HR, et al, "The Seventh Report of the Joint National Committee on Prevention, Detection, Evaluation, and Treatment of High Blood Pressure: The JNC 7 report," *JAMA*, 2003, 289(19):2560-72.
Friedman WF and George BL, "New Concepts and Drugs in the Treatment of Congestive Heart Failure," *Pediatr Clin North Am*, 1984, 31(6):1197-227.
Sinaiko AR, "Pharmacologic Management of Childhood Hypertension," *Pediatr Clin North Am*, 1993, 40(1):195-212.

◆ **Prazosin Hydrochloride** *see* Prazosin *on page 1147*

◆ **Precedex®** *see* Dexmedetomidine *on page 409*

◆ **Precose®** *see* Acarbose *on page 35*

◆ **Pred Forte®** *see* PrednisoLONE *on page 1148*

◆ **Pred-G®** *see* Prednisolone and Gentamicin *on page 1150*

◆ **Pred Mild®** *see* PrednisoLONE *on page 1148*

PrednisoLONE (pred NIS oh lone)

Medication Safety Issues
Sound-alike/look-alike issues:
PrednisoLONE may be confused with predniSONE
Pediapred® may be confused with Pediazole®
Prelone® may be confused with Prozac®

Related Information
Asthma *on page 1697*
Corticosteroids *on page 1487*

U.S. Brand Names Econopred® Plus [DSC]; Millipred™; Omnipred™; Orapred ODT®; Orapred®; Pediapred®; Pred Forte®; Pred Mild®; Prelone®; Veripred™ 20

Canadian Brand Names Diopred®; Hydeltra T.B.A.®; Inflamase® Mild; Novo-Prednisolone; Ophtho-Tate®; Pediapred®; Pred Forte®; Pred Mild®; Sab-Prenase

Therapeutic Category Adrenal Corticosteroid; Anti-inflammatory Agent; Anti-inflammatory Agent, Ophthalmic; Antiasthmatic; Corticosteroid, Ophthalmic; Corticosteroid, Systemic; Glucocorticoid

Generic Available Yes: Excludes orally disintegrating tablet

Use Treatment of endocrine disorders, rheumatic disorders, collagen diseases, dermatologic diseases, allergic states, ophthalmic diseases, respiratory diseases, hematologic disorders, neoplastic diseases, edematous states, and GI diseases

Ophthalmic: Treatment of palpebral and bulbar conjunctivitis; corneal injury from chemical, radiation, thermal burns, or foreign body penetration

Pregnancy Risk Factor C

Pregnancy Considerations Ophthalmic prednisolone was shown to be teratogenic in animal studies and adverse events have been observed with corticosteroids in animal reproduction studies. Prednisolone crosses the placenta; prior to reaching the fetus, prednisolone is converted by placental enzymes to prednisone. As a result, the amount of prednisolone reaching the fetus is ~8-10 times lower than the maternal serum concentration (healthy women at term; similar results observed with preterm pregnancies complicated by HELLP syndrome). Some studies have shown an association between first trimester corticosteroid use and oral clefts; adverse events in the fetus/neonate have been noted in case reports following large doses of systemic corticosteroids during pregnancy. Women exposed to prednisolone during pregnancy for the treatment of an autoimmune disease may contact the OTIS Autoimmune Diseases Study at 877-311-8972.

Lactation Enters breast milk/use caution (AAP rates "compatible")

Breast-Feeding Considerations Prednisolone is excreted into breast milk with peak concentrations occurring ~1 hour after the maternal dose. The milk/plasma ratio was found to be 0.2 with doses ≥30 mg/day and 0.1 with doses <30 mg/day. Following a maternal dose of prednisolone 80 mg/day, a breast-feeding infant would ingest <0.1% of the dose.

Contraindications Hypersensitivity to prednisolone or any component (see Warnings); acute superficial herpes simplex keratitis; systemic fungal infections; varicella infections; live or live, attenuated virus vaccines (with immunosuppressive doses of corticosteroids)

Warnings Hypothalamic-pituitary-adrenal (HPA) suppression may occur; acute adrenal insufficiency (adrenal crisis) may occur with abrupt withdrawal after long term therapy or with stress; withdrawal or discontinuation of corticosteroids should be done carefully; patients with HPA axis suppression may require increased doses of systemic glucocorticosteroids prior to, during, and after unusual stress (eg, surgery). Immunosuppression may occur; patients may be more susceptible to infections; avoid exposure to chickenpox and measles. Corticosteroids may mask signs of infection. Corticosteroids may activate latent opportunistic infections or exacerbate systemic fungal infections. May cause osteoporosis (at any age) or inhibition of bone growth in pediatric patients. Acute myopathy may occur with high doses, elevated IOP may occur (especially with prolonged use), and CNS effects (ranging from euphoria to psychosis) may occur. Rare cases of anaphylactoid reactions have been reported with corticosteroids.

Ophthalmic suspension may contain sodium bisulfite which may cause allergic reactions in susceptible individuals; Orapred® oral solution contains sodium benzoate and Prelone® syrup contains propylene glycol and benzoic acid; benzoic acid (benzoate) is a metabolite of benzyl alcohol; large amounts of benzyl alcohol (≥99 mg/kg/day) have been associated with a potentially fatal toxicity ("gasping syndrome") in neonates; the "gasping syndrome" consists of metabolic acidosis, respiratory distress, gasping respirations, CNS dysfunction (including convulsions, intracranial hemorrhage), hypotension and cardiovascular collapse; use prednisolone products containing sodium benzoate or benzoic acid with caution in neonates; *in vitro* and animal studies have shown that benzoate displaces bilirubin from protein binding sites

Precautions Avoid using higher than recommended doses; suppression of HPA axis, suppression of linear growth (ie, reduction of growth velocity), reduced bone mineral density, hypercorticism (Cushing's syndrome), hyperglycemia, or glucosuria may occur; titrate to lowest effective dose. Reduction in growth velocity may occur when corticosteroids are administered to pediatric patients by any route (monitor growth). Use with extreme caution in patients with respiratory tuberculosis, untreated systemic infections, or ocular herpes simplex; use with caution in patients with thyroid dysfunction, cirrhosis, nonspecific ulcerative colitis, hypertension, renal impairment, osteoporosis, thromboembolic tendencies, CHF, recent MI, convulsive disorders, myasthenia gravis, thrombophlebitis, peptic ulcer, diabetes, glaucoma, cataracts, or hepatic impairment. Prolonged use may result in cataracts or glaucoma.

Adverse Reactions

Cardiovascular: Edema, hypertension, CHF

Central nervous system: Vertigo, seizures, psychoses, pseudotumor cerebri, headache, euphoria, insomnia, intracranial hypertension, nervousness

Dermatologic: Acne, dermal thinning, skin atrophy, impaired wound healing, petechiae, bruising

Endocrine & metabolic: HPA suppression, Cushing's syndrome, growth suppression, glucose intolerance, hyperglycemia, diabetes mellitus, hypokalemia, alkalosis, sodium and water retention, weight gain, appetite increased

Gastrointestinal: Peptic ulcer, nausea, vomiting

Genitourinary: Menstrual irregularities

Neuromuscular & skeletal: Muscle weakness, osteoporosis, fractures, bone mineral density decreased; rare: aseptic necrosis (femoral and humoral heads)

Ocular: Cataracts, IOP elevated, glaucoma

Miscellaneous: Immunosuppression, anaphylactoid reactions (rare)

Drug Interactions

Metabolism/Transport Effects Substrate of CYP3A4 (minor); **Inhibits** CYP3A4 (weak)

Avoid Concomitant Use

Avoid concomitant use of PrednisoLONE with any of the following: Aldesleukin; BCG; Natalizumab; Pimecrolimus; Tacrolimus (Topical); Vaccines (Live)

Increased Effect/Toxicity

PrednisoLONE may increase the levels/effects of: Acetylcholinesterase Inhibitors; Amphotericin B; CycloSPORINE; CycloSPORINE (Systemic); Leflunomide; Loop Diuretics; Natalizumab; NSAID (COX-2 Inhibitor); NSAID (Nonselective); Thiazide Diuretics; Vaccines (Live); Warfarin

The levels/effects of PrednisoLONE may be increased by: Antifungal Agents (Azole Derivatives, Systemic); Aprepitant; Calcium Channel Blockers (Nondihydropyridine); CycloSPORINE; CycloSPORINE (Systemic); Denosumab; Estrogen Derivatives; Fluconazole; Fosaprepitant; Macrolide Antibiotics; Neuromuscular-Blocking Agents (Nondepolarizing); Pimecrolimus; Quinolone Antibiotics; Ritonavir; Salicylates; Tacrolimus (Topical); Trastuzumab

Decreased Effect

PrednisoLONE may decrease the levels/effects of: Aldesleukin; Antidiabetic Agents; BCG; Calcitriol; Corticorelin; Isoniazid; Salicylates; Sipuleucel-T; Vaccines (Inactivated); Vaccines (Live)

The levels/effects of PrednisoLONE may be decreased by: Aminoglutethimide; Antacids; Barbiturates; Bile Acid Sequestrants; Echinacea; Mitotane; Primidone; Rifamycin Derivatives

Food Interactions Systemic use of corticosteroids may require a diet with increased potassium, vitamins A, B_6, C, D, folate, calcium, zinc, and phosphorus and decreased sodium

Stability Dispense oral liquid formulations in tight, light-resistant containers. Storage: Prelone® syrup: Store at room temperature, do not refrigerate; Pediapred® oral solution: Store at 4°C to 24°C (39°F to 77°F), may be refrigerated; Orapred® oral solution: Store in refrigerator [2°C to 8°C (36°F to 46°F)]; Orapred ODT®: Store at controlled room temperature at 20°C to 25°C (68°F to 77°F) in blister pack; protect from moisture

Mechanism of Action Decreases inflammation by suppression of migration of polymorphonuclear leukocytes and reversal of increased capillary permeability; suppresses the immune system by reducing activity and volume of the lymphatic system

Pharmacokinetics (Adult data unless noted)

Absorption: Oral: Well absorbed

Protein binding: 70% to 90% (concentration dependent)

Metabolism: Primarily in the liver, but also metabolized in most tissues, to inactive compounds

Half-life: Adults (serum): 2-4 hours

Elimination: In urine, principally as glucuronide and sulfate-conjugated metabolites

Usual Dosage Dose depends upon condition being treated and response of patient; dosage for infants and children should be based on disease severity and patient response rather than by rigid adherence to dosage guidelines by age, weight, or body surface area. Consider alternate day therapy for long-term therapy. Discontinuation of long-term therapy requires gradual withdrawal by tapering the dose.

NIH Asthma Guidelines (NAEPP, 2007): Oral:

Children <12 years:

Asthma exacerbations (emergency care or hospital doses): 1-2 mg/kg/day in 2 divided doses (maximum: 60 mg/day) until peak expiratory flow is 70% of predicted or personal best

Short-course "burst" (acute asthma): 1-2 mg/kg/day in divided doses 1-2 times/day for 3-10 days; maximum dose: 60 mg/day; **Note:** Burst should be continued until symptoms resolve or patient achieves peak expiratory flow 80% of personal best; usually requires 3-10 days of treatment (~5 days on average); longer treatment may be required

Long-term treatment: 0.25-2 mg/kg/day given as a single dose in the morning or every other day as needed for asthma control; maximum dose: 60 mg/day

Children ≥12 years and Adults:

Asthma exacerbations (emergency care or hospital doses): 40-80 mg/day in divided doses 1-2 times/day until peak expiratory flow is 70% of predicted or personal best

Short-course "burst" (acute asthma): 40-60 mg/day in divided doses 1-2 times/day for 3-10 days; **Note:** Burst should be continued until symptoms resolve and peak expiratory flow is at least 80% of personal best; usually requires 3-10 days of treatment (~5 days on average); longer treatment may be required

Long-term treatment: 7.5-60 mg daily given as a single dose in the morning or every other day as needed for asthma control

Children: Oral:

Anti-inflammatory or immunosuppressive dose: 0.1-2 mg/kg/day in divided doses 1-4 times/day

Nephrotic syndrome:

Pediatric Nephrology Panel recommendations (Hogg, 2000):

Initial: 2 mg/kg/day or 60 mg/m^2/day given every day in 1-3 divided doses (maximum dose: 80 mg/day) until urine is protein free or for 4-6 weeks; followed by maintenance dose: 2 mg/kg/dose or 40 mg/m^2/dose given every other day in the morning; gradually taper and discontinue after 4-6 weeks; **Note:** 6-week daily therapy followed by 6-week alternate day therapy may induce a higher rate of long remission compared to the standard of 4 weeks of daily therapy followed by 4 weeks of alternate day therapy; however, a higher incidence of adverse effects may be seen with the longer regimen and the clinical benefit may be variable

Relapse: Use high-dose daily steroid regimen (listed above) until urine is protein free for 3 days; follow with maintenance-tapering course of alternate day therapy (maintenance dose listed above) for 4-6 weeks; subsequent therapy is determined by individual's response and number of relapses (see Hogg, 2000)

British Pediatric Nephrology Consensus Statement (Report of a Workshop by the British Association for Paediatric Nephrology and Research Unit, 1994):

First 3 episodes: Initial: 2 mg/kg/day or 60 mg/m²/day given every day (maximum dose: 80 mg/day) until urine is protein free for 3 consecutive days (maximum dose: 28 days); followed by 1-1.5 mg/kg/dose or 40 mg/m²/dose (maximum: 60 mg/dose) given every other day for 4 weeks

Frequent relapses (long-term maintenance dose): 0.5-1 mg/kg/dose given every other day for 3-6 months

Adults: Oral: 5-60 mg/day

Children and Adults: Ophthalmic suspension: Instill 1-2 drops into conjunctival sac every hour during day, every 2 hours at night until favorable response is obtained, then use 1 drop every 4 hours

Administration

Oral: Administer after meals or with food or milk to decrease GI upset

Orapred ODT®: Do not cut, split, or break tablets; do not use partial tablets. Remove tablet from blister pack immediately prior to use. May swallow tablet whole or allow to dissolve on tongue

Ophthalmic: Shake suspension well before use; instill drops into affected eye(s); avoid contact of container tip with skin or eye; apply finger pressure to lacrimal sac during and for 1-2 minutes after instillation to decrease risk of absorption and systemic effects

Monitoring Parameters Blood pressure, weight, electrolytes, serum glucose; IOP (use >6 weeks); bone mineral density (long-term use); children's height and growth

Test Interactions Skin tests

Patient Information Avoid alcohol; limit caffeine; do not decrease dose or discontinue without physician's approval; avoid exposure to chicken pox or measles, if exposed, seek medical advice without delay

Dosage Forms Excipient information presented when available (limited, particularly for generics); consult specific product labeling. [DSC] = Discontinued product

Solution, ophthalmic, as sodium phosphate: 1% (5 mL, 10 mL, 15 mL) [contains benzalkonium chloride]

Solution, oral, as base: 15 mg/5 mL (240 mL, 480 mL)

Solution, oral, as sodium phosphate [strength expressed as base]: 5 mg/5 mL (120 mL, 240 mL); 15 mg/5 mL (240 mL)

Millipred™: 10 mg/5 mL (237 mL) [dye free; grape flavor]

Orapred®: 15 mg/5 mL (20 mL, 240 mL) [dye free; contains ethanol 2%, sodium benzoate; grape flavor]

Pediapred®: 5 mg/5 mL (120 mL) [dye free; raspberry flavor]

Veripred™ 20: 20 mg/5 mL (237 mL) [dye free, ethanol free; grape flavor]

Suspension, ophthalmic, as acetate: 1% (5 mL, 10 mL, 15 mL)

Econopred® Plus [DSC], Omnipred™: 1% (5 mL, 10 mL) [contains benzalkonium chloride]

Pred Forte®: 1% (1 mL, 5 mL, 10 mL, 15 mL) [contains benzalkonium chloride and sodium bisulfite]

Pred Mild®: 0.12% (5 mL, 10 mL) [contains benzalkonium chloride and sodium bisulfite]

Syrup, as base: 5 mg/5 mL (120 mL); 15 mg/5 mL (5 mL [DSC], 240 mL, 480 mL)

Prelone®: 15 mg/5 mL (240 mL, 480 mL) [contains ethanol 5%, benzoic acid, propylene glycol; wild cherry flavor]

Tablet, as base: 5 mg

Tablet, orally disintegrating, as sodium phosphate [strength expressed as base]:
Orapred ODT®: 10 mg, 15 mg, 30 mg [grape flavor]

References

Hogg RJ, Portman RJ, Milliner D, et al, "Evaluation and Management of Proteinuria and Nephrotic Syndrome in Children: Recommendations From a Pediatric Nephrology Panel Established at the National Kidney Foundation Conference on Proteinuria, Albuminuria, Risk, Assessment, Detection, and Elimination (PARADE)," *Pediatrics*, 2000, 105(6):1242-9.

National Asthma Education and Prevention Program (NAEPP), "Expert Panel Report 3 (EPR-3): Guidelines for the Diagnosis and Management of Asthma," *Clinical Practice Guidelines*, National Institutes of Health, National Heart, Lung, and Blood Institute, NIH Publication No. 08-4051, prepublication 2007; available at http://www.nhlbi.nih.gov/guidelines/asthma/asthgdln.htm.

Report of a Workshop by the British Association for Paediatric Nephrology and Research Unit, Royal College of Physicians, "Consensus Statement on Management and Audit Potential for Steroid Responsive Nephrotic Syndrome," *Arch Dis Child*, 1994, 70 (2):151-7.

♦ **Prednisolone Acetate** see PrednisoLONE *on page 1148*

♦ **Prednisolone Acetate, Ophthalmic** see PrednisoLONE *on page 1148*

Prednisolone and Gentamicin
(pred NIS oh lone & jen ta MYE sin)

U.S. Brand Names Pred-G®

Therapeutic Category Antibiotic, Ophthalmic; Corticosteroid, Ophthalmic

Generic Available No

Use Treatment of steroid responsive inflammatory conditions and superficial ocular infections due to strains of microorganisms susceptible to gentamicin such as *Staphylococcus*, *E. coli*, *H. influenzae*, *Klebsiella*, *Neisseria*, *Pseudomonas*, *Proteus*, and *Serratia* species

Pregnancy Risk Factor C

Lactation Excretion in breast milk unknown/not recommended

Breast-Feeding Considerations It is unknown if topical use results in sufficient absorption to produce detectable quantities in breast milk.

Contraindications Hypersensitivity to prednisolone, gentamicin, or any component; dendritic keratitis, fungal diseases, vaccinia, varicella, most other viral infections, and mycobacterial infection of the eye. Contraindicated after uncomplicated removal of a corneal foreign body.

Warnings Prolonged use may result in glaucoma, damage to the optic nerve, defects in visual acuity, posterior subcapsular cataract formation, and secondary ocular infections

Adverse Reactions
Local: Burning, stinging, redness
Ocular: Elevation of intraocular pressure, glaucoma, infrequent optic nerve damage, posterior subcapsular cataract formation, superficial punctate keratitis, lacrimation increased
Miscellaneous: Development of secondary infection, allergic sensitization, delayed wound healing

Drug Interactions
Metabolism/Transport Effects Prednisolone: **Substrate** of CYP3A4 (minor); **Inhibits** CYP3A4 (weak)

Avoid Concomitant Use
Avoid concomitant use of Prednisolone and Gentamicin with any of the following: Agalsidase Beta; Aldesleukin; BCG; Gallium Nitrate; Natalizumab; Pimecrolimus; Tacrolimus (Topical); Vaccines (Live)

Increased Effect/Toxicity

Prednisolone and Gentamicin may increase the levels/ effects of: AbobotulinumtoxinA; Acetylcholinesterase Inhibitors; Amphotericin B; Bisphosphonate Derivatives; CARBOplatin; Colistimethate; CycloSPORINE; Cyclo-SPORINE (Systemic); Gallium Nitrate; Leflunomide; Loop Diuretics; Natalizumab; Neuromuscular-Blocking Agents; NSAID (COX-2 Inhibitor); NSAID (Nonselective); OnabotulinumtoxinA; RimabotulinumtoxinB; Thiazide Diuretics; Vaccines (Live); Warfarin

The levels/effects of Prednisolone and Gentamicin may be increased by: Amphotericin B; Antifungal Agents (Azole Derivatives, Systemic); Aprepitant; Calcium Channel Blockers (Nondihydropyridine); Capreomycin; CISplatin; CycloSPORINE; CycloSPORINE (Systemic); Denosumab; Estrogen Derivatives; Fluconazole; Fosaprepitant; Loop Diuretics; Macrolide Antibiotics; Neuromuscular-Blocking Agents (Nondepolarizing); Pimecrolimus; Quinolone Antibiotics; Ritonavir; Salicylates; Tacrolimus (Topical); Trastuzumab; Vancomycin

Decreased Effect

Prednisolone and Gentamicin may decrease the levels/ effects of: Agalsidase Beta; Aldesleukin; Antidiabetic Agents; BCG; Calcitriol; Corticorelin; Isoniazid; Salicylates; Sipuleucel-T; Typhoid Vaccine; Vaccines (Inactivated); Vaccines (Live)

The levels/effects of Prednisolone and Gentamicin may be decreased by: Aminoglutethimide; Antacids; Barbiturates; Bile Acid Sequestrants; Echinacea; Mitotane; Penicillins; Primidone; Rifamycin Derivatives

Mechanism of Action See individual agents.

Usual Dosage Children and Adults: Ophthalmic: Instill 1 drop 2-4 times/day; during the initial 24-48 hours, the dosing frequency may be increased if necessary, up to 1 drop every hour; or small amount (1/2" ribbon) of ointment can be applied into the conjunctival sac 1-3 times/day

Administration Suspension: Shake well before using; instill drop into affected eye; avoid contacting bottle tip with skin or eye; apply finger pressure to lacrimal sac during and for 1-2 minutes after instillation to decrease risk of absorption and systemic effects

Monitoring Parameters With use >10 days, monitor intraocular pressure

Dosage Forms Excipient information presented when available (limited, particularly for generics); consult specific product labeling. [DSC] = Discontinued product

Ointment, ophthalmic:

Pred-G®: Prednisolone acetate 0.6% and gentamicin sulfate 0.3% (3.5 g)

Suspension, ophthalmic:

Pred-G®: Prednisolone acetate 1% and gentamicin sulfate 0.3% (5 mL, 10 mL) [contains benzalkonium chloride] [DSC]

◆ **Prednisolone, Neomycin, and Polymyxin B** *see* Neomycin, Polymyxin B, and Prednisolone *on page 981*

◆ **Prednisolone Sodium Phosphate** *see* PrednisoLONE *on page 1148*

◆ **Prednisolone Sodium Phosphate, Ophthalmic** *see* PrednisoLONE *on page 1148*

PredniSONE (PRED ni sone)

Medication Safety Issues

Sound-alike/look-alike issues:

PredniSONE may be confused with methylPREDNISolone, Pramosone®, prazosin, prednisoLONE, Prilosec®, primidone, promethazine

Related Information

Asthma *on page 1697*
Corticosteroids *on page 1487*

U.S. Brand Names PredniSONE Intensol™; Sterapred® DS [DSC]; Sterapred® [DSC]

Canadian Brand Names Apo-Prednisone®; Novo-Prednisone; Winpred™

Therapeutic Category Adrenal Corticosteroid; Anti-inflammatory Agent; Antiasthmatic; Corticosteroid, Systemic; Glucocorticoid

Generic Available Yes

Use Management of adrenocortical insufficiency; used for its anti-inflammatory or immunosuppressant effects

Pregnancy Considerations Adverse events have been observed with corticosteroids in animal reproduction studies. Prednisone and prednisolone cross the human placenta. In the mother, prednisone is converted to the active metabolite prednisolone by the liver. Prior to reaching the fetus, prednisolone is converted by placental enzymes back to prednisone. As a result, the level of prednisone remaining in the maternal serum and reaching the fetus are similar; however, the amount of prednisolone reaching the fetus is ~8-10 times lower than the maternal serum concentration (healthy women at term). Some studies have shown an association between first trimester prednisone use and oral clefts; adverse events in the fetus/ neonate have been noted in case reports following large doses of systemic corticosteroids during pregnancy. Pregnant women exposed to prednisone for antirejection therapy following a transplant may contact the National Transplantation Pregnancy Registry (NTPR) at 215-955-4820. Women exposed to prednisone during pregnancy for the treatment of an autoimmune disease (eg, rheumatoid arthritis) may contact the OTIS Autoimmune Diseases Study at 877-311-8972.

Lactation Enters breast milk/AAP rates "compatible"

Breast-Feeding Considerations Prednisone and its metabolite prednisolone are found in low concentrations in breast milk. Peak milk concentrations of both were found ~2 hours after the maternal dose in one case report. In a study which included 6 mother/infant pairs, adverse events were not observed in nursing infants (maternal prednisone dose not provided).

Contraindications Hypersensitivity to prednisone or any component; serious infections, except septic shock or tuberculous meningitis; systemic fungal infections; varicella infections; live or live, attenuated virus vaccines (with immunosuppressive doses of corticosteroids)

Warnings Hypothalamic pituitary adrenal (HPA) suppression may occur; acute adrenal insufficiency (adrenal crisis) may occur with abrupt withdrawal after long term therapy or with stress; withdrawal or discontinuation of corticosteroids should be done carefully; patients with HPA axis suppression may require increased doses of systemic glucocorticosteroids prior to, during, and after unusual stress (eg, surgery). Immunosuppression may occur; patients may be more susceptible to infections; avoid exposure to chickenpox and measles. Corticosteroids may mask signs of infection. Corticosteroids may activate latent opportunistic infections or exacerbate systemic fungal infections. May cause osteoporosis (at any age) or inhibition of bone growth in pediatric patients. Acute myopathy may occur with high doses, elevated IOP may occur (especially with prolonged use), CNS effects (ranging from euphoria to psychosis) may occur. Rare cases of anaphylactoid reactions have been reported with corticosteroids.

Oral solution contains sodium benzoate; benzoic acid (benzoate) is a metabolite of benzyl alcohol; large amounts of benzyl alcohol (≥99 mg/kg/day) have been associated with a potentially fatal toxicity ("gasping syndrome") in neonates; the "gasping syndrome" consists of metabolic ▶

acidosis, respiratory distress, gasping respirations, CNS dysfunction (including convulsions, intracranial hemorrhage), hypotension and cardiovascular collapse; use prednisone products containing sodium benzoate with caution in neonates; *in vitro* and animal studies have shown that benzoate displaces bilirubin from protein binding sites

Precautions Avoid using higher than recommended doses; suppression of HPA axis, suppression of linear growth (ie, reduction of growth velocity), reduced bone mineral density, hypercorticism (Cushing's syndrome), hyperglycemia, or glucosuria may occur; titrate to lowest effective dose. Reduction in growth velocity may occur when corticosteroids are administered to pediatric patients by any route (monitor growth). Use with extreme caution in patients with respiratory tuberculosis, untreated systemic infections, or ocular herpes simplex; use with caution in patients with thyroid dysfunction, cirrhosis, nonspecific ulcerative colitis, hypertension, renal impairment, osteoporosis, thromboembolic tendencies, CHF, recent MI, convulsive disorders, myasthenia gravis, thrombophlebitis, peptic ulcer, diabetes, glaucoma, cataracts, or hepatic impairment. Prolonged use may result in cataracts or glaucoma.

Adverse Reactions

Cardiovascular: Edema, hypertension, CHF

Central nervous system: Vertigo, seizures, psychoses, pseudotumor cerebri, headache, euphoria, insomnia, intracranial hypertension, nervousness

Dermatologic: Acne, dermal thinning, skin atrophy, impaired wound healing, petechiae, bruising

Endocrine & metabolic: HPA suppression, Cushing's syndrome, growth suppression, glucose intolerance, hyperglycemia, diabetes mellitus, hypokalemia, alkalosis, sodium and water retention, weight gain, appetite increased

Gastrointestinal: Peptic ulcer, nausea, vomiting

Genitourinary: Menstrual irregularities

Neuromuscular & skeletal: Muscle weakness, osteoporosis, fractures, bone mineral density decreased; rare: aseptic necrosis (femoral and humoral heads)

Ocular: Cataracts, IOP elevated, glaucoma

Miscellaneous: Immunosuppression, anaphylactoid reactions (rare)

Drug Interactions

Metabolism/Transport Effects Substrate of CYP3A4 (minor); **Induces** CYP2C19 (weak), 3A4 (weak)

Avoid Concomitant Use

Avoid concomitant use of PredniSONE with any of the following: Aldesleukin; BCG; Natalizumab; Pimecrolimus; Tacrolimus (Topical); Vaccines (Live)

Increased Effect/Toxicity

PredniSONE may increase the levels/effects of: Acetylcholinesterase Inhibitors; Amphotericin B; CycloSPORINE; CycloSPORINE (Systemic); Leflunomide; Loop Diuretics; Natalizumab; NSAID (COX-2 Inhibitor); NSAID (Nonselective); Thiazide Diuretics; Vaccines (Live); Warfarin

The levels/effects of PredniSONE may be increased by: Antifungal Agents (Azole Derivatives, Systemic); Aprepitant; Calcium Channel Blockers (Nondihydropyridine); CycloSPORINE; CycloSPORINE (Systemic); Denosumab; Estrogen Derivatives; Fluconazole; Fosaprepitant; Macrolide Antibiotics; Neuromuscular-Blocking Agents (Nondepolarizing); Pimecrolimus; Quinolone Antibiotics; Ritonavir; Salicylates; Tacrolimus (Topical); Trastuzumab

Decreased Effect

PredniSONE may decrease the levels/effects of: Aldesleukin; Antidiabetic Agents; BCG; Calcitriol; Corticorelin; Isoniazid; Salicylates; Sipuleucel-T; Vaccines (Inactivated); Vaccines (Live)

The levels/effects of PredniSONE may be decreased by: Aminoglutethimide; Antacids; Barbiturates; Bile Acid Sequestrants; Echinacea; Mitotane; Primidone; Rifamycin Derivatives; Somatropin

Food Interactions Systemic use of corticosteroids may require a diet with increased potassium, vitamins A, B_6, C, D, folate, calcium, zinc, and phosphorus and decreased sodium

Mechanism of Action Decreases inflammation by suppression of migration of polymorphonuclear leukocytes and reversal of increased capillary permeability; suppresses the immune system by reducing activity and volume of the lymphatic system

Pharmacokinetics (Adult data unless noted) Converted rapidly in the liver to prednisolone (active)

Usual Dosage Dose depends upon condition being treated and response of patient; dosage for infants and children should be based on disease severity and patient response rather than by rigid adherence to dosage guidelines by age, weight, or body surface area. Consider alternate day therapy for long-term therapy. Discontinuation of long-term therapy requires gradual withdrawal by tapering the dose. Oral:

NIH Asthma Guidelines (NAEPP, 2007):

Children <12 years:

Asthma exacerbations (emergency care or hospital doses): 1-2 mg/kg/day in 2 divided doses (maximum: 60 mg/day) until peak expiratory flow is 70% of predicted or personal best

Short-course "burst" (acute asthma): 1-2 mg/kg/day in divided doses 1-2 times/day for 3-10 days; maximum dose: 60 mg/day; **Note:** Burst should be continued until symptoms resolve or patient achieves peak expiratory flow 80% of personal best; usually requires 3-10 days of treatment (~5 days on average); longer treatment may be required

Long-term treatment: 0.25-2 mg/kg/day given as a single dose in the morning or every other day as needed for asthma control; maximum dose: 60 mg/day

Children ≥12 years and Adults:

Asthma exacerbations (emergency care or hospital doses): 40-80 mg/day in divided doses 1-2 times/day until peak expiratory flow is 70% of predicted or personal best

Short-course "burst" (acute asthma): 40-60 mg/day in divided doses 1-2 times/day for 3-10 days; **Note:** Burst should be continued until symptoms resolve and peak expiratory flow is at least 80% of personal best; usually requires 3-10 days of treatment (~5 days on average); longer treatment may be required

Long-term treatment: 7.5-60 mg daily given as a single dose in the morning or every other day as needed for asthma control

Children:

Alternative asthma dosing by age:

Short-course "burst" (acute asthma):

<1 year: 10 mg every 12 hours

1-4 years: 20 mg every 12 hours

5-13 years: 30 mg every 12 hours

>13 years: 40 mg every 12 hours

Long-term treatment:

<1 year: 10 mg every other day

1-4 years: 20 mg every other day

5-13 years: 30 mg every other day

>13 years: 40 mg every other day

Anti-inflammatory or immunosuppressive: 0.05-2 mg/kg/day divided 1-4 times/day

Nephrotic syndrome:
Pediatric Nephrology Panel recommendations (Hogg, 2000):
Initial: 2 mg/kg/day or 60 mg/m^2/day given every day in 1-3 divided doses (maximum dose: 80 mg/day) until urine is protein free or for 4-6 weeks; followed by maintenance dose: 2 mg/kg/dose or 40 mg/m^2/dose given every other day in the morning; gradually taper and discontinue after 4-6 weeks; **Note:** 6-week daily therapy followed by 6-week alternate day therapy may induce a higher rate of long remission compared to the standard of 4 weeks of daily therapy followed by 4 weeks of alternate day therapy; however, a higher incidence of adverse effects may be seen with the longer regimen and the clinical benefit may be variable.
Relapse: Use high-dose daily steroid regimen (listed above) until urine is protein free for 3 days; follow with maintenance-tapering course of alternate day therapy (maintenance dose listed above) for 4-6 weeks; subsequent therapy is determined by individual's response and number of relapses (see Hogg, 2000)
British Pediatric Nephrology Consensus Statement (Report of a Workshop by the British Association for Paediatric Nephrology and Research Unit, 1994):
First 3 episodes: Initial: 2 mg/kg/day or 60 mg/m^2/day given every day (maximum dose: 80 mg/day) until urine is protein free for 3 consecutive days (maximum dose: 28 days); followed by 1-1.5 mg/kg/dose or 40 mg/m^2/dose (maximum: 60 mg/dose) given every other day for 4 weeks
Frequent relapses (long-term maintenance dose): 0.5-1 mg/kg/dose given every other day for 3-6 months
Children and Adults: Physiologic replacement: 4-5 mg/m^2/day
Adults: 5-60 mg/day in divided doses 1-4 times/day
Administration Oral: Administer after meals or with food or milk to decrease GI upset
Monitoring Parameters Blood pressure, weight, serum electrolytes, glucose; children's height and growth
Test Interactions Skin tests
Patient Information Avoid alcohol; limit caffeine; do not decrease dose or discontinue without physician's approval
Dosage Forms Excipient information presented when available (limited, particularly for generics); consult specific product labeling. [DSC] = Discontinued product
Solution, oral: 1 mg/mL (5 mL, 120 mL, 500 mL) [contains ethanol 5%, sodium benzoate; peppermint vanilla flavor]
Solution, oral [concentrate]:
PredniSONE Intensol™: 5 mg/mL (30 mL) [dye free, sugar free; contains ethanol 30%, propylene glycol]
Tablet: 1 mg, 2.5 mg, 5 mg, 10 mg, 20 mg, 50 mg
Sterapred®: 5 mg [scored; supplied as 21 tablet 6-day unit-dose package or 48 tablet 12-day unit-dose package] [DSC]
Sterapred® DS: 10 mg [supplied as 21 tablet 6-day unit-dose package or 48 tablet 12-day unit-dose package] [DSC]
References
Hogg RJ, Portman RJ, Milliner D, et al, "Evaluation and Management of Proteinuria and Nephrotic Syndrome in Children: Recommendations From a Pediatric Nephrology Panel Established at the National Kidney Foundation Conference on Proteinuria, Albuminuria, Risk, Assessment, Detection, and Elimination (PARADE)," Pediatrics, 2000, 105(6):1242-9.
Murphy CM, Coonce SL, and Simon PA, "Treatment of Asthma in Children," Clin Pharm, 1991, 10(9):685-703.
National Asthma Education and Prevention Program (NAEPP), "Expert Panel Report 3 (EPR-3): Guidelines for the Diagnosis and Management of Asthma," Clinical Practice Guidelines, National Institutes of Health, National Heart, Lung, and Blood Institute, NIH Publication No. 08-4051, prepublication 2007; available at http://www.nhlbi.nih.gov/guidelines/asthma/asthgdln.htm.

Report of a Workshop by the British Association for Paediatric Nephrology and Research Unit, Royal College of Physicians, "Consensus Statement on Management and Audit Potential for Steroid Responsive Nephrotic Syndrome," Arch Dis Child, 1994, 70 (2):151-7.

◆ **PredniSONE Intensol™** see PredniSONE on page 1151
◆ **Pregnyl®** see Chorionic Gonadotropin on page 305
◆ **Prelone®** see PrednisoLONE on page 1148
◆ **Premarin®** see Estrogens (Conjugated/Equine) on page 539
◆ **Premjact® [OTC]** see Lidocaine on page 818
◆ **Preparation H® [OTC]** see Phenylephrine on page 1102
◆ **Preparation H® Hydrocortisone [OTC]** see Hydrocortisone on page 685
◆ **Pressyn® (Can)** see Vasopressin on page 1410
◆ **Pressyn® AR (Can)** see Vasopressin on page 1410
◆ **Pretz® [OTC]** see Sodium Chloride on page 1270
◆ **Prevacare® [OTC]** see Ethyl Alcohol on page 547
◆ **Prevacid®** see Lansoprazole on page 801
◆ **Prevacid® 24 HR [OTC]** see Lansoprazole on page 801
◆ **Prevacid® FasTab (Can)** see Lansoprazole on page 801
◆ **Prevacid® SoluTab™** see Lansoprazole on page 801
◆ **Prevalite®** see Cholestyramine Resin on page 302
◆ **Prevex® B (Can)** see Betamethasone on page 189
◆ **Prevex® HC (Can)** see Hydrocortisone on page 685
◆ **PreviDent®** see Fluoride on page 595
◆ **PreviDent® 5000 Plus®** see Fluoride on page 595
◆ **Prevnar®** see Pneumococcal Conjugate Vaccine (7-Valent) on page 1121
◆ **Prevnar 13™** see Pneumococcal Conjugate Vaccine (13-Valent) on page 1123
◆ **Prilocaine and Lidocaine** see Lidocaine and Prilocaine on page 823
◆ **Prilosec®** see Omeprazole on page 1016
◆ **Prilosec OTC™ [OTC]** see Omeprazole on page 1016
◆ **Primaclone** see Primidone on page 1154
◆ **Primacor® [DSC]** see Milrinone on page 931
◆ **Primacor® (Can)** see Milrinone on page 931
◆ **Primalev™ [DSC]** see Oxycodone and Acetaminophen on page 1041

Primaquine (PRIM a kween)

Medication Safety Issues
Sound-alike/look-alike issues:
Primaquine may be confused with primidone
Related Information
Malaria on page 1652
Therapeutic Category Antimalarial Agent
Generic Available Yes
Use In conjunction with a blood schizonticidal agent to provide radical cure of P. vivax or P. ovale malaria after a clinical attack has been confirmed by blood smear or serologic titer; prevention of relapse of P. ovale or P. vivax malaria; malaria postexposure prophylaxis
Lactation Excretion in breast milk unknown
Contraindications Acutely ill patients who have a tendency to develop granulocytopenia (rheumatoid arthritis, SLE); patients receiving other drugs capable of depressing the bone marrow; patients receiving quinacrine

◄ **Warnings** Hemolytic reactions may occur in patients with G6PD deficiency. Anemia, methemoglobinemia, and leukopenia have been associated with primaquine use; promptly discontinue with signs of hemolytic anemia (darkening of urine, marked fall in hemoglobin or erythrocyte count).

Precautions Use with caution in patients with G6PD deficiency or NADH methemoglobin reductase deficiency

Adverse Reactions
Cardiovascular: Arrhythmias, hypertension
Central nervous system: Headache
Dermatologic: Pruritus
Gastrointestinal: Nausea, vomiting, abdominal cramps
Hematologic: Hemolytic anemia, methemoglobinemia, leukocytosis, leukopenia, agranulocytosis
Ocular: Interference with visual accommodation

Drug Interactions
Metabolism/Transport Effects Substrate of CYP3A4 (major); **Inhibits** CYP1A2 (strong), 2D6 (weak), 3A4 (weak); **Induces** CYP1A2 (weak)

Avoid Concomitant Use
Avoid concomitant use of Primaquine with any of the following: Artemether; Lumefantrine; Mefloquine

Increased Effect/Toxicity
Primaquine may increase the levels/effects of: Antipsychotic Agents (Phenothiazines); Bendamustine; Beta-Blockers; Cardiac Glycosides; CYP1A2 Substrates; Dapsone; Dapsone (Systemic); Dapsone (Topical); Lumefantrine; Mefloquine

The levels/effects of Primaquine may be increased by: Artemether; Dapsone; Dapsone (Systemic); Mefloquine

Decreased Effect
Primaquine may decrease the levels/effects of: Anthelmintics

The levels/effects of Primaquine may be decreased by: CYP3A4 Inducers (Strong); Deferasirox; Herbs (CYP3A4 Inducers)

Stability Protect from light

Mechanism of Action Eliminates the primary tissue exoerythrocytic forms of *P. falciparum, P. malariae, P. ovale,* and *P. vivax;* interferes with plasmodial DNA

Pharmacokinetics (Adult data unless noted)
Absorption: Oral: Well absorbed
Metabolism: Liver metabolism to carboxyprimaquine, an active metabolite
Half-life: 3.7-9.6 hours
Time to peak serum concentration: Within 6 hours
Elimination: Small amount of unchanged drug excreted in urine

Usual Dosage Oral:
Children: 0.3 mg base/kg/day once daily for 14 days not to exceed 15 mg base/day, or 0.9 mg base/kg once weekly for 8 weeks not to exceed 45 mg base/week
Adults: 15 mg/day (base) once daily for 14 days or 45 mg base once weekly for 8 weeks

Administration Oral: Administer with meals to decrease adverse GI effects; drug has a bitter taste

Monitoring Parameters Periodic CBC, visual color check of urine, methemoglobin

Patient Information Notify physician if a darkening of the urine occurs

Dosage Forms Excipient information presented when available (limited, particularly for generics); consult specific product labeling.
Tablet, as phosphate: 26.3 mg [15 mg base]

References
Lynk A and Gold R, "Review of 40 Children With Imported Malaria," *Pediatr Infect Dis J,* 1989, 8(11):745-50.
Wyler DJ, "Malaria Chemoprophylaxis for the Traveler," *N Engl J Med,* 1993, 329(1):31-7.

◆ **Primaquine Phosphate** *see* Primaquine *on page 1153*

◆ **Primatene® Mist [OTC]** *see* EPINEPHrine *on page 511*

◆ **Primaxin®** *see* Imipenem and Cilastatin *on page 714*

◆ **Primaxin® I.V. (Can)** *see* Imipenem and Cilastatin *on page 714*

Primidone (PRI mi done)

Medication Safety Issues
Sound-alike/look-alike issues:
Primidone may be confused with predniSONE, primaquine, pyridoxine

Related Information
Antiepileptic Drugs *on page 1693*

U.S. Brand Names Mysoline®

Canadian Brand Names Apo-Primidone®

Therapeutic Category Anticonvulsant, Barbiturate; Barbiturate

Generic Available Yes

Use Management of generalized tonic-clonic (grand mal), complex partial and simple partial (focal) seizures

Pregnancy Considerations Crosses the placenta. Dysmorphic facial features; hemorrhagic disease of newborn due to fetal vitamin K depletion, maternal folic acid deficiency may occur. Epilepsy itself, number of medications, genetic factors, or a combination of these probably influence the teratogenicity of anticonvulsant therapy. Benefit:risk ratio usually favors continued use during pregnancy.

Patients exposed to primidone during pregnancy are encouraged to enroll themselves into the NAAED Pregnancy Registry by calling 1-888-233-2334. Additional information is available at www.aedpregnancyregistry.org.

Lactation Enters breast milk/not recommended (AAP recommends use "with caution")

Breast-Feeding Considerations Sedation and feeding problems may occur in nursing infants. AAP recommends USE WITH CAUTION.

Contraindications Hypersensitivity to primidone or any component; porphyria

Warnings Antiepileptic drugs (AEDs) increase the risk of suicidal behavior and ideation in patients receiving these medications for any indication. Pooled analyses of placebo-controlled trials involving 11 different AEDs (regardless of indication) showed a twofold increased risk of suicidal thoughts or behavior (estimated incidence rate 0.43% in AED treated patients compared to 0.24% of patients receiving placebo); increased risk was observed as early as 1 week after initiation of AED and continued through duration of trials (most trials ≤24 weeks); risk did not vary significantly by age (age range: 5–100 years). Consider risks and benefits of AEDs before prescribing. Monitor all patients receiving an AED for emergence of suicidal thoughts or behavior, thoughts of self-harm, any unusual changes in behavior or mood, or the emergence or worsening of depressive symptoms; notify heathcare provider immediately if symptoms or concerning behavior occur. **Note:** The FDA is requiring that a Medication Guide be developed for all antiepileptic drugs informing patients of this risk.

Generic tablet may contain sodium benzoate; benzoic acid (benzoate) is a metabolite of benzyl alcohol; large amounts of benzyl alcohol (≥99 mg/kg/day) have been associated with a potentially fatal toxicity ("gasping syndrome") in neonates; the "gasping syndrome" consists of metabolic acidosis, respiratory distress, gasping respirations, CNS dysfunction (including convulsions, intracranial hemorrhage), hypotension and cardiovascular collapse; avoid use of primidone products containing sodium benzoate in neonates; *in vitro* and animal studies have shown that benzoate displaces bilirubin from protein binding sites

Precautions Use with caution in patients with renal or hepatic impairment. Abrupt discontinuation may precipitate status epilepticus

Adverse Reactions

Central nervous system: Drowsiness, vertigo, lethargy, behavior change, ataxia, suicidal thinking and behavior (see Warnings)

Dermatologic: Rash

Gastrointestinal: Nausea, vomiting

Hematologic: Leukopenia, malignant lymphoma-like syndrome, megaloblastic anemia

Ocular: Diplopia, nystagmus

Miscellaneous: Systemic lupus-like syndrome

Drug Interactions

Metabolism/Transport Effects Metabolized to phenobarbital; **Induces** CYP1A2 (strong), 2B6 (strong), 2C8 (strong), 2C9 (strong), 3A4 (strong)

Avoid Concomitant Use

Avoid concomitant use of Primidone with any of the following: Dienogest; Dronedarone; Everolimus; Nilotinib; Nisoldipine; Pazopanib; Ranolazine; Romidepsin; Tolvaptan

Increased Effect/Toxicity

Primidone may increase the levels/effects of: Alcohol (Ethyl); Barbiturates; CNS Depressants; Methotrimeprazine

The levels/effects of Primidone may be increased by: Carbonic Anhydrase Inhibitors; Divalproex; Felbamate; Methotrimeprazine; Valproic Acid

Decreased Effect

Primidone may decrease the levels/effects of: Bendamustine; Corticosteroids (Systemic); CYP1A2 Substrates; CYP2B6 Substrates; CYP2C8 Substrates (High risk); CYP2C9 Substrates (High risk); CYP3A4 Substrates; Dienogest; Divalproex; Dronedarone; Everolimus; GuanFACINE; LamoTRIgine; Maraviroc; NIFEdipine; Nilotinib; Nisoldipine; Pazopanib; QuiNIDine; Ranolazine; Romidepsin; Rufinamide; Saxagliptin; Sorafenib; Tadalafil; Tolvaptan; Treprostinil; Valproic Acid

The levels/effects of Primidone may be decreased by: Carbonic Anhydrase Inhibitors; Folic Acid; Ketorolac; Ketorolac (Systemic); Leucovorin Calcium-Levoleucovorin; Mefloquine; Methylfolate; Phenytoin

Food Interactions May increase the metabolism of vitamins D and K; dietary requirements of vitamins D, K, B$_{12}$, folate, and calcium may be increased with long-term use

Mechanism of Action Decreases neuron excitability, raises seizure threshold similar to phenobarbital

Pharmacokinetics (Adult data unless noted)

Distribution: V$_d$: Adults: 2-3 L/kg

Protein-binding: 99%

Metabolism: In the liver to phenobarbital (active) and phenylethylmalonamide (PEMA)

Bioavailability: 60% to 80%

Half-life:

Primidone: 10-12 hours

PEMA: 16 hours

Phenobarbital: 52-118 hours (age-dependent)

Time to peak serum concentration: Oral: Within 4 hours

Elimination: Urinary excretion of both active metabolites and unchanged primidone (15% to 25%)

Usual Dosage Oral:

Neonates: 12-20 mg/kg/day in divided doses 2-4 times/day; start with lower dosage and titrate upward

Children <8 years: Initial: 50-125 mg/day given at bedtime; increase by 50-125 mg/day increments every 3-7 days; usual dose: 10-25 mg/kg/day in divided doses 3-4 times/day

Children ≥8 years and Adults: Initial: 125-250 mg/day at bedtime; increase by 125-250 mg/day every 3-7 days;

usual dose: 750-1500 mg/day in divided doses 3-4 times/day with maximum dosage of 2 g/day

Administration Oral: Administer with food to decrease GI upset

Monitoring Parameters Serum primidone and phenobarbital concentrations; CBC with differential; neurological status, seizure frequency, duration, severity; signs and symptoms of suicidality (eg, anxiety, depression, behavior changes) (see Warnings)

Reference Range Monitor both primidone and phenobarbital concentrations (see Phenobarbital on page 1097); Primidone:

Therapeutic: 5-12 mcg/mL (SI: 23-55 micromoles/L)

Toxic effects rarely present with levels <10 mcg/mL (SI: 46 micromoles/L) if phenobarbital concentrations are low

Toxic: >15 mcg/mL (SI: >69 micromoles/L)

Patient Information Avoid alcohol; limit caffeine. May cause drowsiness and impair ability to perform activities requiring mental alertness or physical coordination. Do not abruptly discontinue (an increase in seizure activity may occur) or change dose without physician approval. Antiepileptic agents may increase the risk of suicidal thoughts and behavior; notify physician if you feel more depressed or have thoughts of suicide or self-harm (see Warnings). Report behavioral or CNS changes (increased sedation, lethargy); worsening of seizure activity or loss of seizure control.

Additional Information Mysoline® suspension was discontinued in February 2001

Dosage Forms Excipient information presented when available (limited, particularly for generics); consult specific product labeling.

Tablet: 50 mg, 250 mg [generic tablet may contain sodium benzoate]

Mysoline®: 50 mg, 250 mg

Dosage forms available in Canada: Tablet: 125 mg, 250 mg. **Note:** 50 mg tablet is **not** available in Canada.

◆ **Primlev™** *see* Oxycodone and Acetaminophen *on page 1041*

◆ **Primsol®** *see* Trimethoprim *on page 1386*

◆ **Prinivil®** *see* Lisinopril *on page 832*

◆ **Priorix™ (Can)** *see* Measles, Mumps, and Rubella Vaccines (Combined) *on page 862*

◆ **Pristinamycin** *see* Quinupristin/Dalfopristin *on page 1196*

◆ **Privigen®** *see* Immune Globulin (Intravenous) *on page 719*

◆ **Privine® [OTC]** *see* Naphazoline *on page 966*

◆ **ProAir® HFA** *see* Albuterol *on page 57*

◆ **PRO-Amiodarone (Can)** *see* Amiodarone *on page 84*

◆ **PRO-Azithromycin (Can)** *see* Azithromycin *on page 164*

Probenecid (proe BEN e sid)

Medication Safety Issues

Sound-alike/look-alike issues:

Probenecid may be confused with Procanbid®

Canadian Brand Names Benuryl™

Therapeutic Category Adjuvant Therapy, Penicillin Level Prolongation; Antigout Agent; Uric Acid Lowering Agent; Uricosuric Agent

Generic Available Yes

Use Treatment of hyperuricemia associated with gout and gouty arthritis; adjuvant to therapy with penicillins or cephalosporins to prolong serum levels

Lactation Excretion in breast milk unknown

Contraindications Hypersensitivity to probenecid or any component; children <2 years of age; individuals with blood dyscrasias or uric acid kidney stones

Warnings Salicylates may diminish the therapeutic effect of probenecid; this effect may be more pronounced with high, chronic doses; however, the manufacturer recommends the use of an alternative analgesic even in place of small doses of aspirin; therapy with probenecid should not be initiated until an acute gouty attack has subsided; if an acute attack occurs during probenecid therapy, usage may continue but other appropriate agents (eg, colchicine) should be used to control the acute attack

Precautions Use with caution in patients with peptic ulcer; hematuria, renal colic; formation of uric acid stones associated with the use of probenecid may be prevented by liberal fluid intake and alkalinization of urine; may not be effective when Cl_{cr} <30 mL/minute

Adverse Reactions

Cardiovascular: Flushing

Central nervous system: Dizziness, headache, fever

Dermatologic: Rash, alopecia, dermatitis, pruritus

Gastrointestinal: Anorexia, nausea, vomiting, sore gums

Genitourinary: Urinary frequency, hematuria

Hematologic: Anemia, leukopenia, aplastic anemia, hemolytic anemia (possibly related to G-6-PD deficiency)

Hepatic: Hepatic necrosis

Neuromuscular & skeletal: Costovertebral pain, gouty arthritis (acute)

Renal: Nephrotic syndrome, renal colic, uric acid stones

Miscellaneous: Hypersensitivity reactions

Drug Interactions

Metabolism/Transport Effects Inhibits CYP2C19 (weak)

Avoid Concomitant Use

Avoid concomitant use of Probenecid with any of the following: Doripenem; Ketorolac; Ketorolac (Systemic); Meropenem

Increased Effect/Toxicity

Probenecid may increase the levels/effects of: Cephalosporins; Dapsone; Dapsone (Systemic); Doripenem; Ertapenem; Ganciclovir-Valganciclovir; Gemifloxacin; Imipenem; Ketoprofen; Ketorolac; Ketorolac (Systemic); Loop Diuretics; LORazepam; Meropenem; Methotrexate; Mycophenolate; Nitrofurantoin; Nonsteroidal Anti-Inflammatory Agents; Oseltamivir; Penicillins; Peramivir; Pralatrexate; Quinolone Antibiotics; Sodium Benzoate; Sodium Phenylacetate; Theophylline Derivatives; Zidovudine

Decreased Effect

Probenecid may decrease the levels/effects of: Loop Diuretics

The levels/effects of Probenecid may be decreased by: Salicylates

Mechanism of Action Competitively inhibits the reabsorption of uric acid at the proximal convoluted tubule, thereby promoting its excretion and reducing serum uric acid levels; increases plasma levels of weak organic acids (penicillins, cephalosporins, or other beta-lactam antibiotics) by competitively inhibiting their renal tubular secretion

Pharmacodynamics Exerts maximal effects on penicillin levels after 2 hours; produces maximal renal clearance of uric acid in 30 minutes

Pharmacokinetics (Adult data unless noted)

Absorption: Rapid and complete from GI tract

Protein binding: 85% to 95%

Metabolism: In the liver

Half-life: 6-12 hours

Time to peak serum concentration: Within 2-4 hours

Usual Dosage Oral:

Prolongation of penicillin serum levels:

Children 2-14 years: Initial: 25 mg/kg/dose or 0.7 g/m^2/dose as a single dose; maintenance: 40 mg/kg/day or 1.2 g/m^2/day in 4 divided doses (maximum single dose: 500 mg)

Adults: 500 mg 4 times/day

Hyperuricemia: Adults: Initial: 250 mg twice daily for 1 week; increase to 500 mg twice daily; may increase in 500 mg increments every 4 weeks if needed to a maximum of 2-3 g/day; begin therapy 2-3 weeks after an acute gouty attack

Gonorrhea: Children >45 kg and Adults: CDC guidelines (alternative regimen): 1 g before appropriate antibiotic (eg, cefoxitin)

Pelvic inflammatory disease: CDC guidelines (alternative regimen): 1 g before appropriate antibiotic (eg, cefoxitin)

Neurosyphilis: CDC guidelines (alternative regimen): 500 mg 4 times/day plus procaine penicillin 2.4 million units/day I.M. for 10-14 days

Dosing adjustment in renal impairment: Cl_{cr} <30 mL/minute: Avoid use

Administration Oral: Administer with food or antacids to minimize GI effects

Monitoring Parameters Uric acid, renal function, CBC

Test Interactions False-positive glucosuria with Clinitest®; falsely elevated serum theophylline level (Schack & Waxler technique); inhibits renal excretion of phenosulfonphthalein (PSP), 17-ketosteroids, and sulfobromophthalein (BSP)

Patient Information Drink plenty of fluids to reduce the risk of uric acid stones; the frequency of acute gouty attacks may increase during the first 6-12 months of therapy; avoid taking large doses of aspirin or other salicylates; avoid alcohol

Dosage Forms Excipient information presented when available (limited, particularly for generics); consult specific product labeling.

Tablet: 500 mg

References

Centers for Disease Control and Prevention, "Sexually Transmitted Diseases Treatment Guidelines, 2006," *MMWR Recomm Rep*, 2006, 55(RR-11):1-94.

Procainamide (proe kane A mide)

Medication Safety Issues

Sound-alike/look-alike issues:

Procanbid may be confused with probenecid, Procan SR®

Procan SR® may be confused with procanbid

Pronestyl may be confused with Ponstel®

High alert medication: The Institute for Safe Medication Practices (ISMP) includes this medication among its list of drugs which have a heightened risk of causing significant patient harm when used in error.

Procainamide hydrochloride is available in 10 mL vials of 100 mg/mL and in 2 mL vials with 500 mg/mL. Note that **BOTH** vials contain 1 gram of drug; confusing the strengths can lead to massive overdoses or underdoses.

PCA is an error-prone abbreviation (mistaken as patient controlled analgesia)

Related Information

Adult ACLS Algorithms *on page 1463*

CPR Pediatric Drug Dosages *on page 1455*

Medications for Which A Single Dose May Be Fatal When Ingested By A Toddler *on page 1709*

Pediatric ALS Algorithms *on page 1460*

Canadian Brand Names Apo-Procainamide®; Procainamide Hydrochloride Injection, USP; Procan SR®

Therapeutic Category Antiarrhythmic Agent, Class I-A

Generic Available Yes

Use Treatment of ventricular arrhythmias (eg, sustained ventricular tachycardia) (FDA approved in adults), symptomatic premature ventricular contractions, atrial fibrillation. **Note:** Due to proarrhythmic effects, use should be reserved for life-threatening arrhythmias

Procainamide is recommended in the PALS guidelines for tachycardia with pulses and poor perfusion [SVT (unresponsive to vagal maneuvers and adenosine) and VT (unresponsive to synchronized cardioversion or adenosine)]. It is recommended in the ACLS guidelines as one of several drugs that can be considered for treatment of the following arrhythmias in patients with preserved ventricular function: Stable monomorphic VT; atrial fibrillation or atrial flutter, including pre-excitation syndrome; AV re-entrant narrow complex tachycardias (eg, re-entrant SVT), uncontrolled by adenosine and vagal maneuvers; and stable wide complex regular tachycardia (likely VT).

Pregnancy Risk Factor C

Lactation Enters breast milk/not recommended

Breast-Feeding Considerations Considered compatible by the AAP. However, the AAP stated concern regarding long-term effects and potential for infant toxicity. Use caution and monitor closely if continuing to breast-feed while taking procainamide.

Contraindications Hypersensitivity to procainamide, procaine, related drugs, or any component (see Warnings); complete heart block; second degree heart block or various types of hemiblock without a functional artificial pacemaker; "torsade de pointes" (twisting of the points); SLE

Warnings Antiarrhythmic agents should be reserved for patients with life-threatening ventricular arrhythmias **[U.S. Boxed Warning]**. In the Cardiac Arrhythmia Suppression Trial (CAST), recent (>6 days but <2 years ago) myocardial infarction patients with asymptomatic, nonlife-threatening ventricular arrhythmias did not benefit and may have been harmed by attempts to suppress the arrhythmia with flecainide or encainide. An increased mortality or nonfatal cardiac arrest rate (7.7%) was seen in the active treatment group compared with patients in the placebo group (3%). The applicability of the CAST results to other populations is unknown.

Potentially fatal blood dyscrasias have occurred with therapeutic doses **[U.S. Boxed Warning]**; close monitoring is recommended during the first 3 months of therapy and periodically thereafter (see Adverse Reactions). Long-term administration leads to the development of a positive antinuclear antibody (ANA) test in 50% of patients which may lead to a lupus erythematosus-like syndrome (in 20% to 30% of patients) **[U.S. Boxed Warning]**; assess relative benefits and risks if ANA titer becomes positive and consider alternative agent; discontinue procainamide if SLE symptoms develop and change to alternative agent; injection contains sulfites which may cause allergic reactions in susceptible individuals

Precautions Use with caution in patients with marked A-V conduction disturbances, bundle-branch block or severe cardiac glycoside intoxication, ventricular arrhythmias in patients with organic heart disease or coronary occlusion, CHF, supraventricular tachyarrhythmias unless digitalis glycoside levels are adequate to prevent marked increases in ventricular rates. Use with caution with concurrent use of other antiarrhythmics; may exacerbate or increase the risk of conduction disturbances. Drug may accumulate in patients with renal or hepatic dysfunction; use with caution; dosage adjustment required. Avoid use in myasthenia gravis; may worsen condition. An interruption of procainamide infusion may be required if a significant widening of the QRS complex or marked QT prolongation occurs (this may indicate overdosage). Use with extreme caution in patients with pre-existing QT prolongation; may increase risk for development of torsades de pointes.

Adverse Reactions

Cardiovascular: Arrhythmias, A-V block, flushing, hypotension, QT prolongation, tachycardia, widening QRS complex

Central nervous system: Confusion, depression, disorientation, dizziness, drug fever, hallucinations, psychosis

Dermatologic: Angioneurotic edema, pruritus, rash, urticaria

Gastrointestinal: Abdominal pain, anorexia, diarrhea, nausea, vomiting

Hematologic: Agranulocytosis, hemolytic anemia, neutropenia, thrombocytopenia

Hepatic: Bilirubin increased, hepatomegaly, liver enzymes increased, liver failure

Musculoskeletal: Weakness

Miscellaneous: Lupus-like syndrome (arthralgia, fever, myalgia, pericarditis, pleural effusion, positive Coombs' test, rash, thrombocytopenia)

Drug Interactions

Metabolism/Transport Effects Substrate of CYP2D6 (major)

Avoid Concomitant Use

Avoid concomitant use of Procainamide with any of the following: Artemether; Dronedarone; Lumefantrine; Nilotinib; Pimozide; QuiNINE; Tetrabenazine; Thioridazine; Ziprasidone

Increased Effect/Toxicity

Procainamide may increase the levels/effects of: Dronedarone; Neuromuscular-Blocking Agents; Pimozide; QTc-Prolonging Agents; QuiNINE; Tetrabenazine; Thioridazine; Ziprasidone

The levels/effects of Procainamide may be increased by: Alfuzosin; Amiodarone; Artemether; Chloroquine; Cimetidine; Ciprofloxacin; Ciprofloxacin (Systemic); CYP2D6 Inhibitors (Moderate); CYP2D6 Inhibitors (Strong); Darunavir; Gadobutrol; Lumefantrine; Nilotinib; QuiNINE; Ranitidine; Trimethoprim

Decreased Effect

The levels/effects of Procainamide may be decreased by: Peginterferon Alfa-2b

Stability Use only clear or slightly yellow solutions; stability of parenteral admixture with D_5W at room temperature (25°C) is 24 hours but 7 days at refrigerated temperature (2°C to 8°C)

Mechanism of Action Class IA antiarrhythmic with anticholinergic and local anesthetic effects; decreases myocardial excitability and conduction velocity and depresses myocardial contractility, by increasing the electrical stimulation threshold of ventricle, His-Purkinje system and through direct cardiac effects

Pharmacodynamics Onset of action: I.M. 10-30 minutes

Pharmacokinetics (Adult data unless noted)

Distribution: V_d (decreased with CHF or shock):
  Children: 2.2 L/kg
  Adults: 2 L/kg

Protein binding: 15% to 20%

Metabolism: By acetylation in the liver to produce N-acetyl procainamide (NAPA) (active metabolite)

Half-life:
  Procainamide (dependent upon hepatic acetylator phenotype, cardiac function, and renal function):
    Children: 1.7 hours
    Adults with normal renal function: 2.5-4.7 hours
  NAPA (dependent upon renal function):
    Children: 6 hours
    Adults with normal renal function: 6-8 hours

Time to peak serum concentration: I.M.: 15-60 minutes

Elimination: Urinary excretion (25% as NAPA)

Dialysis: Moderately dialyzable by hemodialysis (20% to 50%), but not dialyzable by peritoneal dialysis

◀ **Usual Dosage** Must be titrated to patient's response
Children:
I.M.: 20-30 mg/kg/day divided every 4-6 hours; maximum: 4 g/day
I.V.:
Loading dose: 3-6 mg/kg/dose over 5 minutes, not to exceed 100 mg/dose; may repeat every 5-10 minutes to maximum total loading dose of 15 mg/kg; do not exceed 500 mg in 30 minutes
Maintenance: Continuous I.V. infusion: 20-80 mcg/kg/minute; maximum dose: 2 g/day
PALS Guidelines 2005 (for perfusing tachycardias): **Note:** Use extreme caution when administering procainamide with other drugs that prolong QT interval (eg, amiodarone); consider consulting with expert
I.V., I.O.: Loading dose: 15 mg/kg infused over 30-60 minutes; monitor ECG and blood pressure; stop the infusion if hypotension occurs or QRS complex widens by >50% of baseline
Adults:
I.M.: 50 mg/kg/day divided every 3-6 hours **or** 0.5-1 g every 4-8 hours (Koch-Weser, 1971)
I.V.:
Loading dose: 15-18 mg/kg administered as slow infusion over 25-30 minutes **or** 100 mg/dose at a rate not to exceed 50 mg/minute repeated every 5 minutes as needed to a total dose of 1 g. Reduce loading dose to 12 mg/kg in severe renal or cardiac impairment.
Maintenance dose: 1-4 mg/minute by continuous infusion. Maintenance infusions should be reduced by one-third in patients with moderate renal or cardiac impairment and by two-thirds in patients with severe renal or cardiac impairment.
ACLS guidelines: Loading dose: Infuse 20 mg/minute (up to 50 mg/minute for more urgent situations) until arrhythmia is controlled, hypotension occurs, QRS complex widens by 50% of its original width, or total of 17 mg/kg is given. **Note:** Not recommended for use in ongoing ventricular fibrillation (VF) or pulseless ventricular tachycardia (VT) due to prolonged administration time and uncertain efficacy. Follow with maintenance dose as continuous infusion.
Dosing interval in renal impairment:
I.V.: Adults:
Loading dose: Reduce dose to 12 mg/kg in severe renal impairment.
Maintenance infusion: Reduce dose by one-third in patients with mild renal impairment. Reduce dose by two-thirds in patients with severe renal impairment.
Dialysis:
Procainamide: Moderately hemodialyzable (20% to 50%): Monitor procainamide/N-acetylprocainamide (NAPA) levels; supplementation may be necessary.
NAPA: Not dialyzable (0% to 5%)
Procainamide/NAPA: Not peritoneal dialyzable (0% to 5%)
Procainamide/NAPA: Replace by blood level during continuous arteriovenous or venovenous hemofiltration
Dosing adjustment in hepatic impairment: Reduce dose by 50%.
Administration I.V.: Do not administer faster than 20-30 mg/minute; severe hypotension can occur with rapid I.V. administration; administer I.V. push over at least 5 minutes; administer I.V. loading doses and intermittent infusions over 25-30 minutes; use concentration of 20-30 mg/mL for loading dose and 2-4 mg/mL for maintenance infusions; rate of infusion (mL/hour) = dose (mcg/kg/minute) x weight (kg) x 60 minutes/hour divided by the concentration
Monitoring Parameters ECG, blood pressure; CBC with differential and platelet counts at weekly intervals for the first 3 months of treatment, periodically thereafter, or if

signs of infection, bruising or bleeding occur; antinuclear antibody test (ANA); renal function; serum drug concentrations (procainamide and NAPA) especially in patients with hepatic impairment, renal failure, or those receiving higher maintenance doses (eg, adults: >3 mg/minute) for >24 hours
Reference Range
Therapeutic:
Procainamide: 4-10 mcg/mL (SI: 15-37 micromoles/L)
Sum of procainamide and N-acetyl procainamide: 10-30 mcg/mL (SI: <110 micromoles/L)
Optimal ranges must be ascertained for individual patients, with ECG monitoring
Toxic (procainamide): >10-12 mcg/mL (SI: >37-44 micromoles/L)
Test Interactions In the presence of propranolol or suprapharmacologic concentrations of lidocaine or meprobamate, tests which depend on fluorescence to measure procainamide/NAPA concentrations may be affected.
Dosage Forms Excipient information presented when available (limited, particularly for generics); consult specific product labeling. [CAN] = Canadian brand name
Injection, solution, as hydrochloride: 100 mg/mL (10 mL); 500 mg/mL (2 mL) [contains sodium metabisulfite]
Tablet, sustained release, oral, as hydrochloride:
Procan SR® [CAN]: 250 mg, 500 mg, 750 mg [not available in U.S.]
References
American Heart Association Emergency Cardiovascular Care Committee, "2005 American Heart Association (AHA) Guidelines for Cardiopulmonary Resuscitation (CPR) and Emergency Cardiovascular Care (ECC), Part 7.2: Management of Cardiac Arrest, Part 7.3: Management of Symptomatic Bradycardia and Tachycardia, and Part 12: Pediatric Advanced Life Support," *Circulation,* 2005, 112(24 Suppl):IV58-77,167-87.
Koch-Weser J and Klein SW, "Procainamide Dosage Schedules, Plasma Concentrations, and Clinical Effects," *JAMA,* 1971, 215 (9):1454-60.
Singh S, Gelband H, Mehta AV, et al, "Procainamide Elimination Kinetics in Pediatric Patients," *Clin Pharmacol Ther,* 1982, 32 (5):607-11.

♦ **Procainamide Hydrochloride** *see* Procainamide *on page 1156*

♦ **Procainamide Hydrochloride Injection, USP (Can)** *see* Procainamide *on page 1156*

Procaine (PROE kane)

Medication Safety Issues
High alert medication: The Institute for Safe Medication Practices (ISMP) includes this medication (epidural administration) among its list of drug classes which have a heightened risk of causing significant patient harm when used in error.
U.S. Brand Names Novocain® [DSC]
Therapeutic Category Local Anesthetic, Injectable
Generic Available No
Use Production of local or regional analgesia and anesthesia by local infiltration and peripheral nerve block techniques
Pregnancy Risk Factor C
Pregnancy Considerations Reproduction studies have not been conducted. Local anesthetics cross the placenta; effects to the fetus depend on procedure and type of administration.
Lactation Excretion in breast milk unknown/use caution
Contraindications Hypersensitivity to procaine, PABA, parabens, any anesthetic of the ester type, or any component; cerebrospinal diseases such as meningitis or syphilis and septicemia (spinal anesthetic use)

Warnings Convulsions and cardiac arrhythmias, due to systemic toxicity leading to cardiac arrest have been reported, presumably following unintentional I.V. injection; should be administered in small incremental doses

Precautions Use with extreme caution as lumbar or caudal anesthesia in patients with existing neurologic disease, spinal deformities, or severe hypertension. Use with caution in patients with cardiac disease, hepatic or renal disease. Use caution in debilitated, elderly, or acutely-ill patients; dose reduction may be required. Some preparations contain metabisulfite which may cause allergic reactions in susceptible individuals. Chondrolysis has been reported following continuous intra-articular infusion; intra-articular administration of local anesthetics is not an FDA-approved route of administration.

Adverse Reactions Degree of adverse effects in the CNS and cardiovascular system is directly related to the blood level of procaine, route of administration, and physical status of the patient. The effects below are more likely to occur after systemic administration rather than infiltration.

Cardiovascular: Bradycardia, cardiac arrest, cardiac output decreased, heart block, hypertension, hypotension, myocardial depression, syncope, tachycardia, ventricular arrhythmias

Central nervous system: Anxiety, chills, depression, dizziness, excitation, fever, headache, restlessness, seizures, tremors

Dermatologic: Angioneurotic edema, erythema, pruritus, urticaria

Gastrointestinal: Fecal incontinence, nausea, vomiting

Genitourinary: Incontinence, urinary retention

Neuromuscular & skeletal: Chondrolysis (continuous intra-articular administration), paralysis, paresthesia, tremors, weakness

Ocular: Blurred vision, pupil constriction

Otic: Tinnitus

Respiratory: Apnea, hypoventilation, sneezing

Miscellaneous: Allergic reaction, anaphylactoid reaction, diaphoresis

Drug Interactions

Avoid Concomitant Use

Avoid concomitant use of Procaine with any of the following: Sulfonamide Derivatives

Increased Effect/Toxicity There are no known significant interactions involving an increase in effect.

Decreased Effect

Procaine may decrease the levels/effects of: Sulfonamide Derivatives

Stability Store at controlled room temperature of 15°C to 30°C (59°F to 86°F); protect from light. Solutions may be sterilized by autoclaving for 15 minutes; reautoclaving increases the likelihood of crystal formation. Stable in dextrose, dextran 6% in NS, D_5LR, $D_51/4NS$, $D_51/2NS$, D_5NS, D_5W, $D_{10}W$, LR, $1/2NS$, NS.

Mechanism of Action Blocks both the initiation and conduction of nerve impulses by decreasing the neuronal membrane's permeability to sodium ions, which results in inhibition of depolarization with resultant blockade of conduction

Pharmacodynamics

Onset of action: 2-5 minutes

Duration (patient, type of block, concentration, and method of anesthesia dependent): 1 hour

Pharmacokinetics (Adult data unless noted)

Metabolism: Rapidly hydrolyzed by plasma enzymes to para-aminobenzoic acid and diethylaminoethanol (80% conjugated before elimination)

Half-life (in vitro):

Neonates: 84 ± 30 seconds

Adults: 40 ± 9 seconds

Elimination: Urine (as metabolites and some unchanged drug)

Usual Dosage Dose varies with procedure, desired depth, and duration of anesthesia, desired muscle relaxation, vascularity of tissues, physical condition, and age of patient. The smallest dose and concentration required to produce the desired effect should be used.

Children: Maximum dose: 15 mg/kg of 0.5% solution

Adults: Maximum dose: 1000 mg per treatment

Infiltration anesthesia: 0.25% to 0.5% solution: 350-600 mg

Peripheral nerve block: 0.5% (up to 200 mL), 1% (up to 100 mL), 2% (up to 50 mL)

Spinal anesthesia: Using 10% (diluted prior to use with NS, SWI, spinal fluid; and for hyperbaric technique, sterile dextrose solution):

Extent of anesthesia: Perineum: 0.5 mL (50 mg) diluent volume 0.5 mL

Perineum and local extremities: 1 mL (100 mg) diluent volume 1 mL

Up to costal margin: 2 mL (200 mg) diluent volume 1 mL

Administration Parenteral: Administer in small incremental doses; when using continuous intermittent catheter techniques, use frequent aspirations before and during the injection to avoid intravascular injection; for spinal anesthesia, inject 1 mL per 5 seconds

Monitoring Parameters Blood pressure, heart rate, respiration, signs of CNS toxicity (lightheadedness, dizziness, tinnitus, restlessness, tremors, twitching, drowsiness, circumoral paresthesia)

Patient Information You will experience decreased sensation to pain, heat, or cold in the area and/or decreased muscle strength (depending on area of application) until effects wear off; use necessary caution to reduce incidence of possible injury until full sensation returns. Report irritation, pain, burning at injection site; chest pain or palpitations; or respiratory difficulty.

Dosage Forms Excipient information presented when available (limited, particularly for generics); consult specific product labeling. [DSC] = Discontinued product

Injection, solution, as hydrochloride:

Novocain®: 10% (2 mL) [contains sodium bisulfite] [DSC]

◆ **Procaine Amide Hydrochloride** see Procainamide on page 1156

◆ **Procaine Benzylpenicillin** see Penicillin G Procaine on page 1081

◆ **Procaine Hydrochloride** see Procaine on page 1158

◆ **Procaine Penicillin G** see Penicillin G Procaine on page 1081

◆ **PRO-Calcitonin (Can)** see Calcitonin on page 227

◆ **Procanbid** see Procainamide on page 1156

◆ **Procan SR® (Can)** see Procainamide on page 1156

Procarbazine (proe KAR ba zeen)

Medication Safety Issues

Sound-alike/look-alike issues:

Procarbazine may be confused with dacarbazine

Matulane® may be confused with Materna®

High alert medication: The Institute for Safe Medication Practices (ISMP) includes this medication among its list of drugs which have a heightened risk of causing significant patient harm when used in error.

Related Information

Emetogenic Potential of Antineoplastic Agents on page 1579

U.S. Brand Names Matulane®

Canadian Brand Names Matulane®; Natulan®

Therapeutic Category Antineoplastic Agent, Miscellaneous

◀ **Generic Available** No

Use Treatment of Hodgkin's disease [FDA approved in pediatrics (age not specified) and adults], has also been used in non-Hodgkin's lymphoma and brain tumors

Pregnancy Risk Factor D

Pregnancy Considerations Animal studies have demonstrated teratogenic effects. There are no adequate and well-controlled studies in pregnant women. There are, however, case reports of fetal malformations in the offspring of pregnant women exposed to procarbazine as part of a combination chemotherapy regimen. Women of childbearing potential should avoid becoming pregnant during treatment.

Lactation Excretion in breast milk unknown/not recommended

Contraindications Hypersensitivity to procarbazine or any component; pre-existing bone marrow aplasia

Warnings Hazardous agent; use appropriate precautions for handling and disposal; procarbazine is a carcinogen which may cause a secondary acute nonlymphocytic leukemia; procarbazine may cause infertility and is potentially teratogenic. Bone marrow suppression may occur 2-8 weeks after treatment initiation; allow ≥1 month interval between radiation therapy or myelosuppressive chemotherapy and initiation of treatment. Withhold treatment for leukopenia (WBC <4000/mm^3) or thrombocytopenia (platelets <100,000/mm^3), hypersensitivity reactions, stomatitis, diarrhea, or hemorrhage or bleeding tendencies.

Precautions May potentiate CNS depression when used with phenothiazine derivatives, barbiturates, narcotics, alcohol, tricyclic antidepressants, methyldopa; use with caution in patients with pre-existing renal or hepatic impairment; renal impairment (serum creatinine >2 mg/dL and/or a blood urea nitrogen >40 mg/dL), or decreased hepatic function (total bilirubin >3 mg/dL)

Adverse Reactions

Central nervous system: Cerebellar ataxia, chills, CNS depression, confusion, dizziness, fever, hallucinations, headache, irritability, nervousness, nightmares, seizures, somnolence

Dermatologic: Alopecia, dermatitis, hypersensitivity, rash, pruritus

Endocrine & metabolic: Amenorrhea, disulfiram-like reaction

Gastrointestinal: Anorexia, diarrhea, nausea, stomatitis, vomiting

Genitourinary: Azoospermia, ovarian failure

Hematologic: Hemolysis, myelosuppression, pancytopenia, thrombocytopenia

Neuromuscular & skeletal: Arthralgia, myalgia, neuropathy, tremor, weakness

Ocular: Diplopia, nystagmus, photophobia

Miscellaneous: Flu-like syndrome

Drug Interactions

Avoid Concomitant Use

Avoid concomitant use of Procarbazine with any of the following: Alpha-/Beta-Agonists (Indirect-Acting); Alpha1-Agonists; Alpha2-Agonists (Ophthalmic); Amphetamines; Anilidopiperidine Opioids; Atomoxetine; BCG; BuPRO-Pion; BusPIRone; CarBAMazepine; Cyclobenzaprine; Dexmethylphenidate; Dextromethorphan; HYDROmorphone; Linezolid; Maprotiline; Meperidine; Methyldopa; Methylphenidate; Mirtazapine; Natalizumab; Pimecrolimus; Propoxyphene; Selective Serotonin Reuptake Inhibitors; Serotonin 5-HT1D Receptor Agonists; Serotonin/Norepinephrine Reuptake Inhibitors; Sibutramine; Tacrolimus (Topical); Tapentadol; Tetrabenazine; Tetrahydrozoline; Tetrahydrozoline (Nasal); Tricyclic Antidepressants; Vaccines (Live)

Increased Effect/Toxicity

Procarbazine may increase the levels/effects of: Alpha-/Beta-Agonists (Direct-Acting); Alpha-/Beta-Agonists (Indirect-Acting); Alpha1-Agonists; Alpha2-Agonists (Ophthalmic); Amphetamines; Antihypertensives; Atomoxetine; Beta2-Agonists; BuPROPion; Dexmethylphenidate; Dextromethorphan; HYDROmorphone; Leflunomide; Linezolid; Lithium; Meperidine; Methadone; Methyldopa; Methylphenidate; Mirtazapine; Natalizumab; Orthostatic Hypotension Producing Agents; Rauwolfia Alkaloids; Selective Serotonin Reuptake Inhibitors; Serotonin 5-HT1D Receptor Agonists; Serotonin Modulators; Serotonin/Norepinephrine Reuptake Inhibitors; Tetrahydrozoline; Tetrahydrozoline (Nasal); Tricyclic Antidepressants; Vaccines (Live); Vitamin K Antagonists

The levels/effects of Procarbazine may be increased by: Altretamine; Anilidopiperidine Opioids; BusPIRone; Car-BAMazepine; COMT Inhibitors; Cyclobenzaprine; Denosumab; Levodopa; MAO Inhibitors; Maprotiline; Pimecrolimus; Propoxyphene; Sibutramine; Tacrolimus (Topical); Tapentadol; Tetrabenazine; TraMADol; Trastuzumab

Decreased Effect

Procarbazine may decrease the levels/effects of: BCG; Cardiac Glycosides; Sipuleucel-T; Vaccines (Inactivated); Vaccines (Live); Vitamin K Antagonists

The levels/effects of Procarbazine may be decreased by: Echinacea

Food Interactions Avoid food with high tyramine content (cheese, tea, dark beer, coffee, cola drinks, wine, bananas) as hypertensive crisis, tremor, excitation, cardiac palpitations, and angina may occur

Stability Unstable in water or aqueous solution; avoid contact of the drug with moisture

Mechanism of Action Inhibits DNA, RNA, and protein synthesis; may damage DNA directly via free-radical formation and suppress mitosis

Pharmacokinetics (Adult data unless noted)

Absorption: Oral: Well absorbed

Distribution: Crosses the blood-brain barrier and distributes into CSF, liver, kidney, intestine, and skin

Metabolism: In the liver; first-pass conversion to cytotoxic metabolites

Half-life: 10 minutes

Time to peak serum concentration: Within 1 hour

Elimination: In urine (<5% as unchanged drug) and 70% as metabolites

Usual Dosage Oral (refer to individual protocols; base dosage on ideal body weight):

Children:

Hodgkin's disease: 50-100 mg/m^2/day once daily for 10-14 days of a 28-day cycle

Brain tumor: 75 mg/m^2 at hour 1 on day 1; repeat cycle every 2-4 weeks if tolerated; **or** 100 mg/m^2 on days 1-14 of a treatment course

Neuroblastoma and medulloblastoma: Doses as high as 100-200 mg/m^2/day once daily have been used

Adults: Initial: 2-4 mg/kg/day in single or divided doses for 7 days then increase dose to 4-6 mg/kg/day until response is obtained or leukocyte count decreases to <4000/mm^3 or the platelet count decreases to <100,000/mm^3; maintenance: 1-2 mg/kg/day

Administration Oral: Administer with food or after meals; total daily dose may be administered at a single time or in divided doses throughout the day to minimize GI toxicity

Monitoring Parameters CBC with differential, platelet count, and reticulocyte count; urinalysis, liver function test, renal function test

Patient Information Notify physician of fever, sore throat, bleeding, or bruising; avoid alcohol (disulfiram-like reaction with nausea, vomiting, headache, sedation, and visual disturbances)

Additional Information Myelosuppressive effects:
WBC: Moderate
Platelets: Moderate
Onset (days): 14
Nadir (days): 21
Recovery (days): 28

Dosage Forms Excipient information presented when available (limited, particularly for generics); consult specific product labeling.
Capsule, as hydrochloride:
Matulane®: 50 mg

References

Longo DL, Young RC, Wesley M, et al, "Twenty Years of MOPP Therapy for Hodgkin's Disease," *J Clin Oncol*, 1986, 4(9):1295-306.
Rodriguez LA, Prados M, Silver P, et al, "Re-evaluation of Procarbazine for the Treatment of Recurrent Malignant Central Nervous System Tumors," *Cancer*, 1989, 64(12):2420-3.

♦ **Procarbazine Hydrochloride** see Procarbazine on page 1159

♦ **Procardia®** see NIFEdipine on page 991

♦ **Procardia XL®** see NIFEdipine on page 991

♦ **PRO-Cefadroxil (Can)** see Cefadroxil on page 261

♦ **PRO-Cefuroxime (Can)** see Cefuroxime on page 277

Prochlorperazine (proe klor PER a zeen)

Medication Safety Issues
Sound-alike/look-alike issues:
Prochlorperazine may be confused with chlorproMAZINE
Compazine® may be confused with Copaxone®, Coumadin®

CPZ (occasional abbreviation for Compazine®) is an error-prone abbreviation (mistaken as chlorpromazine)

Related Information
Compatibility of Chemotherapy and Related Supportive Care Medications on page 1580
Compatibility of Medications Mixed in a Syringe on page 1713

U.S. Brand Names Compro™

Canadian Brand Names Apo-Prochlorperazine®; Nu-Prochlor; Stemetil®

Therapeutic Category Antiemetic; Antipsychotic Agent, Typical, Phenothiazine; Phenothiazine Derivative

Generic Available Yes

Use Management of nonsurgical nausea and vomiting [FDA approved in ages ≥2 years or children >9 kg (20 pounds) and adults]; management of surgery-related nausea and vomiting (FDA approved in adults); acute and chronic psychosis (FDA approved in ages ≥2 years); has also been used for treatment of intractable migraine headaches

Pregnancy Considerations Crosses the placenta. Isolated reports of congenital anomalies, however, some included exposures to other drugs. Jaundice, extrapyramidal signs, hyper-/hyporeflexes have been noted in newborns. Available evidence with use of occasional low doses suggests safe use during pregnancy.

Lactation Excretion in breast milk unknown/use caution

Breast-Feeding Considerations Other phenothiazines are excreted in human milk; excretion of prochlorperazine is not known.

Contraindications Hypersensitivity to prochlorperazine or any component (see Warnings); cross-sensitivity with other phenothiazines may exist; avoid use in patients with narrow-angle glaucoma; severe liver or cardiac disease, severe toxic CNS depression or coma; pediatric surgery

Warnings High incidence of extrapyramidal reactions especially in children, reserve use in children <5 years of age to those who are unresponsive to other antiemetics; incidence of extrapyramidal reactions is increased with acute illnesses such as chicken pox, measles, CNS infections, gastroenteritis, and dehydration; extrapyramidal reactions may also be confused with CNS signs of Reye's syndrome or other encephalopathies; avoid use in these clinical conditions

Lowers seizure threshold, use cautiously in patients with seizure history; discontinue use at least 48 hours before myelography and do not resume therapy until 24 hours post myelography. Use of antipsychotics in combination with lithium has been associated with an encephalopathy syndrome similar to NMS; monitor patients closely and discontinue treatment if encephalopathic symptomatology develops.

Leukopenia, neutropenia, and agranulocytosis (sometimes fatal) have been reported in clinical trials and postmarketing reports with antipsychotic use; presence of risk factors (eg, pre-existing low WBC or history of drug-induced leuko/neutropenia) should prompt periodic blood count assessment. Discontinue therapy at first signs of blood dyscrasias or if absolute neutrophil count <1000/mm^3.

An increased risk of death has been reported with the use of antipsychotics in elderly patients with dementia-related psychosis **[U.S. Boxed Warning]**; most deaths seemed to be cardiovascular (eg, sudden death, heart failure) or infectious (eg, pneumonia) in nature; prochlorperazine is not approved for this indication.

Injection contains benzyl alcohol which may cause allergic reactions in susceptible individuals; large amounts of benzyl alcohol (≥99 mg/kg/day) have been associated with a potentially fatal toxicity ("gasping syndrome") in neonates; the "gasping syndrome" consists of metabolic acidosis, respiratory distress, gasping respirations, CNS dysfunction (including convulsions, intracranial hemorrhage), hypotension and cardiovascular collapse; avoid use of injection in neonates.

Precautions Safety and efficacy have not been established in children <9 kg or <2 years of age.

Adverse Reactions Incidence of extrapyramidal reactions are higher with prochlorperazine than chlorpromazine
Cardiovascular: Arrhythmias, hypotension (especially with I.V. use), orthostatic hypotension, sudden death, tachycardia
Central nervous system: Altered central temperature regulation, anxiety, drowsiness, dyskinesia, neuroleptic malignant syndrome, pseudoparkinsonian signs and symptoms, restlessness, sedation, seizures, tardive dyskinesia; extrapyramidal reactions, which include dystonic reactions, such as extensor rigidity of back muscles, mandibular tics, opisthotonos, spasm of neck muscles, torticollis, and trismus
Dermatologic: Hyperpigmentation, photosensitivity, pruritus, rash
Endocrine & metabolic: Abnormal glucose tolerance, amenorrhea, galactorrhea, gynecomastia, weight gain
Gastrointestinal: Constipation, GI upset, xerostomia
Genitourinary: Impotence, urinary retention
Hematologic: Agranulocytosis, eosinophilia, hemolytic anemia, leukopenia (usually in patients with large doses for prolonged periods), neutropenia, thrombocytopenia
Hepatic: Cholestatic jaundice
Ocular: Blurred vision, retinal pigmentation
Miscellaneous: Anaphylactoid reactions

Drug Interactions

Avoid Concomitant Use
Avoid concomitant use of Prochlorperazine with any of the following: Dofetilide; Metoclopramide

Increased Effect/Toxicity

Prochlorperazine may increase the levels/effects of: Alcohol (Ethyl); Analgesics (Opioid); Anticholinergics; Anti-Parkinson's Agents (Dopamine Agonist); Beta-Blockers; CNS Depressants; Dofetilide; Methotrimeprazine

The levels/effects of Prochlorperazine may be increased by: Acetylcholinesterase Inhibitors (Central); Antimalarial Agents; Beta-Blockers; Lithium formulations; Methotrimeprazine; Metoclopramide; Pramlintide; Tetrabenazine

Decreased Effect

Prochlorperazine may decrease the levels/effects of: Amphetamines; Quinagolide

The levels/effects of Prochlorperazine may be decreased by: Antacids; Anti-Parkinson's Agents (Dopamine Agonist); Lithium formulations

Food Interactions Increase dietary intake of riboflavin

Stability All dosage forms: Store at controlled room temperature; protect from light. With injection, a clear or slightly yellow solution may be used; incompatible with aminophylline, amphotericin B, ampicillin, calcium salts, cephalothin, foscarnet (Y-site), furosemide, hydrocortisone, hydromorphone, methohexital, midazolam, penicillin G, pentobarbital, phenobarbital, thiopental

Mechanism of Action Blocks postsynaptic mesolimbic dopaminergic receptors in the brain, including the medullary chemoreceptor trigger zone; exhibits a strong alpha-adrenergic blocking effect and depresses the release of hypothalamic and hypophyseal hormones

Pharmacodynamics

Onset of action:
Oral: 30-40 minutes
I.M.: Within 10-20 minutes
Rectal: Within 60 minutes

Duration:
I.M., oral extended release: 12 hours
Rectal, oral immediate release: 3-4 hours

Usual Dosage

Antiemetic:
Children >2 years or >9 kg:
Oral, rectal: 0.4 mg/kg/day in 3-4 divided doses; **or** as an alternative:
10-14 kg: 2.5 mg every 12-24 hours as needed; maximum dose: 7.5 mg/day
15-18 kg: 2.5 mg every 8-12 hours as needed; maximum dose: 10 mg/day
19-39 kg: 2.5 mg every 8 hours or 5 mg every 12 hours as needed; maximum dose: 15 mg/day
I.M., I.V.: 0.1-0.15 mg/kg/dose every 8-12 hours; not to exceed 40 mg/day

Adults:
Oral: 5-10 mg 3-4 times/day; usual maximum dose: 40 mg/day
Oral, extended release: 10 mg twice daily or 15 mg once daily
I.M.: 5-10 mg every 3-4 hours; usual maximum dose: 40 mg/day
I.V.: 2.5-10 mg; maximum 10 mg/dose or 40 mg/day; may repeat dose every 3-4 hours as needed
Rectal: 25 mg twice daily

Intractable migraine headaches (limited information available): I.V.: Children: 0.15 mg/kg as a single dose has been studied in 20 children between the ages of 8-17 years combined with I.V. hydration (see Kabbouche, 2001)

Psychoses:
Children 2-12 years:
Oral, rectal: 2.5 mg every 8-12 hours; increase dosage as needed to a maximum dose of 20 mg/day for 2-5 years and 25 mg/day for 6-12 years

I.M.: 0.13 mg/kg/dose, control usually obtained with single dose; change to oral as soon as possible

Adults:
Oral: 5-10 mg 3-4 times/day, increase as needed to a daily maximum dose of 150 mg
I.M.: 10-20 mg every 4 hours as needed, change to oral as soon as possible

Administration

Oral: Administer with food or water
Parenteral: I.M. is preferred; avoid I.V. administration; if necessary, may be administered by direct I.V. injection at a maximum rate of 5 mg/minute; do not administer by SubQ route (tissue damage may occur)

Monitoring Parameters CBC with differential and periodic ophthalmic exams (if chronically used)

Test Interactions False-positives for phenylketonuria, urinary amylase, uroporphyrins, urobilinogen

Patient Information Limit caffeine; may cause drowsiness and impair ability to perform activities requiring mental alertness or physical coordination; may cause dry mouth. May cause photosensitivity reactions (eg, exposure to sunlight may cause severe sunburn, skin rash, redness, or itching); avoid exposure to sunlight and artificial light sources (sunlamps, tanning booth/bed); wear protective clothing, wide-brimmed hats, sunglasses, and lip sunscreen (SPF ≥15); use a sunscreen [broad-spectrum sunscreen or physical sunscreen (preferred) or sunblock with SPF ≥15]; contact physician if reaction occurs.

Nursing Implications Avoid skin contact with injection; contact dermatitis has occurred

Additional Information Use lowest possible dose in pediatric patients to try to decrease incidence of extrapyramidal reactions

Dosage Forms Excipient information presented when available (limited, particularly for generics); consult specific product labeling. **Note:** Strength expressed as base unless otherwise noted.
Injection, solution, as edisylate: 5 mg/mL (2 mL, 10 mL)
Suppository, rectal: 25 mg (12s)
Compro™: 25 mg (12s) [contains coconut and palm oils]
Tablet, oral, as maleate: 5 mg, 10 mg

References

Kabbouche MA, Vockell AL, LeCates SL, et al, "Tolerability and Effectiveness of Prochlorperazine for Intractable Migraine in Children," *Pediatrics*, 2001, 107(4):E62, www.pediatrics.org/cgi/content/full/107/4/e62.

◆ **Prochlorperazine Edisylate** *see* Prochlorperazine *on page 1161*

◆ **Prochlorperazine Maleate** *see* Prochlorperazine *on page 1161*

◆ **PRO-Ciprofloxacin (Can)** *see* Ciprofloxacin *on page 310*

◆ **PRO-Clonazepam (Can)** *see* ClonazePAM *on page 337*

◆ **Procrit®** *see* Epoetin Alfa *on page 513*

◆ **Proctocort®** *see* Hydrocortisone *on page 685*

◆ **ProctoCream® HC** *see* Hydrocortisone *on page 685*

◆ **Procto-Kit™** *see* Hydrocortisone *on page 685*

◆ **Procto-Pak™** *see* Hydrocortisone *on page 685*

◆ **Proctosert** *see* Hydrocortisone *on page 685*

◆ **Proctosol-HC®** *see* Hydrocortisone *on page 685*

◆ **Proctozone-HC™** *see* Hydrocortisone *on page 685*

◆ **Procytox® (Can)** *see* Cyclophosphamide *on page 369*

◆ **PRO-Diclo-Rapide (Can)** *see* Diclofenac *on page 429*

◆ **Prodium® [OTC]** *see* Phenazopyridine *on page 1097*

◆ **PRO-Enalapril (Can)** *see* Enalapril/Enalaprilat *on page 499*

◆ **Profilnine® SD** *see* Factor IX Complex (Human) *on page 558*

◆ **Proflavanol C™ (Can)** *see Ascorbic Acid on page 138*

◆ **PRO-Fluconazole (Can)** *see Fluconazole on page 584*

◆ **PRO-Fluoxetine (Can)** *see FLUoxetine on page 600*

◆ **PRO-Gabapentin (Can)** *see Gabapentin on page 634*

◆ **PRO-Glyburide (Can)** *see GlyBURIDE on page 648*

◆ **Proglycem®** *see Diazoxide on page 427*

◆ **Prograf®** *see Tacrolimus on page 1311*

◆ **Proguanil and Atovaquone** *see Atovaquone and Proguanil on page 154*

◆ **Proguanil Hydrochloride and Atovaquone** *see Atovaquone and Proguanil on page 154*

◆ **PRO-Hydroxyquine (Can)** *see Hydroxychloroquine on page 694*

◆ **Pro-Indo (Can)** *see Indomethacin on page 726*

◆ **Proleukin®** *see Aldesleukin on page 60*

◆ **PRO-Levetiracetam (Can)** *see Levetiracetam on page 808*

◆ **PRO-Lisinopril (Can)** *see Lisinopril on page 832*

◆ **PRO-Lorazepam (Can)** *see LORazepam on page 845*

◆ **PRO-Lovastatin (Can)** *see Lovastatin on page 850*

◆ **PRO-Metformin (Can)** *see MetFORMIN on page 891*

Promethazine (proe METH a zeen)

Medication Safety Issues
Sound-alike/look-alike issues:
Promethazine may be confused with chlorproMAZINE, predniSONE, promazine
Phenergan® may be confused with Phenaphen®, PHENobarbital, Phrenilin®, Theragran®

International issues:
Sominex: Brand name for promethazine in Great Britain, but also is a brand name for diphenhydrAMINE in the U.S.

High alert medication: The Institute for Safe Medication Practices (ISMP) includes this medication (I.V. formulation) among its list of drugs which have a heightened risk of causing significant patient harm when used in error.

Beers Criteria medication: This drug may be inappropriate for use in geriatric patients (high severity risk).

Administration issues:
To prevent or minimize tissue damage during I.V. administration, the Institute for Safe Medication Practices (ISMP) has the following recommendations:
Limit concentration available to the 25 mg/mL product
Consider limiting initial doses to 6.25-12.5 mg
Further dilute the 25 mg/mL strength into 10-20 mL NS
Administer through a large bore vein (not hand or wrist)
Administer via running I.V. line at port farthest from patient's vein
Consider administering over 10-15 minutes
Instruct patients to report immediately signs of pain or burning

Related Information
Compatibility of Chemotherapy and Related Supportive Care Medications *on page 1580*
Compatibility of Medications Mixed in a Syringe *on page 1713*

U.S. Brand Names Phenadoz™; Phenergan®; Promethegan™

Canadian Brand Names Bioniche Promethazine; Histantil; Phenergan®; PMS-Promethazine

Therapeutic Category Antiemetic; Phenothiazine Derivative; Sedative

Generic Available Yes

Use Symptomatic treatment of various allergic conditions and motion sickness; sedative; antiemetic

Pregnancy Risk Factor C

Pregnancy Considerations Teratogenic effects were not observed in animal studies. There are no adequate and well-controlled studies in pregnant women. Crosses the placenta. Use during pregnancy only if benefits outweigh risk. May be used alone or as an adjunct to narcotic analgesics during labor.

Lactation Excretion in breast milk unknown/not recommended

Contraindications Hypersensitivity to promethazine or any component (cross reactivity with other phenothiazines may occur); severe toxic CNS depression or coma; intra-arterial administration; subcutaneous administration; children <2 years (see Warnings)

Warnings Contraindicated in children <2 years of age due to the potential for severe and potentially fatal respiratory depression **[U.S. Boxed Warning]**. A wide range of weight-based doses have resulted in respiratory depression; excessively high doses have been associated with sudden death in children; use with caution and use the lowest effective dose in children ≥2 years of age and avoid concomitant use with other medications having respiratory depressant effects. Injection may contain sodium metabisulfite which may cause allergic reactions in susceptible individuals. Do not give SubQ or intra-arterially due to severe local reactions including necrosis; rapid I.V. administration may produce a transient fall in blood pressure; slow I.V. administration may produce a slightly elevated blood pressure. Neuroleptic malignant syndrome (NMS) has been reported with promethazine when used alone or in combination with antipsychotic drugs. Children with dehydration are at increased risk for development of dystonic reactions. Promethazine injection can cause severe chemical irritation and damage to tissues regardless of the route of administration **[U.S. Boxed Warning]**. Irritation and damage can result from perivascular extravasation, unintentional intra-arterial injection, and intraneuronal or perineural infiltration. Adverse reactions include burning, pain, thrombophlebitis, tissue necrosis, and gangrene.

Precautions Use with caution in patients with cardiovascular disease, narrow-angle glaucoma, prostatic hypertrophy, GI or GU obstruction, bone marrow depression, impaired liver function, asthma, peptic ulcer, sleep apnea, and hypertensive crisis; avoid in patients with suspected Reye's syndrome or other hepatic diseases; promethazine may lower the seizure threshold; use with caution in patients with seizure disorders or receiving other medications which may also lower the seizure threshold; promethazine has been reported to cause cholestatic jaundice

Adverse Reactions
Cardiovascular: Angioneurotic edema, bradycardia, hypotension (rapid I.V. administration), hypertension (slow I.V. administration), palpitations, tachycardia
Central nervous system: Catatonic-like states, confusion, drowsiness, dystonia, excitation (paradoxical), extrapyramidal reactions, fatigue, hallucinations, hysteria, insomnia, NMS, sedation (pronounced), seizures, tardive dyskinesia
Dermatologic: Angioedema, photosensitivity, rash, urticaria
Endocrine & metabolic: Weight gain
Gastrointestinal: Abdominal pain, appetite increased, diarrhea, GI upset, nausea, xerostomia
Genitourinary: Urinary retention
Hematologic: Agranulocytosis (rare), leukopenia, thrombocytopenia
Hepatic: Cholestatic jaundice, hepatitis
Local: Burning, extravasation injury, pain, thrombophlebitis (injection), tissue necrosis

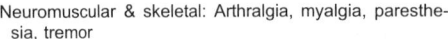

Neuromuscular & skeletal: Arthralgia, myalgia, paresthesia, tremor

Ocular: Blurred vision, diplopia

Otic: Tinnitus

Respiratory: Apnea (particularly severe in children, see Warnings), pharyngitis, respiratory depression, and thickening of bronchial secretions

Miscellaneous: Allergic reactions, gangrene

Drug Interactions

Metabolism/Transport Effects Substrate (major) of CYP2B6, 2D6; **Inhibits** CYP2D6 (weak)

Avoid Concomitant Use

Avoid concomitant use of Promethazine with any of the following: Metoclopramide; Sibutramine

Increased Effect/Toxicity

Promethazine may increase the levels/effects of: Anticholinergics; Serotonin Modulators

The levels/effects of Promethazine may be increased by: CYP2B6 Inhibitors (Moderate); CYP2B6 Inhibitors (Strong); CYP2D6 Inhibitors (Moderate); CYP2D6 Inhibitors (Strong); Darunavir; MAO Inhibitors; Metoclopramide; Pramlintide; Quazepam; Sibutramine

Decreased Effect

Promethazine may decrease the levels/effects of: Acetylcholinesterase Inhibitors (Central)

The levels/effects of Promethazine may be decreased by: Acetylcholinesterase Inhibitors (Central); CYP2B6 Inducers (Strong); Peginterferon Alfa-2b

Food Interactions Increase dietary intake of riboflavin

Stability Protect from light; store injection and tablets at controlled room temperature; refrigerate suppositories; **compatible** (when comixed in the same syringe) with atropine, chlorpromazine, diphenhydramine, droperidol, fentanyl, glycopyrrolate, hydromorphone, hydroxyzine hydrochloride, meperidine, midazolam, nalbuphine, pentazocine, prochlorperazine, scopolamine; **incompatible** when mixed with aminophylline, cefoperazone (Y-site), ceftriaxone (same syringe), chloramphenicol, dexamethasone (same syringe), dimenhydrinate (same syringe), foscarnet (Y-site), furosemide, heparin, hydrocortisone, methohexital, penicillin G, pentobarbital, phenobarbital, thiopental

Mechanism of Action Blocks postsynaptic mesolimbic dopaminergic receptors in the brain; exhibits a strong alpha-adrenergic blocking effect and depresses the release of hypothalamic and hypophyseal hormones; competes with histamine for the H_1-receptor

Pharmacodynamics

Onset of action:

Oral, I.M.: Within 20 minutes

I.V.: 3-5 minutes

Duration: Oral: 4-6 hours

Pharmacokinetics (Adult data unless noted)

Absorption: 88%

Bioavailability: 25% (due to first pass metabolism)

Half-life: 9-16 hours

Metabolism: In the liver

Elimination: Principally as inactive metabolites in the urine and in the feces

Usual Dosage

Children ≥2 years (use with extreme caution utilizing the lowest most effective dose; see Warnings):

Antihistamine: Oral: 0.1 mg/kg/dose (not to exceed 12.5 mg) every 6 hours during the day and 0.5 mg/kg/dose (not to exceed 25 mg) at bedtime as needed

Antiemetic: Oral, I.M., I.V., rectal: 0.25-1 mg/kg (not to exceed 25 mg) 4-6 times/day as needed

Motion sickness: Oral, rectal: 0.5 mg/kg (not to exceed 25 mg) 30 minutes to 1 hour before departure, then every 12 hours as needed

Sedation: Oral, I.M., I.V., rectal: 0.5-1 mg/kg/dose (not to exceed 50 mg) every 6 hours as needed

Adults:

Antihistamine:

Oral, rectal: 6.25-12.5 mg 3 times/day and 25 mg at bedtime

I.M., I.V.: 25 mg, may repeat in 2 hours when necessary; switch to oral route as soon as feasible

Antiemetic: Oral, I.M., I.V., rectal: 12.5-25 mg every 4 hours as needed

Motion sickness: Oral: 25 mg twice daily with the first dose 30 minutes to 1 hour before departure, then repeat 8-12 hours later as needed

Sedation: Oral, I.M., I.V., rectal: 25-50 mg/dose; repeat every 4-6 hours if needed

Administration

Oral: Administer with food, water, or milk to decrease GI distress

Parenteral: Deep I.M. administration is preferred; avoid I.V. use (see Warnings); in selected patients, promethazine has been administered I.V. diluted to a maximum concentration of 25 mg/mL and infused at a maximum rate of 25 mg/minute; to minimize phlebitis, consider administering over 10-15 minutes; consider limiting initial dose to 6.25-12.5 mg; further dilute the 25 mg/mL strength into 10-20 mL NS; administer through a large bore vein (not hand or wrist) or via a running I.V. line at port farthest from patient's vein. Not for SubQ administration; promethazine is a chemical irritant which may produce necrosis.

Test Interactions Alters the flare response in intradermal allergen tests; false negative and positive reactions with pregnancy tests relying on immunological reactions between hCG and anti-hCG

Patient Information May cause drowsiness and impair ability to perform activities requiring mental alertness or physical coordination; notify physician of involuntary movements or feelings of restlessness; may cause dry mouth. May cause photosensitivity reactions (eg, exposure to sunlight may cause severe sunburn, skin rash, redness, or itching; avoid exposure to sunlight and artificial light sources (sunlamps, tanning booth/bed); wear protective clothing, wide-brimmed hats, sunglasses, and lip sunscreen (SPF ≥15); use a sunscreen [broad-spectrum sunscreen or physical sunscreen (preferred) or sunblock with SPF ≥15]; contact physician if reaction occurs.

Additional Information Although promethazine has been used in combination with meperidine and chlorpromazine as a premedication (lytic cocktail), this combination may have a higher rate of adverse effects compared to alternative sedative/analgesics

Dosage Forms Excipient information presented when available (limited, particularly for generics); consult specific product labeling.

Injection, solution, as hydrochloride: 25 mg/mL (1 mL); 50 mg/mL (1 mL)

Phenergan®: 25 mg/mL (1 mL); 50 mg/mL (1 mL) [contains edetate disodium, sodium metabisulfite]

Suppository, rectal, as hydrochloride: 12.5 mg (12s); 25 mg (12s)

Phenadoz™: 12.5 mg (12s); 25 mg (12s)

Promethegan™: 12.5 mg (12s); 25 mg (12s); 50 mg (12s)

Syrup, as hydrochloride: 6.25 mg/5 mL (120 mL, 480 mL)

Tablet, as hydrochloride: 12.5 mg, 25 mg, 50 mg

References

Strenkoski-Nix LC, Ermer J, DeCleene S, et al, "Pharmacokinetics of Promethazine Hydrochloride After Administration of Rectal Suppositories and Oral Syrup to Healthy Subjects," *Am J Health Syst Pharm*, 2000, 57(16):1499-505.

Promethazine and Codeine
(proe METH a zeen & KOE deen)

Therapeutic Category Antitussive; Cough Preparation; Phenothiazine Derivative

Generic Available Yes

Use Temporary relief of coughs and upper respiratory symptoms associated with allergy or the common cold

Restrictions C-V

Pregnancy Risk Factor C

Pregnancy Considerations Reproduction studies have not been conducted with this combination. See individual agents.

Lactation Enters breast milk (codeine)/not recommended

Breast-Feeding Considerations Refer to Codeine monograph.

Contraindications Hypersensitivity to promethazine or other phenothiazines, codeine, or any component; children <6 years of age (see Warnings); lower respiratory tract symptoms, including asthma; coma

Warnings Avoid use in children <6 years of age **[U.S. Boxed Warning]**, due to the potential for severe and potentially fatal respiratory depression associated with the combination of promethazine and other respiratory depressants (eg, codeine); fatalities associated with promethazine use alone in children <2 years of age have also been reported. Use with caution in atopic children. Dose should not be increased if cough does not respond; re-evaluate within 5 days for possible underlying pathology. Codeine is not recommended for cough control in patients with a productive cough. Neuroleptic malignant syndrome (NMS) has been reported with promethazine when used alone or in combination with antipsychotic drugs. May alter temperature regulation or mask toxicity of other drugs due to antiemetic effects. May alter cardiac conduction (life-threatening arrhythmias have occurred with therapeutic doses of phenothiazines).

Precautions Use with caution in patients with cardiovascular disease, narrow-angle glaucoma, prostatic hypertrophy, GI or GU obstruction, bone marrow depression, impaired liver function, peptic ulcer, sleep apnea, and hypertensive crisis; avoid in patients with suspected Reye's syndrome; promethazine may lower the seizure threshold; use with caution in patients with seizure disorders or receiving other medications which may also lower the seizure threshold; use with caution in patients with hypersensitivity reactions to morphine, hydrocodone, hydromorphone, levorphanol, oxycodone, oxymorphone. May cause orthostatic hypotension, use with caution in patients at risk of hypotension or where transient hypotensive episodes would be poorly tolerated (cardiovascular disease or cerebrovascular disease). May cause drowsiness and impair ability to perform hazardous activities requiring mental alertness. Promethazine has been reported to cause cholestatic jaundice. Use with caution in patients with two or more copies of the variant CYP2D6*2 allele (ie, CYP2D6 "ultra-rapid metabolizers"); these patients may have extensive conversion of codeine to morphine with resultant increased opioid-mediated effects.

Adverse Reactions

Promethazine:

Cardiovascular: Tachycardia, bradycardia, palpitations, arrhythmias, orthostatic hypotension

Central nervous system: Sedation (pronounced), confusion, drowsiness, restlessness, anxiety, extrapyramidal reactions, tardive dyskinesia, seizures, hallucinations, NMS

Dermatologic: Rash, photosensitivity

Endocrine & metabolic: Antidiuretic hormone release

Gastrointestinal: GI upset, xerostomia, constipation

Genitourinary: Urinary retention

Hematologic: Agranulocytosis, leukopenia (rare), thrombocytopenia

Hepatic: Cholestatic jaundice, hepatitis

Neuromuscular & skeletal: Arthralgia, tremor, paresthesia, myalgia

Ocular: Blurred vision

Respiratory: Thickening of bronchial secretions, pharyngitis

Miscellaneous: Allergic reactions

Codeine:

Cardiovascular: Palpitations, orthostatic hypotension, tachycardia or bradycardia, peripheral vasodilation

Central nervous system: CNS depression, dizziness, sedation, euphoria, hallucination, seizures

Dermatologic: Pruritus

Gastrointestinal: Nausea, vomiting, constipation, biliary tract spasm

Genitourinary: Urinary tract spasm

Ocular: Miosis

Respiratory: Respiratory depression

Miscellaneous: Physical and psychological dependence, histamine release, allergic reactions

Drug Interactions

Metabolism/Transport Effects Promethazine: **Substrate** (major) of CYP2B6, 2D6; **Inhibits** CYP2D6 (weak)

Avoid Concomitant Use

Avoid concomitant use of Promethazine and Codeine with any of the following: Metoclopramide; Sibutramine

Increased Effect/Toxicity

Promethazine and Codeine may increase the levels/ effects of: Alcohol (Ethyl); Alvimopan; Anticholinergics; CNS Depressants; Desmopressin; Selective Serotonin Reuptake Inhibitors; Serotonin Modulators; Thiazide Diuretics

The levels/effects of Promethazine and Codeine may be increased by: Amphetamines; Antipsychotic Agents (Phenothiazines); CYP2B6 Inhibitors (Moderate); CYP2B6 Inhibitors (Strong); Darunavir; MAO Inhibitors; Metoclopramide; Pramlintide; Quazepam; Sibutramine; Somatostatin Analogs; Succinylcholine

Decreased Effect

Promethazine and Codeine may decrease the levels/ effects of: Acetylcholinesterase Inhibitors (Central); Pegvisomant

The levels/effects of Promethazine and Codeine may be decreased by: Acetylcholinesterase Inhibitors (Central); Ammonium Chloride; CYP2B6 Inducers (Strong); CYP2D6 Inhibitors (Moderate); CYP2D6 Inhibitors (Strong); Mixed Agonist / Antagonist Opioids; Peginterferon Alfa-2b

Food Interactions Increase fluids, fiber intake, and riboflavin in diet

Mechanism of Action See individual agents.

Usual Dosage Oral:

Children <6 years: Use of promethazine/codeine combination is contraindicated in children <6 years of age

Children 6-11 years: 2.5-5 mL every 4-6 hours (maximum: 30 mL/24 hours)

Children ≥12 years and Adults: 5 mL every 4-6 hours (maximum: 30 mL/24 hours)

Administration Oral: Administer with food or water to decrease GI upset. Administer with accurate measuring device; do not use household teaspoon (overdosage may occur).

Test Interactions Alters the flare response in intradermal allergen tests

Codeine: Amylase and lipase plasma levels may by unreliable for 24 hours after codeine administration.

Promethazine: hCG-based pregnancy tests may result in false-negatives or false-positives; increased serum glucose may be seen with glucose tolerance tests.

◄ **Patient Information** May cause drowsiness and impair ability to perform activities requiring mental alertness or physical coordination; may cause dry mouth; may be habit-forming; do not discontinue abruptly. May cause photosensitivity reactions (eg, exposure to sunlight may cause severe sunburn, skin rash, redness, or itching); avoid exposure to sunlight and artificial light sources (sunlamps, tanning booth/bed); wear protective clothing, wide-brimmed hats, sunglasses, and lip sunscreen (SPF ≥15); use a sunscreen [broad-spectrum sunscreen or physical sunscreen (preferred) or sunblock with SPF ≥15]; contact physician if reaction occurs.

Dosage Forms Excipient information presented when available (limited, particularly for generics); consult specific product labeling.

Syrup: Promethazine hydrochloride 6.25 mg and codeine phosphate 10 mg per 5 mL (5 mL, 118 mL, 473 mL)

Promethazine and Phenylephrine
(proe METH a zeen & fen il EF rin)

Related Information
Phenylephrine on page 1102
Promethazine on page 1163

Therapeutic Category Antihistamine/Decongestant Combination

Generic Available Yes

Use Temporary relief of upper respiratory symptoms associated with allergy or the common cold

Pregnancy Risk Factor C

Pregnancy Considerations Reproduction studies have not been conducted with this combination. Refer to Promethazine monograph.

Lactation Excretion in breast milk unknown/not recommended

Contraindications Hypersensitivity to promethazine, phenylephrine, or any component; cross reactivity with other phenothiazines may occur; asthma, peripheral vascular disease, severe hypertension, cardiovascular disease, liver disease, patients receiving MAO inhibitors; children <2 years (see Warnings)

Warnings Avoid use of promethazine in children <2 years of age due to the potential for severe and potentially fatal respiratory depression **[U.S. Boxed Warning]**. A wide range of weight-based doses have resulted in respiratory depression; excessively high doses have been associated with sudden death in children; use with caution and use the lowest effective dose in children >2 years of age and avoid concomitant use with other medications having respiratory depressant effects. Neuroleptic malignant syndrome (NMS) has been reported with promethazine when used alone or in combination with antipsychotic drugs. Children with dehydration are at increased risk for development of dystonic reactions.

Precautions Use with caution in patients with cardiovascular disease, narrow-angle glaucoma, prostatic hypertrophy, GI or GU obstruction, bone marrow depression, impaired liver function, asthma, peptic ulcer, sleep apnea, and hypertensive crisis; avoid in patients with suspected Reye's syndrome; promethazine may lower the seizure threshold; use with caution in patients with seizure disorders or receiving other medications which may also lower the seizure threshold; promethazine has been reported to cause cholestatic jaundice

Adverse Reactions
Promethazine:
Cardiovascular: Hypertension, hypotension, tachycardia
Central nervous system: Sedation (pronounced), drowsiness, confusion, fatigue, excitation, extrapyramidal reactions, dystonia, tardive dyskinesia, hallucinations, NMS

Dermatologic: Photosensitivity, rash, angioedema
Endocrine & metabolic: Weight gain
Gastrointestinal: Xerostomia, GI upset, appetite increased, abdominal pain, diarrhea, nausea
Genitourinary: Urinary retention
Hematologic: Thrombocytopenia, leukopenia, agranulocytosis (rare)
Hepatic: Cholestatic jaundice, hepatitis
Ocular: Blurred vision
Neuromuscular & skeletal: Arthralgia, tremor, paresthesia, myalgia
Respiratory: Thickening of bronchial secretions, pharyngitis
Miscellaneous: Allergic reactions
Phenylephrine:
Cardiovascular: Hypertension, angina, reflex severe bradycardia, arrhythmias, peripheral vasoconstriction
Central nervous system: Restlessness, excitability, headache, anxiety, nervousness, dizziness
Dermatologic: Pilomotor response, skin blanching
Neuromuscular & skeletal: Tremor
Respiratory: Respiratory distress, rebound nasal congestion, sneezing, burning, stinging, dryness

Drug Interactions
Metabolism/Transport Effects Promethazine: **Substrate** (major) of CYP2B6, 2D6; **Inhibits** CYP2D6 (weak)

Avoid Concomitant Use
Avoid concomitant use of Promethazine and Phenylephrine with any of the following: Iobenguane I 123; MAO Inhibitors; Metoclopramide; Sibutramine

Increased Effect/Toxicity
Promethazine and Phenylephrine may increase the levels/effects of: Anticholinergics; Serotonin Modulators; Sympathomimetics

The levels/effects of Promethazine and Phenylephrine may be increased by: Atomoxetine; Cannabinoids; CYP2B6 Inhibitors (Moderate); CYP2B6 Inhibitors (Strong); CYP2D6 Inhibitors (Moderate); CYP2D6 Inhibitors (Strong); Darunavir; MAO Inhibitors; Metoclopramide; Pramlintide; Quazepam; Sibutramine; Tricyclic Antidepressants

Decreased Effect
Promethazine and Phenylephrine may decrease the levels/effects of: Acetylcholinesterase Inhibitors (Central); Iobenguane I 123

The levels/effects of Promethazine and Phenylephrine may be decreased by: Acetylcholinesterase Inhibitors (Central); CYP2B6 Inducers (Strong); Peginterferon Alfa-2b

Food Interactions Increase dietary intake of riboflavin

Usual Dosage Oral:
Children:
2-6 years: 1.25 mL every 4-6 hours, not to exceed 7.5 mL in 24 hours
6-12 years: 2.5 mL every 4-6 hours, not to exceed 15 mL in 24 hours
Children >12 years and Adults: 5 mL every 4-6 hours, not to exceed 30 mL in 24 hours

Administration Oral: Administer with food, water, or milk to decrease GI distress

Test Interactions Alters the flare response in intradermal allergen tests; false negative and positive reactions with pregnancy tests relying on immunological reactions between hCG and anti-hCG

Patient Information May cause drowsiness and impair ability to perform activities requiring mental alertness or physical coordination; may cause dry mouth. May cause photosensitivity reactions (eg, exposure to sunlight may cause severe sunburn, skin rash, redness, or itching); avoid exposure to sunlight and artificial light sources (sunlamps, tanning booth/bed); wear protective clothing, wide-brimmed hats, sunglasses, and lip sunscreen (SPF ≥15); use a sunscreen [broad-spectrum sunscreen or physical sunscreen (preferred) or sunblock with SPF ≥15]; contact physician if reaction occurs.

Dosage Forms Excipient information presented when available (limited, particularly for generics); consult specific product labeling.

Syrup: Promethazine hydrochloride 6.25 mg and phenylephrine hydrochloride 5 mg per 5 mL (473 mL) [contains alcohol]

◆ **Promethazine Hydrochloride** see Promethazine on page 1163

Promethazine, Phenylephrine, and Codeine (proe METH a zeen, fen il EF rin, & KOE deen)

Therapeutic Category Antihistamine/Decongestant Combination; Antitussive; Cough Preparation

Generic Available Yes

Use Temporary relief of coughs and upper respiratory symptoms including nasal congestion

Restrictions C-V

Pregnancy Risk Factor C

Pregnancy Considerations Reproduction studies have not been conducted with this combination. See individual agents.

Lactation Enters breast milk/not recommended

Breast-Feeding Considerations Codeine enters breast milk; excretion of promethazine and phenylephrine is unknown. Also refer to Codeine monograph.

Contraindications Hypersensitivity to promethazine or other phenothiazines, codeine, phenylephrine, or any component; children <6 years of age; asthma, peripheral vascular disease; hypertension; patients receiving MAO inhibitors

Warnings Avoid use in children <6 years of age **[U.S. Boxed Warning]**, due to the potential for severe and potentially fatal respiratory depression associated with the combination of promethazine and other respiratory depressants (eg, codeine); fatalities associated with promethazine use alone in children <2 years of age have also been reported. Dose should not be increased if cough does not respond; re-evaluate within 5 days for possible underlying pathology. Codeine is not recommended for cough control in patients with a productive cough. Neuroleptic malignant syndrome (NMS) has been reported with promethazine when used alone or in combination with antipsychotic drugs. May alter temperature regulation or mask toxicity of other drugs due to antiemetic effects. May alter cardiac conduction (life-threatening arrhythmias have occurred with therapeutic doses of phenothiazines).

Precautions Use with caution in patients with cardiovascular disease, narrow-angle glaucoma, prostatic hypertrophy, GI or GU obstruction, bone marrow depression, impaired liver function, hyperthyroidism, diabetes mellitus, peptic ulcer, sleep apnea, and hypertensive crisis; avoid in patients with suspected Reye's syndrome; promethazine may lower the seizure threshold; use with caution in patients with seizure disorders or receiving other medications which may also lower the seizure threshold; use with caution in patients with hypersensitivity reactions to morphine, hydrocodone, hydromorphone, levorphanol, oxycodone, oxymorphone. May cause orthostatic hypotension, use with caution in patients at risk of hypotension or where transient hypotensive episodes would be poorly tolerated (cardiovascular disease or cerebrovascular disease). May cause drowsiness and impair ability to perform hazardous activities requiring mental alertness. Promethazine has been reported to cause cholestatic jaundice. Use with caution in patients with two or more copies of the variant CYP2D6*2 allele (ie, CYP2D6

"ultra-rapid metabolizers"); these patients may have extensive conversion of codeine to morphine with resultant increased opioid-mediated effects.

Adverse Reactions See individual agents.

Drug Interactions

Metabolism/Transport Effects

Promethazine: **Substrate** (major) of CYP2B6, 2D6; **Inhibits** CYP2D6 (weak)

Codeine: **Substrate** of CYP2D6 (major), 3A4 (minor); **Inhibits** CYP2D6 (weak)

Avoid Concomitant Use

Avoid concomitant use of Promethazine, Phenylephrine, and Codeine with any of the following: Iobenguane I 123; MAO Inhibitors; Metoclopramide; Sibutramine

Increased Effect/Toxicity

Promethazine, Phenylephrine, and Codeine may increase the levels/effects of: Alcohol (Ethyl); Alvimopan; Anticholinergics; CNS Depressants; Desmopressin; Selective Serotonin Reuptake Inhibitors; Serotonin Modulators; Sympathomimetics; Thiazide Diuretics

The levels/effects of Promethazine, Phenylephrine, and Codeine may be increased by: Amphetamines; Antipsychotic Agents (Phenothiazines); Atomoxetine; CYP2B6 Inhibitors (Moderate); CYP2B6 Inhibitors (Strong); Darunavir; MAO Inhibitors; Metoclopramide; Pramlintide; Quazepam; Sibutramine; Somatostatin Analogs; Succinylcholine; Tricyclic Antidepressants

Decreased Effect

Promethazine, Phenylephrine, and Codeine may decrease the levels/effects of: Acetylcholinesterase Inhibitors (Central); Iobenguane I 123; Pegvisomant

The levels/effects of Promethazine, Phenylephrine, and Codeine may be decreased by: Acetylcholinesterase Inhibitors (Central); Ammonium Chloride; CYP2B6 Inducers (Strong); CYP2D6 Inhibitors (Moderate); CYP2D6 Inhibitors (Strong); Mixed Agonist / Antagonist Opioids; Peginterferon Alfa-2b

Food Interactions Increase fluids, fiber intake, and riboflavin in diet

Usual Dosage Oral:

Children <6 years: Use of this combination is contraindicated in children <6 years of age

Children 6-11 years: 2.5-5 mL every 4-6 hours (maximum: 30 mL/24 hours)

Children ≥12 years and Adults: 5 mL every 4-6 hours (maximum: 30 mL/24 hours)

Administration Oral: Administer with food or water to decrease GI upset. Administer with an accurate measuring device; do not use a household teaspoon (overdosage may occur).

Test Interactions

Codeine: Amylase and lipase plasma levels may by unreliable for 24 hours after codeine administration.

Promethazine: hCG-based pregnancy tests may result in false-negatives or false-positives; increased serum glucose may be seen with glucose tolerance tests

Patient Information May cause drowsiness and impair ability to perform activities requiring mental alertness or physical coordination; may cause dry mouth; may be habit-forming; do not discontinue abruptly. May cause photosensitivity reactions (eg, exposure to sunlight may cause severe sunburn, skin rash, redness, or itching); avoid exposure to sunlight and artificial light sources (sunlamps, tanning booth/bed); wear protective clothing, wide-brimmed hats, sunglasses, and lip sunscreen (SPF ≥15); use a sunscreen [broad-spectrum sunscreen or physical sunscreen (preferred) or sunblock with SPF ≥15]; contact physician if reaction occurs.

Dosage Forms Excipient information presented when available (limited, particularly for generics); consult specific product labeling.

Syrup: Promethazine hydrochloride 6.25 mg, phenylephrine hydrochloride 5 mg, and codeine phosphate 10 mg per 5 mL (120 mL, 480 mL)

♦ **Promethegan™** *see* Promethazine *on page 1163*

♦ **PRO-Naproxen EC (Can)** *see* Naproxen *on page 967*

♦ **Pronestyl** *see* Procainamide *on page 1156*

♦ **Propaderm® (Can)** *see* Beclomethasone *on page 176*

Propantheline (proe PAN the leen)

Medication Safety Issues
Beers Criteria medication: This drug may be inappropriate for use in geriatric patients (high severity risk).
Therapeutic Category Anticholinergic Agent; Antispasmodic Agent, Gastrointestinal; Antispasmodic Agent, Urinary
Generic Available Yes
Use Adjunctive treatment of peptic ulcer, irritable bowel syndrome, pancreatitis, ureteral and urinary bladder spasm; to reduce duodenal motility during diagnostic radiologic procedures
Pregnancy Risk Factor C
Lactation Excretion in breast milk unknown
Breast-Feeding Considerations No data reported; however, atropine may be taken while breast-feeding.
Contraindications Hypersensitivity to propantheline or any component; narrow-angle glaucoma; ulcerative colitis; toxic megacolon; obstructive disease of the GI or urinary tract
Warnings Infants, patients with Down's syndrome, and children with spastic paralysis or brain damage may be hypersensitive to antimuscarinic effects
Precautions Use with caution in febrile patients, patients with hyperthyroidism, hepatic, cardiac, or renal disease, hypertension, GI infections, diarrhea, reflux esophagitis
Adverse Reactions
Cardiovascular: Tachycardia, palpitations, flushing
Central nervous system: Insomnia, drowsiness, dizziness, nervousness, headache
Dermatologic: Rash, dry skin
Endocrine & metabolic: Suppression of lactation
Gastrointestinal: Xerostomia, nausea, vomiting, constipation, dry throat, dysphagia
Genitourinary: Impotence, urinary retention
Ocular: Mydriasis, blurred vision
Neuromuscular & skeletal: Weakness
Respiratory: Dry nose
Miscellaneous: Allergic reactions, diaphoresis decreased
Drug Interactions
Avoid Concomitant Use There are no known interactions where it is recommended to avoid concomitant use.
Increased Effect/Toxicity
Propantheline may increase the levels/effects of: AbobotulinumtoxinA; Anticholinergics; Cannabinoids; OnabotulinumtoxinA; Potassium Chloride; RimabotulinumtoxinB

The levels/effects of Propantheline may be increased by: MAO Inhibitors; Pramlintide
Decreased Effect
Propantheline may decrease the levels/effects of: Acetylcholinesterase Inhibitors (Central); Secretin

The levels/effects of Propantheline may be decreased by: Acetylcholinesterase Inhibitors (Central)
Mechanism of Action Competitively blocks the action of acetylcholine at postganglionic parasympathetic receptor sites

Pharmacodynamics
Onset of action: Within 30-45 minutes
Duration: 4-6 hours
Pharmacokinetics (Adult data unless noted)
Metabolism: In the liver and GI tract
Elimination: In urine, bile, and other body fluids
Usual Dosage Oral:
Antisecretory:
Children: 1-2 mg/kg/day in 3-4 divided doses
Adults: 15 mg 3 times/day before meals or food and 30 mg at bedtime; for mild manifestations: 7.5 mg 3 times/day
Antispasmodic:
Children: 2-3 mg/kg/day in divided doses every 4-6 hours and at bedtime
Adults: 15 mg 3 times/day before meals or food and 30 mg at bedtime
Administration Oral: Administer 30 minutes before meals and at bedtime
Patient Information May cause drowsiness and impair ability to perform activities requiring mental alertness or physical coordination; notify physician if skin rash, flushing, or eye pain occurs; or if difficulty in urinating, constipation, or sensitivity to light becomes severe or persists; may cause dry mouth; maintain good oral hygiene habits, because lack of saliva may increase chance of cavities
Dosage Forms Excipient information presented when available (limited, particularly for generics); consult specific product labeling.
Tablet, as bromide: 15 mg [contains lactose 23.2 mg]

♦ **Propantheline Bromide** *see* Propantheline *on page 1168*

Proparacaine (proe PAR a kane)

Medication Safety Issues
Sound-alike/look-alike issues:
Proparacaine may be confused with propoxyphene
U.S. Brand Names Alcaine®; Ophthetic® [DSC]; Parcaine™
Canadian Brand Names Alcaine®; Diocaine®
Therapeutic Category Local Anesthetic, Ophthalmic
Generic Available Yes
Use Local anesthesia for tonometry, gonioscopy; suture removal from cornea; removal of corneal foreign body; cataract extraction, glaucoma surgery; short operative procedure involving the cornea and conjunctiva
Pregnancy Risk Factor C
Contraindications Hypersensitivity to proparacaine or any component
Precautions Use with caution in patients with cardiac disease, hyperthyroidism
Adverse Reactions
Dermatologic: Allergic contact dermatitis
Local: Irritation, stinging, sensitization
Ocular: Keratitis, iritis, erosion of the corneal epithelium, conjunctival congestion and hemorrhage, corneal opacification
Drug Interactions
Avoid Concomitant Use There are no known interactions where it is recommended to avoid concomitant use.
Increased Effect/Toxicity There are no known significant interactions involving an increase in effect.
Decreased Effect There are no known significant interactions involving a decrease in effect.
Stability Refrigerate and protect from light
Mechanism of Action Local anesthetic; prevents initiation and transmission of impulse at the nerve cell membrane by decreasing ion permeability

Pharmacodynamics

Onset of action: Within 20 seconds of instillation

Duration: 15-20 minutes

Usual Dosage Children and Adults:

Ophthalmic surgery: Instill 1 drop of 0.5% solution in eye every 5-10 minutes for 5-7 doses

Tonometry, gonioscopy, suture removal: Instill 1-2 drops of 0.5% solution in eye just prior to procedure

Administration Ophthalmic: Instill drops into affected eye(s); avoid contact of bottle tip with skin or eye

Patient Information Do not rub eye until anesthesia has worn off

Dosage Forms Excipient information presented when available (limited, particularly for generics); consult specific product labeling. [DSC] = Discontinued product

Solution, ophthalmic, as hydrochloride: 0.5% (15 mL) [contains benzalkonium chloride]

Alcaine®: 0.5% (15 mL) [contains benzalkonium chloride]

Ophthetic®: 0.5% (15 mL) [contains benzalkonium chloride] [DSC]

Parcaine™: 0.5% (15 mL) [contains benzalkonium chloride]

◆ **Proparacaine Hydrochloride** *see* Proparacaine *on page 1168*

◆ **Propine® [DSC]** *see* Dipivefrin *on page 461*

◆ **Propine® (Can)** *see* Dipivefrin *on page 461*

◆ **PRO-Piroxicam (Can)** *see* Piroxicam *on page 1118*

Propofol (PROE po fole)

Medication Safety Issues

Sound-alike/look-alike issues:

Diprivan® may be confused with Diflucan®, Ditropan®

Propofol may be confused with fospropofol

High alert medication: The Institute for Safe Medication Practices (ISMP) includes this medication among its list of drugs which have a heightened risk of causing significant patient harm when used in error.

U.S. Brand Names Diprivan®

Canadian Brand Names Diprivan®

Therapeutic Category General Anesthetic

Generic Available Yes

Use Induction of anesthesia in children ≥3 years and adults; maintenance of anesthesia in children ≥2 months and adults; initiation and maintenance of monitored anesthesia care sedation in adults; continuous sedation of intubated, mechanically ventilated adult intensive care unit patients; combined sedation and regional anesthesia in adults

Pregnancy Risk Factor B

Pregnancy Considerations Propofol should only be used in pregnancy if clearly needed. Propofol is not recommended for obstetrics, including cesarean section deliveries. Propofol crosses the placenta and may be associated with neonatal CNS and respiratory depression.

Lactation Enters breast milk/not recommended

Contraindications Hypersensitivity to propofol or any component (see Warnings); hypersensitivity to eggs, egg products, soybeans, or soy products; patients who are not intubated or mechanically ventilated; other contraindications to general anesthesia or sedation apply

Warnings Important Note: In June 2007, the FDA alerted clinicians of several reports of acute febrile reactions occurring in clusters of patients after administration of propofol for sedation in gastrointestinal suites. The FDA is reminding healthcare professionals to strictly adhere to recommendations in product labeling for handling and administering propofol. Clinicians should be vigilant for signs and symptoms of acute febrile reactions and evaluate patients for bacteremia; see Additional Information for further details.

Diprivan® contains egg lecithin, soybean oil, and disodium edetate; generic products may contain egg lecithin, soybean oil, or sodium metabisulfite; any of which may cause allergic reactions in susceptible individuals. Generic products may also contain benzyl alcohol or sodium benzoate; benzoic acid (benzoate) is a metabolite of benzyl alcohol; large amounts of benzyl alcohol (≥99 mg/kg/day) have been associated with a potentially fatal toxicity ("gasping syndrome") in neonates; the "gasping syndrome" consists of metabolic acidosis, respiratory distress, gasping respirations, CNS dysfunction (including convulsions, intracranial hemorrhage), hypotension, and cardiovascular collapse; use propofol products containing benzyl alcohol or sodium benzoate with caution in neonates; *in vitro* and animal studies have shown that benzoate displaces bilirubin from protein binding sites

Not recommended for induction of anesthesia in children <3 years or for maintenance of anesthesia in infants <2 months of age; not recommended for monitored anesthesia care sedation in children; **not recommended for sedation of PICU patients**. An increased number of deaths was observed in a multicenter clinical trial of PICU patients who received propofol (9% mortality) versus patients who received other sedative agents (4% mortality); although causality was not established, propofol is not indicated for sedation in PICU patients until further studies can document its safety in this population. The propofol infusion syndrome, a potentially fatal constellation of metabolic derangements and organ system failures, has been reported in pediatric and adult patients receiving propofol for ICU sedation. This syndrome consists of severe metabolic acidosis, hyperkalemia, lipemia, rhabdomyolysis, hepatomegaly, and cardiac and renal failure. It is usually associated with prolonged, high dose infusions (>5 mg/kg/hour for >48 hours), but may also occur after large-dose, short-term infusions. Alternate sedation therapy should be considered for patients who require prolonged sedation or increasing propofol dosage requirements or in whom the onset of metabolic acidosis is observed. Metabolic acidosis with fatal cardiac failure has occurred in several children (4 weeks to 11 years of age) who received propofol infusions at average rates of infusion of 4.5-10 mg/kg/hour for 66-115 hours (maximum rates of infusion: 6.2-11.5 mg/kg/hour); see Bray, 1995; Parke, 1992; Strickland, 1995. Anecdotal reports of serious adverse events, including death, have been reported in pediatric patients with upper respiratory tract infections receiving propofol for ICU sedation. Concurrent use of fentanyl and propofol in pediatric patients may result in bradycardia.

Patients require continuous monitoring and airway management; cardiovascular and respiratory resuscitation equipment should be available. Use with caution and decrease the dose in ASA III or IV, elderly, debilitated, or hypovolemic patients; do not use rapid bolus dose administration in these patients. Not recommended for use in obstetrics, cesarean deliveries, lactating women, patients with increased ICP, or impaired cerebral circulation. Avoid abrupt discontinuation; abrupt discontinuation may result in rapid awakening, anxiety, agitation, and resistance to mechanical ventilation. Abrupt discontinuation in pediatric patients may cause agitation, hyperirritability, tremulousness, and flushing of hands and feet; increased frequency of bradycardia, jitteriness, and agitation have also been observed.

Although products contain preservatives, rapid growth of micro-organisms can occur; failure to use aseptic technique can result in microbial contamination and fever, sepsis, infection, life-threatening illnesses, or death; **do not use if microbial contamination is suspected; discard unused portions and I.V. tubing within required** time limits (see Stability). Propofol should be administered by qualified healthcare professionals trained in advanced cardiac life support and anesthetic drug use (when used for general anesthesia and monitored anesthesia care sedation) or management of critically ill patients (when used for sedation in intensive care patient). Fatal and life-threatening anaphylactic and anaphylactoid reactions may occur.

Precautions Use with caution in patients with seizures or history of epilepsy, hypotension, hemodynamic instability, or severe cardiac or respiratory disease. Use with caution in patients with hyperlipidemia (propofol may cause hyperlipidemia). I.V. injection may produce transient local pain; perioperative myoclonia may occur. Propofol lacks analgesic properties; pain management requires specific use of analgesic agents, at effective dosages; propofol must be titrated separately from the analgesic agent.

Diprivan® contains disodium edetate which can chelate trace metals, including zinc; as much as 10 mg of elemented zinc may be lost per day when calcium disodium edetate is used in gram doses to treat heavy metal poisonings; no reports of zinc deficiency or low zinc levels have been reported with Diprivan®; mean urinary zinc loss in clinical trials was 1.5-2 mg/day in pediatric patients and 2.5-3 mg/day in adult patients. The manufacturer recommends that Diprivan® not be infused for >5 days without giving a "drug holiday"; during this time off of Diprivan®, replacement of estimated or measured urine zinc losses is recommended.

Adverse Reactions
Cardiovascular: Hypotension (dose related), bradycardia, myocardial depression, flushing
Central nervous system: Fever, headache, dizziness
Dermatologic: Rash, pruritus
Endocrine & metabolic: Hyperlipidemia; fatal metabolic acidosis has been reported; propofol infusion syndrome (see Warnings)
Gastrointestinal: Nausea, vomiting, abdominal cramping
Genitourinary: Discoloration of urine (green)
Local: Pain at injection site (especially when administered via small vein); **Note:** Dilution with D_5W or administration of lidocaine pretreatment may decrease local pain (see Administration)
Neuromuscular & skeletal: Myalgia, twitching, clonic/myoclonic movement
Respiratory: Respiratory acidosis, respiratory depression, apnea
Miscellaneous: Anaphylaxis, anaphylactoid reactions

Drug Interactions
Metabolism/Transport Effects Substrate of CYP1A2 (minor), 2A6 (minor), 2B6 (major), 2C9 (major), 2C19 (minor), 2D6 (minor), 2E1 (minor), 3A4 (minor); **Inhibits** CYP1A2 (moderate), 2C9 (weak), 2C19 (moderate), 2D6 (weak), 2E1 (weak), 3A4 (weak)

Avoid Concomitant Use There are no known interactions where it is recommended to avoid concomitant use.

Increased Effect/Toxicity
Propofol may increase the levels/effects of: Midazolam; Ropivacaine

The levels/effects of Propofol may be increased by: Alfentanil; CYP2B6 Inhibitors (Moderate); CYP2B6 Inhibitors (Strong); Midazolam; Quazepam

Decreased Effect
The levels/effects of Propofol may be decreased by: Peginterferon Alfa-2b

Stability Store at room temperature 4°C to 22°C (40°F to 72°F); refrigeration is not recommended; do not freeze. Protect from light. Do not use if contamination is suspected or if there is evidence of separation of phases of emulsion, particulate matter, or discoloration. Discard unused

portions at end of surgical procedure or at 6 hours (whichever is less). If transferred to a syringe or other container prior to administration, use within 6 hours. If used directly from vial/prefilled syringe, use within 12 hours. For ICU use: Discard tubing and unused portions after 12 hours.

Does not need to be diluted; but may dilute with D_5W only; do not dilute to <2 mg/mL. Diluted emulsion is more stable in glass. Stability in plastic: 95% potency after 2 hours. May administer with D_5W, LR, D_5LR, $D_5^{1/2}NS$, D5/1/4NS. Do not administer with blood or blood products through the same I.V. catheter; do not mix with other drugs (see Administration).

Mechanism of Action Propofol is a hindered phenolic compound with intravenous general anesthetic properties. The drug is unrelated to any of the currently used barbiturate, opioid, benzodiazepine, arylcyclohexylamine, or imidazole intravenous anesthetic agents.

Pharmacodynamics
Onset of anesthesia: Within 30 seconds after bolus infusion
Duration: ~3-10 minutes depending on the dose, rate and duration of administration; with prolonged use (eg, 10 days ICU sedation), propofol accumulates in tissues and redistributes into plasma when the drug is discontinued, so that the time to awakening (duration of action) is increased; however, if dose is titrated on a daily basis, so that the minimum effective dose is utilized, time to awakening may be within 10-15 minutes even after prolonged use

Pharmacokinetics (Adult data unless noted)
Distribution: Large volume of distribution; highly lipophilic
V_d (apparent): Children 4-12 years: 5-10 L/kg
V_{dss}:
  Adults: 170-350 L
  Adults (10-day infusion): 60 L/kg
Protein binding: 97% to 99%
Metabolism: In the liver via glucuronide and sulfate conjugation
Half-life (three-compartment model):
  Alpha: 2-8 minutes
  Beta (second distribution): ~40 minutes
  Terminal: ~200 minutes; range: 300-700 minutes
  Terminal (after 10-day infusion): 1-3 days
Elimination: ~90% excreted in urine as metabolites and <1% as unchanged drug

Usual Dosage Dosage must be individualized based on total body weight and titrated to the desired clinical effect; wait at least 3-5 minutes between dosage adjustments to clinically assess drug effects; smaller doses are required when used with narcotics; the following are general dosing guidelines:

General anesthesia:
I.V. induction: (See "Symbols and Abbreviations Used in This Handbook" in front section of this book for explanation of ASA classes:)
Children (healthy) 3-16 years, ASA I or II: 2.5-3.5 mg/kg over 20-30 seconds; use a lower dose for children ASA III or IV
Adults (healthy), ASA I or II, <55 years: 2-2.5 mg/kg (~40 mg every 10 seconds until onset of induction)
Elderly, debilitated, hypovolemic, or ASA III or IV: 1-1.5 mg/kg (~20 mg every 10 seconds until onset of induction); **do not** use rapid bolus dose (single or repeated)
Cardiac anesthesia: 0.5-1.5 mg/kg (~20 mg every 10 seconds until onset of induction)
Neurosurgical patients: 1-2 mg/kg (~20 mg every 10 seconds until onset of induction)

Maintenance: I.V. infusion:

Infants (healthy) ≥2 months to Children 16 years, ASA I or II: Initial (immediately following induction): 200-300 mcg/kg/minute; decrease dose after 30 minutes if clinical signs of light anesthesia are absent; usual infusion rate: 125-150 mcg/kg/minute; younger pediatric patients may require larger infusion rates compared to older children

Adults (healthy), ASA I or II, <55 years: Initial: 150-200 mcg/kg/minute for 10-15 minutes; decrease by 30% to 50% during first 30 minutes of maintenance; usual infusion rate: 100-200 mcg/kg/minute

Elderly, debilitated, hypovolemic, ASA III or IV: 50-100 mcg/kg/minute

Cardiac anesthesia:

Low dose propofol with primary opioid: 50-100 mcg/kg/minute (see manufacturer's labeling)

Primary propofol with secondary opioid: 100-150 mcg/kg/minute

Neurosurgical patients: 100-200 mcg/kg/minute

Maintenance: I.V. intermittent bolus: Adults, ASA I or II, <55 years: 20-50 mg increments as needed

Monitored Anesthesia Care sedation:

Initiation:

Adults (healthy), ASA I or II, <55 years: Slow I.V. infusion: 100-150 mcg/kg/minute for 3-5 minutes **or** slow injection: 0.5 mg/kg over 3-5 minutes

Elderly, debilitated, neurosurgical, or ASA III or IV patients: Use similar doses to healthy adults; avoid rapid I.V. boluses

Maintenance:

Adults (healthy), ASA I or II, <55 years: I.V. infusion using variable rates (preferred over intermittent boluses): 25-75 mcg/kg/minute **or** incremental bolus doses: 10 mg or 20 mg

Elderly, debilitated, neurosurgical, or ASA III or IV patients: Use 80% of healthy adult dose; **do not** use rapid bolus doses (single or repeated)

ICU sedation in intubated mechanically ventilated patients: Avoid rapid bolus injection; individualize dose and titrate to response

Adults: Continuous infusion: Initial: 0.3 mg/kg/hour; increase by 0.3-0.6 mg/kg/hour every 5-10 minutes until desired sedation level is achieved; usual maintenance: 0.3-3 mg/kg/hour or higher; reduce dose to 80% in elderly, debilitated, and ASA III or IV patients; reduce dose after adequate sedation established and adjust to response (ie, evaluate frequently to use minimum dose for sedation).

Administration Parenteral: I.V.: Strict aseptic technique must be maintained in handling (see Warnings and Stability). Prepare drug for single-patient use only. Shake injection well before use. Administer pediatric induction doses over 20-30 seconds. Do not administer via filter with <5-micron pore size. Do not administer through the same I.V. catheter with blood or plasma. To reduce pain associated with injection, use larger veins of forearm or antecubital fossa; lidocaine I.V. (1 mL of a 1% solution) may also be used prior to administration or it may be added to propofol immediately before administration in a quantity not to exceed 20 mg lidocaine per 200 mg propofol. **Note:** The American College of Critical Care Medicine recommends the use of a central vein for administration in an ICU setting.

Monitoring Parameters Respiratory rate, blood pressure, heart rate, oxygen saturation, ABGs, depth of sedation; serum lipids or triglycerides with use >24 hours; serum potassium; cardiac and renal function; unexplained tachycardia should prompt evaluation of metabolic status (including consideration of acid-base status). In patients at risk for renal impairment, urinalysis and urine sediment should be monitored prior to treatment and every other day of sedation.

Diprivan®: Monitor zinc levels in patients predisposed to deficiency (burns, diarrhea, major sepsis) or after 5 days of treatment.

Nursing Implications Strict aseptic technique must be maintained in handling (see Warnings and Stability). May change urine color to green

Additional Information Due to poor water solubility, the I.V. formulation is an isotonic oil-in-water emulsion and contains soybean oil, glycerol, egg lecithin, and sodium hydroxide (for pH adjustment); the brand name and generic product differ in the preservative used; Diprivan® contains 0.005% disodium edetate, while the generic product contains sodium metabisulfite (0.25 mg/mL); propofol injection contains ~0.1 g of fat/mL (1.1 kcal/mL)

Acute febrile reactions: In June 2007, the FDA alerted clinicians of several reports of chills, fever, and body aches occurring in clusters of patients after administration of propofol for sedation in gastrointestinal suites. These reports were received from several facilities and involved multiple vials and lots. Symptoms appeared 6-18 hours following propofol therapy and persisted for ≤3 days. There is no evidence that any patient had sepsis or that the vials were contaminated. The FDA has tested multiple propofol vials and lots used in these patients and presently have found no evidence of bacterial contamination. Regardless, propofol vials and prefilled syringes have the potential to support the growth of various microorganisms despite product additives intended to suppress microbial growth. To limit the potential for contamination, the FDA is reminding healthcare professionals to strictly adhere to recommendations in product labeling for handling and administering propofol. Clinicians should also be vigilant for signs and symptoms of acute febrile reactions and evaluate patients for bacteremia. The FDA is continuing to work with the Centers for Disease Control and Prevention to investigate factors contributing to these occurrences. Additional information is available at http://www.fda.gov/Drugs/DrugSafety/PostmarketDrugSafetyInformationfor-PatientsandProviders/ucm109357.htm.

Dosage Forms Excipient information presented when available (limited, particularly for generics); consult specific product labeling.

Injection, emulsion: 10 mg/mL (20 mL, 50 mL, 100 mL) [products may contain egg lecithin, and soybean oil; may contain benzyl alcohol, sodium benzoate, or sodium metabisulfite]

Diprivan®: 10 mg/mL (20 mL, 50 mL, 100 mL) [contains egg lecithin, soybean oil, and disodium edetate]

References

Bray RJ, "Fatal Myocardial Failure Associated With a Propofol Infusion in a Child," *Anaesthesia,* 1995, 50(1):94.

Parke TJ, Stevens JE, Rice ASC, et al, "Metabolic Acidosis and Fatal Myocardial Failure After Propofol Infusion in Children: Five Case Reports," *BMJ,* 1992, 305(6854):613-6.

Strickland RA and Murray MJ, "Fatal Metabolic Acidosis in a Pediatric Patient Receiving an Infusion of Propofol in the Intensive Care Unit: Is There a Relationship?" *Crit Care Med,* 1995, 23(2):405-9.

Propoxyphene (proe POKS i feen)

Medication Safety Issues

Sound-alike/look-alike issues:

Propoxyphene may be confused with proparacaine

Darvon® may be confused with Devrom®, Diovan®

Darvon-N® may be confused with Darvocet-N®

High alert medication: The Institute for Safe Medication Practices (ISMP) includes this medication among its list of drug classes which have a heightened risk of causing significant patient harm when used in error.

◄ **Beers Criteria medication:** This drug may be inappropriate for use in geriatric patients (low severity risk).

U.S. Brand Names Darvon-N®; Darvon®

Canadian Brand Names 642® Tablet; Darvon-N®

Therapeutic Category Analgesic, Narcotic

Generic Available Yes: Capsule

Use Management of mild to moderate pain (FDA approved in adults)

Restrictions C-IV

Medication Guide An FDA-approved patient medication guide, which is available with the product information and at http://www.fda.gov/downloads/Drugs/DrugSafety/UCM187068.pdf, must be dispensed with this medication for each new outpatient prescription and refill.

Pregnancy Risk Factor C

Pregnancy Considerations Withdrawal symptoms have been reported in the neonate following propoxyphene use during pregnancy. Teratogenic effects have also been noted in case reports.

Lactation Enters breast milk/use caution (AAP rates "compatible")

Breast-Feeding Considerations Propoxyphene and norpropoxyphene are excreted in breast milk. Based on limited data, a breast-feeding infant would receive ~2% of the maternal weight adjusted dose of propoxyphene. Norpropoxyphene clearance is decreased in neonates. Monitor infant for signs of sedation.

Contraindications Hypersensitivity to propoxyphene or any component; patients with paralytic ileus, acute or severe asthma, hypercarbia, or significant respiratory depression

Warnings Accidental and intentional overdose has occurred (including fatalities) when propoxyphene was used alone or in combination with other CNS depressants (including alcohol) **[U.S. Boxed Warning]**. Fatalities may occur within the first hour of overdosage. Patients with a history of emotional disturbances or suicidal ideation/attempt or who are receiving concurrent sedatives, tranquilizers, muscle relaxants, antidepressants, or other CNS-depressant drugs are at greatest risk of propoxyphene-related deaths **[U.S. Boxed Warning]**. Do not prescribe for patients who are suicidal or for those who have a history of suicidal ideation **[U.S. Boxed Warning]**. Use with caution in patients taking CYP3A4 inhibitors; strong CYP3A4 inhibitors may increase propoxyphene serum concentrations (see Drug Interactions); monitor patients closely; dosage adjustments may be needed **[U.S. Boxed Warning]**.

May cause CNS depression, which may impair physical or mental abilities; warn patient of possible impairment of alertness or physical coordination (see Patient Information). May cause respiratory depression; use with extreme caution in patients with COPD, cor pulmonale, hypoxia, hypercapnia, pre-existing respiratory depression, significantly decreased respiratory reserve; critical respiratory depression may occur, even at therapeutic dosages. Use with extreme caution (and only if essential) in patients with head injury, increased ICP, or other intracranial lesions; exaggerated elevation of ICP may occur. Severe hypotension may occur; use with caution in patients with circulatory shock, hypovolemia, impaired myocardial function or those receiving drugs which may exaggerate hypotensive effects (including phenothiazines or general anesthetics). Orthostatic hypotension may occur in ambulatory patients. Opioids may obscure diagnosis or clinical course of patients with acute abdominal conditions.

Physical and psychological dependence may occur; abrupt discontinuation after prolonged use may result in withdrawal symptoms or seizures. Healthcare provider should be alert to problems of abuse, misuse, and diversion. Do not prescribe to those who are addiction-prone. Infants born to women physically dependent on opioids will also be physically dependent and may experience respiratory difficulties or opioid withdrawal symptoms. Interactions with other CNS depressants, including alcohol, may occur and can result in serious and potentially fatal adverse effects (see Drug Interactions); use with caution in patients receiving sedatives, tranquilizers, muscle relaxants, antidepressants, or other CNS-depressant drugs; warn patients to avoid alcohol use.

Precautions Use with caution and consider dosage reduction in patients with renal or hepatic dysfunction; avoid use in patients with Cl$_{cr}$ <10 mL/minute. Use with caution in patients with biliary tract dysfunction or acute pancreatitis; opioids may cause constriction of sphincter of Oddi or increases in serum amylase.

Adverse Reactions

Central nervous system: CNS depression, dizziness, dysphoria, euphoria, hallucinations, headache, hypotension, intracranial pressure increased, lightheadedness, orthostatic hypotension, sedation

Dermatologic: Rashes

Gastrointestinal: Abdominal pain, biliary tract spasm, constipation, GI upset, nausea, vomiting

Neuromuscular & skeletal: Weakness

Ocular: Visual disturbances

Respiratory: Respiratory depression

Miscellaneous: Physical and psychological dependence, overdose (accidental and intentional, including fatalities; see Warnings)

<1%, postmarketing, and/or case reports: Abnormal behavior, arrhythmia, ataxia, blurred vision, bradycardia, heart failure, cholestatic jaundice (rare), coma, confusion, diarrhea, dyspnea, eye edema, GI bleed, hepatic steatosis, hepatomegaly, hepatocellular injury, histamine release, hypersensitivity reaction, jaundice (rare, reversible), liver dysfunction, liver function tests abnormal, metabolic acidosis, MI, myopathy (associated with overdose), pancreatitis, pruritus, respiratory arrest, seizure, somnolence, suicide, syncope, tachycardia, withdrawal syndrome

Drug Interactions

Metabolism/Transport Effects Substrate of CYP3A4 (major); **Inhibits** CYP2C9 (weak), 2D6 (weak), 3A4 (weak)

Avoid Concomitant Use

Avoid concomitant use of Propoxyphene with any of the following: MAO Inhibitors

Increased Effect/Toxicity

Propoxyphene may increase the levels/effects of: Alcohol (Ethyl); Alvimopan; Beta-Blockers; CarBAMazepine; CNS Depressants; Desmopressin; MAO Inhibitors; Selective Serotonin Reuptake Inhibitors; Thiazide Diuretics; Tricyclic Antidepressants; Vitamin K Antagonists

The levels/effects of Propoxyphene may be increased by: Amphetamines; Antipsychotic Agents (Phenothiazines); CYP3A4 Inhibitors (Moderate); CYP3A4 Inhibitors (Strong); Dasatinib; Succinylcholine

Decreased Effect

Propoxyphene may decrease the levels/effects of: Pegvisomant

The levels/effects of Propoxyphene may be decreased by: Ammonium Chloride; CYP3A4 Inducers (Strong); Deferasirox; Herbs (CYP3A4 Inducers); Mixed Agonist / Antagonist Opioids

Food Interactions Food may decrease rate of absorption, but may slightly increase bioavailability. Avoid grapefruit juice (may increase concentration/effects)

Stability Store at controlled room temperature of 20°C to 25°C (68°F to 77°F).

Mechanism of Action Binds to opiate receptors in the CNS, causing inhibition of ascending pain pathways, altering the perception of and response to pain; produces generalized CNS depression

Pharmacodynamics
Onset of action: Oral: Within 30-60 minutes
Duration: 4-6 hours

Pharmacokinetics (Adult data unless noted)
Distribution: Propoxyphene and norpropoxyphene (major metabolite; active) distribute into breast milk; both cross the placenta
V_d: 16 L/kg
Protein binding: ~80%
Metabolism: In the liver via CYP3A4 mediated N-demethylation to an active metabolite (norpropoxyphene) and inactive metabolites; minor metabolic pathways include ring hydroxylation and glucuronide formation.
Bioavailability: Oral: 30% to 70% due to extensive first-pass effect
Half-life: 6-12 hours
Norpropoxyphene: 30-36 hours
Elimination: Urine [~20% to 25% of dose; primarily as norpropoxyphene (free or conjugated)]
Dialysis: Not dialyzable (8%)

Usual Dosage Oral: Doses should be titrated to appropriate analgesic effect with consideration of severity of pain and patient size.
Children: Dose not well established; doses of propoxyphene hydrochloride of 2-3 mg/kg/day divided every 6 hours have been used
Adults:
Hydrochloride: 65 mg every 4 hours as needed for pain; maximum dose: 390 mg/day
Napsylate: 100 mg every 4 hours as needed for pain; maximum dose: 600 mg/day
Concurrent use with CYP3A4 inhibitors: Monitor closely; dosage adjustment may be necessary
Discontinuation of therapy: In patients on prolonged therapy, gradually discontinue propoxyphene by reducing dose by 25% to 50% daily and carefully monitor for signs/symptoms of withdrawal.

Dosing adjustment in renal impairment: Use with caution; dosage reduction should be considered; however, no specific dosing recommendations are available
Cl_{cr} <10 mL/minute: Avoid use

Dosing adjustment in hepatic impairment: Use with caution; dosage reduction should be considered; however, no specific dosing recommendations are available

Administration Oral: May administer with food to decrease GI upset. Do not administer with grapefruit juice.

Monitoring Parameters Pain relief, respiratory rate, blood pressure, mental status; liver enzymes with long-term use

Test Interactions False-positive methadone test

Patient Information Read the patient Medication Guide that you receive with each prescription and refill of propoxyphene. Take as directed; do not take a larger dose or more often than prescribed. Avoid alcohol; avoid grapefruit juice. Do not use prescription or nonprescription sedatives, tranquilizers, antihistamines, or pain medications without consulting prescriber. May be habit-forming; avoid abrupt discontinuation after prolonged use. May cause dizziness or drowsiness and impair ability to perform activities requiring mental alertness or physical coordination. Report unresolved nausea or vomiting, respiratory difficulty or shortness of breath, or unusual weakness to prescriber.

Additional Information Propoxyphene does not possess any anti-inflammatory or antipyretic actions; it possesses little, if any, antitussive effects. Propoxyphene napsylate 100 mg is equivalent to 65 mg of propoxyphene hydrochloride. Several cases utilizing propoxyphene in children for opioid detoxification have been reported (see References)

Dosage Forms Excipient information presented when available (limited, particularly for generics); consult specific product labeling.
Capsule, as hydrochloride: 65 mg
Darvon®: 65 mg
Tablet, as napsylate:
Darvon-N®: 100 mg

References
Hasday JD and Weintraub M, "Propoxyphene in Children With Iatrogenic Morphine Dependence," *Am J Dis Child,* 1983, 137 (8):745-8.

Propoxyphene and Acetaminophen
(proe POKS i feen & a seet a MIN oh fen)

Medication Safety Issues
Sound-alike/look-alike issues:
Darvocet® may be confused with Percocet®
Darvocet-N® may be confused with Darvon-N®

High alert medication: The Institute for Safe Medication Practices (ISMP) includes this medication among its list of drug classes which have a heightened risk of causing significant patient harm when used in error.

Beers Criteria medication: This drug may be inappropriate for use in geriatric patients (low severity risk).

Duplicate therapy issues: This product contains acetaminophen, which may be a component of other combination products. Do not exceed the maximum recommended daily dose of acetaminophen.

International issues:
Capadex, a brand name for propoxyphene/acetaminophen in Australia and New Zealand, may be confused with Casodex® which is a brand name for bicalutamide in the U.S. or with Kapidex™ which is a brand name for dexlansoprazole in the U.S.

U.S. Brand Names Balacet 325™; Darvocet A500®; Darvocet-N® 100; Darvocet-N® 50

Canadian Brand Names Darvocet-N® 100; Darvocet-N® 50

Therapeutic Category Analgesic, Narcotic

Generic Available Yes

Use Management of mild to moderate pain (FDA approved in adults)

Restrictions C-IV

Medication Guide An FDA-approved patient medication guide, which is available with the product information and at http://www.fda.gov/downloads/Drugs/DrugSafety/UCM187067.pdf, must be dispensed with this medication for each new outpatient prescription and refill.

Pregnancy Risk Factor C

Pregnancy Considerations Teratogenic effects were not observed with propoxyphene in animal reproductive studies. Acetaminophen, propoxyphene, and norpropoxyphene (metabolite) cross the placenta. Withdrawal symptoms have been reported in the neonate following propoxyphene use during pregnancy. Teratogenic effects have also been noted in case reports. Opioid analgesics are considered pregnancy risk factor D if used for prolonged periods or in large doses near term.

Lactation Enters breast milk/use caution

Breast-Feeding Considerations Propoxyphene, norpropoxyphene and acetaminophen are excreted in breast milk. The AAP considers propoxyphene and acetaminophen to be "compatible" with breast-feeding. Based on limited data, a breast-feeding infant would receive ~2% of the maternal weight adjusted dose of propoxyphene. Norpropoxyphene clearance is decreased in neonates. Monitor infant for signs of sedation.

◀ **Contraindications** Hypersensitivity to propoxyphene, acetaminophen, or any component; patients with paralytic ileus, acute or severe asthma, hypercarbia, or significant respiratory depression

Warnings Accidental and intentional overdose has occurred (including fatalities) when propoxyphene was used alone or in combination with other CNS depressants (including alcohol) **[U.S. Boxed Warning]**. Fatalities may occur within the first hour of overdosage. Patients with a history of emotional disturbances or suicidal ideation/ attempt or who are receiving concurrent sedatives, tranquilizers, muscle relaxants, antidepressants, or other CNS-depressant drugs are at greatest risk of propoxyphene-related deaths **[U.S. Boxed Warning]**. Do not prescribe for patients who are suicidal or for those who have a history of suicidal ideation **[U.S. Boxed Warning]**. Use with caution in patients taking CYP3A4 inhibitors; strong CYP3A4 inhibitors may increase propoxyphene serum concentrations (see Drug Interactions); monitor patients closely; dosage adjustments may be needed **[U.S. Boxed Warning]**.

Propoxyphene may cause CNS depression, which may impair physical or mental abilities; warn patient of possible impairment of alertness or physical coordination (see Patient Information). May cause respiratory depression; use with extreme caution in patients with COPD, cor pulmonale, hypoxia, hypercapnia, pre-existing respiratory depression, significantly decreased respiratory reserve; critical respiratory depression may occur, even at therapeutic dosages. Use with extreme caution (and only if essential) in patients with head injury, increased ICP, or other intracranial lesions; exaggerated elevation of ICP may occur. Severe hypotension may occur; use with caution in patients with circulatory shock, hypovolemia, impaired myocardial function or those receiving drugs which may exaggerate hypotensive effects (including phenothiazines or general anesthetics). Orthostatic hypotension may occur in ambulatory patients. Opioids may obscure diagnosis or clinical course of patients with acute abdominal conditions.

Physical and psychological dependence may occur; abrupt discontinuation after prolonged use may result in withdrawal symptoms or seizures. Healthcare provider should be alert to problems of abuse, misuse, and diversion. Do not prescribe to those who are addiction-prone. Infants born to women physically dependent on opioids will also be physically dependent and may experience respiratory difficulties or opioid withdrawal symptoms. Interactions with other CNS depressants, including alcohol, may occur and can result in serious and potentially fatal adverse effects (see Drug Interactions); use propoxyphene with caution in patients receiving sedatives, tranquilizers, muscle relaxants, antidepressants, or other CNS-depressant drugs; warn patients to avoid alcohol use.

Acetaminophen may cause severe hepatic toxicity with acute overdose. Use with caution in patients with alcoholic liver disease (acetaminophen may cause hepatotoxicity and severe liver failure in chronic alcoholics receiving therapeutic doses). Chronic daily dosing of acetaminophen in adults of 5-8 g of acetaminophen over several weeks or 3-4 g/day for 1 year have resulted in liver damage. Do not exceed maximum daily doses; consider acetaminophen content of combination products when evaluating the dose of acetaminophen. Do not use propoxyphene and acetaminophen with other acetaminophen-containing products; hepatotoxicity may occur at higher than recommended doses.

Precautions Use with caution and consider dosage reduction in patients with renal or hepatic dysfunction; propoxyphene should be avoided in patients with Cl$_{cr}$ <10 mL/minute. Use with caution in patients with biliary tract dysfunction or acute pancreatitis; opioids may cause constriction of sphincter of Oddi or increases in serum amylase.

G-6-PD deficiency: Although several case reports of acetaminophen-associated hemolytic anemia have been reported in patients with G-6-PD deficiency, a direct cause and effect relationship has not been well established (concurrent illnesses such as fever or infection may precipitate hemolytic anemia in patients with G-6-PD deficiency); therefore, acetaminophen is generally thought to be safe when given in therapeutic doses to patients with G-6-PD deficiency.

Adverse Reactions

Propoxyphene:
  Central nervous system: CNS depression, dizziness, dysphoria, euphoria, hallucinations, headache, hypotension, intracranial pressure increased, insomnia, lightheadedness, orthostatic hypotension, sedation
  Dermatologic: Rashes
  Gastrointestinal: Abdominal pain, biliary tract spasm, constipation, GI upset, nausea, vomiting
  Neuromuscular & skeletal: Weakness
  Ocular: Visual disturbances
  Respiratory: Respiratory depression
  Miscellaneous: Physical and psychological dependence, overdose (accidental and intentional, including fatalities; see Warnings)
Acetaminophen:
  Dermatologic: Rash
  Hematologic: Blood dyscrasias (leukopenia, neutropenia, pancytopenia)
  Hepatic: Hepatic necrosis with overdose
  Renal: Renal injury with chronic use, renal papillary necrosis (postmarketing reports)
  Miscellaneous: Hypersensitivity reactions (rare)
Propoxyphene and Acetaminophen:
  <1%, postmarketing, and/or case reports: Abnormal behavior, arrhythmia, ataxia, blurred vision, bradycardia, heart failure, cholestatic jaundice (rare), coma, confusion, diarrhea, dyspnea, eye edema, GI bleed, hepatic steatosis, hepatomegaly, hepatocellular injury, histamine release, jaundice (rare, reversible), liver dysfunction, liver function tests abnormal, metabolic acidosis, MI, myopathy (associated with overdose), pancreatitis, pruritus, respiratory arrest, seizure, somnolence, suicide, syncope, tachycardia, withdrawal syndrome

Drug Interactions

Metabolism/Transport Effects

Propoxyphene: **Substrate** of CYP3A4 (major); **Inhibits** CYP2C9 (weak), 2D6 (weak), 3A4 (weak)
Acetaminophen: **Substrate** (minor) of CYP1A2, 2A6, 2C9, 2D6, 2E1, 3A4; **Inhibits** CYP3A4 (weak)

Avoid Concomitant Use

Avoid concomitant use of Propoxyphene and Acetaminophen with any of the following: MAO Inhibitors

Increased Effect/Toxicity

Propoxyphene and Acetaminophen may increase the levels/effects of: Alcohol (Ethyl); Alvimopan; Beta-Blockers; CarBAMazepine; CNS Depressants; Desmopressin; MAO Inhibitors; Selective Serotonin Reuptake Inhibitors; Thiazide Diuretics; Tricyclic Antidepressants; Vitamin K Antagonists

The levels/effects of Propoxyphene and Acetaminophen may be increased by: Amphetamines; Antipsychotic Agents (Phenothiazines); CYP3A4 Inhibitors (Moderate); CYP3A4 Inhibitors (Strong); Dasatinib; Imatinib; Isoniazid; Succinylcholine

Decreased Effect

Propoxyphene and Acetaminophen may decrease the levels/effects of: Pegvisomant

The levels/effects of Propoxyphene and Acetaminophen may be decreased by: Ammonium Chloride; Anticonvulsants (Hydantoin); Barbiturates; CarBAMazepine; Cholestyramine Resin; CYP3A4 Inducers (Strong); Deferasirox; Herbs (CYP3A4 Inducers); Mixed Agonist / Antagonist Opioids; Peginterferon Alfa-2b

Food Interactions Food may decrease rate of absorption of propoxyphene, but may slightly increase bioavailability. The rate of absorption of acetaminophen may be decreased when given with food high in carbohydrates. Avoid grapefruit juice; may increase concentration/effects of propoxyphene.

Stability Store at 25°C (77°F); excursions permitted to 15°C to 30°C (59°F to 86°F).

Mechanism of Action See individual monographs for Propoxyphene on page 1171 and Acetaminophen on page 36

Pharmacodynamics See individual monographs for Propoxyphene on page 1171 and Acetaminophen on page 36

Pharmacokinetics (Adult data unless noted) See individual monographs for Propoxyphene on page 1171 and Acetaminophen on page 36

Usual Dosage Adults: Oral: Doses should be titrated to appropriate analgesic effect with consideration of severity of pain and patient size

Darvocet-N® 50: 1-2 tablets every 4 hours as needed; maximum: 600 mg propoxyphene napsylate/day

Darvocet A500™, Darvocet-N® 100: 1 tablet every 4 hours as needed; maximum: 600 mg propoxyphene napsylate/day

Propoxyphene hydrochloride 65 mg and acetaminophen 650 mg: 1 tablet every 4 hours as needed; maximum: 390 mg/day propoxyphene hydrochloride, 4 g/day acetaminophen)

Note: Formulations contain significant amounts of acetaminophen; adult intake should be limited to <4 g acetaminophen/day (less in patients with hepatic impairment/ethanol abuse) (see Warnings)

Concurrent use with CYP3A4 inhibitors: Monitor closely; dosage adjustment may be necessary

Discontinuation of therapy: In patients on prolonged therapy, gradually discontinue propoxyphene and acetaminophen by reducing dose by 25% to 50% daily and carefully monitor for signs/symptoms of withdrawal.

Dosing adjustment in renal impairment: Serum concentrations of propoxyphene may be increased or elimination may be delayed; consider dosage reduction; specific dosing recommendations not available

Cl$_{cr}$ <10 mL/minute: Avoid use

Dosing adjustment in hepatic impairment: Serum concentrations of propoxyphene and acetaminophen may be increased or elimination may be delayed; consider dosage reduction; specific dosing recommendations not available

Administration Oral: Administer with water on an empty stomach; may administer with food to decrease GI upset. Do not administer with grapefruit juice.

Monitoring Parameters Pain relief, respiratory rate, blood pressure, mental status; liver enzymes with long-term use

Test Interactions False-positive methadone test

Patient Information Read the patient Medication Guide that you receive with each prescription and refill of propoxyphene and acetaminophen. Take as directed; do not take a larger dose or more often than prescribed. Avoid alcohol; avoid grapefruit juice. Do not use prescription or nonprescription sedatives, tranquilizers, antihistamines, or pain medications without consulting prescriber. Do not use other prescription or nonprescription medications that contain acetaminophen. May be habit-forming; avoid abrupt discontinuation after prolonged use. May cause dizziness or drowsiness and impair ability to perform activities requiring mental alertness or physical coordination. Report unresolved nausea or vomiting, respiratory difficulty or shortness of breath, or unusual weakness to prescriber.

Additional Information Propoxyphene napsylate 100 mg is equivalent to 65 mg of propoxyphene hydrochloride.

Dosage Forms Excipient information presented when available (limited, particularly for generics); consult specific product labeling.

Tablet, 50/325:
  Darvocet-N® 50: Propoxyphene napsylate 50 mg and acetaminophen 325 mg
Tablet, 65/650: Propoxyphene hydrochloride 65 mg and acetaminophen 650 mg
Tablet, 100/325: Propoxyphene napsylate 100 mg and acetaminophen 325 mg
  Balacet 325™: Propoxyphene napsylate 100 mg and acetaminophen 325 mg
Tablet, 100/500: Propoxyphene napsylate 100 mg and acetaminophen 500 mg
  Darvocet A500®: Propoxyphene napsylate 100 mg and acetaminophen 500 mg
Tablet, 100/650: Propoxyphene napsylate 100 mg and acetaminophen 650 mg
  Darvocet-N® 100: Propoxyphene napsylate 100 mg and acetaminophen 650 mg

♦ **Propoxyphene Hydrochloride** *see* Propoxyphene *on page 1171*

♦ **Propoxyphene Hydrochloride and Acetaminophen** *see* Propoxyphene and Acetaminophen *on page 1173*

♦ **Propoxyphene Napsylate** *see* Propoxyphene *on page 1171*

♦ **Propoxyphene Napsylate and Acetaminophen** *see* Propoxyphene and Acetaminophen *on page 1173*

Propranolol (proe PRAN oh lole)

Medication Safety Issues

Sound-alike/look-alike issues:

Propranolol may be confused with prasugrel, Pravachol®, Propulsid®

Inderal® may be confused with Adderall®, Enduron®, Enduronyl®, Imdur®, Imuran®, Inderide®, Isordil®, Toradol®

Inderal® 40 may be confused with Enduronyl® Forte

High alert medication: The Institute for Safe Medication Practices (ISMP) includes this medication among its list of drugs which have a heightened risk of causing significant patient harm when used in error.

Significant differences exist between oral and I.V. dosing. Use caution when converting from one route of administration to another.

International issues:

Inderal® may be confused with Indiaral® which is a brand name for loperamide in France

Related Information

Antihypertensive Agents by Class *on page 1481*

U.S. Brand Names Inderal® [DSC]; Inderal® LA; InnoPran XL®

Canadian Brand Names Apo-Propranolol®; Dom-Propranolol; Inderal®; Inderal® LA; Novo-Pranol; Nu-Propranolol; PMS-Propranolol; Propranolol Hydrochloride Injection, USP

Therapeutic Category Antianginal Agent; Antiarrhythmic Agent, Class II; Antihypertensive Agent; Antimigraine Agent; Beta-Adrenergic Blocker

Generic Available Yes

Use

Oral: Management of hypertension (alone or in combination with other agents), angina pectoris, symptomatic treatment of hypertrophic subaortic stenosis, migraine headache prophylaxis, pheochromocytoma, essential tremor, atrial fibrillation, reduction of mortality post-MI (all indications FDA approved in adults); tetralogy of Fallot cyanotic spells; short-term adjunctive therapy of thyrotoxicosis

I.V.: Supraventricular arrhythmias (such as atrial fibrillation and flutter, AV nodal re-entrant tachycardias), ventricular tachycardias (catecholamine-induced arrhythmias, digoxin toxicity) (all indications FDA approved in adults); tetralogy of Fallot cyanotic spells; short-term adjunction therapy of thyrotoxicosis

Pregnancy Risk Factor C

Pregnancy Considerations Adverse events have been observed in some animal reproduction studies; therefore, the manufacturer classifies propranolol as pregnancy category C. Propranolol crosses the placenta and is measurable in the newborn serum following maternal use during pregnancy. Congenital abnormalities have been rarely noted in case reports following maternal use of propranolol in the first trimester. In a cohort study, an increased risk of cardiovascular defects was observed following maternal use of beta-blockers during pregnancy. Intrauterine growth restriction (IUGR), small placentas, bradycardia, hypoglycemia, and/or respiratory depression have been observed in neonates following *in utero* exposure to propranolol at parturition; adequate facilities for monitoring infants at birth should be available. The peak maternal serum concentrations of propranolol and the active metabolite 4-hyrdoxypropranolol do not change during pregnancy; peak serum concentrations of naphthoxylactic acid are lower in the third trimester when compared to postpartum. Propranolol is recommended for use in the management of thyrotoxicosis in pregnancy. Propranolol has been evaluated for the treatment of hypertension in pregnancy, but other beta-blockers may be more appropriate for use. Propranolol has also been used in the management of hypertrophic obstructive cardiomyopathy in pregnancy and has been studied for use as an adjunctive agent in the management of dysfunctional labor (dystocia).

Lactation Enters breast milk/use caution (AAP rates "compatible")

Breast-Feeding Considerations Propranolol is excreted into breast milk with peak concentrations occurring ~2-3 hours after an oral dose. The inactive metabolites of propranolol have also been detected in breast milk. The manufacturer recommends that caution be exercised when administering propranolol to nursing women. The AAP considers propranolol to be "usually compatible with breast-feeding." Due to immature hepatic metabolism in newborns, breast-feeding infants should be monitored for adverse events.

Contraindications Hypersensitivity to propranolol or any component; uncompensated CHF, cardiogenic shock, bradycardia or heart block, asthma, hyperactive airway disease, chronic obstructive lung disease, Raynaud's syndrome

Warnings May depress myocardial activity and precipitate or worsen CHF; use with caution and monitor closely, especially in patients with compensated heart failure. In patients with angina pectoris, exacerbation of angina and, in some cases, MI occurred following abrupt discontinuance of therapy **[U.S. Boxed Warning]**; reduce dose gradually over at least a few weeks when discontinuing therapy. Beta-blockers should generally be avoided in patients with bronchospastic disease (nonallergic bronchospasm, chronic bronchitis, emphysema), as bronchospasm may occur. Hypoglycemia may occur, particularly in infants and children (whether the patient has diabetes mellitus or not), especially during fasting before surgery; hypoglycemia may also occur after prolonged physical exertion and in patients with renal dysfunction. Propranolol decreases the ability of the heart to respond to reflex adrenergic stimuli and may increase the risks of general anesthesia and surgical procedures. Propranolol may mask clinical signs of hyperthyroidism (exacerbation of symptoms of hyperthyroidism, including thyroid storm, may occur following abrupt discontinuation). Severe bradycardia (requiring pacemaker) may occur in patients with Wolff-Parkinson-White syndrome. In patients with pheochromocytoma, adequate alpha-blockade is required prior to use of any beta-blocker. Hypersensitivity reactions (including anaphylactic and anaphylactoid reactions) and serious cutaneous reactions have been reported with propranolol use. Beta-blocker use has been associated with induction or exacerbation of psoriasis, but cause and effect have not been firmly established.

Precautions Propranolol may block hypoglycemia-induced tachycardia and blood pressure changes, use with caution in patients with diabetes mellitus; acute elevations in blood pressure have been reported after insulin-induced hypoglycemia in patients receiving propranolol. Use with caution in patients with peripheral vascular disease (beta-blockers may aggravate arterial insufficiency). Use with caution in patients with renal or hepatic dysfunction; consider dosage reduction in patients with hepatic insufficiency. Avoid I.V. use in patients receiving calcium channel blockers (eg, verapamil) (effects may be potentiated). Patients receiving beta-blockers who have a history of anaphylactic reactions, may be more reactive to a repeated allergen challenge and may not be responsive to the usual epinephrine doses used to treat an allergic reaction

Adverse Reactions

Cardiovascular: Arterial insufficiency, bradycardia, CHF, hypotension, impaired myocardial contractility, mesenteric arterial thrombosis (rare), Raynaud's syndrome, worsening of A-V conduction disturbances

Central nervous system: Amnesia, catatonia, cognitive dysfunction, confusion, depression, dizziness, emotional lability, fatigue, hallucinations, hypersomnolence, insomnia, lethargy, lightheadedness, psychosis, vertigo, vivid dreams

Dermatologic: Alopecia, erythema multiforme, exfoliative dermatitis, psoriasiform eruptions, psoriasis exacerbation, rash, Stevens-Johnson syndrome, toxic epidermal necrolysis, urticaria

Endocrine & metabolic: Hyperglycemia, hyperkalemia, hypoglycemia [also blunts warning signs of hypoglycemia (eg, tachycardia)]

Gastrointestinal: Abdominal cramping, constipation, diarrhea, epigastric distress, ischemic colitis, nausea, vomiting

Genitourinary: Impotence, Peyronie's disease

Hematologic: Agranulocytosis, nonthrombocytopenic purpura, thrombocytopenic purpura

Hepatic: Liver enzymes elevated

Neuromuscular & skeletal: Paresthesia, weakness

Ocular: Visual disturbances

Respiratory: Bronchospasm, dyspnea, laryngospasm, pharyngitis, respiratory distress, wheezing

Miscellaneous: Anaphylactic/anaphylactoid reactions, cold extremities, hypersensitivity reactions, SLE-like syndrome

Drug Interactions

Metabolism/Transport Effects Substrate of CYP1A2 (major), 2C19 (minor), 2D6 (major), 3A4 (minor); **Inhibits** CYP1A2 (weak), CYP2D6 (weak), P-glycoprotein

Avoid Concomitant Use

Avoid concomitant use of Propranolol with any of the following: Dabigatran Etexilate; Methacholine; Topotecan

Increased Effect/Toxicity

Propranolol may increase the levels/effects of: Alpha-/Beta-Agonists (Direct-Acting); Alpha1-Blockers; Alpha2-Agonists; Amifostine; Antihypertensives; Antipsychotic Agents (Phenothiazines); Bupivacaine; Cardiac Glycosides; Colchicine; Dabigatran Etexilate; Hypotensive Agents; Insulin; Lidocaine; Lidocaine (Systemic); Lidocaine (Topical); Mepivacaine; Methacholine; Midodrine; P-Glycoprotein Substrates; RiTUXimab; Rivaroxaban; Rizatriptan; Sulfonylureas; Topotecan; Zolmitriptan

The levels/effects of Propranolol may be increased by: Acetylcholinesterase Inhibitors; Alcohol (Ethyl); Aminoquinolines (Antimalarial); Amiodarone; Anilidopiperidine Opioids; Antipsychotic Agents (Phenothiazines); Calcium Channel Blockers (Nondihydropyridine); CYP1A2 Inhibitors (Moderate); CYP1A2 Inhibitors (Strong); CYP2D6 Inhibitors (Moderate); CYP2D6 Inhibitors (Strong); Darunavir; Diazoxide; Dipyridamole; Disopyramide; Dronedarone; Fluvoxamine; Herbs (Hypotensive Properties); MAO Inhibitors; Pentoxifylline; Phosphodiesterase 5 Inhibitors; Propafenone; Propoxyphene; Prostacyclin Analogues; QuiNIDine; Reserpine; Selective Serotonin Reuptake Inhibitors; Zileuton

Decreased Effect

Propranolol may decrease the levels/effects of: Beta2-Agonists; Theophylline Derivatives

The levels/effects of Propranolol may be decreased by: Alcohol (Ethyl); Barbiturates; Bile Acid Sequestrants; CYP1A2 Inducers (Strong); Herbs (Hypertensive Properties); Methylphenidate; Nonsteroidal Anti-Inflammatory Agents; Peginterferon Alfa-2b; Rifamycin Derivatives; Yohimbine

Food Interactions Avoid natural licorice (causes sodium and water retention and increases potassium loss). Protein-rich foods may increase bioavailability. A change in diet from high carbohydrate/low protein to low carbohydrate/high protein may result in increased oral clearance. A high-fat meal decreases the rate but not the extent of oral absorption of the extended release capsules (InnoPran XL™). Effect of food on bioavailability of sustained release capsule (Inderal® LA) has not been studied.

Stability

Injection: Store at controlled room temperature; protect from freezing or excessive heat; protect from light; injection is compatible in D$_5$W, NS, D$_5$/NS, D$_5$/^{1}/$_2$NS, ^{1}/$_2$NS, LR; incompatible with bicarbonate

Capsule, tablet: Store at 20°C to 25°C (68°F to 77°F). Protect from freezing or excessive heat. Protect from light and moisture. Dispense in tightly closed, light-resistant container.

Mechanism of Action Nonselective beta-adrenergic blocker (class II antiarrhythmic); competitively blocks response to beta$_1$ and beta$_2$-adrenergic stimulation which results in a decrease in heart rate, myocardial contractility, blood pressure, and myocardial oxygen demand. Beta-adrenergic blocking effects are due to the S (-) enantiomer. Propranolol also exerts a quinidine-like or anesthetic-like membrane action at doses higher than those required for beta blockade; this affects the cardiac action potential (clinical significance is uncertain).

Pharmacodynamics Beta blockade: Oral (immediate release):

Onset of action: Within 1-2 hours

Duration: ~6 hours

Pharmacokinetics (Adult data unless noted)

Absorption: Oral: Rapid and complete

Distribution: V$_d$: Adults: 3.9 L/kg; crosses the placenta and blood-brain barrier; small amounts appear in breast milk

Protein-binding (Alpha$_1$-acid glycoprotein and albumin): **Note:** The S-isomer of propranolol preferentially binds to alpha$_1$-acid glycoprotein and the R-isomer preferentially binds to albumin

Newborns: 60% to 68%

Adults: 93%

Metabolism: Extensive first-pass effect, metabolized in the liver to active and inactive compounds; the 3 main metabolic pathways include: Aromatic hydroxylation (primarily 4-hydroxylation), N-dealkylation followed by further side-chain oxidation and direct glucuronidation; the 4 primary metabolites include: Propranolol glucuronide, naphthyloxylactic acid, and sulfate and glucuronic acid conjugates of 4-hydroxy propranolol; **Note:** Aromatic hydroxylation is catalyzed primarily by isoenzyme CYP2D6; side chain oxidation is mainly via CYP1A2, but also CYP2D6; 4-hydroxypropranolol possesses beta-adrenergic receptor blocking activity and is a weak inhibitor of CYP2D6.

Bioavailability: Oral: 26% ± 10%; oral bioavailability may be increased in Down syndrome children; protein-rich foods increase bioavailability of immediate release tablets by ~50%

Half-life, distribution: I.V.: 5-10 minutes

Half-life, elimination (prolonged with hepatic dysfunction): Neonates and Infants: Possible increased half-life

Children: 3.9-6.4 hours

Adults: 4-6 hours

Time to peak serum concentration:

Immediate release: 1-4 hours

Extended release capsule (InnoPran XL™): 12-14 hours

Sustained release capsule (Inderal® LA): 6 hours

Elimination: Metabolites are excreted primarily in urine (96% to 99%); <1% excreted in urine as unchanged drug

Clearance: Decreased in hepatic dysfunction and in chronic renal failure

Dialysis: Not dialyzable: (0% to 5%)

Usual Dosage Note: Dosage should be individualized based on patient response

Neonates:

Oral: Initial: 0.25 mg/kg/dose every 6-8 hours; increase slowly as needed to maximum of 5 mg/kg/day

I.V.: Initial: 0.01 mg/kg slow I.V. push over 10 minutes; may repeat every 6-8 hours as needed; increase slowly to maximum of 0.15 mg/kg/dose every 6-8 hours

Arrhythmias:

Oral:

Children: Initial: 0.5-1 mg/kg/day in divided doses every 6-8 hours; titrate dosage upward every 3-5 days; usual dose: 2-4 mg/kg/day; higher doses may be needed; do not exceed 16 mg/kg/day or 60 mg/day

Adults: Initial: 10-20 mg/dose every 6-8 hours, increase gradually; usual range: 40-320 mg/day

I.V.:

Children: 0.01-0.1 mg/kg slow I.V. over 10 minutes; maximum dose: 1 mg (infants); 3 mg (children)

Adults: 1 mg/dose slow I.V.; repeat every 5 minutes up to a total of 5 mg

Hypertension: Oral:

Children: Initial: 0.5-1 mg/kg/day in divided doses every 6-12 hours; increase gradually every 5-7 days; usual dose: 1-5 mg/kg/day; maximum dose: 8 mg/kg/day

Children and Adolescents 1-17 years: Initial: 1-2 mg/kg/day divided in 2-3 doses/day; titrate dose to effect; maximum dose: 4 mg/kg/day up to 640 mg/day; sustained release formulation may be dosed once daily (National High Blood Pressure Education Program Working Group on High Blood Pressure in Children and Adolescents, 2004)

Adults: Initial: 40 mg twice daily or 60-80 mg once daily as sustained or extended release capsules; increase dosage every 3-7 days; usual dose: Immediate release products: ≤320 mg divided in 2-3 doses/day; sustained or extended release products: 120-160 mg once daily; maximum daily dose: 640 mg; usual dosage range (JNC 7): Immediate release products: 20-80 mg twice daily; sustained or extended release products: 60-180 mg once daily

Migraine headache prophylaxis: Oral:
Children: 0.6-1.5 mg/kg/day divided every 8 hours; maximum dose: 4 mg/kg/day **or**
≤35 kg: 10-20 mg 3 times/day
>35 kg: 20-40 mg 3 times/day
Adults: Initial: 80 mg/day divided every 6-8 hours (or once daily as sustained release capsule); increase by 20-40 mg/dose every 3-4 weeks to a maximum of 160-240 mg/day given in divided doses every 6-8 hours (or once daily as sustained release capsules)

Tetralogy spells: Infants and Children:
Oral: Palliation: Initial: 0.25 mg/kg/dose every 6 hours (1 mg/kg/day); if ineffective within first week of therapy, may increase by 1 mg/kg/day every 24 hours to maximum of 5 mg/kg/day; if patient becomes refractory may increase slowly to a maximum of 10-15 mg/kg/day but must carefully monitor heart rate, heart size, and cardiac contractility; average dose: 2.3 mg/kg/day; range: 0.8-5 mg/kg/day (see Garson, 1981). Some centers use: Initial: 0.5-1 mg/kg/dose every 6 hours; usual: 1-2 mg/kg/dose every 6 hours.
I.V.: 0.01-0.02 mg/kg/dose infused over 10 minutes; maximum initial dose: 1 mg (Committee on Drugs, 1998). Some centers use: 0.15-0.25 mg/kg/dose slow I.V.; may repeat in 15 minutes

Thyrotoxicosis:
Neonates: Oral: 2 mg/kg/day in divided doses every 6-12 hours; occasionally higher doses may be required
Adolescents and Adults: Oral: 10-40 mg/dose every 6 hours
Adults: I.V.: 1-3 mg/dose slow I.V. as a single dose

Administration
Oral: Administer with food; administer extended release capsules consistently either with food or on an empty stomach; do not chew or crush sustained or extended release capsules, swallow whole; mix concentrated oral solution with water, fruit juice, liquid, or semisolid food before administration
Parenteral: I.V. administration should not exceed 1 mg/minute; administer slow I.V. over 10 minutes in children; maximum concentration for injection: 1 mg/mL

Monitoring Parameters ECG, blood pressure, heart rate

Reference Range Therapeutic: 50-100 ng/mL (SI: 190-390 nmol/L) at end of dosing interval

Patient Information Avoid alcohol; do not discontinue abruptly; may mask fast heart rate of hypoglycemia, but sweating will still occur

Nursing Implications The I.V. dose is much smaller than oral dose

Additional Information Not indicated for hypertensive emergencies. Do not abruptly discontinue therapy, taper dosage gradually over 2 weeks. The pH of solution for injection is adjusted with citric acid.

Dosage Forms Excipient information presented when available (limited, particularly for generics); consult specific product labeling. [DSC] = Discontinued product
Capsule, extended release, as hydrochloride: 60 mg, 80 mg, 120 mg, 160 mg
InnoPran XL®: 80 mg, 120 mg
Capsule, sustained release, as hydrochloride:
Inderal® LA: 60 mg, 80 mg, 120 mg, 160 mg
Injection, solution, as hydrochloride: 1 mg/mL (1 mL)
Inderal®: 1 mg/mL (1 mL) [DSC]

Solution, oral, as hydrochloride: 4 mg/mL (500 mL); 8 mg/mL (500 mL)
Tablet, as hydrochloride: 10 mg, 20 mg, 40 mg, 60 mg, 80 mg

References
Brauchli YB, Jick SS, Curtin F, et al, "Association Between Beta-Blockers, Other Antihypertensive Drugs and Psoriasis: Population-Based Case-Control Study," Br J Dermatol, 2008, 158(6):1299-307.
Chobanian AV, Bakris GL, Black HR, et al, "The Seventh Report of the Joint National Committee on Prevention, Detection, Evaluation, and Treatment of High Blood Pressure: The JNC 7 report," JAMA, 2003, 289(19):2560-72.
Committee on Drugs, "Drugs for Pediatric Emergencies," Pediatrics, 1998, 101(1):E13.
Garson A Jr, Gillette PC, and McNamara DG, "Propranolol: The Preferred Palliation for Tetralogy of Fallot," Am J Cardiol, 1981, 47 (5):1098-104.
Gold MH, Holy AK, and Roenigk HH Jr, "Beta-Blocking Drugs and Psoriasis. A Review of Cutaneous Side Effects and Retrospective Analysis of Their Effects on Psoriasis," J Am Acad Dermatol, 1988, 19 (5 Pt 1):837-41.
Lai CW, Ziegler DK, Lansky LL, et al, "Hemiplegic Migraine in Childhood: Diagnostic and Therapeutic Aspects," J Pediatr, 1982, 101(5):696-9.
National High Blood Pressure Education Program Working Group on High Blood Pressure in Children and Adolescents, "The Fourth Report on the Diagnosis, Evaluation, and Treatment of High Blood Pressure in Children and Adolescents," Pediatrics, 2004, 114(2 Suppl 4th Report):555-76.
Pickoff AS, Zies L, Ferrer PL, et al, "High-Dose Propranolol Therapy in the Management of Supraventricular Tachycardia," J Pediatr, 1979, 94(1):144-6.
Rasoulpour M and Marinelli KA, "Systemic Hypertension," Clin Perinatol, 1992, 19(1):121-37.
Schön MP and Boehncke WH, "Psoriasis," N Engl J Med, 2005, 352 (18):1899-912.
Sinaiko AR, "Pharmacologic Management of Childhood Hypertension," Pediatr Clin North Am, 1993, 40(1):195-212.

◆ **Propranolol Hydrochloride** *see* Propranolol *on page 1175*

◆ **Propranolol Hydrochloride Injection, USP (Can)** *see* Propranolol *on page 1175*

◆ **Proprinal [OTC]** *see* Ibuprofen *on page 702*

◆ **Proprinal® Cold and Sinus [OTC]** *see* Pseudoephedrine and Ibuprofen *on page 1184*

◆ **Propulsid®** *see* Cisapride **U.S. - Available Via Limited-Access Protocol Only** *on page 315*

◆ **2-Propylpentanoic Acid** *see* Valproic Acid and Derivatives *on page 1398*

Propylthiouracil (proe pil thye oh YOOR a sil)

Medication Safety Issues
Sound-alike/look-alike issues:
Propylthiouracil may be confused with Purinethol®
PTU is an error-prone abbreviation (mistaken as mercaptopurine [Purinethol®; 6-MP])

Canadian Brand Names Propyl-Thyracil®

Therapeutic Category Antithyroid Agent

Generic Available Yes

Use Palliative treatment of hyperthyroidism (FDA approved in adults); adjunct to ameliorate hyperthyroidism in preparation for surgical treatment or radioactive iodine therapy (FDA approved in adults); has also been used in the management of thyrotoxic crisis

Medication Guide An FDA-approved patient medication guide, which is available with the product information and at http://www.fda.gov/downloads/Drugs/DrugSafety/UCM208533.pdf, must be dispensed with this medication for each new outpatient prescription and refill.

Pregnancy Risk Factor D

Pregnancy Considerations Propylthiouracil crosses the placenta and because adverse events may occur in the fetus following maternal use, it is classified as pregnancy category D. The rate of congenital defects does not appear to be increased with maternal propylthiouracil use; however, fetal thyroid function may be transiently suppressed. Untreated hyperthyroidism may also cause adverse events in the mother (eg, heart failure, miscarriage, preeclampsia, thyroid storm), fetus (eg, goiter, growth restriction, hypo/hyperthyroidism, still birth), and neonate (eg, hyper-/hypothyroidism, neuropsychologic damage). Propylthiouracil is preferred over methimazole for hyperthyroidism during and just prior to the first trimester of pregnancy. However, given hepatotoxicity concerns, switching back to methimazole during the 2nd and 3rd trimesters should be considered. In order to prevent adverse events to the fetus, the lowest effective dose should be used in order to achieve maternal levels of T_4 in the high euthyroid or low hyperthyroid range. Thyroid function should be monitored closely.

Lactation Enters breast milk/AAP rates "compatible"

Breast-Feeding Considerations Propylthiouracil is found in breast milk at levels <0.3% of the weight adjusted maternal dose. Although breast-feeding is contraindicated by the manufacturer, the AAP and other expert analysis have concluded that breast-feeding is generally considered safe. Reviews of thioamide use while breast-feeding have not shown that thyroid function of the breast-fed infant is significantly affected.

Contraindications Hypersensitivity to propylthiouracil or any component; breast-feeding (per manufacturer; however, expert analysis and the AAP state this drug may be used in nursing mothers)

Warnings May cause significant bone marrow depression; the most severe manifestation is agranulocytosis; aplastic anemia, thrombocytopenia, and leukopenia may also occur. Thyroid hyperplasia or carcinoma may occur with prolonged use (>1 year); discontinue in the presence of unexplained fever. Has been associated with a variety of autoimmune reactions, including a lupus-like syndrome; discontinuation may be warranted. Severe liver injury (some fatal) and acute liver failure (some cases requiring transplantation) have been reported **[U.S. Boxed Warning]**. Patients should be counseled to recognize and report symptoms suggestive of hepatic dysfunction (especially in first 6 months of treatment); symptoms suggestive of hepatic dysfunction should prompt immediate discontinuation. Routine liver function test monitoring may not reduce risk due to unpredictable and rapid onset. Has been associated with rare but severe dermatologic reactions; discontinue in the presence of exfoliative dermatitis. Glomerulonephritis and interstitial nephritis with acute renal failure have been reported.

Precautions Use with caution in patients receiving other drugs known to cause myelosuppression, particularly agranulocytosis. Use should be limited to patients unable to tolerate methimazole or in whom surgery or radioactive iodine treatment are not appropriate.

Adverse Reactions
Cardiovascular: ANCA-positive vasculitis, cutaneous vasculitis, edema, leukocytoclastic vasculitis
Central nervous system: Dizziness, drowsiness, drug fever, fever, headache, vertigo
Dermatologic: Alopecia, erythema nodosum, exfoliative dermatitis, pruritus, rash, skin pigmentation, urticaria
Endocrine & metabolic: Goiter, swollen salivary glands, thyroid hyperplasia or carcinoma, weight gain
Gastrointestinal: Ageusia, constipation, nausea, sialoadenopathy, stomach pain, vomiting
Hematologic: Agranulocytosis, bleeding, hypoprothrombinemia, leukopenia, thrombocytopenia
Hepatic: Hepatic necrosis, hepatitis, jaundice
Neuromuscular & skeletal: Arthralgia, neuritis, paresthesia
Renal: Acute renal failure, glomerulonephritis, interstitial nephritis
Respiratory: Alveolar hemorrhage, interstitial pneumonitis
Miscellaneous: SLE-like syndrome

Drug Interactions
Avoid Concomitant Use
Avoid concomitant use of Propylthiouracil with any of the following: Sodium Iodide I131
Increased Effect/Toxicity There are no known significant interactions involving an increase in effect.
Decreased Effect
Propylthiouracil may decrease the levels/effects of: Sodium Iodide I131; Vitamin K Antagonists
Food Interactions Propylthiouracil serum concentrations may be altered if taken with food.
Mechanism of Action Inhibits the synthesis of thyroid hormones by blocking the oxidation of iodine in the thyroid gland; blocks synthesis of thyroxine and triiodothyronine
Pharmacodynamics For significant therapeutic effects 24-36 hours are required; remission of hyperthyroidism usually does not occur before 4 months of continued therapy
Pharmacokinetics (Adult data unless noted)
Distribution: Breast milk to plasma ratio: 0.1
Protein binding: 75% to 80%
Metabolism: Hepatic
Bioavailability: 80% to 95%
Half-life: 1.5-5 hours
End-stage renal disease: 8.5 hours
Time to peak serum concentration: Oral: Within 1 hour; persists for 2-3 hours
Elimination: 35% excreted in urine
Usual Dosage Oral: Adjust dosage to maintain T_3, T_4, and TSH in normal range; elevated T_3 may be sole indicator of inadequate treatment. Elevated TSH indicates excessive antithyroid treatment.
Neonates: 5-10 mg/kg/day in divided doses every 8 hours
Children: 5-7 mg/kg/day in divided doses every 8 hours **or**
6-10 years: 50-150 mg/day divided every 8 hours
≥10 years: 150-300 mg/day divided every 8 hours
Maintenance: Determined by patient response or $1/3$ to $2/3$ of the initial dose in divided doses every 8-12 hours; this begins usually after 2 months on an effective initial dosage
Adults: Initial: 300-400 mg/day in divided doses every 6-8 hours; in patients with severe hyperthyroidism, very large goiters, or both, the dosage is usually 400 mg/day; an occasional patient will require doses of 600-900 mg/day; maintenance: 100-150 mg/day in divided doses every 8-12 hours
Thyrotoxic crisis (recommendations vary widely and have not been evaluated in comparative trials): Dosages of 200-300 mg every 4-6 hours have been recommended for short-term initial therapy (until initial response), followed by gradual reduction to a maintenance dosage (100-150 mg/day in divided doses).
Dosing adjustment in renal impairment: Adjustment is not necessary
Administration Oral: Administer with food
Monitoring Parameters CBC with differential, liver function tests, platelets, thyroid function tests (TSH, T_3, T_4), prothrombin time
Reference Range See normal values for thyroid function in Normal Laboratory Values for Children on page 1672
Patient Information Do not exceed prescribed dosage; take at regular intervals around-the-clock; notify physician or pharmacist if fever, sore throat, unusual bleeding or bruising, headache, nausea, vomiting, loss of appetite, itchiness, dark-colored urine, yellowing of your skin or eyes, tiredness, or general malaise occurs; be aware that severe liver injury has occurred in patients taking propylthiouracil
Dosage Forms Excipient information presented when available (limited, particularly for generics); consult specific product labeling.
Tablet: 50 mg

Extemporaneous Preparations A 5 mg/mL oral suspension may be made by crushing twenty 50 mg propylthiouracil tablets; add by geometric proportions 1:1 mixture of Ora-Plus® and Ora-Sweet® to a final volume of 200 mL; stable 91 days at 4°C and 70 days at 25°C

Nahata MC, Morosco RS, and Trowbridge JM, "Stability of Propylthiouracil in Extemporaneously Prepared Oral Suspensions at 4 and 25 Degrees C," *Am J Health Syst Pharm*, 2000, 57(12):1141-3.

References

American College of Obstetricians and Gynecologists, ACOG Practice Bulletin, Clinical Management Guidelines for Obstetrician-Gynecologists, Number 37, August 2002. (Replaces Practice Bulletin Number 32, November 2001), "Thyroid Disease in Pregnancy," *Obstet Gynecol*, 2002, 100(2):387-96.

Clark SM, Saade GR, Snodgrass WR, et al, "Pharmacokinetics and Pharmacotherapy of Thionamides in Pregnancy," *Ther Drug Monit*, 2006, 28(4):477-83.

Diav-Citrin O and Ornoy A, "Teratogen Update: Antithyroid Drugs – Methimazole, Carbimazole, and Propylthiouracil," *Teratology*, 2002, 65(1):38-44

Lee A, Moretti, ME, Collantes A, et al, "Choice of Breastfeeding and Physicians' Advice: A Cohort Study of Women Receiving Propylthiouracil, *Pediatrics*, 2000, 106(1 Pt 1):27-30.

Lock DR and Sthoeger ZM, "Severe Hepatotoxicity on Beginning Propylthiouracil Therapy," *J Clin Gastroenterol*, 1997, 24(4):267-9.

Mandel SJ and Cooper DS, "The Use of Antithyroid Drugs in Pregnancy and Lactation," *J Clin Endocrinol Metab*, 2001, 86(6):2354-9.

Nayak B and Burman K, "Thyrotoxicosis and Thyroid Storm," *Endocrinol Metab Clin North Am*, 2006, 35(4):663-86.

Raby C, Lagorce JF, Jambut-Absil AC, et al, "The Mechanism of Action of Synthetic Antithyroid Drugs: Iodine Complexation During Oxidation of Iodide," *Endocrinology*, 1990, 126(3):1683-91.

♦ **Propyl-Thyracil® (Can)** *see* Propylthiouracil *on page 1178*

♦ **2-Propylvaleric Acid** *see* Valproic Acid and Derivatives *on page 1398*

♦ **ProQuad®** *see* Measles, Mumps, Rubella, and Varicella Virus Vaccine *on page 864*

♦ **Proquin® XR** *see* Ciprofloxacin *on page 310*

♦ **PRO-Rabeprazole (Can)** *see* Rabeprazole *on page 1197*

♦ **PRO-Risperidone (Can)** *see* Risperidone *on page 1218*

♦ **PRO-Sotalol (Can)** *see* Sotalol *on page 1284*

♦ **Prostacyclin** *see* Epoprostenol *on page 517*

♦ **Prostaglandin E₁** *see* Alprostadil *on page 69*

♦ **Prostigmin®** *see* Neostigmine *on page 982*

♦ **Prostin® VR (Can)** *see* Alprostadil *on page 69*

♦ **Prostin VR Pediatric®** *see* Alprostadil *on page 69*

Protamine (PROE ta meen)

Medication Safety Issues

Sound-alike/look-alike issues:

Protamine may be confused with ProAmatine®, Protonix®, Protopam®, Protropin®

Therapeutic Category Antidote, Heparin

Generic Available Yes

Use Treatment of heparin overdosage; neutralize heparin during surgery or dialysis procedures

Pregnancy Risk Factor C

Lactation Excretion in breast milk unknown

Contraindications Hypersensitivity to protamine or any component

Warnings Anaphylactic reactions may occur; hypotension and other cardiovascular events (including cardiovascular collapse, noncardiogenic pulmonary edema, pulmonary vasoconstriction, and pulmonary hypertension) may occur **[U.S. Boxed Warning]**; risk factors include rapid administration, high doses or overdose, repeated doses, previous protamine administration (including protamine-containing drugs such as NPH insulin), fish allergy, vasectomy, severe left ventricular dysfunction, and abnormal preoperative pulmonary hemodynamics. Heparin rebound associated with anticoagulation and bleeding has been reported to occur occasionally; symptoms typically occur 8-9 hours after protamine administration, but may occur as long as 18 hours later

Precautions Use with caution in patients allergic to fish, with prior history of vasectomy, and patients receiving protamine-containing insulin or previous protamine therapy.

Adverse Reactions

Cardiovascular: Hypotension, bradycardia, flushing, pulmonary hypertension

Central nervous system: Lassitude

Gastrointestinal: Nausea, vomiting

Neuromuscular & skeletal: Back pain

Respiratory: Dyspnea

Miscellaneous: Hypersensitivity reactions

Drug Interactions

Avoid Concomitant Use There are no known interactions where it is recommended to avoid concomitant use.

Increased Effect/Toxicity There are no known significant interactions involving an increase in effect.

Decreased Effect There are no known significant interactions involving a decrease in effect.

Stability Refrigerate; stable for at least 2 weeks at room temperature

Mechanism of Action Combines with strongly acidic heparin to form a stable complex (salt) neutralizing the anticoagulant activity of both drugs

Pharmacodynamics Onset of action: Heparin neutralization occurs within 5 minutes following I.V. injection

Pharmacokinetics (Adult data unless noted) Elimination: Unknown

Usual Dosage I.V.: Protamine dosage is determined by the most recent dosage of heparin or low molecular weight heparin (LMWH); 1 mg of protamine neutralizes 90 USP units of heparin (lung), 115 USP units of heparin (intestinal), and 1 mg (100 units) LMWH; maximum dose: 50 mg

Heparin overdosage: Since blood heparin concentrations decrease rapidly **after** heparin administration, adjust the protamine dosage depending upon the duration of time since heparin administration as follows (see table):

Time Since Last Heparin Dose (min)	Dose of Protamine (mg) to Neutralize 100 units of Heparin
<30	1
30-60	0.5-0.75
60-120	0.375-0.5
>120	0.25-0.375

If heparin is administered by deep SubQ injection, use 1-1.5 mg protamine per 100 units heparin; this may be done by administering a portion of the dose (eg, 25-50 mg) slowly I.V. followed by the remaining portion as a continuous infusion over 8-16 hours (the expected absorption time of the SubQ heparin dose)

LMWH overdosage: If most recent LMWH dose has been administered within the last 4 hours, use 1 mg protamine per 1 mg (100 units) LMWH; a second dose of 0.5 mg protamine per 1 mg (100 units) LMWH may be given if APTT remains prolonged 2-4 hours after the first dose

Administration Parenteral: Reconstitute vial with 5 mL SWI; if using protamine in neonates, reconstitute with preservative free SWI; resulting solution equals 10 mg/mL; inject without further dilution over 10 minutes not to exceed 5 mg/minute; maximum of 50 mg in any 10-minute period

Monitoring Parameters Coagulation tests, APTT or ACT, cardiac monitor, and blood pressure monitor required during administration

Dosage Forms Excipient information presented when available (limited, particularly for generics); consult specific product labeling.

Injection, solution, as sulfate [preservative free]: 10 mg/mL (5 mL, 25 mL)

References

Monagle P, Michelson AD, Bovill E, et al, "Antithrombic Therapy in Children," *Chest*, 2001, 119:344S-70S.

◆ **Protease, Lipase, and Amylase** *see* Pancrelipase *on page 1051*

◆ **Protection Plus® [OTC]** *see* Ethyl Alcohol *on page 547*

◆ **Protein C (Activated), Human, Recombinant** *see* Drotrecogin Alfa (Activated) *on page 484*

◆ **Prothrombin Complex Concentrate** *see* Factor IX Complex (Human) *on page 558*

◆ **Protonix®** *see* Pantoprazole *on page 1054*

◆ **Protopam®** *see* Pralidoxime *on page 1144*

◆ **Protopic®** *see* Tacrolimus *on page 1311*

◆ **PRO-Topiramate (Can)** *see* Topiramate *on page 1360*

Protriptyline (proe TRIP ti leen)

Medication Safety Issues

Sound-alike/look-alike issues:

Vivactil® may be confused with Vyvanse™

Related Information

Antidepressant Agents *on page 1484*

U.S. Brand Names Vivactil®

Therapeutic Category Antidepressant, Tricyclic (Secondary Amine)

Generic Available Yes

Use Treatment of depression

Medication Guide An FDA-approved patient medication guide, which is available with the product information and at http://www.fda.gov/downloads/Drugs/DrugSafety/ucm089820.pdf, must be dispensed with this medication for each new outpatient prescription and refill.

Pregnancy Risk Factor C

Lactation Excretion in breast milk unknown/not recommended

Contraindications Hypersensitivity to protriptyline (cross-reactivity to other cyclic antidepressants may occur) or any component; use of MAO inhibitors within 14 days (potentially fatal reactions may occur, see Drug Interactions); concurrent use of cisapride; use in a patient during the acute recovery phase of MI

Warnings The safety and efficacy of protriptyline have not been established in pediatric patients; however, the FDA-approved labeling contains dosing for adolescent patients. Clinical worsening of depression or suicidal ideation and behavior may occur in children and adults with major depressive disorder **[U.S. Boxed Warning]**. In clinical trials, antidepressants increased the risk of suicidal thinking and behavior (suicidality) in children, adolescents, and young adults (18-24 years of age) with major depressive disorder and other psychiatric disorders. This risk must be considered before prescribing antidepressants for any clinical use. Short-term studies did not show an increased risk of suicidality with antidepressant use in patients >24 years of age and showed a decreased risk in patients ≥65 years.

Patients of all ages who are treated with antidepressants for any indication require appropriate monitoring and close observation for clinical worsening of depression, suicidality, and unusual changes in behavior, especially during the first few months after antidepressant initiation or when the dose is adjusted. Family members and caregivers should be instructed to closely observe the patient (ie, daily) and communicate condition with healthcare provider. Patients should also be monitored for associated behaviors (eg, anxiety, agitation, panic attacks, insomnia, irritability, hostility, aggressiveness, impulsivity, akathisia, hypomania, mania) which may increase the risk for worsening depression or suicidality. Worsening depression or emergence of suicidality (or associated behaviors listed above) that is abrupt in onset, severe, or not part of the presenting symptoms, may require discontinuation or modification of drug therapy.

Do not discontinue abruptly in patients receiving high doses chronically (withdrawal symptoms may occur; see Adverse Reactions). To reduce risk of intentional overdose, write prescriptions for the smallest quantity consistent with good patient care. Screen individuals for bipolar disorder prior to treatment (using antidepressants alone may induce manic episodes in patients with this condition). May worsen psychosis in some patients. Protriptyline is not FDA approved for the treatment of bipolar depression.

Precautions May cause sedation, resulting in impaired performance of tasks requiring alertness (eg, operating machinery or driving). Sedative effects may be additive with other CNS depressants and/or ethanol. The degree of sedation is low relative to other antidepressants. May aggravate aggressive behavior. May increase the risks associated with electroconvulsive therapy; limit such treatment to patients in whom it is essential. Consider discontinuing, when possible, prior to elective surgery. Therapy should not be abruptly discontinued in patients receiving high doses for prolonged periods. May alter glucose regulation; both an increase and decrease in blood glucose has been reported; use with caution in patients with diabetes.

May cause tachycardia and orthostatic hypotension (risk is moderate relative to other antidepressants); use with caution in patients at risk of hypotension or in patients where transient tachycardia and hypotensive episodes would be poorly tolerated (cardiovascular disease or cerebrovascular disease). The degree of anticholinergic blockade produced by this agent is moderate relative to other cyclic antidepressants; however, caution should still be used in patients with urinary retention, benign prostatic hyperplasia, narrow-angle glaucoma, increased IOP, xerostomia, visual problems, constipation, or history of bowel obstruction.

Use with caution in patients with a history of cardiovascular disease (including previous MI, stroke, tachycardia, or conduction abnormalities). The risk of conduction abnormalities with this agent is moderate-high relative to other antidepressants. Use caution in patients with a previous seizure disorder or condition predisposing to seizures such as brain damage, alcoholism, or concurrent therapy with other drugs which lower the seizure threshold. Use with caution in hyperthyroid patients or those receiving thyroid supplementation (cardiac arrhythmias may occur). Use with caution in patients with hepatic or renal dysfunction.

Adverse Reactions

Cardiovascular: Postural hypotension, arrhythmias, tachycardia, hypertension, hypotension, MI, stroke, heart block, palpitation

Central nervous system: Dizziness, drowsiness, headache, confusion, delirium, hallucinations, restlessness, insomnia, nightmares, fatigue, delusions, anxiety, agitation, hypomania, exacerbation of psychosis, panic, seizure, incoordination, ataxia, EPS

Note: Activation is more prevalent in adolescents compared to adults. Somnolence or insomnia is more common in adults compared to adolescents.

Dermatologic: Alopecia, photosensitivity, rash, petechiae, urticaria, itching

Endocrine & metabolic: Breast enlargement, galactorrhea, SIADH, gynecomastia, libido increased or decreased, weight gain or weight loss

Gastrointestinal: Xerostomia, constipation, unpleasant taste, appetite increased, nausea, diarrhea, heartburn, vomiting, anorexia, trouble with gums; decreased lower esophageal sphincter tone may cause GE reflux

Genitourinary: Difficult urination, impotence, testicular edema

Hematologic: Agranulocytosis, leukopenia, eosinophilia, thrombocytopenia, purpura

Hepatic: Cholestatic jaundice, liver enzymes elevated

Neuromuscular & skeletal: Fine muscle tremor, weakness, tremor, numbness, tingling

Ocular: Blurred vision, eye pain, intraocular pressure increased

Otic: Tinnitus

Miscellaneous: Diaphoresis (excessive), allergic reactions; withdrawal symptoms following abrupt discontinuation (headache, nausea, malaise)

Drug Interactions

Metabolism/Transport Effects Substrate of CYP2D6 (major)

Avoid Concomitant Use

Avoid concomitant use of Protriptyline with any of the following: Artemether; Cisapride; Dronedarone; Iobenguane I 123; Lumefantrine; MAO Inhibitors; Metoclopramide; Nilotinib; Pimozide; QuiNINE; Sibutramine; Tetrabenazine; Thioridazine; Ziprasidone

Increased Effect/Toxicity

Protriptyline may increase the levels/effects of: Alcohol (Ethyl); Alpha-/Beta-Agonists (Direct-Acting); Alpha1-Agonists; Amphetamines; Anticholinergics; Beta2-Agonists; Cisapride; CNS Depressants; Desmopressin; Dronedarone; Pimozide; QTc-Prolonging Agents; QuiNIDine; QuiNINE; Serotonin Modulators; Sulfonylureas; Tetrabenazine; Thioridazine; TraMADol; Vitamin K Antagonists; Yohimbine; Ziprasidone

The levels/effects of Protriptyline may be increased by: Alfuzosin; Altretamine; Artemether; Chloroquine; Cimetidine; Cinacalcet; Ciprofloxacin; Ciprofloxacin (Systemic); CYP2D6 Inhibitors (Moderate); CYP2D6 Inhibitors (Strong); Dexmethylphenidate; Divalproex; DULoxetine; Gadobutrol; Lithium; Lumefantrine; MAO Inhibitors; Methylphenidate; Metoclopramide; Nilotinib; Pramlintide; Propoxyphene; Protease Inhibitors; QuiNIDine; QuiNINE; Selective Serotonin Reuptake Inhibitors; Sibutramine; Terbinafine; Terbinafine (Systemic); Valproic Acid

Decreased Effect

Protriptyline may decrease the levels/effects of: Acetylcholinesterase Inhibitors (Central); Alpha2-Agonists; Iobenguane I 123

The levels/effects of Protriptyline may be decreased by: Acetylcholinesterase Inhibitors (Central); Barbiturates; CarBAMazepine; Peginterferon Alfa-2b; St Johns Wort

Food Interactions Grapefruit juice may inhibit the metabolism of some TCAs and clinical toxicity may result.

Mechanism of Action Increases the synaptic concentration of serotonin and/or norepinephrine in the CNS by inhibition of their reuptake by the presynaptic neuronal membrane

Pharmacodynamics

Onset of action: 1-2 weeks

Maximum effect: 4-12 weeks

Duration: 1-2 days

Pharmacokinetics (Adult data unless noted)

Protein binding: 92%

Metabolism: Extensively hepatic via N-oxidation, hydroxylation, and glucuronidation; first-pass effect (10% to 25%)

Half-life: 54-92 hours (average: 74 hours)

Time to peak serum concentration: 24-30 hours

Elimination: Urine

Usual Dosage Oral:

Children: **Note:** Safe and effective use in children has not been established; controlled clinical trials have not shown tricyclic antidepressants to be superior to placebo for the treatment of depression in children and adolescents (see Dopheide, 2006 and Wagner, 2005).

Adolescents: Initial: 5 mg/dose given 2-3 times/day; may increase in 2 weeks as tolerated; slow titration is recommended in order to facilitate monitoring for adverse effects such as behavioral activation; usual dose: 15-20 mg/day in divided doses

Adults: Initial: 10 mg/dose given twice daily; may increase every week as tolerated to a goal of 30-60 mg/day in 3-4 divided doses

Administration Oral: May administer with food to decrease GI upset

Monitoring Parameters Heart rate, blood pressure, mental status, weight. Monitor patient periodically for symptom resolution; monitor for worsening depression, suicidality, and associated behaviors (especially at the beginning of therapy or when doses are increased or decreased; see Warnings).

Reference Range Therapeutic: 70-250 ng/mL (SI: 266-950 nmol/L); Toxic: >500 ng/mL (SI: >1900 nmol/L)

Patient Information Read the patient Medication Guide that you receive with each prescription and refill of protriptyline. An increased risk of suicidal thinking and behavior has been reported with the use of antidepressants in children, adolescents, and young adults (18-24 years of age). Notify physician if you feel more depressed, have thoughts of suicide, or become more agitated or irritable (see Warnings). Avoid alcohol, grapefruit juice, and the herbal medicine St John's wort; limit caffeine intake. This medication may cause drowsiness, lightheadedness, impaired coordination, dizziness, or blurred vision and impair ability to perform activities requiring mental alertness or physical coordination. May cause dry mouth. Do not discontinue abruptly (withdrawal symptoms may occur). May cause photosensitivity reactions (eg, exposure to sunlight may cause severe sunburn, skin rash, redness, or itching); avoid exposure to sunlight and artificial light sources (sunlamps, tanning booth/bed); wear protective clothing, wide-brimmed hats, sunglasses, and lip sunscreen (SPF ≥15); use a sunscreen [broad-spectrum sunscreen or physical sunscreen (preferred) or sunblock with SPF ≥15]; contact physician if reaction occurs.

Do not take any new medication during therapy unless approved by prescriber. Take exactly as directed; do not increase dose or frequency; may take 2-3 weeks to achieve desired results. Maintain adequate hydration unless instructed to restrict fluid intake. May cause nausea, vomiting, loss of appetite, or disturbed taste (small frequent meals, good mouth care, chewing gum, or sucking lozenges may help); constipation; urinary retention (void before taking medication); postural hypotension (use caution climbing stairs or when changing position from lying or sitting to standing). Report chest pain, palpitations, or rapid heartbeat; muscle cramping, weakness, tremors, or rigidity; blurred vision or eye pain; breast enlargement or swelling; or yellowing of skin or eyes.

Nursing Implications Assess other medications patient may be taking for possible interaction (especially MAO inhibitors, P450 inhibitors, and other CNS active agents). Assess mental status for depression, suicidal ideation, and associated behaviors (see Warnings). Periodically evaluate need for continued use. Taper dosage slowly when discontinuing (allow 3-4 weeks between discontinuing this medication and starting another antidepressant). Caution patients with diabetes to monitor glucose levels closely; may increase or decrease serum glucose levels.

Dosage Forms Excipient information presented when available (limited, particularly for generics); consult specific product labeling.

Tablet, as hydrochloride: 5 mg, 10 mg

Vivactil®: 5 mg, 10 mg

References

Dopheide JA, "Recognizing and Treating Depression in Children and Adolescents," *Am J Health Syst Pharm*, 2006, 63(3):233-43.

Larochelle P, Hamet P, and Enjalbert M, "Responses to Tyramine and Norepinephrine After Imipramine and Trazodone," *Clin Pharmacol Ther*, 1979, 26(1):24-30.

Mitchell JR, "Guanethidine and Related Agents. III Antagonism by Drugs Which Inhibit the Norepinephrine Pump in Man," *J Clin Invest*, 1970, 49(8):1596-604.

Pass SE and Simpson RW, "Discontinuation and Reinstitution of Medications During the Perioperative Period," *Am J Health Syst Pharm*, 2004, 61(9):899-912.

Roose SP, Glassman AH, Attia E, et al, "Comparative Efficacy of Selective Serotonin Reuptake Inhibitors and Tricyclics in the Treatment of Melancholia," *Am J Psychiatry*, 1994, 151(12):1735-9.

Rundegren J, van Dijken J, Mörnstad H, et al, "Oral Conditions in Patients Receiving Long-Term Treatment With Cyclic Antidepressant Drugs," *Swed Dent J*, 1985, 9(2):55-64.

Smith IE and Quinnell TG, "Pharmacotherapies for Obstructive Sleep Apnoea: Where Are We Now?" *Drugs*, 2004, 64(13):1385-99.

Svedmyr N, "The Influence of a Tricyclic Antidepressive Agent (Protriptyline) on Some of the Circulatory Effects of Noradrenaline and Adrenalin in Man," *Life Sci*, 1968, 7(1):77-84.

Wagner KD, "Pharmacotherapy for Major Depression in Children and Adolescents," *Prog Neuropsychopharmacol Biol Psychiatry*, 2005, 29 (5):819-26.

◆ **Protriptyline Hydrochloride** *see* Protriptyline *on page 1181*

◆ **PRO-Valacyclovir (Can)** *see* Valacyclovir *on page 1394*

◆ **Proventil® HFA** *see* Albuterol *on page 57*

◆ **Provera®** *see* MedroxyPROGESTERone *on page 870*

◆ **Provera-Pak (Can)** *see* MedroxyPROGESTERone *on page 870*

◆ **PRO-Verapamil SR (Can)** *see* Verapamil *on page 1416*

◆ **Provigil®** *see* Modafinil *on page 940*

◆ **Proxymetacaine** *see* Proparacaine *on page 1168*

◆ **Prozac®** *see* FLUoxetine *on page 600*

◆ **Prozac® Weekly™** *see* FLUoxetine *on page 600*

◆ **PRP-OMP** *see* Haemophilus b Conjugate Vaccine *on page 664*

◆ **PRP-T** *see* Haemophilus b Conjugate Vaccine *on page 664*

◆ **Prudoxin™** *see* Doxepin *on page 475*

◆ **Prymaccone** *see* Primaquine *on page 1153*

◆ **P&S® [OTC]** *see* Salicylic Acid *on page 1241*

◆ **23PS** *see* Pneumococcal Polysaccharide Vaccine (Polyvalent) *on page 1125*

Pseudoephedrine (soo doe e FED rin)

Medication Safety Issues

Sound-alike/look-alike issues:

Sudafed® may be confused with sotalol, Sudafed PE™, Sufenta®

U.S. Brand Names Genaphed® [OTC]; Oranyl [OTC]; Silfedrine Children's [OTC]; Sudafed® 12 Hour [OTC]; Sudafed® 24 Hour [OTC]; Sudafed® Children's [OTC]; Sudafed® Maximum Strength Nasal Decongestant [OTC]; Sudafed® [OTC]; Sudo-Tab® [OTC]; SudoGest Children's [OTC]; SudoGest [OTC]

Canadian Brand Names Balminil Decongestant; Benylin® D for Infants; Contac® Cold 12 Hour Relief Non Drowsy; Drixoral® ND; Eltor®; PMS-Pseudoephedrine; Pseudofrin; Robidrine®; Sudafed® Decongestant

Therapeutic Category Adrenergic Agonist Agent; Decongestant; Sympathomimetic

Generic Available Yes: Excludes extended release products

Use Temporary symptomatic relief of nasal congestion due to common cold, upper respiratory allergies, and sinusitis; also promotes nasal or sinus drainage

Pregnancy Considerations Use during the 1st trimester may be associated with a possible risk of gastroschisis, small intestinal atresia, and hemifacial microsomia due pseudoephedrine's vasoconstrictive effects. However, additional studies are needed to define the magnitude of risk.

Lactation Enters breast milk (AAP rates "compatible")

Breast-Feeding Considerations Pseudoephedrine is excreted in breast milk. The AAP considers it to be "compatible" with breast-feeding.

Contraindications Hypersensitivity to pseudoephedrine or any component; MAO inhibitor therapy, severe hypertension, severe coronary artery disease

Warnings Some products contain sodium benzoate; benzoic acid (benzoate) is a metabolite of benzyl alcohol; large amounts of benzyl alcohol (≥99 mg/kg/day) have been associated with a potentially fatal toxicity ("gasping syndrome") in neonates; *in vitro* and animal studies have shown that benzoate displaces bilirubin from protein binding sites; avoid use of sodium benzoate containing products in neonates

Precautions Use with caution in patients with hyperthyroidism, diabetes mellitus, prostatic hypertrophy, mild-moderate hypertension, arrhythmias. Chewable tablets contain phenylalanine; avoid or use with caution in patients with phenylketonuria.

Adverse Reactions

Cardiovascular: Tachycardia, palpitations, arrhythmias

Central nervous system: Nervousness, excitability, dizziness, insomnia, drowsiness, headache, seizures, hallucinations

Gastrointestinal: Nausea, vomiting

Neuromuscular & skeletal: Tremor, weakness

Miscellaneous: Diaphoresis

Drug Interactions

Avoid Concomitant Use

Avoid concomitant use of Pseudoephedrine with any of the following: Iobenguane I 123; MAO Inhibitors

Increased Effect/Toxicity

Pseudoephedrine may increase the levels/effects of: Bromocriptine; Sympathomimetics

The levels/effects of Pseudoephedrine may be increased by: Antacids; Atomoxetine; Cannabinoids; Carbonic Anhydrase Inhibitors; MAO Inhibitors; Serotonin/Norepinephrine Reuptake Inhibitors

Decreased Effect

Pseudoephedrine may decrease the levels/effects of: Iobenguane I 123

The levels/effects of Pseudoephedrine may be decreased by: Spironolactone

Mechanism of Action Directly stimulates alpha-adrenergic receptors of respiratory mucosa causing vasoconstriction; directly stimulates beta-adrenergic receptors causing bronchial relaxation, increased heart rate and contractility

Pharmacodynamics

Onset of action: Oral: Decongestant effects occur within 15-30 minutes

Duration: 4-6 hours (up to 12 hours with extended release formulation administration)

Pharmacokinetics (Adult data unless noted)

Distribution: Children: V_d: 2.4-2.6 L/kg; breast milk to plasma ratio: 2.6-3.3

Metabolism: Incomplete in the liver to inactive metabolite

Half-life:

Children 3.1 hours

Adults: 9-16 hours

Elimination: 55% to 75% of dose excreted unchanged in urine

Clearance:

Children: 9.2-10.3 mL/minute/kg

Adults: 7.3-7.6 mL/minute/kg

Usual Dosage Oral:

Children:

<2 years: 4 mg/kg/day in divided doses every 6 hours

2-5 years: 15 mg every 6 hours; maximum dose: 60 mg/24 hours

6-12 years: 30 mg every 6 hours; maximum dose: 120 mg/24 hours

Children >12 years and Adults: 60 mg every 6 hours; maximum dose: 240 mg/day; using extended release products: 120 mg every 12 hours or 240 mg once daily

Administration Oral: Administer with water or milk to decrease GI distress; swallow timed release tablets or capsules whole, do not chew or crush

Test Interactions False-positive test for amphetamines by EMIT assay

Dosage Forms Excipient information presented when available (limited, particularly for generics); consult specific product labeling.

Caplet, extended release, oral, as hydrochloride:

Sudafed® 12 Hour: 120 mg

Liquid, oral, as hydrochloride: 30 mg/5 mL (120 mL)

Silfedrine Children's: 15 mg/5 mL (120 mL, 480 mL) [ethanol free, sugar free; grape flavor]

Sudafed® Children's: 15 mg/5 mL (118 mL) [ethanol free, sugar free; contains menthol, sodium 5 mg/5 mL, sodium benzoate; grape flavor]

Syrup, oral, as hydrochloride: 30 mg/5 mL (118 mL, 473 mL)

SudoGest Children's: 15 mg/5 mL (118 mL) [ethanol free, sugar free; contains sodium 5 mg/5 mL, sodium benzoate; grape flavor]

Tablet, oral, as hydrochloride: 30 mg, 60 mg

Genaphed®, Oranyl, Sudafed®, Sudo-Tab®: 30 mg

SudoGest: 30 mg, 60 mg

Tablet, extended release, oral, as hydrochloride:

Sudafed® 24 Hour: 240 mg [contains sodium 10 mg]

References

Simons FE, Gu X, Watson WT, et al, "Pharmacokinetics of the Orally Administered Decongestants Pseudoephedrine and Phenylpropanolamine in Children," *J Pediatr*, 1996, 129(5):729-34.

♦ **Pseudoephedrine and Brompheniramine** *see* Brompheniramine and Pseudoephedrine *on page* 205

♦ **Pseudoephedrine and Carbinoxamine** *see* Carbinoxamine and Pseudoephedrine *on page* 249

Pseudoephedrine and Ibuprofen

(soo doe e FED rin & eye byoo PROE fen)

U.S. Brand Names Advil® Cold & Sinus [OTC]; Advil® Cold, Children's [OTC] [DSC]; Proprinal® Cold and Sinus [OTC]

Canadian Brand Names Advil® Cold & Sinus; Children's Advil® Cold; Sudafed® Sinus Advance

Therapeutic Category Decongestant/Analgesic

Generic Available Yes: Caplet

Use Temporary relief of cold, sinus, and flu symptoms (including nasal congestion, headache, sore throat, minor body aches and pains, and fever)

Pregnancy Risk Factor Ibuprofen: B/D (3rd trimester)

Contraindications Hypersensitivity to pseudoephedrine, ibuprofen, or any component, aspirin, or other NSAIDs; active GI bleeding, ulcer disease; patients with the "aspirin triad" [asthma, rhinitis (with or without nasal polyps), and aspirin intolerance] (fatal asthmatic and anaphylactoid reactions may occur in these patients); MAO inhibitor therapy, severe hypertension, severe coronary artery disease

Warnings Safety and efficacy for the use of cough and cold products in children <2 years of age is limited. Serious adverse effects including death have been reported (in some cases, high blood concentrations of pseudoephedrine were found). The FDA notes that there are no approved OTC uses for these products in children <2 years of age. Healthcare providers are reminded to ask caregivers about the use of OTC cough and cold products in order to avoid exposure to multiple medications containing the same ingredient.

Some products contain sodium benzoate (see Dosage Forms); benzoic acid (benzoate) is a metabolite of benzyl alcohol; large amounts of benzyl alcohol (≥99 mg/kg/day) have been associated with a potentially fatal toxicity ("gasping syndrome") in neonates; the "gasping syndrome" consists of metabolic acidosis, respiratory distress, gasping respirations, CNS dysfunction (including convulsions, intracranial hemorrhage), hypotension and cardiovascular collapse; avoid use of formulations containing sodium benzoate in neonates; *in vitro* and animal studies have shown that benzoate displaces bilirubin from protein binding sites

Precautions Use with caution in patients with mild-moderate hypertension, heart disease, arrhythmias, diabetes mellitus, thyroid disease, asthma, glaucoma, prostatic hypertrophy, CHF, decreased renal or hepatic function, dehydration, history of GI disease (bleeding or ulcers), or those receiving anticoagulants.

Adverse Reactions See individual monographs for Pseudoephedrine on page 1183 and Ibuprofen on page 702.

Drug Interactions

Metabolism/Transport Effects Ibuprofen: **Substrate** (minor) of CYP2C9, 2C19; **Inhibits** CYP2C9 (strong)

Avoid Concomitant Use

Avoid concomitant use of Pseudoephedrine and Ibuprofen with any of the following: Iobenguane I 123; Ketorolac; Ketorolac (Systemic); MAO Inhibitors

Increased Effect/Toxicity

Pseudoephedrine and Ibuprofen may increase the levels/effects of: Aminoglycosides; Anticoagulants; Antiplatelet Agents; Bisphosphonate Derivatives; Bromocriptine; Collagenase (Systemic); CycloSPORINE; CycloSPORINE (Systemic); Desmopressin; Digoxin; Drotrecogin Alfa; Eplerenone; Haloperidol; Ibritumomab; Lithium; Methotrexate; Nonsteroidal Anti-Inflammatory Agents; Pemetrexed; Potassium-Sparing Diuretics; Pralatrexate; Quinolone Antibiotics; Salicylates; Sympathomimetics; Thrombolytic Agents; Tositumomab and Iodine I 131 Tositumomab; Vancomycin; Vitamin K Antagonists

The levels/effects of Pseudoephedrine and Ibuprofen may be increased by: Antacids; Antidepressants (Tricyclic, Tertiary Amine); Atomoxetine; Cannabinoids; Carbonic Anhydrase Inhibitors; Corticosteroids (Systemic); Dasatinib; Glucosamine; Herbs (Anticoagulant/Antiplatelet Properties); Ketorolac; Ketorolac (Systemic); MAO Inhibitors; Nonsteroidal Anti-Inflammatory Agents; Omega-3-Acid Ethyl Esters; Pentosan Polysulfate Sodium; Pentoxifylline; Probenecid; Prostacyclin

Analogues; Selective Serotonin Reuptake Inhibitors; Serotonin/Norepinephrine Reuptake Inhibitors; Treprostinil

Decreased Effect

Pseudoephedrine and Ibuprofen may decrease the levels/effects of: ACE Inhibitors; Angiotensin II Receptor Blockers; Antiplatelet Agents; Beta-Blockers; Eplerenone; HydrALAZINE; Iobenguane I 123; Loop Diuretics; Potassium-Sparing Diuretics; Salicylates; Thiazide Diuretics

The levels/effects of Pseudoephedrine and Ibuprofen may be decreased by: Bile Acid Sequestrants; Nonsteroidal Anti-Inflammatory Agents; Salicylates; Spironolactone

Pharmacodynamics See individual monographs for Pseudoephedrine on page 1183 and Ibuprofen on page 702.

Pharmacokinetics (Adult data unless noted) See individual monographs for Pseudoephedrine on page 1183 and Ibuprofen on page 702.

Usual Dosage Oral:

Manufacturer's recommendations:

Advil® Cold & Sinus (capsules): Children >12 years and Adults: 1 capsule (pseudoephedrine 30 mg/ibuprofen 200 mg) every 4-6 hours; if symptoms do not respond; may use 2 capsules/dose; not to exceed 6 capsules/day

Alternative pediatric dosing: May dose according to the pseudoephedrine component:

Children ≥2 years: 4 mg/kg/day in divided doses every 6 hours or as an alternative:

Children 2-5 years: 15 mg every 6 hours; maximum dose: 60 mg/24 hours

Children 6-12 years: 30 mg every 6 hours or extended release product 60 mg every 12 hours; maximum dose: 120 mg/24 hours

Children >12 years and Adults: 30-60 mg every 6 hours; maximum dose: 240 mg/24 hours

Administration Oral: Administer with food

Test Interactions False-positive test for amphetamines by EMIT assay

Dosage Forms Excipient information presented when available (limited, particularly for generics); consult specific product labeling. [DSC] = Discontinued product

Caplet:

Advil® Cold & Sinus, Proprinal® Cold and Sinus: Pseudoephedrine hydrochloride 30 mg and ibuprofen 200 mg

Capsule, liquid filled:

Advil® Cold & Sinus: Pseudoephedrine hydrochloride 30 mg and ibuprofen 200 mg [solubilized ibuprofen as free acid and potassium salt; contains potassium 20 mg/capsule and coconut oil]

Suspension:

Advil® Cold, Children's: Pseudoephedrine hydrochloride 15 mg and ibuprofen 100 mg per 5 mL (120 mL) [alcohol free; contains sodium 3 mg/5 mL and sodium benzoate; grape flavor] [DSC]

◆ **Pseudoephedrine and Loratadine** *see* Loratadine and Pseudoephedrine *on page 844*

◆ **Pseudoephedrine and Triprolidine** *see* Triprolidine and Pseudoephedrine *on page 1388*

◆ **Pseudoephedrine Hydrochloride** *see* Pseudoephedrine *on page 1183*

◆ **Pseudoephedrine Sulfate** *see* Pseudoephedrine *on page 1183*

◆ **Pseudofrin (Can)** *see* Pseudoephedrine *on page 1183*

◆ **Pseudomonic Acid A** *see* Mupirocin *on page 954*

Psyllium (SIL i yum)

Medication Safety Issues

Sound-alike/look-alike issues:

Fiberall® may be confused with Feverall®

Hydrocil® may be confused with Hydrocet®

U.S. Brand Names Bulk-K [OTC]; Fiberall®; Fibro-Lax [OTC]; Fibro-XL [OTC]; Genfiber™ [OTC]; Hydrocil® Instant [OTC]; Konsyl-D™ [OTC]; Konsyl® Easy Mix™ [OTC]; Konsyl® Orange [OTC]; Konsyl® Original [OTC]; Konsyl® [OTC]; Metamucil® Plus Calcium [OTC]; Metamucil® Smooth Texture [OTC]; Metamucil® [OTC]; Natural Fiber Therapy Smooth Texture [OTC]; Natural Fiber Therapy [OTC]; Reguloid [OTC]

Canadian Brand Names Metamucil®

Therapeutic Category Laxative, Bulk-Producing

Generic Available Yes: Excludes wafers

Use Dietary fiber supplement; treatment of chronic and occasional constipation; management of irritable bowel syndrome; adjunctive treatment with low cholesterol and saturated fat diet to reduce risk of coronary artery disease

Contraindications Hypersensitivity to psyllium or any component; fecal impaction, GI obstruction

Warnings Inhalation of psyllium powder may produce allergic reactions in susceptible individuals

Precautions Use with caution in patients with esophageal strictures, ulcers, stenosis, or intestinal adhesions. Products may contain aspartame which is metabolized to phenylalanine and must be avoided (or used with caution) in patients with phenylketonuria.

Adverse Reactions

Gastrointestinal: Esophageal or bowel obstruction, diarrhea, constipation, abdominal cramps

Respiratory: Bronchospasm

Miscellaneous: Rhinoconjunctivitis, anaphylaxis upon inhalation in susceptible individuals

Drug Interactions

Avoid Concomitant Use There are no known interactions where it is recommended to avoid concomitant use.

Increased Effect/Toxicity There are no known significant interactions involving an increase in effect.

Decreased Effect There are no known significant interactions involving a decrease in effect.

Mechanism of Action Psyllium is a soluble fiber which adsorbs water in the intestine to form a viscous liquid which promotes peristalsis and reduces transit time. Paradoxically, psyllium may also be beneficial in diarrhea as it delays gastric emptying, probably by increasing meal viscosity, and reduces the acceleration of colon transit, possibly by delaying the production of gaseous fermentation products. Postprandial serum glucose and insulin concentrations are reduced with psyllium. Psyllium lowers serum cholesterol. The mechanism for this is considered to be binding bile acids in the intestinal lumen and also by stimulating bile acid synthesis and diverting hepatic cholesterol for bile acid production.

Pharmacodynamics

Onset of action: 12-24 hours

Maximum effect: May take 2-3 days

Pharmacokinetics (Adult data unless noted) Absorption: Oral: Generally not absorbed; small amounts of grain extract present in the preparation have been reportedly absorbed following colonic hydrolysis

Usual Dosage Oral (3.4 g psyllium hydrophilic mucilloid/7 g powder is equivalent to a rounded teaspoonful or 1 packet or 1 wafer):

Adequate intake for total fiber: **Note:** The definition of "fiber" varies; however, the soluble fiber in psyllium is only one type of fiber which makes up the daily recommended intake of total fiber.

Children 1-3 years: 19 g/day

Children 4-8 years: 25 g/day

Children 9-13 years: Male: 31 g/day; Female: 26 g/day

Children 14-18 years: Male: 38 g/day; Female: 26 g/day

Adults 19-50 years: Male: 38 g/day; Female: 25 g/day

Pregnancy: 28 g/day

Lactation: 29 g/day

Constipation:

Children 6-11 years: 1.25-15 g per day in divided doses

Children ≥12 years and Adults: 2.5-30 g per day in divided doses

Reduce risk of CHD: Children ≥12 years and Adults: Soluble fiber ≥7 g (psyllium seed husk ≥10.2 g) per day

Administration Oral: Granules and powder must be mixed in an 8 ounce glass of water or juice; drink an 8 ounce glass of liquid with each dose of wafers or capsules; capsules should be swallowed one at a time. When more than one dose is required, divide throughout the day. Separate dose by at least 2 hours from other drug therapies.

Monitoring Parameters Stool output and frequency

Patient Information Each dose must be taken with an 8 ounce glass of water; inadequate fluid intake may result in throat swelling and choking

Nursing Implications Inhalation of psyllium dust may cause sensitivity to psyllium (runny nose, watery eyes, wheezing)

Dosage Forms Excipient information presented when available (limited, particularly for generics); consult specific product labeling.

Capsule:

Fibro XL: 0.675 g [sugar free; provides dietary fiber 3.8 g and soluble fiber 3 g per 7 capsules]

Genfiber™: 0.52 g [provides dietary fiber 3 g and soluble fiber 2 g per 6 capsules]

Konsyl®: 0.52 g [sugar free; contains calcium 8 mg, potassium <11 mg and sodium 1 mg per capsule; provides dietary fiber 3 g and soluble fiber 2 g per 5 capsules]

Metamucil®: 0.52 g [contains potassium 5 mg/capsule; provides dietary fiber 3 g and soluble fiber 2.1 g per 6 capsules]

Metamucil® Plus Calcium: 0.52 g [contains calcium 60 mg and potassium 6 mg per capsule; provides dietary fiber 3 g and soluble fiber 2.1 g per 5 capsules]

Reguloid: 0.52 g [provides dietary fiber 3 g and soluble fiber 2 g per 6 capsules]

Powder:

Bulk-K: 4.7 g/teaspoon (392 g) [provides dietary fiber 3.8 g and soluble fiber 3 g per teaspoon]

Fiberall®: 0.05 g/tablespoon (454 g) [sugar free; contains phenylalanine; psyllium is in combination with other fiber sources providing total dietary fiber 3.5 g and soluble fiber 2 g per tablespoon; also contains vitamins and minerals; orange flavor]

Fibro-Lax: 4.7 g/teaspoon (140 g, 392 g) [provides dietary fiber 3.8 g and soluble fiber 3 g per teaspoon]

Genfiber®:

3.4 g/teaspoon (397 g, 595 g) [contains sodium ≤5 mg teaspoon; provides dietary fiber 3 g and soluble fiber 2 g per teaspoon; natural flavor]

3.4 g/tablespoon (397 g) [contains sodium ≤5 mg tablespoon; provides dietary fiber 3 g and soluble fiber 2 g per tablespoon; orange flavor]

Hydrocil® Instant:

3.5 g/packet (30s, 500s) [sugar free; provides dietary fiber 3 g and soluble fiber 2.4 g per packet]

3.5 g/teaspoon (300 g) [sugar free; provides dietary fiber 3 g and soluble fiber 2.4 g per teaspoon]

Konsyl®: Original:

6 g/packet (30s, 100s, 500s) [sugar free; contains calcium 10 mg, sodium 5 mg, and potassium 55 mg per packet; provides dietary fiber 5 g and soluble fiber 3 g per packet]

6 g/teaspoon (300 g, 450 g) [sugar free; contains calcium 10 mg, sodium 5 mg, and potassium 55 mg per teaspoon; provides dietary fiber 5 g and soluble fiber 3 g per teaspoon]

Konsyl-D™:

3.4 g/packet (100s, 500s) [contains calcium 6 mg, dextrose 3.1 g, potassium 31 mg and sodium 3 mg per packet; provides dietary fiber 3 g and soluble fiber 2 g per packet]

3.4 g/teaspoon (325 g, 397 g, 500 g) [contains calcium 6 mg, dextrose 3.1 g, potassium 31 mg, and sodium 3 mg per teaspoon; provides dietary fiber 3 g and soluble fiber 2 g per teaspoon]

Konsyl® Easy Mix™:

6 g/packet (500s) [sugar free; contains calcium 10 mg, potassium 55 mg, and sodium 5 mg per packet; provides dietary fiber 5 g and soluble fiber 3 g per packet]

6 g/teaspoon (250 g) [sugar free; contains calcium 10 mg, potassium 55 mg, and sodium 5 mg per teaspoon; provides dietary fiber 5 g and soluble fiber 3 g per teaspoon]

Konsyl® Orange:

3.4 g/packet (30s) [contains calcium 6 mg, potassium 31 mg, sodium 3 mg, and sucrose 8 g per packet; provides dietary fiber 3 g and soluble fiber 2 g per packet; orange flavor]

3.4 g/tablespoon (538 g) [contains calcium 6 mg, potassium 31 mg, sodium 3 mg, and sucrose 8 g per tablespoon; provides dietary fiber 3 g and soluble fiber 2 g per tablespoon; orange flavor]

3.4 g/teaspoon (425 g) [sugar free; contains calcium 6 mg, phenylalanine 21 mg, potassium 31 mg, and sodium 3 mg per teaspoon; provides dietary fiber 3 g and soluble fiber 2 g per teaspoon; orange flavor]

Metamucil®:

3.4 g/teaspoon (390 g, 570 g, 870 g) [contains sodium 5 mg and potassium 30 mg per teaspoon; provides dietary fiber 3 g and soluble fiber ~2 g per teaspoon; unflavored]

3.4g/tablespoon (570 g, 870 g, 1254 g) [contains sodium 5 mg and potassium 30 mg per tablespoon; provides dietary fiber 3 g and soluble fiber ~2 g per tablespoon; orange flavor]

Metamucil® Smooth Texture:

3.3 g/teaspoon (288 g, 432 g, 684 g) [sugar free; contains phenylalanine 19 mg, potassium 35 mg, and sodium 5 mg per teaspoon; provides dietary fiber 3 g and soluble fiber ~2 g per teaspoon; pink lemonade flavor]

3.4 g/packet (30s) [contains sodium 5 mg and potassium 30 mg per packet; provides dietary fiber 3 g and soluble fiber ~2 g per packet; orange flavor]

3.4 g/packet (30s) [sugar free; contains phenylalanine 16 mg, sodium 5 mg, and potassium 30 mg per packet; provides dietary fiber 3 g and soluble fiber ~2 g per packet; berry burst flavor]

3.4 g/packet (30s) [sugar free; contains phenylalanine 25 mg, sodium 5 mg, and potassium 30 mg per packet; provides dietary fiber 3 g and soluble fiber ~2 g per packet; orange flavor]

3.4 g/tablespoon (609 g, 912 g, 1368g 1446 g) [contains sodium 5 mg and potassium 30 mg per dose tablespoon; provides dietary fiber 3 g and soluble fiber ~2 g per tablespoon; orange flavor]

3.4 g/teaspoon (300 g, 450 g, 690 g) [sugar free; contains sodium 5 mg and potassium 30 mg per dose teaspoon; provides dietary fiber 3 g and soluble fiber ~2 g per teaspoon; unflavored]

3.4 g/teaspoon (173 g, 300 g, 450 g, 660 g, 1020 g) [sugar free; contains phenylalanine 25 mg, sodium 5 mg, and potassium 30 mg per teaspoon; provides dietary fiber 3 g and soluble fiber ~2 g per teaspoon; orange flavor]

3.4 g/teaspoon (283 g, 425 g, 660 g) [sugar free; contains potassium 30 mg, sodium 5 mg and phenyl-alanine 16 mg per teaspoon; provides dietary fiber 3 g and soluble fiber ~2 g per teaspoon; berry burst flavor]

Natural Fiber Therapy: 3.4 g/tablespoon (369 g, 539 g) [natural and orange flavors]

Natural Fiber Therapy Smooth Texture: 3.4 g/teaspoon (300 g) [sugar free; orange flavor]

Reguloid:

3.4 g/teaspoon (284 g, 426 g) [sugar free; contains phenylalanine 30 mg and sodium 6 mg per teaspoon; provides dietary fiber 3 g and soluble fiber 3 g per teaspoon; orange flavor]

3.4 g/teaspoon (284 g, 426 g) [sugar free; contains phenylalanine 6 mg and sodium 2 mg per teaspoon; provides dietary fiber 3 g and soluble fiber 2 g per teaspoon; regular flavor]

3.4 g/tablespoon (369 g, 540 g) [contains sodium 9 mg per tablespoon; provides dietary fiber 3 g and soluble fiber 2 g per tablespoon; orange flavor]

3.4 g/tablespoon (369 g, 540 g) [contains sodium 4 mg per tablespoon; provides dietary fiber 2 g and soluble fiber 2 g per tablespoon; regular flavor]

Wafers:

Metamucil®: 3.4 g/2 wafers (24s) [contains soya lecithin, wheat, sodium 20 mg, and potassium 60 mg per 2 wafers; provides dietary fiber 6 g and soluble fiber 3 g per 2 wafers; apple and cinnamon spice flavors]

References

"Dietary Reference Intakes for Energy, Carbohydrate, Fiber, Fat, Fatty Acids, Cholesterol, Protein and Amino Acids," Standing Committee on the Scientific Evaluation of Dietary Reference Intakes, Food and Nutrition Board, Institute of Medicine, National Academy of Sciences, Washington, DC: National Academy Press, 2005. Available at http://www.nap.edu.

James SL, Muir JG, Curtis SL, et al, "Dietary Fibre: A Roughage Guide," *Intern Med J*, 2003, 33(7):291-6.

Singh B, "Psyllium as Therapeutic and Drug Delivery Agent," *Int J Pharm*, 2007, 334(1-2):1-14.

◆ **Psyllium Husk** *see* Psyllium *on page 1185*

◆ **Psyllium Hydrophilic Mucilloid** *see* Psyllium *on page 1185*

◆ **P-Tann** *see* Chlorpheniramine *on page 296*

◆ **Pteroylglutamic Acid** *see* Folic Acid *on page 619*

◆ **PTU (error-prone abbreviation)** *see* Propylthiouracil *on page 1178*

◆ **Pulmicort® (Can)** *see* Budesonide *on page 206*

◆ **Pulmicort Flexhaler™** *see* Budesonide *on page 206*

◆ **Pulmicort Respules®** *see* Budesonide *on page 206*

◆ **Pulmophylline (Can)** *see* Theophylline *on page 1335*

◆ **Pulmozyme®** *see* Dornase Alfa *on page 473*

◆ **Purell® [OTC]** *see* Ethyl Alcohol *on page 547*

◆ **Purell® 2 in 1 [OTC]** *see* Ethyl Alcohol *on page 547*

◆ **Purell® Lasting Care [OTC]** *see* Ethyl Alcohol *on page 547*

◆ **Purell® Moisture Therapy [OTC]** *see* Ethyl Alcohol *on page 547*

◆ **Purell® with Aloe [OTC]** *see* Ethyl Alcohol *on page 547*

◆ **Purified Chick Embryo Cell** *see* Rabies Virus Vaccine *on page 1199*

◆ **Purinethol®** *see* Mercaptopurine *on page 884*

Pyrantel Pamoate (pi RAN tel PAM oh ate)

U.S. Brand Names Pin-X® [OTC]; Reese's® Pinworm Medicine [OTC]

Canadian Brand Names Combantrin™

Therapeutic Category Anthelmintic

Generic Available No

Use Roundworm (*Ascaris lumbricoides*), pinworm (*Enterobius vermicularis*), and hookworm (*Ancylostoma duodenale* and *Necator americanus*) infestations; trichostrongyliasis and moniliformis infections

Pregnancy Risk Factor C

Contraindications Hypersensitivity to pyrantel pamoate or any component

Warnings Pin-X® contains sodium benzoate; benzoic acid (benzoate) is a metabolite of benzyl alcohol; large amounts of benzyl alcohol (≥99 mg/kg/day) have been associated with a potentially fatal toxicity ("gasping syndrome") in neonates; the "gasping syndrome" consists of metabolic acidosis, respiratory distress, gasping respirations, CNS dysfunction (including convulsions, intracranial hemorrhage), hypotension and cardiovascular collapse; avoid use of pyrantel pamoate products containing sodium benzoate in neonates; *in vitro* and animal studies have shown that benzoate displaces bilirubin from protein binding sites

Precautions Use with caution in patients with liver impairment, anemia, malnutrition. The chewable tablet contains aspartame which is metabolized to phenylalanine and must be avoided or used with caution in patients with phenylketonuria.

Adverse Reactions

Central nervous system: Dizziness, drowsiness, insomnia, headache, fever

Dermatologic: Rash

Gastrointestinal: Nausea, vomiting, anorexia, diarrhea, abdominal cramps, tenesmus

Hepatic: Liver enzymes elevated

Neuromuscular & skeletal: Weakness

Drug Interactions

Avoid Concomitant Use There are no known interactions where it is recommended to avoid concomitant use.

Increased Effect/Toxicity There are no known significant interactions involving an increase in effect.

Decreased Effect

The levels/effects of Pyrantel Pamoate may be decreased by: Aminoquinolines (Antimalarial)

Stability Store at room temperature. Protect from light.

Mechanism of Action Promotes release of acetylcholine and inhibits cholinesterase causing neuromuscular paralysis of susceptible helminths

Pharmacokinetics (Adult data unless noted)

Absorption: Oral: Poor

Metabolism: Undergoes partial hepatic metabolism

Time to peak serum concentration: Within 1-3 hours

Elimination: In feces (50% as unchanged drug) and urine (7% as unchanged drug and metabolites)

Usual Dosage Children and Adults: Oral:

Roundworm, pinworm, or trichostrongyliasis: 11 mg pyrantel base/kg administered as a single dose; maximum dose: 1 g; dosage should be repeated after 2 weeks for pinworm infection

Hookworm: 11 mg pyrantel base/kg/day once daily for 3 days

Maximum daily dose: 1 g

Moniliformis infection: 11 mg pyrantel base/kg as a single dose; repeat this dose twice at 2-week intervals

Administration Oral: May mix drug with milk or fruit juice; may administer with or without food; shake suspension well before use. Chewable tablet must be chewed thoroughly before swallowing.

Monitoring Parameters Stool for presence of eggs, worms, and occult blood; serum AST and ALT

Patient Information Hygienic precaution is essential to prevent reinfection. Disinfect toilets; change and wash underclothes, bed linens, towels, and clothes daily. Wash your hands with soap often, especially before eating and after using the toilet. Do not scratch the infected area or place your fingers in your mouth. May cause dizziness or drowsiness and impair ability to perform activities requiring mental alertness or physical coordination.

Nursing Implications Fasting or purgation is not required prior to administration

Dosage Forms Excipient information presented when available (limited, particularly for generics); consult specific product labeling. [DSC] = Discontinued product

Caplet, as pamoate:
Reese's® Pinworm Medicine: 180 mg [equivalent to pyrantel base 62.5 mg/tablet] [DSC]

Suspension, oral as pamoate:
Pin-X®: 144 mg/mL (30 mL, 60 mL) [equivalent to pyrantel base 50 mg/mL; sugar free; contains sodium benzoate; caramel flavor]
Reese's® Pinworm Medicine: 144 mg/mL (30 mL) [equivalent to pyrantel base 50 mg/mL]

Tablet, chewable, as pamoate:
Pin-X®: 720.5 mg [equivalent to pyrantel base 250 mg/tablet; contains aspartame; orange flavor]

Pyrazinamide (peer a ZIN a mide)

Canadian Brand Names Tebrazid™

Therapeutic Category Antitubercular Agent

Generic Available Yes

Use In combination with other antituberculosis agents in the treatment of *Mycobacterium* tuberculosis infection (especially useful in disseminated and meningeal tuberculosis); CDC currently recommends a 3 or 4 multidrug regimen which includes pyrazinamide, rifampin, INH, and at times ethambutol or streptomycin for the treatment of tuberculosis

Pregnancy Risk Factor C

Lactation Enters breast milk/use caution

Contraindications Hypersensitivity to pyrazinamide or any component; severe hepatic damage

Warnings Two-month rifampin-pyrazinamide regimen for the treatment of latent tuberculosis infection (LTBI) has been associated with severe and fatal liver injuries. The IDSA and CDC now recommend that this regimen should not generally be used in patients with LTBI.

Precautions Use with caution in patients with renal failure, gout, diabetes mellitus, patients receiving concurrent medications associated with liver injury (particularly with rifampin), or in patients with a history of alcoholism

Adverse Reactions
Central nervous system: Malaise, fever
Dermatologic: Urticaria, rash, photosensitivity
Endocrine & metabolic: Gout, hyperuricemia
Gastrointestinal: Nausea, vomiting, anorexia, abdominal pain
Hepatic: Hepatotoxicity (increased incidence with doses >30 mg/kg/day), jaundice
Neuromuscular & skeletal: Arthralgia

Drug Interactions

Avoid Concomitant Use There are no known interactions where it is recommended to avoid concomitant use.

Increased Effect/Toxicity
Pyrazinamide may increase the levels/effects of: CycloSPORINE (Systemic); Rifampin

Decreased Effect
Pyrazinamide may decrease the levels/effects of: CycloSPORINE

Mechanism of Action Converted to pyrazinoic acid in susceptible strains of *Mycobacterium* which lowers the pH of the environment

Pharmacokinetics (Adult data unless noted)
Absorption: Oral: Well absorbed
Distribution: Widely distributed into body tissues and fluids including the liver, lung, and CSF
Protein binding: 50%
Metabolism: In the liver
Half-life: 9-10 hours, prolonged with reduced renal or hepatic function
Time to peak serum concentration: Within 2 hours
Elimination: In urine (4% as unchanged drug)

Usual Dosage Oral:
Infants, Children, and Adolescents: 20-40 mg/kg/day in divided doses every 12-24 hours for the first 2 months of active treatment; daily dose not to exceed 2 g; or daily pyrazinamide for 2 weeks followed by directly observed therapy of 50 mg/kg/dose twice weekly to a maximum of 2 g/dose for 6 weeks
Adults: 15-30 mg/kg/day in 1-4 divided doses for the first 2 months of active treatment; maximum daily dose: 3 g/day; or daily pyrazinamide for 2 weeks followed by directly observed therapy of 50-70 mg/kg/dose twice weekly to a maximum of 4 g/dose for 6 weeks

Monitoring Parameters Periodic liver function tests, serum uric acid

Patient Information Notify physician if fatigue, weakness, nausea, abdominal pain, jaundice, vomiting, or joint pain and swelling occur. May cause photosensitivity reactions (eg, exposure to sunlight may cause severe sunburn, skin rash, redness, or itching); avoid exposure to sunlight and artificial light sources (sunlamps, tanning booth/bed); wear protective clothing, wide-brimmed hats, sunglasses, and lip sunscreen (SPF ≥15); use a sunscreen [broad-spectrum sunscreen or physical sunscreen (preferred) or sunblock with SPF ≥15]; contact physician if reaction occurs.

Dosage Forms Excipient information presented when available (limited, particularly for generics); consult specific product labeling.

Tablet: 500 mg

Extemporaneous Preparations
Pyrazinamide suspension can be compounded with simple syrup or 0.5% methylcellulose with simple syrup at a concentration of 100 mg/mL; the suspension is stable for 2 months at 4°C or 25°C when stored in glass or plastic bottles

To prepare pyrazinamide suspension in 0.5% methylcellulose with simple syrup: Crush 200 pyrazinamide 500 mg tablets and mix with a suspension containing 500 mL of 1% methylcellulose and 500 mL simple syrup. Add to this a suspension containing 140 crushed pyrazinamide tablets in 350 mL of 1% methylcellulose and 350 mL of simple syrup to make 1.7 L of suspension containing pyrazinamide 100 mg/mL in 0.5% methylcellulose with simple syrup.

Nahata MC, Morosco RS, and Peritre SP, "Stability of Pyrazinamide in Two Suspensions," *Am J Health-Syst Pharm*, 1995, 52:1558-60.

References
Ad Hoc Committee of the Scientific Assembly on Microbiology, Tuberculosis and Pulmonary Infections, "Treatment of Tuberculosis and Tuberculosis Infection in Adults and Children," *Clin Infect Dis*, 1995, 21:9-27.

American Academy of Pediatrics, Committee on Infectious Diseases, "Chemotherapy for Tuberculosis in Infants and Children," *Pediatrics*, 1992, 89(1):161-5.

Starke JR, "Multidrug Therapy for Tuberculosis in Children," *Pediatr Infect Dis J*, 1990, 9(11):785-93.

Starke JR and Correa AG, "Management of Mycobacterial Infection and Disease in Children," *Pediatr Infect Dis J*, 1995, 14(6):455-70.

"Update: Fatal and Severe Liver Injuries Associated With Rifampin and Pyrazinamide for Latent Tuberculosis Infection, and Revisions in American Thoracic Society/CDC Recommendations - United States, 2001," *MMWR Morb Mortal Wkly Rep*, 2001, 50(34):733-5.

◆ **Pyrazinoic Acid Amide** *see* Pyrazinamide *on page 1188*

◆ **Pyri-500 [OTC]** *see* Pyridoxine *on page 1190*

◆ **2-Pyridine Aldoxime Methochloride** *see* Pralidoxime *on page 1144*

◆ **Pyridium®** *see* Phenazopyridine *on page 1097*

Pyridostigmine (peer id oh STIG meen)

Medication Safety Issues
Sound-alike/look-alike issues:
Pyridostigmine may be confused with physostigmine
Mestinon® may be confused with Metatensin®
Regonol® may be confused with Reglan®, Renagel®

U.S. Brand Names Mestinon®; Mestinon® Timespan®; Regonol®

Canadian Brand Names Mestinon®; Mestinon®-SR

Therapeutic Category Antidote, Neuromuscular Blocking Agent; Cholinergic Agent

Generic Available Yes: Tablet

Use Symptomatic treatment of myasthenia gravis by improving muscle strength; reversal of effects of non-depolarizing neuromuscular blocking agents; pretreatment for Soman nerve gas exposure (military use only)

Pregnancy Risk Factor B

Pregnancy Considerations Safety has not been established for use during pregnancy. The potential benefit to the mother should outweigh the potential risk to the fetus. When pyridostigmine is needed in myasthenic mothers, giving dose parenterally 1 hour before completion of the second stage of labor may facilitate delivery and protect the neonate during the immediate postnatal state.

Lactation Enters breast milk/compatible

Breast-Feeding Considerations Neonates of myasthenia gravis mothers may have difficulty in sucking and swallowing (as well as breathing). Neonatal pyridostigmine may be indicated by symptoms (confirmed by edrophonium test).

Contraindications Hypersensitivity to pyridostigmine, bromides, or any component (see Warnings); GI or GU obstruction

Warnings Overdosage may result in cholinergic crisis, this must be distinguished from myasthenic crisis; adequate facilities should be available for cardiopulmonary resuscitation when testing and adjusting dose for myasthenia gravis; have atropine and epinephrine ready to treat hypersensitivity reactions; neonates of myasthenic mothers may have transient difficulties in swallowing, sucking, and breathing; use of pyridostigmine may be of benefit; use edrophonium test to assess neonate with these symptoms

Some injections contain benzyl alcohol which may cause allergic reactions in susceptible individuals; syrup contains sodium benzoate; large amounts of benzyl alcohol (≥99 mg/kg/day) have been associated with a potentially fatal toxicity ("gasping syndrome") in neonates; the "gasping syndrome" consists of metabolic acidosis, respiratory distress, gasping respirations, CNS dysfunction (including convulsions, intracranial hemorrhage), hypotension and cardiovascular collapse; use injections containing benzyl alcohol with caution in neonates; *in vitro* and animal studies have shown that benzoate, a metabolite of benzyl alcohol, displaces bilirubin from protein binding sites; avoid use of the syrup in neonates

Pretreatment with pyridostigmine alone will not protect against exposure to Soman nerve gas; its efficacy is dependent upon the rapid use of atropine and pralidoxime after exposure. Discontinue use of pyridostigmine after exposure.

Precautions Use with caution in patients with epilepsy, asthma, bradycardia, hyperthyroidism, arrhythmias, recent coronary occlusion, vagotonia, or peptic ulcer; use with caution and modify dosage in patients with renal disease

Adverse Reactions
Cardiovascular: Bradycardia, hypotension, arrhythmias, A-V block, syncope

Central nervous system: Headache, convulsions, drowsiness, dizziness

Dermatologic: Rash, dry skin

Gastrointestinal: Nausea, vomiting, diarrhea, peristalsis increased, abdominal cramps, dysphagia, salivation

Genitourinary: Urinary frequency, dysmenorrhea

Local: Thrombophlebitis (after I.V. administration)

Neuromuscular & skeletal: Muscle cramps, weakness, myalgia

Ocular: Miosis, lacrimation, diplopia, conjunctival hyperemia

Respiratory: Bronchial secretions increased, bronchospasm, laryngospasm, dyspnea, epistaxis

Miscellaneous: Diaphoresis

Drug Interactions
Avoid Concomitant Use There are no known interactions where it is recommended to avoid concomitant use.

Increased Effect/Toxicity
Pyridostigmine may increase the levels/effects of: Beta-Blockers; Cholinergic Agonists; Succinylcholine

The levels/effects of Pyridostigmine may be increased by: Corticosteroids (Systemic)

Decreased Effect
Pyridostigmine may decrease the levels/effects of: Neuromuscular-Blocking Agents (Nondepolarizing)

The levels/effects of Pyridostigmine may be decreased by: Methocarbamol

Stability Protect from light; tablets are extremely moisture sensitive; do not remove desiccant and keep bottle closed tightly. Store 30 mg tablets in refrigerator; stable at room temperature for 3 months

Mechanism of Action Competitively inhibits destruction of acetylcholine by acetylcholinesterase which facilitates transmission of impulses across myoneural junction producing generalized cholinergic responses such as miosis, increased tonus of skeletal and intestinal musculature, bronchial and ureteral constriction, bradycardia, and increased salivary and sweat gland production

Pharmacodynamics
Onset of action:
Oral: 30-45 minutes
I.M.: <15 minutes
I.V.: Within 2-5 minutes
Duration:
Oral: 3-6 hours
I.M., I.V.: 2-3 hours

Pharmacokinetics (Adult data unless noted)
Absorption: Oral: Very poor (10% to 20%) from the GI tract
Distribution: Adults: V_d: 19 ± 12 L
Metabolism: In the liver and at tissue site by cholinesterases
Bioavailability: 10% to 20%
Half-life: Adults: 3 hours
Elimination: Clearance: Adults: 830 mL/minute

Usual Dosage Myasthenia gravis (dosage should be adjusted so patient takes larger doses prior to time of greatest fatigue)

Oral:
Neonates: 5 mg every 4-6 hours
Children: 7 mg/kg/day in 5-6 divided doses
Adults: Initial: 60 mg 3 times/day with maintenance dose ranging from 60 mg to 1.5 g/day (incremental increases every 48 hours or more if needed) or as sustained release tablet (Mestinon® Timespan®) 180-540 mg (1-3 tablets) once or twice daily (the interval between doses should be at least 6 hours)
I.M., I.V.:
Neonates and Children: 0.05-0.15 mg/kg/dose (maximum single dose: 10 mg)
Adults: 2 mg every 2-3 hours (or 1/30th of oral dose)
Reversal of nondepolarizing neuromuscular blocker: I.V.:
Children: 0.1-0.25 mg/kg/dose preceded by atropine or glycopyrrolate
Adults: 10-20 mg preceded by atropine or glycopyrrolate
Pretreatment for Soman nerve gas exposure: Oral: Adults: 30 mg every 8 hours beginning several hours before exposure; discontinue after exposure to nerve gas (treatment with atropine and pralidoxime are indicated after exposure)

Administration
Parenteral: Administer direct I.V. slowly over 2-4 minutes; patients receiving large parenteral doses should be pretreated with atropine
Oral: Swallow sustained release tablets whole, do not chew or crush

Monitoring Parameters Muscle strength, heart rate, vital capacity

Dosage Forms Excipient information presented when available (limited, particularly for generics); consult specific product labeling.
Injection, solution, as bromide:
Regonol®: 5 mg/mL (2 mL) [contains benzyl alcohol]
Syrup, as bromide:
Mestinon®: 60 mg/5 mL (480 mL) [raspberry flavor; contains alcohol 5%, sodium benzoate]
Tablet, as bromide: 60 mg
Mestinon®: 60 mg
Tablet, sustained release, as bromide:
Mestinon® Timespan®: 180 mg

♦ **Pyridostigmine Bromide** see Pyridostigmine on page 1189

Pyridoxine (peer i DOKS een)

Medication Safety Issues
Sound-alike/look-alike issues:
Pyridoxine may be confused with paroxetine, pralidoxime, Pyridium®

International issues:
Doxal® [Brazil] may be confused with Doxil® which is a brand name for doxorubicin in the U.S.
Doxal® [Brazil]: Brand name for doxycycline in Austria; brand name for pyridoxine/thiamine combination in Brazil; brand name for doxepin in Finland

Related Information
Antiepileptic Drugs on page 1693

U.S. Brand Names Aminoxin [OTC]; Pyri-500 [OTC]

Therapeutic Category Antidote, Cycloserine Toxicity; Antidote, Hydrazine Toxicity; Antidote, Mushroom Toxicity; Drug-induced Neuritis, Treatment Agent; Nutritional Supplement; Vitamin, Water Soluble

Generic Available Yes

Use Prevention and treatment of vitamin B_6 deficiency, pyridoxine-dependent seizures in infants; treatment of drug-induced deficiency (eg, isoniazid or hydralazine); treatment of acute intoxication of isoniazid, cycloserine, hydrazine, mushroom (genus *Gyromitra*)

Pregnancy Risk Factor A/C (dose exceeding RDA recommendation)

Pregnancy Considerations Crosses the placenta; available evidence suggests safe use during pregnancy

Lactation Enters breast milk/compatible

Breast-Feeding Considerations Crosses into breast milk; possible inhibition of lactation at doses >600 mg/day. AAP considers **compatible** with breast-feeding.

Contraindications Hypersensitivity to pyridoxine or any component

Adverse Reactions
Central nervous system: Sensory neuropathy (after chronic administration of large doses), seizures (following I.V. administration of very large doses), headache
Gastrointestinal: Nausea
Hematologic: Serum folic acid concentration decreased
Hepatic: AST elevated
Local: Burning or stinging at injection site
Neuromuscular & skeletal: Paresthesia
Respiratory: Respiratory distress
Miscellaneous: Allergic reactions have been reported

Drug Interactions
Avoid Concomitant Use There are no known interactions where it is recommended to avoid concomitant use.

Increased Effect/Toxicity There are no known significant interactions involving an increase in effect.

Decreased Effect
Pyridoxine may decrease the levels/effects of: Altretamine; Barbiturates; Levodopa; Phenytoin

Mechanism of Action Precursor to pyridoxal and pyridoxamine which function as cofactors in the metabolism of proteins, carbohydrates, and fats; also aids in the release of liver and muscle stored glycogen and in the synthesis of GABA (within the CNS) and heme

Pharmacokinetics (Adult data unless noted)
Absorption: Readily from the GI tract; primarily in jejunum
Metabolism: Converted to pyridoxal (active form in liver)
Half-life, biologic: 15-20 days
Elimination: By liver metabolism

Usual Dosage
Adequate intake: Oral: Infants:
<6 months: 0.1 mg (0.01 mg/kg)
6-12 months: 0.3 mg (0.03 mg/kg)
Recommended daily allowance: Oral:
1-3 years: 0.5 mg
4-8 years: 0.6 mg
9-13 years: 1 mg
14-19 years:
Male: 1.3 mg
Female: 1.2 mg
20-50 years: 1.3 mg
>50 years:
Male: 1.7 mg
Female: 1.5 mg
Pyridoxine-dependent seizures: Oral, I.M., I.V.:
Neonates and Infants: Initial: 10-100 mg; maintenance: Oral: 50-100 mg/day
Dietary deficiency: Oral:
Children: 5-25 mg/day for 3 weeks, then 1.5-2.5 mg/day in multivitamin product
Adults: 2.5-10 mg/day until clinical signs are corrected, then 2-5 mg/day (dosage found in multivitamin products)
Drug-induced neuritis (eg, isoniazid, hydralazine, penicillamine, cycloserine): Oral:
Children:
Treatment: 10-50 mg/day
Prophylaxis: 1-2 mg/kg/day

Adults:

Cycloserine: Treatment 100-300 mg/day in divided doses

Isoniazid or penicillamine: Treatment: 100-200 mg/day for 3 weeks; prophylaxis: 25-100 mg/day

Acute intoxication: Children and Adults:

Hydrazine: 25 mg/kg: $^1/_3$ dose I.M. and $^2/_3$ dose I.V. infusion over 3 hours

Isoniazid: Dose equal to isoniazid ingested given as a first dose of 1-4 g I.V., followed by 1 g I.M. every 30 minutes until total dosage completed

Mushroom ingestion (genus *Gyromitra*): I.V.: 25 mg/kg; repeat as necessary to a maximum total dose of 15-20 g

Administration

Parenteral: Administer slow I.V.

Oral: Administer without regard to meals

Monitoring Parameters When administering large I.V. doses, monitor respiratory rate, heart rate, and blood pressure

Reference Range 30-80 ng/mL

Test Interactions False positive urobilinogen spot test using Ehrlich's reagent

Dosage Forms Excipient information presented when available (limited, particularly for generics); consult specific product labeling.

Capsule, as hydrochloride: 50 mg, 250 mg

Aminoxin: 20 mg

Injection, solution, as hydrochloride: 100 mg/mL (1 mL)

Liquid, oral, as hydrochloride: 200 mg/5 mL (120 mL)

Tablet, as hydrochloride: 25 mg, 50 mg, 100 mg, 250 mg, 500 mg

Tablet, sustained release, as hydrochloride:

Pyri-500: 500 mg

Extemporaneous Preparations A 1 mg/mL oral solution has an expected stability of 30 days when refrigerated when compounded as follows: Withdraw 100 mg (1 mL of a 100 mg/mL injection) from a vial with a needle and syringe, add to 99 mL of simple syrup in an amber bottle; keep in refrigerator

Nahata, MC, Pai VB, and Hipple TF, *Pediatric Drug Formulations*, 5th ed, Cincinnati, OH: Harvey Whitney Books Co, 2004.

♦ **Pyridoxine Hydrochloride** see Pyridoxine *on page 1190*

Pyrimethamine (peer i METH a meen)

Medication Safety Issues

Sound-alike/look-alike issues:

Daraprim® may be confused with Dantrium®, Daranide®

U.S. Brand Names Daraprim®

Canadian Brand Names Daraprim®

Therapeutic Category Antimalarial Agent

Generic Available No

Use Used in combination with sulfadiazine for treatment of toxoplasmosis; used in combination with dapsone as primary or secondary prophylaxis for *Pneumocystis jiroveci* in HIV-infected patients; pyrimethamine has been used for chemoprophylaxis of malaria, however, due to severe adverse reactions and reports of resistance to pyrimethamine, other antimalarial agents are now generally preferred

Pregnancy Risk Factor C

Pregnancy Considerations There are no adequate or well-controlled studies in pregnant women. Teratogenicity has been reported in animal studies. If administered during pregnancy (ie, for toxoplasmosis), supplementation of folate is strongly recommended. Pregnancy should be avoided during therapy.

Lactation Enters breast milk/not recommended (AAP rates "compatible")

Breast-Feeding Considerations Pyrimethamine enters breast milk and may result in significant systemic concentrations in breast-fed infants. AAP rates as "compatible" (although the manufacturer does not recommend its use during breast-feeding). The effect of concurrent therapy with sulfonamide or dapsone (frequently used with pyrimethamine as combination treatment) must be considered.

Contraindications Hypersensitivity to pyrimethamine, chloroguanide, or any component; megaloblastic anemia; resistant malaria and patients with seizure disorders

Precautions Use with caution in patients with impaired renal or hepatic function and in patients with possible folate deficiency

Adverse Reactions

Cardiovascular: Shock

Central nervous system: Seizures, fever, fatigue, ataxia, headache

Dermatologic: Rash, photosensitivity

Endocrine & metabolic: Folic acid deficiency

Gastrointestinal: Anorexia, abdominal cramps, vomiting, atrophic glossitis, diarrhea

Hematologic: Megaloblastic anemia, leukopenia, thrombocytopenia, agranulocytosis, pancytopenia, pulmonary eosinophilia

Neuromuscular & skeletal: Tremor

Renal: Hematuria

Respiratory: Respiratory failure

Drug Interactions

Metabolism/Transport Effects Inhibits CYP2C9 (moderate), 2D6 (moderate)

Avoid Concomitant Use

Avoid concomitant use of Pyrimethamine with any of the following: Artemether; Lumefantrine

Increased Effect/Toxicity

Pyrimethamine may increase the levels/effects of: Antipsychotic Agents (Phenothiazines); Carvedilol; CYP2C9 Substrates (High risk); CYP2D6 Substrates; Dapsone; Dapsone (Systemic); Dapsone (Topical); Fesoterodine; Lumefantrine; Nebivolol; Tamoxifen

The levels/effects of Pyrimethamine may be increased by: Artemether; Dapsone; Dapsone (Systemic)

Decreased Effect

Pyrimethamine may decrease the levels/effects of: Codeine; TraMADol

The levels/effects of Pyrimethamine may be decreased by: Methylfolate

Mechanism of Action Inhibits parasitic dihydrofolate reductase resulting in inhibition of tetrahydrofolic acid synthesis

Pharmacokinetics (Adult data unless noted)

Absorption: Oral: Well absorbed

Distribution: V_d: Adults: 2.9 L/kg; appears in breast milk; distributed to the kidneys, lung, liver, and spleen

Protein binding: 80% to 87%

Half-life: 111 hours (range: 54-148 hours)

Time to peak serum concentration: Within 2-6 hours

Elimination: Pyrimethamine and metabolites are excreted in urine

Usual Dosage Oral:

Toxoplasmosis (with sulfadiazine):

Newborns and Infants: Initial: 2 mg/kg/day divided every 12 hours for 2 days, then 1 mg/kg/day once daily given with sulfadiazine for the first 6 months; next 6 months: 1 mg/kg/day 3 times/week with sulfadiazine; oral leucovorin calcium 5-10 mg 3 times/week should be administered to prevent hematologic toxicity

Children: 2 mg/kg/day divided every 12 hours for 3 days followed by 1 mg/kg/day (maximum: 25 mg/day) once daily or divided twice daily for 4 weeks given with sulfadiazine; oral leucovorin calcium 5-10 mg 3 times/week should be administered to prevent hematologic toxicity

Adults: 50-75 mg/day together with 1-4 g of a sulfonamide plus oral leucovorin calcium 5-10 mg 3 times/week for 1-3 weeks depending on patient's tolerance and response, then reduce dose by 50% and continue for 4-5 weeks **or** 25-50 mg/day for 3-4 weeks

Prophylaxis for first episode of *Toxoplasma gondii*:

Children ≥1 month of age: 1 mg/kg/day once daily with dapsone plus oral leucovorin calcium 5 mg every 3 days

Adolescents and Adults: 50 mg once weekly with dapsone plus oral leucovorin calcium 25 mg once weekly

Prophylaxis for recurrence of *Toxoplasma gondii*:

Children ≥1 month of age: 1 mg/kg/day once daily given with sulfadiazine or clindamycin, plus oral leucovorin calcium 5 mg every 3 days

Adolescents and Adults: 25-75 mg once daily in combination with sulfadiazine or clindamycin, plus oral leucovorin calcium 10-25 mg daily

Prophylaxis for first episode or recurrence of *Pneumocystis jiroveci*:

Adolescents and Adults: 50-75 mg once weekly in combination with dapsone plus oral leucovorin calcium 25 mg once weekly

Administration Oral: Administer with meals to minimize vomiting

Monitoring Parameters CBC including platelet counts

Patient Information Notify physician if rash, sore throat, pallor, or glossitis occurs. May cause photosensitivity reactions (eg, exposure to sunlight may cause severe sunburn, skin rash, redness, or itching); avoid exposure to sunlight and artificial light sources (sunlamps, tanning booth/bed); wear protective clothing, wide-brimmed hats, sunglasses, and lip sunscreen (SPF ≥15); use a sunscreen [broad-spectrum sunscreen or physical sunscreen (preferred) or sunblock with SPF ≥15]; contact physician if reaction occurs.

Additional Information Leucovorin calcium may be given in a dosage of 3-9 mg/day for 3 days, or 5 mg every 3 days, or as required to reverse symptoms or to prevent hematologic problems due to pyrimethamine-induced folic acid deficiency

Dosage Forms Excipient information presented when available (limited, particularly for generics); consult specific product labeling.

Tablet: 25 mg

Extemporaneous Preparations Pyrimethamine tablets may be crushed to prepare oral suspensions of the drug in a 1:1 mixture of simple syrup and 1% methylcellulose to yield a suspension with a pyrimethamine concentration of 2 mg/mL; stable for at least 91 days when stored in plastic or glass prescription bottles at 4°C or 25°C

Nahata MC, Morosco RS, and Hipple TF, "Stability of Pyrimethamine in a Liquid Dosage Formulation Stored for Three Months," *Am J Health-Syst Pharm*, 1997, 54:2714-6.

References

"1997 USPHS/IDSA Guidelines for the Prevention of Opportunistic Infections in Persons Infected With Human Immunodeficiency Virus," *MMWR Morb Mortal Wkly Rep*, 1997, 46(RR-12):1-46.

Van Voorhis WC, "Therapy and Prophylaxis of Systemic Protozoan Infections," *Drugs*, 1990, 40(2):176-202.

◆ **Pyrimethamine and Sulfadoxine** *see* Sulfadoxine and Pyrimethamine *on page 1301*

◆ **Q-Tussin [OTC]** *see* GuaiFENesin *on page 656*

◆ **Quadrivalent Human Papillomavirus Vaccine** *see* Papillomavirus (Types 6, 11, 16, 18) Recombinant Vaccine *on page 1057*

◆ **Qualaquin®** *see* QuiNINE *on page 1194*

◆ **Quelicin®** *see* Succinylcholine *on page 1295*

◆ **Questran®** *see* Cholestyramine Resin *on page 302*

◆ **Questran® Light** *see* Cholestyramine Resin *on page 302*

◆ **Questran® Light Sugar Free (Can)** *see* Cholestyramine Resin *on page 302*

◆ **Quinalbarbitone Sodium** *see* Secobarbital *on page 1250*

◆ **Quinate® (Can)** *see* QuiNIDine *on page 1192*

QuiNIDine (KWIN i deen)

Medication Safety Issues

Sound-alike/look-alike issues:

QuiNIDine may be confused with cloNIDine, quiNINE, Quinora®

High alert medication: The Institute for Safe Medication Practices (ISMP) includes this medication (I.V. formulation) among its list of drug classes which have a heightened risk of causing significant patient harm when used in error.

Canadian Brand Names Apo-Quinidine®; BioQuin® Durules™; Novo-Quinidin; Quinate®

Therapeutic Category Antiarrhythmic Agent, Class I-A

Generic Available Yes

Use Prophylaxis after cardioversion of atrial fibrillation and/or flutter to maintain normal sinus rhythm; also used to prevent reoccurrence of paroxysmal supraventricular tachycardia, paroxysmal A-V junctional rhythm, paroxysmal ventricular tachycardia, paroxysmal atrial fibrillation, and atrial or ventricular premature contractions; also has activity against *Plasmodium falciparum* malaria

Pregnancy Risk Factor C

Lactation Enters breast milk/compatible

Contraindications Hypersensitivity to quinidine, any component, or cinchona derivatives; patients who have a history of thrombocytic purpura during prior therapy with quinidine or quinine; patients with complete A-V block with an A-V junctional or idioventricular pacemaker; patients with intraventricular conduction defects (marked widening of QRS complex); patients who might be adversely affected by anticholinergic agents (eg, myasthenia gravis)

Warnings Antiarrhythmic drugs have not been shown to enhance survival in nonlife-threatening ventricular arrhythmias and may increase mortality; the risk is greatest with structural heart disease. Quinidine may increase mortality in treatment of atrial fibrillation/flutter **[U.S. Boxed Warning]**. Quinidine prolongs the QT_c interval, which may lead to torsade de pointes; risk increased by bradycardia, hypokalemia, hypomagnesemia, or high serum levels of quinidine. May increase ventricular response rate in patients with atrial fibrillation or flutter; control AV conduction before initiating. May cause syncope, most likely due to ventricular tachycardia or fibrillation; syncope may subside spontaneously, but occasionally may be fatal; discontinue quinidine if syncope occurs

Precautions Use with caution in patients with myocardial depression, sick sinus syndrome, cardiac glycoside intoxication, hepatic and/or renal insufficiency; hemolysis may occur in patients with G-6-PD deficiency; quinidine-induced hepatotoxicity, including granulomatous hepatitis, increased serum AST and alkaline phosphatase concentrations, and jaundice may occur; use with caution in nursing women; adjust dose with severe renal impairment

Adverse Reactions

Cardiovascular: Syncope, hypotension, tachycardia, heart block, ventricular fibrillation, vascular collapse, severe hypotension with rapid I.V. administration

Central nervous system: Fever, headache

Dermatologic: Angioedema, rash; photosensitivity (rare)

Gastrointestinal: GI disturbances, nausea, vomiting, cramps

Hematologic: Blood dyscrasias, thrombotic thrombocytopenic purpura

Hepatic: AST elevated; alkaline phosphatase elevated, jaundice, granulomatous hepatitis

Respiratory: Respiratory depression

Miscellaneous: Cinchonism (nausea, tinnitus, headache, impaired hearing or vision, vomiting, abdominal pain, vertigo, confusion, delirium, syncope)

Drug Interactions

Metabolism/Transport Effects Substrate of CYP2C9 (minor), CYP2E1 (minor), CYP3A4 (major), P-glycoprotein; **Inhibits** CYP2C9 (weak), CYP2D6 (strong), CYP3A4 (strong), P-glycoprotein

Avoid Concomitant Use

Avoid concomitant use of QuiNIDine with any of the following: Alfuzosin; Antifungal Agents (Azole Derivatives, Systemic); Artemether; Dabigatran Etexilate; Dronedarone; Eplerenone; Everolimus; Halofantrine; Lumefantrine; Mefloquine; Nilotinib; Nisoldipine; Pimozide; Protease Inhibitors; QuiNINE; Ranolazine; Rivaroxaban; Romidepsin; Salmeterol; Silodosin; Tamoxifen; Tamsulosin; Tetrabenazine; Thioridazine; Tolvaptan; Topotecan; Ziprasidone

Increased Effect/Toxicity

QuiNIDine may increase the levels/effects of: Alfuzosin; Almotriptan; Alosetron; Atomoxetine; Beta-Blockers; Bortezomib; Brinzolamide; Cardiac Glycosides; Ciclesonide; Colchicine; CYP2D6 Substrates; CYP3A4 Substrates; Dabigatran Etexilate; Dextromethorphan; Dienogest; Dronedarone; Dutasteride; Eplerenone; Everolimus; FentaNYL; Fesoterodine; GuanFACINE; Halofantrine; Haloperidol; Ixabepilone; Lumefantrine; Maraviroc; Mefloquine; MethylPREDNISolone; Neuromuscular-Blocking Agents; Nilotinib; Nisoldipine; Paricalcitol; Pazopanib; P-Glycoprotein Substrates; Pimecrolimus; Pimozide; QTc-Prolonging Agents; QuiNINE; Ranolazine; Rivaroxaban; Romidepsin; Salmeterol; Saxagliptin; Silodosin; Sorafenib; Tadalafil; Tamoxifen; Tamsulosin; Tetrabenazine; Thioridazine; Tolvaptan; Topotecan; Tricyclic Antidepressants; Verapamil; Vitamin K Antagonists; Ziprasidone

The levels/effects of QuiNIDine may be increased by: Alfuzosin; Amiodarone; Antacids; Antifungal Agents (Azole Derivatives, Systemic); Artemether; Carbonic Anhydrase Inhibitors; Chloroquine; Cimetidine; Ciprofloxacin; Ciprofloxacin (Systemic); CYP3A4 Inhibitors (Moderate); CYP3A4 Inhibitors (Strong); Diltiazem; Fluconazole; Gadobutrol; Lumefantrine; Macrolide Antibiotics; Nilotinib; P-Glycoprotein Inhibitors; Protease Inhibitors; QuiNINE; Selective Serotonin Reuptake Inhibitors; Tricyclic Antidepressants; Verapamil

Decreased Effect

QuiNIDine may decrease the levels/effects of: Codeine; Dihydrocodeine; Hydrocodone; Prasugrel; TraMADol

The levels/effects of QuiNIDine may be decreased by: Barbiturates; Calcium Channel Blockers (Dihydropyridine); CYP3A4 Inducers (Strong); Deferasirox; Herbs (CYP3A4 Inducers); Kaolin; P-Glycoprotein Inducers; Phenytoin; Potassium-Sparing Diuretics; Primidone; Rifamycin Derivatives; Sucralfate

Food Interactions Excessive intake of fruit juices or vitamin C may decrease urine pH and result in increased clearance of quinidine with decreased serum concentration; alkaline foods may result in increased quinidine serum concentrations; food has a variable effect on absorption of extended release formulation. Grapefruit juice delays absorption of quinidine, decreases quinidine clearance, inhibits cytochrome P450 CYP3A4 mediated metabolism of quinidine to 3-hydroxyquinidine (major metabolite of quinidine), and significantly decreases the AUC of 3-hydroxyquinidine (although the clinical significance of the quinidine-grapefruit juice interaction is unknown, grapefruit juice should be avoided). A decrease in dietary salt intake may increase serum quinidine concentrations.

Stability Do not use discolored parenteral solution

Mechanism of Action Class IA antiarrhythmic with anticholinergic, local anesthetic, and mild negative inotropic effects; depresses phase 0 of the action potential; decreases myocardial excitability, conduction velocity, and myocardial contractility by decreasing sodium influx during depolarization and potassium efflux in repolarization; also reduces calcium transport across cell membrane

Pharmacokinetics (Adult data unless noted)

Distribution: V_d: Adults: 2-3.5 L/kg, decreased V_d with CHF, malaria; increased V_d with cirrhosis; crosses the placenta; appears in breast milk

Protein-binding:

Newborns: 60% to 70%

Adults: 80% to 90%

Decreased protein binding with cyanotic congenital heart disease, cirrhosis, or acute MI

Metabolism: Extensive in the liver (50% to 90%) to inactive compounds

Bioavailability:

Gluconate: 70%

Sulfate: 80%

Half-life, plasma (increased half-life with cirrhosis and CHF):

Children: 2.5-6.7 hours

Adults: 6-8 hours

Elimination: In urine (15% to 25% as unchanged drug)

Dialysis: Slightly dialyzable (5% to 20%) by hemodialysis; not removed by peritoneal dialysis

Usual Dosage Note: Dose expressed in terms of the salt: 267 mg of quinidine gluconate = 200 mg of quinidine sulfate

Children: Test dose (for idiosyncratic reaction, intolerance, syncope, thrombocytopenia) (**sulfate**, oral or **gluconate**, I.M.): 2 mg/kg or 60 mg/m^2

Oral (**quinidine sulfate**): Usual: 30 mg/kg/day or 900 mg/m^2/day given in 5 daily doses or 6 mg/kg every 4-6 hours; range: 15-60 mg/kg/day in 4-5 divided doses

I.V. (**quinidine gluconate**): 2-10 mg/kg/dose every 3-6 hours as needed (I.V. route **not** recommended)

Adults: Test dose (for idiosyncratic reaction, intolerance, syncope, thrombocytopenia): 200 mg administered several hours before full dosage

Oral (**sulfate**): 100-600 mg/dose every 4-6 hours; begin at 200 mg/dose and titrate to desired effect

Oral (**gluconate**): 324-972 mg every 8-12 hours

I.M.: 400 mg/dose every 4-6 hours

I.V.: 200-400 mg/dose diluted and given at a rate ≤10 mg/minute

Dosing adjustment in renal impairment: Children and Adults: Cl_{cr} <10 mL/minute: Administer 75% of normal dose

◀ **Administration**

Oral: Administer with water on an empty stomach, but may administer with food or milk to decrease GI upset; best to administer in a consistent manner with regards to meals; avoid administration with grapefruit juice; swallow extended release tablets whole, do not chew or crush

Parenteral: I.V.: Maximum rate of infusion: 10 mg/minute; maximum concentration: 16 mg/mL; I.V. tubing length should be minimized (quinidine may be significantly adsorbed to polyvinyl chloride tubing)

Monitoring Parameters CBC with differential, platelet count, liver and renal function tests, and serum concentrations should be routinely performed during long-term administration

Reference Range Optimal therapeutic level is method dependent

Therapeutic: 2-7 mcg/mL (SI: 6.2-15.4 micromoles/L)

Toxic: >8 mcg/mL (SI: >18 micromoles/L)

Patient Information Notify physician if fever, rash, unusual bruising or bleeding, visual disturbances, or ringing in the ears occurs; avoid grapefruit juice; avoid excessive intake of fruit juices or vitamin C. May rarely cause photosensitivity reactions; avoid exposure to sunlight and artificial light sources (sunlamps, tanning booth/bed); use a sunscreen; contact physician if reaction occurs.

Additional Information Use of extended release products is not recommended in children. Formation of a concretion of tablets or bezoar in the stomach has been reported following tablet ingestion by a 16-month old infant; diagnostic or therapeutic endoscopy may be required in patients with massive overdose and prolonged elevated serum quinidine concentrations

Dosage Forms Excipient information presented when available (limited, particularly for generics); consult specific product labeling.

Injection, solution, as gluconate: 80 mg/mL (10 mL) [equivalent to quinidine base 50 mg/mL]

Tablet, as sulfate: 200 mg, 300 mg

Tablet, extended release, as gluconate: 324 mg [equivalent to quinidine base 202 mg]

Tablet, extended release, as sulfate: 300 mg [equivalent to quinidine base 249 mg]

Extemporaneous Preparations

A 10 mg/mL quinidine sulfate oral liquid preparation made from tablets and 3 different vehicles (cherry syrup, a 1:1 mixture of Ora-Sweet® and Ora-Plus®, or a 1:1 mixture of Ora-Sweet® SF and Ora-Plus®) was stable for 60 days when stored in amber plastic prescription bottles in the dark at room temperature (25°C) or under refrigeration (5°C); Grind six 200 mg tablets in a mortar into a fine powder; add 15 mL of the vehicle and mix well to form a uniform paste; mix while adding the vehicle in geometric proportions to **almost** 120 mL; transfer to a calibrated bottle and qsad to 120 mL; label "shake well" and "protect from light" (Allen, 1998).

Allen LV and Erickson MA, "Stability of Bethanechol Chloride, Pyrazinamide, Quinidine Sulfate, Rifampin, and Tetracycline in Extemporaneously Compounded Oral Liquids," *Am J Health Syst Pharm*, 1998, 55 (17):1804-9.

References

Pickoff AS, Singh S, and Gelband H, *The Medical Management of Cardiac Arrhythmias in Cardiac Arrhythmias in the Neonate, Infant and Child*, Roberts NK and Gelband H, ed, Norwalk, CT: Appleton-Century-Crofts, 1983.

Szefler SJ, Pieroni DR, Gingell RL, et al, "Rapid Elimination of Quinidine in Pediatric Patients," *Pediatrics*, 1982, 70(3):370-5.

◆ **Quinidine Gluconate** *see* QuiNIDine *on page 1192*

◆ **Quinidine Polygalacturonate** *see* QuiNIDine *on page 1192*

◆ **Quinidine Sulfate** *see* QuiNIDine *on page 1192*

QuiNINE (KWYE nine)

Medication Safety Issues

Sound-alike/look-alike issues:

QuiNINE may be confused with quiNIDine

Related Information

Malaria *on page 1652*

Medications for Which A Single Dose May Be Fatal When Ingested By A Toddler *on page 1709*

U.S. Brand Names Qualaquin®

Canadian Brand Names Apo-Quinine®; Novo-Quinine; Quinine-Odan

Therapeutic Category Antimalarial Agent; Skeletal Muscle Relaxant, Miscellaneous

Generic Available No

Use Treatment of chloroquine-resistant, uncomplicated *P. falciparum* malaria infection (inactive against sporozoites, pre-erythrocytic or exoerythrocytic forms of plasmodia) in conjunction with other antimalarial agents [FDA approved in pediatrics (age not specified) and adults]; has also been used for the treatment of uncomplicated chloroquine-resistant *P. vivax* malaria (in conjunction with other antimalarial agents); treatment of *Babesia microti* infection in conjunction with clindamycin

Medication Guide An FDA-approved patient medication guide, which is available with the product information and at http://www.fda.gov/downloads/Drugs/DrugSafety/UCM192698.pdf, must be dispensed with this medication for each new outpatient prescription and refill.

Pregnancy Risk Factor C

Pregnancy Considerations Teratogenic effects have been reported in some animal studies. Quinine crosses the human placenta. Cord plasma to maternal plasma quinine ratios have been reported as 0.18-0.46 and should not be considered therapeutic to the infant. Teratogenic effects, optic nerve hypoplasia, and deafness have been reported in the infant following maternal use of very high doses; however, therapeutic doses used for malaria are generally considered safe. Quinine may also cause significant hypoglycemia when used during pregnancy. Malaria infection in pregnant women may be more severe than in nonpregnant women. Because *P. falciparum* malaria can cause maternal death and fetal loss, pregnant women traveling to malaria-endemic areas must use personal protection against mosquito bites. Quinine may be used for the treatment of malaria in pregnant women; consult current CDC guidelines. Pregnant women should be advised not to travel to areas of *P. falciparum* resistance to chloroquine.

Lactation Enters breast milk/use caution (AAP rate "compatible")

Breast-Feeding Considerations Based on limited data, it is estimated that nursing infants would receive <0.4% of the maternal dose from breast-feeding.

Contraindications Hypersensitivity to quinine or any component or to mefloquine or quinidine (cross sensitivity reported); history of potential hypersensitivity reactions [including black water fever, thrombotic thrombocytopenia purpura (TTP), hemolytic uremic syndrome (HUS), or thrombocytopenia] associated with prior quinine use; prolonged QT interval; myasthenia gravis; optic neuritis; G6PD deficiency

Warnings Quinine is not recommended for the prevention/treatment of nocturnal leg cramps due to the potential for severe and/or life-threatening side effects (eg, cardiac arrhythmias, thrombocytopenia, HUS/TTP, severe hypersensitivity reactions) **[U.S. Boxed Warning]**. These risks, as well as the absence of clinical effectiveness, do not justify its use in the unapproved/unlabeled prevention and/or treatment of leg cramps. Use may cause significant hypoglycemia due to quinine-induced insulin release.

Severe hypersensitivity reactions (eg, Stevens-Johnson syndrome, anaphylactic shock) have occurred; discontinue following any signs of sensitivity. Other events, including acute interstitial nephritis, neutropenia, and granulomatous hepatitis, may also be attributed to hypersensitivity reactions. Immune-mediated thrombocytopenia, including life-threatening cases and hemolytic uremic syndrome/thrombotic thrombocytopenic purpura (HUS/TTP), has occurred with use. Chronic renal failure associated with TTP has also been reported. Thrombocytopenia generally resolves within a week upon discontinuation. Re-exposure may result in increased severity of thrombocytopenia and faster onset.

Precautions Use with caution in patients with clinical conditions or on medications which may prolong the QT interval or cause cardiac arrhythmias (quinine has quinidine-like activity), in patients with myasthenia gravis, and in patients with impaired liver function.

Adverse Reactions

Cardiovascular: Anginal symptoms, conduction disturbances, flushing of the skin, syncope, ventricular tachycardia (see Warnings)

Central nervous system: Confusion, dizziness, fever, headache, restlessness, seizures, vertigo

Dermatologic: Pruritus, rash, Stevens-Johnson syndrome (see Warnings)

Endocrine & metabolic: Hypoglycemia

Gastrointestinal: Diarrhea, epigastric pain, nausea, vomiting

Hematologic: Disseminated intravascular coagulation, hemolysis, leukopenia, thrombocytopenia (see Warnings), thrombotic thrombocytopenic purpura (see Warnings)

Hepatic: Hepatitis

Ocular: Blurred vision, night blindness, optic atrophy, visual disturbances

Otic: Impaired hearing, tinnitus

Renal: Chronic renal failure (associated with TTP), hemolytic uremic syndrome (see Warnings), interstitial nephritis (see Warnings)

Respiratory: Dyspnea

Miscellaneous: Anaphylactic shock (see Warnings); black water fever (see Warnings); cinchonism (abdominal pain, confusion, delirium, headache, impaired hearing or vision, nausea, syncope tinnitus, vertigo, vomiting), hypersensitivity reactions

Drug Interactions

Metabolism/Transport Effects Substrate of CYP1A2 (minor), 2C19 (minor), 3A4 (major); **Inhibits** CYP2C8 (moderate), 2C9 (moderate), 2D6 (moderate), 3A4 (weak)

Avoid Concomitant Use

Avoid concomitant use of QuiNINE with any of the following: Antacids; Artemether; Lumefantrine; Macrolide Antibiotics; Mefloquine; Neuromuscular-Blocking Agents; QTc-Prolonging Agents; Rifampin

Increased Effect/Toxicity

QuiNINE may increase the levels/effects of: Antihypertensives; Antipsychotic Agents (Phenothiazines); Cardiac Glycosides; Carvedilol; CYP2C8 Substrates (High risk); CYP2C9 Substrates (High risk); CYP2D6 Substrates; Dapsone; Dapsone (Systemic); Dapsone (Topical); Fesoterodine; Herbs (Hypotensive Properties); HMG-CoA Reductase Inhibitors; Lumefantrine; Mefloquine; Nebivolol; Neuromuscular-Blocking Agents; QTc-Prolonging Agents; Tamoxifen; Theophylline Derivatives

The levels/effects of QuiNINE may be increased by: Alkalinizing Agents; Artemether; Cimetidine; CYP3A4 Inhibitors (Moderate); CYP3A4 Inhibitors (Strong); Dapsone; Dapsone (Systemic); Macrolide Antibiotics; Mefloquine; QTc-Prolonging Agents

Decreased Effect

QuiNINE may decrease the levels/effects of: Codeine; TraMADol

The levels/effects of QuiNINE may be decreased by: Antacids; CYP3A4 Inducers (Strong); Deferasirox; Herbs (CYP3A4 Inducers); Rifampin

Stability Store at 20°C to 25°C (68°F to 77°F). Protect from light. Do not refrigerate or freeze.

Mechanism of Action Depresses oxygen uptake and carbohydrate metabolism; intercalates into DNA, disrupting the parasite's replication and transcription; affects calcium distribution within muscle fibers and decreases the excitability of the motor end-plate region

Pharmacokinetics (Adult data unless noted)

Absorption: Oral: Readily absorbed, mainly from the upper small intestine

Distribution: Widely distributed to body tissues and fluids including small amounts into bile and CSF (2% to 7% of plasma concentration); crosses the placenta; excreted into breast milk

V_d (children): 0.8 L/kg

V_d (adults): 1.9 L/kg

Protein binding: 70% to 90%

Metabolism: Primarily in the liver via hydroxylation pathways

Half-life:

Children: 6-12 hours

Adults: 8-14 hours

Time to peak serum concentration: Within 2-4 hours

Elimination: In bile and saliva with ~20% excreted unchanged in urine; renal excretion is twofold in the presence of acidic urine

Dialysis: Not effectively removed by peritoneal dialysis; removed by hemodialysis

Usual Dosage Oral: **Note:** Actual duration of quinine treatment for malaria may be dependent upon the geographic region or pathogen. Dosage expressed in terms of the **salt**; 1 capsule Qualaquin® = 324 mg of quinine sulfate = 269 mg of base.

Children:

Treatment of uncomplicated chloroquine-resistant *P. falciparum* malaria: CDC guidelines: 30 mg/kg/day in divided doses every 8 hours for 3-7 days depending on region (maximum dose: 1944 mg/day).Tetracycline, doxycycline, or clindamycin (consider risk versus benefit of using tetracycline or doxycycline in children <8 years of age) should also be given.

Treatment of uncomplicated chloroquine-resistant *P. vivax* malaria: CDC guidelines: 30 mg/kg/day in divided doses every 8 hours for 3-7 days depending on region (maximum dose: 1944 mg/day). Tetracycline or doxycycline (consider risk versus benefit of using tetracycline or doxycycline in children <8 years of age) **plus** primaquine should also be given.

Babesiosis: 30 mg/kg/day, divided every 8 hours for 7-10 days with clindamycin; maximum dose: 648 mg/dose

Adults:

Treatment of uncomplicated chloroquine-resistant *P. falciparum* malaria: CDC guidelines: 648 mg every 8 hours for 3-7 days. Tetracycline, doxycycline, or clindamycin should also be given.

Treatment of uncomplicated chloroquine-resistant *P. vivax* malaria: CDC guidelines: 648 mg every 8 hours for 3-7 days. Tetracycline or doxycycline **plus** primaquine should also be given.

Babesiosis: 648 mg every 8 hours for 7-10 days with clindamycin

Dosing adjustment in renal impairment: Adult:

Cl_{cr} 10-50 mL/minute: Administer every 8-12 hours

Cl_{cr} <10 mL/minute: Administer every 24 hours

Severe chronic renal failure not on dialysis: Initial dose: 648 mg followed by 324 mg every 12 hours

Administration Oral: Do not crush capsule to avoid bitter taste

Monitoring Parameters CBC with platelet count, liver function tests, blood glucose, ophthalmologic examination

Patient Information Report to physician if tinnitus, hearing loss, rash, or visual disturbances occur during therapy

Additional Information Parenteral form of quinine (dihydrochloride) is no longer available from the CDC; quinidine gluconate should be used instead; the FDA has banned over-the-counter (OTC) drug products containing quinine sold for treatment and/or prevention of malaria, as well as, products labeled for treatment or prevention of nocturnal leg cramps

Dosage Forms Excipient information presented when available (limited, particularly for generics); consult specific product labeling.

Capsule, as sulfate:
Qualaquin®: 324 mg

References

Aronoff GR, Berns JS, Brier ME, et al, *Drug Prescribing in Renal Failure: Dosing Guidelines for Adults*, 4th ed. Philadelphia, PA: American College of Physicians; 1999, p 73.

Centers for Disease Control and Prevention (CDC), "Guidelines for Treatment of Malaria in the United States," Treatment Table Update, May 18, 2009. Available at: http://www.cdc.gov/malaria/pdf/treatmenttable.pdf

Centers for Disease Control and Prevention (CDC), "Treatment of Malaria (Guidelines for Clinicians)." Available at: http://www.cdc.gov/malaria/pdf/clinicalguidance.pdf.

"Drugs for Parasitic Infections," *Treatment Guidelines From the Medical Letter*, 2004, 50(Suppl):e1-14.

Schulbe DE, "Quinine Ban Signals Change for Pharmacists, APhA," *Pharmacy Today*, 1995, 1(12):6.

♦ **Quinine-Odan (Can)** *see* QuiNINE *on page 1194*
♦ **Quinine Sulfate** *see* QuiNINE *on page 1194*

Quinupristin/Dalfopristin
(kwi NYOO pris tin/dal FOE pris tin)

U.S. Brand Names Synercid®
Canadian Brand Names Synercid®
Therapeutic Category Antibiotic, Streptogramin
Generic Available No
Use Treatment of serious or life-threatening infections caused by vancomycin-resistant *Enterococcus faecium*; treatment of complicated skin and skin structure infections caused by *Staphylococcus aureus* (methicillin-susceptible) or *Streptococcus pyogenes* (FDA approved in ages ≥16 years and adults)
Pregnancy Risk Factor B
Pregnancy Considerations Because adverse effects were not observed in animal reproduction studies, quinupristin/dalfopristin is classified pregnancy category B. There are no adequate and well-controlled studies of quinupristin/dalfopristin in pregnant women.
Lactation Excretion in breast milk unknown/use caution
Breast-Feeding Considerations It is not known if quinupristin/dalfopristin is excreted in human milk. The manufacturer recommends caution if administering quinupristin/dalfopristin to a nursing woman. The increased molecular weight of quinupristin/dalfopristin may minimize excretion into human milk. Nondose-related effects could include modification of bowel flora.
Contraindications Hypersensitivity to quinupristin, dalfopristin, other streptogramins (pristinamycin or virginiamycin), or to any component
Warnings For the treatment of serious or life-threatening vancomycin-resistant *Enterococcus faecium* infections (VREF) **[U.S. Boxed Warning]**. Quinupristin/dalfopristin inhibit cytochrome P450 3A4 metabolism of cyclosporine, midazolam, nifedipine, and terfenadine. There was a 77% increase in cyclosporine's half-life with a 63% increase in the AUC. Cyclosporine levels should be closely monitored

in patients who are receiving quinupristin/dalfopristin therapy concomitantly. Coadministration of quinupristin/dalfopristin with cytochrome P450 3A4 substrates with narrow therapeutic ranges require serum concentration monitoring of these drugs. Concurrent use with astemizole, terfenadine, and cisapride is not recommended. Drugs metabolized by the cytochrome P450 3A4 system that may prolong the QT$_c$ interval should be avoided. Superinfections and *C. difficile*-associated diarrhea have been reported with the use of quinupristin/dalfopristin. Resistance to quinupristin/dalfopristin has been reported in a few cases of *Enterococcus faecium* infections.

Precautions Use with caution in patients with hepatic or renal dysfunction; dosage reduction may be necessary in patients with hepatic cirrhosis; may cause pain and phlebitis when infused through a peripheral line; episodes of severe arthralgia and myalgia have been reported which improve with a dose frequency reduction to "q12h" or discontinuation of quinupristin/dalfopristin

Adverse Reactions

Central nervous system: Convulsion, headache

Dermatologic: Angioedema, pruritus, rash, urticaria

Gastrointestinal: Diarrhea, nausea, pseudomembranous colitis, vomiting

Hepatic: AST and ALT elevated, hyperbilirubinemia

Local: Pain, edema, inflammation at infusion site; thrombophlebitis

Neuromuscular & skeletal: Arthralgia, myalgia

Miscellaneous: Anaphylaxis, superinfection

Drug Interactions

Metabolism/Transport Effects Quinupristin: **Inhibits** CYP3A4 (weak)

Avoid Concomitant Use There are no known interactions where it is recommended to avoid concomitant use.

Increased Effect/Toxicity
Quinupristin and Dalfopristin may increase the levels/ effects of: Calcium Channel Blockers; CycloSPORINE; CycloSPORINE (Systemic)

Decreased Effect There are no known significant interactions involving a decrease in effect.

Stability Unopened vials should be stored in a refrigerator at 2°C to 8°C (36°F to 46°F); reconstituted drug is stable for 1 hour at room temperature; infusion bag is stable for 5 hours at room temperature and for 54 hours if refrigerated at 2°C to 8°C (36°F to 46°F); incompatible with NS and heparin; compatible with aztreonam, ciprofloxacin, fluconazole, haloperidol, metoclopramide, morphine, and potassium chloride during Y-site administration

Mechanism of Action Inhibits bacterial protein synthesis by binding to the 50S bacterial ribosomal subunit resulting in peptide chain elongation inhibition and peptidyl transferase inhibition

Pharmacokinetics (Adult data unless noted)
Distribution:
V_d: Quinupristin: 0.45 L/kg
V_d: Dalfopristin: 0.24 L/kg
Protein binding:
Quinupristin: 23% to 32%
Dalfopristin: 50% to 56%
Metabolism: Quinupristin is conjugated with glutathione and cysteine to active metabolites; dalfopristin is hydrolyzed to an active metabolite
Half-life:
Quinupristin: 0.85 hour
Dalfopristin: 0.7 hour
Elimination: 75% to 77% excreted in the bile and feces
Dialysis: Not removed by peritoneal dialysis or hemodialysis

Usual Dosage Dosage is expressed in terms of combined "mg" of quinupristin plus dalfopristin: I.V.:

Children: Limited information is available; quinupristin/dalfopristin has been used in a limited number of pediatric patients under a compassionate use protocol

Treatment of vancomycin-resistant *Enterococcus faecium* infection: 7.5 mg/kg/dose every 8 hours

Treatment of vancomycin-resistant *Enterococcus faecium* CNS shunt infection: 7.5 mg/kg/dose every 8 hours (plus 1 mg intrathecal dose daily at the time of shunt tap was used in an 8-month old infant for 28 days in one case report; 1 or 2 mg doses every day for 5-33 days have been administered intrathecally in 6 patients)

Treatment of complicated skin and skin structure infection: 7.5 mg/kg/dose every 12 hours for at least 7 days

Adolescents ≥16 years and Adults:

Treatment of vancomycin-resistant *Enterococcus faecium* infection: 7.5 mg/kg/dose every 8 hours

Treatment of complicated skin and skin structure infection: 7.5 mg/kg/dose every 12 hours

Dosage adjustment in hepatic impairment: Dosage adjustment may be necessary, but exact recommendations cannot be made at this time

Administration Parenteral: Reconstitute vial by slowly adding 5 mL D$_5$W or SWI to make a 100 mg/mL solution; gently swirl the vial contents without shaking to minimize foam formation; further dilute the reconstituted solution with D$_5$W to a final maximum concentration for administration via peripheral line of 2 mg/mL; maximum concentration for administration via a central line is 5 mg/mL; if an injection site reaction occurs, the dose can be further diluted to a final concentration of <1 mg/mL; administer infusion over 60 minutes; following infusion of quinupristin/dalfopristin, the infusion line should be flushed with D$_5$W to minimize venous irritation; **DO NOT FLUSH** with saline or heparin solutions due to incompatibility

Monitoring Parameters CBC, liver function test; monitor infusion site closely; number and type of stools/day for diarrhea

Patient Information Report to physician any venous irritation, arthralgia, myalgia, or the occurrence of persistent watery and bloody stools.

Nursing Implications If moderate to severe venous irritation occurs following peripheral quinupristin/dalfopristin administration, consider increasing the infusion volume, changing infusion sites, or establishing central venous access; administration of hydrocortisone or diphenhydramine did not decrease infusion site reactions

Dosage Forms Excipient information presented when available (limited, particularly for generics); consult specific product labeling.

Injection, powder for reconstitution:

Synercid®: 500 mg: Quinupristin 150 mg and dalfopristin 350 mg

References

Garey KW, Tesoro E, Muggia V, et al, "Cerebrospinal Fluid Concentrations of Quinupristin-Dalfopristin in a Patient With Vancomycin-Resistant *Enterococcus faecium* Ventriculitis," *Pharmacotherapy*, 2001, 21(6):748-50.

Gransden WR, King A, Marossy D, et al, "Quinupristin/Dalfopristin in Neonatal *Enterococcus faecium* Meningitis," *Arch Dis Child Fetal Neonatal Ed*, 1998, 78(3):F235-6.

Gray JW, Darbyshire PJ, Beath SV, et al, "Experience With Quinupristin/Dalfopristin in Treating Infections With Vancomycin-Resistant *Enterococcus faecium* in Children," *Pediatr Infect Dis J*, 2000, 19(3):234-8.

Gupte G, Jyothi S, Graham S, et al, "Synercid Use in Children Is Associated With Arthralgia and Myalgia," *Archives of Disease in Childhood*, 2006, 91(Supp 1):67.

Nachman SA, Verma R, and Egnor M, "Vancomycin-Resistant *Enterococcus faecium* Shunt Infection in an Infant: An Antibiotic Cure," *Microb Drug Resist*, 1995, 1(1):95-6.

◆ **Quixin®** *see* Levofloxacin *on page 813*

◆ **Qutenza™** *see* Capsaicin *on page 241*

◆ **QVAR®** *see* Beclomethasone *on page 176*

◆ **RabAvert®** *see* Rabies Virus Vaccine *on page 1199*

Rabeprazole (ra BE pray zole)

Medication Safety Issues

Sound-alike/look-alike issues:

AcipHex® may be confused with Acephen®, Accupril®, Aricept®, pHisoHex®

Rabeprazole may be confused with aripiprazole, donepezil, lansoprazole, omeprazole, raloxifene

U.S. Brand Names AcipHex®

Canadian Brand Names Novo-Rabeprazole EC; Pariet®; PMS-Rabeprazole EC; PRO-Rabeprazole; Rabeprazole EC; RAN™-Rabeprazole; Riva-Rabeprazole EC; Sandoz-Rabeprazole

Therapeutic Category Gastric Acid Secretion Inhibitor; Gastrointestinal Agent, Gastric or Duodenal Ulcer Treatment; Proton Pump Inhibitor

Generic Available No

Use Treatment of symptomatic gastroesophageal reflux disease (GERD) (FDA approved in ages ≥12 years and adults); short-term treatment (4-8 weeks) and maintenance of erosive or ulcerative GERD (FDA approved in adults); short-term treatment (4 weeks) of duodenal ulcers (FDA approved in adults); long-term treatment of pathological hypersecretory conditions (eg, Zollinger-Ellison syndrome) (FDA approved in adults); in combination with clarithromycin and amoxicillin, adjunctive treatment of duodenal ulcers associated with *Helicobacter pylori* (FDA approved in adults)

Pregnancy Risk Factor B

Pregnancy Considerations Not shown to be teratogenic in animal studies, however, adequate and well-controlled studies have not been done in humans; use during pregnancy only if clearly needed

Lactation Excretion in breast milk unknown/not recommended

Contraindications Hypersensitivity to rabeprazole, substituted benzimidazole proton pump inhibitors (eg, lansoprazole, omeprazole), or any component

Warnings Symptomatic response to therapy with rabeprazole does not preclude the presence of gastric malignancy. Use of gastric acid inhibitors including proton pump inhibitors and H$_2$ blockers has been associated with an increased risk for development of acute gastroenteritis and community-acquired pneumonia (see Canani, 2006).

Precautions Use with caution in patients with severe hepatic impairment

Adverse Reactions

Central nervous system: Headache, pain

Gastrointestinal: Abdominal pain, constipation, diarrhea, flatulence, nausea, vomiting

Respiratory: Pharyngitis

Miscellaneous: Infection

<1%, postmarketing, and/or case reports (limited to important or life-threatening): Agranulocytosis, anaphylaxis, angioedema, bullous drug skin eruptions, coma, delirium, disorientation, erythema multiforme, hemolytic anemia, hyperammonemia, interstitial nephritis, interstitial pneumonia, jaundice, leukopenia, pancytopenia, rhabdomyolysis, Stevens-Johnson syndrome, sudden death, thrombocytopenia, toxic epidermal necrolysis (some fatal), TSH elevation

Drug Interactions

Metabolism/Transport Effects Substrate (major) of CYP2C19, 3A4; **Inhibits** CYP2C8 (moderate), 2C19 (moderate), 2D6 (weak), 3A4 (weak)

Avoid Concomitant Use

Avoid concomitant use of Rabeprazole with any of the following: Delavirdine; Erlotinib; Nelfinavir; Posaconazole

Increased Effect/Toxicity

Rabeprazole may increase the levels/effects of: CYP2C19 Substrates; CYP2C8 Substrates (High risk); Methotrexate; Raltegravir; Saquinavir; Tacrolimus; Tacrolimus (Systemic); Voriconazole

The levels/effects of Rabeprazole may be increased by: Clopidogrel; Fluconazole; Ketoconazole; Ketoconazole (Systemic)

Decreased Effect

Rabeprazole may decrease the levels/effects of: Atazanavir; Cefditoren; Clopidogrel; Dabigatran Etexilate; Dasatinib; Delavirdine; Erlotinib; Indinavir; Iron Salts; Itraconazole; Ketoconazole; Ketoconazole (Systemic); Mesalamine; Mycophenolate; Nelfinavir; Posaconazole

The levels/effects of Rabeprazole may be decreased by: CYP2C19 Inducers (Strong); CYP3A4 Inducers (Strong); Deferasirox; Herbs (CYP3A4 Inducers); Tipranavir

Food Interactions When administered with a high fat meal, absorption may be delayed; however, the extent of absorption (AUC) is not significantly altered.

Stability Store at 25°C (77°F); protect from moisture

Mechanism of Action Suppresses gastric acid secretion by inhibiting the parietal cell membrane enzyme (H^+/K^+)-ATPase or proton pump; demonstrates antimicrobial activity against *Helicobacter pylori*

Pharmacodynamics Onset of action: 1 hour

Pharmacokinetics (Adult data unless noted)

Protein binding: 96.3%

Metabolism: Extensive metabolism in the liver by cytochrome isoenzymes CYP3A and CYP2C19 to inactive metabolites; [CYP2C19 exhibits a known genetic polymorphism due to its deficiency in some subpopulations (3% to 5% of Caucasians and 17% to 20% of Asians) which results in slower metabolism]

Bioavailability: 52%

Half-life:

Adolescents: ~0.55-1 hour (James, 2007)

Adults: 1-2 hours

Time to peak serum concentration:

Adolescents: 3.3-4.1 hours (James, 2007)

Adults: 2-5 hours

Excretion: 90% in urine

Usual Dosage Oral:

Adolescents ≥12 years: GERD: 20 mg/day for up to 8 weeks

Adults:

Erosive/ulcerative GERD: Treatment: 20 mg once daily for 4-8 weeks; if inadequate response, may repeat up to an additional 8 weeks; maintenance: 20 mg once daily

Symptomatic GERD: Treatment: 20 mg once daily for 4 weeks; if inadequate response, may repeat for an additional 4 weeks

Duodenal ulcer: 20 mg/day before breakfast for 4 weeks; additional therapy may be required for some patients

Helicobacter pylori eradication:

Manufacturer labeling: 20 mg twice daily administered with amoxicillin 1000 mg **and** clarithromycin 500 mg twice daily for 7 days

American College of Gastroenterology guidelines (see Chey, 2007):

Nonpenicillin allergy: 20 mg twice daily administered with amoxicillin 1000 mg **and** clarithromycin 500 mg twice daily for 10-14 days

Penicillin allergy: 20 mg twice daily administered with clarithromycin 500 mg **and** metronidazole 500 mg twice daily for 10-14 days **or** 20 mg once or twice daily administered with bismuth subsalicylate 525 mg **and** metronidazole 250 mg **plus** tetracycline 500 mg 4 times/day for 10-14 days

Hypersecretory conditions: 60 mg once daily; dose may need to be adjusted as necessary. Doses as high as 100 mg once daily and 60 mg twice daily have been used and continued as long as necessary (up to 1 year in some patients).

Dosage adjustment in hepatic impairment:

Mild to moderate: No adjustment is necessary

Severe impairment: Use cautiously due to lack of clinical data

Dosage adjustment in renal impairment: No dosage adjustment necessary

Administration Oral: May be administered without regard to food; tablets should be swallowed whole, do not chew, crush, or split. May administer with an antacid.

Patient Information Do not chew or crush tablets; may cause photosensitivity reactions (eg, exposure to sunlight may cause severe sunburn, skin rash, redness, or itching); avoid exposure to sunlight and artificial light sources (sunlamps, tanning booth/bed); wear protective clothing, wide-brimmed hats, sunglasses, and lip sunscreen (SPF ≥15); use a sunscreen [broad-spectrum sunscreen or physical sunscreen (preferred) or sunblock with SPF ≥15]; contact physician if reaction occurs

Dosage Forms Excipient information presented when available (limited, particularly for generics); consult specific product labeling. [CAN] = Canadian brand name

Tablet, delayed release, enteric coated, as sodium:
AcipHex®: 20 mg
Pariet® [CAN]: 10 mg, 20 mg

References

Canani RB, Cirillo P, Roggero P, et al, "Therapy With Gastric Acidity Inhibitors Increases the Risk of Acute Gastroenteritis and Community-Acquired Pneumonia in Children," *Pediatrics*, 2006, 117(5):e817-20.

Chey WD, Wong BC, and Practice Parameters Committee of the American College of Gastroenterology, "American College of Gastroenterology Guideline on the Management of *Helicobacter pylori* Infection," *Am J Gastroenterol*, 2007, 102(8):1808-25.

Gibbons TE and Gold BD, "The Use of Proton Pump Inhibitors in Children: A Comprehensive Review," *Paediatr Drugs*, 2003, 5 (1):25-40.

James L, Walson P, Lomax K, et al, "Pharmacokinetics and Tolerability of Rabeprazole Sodium in Subjects Aged 12 to 16 Years With Gastroesophageal Reflux Disease: An Open-Label, Single- and Multiple-Dose Study," *Clin Ther*, 2007, 29(9):2082-92.

◆ Rabeprazole EC (Can) *see* Rabeprazole *on page 1197*

Rabies Immune Globulin (Human)
(RAY beez i MYUN GLOB yoo lin, HYU man)

U.S. Brand Names HyperRAB™ S/D; Imogam® Rabies-HT

Canadian Brand Names HyperRAB™ S/D; Imogam® Rabies Pasteurized

Therapeutic Category Immune Globulin

Generic Available No

Use Postexposure prophylaxis of persons with suspected rabies exposure who previously have not been vaccinated against rabies; postexposure prophylaxis consists of thorough wound treatment and the administration of rabies vaccine and rabies immune globulin

Pregnancy Risk Factor C

Pregnancy Considerations Reproduction studies have not been conducted. Pregnancy is not a contraindication to postexposure prophylaxis.

Contraindications Persons who have been previously immunized with rabies vaccine and have a confirmed adequate rabies antibody titer should not receive rabies immune globulin as part of the postexposure regimen

Warnings Since rabies immune globulin is made from human plasma, it may potentially transmit an infectious agent. Screening of donors, testing for presence of viruses, and inactivating/removing viruses reduces this risk.

Precautions Use with caution in patients with a history of allergic reactions to human immunoglobulin preparations or with IgA deficiency. Epinephrine should be available for treatment of anaphylaxis. Use caution in patients with thrombocytopenia or coagulation disorders (I.M. injections may be contraindicated).

Adverse Reactions
Central nervous system: Fever, headache, malaise

Dermatologic: Angioneurotic edema, rash, urticaria

Local: Soreness, pain, tenderness, stiffness at injection site

Renal: Nephrotic syndrome

Miscellaneous: Anaphylaxis

Drug Interactions
Avoid Concomitant Use There are no known interactions where it is recommended to avoid concomitant use.

Increased Effect/Toxicity There are no known significant interactions involving an increase in effect.

Decreased Effect

Rabies Immune Globulin (Human) may decrease the levels/effects of: Vaccines (Live)

Stability Store in refrigerator; do not freeze. Solution that has been frozen should be discarded.

Mechanism of Action Provides immediate antibodies to rabies which neutralize rabies virus and inhibit its spread and infective properties.

Pharmacodynamics
Onset of action: Rabies antibody appears in serum within 24 hours

Peak antibody level: 2-13 days

Pharmacokinetics (Adult data unless noted) Half-life: 24 days

Usual Dosage Children and Adults: Local wound infiltration: 20 international units/kg single dose administered as soon as possible after exposure with the first dose of rabies vaccine. If anatomically feasible, the full rabies immune globulin dose should be infiltrated around and into the wound(s); remaining volume should be administered I.M. at a site distant from the vaccine administration site. If rabies vaccine was initiated without rabies immune globulin, rabies immune globulin may be administered through the seventh day after the first vaccine dose. Administration of RIG is not recommended after the seventh day postvaccine since an antibody response to the vaccine is expected during this time period.

Administration Do **not** administer I.V. Do not administer rabies vaccine in the same syringe or at same administration site as RIG.

Wound infiltration: Thoroughly infiltrate in the area around and into the wound(s)

I.M.: Children and Adults: Inject into the deltoid muscle of the upper arm or lateral thigh muscle at a site distant from rabies vaccine administration. The gluteal area should be avoided to reduce the risk of sciatic nerve damage. Children with small muscle mass may require multiple I.M. sites for dose delivery.

Monitoring Parameters Serum rabies antibody titer (if rabies immune globulin is inadvertently administered after the eighth day from the first vaccine dose)

Dosage Forms Excipient information presented when available (limited, particularly for generics); consult specific product labeling.

Injection, solution [preservative free]:

HyperRAB™ S/D: 150 int. units/mL (2 mL, 10 mL) [solvent/detergent treated]

Imogam® Rabies-HT: 150 int. units/mL (2 mL, 10 mL) [heat treated]

References
Atkinson WL, Pickering LK, Schwartz B, et al, "General Recommendations on Immunization. Recommendations of the Advisory Committee on Immunization Practices (ACIP) and the American Academy of Family Physicians (AAFP)," *MMWR Recomm Rep,* 2002, 51(RR-2):1-35.

Manning SE, Rupprecht CE, Fishbein D, et al, "Human Rabies Prevention–United States, 2008: Recommendations of the Advisory Committee on Immunization Practices," *MMWR Recomm Rep,* 2008, 57(RR-3):1-28.

Willoughby RE Jr and Hammarin AL, "Prophylaxis Against Rabies in Children Exposed to Bats," *Pediatr Infect Dis Jp,* 2005, 24 (12):1109-10.

Rabies Virus Vaccine (RAY beez VYE rus vak SEEN)

U.S. Brand Names Imovax® Rabies; RabAvert®

Canadian Brand Names Imovax® Rabies; RabAvert®

Therapeutic Category Vaccine

Generic Available No

Use
Pre-exposure immunization: Vaccinate persons with greater than usual risk due to occupation or avocation including veterinarians, rangers, animal handlers, certain laboratory workers, and persons living in or visiting countries for longer than 1 month where rabies is a constant threat.

Postexposure prophylaxis: If a bite from a carrier animal is unprovoked or if the animal is not captured and rabies is present in that species and area, administer rabies immune globulin (RIG) and the vaccine as indicated

Pregnancy Risk Factor C

Pregnancy Considerations Animal reproduction studies have not been conducted. Pregnancy is not a contraindication to postexposure prophylaxis. Pre-exposure prophylaxis during pregnancy may also be considered if risk of rabies is great.

Lactation Excretion in breast milk unknown

Breast-Feeding Considerations Breast-feeding mothers may be vaccinated.

Contraindications
Pre-exposure treatment: Hypersensitivity to any component of the formulation; (Imovax® Rabies contains albumin and neomycin; RabAvert® contains amphotericin B, bovine gelatin, chicken protein, chlortetracycline, and neomycin); developing febrile illness

Postexposure treatment: Life-threatening allergic reactions to rabies vaccine or any components of the formulation (carefully consider a patient's risk of rabies before continuing therapy)

Warnings Immediate treatment for anaphylactic/anaphylactoid reaction should be available during administration of this vaccine. An immune complex reaction characterized by generalized urticaria, arthralgia, arthritis, angioedema, nausea, vomiting, fever, and malaise has been reported 2-21 days following booster doses of HDCV. Immune response may be decreased in immunocompromised patients. Pre-exposure immunization does not eliminate the need for prompt prophylaxis following an exposure but does reduce the postexposure treatment regimen.

Precautions Administer with caution to patients with thrombocytopenia or any coagulation disorder that would be compromised by I.M. injection. Routine prophylactic administration of acetaminophen to prevent fever due to vaccines has been shown to decrease the immune response of some vaccines; the clinical significance of this reduction in immune response has not been established (see Prymula, 2009).

Adverse Reactions All serious adverse reactions must be reported to the U.S. Department of Health and Human Services (DHHS) Vaccine Adverse Event Reporting System (VAERS) 1-800-822-7967.

◄ Cardiovascular: Edema
Central nervous system: Dizziness, encephalitis, encephalomyelitis, fever, Guillain-Barré syndrome, headache, malaise, meningitis, neuroparalytic reactions, pain, transverse myelitis
Dermatologic: Urticaria pigmentosa
Gastrointestinal: Abdominal pain, nausea,
Local: Erythema, itching, local discomfort, pain at injection site, pain or swelling
Neuromuscular & skeletal: Myalgia, transient paralysis
Miscellaneous: Anaphylaxis

Drug Interactions

Avoid Concomitant Use There are no known interactions where it is recommended to avoid concomitant use.

Increased Effect/Toxicity There are no known significant interactions involving an increase in effect.

Decreased Effect
The levels/effects of Rabies Vaccine may be decreased by: Chloroquine; Immunosuppressants

Stability Store under refrigeration at 2°C to 8°C (36°F to 46°F). Protect from light; do not freeze.

Mechanism of Action Rabies vaccine is an inactivated virus vaccine which promotes immunity by inducing an active immune response. The production of specific antibodies requires about 7-10 days. Rabies immune globulin (RIG) or antirabies serum, equine (ARS) is administered in conjunction with rabies vaccine to provide immune protection until an antibody response can occur.

Pharmacodynamics
Onset of action: I.M.: Rabies antibody: ~7-10 days
Peak effect: ~30-60 days
Duration: ≥1 year

Usual Dosage Children and Adults: I.M.:

Pre-exposure prophylaxis: 1 mL/dose for 3 doses, on days 0, 7, and 21 to 28.

Postexposure prophylaxis: All postexposure treatment should begin with immediate cleansing of the wound with soap and water; immunization should begin as soon as possible after exposure
Persons not previously immunized: 1 mL/dose for 4 doses, on days 0, 3, 7, 14 [Note: Immunocompromised patients should receive a fifth dose on day 28 (ACIP Provisional Recommendations, 2009)]; In addition, administer rabies immune globulin (RIG) 20 units/kg body weight (half of this is infiltrated at bite site if possible, and the remainder is administered I.M. along with rabies vaccine
Persons who have previously received postexposure prophylaxis with rabies vaccine, received a recommended I.M. pre-exposure series of rabies vaccine or have a previously documented rabies antibody titer considered adequate: 1 mL/dose on days 0 and 3; do not administer RIG
Booster (for occupational or other continuing risk): 1 mL/dose every 2-5 years or as indicated by antibody titer measurements

Administration I.M.: Reconstitute with provided diluent; **not for I.V. or SubQ administration;** administer injections in the deltoid muscle, not the gluteal; for younger children the outer aspect of the thigh may be used

Monitoring Parameters Serum rabies antibody titers are not routinely recommended in postexposure patients unless the patient was immunocompromised; to determine the need for repeat booster treatment, titers may be measured every 6 months to 2 years in persons at high risk for exposure

Nursing Implications Federal law requires that the date of administration, the vaccine manufacturer, lot number of vaccine, and the administering person's name, title, and address be entered into the patient's permanent medical record.

Additional Information In order to maximize vaccination rates, the ACIP recommends simultaneous administration of all age-appropriate vaccines (live or inactivated) for which a person is eligible at a single visit, unless contraindications exist. The use of combination vaccines is generally preferred over separate infections, taking into consideration provider assessment, patient preference, and potential adverse events.

For additional information, please refer to the following website: http://www.cdc.gov/vaccines/vpd-vac/.

Dosage Forms Excipient information presented when available (limited, particularly for generics); consult specific product labeling.
Injection, powder for reconstitution [preservative free]:
Imovax® Rabies: ≥2.5 int. units [HDCV; grown in human diploid cell culture; contains albumin (human), neomycin (may have trace amounts)]
RabAvert®: ≥2.5 int. units [contains albumin (human), amphotericin B (may have trace amounts), bovine gelatin, chicken egg protein, chlortetracycline (may have trace amounts), neomycin (may have trace amounts); PCEC; grown in chicken fibroblast culture]

References
ACIP Provisional Recommendations for the Prevention of Human Rabies. Available at: http://www.cdc.gov/vaccines/recs/provisional/downloads/rabies-July2009-508.pdf.
Centers for Disease Control and Prevention (CDC), "General Recommendations on Immunization. Recommendations of the Advisory Committee on Immunization Practices (ACIP)," *MMWR Recomm Rep*, 2006, 55(RR-15):1-48. Available at: http://www.cdc.gov/mmwr/preview/mmwrhtml/rr5515a1.htm.
Manning SE, Rupprecht CE, Fishbein D, et al, "Human Rabies Prevention–United States, 2008: Recommendations of the Advisory Committee on Immunization Practices," *MMWR Recomm Rep*, 2008, 57(RR-3):1-28.
Prymula R, Siegrist CA, Chlibek R, et al, "Effect of Prophylactic Paracetamol Administration at Time of Vaccination on Febrile Reactions and Antibody Responses in Children: Two Open-Label, Randomised Controlled Trials," *Lancet*, 2009, 374(9698):1339-50.

Ranitidine (ra NI ti deen)

Medication Safety Issues
Sound-alike/look-alike issues:
Ranitidine may be confused with amantadine, rimantadine
Zantac® may be confused with Xanax®, Zarontin®, Zofran®, Zyrtec®

International issues:
Antagon®: Brand name for astemizole in Mexico; brand name for ganirelix in the U.S.

U.S. Brand Names Zantac 150® [OTC]; Zantac 75® [OTC]; Zantac®; Zantac® EFFERdose®

Canadian Brand Names Acid Reducer; Acid Reducer Maximum Strength Non Prescription; Apo-Ranitidine®; CO Ranitidine; Dom-Ranitidine; Med-Ranitidine; Mylan-Ranitidine; Novo-Ranidine; Nu-Ranit; PHL-Ranitidine; PMS-Ranitidine; Ranitidine Injection, USP; ratio-Ranitidine; Riva-Ranitidine; Sandoz-Ranitidine; ScheinPharm Ranitidine; Zantac 75®; Zantac Maximum Strength Non-Prescription; Zantac®; ZYM-Ranitidine

Therapeutic Category Gastrointestinal Agent, Gastric or Duodenal Ulcer Treatment; Histamine H_2 Antagonist

Generic Available Yes: Excludes effervescent tablet

Use Short-term treatment of active duodenal ulcers and benign gastric ulcers; long-term prophylaxis of duodenal ulcer and gastric hypersecretory states; gastroesophageal reflux disease (GERD); recurrent postoperative ulcer; treatment and prophylaxis of erosive esophagitis; upper GI bleeding, prevention of acid-aspiration pneumonitis during surgery, and prevention of stress-induced ulcers; over-the-counter (OTC) formulation for use in the relief of heartburn, acid indigestion, and sour stomach

Pregnancy Risk Factor B

Pregnancy Considerations Adverse events were not observed in animal reproduction studies, therefore ranitidine is classified as pregnancy category B. Ranitidine crosses the placenta; available information suggests that it is not teratogenic in humans.

Lactation Enters breast milk/use caution

Contraindications Hypersensitivity to ranitidine or any component or other H_2 antagonists; patients with history of acute porphyria (may precipitate an acute attack)

Warnings Use of gastric acid inhibitors including proton pump inhibitors and H_2 blockers has been associated with an increased risk for development of acute gastroenteritis and community-acquired pneumonia (Canani, 2006). A large epidemiological study has suggested an increased risk for developing pneumonia in patients receiving H_2 receptor antagonists; however, a causal relationship with ranitidine has not been demonstrated. Rapid I.V. administration of ranitidine has been associated with bradycardia, particularly in patients predisposed to cardiac rhythm disturbances.

Zantac® EFFERdose® tablets and granules contain sodium benzoate; benzoic acid (benzoate) is a metabolite of benzyl alcohol; large amounts of benzyl alcohol (≥99 mg/kg/day) have been associated with a potentially fatal toxicity ("gasping syndrome") in neonates; in vitro and animal studies have shown that benzoate displaces bilirubin from protein binding sites; avoid use in neonates

Precautions Use with caution in patients with liver and renal impairment; dosage modification required in patients with renal impairment. Zantac® 150 EFFERdose® tablets and Zantac® 150 EFFERdose® granules contain phenylalanine; use with caution in patients with phenylketonuria.

Adverse Reactions
Cardiovascular: Bradycardia, tachycardia, vasculitis (rare)
Central nervous system: Dizziness, sedation, malaise, mental confusion, headache, hallucinations, anxiety
Dermatologic: Rash, alopecia (rare), erythema multiforme (rare)
Endocrine & metabolic: Gynecomastia
Gastrointestinal: Constipation, nausea, vomiting, abdominal discomfort, pancreatitis (rare)
Hematologic: Thrombocytopenia, aplastic anemia (rare), granulocytopenia, leukopenia
Hepatic: Hepatitis
Local: Transient pain at injection site
Neuromuscular & skeletal: Arthralgias

Renal: Serum creatinine elevated
Respiratory: Pneumonia (causal relationship not established; see Warnings)

Drug Interactions
Metabolism/Transport Effects Substrate of CYP1A2 (minor), CYP2C19 (minor), CYP2D6 (minor), P-glycoprotein; **Inhibits** CYP1A2 (weak), 2D6 (weak)

Avoid Concomitant Use
Avoid concomitant use of Ranitidine with any of the following: Delavirdine; Erlotinib

Increased Effect/Toxicity
Ranitidine may increase the levels/effects of: Procainamide; Saquinavir; Sulfonylureas; Warfarin

The levels/effects of Ranitidine may be increased by: P-Glycoprotein Inhibitors

Decreased Effect
Ranitidine may decrease the levels/effects of: Antifungal Agents (Azole Derivatives, Systemic); Atazanavir; Cefditoren; Cefpodoxime; Cefuroxime; Dasatinib; Delavirdine; Erlotinib; Fosamprenavir; Gefitinib; Indinavir; Iron Salts; Mesalamine; Nelfinavir; Prasugrel

The levels/effects of Ranitidine may be decreased by: Peginterferon Alfa-2b; P-Glycoprotein Inducers

Stability Protect injection from light; stable for 48 hours at room temperature or 30 days when frozen in D_5W or NS; stable for 24 hours in TPN solutions; stable for 24 hours in 3-in-1 total nutrient admixture

Mechanism of Action Competitive inhibition of histamine at H_2-receptors of the gastric parietal cells, which inhibits gastric acid secretion

Pharmacokinetics (Adult data unless noted)
Distribution: Minimally penetrates the blood-brain barrier; breast milk to plasma ratio: 1.9-6.7
V_d:
Children: 1-1.3 L/kg
Adults: 1.4 L/kg
Protein binding: 15%
Metabolism: In the liver
Bioavailability:
Oral: ~50%
I.M.: 90% to 100%
Half-life:
Neonates (receiving ECMO): 6.6 hours
Infants: 3.5 hours
Children 3.5-16 years: 1.8-2 hours
Adults:
Normal renal and hepatic function: 2-2.5 hours
Decreased renal function (Cl_{cr} 25-35 mL/minute): 4.8 hours
Time to peak serum concentration:
Oral: 1-3 hours
I.M.: 15 minutes
Elimination: 30% (oral) or 70% (I.V.) eliminated as unchanged drug in the urine and feces
Dialysis: Hemodialysis: Slightly dialyzable (5% to 20%)

Usual Dosage
Premature and Term Infants <2 weeks:
Oral: 2 mg/kg/day divided every 12 hours
I.V.: 1.5 mg/kg/dose as loading dose, then 12 hours later maintenance dose of 1.5-2 mg/kg/day divided every 12 hours
Continuous infusion: 1.5 mg/kg/dose as loading dose followed by 0.04-0.08 mg/kg/hour infusion (or 1-2 mg/kg/day)
Children ≥1 month to 16 years:
Gastric/duodenal ulcer:
Oral:
Treatment: 4-8 mg/kg/day divided twice daily; maximum: 300 mg/day
Maintenance: 2-4 mg/kg/day once daily; maximum: 150 mg/day

I.V.: 2-4 mg/kg/day divided every 6-8 hours; maximum: 200 mg/day

GERD and erosive esophagitis:

Oral: 4-10 mg/kg/day divided twice daily; maximum: GERD: 300 mg/day; erosive esophagitis: 600 mg/day

I.V.: 2-4 mg/kg/day divided every 6-8 hours; maximum: 200 mg/day **or as an alternative**

Continuous infusion: Initial 1 mg/kg/dose for one dose followed by infusion of 0.08-0.17 mg/kg/hour or 2-4 mg/kg/day

Children ≥16 years and Adults:

Treatment of duodenal or gastric ulcers, GERD, maintenance of erosive esophagitis: Oral: 150 mg/dose twice daily or 300 mg at bedtime

Prophylaxis of recurrent duodenal ulcer: Oral: 150 mg at bedtime

Gastric hypersecretory conditions:

Oral: 150 mg twice daily; maximum: 600 mg/day

I.M., I.V.: 50 mg/dose every 6-8 hours (dose not to exceed 400 mg/day)

Continuous I.V. infusion: Initial 50 mg I.V. followed by 6.25 mg/hour titrated to gastric pH >4.0 for prophylaxis or >7.0 for treatment; **continuous I.V. infusion is preferred in patients with active bleeding**

Erosive esophagitis: Oral: 150 mg 4 times/day

Pathologic hypersecretory conditions (eg, Zollinger-Ellison syndrome):

Continuous I.V. infusion: Initial 50 mg I.V. followed by 1 mg/kg/hour infusion; titrate dosage in 0.5 mg/kg/hour increments to maintain gastric acid output at <10 mEq/hour; doses up to 2.5 mg/kg/hour (220 mg/hour) have been used

Oral: 150 mg twice daily; more frequent administration may be indicated depending upon response; doses up to 6.3 g/day have been used in severe cases

Relief of heartburn, acid indigestion, sour stomach (OTC use): Oral: 75 mg 30-60 minutes before eating; no more than 2 tablets/day

Dosing adjustment in renal impairment:

Children and Adults (Aronoff, 1999):

Cl$_{cr}$ 10-50 mL/minute: Reduce dose to 50% of dose recommended for indication

Cl$_{cr}$ <10 mL/minute: Reduce dose to 25% of dose recommended for indication

or as an alternative per manufacturer's recommendations:

Adults: Cl$_{cr}$ <50 mL/minute:

Oral: 150 mg every 24 hours; adjust dose cautiously if needed

I.V.: 50 mg every 18-24 hours; adjust dose cautiously if needed

Hemodialysis: Adjust dose schedule to administer dose at the end of dialysis

Administration

Oral: Administer with meals and at bedtime; dissolve 25 mg EFFERdose® tablet in 5 mL of water until completely dissolved; dissolve 150 mg EFFERdose® tablet or granules in 6-8 ounces of water before administration

Parenteral: Intermittent I.V. infusion preferred over direct injection to decrease risk of bradycardia; for intermittent infusion, infuse over 15-30 minutes, at a usual concentration of 0.5 mg/mL; for direct I.V. injection, administer over a period of at least 5 minutes, not to exceed 10 mg/minute (4 mL/minute) at a final concentration not to exceed 2.5 mg/mL; For I.M., administer undiluted (25 mg/mL)

Monitoring Parameters AST, ALT, serum creatinine; when used to prevent stress-related GI bleeding, measure the intragastric pH and try to maintain pH >4; gastric acid secretion (<10 mEq/hour)

Reference Range Serum level necessary to inhibit basal acid secretion:

Children: 90% suppression: 40-60 ng/mL

Adults: 50% suppression: 36-94 ng/mL

Test Interactions False-positive urine protein using Multistix®; gastric acid secretion test, skin test allergen extracts

Patient Information Avoid excessive amounts of coffee and aspirin; when self-medicating, if symptoms of heartburn, acid indigestion, or sour stomach persist after 2 weeks of continuous use of the drug, consult a clinician.

Additional Information Causes fewer CNS adverse reactions and drug interactions compared to cimetidine; safety and efficacy of full-dose therapy extending beyond 8 weeks have not been determined; Zantac® EFFERdose® 150 mg tablets and granules contain 7.55 mEq sodium

Dosage Forms Excipient information presented when available (limited, particularly for generics); consult specific product labeling.

Capsule 150 mg, 300 mg

Infusion, premixed in ½NS [preservative free]:

Zantac®: 50 mg (50 mL)

Injection, solution: 25 mg/mL (2 mL, 6 mL, 40 mL)

Zantac®: 25 mg/mL (2 mL, 6 mL, 40 mL) [contains phenol 0.5% as preservative]

Syrup: 15 mg/mL (5 mL, 10 mL, 473 mL)

Zantac®: 15 mg/mL (473 mL) [contains ethanol 7.5%; peppermint flavor]

Tablet: 75 mg [OTC], 150 mg, 300 mg

Zantac®: 150 mg, 300 mg

Zantac 75®: 75 mg

Zantac 150®: 150 mg

Tablet, for solution, oral [effervescent]:

Zantac® EFFERdose®: 25 mg [contains phenylalanine 2.81 mg/tablet, sodium 1.33 mEq/tablet, sodium benzoate]

References

Aronoff GR, Bennett WM, Berns JS, et al, *Drug Prescribing in Renal Failure: Dosing Guidelines for Adults and Children*, 5th ed. Philadelphia, PA: American College of Physicians, 2007.

Blumer JL, Rothstein FC, Kaplan BS, et al, "Pharmacokinetic Determination of Ranitidine Pharmacodynamics in Pediatric Ulcer Disease," *J Pediatr*, 1985, 107(2):301-6.

Canani RB, Cirillo P, Roggero P, et al, "Therapy With Gastric Acidity Inhibitors Increases the Risk of Acute Gastroenteritis and Community-Acquired Pneumonia in Children," *Pediatrics*, 2006, 117(5):e817-20.

Eddleston JM, Booker PD, and Green JR, "Use of Ranitidine in Children Undergoing Cardiopulmonary Bypass," *Crit Care Med*, 1989, 17 (1):26-9.

Fontana M, Massironi E, Rossi A, et al, "Ranitidine Pharmacokinetics in Newborn Infants," *Arch Dis Child*, 1993, 68(5 Spec No):602-3.

Lopez-Herce J, Albajara L, Codoceo R, et al, "Ranitidine Prophylaxis in Acute Gastric Mucosal Damage in Critically Ill Pediatric Patients," *Crit Care Med*, 1988, 16(6):591-93.

Morris DL, Markham SJ, Beechey A, et al, "Ranitidine-Bolus or Infusion Prophylaxis for Stress Ulcer," *Crit Care Med*, 1988, 16(3):229-32.

Roberts CJ, "Clinical Pharmacokinetics of Ranitidine," *Clin Pharmacokinet*, 1984, 9(3):211-21.

◆ **Ranitidine Hydrochloride** *see* Ranitidine *on page 1200*

◆ **Ranitidine Injection, USP (Can)** *see* Ranitidine *on page 1200*

◆ **RAN™-Lisinopril (Can)** *see* Lisinopril *on page 832*

◆ **RAN™-Lovastatin (Can)** *see* Lovastatin *on page 850*

◆ **RAN™-Metformin (Can)** *see* MetFORMIN *on page 891*

◆ **RAN™-Ondansetron (Can)** *see* Ondansetron *on page 1022*

◆ **RAN™-Pantoprazole (Can)** *see* Pantoprazole *on page 1054*

◆ **RAN™-Pravastatin (Can)** *see* Pravastatin *on page 1145*

◆ **RAN™-Rabeprazole (Can)** *see* Rabeprazole *on page 1197*

◆ **RAN™-Risperidone (Can)** *see* Risperidone *on page 1218*

◆ **RAN™-Simvastatin (Can)** *see* Simvastatin *on page 1263*

◆ **Rapamune®** *see* Sirolimus *on page 1265*

◆ **Rapamycin** *see* Sirolimus *on page 1265*

Rasburicase (ras BYOOR i kayse)

U.S. Brand Names Elitek®
Canadian Brand Names Fasturtec®
Therapeutic Category Enzyme; Uric Acid Lowering Agent
Generic Available No
Use Initial management of plasma uric acid levels in patients with leukemia, lymphoma, and solid tumor malignancies who are receiving anticancer therapy expected to result in tumor lysis and subsequent elevation of plasma uric acid (FDA approved in ages ≥1 month and adults)
Pregnancy Risk Factor C
Pregnancy Considerations Adverse effects were observed in animal studies. There are no adequate and well-controlled studies in pregnant women. Use during pregnancy only if the benefit to the mother outweighs the potential risk to the fetus.
Lactation Excretion in breast milk unknown/not recommended
Breast-Feeding Considerations Due to the potential for serious adverse reactions in the nursing infant, breast-feeding should be discontinued during treatment.
Contraindications History of anaphylaxis or severe hypersensitivity to rasburicase or any component; history of hemolytic reaction or methemoglobinemia associated with rasburicase; glucose-6-phosphatase dehydrogenase (G6PD) deficiency
Warnings Rasburicase may cause severe hypersensitivity reactions, including anaphylaxis, at any time during the course of therapy including with the first dose **[U.S. Boxed Warning]; discontinue immediately and permanently** in any patient exhibiting signs and symptoms of severe allergy, including chest pain, dyspnea, hypotension, and/or urticaria

Severe hemolytic reactions may occur in patients with G6PD deficiency (eg, African, Mediterranean, or Southeast Asian ancestry) due to the by-product, hydrogen peroxide **[U.S. Boxed Warning]**; contraindicated in patients with G6PD deficiency; patients at high risk for G6PD deficiency should be screened prior to treatment with rasburicase; **discontinue treatment immediately and permanently** in any patient developing hemolysis (usually develops within 2-4 days of treatment initiation); rasburicase has been associated with methemoglobinemia **[U.S. Boxed Warning]; discontinue treatment immediately** in any patient developing methemoglobinemia; initiate appropriate treatment (eg, transfusion, methylene blue) if methemoglobinemia occurs
Precautions Patients receiving rasburicase should receive I.V. hydration as appropriate for the management of tumor lysis syndrome. Enzymatic degradation of uric acid in blood samples will occur if left at room temperature **[U.S. Boxed Warning]; may interfere with serum uric acid measurements**; specific guidelines for the collection of plasma uric acid samples must be followed (see Test Interactions). Use of alkalinization (with sodium bicarbonate) concurrently with rasburicase is not recommended (Coiffier, 2008). Rasburicase is immunogenic and can elicit an antibody response; administration of more than one course is not recommended.
Adverse Reactions Data suggest that children <2 years of age may experience a higher frequency of adverse effects, particularly vomiting (75% vs 55%), diarrhea (63% vs 20%), fever (50% vs 38%), and rash (38% vs 10%)

Cardiovascular: Arrhythmias, cardiac arrest, cardiac failure, cerebrovascular disorder, chest pain, CHF, cyanosis, fluid overload, flushing, ischemic coronary disorder, MI, peripheral edema, thrombosis, thrombophlebitis
Central nervous system: Anxiety, fever, headache, seizures
Dermatologic: Cellulitis, rash
Endocrine & metabolic: Dehydration, hot flashes, hyperphosphatemia, hypophosphatemia
Gastrointestinal: Abdominal pain, constipation, diarrhea, gastrointestinal/abdominal infection, ileus, intestinal obstruction, mucositis, nausea, vomiting
Hematologic: Hemolysis (see Warnings), hemorrhage, methemoglobinemia (see Warnings), neutropenia, neutropenic fever, pancytopenia
Hepatic: ALT increased, hyperbilirubinemia
Neuromuscular & skeletal: Paresthesia, rigors
Ophthalmic: Retinal hemorrhages
Renal: Acute renal failure
Respiratory: Bronchospasm, pharyngolaryngeal pain, pneumonia, pulmonary edema, pulmonary hemorrhage, pulmonary hypertension, respiratory distress, respiratory failure
Miscellaneous: Antibody formation, infection, sepsis, severe hypersensitivity reactions (including anaphylaxis; see Warnings)
Drug Interactions
Avoid Concomitant Use There are no known interactions where it is recommended to avoid concomitant use.

Increased Effect/Toxicity There are no known significant interactions involving an increase in effect.

Decreased Effect There are no known significant interactions involving a decrease in effect.

Stability Store rasburicase and diluent in the refrigerator; protect from light and do not freeze; reconstituted solution and final dilution (see Administration) are stable refrigerated, but must be used within 24 hours due to the lack of a preservative
Mechanism of Action Rasburicase is a recombinant urate-oxidase enzyme that catalyzes the enzymatic oxidation of uric acid into an inactive and soluble metabolite, allantoin; it does not inhibit the formation of uric acid
Pharmacodynamics Onset: Uric acid levels decrease within 4 hours of initial administration
Pharmacokinetics (Adult data unless noted)
Distribution: V_d: Children: 110-127 mL/kg
Half-life: Children: 18 hours
Usual Dosage I.V.: Hyperuricemia associated with malignancy:
Children and Adults: 0.2 mg/kg/dose once daily for up to 5 days (manufacturer-recommended dose and duration)
  Note: Limited data suggest that a single prechemotherapy dose (versus multiple-day administration) may be sufficiently efficacious. Monitoring electrolytes, hydration status, and uric acid concentrations are necessary to identify the need for additional doses. Other clinical manifestations of tumor lysis syndrome (eg, hyperphosphatemia, hypocalcemia, and hyperkalemia) may occur.
Alternate dosing (Guidelines for the Management of Pediatric and Adult Tumor Lysis Syndrome; Coiffier, 2008): 0.05-0.2 mg/kg once daily for 1-7 days (average of 2-3 days) with the duration of treatment dependant on plasma uric acid levels and clinical judgment (patients with significant tumor burden may require an increase to twice daily); the following dose levels are recommended based on risk of tumor lysis syndrome (TLS):
High risk and baseline uric acid level >7.5 mg/dL: 0.2 mg/kg once daily (duration is based on plasma uric acid levels)

Intermediate risk and baseline uric acid level <7.5 mg/dL: 0.15 mg/kg once daily (duration is based on plasma uric acid levels); may consider managing initially with a single dose

Low risk and baseline uric acid level <7.5 mg/dL: 0.1 mg/kg once daily (duration is based on clinical judgment); a dose of 0.05 mg/kg was used (with good results) in one trial

Single-dose rasburicase (unlabeled use; based on limited data): 0.15 mg/kg; additional doses may be needed based on serum uric acid levels (Liu, 2005)

Administration I.V.: Dilute each 1.5 mg vial with 1 mL or 7.5 mg vial with 5 mL of provided diluent; gently swirl, do not shake; further dilute desired dose in NS to a final volume of 50 mL; infuse over 30 minutes, do not bolus; do not filter or mix with other medications; chemotherapy may be initiated 4 hours after the first dose of rasburicase

Monitoring Parameters Plasma uric acid levels (See Test Interactions); BUN, serum creatinine, phosphorus, urine output, CBC with differential, G6PD deficiency screening (in patients at high risk for deficiency); monitor for hypersensitivity

Test Interactions Rasburicase will cause enzymatic degradation of the uric acid within blood samples when left at room temperature, resulting in spuriously low uric acid levels; to avoid this interaction, blood must be collected into prechilled tubes containing heparin anticoagulant and immediately immersed and maintained in an ice water bath; plasma samples should be assayed within 4 hours of collection

Dosage Forms Excipient information presented when available (limited, particularly for generics); consult specific product labeling.

Injection, powder for reconstitution:

Elitek®: 1.5 mg [packaged with three 1 mL ampuls of diluent]; 7.5 mg [packaged with 5 mL of diluent]

References

Coiffier B, Altman A, Pui CH, et al, "Guidelines for the Management of Pediatric and Adult Tumor Lysis Syndrome: An Evidence-Based Review," *J Clin Oncol*, 2008, 26(16):2767-78.

Coiffier B, Mounier N, Bologna S, et al, "Efficacy and Safety of Rasburicase (Recombinant Urate Oxidase) for the Prevention and Treatment of Hyperuricemia During Induction Chemotherapy of Aggressive Non-Hodgkin's Lymphoma: Results of the GRAAL1 (Groupe d'Etude des Lymphomes de l'Adulte Trial on Rasburicase Activity in Adult Lymphoma) Study," *J Clin Oncol*, 2003, 21 (23):4402-6.

Goldman SC, Holcenberg JS, Finklestein JZ, et al, "A Randomized Comparison Between Rasburicase and Allopurinol in Children With Lymphoma or Leukemia at High Risk for Tumor Lysis," *Blood*, 2001, 97(10):2998-3003.

Jeha S, Kantarjian H, Irwin D, et al, "Efficacy and Safety of Rasburicase, a Recombinant Urate Oxidase (Elitek), in the Management of Malignancy-Associated Hyperuricemia in Pediatric and Adult Patients: Final Results of a Multicenter Compassionate Use Trial," *Leukemia*, 2005, 19(1):34-8.

Liu CY, Sims-McCallum RP, and Schiffer CA, "A Single Dose of Rasburicase Is Sufficient for the Treatment of Hyperuricemia in Patients Receiving Chemotherapy," *Leuk Res*, 2005, 29(4):463-5.

Pui CH, Mahmoud HH, Wiley JM, et al, "Recombinant Urate Oxidase for the Prophylaxis or Treatment of Hyperuricemia in Patients With Leukemia or Lymphoma," *J Clin Oncol*, 2001, 19(3):697-704.

◆ **rATG** *see* Antithymocyte Globulin (Rabbit) *on page 120*

◆ **ratio-Aclavulanate (Can)** *see* Amoxicillin and Clavulanic Acid *on page 98*

◆ **ratio-Acyclovir (Can)** *see* Acyclovir *on page 46*

◆ **ratio-Amiodarone (Can)** *see* Amiodarone *on page 84*

◆ **ratio-Amiodarone I.V. (Can)** *see* Amiodarone *on page 84*

◆ **ratio-Amlodipine (Can)** *see* AmLODIPine *on page 91*

◆ **ratio-Atenolol (Can)** *see* Atenolol *on page 147*

◆ **ratio-Azithromycin (Can)** *see* Azithromycin *on page 164*

◆ **ratio-Baclofen (Can)** *see* Baclofen *on page 171*

◆ **ratio-Brimonidine (Can)** *see* Brimonidine *on page 202*

◆ **ratio-Bupropion SR (Can)** *see* BuPROPion *on page 217*

◆ **ratio-Buspirone (Can)** *see* BusPIRone *on page 222*

◆ **ratio-Carvedilol (Can)** *see* Carvedilol *on page 254*

◆ **ratio-Cefuroxime (Can)** *see* Cefuroxime *on page 277*

◆ **ratio-Ciprofloxacin (Can)** *see* Ciprofloxacin *on page 310*

◆ **ratio-Citalopram (Can)** *see* Citalopram *on page 319*

◆ **ratio-Clarithromycin (Can)** *see* Clarithromycin *on page 324*

◆ **ratio-Clindamycin (Can)** *see* Clindamycin *on page 327*

◆ **ratio-Clobetasol (Can)** *see* Clobetasol *on page 331*

◆ **ratio-Cyclobenzaprine (Can)** *see* Cyclobenzaprine *on page 367*

◆ **ratio-Diltiazem CD (Can)** *see* Diltiazem *on page 443*

◆ **ratio-Emtec (Can)** *see* Acetaminophen and Codeine *on page 39*

◆ **ratio-Enalapril (Can)** *see* Enalapril/Enalaprilat *on page 499*

◆ **ratio-Fentanyl (Can)** *see* FentaNYL *on page 567*

◆ **ratio-Fluoxetine (Can)** *see* FLUoxetine *on page 600*

◆ **ratio-Fluticasone (Can)** *see* Fluticasone *on page 607*

◆ **ratio-Gabapentin (Can)** *see* Gabapentin *on page 634*

◆ **ratio-Glyburide (Can)** *see* GlyBURIDE *on page 648*

◆ **ratio-Indomethacin (Can)** *see* Indomethacin *on page 726*

◆ **ratio-Ipra-Sal (Can)** *see* Albuterol *on page 57*

◆ **ratio-Ketorolac (Can)** *see* Ketorolac *on page 781*

◆ **ratio-Lamotrigine (Can)** *see* LamoTRIgine *on page 795*

◆ **ratio-Lenoltec (Can)** *see* Acetaminophen and Codeine *on page 39*

◆ **ratio-Lisinopril (Can)** *see* Lisinopril *on page 832*

◆ **ratio-Lovastatin (Can)** *see* Lovastatin *on page 850*

◆ **ratio-Metformin (Can)** *see* MetFORMIN *on page 891*

◆ **ratio-Methotrexate (Can)** *see* Methotrexate *on page 900*

◆ **ratio-Methylphenidate (Can)** *see* Methylphenidate *on page 908*

◆ **ratio-Minocycline (Can)** *see* Minocycline *on page 933*

◆ **ratio-Mometasone (Can)** *see* Mometasone Furoate *on page 942*

◆ **ratio-Morphine (Can)** *see* Morphine Sulfate *on page 946*

◆ **ratio-Morphine SR (Can)** *see* Morphine Sulfate *on page 946*

◆ **ratio-Omeprazole (Can)** *see* Omeprazole *on page 1016*

◆ **ratio-Ondansetron (Can)** *see* Ondansetron *on page 1022*

◆ **ratio-Orciprenaline® (Can)** *see* Metaproterenol *on page 890*

◆ **ratio-Pantoprazole (Can)** *see* Pantoprazole *on page 1054*

◆ **ratio-Paroxetine (Can)** *see* PARoxetine *on page 1064*

◆ **ratio-Pentoxifylline (Can)** *see* Pentoxifylline *on page 1090*

◆ **ratio-Pravastatin (Can)** *see* Pravastatin *on page 1145*

◆ **ratio-Ranitidine (Can)** *see* Ranitidine *on page 1200*

◆ **ratio-Risperidone (Can)** *see* Risperidone *on page 1218*

◆ **ratio-Salbutamol (Can)** *see* Albuterol *on page 57*

◆ **ratio-Sertraline (Can)** *see* Sertraline *on page 1254*

◆ **ratio-Simvastatin (Can)** *see* Simvastatin *on page 1263*

◆ **ratio-Sotalol (Can)** *see* Sotalol *on page 1284*

◆ **ratio-Sumatriptan (Can)** *see* SUMAtriptan *on page 1308*

◆ **ratio-Theo-Bronc (Can)** *see* Theophylline *on page 1335*

◆ **ratio-Topiramate (Can)** *see* Topiramate *on page 1360*

◆ **ratio-Trazodone (Can)** *see* TraZODone *on page 1371*

◆ **ratio-Valproic (Can)** *see* Valproic Acid and Derivatives *on page 1398*

◆ **ratio-Valproic ECC (Can)** *see* Valproic Acid and Derivatives *on page 1398*

◆ **ratio-Venlafaxine XR (Can)** *see* Venlafaxine *on page 1412*

◆ **Reactine™ (Can)** *see* Cetirizine *on page 283*

◆ **ReAzo [OTC]** *see* Phenazopyridine *on page 1097*

◆ **Rebetol®** *see* Ribavirin *on page 1210*

◆ **Recombinant α-L-Iduronidase (Glycosaminoglycan α-L-Iduronohydrolase)** *see* Laronidase *on page 803*

◆ **Recombinant Human Deoxyribonuclease** *see* Dornase Alfa *on page 473*

◆ **Recombinant Human Interleukin-2** *see* Aldesleukin *on page 60*

◆ **Recombinant Human Interleukin-11** *see* Oprelvekin *on page 1025*

◆ **Recombinant Interleukin-11** *see* Oprelvekin *on page 1025*

◆ **Recombinant Urate Oxidase** *see* Rasburicase *on page 1203*

◆ **Recombinate** *see* Antihemophilic Factor (Recombinant) *on page 112*

◆ **Recombivax HB®** *see* Hepatitis B Vaccine *on page 675*

◆ **Recothrom™** *see* Thrombin (Topical) *on page 1345*

◆ **Rectacaine [OTC]** *see* Phenylephrine *on page 1102*

◆ **Red Cross™ Canker Sore [OTC]** *see* Benzocaine *on page 182*

◆ **Reese's® Pinworm Medicine [OTC]** *see* Pyrantel Pamoate *on page 1187*

◆ **ReFacto® [DSC]** *see* Antihemophilic Factor (Recombinant) *on page 112*

◆ **ReFacto® (Can)** *see* Antihemophilic Factor (Recombinant) *on page 112*

◆ **Refenesen™ [OTC]** *see* GuaiFENesin *on page 656*

◆ **Refenesen™ 400 [OTC]** *see* GuaiFENesin *on page 656*

◆ **Refenesen™ DM [OTC]** *see* Guaifenesin and Dextromethorphan *on page 658*

◆ **Refissa™** *see* Tretinoin (Topical) *on page 1375*

◆ **Regenecare®** *see* Lidocaine *on page 818*

◆ **Regenecare® HA [OTC]** *see* Lidocaine *on page 818*

◆ **Regitine [DSC]** *see* Phentolamine *on page 1101*

◆ **Regitine® (Can)** *see* Phentolamine *on page 1101*

◆ **Reglan®** *see* Metoclopramide *on page 915*

◆ **Regonol®** *see* Pyridostigmine *on page 1189*

◆ **Regular Insulin** *see* Insulin Regular *on page 748*

◆ **Regulex® (Can)** *see* Docusate *on page 468*

◆ **Reguloid [OTC]** *see* Psyllium *on page 1185*

◆ **Rejuva-A® (Can)** *see* Tretinoin (Topical) *on page 1375*

◆ **Relenza®** *see* Zanamivir *on page 1440*

◆ **Reme-T™ [OTC]** *see* Coal Tar *on page 349*

◆ **Remicade®** *see* InFLIXimab *on page 728*

Remifentanil (rem i FEN ta nil)

Medication Safety Issues
Sound-alike/look-alike issues:
Remifentanil may be confused with alfentanil

High alert medication: The Institute for Safe Medication Practices (ISMP) includes this medication among its list of drug classes which have a heightened risk of causing significant patient harm when used in error.

U.S. Brand Names Ultiva®

Canadian Brand Names Ultiva®

Therapeutic Category Analgesic, Narcotic; General Anesthetic

Generic Available No

Use Analgesic for use during the induction and maintenance of general anesthesia; for continued analgesia into the immediate postoperative period; as the analgesic component of monitored anesthesia

Restrictions C-II

Pregnancy Risk Factor C

Pregnancy Considerations Remifentanil has been shown to cross the placenta. Neonatal respiratory depression and sedation may occur.

Lactation Excretion in breast milk unknown/use caution

Contraindications Hypersensitivity to remifentanil, fentanyl or fentanyl analogs, or any component; **not for intrathecal or epidural administration,** due to the presence of glycine in the formulation

Warnings Remifentanil is not recommended as the sole agent in general anesthesia, because the loss of consciousness cannot be assured and due to the high incidence of apnea, hypotension, tachycardia, and muscle rigidity; it should be administered by individuals specifically trained in the use of anesthetic agents and should not be used in diagnostic or therapeutic procedures outside the monitored anesthesia setting; resuscitative and intubation equipment should be readily available; monitor vital signs and oxygenation continuously during administration.

Rapid I.V. infusion (single doses of >1mcg/kg administered over 30-60 seconds or infusion rates >0.1mcg/kg/minute) may result in skeletal muscle and chest wall rigidity; administer slowly. Interruption of an infusion will result in offset of effects within 5-10 minutes; the discontinuation of remifentanil infusion should be preceded by the establishment of adequate postoperative analgesia orders, especially for patients in whom postoperative pain is anticipated

Precautions Use with caution in the morbidly obese

Adverse Reactions
Cardiovascular: Hypotension (dose dependent), bradycardia (dose dependent), tachycardia, hypertension, asystole, arrhythmias, heart block, syncope, CPK-MB increased

Central nervous system: Dizziness, headache, agitation, fever, hallucinations, anxiety, seizure, amnesia

Dermatologic: Pruritus, erythema, rash

Endocrine & metabolic: Hyperglycemia, electrolyte disorders

Gastrointestinal: Nausea, vomiting, constipation, abdominal discomfort, xerostomia, GERD, dysphagia, diarrhea, heartburn

Hematologic: Thrombocytopenia, anemia, leukocytosis, lymphopenia

Neuromuscular & skeletal: Muscle rigidity (dose and rate of infusion dependent), tremors

Ocular: Visual disturbances, nystagmus

Respiratory: Respiratory depression, apnea, hypoxia, cough, bronchospasm, stridor, pleural effusion, pulmonary edema

Miscellaneous: Shivering, postoperative pain, anaphylactic/anaphylactoid reactions

Drug Interactions

Avoid Concomitant Use
Avoid concomitant use of Remifentanil with any of the following: MAO Inhibitors

Increased Effect/Toxicity

Remifentanil may increase the levels/effects of: Alcohol (Ethyl); Alvimopan; Beta-Blockers; Calcium Channel Blockers (Nondihydropyridine); CNS Depressants; Desmopressin; MAO Inhibitors; Selective Serotonin Reuptake Inhibitors; Thiazide Diuretics

The levels/effects of Remifentanil may be increased by: Amphetamines; Antipsychotic Agents (Phenothiazines); Succinylcholine

Decreased Effect

Remifentanil may decrease the levels/effects of: Pegvisomant

The levels/effects of Remifentanil may be decreased by: Ammonium Chloride; Mixed Agonist / Antagonist Opioids

Stability Prior to reconstitution, store at 2°C to 25°C (36°F to 77°F). Stable for 24 hours at room temperature after reconstitution and further dilution to concentrations of 20-250 mcg/mL in D_5LR, D_5NS, D_5W, 1/2NS, NS, (4 hours if diluted with LR).

Y-site administration: Compatible: Acyclovir, alfentanil, amikacin, aminophylline, ampicillin, ampicillin/sulbactam, aztreonam, bretylium, bumetanide, buprenorphine, butorphanol, calcium gluconate, cefazolin, cefotaxime, cefotetan, cefoxitin, ceftazidime, ceftizoxime, ceftriaxone, cefuroxime, cimetidine, ciprofloxacin, cisatracurium, clindamycin, dexamethasone sodium phosphate, digoxin, diphenhydramine, dobutamine, dopamine, doxycycline, droperidol, enalaprilat, epinephrine, esmolol, famotidine, fentanyl, fluconazole, furosemide, ganciclovir gatifloxacin, gentamicin, haloperidol, heparin, hydrocortisone sodium succinate, hydromorphone, hydroxyzine, imipenem/cilastatin, inamrinone, isoproterenol, ketorolac, lidocaine, linezolid, lorazepam, magnesium sulfate, mannitol, meperidine, methylprednisolone sodium succinate, metoclopramide, metronidazole, midazolam, minocycline, morphine, nalbuphine, netilmicin, nitroglycerin, norepinephrine, ofloxacin, ondansetron, phenylephrine, piperacillin, piperacillin/tazobactam, potassium chloride, procainamide, prochlorperazine, propofol, promethazine, ranitidine, sodium bicarbonate, sufentanil, theophylline, thiopental, ticarcillin, ticarcillin/clavulanate potassium, tobramycin, trimethoprim/sulfamethoxazole, vancomycin, zidovudine.

Mechanism of Action Binds with stereospecific mu-opioid receptors at many sites within the CNS, increases pain threshold, alters pain reception, inhibits ascending pain pathways

Pharmacodynamics

Onset of action: 1-3 minutes

Maximum effect: 3-5 minutes

Duration: 3-10 minutes

Pharmacokinetics (Adult data unless noted)

Distribution: V_d:

Neonates <2 months: 452 ± 144 mL/kg

Children 2-6 years: 240 mL/kg

Children 7-12 years: 249 mL/kg

Adolescents: 223 ± 30.6 mL/kg

Adults: 100-176 mL/kg

Protein binding: ~70% (primarily alpha$_1$ acid glycoprotein)

Metabolism: Rapid via blood and tissue esterases; not metabolized by plasma cholinesterase (pseudocholinesterase) and is not appreciably metabolized by the liver

Half-life (dose dependent): Terminal: 10-20 minutes; effective: 3-10 minutes

Elimination: Clearance:

Neonates <2 months of age: 90.5 ± 36.8 mL/minute/kg

Adolescents: 57.2 ± 21.2 mL/minute/kg

Adults: 41.2 mL/minute/kg

Usual Dosage I.V. continuous infusion: Dose should be based on ideal body weight (IBW) in obese patients (>30% over IBW).

Children birth to 2 months: Maintenance of anesthesia with nitrous oxide (70%): 0.4 mcg/kg/minute (range: 0.4-1 mcg/kg/minute); supplemental bolus dose of 1 mcg/kg may be administered, smaller bolus dose may be required with potent inhalation agents, potent neuraxial anesthesia, significant comorbidities, significant fluid shifts, or without atropine pretreatment. Clearance in neonates is highly variable; dose should be carefully titrated.

Children 1-12 years: Maintenance of anesthesia with halothane, sevoflurane, or isoflurane: 0.25 mcg/kg/minute (range 0.05-1.3 mcg/kg/minute); supplemental bolus dose of 1 mcg/kg may be administered every 2-5 minutes. Consider increasing concomitant anesthetics with infusion rate >1 mcg/kg/minute. Infusion rate can be titrated upward in increments up to 50% or titrated downward in decrements of 25% to 50%. May titrate every 2-5 minutes.

Adults:

Induction of anesthesia: 0.5-1 mcg/kg/minute; if endotracheal intubation is to occur in <8 minutes, an initial dose of 1 mcg/kg may be given over 30-60 seconds; in coronary bypass surgery: 1 mcg/kg/minute

Maintenance of anesthesia: **Note:** Supplemental bolus dose of 1 mcg/kg may be administered every 2-5 minutes. Consider increasing concomitant anesthetics with infusion rate >1 mcg/kg/minute. Infusion rate can be titrated upward in increments of 25% to 100% or downward in decrements of 25% to 50%. May titrate every 2-5 minutes.

With nitrous oxide (66%): 0.4 mcg/kg/minute (range: 0.1-2 mcg/kg/minute)

With isoflurane: 0.25 mcg/kg/minute (range: 0.05-2 mcg/kg/minute)

With propofol: 0.25 mcg/kg/minute (range: 0.05-2 mcg/kg/minute)

Coronary bypass surgery: 1 mcg/kg/minute (range: 0.125-4 mcg/kg/minute); supplemental dose: 0.5-1 mcg/kg

Continuation as an analgesic in immediate postoperative period: 0.1 mcg/kg/minute (range: 0.025-0.2 mcg/kg/minute). Infusion rate may be adjusted every 5 minutes in increments of 0.025 mcg/kg/minute. Bolus doses are not recommended. Infusion rates >0.2 mcg/kg/minute are associated with respiratory depression.

Coronary bypass surgery, continuation as an analgesic into the ICU: 1 mcg/kg/minute (range: 0.05-1 mcg/kg/minute)

Analgesic component of monitored anesthesia care: **Note:** Supplemental oxygen is recommended:

Single I.V. dose given 90 seconds prior to local anesthetic:

Remifentanil alone: 1 mcg/kg over 30-60 seconds

With midazolam: 0.5 mcg/kg over 30-60 seconds

Continuous infusion beginning 5 minutes prior to local anesthetic:

Remifentanil alone: 0.1 mcg/kg/minute

With midazolam: 0.05 mcg/kg/minute

Continuous infusion given after local anesthetic:

Remifentanil alone: 0.05 mcg/kg/minute (range: 0.025-0.2 mcg/kg/minute)

With midazolam: 0.025 mcg/kg/minute (range: 0.025-0.2 mcg/kg/minute)

Note: Following local or anesthetic block, infusion rate should be decreased to 0.05 mcg/kg/minute; rate adjustments of 0.025 mcg/kg/minute may be done at 5-minute intervals

Mechanically-ventilated patients: Acute pain (moderate-to-severe): 0.6-15 mcg/kg/hour

Administration I.V.: Prepare solution by adding 1 mL of diluent per 1 mg of remifentanil. Shake well. Further dilute to a final concentration of 20, 25, 50, or 250 mcg/mL in compatible I.V. solution (see Stability). An infusion device should be used to administer continuous infusions. During the maintenance of general anesthesia, I.V. boluses ≤1 mcg/kg may be administered over 30-60 seconds; for doses >1 mcg/kg, administer over >60 seconds (to reduce the potential to develop skeletal muscle and chest wall rigidity). Injections should be given into I.V. tubing close to the venous cannula; tubing should be cleared after treatment to prevent residual effects when other fluids are administered through the same I.V. line.

Monitoring Parameters Respiratory and cardiovascular status, blood pressure, heart rate

Dosage Forms Excipient information presented when available (limited, particularly for generics); consult specific product labeling.

Injection, powder for reconstitution: 1 mg, 2 mg, 5 mg [contains glycine 15 mg]

References

"Clinical Practice Guidelines for the Sustained Use of Sedatives and Analgesics in the Critically Ill Adult. Task Force of the American College of Critical Care Medicine (ACCM) of the Society of Critical Care Medicine (SCCM), American Society of Health-System Pharmacists (ASHP), American College of Chest Physicians," *Am J Health Syst Pharm*, 2002, 59(2):150-78.

Scott LJ and Perry CM, "Remifentanil: A Review of Its Use During the Induction and Maintenance of General Anaesthesia," *Drugs*, 2005, 65 (13):1793-823.

◆ **Renagel®** *see* Sevelamer *on page 1257*

◆ **Renova®** *see* Tretinoin (Topical) *on page 1375*

◆ **Renvela®** *see* Sevelamer *on page 1257*

◆ **Requa® Activated Charcoal [OTC]** *see* Charcoal, Activated *on page 284*

◆ **Resectisol®** *see* Mannitol *on page 861*

◆ **Respa-DM®** *see* Guaifenesin and Dextromethorphan *on page 658*

◆ **Respahist®** *see* Brompheniramine and Pseudoephedrine *on page 205*

◆ **Restasis®** *see* CycloSPORINE *on page 372*

◆ **Retin-A®** *see* Tretinoin (Topical) *on page 1375*

◆ **Retin-A® Micro** *see* Tretinoin (Topical) *on page 1375*

◆ **Retinoic Acid** *see* Tretinoin (Topical) *on page 1375*

◆ **Retinova® (Can)** *see* Tretinoin (Topical) *on page 1375*

◆ **Retisert®** *see* Fluocinolone *on page 593*

◆ **Retrovir®** *see* Zidovudine *on page 1442*

◆ **Retrovir® (AZT™) (Can)** *see* Zidovudine *on page 1442*

◆ **Revatio®** *see* Sildenafil *on page 1258*

◆ **Revitalose C-1000® (Can)** *see* Ascorbic Acid *on page 138*

◆ **Reyataz®** *see* Atazanavir *on page 144*

◆ **rFVIIa** *see* Factor VIIa (Recombinant) *on page 556*

◆ **R-Gene® 10** *see* Arginine *on page 131*

◆ **rhAPC** *see* Drotrecogin Alfa (Activated) *on page 484*

◆ **rhDNase** *see* Dornase Alfa *on page 473*

◆ **Rheumatrex®** *see* Methotrexate *on page 900*

◆ **rhGAA** *see* Alglucosidase Alfa *on page 64*

◆ **r-h α-GAL** *see* Agalsidase Beta *on page 53*

◆ **RhIG** *see* Rh₀(D) Immune Globulin *on page 1207*

◆ **rhIL-11** *see* Oprelvekin *on page 1025*

◆ **Rhinalar® (Can)** *see* Flunisolide *on page 592*

◆ **Rhinall [OTC]** *see* Phenylephrine *on page 1102*

◆ **Rhinaris-CS Anti-Allergic Nasal Mist (Can)** *see* Cromolyn *on page 363*

◆ **Rhinocort® Aqua®** *see* Budesonide *on page 206*

◆ **Rhinocort® Aqua™ (Can)** *see* Budesonide *on page 206*

◆ **Rhinocort® Turbuhaler® (Can)** *see* Budesonide *on page 206*

◆ **Rho(D) Immune Globulin (Human)** *see* Rh₀(D) Immune Globulin *on page 1207*

◆ **Rho®-Clonazepam (Can)** *see* ClonazePAM *on page 337*

Rh₀(D) Immune Globulin

(ar aych oh (dee) i MYUN GLOB yoo lin)

U.S. Brand Names HyperRHO™ S/D Full Dose; Hyper-RHO™ S/D Mini Dose; MICRhoGAM®; RhoGAM®; Rhophylac®; WinRho® SDF

Canadian Brand Names WinRho® SDF

Therapeutic Category Immune Globulin

Generic Available No

Use

Suppression of Rh isoimmunization: Use in the following situations when an Rh₀(D)-negative individual is exposed to Rh₀(D)-positive blood: During delivery of an Rh₀(D)-positive infant; abortion; amniocentesis; chorionic villus sampling; ruptured tubal pregnancy; abdominal trauma; transplacental hemorrhage. Used when the mother is Rh₀(D) negative, the father of the child is either Rh₀(D) positive or Rh₀(D) unknown, the baby is either Rh₀(D) positive or Rh₀(D) unknown.

Transfusion: Suppression of Rh isoimmunization in Rh₀(D)-negative female children and female adults in their childbearing years transfused with Rh₀(D) antigen-positive RBCs or blood components containing Rh₀(D) antigen-positive RBCs

Treatment of idiopathic thrombocytopenic purpura (ITP): **WinRho® SDF only:** Used in the following nonsplenectomized Rh₀(D) positive individuals: Children with acute or chronic ITP, adults with chronic ITP, children and adults with ITP secondary to HIV infection

Pregnancy Risk Factor C

Pregnancy Considerations Animal studies have not been conducted. Available evidence suggests that Rh₀(D) immune globulin administration during pregnancy does not harm the fetus or affect future pregnancies.

Lactation Does not enter breast milk

Contraindications Hypersensitivity to immune globulin, thimerosal (RhoGAM® formulation) or any component; IgA deficiency; Rh₀(D)-positive mother or pregnant woman; transfusion of Rh₀(D)-positive blood in previous 3 months; prior sensitization to Rh₀(D); mothers whose Rh group or immune status is uncertain

Warnings Rare postmarketing reports of severe, sometimes fatal, intravascular hemolysis including DIC; symptoms including back pain, shaking chills, fever, and discolored urine have occurred in most cases within 4 hours of administration. Serious complications of intravascular hemolysis (anemia, ARF, or DIC) have in some cases been fatal.

Use only WinRho® SDF when treating ITP; when treating ITP, a decrease in hemoglobin concentration as a result of destruction of Rh₀(D)-positive red blood cells can be expected; reduce WinRho® SDF dosage in ITP patients with Hgb <10 g/dL (see Usual Dosage) to minimize the risk of increasing the severity of anemia. These patients should be monitored for signs and/or symptoms of intravascular hemolysis, clinically compromising anemia, and renal insufficiency

When used to suppress Rh isoimmunization, the drug is administered to the mother **not** the infant; anaphylactic hypersensitivity reactions can occur; studies indicate that there is no discernible risk of transmitting HIV or hepatitis B; not intended for use as immunoglobulin replacement therapy for immune deficiency syndromes

Precautions Use with caution in patients with thrombocytopenia or bleeding disorders or in patients with hemoglobin concentrations <8 g/dL; may cause false-positive glucose levels (see Test Interactions)

Adverse Reactions
Cardiovascular: Hypotension, pallor, tachycardia, vasodilation (I.V. formulation), hypertension

Central nervous system: Fever, headache, chills, dizziness, somnolence, lethargy, malaise

Dermatologic: Rash, pruritus

Gastrointestinal: Abdominal pain, diarrhea, splenomegaly, nausea, vomiting

Genitourinary: Hemoglobinuria

Hematologic: Hemoglobin decreased (hemoglobin decrease >2 g/dL in 5% to 10% of ITP patients), intravascular hemolysis (rare; see Warnings), DIC (rare; see Warnings)

Hepatic: Bilirubin elevated, LDH elevated

Local: Discomfort and swelling at injection site

Neuromuscular & skeletal: Back pain, myalgia, hyperkinesia, arthralgia, weakness, hyperkinesia

Renal: Acute renal failure (rare; see Warnings)

Miscellaneous: Hypersensitivity reactions, diaphoresis

Drug Interactions
Avoid Concomitant Use There are no known interactions where it is recommended to avoid concomitant use.

Increased Effect/Toxicity There are no known significant interactions involving an increase in effect.

Decreased Effect
Rho(D) Immune Globulin may decrease the levels/effects of: Vaccines (Live)

Stability Refrigerate, do not freeze; RhoGAM® and BayRho-D® are stable for up to 30 days at room temperature; WinRho® SDF, once reconstituted, is stable for 12 hours at room temperature

Mechanism of Action The Rh_o(D) antigen is responsible for most cases of Rh sensitization, which occurs when Rh-positive fetal RBCs enter the maternal circulation of an Rh-negative woman. Injection of anti-D globulin results in opsonization of the fetal RBCs, which are then phagocytized in the spleen, preventing immunization of the mother. Injection of anti-D into an Rh-positive patient with ITP coats the patient's own D-positive RBCs with antibody and, as they are cleared by the spleen, they saturate the capacity of the spleen to clear antibody-coated cells, sparing antibody-coated platelets. Other proposed mechanisms involve the generation of cytokines following the interaction between antibody-coated RBCs and macrophages.

Pharmacodynamics
Onset of action:

Rh isoimmunization: I.V.: 8 hours

ITP: I.V.: 1-2 days

Maximum effect: ITP: 7-14 days

Duration:

ITP (single dose): I.V.: 30 days

Passive anti-Rh_o(D) antibodies (after 120 mcg dose): I.V.: 6 weeks

Pharmacokinetics (Adult data unless noted)
Distribution: Appears in breast milk, however, not absorbed by the nursing infant

Half-life, elimination:

I.M.: 18-30 days

I.V.: 16-24 days

Time to peak serum concentration:

I.M.: 5-10 days

I.V.: 2 hours

Usual Dosage
ITP: Children and Adults: **WinRho® SDF only:**

Manufacturer's recommendations:

Initial:

Hemoglobin ≥10 g/dL: 50 mcg/kg (250 international units/kg) as single dose or divided into 2 doses given on separate days

Hemoglobin <10 g/dL: 25-40 mcg/kg (125-200 international units/kg) as single dose or divided into 2 doses given on separate days

Hemoglobin <8 g/dL: Use with caution (see Warnings and Precautions)

Maintenance (usage dependent upon clinical response, platelet count, hemoglobin, red blood cell counts, and reticulocyte levels)

Response to initial dose: 25-60 mcg/kg (125-300 international units/kg) as single dose

Nonresponse to initial therapy:

Hemoglobin >10 g/dL: 50-60 mcg/kg (250-300 international units/kg) as single dose

Hemoglobin 8-10 g/dL: 25-40 mcg/kg (125-200 international units/kg) as single dose

Hemoglobin <8 g/dL: Use with caution (see Warnings and Precautions)

Alternative dosing:

New Onset: 75 mcg/kg (375 international units/kg) as a single dose has been used in pediatric patients with platelets of ≤20,000/μL.

Suppression of RH isoimmunization: **Adult female:** I.V., I.M.: See table on next page

Rh₀(D) Immune Globulin Dosage in Pregnancy and Obstetrical Conditions

Condition	WinRho® SDF Dosage I.V. or I.M.	BayRho-D® or RhoGAM® Dosage I.M.	Rhophylac® Dosage I.V. or I.M
Pregnancy	300 mcg (1500 international units) at 28 weeks gestation; repeat every 12 weeks throughout pregnancy	300 mcg at 28 weeks and following delivery, preferably within 72 hours of delivery	300 mcg at 28-30 weeks of gestation
Postpartum (if newborn Rh-positive)	120 mcg (600 international units) as soon as possible, preferably <72 hours, after delivery; if baby's Rh status is not known by 72 hours administer as soon as possible up to 28 days after delivery	300 mcg as soon as possible, preferably within 72 hours of delivery	300 mcg within 72 hours of delivery
Threatened abortion at any time	300 mcg (1500 international units) as soon as possible within 72 hours	300 mcg as soon as possible	300 mcg as soon as possible
Amniocentesis and chronic villus sampling	Before 34 weeks gestation: 300 mcg (1500 international units) administered immediately; repeat every 12 weeks throughout pregnancy After 34 weeks gestation: 120 mcg (600 international units) administered immediately or within 72 hours	At 15-18 weeks gestation or during the 3rd trimester: 300 mcg; if given between 13-18 weeks, repeat at 26-28 weeks and within 72 hours of delivery	300 mcg as soon as possible
Abortion, miscarriage, termination of ectopic pregnancy	After 34 weeks gestation: 120 mcg (600 international units) administered immediately or within 72 hours	<13 weeks gestation: 50 mcg ≥13 weeks gestation: 300 mcg administered immediately or within 72 hours	300 mcg as soon as possible
Abdominal trauma, manipulation	After 34 weeks gestation: 120 mcg (600 international units) administered immediately or within 72 hours	During the 2nd or 3rd trimester: 300 mcg; if given between 13-18 weeks, repeat at 26-28 weeks and within 72 hours of delivery	300 mcg as soon as possible

Note: One "full dose" (300 mcg) provides enough antibody to prevent Rh sensitization if the volume of fetal RBCs entering the maternal circulation is ≤15 mL. When >15 mL is suspected, a fetal red cell count should be performed to determine the appropriate dose.

Treatment of exposure to incompatible blood transfusion or massive fetal hemorrhage, within 72 hours of event:

Exposure to Rh₀(D) positive whole blood: Children and Adults:

WinRho® SDF:

I.M.: 12 mcg (60 international units)/mL blood; administer in 1200 mcg (6000 international units) aliquots every 12 hours until the total calculated dose is administered

I.V.: 9 mcg (45 international units)/mL blood; administer in 600 mcg (3000 international units) aliquots every 8 hours until the total calculated dose is administered

Exposure to Rh₀(D) positive red blood cells:

I.M.: 24 mcg (120 international units)/mL cells administer in 1200 mcg (6000 international units) aliquots every 12 hours until the total calculated dose is administered

I.V.: 18 mcg (90 international units)/mL cells; administer in 600 mcg (3000 international units) aliquots every 8 hours until the total calculated dose is administered

BayRho-D®, RhoGAM®: Adults: I.M.: Multiply the volume of Rh-positive whole blood administered by the hematocrit of the donor unit to equal the volume of RBCs transfused. The volume of RBCs is then divided by 15 mL, resulting in the number of 300 mcg doses to administer. If the dose calculated results in a fraction, round up to the next higher whole 300 mcg dose.

Rhophylac®: Adults: I.M., I.V.: 100 international units (20 mcg) per 2 mL transfused blood or per 1 mL erythrocyte concentrate

Administration Parenteral: WinRho® SDF and Rhophylac® are the only immune globulin products available that can be administered both I.M. and I.V.; however, **for the treatment of ITP, only WinRho SDF® is approved for use and it must be administered I.V.**

I.M.: Administer into the deltoid muscle of upper arm or the anterolateral aspect of the upper thigh; the gluteal region is not recommended for routine administration due to the potential risk of sciatic nerve injury; if gluteal area is used, administer only in the upper, outer quadrant. The total volume can be given in divided doses at different sites at one time or may be divided and given at intervals provided the total dosage is given within 72 hours of the fetomaternal hemorrhage or transfusion

WinRho® SDF: Reconstitute 120 mcg and 300 mcg vials with 1.25 mL NS and the 100 mcg vial with 8.5 mL NS; gently swirl vial; do not shake

I.V.: WinRho® SDF, Rhophylac®: Infuse without further dilution over 3-5 minutes

Monitoring Parameters ITP: Signs and symptoms of intravascular hemolysis, CBC, reticulocytes, UA, renal function, platelets, liver function, DIC-specific tests (eg, FSP, fibrin degradation products, or D-dimer) if applicable

Test Interactions Maltose, present in liquid formulation of Rh₀(D) immune globulin, may cause falsely elevated glucose when using glucose dehydrogenase pyrroloquinolinequinone (GDH-PQQ) or glucose-dye-oxidoreductase methods.

Patient Information Report symptoms of intravascular hemolysis (eg, back pain, shaking chills, fever, discolored urine, decreased urination, sudden weight gain, fluid retention, and shortness of breath) to your healthcare provider immediately.

Additional Information WinRho® SDF 1 mcg = 5 international units

Treatment of ITP in Rh-positive patients with an intact spleen appears to be about as effective as IVIG.

Dosage Forms Excipient information presented when available (limited, particularly for generics); consult specific product labeling. [DSC] = Discontinued product

Injection, solution [preservative free]:

HyperRHO™ S/D Full Dose: 300 mcg [for I.M. use only]

HyperRHO™ S/D Mini Dose: 50 mcg [for I.M. use only]

MICRhoGAM®: 50 mcg [for I.M. use only; contains polysorbate 80]

RhoGAM®: 300 mcg [for I.M. use only; contains polysorbate 80]

Rhophylac®: 300 mcg/2 mL (2 mL) [1500 int. units; for I.M. or I.V. use; contains human albumin]

WinRho® SDF:

120 mcg/~0.5 mL (~0.5 mL) [600 int. units; contains maltose and polysorbate 80; for I.M. or I.V. use] [DSC]

300 mcg/~1.3 mL (~1.3 mL) [1500 int. units; contains maltose and polysorbate 80; for I.M. or I.V. use]

500 mcg/~2.2 mL (~2.2 mL) [2500 int. units; contains maltose and polysorbate 80; for I.M. or I.V. use]

1000 mcg/~4.4 mL (~4.4 mL) [5000 int. units; contains maltose and polysorbate 80; for I.M. or I.V. use]

3000 mcg/~13 mL (~13 mL) [15,000 int. units; contains maltose and polysorbate 80; for I.M. or I.V. use]

References

Gaines AR, "Acute Onset Hemoglobinemia and/or Hemoglobinuria and Sequelae Following Rh(o)(D) Immune Globulin Intravenous Administration in Immune Thrombocytopenic Purpura Patients," *Blood*, 2000, 95(8):2523-9.

Shahgholi E, Vosough P, Sotoudeh K, et al, "Intravenous Immune Globulin Versus Intravenous Anti-D Immune Globulin for the Treatment of Acute Immune Thrombocytopenic Purpura," *Indian J Pediatr*, 2008, 75(12):1231-5.

Tarantino MD, Young G, Bertolone SJ, et al, "Single Dose of Anti-D Immune Globulin at 75 Microg/kg Is as Effective as Intravenous Immune Globulin at Rapidly Raising the Platelet Count in Newly Diagnosed Immune Thrombocytopenic Purpura in Children," *J Pediatr*, 2006, 148(4):489-94.

◆ **RhoGAM®** *see* Rhₒ(D) Immune Globulin *on page 1207*

◆ **RhoIGIV** *see* Rhₒ(D) Immune Globulin *on page 1207*

◆ **RhoIVIM** *see* Rhₒ(D) Immune Globulin *on page 1207*

◆ **Rho®-Loperamine (Can)** *see* Loperamide *on page 838*

◆ **Rho®-Nitro (Can)** *see* Nitroglycerin *on page 996*

◆ **Rhophylac®** *see* Rhₒ(D) Immune Globulin *on page 1207*

◆ **Rhoxal-cyclosporine (Can)** *see* CycloSPORINE *on page 372*

◆ **Rhoxal-fluvoxamine (Can)** *see* Fluvoxamine *on page 615*

◆ **Rhoxal-loperamide (Can)** *see* Loperamide *on page 838*

◆ **Rhoxal-pamidronate (Can)** *see* Pamidronate *on page 1048*

◆ **Rhoxal-sotalol (Can)** *see* Sotalol *on page 1284*

◆ **Rhoxal-sumatriptan (Can)** *see* SUMAtriptan *on page 1308*

◆ **Rhoxal-valproic (Can)** *see* Valproic Acid and Derivatives *on page 1398*

◆ *r*HuEPO-α *see* Epoetin Alfa *on page 513*

◆ **rhuGM-CSF** *see* Sargramostim *on page 1247*

◆ **rhuMAb-E25** *see* Omalizumab *on page 1014*

◆ **rhuMAb-VEGF** *see* Bevacizumab *on page 192*

◆ **RibaPak™ [DSC]** *see* Ribavirin *on page 1210*

◆ **Ribasphere®** *see* Ribavirin *on page 1210*

◆ **Ribasphere® RibaPak®** *see* Ribavirin *on page 1210*

Ribavirin (rye ba VYE rin)

Medication Safety Issues

Sound-alike/look-alike issues:
Ribavirin may be confused with riboflavin, rifampin, Robaxin®

U.S. Brand Names Copegus®; Rebetol®; RibaPak™ [DSC]; Ribasphere®; Ribasphere® RibaPak®; Virazole®

Canadian Brand Names Virazole®

Therapeutic Category Antiviral Agent, Inhalation Therapy

Generic Available Yes: Capsule, tablet

Use

Inhalation: Treatment of patients with RSV infections; specially indicated for treatment of severe lower respiratory tract RSV infections in patients with an underlying compromising condition (prematurity, BPD and other chronic lung conditions, congenital heart disease, immunodeficiency, immunosuppression), and recent transplant recipients; may also be used in other viral infections including influenza A and B and adenovirus

Oral solution: Used in combination with interferon alfa-2b, recombinant injection for the treatment of chronic hepatitic C in patients ≥3 years of age with compensated liver disease who were previously untreated with alpha interferon or patients ≥18 years of age who have relapsed after alpha interferon therapy

Oral capsule: Used in combination with interferon alfa-2b, recombinant injection for the treatment of chronic hepatitis C in patients with compensated liver disease who have relapsed after alpha interferon therapy or were previously untreated with alpha interferon; or used in combination with peginterferon alfa-2b, recombinant injection for the treatment of chronic hepatitis C in patients with compensated liver disease who were previously untreated with alpha interferon

Oral tablet: Used in combination with peginterferon alfa-2a, recombinant injection for the treatment of chronic hepatitis C in patients with compensated liver disease who were previously untreated with alpha interferon

Medication Guide An FDA-approved patient medication guide, which is available with the product information and as follows, must be dispensed with this medication for each new outpatient prescription and refill.

Copegus®: http://www.fda.gov/downloads/Drugs/Drug-Safety/ucm088576.pdf,

Rebetol®: http://www.fda.gov/downloads/Drugs/DrugSafety/ucm089017.pdf

Ribasphere®: http://www.fda.gov/downloads/Drugs/DrugSafety/ucm111342.pdf

Pregnancy Risk Factor X

Pregnancy Considerations [U.S. Boxed Warning]: Significant teratogenic effects have been observed in all animal studies at ~0.01 times the maximum recommended daily human dose. Use is contraindicated in pregnancy. Negative pregnancy test is required before initiation and monthly thereafter. Avoid pregnancy in female patients and female partners of male patients during therapy by using two effective forms of contraception; continue contraceptive measures for at least 6 months after completion of therapy. If patient or female partner becomes pregnant during treatment, she should be counseled about potential risks of exposure. If pregnancy occurs during use or within 6 months after treatment, report to the ribavirin pregnancy registry (800-593-2214).

Lactation Excretion in breast milk unknown/not recommended

Contraindications Hypersensitivity to ribavirin or any component; pregnancy

Additional contraindications for oral formulation: Men whose female partners are pregnant; patients with hemoglobinopathies (ie, thalassemia major, sickle cell anemia); autoimmune hepatitis; as monotherapy for treatment of chronic hepatitis C; pancreatitis; patients with significant or unstable cardiac disease; Cl_{cr} <50 mL/minute; coadministration with didanosine (cases of fatal hepatic failure, peripheral neuropathy, pancreatitis, and hyperlactatemia/lactic acidosis have been reported; see Drug Interactions)

Additional contraindications for ribavirin tablet used in combination with peginterferon alfa-2a: Hepatic impairment (Child-Pugh score >6; class B or C) in cirrhotic chronic hepatitis C monoinfected patients before or during treatment; hepatic impairment (Child-Pugh score ≥6) in cirrhotic chronic hepatitis C patients coinfected with HIV before or during treatment

Warnings Hazardous agent; use appropriate precautions for handling and disposal. Ribavirin is potentially mutagenic, tumor-promoting, and gonadotoxic; ribavirin may cause birth defects and/or death of the exposed fetus **[U.S. Boxed Warning]**. Avoid pregnancy in female patients and female partners of male patients for 6 months after therapy. Pregnant healthcare workers should not be administering aerosolized ribavirin due to risk of exposure. A primary adverse effect of oral ribavirin is hemolytic anemia which may worsen cardiac disease and lead to myocardial infarction **[U.S. Boxed Warning]**. The anemia usually occurs within 1-2 weeks of therapy initiation. Closely monitor hemoglobin or hematocrit pretreatment and during the first 4 weeks of therapy. Patients with underlying cardiac disease should have an ECG performed prior to initiation of oral ribavirin therapy. Severe depression and suicidal ideation have occurred during ribavirin/pegylated interferon alfa-2a therapy (avoid use in patients with a history of depression or psychiatric disorder).

Ribavirin oral solution contains sodium benzoate; benzoic acid (benzoate) is a metabolite of benzyl alcohol; large amounts of benzyl alcohol (≥99 mg/kg/day) have been associated with a potentially fatal toxicity ("gasping syndrome") in neonates; the "gasping syndrome" consists of metabolic acidosis, respiratory distress, gasping respirations, CNS dysfunction (including convulsions, intracranial hemorrhage), hypotension and cardiovascular collapse; avoid use of ribavirin products containing sodium benzoate in neonates; *in vitro* and animal studies have shown that benzoate displaces bilirubin from protein binding sites.

Inhalation: Use with caution in patients requiring assisted ventilation because precipitation of the drug in the respiratory equipment may interfere with safe and effective patient ventilation **[U.S. Boxed Warning]**. Sudden respiratory deterioration has been observed during the initiation of aerosolized ribavirin in infants **[U.S. Boxed Warning]**; carefully monitor infants and carefully monitor patients with COPD and asthma for deterioration of respiratory function

Precautions Oral: Use with caution in patients with pre-existing cardiac disease, patients with evidence of pulmonary infiltrates or pulmonary function impairment (closely monitor), or patients with sarcoidosis (may exacerbate sarcoidosis)

Adverse Reactions

Inhalation:

Cardiovascular: Hypotension, cardiac arrest

Central nervous system: Headache

Dermatologic: Rash, skin irritation

Hematologic: Anemia

Ocular: Conjunctivitis

Respiratory: Mild bronchospasm, worsening of respiratory function, nasal and throat irritation

Oral (documented adverse reactions while receiving combination therapy with interferon alfa-2b):

Cardiovascular: MI, chest pain, arrhythmia

Central nervous system: Depression, suicidal ideation, fever, emotional lability, insomnia, irritability, impaired concentration, headache, fatigue, dizziness, asthenia

Dermatologic: Rash, alopecia, pruritus, urticaria, angioedema

Endocrine & metabolic: Diabetes

Gastrointestinal: Nausea, anorexia, dyspepsia, vomiting, bloody diarrhea, taste perversion, pancreatitis, GI bleeding

Hematologic: Hemolytic anemia (maximum decrease in hemoglobin usually occurs during the first 8 weeks of ribavirin therapy), neutropenia, leukopenia, thrombocytopenia

Hepatic: Hepatic failure

Neuromuscular & skeletal: Myalgia, arthralgia, weakness, pain, peripheral neuropathy

Respiratory: Dyspnea, cough, pharyngitis, nasal congestion, sinusitis, pulmonary infiltrates

Miscellaneous: Flu-like symptoms, anaphylaxis, bacterial infection, autoimmune disorders

Note: Fever, anemia, vomiting, emotional lability, and suicidal ideation occurred more frequently in pediatric patients receiving oral ribavirin with interferon alfa compared to adults.

Drug Interactions

Avoid Concomitant Use

Avoid concomitant use of Ribavirin with any of the following: Didanosine

Increased Effect/Toxicity

Ribavirin may increase the levels/effects of: AzaTHIOprine; Didanosine; Reverse Transcriptase Inhibitors (Nucleoside)

The levels/effects of Ribavirin may be increased by: Interferons (Alfa); Zidovudine

Decreased Effect

Ribavirin may decrease the levels/effects of: Influenza Virus Vaccine (H1N1, Live/Attenuated); Influenza Virus Vaccine (Live/Attenuated)

Food Interactions Fatty meal increases bioavailability of oral ribavirin.

Stability

Inhalation: Reconstituted solution is stable for 24 hours at room temperature; do not mix with other aerosolized medications

Oral: Store capsules, tablets, and solution at room temperature; oral solution may also be refrigerated

Mechanism of Action Inhibits replication of RNA and DNA viruses; inhibits influenza virus RNA polymerase activity and interferes with the expression of messenger RNA resulting in inhibition of viral protein synthesis

Pharmacokinetics (Adult data unless noted)

Absorption: Inhalation: Systemically absorbed from the respiratory tract following nasal and oral inhalation; absorption is dependent upon respiratory factors and method of drug delivery; maximal absorption occurs with the use of the aerosol generator via an endotracheal tube

Distribution: Highest concentrations are found in the respiratory tract and erythrocytes; with chronic oral administration, ribavirin distributes slowly into CSF

Metabolism: Occurs intracellularly and may be necessary for drug action; metabolized by the liver to deribosylated ribavirin (active metabolite)

Bioavailability: Oral: 64%

Half-life:

Respiratory tract secretions: ~2 hours

Plasma:

Children: Inhalation: 6.5-11 hours

Adults: Oral: 24-36 hours after a single dose; half-life is much longer in the erythrocyte (16-40 days), which can be used as a marker for intracellular metabolism; terminal half-life after multiple doses is 151 hours

Time to peak serum concentration: Aerosol inhalation: At the end of the inhalation period

Oral capsule: 3 hours

Tablet: 2 hours

Elimination: Hepatic metabolism is the major route of elimination with 40% of the drug cleared renally as unchanged drug and metabolites

Usual Dosage

Infants, Children, and Adults: Aerosol inhalation:

Use with Viratek® small particle aerosol generator (SPAG-2) at a concentration of 20 mg/mL (6 g reconstituted with 300 mL of sterile water without preservatives); 6 g ribavirin vial has also been diluted with 300 mL of sterile NS solution rather than sterile water to achieve a near isotonic solution.

Note: Dose actually delivered to the patient will depend on patient's minute ventilation

Continuous aerosolization: 12-18 hours/day for 3 days, or up to 7 days in length

Intermittent aerosolization (high-dose, short-duration aerosol): 2 g over 2 hours 3 times/day at a concentration of 60 mg/mL (6 g reconstituted with 100 mL of sterile water without preservatives) in **nonmechanically ventilated** patients for 3-7 days has been used to permit easier accessibility for patient care and limit environmental exposure of healthcare worker. Due to apparent increased potential for crystallization of the high-dose 60 mg/mL solution around areas of turbulent flow such as bends in tubing or connector pieces, use of high-dose therapy in individuals with an endotracheal tube in place is **not** recommended.

Children ≥3 years: Chronic hepatitis C (in combination with interferon alfa-2b):

Oral capsule or solution: 15 mg/kg/day in 2 divided doses (morning and evening)

25-36 kg: 200 mg twice daily

37-49 kg: 200 mg in morning and 400 mg in evening

50-61 kg: 400 mg twice daily

>61 kg: See Adult dosing

Adults:

Oral capsule:

Chronic hepatitis C (in combination with interferon alfa-2b):

≤75 kg: 400 mg in morning and 600 mg in evening

>75 kg: 600 mg twice daily

Chronic hepatitis C (in combination with peginterferon alfa-2b): 400 mg twice daily

Oral tablet:

Chronic hepatitis C, genotype 1,4 (in combination with peginterferon alfa-2a):

<75 kg: 500 mg twice daily for 48 weeks

≥75 kg: 600 mg twice daily for 48 weeks

Chronic hepatitis C, genotype 2,3 (in combination with peginterferon alfa-2a): 400 mg twice daily for 24 weeks

Chronic hepatitis C in HIV coinfected patient (in combination with peginterferon alfa-2a): 400 mg twice daily for 48 weeks, regardless of genotype

Dosage adjustment in renal impairment: Cl_{cr} <50 mL/ minute: Oral route is contraindicated

Dosage adjustment for toxicity: Oral:

Patient without cardiac toxicity:

Hemoglobin <10 g/dL but ≥8.5 g/dL:

Children: 7.5 mg/kg once daily

Adults:

Capsule or solution: 600 mg once daily

Tablet: 200 mg in morning and 400 mg in evening

Hemoglobin <8.5 g/dL: Permanently discontinue treatment

Patient with cardiac toxicity:

≥2 g/dL decrease in hemoglobin during any 4-week period during treatment:

Children: 7.5 mg/kg once daily

Adults:

Capsule or solution: 600 mg once daily

Tablet: 200 mg in morning and 400 mg in evening

Hemoglobin <12 g/dL after 4 weeks of reduced dose: Permanently discontinue treatment

Administration

Inhalation: Ribavirin should be administered in well-ventilated rooms (at least 6 air changes/hour)

Mechanically ventilated patients: Ribavirin can potentially be deposited in the ventilator delivery system depending on temperature, humidity, and electrostatic forces; this deposition can lead to malfunction or obstruction of the expiratory valve, resulting in inadvertently high positive end-expiratory pressures. The use of one-way valves in the inspiratory lines, a breathing circuit filter in the expiratory line, and frequent monitoring and filter replacement have been effective in preventing these problems.

Oral: Administer concurrently with interferon alfa injection. Capsule should not be opened, crushed, chewed, or broken. Use oral solution in children ≤5 years of age, those ≤25 kg, or those who cannot swallow capsules.

Capsule or solution in combination with interferon alfa-2b: May be administered with or without food

Capsule in combination with peginterferon alfa-2b: Administer with food

Tablet: Administer with food

Monitoring Parameters

Inhalation: Respiratory function, hemoglobin, reticulocyte count, CBC, I & O

Oral: Hemoglobin, hematocrit, CBC with differential, platelet count, liver function tests, ECG, pregnancy test (for women of childbearing potential), HCV-RNA after 24 weeks of therapy, TSH

Patient Information

Oral: Read the patient Medication Guide that you receive with each prescription and refill of ribavirin. Avoid pregnancy in female patients and female partners of male patients during therapy by using 2 effective forms of contraception; continue contraceptive measures for at least 6 months after therapy completion. Negative pregnancy test is required before therapy initiation, monthly thereafter during treatment and for 6 months after treatment ends. Avoid alcohol. May cause dizziness, somnolence, fatigue, or impaired concentration decreasing ability to perform activities requiring mental alertness or physical coordination. Inform physician if you feel tired, dizzy, have chest pain, or shortness of breath; hives; suicidal ideation, depression, or a feeling of loss of contact with reality; severe stomach pain or bloody diarrhea; bruising or bleeding. If pregnancy occurs, inform physician immediately.

Nursing Implications

Healthcare workers who are pregnant or who may become pregnant should be advised of the potential risks of exposure and counseled about risk reduction strategies including alternate job responsibilities; limit contact by visitors with patients receiving ribavirin; ribavirin may adsorb to contact lenses

Additional Information

RSV season is usually December to April; viral shedding period for RSV is usually 3-8 days

Dosage Forms

Excipient information presented when available (limited, particularly for generics); consult specific product labeling. [DSC] = Discontinued product

Capsule, oral: 200 mg

Rebetol®, Ribasphere®: 200 mg

Combination package [dose pack]:

RibaPak™ 400/600 [DSC] [each package contains]:

Tablet, oral: 400 mg (7s)

Tablet, oral: 600 mg (7s)

Ribasphere® RibaPak® [each package contains]:

Tablet, oral: 400 mg (7s, 28s)

Tablet, oral: 600 mg (7s, 28s)

Powder for solution, for nebulization:

Virazole®: 6 g (1s) [reconstituted product contains ribavirin 20 mg/mL]

Solution, oral:

Rebetol®: 40 mg/mL (100 mL) [contains propylene glycol and sodium benzoate; bubble-gum flavor]

Tablet, oral: 200 mg

Copegus®: 200 mg

Ribasphere®: 200 mg, 400 mg, 600 mg

Tablet, oral [dose pack]:

RibaPak™ [DSC]: 400 mg (14s); 600 mg (14s)

Ribasphere® RibaPak®: 400 mg (14s, 56s); 600 mg (14s, 56s)

References

American Academy of Pediatrics Committee on Infectious Diseases, "Reassessment of the Indications for Ribavirin Therapy in Respiratory Syncytial Virus Infections," *Pediatrics*, 1996, 97(1):137-40.

Englund JA, Piedra PA, Ahn Y-M, et al, "High-Dose, Short-Duration Ribavirin Aerosol Therapy Compared With Standard Ribavirin Therapy in Children With Suspected Respiratory Syncytial Virus Infection," *J Pediatr*, 1994, 125:635-41.

Janai HK, Marks MI, Zaleska M, et al, "Ribavirin: Adverse Drug Reactions 1986 to 1988," *Pediatr Infect Dis J*, 1990, 9(3):209-11.

Meert KL, Samaik AP, Gelmini MJ, et al, "Aerosolized Ribavirin in Mechanically Ventilated Children With Respiratory Syncytial Virus Lower Respiratory Tract Disease: A Prospective, Double-Blind, Randomized Trial," *Crit Care Med*, 1994, 22(4):566-72.

"NIH Consensus Statement on Management of Hepatitis C: 2002," *NIH Consens State Sci Statements*, 2002, 19(3):1-46.

Smith DW, Frankel LR, Mathers LH, et al, "A Controlled Trial of Aerosolized Ribavirin in Infants Receiving Mechanical Ventilation for Severe Respiratory Syncytial Virus Infection," *N Engl J Med*, 1991, 325(1):24-9.

Wirth S, Lang T, Gehring S, et al, "Recombinant Alfa-Interferon Plus Ribavirin Therapy in Children and Adolescents With Chronic Hepatitis C," *Hepatology*, 2002, 36(5):1280-4.

◆ **Ribo-100** *see* Riboflavin *on page 1213*

Riboflavin (RYE boe flay vin)

Medication Safety Issues
Sound-alike/look-alike issues:
Riboflavin may be confused with ribavirin
U.S. Brand Names Ribo-100
Therapeutic Category Nutritional Supplement; Vitamin, Water Soluble
Generic Available Yes
Use Prevention of riboflavin deficiency and treatment of ariboflavinosis; microcytic anemia associated with gluta-thione reductase deficiency
Pregnancy Risk Factor A/C (dose exceeding RDA recommendation)
Lactation Enters breast milk/compatible
Contraindications Hypersensitivity to riboflavin or any component
Adverse Reactions Genitourinary: Discoloration of urine (bright yellow) with large doses
Drug Interactions
Avoid Concomitant Use There are no known inter-actions where it is recommended to avoid concomitant use.
Increased Effect/Toxicity There are no known signifi-cant interactions involving an increase in effect.
Decreased Effect There are no known significant interactions involving a decrease in effect.
Food Interactions Food increases the extent of GI absorption
Stability Protect from light
Mechanism of Action Converted to coenzymes which act as hydrogen-carrier molecules, which are necessary for normal tissue respiration; also needed for activation of pyridoxine and conversion of tryptophan to niacin
Pharmacokinetics (Adult data unless noted)
Absorption: Readily via GI tract; GI absorption is decreased in patients with hepatitis, cirrhosis, or biliary obstruction
Metabolism: Metabolic fate unknown
Half-life, biologic: 66-84 minutes
Elimination: 9% eliminated unchanged in urine
Usual Dosage Oral:
Riboflavin deficiency:
Children: 3-10 mg/day in divided doses
Adults: 5-30 mg/day in divided doses
Adequate intake: Infants:
<6 months: 0.3 mg (0.04 mg/kg)
6-12 months: 0.4 mg (0.04 mg/kg)
Recommended daily allowance (RDA):
Children:
1-3 years: 0.5 mg
4-8 years: 0.6 mg
9-13 years: 0.9 mg
14-18 years:
Male: 1.3 mg
Female: 1 mg
19-70 years:
Male: 1.3 mg
Female: 1.1 mg
Microcytic anemia associated with glutathione reductase deficiency: Adults: 10 mg daily for 10 days

Administration Oral: Administer with food
Monitoring Parameters CBC and reticulocyte counts (if anemic when treating deficiency)
Test Interactions Large doses may interfere with urinalysis based on spectrometry; may cause false elevations in fluorometric determinations of catechol-amines and urobilinogen
Patient Information Large doses may cause bright yellow urine
Dosage Forms Excipient information presented when available (limited, particularly for generics); consult specific product labeling.
Tablet: 25 mg, 50 mg, 100 mg
Ribo-100: 100 mg

◆ **Rid-A-Pain Dental [OTC]** *see* Benzocaine *on page 182*
◆ **Ridaura®** *see* Auranofin *on page 160*
◆ **Rid® Spray [OTC]** *see* Permethrin *on page 1094*

Rifabutin (rif a BYOO tin)

Medication Safety Issues
Sound-alike/look-alike issues:
Rifabutin may be confused with rifampin
U.S. Brand Names Mycobutin®
Canadian Brand Names Mycobutin®
Therapeutic Category Antibiotic, Miscellaneous; Anti-tubercular Agent
Generic Available No
Use Prevention of disseminated *Mycobacterium avium* complex (MAC) in patients with advanced HIV infection (FDA approved); utilized in multiple drug regimens for treatment of MAC; alternative to rifampin as prophylaxis for latent tuberculosis infection (LTBI) or part of multidrug regimen for treatment active tuberculosis infection; alter-native as agent for prophylaxis of *Mycobacterium avium* complex in children >6 years; add-on therapy for severe *Mycobacterium avium* complex infection
Pregnancy Risk Factor B
Lactation Excretion in breast milk unknown/not recommended
Contraindications Hypersensitivity to rifabutin, any component, or other rifamycin
Warnings Rifabutin as a single agent must not be administered to patients with active tuberculosis since its use may lead to the development of tuberculosis that is resistant to both rifabutin and rifampin; rifabutin should be discontinued in patients with AST >3x ULN (symptomatic) or ≥5x ULN (regardless of symptoms) or if significant bilirubin and/or alkaline phosphatase elevations occur. Tiny, asymptomatic peripheral and central corneal deposits have been observed during routine ophthalmologic exams in HIV-positive patients receiving rifabutin. *C. difficile*-associated diarrhea has been reported with use of rifabutin.
Precautions Use with caution in patients with liver or renal impairment; modify dose in patients with Cl_{cr} <30 mL/minute. Rifabutin is a CYP3A3/4 isoenzyme inducer which may reduce the plasma concentrations of itraconazole, clarithromycin, and saquinavir. CYP3A3/4 isoenzyme inhibitors such as fluconazole and clarithromycin may elevate levels of rifabutin increasing the risk of adverse reactions. Monitor patients, and in some cases, reduce the rifabutin dose when coadministered with fluconazole or clarithromycin (see Drug Interactions). Rifabutin decreases plasma concentrations of delavirdine; delavirdine increases plasma concentrations of rifabutin (coadminis-tration of rifabutin and delavirdine is not recommended; see Drug Interactions). May be associated with neutrope-nia and/or thrombocytopenia (rarely); consider hemato-logic monitoring and discontinue permanently if signs of thrombocytopenia (eg, petechial rash) occur.

◀ **Adverse Reactions**

Central nervous system: Confusion, fever, headache, insomnia, seizures

Dermatologic: Pruritus, rash, staining of skin (brown-orange)

Gastrointestinal: Abdominal pain, anorexia, diarrhea, dysgeusia, dyspepsia, flatulence, nausea, vomiting

Genitourinary: Discoloration of urine (brown-orange)

Hematologic: Anemia, leukopenia, neutropenia, thrombo-cytopenia

Hepatic: Hepatitis, liver enzymes elevated

Neuromuscular & skeletal: Arthralgia, myositis

Ocular: Corneal deposits, uveitis (more common with high-dose rifabutin than in combination with clarithromycin)

Miscellaneous: Discoloration of body fluids (brown-orange)

Drug Interactions

Metabolism/Transport Effects Substrate of CYP3A4 (major); **Induces** CYP3A4 (strong)

Avoid Concomitant Use

Avoid concomitant use of Rifabutin with any of the following: BCG; Dronedarone; Everolimus; Mycopheno-late; Nilotinib; Pazopanib; Ranolazine; Romidepsin; Tolvaptan; Voriconazole

Increased Effect/Toxicity

Rifabutin may increase the levels/effects of: Clopidogrel; HMG-CoA Reductase Inhibitors; Isoniazid

The levels/effects of Rifabutin may be increased by: Antifungal Agents (Azole Derivatives, Systemic); Dela-virdine; Fluconazole; Macrolide Antibiotics; Nevirapine; Protease Inhibitors; Voriconazole

Decreased Effect

Rifabutin may decrease the levels/effects of: Alfentanil; Amiodarone; Angiotensin II Receptor Blockers; Antie-metics (5HT3 Antagonists); Antifungal Agents (Azole Derivatives, Systemic); Aprepitant; Atovaquone; Barbitu-rates; BCG; Benzodiazepines (metabolized by oxidation); BusPIRone; Calcium Channel Blockers; Contraceptives (Estrogens); Contraceptives (Progestins); Corticosteroids (Systemic); CycloSPORINE; CycloSPORINE (Systemic); CYP3A4 Substrates; Dapsone; Dapsone (Systemic); Delavirdine; Disopyramide; Dronedarone; Efavirenz; Etravirine; Everolimus; FentaNYL; Fluconazole; Gefitinib; GuanFACINE; HMG-CoA Reductase Inhibitors; Imatinib; Maraviroc; Morphine (Systemic); Morphine Sulfate; Mycophenolate; Nevirapine; Nilotinib; Pazopanib; Phe-nytoin; Propafenone; Protease Inhibitors; QuiNIDine; Ramelteon; Ranolazine; Repaglinide; Romidepsin; Sax-agliptin; Sorafenib; Sunitinib; Tacrolimus; Tacrolimus (Systemic); Tadalafil; Tamoxifen; Temsirolimus; Terbina-fine; Terbinafine (Systemic); Tolvaptan; Typhoid Vaccine; Vitamin K Antagonists; Voriconazole; Zaleplon; Zolpidem

The levels/effects of Rifabutin may be decreased by: CYP3A4 Inducers (Strong); Deferasirox; Efavirenz; Herbs (CYP3A4 Inducers); Nevirapine

Food Interactions High-fat meal may decrease the rate but not the extent of absorption

Stability Capsules should be stored in a well-closed container at 25°C (77°F) with excursions permitted to 15°C to 30°C (59°F to 86 °F)

Mechanism of Action Inhibits DNA-dependent RNA polymerase at the beta subunit which prevents chain initiation

Pharmacokinetics (Adult data unless noted)

Absorption: Oral: Readily absorbed

Distribution: To body tissues including the lungs, liver, spleen, eyes, and kidneys

V_d: Adults: 9.3 ± 1.5 L/kg

Protein binding: 85%

Metabolism: Hepatically to 5 metabolites; predominantly 25-O-desacetyl-rifabutin (antimicrobial activity equivalent

to parent drug; serum AUC 10% of parent drug) and 31-hydroxy-rifabutin (serum AUC 7% of parent drug)

Bioavailability: 20% in HIV patients

Half-life, terminal: 45 hours (range: 16-69 hours)

Time to peak serum concentration: 2-4 hours

Elimination: Renal and biliary clearance of unchanged drug is 10%; 30% excreted in feces; 53% excreted in urine

Usual Dosage Oral:

Children: Efficacy and safety of rifabutin have not been established in children; a limited number of HIV-positive children with MAC (n=22) have been given rifabutin for MAC prophylaxis; dosages of up to 75 mg/day have been given to children <4 years of age (~5-6 mg/kg/day)

Infants and Children: Prophylaxis for first episode of MAC in HIV-infected patients:

Children <6 years: 5 mg/kg once daily

Children ≥6 years: 300 mg once daily

Infants and Children:

Prophylaxis for recurrence of MAC in HIV-infected patients: 5 mg/kg (maximum dose: 300 mg) once daily as an optional add-on to primary therapy of clarithromycin and ethambutol

Treatment of active TB (as alternative to rifampin): 10-20 mg/kg (maximum dose: 300 mg) once daily or intermittently 2-3 times weekly

Add-on therapy for severe *Mycobacterium avium* complex infection: 10-20 mg/kg once daily (maximum: 300 mg)

Adolescents and Adults:

Prophylaxis for first episode of MAC in HIV-infected patient: 300 mg once daily; for patients who experience GI upset, rifabutin can be administered 150 mg twice daily with food

Prophylaxis for recurrence of MAC in HIV-infected patient: 300 mg once daily as a component of a multiple drug regimen

Treatment of active TB: 300 mg once daily or inter-mittently 2-3 times weekly

Add-on therapy for severe *Mycobacterium avium* com-plex infection: 300 mg once daily

Dosage adjustment for concurrent efavirenz (no concomitant protease inhibitor): Adolescents and Adults: Increase rifabutin dose to 450-600 mg daily, or 600 mg 3 times/week

Dosage adjustment for concurrent nelfinavir, ampre-navir, indinavir: Adolescents and Adults: Reduce rifabutin dose to 150 mg/day; no change in dose if administered twice weekly

Dosage adjustment in renal impairment: Cl_{cr} <30 mL/minute: Reduce dose by 50%

Administration Oral: May administer with or without food or mix with applesauce if patient unable to swallow capsule; administer with food to decrease GI upset

Monitoring Parameters Periodic liver function tests, CBC with differential, platelet count, hemoglobin, hematocrit, ophthalmologic exam, number and type of stools/day for diarrhea

Patient Information May discolor skin, urine, feces, tears, perspiration, or other body fluids to a brown-orange color; soft contact lenses may be permanently stained. Notify physician of any severe flu-like symptoms, nausea, vomiting, persistent diarrhea, dark urine, unusual bleeding or bruising, or any eye problems

Dosage Forms Excipient information presented when available (limited, particularly for generics); consult specific product labeling.

Capsule:

Mycobutin®: 150 mg

Extemporaneous Preparations A 20 mg/mL rifabutin suspension is made by placing the powder from eight 150 mg rifabutin capsules into a glass mortar, levigating with 20 mL of a 1:1 vehicle of Ora-Sweet® and Ora-Plus®

and triturating the mixture to make a paste. Additional vehicle is added in geometric proportion levigating until a uniform mixture is obtained; qsad to 60 mL with vehicle. Stable for 12 weeks at 4°C, 25°C, 30°C, and 40°C. Label "shake well before using."

Haslam JL, Egodage KL, Chen Y, et al, "Stability of Rifabutin in Two Extemporaneously Compounded Oral Liquids," *Am J Health Syst Pharm*, 1999, 56(4):333-6.

References

Adult Prevention and Treatment of Opportunistic Infections Guidelines Working Group, "Guidelines for Prevention and Treatment of Opportunistic Infections in HIV-Infected Adults and Adolescents. March 24, 2009," *MMWR*, 2009; 58 (early release): 1-198. Available at: http://www.cdc.gov/mmwr/preview/mmwrhtml/rr58e324a1.htm. Accessed May 21, 2009.

Krause PJ, Hight DW, Schwartz AN, et al, "Successful Management of *Mycobacterium intracellulare* Pneumonia in a Child," *Pediatr Infect Dis*, 1986, 5(2):269-71.

Levin RH and Bolinger AM, "Treatment of Nontuberculous Mycobacterial Infections in Pediatric Patients," *Clin Pharm*, 1988, 7(7):545-51.

Starke JR and Correa AG, "Management of Mycobacterial Infection and Disease in Children," *Pediatr Infect Dis J*, 1995, 14(6):455-70.

Working Group on Guidelines for the Prevention and Treatment of Opportunistic Infections Among HIV-Exposed and HIV-Infected Children, "Guidelines for Prevention and Treatment of Opportunistic Infections in HIV-Exposed and HIV-Infected Children [DRAFT]. June 20, 2008," 2008, 1-250. Available at: http://aidsinfo.nih.gov/content-files/Pediatric_OI.pdf. Accessed May 21, 2009.

♦ **Rifadin®** *see* Rifampin *on page 1215*

♦ **Rifampicin** *see* Rifampin *on page 1215*

Rifampin (RIF am pin)

Medication Safety Issues
Sound-alike/look-alike issues:
Rifadin® may be confused with Rifater®, Ritalin®
Rifampin may be confused with ribavirin, rifabutin, Rifamate®, rifapentine, rifaximin

U.S. Brand Names Rifadin®

Canadian Brand Names Rifadin®; Rofact™

Therapeutic Category Antibiotic, Miscellaneous; Antitubercular Agent

Generic Available Yes

Use Used in combination with other antitubercular drugs for the treatment of active tuberculosis; elimination of meningococci from asymptomatic carriers; prophylaxis in contacts of patients with *Haemophilus influenzae* type B infection; used in combination with other anti-infectives in the treatment of staphylococcal infections

Pregnancy Risk Factor C

Pregnancy Considerations Teratogenic effects have bee reported in animal studies. Rifampin crosses the human placenta. Due to the risk of tuberculosis to the fetus, treatment is recommended when the probability of maternal disease is moderate to high. Postnatal hemorrhages have been reported in the infant and mother with isoniazid administration during the last few weeks of pregnancy.

Lactation Enters breast milk/not recommended (AAP rates "compatible")

Contraindications Hypersensitivity to rifampin, rifamycins, or any component; concurrent use with amprenavir

Warnings Two month rifampin-pyrazinamide regimen for the treatment of latent tuberculosis infection (LTBI) has been associated with severe and fatal liver injuries. The IDSA and CDC now recommend that this regimen should not generally be used in patients with LTBI.

Precautions Use with caution in patients with liver impairment, patients receiving concurrent medications associated with liver injury (particularly with pyrazinamide), or in patients with a history of alcoholism; modification of dosage should be considered in patients with severe liver impairment

Adverse Reactions
Central nervous system: Drowsiness, fatigue, confusion, ataxia, fever, headache, dizziness

Dermatologic: Rash, pruritus, urticaria

Gastrointestinal: Nausea, vomiting, diarrhea, stomatitis, anorexia

Hematologic: Eosinophilia, blood dyscrasias (leukopenia, thrombocytopenia), hemolytic anemia

Hepatic: Hepatitis, cholestatic jaundice, liver enzymes elevated

Local: Irritation at the I.V. site

Neuromuscular & skeletal: Myalgias, arthralgia, weakness

Renal: Renal failure, interstitial nephritis

Miscellaneous: Flu-like syndrome; discoloration of body fluids (red-orange)

Drug Interactions
Metabolism/Transport Effects Substrate of P-glycoprotein, SLCO1B1; **Induces** CYP1A2 (strong), CYP2A6 (strong), CYP2B6 (strong), CYP2C8 (strong), CYP2C9 (strong), CYP2C19 (strong), CYP3A4 (strong), P-glycoprotein

Avoid Concomitant Use
Avoid concomitant use of Rifampin with any of the following: Atazanavir; BCG; Dronedarone; Etravirine; Everolimus; Mycophenolate; Nilotinib; Pazopanib; Praziquantel; QuiNINE; Ranolazine; Romidepsin; Tolvaptan; Voriconazole

Increased Effect/Toxicity
Rifampin may increase the levels/effects of: Clopidogrel; Gadoxetate; HMG-CoA Reductase Inhibitors; Isoniazid; Leflunomide

The levels/effects of Rifampin may be increased by: Antifungal Agents (Azole Derivatives, Systemic); Delavirdine; Eltrombopag; Fluconazole; Macrolide Antibiotics; P-Glycoprotein Inhibitors; Protease Inhibitors; Pyrazinamide; Voriconazole

Decreased Effect
Rifampin may decrease the levels/effects of: Alfentanil; Amiodarone; Angiotensin II Receptor Blockers; Antidiabetic Agents (Thiazolidinedione); Antiemetics (5HT3 Antagonists); Antifungal Agents (Azole Derivatives, Systemic); Aprepitant; Atazanavir; Atovaquone; Barbiturates; BCG; Bendamustine; Benzodiazepines (metabolized by oxidation); Beta-Blockers; BusPIRone; Calcium Channel Blockers; Caspofungin; Chloramphenicol; Contraceptives (Estrogens); Contraceptives (Progestins); Corticosteroids (Systemic); CycloSPORINE; CycloSPORINE (Systemic); CYP1A2 Substrates; CYP2A6 Substrates; CYP2B6 Substrates; CYP2C19 Substrates; CYP2C8 Substrates (High risk); CYP2C9 Substrates (High risk); CYP3A4 Substrates; Dabigatran Etexilate; Dapsone; Dapsone (Systemic); Deferasirox; Delavirdine; Disopyramide; Divalproex; Dronedarone; Efavirenz; Erlotinib; Etravirine; Everolimus; Exemestane; FentaNYL; Fexofenadine; Fluconazole; Fosaprepitant; Gefitinib; GuanFACINE; HMG-CoA Reductase Inhibitors; Imatinib; LamoTRigine; Maraviroc; Methadone; Morphine (Systemic); Morphine Sulfate; Mycophenolate; Nevirapine; Nilotinib; OxyCODONE; Pazopanib; P-Glycoprotein Substrates; Phenytoin; Prasugrel; Praziquantel; Propafenone; Protease Inhibitors; QuiNIDine; QuiNINE; Raltegravir; Ramelteon; Ranolazine; Repaglinide; Romidepsin; Saxagliptin; Sirolimus; Sorafenib; Sulfonylureas; Sunitinib; Tacrolimus; Tacrolimus (Systemic); Tadalafil; Tamoxifen; Temsirolimus; Terbinafine; Terbinafine (Systemic); Thyroid Products; Tolvaptan; Treprostinil; Typhoid Vaccine; Valproic Acid; Vitamin K Antagonists; Voriconazole; Zaleplon; Zidovudine; Zolpidem

The levels/effects of Rifampin may be decreased by: P-Glycoprotein Inducers

1215

Food Interactions Food may delay and reduce the amount of rifampin absorbed

Stability Reconstituted I.V. solution is stable for 24 hours at room temperature; once the reconstituted rifampin I.V. solution is further diluted, it is stable for 4 hours in D_5W and up to 24 hours in NS. However, 11% to 13% rifampin decomposition has been reported to occur in 24 hours for solutions diluted in NS. Administer rifampin I.V. solution within 4 hours after preparation to avoid potential for precipitation and decomposition beyond this period.

Mechanism of Action Inhibits bacterial RNA synthesis by binding to the beta subunit of DNA-dependent RNA polymerase, blocking RNA transcription

Pharmacokinetics (Adult data unless noted)

Absorption: Oral: Well absorbed

Distribution: Highly lipophilic; crosses the blood-brain barrier and is widely distributed into body tissues and fluids such as the liver, lungs, gallbladder, bile, tears, and breast milk; distributes into CSF when meninges are inflamed

Protein binding: 80%

Metabolism: Undergoes enterohepatic recycling; metabolized in the liver to a deacetylated metabolite (active)

Half-life: 3-4 hours, prolonged with hepatic impairment

Time to peak serum concentration: Oral: Within 2-4 hours

Elimination: Principally in feces (60% to 65%) and urine (~30%)

Dialysis: Plasma rifampin concentrations are not significantly affected by hemodialysis or peritoneal dialysis

Usual Dosage Oral (I.V. infusion dose is the same as for the oral route):

Tuberculosis:

Infants and Children: 10-20 mg/kg/day in divided doses every 12-24 hours

Adults: 10 mg/kg/day administered once daily; maximum dose: 600 mg/day

American Thoracic Society and CDC currently recommend twice weekly therapy as part of a short-course regimen which follows 1-2 months of daily treatment of uncomplicated pulmonary tuberculosis in the compliant patient

Children: 10-20 mg/kg/dose (up to 600 mg) twice weekly under supervision to ensure compliance

Adults: 10 mg/kg (up to 600 mg) twice weekly

H. influenzae prophylaxis:

Neonates <1 month: 10 mg/kg/day every 24 hours for 4 days

Infants and Children: 20 mg/kg/day every 24 hours for 4 days, not to exceed 600 mg/dose

Adults: 600 mg every 24 hours for 4 days

Meningococcal prophylaxis:

<1 month: 10 mg/kg/day in divided doses every 12 hours for 2 days

Infants and Children: 20 mg/kg/day in divided doses every 12 hours for 2 days, not to exceed 600 mg/dose

Adults: 600 mg every 12 hours for 2 days

Nasal carriers of *Staphylococcus aureus*:

Children: 15 mg/kg/day divided every 12 hours for 5-10 days in combination with other antibiotics

Adults: 600 mg once daily for 5-10 days in combination with other antibiotics

Synergy for *Staphylococcus aureus* infections:

Neonates: 5-20 mg/kg/day in divided doses every 12 hours with other antibiotics

Adults: 300-600 mg twice daily with other antibiotics

Administration

Oral: Administer 1 hour before or 2 hours after a meal on an empty stomach; may administer with food to decrease GI distress; may mix contents of capsule with applesauce or jelly

Parenteral: Do not administer I.M. or SubQ; administer I.V. preparation once daily by slow I.V. infusion over 30 minutes to 3 hours at a final concentration not to exceed 6 mg/mL

Monitoring Parameters Periodic monitoring of liver function (AST, ALT); bilirubin, CBC, platelet count

Test Interactions Positive Coombs' reaction [direct], rifampin inhibits standard assay's ability to measure serum folate and vitamin B_{12}

Patient Information May discolor urine, tears, sweat, or other body fluids to a red-orange color; soft contact lenses may be permanently stained. Notify physician of any severe or persistent flu-like symptoms, nausea, vomiting, dark urine, or unusual bleeding or bruising

Nursing Implications The compounded oral suspension must be shaken well before using. Extravasation may cause local irritation and inflammation.

Dosage Forms Excipient information presented when available (limited, particularly for generics); consult specific product labeling.

Capsule: 150 mg, 300 mg

Rifadin®: 150 mg, 300 mg

Injection, powder for reconstitution: 600 mg

Rifadin®: 600 mg

Extemporaneous Preparations Rifampin oral suspension can be compounded with simple syrup or wild cherry syrup at a concentration of 10 mg/mL; the suspension is stable for 4 weeks at room temperature or in a refrigerator when stored in a glass amber prescription bottle. However, there are some experts who do not recommend using rifampin syrup formulated from capsules due to conflicting reports indicating that the product is unstable (14.5% to 68% of labeled potency after preparation). It may be preferable to perform trituration, rather than simple mixing in syrup when preparing rifampin oral suspension.

Nahata MC, Morosco RS, and Hipple TF, "Effect of Preparation Method and Storage on Rifampin Concentration in Suspensions," *Ann Pharmacother*, 1994, 28 (2):182-5.

References

American Academy of Pediatrics Committee on Infectious Diseases, "Chemotherapy for Tuberculosis in Infants and Children," *Pediatrics*, 1992, 89(1):161-5.

Starke JR, "Modern Approach to the Diagnosis and Treatment of Tuberculosis in Children," *Pediatr Clin North Am*, 1988, 35(3):441-64.

Starke JR, "Multidrug Therapy for Tuberculosis in Children," *Pediatr Infect Dis J*, 1990, 9(11):785-93.

Tan TQ, Mason EO Jr, Ou CN, et al, "Use of Intravenous Rifampin in Neonates With Persistent Staphylococcal Bacteremia," *Antimicrob Agents Chemother*, 1993, 37(11):2401-6.

♦ **RIG** *see* Rabies Immune Globulin (Human) *on page 1198*

RimabotulinumtoxinB

(rime uh BOT yoo lin num TOKS in bee)

Medication Safety Issues

Botulinum products are not interchangeable; potency differences may exist between the products.

U.S. Brand Names Myobloc®

Therapeutic Category Muscle Contracture, Treatment

Generic Available No

Use Treatment of cervical dystonia (FDA approved in adults)

Medication Guide An FDA-approved patient medication guide, which is available with the product information and at http://www.fda.gov/downloads/Drugs/DrugSafety/UCM176361.pdf, must be dispensed with this medication for each new outpatient prescription and refill.

Pregnancy Risk Factor C (manufacturer)

Pregnancy Considerations Reproduction studies have not been conducted. Based on limited case reports using onabotulinumtoxinA, adverse fetal effects have not been observed with inadvertent administration during pregnancy. It is currently recommended to ensure adequate contraception in women of childbearing years.

Lactation Excretion in breast milk unknown/use caution

Contraindications Hypersensitivity to botulinum toxin or any component of the formulation

Warnings Use of rimabotulinumtoxinB should be reserved for healthcare providers familiar and experienced in the assessment and management of patients with cervical dystonia

The U.S. Food and Drug Administration (FDA) and Health Canada have issued respective early communications to healthcare professionals alerting them of serious adverse events (including fatalities) in association with the use of onabotulinumtoxinA (Botox®, Botox® Cosmetic) and rimabotulinumtoxinB (Myobloc®). Events reported are suggestive of botulism, indicating systemic spread of the botulinum toxin beyond the site of injection. Reactions were observed in both adult and pediatric patients treated for a variety of conditions with varying doses. However, the most serious outcomes, including respiratory failure and death, were associated with the use in children for cerebral palsy limb spasticity. The FDA has evaluated postmarketing cases and now reports that systemic and potentially fatal toxicity may result from local injection of the botulinum toxins in the treatment of other underlying conditions such as cerebral palsy associated with limb spasticity. Monitor patients closely for signs/symptoms of systemic toxic effects (possibly occurring 1 day to several weeks after treatment) and instruct patients to seek immediate medical attention with worsening symptoms or dysphagia, dyspnea, muscle weakness, or difficulty speaking.

Precautions Use with caution in patients with peripheral motor neuropathic diseases (eg, amyotrophic lateral sclerosis or motor neuropathy) or neuromuscular junction disorders (eg, myasthenia gravis or Lambert-Eaton syndrome) as these patients may be at increased risk for development of significant systemic side effects including severe dysphagia and respiratory compromise; use cautiously if there is inflammation present at the proposed injection site or when excessive weakness or atrophy is present in the target muscles

Adverse Reactions

Cardiovascular: Chest pain, peripheral edema, vasodilation

Central nervous system: Anxiety, chills, confusion, dizziness, fever, headache, malaise, somnolence

Dermatologic: Pruritus

Gastrointestinal: Dyspepsia, dysphagia, glossitis, nausea, stomatitis, taste perversion, xerostomia

Genitourinary: Cystitis, urinary tract infection, vaginal moniliasis

Local: Bruising at injection site, pain

Neuromuscular & skeletal: Arthralgia, back pain, neck pain, tremor, weakness

Ocular: Abnormal vision, amblyopia

Otic: Otitis media, tinnitus

Respiratory: Cough, pneumonia, respiratory failure, rhinitis

Miscellaneous: Abscess, cysts, flu-like syndrome, hypersensitivity reactions, viral infection

Drug Interactions

Avoid Concomitant Use There are no known interactions where it is recommended to avoid concomitant use.

Increased Effect/Toxicity

The levels/effects of RimabotulinumtoxinB may be increased by: AbobotulinumtoxinA; Aminoglycosides; Anticholinergic Agents; Neuromuscular-Blocking Agents; OnabotulinumtoxinA

Decreased Effect There are no known significant interactions involving a decrease in effect.

Stability Store solution in refrigerator at 2°C to 8°C (36°F to 46°F); stable for 4 hours at room temperature after dilution with NS

Mechanism of Action RimabotulinumtoxinB (formerly known as botulinum B toxin) is one of seven neurotoxins produced by *Clostridium botulinum*, a spore-forming anaerobic bacillus; it blocks neuromuscular conduction by binding to receptor sites on motor nerve terminals, entering the nerve terminals and inhibiting the release of acetylcholine. RimabotulinumtoxinB also cleaves synaptic vesicle associated membrane protein (VAMP), a component of the protein complex involved in neurotransmitter release. When injected intramuscularly at therapeutic doses, it produces a localized chemical denervation muscle paralysis. When the muscle is chemically denervated, it atrophies and may develop extrajunctional acetylcholine receptors. There is evidence that the nerve can sprout and reinnervate the muscle, with the weakness being reversible.

Pharmacodynamics Duration of paralysis: 12-16 weeks

Usual Dosage I.M.: Adults: 2500-5000 units divided among affected muscles; patients without a prior history of tolerating botulinum toxin injections should receive a lower initial dose; subsequent doses should be individualized related to the patient's response; doses up to 10,000 units have been used

Administration Parenteral: For I.M. administration only by individuals understanding the relevant neuromuscular anatomy and any alterations to the anatomy due to prior surgical procedures and standard electromyographic techniques; solution may be diluted with NS prior to administration

Monitoring Parameters Monitor patients closely for signs/symptoms of systemic toxic effects (possibly occurring 1 day to several weeks after treatment; see Warnings)

Toronto Western Spasmodic Torticollis Rating Scale (TWSTRS) which evaluates severity, disability, and pain

Patient Information May cause dry mouth

Dosage Forms Excipient information presented when available (limited, particularly for generics); consult specific product labeling.

Injection, solution [preservative free]:

Myobloc®: 5000 units/mL (0.5 mL, 1 mL, 2 mL) [contains albumin 0.05%]

References

"Botulinum Toxin," *NIH Consens Statement*, 1990, 12-14, 8(8):1-20.

Figgitt DP and Noble S, "Botulinum Toxin B: A Review of Its Therapeutic Potential in the Management of Cervical Dystonia," *Drugs*, 2002, 62 (4):705-22.

Rimantadine (ri MAN ta deen)

Medication Safety Issues

Sound-alike/look-alike issues:

Rimantadine may be confused with amantadine, ranitidine, Rimactane®

Flumadine® may be confused with fludarabine, flunisolide, flutamide

U.S. Brand Names Flumadine®

Canadian Brand Names Flumadine®

Therapeutic Category Antiviral Agent, Oral

Generic Available Yes

Use Prophylaxis and treatment of influenza A viral infection (see Warnings)

Pregnancy Risk Factor C

Pregnancy Considerations Animal data suggest embryotoxicity, maternal toxicity, and offspring mortality at doses 7-11 times the recommended human dose. There are no adequate and well-controlled studies in pregnant women.

Lactation Excretion in breast milk unknown/ not recommended

Breast-Feeding Considerations Do not use in nursing mothers due to potential adverse effect in infants.

Contraindications Hypersensitivity to rimantadine, amantadine, or any component

Warnings Resistance of influenza A virus to rimantadine may develop spontaneously or rapidly during treatment; cross-resistance between amantadine and rimantadine occurs. Due to increased resistance, the CDC has recommended that rimantadine and amantadine no longer be used as monotherapy for the treatment or prophylaxis of influenza A in the United States until susceptibility has been re-established. Consult current CDC guidelines for additional information.

Precautions Use with caution in patients with liver disease, epilepsy, history of recurrent eczematoid dermatitis, uncontrolled psychosis, severe psychoneurosis, and in patients receiving CNS stimulant drugs. May increase seizure activity in patients with pre-existing seizure disorders; discontinue use if seizure occurs. Modify dosage in patients with renal impairment, severe hepatic dysfunction, or active seizure disorder; use in patients <1 year of age has not been adequately assessed

Adverse Reactions
Cardiovascular: Orthostatic hypotension, edema
Central nervous system: Dizziness, confusion, headache, insomnia, difficulty in concentrating, anxiety, restlessness, irritability, hallucinations; CNS adverse effects are less than with amantadine
Gastrointestinal: Nausea, vomiting, xerostomia
Genitourinary: Urinary retention

Drug Interactions
Avoid Concomitant Use There are no known interactions where it is recommended to avoid concomitant use.
Increased Effect/Toxicity
The levels/effects of Rimantadine may be increased by: MAO Inhibitors
Decreased Effect
Rimantadine may decrease the levels/effects of: Influenza Virus Vaccine (H1N1, Live/Attenuated); Influenza Virus Vaccine (Live/Attenuated)

Food Interactions Food does not affect rate or extent of absorption

Mechanism of Action Blocks the uncoating of influenza A viral RNA and prevents penetration of the virus into host cell; inhibits M_2 protein in the assembly of progeny virions

Pharmacokinetics (Adult data unless noted)
Absorption: Oral: Well absorbed
Distribution: Adults: 17-25 L/kg
Protein binding: ~40%
Metabolism: Extensively in the liver via hydroxylation and glucuronidation
Half-life:
Children 4-8 years: 13-38 hours
Adults: 24-36 hours
Elimination: <25% excreted unchanged in the urine
Dialysis: Hemodialysis: Negligible effect

Usual Dosage Oral: **Note:** Dosages for prophylaxis and treatment are the same; rimantadine is FDA-approved for prophylaxis in children and adults, and for treatment only in adults; however, it is considered appropriate by certain experts for treatment in children (see AAP, 2000). See Additional Information for duration of therapy.
Children 1-9 years and Children ≥10 years who weigh <40 kg: 5 mg/kg/day in 1-2 divided doses; maximum dose: 150 mg/day
Children ≥10 years who weigh ≥40 kg and Adults: 100 mg twice daily
Dosage adjustment in renal impairment:
Cl_{cr} >10 mL/minute: Dose adjustment not required
Cl_{cr} ≤10 mL/minute: Adults: 100 mg/day
Dosage adjustment in hepatic impairment: Severe dysfunction: Adults: 100 mg/day
Administration Oral: May administer with food

Patient Information May cause dizziness or confusion and impair ability to perform activities requiring mental alertness or physical coordination; may cause dry mouth

Additional Information Not active against influenza B; treatment or prophylaxis in immunosuppressed patients has not been fully evaluated
Duration of treatment: 5-7 days; optimal duration not established
Duration of prophylactic therapy: For at least 10 days after known exposure; usually for 6-8 weeks during influenza A season or local outbreak (or until vaccine produces sufficient antibody titers)
Duration of fever and other symptoms can be reduced if rimantadine therapy is started within the first 48 hours of influenza A illness
During an outbreak of influenza, administer rimantadine prophylaxis for 2-3 weeks after influenza vaccination until vaccine antibody titers are sufficient to provide protection

Dosage Forms Excipient information presented when available (limited, particularly for generics); consult specific product labeling.
Tablet, as hydrochloride: 100 mg
Flumadine®: 100 mg

References
American Academy of Pediatrics, "Influenza," *Red Book®: 2000 Report of the Committee on Infectious Diseases*, 25th ed, Pickering LK, ed, Elk Grove Village, IL: American Academy of Pediatrics, 2000, 354.

◆ **Rimantadine Hydrochloride** *see* Rimantadine *on page 1217*

◆ **Riomet®** *see* MetFORMIN *on page 891*

◆ **RisaQuad™ [OTC]** *see* Lactobacillus *on page 790*

◆ **Risperdal®** *see* Risperidone *on page 1218*

◆ **Risperdal M-Tab** *see* Risperidone *on page 1218*

◆ **Risperdal® M-Tab®** *see* Risperidone *on page 1218*

◆ **Risperdal® Consta®** *see* Risperidone *on page 1218*

Risperidone (ris PER i done)

Medication Safety Issues
Sound-alike/look-alike issues:
Risperidone may be confused with reserpine, ropinirole
Risperdal® may be confused with lisinopril, reserpine, Restoril™

U.S. Brand Names Risperdal®; Risperdal® Consta®; Risperdal® M-Tab®

Canadian Brand Names Apo-Risperidone®; CO Risperidone; Dom-Risperidone; Gen-Risperidone; Mylan-Risperidone; Novo-Risperidone; PHL-Risperidone; PMS-Risperidone ODT; PRO-Risperidone; RAN™-Risperidone; ratio-Risperidone; Risperdal®; Risperdal® Consta®; Risperdal® M-Tab®; Riva-Risperidone; Sandoz-Risperidone; ZYM-Risperidone

Therapeutic Category Antipsychotic Agent, Atypical; Antipsychotic Agent, Benzisoxazole

Generic Available Yes: Excludes injection

Use
Oral: Management of schizophrenia (FDA approved in ages ≥13 years and adults); treatment of acute mania or mixed episodes associated with bipolar I disorder (FDA approved as monotherapy in ages ≥10 years and adults; FDA approved in combination with lithium or valproate in adults); treatment of irritability (including aggression, temper tantrums, self-injurious behavior, and quickly-changing moods) associated with autistic disorder in children and adolescents (FDA approved in ages 5-16 years); has also been used to treat Tourette's syndrome and aggressive behavior in patients with other pervasive developmental disorders or psychiatric diagnoses

I.M.: Management of schizophrenia (FDA approved in adults); maintenance treatment of bipolar I disorder as monotherapy or in combination with lithium or valproate (FDA approved in adults)

Pregnancy Risk Factor C

Pregnancy Considerations Animal studies indicate an increase in fetal mortality. Reversible EPS symptoms were noted in neonates following use of risperidone during the last trimester. Agenesis of the corpus callosum has also been noted in one case report. There are no adequate and well-controlled studies in pregnant women. When using Risperdal® Consta®, patients should notify healthcare provider if they become or intend to become pregnant during therapy or within 12 weeks of last injection. Risperidone may cause hyperprolactinemia, which may decrease reproductive function in both males and females. Healthcare providers are encouraged to enroll women 18-45 years of age exposed to risperidone during pregnancy in the Atypical Antipsychotics Pregnancy Registry (1-866-961-2388).

Lactation Enters breast milk/not recommended

Breast-Feeding Considerations Risperidone and its metabolite are excreted in breast milk; it is recommended that women not breast-feed during therapy or for 12 weeks after the last injection if using Risperdal® Consta®.

Contraindications Hypersensitivity to risperidone or any component (see Warnings)

Warnings May cause neuroleptic malignant syndrome (symptoms include hyperpyrexia, altered mental status, muscle rigidity, autonomic instability, acute renal failure, rhabdomyolysis, and elevated CPK). May cause extrapyramidal reactions, including pseudoparkinsonism, acute dystonic reactions, akathisia, and tardive dyskinesia (risk of these reactions is low relative to other neuroleptics, and is dose-dependent; to decrease risk of tardive dyskinesia: Use smallest dose and shortest duration possible; evaluate continued need periodically; risk of dystonia is increased with the use of high potency and higher doses of conventional antipsychotics and in males and younger patients). May cause hyperglycemia, which may be severe and include potentially fatal ketoacidosis or hyperosmolar coma; use with caution and monitor glucose closely in patients with diabetes mellitus (or with risk factors such as family history or obesity); measure fasting blood glucose at the beginning of therapy and periodically during therapy in these patients; monitor for symptoms of hyperglycemia in all patients treated with risperidone; measure fasting blood glucose in patients who develop symptoms. May alter cardiac conduction (low risk relative to other neuroleptics); QT prolongation and life-threatening arrhythmias have occurred with therapeutic doses of neuroleptics; use with caution in patients with conduction abnormalities.

Leukopenia, neutropenia, and agranulocytosis (sometimes fatal) have been reported in clinical trials and postmarketing reports with antipsychotic use; presence of risk factors (eg, pre-existing low WBC or history of drug-induced leuko/neutropenia) should prompt periodic blood count assessment. Discontinue therapy at first signs of blood dyscrasias or if absolute neutrophil count <1000/mm^3.

An increased risk of death has been reported with the use of antipsychotics in elderly patients with dementia-related psychosis **[U.S. Boxed Warning]**; most deaths seemed to be cardiovascular (eg, sudden death, heart failure) or infectious (eg, pneumonia) in nature; a higher risk of mortality was seen with the use of furosemide plus risperidone (compared to risperidone alone or compared with placebo plus furosemide). An increased incidence of cerebrovascular adverse events (eg, transient ischemic attack, stroke), including fatalities, has been reported with the use of risperidone in elderly patients with dementia-related psychosis. Risperidone is not approved for the treatment of patients with dementia-related psychosis

Oral solution contains benzoic acid; benzoic acid (benzoate) is a metabolite of benzyl alcohol; large amounts of benzyl alcohol (≥99 mg/kg/day) have been associated with a potentially fatal toxicity ("gasping") in neonates; avoid use of risperidone products containing benzoic acid in neonates; *in vitro* and animal studies have shown that benzoate displaces bilirubin from protein binding sites. Vehicle used in injectable product (polylactide-co-glycolide microspheres) has rarely been associated with retinal artery occlusion in patients with abnormal arteriovenous anastomosis (eg, patent foramen ovale).

Precautions Use with caution and decrease the dose in patients with renal or hepatic impairment. Use with caution in patients with breast cancer or other prolactin-dependent tumors; risperidone elevates prolactin levels to a greater degree than other antipsychotic agents; high levels of prolactin may reduce pituitary gonadotropin secretion; galactorrhea, amenorrhea, gynecomastia, impotence, decreased bone density may occur. Use with caution in children and adolescents; adverse effects due to elevated prolactin levels have been observed; long-term effects on growth or sexual maturation have not been evaluated.

Risperidone may cause a higher than normal weight gain in children and adolescents; monitor growth (including weight, height, BMI, and waist circumference) in pediatric patients receiving risperidone; compare weight gain to standard growth curves. Risperidone may cause increases in metabolic indices (eg, serum cholesterol, triglycerides). **Note:** A prospective, nonrandomized cohort study followed 338 antipsychotic naïve pediatric patients (age 4-19 years) for a median 10.8 weeks (range 10.5-11.2 weeks) and reported the following significant mean increases in weight in kg (and % change from baseline): Olanzapine: 8.5 kg (15.2%), quetiapine: 6.1 kg (10.4%), risperidone: 5.3 kg (10.4%), and aripiprazole: 4.4 kg (8.1%) compared to the control cohort: 0.2 kg (0.65%). Increases in metabolic indices (eg, serum cholesterol, triglycerides, glucose) were also reported; a significant increase in serum triglycerides of 9.7 mg/mL was observed for patients receiving risperidone. Biannual monitoring of cardiometabolic indices after the first 3 months of therapy is suggested (see Correll, 2009). Risperidone use in pediatric patients may cause somnolence at a higher incidence than in adults.

Use with caution in patients with seizure disorders (seizures have been rarely reported), concomitant illnesses that may effect hepatic metabolism or hemodynamic responses (eg, unstable cardiac disease, recent MI), Parkinson's disease, or dementia with Lewy Bodies (an increased sensitivity to antipsychotic medications and adverse effects have been reported), in suicidal patients, and in those at risk of aspiration pneumonia (esophageal dysmotility and aspiration have been associated with antipsychotic agents). May cause orthostatic hypotension with resultant dizziness, tachycardia, or syncope (especially during initial dose titration); use with caution in patients with cardiovascular disease (heart failure, past MI, or myocardia ischemia), cerebrovascular disease, dehydration, hypovolemia, or other conditions which may predispose patients to hypotension; may cause hypotension when used with antihypertensive agents. May cause somnolence (dose-related), priapism (rarely), thrombotic thrombocytopenic purpura (case report), alteration of temperature regulation (use with caution in patients exposed to temperature extremes); may mask diseases or toxicity of other drugs due to antiemetic effects.

Orally-disintegrating tablets contain aspartame which is metabolized to phenylalanine and must be avoided (or used with caution) in patients with phenylketonuria.

Adverse Reactions Additional adverse reactions associated with the injectable formulation (I.M. use) are noted below.

Cardiovascular: Arrhythmia, chest pain, edema, hypotension, palpitation, postural hypotension, QT prolongation (see Warnings), syncope, tachycardia; I.M.: Hypertension

Central nervous system: Akathisia, alteration of temperature regulation, anxiety, automatism, confusion, dizziness, dystonia (children 8% to 18%; adults 5% to 11%), fatigue (children 18% to 42%; adults 1% to 3%), fever (children 20%; adults 1% to 2%), neuroleptic malignant syndrome (see Warnings), Parkinsonism, seizures, somnolence (children 12% to 67%; adults 5% to 14%), tardive dyskinesia; I.M.: Attention disturbances, headache, hypoesthesia

Dermatologic: Acne, angioedema, photosensitivity, pigmentation increased, rash, seborrhea; I.M.: Dry skin

Endocrine & metabolic: Amenorrhea, galactorrhea, gynecomastia, hyperglycemia (see Warnings), lactation non-puerperal (children 2% to 5%; adults 1%), serum prolactin increased (see Precautions), weight gain (see Precautions); I.M.: Weight decrease

Gastrointestinal: Abdominal pain (children 15% to 18%; adults 3% to 4%), anorexia, appetite increased, constipation (children 21%; adults 8% to 9%), diarrhea, dyspepsia, nausea, salivation increased (children ≤ 22%; adults 1% to 3%), vomiting, xerostomia (children 13%; adults ≤4%); I.M.: Appetite decreased

Genitourinary: Priapism (see Precautions), urinary incontinence (children ≤22%), urinary tract infection

Hematologic: Agranulocytosis, leukopenia, neutropenia (see Warnings), thrombotic thrombocytopenic purpura

Hepatic: Hepatotoxicity (rare) (see Kumra, 1997; McDougle, 2000), transaminases increased

Local: I.M.: Pain, redness, and swelling at injection site

Neuromuscular & skeletal: Arthralgia, back pain, CPK increased, dyskinesia, myalgia, skeletal pain, tremor; I.M.: Abnormal gait

Ocular: Abnormal vision, blurred vision; I.M.: Retinal artery occlusion in the presence of abnormal arteriovenous anastomosis (rare) (see Warnings)

Respiratory: Cough, dyspnea, epistaxis, pharyngitis, rhinitis, upper respiratory infection

Miscellaneous: Anaphylactic reactions

<2%, postmarketing, and/or case reports (limited to important or life-threatening): Abscess, accommodation disturbances, agitation, allergic reaction, allergy, allergy aggravated, akinesia, alopecia, anaphylactoid reaction, anemia, angioedema, anorexia, apathy, ataxia, atrial fibrillation, AV block, bronchitis, bundle branch block, cardiopulmonary arrest, cellulitis, cerebrovascular disorder, chest discomfort, coma, concentration impaired, conjunctivitis, coordination abnormal, crying abnormal, cyst, cystitis, depression, diabetes mellitus aggravated, diabetic coma, diabetic ketoacidosis, drooling, dysarthria, dysphagia, dysphonia, earache, ear infection, ear pain, eczema, edema peripheral, ejaculation disorder/failure, emotional lability, erectile dysfunction, erythema multiforme, facial edema, fall, flatulence, flu-like symptoms, gastritis, gastroenteritis, hematoma, hypoesthesia, hypokinesia, hypothermia, impotence, inappropriate ADH secretion, insomnia, intestinal obstruction, jaundice, leg cramps/pain, libido decreased, malaise, mania, menstrual disorder, muscle weakness, nervousness, nodule, oligomenorrhea, otitis media, pain, pancreatitis, paresthesia, pharyngolaryngeal pain, pituitary adenoma, pneumonia, posture abnormal, precocious puberty, procedural pain, pruritus generalized, pulmonary embolism, rash maculopapular, respiratory disorder, rhabdomyolysis, rigors, sexual dysfunction, skin discoloration, skin exfoliation, skin necrosis, skin ulceration, sleep apnea, sleep disorder, sluggishness, speech disorder, stomach discomfort, stupor, subcutaneous abscess, sudden death, thirst, urinary frequency, urinary retention, vertigo, viral infection, visual acuity reduced, water intoxication, weakness, xerophthalmia

Drug Interactions

Metabolism/Transport Effects Substrate of CYP2D6 (major), 3A4 (minor); **Inhibits** CYP2D6 (weak), 3A4 (weak)

Avoid Concomitant Use

Avoid concomitant use of Risperidone with any of the following: Artemether; Dronedarone; Lumefantrine; Metoclopramide; Nilotinib; Pimozide; QuiNINE; Tetrabenazine; Thioridazine; Ziprasidone

Increased Effect/Toxicity

Risperidone may increase the levels/effects of: Alcohol (Ethyl); Anticholinergics; CNS Depressants; Dronedarone; Paliperidone; Pimozide; QTc-Prolonging Agents; QuiNINE; Tetrabenazine; Thioridazine; Ziprasidone

The levels/effects of Risperidone may be increased by: Acetylcholinesterase Inhibitors (Central); Alfuzosin; Artemether; Chloroquine; Ciprofloxacin; Ciprofloxacin (Systemic); CYP2D6 Inhibitors (Moderate); CYP2D6 Inhibitors (Strong); Darunavir; Divalproex; Gadobutrol; Lithium formulations; Lumefantrine; Metoclopramide; Nilotinib; Pramlintide; QuiNINE; Selective Serotonin Reuptake Inhibitors; Tetrabenazine; Valproic Acid; Verapamil

Decreased Effect

Risperidone may decrease the levels/effects of: Amphetamines; Anti-Parkinson's Agents (Dopamine Agonist); Quinagolide

The levels/effects of Risperidone may be decreased by: CarBAMazepine; Lithium formulations; Peginterferon Alfa-2b

Food Interactions Food does not affect rate or extent of oral absorption; oral solution is not compatible with cola or tea

Stability

Oral solution, tablet: Store at controlled room temperature 15°C to 25°C (59°F to 77°F); protect from light; protect tablets from moisture; protect oral solution from freezing; do not store orally-disintegrating tablets once removed from blister unit.

Injection: Store undiluted vials and diluent at 2°C to 8°C (36°F to 46°F); protect from light; may store at room temperature ≤77°F (25°C) for ≤7 days prior to reconstitution; reconstituted suspension must be used within 6 hours.

Mechanism of Action Atypical antipsychotic (benzisoxazole derivative); highly potent serotonin and dopamine receptor antagonist; binds to 5-HT$_2$-receptors in the CNS and in the periphery with a very high affinity; binds to dopamine-D$_2$ receptors, but with less affinity (~20 times lower). The addition of serotonin antagonism to dopamine antagonism (classic neuroleptic mechanism) is thought to improve negative symptoms of psychoses and reduce the incidence of extrapyramidal side effects. Alpha$_1$, alpha$_2$ adrenergic, and histaminergic receptors are also antagonized with high affinity. Risperidone has low to moderate affinity for 5-HT$_{1c}$, 5-HT$_{1D}$, and 5-HT$_{1A}$ receptors, weak affinity for D$_1$ and no affinity for cholinergic muscarinic or beta$_1$ and beta$_2$ receptors

Pharmacokinetics (Adult data unless noted) Note: Following oral administration, the pharmacokinetics of risperidone and 9-hydroxyrisperidone in children were found to be similar to values in adults (after adjusting for differences in body weight).

Absorption:

Oral: Well absorbed

I.M.: Initial: <1% of dose released from microspheres; main release starts at ≥3 weeks; release is maintained from 4-6 weeks; release ends by 7 weeks

Distribution: Distributes into breast milk; breast milk to plasma ratio (n=1): Risperidone: 0.42; 9-hydroxyrisperidone: 0.24 (see Hill, 2000)

V_d: Risperidone: 1-2 L/kg

Protein binding: Risperidone: 90%, plasma protein binding increases with increasing concentrations of alpha$_1$-acid glycoprotein; 9-hydroxyrisperidone: 77%; **Note:** Risperidone free fraction may be increased by ~35% in patients with hepatic impairment due to decreased concentrations of albumin and alpha$_1$-acid glycoprotein

Metabolism: Extensive in the liver via cytochrome P450 CYP2D6 to 9-hydroxyrisperidone (major active metabolite); also undergoes N-dealkylation (minor pathway); **Note:** 9-hydroxyrisperidone is the predominant circulating form and is approximately equal to risperidone in receptor binding activity; clinical effects are from combined concentrations of risperidone and 9-hydroxyrisperidone; clinically important differences between CYP2D6 poor and extensive metabolizers are not expected (pharmacokinetics of the sum of risperidone and 9-hydroxyrisperidone were similar in poor and extensive metabolizers)

Bioavailability:

Oral: 70%; tablet (relative to solution): 94%; **Note:** Orally-disintegrating tablets and oral solution are bioequivalent to tablets.

IM: Deltoid I.M. injection is bioequivalent to gluteal I.M. injection

Half-life (apparent):

Oral:

Risperidone: Extensive metabolizers: 3 hours; poor metabolizers: 20 hours

9-hydroxyrisperidone: Extensive metabolizers: 21 hours; poor metabolizers: 30 hours

Sum of risperidone and 9-hydroxyrisperidone: Overall mean: 20 hours

I.M.: 3-6 days (due to extended release of drug from microspheres and subsequent absorption)

Time to peak serum concentration: Oral: Solution or tablet: Risperidone: 1 hour

9-hydroxyrisperidone: Extensive metabolizers: 3 hours; poor metabolizers: 17 hours

Elimination: Excreted as risperidone and metabolites in urine (70%) and feces (14%)

Clearance: Moderate to severe renal impairment (sum of risperidone and 9-hydroxyrisperidone): Decreased by 60%

Usual Dosage

Oral:

Children and Adolescents:

Autism: Treatment of irritability associated with autistic disorder, including aggression, temper tantrums, self-injurious behavior, and quickly changing moods:

Children ≥5 years and Adolescents: Manufacturer's recommendation: **Note:** Individualize dose according to patient response and tolerability:

<15 kg: Use with caution; specific dosing recommendations not available

<20 kg: Initial: 0.25 mg/day; after ≥4 days may increase dose to 0.5 mg/day; maintain this dose for ≥14 days. In patients not achieving sufficient clinical response, may increase dose in increments of 0.25 mg/day at ≥2-week intervals. Therapeutic effect reached plateau at 1 mg/day in clinical trials. Following clinical response, consider gradually decreasing dose to lowest effective dose. May be administered once daily or in divided doses twice daily.

≥20 kg: Initial: 0.5 mg/day; after ≥4 days may increase dose to 1 mg/day; maintain this dose for ≥14 days. In patients not achieving sufficient clinical response, may increase dose in increments of 0.5 mg/day at ≥2-week intervals. Therapeutic effect reached plateau at 2.5 mg/day (3 mg/day in children >45 kg) in clinical trials. Following clinical response, consider gradually decreasing to lowest effective dose. May be administered once daily or in divided doses twice daily.

Note: See Additional Information for doses used in studies to treat aggressive behavior and serious behavioral problems in pediatric patients with pervasive developmental disorders and other various psychiatric diagnoses.

Bipolar disorder: Children and Adolescents 10-17 years: Initial: 0.5 mg once daily; dose may be adjusted if needed, in increments of 0.5-1 mg/day at intervals ≥24 hours, as tolerated, to a dose of 2.5 mg/day. Doses ranging from 0.5-6 mg/day have been evaluated; however, doses >2.5 mg/day do not confer additional benefit and are associated with increased adverse events. Doses >6 mg/day have not been studied. **Note:** May administer 1/2 the daily dose twice daily in patients who experience persistent somnolence.

Schizophrenia: Adolescents 13-17 years: Initial: 0.5 mg once daily; dose may be adjusted if needed, in increments of 0.5-1 mg/day at intervals ≥24 hours, as tolerated, to a dose of 3 mg/day. Doses ranging from 1-6 mg/day have been evaluated; however, doses >3 mg/day do not confer additional benefit and are associated with increased adverse events. Doses >6 mg/day have not been studied. **Note:** May administer 1/2 the daily dose twice daily in patients who experience persistent somnolence.

Tourette's syndrome: Limited information is available: In a multicenter, double-blind, parallel-group comparative study, 50 patients 11-50 years of age were treated for Tourette's syndrome with risperidone (n=26; median age: 20 years; 10 patients <18 years of age) versus pimozide (n=24); a fixed-dose titration of risperidone from 0.5 mg/day to 2 mg/day was used for the first week of therapy; this was followed by a flexible dosing period of 7 weeks; doses were increased by ≤1 mg/week up to a maximum of 6 mg/day and were given once daily; final dose: 0.5-6 mg/day (mean: 3.8 mg/day); both drugs significantly improved tics; although there was no difference in efficacy between drugs, risperidone was better tolerated; the authors suggest that the average dose in this study is high compared to their clinical experience and that the fixed-dose titration during the first week may have been too rapid; a slower dosing schedule and lower long-term doses (eg, 1-2 mg/day) may be needed (see Bruggeman, 2001).

Seven patients 11-16 years of age (mean: 12.9 ± 1.9 years) were treated in a prospective open-labeled trial for chronic tic disorders (5 with Tourette's syndrome) with initial doses of 0.5 mg at bedtime; doses were increased in 5 of the 7 patients by 0.5 mg/day increments every 5 days as tolerated to a maximum of 2.5 mg/day and given in twice daily doses (doses were increased more rapidly in 2 patients); final dose: 1-2.5 mg/day; a decrease in tic severity was seen in all patients; the authors recommend initial doses of 0.5 mg/day and increases of 0.5 mg/day every 5-7 days (see Lombroso, 1995). In a retrospective review, 28 patients 5-18 years of age (mean 11.1 ± 3.6 years) with Tourette's syndrome and aggressive behavior were treated with risperidone; final dose: 0.5-9 mg/day (mean: 2 mg/day); a decrease in aggression scores occurred in 22 of 28 patients (78.5%); frequency and severity of tics were decreased in 17 patients (61.7%) (see Sandor, 2000). Further studies are needed.

Adults: **Note:** Patients predisposed to hypotension or in whom hypotension would be a risk, and debilitated patients should use the dose listed below for renal or hepatic impairment; monitor carefully; debilitated patients should receive twice daily dosing for 2-3 days at the target dose before switching to once daily dosing.
Schizophrenia: Initial: 1 mg twice daily; increase dose in increments of 1-2 mg/day at intervals ≥24 hours, as tolerated, to a recommended dosage range of 4-8 mg/day; some patients may require a slower titration; dose may be given as a single daily dose once maintenance dose is achieved; for twice daily dosing, doses >6 mg/day did not appear to be more effective than lower doses and were associated with more adverse effects (eg, extrapyramidal symptoms). Further dose adjustments should be made in increments/decrements of 1-2 mg/day on a weekly basis. For once-daily dosing, efficacy was stronger for 8 mg/day versus 4 mg/day in one study. Dose range studied in clinical trials: 4-16 mg/day; safety of doses >16 mg/day has not been assessed. Use lowest effective dose; reassess periodically for continued need.
Maintenance therapy: Recommended dosage range: 2-8 mg/day
Bipolar mania: Initial: 2-3 mg/dose once daily; adjust dose as needed, by 1 mg/day increments at intervals ≥24 hours; dosing range: 1-6 mg/day

I.M.:
Adults: **Schizophrenia, Bipolar I maintenance:** (Risperdal® Consta®): 25 mg every 2 weeks; some patients may benefit from larger doses; maximum dose: 50 mg every 2 weeks; do not increase dose more often than every 4 weeks. A lower initial dose of 12.5 mg may be appropriate in some patients (eg, those with hepatic or renal impairment; certain drug interactions which increase risperidone levels; patients with a history of poor tolerance to psychotropic medications). **Note:** The efficacy of the 12.5 mg dose has not been assessed in clinical trials.
Note: Oral risperidone (or other antipsychotic) should be administered with the initial I.M. injection of Risperdal® Consta® and continued for 3 weeks (then discontinued) to maintain adequate therapeutic plasma concentrations before the main release phase of risperidone from the injection site (see Pharmacokinetics, Absorption). When switching from depot administration to short-acting formulation, administer short-acting agent in place of the next regularly-scheduled depot injection.
Dosing adjustment in renal impairment: Adults:
Oral: Initial: 0.5 mg twice daily; increase (as tolerated) in increments of ≤0.5 mg twice daily; increases to dosages >1.5 mg twice daily should be made at intervals of ≥7 days; slower titration may be required in some patients. Clearance of the active moiety (sum of parent drug and active metabolite) is decreased by 60% in patients with moderate-to-severe renal disease compared to healthy subjects.
I.M.: Carefully titrate with oral risperidone, first; then may transition to I.M therapy; consider initial I.M. dose of 12.5 mg.
Dosing adjustment in hepatic impairment: Adults:
Oral: Initial: 0.5 mg twice daily; increase (as tolerated) in increments of ≤0.5 mg twice daily; increases to dosages >1.5 mg twice daily should be made at intervals of ≥7 days; slower titration may be required in some patients. The mean free fraction of risperidone in plasma was increased by 35% in patients with hepatic impairment compared to healthy subjects.
I.M.: Carefully titrate with oral risperidone, first; then may transition to I.M therapy; consider initial I.M. dose of 12.5 mg.

Administration
Oral: May be administered without regard to meals.
Oral solution: May administer directly from the manufacturer provided calibrated pipette or may mix with water, coffee, orange juice, or low-fat milk; do not mix with cola or tea; **Note:** Manufacturer provided calibrated pipette is calibrated in milligrams and milliliters; minimum calibrated volume: 0.25 mL; maximum calibrated volume: 3 mL
Orally-disintegrating tablets: Do not remove tablet from blister pack until ready to administer; do not push tablet through foil (tablet may become damaged); peel back foil to expose tablet; use dry hands to remove tablet and place immediately on tongue; tablet will dissolve within seconds and may be swallowed with or without liquid; do not split or chew tablet
I.M.: Before reconstitution, bring injection and diluent to room temperature; reconstitute with provided diluent only; shake vial vigorously for a minimum of 10 seconds to properly mix; suspension should appear thick, milky, and uniform; use immediately (or within 6 hours of reconstitution); if suspension settles prior to use, shake vigorously to resuspend
Adults: Administer deep I.M. into either the deltoid muscle or the upper-outer quadrant of the gluteal area; avoid inadvertent injection into blood vessel; **do not administer I.V.;** alternate injection site between the two arms or buttocks; do not combine two different dosage strengths into one single administration; administer with needle provided (1-inch needle for deltoid administration or 2-inch needle for gluteal administration); do not substitute any components of the dose pack

Monitoring Parameters Orthostatic blood pressure and heart rate, especially during dosage titration; weight, growth, BMI, and waist circumference, especially in children (see Precautions); CBC with differential; liver enzymes in children (especially obese children or those who are rapidly gaining weight while receiving therapy); lipid profile; serum glucose; fasting blood glucose at the beginning of therapy and periodically in patients with diabetes mellitus (or with risk factors such as family history or obesity); fasting blood glucose in patients who develop symptoms of hyperglycemia

Patient Information May cause dizziness or drowsiness and impair ability to perform activities requiring mental alertness or physical coordination; may cause dry mouth; may cause postural hypotension, especially during initial dose titration (use caution when changing position from lying or sitting to standing). May cause photosensitivity reactions (eg, exposure to sunlight may cause severe sunburn, skin rash, redness, or itching); avoid exposure to sunlight and artificial light sources (sunlamps, tanning booth/bed); wear protective clothing, wide-brimmed hats, sunglasses, and lip sunscreen (SPF ≥15); use a sunscreen [broad-spectrum sunscreen or physical sunscreen (preferred) or sunblock with SPF ≥15]; contact physician if reaction occurs.

Report the use of other medications, nonprescription medications and herbal or natural products to your physician and pharmacist; avoid alcohol and the herbal medicine, St John's wort. Report persistent CNS effects (eg, trembling fingers, altered gait or balance, excessive sedation, seizures, unusual muscle or skeletal movements), rapid heartbeat, palpitations, severe dizziness, fainting, swelling or pain in breasts (male and female), altered menstrual pattern, changes in urinary patterns, vision changes, skin rash, difficulty breathing, or worsening of condition to your physician

Nursing Implications May need to assist patient in rising slowly from lying or sitting to standing position [orthostatic blood pressure changes, tachycardia and syncope (rare) may occur (see Warnings and Monitoring Parameters)]

Additional Information Long-term usefulness of risperidone should be periodically re-evaluated in patients receiving the drug for extended periods of time. Risperdal® Consta® is a long-acting injection comprised of an extended release microsphere formulation; prior to injection, the microspheres are suspended in the provided diluent; the small polymeric microspheres degrade slowly, releasing the medication at a controlled rate (see Pharmacokinetics, Absorption). Lactating women receiving oral risperidone should **not** breast-feed an infant; lactating women receiving I.M. risperidone should **not** breast-feed an infant during therapy and for at least 12 weeks after her last injection.

Additional detailed risperidone dosing information for Children and Adolescents: Oral:

Aggressive behavior in patients with various psychiatric diagnoses: Limited information is available: In a randomized, double-blind, placebo-controlled study, 10 patients 6-14 years of age (mean: 9.2 ± 2.9 years) with conduct disorder and prominent aggressive behavior received risperidone in the following doses: Patients <50 kg: Initial: 0.25 mg once daily; doses were increased as needed by 0.25 mg/day increments each week to a maximum of 1.5 mg/day; patients ≥50 kg: Initial: 0.5 mg once daily; doses were increased as needed by 0.5 mg/day increments each week to a maximum of 3 mg/day; doses were given once daily in the morning; 6 of 10 patients completed the 10-week study; final dose: 0.75-1.5 mg/day; mean: 0.028 ± 0.004 mg/kg/day; risperidone was more effective than placebo in decreasing aggressive behavior (see Findling, 2000). In another randomized, double-blind, placebo-controlled study, 19 adolescents (mean age: 14 ± 1.5 years; 7 with borderline IQ and 6 with mild mental retardation) who were hospitalized for treatment of psychiatric disorders associated with aggressive behavior, received initial risperidone doses of 0.5 mg twice daily; doses were increased as needed by 1 mg/day increments up to a planned maximum of 5 mg twice daily; final doses: Range: 1.5-4 mg/day (0.019-0.08 mg/kg/day); mean: 2.9 mg/day (0.044 mg/kg/day); risperidone was more effective than placebo in decreasing aggressive behavior; although the initial dose was well tolerated by all patients, the authors recommend the following initial doses for clinical practice: Patients <25 kg: 0.25 mg/day; patients ≥25 kg: 0.5 mg/day (see Buitelaar, 2001).

In an open trial, 26 patients 10-18 years of age (mean: 15 ± 1.9 years) with a borderline IQ (n=19) or mild mental retardation (n=5), who were hospitalized for treatment of psychiatric disorders associated with aggressive behavior, received initial risperidone doses of 0.5 mg/day; doses were increased by 0.5-1 mg/day increments every 3 days up to a planned maximum of 6 mg/day and given in twice daily doses; final dose: 0.5-4 mg/day; mean: 2.1 ± 1 mg/day; a marked reduction in aggressive behavior was observed in 14 of 26 patients (54%); **Note:** Four subjects who discontinued therapy after 8 weeks received higher doses (mean: 3.3 ± 1 mg/day) than those who continued on medication (mean: 1.9 ± 0.9 mg/day) (see Buitelaar, 2000). Eleven patients 5.5-16 years of age (mean: 9.8 years) with mood disorders and aggressive behavior received risperidone in titrated doses in an open trial; final dose: 0.75-2.5 mg/day given in 2-3 divided doses; a decrease in aggressive behavior was observed in 8 of 11 patients (see Schreier, 1998).

Pervasive developmental disorders (PDDs): Limited information is available: In a prospective open-labeled study, 18 patients 5-18 years of age (mean: 10.2 ± 3.7 years) were treated for PDDs (11 with autistic disorder) with initial doses of 0.5 mg at night; doses were increased as needed by 0.5 mg/day increments every week and dosed twice daily; optimal dose: 1-4 mg/day (mean: 1.8 ± 1 mg/day); 12 of 18 patients responded (see McDougle, 1997). Fourteen patients 9-17 years of age (mean: 12.7 ± 4 years) were treated in an open case series, for PDDs (4 with autistic disorder) with initial doses of 0.25 mg twice daily; doses were increased as needed by 0.25 mg/day increments every 5-7 days; optimal dose: 0.75-1.5 mg/day given in divided doses; 13 of 14 patients showed a beneficial response (see Fisman, 1996). In an open trial, 6 patients 7-14 years of age (mean: 10.7 ± 3.3 years) were treated for PDDs (5 with autistic disorder; all 6 with severe behavioral problems) with initial doses of 0.5 mg once or twice daily; doses were increased as needed by 0.5 mg/day increments every few days; optimal dose: 1-6 mg/day (mean: 2.7 ± 2.2 mg/day); significant benefit was seen in 5 of the 6 patients (see Perry, 1997). Twenty patients (age: 8-17 years) with developmental disorders refractory to previous psychotropic agents were treated in an open clinical trial with risperidone; doses were increased as needed slowly over several weeks; final doses (n=20): 1.5-10 mg/day; responders (n=13): 1-4 mg/day; nonresponders: 4.5-10 mg/day (see Hardan, 1996). Further studies are needed.

Dosage Forms Excipient information presented when available (limited, particularly for generics); consult specific product labeling.

Injection, microspheres for reconstitution, extended release:

Risperdal® Consta®: 12.5 mg, 25 mg, 37.5 mg, 50 mg [contains polylactide-co-glycolide; supplied in a dose-pack containing vial with active ingredient in microsphere formulation, prefilled syringe with diluent, needle-free vial access device, and 2 safety needles (a 21 G UTW 1-inch and a 20 G TW 2-inch)]

Solution, oral: 1 mg/mL (30 mL)

Risperdal®: 1 mg/mL (30 mL) [contains benzoic acid]

Tablet: 0.25 mg, 0.5 mg, 1 mg, 2 mg, 3 mg, 4 mg

Risperdal®: 0.25 mg, 0.5 mg, 1 mg, 2 mg, 3 mg, 4 mg

Tablet, orally disintegrating: 0.25 mg, 0.5 mg, 1 mg, 2 mg, 3 mg, 4 mg

Risperdal® M-Tab®: 0.5 mg [contains phenylalanine 0.14 mg]; 1 mg [contains phenylalanine 0.28 mg]; 2 mg [contains phenylalanine 0.42 mg]; 3 mg [contains phenylalanine 0.63 mg]; 4 mg [contains phenylalanine 0.84 mg]

References

American Diabetes Association, American Psychiatric Association, American Association of Clinical Endocrinologists, and North American Association for the Study of Obesity, "Consensus Development Conference on Antipsychotic Drugs and Obesity and Diabetes," *Diabetes Care*, 2004, 27(2):596-601.

Armenteros JL, Whitaker AH, Welikson M, et al, "Risperidone in Adolescents With Schizophrenia: An Open Pilot Study," *J Am Acad Child Adolesc Psychiatry*, 1997, 36(5):694-700.

Bruggeman R, van der Linden C, Buitelaar JK, et al, "Risperidone Versus Pimozide in Tourette's Disorder: A Comparative Double-Blind Parallel-Group Study," *J Clin Psychiatry*, 2001, 62(1):50-6.

Buitelaar JK, "Open-Label Treatment With Risperidone of 26 Psychiatrically-Hospitalized Children and Adolescents With Mixed Diagnoses and Aggressive Behavior," *J Child Adolesc Psychopharmacol*, 2000, 10(1):19-26.

Buitelaar JK, van der Gaag RJ, Cohen-Kettenis P, et al, "A Randomized Controlled Trial of Risperidone in the Treatment of Aggression in Hospitalized Adolescents With Subaverage Cognitive Abilities," *J Clin Psychiatry*, 2001, 62(4):239-48.

Correll CU, Manu P, Olshanskiy V, et al, "Cardiometabolic Risk of Second-Generation Antipsychotic Medications During First-Time Use in Children and Adolescents," *JAMA*, 2009, 302(16):1765-73.

Findling RL, Maxwell K, and Wiznitzer M, "An Open Clinical Trial of Risperidone Monotherapy in Young Children With Autistic Disorder," *Psychopharmacol Bull*, 1997, 33(1):155-9.

Findling RL, McNamara NK, Branicky LA, et al, "A Double-Blind Pilot Study of Risperidone in the Treatment of Conduct Disorder," *J Am Acad Child Adolesc Psychiatry*, 2000, 39(4):509-16.

Fisman S and Steele M, "Use of Risperidone in Pervasive Developmental Disorders: A Case Series," *J Child Adolesc Psychopharmacol*, 1996, 6(3):177-90.

Frazier JA, Meyer MC, Biederman J, et al, "Risperidone Treatment for Juvenile Bipolar Disorder: A Retrospective Chart Review," *J Am Acad Child Adolesc Psychiatry*, 1999, 38(8):960-5.

Fu-I L, Boarati MA, Stravogiannis A, et al, "Use of Risperidone Long-Acting Injection to Support Treatment Adherence and Mood Stabilization in Pediatric Bipolar Patients: A Case Series," *J Clin Psychiatry*, 2009, 70(4):604-6.

Grcevich SJ, Findling RL, Rowane WA, et al, "Risperidone in the Treatment of Children and Adolescents With Schizophrenia: A Retrospective Study," *J Child Adolesc Psychopharmacol*, 1996, 6 (4):251-7.

Hardan A, Johnson K, Johnson C, et al, "Case Study: Risperidone Treatment of Children and Adolescents With Developmental Disorders," *J Am Acad Child Adolesc Psychiatry*, 1996, 35 (11):1551-6.

Hill RC, McIvor RJ, Wojnar-Horton RE, et al, "Risperidone Distribution and Excretion Into Human Milk: Case Report and Estimated Infant Exposure During Breast-Feeding," *J Clin Psychopharmacol*, 2000, 20 (2):285-6.

Kumra S, Herion D, Jacobsen LK, et al, "Case Study: Risperidone-Induced Hepatotoxicity in Pediatric Patients," *J Am Acad Child Adolesc Psychiatry*, 1997, 36(5):701-5.

Lombroso PJ, Scahill L, King RA, et al, "Risperidone Treatment of Children and Adolescents With Chronic Tic Disorders: A Preliminary Report," *J Am Acad Child Adolesc Psychiatry*, 1995, 34(9):1147-52.

McCracken JT, McGough J, Shah B, et al, "Risperidone in Children With Autism and Serious Behavioral Problems," *N Engl J Med*, 2002, 347 (5):314-21.

McDougle CJ, Holmes JP, Bronson MR, et al, "Risperidone Treatment of Children and Adolescents With Pervasive Developmental Disorders: A Prospective Open-Label Study," *J Am Acad Child Adolesc Psychiatry*, 1997, 36(5):685-93.

McDougle CJ, Scahill L, McCracken JT, et al, "Research Units on Pediatric Psychopharmacology (RUPP) Autism Network. Background and Rationale for an Initial Controlled Study of Risperidone," *Child Adolesc Psychiatr Clin N Am*, 2000, 9(1):201-24.

Nicolson R, Awad G, and Sloman L, "An Open Trial of Risperidone in Young Autistic Children," *J Am Acad Child Adolesc Psychiatry*, 1998, 37(4):372-6.

Perry R, Pataki C, Munoz-Silva DM, et al, "Risperidone in Children and Adolescents With Pervasive Developmental Disorder: Pilot Trial and Follow-Up," *J Child Adolesc Psychopharmacol*, 1997, 7(3):167-79.

Sandor P and Stephens RJ, "Risperidone Treatment of Aggressive Behavior in Children With Tourette Syndrome," *J Clin Psychopharmacol*, 2000, 20(6):710-2.

Schreier HA, "Risperidone for Young Children With Mood Disorders and Aggressive Behavior," *J Child Adolesc Psychopharmacol*, 1998, 8 (1):49-59.

◆ **Ritalin®** *see* Methylphenidate *on page 908*

◆ **Ritalin LA®** *see* Methylphenidate *on page 908*

◆ **Ritalin-SR®** *see* Methylphenidate *on page 908*

◆ **Ritalin® SR (Can)** *see* Methylphenidate *on page 908*

Ritonavir (rit ON uh veer)

Medication Safety Issues
Sound-alike/look-alike issues:
Ritonavir may be confused with Retrovir®
Norvir® may be confused with Norvasc®

Related Information
Adult and Adolescent HIV *on page 1620*
Management of Healthcare Worker Exposures to HBV, HCV, and HIV *on page 1661*
Pediatric HIV *on page 1613*
Perinatal HIV *on page 1628*

U.S. Brand Names Norvir®

Canadian Brand Names Norvir®; Norvir® SEC

Therapeutic Category Antiretroviral Agent; HIV Agents (Anti-HIV Agents); Protease Inhibitor

Generic Available No

Use Treatment of HIV infection in combination with other antiretroviral agents (FDA approved in ages >1 month and adults). (**Note:** HIV regimens consisting of **three** antiretroviral agents are strongly recommended)

Pregnancy Risk Factor B

Pregnancy Considerations Ritonavir crosses the placenta in minimal amounts; no increased risk of overall birth defects has been observed following 1st trimester exposure according to data collected by the antiretroviral pregnancy registry. Early studies have shown lower plasma levels during pregnancy compared to postpartum. If needed during pregnancy, use in combination with another PI to boost levels of second PI. Pregnancy and protease inhibitors are both associated with an increased risk of hyperglycemia. Glucose levels should be closely monitored. The Perinatal HIV Guidelines Working Group considers ritonavir to be an alternative PI for use during pregnancy. Healthcare professionals are encouraged to contact the antiretroviral pregnancy registry to monitor outcomes of pregnant women exposed to antiretroviral medications (1-800-258-4263 or www.APRegistry.com).

Lactation Excretion in breast milk unknown/not recommended

Breast-Feeding Considerations In infants born to mothers who are HIV positive, HAART while breast-feeding may decrease postnatal infection. However, maternal or infant antiretroviral therapy does not completely eliminate the risk of postnatal HIV transmission.

In the United States where formula is accessible, affordable, safe, and sustainable, complete avoidance of breast-feeding by HIV-infected women is recommended to decrease potential transmission of HIV.

Contraindications Hypersensitivity to ritonavir or any component; concurrent therapy with alfuzosin, amiodarone, bepridil, cisapride, dihydroergotamine, ergotamine, ergonovine, flecainide, lovastatin, methylergonovine, midazolam (oral), pimozide, propafenone, quinidine, sildenafil (when used for the treatment of pulmonary arterial hypertension), simvastatin, St John's wort, triazolam; concurrent therapy with voriconazole [when ritonavir dose is ≥800 mg/day; **Note:** The ≥800 mg/day is based on adult studies; the pediatric dose of ritonavir which requires voriconazole be contraindicated is not known; pediatric clinicians consider voriconazole to be contraindicated when using therapeutic doses of ritonavir; it should be noted that booster doses of ritonavir (in pediatric patients and adults) should be avoided in patients receiving voriconazole, unless benefit outweighs the risk] (see Drug Interactions)

Warnings Ritonavir is a potent CYP3A enzyme inhibitor that interacts with numerous drugs **[U.S. Boxed Warnings]**. Due to potential serious and/or life-threatening drug interactions, some drugs are contraindicated (see Contraindications and Drug Interactions). Concomitant use with fluticasone, salmeterol, high-dose ketoconazole, high-dose itraconazole, or high-dose or long-term use of meperidine is **not** recommended. Alteration of dose or serum concentration monitoring may be required with other medications (see Drug Interactions). Use of ritonavir with other antiretroviral agents (eg, certain protease inhibitors) may require dosage adjustment of both agents (see individual monographs for specific dosage recommendations).

Potentially fatal pancreatitis may occur; advanced HIV disease and elevated serum triglycerides may place patient at increased risk; discontinue ritonavir in patients with pancreatitis. Hepatic reactions, including elevated liver enzymes, hepatitis, and jaundice may occur; coinfection with hepatitis B or C may increase risk; hepatic dysfunction with fatalities has also been reported. Significant elevations of serum triglycerides and cholesterol may occur (monitor and manage appropriately). Allergic reactions may also occur (see Adverse Reactions); discontinue ritonavir if severe allergic reaction occurs.

New onset diabetes mellitus, exacerbation of diabetes, and hyperglycemia have been reported in HIV-infected patients receiving protease inhibitors.

Precautions Use with caution in patients with hepatic insufficiency, elevated liver enzymes, or hepatitis. Ritonavir may prolong the PR interval; cases of second- or third-degree AV block have been reported; use with caution in patients with cardiomyopathy, ischemic heart disease, pre-existing conduction abnormalities, or structural heart disease [these patients may be at increased risk of conduction abnormalities (eg, second- or third-degree AV block)]; use with caution with drugs that prolong the PR interval. Spontaneous bleeding episodes have been reported in patients with hemophilia type A and B receiving protease inhibitors. Fat redistribution and accumulation [ie, central obesity, peripheral wasting, facial wasting, breast enlargement, dorsocervical fat enlargement (buffalo hump), and cushingoid appearance] have been observed in patients receiving antiretroviral agents (causal relationship not established). Immune reconstitution syndrome (an acute inflammatory response to residual or indolent opportunistic infections) may occur in HIV patients during initial treatment with combination antiretroviral agents, including ritonavir; this syndrome may require further patient assessment and therapy. Ritonavir oral solution contains 43% alcohol by volume; accidental ingestion could result in alcohol-related toxicity. Safety and efficacy of ritonavir in patients <1 month of age have not been established.

Adverse Reactions Note: In pediatric clinical trials, adverse event profiles were similar to adults.

Cardiovascular: AV block, PR prolongation (see Warnings), right bundle branch block, vasodilation

Central nervous system: Confusion, dizziness, fever, headache, insomnia, somnolence, syncope

Endocrine & metabolic: Creatine phosphokinase increased; fat redistribution and accumulation (see Precautions); triglycerides and cholesterol increased (see Warnings); Rare: Exacerbation of diabetes, hyperglycemia, ketoacidosis, new-onset diabetes mellitus (see Warnings)

Gastrointestinal: Abdominal pain, anorexia, diarrhea, nausea, pancreatitis (see Warnings), taste perversion, vomiting; **Note:** Patients taking the soft gel capsule may experience more GI side effects when switching to the tablet due to higher peak concentrations.

Hematologic: Rare: Spontaneous bleeding episodes in hemophiliacs (see Warnings)

Hepatic: Hepatitis (may be life-threatening in rare cases) (see Warnings), liver enzymes increased, worsening of chronic liver disease

Neuromuscular & skeletal: Circumoral and peripheral paresthesias, weakness

Miscellaneous: Allergic reaction (angioedema, bronchospasm, rash, urticaria; see Warnings), anaphylaxis, immune reconstitution syndrome (see Precautions)

<2%, postmarketing, and/or case reports (limited to important or life-threatening): Abnormal vision, acute myeloblastic leukemia, adrenal cortex insufficiency, amnesia, anemia, aphasia, asthma, cachexia, cerebral ischemia, cerebral venous thrombosis, chest pain, cholestatic jaundice, coma, dehydration, dementia, depersonalization, dyspnea, edema, esophageal ulcer, gastroenteritis, GI hemorrhage, hallucinations, hepatic coma, hepatomegaly, hepatosplenomegaly, hyper-/hypotension, hypothermia, hypoventilation, ileus, interstitial pneumonia, kidney failure, larynx edema, leukopenia, lymphadenopathy, lymphocytosis, manic reaction, MI, myeloproliferative disorder, neuropathy, orthostatic hypotension, palpitation, paralysis, postural hypotension, pseudomembranous colitis, rectal hemorrhage, seizure, skin melanoma, Stevens-Johnson syndrome, subdural

hematoma, tachycardia, thrombocytopenia, tongue edema, ulcerative colitis, vasospasm

Drug Interactions

Metabolism/Transport Effects Substrate of CYP1A2 (minor), CYP2B6 (minor), CYP2D6 (major), CYP3A4 (major), P-glycoprotein; **Inhibits** CYP2C8 (strong), CYP2C9 (weak), CYP2C19 (weak), CYP2D6 (strong), CYP2E1 (weak), CYP3A4 (strong), P-glycoprotein; **Induces** CYP1A2 (weak), 2C8 (weak), 2C9 (weak), 3A4 (weak)

Avoid Concomitant Use

Avoid concomitant use of Ritonavir with any of the following: Alfuzosin; Amiodarone; Cisapride; Dabigatran Etexilate; Disulfiram; Dronedarone; Eplerenone; Ergot Derivatives; Etravirine; Everolimus; Flecainide; Fluticasone (Nasal); Halofantrine; Lovastatin; Midazolam; Nilotinib; Nisoldipine; Pimozide; Pitavastatin; Propafenone; QuiNIDine; Ranolazine; Rivaroxaban; Romidepsin; Salmeterol; Silodosin; Simvastatin; St Johns Wort; Tamoxifen; Tamsulosin; Thioridazine; Tolvaptan; Topotecan; Triazolam; Voriconazole

Increased Effect/Toxicity

Ritonavir may increase the levels/effects of: Alfuzosin; Almotriptan; Alosetron; ALPRAZolam; Amiodarone; Antifungal Agents (Azole Derivatives, Systemic); Atomoxetine; Bortezomib; Bosentan; Brinzolamide; Calcium Channel Blockers (Dihydropyridine); Calcium Channel Blockers (Nondihydropyridine); CarBAMazepine; Ciclesonide; Cisapride; Clarithromycin; Clorazepate; Colchicine; Corticosteroids (Orally Inhaled); CycloSPORINE; CycloSPORINE (Systemic); CYP2C8 Substrates (High risk); CYP2D6 Substrates; CYP3A4 Substrates; Dabigatran Etexilate; Diazepam; Dienogest; Digoxin; Dronabinol; Dronedarone; Dutasteride; Enfuvirtide; Eplerenone; Ergot Derivatives; Estazolam; Everolimus; FentaNYL; Fesoterodine; Flecainide; Flurazepam; Fluticasone (Nasal); Fusidic Acid; GuanFACINE; Halofantrine; HMG-CoA Reductase Inhibitors; Ixabepilone; Lovastatin; Lumefantrine; Maraviroc; Meperidine; MethylPREDNISolone; Midazolam; Nebivolol; Nefazodone; Nilotinib; Nisoldipine; Paricalcitol; Pazopanib; P-Glycoprotein Substrates; Pimecrolimus; Pimozide; Pitavastatin; PredniSOLONE; PredniSONE; Propafenone; Protease Inhibitors; QuiNIDine; Ranolazine; Rifamycin Derivatives; Rivaroxaban; Romidepsin; Salmeterol; Saxagliptin; Sildenafil; Silodosin; Simvastatin; Sirolimus; Sorafenib; Tacrolimus; Tacrolimus (Systemic); Tacrolimus (Topical); Tadalafil; Tamoxifen; Tamsulosin; Temsirolimus; Tenofovir; Tetrabenazine; Thioridazine; Tolvaptan; Topotecan; TraZODone; Treprostinil; Triazolam; Tricyclic Antidepressants; Vardenafil; VinBLAStine; VinCRIStine

The levels/effects of Ritonavir may be increased by: Antifungal Agents (Azole Derivatives, Systemic); Clarithromycin; CycloSPORINE; CycloSPORINE (Systemic); Delavirdine; Disulfiram; Efavirenz; Enfuvirtide; Fusidic Acid; MetroNIDAZOLE (Topical); P-Glycoprotein Inhibitors

Decreased Effect

Ritonavir may decrease the levels/effects of: Abacavir; Atovaquone; BuPROPion; Clarithromycin; Codeine; Contraceptives (Estrogens); Deferasirox; Delavirdine; Divalproex; Etravirine; LamoTRIgine; Meperidine; Methadone; Phenytoin; Prasugrel; Theophylline Derivatives; TraMADol; Valproic Acid; Voriconazole; Warfarin; Zidovudine

The levels/effects of Ritonavir may be decreased by: Antacids; CarBAMazepine; Contraceptives (Estrogens); CYP3A4 Inducers (Strong); Efavirenz; Garlic; Nevirapine; Peginterferon Alfa-2b; P-Glycoprotein Inducers; Phenytoin; Rifamycin Derivatives; St Johns Wort; Tenofovir

Food Interactions

Oral solution: Food decreases peak concentrations by 23% and AUC by 7%.

Tablets: Food decreases the bioavailability of ritonavir tablets; however, no difference occurs between a high-fat meal versus a moderate-fat meal. A high fat meal decreases peak concentrations by 23% and AUC by 23%. A moderate-fat meal decreases peak concentrations by 22% and AUC by 21%.

Stability

Capsules: Refrigerate; stable for 30 days at room temperature <77°F (25°C); protect from light; avoid exposure to excessive heat

Tablets: Store at 20°C to 25°C (68°F to 77°F); excursions permitted to 15°C to 30°C (59°F to 86°F). Dispense in original container or USP equivalent tight container (60 mL or less). Exposure to high humidity outside the original or USP equivalent tight container for >2 weeks is **not** recommended.

Oral solution: Dispense and store in original container; store at room temperature 20°C to 25°C (68°F to 77°F); do not refrigerate; avoid exposure to excessive heat; keep bottle tightly closed; use by product expiration date (limited shelf life of 6 months)

Mechanism of Action A protease inhibitor which acts on an enzyme (protease) late in the HIV replication process after the virus has entered into the cell's nucleus; ritonavir binds to the protease activity site and inhibits the activity of the enzyme, thus preventing cleavage of viral polyprotein precursors (gag-pol protein precursors) into individual functional proteins found in infectious HIV; this results in the formation of immature, noninfectious viral particles

Pharmacokinetics (Adult data unless noted)

Absorption: Well absorbed

Distribution: High concentrations in serum and lymph nodes; V_d (apparent): 0.41 ± 0.25 L/kg

Protein binding: 98% to 99%

Metabolism: In the liver by cytochrome P450 isoenzyme CYP3A and (to a lesser extent) CYP2D6; five metabolites have been identified; the major metabolite (M-2), an isopropylthiazole oxidation metabolite, is active at a level similar to ritonavir, but is found in low concentrations in the plasma

Bioavailability: Absolute bioavailability unknown; tablets are **not** bioequivalent to capsules; mean peak concentration of tablet was found to be 26% higher than capsule in a single dose study, in patients fed a moderate-fat meal

Half-life:

Children: 2-4 hours

Adults: 3-5 hours

Time to peak serum concentration: Oral solution: Fasting: 2 hours; nonfasting: 4 hours

Elimination: Renal clearance is negligible; 3.5% of dose is excreted as unchanged drug in the urine; 34% excreted as unchanged drug in the feces

Clearance: Pediatric patients: 1.5 to 1.7 times faster than adults

Usual Dosage Oral (use in combination with other antiretroviral agents):

Ritonavir as sole protease inhibitor:

Neonates: Not approved for use; dose not established; further studies are needed; **Note:** Investigational dose of 450 mg/m²/dose twice daily resulted in lower ritonavir serum concentrations than those seen in adults receiving the standard adult dose.

Infants >1 month and Children: Initial: 250 mg/m²/dose twice daily (every 12 hours); titrate upward at 2-3 day intervals by 50 mg/m²/dose twice daily increments to 350-400 mg/m²/dose twice daily; maximum dose: 600 mg/dose twice daily; **Note:** Patients who do not tolerate 400 mg/m² twice daily (due to adverse effects) may be treated with the highest tolerated dose; however, an alternative antiretroviral agent should be considered. Serum concentrations comparable to those seen in adults receiving standard doses were obtained in children >2 years of age who received 350-400 mg/m²

twice daily. In younger patients (1 month to 2 years of age), who received 350 or 450 mg/m²/dose twice daily, ritonavir AUCs were 16% lower and trough concentrations were 60% lower than those observed in adults receiving standard doses; higher ritonavir AUCs were not observed with the 450 mg/m²/dose twice daily compared to the 350 mg/m²/dose twice daily dosing.

Adolescents and Adults: 600 mg twice daily; may use a dose titration schedule to reduce adverse events (nausea/vomiting) by initiating therapy at 300 mg twice daily; increase dose at 2-3 day intervals by 100 mg twice daily increments up to a maximum dose of 600 mg twice daily

Ritonavir as pharmacokinetic enhancer ("booster doses" of ritonavir): Note: Ritonavir is used at lower doses to increase the serum concentrations of other protease inhibitors; the recommended dose of ritonavir varies when used with different protease inhibitors; see monographs for individual protease inhibitors for recommended doses; appropriate pediatric "booster doses" of ritonavir have not been established for use with every protease inhibitor or for all pediatric age groups.

Adults: Usual dose: 100-400 mg/day, usually as 100-200 mg once or twice daily; range: 100-800 mg/day; dose depends on the protease inhibitor (see **Note** above)

Dosage adjustment in renal impairment: No adjustment recommended (renal clearance is negligible)

Dosage adjustment in hepatic impairment:

Mild to moderate hepatic impairment: No adjustment recommended; lower ritonavir serum concentrations have been reported in patients with moderate hepatic impairment (use with caution; monitor closely for adequate response)

Severe hepatic impairment: Use with caution; pharmacokinetics of ritonavir has not been studied in these patients

Administration Administer with meals. Swallow tablets whole; do not chew, break, or crush. Consider reserving liquid formulation for use in patients receiving tube feeding due to its bad taste. Shake liquid well before use. May mix liquid formulation with milk, chocolate milk, vanilla or chocolate pudding or ice cream, or a liquid nutritional supplement. Other techniques used to increase tolerance in children include dulling the taste buds by chewing ice, giving popsicles or spoonfuls or partially frozen orange or grape juice concentrates before administration of ritonavir; coating the mouth with peanut butter to eat before the dose; administration of strong-tasting foods such as maple syrup, cheese, or strong-flavored chewing gum immediately after a dose. Oral solution is highly concentrated; use a calibrated oral dosing syringe to measure and administer. Separate administration of ritonavir and didanosine by 2.5 hours.

Monitoring Parameters Liver function tests, blood glucose concentrations, serum triglycerides, cholesterol, CPK, uric acid, CD4 cell count, plasma concentrations of HIV RNA

Patient Information Ritonavir is not a cure for HIV. Some medicines should not be taken with ritonavir; report the use of other medications, nonprescription medications, and herbal or natural products to your physician and pharmacist; avoid the herbal medicine St John's wort. Take ritonavir every day as prescribed; do not change dose or discontinue without physician's advice; if dose is missed, take it as soon as possible, then return to normal dosing schedule; if a dose is skipped, do not double the next dose. Notify physician if you have an increase in thirst and/or frequent urination, nausea, vomiting, or abdominal pain, muscle numbness or tingling, respiratory difficulty or chest pain, unusual skin rash, change in color of stool or urine, or any persistent adverse effects.

Ritonavir may cause changes in the electrocardiogram (ECG); notify physician before starting ritonavir if you have a heart defect or conduction defect (these patients should avoid ritonavir); once taking ritonavir, notify physician if you develop lightheadedness, dizziness, an abnormal heart beat, or fainting spells. HIV medications may cause changes in body fat, including an increase in fat in the upper back and neck, breasts, and trunk; a loss of fat from the face, arms, and legs may also occur.

Patients taking the soft gel capsule may experience more GI side effects when switching to the tablet due to higher peak concentrations; these side effects may decrease as the medication is continued. Exposure of the tablets to high humidity outside the original container (or container given to you by the pharmacist) for longer than 2 weeks is **not** recommended.

Nursing Implications Ritonavir is started at lower initial doses and titrated upwards to minimize nausea and vomiting.

Dosage Forms Excipient information presented when available (limited, particularly for generics); consult specific product labeling.

Capsule, soft gelatin, oral:

Norvir®: 100 mg [contains ethanol and polyoxyl 35 castor oil]

Solution, oral:

Norvir®: 80 mg/mL (240 mL) [contains ethanol, polyoxyl 35 castor oil, and propylene glycol; peppermint and caramel flavor]

Tablet, oral:

Norvir®: 100 mg

References

Briars LA, Hilao JJ, and Kraus DM, "A Review of Pediatric Human Immunodeficiency Virus Infection," *Journal of Pharmacy Practice*, 2004, 17(6):407-31.

Danner SA, Carr A, Leonard JM, et al, "A Short-Term Study of the Safety, Pharmacokinetics, and Efficacy of Ritonavir, an Inhibitor of HIV-1 Protease. European-Australian Collaborative Ritonavir Study Group," *N Engl J Med*, 1995, 333(23):1528-33.

DeSilva KE, Le Flore DB, Marston BJ, et al, "Serotonin Syndrome in HIV-Infected Individuals Receiving Antiretroviral Therapy and Fluoxetine," *AIDS*, 2001, 15(10)1281-5.

Gatti G, Pontali E, Boni S, et al, "The Relationship Between Ritonavir Plasma Trough Concentration and Virological and Immunological Response in HIV-Infected Children," *HIV Med*, 2002, 3(2):125-8.

Mueller BU, Nelson RP Jr, Sleasman J, et al, "A Phase I/II Study of the Protease Inhibitor Ritonavir in Children With Human Immunodeficiency Virus Infection," *Pediatrics*, 1998, 101(3 Pt 1):335-43.

Nachman SA, Lindsey JC, Pelton S, et al, "Growth in Human Immunodeficiency Virus-Infected Children Receiving Ritonavir-Containing Antiretroviral Therapy," *Arch Pediatr Adolesc Med*, 2002, 156 (5):497-503.

Nachman SA, Stanley K, Yogev R, et al, "Nucleoside Analogs Plus Ritonavir in Stable Antiretroviral Therapy-Experienced HIV-Infected Children: A Randomized Controlled Trial. Pediatric AIDS Clinical Trials Group 338 Study Team," *JAMA*, 2000, 283(4):492-8.

Panel on Antiretroviral Guidelines for Adults and Adolescents, "Guidelines for the Use of Antiretroviral Agents in HIV-Infected Adults and Adolescents," December 1, 2009. Available at: http://www.aidsinfo.nih.gov.

Working Group on Antiretroviral Therapy and Medical Management of HIV-Infected Children, "Guidelines for the Use of Antiretroviral Agents in Pediatric HIV Infection," February 23, 2009. Available at http://www.aidsinfo.nih.gov.

◆ **Ritonavir and Lopinavir** see Lopinavir and Ritonavir on page 839

◆ **Rituxan®** see RiTUXimab on page 1227

RiTUXimab (ri TUK si mab)

Medication Safety Issues

Sound-alike/look-alike issues:

Rituxan® may be confused with Remicade®

RiTUXimab may be confused with bevacizumab, inFLIXimab

High alert medication: The medication is in a class the Institute for Safe Medication Practices (ISMP) includes among its list of drug classes which have a heightened risk of causing significant patient harm when used in error.

The rituximab dose for rheumatoid arthritis is a flat dose (1000 mg) and is not based on body surface area (BSA).

Related Information

Emetogenic Potential of Antineoplastic Agents on page 1579

U.S. Brand Names Rituxan®

Canadian Brand Names Rituxan®

Therapeutic Category Antineoplastic Agent, Monoclonal Antibody; Monoclonal Antibody

Generic Available No

Use Treatment of relapsed or refractory low-grade or follicular, CD20 positive, B-cell non-Hodgkin's lymphoma; first-line treatment of diffuse large B-cell, CD20-positive, non-Hodgkin's lymphoma in combination with CHOP or other anthracycline-based chemotherapy regimen; systemic autoimmune disorders (ie, autoimmune hemolytic anemia); post-transplant lymphoproliferative disorder (PTLD); rheumatoid arthritis; refractory systemic lupus erythematosus; refractory chronic graft-versus-host disease (GVHD)

Medication Guide An FDA-approved patient medication guide, which is available with the product information and at http://www.fda.gov/downloads/Drugs/DrugSafety/UCM169892.pdf, must be dispensed with this medication for each new outpatient prescription and refill.

Pregnancy Risk Factor C

Pregnancy Considerations Animal studies have demonstrated adverse effects including decreased (reversible) B-cells and immunosuppression. There are no adequate and well-controlled studies in pregnant women. IgG molecules are known to cross the placenta (rituximab is an engineered IgG molecule) and rituximab has been detected in the serum of infants exposed in utero. B-Cell lymphocytopenia lasting <6 months may occur in exposed infants. Use during pregnancy only if clearly needed.

Lactation Excretion in breast milk unknown/not recommended

Breast-Feeding Considerations It is not known if rituximab is excreted in human milk. However, human IgG is excreted in breast milk, and therefore, rituximab may also be excreted in milk. The manufacturer recommends discontinuing breast-feeding until circulating levels of rituximab are no longer detectable.

Contraindications There are no contraindications listed in the manufacturer's labeling.

Warnings Progressive multifocal leukoencephalopathy (PML) due to JC virus has been reported with rituximab use **[U.S. Boxed Warning]**. Cases were reported in patients with hematologic malignancies or autoimmune diseases receiving rituximab either with combination chemotherapy or with hematopoietic stem cell transplant. Cases were also reported in patients receiving rituximab for autoimmune disease (not an approved use) and may have received concurrent or prior immunosuppressant therapy. Onset may be delayed. Evaluate any neurological change promptly.

Fatal infusion reactions which may include hypotension, angioedema, hypoxia, bronchospasm, pulmonary infiltrates, acute respiratory distress syndrome, MI, ventricular fibrillation, and cardiogenic shock have occurred within 24 hours of rituximab administration **[U.S. Boxed Warning]**. Most of these reactions occurred during the first infusion with time to onset of 30-120 minutes. Fatal infusion reactions were more frequently associated with female gender, pulmonary infiltrates, CLL, or mantle cell lymphoma. Close monitoring required during first and subsequent infusions of patients with pre-existing cardiac and pulmonary conditions, patients with prior cardiopulmonary adverse events, and those with high levels of circulating malignant cells ($\geq 25,000/mm^3$). In the event of a severe reaction, interrupt the rituximab infusion and institute supportive care measures (eg, I.V. fluids, vasopressors, oxygen, bronchodilators, diphenhydramine, and acetaminophen). When symptoms completely resolve, may resume rituximab at a 50% reduction from the previous infusion rate. Discontinue rituximab in the event of serious or life-threatening cardiac arrhythmias.

Tumor lysis syndrome leading to acute renal failure requiring dialysis may occur 12-24 hours following the first dose **[U.S. Boxed Warning]**. Prophylaxis for tumor lysis syndrome should be considered for patients at risk (patients with high tumor burden or with high numbers of circulating malignant cells). Severe and sometimes fatal mucocutaneous reactions (lichenoid dermatitis, paraneoplastic pemphigus, Stevens-Johnson syndrome, toxic epidermal necrolysis and vesiculobullous dermatitis) have been reported, occurring from 1-13 weeks following exposure **[U.S. Boxed Warning]**. Patients experiencing severe mucocutaneous skin reactions should not receive further infusions and should seek prompt medical evaluation. Bowel obstruction and perforation have been reported; complaints of abdominal pain should be evaluated.

Reactivation of hepatitis B has been reported in association with use (rare); consider screening in high-risk patients. Other serious and potentially fatal viral infections, either new or reactivated, associated with use include cytomegalovirus, herpes simplex virus, parvovirus B19, varicella zoster virus, West Nile virus, and hepatitis C. Viral infections may be delayed, occurring up to 1 year after discontinuation of therapy.

Precautions Use with caution in patients with pre-existing cardiac or pulmonary conditions, renal impairment, and patients at risk for developing tumor lysis syndrome.

Adverse Reactions

Cardiovascular: Hypotension, angina, arrhythmia, MI, peripheral edema, flushing, syncope, cardiogenic shock, hypertension

Central nervous system: Fever, chills, headache, dizziness, anxiety, progressive multifocal leukoencephalopathy (PML), agitation, insomnia, somnolence, vertigo, malaise, depression

Dermatologic: Angioedema, pruritus, rash, urticaria, Stevens-Johnson syndrome, toxic epidermal necrolysis

Endocrine & metabolic: Hyperglycemia, tumor lysis syndrome, hypoglycemia

Gastrointestinal: Nausea, vomiting, abdominal pain, diarrhea, bowel obstruction and perforation, dyspepsia, anorexia

Hematologic: Lymphopenia, leukopenia, thrombocytopenia, neutropenia (up to 30 days after last dose), aplastic anemia, hemolytic anemia

Hepatic: Hepatitis

Local: Pain at injection site

Neuromuscular & skeletal: Myalgia, asthenia, arthralgia, back pain, weakness, paresthesia, hypertonia

Ocular: Optic neuritis, conjunctivitis, lacrimation disorder

Renal: Acute renal failure

Respiratory: Bronchospasm, dyspnea, rhinitis, throat irritation, cough, pneumonitis, bronchiolitis obliterans, sinusitis

Miscellaneous: Immunosuppression, infection, hepatitis B virus reactivation, anaphylaxis, infusion related reaction (fever, chills, rigors occur in 80% of patients after first infusion, decreasing to 40% in subsequent infusions), lupus-like syndrome, serum sickness

Drug Interactions

Avoid Concomitant Use
Avoid concomitant use of RiTUXimab with any of the following: BCG; Certolizumab Pegol; Natalizumab; Pimecrolimus; Tacrolimus (Topical); Vaccines (Live)

Increased Effect/Toxicity
RiTUXimab may increase the levels/effects of: Certolizumab Pegol; Hypoglycemic Agents; Leflunomide; Natalizumab; Vaccines (Live)

The levels/effects of RiTUXimab may be increased by: Abciximab; Antihypertensives; Denosumab; Herbs (Hypoglycemic Properties); Pimecrolimus; Tacrolimus (Topical); Trastuzumab

Decreased Effect
RiTUXimab may decrease the levels/effects of: BCG; Sipuleucel-T; Vaccines (Inactivated); Vaccines (Live)

The levels/effects of RiTUXimab may be decreased by: Echinacea

Stability Store vials in refrigerator at 2°C to 8°C; do not freeze or shake; protect vials from direct sunlight; dilution of rituximab to a final concentration of 1-4 mg/mL in NS or D_5W is stable for 24 hours if refrigerated or stored at room temperature

Mechanism of Action Rituximab is a monoclonal antibody directed against the CD20 antigen on B-lymphocytes. Rituximab binds to the antigen on the cell surface, activating complement-dependent cytotoxicity; binds to human Fc receptors mediating cell killing through an antibody-dependent cellular toxicity.

Pharmacodynamics Duration: B-cell recovery begins ~6 months following completion of treatment; medium B-cell levels return to normal by 12 months

Pharmacokinetics (Adult data unless noted)
Distribution: Binds to lymphoid cells in the thymus, spleen, and B lymphocytes in peripheral blood and lymph nodes
Half-life: Adults:
  Cancer: Proportional to dose; range in half-life may reflect variable tumor burden among patients and changes in CD20 positive B-cell population with repeat doses:
    1st infusion: 76.3 hours (range: 31.5-152.6 hours)
    4th infusion: 205.8 hours (range: 83.9-407 hours)
  Rheumatoid arthritis: 19 days

Usual Dosage Refer to individual protocols
Children and Adults: I.V. infusion:
  CD20 positive B-cell, non-Hodgkin's lymphoma: Initial: 375 mg/m^2 once weekly for 4-8 doses as single drug therapy or in combination with CHOP (cyclophosphamide, doxorubicin, vincristine, and prednisone)
  Retreatment (patients who subsequently develop progressive disease may receive an additional course): 375 mg/m^2 once weekly for 4 doses or retreatment for refractory cases: 375 mg/m^2 once weekly for 4 doses given every 6 months for up to 2 years
  Refractory CD20 positive non-Hodgkin's lymphoma or B-cell ALL: 375 mg/m^2 on days 1 and 3 in combination with ifosfamide with mesna, carboplatin and etoposide (ICE)
  Relapsed or refractory low-grade, follicular or transformed B-cell non-Hodgkin's lymphoma: Radioimmunotherapy with Ibritumomab: 250 mg/m^2 infused within 4 hours prior to administration of indium ibritumomab; 7-9 days later, 250 mg/m^2 infused within 4 hours prior to yttrium Y90 ibritumomab
  Refractory chronic GVHD, post-transplant lymphoproliferative disorder: 375 mg/m^2 once weekly for 3-4 doses
  Refractory SLE: 375 mg/m^2 once weekly for 2-4 doses; or 750 mg/m^2 on days 1 and 15 (maximum dose: 1000 mg)
  Autoimmune hemolytic anemia, chronic ITP: 375 mg/m^2 once weekly for 3-6 doses

Adults: Rheumatoid arthritis: 1000 mg on days 1 and 15; premedication with a corticosteroid (eg, methylprednisolone 100 mg I.V.) prior to each rituximab dose is recommended.

Administration DO NOT ADMINISTER UNDILUTED NOR as an I.V. Push or rapid injection: I.V. infusion: Administer first infusion at an initial rate of 50 mg/hour at a final concentration for administration of 1-4 mg/mL in NS or D_5W. If no hypersensitivity or infusion-related reactions occur, increase infusion rate in 50 mg/hour increments every 30 minutes to a maximum infusion rate of 400 mg/hour as tolerated. Subsequent rituximab doses can be administered at an initial rate of 100 mg/hour and increased by 100 mg/hour increments at 30 minute intervals to a maximum infusion rate of 400 mg/hour. If hypersensitivity or infusion-related reactions occur, slow or interrupt the infusion. If symptoms completely resolve, resume infusion at $\frac{1}{2}$ the previous rate.

Monitoring Parameters Vital signs, CBC with differential and platelet counts, serum electrolytes, renal function tests, liver function tests, fluid balance; cardiac monitoring for patients with pre-existing cardiac condition; peripheral CD20+ cells; human antimurine antibody and human antichimeric antibody titers; screening for hepatitis B

Reference Range Peripheral CD20+ cells: High pretreatment level (500-1600 cells/microliter) may indicate risk for severe infusion reactions

Patient Information Notify physician if fever, sore throat, rash, dizziness, chest pain, abdominal pain, yellowing of skin or eyes, feeling of weakness, bruising, bleeding, or shortness of breath occurs. Inform physician if you experience any new neurological signs or symptoms including major changes in vision, unusual movements, loss of balance or coordination, disorientation, or confusion. Advise individuals of childbearing potential to use effective contraceptive methods and avoid becoming pregnant during and for 12 months following treatment with rituximab.

Nursing Implications Maintain adequate patient hydration during therapy unless instructed to restrict fluid intake. Hold antihypertensive medications for 12 hours prior to infusion; patient may need to be premedicated with acetaminophen and diphenhydramine prior to each dose to prevent infusion-related reactions. Epinephrine, diphenhydramine, and corticosteroids should be available for immediate use in case of a hypersensitivity reaction.

Dosage Forms Excipient information presented when available (limited, particularly for generics); consult specific product labeling.

Injection, solution [preservative free]:
  Rituxan®: 10 mg/mL (10 mL, 50 mL) [contains polysorbate 80]

References
Edwards JC, Szczepanski L, Szechinski J, et al, "Efficacy of B-Cell-Targeted Therapy With Rituximab in Patients With Rheumatoid Arthritis," *N Engl J Med*, 2004, 350(25):2572-81.

Marks SD, Patey S, Brogan PA, et al, "B Lymphocyte Depletion Therapy in Children With Refractory Systemic Lupus Erythematosus," *Arthritis Rheum*, 2005, 52(10):3168-74.

Serinet MO, Jacquenin E, Habes D, et al, "Anti-CD20 Monoclonal Antibody (Rituximab) Treatment for Epstein-Barr Virus-Associated, B-Cell Lymphoproliferative Disease in Pediatric Liver Transplant Recipients," *J Ped Gastroenterology & Nutrition*, 2002, 34(4):389-93.

Wang J, Wiley JM, Luddy R, et al, "Chronic Immune Thrombocytopenic Purpura in Children: Assessment of Rituximab Treatment," *J Pediatr*, 2005, 146(2):217-21.

Zecca M, Nobili B, Ramenghi U, et al, "Rituximab for the Treatment of Refractory Autoimmune Hemolytic Anemia in Children," *Blood*, 2003, 101(10):3857-61.

♦ **Riva-Amiodarone (Can)** *see* Amiodarone *on page 84*

♦ **Riva-Amlodipine (Can)** *see* AmLODIPine *on page 91*

♦ **Riva-Atenolol (Can)** *see* Atenolol *on page 147*

♦ **Riva-Azithromycin (Can)** *see* Azithromycin *on page 164*

♦ **Riva-Baclofen (Can)** *see* Baclofen *on page 171*

♦ **Riva-Buspirone (Can)** *see* BusPIRone *on page 222*

♦ **Riva-Ciprofloxacin (Can)** *see* Ciprofloxacin *on page 310*

♦ **Riva-Citalopram (Can)** *see* Citalopram *on page 319*

♦ **Riva-Clindamycin (Can)** *see* Clindamycin *on page 327*

♦ **Riva-Cycloprine (Can)** *see* Cyclobenzaprine *on page 367*

♦ **Riva-Dicyclomine (Can)** *see* Dicyclomine *on page 433*

♦ **Riva-Enalapril (Can)** *see* Enalapril/Enalaprilat *on page 499*

♦ **Riva-Fluconazole (Can)** *see* Fluconazole *on page 584*

♦ **Riva-Fluoxetine (Can)** *see* FLUoxetine *on page 600*

♦ **Riva-Fluvox (Can)** *see* Fluvoxamine *on page 615*

♦ **Riva-Fosinopril (Can)** *see* Fosinopril *on page 627*

♦ **Riva-Gabapentin (Can)** *see* Gabapentin *on page 634*

♦ **Riva-Glyburide (Can)** *see* GlyBURIDE *on page 648*

♦ **Riva-Lisinopril (Can)** *see* Lisinopril *on page 832*

♦ **Riva-Loperamide (Can)** *see* Loperamide *on page 838*

♦ **Riva-Lovastatin (Can)** *see* Lovastatin *on page 850*

♦ **Riva-Metformin (Can)** *see* MetFORMIN *on page 891*

♦ **Riva-Metoprolol (Can)** *see* Metoprolol *on page 918*

♦ **Riva-Minocycline (Can)** *see* Minocycline *on page 933*

♦ **Riva-Naproxen (Can)** *see* Naproxen *on page 967*

♦ **Rivanase AQ (Can)** *see* Beclomethasone *on page 176*

♦ **Riva-Oxybutynin (Can)** *see* Oxybutynin *on page 1037*

♦ **Riva-Pantoprazole (Can)** *see* Pantoprazole *on page 1054*

♦ **Riva-paroxetine (Can)** *see* PARoxetine *on page 1064*

♦ **Riva-Pravastatin (Can)** *see* Pravastatin *on page 1145*

♦ **Riva-Rabeprazole EC (Can)** *see* Rabeprazole *on page 1197*

♦ **Riva-Ranitidine (Can)** *see* Ranitidine *on page 1200*

♦ **Riva-Risperidone (Can)** *see* Risperidone *on page 1218*

♦ **Riva-Sertraline (Can)** *see* Sertraline *on page 1254*

♦ **Riva-Simvastatin (Can)** *see* Simvastatin *on page 1263*

♦ **Riva-Sotalol (Can)** *see* Sotalol *on page 1284*

♦ **Riva-Sumatriptan (Can)** *see* SUMAtriptan *on page 1308*

♦ **Riva-Terbinafine (Can)** *see* Terbinafine *on page 1322*

♦ **Riva-Valacyclovir (Can)** *see* Valacyclovir *on page 1394*

♦ **Riva-Venlafaxine XR (Can)** *see* Venlafaxine *on page 1412*

♦ **Riva-Verapamil SR (Can)** *see* Verapamil *on page 1416*

♦ **Rivotril® (Can)** *see* ClonazePAM *on page 337*

♦ **rLFN-α2** *see* Interferon Alfa-2b *on page 751*

♦ **Ro 5488** *see* Tretinoin (Systemic) *on page 1373*

♦ **Robafen AC** *see* Guaifenesin and Codeine *on page 657*

♦ **Robafen Cough [OTC]** *see* Dextromethorphan *on page 421*

♦ **Robafen DM [OTC]** *see* Guaifenesin and Dextromethorphan *on page 658*

♦ **Robafen DM Clear [OTC]** *see* Guaifenesin and Dextromethorphan *on page 658*

♦ **Robaxin®** *see* Methocarbamol *on page 898*

♦ **Robaxin®-750** *see* Methocarbamol *on page 898*

♦ **Robidrine® (Can)** *see* Pseudoephedrine *on page 1183*

♦ **Robinul®** *see* Glycopyrrolate *on page 651*

♦ **Robinul® Forte** *see* Glycopyrrolate *on page 651*

♦ **Robitussin® (Can)** *see* GuaiFENesin *on page 656*

♦ **Robitussin AC** *see* Guaifenesin and Codeine *on page 657*

♦ **Robitussin® Chest Congestion [OTC]** *see* GuaiFENesin *on page 656*

♦ **Robitussin® Children's Cough Long Acting [OTC]** *see* Dextromethorphan *on page 421*

♦ **Robitussin® Cough and Congestion [OTC]** *see* Guaifenesin and Dextromethorphan *on page 658*

♦ **Robitussin® CoughGels™ [OTC]** *see* Dextromethorphan *on page 421*

♦ **Robitussin® Cough Long-Acting [OTC]** *see* Dextromethorphan *on page 421*

♦ **Robitussin® DM [OTC]** *see* Guaifenesin and Dextromethorphan *on page 658*

♦ **Robitussin® DM (Can)** *see* Guaifenesin and Dextromethorphan *on page 658*

♦ **Robitussin® DM Infant [OTC] [DSC]** *see* Guaifenesin and Dextromethorphan *on page 658*

♦ **Robitussin® Pediatric Cough [OTC] [DSC]** *see* Dextromethorphan *on page 421*

♦ **Robitussin® Sugar Free Cough [OTC]** *see* Guaifenesin and Dextromethorphan *on page 658*

♦ **Rocaltrol®** *see* Calcitriol *on page 229*

♦ **Rocephin®** *see* CefTRIAXone *on page 275*

Rocuronium (roe kyoor OH nee um)

Medication Safety Issues
Sound-alike/look-alike issues:
Zemuron® may be confused with Remeron®

High alert medication: The Institute for Safe Medication Practices (ISMP) includes this medication among its list of drugs which have a heightened risk of causing significant patient harm when used in error.

United States Pharmacopeia (USP) 2006: The Interdisciplinary Safe Medication Use Expert Committee of the USP has recommended the following:
- Hospitals, clinics, and other practice sites should institute special safeguards in the storage, labeling, and use of these agents and should include these safeguards in staff orientation and competency training.
- Healthcare professionals should be on high alert (especially vigilant) whenever a neuromuscular-blocking agent (NMBA) is stocked, ordered, prepared, or administered.

U.S. Brand Names Zemuron®
Canadian Brand Names Rocuronium Bromide Injection; Zemuron®
Therapeutic Category Neuromuscular Blocker Agent, Nondepolarizing; Skeletal Muscle Relaxant, Paralytic
Generic Available Yes
Use Produces skeletal muscle relaxation during surgery after induction of general anesthesia, increases pulmonary compliance during assisted mechanical respiration, facilitates endotracheal intubation
Pregnancy Risk Factor C
Pregnancy Considerations Teratogenic effects were not observed in animal studies. Rocuronium crosses the placenta; umbilical venous plasma levels are ~18% of the maternal concentration. The manufacturer does not recommend use for rapid sequence induction during cesarean section.
Lactation Excretion in breast milk unknown/use caution
Contraindications Hypersensitivity to rocuronium, other neuromuscular blocking agents, or any component
Warnings Dosage adjustment needed in patients with severe hepatic disease; ventilation must be supported during neuromuscular blockade; rocuronium should only be used by individuals who are experienced in the maintenance of an adequate airway and respiratory support. Some patients may experience prolonged recovery of neuromuscular function after administration (especially after prolonged use); patients should be adequately recovered prior to extubation.

Precautions Many clinical conditions may potentiate or antagonize neuromuscular blockade, see table.

Clinical Conditions Affecting Neuromuscular Blockade

Potentiation	Antagonism
Electrolyte abnormalities	Alkalosis
Severe hyponatremia	Hypercalcemia
Severe hypocalcemia	Demyelinating lesions
Severe hypokalemia	Peripheral neuropathies
Hypermagnesemia	Diabetes mellitus
Neuromuscular diseases	
Acidosis	
Acute intermittent porphyria	
Renal failure	
Hepatic failure	

Increased sensitivity in patients with myasthenia gravis, Eaton-Lambert syndrome; resistance to neuromuscular blockade in burn patients (>30% of body) for period of 5-70 days postinjury; resistance to neuromuscular blockade in patients with muscle trauma, denervation, immobilization, infection

Adverse Reactions Most frequent adverse reactions are associated with prolongation of its pharmacologic actions
Cardiovascular: Hypotension, hypertension, arrhythmias, tachycardia
Dermatologic: Rash, pruritus
Gastrointestinal: Vomiting
Local: Injection site edema
Neuromuscular & skeletal: Muscle weakness
Respiratory: Bronchospasm
Miscellaneous: Hiccups, hypersensitivity reactions including anaphylaxis

Drug Interactions
Avoid Concomitant Use
Avoid concomitant use of Rocuronium with any of the following: QuiNINE

Increased Effect/Toxicity
Rocuronium may increase the levels/effects of: Cardiac Glycosides; Corticosteroids (Systemic); OnabotulinumtoxinA; RimabotulinumtoxinB

The levels/effects of Rocuronium may be increased by: AbobotulinumtoxinA; Aminoglycosides; Calcium Channel Blockers; Capreomycin; Colistimethate; Inhalational Anesthetics; Ketorolac; Ketorolac (Systemic); Lincosamide Antibiotics; Lithium; Loop Diuretics; Magnesium Salts; Polymyxin B; Procainamide; QuiNIDine; QuiNINE; Spironolactone; Tetracycline Derivatives; Vancomycin

Decreased Effect
The levels/effects of Rocuronium may be decreased by: Acetylcholinesterase Inhibitors; Loop Diuretics

Stability Refrigerate; unopened vials are stable 60 days at room temperature; open vials are stable for 30 days at room temperature; compatible with NS and D_5W; do not mix with alkaline solutions

Mechanism of Action Nondepolarizing neuromuscular blocking agent which blocks neural transmission at the myoneural junction by binding with cholinergic receptor sites

Pharmacodynamics
Maximum effect:
Children: 30 seconds to 1 minute
Adults: 1-3.7 minutes

Duration:
Children:
3-12 months: 40 minutes
1-12 years: 26-30 minutes
Adults: 20-94 minutes (dose-related) (most prolonged in elderly ≥65 years of age)

Pharmacokinetics (Adult data unless noted)
Distribution: V_d:
Children: 0.21-0.3 L/kg
Adults: 0.22-0.26 L/kg
Hepatic dysfunction: 0.53 L/kg
Renal dysfunction: 0.34 L/kg
Protein binding: ~30%
Half-life:
Alpha elimination: 1-2 minutes
Beta elimination:
Children:
3-12 months: 1.3 ± 0.5 hours
1 to <3 years: 1.1 ± 0.7 hours
3 to <8 years: 0.8 ± 0.3 hours
Adults: 1.4-2.4 hours
Hepatic dysfunction: 4.3 hours
Renal dysfunction: 2.4 hours
Elimination: Primarily biliary excretion (70%); up to 30% of dose excreted unchanged in urine
Clearance: Children:
3 to <12 months: 0.35 L/kg/hour
1 to <3 years: 0.32 L/kg/hour
3 to <8 years: 0.44 L/kg/hour

Usual Dosage I.V. (dosage based upon actual body weight even if the patient is obese): **Note:** In general, the onset of effect is shortened and duration is prolonged as the dose increases. The time to maximum nerve block is longest in neonates <28 days and shortest in infants 28 days to 3 months; the duration of relaxation is shortest in children 2-11 years and longest in infants

Suggested Dosing Based on Indication

Indication	Dose
Rapid sequence intubation (unlabeled use)[1]	0.6-1.2 mg/kg
Tracheal intubation	0.45-0.6 mg/kg
Maintenance for continued surgical relaxation, bolus[2]	0.075-0.125 mg/kg
Maintenance for continued surgical relaxation, continuous infusion[3]	7-12 mcg/kg/min

[1]Not recommended, per the manufacturer, for rapid sequence intubation in pediatric patients; however, it has been used successfully in clinical trials for this indication in children >1 year of age (Cheng, 2002; Fuchs-Buder, 1996; Mazurek, 1998; Naguib, 1997). An alternative dose of 1 mg/kg may also be used.

[2]Redosing interval is guided by monitoring with a peripheral nerve stimulator.

[3]Use lower end of the continuous infusion dosing range for neonates and infants up to age 28 days and the upper end for children >2 to ≤11 years of age.

Note: While I.V. administration is preferred, I.M. administration in single doses of 1 mg/kg (infants) and 1.8 mg/kg (children) has been used successfully (Kaplan, 1999).

Administration Parenteral: May be administered undiluted by rapid I.V. injection; for continuous infusion, dilute with NS, D_5W, or LR to a concentration of 0.5-1 mg/mL

Monitoring Parameters Peripheral nerve stimulator measuring twitch response, heart rate, blood pressure, assisted ventilation status

Nursing Implications Does not alter the patient's state of consciousness; addition of sedation and analgesia are recommended

Dosage Forms Excipient information presented when available (limited, particularly for generics); consult specific product labeling.

Injection, solution, as bromide: 10 mg/mL (5 mL, 10 mL)
Zemuron®: 10 mg/mL (5 mL, 10 mL)

References
Cheng CA, Aun CST, and Gin T, "Comparison of Rocuronium and Suxamethonium for Rapid Tracheal Intubation in Children," *Paediatr Anaesth*, 2002, 12(2):140-5.

Fuchs-Buder T and Tassonyi E, "Intubating Conditions and Time Course of Rocuronium-Induced Neuromuscular Block in Children," *Br J Anaesth*, 1996, 77(3):335-8.

Kaplan RF, Uejima T, Lobel G, et al, "Intramuscular Rocuronium in Infants and Children: A Multicenter Study to Evaluate Tracheal Intubating Conditions, Onset, and Duration of Action," *Anesthesiology*, 1999, 91(3):633-8.

Martin LD, Bratton SL, and O'Rourke PP, "Clinical Uses and Controversies of Neuromuscular Blocking Agents in Infants and Children," *Crit Care Med*, 1999, 27(7):1358-68.

Mazurek AJ, Rae B, Hann S, et al, "Rocuronium Versus Succinylcholine: Are They Equally Effective During Rapid-Sequence Induction of Anesthesia?" *Anesth Analg*, 1998, 87:1259-62.

Naguib M, Samarkandi AH, Ammar A, et al, "Comparison of Suxamethonium and Different Combinations of Rocuronium and Mivacurium for Rapid Tracheal Intubation in Children," *Br J Anaesth*, 1997, 79(4):450-5.

Reynolds LM, Lau M, Brown R, et al, "Bioavailability of Intramuscular Rocuronium in Infants and Children," *Anesthesiology*, 1997, 87 (5):1096-105.

Willets LS, "Rocuronium for Tracheal Intubation," *Ped Pharmacotherapy*, 2000, 6(10):1-6.

♦ **Rocuronium Bromide** *see* Rocuronium *on page 1230*

♦ **Rocuronium Bromide Injection (Can)** *see* Rocuronium *on page 1230*

♦ **Rofact™ (Can)** *see* Rifampin *on page 1215*

♦ **Rogaine® (Can)** *see* Minoxidil *on page 935*

♦ **Rogaine® Extra Strength for Men [OTC]** *see* Minoxidil *on page 935*

♦ **Rogaine® for Men [OTC]** *see* Minoxidil *on page 935*

♦ **Rogaine® for Women [OTC]** *see* Minoxidil *on page 935*

♦ **Rogitine® (Can)** *see* Phentolamine *on page 1101*

♦ **Rolaids® Softchews [OTC]** *see* Calcium Carbonate *on page 232*

♦ **Rolaids® Softchews [OTC]** *see* Calcium Supplements *on page 239*

♦ **Romazicon®** *see* Flumazenil *on page 590*

♦ **Romilar® AC [DSC]** *see* Guaifenesin and Codeine *on page 657*

♦ **Romycin® [DSC]** *see* Erythromycin *on page 525*

Ropivacaine (roe PIV a kane)

Medication Safety Issues
Sound-alike/look-alike issues:
Ropivacaine may be confused with bupivacaine, ropinirole

High alert medication: The Institute for Safe Medication Practices (ISMP) includes this medication (epidural administration) among its list of drug classes which have a heightened risk of causing significant patient harm when used in error.

U.S. Brand Names Naropin®
Canadian Brand Names Naropin®
Therapeutic Category Local Anesthetic, Injectable
Generic Available No
Use Production of local or regional anesthesia for surgery, obstetrical procedures, and for acute pain management: peripheral nerve block, local infiltration, sympathetic block, caudal or epidural block
Pregnancy Risk Factor B
Pregnancy Considerations Teratogenic events were not observed in animal studies. When used for epidural block during labor and delivery, systemically absorbed ropivacaine may cross the placenta, resulting in varying degrees of fetal or neonatal effects (eg, CNS or cardiovascular

depression). Fetal or neonatal adverse events include fetal bradycardia (12%), neonatal jaundice (8%), low Apgar scores (3%), fetal distress (2%), neonatal respiratory disorder (3%). Maternal hypotension may also result from systemic absorption. In cases of hypotension, position pregnant woman in left lateral decubitus position to prevent aortocaval compression by the gravid uterus. Epidural anesthesia may prolong the second stage of labor.

Lactation Excretion in breast milk unknown/use caution

Contraindications Hypersensitivity to ropivacaine hydrochloride, any anesthetic of the amide type (eg, bupivacaine, lidocaine, mepivacaine), or any component; not recommended for I.V. regional anesthesia (Bier block)

Warnings Convulsions and cardiac arrhythmias, due to systemic toxicity leading to cardiac arrest have been reported, presumably following unintentional I.V. injection; should be administered in small incremental doses; not for use in emergency situations when rapid onset of surgical anesthesia is necessary; not for use for the production of obstetrical paracervical block anesthesia, retrobulbar block, or spinal anesthesia (subarachnoid block); unlike other local anesthetics, administration with epinephrine does not affect onset, duration of action, or the systemic absorption of ropivacaine. Supraclavicular brachial plexus blocks may be associated with a higher frequency of serious adverse effects; major peripheral nerve blocks, often close to large blood vessels pose an increased risk of intravenous systemic absorption due to the proximity and large volume of dosage. Chondrolysis has been reported following continuous intra-articular infusion; intra-articular administration of local anesthetics is not an FDA-approved route of administration.

Precautions Use with caution in patients with liver disease, impaired cardiovascular function, particularly CHF, hypotension, hypovolemia, heart block, and neurological or psychiatric disorders. Patients treated with class III antiarrhythmics may be at increased risk for additive cardiac effects and should be monitored closely (consider ECG monitoring). For epidural use, it is recommended that a test dose of either a local anesthetic with rapid onset alone or in combination with epinephrine be administered prior to ropivacaine to detect unintentional intravascular or intrathecal injection which would result in systemic toxicity (CNS or cardiovascular)

Adverse Reactions

Cardiovascular: Cardiac arrest, hypotension, bradycardia, fetal bradycardia (during epidural anesthesia for cesarean section), arrhythmias, hypertension, tachycardia, chest pain

Central nervous system: Headache, restlessness, anxiety, agitation, lightheadedness, dizziness, tinnitus, seizures, fever, incoherent speech, depression, drowsiness

Dermatologic: Pruritus, rash

Endocrine & metabolic: Hypomagnesemia, hypokalemia

Gastrointestinal: Nausea, vomiting, fecal incontinence, tenesmus

Genitourinary: Urinary retention

Hepatic: Jaundice

Local: Pain at injection site

Neuromuscular & skeletal: Back pain, chondrolysis (continuous intra-articular administration), paresthesia (particularly of the mouth and lips), tremors, twitching, weakness

Ocular: Vision abnormalities

Otic: Tinnitus

Respiratory: Dyspnea, rhinitis

Miscellaneous: Chills, fetal disorders including tachycardia, fetal distress, fever, jaundice, rigor, shivering, tachypnea, vomiting

Drug Interactions

Metabolism/Transport Effects Substrate of CYP1A2 (major), 2B6 (minor), 2D6 (minor), 3A4 (minor)

Avoid Concomitant Use There are no known interactions where it is recommended to avoid concomitant use.

Increased Effect/Toxicity
The levels/effects of Ropivacaine may be increased by: Ciprofloxacin; Ciprofloxacin (Systemic); CYP1A2 Inhibitors (Moderate); CYP1A2 Inhibitors (Strong); Fluvoxamine; Fospropofol; Propofol

Decreased Effect
The levels/effects of Ropivacaine may be decreased by: Peginterferon Alfa-2b

Stability Store at controlled room temperature; preservative-free, discard promptly after use; do not mix with alkaline solutions as precipitation will occur

Mechanism of Action Blocks both the initiation and conduction of nerve impulses by decreasing the neuronal membrane's permeability to sodium ions, which results in inhibition of depolarization with resultant blockade of conduction

Pharmacodynamics

Onset of anesthetic action (dependent on dose and route of administration):

Epidural block (100-200 mg): T10 sensory block: 10 minutes (range: 5-13 minutes)

Epidural block, Cesarean section (up to 150 mg): T6 sensory block: 11-26 minutes

Duration (dependent upon dose and route of administration):

Epidural block (100-200 mg): 4 hours (range: 3-5 hours)

Epidural block, Cesarean section (up to 150 mg):
Sensory block: 1.7-3.2 hours
Motor block: 1.4-2.9 hours

Pharmacokinetics (Adult data unless noted)

Absorption: Well absorbed systemically in a biphasic manner following epidural administration; addition of epinephrine has no affect on the absorption of ropivacaine

Distribution: Distributes into breast milk

V_d (after intravascular infusion):
Children: 2.1-4.2 L/kg
Adults: 41 ± 7 L

Protein binding: 94%

Metabolism: In the liver via cytochrome P450 isoenzyme, predominantly CYP1A2 and CYP3A4 (10 metabolites with 2 active)

Bioavailability: 87% to 98% (epidural)

Half-life:
Epidural: Terminal phase:
Children: 4.9 hours (range: 3-6.7 hours)
Adults: 4.2 ± 1 hour
I.V.: Adults: 1.9 ± 0.5 hours

Time to peak serum concentration (dose and route dependent):
Caudal (children): 0.33-2.05 hours
Cesarean section: 14-65 minutes
Epidural (adults): 17-97 minutes

Elimination: 1% to 2% excreted unchanged in urine

Usual Dosage Dose varies with procedure, depth of anesthesia, vascularity of tissues, duration of anesthesia, and condition of patient

Caudal block: Children (limited data): 2 mg/kg

Epidural block (other than caudal block): Children: 1.7 mg/kg

Lumbar epidural surgery: Adults: 75-150 mg (15-30 mL 0.5%); maximum: 200 mg (40 mL 0.5%)

Lumbar epidural Cesarean section: Adults: 100-150 mg (20-30 mL 0.5% **or** 15-20 mL 0.75%)

Thoracic epidural surgery: Adults: 25-75 mg (5-15 mL 0.5%)

Epidural continuous infusion:
Children 4 months to 7 years (limited data) (Hansen, 2000): 1 mg/kg loading dose followed by 0.4 mg/kg/hour continuous **epidural** infusion

Adults: 10-14 mg loading dose (5-7 mL 0.2%) followed by 12-28 mg/hour (6-14 mL/hour 0.2%) continuous **epidural** infusion

Major nerve block (eg, brachial plexus block): Adults: 75-300 mg (10-40 mL 0.75%)

Minor nerve block and infiltration: Adults: 5-200 mg (1-40 mL 0.5%)

Administration Parenteral: Administer in small incremental doses; when using continuous intermittent catheter techniques, use frequent aspirations before and during the injection to avoid intravascular injection

Monitoring Parameters After epidural or subarachnoid administration: Blood pressure, heart rate, respiration, signs of CNS toxicity (lightheadedness, dizziness, tinnitus, restlessness, tremors, twitching, drowsiness, circumoral paresthesia)

Patient Information Temporary loss of sensation and motor activity in the anesthetized part of the body may occur following proper administration of lumbar epidural anesthesia.

Dosage Forms Excipient information presented when available (limited, particularly for generics); consult specific product labeling.

Infusion, as hydrochloride:

Naropin®: 2 mg/mL (100 mL, 200 mL)

Injection, solution, as hydrochloride [preservative free]:

Naropin®: 2 mg/mL (10 mL, 20 mL); 5 mg/mL (20 mL, 30 mL); 7.5 mg/mL (20 mL); 10 mg/mL (10 mL, 20 mL)

References

Hansen TG, Ilett KF, Lim SI, et al, "Pharmacokinetics and Clinical Efficacy of Long-Term Epidural Ropivacaine Infusion in Children," *Br J Anaesth*, 2000, 85(3):347-53.

Hansen TG, Ilett KF, Reid C, et al, "Caudal Ropivacaine in Infants: Population Pharmacokinetics and Plasma Concentrations," *Anesthesiology*, 2001, 94(4):579-84.

Lonnqvist PA, Westrin P, Larsson BA, et al, "Ropivacaine Pharmacokinetics After Caudal Block in 1-8 Year Old Children," *Br J Anaesth*, 2000, 85(4):506-11.

Wulf H, Peters C, and Behnke H, "The Pharmacokinetics of Caudal Ropivacaine 0.2% in Children. A Study of Infants Aged Less Than 1 Year and Toddlers Aged 1-5 Years Undergoing Inguinal Hernia Repair," *Anaesthesia*, 2000, 55(8):757-60.

◆ **Ropivacaine Hydrochloride** *see* Ropivacaine on page 1231

Rosiglitazone (ROSE i gli ta zone)

Medication Safety Issues

Sound-alike/look-alike issues:

Avandia® may be confused with Avalide®, Coumadin®, Prandin®

International issues:

Avandia® may be confused with Avanza® which is a brand name for mirtazapine in Australia

U.S. Brand Names Avandia®

Canadian Brand Names Avandia®

Therapeutic Category Antidiabetic Agent, Oral; Antidiabetic Agent, Thiazolidinedione

Generic Available No

Use Type 2 diabetes mellitus (noninsulin-dependent, NIDDM) when diet and exercise alone do not result in adequate glycemic control; may be used in combination with metformin, sulfonylurea, or insulin

Medication Guide An FDA-approved patient medication guide, which is available with the product information and at http://www.fda.gov/downloads/Drugs/DrugSafety/ucm085922.pdf, must be dispensed with this medication for each new outpatient prescription and refill.

Pregnancy Risk Factor C

Pregnancy Considerations Rosiglitazone is classified as pregnancy category C due to adverse effects observed in initial animal studies. Rosiglitazone has been found to cross the placenta during the first trimester of pregnancy.

Inadvertent use early in pregnancy has not shown adverse fetal effects although in the majority of cases, the medication was stopped as soon as pregnancy was detected. Thiazolidinediones may cause ovulation in anovulatory premenopausal women, increasing the risk of pregnancy; adequate contraception in premenopausal women is recommended. Maternal hyperglycemia can be associated with adverse effects in the fetus, including macrosomia, neonatal hypoglycemia, and hyperbilirubinemia; the risk of congenital malformations is increased when the Hb A_{1c} is above the normal range. Diabetes can also be associated with adverse effects in the mother. Poorly-treated diabetes may cause end-organ damage that may in turn negatively affect obstetric outcomes. Physiologic glucose levels should be maintained prior to and during pregnancy to decrease the risk of adverse events in the mother and the fetus. Until additional safety and efficacy data are obtained, the use of oral agents is generally not recommended as routine management of GDM or type 2 diabetes mellitus during pregnancy. Insulin is the drug of choice for the control of diabetes mellitus during pregnancy.

Lactation Excretion in breast milk unknown/not recommended

Breast-Feeding Considerations It is not known if rosiglitazone is excreted in breast milk. Breast-feeding is not recommended by the manufacturer.

Contraindications Hypersensitivity to rosiglitazone or any component; NYHA Class III/IV heart failure (initiation of therapy)

Warnings Used alone or in combination with insulin, rosiglitazone can cause fluid retention which can exacerbate or lead to CHF **[U.S. Boxed Warning]**; patients should be closely monitored for signs and symptoms of CHF; discontinue use if any deterioration of cardiac function occurs; avoid use in patients with NYHA class 3 or 4 heart failure. May be associated with an increased risk of MI and cardiovascular death. FDA evaluating evidence; future trials may clarify; use caution and monitor closely. Use in combination with insulin is not indicated. Concomitant use with nitrates is not recommended. An increased risk of MI has been observed in nitrate users vs non-nitrate users in clinical trials.

A dose-related weight gain has been reported with rosiglitazone which may be due to a combination of fluid retention and fat accumulation over time; a more rapid onset of weight gain may be suggestive of excessive edema and heart failure.

Idiosyncratic hepatotoxicity has been reported with another thiazolidinedione agent (troglitazone); two cases of hepatocellular injury (Al-Salman, 2000; Forman, 2000) have been reported occurring within 2-3 weeks after initiation of rosiglitazone therapy; LFTs in these patients revealed severe hepatocellular injury which responded with rapid improvement of liver function and resolution of symptoms upon discontinuation of rosiglitazone; monitoring should include periodic determinations of liver function. Use with caution in patients with elevated transaminases (AST or ALT); do not initiate in patients with active liver disease or ALT >2.5 times the upper limit of normal (ULN) at baseline; evaluate patients with ALT ≤2.5 times ULN at baseline or during therapy for cause of enzyme elevation; during therapy, if ALT >3 times ULN, re-evaluate levels promptly and discontinue if elevation persists or if jaundice occurs at any time during use. Avoid use in patients who previously experienced jaundice during troglitazone therapy; discontinue use in patients who develop jaundice during therapy.

A significant increase in fractures (primarily in the upper arm, hand, or foot) was noted in women taking rosiglitazone monotherapy when compared with metformin or glyburide (Kahn, 2006); the etiology for this is undetermined.

Not for use in Type 1 diabetes mellitus or diabetic ketoacidosis as the mechanism of action of rosiglitazone requires the presence of insulin.

Precautions Use with extreme caution in patients with heart failure or edema (see Warnings); use with caution in patients with elevated transaminases (AST or ALT) and in patients with anemia or depressed leukocyte counts (may reduce hemoglobin, hematocrit, and/or WBC); may induce ovulation in premenopausal anovulatory women; adequate contraception in premenopausal women is recommended. Use with caution in patients with pre-existing macular edema or diabetic retinopathy; postmarketing events of new-onset or worsening diabetic macular edema with decreased visual acuity have been reported; most patients had peripheral edema at the time of diagnosis; regular ophthalmic exams are recommended.

Adverse Reactions
Cardiovascular: Angina, CHF, edema, MI
Central nervous system: Headache, fatigue
Dermatologic: Urticaria, Stevens-Johnson syndrome
Endocrine & metabolic: Weight gain, total LDL and HDL cholesterol elevated, hyperglycemia, hypoglycemia, ovulation
Gastrointestinal: Diarrhea
Hematologic: Anemia, thrombocytopenia
Hepatic: Transaminases elevated, bilirubin elevated, hepatitis, hepatic failure, jaundice (reversible)
Neuromuscular & skeletal: Back pain, fractures (see Warnings)
Ocular: Macular edema, blurred vision, visual acuity decreased
Respiratory: Upper respiratory tract infection, sinusitis, pleural effusion, pulmonary edema
Miscellaneous: Hypersensitivity reactions including anaphylaxis

Drug Interactions
Metabolism/Transport Effects Substrate of CYP2C8 (major), 2C9 (minor); **Inhibits** CYP2C8 (moderate), 2C9 (weak), 2C19 (weak)
Avoid Concomitant Use There are no known interactions where it is recommended to avoid concomitant use.

Increased Effect/Toxicity
Rosiglitazone may increase the levels/effects of: CYP2C8 Substrates (High risk); Hypoglycemic Agents

The levels/effects of Rosiglitazone may be increased by: CYP2C8 Inhibitors (Moderate); CYP2C8 Inhibitors (Strong); Deferasirox; Gemfibrozil; Herbs (Hypoglycemic Properties); Insulin; Pegvisomant; Pregabalin; Trimethoprim; Vasodilators (Organic Nitrates)

Decreased Effect
The levels/effects of Rosiglitazone may be decreased by: Bile Acid Sequestrants; Corticosteroids (Orally Inhaled); Corticosteroids (Systemic); CYP2C8 Inducers (Highly Effective); Luteinizing Hormone-Releasing Hormone Analogs; Rifampin; Somatropin; Thiazide Diuretics

Food Interactions Peak concentrations are lower by 28% and delayed when administered with food; these effects are not believed to be clinically significant; avoid alfalfa, aloe, bilberry, bitter melon, burdock, celery, damiana, fenugreek, garcinia, garlic, ginger, ginseng (American), bymnema, marshmallow, stinging nettle (may cause hypoglycemia)

Stability Store at room temperature; protect from light

Mechanism of Action Thiazolidinedione antidiabetic agent that lowers blood glucose by improving target cell response to insulin, without increasing pancreatic insulin secretion; this mechanism of action is dependent on the presence of insulin for activity

Pharmacodynamics Maximum effect: Up to 12 weeks
Pharmacokinetics (Adult data unless noted)
Distribution: V_{dss} (apparent): Adults: 17.6 L
Protein binding: Adults: 99%
Metabolism: Hepatic (99%), metabolism by cytochrome P450 isoenzyme CYP2C8, minor metabolism via CYP2C9
Bioavailability: 99%
Half-life: 3-4 hours
Time to peak serum concentration: 1 hour
Elimination: As metabolites, in urine (64%) and feces (23%)

Usual Dosage Adults: Oral: All patients should be initiated at the lowest recommended dose:
Monotherapy: Initial: 4 mg in single or divided doses twice daily; after 8-12 weeks of treatment the dosage may be increased to 8 mg daily in single or divided doses twice daily. **Note:** When changing patients from troglitazone to rosiglitazone, a 1-week washout is recommended before initiating therapy with rosiglitazone.
Combination therapy: When adding rosiglitazone to existing therapy, continue current dose(s) of previous agents:
With sulfonylureas: Initial: 4 mg daily as a single daily dose or in divided doses twice daily; dose of sulfonylurea should be reduced if the patient reports hypoglycemia. Doses of rosiglitazone >4 mg/day are not indicated in combination with sulfonylureas.
With metformin: Initial: 4 mg daily as a single daily dose or in divided doses twice daily. If response is inadequate after 12 weeks of treatment, the dosage may be increased to 8 mg daily as a single daily dose or in divided doses twice daily. It is unlikely that the dose of metformin will need to be reduced due to hypoglycemia

Dosage adjustment in renal impairment: No dosage adjustment is required

Dosage comment in hepatic impairment: Clearance is significantly lower in hepatic impairment. Therapy should not be initiated if the patient exhibits active liver disease with increased transaminases (>2.5 times the upper limit of normal) at baseline (see Contraindications and Warnings)

Administration Oral: May be taken without regard to meals

Monitoring Parameters Signs and symptoms of hypoglycemia, fluid retention, or heart failure, fasting blood glucose, hemoglobin A_{1c}; liver enzymes: Baseline, every 2 months for the first 12 months of therapy, and periodically thereafter; patients with an elevation in ALT >3 times the upper limit of normal should be rechecked as soon as possible; if the ALT levels remain >3 times the upper limit of normal, therapy with rosiglitazone should be discontinued; ophthalmic exams

Reference Range Target range:
Blood glucose: Fasting and preprandial: 80-120 mg/dL; bedtime: 100-140 mg/dL
Glycosylated hemoglobin (hemoglobin A_{1c}): <7%

Patient Information Follow directions of prescriber; if dose is missed at the usual meal, take it with next meal; do not double dose if daily dose is missed completely; more frequent monitoring is required during periods of stress, trauma, surgery, pregnancy, increased activity, or exercise; avoid alcohol; report an unusually rapid increase in weight, edema, or shortness of breath immediately to your physician; also report chest pain, rapid heartbeat or palpitations, abdominal pain, fever, rash, hypoglycemic reactions, yellowing of skin or eyes, dark urine or light stool, or unusual fatigue or nausea/vomiting.

Dosage Forms Excipient information presented when available (limited, particularly for generics); consult specific product labeling.
Tablet:
Avandia®: 2 mg, 4 mg, 8 mg

References

Al-Salman J, Arjomand H, Kemp DG, et al, "Hepatocellular Injury in a Patient Receiving Rosiglitazone. A Case Report," *Ann Intern Med*, 2000, 132(2):121-4.

DeFronzo RA, "Pharmacologic Therapy for Type 2 Diabetes Mellitus," *Ann Intern Med*, 1999, 131(4):281-303.

Forman LM, Simmons DA, and Diamond RH, "Hepatic Failure in a Patient Taking Rosiglitazone," *Ann Intern Med*, 2000, 132(2):118-21.

Kahn SE, Haffner SM, Heise MA, et al, "Glycemic Durability of Rosiglitazone, Metformin, or Glyburide Monotherapy," *N Engl J Med*, 2006, 355(23):2427-43.

◆ **Rosula® NS** *see* Sulfacetamide *on page 1298*

Rosuvastatin (roe SOO va sta tin)

Medication Safety Issues

Sound-alike/look-alike issues:

Rosuvastatin may be confused with atorvastatin, nystatin, pitavastatin

Related Information

Normal Laboratory Values for Children *on page 1672*

U.S. Brand Names Crestor®

Canadian Brand Names Crestor®

Therapeutic Category Antilipemic Agent, HMG-CoA Reductase Inhibitor

Generic Available No

Use Adjunct to dietary therapy to reduce elevated total-C, LDL-C, and apo-B levels in patients with heterozygous familial hypercholesterolemia (HFH) [FDA approved in ages 10-17 years (girls ≥1 year postmenarche)] (see Additional Information for recommendations for initiating treatment in children ≥8 years). Adjunct to dietary therapy for hyperlipidemias to reduce elevations in total cholesterol (TC), LDL-C, apo-B, nonHDL-C, and triglycerides (TG) in patients with primary hypercholesterolemia (elevations of 1 or more components are present in Fredrickson type IIa, IIb, and IV hyperlipidemias) (FDA approved in adults); treatment of primary dysbetalipoproteinemia (Fredrickson type III hyperlipidemia) (FDA approved in adults); treatment of homozygous familial hypercholesterolemia (FH) (FDA approved in adults); to slow progression of atherosclerosis as an adjunct to diet to lower TC and LDL-C (FDA approved in adults)

Pregnancy Risk Factor X

Pregnancy Considerations Cholesterol biosynthesis may be important in fetal development. Contraindicated in pregnancy. Administer to women of childbearing potential only when conception is highly unlikely and patients have been informed of potential hazards.

Lactation Excretion in breast milk unknown/contraindicated

Contraindications Hypersensitivity to rosuvastatin or any component; active liver disease; unexplained persistent elevations of hepatic serum transaminases (>3 times ULN); pregnancy; breast-feeding

Warnings Rhabdomyolysis with acute renal failure and myopathy secondary to myoglobinuria has been reported; discontinue if myopathy suspected or creatinine kinase levels become markedly increased. Risk increased with higher doses (eg, 40 mg, although can occur at any dose level) and concurrent use of other lipid-lowering agents (eg, niacin and fibric acid derivatives), or medications that can increase rosuvastatin levels (amiodarone, atazanavir/ritonavir, cyclosporine, gemfibrozil, indinavir, or lopinavir/ritonavir). Advise patients to promptly report any unexplained muscle pain, tenderness, or weakness.Temporarily discontinue rosuvastatin for elective major surgery, acute medical or surgical conditions, or in any patient experiencing an acute or serious condition predisposing to renal failure (eg, sepsis, hypotension, trauma, uncontrolled seizures).

Precautions Use with caution in patients with predisposing factors for the development of myopathy, including hypothyroidism, renal impairment, or age ≥65 years. Elevations in serum transaminases have been reported; elevations are typically transient and improve with continued therapy or following a brief interruption of therapy. Liver function should be monitored at baseline and periodically thereafter, or following any dose increase. If ALT or AST exceeds >3 times ULN, decrease dose or discontinue therapy. Use with caution in patients who consume substantial quantities of alcohol or have a history of chronic liver disease. Rosuvastatin significantly increases INR in patients on warfarin. INR should be monitored before starting rosuvastatin and frequently during therapy. Transient proteinuria and hematuria have been reported; consider dose reduction if finding persists. Use caution in patients with conditions or on medications that reduce steroidogenesis (eg, ketoconazole, spironolactone, cimetidine).

Adverse Reactions

Central nervous system: Dizziness, headache

Gastrointestinal: Abdominal pain, constipation, nausea

Hepatic: ALT increased (>3 times ULN)

Neuromuscular & skeletal: Arthralgia, CPK increased, myalgia, myopathy (see Warnings), rhabdomyolysis (see Warnings), weakness (see Warnings)

Miscellaneous: Hypersensitivity reactions (including angioedema, pruritus, rash, urticaria) (see Warnings)

<2%, postmarketing, and/or case reports: Alkaline phosphatase increased, AST increased, bilirubin increased, GGT increased, hematuria (microscopic), hepatic failure, hepatitis, hyperglycemia, memory deficits, myoglobinuria, myositis, pancreatitis, proteinuria (dose related), renal failure, thyroid function test abnormalities

Drug Interactions

Metabolism/Transport Effects Substrate (minor) of CYP2C9, 3A4

Avoid Concomitant Use There are no known interactions where it is recommended to avoid concomitant use.

Increased Effect/Toxicity Cyclosporine may increase serum concentrations of rosuvastatin (up to 10-fold); limit dose to 5 mg/day. Serum concentrations of rosuvastatin may be increased (doubled) during concurrent administration of gemfibrozil; combination should be avoided; limit dose to 10 mg/day. Clofibrate, fenofibrate, or niacin may increase the risk of myopathy and rhabdomyolysis with HMG-CoA reductase inhibitors; the effects on lipids may be additive. The anticoagulant effects of warfarin may be increased by rosuvastatin (monitor). Rosuvastatin increases serum concentrations of hormonal contraceptives (ethinyl estradiol and norgestrel).

Decreased Effect Plasma concentrations of rosuvastatin may be decreased when given with magnesium/aluminum hydroxide-containing antacids; antacids should be administered at least 2 hours after rosuvastatin. Cholestyramine and colestipol (bile acid sequestrants) may reduce absorption of several HMG-CoA reductase inhibitors; separate administration times by at least 4 hours; cholesterol-lowering effects are additive.

Food Interactions Food does not affect AUC; excessive ethanol consumption should be avoided.

Stability Store between 20°C and 25°C (68°F to 77°F). Protect from moisture.

Mechanism of Action Acts as a selective, competitive inhibitor of 3-hydroxy-3-methylglutaryl-coenzyme A (HMG-CoA) reductase, the enzyme that catalyzes the rate-limiting step in cholesterol biosynthesis

Pharmacodynamics

Onset of action: Within 1 week

Maximum effect: 4 weeks

◄ **Pharmacokinetics (Adult data unless noted) Note:** In pediatric patients (10-17 years of age), maximum serum concentration and AUC have been shown to be similar to adult values.

Distribution: V_d: 134 L

Protein binding: 88%, mostly to albumin

Metabolism: Hepatic (10%), via CYP2C9 (1 active metabolite identified); N-desmethyl rosuvastatin, one-sixth to one-half the HMG-CoA reductase activity of the parent compound)

Bioavailability: ~20% (high first-pass extraction by liver); increased in Asian patients (twofold increase in median exposure)

Half-life elimination: ~19 hours

Time to peak serum concentration: 3-5 hours

Elimination: Feces (90%), primarily as unchanged drug

Usual Dosage Oral:

Children:

Heterozygous familial hypercholesterolemia: Children and Adolescents 10-17 years: 5-20 mg once daily; maximum dose: 20 mg; dosage adjustment should be made at 4-week intervals and individualized according to therapy goals

Homozygous familial hypercholesterolemia: Limited data available; dose not established. Initial dose (≥8 years and ≥32 kg): 20 mg once daily; titrate at 6-week intervals to 40 mg once daily. Although higher doses have been used (ie, 80 mg/day), additional benefit has not been reported. Dosing based on an open-label, forced-titration study of 44 patients (n=8 pediatric patients ≥8 years) which reported 72% of patients responded to rosuvastatin treatment (see Marias, 2008).

Note: A lower, conservative dosing regimen may be necessary in patient populations predisposed to myopathy, including patients of Asian descent or concurrently receiving other lipid-lowering agents (eg, gemfibrozil, niacin, fibric acid derivatives), amiodarone, atazanavir/ritonavir, cyclosporine, lopinavir/ritonavir, or indinavir (see conservative, maximum adult doses below).

Adults:

Hyperlipidemia, mixed dyslipidemia, hypertriglyceride-mia, primary dysbetalipoproteinemia, slowing progression of atherosclerosis:

Initial dose:

General dosing: 10 mg once daily; 20 mg once daily may be used in patients with severe hyperlipidemia (LDL >190 mg/dL) and aggressive lipid targets

Conservative dosing: Patients requiring less aggressive treatment or predisposed to myopathy (including patients of Asian descent): 5 mg once daily

Titration: After 2 weeks, may be increased by 5-10 mg once daily; dosing range: 5-40 mg/day (maximum dose: 40 mg/day)

Note: The 40 mg dose should be reserved for patients who have not achieved goal cholesterol levels on a dose of 20 mg/day, including patients switched from another HMG-CoA reductase inhibitor.

Homozygous familial hypercholesterolemia (FH): Initial: 20 mg once daily; maximum dose: 40 mg/day

Dosage adjustment with concomitant medications: Adults:

Cyclosporine: Rosuvastatin dose should not exceed 5 mg/day

Atazanavir/ritonavir, gemfibrozil, or lopinavir/ritonavir: Rosuvastatin dose should not exceed 10 mg/day

Dosage adjustment in renal impairment: Adults:

Mild to moderate impairment: No dosage adjustment required

Cl_{cr} <30 mL/minute/1.73 m^2: Initial: 5 mg/day; do not exceed 10 mg once daily

Administration May be taken with or without food; dosing time of day has not been shown to affect efficacy.

Monitoring Parameters Total cholesterol, LDL, and HDL cholesterol within 2-4 weeks of treatment initiation or dose change; liver function tests should be determined at baseline (prior to initiation), 3 months following initiation, 3 months after any increase in dose, and periodically thereafter (eg, semiannually); baseline CPK (recheck CPK in any patient with symptoms suggestive of myopathy).

Reference Range See Related Information for age- and gender-specific serum cholesterol, LDL-C, TG, and HDL concentrations.

Patient Information Report severe and unresolved gastric upset, any vision changes, muscle pain and weakness, changes in color of urine or stool, yellowing of skin or eyes, and any unusual bruising. Avoid alcohol consumption. Female patients of childbearing age must be counseled to use two effective forms of contraception simultaneously, unless absolute abstinence is the chosen method; this drug may cause severe fetal defects.

Additional Information The current recommendation for pharmacologic treatment of hypercholesterolemia in children is limited to children ≥8 years of age and is based on LDL-C concentrations and the presence of coronary vascular disease (CVD) risk factors (see table and Daniels, 2008). In adults, for each 1% lowering in LDL-C, the relative risk for major cardiovascular events is reduced by ~1%. For more specific risk assessment and treatment recommendations for adults, see NCEP ATPIII, 2001.

Recommendations for Initiating Pharmacologic Treatment in Children ≥8 Years[1]

No risk factors for CVD	LDL ≥190 mg/dL despite 6-month to 1-year diet therapy
Family history of premature CVD or ≥2 CVD risk factors present, including obesity, hypertension, or cigarette smoking	LDL ≥160 mg/dL despite 6-month to 1-year diet therapy
Diabetes mellitus present	LDL ≥130 mg/dL

[1]Adapted from Daniels SR, Greer FR, and Committee on Nutrition, "Lipid Screening and Cardiovascular Health in Childhood," *Pediatrics*, 2008, 122(1):198-208.

Dosage Forms Excipient information presented when available (limited, particularly for generics); consult specific product labeling.

Tablet:

Crestor®: 5 mg, 10 mg, 20 mg, 40 mg

References

American Academy of Pediatrics Committee on Nutrition, "Cholesterol in Childhood," *Pediatrics*, 1998, 101(1 Pt 1):141-7.

American Academy of Pediatrics, "National Cholesterol Education Program: Report of the Expert Panel on Blood Cholesterol Levels in Children and Adolescents," *Pediatrics*, 1992, 89(3 Pt 2):525-84.

Daniels SR, Greer FR, and Committee on Nutrition, "Lipid Screening and Cardiovascular Health in Childhood," *Pediatrics*, 2008, 122 (1):198-208.

"Executive Summary of the Third Report of the National Cholesterol Education Program (NCEP) Expert Panel on Detection, Evaluation, and Treatment of High Blood Cholesterol in Adults (Adult Treatment Panel III)," *JAMA*, 2001, 285(19):2486-97.

Grundy SM, Cleeman JI, Merz CN, et al, "Implications of Recent Clinical Trials for the National Cholesterol Education Program Adult Treatment Panel III Guidelines," *Circulation*, 2004, 110(2):227-39.

Marais AD, Raal FJ, Stein EA, et al, "A Dose-Titration and Comparative Study of Rosuvastatin and Atorvastatin in Patients With Homozygous Familial Hypercholesterolaemia," *Atherosclerosis*, 2008, 197 (1):400-6.

McCrindle BW, Urbina EM, Dennison BA, et al, "Drug Therapy of High-Risk Lipid Abnormalities in Children and Adolescents: A Scientific Statement From the American Heart Association Atherosclerosis, Hypertension, and Obesity in Youth Committee, Council of Cardiovascular Disease in the Young, With the Council on Cardiovascular Nursing," *Circulation*, 2007, 115(14):1948-67.

◆ **Rosuvastatin Calcium** see Rosuvastatin on page 1235
◆ **Rotarix®** see Rotavirus Vaccine on page 1237
◆ **RotaTeq®** see Rotavirus Vaccine on page 1237

Rotavirus Vaccine
(ROE ta vye us vak SEEN live pen ta VAY lent)

U.S. Brand Names Rotarix®; RotaTeq®
Canadian Brand Names Rotarix®; RotaTeq®
Therapeutic Category Vaccine, Live Virus
Generic Available No
Use Routine immunization to prevent rotavirus gastro-enteritis caused by serotypes G1, G2, G3, and G4 (RotaTeq®) or serotypes G1, G3, G4, and G9 (Rotarix®) (Rotarix®: FDA approved in ages 6-24 weeks; RotaTeq®: FDA approved in ages 6-32 weeks)
Pregnancy Risk Factor C
Pregnancy Considerations Reproduction studies have not been conducted. Not indicated for use in women of reproductive age. Infants living in households with pregnant women may be vaccinated.
Lactation Infants receiving vaccine may be breast-fed.
Breast-Feeding Considerations Infants receiving vaccine may be breast fed.
Contraindications Hypersensitivity to rotavirus vaccine or any component; infants with severe combined immunode-ficiency disease (SCID). Rotarix® is contraindicated in patients with a history of uncorrected congenital GI malformations (including Meckel's diverticulum) that may predispose them to intussusception.
Warnings Rotavirus vaccine should not be administered to infants with acute, moderate-to-severe gastroenteritis until the condition improves. Rotavirus vaccine administration may be delayed in patients with febrile illness except when the physician decides that withholding the vaccine entails a greater risk. Patients with mild low-grade fever (<38.1°C), mild gastroenteritis, or mild upper respiratory infection may receive vaccine. Information is not available for use of rotavirus vaccine in postexposure prophylaxis. Live virus vaccines may be transmitted to nonvaccinated contacts. Postmarketing cases of intussusception asso-ciated with rotavirus vaccine administration have been reported. The oral applicator of Rotarix® contains latex. The RotaTeq® dosing tube is latex-free.
Precautions Use with caution in infants with a history of gastrointestinal disorders (eg, active acute gastrointestinal disorders, chronic diarrhea, failure to thrive, history of congenital abdominal disorders, abdominal surgery and intussusception), infants with immunodeficient close contacts, such as immunocompromised individuals with malignancies or individuals receiving immunosuppressive therapy. No safety or efficacy data available for admin-istration of rotavirus vaccine to immunodeficient or immunocompromised infants or infants receiving immuno-suppressive therapy. Rotavirus vaccine may be adminis-tered at any time before, concurrent with, or after administration of any blood product, including antibody-containing products. Routine prophylactic administration of acetaminophen to prevent fever due to vaccines has been shown to decrease the immune response of some vaccines; the clinical significance of this reduction in immune response has not been established (see Prymula, 2009).
Adverse Reactions All serious adverse reactions must be reported to the U.S. Department of Health and Human Services (DHHS) Vaccine Adverse Event Reporting System (VAERS) 1-800-822-7967 or report online to www.vaers.hhs.gov.
Central nervous system: Fever, irritability
Gastrointestinal: Anorexia, diarrhea, flatulence, gastro-enteritis, intussusceptions (see Warnings), vomiting
Genitourinary: Urinary tract infection

Otic: Otitis media
Respiratory: Bronchiolitis, pneumonia, bronchospasm, nasopharyngitis
Miscellaneous: Gastroenteritis with severe diarrhea and prolonged vaccine viral shedding in infants with SCID (see Contraindications)
<1%, postmarketing, and/or case reports: Hematochezia, idiopathic thrombocytopenia purpura, Kawasaki disease, seizure, urticaria
Drug Interactions
Avoid Concomitant Use
Avoid concomitant use of Rotavirus Vaccine with any of the following: Immunosuppressants
Increased Effect/Toxicity
The levels/effects of Rotavirus Vaccine may be increased by: Immunosuppressants
Decreased Effect
Rotavirus Vaccine may decrease the levels/effects of: Tuberculin Tests

The levels/effects of Rotavirus Vaccine may be decreased by: Immune Globulins; Immunosuppressants
Stability
Rotarix®: Prior to reconstitution, store powder under refrigeration at 2°C to 8°C (36°F to 46°F); diluent may be stored at room temperature 20°C to 25°C (68°F to 77°F). Protect from light; discard if frozen. Following reconstitution, may be refrigerated or stored at room temperature for up to 24 hours. Discard if frozen.
RotaTeq®: Store and transport under refrigeration at 2°C to 8°C (36°F to 46°F). Administer as soon as possible once removed from refrigerator. Protect from light.
Mechanism of Action Live viral vaccine that replicates in the small intestine and induces active immunity.
Usual Dosage Oral: **Note:** The ACIP Provisional Recom-mendations for vaccination state to complete the vaccine series with the same product whenever possible. If continuing with same product causes vaccination to be deferred or if product used previously is unknown, vaccination should be completed with the product available. If RotaTeq® was used in any previous doses or if the specific product used was unknown, a total of 3 doses should be given. Vaccination should not be initiated in infants ≥15 weeks. The final dose in the series should be administered by 8 months 0 days of age. If Rotarix® is used at ages 2 and 4 months, a dose at 6 months is not indicated.
Infants 6-24 weeks of age (Rotarix®): 1 mL per dose; a 2-dose series at 2 and 4 months of age. Initial dose should be administered from 6 weeks through 14 weeks 6 days of age; the first and second dose should be separated by ≥4 weeks. The 2-dose series should be completed by 24 weeks of age.
Infants 6-32 weeks (RotaTeq®): 2 mL per dose; a 3-dose series at 2, 4, and 6 months of age. Initial dose should be administered from 6 weeks through 14 weeks 6 days of age; subsequent 2 doses administered at ≥4 week intervals (final third dose should not be given after 8 months and 0 days of age).
Administration Oral use only; **not for injection**:
Rotarix®: Connect transfer adapter onto vial and push downwards until transfer adapter is in place. Shake oral applicator containing liquid diluent (suspension will be a turbid liquid). Connect oral applicator to transfer adapter and transfer entire contents of oral applicator into the lyophilized vaccine. With transfer adapter in place, shake vigorously. Withdraw entire mixture back into oral applicator. Infant should be in reclining position. Using oral applicator, administer contents into infant's inner cheek. If most of dose is spit out or regurgitated, may administer a replacement dose at the same visit. Dispose of applicator and vaccine vial in biologic waste container.

RotaTeq®: Clear fluid from the dispensing tip by holding dosing tube vertically and tapping cap; puncture dispensing tip by screwing cap clockwise; remove cap by turning counterclockwise; gently squeeze liquid dose into infant's mouth toward the inner cheek until dosing tube is empty. If an incomplete dose is given (eg, infant spits or regurgitates dose), do not administer replacement dose. The infant can continue to receive any remaining doses of the series at the designated time interval. Do not mix or dilute vaccine with any other vaccine or solution.

Test Interactions Rotavirus vaccine may diminish the diagnostic effect of tuberculin tests (see Drug Interactions).

Patient Information Infants living in households with pregnant women may be vaccinated. Inform healthcare provider if there has been a previous reaction to rotavirus vaccine. Advise parents to contact the child's physician immediately if stomach pain, vomiting, diarrhea, blood in stool, or change in bowel movements occur after vaccine administration.

Nursing Implications
Due to fecal shedding of vaccine virus for up to 15 days after administration, vaccine should not be administered to hospitalized infants until the time prior to discharge. Discard empty tube and cap in approved biological waste container. Federal law requires that the date of administration, the vaccine manufacturer, lot number of vaccine, and the administering person's name, title, and address be entered into the patient's permanent medical record.

Additional Information Diphtheria and tetanus antigens in DTaP, HIB, IPV, hepatitis B vaccine, and pneumococcal conjugate vaccine may be given concurrently with rotavirus vaccine.

In the United States, rotavirus outbreaks occur from late fall to early spring. In the Southwest, the peak rotavirus season is November through December; the peak epidemic travels across the United States from west to east terminating in April through May in the Northeast.

In order to maximize vaccination rates, the ACIP recommends simultaneous administration of all age-appropriate vaccines (live or inactivated) for which a person is eligible at a single visit, unless contraindications exist. The use of combination vaccines is generally preferred over separate infections, taking into consideration provider assessment, patient preference, and potential adverse events.

For additional information, please refer to the following website: http://www.cdc.gov/vaccines/vpd-vac/.

Dosage Forms Excipient information presented when available (limited, particularly for generics); consult specific product labeling.

Powder, for suspension, oral [preservative free; human derived]:

Rotarix®: G1P[8] $\geq 10^6$ infectious units per 1 mL [oral applicator contains natural latex/natural rubber]

Suspension, oral [preservative free; bovine and human derived]:

RotaTeq®: G1 $\geq 2.2 \ 10^6$ infectious units, G2 $\geq 2.8 \ 10^6$ infectious units, G3 $\geq 2.2 \ 10^6$ infectious units, G4 $\geq 2 \ 10^6$ infectious units, and P1 [8] $\geq 2.3 \ 10^6$ infectious units per 2 mL (2 mL)

References
American Academy of Pediatrics Committee on Infectious Diseases, "Prevention of Rotavirus Disease: Guidelines for Use of Rotavirus Vaccine," *Pediatrics*, 2007, 119(1):171-82.

Centers for Disease Control and Prevention (CDC), "General Recommendations on Immunization. Recommendations of the Advisory Committee on Immunization Practices (ACIP)," *MMWR Recomm Rep*, 2006, 55(RR-15):1-48. Available at: http://www.cdc.gov/mmwr/preview/mmwrhtml/rr5515a1.htm.

Cortese MM, Parashar UD, and Centers for Disease Control and Prevention (CDC), "Prevention of Rotavirus Gastroenteritis Among Infants and Children: Recommendations of the Advisory Committee on Immunization Practices (ACIP)," *MMWR Recomm Rep*, 2009, 58 (RR-2):1-25.

Prymula R, Siegrist CA, Chlibek R, et al, "Effect of Prophylactic Paracetamol Administration at Time of Vaccination on Febrile Reactions and Antibody Responses in Children: Two Open-Label, Randomised Controlled Trials," *Lancet*, 2009, 374(9698):1339-50.

Vesikari T, Matson DO, Dennehy P, et al, "Safety and Efficacy of a Pentavalent Human-Bovine (WC3) Reassortant Rotavirus Vaccine," *N Engl J Med*, 2006, 354(1):23-33.

◆ **Rotavirus Vaccine, Pentavalent** *see* Rotavirus Vaccine *on page 1237*

◆ **Rowasa®** *see* Mesalamine *on page 887*

◆ **Roxanol™ [DSC]** *see* Morphine Sulfate *on page 946*

◆ **Roxicet™** *see* Oxycodone and Acetaminophen *on page 1041*

◆ **Roxicet™ 5/500** *see* Oxycodone and Acetaminophen *on page 1041*

◆ **Roxicodone®** *see* OxyCODONE *on page 1038*

◆ **Roychlor® (Can)** *see* Potassium Chloride *on page 1136*

◆ **RP-6976** *see* Docetaxel *on page 465*

◆ **RP-59500** *see* Quinupristin/Dalfopristin *on page 1196*

◆ **RS-25259** *see* Palonosetron *on page 1047*

◆ **RS-25259-197** *see* Palonosetron *on page 1047*

◆ **RTCA** *see* Ribavirin *on page 1210*

◆ **Rubella, Measles and Mumps Vaccines** *see* Measles, Mumps, and Rubella Vaccines (Combined) *on page 862*

◆ **Rubella, Varicella, Measles, and Mumps Vaccine** *see* Measles, Mumps, Rubella, and Varicella Virus Vaccine *on page 864*

Rubella Virus Vaccine (Live)
(rue BEL a VYE rus vak SEEN, live)

Medication Safety Issues
Sound-alike/look-alike issues:
Meruvax® II may be confused with Attenuvax®
Related Information
Immunization Guidelines *on page 1636*
U.S. Brand Names Meruvax® II [DSC]
Therapeutic Category Vaccine, Live Virus
Generic Available No
Use Provide active immunity against rubella (FDA approved in ages ≥ 12 months and adults); **Note**: Trivalent measles-mumps-rubella (MMR) vaccine is the preferred agent for most children and many adults.

Pregnancy Risk Factor C
Pregnancy Considerations Animal reproduction studies have not been conducted. Rubella infection during pregnancy may cause miscarriage, stillbirth or congenital rubella syndrome (CRS) in the infant. Evidence of rubella immunity should be determined in women of childbearing potential. Women born prior to 1957 and who may become pregnant are not considered immune and should be vaccinated. Vaccine should not be administered to pregnant women and the ACIP recommends that pregnancy be avoided for 1 month following vaccination. Women who are pregnant when vaccinated or who become pregnant within 1 month of vaccination should be counseled on the theoretical risks to the fetus. The theoretical risk of rubella-associated malformations in children born to women following vaccination while pregnant is 1.3%. In comparison, the risk of CRS associated with maternal infection during the first 20 weeks of pregnancy is $\geq 20\%$. MMR is the vaccine of choice if recipients are likely to be susceptible to measles or mumps as well as to rubella.
Lactation Enters breast milk/use caution

Breast-Feeding Considerations Following vaccination in the mother, rubella virus may be transmitted to the nursing infant via breast milk. Infants may show serologic evidence of infection, however, severe disease is not expected.

Contraindications Hypersensitivity to gelatin or any other component of the vaccine; history of anaphylactic reactions to neomycin; individuals with blood dyscrasias, leukemia, lymphomas, or other malignant neoplasms affecting the bone marrow or lymphatic systems; concurrent immunosuppressive therapy; primary and acquired immunodeficiency states; family history of congenital or hereditary immunodeficiency; active/untreated tuberculosis; current febrile illness or active febrile infection; pregnancy

Warnings Women who are pregnant when vaccinated or who become pregnant within 28 days of vaccination should be counseled on the theoretical risks to the fetus. Immediate treatment for anaphylactic/anaphylactoid reaction should be available during vaccine use. Defer vaccination at least 3 months after receiving blood and plasma transfusions or immune globulin (See Appendix Immunization Guidelines, "Suggested Intervals Between Administration of Antibody-Containing Products for Different Indications and Measles-Containing Vaccine and Varicella-Containing Vaccine").

Children with HIV infection, who are asymptomatic and not immunosuppressed may be vaccinated. Patients with minor illnesses (diarrhea, mild upper respiratory tract infection with or without low-grade fever or other illnesses with low-grade fever) may receive vaccine.

Precautions Use with caution in patients with thrombocytopenia and those who develop thrombocytopenia after first dose; thrombocytopenia may worsen; excretion of small amounts of the live attenuated rubella virus from the nose or throat occurs 7-28 days after vaccination; however, transmission to a susceptible individual is not considered a significant risk. Routine prophylactic administration of acetaminophen to prevent fever due to vaccines has been shown to decrease the immune response of some vaccines; the clinical significance of this reduction in immune response has not been established (see Prymula, 2009).

Adverse Reactions All serious adverse reactions must be reported to the U.S. Department of Health and Human Services (DHHS) Vaccine Adverse Event Reporting System (VAERS) 1-800-822-7967.

Cardiovascular: Syncope, vasculitis

Central nervous system: Dizziness, encephalitis, fever, Guillain-Barré syndrome, headache, irritability, malaise, polyneuritis, polyneuropathy

Dermatologic: Angioneurotic edema, erythema multiforme, purpura, rash, Stevens-Johnson syndrome, urticaria

Gastrointestinal: Diarrhea, nausea, sore throat, vomiting

Hematologic: Leukocytosis, thrombocytopenia

Local: Injection site reactions which include burning, induration, pain, redness, stinging, wheal, and flare

Neuromuscular & skeletal: Arthralgia/arthritis (variable; highest rates in women, 12% to 26% versus children, up to 3%), myalgia, paresthesia

Ocular: Conjunctivitis, optic neuritis, papillitis, retrobulbar neuritis

Otic: Nerve deafness, otitis media

Respiratory: Bronchial spasm, cough, rhinitis

Miscellaneous: Anaphylactoid reactions, anaphylaxis, regional lymphadenopathy

Drug Interactions

Avoid Concomitant Use

Avoid concomitant use of Rubella Virus Vaccine (Live) with any of the following: Immunosuppressants

Increased Effect/Toxicity

The levels/effects of Rubella Virus Vaccine (Live) may be increased by: Immunosuppressants

Decreased Effect

Rubella Virus Vaccine (Live) may decrease the levels/effects of: Tuberculin Tests

The levels/effects of Rubella Virus Vaccine (Live) may be decreased by: Immune Globulins; Immunosuppressants

Stability Refrigerate, discard reconstituted vaccine after 8 hours; store at 2°C to 8°C (36°F to 46°F); ship vaccine at 10°C; may use dry ice; protect from light.

Mechanism of Action Rubella vaccine is a live attenuated vaccine that contains the Wistar Institute RA 27/3 strain, which is adapted to and propagated in human diploid cell culture. Promotes active immunity by inducing rubella hemagglutination-inhibiting antibodies.

Pharmacodynamics Onset of action: Antibodies to vaccine: 2-4 weeks

Pharmacokinetics (Adult data unless noted) Distribution: Rubella virus distributes into breast milk. Infants of recently immunized mothers may show serologic evidence of infection; however, severe disease is not expected.

Usual Dosage SubQ: 0.5 mL

Infants and Children: First dose at 12-15 months of age and a second dose 4-6 years of age

Adults: One dose for women of childbearing age whose immunization history is unreliable, young adults who work in or congregate in hospitals, colleges, or military bases, and susceptible travelers

Note: MMR (trivalent vaccine for measles, mumps, and rubella) is the vaccine of choice if recipients are likely to be susceptible to measles and/or mumps as well as to rubella.

Administration Reconstitute only with provided diluent and agitate to mix thoroughly; administer subcutaneously into the anterolateral aspect of the thigh or the outer aspect of upper arm; avoid injection into blood vessel; **not for I.V. administration**

Monitoring Parameters Monitor for syncope for ≥15 minutes following vaccination.

Test Interactions May depress tuberculin skin test sensitivity

Patient Information This medication is only given by subcutaneous injection. You may experience burning or stinging at the injection site; joint pain usually occurs 1-10 weeks after vaccination and persists 1-3 days. Notify your healthcare provider immediately if these effects continue or are severe, or for a high fever, seizures or allergic reaction (respiratory difficulty, hives, weakness, dizziness, fast heartbeat). Not to be used during pregnancy; do not get pregnant for 28 days after getting the vaccine. Pregnant women should wait until after giving birth to get the vaccine. Consult healthcare provider if breast-feeding.

Nursing Implications Federal law requires that the date of administration, the vaccine manufacturer, lot number of vaccine, and the administering person's name, title, and address be entered into the patient's permanent record.

Additional Information Live attenuated virus vaccine. Using separate sites and syringes, rubella virus vaccine may be administered concurrently with DTaP, Haemophilus b conjugate vaccine (PedvaxHIB®), or hepatitis B vaccine. Unless otherwise specified, rubella virus vaccine should be given 1 month before or 1 month after other live viral vaccines. Rubella virus vaccine and varicella virus vaccine may be administered together (using separate sites and syringes); however, if vaccines are not administered simultaneously, doses should be separated by at least 30 days.

In order to maximize vaccination rates, the ACIP recommends simultaneous administration of all age-appropriate vaccines (live or inactivated) for which a

◀

persón is eligible at a single visit, unless contraindications exist. The use of combination vaccines is generally preferred over separate infections, taking into consideration provider assessment, patient preference, and potential adverse events.

For additional information, please refer to the following website: http://www.cdc.gov/vaccines/vpd-vac/.

Dosage Forms Excipient information presented when available (limited, particularly for generics); consult specific product labeling. [DSC] = Discontinued product

Injection, powder for reconstitution [preservative free]:
Meruvax® II: ≥1000 $TCID_{50}$ (Wistar RA 27/3 Strain) [contains gelatin, human albumin, sorbitol, sucrose, and neomycin] [DSC]

References

Centers for Disease Control and Prevention (CDC), "General Recommendations on Immunization. Recommendations of the Advisory Committee on Immunization Practices (ACIP)," *MMWR Recomm Rep*, 2006, 55(RR-15):1-48. Available at: http://www.cdc.gov/mmwr/preview/mmwrhtml/rr5515a1.htm.

Centers for Disease Control and Prevention (CDC), "Recommended Adult Immunization Schedule – United States, 2009" *MMWR Morb Mortal Wkly Rep*, 2009, 57(53):Q1-4.

Centers for Disease Control and Prevention (CDC), "Recommended Immunization Schedules for Persons Aged 0 Through 18 Years – United States, 2009," *MMWR Morb Mortal Wkly Rep*, 2009, 57 (51 and 52):Q1-4.

Centers for Disease Control and Prevention (CDC), "Revised ACIP Recommendation for Avoiding Pregnancy After Receiving a Rubella-Containing Vaccine," *MMWR Morb Mortal Wkly Rep*, 2001, 50 (49):1117.

Centers for Disease Control and Prevention (CDC), "Simultaneous Administration of Varicella Vaccine and Other Recommended Childhood Vaccines - United States, 1995-1999," *MMWR Morb Mortal Wkly Rep*, 2001, 50(47):1058-61.

Centers for Disease Control and Prevention (CDC), "Syncope After Vaccination – United States, January 2005-July 2007," *MMWR Morb Mortal Wkly Rep*, 2008, 57(17):457-60.

Prymula R, Siegrist CA, Chlibek R, et al, "Effect of Prophylactic Paracetamol Administration at Time of Vaccination on Febrile Reactions and Antibody Responses in Children: Two Open-Label, Randomised Controlled Trials," *Lancet*, 2009, 374(9698):1339-50.

Watson JC, Hadler SC, Dykewicz CA, et al, "Measles, Mumps, and Rubella–Vaccine Use and Strategies for Elimination of Measles, Rubella, and Congenital Rubella Syndrome and Control of Mumps: Recommendations of the Advisory Committee on Immunization Practices (ACIP)," *MMWR Recomm Rep*, 1998, 47(RR-8):1-57.

◆ **Rubeola Vaccine** *see* Measles Virus Vaccine (Live) *on page 866*

◆ **Rubidomycin Hydrochloride** *see* DAUNOrubicin *on page 394*

◆ **RV1 (Rotarix®)** *see* Rotavirus Vaccine *on page 1237*

◆ **RV5 (RotaTeq®)** *see* Rotavirus Vaccine *on page 1237*

◆ **RWJ-270201** *see* Peramivir *on page 1092*

◆ **Rylosol (Can)** *see* Sotalol *on page 1284*

◆ **Rythmodan® (Can)** *see* Disopyramide *on page 462*

◆ **Rythmodan®-LA (Can)** *see* Disopyramide *on page 462*

◆ **Ryzolt™** *see* TraMADol *on page 1367*

◆ **S2® [OTC]** *see* EPINEPHrine *on page 511*

◆ **7432-S** *see* Ceftibuten *on page 273*

◆ **Sab-Prenase (Can)** *see* PrednisoLONE *on page 1148*

◆ **Sabril®** *see* Vigabatrin *on page 1420*

Sacrosidase (sak RO se dase)

U.S. Brand Names Sucraid®
Canadian Brand Names Sucraid®
Therapeutic Category Sucrase Deficiency, Treatment Agent
Generic Available No
Use Oral replacement therapy in congenital sucrase-isomaltase deficiency (CSID)

Restrictions Sucraid® is not available in retail pharmacies or via mail-order pharmacies. To obtain the product, please refer to http://www.sucraid.net/or call 1-866-740-2743.
Pregnancy Risk Factor C
Pregnancy Considerations Animal studies have not been conducted. Should be administered to a pregnant woman only when indicated.
Lactation Enters breast milk/compatible
Contraindications Hypersensitivity to sacrosidase or any component, yeast and yeast products and glycerol
Warnings Hypersensitivity reactions to sacrosidase, including bronchospasm, have been reported; administer initial doses in a setting where acute hypersensitivity reactions may be treated within a few minutes; skin testing may be performed prior to administration to potentially identify patients at risk for hypersensitivity reactions.
Precautions Use with caution in CSID patients with diabetes mellitus, as Sucraid® will improve absorption of the products of sucrose hydrolysis (glucose and fructose); diet and/or insulin dosage may need to be adjusted. Product may contain papain. Severe hypersensitivity reactions, including anaphylaxis, have been observed with papain exposure. Tachycardia and hypotension, in association with some papain-induced hypersensitivity reactions, have also been observed. In addition, inconclusive data suggests a possible cross-sensitivity may exist between patients with natural rubber latex hypersensitivity and papaya, the source of papain.
Adverse Reactions
Central nervous system: Insomnia, headache, nervousness
Endocrine & metabolic: Dehydration
Gastrointestinal: Abdominal pain, vomiting, nausea, diarrhea, constipation
Respiratory: Bronchospasm
Miscellaneous: Hypersensitivity reactions (see Warnings)
Drug Interactions
Avoid Concomitant Use There are no known interactions where it is recommended to avoid concomitant use.
Increased Effect/Toxicity There are no known significant interactions involving an increase in effect.
Decreased Effect There are no known significant interactions involving a decrease in effect.
Food Interactions May be inactivated or denatured if administered with fruit juice, warm or hot food or liquids; since isomaltase deficiency is not affected by sacrosidase, adherence to a low-starch diet may be required to decrease symptomatology
Stability Refrigerate at 2°C to 8°C (36°F to 46°F); protect from light; discard 4 weeks after opening
Mechanism of Action Sacrosidase is a naturally occurring GI enzyme which breaks down the disaccharide sucrose into its monosaccharide components; this hydrolysis is necessary to allow absorption of these nutrients
Pharmacokinetics (Adult data unless noted) Metabolism: Sacrosidase is metabolized in the GI tract to individual amino acids which are systemically absorbed
Usual Dosage Oral:
Infants and Children ≤15 kg: 8500 international units (1 mL) per meal or snack
Children >15 kg and Adults: 17,000 international units (2 mL) per meal or snack
Administration Oral: Dilute in 2-4 ounces of water, milk, or formula; approximately $1/2$ of the dose may be taken before, and the remainder of the dose at the completion of, each meal or snack; do not administer with fruit juices, warm or hot food or liquids (see Food Interactions)
Monitoring Parameters Breath hydrogen test, oral sucrose tolerance test, urinary disaccharides, intestinal disaccharidases (measured from small bowel biopsy)

CSID symptomatology: Diarrhea, abdominal pain, gas and bloating

Additional Information 1 mL = 22 drops from sacrosidase container tip

Oral solution contains 50% glycerol. Oral solution may contain papain, an enzyme used during the manufacturing process to obtain sacrosidase.

Dosage Forms Excipient information presented when available (limited, particularly for generics); consult specific product labeling.

Solution, oral:

Sucraid®: 8500 int. units per mL (118 mL)

References

Treem WR, McAdams L, Stanford L, et al, "Sacrosidase Therapy for Congenital Sucrose-Isomaltase Deficiency," *J Pediatr Gastroenterol Nutr*, 1999, 28(2):137-42.

◆ **Safe Tussin® DM [OTC]** *see* Guaifenesin and Dextromethorphan *on page 658*

◆ **Saizen®** *see* Somatropin *on page 1281*

◆ **SalAc® [OTC] [DSC]** *see* Salicylic Acid *on page 1241*

◆ **Sal-Acid® [OTC] [DSC]** *see* Salicylic Acid *on page 1241*

◆ **Salactic® [OTC]** *see* Salicylic Acid *on page 1241*

◆ **Salagen®** *see* Pilocarpine *on page 1110*

◆ **Salazopyrin® (Can)** *see* Sulfasalazine *on page 1304*

◆ **Salazopyrin En-Tabs® (Can)** *see* Sulfasalazine *on page 1304*

◆ **Salbu-2 (Can)** *see* Albuterol *on page 57*

◆ **Salbu-4 (Can)** *see* Albuterol *on page 57*

◆ **Salbutamol** *see* Albuterol *on page 57*

◆ **Salbutamol Sulphate** *see* Albuterol *on page 57*

◆ **Salex®** *see* Salicylic Acid *on page 1241*

◆ **Salicylazosulfapyridine** *see* Sulfasalazine *on page 1304*

Salicylic Acid (sal i SIL ik AS id)

Medication Safety Issues

Sound-alike/look-alike issues:

Occlusal®-HP may be confused with Ocuflox®

Transdermal patch may contain conducting metal (eg, aluminum); remove patch prior to MRI.

U.S. Brand Names Akurza [DSC]; Aliclen™; Beta Sal® [OTC]; Compound W® One-Step Wart Remover for Feet [OTC]; Compound W® One-Step Wart Remover for Kids [OTC]; Compound W® One-Step Wart Remover [OTC]; Compound W® [OTC]; Dermarest® Psoriasis Medicated Moisturizer [OTC]; Dermarest® Psoriasis Medicated Scalp Treatment [OTC]; Dermarest® Psoriasis Medicated Shampoo/Conditioner [OTC]; Dermarest® Psoriasis Medicated Skin Treatment [OTC]; Dermarest® Psoriasis Overnight Treatment [OTC]; Dermarest® Psoriasis Scalp Treatment Mousse [OTC] [DSC]; DHS™ Sal [OTC]; Durasal™; Freezone® [OTC]; Fung-O® [OTC]; Gordofilm® [OTC]; Hydrisalic™ [OTC]; Ionil Plus® [OTC]; Ionil® [OTC]; Keralyt® [OTC]; LupiCare® Dandruff [OTC]; LupiCare® Psoriasis Scalp [OTC] [DSC]; LupiCare® Psoriasis [OTC]; Mosco® Callus & Corn Remover [OTC]; Neutrogena® Advanced Solutions™ [OTC]; Neutrogena® Blackhead Eliminating™ 2-in-1 Foaming Pads [OTC]; Neutrogena® Blackhead Eliminating™ Astringent [OTC] [DSC]; Neutrogena® Blackhead Eliminating™ Daily Scrub [OTC]; Neutrogena® Blackhead Eliminating™ Treatment Mask [OTC] [DSC]; Neutrogena® Body Clear® [OTC]; Neutrogena® Clear Pore™ Oil-Controlling Astringent [OTC]; Neutrogena® Oil-Free Acne Wash 60 Second Mask Scrub [OTC]; Neutrogena® Oil-Free Acne Wash Cream Cleanser [OTC]; Neutrogena® Oil-Free Acne Wash Foam Cleanser [OTC]; Neutrogena® Oil-Free Acne Wash [OTC]; Neutrogena® Rapid Clear® Acne Defense [OTC]; Neutrogena® Rapid Clear® Acne Eliminating [OTC]; Occlusal®-HP [OTC] [DSC]; Off-Ezy® Wart Remover [OTC] [DSC]; P&S® [OTC]; Palmer's® Skin Success Acne Cleanser [OTC]; Sal-Acid® [OTC] [DSC]; Sal-Plant® [OTC]; Salactic® [OTC]; SalAc® [OTC] [DSC]; Salex®; Salitop™; Salvax; Stridex® Essential Care® [OTC]; Stridex® Facewipes To Go® [OTC]; Stridex® Maximum Strength [OTC]; Stridex® Sensitive Skin [OTC]; Tinamed® Corn and Callus Remover [OTC]; Tinamed® Wart Remover [OTC]; Trans-Ver-Sal® [OTC]; Wart-Off® Maximum Strength [OTC]

Canadian Brand Names Duofilm®; Duoforte® 27; Occlusal™-HP; Sebcur®; Soluver®; Soluver® Plus; Trans-Plantar®; Trans-Ver-Sal®

Therapeutic Category Keratolytic Agent

Generic Available Yes: Cream, gel, lotion, soap

Use Topically for its keratolytic effect in controlling seborrheic dermatitis or psoriasis of body and scalp, dandruff, and other scaling dermatoses; removing excessive keratin in hyperkeratotic skin disorders (eg, verrucae, ichthyoses, keratosis palmaris and plantaris, keratosis pilaris, and pityriasis rubra pilaris); removing warts, corns, calluses; used in the treatment of acne

Pregnancy Risk Factor C

Contraindications Hypersensitivity to salicylic acid or any component (see Warnings); children <2 years of age

Warnings Should not be used systemically due to severe irritating effect on GI mucosa; prolonged use over large areas, especially in children, may result in salicylate toxicity; do not apply on irritated, reddened, or infected skin; do not use on moles, birthmarks, warts with hair growing from them, or genital warts; topical liquid may contain tartrazine which may cause allergic reactions in susceptible individuals

Precautions For external use only; avoid contact with eyes, face, lips, and other mucous membranes

Adverse Reactions

Dermatologic: Facial scarring, erythema, scaling, pruritus

Local: Irritation, burning, stinging

Drug Interactions

Avoid Concomitant Use There are no known interactions where it is recommended to avoid concomitant use.

Increased Effect/Toxicity There are no known significant interactions involving an increase in effect.

Decreased Effect There are no known significant interactions involving a decrease in effect.

Mechanism of Action Produces desquamation of hyperkeratotic epithelium; increases hydration of the stratum corneum causing the skin to swell, soften, and desquamate

Pharmacokinetics (Adult data unless noted)

Absorption: Topical: Readily absorbed

Time to peak serum concentration: Within 5 hours when applied with an occlusive dressing

Elimination: Salicyluric acid (52%), salicylate glucuronides (42%), and salicylic acid (6%) are the major metabolites identified in urine after percutaneous absorption

Usual Dosage Children ≥2 years and Adults: Topical:

Foam: Apply to the affected area twice daily. Rub into skin until completely absorbed.

Lotion, cream, gel: Apply a thin layer to the affected area once or twice daily

Plaster: Cut to size that covers the corn or callus, apply and leave in place for 48 hours; do not exceed 5 applications over a 14-day period

Shampoo: Initial: Use daily or every other day; apply to wet hair and massage vigorously into the scalp; rinse hair thoroughly after shampooing; 1-2 treatments/week will usually maintain control

Solution: Apply a thin layer directly to wart using brush applicator once daily as directed for 1 week or until the wart is removed

Administration Topical: For external use only. Not for ophthalmic, oral, anal, or intravaginal use. When applying in concentrations >10%, protect surrounding normal tissue with petrolatum

Monitoring Parameters Signs and symptoms of salicylate toxicity: Nausea, vomiting, dizziness, tinnitus, loss of hearing, lethargy, diarrhea, psychic disturbances

Patient Information Inform physician if redness or irritation occurs. Nursing mothers should not apply salicylic acid to the chest area or any area with which the nursing child's mouth may come in contact.

Nursing Implications For warts: Before applying product, soak area in warm water for 5 minutes; dry area thoroughly, then apply medication

Dosage Forms Excipient information presented when available (limited, particularly for generics); consult specific product labeling. [DSC] = Discontinued product
Aerosol, topical [foam]:
Dermarest® Psoriasis Scalp Treatment Mousse: 3% (90 mL) [DSC]
Salvax: 6% (70 g, 200 g) [ethanol free]
Bar, topical [soap]: 2%
Cloth, topical:
Neutrogena® Oil-Free Acne Wash: 2% (30s)
Cream, topical: 6% (400 g)
Akurza: 6% (340 g) [DSC]
LupiCare® Psoriasis Scalp: 2% (113 g, 227 g) [DSC]
LupiCare™ Psoriasis: 2% (56 g [DSC]; 227 g)
Neutrogena® Oil-Free Acne Wash Cream Cleanser: 2% (200 mL) [contains ethanol]
Salex®: 6% (400 g [DSC]; 454 g)
Salitop™: 6% (400 g) [contains ethanol]
Gel, topical:
Compound W®: 17.6% (7 g) [contains ethanol 67.5%]
Dermarest® Psoriasis Medicated Scalp Treatment: 3% (118 mL)
Dermarest® Psoriasis Medicated Skin Treatment: 3% (118 mL)
Dermarest® Psoriasis Overnight Treatment: 3% (56.7 g)
Hydrisalic®: 6% (28 g) [contains ethanol]
Keralyt®: 3% (30 g); 6% (40 g, 100 g) [contains ethanol 21%]
Neutrogena® Oil-Free Acne Wash: 2% (177 mL) [contains tartrazine]
Neutrogena® Rapid Clear® Acne Eliminating: 2% (15L) [contains ethanol 38%]
Sal-Plant®: 17% (14 g) [contains isopropyl alcohol]
Gel, topical [mask]:
Neutrogena® Blackhead Eliminating™ Treatment Mask: 0.5% (56 g) [DSC]
Gel, topical [peel]:
Neutrogena® Advanced Solutions™: 2% (40 g)
Liquid, topical: 17% (14.8 mL)
Compound W®: 17.6% (9 mL) [contains ethanol 21.2%]
Durasal™: 26% (10 mL) [contains isopropyl alcohol]
Freezone®: 17.6% (9.3 mL) [contains ethanol]
Fung-O®: 17% (15 mL) [contains ethanol 2%]
Gordofilm: 16.7% (15 mL)
Mosco® Callus & Corn Remover: 17.6% (9 mL) [contains ethanol 27%]
Neutrogena® Blackhead Eliminating™ Astringent: 0.5% (250 mL) [contains ethanol 35%] [DSC]
Neutrogena® Blackhead Eliminating™ Daily Scrub: 2% (125 mL)
Neutrogena® Clear Pore™ Oil-Controlling Astringent: 2% (236 mL) [contains ethanol 45%]
Occlusal®-HP: 17% (10 mL) [DSC]
Off-Ezy® Wart Remover: 17% (13.3 mL) [DSC]
Palmer's® Skin Success Acne Cleanser: 0.5% (240 mL) [contains aloe, vitamin E]

Salactic®: 17% (15 mL) [contains isopropyl alcohol]
Tinamed® Corn and Callus Remover: 17% (15 mL)
Tinamed® Wart Remover: 17% (15 mL)
Wart-Off® Maximum Strength: 17% (13 mL [DSC]),17.5% (14.8 mL) [contains ethanol]
Liquid, topical [body scrub with microbeads]:
Neutrogena® Body Clear®: 2% (250 mL) [contains tartrazine]
Liquid, topical [body wash]:
Neutrogena® Body Clear®: 2% (250 mL) [contains tartrazine]
Liquid, topical [cleanser]:
SalAc®: 2% (177 mL) [contains benzyl alcohol] [DSC]
Liquid, topical [foam]:
Neutrogena® Oil-Free Acne Wash Foam Cleanser: 2% (150 mL)
Liquid, topical [mask/wash]:
Neutrogena® Oil-Free Acne Wash 60 Second Mask Scrub: 1% (170 g) [ethanol free]
Lotion, topical: 6% (414 mL, 420 mL)
Akurza: 6% (355 mL) [DSC]
Dermarest® Psoriasis Medicated Moisturizer: 2% (118 mL)
Neutrogena® Rapid Clear® Acne Defense: 2% (50 mL) [contains ethanol]
Salex®: 6% (237 mL; 414 mL [DSC])
Salitop™: 6% (414 mL) [contains ethanol]
Pad, topical:
Neutrogena® Blackhead Eliminating™ 2-in-1 Foaming Pads: 0.5% (28s)
Stridex® Essential Care®: 1% (55s) [ethanol free; contains vitamin A, vitamin E]
Stridex® Facewipes To Go™: 0.5% (32s) [contains aloe, ethanol 28%]
Stridex® Maximum Strength: 2% (55s, 90s) [ethanol free]
Stridex® Sensitive Skin: 0.5% (55s, 90s) [ethanol free]
Patch, topical:
Compound W® One-Step Wart Remover for Feet: 40% (20s)
Compound W® One-Step Wart Remover: 40% (14s)
Compound W® One-Step Wart Remover for Kids: 40% (12s)
Trans-Ver-Sal®: 15% (10s, 25s) [20 mm PlantarPatch]
Trans-Ver-Sal®: 15% (15s, 40s) [contains propylene glycol]
Trans-Ver-Sal®: 15% (12s, 40s) [contains propylene glycol; 12 mm AdultPatch]
Plaster, topical:
Sal-Acid®: 40% (14s) [applied as plaster-impregnated bandages] [DSC]
Shampoo, topical: 6% (177 mL)
Aliclen™, Salex®: 6% (177 mL)
Beta Sal®: 3% (480 mL)
DHS™ Sal: 3% (120 mL)
Ionil Plus®: 2% (240 mL) [conditioning shampoo]
Ionil®: 2% (120 mL; 240 mL, 480 mL, 960 mL [DSC])
LupiCare® Dandruff: 2% (237 mL)
LupiCare® Psoriasis: 2% (118 mL [DSC]; 237 mL)
P&S®: 2% (118 mL, 236 mL)
Shampoo/conditioner, topical:
Dermarest® Psoriasis Medicated Shampoo/Conditioner: 3% (236 mL)

◆ **Salicylic Acid and Sulfur** see Sulfur and Salicylic Acid on page 1306
◆ **Saline** see Sodium Chloride on page 1270
◆ **Saline Mist [OTC]** see Sodium Chloride on page 1270
◆ **SalineX® [OTC] [DSC]** see Sodium Chloride on page 1270
◆ **Salitop™** see Salicylic Acid on page 1241
◆ **Salk Vaccine** see Poliovirus Vaccine (Inactivated) on page 1127

Salmeterol (sal ME te role)

Medication Safety Issues
Sound-alike/look-alike issues:

Salmeterol may be confused with Salbutamol, Solu-Medrol®

Serevent® may be confused with Atrovent®, Combivent®, Serentil®, sertraline, Sinemet®, Spiriva®, Zoloft®

Related Information
Asthma *on page 1697*

U.S. Brand Names Serevent® Diskus®

Canadian Brand Names Serevent® Diskhaler® Disk; Serevent® Diskus®

Therapeutic Category Adrenergic Agonist Agent; Antiasthmatic; Beta$_2$-Adrenergic Agonist Agent; Bronchodilator

Generic Available No

Use Maintenance treatment of asthma and prevention of bronchospasm in patients with reversible obstructive airway disease, including patients with nocturnal symptoms (FDA approved in ages >4 years and adults); prevention of exercise-induced bronchospasm (FDA approved in ages >4 years and adults)

Medication Guide An FDA-approved patient medication guide, which is available with the product information and at http://www.fda.gov/downloads/Drugs/DrugSafety/ucm089125.pdf, must be dispensed with this medication for each new outpatient prescription and refill.

Pregnancy Risk Factor C

Pregnancy Considerations Animal studies have demonstrated (dose-dependent) teratogenicity. There are no adequate and well-controlled studies in pregnant women. Beta-agonists may interfere with uterine contractility if administered during labor. Use only if clearly needed.

Lactation Enters breast milk/use caution

Contraindications Hypersensitivity to salmeterol, adrenergic amines, or any component

Warnings Long-acting beta$_2$-adrenergic agents (eg, salmeterol) have been associated with an increased risk of asthma-related death **[U.S. Boxed Warning]**. Salmeterol should only be prescribed in patients not adequately controlled on other asthma-controller medications, such as inhaled corticosteroids, or patients whose disease severity clearly warrants treatment with two maintenance therapies; should not be used as monotherapy. Salmeterol should not be used to relieve acute asthmatic symptoms. Acute episodes should be treated with short-acting beta$_2$-agonist. Do not increase the frequency of salmeterol use. Paroxysmal bronchospasm (which can be fatal) has been reported with this and other inhaled agents. If this occurs, discontinue treatment; most commonly occurs with first use of a new canister or vial. A medication guide is available to provide information to patients covering the risk of use. Because long-acting beta$_2$-agonists (LABAs) may disguise poorly-controlled persistent asthma, frequent or chronic use of LABAs for exercise-induced bronchospasm is discouraged by the NIH Asthma Guidelines (NIH, 2007).

Precautions Use with caution in patients with cardiovascular disorders (especially coronary insufficiency, arrhythmias, hypertension, heart failure), although uncommon at recommended doses, beta-agonists may cause elevation in BP and HR and result in CNS stimulation and excitation. Caution should also be used in patients with thyrotoxicosis, convulsive disorders, or conditions that are unusually sensitive to sympathomimetic amines. Transient hypokalemia from intracellular shunting may occur and produce adverse cardiovascular effects. Use with caution in patients with diabetes mellitus (DM); beta$_2$-agonists can increase serum glucose aggravating pre-existing DM and ketoacidosis. Use caution in patients with hepatic impairment. Powder for oral inhalation contains lactose; very rare anaphylactic reactions have been reported in patients with severe milk protein allergy.

Adverse Reactions
Cardiovascular: Hypertension, pallor, edema, arrhythmias (atrial fibrillation, SVT, extrasystoles, prolonged QT$_c$ interval with large doses)

Central nervous system: Headache, dizziness, anxiety, fever, migraine, sleep disturbance

Dermatologic: Rash, urticaria, photodermatitis, contact dermatitis, eczema

Endocrine & metabolic: Hyperglycemia, hypokalemia

Gastrointestinal: Oropharyngeal irritation, nausea, vomiting, dental pain, dyspepsia, GI infection, oropharyngeal candidiasis, xerostomia

Neuromuscular & skeletal: Musculoskeletal pain, muscular cramps/spasm, articular rheumatism, arthralgia, joint pain, muscular stiffness, paresthesia, rigidity

Respiratory: Nasal congestion, tracheitis/bronchitis, pharyngitis, cough, influenza, viral respiratory infections, sinusitis, rhinitis, asthma, respiratory arrest, paradoxical bronchospasm (see Warnings)

Miscellaneous: Hypersensitivity reactions, anaphylaxis, tachyphylaxis

Drug Interactions
Metabolism/Transport Effects Substrate of CYP3A4 (major)

Avoid Concomitant Use

Avoid concomitant use of Salmeterol with any of the following: CYP3A4 Inhibitors (Strong); Iobenguane I 123

Increased Effect/Toxicity

Salmeterol may increase the levels/effects of: Sympathomimetics

The levels/effects of Salmeterol may be increased by: Atomoxetine; Cannabinoids; CYP3A4 Inhibitors (Moderate); CYP3A4 Inhibitors (Strong); MAO Inhibitors; Tricyclic Antidepressants

Decreased Effect

Salmeterol may decrease the levels/effects of: Iobenguane I 123

The levels/effects of Salmeterol may be decreased by: Alpha-/Beta-Blockers; Beta-Blockers (Beta1 Selective); Beta-Blockers (Nonselective); Betahistine

Stability Store at controlled room temperature in a dry place; stable for 6 weeks after protective foil is removed

Mechanism of Action Relaxes bronchial smooth muscle by selective action on beta$_2$-receptors with little effect on heart rate; acts locally in the lung

Pharmacodynamics
Onset of action: Asthma: 30-48 minutes; COPD: 2 hours

Peak effect: Asthma: 3 hours; COPD: 2-5 hours

Duration: Up to 12 hours

Pharmacokinetics (Adult data unless noted)
Protein binding: 96%

Metabolism: Extensive hydroxylation via CYP3A4

Half-life: 5.5 hours

Elimination: 60% in feces and 25% in urine over a 7-day period

Usual Dosage Children >4 years and Adults:

Maintenance and prevention of asthma: Inhalation, oral: 50 mcg (1 actuation/puff) twice daily, 12 hours apart; **Note:** For long-term asthma control, long-acting beta$_2$-agonists should be used in combination with inhaled corticosteroids and **not** as monotherapy.

Prevention of exercise-induced asthma: Inhalation: 50 mcg (1 inhalation/puff) 30 minutes prior to exercise; additional doses should not be used for 12 hours; patients who are using salmeterol twice daily should **not** use an additional salmeterol dose prior to exercise; if twice daily use is not effective during exercise, consider other appropriate therapy; **Note:** Because long-acting beta$_2$-agonists

(LABAs) may disguise poorly-controlled persistent asthma, frequent or chronic use of LABAs for exercise-induced bronchospasm is discouraged by the NIH Asthma Guidelines (NIH, 2007).

COPD maintenance: Adults: 50 mcg (1 inhalation/puff) twice daily (~12 hours apart); maximum: 1 inhalation twice daily

Administration Inhalation: Not for use with a spacer

Monitoring Parameters Pulmonary function tests

Patient Information Do not use to treat acute symptoms; do not exceed the prescribed dose of salmeterol; do not stop using inhaled or oral corticosteroids without medical advice even if feeling better; do not exhale into the Diskus®; do not wash the mouthpiece or any part of the diskus; keep it dry; never attempt to take Diskus® apart; may cause dry mouth

Additional Information When salmeterol is initiated in patients previously receiving a short-acting beta agonist, instruct the patient to discontinue the regular use of the short-acting beta agonist and to utilize the shorter-acting agent for symptomatic or acute episodes only.

Dosage Forms Excipient information presented when available (limited, particularly for generics); consult specific product labeling. [CAN] = Canadian brand name

Powder for oral inhalation:
Serevent® Diskus®: Salmeterol xinafoate 50 mcg (28s, 60s) [delivers 50 mcg/inhalation; contains lactose]
Serevent® Diskhaler® Disk [CAN]: Salmeterol xinafoate 50 mcg (60s) [delivers 50 mcg/inhalation; contains lactose] [not available in U.S]

References

"Guidelines for the Diagnosis and Management of Asthma. NAEPP Expert Panel Report 3," August 2007, www.nhlbi.nih.gov/guidelines/asthma/asthgdln.pdf.

Meyer JM, Wenzel CL, and Kradjan WA, "Salmeterol: A Novel, Long-Acting Beta₂-Agonist," *Ann Pharmacother*, 1993, 27(12):1478-87.

"National Asthma Education and Prevention Program. Expert Panel Report: Guidelines for the Diagnosis and Management of Asthma Update on Selected Topics–2002," *J Allergy Clin Immunol*, 2002, 110 (5 Suppl):S141-219.

◆ **Sandoz-Rabeprazole (Can)** *see* Rabeprazole *on page 1197*

◆ **Sandoz-Ranitidine (Can)** *see* Ranitidine *on page 1200*

◆ **Sandoz-Risperidone (Can)** *see* Risperidone *on page 1218*

◆ **Sandoz-Salbutamol (Can)** *see* Albuterol *on page 57*

◆ **Sandoz-Sertraline (Can)** *see* Sertraline *on page 1254*

◆ **Sandoz-Simvastatin (Can)** *see* Simvastatin *on page 1263*

◆ **Sandoz-Sotalol (Can)** *see* Sotalol *on page 1284*

◆ **Sandoz-Sumatriptan (Can)** *see* SUMAtriptan *on page 1308*

◆ **Sandoz-Terbinafine (Can)** *see* Terbinafine *on page 1322*

◆ **Sandoz-Timolol (Can)** *see* Timolol *on page 1351*

◆ **Sandoz-Tobramycin (Can)** *see* Tobramycin *on page 1354*

◆ **Sandoz-Topiramate (Can)** *see* Topiramate *on page 1360*

◆ **Sandoz-Trifluridine (Can)** *see* Trifluridine *on page 1384*

◆ **Sandoz-Valproic (Can)** *see* Valproic Acid and Derivatives *on page 1398*

◆ **Sandoz-Venlafaxine XR (Can)** *see* Venlafaxine *on page 1412*

◆ **Sani-Supp® [OTC]** *see* Glycerin *on page 650*

◆ **Sans Acne® (Can)** *see* Erythromycin *on page 525*

Saquinavir (sa KWIN a veer)

Medication Safety Issues
Sound-alike/look-alike issues:
Saquinavir may be confused with Sinequan®
Related Information
Adult and Adolescent HIV *on page 1620*
Management of Healthcare Worker Exposures to HBV, HCV, and HIV *on page 1661*
Pediatric HIV *on page 1613*
Perinatal HIV *on page 1628*
U.S. Brand Names Invirase®
Canadian Brand Names Invirase®
Therapeutic Category Antiretroviral Agent; HIV Agents (Anti-HIV Agents); Protease Inhibitor
Generic Available No
Use Treatment of HIV infection in combination with other antiretroviral agents (FDA approved in ages ≥16 years and adults); (**Note:** HIV regimens consisting of three antiretroviral agents are strongly recommended; due to its low bioavailability, Invirase® must be used in combination regimens that include ritonavir "booster doses" so that adequate plasma saquinavir concentrations are attained); postexposure chemoprophylaxis following occupational exposure to HIV
Pregnancy Risk Factor B
Pregnancy Considerations Adverse events were not observed in animal studies and saquinavir crosses the human placenta in minimal amounts. Based on limited data, Invirase® 1000 mg (capsules and tablets) administered twice daily with ritonavir 100 mg twice daily provide adequate levels in pregnant women. The Perinatal HIV Guidelines Working Group considers Invirase® capsules and ritonavir to be an alternative combination for use during pregnancy. Pregnancy and protease inhibitors are both associated with an increased risk of hyperglycemia. Glucose levels should be closely monitored. Health professionals are encouraged to contact the antiretroviral pregnancy registry to monitor outcomes of pregnant women exposed to antiretroviral medications (1-800-258-4263 or www.APRegistry.com).

Lactation Excretion in breast milk unknown/contraindicated

Breast-Feeding Considerations In infants born to mothers who are HIV positive, HAART while breast-feeding may decrease postnatal infection. However, maternal or infant antiretroviral therapy does not completely eliminate the risk of postnatal HIV transmission.

In the United States where formula is accessible, affordable, safe, and sustainable, complete avoidance of breast-feeding by HIV-infected women is recommended to decrease potential transmission of HIV.

Contraindications Hypersensitivity (eg, anaphylaxis, Stevens-Johnson syndrome) to saquinavir, saquinavir mesylate, or any component; patients with severe hepatic impairment; concurrent therapy with amiodarone, astemizole, bepridil, cisapride, dihydroergotamine, ergonovine, ergotamine, flecainide, lovastatin, methylergonovine, midazolam (oral), pimozide, propafenone, quinidine, rifampin, simvastatin, terfenadine, triazolam (see Drug Interactions)

Warnings Saquinavir must be used in combination with ritonavir. Saquinavir is a potent CYP3A4 isoenzyme inhibitor that interacts with numerous drugs. Due to potential serious and/or life-threatening drug interactions, some drugs are contraindicated (see Contraindications and Drug Interactions). Concurrent use with St John's wort or garlic capsules is **not** recommended. Alteration of dose or serum concentration monitoring may be required with other medications (see Drug Interactions).

Spontaneous bleeding episodes have been reported in patients with hemophilia receiving an HIV protease inhibitor. New onset diabetes mellitus, exacerbation of diabetes and hyperglycemia has been reported in HIV-infected patients receiving protease inhibitors. Significant elevations of serum triglycerides and cholesterol may occur (monitor and manage appropriately).

Preliminary data suggest that the combined use of saquinavir with ritonavir may cause a dose-dependent prolongation of the QT and PR intervals, potentially increasing the risk for torsade de pointes, heart block, or other arrhythmias. Do not use saquinavir combined with ritonavir in patients with a history of QT interval prolongation, cardiomyopathy, pre-existing conduction system disease, ischemic heart disease, uncorrected hypokalemia, hypomagnesemia, or underlying structural heart disease. In addition, avoid this combination in patients currently using Class IA (eg, quinidine) or Class III (eg, amiodarone) antiarrhythmic drugs or other drugs that may prolong the QT or PR interval (eg, verapamil).

Precautions Use with caution in patients with hepatic impairment; increased saquinavir concentrations, increased liver enzymes, or worsening liver disease may occur. Fat redistribution and accumulation [ie, central obesity, peripheral wasting, facial wasting, breast enlargement, dorsocervical fat enlargement (buffalo hump), and cushingoid appearance] have been observed in patients receiving antiretroviral agents (causal relationship not established). Immune reconstitution syndrome (an acute inflammatory response to residual or indolent opportunistic infections) may occur in HIV patients during initial treatment with combination antiretroviral agents, including saquinavir; this syndrome may require further patient assessment and therapy.

Adverse Reactions
Cardiovascular: Prolongation of QT and PR intervals (see Warnings), thrombophlebitis
Central nervous system: Agitation, asthenia, ataxia, confusion, dizziness, fatigue, fever, hallucinations, headache, seizures
Dermatologic: Acne, dry lips/skin, eczema, photosensitivity, pruritus, rash

Endocrine & metabolic: Creatine phosphokinase increased, hypoglycemia, fat redistribution (see Precautions), hyperlipidemia (see Warnings); rare: Diabetes, hyperglycemia, ketoacidosis

Gastrointestinal: Abdominal discomfort, abdominal pain, constipation, diarrhea, GI intolerance, nausea, stomatitis, vomiting; rare: Pancreatitis

Hematologic: Hemolytic anemia, microhemorrhages, pancytopenia, thrombocytopenia; rare: Spontaneous bleeding episodes in hemophiliacs

Hepatic: ALT, AST, bilirubin, and amylase increased; worsening of chronic liver disease

Neuromuscular & skeletal: Arthralgia, back pain, parethesias, peripheral neuropathy, tremor

Respiratory: Cough

Drug Interactions

Metabolism/Transport Effects Substrate of CYP2D6 (minor), CYP3A4 (major), P-glycoprotein; **Inhibits** CYP2C9 (weak), CYP2C19 (weak), CYP2D6 (weak), CYP3A4 (moderate), P-glycoprotein

Avoid Concomitant Use

Avoid concomitant use of Saquinavir with any of the following: Alfuzosin; Amiodarone; Cisapride; Dabigatran Etexilate; Darunavir; Dronedarone; Eplerenone; Ergot Derivatives; Everolimus; Halofantrine; Lovastatin; Midazolam; Nilotinib; Nisoldipine; Pimozide; QuiNIDine; Ranolazine; Rivaroxaban; Romidepsin; Salmeterol; Silodosin; Simvastatin; St Johns Wort; Tamsulosin; Tolvaptan; Topotecan; Triazolam

Increased Effect/Toxicity

Saquinavir may increase the levels/effects of: Alfuzosin; Almotriptan; Alosetron; ALPRAZolam; Amiodarone; Antifungal Agents (Azole Derivatives, Systemic); Bortezomib; Brinzolamide; Calcium Channel Blockers (Dihydropyridine); Calcium Channel Blockers (Nondihydropyridine); CarBAMazepine; Ciclesonide; Cisapride; Clarithromycin; Clorazepate; Colchicine; Corticosteroids (Orally Inhaled); CycloSPORINE; CycloSPORINE (Systemic); CYP3A4 Substrates; Dabigatran Etexilate; Diazepam; Dienogest; Digoxin; Dronedarone; Dutasteride; Enfuvirtide; Eplerenone; Ergot Derivatives; Etravirine; Everolimus; FentaNYL; Fesoterodine; Flurazepam; Fusidic Acid; GuanFACINE; Halofantrine; HMG-CoA Reductase Inhibitors; Ixabepilone; Lovastatin; Lumefantrine; Maraviroc; Meperidine; MethylPREDNISolone; Midazolam; Nefazodone; Nilotinib; Nisoldipine; Paricalcitol; Pazopanib; P-Glycoprotein Substrates; Pimecrolimus; Pimozide; Protease Inhibitors; QuiNIDine; Ranolazine; Rifamycin Derivatives; Rivaroxaban; Romidepsin; Salmeterol; Saxagliptin; Sildenafil; Silodosin; Simvastatin; Sirolimus; Sorafenib; Tacrolimus; Tacrolimus (Systemic); Tacrolimus (Topical); Tadalafil; Tamsulosin; Temsirolimus; Tolvaptan; Topotecan; TraZODone; Triazolam; Tricyclic Antidepressants; Vardenafil

The levels/effects of Saquinavir may be increased by: Antifungal Agents (Azole Derivatives, Systemic); Clarithromycin; CycloSPORINE; CycloSPORINE (Systemic); Delavirdine; Efavirenz; Enfuvirtide; Etravirine; Fusidic Acid; H2-Antagonists; P-Glycoprotein Inhibitors; Proton Pump Inhibitors

Decreased Effect

Saquinavir may decrease the levels/effects of: Abacavir; Clarithromycin; Contraceptives (Estrogens); Darunavir; Delavirdine; Divalproex; Etravirine; Meperidine; Methadone; Prasugrel; Theophylline Derivatives; Valproic Acid; Zidovudine

The levels/effects of Saquinavir may be decreased by: Antacids; CarBAMazepine; Contraceptives (Estrogens); CYP3A4 Inducers (Strong); Deferasirox; Efavirenz; Garlic; Nevirapine; Peginterferon Alfa-2b; P-Glycoprotein Inducers; Rifamycin Derivatives; St Johns Wort

Food Interactions Presence of a high fat meal maximizes bioavailability of saquinavir; grapefruit juice may increase saquinavir concentrations. No information about the effect of food on the bioavailability of Invirase® in combination with ritonavir is available.

Stability Invirase® capsules and tablets: Store at controlled room temperature of 25°C (77°F); excursions permitted to 15°C to 30°C (59°F to 86°F); store in tightly closed bottles

Mechanism of Action A protease inhibitor which acts on an enzyme (protease) late in the HIV replication process after the virus has entered into the cell's nucleus; saquinavir binds to the protease activity site and inhibits the activity of the enzyme, thus preventing cleavage of viral polyprotein precursors (gag-pol protein precursors) into individual functional proteins found in infectious HIV; this results in the formation of immature, noninfectious viral particles

Pharmacokinetics (Adult data unless noted)

Distribution: CSF concentration is negligible when compared to concentrations from matched plasma samples; partitions into tissues

V_d: Adults: 700 L

Protein binding: 98%

Metabolism: Extensive first-pass effect; hepatic metabolism by cytochrome P450 3A system to inactive mono- and dihydroxylated metabolites

Bioavailability:

Invirase® capsules: 4% (increased in the presence of food); bioavailability of Invirase® capsules and tablets are similar when administered with low dose ritonavir (ie, booster doses of ritonavir)

Half-life, serum: Adults: 1-2 hours

Elimination: 81% to 88% of dose eliminated in feces; 1% to 3% excreted in urine within 5 days

Clearance: Children: Significantly higher than adults

Usual Dosage Oral (use in combination with other antiretroviral agents): **Note:** Invirase® must only be used in regimens that include ritonavir "booster doses" so that adequate saquinavir serum concentrations are attained; do **not** use without ritonavir booster doses

Neonates and Infants: Not approved for use; appropriate dose is unknown.

Children: Not approved for use; appropriate dose is unknown; Fortovase® 50 mg/kg/dose every 8 hours did **not** provide adequate saquinavir serum concentrations in children; ongoing studies are evaluating saquinavir in combination with ritonavir, nelfinavir, or lopinavir/ritonavir; do **not** use saquinavir as sole protease inhibitor in pediatric patients <16 years of age

Adolescents ≥16 years and Adults:

Ritonavir boosted regimen: **Note:** Take ritonavir at the same time as saquinavir

Invirase®: 1000 mg twice daily with ritonavir 100 mg twice daily

Lopinavir/ritonavir boosted regimen: **Note:** Take lopinavir/ritonavir at the same time as saquinavir

Invirase®: 1000 mg twice daily with lopinavir 400 mg/ritonavir 100 mg twice daily

Administration Oral: Administer saquinavir (along with ritonavir) within 2 hours after a full meal to increase absorption; avoid taking saquinavir with grapefruit juice

Monitoring Parameters Liver function tests, serum cholesterol and triglyceride concentrations, blood glucose concentrations, CD4 cell count, plasma concentrations of HIV RNA

Patient Information Saquinavir is not a cure for HIV infection. Notify physician if numbness, tingling, persistent severe abdominal pain, nausea, or vomiting occurs. Saquinavir must be taken with ritonavir, in order to "boost" (increase) saquinavir concentrations to the correct concentration. Some medicines should not be taken with saquinavir; report the use of other medications, non-prescription medications, and herbal or natural products to your physician and pharmacist; avoid the herbal medicine St John's wort and garlic capsules. Take saquinavir every day as prescribed; do not change dose or discontinue without physician's advice; if a dose is missed, take it as soon as possible, then return to normal dosing schedule; if a dose is skipped, do not double the next dose. May cause photosensitivity reactions (eg, exposure to sunlight may cause severe sunburn, skin rash, redness, or itching); avoid exposure to sunlight and artificial light sources (sunlamps, tanning booth/bed); wear protective clothing, wide-brimmed hats, sunglasses, and lip sunscreen (SPF ≥15); use a sunscreen [broad-spectrum sunscreen or physical sunscreen (preferred) or sunblock with SPF ≥15]; contact physician if reaction occurs.

HIV medications may cause changes in body fat, including an increase in fat in the upper back and neck, breasts, and trunk; a loss of fat from the face, arms, and legs may also occur.

Additional Information Fortovase® (saquinavir soft gel capsules) has been discontinued in the U.S. because ritonavir-boosted Invirase® tablet-containing regimens result in fewer GI side effects and a lower pill burden compared to ritonavir-boosted Fortovase® regimens.

Dosage Forms Excipient information presented when available (limited, particularly for generics); consult specific product labeling.

Capsule:
Invirase®: 200 mg [contains lactose 63.3 mg/capsule]
Tablet:
Invirase®: 500 mg

References

Briars LA, Hilao JJ, and Kraus DM, "A Review of Pediatric Human Immunodeficiency Virus Infection," *Journal of Pharmacy Practice*, 2004, 17(6):407-31.

Collier AC, Coombs RW, Schoenfeld DA, et al, "Treatment of Human Immunodeficiency Virus Infection With Saquinavir, Zidovudine, and Zalcitabine," *N Engl J Med*, 1996, 334(16):1011-7.

Mueller BU, "Antiviral Chemotherapy," *Curr Opin Pediatr*, 1997, 9 (2):178-83.

Panel on Antiretroviral Guidelines for Adults and Adolescents, "Guidelines for the Use of Antiretroviral Agents in HIV-Infected Adults and Adolescents," December 1, 2009. Available at: http://www.aidsinfo.nih.gov.

Singh M, Arora R, and Jawad E, "HIV Protease Inhibitors Induced Prolongation of the QT Interval: Electrophysiology and Clinical Implications," *Am J Ther*, 2009.

Working Group on Antiretroviral Therapy and Medical Management of HIV-Infected Children, "Guidelines for the Use of Antiretroviral Agents in Pediatric HIV Infection," February 23, 2009. Available at http://www.aidsinfo.nih.gov.

◆ **Saquinavir Mesylate** see Saquinavir on page *1245*

◆ **Sarafem®** see FLUoxetine on page *600*

Sargramostim (sar GRAM oh stim)

Medication Safety Issues
Sound-alike/look-alike issues:
Leukine® may be confused with Leukeran®, leucovorin
Related Information
Compatibility of Chemotherapy and Related Supportive Care Medications on page *1580*
U.S. Brand Names Leukine®
Canadian Brand Names Leukine®
Therapeutic Category Colony-Stimulating Factor
Generic Available No
Use Accelerates myeloid recovery in patients undergoing autologous or allogeneic BMT; mobilize hematopoietic progenitor cells into peripheral blood for collection by leukapheresis; accelerate myeloid engraftment following autologous peripheral blood progenitor cell transplantation; increase neutrophil counts in patients with malignancies receiving myelosuppressive chemotherapy; neonatal neutropenia

Pregnancy Risk Factor C

Pregnancy Considerations Clinical effects to the fetus: Animal reproduction studies have not been conducted. It is not known whether sargramostim can cause fetal harm when administered to a pregnant woman or can affect reproductive capability. Sargramostim should be given to a pregnant woman only if clearly needed.

Lactation Excretion in breast milk unknown/use caution

Contraindications Hypersensitivity to GM-CSF, yeast-derived products, or any component (see Warnings); excessive leukemic myeloid blasts in bone marrow or peripheral blood ≥10%; history of idiopathic thrombocytopenic purpura

Warnings Injection solution contains benzyl alcohol which may cause allergic reactions in susceptible individuals; large amounts of benzyl alcohol (≥99 mg/kg/day) have been associated with a potentially fatal toxicity ("gasping syndrome") in neonates; the "gasping syndrome" consists of metabolic acidosis, respiratory distress, gasping respirations, CNS dysfunction (including convulsions, intracranial hemorrhage), hypotension and cardiovascular collapse; use sargramostim injection products containing benzyl alcohol with caution in neonates; *in vitro* and animal studies have shown that benzoate, a metabolite of benzyl alcohol, displaces bilirubin from protein binding sites

Precautions Use with caution in patients with autoimmune or chronic inflammatory disease, hypertension, cardiovascular disease, pulmonary disease, or renal or hepatic impairment

Rapid increase in peripheral blood counts: If ANC is >20,000/mm^3 or platelets >500,000/mm^3, decrease dose by 50% or discontinue drug (counts will fall to normal within 3-7 days after discontinuing drug)

Growth factor potential: Caution with myeloid malignancies; do **not** administer within 24 hours prior to or after chemotherapy or 12 hours prior to or after radiation therapy

Adverse Reactions
Cardiovascular: Hypotension, tachycardia, flushing, pericardial effusion, fluid retention, venous thrombosis
Central nervous system: Malaise, fever, headache, chills
Dermatologic: Rash
Endocrine & metabolic: Polydipsia
Gastrointestinal: Nausea, vomiting, diarrhea, stomatitis, GI hemorrhage
Hepatic: Liver function tests elevated
Neuromuscular & skeletal: Bone pain, myalgia, rigors, weakness
Respiratory: Dyspnea
Miscellaneous: "First dose" reaction (fever, hypotension, tachycardia, rigors, flushing, nausea, vomiting, dyspnea)

Drug Interactions
Avoid Concomitant Use There are no known interactions where it is recommended to avoid concomitant use.

Increased Effect/Toxicity
Sargramostim may increase the levels/effects of: Bleomycin

Decreased Effect There are no known significant interactions involving a decrease in effect.

Stability Store vial in the refrigerator; stable after reconstitution for 6 hours at room temperature; use only NS to prepare I.V. infusion solution; GM-CSF at a concentration ≥10 mcg/mL is compatible with TPN during Y-site administration

Mechanism of Action Stimulates proliferation, differentiation and functional activity of neutrophils, eosinophils, monocytes and macrophages

Pharmacodynamics
Onset of action: Increase in WBC in 7-14 days

◄ Duration: WBC will return to baseline within 1 week after discontinuing drug

Pharmacokinetics (Adult data unless noted)
Half-life: 2 hours
Time to peak serum concentration: SubQ: Within 3 hours
Usual Dosage I.V., SubQ:
Neonates: 10 mcg/kg/day once daily for 5 days has been administered to preterm neonates at high risk of both neutropenia and sepsis
Children (no dosing for children has been FDA approved): 250 mcg/m²/day once daily for 21 days to begin 2-4 hours after the marrow infusion on day 0 of BMT or not less than 24 hours after chemotherapy. If significant adverse effects or "first dose" reaction is seen at this dose, discontinue the drug until toxicity resolves, then restart at a reduced dose of 125 mcg/m²/day
Adults: 250 mcg/m²/day once daily for 21 days to begin 2-4 hours after BMT, or not less than 24 hours after chemotherapy (to minimize first dose reaction, start with low doses and increase gradually)
Administration Parenteral:
I.V.: Administer as a 30-minute, 2-hour, or 6-hour I.V. infusion or by continuous I.V. infusion. Do not shake solution to avoid foaming. Dilute in NS; if the final concentration of GM-CSF in NS is <10 mcg/mL, then add 1 mg albumin per mL of I.V. fluid. Albumin acts as a carrier molecule to prevent drug adsorption to the I.V. tubing. Albumin should be added to NS prior to addition of GM-CSF. An in-line membrane filter should **not** be used for intravenous administration.
SubQ: Reconstituted 250 mcg/mL or 500 mcg/mL solution may be administered without further dilution; rotate injection sites
Monitoring Parameters CBC with differential, platelets; renal/liver function tests, especially with previous dysfunction; vital signs, weight; pulmonary function
Reference Range Excessive leukocytosis (WBC >50,000 cells/mm³, ANC >20,000 cells/mm³)
Patient Information Possible bone pain may occur
Nursing Implications Can premedicate with analgesics and antipyretics; control bone pain with non-narcotic analgesics
Additional Information Produced by recombinant DNA technology using a yeast-derived expression system
Dosage Forms Excipient information presented when available (limited, particularly for generics); consult specific product labeling.
Injection, powder for reconstitution:
Leukine®: 250 mcg [contains sucrose 10 mg/mL]
Injection, solution:
Leukine®: 500 mcg/mL (1 mL) [contains benzyl alcohol and sucrose 10 mg/mL]

References
Carr R, Modi N, Dore CJ, et al, "A Randomized, Controlled Trial of Prophylactic Granulocyte-Macrophage Colony-Stimulating Factor in Human Newborns Less Than 32 Weeks Gestation," *Pediatrics*, 1999, 103(4 Pt 1):796-802.
Lieschke GJ and Burgess AW, "Granulocyte Colony-Stimulating Factor and Granulocyte-Macrophage Colony-Stimulating Factor," (1) *N Engl J Med*, 1992, 327(1):28-35.
Lieschke GJ and Burgess AW, "Granulocyte Colony-Stimulating Factor and Granulocyte-Macrophage Colony-Stimulating Factor," (2) *N Engl J Med*, 1992, 327(2):99-106.
Stute N, Furman WL, Schell M, et al, "Pharmacokinetics of Recombinant Human Granulocyte - Macrophage Colony - Stimulating Factor in Children After Intravenous and Subcutaneous Administration," *J Pharm Sci*, 1995, 84(7):824-8.
Trissel LA, Bready BB, Kwan JW, et al, "Visual Compatibility of Sargramostim With Selected Antineoplastic Agents, Anti-infectives, or Other Drugs During Simulated Y-Site Injection," *Am J Hosp Pharm*, 1992, 49(2):402-6.

♦ **Sarna® HC (Can)** see Hydrocortisone *on page 685*
♦ **Sarnol®-HC [OTC]** see Hydrocortisone *on page 685*
♦ **SC 33428** see IDArubicin *on page 707*

♦ **S-Caine** see Lidocaine and Tetracaine *on page 824*
♦ **Scandonest® 3% Plain** see Mepivacaine *on page 883*
♦ **SCH 39720** see Ceftibuten *on page 273*
♦ **SCH 56592** see Posaconazole *on page 1132*
♦ **ScheinPharm Ranitidine (Can)** see Ranitidine *on page 1200*
♦ **S-Citalopram** see Escitalopram *on page 529*
♦ **Scopace™** see Scopolamine *on page 1248*

Scopolamine (skoe POL a meen)

Medication Safety Issues
Transdermal patch may contain conducting metal (eg, aluminum); remove patch prior to MRI.
U.S. Brand Names Isopto® Hyoscine; Scopace™; Transderm Scōp®
Canadian Brand Names Buscopan®; Transderm-V®
Therapeutic Category Anticholinergic Agent; Anticholinergic Agent, Ophthalmic; Anticholinergic Agent, Transdermal; Ophthalmic Agent, Mydriatic
Generic Available Yes: Injection
Use Preoperative medication to produce amnesia and decrease salivary and respiratory secretions; to produce cycloplegia and mydriasis (ophthalmic formulation); treatment of iridocyclitis (ophthalmic formulation); prevention of motion sickness (oral and transdermal formulations) and prevention of postoperative nausea and vomiting (transdermal formulation); inhibits excessive motility and hypertonus of the GI tract in such conditions as the irritable colon syndrome, mild dysentery, diverticulitis, and pylorospasm (oral formulation)
Pregnancy Risk Factor C
Pregnancy Considerations Teratogenic effects were not observed in animal studies; embryotoxic events were observed in some studies. Scopolamine crosses the placenta; may cause respiratory depression and/or neonatal hemorrhage when used during pregnancy. Transdermal scopolamine has been used as an adjunct to epidural anesthesia for cesarean delivery without adverse CNS effects on the newborn. Except when used prior to cesarean section, use during pregnancy only if the benefit to the mother outweighs the potential risk to the fetus.
Lactation Enters breast milk/use caution (AAP rates "compatible")
Contraindications Hypersensitivity to scopolamine or any component; patients hypersensitive to belladonna or barbiturates may be hypersensitive to scopolamine; narrow-angle glaucoma, GI or GU obstruction, thyrotoxicosis, tachycardia secondary to cardiac insufficiency, paralytic ileus, myasthenia gravis
Warnings Drug withdrawal symptoms such as nausea, vomiting, headache, dizziness, and equilibrium disturbance have been reported following removal of transdermal system, primarily in patients using the system for more than 3 days; discontinue if patient reports unusual visual disturbances or pain within the eye. Patients with idiosyncratic reactions to anticholinergics, including scopolamine, may experience disorientation, delirium, and/or marked somnolence; may be accompanied by dilated pupils, rapid pulse, and xerostomia. Safety and efficacy have not been established for use of transdermal and oral scopolamine in children.

Transdermal patch may contain conducting metal (eg, aluminum); remove patch prior to MRI. Scopolamine (hyoscine) hydrobromide should not be interchanged with scopolamine butylbromide formulations; dosages are not equivalent.
Precautions Use with caution with hepatic or renal dysfunction since adverse CNS effects occur more often in these patients; use with caution in infants and children

since they may be more susceptible to adverse effects of scopolamine; use with caution in patients with cardiac disease, seizures, or psychoses

Adverse Reactions

Cardiovascular: Tachycardia, palpitations

Central nervous system: Disorientation, drowsiness, hallucinations, confusion, psychosis, delirium, excitement, restlessness, dizziness

Gastrointestinal: Xerostomia, constipation, nausea, vomiting, dysphagia, dysgeusia

Genitourinary: Urinary retention

Ocular: Blurred vision, cycloplegia, mydriasis, photophobia, intraocular pressure elevated

Miscellaneous: Anaphylaxis, allergic reactions

Note: Systemic adverse effects have been reported with both the topical and ophthalmic preparations

Drug Interactions

Avoid Concomitant Use There are no known interactions where it is recommended to avoid concomitant use.

Increased Effect/Toxicity

Scopolamine Derivatives may increase the levels/effects of: AbobotulinumtoxinA; Alcohol (Ethyl); Anticholinergics; Cannabinoids; CNS Depressants; Methotrimeprazine; OnabotulinumtoxinA; Potassium Chloride; RimabotulinumtoxinB

The levels/effects of Scopolamine Derivatives may be increased by: Methotrimeprazine; Pramlintide

Decreased Effect

Scopolamine Derivatives may decrease the levels/effects of: Acetylcholinesterase Inhibitors (Central); Secretin

The levels/effects of Scopolamine Derivatives may be decreased by: Acetylcholinesterase Inhibitors (Central)

Stability

Injection and tablet: Store at room temperature 15°C to 30°C (58°F to 86°F)

Ophthalmic solution: Store at 8°C to 27°C (46°F to 80°F); protect from light

Transdermal system: Store at 20°C to 25°C (68°F to 77°F)

Physically compatible when mixed in the same syringe with atropine, butorphanol, chlorpromazine, dimenhydrinate, diphenhydramine, droperidol, fentanyl, glycopyrrolate, hydromorphone, hydroxyzine, meperidine, metoclopramide, morphine, pentazocine, pentobarbital, perphenazine, prochlorperazine, promazine, promethazine, or thiopental

Mechanism of Action Blocks the action of acetylcholine at parasympathetic sites in smooth muscle, secretory glands and the CNS, resulting in anticholinergic activity (inhibition of secretion of saliva and sweat, decreased GI motility and secretions, dilated pupils, increased heart rate, drowsiness, depressed motor function); antagonizes histamine and serotonin

Pharmacodynamics

Onset of action:

Oral, I.M.: 30 minutes to 1 hour

I.V.: 10 minutes

Transdermal: 4 hours

Duration:

Oral, I.M.: 4-6 hours

I.V.: 2 hours

Transdermal: 72 hours

Pharmacokinetics (Adult data unless noted)

Absorption: Well absorbed by all routes of administration

Metabolism: In the liver

Half-life: 9.5 hours

Excretion: <5% excreted unchanged in the urine

Usual Dosage

Preoperatively and antiemetic:

I.M., I.V., SubQ:

Children: 6 mcg/kg/dose (maximum dose: 0.3 mg/dose); may be repeated every 6-8 hours

Adults: 0.3-0.65 mg; may be repeated 3-4 times/day

Transdermal: Adults: Apply 1 disc behind the ear the evening before surgery; if prior to cesarean section, apply 1 hour prior to minimize exposure to infant

Motion sickness:

Oral: Children >12 years and Adults: 1-2 tablets 1 hour prior to exposure; may repeat after 8 hours of continued exposure

Transdermal: Children >12 years and Adults: Apply 1 disc behind the ear at least 4 hours prior to exposure every 3 days as needed

Ophthalmic:

Refraction:

Children: Instill 1 drop of 0.25% to eye(s) twice daily for 2 days before procedure

Adults: Instill 1-2 drops of 0.25% to eye(s) 1 hour before procedure

Iridocyclitis:

Children: Instill 1 drop of 0.25% to eye(s) up to 3 times/day

Adults: Instill 1-2 drops of 0.25% to eye(s) up to 3 times/day

Administration

Oral: May be administered without regard to food

Parenteral: I.V.: Dilute with an equal volume of SWI and administer by direct I.V. injection over 2-3 minutes

Transdermal: Transdermal patch is programmed to deliver 1 mg over 3 days. Once applied, do not remove the patch for 3 full days. Apply patch to hairless area behind one ear; wash hands before and after application; if becomes dislodged, replace with fresh patch

Ophthalmic: Instill drops to conjunctival sac of affected eye(s); avoid contact of bottle tip with skin or eye; finger pressure should be applied to lacrimal sac during and for 1-2 minutes after instillation to decrease risk of absorption and systemic reactions. Remove contact lenses prior to administration; wait 15 minutes before reinserting if using products containing benzalkonium chloride. Wash hands following administration.

Patient Information May cause drowsiness and impair ability to perform activities requiring mental alertness or physical coordination; may cause dry mouth; avoid alcohol; wash hands thoroughly with soap and water after handling the patch as dilation of pupils and blurred vision may occur if contact with eye; dispose of patches properly to avoid contact with children or pets; remove patch immediately if experiencing difficulty urinating or pain and reddening of eyes accompanied by dilated pupils

Additional Information Transdermal disc is programmed to deliver *in vivo* 0.5 mg over 3 days

Dosage Forms Excipient information presented when available (limited, particularly for generics); consult specific product labeling. [CAN] = Canadian brand name

Injection, solution, as hydrobromide: 0.4 mg/mL (1 mL)

Injection, solution, as hyoscine-N-butylbromide:

Buscopan® [CAN]: 20 mg/mL [not available in U.S.]

Patch, transdermal:

Transderm Scōp®: 1.5 mg (4s, 10s, 24s) [releases ~1 mg over 72 hours]

Solution, ophthalmic, as hydrobromide:

Isopto® Hyoscine: 0.25% (5 mL) [contains benzalkonium chloride]

Tablet, as hyoscine-N-butylbromide:

Buscopan® [CAN]: 10 mg [not available in U.S.]

Tablet, soluble, as hydrobromide:

Scopace™: 0.4 mg

◆ **Scopolamine Base** *see* Scopolamine *on page 1248*

◆ **Scopolamine Butylbromide** *see* Scopolamine *on page 1248*

◆ **Scopolamine Hydrobromide** *see* Scopolamine *on page 1248*

◆ **Scopolamine, Hyoscyamine, Atropine, and Phenobarbital** *see* Hyoscyamine, Atropine, Scopolamine, and Phenobarbital *on page 700*

◆ **Scot-Tussin® Diabetes [OTC]** *see* Dextromethorphan *on page 421*

◆ **Scot-Tussin® Expectorant [OTC]** *see* GuaiFENesin *on page 656*

◆ **Scot-Tussin® Senior [OTC]** *see* Guaifenesin and Dextromethorphan *on page 658*

◆ **Scytera™ [OTC]** *see* Coal Tar *on page 349*

◆ **SD/01** *see* Pegfilgrastim *on page 1070*

◆ **SDZ ASM 981** *see* Pimecrolimus *on page 1111*

◆ **Sebcur® (Can)** *see* Salicylic Acid *on page 1241*

◆ **Seb-Prev™** *see* Sulfacetamide *on page 1298*

Secobarbital (see koe BAR bi tal)

Medication Safety Issues
Sound-alike/look-alike issues:
Seconal® may be confused with Sectral®

Beers Criteria medication: This drug may be inappropriate for use in geriatric patients (high severity risk).

Related Information
Laboratory Detection of Drugs in Urine *on page 1706*

U.S. Brand Names Seconal®

Therapeutic Category Barbiturate; Hypnotic; Sedative

Generic Available No

Use Short-term treatment of insomnia; preanesthetic agent

Restrictions C-II

Pregnancy Risk Factor D

Lactation Enters breast milk/use caution (AAP rates "compatible")

Contraindications Hypersensitivity to secobarbital or any component; pre-existing CNS depression, severe uncontrolled pain, porphyria, severe respiratory disease with dyspnea or obstruction

Warnings Hypersensitivity reactions including anaphylaxis and angioedema may occur. Hazardous sleep-related activities, such as sleep-driving (driving while not fully awake without any recollection of driving), preparing and eating food, and making phone calls while asleep have also been reported. Effects with other sedative drugs or ethanol may be potentiated.

Precautions Use with caution in patients with hypovolemic shock, CHF, hepatic impairment, respiratory dysfunction or depression, previous addiction to the sedative/hypnotic group, chronic or acute pain, renal dysfunction; tolerance or psychological and physical dependence may occur with prolonged use; abrupt discontinuation after prolonged use may result in withdrawal symptoms

Adverse Reactions
Cardiovascular: Hypotension, cardiac arrhythmias, bradycardia

Central nervous system: Dizziness, lightheadedness, drowsiness, "hangover" effect, lethargy, impaired judgment, CNS depression or paradoxical excitation, hypothermia, nightmares, hallucinations

Dermatologic: Rash, exfoliative dermatitis, Stevens-Johnson syndrome

Gastrointestinal: Nausea, vomiting, constipation

Hematologic: Megaloblastic anemia, thrombocytopenia, agranulocytosis

Respiratory: Respiratory depression, apnea

Miscellaneous: Psychological and physical dependence with prolonged use; hypersensitivity reactions, anaphylaxis, angioedema; hazardous sleep-related activities (see Warnings)

Drug Interactions
Metabolism/Transport Effects Induces CYP2A6 (strong), 2C8 (strong), 2C9 (strong)

Avoid Concomitant Use There are no known interactions where it is recommended to avoid concomitant use.

Increased Effect/Toxicity
Secobarbital may increase the levels/effects of: Alcohol (Ethyl); CNS Depressants; Meperidine; Thiazide Diuretics

The levels/effects of Secobarbital may be increased by: Chloramphenicol; Divalproex; Felbamate; Primidone; Valproic Acid

Decreased Effect
Secobarbital may decrease the levels/effects of: Acetaminophen; Beta-Blockers; Calcium Channel Blockers; Chloramphenicol; Contraceptives (Estrogens); Contraceptives (Progestins); Corticosteroids (Systemic); CycloSPORINE; CycloSPORINE (Systemic); CYP2A6 Substrates; CYP2C8 Substrates (High risk); CYP2C9 Substrates (High risk); Disopyramide; Divalproex; Doxycycline; Etoposide; Etoposide Phosphate; Griseofulvin; LamoTRIgine; Methadone; Propafenone; QuiNIDine; Teniposide; Theophylline Derivatives; Treprostinil; Tricyclic Antidepressants; Valproic Acid; Vitamin K Antagonists

The levels/effects of Secobarbital may be decreased by: Pyridoxine; Rifamycin Derivatives

Food Interactions High doses of pyridoxine may decrease drug effect; barbiturates may increase the metabolism of vitamins D and K

Mechanism of Action Depresses CNS activity by binding to barbiturate site at GABA-receptor complex enhancing GABA activity; depresses reticular activating system; higher doses may be gabamimetic

Pharmacodynamics
Onset of action: Hypnosis: Oral: 15-30 minutes
Duration: Hypnosis: Oral: 3-4 hours with 100 mg dose

Pharmacokinetics (Adult data unless noted)
Absorption: Oral: Well absorbed (90%)
Distribution: V_d: Adults: 1.5 L/kg; crosses the placenta; appears in breast milk
Protein binding: 45% to 60%
Metabolism: In the liver by the microsomal enzyme system
Half-life:
Children: 2-13 years: 2.7-13.5 hours
Adults: 15-40 hours; mean 28 hours
Time to peak serum concentration: Oral: Within 2-4 hours
Elimination: Renally as inactive metabolites and small amounts as unchanged drug
Dialysis: Hemodialysis: Slightly dialyzable (5% to 20%)

Usual Dosage Oral:
Children:
Preoperative sedation: 2-6 mg/kg (maximum dose: 100 mg/dose) 1-2 hours before procedure
Sedation: 6 mg/kg/day divided every 8 hours
Adults:
Hypnotic: Usual: 100 mg/dose at bedtime; range 100-200 mg/dose
Preoperative sedation: 100-300 mg 1-2 hours before procedure

Monitoring Parameters Blood pressure, heart rate, respiratory rate, pulse oximetry, CNS status

Patient Information Avoid alcohol and other CNS depressants. May be habit-forming; avoid abrupt discontinuation after prolonged use. May cause dizziness or drowsiness and impair ability to perform activities requiring mental alertness or physical coordination. May cause hypersensitivity reactions. May cause hazardous sleep-related activities (ie, driving, preparing and eating foods, and making phone calls while not fully awake).

Additional Information Effectiveness for insomnia decreases greatly after 2 weeks of use; alkalinization of urine does not significantly increase excretion; withdraw slowly over 5-6 days after prolonged use to avoid sleep disturbances and rapid eye movement (REM) rebound

In March 2007, the FDA requested that all manufacturers of sedative-hypnotic drug products, including Seconal® (secobarbital), revise the labeling to include a greater emphasis on the risks of adverse events. The events include severe hypersensitivity reactions including anaphylaxis and/or angioedema, as well as hazardous sleep-related activities (eg, sleep-driving - driving while not fully awake after consumption of sedative-hypnotic drug, with no recollection of the event). Other activities may include preparing and ingesting food, and the use of the telephone, while asleep. These events may occur at any time during therapy including with the first dose administered.

Manufacturers must provide written notification to health-care providers regarding the new warnings. In addition, manufacturers are to develop "Patient Medication Guides" designed to educate consumers about the potential risks and to advise them of precautionary measures that can be taken. This advice will contain recommendations on correct utilization of the medication as well as the avoidance of the consumption of ethanol and/or other CNS-depressant agents. The FDA is also recommending manufacturers conduct studies evaluating the frequencies of sleep-driving (and other sleep-related behaviors) with the individual products.

Patients should be instructed not to discontinue these medications without first speaking with their healthcare provider. Patients should also be informed of the potential for an allergic reaction, the signs and symptoms of anaphylaxis, and the appropriate emergency self-treatment of an anaphylactic reaction.

Additional information on the sedative-hypnotic products and sleep disorders is available at http://www.fda.gov/NewsEvents/Newsroom/PressAnnouncements/2007/ucm108868.htm

Dosage Forms Excipient information presented when available (limited, particularly for generics); consult specific product labeling.

Capsule, as sodium: 100 mg

References

Levine HL, Cohen ME, Duffner PK, et al, "Rectal Absorption and Disposition of Secobarbital in Epileptic Children," *Pediatr Pharmacol (New York)*, 1982, 2(1):33-8.

Nahata MC, Starling S, and Edwards RC, "Prolonged Sedation Associated With Secobarbital in Newborn Infants Receiving Ventilatory Support," *Am J Perinatol*, 1991, 8(1):35-6.

Wolfert RR and Cox RM, "Room Temperature Stability of Drug Products Labeled for Refrigerated Storage," *Am J Hosp Pharm*, 1975, 32(6):585-7.

♦ **Secobarbital Sodium** *see* Secobarbital *on page 1250*

♦ **Seconal®** *see* Secobarbital *on page 1250*

♦ **SecreFlo™ [DSC]** *see* Secretin *on page 1251*

Secretin (SEE kre tin)

U.S. Brand Names ChiRhoStim®; SecreFlo™ [DSC]

Therapeutic Category Diagnostic Agent, Gastrinoma (Zollinger-Ellison Syndrome); Diagnostic Agent, Pancreatic Exocrine Insufficiency

Generic Available No

Use Diagnosis of gastrinoma (Zollinger-Ellison syndrome) and diagnosis of pancreatic exocrine dysfunction (chronic pancreatitis); facilitation of endoscopic retrograde cholangiopancreatography (ERCP) visualization

Pregnancy Risk Factor C

Pregnancy Considerations Reproduction studies have not been conducted.

Lactation Excretion in breast milk unknown/use caution

Contraindications Hypersensitivity to secretin or any component; do not give to patients with acute pancreatitis until attack has subsided

Precautions Administer an I.V. test dose of 0.2 mcg (0.1 mL) particularly in patients with a history of hypersensitivity, allergy or asthma; use with caution in patients who are highly nervous or have an excessive gag reflex; patients receiving anticholinergics, patients who have had a vagotomy, or patients with inflammatory bowel disease may have a reduced response to secretin; patients with alcoholic or other liver diseases may have an increased response to secretin

Adverse Reactions

Cardiovascular: Hypotension, bradycardia (mild), flushing, tachycardia

Central nervous system: Headache, fever, anxiety, faintness, sedation

Gastrointestinal: Abdominal discomfort and cramps, vomiting, diarrhea, nausea, oral secretions increased

Neuromuscular & skeletal: Tingling in legs

Respiratory: Transient decrease in oxygen saturation, respiratory distress

Miscellaneous: Hypersensitivity reactions, diaphoresis

Drug Interactions

Avoid Concomitant Use There are no known interactions where it is recommended to avoid concomitant use.

Increased Effect/Toxicity There are no known significant interactions involving an increase in effect.

Decreased Effect

The levels/effects of Secretin may be decreased by: Anticholinergic Agents

Stability Store in freezer (-20°C); SecreFlo™ should be used immediately after reconstitution; human secretin is also stable for 1 year refrigerated and 6 months at room temperature

Mechanism of Action Secretin is a naturally-occurring hormone secreted by cells in the duodenal and upper jejunal mucosa which increases the volume and bicarbonate content of pancreatic juice; when used as a diagnostic agent, synthetic porcine secretin stimulates an increase in gastrin release in patients with Zollinger-Ellison syndrome when compared with normal patients; gastrin bicarbonate concentration is reduced in patients with chronic pancreatitis when compared with a normal patient's response to secretin

Pharmacodynamics

Maximum output of pancreatic secretions: Within 30 minutes

Duration: At least 2 hours

Pharmacokinetics (Adult data unless noted)

Distribution: V_d: Porcine formulation: 2 L (approximately); human formulation: 2.7 L

Protein binding: 40%

Inactivated by proteolytic enzymes if administered orally

Metabolism: Metabolic fate is thought to be hydrolysis to smaller peptides

Half-life: Porcine formulation: 27 minutes; human formulation: 45 minutes

Elimination: Clearance: Porcine formulation: 487 ± 136 mL/minute; human formulation: 580.9 ± 51.3 mL/minute

Usual Dosage Children and Adults: I.V.:

Diagnostic agent for pancreatic function: 0.2 mcg/kg as single dose

Diagnostic agent for gastrinoma (Zollinger-Ellison): 0.4 mcg/kg as single dose

Facilitation of ERCP visualization: 0.2 mcg/kg as a single dose

Administration Parenteral: Reconstitute with 8 mL of NS resulting in a 2 mcg/mL solution; shake vigorously to ensure dissolution; use immediately by direct I.V. injection slowly over 1 minute

Monitoring Parameters Peak bicarbonate concentration of duodenal fluid aspirate (chronic pancreatitis); serum gastrin (gastrinoma)

Reference Range

Peak gastric bicarbonate concentration:

Normal: 94-134 mEq/L

Chronic pancreatitis: <80 mEq/L

Severe pancreatitis: <50 mEq/L

Serum gastrin:

Normal: ≤110 pg/mL

Gastrinoma: >110 pg/mL

Nursing Implications Patients should fast at least 12 hours before testing for Zollinger-Ellison syndrome

Additional Information SecreFlo™ is available currently as an orphan drug by contacting the manufacturer Repligen; a double-blind crossover study of secretin 0.2 clinical units/kg versus placebo in 56 autistic children revealed no significant differences between the 2 groups (1 clinical unit is equivalent to 0.2 mcg) (Owley, 2001)

Dosage Forms Excipient information presented when available (limited, particularly for generics); consult specific product labeling. [DSC] = Discontinued product

Injection, powder for reconstitution [human derived]:

ChiRhoStim®: 16 mcg

Injection, powder for reconstitution [porcine derived]:

SecreFlo™: 16 mcg [DSC]

References

Owley T, McMahon W, Cook EH, et al, "Multisite, Double-Blind, Placebo-Controlled Trial of Porcine Secretin in Autism," *J Am Acad Child Adolesc Psychiatry*, 2001, 40(11):1293-9.

♦ **Secretin, Human** *see* Secretin *on page 1251*

♦ **Secretin, Porcine** *see* Secretin *on page 1251*

♦ **Secura® Antifungal Extra Thick [OTC]** *see* Miconazole *on page 927*

♦ **Secura® Antifungal Greaseless [OTC]** *see* Miconazole *on page 927*

♦ **Selax® (Can)** *see* Docusate *on page 468*

♦ **Selenium** *see* Trace Metals *on page 1366*

Selenium Sulfide (se LEE nee um SUL fide)

U.S. Brand Names Dandrex [OTC]; Head & Shoulders® Intensive Treatment [OTC]; Selseb®; Selsun blue® 2-in-1 Treatment [OTC]; Selsun blue® Daily Treatment [OTC]; Selsun blue® Medicated Treatment [OTC]; Selsun blue® Moisturizing Treatment [OTC]; Tersi

Canadian Brand Names Versel®

Therapeutic Category Antiseborrheic Agent, Topical; Shampoos

Generic Available Yes: Excludes foam

Use To treat itching and flaking of the scalp associated with dandruff; to control scalp seborrheic dermatitis; treatment of tinea versicolor

Pregnancy Risk Factor C

Pregnancy Considerations Animal studies have not been conducted. Avoid use in pregnant women unless the potential benefit justifies the potential risk to the fetus.

Lactation Excretion in breast milk unknown/use caution

Contraindications Hypersensitivity to selenium or any component

Warnings Safety in infants has not been established; avoid use in children <2 years of age

Precautions Do not use on damaged skin to avoid any systemic toxicity

Adverse Reactions

Central nervous system: Lethargy

Dermatologic: Alopecia, discoloration of hair

Gastrointestinal: Vomiting following long-term use on damaged skin, abdominal pain, garlic breath

Local: Local irritation

Neuromuscular & skeletal: Tremor

Miscellaneous: Perspiration

Drug Interactions

Avoid Concomitant Use There are no known interactions where it is recommended to avoid concomitant use.

Increased Effect/Toxicity There are no known significant interactions involving an increase in effect.

Decreased Effect There are no known significant interactions involving a decrease in effect.

Mechanism of Action May block the enzymes involved in growth of epithelial tissue

Pharmacokinetics (Adult data unless noted) Absorption: Not absorbed topically through intact skin, but can be absorbed topically through damaged skin

Usual Dosage Children ≥2 years and Adults: Topical:

Dandruff, seborrhea: Massage 5-10 mL into wet scalp, leave on scalp 2-3 minutes, rinse thoroughly and repeat application; alternatively, 5-10 mL of shampoo is applied and allowed to remain on scalp for 5-10 minutes before being rinsed off thoroughly without a repeat application; shampoo twice weekly for 2 weeks initially, then use once every 1-4 weeks as indicated depending upon control

Tinea versicolor: Apply the 2.5% lotion in a thin layer covering the body surface from the face to the knees; leave on skin for 10 minutes, then rinse thoroughly; apply every day for 7 days; then follow with monthly applications for 3 months to prevent recurrences

Administration Topical: For external use only; avoid contact with eyes or acutely inflamed skin

Patient Information Remove all jewelry before using the lotion; wash hands thoroughly following application of the lotion; may discolor hair

Dosage Forms Excipient information presented when available (limited, particularly for generics); consult specific product labeling.

Aerosol, topical [foam]:

Tersi: 2.25% (70 g)

Lotion, topical: 2.5% (120 mL)

Shampoo, topical: 1% (210 mL)

Dandrex: 1% (240 mL)

Head & Shoulders® Intensive Treatment: 1% (420 mL)

Selseb®: 2.25% (180 mL)

Selsun blue® Daily Treatment: 1% (207 mL, 325 mL)

Selsun blue® Medicated Treatment: 1% (120 mL, 207 mL, 325 mL) [contains menthol]

Selsun blue® Moisturizing Treatment: 1% (207 mL, 325 mL) [contains aloe and moisturizers]

Selsun blue® 2-in-1 Treatment: 1% (207 mL, 325 mL) [contains conditioner]

References

Lester RS, "Topical Formulary for the Pediatrician," *Pediatr Clin North Am*, 1983, 30(4):749-65.

♦ **Selfemra®** *see* FLUoxetine *on page 600*

♦ **Selseb®** *see* Selenium Sulfide *on page 1252*

♦ **Selsun blue® 2-in-1 Treatment [OTC]** *see* Selenium Sulfide *on page 1252*

♦ **Selsun blue® Daily Treatment [OTC]** *see* Selenium Sulfide *on page 1252*

♦ **Selsun blue® Medicated Treatment [OTC]** *see* Selenium Sulfide *on page 1252*

♦ **Selsun blue® Moisturizing Treatment [OTC]** *see* Selenium Sulfide *on page 1252*

◆ **Senexon® [OTC]** *see* Senna *on page 1253*

Senna (SEN na)

Medication Safety Issues
Sound-alike/look-alike issues:
Perdiem® may be confused with Pyridium®
Senexon® may be confused with Cenestin®
Senokot® may be confused with Depakote®

U.S. Brand Names Black-Draught™ Tablets [OTC]; Evac-U-Gen [OTC]; ex-lax® Maximum Strength [OTC]; ex-lax® [OTC]; Fleet® Pedia-Lax™ Quick Dissolve [OTC]; Fletcher's® [OTC]; Little Tummys® Laxative [OTC]; Perdiem® Overnight Relief [OTC]; Senexon® [OTC]; Senna-Gen® [OTC]; SenokotXTRA® [OTC]; Senokot® [OTC]; Seno-Sol™ [OTC] [DSC]; SenoSol™-X [OTC] [DSC]; Uni-Cenna [OTC] [DSC]

Therapeutic Category Laxative, Stimulant

Generic Available Yes

Use Short-term treatment of constipation; evacuate the colon for bowel or rectal examinations

Contraindications Hypersensitivity to senna or any component; nausea and vomiting; undiagnosed abdominal pain, appendicitis, intestinal obstruction or perforation

Warnings Concentrated liquid contains sodium benzoate which may cause allergic reactions in susceptible individuals; use products containing sodium benzoate with caution in neonates; *in vitro* and animal studies have shown that benzoate displaces bilirubin from protein binding sites

Precautions Avoid prolonged use (>1 week); chronic use may lead to dependency, fluid and electrolyte imbalance, vitamin and mineral deficiencies

Adverse Reactions
Endocrine & metabolic: Electrolyte and fluid imbalance
Gastrointestinal: Nausea, vomiting, diarrhea, abdominal cramps, perianal irritation, discoloration of feces
Genitourinary: Discoloration of urine

Drug Interactions
Avoid Concomitant Use There are no known interactions where it is recommended to avoid concomitant use.
Increased Effect/Toxicity There are no known significant interactions involving an increase in effect.
Decreased Effect There are no known significant interactions involving a decrease in effect.

Mechanism of Action Active metabolite (aglycone) acts as a local irritant on the colon, stimulates Auerbach's plexus to produce peristalsis

Pharmacodynamics Onset of action:
Oral: Within 6-24 hours
Rectal: Evacuation occurs in 30 minutes to 2 hours

Pharmacokinetics (Adult data unless noted)
Metabolism: In the liver
Elimination: In the feces (via bile) and in urine

Usual Dosage Oral:
Constipation:
Infants 1 month to 2 years: Syrup: 1.25-2.5 mL (2.2-4.4 mg sennosides) at bedtime, not to exceed 5 mL (8.8 mg sennosides)/day
Children:
Syrup:
2 to <6 years: 2.5-3.75 mL (4.4-6.6 mg sennosides) at bedtime, not to exceed 3.75 mL (6.6 mg sennosides) twice daily
6-12 years: 5-7.5 mL (8.8-13.2 mg sennosides) at bedtime, not to exceed 7.5 mL (13.2 mg sennosides) twice daily
Tablet:
2 to <6 years: 1/2 tablet (4.3 sennosides) at bedtime, not to exceed 1 tablet (8.6 mg sennosides) twice daily

6-12 years: 1 tablet (8.6 mg sennosides) at bedtime, not to exceed 2 tablets (17.2 mg sennosides) twice daily
Children ≥12 years and Adults:
Syrup: 10-15 mL (17.6-26.4 mg sennosides) at bedtime, not to exceed 15 mL (26.4 mg sennosides) twice daily
Tablet: 2 tablets (17.2 mg sennosides) at bedtime, not to exceed 4 tablets (34.4 mg sennosides) twice daily
Bowel evacuation: Children ≥12 years and Adults: 130 mg sennosides (X-Prep® 75 mL) between 2:00 PM to 4:00 PM on the day prior to procedure

Administration Oral: Administer with water; syrup can be taken with juice or milk or mixed with ice cream to mask taste.

Monitoring Parameters I & O, frequency of bowel movements, serum electrolytes if severe diarrhea occurs

Patient Information May discolor urine or feces; drink plenty of fluids

Dosage Forms Excipient information presented when available (limited, particularly for generics); consult specific product labeling. [DSC] = Discontinued product
Liquid:
Senexon®: Sennosides 8.8 mg/5 mL (240 mL) [contains propylene glycol]
Liquid [concentrate]:
Fletcher's®: Senna concentrate 33.3 mg/mL (75 mL) [alcohol free; contains sodium benzoate; root beer flavor]
Liquid [concentrate; drops]:
Little Tummys® Laxative: Sennosides 8.8 mg/1 mL (30 mL) [alcohol free, dye free; contains propylene glycol and soya lecithin; chocolate flavor]
Strip, orally disintegrating:
Fleet® Pedia-Lax™ Quick Dissolve: Sennosides 8.6 mg (12s) [grape flavor]
Syrup: Sennosides 8.8 mg/5 mL (240 mL)
Tablet: Sennosides 8.6 mg
ex-lax®: Sennosides USP 15 mg
ex-lax® Maximum Strength: Sennosides USP 25 mg
Perdiem® Overnight Relief: Sennosides USP 15 mg
Senokot®, Senexon®, Senna-Gen®, SenoSol™ [DSC], Uni-Cenna [DSC]: Sennosides 8.6 mg
SenokotXTRA®, SenoSol™-X [DSC]: Sennosides 17 mg
Tablet, chewable:
Black-Draught™: Sennosides 10 mg
ex-lax®: Sennosides USP 15 mg [chocolate flavor]
Evac-U-Gen: Sennosides 10 mg

References
Perkin JM, "Constipation in Childhood: A Controlled Comparison Between Lactulose and Standardized Senna," *Curr Med Res Opin*, 1977, 4(8):540-3.

◆ **Senna and Docusate** *see* Docusate and Senna *on page 469*

◆ **Senna-Gen® [OTC]** *see* Senna *on page 1253*

◆ **Senna-S** *see* Docusate and Senna *on page 469*

◆ **Sennosides** *see* Senna *on page 1253*

◆ **Senokot® [OTC]** *see* Senna *on page 1253*

◆ **Senokot-S® [OTC]** *see* Docusate and Senna *on page 469*

◆ **SenokotXTRA® [OTC]** *see* Senna *on page 1253*

◆ **SenoSol™ [OTC] [DSC]** *see* Senna *on page 1253*

◆ **SenoSol™-X [OTC] [DSC]** *see* Senna *on page 1253*

◆ **SenoSol™-SS [OTC]** *see* Docusate and Senna *on page 469*

◆ **Sensorcaine®** *see* Bupivacaine *on page 213*

◆ **Sensorcaine®-MPF** *see* Bupivacaine *on page 213*

◆ **Sensorcaine®-MPF Spinal** *see* Bupivacaine *on page 213*

◆ **Sepasoothe®** *see* Benzocaine *on page 182*

◆ **Septra®** *see* Sulfamethoxazole and Trimethoprim *on page 1302*

◆ **Septra® DS** *see* Sulfamethoxazole and Trimethoprim *on page 1302*

◆ **Septra® Injection (Can)** *see* Sulfamethoxazole and Trimethoprim *on page 1302*

◆ **Serevent® Diskhaler® Disk (Can)** *see* Salmeterol *on page 1243*

◆ **Serevent® Diskus®** *see* Salmeterol *on page 1243*

◆ **Seromycin®** *see* CycloSERINE *on page 371*

◆ **Serostim®** *see* Somatropin *on page 1281*

Sertraline (SER tra leen)

Medication Safety Issues
Sound-alike/look-alike issues:
Sertraline may be confused with selegiline, Serentil®, Serevent®, Soriatane®
Zoloft® may be confused with Zocor®

Related Information
Antidepressant Agents *on page 1484*
Serotonin Syndrome *on page 1695*

U.S. Brand Names Zoloft®

Canadian Brand Names Apo-Sertraline®; CO Sertraline; Dom-Sertraline; Mylan-Sertraline; Novo-Sertraline; Nu-Sertraline; PHL-Sertraline; PMS-Sertraline; ratio-Sertraline; Riva-Sertraline; Sandoz-Sertraline; Zoloft®

Therapeutic Category Antidepressant, Selective Serotonin Reuptake Inhibitor (SSRI)

Generic Available Yes

Use Treatment of major depression, obsessive-compulsive disorder, panic disorder (with or without agoraphobia), post-traumatic stress disorder, premenstrual dysphoric disorder, social anxiety disorder

Medication Guide An FDA-approved patient medication guide, which is available with the product information and at http://www.fda.gov/downloads/Drugs/DrugSafety/ucm089832.pdf, must be dispensed with this medication for each new outpatient prescription and refill.

Pregnancy Risk Factor C

Pregnancy Considerations Due to adverse effects observed in animal studies, sertraline is classified as pregnancy category C. Sertraline crosses the human placenta. Nonteratogenic effects in the newborn following SSRI exposure late in the third trimester include respiratory distress, cyanosis, apnea, seizures, temperature instability, feeding difficulty, vomiting, hypoglycemia, hypo- or hypertonia, hyper-reflexia, jitteriness, irritability, constant crying, and tremor. An increased risk of low birth weight, lower Apgar scores, and blunted behavioral response to pain for a prolonged period after delivery has also been reported. Exposure to SSRIs after the twentieth week of gestation has been associated with persistent pulmonary hypertension of the newborn (PPHN). Adverse effects may be due to toxic effects of the SSRI or drug discontinuation. The long-term effects of *in utero* SSRI exposure on infant development and behavior are not known.

Due to pregnancy-induced physiologic changes, women who are pregnant may require increased doses of sertraline to achieve euthymia. Women treated for major depression and who are euthymic prior to pregnancy are more likely to experience a relapse when medication is discontinued as compared to pregnant women who continue taking antidepressant medications. The ACOG recommends that therapy with SSRIs or SNRIs during pregnancy be individualized; treatment of depression during pregnancy should incorporate the clinical expertise of the mental health clinician, obstetrician, primary healthcare provider, and pediatrician. If treatment during pregnancy is required, consider tapering therapy during the third trimester in order to prevent withdrawal symptoms in the infant. If this is done and the woman is considered to be at risk of relapse from her major depressive disorder, the medication can be restarted following delivery, although the dose should be readjusted to that required before pregnancy. Treatment algorithms have been developed by the ACOG and the APA for the management of depression in women prior to conception and during pregnancy (Yonkers, 2009).

Lactation Enters breast milk/use caution (AAP rates "of concern")

Breast-Feeding Considerations Sertraline and desmethylsertraline are excreted in breast milk. Infants exposed to sertraline while breast-feeding generally receive a low relative dose and serum concentrations are not detectable in most infants. Adverse reactions have not been reported in nursing infants. Sertraline concentrations in the hindmilk are higher than in foremilk. If the benefits of the mother receiving the sertraline and breast-feeding outweigh the risks, the mother may consider pumping and discarding breast milk with the feeding 7-9 hours after the daily dose to decrease sertraline exposure to the infant. The long-term effects on development and behavior have not been studied. The manufacturer recommends that caution be exercised when administering sertraline to nursing women. The AAP recommends sertraline be considered "a drug for which the effect on nursing infants is unknown but may be of concern."

Contraindications Hypersensitivity to sertraline or any component; use of MAO inhibitors within 14 days (potentially fatal reactions may occur, see Drug Interactions); concurrent use of pimozide; oral concentrate is contraindicated in patients receiving disulfiram (contains 12% alcohol)

Warnings Safety and efficacy in pediatric patients ≥6 years of age have been established only for the treatment of obsessive compulsive disorder; sertraline is not approved for the treatment of depression in pediatric patients. Clinical worsening of depression or suicidal ideation and behavior may occur in children and adults with major depressive disorder **[U.S. Boxed Warnings]**. In clinical trials, antidepressants increased the risk of suicidal thinking and behavior (suicidality) in children, adolescents, and young adults (18-24 years of age) with major depressive disorder and other psychiatric disorders. This risk must be considered before prescribing antidepressants for any clinical use. Short-term studies did **not** show an increased risk of suicidality with antidepressant use in patients >24 years of age and showed a decreased risk in patients ≥65 years.

Patients of all ages who are treated with antidepressants for any indication require appropriate monitoring and close observation for clinical worsening of depression, suicidality, and unusual changes in behavior, especially during the first few months after antidepressant initiation or when the dose is adjusted. Family members and caregivers should be instructed to closely observe the patient (ie, daily) and communicate condition with healthcare provider. Patients should also be monitored for associated behaviors (eg, anxiety, agitation, panic attacks, insomnia, irritability, hostility, aggressiveness, impulsivity, akathisia, hypomania, mania) which may increase the risk for worsening depression or suicidality. Worsening depression or emergence of suicidality (or associated behaviors listed above) that is abrupt in onset, severe, or not part of the presenting symptoms, may require discontinuation or modification of drug therapy.

Avoid abrupt discontinuation; discontinuation symptoms (including agitation, dysphoria, anxiety, confusion, dizziness, hypomania, nightmares, and other symptoms) may occur if therapy is abruptly discontinued or dose reduced; taper the dose to minimize risks of discontinuation symptoms; if intolerable symptoms occur following a decrease in dosage or upon discontinuation of therapy, consider resuming the previous dose with a more gradual taper. To reduce risk of intentional overdose, write prescriptions for the smallest quantity consistent with good patient care. Screen individuals for bipolar disorder prior to treatment (using antidepressants alone may induce manic episodes in patients with this condition). Potentially fatal serotonin syndrome may occur when SSRIs are used in combination with serotonergic drugs (eg, triptans) or drugs that impair the metabolism of serotonin (eg, MAO inhibitors); see Drug Interactions.

Dropper for oral concentrate contains natural rubber latex which may cause allergic reactions in susceptible individuals; avoid use in patients with allergy to latex.

Precautions Use with caution in patients with seizure disorders, concomitant illnesses that may effect hepatic metabolism or hemodynamic responses (eg, unstable cardiac disease, recent MI), and in suicidal patients; use with caution and decrease dose in patients with hepatic dysfunction; may result in hyponatremia, SIADH, significant weight loss (monitor weight and growth in pediatric patients), decrease in serum uric acid (mild uricosuric effect, use with caution in patient at risk of uric acid nephropathy), activation of mania/hypomania, or abnormal bleeding; SSRIs may increase risk of bleeding (eg, upper GI bleeding) especially in patients receiving nonselective NSAIDs, aspirin, or other drugs that affect coagulation. Use with caution during late third trimester of pregnancy [newborns may experience adverse effects or withdrawal symptoms (consider risk and benefits); see Additional Information; exposure to SSRIs late in pregnancy may also be associated with an increased risk for persistent pulmonary hypertension of the newborn (see Chambers, 2006)].

Adverse Reactions

Central nervous system: Agitation, dizziness, headache, insomnia, nervousness, fatigue, somnolence, fever, impaired concentration, activation of mania or hypomania, emotional lability, aggressive reaction, abnormal thinking, seizures, hyperkinesia; suicidal thinking and behavior (see Warnings)

Note: SSRI-associated behavioral activation (ie, restlessness, hyperkinesis, hyperactivity, agitation) is 2- to 3-fold more prevalent in children compared to adolescents; it is more prevalent in adolescents compared to adults. Somnolence (including sedation and drowsiness) is more common in adults compared to children and adolescents (see Safer, 2006).

Dermatologic: Rash

Endocrine & metabolic: Weight loss; SIADH, hyponatremia (volume-depleted patients); serum uric acid decreased, sexual dysfunction, libido decreased; weight gain has also been reported

Gastrointestinal: Nausea, vomiting, diarrhea, loose stools, xerostomia, constipation, anorexia, dyspepsia

Note: SSRI-associated vomiting is 2- to 3-fold more prevalent in children compared to adolescents; it is more prevalent in adolescents compared to adults.

Genitourinary: Urinary incontinence

Hematologic: Altered platelet function, purpura

Neuromuscular & skeletal: Tremor, paresthesia, hyperkinesia, twitching, malaise

Ocular: Abnormal vision

Respiratory: Epistaxis

Miscellaneous: Diaphoresis; withdrawal symptoms following abrupt discontinuation (see Warnings)

Drug Interactions

Metabolism/Transport Effects Substrate of CYP2B6 (minor), 2C9 (minor), 2C19 (major), 2D6 (major), 3A4 (minor); **Inhibits** CYP1A2 (weak), 2B6 (moderate), 2C8 (weak), 2C9 (weak), 2C19 (moderate), 2D6 (moderate), 3A4 (moderate)

Avoid Concomitant Use

Avoid concomitant use of Sertraline with any of the following: Clopidogrel; Disulfiram; Iobenguane I 123; MAO Inhibitors; Metoclopramide; Pimozide; Sibutramine; Thioridazine; Tolvaptan

Increased Effect/Toxicity

Sertraline may increase the levels/effects of: Alcohol (Ethyl); Alpha-/Beta-Blockers; Anticoagulants; Antidepressants (Serotonin Reuptake Inhibitor/Antagonist); Antiplatelet Agents; Aspirin; Beta-Blockers; BusPIRone; CarBAMazepine; Clozapine; CNS Depressants; Colchicine; Collagenase (Systemic); CYP2B6 Substrates; CYP2C19 Substrates; CYP2D6 Substrates; CYP3A4 Substrates; Desmopressin; Dextromethorphan; Drotrecogin Alfa; Eplerenone; Everolimus; Fesoterodine; Galantamine; Halofantrine; Haloperidol; Ibritumomab; Lithium; Methadone; Methotrimeprazine; NSAID (COX-2 Inhibitor); NSAID (Nonselective); Phenytoin; Pimecrolimus; Pimozide; Ranolazine; Risperidone; Salicylates; Salmeterol; Saxagliptin; Serotonin Modulators; Tamoxifen; Thioridazine; Thrombolytic Agents; Tolvaptan; Tositumomab and Iodine I 131 Tositumomab; TraMADol; Tricyclic Antidepressants; Vitamin K Antagonists

The levels/effects of Sertraline may be increased by: Analgesics (Opioid); BusPIRone; Cimetidine; CYP2D6 Inhibitors (Moderate); CYP2D6 Inhibitors (Strong); Dasatinib; Disulfiram; Glucosamine; Herbs (Anticoagulant/ Antiplatelet Properties); Macrolide Antibiotics; MAO Inhibitors; Methotrimeprazine; Metoclopramide; Omega-3-Acid Ethyl Esters; Pentosan Polysulfate Sodium; Pentoxifylline; Prostacyclin Analogues; Sibutramine; TraMADol; Tryptophan

Decreased Effect

Sertraline may decrease the levels/effects of: Clopidogrel; Iobenguane I 123

The levels/effects of Sertraline may be decreased by: CarBAMazepine; Cyproheptadine; Darunavir; Efavirenz; Peginterferon Alfa-2b

Food Interactions Tryptophan supplements may increase serious side effects; its use is **not recommended**. Grapefruit juice may significantly increase sertraline serum concentrations

Tablets: Food may slightly increase AUC, increase peak concentrations by 25% and shorten the time to peak plasma concentrations

Oral concentrate: Food may prolong the rate, but does not effect the extent of absorption

Stability Store at room temperature

Mechanism of Action Selective inhibitor of CNS neuronal serotonin uptake; minimal effects on reuptake of norepinephrine or dopamine; does not significantly bind to alpha-adrenergic, benzodiazepine, cholinergic, dopamine, GABA, histamine, or serotonin receptors; may therefore be useful in patients at risk from sedation, hypotension and anticholinergic effects of tricyclic antidepressants; does not inhibit monoamine oxidase

Pharmacodynamics Maximum effect may take several weeks

Pharmacokinetics (Adult data unless noted)

Protein binding: 98%

Metabolism: Significant first pass effect; undergoes N-demethylation to N-desmethylsertraline (significantly less active than sertraline); both parent and metabolite undergo oxidative deamination, followed by reduction, hydroxylation and conjugation with glucuronide (**Note:** Children 6-17 years may metabolize sertraline slightly better than adults, as pediatric AUCs and peak concentrations were 22% lower than adults when

◄ adjusted for weight; however, lower doses are recommended for younger pediatric patients to avoid excessive drug levels)

Bioavailability: Tablets approximately equal to oral solution

Half-life: Parent: Mean: 26 hours; metabolite (N-desmethylsertraline): 62-104 hours

Children: 6-12 years: Mean: 26.2 hours

Children: 13-17 years: Mean: 27.8 hours

Adults: 18-45 years: Mean: 27.2 hours

Elimination: 40% to 45% of dose eliminated in urine (none as unchanged drug); 40% to 45% eliminated in feces (12% to 14% as unchanged drug)

Clearance: May be decreased in patients with hepatic impairment

Dialysis: Not likely to remove significant amount of drug due to large V_d

Usual Dosage Oral: (**Note:** See Additional Information)

Children 6-12 years:

Depression: **Note:** Not FDA approved; see Warnings: Initial: 12.5-25 mg once daily; titrate dose upwards if clinically needed; may increase by 25-50 mg/day increments at intervals of at least 1 week; mean final dose in 21 children (8-18 years of age) was 100 ± 53 mg or 1.6 mg/kg/day (n=11); range: 25-200 mg/day; maximum dose: 200 mg/day (see Tierney, 1995 and Dopheide, 2006); avoid excessive dosing

Obsessive-compulsive disorder: Initial: 25 mg once daily; titrate dose upwards if clinically needed; increase by 25-50 mg/day increments at intervals of at least 1 week; range: 25-200 mg/day; maximum dose: 200 mg/day; avoid excessive dosing

Adolescents 13-17 years:

Depression: Initial 25-50 mg once daily; titrate dose upwards if clinically needed; may increase by 50 mg/day increments at intervals of at least 1 week; mean final dose in 13 adolescents was 110 ± 50 mg or about 2 mg/kg/day (see McConville, 1996); in another study using a slower titration, the mean dose at week 6 was 93 mg (n=41) and at week 10 was 127 mg (n=34) (see Ambrosini, 1999); range: 25-200 mg/day; maximum dose: 200 mg/day (see Dopheide, 2006).

Obsessive-compulsive disorder: Initial: 50 mg once daily; titrate dose upwards if clinically needed; increase by 50 mg/day increments at intervals of at least 1 week; range: 25-200 mg/day; maximum dose: 200 mg/day

Adults:

Depression and obsessive-compulsive disorder: Initial: 50 mg once daily; titrate dose upwards if clinically needed; increase by 50 mg/day increments at intervals of at least 1 week; range: 50-200 mg/day; maximum dose: 200 mg/day

Panic disorder, post-traumatic stress disorder, and social anxiety disorder: Initial: 25 mg once daily; increase dose after 1 week to 50 mg once daily; titrate dose further if clinically needed; increase by 50 mg/day increments at intervals of at least 1 week; range: 50-200 mg/day; maximum dose: 200 mg/day

Premenstrual dysphoric disorder: Initial: 50 mg/day given daily throughout the menstrual cycle **or** only during the luteal phase of the menstrual cycle (depending on assessment of physician); may increase if needed by 50 mg increments per menstrual cycle; maximum dose when using daily dosing throughout the menstrual cycle: 150 mg/day; maximum dose when dosing only during the luteal phase of the menstrual cycle: 100 mg/day. **Note:** If using a 100 mg/day dose with luteal phase dosing, use a 50 mg/day titration step for 3 days at the beginning of each luteal phase dosing period.

Dosing adjustment in renal impairment: None needed

Dosing adjustment in hepatic impairment: Use with caution and in reduced doses

Administration Oral: May be administered without regard to food; avoid administration with grapefruit juice;

administer once daily dosage in morning or evening. Must dilute oral concentrate before use; measure dose with dropper provided and mix with 4 ounces of water, orange juice, lemonade, ginger ale, or lemon/lime soda; do not mix with other liquids; take dose immediately after mixing, do not mix ahead of time; sometimes a slight haze may be seen after mixing (this is normal)

Monitoring Parameters Weight and growth in children if long-term therapy; uric acid, CBC, liver function, serum sodium, urine output. Monitor patient periodically for symptom resolution; monitor for worsening depression, suicidality, and associated behaviors (especially at the beginning of therapy or when doses are increased or decreased; see Warnings)

Patient Information Read the Patient Medication Guide that you receive with each prescription and refill of sertraline. An increased risk of suicidal thinking and behavior has been reported with the use of antidepressants in children, adolescents, and young adults (18-24 years of age). Notify physician if you feel depressed, have thoughts of suicide, or become more agitated or irritable (see Warnings). May cause dizziness or drowsiness and impair ability to perform activities requiring mental alertness or physical coordination; may cause dry mouth. Take as directed; do not alter dose or frequency without consulting prescriber; avoid abrupt discontinuation. Some medicines should not be taken with sertraline or should not be taken for a while after sertraline has been discontinued; report the use of other medications, nonprescription medications, and herbal or natural products to your physician and pharmacist; avoid alcohol, grapefruit juice, tryptophan supplements, and the herbal medicine St John's wort; avoid aspirin, NSAIDs, or other drugs that affect coagulation (may increase risks of bleeding).

Nursing Implications If patient experiences somnolence, administer dose at bedtime; if patient experiences insomnia, administer dose in morning. Assess other medications patient may be taking for possible interaction (especially MAO inhibitors, P450 inhibitors, and other CNS active agents). Assess mental status for depression, suicidal ideation, anxiety, social functioning, mania, or panic attack.

Additional Information Two larger studies of children and adolescents with depression and obsessive-compulsive disorder utilized a forced upward dosage titration of sertraline to 200 mg/day; these studies conclude that the adult dosage titration regimen can be used in children ≥6 years and adolescents (see Alderman, 1998 and March, 1998); however, other studies in adults (see Fabre, 1995) demonstrate that lower sertraline doses (50 mg/day) are as effective as higher doses with fewer adverse effects and discontinuations of therapy. Further studies are needed in pediatric patients to identify optimal doses; clinically, doses should be individually titrated based on patient response and adverse effects.

A recent report (Lake, 2000) describes 5 children (age 8-15 years) who developed epistaxis (n=4) or bruising (n=1) while receiving sertraline therapy. Another recent report describes the SSRI discontinuation syndrome in 6 children; the syndrome was similar to that reported in adults (see Diler, 2002). Due to limited long-term studies, the clinical usefulness of sertraline should be periodically re-evaluated in patients receiving the drug for extended intervals; effects of long term use of sertraline on pediatric growth, development, and maturation have not been directly assessed.

Neonates born to women receiving SSRIs late during the third trimester may experience respiratory distress, apnea, cyanosis, temperature instability, vomiting, feeding difficulty, hypoglycemia, constant crying, irritability, hypotonia, hypertonia, hyper-reflexia, tremor, jitteriness, and seizures; these symptoms may be due to a direct toxic effect, withdrawal syndrome, or (in some cases) serotonin syndrome. Withdrawal symptoms occur in 30% of neonates exposed to SSRIs *in utero*; monitor newborns for at least 48 hours after birth; long-term effects of *in utero* exposure to SSRIs are unknown (see Levinson-Castiel, 2006).

Dosage Forms Excipient information presented when available (limited, particularly for generics); consult specific product labeling.

Solution, oral [concentrate]: 20 mg/mL (60 mL)
  Zoloft®: 20 mg/mL (60 mL) [contains ethanol 12%; natural rubber/natural latex in packaging]
Tablet: 25 mg, 50 mg, 100 mg
  Zoloft®: 25 mg, 50 mg, 100 mg

References

Alderman J, Wolkow R, Chung M, et al, "Sertraline Treatment of Children and Adolescents With Obsessive-Compulsive Disorder or Depression: Pharmacokinetics, Tolerability, and Efficacy," *J Am Acad Child Adolesc Psychiatry*, 1998, 37(4):386-94.

Ambrosini PJ, Wagner KD, Biederman J, et al, "Multicenter Open-Label Sertraline Study in Adolescent Outpatients With Major Depression," *J Am Acad Child Adolesc Psychiatry*, 1999, 38(5):566-72.

Chambers CD, Hernandez-Diaz S, Van Marter LJ, et al, "Selective Serotonin-Reuptake Inhibitors and Risk of Persistent Pulmonary Hypertension of the Newborn," *N Engl J Med*, 2006, 354(6):579-87.

Diler R and Avci A, "Selective Serotonin Reuptake Inhibitor Discontinuation Syndrome in Children: Six Case Reports," *Current Therapeutic Research*, 2002, 63(3):188-97.

Dopheide JA, "Recognizing and Treating Depression in Children and Adolescents," *Am J Health Syst Pharm*, 2006, 63(3):233-43.

Fabre LF, Abuzzahab FS, Amin M, et al, "Sertraline Safety and Efficacy in Major Depression: A Double-Blind Fixed-Dose Comparison With Placebo," *Biol Psychiatry*, 1995, 38(9):592-602.

Findling RL, Reed MD, and Blumer JL, "Pharmacological Treatment of Depression in Children and Adolescents," *Paediatr Drugs*, 1999, 1 (3):161-82.

Lake MB, Birmaher B, Wassick S, et al, "Bleeding and Selective Serotonin Reuptake Inhibitors in Childhood and Adolescence," *J Child Adolesc Psychopharmacol*, 2000, 10(1):35-8.

Levinson-Castiel R, Merlob P, Linder N, et al, "Neonatal Abstinence Syndrome After *in utero* Exposure to Selective Serotonin Reuptake Inhibitors in Term Infants," *Arch Pediatr Adolesc Med*, 2006, 160 (2):173-6.

March JS, Biederman J, Wolkow R, et al, "Sertraline in Children and Adolescents With Obsessive-Compulsive Disorder: A Multicenter Randomized Controlled Trial," *JAMA*, 1998, 280(20):1752-6.

McConville BJ, Minnery KL, Sorter MT, et al, "An Open Study of the Effects of Sertraline on Adolescent Major Depression," *J Child Adolesc Psychopharmacol*, 1996, 6(1):41-51.

Safer DJ and Zito JM, "Treatment Emergent Adverse Effects of Selective Serotonin Reuptake Inhibitors by Age Group: Children vs. Adolescents," *J Child Adolesc Psychopharmacol*, 2006, 16(1/2):159-69.

Sharp SC and Hellings JA, "Efficacy and Safety of Selective Serotonin Reuptake Inhibitors in the Treatment of Depression in Children and Adolescents: Practitioner Review," *Clin Drug Investig*, 2006, 26 (5):247-55.

Thomsen PH, "Obsessive-Compulsive Disorder: Pharmacological Treatment," *Eur Child Adolesc Psychiatry*, 2000, 9(Suppl 1):I76-84.

Tierney E, Joshi PT, Llinas JF, et al, "Sertraline for Major Depression in Children and Adolescents: Preliminary Clinical Experience," *J Child Adolesc Psychopharmacol*, 1995; 5(1):13-27.

Wagner KD, "Pharmacotherapy for Major Depression in Children and Adolescents," *Prog Neuropsychopharmacol Biol Psychiatry*, 2005, 29 (5):819-26.

◆ **Sertraline Hydrochloride** *see* Sertraline *on page 1254*

◆ **Serzone** *see* Nefazodone *on page 971*

Sevelamer *(se VEL a mer)*

Medication Safety Issues
Sound-alike/look-alike issues:
Renagel® may be confused with Reglan®, Regonol®, Renal Caps, Renvela®
Renvela® may be confused with Reglan®, Regonol®, Renagel®, Renal Caps
Sevelamer may be confused with Savella™

International issues:
Renagel® may be confused with Remegel® which is a brand name for calcium carbonate in Ireland, Italy, and Great Britain

U.S. Brand Names Renagel®; Renvela®
Canadian Brand Names Renagel®
Therapeutic Category Phosphate Binder
Generic Available No

Use Reduction of serum phosphorus in patients with chronic kidney disease on hemodialysis (FDA approved in adults)

Pregnancy Risk Factor C

Pregnancy Considerations Animal studies have shown reduced or irregular ossification of fetal bones. Because sevelamer may cause a reduction in the absorption of some vitamins, it should be used with caution in pregnant women.

Lactation Excretion in breast milk unknown/use caution (not absorbed systemically but may alter maternal nutrition)

Breast-Feeding Considerations It is not known whether sevelamer is excreted in human milk. Because sevelamer may cause a reduction in the absorption of some vitamins, it should be used with caution in nursing women.

Contraindications Hypersensitivity to sevelamer or any component; hypophosphatemia, bowel obstruction

Warnings In preclinical animal studies, sevelamer (at doses of 6-100 times the recommended human dose) reduced the levels of vitamin D, E, K, and folic acid; no evidence of decreased vitamin levels has been shown in human trials, however, most patients were receiving vitamin supplements

Precautions Use with caution in patients with GI disorders including dysphagia, swallowing disorders, severe GI motility disorders, or major GI surgery; bowel obstruction and perforation have been reported

Adverse Reactions
Cardiovascular: Hypertension, hypotension, thrombosis
Central nervous system: Fatigue, headache
Dermatologic: Pruritus
Endocrine & metabolic: Hypercalcemia, metabolic acidosis
Gastrointestinal: Abdominal pain, anorexia, bowel obstruction, constipation, diarrhea, dyspepsia, fecal impaction, flatulence, intestinal perforation, nausea, peritonitis, vomiting
Neuromuscular & skeletal: Arthralgia, pain
Respiratory: Cough
<5%, postmarketing, and/or case reports: Fecal impaction, rash

Drug Interactions
Avoid Concomitant Use There are no known interactions where it is recommended to avoid concomitant use.

Increased Effect/Toxicity There are no known significant interactions involving an increase in effect.

Decreased Effect
Sevelamer may decrease the levels/effects of: Levothyroxine; Mycophenolate; Quinolone Antibiotics

Stability Store at controlled room temperature; protect from moisture

Mechanism of Action Sevelamer is a cationic polymeric compound that binds phosphate in the intestinal lumen, limiting absorption and decreasing serum phosphate concentrations without altering calcium, aluminum, or bicarbonate concentrations. It may also lower low-density lipoprotein (LDL) and total serum cholesterol levels.

Pharmacokinetics (Adult data unless noted)
Absorption: Not systemically absorbed
Elimination: Feces 100%

◀ **Usual Dosage** Oral:

Children: In a small pilot study of 17 pediatric patients aged 11.8 ± 3.7 years on hemodialysis (n=3) or peritoneal dialysis (n=14), initial doses of 121 ± 50 mg/kg/day (4.5 ± 5 g/day) were used. Doses were adjusted based on the serum phosphorus with final doses of 163 ± 46 mg/kg (6.7 ± 2.4 g/day) without any adverse effects (see Mahdavi, 2003). In a study of 18 patients aged 0.9-18 years with chronic kidney disease, a mean dose of 140 ± 86 mg/kg/day (5.38 ± 3.24 g/day) resulted in good phosphorus control with minimal adverse effects. Initial doses were based on prior phosphate-binder dose and were adjusted based on the serum phosphorus (see Pieper, 2006).

Adults (not taking another phosphate binder, eg, calcium acetate): 800-1600 mg with each meal; the initial dose may be based on the serum phosphorus: See table:

Serum Phosphorus (mg/dL)	Initial Sevelamer Dose[1] (mg)
>5.5 and <7.5	800
≥7.5 and <9	1200-1600
≥9	1600

[1] Administered 3 times/day.

Adjust the daily dosage by 400-800 mg per meal at 2-week intervals depending upon the serum phosphorus. The manufacturer recommends the following titration schedule:

Serum Phosphorus (mg/dL)	Sevelamer Dosage Adjustment
>5.5	Increase by 400-800 mg per meal at 2-week intervals
3.5-5.5	Maintain current dose
<3.5	Decrease by 400-800 mg per meal

Patients changing from calcium acetate to sevelamer may use the following conversions:

Calcium Acetate Dosage (mg)	Initial Sevelamer Dose[1] (mg)
667 (1 tablet)	800
1334 (2 tablets)	1200-1600
2001 (3 tablets)	2000-2400

[1] Administer 3 times/day.

Administration

Oral: Administer with meals, at least 1 hour before or 3 hours after other medications.

Tablets: Because the contents will expand with water, swallow tablets whole; do not chew or crush.

Packets for oral suspension: Mix powder with water prior to administration. The 0.8 g packet should be mixed with 30 mL of water and the 2.4 g packet should be mixed with 60 mL of water (multiple packets may be mixed together using the appropriate amount of water). Stir vigorously to suspend mixture just prior to drinking; powder does not dissolve. Drink within 30 minutes of preparing or resuspend just prior to drinking.

Monitoring Parameters Serum electrolytes

Product Availability Renvela® powder of oral suspension: FDA approved August 2009; availability of the 0.8 g packet size is expected Spring 2010

Dosage Forms Excipient information presented when available (limited, particularly for generics); consult specific product labeling.

Powder for suspension, oral, as carbonate:

Renvela®: 2.4 g/packet (90s) [contains propylene glycol; citrus-cream flavor]

Tablet, oral, as carbonate:

Renvela®: 800 mg

Tablet, oral, as hydrochloride:

Renagel®: 400 mg, 800 mg

References

Mahdavi H, Kuizon BD, Gales B, et al, "Sevelamer Hydrochloride: An Effective Phosphate Binder in Dialyzed Children," *Pediatr Nephrol*, 2003, 18(12):1260-4.

Pieper AK, Haffner D, Hoppe B, et al, "A Randomized Crossover Trial Comparing Sevelamer With Calcium Acetate in Children With CKD," *Am J Kidney Dis*, 2006, 47(4):625-35.

◆ **Sevelamer Carbonate** see Sevelamer on page 1257

◆ **Sevelamer Hydrochloride** see Sevelamer on page 1257

◆ **sfRowasa™** see Mesalamine on page 887

◆ **Shohl's Solution, Modified** see Citrate and Citric Acid on page 322

◆ **Sig-Enalapril (Can)** see Enalapril/Enalaprilat on page 499

◆ **Silace [OTC]** see Docusate on page 468

◆ **Siladryl Allergy [OTC]** see DiphenhydrAMINE on page 448

◆ **Silafed [OTC]** see Triprolidine and Pseudoephedrine on page 1388

◆ **Silapap Children's [OTC]** see Acetaminophen on page 36

◆ **Silapap Infant's [OTC]** see Acetaminophen on page 36

◆ **Sildec [DSC]** see Carbinoxamine and Pseudoephedrine on page 249

◆ **Sildec Syrup** see Brompheniramine and Pseudoephedrine on page 205

Sildenafil (sil DEN a fil)

Medication Safety Issues

Sound-alike/look-alike issues:

Revatio® may be confused with ReVia®

Sildenafil may be confused with silodosin, tadalafil, vardenafil

Viagra® may be confused with Allegra®, Vaniqa®

U.S. Brand Names Revatio®; Viagra®

Canadian Brand Names Revatio®; Viagra®

Therapeutic Category Phosphodiesterase Type-5 (PDE5) Inhibitor

Generic Available No

Use Treatment of pulmonary arterial hypertension (PAH) (Revatio®); primary pulmonary hypertension; persistent pulmonary hypertension of the newborn (PPHN) refractory to treatment with inhaled nitric oxide; to facilitate weaning from nitric oxide (ie, to attenuate rebound effects after discontinuing inhaled nitric oxide); secondary pulmonary hypertension following cardiac surgery; treatment of erectile dysfunction in adult males (Viagra®)

Pregnancy Risk Factor B

Pregnancy Considerations Teratogenic effects were not observed in animal studies. There are no adequate and well-controlled studies in pregnant women. Less than 0.001% appears in the semen.

Lactation Excretion in breast milk unknown/use caution

Contraindications Hypersensitivity to sildenafil or any component; concurrent use of organic nitrates (eg, nitroglycerin, isosorbide dinitrate) in any form (potentiates the hypotensive effects)

Warnings Decreases in blood pressure may occur due to vasodilator effects; the cardiovascular status of the patient should be considered prior to initiating treatment; certain patients may be adversely affected by vasodilator effects (eg, patients with resting hypotension, fluid depletion, severe left ventricular outflow obstruction, or autonomic dysfunction). Sildenafil is not recommended for use in patients with pulmonary veno-occlusive disease; consider diagnosis of pulmonary veno-occlusive disease in patients who develop pulmonary edema when receiving sildenafil. Sildenafil may cause transient dose-related impairment of blue/green color discrimination.

A sudden decrease or loss of hearing has been reported rarely, in patients receiving sildenafil for the treatment of pulmonary arterial hypertension and for erectile dysfunction. Hearing changes may be accompanied by vestibular symptoms (eg, tinnitus, vertigo, dizziness). It is not known if PDE5 inhibitors cause this condition or if other related factors are responsible. Patients receiving sildenafil for the treatment of pulmonary arterial hypertension who experience sudden hearing changes should **not** stop taking the medication, but should contact their healthcare provider immediately. Patients receiving sildenafil for erectile dysfunction who experience a sudden hearing change should discontinue the drug and notify a healthcare provider immediately.

Additional warnings for patients treated for erectile dysfunction: Rare cases of sudden vision loss attributed to nonarteritic ischemic optic neuropathy (NAION) have been reported with the use of phosphodiesterase type-5 (PDE5) inhibitors when used for the treatment of male erectile dysfunction; NAION is a condition where blood flow is blocked to the optic nerve. NAION is more common in individuals with heart disease, diabetes, hypertension, certain eye problems, smokers, or those >50 years of age. Vision loss in one eye has been reported in some men after taking PDE5 inhibitors. It is not known if PDE5 inhibitors cause this condition or if other related factors are responsible. Patients taking a PDE5 inhibitor and who experience vision loss should stop taking the drug and notify a healthcare provider immediately.

A degree of cardiac risk is associated with sexual activity in patients with pre-existing cardiovascular disease; sildenafil should not generally be used to treat erectile dysfunction in men with underlying cardiovascular disease which would deem sexual activity inadvisable. Prolonged or painful erections may occur; patients should seek immediate medical assistance if erection lasts >4 hours; permanent damage to the penis may occur without immediate treatment. The safety and efficacy of sildenafil with other treatments for erectile dysfunction have not been established; concurrent use is not recommended.

Precautions Use with caution in patients with resting hypotension or hypertension; cardiovascular disease, including cardiac failure, unstable angina, or a recent history (within the last 6 months) of MI, stroke, or life-threatening arrhythmia; patients with retinitis pigmentosa (subpopulation of these patients have a retinal phosphodiesterase disorder); patients receiving concurrent bosentan (efficacy has not been evaluated; bosentan decreases sildenafil serum concentrations); patients receiving alpha-blockers or other antihypertensive agents (additive hypotensive effects; symptomatic hypotension may occur). Use with caution in patients with hepatic or renal impairment; dosage adjustment may be needed.

Use with caution in patients with anatomical deformation of the penis (angulation, cavernosal fibrosis, Peyronie's disease); conditions which may predispose patients to priapism (sickle cell anemia, multiple myeloma, leukemia). Epistaxis may occur and at a higher incidence in patients with pulmonary arterial hypertension due to connective tissue disorders or in patients receiving concurrent oral vitamin K antagonists. Safety of sildenafil is not known in patients with bleeding disorders or with active peptic ulcer disease. Safety and efficacy in pediatric patients have not been established.

Adverse Reactions Note: Adverse effects such as flushing, diarrhea, myalgia, and visual disturbances may be increased with higher doses (eg, adult doses >100 mg/24 hours).

Cardiovascular: Flushing, hypotension, tachycardia, MI, ventricular arrhythmia, cerebrovascular hemorrhage, pulmonary hemorrhage

Central nervous system: Headache, insomnia, pyrexia, dizziness, seizure, anxiety

Dermatologic: Erythema, rash

Gastrointestinal: Nausea, diarrhea, dyspepsia, gastritis

Genitourinary: Prolonged erection, priapism, hematuria, urinary tract infection

Hematologic: Platelet dysfunction (*in vitro* study with human platelets indicates that sildenafil potentiates the antiaggregatory effect of nitric oxide)

Neuromuscular & skeletal: Myalgia, paresthesia

Ocular: Blurred vision, sensitivity to light increased, change in color vision; nonarteritic ischemic optic neuropathy (NAION; see Warnings); retinopathy of prematurity (1 possible case reported after treatment with IV sildenafil; see Marsh, 2004 and Pierce, 2005)

Otic: Sudden decrease or loss of hearing (see Warnings)

Respiratory: Epistaxis, dyspnea, rhinitis, sinusitis, nasal congestion

Drug Interactions

Metabolism/Transport Effects Substrate of CYP2C9 (minor), 3A4 (major); **Inhibits** CYP1A2 (weak), 2C9 (weak), 2C19 (weak), 2D6 (weak), 2E1 (weak), 3A4 (weak)

Avoid Concomitant Use

Avoid concomitant use of Sildenafil with any of the following: Phosphodiesterase 5 Inhibitors; Vasodilators (Organic Nitrates)

Increased Effect/Toxicity

Sildenafil may increase the levels/effects of: Alpha1-Blockers; Antihypertensives; Bosentan; HMG-CoA Reductase Inhibitors; Phosphodiesterase 5 Inhibitors; Vasodilators (Organic Nitrates)

The levels/effects of Sildenafil may be increased by: Antifungal Agents (Azole Derivatives, Systemic); CYP3A4 Inhibitors (Moderate); CYP3A4 Inhibitors (Strong); Dasatinib; Macrolide Antibiotics; Protease Inhibitors; Sapropterin

Decreased Effect

The levels/effects of Sildenafil may be decreased by: Bosentan; CYP3A4 Inducers (Strong); Deferasirox; Etravirine; Herbs (CYP3A4 Inducers); Peginterferon Alfa-2b

Food Interactions A high fat meal decreases the rate of absorption and peak concentration. Grapefruit juice may increase serum concentrations or toxicity of sildenafil (avoid concurrent use).

Stability Store tablets at controlled room temperature.

Mechanism of Action Selective phosphodiesterase-type 5 (PDE-5) inhibitor. PDE-5 is found in the pulmonary vascular smooth muscle, vascular and visceral smooth muscle, corpus cavernosum, and platelets. PDE-5 is responsible for the degradation of cyclic guanosine monophosphate (cGMP). Normally, nitric oxide (NO) activates the enzyme guanylate cyclase, which increases the levels of cGMP; cGMP produces smooth muscle relaxation. Inhibition of PDE-5 by sildenafil increases the cellular levels of cGMP.

Increased levels of cGMP potentiate vascular smooth muscle relaxation, particularly in the lung where PDE5 is found in high concentrations. In patients with pulmonary arterial hypertension, sildenafil causes vasodilation in the pulmonary vasculature and, to a lesser extent, in the systemic circulation. Clinically, the drug decreases pulmonary arterial pressure and increases exercise capacity in these patients.

In patients with erectile dysfunction, sildenafil does not directly cause penile erections, but affects the response to sexual stimulation. Normally, NO is released in the corpus cavernosum during sexual stimulation. NO then activates the enzyme guanylate cyclase, which increases the levels of cGMP; cGMP produces smooth muscle relaxation and allows an inflow of blood to the corpus cavernosum producing an erection. Sildenafil enhances the effect of NO by inhibiting PDE-5 and increasing the levels of cGMP in the corpus cavernosum. At recommended doses, sildenafil has no effect on erection in the absence of sexual stimulation.

Pharmacokinetics (Adult data unless noted)

Absorption: Oral: Rapid; slower with a high-fat meal

Distribution: Distributes into tissues

V_{dss}: Adults: 105 L

Protein binding: 96%

Metabolism: Via the liver via cytochrome P450 isoenzyme CYP3A4 (major route) and CYP2C9 (minor route). Major metabolite is formed via N-desmethylation pathway and has 50% of the activity as sildenafil.

Bioavailability: Oral: 40% (may be higher in patients with PAH compared to healthy volunteers)

Half-life: Sildenafil: 4 hours; active N-desmethyl metabolite: 4 hours

Time to peak serum concentration: Oral: Fasting: 30-120 minutes (median 60 minutes); delayed by 60 minutes with a high-fat meal

Elimination: Excreted as metabolites; 80% of dose excreted in feces, 13% in urine

Clearance: Decreased in patients with hepatic cirrhosis or severe renal impairment; clearance may be lower in patients with PAH compared to normal volunteers

Dialysis: Not likely to be beneficial due to high protein binding

Usual Dosage Oral: Note: Limited pediatric information exists; most pediatric literature consists of case reports or small studies; further studies are needed.

Neonates: Pulmonary hypertension: A wide range of doses has been reported: Initial: 0.3 mg/kg/dose every 8-12 hours; doses of 0.25-1 mg/kg/dose every 6-12 hours have been used; Note: Individual doses of 0.3 mg/kg/dose given only one time have been used in select patients to facilitate weaning from inhaled nitric oxide (see Atz, 1999).

One randomized placebo controlled study of 13 neonates (>35.5 weeks GA and <3 days old) with severe PPHN and an oxygenation index (OI) of >25 received placebo (n=6) or sildenafil (n=7) at initial doses of 1 mg/kg every 6 hours; Note: OI = (fraction of inspired oxygen x mean airway pressure) / PaO_2; the sildenafil dose was doubled if the OI did not improve and the mean blood pressure remained stable; therapy was discontinued if the OI became <20 or the patient received a maximum of 8 doses; 5 of 7 neonates received 1 mg/kg every 6 hours for all doses; 2 neonates required a dosage increase to 2 mg/kg every 6 hours; overall, 2 patients required 6 doses and 5 patients required 7 doses; the median total amount of sildenafil was 7 mg/kg/course of therapy (see Baquero, 2006).

Infants and Children: Pulmonary hypertension: A wide range of doses has been reported: Initial: 0.25-0.5 mg/kg/dose every 4-8 hours; increase if needed and if tolerated to 1 mg/kg/dose every 4-8 hours; doses as high as 2 mg/kg/dose every 4 hours have been used in several case reports (see Karatza 2004, Karatza 2005).

One 12 month, open-label, pilot study of sildenafil in 14 children, 5-18 years of age (median 9.8 years) used initial doses of 0.25 mg/kg/dose given 4 times daily for 2 doses; if this dose was tolerated, it was increased to 0.5 mg/kg/dose given 4 times daily; doses were adjusted so that easily divisible fractions of the commercially available tablets could be administered;

the first 4 doses were administered in the hospital; at 12 months, the median dose was 0.5 mg/kg/dose (range: 0.3-1 mg/kg/dose) given 4 times daily (see Humpl, 2005).

Adults:

Erectile dysfunction (Viagra®): Usual: 50 mg taken as needed, ~1 hour before sexual activity (dose may be taken 30 minutes to 4 hours before sexual activity). Based on effectiveness and tolerance, may increase dose to a maximum of 100 mg or decrease to 25 mg. Maximum recommended dosing frequency: Once daily

Pulmonary arterial hypertension (Revatio®): 20 mg 3 times/day; no evidence for additional efficacy was observed with higher doses; treatment with higher doses is not recommended

Dosage adjustment in hepatic impairment: Adults:

Revatio®:

Mild to moderate hepatic impairment (Child Pugh class A and B): No dosage adjustment needed

Severe hepatic impairment (Child Pugh class C): Has not been studied

Viagra®: Cirrhosis: Starting dose of 25 mg should be considered

Dosage adjustment in renal impairment: Adults:

Revatio®: No dosage adjustments needed

Viagra®: Severe renal impairment (creatinine clearance <30 mL/minute): Starting dose of 25 mg should be considered

Dosage considerations for patients taking alpha blockers: Adults: Viagra®: Initial: 25 mg

Dosage adjustment for concomitant use of potent CYP34A inhibitors: Adults:

Revatio®:

Erythromycin, saquinavir: No dosage adjustment needed

Bosentan, barbiturates, carbamazepine, efavirenz, nevirapine, phenytoin, rifabutin, rifampin: Dosage adjustments may be needed; specific guidelines are not available; see Drug Interactions

Itraconazole, ketoconazole, ritonavir: Use is not recommended

Viagra®:

Erythromycin, itraconazole, ketoconazole, saquinavir: Starting dose of 25 mg should be considered

Ritonavir: Maximum: 25 mg every 48 hours

Administration Oral:

Revatio®: Administer doses at least 4-6 hours apart; may be administered without regard to meals

Viagra®: Administer dose ~1 hour before sexual activity (may be administered 30 minutes to 4 hours before sexual activity).

Monitoring Parameters Heart rate, blood pressure, oxygen saturation, PaO_2

Patient Information Do not take nitroglycerin or other nitrate medications while using sildenafil (serious side effects may occur). Avoid grapefruit juice and the herbal medicine, St John's wort. Certain other medications should not be taken with sildenafil or may require a dosage adjustment of sildenafil; report the use of other medications, nonprescription medications, and herbal or natural products to your physician and pharmacist.

Headache, flushing, or abnormal vision (color changes, blurred or increased sensitivity to light) may occur; use caution when driving at night or in poorly lit environments. Seek immediate medical attention if a sudden vision loss in one or both eyes occurs or if a sudden decrease or loss of hearing occurs (see Warnings). Report immediately acute allergic reactions; chest pain or palpitations; persistent dizziness; signs of urinary tract infection; skin rash; respiratory difficulty; genital swelling; or other adverse reactions.

Do not combine sildenafil with other approaches to treating erectile dysfunction without consulting prescriber. If erection lasts longer than 4 hours, contact prescriber immediately; permanent damage to the penis can occur. **Note:** Sildenafil provides no protection against sexually-transmitted diseases, including HIV.

Nursing Implications Do not administer sildenafil to patients receiving nitroglycerin or other organic nitrates; be aware of other drug interactions. Instruct patient to seek immediate medical attention if a sudden loss of vision occurs in one or both eyes, or if erection lasts longer than 4 hours.

Additional Information Sildenafil is ~10 times more selective for PDE-5 as compared to PDE-6. PDE-6 is found in the retina and is involved in phototransduction. At higher plasma levels, inhibition of PDE-6 may occur and may account for the abnormalities in color vision noted in some patients.

Dosage Forms Excipient information presented when available (limited, particularly for generics); consult specific product labeling.

Injection, solution:
Revatio®: 0.8 mg/mL (12.5 mL)
Tablet:
Revatio®: 20 mg
Viagra®: 25 mg, 50 mg, 100 mg

Extemporaneous Preparations A 2.5 mg/mL oral suspension made from sildenafil citrate (Viagra®) and 2 different vehicles (a 1:1 mixture of Ora-Sweet® and Ora-Plus® or a 1:1 mixture of methylcellulose 1% and Simple Syrup, NF) was stable for 91 days when stored in amber plastic prescription bottles at room temperature (25°C) or under refrigeration (5°C); grind thirty 25 mg tablets in a mortar into a fine powder; add a small amount of the vehicle and mix well to form a uniform paste; mix while adding the vehicle in geometric proportions to almost 300 mL; transfer to a graduated cylinder and qsad with vehicle to 300 mL while mixing; place in amber plastic prescription bottles; label "shake well."

Nahata MC, Morosco RS, and Brady M, "Extemporaneous Sildenafil Citrate Oral Suspensions for the Treatment of Pulmonary Hypertension in Children," *Am J Health Syst Pharm*, 2006, 63(3):254-7.

References

Atz AM and Wessel DL, "Sildenafil Ameliorates Effects of Inhaled Nitric Oxide Withdrawal," *Anesthesiology*, 1999, 91(1):307-10.

Baquero H, Soliz A, Neira F, et al, "Oral Sildenafil in Infants With Persistent Pulmonary Hypertension of the Newborn: A Pilot Randomized Blinded Study," *Pediatrics*, 2006, 117(4):1077-83.

Carroll WD and Dhillon R, "Sildenafil as a Treatment for Pulmonary Hypertension," *Arch Dis Child*, 2003, 88(9):827-8.

Erickson S, Reyes J, Bohn D, et al, "Sildenafil (Viagra) in Childhood and Neonatal Pulmonary Hypertension," *J Am Coll Cardiol*, 2002, 39 (Suppl):S402.

Humpl T, Reyes JT, Holtby H, et al, "Beneficial Effect of Oral Sildenafil Therapy on Childhood Pulmonary Arterial Hypertension: Twelve-Month Clinical Trial of a Single-Drug, Open-Label, Pilot Study," *Circulation*, 2005, 111(24):3274-80.

Karatza AA, Bush A, and Magee AG, "Safety and Efficacy of Sildenafil Therapy in Children With Pulmonary Hypertension," *Int J Cardiol*, 2005, 100(2):267-73.

Karatza AA, Narang I, Rosenthal M, et al, "Treatment of Primary Pulmonary Hypertension With Oral Sildenafil," *Respiration*, 2004, 71 (2):192-4.

Kothari SS and Duggal B, "Chronic Oral Sildenafil Therapy in Severe Pulmonary Artery Hypertension," *Indian Heart J*, 2002, 54(4):404-9.

Marsh CS, Marden B, and Newsom R, "Severe Retinopathy of Prematurity (ROP) in a Premature Baby Treated With Sildenafil Acetate (Viagra) for Pulmonary Hypertension," *Br J Ophthalmol*, 2004, 88(2):306-7.

Pierce CM, Petros AJ, and Fielder AR, "No Evidence for Severe Retinopathy of Prematurity Following Sildenafil," *Br J Ophthalmol*, 2005, 89(2):250.

◆ **Sildenafil Citrate** *see* Sildenafil *on page 1258*

◆ **Silexin [OTC]** *see* Guaifenesin and Dextromethorphan *on page 658*

◆ **Silfedrine Children's [OTC]** *see* Pseudoephedrine *on page 1183*

◆ **Silphen Cough [OTC]** *see* DiphenhydrAMINE *on page 448*

◆ **Silphen DM® [OTC]** *see* Dextromethorphan *on page 421*

◆ **Siltussin DAS [OTC]** *see* GuaiFENesin *on page 656*

◆ **Siltussin DM [OTC]** *see* Guaifenesin and Dextromethorphan *on page 658*

◆ **Siltussin DM DAS [OTC]** *see* Guaifenesin and Dextromethorphan *on page 658*

◆ **Siltussin SA [OTC]** *see* GuaiFENesin *on page 656*

◆ **Silvadene®** *see* Silver Sulfadiazine *on page 1262*

Silver Nitrate (SIL ver NYE trate)

Therapeutic Category Ophthalmic Agent, Miscellaneous; Topical Skin Product

Generic Available Yes

Use Cauterization of wounds and sluggish ulcers, removal of granulation tissue and warts

Pregnancy Risk Factor C

Contraindications Hypersensitivity to silver nitrate or any component; not for use on broken skin or cuts

Warnings Do not use applicator sticks on the eyes

Adverse Reactions
Dermatologic: Staining of the skin
Hematologic: Methemoglobinemia
Local: Burning and skin irritation
Ocular: Cauterization of the cornea, blindness, chemical conjunctivitis

Drug Interactions
Avoid Concomitant Use
Avoid concomitant use of Silver Nitrate with any of the following: BCG
Increased Effect/Toxicity There are no known significant interactions involving an increase in effect.
Decreased Effect
Silver Nitrate may decrease the levels/effects of: BCG

Stability Store applicator sticks in a dry place since moisture causes the oxidized film to dissolve; protect from light

Mechanism of Action Free silver ions precipitate bacterial proteins by combining with chloride in tissue forming silver chloride; coagulates cellular protein to form an eschar

Pharmacokinetics (Adult data unless noted) Absorption: Not readily absorbed from mucous membranes

Usual Dosage Children and Adults:
Sticks: Apply to mucous membranes and other moist skin surfaces only on area to be treated 2-3 times/week for 2-3 weeks
Topical solution: Apply a cotton applicator dipped in solution on the affected area 2-3 times/week for 2-3 weeks

Monitoring Parameters With prolonged use, monitor methemoglobin levels

Patient Information Discontinue topical preparation if redness or irritation develop; silver nitrate solution may stain skin

Nursing Implications Silver nitrate solutions stain skin and utensils

Dosage Forms Excipient information presented when available (limited, particularly for generics); consult specific product labeling.

Applicator sticks, topical: Silver nitrate 75% and potassium nitrate 25% (6", 12", 18")
Solution, topical: 0.5% (960 mL); 10% (30 mL); 25% (30 mL); 50% (30 mL)

References
Cushing AH and Smith S, "Methemoglobinemia With Silver Nitrate Therapy of a Burn: Report of a Case," *J Pediatr*, 1969, 74(4):613-5.

Silver Sulfadiazine (SIL ver sul fa DYE a zeen)

U.S. Brand Names Silvadene®; SSD®; SSD® AF; Thermazene®

Canadian Brand Names Flamazine®

Therapeutic Category Antibiotic, Topical

Generic Available Yes

Use Adjunct in the prevention and treatment of infection in second and third degree burns

Pregnancy Risk Factor B

Pregnancy Considerations Adverse events were not observed in animal reproduction studies. Because of the theoretical increased risk for hyperbilirubinemia and kernicterus, sulfadiazine is contraindicated for use near term, on premature infants, or on newborn infants during the first 2 months of life (refer to Sulfadiazine monograph).

Lactation Excretion unknown/not recommended

Breast-Feeding Considerations It is not known if sulfadiazine is found in breast milk following topical application; however, sulfonamide serum concentrations may reach therapeutic levels following application to extensive areas. Oral sulfadiazine is contraindicated in nursing mothers since sulfonamides cross into the milk and may cause kernicterus in the newborn (refer to Sulfadiazine monograph).

Contraindications Hypersensitivity to silver sulfadiazine or any component; premature infants or neonates <2 months of age since sulfas may displace bilirubin from protein binding sites and cause kernicterus

Precautions Use with caution in patients with G-6-PD deficiency and renal impairment; sulfadiazine may accumulate in patients with impaired hepatic or renal function

Adverse Reactions
Dermatologic: Itching, rash, erythema multiforme, discoloration of skin
Hematologic: Hemolytic anemia, leukopenia, agranulocytosis, aplastic anemia, thrombocytopenia
Hepatic: Hepatitis
Local: Pain, burning
Renal: Interstitial nephritis
Miscellaneous: Serum hyperosmolality (due to propylene glycol component in the cream), hypersensitivity reactions to sulfas

Drug Interactions
Avoid Concomitant Use
Avoid concomitant use of Silver Sulfadiazine with any of the following: BCG
Increased Effect/Toxicity There are no known significant interactions involving an increase in effect.
Decreased Effect
Silver Sulfadiazine may decrease the levels/effects of: BCG

Stability Discard if cream is darkened (reacts with heavy metals resulting in release of silver)

Mechanism of Action Acts upon the bacterial cell wall and cell membrane

Pharmacokinetics (Adult data unless noted)
Absorption: Significant percutaneous absorption of sulfadiazine can occur especially when applied to extensive burns
Half-life: 10 hours and is prolonged in patients with renal insufficiency
Time to peak serum concentration: Within 3-11 days of continuous topical therapy
Elimination: ~50% excreted unchanged in urine

Usual Dosage Children and Adults: Topical: Apply once or twice daily with a sterile gloved hand; apply to a thickness of $^1/_{16}$"; burned area should be covered with cream at all times

Administration Topical: Apply to cleansed, debrided burned areas

Monitoring Parameters Serum electrolytes, UA, renal function test, CBC in patients with extensive burns on long-term treatment

Patient Information For external use only; may discolor skin

Additional Information Contains methylparaben

Dosage Forms Excipient information presented when available (limited, particularly for generics); consult specific product labeling.
Cream, topical: 1% (25 g, 50 g, 85 g, 400 g)
Silvadene®, Thermazene®: 1% (20 g, 50 g, 85 g, 400 g, 1000 g)
SSD®: 1% (25 g, 50 g, 85 g, 400 g)
SSD® AF: 1% (50 g, 400 g)

References
Kulick MI, Wong R, Okarma TB, et al, "Prospective Study of Side Effects Associated With the Use of Silver Sulfadiazine in Severely Burned Patients," *Ann Plast Surg*, 1985, 14(5):407-18.
Lockhart SP, Rushworth A, Azmy AA, et al, "Topical Silver Sulfadiazine: Side Effects and Urinary Excretion," *Burns Incl Therm Inj*, 1983, 10 (1):9-12.

Simethicone (sye METH i kone)

Medication Safety Issues
Sound-alike/look-alike issues:
Simethicone may be confused with cimetidine
Mylanta® may be confused with Mynatal®
Mylicon® may be confused with Modicon®, Myleran®
Phazyme® may be confused with Pherazine®

U.S. Brand Names Equalizer Gas Relief [OTC]; Gas-X® Extra Strength [OTC]; Gas-X® Infant [OTC]; Gas-X® Maximum Strength [OTC]; Gas-X® Thin Strips™ [OTC]; Gas-X® [OTC]; Gas-X®, Children's Tongue Twisters™ [OTC]; Genasyme® [OTC] [DSC]; Infantaire Gas Drops [OTC]; Little Tummys® Gas Relief [OTC]; Mylanta® Gas Maximum Strength [OTC]; Mylicon® Infants [OTC]; Phazyme® Ultra Strength [OTC]

Canadian Brand Names Ovol®; Phazyme™

Therapeutic Category Antiflatulent

Generic Available Yes

Use Relieve flatulence, functional gastric bloating, and postoperative gas pains

Contraindications Hypersensitivity to simethicone or any component

Warnings Mylicon® Infant drops contain sodium benzoate; benzoic acid (benzoate) is a metabolite of benzyl alcohol; large amounts of benzyl alcohol (≥99 mg/kg/day) have been associated with a potentially fatal toxicity ("gasping syndrome") in neonates; *in vitro* and animal studies have shown that benzoate displaces bilirubin from protein binding sites; avoid use of Mylicon® Infant drops in neonates.

Precautions Phazyme® Quick Dissolve contains phenylalanine; avoid use or use with caution in phenylketonurics

Drug Interactions
Avoid Concomitant Use There are no known interactions where it is recommended to avoid concomitant use.
Increased Effect/Toxicity There are no known significant interactions involving an increase in effect.
Decreased Effect There are no known significant interactions involving a decrease in effect.
Food Interactions Avoid gas-forming foods

Mechanism of Action Spreads on surface of aqueous liquids forming a film of low surface tension which collapses foam bubbles; allows mucous-surrounded gas bubbles to coalesce and be expelled

Pharmacokinetics (Adult data unless noted) Elimination: In feces

Usual Dosage Oral:
Infants and Children <2 years: 20 mg 4 times/day
Children 2-12 years: 40 mg 4 times/day
Children >12 years and Adults: 40-250 mg after meals and at bedtime as needed, not to exceed 500 mg/day

Administration Oral: Administer after meals or at bedtime; chew tablets thoroughly before swallowing; mix with water, infant formula or other liquid; place strips (Gas-X® Children's Tongue Twisters™ or Gas-X® Thin Strips™) directly on the tongue

Patient Information Avoid carbonated beverages

Dosage Forms Excipient information presented when available (limited, particularly for generics); consult specific product labeling. [DSC] = Discontinued product
Softgels: 125 mg
Gas-X® Extra Strength, Mylanta® Gas Maximum Strength: 125 mg
Gas-X® Maximum Strength: 166 mg
Phazyme® Ultra Strength: 180 mg
Strips, oral:
Gas-X®, Children's Tongue Twisters™: 40 mg (16s) [sweet cinnamon flavor]
Gas-X® Thin Strips™: 62.5 mg (18s, 32s) [peppermint flavor]; 62.5 mg (18s) [cinnamon flavor]
Suspension, oral [drops]: 40 mg/0.6 mL (30 mL)
Equalizer Gas Relief, Genasyme® [DSC], Infantaire Gas Drops: 40 mg/0.6 mL (30 mL)
Gas-X® Infant: 40 mg/0.6 mL (30 mL) [alcohol free; contains sodium benzoate]
Little Tummys® Gas Relief: 40 mg/0.6 mL (30 mL, 45 mL) [contains sodium benzoate; strawberry flavor]
Mylicon® Infants: 40 mg/0.6 mL (15 mL, 30 mL) [alcohol free; contains sodium benzoate; available in a non-staining formula]
Tablet, chewable: 80 mg, 125 mg
Gas-X®: 80 mg [sodium free; contains calcium 30 mg/tablet; peppermint creme or cherry creme flavor]
Gas-X® Extra Strength: 125 mg [contains calcium 45 mg/tablet; peppermint creme or cherry creme flavor]
Genasyme®: 80 mg [DSC]
Mylanta® Gas Maximum Strength: 125 mg [cherry and mint flavors]

◆ **Similac® Glucose** see Dextrose on page 422

◆ **Simply Saline® [OTC]** see Sodium Chloride on page 1270

◆ **Simply Saline® Baby [OTC]** see Sodium Chloride on page 1270

◆ **Simply Saline® Nasal Moist® [OTC]** see Sodium Chloride on page 1270

◆ **Simply Sleep™ [OTC]** see DiphenhydrAMINE on page 448

◆ **Simply Sleep® (Can)** see DiphenhydrAMINE on page 448

◆ **Simuc-DM** see Guaifenesin and Dextromethorphan on page 658

◆ **Simulect®** see Basiliximab on page 174

Simvastatin (SIM va stat in)

Medication Safety Issues
Sound-alike/look-alike issues:
Simvastatin may be confused with atorvastatin, nystatin, pitavastatin

Zocor® may be confused with Cozaar®, Lipitor®, Yocon®, Zoloft®, Zyrtec®

International issues:
Cardin® [Poland] may be confused with Cardene® which is a brand name for nicardipine in the U.S.
Cardin® [Poland] may be confused with Cardem® which is a brand name for celiprolol in Spain

Related Information
Normal Laboratory Values for Children on page 1672

U.S. Brand Names Zocor®

Canadian Brand Names Apo-Simvastatin®; CO Simvastatin; Dom-Simvastatin; JAMP-Simvastatin; Mylan-Simvastatin; Nu-Simvastatin; PHL-Simvastatin; PMS-Simvastatin; RAN™-Simvastatin; ratio-Simvastatin; Riva-Simvastatin; Sandoz-Simvastatin; Taro-Simvastatin; Teva-Simvastatin; Zocor®; ZYM-Simvastatin

Therapeutic Category Antilipemic Agent; HMG-CoA Reductase Inhibitor

Generic Available Yes

Use Hyperlipidemia: Adjunct to dietary therapy to decrease elevated serum total (total-C) and low density lipoprotein cholesterol (LDL-C), and apolipoprotein B (apo-B) in pediatric patients with heterozygous familial hypercholesterolemia (FDA approved in boys and postmenarchal girls 10-17 years) (see Additional Information for recommendations on initiating hypercholesterolemia pharmacologic treatment in children ≥8 years); adjunct to dietary therapy to decrease elevated serum total-C, LDL-C, apo-B, and triglyceride (TG) levels and to increase high-density lipoprotein cholesterol (HDL-C) in patients with primary hypercholesterolemia (heterozygous, familial, and nonfamilial) and mixed dyslipidemia (Fredrickson types IIa and IIb) (FDA approved in adults); reduce elevated TG in patients with hypertriglyceridemia (Fredrickson type IV) (FDA approved in adults); reduce elevated TG and VLDL-C in patients with primary dysbetalipoproteinemia (Fredrickson Type III) (FDA approved in adults); reduce elevated total-C and LDL-C in patients with homozygous familial hypercholesterolemia (FDA approved in adults)

Secondary prevention of cardiovascular events in hypercholesterolemic patients with established coronary heart disease (CHD) or at high risk for CHD: To reduce cardiovascular morbidity (myocardial infarction, coronary/noncoronary revascularization procedures) and mortality; to reduce the risk of stroke (FDA approved in adults)

Pregnancy Risk Factor X

Pregnancy Considerations Cholesterol biosynthesis may be important in fetal development. Contraindicated in pregnancy. Administer to women of childbearing potential only when conception is highly unlikely and patients have been informed of potential hazards. If pregnancy occurs during treatment, discontinue simvastatin immediately.

Lactation Excretion in breast milk unknown/contraindicated

Breast-Feeding Considerations Excretion in breast milk is unknown, but would be expected; other medications in this class are excreted in human milk. Breast-feeding is contraindicated.

Contraindications Hypersensitivity to simvastatin or any component; active liver disease; unexplained persistent elevations of serum transaminases; pregnancy; breast-feeding

Warnings Rhabdomyolysis with acute renal failure has occurred. Risk is dose-related and is increased with concurrent use of lipid-lowering agents which may also cause rhabdomyolysis (gemfibrozil, other fibric acid derivatives, or niacin at doses ≥1 g/day), and concurrent use with danazol or moderate to strong CYP3A4 inhibitors (including amiodarone, cyclosporine, grapefruit juice in large quantities, or verapamil). Avoid use with strong

CYP3A4 inhibitors (eg, itraconazole, ketoconazole, erythromycin, clarithromycin, telithromycin, nefazodone, and HIV protease inhibitors). Monitor closely if used with other drugs associated with myopathy (eg, colchicine). Assess the risk versus benefit when combining any of these drugs with simvastatin. Concomitant use of high-dose simvastatin (80 mg) with niacin ≥1 g/day may increase risk of myopathy in Chinese patients. A lowered dosage of simvastatin is recommended when used with medications which may increase risk of rhabdomyolysis (see Usual Dosage). Advise patients to promptly report any unexplained muscle pain, tenderness, or weakness. Temporarily discontinue simvastatin in any patient experiencing an acute or serious condition predisposing to renal failure due to the potential risk of developing rhabdomyolysis.

Precautions Persistent increases in serum transaminases have occurred; liver function must be monitored by laboratory assessment at the initiation of therapy and periodically thereafter for the first year of treatment or until one year after the last elevation in dose. Patients titrated to the 80 mg dose should receive an additional test at 3 months of therapy. Use with caution in patients who consume substantial quantities of alcohol or have a previous history of liver disease. Use with caution in patients with diabetes mellitus and renal impairment (may be at increased risk for developing rhabdomyolysis)

Adverse Reactions

Cardiovascular: Atrial fibrillation, edema

Central nervous system: Headache, insomnia, vertigo

Dermatologic: Eczema

Endocrine & metabolic: Diabetes mellitus

Gastrointestinal: Abdominal pain, constipation, gastritis, nausea

Genitourinary: Urinary tract infection

Hepatic: Serum transaminases increased (>3 x ULN)

Neuromuscular & skeletal: Arthralgias, CPK increased, muscle cramps, myalgia, myopathy, rhabdomyolysis (see Warnings)

Renal: Acute renal failure (see Warnings)

Respiratory: Bronchitis, sinusitis, upper respiratory infections

<1%, postmarketing, and/or case reports: Alkaline phosphatase increased, alopecia, anaphylaxis, anemia, angioedema, arthritis, chills, depression, dermatomyositis, diarrhea, dizziness, dryness of skin/mucous membranes, dyspepsia, dyspnea, eosinophilia, erythema multiforme, ESR increased, fever, flatulence, flushing, GGT increased, hemolytic anemia, hepatic failure, hepatitis, hypersensitivity reaction, jaundice, leukopenia, malaise, memory loss, muscle cramps, nail changes, nodules, pancreatitis, paresthesia, peripheral neuropathy, photosensitivity, polymyalgia rheumatica, positive ANA, pruritus, purpura, rash, rhabdomyolysis, skin discoloration, Stevens-Johnson syndrome, systemic lupus erythematosus-like syndrome, thrombocytopenia, toxic epidermal necrolysis, urticaria, vasculitis, vomiting, weakness

Additional class-related events or case reports (not necessarily reported with simvastatin therapy): Alteration in taste, anorexia, anxiety, bilirubin increased, cataracts, cholestatic jaundice, cirrhosis, CPK (>10x normal) increased, erectile dysfunction/impotence, facial paresis, fatty liver, fulminant hepatic necrosis, gynecomastia, hepatoma, hyperbilirubinemia, impaired extraocular muscle movement libido decreased, ophthalmoplegia, peripheral nerve palsy, psychic disturbance, thyroid dysfunction, tremor

Drug Interactions

Metabolism/Transport Effects Substrate of CYP3A4 (major), SLCO1B1; **Inhibits** CYP2C8 (weak), 2C9 (weak), 2D6 (weak)

Avoid Concomitant Use

Avoid concomitant use of Simvastatin with any of the following: Protease Inhibitors

Increased Effect/Toxicity

Simvastatin may increase the levels/effects of: DAPTOmycin; Diltiazem; Vitamin K Antagonists

The levels/effects of Simvastatin may be increased by: Amiodarone; Antifungal Agents (Azole Derivatives, Systemic); Colchicine; CycloSPORINE; CycloSPORINE (Systemic); CYP3A4 Inhibitors (Moderate); CYP3A4 Inhibitors (Strong); Danazol; Dasatinib; Diltiazem; Dronedarone; Eltrombopag; Fenofibrate; Fenofibric Acid; Fluconazole; Fusidic Acid; Gemfibrozil; Grapefruit Juice; Imatinib; Macrolide Antibiotics; Nefazodone; Niacin; Niacinamide; Protease Inhibitors; QuiNINE; Ranolazine; Rifamycin Derivatives; Sildenafil; Verapamil

Decreased Effect

The levels/effects of Simvastatin may be decreased by: Antacids; Bosentan; CYP3A4 Inducers (Strong); Deferasirox; Etravirine; Phenytoin; Rifamycin Derivatives; St Johns Wort

Food Interactions Simvastatin serum concentration may be increased when taken with large quantities (>1 quart/day) of grapefruit juice; avoid concurrent use

Stability Tablets should be stored in well closed containers at temperatures between 5°C to 30°C (41°F to 86°F)

Mechanism of Action Simvastatin is a methylated derivative of lovastatin that acts by competitively inhibiting 3-hydroxy-3-methylglutaryl-coenzyme A (HMG-CoA) reductase, the enzyme that catalyzes the rate-limiting step in cholesterol biosynthesis

Pharmacodynamics

Onset of action: >3 days

Maximum effect: After 2 weeks

LDL-C reduction: 20-40 mg/day: 35% to 41% (for each doubling of this dose, LDL-C is lowered ~6%)

Average HDL-C increase: 5% to 15%

Average triglyceride reduction: 7% to 30%

Pharmacokinetics (Adult data unless noted)

Absorption: Oral: Although 85% is absorbed following administration, <5% reaches the general circulation due to an extensive first-pass effect

Time to peak serum concentration: 1.3-2.4 hours

Protein binding: ~95%

Elimination: 13% excreted in urine and 60% in feces

Usual Dosage Oral:

Children and Adolescents:

Heterozygous familial hypercholesterolemia: Adolescents 10-17 years: 10 mg once daily in the evening; may increase dose in intervals of 4 weeks or more to a maximum of 40 mg/day

Hyperlipidemia: Limited data in 32 children (<17 years of age) enrolled in compassionate use study (see Ducobu, 1992):

Children <10 years: 5 mg once daily in the evening increasing to 10 mg once daily after 4 weeks and to 20 mg once daily after 8 weeks as tolerated

Children ≥10 years: 10 mg once daily in the evening increasing to 20 mg once daily after 6 weeks and to 40 mg once daily after 12 weeks as tolerated

Note: A lower, conservative dosing regimen may be necessary in patient populations predisposed to myopathy including patients of Chinese descent or those concurrently receiving other lipid-lowering agents (eg, gemfibrozil, niacin, fibric acid derivatives), amiodarone, verapamil, cyclosporine, danazol (see the following conservative, maximum adult doses)

Adults:

Initial: 20 mg once daily in the evening; patients who require only a moderate reduction of LDL-C may be started at 10 mg once daily; patients who require a reduction of >45% in LDL-C may be started at 40 mg once daily

Maintenance: Recommended dosage range: 5-80 mg/day as a single dose in the evening; doses should be adjusted at intervals of at least 4 weeks

Homozygous familial hypercholesterolemia: Adults: 40 mg in the evening or 80 mg/day in 3 divided doses of 20 mg, 20 mg, and an evening dose of 40 mg.

Dosage adjustment in patients who are concomitantly receiving cyclosporine or danazol: Adults: Initial: 5 mg, not to exceed 10 mg/day

Dosage adjustment in patients receiving concomitant fibrates or niacin: Adults: Dose should not exceed 10 mg/day

Dosage adjustment in patients receiving concomitant amiodarone or verapamil: Adults: Dose should not exceed 20 mg/day

Dosage adjustment in patients receiving concomitant diltiazem: Adults: Dose should not exceed 40 mg/day

Dosage adjustment in Chinese patients on niacin ≥1 g/day: Because of an increased risk of myopathy, do not increase simvastatin dose to 80 mg.

Dosing adjustment in renal impairment: Adults: Because simvastatin does not undergo significant renal excretion, modification of dose should only be necessary in patients with severe renal impairment: Cl_{cr} <10 mL/minute: Initial: 5 mg/day

Administration Oral: May be taken without regard to meals. Administration with the evening meal or at bedtime has been associated with somewhat greater LDL-C reduction

Monitoring Parameters Serum cholesterol (total and fractionated), CPK; liver function tests (see Precautions)

Reference Range See Related Information for age- and gender-specific serum cholesterol, LDL-C, TG, and HDL concentrations.

Patient Information May rarely cause photosensitivity reactions (eg, exposure to sunlight may cause severe sunburn, skin rash, redness, or itching); avoid direct exposure to sunlight. Report severe and unresolved gastric upset, any vision changes, muscle pain and weakness, changes in color of urine or stool, yellowing of skin or eyes, and any unusual bruising. Female patients of childbearing age must be counseled to use 2 effective forms of contraception simultaneously, unless absolute abstinence is the chosen method; this drug may cause severe fetal defects.

Additional Information The current recommendation for pharmacologic treatment of hypercholesterolemia in children is limited to children ≥8 years of age and is based on LDL-C concentrations and the presence of coronary vascular disease (CVD) risk factors (see table and Daniels, 2008). In adults, for each 1% lowering in LDL-C, the relative risk for major cardiovascular events is reduced by ~1%. For more specific risk assessment and treatment recommendations for adults, see NCEP ATPIII, 2001.

Recommendations for Initiating Pharmacologic Treatment in Children ≥8 Years[1]

No risk factors for CVD	LDL ≥190 mg/dL despite 6-month to 1-year diet therapy
Family history of premature CVD or ≥2 CVD risk factors present, including obesity, hypertension, or cigarette smoking	LDL ≥160 mg/dL despite 6-month to 1-year diet therapy
Diabetes mellitus present	LDL ≥130 mg/dL

[1]Adapted from Daniels SR, Greer FR, and Committee on Nutrition, "Lipid Screening and Cardiovascular Health in Childhood," *Pediatrics*, 2008, 122(1):198-208.

Dosage Forms Excipient information presented when available (limited, particularly for generics); consult specific product labeling.

Tablet: 5 mg, 10 mg, 20 mg, 40 mg, 80 mg

Zocor®: 5 mg, 10 mg, 20 mg, 40 mg, 80 mg

References

American Academy of Pediatrics Committee on Nutrition, "Cholesterol in Childhood," *Pediatrics*, 1998, 101(1 Pt 1):141-7.

American Academy of Pediatrics, "National Cholesterol Education Program: Report of the Expert Panel on Blood Cholesterol Levels in Children and Adolescents," *Pediatrics*, 1992, 89(3 Pt 2):525-84.

Daniels SR, Greer FR, and Committee on Nutrition, "Lipid Screening and Cardiovascular Health in Childhood," *Pediatrics*, 2008, 122 (1):198-208.

DeJongh S, et al, "Efficacy, Safety, and Tolerability of Simvastatin in Children With Familial Hypercholesterolemia," *Clin Drug Invest*, 2002, 22(8): 533-40.

Ducobu J, Brasseur D, Chaudron JM, et al, "Simvastatin Use in Children," *Lancet*, 1992, 339(8807):1488.

Duplaga BA, "Treatment of Childhood Hypercholesterolemia With HMG-CoA Reductase Inhibitors," *Ann Pharmacother*, 1999, 33 (11):1224-7.

Grundy SM, Cleeman JI, Merz CN, et al, "Implications of Recent Clinical Trials for the National Cholesterol Education Program Adult Treatment Panel III Guidelines," *Circulation*, 2004, 110(2):227-39.

McCrindle BW, Urbina EM, Dennison BA, et al, "Drug Therapy of High-Risk Lipid Abnormalities in Children and Adolescents: A Scientific Statement from the American Heart Association Atherosclerosis, Hypertension, and Obesity in Youth Committee, Council of Cardiovascular Disease in the Young, With the Council on Cardiovascular Nursing," *Circulation*, 2007, 115(14):1948-67.

"Third Report of the National Cholesterol Education Program Expert Panel on Detection, Evaluation, and Treatment of High Blood Cholesterol in Adults (Adult Treatment Panel III)," May 2001, www.nhlbi.nih.gov/guidelines/cholesterol.

◆ **Simvastatin and Ezetimibe** *see* Ezetimibe and Simvastatin *on page 554*

◆ **Sinequan® [DSC]** *see* Doxepin *on page 475*

◆ **Sinequan® (Can)** *see* Doxepin *on page 475*

◆ **Singulair®** *see* Montelukast *on page 945*

Sirolimus (sir OH li mus)

Medication Safety Issues

Sound-alike/look-alike issues:

Rapamune® may be confused with Rapaflo™

Sirolimus may be confused with everolimus, tacrolimus, temsirolimus

U.S. Brand Names Rapamune®

Canadian Brand Names Rapamune®

Therapeutic Category Immunosuppressant Agent

Generic Available No

Use Prophylaxis of organ rejection in renal transplant patients at low-moderate immunologic risk in combination with corticosteroids and cyclosporine (cyclosporine may be withdrawn after 2-4 months in conjunction with an increase in sirolimus dosage) (FDA approved in ages ≥13 years and adults); prophylaxis of organ rejection in renal transplant patients at high immunologic risk in combination with cyclosporine and corticosteroids for the first year (FDA approved in ages ≥18 years and adults); studied as primary immunosuppression in heart and intestinal transplantation (given in conjunction with a calcineurin inhibitor, as a substitute for a calcineurin inhibitor to reduce side effects, or to eliminate steroid use); rescue agent for acute and chronic organ rejection (rescue due to calcineurin toxicity or to treat resistant acute or chronic rejection despite calcineurin inhibitor therapy; GVHD prophylaxis in BMT or hematopoietic stem cell transplant patients

Pregnancy Risk Factor C

Pregnancy Considerations Animal studies have demonstrated embryotoxicity and fetotoxicity, as evidenced by increased mortality, reduced fetal weights and delayed ossification. There are no adequate and well-controlled studies in pregnant women. Effective contraception must be initiated before therapy with sirolimus and continued for 12 weeks after discontinuation.

The National Transplantation Pregnancy Registry (NTPR, Temple University) is a registry for pregnant women taking immunosuppressants following any solid organ transplant. The NTPR encourages reporting of all immunosuppressant exposures during pregnancy in transplant recipients at 877-955-6877.

Lactation Excretion in breast milk unknown/not recommended

Breast-Feeding Considerations Due to the potential for adverse reactions in the breast-fed infant, including possible immunosuppression, breast-feeding is not recommended.

Contraindications Hypersensitivity to sirolimus, its derivatives, or any component

Warnings Immunosuppression with sirolimus may result in increased susceptibility to infection **[U.S Boxed Warning]**. Immunosuppressive agents, including sirolimus, may be associated with the development of lymphoma or other malignancies **[U.S. Boxed Warning]**. Immunosuppressant therapy is associated with an increased risk of skin cancer; limit sun and ultraviolet light exposure; use appropriate sun protection. Hypersensitivity reactions, anaphylaxis, angioedema, exfoliative dermatitis, and hypersensitivity vasculitis have been reported following administration of sirolimus. Sirolimus is not recommended for use in *de novo* lung transplant patients **[U.S. Boxed Warning]**. Cases of fatal bronchial anastomotic dehiscence have been reported in lung transplant patients who received sirolimus in combination with other immunosuppressants. Sirolimus is not recommended for use in *de novo* liver transplant patients **[U.S. Boxed Warning]**. Hepatic artery thrombosis, graft loss, and death have been reported in liver transplant patients who received sirolimus in combination with other immunosuppressants. Increased urinary protein excretion has been observed when converting renal transplant patients from calcineurin inhibitors to sirolimus during maintenance therapy. A higher level of proteinuria prior to sirolimus conversion correlates with a higher degree of proteinuria after conversion. In some patients, proteinuria may reach nephrotic levels. Increased risk of BK viral-associated nephropathy which may impair renal function and cause graft loss; consider decreasing immunosuppressive burden if evidence of deteriorating renal function. Use has been associated with an increased risk of fluid accumulation, impaired wound healing, and lymphocele. Peripheral edema, lymphedema, and pleural and pericardial effusions (including significant effusions and tamponade) were reported; use with caution in patients in whom fluid accumulation may be poorly tolerated, such as in cardiovascular disease (heart failure or hypertension) and pulmonary disease. Cases of interstitial lung disease [eg, pneumonitis, bronchiolitis obliterans organizing pneumonia (BOOP), pulmonary fibrosis] have been observed (some fatal); risk may be increased with higher trough concentrations.

Concurrent use with strong inhibitors of CYP3A4 and/or p-glycoprotein (ie, erythromycin, ketoconazole, voriconazole, itraconazole, telithromycin, or clarithromycin) or strong inducers of CYP3A4 and/or p-glycoprotein (rifampin or rifabutin) is not recommended. Concurrent use with a calcineurin inhibitor (cyclosporine, tacrolimus) may increase the risk of calcineurin inhibitor-induced hemolytic uremic syndrome/thrombotic thrombocytopenic purpura/thrombotic microangiopathy (HUS/TTP/TMA).

Precautions Use with caution in patients with hepatic impairment; a reduction in the maintenance dose is recommended. Use with caution in patients with hyperlipidemia (sirolimus may increase serum cholesterol and triglycerides), renal impairment, or when used concurrently with medications which alter renal function (sirolimus may

decrease GFR and increase serum creatinine). In renal transplant patients, *de novo* use without cyclosporine has been associated with higher rates of acute rejection. Sirolimus should be used in combination with cyclosporine initially. Sirolimus may delay recovery of renal function in patients with delayed allograft function. Monitor renal function closely when combined with cyclosporine; consider dosage adjustment or discontinue in patients with increasing serum creatinine. Separate dosing; sirolimus should be administered 4 hours after oral cyclosporine doses.

Use caution in the perioperative period due to increased chance of surgical complications from wound dehiscence and impaired wound and tissue healing (patients with a body mass index >30 kg/m^2 are at increased risk for abnormal wound healing). Antimicrobial prophylaxis for *Pneumocystis jiroveci* pneumonia should be administered for 1 year following transplantation; CMV prophylaxis is recommended for 3 months after transplantation.

Adverse Reactions

Cardiovascular: Atrial fibrillation, chest pain, edema, heart failure, hepatic artery thrombosis, hypertension, hypervolemia, hypotension, pericardial effusion, peripheral edema, postural hypotension, syncope, tachycardia, tamponade, thrombosis, thrombotic microangiopathy, venous thromboembolism

Central nervous system: Anxiety, chills, confusion, depression, dizziness, emotional lability, headache, hypoesthesia, hypotonia, insomnia, malaise, neuropathy, pain, somnolence

Dermatologic: Acne, angioedema, cellulitis, dermatitis (fungal), ecchymosis, exfoliative dermatitis, hirsutism, pruritus, rash, skin cancer, skin hypertrophy

Endocrine & metabolic: Acidosis, Cushing's syndrome, dehydration, diabetes mellitus, hypercalcemia, hypercholesterolemia, hyperglycemia, hyperphosphatemia, hypertriglyceridemia, hypocalcemia, hypoglycemia, hypokalemia, hypomagnesemia, hyponatremia, hypophosphatemia, weight gain

Gastrointestinal: Abdominal pain, anorexia, aphthous ulcers, constipation, diarrhea, dysphagia, eructation, esophagitis, flatulence, gastritis, gingival hyperplasia, ileus, incisional hernia, nausea, pancreatitis, stomatitis, vomiting

Genitourinary: Azoospermia, bladder pain, dysuria, impotence, nocturia, pelvic pain, pyuria, scrotal edema, urinary frequency, urinary incontinence, urinary retention, urinary tract infection

Hematologic: Anemia, hemolytic-uremic syndrome, hemorrhage, leukocytosis, leukopenia, neutropenia, pancytopenia, polycythemia, thrombocytopenia, thrombotic microangiopathy, thrombotic thrombocytopenic purpura

Hepatic: Alkaline phosphatase increased, ascites, AST and ALT increased, hepatic artery thrombosis, hepatic necrosis, hepatotoxicity, LDH increased

Neuromuscular & skeletal: Arthralgia, arthrosis, back pain, bone necrosis, bone pain, CPK increased, leg cramps, myalgia, osteoporosis, paresthesia, tetany, tremor, weakness

Ocular: Abnormal vision, cataract, conjunctivitis

Otic: Ear pain, otitis media, tinnitus

Renal: Albuminuria, BK viral-associated nephrology (see Warnings), BUN and serum creatinine increased, focal segmental glomerulosclerosis, hematuria, hydronephrosis, kidney pain, nephropathy (toxic), nephrotic syndrome, oliguria, proteinuria, pyelonephritis, tubular necrosis.

Respiratory: Alveolar proteinosis, asthma, atelectasis, bronchial anastomotic dehiscence, bronchitis, cough, dyspnea, epistaxis, hypoxia, interstitial lung disease [dose related; includes pneumonitis, pulmonary fibrosis, and bronchiolitis obliterans organizing pneumonia

SIROLIMUS

(BOOP) with no identified infectious etiology], lung edema, pleural effusion, *pneumocystis* pneumonia, pneumonia, pulmonary embolism, pulmonary hemorrhage, rhinitis, sinusitis, tuberculosis, upper respiratory infection

Miscellaneous: Abscess, anaphylactoid reaction, anaphylaxis, diaphoresis, flu-like syndrome, graft failure, hernia, hypersensitivity vasculitis, infection (including opportunistic), interference with wound and tissue healing, lymphadenopathy, lymphedema, lymphocele, lymphoproliferative disease/lymphoma (1% to 3%), peritonitis, sepsis

Drug Interactions

Metabolism/Transport Effects Substrate of CYP3A4 (major), P-glycoprotein; **Inhibits** CYP3A4 (weak)

Avoid Concomitant Use

Avoid concomitant use of Sirolimus with any of the following: BCG; Natalizumab; Pimecrolimus; Posaconazole; Tacrolimus; Tacrolimus (Systemic); Tacrolimus (Topical); Vaccines (Live); Voriconazole

Increased Effect/Toxicity

Sirolimus may increase the levels/effects of: ACE Inhibitors; CycloSPORINE; CycloSPORINE (Systemic); Hypoglycemic Agents; Leflunomide; Natalizumab; Tacrolimus; Tacrolimus (Systemic); Tacrolimus (Topical); Vaccines (Live)

The levels/effects of Sirolimus may be increased by: CycloSPORINE; CycloSPORINE (Systemic); CYP3A4 Inhibitors (Moderate); CYP3A4 Inhibitors (Strong); Dasatinib; Denosumab; Fluconazole; Herbs (Hypoglycemic Properties); Itraconazole; Ketoconazole; Ketoconazole (Systemic); Macrolide Antibiotics; P-Glycoprotein Inhibitors; Pimecrolimus; Posaconazole; Protease Inhibitors; Tacrolimus; Tacrolimus (Systemic); Tacrolimus (Topical); Trastuzumab; Voriconazole

Decreased Effect

Sirolimus may decrease the levels/effects of: BCG; Sipuleucel-T; Tacrolimus; Tacrolimus (Systemic); Vaccines (Inactivated); Vaccines (Live)

The levels/effects of Sirolimus may be decreased by: CYP3A4 Inducers (Strong); Deferasirox; Echinacea; Efavirenz; Herbs (CYP3A4 Inducers); P-Glycoprotein Inducers; Phenytoin; Rifampin

Food Interactions Avoid administration with grapefruit juice (may reduce metabolism of sirolimus); ingestion with a high fat meal decreases peak concentration but increases AUC by 35% (take sirolimus consistently either with or without food to minimize variability)

Stability Store tablets at controlled room temperature [20°C to 25°C (68°F to 77°F)] and protect from light. Refrigerate oral solution and protect from light; store oral solution in original container and use contents within one month after opening. Oral solution bottle may be stored at room temperature for a short period of time not to exceed 15 days; amber syringe containing solution may be stored at room temperature or in the refrigerator for a maximum of 24 hours.

Mechanism of Action Sirolimus reduces T-cell activation and proliferation by inhibiting cytokine-induced signal transduction pathways resulting in the suppression of IL-2 or IL-4 driven T-cell proliferation. Sirolimus inhibits antibody production. Sirolimus binds to FKBP-12, an intracellular protein, to form an immunosuppressive complex which inhibits the regulatory kinase, mTOR (mammalian target of rapamycin). This inhibition suppresses cytokine mediated T-cell proliferation, halting progression from the G1 to the S phase of the cell cycle. It inhibits acute rejection of allografts and prolongs graft survival.

Pharmacokinetics (Adult data unless noted)

Absorption: Rapid

Distribution: V_{dss}: 12 ± 8 L/kg

Protein binding: ~92%

Metabolism: By liver and intestinal cytochrome P450 enzyme CYP3A4; undergoes counter-transport from enterocytes of the small intestine into the gut lumen by the p-glycoprotein drug efflux pump; metabolized by O-demethylation and/or hydroxylation

Bioavailability: Oral solution: 14%; tablet: 18%

Half-life:
Children: 13.7 ± 6.2 hours
Adults: 62 ± 16 hours

Time to peak serum concentration: Oral solution: 1-3 hours; tablet: 1-6 hours

Elimination: Primarily eliminated via feces (91%) and urine (2.2%)

Usual Dosage Oral: **Note:** Sirolimus tablets and oral solution are not bioequivalent due to differences in absorption; however, clinical equivalence has been demonstrated at the 2 mg dose level

Children ≥13 years of age and <40 kg: Loading dose: 3 mg/m^2 on day 1; initial maintenance dose: 1 mg/m^2/day divided every 12 hours or once daily; adjust dose to achieve target sirolimus trough blood concentration

Adults:

Low- to moderate-immunologic risk renal transplant patients: Dosing by body weight:
<40 kg: Loading dose: 3 mg/m^2 on day 1, followed by maintenance dosing of 1 mg/m^2 once daily
≥40 kg: Loading dose: 6 mg on day 1; maintenance: 2 mg once daily

High-immunologic risk renal transplant patients: Adults: Loading dose: Up to 15 mg on day 1; maintenance: 5 mg/day; obtain trough concentration between days 5-7 and adjust accordingly. Continue concurrent cyclosporine/sirolimus therapy for 1 year following transplantation. Further adjustment of the regimen must be based on clinical status.

Intestinal transplant: Initial loading dose: 2-3 mg/m^2; maintenance dose: 1 mg/m^2 once daily to achieve blood concentrations of 8-10 ng/mL

Dosage adjustment: Sirolimus dosages should be adjusted to maintain trough concentrations within desired range based on risk and concomitant therapy. Maximum daily dose: 40 mg. Dosage should be adjusted at intervals of 7-14 days to account for the long half-life of sirolimus. In general, dose proportionality may be assumed. New sirolimus dose **equals** current dose **multiplied by** (target concentration/current concentration). **Note:** If large dose increase is required, consider loading dose calculated as:
Loading dose **equals** (new maintenance dose) **minus** current maintenance dose) **multiplied by** 3
Maximum dose in 1 day: 40 mg; if required dose is >40 mg (due to loading dose), divide over 2 days. Serum concentrations should not be used as the sole basis for dosage adjustment (monitor clinical signs/symptoms, tissue biopsy, and laboratory parameters).

Maintenance therapy after withdrawal of cyclosporine: Cyclosporine withdrawal is not recommended in high-immunological risk patients. Following 2-4 months of combined therapy, withdrawal of cyclosporine may be considered in low-to-moderate risk patients. Cyclosporine should be discontinued over 4-8 weeks, and a necessary increase in the dosage of sirolimus (up to fourfold) should be anticipated due to removal of metabolic inhibition by cyclosporine and to maintain adequate immunosuppressive effects. Dose-adjusted trough target concentrations are typically 16-24 ng/mL for the first year post-transplant and 12-20 ng/mL thereafter (measured by chromatographic methodology).

Dosage adjustment in renal impairment: No dosage adjustment necessary (in loading or maintenance dose); however, adjustment of regimen (including discontinuation of therapy) should be considered when used concurrently with cyclosporine and elevated or increasing serum creatinine is noted.

Dosage adjustment in hepatic impairment:

Loading dose: No adjustment required

Maintenance dose:

Mild-to-moderate hepatic impairment: Reduce maintenance dose by ~33%

Severe hepatic impairment: Reduce maintenance dose by ~50%

Administration May be taken with or without food, but take medication consistently with respect to meals to minimize absorption variability. Initial dose should be administered as soon as possible after transplant. Sirolimus should be taken 4 hours after oral cyclosporine (Neoral® or Gengraf®). Tablets should not be crushed, split, or chewed.

Oral solution: Use amber oral syringe to withdraw solution from the bottle. Empty dose from syringe into a glass or plastic cup and mix with at least 2 ounces of water or orange juice. No other liquids should be used for dilution. Patient should stir vigorously and drink the diluted sirolimus solution immediately. Then refill cup with an additional 4 ounces of water or orange juice; stir contents vigorously and have patient drink solution at once.

Monitoring Parameters Whole blood sirolimus trough concentration, serum cholesterol and triglycerides, serum creatinine; blood pressure, CBC with differential, hemoglobin, platelet count, liver function, urinary protein

Reference Range Results from whole blood sirolimus concentrations measured by HPLC vs immunoassay methodologies are not interchangeable. Chromatographic methods yield results ~20% lower than immunoassay results.

Serum trough concentrations (HPLC):

Concomitant cyclosporine: 4-12 ng/mL

After cyclosporine withdrawal: 16-24 ng/mL for the first year after transplant; after 1 year: 12-20 ng/mL

Patient Information Due to the increased risk for skin cancer, avoid exposure to sunlight and artificial light sources (sunlamps, tanning booth/bed); wear protective clothing, wide-brimmed hats, sunglasses, and lip sunscreen (SPF ≥15); use a sunscreen [broad-spectrum sunscreen or physical sunscreen (preferred) or sunblock with SPF ≥15]. Advise women of childbearing potential to avoid becoming pregnant; use effective contraception prior to starting sirolimus therapy, during therapy and for 12 weeks after sirolimus has been stopped.

Dosage Forms Excipient information presented when available (limited, particularly for generics); consult specific product labeling.

Solution, oral:

Rapamune®: 1 mg/mL (60 mL) [contains ethanol 1.5% to 2.5%; packaged with oral syringes and a carrying case]

Tablet:

Rapamune®: 1 mg, 2 mg

References

Balfour IC, Srun SW, Wood EG, et al, "Early Renal Benefit of Rapamycin Combined With Reduced Calcineurin Inhibitor Dose in Pediatric Heart Transplantation Patients," *J Heart Lung Transplant*, 2006, 25(5):518-22.

Castillo RO, Zarge R, Cox K, et al, "Pediatric Intestinal Transplantation at Packard Children's Hospital/Stanford University Medical Center: Report of a Four-Year Experience," *Transplant Proc*, 2006, 38 (6):1716-7.

Ettenger RB and Grimm EM, "Safety and Efficacy of TOR Inhibitors in Pediatric Renal Transplant Recipients," *Am J Kidney Dis*, 2001, 38(4 Suppl 2):S22-8.

Gupta P, Kaufman S, and Fishbein TM, "Sirolimus for Solid Organ Transplantation in Children," *Pediatr Transplant*, 2005, 9(3):269-76.

Lobach NE, Pollock-Barziv SM, West LJ, et al, "Sirolimus Immunosuppression in Pediatric Heart Transplant Recipients: A Single-Center Experience," *J Heart Lung Transplant*, 2005, 24(2):184-9.

Sarwal M and Pascual J, "Immunosuppression Minimization in Pediatric Transplantation," *Am J Transplant*, 2007, 7(10):2227-35.

Schubert M, Venkataramanan R, Holt DW, et al, "Pharmacokinetics of Sirolimus and Tacrolimus in Pediatric Transplant Patients," *Am J Transplant*, 2004, 4(5):767-73.

◆ **Skeeter Stik [OTC]** *see* Benzocaine *on page 182*

◆ **SKF 104864** *see* Topotecan *on page 1363*

◆ **SKF 104864-A** *see* Topotecan *on page 1363*

◆ **Sleep-ettes D [OTC]** *see* DiphenhydrAMINE *on page 448*

◆ **Sleepinal® [OTC]** *see* DiphenhydrAMINE *on page 448*

◆ **Sleep-Tabs [OTC]** *see* DiphenhydrAMINE *on page 448*

◆ **Slo-Niacin® [OTC]** *see* Niacin *on page 986*

◆ **Slo-Pot (Can)** *see* Potassium Chloride *on page 1136*

◆ **Slow FE® [OTC]** *see* Ferrous Sulfate *on page 577*

◆ **Slow-K® (Can)** *see* Potassium Chloride *on page 1136*

◆ **Slow-Mag® [OTC]** *see* Magnesium Chloride *on page 853*

◆ **Slow-Mag® [OTC]** *see* Magnesium Supplements *on page 859*

◆ **SM-7338** *see* Meropenem *on page 885*

◆ **SMZ-TMP** *see* Sulfamethoxazole and Trimethoprim *on page 1302*

◆ **Sodium 2-Mercaptoethane Sulfonate** *see* Mesna *on page 888*

◆ **Sodium L-Triiodothyronine** *see* Liothyronine *on page 828*

Sodium Acetate (SOW dee um AS e tate)

Therapeutic Category Alkalinizing Agent, Parenteral; Electrolyte Supplement, Parenteral; Sodium Salt

Generic Available Yes

Use Sodium salt replacement; correction of acidosis through conversion of acetate to bicarbonate

Pregnancy Risk Factor C

Contraindications Hypersensitivity to sodium acetate or any component; alkalosis, hypocalcemia, edema, cirrhosis, excessive chloride losses, hypernatremia

Warnings Avoid extravasation

Precautions Use with caution in patients with hepatic failure, CHF or other sodium-retaining conditions

Adverse Reactions

Cardiovascular: Thrombosis, hypervolemia, edema, cerebral hemorrhage

Endocrine & metabolic: Hypernatremia, hypokalemic metabolic alkalosis, hypocalcemia

Local: Extravasant, local cellulitis

Respiratory: Pulmonary edema

Drug Interactions

Avoid Concomitant Use There are no known interactions where it is recommended to avoid concomitant use.

Increased Effect/Toxicity There are no known significant interactions involving an increase in effect.

Decreased Effect There are no known significant interactions involving a decrease in effect.

Stability Protect from light, heat, and from freezing; **incompatible** with acids, acidic salts, catecholamines, atropine

Mechanism of Action Sodium is the principal extracellular cation; functions in fluid and electrolyte balance, osmotic pressure control, and water distribution; acetate is metabolized to bicarbonate which neutralizes hydrogen ion concentration and raises blood and urinary pH

Usual Dosage Sodium acetate is metabolized to bicarbonate on an equimolar basis outside the liver; administer in large volume I.V. fluids as a sodium source. Dosage is dependent upon the clinical condition, fluid, electrolytes and acid-base balance of the patient.

Maintenance sodium requirements: I.V.:
Neonates, Infants, and Children: 3-4 mEq/kg/day; maximum dose: 100-150 mEq/day
Adults: 154 mEq/day
Metabolic acidosis: If sodium acetate is desired over sodium bicarbonate, the amount of acetate may be dosed utilizing the equation found in the sodium bicarbonate monograph as each mEq acetate is converted to a mEq of HCO_3; see Sodium Bicarbonate on page 1269

Administration Parenteral: Must be diluted prior to I.V. administration; infuse hypertonic solutions (>154 mEq/L) via a central line; maximum rate of administration: 1 mEq/kg/hour

Monitoring Parameters Serum electrolytes including calcium, arterial blood gases (if indicated)

Additional Information Sodium and acetate content of 1 g: 7.3 mEq

Dosage Forms Excipient information presented when available (limited, particularly for generics); consult specific product labeling. [DSC] = Discontinued product
Injection, solution, as anhydrous [concentrate]: 2 mEq/mL (20 mL, 50 mL, 100 mL; 250 mL [DSC]); 4 mEq/mL (50 mL, 100 mL)

◆ **Sodium Acid Carbonate** see Sodium Bicarbonate on page 1269

◆ **Sodium Aurothiomalate** see Gold Sodium Thiomalate on page 652

Sodium Benzoate (SOW dee um BENZ oh ate)

Therapeutic Category Ammonium Detoxicant; Hyperammonemia Agent; Urea Cycle Disorder (UCD) Treatment Agent

Use Adjunctive therapy for the prevention and treatment of hyperammonemia due to suspected or proven urea cycle disorders

Precautions Use with caution in patients with Reye's syndrome, propionic or methylmalonic acidemia. *In vitro* and animal studies have shown that benzoate, a metabolite of benzyl alcohol, displaces bilirubin from protein binding sites; use cautiously in neonates, particularly those with hyperbilirubinemia.

Adverse Reactions

Endocrine & metabolic: Metabolic acidosis
Gastrointestinal: Nausea, vomiting

Drug Interactions

Avoid Concomitant Use There are no known interactions where it is recommended to avoid concomitant use.

Increased Effect/Toxicity

The levels/effects of Sodium Benzoate may be increased by: Probenecid

Decreased Effect There are no known significant interactions involving a decrease in effect.

Mechanism of Action Assists in lowering serum ammonia levels by activation of a nonurea cycle pathway (the benzoate-hippurate pathway); ammonia in the presence of benzoate will conjugate with glycine to form hippurate which is excreted by the kidney

Pharmacokinetics (Adult data unless noted)

Half-life: 0.75-7.4 hours
Elimination: Clearance is largely attributable to metabolism with urinary excretion of hippurate, the major metabolite

Usual Dosage Investigational use (not FDA approved): Oral, I.V.:
Infants and Children: 0.25 g/kg bolus followed by 0.25 g/kg/day as continuous infusion or divided every 6-8 hours
Adolescents and Adults: Initial 5.5 g/m^2 bolus followed by 5.5 g/m^2/day as continuous I.V. infusion or divided every 6-8 hours

Administration Not available commercially
Oral: Must be compounded using chemical powder
I.V.: I.V. solutions must also be compounded and tested for sterility and pyrogenicity prior to use; infuse bolus (with sodium phenylacetate) over 90 minutes in 25-35 mL/kg $D_{10}W$

Monitoring Parameters Plasma ammonia and amino acids

Additional Information Used to treat urea cycle enzyme deficiency in combination with arginine; a maximum of 1 mole nitrogen is removed for every 1 mole of benzoate administered

Dosage Forms Powder: 454 g

References

Batshaw ML, "Hyperammonemia," *Curr Probl Pediatr*, 1984, 14 (11):1-69.
Batshaw ML and Brusilow SW, "Treatment of Hyperammonemic Coma Caused by Inborn Errors of Urea Synthesis," *J Pediatr*, 1980, 97 (6):893-900.
Batshaw ML, MacArthur RB, and Tuchman M, "Alternative Pathway Therapy for Urea Cycle Disorders: Twenty Years Later," *J Pediatr*, 2001, 138(1 Suppl):S46-54.
Green TP, Marchessault RP, and Freese DK, "Disposition of Sodium Benzoate in Newborn Infants With Hyperammonemia," *J Pediatr*, 1983, 102(5):785-90.
Maestri NE, Hauser ER, Bartholomew D, et al, "Prospective Treatment of Urea Cycle Disorders," *J Pediatr*, 1991, 119(6):923-8.
Summar M, "Current Strategies for the Management of Neonatal Urea Cycle Disorders," *J Pediatr*, 2001, 138(1 Suppl):S30-9.

◆ **Sodium Benzoate and Caffeine** see Caffeine on page 225

◆ **Sodium Benzoate and Sodium Phenylacetate** see Sodium Phenylacetate and Sodium Benzoate on page 1274

Sodium Bicarbonate (SOW dee um bye KAR bun ate)

Related Information

Adult ACLS Algorithms on page 1463
CPR Pediatric Drug Dosages on page 1455

U.S. Brand Names Brioschi® [OTC]; Neut®

Therapeutic Category Alkalinizing Agent, Oral; Alkalinizing Agent, Parenteral; Antacid; Electrolyte Supplement, Oral; Electrolyte Supplement, Parenteral; Sodium Salt

Generic Available Yes: Excludes granules

Use Management of metabolic acidosis; antacid; alkalinization of urine; stabilization of acid base status in cardiac arrest (see Warnings) and treatment of life-threatening hyperkalemia

Pregnancy Risk Factor C

Lactation Enters breast milk/compatible

Contraindications Hypersensitivity to sodium bicarbonate or any component; alkalosis, hypocalcemia, hypernatremia; unknown abdominal pain, inadequate ventilation during cardiopulmonary resuscitation; excessive chloride losses

Warnings Avoid extravasation, tissue necrosis can occur due to the hypertonicity of $NaHCO_3$; use of I.V. $NaHCO_3$ should be reserved for documented metabolic acidosis and for life-threatening hyperkalemia; routine use in cardiac arrest is not recommended; patient should be adequately ventilated before administering in cardiac arrest; administration of excessive amounts of sodium bicarbonate may result in metabolic alkalosis which decreases the delivery of oxygen to tissues; monitor use closely

Precautions Use with caution in patients with CHF or other sodium-retaining conditions, renal insufficiency

Adverse Reactions
Cardiovascular: Edema, cerebral hemorrhage (especially with rapid injection of the hyperosmotic $NaHCO_3$ solution in infants)
Central nervous system: Tetany, intracranial acidosis
Endocrine & metabolic: Metabolic alkalosis, hypernatremia, hypokalemia, hypocalcemia, hyperosmolality
Gastrointestinal: Gastric distention, flatulence may occur with oral administration
Local: Tissue necrosis, ulceration after I.V. extravasation
Respiratory: Pulmonary edema

Drug Interactions
Avoid Concomitant Use There are no known interactions where it is recommended to avoid concomitant use.

Increased Effect/Toxicity
Sodium Bicarbonate may increase the levels/effects of: Alpha-/Beta-Agonists; Amphetamines; Flecainide; Memantine; QuiNIDine; QuiNINE

The levels/effects of Sodium Bicarbonate may be increased by: Calcium Polystyrene Sulfonate

Decreased Effect
Sodium Bicarbonate may decrease the levels/effects of: ACE Inhibitors; Anticonvulsants (Hydantoin); Antifungal Agents (Azole Derivatives, Systemic); Antipsychotic Agents (Phenothiazines); Atazanavir; Bisacodyl; Cefditoren; Cefpodoxime; Cefuroxime; Chloroquine; Corticosteroids (Oral); Dabigatran Etexilate; Dasatinib; Delavirdine; Erlotinib; Flecainide; HMG-CoA Reductase Inhibitors; Iron Salts; Isoniazid; Lithium; Mesalamine; Methenamine; Penicillamine; Phosphate Supplements; Protease Inhibitors; Tetracycline Derivatives; Trientine; Ursodiol

Stability Do not mix $NaHCO_3$ with calcium salts, catecholamines, atropine

Mechanism of Action Dissociates to provide bicarbonate ion which neutralizes hydrogen ion concentration and raises blood and urinary pH

Pharmacodynamics
Onset of action:
Oral, as antacid: 15 minutes
I.V.: Rapid
Duration:
Oral: 1-3 hours
I.V.: 8-10 minutes

Pharmacokinetics (Adult data unless noted)
Absorption: Oral: Well absorbed
Elimination: Reabsorbed by kidney and <1% is excreted in urine

Usual Dosage
Cardiac arrest: See Warnings; patient should be adequately ventilated before administering $NaHCO_3$
Infants: 1 mEq/kg slow IVP initially; may repeat with 0.5 mEq/kg in 10 minutes one time, or as indicated by the patient's acid-base status
Children and Adults: 1 mEq/kg IVP initially; may repeat with 0.5 mEq/kg in 10 minutes one time, or as indicated by the patient's acid-base status
Metabolic acidosis: Dosage should be based on the following formula if blood gases and pH measurements are available:
Neonates, Infants and Children: $HCO_3^-(mEq) = 0.3 \times$ weight (kg) $\times$ base deficit (mEq/L) **or** $HCO_3^-(mEq) = 0.5 \times$ weight (kg) $\times$ [24 - serum $HCO_3^-(mEq/L)$]
Adults: $HCO_3^-(mEq) = 0.2 \times$ weight (kg) $\times$ base deficit (mEq/L) **or** $HCO_3^-(mEq) = 0.5 \times$ weight (kg) $\times$ [24 - serum $HCO_3^-(mEq/L)$]
If acid-base status is not available: Dose for older Children and Adults: 2-5 mEq/kg I.V. infusion over

4-8 hours; subsequent doses should be based on patient's acid-base status
Prevention of hyperuricemia secondary to tumor lysis syndrome (urinary alkalinization) (refer to individual protocols):
Infants and Children:
I.V.: 120-200 $mEq/m^2/day$ diluted in maintenance I.V. fluids of 3000 $mL/m^2/day$; titrate to maintain urine pH between 6-7
Oral: 12 $g/m^2/day$ divided into 4 doses; titrate to maintain urine pH between 6-7
Chronic renal failure: Oral: Initiate when plasma HCO_3^- <15 mEq/L:
Children: 1-3 mEq/kg/day in divided doses
Adults: 20-36 mEq/day in divided doses
Renal tubular acidosis: Oral:
Distal:
Children: 2-3 mEq/kg/day in divided doses
Adults: 0.5-2 mEq/kg/day given in 4-5 divided doses
Proximal: Children and Adults: Initial: 5-10 mEq/kg/day in divided doses; maintenance: Increase as required to maintain serum bicarbonate in the normal range
Urine alkalinization: Oral:
Children: 1-10 mEq (84-840 mg)/kg/day in divided doses; dose should be titrated to desired urinary pH
Adults: 48 mEq (4 g) initially, then 12-24 mEq (1-2 g) every 4 hours; dose should be titrated to desired urinary pH; doses up to 16 g/day have been used
Antacid: Oral: Adults: 325 mg to 2 grams 1-4 times/day

Administration
Oral: Administer 1-3 hours after meals
Parenteral: For direct I.V. administration: in neonates and infants, use the 0.5 mEq/mL solution or dilute the 1 mEq/mL solution 1:1 with **SWI**; in children and adults, the 1 mEq/mL solution may be used; administer slowly (maximum rate in neonates and infants: 10 mEq/minute); for infusion, dilute to a maximum concentration of 0.5 mEq/mL in dextrose solution and infuse over 2 hours (maximum rate of administration: 1 mEq/kg/hour)

Monitoring Parameters Serum electrolytes including calcium, urinary pH, arterial blood gases (if indicated)

Additional Information 1 mEq $NaHCO_3$ is equivalent to 84 mg; each g of $NaHCO_3$ provides 12 mEq each of sodium and bicarbonate ions; the osmolarity of 0.5 mEq/mL is 1000 mOsm/L and 1 mEq/mL is 2000 mOsm/L

Dosage Forms Excipient information presented when available (limited, particularly for generics); consult specific product labeling.
Granules, for solution, oral [effervescent]:
Brioschi®: 2.69 g/packet (12s) [contains sodium 770 mg/packet; lemon flavor]; 2.69 g/capful (120 g, 240 g) [contains sodium 770 mg/capful; lemon flavor]
Infusion [premixed in water for injection]: 5% (500 mL) [5.95 mEq/10 mL]
Injection, solution:
4.2% (10 mL) [5 mEq/10 mL]
7.5% (50 mL) [8.92 mEq/10 mL]
8.4% (10 mL, 50 mL, 250 mL, 500 mL) [10 mEq/10 mL]
Neut®: 4% (5 mL) [2.4 mEq/5 mL; contains edetate disodium]
Powder, oral: USP: 100% (120 g, 480 g) [contains sodium 30 mEq per 1/2 teaspoon]
Tablet, oral: 325 mg [3.8 mEq]; 650 mg [7.6 mEq]

◆ **Sodium Bicarbonate and Omeprazole** *see* Omeprazole and Sodium Bicarbonate *on page 1018*

Sodium Chloride (SOW dee um KLOR ide)

Medication Safety Issues
Per The Joint Commission (TJC) recommendations, concentrated electrolyte solutions (eg, NaCl >0.9%) should not be available in patient care areas.

High alert medication: The Institute for Safe Medication Practices (ISMP) includes this medication (I.V. formulation >0.9% concentration) among its list of drugs which have a heightened risk of causing significant patient harm when used in error.

Inappropriate use of low sodium or sodium-free intravenous fluids (eg, D$_5$W, hypotonic saline) in pediatric patients can lead to significant morbidity and mortality due to hyponatremia (ISMP, 2009).

Related Information

Laboratory Calculations *on page 1680*
Normal Laboratory Values for Children *on page 1672*

U.S. Brand Names
4-Way® Saline Moisturizing Mist [OTC]; Altachlore [OTC]; Altamist [OTC]; Ayr® Allergy Sinus [OTC]; Ayr® Baby Saline [OTC]; Ayr® Saline No-Drip [OTC]; Ayr® Saline [OTC]; Breathe Free® [OTC]; Deep Sea [OTC]; Entsol® [OTC]; Humist® for Kids [OTC]; Humist® [OTC]; Hyper-Sal™; Little Noses® Saline [OTC]; Little Noses® Stuffy Nose Kit [OTC]; Muro 128® [OTC]; Mycinaire™ [OTC] [DSC]; Na-Zone® [OTC]; Nasal Moist® Saline [OTC]; Nasal Spray [OTC]; NãSal™ [OTC]; Ocean® for Kids [OTC]; Ocean® [OTC]; Pretz® [OTC]; Saline Mist [OTC]; SalineX® [OTC] [DSC]; Simply Saline® Baby [OTC]; Simply Saline® Nasal Moist® [OTC]; Simply Saline® [OTC]; Syrex; Wound Wash Saline™ [OTC]

Therapeutic Category
Electrolyte Supplement, Oral; Electrolyte Supplement, Parenteral; Lubricant, Ocular; Sodium Salt

Generic Available
Yes

Use
Restoration of sodium ion in hyponatremia [FDA approved in pediatric patients (age not specified) and adults], restores moisture to nasal membranes [FDA approved in pediatric patients (age not specified) and adults], source of electrolytes and water for expansion of the extracellular fluid compartment [FDA approved in pediatric patients (age not specified) and adults], diluent and delivery system of compatible drug additives [FDA approved in pediatric patients (age not specified) and adults]; has also been used for reduction of intracranial pressure (ICP) in head trauma patients, improvement of mucociliary clearance and airway hydration in CF and acute viral bronchiolitis, reduction of corneal edema, prevention of muscle cramps and heat prostration

Pregnancy Risk Factor
C

Contraindications
Hypersensitivity to sodium chloride or any component; hypertonic uterus, hypernatremia (except when used for increased intracranial pressure), fluid retention

Warnings
Sodium toxicity is almost exclusively related to how fast a sodium deficit is corrected; both rate and magnitude of correction are extremely important; administration of low sodium or sodium free I.V. solutions may result in significant hyponatremia or water intoxication in pediatric patients; monitor serum sodium concentration

Precautions
Use with caution in patients with heart failure, renal insufficiency, cirrhosis, hypertension

Adverse Reactions
Cardiovascular: Edema, hypervolemia, thrombosis
Endocrine & metabolic: Dilution of serum electrolytes, hypernatremia, overhydration
Gastrointestinal: Nausea, vomiting (oral use)
Local: Phlebitis (with concentrations >0.9%)
Respiratory: Bronchospasm (inhalation with hypertonic solutions), pulmonary edema

Drug Interactions

Avoid Concomitant Use
Avoid concomitant use of Sodium Chloride with any of the following: Tolvaptan

Increased Effect/Toxicity
Sodium Chloride may increase the levels/effects of: Tolvaptan

Decreased Effect
Sodium Chloride may decrease the levels/effects of: Lithium

Mechanism of Action
Principal extracellular cation; functions in fluid and electrolyte balance, osmotic pressure control, and water distribution

Pharmacokinetics (Adult data unless noted)
Absorption: Oral, I.V.: Rapid
Distribution: Widely distributed
Elimination: Mainly in urine but also in sweat, tears, and saliva

Usual Dosage
Dosage depends upon clinical condition, fluid, electrolyte, and acid-base balance of patient; systemic hypertonic solutions (>0.9%) should only be used for the initial treatment of acute serious symptomatic hyponatremia or increased intracranial pressure; see Fluid and Electrolyte Requirements in Children on page 1556
Oral, I.V: Maintenance sodium requirements:
Premature neonates: 2-8 mEq/kg/day; infants born at ≤32 weeks gestation may require higher range in dosage for the first 2 weeks of life (see Al-Dahhan, 2002)
Term neonates: 1-4 mEq/kg/day
Infants and Children: 3-4 mEq/kg/day; maximum dose: 100-150 mEq/day
Adults: 154 mEq/day
To correct acute, serious hyponatremia: mEq sodium = [desired sodium (mEq/L) - actual sodium (mEq/L)] x 0.6 x wt (kg); for acute correction use 125 mEq/L as the desired serum sodium; acutely correct serum sodium in 5 mEq/L/dose increments; more gradual correction in increments of 10 mEq/L/day is indicated in the asymptomatic patient
I.V.: Children:
Dehydration: Initial: 0.9%: 20 mL/kg/dose; maximum: 1000 mL followed by remaining replacement using sodium chloride concentration appropriate for age over 24 hours for dehydration (see Meyers, 2009)
Hypovolemic shock: 0.9%: 20 mL/kg/dose; may repeat up to ≥60 mL/kg until capillary perfusion improves or signs of fluid overload occur (see Ceneviva, 1998; Parker, 2004)
Increased intracranial pressure: 3%: 0.1-1 mL/kg/hour continuous infusion titrated to maintain ICP <20 mm Hg (see Adleson, 2003); monitor serum sodium concentration closely; some centers utilize titration protocols with rate adjustments varying with serum sodium concentration
Inhalation:
Cystic fibrosis: Children ≥6 years and Adults: 7%: 4 mL inhaled twice daily. **Note:** Clinically, some CF centers are using 3% or 3.5% inhaled solutions if patients cannot tolerate 7%; pretreatment with a bronchodilator is recommended to prevent potential bronchospam
Inpatient viral bronchiolitis: Infants and Children 1-24 months: 3%: 4 mL inhaled every 2 hours for 3 doses followed by every 4 hours for 5 doses and continued every 6 hours until discharge (see Kuzik, 2007); pretreatment with a bronchodilator may be necessary to prevent potential bronchospam
Nasal: Children and Adults: Use as often as needed
Ophthalmic, ointment: Children and Adults: Apply once daily or more often as needed

Administration
Inhalation: Nebulization; studies administering hypertonic saline utilized varying types of nebulizers, including jet and ultrasonic
Nasal: Spray into 1 nostril while gently occluding other
Ophthalmic: Apply to affected eye(s); avoid contact of bottle tip with eye or skin
Oral: Administer with full glass of water
Parenteral: Infuse hypertonic solutions (>0.9% saline) via central line only; maximum rate of administration: 1 mEq/kg/hour

◀ **Monitoring Parameters** Serum sodium, chloride, I & O, weight; ICP (head trauma), capillary perfusion, MAP, CVP (fluid resuscitation)

Reference Range Serum/plasma sodium concentration:
Premature neonates: 132-140 mEq/L
Full-term neonates: 133-142 mEq/L
Infants ≥2 months to Adults: 135-145 mEq/L

Nursing Implications Bacteriostatic NS should not be used for diluting or reconstituting drugs for administration in neonates

Additional Information Normal saline (0.9%) = 154 mEq/L; 3% NaCl = 513 mEq/L; 5% NaCl = 856 mEq/L

Dosage Forms Excipient information presented when available (limited, particularly for generics); consult specific product labeling. [DSC] = Discontinued product

Aerosol, intranasal [spray; preservative free]:
Entsol®: 3% (100 mL) [chlorofluorocarbon free]

Gel, intranasal:
Ayr® Saline: <0.5% (14 g) [contains soybean oil and aloe]
Entsol®: 3% (20 g) [contains benzalkonium chloride; with aloe and vitamin E]
Simply Saline® Nasal Moist®: 0.65% (30 g) [contains aloe]

Gel, intranasal [spray]:
Ayr® Saline No-Drip: <0.5% (22 mL) [contains benzalkonium chloride, benzyl alcohol, and soybean oil]

Injection, solution: 0.45% (25 mL, 50 mL, 100 mL, 250 mL, 500 mL, 1000 mL); 0.9% (25 mL, 50 mL, 100 mL, 150 mL, 250 mL, 500 mL, 1000 mL, 1 g); 3% (500 mL); 5% (500 mL)

Injection, solution [preservative free]: 0.9% (2 mL, 3 mL, 5 mL, 10 mL, 20 mL, 50 mL, 100 mL)

Injection, solution [I.V. flush]: 0.9% (10 mL)

Injection, solution [I.V. flush; preservative free]: 0.9% (1 mL, 2 mL, 2.5 mL, 3 mL, 5 mL, 10 mL)
Syrex: 0.9% (2.5 mL, 3 mL, 5 mL, 10 mL)

Injection, solution [bacteriostatic]: 0.9% (10 mL, 20 mL, 30 mL)

Injection, solution [concentrate]: 14.6% (40 mL); 23.4% (100 mL, 250 mL)

Injection, solution [concentrate; preservative free]: 14.6% (20 mL, 40 mL); 23.4% (30 mL, 100 mL, 200 mL)

Ointment, ophthalmic: 5% (3.5 g)
Altachlore: 5% (3.5 g)

Ointment, ophthalmic [preservative free]:
Muro 128®: 5% (3.5 g)

Powder for solution, intranasal [preservative free]:
Entsol®: 3% (10.5 g)

Solution for blood processing [not for injection]: 0.9% (3000 mL)

Solution for inhalation [preservative free]: 0.9% (3 mL, 5 mL [DSC], 15 mL [DSC]); 3% (15 mL [DSC])

Solution for inhalation [hypertonic; preservative free]: 10% (15 mL) [DSC]

Solution for inhalation [hypotonic; preservative free]: 0.45% (5 mL) [DSC]

Solution for injection [I.V. flush; preservative free]: 0.9% (2.5 mL, 5 mL, 10 mL)

Solution for irrigation: 0.45% (2000 mL); 0.9% (250 mL, 500 mL, 1000 mL, 1500 mL, 2000 mL, 3000 mL, 4000 mL, 5000 mL)

Solution for irrigation [preservative free]: 0.45% (1500 mL [DSC]; 2000 mL); 0.9% (250 mL, 500 mL, 1000 mL, 1500 mL, 2000 mL, 3000 mL)

Solution for irrigation [slush solution]: 0.9% (1000 mL)

Solution for nebulization [preservative free]:
Hyper-Sal™: 7% (4 mL)

Solution, intranasal [preservative free]:
Simply Saline®: 3% (44 mL)

Solution, intranasal [drops]:
Ayr® Saline: 0.65% (50 mL) [alcohol free; contains benzalkonium chloride]
NāSal™: 0.65% (15 mL) [alcohol free; contains benzalkonium chloride]
SalineX®: 0.4% (15 mL) [contains benzalkonium chloride] [DSC]

Solution, intranasal [drops, mist, spray]:
Humist®: 0.65% (45 mL) [ethanol free]
Humist® for Kids: 0.65% (30 mL) [ethanol free; bubblegum flavor]
Ocean®: 0.65% (45 mL, 473 mL) [gluten free; contains benzalkonium chloride and benzyl alcohol]
Ocean® for Kids: 0.65% (37.5 mL) [alcohol free; contains benzalkonium chloride]

Solution, intranasal [drops, spray]:
Ayr® Baby Saline: 0.65% (30 mL) [ethanol free; contains benzalkonium chloride]
Little Noses® Saline: 0.65% (30 mL) [contains benzalkonium chloride]
Little Noses® Stuffy Nose Kit: 0.65% (15 mL) [contains benzalkonium chloride]

Solution, intranasal [drops, spray, stream]:
Saline Mist: 0.65% (45 mL) [contains benzalkonium chloride] [DSC]

Solution, intranasal [irrigation]:
Pretz®: 0.75% (237 mL, 960 mL) [contains benzalkonium chloride and sodium benzoate; with yerba santa]

Solution, intranasal [mist]:
Ayr® Allergy Sinus: 2.65% (50 mL)
Ayr® Saline: 0.65% (50 mL) [ethanol free; contains benzalkonium chloride]
Entsol®: 3% (30 mL) [contains benzalkonium chloride]
Mycinaire™: 0.65% (30 mL) [contains benzalkonium chloride] [DSC]
Saline Mist: 0.65% (45 mL) [contains benzalkonium chloride]
SalineX®: 0.4% (50 mL) [contains benzalkonium chloride] [DSC]
4-Way® Moisturizing Mist: 0.74% (29.6 mL) [ethanol free; contains benzalkonium chloride and menthol]

Solution, intranasal [mist, preservative free]:
Simply Saline®: 0.9% (44 mL, 90 mL)
Simply Saline® Baby: 0.9% (45 mL)

Solution, intranasal [nasal wash; preservative free]:
Entsol®: 3% (240 mL)

Solution, intranasal [spray]:
Altamist: 0.65% (60 mL) [contains benzalkonium chloride]
Breathe Free®: 0.65% (44.3 mL) [contains benzalkonium chloride]
Deep Sea: 0.65% (45 mL) [contains benzalkonium chloride and benzyl alcohol]
Na-Zone®: 0.65% (60 mL) [contains benzalkonium chloride]
Nasal Moist® Saline: 0.65% (45 mL)
Nasal Spray: 0.65% (45 mL) [contains benzalkonium chloride and benzyl alcohol]
NāSal™: 0.65% (30 mL) [ethanol free; contains benzalkonium chloride and thimerosal]

Solution, intranasal [spray, isotonic, buffered]:
Pretz®: 0.75% (50 mL) [contains benzalkonium chloride and sodium benzoate; with yerba santa]

Solution, ophthalmic: 5% (15 mL)

Solution, ophthalmic [drops]: 5% (15 mL)
Altachlore: 5% (15 mL, 30 mL)
Muro 128®: 2% (15 mL); 5% (15 mL, 30 mL)

Solution, topical [preservative free]:
Wound Wash Saline™: 0.9% (90 mL, 210 mL)

Swab, intranasal:
Ayr® Saline: <0.5% (20) [contains aloe and soybean oil]

Tablet, oral: 1 g

Tablet for solution, topical: 1000 mg

References

Adelson PD, Bratton SL, Carney NA, et al, "Guidelines for the Acute Medical Management of Severe Traumatic Brain Injury in Infants, Children, and Adolescents. Chapter 11. Use of Hyperosmolar Therapy in the Management of Severe Pediatric Traumatic Brain Injury," *Pediatr Crit Care Med*, 2003, 4(3 Suppl):S40-4.

Al-Dahhan J, Jannoun L, and Haycock GB, "Effect of Salt Supplementation of Newborn Premature Infants on Neurodevelopmental Outcome at 10-13 Years of Age," *Arch Dis Child Fetal Neonatal Ed*, 2002, 86(2):F120-3.

Ceneviva G, Paschall JA, Maffei F, et al, "Hemodynamic Support in Fluid-Refractory Pediatric Septic Shock," *Pediatrics*, 1998, 102(2):e19.

Dellon EP, Donaldson SH, Johnson R, et al, "Safety and Tolerability of Inhaled Hypertonic Saline in Young Children With Cystic Fibrosis," *Pediatr Pulmonol*, 2008, 43(11):1100-6.

Elkins MR, Robinson M, Rose BR, et al, "A Controlled Trial of Long-Term Inhaled Hypertonic Saline in Patients With Cystic Fibrosis," *N Engl J Med*, 2006, 354(3):229-40.

Fisher B, Thomas D, and Peterson B, "Hypertonic Saline Lowers Raised Intracranial Pressure in Children After Head Trauma," *J Neurosurg Anesthesiol*, 1992, 4(1):4-10.

Institute for Safe Medication Practice, "Plain D$_5$W or Hypotonic Saline Solutions Post-Op Could Result in Acute Hyponatremia and Death in Healthy Children," ISMP Medication Safety Alert, August 13, 2009. Available online at http://www.ismp.org/Newsletters/acutecare/articles/20090813.asp.

Khanna S, Davis D, Peterson B, et al, "Use of Hypertonic Saline in the Treatment of Severe Refractory Posttraumatic Intracranial Hypertension in Pediatric Traumatic Brain Injury," *Crit Care Med*, 2000, 28 (4):1144-51.

Kuzik BA, Al-Qadhi SA, Kent S, et al, "Nebulized Hypertonic Saline in the Treatment of Viral Bronchiolitis in Infants," *J Pediatr*, 2007, 151 (3):266-70, 270.e1.

Meyers R, "Pediatric Fluid and Electrolyte Therapy," *J Pediatr Pharmacol Ther*, 2009, 14:204–11

Parker MM, Hazelzet JA, and Carcillo JA, "Pediatric Considerations," *Crit Care Med*, 2004, 32(11 Suppl):S591-4.

Subbarao P, Balkovec S, Solomon M, et al, "Pilot Study of Safety and Tolerability of Inhaled Hypertonic Saline in Infants With Cystic Fibrosis," *Pediatr Pulmonol*, 2007, 42(5):471-6.

◆ **Sodium Diuril®** *see* Chlorothiazide *on page 295*

◆ **Sodium Edecrin®** *see* Ethacrynic Acid *on page 543*

◆ **Sodium Edetate** *see* Edetate Disodium *on page 489*

◆ **Sodium Etidronate** *see* Etidronate Disodium *on page 549*

◆ **Sodium Ferric Gluconate** *see* Ferric Gluconate *on page 574*

◆ **Sodium Fluoride** *see* Fluoride *on page 595*

◆ **Sodium Hydrogen Carbonate** *see* Sodium Bicarbonate *on page 1269*

◆ **Sodium Hyposulfate** *see* Sodium Thiosulfate *on page 1280*

◆ **Sodium Nafcillin** *see* Nafcillin *on page 962*

Sodium Nitrite, Sodium Thiosulfate, and Amyl Nitrite

(AM il NYE trate, SOW dee um NYE trate, & SOW dee um thye oh SUL fate)

U.S. Brand Names Cyanide Antidote Package

Therapeutic Category Antidote, Cyanide

Generic Available No

Use Treatment agents for cyanide poisoning

Pregnancy Risk Factor C (sodium thiosulfate and sodium nitrite); C (amyl nitrite)

Contraindications Hypersensitivity to amyl nitrite, sodium nitrite, sodium thiosulfate, or any component

Warnings Excessive methemoglobin results when sodium nitrite dosage is exceeded; use only enough sodium nitrite to achieve a satisfactory clinical response; avoid methemoglobin levels >30%; patients with malignancy and G6PD deficiency have increased sensitivity to the methemoglobin-generating activities of sodium nitrite

Precautions When cyanide poisoning is related to smoke inhalation, if possible, the patient should be at pressure in a hyperbaric chamber before the kit is administered; the methemoglobin initially produced by sodium nitrite injection may otherwise exacerbate concomitant carbon monoxide poisoning that has already severely diminished oxygen-carrying capacity in red cells

Adverse Reactions Reactions listed are those of sodium nitrite; see individual monographs for Amyl Nitrite and Sodium Thiosulfate

Cardiovascular: Tachycardia, syncope, cyanosis, hypotension (associated with rapid infusion), flushing

Central nervous system: Dizziness, headache

Gastrointestinal: Nausea, vomiting

Miscellaneous: Methemoglobin formation

Drug Interactions

Avoid Concomitant Use There are no known interactions where it is recommended to avoid concomitant use.

Increased Effect/Toxicity

Sodium Nitrite, Sodium Thiosulfate, and Amyl Nitrite may increase the levels/effects of: Hypotensive Agents

Decreased Effect There are no known significant interactions involving a decrease in effect.

Stability Sodium nitrite is stable at room temperature; do not mix with other medications; see individual monographs Amyl Nitrite and Sodium Thiosulfate

Mechanism of Action Amyl nitrite and sodium nitrite promote the formation of methemoglobin which binds with cyanide to form cyanomethemoglobin (nontoxic); sodium thiosulfate, by providing an extra sulfur group to the enzyme rhodanase, increases the rate of detoxification of cyanide

Usual Dosage Administer in sequential order:

Amyl nitrite: Infants, Children, and Adults: Inhale vapors from 1 ampul continuously for 15-30 seconds, followed by a rest for 15 seconds (this interrupted schedule is important because continuous use of amyl nitrite may prevent adequate oxygenation); reapply until sodium nitrite can be administered

Sodium nitrite: I.V.: Note: There are limited case reports of use in children. Below are manufacturer's guidelines. Infants and Children: 6 mg/kg/dose (maximum: 300 mg) or 6-8 mL/m^2 (180-240 mg/m^2) (maximum: 10 mL)

Variation of Sodium Nitrite and Sodium Thiosulfate Dose With Hemoglobin Concentration[1]

Hemoglobin (g/dL)	Initial Dose Sodium Nitrite (mg/kg)	Initial Dose Sodium Nitrite 3% (mL/kg)	Initial Dose Sodium Thiosulfate 25% (mL/kg)
7	5.8	0.19	0.95
8	6.6	0.22	1.10
9	7.5	0.25	1.25
10	8.3	0.27	1.35
11	9.1	0.30	1.50
12	10.0	0.33	1.65
13	10.8	0.36	1.80
14	11.6	0.39	1.95

[1]Adapted from Berlin DM Jr, "The Treatment of Cyanide Poisoning in Children," *Pediatrics*, 1970, 46:793.

Adolescents and Adults: 300 mg; follow immediately with sodium thiosulfate

Sodium thiosulfate: I.V.: Note: There are limited case reports of use in children. Below are manufacturer's guidelines.

Infants and Children: 7 g/m^2 (maximum: 12.5 g) over ~10 minutes, if needed; injection of both may be repeated at $^1/_2$ the original dose

Adolescents and Adults: 12.5 g

Patients should be watched for at least 24-48 hours; if signs of poisoning reappear, injection of both sodium nitrite and sodium thiosulfate should be repeated, but each in ¹/₂ of the original dose; even if the patient is asymptomatic, repeat ¹/₂ doses of both sodium nitrite and sodium thiosulfate may be given for prophylactic purposes 2 hours after the first injection

Administration

Inhalation: **Amyl nitrite:** Crush ampul in cloth and hold under patient's nares for 15-30 seconds; remove for 15 seconds; repeat

Parenteral: I.V.:

Sodium nitrite: Administer undiluted at a rate of 2.5-5 mL/minute

Sodium thiosulfate: Administer undiluted over at least 10 minutes; rapid administration may cause hypotension

Monitoring Parameters Blood cyanide levels, methemoglobin levels, arterial blood gases, oxygen saturation, vital signs

Reference Range Symptoms associated with blood cyanide levels:

Flushing and tachycardia: 0.5-1 mcg/mL

Obtundation: 1-2.5 mcg/mL

Coma and respiratory depression: >2.5 mcg/mL

Death: >3 mcg/mL

Dosage Forms Excipient information presented when available (limited, particularly for generics); consult specific product labeling.

Kit [each kit contains] (Cyanide Antidote Package):

Injection, solution:

Sodium nitrite 300 mg/10 mL (2)

Sodium thiosulfate 12.5 g/50 mL (2)

Inhalant: Amyl nitrite 0.3 mL (12)

[kit also includes disposable syringes, stomach tube, tourniquet, and instructions]

References

Berlin CM Jr, "The Treatment of Cyanide Poisoning in Children," *Pediatrics*, 1970, 46(5):793-6.

Geller RJ, Barthold C, Saiers JA, et al, "Pediatric Cyanide Poisoning: Causes, Manifestations, Management, and Unmet Needs," *Pediatrics*, 2006, 118(5):2146-58.

◆ **Sodium Nitroferricyanide** *see* Nitroprusside *on page 998*

◆ **Sodium Nitroprusside** *see* Nitroprusside *on page 998*

Sodium Phenylacetate and Sodium Benzoate

(SOW dee um fen il AS e tate & SOW dee um BENZ oh ate)

U.S. Brand Names Ammonul®

Therapeutic Category Ammonium Detoxicant; Hyperammonemia Agent; Urea Cycle Disorder (UCD) Treatment Agent

Generic Available No

Use Adjunct to treatment of acute hyperammonemia and encephalopathy in patients with urea cycle disorders involving partial or complete deficiencies of carbamylphosphate synthetase (CPS), ornithine transcarbamoylase (OTC), argininosuccinate lyase (ASL), or argininosuccinate synthetase (ASS); for use with hemodialysis in acute neonatal hyperammonemic coma, moderate-to-severe hyperammonemic encephalopathy and hyperammonemia which fails to respond to initial therapy

Pregnancy Risk Factor C

Pregnancy Considerations In animal studies, phenylacetate was shown to cause neurological toxicity. Reproduction studies have not been conducted with this combination.

Lactation Excretion in breast milk unknown/use caution

Contraindications Hypersensitivity to sodium phenylacetate, sodium benzoate, or any component of the formulation

Warnings Severity of hyperammonemia may require hemodialysis, as well as nutritional management and medical support; due to enhanced potassium excretion, monitor potassium level closely; potential tissue extravasant which may result in skin necrosis, administer only through central I.V. line. Repeat loading doses are not indicated due to prolonged plasma levels noted in pharmacokinetic studies.

Precautions Due to high sodium content use with caution in patients with congestive heart failure, renal or hepatic dysfunction, or sodium retention associated with edema; maintain caloric intake at 80 cal/kg/day

Adverse Reactions Patients ≤30 days of age reported more blood, lymphatic system, and vascular disorders; patients >30 days of age reported more gastrointestinal disorders.

Cardiovascular: Hypotension, edema, cardiac arrest, cardiomyopathy, chest pain, hypertension

Central nervous system: Fever, agitation, coma, acute psychosis, confusion, hallucinations, ataxia, intracranial pressure increased

Dermatologic: Pruritus, maculo-papular rash, urticaria, hemangioma

Endocrine & metabolic: Hyperglycemia, hypoglycemia, hypokalemia, hyperammonemia, metabolic acidosis, hypocalcemia, hypernatremia

Gastrointestinal: Vomiting, diarrhea, nausea, GI hemorrhage

Genitourinary: Urinary tract infection, urinary retention, renal failure, anuria

Hematologic: Anemia, DIC, thrombocytopenia, thrombosis, pancytopenia

Hepatic: Hepatotoxicity, jaundice, cholestasis

Local: Injection site reaction, extravasation, skin necrosis

Neuromuscular & skeletal: Areflexia, weakness, tremor, clonus

Ophthalmic: Blindness

Respiratory: Respiratory distress, dyspnea, ARDS, pneumonia, pulmonary edema, pulmonary hemorrhage, hyperventilation, pneumothorax

Drug Interactions

Avoid Concomitant Use There are no known interactions where it is recommended to avoid concomitant use.

Increased Effect/Toxicity

The levels/effects of Sodium Phenylacetate and Sodium Benzoate may be increased by: Probenecid

Decreased Effect There are no known significant interactions involving a decrease in effect.

Stability Prior to dilution, store at room temperature of 25°C (77°F). Following dilution in D₁₀W, solution for infusion may be stored at room temperature for up to 24 hours. Stable when mixed with arginine HCl 10% injection

Mechanism of Action Sodium phenylacetate and sodium benzoate provide alternate pathways for the removal of ammonia through the formation of their metabolites. One mole of sodium phenylacetate removes two moles of nitrogen; one mole of sodium benzoate removes one mole of nitrogen.

Pharmacokinetics (Adult data unless noted)

Metabolism: Hepatic and renal; sodium phenylacetate conjugates with glutamine, forming the active metabolite, phenylacetylglutamine (PAG); sodium benzoate combines with glycine to form the active metabolite hippuric acid (HIP)

Excretion: Urine

Usual Dosage IV: Administer as a loading dose over 90-120 minutes, followed by an equivalent dose as a maintenance infusion over 24 hours. Arginine HCl is administered concomitantly. Dosage based on weight and specific enzyme deficiency; therapy should continue until ammonia levels are in normal range. Do not repeat loading dose.

Infants and Children ≤20 kg:

CPS and OTC deficiency: Ammonul® 2.5 mL/kg and arginine 10% 2 mL/kg (provides sodium phenylacetate 250 mg/kg, sodium benzoate 250 mg/kg, and arginine hydrochloride 200 mg/kg)

ASS and ASL deficiency: Ammonul® 2.5 mL/kg and arginine 10% 6 mL/kg (provides sodium phenylacetate 250 mg/kg, sodium benzoate 250 mg/kg, and arginine hydrochloride 600 mg/kg)

Note: Pending a specific diagnosis in infants, the bolus and maintenance dose of arginine should be 6 mL/kg. If ASS or ASL are excluded as diagnostic possibilities, reduce dose of arginine to 2 mL/kg/day.

Children >20 kg:

CPS and OTC deficiency: Ammonul® 55 mL/m^2 and arginine 10% 2 mL/kg (provides sodium phenylacetate 5.5 g/m^2, sodium benzoate 5.5 g/m^2, and arginine hydrochloride 200 mg/kg)

ASS and ASL deficiency: Ammonul® 55 mL/m^2 and arginine 10% 6 mL/kg (provides sodium phenylacetate 5.5 g/m^2, sodium benzoate 5.5 g/m^2, and arginine hydrochloride 600 mg/kg)

Dosage adjustment in renal impairment: Use with caution; monitor closely

Dialysis: Ammonia clearance is ~10 times greater with hemodialysis than by peritoneal dialysis or hemofiltration. Exchange transfusion is ineffective.

Dosage adjustment in hepatic impairment: Use with caution

Administration I.V.: Must be administered via central line; administration via peripheral line may cause burns. Dilute in D$_{10}$W at ≥25 mL/kg prior to administration. May mix with arginine HCl. In case of extravasation, discontinue infusion and resume at new injection site.

Monitoring Parameters Neurologic status, plasma ammonia, plasma glutamine, clinical response, serum electrolytes (potassium or bicarbonate supplementation may be required), acid-base balance, infusion site

Reference Range Long-term target levels (may not be appropriate for every patient):

Plasma ammonia: <40 µmol/L

Plasma glutamine: <1000 µmol/L

Normal plasma levels of alanine, glycine, lysine, arginine (except in arginase deficiency); normal urinary orotate excretion; normal plasma protein concentration

Nursing Implications Extravasation may cause skin necrosis; administer through central line only. Treatment of extravasation may include aspiration of residual mediation from catheter, limb elevation, intermittent cooling with cold packs. Due to its lingering odor, exercise care in mixing to minimize contact with skin and clothing.

Additional Information Ucephan® (sodium phenylacetate and sodium benzoate), was previously available as an oral liquid for chronic treatment of urea cycle disorders. Although no longer commercially available, this combination may be compounded for patients not responsive to or tolerant of other treatments.

Dosage Forms Excipient information presented when available (limited, particularly for generics); consult specific product labeling.

Injection, solution [concentrate]:

Ammonul®: Sodium phenylacetate 100 mg and sodium benzoate 100 mg per 1 mL (50 mL)

References

Batshaw ML, MacArthur RB, and Tuchman M, "Alternative Pathway Therapy for Urea Cycle Disorders: Twenty Years Later," *J Pediatr*, 2001, 138(1 Suppl):46-54.

Berry GT and Steiner RD, "Long-Term Management of Patients With Urea Cycle Disorders," *J Pediatr*, 2001, 138(1 Suppl):56-60.

Brusilow SW, Danney M, Waber LJ, et al, "Treatment of Episodic Hyperammonemia in Children With Inborn Errors of Urea Synthesis," *N Engl J Med*, 1984, 310(25):1630-4.

"Consensus Statement From a Conference for the Management of Patients With Urea Cycle Disorders. Urea Cycle Disorders Conference Group," *J Pediatr*, 2001, 138(1 Suppl):1-5.

Gutteridge C and Kuhn RJ, "Compatibility of 10% Sodium Benzoate Plus 10% Sodium Phenylacetate With Various Flavored Vehicles," *Am J Hosp Pharm*, 1994, 51(19):2508, 2510.

Sodium Phenylbutyrate

(SOW dee um fen il BYOO ti rate)

U.S. Brand Names Buphenyl®

Therapeutic Category Ammonium Detoxicant; Hyperammonemia Agent; Urea Cycle Disorder (UCD) Treatment Agent

Generic Available No

Use Adjunctive therapy in the chronic management of patients with urea cycle disorder involving deficiencies of carbamoylphosphate synthetase, ornithine transcarbamylase, or argininosuccinic acid synthetase; provides an alternative pathway for waste nitrogen excretion

Pregnancy Risk Factor C

Pregnancy Considerations Animal reproduction studies have not been conducted.

Lactation Excretion in breast milk unknown/use caution

Contraindications Hypersensitivity to phenylbutyrate, or any component; patients with severe hypertension, heart failure or renal dysfunction; **phenylbutyrate is not indicated in the treatment of acute hyperammonemia**

Precautions Use cautiously in patients with renal or hepatic dysfunction and in patients who must maintain a low sodium diet as each gram of drug contains 125 mg sodium

Adverse Reactions

Cardiovascular: Edema, arrhythmias, syncope

Central nervous system: Headache, depression

Dermatologic: Rash

Endocrine & metabolic: Amenorrhea, menstrual dysfunction, acidosis, alkalosis, hyperchloremia, hyperuricemia, hypokalemia, hypernatremia, hyperphosphatemia, weight gain

Gastrointestinal: Anorexia, abnormal taste, abdominal pain, nausea, vomiting, gastritis; rare: peptic ulcer, rectal bleeding, pancreatitis

Hematologic: Anemia, leukopenia, leukocytosis, thrombocytopenia, aplastic anemia

Hepatic: Hypoalbuminemia, liver enzymes elevated, bilirubin elevated

Renal: Renal tubular acidosis

Miscellaneous: Offensive body odor

Drug Interactions

Avoid Concomitant Use There are no known interactions where it is recommended to avoid concomitant use.

Increased Effect/Toxicity There are no known significant interactions involving an increase in effect.

Decreased Effect There are no known significant interactions involving a decrease in effect.

Food Interactions Avoid mixing with acidic-type beverages (eg, colas, lemonade, grape juice) since drug may precipitate

Stability Store at room temperature (59°F to 86°F); after opening, containers should be kept tightly closed

Mechanism of Action Sodium phenylbutyrate is a prodrug that, when given orally, is rapidly converted to phenylacetate. Phenylacetate is conjugated with glutamine to form the active compound phenylacetyglutamine. Phenylacetyglutamine serves as a substitute for urea and is excreted in the urine carrying with it 2 moles nitrogen (equivalent to urea) per mole of phenylacetyglutamine thus assisting in the clearance of nitrogenous waste in patients with urea cycle disorders.

Pharmacokinetics (Adult data unless noted)
Distribution: V_d: 0.2 L/kg

Metabolism: conjugation to phenylacetylglutamine (active form); undergoes nonlinear Michaelis-Menten elimination kinetics

Half-life: 0.8 hours (parent compound); 1.2 hours (phenylacetate)

Time to peak serum concentration:

Powder: 1 hour

Tablet: 1.35 hours

Elimination: 80% of metabolite excreted in urine in 24 hours

Usual Dosage Oral:
Neonates, Infants, and Children <20 kg: 450-600 mg/kg/day divided 4-6 times daily; maximum daily dose: 20 g/day

Children >20 kg and Adults: 9.9-13 g/m^2/day, divided four to six times daily; maximum daily dose 20 g/day

Administration Oral: Administer with meals or feedings; mix powder with food or drink; avoid mixing with acidic beverages (eg, most fruit juices or colas)

Monitoring Parameters Plasma ammonia and glutamine concentrations, serum electrolytes, proteins, hepatic and renal function tests, physical signs/symptoms of hyperammonemia (ie, lethargy, ataxia, confusion, vomiting, seizures, and memory impairment)

Patient Information It is important to follow the dietary restrictions required when treating this disorder, the medication must be taken in strict accordance with the prescribed regimen; avoid altering the dosage without the prescriber's knowledge; the powder formulation has a very salty taste

Additional Information Teaspoon and tablespoon measuring devices are provided with the powder; each 1 g powder contains 0.94 g sodium phenylbutyrate = 125 mg sodium; each tablet contains 0.5 g sodium phenylbutyrate = 62 mg sodium

Dosage Forms Excipient information presented when available (limited, particularly for generics); consult specific product labeling.

Powder, for oral solution:

Buphenyl®: 3 g/level teaspoon (250 g) [contains sodium 125 mg/g; packaged with measuring devices]

Tablet:

Buphenyl®: 500 mg [contains sodium 124 mg/g]

References
Batshaw ML, MacArthur RB, and Tuchman M, "Alternative Pathway Therapy for Urea Cycle Disorders: Twenty Years Later," *J Pediatr*, 2001, 138(1 Suppl):S46-S55.

Berry GT and Steiner RD, "Long-Term Management of Patients With Urea Cycle Disorders," *J Pediatr*, 2001, 138(1 Suppl):S56-60.

Brusilow SW, "Phenylacetylglutamine May Replace Urea as a Vehicle for Waste Nitrogen Excretion," *Pediatr Res*, 1991, 29(2):147-50.

Maestri NE, Brusilow SW, Clissold DB, et al, "Long-Term Treatment of Girls With Ornithine Transcarbamylase Deficiency," *N Engl J Med*, 1996, 335(12):855-9.

Sodium Phosphate (SOW dee um FOS fates)

Medication Safety Issues
Sound-alike/look-alike issues:

Visicol® may be confused with Asacol®, VESIcare®

Enemas and oral solution are available in pediatric and adult sizes; prescribe by "volume" not by "bottle."

Safe Prescribing: Because inorganic phosphate exists as monobasic and dibasic anions, with the mixture of valences dependent on pH, ordering by mEq amounts is unreliable and may lead to large dosing errors. In addition, I.V. phosphate is available in the sodium and potassium salt; therefore, the content of these cations must be considered when ordering phosphate. The most reliable method of ordering I.V. phosphate is by millimoles, then specifying the potassium or sodium salt.

U.S. Brand Names Fleet® Enema Extra® [OTC]; Fleet® Enema [OTC]; Fleet® Pedia-Lax™ Enema [OTC]; Fleet® Phospho-soda® EZ-Prep™ [OTC] [DSC]; Fleet® Phospho-soda® [OTC] [DSC]; LaCrosse Complete [OTC]; OsmoPrep®; Visicol®

Canadian Brand Names Fleet Enema®

Therapeutic Category Electrolyte Supplement, Oral; Electrolyte Supplement, Parenteral; Laxative, Saline; Sodium Salt

Generic Available Yes: Enema, injection, oral solution

Use Treatment and prevention of hypophosphatemia; short-term treatment of constipation (oral/rectal); evacuation of the colon for rectal and bowel exams; source of phosphate in large volume I.V. fluids

Medication Guide An FDA-approved patient medication guide, which is available with the product information and as follows, must be dispensed with each new outpatient prescription and refill.

OsmoPrep®:http://www.fda.gov/downloads/Drugs/DrugSafety/UCM135936.pdf

Visicol®:http://www.fda.gov/downloads/Drugs/DrugSafety/UCM134684.pdf

Pregnancy Risk Factor C

Pregnancy Considerations Reproduction studies have not been conducted with these products. Use with caution in pregnant women.

Lactation Use caution in nursing women.

Breast-Feeding Considerations Phosphorus, sodium, and potassium are normal constituents of human milk.

Contraindications Hypersensitivity to phosphate (salts) or any component; hyperphosphatemia, hypocalcemia, hypomagnesemia, hypernatremia, severe renal impairment (Cl_{cr} <30 mL/minute), severe tissue trauma, heat cramps, abdominal pain (rectal forms), fecal impaction (rectal forms)

Warnings Administration of sodium phosphate products (OsmoPrep™, Visicol®, >45 mL/day oral sodium phosphate solution) as a bowel preparation in adults has been associated with significant fluid shifts, severe electrolyte abnormalities, and cardiac arrhythmias resulting in symptomatic dehydration, renal failure, metabolic acidosis, tetany, and death; fatalities have been observed in patients with renal insufficiency, bowel perforation, and in patients who misused or overdosed sodium phosphate products. Consider obtaining baseline and post-treatment electrolytes particularly in patients who may be at increased risk for serious adverse events, including patients with history of acute phosphate nephropathy, known or suspected electrolyte disorders, seizures, arrhythmias, cardiomyopathy, prolonged QT, or recent history of MI. Patients should be adequately hydrated before, during, and after use. Hypovolemia, kidney disease, bowel obstruction, acute colitis, increased age, and medications affecting renal perfusion or function such as diuretics, ACE inhibitors, ARBs, and NSAIDs have been associated with the development of renal failure and acute phosphate nephropathy in patients receiving sodium phosphate for colon cleansing; some cases have resulted in permanent renal impairment (some requiring dialysis). Acute phosphate nephropathy has also been reported in patients without apparent risk factors. Correct dehydration and avoid exceeding the maximum recommended doses and concurrent use of other laxatives containing sodium phosphate.

Precautions Use with considerable caution in patients with renal impairment, CHF, unstable angina, gastric retention, ileus, acute bowel obstruction, pseudo-obstruction of the bowel, severe chronic constipation, bowel perforation, acute colitis, toxic megacolon, gastric bypass or stapling surgery, hypomotility syndrome, and ascites; use with caution in patients with adrenal insufficiency, chronic inflammatory bowel disease, and cirrhosis. Some products contain phenylalanine; use with caution in patients with phenylketonuria.

Adverse Reactions Cardiovascular: Hypotension, cardiac arrhythmias, edema

Central nervous system: Mental confusion, seizures, dizziness, headache

Dermatologic: Rash, pruritus, urticaria

Endocrine & metabolic: Hyperphosphatemia, hypocalcemia, hypernatremia, hypomagnesemia, metabolic acidosis

Gastrointestinal: Nausea, vomiting, diarrhea, flatulence (oral use); colonic mucosal aphthous ulceration, abdominal bloating, and abdominal pain (oral forms); throat tightness, pharyngeal edema, dysphagia

Local: Phlebitis (parenteral forms)

Neuromuscular & skeletal: Paresthesia, bone and joint pain, arthralgia, weakness, muscle cramps, tetany

Renal: Acute renal failure, nephrocalcinosis, acute phosphate nephropathy

Respiratory: Bronchospasm, dyspnea

Miscellaneous: Hypersensitivity reactions including anaphylaxis, lip and facial swelling

Clinical manifestations of hypophosphatemia by systems:

Neuromuscular: Muscle weakness, anorexia, tremor, paresthesia, convulsions, coma, hyporeflexia, irritability, numbness, abnormal EEG, cardiomyopathy, respiratory failure, inability to wean from ventilator

Hematologic: Rhabdomyolysis, hemolytic anemia, oxygen release decreased, chemotaxis decreased, phagocytosis decreased, platelet survival decreased, myoglobinuria, thrombocytopenia

Skeletal: Osteomalacia, joint arthralgias, pathologic fractures

Drug Interactions

Avoid Concomitant Use There are no known interactions where it is recommended to avoid concomitant use.

Increased Effect/Toxicity

The levels/effects of Sodium Phosphates may be increased by: Bisphosphonate Derivatives

Decreased Effect

The levels/effects of Sodium Phosphates may be decreased by: Antacids; Calcium Salts; Iron Salts; Magnesium Salts; Sucralfate

Food Interactions

Avoid giving with oxalate (ie, berries, nuts, chocolate, beans, celery, tomatoes) or phytate-containing foods (ie, bran, whole wheat).

Stability Store at room temperature; phosphate salts may precipitate when mixed with calcium salts; solubility is improved in parenteral nutrition solutions which contain amino acids; check with a pharmacist to determine compatibility

Mechanism of Action Phosphorus is an essential mineral that is usually found in nature combined with oxygen as phosphate. It participates in bone deposition, calcium metabolism, as part of molecules that regulate many coenzymes, steps in the clotting cascade, and functions of the immune system. It is a component of the lipid bilayer of cell membranes in the form of phospholipids and of other intracellular compounds like nucleic acids and nucleoproteins. It acts as a buffer for the maintenance of plasma and urinary pH. When administered orally or rectally as a laxative, it exerts osmotic effect in the small intestine by drawing water into the lumen of the gut, producing distension, promoting peristalsis, and evacuation of the bowel.

Pharmacodynamics Onset of action (catharsis):

Oral: 3-6 hours

Rectal: 2-5 minutes

Pharmacokinetics (Adult data unless noted)

Absorption: Oral: 1% to 20%

Elimination: Oral forms excreted in feces; I.V. forms are excreted in the urine with over 80% to 90% of dose reabsorbed by the kidney

Usual Dosage Note: Consider the contribution of sodium when determining the appropriate phosphate replacement. Phosphorus: Oral: See table.

Phosphorus − Recommended Daily Allowance (RDA) and Estimated Average Requirement (EAR)

Age	RDA (mmol/day)	EAR (mmol/day)
0-6 mo	–	3.2[1]
7-12 mo	–	8.9[1]
1-3 y	14.8	12.3
4-8 y	16.1	13.1
9-18 y	40.3	34
19-30 y	22.6	18.7

[1]Adequate intake (AI)

Hypophosphatemia: Hypophosphatemia does not necessarily equate with phosphate depletion. Hypophosphatemia may occur in the presence of low, normal, or high total body phosphate and conversely, phosphate depletion may exist with normal, low, or elevated levels of serum phosphate (Gaasbeek, 2005). It is difficult to provide concrete guidelines for the treatment of severe hypophosphatemia because the extent of total body deficits and response to therapy are difficult to predict. Aggressive doses of phosphate may result in a transient serum elevation followed by redistribution into intracellular compartments or bone tissue. Various regimens for replacement of phosphate in adults have been studied. The regimens below have only been studied in adult patients; however, many institutions have used them in children safely and successfully.

I.V. doses may be incorporated into the patient's maintenance I.V. fluids; intermittent I.V. infusion should be reserved for severe depletion situations. **Note:** Doses listed as mmol of **phosphate** (see also Additional Information).

Intermittent I.V. infusion: It is recommended that repletion of severe hypophosphatemia be done I.V. because large doses of oral phosphate may cause diarrhea and intestinal absorption may be unreliable.

Children and Adults: **Note:** There are no prospective studies of parenteral phosphate replacement in children. The following weight-based guidelines for adult dosing may be cautiously employed in pediatric patients. Guidelines differ based on degree of illness, use of TPN, and severity of hypophosphatemia.

General replacement guidelines (Lentz, 1978): **Note:** The initial dose may be increased by 25% to 50% if the patient is symptomatic secondary to hypophosphatemia and lowered by 25% to 50% if the patient is hypercalcemic.

Low dose: 0.08 mmol/kg over 6 hours; use if losses are recent and uncomplicated

Intermediate dose: 0.16-0.24 mmol/kg over 4-6 hours; use if serum phosphorus level 0.5-1 mg/dL (0.16-0.32 mmol/L)

High dose: 0.36 mmol/kg over 6 hours; use if serum phosphorus <0.5 mg/dL (<0.16 mmol/L)

Patients receiving TPN (Clark, 1995):

Low dose: 0.16 mmol/kg over 4-6 hours; use if serum phosphorus level 2.3-3 mg/dL (0.73- 0.96 mmol/L)

Intermediate dose: 0.32 mmol/kg over 4-6 hours; use if serum phosphorus level 1.6-2.2 mg/dL (0.51-0.72 mmol/L)

High dose: 0.64 mmol/kg over 8-12 hours; use if serum phosphorus <1.5 mg/dL (< 0.5 mmol/L)

Critically ill adult trauma patients receiving TPN (Brown, 2006):

Low dose: 0.32 mmol/kg over 4-6 hours; use if serum phosphorus level 2.3-3 mg/dL (0.73-0.96 mmol/L)

Intermediate dose: 0.64 mmol/kg over 4-6 hours; use if serum phosphorus level 1.6-2.2 mg/dL (0.51-0.72 mmol/L)

High dose: 1 mmol/kg over 8-12 hours; use if serum phosphorus <1.5 mg/dL (< 0.5 mmol/L)

Alternative method in critically ill patients (Kingston, 1985):

Low dose: 0.25 mmol/kg over 4 hours; use if serum phosphorus level 0.5-1 mg/dL (0.16-0.32 mmol/L)

Moderate dose: 0.5 mmol/kg over 4 hours; use if serum phosphorus level <0.5 mg/dL (<0.16 mmol/L)

Adults: 15 mmol/dose over 2 hours; use if serum phosphorus <2 mg/dL (0.65 mmol/L); may repeat in 6- to 8-hour intervals if repeat serum phosphorus (at least 6 hours postdose) <2 mg/dL (0.65 mmol/L); not to exceed 45 mmol/24 hours (Rosen, 1995)

Maintenance:

I.V.:

Neonates: 0.8-1.5 mmol/kg/day

Infants and Children <25 kg: 0.5-1.5 mmol/kg/day

Children 25-45 kg: 0.5-1 mmol/kg/day

Oral: 2-3 mmol/kg/day in divided doses (including dietary intake: See Additional Information)

Adults:

I.V.: 50-70 mmol/day

Oral: 50-150 mmol/day in divided doses (including dietary intake; see Additional Information)

Laxative:

Oral:

Fleet® Phospho-Soda®: Oral:

Children 5-9 years: 5 mL as a single dose

Children 10-12 years: 10 mL as a single dose

Children ≥12 years and Adults: 20-30 mL as a single dose

Visicol®: Oral: Must be administered with a full glass of water

Children 5-9 years: 2-4 tablets (~0.9-1.8 g dibasic sodium phosphate and 2.4-4.8 g monobasic sodium phosphate) daily as a single dose

Children 10-11 years: 4-9 tablets (~1.8-3.6 g dibasic sodium phosphate and 4.8-9.6 g monobasic sodium phosphate) daily as a single dose

Children ≥12 years and Adults: 9-20 tablets (~3.6-8.1 g dibasic sodium phosphate and 9.6-21.6 g monobasic sodium phosphate) daily as a single dose

Evacuation of colon prior to colonoscopy: Adults ≥18 years: Administer each 4 tablets with 8 ounces of water:

OsmoPrep™: Prior to colonoscopy per manufacturer: The night before the procedure: 4 tablets every 15 minutes until a total dose of 20 tablets; repeat starting 3-5 hours before the procedure with 4 tablets every 15 minutes for a total of 12 tablets

Visicol®: Prior to colonoscopy per manufacturer: The night before the procedure: 4 tablets every 15 minutes until a total dose of 20 tablets; repeat 3-5 hours before the procedure with 4 tablets every 15 minutes until a total dose of 40 tablets has been administered

Rectal: Fleet® Enema:

Children 2-11 years: Contents of one 2.25 oz pediatric enema as a single dose, may repeat

Children ≥12 years and Adults: Contents of one 4.5 oz enema as a single dose, may repeat

Administration

Oral: Administer with food to reduce the risk of diarrhea; contents of 1 packet should be diluted in 75 mL water before administration; administer tablets with a full glass of water; maintain adequate fluid intake; dilute oral solution with an equal volume of cool water. Products used as preparation for colonoscopy (OsmoPrep™, Visicol®) should be administered with at least 8 ounces water for each dose.

Parenteral: For intermittent I.V. infusion: Peripheral line: Dilute to a maximum concentration of 0.05 mmol/mL; Central line: Dilute to a maximum concentration of 0.12 mmol/mL (maximum concentrations were determined with consideration for maximum sodium concentration); maximum rate of infusion: 0.06 mmol/kg/hour; do **not** infuse with calcium-containing I.V. fluids

Monitoring Parameters

Serum sodium, calcium, phosphorus, renal function, reflexes, stool output (laxative use)

Reference Range Note: There is a diurnal variation with the nadir at 1100, plateau at 1600, and peak in the early evening (Gaasbeek, 2005); 1 mmol/L phosphate = 3.1 mg/dL phosphorus

Newborns: 4.2-9 mg/dL phosphorus (1.36-2.91 mmol/L phosphate)

6 weeks to 18 months: 3.8-6.7 mg/dL phosphorus (1.23-2.16 mmol/L phosphate)

18 months to 3 years: 2.9-5.9 mg/dL phosphorus (0.94-1.91 mmol/L phosphate)

3-15 years: 3.6-5.6 mg/dL phosphorus (1.16-1.81 mmol/L phosphate)

>15 years: 2.5-5 mg/dL phosphorus (0.81-1.62 mmol/L phosphate)

Hypophosphatemia:

Moderate: 1-2 mg/dL phosphorus (0.32-0.65 mmol/L phosphate)

Severe: <1 mg/dL phosphorus (<0.32 mmol/L phosphate)

Additional Information Each mmol of phosphate contains 31 mg elemental phosphorus; 1 mmol/L phosphate = 3.1 mg/dL phosphorus; cow's milk is a good source of phosphate with 1 mg elemental (0.032 mmol) elemental phosphate per mL

With orders for I.V. phosphate, there is considerable confusion associated with the use of millimoles (mmol) versus milliequivalents (mEq) to express the phosphate requirement. Because inorganic phosphate exists as monobasic and dibasic anions, with the mixture of valences dependent on pH, ordering by mEq amounts is unreliable and may lead to large dosing errors. In addition, I.V. phosphate is available in the sodium and potassium salt; therefore, the content of these cations must be considered when ordering phosphate. The most reliable method of ordering I.V. phosphate is by millimoles, then specifying the potassium or sodium salt.

Dosage Forms Excipient information presented when available (limited, particularly for generics); consult specific product labeling. [DSC] = Discontinued product

Kit [packaged as a two-dose kit which contains]:

Fleet® Phospho-soda® EZ-Prep™ [DSC]:

Solution, oral: Monobasic sodium phosphate monohydrate 2.4 g and dibasic sodium phosphate heptahydrate 0.9 g per 5 mL (30 mL) [sugar-free; contains sodium 556 mg/5 mL and phosphate 62.25 mEq/5 mL; packaged with lemonade flavor packets which contain phenylalanine]

Solution, oral: Monobasic sodium phosphate monohydrate 2.4 g and dibasic sodium phosphate heptahydrate 0.9 g per 5 mL (45 mL) [sugar-free; contains sodium 556 mg/5 mL and phosphate 62.25 mEq/5mL; packaged with lemonade flavor packets which contain phenylalanine]

Injection, solution [concentrate; preservative free]: Phosphorus 3 mmol and sodium 4 mEq per 1 mL (5 mL, 15 mL, 50 mL) [equivalent to phosphorus 93 mg and sodium 92 mg per 1 mL; source of electrolytes; monobasic and dibasic sodium phosphate]

Solution, oral: Monobasic sodium phosphate monohydrate 2.4 g and dibasic sodium phosphate heptahydrate 0.9 g per 5 mL (45 mL)

Fleet® Phospho-soda®: Monobasic sodium phosphate monohydrate 2.4 g and dibasic sodium phosphate heptahydrate 0.9 g per 5 mL (45 mL) [sugar free; contains sodium 556 mg/5 mL, sodium benzoate, and phosphate 62.25 mEq/5 mL; unflavored or ginger-lemon flavor] [DSC]

Solution, rectal [enema]: Monobasic sodium phosphate monohydrate 19 g and dibasic sodium phosphate heptahydrate 7 g per 118 mL delivered dose (133 mL)

Fleet® Enema: Monobasic sodium phosphate monohydrate 19 g and dibasic sodium phosphate heptahydrate 7 g per 118 mL delivered dose (133 mL) [contains sodium 4.4 g/118 mL]

Fleet® Enema Extra®: Monobasic sodium phosphate monohydrate 19 g and dibasic sodium phosphate heptahydrate 7 g per 197 mL delivered dose (230 mL) [contains sodium 4.4 g/197 mL]

Fleet® Pedia-Lax™ Enema: Monobasic sodium phosphate monohydrate 9.5 g and dibasic sodium phosphate heptahydrate 3.5 g per 59 mL delivered dose (66 mL) [contains sodium 2.2 g/59 mL]

LaCrosse Complete: Monobasic sodium phosphate monohydrate 19 g and dibasic sodium phosphate heptahydrate 7 g per 118 mL delivered dose (133 mL) [contains sodium 4.4 g/118 mL]

Tablet, oral [scored]:

OsmoPrep®, Visicol®: Monobasic sodium phosphate monohydrate 1.102 g and dibasic sodium phosphate anhydrous 0.398 g [sodium phosphate 1.5 g per tablet; gluten free]

References

Brown KA, Dickerson RN, Morgan LM, et al, "A New Graduated Dosing Regimen for Phosphorus Replacement in Patients Receiving Nutrition Support," *JPEN*, 2006, 30(3):209-14.

Clark CL, Sacks GS, Dickerson RN, et al, "Treatment of Hypophosphatemia in Patients Receiving Specialized Nutrition Support Using a Graduated Dosing Scheme: Results From a Prospective Clinical Trial," *Crit Care Med*, 1995, 23(9):1504-11.

"Dietary Reference Intakes for Calcium, Phosphorus, Magnesium, Vitamin D, and Fluoride. Standing Committee on the Scientific Evaluation of Dietary Reference Intakes, Food and Nutrition Board, Institute of Medicine," National Academy of Sciences, Washington, DC: National Academy Press, 1997.

Gaasbeek A and Meinders AE, "Hypophosphatemia: An Update on Its Etiology and Treatment", *Am J Med*, 2005, 118(10):1094-101.

Kingston M and Al-Siba'i MB, "Treatment of Severe Hypophosphatemia," *Crit Care Med*, 1985, 13(1):16-8

Lentz RD, Brown BM, and Kjellstrand CM, "Treatment of Severe Hypophosphatemia," *Ann Intern Med*, 1978, 89(6):941-4.

Lloyd CW and Johnson CE, "Management of Hypophosphatemia," *Clin Pharm*, 1988, 7(2):123-8.

Rosen GH, Boullata JI, O'Rangers EA, et al, "Intravenous Phosphate Repletion Regimen for Critically Ill Patients With Moderate Hypophosphatemia," *Crit Care Med*, 1995, 23(7):1204-10.

◆ **Sodium Phosphate and Potassium Phosphate** *see* Potassium Phosphate and Sodium Phosphate *on page 1143*

Sodium Polystyrene Sulfonate
(SOW dee um pol ee STYE reen SUL fon ate)

Medication Safety Issues

Sound-alike/look-alike issues:

Kayexalate® may be confused with Kaopectate®

Sodium polystyrene sulfonate may be confused with calcium polystyrene sulfonate

Always prescribe either one-time doses or as a specific number of doses (eg, 15 g q6h x 2 doses). Scheduled doses with no dosage limit could be given for days leading to dangerous hypokalemia.

International issues:

Kionex™ may be confused with Kinex® which is a brand name for biperiden in Mexico

U.S. Brand Names Kalexate; Kayexalate®; Kionex®; SPS®

Canadian Brand Names Kayexalate®; PMS-Sodium Polystyrene Sulfonate

Therapeutic Category Antidote, Hyperkalemia

Generic Available No

Use Treatment of hyperkalemia

Pregnancy Risk Factor C

Lactation Excretion in breast milk unknown/use caution

Contraindications Hypersensitivity to sodium polystyrene sulfonate or any component; hypernatremia; hypokalemia; intestinal obstruction or perforation (oral use)

Warnings Treatment with this drug alone may be insufficient to rapidly correct severe hyperkalemia; other more rapidly effective appropriate measures should be used; enema will reduce the serum potassium faster than oral administration, but the oral route will result in a greater reduction over several hours; systemic alkalosis has been reported when administered in conjunction with non-absorbable cation-donating antacids and laxatives such as magnesium hydroxide and aluminum carbonate. Intestinal obstructions due to concretions of aluminum hydroxide have been reported when administered with sodium polystyrene sulfonate.

Precautions Use with caution in patients with severe CHF, hypertension, or edema; small amounts of magnesium and calcium may also be lost in binding

Adverse Reactions

Endocrine & metabolic: Hypokalemia, hypocalcemia, hypomagnesemia, hypernatremia

Gastrointestinal: Anorexia, nausea, vomiting, constipation, intestinal colonic necrosis (rare), diarrhea

Drug Interactions

Avoid Concomitant Use

Avoid concomitant use of Sodium Polystyrene Sulfonate with any of the following: Laxatives; Sorbitol

Increased Effect/Toxicity

Sodium Polystyrene Sulfonate may increase the levels/effects of: Aluminum Hydroxide; Antacids; Digoxin; Laxatives; Sorbitol

Decreased Effect

Sodium Polystyrene Sulfonate may decrease the levels/effects of: Lithium; Thyroid Products

Food Interactions Never mix in orange juice

Stability Store at room temperature; suspensions made from powder should be freshly prepared and used within 24 hours of preparation

Mechanism of Action Removes potassium by exchanging sodium ions for potassium ions in the intestine before the resin is passed from the body

Pharmacodynamics Onset of action: Within 2-24 hours

Pharmacokinetics (Adult data unless noted) Elimination: Remains in the GI tract to be completely excreted in the feces (primarily as potassium polystyrene sulfonate)

Usual Dosage

Children:
Oral: 1 g/kg/dose every 6 hours
Rectal: 1 g/kg/dose every 2-6 hours
Adults:
Oral: 15 g 1-4 times/day
Rectal: 30-50 g every 6 hours

Administration

Oral or NG: Shake commercially available suspension well before use; when using powder, dilute in 3-4 mL fluid per g of resin; 10% sorbitol, water, or syrup may be used as diluent

Enema: Shake commercially available suspension well before use; when using powder, dilute in water or 25% sorbitol at a concentration of 0.3-0.5 g/mL; retain enema in colon for at least 30-60 minutes or several hours, if possible

Monitoring Parameters Serum sodium, potassium, calcium, magnesium, ECG (if applicable)

Additional Information 1 g of resin binds ~1 mEq of potassium; 4.1 mEq sodium per g of powder; 1 level teaspoon contains 3.5 g polystyrene sulfonate

Dosage Forms Excipient information presented when available (limited, particularly for generics); consult specific product labeling.

Powder for suspension, oral/rectal:
Kalexate: 15 g/4 level teaspoons (454 g) [contains sodium 100 mg (4.1 mEq)/g]
Kayexalate®: 15 g/4 level teaspoons (480 g) [contains sodium 100 mg (4.1 mEq)/g]
Kionex®: 15 g/4 level teaspoons (454 g) [contains sodium 100 mg (4.1 mEq)/g]
Suspension, oral/rectal:
SPS®: 15 g/60 mL (60 mL, 120 mL, 480 mL) [contains alcohol 0.3%, sodium 1500 mg (65 mEq)/60 mL, propylene glycol, and sorbitol; cherry flavor]

◆ **Sodium Sulamyd (Can)** see Sulfacetamide on page 1298

◆ **Sodium Sulfacetamide** see Sulfacetamide on page 1298

Sodium Thiosulfate (SOW dee um thye oh SUL fate)

U.S. Brand Names Versiclear™

Therapeutic Category Antidote, Cisplatin; Antidote, Cyanide; Antidote, Extravasation; Antifungal Agent, Topical

Generic Available Yes: Injection

Use

Parenteral: Used alone or with sodium nitrite or amyl nitrite in cyanide poisoning; treatment of cyanide poisoning due to nitroprusside; reduce the risk of nephrotoxicity associated with cisplatin therapy; local infiltration (in diluted form) of selected chemotherapy extravasation

Topical: Treatment of tinea versicolor, acne

Pregnancy Risk Factor C

Pregnancy Considerations Safety has not been established in pregnant women. Use only when potential benefit to the mother outweighs the possible risk to the fetus.

Contraindications Hypersensitivity to sodium thiosulfate or any component

Precautions Discontinue if irritation or sensitivity occurs; rapid I.V. infusion has caused transient hypotension and ECG changes in dogs

Fire victims may present with both cyanide and carbon monoxide poisoning. In this scenario, sodium thiosulfate may be used alone to promote the clearance of cyanide; however, it does have a slow onset of action.

Adverse Reactions

Cardiovascular: Hypotension (infusion rate-dependent)
Dermatologic: Contact dermatitis, local irritation

Gastrointestinal: Nausea, vomiting
Miscellaneous: Hypersensitivity reactions

Drug Interactions

Avoid Concomitant Use There are no known interactions where it is recommended to avoid concomitant use.

Increased Effect/Toxicity There are no known significant interactions involving an increase in effect.

Decreased Effect There are no known significant interactions involving a decrease in effect.

Stability Store at 15°C to 30°C (59°F to 86°F); stable diluted in NS, D_5W, or $D_5^{1/2}NS$ at concentrations of 1.5% and 9.76% sodium thiosulfate for 24 hours (Redkar, 1986)

Mechanism of Action

Cyanide toxidity: Accelerates the clearance of cyanide via the rhodanase-catalyzed detoxification of cyanide to thiocyanate (much less toxic than cyanide). The accelerated action of rhodanase is a result of the exogenous sulfur provided by sodium thiosulfate.

Prevention of cisplatin nephrotoxicity: Complexes with cisplatin to form a compound that is nontoxic to either normal or cancerous cells

Pharmacokinetics (Adult data unless noted)

Half-life, elimination: 0.65 hours
Elimination: 28.5% excreted unchanged in the urine

Usual Dosage

Cyanide and nitroprusside antidote: I.V.: See Usual Dosage in Sodium Nitrite, Sodium Thiosulfate, and Amyl Nitrite on page 1273

Prevention of cisplatin nephrotoxicity: Adults: I.V.: 12 g over 6 hours in association with cisplatin **or** 9 g/m² I.V. bolus then 1.2 g/m²/hour for 6 hours; should be administered before or during cisplatin administration

Chemotherapy infiltration: Children and Adults: Dilute 10% sodium thiosulfate 4-8 mL with 6 mL SWI to make 1/6 to 1/3 molar solution; as local infiltration for the following chemotherapy agents:
Mechlorethamine: Use 2 mL for each mg infiltrated
Cisplatin: 1/6 (~4%) molar solution: Inject into the affected area; various volumes have also been suggested for direct injection into existing I.V. line; however, the optimal volume and efficacy of such practices have not been thoroughly evaluated. **Note:** Use only for large cisplatin infiltrates (>20 mL) and cisplatin concentrations >0.5 mg/mL.

Topical use (antifungal, acne): Children and Adults: 25% solution: Apply thin film twice daily to affected areas for several weeks to months

Administration

Parenteral: I.V.: Inject slowly, over at least 10 minutes; rapid administration may cause hypotension

Topical: Do not apply topically to or near eyes; thoroughly cleanse and dry affects areas prior to application

Dosage Forms Excipient information presented when available (limited, particularly for generics); consult specific product labeling.

Injection, solution [preservative free]: 100 mg/mL (10 mL); 250 mg/mL (50 mL)

Lotion: Sodium thiosulfate 25% and salicylic acid 1% (120 mL) [contains isopropyl alcohol 10%]

References

Berlin CM Jr, "The Treatment of Cyanide Poisoning in Children," Pediatrics, 1970, 46(5):793-6.
Bertelli G, "Prevention and Management of Extravasation of Cytotoxic Drugs," Drug Saf, 1995, 12(4):245-55.
Dorr RT, "Antidotes to Vesicant Chemotherapy Extravasations," Blood Rev, 1990, 4(1):41-60.
Ener RA, Meglathery SB, and Styler M, "Extravasation of Systemic Hemato-Oncological Therapies," Ann Oncol, 2004, 15(6):858-62.
Geller RJ, Barthold C, Saiers JA, et al, "Pediatric Cyanide Poisoning: Causes, Manifestations, Management, and Unmet Needs," Pediatrics, 2006, 118(5):2146-58.
Hall AH, Dart R, and Bogdan G, "Sodium Thiosulfate or Hydroxocobalamin for the Empiric Treatment of Cyanide Poisoning?" Ann Emerg Med, 2007, 49(6):806-13.

Naughton M, "Acute Cyanide Poisoning," *Anaesth Intensive Care,* 1974, 2(4):351-6.

Redkar S and Dave N, "Stability of Sodium Thiosulfate Injection Solutions in Different Diluents," Technical Information, Skin-T-Gens International Inc, Canoga Park, CA, 1986.

◆ **Sodium Thiosulfate, Sodium Nitrite, and Amyl Nitrite** *see* Sodium Nitrite, Sodium Thiosulfate, and Amyl Nitrite *on page 1273*

◆ **Sodium Thiosulphate** *see* Sodium Thiosulfate *on page 1280*

◆ **Soflax™ (Can)** *see* Docusate *on page 468*

◆ **Solaraze®** *see* Diclofenac *on page 429*

◆ **Solarcaine® Aloe Extra Burn Relief [OTC] [DSC]** *see* Lidocaine *on page 818*

◆ **Solarcaine® cool aloe Burn Relief [OTC]** *see* Lidocaine *on page 818*

◆ **Solodyn®** *see* Minocycline *on page 933*

◆ **Solu-Cortef®** *see* Hydrocortisone *on page 685*

◆ **Solugel® (Can)** *see* Benzoyl Peroxide *on page 184*

◆ **Solumedrol** *see* MethylPREDNISolone *on page 912*

◆ **Solu-Medrol®** *see* MethylPREDNISolone *on page 912*

◆ **Soluver® (Can)** *see* Salicylic Acid *on page 1241*

◆ **Soluver® Plus (Can)** *see* Salicylic Acid *on page 1241*

Somatropin (soe ma TROE pin)

Medication Safety Issues
Sound-alike/look-alike issues:
Humatrope® may be confused with homatropine
Somatrem may be confused with somatropin
Somatropin may be confused with homatropine, somatrem, sumatriptan

International issues:
Genotropin® may be confused with Genatropine® which is a brand name for atropine in France

U.S. Brand Names Genotropin Miniquick®; Genotropin®; Humatrope®; Norditropin NordiFlex®; Norditropin®; Norditropin® FlexPro®; Nutropin AQ®; Nutropin®; Omnitrope®; Saizen®; Serostim®; Tev-Tropin®; Zorbtive®

Canadian Brand Names Humatrope®; Nutropin®; Nutropin® AQ; Omnitrope®; Saizen®; Serostim®

Therapeutic Category Growth Hormone

Generic Available No

Use
Children: Long-term treatment of growth failure as a result of lack or inadequate endogenous growth hormone secretion (FDA approved in children and adults), Prader-Willi syndrome, birth at small for gestational age (SGA) with failure to catch-up growth by 2-4 years of age (FDA approved in ages >2 years); chronic renal insufficiency (up until the time of renal transplantation) (FDA approved in children); short stature associated with Turner syndrome (in patients whose epiphyses are not closed) (FDA approved in children), Noonan syndrome or short stature homeobox gene (SHOX) deficiency (FDA approved in children); idiopathic short stature (also known as nongrowth hormone-deficient short stature) defined by height more than 2.25 standard deviations below the mean for age and sex (FDA approved in children)

Adults: Growth hormone deficiency as a result of pituitary disease, hypothalamic disease, surgery, radiation, or trauma
Genotropin®, Norditropin®, Saizen®: Adults with growth hormone deficiency during childhood who have this deficiency confirmed as an adult prior to growth hormone replacement (FDA approved in adults)
Serostim®: Treatment of AIDS-related wasting or cachexia (FDA approved in adults)

Zorbtive™: Treatment of short-bowel syndrome (in conjunction with nutritional support) (FDA approved in adults)

Pregnancy Risk Factor B/C (depending upon manufacturer)

Pregnancy Considerations Teratogenic effects were not observed in animal studies. Reproduction studies have not been conducted with all agents. During normal pregnancy, maternal production of endogenous growth hormone decreases as placental growth hormone production increases. Data with somatropin use during pregnancy is limited.

Lactation Excretion in breast milk unknown/use caution

Contraindications Hypersensitivity to human growth hormone or any component (see Warnings); patients with Prader-Willi syndrome who are severely obese or have severe respiratory impairment; do not use for growth promotion in pediatric patients with closed epiphyses; patients with acute critical illness due to complications following open heart or abdominal surgery, multiple accidental trauma, or acute respiratory failure; patients with active neoplasia, patients with proliferative or preproliferative diabetic retinopathy

Warnings Fatalities in pediatric patients with Prader-Willi syndrome following the use of growth hormone have been reported; these fatalities occurred in patients with one or more risk factors, including severe obesity, sleep apnea, respiratory impairment, or unidentified respiratory infection. In addition, male patients may be at increased risk. Treatment interruption is recommended in patients who show signs of upper airway obstruction, including the onset of or increased snoring. In addition, evaluation of and/or monitoring for sleep apnea and respiratory infections are recommended. 35% of childhood-onset adult GH-deficient subjects treated with growth hormone 0.025 mg/kg/day for 2 years had supraphysiologic levels of insulin-like growth factor-1 (IGF-1) identified during research studies, the risks of this elevation are unknown at this time; the manufacturer recommends reduction in dosage if IGF-1 levels are excessive.

Diluents for Nutropin®, Saizen®, and Zorbtive™ contain benzyl alcohol which may cause allergic reactions in susceptible individuals; large amounts of benzyl alcohol (≥99 mg/kg/day) have been associated with a potentially fatal toxicity ("gasping syndrome") in neonates; the "gasping syndrome" consists of metabolic acidosis, respiratory distress, gasping respirations, CNS dysfunction (including convulsions, intracranial hemorrhage), hypotension and cardiovascular collapse; *in vitro* and animal studies have shown that benzoate, a metabolite of benzyl alcohol, displaces bilirubin from protein-binding sites; avoid use of benzyl alcohol containing diluents in neonates.

Intracranial hypertension with papilledema, visual changes, headache, nausea, and/or vomiting has been reported; this has occurred during the first 8 weeks of therapy; all reported cases were reversible upon discontinuation of therapy; baseline and regular fundoscopic exams are recommended for assistance in recognizing this potential adverse effect.

Precautions Use with caution in patients with diabetes or family history of diabetes; use with caution in patients with evidence of active malignancy, progression of any underlying intracranial lesion, or actively growing intracranial tumor; monitor these patients closely for progression or recurrence of the underlying disease process; insulin dosage may require adjustment when growth hormone therapy is instituted; patients with hypopituitarism may develop hypothyroidism during growth hormone therapy; children may develop slipped capital epiphyses during therapy; progression of scoliosis may occur in patients with a history of scoliosis

Adverse Reactions

Cardiovascular: Hypertension, mild transient edema

Central nervous system: Headache, insomnia, intracranial hypertension; Zorbtive™: Dizziness, fever, malaise

Dermatologic: Growth of pre-existing nevi increased, rash; local lipoatrophy or lipodystrophy (SubQ administration); Zorbtive™: Swelling of hands and feet; Saizen®: Exacerbation of pre-existing psoriasis

Endocrine & metabolic: Mild hyperglycemia, reversible hypothyroidism (reported in pituitary-derived growth hormone); gynecomastia (rare), hyperlipidemia

Gastrointestinal: Pancreatitis (rare); Zorbtive™: Abdominal pain, flatulence, gastritis, gastroenteritis, nausea, pharyngitis, vomiting

Hematologic: Small risk for developing leukemia

Local: Pain at injection site

Neuromuscular & skeletal: Carpal tunnel syndrome (rare); pain in hip, knee, and back; scoliosis; myalgia, weakness; Saizen® and Zorbtive™: Arthralgia, musculoskeletal pain, stiffness, swelling

Otic: Otitis media

Renal: Glucosuria

Respiratory: Rhinitis

Miscellaneous: Flu-like syndrome, hypersensitivity reactions

Drug Interactions

Avoid Concomitant Use There are no known interactions where it is recommended to avoid concomitant use.

Increased Effect/Toxicity There are no known significant interactions involving an increase in effect.

Decreased Effect

Somatropin may decrease the levels/effects of: Antidiabetic Agents; Cortisone; PredniSONE

The levels/effects of Somatropin may be decreased by: Estrogen Derivatives

Stability For long-term storage, refrigerate all products except Zorbtive™, do not freeze; Zorbtive™ is stable at room temperature prior to reconstitution; once reconstituted with diluents containing preservatives and refrigerated, Humatrope®, Nutropin®, Saizen®, Tev-Tropin™, and Zorbtive™ are stable for 14 days, Genotropin® is stable for 21 days, and Humotrope® cartridges are stable for 28 days; Nutropin® AQ (aqueous form) is stable for 28 days after initial entry; Nutropin Depot® must be used immediately after reconstitution. Genotropin MiniQuick® is stable prior to reconstitution for up to 3 months at room temperature. If diluents without preservatives are used, stability is 24 hours refrigerated. Zorbtive™ should be used immediately after reconstitution. After a Norditropen® cartridge has been inserted into the NordiPen® injector, it is stable (in the pen) refrigerated for 4 weeks. Humatrope® cartridges may only be reconstituted with provided diluent; do not substitute with diluent provided with Humatrope® multiuse vials.

Mechanism of Action Somatropin and somatrem are purified polypeptide hormones of recombinant DNA origin; somatropin contains the identical sequence of amino acids found in human growth hormone while somatrem's amino acid sequence is identical plus an additional amino acid, methionine; human growth hormone stimulates growth of linear bone, skeletal muscle, and organs; stimulates erythropoietin which increases red blood cell mass; exerts both insulin-like and diabetogenic effects; in short-bowel syndrome, growth hormone may directly stimulate receptors in the intestinal mucosa or indirectly stimulate the production of insulin-like growth factor-I which is known to mediate many of the cellular actions of growth hormone

Pharmacokinetics (Adult data unless noted)

Absorption: I.M., SubQ: Well absorbed

Distribution: V_d:

Somatrem: 50 mL/kg

Somatropin: 70 mL/kg

Metabolism: ~90% of dose metabolized in the liver and kidney cells

Bioavailability:

SubQ:

Somatrem: 81% ± 20%

Somatropin: 75%

I.M.: Somatropin: 63%

Half-life:

SubQ:

Somatrem: 2.3 ± 0.42 hours

Somatropin: 3.8 hours

I.M.: Somatropin: 4.9 hours

Elimination: 0.1% of dose excreted in urine unchanged

Usual Dosage

I.M., SubQ (preferred route); not for I.V. injection: **Note:** Human growth hormone therapy should be individualized; discontinue therapy when the patient has reached satisfactory adult height, when epiphyses have fused, or when the patient ceases to respond. Growth ≥5 cm/year is expected, if growth rate does not exceed 2.5 cm in a 6-month period, double the dose for the next 6 months, if there is still no satisfactory response, discontinue therapy.

Growth hormone inadequacy:

Children: Somatropin:

Genotropin®, Omnitrope®: 0.16-0.24 mg/kg **weekly** divided into daily doses (6-7 doses)

Humatrope®: 0.18-0.3 mg/kg (0.54-0.9 international units/kg) **weekly** divided into equal doses 6-7 days/week

Norditropin®: 0.024-0.034 mg/kg/dose (0.07-0.1 international units/kg/dose) 6-7 times per week

Nutropin®, Nutropin® AQ: 0.3 mg/kg (0.9 international units/kg) **weekly** divided into daily doses; in pubertal patients, dosage may be increased to 0.7 mg/kg (2.1 international units/kg) **weekly** divided into daily doses

Saizen®: 0.18 mg/kg weekly (0.54 international units/kg) divided 3 times per week

Tev-Tropin™: 0.3 mg/kg (0.9 international units/kg) divided 3 times per week

Nutropin® Depot™: SubQ only:

Once-monthly injection: 1.5 mg/kg body weight administered on the same day of each month; patients >15 kg will require more than one injection per dose

Twice-monthly injection: 0.75 mg/kg body weight administered twice each month on the same days of each month (eg, days 1 and 15 of each month); patients >30 kg will require more than one injection per dose; twice monthly dosing is recommended in patients >45 kg

Adults: **Note:** To minimize adverse events in older or overweight patients, reduced dosages may be necessary. During therapy, dosage should be decreased if required by the occurrence of side effects or excessive IGF-1 levels.

Weight-based dosing:

Norditropin®: SubQ: Initial dose ≤0.028 mg/kg weekly divided into equal doses 7 days/week; after 6 weeks of therapy, may increase dose to 0.112 mg/kg weekly divided into equal doses 7 days/week

Nutropin®, Nutropin® AQ: SubQ: ≤0.006 mg/kg/day; dose may be increased according to individual requirements, up to a maximum of 0.025 mg/kg/day in patients <35 years of age, or up to a maximum of 0.0125 mg/kg/day in patients ≥35 years of age

Humatrope®: SubQ: ≤0.006 mg/kg/day; dose may be increased according to individual requirements, up to a maximum of 0.0125 mg/kg/day

Genotropin®, Omnitrope®: SubQ: Weekly dosage: ≤0.04 mg/kg divided into 6-7 doses; dose may be increased at 4- to 8-week intervals according to individual requirements, to a maximum of 0.08 mg/kg/week

Saizen®: SubQ: ≤0.005 mg/kg/day; dose may be increased to not more than 0.01 mg/kg/day after 4 weeks, based on individual requirements.

Nonweight-based dosing: Initial: 0.2 mg/day (range: 0.15-0.3 mg/day); may increase every 1-2 months by 0.1-0.2 mg/day based on response and/or serum IGF-I levels

Dosage adjustment with estrogen supplementation (growth hormone deficiency): Larger doses of somatropin may be needed for women taking oral estrogen replacement products; dosing not affected by topical products

Idiopathic short stature: Children:

Genotropin®: 0.47 mg/kg **weekly** divided into equal doses 6-7 days/week

Humatrope®: 0.37 mg/kg **weekly** divided into daily doses (6-7 doses)

Nutropin®, Nutropin® AQ: Up to 0.3 mg/kg **weekly** divided into daily doses

Chronic renal insufficiency: Children: Nutropin®, Nutropin® AQ: 0.35 mg/kg **weekly** divided into daily injections; continue until the time of renal transplantation

Dosage recommendations in patients treated for CRI who require dialysis:

Hemodialysis: Administer dose at night prior to bedtime or at least 3-4 hours after hemodialysis to prevent hematoma formation from heparin

CCPD: Administer dose in the morning following dialysis

CAPD: Administer dose in the evening at the time of overnight exchange

Prader-Willi syndrome: Children: Genotropin®: 0.24 mg/kg **weekly** divided daily into 6-7 doses per week

Children SGA at birth:

Genotropin®: 0.48 mg/kg **weekly** divided daily into 6-7 doses per week

Humatrope®: SubQ: Weekly dosage: 0.47 mg/kg divided into equal doses 6-7 days/week

Norditropin®: SubQ: Up to 0.469 mg/kg weekly divided into equal doses 7 days/week

Alternate dosing (small for gestational age): In older/early pubertal children or children with very short stature, consider initiating therapy at higher doses (0.469 mg/kg weekly divided into equal doses 7 days/week) and then consider reducing the dose (0.231 mg/kg weekly) if substantial catch-up growth observed. In younger children (<4 years) with less severe short stature, consider initiating therapy with lower doses (0.231 mg/kg weekly) and then titrating the dose upwards as needed.

Turner syndrome: Children:

Genotropin®: Weekly dosage 0.33 mg/kg divided into 6-7 doses/week

Humatrope®: Weekly dosage: 0.375 mg/kg divided into equal doses 6-7 days/week

Nutropin®, Nutropin® AQ: Weekly dosage of up to 0.375 mg/kg divided into equal doses 3-7 times/week

AIDS-related wasting or cachexia: Serostim®:

Children (limited information): 0.04-0.07 mg/kg/day for 4 weeks

Adults: Administered once daily at bedtime:

<35 kg: 0.1 mg/kg

35-44 kg: 4 mg

45-55 kg: 5 mg

>55 kg: 6 mg

Short-bowel syndrome: Adults: Zorbtive™: SubQ: 0.1 mg/kg daily not to exceed 8 mg/day; treatment >4 weeks has not been studied adequately. Excessive fluid retention or arthralgias may be treated symptomatically or by a 50% dosage reduction; stop therapy for up to 5 days prior to lowering dosage if symptoms are severe; if symptoms do not resolve after 5 days or recur with the lowered dosage, discontinue treatment.

Administration Parenteral: Administer SubQ (preferred route) or I.M.; not for I.V. injection; do not shake vial; rotate injection site; administer into the thigh, buttock, or abdomen; limit SubQ injection volume to 1 mL per site; Somatropin:

Genotropin® cartridges: Reconstitute with provided diluent resulting in the following concentrations: 1.5 mg cartridge = 1.3 mg/mL (4 international units/mL), 5.8 mg cartridge = 5 mg/mL (15 international units/mL), and 13.8 mg cartridge = 12 mg/mL (36 international units/mL)

Nutropin®: Reconstitute each 5 mg vial with 1.5-5 mL diluent

Norditropin® Cartridges: Must be used with the NordiPen® injection pen (each cartridge has a color-coded injection pen which is graduated to deliver the appropriate dose); do not interchange

Nutropin® Depot™: Reconstitute vials with provided diluent only, resulting in 19 mg/mL concentration; swirl vigorously for 2 minutes until all the powder is fully dispersed; withdraw measured dose, change to a new needle, and administer immediately to avoid settling of the suspension in the syringe; inject SubQ at a continuous rate over no more than 5 seconds

Saizen®: Reconstitute 5 mg vial with 1-3 mL provided diluent and 8.8 mg vial with 2-3 mL provided diluent (diluent contains benzyl alcohol); swirl vial with gentle rotary motion; do not shake

Tev-Tropin™: Reconstitute with 1-5 mL NS (bacteriostatic NS is provided; NS without preservative may be used in neonates); swirl gently; do not shake. Cloudiness may occur when stored in the refrigerator after reconstitution. Allow solution to warm to room temperature. If cloudiness persists, do not use.

Zorbtive™: Reconstitute each 4 mg, 5 mg, or 6 mg vial with 0.5 mL or 1 mL preservative free SWI; reconstitute 8.8 mg vial with 1 mL or 2 mL diluent (contains benzyl alcohol)

Note: When treating chronic renal insufficiency patients, growth hormone should be administered as follows: in hemodialysis patients, administer injection at night just prior to sleeping and at least 3-4 hours after dialysis; in chronic cycling peritoneal dialysis patients, administer injection in the morning after dialysis; in chronic ambulatory peritoneal dialysis patients administer injection in the evening at the time of the overnight exchange.

Monitoring Parameters Growth curve, periodic thyroid function tests, bone age (annually), periodical urine testing for glucose, somatomedin C levels; fundoscopic exams (see Warnings); progression of scoliosis and clinical evidence of slipped capital femoral epiphysis such as a limp or hip or knee pain

Patient Information Report the development of a severe headache, acute visual changes, a limp or complaints of hip or knee pain to your physician

Additional Information SubQ administration can cause local lipoatrophy or lipodystrophy and may enhance the development of neutralizing antibodies

Dosage Forms Excipient information presented when available (limited, particularly for generics); consult specific product labeling. [DSC] = Discontinued product

Injection, powder for reconstitution [rDNA origin]:

Genotropin®: 5.8 mg [~15 int. units/mL; delivers 5 mg/mL; contains m-cresol]; 13.8 mg [~36 int. units/mL; delivers 12 mg/mL; contains m-cresol]

Genotropin Miniquick® [preservative free]: 0.2 mg, 0.4 mg, 0.6 mg, 0.8 mg, 1 mg, 1.2 mg, 1.4 mg, 1.6 mg, 1.8 mg, 2 mg [each strength delivers 0.25 mL]

Humatrope®: 5 mg [15 int. units], 6 mg [18 int. units], 12 mg [36 int. units], 24 mg [72 int. units]

Nutropin®: 5 mg [~15 int. units; packaged with diluent containing benzyl alcohol]; 10 mg [~30 int. units; packaged with diluent containing benzyl alcohol]

Omnitrope®: 5.8 mg [~17.4 int. units; packaged with diluent containing benzyl alcohol]

Saizen®: 5 mg [~15 int. units; contains sucrose 34.2 mg; packaged with diluent containing benzyl alcohol]; 8.8 mg [~26.4 int. units; contains sucrose 60.2 mg; packaged with diluent containing benzyl alcohol]

Serostim®: 4 mg [~12 int. units; contains sucrose 27.3 mg; packaged with diluent containing benzyl alcohol; 5 mg [~15 int. units; contains sucrose 34.2 mg]; 6 mg [~18 int. units; contains sucrose 41 mg]; 8.8 mg [DSC] [~26.4 int. units; contains sucrose 60.19 mg; packaged with diluent containing benzyl alcohol]

Tev-Tropin®: 5 mg [15 int. units/mL; packaged with diluent containing benzyl alcohol]

Zorbtive®: 8.8 mg [~26.4 int. units; contains sucrose 60.19 mg; packaged with diluent containing benzyl alcohol]

Injection, solution [rDNA origin]:

Norditropin®: 5 mg/1.5 mL (1.5 mL); 15 mg/1.5 mL (1.5 mL)

Norditropin® FlexPro®: 5 mg/1.5 mL (1.5 mL); 10 mg/1.5 mL (1.5 mL); 15 mg/1.5 mL (1.5 mL)

Norditropin NordiFlex®: 5 mg/1.5 mL (1.5 mL); 10 mg/1.5 mL (1.5 mL); 15 mg/1.5 mL (1.5 mL); 30 mg/3 mL (3 mL)

Nutropin AQ®: 5 mg/mL (2 mL) [~15 int. units/mL]

Omnitrope®: 5 mg/1.5 mL (1.5 mL); 10 mg/1.5 mL (1.5 mL)

References

Cohen P, Rogol AD, Deal CL, et al, "Consensus Statement on the Diagnosis and Treatment of Children With Idiopathic Short Stature: A Summary of the Growth Hormone Research Society, the Lawson Wilkins Pediatric Endocrine Society, and the European Society for Paediatric Endocrinology Workshop," *J Clin Endocrinol Metab*, 2008, 93(11):4210-7.

Gharib H, Cook DM, Saenger PH, et al, "American Association of Clinical Endocrinologists Medical Guidelines for Clinical Practice for Growth Hormone Use in Adults and Children - 2003 Update," *Endocr Pract*, 2003, 9(1):64-76.

Howrie DL, "Growth Hormone for the Treatment of Growth Failure in Children," *Clin Pharm*, 1987, 6(4):283-91.

Molitch ME, Clemmons DR, Malozowski S, et al, "Evaluation and Treatment of Adult Growth Hormone Deficiency: An Endocrine Society Clinical Practice Guideline," *J Clin Endocrinol Metab*, 2006, 91(5):1621-34.

◆ **Sominex® [OTC]** see DiphenhydrAMINE *on page 448*

◆ **Sominex® Maximum Strength [OTC]** see Diphenhydr-AMINE *on page 448*

◆ **Somnote®** see Chloral Hydrate *on page 286*

◆ **Som Pam (Can)** see Flurazepam *on page 604*

Sorbitol (SOR bi tole)

Therapeutic Category Laxative, Hyperosmolar; Laxative, Osmotic

Generic Available Yes

Use Humectant; sweetening agent; hyperosmotic laxative; facilitates the passage of sodium polystyrene sulfonate or a charcoal-toxin complex through the intestinal tract

Pregnancy Risk Factor C

Lactation Excretion in breast milk unknown

Contraindications Anuria

Adverse Reactions

Endocrine & metabolic: Fluid and electrolyte losses, lactic acidosis

Gastrointestinal: Diarrhea, abdominal distress, nausea, vomiting

Drug Interactions

Avoid Concomitant Use

Avoid concomitant use of Sorbitol with any of the following: Calcium Polystyrene Sulfonate; Sodium Polystyrene Sulfonate

Increased Effect/Toxicity

The levels/effects of Sorbitol may be increased by: Calcium Polystyrene Sulfonate; Sodium Polystyrene Sulfonate

Decreased Effect There are no known significant interactions involving a decrease in effect.

Mechanism of Action A polyalcoholic sugar with osmotic cathartic actions

Pharmacodynamics

Onset of action: Oral: Mean time to first stool in patients receiving a charcoal-sorbitol slurry:

Children (ingestions):

6.4 hours (dose: 1.5 g/kg in 4 patients)

8.48 hours (dose: 2 g/kg in 33 patients)

Adults:

Nonpoisoned volunteers: 1.6 hours (dose: 2 g/kg)

Ingestion: 7.2 hours (14 adults; dose not specified)

Pharmacokinetics (Adult data unless noted)

Absorption: Oral, rectal: Poor

Metabolism: Mainly in the liver to fructose

Usual Dosage Hyperosmotic laxative (as single dose, at infrequent intervals):

Children 2-11 years:

Oral: 2 mL/kg (as 70% solution)

Rectal enema: 30-60 mL as 25% to 30% solution

Children ≥12 years and Adults:

Oral: 30-150 mL (as 70% solution)

Rectal enema: 120 mL as 25% to 30% solution

Adjunct to sodium polystyrene sulfonate: 15 mL as 70% solution orally until diarrhea occurs (10-20 mL/2 hours) or 20-100 mL as an oral vehicle for the sodium polystyrene sulfonate resin

When administered with charcoal: Oral:

Children: 4.3 mL/kg of 35% sorbitol with 1 g/kg of activated charcoal or maximum dose: 2 g/kg sorbitol with activated charcoal

Adults: 4.3 mL/kg of 70% sorbitol with 1 g/kg of activated charcoal

Monitoring Parameters Serum electrolytes, I & O

Dosage Forms Excipient information presented when available (limited, particularly for generics); consult specific product labeling.

Solution, genitourinary irrigation: 3% (3000 mL, 5000 mL); 3.3% (2000 mL, 4000 mL)

Solution, oral: 70% (30 mL, 480 mL, 3840 mL)

References

Charney EB and Bodurtha JN, "Intractable Diarrhea Associated With the Use of Sorbitol," *J Pediatr*, 1981, 98:157-8.

James LP, Nichols MH, and King WD, "A Comparison of Cathartics in Pediatric Ingestions," *Pediatrics*, 1995, 96(2 Pt 1):235-8.

Kumar A, Weatherly MR, and Beaman DC, "Sweeteners, Flavorings, and Dyes in Antibiotic Preparations," *Pediatrics*, 1991, 87(3):352-60.

◆ **Sorine®** see Sotalol *on page 1284*

Sotalol (SOE ta lol)

Medication Safety Issues

Sound-alike/look-alike issues:

Sotalol may be confused with Stadol®, Sudafed®

Betapace® may be confused with Betapace AF®

Betapace AF® may be confused with Betapace®

Related Information

Adult ACLS Algorithms *on page 1463*

U.S. Brand Names Betapace AF®; Betapace®; Sorine®

Canadian Brand Names Apo-Sotalol®; CO Sotalol; Dom-Sotalol; Med-Sotalol; Mylan-Sotalol; Novo-Sotalol; Nu-Sotalol; PHL-Sotalol; PMS-Sotalol; PRO-Sotalol; ratio-Sotalol; Rhoxal-sotalol; Riva-Sotalol; Rylosol; Sandoz-Sotalol; ZYM-Sotalol

Therapeutic Category Antiarrhythmic Agent, Class II; Antiarrhythmic Agent, Class III; Beta-Adrenergic Blocker

Generic Available Yes

Use

Betapace®, Sorine®, generic: Treatment of life-threatening ventricular arrhythmias (eg, sustained ventricular tachycardia) (Betapace®: FDA approved in ages ≥3 days and adults; Sorine®, generic: FDA approved in adults)

Betapace AF®: Maintenance of normal sinus rhythm in patients who have highly symptomatic atrial fibrillation and atrial flutter, but who are currently in normal sinus rhythm [not usually for use in patients with paroxysmal atrial fibrillation/flutter that is easily reversed (eg, by Valsalva maneuver)] (FDA approved in ages ≥3 days and adults)

Note: Do not substitute Betapace AF® for other products (and vice versa); significant differences in FDA approved labeling exist [eg, dosage and administration, safety information and patient package insert (Betapace AF® labeling contains a patient package insert specific for atrial fibrillation/flutter)]

Injection: Substitution for oral sotalol in those who are unable to take sotalol orally (FDA approved in ages ≥3 years and adults)

Pregnancy Risk Factor B

Pregnancy Considerations Adverse events were not observed in the initial animal reproduction studies; therefore, the manufacturer classifies sotalol as pregnancy category B. Sotalol crosses the placenta and is found in amniotic fluid. In a cohort study, an increased risk of cardiovascular defects was observed following maternal use of beta-blockers during pregnancy. Intrauterine growth restriction (IUGR), small placentas, bradycardia, hypoglycemia, and/or respiratory depression have been observed in neonates following *in utero* exposure to nonselective beta-blockers at parturition; adequate facilities for monitoring infants at birth should be available. Because sotalol crosses the placenta in concentrations similar to the maternal serum, it has been used for the treatment of fetal atrial flutter or fetal supraventricular tachycardia without hydrops. The clearance of sotalol is increased during the third trimester of pregnancy, but other pharmacokinetic parameters do not significantly differ from nonpregnant values. Severe, untreated chronic hypertension during pregnancy may be associated with maternal and fetal adverse events; however, sotalol is currently not recommended for the initial treatment of hypertension in pregnancy. Also refer to the Propranolol monograph for additional information on a nonselective beta-blocking agent.

Lactation Enters breast milk/consider risk:benefit (AAP rates "compatible")

Breast-Feeding Considerations Sotalol is excreted into breast milk in concentrations higher than those found in the maternal serum. Although adverse events in nursing infants have not been observed in case reports, close monitoring for bradycardia, hypotension, respiratory distress, and hypoglycemia is advised. According to the manufacturer, the decision to continue or discontinue breast-feeding during therapy should take into account the risk of exposure to the infant and the benefits of treatment to the mother. The AAP considers sotalol to be "usually compatible" with breast-feeding.

Contraindications Hypersensitivity to sotalol or any component; sinus bradycardia; second or third degree AV heart block (except in patients with a functioning artificial pacemaker); congenital or acquired long QT syndromes; uncontrolled heart failure; cardiogenic shock; asthma

Additional contraindications: Betapace AF® and the injectable formulation: Baseline QT_c interval >450 msec; bronchospastic conditions; Cl_{cr} <40 mL/minute; serum potassium <4 mEq/L; sick sinus syndrome (except in patients with a functioning artificial pacemaker)

Warnings Initiation, reinitiation, and dosage increases of sotalol must occur in a facility that can provide continuous ECG monitoring, recognition and treatment of life-threatening arrhythmias, and CPR **[U.S. Boxed Warning]** Patients must be monitored with continuous ECG for a minimum of 3 days (on their maintenance dose). Use with caution and adjust the dose in patients with renal impairment; creatinine clearance must be calculated prior to dosing.

May cause serious and life-threatening proarrhythmias [may cause or worsen ventricular arrhythmias (eg, sustained ventricular tachycardia, torsade de pointes, ventricular fibrillation)] **[U.S. Boxed Warning]**; risk factors for torsade de pointes include: Higher sotalol doses, presence of sustained VT, female gender, excessive prolongation of the QT_c interval, history of heart failure or cardiomegaly, decreased renal function, hypokalemia, hypomagnesemia, and bradycardia; monitor ECG for proarrhythmic effects; adjust dose to prevent QT prolongation; correct electrolyte imbalances (especially hypokalemia and hypomagnesemia) before initiating sotalol. Do not initiate I.V. therapy if baseline QT_c interval is >450 msec; if QT_c exceeds 500 msec during therapy, reduce the dose, prolong the infusion duration, or discontinue use **[U.S. Boxed Warning]**.

Bradycardia, heart block, or hypotension may occur. Use oral formulation only with extreme caution in patients with sick sinus syndrome; do not use I.V. product in patients with sick sinus syndrome unless functioning artificial pacemaker is present. May cause or worsen heart failure (use with caution in patients with compensated heart failure); use with caution and titrate dose carefully within the first 2 weeks post-MI (experience is limited); use with caution in patients with peripheral vascular disease (may aggravate arterial insufficiency). Concomitant use with other drugs that prolong the QT interval (eg, Class I and Class III antiarrhythmics, phenothiazines, tricyclic antidepressants, and certain oral macrolide and quinolone antibiotics) or prolong refractoriness (eg, disopyramide, quinidine, procainamide, and amiodarone) is not recommended (see Drug Interactions); Class I or Class III antiarrhythmic agents should be withheld for at least three half-lives prior to starting sotalol.

Exacerbation of angina, arrhythmias, and in some cases MI may occur following abrupt discontinuation of beta-blockers; avoid abrupt discontinuation, wean slowly, monitor for signs and symptoms of ischemia. Beta-blockers should generally be avoided in patients with bronchospastic disease; if administered, use the lowest possible dose and monitor patients carefully. Patients receiving beta-blockers, who have a history of anaphylactic reactions, may be more reactive to a repeated allergen challenge and may not be responsive to the usual epinephrine doses used to treat an allergic reaction. Beta-blockers may block hypoglycemia-induced tachycardia and blood pressure changes; use with caution in patients with diabetes mellitus. May mask signs of thyrotoxicosis. Use caution with anesthetic agents that decrease myocardial function.

Precautions Use with caution in patients receiving calcium channel blockers (see Drug Interactions).

Adverse Reactions Note: No data are currently available for I.V. sotalol; however, based on similar systemic exposure between I.V. and oral products, adverse reactions for I.V. route are expected to be similar to oral.

Cardiovascular: Abnormal ECG, bradycardia, chest pain, edema, heart block, heart failure, hypotension, palpitations, peripheral vascular disorders, proarrhythmias, QT interval prolongation, sinus pauses, syncope, torsade de pointes (see Warnings)

Central nervous system: Anxiety, confusion, depression, dizziness, fatigue, headache, insomnia, lightheadedness, mood change

Dermatologic: Rash

Endocrine & metabolic: Hyperglycemia in diabetic patients, sexual dysfunction, weight change

Gastrointestinal: Abdominal distention, abdominal pain, appetite disorder, diarrhea, dyspepsia, flatulence, nausea, vomiting

Hematologic: Bleeding

Neuromuscular & skeletal: Back pain, extremity pain, paresthesia, weakness

Ocular: Vision problems

Respiratory: Asthma, cough, dyspnea, upper respiratory tract problems

Miscellaneous: Sweating

<1%, postmarketing, and/or case reports: Alopecia, bronchiolitis obliterans with organized pneumonia, clouded sensorium, cold extremities, emotional lability, eosinophilia, fever, hyperlipidemia, incoordination, leukocytoclastic vasculitis, leukopenia, myalgia, paralysis, phlebitis, photosensitivity reaction, pruritus, pulmonary edema, Raynaud's phenomenon, red crusted skin, retroperitoneal fibrosis, serum transaminases increased, skin necrosis after extravasation, thrombocytopenia, vertigo, xerostomia

Drug Interactions

Avoid Concomitant Use

Avoid concomitant use of Sotalol with any of the following: Artemether; Dronedarone; Lumefantrine; Methacholine; Nilotinib; Pimozide; QuiNINE; Tetrabenazine; Thioridazine; Ziprasidone

Increased Effect/Toxicity

Sotalol may increase the levels/effects of: Alpha-/Beta-Agonists (Direct-Acting); Alpha1-Blockers; Alpha2-Agonists; Amifostine; Antihypertensives; Antipsychotic Agents (Phenothiazines); Bupivacaine; Cardiac Glycosides; Dronedarone; Hypotensive Agents; Insulin; Lidocaine; Lidocaine (Systemic); Lidocaine (Topical); Mepivacaine; Methacholine; Midodrine; Pimozide; QTc-Prolonging Agents; QuiNINE; RiTUXimab; Sulfonylureas; Tetrabenazine; Thioridazine; Ziprasidone

The levels/effects of Sotalol may be increased by: Acetylcholinesterase Inhibitors; Alfuzosin; Aminoquinolines (Antimalarial); Amiodarone; Anilidopiperidine Opioids; Antipsychotic Agents (Phenothiazines); Artemether; Calcium Channel Blockers (Nondihydropyridine); Chloroquine; Ciprofloxacin; Ciprofloxacin (Systemic); Diazoxide; Dipyridamole; Disopyramide; Dronedarone; Gadobutrol; Herbs (Hypotensive Properties); Lumefantrine; MAO Inhibitors; Nilotinib; Pentoxifylline; Phosphodiesterase 5 Inhibitors; Propafenone; Propoxyphene; Prostacyclin Analogues; QuiNIDine; QuiNINE; Reserpine; Selective Serotonin Reuptake Inhibitors

Decreased Effect

Sotalol may decrease the levels/effects of: Beta2-Agonists; Theophylline Derivatives

The levels/effects of Sotalol may be decreased by: Barbiturates; Herbs (Hypertensive Properties); Methylphenidate; Nonsteroidal Anti-Inflammatory Agents; Rifamycin Derivatives; Yohimbine

Food Interactions Food decreases oral absorption by ~20% compared to fasting

Stability

Tablets and injection: Store at controlled room temperature 25°C (77°F); excursions permitted to 15°C to 30°C (59°F to 86°F)

Tablets: Dispense in tight, light-resistant container

Injection: Protect from light; do not freeze. Stable in D_5W, NS, or lactated ringers.

Mechanism of Action Beta-blocker with both class II antiarrhythmic (beta-adrenergic blockade) and class III antiarrhythmic (prolongation of the cardiac action potential duration) properties; does not possess partial agonist or membrane stabilizing activity. Class II effects: Nonselective beta-blockade; competitively blocks response to $beta_1$- and $beta_2$-adrenergic stimulation; decreases heart rate and AV nodal conduction; increases AV nodal refractoriness. Class III effects: Prolongs atrial and ventricular monophasic action potentials; prolongs the effective refractory period of atrial muscle, ventricular muscle, and AV accessory pathways (if present) in both antegrade and retrograde directions. Significant beta-blocking effects may be seen at lower doses (children: ≥90 mg/m^2/day; adults: 25 mg); class III electrophysiologic effects are seen at higher doses (children: 210 mg/m^2/day; adults: ≥160 mg/day). Sotalol is available as a racemic mixture; both isomers (d- and l-sotalol) have similar class III antiarrhythmic effects; the l-isomer is responsible for almost all of the beta-adrenergic blocking activity

Pharmacokinetics (Adult data unless noted)

Distribution: Poor penetration across blood-brain barrier; distributes into breast milk; breast milk to plasma ratio: 2.2-8.8 (mean: 5.4) (O'Hare, 1980)

Protein binding: Sotalol is not protein bound

Metabolism: Sotalol is not metabolized

Bioavailability: Oral: 90% to 100%

Half-life (mean):

Neonates ≤1 month: 8.4 hours

Infants and children >1 month to 24 months: 7.4 hours

Children >2 years to <7 years: 9.1 hours

Children 7-12 years: 9.2 hours

Adults: 12 hours

Adults with renal failure (anuric): Up to 69 hours

Time to peak serum concentration: Oral:

Children 4 days to 12 years: Mean: 2-3 hours

Adults: 2.5-4 hours

Elimination: Primarily as unchanged drug via the kidney

Clearance (apparent):

Neonates ≤1 month: 11 mL/minute

Infants and children >1 month to 24 months: 32 mL/minute

Children >2 years to <7 years: 63 mL/minute

Children 7-12 years: 95 mL/minute

Dialysis: Partially removed by hemodialysis; partial rebound in serum concentrations may occur following dialysis

Usual Dosage

Oral: **Note:** Baseline QT$_c$ interval and Cl$_{cr}$ must be determined prior to initiation. Dosage must be adjusted to individual response and tolerance; doses should be initiated or increased in a hospital facility that can provide continuous ECG monitoring, recognition and treatment of life-threatening arrhythmias, and CPR (see Warnings):

Neonates, Infants, and Children: **Note:** Safety and efficacy in pediatric patients have not been established; manufacturer's dosing recommendations are based on doses per m^2 (that are equivalent to the doses recommended in adults) and on pediatric pharmacokinetic and pharmacodynamic studies (see Saul, 2001 and Saul, 2001a). BSA, rather than body weight, better predicted apparent clearance of sotalol; however, for a given dose per m^2, a larger drug exposure (larger AUC) and greater pharmacologic effects were observed in smaller subjects (ie, those with BSA <0.33 m^2 versus those with BSA ≥0.33 m^2). For infants and children ≤2 years of age, the manufacturer recommends a dosage reduction based on an age factor determined from a graph (see graph on next page).

Manufacturer's recommendations: **Note:** Use with extreme caution if QT_c is >500 msec while receiving sotalol; reduce the dose or discontinue drug if QT_c >550 msec.

Neonates, infants, and children ≤2 years: The pediatric dosage listed below must be reduced by an age-related factor that is obtained from the graph (see graph). First, obtain the patient's age in months; use the graph to determine where the patient's age (on the logarithmic scale) intersects the age factor curve; read the age factor from the Y-axis; then multiply the age factor by the pediatric dose listed below (ie, the dose for children >2 years); this will result in the proper reduction in dose for age. For example, the age factor for an infant 1 month of age is 0.68, so the initial dosage would be (0.68 x 30 mg/ m^2/dose) = 20 mg/m^2/dose given 3 times daily. Similar calculations should be made for dosage titrations; increase dosage gradually, if needed; allow adequate time between dosage increments to achieve new steady-state and to monitor clinical response, heart rate and QT_c intervals; half-life is prolonged with decreasing age (<2 years), so time to reach new steady-state will increase; for example, the time to reach steady-state in a neonate may be ≥1 week

Sotalol Age Factor Nomogram for Patients ≤2 Years of Age

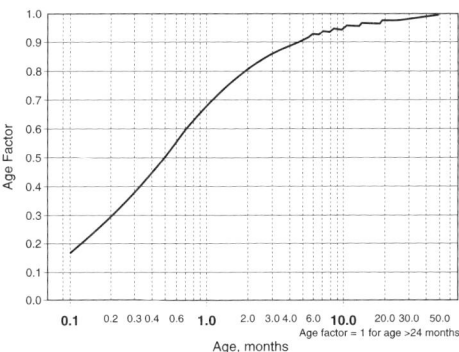

Age, months

Adapted from U.S. Food and Drug Administration.
http://www.fda.gov/cder/foi/label/2001/2115s3lbl.PDF

Children >2 years: Initial: 30 mg/m^2/dose given 3 times daily; increase dosage gradually if needed; allow at least 36 hours between dosage increments to achieve new steady-state and to monitor clinical response, heart rate, and QT_c intervals; may increase gradually to a maximum of 60 mg/m^2/dose given 3 times daily

Alternative pediatric dosing:

Initial: 2 mg/kg/day divided every 8 hours; if needed, increase dosage gradually by 1-2 mg/kg/day increments; allow 3 days between dosage increments to achieve new steady-state and to monitor clinical response, heart rate, and QT_c intervals; maximum: 10 mg/kg/day (if no limiting side effects occur) (see Beaufort-Krol, 1997; Colloridi, 1992; Läer, 2005; Maragnes, 1992; Pfammatter, 1995; Pfammatter, 1997; Tipple, 1991); do not exceed adult doses

Proposed required doses: **Note:** It is not necessary to increase to required dosage if desired clinical effect has been achieved at a lower dosage.

Neonates: 4 mg/kg/day divided every 8 hours

Infants and children 1 month to 6 years: 6 mg/kg/day divided every 8 hours

Children >6 years: 4 mg/kg/day divided every 8 hours

Adults:

Ventricular arrhythmias (Betapace®, Sorine®, generic) (**Note:** Use with extreme caution if QT_c is >500 msec while receiving sotalol; reduce the dose or discontinue drug if QT_c >550 msec): Initial: 80 mg twice daily; increase dosage gradually if needed; allow 3 days between dosage increments to achieve new steady-state and to determine maximum effects on QT interval; may increase gradually to 240-320 mg/day in 2 divided doses; usual effective dose: 160-320 mg/day given in 2-3 divided doses; **Note:** Doses as high as 480-640 mg/day may be required in some patients with life-threatening refractory ventricular arrhythmias; however, potential benefit must outweigh increased risk of adverse effects (eg, proarrhythmias).

Atrial fibrillation or atrial flutter (Betapace AF®): [**Note:** If baseline QT interval is >450 msec, do not initiate therapy (see Contraindications). During initiation and dose titration, if the QT interval is ≥500 msec, reduce the dose or discontinue the drug. During maintenance therapy, monitor the QT interval regularly; if the QT interval is ≥520 msec, reduce the dose or discontinue the drug]: Initial: 80 mg twice daily; increase dosage gradually after 3 days, if needed [ie, if frequency of relapses of atrial fibrillation/flutter is not reduced and the dose is tolerated without excessive QT prolongation (ie, if QT interval is <520 msec)]; allow 3 days between dosage increments to achieve new steady-state and to determine maximum effects on QT interval; reduce the dose or discontinue the drug if the QT interval is ≥500 msec; dose may be increased to 120 mg twice daily (usual effective dose); the dosage may be further increased to 160 mg twice daily if response is inadequate and the dose is tolerated without excessive QT prolongation; maximum dose: 160 mg twice daily.

I.V.: Adults: **Note:** Baseline QT_c interval and Cl_{cr} must be determined prior to initiation. The effects of the initial I.V. dose must be monitored and the dose titrated either upward or downward, if needed, based on clinical effect, QT_c interval, or adverse reactions. Doses should be initiated or increased in a hospital facility that can provide continuous ECG monitoring, recognition, and treatment of life-threatening arrhythmias, and CPR (see Warnings):

Conversion from oral sotalol to I.V. sotalol:
80 mg oral equivalent to 75 mg I.V.
120 mg oral equivalent to 112.5 mg I.V.
160 mg oral equivalent to 150 mg I.V.

Ventricular arrhythmias:
Substitution for oral sotalol: Initial dose: 75 mg infused over 5 hours twice daily

Dose adjustment: If the frequency of relapse does not reduce and excessive QT_c prolongation does not occur, may increase to 112.5 mg twice daily. For ventricular arrhythmias, may increase dose every 3 days in increments of 75 mg/day.

Dose range: Usual therapeutic dose: 75-150 mg twice daily; maximum dose: 300 mg twice daily

Atrial fibrillation or atrial flutter:
Substitution for oral sotalol: Initial dose: 75 mg infused over 5 hours twice daily

Dose adjustment: If the frequency of relapse does not reduce and excessive QT_c prolongation does not occur, may increase to 112.5 mg twice daily. For ventricular arrhythmias, may increase dose every 3 days in increments of 75 mg/day.

Dose range: Usual therapeutic dose: 112.5 mg twice daily; maximum dose: 150 mg twice daily

Dosing adjustment in renal impairment:

Children: Dosing in children with renal impairment has not been investigated; use lower doses or increased dosing intervals; closely monitor clinical response, heart rate and QT$_c$ interval; allow adequate time between dosage increments to achieve new steady-state, since half-life will be prolonged with renal impairment

Adults: Administer the initial dose (ie, 80 mg) and subsequent doses at the following intervals:

Ventricular arrhythmias (Betapace®, Sorine®, generic):

Cl$_{cr}$ >60 mL/minute: Administer every 12 hours

Cl$_{cr}$ 30-60 mL/minute: Administer every 24 hours

Cl$_{cr}$ 10-29 mL/minute: Administer every 36-48 hours

Cl$_{cr}$ <10 mL/minute: Individualize dose

Atrial fibrillation/flutter (Betapace AF®):

Cl$_{cr}$ >60 mL/minute: Administer every 12 hours

Cl$_{cr}$ 40-60 mL/minute: Administer every 24 hours

Cl$_{cr}$ <40 mL/minute: Use is contraindicated (per product labeling)

Note: The manufacturer of the injectable formulation recommends adjustment similar to that used for Betapace AF®; however, the injectable formulation may be used for either indication.

Note: Due to the prolonged half-life in patients with renal dysfunction, allow at least 5-6 doses (at the above recommended interval) between dosage increments to achieve a new steady-state and to monitor QT intervals

Dosing adjustment in hepatic impairment: Not needed

Administration

Oral: May be administered without regard to meals, but should be administered at the same time each day

I.V.: Dilute in NS, D$_5$W, or LR to final concentration of 0.75-1.5 mg/mL and infuse over 5 hours

Monitoring Parameters Continuous ECG for a minimum of 3 days with initiation of therapy or dosage increase, QT interval, heart rate, renal function, serum potassium, and magnesium

Betapace AF®: In addition, during initiation and dosage titration, monitor the QT interval 2-4 hours after each dose.

Injectable formulation: Monitor QT interval after completion of each infusion.

Test Interactions May falsely increase urinary metanephrine values when fluorimetric or photometric methods are used; does not interact with HPLC assay with solid phase extraction for determination of urinary catecholamines

Patient Information Take sotalol every day as prescribed; do not change dose or discontinue without physician's advice; if a dose is missed, do not double the next dose, take the next dose at the usual time. Avoid abrupt discontinuation; if sotalol is to be discontinued, physician will advise how to slowly taper the dose over 1-2 weeks. May cause drowsiness and impair ability to perform activities requiring mental alertness or physical coordination. Regular cardiac checkups, ECGs, and blood tests will be needed while taking this medication. Report the use of other medications, nonprescription medications, and herbal or natural products to your physician and pharmacist; do not start new medications without checking with your physician and pharmacist; tell your dentist and physician that you are taking sotalol before you have dental surgery or an operation (sotalol may interact with certain anesthetic agents). Report fast heartbeats, dizziness, or fainting immediately to your physician or go to an emergency room (these may be signs of an abnormal heartbeat); report severe diarrhea, unusual sweating, vomiting, increased thirst, or decreased appetite immediately to your physician (these may be things that make an abnormal heartbeat more likely to occur); report chest pain, fast heartbeat, swelling of ankles or legs, difficulty breathing or unusual cough to your physician (these may be serious side effects of the medication).

Nursing Implications Be prepared to recognize and treat cardiac arrhythmias; lidocaine and other resuscitative measures should be available (see Warnings)

Additional Information Betapace AF®: Do not discharge patients from the hospital within 12 hours of electrical or pharmacological conversion from atrial fibrillation/flutter to normal sinus rhythm.

Dosage Forms Excipient information presented when available (limited, particularly for generics); consult specific product labeling.

Injection, solution, as hydrochloride: 15 mg/mL (10 mL)

Tablet, as hydrochloride: 80 mg, 80 mg [atrial fibrillation], 120 mg, 120 mg [atrial fibrillation], 160 mg, 160 mg [atrial fibrillation], 240 mg

Betapace®: 80 mg, 120 mg, 160 mg, 240 mg

Betapace AF®: 80 mg, 120 mg, 160 mg [atrial fibrillation]

Sorine®: 80 mg, 120 mg, 160 mg, 240 mg

Extemporaneous Preparations A 5 mg/mL syrup of sotalol hydrochloride made from Betapace® or Betapace AF® tablets and Simple Syrup containing 0.1% sodium benzoate (Syrup, NF) is stable for 3 months when stored at controlled room temperature (15°C to 30°C; 59°F to 86°F) and ambient humidity; place 120 mL of Syrup, NF into a 6 ounce amber plastic (polyethylene terephthalate) prescription bottle; add five Betapace® or Betapace AF® 120 mg tablets; shake the bottle to wet the tablets; allow tablets to hydrate for at least 2 hours; then shake intermittently over ≥2 hours until the tablets are completely disintegrated; a dispersion of fine particles (water-insoluble inactive ingredients) in syrup should be obtained (**Note:** To simplify the disintegration process, tablets can hydrate overnight; tablets may also be crushed, carefully transferred into the bottle and shaken well until a dispersion of fine particles in syrup is obtained); label "shake well" [Betapace® and Betapace AF® tablets (package inserts), 2007 and 2009].

A 5 mg/mL liquid formulation of sotalol hydrochloride made from 160 mg tablets [Sotocor® (from Canada)] and a suspending vehicle (300 mL of Simple Syrup and 700 mL of a methylcellulose 1% gel containing sodium benzoate) was stable and had no evidence of microbial growth for 8 weeks when stored in amber glass bottles under refrigeration (4°C); **Note:** Microbial growth was observed in samples stored at room temperature; to prepare the methylcellulose 1% gel and the suspending vehicle, see reference; label "shake well" and "refrigerate" (Dupuis, 1988).

Betapace® and Betapace AF® (package inserts), Wayne, NJ: Bayer HealthCare Pharmaceuticals Inc.; 2007 and 2009.

Dupuis LL, James G, and Bacola G, "Stability of Sotalol Hydrochloride Oral Liquid Formulation," *Canadian Journal of Hospital Pharmacy*, 1988, 41(3):121-3.

References

Beaufort-Krol GC and Bink-Boelkens MT, "Effectiveness of Sotalol for Atrial Flutter in Children After Surgery for Congenital Heart Disease," *Am J Cardiol*, 1997, 79(1):92-4.

Colloridi V, Perri C, Ventriglia F, et al, "Oral Sotalol in Pediatric Atrial Ectopic Tachycardia," *Am Heart J*, 1992, 123(1):254-6.

Läer S, Elshoff JP, Meibohm B, et al, "Development of a Safe and Effective Pediatric Dosing Regimen for Sotalol Based on Population Pharmacokinetics and Pharmacodynamics in Children With Supraventricular Tachycardia," *J Am Coll Cardiol*, 2005, 46(7):1322-30.

Maragnes P, Tipple M, and Fournier A, "Effectiveness of Oral Sotalol for Treatment of Pediatric Arrhythmias," *Am J Cardiol*, 1992, 69(8):751-4.

O'Hare MF, Murnaghan GA, Russell CJ, et al, "Sotalol as a Hypotensive Agent in Pregnancy," *Br J Obstet Gynaecol*, 1980, 87(9):814-20.

Pfammatter JP and Paul T, "New Antiarrhythmic Drug in Pediatric Use: Sotalol," *Pediatr Cardiol*, 1997, 18(1):28-34.

Pfammatter JP, Paul T, Lehmann C, et al, "Efficacy and Proarrhythmia of Oral Sotalol in Pediatric Patients," *J Am Coll Cardiol*, 1995, 26 (4):1002-7.

Saul JP, Ross B, Schaffer MS, et al, "Pharmacokinetics and Pharmacodynamics of Sotalol in a Pediatric Population With Supraventricular and Ventricular Tachyarrhythmia," *Clin Pharmacol Ther*, 2001, 69(3):145-57.

Saul JP, Schaffer MS, Karpawich PP, et al, "Single-Dose Pharmaco-kinetics of Sotalol in a Pediatric Population With Supraventricular and/or Ventricular Tachyarrhythmia," *J Clin Pharmacol*, 2001, 41(1):35-43.

Tanel RE, Walsh EP, Lulu JA, et al, "Sotalol for Refractory Arrhythmias in Pediatric and Young Adult Patients: Initial Efficacy and Long-Term Outcome," *Am Heart J*, 1995, 130(4):791-7.

Tipple M and Sandor G, "Efficacy and Safety of Oral Sotalol in Early Infancy," *Pacing Clin Electrophysiol*, 1991, 14(11 Pt 2):2062-5.

◆ **Sotalol Hydrochloride** *see* Sotalol *on page 1284*

◆ **Sotret®** *see* Isotretinoin *on page 769*

◆ **SPA** *see* Albumin *on page 55*

◆ **SPD417** *see* CarBAMazepine *on page 244*

◆ **Spiriva® (Can)** *see* Tiotropium *on page 1353*

◆ **Spiriva® HandiHaler®** *see* Tiotropium *on page 1353*

Spironolactone (speer on oh LAK tone)

Medication Safety Issues
Sound-alike/look-alike issues:
Aldactone® may be confused with Aldactazide®

International issues:
Aldactone®: Brand name for spironolactone [U.S., Canada], but also the brand name for potassium canrenoate [Austria, Czech Republic, Germany, Hungary, Poland]

Related Information
Antihypertensive Agents by Class *on page 1481*

U.S. Brand Names Aldactone®

Canadian Brand Names Aldactone®; Novo-Spiroton

Therapeutic Category Antihypertensive Agent; Diuretic, Potassium Sparing

Generic Available Yes

Use Management of edema associated with CHF, cirrhosis of the liver accompanied by edema or ascites, and nephrotic syndrome; treatment of essential hypertension, primary hyperaldosteronism, hypokalemia, and hirsutism; treatment of severe heart failure (NYHA class III-IV) to increase survival and reduce hospitalizations when used in addition to standard therapy

Pregnancy Risk Factor C/D in pregnancy-induced hypertension (per expert analysis)

Pregnancy Considerations Teratogenic effects were not observed in animal studies; however, doses used were less than or equal to equivalent doses in humans. The antiandrogen effects of spironolactone have been shown to cause feminization of the male fetus in animal studies. Two case reports did not demonstrate this effect in humans however, the authors caution that adequate data is lacking. Diuretics are generally avoided in pregnancy due to the theoretical risk that decreased plasma volume may cause placental insufficiency. Diuretics should not be used during pregnancy in the presence of reduced placental perfusion (eg, pre-eclampsia, intrauterine growth restriction).

Lactation Enters breast milk/not recommended (AAP rates "compatible")

Breast-Feeding Considerations The active metabolite of spironolactone has been found in breast milk. Effects to humans are not known; however, this metabolite was found to be carcinogenic in rats. The manufacturer recommends discontinuing spironolactone or using an alternative method of feeding.

Contraindications Hypersensitivity to spironolactone or any component; renal dysfunction, anuria, hyperkalemia

Warnings Spironolactone has been shown to be tumorigenic in toxicity studies using 25-250 times the usual human dose in rats **[U.S. Boxed Warning]**.

Precautions Concomitant administration of potassium-sparing diuretics (eg, amiloride and triamterene) and ACE inhibitors or NSAIDs has been associated with severe hyperkalemia; may cause transient elevation of BUN, possibly due to a concentration effect; sustained elevations should be evaluated; monitor potassium levels closely; in CHF, potassium levels and renal function should be checked in 3 days and 1 week after beginning therapy, then every 2-4 weeks for 3-12 months, then every 3-6 months. Discontinue or interrupt therapy for serum potassium >5 mEq/L or for serum creatinine >4 mg/dL in patients with heart failure. Use with caution in patients with dehydration, hyponatremia, impaired renal clearance (Cl_{cr} <50 mL/minute) or hepatic dysfunction

Adverse Reactions
Cardiovascular: Arrhythmia

Central nervous system: Lethargy, headache, mental confusion, fever, ataxia

Dermatologic: Rash, urticaria

Endocrine & metabolic: Hyperkalemia, dehydration, hypo-natremia, hyperchloremic metabolic acidosis, postmeno-pausal bleeding, amenorrhea, gynecomastia (in males); breast tenderness, deepening of voice, and hair growth increased (in females)

Gastrointestinal: Anorexia, nausea, vomiting, diarrhea, gastritis, cramping, gastric bleeding

Genitourinary: Dysuria

Hematologic: Agranulocytosis

Neuromuscular & skeletal: Weakness, numbness or paresthesia in hands, feet or lips, lower back or side pain

Renal: Renal function decreased (including renal failure)

Respiratory: Cough, shortness of breath, dyspnea, hoarseness

Drug Interactions
Avoid Concomitant Use There are no known inter-actions where it is recommended to avoid concomitant use.

Increased Effect/Toxicity
Spironolactone may increase the levels/effects of: ACE Inhibitors; Amifostine; Ammonium Chloride; Antihyper-tensives; Cardiac Glycosides; Digoxin; Hypotensive Agents; Neuromuscular-Blocking Agents (Nondepolariz-ing); RiTUXimab

The levels/effects of Spironolactone may be increased by: Angiotensin II Receptor Blockers; Diazoxide; Drospir-enone; Eplerenone; Herbs (Hypotensive Properties); MAO Inhibitors; Nonsteroidal Anti-Inflammatory Agents; Pentoxifylline; Phosphodiesterase 5 Inhibitors; Potas-sium Salts; Prostacyclin Analogues; Tolvaptan

Decreased Effect
Spironolactone may decrease the levels/effects of: Alpha-/Beta-Agonists; Cardiac Glycosides; Mitotane; QuiNIDine

The levels/effects of Spironolactone may be decreased by: Herbs (Hypertensive Properties); Methylphenidate; Nonsteroidal Anti-Inflammatory Agents; Yohimbine

Food Interactions Avoid natural licorice (causes sodium and water retention and increases potassium loss) and salt substitutes; avoid diets high in potassium

Mechanism of Action Competes with aldosterone for receptor sites in the distal renal tubules, increasing sodium chloride and water excretion while conserving potassium and hydrogen ions; may block the effect of aldosterone on arteriolar smooth muscle as well

Pharmacokinetics (Adult data unless noted)
Distribution: V_d: Breast milk to plasma ratio: 0.51-0.72

Protein binding: 91% to 98%

Metabolism: In the liver to multiple metabolites, including canrenone (active)

Half-life:
Spironolactone: 78-84 minutes
Canrenone: 13-24 hours

Time to peak serum concentration: Within 1-3 hours (primarily as the active metabolite)

Elimination: Urinary and biliary

◀ **Usual Dosage** Oral:

Neonates: Diuretic: 1-3 mg/kg/day every 12-24 hours

Children:

Diuretic, hypertension: 1-3.3 mg/kg/day or 60 mg/m^2/day in divided doses every 6-12 hours; not to exceed 100 mg/day

Diagnosis of primary aldosteronism: 100-400 mg/m^2/day in 1-2 divided doses

Adults:

Edema, hypokalemia: 25-200 mg/day in 1-2 divided doses

Hypertension (JCN 7): 25-50 mg/day divided once or twice daily

Diagnosis of primary aldosteronism: 100-400 mg/day in 1-2 divided doses

Acne in women: 25-200 mg once daily

Hirsutism in women: 50-200 mg/day in 1-2 divided doses

CHF: Patients with severe heart failure already using an ACE inhibitor and a loop diuretic ± digoxin: 12.5-25 mg/day, increase or reduce depending on individual response and evidence of hyperkalemia; maximum daily dose: 50 mg

Dosing interval in renal impairment:

Cl_{cr} 10-50 mL/minute: Administer every 12-24 hours

Cl_{cr} <10 mL/minute: Avoid use

Administration Oral: Administer with food

Monitoring Parameters Serum potassium, sodium, and renal function

Test Interactions May cause false elevation in serum digoxin concentrations measured by RIA

Patient Information May cause drowsiness and impair ability to perform activities requiring mental alertness or physical coordination

Dosage Forms Excipient information presented when available (limited, particularly for generics); consult specific product labeling.

Tablet: 25 mg, 50 mg, 100 mg

Aldactone®: 25 mg

Aldactone®: 50 mg, 100 mg [scored]

Extemporaneous Preparations

A 1 mg/mL suspension may be compounded by crushing ten 25 mg tablets, add a small amount of water and soak for 5 minutes; add 50 mL 1.5% carboxymethylcellulose, 100 mL syrup NF, and mix; use a sufficient quantity of purified water to a total volume of 250 mL; stable at room temperature or refrigerated for 3 months (Nahata, 1993)

A 2.5 mg/mL suspension may be made by crushing twelve 25 mg tablets, levigating with a small amount of distilled water or glycerin; dilute with cherry syrup to make a final volume of 120 mL; stable 28 days when refrigerated (Mathur, 1989)

A 5 mg/mL suspension may be made by crushing twenty-four 25 mg tablets, levigating with a small amount of distilled water or glycerin; dilute with cherry syrup to a total volume of 120 mL; stable 28 days refrigerated (Mathur, 1989)

A 25 mg/mL suspension may be made by crushing one-hundred twenty (120) 25 mg tablets, add in geometric proportions a 1:1 mixture of Ora-Sweet® and Ora-Plus® or Ora-Sweet® SF and Ora-Plus® to a total volume of 120 mL; stable 60 days refrigerated stored in amber bottles; shake well (Allen, 1996)

Allen LV and Erickson MA, "Stability of Labetalol Hydrochloride, Metoprolol Tartrate, Verapamil Hydrochloride, and Spironolactone With Hydrochlorothiazide in Extemporaneously Compounded Oral Liquids," *Am J Health Syst Pharm*, 1996, 53(19):2304-9.

Mathur LK and Wickman A, "Stability of Extemporaneously Compounded Spironolactone Suspensions," *Am J Hosp Pharm*, 1989, 46(10):2040-2.

Nahata MC, Morosco RS, and Hipple TF, "Stability of Spironolactone in an Extemporaneously Prepared

Suspension at Two Temperatures," *Ann Pharmacother*, 1993, 27:1198-9.

References

Chobanian AV, Bakris GL, Black HR, et al, "The Seventh Report of the Joint National Committee on Prevention, Detection, Evaluation, and Treatment of High Blood Pressure: The JNC 7 Report," *JAMA*, 2003, 289(19):2560-72.

Hunt SA, Abraham WT, Chin MH, et al, "ACC/AHA 2005 Guideline Update for the Diagnosis and Management of Chronic Heart Failure in the Adult-Summary Article: A Report of the American College of Cardiology/American Heart Association Task Force on Practice Guidelines (Writing Committee to Update the 2001 Guidelines for the Evaluation and Management of Heart Failure)," *J Am Coll Cardiol*, 2005, 46(6):1116-43.

Juurlink DN, Mamdani MM, Lee DS, et al, "Rates of Hyperkalemia After Publication of the Randomized Aldactone Evaluation Study," *N Engl J Med*, 2004, 351(6):543-51.

National High Blood Pressure Education Program Working Group on High Blood Pressure in Children and Adolescents, "The Fourth Report on the Diagnosis, Evaluation, and Treatment of High Blood Pressure in Children and Adolescents," *Pediatrics*, 2004, 114(2 Suppl):555-76.

Pitt B, Zannad F, Remme WJ, et al, "The Effect of Spironolactone on Morbidity and Mortality in Patients With Severe Heart Failure. Randomized Aldactone Evaluation Study Investigators," *N Engl J Med*, 1999, 341(10):709-17.

van der Vorst MM, Kist JE, van der Heijden AJ, et al, "Diuretics in Pediatrics: Current Knowledge and Future Prospects," *Paediatr Drugs*, 2006, 8(4):245-64.

◆ **Spironolactone and Hydrochlorothiazide** *see* Hydrochlorothiazide and Spironolactone *on page 683*

◆ **Sporanox®** *see* Itraconazole *on page 773*

◆ **Sprix™** *see* Ketorolac *on page 781*

◆ **SPS®** *see* Sodium Polystyrene Sulfonate *on page 1279*

◆ **SS734** *see* Besifloxacin *on page 187*

◆ **SSD®** *see* Silver Sulfadiazine *on page 1262*

◆ **SSD® AF** *see* Silver Sulfadiazine *on page 1262*

◆ **SSKI®** *see* Potassium Iodide *on page 1138*

◆ **Stagesic™** *see* Hydrocodone and Acetaminophen *on page 684*

◆ **StanGard®** *see* Fluoride *on page 595*

◆ **StanGard® Perio** *see* Fluoride *on page 595*

◆ **Stannous Fluoride** *see* Fluoride *on page 595*

◆ **Statex® (Can)** *see* Morphine Sulfate *on page 946*

Stavudine (STAV yoo deen)

Medication Safety Issues

Sound-alike/look-alike issues:

Zerit® may be confused with Zestril®, Ziac®, Zyrtec®

Related Information

Adult and Adolescent HIV *on page 1620*

Management of Healthcare Worker Exposures to HBV, HCV, and HIV *on page 1661*

Pediatric HIV *on page 1613*

Perinatal HIV *on page 1628*

U.S. Brand Names Zerit®

Canadian Brand Names Zerit®

Therapeutic Category Antiretroviral Agent; HIV Agents (Anti-HIV Agents); Nucleoside Reverse Transcriptase Inhibitor (NRTI)

Generic Available Yes: Capsule

Use Treatment of HIV infection in combination with other antiretroviral agents (FDA approved in ages ≥0 days and adults). (**Note:** HIV regimens consisting of **three** antiretroviral agents are strongly recommended)

Pregnancy Risk Factor C

Pregnancy Considerations Adverse events were observed in some animal reproduction studies. No increased risk of overall birth defects has been observed following 1st trimester exposure according to data collected by the antiretroviral pregnancy registry. Cases of fatal and nonfatal lactic acidosis, with or without pancreatitis, have been reported in pregnant women. It is not known if pregnancy itself potentiates this known side effect; however, pregnant women may be at increased risk of lactic acidosis and liver damage. Combination treatment with didanosine may also contribute to the risk of lactic acidosis, and should be considered only if benefit outweighs risk. Hepatic enzymes and electrolytes should be monitored frequently during the third trimester of pregnancy. Pharmacokinetics of stavudine are not significantly altered during pregnancy; dose adjustments are not needed. There are no adequate and well-controlled studies in pregnant women; however, the Perinatal HIV Guidelines Working Group considers stavudine to be an alternative NRTI in dual nucleoside combination regimens; use with didanosine only if no alternatives are available, do not use with zidovudine. Health professionals are encouraged to contact the antiretroviral pregnancy registry to monitor outcomes of pregnant women exposed to antiretroviral medications (1-800-258-4263 or www.-APRegistry.com).

Lactation Excretion in breast milk unknown/contra-indicated

Breast-Feeding Considerations In infants born to mothers who are HIV positive, HAART while breast-feeding may decrease postnatal infection. However, maternal or infant antiretroviral therapy does not completely eliminate the risk of postnatal HIV transmission.

In the United States where formula is accessible, affordable, safe, and sustainable, complete avoidance of breast-feeding by HIV-infected women is recommended to decrease potential transmission of HIV.

Contraindications Hypersensitivity to stavudine or any component

Warnings The major clinical toxicity of stavudine is peripheral neuropathy which has occurred in 8% to 21% of patients in controlled trials; it can be dose-limiting and occurs more frequently in patients with a history of neuropathy, advanced HIV, and in patients receiving other drugs known to cause neuropathy (eg, didanosine). Lactic acidosis and severe hepatomegaly with steatosis, including fatal cases, have been reported with the use of NRTIs **[U.S. Boxed Warning]**; it may be more common with antiretroviral regimens containing stavudine. Risk may be increased in obesity, prolonged nucleoside exposure, prior liver disease, or in female patients. Increased risk of hepatotoxicity also occurs with combined use of stavudine with didanosine and hydroxyurea (avoid this combination). Fatal lactic acidosis has occurred in pregnant women who received stavudine plus didanosine with other antiretroviral agents; use stavudine plus didanosine with caution during pregnancy (and in other patients) and only if benefit clearly outweighs risks. Severe motor weakness (resembling Guillain-Barré syndrome) has been reported, usually in association with lactic acidosis. Manufacturer recommends prompt suspension of all antiretroviral therapy in suspected cases of symptomatic hyperlactatemia, lactic acidosis (with or without neuromuscular weakness), or pronounced hepatotoxicity (see also Additional Information).

Fatal and nonfatal pancreatitis has occurred during combination antiretroviral therapy which included stavudine and didanosine **[U.S. Boxed Warning]**; avoid the use of stavudine with didanosine; discontinue these drugs (and any other drugs that are toxic to the pancreas) if pancreatitis is suspected; use extreme caution and closely monitor patient if stavudine is restarted in patients with confirmed pancreatitis; the new medication regimen should **not** contain didanosine. **Note:** The incidence of stavudine-associated toxicities may be increased when stavudine is used in combination with other medications that have similar toxicities. An increased risk of pancreatitis and hepatotoxicity (either of which may be fatal) and

severe peripheral neuropathy may occur when patients are treated with stavudine in combination with didanosine (with or without hydroxyurea). The combined use of stavudine and hydroxyurea (with or without didanosine) should be avoided. The combined use of stavudine and didanosine is **not** recommended, unless the potential benefit clearly outweighs the risks (Panel on Antiretroviral Guidelines for Adults and Adolescents, 2009; Working Group on Antiretroviral Therapy and Medical Management of HIV-Infected Children, 2009)

Safety and efficacy have not been established in patients with significant liver disease; patients with liver impairment, including chronic active hepatitis, may be at increased risk for liver function abnormalities, including hepatic adverse events that may be severe and potentially fatal; monitor patients carefully; if liver function worsens, consider interruption or discontinuation of therapy. Concomitant use of combination antiretroviral therapy with interferon alfa (with or without ribavirin) has resulted in hepatic decompensation (with some fatalities) in patients coinfected with HIV and HCV; monitor patients closely, especially for hepatic decompensation, neutropenia, and anemia; consider discontinuation of stavudine if needed; consider dose reduction or discontinuation of interferon alfa, ribavirin, or both if clinical toxicities, including hepatic decompensation, worsen (see Drug Interactions). Use of stavudine with zidovudine is **not** recommended due to antagonistic effects (see Drug Interactions).

Precautions Use with caution in patients with a history of peripheral neuropathy, or hepatic or renal impairment; dosage adjustment required in patients with impaired renal function. Fat redistribution and accumulation [ie, central obesity, peripheral wasting, facial wasting, breast enlargement, dorsocervical fat enlargement (buffalo hump), and cushingoid appearance] have been observed in patients receiving antiretroviral agents (causal relationship not established). Immune reconstitution syndrome (an acute inflammatory response to residual or indolent opportunistic infections) may occur in HIV patients during initial treatment with combination antiretroviral agents; this syndrome may require further patient assessment and therapy.

Adverse Reactions

Central nervous system: Headache

Dermatologic: Rash

Endocrine & metabolic: Fat redistribution and accumulation (see Precautions), hyperlactatemia (symptomatic), lactic acidosis

Gastrointestinal: Amylase increased, anorexia, diarrhea, lipase increased, nausea, pancreatitis (see Warnings), vomiting

Hepatic: AST and ALT increased, bilirubin increased, GGT increased, hepatic steatosis, hepatomegaly

Neuromuscular & skeletal: Motor weakness (may resemble Guillain-Barré syndrome), peripheral neuropathy (burning, numbness of hands or feet, pain, tingling)

Miscellaneous: Immune reconstitution syndrome (see Precautions)

<1%, postmarketing, and/or case reports: Abdominal pain, allergic reaction, anemia, chills, diabetes mellitus, fever, hepatitis, hyperglycemia, insomnia, leukopenia, macrocytosis, myalgia, thrombocytopenia

Drug Interactions

Avoid Concomitant Use

Avoid concomitant use of Stavudine with any of the following: Hydroxyurea; Zidovudine

Increased Effect/Toxicity

Stavudine may increase the levels/effects of: Didanosine; Hydroxyurea

The levels/effects of Stavudine may be increased by: Hydroxyurea; Ribavirin

Decreased Effect

The levels/effects of Stavudine may be decreased by:
DOXOrubicin; DOXOrubicin (Liposomal); Zidovudine

Stability

Capsules: Store in tightly closed containers at room temperature

Oral solution: Reconstitute powder for oral solution according to manufacturer's instructions; dispense in original container; keep refrigerated; solution is stable for 30 days

Mechanism of Action Antiviral activity is dependent on intracellular conversion of stavudine to the active metabolite d4-triphosphate; Inhibits replication of retroviruses by competing with thymidine triphosphate for viral RNA-directed DNA polymerase and incorporation into viral DNA

Pharmacokinetics (Adult data unless noted)

Absorption: Rapid

Distribution: Penetrates into the CSF achieving 16% to 97% (mean: 59%) of concomitant plasma concentrations; distributes into extravascular spaces and equally between RBCs and plasma

V_d:

Children: 0.73 ± 0.32 L/kg

Adults: 46 ± 21 L

Protein binding: Negligible

Metabolism: Converted intracellularly to active triphosphate form; metabolism of stavudine plays minimal role in its clearance; minor metabolites include oxidized stavudine and its glucuronide conjugate, glucuronide conjugate of stavudine, N-acetylcysteine conjugate of the ribose after glycosidic cleavage

Bioavailability: Capsule and solution are bioequivalent

Children: 77%

Adults: 86%

Half-life, elimination:

Newborns (at birth): 5.3 ± 2 hours

Neonates 14-28 days old: 1.6 ± 0.3 hours

Infants 5 weeks to Children 15 years: 0.9 ± 0.3 hours

Adults: 1.6 ± 0.2 hours

Note: Half-life is prolonged with renal dysfunction

Half-life, intracellular: Adults: 3.5-7 hours

Time to peak serum concentration: Within 1 hour

Elimination: Urine: 95% of dose (74% as unchanged drug); feces: 3% (62% as unchanged drug); undergoes glomerular filtration and active tubular secretion

Dialysis: 31 ± 5% of the dose is removed by hemodialysis; hemodialysis clearance (n=12) (mean ± SD): 120 ± 18 mL/minute

Usual Dosage Oral (use in combination with other antiretroviral agents):

Neonates 0-13 days old: 0.5 mg/kg/dose every 12 hours

Neonates ≥14 days old, Infants, and Children <30 kg: 1 mg/kg/dose every 12 hours; maximum: 30 mg every 12 hours

Children, Adolescents, and Adults:

30-59 kg: 30 mg every 12 hours

≥60 kg: 40 mg every 12 hours

Dosing adjustment in renal impairment:

Cl_{cr} 26-50 mL/minute: Decrease daily dose by 50% (eg, Adults ≥60 kg: Administer 20 mg every 12 hours; Adults <60 kg: Administer 15 mg every 12 hours)

Cl_{cr} <10-25 mL/minute: Decrease daily dose by 75% (eg, Adults ≥60 kg: Administer 20 mg every 24 hours; Adults <60 kg: Administer 15 mg every 24 hours)

Hemodialysis: Decrease daily dose by 75% (see Cl_{cr} <10-25 mL/minute); administer dose after hemodialysis on dialysis days and at same time of day on nondialysis days

Dosing adjustment in hepatic impairment: No data

Administration Oral: Administer with or without food; shake solution well before using

Monitoring Parameters Periodic CBC with differential, hemoglobin, renal function, liver enzymes, serum amylase and lipase, CD4 cell count, HIV RNA plasma levels, signs/symptoms of peripheral neuropathy

Patient Information Stavudine is not a cure for HIV. Take stavudine every day as prescribed; do not change dose or discontinue without physician's advice. If a dose is missed, take it as soon as possible, then return to normal dosing schedule; if a dose is skipped, do **not** double the next dose. Avoid alcohol. Notify physician if tingling, burning, pain, numbness of hands or feet, unexplained weight loss, abdominal discomfort, nausea, vomiting, fatigue, dyspnea, or motor weakness occurs

HIV medications may cause changes in body fat, including an increase in fat in the upper back and neck, breasts, and trunk; a loss of fat from the face, arms, and legs may also occur.

Additional Information Signs and symptoms of symptomatic hyperlactemia or lactic acidosis syndrome may include generalized fatigue, GI symptoms (nausea, vomiting, abdominal pain, unexplained weight loss), respiratory symptoms (tachypnea, dyspnea), or neurologic symptoms (motor weakness, Guillain-Barré type syndrome)

Dosage Forms Excipient information presented when available (limited, particularly for generics); consult specific product labeling.

Capsule: 15 mg, 20 mg, 30 mg, 40 mg

Zerit®: 15 mg, 20 mg, 30 mg, 40 mg

Powder for solution, oral:

Zerit®: 1 mg/mL (200 mL) [dye free; contains sucrose 50 mg/mL; fruit flavor]

References

Briars LA, Hilao JJ, and Kraus DM, "A Review of Pediatric Human Immunodeficiency Virus Infection," *Journal of Pharmacy Practice*, 2004, 17(6):407-31.

Kline MW, Dunkle LM, Church JA, et al, "A Phase I/II Evaluation of Stavudine (d4T) in Children With Human Immunodeficiency Virus Infection," *Pediatrics*, 1995, 96(2 Pt 1):247-52.

Panel on Antiretroviral Guidelines for Adults and Adolescents, "Guidelines for the Use of Antiretroviral Agents in HIV-Infected Adults and Adolescents," December 1, 2009, http://www.aidsinfo.nih.gov.

Working Group on Antiretroviral Therapy and Medical Management of HIV-Infected Children, "Guidelines for the Use of Antiretroviral Agents in Pediatric HIV Infection," February 23, 2009. Available at http://www.aidsinfo.nih.gov.

◆ **Stavzor™** *see* Valproic Acid and Derivatives *on page 1398*

◆ **Stelazine** *see* Trifluoperazine *on page 1382*

◆ **Stemetil® (Can)** *see* Prochlorperazine *on page 1161*

◆ **Sterapred® [DSC]** *see* PredniSONE *on page 1151*

◆ **Sterapred® DS [DSC]** *see* PredniSONE *on page 1151*

◆ **STI-571** *see* Imatinib *on page 710*

◆ **Stieprox® (Can)** *see* Ciclopirox *on page 306*

◆ **Stimate®** *see* Desmopressin *on page 404*

◆ **Sting-Kill [OTC]** *see* Benzocaine *on page 182*

◆ **St. Joseph® Adult Aspirin [OTC]** *see* Aspirin *on page 141*

◆ **Stop®** *see* Fluoride *on page 595*

◆ **Strattera®** *see* Atomoxetine *on page 149*

Streptomycin (strep toe MYE sin)

Medication Safety Issues

Sound-alike/look-alike issues:

Streptomycin may be confused with streptozocin

Therapeutic Category Antibiotic, Aminoglycoside; Antitubercular Agent

Generic Available Yes

Use Combination therapy of active tuberculosis; used in combination with other agents for treatment of streptococcal or enterococcal endocarditis, mycobacterial infections, plague, tularemia, and brucellosis

Pregnancy Risk Factor D

Pregnancy Considerations Streptomycin crosses the placenta. Many case reports of hearing impairment in children exposed *in utero* have been published. Impairment has ranged from mild hearing loss to bilateral deafness. Because of several reports of total irreversible bilateral congenital deafness in children whose mothers received streptomycin during pregnancy, the manufacturer classifies streptomycin as pregnancy risk factor D.

Lactation Enters breast milk/not recommended (AAP rates "compatible")

Breast-Feeding Considerations Streptomycin is excreted into breast milk; however, it is not well absorbed when taken orally. This limited oral absorption may minimize exposure to the nursing infant. Nondose-related effects could include modification of bowel flora. The AAP considers streptomycin to be "usually compatible with breast-feeding." Breast-feeding is not recommended by the manufacturer.

Contraindications Hypersensitivity to streptomycin or any component

Warnings Aminoglycosides are associated with significant nephrotoxicity; risk of nephrotoxicity is increased in patients with impaired renal function, high dose therapy, or prolonged therapy. Risk of nephrotoxicity increases when used concurrently with other potentially nephrotoxic drugs **[U.S. Boxed Warning]**; renal damage is usually reversible. May cause severe neurotoxic reactions; risk of neurotoxic reactions increased in patients with impaired renal function **[U.S. Boxed Warning]**; neurotoxicity is manifested as disturbances in vestibular and cochlear function, optic nerve dysfunction, peripheral neuritis, arachnoiditis, and encephalopathy. Headache, nausea, vomiting, and disequilibrium may be indications of vestibular injury. Loss of high frequency hearing is indicative of cochlear toxicity. Risk of ototoxicity increases with use of potent diuretics. May cause neuromuscular blockade and respiratory paralysis **[U.S. Boxed Warning]**; especially when given soon after anesthesia or muscle relaxants. Aminoglycosides can cause fetal harm when administered to a pregnant woman aminoglycosides have been associated with several reports of total irreversible bilateral congenital deafness in pediatric patients exposed *in utero*.

Precautions Use with caution in patients with pre-existing vertigo, tinnitus, hearing loss, or neuromuscular disorders. Use with caution in patients with renal impairment; modify dosage in patients with renal impairment; monitor renal function carefully during therapy **[U.S. Boxed Warning]**. Parenteral form should be used only where appropriate audiometric and laboratory testing facilities are available **[U.S. Boxed Warning]**.

Adverse Reactions

Cardiovascular: Myocarditis, cardiovascular collapse

Central nervous system: Dizziness, vertigo, headache, ataxia

Dermatologic: Toxic epidermal necrolysis

Gastrointestinal: Vomiting

Hematologic: Bone marrow suppression

Neuromuscular & skeletal: Neuromuscular blockade

Otic: Ototoxicity, hearing loss

Renal: Nephrotoxicity

Miscellaneous: Hypersensitivity reactions, serum sickness

Drug Interactions

Avoid Concomitant Use

Avoid concomitant use of Streptomycin with any of the following: BCG; Gallium Nitrate

Increased Effect/Toxicity

Streptomycin may increase the levels/effects of: AbobotulinumtoxinA; Bisphosphonate Derivatives; CARBOplatin; Colistimethate; CycloSPORINE; CycloSPORINE (Systemic); Gallium Nitrate; Neuromuscular-Blocking Agents; OnabotulinumtoxinA; RimabotulinumtoxinB

The levels/effects of Streptomycin may be increased by: Amphotericin B; Capreomycin; CISplatin; Loop Diuretics; Nonsteroidal Anti-Inflammatory Agents; Vancomycin

Decreased Effect

Streptomycin may decrease the levels/effects of: BCG; Typhoid Vaccine

The levels/effects of Streptomycin may be decreased by: Penicillins

Stability Streptomycin injection should be stored in the refrigerator

Mechanism of Action Inhibits bacterial protein synthesis by binding directly to the 30S ribosomal subunits causing faulty peptide sequence to form in the protein chain

Pharmacokinetics (Adult data unless noted)

Distribution: Distributes into most body tissues and fluids except the brain; small amounts enter the CSF only with inflamed meninges; crosses the placenta; small amounts appear in breast milk

Protein binding: 34%

Half-life (prolonged with renal impairment):

Newborns: 4-10 hours

Adults: 2-4.7 hours

Time to peak serum concentration: I.M.: Within 1-2 hours

Elimination: 30% to 90% of dose excreted as unchanged drug in urine, with small amount (1%) excreted in bile, saliva, sweat, and tears

Usual Dosage I.M. (I.V. in patients who cannot tolerate I.M. injections):

Newborns: 10-20 mg/kg/day once daily

Infants: 20-30 mg/kg/day in divided doses every 12 hours

Children:

Tuberculosis: 20-40 mg/kg/day once daily, not to exceed 1 g/day; **or** 20-40 mg/kg/dose twice weekly under direct observation, not to exceed 1.5 g/dose; usually discontinued after 2-3 months of therapy or as soon as isoniazid and rifampin susceptibility is established

Other infections: 20-40 mg/kg/day in combination with other antibiotics divided every 6-12 hours

Plague: 30 mg/kg/day divided every 8-12 hours

Adults:

Tuberculosis: 15 mg/kg/day once daily, not to exceed 1 g/day; **or** 25-30 mg/kg/dose twice weekly under direct observation, not to exceed 1.5 g/dose

Enterococcal endocarditis: 1 g every 12 hours for 2 weeks, then 500 mg every 12 hours for 4 weeks in combination with penicillin

Streptococcal endocarditis: 1 g every 12 hours for 1 week, then 500 mg every 12 hours for 1 week

Tularemia: 1-2 g/day in divided doses for 7-10 days or until patient is afebrile for 5-7 days

Plague: 2 g/day in divided doses until the patient is afebrile for at least 3 days

Dosing adjustment in renal impairment:

Cl_{cr} 50-80 mL/minute: Administer 7.5 mg/kg/dose every 24 hours

Cl_{cr} 10-50 mL/minute: Administer 7.5 mg/kg/dose every 24-72 hours

Cl_{cr} <10 mL/minute: Administer 7.5 mg/kg/dose every 72-96 hours

Administration Parenteral:

I.M.: Inject deep I.M. into a large muscle mass; administer at a concentration not to exceed 500 mg/mL; rotate injection sites

I.V.: I.V. infusion through a peripheral or central line; 12-15 mg/kg/dose is diluted in 100 mL of NS; infuse over 30-60 minutes

◀ **Monitoring Parameters** Hearing (audiogram), BUN, creatinine; serum concentration of the drug should be monitored in patients with renal impairment; eighth cranial nerve damage is usually preceded by high-pitched tinnitus, roaring noises, sense of fullness in ears, or impaired hearing and may persist for weeks after drug is discontinued

Reference Range Therapeutic serum concentrations: Peak: 15-40 mcg/mL; trough: <5 mcg/mL

Test Interactions False-positive urine glucose with Benedict's solution

Additional Information For use by patients with active tuberculosis that is resistant to isoniazid and rifampin or patients with active tuberculosis in areas where resistance is common and whose drug susceptibility is not yet known. Pfizer will distribute streptomycin directly to physicians and health clinics at no charge. Call Pfizer at 1-800-254-4445.

Dosage Forms Excipient information presented when available (limited, particularly for generics); consult specific product labeling.

Injection, powder for reconstitution: 1 g

References

Ad Hoc Committee of the Scientific Assembly on Microbiology, Tuberculosis, and Pulmonary Infections, "Treatment of Tuberculosis and Tuberculosis Infection in Adults and Children," *Clin Infect Dis*, 1995, 21:9-27.

American Academy of Pediatrics Committee on Infectious Diseases, "Chemotherapy for Tuberculosis in Infants and Children," *Pediatrics* 1992, 89(1):161-5.

Arguedas AG and Wehrle PP, "New Concepts for Antimicrobial Use in Central Nervous System Infections," *Semin Pediatr Infect Dis*, 1991, 2 (1):36-42.

Lorin MI, Hsu KH, and Jacob SC, "Treatment of Tuberculosis in Children," *Pediatr Clin North Am*, 1983, 30(2):333-48.

◆ **Streptomycin Sulfate** *see* Streptomycin *on page 1292*

◆ **Striant®** *see* Testosterone *on page 1325*

◆ **Stridex® Essential Care® [OTC]** *see* Salicylic Acid *on page 1241*

◆ **Stridex® Facewipes To Go® [OTC]** *see* Salicylic Acid *on page 1241*

◆ **Stridex® Maximum Strength [OTC]** *see* Salicylic Acid *on page 1241*

◆ **Stridex® Sensitive Skin [OTC]** *see* Salicylic Acid *on page 1241*

◆ **Strifon Forte® (Can)** *see* Chlorzoxazone *on page 300*

◆ **Stromectol®** *see* Ivermectin *on page 775*

◆ **Strong Iodine Solution** *see* Potassium Iodide and Iodine *on page 1140*

◆ **Sublimaze® [DSC]** *see* FentaNYL *on page 567*

◆ **Suboxone®** *see* Buprenorphine and Naloxone *on page 216*

◆ **Subutex®** *see* Buprenorphine *on page 214*

Succimer (SUKS i mer)

U.S. Brand Names Chemet®

Canadian Brand Names Chemet®

Therapeutic Category Antidote, Lead Toxicity; Chelating Agent, Oral

Generic Available No

Use Treatment of lead poisoning in children with blood levels >45 mcg/dL; not indicated for prophylaxis of lead poisoning in a lead-containing environment

Pregnancy Risk Factor C

Pregnancy Considerations Adverse events were observed in animal reproduction studies. Following maternal occupational exposure, lead crosses the placenta in amounts related to maternal plasma levels. Possible outcomes of maternal lead exposure >10 mcg/dL includes spontaneous abortion, postnatal developmental delay, and reduced birth weight. Chelation therapy during pregnancy is for maternal benefit only and should be limited to the treatment of severe, symptomatic lead poisoning.

Lactation Excretion in breast milk unknown/not recommended

Breast-Feeding Considerations It is not known if succimer is found in breast milk. The amount of lead in breast milk may range from 0.6% to 3% of the maternal serum concentration. Calcium supplementation may reduce the amount of lead in breast milk.

Contraindications Hypersensitivity to succimer or any component

Warnings Elevated blood lead levels and associated symptoms may return rapidly after discontinuation due to redistribution of lead from bone stores to soft tissues and blood; monitor blood lead levels for "rebound" after therapy; mild to moderate neutropenia has been reported; monitor CBC with differential prior to and during therapy; discontinue treatment if ANC <1200/microliter

Precautions Use with caution in patients with renal or hepatic impairment; adequate hydration should be maintained during therapy

Adverse Reactions The most common events attributable to succimer have been observed in about 10% of patients treated

Central nervous system: Headache, fatigue, dizziness

Dermatologic: Rash, pruritus

Gastrointestinal: Nausea, vomiting, diarrhea, appetite loss, metallic taste, hemorrhoidal symptoms, sulfurous odor to breath, sore throat

Hematologic: Thrombocytosis, eosinophilia, reversible neutropenia

Hepatic: AST, ALT, alkaline phosphatase, and serum cholesterol elevated (transient)

Neuromuscular & skeletal: Paresthesia, sensorimotor neuropathy, back, rib, kneecap, and leg pains

Ocular: Watery eyes, cloudy film in eye

Renal: Sulfurous odor to urine, urination decreased, proteinuria

Respiratory: Rhinorrhea, nasal congestion

Miscellaneous: Flu-like symptoms, mucocutaneous hypersensitivity reactions (with repeat administration)

Drug Interactions

Avoid Concomitant Use There are no known interactions where it is recommended to avoid concomitant use.

Increased Effect/Toxicity There are no known significant interactions involving an increase in effect.

Decreased Effect There are no known significant interactions involving a decrease in effect.

Mechanism of Action Forms stable water-soluble complexes with lead resulting in increased urinary excretion; also chelates other toxic heavy metals such as arsenic and mercury

Pharmacokinetics (Adult data unless noted)

Absorption: Oral: Rapid, variable

Metabolism: Extensive to mixed succimer-cysteine disulfides

Half-life, elimination: 2 days

Time to peak serum concentration: ~1-2 hours

Elimination: ~25% in urine with peak urinary excretion occurring between 2-4 hours after dosing; of the total amount of succimer eliminated in urine, 90% is eliminated as mixed succimer-cysteine disulfide conjugates; 10% is excreted unchanged; fecal excretion of succimer probably represents unabsorbed drug

Dialysis: Succimer is dialyzable but lead chelates are not

Usual Dosage Children and Adults: Oral: 10 mg/kg/dose (or 350 mg/m^2/dose) every 8 hours for 5 days followed by 10 mg/kg/dose (or 350 mg/m^2/dose) every 12 hours for 14 days

Succimer Dosing

Weight		Dosage[1] (mg)
18-35 lbs	8-15 kg	100
36-55 lbs	16-23 kg	200
56-75 lbs	24-34 kg	300
76-100 lbs	35-44 kg	400
>100 lbs	>45 kg	500

[1]To be administered every 8 hours.

Note: Concomitant iron therapy has been reported in a small number of children without the formation of a toxic complex with iron (as seen with dimercaprol); courses of therapy may be repeated if indicated by weekly monitoring of blood lead levels; lead levels should be stabilized to <15 mcg/dL; 2 weeks between courses is recommended unless more timely treatment is indicated by lead levels; patients who have received calcium disodium EDTA with or without BAL may be treated with succimer after at least 4 weeks have passed since treatment

Dosing adjustment in renal/hepatic impairment: Administer with caution and monitor closely

Administration Oral: Ensure adequate patient hydration; for patients who cannot swallow the capsule, sprinkle the medicated beads on a small amount of soft food or administer with a fruit juice to mask the odor

Monitoring Parameters Blood lead levels; liver enzymes and CBC with differential (prior to therapy and weekly during therapy)

Test Interactions Falsely decreased CPK; false-positive urine ketones with Ketostix®, falsely decreased uric acid measurements

Dosage Forms Excipient information presented when available (limited, particularly for generics); consult specific product labeling.

Capsule:

Chemet®:100 mg

References

American Academy of Pediatrics Committee on Environmental Health, "Lead Exposure in Children: Prevention, Detection, and Management," *Pediatrics*, 2005, 116(4):1036-46.

Binns HJ, Campbell C, Brown MJ, et al, "Interpreting and Managing Blood Lead Levels of Less Than 10 micrograms/dL in Children and Reducing Childhood Exposure to Lead: Recommendations of the Centers for Disease Control and Prevention Advisory Committee on Childhood Lead Poisoning Prevention," *Pediatrics*, 2007, 120(5):e1285-98.

Gracia RC and Snodgrass WR, "Lead Toxicity and Chelation Therapy," *Am J Health Syst Pharm*, 2007, 64(1):45-53.

Mann KV and Travers JD, "Succimer, An Oral Lead Chelator," *Clin Pharm*, 1991, 10(12):914-22.

Succinylcholine (suks in il KOE leen)

Medication Safety Issues

International issues:

Quelicin® [U.S., Brazil, Canada, Indonesia] may be confused with Keflin, a brand name for cefalotin [Argentina, Brazil, Mexico, Netherlands, Norway]

High alert medication: The Institute for Safe Medication Practices (ISMP) includes this medication among its list of drugs which have a heightened risk of causing significant patient harm when used in error.

United States Pharmacopeia (USP) 2006: The Interdisciplinary Safe Medication Use Expert Committee of the USP has recommended the following:

- Hospitals, clinics, and other practice sites should institute special safeguards in the storage, labeling, and use of these agents and should include these safeguards in staff orientation and competency training.
- Healthcare professionals should be on high alert (especially vigilant) whenever a neuromuscular-blocking agent (NMBA) is stocked, ordered, prepared, or administered.

U.S. Brand Names Anectine®; Quelicin®

Canadian Brand Names Quelicin®

Therapeutic Category Neuromuscular Blocker Agent, Depolarizing; Skeletal Muscle Relaxant, Paralytic

Generic Available No

Use Used to produce skeletal muscle relaxation in procedures of short duration such as endotracheal intubation or endoscopic exams

Pregnancy Risk Factor C

Pregnancy Considerations Reproduction studies have not been conducted. Small amounts cross the placenta. Sensitivity to succinylcholine may be increased due to a ~24% decrease in plasma cholinesterase activity during pregnancy and several days postpartum.

Lactation Excretion in breast milk unknown/use caution

Contraindications Hypersensitivity to succinylcholine chloride, or any component; personal or familial history of malignant hyperthermia; skeletal muscle myopathies; acute phase injury following major burns, multiple trauma, extensive denervation of skeletal muscle, or upper motor neuron injury (see Precautions); narrow-angle glaucoma; penetrating eye injuries (increased intraocular pressure)

Warnings Malignant hyperthermia may be triggered by succinylcholine use; risk increases with the concomitant administration of volatile anesthetics; monitor closely for signs/symptoms. Use with caution in children and adolescents; rare reports of acute rhabdomyolysis with hyperkalemia followed by ventricular dysrhythmias, cardiac arrest, and death have been reported in children with undiagnosed skeletal muscle myopathy, most frequently Duchenne's muscular dystrophy **[U.S. Boxed Warning]**. This syndrome presents as peaked T-waves and sudden cardiac arrest within minutes after the administration of succinylcholine. Also, if sudden cardiac arrest occurs immediately after administration of succinylcholine, consider hyperkalemia as potential etiology and manage accordingly. Since it is difficult to predict which patients may develop this reaction, it is recommended that the use of succinylcholine be limited to emergency intubation or instances where immediate securing of the airway is necessary (eg, laryngospasm, difficult airway, full stomach, or for intramuscular use when a suitable vein is inaccessible). Avoid use in patients with serum potassium >5.5 mEq/L. Metabolized by plasma cholinesterase; use with caution (if at all) in patients suspected of being homozygous for the atypical plasma cholinesterase gene. Plasma cholinesterase activity may also be reduced by burns, decompensated heart disease, infections, malignant tumors, myxedema, pregnancy, severe hepatic or renal dysfunction, ulcer, and certain medications and chemicals. May increase IOP; use caution with narrow-angle glaucoma or penetrating eye injuries; do not use when increase in intraocular pressure is undesirable unless benefit outweighs the risk.

Precautions Use with extreme caution in patients recovering from severe trauma, extensive or severe burns, extensive denervation of skeletal muscle because of disease or injury to the CNS, or with degenerative or dystrophic neuromuscular disease due to increased risk for development of hyperkalemia; risk for hyperkalemia in these patients increases over time and usually peaks at

◀ 7-10 days after the injury; risk is dependent upon the extent and location of the injury. Use with caution in patients with fractures or muscle spasms as initial muscle fasciculations from succinylcholine may cause additional trauma. Tachyphylaxis occurs with repeated administration. As succinylcholine has no effects on consciousness, pain threshold, or cerebration, it should be used with adequate sedation. Neuromuscular blockade may be prolonged in patients with severe hypokalemia, severe hypocalcemia, severe hyponatremia, hypermagnesemia, neuromuscular diseases, acidosis, acute intermittent porphyria, Eaton-Lambert syndrome, myasthenia gravis, renal failure, and hepatic failure.

Adverse Reactions
Cardiovascular: Bradycardia and rarely asystole (incidence higher in children than adults, with doses >1.5 mg/kg in children, and following a second dose in both children and adults), hypotension, cardiac arrhythmias, flushing, cardiac arrest, hypertension, tachycardia
Central nervous system: Malignant hyperthermia
Dermatologic: Rash
Endocrine & metabolic: Hyperkalemia, myoglobinemia
Gastrointestinal: Intragastric pressure elevated, salivation
Neuromuscular & skeletal: Myalgia due to muscle fasciculations, muscle weakness
Ocular: Intraocular pressure elevated
Renal: Myoglobinuria
Respiratory: Apnea, bronchospasm, respiratory depression

Drug Interactions
Avoid Concomitant Use
Avoid concomitant use of Succinylcholine with any of the following: QuiNINE

Increased Effect/Toxicity
Succinylcholine may increase the levels/effects of: Analgesics (Opioid); Cardiac Glycosides; OnabotulinumtoxinA; RimabotulinumtoxinB

The levels/effects of Succinylcholine may be increased by: AbobotulinumtoxinA; Acetylcholinesterase Inhibitors; Aminoglycosides; Capreomycin; Colistimethate; Cyclophosphamide; Echothiophate Iodide; Lincosamide Antibiotics; Lithium; Loop Diuretics; Magnesium Salts; Phenelzine; Polymyxin B; Procainamide; QuiNIDine; QuiNINE; Tetracycline Derivatives; Vancomycin

Decreased Effect
The levels/effects of Succinylcholine may be decreased by: Loop Diuretics

Stability Refrigerate; stability at room temperature is product specific; check with each manufacturer; injection is incompatible with alkaline solutions

Mechanism of Action Acts similarly to acetylcholine, produces depolarization of the motor endplate at the myoneural junction which causes sustained flaccid skeletal muscle paralysis

Pharmacodynamics
I.M.:
Onset of action: 2-3 minutes
Duration: 10-30 minutes
I.V.:
Onset of action: Within 30-60 seconds
Duration: ~4-6 minutes

Pharmacokinetics (Adult data unless noted)
Metabolism: Succinylcholine is rapidly hydrolyzed by plasma pseudocholinesterase to inactive metabolites
Elimination: 10% excreted unchanged in urine

Usual Dosage
Children: **Note:** Because of the risk of malignant hyperthermia, use of continuous infusion is **not** recommended in infants and children.
I.M.: 3-4 mg/kg

I.V.:
Infants: Initial: 2 mg/kg; maintenance: 0.3-0.6 mg/kg every 5-10 minutes as needed
Children: Initial: 1 mg/kg; maintenance: 0.3-0.6 mg/kg every 5-10 minutes as needed
Adults: I.M., I.V.: 0.6 mg/kg (range: 0.3-1.1 mg/kg); maintenance: 0.04-0.07 mg/kg every 5-10 minutes as needed
Continuous infusion: 2.5 mg/minute (range: 0.5-10 mg/minute)
Note: Pretreatment with atropine may reduce occurrence of bradycardia

Dosing adjustment in hepatic impairment: Dose should be decreased in patients with severe liver disease

Administration Parenteral: I.M.: May be administered by rapid I.V. injection without further dilution; continuous infusion: Dilute 1-2 mg/mL in NS or D_5W; I.M.: Injection should be made deeply

Monitoring Parameters Heart rate, serum potassium, assisted ventilator status, peripheral nerve stimulator measuring twitch response

Dosage Forms Excipient information presented when available (limited, particularly for generics); consult specific product labeling.
Injection, solution, as chloride:
Anectine®: 20 mg/mL (10 mL)
Quelicin®: 20 mg/mL (10 mL)
Injection, solution, as chloride [preservative free]:
Quelicin®: 100 mg/mL (10 mL)

◆ **Succinylcholine Chloride** see Succinylcholine on page 1295

◆ **Sucraid**® see Sacrosidase on page 1240

Sucralfate (soo KRAL fate)

Medication Safety Issues
Sound-alike/look-alike issues:
Sucralfate may be confused with salsalate
Carafate® may be confused with Cafergot®
U.S. Brand Names Carafate®
Canadian Brand Names Novo-Sucralate; Nu-Sucralate; PMS-Sucralate; Sulcrate®; Sulcrate® Suspension Plus
Therapeutic Category Gastrointestinal Agent, Gastric or Duodenal Ulcer Treatment
Generic Available Yes
Use Short-term management of duodenal ulcers; gastric ulcers; suspension may be used topically for treatment of stomatitis due to cancer chemotherapy or other causes of esophageal, gastric, and rectal erosions; treatment of NSAID mucosal damage; prevention of stress ulcers
Pregnancy Risk Factor B
Pregnancy Considerations Teratogenic effects were not observed in animal studies. Sucralfate is only minimally absorbed following oral administration.
Lactation Excretion in breast milk unknown/use caution
Contraindications Hypersensitivity to sucralfate or any component
Warnings Because of the potential for sucralfate to alter the absorption of some drugs, separate administration times (administer other medications 2 hours before or after sucralfate) should be considered when alterations in bioavailability are believed to be critical
Precautions Use with caution in renal failure due to accumulation of aluminum
Adverse Reactions
Cardiovascular: Facial edema
Central nervous system: Dizziness, sleepiness, vertigo, headache
Dermatologic: Rash, pruritus, angioedema
Gastrointestinal: Constipation, diarrhea, nausea, gastric discomfort, indigestion, xerostomia, flatulence

Neuromuscular & skeletal: Back pain

Respiratory: Laryngospasm, rhinitis, respiratory difficulty

Drug Interactions

Avoid Concomitant Use There are no known interactions where it is recommended to avoid concomitant use.

Increased Effect/Toxicity There are no known significant interactions involving an increase in effect.

Decreased Effect

Sucralfate may decrease the levels/effects of: Antifungal Agents (Azole Derivatives, Systemic); Digoxin; Eltrombopag; Levothyroxine; Phosphate Supplements; QuiNIDine; Quinolone Antibiotics; Tetracycline Derivatives; Vitamin K Antagonists

Food Interactions Interferes with absorption of vitamin A, vitamin D, vitamin E, and vitamin K

Mechanism of Action Aluminum salt of sulfated sucrose which in the presence of acid pH (gastric acid) forms a complex, paste-like substance that adheres to the damaged mucosal area. This selectively forms a protective coating that protects the lining against peptic acid, pepsin, and bile salts.

Pharmacodynamics GI protection effect:

Acid neutralizing capacity: 14-17 mEq/1 g dose of sucralfate

Onset of action: 1-2 hours

Duration: Up to 6 hours

Pharmacokinetics (Adult data unless noted)

Absorption: Oral: <5%

Metabolism: Not metabolized

Elimination: 90% excreted in stool; small amounts that are absorbed are excreted in the urine as unchanged compounds

Usual Dosage Oral:

Children: Dose not established; doses of 40-80 mg/kg/day divided every 6 hours have been used

Stomatitis: 5-10 mL (1 g/10 mL); swish and spit or swish and swallow 4 times/day

Adults:

Stress ulcer prophylaxis: 1 g 4 times/day

Stress ulcer treatment: 1 g every 4 hours

Duodenal ulcer:

Treatment: 1 g 4 times/day for 4-8 weeks, or alternatively 2 g twice daily; treatment is recommended for 4-8 weeks in adults

Maintenance: Prophylaxis: 1 g twice daily

Stomatitis: 1 g/10 mL suspension, swish and spit or swish and swallow 4 times/day

Proctitis: Rectal enema: 2 g/20 mL once or twice daily

Dosage comment in renal impairment: Aluminum salt is minimally absorbed (<5%), however, may accumulate in renal failure

Administration

Oral: Administer on an empty stomach 1 hour before meals and at bedtime (see Warnings); tablet may be broken or dissolved in water before ingestion; do not administer antacids within 30 minutes of administration; shake suspension well before use

Rectal: May administer oral suspension as rectal enema; shake suspension well before use

Patient Information May cause dry mouth; separate times of administration with other medications (see Drug Interactions) by at least 2 hours

Additional Information There is approximately 14-16 mEq acid neutralizing capacity per 1 g sucralfate

Dosage Forms Excipient information presented when available (limited, particularly for generics); consult specific product labeling.

Suspension, oral: 1 g/10 mL (10 mL)

Carafate®: 1 g/10 mL (420 mL)

Tablet: 1 g

Carafate®: 1 g

References

Melko GP, Turco TF, Phelan TF, et al, "Treatment of Radiation-Induced Proctitis With Sucralfate Enemas," *Ann Pharmacother*, 1999, 33 (12):1274-6.

◆ **Sucrets® [OTC]** *see* Dyclonine *on page 486*

◆ **Sudafed® [OTC]** *see* Pseudoephedrine *on page 1183*

◆ **Sudafed® 12 Hour [OTC]** *see* Pseudoephedrine *on page 1183*

◆ **Sudafed® 24 Hour [OTC]** *see* Pseudoephedrine *on page 1183*

◆ **Sudafed® Children's [OTC]** *see* Pseudoephedrine *on page 1183*

◆ **Sudafed® Decongestant (Can)** *see* Pseudoephedrine *on page 1183*

◆ **Sudafed® Maximum Strength Nasal Decongestant [OTC]** *see* Pseudoephedrine *on page 1183*

◆ **Sudafed OM® Sinus Congestion [OTC]** *see* Oxymetazoline *on page 1043*

◆ **Sudafed PE® Children's [OTC]** *see* Phenylephrine *on page 1102*

◆ **Sudafed PE® Congestion [OTC]** *see* Phenylephrine *on page 1102*

◆ **Sudafed PE® Nasal Decongestant [OTC]** *see* Phenylephrine *on page 1102*

◆ **Sudafed® Sinus Advance (Can)** *see* Pseudoephedrine and Ibuprofen *on page 1184*

◆ **SudoGest [OTC]** *see* Pseudoephedrine *on page 1183*

◆ **SudoGest Children's [OTC]** *see* Pseudoephedrine *on page 1183*

◆ **Sudogest™ PE [OTC]** *see* Phenylephrine *on page 1102*

◆ **Sudo-Tab® [OTC]** *see* Pseudoephedrine *on page 1183*

◆ **Sufenta®** *see* SUFentanil *on page 1297*

SUFentanil (soo FEN ta nil)

Medication Safety Issues

Sound-alike/look-alike issues:

SUFentanil may be confused with alfentanil, fentaNYL

Sufenta® may be confused with Alfenta®, Sudafed®, Survanta®

High alert medication: The Institute for Safe Medication Practices (ISMP) includes this medication among its list of drugs which have a heightened risk of causing significant patient harm when used in error.

U.S. Brand Names Sufenta®

Canadian Brand Names Sufentanil Citrate Injection, USP; Sufenta®

Therapeutic Category Analgesic, Narcotic; General Anesthetic

Generic Available Yes

Use Analgesia; analgesia adjunct; anesthetic agent

Restrictions C-II

Pregnancy Risk Factor C

Pregnancy Considerations Animal studies suggest embryocidal effects when given I.V. for a period of 10 days to >30 days. No evidence of teratogenic effects observed in animals. Administration of epidural sufenanil with bupivacaine with or without epinephrine is indicated in labor and delivery. Intravenous use or larger epidural doses are not recommended in pregnant women.

Contraindications Hypersensitivity to sufentanil or any component; increased intracranial pressure; severe respiratory depression

Warnings May cause severe respiratory depression; rapid I.V. infusion may result in skeletal muscle and chest wall rigidity, impaired ventilation, respiratory distress, apnea, bronchoconstriction, laryngospasm, arrest; inject slowly over 3-5 minutes; nondepolarizing skeletal muscle relaxant may be required; abrupt discontinuation after prolonged use may result in withdrawal symptoms

Precautions Use with caution in patients with head injuries, hepatic impairment, pulmonary disease, or with use of MAO inhibitors within past 14 days; sufentanil shares the toxic potential of opiate agonists, precautions of opiate agonist therapy should be observed

Adverse Reactions
Cardiovascular: Bradycardia, hypotension, peripheral vasodilation
Central nervous system: CNS depression, drowsiness, dizziness, sedation
Dermatologic: Erythema, pruritus, rash
Endocrine & metabolic: ADH release
Gastrointestinal: Nausea, vomiting, constipation, biliary tract spasm
Genitourinary: Urinary tract spasm
Neuromuscular & skeletal: Skeletal and thoracic muscle rigidity, especially after rapid I.V. administration
Ocular: Miosis, blurred vision
Respiratory: Respiratory depression, apnea
Miscellaneous: Physical and psychological dependence with prolonged use

Drug Interactions
Metabolism/Transport Effects Substrate of CYP3A4 (major)
Avoid Concomitant Use
Avoid concomitant use of SUFentanil with any of the following: MAO Inhibitors
Increased Effect/Toxicity
SUFentanil may increase the levels/effects of: Alcohol (Ethyl); Alvimopan; Beta-Blockers; Calcium Channel Blockers (Nondihydropyridine); CNS Depressants; Desmopressin; MAO Inhibitors; Selective Serotonin Reuptake Inhibitors; Thiazide Diuretics

The levels/effects of SUFentanil may be increased by: Amphetamines; Antipsychotic Agents (Phenothiazines); CYP3A4 Inhibitors (Moderate); CYP3A4 Inhibitors (Strong); Dasatinib; Succinylcholine

Decreased Effect
SUFentanil may decrease the levels/effects of: Pegvisomant

The levels/effects of SUFentanil may be decreased by: Ammonium Chloride; Mixed Agonist / Antagonist Opioids
Mechanism of Action Binds with stereospecific receptors at many sites within the CNS, increases pain threshold, alters pain reception, inhibits ascending pain pathways; ultra short-acting narcotic

Pharmacodynamics
Onset of action: 1-3 minutes
Duration: Dose dependent; anesthesia adjunct doses: 5 minutes

Pharmacokinetics (Adult data unless noted)
Distribution: V_{dss}:
Children 2-8 years: 2.9 ± 0.6 L/kg
Adults: 1.7 ± 0.2 L/kg
Protein binding (alpha$_1$acid glycoprotein):
Neonates: 79%
Adults:
Male: 93%
Postpartum women: 91%
Metabolism: Primarily by the liver via demethylation and dealkylation
Half-life, elimination:
Neonates: 382-1162 minutes
Children 2-8 years: 97 ± 42 minutes
Adolescents 10-15 years: 76 ± 33 minutes
Adults: 164 ± 22 minutes

Elimination: ~2% excreted unchanged in the urine; 80% of dose excreted in urine (mostly as metabolites) within 24 hours
Clearance:
Children 2-8 years: 30.5 ± 8.8 mL/minute/kg
Adolescents: 12.8 ± 12 mL/minute/kg
Adults: 12.7 ± 0.8 mL/minute/kg

Usual Dosage Doses should be titrated to appropriate effects; wide range of doses, dependent upon desired degree of analgesia or anesthesia; use lean body weight to dose patients who are >20% above ideal body weight

Children <12 years: Anesthesia: I.V.: Initial: 10-25 mcg/kg; maintenance: Up to 25-50 mcg as needed
Adults: I.V.:
Adjunct to general anesthesia:
Low dose: Initial: 0.5-1 mcg/kg; maintenance: 10-25 mcg as needed
Moderate dose: Initial: 2-8 mcg/kg; maintenance: 10-50 mcg as needed
Anesthesia: Initial: 8-30 mcg/kg; maintenance: 10-50 mcg as needed

Administration Parenteral: I.V.: Slow I.V. injection or by infusion
Monitoring Parameters Respiratory rate, blood pressure, heart rate, oxygen saturation, neurological status (for degree of analgesia/anesthesia)
Patient Information May be habit-forming; avoid abrupt discontinuation after prolonged use
Nursing Implications Patient may develop rebound respiratory depression postoperatively
Dosage Forms Excipient information presented when available (limited, particularly for generics); consult specific product labeling.
Injection, solution [preservative free]: 50 mcg/mL (1 mL, 2 mL, 5 mL)
Sufenta®: 50 mcg/mL (1 mL, 2 mL, 5 mL)

References
Guay J, Gaudreault P, Tang A, et al, "Pharmacokinetics of Sufentanil in Normal Children," *Can J Anaesth*, 1992, 39(1):14-20.
Seguin JH, Erenberg A, and Leff RD, "Safety and Efficacy of Sufentanil Therapy in the Ventilated Infant," *Neonatal Netw*, 1994, 13(4):37-40.

♦ **Sufentanil Citrate** *see* SUFentanil *on page 1297*
♦ **Sufentanil Citrate Injection, USP (Can)** *see* SUFentanil *on page 1297*
♦ **Sulamyd** *see* Sulfacetamide *on page 1298*
♦ **Sulbactam and Ampicillin** *see* Ampicillin and Sulbactam *on page 106*
♦ **Sulcrate® (Can)** *see* Sucralfate *on page 1296*
♦ **Sulcrate® Suspension Plus (Can)** *see* Sucralfate *on page 1296*

Sulfacetamide (sul fa SEE ta mide)

Medication Safety Issues
Sound-alike/look-alike issues:
Bleph®-10 may be confused with Blephamide®
Klaron® may be confused with Klor-Con®
U.S. Brand Names Bleph®-10; Carmol® Scalp Treatment; Klaron®; Ovace®; Ovace® Plus; Rosula® NS; Seb-Prev™
Canadian Brand Names AK Sulf Liq; Bleph 10 DPS; Diosulf™; PMS-Sulfacetamide; Sodium Sulamyd; Sulfacet-R
Therapeutic Category Antibiotic, Ophthalmic; Antibiotic, Sulfonamide Derivative
Generic Available Yes: Ointment, solution, suspension
Use
Ophthalmic: Treatment and prophylaxis of conjunctivitis, corneal ulcers, and other superficial ocular infections due to susceptible organisms

Dermatologic: Scaling dermatosis (seborrheic); bacterial infections of the skin due to organisms susceptible to sulfonamides; acne vulgaris

Pregnancy Risk Factor C

Pregnancy Considerations Animal reproduction studies have not been conducted. Use of systemic sulfonamides during pregnancy may cause kernicterus in the newborn; the amount of systemic absorption following topical administration is not known. Use during pregnancy only if clearly needed.

Lactation Excretion in breast milk unknown/use caution

Breast-Feeding Considerations The amount of systemic absorption following topical administration is not known. Use of systemic sulfonamides while breast-feeding may cause kernicterus in the newborn; the amount of systemic absorption following topical administration is not known.

Contraindications Hypersensitivity to sulfacetamide, any component (see Warnings), or sulfonamides; infants <2 months of age; epithelial herpes simplex keratitis, vaccinia, varicella, and other viral diseases of the cornea and conjunctiva; fungal diseases of the ocular structures

Warnings Antibacterial activity may be decreased in the presence of purulent exudates containing para-amino-benzoic acid (PABA); nonsusceptible organisms such as fungi may proliferate with prolonged or repeated use of sulfonamide preparations; hemolysis may occur in patients with G-6-PD deficiency. Hypersensitivity reactions may occur when a sulfonamide is readministered, irrespective of the route of administration. Stevens-Johnson syndrome has been reported following the use of sulfacetamide topically. At the first sign of hypersensitivity, skin rash, or other reactions, inform physician and discontinue use. Some products contain sulfites which may cause allergic reactions in susceptible individuals

Precautions Use with caution in patients with severe dry eye or G-6-PD deficiency

Adverse Reactions

Central nervous system: Headache, fever

Dermatologic: Stevens-Johnson syndrome, exfoliative dermatitis, toxic epidermal necrolysis, rash, photosensitivity, erythema, pruritus, scaling of the skin

Hematologic: Bone marrow suppression

Local: Irritation, stinging and burning (especially with 30% solution)

Ocular: Blurred vision, transient epithelial keratitis, reactive hyperemia, conjunctival edema

Miscellaneous: Hypersensitivity reactions, syndrome resembling systemic lupus erythematosus

Drug Interactions

Avoid Concomitant Use

Avoid concomitant use of Sulfacetamide with any of the following: BCG; Methenamine; Procaine

Increased Effect/Toxicity

Sulfacetamide may increase the levels/effects of: Methotrexate; Phenytoin; Vitamin K Antagonists

The levels/effects of Sulfacetamide may be increased by: Methenamine

Decreased Effect

Sulfacetamide may decrease the levels/effects of: BCG; Typhoid Vaccine

The levels/effects of Sulfacetamide may be decreased by: Procaine

Stability Protect from light; discolored or cloudy solutions should not be used; incompatible with silver and zinc sulfate; sulfacetamide is inactivated by blood or purulent exudates

Mechanism of Action Interferes with bacterial growth by inhibiting bacterial folic acid synthesis through competitive antagonism of PABA

Pharmacodynamics Onset of action: Improvement of conjunctivitis is usually seen within 3-6 days

Pharmacokinetics (Adult data unless noted)

Distribution: Excreted in breast milk

Half-life: 7-13 hours

Elimination: When absorbed, excreted primarily in urine as unchanged drug

Usual Dosage Children >2 months and Adults:

Ophthalmic:

Ointment: Apply to lower conjunctival sac 1-4 times/day and at bedtime or apply 1/2" to 1" into the conjunctival sac at night in conjunction with the use of drops during the day

Solution: Instill 1-2 drops into the lower conjunctival sac every 1-3 hours according to severity of infection during the waking hours and less frequently at night; increase dosing interval as condition responds. Usual duration of treatment: 7-10 days

Topical: Children and Adults:

Lotion: Apply to affected areas twice daily

Scalp lotion: Apply at bedtime. For severe cases with crusting, heavy scaling and inflammation, apply twice daily. Once eruption subsides, apply once or twice weekly or every other week to prevent reoccurrence.

Wash: Wash affected areas twice daily. If skin dryness occurs, use less frequently.

Medicated pads: Gently apply to affected areas 1-2 times/day

Administration

Ophthalmic: Avoid contact of tube or bottle tip with skin or eye; solution: Apply finger pressure to lacrimal sac during and for 1-2 minutes after instillation to decrease risk of absorption and systemic effects

Topical: For external use only

Lotion: Shake lotion well before using; apply a thin film to affected area.

Scalp lotion: Wash hair and scalp prior to application. Part hair a section at a time and apply a small quantity of lotion. Completely moisten scalp and gently rub in lotion with the fingertips. Then brush hair thoroughly for 2-3 minutes.

Wash: Wet skin and apply wash liberally to areas to be cleansed. Massage gently into skin working into a lather; rinse thoroughly and pat dry.

Monitoring Parameters Response to therapy

Patient Information Eye drops may burn and sting when first instilled; may cause sensitivity to bright light.

Dosage Forms Excipient information presented when available (limited, particularly for generics); consult specific product labeling. [DSC] = Discontinued product

Aerosal, topical, as sodium [foam]:

Ovace®: 10% (50 g [DSC], 70 g, 100 g [DSC])

Cream, topical, as sodium:

Ovace®: 10% (30 g, 60 g) [DSC]

Seb-Prev™: 10% (30 g, 60 g) [contains benzyl alcohol]

Gel, topical, as sodium:

Ovace® [DSC], Seb-Prev™: 10% (30 g, 60 g)

Lotion, topical, as sodium: 10% (120 mL)

Carmol® Scalp Treatment: 10% (85 g) [contains urea 10%]

Klaron®: 10% (120 mL) [contains sodium metabisulfite]

Lotion, topical, as sodium [wash]:

Ovace®: 10% (180 mL, 360 mL)

Lotion, topical, as sodium [emulsion-based wash]:

Ovace® Plus: 10% (180 mL [DSC], 360 mL [DSC], 480 mL)

Pad, topical, as sodium:

Rosula® NS: 10% (30s) [contains urea 10%]

Soap, topical, as sodium [wash]:

Seb-Prev™: 10% (170 mL, 340 mL)

Solution, ophthalmic, as sodium [drops]: 10% (15 mL)

Bleph®-10: 10% (5 mL) [contains benzalkonium chloride]

Suspension, topical, as sodium: 10% (118 mL)

References

Lohr JA, Austin RD, Grossman M, et al, "Comparison of Three Topical Antimicrobials for Acute Bacterial Conjunctivitis," *Pediatr Infect Dis J*, 1988, 7(9):626-9.

◆ **Sulfacetamide Sodium** *see* Sulfacetamide *on page 1298*

◆ **Sulfacet-R (Can)** *see* Sulfacetamide *on page 1298*

SulfADIAZINE (sul fa DYE a zeen)

Medication Safety Issues
Sound-alike/look-alike issues:
SulfaDIAZINE may be confused with sulfasalazine, sulfiSOXAZOLE

Therapeutic Category Antibiotic, Sulfonamide Derivative

Generic Available Yes

Use Adjunctive treatment in toxoplasmosis; treatment of urinary tract infections and nocardiosis; rheumatic fever prophylaxis in penicillin-allergic patient; uncomplicated attack of malaria

Pregnancy Risk Factor C

Pregnancy Considerations Adverse events have been observed in animal reproduction studies; therefore, the manufacturer classifies sulfadiazine as pregnancy category C. Sulfadiazine crosses the placenta. Available studies and case reports have failed to show an increased risk for congenital malformations after use. Sulfadiazine is indicated for use in children <2 months of age for the treatment of congenital toxoplasmosis and may be used in pregnancy for the maternal treatment of *Toxoplasmic gondii* encephalitis and as an alternative agent for the secondary prevention of rheumatic fever. Because of the theoretical increased risk for hyperbilirubinemia and kernicterus, sulfadiazine is contraindicated by the manufacturer for use near term. Neonatal healthcare providers should be informed if maternal sulfonamide therapy is used near the time of delivery.

Lactation Enters breast milk/contraindicated

Breast-Feeding Considerations Sulfadiazine distributes into human milk. Per the manufacturer, sulfadiazine is contraindicated in nursing mothers since sulfonamides cross into the milk and may cause kernicterus in the newborn. Because sulfadiazine has therapeutic indications for infants ≥2 months of age, kernicterus after exposure via breast-feeding would not be expected in healthy infants of this age group; however, sulfonamides should not be used while nursing an infant with G6PD deficiency or hyperbilirubinemia. Nondose-related effects could include modification of bowel flora.

Contraindications Hypersensitivity to any sulfa drug or any component; porphyria; infants <2 months of age due to competition with bilirubin for protein-binding sites (unless indicated for the treatment of congenital toxoplasmosis); pregnant women during third trimester

Precautions Use with caution in patients with impaired hepatic function or impaired renal function, urinary obstruction, blood dyscrasia, G-6-PD deficiency; dosage modification required in patients with renal impairment

Adverse Reactions
Cardiovascular: Vasculitis

Central nervous system: Dizziness, fever, headache

Dermatologic: Rash, exfoliative dermatitis, Stevens-Johnson syndrome, photosensitivity, urticaria

Gastrointestinal: Nausea, vomiting, abdominal pain

Genitourinary: Crystalluria

Hematologic: Granulocytopenia, leukopenia, thrombocytopenia, aplastic anemia, hemolytic anemia

Hepatic: Jaundice, hepatitis

Renal: Acute nephropathy, hematuria

Miscellaneous: Serum sickness-like reactions

Drug Interactions
Metabolism/Transport Effects Substrate of CYP2C9 (major), 2E1 (minor), 3A4 (minor); **Inhibits** CYP2C9 (strong)

Avoid Concomitant Use
Avoid concomitant use of SulfADIAZINE with any of the following: BCG; Methenamine; Procaine

Increased Effect/Toxicity
SulfADIAZINE may increase the levels/effects of: Carvedilol; CycloSPORINE; CycloSPORINE (Systemic); CYP2C9 Substrates (High risk); Methotrexate; Phenytoin; Sulfonylureas; Vitamin K Antagonists

The levels/effects of SulfADIAZINE may be increased by: CYP2C9 Inhibitors (Moderate); CYP2C9 Inhibitors (Strong); Methenamine

Decreased Effect
SulfADIAZINE may decrease the levels/effects of: BCG; CycloSPORINE; CycloSPORINE (Systemic); Typhoid Vaccine

The levels/effects of SulfADIAZINE may be decreased by: CYP2C9 Inducers (Highly Effective); Peginterferon Alfa-2b; Procaine

Food Interactions Supplemental leucovorin calcium should be administered to reverse symptoms or prevent problems due to folic acid deficiency; avoid large quantities of vitamin C or acidifying agents (cranberry juice) to prevent crystalluria

Stability Protect from light

Mechanism of Action Interferes with bacterial growth by inhibiting bacterial folic acid synthesis through competitive antagonism of PABA

Pharmacokinetics (Adult data unless noted)
Absorption: Oral: Well absorbed

Distribution: Excreted in breast milk; diffuses into CSF with higher concentrations reached when meninges are inflamed; distributed into most body tissues

Protein binding: 32% to 56%

Metabolism: Metabolized by N-acetylation

Half-life: 10 hours

Time to peak serum concentration: Within 4 hours

Elimination: In urine as metabolites (15% to 40%) and as unchanged drug (43% to 60%)

Usual Dosage Oral:
Congenital toxoplasmosis: Newborns: 100 mg/kg/day divided every 12 hours for 12 months in conjunction with pyrimethamine 1 mg/kg/day once daily and supplemental leucovorin calcium 5 mg every 3 days for first 6 months, then pyrimethamine 1 mg/kg/day 3 times/week and leucovorin calcium 10 mg 3 times/week for the next 6 months

Toxoplasmosis:
Children: 120-200 mg/kg/day divided every 6 hours in conjunction with pyrimethamine 2 mg/kg/day divided every 12 hours for 3 days followed by 1 mg/kg/day once daily (maximum dose: 25 mg/day) with supplemental leucovorin calcium 5-10 mg every 3 days

Adults: 2-8 g/day divided every 6 hours in conjunction with pyrimethamine 25 mg/day and with supplemental leucovorin calcium 5-10 mg every 3 days

Prophylaxis of recurrent rheumatic fever:
≤30 kg: 500 mg once daily
>30 kg: 1 g once daily

Administration Oral: Administer with water on an empty stomach

Monitoring Parameters CBC, renal function tests, urinalysis

Patient Information Drink plenty of fluids; limit alcohol; notify physician if rash, sore throat, fever, arthralgia, shortness of breath, or jaundice occurs. May cause photosensitivity reactions (eg, exposure to sunlight may cause severe sunburn, skin rash, redness, or itching);

avoid exposure to sunlight and artificial light sources (sunlamps, tanning booth/bed); wear protective clothing, wide-brimmed hats, sunglasses, and lip sunscreen (SPF ≥15); use a sunscreen [broad-spectrum sunscreen or physical sunscreen (preferred) or sunblock with SPF ≥15]; contact physician if reaction occurs.

Dosage Forms Excipient information presented when available (limited, particularly for generics); consult specific product labeling.

Tablet: 500 mg

Extemporaneous Preparations Tablets may be crushed to prepare oral suspension of the drug in water or with a sucrose-containing solution; aqueous suspension with concentrations of 100 mg/mL should be stored in the refrigerator and used within 7 days

References

Frenkel JK, "Toxoplasmosis," *Pediatr Clin North Am*, 1985, 32 (4):917-32.

Sulfadoxine and Pyrimethamine
(sul fa DOKS een & peer i METH a meen)

U.S. Brand Names Fansidar® [DSC]

Therapeutic Category Antimalarial Agent

Generic Available No

Use Treatment of *Plasmodium falciparum* malaria in patients in whom chloroquine resistance is suspected; malaria prophylaxis for travelers to areas where chloroquine-resistant malaria is endemic

Pregnancy Risk Factor C/D (at term)

Contraindications Hypersensitivity to any sulfa drug, pyrimethamine, or any component; megaloblastic anemia due to folate deficiency; children <2 months of age (due to competition with bilirubin for protein binding sites); pregnant women at term; breast-feeding; repeated prophylactic use in patients with renal or hepatic failure or with blood dyscrasias

Warnings Fatalities associated with sulfonamides, although rare, have occurred due to severe reactions including Stevens-Johnson syndrome, toxic epidermal necrolysis, hepatic necrosis, agranulocytosis, aplastic anemia and other blood dyscrasias [U.S. Boxed Warning]; discontinue use at first sign of rash or any sign of adverse reaction; hemolysis may occur in patients with G-6-PD deficiency

Precautions Use with caution in patients with renal or hepatic impairment, patients with possible folate deficiency, patients with bronchial asthma, and patients with seizure disorders. Avoid excess sun exposure.

Adverse Reactions

Cardiovascular: Vasculitis

Central nervous system: Seizures, headache, insomnia, ataxia, fatigue, hyperesthesia

Dermatologic: Erythema multiforme, Stevens-Johnson syndrome, toxic epidermal necrolysis, rash, photosensitivity, urticaria, pruritus

Endocrine & metabolic: Folic acid deficiency

Gastrointestinal: Anorexia, vomiting, gastritis, glossitis, diarrhea, abdominal cramps

Hematologic: Megaloblastic anemia, leukopenia, thrombocytopenia, pancytopenia, agranulocytosis, pulmonary eosinophilia

Hepatic: Hepatic necrosis; jaundice; ALT, AST elevated

Neuromuscular & skeletal: Tremor

Respiratory: Respiratory failure

Drug Interactions

Metabolism/Transport Effects Pyrimethamine: **Inhibits** CYP2C9 (moderate), 2D6 (moderate)

Avoid Concomitant Use

Avoid concomitant use of Sulfadoxine and Pyrimethamine with any of the following: Artemether; BCG; Lumefantrine; Methenamine; Procaine

Increased Effect/Toxicity

Sulfadoxine and Pyrimethamine may increase the levels/ effects of: Antipsychotic Agents (Phenothiazines); Carvedilol; CycloSPORINE; CycloSPORINE (Systemic); CYP2C9 Substrates (High risk); CYP2D6 Substrates; Dapsone; Dapsone (Systemic); Dapsone (Topical); Fesoterodine; Lumefantrine; Methotrexate; Nebivolol; Phenytoin; Sulfonylureas; Tamoxifen; Vitamin K Antagonists

The levels/effects of Sulfadoxine and Pyrimethamine may be increased by: Artemether; Dapsone; Dapsone (Systemic); Methenamine

Decreased Effect

Sulfadoxine and Pyrimethamine may decrease the levels/effects of: BCG; Codeine; CycloSPORINE; CycloSPORINE (Systemic); TraMADol; Typhoid Vaccine

The levels/effects of Sulfadoxine and Pyrimethamine may be decreased by: Methylfolate; Procaine

Stability Protect from light

Mechanism of Action Sulfadoxine interferes with bacterial folic acid synthesis and growth via competitive inhibition of para-aminiobenzoic acid; pyrimethamine inhibits microbial dihydrofolate reductase, resulting in inhibition of tetrahydrofolic acid synthesis

Pharmacokinetics (Adult data unless noted)

Absorption: Oral: Well absorbed

Distribution: Excreted in breast milk; pyrimethamine is distributed to kidneys, lungs, liver, and spleen; sulfadoxine is widely distributed in the body

Protein binding:

Pyrimethamine: 80% to 87%

Sulfadoxine: 90% to 95%

Half-life:

Pyrimethamine: 111 hours

Sulfadoxine: 169 hours

Time to peak serum concentration: Within 2-8 hours

Elimination: In urine as parent compounds and several unidentified metabolites

Usual Dosage Children ≥ 2 months and Adults: Oral:

Treatment of acute attack of malaria: A single dose of the following number of Fansidar® tablets is used in sequence with quinine on last day of quinine therapy:

2-11 months: 1/4 tablet

1-3 years: 1/2 tablet

4-8 years: 1 tablet

9-14 years: 2 tablets

>14 years: 3 tablets

Adults: 3 tablets on last day of quinine therapy

Malaria prophylaxis (for areas where chloroquine-resistant *P. falciparum* exists):

Short-term travel (≤3 weeks): Travelers should carry pyrimethamine-sulfadoxine for use as presumptive self-treatment if a febrile illness develops while taking chloroquine for prophylaxis. Take single dose in the event of febrile illness when medical attention is not immediately available:

2-11 months: 1/4 tablet

1-3 years: 1/2 tablet

4-8 years: 1 tablet

9-14 years: 2 tablets

>14 years and Adults: 3 tablets

Administration Oral: Administer with meals

Monitoring Parameters Liver function tests, CBC including platelet counts, renal function tests and urinalysis should be performed periodically

Patient Information Drink plenty of fluids; notify physician if rash, sore throat, pallor, glossitis, fever, arthralgia, cough, shortness of breath, or jaundice occurs; limit alcohol. May cause photosensitivity reactions (eg, exposure to sunlight may cause severe sunburn, skin rash, redness, or itching); avoid exposure to sunlight and artificial light sources (sunlamps, tanning booth/bed); wear protective clothing, wide-brimmed hats, sunglasses, and lip sunscreen (SPF ≥15); use a sunscreen [broad-spectrum sunscreen or physical sunscreen (preferred) or sunblock with SPF ≥15]; contact physician if reaction occurs.

Additional Information Leucovorin calcium should be administered to reverse signs and symptoms of folic acid deficiency

Dosage Forms Excipient information presented when available (limited, particularly for generics); consult specific product labeling. [DSC] = Discontinued product

Tablet:

Fansidar®: Sulfadoxine 500 mg and pyrimethamine 25 mg [DSC]

References

Lynk A and Gold R, "Review of 40 Children With Imported Malaria," *Pediatr Infect Dis J*, 1989, 8(11):745-50.

Randall G and Seidel JS, "Malaria," *Pediatr Clin North Am*, 1985, 32 (4):893-916.

Sulfamethoxazole and Trimethoprim
(sul fa meth OKS a zole & trye METH oh prim)

Medication Safety Issues
Sound-alike/look-alike issues:
Bactrim™ may be confused with bacitracin, Bactine®, Bactroban®
Co-trimoxazole may be confused with clotrimazole
Septra® may be confused with Ceptaz®, Sectral®
Septra® DS may be confused with Semprex®-D

U.S. Brand Names Bactrim™; Bactrim™ DS; Septra®; Septra® DS; Sulfatrim®

Canadian Brand Names Apo-Sulfatrim®; Apo-Sulfatrim® DS; Apo-Sulfatrim® Pediatric; Novo-Trimel; Novo-Trimel D.S.; Nu-Cotrimox; Septra® Injection

Therapeutic Category Antibiotic, Sulfonamide Derivative

Generic Available Yes

Use Treatment of urinary tract infections caused by susceptible *E. coli*, *Klebsiella*, *Enterobacter*, *Proteus mirabilis*, *Proteus* (indole positive); acute otitis media due to amoxicillin-resistant *H. influenzae*, *S. pneumoniae*, and *M. catarrhalis*; acute exacerbations of chronic bronchitis; prophylaxis and treatment of *Pneumocystis jiroveci* pneumonitis (PCP); treatment of susceptible shigellosis, typhoid fever, *Nocardia asteroides* infection, and *Xanthomonas maltophilia* infection; the I.V. preparation is used for treatment of *Pneumocystis jiroveci* pneumonia, *Shigella*, and severe urinary tract infections

Pregnancy Risk Factor C

Pregnancy Considerations Adverse events have been observed in animal reproduction studies; therefore, the manufacturer classifies TMP-SMX as pregnancy category C. TMP-SMX crosses the placenta and distributes to amniotic fluid. Due to trimethoprim's potential effect on folic acid metabolism, TMP-SMX should only be used during pregnancy if the benefit justifies the potential risk. The use of dihydrofolate reductase inhibitors, including trimethoprim, during pregnancy may increase the risk of congenital anomalies including cardiovascular defects, oral clefts, urinary tract anomalies, and neural tube defects. Folic acid supplementation may decrease this risk. A few case reports have described additional congenital anomalies after TMP-SMX exposure, but none of these have proven causality. Most studies and case reports have failed to show an increased risk for congenital malformations after use of TMP-SMX. Per the manufacturer, TMP-SMX is contraindicated in late pregnancy because sulfonamides pass the placenta and may cause kernicterus in the newborn, but this has not been observed specifically with SMX. Neonatal healthcare providers should be informed if maternal sulfonamide therapy is used near the time of delivery. TMP-SMX may be used in pregnancy for prophylaxis or treatment of *Pneumocystis jirovecii*

pneumonia (PCP), the prophylaxis of *Toxoplasmic gondii* encephalitis (TE), and may prevent fetal loss in patients with Q fever (*Coxiella burnetii*). The pharmacokinetics of TMP-SMX are similar to nonpregnant values in early pregnancy.

Lactation Enters breast milk/contraindicated (AAP rates "compatible")

Breast-Feeding Considerations Small amounts of TMP and SMX are transferred to breast milk. The AAP considers TMP-SMX "usually compatible with breast-feeding." Per the manufacturer, TMP-SMX is contraindicated in nursing mothers since sulfonamides cross into the milk and may cause kernicterus in the newborn. Because TMP-SMX has therapeutic indications for infants ≥2 months of age, kernicterus after exposure via breast-feeding would not be expected in healthy infants of this age group; however, sulfonamides should not be used while nursing an infant with G6PD deficiency or hyperbilirubinemia. Nondose related effects could include modification of bowel flora.

Contraindications Hypersensitivity to any sulfa drug, trimethoprim, or any component (see Warnings); porphyria; megaloblastic anemia due to folate deficiency; infants <2 months of age (for exception, see Additional Information)

Warnings Fatalities associated with sulfonamides, although rare, have occurred due to severe reactions including Stevens-Johnson syndrome, toxic epidermal necrolysis, hepatic necrosis, agranulocytosis, aplastic anemia, and other blood dyscrasias; discontinue use at first sign of rash or any sign of adverse reaction

Oral suspension and tablets may contain sodium benzoate; injection contains propylene glycol, benzyl alcohol, and sodium metabisulfites; propylene glycol may be toxic to newborns in high doses; sodium benzoate, benzyl alcohol and sodium metabisulfites may cause allergic reactions in susceptible individuals; large amounts of benzyl alcohol (≥99 mg/kg/day) have been associated with a potentially fatal toxicity ("gasping syndrome") in neonates; the "gasping syndrome" consists of metabolic acidosis, respiratory distress, gasping respirations, CNS dysfunction (including convulsions, intracranial hemorrhage), hypotension and cardiovascular collapse; use products containing benzyl alcohol with caution in neonates; *in vitro* and animal studies have shown that benzoate, a metabolite of benzyl alcohol, displaces bilirubin from protein binding sites

Precautions Use with caution in patients with G-6-PD deficiency, impaired renal or hepatic function; adjust dosage in patients with renal impairment

Adverse Reactions
Cardiovascular: Allergic myocarditis, hypotension

Central nervous system: Confusion, depression, hallucinations, seizures, fever, ataxia, kernicterus in neonates, aseptic meningitis, headache, insomnia

Dermatologic: Rash (more common in patients taking large dosages or in patients with AIDS), erythema multiforme, epidermal necrolysis, Stevens-Johnson syndrome, pruritus, urticaria

Endocrine & metabolic: Hyperkalemia

Gastrointestinal: Nausea, vomiting, glossitis, stomatitis, diarrhea, pseudomembranous colitis, pancreatitis, splenomegaly, anorexia

Hematologic: Thrombocytopenia, megaloblastic anemia, granulocytopenia, aplastic anemia, hemolysis (with G-6-PD deficiency)

Hepatic: Hepatitis, cholestatic jaundice

Local: Local irritation, pain, phlebitis

Neuromuscular & skeletal: Arthralgia, myalgia, rhabdomyolysis

Renal: Interstitial nephritis, renal tubular acidosis

Respiratory: Shortness of breath, cough, pulmonary infiltrates

Miscellaneous: Serum sickness, angioedema

Drug Interactions

Metabolism/Transport Effects

Sulfamethoxazole: **Substrate** of CYP2C9 (major), 3A4 (minor); **Inhibits** CYP2C9 (moderate)

Trimethoprim: **Substrate** (major) of CYP2C9, 3A4; **Inhibits** CYP2C8 (moderate), 2C9 (moderate)

Avoid Concomitant Use

Avoid concomitant use of Sulfamethoxazole and Trimethoprim with any of the following: BCG; Dofetilide; Methenamine; Procaine

Increased Effect/Toxicity

Sulfamethoxazole and Trimethoprim may increase the levels/effects of: ACE Inhibitors; Amantadine; Angiotensin II Receptor Blockers; Antidiabetic Agents (Thiazolidinedione); AzaTHIOprine; Carvedilol; CycloSPORINE; CycloSPORINE (Systemic); CYP2C8 Substrates (High risk); CYP2C9 Substrates (High risk); Dapsone; Dapsone (Systemic); Dapsone (Topical); Dofetilide; LamiVUDine; Memantine; Methotrexate; Phenytoin; Pralatrexate; Procainamide; Repaglinide; Sulfonylureas; Vitamin K Antagonists

The levels/effects of Sulfamethoxazole and Trimethoprim may be increased by: Amantadine; CYP2C9 Inhibitors (Moderate); CYP2C9 Inhibitors (Strong); Dapsone; Dapsone (Systemic); Memantine; Methenamine

Decreased Effect

Sulfamethoxazole and Trimethoprim may decrease the levels/effects of: BCG; CycloSPORINE; CycloSPORINE (Systemic); Typhoid Vaccine

The levels/effects of Sulfamethoxazole and Trimethoprim may be decreased by: CYP2C9 Inducers (Highly Effective); CYP3A4 Inducers (Strong); Deferasirox; Herbs (CYP3A4 Inducers); Leucovorin Calcium-Levoleucovorin; Peginterferon Alfa-2b; Procaine

Stability Do not refrigerate concentrate for injection; protect from light. For I.V. administration, a 1:25 dilution in D_5W (5 mL drug to 125 mL D_5W) is stable for 6 hours or a 1:20 dilution in D_5W (5 mL drug to 100 mL D_5W) is stable for 4 hours at room temperature; in patients who require fluid restriction, 1:15 dilution (5 mL drug to 75 mL D_5W) is stable for 2 hours. 1:10 highly concentrated admixture (5 mL drug to 50 mL D_5W) may precipitate in 1-2 hours; do not mix with other drugs or solutions.

Mechanism of Action Sulfamethoxazole interferes with bacterial folic acid synthesis and growth via inhibition of dihydrofolic acid formation from para-aminobenzoic acid; trimethoprim inhibits dihydrofolic acid reduction to tetrahydrofolate resulting in sequential inhibition of enzymes of the folic acid pathway

Pharmacokinetics (Adult data unless noted)

Absorption: Oral: Almost completely (90% to 100%)

Distribution: Crosses the placenta; distributes into breast milk, joint fluid, sputum, middle ear fluid, bile, and CSF

Protein binding:

TMP: 45%

SMX: 68%

Metabolism:

TMP: Metabolized to oxide and hydroxylated metabolites

SMX: N-acetylated and glucuronidated

Half-life:

TMP: 6-11 hours, prolonged in renal failure

SMX: 9-12 hours, prolonged in renal failure

Time to peak serum concentration: Oral: Within 1-4 hours

Elimination: Both excreted in urine as metabolites and unchanged drug

Usual Dosage Oral, I.V. **(dosage recommendations are based on the trimethoprim (TMP) component)**:

Children >2 months and Adults:

Mild-moderate infections: 6-12 mg TMP/kg/day in divided doses every 12 hours

Serious infection/*Pneumocystis*: 15-20 mg TMP/kg/day in divided doses every 6-8 hours

Prophylaxis of *Pneumocystis* (see **Note** in Additional Information): 150 mg TMP/m²/day in divided doses every 12 hours 3 days/week on consecutive days; acceptable alternative dosage schedules include 150 mg TMP/m²/day as a single daily dose 3 times/week on consecutive days or 150 mg TMP/m²/day in divided doses every 12 hours administered 7 days/week, or 150 mg TMP/m²/day in divided doses every 12 hours administered 3 times/week on alternate days; dose should not exceed 320 mg trimethoprim and 1600 mg sulfamethoxazole/day

Urinary tract infection prophylaxis: 2 mg TMP/kg/dose daily or 5 mg TMP/kg/dose twice weekly

Adults:

Urinary tract infection/chronic bronchitis: 1 double strength tablet every 12 hours for 10-14 days

Prophylaxis of *Pneumocystis*: One double-strength tablet daily or an acceptable alternative is 1 single-strength tablet daily

Dosing adjustment in renal impairment (frequency may need to be adjusted):

Cl_{cr} 15-30 mL/minute: Reduce dose by 50%

Cl_{cr} <15 mL/minute: Not recommended

Administration

Oral: May administer with water on an empty stomach; shake suspension well before use

Parenteral: **Do not administer I.M.**

I.V. infusion: Inspect solution for evidence of cloudiness or precipitation prior to administration; infuse I.V. sulfamethoxazole and trimethoprim over 60-90 minutes; must be further diluted 1:25 (5 mL drug to 125 mL diluent, ie, D_5W); in patients who require fluid restriction, a 1:15 dilution (5 mL drug to 75 mL diluent, ie, D_5W) or a 1:10 dilution (5 mL drug to 50 mL diluent, ie, D_5W) may be administered; see Stability

Monitoring Parameters CBC, renal function test, liver function test, urinalysis; observe for change in bowel frequency

Patient Information Maintain adequate fluid intake

Additional Information Note: Guidelines for prophylaxis of *Pneumocystis jiroveci* pneumonia: Initiate PCP prophylaxis in the following patients: Children born to HIV-infected mothers should be given prophylaxis with TMP/SMZ beginning at 4-6 weeks of age and continue through the first year of life or until HIV infection has been reasonably excluded; children 1-5 years of age with CD4+ count <500 or CD4+ percentage <15%; children 6-12 years of age with CD4+ count <200 or CD4+ percentage <15%; adolescents and adults with CD4+ count <200 or oropharyngeal candidiasis. Leucovorin calcium should be given if bone marrow suppression occurs.

Dosage Forms Excipient information presented when available (limited, particularly for generics); consult specific product labeling. **Note:** The 5:1 ratio (SMX:TMP) remains constant in all dosage forms.

Injection, solution: Sulfamethoxazole 80 mg and trimethoprim 16 mg per mL (5 mL, 10 mL, 30 mL) [contains benzyl alcohol, ethanol 12.2%, propylene glycol 400 mg/mL, sodium metabisulfite]

Suspension, oral: Sulfamethoxazole 200 mg and trimethoprim 40 mg per 5 mL (480 mL)

Sulfatrim®: Sulfamethoxazole 200 mg and trimethoprim 40 mg per 5 mL (100 mL, 480 mL) [contains alcohol ≤0.5% propylene glycol; cherry flavor]

Tablet: Sulfamethoxazole 400 mg and trimethoprim 80 mg

Bactrim™: Sulfamethoxazole 400 mg and trimethoprim 80 mg

Septra®: Sulfamethoxazole 400 mg and trimethoprim 80 mg

Tablet, double strength: Sulfamethoxazole 800 mg and trimethoprim 160 mg

Bactrim™ DS: Sulfamethoxazole 800 mg and trimethoprim 160 mg

Septra® DS: Sulfamethoxazole 800 mg and trimethoprim 160 mg

References

Hughes WT, "*Pneumocystis carinii* Pneumonia: New Approaches to Diagnosis, Treatment, and Prevention," *Pediatr Infect Dis J*, 1991, 10 (5):391-9.

Jarosinki PF, Kennedy PE, and Gallelli JF, "Stability of Concentrated Trimethoprim-Sulfamethoxazole Admixtures," *AJHP*, 1989, 46 (4):732-7.

"1999 USPHS/IDSA Guidelines for the Prevention of Opportunistic Infections in Persons Infected With Human Immunodeficiency Virus. USPHS/IDSA Prevention of Opportunistic Infections Working Group," *MMWR Morb Mortal Wkly Rep*, 1999, 48(RR-10):1-66.

◆ **Sulfamylon®** *see Mafenide on page 852*

Sulfasalazine (sul fa SAL a zeen)

Medication Safety Issues

Sound-alike/look-alike issues:

Sulfasalazine may be confused with salsalate, sulfaDIAZINE, sulfiSOXAZOLE

Azulfidine® may be confused with Augmentin®, azaTHIOprine

U.S. Brand Names Azulfidine®; Azulfidine® EN-tabs®

Canadian Brand Names Alti-Sulfasalazine; Salazopyrin En-Tabs®; Salazopyrin®

Therapeutic Category 5-Aminosalicylic Acid Derivative; Anti-inflammatory Agent

Generic Available Yes

Use Management of ulcerative colitis (FDA approved in ages ≥2 years and adults); treatment of active Crohn's disease and juvenile rheumatoid arthritis

Pregnancy Risk Factor B

Pregnancy Considerations Adverse events have not been observed in animal reproduction studies. Sulfasalazine and sulfapyridine cross the placenta; a potential for kernicterus in the newborn exists. Agranulocytosis was noted in an infant following maternal use of sulfasalazine during pregnancy.

Lactation Enters breast milk/use caution (AAP recommends use "with caution")

Breast-Feeding Considerations Sulfonamides are excreted in human breast milk and may cause kernicterus in the newborn. Although sulfapyridine has poor bilirubin-displacing ability, use with caution in women who are breast-feeding. The AAP classifies this agent to be used with caution since adverse effects have been reported in nursing infants.

Contraindications Hypersensitivity to sulfasalazine, sulfa drugs, salicylates, or any component; porphyria, GI or GU obstruction

Warnings Deaths from irreversible neuromuscular and central nervous system changes have been reported. Fatalities associated with severe reactions including Stevens-Johnson syndrome and toxic epidermal necrolysis have occurred with sulfonamides; discontinue use at first sign of rash. Deaths from fibrosing alveolitis have been reported. May cause folate deficiency; consider providing folate supplement. Nausea, vomiting, and abdominal discomfort commonly occur; titration of dose and/or using the enteric coated formulation may decrease GI adverse effects. Fatalities associated with hepatic damage have occurred; discontinue use at first sign of jaundice or hepatotoxicity. In males, oligospermia (rare) has been reported; usually reverses upon discontinuation. Chemical

similarities are present among sulfonamides, sulfonylureas, carbonic anhydrase inhibitors, thiazides, and loop diuretics (except ethacrynic acid). Use in patients with sulfonamide allergy is specifically contraindicated in product labeling, however, a risk of cross-reaction exists in patients with allergy to any of these compounds; avoid use when previous reaction has been severe.

Precautions Use with caution in patients with renal impairment, liver impairment, G-6-PD deficiency, blood dyscrasias, slow acetylators, severe allergies, or bronchial asthma

Adverse Reactions Incidence of adverse effects increase with dosage >4 g/day and in slow acetylators of sulfapyridine

Cardiovascular: Cyanosis, vasculitis

Central nervous system: Dizziness, fever, headache, malaise, mood changes

Dermatologic: Photosensitivity, pruritus, rash, Stevens-Johnson syndrome, toxic epidermal necrolysis (see Warnings), urticaria

Gastrointestinal: Abdominal pain, anorexia, dyspepsia, gastric distress, nausea, pancreatitis, stomatitis, vomiting

Genitourinary: Crystalluria, discoloration of urine (orange-yellow), infertility (oligospermia)

Hematologic: Heinz body anemia, hemolytic anemia, leukopenia, neutropenia, thrombocytopenia

Hepatic: Liver enzymes increased, liver necrosis/failure

Renal: Nephrotoxicity

Respiratory: Fibrosing alveolitis (see Warnings), pulmonary eosinophilia

Miscellaneous: Anaphylaxis, serum sickness-like reaction

<1%, postmarketing, and/or case reports (includes reactions reported with mesalamine or other sulfonamides): Agranulocytosis, alopecia, aplastic anemia, arthralgia, ataxia, cholestatic jaundice, cirrhosis, crystalluria, depression, diarrhea, drowsiness, drug rash with eosinophilia and systemic symptoms (DRESS), eosinophilia, epidermal necrolysis, exfoliative dermatitis, fulminant hepatitis, Guillain-Barré syndrome, hallucinations, hearing loss, hemolytic-uremic syndrome, hematuria, hepatitis, hypoprothrombinemia, insomnia, interstitial lung disease, interstitial nephritis, jaundice, Kawasaki-like syndrome (single case report), lupus-like syndrome, megaloblastic anemia, meningitis, methemoglobinemia, myelitis, myelodysplastic syndrome, myocarditis (allergic), nephropathy (acute), nephrotic syndrome, neutropenia (congenital), neutropenic enterocolitis, pericarditis, periorbital edema, pancreatitis, peripheral neuropathy, photosensitization, pleuritis, pneumonitis, polyarteritis nodosa, proteinuria, purpura, rhabdomyolysis, seizure, skin discoloration, thyroid function disturbance, tinnitus, urine discoloration, vasculitis, vertigo

Drug Interactions

Avoid Concomitant Use There are no known interactions where it is recommended to avoid concomitant use.

Increased Effect/Toxicity

Sulfasalazine may increase the levels/effects of: Heparin; Heparin (Low Molecular Weight); Thiopurine Analogs; Varicella Virus-Containing Vaccines

Decreased Effect

Sulfasalazine may decrease the levels/effects of: Cardiac Glycosides; Methylfolate

Food Interactions Need to increase dietary intake of iron; since sulfasalazine impairs folate absorption, consider providing 1 mg/day folate supplement

Mechanism of Action Acts locally in the colon to decrease the inflammatory response and interfere with secretion by inhibiting prostaglandin synthesis; therapeutic effect may result from antibacterial action with change in intestinal flora

Pharmacodynamics Onset of action:
JRA: Minimum trial of 3 months is necessary
Ulcerative colitis: >3-4 weeks

Pharmacokinetics (Adult data unless noted)
Absorption: Oral: 10% to 15% as unchanged drug from the small intestine; upon administration, the drug is split into sulfapyridine and 5-aminosalicylic acid (5-ASA) in the colon
Bioavailability: Sulfasalazine: <15%; sulfapyridine: ~60%; 5-aminosalicylic acid: ~10% to 30%
Distribution: Breast milk to plasma ratio: 0.09-0.17
Metabolism: Both components are metabolized in the liver; slow acetylators have higher plasma sulfapyridine concentrations
Half-life:
Sulfasalazine:
Single dose: 5.7 hours
Multiple doses: 7.6 hours
Sulfapyridine:
Single dose: 8.4 hours
Multiple doses: 10.4 hours
Time to peak serum concentration:
Serum sulfasalazine: Within 1.5-6 hours
Serum sulfapyridine (active metabolite): Within 6-24 hours
Elimination: Primarily in urine (as unchanged drug, components, and acetylated metabolites); small amounts appear in feces

Usual Dosage Oral:
Children ≥2 years:
Ulcerative colitis:
Mild exacerbation: 40-50 mg/kg/day divided every 6 hours
Moderate-severe exacerbation: 50-60 mg/kg/day divided every 4-6 hours, not to exceed 4 g/day
Maintenance dose: 30-50 mg/kg/day divided every 4-8 hours; not to exceed 2 g/day
Juvenile rheumatoid arthritis (JRA): Initial: 10 mg/kg/day; increase weekly by 10 mg/kg/day; usual dose: 30-50 mg/kg/day in 2 divided doses; maximum dose: 2 g/day
Adults:
Ulcerative colitis: 3-4 g/day in evenly divided doses at intervals less than or equal to every 8 hours; maintenance: 2 g/day evenly divided doses at intervals less than or equal to every 8 hours; may initiate therapy with 1-2 g/day to reduce GI intolerance
Rheumatoid arthritis: Enteric coated tablet: Initial: 0.5-1 g/day; increase weekly to maintenance dose of 2 g/day in 2 divided doses; maximum: 3 g/day (if response to 2 g/day is inadequate after 12 weeks of treatment)

Administration Administer after meals or with food; do not administer with antacids. Do not crush enteric coated tablets.

Monitoring Parameters CBC, liver function tests (prior to therapy, then every other week for first 3 months of therapy, followed by every month for the second 3 months, then once every 3 months thereafter), urinalysis, renal function tests, liver function tests, stool frequency, hematocrit, reticulocyte count

Patient Information Maintain adequate fluid intake; may cause orange-yellow discoloration of urine and skin; may stain soft contact lenses yellow. May cause photosensitivity reactions (eg, exposure to sunlight may cause severe sunburn, skin rash, redness, or itching); avoid exposure to sunlight and artificial light sources (sunlamps, tanning booth/bed); wear protective clothing, wide-brimmed hats, sunglasses, and lip sunscreen (SPF ≥15); use a sunscreen [broad-spectrum sunscreen or physical sunscreen (preferred) or sunblock with SPF ≥15]; contact physician if reaction occurs.

Additional Information Good response to sulfasalazine for JRA is most likely to occur in HLA B27-positive boys who are older than 9 years of age at onset of arthritis

Dosage Forms Excipient information presented when available (limited, particularly for generics); consult specific product labeling.
Tablet: 500 mg
Azulfidine®: 500 mg
Tablet, delayed release, enteric coated: 500 mg
Azulfidine® EN-tabs®: 500 mg

References
American College of Rheumatology Ad Hoc Committee on Clinical Guidelines, "Guidelines for the Management of Rheumatoid Arthritis," *Arthritis Rheum*, 1996, 39(5):713-22.

Giannini EH and Cawkwell GD, "Drug Treatment in Children With Juvenile Rheumatoid Arthritis," *Pediatr Clin North Am*, 1995, 42 (5):1099-125.

Kirschner BS, "Inflammatory Bowel Disease in Children," *Pediatr Clin North Am*, 1988, 35(1):189-208.

◆ **Sulfatrim** *see* Sulfamethoxazole and Trimethoprim *on page 1302*

◆ **Sulfatrim®** *see* Sulfamethoxazole and Trimethoprim *on page 1302*

SulfiSOXAZOLE (sul fi SOKS a zole)

Medication Safety Issues
Sound-alike/look-alike issues:
SulfiSOXAZOLE may be confused with sulfaDIAZINE, sulfamethoxazole, sulfasalazine
Gantrisin® may be confused with Gastrosed™

U.S. Brand Names Gantrisin® [DSC]

Canadian Brand Names Novo-Soxazole; Sulfizole®

Therapeutic Category Antibiotic, Sulfonamide Derivative

Generic Available No

Use Treatment of uncomplicated urinary tract infections, otitis media, *Chlamydia*; nocardiosis; treatment of acute pelvic inflammatory disease in prepubertal children

Pregnancy Risk Factor C

Pregnancy Considerations Adverse events have been observed in animal reproduction studies; therefore, the manufacturer classifies sulfisoxazole as pregnancy category C. Based on available information, an increased risk for congenital malformations has not been observed after use of sulfisoxazole during pregnancy. Per the manufacturer, sulfisoxazole is contraindicated in late pregnancy because sulfonamides may cause kernicterus in the newborn. One case has been reported of fetal death after sulfisoxazole was administered to a G6PD deficient mother. Neonatal healthcare providers should be informed if maternal sulfonamide therapy is used near the time of delivery. Maternal serum protein binding of sulfisoxazole decreases during the second and third trimesters of pregnancy.

Lactation Enters breast milk/not recommended (contraindicated in infants <2 months of age)

Breast-Feeding Considerations Small amounts of sulfisoxazole are transferred to breast milk. Per the manufacturer, sulfisoxazole is contraindicated in mothers nursing infants <2 months of age because sulfonamides cross into milk and may cause kernicterus in the newborn. The AAP considers use during breast-feeding "compatible" in full-term neonates; however, breast-feeding is not recommended if the infant is ill, stressed, or premature or if the infant has G6PD deficiency or hyperbilirubinemia. Nondose-related effects could include modification of bowel flora.

Contraindications Hypersensitivity to any sulfa drug or any component; porphyria; infants <2 months of age (sulfas compete with bilirubin for protein binding sites which may result in kernicterus in newborns); patients with urinary obstruction; pregnant women during third trimester; nursing mothers

Precautions Use with caution in patients with G-6-PD deficiency (hemolysis may occur), hepatic or renal impairment; dosage modification required in patients with renal impairment; risk of crystalluria should be considered in patients with impaired renal function

Adverse Reactions
Cardiovascular: Vasculitis
Central nervous system: Dizziness, headache, fever, vertigo, disorientation
Dermatologic: Rash, Stevens-Johnson syndrome, photosensitivity, exfoliative dermatitis
Gastrointestinal: Nausea, vomiting, anorexia, stomatitis, pseudomembranous colitis
Genitourinary: Crystalluria (rare)
Hematologic: Thrombocytopenia, leukopenia, agranulocytosis, aplastic anemia, hemolytic anemia, neutropenia
Hepatic: Jaundice, hepatitis
Renal: Nephrotoxicity
Miscellaneous: Hypersensitivity reactions

Drug Interactions
Metabolism/Transport Effects Substrate of CYP2C9 (major); **Inhibits** CYP2C9 (strong)
Avoid Concomitant Use
Avoid concomitant use of SulfiSOXAZOLE with any of the following: BCG; Methenamine; Procaine
Increased Effect/Toxicity
SulfiSOXAZOLE may increase the levels/effects of: Carvedilol; CycloSPORINE; CycloSPORINE (Systemic); CYP2C9 Substrates (High risk); Methotrexate; Phenytoin; Sulfonylureas; Vitamin K Antagonists

The levels/effects of SulfiSOXAZOLE may be increased by: CYP2C9 Inhibitors (Moderate); CYP2C9 Inhibitors (Strong); Methenamine
Decreased Effect
SulfiSOXAZOLE may decrease the levels/effects of: BCG; CycloSPORINE; CycloSPORINE (Systemic); Typhoid Vaccine

The levels/effects of SulfiSOXAZOLE may be decreased by: CYP2C9 Inducers (Highly Effective); Peginterferon Alfa-2b; Procaine
Food Interactions Interferes with folate absorption
Stability Protect from light
Mechanism of Action Interferes with bacterial growth by inhibiting bacterial folic acid synthesis through competitive antagonism of PABA
Pharmacokinetics (Adult data unless noted)
Absorption: Sulfisoxazole acetyl is hydrolyzed in the GI tract to sulfisoxazole which is readily absorbed
Distribution: Crosses the placenta; excreted into breast milk; distributes into extracellular space; CSF concentration ranges from 8% to 57% of blood concentration in patients with normal meninges
Protein binding: 85% to 88%
Metabolism: In the liver by acetylation and glucuronide conjugation to inactive compounds
Half-life: 4-8 hours, prolonged with renal impairment
Time to peak serum concentration: Within 2-4 hours
Elimination: Primarily in urine (95% within 24 hours), 40% to 60% as unchanged drug
Dialysis: >50% removed by hemodialysis
Usual Dosage
Infants ≥2 months and Children: Oral: Initial: 75 mg/kg for 1 dose, followed by 120-150 mg/kg/day in divided doses every 4-6 hours; not to exceed 6 g/day

Pelvic inflammatory disease: 100 mg/kg/day in divided doses every 6 hours; used in combination with ceftriaxone
Chlamydia trachomatis: 100 mg/kg/day divided every 6 hours; maximum dose: 2 g/day
Prophylaxis of UTI: 10-20 mg/kg/day divided every 12 hours
Prophylaxis of recurrent acute otitis media: 35-75 mg/kg/day once daily at bedtime
Adults: Oral: 2-4 g stat, followed by 4-8 g/day in divided doses every 4-6 hours
Children and Adults: Ophthalmic: Solution: Instill 1-2 drops to conjunctiva of affected eye every 2-3 hours
Dosing interval in renal impairment:
Cl_{cr} 10-50 mL/minutes: Administer every 8-12 hours
Cl_{cr} <10 mL/minute: Administer every 12-24 hours
Administration
Ophthalmic: Avoid contact of bottle tip with skin or eye; apply finger pressure to lacrimal sac during and for 1-2 minutes after instillation of drops to decrease risk of absorption and systemic effects
Oral: Administer with a glass of water on an empty stomach; shake suspension well before use
Monitoring Parameters CBC, urinalysis, renal function tests
Test Interactions False-positive protein in urine; false-positive urine glucose with Clinitest®
Patient Information Report to physician any sore throat, mouth sores, rash, unusual bleeding, or fever; limit alcohol. May cause photosensitivity reactions (eg, exposure to sunlight may cause severe sunburn, skin rash, redness, or itching); avoid exposure to sunlight and artificial light sources (sunlamps, tanning booth/bed); wear protective clothing, wide-brimmed hats, sunglasses, and lip sunscreen (SPF ≥15); use a sunscreen [broad-spectrum sunscreen or physical sunscreen (preferred) or sunblock with SPF ≥15]; contact physician if reaction occurs.
Nursing Implications Maintain adequate patient fluid intake
Dosage Forms Excipient information presented when available (limited, particularly for generics); consult specific product labeling. [DSC] = Discontinued product
Suspension, oral [pediatric]
Gantrisin®: 500 mg/5 mL (480 mL) [contains alcohol 0.3%; raspberry flavor] [DSC]

References
Erramouspe J and Heyneman CA, "Treatment and Prevention of Otitis Media," Ann Pharmacother, 2000, 34(12):1452-68.
Klein JO, "Protecting the Therapeutic Advantage of Antimicrobial Agents Used for Otitis Media," Pediatr Infect Dis J, 1998, 17(6):571-5.
"Practice Parameter: The Diagnosis, Treatment, and Evaluation of the Initial Urinary Tract Infection in Febrile Infants and Young Children. American Academy of Pediatrics. Committee on Quality Improvement. Subcommittee on Urinary Tract Infection," Pediatrics, 1999, 103 (4 Pt 1):843-52.
Thoene DE and Johnson CE, "Pharmacotherapy of Otitis Media," Pharmacotherapy, 1991, 11(3):212-21.

♦ **Sulfisoxazole Acetyl** see SulfiSOXAZOLE on page 1305

♦ **Sulfisoxazole and Erythromycin** see Erythromycin and Sulfisoxazole on page 528

♦ **Sulfizole® (Can)** see SulfiSOXAZOLE on page 1305

Sulfur and Salicylic Acid
(SUL fur & sal i SIL ik AS id)

Therapeutic Category Antiseborrheic Agent, Topical
Use Therapeutic shampoo for dandruff and seborrheal dermatitis; acne skin cleanser
Pregnancy Risk Factor C
Contraindications Hypersensitivity to sulfur, salicylic acid, or any component

Warnings For external use only; avoid contact with eyes; discontinue use if skin irritation develops

Precautions Infants are more sensitive to sulfur than adults; do not use in children <2 years of age

Adverse Reactions Topical preparations containing 2% to 5% sulfur generally are well tolerated; concentration >15% is very irritating to the skin; higher concentrations (eg, 10% or higher) may cause systemic toxicity

Cardiovascular: Collapse (with sulfur concentration >10%)
Central nervous system: Dizziness, headache
Gastrointestinal: Vomiting
Local: Irritation
Neuromuscular & skeletal: Muscle cramps

Stability Preparations containing sulfur may react with metals including silver and copper, resulting in discoloration of the metal

Mechanism of Action Salicylic acid works synergistically with sulfur in its keratolytic action to break down keratin and promote skin peeling

Pharmacokinetics (Adult data unless noted) Absorption: 1% of topically applied sulfur is absorbed; sulfur is reduced to hydrogen sulfide

Usual Dosage Children ≥2 years and Adults: Topical:
Shampoo: Initial: Massage onto wet scalp; leave lather on scalp for 5 minutes, rinse, repeat application, then rinse thoroughly; use daily or every other day; 1-2 treatments/ week will usually maintain control
Soap: Use daily or every other day

Administration Topical: Avoid contact with the eyes; for external use only

Patient Information Contact physician if condition worsens or rash or irritation develops

Dosage Forms
Cake: Sulfur 2% and salicylic acid 2% (123 g)
Cleanser: Sulfur 2% and salicylic acid 1.5% (60 mL, 120 mL)
Shampoo: Micropulverized sulfur 2% and salicylic acid 2% (120 mL, 240 mL)
Soap: Micropulverized sulfur 2% and salicylic acid 2% (113 g)
Wash: Sulfur 1.6% and salicylic acid 1.6% (75 mL)

Sulindac (sul IN dak)

Medication Safety Issues
Sound-alike/look-alike issues:
Clinoril® may be confused with Cleocin®, Clozaril®
U.S. Brand Names Clinoril®
Canadian Brand Names Apo-Sulin®; Novo-Sundac; Nu-Sundac
Therapeutic Category Analgesic, Non-narcotic; Anti-inflammatory Agent; Nonsteroidal Anti-inflammatory Drug (NSAID), Oral
Generic Available Yes
Use Management of inflammatory disease, rheumatoid disorders; acute gouty arthritis
Medication Guide An FDA-approved patient medication guide, which is available with the product information and at http://www.fda.gov/downloads/Drugs/DrugSafety/ucm088573.pdf, must be dispensed with this medication for each new outpatient prescription and refill.
Pregnancy Risk Factor C
Pregnancy Considerations Adverse events were not observed in the initial animal reproduction studies; therefore, the manufacturer classifies sulindac as pregnancy category C. Sulindac and the sulfide metabolite have been found to cross the placenta. NSAID exposure during the first trimester is not strongly associated with congenital malformations; however, cardiovascular anomalies and cleft palate have been observed following NSAID exposure in some studies. The use of an NSAID in the first trimester may be associated with an increased risk of miscarriage. Nonteratogenic effects have been observed following NSAID administration during the third trimester including myocardial degenerative changes, prenatal constriction of the ductus arteriosus, failure of the ductus arteriosus to close postnatally, and fetal tricuspid regurgitation; renal dysfunction or failure, oligohydramnios; gastrointestinal bleeding or perforation, increased risk of necrotizing enterocolitis; intracranial bleeding, platelet dysfunction with resultant bleeding; or pulmonary hypertension. Because they may cause premature closure of the ductus arteriosus, use of NSAIDs late in pregnancy should be avoided (use after 31-32 weeks gestation is not recommended by some clinicians). Sulindac has been used in the management of preterm labor. The chronic use of NSAIDs in women of reproductive age may be associated with infertility that is reversible upon discontinuation of the medication. A registry is available for pregnant women exposed to autoimmune medications including sulindac. For additional information contact the Organization of Teratology Information Specialists, OTIS Autoimmune Diseases Study, at (877) 311-8972.

Lactation Excretion in breast milk unknown/not recommended

Breast-Feeding Considerations It is not known if sulindac is excreted into breast milk. Breast-feeding is not recommended by the manufacturer.

Contraindications Hypersensitivity to sulindac or any component; history of asthma, urticaria, or allergic-type reaction to aspirin, or other NSAIDs; patients with the "aspirin triad" [asthma, rhinitis (with or without nasal polyps), and aspirin intolerance] (fatal asthmatic and anaphylactoid reactions may occur in these patients); perioperative pain in the setting of coronary artery bypass graft (CABG)

Warnings NSAIDs are associated with an increased risk of adverse cardiovascular thrombotic events, including potentially fatal MI and stroke **[U.S. Boxed Warning]**; risk may be increased with duration of use or pre-existing cardiovascular risk factors or disease; carefully evaluate cardiovascular risk profile prior to prescribing; use the lowest effective dose for the shortest duration of time, taking into consideration individual patient treatment goals; alternate therapies should be considered for patients at high risk. Use is contraindicated for treatment of perioperative pain in the setting of CABG surgery **[U.S. Boxed Warning]**; an increased incidence of MI and stroke was found in patients receiving COX-2 selective NSAIDs for the treatment of pain within the first 10-14 days after CABG surgery. NSAIDs may cause fluid retention, edema, and new onset or worsening of pre-existing hypertension; use with caution in patients with hypertension, CHF, or fluid retention. Concurrent administration of ibuprofen, with potentially other nonselective NSAIDs, may interfere with aspirin's cardioprotective effect.

NSAIDs may increase the risk of GI inflammation, ulceration, bleeding, and perforation **[U.S. Boxed Warning]**. These events, which can be potentially fatal, may occur at any time during therapy and without warning. Avoid the use of NSAIDs in patients with active GI bleeding or ulcer disease. Use NSAIDs with extreme caution in patients with a history of GI bleeding or ulcers (these patients have a 10-fold increased risk for developing a GI bleed). Use NSAIDs with caution in patients with other risk factors which may increase GI bleeding (eg, concurrent therapy with aspirin, anticoagulants, and/or corticosteroids, longer duration of NSAID use, smoking, use of alcohol, and poor general health). Use the lowest effective dose for the shortest duration of time, taking into consideration individual patient treatment goals; alternate therapies should be considered for patients at high risk.

NSAIDs may compromise existing renal function. Renal toxicity may occur in patients with impaired renal function, dehydration, heart failure, liver dysfunction, or those taking diuretics and ACE inhibitors; use with caution in these patients; monitor renal function closely. NSAIDs are not recommended for use in patients with advanced renal disease. Long-term use of NSAIDs may cause renal papillary necrosis and other renal injury. Use caution in patients with renal lithiasis; sulindac metabolites have been reported as components of renal stones; use hydration in patients with a history of renal stones. Use with caution in patients with decreased hepatic function. Closely monitor patients with any abnormal LFT. Severe hepatic reactions (eg, fulminant hepatitis, liver failure) have occurred with NSAID use, rarely; discontinue if signs or symptoms of liver disease develop or if systemic manifestations occur. May require dosage adjustment in hepatic dysfunction; sulfide and sulfone metabolites may accumulate. Pancreatitis has been reported; discontinue with suspected pancreatitis. May increase the risk of aseptic meningitis, especially in patients with systemic lupus erythematosus (SLE) and mixed connective tissue disorders.

Fatal asthmatic and anaphylactoid reactions may occur in patients with the "aspirin triad" who receive NSAIDs (see Contraindications). NSAIDs may cause serious dermatologic adverse reactions including exfoliative dermatitis, Stevens-Johnson syndrome, and toxic epidermal necrolysis. Avoid use of NSAIDs in late pregnancy as they may cause premature closure of the ductus arteriosus.

Precautions Use with caution in patients with peptic ulcer disease, GI bleeding, bleeding abnormalities, impaired renal or hepatic function, CHF, hypertension, and patients receiving anticoagulants

Adverse Reactions

Cardiovascular: Edema

Central nervous system: Dizziness, nervousness, headache

Dermatologic: Rash, pruritus

Gastrointestinal: Abdominal pain; GI bleeding, ulcer, perforation; nausea; vomiting; diarrhea; constipation

Hematologic: Thrombocytopenia, agranulocytosis, inhibition of platelet aggregation, bone marrow suppression

Hepatic: Hepatitis

Otic: Tinnitus

Renal: Renal impairment

Respiratory: Bronchospasm

Drug Interactions

Avoid Concomitant Use

Avoid concomitant use of Sulindac with any of the following: Ketorolac; Ketorolac (Systemic)

Increased Effect/Toxicity

Sulindac may increase the levels/effects of: Aminoglycosides; Anticoagulants; Antiplatelet Agents; Bisphosphonate Derivatives; Collagenase (Systemic); CycloSPORINE; CycloSPORINE (Systemic); Desmopressin; Digoxin; Drotrecogin Alfa; Eplerenone; Haloperidol; Ibritumomab; Methotrexate; Nonsteroidal Anti-Inflammatory Agents; Pemetrexed; Potassium-Sparing Diuretics; Pralatrexate; Quinolone Antibiotics; Salicylates; Thrombolytic Agents; Tositumomab and Iodine I 131 Tositumomab; Vancomycin; Vitamin K Antagonists

The levels/effects of Sulindac may be increased by: Antidepressants (Tricyclic, Tertiary Amine); Corticosteroids (Systemic); Dasatinib; Dimethyl Sulfoxide; Glucosamine; Herbs (Anticoagulant/Antiplatelet Properties); Ketorolac; Ketorolac (Systemic); Nonsteroidal Anti-Inflammatory Agents; Omega-3-Acid Ethyl Esters; Pentosan Polysulfate Sodium; Pentoxifylline; Probenecid; Prostacyclin Analogues; Selective Serotonin Reuptake Inhibitors; Serotonin/Norepinephrine Reuptake Inhibitors; Treprostinil

Decreased Effect

Sulindac may decrease the levels/effects of: ACE Inhibitors; Angiotensin II Receptor Blockers; Antiplatelet Agents; Beta-Blockers; Eplerenone; HydrALAZINE; Loop Diuretics; Potassium-Sparing Diuretics; Salicylates; Thiazide Diuretics

The levels/effects of Sulindac may be decreased by: Bile Acid Sequestrants; Nonsteroidal Anti-Inflammatory Agents; Salicylates

Food Interactions Food may decrease rate and extent of absorption

Mechanism of Action Inhibits prostaglandin synthesis by decreasing the activity of the enzyme, cyclooxygenase, which results in decreased formation of prostaglandin precursors

Usual Dosage Oral:

Children: Limited information exists; some centers use the following: 2-4 mg/kg/day in 2 divided doses; maximum: 6 mg/kg/day; do not exceed 400 mg/day (Giannini, 1995; Skeith, 1991)

Adults: 150-200 mg twice daily; not to exceed 400 mg/day

Administration Oral: Administer with food or milk to decrease GI upset

Monitoring Parameters Liver enzymes, BUN, serum creatinine, CBC with differential, platelet count; periodic ophthalmologic exams with chronic use

Patient Information Avoid alcohol; may cause dizziness; do not take with aspirin

Dosage Forms Excipient information presented when available (limited, particularly for generics); consult specific product labeling.

Tablet: 150 mg, 200 mg

Clinoril®: 200 mg

References

Giannini EH and Cawkwell GD, "Drug Treatment in Children With Juvenile Rheumatoid Arthritis. Past, Present, and Future," *Pediatr Clin North Am*, 1995, 42(5):1099-125.

Skeith KJ and Jamali F, "Clinical Pharmacokinetics of Drugs Used in Juvenile Arthritis," *Clin Pharmacokinet*, 1991, 21(2):129-49.

◆ **Sulphafurazole** see SulfiSOXAZOLE *on page 1305*

SUMAtriptan (SOO ma trip tan)

Medication Safety Issues

Sound-alike/look-alike issues:

SUMAtriptan may be confused with saxagliptin, sitaGLIPtin, somatropin, zolmitriptan

International issues:

Imitrex® may be confused with Nitrex® which is a brand name for isosorbide mononitrate in Italy

Related Information

Serotonin Syndrome *on page 1695*

U.S. Brand Names Imitrex®; Sumavel™ DosePro™

Canadian Brand Names Apo-Sumatriptan®; CO Sumatriptan; Dom-Sumatriptan; Gen-Sumatriptan; Imitrex®; Imitrex® DF; Imitrex® Nasal Spray; Mylan-Sumatriptan; Novo-Sumatriptan; PHL-Sumatriptan; PMS-Sumatriptan; ratio-Sumatriptan; Rhoxal-sumatriptan; Riva-Sumatriptan; Sandoz-Sumatriptan; Sumatryx

Therapeutic Category Antimigraine Agent

Generic Available Yes

Use

Injection, intranasal, and tablets: Acute treatment of migraine with or without aura

Injection: Acute treatment of cluster headaches

Pregnancy Risk Factor C

Pregnancy Considerations There are no adequate and well-controlled studies using sumatriptan in pregnant women. Use only if potential benefit to the mother outweighs the potential risk to the fetus. A pregnancy registry has been established to monitor outcomes of women exposed to sumatriptan during pregnancy (800-336-2176). Preliminary data from the registry do not suggest a greater risk of birth defects than the general population and so far a specific pattern of malformations has not been identified. However, sample sizes are small and studies are ongoing. In some (but not all) animal studies, administration was associated with embryolethality, fetal malformations and pup mortality.

Lactation Enters breast milk/use caution (AAP rates "compatible")

Breast-Feeding Considerations The amount of sumatriptan an infant would be exposed to following breastfeeding is considered to be small (although the mean milk-to-plasma ratio is ~4.9, weight adjusted doses estimates suggest breast-fed infants receive 3.5% of a maternal dose). Expressing and discarding the milk for 8-12 hours after a single dose is suggested to reduce the amount present even further. The half-life of sumatriptan in breast milk is 2.22 hours.

Contraindications Hypersensitivity to sumatriptan or any component; I.V. administration (coronary vasospasm may occur); ischemic heart disease, Prinzmetal angina, cerebrovascular or peripheral vascular syndromes (eg, stroke, TIA, ischemic bowel disease), severe hepatic impairment, patients with signs or symptoms of ischemic heart disease, MI, silent MI, uncontrolled hypertension; concomitant use of ergotamine derivatives (within last 24 hours), vasoconstrictive drugs, methysergide, or MAO inhibitors; use of MAO inhibitors within past 2 weeks; management of hemiplegic or basilar migraine

Warnings Life-threatening or fatal hypersensitivity reactions may occur; rarely, serious coronary events including acute MI, life-threatening arrhythmias, and death, may occur; avoid use in patients with risk factors for coronary artery disease, unless cardiovascular disease can be ruled out; consider administering first dose under first supervision to patients at high risk for coronary disease; ECG should be performed if angina-like symptoms occur; periodically evaluate cardiovascular system in patients with risk factors for coronary artery disease

Precautions Temporary increases in peripheral vascular resistance and blood pressure may occur; use with caution in patients with impaired hepatic or renal function, history of seizure disorder or conditions associated with a decrease in the seizure threshold; cross-hypersensitivity to sulfonamides is possible; other potentially serious neurological conditions should be ruled out prior to acute migraine therapy; sumatriptan (given at five times the maximum oral single dose) has caused corneal opacities in dogs; other animal studies suggest it may bind to the melanin of the eye; human studies are not available

Serious adverse effects, such as MI, stroke, visual loss, and death have been reported in pediatric patients after sumatriptan use by the oral, intranasal, and/or SubQ route; frequency of such adverse effects cannot currently be determined, thus the use of sumatriptan in patients <18 years of age is not recommended.

Adverse Reactions

Cardiovascular: Hypertension; flushing; chest tightness, pressure, pain; coronary artery vasospasm; vascular ischemia; colonic ischemia; rarely: acute MI, life-threatening arrhythmias

Central nervous system: Dizziness, drowsiness, headache; seizures (rare)

Gastrointestinal: Nausea, vomiting, abdominal discomfort; bad or unusual taste (with intranasal use)

Local: Injection site reaction (59%), pain, redness at injection site

Neuromuscular & skeletal: Weakness, myalgia, neck pain with stiffness

Miscellaneous: Atypical sensations of tingling, heat, flushing, burning, heaviness, pressure, tightness, numbness; jaw, mouth, tongue discomfort; diaphoresis; rarely: hypersensitivity reactions (potentially fatal anaphylaxis or anaphylactoid reactions)

Drug Interactions

Avoid Concomitant Use

Avoid concomitant use of SUMAtriptan with any of the following: Ergot Derivatives; MAO Inhibitors; Sibutramine

Increased Effect/Toxicity

SUMAtriptan may increase the levels/effects of: Ergot Derivatives; Serotonin Modulators

The levels/effects of SUMAtriptan may be increased by: Ergot Derivatives; MAO Inhibitors; Sibutramine

Decreased Effect There are no known significant interactions involving a decrease in effect.

Food Interactions Food slightly delays the rate but not the extent of oral absorption

Stability Store at 2°C to 20°C (36°F to 86°F); protect from light

Mechanism of Action Selective agonist for serotonin ($5\text{-}HT_1$) receptor in cranial arteries; causes vasoconstriction and reduces sterile inflammation associated with antidromic neuronal transmission correlating with relief of migraine

Pharmacodynamics Migraine pain relief:

Onset of action:

Oral: 1-1.5 hours

SubQ: 10 minutes to 2 hours

Maximum effect: Oral: 2-4 hours

Pharmacokinetics (Adult data unless noted)

Distribution: Adults:

V_d (central): 50 L

V_d (apparent): 2.4 L/kg

Protein binding: 14% to 21%

Metabolism: In the liver to an indole acetic acid metabolite (inactive) which then undergoes ester glucuronide conjugation; may be metabolized by monoamine oxidase (MAO)

Bioavailability:

Oral: ~15%; may be significantly increased with liver disease

Intranasal: 17% (compared to SubQ)

SubQ: 97%

Half-life:

Distribution: 15 minutes

Terminal: 2 hours; range: 1-4 hours

Time to peak serum concentration:

Oral: Healthy adults: 2 hours; during migraine attacks: 2.5 hours

SubQ: Range: 5-20 minutes; mean: 12 minutes

Elimination: 60% of an oral dose is renally excreted (primarily as metabolites), 40% is eliminated via the feces, and only 3% as unchanged drug; 42% of an intranasal dose is excreted as the indole acetic acid metabolite with 3% excreted in the urine unchanged; 22% of a SubQ dose is excreted in urine unchanged and 38% as the indole acetic acid metabolite

Usual Dosage

Children and Adolescents <18 years: Use not recommended (see Precautions):

Intranasal: Efficacy of intranasal sumatriptan was **not** established in 2 controlled clinical trials in migraine patients 12-17 years of age (n=1248) with doses of 5-20 mg; adverse events were similar to adults (see also Additional Information)

Oral: Efficacy of oral sumatriptan was **not** established in placebo-controlled trials in patients 12-17 years of age (n=701) with doses of 25-100 mg; adverse events were similar to adults; frequency of adverse events was dose- and age-dependent (increased frequency of adverse events in younger patients); postmarketing reports include the occurrence of MI in a 14-year-old male after oral sumatriptan with symptoms occurring within 1 day of drug use

SubQ: An open-labeled prospective trial in 17 children 6-16 years of age with juvenile migraine used SubQ doses of 6 mg in 15 children 30-70 kg, and 3 mg/dose in two children who weighed 22 kg and 30 kg (MacDonald, 1994); additional studies are needed

Adults:

Intranasal: Initial single dose: 5 mg, 10 mg, or 20 mg administered in one nostril, given as soon as possible after the onset of migraine; 10 mg dose may be administered as 5 mg in each nostril; may repeat after 2 hours; maximum: 40 mg/day

Oral: Initial single dose: 25 mg given as soon as possible after the onset of a migraine; range: 25-100 mg/dose; maximum single dose: 100 mg; may repeat after 2 hours; maximum: 200 mg/day

SubQ: 6 mg given as soon as possible after the onset of a migraine; a second injection (≤6 mg) may be administered at least 1 hour after the initial dose; maximum dose: 12 mg/24 hours

Dosing adjustment in hepatic dysfunction: Adults: Oral: Maximum single dose: 50 mg

Administration

Intranasal: Each nasal spray unit is preloaded with 1 dose; **do not** test the spray unit before use; remove unit from plastic pack when ready to use; while sitting down, gently blow nose to clear nasal passages; keep head upright and close one nostril gently with index finger; hold container with other hand, with thumb supporting bottom and index and middle fingers on either side of nozzle; insert nozzle into nostril about 1/2 inch; close mouth; take a breath through nose while releasing spray into nostril by pressing firmly on blue plunger; remove nozzle from nostril; keep head level for 10-20 seconds and gently breathe in through nose and out through mouth; **do not breathe deeply**

Oral: Administer with fluids

Parenteral: SubQ use only; do **not** administer I.M.; do **not** administer I.V. (may cause coronary vasospasm)

Patient Information If pain or tightness in chest or throat occurs, notify physician; females should avoid pregnancy; pain at injection site lasts <1 hour

Additional Information Safety of treating >4 headaches per month is not established; sumatriptan is **not** indicated for migraine prophylaxis

A randomized, double-blind, placebo-controlled, single-attack study in adolescent migraine patients (12-17 years of age) used sumatriptan nasal spray in doses of 5 mg (n=128), 10 mg (n=133), and 20 mg (n=118). Compared to placebo, the percent of patients with headache relief (reduction in headache pain) at 1 hour postdose was significantly greater for the 10 mg and 20 mg group and at 2 hours postdose was significantly greater for the 5 mg group. The percent of patients with **complete** headache relief at 2 hours was significantly greater for the 20 mg group. Younger patients (12-14 years of age) had higher efficacy rates at lower doses, but patients 15-17 years of age had the highest efficacy with the 20 mg doses (Winner, 2000); a small retrospective review of 10 younger children, 5-12 years of age (mean: 9.9 years) used intranasal doses of 5 mg (n=2) or 20 mg (n=8) to treat 57 headaches; 82.5% of headaches responded to sumatriptan (Hershey, 2001); additional studies are needed

Dosage Forms Excipient information presented when available (limited, particularly for generics); consult specific product labeling. **Note:** Strength expressed as sumatriptan base

Injection, solution, as succinate: 4 mg/0.5 mL (0.5 mL); 6 mg/0.5 mL (0.5 mL)

Imitrex®: 4 mg/0.5 mL (0.5 mL); 6 mg/0.5 mL (0.5 mL) Sumavel™ DosePro™: 6 mg/0.5 mL (0.5 mL)

Solution, intranasal [spray]: 5 mg/0.1 mL (6s); 20 mg/0.1 mL (6s)

Imitrex®: 5 mg/0.1 mL (6s); 20 mg/0.1 mL (6s)

Tablet, as succinate: 25 mg, 50 mg, 100 mg

Imitrex®: 25 mg, 50 mg, 100 mg

Extemporaneous Preparations A 5 mg/mL oral liquid preparation made from tablets and 3 different vehicles (Ora-Sweet®, Ora-Sweet® SF, or Syrpalta® syrups) was stable for 21 days when stored in amber glass bottles in the dark under refrigeration (4°C); **Note:** Preparations with Ora-Sweet® and Ora-Sweet® SF used Ora-Plus® as a suspending vehicle; grind nine 100 mg tablets in a mortar into a fine powder; add 40 mL of Ora-Plus® Suspending Vehicle, 5 mL at a time, and mix thoroughly between each addition; **Note:** The suspending vehicle helps to facilitate dispersion of the tablets and is used only if Ora-Sweet® or Ora-Sweet® SF is the vehicle to be used (ie, suspending vehicle is not used if preparation uses Syrpalta® syrup as the vehicle); transfer to a calibrated amber glass bottle; rinse mortar and pestle 5 times with 10 mL of Ora-Plus® suspension vehicle pouring into bottle each time; qsad with appropriate syrup (Ora-Sweet® or Ora-Sweet® SF) to 180 mL; label "shake well," "refrigerate," and "protect from light"; (**Note:** This study also tested microbial growth on days 0 and 28; no growth of bacteria or fungus occurred) (Fish, 1997)

Fish DN, Beall HD, Goodwin SD, et al, "Stability of Sumatriptan Succinate in Extemporaneously Prepared Oral Liquids," *Am J Health Syst Pharm*, 1997, 54 (14):1619-22.

References

Hershey AD, Powers SW, LeCates S, et al, "Effectiveness of Nasal Sumatriptan in 5- to 12-Year-Old Children," *Headache*, 2001, 41 (7):693-7.

MacDonald JT, "Treatment of Juvenile Migraine With Subcutaneous Sumatriptan," *Headache*, 1994, 34(10):581-2.

Scott AK, "Sumatriptan Clinical Pharmacokinetics," *Clin Pharmacokinet*, 1994, 27(5):337-44.

Winner P, Rothner AD, Saper J, et al, "A Randomized, Double-Blind, Placebo-Controlled Study of Sumatriptan Nasal Spray in the Treatment of Acute Migraine in Adolescents," *Pediatrics*, 2000, 106 (5):989-97.

♦ **Symbicort®** *see* Budesonide and Formoterol *on page 210*

♦ **Symmetrel®** *see* Amantadine *on page 77*

♦ **Synacthen** *see* Cosyntropin *on page 362*

♦ **Synagis®** *see* Palivizumab *on page 1046*

♦ **Synalar® (Can)** *see* Fluocinolone *on page 593*

♦ **Synera™** *see* Lidocaine and Tetracaine *on page 824*

♦ **Synercid®** *see* Quinupristin/Dalfopristin *on page 1196*

♦ **Synthroid®** *see* Levothyroxine *on page 816*

♦ **Syrex** *see* Sodium Chloride *on page 1270*

♦ **Syrup of Ipecac** *see* Ipecac Syrup *on page 756*

♦ **T_3 Sodium (error-prone abbreviation)** *see* Liothyronine *on page 828*

♦ **T_4** *see* Levothyroxine *on page 816*

♦ **T-20** *see* Enfuvirtide *on page 503*

♦ **642® Tablet (Can)** *see* Propoxyphene *on page 1171*

♦ **Tabloid®** *see* Thioguanine *on page 1339*

Tacrolimus (ta KROE li mus)

Medication Safety Issues
Sound-alike/look-alike issues:
Prograf® may be confused with Gengraf®, Prozac®
Tacrolimus may be confused with everolimus, pimcrolimus, sirolimus, temsirolimus

U.S. Brand Names Prograf®; Protopic®

Canadian Brand Names Advagraf™; Prograf®; Protopic®

Therapeutic Category Immunosuppressant Agent

Generic Available Yes: Capsule

Use
Oral/injection: Prevention of organ rejection in solid organ transplantation patients (FDA approved in children and adults) or prevention and treatment of graft versus host disease (GVHD) in allogeneic stem cell transplantation patients

Topical: Second-line agent for short-term and intermittent treatment of moderate to severe atopic dermatitis in nonimmunocompromised patients not responsive to conventional therapy or when conventional therapy is not appropriate (0.03% ointment: FDA approved in ages 2-15 years and adults; 0.1% ointment: FDA approved in ages ≥18 years)

Medication Guide An FDA-approved patient medication guide, which is available with the product information and at http://www.fda.gov/downloads/Drugs/DrugSafety/ucm088996.pdf, must be dispensed with this medication for each new outpatient prescription and refill.

Pregnancy Risk Factor C

Pregnancy Considerations Adverse events were observed in animal reproduction studies. Tacrolimus crosses the human placenta and is measurable in the cord blood, amniotic fluid, and newborn serum. Tacrolimus concentrations in the placenta may be higher than the maternal serum. No consistent pattern of congenital anomalies has been observed. Transient neonatal hyperkalemia and renal dysfunction have been reported.

The National Transplantation Pregnancy Registry (NTPR, Temple University) is a registry for pregnant women taking immunosuppressants following any solid organ transplant. The NTPR encourages reporting of all immunosuppressant exposures during pregnancy in transplant recipients at 877-955-6877.

Lactation Enters breast milk/not recommended

Breast-Feeding Considerations Concentrations of tacrolimus in breast milk are lower than that of the maternal serum. The low bioavailability of tacrolimus following oral absorption may also decrease the amount of exposure to a nursing infant.

Contraindications Hypersensitivity to tacrolimus, polyoxyl 60 hydrogenated castor oil, or any component

Warnings
Systemic therapy: Immunosuppression with tacrolimus may result in increased susceptibility to infection and the possible development of lymphoma **[U.S. Boxed Warning]**. Increased risk of other malignancies, including skin malignancies; risk is related to intensity and duration of immunosuppression. Lymphoproliferative disorder related to EBV infection has been reported in immunosuppressed organ transplant patients; risk highest in young children; use combination immunosuppressant therapy with caution. Insulin-dependent post-transplant diabetes mellitus has been reported with use; risk increases in African-American and Hispanic kidney transplant patients. Neurotoxicity and nephrotoxicity have been reported especially when used in high doses. To avoid excess nephrotoxicity, do not administer simultaneously with cyclosporine; 24 hours should elapse before one is given after the other. Monitor serum potassium levels during therapy; hyperkalemia and hypokalemia have been reported. May cause hypertension; antihypertensive therapy may be required. Myocardial hypertrophy has been reported; ECG evaluation should be considered in any patient who develops renal failure or clinical manifestations of ventricular dysfunction. Closely monitor tacrolimus levels to assist in dose adjustment, monitor compliance, prevent organ rejection, and reduce drug-related toxicity.

Each mL of injection contains polyoxyl 60 hydrogenated castor oil (HCO-60) (200 mg) and dehydrated alcohol USP 80% v/v. Anaphylaxis has been reported with the injection; use should be reserved for those patients not able to take oral medication. Adequate airway, supportive measures, and agents for treating anaphylaxis should be available when tacrolimus is administered I.V.

Topical therapy: Topical calcineurin inhibitors have been associated with rare cases of malignancy **[U.S. Boxed Warning]**. Avoid use on malignant or premalignant skin conditions (eg, cutaneous T-cell lymphoma). Should not be used in immunocompromised patients. Do not apply to areas of active bacterial or viral infection; infections at the treatment site should be cleared prior to therapy. Patients with atopic dermatitis are predisposed to skin infections and tacrolimus therapy has been associated with risk of developing eczema herpeticum, varicella zoster, and herpes simplex. May be associated with development of lymphadenopathy; possible infectious causes should be investigated. Discontinue use in patients with unknown cause of lymphadenopathy or acute infectious mononucleosis. Use should be limited to short-term and intermittent treatment using the minimum amount necessary for the control of symptoms **[U.S. Boxed Warning]**. Application should be limited to involved areas. If symptoms of atopic dermatitis not improved within 6 weeks; re-evaluate to confirm diagnosis. Not recommended for use in patients with skin disease which may increase systemic absorption (eg, Netherton's syndrome). Safety of intermittent use for >1 year has not been established. The use of Protopic® in children <2 years of age is not recommended **[U.S. Boxed Warning]**; only 0.03% ointment is indicated for children 2-15 years. Acute renal failure has been reported (rarely) with topical tacrolimus therapy.

Precautions Use with caution and modify dosage in patients with hepatic or renal impairment. Minimize exposure to sunlight while on topical therapy.

Adverse Reactions

Systemic therapy:

Cardiovascular: Angina pectoris, arrhythmias, chest pain, CHF, hypertension, hypertrophic obstructive cardiomyopathy, hypotension, myocardial hypertrophy, palpitations, peripheral edema, thrombosis

Central nervous system: Agitation, altered mental status, depression, dizziness, encephalopathy, fever, hallucinations, headache, insomnia, pain, seizures

Dermatologic: Photosensitivity, pruritus, rash, skin cancer, Stevens-Johnson syndrome

Endocrine & metabolic: Cushing's syndrome, hypercalcemia, hypercholesterolemia, hyperglycemia, hyperkalemia, hypokalemia, hypomagnesemia, hypophosphatemia

Gastrointestinal: Constipation, diarrhea, dyspepsia, GI hemorrhage, nausea, pancreatitis, vomiting

Genitourinary: Albuminuria, cystitis, dysuria, hematuria, nocturia

Hematologic: Anemia, eosinophilia, leukocytosis, thrombocytopenia

Hepatic: AST, ALT, and LDH elevated; hepatotoxicity

Neuromuscular & skeletal: Arthralgia, back pain, myalgia, paresthesia, tremor

Ocular: Abnormal vision

Otic: Deafness, tinnitus

Renal: BUN and serum creatinine elevated, nephrotoxicity, oliguria

Respiratory: Cough, pleural effusion, respiratory distress

Miscellaneous: Anaphylaxis (may be due to polyoxyl 60 hydrogenated castor oil injectable vehicle), hemolytic-uremic syndrome, lymphoproliferative disorders, susceptibility to infections increased

Topical therapy:

Cardiovascular: Peripheral edema

Central nervous system: Fever, headache, hyperesthesia, pain

Dermatologic: Acne, erythema, pruritus, rash, skin burning, skin cancer, urticaria

Endocrine & metabolic: Dysmenorrhea

Gastrointestinal: Abdominal pain, diarrhea, nausea

Respiratory: Cough, rhinitis

Miscellaneous: Lymphoma

Drug Interactions

Metabolism/Transport Effects Substrate of CYP3A4 (major), P-glycoprotein; **Inhibits** CYP3A4 (weak), P-glycoprotein

Avoid Concomitant Use

Avoid concomitant use of Tacrolimus with any of the following: Artemether; BCG; CycloSPORINE; CycloSPORINE (Systemic); Dabigatran Etexilate; Dronedarone; Grapefruit Juice; Lumefantrine; Natalizumab; Nilotinib; Pimecrolimus; Pimozide; QuiNINE; Silodosin; Sirolimus; Tacrolimus (Topical); Temsirolimus; Tetrabenazine; Thioridazine; Topotecan; Vaccines (Live); Ziprasidone

Increased Effect/Toxicity

Tacrolimus may increase the levels/effects of: Alcohol (Ethyl); Colchicine; CycloSPORINE; CycloSPORINE (Systemic); Dabigatran Etexilate; Dronedarone; Leflunomide; Natalizumab; P-Glycoprotein Substrates; Phenytoin; Pimozide; QTc-Prolonging Agents; QuiNINE; Rivaroxaban; Silodosin; Sirolimus; Temsirolimus; Tetrabenazine; Thioridazine; Topotecan; Vaccines (Live); Ziprasidone

The levels/effects of Tacrolimus may be increased by: Alfuzosin; Antidepressants (Serotonin Reuptake Inhibitor/Antagonist); Antifungal Agents (Azole Derivatives, Systemic); Artemether; Calcium Channel Blockers (Dihydropyridine); Calcium Channel Blockers (Nondihydropyridine); Chloroquine; Ciprofloxacin; Ciprofloxacin (Systemic); CycloSPORINE; CycloSPORINE (Systemic);

CYP3A4 Inhibitors (Moderate); CYP3A4 Inhibitors (Strong); Denosumab; Fluconazole; Gadobutrol; Grapefruit Juice; Lumefantrine; Macrolide Antibiotics; MetroNIDAZOLE; MetroNIDAZOLE (Systemic); Nilotinib; P-Glycoprotein Inhibitors; Pimecrolimus; Protease Inhibitors; Proton Pump Inhibitors; QuiNINE; Sirolimus; Tacrolimus (Topical); Temsirolimus; Trastuzumab

Decreased Effect

Tacrolimus may decrease the levels/effects of: BCG; Sipuleucel-T; Vaccines (Inactivated); Vaccines (Live)

The levels/effects of Tacrolimus may be decreased by: Caspofungin; Cinacalcet; CYP3A4 Inducers (Strong); Deferasirox; Echinacea; Efavirenz; P-Glycoprotein Inducers; Phenytoin; Rifamycin Derivatives; Sirolimus; St Johns Wort; Temsirolimus

Food Interactions Food reduces the rate and extent of absorption by ~27%; grapefruit juice may increase tacrolimus blood concentration

Stability Reconstitution: Stable for 24 hours when mixed in D_5W or NS in glass or polyolefin containers; 24-hour stability in plastic syringes stored at 24°C; no need to protect from light; do not store in polyvinyl chloride containers since the polyoxyl 60 hydrogenated castor oil injectable vehicle may leach phthalates from polyvinyl chloride containers; polyvinyl-containing administration sets adsorb drug and may lead to a lower dose being delivered to the patient; tacrolimus is unstable in alkaline media; do not mix with acyclovir or ganciclovir

Mechanism of Action Binds to an intracellular protein forming a complex which inhibits phosphatase activity of calcineurin resulting in the inhibition of T-cell activation

Pharmacokinetics (Adult data unless noted)

Absorption: Erratic and incomplete oral absorption (5% to 67%); food within 15 minutes of administration decreases absorption (27%)

Distribution: Distributes to erythrocytes, breast milk, lung, kidneys, pancreas, liver, placenta, heart, and spleen

Children: 2.6 L/kg (mean)

Adults: 0.85-1.41 L/kg (mean) in liver and renal transplant patients

Protein binding: 99% to alpha-acid glycoprotein (some binding to albumin)

Metabolism: Hepatic metabolism through the cytochrome P450 system (CYP3A) to eight possible metabolites (major metabolite: 31-demethyl tacrolimus has same activity as tacrolimus *in vitro*)

Bioavailability:

Oral:

Children: 7% to 55%

Adults: 7% to 32%

Topical: <0.5%

Half-life:

Children: 7.7-15.3 hours

Adults: 23-46 hours (in healthy volunteers)

Time to peak serum concentration: Oral: 0.5-6 hours

Elimination: Primarily in bile; <1% excreted unchanged in urine

Clearance: 7-103 mL/minute/kg (average: 30 mL/minute/kg); clearance higher in children

Usual Dosage

Children: **Note:** Younger children generally require higher maintenance doses on a mg/kg basis than older children, adolescents, or adults (see Kim, 2005; Montini, 2006)

Oral:

Liver transplant: Initial: 0.15-0.2 mg/kg/day divided every 12 hours

Heart transplant: Initial: 0.1-0.3 mg/kg/day divided every 12 hours (see Pollock-Barziv, 2005; Swenson, 1995)

Kidney transplant: Initial: 0.2-0.3 mg/kg/day divided every 12 hours (see Filler, 2005; Kim, 2005; Montini, 2006)

Prevention of graft-vs-host disease (unlabeled use): Convert from I.V. to oral dose (1:4 ratio): Multiply total daily I.V. dose times 4 and administer in 2 divided oral doses per day, every 12 hours (Yanik, 2000)

I.V.:

Liver transplant: 0.03-0.05 mg/kg/day as a continuous infusion

Heart transplant: 0.01-0.03 mg/kg/day as a continuous infusion (see Groetzner, 2005)

Kidney transplant: 0.06 mg/kg/day as a continuous infusion (see Trompeter, 2002)

Prevention of graft-vs-host disease (unlabeled use): Initial: 0.03 mg/kg/day (based on lean body weight) as continuous infusion. Treatment should begin at least 24 hours prior to stem cell infusion and continued only until oral medication can be tolerated (Yanik, 2000).

Topical: Children ≥2 years: Moderate-to-severe atopic dermatitis: Apply 0.03% ointment to affected area twice daily; continue applications for 1 week after symptoms have cleared

Adults:

Oral: 0.075-0.2 mg/kg/day divided every 12 hours

Liver transplant: Initial: 0.1-0.15 mg/kg/day divided every 12 hours

Heart transplant: Initial: 0.075 mg/kg/day divided every 12 hours

Kidney transplant: Initial: 0.2 mg/kg/day in combination with azathioprine or 0.1 mg/kg/day in combination with mycophenoplate mofetil. Administer in 2 divided doses every 12 hours.

Prevention of graft-vs-host disease (unlabeled use): Convert from I.V. to oral dose (1:4 ratio): Multiply total daily I.V. dose times 4 and administer in 2 divided oral doses per day, every 12 hours (Uberti, 1999)

I.V. continuous infusion: 0.01-0.05 mg/kg/day

Liver or kidney transplant: Initial: 0.03-0.05 mg/kg/day

Heart transplant: Initial: 0.01 mg/kg/day

Graft-vs-host disease (unlabeled use):

Prevention: 0.03 mg/kg/day (based on lean body weight) as continuous infusion. Treatment should begin at least 24 hours prior to stem cell infusion and continued only until oral medication can be tolerated (Przepiorka, 1999).

Treatment: Initial: 0.03 mg/kg/day (based on lean body weight) as continuous infusion (Furlong, 2000; Przepiorka, 1999)

Topical: Moderate-to-severe atopic dermatitis: Apply 0.03% or 0.1% ointment to affected area twice daily; rub in gently and completely

Dosing adjustment in renal or hepatic impairment: Patients with renal or hepatic impairment should receive the lowest dose in the recommended dosage range; further reductions in dose below these ranges may be required

Hemodialysis: Not removed by hemodialysis

Administration

Oral: Administer on an empty stomach; use oral syringe or glass container (not plastic or foam cup) when administering this medication; do not administer with grapefruit juice; do not administer within 2 hours before or after antacids

Parenteral: May administer by I.V. continuous infusion; I.V. concentrate for injection must be diluted to 0.004-0.02 mg/mL in NS or D$_5$W prior to administration; PVC-free administration tubing should be used to minimize the potential for significant drug absorption onto the tubing; begin no sooner than 6-hours post-transplant; continue only until oral medication can be tolerated

Topical: For external use only; do not cover with occlusive dressings; apply thin layer and rub ointment in gently and completely onto clean, dry skin

Monitoring Parameters Liver enzymes, BUN, serum creatinine, glucose, potassium, magnesium, phosphorus, blood tacrolimus concentrations, CBC with differential; blood pressure, neurologic status, ECG

Reference Range Limited data correlating serum concentration to therapeutic efficacy/toxicity:

Trough (whole blood ELISA): 5-20 ng/mL

Trough (HPLC): 0.5-1.5 ng/mL

Heart: Typical whole blood trough concentrations:

Months 1-3: 10-20 ng/mL

Months ≥4: 6-18 ng/mL

Kidney transplant: Whole blood trough concentrations:

In combination with azathioprine:

Months 1-3: 7-20 ng/mL

Months 4-12: 5-15 ng/mL

In combination with mycophenolate mofetil/IL-2 receptor antagonist (eg, daclizumab): Months 1-2: 4-11 ng/mL

Liver transplant: Whole blood trough concentrations:

Months 1-12: 5-20 ng/mL

Prevention of graft-vs-host disease (unlabeled use): 10-20 ng/mL (Uberti, 1999); although some institutions use a lower limit of 5 ng/mL and an upper limit of 15 ng/mL (Przepiorka, 1999; Yanik, 2000)

Patient Information Administer dose at the same time each day; you will be susceptible to infection (avoid crowds and people with infections); notify physician if you develop increased urination, thirst, chest pain, acute headache or dizziness, symptoms of respiratory infection, rash, unusual bruising or bleeding. May cause photosensitivity reactions (eg, exposure to sunlight may cause severe sunburn, skin rash, redness, or itching); avoid exposure to sunlight and artificial light sources (sunlamps, tanning booth/bed); wear protective clothing, wide-brimmed hats, sunglasses, and lip sunscreen (SPF ≥15); use a sunscreen [broad-spectrum sunscreen or physical sunscreen (preferred) or sunblock with SPF ≥15]; contact physician if reaction occurs.

Nursing Implications Patients receiving I.V. tacrolimus should be under continuous observation for at least the first 30 minutes following dosage initiation; adequate airway, supportive measures, and agents for treating anaphylaxis should be available when tacrolimus is administered I.V.

Additional Information Tacrolimus should be initiated no sooner than 6 hours after transplant; convert I.V. tacrolimus to oral form as soon as possible or within 2-3 days (the oral formulation should be started 8-12 hours after stopping the I.V. infusion); when switching a patient from cyclosporine to tacrolimus, allow at least 24 hours after discontinuing cyclosporine before initiating tacrolimus therapy to minimize the risk of nephrotoxicity

Additional dosing considerations:

Switch from I.V. to oral therapy: Approximately threefold increase in dose compared to I.V.

Pediatric patients: Approximately two times higher dose compared to adults

Dosage Forms Excipient information presented when available (limited, particularly for generics); consult specific product labeling.

Capsule: 0.5 mg, 1 mg, 5 mg

Prograf®: 0.5 mg, 1 mg, 5 mg

Injection, solution:

Prograf®: 5 mg/mL (1 mL) [contains dehydrated alcohol 80% and polyoxyl 60 hydrogenated castor oil]

Ointment, topical:

Protopic®: 0.03% (30 g, 60 g, 100 g); 0.1% (30 g, 60 g, 100 g)

Extemporaneous Preparations A 0.5 mg/mL suspension has been prepared by mixing the contents of six 5 mg tacrolimus capsules with equal amounts of Ora-Plus® and Simple Syrup, NF to make a final volume of 60 mL. When compounding tacrolimus oral suspension, protect hands with latex gloves. The suspension is stable for 56 days when stored at room temperature in either glass or plastic amber prescription bottles. Label "shake well before using."

Jacobson PA, Johnson CE, West NJ, et al, "Stability of Tacrolimus in an Extemporaneously Compounded Oral Liquid," *Am J Health Sys Pharm*, 1997, 54(2):178-80.

References

Asante-Korang A, Boyle GJ, Webber SA, et al, "Experience of FK506 Immune Suppression in Pediatric Heart Transplantation: A Study of Long-Term Adverse Effects," *J Heart Lung Transplant*, 1996, 15 (4):415-22.

Filler G, Webb NJ, Milford DV, et al, "Four-Year Data After Pediatric Renal Transplantation: A Randomized Trial of Tacrolimus Vs Cyclosporin Microemulsion," *Pediatr Transplant*, 2005, 9(4):498-503.

Furlong T, Storb R, Anasetti C, et al, "Clinical Outcome After Conversion to FK 506 (Tacrolimus) Therapy for Acute Graft-Versus-Host Disease Resistant to Cyclosporine or for Cyclosporine-Associated Toxicities," *Bone Marrow Transplant*, 2000, 26(9):985-91.

Groetzner J, Reichart B, Roemer U, et al, "Cardiac Transplantation in Pediatric Patients: Fifteen-Year Experience of a Single Center," *Ann Thorac Surg*, 2005, 79(1):53-60.

Kim JS, Aviles DH, Silverstein DM, et al, "Effect of Age, Ethnicity, and Glucocorticoid Use on Tacrolimus Pharmacokinetics in Pediatric Renal Transplant Patients," *Pediatr Transplant*, 2005, 9(2):162-9.

McDiarmid SV, Colonna JO, Shaked A, et al, "Differences in Oral FK506 Dose Requirements Between Adults and Pediatric Liver Transplant Patients," *Transplantation*, 1993, 55(6):1328-32.

Menegaux F, Keeffe EB, Andrews BT, et al, "Neurological Complications of Liver Transplantation in Adult Versus Pediatric Patients," *Transplantation*, 1994, 58(4):447-50.

Montini G, Ujka F, Varagnolo C, et al, "The Pharmacokinetics and Immunosuppressive Response of Tacrolimus in Paediatric Renal Transplant Recipients," *Pediatr Nephrol*, 2006, 21(5):719-24.

Pollock-Barziv SM, Dipchand AI, McCrindle BW, et al, "Randomized Clinical Trial of Tacrolimus- Vs Cyclosporine-Based Immunosuppression in Pediatric Heart Transplant: Preliminary Results at 15-Month Follow-Up," *J Heart Lung Transplant*, 2005, 24(2):190-4.

Przepiorka D, Devine S, Fay J, et al, "Practical Considerations in the Use of Tacrolimus for Allogeneic Marrow Transplantation," *Bone Marrow Transplant*, 1999, 24(10):1053-6.

Swenson JM, Fricker FJ, and Armitage JM, "Immunosuppression Switch in Pediatric Heart Transplant Recipients: Cyclosporine to FK 506," *J Am Coll Cardiol*, 1995, 25(5):1183-8.

Trompeter R, Filler G, Webb NJ, et al, "Randomized Trial of Tacrolimus Versus Cyclosporin Microemulsion in Renal Transplantation," *Pediatr Nephrol*, 2002, 17(3):141-9.

Uberti JP, Cronin S, and Ratanatharathorn V, "Optimum Use of Tacrolimus in the Prophylaxis of Graft Versus Host Disease," *BioDrugs*, 1999, 11(5):343-58.

Yanik G, Levine JE, Ratanatharathorn V, et al, "Tacrolimus (FK506) and Methotrexate as Prophylaxis for Acute Graft-Versus-Host Disease in Pediatric Allogeneic Stem Cell Transplantation," *Bone Marrow Transplant*, 2000, 26(2):161-7.

◆ **Tagamet® HB (Can)** *see* Cimetidine *on page 309*

◆ **Tagamet® HB 200 [OTC]** *see* Cimetidine *on page 309*

◆ **Talwin®** *see* Pentazocine *on page 1085*

◆ **Tambocor™** *see* Flecainide *on page 582*

◆ **Tamiflu®** *see* Oseltamivir *on page 1027*

◆ **Tanac® [OTC]** *see* Benzocaine *on page 182*

◆ **Tanta-Orciprenaline® (Can)** *see* Metaproterenol *on page 890*

◆ **TAP-144** *see* Leuprolide *on page 805*

◆ **Tapazole®** *see* Methimazole *on page 897*

◆ **Targel® (Can)** *see* Coal Tar *on page 349*

◆ **Taro-Carbamazepine Chewable (Can)** *see* CarBAMazepine *on page 244*

◆ **Taro-Ciprofloxacin (Can)** *see* Ciprofloxacin *on page 310*

◆ **Taro-Clindamycin (Can)** *see* Clindamycin *on page 327*

◆ **Taro-Clobetasol (Can)** *see* Clobetasol *on page 331*

◆ **Taro-Enalapril (Can)** *see* Enalapril/Enalaprilat *on page 499*

◆ **Taro-Fluconazole (Can)** *see* Fluconazole *on page 584*

◆ **Taro-Mometasone (Can)** *see* Mometasone Furoate *on page 942*

◆ **Taro-Simvastatin (Can)** *see* Simvastatin *on page 1263*

◆ **Taro-Sone (Can)** *see* Betamethasone *on page 189*

◆ **Taro-Warfarin (Can)** *see* Warfarin *on page 1432*

◆ **Tavist® Allergy [OTC]** *see* Clemastine *on page 327*

◆ **Tavist® ND Allergy [OTC]** *see* Loratadine *on page 842*

◆ **Taxol® [DSC]** *see* Paclitaxel *on page 1044*

◆ **Taxol® (Can)** *see* Paclitaxel *on page 1044*

◆ **Taxotere®** *see* Docetaxel *on page 465*

Tazarotene (taz AR oh teen)

U.S. Brand Names Avage™; Tazorac®

Canadian Brand Names Tazorac®

Therapeutic Category Acne Products; Keratolytic Agent

Generic Available No

Use Topical treatment of facial acne vulgaris; topical treatment of stable plaque psoriasis of up to 20% body surface area involvement; mitigation (palliation) of facial skin wrinkling, facial mottled hyper/hypopigmentation, and benign facial lentigines

Pregnancy Risk Factor X

Pregnancy Considerations May cause fetal harm if administered to a pregnant woman. A negative pregnancy test should be obtained 2 weeks prior to treatment; treatment should begin during a normal menstrual period.

Lactation Excretion in breast milk unknown/use caution

Contraindications Hypersensitivity to tazarotene, other retinoids, or vitamin A derivatives (eg, isotretinoin, tretinoin), or any component; pregnancy; use in women of childbearing potential who are unable to comply with birth control requirements; sunburn

Warnings Retinoids should not be used on eczematous skin as they may cause severe irritation; may cause photosensitivity; avoid excessive exposure to sunlight or sunlamps; women of childbearing potential should use adequate birth control measures; a negative pregnancy test within 2 weeks prior to beginning treatment is recommended; begin treatment during a normal menstrual period

Precautions Administer with caution to patients receiving medications known to be photosensitizing (see Drug Interactions) as they may potentiate photosensitivity reactions

Adverse Reactions Dermatologic: Pruritus, burning/stinging, erythema, worsening of psoriasis, irritation, skin pain, rash, desquamation, irritant contact dermatitis, skin inflammation, dry skin, skin fissures, localized edema, skin discoloration

Drug Interactions

Avoid Concomitant Use There are no known interactions where it is recommended to avoid concomitant use.

Increased Effect/Toxicity There are no known significant interactions involving an increase in effect.

Decreased Effect There are no known significant interactions involving a decrease in effect.

Stability Store at room temperature

Mechanism of Action A retinoid prodrug which is converted to its active form by rapid de-esterification; its mechanism of action for treatment of acne and psoriasis is not well defined

Pharmacodynamics

Onset of action: Psoriasis: 1 week

Duration: Psoriasis: Up to 12 weeks after discontinuation when initially treated for 2-3 months (duration may be less if initial treatment was shorter)

Pharmacokinetics (Adult data unless noted)

Absorption (without occlusion): Adults: Psoriatic patients: <1%; normal controls: <5%

Protein binding: Metabolite: >99%

Metabolism: Following topical application, undergoes esterase hydrolysis to form its active metabolite, AGN 190299

Half-life: Metabolite: 18 hours

Excretion: Urine and feces as metabolites

Usual Dosage Topical:

Acne vulgaris: Children ≥12 years and Adults: Tazorac®: 0.1% cream or gel applied as a thin film (2 mg/cm^2) to affected areas once daily in the evening

Psoriasis: Children ≥12 years and Adults: Tazorac®: 0.05% to 0.1% cream or gel applied as a thin film (2 mg/cm^2) to affected area once daily in the evening; apply to no more than 20% of the body surface area

Palliation of fine facial wrinkles, facial mottled hyper/hypopigmentation, benign facial lentigines: Adolescents ≥17 years and Adults: Avage™: Apply a pea-sized amount once daily at bedtime; lightly cover entire face including eyelids if desired

Administration Topical: Apply thin film to affected areas; avoid eyes and mouth; skin should be dry before applying

Monitoring Parameters Disease severity in plaque psoriasis (reduction in erythema, scaling, induration); pregnancy test prior to treatment of females of childbearing age

Patient Information May cause photosensitivity reactions (eg, exposure to sunlight may cause severe sunburn, skin rash, redness, or itching); avoid exposure to sunlight and artificial light sources (sunlamps, tanning booth/bed); wear protective clothing, wide-brimmed hats, sunglasses, and lip sunscreen (SPF ≥15); use a sunscreen [broad-spectrum sunscreen or physical sunscreen(preferred) or sunblock with SPF ≥15]; contact physician if reaction occurs. Avoid washing face more frequently than 2-3 times/day; avoid using topical preparations with high alcoholic content during treatment period.

Dosage Forms Excipient information presented when available (limited, particularly for generics); consult specific product labeling.

Cream:

Avage™: 0.1% (30 g) [contains benzyl alcohol]

Tazorac®: 0.05% (30 g, 60 g); 0.1% (30 g, 60 g) [contains benzyl alcohol]

Gel (Tazorac®): 0.05% (30 g, 100 g); 0.1% (30 g, 100 g) [contains benzyl alcohol]

◆ **Tazicef®** see Ceftazidime on page 272

◆ **Tazobactam and Piperacillin** see Piperacillin and Tazobactam on page 1116

◆ **Tazocin® (Can)** see Piperacillin and Tazobactam on page 1116

◆ **Tazorac®** see Tazarotene on page 1314

◆ **Taztia XT®** see Diltiazem on page 443

◆ **3TC** see LamiVUDine on page 791

◆ **3TC® (Can)** see LamiVUDine on page 791

◆ **3TC, Abacavir, and Zidovudine** see Abacavir, Lamivudine, and Zidovudine on page 31

◆ **3TC and Abacavir** see Abacavir and Lamivudine on page 29

◆ **3TC and ABC** see Abacavir and Lamivudine on page 29

◆ **3TC and AZT** see Lamivudine and Zidovudine on page 794

◆ **3TC and ZDV** see Lamivudine and Zidovudine on page 794

◆ **T-Cell Growth Factor** see Aldesleukin on page 60

◆ **TCGF** see Aldesleukin on page 60

◆ **TCN** see Tetracycline on page 1331

◆ **Td** see Diphtheria and Tetanus Toxoid on page 452

◆ **Td Adsorbed (Can)** see Diphtheria and Tetanus Toxoid on page 452

◆ **Tdap** see Diphtheria, Tetanus Toxoids, and Acellular Pertussis Vaccine on page 458

◆ **TDF** see Tenofovir on page 1319

◆ **TDF and FTC** see Emtricitabine and Tenofovir on page 498

◆ **TDF, Efavirenz, and FTC** see Efavirenz, Emtricitabine, and Tenofovir on page 493

◆ **TDF, FTC, and Efavirenz** see Efavirenz, Emtricitabine, and Tenofovir on page 493

◆ **Tebrazid™ (Can)** see Pyrazinamide on page 1188

◆ **Tecta™ (Can)** see Pantoprazole on page 1054

◆ **Tegretol®** see CarBAMazepine on page 244

◆ **Tegretol®-XR** see CarBAMazepine on page 244

◆ **Teldrin® HBP [OTC]** see Chlorpheniramine on page 296

◆ **Telzir® (Can)** see Fosamprenavir on page 623

◆ **Temodal® (Can)** see Temozolomide on page 1315

◆ **Temodar®** see Temozolomide on page 1315

◆ **Temovate®** see Clobetasol on page 331

◆ **Temovate E®** see Clobetasol on page 331

Temozolomide (te mo ZOLE oh mide)

Medication Safety Issues

Sound-alike/look-alike issues:

Temodar® may be confused with Tambocor®

High alert medication: The Institute for Safe Medication Practices (ISMP) includes this medication among its list of drug classes which have a heightened risk of causing significant patient harm when used in error.

Related Information

Emetogenic Potential of Antineoplastic Agents on page 1579

U.S. Brand Names Temodar®

Canadian Brand Names Temodal®

Therapeutic Category Antineoplastic Agent, Alkylating Agent

Generic Available No

Use Treatment of refractory anaplastic astrocytoma with relapse after initial therapy with a nitrosourea and procarbazine (FDA approved in adults); treatment of newly-diagnosed glioblastoma multiforme (initially in combination with radiotherapy, then as maintenance treatment) (FDA approved in adults)

Active against recurrent glioblastoma multiforme, metastatic melanoma, anaplastic oligodendroglioma, ependymoma, recurrent brain stem glioma, medulloblastoma/PNET, neuroblastoma, cutaneous T-Cell lymphomas (mycosis fungoides [MF] and Sezary Syndrome [SS]), carcinoid tumors

Pregnancy Risk Factor D

Pregnancy Considerations May cause fetal harm when administered to pregnant women. Animal studies, at doses less than used in humans, resulted in numerous birth defects. Testicular toxicity was demonstrated in animal studies using smaller doses than recommended for cancer treatment. There are no adequate and well-controlled studies in pregnant women. Male and female patients should avoid pregnancy while receiving drug.

Lactation Excretion in breast milk unknown/not recommended

Breast-Feeding Considerations Due to the potential for serious adverse reactions in the nursing infant, breast-feeding is not recommended.

Contraindications Hypersensitivity to temozolomide, dacarbazine, or any component

Warnings Hazardous agent; use appropriate precautions for handling and disposal. Thrombocytopenia and neutropenia are dose-limiting toxicities which occur late in the treatment cycle and usually resolve within 14 days; prior to therapy initiation patients must have an absolute neutrophil count (ANC) ≥1.5 x 10^9/L and a platelet count ≥100 x 10^9/L; obtain a CBC on day 22 and weekly until the ANC >1.5 x 10^9/L and platelet count >100 x 10^9/L. Prolonged pancytopenia resulting in aplastic anemia has been reported; concurrent use of temozolomide with medications associated with aplastic anemia (eg, carbamazepine, sulfamethoxazole and trimethoprim, phenytoin) may obscure assessment for development of aplastic anemia. *Pneumocystis jiroveci* pneumonia (PCP) may occur; risk is increased in those patients receiving steroids or longer dosing regimens; PCP prophylaxis is required in patients receiving radiotherapy in combination with the 42-day temozolomide regimen. Rare cases of myelodysplastic syndrome and secondary malignancies, including myeloid leukemia, have been reported. May cause fetal harm; pregnancy should be avoided during therapy.

Precautions Use with caution in patients with severe renal or hepatic impairment.

Adverse Reactions

Cardiovascular: Peripheral edema, pulmonary embolism, thromboembolism

Central nervous system: Amnesia, anxiety, confusion, convulsions, depression, dizziness, fatigue, fever, headache, hemiparesis, insomnia, lethargy, memory impairment, somnolence

Dermatologic: Alopecia, dry skin, erythema, petechiae, pruritus, rash

Endocrine & metabolic: Breast pain, hypercorticism, hyperglycemia, weight gain,

Gastrointestinal: Abdominal pain, anorexia, constipation, diarrhea, dysphagia, mucositis, nausea, oral candidiasis, stomatitis, taste perversion, vomiting

Genitourinary: Incontinence, urinary frequency, urinary tract infection

Hematologic: Anemia, aplastic anemia, hemorrhage, leukopenia, lymphopenia, neutropenia, pancytopenia, thrombocytopenia

Hepatic: Hepatotoxicity, liver enzymes increased

Local: Injection site reactions (erythema, irritation, pain, pruritus, swelling, warmth)

Neuromuscular & skeletal: Abnormal gait, arthralgia, ataxia, back pain, coordination problems, myalgia, neuropathy, paresthesia, weakness

Ocular: Blurred vision, diplopia, visual changes, visual deficit

Respiratory: Cough, dyspnea, pharyngitis, sinusitis, upper respiratory tract infection

Miscellaneous: Allergic reaction, anaphylaxis (rare), myelodysplastic syndrome, opportunistic infections [including *Pneumocystis jiroveci* pneumonia (see Warnings)], secondary malignancies (including myeloid leukemia), viral infection

<1%, postmarketing, and/or case reports: Agitation, alkaline phosphatase increased, apathy, emotional lability, erythema multiforme, flu-like syndrome, hallucination, hematoma, herpes simplex, herpes zoster, hypokalemia, interstitial pneumonitis, oral candidiasis, peripheral neuropathy, pneumonitis, Stevens-Johnson syndrome, thrombophlebitis, toxic epidermal necrolysis, weight loss

Drug Interactions

Avoid Concomitant Use

Avoid concomitant use of Temozolomide with any of the following: BCG; Natalizumab; Pimecrolimus; Tacrolimus (Topical); Vaccines (Live)

Increased Effect/Toxicity

Temozolomide may increase the levels/effects of: Leflunomide; Natalizumab; Vaccines (Live)

The levels/effects of Temozolomide may be increased by: Denosumab; Divalproex; Pimecrolimus; Tacrolimus (Topical); Trastuzumab; Valproic Acid

Decreased Effect

Temozolomide may decrease the levels/effects of: BCG; Sipuleucel-T; Vaccines (Inactivated); Vaccines (Live)

The levels/effects of Temozolomide may be decreased by: Echinacea

Food Interactions Food reduces the rate and extent of absorption

Stability Store capsules at 25°C (77°F); excursions permitted to 15°C to 30°C (59°F to 86°F). Refrigerate intact vials for injection at 2°C to 8°C (36°F to 46°F). Reconstituted vials may be stored for up to 14 hours at room temperature (25°C or 77°F). Infusion must be completed within 14 hours of reconstitution.

Mechanism of Action Prodrug which is hydrolyzed to MTIC and exerts its effect by site-specific DNA cross-linking resulting from the methylation of the O^6 and N^7 positions of guanine.

Pharmacokinetics (Adult data unless noted)

Absorption: Oral: Adults: Rapidly and completely absorbed

Distribution: Extensive tissue distribution; crosses the blood brain barrier; V_d: 0.4 L/kg

Protein binding: 14%

Bioavailability: Oral: 100% (on a mg-per-mg basis, I.V. temozolomide, infused over 90 minutes, is bioequivalent to an oral dose)

Metabolism: At a neutral or alkaline pH, hydrolyzes to active MTIC (3-methyl-(triazen-1-yl) imidazole-4-carboxamide) and temozolomide acid metabolite; MTIC is further metabolized to 5-amino-imidazole-4-carboxamide (AIC) and methylhydrazine (active alkylating agent); CYP isoenzymes play only a minor role in metabolism (of temozolomide and MTIC)

Half-life:

Children: 1.7 hours

Adults: 1.6-1.8 hours

Time to peak serum concentration: Oral: 1 hour; 2.3 hours after high fat meal

Elimination: <1% excreted in feces; 5% to 7% of unchanged temozolomide excreted renally

Clearance: 5.5 L/hour/m²; women have a ~5% lower clearance than men (adjusted for body surface area); children 3-17 years have similar temozolomide clearance as adults

Usual Dosage Oral, I.V. (refer to individual protocols):

Children: 100-200 mg/m² once daily for 5 days every 28 days

In a Phase I study to determine the maximum tolerated dose of temozolomide in pediatric solid tumor patients with prior craniospinal irradiation (CSI) therapy and those without prior CSI (n=53; age range: 1-19 years), 100-240 mg/m²/day was administered; the maximum tolerated dose was 215 mg/m²/day for 5 days in patients without prior CSI and 180 mg/m²/day for 5 days in patients with prior CSI with subsequent courses to begin on day 28 (Nicholson, 1998)

Adults:

Anaplastic astrocytoma (refractory): Initial dose: 150 mg/m²/dose once daily for 5 days; repeat every 28 days. Subsequent doses of 100-200 mg/m²/dose once daily for 5 days per treatment cycle; based upon hematologic tolerance

Dosage modification for toxicity:

ANC <1000/mm³ or platelets <50,000/mm³ on day 22 or day 29 (day 1 of next cycle): Postpone therapy until ANC >1500/mm³ and platelets >100,000/mm³; reduce dose by 50 mg/m²/day for subsequent cycle

ANC 1000-1500/mm^3 or platelets 50,000-100,000/mm^3 on day 22 or day 29 (day 1 of next cycle): Postpone therapy until ANC >1500/mm^3 and platelets >100,000/mm^3; maintain initial dose

ANC >1500/mm^3 and platelets >100,000/mm^3 on day 22 or day 29 (day 1 of next cycle): Increase dose to or maintain dose at 200 mg/m^2/day for 5 days for subsequent cycle

Glioblastoma multiforme (newly diagnosed, high-grade glioma):

Concomitant phase: 75 mg/m^2/dose once daily for 42 days with focal radiotherapy (60 Gy administered in 30 fractions). **Note:** PCP prophylaxis is required during concomitant phase and should continue in patients who develop lymphocytopenia until lymphocyte recovery to ≤grade 1. Obtain weekly CBC.

ANC ≥1500/mm^3, platelet count ≥100,000/mm^3, and nonhematologic toxicity ≤grade 1 (excludes alopecia, nausea/vomiting): Temozolomide 75 mg/m^2/dose once daily may be continued throughout the 42-day concomitant period up to 49 days

Dosage modification for toxicity:

ANC ≥500/mm^3 but <1500/mm^3 **or** platelet count ≥10,000/mm^3 but <100,000/mm^3 **or** grade 2 nonhematologic toxicity (excludes alopecia, nausea/vomiting): **Interrupt therapy**

ANC <500/mm^3 **or** platelet count <10,000/mm^3 **or** grade 3/4 nonhematologic toxicity (excludes alopecia, nausea/vomiting): **Discontinue therapy**

Maintenance phase (consists of 6 treatment cycles): Begin 4 weeks after concomitant phase completion. **Note:** Each subsequent cycle is 28 days (consisting of 5 days of drug treatment followed by 23 days without treatment). Draw CBC within 48 hours of day 22; hold next cycle and do weekly CBC until ANC >1500/mm^3 and platelet count >100,000/mm^3; dosing modification should be based on lowest blood counts and worst nonhematologic toxicity during the previous cycle.

Cycle 1: 150 mg/m^2/dose once daily for 5 days; repeat every 28 days of a 28-day treatment cycle

Cycles 2-6: May increase to 200 mg/m^2/dose once daily for 5 days every 28 days (if ANC ≥1500/mm^3, platelets ≥100,000/mm^3, and nonhematologic toxicities for cycle 1 are ≤grade 2; if dose was not escalated at the onset of cycle 2, do not increase for cycles 3-6)

Dosage modification (during maintenance phase) for toxicity:

ANC <1000/mm^3, platelet count <50,000/mm^3, or grade 3 nonhematologic toxicity (excludes alopecia, nausea/vomiting) during previous cycle: Decrease dose by 1 dose level (50 mg/m^2/day for 5 days), unless dose has already been lowered to 100 mg/m^2/day, then discontinue therapy.

If dose reduction <100 mg/m^2/day is required or grade 4 nonhematologic toxicity (excludes alopecia, nausea/vomiting), or if the same grade 3 nonhematologic toxicity occurs after dose reduction: Discontinue therapy.

Metastatic melanoma (unlabeled use): Oral: 200 mg/m^2/dose once daily for 5 days every 28 days (for up to 12 cycles). For subsequent cycles, reduce dose to 75% of the original dose for grade 3/4 hematologic toxicity and reduce the dose to 50% of the original dose for grade 3/4 nonhematologic toxicity (Middleton, 2000).

Administration Standard antiemetics may be administered if needed.

Oral: Swallow capsule intact with a glass of water; do not chew; if patient is unable to swallow capsule, open capsule and dissolve in apple juice or applesauce taking precautions to avoid exposure to the cytotoxic agent; administer on an empty stomach or at bedtime to reduce the incidence of nausea and vomiting; may administer with food as long as food intake and administration time are performed at the same time each day to ensure consistent bioavailability. Do not repeat if vomiting occurs after dose is administered; wait until the next scheduled dose.

Parenteral: I.V.: Bring to room temperature prior to reconstitution. Reconstitute each 100 mg vial with 41 mL sterile water for injection to a final concentration of 2.5 mg/mL. Swirl gently; do not shake. Place dose without further dilution into a 250 mL empty sterile PVC infusion bag. Infuse over 90 minutes. Infusion must be completed within 14 hours of reconstitution. Do not administer other medications through the same I.V. line. Flush line before and after administration.

Monitoring Parameters CBC with ANC (absolute neutrophil count) and platelet count

Patient Information Inform physician of any unusual bruising or bleeding, shortness of breath, fever, chills or cough. Instruct patient that temozolomide comes in different strengths and that you may need to take more than one strength of capsule each day during treatment. Women of childbearing potential should be advised to avoid becoming pregnant. Male and female patients should use appropriate contraceptive measures.

Nursing Implications Avoid opening capsules; if capsules are accidentally opened, avoid inhalation or contact with skin or mucous membranes

Additional Information To minimize the risk of a wrong dose error, each strength of temozolomide must be packaged and dispensed in a separate vial or in its original glass bottle. Label each container with the appropriate number of capsules to be taken each day.

Increased MGMT (O-6-methylguanine-DNA methyltransferase) activity/levels within tumor tissue is associated with temozolomide resistance. Glioblastoma patients with decreased levels (due to methylated MGMT promoter) may be more likely to benefit from the combination of radiation therapy and temozolomide (Hegi, 2008; Stupp, 2009). Determination of MGMT status may be predictive for response to alklylating agents.

Dosage Forms Excipient information presented when available (limited, particularly for generics); consult specific product labeling.

Capsule:

Temodar®: 5 mg, 20 mg, 100 mg, 140 mg, 180 mg, 250 mg

Injection, powder for reconstitution:

Temodar®: 100 mg [contains polysorbate 80]

Extemporaneous Preparations

A 10 mg/mL oral suspension of temozolomide may be compounded in a vertical flow hood mixing the contents of ten 100-mg capsules and 500 mg of povidone K-30 powder in a glass mortar; add 25 mg anhydrous citric acid dissolved in 1.5 mL purified water to form a paste; add 50 mL Ora-Plus® (add a small amount at first, mix, add balance); transfer to amber plastic bottle; add Ora-Sweet® or Ora-Sweet® SF to a final volume of 100 mL by rinsing the mortar with small aliquots of Ora-Sweet®; repeat rinsing 3 more times. The suspension is stable for 7 days at room temperature or 60 days refrigerated in plastic amber prescription bottles. Label "Shake well," "Refrigerate," and include the beyond-use date. **Note:** Use appropriate handling precautions during preparation.

Trissel LA, Yanping Z, and Koontz SE, "Temozolomide Stability in Extemporaneously Compounded Oral Suspension," *Int J Pharm Compounding*, 2006, 10 (5):396-9.

References

Bazatell R, Wagner LM, Cohn SL, et al, "Irinotecan Plus Temozolomide in Children With Recurrent or Refractory Neuroblastoma: A Phase II Children's Oncology Group Study," *J Clin Oncol*, 2009, 27(15S) (abstract).

Hegi ME, Diserens AC, Gorlia T, et al, "MGMT Gene Silencing and Benefit From Temozolomide in Glioblastoma," *N Engl J Med*, 2005, 352(10):997-1003.

Hegi ME, Liu L, Herman JG, et al, "Correlation of O6-Methylguanine Methyltransferase (MGMT) Promoter Methylation With Clinical Outcomes in Glioblastoma and Clinical Strategies to Modulate MGMT Activity," *J Clin Oncol*, 2008, 26(25):4189-99.

Horton TM, Thompson PA, Berg SL, et al, "Phase I Pharmacokinetic and Pharmacodynamic Study of Temozolomide in Pediatric Patients With Refractory or Recurrent Leukemia: A Children's Oncology Group Study," *J Clin Oncol*, 2007, 25(31):4922-8.

Loh KC, Willert J, Meltzer H, et al, "Temozolomide and Radiation for Aggressive Pediatric Central Nervous System Malignancies," *J Pediatr Hematol Oncol*, 2005, 27(5):254-8.

Middleton MR, Grob JJ, Aaronson N, et al, "Randomized Phase III Study of Temozolomide Versus Dacarbazine in the Treatment of Patients With Advanced Metastatic Malignant Melanoma," *J Clin Oncol*, 2000, 18(1):158-66.

National Comprehensive Cancer Network (NCCN)®, "Clinical Practice Guidelines in Oncology™: Non-Hodgkin's Lymphomas," Version 1, 2009. Available at http://www.nccn.org/professionals/physician_gls/PDF/nhl.pdf.

National Comprehensive Cancer Network (NCCN)®, "Practice Guidelines in Oncology™: Central Nervous System Cancers," Version 1, 2008. Available at http://www.nccn.org/professionals/physician_gls/PDF/cns.pdf.

Nicholson HS, Krailo M, Ames MM, et al, "Phase I Study of Temozolomide in Children and Adolescents With Recurrent Solid Tumors: A Report From the Children's Cancer Group," *J Clin Oncol*, 1998, 16(9):3037-43.

Stupp R, Hegi ME, Mason WP, et al, "Effects of Radiotherapy With Concomitant and Adjuvant Temozolomide Versus Radiotherapy Alone on Survival in Glioblastoma in a Randomised Phase III Study: 5-Year Analysis of the EORTC-NCIC Trial," *Lancet Oncol*, 2009, 10 (5):459-66.

◆ **Tempra® (Can)** see Acetaminophen *on page 36*

◆ **Tenex®** see GuanFACINE *on page 660*

Teniposide (ten i POE side)

Medication Safety Issues

Sound-alike/look-alike issues:
Teniposide may be confused with etoposide

High alert medication: The Institute for Safe Medication Practices (ISMP) includes this medication among its list of drug classes which have a heightened risk of causing significant patient harm when used in error.

U.S. Brand Names Vumon®

Canadian Brand Names Vumon®

Therapeutic Category Antineoplastic Agent, Podophyllotoxin Derivative

Generic Available No

Use Treatment of childhood acute lymphoblastic leukemia (ALL) refractory to induction with other therapy (FDA approved in pediatric patients ages ≥2 weeks); has also been used in the treatment of refractory ALL in adults

Pregnancy Risk Factor D

Pregnancy Considerations Adverse effects were observed in animal studies. There are no adequate and well-controlled studies in pregnant women. May cause fetal harm if administered during pregnancy. Women of childbearing potential should avoid becoming pregnant during teniposide treatment.

Lactation Excretion in breast milk unknown/not recommended

Breast-Feeding Considerations Due to the potential for serious adverse reactions in the nursing infant, breast-feeding is not recommended.

Contraindications Hypersensitivity to teniposide, polyoxyethylated castor oil, or any component

Warnings Hazardous agent; use appropriate precautions for handling and disposal. Teniposide should be administered under the supervision of a physician experienced in the use of cancer chemotherapy agents. Severe, dose-related myelosuppression with resulting infection or bleeding may occur **[U.S. Boxed Warning]**; monitor for infection and bleeding. Hypersensitivity reactions, including anaphylaxis-like reactions have been reported with initial dosing or with repeated dosing **[U.S. Boxed Warning]**; risk for hypersensitivity reactions appears to increase with previous reactions and in patients with neuroblastoma or brain tumors; stop infusion for signs of anaphylaxis; medications for treatment of hypersensitivity reactions (epinephrine, I.V. fluids, corticosteroids, and antihistamines) must be readily available for use in case of a reaction.

Teniposide injection contains benzyl alcohol which may cause allergic reactions in susceptible individuals; large amounts of benzyl alcohol (≥99 mg/kg/day) have been associated with a potentially fatal toxicity ("gasping syndrome") in neonates; use teniposide injection with caution in neonates. The injection contains polyoxyl 35 castor oil which may cause hypotension and increase the frequency of hypersensitivity reactions. If hypotension occurs during administration, discontinue infusion and administer I.V. fluids and supportive therapy as needed. The teniposide formulation contains ~43% alcohol and may contribute to adverse effects such as CNS depression, somnolence, lethargy, hypotension, and metabolic acidosis. Teniposide may cause local tissue necrosis or thrombophlebitis if extravasation occurs. Teniposide is a potential carcinogen; may cause fetal harm when administered to pregnant women; may induce a secondary leukemia.

Precautions Use with caution in patients with renal or hepatic impairment (may require a dosage adjustment with significant impairment); use with caution and adjust dosage in patients with Down's syndrome who may be more sensitive to myelosuppressive effects of teniposide

Adverse Reactions

Cardiovascular: Flushing, hypertension, hypotension (associated with rapid infusions <30 minutes), tachycardia

Central nervous system: Chills, fever, lethargy, somnolence

Dermatologic: Alopecia, rash

Endocrine & metabolic: Metabolic acidosis

Gastrointestinal: Anorexia, diarrhea, mucositis, nausea, vomiting

Hematologic: Anemia, bleeding, leukopenia, myelosuppression, neutropenia, thrombocytopenia

Hepatic: Hepatic impairment

Local: Thrombophlebitis, tissue necrosis upon extravasation

Renal: Renal impairment

Respiratory: Bronchospasm, dyspnea

Miscellaneous: Hypersensitivity reactions, secondary leukemia

<1%, postmarketing, and/or case reports: Arrhythmia, CNS depression, hepatic dysfunction, metabolic abnormality, neurotoxicity, renal dysfunction

Drug Interactions

Metabolism/Transport Effects Substrate of CYP3A4 (major), P-glycoprotein; **Inhibits** CYP2C9 (weak), 3A4 (weak)

Avoid Concomitant Use

Avoid concomitant use of Teniposide with any of the following: BCG; Natalizumab; Pimecrolimus; Tacrolimus (Topical); Vaccines (Live)

Increased Effect/Toxicity

Teniposide may increase the levels/effects of: Leflunomide; Natalizumab; Vaccines (Live)

The levels/effects of Teniposide may be increased by: CYP3A4 Inhibitors (Moderate); CYP3A4 Inhibitors (Strong); Dasatinib; Denosumab; P-Glycoprotein Inhibitors; Pimecrolimus; Tacrolimus (Topical); Trastuzumab

Decreased Effect

Teniposide may decrease the levels/effects of: BCG; Sipuleucel-T; Vaccines (Inactivated); Vaccines (Live)

The levels/effects of Teniposide may be decreased by: Barbiturates; CYP3A4 Inducers (Strong); Deferasirox; Echinacea; Herbs (CYP3A4 Inducers); P-Glycoprotein Inducers; Phenytoin

Stability Store ampuls in refrigerator at 2°C to 8°C (36°F to 46°F). Protect from light. Solutions diluted for infusion to a concentration of 0.1, 0.2, or 0.4 mg/mL are stable at room temperature for up to 24 hours after preparation; solutions diluted to 1 mg/mL should be used within 4 hours of preparation. Refrigeration of diluted solutions is not recommended. Because precipitation may occur at any concentration, the manufacturer recommends administrating as soon as possible after preparation. Use appropriate precautions for handling and disposal. Teniposide must be diluted with either D_5W or 0.9% sodium chloride solutions to a final concentration of 0.1, 0.2, 0.4 or 1 mg/mL. In order to prevent extraction of the plasticizer DEHP, **solutions should be prepared in non-DEHP-containing containers, such as glass or polyolefin containers**. The use of polyvinyl chloride (PVC) containers is not recommended.

Mechanism of Action Type II topoisomerase inhibitor that induces single-stranded DNA breaks, double-stranded DNA breaks, and DNA-protein cross-links; induces late S phase or early G2-phase arrest resulting in inhibition of DNA synthesis

Pharmacokinetics (Adult data unless noted)

Distribution: Mainly into liver, kidneys, small intestine, and adrenals; limited distribution into CSF <1%
Children: V_d: 3-11 L/m^2
Adults: V_d: 8-44 L/m^2
Protein binding: >99%
Metabolism: Hepatic
Half-life: Children: 5 hours
Elimination: 0% to 10% excreted in feces; 4% to 12% excreted unchanged in urine
Clearance: Renal: 10% of total body clearance

Usual Dosage Note: Patients with Down syndrome and leukemia may be more sensitive to the myelosuppressive effects; administer the first course at half the usual dose and adjust dose in subsequent cycles upward based on degree of toxicities (myelosuppression and mucositis) in the previous course(s).

Children: I.V.: Acute lymphoblastic leukemia (ALL): 165 mg/m^2 twice weekly for 8-9 doses or 250 mg/m^2 weekly for 4-8 weeks **or** 165 mg/m^2/dose days 1 and 2 of weeks 3, 13, and 23 (see Lauer, 2001)

Dosing adjustment in renal or hepatic impairment: No specific recommendation (insufficient data). Dose adjustments may be necessary in patient with significant renal or hepatic impairment.

Administration Parenteral: I.V. infusion: Do not administer by rapid I.V. injection. Administer by I.V. infusion over at least 30-60 minutes to minimize the risk of hypotensive reactions; administer at a final concentration of 0.1, 0.2, 0.4, or 1 mg/mL diluted in D_5W or NS. Inspect infusion solution for particulate matter since precipitation may occur at any concentration. Administer 1 mg/mL solutions within 4 hours of preparation to reduce the potential for precipitation. Administer through non-DEHP-containing administration sets. Incompatible with heparin; flush infusion line with D_5W or NS before and after infusion. Precipitation may occur at any concentration; administer as soon as possible after preparation; inspect solution prior to administration

Monitoring Parameters Vital signs (blood pressure), CBC with differential, hemoglobin, platelet count, renal and hepatic function tests; observe for possible hypersensitivity reactions. Inspect solution and tubing for precipitation before and during infusion.

Patient Information Notify physician if fever, sore throat, painful/burning urination, bleeding problems, tiredness or weakness, skin rash, pain or numbness in extremities, or shortness of breath occur. Advise women of childbearing potential to avoid becoming pregnant while receiving teniposide.

Nursing Implications Agents for treating hypotension or anaphylactoid reactions should be present when I.V. teniposide is being administered; avoid extravasation.

Dosage Forms Excipient information presented when available (limited, particularly for generics); consult specific product labeling.

Injection, solution:
Vumon®: 10 mg/mL (5 mL) [contains benzyl alcohol, dehydrated ethanol 42.7%, and polyoxyethylated castor oil]

References

Clark PI and Slevin ML, "The Clinical Pharmacology of Etoposide and Teniposide," *Clin Pharmacokinet*, 1987, 12(4):223-52.

Lauer SJ, Shuster JJ, Mahoney DH Jr, et al, "A Comparison of Early Intensive Methotrexate/Mercaptopurine With Early Intensive Alternating Combination Chemotherapy for High-Risk B-Precursor Acute Lymphoblastic Leukemia: A Pediatric Oncology Group Phase III Randomized Trial," *Leukemia*, 2001, 15(7):1038-45.

Sinkule JA, Stewart CF, Crom WR, et al, "Teniposide (VM26) Disposition in Children With Leukemia," *Cancer Res*, 1984, 44 (3):1235-7.

Tenofovir (te NOE fo veer)

Related Information

Adult and Adolescent HIV *on page 1620*
Management of Healthcare Worker Exposures to HBV, HCV, and HIV *on page 1661*`
Pediatric HIV *on page 1613*
Perinatal HIV *on page 1628*

U.S. Brand Names Viread®

Canadian Brand Names Viread®

Therapeutic Category Antiretroviral Agent; HIV Agents (Anti-HIV Agents); Nucleotide Reverse Transcriptase Inhibitor (NRTI)

Generic Available No

Use Treatment of HIV-1 infection in combination with other antiretroviral agents. (**Note:** HIV regimens consisting of **three** antiretroviral agents are strongly recommended); treatment of chronic hepatitis B virus (HBV)

Pregnancy Risk Factor B

Pregnancy Considerations Animal studies have shown decreased fetal growth and reduced fetal bone porosity. Clinical studies in children have shown bone demineralization with chronic use. Tenofovir crosses the human placenta; limited data indicate decreased maternal bioavailability during the third trimester. Due to the potential for bone effects and limited data in pregnancy, use in pregnancy only in special circumstances after considering use of other alternatives. Cases of lactic acidosis/hepatic steatosis syndrome have been reported in pregnant women receiving nucleoside analogues. It is not known if pregnancy itself potentiates this known side effect; however, pregnant women may be at increased risk of lactic acidosis and liver damage. Hepatic enzymes and electrolytes should be monitored frequently during the third trimester of pregnancy in women receiving nucleoside analogues. Renal function should also be monitored. Use caution with hepatitis B coinfection; hepatitis B flare may occur if tenofovir is discontinued postpartum. Health professionals are encouraged to contact the Antiretroviral Pregnancy Registry to monitor outcomes of pregnant women exposed to antiretroviral medications (1-800-258-4263 or www.APRegistry.com).

Lactation Excretion in breast milk unknown/contraindicated

Breast-Feeding Considerations In infants born to mothers who are HIV positive, HAART while breast-feeding may decrease postnatal infection. However, maternal or infant antiretroviral therapy does not completely eliminate the risk of postnatal HIV transmission.

In the United States where formula is accessible, affordable, safe, and sustainable, complete avoidance of breast-feeding by HIV-infected women is recommended to decrease potential transmission of HIV.

Contraindications Hypersensitivity to tenofovir or any component

Warnings Cases of lactic acidosis, severe hepatomegaly with steatosis and death have been reported in patients receiving tenofovir and other nucleoside analogues **[U.S. Boxed Warning]**; most of these cases have been in women; prolonged nucleoside use, obesity, and prior liver disease may be risk factors; use with extreme caution in patients with other risk factors for liver disease; discontinue therapy in patients who develop laboratory or clinical evidence of lactic acidosis or pronounced hepatotoxicity. Use with caution and adjust dose in patients with renal dysfunction (Cl_{cr} <50 mL/minute); monitor renal function closely; renal dysfunction, including acute renal failure and Fanconi syndrome (renal tubular injury with severe hypophosphatemia) may occur (especially in patients with renal disease, underlying systemic disease, or those taking nephrotoxic medications); adults with a low body weight and those taking medications that increase tenofovir serum concentration may also be at increased risk for tenofovir-associated nephrotoxicity; avoid tenofovir in patients with concomitant or recent use of nephrotoxic agents; cases of nephrotoxicity have been reported in adolescents receiving tenofovir-containing regimens; evaluate and monitor renal function in all patients receiving tenofovir (regardless of age).

Severe acute exacerbations of HBV have occurred after tenofovir discontinuation in patients infected with HBV **[U.S. Boxed Warning]**; follow hepatic function of HBV-infected patients closely (clinically and with laboratory tests) for at least several months after discontinuing tenofovir therapy; initiate antihepatitis B therapy if needed. Testing for HBV and HIV is recommended prior to the initiation of tenofovir therapy (treatment of HBV in patients with unrecognized/untreated HIV may lead to HIV resistance; treatment of HIV in patients with unrecognized/untreated HBV may lead to rapid HBV resistance). In patients who are coinfected with HIV and HBV, tenofovir should only be used as part of an appropriate combination antiretroviral regimen.

Immune reconstitution syndrome (an acute inflammatory response to residual or indolent opportunistic infections) may occur in HIV patients during initial treatment with combination antiretroviral agents including tenofovir; this syndrome may require further patient assessment and therapy. Do not use Viread® (tenofovir) with other tenofovir-containing combination formulations (ie, Truvada®, Atripla®). Do not use tenofovir or tenofovir-containing products with adefovir for the treatment of chronic HBV.

Precautions Use with caution in patients with hepatic impairment. Significant drug interactions may occur (see Drug Interactions). Fat redistribution and accumulation [ie, central obesity, peripheral wasting, facial wasting, breast enlargement, dorsocervical fat enlargement (buffalo hump), and cushingoid appearance] have been observed in patients receiving antiretroviral agents (causal relationship not established).

Bone toxicity (osteomalacia and reduced bone mineral density) may occur; long-term effects in humans are not known (see also Adverse Reactions); monitor for potential bone toxicities during therapy; supplementation with calcium and vitamin D may be beneficial (but has not been studied). **Note:** Postmarketing cases of osteomalacia (which may increase risk of bone fractures) have also been reported in association with proximal renal tubulopathy. Safety and efficacy have not been established in patients <18 years of age. Recent studies suggest that tenofovir-related bone loss may be greater in children who are less mature (eg, Tanner stage 1-2) than in those who are more physically mature (Tanner ≥3). Thus, tenofovir-associated bone mineral density loss may limit the usefulness of tenofovir in prepubertal children (see Adverse Reactions; Giacomet, 2005; Hazra, 2005; Purdy, 2008, Working Group, 2008).

The use of antiretroviral regimens that only contain triple nucleoside reverse transcriptase inhibitors (NRTIs) are generally less effective than regimens containing 2 NRTIs and either an NNRTI or protease inhibitor; use triple NRTI-containing regimens with great caution; early virological failure and high rates of resistance may occur; closely monitor for virologic failure and consider treatment modification (see Additional Information)

Adverse Reactions

Cardiovascular: Chest pain

Central nervous system: Headache, dizziness, fever, pain, depression, insomnia, anxiety, fatigue

Dermatologic: Rash

Endocrine & metabolic: Hypophosphatemia, lactic acidosis, weight loss, fat redistribution and accumulation (see Precautions), hypercholesterolemia, hypertriglyceridemia, amylase elevated, hypokalemia (postmarketing reports)

Gastrointestinal: Nausea, diarrhea, vomiting, dyspepsia, abdominal pain, flatulence, anorexia, pancreatitis

Hematologic: Neutropenia

Hepatic: Liver enzymes elevated

Neuromuscular & skeletal: Asthenia, peripheral neuropathy, arthralgia, myalgia, back pain, reduction in bone mineral density, osteomalacia, elevations in biochemical markers of bone metabolism (eg, serum bone-specific alkaline phosphatase); **Note:** A significant decrease in lumbar spine bone mineral density (>6%) was reported in 5 of 15 pediatric patients who received a tenofovir-containing regimen for 48 weeks. No orthopedic fractures occurred, but 2 patients required discontinuation of tenofovir. All 5 patients with a decrease in bone mineral density were virologic responders and prepubertal (Tanner Stage 1). This study found a moderately strong correlation between decreases in bone mineral density z scores at week 48 and age at baseline. No correlation between decreases in bone mineral density z scores and tenofovir dose or pharmacokinetics was observed. The authors conclude that bone mineral density loss may limit the usefulness of tenofovir in prepubertal children (see Hazra, 2005). Postmarketing cases of osteomalacia and myopathy have also been reported, both in association with proximal renal tubulopathy.

Renal: Glycosuria, renal impairment, serum creatinine elevated, acute renal failure, Fanconi syndrome, acute tubular necrosis; postmarketing cases of proximal renal tubulopathy

Respiratory: Dyspnea

Miscellaneous: Sweating, immune reconstitution syndrome (see Warnings)

Drug Interactions

Metabolism/Transport Effects Inhibits CYP1A2 (weak)

Avoid Concomitant Use There are no known interactions where it is recommended to avoid concomitant use.

Increased Effect/Toxicity

Tenofovir may increase the levels/effects of: Adefovir; Didanosine

The levels/effects of Tenofovir may be increased by: Acyclovir-Valacyclovir; Atazanavir; Ganciclovir-Valganciclovir; Lopinavir; Protease Inhibitors

Decreased Effect

Tenofovir may decrease the levels/effects of: Atazanavir; Didanosine; Protease Inhibitors

The levels/effects of Tenofovir may be decreased by: Adefovir

Food Interactions A high-fat meal increases oral bioavailability (AUC) by 40% and increases peak serum concentrations by 14%; a light meal had no significant effect on tenofovir pharmacokinetics compared to administration while fasting; food delays the time to peak concentrations by 1 hour

Stability Store at controlled room temperature at 25°C (77°F); excursions permitted to 15°C to 30°C (59°F to 86°F).

Mechanism of Action Tenofovir disoproxil fumarate (TDF) is a prodrug of tenofovir; *in vivo*, TDF undergoes diester hydrolysis to tenofovir; tenofovir is an acyclic nucleoside phosphate (nucleotide) analog of adenosine 5'-monophosphate; tenofovir undergoes phosphorylation by cellular enzymes to the active tenofovir diphosphate, which serves as an alternative substrate to deoxyadenosine 5'-triphosphate, a natural substrate for cellular DNA polymerase and reverse transcriptase; tenofovir diphosphate inhibits HIV viral reverse transcriptase and HBV polymerase by competing with natural deoxyadenosine 5'-triphosphate and by becoming incorporated into viral DNA causing DNA chain termination.

Pharmacokinetics (Adult data unless noted)

Distribution: Mean V_d: Adults: 1.2-1.3 L/kg

Protein binding: Minimal (7.2% to serum proteins)

Metabolism: Not metabolized by CYP isoenzymes; tenofovir disoproxil fumarate (a prodrug) undergoes diester hydrolysis to tenofovir; tenofovir undergoes phosphorylation to the active tenofovir diphosphate

Bioavailability: Adults: 25% (fasting); high-fat meals will increase AUC by 40%

Half-life: Adults: Serum: 17 hours; intracellular: 10-50 hours

Time to peak serum concentration: Fasting: 1 hour

Elimination: Excreted via glomerular filtration and active tubular secretion; after I.V. administration: 70% to 80% is excreted in the urine as unchanged drug within 72 hours; after multiple oral doses (administered with food): 32% ± 10% is excreted in the urine within 24 hours

Clearance: Total body clearance is decreased in patients with renal impairment

Dialysis:

Hemodialysis: Efficiently removes tenofovir; 4 hours of hemodialysis removed ~10% of a single 300 mg dose

Peritoneal dialysis: Effects unknown

Usual Dosage Oral:

HIV (use in combination with other antiretroviral agents):

Neonates and Infants: Not approved for use; dose is unknown

Children: Clinical trials previously excluded patients <18 years of age; current pediatric studies are assessing the following doses using investigational formulations:

Children 2-8 years: 8 mg/kg/dose once daily; maximum: 300 mg/day

Children >8 years: Median dose: 210 mg/m^2/dose once daily; maximum: 300 mg/day

Note: A phase III study in children >8 years of age will use a dose of 175 mg/m^2 once daily. This target dose was used in a pharmacokinetic study of 18 children 6.2-16.2 years of age (mean ± SD: 12 ± 2.5 years of age). The actual dose administered was 208 mg/m^2 (range: 161-256 mg/m^2) once daily, due to constraints of using a 75 mg investigational tablet. Tenofovir exposure at steady state in 16 subjects receiving

combination antiretroviral therapy [that included a protease inhibitor plus low-dose ritonavir ("Booster doses")] approached values observed in adult patients treated with tenofovir disoproxil fumarate 300 mg once daily (see Hazra, 2004). Further pediatric studies are needed.

Adolescents ≥18 years and Adults: 300 mg once daily

Adults:

Coadministration with atazanavir: Tenofovir 300 mg is recommended to be given with atazanavir 300 mg plus ritonavir 100 mg (all as a single daily dose); administer with food; do **not** use tenofovir and atazanavir without booster doses of ritonavir (see Drug Interactions)

Coadministration with didanosine: Reduce dose of didanosine when used in combination with tenofovir; use didanosine delayed release capsule formulation (Videx EC®):

Adults <60 kg: Videx EC® 200 mg once daily with tenofovir 300 mg once daily

Adults ≥60 kg: Videx EC® 250 mg once daily with tenofovir 300 mg once daily

Chronic hepatitis B infection: Adolescents ≥18 years and Adults: 300 mg once daily (**Note:** Optimal duration of therapy is unknown)

Dosing adjustment in renal impairment: Adolescents ≥18 years and Adults: Oral: **Note:** Closely monitor clinical response and renal function in these patients (clinical effectiveness and safety of these guidelines have not been evaluated)

Cl$_{cr}$ ≥50 mL/minute: No adjustment necessary

Cl$_{cr}$ 30-49 mL/minute: 300 mg every 48 hours

Cl$_{cr}$ 10-29 mL/minute: 300 mg every 72-96 hours

Cl$_{cr}$ <10 mL/minute without dialysis: No dosing recommendation available

Hemodialysis: 300 mg every 7 days or after a total of ~12 hours of dialysis (eg, once weekly with 3 hemodialysis sessions of ~4 hours in length); administer dose after completion of dialysis

Dosing adjustment in hepatic impairment: No dosage adjustment required; **Note:** Tenofovir has not been evaluated for the treatment of HBV in patients with decompensated liver disease.

Administration May be administered without regard to meals

Monitoring Parameters CBC with differential, hemoglobin, MCV, reticulocyte count, liver enzymes, bilirubin, renal and hepatic function tests, CD4 cell count and HIV RNA plasma levels (patients with HIV), and HBV RNA plasma levels (patients with HBV). Monitor for potential bone and renal abnormalities. Calculate creatinine clearance in all patients prior to starting tenofovir therapy and as clinically needed; monitor for alterations in calculated creatinine clearance and serum phosphorus in patients at risk or with a history of renal dysfunction and patients receiving concurrent nephrotoxic agents. Test patients for hepatitis B (HBV) and HIV prior to starting therapy; in patients infected with HBV, monitor hepatic function closely (clinically and with laboratory tests) for at least several months after discontinuing tenofovir therapy (see Warnings).

Patient Information Tenofovir is not a cure for HIV or HBV; take tenofovir every day as prescribed; do not change dose or discontinue without physician's advice; if a dose is missed, take it as soon as possible, then return to normal dosing schedule; if a dose is skipped, do **not** double the next dose; report the use of other medications, nonprescription medications and herbal or natural products to your physician and pharmacist; long-term effects are not known; notify physician if persistent severe abdominal pain, nausea, or vomiting occurs

HIV medications may cause changes in body fat, including an increase in fat in the upper back and neck, breasts, and trunk; a loss of fat from the face, arms, and legs may also occur. Some HIV medications (including tenofovir) may cause a serious, but rare, condition called lactic acidosis with an increase in liver size (hepatomegaly). Before starting tenofovir, inform your physician about your medical conditions, including any liver or kidney problems. Do not take Viread® with other tenofovir-containing medications (eg, Truvada®, Atripla®).

Additional Information A powder formulation is in development; 75 mg investigational tablets are currently being studied in children; an investigational liquid formulation has been studied in children 2-8 years of age (Working Group, 2008).

Long term studies demonstrating a decrease of clinical progression of HIV in patients receiving tenofovir are needed. Consider tenofovir in patients with HIV strains that would be susceptible as assessed by treatment history or laboratory tests. Mutation of reverse transcriptase at the 65 codon (K65R mutation) confers *in vitro* resistance to tenofovir; the K65R mutation is selected in some patients after treatment with didanosine, zalcitabine, or abacavir; thus, cross-resistance may occur. Multiple nucleoside mutations with a T69S double insertion showed decreased *in vitro* susceptibility to tenofovir; patients with HIV strains that had ≥3 zidovudine-associated mutations that included M41L or L210W showed decreased responses to tenofovir (but these responses were still better than placebo); patients with mutations at K65R, or L74V without zidovudine-associated mutations seemed to have a decreased response to tenofovir

A high rate of early virologic failure in therapy-naive adult HIV patients has been observed with the once-daily three-drug combination therapy of didanosine enteric-coated beadlets (Videx® EC), lamivudine, and tenofovir and the once-daily three-drug combination therapy of abacavir, lamivudine, and tenofovir. These combinations should not be used as a new treatment regimen for naive or pretreated patients. Any patient currently receiving either of these regimens should be closely monitored for virologic failure and considered for treatment modification. Early virologic failure was also observed in therapy-naive adult HIV patients treated with tenofovir, didanosine enteric-coated beadlets (Videx® EC) and either efavirenz or nevirapine; rapid emergence of resistant mutations has also been reported with this combination; the combination of tenofovir, didanosine, and any non-nucleoside reverse transcriptase inhibitor is **not** recommended as initial antiretroviral therapy.

Dosage Forms Excipient information presented when available (limited, particularly for generics); consult specific product labeling.

Tablet, as disoproxil fumarate:
Viread®: 300 mg [equivalent to 245 mg tenofovir disoproxil]

References

Briars LA, Hilao JJ, and Kraus DM, "A Review of Pediatric Human Immunodeficiency Virus Infection," *Journal of Pharmacy Practice*, 2004, 17(6):407-31.

Giacomet V, Mora S, Martelli L, et al, "A 12-Month Treatment With Tenofovir Does Not Impair Bone Mineral Accrual in HIV-Infected Children," *J Acquir Immune Defic Syndr*, 2005, 40(4):448-50.

Hazra R, Balis FM, Tullio AN, et al, "Single-Dose and Steady-State Pharmacokinetics of Tenofovir Disoproxil Fumarate in Human Immunodeficiency Virus-Infected Children," *Antimicrob Agents Chemother*, 2004, 48(1):124-9.

Hazra R, Gafni RI, Maldarelli F, et al, "Tenofovir Disoproxil Fumarate and an Optimized Background Regimen of Antiretroviral Agents as Salvage Therapy for Pediatric HIV Infection," *Pediatrics*, 2005, 116(6):e846-54.

Lyseng-Williamson KA, Reynolds NA, and Plosker GL, "Tenofovir Disoproxil Fumarate: A Review of Its Use in the Management of HIV Infection," *Drugs*, 2005, 65(3):413-32.

Morris JL and Kraus DM, "New Antiretroviral Therapies for Pediatric HIV Infection," *J Pediatr Pharmacol Ther*, 2005, 10:215-47.

Panel on Antiretroviral Guidelines for Adults and Adolescents, "Guidelines for the Use of Antiretroviral Agents in HIV-Infected Adults and Adolescents," December 1, 2009, http://www.aidsinfo.nih.gov.

Purdy JB, Gafni RI, Reynolds JC, et al, "Decreased Bone Mineral Density With Off-Label Use of Tenofovir in Children and Adolescents Infected With Human Immunodeficiency Virus," *J Pediatr*, 2008, 152 (4):582-4.

Working Group on Antiretroviral Therapy and Medical Management of HIV-Infected Children, "Guidelines for the Use of Antiretroviral Agents in Pediatric HIV Infection," February 23, 2009. Available at http://www.aidsinfo.nih.gov.

◆ **Tenofovir and Emtricitabine** *see* Emtricitabine and Tenofovir *on page 498*

◆ **Tenofovir Disoproxil Fumarate** *see* Tenofovir *on page 1319*

◆ **Tenofovir Disoproxil Fumarate and Emtricitabine** *see* Emtricitabine and Tenofovir *on page 498*

◆ **Tenofovir Disoproxil Fumarate, Efavirenz, and Emtricitabine** *see* Efavirenz, Emtricitabine, and Tenofovir *on page 493*

◆ **Tenofovir Disoproxil Fumarate, Emtricitabine, and Efavirenz** *see* Efavirenz, Emtricitabine, and Tenofovir *on page 493*

◆ **Tenofovir, Efavirenz, and Emcitrabine** *see* Efavirenz, Emtricitabine, and Tenofovir *on page 493*

◆ **Tenofovir, Emcitrabine, and Efavirenz** *see* Efavirenz, Emtricitabine, and Tenofovir *on page 493*

◆ **Tenormin®** *see* Atenolol *on page 147*

◆ **Tensilon® (Can)** *see* Edrophonium *on page 490*

◆ **Tera-Gel™ [OTC]** *see* Coal Tar *on page 349*

Terbinafine (TER bin a feen)

Medication Safety Issues

Sound-alike/look-alike issues:
Terbinafine may be confused with terbutaline
Lamisil® may be confused with Lamictal®, Lomotil®

International issues:
Lamisil® may be confused with Lemesil® which is a brand name for nimesulide in Greece and Romania

U.S. Brand Names Lamisil AT® [OTC]; Lamisil®

Canadian Brand Names Apo-Terbinafine®; CO Terbinafine; Gen-Terbinafine; Lamisil®; Mylan-Terbinafine; Novo-Terbinafine; PHL-Terbinafine; PMS-Terbinafine; Riva-Terbinafine; Sandoz-Terbinafine; Terbinafine-250

Therapeutic Category Antifungal Agent, Oral; Antifungal Agent, Topical

Generic Available Yes: Excludes gel, granules, and solution

Use

Oral: Onychomycosis of the toenail or fingernail due to susceptible dermatophytes; treatment of tinea capitis in children >4 years and adults

Topical: Antifungal for the treatment of tinea pedis (athlete's foot), tinea cruris (jock itch), and tinea corporis (ringworm) (OTC/prescription formulations); tinea versicolor (prescription formulations)

Pregnancy Risk Factor B

Pregnancy Considerations Adverse events were not observed in animal reproduction studies. Avoid use in pregnancy since treatment of onychomycosis is postponable.

Lactation Enters breast milk/not recommended

Breast-Feeding Considerations Terbinafine is found in breast milk following oral administration. The milk/plasma ratio is 7:1.

Contraindications Hypersensitivity to terbinafine or any component

Warnings Topical formulations (gel, cream, or solution) are not for ophthalmic, oral, or intravaginal use. Although rare, Stevens-Johnson syndrome and toxic epidermal necrolysis have been reported with oral use; discontinue therapy if progressive skin rash occurs. Pancytopenia and neutropenia have been reported rarely with oral use; discontinuation of therapy may be required. Monitor CBCs in patients with pre-existing immunosuppression if use to continue >6 weeks. Rare cases of hepatic failure (including fatal cases) have been reported following oral treatment; not recommended for use in patients with active or chronic liver disease. Pretreatment hepatic enzymes tests are recommended for patients receiving oral therapy. Discontinue if symptoms or signs of hepatobiliary dysfunction or cholestatic hepatitis develop. Changes in the ocular lens and retina have been reported with oral use; discontinuation of therapy may be required.

Use of oral therapy not recommended in patients with hepatic cirrhosis; clearance is reduced. Precipitation or exacerbation of cutaneous or systemic lupus erythematosus has been observed with oral therapy; discontinue if signs and/or symptoms develop. Use of oral therapy not recommended in patients with renal dysfunction (Cl_{cr} ≤50 mL/minute); clearance is reduced by approximately 50%.

Precautions Use with caution in patients sensitive to allylamine antifungals (eg, naftifine, butenafine); cross sensitivity to terbinafine may exist

Adverse Reactions Oral: Adverse events listed for tablets unless otherwise specified. Oral granules were studied in patients 4-12 years of age.

Cardiovascular: Angioedema

Central nervous system: Headache (13%; granules 7%), fever (granules 7%), dizziness, fatigue, malaise

Dermatologic: Rash (6%; granules 2%), pruritus (3%; granules 1%), urticaria (1%), burning, contact dermatitis, dryness, exfoliation, irritation, skin discoloration (hyperpigmentation), Stevens-Johnson syndrome, toxic epidermal necrolysis, alopecia, generalized exanthematous pustulosis (acute), psoriaform eruption, psoriasis exacerbation

Gastrointestinal: Diarrhea (6%; granules 3%), vomiting (granules 5%), dyspepsia (4%), nausea (3%; granules 2%), taste disturbance (3%), abdominal pain (2%; granules 2% to 4%), toothache (granules 1%), acute pancreatitis, appetite decreased

Hematologic: Anemia, agranulocytosis, neutropenia (rare), pancytopenia, thrombocytopenia

Hepatic: Liver enzyme abnormalities (3%), hepatic failure, cholestatic hepatitis

Local: Irritation, stinging

Neuromuscular & skeletal: Arthralgia, myalgia, rhabdomyolysis

Ocular: Lens and retinal changes, visual field acuity decreased, visual field defects

Respiratory: Nasopharyngitis (granules 10%), cough (granules 6%), nasal congestion (granules 2%), pharyngeal pain (granules 2%), rhinorrhea (granules 2%)

Miscellaneous: Allergic hypersensitivity reactions including anaphylaxis, precipitation/exacerbation of cutaneous and systemic lupus erythematosus

Drug Interactions

Metabolism/Transport Effects Substrate (minor) of 1A2, 2C9, 2C19, 3A4; **Inhibits** CYP2D6 (strong); **Induces** CYP3A4 (weak)

Avoid Concomitant Use

Avoid concomitant use of Terbinafine with any of the following: Tamoxifen; Thioridazine

Increased Effect/Toxicity

Terbinafine may increase the levels/effects of: Atomoxetine; CYP2D6 Substrates; Fesoterodine; Nebivolol; Tamoxifen; Tetrabenazine; Thioridazine; Tricyclic Antidepressants

Decreased Effect

Terbinafine may decrease the levels/effects of: Codeine; CycloSPORINE; CycloSPORINE (Systemic); Saccharomyces boulardii; Saxagliptin; TraMADol

The levels/effects of Terbinafine may be decreased by: Rifamycin Derivatives

Stability

Cream: Store at 5°C to 30°C (41°F to 86°F).

Granules: Store at controlled room temperature of 15°C to 30°C (59°F to 86°F).

Solution: Store at 5°C to 25°C (41°F to 77°F); do not refrigerate.

Tablet: Store below 25°C (77°F); protect from light.

Mechanism of Action Synthetic allylamine derivative which inhibits squalene epoxidase, a key enzyme in sterol biosynthesis in fungi. This results in a deficiency in ergosterol within the fungal cell wall and results in fungal cell death. Active against most strains of *Trichophyton mentagrophytes*, *Trichophyton rubrum*; may be effective for infections of *Microsporum gypseum* and *M. nanum*, *Trichophyton verrucosum*, *Epidermophyton floccosum*, *Candida albicans*, and *Scopulariopsis brevicaulis*.

Pharmacokinetics (Adult data unless noted)

Absorption: Children and Adults: Topical: Limited (<5%); Oral: >70%

Distribution: Distributed to sebum and skin predominantly

Protein binding: Plasma: >99%

Metabolism: Hepatic; no active metabolites; first-pass effect

Bioavailability: Oral:

Children: 36% to 64%

Adults: 40%

Half-life:

Topical: Adults: 14-35 hours

Oral: Terminal half-life: 200-400 hours; very slow release of drug from skin and adipose tissues occurs; effective half-life: ~36 hours (children: 27-31 hours)

Time to peak serum concentration: Children and Adults: 1-2 hours

Elimination: Children and Adults: 70% in urine

Clearance: Children (14-68 kg): 15.6-26.7 L/hour

Usual Dosage

Oral:

Granules: Tinea capitis: Children ≥4 years:

<25 kg: 125 mg once daily for 6 weeks

25-35 kg: 187.5 mg once daily for 6 weeks

>35 kg: 250 mg once daily for 6 weeks

Tablet: Onychomycosis:

Children:

10-20 kg: 62.5 mg once daily for 6 weeks (fingernails) **or** 12 weeks (toenails)

20-40 kg: 125 mg once daily for 6 weeks (fingernails) **or** 12 weeks (toenails)

>40 kg: 250 mg once daily for 6 weeks (fingernails) **or** 12 weeks (toenails)

Adults:

Superficial mycoses: Fingernail: 250 mg/day for up to 6 weeks; toenail: 250 mg/day for 12 weeks; doses may be given in 2 divided doses

Systemic mycosis: 250-500 mg/day for up to 16 months

Topical:

Cream, gel, solution: Children ≥12 years and Adults:

Athlete's foot (tinea pedis): OTC/prescription formulations: Apply to affected area twice daily for at least 1 week, not to exceed 4 weeks

Ringworm (tinea corporis) and jock itch (tinea cruris): OTC formulations: Apply cream to affected area once or twice daily for at least 1 week, not to exceed 4 weeks; apply gel or solution once daily for 7 days

Cream, solution: Adults: Tinea versicolor: Prescription formulation: Apply to affected area twice daily for 1 week

Dosing adjustment in renal impairment: Cl_{cr} <50 mL/ minute: Clearance decreased by ~50%; oral administration is not recommended

Dosing adjustment in hepatic impairment: Clearance is decreased by ~50% with hepatic cirrhosis; oral administration is not recommended

Administration

Oral: Tablets may be administered without regard to meals. Granules should be taken with food; sprinkle on a spoonful of nonacidic food (eg, pudding, mashed potatoes); do not use applesauce or fruit-based foods; swallow granules whole without chewing.

Topical: Apply to clean, dry affected area in sufficient quantity to cover; avoid contact with eyes, nose, mouth, or other mucous membranes. Do not use occlusive dressings.

Monitoring Parameters Oral therapy: AST/ALT prior to initiation, repeat if used >6 weeks; CBC

Patient Information Do not take any new medication during therapy without consulting prescriber. Use exactly as directed. Finish all of the prescription even if symptoms appear resolved, may take several months for full treatment (inadequate treatment may result in reinfection). May cause altered taste (normal). Report unusual fatigue; persistent loss of appetite, nausea or vomiting; dark urine/ pale stool; or other persistent adverse response.

Topical (cream or spray): For topical use only. Wash and dry nails thoroughly before applying. Avoid contact with eyes, nose, or mouth. Report irritation, itching, or burning of skin around nail. Full clinical effect may require several months due to the time required for a new nail to grow.

Additional Information Due to potential toxicity, the manufacturer recommends confirmation of diagnosis testing of nail specimens prior to treatment of onychomycosis. Patients should not be considered therapeutic failures until they have been symptom-free for 2-4 weeks following a course of treatment; GI complaints usually subside with continued administration.

A meta-analysis of efficacy studies for toenail infections revealed that weighted average mycological cure rates for continuous therapy were 36.7% (griseofulvin), 54.7% (itraconazole), and 77% (terbinafine). Cure rate for 4-month pulse therapy for itraconazole and terbinafine were 73.3% and 80%. Additionally, the final outcome measure of final costs per cured infections for continuous therapy was significantly lower for terbinafine (De Backer, 1998).

Dosage Forms Excipient information presented when available (limited, particularly for generics); consult specific product labeling.

Cream, topical, as hydrochloride: 1% (12 g, 24 g)

Lamisil AT®: 1% (12 g, 15 g, 24 g, 30 g, 36 g) [contains benzyl alcohol]

Gel, topical:

Lamisil AT®: 1% (6 g, 12 g) [contains benzyl alcohol]

Granules, oral:

Lamisil®: 125 mg/packet (42s); 187.5 mg/packet (42s)

Solution, topical, as hydrochloride [spray]:

Lamisil AT®: 1% (30 mL) [contains ethanol]

Tablet, oral: 250 mg

Lamisil®: 250 mg

References

Abdel-Rahman SM and Nahata MC, "Oral Terbinafine: A New Antifungal Agent," *Ann Pharmacother*, 1997, 31(4):445-56.

Abdel-Rahman SM, Herron J, Fallon-Friedlander S, et al, "Pharmacokinetics of Terbinafine in Young Children Treated for Tinea Capitis," *Pediatr Infect Dis J*, 2005, 24(10):886-91.

Amichai B and Grunwald MH, "Adverse Drug Reactions of the New Oral Antifungal Agents - Terbinafine, Fluconazole, and Itraconazole," *Int J Dermatol*, 1998, 37(6):410-5.

Angello JT, Voytovich RM, and Jan SA, "A Cost/Efficacy Analysis of Oral Antifungals Indicated for the Treatment of Onychomycosis: Griseofulvin, Itraconazole, and Terbinafine," *Am J Manag Care*, 1997, 3(3):443-50.

De Backer M, De Vroey C, Lesaffre E, et al, "Twelve Weeks of Continuous Oral Therapy for Toenail Onychomycosis Caused by Dermatophytes: A Double-Blind Comparative Trial of Terbinafine 250 mg/day Versus Itraconazole 200 mg/day," *J Am Acad Dermatol*, 1998, 38(5 Pt 3):S57-63.

Dwyer CM, White MI, and Sinclair TS, "Cholestatic Jaundice Due to Terbinafine," *Br J Dermatol*, 1997, 136(6):976-7.

Friedlander SF, Aly R, Krafchik B, et al, "Terbinafine in the Treatment of *Trichophyton* Tinea Capitis: A Randomized, Double-Blind, Parallel-Group, Duration-Finding Study," *Pediatrics*, 2002, 109(4):602-7.

Gupta AK and Shear NH, "Terbinafine: An Update," *J Am Acad Dermatol*, 1997, 37(6):979-88.

Gupta AK, Sibbald RG, Knowles SR, et al, "Terbinafine Therapy May Be Associated With the Development of Psoriasis De Novo or Its Exacerbation: Four Case Reports and a Review of Drug Induced Psoriasis," *J Am Acad Dermatol*, 1997, 36(5 Part 2):858-62.

Gupta AK, Sibbald RG, Lynde CW, et al, "Onychomycosis in Children: Prevalence and Treatment Strategies," *J Am Acad Dermatol*, 1997, 36(3 Pt 1):395-402.

Jones TC, "Overview of the Use of Terbinafine in Children," *Br J Dermatol*, 1995, 132(5):683-9.

Trepanier EF and Amsden GW, "Current Issues in Onychomycosis," *Ann Pharmacother*, 1998, 32(2):204-14.

Vickers AE, Sinclair JR, Zollinger M, et al, "Multiple Cytochrome P-450s Involved in the Metabolism of Terbinafine Suggest a Limited Potential for Drug-Drug Interactions," *Drug Metab Dispos*, 1999, 27(9):1029-38.

♦ **Terbinafine-250 (Can)** *see* Terbinafine *on page 1322*

♦ **Terbinafine Hydrochloride** *see* Terbinafine *on page 1322*

Terbutaline (ter BYOO ta leen)

Medication Safety Issues

Sound-alike/look-alike issues:

Brethine may be confused with Methergine®

Terbutaline may be confused with terbinafine, TOLBUTamide

Terbutaline and methylergonovine parenteral dosage forms look similar. Due to their contrasting indications, use care when administering these agents.

Related Information

Asthma *on page 1697*

Canadian Brand Names Bricanyl®

Therapeutic Category Adrenergic Agonist Agent; Anti-asthmatic; Beta$_2$-Adrenergic Agonist Agent; Bronchodilator; Sympathomimetic; Tocolytic Agent

Generic Available Yes

Use Bronchodilator for relief of reversible bronchospasm in patients with asthma, bronchitis, and emphysema

Pregnancy Risk Factor B

Lactation Enters breast milk/compatible

Contraindications Hypersensitivity to terbutaline, other sympathomimetic amines, or any component

Warnings Paradoxical bronchoconstriction may occur with excessive use; if it occurs, discontinue terbutaline immediately

Precautions Use with caution in patients with diabetes mellitus, hypertension, hyperthyroidism, history of seizures, or cardiac disease; excessive or prolonged use may lead to tolerance

Adverse Reactions

Cardiovascular: Tachycardia, hypertension, arrhythmias, flushing, prolonged QT_c interval, CPK isoenzyme elevated

Central nervous system: Drowsiness, headache, nervousness, seizures, dizziness

Endocrine & metabolic: Hyperglycemia, hypokalemia

Gastrointestinal: Nausea, vomiting, dysgeusia

Neuromuscular & skeletal: Tremor

Otic: Tinnitus

Respiratory: Dyspnea, bronchospasm (with excessive use), pharyngitis, dry throat, chest tightness

Miscellaneous: Diaphoresis

Drug Interactions

Avoid Concomitant Use

Avoid concomitant use of Terbutaline with any of the following: Iobenguane I 123

Increased Effect/Toxicity

Terbutaline may increase the levels/effects of: Sympathomimetics

The levels/effects of Terbutaline may be increased by: Atomoxetine; Cannabinoids; MAO Inhibitors; Tricyclic Antidepressants

Decreased Effect

Terbutaline may decrease the levels/effects of: Iobenguane I 123

The levels/effects of Terbutaline may be decreased by: Alpha-/Beta-Blockers; Beta-Blockers (Beta1 Selective); Beta-Blockers (Nonselective); Betahistine

Mechanism of Action Relaxes bronchial smooth muscle and muscles of peripheral vasculature by action on beta$_2$-receptors with less effect on heart rate

Pharmacodynamics

Onset of action:

Oral: 30 minutes

Oral inhalation: 5-30 minutes

SubQ: 6-15 minutes

Duration:

Oral: 4-8 hours

Oral inhalation: 3-6 hours

SubQ: 1.5-4 hours

Pharmacokinetics (Adult data unless noted)

Absorption: 33% to 50%

Distribution: Breast milk to plasma ratio: <2.9

Metabolism: Possible first-pass metabolism after oral use

Half-life: 5.7 hours (range: 2.9-14 hours)

Time to peak serum concentration: SubQ: 0.5 hours

Elimination: Primarily (60%) unchanged in urine after parenteral use

Usual Dosage

Children <12 years:

Oral: Initial: 0.05 mg/kg/dose every 8 hours, increase gradually, up to 0.15 mg/kg/dose; maximum daily dose: 5 mg

SubQ: 0.005-0.01 mg/kg/dose to a maximum of 0.4 mg/dose every 15-20 minutes for 3 doses; may repeat every 2-6 hours as needed

Note: Continuous I.V. infusion has been used successfully in children with asthma; a 2-10 mcg/kg loading dose followed by an 0.08-0.4 mcg/kg/minute continuous infusion; depending upon the clinical response, the dosage may require titration in increments of 0.1-0.2 mcg/kg/minute every 30 minutes; doses as high as 10 mcg/kg/minute have been used.

Children ≥12 years and Adults:

Oral: 2.5-5 mg/dose every 6-8 hours; maximum daily dose:

12-15 years: 7.5 mg

>15 years: 15 mg

SubQ: 0.25 mg/dose repeated in 20 minutes for 3 doses; a total dose of 0.75 mg should not be exceeded

Nebulization: Children and Adults: 0.01-0.03 mL/kg (1 mg = 1 mL using injection); minimum dose: 0.1 mL; maximum dose: 2.5 mL every 4-6 hours

Administration

Oral: May administer without regard to food

Parenteral: May administer undiluted, direct I.V. over 5-10 minutes; for continuous infusion, dilute to a maximum concentration of 1 mg/mL in D$_5$W or NS

Inhalation: Nebulization: Dilute dose with 1-2 mL NS

Monitoring Parameters Heart rate, blood pressure, respiratory rate, serum potassium, arterial or capillary blood gases (if applicable)

Dosage Forms Excipient information presented when available (limited, particularly for generics); consult specific product labeling. [CAN] = Canadian brand name

Injection, solution, as sulfate: 1 mg/mL (1 mL)

Powder for oral inhalation:

Bricanyl® Turbuhaler [CAN]: 500 mcg/actuation [50 or 200 metered actuations] [not available in U.S.]

Tablet, as sulfate: 2.5 mg, 5 mg

Extemporaneous Preparations A 1 mg/mL suspension made from terbutaline tablets in simple syrup NF is stable 30 days when refrigerated

Horner RK and Johnson CE, "Stability of An Extemporaneously Compounded Terbutaline Sulfate Oral Liquid," *Am J Hosp Pharm*, 1991, 48(2):293-5.

References

Bohn D, Kalloghlian A, Jenkins J, et al, "Intravenous Salbutamol in the Treatment of Status Asthmaticus in Children," *Crit Care Med*, 1984, 12(10):892-6.

Canny GJ and Levison H, "Aerosols - Therapeutic Use and Delivery in Childhood Asthma," *Ann Allergy*, 1988, 60(1):11-9.

Expert Panel Report 2, "Guidelines for the Diagnosis and Management of Asthma," *Clinical Practice Guidelines*, National Institutes of Health, National Heart, Lung, and Blood Institute, NIH Publication No. 94-4051, April, 1997.

Fuglsang G, Pedersen S, and Borgstrom L, "Dose-Response Relationships of I.V. Administered Terbutaline in Children With Asthma," *J Pediatr*, 1989, 114(2):315-20.

Goldenhersh N and Rachelefsky GS, "Childhood Asthma: Management," *Pediatr Rev*, 1989, 10(9):259-67.

"Guidelines for the Diagnosis and Management of Asthma. NAEPP Expert Panel Report 3," August 2007, www.nhlbi.nih.gov/guidelines/asthma/asthgdln.pdf.

National Asthma Education and Prevention Program (NAEPP), "Expert Panel Report 3 (EPR-3): Guidelines for the Diagnosis and Management of Asthma," *Clinical Practice Guidelines*, National Institutes of Health, National Heart, Lung, and Blood Institute, NIH Publication No. 08-4051, prepublication 2007; available at http://www.nhlbi.nih.gov/guidelines/asthma/asthgdln.htm.

Rachelefsky GS and Siegel SC, "Asthma in Infants and Children - Treatment of Childhood Asthma: Part II," *J Allergy Clin Immunol*, 1985, 76(3):409-25.

Tipton WR and Nelson HS, "Frequent Parenteral Terbutaline in the Treatment of Status Asthmaticus in Children," *Ann Allergy*, 1987, 58 (4):252-6.

◆ **Terfluzine (Can)** *see* Trifluoperazine *on page 1382*

◆ **Tersi** *see* Selenium Sulfide *on page 1252*

◆ **TESPA** *see* Thiotepa *on page 1342*

◆ **Testim®** *see* Testosterone *on page 1325*

◆ **Testopel®** *see* Testosterone *on page 1325*

Testosterone (tes TOS ter one)

Medication Safety Issues

Sound-alike/look-alike issues:

Testosterone may be confused with testolactone

Testoderm® may be confused with Estraderm®

Transdermal patch may contain conducting metal (eg, aluminum); remove patch prior to MRI.

U.S. Brand Names Androderm®; AndroGel®; Delatestryl®; Depo®-Testosterone; First®-Testosterone; First®-Testosterone MC; Striant®; Testim®; Testopel®

Canadian Brand Names Andriol®; Androderm®; AndroGel®; Andropository; Delatestryl®; Depotest® 100; Everone® 200; PMS-Testosterone; Testim®

Therapeutic Category Androgen

Generic Available Yes: Injection

Use Testosterone replacement therapy in males for conditions associated with a deficiency or absence of endogenous testosterone; primary hypogonadism (congenital or acquired) and hypogonadotropic hypogonadism (congenital or acquired) (FDA approved in adults)

Restrictions C-III

Medication Guide An FDA-approved patient medication guide, which is available with the product and as follows, must be dispensed with this medication for each new outpatient prescription and refill.

Androgel®: http://www.fda.gov/downloads/Drugs/Drug-Safety/UCM188474.pdf

Testim®: http://www.fda.gov/downloads/Drugs/DrugSafety/UCM188475.pdf

Pregnancy Risk Factor X

Pregnancy Considerations Testosterone may cause adverse effects, including masculinization of the female fetus, if used during pregnancy. Females who are or may become pregnant should also avoid skin-to-skin contact to areas where testosterone has been applied topically on another person.

Lactation Enters breast milk/contraindicated

Breast-Feeding Considerations High levels of endogenous maternal testosterone, such as those caused by certain ovarian cysts, suppress milk production. Maternal serum testosterone levels generally fall following pregnancy and return to normal once breast-feeding is stopped. The amount of testosterone present in breast milk or the effect to the nursing infant following maternal supplementation is not known. Some products are contraindicated while breast-feeding.

Contraindications Hypersensitivity to testosterone or any component including testosterone USP that is chemically synthesized from soy (see Warnings); severe renal, hepatic, or cardiac disease; male patients with prostatic or breast cancer, hypercalcemia, pregnancy; use in women

Warnings May accelerate bone maturation without producing compensating gain in linear growth; perform radiographic examination of the hand and wrist every 6 months to determine the rate of bone maturation (when using in prepubertal children). Depo®-Testosterone contains benzyl alcohol which may cause allergic reactions in susceptible individuals; large amounts of benzyl alcohol (≥99 mg/kg/day) have been associated with a potentially fatal toxicity ("gasping syndrome") in neonates; the "gasping syndrome" consists of metabolic acidosis, respiratory distress, gasping respirations, CNS dysfunction (including convulsions, intracranial hemorrhage), hypotension, and cardiovascular collapse; *in vitro* and animal studies have shown that benzoate, a metabolite of benzyl alcohol, displaces bilirubin from protein binding sites; avoid use of Depo®-Testosterone in neonates. Virilization in children has been reported following contact with unwashed or unclothed application sites of men using the topical gel **[U.S. Boxed Warning]**. Patients should strictly adhere to instructions for use in order to prevent secondary exposure. Virilization of female sexual partners has also been reported with male use of the topical gel. Symptoms of virilization generally regress following removal of exposure; however, some children did not fully return to age appropriate normal. Signs of inappropriate virilization in women or children following secondary exposure to testosterone gel should be brought to the attention of a healthcare provider. In the event that unwashed or unclothed skin comes in direct contact with testosterone gel following secondary exposure, wash with soap and water. Long-term therapy has been associated with serious hepatic adverse effects (hepatitis, hepatic neoplasms, cholestatic hepatitis, jaundice).

Precautions Use with caution in patients with hepatic, cardiac, or renal dysfunction; may decrease blood glucose and insulin requirements in diabetics; may cause fluid retention. Use with caution in patients with mild to moderate cardiovascular disease or other edematous conditions; use in hypogonadal men may potentiate sleep apnea especially those with risk factors such as obesity or chronic lung disease; use in men with benign prostatic

hyperplasia (BPH) may have worsening of BPH symptoms. Long-term effects on gum safety when using the buccal formulation are not available; instruct patients to regularly inspect gum region where buccal formulation has been applied

Adverse Reactions

Cardiovascular: Edema, flushing, hypertension, tachycardia

Central nervous system: Aggressive behavior, anxiety, excitation, headache, mental depression, nervousness, sleeplessness

Dermatologic: Acne, hirsutism, urticaria

Endocrine & metabolic: Breast pain, gynecomastia, hypercalcemia, hyperlipemia, hypoglycemia, hyponatremia, libido increased or decreased, serum cholesterol increased, virilization of children following secondary exposure to topical gel (advanced bone age, aggressive behavior, enlargement of clitoris requiring surgery, enlargement of penis, erections increased, libido increased, pubic hair development)

Gastrointestinal: Abdominal pain, diarrhea, nausea; bitter taste, gum edema, gum or mouth irritation or pain, taste perversion (buccal formulation)

Genitourinary: Bladder irritability, epididymitis, priapism

Hematologic: Leukopenia, polycythemia, suppression of clotting factors

Hepatic: Cholestatic hepatitis, hepatocellular carcinoma (high doses), liver function tests increased, peliosis hepatitis

Local: Inflammation and itching at injection site

Neuromuscular & skeletal: Myalgia

Respiratory: Sleep apnea

Drug Interactions

Metabolism/Transport Effects Substrate (minor) of CYP2B6, 2C9, 2C19, 3A4; **Inhibits** CYP3A4 (weak)

Avoid Concomitant Use There are no known interactions where it is recommended to avoid concomitant use.

Increased Effect/Toxicity

Testosterone may increase the levels/effects of: CycloSPORINE; CycloSPORINE (Systemic); Vitamin K Antagonists

Decreased Effect There are no known significant interactions involving a decrease in effect.

Stability Store at room temperature; protect from light; drug reservoirs for transdermals may burst due to excessive pressure or heat; do not store transdermal formulations outside of protective pouches

Mechanism of Action Principal endogenous androgen responsible for promoting the growth and development of the male sex organs and maintaining secondary sex characteristics in androgen-deficient males

Pharmacodynamics Duration: Based upon the route of administration and the specific testosterone ester used; the cypionate and enanthate esters have the longest duration, up to 2-4 weeks after I.M. administration; pellets 3-4 months; gel: 24-48 hours

Pharmacokinetics (Adult data unless noted)

Absorption: Transdermal gel: 10%

Protein binding: 98%

Metabolism: In the liver to various 17-keto steroids; major active metabolites are estradiol and dihydrotestosterone

Half-life: Cypionate: I.M.: 8 days

Time to peak serum concentration: Buccal: 10-12 hours

Elimination: 90% excreted in urine as metabolites, 6% unconjugated in the feces

Usual Dosage

Children: I.M.:

Male hypogonadism: Testosterone cypionate or enanthate: Dosage and duration of therapy depends upon age, sex, diagnosis, patient's response to therapy, and appearance of adverse effects; in general total doses

>400 mg/month are not required due to the prolonged action of the drug

Initiation of pubertal growth: 40-50 mg/m^2/dose monthly until the growth rate falls to prepubertal levels

Terminal growth phase: 100 mg/m^2/dose monthly until growth ceases

Maintenance virilizing dose: 100 mg/m^2/dose twice monthly

Delayed puberty: 40-50 mg/m^2/dose monthly for 6 months or per manufacturer: 50-200 mg every 2-4 weeks

Adults: Hypogonadism:

Buccal (Striant™): Apply one mucoadhesive dose (30 mg) twice daily every 12 hours in the morning and evening

Testosterone cypionate or enanthate: I.M.: 50-400 mg every 2-4 weeks

Transdermal: Androderm®: 5 mg/day initially (as one 5 mg or two 2.5 mg systems applied at night); adjust dosage in 3-4 weeks depending upon testosterone concentration to a maximum of 7.5 mg/day

Testosterone pellets: SubQ: Dosage depends on the minimum daily requirements of testosterone propionate [each 25 mg testosterone propionate weekly equals 150 mg (2 pellets)]; usual dose (testosterone pellets): 150-450 mg (2-6 pellets) every 3 months

AndroGel®, Testim®: Transdermal gel: Males >18 years: Initial: 5 g of gel (contains 50 mg testosterone) applied once daily (preferably in the morning); may increase as needed to a maximum of 10 g once daily

Adults: Postpubertal cryptorchism: Testosterone or testosterone propionate: I.M.: 10-25 mg 2-3 times/week

Administration

Buccal: Striant™: One mucoadhesive for buccal application (buccal system) should be applied to a comfortable area above the incisor tooth. Apply flat side of system to gum. Rotate to alternate sides of mouth with each application. Hold buccal system firmly in place for 30 seconds to ensure adhesion. The buccal system should adhere to gum for 12 hours. If the buccal system falls out, replace with a new system. If the system falls out within 4 hours of next dose, the new buccal system should remain in place until the time of the following scheduled dose. System will soften and mold to shape of gum as it absorbs moisture from mouth. Do not chew or swallow the buccal system; check to ensure buccal system is in place following toothbrushing, use of mouthwash, and consumption of food or beverages. The buccal system will not dissolve; gently remove by sliding downwards from gum; avoid scratching gum.

Parenteral: Administer deep I.M.; not for I.V. administration; pellets only are for SubQ administration

Topical:

Androderm®: The adhesive side of system should be applied to clean, dry area of the skin on the back, abdomen, upper arms or thighs at night; avoid application over boney prominences or on a part of the body that may be subject to prolonged pressure; **do not apply to the scrotum**; rotate sites every 7 days

AndroGel®: Apply AndroGel® to clean, dry, intact skin of the shoulder and upper arms and/or abdomen. Upon opening the packet(s), the entire contents should be squeezed into the palm of the hand and immediately applied to the application site(s). Area of application should be limited to what will be covered by a short sleeve t-shirt. Application sites should be allowed to dry for a few minutes prior to dressing. Hands should be washed with soap and water after application. Wait at least 1 hour, preferably 5-6 hours, after application before showering or swimming. **Do not apply Andro-Gel® to the genitals.** Strict adherence to application instructions is needed in order to decrease secondary exposure. Secondary exposure has also been reported

following exposure to secondary items (eg, towel, shirt, sheets). If secondary exposure occurs, the other person should thoroughly wash the skin with soap and water as soon as possible.

Androgel® metered dose pump: Apply topically as described for Androgel®; each actuation delivers 1.25 g of gel (4 actuations = 5 g; 6 actuations = 7.5 g; 8 actuations = 10 g); pump must be primed prior to initial use by fully depressing pump mechanism 3 times and discarding any portion delivered; each actuation may be applied individually or all at the same time.

Testim®: Apply (preferably in the morning) to clean, dry, intact skin of the shoulder and upper arms; do not apply to abdomen. Area of application should be limited to what will be covered by a short sleeve t-shirt. Upon opening the packet(s), the entire contents should be squeezed into the palm of the hand and immediately applied to the application site(s). Application sites should be allowed to dry for a few minutes prior to dressing. Hands should be washed with soap and water after application. Application site should not be washed for ≥2 hours following application of Testim®. Strict adherence to application instructions is needed in order to decrease secondary exposure. Secondary exposure has also been reported following exposure to secondary items (eg, towel, shirt, sheets). If secondary exposure occurs, the other person should thoroughly wash the skin with soap and water as soon as possible.

Monitoring Parameters Periodic liver function tests, radiologic examination of wrist and hand every 6 months (when using in prepubertal children); hemoglobin, hematocrit, serum electrolytes, HDL cholesterol, prostate-specific antigen (PSA); testosterone concentration; (when using buccal formulation, measure testosterone concentration prior to morning dose and when using the transdermal formulation, in the morning following application the night before), measure testosterone concentration 4-12 weeks after initiating treatment

Reference Range Normal physiologic: Male:
Testosterone, urine: 100-1500 ng/24 hours
Testosterone, serum: 300-1050 ng/dL

Patient Information See Administration. Notify healthcare provider if penile erections are too frequent or prolonged, if nausea, vomiting, yellow skin (jaundice), ankle swelling, or breathing problems develop and in particular if sleeping or difficulty with urination occurs; if using buccal formulation, regularly inspect gum region where it is applied; gum irritation or tenderness should resolve in 1-14 days; notify healthcare provider if persists beyond this time

Nursing Implications 0.1% triamcinolone cream may be applied to skin under Androderm® to decrease irritation; do not use ointment formulations for pretreatment; they may significantly reduce testosterone absorption

Additional Information Testosterone 5% cream, not available commercially (must be compounded), has been effective in the treatment of microphallus when applied topically for 21 days

Dosage Forms Excipient information presented when available (limited, particularly for generics); consult specific product labeling. [CAN] = Canadian brand name

Capsule, gelatin, as undecanoate:
Andriol™ [CAN]: 40 mg (10s) [not available in U.S.]

Gel, topical:
AndroGel®: 1% [1.25 g gel/actuation] (75 g) [contains ethanol 67%; may be chemically synthesized for soy]
AndroGel®: 1% [2.5 g gel/packet] (30s) [contains ethanol 67%; may be chemically synthesized from soy]
AndroGel®: 1% [5 g gel/packet] (30s) [contains ethanol 67%; may be chemically synthesized from soy]
Testim®: 1% [5 g gel/tube] (30s) [contains ethanol 74%; may be chemically synthesized from soy]

Implant, subcutaneous:
Testopel®: 75 mg (10s, 100s)

Injection, in oil, as cypionate: 100 mg/mL (10 mL); 200 mg/mL (1 mL, 10 mL)
Depo®-Testosterone: 100 mg/mL (10 mL); 200 mg/mL (1 mL, 10 mL) [contains benzyl alcohol, benzyl benzoate, and cottonseed oil]
Injection, in oil, as enanthate: 200 mg/mL (5 mL)
Delatestryl®: 200 mg/mL (1 mL, 5 mL) [contains sesame oil]
Kit [for prescription compounding; testosterone 2%]:
First®-Testosterone:
Injection, in oil: Testosterone propionate 100 mg/mL (12 mL) [contains sesame oil and benzyl alcohol]
Ointment: White petrolatum (48 g)
First®-Testosterone MC:
Injection, in oil: Testosterone propionate 100 mg/mL (12 mL) [contains sesame oil and benzyl alcohol]
Cream: Moisturizing cream (48 g)
Mucoadhesive, for buccal application [buccal system]:
Striant®: 30 mg (10s) [may be chemically synthesized from soy]
Patch, transdermal:
Androderm®: 2.5 mg/day (60s) [contains ethanol]; 5 mg/day (30s) [contains ethanol]

◆ **Testosterone Cypionate** see Testosterone on page 1325

◆ **Testosterone Enanthate** see Testosterone on page 1325

◆ **Tetanus and Diphtheria Toxoid** see Diphtheria and Tetanus Toxoid on page 452

Tetanus Immune Globulin (Human)
(TET a nus i MYUN GLOB yoo lin HYU man)

Related Information
Immunization Guidelines on page 1636
U.S. Brand Names HyperTET™ S/D
Canadian Brand Names HyperTET™ S/D
Therapeutic Category Immune Globulin
Generic Available No
Use Prophylaxis for tetanus following injury in patients whose immunization for tetanus is incomplete or uncertain
Pregnancy Risk Factor C
Pregnancy Considerations Animal reproduction studies have not been conducted. Tetanus immune globulin and a tetanus toxoid containing vaccine are recommended by the ACIP as part of the standard wound management to prevent tetanus in pregnant women.
Contraindications Hypersensitivity to tetanus immune globulin, thimerosal, or any component
Warnings As a product of human plasma, this product may potentially transmit infectious agents such as viruses; screening of donors, as well as testing and/or inactivation of certain viruses has reduced this risk. Although extremely rare, severe hypersensitivity reactions including anaphylaxis may occur; epinephrine and other anaphylactic treatment agents should be readily available. Not for I.V. administration; serious systemic reactions including hypotension have occurred with inadvertent I.V. administration
Precautions Administer with caution to patients with thrombocytopenia or any coagulation disorder that would be compromised by I.M. injection; administer with caution in patients with IgA deficiency or a prior history of systemic allergic reactions following the administration of human immunoglobulin preparations.
Adverse Reactions
Central nervous system: Fever (mild)
Dermatologic: Urticaria, angioedema
Local: Pain, tenderness, erythema at injection site
Neuromuscular & skeletal: Muscle stiffness
Renal: Nephrotic syndrome (rare)
Miscellaneous: Anaphylaxis reaction (rare)

Drug Interactions
Avoid Concomitant Use There are no known interactions where it is recommended to avoid concomitant use.
Increased Effect/Toxicity There are no known significant interactions involving an increase in effect.
Decreased Effect
Tetanus Immune Globulin (Human) may decrease the levels/effects of: Vaccines (Live)
Stability Refrigerate; do not freeze
Mechanism of Action Passive immunity toward tetanus
Pharmacodynamics
A single dose may provide protection for up to 14 weeks
Pharmacokinetics (Adult data unless noted)
Absorption: Well absorbed
Time to peak serum concentration: 2 days
Usual Dosage I.M.:
Prophylaxis of tetanus:
Children <7 years: 4 units/kg as a single dose; some experts recommend administering 250 units regardless of weight or age
Children ≥7 years and Adults: 250 units as a single dose; may be increased to 500 units if there has been a delay in initiating prophylaxis or when the wound is considered very tetanus prone
Note: Additional doses of TIG can be given at 4-week intervals in situations where the risk of tetanus infection persists.
Treatment of tetanus:
Neonates: 500 units
Children and Adults: 3000-6000 units

Tetanus Immune Globulin (TIG) and/or Tetanus Toxoid (Td) Wound Management				
Number of Prior Tetanus Toxoid Doses	Clean, Minor Wounds		All Other Wounds	
	DT or Td[1]	TIG[2]	DT or Td[1]	TIG[2]
Unknown or <3	Yes	No	Yes	Yes
≥3[3]	No[4]	No	No[5]	No

[1] Use of combined antigen immunization (DT, Td, or DTaP) is preferred. Use tetanus and diphtheria toxoids formulation based upon age; use pediatric preparations (DT or DTaP) if the patient is <7 years old and Td if ≥7 years

[2] Tetanus immune globulin.

[3] If only three doses of fluid tetanus toxoid have been received, a fourth dose of toxoid, preferably an adsorbed toxoid, should be given.

[4] Yes, if >10 years since last dose.

[5] Yes, if >5 years since last dose.

Adapted from Report of the Committee on Infectious Diseases, American Academy of Pediatrics, Elk Grove Village, IL: American Academy of Pediatrics, 1986.

Administration I.M.: Administer into lateral aspect of midthigh or deltoid muscle of upper arm; **not for I.V. administration.** When administered for treatment of tetanus, may be infiltrated locally around the wound site. Do not administer tetanus toxoid and TIG in same syringe (toxoid will be neutralized); tetanus toxoid may be administered at the same time at a separate site
Dosage Forms Excipient information presented when available (limited, particularly for generics); consult specific product labeling.
Injection, solution [preservative free]:
HyperTET™ S/D: 250 units/mL (1 mL) [prefilled syringe]

◆ **Tetanus Toxoid** see Diphtheria and Tetanus Toxoids, Acellular Pertussis, Poliovirus and *Haemophilus* b Conjugate Vaccine on page 455

Tetanus Toxoid (Adsorbed)
(TET a nus TOKS oyd, ad SORBED)

Medication Safety Issues
Sound-alike/look-alike issues:
Tetanus toxoid products may be confused with influenza virus vaccine and tuberculin products. Medication errors have occurred when tetanus toxoid products have been inadvertently administered instead of tuberculin skin tests (PPD) and influenza virus vaccine. These products are refrigerated and often stored in close proximity to each other.

Related Information
Immunization Guidelines *on page 1636*

Therapeutic Category Vaccine

Generic Available No

Use
Indicated as booster dose in the active immunization against tetanus in children >7 years or adults when combined antigen preparations are not indicated

Pregnancy Risk Factor C

Pregnancy Considerations
Animal studies have not been conducted. The ACIP recommends vaccination in previously unvaccinated women or in women with an incomplete vaccination series, whose child may be born in unhygienic conditions. Tetanus immune globulin and a tetanus toxoid-containing vaccine are recommended by the ACIP as part of the standard wound management to prevent tetanus in pregnant women. Vaccination using Td is preferred.

Lactation
Excretion in breast milk unknown/use caution

Contraindications
Hypersensitivity to tetanus toxoid or any component of the formulation

Warnings
Patients with a history of severe local reaction (Arthus-type) or temperature of >39.4°C (103°F) following a previous dose should not be given further routine or emergency doses of tetanus toxoid more frequently than every 10 years. Guillain-Barré syndrome occurring within 6 weeks of tetanus toxoid vaccination has been reported. Defer administration during moderate or severe illness (with or without fever). Immune response may be decreased in immunocompromised patients; may be used in patients with HIV infection. Contains thimerosal; vial stopper contains natural latex rubber. Safety and efficacy in children <6 weeks of age have not been established; this product is not indicated for use in children <7 years of age; see diphtheria, pertussis, and tetanus vaccine and diphtheria and tetanus vaccine

Precautions
Administer with caution to patients with thrombocytopenia or any coagulation disorder that would be compromised by an I.M. injection; if the patient receives antihemophilia or other similar therapy, I.M. injection can be scheduled shortly after such therapy is administered; immediate treatment for anaphylactoid or acute hypersensitivity reactions should be available during vaccine use. Routine prophylactic administration of acetaminophen to prevent fever due to vaccines has been shown to decrease the immune response of some vaccines; the clinical significance of this reduction in immune response has not been established (see Prymula, 2009).

Adverse Reactions All serious adverse reactions must be reported to the U.S. Department of Health and Human Services (DHHS) Vaccine Adverse Event Reporting System (VAERS) 1-800-822-7967.
Cardiovascular: Hypotension

Central nervous system: Brachial neuritis, fever, malaise

Dermatologic: Rash, urticaria

Gastrointestinal: Nausea

Local: Edema, induration (with or without tenderness), redness, warmth

Neuromuscular & skeletal: Arthralgia, Guillain-Barré syndrome, brachial neuritis

Miscellaneous: Anaphylaxis, Arthus-type hypersensitivity reactions (severe local reaction developing 2-8 hours following injection)

Drug Interactions
Avoid Concomitant Use There are no known interactions where it is recommended to avoid concomitant use.

Increased Effect/Toxicity There are no known significant interactions involving an increase in effect.

Decreased Effect
The levels/effects of Tetanus Toxoid (Adsorbed) may be decreased by: Immunosuppressants

Stability
Refrigerate 2°C to 8°C (35°F to 46°F). Do not freeze.

Mechanism of Action
Tetanus toxoid preparations contain the toxin produced by virulent tetanus bacilli (detoxified growth products of *Clostridium tetani*). The toxin has been modified by treatment with formaldehyde so that is has lost toxicity but still retains ability to act as antigen and produce active immunity.

Usual Dosage
Primary immunization: Not indicated for this use; combined antigen vaccines are recommended

Booster doses: I.M.: 0.5 mL every 10 years

Tetanus prophylaxis in wound management: Use of tetanus toxoid and/or tetanus immune globulin (TIG) depends upon the number of prior tetanus toxoid doses and type of wound: See table.

Tetanus Immune Globulin (TIG) and/or Tetanus Toxoid (Td) Wound Management

Number of Prior Tetanus Toxoid Doses	Clean, Minor Wounds		All Other Wounds	
	DT or Td[1]	TIG[2]	DT or Td[1]	TIG[2]
Unknown or <3	Yes	No	Yes	Yes
≥3[3]	No[4]	No	No[5]	No

[1]Use of combined antigen immunization (DT, Td, or DTaP) is preferred. Use tetanus and diphtheria toxoids formulation based upon age; use pediatric preparations (DT or DTaP) if the patient is <7 years old and Td if ≥7 years

[2]Tetanus immune globulin.

[3]If only three doses of fluid tetanus toxoid have been received, a fourth dose of toxoid, preferably an adsorbed toxoid, should be given.

[4]Yes, if >10 years since last dose.

[5]Yes, if >5 years since last dose.

Adapted from Report of the Committee on Infectious Diseases, American Academy of Pediatrics, Elk Grove Village, IL: American Academy of Pediatrics, 1986.

Administration
I.M. Shake well prior to use. Administer into lateral aspect of midthigh or deltoid muscle of upper arm; **not for I.V. or SubQ administration**

Patient Information
May experience mild fever or soreness, swelling, and redness/knot at the injection site usually lasting 1-2 days

Nursing Implications
Federal law requires that the date of administration, the vaccine manufacturer, lot number of vaccine, and the administering person's name, title, and address be entered into the patient's permanent medical record.

Additional Information
In order to maximize vaccination rates, the ACIP recommends simultaneous administration of all age-appropriate vaccines (live or inactivated) for which a person is eligible at a single visit, unless contraindications exist. The use of combination vaccines is generally preferred over separate infections, taking into consideration provider assessment, patient preference, and potential adverse events.

For additional information, please refer to the following website: http://www.cdc.gov/vaccines/vpd-vac/.

Dosage Forms Excipient information presented when available (limited, particularly for generics); consult specific product labeling.

Injection, suspension: Tetanus 5 Lf units per 0.5 mL (0.5 mL) [contains trace amounts of thimerosal]

References

American Academy of Pediatrics Committee on Infectious Diseases, "Recommended Childhood and Adolescent Immunization Schedule – United States, January-June 2004," *Pediatrics*, 2004, 113(1 Pt 1):142-3.

Atkinson WL, Pickering LK, Schwartz B, et al, "General Recommendations on Immunization. Recommendations of the Advisory Committee on Immunization Practices (ACIP) and the American Academy of Family Physicians (AAFP)," *MMWR Recomm Rep*, 2002, 51(RR-2):18.

Centers for Disease Control and Prevention (CDC), "General Recommendations on Immunization. Recommendations of the Advisory Committee on Immunization Practices (ACIP)," *MMWR Recomm Rep*, 2006, 55(RR-15):1-48. Available at: http://www.cdc.gov/mmwr/preview/mmwrhtml/rr5515a1.htm.

Prymula R, Siegrist CA, Chlibek R, et al, "Effect of Prophylactic Paracetamol Administration at Time of Vaccination on Febrile Reactions and Antibody Responses in Children: Two Open-Label, Randomised Controlled Trials," *Lancet*, 2009, 374(9698):1339-50.

◆ **Tetanus Toxoid Plain** *see* Tetanus Toxoid (Adsorbed) *on page 1329*

◆ **Tetanus Toxoid, Reduced Diphtheria Toxoid, and Acellular Pertussis, Adsorbed** *see* Diphtheria, Tetanus Toxoids, and Acellular Pertussis Vaccine *on page 458*

Tetracaine (TET ra kane)

U.S. Brand Names Pontocaine® Niphanoid®; Pontocaine® [DSC]

Canadian Brand Names Ametop™; Pontocaine®

Therapeutic Category Analgesic, Topical; Local Anesthetic, Injectable; Local Anesthetic, Ophthalmic; Local Anesthetic, Oral; Local Anesthetic, Topical

Generic Available Yes: Ophthalmic solution, solution for injection

Use Local anesthesia in the eye for various diagnostic and examination purposes; spinal anesthesia; local anesthesia for mucous membranes

Pregnancy Risk Factor C

Pregnancy Considerations Animal reproduction studies have not been conducted.

Lactation Excretion in breast milk unknown/use caution

Contraindications Hypersensitivity to tetracaine or any component (see Warnings); patients with liver disease; CNS disease, meningitis (if used for epidural or spinal anesthesia); myasthenia gravis, impaired cardiac conduction; eye infection (ophthalmic) formulation

Warnings Topical use prior to cosmetic procedures can result in high systemic levels and lead to toxic effects (eg, arrhythmias, seizures, coma, respiratory depression, and death), particularly when applied in large amounts to cover large areas and/or left on for long periods of time or used with materials, wraps, or dressings to cover the skin after anesthetic application. These practices may increase the degree of systemic absorption and should be avoided. The FDA is recommending consumers consult their healthcare provider for instructions on safe use prior to applying topical anesthetics for medical or cosmetic purposes. Use of products with the lowest amount of anesthetic with the least amount of application possible to relieve pain is also recommended.

Parenteral form may contain sulfites which may cause allergic reactions in susceptible individuals

Precautions Use with caution in patients with cardiac disease and hyperthyroidism

Adverse Reactions

Cardiovascular: Cardiac arrest, bradycardia, myocardial depression, cardiac arrhythmias, hypotension

Central nervous system: Anxiety, apprehension, nervousness, disorientation, seizures, drowsiness, unconsciousness

Dermatologic: Urticaria

Gastrointestinal: Nausea, vomiting

Local: Stinging, burning at injection site

Ocular: Lacrimation, photophobia, corneal epithelial erosion, keratitis, corneal opacification, miosis

Otic: Tinnitus

Respiratory: Respiratory arrest

Drug Interactions

Avoid Concomitant Use There are no known interactions where it is recommended to avoid concomitant use.

Increased Effect/Toxicity There are no known significant interactions involving an increase in effect.

Decreased Effect There are no known significant interactions involving a decrease in effect.

Mechanism of Action Blocks both the generation and conduction of sensory, motor, and autonomic nerve fibers by decreasing the neuronal membrane's permeability to sodium ions, which results in decreasing the rate of depolarization of the nerve membrane

Pharmacodynamics

Onset of action:

Ophthalmic instillation: Anesthetic effects occur within 60 seconds

Topical: Within 3 minutes when applied to mucous membranes

Duration: 1.5-3 hours

Pharmacokinetics (Adult data unless noted)

Metabolism: By the liver

Elimination: Metabolites are renally excreted

Usual Dosage

Children: Safety and efficacy have not been established

Adults:

Cream: Apply to affected area as needed

Injection: Dosage varies with the anesthetic procedure, the degree of anesthesia required, and the individual patient response; it is administered by subarachnoid injection for spinal anesthesia. High, medium, low, or saddle blocks use 0.2% or 0.3% solution. Prolonged effect (2-3 hours): Use 1% solution (a 1% solution should be diluted with an equal volume of CSF before administration)

Perineal anesthesia: 5 mg

Perineal and lower extremities: 10 mg

Anesthesia extending up to the costal margin: 15-20 mg

Low spinal anesthesia (saddle block): 2-5 mg

Ophthalmic: Solution: Instill 1-2 drops

Topical solution (mucous membranes): Apply 2% solution as needed; do not exceed 20 mg (1 mL) per application

Administration

Ophthalmic: Apply drops to conjunctiva of affected eye(s); avoid contact of bottle tip with skin or eye; finger pressure should be applied to lacrimal sac during and for 1-2 minutes after instillation to decrease risk of absorption and systemic reactions

Parenteral: Subarachnoid administration by experienced individuals only

Patient Information Do not touch or rub eye until anesthesia (if ophthalmic) has worn off

Nursing Implications Not for prolonged use topically

Dosage Forms Excipient information presented when available (limited, particularly for generics); consult specific product labeling. [DSC] = Discontinued product

Injection, powder for reconstitution, as hydrochloride [preservative free]:

Pontocaine® Niphanoid®: 20 mg

Injection, solution, as hydrochloride [preservative free]: 1% [10 mg/mL] (2 mL)

Pontocaine® [DSC]: 1% [10 mg/mL] (2 mL) [contains sodium bisulfite]

Solution, ophthalmic, as hydrochloride: 0.5% [5 mg/mL] (2 mL, 15 mL)

Solution, topical, as hydrochloride:
Pontocaine®: 2% [20 mg/mL] (30 mL, 118 mL) [for rhinolaryngology]

◆ **Tetracaine and Lidocaine** *see* Lidocaine and Tetracaine *on page 824*

◆ **Tetracaine Hydrochloride** *see* Tetracaine *on page 1330*

◆ **Tetracosactide** *see* Cosyntropin *on page 362*

Tetracycline (tet ra SYE kleen)

Medication Safety Issues
Sound-alike/look-alike issues:
Tetracycline may be confused with tetradecyl sulfate
Achromycin may be confused with actinomycin, Adriamycin PFS®

Related Information
Malaria *on page 1652*

Canadian Brand Names Apo-Tetra®; Nu-Tetra

Therapeutic Category Acne Products; Antibiotic, Ophthalmic; Antibiotic, Tetracycline Derivative; Antibiotic, Topical

Generic Available Yes: Capsule

Use
Children, Adolescents and Adults: Treatment of Rocky Mountain spotted fever caused by susceptible *Rickettsia* or brucellosis

Adolescents and Adults: Presumptive treatment of chlamydial infection in patients with gonorrhea

Children >8 years, Adolescents and Adults: Treatment of moderate to severe inflammatory acne vulgaris, Lyme disease, mycoplasmal disease or *Legionella*

Pregnancy Risk Factor D

Pregnancy Considerations Tetracyclines cross the placenta, enter fetal circulation, and may cause permanent discoloration of teeth if used during the second or third trimester. Maternal hepatic toxicity has been associated with the use of tetracycline during pregnancy, especially in patients with azotemia or pyelonephritis. Because use during pregnancy may cause fetal harm, tetracycline is classified as pregnancy category D.

Lactation Enters breast milk/not recommended (AAP rates "compatible")

Breast-Feeding Considerations Tetracyclines are excreted in breast milk. Tetracycline binds to calcium. The calcium in the maternal milk will decrease the amount of tetracycline absorbed by the breast-feeding infant. Because of this "negligible absorption by the neonate," the AAP considers tetracycline to be "usually compatible with breast-feeding." Nondose-related effects could include modification of bowel flora.

Contraindications Hypersensitivity to tetracycline or any component; pregnancy; children ≤8 years; use of tetracyclines during tooth development may cause permanent discoloration of the teeth, enamel hypoplasia and retardation of skeletal development and bone growth with risk being greatest for children <4 years and in those receiving high doses

Warnings Photosensitivity reaction may occur with this drug; avoid prolonged exposure to sunlight or tanning equipment; prolonged use may result in superinfection

Precautions Use with caution in patients with renal and liver impairment; dosage modification required in patients with renal impairment

Adverse Reactions
Central nervous system: Pseudotumor cerebri, fever
Dermatologic: Rash, exfoliative dermatitis, photosensitivity, angioedema, discoloration of nails

Gastrointestinal: Nausea, vomiting, diarrhea, stomatitis, glossitis, antibiotic-associated pseudomembranous colitis, esophagitis, oral candidiasis

Hematologic: Hemolytic anemia

Hepatic: Hepatotoxicity

Neuromuscular & skeletal: Injury to growing bones and teeth

Renal: Renal damage, Fanconi-like syndrome

Respiratory: Pulmonary infiltrates with eosinophilia

Miscellaneous: Hypersensitivity reactions, candidal superinfection

Drug Interactions
Metabolism/Transport Effects Substrate of CYP3A4 (major); **Inhibits** CYP3A4 (moderate)

Avoid Concomitant Use
Avoid concomitant use of Tetracycline with any of the following: BCG; Retinoic Acid Derivatives; Tolvaptan

Increased Effect/Toxicity
Tetracycline may increase the levels/effects of: Colchicine; CYP3A4 Substrates; Eplerenone; Everolimus; FentaNYL; Halofantrine; Neuromuscular-Blocking Agents; Pimecrolimus; Ranolazine; Retinoic Acid Derivatives; Salmeterol; Saxagliptin; Tolvaptan; Vitamin K Antagonists

Decreased Effect
Tetracycline may decrease the levels/effects of: Atovaquone; BCG; Penicillins; Typhoid Vaccine

The levels/effects of Tetracycline may be decreased by: Antacids; Bile Acid Sequestrants; Bismuth; Bismuth Subsalicylate; CYP3A4 Inducers (Strong); Deferasirox; Herbs (CYP3A4 Inducers); Iron Salts; Magnesium Salts; Quinapril; Sucralfate; Zinc Salts

Food Interactions Tetracyclines decrease absorption of magnesium, zinc, calcium, dairy products, iron, and amino acids; calcium, dairy products, iron supplements decrease tetracycline absorption

Stability Protect from light; outdated tetracyclines have caused a Fanconi-like syndrome

Mechanism of Action Inhibits bacterial protein synthesis by binding to the 30S and possibly the 50S ribosomal subunit(s) of susceptible bacteria preventing additions of amino acids to the growing peptide chain; may also cause alterations in the cytoplasmic membrane

Pharmacokinetics (Adult data unless noted)
Distribution: Widely distributed to most body fluids and tissues including ascitic, synovial and pleural fluids; bronchial secretions; appears in breast milk; poor penetration into CSF

Absorption:
Oral: 75%
I.M.: Poor, with less than 60% of dose absorbed

Protein binding: 30% to 60%

Half-life: 6-12 hours with normal renal function and is prolonged with renal impairment

Time to peak serum concentration: Within 2-4 hours

Elimination: Primary route is the kidney, with 60% of a dose excreted as unchanged drug in urine, small amounts appear in bile

Dialysis: Slightly dialyzable (5% to 20%)

Usual Dosage
Children >8 years: Oral: 25-50 mg/kg/day in divided doses every 6 hours; not to exceed 3 g/day

Adolescents and Adults:
Oral: 250-500 mg/dose every 6-12 hours
Topical: Ointment: Apply small amount of ointment to cleansed area 2-3 times daily

Dosing adjustment in renal impairment:
Cl_{cr} 50-80 mL/minute: Administer every 8-12 hours
Cl_{cr} 10-50 mL/minute: Administer every 12-24 hours
Cl_{cr} <10 mL/minute: Administer every 24 hours

Administration

Oral: Administer 1 hour before or 2 hours after meals with adequate amounts of fluid; avoid taking antacids, calcium, iron, dairy products, or milk formulas within 3 hours of tetracyclines

Topical: Small amount of ointment should be applied to cleansed affected area.

Monitoring Parameters Renal, hepatic, and hematologic function tests

Test Interactions False-negative urine glucose with Clinistix®

Patient Information May discolor nails. May cause photosensitivity reactions (eg, exposure to sunlight may cause severe sunburn, skin rash, redness, or itching); avoid exposure to sunlight and artificial light sources (sunlamps, tanning booth/bed); wear protective clothing, wide-brimmed hats, sunglasses, and lip sunscreen (SPF ≥15); use a sunscreen [broad-spectrum sunscreen or physical sunscreen (preferred) or sunblock with SPF ≥15]; contact physician if reaction occurs.

Dosage Forms Excipient information presented when available (limited, particularly for generics); consult specific product labeling.

Capsule, as hydrochloride: 250 mg, 500 mg

References

American Academy of Pediatrics. Committee on Drugs. "Requiem for Tetracyclines," *Pediatrics*, 1975, 55(1):142-3.

◆ **Tetracycline Hydrochloride** *see* Tetracycline *on page 1331*

◆ **Tetrahydrocannabinol** *see* Dronabinol *on page 482*

◆ **Teva-Atenolol (Can)** *see* Atenolol *on page 147*

◆ **Teva-Azathioprine (Can)** *see* AzaTHIOprine *on page 161*

◆ **Teva-Fosinopril (Can)** *see* Fosinopril *on page 627*

◆ **Teva-Gabapentin (Can)** *see* Gabapentin *on page 634*

◆ **Teva-Simvastatin (Can)** *see* Simvastatin *on page 1263*

◆ **Teva-Venlafaxine XR (Can)** *see* Venlafaxine *on page 1412*

◆ **Tev-Tropin®** *see* Somatropin *on page 1281*

◆ **Texacort®** *see* Hydrocortisone *on page 685*

◆ **TG** *see* Thioguanine *on page 1339*

◆ **6-TG (error-prone abbreviation)** *see* Thioguanine *on page 1339*

Thalidomide (tha LI doe mide)

Medication Safety Issues

Sound-alike/look-alike issues:

Thalidomide may be confused with flutamide, lenalidomide

Thalomid® may be confused with thiamine

High alert medication: The Institute for Safe Medication Practices (ISMP) includes this medication among its list of drugs which have a heightened risk of causing significant patient harm when used in error.

International issues:

Thalomid® may be confused with Thilomide® which is a brand name for Iodoxamide in Greece and Turkey

Related Information

Emetogenic Potential of Antineoplastic Agents *on page 1579*

U.S. Brand Names Thalomid®

Canadian Brand Names Thalomid®

Therapeutic Category Angiogenesis Inhibitor; Immunosuppressant Agent; Tumor Necrosis Factor (TNF) Blocking Agent

Generic Available No

Use Treatment of multiple myeloma in combination with dexamethasone; treatment and maintenance of cutaneous manifestations of erythema nodosum leprosum (ENL). Currently under investigation for use in children when other therapies have failed for treatment of Crohn's disease; chronic graft-versus-host disease (CGVHD); AIDS-related aphthous stomatitis; systemic-onset juvenile idiopathic arthritis (SOJIA); various malignancies.

Restrictions Thalidomide is only available for marketing through a special distribution program, "System for Thalidomide Education and Prescribing Safety" [S.T.E.P.S.® (888) 423-5436], which has been approved by the FDA. Prescribers and pharmacists must be registered with the program; patients (or legal guardians if patient <18 years of age) must be advised, agree to, and comply with program requirements. No more than a 4-week supply should be dispensed. Blister packs should be dispensed intact (do not repackage capsules). Prescriptions must be filled within 7 days. Subsequent prescriptions may be filled only if fewer than 7 days of therapy remain on the previous prescription. A new prescription is required for further dispensing (a telephone prescription may not be accepted).

Pregnancy Risk Factor X

Pregnancy Considerations [U.S. Boxed Warning]: Thalidomide is a known teratogen; effective contraception must be used for at least 4 weeks before initiating therapy, during therapy, and for 4 weeks following discontinuation of thalidomide for women of childbearing potential. Embryotoxic with limb defects noted from the 27th to 40th gestational day of exposure; all cases of phocomelia occur from the 27th to 42nd gestational day; fetal cardiac, gastrointestinal, bone, external ear, eye, and genitourinary tract abnormalities have also been described. Mortality at or shortly after birth has also been reported. Either abstinence or two forms of effective contraception must be used for at least 4 weeks before initiating therapy, during therapy, and for 4 weeks following discontinuation of thalidomide. A negative pregnancy test (sensitivity of at least 50 mIU/mL) within 24 hours prior to beginning therapy, weekly during the first 4 weeks, and every 4 weeks (every 2 weeks for women with irregular menstrual cycles) thereafter is required for women of childbearing potential. Males (even those vasectomized) must use a latex condom during any sexual contact with women of childbearing age. Risk to the fetus from semen of male patients is unknown. Thalidomide must be immediately discontinued and the patient referred to a reproductive toxicity specialist if pregnancy occurs during treatment. Any suspected fetal exposure to thalidomide must be reported to the FDA via the MedWatch program (1-800-FDA-1088) and to Celgene Corporation (1-888-423-5436).

Lactation Excretion in breast milk unknown/not recommended

Breast-Feeding Considerations Due to the potential for serious adverse reactions in the infant, a decision should be made to discontinue nursing or discontinue treatment with thalidomide.

Contraindications Hypersensitivity to thalidomide or any component; pregnancy; women of childbearing potential, unless alternative therapies are inappropriate and adequate precautions are taken to avoid pregnancy; patients unable to comply with S.T.E.P.S.® program (including males)

Warnings Hazardous agent; use appropriate precautions for handling and disposal. Thalidomide is a known teratogen, even following a single dose **[U.S. Boxed Warning]**; embryotoxic with limb defects noted from the 27th to 40th gestational day of exposure; all cases of phocomelia occur from the 27th to 42nd gestational day; fetal cardiac, gastrointestinal, bone, external ear, eye, and genitourinary tract abnormalities have also been described. Mortality at or shortly after birth has also been reported. Two reliable forms of contraception or abstinence must be used for at least 4 weeks before initiating therapy, during therapy, and for 4 weeks following discontinuation of thalidomide for women of childbearing potential. A negative pregnancy test (sensitivity of at least 50 mIU/mL) within 24 hours prior to beginning therapy, weekly during the first 4 weeks, and every 4 weeks (every 2 weeks for women with irregular menstrual cycles) thereafter is required. Males (even those vasectomized) must use a latex condom during any sexual contact with women of childbearing age. Risk to the fetus from semen of male patients is unknown. Thalidomide must be immediately discontinued and the patient referred to a reproductive toxicity specialist if pregnancy occurs during treatment. Any suspected fetal exposure to thalidomide must be reported to the FDA via the MedWatch program (800) FDA-1088 and to Celgene Corporation (888) 423-5436.

Use in multiple myeloma patients results in an increased risk of thrombotic events such as deep vein thrombosis and pulmonary embolism **[U.S. Boxed Warning]**. Risk significantly increases when used in combination with standard chemotherapeutic agents, including dexamethasone. Monitor for signs and symptoms of thromboembolism; some patients at risk may benefit from prophylactic anticoagulation or aspirin therapy.

Frequently causes drowsiness and somnolence. Patients must be cautioned about performing tasks which require mental alertness (eg, operating machinery or driving). May cause peripheral neuropathy which may be irreversible; usually associated with chronic use, but has been seen following short-term therapy; no correlation with cumulative dose identified in adults. In children, significant correlations with cumulative dose (>20 g) and duration of therapy (>10 months) have been reported (Priolo, 2008). Patients should be monitored for signs and symptoms of peripheral neuropathy; consider immediate discontinuation (if clinically appropriate) in patients who develop neuropathy.

May cause dizziness and orthostatic hypotension. May cause neutropenia; discontinue therapy if absolute neutrophil count decreases to <750/mm^3. Increase HIV viral load has been reported in clinical trials; clinical significance is unknown.

Precautions Hypersensitivity reactions, Stevens-Johnson syndrome (SJS), and toxic epidermal necrolysis (TEN) have been reported; withhold therapy and evaluate skin rashes; permanently discontinue if rash is exfoliative, purpuric, bullous, or if SJS or TEN is suspected. May cause bradycardia; in some cases, medical intervention may be required; use with caution in patients with cardiovascular disease. May cause seizures; use with caution in patients with a history of seizures, concurrent therapy with drugs which alter seizure threshold, or conditions which predispose to seizures.

Adverse Reactions

Cardiovascular: Bradycardia, edema, hypotension, thrombosis/embolism

Central nervous system: Anxiety/agitation, confusion, dizziness, fatigue, fever, headache, insomnia, malaise, motor neuropathy, nervousness, pain, seizures, sensory neuropathy, somnolence, vertigo

Dermatologic: Acne, dry skin, fungal dermatitis, maculopapular rash, nail disorder, pruritus, rash, Stevens-Johnson syndrome, toxic epidermal necrolysis

Endocrine & metabolic: Hyperlipemia, hypocalcemia, weight gain, weight loss

Gastrointestinal: Anorexia, constipation, diarrhea, flatulence, nausea, oral moniliasis, tooth pain, xerostomia

Hematologic: Anemia, leukopenia, lymphadenopathy, neutropenia

Hepatic: AST elevated, bilirubin elevated

Neuromuscular & skeletal: Arthralgia, back pain, muscle weakness, myalgia, neck pain, neck rigidity, paresthesia, peripheral neuropathy, tremor, weakness

Renal: Albuminuria, hematuria

Respiratory: Dyspnea, pharyngitis, pulmonary embolus, rhinitis, sinusitis

Miscellaneous: Diaphoresis, hypersensitivity reactions, infection

Drug Interactions

Avoid Concomitant Use

Avoid concomitant use of Thalidomide with any of the following: Abatacept; Anakinra; BCG; Canakinumab; Certolizumab Pegol; Natalizumab; Pimecrolimus; Rilonacept; Tacrolimus (Topical); Vaccines (Live)

Increased Effect/Toxicity

Thalidomide may increase the levels/effects of: Abatacept; Alcohol (Ethyl); Anakinra; Canakinumab; Certolizumab Pegol; CNS Depressants; Leflunomide; Methotrimeprazine; Natalizumab; Pamidronate; Rilonacept; Vaccines (Live); Zoledronic Acid

The levels/effects of Thalidomide may be increased by: Denosumab; Dexamethasone; Dexamethasone (Systemic); Methotrimeprazine; Pimecrolimus; Tacrolimus (Topical); Trastuzumab

Decreased Effect

Thalidomide may decrease the levels/effects of: BCG; Sipuleucel-T; Vaccines (Inactivated); Vaccines (Live)

The levels/effects of Thalidomide may be decreased by: Echinacea

Stability Store at 15°C to 30°C (50°F to 86°F). Protect from light. Keep in original package.

Mechanism of Action The exact mechanism of action is unknown. Thalidomide has immunomodulatory, anti-inflammatory, and antiangiogenic characteristics; may suppress excessive tumor necrosis factor-alpha production in patients with ENL, yet may increase plasma tumor necrosis factor-alpha levels in HIV-positive patients. In multiple myeloma, thalidomide is associated with an increase in natural killer cells and increased levels of interleukin-2 and interferon gamma. Other proposed mechanisms of action include suppression of angiogenesis, prevention of free-radical-mediated DNA damage, increased cell mediated cytotoxic effects, and altered expression of cellular.

Pharmacokinetics (Adult data unless noted)

Distribution: Adults: V_d: 70-120 L

Protein binding: 55% to 66%

Metabolism: Nonenzymatic hydrolysis in plasma; forms multiple metabolites

Half-life elimination: Adults: 5-7 hours

Time to peak, plasma: 3-6 hours

Excretion: Urine (<1% as unchanged drug)

Usual Dosage Oral:

Children and Adolescents (information based on small clinical trials):

Chronic graft-vs-host disease (CGVHD): Children ≥2 years: Initial 3-6 mg/kg/day divided into 2 or 4 doses before meals; may be adjusted every 2 weeks based on patient response (Browne, 2000; Rovelli, 1998; Vogelsang, 1992).

Data based on clinical trials:

(Vogelsang, 1992): n=23, age: 3-50 years, median: 28 years; dose adjusted to goal thalidomide concentration of 5 mcg/mL 2 hours postdose, 30% of patients with refractory CGVHD showed complete response and 47% showed partial; in patients with high-risk GVHD, 33% of patients had complete response

(Rovell, 1998): n=14, age: 2-19 years, showed partial or complete response in 10 of 14 patients

(Browne, 2000): n=37, age: 2-47 years, n=21 of <18 years, 46% of children in study population responded, and of all partial responders 77% were children.

Crohn's disease/ulcerative colitis: Children ≥1 year: 1.5-2 mg/kg/day, usually dosed once daily in the evening

Data based on clinical trials:

(Lazzerini, 2007): n=28, age: 2-20 years, 75% of patients achieved remission

(Martelossi, 2004): n=23, age: 1-17 years, 78% response rate

(Facchini, 2001): n=5, age: 14-22 years, 4 of 5 patients had clinical response and achieved remission, fifth patient stopped therapy after one week

Systemic-onset juvenile idiopathic arthritis: Children ≥3 years: Initial 2 mg/kg/day, if necessary may increase at 2-week intervals to 3-5 mg/kg/day; all doses should be rounded to nearest 50 mg increment. Data based on a multicenter, open-labeled prospective study (n=13, age: 3-23 years); within 4 weeks, 11 of 13 patients showed improvement in JRA scores, significant decreases in ESR, and significant increase in hemoglobin (Lehman, 2004).

Cutaneous erythema nodosum leprosum (ENL): Adolescents ≥12 years: Initial: 100-300 mg once daily at bedtime (400 mg/day in severe cases); for patients <50 kg, initiate at lower end of dosage range. Maintenance: Continue initial dose until active reaction subsides then taper in 50 mg decrements every 2-4 weeks. If used for severe cutaneous reaction or in patients who had previously required a high dose for treatment, may initiate at 400 mg/day; doses may be divided and taken 1 hour after meals. Patients who flare during tapering or with a history of requiring prolonged maintenance should be maintained on the minimum dosage necessary to control the reaction. Efforts to taper should be repeated every 3-6 months, in increments of 50 mg every 2-4 weeks.

AIDS-related aphthous stomatitis: Adolescents ≥13 years: 200 mg once daily at bedtime for 4 weeks or sooner if resolution. May be increased to 200 mg twice daily if no improvement after 4 weeks (Jacobson, 1997). Data based on double-blind, placebo-controlled trial by AIDS Clinical Trials Group (n=57, age: ≥13 years) which showed 55% healing in treatment group vs 7% in placebo (Jacobson, 1997).

Adults:

Multiple myeloma: 200 mg once daily (with dexamethasone 40 mg daily on days 1-4, 9-12, and 17-20 of a 28-day treatment cycle)

Cutaneous erythema nodosum leprosum (ENL): Initial: 100-300 mg once daily at bedtime (400 mg/day in severe cases); for patients <50 kg, initiate at lower end of dosage range. Maintenance: Continue initial dose until active reaction subsides then taper in 50 mg decrements every 2-4 weeks. If severe cutaneous reaction or in patients who had previously required a high dose for treatment, may initiate at 400 mg/day; doses may be divided, and taken 1 hour after meals. Patients who flare during tapering or with a history of requiring prolonged maintenance should be maintained on the minimum dosage necessary to control the reaction. Efforts to taper should be repeated every 3-6 months, in increments of 50 mg every 2-4 weeks.

Behçet's syndrome: 100-400 mg/day

Graft-vs-host reactions: 100-1600 mg/day; usual initial dose: 200 mg 4 times/day for use up to 700 days

AIDS-related aphthous stomatitis: 200 mg twice daily for 5 days, then 200 mg/day for up to 8 weeks

Discoid lupus erythematosus: 100-400 mg/day; maintenance dose: 25-50 mg

Administration Administer with water, preferably at bedtime, once daily on an empty stomach, at least 1 hour after the evening meal. Doses >400 mg/day may be given in 2-3 divided doses. Avoid extensive handling of capsules; capsules should remain in blister pack until ingestion. If exposed to the powder content from broken capsules or body fluids from patients receiving thalidomide, the exposed area should be washed with soap and water.

Monitoring Parameters Pregnancy testing (sensitivity of at least 50 mIU/mL) is required within 24 hours prior to initiation of therapy, weekly during the first 4 weeks, then every 4 weeks in women with regular menstrual cycles or every 2 weeks in women with irregular menstrual cycles. Signs of neuropathy monthly for the first 3 months, then periodically during treatment; consider monitoring of sensory nerve application potential amplitudes (at baseline and every 6 months) to detect asymptomatic neuropathy. In HIV-seropositive patients: Viral load after 1 and 3 months, then every 3 months.

Reference Range One study suggests that therapeutic plasma thalidomide concentrations in graft-vs-host reactions are 5-8 mcg/mL 2 hours postdose (Vogelsang, 1992).

Patient Information Birth defects may occur; oral and written instructions about the necessity of using two methods of contraception and the necessity of keeping return visits for pregnancy testing will be provided. Do not donate blood or sperm (male patients) while taking this medicine. Avoid extensive handling of capsules; capsules should remain in blister pack until ingestion. If exposed to the powder content from broken capsules or body fluids from patients receiving thalidomide, the exposed area should be washed with soap and water. Avoid alcohol. May experience sleepiness; dizziness; fatigue; fever; headaches; lack of concentration (use caution when driving, climbing stairs, or engaging in tasks requiring alertness until response to drug is known); nausea or vomiting; constipation or diarrhea; or dry mouth. Report any of the above if persistent or severe. Report chest pain or palpitations or swelling of extremities; respiratory difficulty; back, neck, muscle pain, muscle weakness, or stiffness; numbness or pain in extremities; significant weight loss or gain; skin rash or eruptions; increased nervousness, anxiety, confusion, or insomnia; or any other symptom of adverse reactions.

Additional Information Thalidomide-associated birth defects have only been reported as a result of direct oral ingestion of drug; data is not available regarding cutaneous absorption or inhalation exposures and whether these exposures may result in birth defects.

Dosage Forms Excipient information presented when available (limited, particularly for generics); consult specific product labeling.

Capsule:

Thalomid®: 50 mg, 100 mg, 150 mg, 200 mg

References

Bessmertniy O and Pham T, "Thalidomide Use in Pediatric Patients," *Ann Pharmacother*, 2002, 36(3):521-5.

Britton WJ and Lockwood DN, "Leprosy," *Lancet*, 2004, 363 (9416):1209-19.

Browne PV, Weisdorf DJ, DeFor T, et al, "Response to Thalidomide Therapy in Refractory Chronic Graft-Versus-Host Disease," *Bone Marrow Transplant*, 2000, 26(8):865-9.

Facchini S, Candusso M, Martelossi S, et al, "Efficacy of Long-Term Treatment With Thalidomide in Children and Young Adults With Crohn Disease: Preliminary Results," *J Pediatr Gastroenterol Nutr*, 2001, 32 (2):178-81.

Jacobson JM, Greenspan JS, Spritzler J, et al, "Thalidomide for the Treatment of Oral Aphthous Ulcers in Patients With Human Immunodeficiency Virus Infection. National Institute of Allergy and Infectious Diseases AIDS Clinical Trials Group," *N Engl J Med*, 1997, 336(21):1487-93.

Lazzerini M, Martelossi S, Marchetti F, et al, "Efficacy and Safety of Thalidomide in Children and Young Adults With Intractable Inflammatory Bowel Disease: Long-Term Results," *Aliment Pharmacol Ther*, 2007, 25(4):419-27.

Lehman TJ, Schechter SJ, Sundel RP, et al, "Thalidomide for Severe Systemic Onset Juvenile Rheumatoid Arthritis: A Multicenter Study," *J Pediatr*, 2004, 145(6):856-7.

Martelossi S, Marchetti F, Lenhard A, et al, "Treatment With Thalidomide in Children and Adolescents With Inflammatory Bowel Disease," *J Pediatr Gastroenterol Nutr*, 2004, 39(1):S282-3.

Matthews SJ and McCoy C, "Thalidomide: A Review of Approved and Investigational Uses," *Clin Ther*, 2003, 25(2):342-95.

Mehta P, Kedar A, Graham-Pole J, et al, "Thalidomide in Children Undergoing Bone Marrow Transplantation: Series at a Single Institution and Review of the Literature," *Pediatrics*, 1999, 103(4):e44.

Okafor MC, "Thalidomide for Erythema Nodosum Leprosum and Other Applications," *Pharmacotherapy*, 2003, 23(4):481-93.

Priolo T, Lamba LD, Giribaldi G, et al, "Childhood Thalidomide Neuropathy: A Clinical and Neurophysiologic Study," *Pediatr Neurol*, 2008, 38(3):196-9.

Rovelli A, Arrigo C, Nesi F, et al, "The Role of Thalidomide in the Treatment of Refractory Chronic Graft-Versus-Host Disease Following Bone Marrow Transplantation in Children," *Bone Marrow Transplant*, 1998, 21(6):577-81.

Teo SK, Colburn WA, Tracewell WG, et al, "Clinical Pharmacokinetics of Thalidomide," *Clin Pharmacokinet*, 2004, 43(5):311-27.

Thompson JL and Hansen LA, "Thalidomide Dosing in Patients With Relapsed or Refractory Multiple Myeloma," *Ann Pharmacother*, 2003, 37(4):571-6.

Vogelsang GB, Farmer ER, Hess AD, et al, "Thalidomide for the Treatment of Chronic Graft-Versus-Host Disease," *N Engl J Med*, 1992, 326(16):1055-8.

◆ **Thalomid®** *see* Thalidomide *on page 1332*

◆ **THAM®** *see* Tromethamine *on page 1389*

◆ **THC** *see* Dronabinol *on page 482*

◆ **Theo-24®** *see* Theophylline *on page 1335*

◆ **Theochron™** *see* Theophylline *on page 1335*

◆ **Theochron® SR (Can)** *see* Theophylline *on page 1335*

Theophylline (thee OF i lin)

Related Information
Asthma *on page 1697*
Medications for Which A Single Dose May Be Fatal When Ingested By A Toddler *on page 1709*
Therapeutic Drug Monitoring: Blood Sampling Time Guidelines *on page 1704*

U.S. Brand Names Elixophyllin®; Theo-24®; Theochron™; Uniphyl® [DSC]

Canadian Brand Names Apo-Theo LA®; Novo-Theophyl SR; PMS-Theophylline; Pulmophylline; ratio-Theo-Bronc; Theochron® SR; Uniphyl® SRT

Therapeutic Category Antiasthmatic; Bronchodilator; Respiratory Stimulant; Theophylline Derivative

Generic Available Yes: Extended release tablet, infusion

Use Treatment of symptoms and reversible airway obstruction due to chronic asthma, chronic bronchitis, or COPD; treatment of idiopathic apnea of prematurity in neonates

Pregnancy Risk Factor C

Pregnancy Considerations Adverse events were observed in animal reproduction studies. Theophylline crosses the placenta; adverse effects may be seen in the newborn. Use is generally safe when used at the recommended doses (serum concentrations 5-12 mcg/mL) however maternal adverse events may be increased and efficacy may be decreased in pregnant women. Theophylline metabolism may change during pregnancy; the half-life is similar to that observed in otherwise healthy, nonsmoking adults with asthma during the first and second trimesters (~8.7 hours), but may increase to 13 hours (range: 8-18 hours) during the third trimester. The volume of distribution is also increased during the third trimester. Monitor serum levels. The recommendations for the use of theophylline in pregnant women with asthma are similar to those used in nonpregnant adults (National Heart, Lung, and Blood Institute Guidelines, 2004).

Lactation Enters breast milk/compatible (AAP rates "compatible")

Breast-Feeding Considerations The concentration of theophylline in breast milk is similar to the maternal serum concentration. Irritability may be observed in the nursing infant. Serious adverse events in the infant are unlikely unless toxic serum levels are present in the mother.

Contraindications Hypersensitivity to theophylline or any component

Warnings If a patient develops signs and symptoms of theophylline toxicity (eg, persistent, repetitive vomiting), a serum theophylline level should be measured and subsequent doses held; due to potential saturation of theophylline clearance at serum levels within or (in some patients) less than the therapeutic range, dosage adjustments should be made in small increments (maximum dosage adjustment: 25%); due to wide interpatient variability, theophylline serum level measurements must be used to optimize therapy and prevent serious toxicity

Precautions Use with caution in patients with peptic ulcer, hyperthyroidism, seizure disorders, hypertension, and patients with cardiac arrhythmias (excluding bradyarrhythmias)

Adverse Reactions See table.

Theophylline Serum Levels (mcg/mL)[1]	Adverse Reactions
15-25	GI upset, GE reflux, diarrhea, nausea, vomiting, abdominal pain, nervousness, headache, insomnia, agitation, dizziness, muscle cramp, tremor
25-35	Tachycardia, occasional PVC
>35	Ventricular tachycardia, frequent PVC, seizure

[1]Adverse effects do not necessarily occur according to serum levels. Arrhythmia and seizure can occur without seeing the other adverse effects.

Drug Interactions
Metabolism/Transport Effects Substrate of CYP1A2 (major), 2C9 (minor), 2D6 (minor), 2E1 (major), 3A4 (major); **Inhibits** CYP1A2 (weak)

Avoid Concomitant Use
Avoid concomitant use of Theophylline with any of the following: Febuxostat; Iobenguane I 123

Increased Effect/Toxicity
Theophylline may increase the levels/effects of: Sympathomimetics

The levels/effects of Theophylline may be increased by: Allopurinol; Atomoxetine; Cannabinoids; Cimetidine; CYP1A2 Inhibitors (Moderate); CYP1A2 Inhibitors (Strong); CYP3A4 Inhibitors (Moderate); CYP3A4 Inhibitors (Strong); Dasatinib; Disulfiram; Febuxostat; Fluvoxamine; Interferons; Isoniazid; Macrolide Antibiotics; Mexiletine; Pentoxifylline; QuiNINE; Quinolone Antibiotics; Thiabendazole; Ticlopidine; Zileuton

Decreased Effect
Theophylline may decrease the levels/effects of: Adenosine; Benzodiazepines; Iobenguane I 123; Lithium; Phenytoin; Regadenoson; Zafirlukast

The levels/effects of Theophylline may be decreased by: Aminoglutethimide; Barbiturates; Beta-Blockers (Beta1 Selective); Beta-Blockers (Nonselective); CarBAMazepine; CYP1A2 Inducers (Strong); CYP3A4 Inducers (Strong); Deferasirox; Herbs (CYP3A4 Inducers); Phenytoin; Protease Inhibitors; Thyroid Products

Food Interactions Food does not appreciably affect the absorption of liquid, fast-release products and most sustained release products; however, food may induce a sudden release (dose-dumping) of once-daily sustained release products resulting in an increase in serum drug levels and potential toxicity; avoid excessive amounts of caffeine; avoid extremes of dietary protein and carbohydrate intake; limit charcoal-broiled foods and caffeinated beverages

◄ **Mechanism of Action** Competitively inhibits two iso-enzymes of the enzyme phosphodiesterase resulting in increased levels of cyclic adenine monophosphate (cAMP) which may be responsible for most of theophylline's effects; effects on the myocardium and neuromuscular transmission may be due to the intracellular translocation of ionized calcium; overall, theophylline produces the following effects: relaxation of the smooth muscle of the respiratory tract, suppression of the response of airways to stimuli, increases the force of contraction of diaphragmatic muscles; pulmonary, coronary, and renal artery dilation; CNS stimulation, diuresis, stimulation of catecholamine release, gastric acid secretion, and relaxation of biliary and GI smooth muscle

Pharmacokinetics (Adult data unless noted)

Absorption: Oral: Rapid and complete with up to 100% absorption depending upon the formulation used

Distribution: V_d: 0.45 L/kg; distributes into breast milk; breast milk to plasma ratio: 0.67; crosses the placenta and into the CSF

Protein binding: 40%; decreased protein binding in neonates (due to a greater percentage of fetal albumin), hepatic cirrhosis, uncorrected acidemia, women in third trimester of pregnancy, and geriatric patients

Metabolism: In the liver by demethylation and oxidation; theophylline is metabolized to caffeine (active); in neonates this theophylline-derived caffeine accumulates (due to decreased hepatic metabolism) and significant concentrations of caffeine may occur; a substantial decrease in serum caffeine concentrations occurs after 40 weeks postconceptional age

Half-life: See table.

Theophylline Clearance and Half-Life With Respect to Age and Altered Physiological States[1]

Patient Group	Mean Clearance (mL/kg/min)	Mean Half-life (h)
Premature infants		
postnatal age 3-15 d	0.29	30
postnatal age 25-57 d	0.64	20
Term infants		
postnatal age 1-2 d	Not reported[2]	25
postnatal age 3-30 wk[3]	Not reported[2]	11
Children		
1-4 y	1.7	3.4
4-12 y	1.6	Not reported[2]
13-15 y	0.9	Not reported[2]
16-17 y	1.4	3.7 (range: 1.5-5.9)
Adults		
16-60 (nonsmoking)	0.65	8.2
>60 y (nonsmoking, healthy)	0.41	9.8
Acute pulmonary edema	0.33	19
Cystic fibrosis (14-28 y)	1.25	6
Liver disease		
acute hepatitis	0.35	19.2
cholestasis	0.65	14.4
cirrhosis	0.31	32
Sepsis with multiorgan failure	0.46	18.8
Hypothyroid	0.38	11.6
Hyperthyroid	0.8	4.5
COPD >60 y, nonsmoking >1 y	0.54	11

[1]From Hendeles L, 1995.

[2]Either not reported or not reported in a comparable format.

[3]Maturation of clearance in premature infants and term infants is most closely related to postconceptional age (PCA); adult clearance values are reached at approximately 55 weeks PCA and higher pediatric values at approximately 60 weeks PCA (Kraus, 1993).

Elimination: In urine; children >3 months and adults excrete 10% in urine as unchanged drug; neonates excrete approximately 50% of the dose unchanged in urine

Usual Dosage Oral (see Aminophylline on page 83 for I.V. doses):

Loading dose:

Neonates: Apnea of prematurity: 4 mg/kg/dose

Infants and Children: Treatment of acute bronchospasm: (to achieve a serum level of about 10 mcg/mL; loading doses should be given using a rapidly absorbed oral product **not** a sustained release product):

If no theophylline has been administered in the previous 24 hours: 5 mg/kg theophylline

If theophylline has been administered in the previous 24 hours: 2.5 mg/kg theophylline may be given in emergencies when serum levels are not available

A modified loading dose (mg/kg) may be calculated (when the serum level is known) by: [Blood level desired - blood level measured] divided by 2 (for every 1 mg/kg theophylline given, the blood level will rise by approximately 2 mcg/mL)

Maintenance dose: See table.

Maintenance Dose for Acute Symptoms

Population Group	Oral Theophylline (mg/kg/day)
Premature infant or newborn to 6 wk (for apnea/bradycardia)	4[1]
6 wk to 6 mo	10[1]
Infants 6 mo to 1 y	12-18[1]
Children 1-9 y	20-24
Children 9-12 y, adolescent daily smokers of cigarettes or marijuana, and otherwise healthy adult smokers <50 y	16
Adolescents 12-16 y (nonsmokers)	13
Otherwise healthy nonsmoking adults (including elderly patients)	10 (not to exceed 900 mg/day)
Cardiac decompensation, cor pulmonale, and/or liver dysfunction	5 (not to exceed 400 mg/day)

[1] **Alternative dosing regimen for full-term infants <1 year of age:**

Total daily dose (mg) = [(0.2 x age in weeks) + 5] x weight (kg).

Postnatal age <26 weeks: Total daily dose divided every 8 hours.

Postnatal age >26 weeks: Total daily dose divided every 6 hours.

These recommendations, based on mean clearance rates for age or risk factors, were calculated to achieve a serum level of 10 mcg/mL (5 mcg/mL for newborns with apnea/bradycardia). In newborns and infants, a fast-release oral product can be used. The total daily dose can be divided every 12 hours in newborns and every 6-8 hours in infants. In children and healthy adults, a slow-release product can be used. The total daily dose can be divided every 8-12 hours.

Use ideal body weight for obese patients

Dose should be further adjusted based on serum levels. Guidelines for drawing theophylline serum levels are shown in the table on the next page.

1336

THIABENDAZOLE

Guidelines for Drawing Theophylline Serum Levels

Dosage Form	Time to Draw Level[1]
I.V. bolus	30 min after end of 30-min infusion
I.V. continuous infusion	12-24 h after initiation of infusion
P.O. liquid, fast-release formulation	Peak: 1 h postdose after at least 1 day of therapy Trough: Just before a dose after at least 1 day of therapy

[1]The time to achieve steady-state serum levels is prolonged in patients with longer half-lives (eg, premature neonates, infants, and adults with cardiac or liver failure (see theophylline half-life table). In these patients, serum theophylline levels should be drawn after 48-72 hours of therapy; serum levels may need to be done prior to steady-state to assess the patient's current progress or evaluate potential toxicity.

Administration
Oral: Sustained release preparations should be administered with a full glass of water, whole or cut by half only; do not crush; sustained release capsule forms may be opened and sprinkled on soft foods; do not chew or crush beads

Parenteral: Premade I.V. infusion bags for continuous infusion usage; rate of infusion dependent upon dosage; loading doses using I.V. infusion should be administered over 20-30 minutes

Monitoring Parameters Respiratory rate, heart rate, serum theophylline level, arterial or capillary blood gases (if applicable); number and severity of apnea spells (apnea of prematurity)

Reference Range
Therapeutic levels:
Asthma: 10-15 mcg/mL (peak level)
Apnea of prematurity: 6-14 mcg/mL
Toxic concentration: >20 mcg/mL

Test Interactions May elevate uric acid levels

Patient Information Contact physician whenever nausea, vomiting, persistent headache, or irregular heartbeats occur; notify physician if a new illness develops (especially if high fevers); do not alter time, dose, or frequency of administration without physician knowledge; avoid drinking or eating of large quantities of caffeine-containing beverages or food

Additional Information Due to improved theophylline clearance during the first year of life, serum concentration determinations and dosage adjustments may be needed to optimize therapy

Dosage Forms Excipient information presented when available (limited, particularly for generics); consult specific product labeling. [DSC] = Discontinued product
Capsule, extended release:
Theo-24®: 100 mg, 200 mg, 300 mg, 400 mg [24 hours]
Elixir:
Elixophyllin®: 80 mg/15 mL (473 mL) [contains alcohol 20%; mixed fruit flavor]
Infusion [premixed in D$_5$W]: 200 mg (50 mL [DSC]; 100 mL); 400 mg (250 mL, 500 mL); 800 mg (250 mL, 500 mL, 1000 mL)
Tablet, controlled release:
Uniphyl®: 400 mg, 600 mg [24 hours] [DSC]
Tablet, extended release: 100 mg, 200 mg, 300 mg, 400 mg, 450 mg, 600 mg
Theochron™: 100 mg, 200 mg, 300 mg, 450 mg [12-24 hours]

References
Bhatt-Mehta V and Schumacher RE, "Treatment of Apnea of Prematurity," *Paediatr Drugs*, 2003, 5(3):195-210.
Hendeles L, Jenkins J, and Temple R, "Revised FDA Labeling Guideline for Theophylline Oral Dosage Forms," *Pharmacotherapy*, 1995, 15(4):409-427.
Kearney TE, Manoguerra AS, Curtis GP, et al, "Theophylline Toxicity and the Beta-Adrenergic System," *Ann Intern Med*, 1985, 102 (6):766-9.
Kraus DM, Fischer JH, Reitz SJ, et al, "Alterations in Theophylline Metabolism During the First Year of Life," *Clin Pharmacol Ther*, 1993, 54(4):351-9.
National Asthma Education and Prevention Program (NAEPP), "Expert Panel Report 3 (EPR-3): Guidelines for the Diagnosis and Management of Asthma," *Clinical Practice Guidelines*, National Institutes of Health, National Heart, Lung, and Blood Institute, NIH Publication No. 08-4051, prepublication 2007; available at http://www.nhlbi.nih.gov/guidelines/asthma/asthgdln.htm.
Upton RA, "Pharmacokinetic Interactions Between Theophylline and Other Medication (Part I)," *Clin Pharmacokinet*, 1991, 20(1):66-80.

◆ **Theophylline Anhydrous** *see* Theophylline *on page 1335*

◆ **Theophylline Ethylenediamine** *see* Aminophylline *on page 83*

◆ **Thera-Flur-N® [DSC]** *see* Fluoride *on page 595*

◆ **Theraflu® Thin Strips® Multi Symptom [OTC]** *see* DiphenhydrAMINE *on page 448*

◆ **Thermazene®** *see* Silver Sulfadiazine *on page 1262*

Thiabendazole (thye a BEN da zole)

U.S. Brand Names Mintezol®
Therapeutic Category Anthelmintic
Generic Available No
Use Treatment of strongyloidiasis, cutaneous larva migrans, visceral larva migrans, dracunculosis, trichinosis, and mixed helminthic infections
Pregnancy Risk Factor C
Pregnancy Considerations Cleft palate and skeletal defects were observed in some animal studies. There are no adequate and well-controlled studies in pregnant women.
Lactation Excretion in breast milk unknown/not recommended
Contraindications Hypersensitivity to thiabendazole or any component; pregnancy. Contraindicated as prophylactic treatment for pinworm infestation.
Warnings Abnormal sensation in eyes, blurred vision, xanthopsia, drying of mucous membranes, and Sicca syndrome have been reported in patients receiving thiabendazole; ocular adverse effect may persist beyond one year in some cases
Precautions Use with caution in patients with renal or hepatic impairment, malnutrition, anemia, or dehydration
Adverse Reactions
Cardiovascular: Flushing, hypotension, bradycardia
Central nervous system: Dizziness, drowsiness, vertigo, seizures, fever, malaise, headache, chills, hallucinations
Dermatologic: Rash, Stevens-Johnson syndrome, erythema multiforme, pruritus
Endocrine & metabolic: Hyperglycemia
Gastrointestinal: Nausea, vomiting, diarrhea, anorexia, abdominal pain
Genitourinary: Malodor of the urine
Hematologic: Leukopenia
Hepatic: Hepatotoxicity, jaundice, cholestasis
Neuromuscular & skeletal: Paresthesia, numbness
Ocular: Blurred vision, Sicca syndrome
Otic: Tinnitus
Renal: Nephrotoxicity, hematuria
Miscellaneous: Hypersensitivity reactions, lymphadenopathy
Drug Interactions
Metabolism/Transport Effects Substrate of CYP1A2 (minor); **Inhibits** CYP1A2 (strong)
Avoid Concomitant Use There are no known interactions where it is recommended to avoid concomitant use.

◀

Increased Effect/Toxicity
Thiabendazole may increase the levels/effects of:
Bendamustine; CYP1A2 Substrates; Theophylline Derivatives

Decreased Effect
The levels/effects of Thiabendazole may be decreased by: Aminoquinolines (Antimalarial)

Mechanism of Action Inhibits helminth-specific mitochondrial fumarate reductase

Pharmacokinetics (Adult data unless noted)
Absorption: From the GI tract and through the skin
Metabolism: Extensive in the liver via hydroxylation and conjugation with sulfuric and/or glucuronic acid
Time to peak serum concentration: Within 1-2 hours
Elimination: In feces (5%) and urine (87%), primarily as conjugated metabolites

Usual Dosage
Oral:
Children and Adults: 50 mg/kg/day divided every 12 hours (maximum dose: 3 g/day)
Strongyloidiasis: For 2 consecutive days (5 days or longer for disseminated disease)
Cutaneous larva migrans: For 2-5 consecutive days
Visceral larva migrans: For 5-7 consecutive days
Trichinosis: For 2-4 consecutive days
Angiostrongylosis: 50-75 mg/kg/day divided every 8-12 hours for 3 days
Dracunculosis: 50-75 mg/kg/day divided every 12 hours for 3 days
Topical: Cutaneous larva migrans: Instead of oral therapy, thiabendazole 10% to 15% suspension or a 10% ointment in white petrolatum has been applied topically to lesions 4-6 times/day

Administration Oral: Administer after meals; chew tablet well before swallowing

Monitoring Parameters Periodic renal and hepatic function tests, serum glucose

Patient Information May cause drowsiness and impair ability to perform activities requiring mental alertness or physical coordination

Nursing Implications Purgation is not required prior to use

Dosage Forms Excipient information presented when available (limited, particularly for generics); consult specific product labeling. [DSC] = Discontinued product
Suspension, oral: 500 mg/5 mL (120 mL) [DSC]
Tablet, chewable: 500 mg [orange flavor]

References
Walden J, "Parasitic Diseases. Other Roundworms. *Trichuris*, Hookworm, and *Strongyloides*," *Prim Care*, 1991, 18(1):53-74.
Zygmunt DJ, "*Strongyloides stearcoralis*," *Infect Control Hosp Epidemiol*, 1990, 11(9):495-7.

◆ **Thiamazole** *see* Methimazole *on page 897*

◆ **Thiamin** *see* Thiamine *on page 1338*

Thiamine (THYE a min)

Medication Safety Issues
Sound-alike/look-alike issues:
Thiamine may be confused with Tenormin®, Thalomid®, Thorazine®

International issues:
Doxal® [Brazil] may be confused with Doxil® which is a brand name for doxorubicin in the U.S.
Doxal® [Brazil]: Brand name for doxycycline in Austria; brand name for pyridoxine/thiamine combination in Brazil; brand name for doxepin in Finland

Canadian Brand Names Betaxin®

Therapeutic Category Nutritional Supplement; Vitamin, Water Soluble

Generic Available Yes

Use Treatment of thiamine deficiency including beriberi, Wernicke's encephalopathy syndrome, and peripheral neuritis associated with pellagra; alcoholic patients with altered sensorium; various genetic metabolic disorders

Pregnancy Risk Factor A/C (dose exceeding RDA recommendation)

Pregnancy Considerations
Thiamine requirements are increased during pregnancy. Severe nausea and vomiting (hyperemesis gravidarum) may lead to thiamine deficiency manifested as Wernicke's encephalopathy.

Lactation Enters breast milk/use caution (AAP rates "compatible")

Contraindications Hypersensitivity to thiamine or any component

Warnings Large doses should be given in divided doses for better oral absorption

Precautions Use parenteral route cautiously, see Adverse Reactions

Adverse Reactions
Cardiovascular: Cardiovascular collapse and death (primarily following repeated I.V. administration), warmth
Dermatologic: Rash, angioedema
Genitourinary: Discoloration of urine (bright yellow) with large doses
Neuromuscular & skeletal: Paresthesia

Drug Interactions
Avoid Concomitant Use There are no known interactions where it is recommended to avoid concomitant use.
Increased Effect/Toxicity There are no known significant interactions involving an increase in effect.
Decreased Effect There are no known significant interactions involving a decrease in effect.

Food Interactions High carbohydrate diets may increase thiamine requirement

Stability Unstable with alkaline or neutral solutions

Mechanism of Action An essential coenzyme in carbohydrate metabolism; combines with adenosine triphosphate to form thiamine pyrophosphate

Pharmacokinetics (Adult data unless noted)
Absorption:
Oral: Poor
I.M.: Rapid and complete
Metabolism: In the liver
Elimination: Renally as unchanged drug only after body storage sites become saturated

Usual Dosage
Adequate intake: Oral: Infants:
<6 months: 0.2 mg (0.03 mg/kg)
6-12 months: 0.3 mg (0.03 mg/kg)
Recommended daily allowance (RDA): Oral:
1-3 years: 0.5 mg
4-8 years: 0.6 mg
9-13 years: 0.9 mg
14-18 years:
Male: 1.2 mg
Female: 1 mg
≥19 years:
Male: 1.2 mg
Female: 1.1 mg
Dietary supplement (depends on caloric or carbohydrate content of the diet)
Oral:
Infants: 0.3-0.5 mg/day
Children: 0.5-1 mg/day
Adults: 1-2 mg/day
Note: The above doses can be found in multivitamin preparations

Thiamine deficiency (beriberi):
Children: 10-25 mg/dose I.M. or I.V. daily (if critically ill), or 10-50 mg/dose orally every day for 2 weeks, then 5-10 mg/dose orally daily for 1 month
Adults: 5-30 mg/dose I.M. or I.V. 3 times/day (if critically ill); then orally 5-30 mg/day in single or divided doses 3 times/day for 1 month
Wernicke's encephalopathy: Adults: Initial: 100 mg I.V., then 50-100 mg/day I.M. or I.V. until consuming a regular, balanced diet
Metabolic disorders: Oral: Adults: 10-20 mg/day (dosages up to 4 g/day in divided doses have been used)

Administration
Oral: May administer with or without food
Parenteral: Administer by slow I.V. injection or I.M.

Reference Range Normal values: 1.6-4 mg/dL

Test Interactions False-positive for uric acid using the phosphotungstate method and for urobilinogen using the Ehrlich's reagent; large doses may interfere with the spectrophotometric determination of serum theophylline concentration

Patient Information May color urine bright yellow

Additional Information Dietary sources include legumes, pork, beef, whole grains, yeast, fresh vegetables; a deficiency state can occur in as little as 3 weeks following total dietary absence

Dosage Forms Excipient information presented when available (limited, particularly for generics); consult specific product labeling.
Injection, solution, as hydrochloride: 100 mg/mL (2 mL)
Tablet, as hydrochloride: 50 mg, 100 mg, 250 mg, 500 mg

♦ **Thiamine Hydrochloride** see Thiamine on page 1338
♦ **Thiaminium Chloride Hydrochloride** see Thiamine on page 1338

Thioguanine (thye oh GWAH neen)

Medication Safety Issues
International issues:
Lanvis® [Canada and multiple international markets] may be confused with Lantus® brand name for insulin glargine [U.S., Canada, and multiple international markets]

High alert medication: The Institute for Safe Medication Practices (ISMP) includes this medication among its list of drugs which have a heightened risk of causing significant patient harm when used in error.

6-thioguanine and 6-TG are error-prone abbreviations (associated with sixfold overdoses of thioguanine)

Related Information
Emetogenic Potential of Antineoplastic Agents on page 1579

U.S. Brand Names Tabloid®
Canadian Brand Names Lanvis®
Therapeutic Category Antineoplastic Agent, Antimetabolite
Generic Available No
Use Remission induction and remission consolidation treatment of acute myelogenous (nonlymphocytic) leukemia [FDA approved in pediatrics (age not specified) and adults]

Pregnancy Risk Factor D
Lactation Excretion in breast milk unknown
Contraindications Hypersensitivity to thioguanine or any component; pregnancy; history of previous therapy resistance with thioguanine and in patients resistant to mercaptopurine (usual to find cross-resistance between thioguanine and mercaptopurine)
Warnings The FDA currently recommends that procedures for proper handling and disposal of antineoplastic agents

be considered; thioguanine is potentially carcinogenic and teratogenic. Liver toxicity associated with vascular endothelial damage has been reported in patients receiving long-term thioguanine maintenance therapy. The liver toxicity is particularly prevalent in children receiving maintenance therapy for acute lymphoblastic leukemia and in males; liver toxicity usually presents as the clinical syndrome of hepatic veno-occlusive disease or portal hypertension. Discontinue thioguanine therapy in patients with signs and symptoms of liver toxicity.

Precautions Use with caution and reduce dose of thioguanine in patients with renal or hepatic impairment. Substantial dosage reductions may be required in patients with an inherited deficiency of the enzyme thiopurine methyltransferase (TPMT).

Adverse Reactions
Central nervous system: Headache, neurotoxicity
Dermatologic: Photosensitivity, skin rash, staining of skin or eyes (yellow)
Endocrine & metabolic: Hyperuricemia
Gastrointestinal: Anorexia, diarrhea, intestinal necrosis and perforation, mild nausea or vomiting, splenomegaly, stomatitis
Hematologic: Myelosuppression (anemia, granulocytopenia, leukopenia, thrombocytopenia)
Hepatic: Ascites, hepatitis, hyperbilirubinemia, jaundice, liver transaminases increased, portal hypertension, veno-occlusive hepatic disease
Neuromuscular & skeletal: Unsteady gait

Drug Interactions
Avoid Concomitant Use
Avoid concomitant use of Thioguanine with any of the following: BCG; Natalizumab; Pimecrolimus; Tacrolimus (Topical); Vaccines (Live)

Increased Effect/Toxicity
Thioguanine may increase the levels/effects of: Leflunomide; Natalizumab; Vaccines (Live)

The levels/effects of Thioguanine may be increased by: 5-ASA Derivatives; Denosumab; Pimecrolimus; Tacrolimus (Topical); Trastuzumab

Decreased Effect
Thioguanine may decrease the levels/effects of: BCG; Sipuleucel-T; Vaccines (Inactivated); Vaccines (Live)

The levels/effects of Thioguanine may be decreased by: Echinacea

Food Interactions Enhanced absorption if administered between meals

Stability Store at room temperature in a dry location.

Mechanism of Action Purine analog that is incorporated into DNA and RNA resulting in the inhibition of synthesis and utilization of purine nucleotides

Pharmacokinetics (Adult data unless noted)
Absorption: Oral: 30% (variable and incomplete)
Distribution: Crosses the placenta; does not appear to cross into CSF
Metabolism: Rapid and extensive hepatic metabolism by methylation of thioguanine to 2-amino-6-methylthioguanine (active) and inactive compounds
Half-life, terminal: 11 hours
Time to peak serum concentration: Within 8-12 hours
Elimination: Metabolites excreted in urine

Usual Dosage Oral (refer to individual protocols):
Infants <3 years: Combination drug therapy for ANLL: 3.3 mg/kg/day in divided doses twice daily for 4 days
Children and Adults:
Single agent chemotherapy for ANLL: 2-3 mg/kg/day once daily calculated to nearest 20 mg
Induction of remission in patients with acute leukemia (combination therapy): 75-200 mg/m^2/day in 1-2 divided doses for 5-7 days or until remission is attained

Note: Lower dose maintenance therapy is no longer recommended in the U.S. Instead, shorter period induction and consolidation therapy at higher doses is employed.

Administration Oral: Administer between meals on an empty stomach

Monitoring Parameters CBC with (differential, platelet count), liver function tests (serum transaminases, alkaline phosphatase, bilirubin), hemoglobin, hematocrit, serum uric acid; testing for thiopurine methyltransferase (TPMT) deficiency; clinical signs of portal hypertension or veno-occlusive disease

Patient Information Notify physician if fever, sore throat, bleeding, bruising, nausea, vomiting, yellow discoloration of skin or eyes, or leg swelling occurs. May cause photosensitivity reactions (eg, exposure to sunlight may cause severe sunburn, skin rash, redness, or itching); avoid exposure to sunlight and artificial light sources (sunlamps, tanning booth/bed); wear protective clothing, wide-brimmed hats, sunglasses, and lip sunscreen (SPF ≥15); use a sunscreen [broad-spectrum sunscreen or physical sunscreen (preferred) or sunblock with SPF ≥15]; contact physician if reaction occurs. Women of child-bearing potential should be advised to avoid becoming pregnant.

Nursing Implications Ensure adequate patient hydration, alkalinization of the urine, and/or administration of allopurinol to prevent hyperuricemia

Additional Information Myelosuppressive effects:
WBC: Moderate
Platelets: Moderate
Onset (days): 7-10
Nadir (days): 14
Recovery (days): 21

Dosage Forms Excipient information presented when available (limited, particularly for generics); consult specific product labeling.
Tablet [scored]:
Tabloid®: 40 mg

Extemporaneous Preparations A 20 mg/mL oral suspension can be made by crushing fifteen 40 mg tablets in a mortar. Add 10 mL of methylcellulose 1% in small amounts and mix. Transfer to a graduate and add a sufficient quantity of syrup to make 30 mL. Stable for 60 days at room temperature. Label "shake well."
Nahata MC and Hipple TF, *Pediatric Drug Formulations*, 4th ed, Cincinnati, OH: Harvey Whitney Books Co, 2000.

References
Broxson EH, Dole M, Wong R, et al, "Portal Hypertension Develops in a Subset of Children With Standard Risk Acute Lymphoblastic Leukemia Treated With Oral 6-Thioguanine During Maintenance Therapy," *Pediatr Blood Cancer*, 2005, 44(3):226-31.
Culbert SJ, Shuster JJ, Land VJ, et al, "Remission Induction and Continuation Therapy in Children With Their First Relapse of Acute Lymphoid Leukemia: A Pediatric Oncology Group Study," *Cancer*, 1991, 67(1):37-42.
Steuber CP, Civin C, Krischer J, et al, "A Comparison of Induction and Maintenance Therapy for Acute Nonlymphocytic Leukemia in Childhood: Results of a Pediatric Oncology Group Study," *J Clin Oncol*, 1991, 9(2):247-58.

◆ **6-Thioguanine (error-prone abbreviation)** *see* Thioguanine *on page 1339*

Thiopental (thye oh PEN tal)

Medication Safety Issues
High alert medication: The Institute for Safe Medication Practices (ISMP) includes this medication among its list of drugs which have a heightened risk of causing significant patient harm when used in error.

Related Information
Preprocedure Sedatives in Children *on page 1688*

U.S. Brand Names Pentothal®

Canadian Brand Names Pentothal®

Therapeutic Category Anticonvulsant, Barbiturate; Barbiturate; General Anesthetic; Hypnotic; Sedative

Generic Available No

Use Induction of anesthesia; adjunct for intubation in head injury patients; control of convulsive states; treatment of elevated intracranial pressure

Restrictions C-III

Pregnancy Risk Factor C

Contraindications Hypersensitivity to thiopental, pentobarbital, any component, or other barbiturates; porphyria (variegate or acute intermittent)

Precautions Use with caution in patients with asthma or pharyngeal infections because cough, laryngospasm, or bronchospasms may occur; use with caution in patients with hypotension, severe cardiovascular disease, hepatic or renal dysfunction; avoid extravasation or intra-arterial injection which may cause necrosis due to pH of 10.6; ensure patient has intravenous access

Adverse Reactions
Cardiovascular: Cardiac output decreased, hypotension
Local: Necrosis with I.V. extravasation
Renal: Urine output decreased
Respiratory: Cough, laryngospasm, bronchospasm, respiratory depression, apnea
Miscellaneous: Anaphylaxis

Drug Interactions
Avoid Concomitant Use There are no known interactions where it is recommended to avoid concomitant use.

Increased Effect/Toxicity
Thiopental may increase the levels/effects of: Alcohol (Ethyl); CNS Depressants; Meperidine; Thiazide Diuretics

The levels/effects of Thiopental may be increased by: Carbonic Anhydrase Inhibitors; Chloramphenicol; Divalproex; Felbamate; Primidone; Valproic Acid

Decreased Effect
Thiopental may decrease the levels/effects of: Acetaminophen; Beta-Blockers; Calcium Channel Blockers; Chloramphenicol; Contraceptives (Estrogens); Contraceptives (Progestins); Corticosteroids (Systemic); Cyclo-SPORINE; CycloSPORINE (Systemic); Disopyramide; Divalproex; Doxycycline; Etoposide; Etoposide Phosphate; LamoTRIgine; Methadone; Propafenone; QuiNIDine; Teniposide; Theophylline Derivatives; Tricyclic Antidepressants; Valproic Acid; Vitamin K Antagonists

The levels/effects of Thiopental may be decreased by: Ketorolac; Ketorolac (Systemic); Mefloquine; Pyridoxine; Rifamycin Derivatives

Stability Solutions are alkaline and incompatible with drugs with acidic pH, such as succinylcholine, atropine sulfate

Mechanism of Action Ultra-short-acting barbiturate; depresses CNS activity by binding to barbiturate site at GABA-receptor complex enhancing GABA activity; depresses reticular activating system; higher doses may be gabamimetic

Pharmacodynamics Anesthesia effects:
Onset of action: I.V.: 30-60 seconds
Duration: 5-30 minutes

Pharmacokinetics (Adult data unless noted)
Distribution: V_d: Adults: 1.4 L/kg
Protein binding: 72% to 86%
Metabolism: In the liver primarily to inactive metabolites but pentobarbital is also formed
Half-life, adults: 3-11.5 hours (shorter half-life in children)

Usual Dosage

Induction anesthesia: I.V.:
  Neonates: 3-4 mg/kg
  Infants: 5-8 mg/kg
  Children 1-12 years: 5-6 mg/kg
  Children >12 years and Adults: 3-5 mg/kg
Maintenance anesthesia: I.V.:
  Children: 1 mg/kg as needed
  Adults: 25-100 mg as needed
Increased intracranial pressure: Children: I.V.: 1.5-5 mg/kg/dose; repeat as needed to control intracranial pressure; larger doses (30 mg/kg) to induce coma after hypoxic-ischemic injury do not appear to improve neurologic outcome
Seizures: I.V.:
  Children: 2-3 mg/kg/dose, repeat as needed
  Adults: 75-250 mg/dose, repeat as needed
Sedation: Rectal:
  Children: 5-10 mg/kg/dose
  Adults: 3-4 g/dose

Administration Parenteral: Avoid rapid I.V. injection (may cause hypotension or decreased cardiac output); may administer by intermittent infusion over 10-60 minutes at a maximum concentration of 50 mg/mL

Monitoring Parameters Respiratory rate, heart rate, blood pressure

Reference Range
Therapeutic:
  Hypnotic: 1-5 mcg/mL (SI: 4.1-20.7 micromoles/L)
  Coma: 30-100 mcg/mL (SI: 124-413 micromoles/L)
  Anesthesia: 7-130 mcg/mL (SI: 29-536 micromoles/L)

Nursing Implications Avoid extravasation, necrosis may occur

Additional Information Accumulation may occur with chronic dosing due to lipid solubility; prolonged recovery occurs due to redistribution of thiopental from fat stores; therefore, thiopental is usually not used for procedures lasting >15-20 minutes; sodium content, injection: 4.9 mEq/g

Dosage Forms Excipient information presented when available (limited, particularly for generics); consult specific product labeling.
Injection, powder for reconstitution, as sodium:
  Pentothal®: 250 mg [DSC]; 400 mg, 500 mg, 1 g [contains sodium 105 mg/g]

◆ **Thiopental Sodium** see Thiopental on page 1340
◆ **Thiophosphoramide** see Thiotepa on page 1342
◆ **Thioplex** see Thiotepa on page 1342

Thioridazine (thye oh RID a zeen)

Medication Safety Issues
Sound-alike/look-alike issues:
  Thioridazine may be confused with thiothixene, Thorazine®
  Mellaril® may be confused with Elavil®, Mebaral®

Beers Criteria medication: This drug may be inappropriate for use in geriatric patients (high severity risk).

Related Information
Medications for Which A Single Dose May Be Fatal When Ingested By A Toddler on page 1709

Canadian Brand Names Mellaril®

Therapeutic Category Antipsychotic Agent, Typical, Phenothiazine; Phenothiazine Derivative

Generic Available Yes

Use Due to prolongation of the QT_c interval (see Warnings), thioridazine is currently indicated only for the treatment of refractory schizophrenic patients [FDA approved in pediatric patients (age not specified) and adults]; in the past, the drug had been used for management of psychotic disorders; depressive neurosis; dementia in elderly; severe behavioral problems in children

Pregnancy Risk Factor C

Lactation Excretion in breast milk unknown/not recommended

Contraindications Hypersensitivity to thioridazine or any component; cross-sensitivity to other phenothiazines may exist; concurrent therapy with propranolol, pindolol, fluvoxamine, fluoxetine, paroxetine, drugs that inhibit cytochrome P450 isoenzyme CYP2D6, drugs that prolong the QT_c interval, and patients with reduced levels of CYP2D6, a history of cardiac arrhythmias, congenital long QT syndrome, or a QT_c interval >450 msec (adults); severe CNS depression; avoid use in patients with narrow-angle glaucoma, blood dyscrasias, severe liver or cardiac disease

Warnings Dose-related prolongation of the QT_c interval may occur and may be associated with torsade de pointes arrhythmias and sudden death **[U.S. Boxed Warning]**; reserve use for schizophrenic patients who do not respond to adequate treatment with other antipsychotic agents. May cause extrapyramidal symptoms, including pseudoparkinsonism, acute dystonic reactions, akathisia, and tardive dyskinesia (risk of these reactions is low relative to other neuroleptics, and is dose-dependent; to decrease risk of tardive dyskinesia: Use smallest dose and shortest duration possible; evaluate continued need periodically; risk of dystonia is increased with the use of high potency and higher doses of conventional antipsychotics and in males and younger patients). May cause neuroleptic malignant syndrome; monitor for mental status changes, fever, muscle rigidity, and/or autonomic instability (risk may be increased in patients with Parkinson's disease or Lewy body dementia).

Leukopenia, neutropenia, and agranulocytosis (sometimes fatal) have been reported in clinical trials and postmarketing reports with antipsychotic use; presence of risk factors (eg, pre-existing low WBC or history of drug-induced leuko/neutropenia) should prompt periodic blood count assessment. Discontinue therapy at first signs of blood dyscrasias or if absolute neutrophil count <1000/mm³.

An increased risk of death has been reported with the use of antipsychotics in elderly patients with dementia-related psychosis **[U.S. Boxed Warning]**; most deaths seemed to be cardiovascular (eg, sudden death, heart failure) or infectious (eg, pneumonia) in nature; thioridazine is not approved for this indication.

Precautions Use with caution in patients with severe cardiovascular disorder or seizures

Adverse Reactions Sedation and anticholinergic effects are more pronounced than extrapyramidal effects; ECG changes and retinal pigmentation are more common than with chlorpromazine

Cardiovascular: Arrhythmias, hypotension, orthostatic hypotension, tachycardia

Central nervous system: Altered central temperature regulation, anxiety, drowsiness, extrapyramidal reactions, neuroleptic malignant syndrome, pseudoparkinsonian signs and symptoms, restlessness, sedation, seizures, tardive dyskinesia

Dermatologic: Contact dermatitis, hyperpigmentation, photosensitivity (rare), pruritus, rash

Endocrine & metabolic: Amenorrhea, galactorrhea, gynecomastia, weight gain

Gastrointestinal: Constipation, GI upset, xerostomia

Genitourinary: Urinary retention

Hematologic: Agranulocytosis, leukopenia (usually in patients with large doses for prolonged periods), neutropenia

Hepatic: Cholestatic jaundice

Ocular: Blurred vision, brownish coloring of vision, night vision decreased, retinal pigmentation (usually in patients receiving larger than recommended doses); visual acuity decreased (may be irreversible)

Miscellaneous: Anaphylactoid reactions

Drug Interactions

Metabolism/Transport Effects Substrate of CYP2C19 (minor), 2D6 (major); **Inhibits** CYP1A2 (weak), 2C9 (weak), 2D6 (moderate), 2E1 (weak)

Avoid Concomitant Use

Avoid concomitant use of Thioridazine with any of the following: Artemether; CYP2D6 Inhibitors; Dronedarone; Fluvoxamine; Lumefantrine; Metoclopramide; Nilotinib; Pimozide; QTc-Prolonging Agents; QuiNINE; Tamoxifen; Tetrabenazine; Ziprasidone

Increased Effect/Toxicity

Thioridazine may increase the levels/effects of: Alcohol (Ethyl); Analgesics (Opioid); Anticholinergics; Anti-Parkinson's Agents (Dopamine Agonist); Atomoxetine; Beta-Blockers; CNS Depressants; CYP2D6 Substrates; Dronedarone; Fesoterodine; Pimozide; QTc-Prolonging Agents; QuiNINE; Tamoxifen; Tetrabenazine; Ziprasidone

The levels/effects of Thioridazine may be increased by: Acetylcholinesterase Inhibitors (Central); Alfuzosin; Antimalarial Agents; Artemether; Beta-Blockers; Chloroquine; Ciprofloxacin; Ciprofloxacin (Systemic); CYP2D6 Inhibitors; Darunavir; Fluvoxamine; Gadobutrol; Lithium formulations; Lumefantrine; Metoclopramide; Nilotinib; Pramlintide; QTc-Prolonging Agents; QuiNINE; Tetrabenazine

Decreased Effect

Thioridazine may decrease the levels/effects of: Amphetamines; Quinagolide; TraMADol

The levels/effects of Thioridazine may be decreased by: Antacids; Anti-Parkinson's Agents (Dopamine Agonist); Lithium formulations; Peginterferon Alfa-2b

Food Interactions May increase dietary requirements for riboflavin; liquid thioridazine formulations may precipitate with enteral formulas

Mechanism of Action Blocks postsynaptic mesolimbic dopaminergic receptors in the brain; exhibits a strong alpha-adrenergic blocking effect and depresses the release of hypothalamic and hypophyseal hormones

Pharmacokinetics (Adult data unless noted)

Protein binding: 99%

Metabolism: In the liver to active and inactive metabolites

Bioavailability: 25% to 33%

Half-life: Adults: 9-30 hours

Dialysis: Not dialyzable: (0% to 5%)

Usual Dosage Oral:

Children >2 years: Initial: 0.5 mg/kg/day in 2-3 divided doses; range: 0.5-3 mg/kg/day; usual: 1 mg/kg/day in 2-3 divided doses; maximum dose: 3 mg/kg/day

Behavior problems: Initial: 10 mg 2-3 times/day, increase gradually

Severe psychoses: Initial: 25 mg 2-3 times/day, increase gradually

Children >12 years and Adults:

Schizophrenia/psychoses: Initial: 25-100 mg 3 times/day with gradual increments as needed and tolerated; maximum daily dose: 800 mg/day in 2-4 divided doses; maintenance: 10-200 mg/dose 2-4 times/day

Depressive disorders, dementia: Initial: 25 mg 3 times/day; maintenance dose: 20-200 mg/day

Administration Oral: Administer with water, food, or milk to decrease GI upset; dilute the oral concentrate with water or juice before administration; do not administer liquid thioridazine simultaneously with carbamazepine suspension (see Drug Interactions); do not mix liquid thioridazine with enteric formulas (see Food Interactions)

Monitoring Parameters Baseline and periodic ECG and serum potassium; periodic eye exam, CBC with differential, blood pressure, liver enzyme tests

Test Interactions False-positives for phenylketonuria, urinary amylase, uroporphyrins, urobilinogen

Patient Information Avoid alcohol; may cause drowsiness and impair ability to perform activities requiring mental alertness or physical coordination; may cause dry mouth; avoid skin contact with oral liquid preparations, may cause contact dermatitis; do not discontinue or alter dose without physician approval. May rarely cause photosensitivity reactions; avoid exposure to sunlight and artificial light sources (sunlamps, tanning booth/bed); use a sunscreen; contact physician if reaction occurs

Additional Information In cases of overdoses, cardiovascular monitoring and continuous ECG monitoring should be performed; avoid drugs (such as quinidine, disopyramide, and procainamide) that may further prolong the QT interval

Note: All Mellaril® (brand name) products have been discontinued; Mellaril® suspension was discontinued October, 2000; oral concentrate 100 mg/mL was discontinued March 2001; tablets and 30 mg/mL oral concentrate were discontinued in January 2002.

Dosage Forms Excipient information presented when available (limited, particularly for generics); consult specific product labeling. [DSC] = Discontinued product

Tablet, as hydrochloride: 10 mg, 15 mg [DSC], 25 mg, 50 mg, 100 mg, 150 mg [DSC], 200 mg [DSC]

References

Aman MG, Marks RE, Turbott SH, et al, "Clinical Effects of Methylphenidate and Thioridazine in Intellectually Subaverage Children," *J Am Acad Child Adolesc Psychiatry*, 1991, 30(2):246-56.

◆ **Thioridazine Hydrochloride** *see* Thioridazine *on page 1341*

◆ **Thiosulfuric Acid Disodium Salt** *see* Sodium Thiosulfate *on page 1280*

Thiotepa (thye oh TEP a)

Medication Safety Issues

Sound-alike/look-alike issues:

Thiotepa may be confused with thioguanine

High alert medication: This medication is in a class the Institute for Safe Medication Practices (ISMP) includes among its list of drugs which have a heightened risk of causing significant patient harm when used in error.

Intrathecal medication safety: The American Society of Clinical Oncology (ASCO)/Oncology Nursing Society (ONS) chemotherapy administration safety standards (Jacobson, 2009) encourage the following safety measures for intrathecal chemotherapy:

• Intrathecal medication should not be prepared during the preparation of any other agents

• After preparation, store in an isolated location or container clearly marked with a label identifying as "intrathecal" use only

• Delivery to the patient should only be with other medications intended for administration into the central nervous system

Related Information

Compatibility of Chemotherapy and Related Supportive Care Medications *on page 1580*

Emetogenic Potential of Antineoplastic Agents *on page 1579*

Therapeutic Category Antineoplastic Agent, Alkylating Agent

Generic Available Yes

Use Treatment of superficial tumors of the bladder; palliative treatment of adenocarcinoma of breast or ovary;

control of pleural, pericardial, or peritoneal effusions caused by metastatic tumors (FDA approved in adults); has also been used as intrathecal treatment of neoplastic meningitis and high-dose regimens with autologous bone marrow transplantation

Pregnancy Risk Factor D

Pregnancy Considerations Animal studies have demonstrated teratogenicity and fetal loss. There are no adequate and well-controlled studies in pregnant women. May cause harm if administered during pregnancy. Effective contraception is recommended for men and women of childbearing potential.

Lactation Excretion in breast milk unknown/not recommended

Breast-Feeding Considerations Due to the potential for serious adverse reactions in the nursing infant, breast-feeding is not recommended.

Contraindications Hypersensitivity to thiotepa or any component; severe myelosuppression with leukocyte count <3000/mm^3 or platelet count <150,000 mm^3; pregnancy

Warnings The FDA currently recommends that procedures for proper handling and disposal of antineoplastic agents be considered. The drug is potentially mutagenic, carcinogenic, teratogenic, and may cause fertility impairment. Death due to bone marrow depression has been reported after intravesical administration. Death due to sepsis and hemorrhage as a result of thiotepa administration has also been reported.

Precautions Reduce dosage in patients with hepatic, renal, or bone marrow dysfunction

Adverse Reactions

Central nervous system: Confusion, dizziness, fatigue, fever, headache, somnolence

Dermatologic: Alopecia, contact dermatitis, hyperpigmentation of skin with high-dose therapy, pruritus, rash, urticaria

Endocrine & metabolic: Amenorrhea, azoospermia, hyperuricemia

Gastrointestinal: Abdominal pain, anorexia, esophagitis, mucositis, nausea, vomiting

Genitourinary: Rarely hemorrhagic cystitis, urinary retention

Hematologic: Anemia, granulocytopenia, leukopenia (nadir: 7-10 days), thrombocytopenia (nadir: 3 weeks)

Hepatic: Liver transaminase and bilirubin increased (high-dose therapy)

Local: Pain at injection site

Ocular: Blurred vision, conjunctivitis

Renal: Hematuria

Respiratory: Laryngeal edema, wheezing

Miscellaneous: Anaphylaxis

<1%, postmarketing, and/or case reports: Like other alkylating agents, this drug is carcinogenic; stomatitis

Drug Interactions

Metabolism/Transport Effects Inhibits CYP2B6 (strong)

Avoid Concomitant Use

Avoid concomitant use of Thiotepa with any of the following: BCG; Natalizumab; Pimecrolimus; Tacrolimus (Topical); Vaccines (Live)

Increased Effect/Toxicity

Thiotepa may increase the levels/effects of: CYP2B6 Substrates; Leflunomide; Natalizumab; Vaccines (Live)

The levels/effects of Thiotepa may be increased by: Denosumab; Pimecrolimus; Tacrolimus (Topical); Trastuzumab

Decreased Effect

Thiotepa may decrease the levels/effects of: BCG; Sipuleucel-T; Vaccines (Inactivated); Vaccines (Live)

The levels/effects of Thiotepa may be decreased by: Echinacea

Stability Refrigerate, protect from light; the reconstituted 10 mg/mL solution is chemically stable for 5 days when stored in the refrigerator; since it contains no preservatives use within 8 hours; unstable in acid medium. Thiotepa is stable for 24 hours at a concentration of 1-5 mg/mL in NS when stored at room temperature; at 0.5 mg/mL, thiotepa is stable for 8 hours at room temperature; stability decreases significantly at concentrations <0.5 mg/mL (1 hour).

Mechanism of Action Polyfunctional alkylating agent that reacts with DNA phosphate groups to produce cross-linking of DNA strands leading to inhibition of DNA, RNA, and protein synthesis

Pharmacokinetics (Adult data unless noted)

Absorption: Variable absorption through serous membranes and from I.M. injection sites; bladder mucosa: 10% to 100% and is increased with mucosal inflammation or tumor infiltration

Distribution: V_{dss}: 0.7-1.6 L/kg; distributes into CSF

Protein binding: 8% to 13%

Metabolism: In the liver via oxidative desulfuration (cytochrome P450 microsomal enzyme system) primarily to TEPA (active metabolite)

Half-life, terminal:

Thiotepa: 109 minutes (51.6-212 minutes) with dose-dependent clearance

TEPA: 10-21 hours

Elimination: Very little thiotepa or active metabolite are excreted unchanged in urine (1.5% of thiotepa dose)

Usual Dosage Refer to individual protocols

Children:

I.V.: ABMT: One regimen uses 300 mg/m^2/dose; repeat every 24 hours for a total of 3 doses (see Finlay, 2008); maximum tolerated dose over 3 days: 900-1125 mg/m^2

Intrathecal: 5-11.5 mg/m^2 per dose weekly for 2-7 doses

Adults:

I.V.: Ovarian, breast cancer: 0.3-0.4 mg/kg by rapid I.V. administration every 1-4 weeks

Intracavitary: Effusions: 0.6-0.8 mg/kg

Intrathecal: Neoplastic meningitis: 10 mg twice a week for 4 weeks, then weekly for 4 weeks, then monthly for 4 doses (NCCN CNS cancer guidelines v.1.2009)

Intravesical: Bladder cancer: 60 mg in 30-60 mL NS retained for 2 hours once weekly for 4 weeks

Administration

Bladder instillation: Prepare with 60 mg diluted in 30-60 mL sterile water and instill by catheter and retain for 2 hours

Intrapleural or pericardial: Dose is further diluted to a volume of 10-20 mL in NS or D$_5$W

Intraperitoneal: Administration requires dilution in larger volumes (up to 2 L)

Intrathecal: Reconstitute drug with preservative-free SWI then dilute to a final concentration of 1 mg/mL with NS

I.V.: Filter through a 0.22 micron filter (Millex-GS or Gelman Sterile Acrodisc®) prior to administration; administer direct I.V. over 5 minutes at a final concentration of about 10 mg/mL; administer I.V. intermittent or continuous infusion at a final concentration for administration of 1 mg/mL (thiotepa may be further diluted in D$_5$W, NS, or LR)

Monitoring Parameters CBC with differential and platelet count, uric acid, urinalysis, renal and hepatic function tests

Patient Information Notify physician if fever, sore throat, urine color change, bleeding, or bruising occurs. Patients of childbearing potential should avoid becoming pregnant while on thiotepa therapy. Effective contraception should be used if either the patient or partner is of childbearing potential.

Nursing Implications Wear protective gloves during handling of thiotepa solution; if thiotepa solution comes in contact with skin or mucosa, the affected area should be washed with soap and water immediately or affected mucosa should be rinsed thoroughly with water.

Additional Information Myelosuppressive effects:

WBC: Moderate

Platelets: Severe

Onset (days): 7-10

Nadir (days): 14-20

Recovery (days): 28

Dosage Forms Excipient information presented when available (limited, particularly for generics); consult specific product labeling. [DSC] = Discontinued product

Injection, powder for reconstitution: 15 mg; 30 mg [DSC]

References

Fagioli F, Biasin E, Mastrodicasa L, et al, "High-Dose Thiotepa and Etoposide in Children With Poor-Prognosis Brain Tumors," *Cancer*, 2004, 100(10):2215-21.

Finlay JL, Dhall G, Boyett JM, et al, "Myeloablative Chemotherapy With Autologous Bone Marrow Rescue in Children and Adolescents With Recurrent Malignant Astrocytoma: Outcome Compared With Conventional Chemotherapy: A Report From the Children's Oncology Group," *Pediatr Blood Cancer*, 2008, 51(6):806-11.

Fisher PG, Kadan-Lottick NS, and Korones DN, "Intrathecal Thiotepa: Reappraisal of an Established Therapy," *J Pediatr Hematol Oncol*, 2002, 24(4):274-8.

Grovas AC, Boyett JM, Lindsley K, et al, "Regimen-Related Toxicity of Myeloablative Chemotherapy With BCNU, Thiotepa, and Etoposide Followed by Autologous Stem Cell Rescue for Children With Newly Diagnosed Glioblastoma Multiforme: Report From the Children's Cancer Group," *Med Pediatr Oncol*, 1999, 33(2):83-7.

Heideman R, Cole D, Balis F, et al, "Phase I and Pharmacokinetic Evaluation of Thiotepa in the Cerebrospinal Fluid and Plasma of Pediatric Patients: Evidence for Dose-Dependent Plasma Clearance of Thiotepa," *Cancer Res*, 1989, 49(3):736-41.

Herzig GP, "Phase I-II Studies of High-Dose Thiotepa and Autologous BMT in Patients With Refractory Malignancies," *Adv Cancer Chemotherapy*, 1987, 17-29 (proceedings of a symposium, Oct 1986)

National Comprehensive Cancer Network® (NCCN), "Clinical Practice Guidelines in Oncology™: Central Nervous System Cancers," Version 2.2009. Available at: http://www.nccn.org/professionals/physician_gls/PDF/cns.pdf.

Saarinen UM, Hovi L, and Makipern CA, "High Dose Thiotepa With Autologous Bone Marrow Rescue in Pediatric Solid Tumors," *Proc Am Soc Clin Oncol*, 1989, 8:303.

Thiothixene (thye oh THIKS een)

Medication Safety Issues

Sound-alike/look-alike issues:

Thiothixene may be confused with FLUoxetine, thioridazine

Navane® may be confused with Norvasc®, Nubain®

U.S. Brand Names Navane®

Canadian Brand Names Navane®

Therapeutic Category Antipsychotic Agent, Typical, Phenothiazine; Phenothiazine Derivative

Generic Available Yes

Use Management of schizophrenia (FDA approved in ages ≥12 years and adults); also used for management of psychotic disorders

Pregnancy Risk Factor C

Lactation Excretion in breast milk unknown/not recommended

Contraindications Hypersensitivity to thiothixene or any component; cross-sensitivity with other phenothiazines may exist; patients with CNS depression, comatose states, circulatory collapse, or blood dyscrasias; avoid use in patients with narrow-angle glaucoma, bone marrow suppression, severe liver or cardiac disease

Warnings May alter cardiac conduction; life-threatening arrhythmias have occurred with therapeutic doses of neuroleptics. May mask toxicity of other drugs or conditions (eg, intestinal obstruction, Reye's syndrome, brain tumor) due to antiemetic effects. Elevates prolactin levels; use with caution in patients with breast cancer or other prolactin-dependent tumors.

May cause extrapyramidal symptoms (EPS), including pseudoparkinsonism, acute dystonic reactions, akathisia, and tardive dyskinesia (risk of these reactions is high relative to other neuroleptics, and is dose-dependent; to decrease risk of tardive dyskinesia: Use smallest dose and shortest duration possible; evaluate continued need periodically; risk of dystonia is increased with the use of high potency and higher doses of conventional antipsychotics and in males and younger patients). Use may be associated with neuroleptic malignant syndrome (NMS); monitor for mental status changes, fever, muscle rigidity, and/or autonomic instability; risk may be increased in patients with Parkinson's disease or Lewy body dementia.

May cause pigmentary retinopathy, and lenticular and corneal deposits, particularly with prolonged therapy. May be sedating, use with caution in disorders in which CNS depression is a feature; patients must be cautioned about performing tasks which require mental alertness (eg, operating machinery or driving). Impaired core body temperature regulation may occur; caution with strenuous exercise, heat exposure, dehydration, and concomitant medication possessing anticholinergic effects. Thiothixene has not been evaluated for the treatment of behavioral complications in patients with mental retardation. Safety and efficacy have not been established in children <12 years of age.

Leukopenia, neutropenia, and agranulocytosis (sometimes fatal) have been reported in clinical trials and postmarketing reports with antipsychotic use; presence of risk factors (eg, pre-existing low WBC or history of drug-induced leuko/neutropenia) should prompt periodic blood count assessment. Discontinue therapy at first signs of blood dyscrasias or if absolute neutrophil count <1000/mm^3. Use is contraindicated in patients with blood dyscrasias.

An increased risk of death has been reported with the use of antipsychotics in elderly patients with dementia-related psychosis **[U.S. Boxed Warning]**; most deaths seemed to be cardiovascular (eg, sudden death, heart failure) or infectious (eg, pneumonia) in nature; thiothixene is not approved for this indication.

Precautions Use with caution in patients with cardiovascular disease or seizures

Adverse Reactions Sedation and extrapyramidal effects occur more often.

Cardiovascular: Arrhythmias, hypotension (especially with parenteral use), orthostatic hypotension, tachycardia

Central nervous system: Altered central temperature regulation, anxiety, drowsiness, extrapyramidal reactions, insomnia, neuroleptic malignant syndrome, restlessness, sedation, seizures, tardive dyskinesia

Dermatologic: Photosensitivity, rash

Endocrine & metabolic: Amenorrhea, galactorrhea, gynecomastia, weight gain

Gastrointestinal: Constipation, GI upset, xerostomia

Genitourinary: Urinary retention

Hematologic: Agranulocytosis, leukopenia, leukocytosis (usually transient), neutropenia

Ocular: Blurred vision, retinal pigmentation

Drug Interactions

Metabolism/Transport Effects Substrate of CYP1A2 (major); **Inhibits** CYP2D6 (weak)

Avoid Concomitant Use

Avoid concomitant use of Thiothixene with any of the following: Artemether; Dronedarone; Lumefantrine; Metoclopramide; Nilotinib; Pimozide; QuiNINE; Tetrabenazine; Thioridazine; Ziprasidone

Increased Effect/Toxicity

Thiothixene may increase the levels/effects of: Alcohol (Ethyl); Anticholinergics; Anti-Parkinson's Agents (Dopamine Agonist); CNS Depressants; Dronedarone; Pimozide; QTc-Prolonging Agents; QuiNINE; Tetrabenazine; Thioridazine; Ziprasidone

The levels/effects of Thiothixene may be increased by: Acetylcholinesterase Inhibitors (Central); Alfuzosin; Artemether; Chloroquine; Ciprofloxacin; Ciprofloxacin (Systemic); CYP1A2 Inhibitors (Moderate); CYP1A2 Inhibitors (Strong); Gadobutrol; Lithium formulations; Lumefantrine; Metoclopramide; Nilotinib; Pramlintide; QuiNINE; Tetrabenazine

Decreased Effect

Thiothixene may decrease the levels/effects of: Amphetamines; Quinagolide

The levels/effects of Thiothixene may be decreased by: Anti-Parkinson's Agents (Dopamine Agonist); CYP1A2 Inducers (Strong); Lithium formulations

Food Interactions May cause increase in dietary riboflavin requirements

Mechanism of Action Elicits antipsychotic activity by postsynaptic blockade of CNS dopamine receptors resulting in inhibition of dopamine-mediated effects; also has alpha-adrenergic blocking activity

Usual Dosage Oral:

Children <12 years: Dose not well established (use not recommended); 0.25 mg/kg/day in divided doses
Children ≥12 years and Adults: Initial: 2 mg 3 times/day, up to 20-30 mg/day; maximum dose: 60 mg/day

Administration Oral: Administer with food or water

Monitoring Parameters Periodic eye exam, CBC with differential, blood pressure, liver enzyme tests

Patient Information Avoid alcohol; limit caffeine; may cause drowsiness and impair ability to perform activities requiring mental alertness or physical coordination; may cause dry mouth. May cause photosensitivity reactions (eg, exposure to sunlight may cause severe sunburn, skin rash, redness, or itching); avoid exposure to sunlight and artificial light sources (sunlamps, tanning booth/bed); wear protective clothing, wide-brimmed hats, sunglasses, and lip sunscreen (SPF ≥15); use a sunscreen [broad-spectrum sunscreen or physical sunscreen (preferred) or sunblock with SPF ≥15]; contact physician if reaction occurs.

Dosage Forms Excipient information presented when available (limited, particularly for generics); consult specific product labeling. [DSC] = Discontinued product

Capsule: 1 mg, 2 mg, 5 mg, 10 mg
Navane®: 1 mg [DSC], 2 mg, 5 mg, 10 mg, 20 mg

References

Wiener JM, "Psychopharmacology in Childhood Disorders," *Psychiatr Clin North Am*, 1984, 7(4):831-43.

♦ **Thorazine** *see* ChlorproMAZINE *on page 298*

♦ **Thorets [OTC]** *see* Benzocaine *on page 182*

♦ **Thrombi-Gel®** *see* Thrombin (Topical) *on page 1345*

♦ **Thrombin-JMI®** *see* Thrombin (Topical) *on page 1345*

♦ **Thrombin-JMI® Epistaxis Kit** *see* Thrombin (Topical) *on page 1345*

♦ **Thrombin-JMI® Spray Kit** *see* Thrombin (Topical) *on page 1345*

♦ **Thrombin-JMI® Syringe Spray Kit** *see* Thrombin (Topical) *on page 1345*

Thrombin (Topical) (THROM bin, TOP i kal)

Medication Safety Issues

Administration: For topical use only. Do not administer intravenously or intra-arterially.

To reduce the risk of intravascular administration, the Institute for Safe Medication Practices (ISMP) has the following recommendations:

• Prepare, label, and dispense topical thrombin from the pharmacy department (including doses used in the operating room).

• Do not leave vial or syringe at bedside.

• Add auxiliary label to all labels and syringes stating "For topical use only - do not inject".

• When appropriate, use solutions which can be applied with an absorbable gelatin sponge or use a dry form on oozing surfaces.

• When appropriate, use spray kits to help differentiate between parenteral products.

U.S. Brand Names Evithrom™; Recothrom™; Thrombi-Gel®; Thrombi-Pad®; Thrombin-JMI®; Thrombin-JMI® Epistaxis Kit; Thrombin-JMI® Spray Kit; Thrombin-JMI® Syringe Spray Kit

Therapeutic Category Hemostatic Agent

Generic Available No

Use Hemostasis whenever minor bleeding from capillaries and small venules is accessible

Thrombi-Gel®; Thrombi-Pad®: Temporary control as trauma dressing for moderate-to-severe bleeding wounds; control of surface bleeding from vascular access sites and percutaneous catheter/ tubes

Pregnancy Risk Factor C

Pregnancy Considerations Adequate reproduction studies have not been conducted. Reproduction studies conducted with the solvent/detergent used in processing the human-derived product showed adverse events in animals. Only residual levels of the solvent/detergent would be expected to remain in the finished product.

Contraindications Hypersensitivity to thrombin or any component; not to be injected directly into circulatory system; Evithrom™ is contraindicated for the treatment of massive or brisk arterial bleeding and in patients with a known anaphylactic or severe systemic reaction to blood products; Recothrom™ is contraindicated for the treatment of severe or brisk arterial bleeding and in patients with hypersensitivity to hamster or snake proteins; Thrombin-JMI® and Thrombi-Pad® are contraindicated in patients with hypersensitivity to material of bovine origin; Thrombi-Gel® should not be used in closure of skin incisions due to possible interference with healing of skin edges

Warnings For topical use only - do not inject; injection may result in extensive intravascular clotting and death. Use of bovine-source topical thrombin has been associated with abnormalities in hemostasis ranging from asymptomatic alterations in PT and PTT to severe bleeding or thrombosis which have rarely been fatal **[U.S. Boxed Warning]**. These hemostatic effects may be related to formation of antibodies against bovine thrombin and/or factor V which in some cases may cross react with human factor V resulting in factor V deficiency; patients with antibodies to bovine thrombin should not receive topical thrombin again. Thrombi-Gel®, Thrombi-Pad® should not be used in the presence of infection; use caution in areas of contamination. Thrombi-Pad® is nonabsorbable and should not be left in the body.

Adverse Reactions

Central nervous system: Fever
Local: Incision site complication
Miscellaneous: Allergic reactions

Drug Interactions

Avoid Concomitant Use There are no known interactions where it is recommended to avoid concomitant use.

Increased Effect/Toxicity There are no known significant interactions involving an increase in effect.

Decreased Effect There are no known significant interactions involving a decrease in effect.

Stability

Evithrom™: Store frozen vials at -18°C for up to 2 years; unopened vials may be stored at 2°C to 8°C for up to 30 days; stable at room temperature for 24 hours; do not refreeze after thawing; do not refrigerate once at room temperature.

Recothrom™: Store at room temperature; reconstituted solutions may be stored refrigerated for 24 hours.

Thrombi-Gel®: Store at 2°C to 25°C (36°F to 77°F). After wetting with SWI or 0.9% sodium chloride, use within 3 hours.

Thrombi-Pad®: Store at 2°C to 25°C (36°F to 77°F). If pad is wetted with 0.9% sodium chloride, use within 1 hour.

Thrombi-JMI®: Store vials at room temperature; reconstituted vials may be stored in refrigerator for 24 hours or at room temperature for 8 hours.

Mechanism of Action Activates platelets and catalyzes the conversion of fibrinogen to fibrin

Usual Dosage Topical: Hemostasis:

Powder or solution formulations: Apply 1000-2000 units/mL solution directly or via absorbable gelatin sponge to the site of bleeding or oozing surface; Thrombin-JMI® may also be applied in dry powder form directly to the site. For general use in plastic surgery, dental extractions, skin grafting, etc, solutions containing approximately 100 units/mL are frequently used.

Thrombi-Gel®10, 40, 100: Adults: Wet product with up to 3 mL, 10 mL, or 20 mL, respectively, of 0.9% sodium chloride or SWI; apply directly over source of the bleeding with manual pressure

Thrombi-Pad®: Adults: Apply pad directly over source of bleeding. May apply dry or wetted with up to 10 mL of 0.9% sodium chloride. If desired, product may be left in place for up to 24 hours; do not leave in the body

Administration Not for injection

Topical: Powder or solution formulations: May be applied directly as a powder (Thrombin-JMI®) or as reconstituted solution; the most effective hemostasis results when the thrombin mixes freely with blood as it appears; use NS to reconstitute powder to 1000-2000 units/mL concentration; (Evithrom™ must be thawed prior to use and requires no further dilution). The recipient surface should be sponged (not wiped) free of blood before application; do not sponge **treated** surfaces to assure that clot remains securely in place. Refer to manufacturer's information for more specific application information.

Pad or sponge formulations: May cut or roll Thrombi-Gel® to desired shape prior to wetting; once wetted and prior to applying, knead thoroughly to saturate the pad remove trapped air bubbles. Thrombi-Pad® may be applied dry or wet.

Additional Information One unit is amount required to clot 1 mL of standardized fibrinogen solution in 15 seconds

Dosage Forms Excipient information presented when available (limited, particularly for generics); consult specific product labeling.

Pad, topical [preservative free; bovine derived]:
Thrombi-Pad® 3x3: ≥200 units

Powder for reconstitution, topical [bovine derived]:
Thrombi-JMI®: 5000 int. units, 20,000 int. units
Thrombi-JMI® Epistaxis kit: 5000 int. units
Thrombi-JMI® Spray Kit: 20,000 int. units
Thrombi-JMI® Syringe Spray Kit: 20,000 int. units

Powder for reconstitution, topical [preservative free; recombinant]:
Recothrom™: 5000 int. units; 20,000 int. units

Solution, topical [human derived]:
Evithrom™: 800-1200 int. units/mL (2 mL, 5 mL, 20 mL)

Sponge, topical [preservative free; bovine derived]:
Thrombi-Gel® 10: ≥1000 units (10s)
Thrombi-Gel® 40: ≥1000 units (5s)
Thrombi-Gel® 100: ≥2000 units (5s)

◆ **Thrombi-Pad®** *see* Thrombin (Topical) *on page 1345*

◆ **Thymocyte Stimulating Factor** *see* Aldesleukin *on page 60*

◆ **Thymoglobulin®** *see* Antithymocyte Globulin (Rabbit) *on page 120*

◆ **ThyroSafe™ [OTC]** *see* Potassium Iodide *on page 1138*

◆ **ThyroShield™ [OTC]** *see* Potassium Iodide *on page 1138*

◆ **Tiabendazole** *see* Thiabendazole *on page 1337*

TiaGABine (tye AG a bene)

Medication Safety Issues
Sound-alike/look-alike issues:
TiaGABine may be confused with tiZANidine

U.S. Brand Names Gabitril®

Canadian Brand Names Gabitril®

Therapeutic Category Anticonvulsant, Miscellaneous

Generic Available No

Use Adjunctive therapy in the treatment of partial seizures (FDA approved in ages ≥12 years and adults)

Pregnancy Risk Factor C

Pregnancy Considerations Patients exposed to tiagabine during pregnancy are encouraged to enroll themselves into the AED Pregnancy Registry by calling 1-888-233-2334. Additional information is available at www.aedpregnancyregistry.org.

Lactation Enters breast milk/not recommended

Contraindications Hypersensitivity to tiagabine or any component

Warnings Current tiagabine dosing recommendations are based on studies in which most patients also received enzyme-inducing AEDs. Use of recommended tiagabine doses in patients **not** receiving enzyme-inducing AEDs may result in serum concentrations more than twice that of patients receiving enzyme-inducing AEDs. Use with caution and decrease the dose in patients who are **not** receiving enzyme-inducing AEDs; a slower titration of the drug may also be required in these patients.

New-onset seizures and status epilepticus have been reported with tiagabine use (for unlabeled indications) in patients without epilepsy. Higher doses may be a risk factor, but seizures have occurred in patients taking doses as low as 4 mg/day. Seizures have also occurred shortly after a dosage increase. In most cases, patients were also receiving concomitant medications that are thought to lower the seizure threshold (eg, antidepressants, antipsychotics, stimulants, narcotics). Discontinue tiagabine and evaluate patients for an underlying seizure disorder in nonepileptic patients who develop seizures while receiving tiagabine.

When used to treat epilepsy, do not abruptly discontinue therapy; withdraw gradually to lessen chance for increased seizure frequency (unless a more rapid withdrawal is required due to safety concerns). Cognitive and neuropsychiatric adverse effects may occur (see Adverse Reactions). Exacerbation of EEG abnormalities associated with CNS adverse events (cognitive and neuropsychiatric) may occur in patients with an EEG history of spike and wave discharges and may require dosage adjustment.

Nonconvulsant status epilepticus has also been reported and may respond to dosage reduction or discontinuation. Seizures and status epilepticus may also occur with tiagabine overdose.

Antiepileptic drugs (AEDs) increase the risk of suicidal behavior and ideation in patients receiving these medications for any indication. Pooled analyses of placebo-controlled trials involving 11 different AEDs (regardless of indication) showed a twofold increased risk of suicidal thoughts or behavior (estimated incidence rate: 0.43% in AED treated patients compared to 0.24% of patients receiving placebo); increased risk was observed as early as 1 week after initiation of AED and continued through duration of trials (most trials ≤24 weeks); risk did not vary significantly by age (age range: 5–100 years). Consider risks and benefits of AEDs before prescribing. Monitor all patients receiving an AED for emergence of suicidal thoughts or behavior, thoughts of self-harm, any unusual changes in behavior or mood, or the emergence or worsening of depressive symptoms; notify healthcare provider immediately if symptoms or concerning behavior occur. **Note:** The FDA is requiring that a Medication Guide be developed for all antiepileptic drugs informing patients of this risk.

Precautions Use with caution in patients with hepatic impairment. Possible long-term ophthalmologic effects exist (more studies are needed). Use with caution with alcohol or other CNS depressants. Safety and effectiveness have not been established in children <12 years of age or for any indication other than as adjunctive therapy for partial seizures.

Adverse Reactions

Central nervous system: Impaired concentration, speech/language problems, confusion, somnolence, fatigue, dizziness, nervousness, depression, ataxia, insomnia, emotional lability, headache; suicidal thinking and behavior (see Warnings)

Gastrointestinal: Nausea, abdominal pain, diarrhea

Neuromuscular & skeletal: Asthenia, tremor

Drug Interactions

Metabolism/Transport Effects Substrate of 3A4 (major)

Avoid Concomitant Use There are no known interactions where it is recommended to avoid concomitant use.

Increased Effect/Toxicity

TiaGABine may increase the levels/effects of: Alcohol (Ethyl); CNS Depressants; Methotrimeprazine

The levels/effects of TiaGABine may be increased by: CYP3A4 Inhibitors (Moderate); CYP3A4 Inhibitors (Strong); Dasatinib; Methotrimeprazine

Decreased Effect

The levels/effects of TiaGABine may be decreased by: CYP3A4 Inducers (Strong); Deferasirox; Herbs (CYP3A4 Inducers); Ketorolac; Ketorolac (Systemic); Mefloquine

Food Interactions Food may decrease the rate but not the extent of absorption

Stability Protect from moisture and light; store at room temperature

Mechanism of Action Exact mechanism unknown; thought to potentiate the action of GABA (an inhibitory neurotransmitter) by selectively binding to the GABA uptake carrier and blocking GABA uptake into presynaptic neurons. This allows more GABA to be available at its site of action to bind to postsynaptic neuronal receptors.

Pharmacokinetics (Adult data unless noted)

Absorption: Rapid and nearly complete (>95%)

Distribution: Mean V_d:

Children 3-10 years: 2.4 L/kg

Adults: 1.3-1.6 L/kg

Note: V_d values are more similar between children and adults when expressed as L/m^2 (see Gustavson, 1997)

Protein binding: 96%, mainly to albumin and alpha$_1$-acid glycoprotein

Metabolism: Extensive in the liver via oxidation and glucuronidation; undergoes enterohepatic recirculation

Bioavailability: Oral: 90%

Diurnal effect: Trough concentrations and AUC are lower in the evening versus morning

Half-life:

Children 3-10 years: Mean: 5.7 hours (range: 2-10 hours)

Children 3-10 years receiving enzyme-inducing AEDs: Mean: 3.2 hours (range: 2-7.8 hours)

Adults (normal volunteers): 7-9 hours

Adult patients receiving enzyme-inducing AEDs: 2-5 hours

Time to peak serum concentration: Fasting state: ~45 minutes

Elimination: ~2% excreted unchanged in urine; 25% excreted in urine and 63% excreted in feces as metabolites

Clearance:

Children 3-10 years: 4.2 ± 1.6 mL/minute/kg

Children 3-10 years receiving enzyme-inducing AEDs: 8.6 ± 3.3 mL/minute/kg

Adults (normal volunteers): 109 mL/minute

Adult patients: 1.9 ± 0.5 mL/minute/kg

Adult patients receiving enzyme-inducing AEDs: 6.3 ± 3.5 mL/minute/kg

Note: Clearance values are more similar between children and adults when expressed as $mL/minute/m^2$ (see Gustavson, 1997)

Hepatic impairment: Clearance of unbound drug is decreased by 60%

Usual Dosage Oral: **Note:** Doses were determined in patients receiving enzyme-inducing AEDs; use of these doses in patients **not** receiving enzyme-inducing AEDs may result in serum concentrations more than twice those of patients receiving enzyme-inducing AEDS; **lower doses are required in patients not receiving enzyme-inducing agents;** a slower titration may also be necessary in these patients. Consider tiagabine dosage adjustment if enzyme-inducing agent is added, discontinued, or dose is changed. Do **not** use loading doses of tiagabine in any patient; do **not** use a rapid dosage escalation or increase the dose in large increments.

Children <12 years: Only limited preliminary information is available; dosing guidelines are not established (see Adkins, 1998 and Pellock, 1999)

Children 12-18 years: Initial: 4 mg once daily for 1 week, then 8 mg/day given in 2 divided doses for 1 week, then increase weekly by 4-8 mg/day; administer in 2-4 divided doses per day; titrate dose to response; maximum dose: 32 mg/day (doses >32 mg/day have been used in select adolescent patients for short periods of time)

Adults: Initial: 4 mg once daily for 1 week, then increase weekly by 4-8 mg/day; administer in 2-4 divided doses per day; titrate dose to response; usual maintenance: 32-56 mg/day in 2-4 divided doses; maximum dose: 56 mg/day. **Note:** Twice daily dosing may not be well tolerated and dosing 3 times/day is the currently favored dosing frequency (see Kalviainen, 1998).

Dosing adjustment in renal impairment: None needed

Dosing adjustment in hepatic impairment: Reduced doses and longer dosing intervals may be required

Administration Oral: Administer with food (to avoid rapid increase in plasma concentrations and adverse CNS effects)

Monitoring Parameters Seizure frequency, duration, and severity; signs and symptoms of suicidality (eg, anxiety, depression, behavior changes) (see Warnings)

Reference Range Not established

Patient Information May cause dizziness or drowsiness and impair ability to perform activities requiring mental alertness or physical coordination. If a dose is missed, do not increase or double the next dose; if multiple doses are missed, contact your healthcare provider for possible retitration of the dose as clinically needed. Do not discontinue abruptly (an increase in seizure activity may result). Antiepileptic agents may increase the risk of suicidal thoughts and behavior; notify physician if you feel more depressed or have thoughts of suicide or self-harm (see Warnings). Report worsening of seizure activity or loss of seizure control.

Additional Information Population pharmacokinetic analysis suggests that tiagabine may be administered at similar doses without adjustment for age, gender, or body weight in epilepsy patients ≥11 years of age (see Samara, 1998)

Dosage Forms Excipient information presented when available (limited, particularly for generics); consult specific product labeling.

Tablet, as hydrochloride:
Gabitril®: 2 mg, 4 mg, 12 mg, 16 mg

Extemporaneous Preparations

A 1 mg/mL tiagabine hydrochloride oral suspension made from tablets and a 1:1 mixture of Ora-Sweet® and Ora-Plus® was stable for 10 weeks when stored at room temperature (25°C) or for 13 weeks when stored under refrigeration (4°C) in amber plastic prescription bottles (Nahata, 2003). Grind ten 12 mg tablets in a mortar into a fine powder; add a small amount of the vehicle and mix well to form a uniform paste; mix while adding the vehicle in geometric proportions to **almost** 120 mL; transfer to a graduate; rinse the mortar with the vehicle and transfer to the graduate; qsad with vehicle to make 120 mL; label "shake well" and "refrigerate" (Nahata, 2004).

A 1 mg/mL suspension made from tablets and a 6:1 mixture of simple syrup, NF and 1% methylcellulose was stable for 6 weeks when stored at room temperature (25°C) and for 13 weeks when stored under refrigeration (4°C) in amber prescription bottles (Nahata, 2003). Grind ten 12 mg tablets in a mortar into a fine powder; add 17 mL of 1% methylcellulose gel and mix well to obtain a uniform paste; mix while adding simple syrup, NF in geometric proportions to **almost** 120 mL; transfer to a graduate; rinse the mortar with syrup and transfer to the graduate; qsad with syrup to 120 mL; label "shake well" and "refrigerate" (Nahata, 2004).

Nahata MC and Morosco RS, "Stability of Tiagabine in Two Oral Liquid Vehicles," *Am J Health-Syst Pharm*, 2003, 60: 75-77.

Nahata MC, Pai VB, and Hipple TF, *Pediatric Drug Formulations*, 5th ed, Cincinnati, OH: Harvey Whitney Books Co, 2004.

References
Adkins JC and Noble S, "Tiagabine. A Review of Its Pharmacodynamic and Pharmacokinetic Properties and Therapeutic Potential in the Management of Epilepsy," *Drugs*, 1998, 55(3):437-60.
Gustavson LE, Boellner SW, Granneman GR, et al, "A Single-Dose Study to Define Tiagabine Pharmacokinetics in Pediatric Patients With Complex Partial Seizures," *Neurology*, 1997, 48(4):1032-7.
Kalviainen R, Brodie MJ, Duncan J, et al, "A Double-Blind, Placebo-Controlled Trial of Tiagabine Given Three-Times Daily as Add-On Therapy for Refractory Partial Seizures. Northern European Tiagabine Study Group," *Epilepsy Res*, 1998, 30(1):31-40.
Leach JP and Brodie MJ, "Tiagabine," *Lancet*, 1998, 351(9097):203-7.
Pellock JM, "Managing Pediatric Epilepsy Syndromes With New Antiepileptic Drugs," *Pediatrics*, 1999, 104(5 Pt 1):1106-16.
Samara EE, Gustavson LE, El-Shourbagy T, et al, "Population Analysis of the Pharmacokinetics of Tiagabine in Patients With Epilepsy," *Epilespy*, 1998, 39(8):868-73.

♦ **Tiagabine Hydrochloride** *see* TiaGABine *on page 1346*

♦ **Tiamol® (Can)** *see* Fluocinonide *on page 595*

♦ **Tiazac®** *see* Diltiazem *on page 443*

♦ **Tiazac® XC (Can)** *see* Diltiazem *on page 443*

Ticarcillin and Clavulanate Potassium

(tye kar SIL in & klav yoo LAN ate poe TASS ee um)

U.S. Brand Names Timentin®
Canadian Brand Names Timentin®
Therapeutic Category Antibiotic, Beta-lactam and Beta-lactamase Combination; Antibiotic, Penicillin (Antipseudomonal)
Generic Available No
Use Treatment of infections caused by susceptible organisms involving the lower respiratory tract, urinary tract, skin and skin structures, bone and joint, gynecologic, intra-abdominal infections, and septicemia (FDA approved in ages ≥3 months and adults). Clavulanate expands activity of ticarcillin to include beta-lactamase producing strains of *S. aureus*, *H. influenzae*, *Moraxella catarrhalis*, *B. fragilis*, *Klebsiella*, *Prevotella*, *P. aeruginosa*, *Stenotrophomonas maltophilia*, *E. coli*, and *Proteus* species
Pregnancy Risk Factor B
Pregnancy Considerations Adverse events were not observed in animal reproduction studies; therefore, ticarcillin/clavulanate is classified as pregnancy category B. Ticarcillin and clavulanate cross the placenta. Human experience with the penicillins during pregnancy has shown no evidence of adverse effects to the fetus. Ticarcillin/clavulanate is approved for the treatment of postpartum gynecologic infections, including endometritis, caused by susceptible organisms.
Lactation Enters breast milk/use caution
Breast-Feeding Considerations Small amounts of ticarcillin are found in breast milk; however, it is not orally-absorbed. The AAP considers ticarcillin alone to be "usually compatible with breast-feeding."

Based on available data for ticarcillin, ticarcillin/clavulanate is generally considered compatible (low risk to infant) while breast-feeding [human data].
Contraindications Hypersensitivity to ticarcillin, clavulanate, any of the penicillins, or any component
Warnings Seizures, abnormal platelet aggregation, and prolonged bleeding have been reported in patients with renal impairment receiving high doses; prolonged use may result in superinfection including *C. difficile*-associated diarrhea and pseudomembranous colitis. Severe anaphylactic reactions have been reported in patients receiving ticarcillin and clavulanate; be prepared to treat anaphylaxis when administering Timentin®
Precautions Use with caution and modify dosage in patients with renal impairment; use with caution in patients with heart failure due to high sodium content of the formulation and in patients with pre-existing seizure disorder. Use an alternative agent in patients with meningeal seeding from a distant infection site, in whom meningitis is suspected or documented, or in patients who require prophylaxis against central nervous system infection.

Adverse Reactions

Central nervous system: Chills, fever, headache, seizures (see Warnings)

Dermatologic: Erythema multiforme, pruritus, rash, Stevens-Johnson syndrome, toxic epidermal necrolysis, urticaria

Endocrine & metabolic: Hypernatremia, hypokalemia, metabolic alkalosis

Gastrointestinal: Diarrhea, epigastric pain, nausea, pseudomembranous colitis, stomatitis, vomiting

Genitourinary: Cystitis, hematuria, hemorrhagic cystitis (rare)

Hematologic: Eosinophilia, hemoglobin and hematocrit decreased, hemolytic anemia, inhibition of platelet aggregation (see Warnings), leukopenia, neutropenia, prolongation of bleeding time, thrombocytopenia

Hepatic: ALT and AST increased, cholestatic jaundice, hepatitis, serum bilirubin and alkaline phophatase increased

Local: Burning, pain, swelling, thrombophlebitis

Neuromuscular & skeletal: Arthralgia, myalgia

Renal: BUN increased, serum creatinine increased

Miscellaneous: Hypersensitivity reactions including anaphylaxis, superinfection (see Warnings)

Drug Interactions

Avoid Concomitant Use

Avoid concomitant use of Ticarcillin and Clavulanate Potassium with any of the following: BCG

Increased Effect/Toxicity

Ticarcillin and Clavulanate Potassium may increase the levels/effects of: Methotrexate

The levels/effects of Ticarcillin and Clavulanate Potassium may be increased by: Probenecid

Decreased Effect

Ticarcillin and Clavulanate Potassium may decrease the levels/effects of: Aminoglycosides; BCG; Mycophenolate; Typhoid Vaccine

The levels/effects of Ticarcillin and Clavulanate Potassium may be decreased by: Fusidic Acid; Tetracycline Derivatives

Stability Reconstituted 200 mg/mL solution is stable for 6 hours at room temperature and 72 hours when refrigerated; reconstituted 200 mg/mL solution further diluted in D_5W or NS to 10-100 mg/mL is stable for 24 hours at room temperature. Solution diluted in D_5W is stable 3 days if refrigerated; solution diluted in NS is stable 7 days if refrigerated; darkening of drug indicates loss of potency of clavulanate potassium; incompatible with sodium bicarbonate and aminoglycosides

Premixed solution: Store frozen; thawed solution is stable for 24 hours at room temperature or 7 days under refrigeration; do not refreeze

Mechanism of Action Ticarcillin inhibits bacterial cell wall synthesis by binding to one or more of the penicillin-binding proteins; inhibits the final transpeptidation step of peptidoglycan synthesis in bacterial cell walls; clavulanic acid inhibits degradation of ticarcillin by binding to beta-lactamases

Pharmacokinetics (Adult data unless noted)

Distribution: Ticarcillin is distributed into tissue, interstitial fluid, pleural fluid, bile, and breast milk; low concentrations of ticarcillin distribute into the CSF but increase when meninges are inflamed

V_{dss} ticarcillin: 0.22 L/kg

V_{dss} clavulanic acid: 0.4 L/kg

Protein binding:

Ticarcillin: 45% to 65%

Clavulanic acid: 9% to 30%

Metabolism: Clavulanic acid is metabolized in the liver

Half-life: In patients with normal renal function

Neonates:

Clavulanic acid: 1.9 hours

Ticarcillin: 4.4 hours

Children (1 month to 9.3 years):

Clavulanic acid: 54 minutes

Ticarcillin: 66 minutes

Adults:

Clavulanic acid: 66-90 minutes

Ticarcillin: 66-72 minutes; 13 hours (in patients with renal failure)

Clavulanic acid does not affect the clearance of ticarcillin

Elimination:

Children: 71% of the ticarcillin and 50% of the clavulanic acid dose are excreted unchanged in the urine over 4 hours

Adults: 35% to 45% of clavulanate is excreted unchanged in urine, whereas 60% to 70% of ticarcillin is excreted unchanged in urine over 6 hours

Dialysis: Removed by hemodialysis

Usual Dosage I.V.: (**Note:** Timentin® (ticarcillin/clavulanate) is a combination product; each 3.1 g vial contains 3 g ticarcillin disodium and 0.1 g clavulanic acid. Dosage recommendations are based on **ticarcillin** component):

Neonates 0-4 weeks: <1200 g: 150 mg/kg/day divided every 12 hours

Postnatal age <1 week:

1200-2000 g: 150 mg/kg/day divided every 12 hours

>2000 g: 225 mg/kg/day divided every 8 hours

Postnatal age ≥1 week:

1200-2000 g: 225 mg/kg/day divided every 8 hours

>2000 g: 300 mg/kg/day divided every 8 hours

Infants ≥3 months and Children <60 kg:

Mild to moderate infection: 200 mg/kg/day divided every 6 hours

Severe infections that occur outside the CNS: 200-300 mg/kg/day in divided doses every 4-6 hours; maximum dose: 400 mg/kg/day not to exceed 18-24 g/day

Adults ≥60 kg: 3 g every 4-6 hours; maximum dose: 18-24 g/day. Usual duration of therapy is 10-14 days; however, more prolonged therapy may be required in the treatment of complicated infections.

Urinary tract infections: 3 g every 6-8 hours

Dosing adjustment in renal impairment: Adults: (**Note:** Dosage recommendations are based on **ticarcillin** component):

Cl_{cr} 30-60 mL/minute: 2 g every 4 hours or 3 g every 8 hours

Cl_{cr} 10-30 mL/minute: 2 g every 8 hours or 3 g every 12 hours

Cl_{cr} <10 mL/minute: 2 g every 12 hours

CVVH: Dose as for Cl_{cr} 10-50 mL/minute

Hemodialysis: 2 g every 12 hours; supplement with 3 g after each dialysis

Peritoneal Dialysis: 3 g every 12 hours

Dosing in hepatic impairment and a Cl_{cr} <10 mL/minute: Administer 2 g every 24 hours

Administration Parenteral: Administer by I.V. intermittent infusion over 30 minutes; final concentration for administration should not exceed 100 mg/mL of ticarcillin; however, concentrations ≤50 mg/mL are preferred; if the patient is on concurrent aminoglycoside therapy, separate ticarcillin and clavulanate potassium administration from the aminoglycoside by at least 30-60 minutes (mixing of Timentin® with an aminoglycoside can result in inactivation of the aminoglycoside)

Monitoring Parameters Serum electrolytes, periodic renal, hepatic and hematologic function tests; observe I.V. injection site for signs of extravasation

Test Interactions Positive Coombs' [direct], false-positive urinary and serum proteins

Patient Information Notify physician if watery and bloody stools occur.

Additional Information

Sodium content of 1 g: 4.51 mEq

Potassium content of 1 g: 0.15 mEq

Dosage Forms Excipient information presented when available (limited, particularly for generics); consult specific product labeling.

Infusion [premixed, frozen]: Ticarcillin 3 g and clavulanic acid 0.1 g (100 mL) [contains sodium 4.51 mEq and potassium 0.15 mEq per g]

Injection, powder for reconstitution: Ticarcillin 3 g and clavulanic acid 0.1 g (3.1 g, 31 g) [contains sodium 4.51 mEq and potassium 0.15 mEq per g]

References

Begue P, Quiniou F, Quinet B, "Efficacy and Pharmacokinetics of Timentin® in Paediatric Infections," *J Antimicrob Chemother*, 1986, 17 (Suppl C):81-91.

Krueger TS, Clark EA, and Nix DE, "*In vitro* Susceptibility of *Stenotrophomonas maltophilia* to Various Antimicrobial Combinations," *Diagn Microbiol Infect Dis*, 2001, 41(1-2):71-8.

Nicodemo AC and Paez JI, "Antimicrobial Therapy for *Stenotrophomonas maltophilia* Infections," *Eur J Clin Microbiol Infect Dis*, 2007, 26 (4):229-37.

Reed MD, Yamashita TS, and Blumer JL, "Pharmacokinetic-Based Ticarcillin/Clavulanic Acid Dose Recommendations for Infants and Children," *J Clin Pharmacol*, 1995, 35(7):658-65.

Stutman HR and Marks MI, "Review of Pediatric Antimicrobial Therapies," *Semin Pediatr Infect Dis*, 1991, 2:3-17.

◆ **Ticarcillin and Clavulanic Acid** *see* Ticarcillin and Clavulanate Potassium *on page 1348*

◆ **Ticarcillin Disodium and Clavulanate Potassium** *see* Ticarcillin and Clavulanate Potassium *on page 1348*

◆ **TIG** *see* Tetanus Immune Globulin (Human) *on page 1328*

◆ **Tigan®** *see* Trimethobenzamide *on page 1385*

Tigecycline (tye ge SYE kleen)

U.S. Brand Names Tygacil®
Canadian Brand Names Tygacil®
Therapeutic Category Antibiotic, Glycylcycline
Generic Available No
Use Treatment of complicated skin and skin structure infections caused by susceptible organisms, including *E. coli, S. agalactiae, S. anginosus* group, *S. pyogenes, B. fragilis*, methicillin-resistant *S. aureus*, vancomycin-susceptible *E. faecalis, E. cloacae, K. pneumoniae*, and rapidly-growing mycobacteria; treatment of complicated intra-abdominal infections (eg, appendicitis, cholecystitis, peritonitis, liver abscess) caused by susceptible organisms; treatment of community-acquired pneumonia caused by susceptible organisms, including *S. pneumoniae* (penicillin-susceptible isolates), *H. influenzae* (beta-lactamase negative isolates), and *L. pneumophila* (FDA approved in ages >18 years and adults). **Note:** Not indicated for the treatment of hospital-acquired pneumonia (HAP), including ventilator-associated pneumonia (VAP). Subgroup of patients with ventilator-associated pneumonia who received tigecycline demonstrated inferior efficacy, including lower cure rates and increased mortality than the comparator group.
Pregnancy Risk Factor D
Pregnancy Considerations Because adverse effects were observed in animals and because of the potential for permanent tooth discoloration, tigecycline is classified pregnancy category D. Tigecycline frequently causes nausea and vomiting and, therefore, may not be ideal for use in a patient with pregnancy-related nausea.
Lactation Excretion in breast milk unknown/use caution
Breast-Feeding Considerations It is not known if tigecycline is found in breast milk. The manufacturer recommends caution if giving tigecycline to a nursing woman. Nondose-related effects could include modification of bowel flora.
Contraindications Hypersensitivity to tigecycline or any component
Warnings Life-threatening anaphylaxis/anaphylactoid reactions have been reported; use caution in patients with known tetracycline hypersensitivity. May cause fetal harm if used during pregnancy; patients should be advised of potential risks associated with use. Due to structural similarity with tetracyclines, permanent discoloration of teeth (brown-yellow-gray) may occur if used during tooth development (fetal stage through children up to 8 years of age); use may be associated with photosensitivity, pseudotumor cerebri, pancreatitis, and antianabolic effects

(including increased BUN, azotemia, acidosis, and hyperphosphatemia). Prolonged use may result in fungal or bacterial superinfection, including *C. difficile*-associated diarrhea or pseudomembranous colitis.
Precautions Use with caution in patients with hepatic impairment; cases of significant hepatic dysfunction and hepatic failure have been reported with tigecycline use; monitor patients for abnormal liver function tests; may need to modify dose with severe hepatic impairment. Due to structural similarity with tetracyclines, use caution in patients with prior hypersensitivity and/or severe adverse reactions associated with tetracycline use. Use caution in patients with intestinal perforation (septic shock occurred more frequently than in patients treated with imipenem/cilastatin).
Adverse Reactions
Central nervous system: Chills, dizziness, headache, pseudotumor cerebri
Dermatologic: Photosensitivity, pruritus, rash
Endocrine & metabolic: Hypocalcemia, hypoglycemia, hyponatremia, hypoproteinemia
Gastrointestinal: Abdominal pain, abnormal stools, anorexia, *C. difficile*-associated diarrhea, diarrhea, dyspepsia, nausea, pancreatitis, pseudomembranous colitits, taste perversion, vomiting
Genitourinary: Leukorrhea, vaginal moniliasis, vaginitis
Hematologic: Anemia, eosinophilia, INR elevated, prolonged PT and aPTT, thrombocytopenia
Hepatic: ALT, AST, alkaline phosphatase elevated; amylase elevated; bilirubin elevated; hepatic cholestasis; jaundice
Local: Injection site reaction (eg, edema, inflammation, pain, phlebitis), thrombophlebitis
Neuromuscular & skeletal: Weakness
Renal: Serum creatinine and BUN elevated
Miscellaneous: Abnormal healing, abscess, allergic reaction, anaphylaxis/anaphylactoid reactions, septic shock, tooth discoloration
Drug Interactions
Avoid Concomitant Use There are no known interactions where it is recommended to avoid concomitant use.
Increased Effect/Toxicity
Tigecycline may increase the levels/effects of: Warfarin
Decreased Effect There are no known significant interactions involving a decrease in effect.
Stability Store vial at controlled room temperature at 20°C to 25°C (68°F to 77°F). Reconstituted solution may be stored at room temperature for up to 6 hours or up to 24 hours if further diluted in a compatible I.V. solution. Alternatively, may be stored refrigerated at 2°C to 8°C (36°F to 46°F) for up to 48 hours following immediate transfer of the reconstituted solution into NS or D$_5$W. Reconstituted solution is red-orange.
Mechanism of Action Inhibits protein synthesis by binding to the 30S ribosomal subunit of susceptible bacteria, inhibiting protein translation and blocking entry of amino-acyl tRNA into the A site of the ribosome. Generally considered bacteriostatic; however, bactericidal activity has been demonstrated against isolates of *S. pneumoniae* and *L. pneumophila*. Tigecycline is a derivative of minocycline (9-t-butylglycylamido minocycline), and while not classified as a tetracycline, it may share some class-associated adverse effect. Tigecycline has demonstrated activity against a variety of gram-positive and gram-negative bacterial pathogens including methicillin-resistant staphylococci.
Pharmacokinetics (Adult data unless noted)
Distribution: Extensive tissue distribution; distributes into gallbladder, lung, and colon
V$_d$: 7-9 L/kg
Protein binding: 71% to 89%

Metabolism: Hepatic, via glucuronidation, N-acetylation, and epimerization to several metabolites, each <10% of the dose. Clearance is reduced by 55% and half-life increased by 43% in moderate hepatic impairment.

Half-life elimination: Single dose: 27 hours; Multiple doses: 42 hours

Elimination: 22% excreted in urine as unchanged drug; 59% in feces, primarily as unchanged drug

Dialysis: Not dialysable

Usual Dosage I.V.:

Children ≥12 years: Safety and efficacy in children <18 years of age has not been established; use in patients <8 years is not recommended due to effects on tooth development; use only in highly selective cases. (Limited experience, Wyeth Pharmaceuticals; data on file; CSR-53874): Initial: 1.5 mg/kg as a single dose (maximum: 100 mg/dose). Maintenance dose: 1 mg/kg/dose (maximum: 50 mg/dose) every 12 hours

Adults: Initial: 100 mg as a single dose. Maintenance dose:

Complicated skin and skin structure infection or intra-abdominal infection: 50 mg every 12 hours for 5-14 days

Community-acquired pneumonia: 50 mg every 12 hours for 7-14 days

Note: Duration dependant on severity/site of infection and clinical status and response to therapy

Dosage adjustment in hepatic impairment: (Child-Pugh class C): Initial dose of 100 mg should be followed with a maintenance dose of 25 mg every 12 hours

Administration Parenteral: I.V.: Infuse over 30-60 minutes at a maximum concentration of 1 mg/mL

Monitoring Parameters Periodic hepatic function tests; resolution of infection; observe patient for diarrhea

Patient Information May discolor teeth if <8 years of age; may cause photosensitivity reactions (eg, exposure to sunlight may cause severe sunburn, skin rash, redness, or itching); avoid exposure to sunlight, sunlamps, and tanning booths; wear protective clothing, wide-brimmed hats, sunglasses, and lip sunscreen. May cause lightheadedness/dizziness and impair ability to perform activities requiring mental alertness or physical coordination. Women of childbearing potential should be advised to avoid becoming pregnant.

Nursing Implications Nausea and vomiting with tigecycline is not decreased by slowing the rate of infusion; pretreatment with antiemetics may improve tolerability

Dosage Forms Excipient information presented when available (limited, particularly for generics); consult specific product labeling.

Injection, powder for reconstitution:

Tygacil®: 50 mg [contains lactose 100 mg]

References

Pankey GA and Steele RW, "Tigecycline: A Single Antibiotic for Polymicrobial Infections," *Pediatr Infect Dis J*, 2007, 26(1):77-8.

Zhanel GG, Homenuik K, Nichol K, et al, "The Glycylcyclines: A Comparative Review With the Tetracyclines," *Drugs*, 2004, 64 (1):63-88.

◆ **Tilade® [DSC]** see Nedocromil on page 970

◆ **Tilade® (Can)** see Nedocromil on page 970

◆ **Tim-AK (Can)** see Timolol on page 1351

◆ **Time-C [OTC]** see Ascorbic Acid on page 138

◆ **Time-C-Bio [OTC]** see Ascorbic Acid on page 138

◆ **Timentin®** see Ticarcillin and Clavulanate Potassium on page 1348

Timolol (TYE moe lole)

Medication Safety Issues

Sound-alike/look-alike issues:

Timolol may be confused with atenolol, Tylenol®

Timoptic® may be confused with Betoptic® S, Talacen®, Viroptic®

Bottle cap color change:

Timoptic®: Both the 0.25% and 0.5% strengths are now packaged in bottles with yellow caps; previously, the color of the cap on the product corresponded to different strengths.

International issues:

Betimol® may be confused with Betanol® which is a brand name for metipranolol in Monaco

Related Information

Antihypertensive Agents by Class on page 1481

U.S. Brand Names Betimol®; Istalol®; Timolol GFS; Timoptic-XE®; Timoptic®; Timoptic® in OcuDose®

Canadian Brand Names Alti-Timolol; Apo-Timol®; Apo-Timop®; Gen-Timolol; Mylan-Timolol; Nu-Timolol; Phoxal-timolol; PMS-Timolol; Sandoz-Timolol; Tim-AK; Timoptic-XE®; Timoptic®

Therapeutic Category Antihypertensive Agent; Antimigraine Agent; Beta-Adrenergic Blocker; Beta-Adrenergic Blocker, Ophthalmic

Generic Available Yes: Excludes hemihydrate ophthalmic solutions. gel-forming ophthalmic solutions, and preservative free maleate ophthalmic solutions

Use

Ophthalmic: Treatment of elevated intraocular pressure in patients with open-angle glaucoma or ocular hypertension (FDA approved in adults)

Oral: Treatment of hypertension, alone or in combination with other agents (FDA approved in adults); reduction of cardiovascular mortality and risk of reinfarction in stable post-MI patients (FDA approved in adults); prevention of migraine headaches (FDA approved in adults); treatment of angina

Pregnancy Risk Factor C

Pregnancy Considerations Adverse events were not observed in the initial animal reproduction studies; therefore, the manufacturer classifies timolol as pregnancy category C. Timolol crosses the placenta and decreased fetal heart rate has been observed following maternal use of oral and ophthalmic timolol during pregnancy. In a cohort study, an increased risk of cardiovascular defects was observed following maternal use of beta-blockers during pregnancy. In addition, intrauterine growth restriction (IUGR), small placentas, hypoglycemia, and/or respiratory depression have been observed in neonates following in utero exposure to nonselective beta-blockers at parturition; adequate facilities for monitoring infants at birth should be available. Severe, untreated chronic hypertension during pregnancy may be associated with maternal and fetal adverse events; however, timolol is currently not recommended for the initial treatment of hypertension in pregnancy. If timolol is required for the treatment of glaucoma during pregnancy, the minimum effective dose should be used in combination with punctual occlusion to decrease exposure to the fetus. Also refer to the Propranolol monograph for additional information on a nonselective beta-blocking agent.

Lactation Enters breast milk/ consider risk:benefit (AAP rates "compatible")

Breast-Feeding Considerations Timolol is excreted into breast milk. According to the manufacturer, the decision to continue or discontinue breast-feeding during therapy should take into account the risk of exposure to the infant and the benefits of treatment to the mother. The AAP considers timolol to be "usually compatible with breast-feeding." Due to the potential for adverse events, nursing infants (especially those with cardiorespiratory problems) should be monitored.

Contraindications Hypersensitivity to timolol or any component; uncompensated CHF, cardiogenic shock, bradycardia or heart block, bronchial asthma, severe chronic obstructive pulmonary disease or history of asthma, CHF or bradycardia

Warnings

Systemic therapy: Exacerbation of angina, arrhythmias, and in some cases MI may occur following abrupt discontinuation of beta-blockers **[U.S. Boxed Warning]**; avoid abrupt discontinuation, wean slowly, monitor for signs and symptoms of ischemia. Timolol decreases the ability of the heart to respond to reflex adrenergic stimuli and may increase the risk of general anesthesia and surgical procedures; beta-blockers should generally be avoided in patients with bronchospastic disease; if administered, use the lowest possible dose and monitor patients carefully. Patients receiving beta-blockers, who have a history of anaphylactic reactions, may be more reactive to a repeated allergen challenge and may not be responsive to the usual epinephrine doses used to treat an allergic reaction. Beta-blockers may block hypoglycemia-induced tachycardia and blood pressure changes; use with caution in patients with diabetes mellitus. May mask signs of thyrotoxicosis (exacerbation of symptoms of hyper-thyroidism, including thyroid storm, may occur following abrupt discontinuation). Use caution with anesthetic agents that decrease myocardial function. Beta-blocker use has been associated with induction or exacerbation of psoriasis, but cause and effect have not been firmly established.

Ocular therapy: Severe CNS, cardiovascular and respiratory adverse effects have been seen following ophthalmic use; same adverse reactions seen with systemic therapy may occur with ocular therapy. Some products do contain benzalkonium chloride which may be absorbed by soft contact lenses; remove lens prior to administration and wait 15 minutes before reinserting.

Precautions Similar to other beta-blockers; use with caution in patients with decreased renal or hepatic function (dosage adjustment required); use with a miotic in angle-closure or narrow-angle glaucoma; use with caution in patients with diabetes mellitus, may block hypoglycemia-induced tachycardia and blood pressure changes. Use with caution in patients with myasthenia gravis or myasthenic symptoms; may potentiate muscle weakness. Multi-use ocular products have been associated with bacterial keratitis; avoid touching tip of applicator to eye or other surfaces.

Adverse Reactions

Cardiovascular: Arrhythmia, bradycardia, hypertension after ophthalmic use, hypotension, syncope

Central nervous system: Dizziness, headache

Dermatologic: Psoriasiform rash, psoriasis exacerbation, rash

Gastrointestinal: Diarrhea, nausea

Local (ocular): Blurred vision, burning, cataract, conjunctivitis, irritation, itching, keratitis, stinging, visual acuity decreased, visual disturbances

Respiratory: Bronchospasm, dyspnea

Miscellaneous: Anaphylaxis, hypersensitivity reactions

Drug Interactions

Metabolism/Transport Effects Substrate of CYP2D6 (major); **Inhibits** CYP2D6 (weak)

Avoid Concomitant Use

Avoid concomitant use of Timolol with any of the following: Methacholine

Increased Effect/Toxicity

Timolol may increase the levels/effects of: Alpha-/Beta-Agonists (Direct-Acting); Alpha1-Blockers; Alpha2-Agonists; Amifostine; Antihypertensives; Antipsychotic Agents (Phenothiazines); Bupivacaine; Cardiac Glycosides; Hypotensive Agents; Insulin; Lidocaine; Lidocaine (Systemic); Lidocaine (Topical); Mepivacaine; Methacholine; Midodrine; RiTUXimab; Sulfonylureas

The levels/effects of Timolol may be increased by: Acetylcholinesterase Inhibitors; Aminoquinolines (Antimalarial); Amiodarone; Anilidopiperidine Opioids; Antipsychotic Agents (Phenothiazines); Calcium Channel Blockers (Nondihydropyridine); CYP2D6 Inhibitors (Moderate); CYP2D6 Inhibitors (Strong); Darunavir; Diazoxide; Dipyridamole; Disopyramide; Dronedarone; Herbs (Hypotensive Properties); MAO Inhibitors; Pentoxifylline; Phosphodiesterase 5 Inhibitors; Propafenone; Propoxyphene; Prostacyclin Analogues; QuiNIDine; Reserpine; Selective Serotonin Reuptake Inhibitors

Decreased Effect

Timolol may decrease the levels/effects of: Beta2-Agonists; Theophylline Derivatives

The levels/effects of Timolol may be decreased by: Barbiturates; Herbs (Hypotensive Properties); Methylphenidate; Nonsteroidal Anti-Inflammatory Agents; Peginterferon Alfa-2b; Rifamycin Derivatives; Yohimbine

Stability Ophthalmic: Store at room temperature; do not freeze; protect from light

Timoptic® OcuDose®: Store in protective foil wrap; use within 1 month after opening foil package

Mechanism of Action Blocks both beta$_1$- and beta$_2$-adrenergic receptors; reduces intraocular pressure by reducing aqueous humor production or possibly outflow; reduces blood pressure by blocking adrenergic receptors and decreasing sympathetic outflow; produces negative chronotropic and negative inotropic activity

Pharmacodynamics

Hypotensive effects: Oral:

Onset of action: Within 15-45 minutes

Maximum effect: 30-150 minutes

Duration: 4 hours

Intraocular pressure reduction: Ophthalmic:

Onset of action: Within 30 minutes

Maximum effect: 1-2 hours

Duration: 24 hours

Pharmacokinetics (Adult data unless noted)

Distribution: Oral and Ophthalmic: Distributes into human breast milk

Protein binding: <10%

Metabolism: Extensively in the liver, extensive first-pass effect

Bioavailability: Oral: ~60%

Half-life: Adults: 2-4 hours; prolonged with reduced renal function

Elimination: Urinary excretion (15% to 20% as unchanged drug)

Dialysis: Not readily dialyzable

Usual Dosage

Ophthalmic:

Gel (Timoptic-XE®): Adults: 0.25% or 0.5% gel, instill 1 drop once daily; do not exceed 1 drop once daily of 0.5% gel

Solution (Timoptic®): Children and Adults: Initial: 0.25% solution, instill 1 drop twice daily; increase to 0.5% solution if response not adequate; decrease to 1 drop/day if controlled; do not exceed 1 drop twice daily of 0.5% solution (see Additional Information)

Solution (Istalol™): Adults: Initial: 0.5% solution: Instill 1 drop once daily in the morning

Oral:

Children: No information regarding pediatric dose is currently available in literature

Adults:

Hypertension: Initial: 10 mg twice daily, increase gradually every 7 days, usual dosage: 20-40 mg/day in 2 divided doses; maximum dose: 60 mg/day; usual dosage range (JNC 7): 20-40 mg/day in 2 divided doses

Prevention of MI: 10 mg twice daily initiated within 1-4 weeks after infarction

Migraine headache: Initial: 10 mg twice daily, increase to maximum of 30 mg/day

Administration

Ophthalmic: Apply gentle pressure to lacrimal sac during and immediately following instillation (1 minute) or instruct patient to gently close eyelid after administration, to decrease systemic absorption of ophthalmic drops; avoid contact of bottle tip with skin or eye. Remove contact lenses prior to administration (ophthalmic solution contains benzalkonium chloride which may adsorb to soft contact lenses); lenses may be inserted 15 minutes after administration. Gel: Invert container, shake once before use; administer other topical ophthalmic medications at least 10 minutes before Timoptic-XE®

Oral: May be administered without regard to food

Monitoring Parameters Heart rate, blood pressure; liver enzymes, BUN, serum creatinine with long-term oral use; monitor IOP with ophthalmic use; monitor respiratory rate, CNS status, and cardiovascular status with ophthalmic use in patients at risk for adverse effects (eg, asthmatics, CHF patients, etc)

Patient Information Potential visual disturbances from ophthalmic use may impair ability to perform hazardous duties such as driving or operating machinery

Nursing Implications Discontinue medication if breathing difficulty occurs

Additional Information Ophthalmic: Use lowest effective dose in pediatric patients. Children had higher plasma concentrations vs adults following ophthalmic use; some achieved therapeutic levels; this may result in increased adverse systemic effects. The concurrent use of 2 ophthalmic beta blockers is not recommended.

Dosage Forms Excipient information presented when available (limited, particularly for generics); consult specific product labeling. [DSC] = Discontinued product

Gel-forming solution, ophthalmic, as maleate [strength expressed as base]:
Timolol GFS: 0.25% (2.5 mL [DSC], 5 mL); 0.5% (2.5 mL [DSC], 5 mL)
Timoptic-XE®: 0.25% (5 mL); 0.5% (5 mL)

Solution, ophthalmic, as hemihydrate [strength expressed as base]:
Betimol®: 0.25% (5 mL, 10 mL [DSC], 15 mL [DSC]); 0.5% (5 mL, 10 mL, 15 mL) [contains benzalkonium chloride]

Solution, ophthalmic, as maleate [strength expressed as base]: 0.25% (5 mL, 10 mL, 15 mL); 0.5% (5 mL, 10 mL, 15 mL)
Istalol®: 0.5% (10 mL) [contains benzalkonium chloride and potassium sorbate]
Timoptic®: 0.25% (5 mL); 0.5% (5 mL, 10 mL) [contains benzalkonium chloride]

Solution, ophthalmic, as maleate [strength expressed as base; preservative free]:
Timoptic® in OcuDose®: 0.25% (0.2 mL); 0.5% (0.2 mL)

Tablet, as maleate: 5 mg, 10 mg, 20 mg [strength expressed as salt]

References

Brauchli YB, Jick SS, Curtin F, et al, "Association Between Beta-Blockers, Other Antihypertensive Drugs and Psoriasis: Population-Based Case-Control Study," Br J Dermatol, 2008, 158(6):1299-307.
Chobanian AV, Bakris GL, Black HR, et al, "The Seventh Report of the Joint National Committee on Prevention, Detection, Evaluation, and Treatment of High Blood Pressure: The JNC 7 report," JAMA, 2003, 289(19):2560-72.
Gold MH, Holy AK, and Roenigk HH Jr, "Beta-Blocking Drugs and Psoriasis. A Review of Cutaneous Side Effects and Retrospective Analysis of Their Effects on Psoriasis," J Am Acad Dermatol, 1988, 19 (5 Pt 1):837-41.
Hoskins HD, Hetherington J Jr, Magee SD, et al, "Clinical Experience With Timolol in Childhood Glaucoma," Arch Ophthalmol, 1985, 103 (8):1163-5.
Passo MS, Palmer EA, and Van Buskirk EM, "Plasma Timolol in Glaucoma Patients," Ophthalmology, 1984, 91(11):1361-3.

Schön MP and Boehncke WH, "Psoriasis," N Engl J Med, 2005, 352 (18):1899-912.

◆ **Timolol GFS** see Timolol on page 1351

◆ **Timolol Hemihydrate** see Timolol on page 1351

◆ **Timolol Maleate** see Timolol on page 1351

◆ **Timoptic®** see Timolol on page 1351

◆ **Timoptic® in OcuDose®** see Timolol on page 1351

◆ **Timoptic-XE®** see Timolol on page 1351

◆ **Tinactin® Antifungal [OTC]** see Tolnaftate on page 1358

◆ **Tinactin® Antifungal Deodorant [OTC]** see Tolnaftate on page 1358

◆ **Tinactin® Antifungal Jock Itch [OTC]** see Tolnaftate on page 1358

◆ **Tinaderm [OTC]** see Tolnaftate on page 1358

◆ **Tinamed® Corn and Callus Remover [OTC]** see Salicylic Acid on page 1241

◆ **Tinamed® Wart Remover [OTC]** see Salicylic Acid on page 1241

◆ **Ting® Cream [OTC]** see Tolnaftate on page 1358

◆ **Ting® Spray Liquid [OTC]** see Tolnaftate on page 1358

◆ **Tioguanine** see Thioguanine on page 1339

◆ **Tiotixene** see Thiothixene on page 1344

Tiotropium (ty oh TRO pee um)

Medication Safety Issues
Sound-alike/look-alike issues:
Spiriva® may be confused with Inspra™, Serevent®
Tiotropium may be confused with ipratropium
Spiriva® capsules for inhalation are for administration via HandiHaler® device and are **not** for oral use

U.S. Brand Names Spiriva® HandiHaler®

Canadian Brand Names Spiriva®

Therapeutic Category Antiasthmatic; Anticholinergic Agent; Bronchodilator

Generic Available No

Use Maintenance treatment of bronchospasm associated with COPD, including chronic bronchitis and emphysema (FDA approved in adults); reduction of COPD exacerbations (FDA approved in adults)

Pregnancy Risk Factor C

Pregnancy Considerations Adverse events (fetal loss, decreased birth weights, delayed sexual maturation) were observed in some animal studies. There are no adequate and well-controlled studies in pregnant women. Use only when expected benefit to mother outweighs potential risk to the fetus.

Lactation Excretion in breast milk unknown/use caution

Contraindications Hypersensitivity to tiotropium, ipratropium, or any component of the formulation (contains lactose); not for use as an acute ("rescue") bronchodilator

Warnings Not indicated for the initial treatment of acute episodes of bronchospasm. Immediate hypersensitivity reactions including angioedema may occur. Use with caution in patients with a history of hypersensitivity to atropine. May cause paradoxical bronchospasm. Safety and efficacy have not been established in pediatric patients.

Precautions Use with caution in patients with myasthenia gravis, narrow-angle glaucoma, prostatic hyperplasia, or bladder neck obstruction; use with caution and monitor use closely in patients with moderate to severe renal impairment ($Cl_{cr} \leq 50$ mL/minute). Avoid inadvertent instillation of powder into the eyes. Explain administration carefully; capsules are not for oral use and must only be administered using HandiHaler® inhalation device. Contains lactose; use with caution in patients with severe milk protein allergy.

◀ **Adverse Reactions**

Cardiovascular: Angina, chest pain, edema, tachycardia

Central nervous system: Depression, headache, insomnia

Dermatologic: Rash

Endocrine & metabolic: Hypercholesterolemia, hyperglycemia

Gastrointestinal: Abdominal pain, constipation, dyspepsia, reflux, stomatitis (including ulcerative), vomiting, xerostomia

Genitourinary: Urinary tract infection

Neuromuscular & skeletal: Arthritis, leg pain, myalgia, paresthesia, skeletal pain

Ocular: Blurred vision, cataract, glaucoma, intraocular pressure increased, pupil dilation (powder contact with eyes)

Respiratory: Cough, dysphonia, epistaxis, laryngitis, paradoxical bronchospasm, pharyngitis, rhinitis, sinusitis, upper respiratory tract infection

Miscellaneous: Allergic reaction, flu-like syndrome, herpes zoster, hypersensitivity reactions, infection, moniliasis

<1%, postmarketing, and/or case reports: Angioedema, atrial fibrillation, dehydration, dry skin, dysphagia, hoarseness, intestinal obstruction, joint swelling, oral irritation, palpitation, paralytic ileus, pruritus, skin ulceration, supraventricular tachycardia, tachycardia, throat irritation, urinary retention, urticaria

Drug Interactions

Metabolism/Transport Effects Substrate (minor) of CYP2D6, 3A4

Avoid Concomitant Use There are no known interactions where it is recommended to avoid concomitant use.

Increased Effect/Toxicity

Tiotropium may increase the levels/effects of: AbobotulinumtoxinA; Anticholinergics; Cannabinoids; OnabotulinumtoxinA; Potassium Chloride; RimabotulinumtoxinB

The levels/effects of Tiotropium may be increased by: Pramlintide

Decreased Effect

Tiotropium may decrease the levels/effects of: Acetylcholinesterase Inhibitors (Central); Secretin

The levels/effects of Tiotropium may be decreased by: Acetylcholinesterase Inhibitors (Central); Peginterferon Alfa-2b

Stability Store between 15°C and 25°C. Avoid excessive temperatures and moisture. Do not store capsules in HandiHaler® device. Capsules should be stored in the blister pack and only removed immediately before use. After first capsule in the strip is used, the 2 remaining capsules should be used over the next 2 days.

Mechanism of Action Blocks the action of acetylcholine at parasympathetic sites in bronchial smooth muscle causing bronchodilation

Pharmacokinetics (Adult data unless noted)

Absorption: Poorly absorbed from GI tract; systemic absorption may occur from lung

Distribution: V_d: 32 L/kg

Protein binding: 72%

Metabolism: Hepatic (minimal), via CYP2D6 and CYP3A4

Bioavailability: Absolute: 19.5%

Half-life: 5-6 days

Time to peak serum concentration: 5 minutes (following inhalation)

Elimination: Urine (74% as unchanged drug)

Usual Dosage Inhalation: Adults: Contents of 1 capsule (18 mcg) inhaled once daily using HandiHaler® device (see Administration)

Dosage adjustment in renal impairment: Plasma concentrations may increase in renal impairment (Cl_{cr} ≤50 mL/minute). Use caution; no specific dosage adjustment recommended.

Administration Inhalation: **Not for oral use.** Remove capsule from foil blister immediately before use. Place capsule in the capsule-chamber in the base of the HandiHaler® Inhaler. Must only use the HandiHaler® Inhaler. Close mouthpiece until a click is heard, leaving dustcap open. Exhale fully. Do not exhale into inhaler. Tilt head slightly back and inhale (rapidly, steadily, and deeply); the capsule vibration may be heard within the device. Hold breath as long as possible. If any powder remains in capsule, exhale and inhale again. Repeat until capsule is empty. Throw away empty capsule; do not leave in inhaler. Do not use a spacer with the HandiHaler® Inhaler. Always keep capsules and inhaler dry.

Delivery of dose: Instruct patient to place mouthpiece gently between teeth, closing lips around inhaler. Instruct patient to inhale deeply and hold breath for 5-10 seconds. The amount of drug delivered is small, and the individual will not sense the medication as it is inhaled. Remove mouthpiece prior to exhalation. Patient should not breathe out through the mouthpiece. After use of the inhaler, patient should rinse mouth/oropharynx with water and spit out rinse solution.

Monitoring Parameters FEV_1, peak flow (or other pulmonary function studies)

Patient Information Use inhaler and medication as instructed - once daily, at same time each day. Do not use more often than prescribed. Do not use as an acute "rescue" bronchodilator. Report swelling of face, mouth, or tongue; skin rash; chest pain or palpitations; persistent gastrointestinal effects; muscle or skeletal pain or weakness; change in vision; respiratory changes, sore throat, or flu-like symptoms. May cause dry mouth.

Dosage Forms Excipient information presented when available (limited, particularly for generics); consult specific product labeling.

Powder for oral inhalation [capsule]:

Spiriva® HandiHaler®: 18 mcg/capsule (5s, 30s, 90s) [contains lactose]

♦ **Tiotropium Bromide Monohydrate** *see* Tiotropium *on page 1353*

♦ **Titralac™ [OTC]** *see* Calcium Carbonate *on page 232*

♦ **Titralac® [OTC]** *see* Calcium Supplements *on page 239*

♦ **Titralac® Extra Strength [OTC]** *see* Calcium Supplements *on page 239*

♦ **TMP** *see* Trimethoprim *on page 1386*

♦ **TMP-SMZ** *see* Sulfamethoxazole and Trimethoprim *on page 1302*

♦ **TMZ** *see* Temozolomide *on page 1315*

♦ **TOBI®** *see* Tobramycin *on page 1354*

Tobramycin (toe bra MYE sin)

Medication Safety Issues

Sound-alike/look-alike issues:

Tobramycin may be confused with Trobicin®, vancomycin

Nebcin® may be confused with Inapsine®, Naprosyn®, Nubain®

Tobrex® may be confused with TobraDex®

High alert medication: The Institute for Safe Medication Practices (ISMP) includes this medication (intrathecal administration) among its list of drug classes which have a heightened risk of causing significant patient harm when used in error.

Related Information

Therapeutic Drug Monitoring: Blood Sampling Time Guidelines *on page 1704*

U.S. Brand Names AK-Tob™; TOBI®; Tobrex®

Canadian Brand Names PMS-Tobramycin; Sandoz-Tobramycin; TOBI®; Tobramycin Injection, USP; Tobrex®

Therapeutic Category Antibiotic, Aminoglycoside; Antibiotic, Ophthalmic

Generic Available Yes: Excludes ophthalmic ointment, solution for nebulization

Use Treatment of documented or suspected infections caused by susceptible gram-negative bacilli including *Pseudomonas aeruginosa*; nonpseudomonal enteric bacillus infection which is more sensitive to tobramycin than gentamicin based on susceptibility tests; susceptible organisms in lower respiratory tract infections, septicemia; intra-abdominal, skin, bone, and urinary tract infections; empiric therapy in cystic fibrosis and immunocompromised patients; used topically to treat superficial ophthalmic infections caused by susceptible bacteria; inhalation therapy management of cystic fibrosis patients with *P. aeruginosa*

Pregnancy Risk Factor D (injection, inhalation); B (ophthalmic)

Pregnancy Considerations [U.S. Boxed Warning]: Aminoglycosides may cause fetal harm if administered to a pregnant woman. There are several reports of total irreversible bilateral congenital deafness in children whose mothers received another aminoglycoside (streptomycin) during pregnancy; therefore, tobramycin is classified as pregnancy category D. Tobramycin crosses the placenta and produces detectable serum levels in the fetus. Although serious side effects to the fetus have not been reported following maternal use of tobramycin, a potential for harm exists.

Due to pregnancy induced physiologic changes, some pharmacokinetic parameters of tobramycin may be altered. Pregnant women have an average-to-larger volume of distribution which may result in lower serum peak levels than for the same dose in nonpregnant women. Serum half-life is also shorter.

Lactation Enters breast milk/not recommended

Breast-Feeding Considerations Tobramycin is excreted into breast milk and breast-feeding is not recommended by the manufacturer; however, tobramycin is not well absorbed when taken orally. This limited oral absorption may minimize exposure to the nursing infant. Nondose-related effects could include modification of bowel flora.

Contraindications Hypersensitivity to tobramycin, any component (see Warnings), or aminoglycosides

Warnings Aminoglycosides are associated with significant nephrotoxicity **[U.S. Boxed Warning]**; neurotoxicity, manifested as vestibular and permanent bilateral auditory ototoxicity, can occur **[U.S. Boxed Warning]**. Tinnitus or vertigo are indications of vestibular injury and impending bilateral irreversible deafness. Risk of nephrotoxicity and ototoxicity is increased in patients with impaired renal function, high dose therapy, or prolonged therapy. Risk of nephrotoxicity increases when used concurrently with other potentially nephrotoxic drugs **[U.S. Boxed Warning]**; renal damage is usually reversible. Risk of ototoxicity increases with use of potent diuretics **[U.S. Boxed Warning]**. Aminoglycosides can cause fetal harm when administered to a pregnant woman **[U.S. Boxed Warning]**; aminoglycosides have been associated with several reports of total irreversible bilateral congenital deafness in pediatric patients exposed *in utero*. Use with caution in premature infants and neonates **[U.S. Boxed Warning]**; immature renal function may increase risk of accumulation and related toxicity. Some formulations contain sulfites which may cause allergic reactions in susceptible individuals. Prolonged use may result in superinfection.

Inhalation: Transient tinnitus and hearing loss have been reported in tobramycin inhalation-treated patients; bronchospasm can occur with inhalation of tobramycin.

Precautions Use with caution in patients with pre-existing renal impairment, auditory or vestibular impairment, hypocalcemia, myasthenia gravis, and in conditions which depress neuromuscular transmission. May cause neuromuscular blockade and respiratory paralysis; risk increased with concomitant use of anesthesia or muscle relaxants; modify dosage in patients with renal impairment and in neonates on extracorporeal membrane oxygenation (ECMO). Monitor renal and eighth nerve function in patients with known or suspected renal impairment **[U.S. Boxed Warning]**; cross-allergenicity with other aminoglycosides has been observed

Adverse Reactions

Central nervous system: Ataxia, dizziness, fever, gait instability, headache, vertigo

Dermatologic: Allergic contact dermatitis, rash

Endocrine & metabolic: Hypomagnesemia

Gastrointestinal: Nausea, vomiting

Hematologic: Eosinophilia, granulocytopenia, thrombocytopenia

Hepatic: ALT and AST elevated

Local: Thrombophlebitis

Neuromuscular & skeletal: Neuromuscular blockade, paresthesia, tremor, weakness

Ocular: Ophthalmic use: Edema of the eyelid, itching, keratitis, lacrimation

Otic: Ototoxicity (may be associated with high serum aminoglycoside concentrations persisting for prolonged periods or with high peak serum concentrations following rapid I.V. bolus administration) with tinnitus, hearing loss; early toxicity usually affects high-pitched sound

Renal: Casts in urine and possible electrolyte wasting, decrease in urine specific gravity, nephrotoxicity (high trough levels) with proteinuria, reduction in glomerular filtration rate, serum creatinine elevated

Respiratory: With inhalation therapy: Bronchospasm, cough increased, dyspnea, hoarseness, pharyngitis, voice alteration

Drug Interactions

Avoid Concomitant Use

Avoid concomitant use of Tobramycin with any of the following: BCG; Gallium Nitrate

Increased Effect/Toxicity

Tobramycin may increase the levels/effects of: AbobotulinumtoxinA; Bisphosphonate Derivatives; CARBOplatin; Colistimethate; CycloSPORINE; CycloSPORINE (Systemic); Gallium Nitrate; Neuromuscular-Blocking Agents; OnabotulinumtoxinA; RimabotulinumtoxinB

The levels/effects of Tobramycin may be increased by: Amphotericin B; Capreomycin; CISplatin; Loop Diuretics; Nonsteroidal Anti-Inflammatory Agents; Vancomycin

Decreased Effect

Tobramycin may decrease the levels/effects of: BCG; Typhoid Vaccine

The levels/effects of Tobramycin may be decreased by: Penicillins

Stability Incompatible with penicillins, cephalosporins, heparin

Inhalation solution: Store in refrigerator; upon removal from the refrigerator, the solution may be stored at room temperature for up to 28 days; do not use solution if it is cloudy or contains particles; a darkened yellow solution does not indicate loss of potency; protect from intense light; incompatible with dornase alfa (may precipitate)

Mechanism of Action Inhibits cellular initiation of bacterial protein synthesis by binding to 30S and 50S ribosomal subunits resulting in a defective bacterial cell membrane

Pharmacokinetics (Adult data unless noted)
Absorption:
Oral: Poor
I.M.: Rapid and complete
Inhalation: Low systemic bioavailability although peak tobramycin serum concentration 1 hour after inhalation ranges between 0.95-1.05 mg/mL
Distribution: Crosses the placenta; distributes primarily in the extracellular fluid volume; poor penetration into the CSF and into bronchial secretions; drug accumulates in the renal cortex; small amounts distribute into bile, sputum, saliva, tears, and breast milk
V_d: Increased by fever, edema, ascites, fluid overload, and in neonates; V_d is decreased in patients with dehydration
Neonates: 0.45 ± 0.1 L/kg
Infants: 0.4 ± 0.1 L/kg
Children: 0.35 ± 0.15 L/kg
Adolescents: 0.3 ± 0.1 L/kg
Adults: 0.2-0.3 L/kg
Protein binding: <30%
Half-life:
Neonates:
≤1200 g: 11 hours
>1200 g: 2-9 hours
Infants: 4 ± 1 hour
Children: 2 ± 1 hour
Adolescents: 1.5 ± 1 hour
Adults with normal renal function: 2-3 hours, directly dependent upon glomerular filtration rate; impaired renal function: 5-70 hours
Time to peak serum concentration:
I.M.: Within 30-60 minutes
I.V.: 30 minutes after a 30-minute infusion
Elimination: With normal renal function, ~90% to 95% of dose excreted in urine within 24 hours
Dialysis: Dialyzable (50% to 100%)
Usual Dosage Dosage should be based on an estimate of ideal body weight except in neonates (neonatal dosage should be based on actual weight unless the patient has hydrocephalus or hydrops fetalis)
Neonates: I.M., I.V.:
Preterm neonates <1000 g: 3.5 mg/kg/dose every 24 hours
0-4 weeks, <1200 g: 2.5 mg/kg/dose every 18 hours
Postnatal age ≤7 days:
1200-2000 g: 2.5 mg/kg/dose every 12 hours
>2000 g: 2.5 mg/kg/dose every 12 hours
Postnatal age >7 days:
1200-2000 g: 2.5 mg/kg/dose every 8-12 hours
>2000 g: 2.5 mg/kg/dose every 8 hours
Infants and Children <5 years: I.M., I.V.: 2.5 mg/kg/dose every 8 hours*
Pulmonary infection in cystic fibrosis: 2.5-3.3 mg/kg/dose every 6-8 hours
Patients on hemodialysis: 1.25-1.75 mg/kg/dose postdialysis
Children ≥5 years: I.M., I.V.: 2-2.5 mg/kg/dose every 8 hours*
Pulmonary infection in cystic fibrosis: 2.5-3.3 mg/kg/dose every 6-8 hours
Patients on hemodialysis: 1.25-1.75 mg/kg/dose postdialysis
*Note: Some patients may require larger or more frequent doses if serum levels document the need (ie, cystic fibrosis, patients undergoing continuous hemofiltration, patients with major burns, or febrile granulocytopenic patients); modify dose based on individual patient requirements as determined by renal function, serum drug concentrations, and patient-specific clinical parameters.

Children ≥2 months and Adults:
Ophthalmic:
Ointment: Apply 0.5" ribbon into the affected eye 2-3 times/day; for severe infections, apply ointment every 3-4 hours
Solution:
Mild to moderate infections: Instill 1-2 drops every 4 hours
Severe infections: instill 2 drops every 30-60 minutes initially, then reduce to less frequent intervals
Inhalation:
High dose regimen (cystic fibrosis patients): Children ≥6 years and Adults: 300 mg every 12 hours (do not administer doses less than 6 hours apart); administer in repeated cycles of 28 days on drug followed by 28 days off drug
Low dose regimen (noncystic fibrosis patients; **Note:** Used by some centers; no published data are available): Children: 40-80 mg/dose 2-3 times/day
Adults: I.M., I.V.: 3-6 mg/kg/day in 3 divided doses; studies of once daily dosing have used I.V. doses of 4-6.6 mg/kg once daily
Patients on hemodialysis: 0.5-0.7 mg/kg/dose postdialysis
Dosing in Renal Impairment:
Children and Adults: 2.5 mg/kg (2-3 serum level measurements should be obtained after the initial dose to measure the half-life in order to determine the frequency of subsequent doses)

Administration
Inhalation (high-dose regimen): Use a PARI LC Plus™ reusable nebulizer and a DeVilbiss Pulmo-Aide® air compressor for administration of tobramycin by inhalation; patient should be sitting or standing upright and breathing normally through the mouthpiece of the nebulizer. Nebulizer treatment period is usually over 15 minutes.
Ophthalmic: Avoid contact of tube or bottle tip with skin or eye; apply finger pressure to lacrimal sac during and for 1-2 minutes after instillation of drops to decrease risk of absorption and systemic effects
Parenteral: Administer by I.M., I.V. slow intermittent infusion over 30-60 minutes or by direct injection over 15 minutes; final I.V. concentration for administration should not exceed 10 mg/mL; administer other antibiotics such as penicillins and cephalosporins at least 1 hour before or after tobramycin

Monitoring Parameters Urinalysis, urine output, BUN, serum creatinine, peak and trough serum tobramycin levels; be alert to ototoxicity, audiograms

Not all pediatric patients who receive aminoglycosides require monitoring of serum aminoglycoside concentrations. Indications for use of aminoglycoside serum concentration monitoring include:
Treatment course >5 days
Patients with decreased or changing renal function
Patients with a poor therapeutic response
Infants <3 months of age
Atypical body constituency (obesity, expanded extracellular fluid volume)
Clinical need for higher doses or shorter intervals (cystic fibrosis, burns, endocarditis, meningitis, relatively resistant organism)
Patients on hemodialysis or chronic ambulatory peritoneal dialysis
Signs of nephrotoxicity or ototoxicity
Concomitant use of other nephrotoxic agents
Patients on high-dose aerosolized tobramycin: Peak tobramycin level obtained 1 hour following inhalation to identify patients who are significant absorbers

Reference Range

Peak: 4-12 mcg/mL; peak values are 2-3 times greater with once daily dosing regimens

Trough: 0.5-2 mcg/mL

Test Interactions Aminoglycoside serum levels measured in blood taken from Silastic® central line catheters can sometimes give falsely high readings

Patient Information Report any dizziness or sensation of ringing or fullness in ears to the physician

Nursing Implications Obtain serum concentration after the third dose except in neonates or patients with rapidly changing renal function in whom levels need to be measured sooner; peak tobramycin serum concentrations are drawn 30 minutes after the end of a 30-minute infusion, immediately on completion of a 1-hour I.V. infusion or 1 hour after an intramuscular injection; the trough is drawn just before the next dose; provide optimal patient hydration and perfusion

Dosage Forms Excipient information presented when available (limited, particularly for generics); consult specific product labeling.

Infusion [premixed in NS]: 60 mg (50 mL); 80 mg (100 mL)

Injection, powder for reconstitution: 1.2 g

Injection, solution: 10 mg/mL (2 mL, 8 mL); 40 mg/mL (2 mL, 30 mL, 50 mL) [may contain sodium metabisulfite]

Ointment, ophthalmic:

Tobrex®: 0.3% (3.5 g)

Solution for nebulization [preservative free]

TOBI®: 60 mg/mL (5 mL)

Solution, ophthalmic: 0.3% (5 mL)

AK-Tob™, Tobrex®: 0.3% (5 mL) [contains benzalkonium chloride]

References

Gilbert DN, "Once-Daily Aminoglycoside Therapy," *Antimicrob Agents Chemother*, 1991, 35(3):399-405.

Green TP, Mirkin BL, Peterson PK, et al, "Tobramycin Serum Level Monitoring in Young Patients With Normal Renal Function," *Clin Pharmacokinet*, 1984, 9(5):457-68.

Nahata MC, Powell DA, Durrell DE, et al, "Effect of Gestational Age and Birth Weight on Tobramycin Kinetics in Newborn Infants," *J Antimicrob Chemother*, 1984, 14(1):59-65.

Ramsey BW, Burns J, Smith A, et al, "Safety and Efficacy of Tobramycin for Inhalation in Patients With Cystic Fibrosis: The Results of Two Phase III Placebo Controlled Clinical Trials," *Pediatr Pulmonol*, 1997, (Suppl 14):137-8, S10.3.

Ramsey BW, Dorkin HL, Eisenberg JD, et al, "Efficacy of Aerosolized Tobramycin in Patients With Cystic Fibrosis," *N Engl J Med*, 1993, 328 (24):1740-6.

Shaw PK, Braun TL, Liebergen A, et al, "Aerosolized Tobramycin Pharmacokinetics in Cystic Fibrosis Patients," *J Pediatr Pharm Pract*, 1997, 2(1):23-6.

◆ **Tobramycin Injection, USP (Can)** see Tobramycin on page 1354

◆ **Tobramycin Sulfate** see Tobramycin on page 1354

◆ **Tobrex®** see Tobramycin on page 1354

◆ **Tofranil®** see Imipramine on page 716

◆ **Tofranil-PM®** see Imipramine on page 716

◆ **Tolectin** see Tolmetin on page 1357

Tolmetin (TOLE met in)

Therapeutic Category Analgesic, Non-narcotic; Non-steroidal Anti-inflammatory Drug (NSAID), Oral

Generic Available Yes

Use Treatment of inflammatory and rheumatoid disorders, including juvenile rheumatoid arthritis

Medication Guide An FDA-approved patient medication guide, which is available with the product information and at http://www.fda.gov/downloads/Drugs/DrugSafety/ucm089162.pdf, must be dispensed with this medication for each new outpatient prescription and refill.

Pregnancy Risk Factor C

Pregnancy Considerations Adverse events were not observed in the initial animal reproduction studies; therefore, the manufacturer classifies tolmetin as pregnancy category C. NSAID exposure during the first trimester is not strongly associated with congenital malformations; however, cardiovascular anomalies and cleft palate have been observed following NSAID exposure in some studies. The use of an NSAID close to conception may be associated with an increased risk of miscarriage. Non-teratogenic effects have been observed following NSAID administration during the third trimester including myocardial degenerative changes, prenatal constriction of the ductus arteriosus, fetal tricuspid regurgitation, failure of the ductus arteriosus to close postnatally; renal dysfunction or failure, oligohydramnios; gastrointestinal bleeding or perforation, increased risk of necrotizing enterocolitis; intracranial bleeding (including intraventricular hemorrhage), platelet dysfunction with resultant bleeding; pulmonary hypertension. Because they may cause premature closure of the ductus arteriosus, use of NSAIDs late in pregnancy should be avoided (use after 31 or 32 weeks gestation is not recommended by some clinicians). The chronic use of NSAIDs in women of reproductive age may be associated with infertility that is reversible upon discontinuation of the medication.

Lactation Enters breast milk/not recommended (AAP rates "compatible")

Breast-Feeding Considerations Tolmetin is found in breast milk and breast-feeding is not recommended by the manufacturer. The AAP considers tolmetin to be "usually compatible with breast-feeding."

Contraindications Hypersensitivity to tolmetin or any component; history of asthma, urticaria, or allergic-type reaction to aspirin, or other NSAIDs; patients with the "aspirin triad" [asthma, rhinitis (with or without nasal polyps), and aspirin intolerance] (fatal asthmatic and anaphylactoid reactions may occur in these patients); perioperative pain in the setting of coronary artery bypass graft (CABG)

Warnings NSAIDs are associated with an increased risk of adverse cardiovascular thrombotic events, including potentially fatal MI and stroke **[U.S. Boxed Warning]**; risk may be increased with duration of use or pre-existing cardiovascular risk factors or disease; carefully evaluate cardiovascular risk profile prior to prescribing; use the lowest effective dose for the shortest duration of time, taking into consideration individual patient treatment goals; alternate therapies should be considered for patients at high risk. Use is contraindicated for treatment of perioperative pain in the setting of CABG surgery **[U.S. Boxed Warning]**; an increased incidence of MI and stroke was found in patients receiving COX-2 selective NSAIDs for the treatment of pain within the first 10-14 days after CABG surgery. NSAIDs may cause fluid retention, edema, and new onset or worsening of pre-existing hypertension; use with caution in patients with hypertension, CHF, or fluid retention. Concurrent administration of ibuprofen and potentially other nonselective NSAIDs may interfere with aspirin's cardioprotective effect.

NSAIDs may increase the risk of gastrointestinal inflammation, ulceration, bleeding, and perforation **[U.S. Boxed Warning]**. These events, which can be potentially fatal, may occur at any time during therapy and without warning. Avoid the use of NSAIDs in patients with active GI bleeding or ulcer disease. Use NSAIDs with extreme caution in patients with a history of GI bleeding or ulcers (these patients have a 10-fold increased risk for developing a GI bleed). Use NSAIDs with caution in patients with other risk factors which may increase GI bleeding (eg, concurrent therapy with aspirin, anticoagulants, and/or corticosteroids, longer duration of NSAID use, smoking, use of alcohol, and poor general health). Use the lowest effective dose for the shortest duration of time, taking into consideration individual patient treatment goals; alternate therapies should be considered for patients at high risk

NSAIDs may compromise existing renal function. Renal toxicity may occur in patients with impaired renal function, dehydration, heart failure, liver dysfunction, those taking diuretics and ACE inhibitors; use with caution in these patients; monitor renal function closely. NSAIDs are not recommended for use in patients with advanced renal disease. Long-term use of NSAIDs may cause renal papillary necrosis and other renal injury. Rare cases of severe hepatic reactions (eg, fulminant hepatitis, liver failure) have occurred with NSAID use; closely monitor patients with any abnormal LFT; discontinue if signs or symptoms of liver disease develop or if systemic manifestations occur

Fatal asthmatic and anaphylactoid reactions may occur in patients with the "aspirin triad" who receive NSAIDs (see Contraindications). NSAIDs may cause serious dermatologic adverse reactions including exfoliative dermatitis, Stevens-Johnson syndrome, and toxic epidermal necrolysis. Avoid use of NSAIDs in late pregnancy as they may cause premature closure of the ductus arteriosus.

Precautions Use with caution in patients with upper GI disease, impaired renal function, CHF, hypertension, and patients receiving anticoagulants; although rare, anaphylactoid reactions occur more commonly with tolmetin than other NSAIDs

Adverse Reactions

Cardiovascular: Edema

Central nervous system: Dizziness, nervousness, drowsiness, headache

Dermatologic: Rash, urticaria

Gastrointestinal: Nausea, abdominal pain, dyspepsia, diarrhea, constipation, GI bleeding, ulcer, perforation

Hematologic: Anemia, leukopenia, prolongation of bleeding time

Hepatic: Hepatitis

Otic: Tinnitus

Renal: Acute renal failure, renal dysfunction

Drug Interactions

Avoid Concomitant Use

Avoid concomitant use of Tolmetin with any of the following: Ketorolac; Ketorolac (Systemic)

Increased Effect/Toxicity

Tolmetin may increase the levels/effects of: Aminoglycosides; Anticoagulants; Antiplatelet Agents; Bisphosphonate Derivatives; Collagenase (Systemic); CycloSPORINE; CycloSPORINE (Systemic); Desmopressin; Digoxin; Drotrecogin Alfa; Eplerenone; Haloperidol; Ibritumomab; Lithium; Methotrexate; Nonsteroidal Anti-Inflammatory Agents; Pemetrexed; Potassium-Sparing Diuretics; Pralatrexate; Quinolone Antibiotics; Salicylates; Thrombolytic Agents; Tositumomab and Iodine I 131 Tositumomab; Vancomycin; Vitamin K Antagonists

The levels/effects of Tolmetin may be increased by: Antidepressants (Tricyclic, Tertiary Amine); Corticosteroids (Systemic); Dasatinib; Glucosamine; Herbs (Anticoagulant/Antiplatelet Properties); Ketorolac; Ketorolac (Systemic); Nonsteroidal Anti-Inflammatory Agents; Omega-3-Acid Ethyl Esters; Pentosan Polysulfate Sodium; Pentoxifylline; Probenecid; Prostacyclin Analogues; Selective Serotonin Reuptake Inhibitors; Serotonin/Norepinephrine Reuptake Inhibitors; Treprostinil

Decreased Effect

Tolmetin may decrease the levels/effects of: ACE Inhibitors; Angiotensin II Receptor Blockers; Antiplatelet Agents; Beta-Blockers; Eplerenone; HydrALAZINE; Loop Diuretics; Potassium-Sparing Diuretics; Salicylates; Thiazide Diuretics

The levels/effects of Tolmetin may be decreased by: Bile Acid Sequestrants; Nonsteroidal Anti-Inflammatory Agents; Salicylates

Food Interactions Food or milk may decrease the extent of oral absorption

Mechanism of Action Inhibits prostaglandin synthesis by decreasing the activity of the enzyme, cyclooxygenase, which results in decreased formation of prostaglandin precursors

Pharmacokinetics (Adult data unless noted)

Absorption: Oral: Well absorbed

Protein binding: 99%

Metabolism: In the liver via oxidation and conjugation

Half-life, elimination: 5 hours

Time to peak serum concentration: Within 30-60 minutes

Elimination: Excreted in the urine as metabolites or conjugates

Usual Dosage Oral:

Children ≥2 years:

Anti-inflammatory: Initial: 20 mg/kg/day in 3-4 divided doses, then 15-30 mg/kg/day in 3-4 divided doses; maximum dose: 30 mg/kg/day in 4 divided doses; do not exceed 1800 mg/day

Analgesic: 5-7 mg/kg/dose every 6-8 hours

Adults: 400 mg 3 times/day; usual dose: 600 mg to 1.8 g/day; maximum dose: 2 g/day

Administration Oral: May administer with food, milk, or antacids to decrease GI adverse effects

Monitoring Parameters CBC with differential, liver enzymes, occult blood loss, BUN, serum creatinine; periodic ophthalmologic exams

Patient Information Avoid alcohol; may cause dizziness or drowsiness and impair ability to perform activities requiring mental alertness or physical coordination

Dosage Forms Excipient information presented when available (limited, particularly for generics); consult specific product labeling.

Capsule: 400 mg

Tablet: 200 mg, 600 mg

References

Berde C, Ablin A, Glazer J, et al, "American Academy of Pediatrics Report of the Subcommittee on Disease-Related Pain in Childhood Cancer," Pediatrics, 1990, 86(5 Pt 2):818-25.

Giannini EH and Cawkwell GD, "Drug Treatment in Children With Juvenile Rheumatoid Arthritis. Past, Present, and Future," Pediatr Clin North Am, 1995, 42(5):1099-125.

Hollingworth P, "The Use of Non-Steroidal Anti-inflammatory Drugs in Paediatric Rheumatic Diseases," Br J Rheumatol, 1993, 32(1):73-7.

Rose CD and Doughty RA, "Pharmacological Management of Juvenile Rheumatoid Arthritis," Drugs, 1992, 43(6):849-63.

◆ **Tolmetin Sodium** see Tolmetin on page 1357

Tolnaftate (tole NAF tate)

Medication Safety Issues

Sound-alike/look-alike issues:

Tolnaftate may be confused with Tornalate®

Tinactin® may be confused with Talacen®

U.S. Brand Names Blis-To-Sol® [OTC]; FungiGuard [OTC]; Mycocide® NS [OTC]; Podactin Powder [OTC]; Tinactin® Antifungal Deodorant [OTC]; Tinactin® Antifungal Jock Itch [OTC]; Tinactin® Antifungal [OTC]; Tinaderm [OTC]; Ting® Cream [OTC]; Ting® Spray Liquid [OTC]

Canadian Brand Names Pitrex

Therapeutic Category Antifungal Agent, Topical

Generic Available Yes: Cream, powder, solution

Use Treatment of tinea pedis, tinea cruris, tinea corporis, tinea manuum caused by *Trichophyton rubrum*, *T. mentagrophytes*, *T. tonsurans*, *M. canis*, *M. audouinii*, and *E. floccosum*; also effective in the treatment of tinea versicolor infections due to *Malassezia furfur*

Pregnancy Risk Factor C

Contraindications Hypersensitivity to tolnaftate or any component; nail and scalp infections

Adverse Reactions
Dermatologic: Pruritus, contact dermatitis
Local: Irritation, stinging
Miscellaneous: Hypersensitivity reaction, sensitization to butylated hydroxytoluene component of cream, solution, and aerosol powder

Drug Interactions
Avoid Concomitant Use There are no known interactions where it is recommended to avoid concomitant use.
Increased Effect/Toxicity There are no known significant interactions involving an increase in effect.
Decreased Effect There are no known significant interactions involving a decrease in effect.

Mechanism of Action Distorts the hyphae and stunts mycelial growth in susceptible fungi

Pharmacodynamics Onset of action: Response may be seen 24-72 hours after initiation of therapy

Usual Dosage Children and Adults: Topical: Apply 1-3 drops of solution or a small amount of cream or powder and rub into the affected areas 2-3 times/day for 2-4 weeks

Administration Topical: Wash and dry affected area before drug application; avoid contact with eyes

Monitoring Parameters Resolution of skin infection

Patient Information Avoid contact with the eyes; apply to clean dry area; consult the physician if a skin irritation develops or if the skin infection worsens or does not improve after 10 days of therapy

Additional Information Usually not effective alone for the treatment of infections involving hair follicles or nails

Dosage Forms Excipient information presented when available (limited, particularly for generics); consult specific product labeling. [DSC] = Discontinued product
Aerosol, topical [spray]:
Tinactin® Antifungal: 1% (150 g) [contains ethanol 29% v/v]
Ting®: 1% (128 g) [contains ethanol 41% v/v]
Aerosol, topical [powder, spray]:
Tinactin® Antifungal Deodorant: 1% (133 g) [contains ethanol 11% v/v, talc]
Tinactin® Antifungal: 1% (133 g) [contains ethanol 11% v/v, talc]
Tinactin® Antifungal Jock Itch: 1% (133 g) [contains ethanol 11%, talc]
Cream, topical: 1% (15 g, 30 g)
FungiGuard, Tinactin® Antifungal Jock Itch, Ting®: 1% (15 g)
Tinactin® Antifungal: 1% (15 g, 30 g)
Liquid, topical:
Blis-To-Sol®: 1% (30 mL, 55 mL)
FungiGuard: 1% (30 mL) [contains vitamin E and aloe]
Liquid, topical [spray]:
Tinactin® Antifungal: 1% (59 mL) [contains ethanol 70% v/v]
Powder, topical: 1% (45 g)
Podactin: 1% (45 g)
Tinactin® Antifungal: 1% (108 g)
Solution, topical: 1% (10 mL)
Mycocide® NS: 1% (30 mL)
Tinaderm: 1% (10 mL)

◆ **Toloxin® (Can)** see Digoxin on page 437

Tolterodine (tole TER oh deen)

Medication Safety Issues
Sound-alike/look-alike issues:
Tolterodine may be confused with fesoterodine
Detrol® may be confused with Ditropan®

International issues:
Detrol® may be confused with Desurol® which is a brand name for oxolinic acid in the Czech Republic

U.S. Brand Names Detrol®; Detrol® LA
Canadian Brand Names Detrol®; Detrol® LA; Unidet®
Therapeutic Category Anticholinergic Agent
Generic Available No

Use Treatment of patients with an overactive bladder with symptoms of urinary frequency, urgency, or urge incontinence

Pregnancy Risk Factor C

Pregnancy Considerations Teratogenic effects were observed in one animal studies. There are no adequate and well-controlled studies in pregnant women. Use during pregnancy only if the potential benefit to the mother outweighs the possible risk to the fetus.

Lactation Excretion in breast milk unknown/not recommended

Contraindications Hypersensitivity to tolterodine or any component; urinary retention; gastric retention; uncontrolled narrow-angle glaucoma; myasthenia gravis

Warnings May cause drowsiness and/or blurred vision, which may impair physical or mental abilities; patients must be cautioned about performing tasks which require mental alertness (eg, operating machinery or driving). Use been associated with QT_c prolongation at high (supratherapeutic) doses. The manufacturer recommends caution in patients with congenital prolonged QT or in patients receiving concurrent therapy with QT_c-prolonging drugs (class IA or III antiarrhythmics). However, the extent of QT_c prolongation even at supratherapeutic dosages was <15 msec. Individuals who are poor metabolizers via CYP2D6 or in the presence of inhibitors of CYP2D6 and CYP3A4 may be more likely to exhibit prolongation.

Dosage adjustment is recommended in patients receiving CYP3A4 inhibitors; a lower dose of tolterodine is recommended. Also see QT prolongation in "Concerns related to adverse effects."

Precautions Use with caution in patients with bladder flow obstruction; may increase the risk of urinary retention. Use with caution in patients with gastrointestinal obstructive disorders (ie, pyloric stenosis); may increase the risk of gastric retention. Use with caution in patients with controlled (treated) narrow-angle glaucoma, hepatic impairment (dosage adjustment is required), and renal impairment (dosage adjustment is required).

Adverse Reactions As reported with immediate release tablet, unless otherwise specified
Cardiovascular: Chest pain (2%), angioedema, palpitation, peripheral edema, QT_c prolongation, tachycardia
Central nervous system: Headache (7%; extended release capsules 6%), somnolence (3%; extended release capsules 3%), fatigue (4%; extended release capsules 2%), dizziness (5%; extended release capsules 2%), anxiety (extended release capsules 1%), confusion, disorientation, hallucinations, memory impairment, aggressive abnormal and hyperactive behavior (children 3%)
Dermatologic: Dry skin (1%)
Endocrine & metabolic: Weight gain (1%)
Gastrointestinal: Dry mouth (35%; extended release capsules 23%), abdominal pain (5%; extended release capsules 4%), constipation (7%; extended release capsules 6%), dyspepsia (4%; extended release capsules 3%), diarrhea (4%)
Genitourinary: Dysuria (2%; extended release capsules 1%)
Neuromuscular & skeletal: Arthralgia (2%)
Ocular: Abnormal vision (2%; extended release capsules 1%), dry eyes (3%; extended release capsules 3%)
Renal: Urinary tract infections (children: 6.6%)

Respiratory: Bronchitis (2%), sinusitis (extended release capsules 2%)

Miscellaneous: Flu-like syndrome (3%), infection (1%), hypersensitivity reactions

Drug Interactions

Metabolism/Transport Effects Substrate of CYP2C9 (minor), 2C19 (minor), 2D6 (major), 3A4 (major)

Avoid Concomitant Use There are no known interactions where it is recommended to avoid concomitant use.

Increased Effect/Toxicity

Tolterodine may increase the levels/effects of: AbobotulinumtoxinA; Anticholinergics; Cannabinoids; OnabotulinumtoxinA; Potassium Chloride; RimabotulinumtoxinB; Warfarin

The levels/effects of Tolterodine may be increased by: Antifungal Agents (Azole Derivatives, Systemic); CYP2D6 Inhibitors (Moderate); CYP2D6 Inhibitors (Strong); CYP3A4 Inhibitors (Moderate); CYP3A4 Inhibitors (Strong); Darunavir; Dasatinib; Fluconazole; Pramlintide; VinBLAStine

Decreased Effect

Tolterodine may decrease the levels/effects of: Acetylcholinesterase Inhibitors (Central); Secretin

The levels/effects of Tolterodine may be decreased by: Acetylcholinesterase Inhibitors (Central); CYP3A4 Inducers (Strong); Deferasirox; Herbs (CYP3A4 Inducers); Peginterferon Alfa-2b

Food Interactions Food increases bioavailability (~53% increase) of tolterodine immediate release tablets, but does not affect the pharmacokinetics of tolterodine extended release capsules; adjustment of dose is not needed. As a CYP3A4 inhibitor, grapefruit juice may increase the serum level and/or toxicity of tolterodine, but unlikely secondary to high oral bioavailability. The herbal medicine St John's wort (*Hypericum perforatum*) appears to induce CYP3A enzymes and could decrease tolterodine levels/effects.

Stability Store at 15°C to 30°C (59°F to 86°F); protect from light.

Mechanism of Action Tolterodine is a competitive antagonist of muscarinic receptors. In animal models, tolterodine demonstrates selectivity for urinary bladder receptors over salivary receptors. Urinary bladder contraction is mediated by muscarinic receptors. Tolterodine increases residual urine volume and decreases detrusor muscle pressure.

Pharmacokinetics (Adult data unless noted)

Absorption: Immediate release tablet: Rapid; ≥77%

Distribution: I.V.: V_d: Adults: 113 ± 27 L

Protein binding: >96% (primarily bound to alpha$_1$-acid glycoprotein)

Metabolism: Extensively hepatic, primarily via CYP2D6 (some metabolites share activity) and CYP3A4 usually (minor pathway). In patients with a genetic deficiency of CYP2D6, metabolism via CYP3A4 predominates. Forms three active metabolites.

Half-life elimination:

Immediate release tablet: Extensive metabolizers: ~2 hours; poor metabolizers: ~10 hours

Extended release capsule: Extensive metabolizers: ~7 hours; poor metabolizers: ~18 hours

Time to peak serum concentration:

Immediate release tablet: 1-2 hours

Extended release tablet: 2-6 hours

Excretion: Urine (77%); feces (17%); excreted primarily as metabolites (<1% unchanged drug) of which the active 5-hydroxymethyl metabolite accounts for 5% to 14% (<1% in poor metabolizers)

Usual Dosage Oral: Adults: Treatment of overactive bladder:

Immediate release tablet: 2 mg twice daily; the dose may be lowered to 1 mg twice daily based on individual response and tolerability

Dosing adjustment in patients concurrently taking CYP3A4 inhibitors: 1 mg twice daily

Extended release capsule: 4 mg once daily; dose may be lowered to 2 mg once daily based on individual response and tolerability

Dosing adjustment in patients concurrently taking CYP3A4 inhibitors: 2 mg once daily

Dosing adjustment in renal impairment: Use with caution (studies conducted in patients with Cl_{cr} 10-30 mL/minute):

Immediate release tablet: 1 mg twice daily

Extended release capsule: 2 mg once daily

Dosing adjustment in hepatic impairment:

Immediate release tablet: 1 mg twice daily

Extended release capsule: 2 mg once daily

Administration Oral: Administer without regard to food; do not break, crush, or chew extended release capsules.

Patient Information May cause headache, dry mouth, dizziness, nervousness, or sleepiness; use caution when driving, climbing stairs, or engaging in tasks requiring alertness until response to drug is known; or abdominal discomfort, diarrhea, constipation, nausea, or vomiting; small frequent meals, increased exercise, adequate hydration may help. Report back pain, muscle spasms, alteration in gait, or numbness of extremities; unresolved or persistent constipation, diarrhea, or vomiting; or symptoms of upper respiratory infection or flu. Report immediately any chest pain or palpitations, difficulty urinating, or pain on urination.

Dosage Forms Excipient information presented when available (limited, particularly for generics); consult specific product labeling.

Capsule, extended release, oral, as tartrate:

Detrol® LA: 2 mg, 4 mg

Tablet, oral, as tartrate:

Detrol®: 1 mg, 2 mg

◆ **Tolterodine Tartrate** *see* Tolterodine *on page 1359*

◆ **Tomoxetine** *see* Atomoxetine *on page 149*

◆ **Topactin (Can)** *see* Fluocinonide *on page 595*

◆ **Topamax®** *see* Topiramate *on page 1360*

◆ **Topicaine® [OTC]** *see* Lidocaine *on page 818*

◆ **Topilene® (Can)** *see* Betamethasone *on page 189*

Topiramate (toe PYE ra mate)

Medication Safety Issues

Sound-alike/look-alike issues:

Topamax® may be confused with Sporanox®, Tegretol®, Tegretol®-XR, Toprol-XL®

Related Information

Antiepileptic Drugs *on page 1693*

U.S. Brand Names Topamax®

Canadian Brand Names Apo-Topiramate®; CO Topiramate; Dom-Topiramate; Mint-Topiramate; Mylan-Topiramate; Novo-Topiramate; PHL-Topiramate; PMS-Topiramate; PRO-Topiramate; ratio-Topiramate; Sandoz-Topiramate; Topamax®; ZYM-Topiramate

Therapeutic Category Anticonvulsant, Miscellaneous

Generic Available Yes

Use Initial monotherapy of primary generalized tonic-clonic seizures or partial onset seizures (FDA approved in ages ≥10 years and adults); adjunctive treatment of primary generalized tonic-clonic seizures or partial onset seizures (FDA approved in ages ≥2 years and adults); adjunctive treatment of seizures associated with Lennox-Gastaut syndrome (FDA approved in ages ≥2 years); prophylaxis of migraine headache (FDA approved in adults); may potentially be useful in infantile spasms

Medication Guide An FDA-approved patient medication guide, which is available with the product information and at http://www.fda.gov/downloads/Drugs/DrugSafety/UCM152837.pdf, must be dispensed with this medication for each new outpatient prescription and refill.

Pregnancy Risk Factor C

Pregnancy Considerations Topiramate was found to be teratogenic in animal studies. Based on limited data, topiramate was found to cross the placenta. Although not evaluated during pregnancy, metabolic acidosis may be induced by topiramate. In general, metabolic acidosis during pregnancy may result in adverse effects and fetal death.

Patients exposed to topiramate during pregnancy are encouraged to enroll themselves into the AED Pregnancy Registry by calling 1-888-233-2334. Additional information is available at www.aedpregnancyregistry.org.

Lactation Enters breast milk/use caution

Breast-Feeding Considerations Based on limited data, topiramate was found in breast milk. Infant plasma concentrations of topiramate have been reported as 10% to 20% of the maternal plasma concentration.

Contraindications Hypersensitivity to topiramate or any component

Warnings Hyperchloremic metabolic acidosis may occur in patients receiving topiramate. Topiramate may decrease serum bicarbonate concentrations, due to inhibition of carbonic anhydrase and increased renal bicarbonate loss. In pediatric clinical trials for adjunctive treatment of seizures, persistent decreases in serum bicarbonate occurred in 67% of patients receiving topiramate (versus 10% of those receiving placebo). Markedly low serum bicarbonate values were reported in 11% of pediatric patients receiving topiramate (versus 0% of those receiving placebo). In pediatric monotherapy trials, persistent decreases in serum bicarbonate occurred in 7% of patients receiving 50 mg/day and 20% of patients receiving 400 mg/day. Markedly low serum bicarbonate values were reported in 4% of pediatric patients receiving topiramate monotherapy. The risk of topiramate-induced metabolic acidosis may be increased in patients with predisposing conditions (eg, diarrhea, status epilepticus, renal dysfunction, severe respiratory disorders, ketogenic diet, surgery) or concurrent treatment with other drugs that may cause acidosis.

Serum bicarbonate should be monitored at baseline and periodically during topiramate therapy. Patients should also be monitored for symptoms of metabolic acidosis (eg, hyperventilation, fatigue, anorexia, stupor, cardiac arrhythmias) and for potential complications of chronic acidosis (eg, nephrolithiasis, rickets, and reduced growth rates). Dose reduction or discontinuation (by tapering the dose) should be considered in patients with persistent or severe metabolic acidosis. If treatment is continued, alkali supplementation should be considered.

An ocular syndrome (characterized by secondary acute angle closure glaucoma and acute myopia) has been reported in adult and pediatric patients. Symptoms generally occur within 1 month of treatment initiation and include an acute decrease in visual acuity and/or ocular pain. Ophthalmologic findings may include increased IOP, anterior chamber shallowing, ocular hyperemia, mydriasis, and supracilliary effusion with anterior displacement of lens and iris. Patients experiencing blurred vision and/or eye pain should contact their physician immediately. Primary treatment of this syndrome is discontinuation of topiramate as soon as possible, based on physician judgment. If left untreated, this syndrome may cause serious damage to the eye, including permanent vision loss.

Rare, but significant, reports of oligohydrosis (decreased sweating) and hyperthermia have occurred in patients receiving topiramate. Most cases occurred in children, and were associated with vigorous exercise and/or high environmental temperatures. Due to the potential for serious sequelae, the use of preventative strategies (hydration before and during exercise or exposure to warm temperatures) is recommended. Monitor patients, especially pediatric patients, for decreased sweating and hyperthermia, especially in warm or hot weather. Use topiramate with caution in patients receiving drugs that predispose to heat-related disorders (eg, anticholinergic agents, carbonic anhydrase inhibitors).

Do not abruptly discontinue therapy in patients with or without a history of epilepsy or seizures; withdraw gradually to lessen the chance for seizures or increased seizure frequency; in pediatric epilepsy clinical trials, doses were gradually withdrawn over 2-8 weeks; in adult trials, daily doses were decreased in weekly intervals by 50-100 mg in epilepsy patients and by 25-50 mg in adult patients with migraines; monitor patients carefully if rapid withdrawal of topiramate is medically required. CNS adverse effects are common (see Adverse Reactions); nephrolithiasis (kidney stones) or paresthesia (usually tingling of extremities) may occur; avoid use with alcohol, CNS depressants, or carbonic anhydrase inhibitors (see Drug Interactions); avoid use of ketogenic diet (may increase risk of nephrolithiasis).

Antiepileptic drugs (AEDs) increase the risk of suicidal behavior and ideation in patients receiving these medications for any indication. Pooled analyses of placebo-controlled trials involving 11 different AEDs (regardless of indication) showed a twofold increased risk of suicidal thoughts or behavior (estimated incidence rate: 0.43% in AED treated patients compared to 0.24% of patients receiving placebo); increased risk was observed as early as 1 week after initiation of AED and continued through duration of trials (most trials ≤24 weeks); risk did not vary significantly by age (age range: 5–100 years). Consider risks and benefits of AEDs before prescribing. Monitor all patients receiving an AED for emergence of suicidal thoughts or behavior, thoughts of self-harm, any unusual changes in behavior or mood, or the emergence or worsening of depressive symptoms; notify heathcare provider immediately if symptoms or concerning behavior occur. **Note:** The FDA is requiring that a Medication Guide be developed for all antiepileptic drugs informing patients of this risk.

Precautions Use with caution and decrease the dose in patients with renal dysfunction; use with caution in patients allergic to sulfa drugs and in patients with hepatic impairment. Concurrent use with valproic acid may result in hyperammonemia with or without encephalopathy; use with caution in patients with inborn errors of metabolism or decreased hepatic mitochondrial activity; these patients may be at increased risk.

Adverse Reactions

Central nervous system: Ataxia, difficulty in concentrating, dizziness, memory difficulties, fatigue, nervousness, somnolence, psychomotor slowing, speech/language problems, confusion, depression, mood problems, anxiety, cognitive problems; fever, irritability, and sleep disturbances (reported in children); suicidal thinking and behavior (see Warnings); **Note:** Somnolence and fatigue are the most common neuropsychiatric adverse effects in children

Dermatologic: Alopecia, rash, pruritus, acne

Endocrine & metabolic: Weight loss; serum bicarbonate decreased, hyperchloremic metabolic acidosis (non-anion gap) (see Warnings); dehydration, hypokalemia

Gastrointestinal: Anorexia, nausea, diarrhea

Hematologic: Purpura

Neuromuscular & skeletal: Paresthesia, tremor

Ocular: Nystagmus, diplopia, abnormal vision, ocular syndrome (see Warnings)

Otic: Tinnitus

Renal: Nephrolithiasis

Respiratory: Epistaxis

Miscellaneous: Oligohydrosis (sweating decreased) and hyperthermia [pediatric patients may be at increased risk (see Warnings)]

Drug Interactions

Metabolism/Transport Effects Inhibits CYP2C19 (weak); **Induces** CYP3A4 (weak)

Avoid Concomitant Use There are no known interactions where it is recommended to avoid concomitant use.

Increased Effect/Toxicity

Topiramate may increase the levels/effects of: Alcohol (Ethyl); CNS Depressants; Divalproex; Lithium; Methotrimeprazine; Phenytoin; Valproic Acid

The levels/effects of Topiramate may be increased by: Methotrimeprazine

Decreased Effect

Topiramate may decrease the levels/effects of: Contraceptives (Estrogens); Contraceptives (Progestins); Saxagliptin

The levels/effects of Topiramate may be decreased by: CarBAMazepine; Ketorolac; Ketorolac (Systemic); Mefloquine; Phenytoin

Food Interactions Food may decrease the rate but not the extent of absorption; ketogenic diet may increase risk of nephrolithiasis

Stability Protect from moisture; store at room temperature

Mechanism of Action Exact mechanism unknown; efficacy for epilepsy and migraine prophylaxis may be due to blockade of voltage-dependent sodium channels, potentiation of GABA (an inhibitory neurotransmitter) and antagonism of kainate activation of glutamate (an excitatory amino acid) subtype receptors; also inhibits carbonic anhydrase (minor effect)

Pharmacokinetics (Adult data unless noted) Note: Sprinkle capsule is bioequivalent to tablet

Absorption: Rapid

Distribution: Distributes extensively into breast milk

V_d: Adults: 0.6-0.8 L/kg

Protein binding: 15% to 41%; percent protein bound decreases as blood concentrations increase

Metabolism: Minor amounts metabolized in liver via hydroxylation, hydrolysis, and glucuronidation; percentage of dose metabolized in liver and clearance are increased in patients receiving enzyme inducers

Bioavailability: Tablet: 80% (relative to a prepared solution)

Half-life:

Adults: 19-23 hours (mean 21 hours)

Adults with renal impairment: 59 ± 11 hours (n=7)

Time to peak serum concentration: 2 hours; range: 1.4-4.3 hours

Elimination: 70% of dose excreted unchanged in urine; may undergo renal tubular reabsorption

Clearance:

Children 4-17 years: ~50% higher than adults (per kg)

Adults: 20-30 mL/minute

Renal impairment: Reduced

Hepatic impairment: May be reduced

Dialysis: Significantly hemodialyzed; dialysis clearance: 120 mL/minute (4-6 times higher than in adults with

normal renal function); supplemental doses may be required

Usual Dosage Oral:

Anticonvulsant, adjunctive therapy:

Children 2-16 years:

Partial onset seizures or Lennox-Gastaut syndrome: Initial: 1-3 mg/kg/day (maximum: 25 mg) given nightly for 1 week; increase at 1- to 2-week intervals by 1-3 mg/kg/day given in 2 divided doses; titrate dose to response; usual maintenance: 5-9 mg/kg/day given in 2 divided doses

Primary generalized tonic-clonic seizures: Use initial dose as listed above, but use slower initial titration rate; titrate to 6 mg/kg/day by the end of 8 weeks

Adolescents ≥17 years and Adults:

Partial onset seizures: Initial: 25-50 mg/day given daily for 1 week; increase at weekly intervals by 25-50 mg/day; give in 2 divided doses; titrate dose to response; usual maintenance: 100-200 mg twice daily; maximum dose: 1600 mg/day

Primary generalized tonic-clonic seizures: Use initial dose as listed above, but use slower initial titration rate; give in 2 divided doses; titrate upwards to recommended dose by the end of 8 weeks; usual maintenance: 200 mg twice daily; maximum dose: 1600 mg/day

Anticonvulsant, monotherapy: Partial onset seizures or primary generalized tonic-clonic seizures: Children ≥10 years and Adults: Initial: 25 mg twice daily; increase at weekly intervals by 50 mg/day up to a dose of 100 mg twice daily (week 4 dose); thereafter, may further increase at weekly intervals by 100 mg/day up to the recommended maximum dose of 200 mg twice daily

Migraine prophylaxis: Adults: Initial: 25 mg/day; increase at weekly intervals by 25 mg/day; give in 2 divided doses; titrate dose to response; recommended dose: 50 mg twice daily; **Note:** A randomized controlled trial that included adolescent patients, titrated doses based on response, up to a maximum dose of 100 mg twice daily (see Brandes, 2004)

Dosing adjustment in renal impairment: Cl_{cr} <70 mL/minute/1.73 m²: Administer 50% of the usual dose; titrate more slowly due to prolonged half-life; supplemental doses may be required in patients undergoing hemodialysis (see Pharmacokinetics)

Dosing adjustment in hepatic impairment: Carefully adjust dose as plasma concentrations may be increased if normal dosing is used

Administration May be administered without regard to food; broken tablets have a bitter taste; tablets may be crushed, mixed with water, and administered immediately. Swallow sprinkle capsules whole or open and sprinkle contents on small amount of soft food (eg, 1 teaspoonful of applesauce, oatmeal, ice cream, pudding, custard, or yogurt); swallow sprinkle/food mixture immediately; do not chew; do not store for later use; drink fluids after dose to make sure mixture is completely swallowed

Monitoring Parameters Frequency, duration, and severity of seizure episodes or migraine headaches; renal function; monitor serum electrolytes including baseline and periodic serum bicarbonate, symptoms of metabolic acidosis (see Warnings), complications of chronic acidosis (eg, nephrolithiasis, rickets, and reduced growth rates); monitor body temperature and for decreased sweating, especially in warm or hot weather; monitor serum ammonia concentration in patients with unexplained lethargy, vomiting, or mental status changes; intraocular pressure, symptoms of secondary angle closure glaucoma (see Warnings); signs and symptoms of suicidality (eg, anxiety, depression, behavior changes) (see Warnings)

Reference Range Not applicable; plasma topiramate concentrations have not been shown to correlate with clinical efficacy

Patient Information Read the patient Medication Guide that you receive with each prescription and refill of topiramate. Antiepileptic agents may increase the risk of suicidal thoughts and behavior; notify physician if you feel more depressed or have thoughts of suicide or self harm (see Warnings). Before taking this medication, inform physician if you have any of the following conditions: Liver or kidney problems, kidney stones, lung or breathing problems, eye problems, glaucoma, bone problems, growth problems, diarrhea, history of metabolic acidosis, depression, mood problems, suicidal thoughts or behavior, are receiving a ketogenic diet, or will be having surgery. Report the use of other medications, nonprescription medications, and herbal or natural products to your physician and pharmacist. Topiramate may decrease the effectiveness of birth control pills; talk to your doctor about using an alternative, nonhormonal form of contraception.

Take topiramate everyday as prescribed; do not change dose or discontinue without physician's advice; if a dose is missed, take it as soon as possible; however, if you are within 6 hours of your next dose, skip the missed dose and take your scheduled dose as usual; if a dose is skipped, do **not** double the next dose. Do not abruptly discontinue therapy (an increase in seizure activity may result). Contact physician immediately if blurred vision or eye pain occur, as these can lead to blindness if not treated right away. Ensure adequate fluid intake to avoid kidney stone formation and to help prevent dehydration and hyperthermia before and during exercise or exposure to warm temperatures. May cause dizziness or drowsiness and impair ability to perform activities requiring mental alertness or physical coordination. Avoid alcohol. Report worsening of seizure activity or loss of seizure control.

Dosage Forms Excipient information presented when available (limited, particularly for generics); consult specific product labeling.

Capsule, sprinkle: 15 mg, 25 mg
  Topamax®: 15 mg, 25 mg
Tablet: 25 mg, 50 mg, 100 mg, 200 mg
  Topamax®: 25 mg, 50 mg, 100 mg, 200 mg

Extemporaneous Preparations A 6 mg/mL topiramate oral suspension made from tablets and 2 different vehicles (a 1:1 mixture of Ora-Sweet® and Ora-Plus®, or a mixture of Simple Syrup, NF and methylcellulose 1% with parabens) was stable for 90 days when stored in plastic prescription bottles under refrigeration (preferred) or at room temperature; grind six 100 mg tablets in a mortar into a fine powder; add a small amount of methylcellulose gel and mix well to form a uniform paste (**Note:** Use a small amount of methylcellulose gel when using the 1:1 Ora-Sweet® and Ora-Plus® mixture as the vehicle; use 10 mL of methylcellulose 1% with parabens when using Simple Syrup, NF as the vehicle; mix while adding the vehicle in geometric proportions to **almost** 100 mL; transfer to a graduate; rinse the mortar with the vehicle and transfer to the graduate; qsad with vehicle to make 100 mL; label "shake well" and "refrigerate" (Nahata, 2004).

Nahata MC, Pai VB, and Hipple TF, *Pediatric Drug Formulations*, 5th ed, Cincinnati, OH: Harvey Whitney Books Co, 2004.

References
Brandes JL, Saper JR, Diamond M, et al, "Topiramate for Migraine Prevention: A Randomized Controlled Trial," *JAMA*, 2004, 291 (8):965-73.
Doose DR, Walker SA, Gisclon LG, et al, "Single-Dose Pharmacokinetics and Effect of Food on the Bioavailability of Topiramate, a Novel Antiepileptic Drug," *J Clin Pharmacol*, 1996, 36(10):884-91.
Glauser TA, "Preliminary Observations on Topiramate in Pediatric Epilepsies," *Epilepsia*, 1997, 38(Suppl 1):S37-41.
Glauser TA, "Topiramate Use in Pediatric Patients," *Can J Neurol Sci*, 1998, 25(3):S8-12.
Glauser TA, Clark PO, and Strawsburg R, "A Pilot Study of Topiramate in the Treatment of Infantile Spasms," *Epilepsia*, 1998, 39(12):1324-8.
Hershey AD, Powers SW, Vockell AL, et al, "Effectiveness of Topiramate in the Prevention of Childhood Headaches," *Headache*, 2002, 42(8):810-8.
Pellock JM, "Managing Pediatric Epilepsy Syndromes With New Antiepileptic Drugs," *Pediatrics*, 1999, 104(5 Pt 1):1106-16.
Sachdeo RC, "Topiramate. Clinical Profile in Epilepsy," *Clin Pharmacokinet*, 1998, 34(5):335-46.

◆ **Topisone® (Can)** *see* Betamethasone *on page* 189
◆ **Toposar™** *see* Etoposide *on page* 551

Topotecan (toe poe TEE kan)

Medication Safety Issues
Sound-alike/look-alike issues:
  Hycamtin® may be confused with Hycomine®, Mycamine®

High alert medication: The Institute for Safe Medication Practices (ISMP) includes this medication among its list of drugs which have a heightened risk of causing significant patient harm when used in error.

Related Information
Emetogenic Potential of Antineoplastic Agents *on page* 1579

U.S. Brand Names Hycamtin®

Canadian Brand Names Hycamtin®; Topotecan For Injection

Therapeutic Category Antineoplastic Agent, Camptothecin; Antineoplastic Agent, Topoisomerase Inhibitor

Generic Available No

Use Treatment of ovarian cancer after failure of first-line chemotherapy; second-line treatment of small cell lung cancer; cervical cancer (FDA approved in adults); has also been used in nonsmall cell lung cancer, myelodysplastic syndrome, pediatric solid tumor, including sarcoma and neuroblastoma

Pregnancy Risk Factor D

Pregnancy Considerations Animal studies found reduced fetal body weight, eye, brain, skull, and vertebrae malformations. May cause fetal harm in pregnant women. Use during pregnancy is contraindicated.

Lactation Excretion in breast milk unknown/contraindicated

Breast-Feeding Considerations Breast-feeding should be discontinued in women who are receiving topotecan.

Contraindications Hypersensitivity to topotecan or any component; severe bone marrow depression (patients with baseline neutrophil counts <1,500 cells/mm^3 and platelet count <100,000/mm^3); pregnancy; breast-feeding

Warnings Hazardous agent; use appropriate precautions for handling and disposal. The dose-limiting toxicity is bone marrow suppression, primarily neutropenia (may also cause thrombocytopenia and anemia); monitor bone marrow function. Neutropenia is not cumulative over time. Should only administer to patients with adequate bone marrow reserves, baseline neutrophils at least 1500 cells/mm^3 and platelet counts at least 100,000/mm^3 **[U.S. Boxed Warning]**. Topotecan-induced neutropenia may lead to neutropenic colitis; should be considered in patients presenting with neutropenia, fever, and abdominal pain. Severe diarrhea, including cases requiring hospitalization, have been reported with oral topotecan; dose adjustment may be needed. May cause fetal harm when administered to pregnant women.

Precautions Use caution in patients with renal or hepatic impairment; modify dosage in patients with renal impairment

Adverse Reactions
Cardiovascular: Hypotension
Central nervous system: Asthenia, fatigue, fever, headache, pain
Dermatologic: Alopecia, rash
Genitourinary: Hematuria

Gastrointestinal: Anorexia, colitis, constipation, diarrhea, mucositis, nausea, vomiting

Hematologic: Anemia, fibrinogen level decreased, hemorrhage, leukopenia, neutropenia, thrombocytopenia

Hepatic: Bilirubin and alkaline phosphatase increased, liver enzymes increased

Neuromuscular & skeletal: Arthralgia, myalgia, paresthesia

Respiratory: Cough, dyspnea

Miscellaneous: Anaphylactoid reactions, sepsis

<1%, postmarketing, and/or case reports: Abdominal pain, allergic reactions, angioedema, bleeding (severe, associated with thrombocytopenia), dermatitis (severe), injection site reactions (mild erythema, bruising), neutropenic colitis, pancytopenia, pruritus (severe)

Drug Interactions

Avoid Concomitant Use

Avoid concomitant use of Topotecan with any of the following: BCG; Natalizumab; P-Glycoprotein Inhibitors; Pimecrolimus; Tacrolimus (Topical); Vaccines (Live)

Increased Effect/Toxicity

Topotecan may increase the levels/effects of: Leflunomide; Natalizumab; Vaccines (Live)

The levels/effects of Topotecan may be increased by: BCRP/ABCG2 Inhibitors; Denosumab; Filgrastim; P-Glycoprotein Inhibitors; Pimecrolimus; Platinum Derivatives; Tacrolimus (Topical); Trastuzumab

Decreased Effect

Topotecan may decrease the levels/effects of: BCG; Sipuleucel-T; Vaccines (Inactivated); Vaccines (Live)

The levels/effects of Topotecan may be decreased by: Echinacea

Stability Store capsules in refrigerator. Store intact vials containing lyophilized powder at room temperature; protect from light. Reconstituted solution for injection is stable for 24 hours at room temperature or up to 7 days if refrigerated; if topotecan is further diluted in D_5W or NS, it is stable for 24 hours at room temperature or up to 7 days under refrigeration. Do **not** dilute in alkaline solutions.

Mechanism of Action Topoisomerase I inhibitor which stabilizes the covalent complex between topoisomerase I and DNA preventing religation of DNA single-strand breaks resulting in interference with DNA replication, RNA transcription, and DNA repair.

Pharmacokinetics (Adult data unless noted)

Distribution: V_d: Adults: 87.3 L/m^2; distributes into tissues and CSF

Protein binding: 35%

Metabolism: Undergoes pH dependent hydrolysis of its active lactone moiety to yield a relatively inactive open-ring hydroxy acid form in plasma; active metabolite, N-demethylated topotecan, formed in the liver

Bioavailability: Oral: ~40%

Half-life: Adults:

I.V.: 2-3 hours; 5 hours with renal impairment

Oral: 3-6 hours

Time to peak serum concentration: Oral: 1-2 hours

Elimination:

I.V.: Urine: 51%; feces: 18%

Oral: Urine: 20%; feces: 33%

Clearance: Topotecan plasma clearance is 24% higher in males than in female patients

Children:

No previous radiation therapy and no bone marrow involvement: 12.2 ± 3.5 $L/hour/m^2$ (range: 6.8-17.4 $L/hour/m^2$)

Previous radiation without bone marrow involvement: 9.8 ± 4.1 $L/hour/m^2$ (range: 4.8-17.4 $L/hour/m^2$)

Adults: 6.5-30 $L/hour/m^2$

Usual Dosage Refer to Individual Protocols:

Children: I.V.:

Pediatric solid tumors: 1 mg/m^2/day (range: 0.75-1.9 mg/m^2/day) for 3 days as a continuous infusion, repeated every 3 weeks

Single-agent therapy for refractory solid tumors or hematologic malignancies: 2.4 mg/m^2/day once daily for 5 days of a 21 day course.

Combination therapy for solid tumors: 0.75 mg/m^2/dose once daily for 5 days every 21 days in combination with cyclophosphamide.

Adults:

I.V.: Intermittent infusion:

Ovarian cancer and small cell lung cancer: 1.5 mg/m^2/day once daily for 5 days followed by a 16 day rest period; repeat course every 21 days for 4 courses. If neutrophil count falls to <500/mm^3 or if platelets decrease to <25,000 cells/mm^3, reduce dose by 0.25 mg/m^2 for subsequent courses. Alternatively for severe neutropenia, administer G-CSF 24 hours after completion of topotecan infusion following subsequent courses

Cervical cancer: 0.75 mg/m^2/day once daily on days 1, 2, and 3; repeat every 21 days in combination with cisplatin

I.V.: Continuous infusion: Ovarian cancer: 0.2-0.7mg/m^2/day for 7-21 days

Oral: Small cell lung cancer: 2.3 mg/m^2/day for 5 days; repeat every 21 days. If patient vomits after dose is administered, do not give a replacement dose.

Dosing adjustment in renal impairment: Adults:

I.V.:

Cl_{cr} 20-39 mL/minute: Reduce dosage by 50% or by 0.75 mg/m^2/dose

Cl_{cr} <20 mL/minute: Insufficient data available to recommend dosage adjustment guidelines

Oral:

Cl_{cr} 30-49 mL/minute: Reduce dose to 1.8 mg/m^2/day

Cl_{cr} <30 mL/minute: Insufficient data available for dosing recommendation

Dosing adjustment in hepatic impairment:

I.V.: Bilirubin 1.5-10 mg/dL: No adjustment necessary.

Oral: Bilirubin >1.5 mg/dL: No adjustment necessary.

Dosing adjustment for toxicity:

I.V.:

Ovarian and small cell lung cancer: Dosage adjustment for hematological effects: Severe neutropenia or platelet count <25,000/mm^3: Reduce dose to 1.25 mg/m^2/day for subsequent cycles (may consider G-CSF support [beginning on day 6] prior to instituting dose reduction for neutropenia

Cervical cancer: Severe febrile neutropenia (ANC <1000/mm^3 with temperature of 38° C) or platelet count <10,000/mm^3: Reduce topotecan to 0.6 mg/m^2/day for subsequent cycles (may consider C-CSF support [beginning on day 4] prior to instituting dose reduction for neutropenic fever.

For neutropenic fever despite G-SCF use, reduce dose to 0.45 mg/m^2/day for subsequent cycles. **Note:** Cisplatin may also require dose adjustment.

Oral: Small cell lung cancer: Severe neutropenia (neutrophils <500/mm^3 associated with fever or infection or lasting >7 days) or prolonged neutropenia (neutrophils ≥500/mm^3 to ≤1000/mm^3 lasting beyond day 21) or platelets <25,000/mm^3 or grades 3/4 diarrhea: Reduce dose to 1.9 mg/m^2/day for subsequent cycles (may consider same dosage reduction for grade 2 diarrhea if clinically indicated.)

Administration

Parenteral: May administer by intermittent infusion over 30 minutes or by continuous infusion at a final concentration not to exceed 0.5 mg/mL in D_5W or NS.

Oral: May administer with or without food. Swallow capsule whole; do not crush, chew, or divide capsule.

Monitoring Parameters CBC with differential and platelet count; renal and hepatic function tests; blood pressure during infusion

Patient Information Inform physician of persistent fever, chills, bruising, bleeding, abdominal pain, diarrhea, yellowing of eyes or skin, or pain at infusion site. Avoid alcohol; may cause fatigue and impair ability to perform activities requiring mental alertness or physical coordination. Topotecan may cause birth defects; contraceptive measures are recommended during therapy. If vomiting occurs after oral topotecan dose, do not take replacement dose.

Nursing Implications Care should be taken to avoid extravasation. Extravasation of topotecan has been associated with local reactions such as erythema and bruising. If a topotecan solution comes in contact with skin or mucous membranes, wash skin immediately and thoroughly with soap and water; flush mucosa thoroughly with water.

Additional Information
Myelosuppressive effects:
WBC (nadir): 8-11 days; recovery: 21 days
Neutrophils (nadir): 12 days
Platelets (nadir): 15 days

Dosage Forms Excipient information presented when available (limited, particularly for generics); consult specific product labeling.
Capsule:
Hycamtin®: 0.25 mg, 1 mg
Injection, powder for reconstitution:
Hycamtin®: 4 mg

References

Furman WL, Stewart CF, Kirstein M, et al, "Protracted Intermittent Schedule of Topotecan in Children With Refractory Acute Leukemia: A Pediatric Oncology Group Study," *J of Clin Oncology*, 2002, 20 (6):1617-24.

Santana VM, Zamboni WC, Kirstein MN, et al, "A Pilot Study of Protracted Topotecan Dosing Using a Pharmacokinetically Guided Dosing Approach in Children With Solid Tumors," *Clin Cancer Res*, 2003, 9(2):633-40.

Saylors RL 3rd, Stine KC, Sullivan J, et al, "Cyclophosphamide Plus Topotecan in Children With Recurrent or Refractory Solid Tumors: A Pediatric Oncology Group Phase II Study," *J Clin Oncol*, 2001, 19 (15):3463-9.

Walterhouse DO, Lyden ER, Breitfeld PP, et al, "Efficacy of Topotecan and Cyclophosphamide Given in a Phase II Window Trial in Children With Newly Diagnosed Metastatic Rhabdomyosarcoma: A Children's Oncology Group Study," *J Clin Oncol*, 2004, 22(8):1398-403.

Wells RJ, Reid JM, Ames MM, et al, "Phase I Trial of Cisplatin and Topotecan in Children With Recurrent Solid Tumors: Children's Cancer Group Study 0942," *J Pediatr Hematol Oncol*, 2002, 24 (2):89-93.

♦ **Topotecan For Injection (Can)** *see* Topotecan *on page 1363*

♦ **Topotecan Hydrochloride** *see* Topotecan *on page 1363*

♦ **Toprol-XL®** *see* Metoprolol *on page 918*

♦ **Topsyn® (Can)** *see* Fluocinonide *on page 595*

♦ **Toradol** *see* Ketorolac *on page 781*

♦ **Toradol® (Can)** *see* Ketorolac *on page 781*

♦ **Toradol® IM (Can)** *see* Ketorolac *on page 781*

Torsemide (TOR se mide)

Medication Safety Issues
Sound-alike/look-alike issues:
Torsemide may be confused with furosemide
Demadex® may be confused with Denorex®

Related Information
Antihypertensive Agents by Class *on page 1481*

U.S. Brand Names Demadex®

Therapeutic Category Antihypertensive Agent; Diuretic, Loop

Generic Available Yes

Use Management of edema associated with CHF and hepatic or renal disease; used alone or in combination with antihypertensives in treatment of hypertension

Pregnancy Risk Factor B

Pregnancy Considerations A decrease in fetal weight, an increase in fetal resorption, and delayed fetal ossification has occurred in animal studies.

Lactation Excretion in breast milk unknown/use caution

Contraindications Hypersensitivity to torsemide, any component, or other sulfonylureas; anuria

Warnings Loop diuretics are potent diuretics, excess amounts can lead to profound diuresis with fluid and electrolyte loss; close medical supervision and dose evaluation is required

Adverse Reactions
Cardiovascular: Orthostatic hypotension, ECG abnormality, chest pain, atrial fibrillation, ventricular tachycardia, syncope

Central nervous system: Headache, dizziness, insomnia, nervousness

Dermatologic: Rash, photosensitivity

Endocrine & metabolic: Hyponatremia, hypokalemia, hypochloremia, alkalosis, hypocalcemia, dehydration, hyperuricemia, gout

Gastrointestinal: Diarrhea, nausea, constipation, dyspepsia, GI hemorrhage, stomach cramps, pancreatitis

Genitourinary: Excessive urination

Hematologic: Agranulocytosis, anemia

Neuromuscular & skeletal: Myalgia, arthralgia, weakness

Otic: Ototoxicity

Renal: Prerenal azotemia, interstitial nephritis, nephrocalcinosis

Drug Interactions

Metabolism/Transport Effects Substrate of CYP2C8 (minor), CYP2C9 (major), SLCO1B1; **Inhibits** CYP2C19 (weak)

Avoid Concomitant Use There are no known interactions where it is recommended to avoid concomitant use.

Increased Effect/Toxicity
Torsemide may increase the levels/effects of: ACE Inhibitors; Allopurinol; Amifostine; Aminoglycosides; Antihypertensives; CISplatin; Dofetilide; Hypotensive Agents; Lithium; Neuromuscular-Blocking Agents; RiTUXimab; Salicylates; Warfarin

The levels/effects of Torsemide may be increased by: Corticosteroids (Orally Inhaled); Corticosteroids (Systemic); CYP2C9 Inhibitors (Moderate); CYP2C9 Inhibitors (Strong); Diazoxide; Eltrombopag; Herbs (Hypotensive Properties); MAO Inhibitors; Pentoxifylline; Phosphodiesterase 5 Inhibitors; Probenecid; Prostacyclin Analogues

Decreased Effect
Torsemide may decrease the levels/effects of: Lithium; Neuromuscular-Blocking Agents

The levels/effects of Torsemide may be decreased by: Bile Acid Sequestrants; CYP2C9 Inducers (Highly Effective); Herbs (Hypotensive Properties); Methylphenidate; Nonsteroidal Anti-Inflammatory Agents; Peginterferon Alfa-2b; Phenytoin; Probenecid; Salicylates; Yohimbine

Stability Stable for 24 hours at room temperature when mixed with D_5W or NS

Mechanism of Action Inhibits reabsorption of sodium and chloride in the ascending loop of Henle and distal renal tubule, interfering with the chloride-binding cotransport system, thus causing increased excretion of water, sodium, chloride, magnesium, and calcium

Pharmacodynamics

Onset of action:
Oral: 60 minutes
I.V.: 10 minutes
Maximum effect:
Oral: 60-120 minutes
I.V.: Within 60 minutes
Duration: Oral, I.V.: 6-8 hours

Pharmacokinetics (Adult data unless noted)

Absorption: Oral: Rapid
Distribution: V_d: 12-15 L (adults)
Protein binding: Plasma: ~97% to 99%
Metabolism: Hepatic by cytochrome P450, 80%
Bioavailability: 80% to 90%
Half-life: 3.5 hours (range 2-4 hours); 7-8 hours in cirrhosis (dose modification appears unnecessary)
Time to peak serum concentration: Oral: 1 hour
Elimination: 20% eliminated unchanged in urine

Usual Dosage Adults: Oral, I.V.:

Edema: 10-20 mg once daily; titrate upward as needed (maximum dose: 200 mg/day)
Hepatic cirrhosis: 5-10 mg once daily
Hypertension: Initial: 5 mg once daily; increase to 10 mg if ineffective after 4-6 weeks of therapy

Administration

Oral: May be administered with food or milk
Parenteral: May be administered undiluted direct I.V. over 3-5 minutes

Monitoring Parameters Renal function, serum electrolytes, fluid balance, blood pressure, body weight

Patient Information Rise slowly from a lying or sitting position to minimize dizziness, lightheadedness or fainting; also use extra care when exercising, standing for long periods of time. Take last dose of day early in the evening to prevent nocturia. May cause photosensitivity reactions (eg, exposure to sunlight may cause severe sunburn, skin rash, redness, or itching); avoid exposure to sunlight and artificial light sources (sunlamps, tanning booth/bed); wear protective clothing, wide-brimmed hats, sunglasses, and lip sunscreen (SPF ≥15); use a sunscreen [broadspectrum sunscreen or physical sunscreen (preferred) or sunblock with SPF ≥15]; contact physician if reaction occurs.

Additional Information 10-20 mg torsemide is approximately equivalent to:
Furosemide 40 mg
Bumetanide 1 mg

Dosage Forms Excipient information presented when available (limited, particularly for generics); consult specific product labeling. [DSC] = Discontinued product
Injection, solution: 10 mg/mL (2 mL, 5 mL)
Demadex®: 10 mg/mL (2 mL [DSC], 5 mL [DSC])
Tablet: 5 mg, 10 mg, 20 mg, 100 mg
Demadex®: 5 mg, 10 mg, 20 mg, 100 mg [scored]

References

Chobanian AV, Bakris GL, Black HR, et al, "The Seventh Report of the Joint National Committee on Prevention, Detection, Evaluation, and Treatment of High Blood Pressure: The JNC 7 Report," *JAMA*, 2003, 289(19):2560-72.

◆ **Totect®** *see* Dexrazoxane *on page 413*

◆ **tPA** *see* Alteplase *on page 71*

◆ **tRA** *see* Tretinoin (Systemic) *on page 1373*

◆ **Trace Elements** *see* Trace Metals *on page 1366*

◆ **4 Trace Elements** *see* Trace Metals *on page 1366*

◆ **Trace Elements 4 Pediatric** *see* Trace Metals *on page 1366*

Trace Metals (trase MET als)

Related Information

Parenteral Nutrition (PN) *on page 1559*

U.S. Brand Names 4 Trace Elements; Multitrace®-4; Multitrace®-4 Concentrate; Multitrace®-4 Neonatal; Multitrace®-4 Pediatric; Multitrace®-5; Multitrace®-5 Concentrate; Trace Elements 4 Pediatric

Therapeutic Category Mineral, Parenteral; Trace Element, Multiple, Neonatal; Trace Element, Parenteral

Generic Available Yes

Use Prevent and correct trace metal deficiencies

Pregnancy Risk Factor C

Contraindications Hypersensitivity to a specific trace metal or component of the trace metal solution (see Warnings); do not give by direct injection because of potential for phlebitis, tissue irritation, and potential to increase renal loss of minerals from a bolus injection

Warnings Metals may accumulate in conditions of renal failure or biliary obstruction; consider reduction in dosage or deletion of copper and manganese in patients with biliary obstruction; avoid copper use in patients with Wilson's disease; administration of copper in the absence of zinc or zinc in the absence of copper may cause decreases in their respective plasma levels; molybdenum promotes the utilization of copper and increases its excretion; excessive amounts of molybdenum may produce copper deficiency; multiple trace metal solutions present a risk of overdosage when the need for one trace element is appreciably higher than for others in the formulation; utilization of individual trace metal solutions may be needed. Consider reduction in dosage or deletion of selenium and chromium in patients with renal dysfunction.

Some products contain benzyl alcohol which may cause allergic reactions in susceptible individuals; large amounts of benzyl alcohol (≥99 mg/kg/day) have been associated with a potentially fatal toxicity ("gasping syndrome") in neonates; the "gasping syndrome" consists of metabolic acidosis, respiratory distress, gasping respirations, CNS dysfunction (including convulsions, intracranial hemorrhage), hypotension and cardiovascular collapse; *in vitro* and animal studies have shown that benzoate, a metabolite of benzyl alcohol, displaces bilirubin from protein-binding sites; use benzyl alcohol-containing products with caution in neonates.

Precautions Chromic chloride contains aluminum which may accumulate with prolonged use, particularly in patients with decreased renal function; use cautiously in neonates and other patients with decreased renal function

Adverse Reactions The following describe the symptomatology associated with excess trace metals:

Chromium: Nausea, vomiting, GI ulcers, renal and hepatic dysfunction, convulsions, coma
Copper: Prostration, behavioral changes, diarrhea, progressive marasmus, hypotonia, photophobia, hepatic dysfunction, peripheral edema
Manganese: Irritability, speech disturbances, abnormal gait, headache, anorexia, apathy, impotence, cholestatic jaundice, movement disorders
Molybdenum: Gout-like syndrome with elevated blood levels of uric acid and xanthine oxidase
Selenium: Alopecia, weak nails, dermatitis, dental defects, GI disorders, nervousness, mental depression, metallic taste, garlic odor of breath and sweat
Zinc: Profuse diaphoresis, consciousness decreased, blurred vision, tachycardia, hypothermia

Mechanism of Action

Chromium: Part of glucose tolerance factor, an essential activator of insulin-mediated reactions; helps maintain normal glucose metabolism and peripheral nerve function

Copper: Cofactor for serum ceruloplasmin, helps maintain normal rates of red and white cell formation

Manganese: Activator for several enzymes including manganese-dependent superoxide dismutase and pyruvate carboxylase; activates glycosyl transferases involved in mucopolysaccharide synthesis

Molybdenum: Constituent of the enzymes xanthine oxidase, sulfite oxidase, and aldehyde oxidase

Selenium: Part of glutathione peroxidase which protects cell components from oxidative damage due to peroxides produced in cellular metabolism

Zinc: A cofactor for >70 different enzymes; facilitates wound healing, helps maintain normal growth rates, normal skin hydration, and the senses of taste and smell

Pharmacokinetics (Adult data unless noted)

Chromium: 10% to 20% oral absorption; excretion primarily via kidneys and bile

Copper: 30% oral absorption; 80% elimination via bile; intestinal wall 16% and urine 4%

Manganese: 10% oral absorption; excretion primarily via bile; ancillary routes via pancreatic secretions or reabsorption into the intestinal lumen occur during periods of biliary obstruction

Molybdenum: 30% to 70% oral absorption; primarily renal excretion; some biliary excretion associated with an enterohepatic cycle

Selenium: Very poor oral absorption; 75% excretion via kidneys, remainder via feces, lung, and skin

Zinc: 20% to 30% oral absorption; 90% excretion in stools, remainder via urine and perspiration

Usual Dosage See table.

Trace Mineral Daily Requirements[1]

	Infants	Children (≥3 mo to ≤5 y)	Older Children, Adolescents, and Adults
Chromium[2]	0.2 mcg/kg	0.14-0.2 mcg/kg (max: 5 mcg)	10-15 mcg
Copper[3]	20 mcg/kg	20 mcg/kg (max: 300 mcg)	0.3-0.5 mg
Iodide[4]	1 mcg/kg	1 mcg/kg	1 mcg/kg
Manganese[3]	1 mcg/kg	2-10 mcg/kg (max: 50 mcg)	60-150 mcg
Selenium[2,5]	2-3 mcg/kg	2-3 mcg/kg (max: 30 mcg)	20-60 mcg
Zinc	Preterm: 400 mcg/kg Term <3 mo: 300 mcg/kg	100 mcg/kg (max: 5 mg)	2.5-5 mg

[1]Recommended intakes of trace elements cannot be achieved through the use of a commercially available combination trace element product. Only through the use of individualized trace element products can recommended intakes be achieved.

[2]Omit in patients with renal dysfunction.

[3]Omit in patients with impaired biliary excretion or cholestatic liver disease.

[4]Percutaneous absorption from protein-bound iodine may be adequate.

[5]Indicated for use in long-term parenteral nutrition patients.

Administration Parenteral: Must be diluted prior to use and infused as component of parenteral nutrition or parenteral solutions

Reference Range

Chromium: 0.18-0.47 ng/mL (SI: 35-90 nmol/L); some laboratories report much higher

*Copper: ~0.7-1.5 mcg/mL (SI: 11-24 micromoles/L); levels are higher in pregnant women and children

Manganese: 18-30 mcg/dL (SI: 2.3-3.8 micromoles/L)

Selenium: 95-165 ng/mL (SI: 120-209 nmol/L)

Zinc: 70-120 mcg/dL (SI: 10-18.4 micromoles/L)

*May not be a meaningful measurement of body stores

Additional Information Persistent diarrhea or excessive GI fluid losses from ostomy sites may grossly increase zinc losses

Dosage Forms Excipient information presented when available (limited, particularly for generics); consult specific product labeling.

Injection, solution [combination products]:

Multitrace®-4: Chromium 4 mcg, copper 0.4 mg, manganese 0.1 mg, and zinc 1 mg per 1 mL (10 mL) [contains aluminum, benzyl alcohol]

Multitrace®-4 Concentrate: Chromium 10 mcg, copper 1 mg, manganese 0.5 mg, and zinc 5 mg per 1 mL (1 mL) [contains aluminum]; chromium 10 mcg, copper 1 mg, manganese 0.5 mg, and zinc 5 mg per 1 mL (10 mL) [contains benzyl alcohol]

Multitrace®-4 Neonatal: Chromium 0.85 mcg, copper 0.1 mg, manganese 0.025 mg, and zinc 1.5 mg per 1 mL (2 mL) [contains aluminum]

Multitrace®-5: Chromium 4 mcg, copper 0.4 mg, manganese 0.1 mg, selenium 20 mcg, and zinc 1 mg per 1 mL (10 mL) [contains aluminum, benzyl alcohol]

Multitrace®-5 Concentrate: Chromium 10 mcg, copper 1 mg, manganese 0.5 mg, selenium 60 mcg, and zinc 5 mg per 1 mL (1 mL) [contains aluminum]; chromium 10 mcg, copper 1 mg, manganese 0.5 mg, selenium 60 mcg, and zinc 5 mg per 1 mL (10 mL) [contains benzyl alcohol]

Trace Elements 4 Pediatric: Chromium 1 mcg, copper 0.1 mg, manganese 0.03 mg, and zinc 0.5 mg per 1 mL (10 mL) [contains aluminum, benzyl alcohol]

Injection, solution [combination products, preservative free]:

4 Trace Elements: Chromium 2 mcg, copper 0.2 mg, manganese 0.16 mg, and zinc 0.8 mg per 1 mL (5 mL, 50 mL) [contains aluminum]

Multitrace®-4 Pediatric: Chromium 1 mcg, copper 0.1 mg, manganese 0.025 mg, and zinc 1 mg per 1 mL (3 mL) [contains aluminum]

References

Dahlstrom KA, Ament ME, Medhin MG, et al, "Serum Trace Elements in Children Receiving Long-Term Parenteral Nutrition," J Pediatr, 1986, 109(4):625-30.

Fell JM, Reynolds AP, Meadows N, et al, "Manganese Toxicity in Children Receiving Long-Term Parenteral Nutrition," Lancet, 1996, 347(9010):1218-21.

Greene HL, Hambridge KM, Schanler R, et al, "Guidelines for the Use of Vitamins, Trace Elements, Calcium, Magnesium and Phosphorus in Infants and Children Receiving Total Parenteral Nutrition: Report of the Subcommittee on Pediatric Nutrient Requirements From the Committee on Clinical Practice Issues of The American Society for Clinical Nutrition," Am J Clin Nutr, 1988, 48(5):1324-42.

"Guidelines for the Use of Parenteral and Enteral Nutrition in Adult and Pediatric Patients. ASPEN Board of Directors and The Clinical Guidelines Task Force," JPEN J Parenter Enteral Nutr, 2002, 26(1 Suppl):1-138SA.

Litov RE, and Combs GF Jr, "Selenium in Pediatric Nutrition," Pediatrics, 1991, 87(3):339-51.

◆ **Tracleer®** see Bosentan on page 197

TraMADol (TRA ma dole)

Medication Safety Issues

Sound-alike/look-alike issues:

TraMADol may be confused with tapentadol, Toradol®, Trandate®, traZODone, Voltaren®

Ultram® may be confused with Ultane®, Ultracet®, Voltaren®

International issues:

Theradol® [Netherlands] may be confused with Foradil® which is a brand name for formoterol in the U.S.

Theradol® [Netherlands] may be confused with Terazol® which is a brand name for terconazole in the U.S. Theradol® [Netherlands] may be confused with Toradol® which is a brand name for ketorolac in the U.S.

U.S. Brand Names Ryzolt™; Ultram®; Ultram® ER

Canadian Brand Names Ralivia™ ER; Tridural™; Zytram® XL

Therapeutic Category Analgesic, Opioid

Generic Available Yes

Use

Immediate release formulation: Relief of moderate to moderately-severe acute or chronic pain, including postoperative, cancer, neuropathic, low back pain, and pain associated with orthopedic disorders (FDA approved in ages ≥17 years)

Extended release formulations: For patients requiring around-the-clock management of moderate to moderately-severe pain for an extended period of time (Ryzolt™: FDA approved in ages ≥16 years; Ultram® ER: FDA approved in ages ≥18 years)

Pregnancy Risk Factor C

Pregnancy Considerations Adverse events were observed in animal studies. Tramadol has been shown to cross the human placenta when administered during labor. Postmarketing reports following tramadol use during pregnancy include neonatal seizures, withdrawal syndrome, fetal death, and stillbirth. Not recommended for use during labor and delivery.

Lactation Enters breast milk/not recommended

Breast-Feeding Considerations Sixteen hours following a single 100 mg I.V. dose, the amount of tramadol found in breast milk was 0.1% of the maternal dose. Use is not recommended by the manufacturer for postdelivery analgesia in nursing mothers.

Contraindications Hypersensitivity to tramadol, opioids, or any component; opioid-dependent patients; acute intoxication with alcohol, hypnotics, centrally-acting analgesics, opioids, or psychotropic drugs

Tramadol extended release tablets: Patients with severe renal impairment (Cl_{cr} <30 mL/minute) or severe hepatic impairment (Child-Pugh Class C) since the extended release dosage form does not permit dosing flexibility required in this patient population; patients with severe/acute bronchial asthma, hypercapnia, or significant respiratory depression in the absence of an appropriately monitored setting and resuscitation equipment

Warnings Should only be used with **EXTREME** caution in patients receiving MAO inhibitors. Not recommended for use during pregnancy or in nursing mothers. Tolerance or drug dependence may result from extended use (withdrawal symptoms have been reported); abrupt discontinuation should be avoided. Tapering of dose at the time of discontinuation reduces the risk of withdrawal symptoms.

Serotonin syndrome (eg, agitation, hallucinations, coma, tachycardia, labile blood pressure, hyperthermia, hyperreflexia, incoordination, nausea, vomiting, diarrhea) may occur with concomitant use of tramadol and SSRIs, tricyclic antidepressants, MAOIs, triptans, linezolid, SNRIs, or drugs which impair tramadol metabolism (CYP2D6 and CYP3A4 inhibitors).

Precautions Use with caution and reduce dosage when administered to patients receiving other CNS depressants (may cause CNS depression and/or respiratory depression when combined with other CNS depressants). Use with caution in patients with a history or with an increased risk of seizures (head trauma, increased intracranial pressure, metabolic disorders, CNS infection, malignancy, or drug withdrawal). An increased risk of seizures may occur in patients receiving serotonin reuptake inhibitors (SSRIs) or anorectics, tricyclic antidepressants, cyclobenzaprine, promethazine, neuroleptics, MAO inhibitors, other opioids, or drugs which lower seizure threshold. The risk of

seizures increases with doses above the recommended range and if naloxone administration is used to treat tramadol overdose. Use with caution in patients with increased intracranial pressure or head injury. Use with caution and reduce dosage in patients with liver disease, renal impairment, myxedema, hypothyroidism, or hypoadrenalism. Avoid use in patients who are suicidal or addiction prone. Avoid use during pregnancy (neonatal seizures, neonatal withdrawal syndrome, and fetal death have been reported).

Adverse Reactions

Cardiovascular: Vasodilation, syncope, tachycardia, flushing, chest pain, orthostatic hypotension, bradycardia, palpitations

Central nervous system: Dizziness, headache, somnolence, vertigo, agitation, anxiety, confusion, seizure, emotional lability, euphoria, hallucinations, malaise, nervousness, sleep disorder, amnesia, depression, suicidal tendency, fever, insomnia

Dermatologic: Pruritus, rash, angioedema, Stevens-Johnson syndrome, toxic epidermal necrolysis

Endocrine & metabolic: Menopausal symptoms

Gastrointestinal: Constipation, nausea, abdominal pain, anorexia, diarrhea, dry mouth, dyspepsia, vomiting, GI bleeding, pancreatitis

Genitourinary: Urinary frequency, urinary retention

Hematologic: Thrombocytopenia

Hepatic: Liver failure, hepatitis, cholelithiasis

Neuromuscular & skeletal: Tremor, impaired coordination, hypertonia, spasticity, weakness, arthralgia

Ocular: Miosis, visual disturbance

Renal: Serum creatinine elevated

Respiratory: Bronchospasm, dyspnea, respiratory depression, cough, nasal congestion

Miscellaneous: Diaphoresis, anaphylaxis, withdrawal syndrome, serotonin syndrome, anaphylactoid reaction

Drug Interactions

Metabolism/Transport Effects Substrate of CYP2D6 (major), 3A4 (major)

Avoid Concomitant Use

Avoid concomitant use of TraMADol with any of the following: Sibutramine

Increased Effect/Toxicity

TraMADol may increase the levels/effects of: Alcohol (Ethyl); CNS Depressants; MAO Inhibitors; Methotrimeprazine; Selective Serotonin Reuptake Inhibitors; Serotonin Modulators

The levels/effects of TraMADol may be increased by: CYP3A4 Inhibitors (Moderate); CYP3A4 Inhibitors (Strong); Dasatinib; Methotrimeprazine; Selective Serotonin Reuptake Inhibitors; Sibutramine; Tricyclic Antidepressants

Decreased Effect

The levels/effects of TraMADol may be decreased by: CYP2D6 Inhibitors (Moderate); CYP2D6 Inhibitors (Strong); CYP3A4 Inducers (Strong); Deferasirox

Stability Store tablets at room temperature; protect from light

Mechanism of Action Tramadol and its O-desmethyl metabolite bind to μ-opiate receptors in the CNS causing inhibition of ascending pain pathways, altering the perception of and response to pain; inhibits the reuptake of norepinephrine and serotonin which also modifies the ascending pain pathway

Pharmacodynamics Immediate release formulation:

Onset of action: ~1 hour

Maximum effect: 2-4 hours

Duration: 3-6 hours

Pharmacokinetics (Adult data unless noted)

Absorption: Rapid and complete

Distribution: Crosses the placenta; distributes to breast milk

V_d: Adults: 2.5-3 L/kg

Protein binding: 20%

Metabolism: Primarily hepatic via demethylation, glucuronidation, and sulfation; N-demethylation via CYP3A4; active O-desmethyltramadol metabolite formed by CYP2D6

Bioavailability: Immediate release: 75%; extended release: 85% to 95% as compared to the immediate-release dosage form

Half-life:

Tramadol: ~6-8 hours

Active metabolite: 7-9 hours (prolonged in hepatic or renal impairment)

Time to peak serum concentration: Immediate release: 2 hours; extended release (formulation specific):

Ultram® ER: ~12 hours

Ryzolt™: ~4-5 hours

Elimination: Excreted in urine as unchanged drug (30%) and metabolites (60%)

Dialysis: <7% removed in a 4-hour hemodialysis period

Usual Dosage Oral:

Immediate release formulation:

Children: 1-2 mg/kg/dose every 4-6 hours; maximum: 400 mg/day

Adolescents and Adults: 50-100 mg every 4-6 hours; maximum: 400 mg/day

For patients not requiring rapid onset of effect, tolerability to adverse effects may be improved by initiating therapy at 25 mg/day and titrating dose by 25 mg every 3 days until 25 mg 4 times/day is reached. Dose may then be increased by 50 mg every 3 days as tolerated to reach 50 mg 4 times/day.

Extended release formulation:

Ultram® ER: Adults ≥18 years: 100 mg once daily; titrate by 100 mg increments every 5 days if needed for pain relief; maximum: 300 mg/day

Ryzolt™: Adolescents ≥16 years and Adults: Initial: 100 mg once daily; titrate by 100 mg increments every 2-3 days if needed for pain control; maximum: 300 mg/day

Dosing adjustment in hepatic impairment:

Immediate release formulation: Adults: Cirrhosis: Recommended dose: 50 mg every 12 hours

Extended release formulation:

Ultram® ER: Do not use in patients with severe (Child-Pugh Class C) hepatic impairment

Ryzolt™: Do not use in patients with any degree of hepatic impairment

Dosing adjustment in renal impairment:

Immediate release formulation: Adults: Cl_{cr} <30 mL/minute: Administer 50-100 mg dose every 12 hours (maximum: 200 mg/day)

Extended release formulation: Do not use in patients with Cl_{cr} <30 mL/minute

Administration Oral: May administer with or without food, but it is recommended that it be administered in a consistent manner.

Extended release tablet: Swallow whole with a sufficient amount of liquid. Do not crush, cut, dissolve, or chew extended release tablet; tablet should be taken once daily at approximately the same time each day.

Monitoring Parameters Pain relief, respiratory rate, blood pressure, and pulse; signs of tolerance, oversedation, or withdrawal; renal and hepatic function

Patient Information Avoid alcohol and medications such as sedatives, hypnotics, or other narcotic-containing preparations; may cause drowsiness and impair ability to perform activities requiring mental alertness or physical coordination; may be habit-forming; avoid abrupt discontinuation after prolonged use

Dosage Forms Excipient information presented when available (limited, particularly for generics); consult specific product labeling. [CAN] = Canadian brand name

Tablet, as hydrochloride: 50 mg

Ultram®: 50 mg

Tablet, extended release, as hydrochloride: 100 mg, 200 mg

Ultram® ER: 100 mg, 200 mg, 300 mg

Ralivia™ ER [CAN]: 100 mg, 200 mg, 300 mg [not available in the U.S.]

Ryzolt™: 100 mg, 200 mg, 300 mg

Tridural™ [CAN]: 100 mg, 200 mg, 300 mg [not available in the U.S.]

Zytram® XL [CAN]: 150 mg, 200 mg, 300 mg, 400 mg [not available in the U.S.]

Extemporaneous Preparations A 5 mg/mL oral liquid may be made by crushing six 50 mg tramadol tablets; add 30 mL of Oral-Plus® with 30 mL of strawberry syrup or Ora-Sweet® SF to total volume of 60 mL. Label "shake well before use"; stable for 90 days when stored at 3°C to 5°C or 23°C to 25°C.

Wagner DS, Johnson CE, Cichon-Hensley BK, et al, "Stability of Oral Liquid Preparations of Tramadol in Strawberry Syrup and a Sugar-Free Vehicle," *Am J Health Syst Pharm*, 2003, 60(12):1268-70.

References

Finkel JC, Rose JB, Schmitz ML, et al, "An Evaluation of the Efficacy and Tolerability of Oral Tramadol Hydrochloride Tablets for the Treatment of Postsurgical Pain in Children," *Anesth Analg*, 2002, 94 (6):1469-73.

Rose JB, Finkel JC, Arquedas-Mohs A, et al, "Oral Tramadol for the Treatment of Pain of 7-30 Days' Duration in Children," *Anesth Analg*, 2003, 96(1):78-81.

◆ **Tramadol Hydrochloride** see TraMADol on page 1367

◆ **Trandate®** see Labetalol on page 787

Tranexamic Acid (tran eks AM ik AS id)

Medication Safety Issues

Sound-alike/look-alike issues:

Cyklokapron® may be confused with cycloSPORINE

U.S. Brand Names Cyklokapron®; Lysteda™

Canadian Brand Names Cyklokapron®; Tranexamic Acid Injection BP

Therapeutic Category Antifibrinolytic Agent; Antihemophilic Agent; Hemostatic Agent

Generic Available No

Use

Injection: Short-term use (2-8 days) in hemophilia patients to reduce or prevent hemorrhage and reduce need for blood factor replacement therapy during and following tooth extraction [FDA approved in pediatric patients (age not specified) and adults]; primary menorrhagia; prevention of GI hemorrhage and hemorrhage following ocular trauma; recurrent epistaxis; hereditary angioneurotic edema; prophylactic use to decrease perioperative blood loss and the need for transfusion in patients undergoing congenital heart disease or scoliosis-related surgery

Tablet: Treatment of cyclic heavy menstrual bleeding (FDA approved in postmenarcheal women >18 years)

Pregnancy Risk Factor B

Pregnancy Considerations Adverse events were not observed in animal reproduction studies. There are no adequate and well-controlled studies in pregnant women. Tranexamic acid crosses the placenta and concentrations within cord blood are similar to maternal concentrations.

Use only if the potential benefit justifies the potential risk to the fetus. Lysteda™ is not indicated for use in pregnant women.

Lactation Enters breast milk/not recommended

Contraindications Hypersensitivity to tranexamic acid or any component; subarachnoid hemorrhage; acquired defective color vision, active intravascular clotting process; active thromboembolic disease (eg, cerebral thrombosis, DVT, or PE); history of thrombosis or thromboembolism, including retinal vein or retinal artery occlusion; intrinsic risk of thrombosis or thromboembolism (eg, hypercoagulopathy, thrombogenic cardiac rhythm disease, thrombogenic valvular disease)

Warnings Do not administer concomitantly with factor IX complex concentrates or anti-inhibitor coagulant concentrates due to increased risk of thrombosis. Concomitant use with combination hormonal contraception may further increase risk of thromboembolism; patients taking hormonal contraceptives were excluded from clinical trials. Visual defects (eg, color vision change, visual loss), and retinal venous and arterial occlusions have been reported; discontinue treatment if changes in vision occur; prompt ophthalmic examination should be performed by an ophthalmologist. Avoid use in patients with acquired defective color vision since this would prohibit monitoring one endpoint as a measure of ophthalmic toxicity. Ligneous conjunctivitis has been reported with the tablet, but usually resolves upon discontinuation of therapy. Severe hypersensitivity reactions have been reported rarely.

Precautions Dosage modification required in patients with renal impairment; use with caution in patients with cardiovascular, renal, cerebrovascular disease, or transurethral prostatectomy. Use with caution in patients with upper urinary tract bleeding; ureteral obstruction due to clot formation has been reported. Use with extreme caution in patients with DIC requiring antifibrinolytic therapy; patients should be under strict supervision of a physician experienced in treating this disorder. Use with caution with concurrent tretinoin use; may exacerbate procoagulant effects.

Adverse Reactions

Injection:

Cardiovascular: Hypotension (with rapid I.V. administration), thromboembolic events (eg, deep vein thrombosis, pulmonary embolism, acute renal cortical necrosis) (see Warnings)

Central nervous system: Cerebral ischemia and infarction (when used in the treatment of subarachnoid hemorrhage), fatigue, giddiness, headache (50%)

Gastrointestinal: Abdominal pain (20%), diarrhea, nausea, vomiting

Hematologic: Abnormal bleeding times, anemia, coagulation defects

Neuromuscular & skeletal: Arthralgia, back pain (21%), muscle cramps, muscle pain, spasms

Ocular: Central venous stasis retinopathy (see Warnings), visual abnormalities (focal areas of retinal degeneration have been seen in animals)

Respiratory: Nasal/sinus symptoms (25%)

Miscellaneous: Allergic skin reaction, anaphylactic shock, anaphylactoid reactions (rare)

Drug Interactions

Avoid Concomitant Use

Avoid concomitant use of Tranexamic Acid with any of the following: Anti-inhibitor Coagulant Complex

Increased Effect/Toxicity

Tranexamic Acid may increase the levels/effects of: Anti-inhibitor Coagulant Complex; Fibrinogen Concentrate (Human)

The levels/effects of Tranexamic Acid may be increased by: Contraceptives (Estrogens); Contraceptives (Progestins); Fibrinogen Concentrate (Human); Tretinoin (Systemic)

Decreased Effect There are no known significant interactions involving a decrease in effect.

Stability Store vials at controlled room temperature; prepare on same day of infusion. Incompatible with solutions containing penicillin; compatible with dextrose, saline, and heparin, as well as with electrolyte, amino acid, or dextran solutions

Mechanism of Action Forms a reversible complex that displaces plasminogen from fibrin resulting in inhibition of fibrinolysis; it also inhibits the proteolytic activity of plasmin

Pharmacokinetics (Adult data unless noted)

Distribution: Breast milk levels are 1% of serum; CSF levels are 10% of plasma

V_d: Adults: 9-27 L

Protein binding: 3%

Bioavailability: I.M.: 100%; oral: ~45%

Half-life: 2 hours

Time to peak serum concentration:

I.M.: 1 hour

I.V.: 5 minutes

Oral: ~3 hours

Elimination: Elimination characteristics differ by route of administration: after I.V. administration 95% excreted as unchanged drug in urine vs 39% after oral administration

Usual Dosage Children: IV:

Tooth extraction in patients with hemophilia (in combination with replacement therapy): 10 mg/kg immediately before surgery, then 10 mg/kg/dose 3-4 times/day; may be used for 2-8 days

Surgery for congenital heart disease (to reduce perioperative blood loss and need for transfusions): 2 months to 15 years: (Limited data available; dose not established): Reported dosing regimens variable; ideal dose-response not established: Loading dose: 100 mg/kg, followed by 10 mg/kg/hour infusion (continued until ICU transport) and 100 mg/kg priming dose when by-pass initiated (see Reid, 1997); also reported: Loading dose: 10 mg/kg, priming dose: 10 mg/kg and 10 mg/kg after protamine (see Chauhan, 2004; Chauhan, 2004; Eaton, 2008)

Surgery for scoliosis (to reduce perioperative blood loss and need for transfusions): 8-18 years: (Limited data available; dose not established): Reported dosing regimens variable; ideal dose-response not established: Loading dose: 100 mg/kg, followed by infusion: 10 mg/kg/hour until skin closure (see Sethna, 2005; Shapiro 2007). Other regimens reported with positive results: Loading dose: 20 mg/kg, followed by 10 mg/kg/hour infusion (see Grant, 2009) or loading dose: 10 mg/kg and 1 mg/kg/hour infusion (see Grant, 2009; Neilipovitz, 2001)

Adults:

Tooth extraction in patients with hemophilia (in combination with replacement therapy): I.V.: 10 mg/kg immediately before surgery, then 10 mg/kg/dose 3-4 times/day; may be used for 2-8 days

Menorrhagia: Oral: 1300 mg 3 times daily (3900 mg/day) for up to 5 days during monthly menstruation

Dosing adjustment in renal impairment: Adults: See table.

Serum Creatinine (mg/dL)	I.V. Dose
1.36-2.83	10 mg/kg twice daily
>2.83-5.66	10 mg/kg once daily
>5.66	10 mg/kg every 48 h or 5 mg/kg every 24 h

Oral: Adult:
Serum creatinine >1.4-2.8 mg/dL: 1300 mg twice daily (2600 mg/day) for up to 5 days
Serum creatinine 2.9-5.7 mg/dL: 1300 mg once daily for up to 5 days
Serum creatinine >5.7 mg/dL: 650 mg once daily for up to 5 days

Administration
Oral: Administer without regard to meals. Should be swallowed whole; do not break, chew, or crush.

Parenteral: May be administered by direct I.V. injection at a maximum rate of 100 mg/minute (1 mL/minute); in pediatric scoliosis studies, loading dose infused over 15 minutes

Monitoring Parameters Ophthalmologic exams (baseline and at regular intervals) of chronic therapy

Reference Range 5-10 mcg/mL is required to decrease fibrinolysis

Patient Information
Report any unusual bruising, bleeding, sudden change in vision, eye pain or irritation, or rash to your physician.

Dosage Forms Excipient information presented when available (limited, particularly for generics); consult specific product labeling.
Injection, solution:
Cyklokapron®: 100 mg/mL (10 mL)
Tablet, oral:
Lysteda™: 650 mg

References
Chauhan S, Bisoi A, Kumar N, et al, "Dose Comparison of Tranexamic Acid in Pediatric Cardiac Surgery," Asian Cardiovasc Thorac Ann, 2004, 12(2):121-4.
Chauhan S, Das SN, Bisoi A, et al, "Comparison of Epsilon Aminocaproic Acid and Tranexamic Acid in Pediatric Cardiac Surgery," J Cardiothorac Vasc Anesth, 2004, 18(2):141-3.
Eaton MP, "Antifibrinolytic Therapy in Surgery for Congenital Heart Disease," Anesth Analg, 2008, 106(4):1087-100.
Grant JA, Howard J, Luntley J, et al, "Perioperative Blood Transfusion Requirements in Pediatric Scoliosis Surgery: The Efficacy of Tranexamic Acid," J Pediatr Orthop, 2009, 29(3):300-4.
Neilipovitz DT, Murto K, Hall L, et al, "A Randomized Trial of Tranexamic Acid to Reduce Blood Transfusion for Scoliosis Surgery," Anesth Analg, 2001, 93(1):82-7.
Reid RW, Zimmerman AA, Laussen PC, et al, "The Efficacy of Tranexamic Acid Versus Placebo in Decreasing Blood Loss in Pediatric Patients Undergoing Repeat Cardiac Surgery," Anesth Analg, 1997, 84(5):990-6.
Sethna NF, Zurakowski D, Brustowicz RM, et al, "Tranexamic Acid Reduces Intraoperative Blood Loss in Pediatric Patients Undergoing Scoliosis Surgery," Anesthesiology, 2005, 102(4):727-32.
Shapiro F, Zurakowski D, and Sethna NF, "Tranexamic Acid Diminishes Intraoperative Blood Loss and Transfusion in Spinal Fusions for Duchenne Muscular Dystrophy Scoliosis," Spine (Phila Pa 1976), 2007, 32(20):2278-83.

◆ **Tranexamic Acid Injection BP (Can)** see Tranexamic Acid on page 1369

◆ **transAMCA** see Tranexamic Acid on page 1369

◆ **Transderm-V® (Can)** see Scopolamine on page 1248

◆ **Transderm-Nitro® (Can)** see Nitroglycerin on page 996

◆ **Transderm Scōp®** see Scopolamine on page 1248

◆ **Trans-Plantar® (Can)** see Salicylic Acid on page 1241

◆ **trans-Retinoic Acid** see Tretinoin (Systemic) on page 1373

◆ **trans-Retinoic Acid** see Tretinoin (Topical) on page 1375

◆ **Trans-Ver-Sal® [OTC]** see Salicylic Acid on page 1241

◆ **Trans-Ver-Sal® (Can)** see Salicylic Acid on page 1241

◆ **trans Vitamin A Acid** see Tretinoin (Systemic) on page 1373

◆ **Tranxene T-Tab** see Clorazepate on page 343

◆ **Tranxene® T-Tab®** see Clorazepate on page 343

◆ **Trasylol®** see Aprotinin on page 126

◆ **Trav-L-Tabs® [OTC]** see Meclizine on page 869

TraZODone (TRAZ oh done)

Medication Safety Issues
Sound-alike/look-alike issues:
Desyrel® may be confused with Demerol®, Delsym®, Zestril®
TraZODone may be confused with traMADol

International issues:
Desyrel® may be confused with Deseril® which is a brand name for methysergide in multiple international markets

Related Information
Antidepressant Agents on page 1484
Serotonin Syndrome on page 1695

U.S. Brand Names Oleptro™

Canadian Brand Names Apo-Trazodone D®; Apo-Trazodone®; Desyrel®; Dom-Trazodone; Mylan-Trazodone; Novo-Trazodone; Nu-Trazodone; PHL-Trazodone; PMS-Trazodone; ratio-Trazodone; Trazorel®; ZYM-Trazodone

Therapeutic Category Antidepressant, Serotonin Reuptake Inhibitor/Antagonist

Generic Available Yes

Use Treatment of depression

Medication Guide
An FDA-approved patient medication guide, which is available with the product information and at http://www.fda.gov/downloads/Drugs/DrugSafety/ucm089021.pdf, must be dispensed with this medication for each new outpatient prescription and refill.

Pregnancy Risk Factor C

Pregnancy Considerations Trazodone is classified as pregnancy category C due to adverse effects observed in animal studies. When trazodone is taken during pregnancy, an increased risk of major malformations has not been observed in the small number of pregnancies studied. The long-term effects on neurobehavior have not been evaluated.

Women treated for major depression and who are euthymic prior to pregnancy are more likely to experience a relapse when medication is discontinued as compared to pregnant women who continue taking antidepressant medications. Therapy during pregnancy should be individualized; treatment of depression during pregnancy should incorporate the clinical expertise of the mental health clinician, obstetrician, primary healthcare provider, and pediatrician. If treatment during pregnancy is required, consider tapering therapy during the third trimester to prevent potential withdrawal symptoms in the infant. If this is done and the woman is considered to be at risk of relapse from her major depressive disorder, the medication can be restarted following delivery. Treatment algorithms have been developed by the ACOG and the APA for the management of depression in women prior to conception and during pregnancy (Yonkers, 2009).

Lactation Enters breast milk/use caution (AAP rates "of concern")

Breast-Feeding Considerations Trazodone is excreted into breast milk; breast milk concentrations peak ~2 hours following administration. It is not known if the trazodone metabolite is found in breast milk. The long-term effects on neurobehavior have not been studied. The manufacturer recommends that caution be exercised when administering trazodone to nursing women. The AAP considers trazodone to be a "drug for which the effect on the nursing infant is unknown, but may be of concern."

Contraindications Hypersensitivity to trazodone or any component

Warnings Trazodone is not approved for use in pediatric patients. Clinical worsening of depression or suicidal ideation and behavior may occur in children and adults with major depressive disorder **[U.S. Boxed Warning]**. In clinical trials, antidepressants increased the risk of suicidal thinking and behavior (suicidality) in children, adolescents, and young adults (18-24 years of age) with major depressive disorder and other psychiatric disorders. This risk must be considered before prescribing antidepressants for any clinical use. Short-term studies did **not** show an increased risk of suicidality with antidepressant use in patients >24 years of age and showed a decreased risk in patients ≥65 years.

Patients of all ages who are treated with antidepressants for any indication require appropriate monitoring and close observation for clinical worsening of depression, suicidality, and unusual changes in behavior, especially during the first few months after antidepressant initiation or when the dose is adjusted. Family members and caregivers should be instructed to closely observe the patient (ie, daily) and communicate condition with healthcare provider. Patients should also be monitored for associated behaviors (eg, anxiety, agitation, panic attacks, insomnia, irritability, hostility, aggressiveness, impulsivity, akathisia, hypomania, mania) which may increase the risk for worsening depression or suicidality. Worsening depression or emergence of suicidality (or associated behaviors listed above) that is abrupt in onset, severe, or not part of the presenting symptoms, may require discontinuation or modification of drug therapy.

To reduce risk of intentional overdose, write prescriptions for the smallest quantity consistent with good patient care. Screen individuals for bipolar disorder prior to treatment (using antidepressants alone may induce manic episodes in patients with this condition).

Monitor closely and use with extreme caution in patients with cardiac disease or arrhythmias; not recommended for use during post-MI initial recovery phase. Trazodone may cause prolonged priapism requiring surgical intervention; discontinue use immediately if prolonged or inappropriate erections occur.

Precautions Hypotension and syncope may occur; use with caution in patients receiving antihypertensive agents. Discontinue use prior to elective surgery (unknown interactions with general anesthetics may exist).

Adverse Reactions Possesses fewer anticholinergic and cardiac adverse effects than tricyclic antidepressants

Cardiovascular: Postural hypotension (5%), arrhythmias, syncope

Central nervous system: Drowsiness (20% to 50%), sedation, dizziness, insomnia, confusion, agitation, seizures, extrapyramidal reactions, headache; suicidal thinking and behavior (see Warnings)

Gastrointestinal: Xerostomia, constipation, nausea, vomiting

Genitourinary: Prolonged priapism (1:6000), urinary retention (rare)

Hepatic: Hepatitis

Neuromuscular & skeletal: Weakness

Ocular: Blurred vision (15% to 30%)

Drug Interactions

Metabolism/Transport Effects Substrate of CYP2D6 (minor), 3A4 (major); **Inhibits** CYP2D6 (moderate), 3A4 (weak); **Induces** P-glycoprotein

Avoid Concomitant Use

Avoid concomitant use of TraZODone with any of the following: Sibutramine

Increased Effect/Toxicity

TraZODone may increase the levels/effects of: Alcohol (Ethyl); CNS Depressants; Serotonin Modulators

The levels/effects of TraZODone may be increased by: BusPIRone; CYP3A4 Inhibitors (Moderate); CYP3A4 Inhibitors (Strong); Dasatinib; MAO Inhibitors; Protease Inhibitors; Selective Serotonin Reuptake Inhibitors; Sibutramine; Venlafaxine

Decreased Effect

TraZODone may decrease the levels/effects of: Dabigatran Etexilate; P-Glycoprotein Substrates

The levels/effects of TraZODone may be decreased by: CYP3A4 Inducers (Strong); Deferasirox; Peginterferon Alfa-2b

Food Interactions Food may decrease the rate but increase the extent of absorption

Stability Store tablets at room temperature; avoid temperatures >104°F (40°C); dispense in tight, light-resistant container

Mechanism of Action Inhibits reuptake of serotonin; minimal or no effect on reuptake of norepinephrine or dopamine; possesses little if any anticholinergic effects; alpha-adrenergic blockade thought to be responsible for orthostatic hypotension and dry mouth

Pharmacodynamics Maximum antidepressant effect: 2-4 weeks

Pharmacokinetics (Adult data unless noted)

Protein binding: 85% to 95%

Metabolism: In the liver via hydroxylation and oxidation; metabolized by cytochrome P450 isoenzyme CYP3A4 to active metabolite, m-chlorophenylpiperazine (mCPP)

Half-life, elimination: 5-9 hours, prolonged in obese patients

Time to peak serum concentration:

Administration on empty stomach: 1 hour

Administration with food: 2 hours

Elimination: Primarily in urine (74%) with ~21% excreted in feces

Usual Dosage Oral: **Note:** Not FDA approved for the treatment of depression in pediatric patients (see Warnings)

Children 6-18 years: Initial: 1.5-2 mg/kg/day in divided doses; increase gradually every 3-4 days as needed; maximum dose: 6 mg/kg/day in 3 divided doses

Adolescents: Initial: 25-50 mg/day; increase to 100-150 mg/day in divided doses

Adults: Initial: 150 mg/day in 3 divided doses (may increase by 50 mg/day every 3-7 days); maximum dose: 600 mg/day

Administration Oral: Administer after meals or a snack to decrease lightheadedness, sedation, and postural hypotension

Monitoring Parameters Blood pressure, mental status, liver enzymes. Monitor patient periodically for symptom resolution; monitor for worsening depression, suicidality, and associated behaviors (especially at the beginning of therapy or when doses are increased or decreased; see Warnings).

Reference Range

Therapeutic: 0.5-2.5 mcg/mL (SI: 1-6 micromoles/L)

Potentially toxic: >2.5 mcg/mL (SI: >6 micromoles/L)

Toxic: >4 mcg/mL (SI: >10 micromoles/L)

Patient Information Read the patient Medication Guide that you receive with each prescription and refill of trazodone. An increased risk of suicidal thinking and behavior has been reported with the use of antidepressants in children, adolescents, and young adults (18-24 years of age). Notify physician if you feel more depressed, have thoughts of suicide, or become more agitated or irritable (see Warnings). Avoid alcohol; may cause drowsiness and impair ability to perform activities requiring mental alertness or physical coordination; may cause dry mouth; discontinue use and consult physician immediately if prolonged or inappropriate erections occur

Additional Information Mean doses of ~5 mg/kg/day were used in 22 children 5-12 years of age to treat severe behavioral disorders (Zubieta, 1992). Doses of 1 mg/kg/day given in 3 divided doses were used for migraine prophylaxis in 40 patients 7-18 years of age (Battistella, 1993). Further studies are needed before trazodone can be recommended in children for these indications.

Product Availability

Oleptro™: FDA approved January 2010; availability expected later in 2010

Oleptro™ is a once-daily formulation of trazodone indicated for the treatment of major depressive disorder in adults.

Dosage Forms Excipient information presented when available (limited, particularly for generics); consult specific product labeling.

Tablet, as hydrochloride: 50 mg, 100 mg, 150 mg, 300 mg

References

Battistella PA, Ruffilli R, Cernetti R, et al, "A Placebo-Controlled Crossover Trial Using Trazodone in Pediatric Migraine," *Headache*, 1993, 33(1):36-9.

Zubieta JK and Alessi NE, "Acute and Chronic Administration of Trazodone in the Treatment of Disruptive Behavior Disorders in Children," *J Clin Psychopharmacol*, 1992, 12(5):346-51.

♦ **Trazodone Hydrochloride** *see* TraZODone *on page 1371*

♦ **Trazorel® (Can)** *see* TraZODone *on page 1371*

♦ **Trecator®** *see* Ethionamide *on page 545*

♦ **Trental®** *see* Pentoxifylline *on page 1090*

♦ **Tretin-X™** *see* Tretinoin (Topical) *on page 1375*

Tretinoin (Systemic) (TRET i noyn, oral)

Related Information

Emetogenic Potential of Antineoplastic Agents *on page 1579*

U.S. Brand Names Vesanoid® [DSC]

Canadian Brand Names Vesanoid®

Therapeutic Category Antineoplastic Agent, Miscellaneous; Retinoic Acid Derivative

Generic Available Yes

Use Induction of remission in patients with acute promyelocytic leukemia (APL), French American British (FAB) classification M3 (including the M3 variant) characterized by t(15;17) translocation and/or PML/RARα gene presence (FDA approved in adults); has also been used in post consolidation and maintenance therapy in APL and combination therapy (with arsenic trioxide) for remission induction in APL

Pregnancy Risk Factor D

Pregnancy Considerations [U.S. Boxed Warning]: High risk of teratogenicity; if treatment with tretinoin is required in women of childbearing potential, two reliable forms of contraception should be used during and for 1 month after treatment. Within 1 week prior to starting therapy, serum or urine pregnancy test (sensitivity 50 mIU/mL) should be collected. If possible, delay therapy until results are available. Repeat pregnancy testing and contraception counseling monthly throughout the period of treatment. An increase in fetal resorptions and a decrease in live fetuses were observed in all animal studies; teratogenic effects have also been observed. Use in humans is limited, however, major fetal abnormalities and spontaneous abortions have been reported with other retinoids. If the clinical condition of a patient presenting with APL during pregnancy warrants immediate treatment, tretinoin use should be avoided in the first trimester; treatment with tretinoin may be considered in the second and third trimester with careful fetal cardiac monitoring.

Lactation Excretion in breast milk unknown/not recommended

Contraindications Hypersensitivity to tretinoin, other retinoids, parabens, or any component

Warnings About 25% of patients with APL treated with tretinoin have experienced APL differentiation syndrome (DS); formerly called retinoic acid-APL [RA-APL] syndrome, which is characterized by fever, dyspnea, acute respiratory distress, weight gain, radiographic pulmonary infiltrates, and pleural or pericardial effusions, edema, and hepatic, renal, and/or multiorgan failure **[U.S. Boxed Warning]**. DS usually occurs during the first month of treatment with some cases reported following the first dose. DS has been observed with or without concomitant leukocytosis and has occasionally been accompanied by impaired myocardial contractility and episodic hypotension. Endotracheal intubation and mechanical ventilation have been required in some cases due to progressive hypoxemia and several patients have expired with multiorgan failure. About one half of DS cases are severe, which is associated with increased mortality. Management has not been defined, although high-dose steroids given at the first suspicion appear to reduce morbidity and mortality. Regardless of the leukocyte count, at the first signs suggestive of DS, immediately initiate steroid therapy with dexamethasone (10 mg I.V. every 12 hours for 3-5 days); taper off over 2 weeks. Most patients do not require termination of tretinoin therapy during treatment of DS. Tretinoin should only be administered under the supervision of a physician who is experienced in the management of patients with acute leukemia, including assessment of possible benefit outweighing risks of known adverse effects **[U.S. Boxed Warning]**.

During treatment, ~40% of patients will develop rapidly evolving leukocytosis **[U.S. Boxed Warning]**. A high WBC at diagnosis increases the risk for further leukocytosis and may be associated with a higher risk of life-threatening complications. If signs and symptoms of the APL-DS syndrome are present together with leukocytosis, initiate treatment with high-dose steroids immediately. Consider adding full-dose chemotherapy (including an anthracycline if not contraindicated) to the tretinoin therapy on day 1 or 2 for patients presenting with a WBC count of >5 x 10⁹/L; or start immediately if WBC is <5 x 10⁹/L at presentation or reaches ≥6 x 10⁹/L by day 5 or ≥10 x 10⁹/L by day 10 or ≥15 x 10⁹/L by day 28.

Retinoids have been associated with pseudotumor cerebri (benign intracranial hypertension), especially in children. Concurrent use of other drugs associated with this effect (eg, tetracyclines) may increase risk. Early signs and symptoms include papilledema, headache, nausea, vomiting, visual disturbances, intracranial noises, or pulsate tinnitus.

There is a high risk of teratogenicity **[U.S. Boxed Warning]**. Increased risk of spontaneous abortion and major fetal abnormalities have been reported with use of other retinoids. If treatment with tretinoin is required in women of childbearing potential, two reliable forms of contraception should be used during and for 1 month after treatment. Microdosed progesterone preparations (eg, "minipill") may be inadequate during tretinoin treatment. Pregnancy testing and contraception counseling should be repeated monthly throughout the period of treatment. If possible, initiation of treatment with tretinoin should be delayed until negative pregnancy test result is confirmed.

Tretinoin treatment for APL should be initiated early; discontinue and consider alternate therapy if pending cytogenetic analysis does not confirm APL by t(15;17) translocation or the presence of the PML/RARα fusion protein (caused by translocation of the promyelocytic [PML] gene on chromosome 15 and retinoic acid receptor [RAR] alpha gene on chromosome 17).

Hypercholesterolemia and hypertriglyceridemia have been reported in up to 60% of patients, which was reversible upon completion of treatment. Elevated liver function test results occur in 50% to 60% of patients during treatment. Carefully monitor liver function test results during treatment and give consideration to a temporary withdrawal of tretinoin if test results reach >5 times the upper limit of normal. Most liver function test abnormalities will resolve without interruption of treatment or after therapy completion.

Precautions Hazardous agent; use appropriate precautions for handling and disposal. The risk for thrombosis (arterial and venous) is increased during the first month of treatment. Use with caution with antifibrinolytic agents (eg, tranexamic acid, aminocaproic acid, aprotinin); thrombotic complications have been reported (rarely) with concomitant use. May cause headache, malaise, and/or dizziness; caution patients about performing tasks which require mental alertness (eg, operating machinery or driving). Avoid additional vitamin A supplementation; may lead to vitamin A toxicity.

Adverse Reactions Most patients will experience drug-related toxicity, especially headache, fever, weakness, and fatigue. These are seldom permanent or irreversible and do not typically require therapy interruption.

Cardiovascular: Arrhythmias, cerebral hemorrhage, chest discomfort, edema, facial edema, flushing, heart failure, hyper-/hypotension, pallor, peripheral edema

Central nervous system: Agitation, anxiety, confusion, depression, dizziness, fever, forgetfulness, hallucination, headache, insomnia, intracranial hypertension, malaise, pain, pseudotumor cerebri (see Warnings)

Dermatologic: Alopecia, cellulitis, pruritus, rash, skin changes, skin/mucous membrane dryness

Endocrine & metabolic: Fluid imbalance, hypercholesterolemia, hypertriglyceridemia (see Warnings), weight gain/loss

Gastrointestinal: Abdominal distention, abdominal pain, anorexia, constipation, diarrhea, dyspepsia, GI hemorrhage, hepatosplenomegaly, mucositis, nausea, vomiting

Genitourinary: Dysuria

Hematologic: Disseminated intravascular coagulation, hemorrhage, leukocytosis (see Warnings)

Hepatic: Liver function tests increased

Local: Phlebitis

Neuromuscular & skeletal: Bone pain, flank pain, myalgia, paresthesia

Ocular: Ocular disorder, visual acuity change, visual disturbance

Otic: Earache, ear fullness, hearing loss (reversible)

Renal: Renal insufficiency

Respiratory: Dyspnea, expiratory wheezing, pleural effusion, pneumonia, pulmonary infiltration, rales, respiratory insufficiency, respiratory tract disorders (lower/upper)

Miscellaneous: Diaphoresis, infection, lymph disorder, RA-APL differentiation syndrome (see Warnings), shivering

≤3%, rare but important, or life-threatening: Abnormal gait, acidosis, acute renal failure, agnosia, aphasia, arterial thrombosis, asterixis, basophilia, bone inflammation, cardiac arrest, cardiomyopathy (secondary), cerebellar disorders, cerebellar edema, CNS depression, coma, convulsions, dementia, dysarthria, encephalopathy, enlarged heart, erythema nodosum, facial paralysis, forgetfulness, genital ulceration, hearing loss (irreversible), heart murmur, hemiplegia, hepatitis, hypercalcemia, hyperhistaminemia, hyporeflexia, hypotaxia, hypothermia, ischemia, larynx edema, leg weakness, liver disorder (unspecified), MI, micturition frequency, myocarditis, myositis, neurologic reaction, no light reflex, organomegaly, pancreatitis, pericarditis, prostate enlarged, pulmonary disease (unspecified), pulmonary hypertension, renal infarct, renal tubular necrosis, sepsis, slow speech, somnolence, spinal cord disorder, stroke,

Sweet's syndrome, thrombocytosis, tremor, ulcer, unconsciousness, vasculitis (skin), venous thrombosis, visual field defects

Drug Interactions

Metabolism/Transport Effects Substrate (minor) of CYP2A6, 2B6, 2C8/9; **Inhibits** CYP2C8/9 (weak); **Induces** CYP2E1 (weak)

Avoid Concomitant Use

Avoid concomitant use of Tretinoin (Systemic) with any of the following: BCG; Natalizumab; Pimecrolimus; Tacrolimus (Topical); Tetracycline Derivatives; Vaccines (Live); Vitamin A

Increased Effect/Toxicity Ketoconazole increases the mean plasma AUC of tretinoin. Concurrent use with antifibrinolytic agents (eg, aminocaproic acid, aprotinin, tranexamic acid) may increase risk of thrombosis. Concurrent use with tetracyclines may increase risk of pseudotumor cerebri.

Decreased Effect

Tretinoin (Systemic) may decrease the levels/effects of: BCG; Contraceptives (Estrogens); Contraceptives (Progestins); Sipuleucel-T; Vaccines (Inactivated); Vaccines (Live)

The levels/effects of Tretinoin (Systemic) may be decreased by: CYP2C8 Inducers (Highly Effective); Echinacea

Food Interactions The absorption of retinoids (as a class) is enhanced when taken with food.

Stability Store at 15°C to 30°C (59°F to 86°F); protect from light

Mechanism of Action Tretinoin appears to bind one or more nuclear receptors and decrease proliferation and induce differentiation of APL cells; initially producing maturation of primitive promyelocytes and repopulation of the marrow and peripheral blood with normal hematopoietic cells to achieve complete remission.

Pharmacokinetics (Adult data unless noted) Note: Reported pediatric values similar to adult (see Smith, 1992; Takitani, 2004)

Absorption: Well-absorbed

Protein binding: >95%, predominantly to albumin

Metabolism: Hepatic via CYP; primary metabolite: 4-oxo-all-*trans*-retinoic acid; displays autometabolism

Half-life: 0.5-2 hours

Time to peak serum concentration: 1-2 hours

Elimination: Urine (63%); feces (30%)

Usual Dosage Oral (refer to individual protocols): Note: Induction treatment of APL with tretinoin should be initiated early; discontinue if pending cytogenetic analysis does not confirm t(15;17) translocation or the presence of the PML/RARα fusion protein.

Acute promyelocytic leukemia (APL):

Children: Limited data available (see de Botton, 2004; Gregory, 2009; Mann, 2001; Ortega, 2005; Sanz, 2009; Testi, 2005):

Remission induction: 45 mg/m^2/day in two equally divided doses until documentation of complete remission (CR); discontinue after CR or after 90 days of treatment, whichever occurs first

Remission induction (in combination with an anthracycline): 25 mg/m^2/day in two equally divided doses until complete remission or 90 days

Consolidation therapy, intermediate- and high-risk patients: 25 mg/m^2/day in two equally divided doses for 15 days each month for 3 months

Maintenance therapy, intermediate- and high-risk patients: 25 mg/m^2/day in two equally divided doses for 15 days every 3 months for 2 years

Adults:

Remission induction: 45 mg/m^2/day in two equally divided doses until documentation of complete remission (CR); discontinue 30 days after CR or after 90 days of treatment, whichever occurs first

Remission induction (in combination with an anthracycline): 45 mg/m^2/day in two equally divided doses until complete remission or 90 days (see Sanz, 2004; Sanz, 2008)

Consolidation therapy, intermediate- and high-risk patients: 45 mg/m^2/day in two equally divided doses for 15 days each month for 3 months (see Sanz, 2004)

Maintenance therapy, intermediate- and high-risk patients: 45 mg/m^2/day in two equally divided doses for 15 days every 3 months for 2 years (see Sanz, 2004)

Administration Administer with a meal; do not crush capsules.

It is not recommended to use the capsule contents to extemporaneously prepare tretinoin suspension; however, there are limited case reports of use in patients who are unable to swallow the capsules whole. In a patient with a nasogastric (NG) tube, tretinoin capsules were cut open, with partial aspiration of the contents into a glass syringe, the residual capsule contents were mixed with soy bean oil and aspirated into the same syringe and administered (see Shaw, 1995). Tretinoin capsules have also been mixed with sterile water (~20 mL) and heated in a water bath (37°C) to melt the capsules and create an oily suspension for NG tube administration (see Bargetzi, 1996). Tretinoin has also been administered sublingually by squeezing the capsule contents beneath the tongue (see Kueh, 1999). Low plasma levels have been reported when contents of tretinoin capsules were administered directly through a feeding tube, although patient-specific impaired absorption may have been a contributing factor (see Takitani, 2004).

Monitoring Parameters Bone marrow cytology to confirm t(15;17) translocation or the presence of the PML/RARα fusion protein (do not withhold treatment initiation for results); monitor CBC with differential, coagulation profile, liver function test results, and triglyceride and cholesterol levels frequently; monitor closely for signs of APL differentiation syndrome (eg, monitor volume status, pulmonary status, temperature, respiration)

Patient Information Do not take any new medication during therapy unless approved by prescriber. Take with food. Do not crush, chew, or dissolve capsules. Maintain adequate hydration unless instructed to restrict fluid intake. Avoid alcohol and foods containing vitamin A, as well as foods with high fat content. May cause lethargy, dizziness, visual changes, confusion, and anxiety (avoid driving or engaging in tasks requiring alertness until response to drug is known); nausea, vomiting, loss of appetite, or dry mouth (small, frequent meals, chewing gum, or sucking lozenges may help); photosensitivity (use sunscreen, wear protective clothing and eyewear, and avoid direct sunlight); dry, itchy skin; or dry or irritated eyes (avoid contact lenses). Report persistent vomiting or diarrhea, respiratory difficulty, unusual bleeding or bruising, acute GI pain, bone pain, swelling of extremities, unusual weight gain, or vision changes immediately. **Pregnancy/Breast-Feeding Precautions:** Do not get pregnant (females) or cause a pregnancy (males) while taking this medication and for 1 month following completion of therapy. Consult prescriber for appropriate barrier contraceptive measures if necessary or if you suspect you might be pregnant. This drug should not be used in the first trimester of pregnancy. Breast-feeding is not recommended.

Additional Information For management of APL differentiation syndrome, initiate at first signs of DS: Dexamethasone 10 mg I.V. every 12 hours for 3-5 days; consider interrupting tretinoin until resolution of hypoxia

Dosage Forms Excipient information presented when available (limited, particularly for generics); consult specific product labeling.

Capsule: 10 mg
Vesanoid®: 10 mg [contains soybean oil and parabens] [DSC]

References

Bargetzi MJ, Tichelli A, Gratwohl A, et al, "Oral All-transretinoic Acid Administration in Intubated Patients With Acute Promyelocytic Leukemia," *Schweiz Med Wochenschr*, 1996, 126(45):1944-5.

de Botton S, Coiteux V, Chevret S, et al, "Outcome of Childhood Acute Promyelocytic Leukemia With All-*Trans*-Retinoic Acid and Chemotherapy," *J Clin Oncol*, 2004, 22(8):1404-12.

Gregory J, Kim H, Alonzo T, et al, "Treatment of Children With Acute Promyelocytic Leukemia: Results of the First North American Intergroup Trial INT0129," *Pediatr Blood Cancer*, 2009, 53 (6):1005-10.

Kueh YK, Liew PP, Ho PC, et al, "Sublingual Administration of All-*Trans*-retinoic Acid to a Comatose Patient With Acute Promyelocytic Leukemia," *Ann Pharmacother*, 1999, 33(4):503-5.

Mann G, Reinhardt D, Ritter J, et al, "Treatment With All-trans Retinoic Acid in Acute Promyelocytic Leukemia Reduces Early Deaths in Children," *Ann Hematol*, 2001, 80(7):417-22.

National Comprehensive Cancer Network® (NCCN), "Practice Guidelines in Oncology™: Acute Myeloid Leukemia," Version 1, 2010. Available at http://www.nccn.org/professionals/physician_gls/PDF/aml.pdf.

Ortega JJ, Madero L, Martín G, et al, "Treatment With All-*trans* Retinoic Acid and Anthracycline Monochemotherapy for Children With Acute Promyelocytic Leukemia: A Multicenter Study by the PETHEMA Group," *J Clin Oncol*, 2005, 23(30):7632-40.

Sanz MA, Grimwade D, Tallman MS, et al, "Management of Acute Promyelocytic Leukemia: Recommendations From an Expert Panel on Behalf of the European LeukemiaNet," *Blood*, 2009, 113 (9):1875-91.

Sanz MA, Martín G, González M, et al, "Risk-Adapted Treatment of Acute Promyelocytic Leukemia With All-*trans*-retinoic Acid and Anthracycline Monochemotherapy: A Multicenter Study by the PETHEMA Group," *Blood*, 2004, 103(4):1237-43.

Sanz MA, Montesinos P, Vellenga E, et al, "Risk-Adapted Treatment of Acute Promyelocytic Leukemia With All-trans Retinoic Acid and Anthracycline Monochemotherapy: Long-Term Outcome of the LPA 99 Multicenter Study by the PETHEMA Group," *Blood*, 2008, 112 (8):3130-4.

Shaw PJ, Atkins MC, Nath CE, et al, "ATRA Administration in the Critically Ill Patient," *Leukemia*, 1995, 9(7):1288.

Takitani K, Koh M, Inoue A, et al, "Pharmacokinetics of All-*Trans* Retinoic Acid in Adults and Children With Acute Promyelocytic Leukemia," *Am J Hematol*, 2006, 81(9):720-1.

Takitani K, Nakao Y, Kosaka Y, et al, "Low Plasma Level of All-*trans* Retinoic Acid After Feeding Tube Administration for Acute Promyelocytic Leukemia," *Am J Hematol*, 2004, 76(1):97-8.

Testi AM, Biondi A, Lo Coco F, et al, "GIMEMA-AIEOPAIDA Protocol for the Treatment of Newly Diagnosed Acute Promyelocytic Leukemia (APL) in Children," *Blood*, 2005, 106(2):447-53.

Vesanoid® data on file, Roche Pharmaceuticals.

Tretinoin (Topical) (TRET i noyn, TOP i kal)

Medication Safety Issues

Sound-alike/look-alike issues:
Tretinoin may be confused with isotretinoin, Tenormin®, triamcinolone, trientine

International issues:
Renova® may be confused with Remov® which is a brand name for nimesulide in Italy

U.S. Brand Names Atralin™; Avita®; Refissa™; Renova®; Retin-A®; Retin-A® Micro; Tretin-X™

Canadian Brand Names Rejuva-A®; Renova®; Retin-A®; Retin-A® Micro; Retinova®

Therapeutic Category Acne Products; Retinoic Acid Derivative; Vitamin, Topical

Generic Available Yes

Use Treatment of acne vulgaris, photodamaged skin, and some skin cancers

Pregnancy Risk Factor C

Pregnancy Considerations Oral tretinoin is teratogenic and fetotoxic in rats at doses 1000 and 500 times the topical human dose, respectively. Tretinoin does not appear to be teratogenic when used topically since it is rapidly metabolized by the skin; however, there are rare reports of fetal defects. Use for acne only if benefit to mother outweighs potential risk to fetus. During pregnancy, do not use for palliation of fine wrinkles, mottled hyper-pigmentation, and tactile roughness of facial skin.

Lactation Enters breast milk/compatible

Contraindications Hypersensitivity to tretinoin or any component; sunburn

Warnings Avoid contact with abraded skin, mucous membranes, eyes, mouth, angles of the nose; avoid excessive exposure to sunlight or sunlamps

Precautions Use with caution in patients with eczema

Adverse Reactions

Cardiovascular: Edema

Dermatologic: Excessive dryness, erythema, scaling of the skin, hyperpigmentation or hypopigmentation, photo-sensitivity, initial acne flare-up

Local: Stinging, blistering

Drug Interactions

Metabolism/Transport Effects Substrate of CYP2A6 (minor), 2B6 (minor), 2C8 (major), 2C9 (minor); **Inhibits** CYP2C9 (weak); **Induces** CYP2E1 (weak)

Avoid Concomitant Use There are no known inter-actions where it is recommended to avoid concomitant use.

Increased Effect/Toxicity There are no known signifi-cant interactions involving an increase in effect.

Decreased Effect

Tretinoin (Topical) may decrease the levels/effects of:
Contraceptives (Progestins)

Food Interactions Avoid excessive intake of vitamin A

Mechanism of Action Keratinocytes in the sebaceous follicle become less adherent which allows for easy removal; inhibits microcomedone formation and eliminates lesions already present

Pharmacodynamics

Onset of action: 2-3 weeks

Maximum effect: May require 6 weeks or longer ·

Pharmacokinetics (Adult data unless noted)

Absorption: Topical: Minimum absorption

Metabolism: In the liver

Elimination: In bile and urine

Usual Dosage Children >12 years and Adults: Topical: Begin therapy with a weaker formulation of tretinoin (0.025% cream or 0.01% gel) and increase the concen-tration as tolerated; apply once daily before retiring or on alternate days; if stinging or irritation develop, decrease frequency of application

Administration Topical: Apply to dry skin (wait at least 15-30 minutes to apply after cleansing); avoid contact with eyes, mucous membranes, mouth, or open wounds

Patient Information May cause photosensitivity reactions (eg, exposure to sunlight may cause severe sunburn, skin rash, redness, or itching); avoid exposure to sunlight and artificial light sources (sunlamps, tanning booth/bed); wear protective clothing, wide-brimmed hats, sunglasses, and lip sunscreen (SPF ≥15); use a sunscreen [broad-spectrum sunscreen or physical sunscreen (preferred) or sunblock with SPF ≥15]; contact physician if reaction occurs. Avoid washing face more frequently than 2-3 times/day; avoid using topical preparations with high alcoholic content during treatment period.

Additional Information Liquid preparation generally is more irritating

Dosage Forms Excipient information presented when available (limited, particularly for generics); consult specific product labeling. [DSC] = Discontinued product

Cream, topical: 0.025% (20 g, 45 g); 0.05% (20 g, 45 g); 0.1% (20 g, 45 g)

Avita®: 0.025% (20 g, 45 g)

Refissa™: 0.05% (40 g)

Renova®: 0.02% (40 g, 44 g, 60 g) [contains benzyl alcohol]

Retin-A®: 0.025% (20 g, 45 g); 0.05% (20 g, 45 g); 0.1% (20 g, 45 g)

Tretin-X™: 0.025% (35 g); 0.05% (35 g); 0.1% (35 g)

Gel, topical: 0.01% (15 g, 45 g); 0.025% (15 g, 45 g)

Atralin™: 0.05% (45 g) [contains benzyl alcohol and fish collagen]

Avita®: 0.025% (20 g, 45 g) [contains ethanol 83%]

Retin-A®: 0.01% (15 g, 45 g); 0.025% (15 g, 45 g) [contains ethanol 90%]

Tretin-X™: 0.025% (35 g); 0.01% (35 g) [contains ethanol 90%]

Gel, topical [microsphere gel]:

Retin-A® Micro: 0.04% (20 g, 45 g, 50 g); 0.1% (20 g, 45 g, 50 g) [contains benzyl alcohol]

References

Winston MH, Shalita AR, "Acne Vulgaris, Pathogenesis and Treat-ment," *Pediatr Clin North Am*, 1991, 38(4):889-903.

♦ **Tretinoinum** *see* Tretinoin (Systemic) *on page 1373*

♦ **Trexall™** *see* Methotrexate *on page 900*

♦ **Triaderm (Can)** *see* Triamcinolone *on page 1376*

Triamcinolone (trye am SIN oh lone)

Medication Safety Issues

Sound-alike/look-alike issues:

Kenalog® may be confused with Ketalar®

Nasacort® may be confused with NasalCrom®

TAC (occasional abbreviation for triamcinolone) is an error-prone abbreviation (mistaken as tetracaine-adrenaline-cocaine)

Related Information

Asthma *on page 1697*

Corticosteroids *on page 1487*

U.S. Brand Names Aristospan®; Azmacort® [DSC]; Kenalog®; Kenalog®-10; Kenalog®-40; Nasacort® AQ; Oralone®; Triderm®; Triesence™; Zytopic™ [DSC]

Canadian Brand Names Aristospan®; Kenalog®; Nasa-cort® AQ; Oracort; Triaderm; Trinasal®

Therapeutic Category Adrenal Corticosteroid; Anti-inflammatory Agent; Antiasthmatic; Corticosteroid, Inha-lant (Oral); Corticosteroid, Intranasal; Corticosteroid, Ophthalmic; Corticosteroid, Systemic; Corticosteroid, Top-ical; Glucocorticoid

Generic Available Yes: Cream, lotion, ointment, paste, powder

Use

Oral inhalation: Long-term (chronic) control of persistent bronchial asthma; **NOT** indicated for the relief of acute bronchospasm. Also used to help reduce or discontinue oral corticosteroid therapy for asthma.

Intra-articular (soft tissue): Acute gouty arthritis, acute/subacute bursitis, acute tenosynovitis, epicondylitis, rheumatoid arthritis, synovitis of osteoarthritis

Intralesional (injectable suspension): Alopecia areata; discoid lupus erythematosus; infiltrated, inflammatory lesions associated with granuloma annulare, lichen planus, neurodermatitis, and psoriatic plaques; keloids; necrobiosis lipoidica diabeticorum; possibly helpful in cystic tumors of an aponeurosis or tendon (ganglia)

Intranasal: Management of seasonal and perennial allergic rhinitis

Ophthalmic: Intravitreal: Treatment of sympathetic oph-thalmia, temporal arteritis, uveitis, ocular inflammatory conditions unresponsive to topical corticosteroids

Triesence™: Visualization during vitrectomy

Systemic: Immunosuppression; relief of severe inflam-mation

Topical: Relief of inflammation and pruritus associated with corticosteroid-responsive dermatoses

Topical (dental paste): Adjunctive treatment and temporary relief of symptoms related to oral inflammatory lesions and ulcerative lesions due to trauma

Pregnancy Risk Factor C/D (ophthalmic suspension)

Pregnancy Considerations Triamcinolone was shown to be teratogenic in animal reproduction studies. Some studies have shown an association between first trimester corticosteroid use and oral clefts; adverse events in the fetus/neonate have been noted in case reports following large doses of systemic corticosteroids during pregnancy. Inhaled corticosteroids are recommended for the treatment of asthma (most information available using budesonide) and allergic rhinitis during pregnancy. In general, the use of topical corticosteroids during pregnancy is not considered to have significant risk, however, intrauterine growth retardation in the infant has been reported (rare). The use of large amounts or for prolonged periods of time should be avoided.

Lactation Excretion in breast milk unknown/use caution

Breast-Feeding Considerations Corticosteroids are excreted in human milk; information specific to triamcinolone has not been located. The use of inhaled corticosteroids is not considered a contraindication to breast-feeding.

Contraindications Hypersensitivity to triamcinolone or any component (see Warnings); primary treatment of status asthmaticus or other acute episodes of asthma; systemic fungal infections; cerebral malaria; serious infections (except septic shock or tuberculous meningitis). Immunosuppressive doses: Contraindicated with immunization with live or live-attenuated vaccines

Topical: Contraindicated with local fungal, viral, or bacterial infections

I.M.: Contraindicated with idiopathic thrombocytopenic purpura

Warnings Fatalities have occurred due to adrenal insufficiency in asthmatic patients during and after switching from systemic corticosteroids to aerosol steroids; several months may be required for full recovery of hypothalamic-pituitary-adrenal (HPA) function; patients receiving higher doses of systemic corticosteroids (eg, adults receiving ≥20 mg of prednisone per day) may be at greater risk; during this period of HPA suppression, aerosol steroids do **not** provide the systemic glucocorticoid or mineralocorticoid activity needed to treat patients requiring stress doses (ie, patients with major stress such as trauma, surgery, infections, or other conditions associated with severe electrolyte loss). When used at high doses or for a prolonged time, hypocorticism and HPA suppression (including adrenal crisis) may occur; use with inhaled or systemic corticosteroids (even alternate-day dosing) may increase risk of HPA suppression; withdrawal and discontinuation of corticosteroids should be done carefully; patients with HPA axis suppression may require doses of systemic glucocorticosteroids prior to, during, and after unusual stress (eg, surgery). Immunosuppression may occur; patients may be more susceptible to infections; avoid exposure to chickenpox and measles. Switching patients from systemic corticosteroids to aerosol steroids may unmask allergic conditions previously treated by the systemic steroid. Bronchospasm may occur after use of inhaled asthma medications (see Additional Information).

High-dose corticosteroids should not be used for the management of traumatic brain injury (an increase in mortality was observed in patients with cranial trauma who received high-dose methylprednisolone).

Injectable ocular products: Intravitreal (Triesence™, Trivaris™) injection has been associated with endophthalmitis and visual disturbances. Blindness has been reported following injection into nasal turbinates and intralesional injections into the head. Safety of intraturbinal, subconjunctival, subtenons, or retrobulbar injection has not been demonstrated. Some injectable formulations should not be administered intravitreally.

Injection and cream may contain benzyl alcohol which may cause allergic reactions in susceptible individuals; large amounts of benzyl alcohol (≥99 mg/kg/day) have been associated with a potentially fatal toxicity ("gasping syndrome") in neonates; the "gasping syndrome" consists of metabolic acidosis, respiratory distress, gasping respirations, CNS dysfunction (including convulsions, intracranial hemorrhage), hypotension and cardiovascular collapse; avoid use of triamcinolone products containing benzyl alcohol or sodium benzoate in neonates; *in vitro* and animal studies have shown that benzoate displaces bilirubin from protein binding sites

Precautions Avoid using higher than recommended doses; suppression of HPA axis function, suppression of linear growth (ie, reduction of growth velocity), reduced bone mineral density, hypercorticism (Cushing's syndrome), hyperglycemia, or glucosuria may occur; titrate to lowest effective dose. Use with extreme caution in patients with respiratory tuberculosis or untreated systemic infections. Use with caution in patients with thyroid dysfunction, peptic ulcer disease, osteoporosis, myasthenia gravis, hypertension, CHF, nonspecific ulcerative colitis, fresh intestinal anastomoses, thromboembolic disorders, renal dysfunction, recent MI (left ventricular free wall rupture has been reported). Avoid injection into an infected site. Response to killed or inactivated vaccines cannot be predicted in patients receiving immunosuppressive doses of corticosteroids.

Use with caution in patients with cataracts and/or glaucoma; increased intraocular pressure, open-angle glaucoma, and cataracts have occurred with prolonged use. Corticosteroids should not be used in active ocular herpes simplex. Oral use is not recommended in the treatment of optic neuritis; an increased risk of new episodes may occur.

Epistaxis and nasal ulceration may occur with intranasal use. Nasal septum perforation has been reported with intranasal use of corticosteroids. Corticosteroids impair wound healing; do not use intranasal triamcinolone in patients with recent nasal ulcers, nasal surgery, or nasal trauma; allow healing to occur before use.

Adverse Reactions

Cardiovascular: CHF, edema, hypertension

Central nervous system: Depression, dizziness, euphoria, fatigue, headache (intranasal use) insomnia, malaise

Dermatologic: Acne, dermal thinning, hyperpigmentation, hypopigmentation, hypertrichosis, itching, skin atrophy

Endocrine & metabolic: Appetite increased, calcium absorption decreased, calcium excretion increased, Cushing's syndrome, diabetes mellitus, glucose intolerance, growth suppression, HPA suppression, hyperglycemia, hypokalemia, sodium and water retention, weight gain

Gastrointestinal: Dry throat, nausea, oral candidiasis, peptic ulcer, vomiting, xerostomia

Local: Burning, injection site atrophy, sterile abscesses

Neuromuscular & skeletal: Aseptic necrosis (femoral and humeral heads; rare), bone mineral density decreased, muscle weakness, osteoporosis

Ocular: Cataracts, glaucoma, IOP elevated

Ophthalmic use (intravitreal injection): Blurred vision, conjunctival hemorrhage, discomfort (transient), endophthalmitis, glaucoma, hypopyon, inflammation, optic disc vascular disorder, retinal detachment, vitreous floaters, visual acuity decreased

Respiratory: Cough, dysphonia, hoarseness, wheezing

Intranasal use: Cough increased, epistaxis, local *Candida* infections (nose and pharynx), nasal septal perforation, pharyngitis

Miscellaneous: Anaphylactoid reactions (rare); fungal infection exacerbation, infection symptoms masked, Kaposi's sarcoma (with prolonged systemic use), susceptibility to infection increased, tuberculosis reactivation

Drug Interactions

Avoid Concomitant Use

Avoid concomitant use of Triamcinolone with any of the following: Aldesleukin; BCG; Natalizumab; Pimecrolimus; Tacrolimus (Topical); Vaccines (Live)

Increased Effect/Toxicity

Triamcinolone may increase the levels/effects of: Acetylcholinesterase Inhibitors; Amphotericin B; Leflunomide; Loop Diuretics; Natalizumab; NSAID (COX-2 Inhibitor); NSAID (Nonselective); Thiazide Diuretics; Vaccines (Live); Warfarin

The levels/effects of Triamcinolone may be increased by: Antifungal Agents (Azole Derivatives, Systemic); Aprepitant; Calcium Channel Blockers (Nondihydropyridine); Denosumab; Estrogen Derivatives; Fluconazole; Fosaprepitant; Macrolide Antibiotics; Neuromuscular-Blocking Agents (Nondepolarizing); Pimecrolimus; Quinolone Antibiotics; Salicylates; Tacrolimus (Topical); Trastuzumab

Decreased Effect

Triamcinolone may decrease the levels/effects of: Aldesleukin; Antidiabetic Agents; BCG; Calcitriol; Corticorelin; Isoniazid; Salicylates; Sipuleucel-T; Vaccines (Inactivated); Vaccines (Live)

The levels/effects of Triamcinolone may be decreased by: Aminoglutethimide; Barbiturates; Echinacea; Mitotane; Primidone; Rifamycin Derivatives

Food Interactions Systemic use of corticosteroids may require a diet with increased potassium, vitamins A, B_6, C, D, folate, calcium, zinc, and phosphorus and decreased sodium

Stability

Injection, suspension:

Acetonide injectable suspension: All products: Avoid freezing, protect from light

Kenalog®: Store at 20°C to 25°C (68°F to 77°F)

Triesence™: Store at 4°C to 25°C (39°F to 77°F)

Trivaris™: Store at 2°C to 8°C (36°F to 46°F)

Hexacetonide injectable suspension: Store at 20°C to 25°C (68°F to 77°F); avoid freezing. Protect from light. Avoid diluents containing parabens, phenol, or other preservatives (may cause flocculation). Diluted suspension stable up to 1 week. Suspension for intralesional use may be diluted with D_5NS, D_{10}NS, NS, or SWI to a 1:1, 1:2, or 1:4 concentration. Solutions for intra-articular use may be diluted with lidocaine 1% or 2%.

Intranasal: Store at controlled room temperature of 20°C to 25°C (68°F to 77°F); do not freeze

Oral inhalation: Azmacort®: Store at controlled room temperature of 20°C to 25°C (68°F to 77°F); do not expose to temperatures >120°F (may cause bursting); do not puncture or incinerate. Do not use or store near open flame or heat.

Topical:

Ointment: Store at room temperature.

Spray: Store at room temperature; avoid excessive heat

Mechanism of Action Controls the rate of protein synthesis, depresses the migration of polymorphonuclear leukocytes and fibroblasts, reverses capillary permeability, and stabilizes lysosomal membranes at the cellular level to prevent or control inflammation

Pharmacokinetics (Adult data unless noted)

Distribution: V_d: Adults: 99.5 ± 27.5 L

Protein binding: ~68%

Metabolism: Hepatic to 3 identified metabolites (significantly less active than parent drug)

Half-life: Elimination: 88 minutes; Biologic: 18-36 hours

Time to peak serum concentration: I.M.: Within 8-10 hours

Elimination: 40% of dose is excreted in urine; 60% in feces

Usual Dosage Adjust dose depending upon condition being treated and response of patient. The lowest possible dose should be used to control the condition; when dose reduction is possible, the dose should be reduced gradually. In life-threatening situations, parenteral doses larger than the oral dose may be needed.

I.M. (as **acetonide**):

Children: Initial: 0.11–1.6 mg/kg/day (or 3.2–48 mg/m²/day) in 3–4 divided doses

Children 6-12 years: Initial: 40 mg; some centers use 0.03-0.2 mg/kg at 1- to 7-day intervals

Adolescents >12 years and Adults: Initial: 60 mg; usual dose: 40–80 mg; some patients may respond to 20 mg/dose

Hay fever/pollen asthma: 40-100 mg as a single injection/season

Multiple sclerosis (acute exacerbation): 160 mg daily for 1 week, followed by 64 mg every other day for 1 month

Intra-articular (as **hexacetonide**): Children >12 years and Adults: Large joints: 10-20 mg; small joints: 2-6 mg; usual frequency: Every 3-4 weeks; more frequent administration is not recommended

Intra-articular, intrabursal, tendon-sheath injection (as **acetonide**): Adults: Initial: Smaller joints: 2.5-5 mg, larger joints: 5-15 mg; may require up to 10 mg for small joints and up to 40 mg for large joints; maximum dose/treatment (several joints at one time): 20-80 mg

Intra-articular, intrasynovial (as **acetonide**): Children >12 years and Adults: 2.5-40 mg, repeat as needed when signs and symptoms recur

Intradermal (as **acetonide**): Adults: Initial: 1 mg

Intralesional, sublesional (as **acetonide**): Children >12 years and Adults: Up to 1 mg per injection site and may be repeated 1 or more times weekly; multiple sites may be injected if they are 1 cm or more apart, not to exceed 30 mg

Intralesional, sublesional (as **hexacetonide**): Children >12 years and Adults: Up to 0.5 mg/square inch of affected skin; initial range: 2-48 mg; frequency of dose is determined by clinical response

Intranasal:

Nasacort® AQ: 55 mcg/spray; **Note:** Doses should be titrated to the lowest effective dose once symptoms are controlled; discontinue treatment if adequate control of symptoms has not occurred after 3 weeks of use

Children <2 years: Not recommended

Children 2-5 years: 110 mcg/day as 1 spray in each nostril once daily [maximum: 2 sprays/day (110 mcg/day)]

Children 6-11 years: Initial: 110 mcg/day as 1 spray in each nostril once daily; may increase to 220 mcg/day as 2 sprays in each nostril once daily if response not adequate; once symptoms are controlled may reduce to 110 mcg/day as 1 spray in each nostril once daily

Children >12 years and Adults: Initial: 220 mcg/day as 2 sprays in each nostril once daily; titrate to lowest effective dose once symptoms are controlled; usual maintenance dose: 110 mcg/day as 1 spray in each nostril once daily

Tri-Nasal®: Children >12 years and Adults: Initial: 2 sprays in each nostril once daily; may increase to maximum dose of 4 sprays in each nostril once daily or 2 sprays in each nostril twice daily; may initiate at maximum doses if faster relief of symptoms is required; titrate to lowest effective dose once symptoms are controlled

Ophthalmic injection: Intravitreal: Children and Adults
Ocular disease: Initial: 4 mg as a single dose; additional doses may be given as needed over the course of treatment
Visualization during vitrectomy (Triesence™): 1-4 mg
Oral: Children >12 years and Adults: 4-100 mg/day in 1-4 divided doses
Oral inhalation: Doses should be titrated to the lowest effective dose once asthma is controlled; maintenance doses may be given twice daily. Manufacturer recommendation:
Children: 6-12 years: 1-2 puffs given 3-4 times/day **or** 2-4 puffs given twice daily; maximum dose: 12 puffs/day
Children >12 years and Adults: 2 puffs given 3-4 times/day **or** 4 puffs given twice daily; for severe asthma may initiate at initial dose of 12-16 puffs/day divided into 3-4 doses/day; maximum dose: 16 puffs/day
NIH Asthma Guidelines (NAEPP, 2007) [give in divided doses 3-4 times/day]:
Children 5-11 years:
"Low" dose: 300-600 mcg/day (4-8 puffs/day)
"Medium" dose: >600-900 mcg/day (>8-12 puffs/day)
"High" dose: >900 mcg/day (>12 puffs/day)
Children ≥12 years and Adults:
"Low" dose: 300-750 mcg/day (4-10 puffs/day)
"Medium" dose: >750-1500 mcg/day (>10-20 puffs/day)
"High" dose: >1500 mcg/day (>20 puffs/day)
Topical: Children and Adults: Apply a thin film 2-3 times/day
Topical (dental): Adults: Press a small amount (~1/4 inch) to the lesion until a thin film develops; some lesions may require a larger quantity; apply once daily at bedtime; more severe lesions may require application 2-3 times/day (preferably after meals)

Administration

Oral: May administer with meals to decrease GI upset
Oral inhalant: Shake canister well before use; use at room temperature. Rinse mouth with water (without swallowing) after inhalation to decrease chance of oral candidiasis. Use a spacer device for children <8 years of age. Do not spray in eyes. To prime canister prior to first use, shake inhaler well, then press canister to release 2 puffs; inhaler will need to be reprimed if not used for >3 days.
Intranasal: Shake container well before use; clear nasal passages by blowing nose prior to use; do not spray in eyes; Nasacort® AQ: Prime prior to first use, by shaking container well and releasing 5 sprays into the air; if product is not used for more than 2 weeks, reprime with one spray.
Ophthalmic injection (intravitreal): Triesence™: **Not for I.V. use.** Shake vial well prior to use. Administer under controlled aseptic conditions (eg, sterile gloves, sterile drape, sterile eyelid speculum). Adequate anesthesia and a broad-spectrum bactericidal agent should be administered prior to injection. Inject immediately after withdrawing from vial. If administration is required in the second eye, a new vial should be used. Do not use if agglomerated (clumpy or granular appearance); Trivaris™ (see parenteral below).
Parenteral: Avoid SubQ use; **do not inject I.V.;** shake well prior to use; acetonide or hexacetonide may be administered I.M.; for I.M. administration: Inject deep in large muscle mass, avoid deltoid. See Usual Dosage for other parenteral routes of administration.
Trivaris™: Can be administered I.M., intra-articular and intravitreal; **not for I.V. use.** Bring to room temperature prior to administration. A 27 gauge1/2-inch needle is recommended for intravitreal administration.
Topical: Apply sparingly to affected area, gently rub in until disappears; avoid application on face; do not occlude area unless directed; do not use on open skin; avoid contact with eyes
Topical (dental): Apply sparingly; do not rub in; spreading the paste may result in a granular, gritty sensation and crumbling; apply at bedtime to allow contact of the medication with the lesion overnight.

Monitoring Parameters

Oral inhalation and intranasal use: Check mucus membranes for signs of fungal infection; monitor growth in pediatric patients. Assess HPA suppression in patients using potent topical steroids applied to a large surface area or to areas under occlusion. Monitor IOP with therapy >6 weeks. Monitor blood pressure and for clinical presence of adverse effects.
Ophthalmic injection (intravitreal): Following injection, monitor for increased intraocular pressure and endophthalmitis; check for perfusion of optic nerve head immediately after injection, tonometry within 30 minutes; biomicroscopy between 2-7 days after injection.
Systemic: Intraocular pressure (if therapy > 6 weeks), linear growth of pediatric patients (with chronic use), assess HPA suppression. Monitor blood pressure, serum glucose, potassium, and calcium and clinical presence of adverse effects.

Patient Information Notify physician if condition being treated persists or worsens; do not decrease dose or discontinue without physician approval; avoid exposure to chicken pox or measles, if exposed seek medical advice without delay; may cause dry mouth; avoid alcohol
Oral inhalant: Rinse mouth with water without swallowing to decrease chance of oral candidiasis; report sore mouth or mouth lesions to physician

Nursing Implications Once daily oral doses should be given in the morning

Additional Information Oral inhalation: If bronchospasm with wheezing occurs after use, a fast-acting bronchodilator may be used; discontinue orally inhaled corticosteroid and initiate alternative chronic therapy. Azmacort® contains dichlorodifluoromethane as a propellant and dehydrated alcohol 1%. The FDA, in accordance with the Montreal Protocol on Substances that Deplete the Ozone Layer, has issued a phase out of seven metered-dose inhalers (MDIs) that contain ozone-depleting chlorofluorocarbons (CFCs). The CFC-propelled Azmacort® inhalation aerosol (triamcinolone) will not be manufactured, sold, or dispensed in the U.S. after December 31, 2010, and patients should be transitioned to another therapy.

Product Availability

Dosage Forms Excipient information presented when available (limited, particularly for generics); consult specific product labeling. [DSC] = Discontinued product
Aerosol for oral inhalation, as acetonide:
Azmacort®: 75 mcg per actuation (20 g) [contains chlorofluorocarbon; 240 actuations] [DSC]
Aerosol, topical, as acetonide:
Kenalog®: 0.2 mg/2-second spray (63 g) [contains dehydrated ethanol 10.3%]
Cream, topical, as acetonide: 0.025% (15 g, 80 g, 454 g); 0.1% (15 g, 30 g, 80 g, 454 g; 2270 g [DSC]); 0.5% (15 g)
Triderm®: 0.1% (30 g, 85 g)
Zytopic™: 0.1% (85 g) [DSC]
Injection, suspension, as acetonide:
Kenalog®-10: 10 mg/mL (5 mL) [contains benzyl alcohol, polysorbate 80; not for I.V. or I.M. use]
Kenalog®-40: 40 mg/mL (1 mL, 5 mL, 10 mL) [contains benzyl alcohol, polysorbate 80; not for I.V. or intradermal use]
Injection, suspension, as hexacetonide:
Aristospan®: 5 mg/mL (5 mL); 20 mg/mL (1 mL, 5 mL) [contains benzyl alcohol, polysorbate 80; not for I.V. use]

Injection, suspension, ophthalmic, as acetonide: Triesence™: 40 mg/mL (1 mL) [contains polysorbate 80; not for I.V. use]

Lotion, topical, as acetonide: 0.025% (60 mL); 0.1% (60 mL)

Ointment, topical, as acetonide: 0.025% (15 g, 80 g, 454 g); 0.05% (430 g); 0.1% (15 g, 80 g, 454 g); 0.5% (15 g)

Paste, oral, topical, as acetonide: 0.1% (5 g) Oralone®: 0.1% (5 g)

Powder, topical, as acetonide [micronized]: USP: 100% (5 g)

Suspension, intranasal, as acetonide [spray]: Nasacort® AQ: 55 mcg/inhalation (16.5 g) [chlorofluorocarbon free; contains benzalkonium chloride; 120 actuations]

References
National Asthma Education and Prevention Program (NAEPP), "Expert Panel Report 3 (EPR-3): Guidelines for the Diagnosis and Management of Asthma," *Clinical Practice Guidelines*, National Institutes of Health, National Heart, Lung, and Blood Institute, NIH Publication No. 08-4051, prepublication 2007; available at http://www.nhlbi.nih.gov/guidelines/asthma/asthgdln.htm.

♦ **Triamcinolone Acetonide, Aerosol** *see* Triamcinolone *on page 1376*

♦ **Triamcinolone Acetonide, Parenteral** *see* Triamcinolone *on page 1376*

♦ **Triamcinolone Hexacetonide** *see* Triamcinolone *on page 1376*

♦ **Triamcinolone, Oral** *see* Triamcinolone *on page 1376*

♦ **Triaminic® Children's Cough Long Acting [OTC]** *see* Dextromethorphan *on page 421*

♦ **Triaminic Thin Strips® Children's Cough and Runny Nose [OTC]** *see* DiphenhydrAMINE *on page 448*

♦ **Triaminic® Thin Strips® Children's Long Acting Cough [OTC]** *see* Dextromethorphan *on page 421*

♦ **Triaminic Thin Strips® Children's Cold with Stuffy Nose [OTC]** *see* Phenylephrine *on page 1102*

♦ **Triaminic Thin Strips® Cold [OTC] [DSC]** *see* Phenylephrine *on page 1102*

Triamterene (trye AM ter een)

Medication Safety Issues
Sound-alike/look-alike issues:
Triamterene may be confused with trimipramine
Dyrenium® may be confused with Pyridium®

Related Information
Antihypertensive Agents by Class *on page 1481*

U.S. Brand Names Dyrenium®

Therapeutic Category Antihypertensive Agent; Diuretic, Potassium Sparing

Generic Available No

Use Used alone or in combination with other diuretics to treat edema and hypertension; decreases potassium excretion caused by kaliuretic diuretics

Pregnancy Risk Factor C

Pregnancy Considerations No data available. Generally, use of diuretics during pregnancy is avoided due to risk of decreased placental perfusion.

Lactation Excretion in breast milk unknown

Breast-Feeding Considerations No data available.

Contraindications Hypersensitivity to triamterene or any component; severe renal or hepatic impairment, hyperkalemia; patients receiving other potassium-sparing diuretics

Warnings Hyperkalemia (serum potassium ≥5.5 mEq/L) can occur; patients at risk include those with renal impairment, diabetes, the elderly, and the severely ill [U.S. Boxed Warning]. Serum potassium levels must be monitored at frequent intervals especially when dosages are changed or with any illness that may cause renal dysfunction. Hypersensitivity reactions have been reported; monitor for possible occurrence of blood dyscrasias, liver damage, or other idiosyncratic reactions.

Precautions Use with caution in patients with impaired hepatic or renal function, history of renal calculi, diabetes mellitus; patients receiving other potassium-sparing diuretics or potassium supplements may cause uric acid elevations; use with caution in patients with gouty arthritis

Adverse Reactions
Cardiovascular: Hypotension

Central nervous system: Dizziness, headache

Endocrine & metabolic: Hyperkalemia, hyponatremia, hypomagnesemia, hyperchloremia, hyperuricemia, metabolic acidosis

Dermatologic: Photosensitivity

Gastrointestinal: Nausea, vomiting, diarrhea, xerostomia

Genitourinary: Slight alkalinization of urine

Hematologic: Blood dyscrasias, thrombocytopenia, megaloblastic anemia

Hepatic: Abnormal liver function

Neuromuscular & skeletal: Muscle cramps, weakness

Renal: Prerenal azotemia, nephrolithiasis (rare), reversible acute renal failure

Miscellaneous: Allergic reactions have been reported

Drug Interactions

Avoid Concomitant Use There are no known interactions where it is recommended to avoid concomitant use.

Increased Effect/Toxicity
Triamterene may increase the levels/effects of: ACE Inhibitors; Amifostine; Ammonium Chloride; Antihypertensives; Cardiac Glycosides; Hypotensive Agents; RiTUXimab

The levels/effects of Triamterene may be increased by: Angiotensin II Receptor Blockers; Diazoxide; Drospirenone; Eplerenone; Herbs (Hypotensive Properties); Indomethacin; MAO Inhibitors; Nonsteroidal Anti-Inflammatory Agents; Pentoxifylline; Phosphodiesterase 5 Inhibitors; Potassium Salts; Prostacyclin Analogues; Tolvaptan

Decreased Effect
Triamterene may decrease the levels/effects of: Cardiac Glycosides; QuiNIDine

The levels/effects of Triamterene may be decreased by: Herbs (Hypertensive Properties); Methylphenidate; Nonsteroidal Anti-Inflammatory Agents; Yohimbine

Food Interactions Avoid salt substitutes and diets with increased potassium

Mechanism of Action Interferes with potassium/sodium exchange (active transport) in the distal tubule, cortical collecting tubule and collecting duct by inhibiting sodium, potassium-ATPase; decreases calcium excretion; increases magnesium loss

Pharmacodynamics
Onset of action: Diuresis occurs within 2-4 hours

Duration: 7-9 hours

Note: Maximum therapeutic effect may not occur until after several days of therapy

Pharmacokinetics (Adult data unless noted)
Absorption: Oral: Unreliably absorbed

Metabolism: Hepatic conjugation

Half-life: 100-150 minutes

Elimination: 21% excreted unchanged in urine

Usual Dosage Oral:
Children: 1-2 mg/kg/day in 1-2 divided doses; maximum dose: 3-4 mg/kg/day and not to exceed 300 mg/day
Adults: 100-300 mg/day in 1-2 divided doses; usual dosage range (JNC 7): 50-100 mg/day

Dosage adjustment in renal impairment: Cl_{cr} <10 mL/minute: Avoid use

Dosage adjustment in hepatic impairment: Dose reduction is recommended in patients with cirrhosis

Administration Oral: Administer with food to avoid GI upset

Monitoring Parameters Electrolytes (sodium, potassium, magnesium, HCO_3, chloride), CBC, BUN, creatinine, platelets

Test Interactions Interferes with fluorometric assay of quinidine

Patient Information May cause dry mouth. May cause photosensitivity reactions (eg, exposure to sunlight may cause severe sunburn, skin rash, redness, or itching); avoid exposure to sunlight and artificial light sources (sunlamps, tanning booth/bed); wear protective clothing, wide-brimmed hats, sunglasses, and lip sunscreen (SPF ≥15); use a sunscreen [broad-spectrum sunscreen or physical sunscreen (preferred) or sunblock with SPF ≥15]; contact physician if reaction occurs.

Additional Information Abrupt discontinuation of therapy may result in rebound kaliuresis; taper off gradually

Dosage Forms Excipient information presented when available (limited, particularly for generics); consult specific product labeling.

Capsule: 50 mg, 100 mg [contains benzyl alcohol]

References

Chobanian AV, Bakris GL, Black HR, et al, "The Seventh Report of the Joint National Committee on Prevention, Detection, Evaluation, and Treatment of High Blood Pressure: The JNC 7 Report.," *JAMA*, 2003, 289(19):2560-72.

National High Blood Pressure Education Program Working Group on High Blood Pressure in Children and Adolescents, "The Fourth Report on the Diagnosis, Evaluation, and Treatment of High Blood Pressure in Children and Adolescents," *Pediatrics*, 2004, 114(2 Suppl):555-76.

van der Vorst MM, Kist JE, van der Heijden AJ, et al, "Diuretics in Pediatrics: Current Knowledge and Future Prospects," *Paediatr Drugs*, 2006, 8(4):245-64.

♦ **Triatec-8 (Can)** *see* Acetaminophen and Codeine *on page 39*

♦ **Triatec-8 Strong (Can)** *see* Acetaminophen and Codeine *on page 39*

♦ **Triatec-30 (Can)** *see* Acetaminophen and Codeine *on page 39*

♦ **Triaz®** *see* Benzoyl Peroxide *on page 184*

Triazolam (trye AY zoe lam)

Medication Safety Issues

Sound-alike/look-alike issues:

Triazolam may be confused with alPRAZolam

Halcion® may be confused with halcinonide, Haldol®

Beers Criteria medication: This drug may be inappropriate for use in geriatric patients (high severity risk).

U.S. Brand Names Halcion®

Canadian Brand Names Apo-Triazo®; Gen-Triazolam; Halcion®; Mylan-Triazolam

Therapeutic Category Benzodiazepine; Hypnotic; Sedative

Generic Available Yes

Use Short-term treatment of insomnia

Restrictions C-IV

Medication Guide An FDA-approved patient medication guide, which is available with the product information and at http://www.fda.gov/downloads/Drugs/DrugSafety/ucm088610.pdf, must be dispensed with this medication for each new outpatient prescription and refill.

Pregnancy Risk Factor X

Pregnancy Considerations Other benzodiazepines are known to cross the placenta and accumulate in the fetus. Teratogenic effects have been reported. Use of triazolam is contraindicated in pregnancy.

Lactation Excretion in breast milk unknown/not recommended

Breast-Feeding Considerations It is not known if triazolam is excreted in breast milk; however, other benzodiazepines are known to be excreted in breast milk. The AAP rates use of related agents as "of concern" and breast-feeding is not recommended.

Contraindications Hypersensitivity to triazolam or any component; cross-sensitivity with other benzodiazepines may occur; severe uncontrolled pain; pre-existing CNS depression; narrow-angle glaucoma; pregnancy; concomitant use with ketoconazole, itraconazole, or nefazodone (see Drug Interactions)

Warnings Evaluate patient carefully for medical or psychiatric causes of insomnia prior to initiation of drug treatment; failure of triazolam to treat insomnia (after 7-10 days of therapy), a worsening of insomnia, or the emergence of behavioral changes or thinking abnormalities, may indicate a medical or psychiatric illness requiring evaluation; these effects also have been reported with triazolam use. Due to possible adverse effects, use lowest effective dose. Abrupt discontinuation after prolonged use may result in withdrawal symptoms or rebound insomnia. Triazolam is a substrate of cytochrome P450 isoenzyme CYP3A4; serious drug interactions may occur (see Drug Interactions).

Hypersensitivity reactions including anaphylaxis and angioedema may occur. Hazardous sleep-related activities, such as sleep-driving (driving while not fully awake without any recollection of driving), preparing and eating food, and making phone calls while asleep have also been reported. Effects with other sedative drugs or ethanol may be potentiated.

Precautions Use with caution in patients with depression, renal or hepatic dysfunction, chronic pulmonary insufficiency, or sleep apnea; use in lactating women is not recommended

Adverse Reactions

Central nervous system: Drowsiness, anterograde amnesia, confusion, bizarre behavior, agitation, dizziness, hallucinations, nightmares, headache, ataxia

Gastrointestinal: Xerostomia, nausea, vomiting

Hepatic: Cholestatic jaundice

Miscellaneous: Physical and psychological dependence; hypersensitivity reactions, anaphylaxis, angioedema; hazardous sleep-related activities (see Warnings)

Drug Interactions

Metabolism/Transport Effects Substrate of CYP3A4 (major); **Inhibits** CYP2C8 (weak), 2C9 (weak)

Avoid Concomitant Use

Avoid concomitant use of Triazolam with any of the following: Efavirenz; Protease Inhibitors

Increased Effect/Toxicity

Triazolam may increase the levels/effects of: Alcohol (Ethyl); Clozapine; CNS Depressants; Methotrimeprazine; Phenytoin

The levels/effects of Triazolam may be increased by: Antifungal Agents (Azole Derivatives, Systemic); Aprepitant; Calcium Channel Blockers (Nondihydropyridine); Cimetidine; Contraceptives (Estrogens); Contraceptives (Progestins); CYP3A4 Inhibitors (Moderate); CYP3A4 Inhibitors (Strong); Dasatinib; Efavirenz; Fluconazole; Fosaprepitant; Grapefruit Juice; Isoniazid; Macrolide Antibiotics; Methotrimeprazine; Nefazodone; Protease Inhibitors; Proton Pump Inhibitors; Selective Serotonin Reuptake Inhibitors

Decreased Effect

The levels/effects of Triazolam may be decreased by: CarBAMazepine; CYP3A4 Inducers (Strong); Deferasirox; Rifamycin Derivatives; St Johns Wort; Theophylline Derivatives; Yohimbine

Food Interactions Food may decrease the rate, but not the extent of absorption; grapefruit juice significantly increases the bioavailability of oral triazolam

Mechanism of Action Depresses all levels of the CNS, including the limbic and reticular formation, by binding to the benzodiazepine site on the gamma-aminobutyric acid (GABA) receptor complex and modulating GABA, which is a major inhibitory neurotransmitter in the brain

Pharmacodynamics Hypnotic effects:
Onset of action: Within 15-30 minutes
Duration: 6-7 hours

Pharmacokinetics (Adult data unless noted)
Distribution: Drug and metabolites distribute into breast milk
V_d: Adults: 0.8-1.8 L/kg
Protein binding: 89%
Metabolism: Extensive in the liver; primary metabolites are conjugated glucuronides
Half-life: Adults: 1.5-5.5 hours
Time to peak serum concentration: Within 2 hours
Elimination: In urine as unchanged drug (minor amounts) and metabolites

Usual Dosage Oral:
Children <18 years: Dosage not established; investigational doses of 0.02 mg/kg given as an elixir have been used in children (n=20) for sedation prior to dental procedures; further studies are needed before this dose can be recommended
Adolescents ≥18 years and Adults: Usual: 0.125-0.25 mg at bedtime; dose may be increased to 0.5 mg at bedtime in patients who do not respond to lower doses; maximum dose: 0.5 mg/day

Administration Oral: Administer dose in bed, since onset of hypnotic effect is rapid; do not administer with grapefruit juice

Monitoring Parameters Liver enzymes with prolonged use

Patient Information Read the patient Medication Guide that you receive with each prescription and refill of triazolam. Avoid alcohol, other CNS depressants, and grapefruit juice. May be habit-forming; avoid abrupt discontinuation with prolonged use. May cause drowsiness and impair ability to perform activities requiring mental alertness or physical coordination. Take dose in bed at bedtime. May also cause daytime drowsiness. May cause dry mouth. May cause hypersensitivity reactions. May cause hazardous sleep-related activities (ie, driving, preparing and eating foods, and making phone calls while not fully awake).

Additional Information Onset of action is rapid; patient should be in bed when taking medication

Dosage Forms Excipient information presented when available (limited, particularly for generics); consult specific product labeling. [DSC] = Discontinued product
Tablet: 0.125 mg, 0.25 mg
Halcion®: 0.125 mg [DSC], 0.25 mg

References

Meyer ML, Mourino AP, and Farrington FH, "Comparison of Triazolam to a Chloral Hydrate/Hydroxyzine Combination in the Sedation of Pediatric Dental Patients," *Pediatr Dent*, 1990, 12(5):283-7.

◆ **Tribavirin** *see* Ribavirin *on page 1210*

◆ **Tricalcium Phosphate** *see* Calcium Phosphate (Tribasic) *on page 238*

◆ **Trichloroacetaldehyde Monohydrate** *see* Chloral Hydrate *on page 286*

◆ **Tricosal** *see* Choline Magnesium Trisalicylate *on page 304*

◆ **Triderm®** *see* Triamcinolone *on page 1376*

◆ **Tridil** *see* Nitroglycerin *on page 996*

◆ **Tridural™ (Can)** *see* TraMADol *on page 1367*

◆ **Triesence™** *see* Triamcinolone *on page 1376*

◆ **Triethylenethiophosphoramide** *see* Thiotepa *on page 1342*

Trifluoperazine (trye floo oh PER a zeen)

Medication Safety Issues

Sound-alike/look-alike issues:
Trifluoperazine may be confused with triflupromazine, trihexyphenidyl
Stelazine® may be confused with selegiline

International issues:
Eskazine [Spain] may be confused with Ecazide, a brand name for captopril/hydrochlorothiazide [France, Spain]

Canadian Brand Names Apo-Trifluoperazine®; Novo-Trifluzine; PMS-Trifluoperazine; Terfluzine

Therapeutic Category Antipsychotic Agent, Typical, Phenothiazine; Phenothiazine Derivative

Generic Available Yes

Use Treatment of schizophrenia (FDA approved in ages ≥6 years and adults); short-term treatment of generalized nonpsychotic anxiety (not a drug of choice) (FDA approved in adults); also used for management of psychotic disorders

Pregnancy Risk Factor C

Lactation Enters breast milk/not recommended (AAP rates "of concern")

Contraindications Hypersensitivity to trifluoperazine or any component; cross-sensitivity with other phenothiazines may exist; severe CNS depression; bone marrow suppression; blood dyscrasias; severe hepatic disease; coma

Warnings May cause extrapyramidal symptoms, including pseudoparkinsonism, acute dystonic reactions, akathisia, and tardive dyskinesia (risk of these reactions is high relative to other typical antipsychotics, and is dose-dependent; to decrease risk of tardive dyskinesia: Use smallest dose and shortest duration possible; evaluate continued need periodically; risk of dystonia is increased with the use of high potency and higher doses of conventional antipsychotics and in males and younger patients). May be associated with neuroleptic malignant syndrome (NMS); monitor for mental status changes, fever, muscle rigidity, and/or autonomic instability (risk may be increased in patients with Parkinson's disease or Lewy body dementia). Safety for use during pregnancy has not been established; prolonged jaundice, hyper-reflexia, hyporeflexia, or extrapyramidal signs may occur in newborn infants of mothers who received phenothiazines; clinical benefits should clearly outweigh risks before initiating use during pregnancy. May cause pigmentary retinopathy (discontinue drug if ophthalmoscopic or visual field exam demonstrates retinal changes).

Leukopenia, neutropenia, and agranulocytosis (sometimes fatal) have been reported in clinical trials and postmarketing reports with antipsychotic use; presence of risk factors (eg, pre-existing low WBC or history of drug-induced leuko/neutropenia) should prompt periodic blood count assessment. Thrombocytopenia, anemia, agranulocytosis, and pancytopenia have been reported with trifluoperazine use. Discontinue therapy at first signs of blood dyscrasias or if absolute neutrophil count <1000/mm^3. Use is contraindicated in patients with existing blood dyscrasias or bone marrow suppression.

An increased risk of death has been reported with the use of antipsychotics in elderly patients with dementia-related psychosis **[U.S. Boxed Warning]**; most deaths seemed to be cardiovascular (eg, sudden death, heart failure) or infectious (eg, pneumonia) in nature; trifluoperazine is not approved for this indication.

Precautions Use with caution in patients with hemodynamic instability; predisposition to seizures; subcortical brain damage; hepatic impairment; severe cardiac, renal, or respiratory disease. May cause sedation, which may impair physical or mental abilities; patients must be cautioned about performing tasks which require mental alertness (eg, operating machinery or driving); use with caution in disorders where CNS depression is a feature. Use with caution in Parkinson's disease. Esophageal dysmotility and aspiration have been associated with antipsychotic use; use with caution in patients at risk of pneumonia. Use with caution in breast cancer or other prolactin-dependent tumors (may elevate prolactin levels). May alter temperature regulation (use with caution with strenuous exercise, heat exposure, dehydration, and concomitant medication possessing anticholinergic effects). May mask toxicity of other drugs due to antiemetic effects. May alter cardiac conduction; life-threatening arrhythmias have occurred with therapeutic doses of phenothiazines. May cause orthostatic hypotension; use with caution in patients at risk of this effect or those who would not tolerate transient hypotensive episodes (cerebrovascular disease, cardiovascular disease, or other medications which may predispose). Trifluoperazine has not been shown to be effective for the treatment of behavioral complications in patients with mental retardation. Safety and efficacy in children <6 years of age have not been established.

Cholestatic jaundice, liver damage, and hepatitis may occur; obtain appropriate liver tests if patient develops fever with grippe-like symptoms; discontinue treatment if liver tests are abnormal. Phenothiazines may cause anticholinergic effects (confusion, agitation, constipation, xerostomia, blurred vision, urinary retention); therefore, they should be used with caution in patients with decreased GI motility, urinary retention, benign prostatic hypertrophy, xerostomia, or visual disturbances. Conditions which also may be exacerbated by cholinergic blockade include narrow-angle glaucoma (screening is recommended) and worsening of myasthenia gravis. Relative to other antipsychotics, trifluoperazine has a low potency of cholinergic blockade.

Adverse Reactions

Cardiovascular: Cardiac arrest, hypotension, orthostatic hypotension

Central nervous system: Dizziness, drowsiness, extrapyramidal symptoms (akathisia, dystonias, pseudoparkinsonism, tardive dyskinesia), fatigue, headache, impairment of temperature regulation, insomnia, lowering of seizure threshold, NMS

Dermatologic: Discoloration of skin (blue-gray), photosensitivity, rash, skin reactions

Endocrine & metabolic: Amenorrhea, breast pain, changes in menstrual cycle, galactorrhea, gynecomastia, hyperglycemia, hypoglycemia, lactation, libido (changes in), weight gain

Gastrointestinal: Anorexia, constipation, nausea, stomach pain, vomiting, xerostomia

Genitourinary: Difficulty in urination, ejaculatory disturbances, priapism, urinary retention

Hematologic: Agranulocytosis, aplastic anemia, eosinophilia, hemolytic anemia, leukopenia, neutropenia, pancytopenia, thrombocytopenic purpura

Hepatic: Cholestatic jaundice, hepatotoxicity

Neuromuscular & skeletal: Muscular weakness, tremor

Ocular: Blurred vision, cornea and lens changes, pigmentary retinopathy

Respiratory: Nasal congestion

Drug Interactions

Metabolism/Transport Effects Substrate of CYP1A2 (major)

Avoid Concomitant Use

Avoid concomitant use of Trifluoperazine with any of the following: Metoclopramide

Increased Effect/Toxicity

Trifluoperazine may increase the levels/effects of: Alcohol (Ethyl); Analgesics (Opioid); Anticholinergics; Anti-Parkinson's Agents (Dopamine Agonist); Beta-Blockers; CNS Depressants; Methotrimeprazine

The levels/effects of Trifluoperazine may be increased by: Acetylcholinesterase Inhibitors (Central); Antimalarial Agents; Beta-Blockers; CYP1A2 Inhibitors (Moderate); CYP1A2 Inhibitors (Strong); Lithium formulations; Methotrimeprazine; Metoclopramide; Pramlintide; Tetrabenazine

Decreased Effect

Trifluoperazine may decrease the levels/effects of: Amphetamines; Quinagolide

The levels/effects of Trifluoperazine may be decreased by: Antacids; Anti-Parkinson's Agents (Dopamine Agonist); CYP1A2 Inducers (Strong); Lithium formulations

Food Interactions May cause increase in dietary riboflavin requirements

Stability Store at controlled room temperature at 20°C to 25°C (68°F to 77°F); dispense in tight, light-resistant container

Mechanism of Action Trifluoperazine is a piperazine phenothiazine antipsychotic which is thought to improve psychosis by blocking postsynaptic mesolimbic dopaminergic receptors in the brain; adverse effects are associated with postsynaptic dopaminergic blockade in nigrostriatal and tuberoinfundibular dopaminergic tracts. It depresses the release of hypothalamic and hypophyseal hormones and exhibits alpha-adrenergic blocking effect. Blockade of muscarinic cholinergic receptors is low but may be significant for some patients.

Pharmacodynamics

Onset of action: For control of agitation, aggression, hostility: 2-4 weeks; for control of psychotic symptoms (hallucinations, disorganized thinking or behavior, delusions): Within 1 week

Adequate trial: 6 weeks at moderate to high dose based on tolerability

Duration: Variable

Pharmacokinetics (Adult data unless noted)

Metabolism: Extensively hepatic

Half-life: >24 hours with chronic use

Dialysis: Not dialyzable (0% to 5%)

Usual Dosage Oral:

Schizophrenia/psychoses (**Note:** Dosage should be individualized; use lowest effective dose and shortest effective duration; periodically reassess the need for continued treatment):

Children <6 years: Dosage not established

Children 6-12 years: Hospitalized or well-supervised patients: Initial: 1 mg 1-2 times/day; gradually increase dose until symptoms are controlled or adverse effects have become troublesome; maintenance: 1-15 mg/day in 1-2 divided doses (maximum: 15 mg/day)

Children >12 years:

Inpatient: Initial: 2-5 mg twice daily; gradually increase dose; usual maintenance: 15-20 mg/day in 2 divided doses (maximum: 40 mg/day)

Outpatient: Initial: 1-3 mg twice daily (maximum: 6 mg/day)

Adults:

Inpatient: Initial: 2-5 mg twice daily; gradually increase dose; usual maintenance: 15-20 mg/day in 2 divided doses (maximum dose: 40 mg/day)

Outpatient: Initial: 1-3 mg twice daily (maximum: 40 mg/day); exceptions occur-indication specific)

Nonpsychotic anxiety: Adults: 1-2 mg twice daily; maximum: 6 mg/day; therapy for anxiety should not exceed 12 weeks; do not exceed 6 mg/day for longer than 12 weeks when treating anxiety; agitation, jitteriness, or insomnia may be confused with original neurotic or psychotic symptoms

Administration May be taken with food to decrease GI upset; do not take within 2 hours of any antacids

Monitoring Parameters Vital signs; periodic eye exam, CBC with differential, liver enzyme tests; fasting blood glucose/Hgb A_{1c}; BMI; therapeutic response (mental status, mood, affect, gait), and adverse reactions at beginning of therapy and periodically with long-term use [eg, excess sedation, extrapyramidal symptoms, tardive dyskinesia, CNS changes, abnormal involuntary movement scale (AIMS)]

Test Interactions False-positive for phenylketonuria

Patient Information Use exactly as directed; do not increase dose or frequency. Do not discontinue without consulting prescriber. Avoid alcohol, caffeine, and other prescription or nonprescription medications not approved by prescriber. May cause drowsiness, dizziness, light-headedness, or blurred vision, and impair ability to perform activities requiring mental alertness or physical coordination (use caution driving or when engaging in tasks requiring alertness until response to drug is known). May cause dry mouth. May cause photosensitivity reactions (eg, exposure to sunlight may cause severe sunburn, skin rash, redness, or itching); avoid exposure to sunlight and artificial light sources (sunlamps, tanning booth/bed); wear protective clothing, wide-brimmed hats, sunglasses, and lip sunscreen (SPF ≥15); use a sunscreen (broad-spectrum sunscreen or physical sunscreen [preferred] or sunblock with SPF ≥15); contact physician if reaction occurs.

Maintain adequate hydration unless instructed to restrict fluid intake. May cause nausea or vomiting (small frequent meals, frequent mouth care, chewing gum, or sucking lozenges may help); constipation; postural hypotension (use caution climbing stairs or when changing position from lying or sitting to standing); urinary retention (void before taking medication); or decreased perspiration (avoid strenuous exercise in hot environments). Report persistent CNS effects (eg, trembling fingers, altered gait or balance, excessive sedation, seizures, unusual movements, anxiety, abnormal thoughts, confusion, personality changes); chest pain, palpitations, rapid heartbeat, severe dizziness; unresolved urinary retention or changes in urinary pattern; altered menstrual pattern, changes in libido, swelling or pain in breasts (male or female); vision changes; skin rash, irritation, or changes in color of skin (gray-blue); or worsening of condition.

Nursing Implications Review ophthalmic exam and monitor laboratory results, therapeutic effectiveness (according to rationale for therapy), and adverse reactions at beginning of therapy and periodically with long-term use. Initiate at lower doses and taper dosage slowly when discontinuing.

Additional Information Long-term usefulness of trifluoperazine should be periodically re-evaluated in patients receiving the drug for extended periods; consideration should be given whether to decrease the maintenance dose or discontinue drug therapy

Dosage Forms Excipient information presented when available (limited, particularly for generics); consult specific product labeling.
Tablet: 1 mg, 2 mg, 5 mg, 10 mg

References
"American Academy of Pediatrics Committee on Drugs. The Transfer of Drugs and Other Chemicals Into Human Milk," *Pediatrics*, 2001, 108 (3):776-89.
Miyamoto S, Duncan GE, Marx CE, et al, "Treatments for Schizophrenia: A Critical Review of Pharmacology and Mechanisms of Action of Antipsychotic Drugs," *Mol Psychiatry*, 2005, 10(1):79-104.
Remington G, "Tardive Dyskinesia: Eliminated, Forgotten, or Overshadowed?" *Curr Opin Psychiatry*, 2007, 20(2):131-7.

◆ **Trifluoperazine Hydrochloride** *see* Trifluoperazine *on page 1382*

◆ **Trifluorothymidine** *see* Trifluridine *on page 1384*

Trifluridine (trye FLURE i deen)

Medication Safety Issues
Sound-alike/look-alike issues:
Viroptic® may be confused with Timoptic®
U.S. Brand Names Viroptic®
Canadian Brand Names Sandoz-Trifluridine; Viroptic®
Therapeutic Category Antiviral Agent, Ophthalmic
Generic Available Yes
Use Treatment of primary keratoconjunctivitis and recurrent epithelial keratitis caused by herpes simplex virus types I and II
Pregnancy Risk Factor C
Lactation Excretion in breast milk unknown
Contraindications Hypersensitivity to trifluridine or any component
Adverse Reactions
Cardiovascular: Hyperemia
Local: Burning, stinging
Ocular: Palpebral edema, epithelial keratopathy, keratitis, stromal edema, intraocular pressure elevated
Miscellaneous: Hypersensitivity reactions
Drug Interactions
Avoid Concomitant Use There are no known interactions where it is recommended to avoid concomitant use.
Increased Effect/Toxicity There are no known significant interactions involving an increase in effect.
Decreased Effect There are no known significant interactions involving a decrease in effect.
Stability Store in refrigerator; storage at room temperature may result in a solution with altered pH which could result in ocular discomfort upon administration and/or decreased potency
Mechanism of Action Interferes with viral replication by incorporating into viral DNA in place of thymidine, inhibiting thymidylate synthetase resulting in the formation of defective proteins
Pharmacodynamics Onset of action: Response to treatment occurs within 2-7 days; epithelial healing is complete in 1-2 weeks
Pharmacokinetics (Adult data unless noted) Absorption: Ophthalmic: Systemic absorption is negligible, while corneal penetration is adequate
Usual Dosage Children and Adults: Ophthalmic: Instill 1 drop into affected eye every 2 hours while awake, to a maximum of 9 drops/day, until re-epithelialization of corneal ulcer occurs; then use 1 drop every 4 hours for another 7 days; do **not** exceed 21 days of treatment
Administration Ophthalmic: Avoid contact of bottle tip with skin or eye; instill drops onto the cornea of the affected eye(s); apply finger pressure to lacrimal sac during and for 1-2 minutes after instillation to decrease risk of absorption and systemic effects

Monitoring Parameters Ophthalmologic exam (test for corneal staining with fluorescein or rose Bengal)

Additional Information Found to be effective in 138 of 150 patients unresponsive or intolerant to idoxuridine or vidarabine

Dosage Forms Excipient information presented when available (limited, particularly for generics); consult specific product labeling.
Solution, ophthalmic: 1% (7.5 mL)
Viroptic®: 1% (7.5 mL)

♦ **Triglycerides, Medium Chain** see Medium Chain Triglycerides *on page 870*

♦ **Trihexyphen (Can)** see Trihexyphenidyl *on page 1385*

Trihexyphenidyl (trye heks ee FEN i dil)

Medication Safety Issues
Sound-alike/look-alike issues:
Trihexyphenidyl may be confused with trifluoperazine

Canadian Brand Names PMS-Trihexyphenidyl; Trihexyphen; Trihexyphenidyl

Therapeutic Category Anti-Parkinson's Agent; Anticholinergic Agent; Antidote, Drug-induced Dystonic Reactions

Generic Available Yes

Use Adjunctive treatment of Parkinson's disease; also used in treatment of drug-induced extrapyramidal effects and acute dystonic reactions

Lactation Excretion in breast milk unknown/use caution

Breast-Feeding Considerations Anticholinergic agents may suppress lactation.

Contraindications Hypersensitivity to trihexyphenidyl or any component; children younger than 3 years of age; patients with narrow-angle glaucoma, GI or GU obstruction; myasthenia gravis, achalasia

Precautions Use with caution in patients with hyperthyroidism, renal or hepatic dysfunction, hypertension, hiatal hernia, tachycardia, cardiac arrhythmias, peptic ulcer, esophageal reflux; use with caution in hot weather or during exercise

Adverse Reactions
Cardiovascular: Tachycardia
Central nervous system: Dizziness, nervousness, drowsiness, agitation, delirium, headache
Dermatologic: Rash
Gastrointestinal: Xerostomia, nausea, constipation
Genitourinary: Urinary hesitancy or retention
Neuromuscular & skeletal: Weakness
Ocular: Blurred vision, mydriasis, intraocular tension elevated

Drug Interactions
Avoid Concomitant Use There are no known interactions where it is recommended to avoid concomitant use.

Increased Effect/Toxicity
Trihexyphenidyl may increase the levels/effects of: AbobotulinumtoxinA; Anticholinergics; Cannabinoids; OnabotulinumtoxinA; Potassium Chloride; RimabotulinumtoxinB

The levels/effects of Trihexyphenidyl may be increased by: Pramlintide

Decreased Effect
Trihexyphenidyl may decrease the levels/effects of: Acetylcholinesterase Inhibitors (Central); Secretin

The levels/effects of Trihexyphenidyl may be decreased by: Acetylcholinesterase Inhibitors (Central)

Mechanism of Action Presumed to act by blocking excess acetylcholine at cerebral synapses; many of its effects are due to its pharmacologic similarities with atropine

Pharmacodynamics
Onset of action: 1 hour
Maximum effect: 2-3 hours
Duration: 6-12 hours

Pharmacokinetics (Adult data unless noted)
Metabolism: Metabolic fate undetermined
Bioavailability: 100%
Half-life: 5.6-10.2 hours
Elimination: Some urinary excretion

Usual Dosage Adults: Oral:
Extrapyramidal: 5-15 mg/day in 3-4 divided doses
Parkinsonism: 1 mg daily; increase by 2 mg increments every 3-5 days to 6-10 mg/day (maximum daily dosage: 12-15 mg); doses >10 mg/day should be divided into 3-4 doses

Administration Oral: Administer with food or water to decrease GI irritation

Monitoring Parameters Intraocular pressure monitoring (baseline and at regular intervals)

Patient Information May cause drowsiness and impair ability to perform activities requiring mental alertness or physical coordination; may cause dry mouth

Dosage Forms Excipient information presented when available (limited, particularly for generics); consult specific product labeling.
Elixir, as hydrochloride: 2 mg/5 mL (480 mL)
Tablet, as hydrochloride: 2 mg, 5 mg

♦ **Trihexyphenidyl Hydrochloride** see Trihexyphenidyl *on page 1385*

♦ **TriHIBit®** see Diphtheria, Tetanus Toxoids, and Acellular Pertussis Vaccine and *Haemophilus influenzae* b Conjugate Vaccine *on page 460*

♦ **Trikacide (Can)** see MetroNIDAZOLE *on page 921*

♦ **Trilafon** see Perphenazine *on page 1094*

♦ **Trileptal®** see OXcarbazepine *on page 1035*

♦ **Trilisate** see Choline Magnesium Trisalicylate *on page 304*

♦ **TriLyte®** see Polyethylene Glycol-Electrolyte Solution *on page 1129*

Trimethobenzamide (trye meth oh BEN za mide)

Medication Safety Issues
Sound-alike/look-alike issues:
Tigan® may be confused with Tiazac®, Ticar®, Ticlid®
Trimethobenzamide may be confused with metoclopramide, trimethoprim

Beers Criteria medication: This drug may be inappropriate for use in geriatric patients (high severity risk).

Related Information
Compatibility of Medications Mixed in a Syringe *on page 1713*

U.S. Brand Names Tigan®

Canadian Brand Names Tigan®

Therapeutic Category Antiemetic

Generic Available Yes

Use Treatment of postoperative nausea and vomiting; treatment of nausea and vomiting associated with gastroenteritis

Pregnancy Considerations Teratogenic effects were not observed in animal studies. Safety and efficacy have not been established in pregnant patients. Trimethobenzamide has been used to treat nausea and vomiting of pregnancy.

Lactation Excretion in breast milk unknown

Contraindications Hypersensitivity to trimethobenzamide or any component; injection is contraindicated in children

Warnings Use cautiously in infants and children; antiemetics are not recommended for uncomplicated vomiting in children; limit antiemetic use to prolonged vomiting of known etiology; may mask emesis due to Reye's syndrome, may mimic CNS effects of Reye's syndrome in patients with emesis of other etiologies, and may cause extrapyramidal symptoms (EPS) which may be confused with CNS symptoms of primary disease responsible for emesis. May produce drowsiness and concomitant use with alcohol may result in an adverse interaction.

Precautions Risk of adverse effects (eg, EPS, seizure) may be increased in patients with acute febrile illness, dehydration, electrolyte imbalance, encephalitides, or gastroenteritis; use with caution. Allergic-type skin reactions have been reported with use; discontinue with signs of sensitization. Trimethobenzamide clearance is predominantly renal; consider dosage reductions in patients with renal impairment.

Adverse Reactions

Cardiovascular: Hypotension (especially after I.M. use)

Central nervous system: Coma, disorientation, dizziness, depression, drowsiness, EPS, headache, opisthotonos, Parkinson-like symptoms, sedation, seizure

Dermatologic: Hypersensitivity (allergic-type) skin reactions

Gastrointestinal: Diarrhea

Hematologic: Blood dyscrasias

Hepatic: Jaundice

Local: Burning, pain, redness, swelling, stinging at I.M. injection site

Neuromuscular & skeletal: Muscle cramps

Ocular: Blurred vision

Miscellaneous: Hypersensitivity reactions

Drug Interactions

Avoid Concomitant Use There are no known interactions where it is recommended to avoid concomitant use.

Increased Effect/Toxicity

Trimethobenzamide may increase the levels/effects of: AbobotulinumtoxinA; Anticholinergics; Cannabinoids; OnabotulinumtoxinA; Potassium Chloride; RimabotulinumtoxinB

The levels/effects of Trimethobenzamide may be increased by: Pramlintide

Decreased Effect

Trimethobenzamide may decrease the levels/effects of: Acetylcholinesterase Inhibitors (Central); Secretin

The levels/effects of Trimethobenzamide may be decreased by: Acetylcholinesterase Inhibitors (Central)

Stability Store at room temperature.

Mechanism of Action Acts centrally to inhibit stimulation of the medullary chemoreceptor trigger zone

Pharmacodynamics

Onset of action:

Oral: 10-40 minutes

I.M.: 15-35 minutes

Duration:

Oral: 3-4 hours

I.M.: 2-3 hours

Pharmacokinetics (Adult data unless noted)

Metabolism: Via oxidation, forms metabolite trimethobenzamide N-oxide

Bioavailability: Oral dose is 100% of I.M. dose

Half-life: Adults: 7-9 hours

Time to peak serum concentration:

Oral: 45 minutes

I.M.: 30 minutes

Elimination: 30% to 50% excreted unchanged in urine in 24 hours

Usual Dosage

Children:

Oral: 15-20 mg/kg/day (400-500 mg/m^2/day) divided into 3-4 doses; **or as an alternative**

<13.6 kg: 100 mg 3-4 times/day

13.6-40 kg: 100-200 mg 3-4 times/day

>40 kg: 300 mg 3-4 times/day

I.M.: Not recommended

Adults:

Oral: 300 mg 3-4 times/day

I.M.: 200 mg 3-4 times/day

Postoperative nausea and vomiting (PONV): I.M.: 200 mg, followed 1 hour later by a second 200 mg dose

Dosage adjustment in renal impairment: Cl$_{cr}$ ≤70 mL/minute: Consider dosage reduction or increasing dosing interval (specific adjustment guidelines are not provided in the manufacturer's labeling)

Administration

Oral: May administer without regard to food

Parenteral: I.M. use only by deep injection into upper outer quadrant of gluteal region; **not** for I.V. use

Patient Information May cause drowsiness and impair ability to perform activities requiring mental alertness or physical coordination

Additional Information Note: Less effective than phenothiazines but may be associated with fewer side effects

Dosage Forms Excipient information presented when available (limited, particularly for generics); consult specific product labeling.

Capsule, as hydrochloride: 300 mg

Tigan®: 300 mg

Injection, solution, as hydrochloride: 100 mg/mL (2 mL)

Tigan®: 100 mg/mL (20 mL)

Injection, solution, as hydrochloride [preservative free]:

Tigan®: 100 mg/mL (2 mL)

References

Leung AK and Robson WL, "Acute Gastroenteritis in Children: Role of Anti-Emetic Medication for Gastroenteritis-Related Vomiting," *Paediatr Drugs*, 2007, 9(3):175-84.

♦ **Trimethobenzamide Hydrochloride** *see* Trimethobenzamide *on page 1385*

Trimethoprim (trye METH oh prim)

Medication Safety Issues

Sound-alike/look-alike issues:

Trimethoprim may be confused with trimethaphan

Related Information

Therapeutic Drug Monitoring: Blood Sampling Time Guidelines *on page 1704*

U.S. Brand Names Primsol®

Canadian Brand Names Apo-Trimethoprim®

Therapeutic Category Antibiotic, Miscellaneous

Generic Available Yes: Tablet

Use Treatment of urinary tract infections caused by susceptible *Escherichia coli*, *Proteus mirabilis*, *Klebsiella pneumoniae*, *Enterobacter* species, and coagulase-negative *Staphylococcus* (including *S. saprophyticus*); prophylaxis of urinary tract infections; in combination with other agents for treatment of *Pneumocystis jiroveci* pneumonia; treatment of otitis media caused by susceptible *Streptococcus pneumoniae* and *Haemophilus influenzae* (not indicated for *Moraxella catarrhalis* due to consistent resistance); not indicated for prolonged administration or prophylaxis of otitis media

Pregnancy Risk Factor C

Pregnancy Considerations Because adverse effects have been observed in animals, trimethoprim is classified pregnancy category C. Trimethoprim crosses the placenta and can be detected in the fetal serum and amniotic fluid. Due to trimethoprim's potential effect on folic acid metabolism, TMP should only be used during pregnancy if the benefit justifies the potential risk. The use of dihydrofolate reductase inhibitors, including trimethoprim, during pregnancy may increase the risk of congenital anomalies including cardiovascular defects, oral clefts, urinary tract anomalies, and neural tube defects. Folic acid supplementation may decrease this risk. The majority of studies evaluating the effects of trimethoprim administration in pregnancy have been conducted with sulfamethoxazole/trimethoprim. Trimethoprim in combination with sulfamethoxazole is used in pregnancy for various indications (see the sulfamethoxazole/trimethoprim monograph for details).

Lactation Enters breast milk/use caution

Breast-Feeding Considerations Trimethoprim is excreted in breast milk. The manufacturer recommends caution while using trimethoprim in a breast-feeding woman because trimethoprim may interfere with folic acid metabolism. The American Academy of Pediatrics considers trimethoprim in combination with sulfisoxazole to be "usually compatible with breast-feeding." Nondose-related effects could include modification of bowel flora. Also see the sulfamethoxazole/trimethoprim monograph for additional information.

Contraindications Hypersensitivity to trimethoprim or any component; megaloblastic anemia due to folate deficiency

Warnings May cause folate deficiencies with subsequent bone marrow suppression and blood dyscrasias; monitor patients for fever, sore throat, purpura, or pallor; discontinue trimethoprim if bone marrow depression occurs; leucovorin calcium may be needed to restore normal hematopoiesis

Oral solution contains propylene glycol and sodium benzoate; benzoic acid (benzoate) is a metabolite of benzyl alcohol; large amounts of benzyl alcohol (≥99 mg/kg/day) have been associated with a potentially fatal toxicity ("gasping syndrome") in neonates; the "gasping syndrome" consists of metabolic acidosis, respiratory distress, gasping respirations, CNS dysfunction (including convulsions, intracranial hemorrhage), hypotension and cardiovascular collapse; avoid use of trimethoprim products containing sodium benzoate in neonates; *in vitro* and animal studies have shown that benzoate displaces bilirubin from protein binding sites

Precautions Use with caution in patients with impaired renal or hepatic function or with possible folate deficiency; decrease dose in patients with renal dysfunction; safety is not established in infants <2 months of age; effectiveness for treatment of acute otitis media is not established in infants <6 months of age

Adverse Reactions

Central nervous system: Fever, headache, aseptic meningitis (rare)

Dermatologic: Rash, pruritus, phototoxic skin eruptions, exfoliative dermatitis (rare), erythema multiforme (rare), Stevens-Johnson syndrome (rare), toxic epidermal necrolysis (rare)

Endocrine & metabolic: Hyperkalemia, hyponatremia

Hematologic: Megaloblastic anemia, neutropenia, leukopenia, thrombocytopenia, methemoglobinemia

Hepatic: Liver enzymes elevated, cholestatic jaundice

Gastrointestinal: Nausea, vomiting, epigastric distress, glossitis

Renal: Elevated BUN and serum creatinine

Miscellaneous: Anaphylaxis, hypersensitivity reactions

Drug Interactions

Metabolism/Transport Effects Substrate (major) of CYP2C9, 3A4; **Inhibits** CYP2C8 (moderate), 2C9 (moderate)

Avoid Concomitant Use

Avoid concomitant use of Trimethoprim with any of the following: BCG; Dofetilide

Increased Effect/Toxicity

Trimethoprim may increase the levels/effects of: ACE Inhibitors; Amantadine; Angiotensin II Receptor Blockers; Antidiabetic Agents (Thiazolidinedione); AzaTHIOprine; Carvedilol; CYP2C8 Substrates (High risk); CYP2C9 Substrates (High risk); Dapsone; Dapsone (Systemic); Dapsone (Topical); Dofetilide; LamiVUDine; Memantine; Methotrexate; Phenytoin; Pralatrexate; Procainamide; Repaglinide

The levels/effects of Trimethoprim may be increased by: Amantadine; CYP2C9 Inhibitors (Moderate); CYP2C9 Inhibitors (Strong); Dapsone; Dapsone (Systemic); Memantine

Decreased Effect

Trimethoprim may decrease the levels/effects of: BCG; Typhoid Vaccine

The levels/effects of Trimethoprim may be decreased by: CYP2C9 Inducers (Highly Effective); CYP3A4 Inducers (Strong); Deferasirox; Herbs (CYP3A4 Inducers); Leucovorin Calcium-Levoleucovorin; Peginterferon Alfa-2b

Food Interactions May cause folic acid deficiency, supplements may be needed

Stability Store tablets and solution at 15°C to 25°C (59°F to 77°F); protect from light

Mechanism of Action Binds to the enzyme dihydrofolate reductase in bacteria and inhibits conversion of dihydrofolic acid to tetrahydrofolate (functional form of folic acid). This results in depletion of folic acid, interference with bacterial biosynthesis of nucleic acids and protein production, and inhibition of microbial growth.

Pharmacokinetics (Adult data unless noted)

Absorption: Oral: Readily and extensively absorbed (90% to 100%)

Distribution: Penetrates into middle ear fluid with a mean peak middle ear fluid concentration in children 1-12 years of 2 mcg/mL after a single 4 mg/kg dose; crosses the placenta; excreted in breast milk

V_d:

Newborns: ~2.7 L/kg

Infants: 1.5 L/kg

Children 1-10 years: ~1 L/kg

Adults: 1.3-1.8 L/kg

Protein binding: 42% to 46%

Metabolism: Partially (10% to 20%) metabolized in the liver via demethylation, oxidation, and hydroxylation

Bioavailability: Similar for tablets and solution

Half-life (prolonged in renal dysfunction):

Newborns: ~19 hours

Infants 2 months to 1 year: 3-6 hours; mean: 4.6 hours

Children 1-10 years: 3-5.5 hours

Adults, normal renal function: 8-11 hours

Adults, anuric: 20-50 hours

Time to peak serum concentration: Within 1-4 hours

Elimination: Significantly excreted in urine (60% to 80%) as unchanged drug via glomerular filtration and tubular secretion; increased renal excretion with acidic urine

Dialysis: Moderately dialyzable (20% to 50%)

Usual Dosage Oral:

Infants ≥6 months and Children: Acute otitis media: 10 mg/kg/day in divided doses every 12 hours for 10 days

Infants and Children <12 years: Urinary tract infection: Treatment: 4-6 mg/kg/day in divided doses every 12 hours for 10 days

Children ≥12 years and Adults:

Urinary tract infection: Treatment: 100 mg every 12 hours or 200 mg every 24 hours for 10 days

Prophylaxis: 100 mg once daily

Pneumocystis jiroveci pneumonia treatment (given with dapsone): 15-20 mg/kg/day in 4 divided doses for 21 days

Dosing adjustment in renal impairment:

Cl_{cr} 15-30 mL/minute: Administer 50% of normal dose

Cl_{cr} <15 mL/minute: Avoid use

Administration Oral: Administer on an empty stomach; may administer with milk or food if GI upset occurs

Monitoring Parameters CBC with differential, platelet count, liver enzyme tests, bilirubin, serum creatinine and BUN

Reference Range Therapeutic:
Peak: 5-15 mg/L
Trough: 2-8 mg/L

Test Interactions May falsely increase creatinine determination measured by the Jaffé alkaline picrate assay; may interfere with determination of serum methotrexate when measured by methods that use a bacterial dihydrofolate reductase as the binding protein (eg, the competitive binding protein technique); does **not** interfere with RIA for methotrexate

Patient Information Report any skin rash, persistent or severe fatigue, fever, sore throat, or unusual bleeding or bruising; complete full course of therapy

Additional Information Not effective versus *Pseudomonas* or *B. fragilis*; discontinue if bone marrow suppression occurs

Dosage Forms Excipient information presented when available (limited, particularly for generics); consult specific product labeling.
Solution, oral:
Primsol®: 50 mg (base)/5 mL (473 mL) [dye free, ethanol free; contains propylene glycol, sodium benzoate; bubble gum flavor]
Tablet: 100 mg

References
Hoppu K, "Age Differences in Trimethoprim Pharmacokinetics: Need for Revised Dosing in Children?" *Clin Pharmacol Ther*, 1987, 41 (3):336-43.
Hoppu K, Koskimies O, and Vilska J, "Trimethoprim in the Treatment of Acute Urinary Tract Infections in Children," *Int J Clin Pharmacol Ther Toxicol*, 1988, 26(2):65-8.
Leff RD, Cho CT, and Reed MD, "Safety and Efficacy of Trimethoprim Hydrochloride Solution for the Treatment of Children With Otitis Media," *Journal of Pediatric Pharmacy Practice*, 1998, 3(1): 33-9.

◆ **Trimethoprim and Sulfamethoxazole** *see* Sulfamethoxazole and Trimethoprim *on page 1302*

◆ **Trinasal® (Can)** *see* Triamcinolone *on page 1376*

◆ **Trinipatch® 0.2 (Can)** *see* Nitroglycerin *on page 996*

◆ **Trinipatch® 0.4 (Can)** *see* Nitroglycerin *on page 996*

◆ **Trinipatch® 0.6 (Can)** *see* Nitroglycerin *on page 996*

◆ **Triostat®** *see* Liothyronine *on page 828*

◆ **Tripedia®** *see* Diphtheria, Tetanus Toxoids, and Acellular Pertussis Vaccine *on page 458*

◆ **Triple Antibiotic** *see* Bacitracin, Neomycin, and Polymyxin B *on page 170*

◆ **Tripohist™ D** *see* Triprolidine and Pseudoephedrine *on page 1388*

Triprolidine and Pseudoephedrine
(trye PROE li deen & soo doe e FED rin)

Medication Safety Issues
Sound-alike/look-alike issues:
Aprodine® may be confused with Aphrodyne®

U.S. Brand Names Allerfrim [OTC]; Aprodine [OTC]; Genac™ [OTC]; Pediatex® TD; Silafed [OTC]; Tripohist™ D

Canadian Brand Names Actifed®

Therapeutic Category Antihistamine/Decongestant Combination; Sympathomimetic

Generic Available Yes

Use Temporary relief of nasal congestion, running nose, sneezing, itching of nose or throat and itchy, watery eyes due to common cold, hay fever or other upper respiratory allergies (FDA approved in ages ≥6 years and adults)

Pregnancy Risk Factor C

Contraindications Hypersensitivity to triprolidine, pseudoephedrine, or any component; severe hypertension or coronary artery disease; MAO inhibitor therapy, GI or GU obstruction, narrow-angle glaucoma

Warnings Safety and efficacy for the use of cough and cold products in children <4 years of age is limited. Serious adverse effects including death have been reported (in some cases, high blood concentrations of pseudoephedrine were found). The FDA notes that there are no approved OTC uses for these products in children <4 years of age. Healthcare providers are reminded to ask caregivers about the use of OTC cough and cold products in order to avoid exposure to multiple medications containing the same ingredient.

Precautions Use with caution in patients with mild to moderate high blood pressure, heart disease, diabetes mellitus, asthma, thyroid disease, or prostatic hypertrophy

Adverse Reactions
Cardiovascular: Hypertension, tachycardia
Central nervous system: CNS stimulation, headache, sedation
Gastrointestinal: Anorexia, nausea, vomiting, xerostomia

Drug Interactions
Metabolism/Transport Effects Triprolidine: **Inhibits** CYP2D6 (weak)

Avoid Concomitant Use
Avoid concomitant use of Triprolidine and Pseudoephedrine with any of the following: Iobenguane I 123; MAO Inhibitors

Increased Effect/Toxicity
Triprolidine and Pseudoephedrine may increase the levels/effects of: Alcohol (Ethyl); Anticholinergics; Bromocriptine; CNS Depressants; Sympathomimetics

The levels/effects of Triprolidine and Pseudoephedrine may be increased by: Antacids; Atomoxetine; Cannabinoids; Carbonic Anhydrase Inhibitors; MAO Inhibitors; Pramlintide; Serotonin/Norepinephrine Reuptake Inhibitors

Decreased Effect
Triprolidine and Pseudoephedrine may decrease the levels/effects of: Acetylcholinesterase Inhibitors (Central); Betahistine; Iobenguane I 123

The levels/effects of Triprolidine and Pseudoephedrine may be decreased by: Acetylcholinesterase Inhibitors (Central); Amphetamines; Spironolactone

Usual Dosage Oral:
≥2 years: May dose according to **pseudoephedrine** component: 4 mg/kg/day in divided doses 3-4 times/day not to exceed a maximum of 60 mg pseudoephedrine per dose
Liquid:
Children 6-12 years: Pediatex® TD: 1.33 mL every 6 hours (maximum: 4 doses/24 hours); Tripohist™ D: 2.5-5 mL every 4-6 hours (maximum pseudoephedrine: 120 mg/24 hours)
Children ≥12 years and Adults: Pediatex® TD: 2.67 mL every 6 hours (maximum: 4 doses/24 hours); Tripohist™ D: 5-10 mL every 4-6 hours (maximum pseudoephedrine: 240 mg/24 hours)
Syrup (Allerfrim, Aprodine):
Children 6-12 years: 5 mL every 4-6 hours; do not exceed 4 doses in 24 hours
Children >12 years and Adults: 10 mL every 4-6 hours; do not exceed 4 doses in 24 hours
Tablet (Aprodine):
Children 6-12 years: 1/2 tablet every 4-6 hours; do not exceed 4 doses in 24 hours
Children >12 years and Adults: One tablet every 4-6 hours; do not exceed 4 doses in 24 hours

Administration Oral: Administer with food or milk to decrease GI irritation

Patient Information May cause drowsiness and impair ability to perform activities requiring mental alertness or physical coordination; may cause dry mouth

Dosage Forms Excipient information presented when available (limited, particularly for generics); consult specific product labeling. [DSC] = Discontinued product

Liquid, oral:

Pediatex® TD: Triprolidine hydrochloride 0.938 mg and pseudoephedrine hydrochloride 10 mg per 1 mL (30 mL) [cotton candy flavor]

Tripohist™ D: Triprolidine hydrochloride 1.25 mg and pseudoephedrine hydrochloride 45 mg per 5 mL (473 mL) [ethanol free, sugar free; contains sodium benzoate; blueberry flavor]

Syrup, oral: Triprolidine hydrochloride 1.25 mg and pseudoephedrine hydrochloride 30 mg per 5 mL (120 mL) [DSC]

Allerfrim: Triprolidine hydrochloride 1.25 mg and pseudoephedrine hydrochloride 30 mg per 5 mL (118 mL, 473 mL) [contains sodium benzoate]

Aprodine: Triprolidine hydrochloride 1.25 mg and pseudoephedrine hydrochloride 30 mg per 5 mL (120 mL)

Silafed: Triprolidine hydrochloride 1.25 mg and pseudoephedrine hydrochloride 30 mg per 5 mL (120 mL, 240 mL)

Tablet, oral:

Allerfrim, Aprodine, Genac™: Triprolidine hydrochloride 2.5 mg and pseudoephedrine hydrochloride 60 mg

◆ **TripTone® [OTC]** see DimenhyDRINATE on page 446

◆ **Tris Buffer** see Tromethamine on page 1389

◆ **Tris(hydroxymethyl)aminomethane** see Tromethamine on page 1389

◆ **Trivagizole-3® (Can)** see Clotrimazole on page 344

◆ **Trivalent Inactivated Influenza Vaccine (TIV)** see Influenza Virus Vaccine (H1N1, Inactivated) on page 731

◆ **Trivalent Inactivated Influenza Vaccine (TIV)** see Influenza Virus Vaccine (Inactivated) on page 734

◆ **Trizivir®** see Abacavir, Lamivudine, and Zidovudine on page 31

◆ **Trocaine® [OTC]** see Benzocaine on page 182

◆ **Trocal® [OTC]** see Dextromethorphan on page 421

Tromethamine (troe METH a meen)

Medication Safety Issues
Sound-alike/look-alike issues:
Tromethamine may be confused with TrophAmine®

U.S. Brand Names THAM®

Therapeutic Category Alkalinizing Agent, Parenteral

Generic Available No

Use Correction of metabolic acidosis associated with cardiac bypass surgery or cardiac arrest; to correct excess acidity of stored blood that is preserved with acid citrate dextrose (ACD); to prime the pump-oxygenator during cardiac bypass surgery; indicated in severe metabolic acidosis in patients in whom sodium or carbon dioxide elimination is restricted [eg, infants needing alkalinization after receiving maximum sodium bicarbonate (8-10 mEq/kg/24 hours)]

Pregnancy Risk Factor C

Pregnancy Considerations Animal studies have not been conducted. There are no adequate and well-controlled studies in pregnant women. Use only if potential benefit outweighs possible risk to the fetus.

Lactation Excretion in breast milk unknown/use caution

Contraindications Hypersensitivity to tromethamine or any component; uremia or anuria; chronic respiratory acidosis (neonates); salicylate intoxication (neonates)

Warnings Avoid infusion via low-lying umbilical venous catheters due to associated risk of hepatocellular necrosis; severe local tissue necrosis and sloughing may occur if solution extravasates; administer via central line or large vein slowly. Due to tromethamine's greater osmotic effects, use of sodium bicarbonate for the treatment of acidotic neonates and infants with RDS may be preferred; rapid I.V. infusion and overdosage may cause prolonged hypoglycemia. Monitor pH carefully as large doses may increase blood pH greater than normal which may result in depressed respiration.

Precautions Reduce dose and monitor pH and serum potassium carefully in renal impairment.

Adverse Reactions

Cardiovascular: Venospasm

Central nervous system: Fever

Endocrine & metabolic: Hyperosmolality of serum, hyperkalemia, hypoglycemia (rapid administration and use in neonates)

Hepatic: Liver cell destruction from direct contact with tromethamine, hemorrhagic hepatic necrosis (when administered through umbilical vein at concentrations ≥1.2 M)

Local: Tissue irritation, necrosis with extravasation

Respiratory: Respiratory depression, apnea

Drug Interactions

Avoid Concomitant Use There are no known interactions where it is recommended to avoid concomitant use.

Increased Effect/Toxicity

Tromethamine may increase the levels/effects of: Amphetamines; Flecainide; QuiNINE

Decreased Effect There are no known significant interactions involving a decrease in effect.

Stability Store at room temperature; protect from freezing

Mechanism of Action Acts as a proton acceptor, which combines with hydrogen ions to form bicarbonate and buffer to correct acidosis; buffers both metabolic and respiratory acids, limiting carbon dioxide generation; also acts as an osmotic diuretic

Pharmacokinetics (Adult data unless noted) 30% of dose is not ionized; rapidly eliminated by kidneys

Usual Dosage I.V.: Dose depends on severity and progression of acidosis:

Neonates: Manufacturer's recommendation: 1 mL/kg for each pH unit below 7.4; additional doses to be determined by changes in PaO_2, pH, and pCO_2

Infants, Children, and Adults:

Empiric dosage based upon base deficit: Tromethamine mL of 0.3 M solution = body weight (kg) x base deficit (mEq/L) x 1.1*; maximum: 500 mg/kg/dose = 13.9 mL/kg/dose using 0.3 M solution

*Factor of 1.1 accounts for an approximate reduction of 10% in buffering capacity due to the presence of sufficient acetic acid to lower the pH of the 0.3 M solution to approximately 8.6

Metabolic acidosis with cardiac arrest: Tromethamine mL of 0.3 M solution: 3.5-6 mL/kg/dose (126-216 mg/kg/dose); maximum: 500 mg/kg/dose = 13.9 mL/kg/dose

Metabolic acidosis with cardiac arrest: Direct instillation to ventricle: Adults: Tromethamine 0.3 M solution: 2-6 g (62-185 mL); do not inject into cardiac muscle

Excess acidity of acid citrate dextrose priming blood: Tromethamine mL of 0.3 M solution: 15-77 mL added to each 500 mL of ACD blood used for priming the pump-oxygenator

Acidosis during cardiac bypass surgery: Tromethamine mL of 0.3 M solution: 9 mL/kg (324 mg/kg/dose); maximum: 1000 mL (36 g) as single dose in severe cases and not to exceed 500 mg/kg over a period of 1 hour (eg, for 70 kg patient, not to exceed 35 g/hour)

◀ **Administration** Parenteral: Maximum concentration: 0.3 molar; infuse slowly over at least 1 hour or 3-16 mL/kg/hour up to 33-40 mL/kg/day; administer into a central venous line and avoid administration into low-lying umbilical venous lines

Monitoring Parameters Serum electrolytes, arterial blood gases, serum pH, blood sugar, ECG monitoring, renal function tests

Additional Information 1 mM = 120 mg = 3.3 mL = 1 mEq of THAM®

Dosage Forms Excipient information presented when available (limited, particularly for generics); consult specific product labeling.

Injection, solution:
   THAM®: 18 g [0.3 molar] (500 mL)

♦ **Tronolane® Suppository [OTC]** *see* Phenylephrine *on page 1102*

♦ **Tropicacyl®** *see* Tropicamide *on page 1390*

Tropicamide (troe PIK a mide)

U.S. Brand Names Mydral™; Mydriacyl®; Tropicacyl®
Canadian Brand Names Diotrope®; Mydriacyl®
Therapeutic Category Ophthalmic Agent, Mydriatic
Generic Available Yes
Use Short-acting mydriatic used in diagnostic procedures; as well as preoperatively and postoperatively; treatment of some cases of acute iritis, iridocyclitis, and keratitis
Pregnancy Risk Factor C
Contraindications Hypersensitivity to tropicamide or any component; glaucoma, adhesions between the iris and the lens
Warnings Tropicamide may cause an increase in intraocular pressure
Precautions Use with caution in infants and children since tropicamide may cause potentially dangerous CNS disturbances and psychotic reactions

Adverse Reactions
Cardiovascular: Tachycardia, flushing
Central nervous system: Parasympathetic stimulation, drowsiness, headache, behavioral disturbances, psychotic reactions
Gastrointestinal: Xerostomia
Local: Transient stinging
Ocular: Blurred vision, photophobia, intraocular pressure elevated, follicular conjunctivitis
Miscellaneous: Allergic reactions

Drug Interactions
Avoid Concomitant Use There are no known interactions where it is recommended to avoid concomitant use.
Increased Effect/Toxicity There are no known significant interactions involving an increase in effect.
Decreased Effect There are no known significant interactions involving a decrease in effect.

Stability Store at room temperature; do not refrigerate
Mechanism of Action Prevents the sphincter muscle of the iris and the muscle of the ciliary body from responding to cholinergic stimulation producing pupillary dilation and paralysis of accommodation

Pharmacodynamics
Maximum mydriatic effect: ~20-40 minutes
   Duration: ~6-7 hours
Maximum cycloplegic effect:
   Peak: 20-35 minutes
   Duration: <6 hours

Usual Dosage Children and Adults: Ophthalmic:
Cycloplegia: Instill 1-2 drops (1%); may repeat in 5 minutes. The exam must be performed within 30 minutes after the repeat dose; if the patient is not examined within 20-30 minutes, instill an additional drop. Concentrations

<1% are inadequate for producing satisfactory cycloplegia.
Mydriasis: Instill 1-2 drops (0.5%) 15-20 minutes before exam; may repeat every 30 minutes as needed

Administration Ophthalmic: To minimize systemic absorption, apply finger pressure on the lacrimal sac for 1-2 minutes following instillation of the ophthalmic solution; avoid contact of bottle tip with skin or eye

Patient Information May cause blurred vision; do not drive or engage in hazardous activities while the pupils are dilated; may cause sensitivity to light; may cause dry mouth

Dosage Forms Excipient information presented when available (limited, particularly for generics); consult specific product labeling.

Solution, ophthalmic [drops]: 0.5% (15 mL); 1% (2 mL, 3 mL, 15 mL)
   Mydriacyl®: 1% (3 mL, 15 mL) [contains benzalkonium chloride]
   Mydral™, Tropicacyl®: 0.5% (15 mL); 1% (15 mL) [contains benzalkonium chloride]

References
Caputo AR and Schnitzer RE, "Systemic Response to Mydriatic Eyedrops in Neonates: Mydriatics in Neonates," *J Pediatr Ophthalmol Strabismus*, 1978, 15(2):109-22.

♦ **Trusopt®** *see* Dorzolamide *on page 473*

♦ **Truvada®** *see* Emtricitabine and Tenofovir *on page 498*

♦ **TSPA** *see* Thiotepa *on page 1342*

♦ **Tucks® Anti-Itch [OTC]** *see* Hydrocortisone *on page 685*

♦ **Tums® [OTC]** *see* Calcium Carbonate *on page 232*

♦ **Tums® [OTC]** *see* Calcium Supplements *on page 239*

♦ **Tums® E-X [OTC]** *see* Calcium Carbonate *on page 232*

♦ **Tums® E-X [OTC]** *see* Calcium Supplements *on page 239*

♦ **Tums® Extra Strength Sugar Free [OTC]** *see* Calcium Carbonate *on page 232*

♦ **Tums® Extra Strength Sugar Free [OTC]** *see* Calcium Supplements *on page 239*

♦ **Tums® Smoothies™ [OTC]** *see* Calcium Carbonate *on page 232*

♦ **Tums® Smoothies™ [OTC]** *see* Calcium Supplements *on page 239*

♦ **Tums® Ultra [OTC]** *see* Calcium Carbonate *on page 232*

♦ **Tums® Ultra® [OTC]** *see* Calcium Supplements *on page 239*

♦ **Tussi-Bid®** *see* Guaifenesin and Dextromethorphan *on page 658*

♦ **Tussi-Organidin® DM NR [DSC]** *see* Guaifenesin and Dextromethorphan *on page 658*

♦ **Tussi-Organidin® DM-S NR [DSC]** *see* Guaifenesin and Dextromethorphan *on page 658*

♦ **Tussi-Organidin® NR [DSC]** *see* Guaifenesin and Codeine *on page 657*

♦ **Tussi-Organidin® S-NR [DSC]** *see* Guaifenesin and Codeine *on page 657*

♦ **Tusso-C™** *see* Guaifenesin and Codeine *on page 657*

♦ **Twelve Resin-K [OTC]** *see* Cyanocobalamin *on page 365*

♦ **Twilite® [OTC]** *see* DiphenhydrAMINE *on page 448*

♦ **Twinject®** *see* EPINEPHrine *on page 511*

♦ **Ty21a Vaccine** *see* Typhoid Vaccine *on page 1391*

♦ **Tycolene [OTC] [DSC]** *see* Acetaminophen *on page 36*

♦ **Tycolene Maximum Strength [OTC]** *see* Acetaminophen *on page 36*

◆ **Tygacil®** *see* Tigecycline *on page 1350*

◆ **Tylenol® [OTC]** *see* Acetaminophen *on page 36*

◆ **Tylenol® (Can)** *see* Acetaminophen *on page 36*

◆ **Tylenol #2** *see* Acetaminophen and Codeine *on page 39*

◆ **Tylenol #3** *see* Acetaminophen and Codeine *on page 39*

◆ **Tylenol® 8 Hour [OTC]** *see* Acetaminophen *on page 36*

◆ **Tylenol® Arthritis Pain Extended Relief [OTC]** *see* Acetaminophen *on page 36*

◆ **Tylenol® Children's [OTC]** *see* Acetaminophen *on page 36*

◆ **Tylenol® Children's Meltaways [OTC]** *see* Acetaminophen *on page 36*

◆ **Tylenol Elixir with Codeine (Can)** *see* Acetaminophen and Codeine *on page 39*

◆ **Tylenol® Extra Strength [OTC]** *see* Acetaminophen *on page 36*

◆ **Tylenol® Infant's Concentrated [OTC]** *see* Acetaminophen *on page 36*

◆ **Tylenol® Jr. Meltaways [OTC]** *see* Acetaminophen *on page 36*

◆ **Tylenol No. 1 (Can)** *see* Acetaminophen and Codeine *on page 39*

◆ **Tylenol No. 1 Forte (Can)** *see* Acetaminophen and Codeine *on page 39*

◆ **Tylenol No. 2 with Codeine (Can)** *see* Acetaminophen and Codeine *on page 39*

◆ **Tylenol No. 3 with Codeine (Can)** *see* Acetaminophen and Codeine *on page 39*

◆ **Tylenol No. 4 with Codeine (Can)** *see* Acetaminophen and Codeine *on page 39*

◆ **Tylenol® with Codeine No. 3** *see* Acetaminophen and Codeine *on page 39*

◆ **Tylenol® with Codeine No. 4** *see* Acetaminophen and Codeine *on page 39*

◆ **Tylox®** *see* Oxycodone and Acetaminophen *on page 1041*

◆ **Typherix® (Can)** *see* Typhoid Vaccine *on page 1391*

◆ **Typhim Vi®** *see* Typhoid Vaccine *on page 1391*

Typhoid Vaccine (TYE foid vak SEEN)

Related Information
Immunization Guidelines *on page 1636*
U.S. Brand Names Typhim Vi®; Vivotif®
Canadian Brand Names Typherix®; Typhim Vi®; Vivotif®
Therapeutic Category Vaccine
Generic Available No
Use Immunization to prevent disease from exposure to *Salmonella typhi*; use is not routinely recommended in the U.S. but is reserved for selected individuals who are either traveling to an area in which there is a recognized risk of exposure to *S. typhi*, who have intimate exposure (eg, household contact) to a *S. typhi* carrier, or who work frequently with *S. typhi* in laboratory settings
Parenteral: Typhim Vi®: Approved for use in children ≥2 years and adults
Oral: Live attenuated Ty21a vaccine (Vivotif Berna®): Approved for use in children ≥6 years and adults
Pregnancy Risk Factor C
Pregnancy Considerations Reproduction studies have not been conducted. The manufacturer of the Typhim Vi® injection suggests delaying vaccination until the 2nd or 3rd trimester if possible. Untreated typhoid fever may lead to miscarriage or vertical intrauterine transmission causing neonatal typhoid (rare).
Lactation Excretion in breast milk unknown/use caution

Contraindications Hypersensitivity to the vaccine or any component; individuals with blood dyscrasias, leukemia, lymphomas, or other malignant neoplasms affecting the bone marrow or lymphatic systems; concurrent immunosuppressive therapy; primary and acquired immunodeficiency states; family history of congenital or hereditary immunodeficiency; current febrile illness or active febrile infection, oral formulation use: Acute GI illness, persistent diarrhea or vomiting, concurrent systemic antibiotics

Warnings Not all recipients of typhoid vaccine will be fully protected against typhoid fever; demonstrated efficacy ranges from 50% to 80%. Travelers should take all necessary precautions to avoid contact or ingestion of potentially contaminated food or water sources. Unless a complete immunization schedule with oral live attenuated Ty21a vaccine (Vivotif Berna®) is followed, an optimum immune response may not be achieved. Vivotif Berna® should not be administered to immunocompromised persons, including those known to be infected with HIV. Parenteral inactivated vaccine may be an alternative for these individuals.

Precautions Administer Typhim Vi® with caution to patients with thrombocytopenia or any coagulation disorder that would be compromised by I.M. injection. Routine prophylactic administration of acetaminophen to prevent fever due to vaccines has been shown to decrease the immune response of some vaccines; the clinical significance of this reduction in immune response has not been established (see Prymula, 2009).

Adverse Reactions All serious adverse reactions must be reported to the U.S. Department of Health and Human Services (DHHS) Vaccine Adverse Event Reporting System (VAERS) 1-800-822-7967.
Injection: Typhim Vi®:
Cardiovascular: Hypotension
Central nervous system: Headache (20%), fever, malaise (4% to 24%)
Gastrointestinal: Nausea, diarrhea, vomiting
Local at injection site: Erythema, pain (27% to 41%), tenderness (98%), induration (5% to 15%)
Neuromuscular & skeletal: Myalgia
Miscellaneous: Allergic reactions
Oral: Vivotif Berna®:
Central nervous system: Headache (4.8%), fever (3.3%)
Dermatologic: Rash, urticaria
Gastrointestinal: Abdominal pain (6.4%), diarrhea (2.9%), nausea, vomiting
Miscellaneous: Anaphylactic reaction

Drug Interactions
Avoid Concomitant Use
Avoid concomitant use of Typhoid Vaccine with any of the following: Immunosuppressants
Increased Effect/Toxicity
The levels/effects of Typhoid Vaccine may be increased by: Immunosuppressants; Mefloquine
Decreased Effect
Typhoid Vaccine may decrease the levels/effects of: Tuberculin Tests

The levels/effects of Typhoid Vaccine may be decreased by: Antibiotics; Immune Globulins; Immunosuppressants
Stability Refrigerate at 2°C to 8°C (35°F to 46°F); do not freeze
Mechanism of Action Each vaccine formulation promotes immunity to disease caused by *Salmonella typhi.* I.M. formulation (Typhim Vi®) is an inactivated vaccine which contains the cell surface Vi polysaccharide extracted from *Salmonella enterica serovar typhi, S typhi* Ty2 strain. Oral formulation (Vivotif Berna®) is a live attenuated virus vaccine which confers immunity by provoking a local immune response in the intestinal tract.

Pharmacokinetics (Adult data unless noted)
Onset of action: Immunity to *Salmonella typhi*: Oral: ~1 week; I.M.: ~2 weeks
Duration: Immunity: Oral: ~5 years; Parenteral: ~3 years
Usual Dosage Immunization:
Oral (Vivotif Berna®): Children ≥6 years and Adults:
Primary immunization: One capsule on alternate days (day 1, 3, 5, and 7) for a total of 4 doses; all doses should be completed at least 1 week prior to potential exposure
Reimmunization: Repeat full course of primary immunization every 5 years
I.M. (Typhim Vi®): Children ≥2 years and Adults:
Primary immunization: 0.5 mL given at least 2 weeks prior to expected exposure
Reimmunization: 0.5 mL; optimal schedule has not been established; a single dose every 2 years is currently recommended for repeated or continued exposure
Note: There is no data concerning using one vaccine (oral vs. I.M.) as a booster after primary immunization with the other vaccine.
Administration
Parenteral: Administer by I.M. injection into the anterolateral aspect of the thigh or arm; **not for I.V. or SubQ** administration
Oral: Oral capsule should be taken 1 hour before a meal with cold or lukewarm drink on alternate days (days 1, 3, 5, and 7); swallow capsule whole, do not chew
Nursing Implications Federal law requires that the date of administration, the vaccine manufacturer, lot number of vaccine, and the administering person's name, title, and address be entered into the patient's permanent medical record.
Additional Information In order to maximize vaccination rates, the ACIP recommends simultaneous administration of all age-appropriate vaccines (live or inactivated) for which a person is eligible at a single visit, unless contraindications exist. The use of combination vaccines is generally preferred over separate infections, taking into consideration provider assessment, patient preference, and potential adverse events.

For additional information, please refer to the following website: http://www.cdc.gov/vaccines/vpd-vac/.
Dosage Forms Excipient information presented when available (limited, particularly for generics); consult specific product labeling. [CAN] = Canadian brand name
Capsule, enteric coated:
Vivotif®: Viable *S. typhi* Ty21a 2-6.8 x 10^9 colony-forming units and nonviable *S. typhi* Ty21a 5-50 x 10^9 bacterial cells [contains lactose 100-180 mg/capsule and sucrose 26-130 mg/capsule]
Injection, solution:
Typherix® [CAN]: Vi capsular polysaccharide 25 mcg/0.5 mL (0.5 mL) [derived from *S. typhi* Ty2 strain] [not available in U.S.]
Typhim Vi®: Purified Vi capsular polysaccharide 25 mcg/0.5 mL (0.5 mL, 10 mL) [derived from *S. typhi* Ty2 strain]
References
Centers for Disease Control and Prevention (CDC), "General Recommendations on Immunization. Recommendations of the Advisory Committee on Immunization Practices (ACIP)," *MMWR Recomm Rep*, 2006, 55(RR-15):1-48. Available at: http://www.cdc.gov/mmwr/preview/mmwrhtml/rr5515a1.htm.
Prymula R, Siegrist CA, Chlibek R, et al, "Effect of Prophylactic Paracetamol Administration at Time of Vaccination on Febrile Reactions and Antibody Responses in Children: Two Open-Label, Randomised Controlled Trials," *Lancet*, 2009, 374(9698):1339-50.
Red Book: 2006 Report of the Committee on Infectious Diseases, 27th ed, Pickering LK,ed, Elk Grove Village, IL: American Academy of Pediatrics, 2006.

◆ **Typhoid Vaccine Live Oral Ty21a** *see* Typhoid Vaccine *on page 1391*

◆ **506U78** *see* Nelarabine *on page 974*

◆ **UCB-P071** *see* Cetirizine *on page 283*
◆ **U-Cort™** *see* Hydrocortisone *on page 685*
◆ **UK92480** *see* Sildenafil *on page 1258*
◆ **UK109496** *see* Voriconazole *on page 1429*
◆ **Ulcidine (Can)** *see* Famotidine *on page 561*
◆ **Ulesfia™** *see* Benzyl Alcohol *on page 186*
◆ **Ultiva®** *see* Remifentanil *on page 1205*
◆ **Ultram®** *see* TraMADol *on page 1367*
◆ **Ultram® ER** *see* TraMADol *on page 1367*
◆ **Ultraprin [OTC]** *see* Ibuprofen *on page 702*
◆ **Ultrase® [DSC]** *see* Pancrelipase *on page 1051*
◆ **Ultrase® (Can)** *see* Pancrelipase *on page 1051*
◆ **Ultrase® MT [DSC]** *see* Pancrelipase *on page 1051*
◆ **Ultrase® MT (Can)** *see* Pancrelipase *on page 1051*
◆ **Ultravate®** *see* Halobetasol *on page 665*
◆ **Unasyn®** *see* Ampicillin and Sulbactam *on page 106*
◆ **Unburn®** *see* Lidocaine *on page 818*

Undecylenic Acid and Derivatives
(un de sil EN ik AS id & dah RIV ah tivs)

U.S. Brand Names Fungi-Nail® [OTC]
Therapeutic Category Antifungal Agent, Topical
Generic Available No
Use Treatment of athlete's foot (tinea pedis), ringworm (except nails and scalp), prickly heat, jock itch (tinea cruris), diaper rash, and other minor skin irritations due to superficial dermatophytes
Contraindications Hypersensitivity to undecylenic acid and derivatives or any component; fungal infections of the scalp or nails
Warnings Do not apply to blistered, raw, or oozing areas of skin or over deep wounds or puncture wounds
Adverse Reactions
Dermatologic: Rash
Local: Skin irritation, stinging, sensitization
Drug Interactions
Avoid Concomitant Use There are no known interactions where it is recommended to avoid concomitant use.
Increased Effect/Toxicity There are no known significant interactions involving an increase in effect.
Decreased Effect There are no known significant interactions involving a decrease in effect.
Mechanism of Action Undecylenic acid is a fatty acid with fungistatic activity that retards proliferation of the fungus by altering the conditions of growth; zinc undecylenate provides an astringent action that aids in the reduction of inflammation and irritation
Pharmacodynamics Onset of action: Improvement in erythema and pruritus may be seen within 1 week after initiation of therapy
Usual Dosage Children and Adults: Topical: Apply as needed twice daily for 2-4 weeks
Administration Topical: Clean and dry the affected area before topical application; if the solution is sprayed or applied onto the affected area, allow area to air dry; ointment or cream should be applied at night, the powder may be applied during the day or used alone when a drying effect is needed
Monitoring Parameters Resolution of skin infection
Patient Information For external use only; avoid contact with the eye; do not inhale the powder
Dosage Forms Excipient information presented when available (limited, particularly for generics); consult specific product labeling.
Solution, topical:
Fungi-Nail®: Undecylenic acid 25% (29.57 mL)

◆ **Uni-Cenna [OTC] [DSC]** *see* Senna *on page 1253*

◆ **Unidet® (Can)** *see* Tolterodine *on page 1359*

◆ **Unipen® (Can)** *see* Nafcillin *on page 962*

◆ **Uniphyl® [DSC]** *see* Theophylline *on page 1335*

◆ **Uniphyl® SRT (Can)** *see* Theophylline *on page 1335*

◆ **Unisom® SleepGels® Maximum Strength [OTC]** *see* DiphenhydrAMINE *on page 448*

◆ **Unisom® SleepMelts™ [OTC]** *see* DiphenhydrAMINE *on page 448*

◆ **Unithroid®** *see* Levothyroxine *on page 816*

◆ **Urasal® (Can)** *see* Methenamine *on page 896*

◆ **Urate Oxidase** *see* Rasburicase *on page 1203*

◆ **Urea Peroxide** *see* Carbamide Peroxide *on page 248*

◆ **Urecholine®** *see* Bethanechol *on page 191*

◆ **Urex™** *see* Methenamine *on page 896*

◆ **Uro-KP-Neutral®** *see* Potassium Phosphate and Sodium Phosphate *on page 1143*

◆ **Uro-Mag® [OTC]** *see* Magnesium Oxide *on page 857*

◆ **Uro-Mag® [OTC]** *see* Magnesium Supplements *on page 859*

◆ **Uromax® (Can)** *see* Oxybutynin *on page 1037*

◆ **Uromitexan (Can)** *see* Mesna *on page 888*

◆ **Urso® (Can)** *see* Ursodiol *on page 1393*

◆ **Urso 250®** *see* Ursodiol *on page 1393*

◆ **Ursodeoxycholic Acid** *see* Ursodiol *on page 1393*

Ursodiol (ER soe dye ole)

U.S. Brand Names Actigall®; Urso 250®; Urso Forte®
Canadian Brand Names Dom-Ursodiol C; PHL-Ursodiol C; PMS-Ursodiol C; Urso®; Urso® DS
Therapeutic Category Gallstone Dissolution Agent
Generic Available Yes
Use Gallbladder stone dissolution (FDA approved in adults); prevention of gallstone formation (obese patients experiencing rapid weight loss) (FDA approved in adults); primary biliary cirrhosis (Urso®) (FDA approved in adults). Other uses include facilitate bile excretion in infants with biliary atresia; treatment of cholestasis secondary to PN; improve the hepatic metabolism of essential fatty acids in patients with cystic fibrosis
Pregnancy Risk Factor B
Lactation Excretion in breast milk unknown/use caution
Contraindications Hypersensitivity to ursodiol, bile acids, or any component; not to be used with calcified cholesterol stones, radiopaque stones, or bile pigment stones; patients with compelling reasons for cholecystectomy (eg, unremitting acute cholecystitis, cholangitis, biliary obstruction)
Warnings Gallbladder stone dissolution may take several months of therapy; complete dissolution may not occur and recurrence of stones within 5 years has been observed in 50% of patients; use with caution in patients with a reduced metabolic capacity to detoxify via sulfation as lithocholic acid (a naturally occurring bile acid) is a known hepatotoxic metabolite that is cleared via sulfation
Precautions Use with caution in patients with a non-visualizing gallbladder and those with chronic liver disease
Adverse Reactions
Central nervous system: Anxiety, depression, dizziness, fatigue, headache, sleep disorder
Dermatologic: Hair thinning, rash
Endocrine & metabolic: Hyperglycemia
Gastrointestinal: Abdominal pain, biliary pain, constipation, diarrhea, dyspepsia, flatulence, nausea, stomatitis, vomiting
Genitourinary: Urinary tract infection

Hematologic: Leukopenia, thrombocytopenia
Hepatic: Cholecystitis, liver enzymes increased (see Warnings)
Neuromuscular & skeletal: Arthralgias, back pain, myalgia
Respiratory: Bronchitis, cough, pharyngitis, rhinitis, upper respiratory tract infection
Miscellaneous: Allergy, flu-like symptoms, viral infection
<1%, postmarketing, and/or case reports: Angioedema, anorexia, esophagitis, fever, malaise, metallic taste, peripheral edema, pruritus, weakness
Drug Interactions
Avoid Concomitant Use There are no known interactions where it is recommended to avoid concomitant use.
Increased Effect/Toxicity There are no known significant interactions involving an increase in effect.
Decreased Effect
Ursodiol may decrease the levels/effects of: Nitrendipine

The levels/effects of Ursodiol may be decreased by: Antacids; Bile Acid Sequestrants; Estrogen Derivatives; Fibric Acid Derivatives
Stability Store at 20°C to 25°C (68°F to 77°F). Half-tablets (scored URSO Forte 500 mg tablets broken in half) maintain acceptable quality for up to 28 days when stored in the current packaging (bottles) at 20°C to 25°C (68°F to 77°F). Due to the bitter taste, the halved segments should be stored separately from the whole tablets.
Mechanism of Action Decreases the cholesterol content of bile and bile stones by reducing the secretion of cholesterol from the liver and the fractional reabsorption of cholesterol by the intestines; mechanism of action in primary biliary cirrhosis is not clearly defined
Pharmacokinetics (Adult data unless noted)
Absorption: 90%
Protein binding: 70%
Metabolism: Undergoes extensive enterohepatic recycling; following hepatic conjugation and biliary secretion, the drug is hydrolyzed to active ursodiol, where it is recycled or transformed to lithocholic acid by colonic microbial flora; during chronic administration, ursodiol becomes a major biliary and plasma bile acid constituting 30% to 50% of biliary and plasma bile acids
Elimination: In feces via bile
Usual Dosage Oral:
Biliary atresia: Infants: 10-15 mg/kg/day once daily
Improvement in the hepatic metabolism of essential fatty acids in cystic fibrosis: Children: 30 mg/kg/day in 2 divided doses
TPN-induced cholestasis: Infants and Children: 30 mg/kg/day in 3 divided doses
Gallstone dissolution: Adults: 8-10 mg/kg/day in 2-3 divided doses; maintenance therapy: 250 mg/day at bedtime for 6 months to 1 year; use beyond 24 months is not established
Gallstone prevention: Adults: 300 mg twice daily
Primary biliary cirrhosis: Adults: 13-15 mg/kg/day in 4 divided doses
Administration Oral: Administer with food or, if a single dosage, at bedtime
Monitoring Parameters ALT, AST, sonogram, oral cholecystogram before therapy and every 6 months during therapy; obtain ultrasound images of gallbladder at 6-month intervals for the first year of therapy
Patient Information Frequent blood work necessary to follow drug effects; report any persistent nausea, vomiting, abdominal pain
Additional Information 30% to 50% of patients have stone recurrence after dissolution
Dosage Forms Excipient information presented when available (limited, particularly for generics); consult specific product labeling.

Capsule: 300 mg
  Actigall®: 300 mg
Tablet: 250 mg, 500 mg
  Urso 250®: 250 mg
  Urso Forte®: 500 mg

Extemporaneous Preparations
A 20 mg/mL ursodiol suspension may be made by opening seventeen 300 mg capsules; add in geometric proportions a 1:1 mixture of Ora-Sweet®:Ora-Plus® or 1% methylcellulose:syrup NF to a total volume of 255 mL; stable 91 days refrigerated. (Nahata, 1999)

A 25 mg/mL ursodiol suspension may be made by opening ten 300 mg capsules; mix with 10 mL Glycerin, USP until smooth mixture is obtained. Add 60 mL Ora-Plus® and continue to levigate until a smooth mixture is achieved. Transfer mixture to a light-resistant bottle; add a small amount of Orange Syrup, NF to wash remaining drug from the mortar to bottle. Add additional syrup to make final volume of 120 mL. Label "shake well"; stable 60 days at room temperature or refrigerated. (Mallett MS)

A 50 mg/mL ursodiol suspension may be made by crushing twelve 250 mg tablets, add 30 mL Ora-Plus® and 30 mL either strawberry syrup or Ora-Sweet® SF; final volume 60 mL. Stable 90 days refrigerated (Johnson, 2002)

A 60 mg/mL ursodiol suspension may be made in a similar method by opening twelve 300 mg capsules and wetting with sufficient glycerin and triturating to make a fine paste; gradually add simple syrup to make a final volume of 60 mL. Label "shake well"; stable 35 days in refrigerator. (Johnson, 1995)

Johnson CE and Nesbitt J, "Stability of Ursodiol in an Extemporaneously Compounded Oral Liquid," *Am J Health Syst Pharm*, 1995, 52(16):1798-800.

Johnson CE and Streetman DD, "Stability of Oral Suspension of Ursodiol Made From Tablets," *Am J Health Syst Pharm*, 2002, 59(4):361-3.

Mallett MS, Hagan RL, and Peters DA, "Stability of Ursodiol 25 mg/mL in an Extemporaneously Prepared Oral Liquid," *Am J Health-Syst Pharm*, 1997, 54 (12):1401-4.

Nahata MC, Morosco RS, and Hipple TF, "Stability of Ursodiol in Two Extemporaneously Prepared Oral Suspensions," *J Appl Ther Res*, 1999, 3:221-4.

References
Colombo C, Setchell KD, Podda M, et al, "Effect of Ursodeoxycholic Acid Therapy for Liver Disease Associated With Cystic Fibrosis," *J Pediatr*, 1990, 117(3):482-9.

Lepage G, Paradis K, Lacaille F, et al, "Ursodeoxycholic Acid Improves the Hepatic Metabolism of Essential Fatty Acids and Retinol in Children With Cystic Fibrosis," *J Pediatr*, 1997, 130(1)52-8.

Spagnuolo MI, Iorio R, Vegnente A, et al, "Ursodeoxycholic Acid for Treatment of Cholestasis in Children on Long-Term Total Parenteral Nutrition - A Pilot Study," *Gastroenterology*, 1996, 111(3):716-9.

Ullrich D, Rating D, Schroter W, et al, "Treatment With Ursodeoxycholic Acid Renders Children With Biliary Atresia Suitable for Liver Transplantation," *Lancet*, 1987, 2(8571):1324.

◆ **Urso® DS (Can)** see Ursodiol on page 1393
◆ **Urso Forte®** see Ursodiol on page 1393
◆ **UTI Relief® [OTC]** see Phenazopyridine on page 1097
◆ **Vagifem®** see Estradiol on page 536

Valacyclovir (val ay SYE kloe veer)

Medication Safety Issues
Sound-alike/look-alike issues:
  Valtrex® may be confused with Keflex®, Valcyte®, Zovirax®
  ValACYclovir may be confused with acyclovir, valGAN-Clclovir, vancomycin

U.S. Brand Names Valtrex®

Canadian Brand Names Apo-Valacyclovir®; Mylan-Valacyclovir; PHL-Valacyclovir; PMS-Valacyclovir; PRO-Valacyclovir; Riva-Valacyclovir; Valtrex®

Therapeutic Category Antiviral Agent, Oral

Generic Available Yes

Use Treatment of herpes zoster (shingles) in immunocompetent patients; treatment of initial and recurrent episodes of genital herpes; suppression of recurrent genital herpes and reduction of heterosexual transmission of genital herpes in immunocompetent patients; suppression of genital herpes in HIV-infected individuals; treatment of herpes labialis (cold sores) in adults and children >12 years; treatment of chickenpox in immunocompetent children >2 years and <18 years; suppression and prevention of vertical transmission of recurrent genital herpes during labor and delivery; used investigationally for prevention and treatment of herpes infections in both immunocompromised and immunocompetent patients

Pregnancy Risk Factor B

Pregnancy Considerations Teratogenic events were not observed in animal studies. Data from a pregnancy registry has shown no increased rate of birth defects than that of the general population; however, the registry is small and use during pregnancy is only warranted if the potential benefit to the mother justifies the risk of the fetus.

Lactation Enters breast milk/use caution

Breast-Feeding Considerations Peak concentrations in breast milk range from 0.5-2.3 times the corresponding maternal acyclovir serum concentration. This is expected to provide a nursing infant with a dose of acyclovir equivalent to ~0.6 mg/kg/day following ingestion of valacyclovir 500 mg twice daily by the mother. Use with caution while breast-feeding.

Contraindications Hypersensitivity to valacyclovir, acyclovir, or any component

Warnings Thrombotic thrombocytopenic purpura/hemolytic uremic syndrome (TTP/HUS) has occurred in immunocompromised patients (bone marrow or renal transplant or advanced HIV disease) receiving 8 g/day.

Precautions Use with caution in patients with renal impairment or patients receiving concomitant nephrotoxic drugs; modify dose in patients with renal impairment.

Adverse Reactions
Cardiovascular: Hypertension, tachycardia, facial edema
Central nervous system: Headache, dizziness, fever
Dermatologic: Rash
Endocrine & metabolic: Dysmenorrhea, dehydration
Gastrointestinal: Nausea, abdominal pain, vomiting, diarrhea
Hematologic: Neutropenia, thrombocytopenia, TTP/HUS (rare)
Hepatic: ALT, AST, alkaline phosphatase elevated; hepatitis
Neuromuscular & skeletal: Arthralgia
Renal: Creatinine elevated, renal failure
Respiratory: Nasopharyngitis, rhinorrhea
Miscellaneous: Anaphylaxis

Drug Interactions
  Avoid Concomitant Use
  Avoid concomitant use of ValACYclovir with any of the following: Zoster Vaccine
  Increased Effect/Toxicity
  ValACYclovir may increase the levels/effects of: Mycophenolate; Tenofovir; Zidovudine

  The levels/effects of ValACYclovir may be increased by: Mycophenolate
  Decreased Effect
  ValACYclovir may decrease the levels/effects of: Zoster Vaccine

Food Interactions Food does not appear to affect absorption.

Stability Store at room temperature.

Mechanism of Action Valacyclovir is rapidly and nearly completely converted to acyclovir by intestinal and hepatic metabolism. Acyclovir is converted to acyclovir monophosphate by virus-specific thymidine kinase then further converted to acyclovir triphosphate by other cellular enzymes. Acyclovir triphosphate inhibits DNA synthesis and viral replication by competing with deoxyguanosine triphosphate for viral DNA polymerase and being incorporated into viral DNA.

Pharmacokinetics (Adult data unless noted)

Absorption: Rapid

Distribution: Acyclovir is widely distributed throughout the body including brain, kidney, lungs, liver, spleen, muscle, uterus, vagina, and CSF; CSF acyclovir concentration is 50% of serum concentration; crosses the placenta; excreted into breast milk

Protein binding: 13.5% to 17.9%

Metabolism: Valacyclovir is converted to acyclovir and L-valine by first-pass intestinal and/or hepatic metabolism; acyclovir is metabolized to a small extent by aldehyde oxidase, alcohol, and aldehyde dehydrogenase to inactive metabolites

Bioavailability: ~42% to 64%, decreased bioavailability with higher doses in children

Half-life:

Normal renal function:

Acyclovir:

Children: 1.3-2.5 hours, slower clearance with increased age

Adults: 2-3.5 hours

Valacyclovir: Adults: ~30 minutes

End-stage renal disease: Acyclovir: 14-20 hours

Time to peak serum concentration:

Children: 1.4-2.6 hours

Adults: 1.5 hours

Elimination: 88% as acyclovir in the urine. **Note:** Following oral radiolabeled valacyclovir administration, 46% of the label is eliminated in feces and 47% is eliminated in urine.

Dialysis: 33% removed during 4-hour hemodialysis session; administer dose postdialysis

Usual Dosage Oral:

Children:

Chickenpox (immunocompetent patients): 2 years to <18 years: 20 mg/kg/dose 3 times/day for 5 days (maximum: 1 g 3 times/day), initiate within 24 hours of rash onset

Herpes labialis (cold sores): >12 years: 2 g every 12 hours for 1 day (2 doses), initiated at earliest symptoms

Immunocompromised children at risk for HSV or VZV infection with normal renal function (limited study data available): 15-30 mg/kg/dose given 3 times/day have been reported in pharmacokinetic studies (maximum dose: 2 g/dose)

Adults:

CMV prophylaxis in allogeneic HSCT recipients: 2 g 4 times/day

Herpes zoster (shingles): 1 g 3 times/day for 7 days

HSV, VZV in cancer patients: Prophylaxis: 500 mg 2-3 times/day; treatment: 1 g 3 times/day

Genital herpes:

Initial episode: 1 g twice daily for 10 days

Recurrent episode: 500 mg twice daily for 3 days

Reduction of transmission: 500 mg once daily (source partner)

Suppressive therapy:

Immunocompetent patients: 1 g once daily (500 mg once daily in patients with <9 recurrences/year)

HIV-infected patients (CD4 ≥100 cells/mm^3): 500 mg twice daily

Suppressive therapy during pregnancy: 500 mg twice daily from 36 weeks estimated gestational age until delivery

Dosing interval in renal impairment:

Herpes labialis: Adolescents and Adults:

Cl_{cr} 30-49 mL/minute: 1 g every 12 hours for 2 doses

Cl_{cr} 10-29 mL/minute: 500 mg every 12 hours for 2 doses

Cl_{cr} <10 mL/minute: 500 mg as a single dose

Herpes zoster: Adults:

Cl_{cr} 30-49 mL/minute: 1 g every 12 hours

Cl_{cr} 10-29 mL/minute: 1 g every 24 hours

Cl_{cr} <10 mL/minute: 500 mg every 24 hours

Genital herpes: Adolescents and Adults:

Initial episode:

Cl_{cr} 10-29 mL/minute: 1 g every 24 hours

Cl_{cr} <10 mL/minute: 500 mg every 24 hours

Recurrent episode: Cl_{cr} ≤10-29 mL/minute: 500 mg every 24 hours

Suppressive therapy: Cl_{cr} ≤10-29 mL/minute:

For usual dose of 1 g every 24 hours, decrease dose to 500 mg every 24 hours

For usual dose of 500 mg every 24 hours, decrease dose to 500 mg every 48 hours

HIV-infected patients: 500 mg every 24 hours

Administration Oral: May administer with or without food

Monitoring Parameters Urinalysis, BUN, serum creatinine, liver enzymes, CBC

Patient Information Report any rash, headache, nausea, vomiting, problems with vision, behavioral changes, unusual bleeding or bruising, or blood in urine or stool.

Additional Information

Nadal (2002) suggests the following dosage equivalency: 30 mg/kg/dose 3 times/day valacyclovir corresponds to I.V. acyclovir 250 mg/m^2 or 10 mg/kg/dose 3 times/day 20 mg/kg/dose 3 times/day valacyclovir corresponds to oral acyclovir 20 mg/kg 4-5 times/day

Eksborg, et al (2002) suggests the following dosage equivalency: 500 mg valacyclovir equivalent to 349 mg of I.V. acyclovir

Dosage Forms Excipient information presented when available (limited, particularly for generics); consult specific product labeling.

Caplet, oral: 500 mg, 1 g

Valtrex®: 500 mg

Valtrex®: 1 g [scored]

Extemporaneous Preparations To prepare a valacyclovir 25 mg/mL oral suspension, crush 5 valacyclovir 500 mg caplets (10 caplets for 50 mg/mL suspension) into a fine powder in a mortar. Gradually add 5 mL aliquots of Suspension Structured Vehicle USP-NF (SSV) to powder and triturate until a paste is formed. Continue adding 5 mL aliquots of SSV to the mortar until a suspension is formed (minimum: 20 mL SSV and maximum: 40 mL SSV). Transfer to 100 mL bottle. Add the cherry flavor (amount recommended on package) to the mortar and dissolve in ~5 mL of SSV. Add to bottle once dissolved. Rinse the mortar at least 3 times with ~5 mL of SSV, transferring contents between additions of SSV. Continue to add the SSV to bring final volume to 100 mL. The preparation is stable for 28 days under refrigeration; shake well before using.

A 50 mg/mL oral suspension can be prepared using 2 different vehicles (Ora-Sweet® or Ora-Sweet SF®); crush eighteen 500 mg valacyclovir hydrochloride caplets into a fine powder in a mortar; add 40 mL of the vehicle, 5 mL at a time and mix thoroughly; transfer to a 180 mL amber glass bottle; rinse mortar with 10 mL of vehicle and transfer into bottle; repeat rinsing process for a total of five rinses, 10 mL each; qsad with vehicle to 180 mL; suspension is stable for 21 days when stored in an amber glass bottle under refrigeration (4°C); label "shake well" and "refrigerate."

References

ACOG Committee on Practice Bulletins, "ACOG Practice Bulletin. Clinical Management Guidelines for Obstetrician-Gynecologists. No. 82 June 2007. Management of Herpes in Pregnancy," *Obstet Gynecol*, 2007, 109(6):1489-98.

Balfour HH Jr, Hokanson KM, Schacherer RM, et al, "A Virologic Pilot Study of Valacyclovir in Infectious Mononucleosis," *J Clin Virol*, 2007, 39(1):16-21.

Bomgaars L, Thompson P, Berg S, et al, "Valacyclovir and Acyclovir Pharmacokinetics in Immunocompromised Children," *Pediatr Blood Cancer*, 2008, 51(4):504-8.

Eksborg S, Pal N, Kalin M, et al, "Pharmacokinetics of Acyclovir in Immunocompromised Children With Leukopenia and Mucositis After Chemotherapy: Can Intravenous Acyclovir Be Substituted by Oral Valacyclovir?" *Med Pediatr Oncol*, 2002, 38(4):240-6.

Fish DN, Vidaurri VA, and Deeter RG, "Stability of Valacyclovir Hydrochloride in Extemporaneously Prepared Oral Liquids," *Am J Health Syst Pharm*, 1999, 56(19):1957-60.

Nadal D, Leverger G, Sokal EM, et al, "An Investigation of the Steady-State Pharmacokinetics of Oral Valacyclovir in Immunocompromised Children," *J Infect Dis*, 2002, 186(Suppl 1):S123-30.

Simon MW, Fish DN, and Deeter RG, "Pharmacokinetics and Safety of Valacyclovir in Children With Epstein-Barr Virus Illness," *Drugs R D*, 2002, 3(6):365-73.

♦ **Valacyclovir Hydrochloride** *see* Valacyclovir *on page 1394*

♦ **Valcyte®** *see* Valganciclovir *on page 1396*

♦ **23-Valent Pneumococcal Polysaccharide Vaccine** *see* Pneumococcal Polysaccharide Vaccine (Polyvalent) *on page 1125*

Valganciclovir (val gan SYE kloh veer)

Medication Safety Issues
Sound-alike/look-alike issues:
Valcyte® may be confused with Valium®, Valtrex®
ValGANCIclovir may be confused with valACYclovir

U.S. Brand Names Valcyte®
Canadian Brand Names Valcyte®
Therapeutic Category Antiviral Agent
Generic Available No
Use Prevention of CMV disease in high-risk patients undergoing heart or kidney transplantation (FDA approved in ages 4 months to 16 years and adults); treatment of cytomegalovirus (CMV) retinitis in patients with acquired immunodeficiency syndrome (AIDS) (FDA approved in adults); prevention of CMV disease in high-risk patients (donor CMV positive/recipient CMV negative) undergoing kidney/pancreas transplantation (FDA approved in adults); has also been used for prevention of CMV disease in high-risk pediatric patients undergoing BMT or hematopoietic stem cell transplant, solid organ transplants other than those indicated above, and congenital CMV disease (see Acosta, 2007; Galli, 2007; Lombardi, 2009)

Pregnancy Risk Factor C
Pregnancy Considerations Valganciclovir is converted to ganciclovir and shares its reproductive toxicity. **[U.S. Boxed Warning]: Ganciclovir may be teratogenic and cause aspermatogenesis.** Based on animal data, temporary or permanent impairment of fertility may occur in males and females. Ganciclovir is also teratogenic in animals. Females should use effective contraception during treatment and for 30 days after; males should use barrier contraception during treatment and for 90 days after.

Lactation Excretion in breast milk unknown/not recommended
Breast-Feeding Considerations HIV-infected mothers are discouraged from breast-feeding to decrease the potential transmission of HIV.
Contraindications Hypersensitivity to valganciclovir, ganciclovir, or any component

Warnings Hazardous agent; use appropriate precautions for handling and disposal. May cause dose- or therapy-limiting granulocytopenia, anemia, and/or thrombocytopenia **[U.S. Boxed Warning]**; do not use if ANC <500 cells/mm^3, platelets <25,000/mm^3, or hemoglobin <8 g/dL. Valganciclovir is converted to ganciclovir and shares its reproductive toxicity. Animal studies have demonstrated carcinogenic and teratogenic effects, inhibition of spermatogenesis, and impairment of fertility with ganciclovir **[U.S. Boxed Warning]**. Due to its teratogenic potential, contraceptive precautions need to be followed during and for at least 30 days after therapy for women and 90 days after therapy for men. Studies in liver transplant patients reported a higher incidence of tissue-invasive CMV with valganciclovir relative to oral ganciclovir.

Precautions The bioavailability of ganciclovir from valganciclovir tablets is significantly higher than with ganciclovir capsules; valganciclovir tablets cannot be substituted for ganciclovir capsules on a one-to-one basis. In pediatric patients, the preferred dosage form is oral solution; however, if calculated dose is within 10% of the lowest tablet strength (450 mg), then valganciclovir tablets may be used for doses. Use with caution in patients with pre-existing bone marrow suppression, cytopenias, or in those patients receiving myelosuppressive drugs or irradiation; adjust dose or interrupt valganciclovir therapy in patients with neutropenia and/or thrombocytopenia. Use with caution and modify dosage in patients with impaired renal function or in patients receiving concomitant nephrotoxic drugs; maintain adequate hydration.

Oral solution contains sodium benzoate; benzoic acid (benzoate) is a metabolite of benzyl alcohol; large amounts of benzyl alcohol (≥99 mg/kg/day) have been associated with a potentially fatal toxicity ("gasping syndrome") in neonates; the "gasping syndrome" consists of metabolic acidosis, respiratory distress, gasping respirations, CNS dysfunction (including convulsions, intracranial hemorrhage), hypotension, and cardiovascular collapse; use oral solution containing sodium benzoate with caution in neonates; *in vitro* and animal studies have shown that benzoate displaces bilirubin from protein binding sites.

Adverse Reactions
Cardiovascular: Edema, hypertension, hypotension, peripheral edema
Central nervous system: Agitation, confusion, depression, dizziness, fatigue, fever, hallucinations, headache, insomnia, pain, paresthesia, peripheral neuropathy, psychosis, seizure
Dermatologic: Acne, dermatitis, pruritus
Gastrointestinal: Abdominal distention, abdominal pain, appetite decreased, constipation, diarrhea, dyspepsia, nausea, vomiting
Endocrine & metabolic: Dehydration, hyperglycemia, hyper/hypokalemia, hypocalcemia, hypomagnesemia, hypophosphatemia
Hematologic: Anemia, aplastic anemia, bleeding, bone marrow suppression, granulocytopenia, leukopenia, neutropenia, pancytopenia, thrombocytopenia
Hepatic: Ascites
Neuromuscular & skeletal: Arthralgia, back pain, limb pain, muscle cramps, paresthesia, peripheral neuropathy, tremors, weakness
Ocular: Retinal detachment
Renal: Acute renal failure, dysuria, renal function decreased, serum creatinine increased
Respiratory: Cough, dyspnea, nasopharyngitis, pharyngitis, pleural effusion, rhinorrhea, upper respiratory tract infection
Miscellaneous: Allergic reactions, infections including sepsis
<1%, postmarketing, and/or case reports: Valganciclovir is expected to share the toxicities which may occur at a low incidence or due to idiosyncratic reactions which have been associated with ganciclovir.

Drug Interactions
Avoid Concomitant Use
Avoid concomitant use of ValGANClclovir with any of the following: Imipenem
Increased Effect/Toxicity
ValGANClclovir may increase the levels/effects of: Imipenem; Mycophenolate; Reverse Transcriptase Inhibitors (Nucleoside); Tenofovir

The levels/effects of ValGANClclovir may be increased by: Mycophenolate; Probenecid

Decreased Effect There are no known significant interactions involving a decrease in effect.

Food Interactions High fat meal may increase AUC by 30%.

Stability
Oral solution: Store dry powder at 25°C (77°F); excursions permitted to 15°C to 30°C (59°F to 86°F). Prior to dispensing, prepare the oral solution by adding 91 mL of purified water to the bottle; shake well. Store oral solution under refrigeration at 2°C to 8°C (36°F to 46°F); do not freeze. Discard any unused medication after 49 days. A reconstituted 100 mL bottle will only provide 88 mL of solution for administration.

Tablets: Store at 25°C (77°F); excursions permitted to 15°C to 30°C (59°F to 86°F).

Mechanism of Action
Valganciclovir is rapidly converted to ganciclovir in the body. The bioavailability of ganciclovir from valganciclovir is increased 10-fold compared to oral ganciclovir. A dose of 900 mg achieved systemic ganciclovir exposure comparable to that achieved with the recommended 5 mg/kg doses of intravenous ganciclovir. Ganciclovir is phosphorylated to a substrate which competitively inhibits the binding of deoxyguanosine triphosphate to DNA polymerase resulting in inhibition of viral DNA synthesis.

Pharmacokinetics (Adult data unless noted)
Absorption: Well absorbed; high-fat meal increases AUC by 30%

Distribution: V_{dss}: Ganciclovir: 0.7 L/kg; distributes to most body fluids, tissues, and organs including CSF, ocular tissue, and brain

Protein binding: Ganciclovir: 1% to 2%

Metabolism: Prodrug converted to ganciclovir by intestinal mucosal cells and hepatocytes

Bioavailability: 60% (with food)

Half-life: Ganciclovir:
  In either healthy or HIV-positive/CMV-positive patients: 4.08 hours; prolonged with renal impairment (up to 68 hours with severe renal impairment): 4.08 hours
  In heart, kidney, kidney-pancreas, or liver transplant patients: 6.48 hours

Time to peak serum concentration: Ganciclovir: 1-3 hours

Elimination: Majority (80% to 90%) excreted as ganciclovir in the urine

Dialysis: 50% removed by a 4-hour hemodialysis

Usual Dosage
Oral: **Note:** Valganciclovir tablets and ganciclovir capsules cannot be substituted on a mg-per-mg basis since they are **NOT BIOEQUIVALENT.**

Neonates >7 days to 3 months of age: 16 mg/kg/dose every 12 hours; a pharmacokinetic study of 24 neonates demonstrated that 16 mg/kg/dose twice daily produced similar serum concentrations to ganciclovir 6 mg/kg intravenously twice daily (see Acosta, 2007; Kimberlin, 2008)

Children 4 months to 16 years:
  Manufacturer's recommendations:
    Prevention of CMV disease following kidney or heart transplantation:
      Dose (mg) = 7 x body surface area x creatinine clearance* once daily beginning within 10 days of transplantation; continue therapy until 100 days post-transplantation. Doses should be rounded to the nearest 25 mg increment; maximum dose: 900 mg/day
      * Cl_{cr} (mL/minute/1.73 m^2) = [k x height (cm)] ÷ serum creatinine (mg/dL)
      Note: Calculated using a *modified* Schwartz formula where k =
        • 0.45 in patients <2 years
        • 0.55 in boys age 2 to <13 years
        • 0.55 in girls age 2-16 years
        • 0.7 in boys age 13-16 years
    Alternate dosing: Limited information available: 15-18 mg/kg/day once daily for the first 100 days post liver transplant in patients considered low-risk for CMV disease reported by one center for the prevention of CMV disease following transplantation (see Clark, 2004)

Children >16 years and Adults:
  CMV retinitis:
    Induction: 900 mg twice daily for 21 days
    Maintenance: Following induction treatment or for patients with inactive CMV retinitis who require maintenance therapy: 900 mg once daily
  Prevention of CMV disease following transplantation: 900 mg once daily beginning within 10 days of transplantation; continue therapy until 100 days post-transplantation

Dosage adjustment in renal impairment:
Children 4 months to 16 years: No additional dosage adjustments required; use of equation adjusts for renal function
Children >16 years and Adults (tablet formulation):
  Induction dose:
    Cl_{cr} 40-59 mL/minute: 450 mg twice daily
    Cl_{cr} 25-39 mL/minute: 450 mg once daily
    Cl_{cr} 10-24 mL/minute: 450 mg every 2 days
  Maintenance dose:
    Cl_{cr} 40-59 mL/minute: 450 mg once daily
    Cl_{cr} 25-39 mL/minute: 450 mg every 2 days
    Cl_{cr} 10-24 mL/minute: 450 mg twice weekly
  Note: Valganciclovir is not recommended in patients receiving hemodialysis. For patients on hemodialysis (Cl_{cr} <10 mL/minute), it is recommended that ganciclovir be used instead of valganciclovir with dose adjusted as specified for ganciclovir.

Administration Oral: Administer with meals.

Monitoring Parameters Retinal exam at least every 4-6 weeks; CBC with differential, platelet count, serum creatinine

Patient Information Valganciclovir is not a cure for CMV retinitis. Regular follow-up ophthalmologic exams are necessary. For oral administration, take with food and maintain adequate fluid hydration. Swallow tablets whole; do not break or crush. Avoid handling broken or crushed tablets and oral solution. Wash area thoroughly if contact occurs. Report fever, chills, unusual bleeding or bruising, infection, or unhealed sores or white plaques in mouth. Male patients and female patients of childbearing potential need to follow contraceptive precautions during and for at least 3 months after therapy with valganciclovir.

Nursing Implications Ensure adequate patient hydration. Consideration should be given to handling and disposal of valganciclovir according to guidelines issued for antineoplastic agents. Avoid direct contact of skin or mucous membranes with broken or crushed tablets or oral solution.

Dosage Forms Excipient information presented when available (limited, particularly for generics); consult specific product labeling.
Powder for solution, oral:
  Valcyte®: 50 mg/mL (100 mL) [contains sodium benzoate; tutti-frutti flavor]
Tablet, oral:
  Valcyte®: 450 mg

Extemporaneous Preparations Note: A commercial preparation is available. A 60 mg/mL oral liquid preparation made from valganciclovir 450 mg tablets and a 1:1 mixture of Ora-Sweet® and Ora-Plus® was stable for 35 days when stored in an amber glass bottle under refrigeration at 4°C; grind sixteen 450 mg tablets in a mortar into a fine powder; add 10 mL of the vehicle in 1 mL increments and triturate to a paste; mix while adding the vehicle in geometric proportions to almost 120 mL. Pour the resulting mixture into a 120 mL amber glass bottle; rinse mortar with vehicle and transfer to bottle; qsad with vehicle to 120 mL; label "shake well" and "refrigerate".

Henkin CC, Griener JC, and Ten Eick AP, "Stability of Valganciclovir in Extemporaneously Compounded Liquid Formulations," *Am J Health-Syst Pharm*, 2003, 60:687-90.

References

Acosta EP, Brundage RC, King JR, et al, "Ganciclovir Population Pharmacokinetics in Neonates Following Intravenous Administration of Ganciclovir and Oral Administration of a Liquid Valganciclovir Formulation," *Clin Pharmacol Ther*, 2007, 81(6):867-72.

Burri M, Wiltshire H, Kahlert C, et al, "Oral Valganciclovir in Children: Single Dose Pharmacokinetics in a Six-Year-Old Girl," *Pediatr Infect Dis J*, 2004, 23(3):263-6.

Clark BS, Chang IF, Karpen SJ, et al, "Valganciclovir for the Prophylaxis of Cytomegalovirus Disease in Pediatric Liver Transplant Recipients," *Transplantation*, 2004, 77(9):1480.

Galli L, Novelli A, Chiappini E, et al, "Valganciclovir for Congenital CMV Infection: A Pilot Study on Plasma Concentration in Newborns and Infants," *Pediatr Infect Dis J*, 2007, 26(5):451-3.

Kimberlin DW, Acosta EP, Sánchez PJ, et al, "Pharmacokinetic and Pharmacodynamic Assessment of Oral Valganciclovir in the Treatment of Symptomatic Congenital Cytomegalovirus Disease," *J Infect Dis*, 2008, 197(6):836-45.

Lombardi G, Garofoli F, Villani P, et al, "Oral Valganciclovir Treatment in Newborns With Symptomatic Congenital Cytomegalovirus Infection," *Eur J Clin Microbiol Infect Dis*, 2009, 28(12):1465-70.

Peyriere H, Jeziorsky E, Jalabert A, et al, "Neurotoxicity Related to Valganciclovir in a Child With Impaired Renal Function: Usefulness of Therapeutic Drug Monitoring," Ann Pharmacother, 2006, 40(1):143-6.

◆ **Valganciclovir Hydrochloride** *see* Valganciclovir *on page 1396*

◆ **Valisone® Scalp Lotion (Can)** *see* Betamethasone *on page 189*

◆ **Valium®** *see* Diazepam *on page 424*

◆ **Valorin [OTC]** *see* Acetaminophen *on page 36*

◆ **Valorin Extra [OTC]** *see* Acetaminophen *on page 36*

◆ **Valproate Semisodium** *see* Valproic Acid and Derivatives *on page 1398*

◆ **Valproate Sodium** *see* Valproic Acid and Derivatives *on page 1398*

◆ **Valproic Acid** *see* Valproic Acid and Derivatives *on page 1398*

Valproic Acid and Derivatives
(val PROE ik AS id & dah RIV ah tivs)

Medication Safety Issues
Sound-alike/look-alike issues:
Depakene® may be confused with Depakote®
Depakote® may be confused with Depakene®, Depakote® ER, Senokot®
Depakote® ER may be confused with Depakote®, divalproex enteric coated
Valproate sodium may be confused with vecuronium

Related Information
Antiepileptic Drugs *on page 1693*
Febrile Seizures *on page 1690*
Serotonin Syndrome *on page 1695*
Therapeutic Drug Monitoring: Blood Sampling Time Guidelines *on page 1704*

U.S. Brand Names Depacon®; Depakene®; Depakote®; Depakote® ER; Depakote® Sprinkle; Stavzor™

Canadian Brand Names Alti-Divalproex; Apo-Divalproex®; Apo-Valproic®; Depakene®; Dom-Divalproex; Epival® I.V.; Gen-Divalproex; Mylan-Divalproex; Mylan-Valproic; Novo-Divalproex; Nu-Divalproex; PHL-Divalproex; PHL-Valproic Acid; PHL-Valproic Acid E.C.; PMS-Valproic Acid; PMS-Valproic Acid E.C.; ratio-Valproic; ratio-Valproic ECC; Rhoxal-valproic; Sandoz-Valproic

Therapeutic Category Anticonvulsant, Miscellaneous; Infantile Spasms, Treatment

Generic Available Yes: Excludes capsule (softgel/delayed release)

Use All products: Monotherapy and adjunctive therapy in the treatment of patients with complex partial seizures; monotherapy and adjunctive therapy of simple and complex absence seizures; adjunctive therapy in patients with multiple seizure types that include absence seizures; has also been used to treat mixed seizure types, myoclonic and generalized tonic-clonic (grand mal) seizures; may be effective in infantile spasms. **Note:** I.V. formulation is indicated for patients in whom oral administration of valproate is temporarily not feasible; has also been used in patients with absence status epilepticus.

Divalproex sodium delayed-release tablets (Depakote®) are also indicated in adults for the treatment of manic episodes of bipolar disorders and the prevention of migraine headaches. Divalproex extended-release tablets (Depakote®-ER) are also indicated in adults for the treatment of acute manic or mixed episodes associated with bipolar disorder and for the prevention of migraine headaches.

Pregnancy Risk Factor D

Pregnancy Considerations [U.S. Boxed Warning]: May cause teratogenic effects such as neural tube defects (eg, spina bifida). Teratogenic effects have been reported in animals and humans. Valproic acid crosses the placenta. Neural tube, cardiac, facial (characteristic pattern of dysmorphic facial features), skeletal, multiple other defects reported. Epilepsy itself, number of medications, genetic factors, or a combination of these probably influence the teratogenicity of anticonvulsant therapy. Information from the North American Antiepileptic Drug Pregnancy Registry notes a fourfold increase in congenital malformations with exposure to valproic acid monotherapy during the 1st trimester of pregnancy when compared to monotherapy with other antiepileptic drugs (AED). The risk of neural tube defects is ~1% to 2% (general population risk estimated to be 0.14% to 0.2%). The effect of folic acid supplementation to decrease this risk is unknown, however, folic acid supplementation is recommended for all women contemplating pregnancy. An information sheet describing the teratogenic potential is available from the manufacturer.

Nonteratogenic effects have also been reported. Afibrinogenemia leading to fatal hemorrhage and hepatotoxicity have been noted in case reports of infants following *in utero* exposure to valproic acid. Developmental delay, autism and/or autism spectrum disorder have also been reported. Use in women of childbearing potential requires that benefits of use in mother be weighed against the potential risk to fetus, especially when used for conditions not associated with permanent injury or risk of death (eg, migraine).

Patients exposed to valproic acid during pregnancy are encouraged to enroll themselves into the AED Pregnancy Registry by calling 1-888-233-2334. Additional information is available at www.aedpregnancyregistry.org.

Lactation Enters breast milk/not recommended (AAP considers "compatible")

Breast-Feeding Considerations Breast milk concentrations of valproic acid have been reported as 1% to 10% of maternal concentration. The weight-adjusted dose to the infant has been calculated to be ~4%.

Contraindications Hypersensitivity to valproic acid or derivatives or any component; hepatic disease or significant hepatic dysfunction; urea cycle disorders

Warnings Hepatic failure resulting in death may occur **[U.S. Boxed Warning]**; children <2 years of age (especially those on polytherapy, with congenital metabolic disorders, with seizure disorders and mental retardation, or with organic brain disease) are at considerable risk; monitor patients closely for appearance of malaise, loss of seizure control, weakness, facial edema, anorexia, jaundice and vomiting; hepatotoxicity has been reported after 3 days to 6 months of therapy; discontinue valproate if hepatotoxicity occurs. Cases of life-threatening pancreatitis (including fatalities) have been reported in children and adults **[U.S. Boxed Warning]**; pancreatitis may be hemorrhagic and rapidly progress to death; onset has occurred shortly after starting therapy and after several years of treatment; monitor patients closely for nausea, vomiting, anorexia, and abdominal pain and evaluate promptly; discontinue valproate if pancreatitis occurs. Dose-related thrombocytopenia may occur. I.V. valproate is not recommended for the prophylaxis of post-traumatic seizures in patients with acute head trauma.

Hyperammonemic encephalopathy, which was sometimes fatal, has been reported following initiation of valproate therapy in patients with known or suspected urea cycle disorders (UCD) (particularly ornithine transcarbamylase deficiency). Before valproate therapy is started, evaluation for UCD should be considered in patients with 1) a history of unexplained coma or encephalopathy, encephalopathy associated with a protein load, unexplained mental retardation, pregnancy-related encephalopathy, postpartum encephalopathy, or history of increased plasma ammonia or glutamine; 2) cyclical vomiting and lethargy, episodic extreme irritability, ataxia, low BUN, or protein avoidance; 3) family history of UCD or family history of unexplained infant deaths (especially males); 4) other signs and symptoms of UCD. Patients who develop symptoms of hyperammonemic encephalopathy during therapy with valproate should receive prompt treatment; valproate therapy should be discontinued, and patients should be evaluated for UCD.

Congenital malformations such as neural tube defects (eg, spina bifida), craniofacial defects, cardiovascular malformations, and anomalies of other body systems may occur **[U.S. Boxed Warning]**. Use in women of childbearing potential requires that benefits of use in mother be weighed against the potential risk to fetus, especially when used for conditions not associated with permanent injury or risk of death (eg, migraine). Maternal use of valproate during pregnancy may result in clotting abnormalities or hepatic failure in the newborn.

Antiepileptic drugs (AEDs) increase the risk of suicidal behavior and ideation in patients receiving these medications for any indication. Pooled analyses of placebo-controlled trials involving 11 different AEDs (regardless of indication) showed a twofold increased risk of suicidal thoughts or behavior (estimated incidence rate: 0.43% in AED-treated patients compared to 0.24% of patients receiving placebo); increased risk was observed as early as 1 week after initiation of AED and continued through duration of trials (most trials ≤24 weeks); risk did not vary significantly by age (age range: 5-100 years). Consider risks and benefits of AEDs before prescribing. Monitor all patients receiving an AED for emergence of suicidal thoughts or behavior, thoughts of self-harm, any unusual changes in behavior or mood, or the emergence or worsening of depressive symptoms; notify healthcare provider immediately if symptoms or concerning behavior occur. **Note:** The FDA is requiring that a Medication Guide be developed for all antiepileptic drugs, informing patients of this risk.

Precautions Hyperammonemia may occur, even in the absence of liver enzyme abnormalities; asymptomatic elevations of ammonia require continued monitoring; discontinuation of valproate should be considered if elevations persist. Hyperammonemic encephalopathy should be considered in patients with unexplained lethargy, vomiting, or changes in mental status and serum ammonia should be measured; valproate should be discontinued in symptomatic patients with elevated serum ammonia; hyperammonemia should be treated and patients should be evaluated for UCD. Concurrent use of valproic acid with topiramate may result in hyperammonemia with or without encephalopathy; use with caution in patients with inborn errors of metabolism or decreased hepatic mitochondrial activity; these patients may be at increased risk.

Multiorgan hypersensitivity reactions have been rarely reported in adults and pediatric patients in association with initiation of valproic acid use; at least one death has been reported; patient may present with fever and rash in association with symptoms of organ system dysfunction [eg, lymphadenopathy, hepatitis, abnormalities in liver function tests, hematologic abnormalities (eosinophilia, neutropenia, thrombocytopenia), pruritus, oliguria, nephritis, arthralgia, asthenia]; valproate should be discontinued in patients suspected of having multiorgan hypersensitivity reactions.

Valproate may stimulate the replication of HIV and CMV *in vitro*; clinical effects are unknown. CNS depression may occur with valproic acid use. Patients must be cautioned about performing tasks which require mental alertness (operating machinery or driving). Effects with other sedative drugs or ethanol may be potentiated. Anticonvulsants should not be discontinued abruptly because of the possibility of increasing seizure frequency; valproic acid should be withdrawn gradually to minimize the potential of increased seizure frequency, unless safety concerns require a more rapid withdrawal. Patients treated for bipolar disorder should be monitored closely for clinical worsening or suicidality; prescriptions should be written for the smallest quantity consistent with good patient care.

Adverse Reactions

Cardiovascular: Chest pain, hypertension, palpitation, peripheral edema, tachycardia

Central nervous system: Drowsiness, somnolence, irritability, confusion, restlessness, nervousness, hyperactivity, malaise, headache, ataxia, dizziness, abnormal dreams, amnesia, anxiety, abnormal coordination, depression, personality disorder; hyperammonemic encephalopathy (in patients with UCD; see Warnings); suicidal thinking and behavior (see Warnings)

Dermatologic: Alopecia, erythema multiforme, bruising, dry skin, petechia, pruritus, rash

Endocrine & metabolic: Hyperammonemia, impaired fatty-acid oxidation, carnitine deficiency, weight gain, amenorrhea, dysmenorrhea

Gastrointestinal: Nausea, vomiting, diarrhea, dyspepsia, constipation, abdominal pain, anorexia, increase appetite, eructation, flatulence, hematemesis, pancreatitis (potentially fatal), taste perversion (I.V.)

Genitourinary: Urinary frequency, urinary incontinence, vaginitis

Hematologic: Thrombocytopenia [risk increases significantly with serum levels ≥110 mcg/mL (females) or ≥135 mcg/mL (males)], prolongation of bleeding time

Hepatic: Liver enzymes elevated (transient), liver failure (can be fatal; see Warnings)

Local: I.V.: Pain and local reaction at injection site

Neuromuscular & skeletal: Tremor, asthenia, abnormal gait, arthralgia, back pain, hypertonia, leg cramps, myalgia, myasthenia, paresthesia, twitching

Ocular: Diplopia, blurred vision, nystagmus

Otic: Deafness, otitis media, tinnitus

Respiratory: Cough increased, dyspnea, epistaxis, pharyngitis, pneumonia, sinusitis

Miscellaneous: Multiorgan hypersensitivity reactions (rare, but potentially fatal; see Precautions)

Drug Interactions

Metabolism/Transport Effects For valproic acid: **Substrate** (minor) of CYP2A6, 2B6, 2C9, 2C19, 2E1; **Inhibits** CYP2C9 (weak), 2C19 (weak), 2D6 (weak), 3A4 (weak); **Induces** CYP2A6 (weak)

Avoid Concomitant Use There are no known interactions where it is recommended to avoid concomitant use.

Increased Effect/Toxicity

Valproic Acid and Derivatives may increase the levels/ effects of: Barbiturates; Ethosuximide; LamoTRIgine; LORazepam; Paliperidone; Primidone; Risperidone; Rufinamide; Temozolomide; Tricyclic Antidepressants; Vorinostat; Zidovudine

The levels/effects of Valproic Acid and Derivatives may be increased by: ChlorproMAZINE; Felbamate; GuanFA-CINE; Salicylates; Topiramate

Decreased Effect

Valproic Acid and Derivatives may decrease the levels/ effects of: CarBAMazepine; OXcarbazepine; Phenytoin

The levels/effects of Valproic Acid and Derivatives may be decreased by: Barbiturates; CarBAMazepine; Carbapenems; Ethosuximide; Methylfolate; Phenytoin; Primidone; Protease Inhibitors; Rifampin

Food Interactions Dietary carnitine requirements may be increased; food may decrease the rate but not the extent of absorption

Stability

Depakote® tablets and Depakene® solution: Store below 30°C (86°F)

Depakote® Sprinkles: Store below 25°C (77°F)

Depakote® ER: Store at controlled room temperature of 25°C (77°F); excursions permitted to 15°C to 30°C (59°F to 86°F)

Depakene® capsule: Store at 15°C to 25°C (59°F to 77°F)

Depacon® injection: Store vials at controlled room temperature of 15°C to 30°C (59°F to 86°F). Stable for at least 24 hours at room temperature when diluted in D₅W, NS, or LR and stored in glass or polyvinyl chloride bags. Discard unused portion of vial (does not contain preservative).

Mechanism of Action Causes increased availability of gamma-aminobutyric acid (GABA), an inhibitory neurotransmitter, to brain neurons or may enhance the action of GABA or mimic its action at postsynaptic receptor sites

Pharmacokinetics (Adult data unless noted)

Protein binding: 80% to 90% (dose dependent); decreased protein binding in neonates and patients with renal impairment or chronic hepatic disease

Distribution: Distributes into CSF at concentrations similar to unbound concentration in plasma (ie, ~10% of total plasma concentration)

Metabolism: Extensive in liver via glucuronide conjugation and oxidation

Bioavailability: Oral (all products except Depakote®-ER): Equivalent to I.V.; **Depakote®-ER tablets are not bioequivalent to Depakote® delayed release tablets**; mean bioavailability of Depakote®-ER tablets is 81% to 89%, relative to Depakote® delayed release tablets; recent studies in adults show that when Depakote®-ER is administered in doses 8% to 20% higher than the total

daily dose of Depakote®, then the 2 products are bioequivalent. In patients 10-17 years of age, once-daily administration of Depakote®-ER produced valproic acid plasma concentration-time profiles similar to adults.

Half-life: Increased with liver disease

Newborns (exposed to VPA *in utero*): 30-60 hours

Newborns 1st week of life: 40-45 hours

Newborns <10 days: 10-67 hours

Children >2 months: 7-13 hours

Children 2-14 years: Mean: 9 hours; range: 3.5-20 hours

Adults: 8-17 hours

Time to peak serum concentration:

Oral: 1-4 hours; divalproex (enteric coated): 3-5 hours

I.V.: At the end of the infusion

Elimination: 2% to 3% excreted unchanged in urine; faster clearance in children who receive other antiepileptic drugs and those who are younger; age and polytherapy explain 80% of interpatient variability in total clearance; children >10 years of age have pharmacokinetic parameters similar to adults

Usual Dosage Note: Use of Depakote®-ER in pediatric patients <10 years of age is not recommended; do not confuse Depakote®-ER with Depakote®. **Erroneous substitution of Depakote® (delayed release tablets) for Depakote®-ER has resulted in toxicities; only Depakote®-ER is intended for once daily administration.**

Seizures disorders: Children and Adults:

Oral: Initial: 10-15 mg/kg/day in 1-3 divided doses; increase by 5-10 mg/kg/day at weekly intervals until therapeutic levels are achieved; maintenance: 30-60 mg/kg/day in 2-3 divided doses; Depakote® and Depakote® Sprinkle can be given twice daily

Note: Children receiving more than 1 anticonvulsant (ie, polytherapy) may require doses up to 100 mg/kg/day in 3-4 divided doses. Due to differences in bioavailability, children ≥10 years of age and adult epilepsy patients receiving Depakote® may be switched to Depakote®-ER by using a once-daily Depakote®-ER dose that is 8% to 20% higher than the total daily dose of Depakote® (see Depakote®-ER package insert for details)

I.V.: Total daily I.V. dose is equivalent to the total daily oral dose, however, I.V. dose should be divided with a frequency of every 6 hours; if I.V. form is administered 2-3 times/day, close monitoring of trough levels is recommended; switch patients to oral product as soon as clinically possible (I.V. use has not been studied for >14 days)

Rectal: Dilute syrup 1:1 with water for use as a retention enema; loading dose: 17-20 mg/kg one time; maintenance: 10-15 mg/kg/dose every 8 hours

Refractory status epilepticus:

Infants and Children:

I.V.: Loading dose: Initial: Optimal dosage is not established; pediatric studies have used initial loading doses of 20-40 mg/kg.

Note: In one retrospective study, an initial loading dose of 25 mg/kg (administered at ~3 mg/kg/minute) was effective in stopping seizure activity within 20 minutes after the end of the infusion in all 18 patients treated for status epilepticus (see Yu, 2003). A separate retrospective trial found a higher efficacy rate in pediatric patients (n=41) who received an initial loading dose of 30-40 mg/kg (compared to 20-30 mg/kg or >40 mg/kg) (see Uberall, 2000). In an open-label, randomized comparative trial, an initial loading dose of 30 mg/kg was administered (n=20; age range: 7 months-10 years of age; mean age: 3 years); a repeat bolus of 10 mg/kg could be administered if seizures were not controlled within 10 minutes; mean required dose: 37.5 ± 4.4 mg/kg;

median required dose: 40 mg/kg (see Mehta, 2007). Further studies are needed.

I.V.: Maintenance dose: I.V. infusion: Optimal dosage is not established; pediatric studies used continuous infusions of 5 mg/kg/hour after the loading dose (see Mehta, 2007; Uberall, 2000); once patients were seizure-free for 6 hours, the infusion rate was decreased by 1 mg/kg/hour every 2 hours (see Mehta, 2007). Further studies are needed.

Adults:

I.V.: Loading dose: Recommendations from the European Federation of Neurological Societies (AFNS): Initial: 25-45 mg/kg administered at ≤6 mg/kg/minute (see Meierkord, 2006); range: 15-45 mg/kg

I.V.: Maintenance dose: I.V. infusion: 1-4 mg/kg/hour; titrate dose as needed based upon patient response and evaluation of drug-drug interactions

Prophylaxis of migraine headaches: Adults: Oral:

Depakote®: Initial: 250 mg twice daily; increase dose based on patient response; maximum dose: 1000 mg/day

Depakote®-ER: Initial: 500 mg once daily for 7 days; may increase if needed to 1000 mg once daily; range: 500-1000 mg/day; dose should be individualized; if smaller dosage adjustments are needed, use Depakote® delayed release tablets; may initiate treatment with lower dose of Depakote® delayed release tablet in patients who have GI upset

Mania: Adults: Oral:

Depakote®: Initial: 750 mg/day in divided doses; adjust dose as rapidly as possible to desired clinical effect or plasma concentration; maximum recommended dose: 60 mg/kg/day

Depakote®-ER: Initial 25 mg/kg/day given once daily; increase dose rapidly to achieve lowest therapeutic dose (based on clinical effects) or target range of serum concentrations; maximum recommended dose: 60 mg/kg/day

Dosing adjustment in renal impairment: Cl_{cr} <10 mL/minute: No dosage adjustment is needed for patients on hemodialysis (unbound clearance of valproate is reduced (27%) in these patients, but hemodialysis reduces valproate concentrations by ~20%). Protein binding is reduced in patients with renal impairment; monitoring only total valproate serum concentrations may be misleading.

Dosing adjustment in hepatic impairment: Valproic acid is contraindicated in patients with hepatic disease or significant hepatic dysfunction. Potentially fatal hepatotoxicity may occur with valproic acid use (see Warnings). Clearance is decreased in patients with liver impairment. Hepatic disease is also associated with decreased albumin concentrations and 2- to 2.6-fold increase in the unbound fraction of valproate. Free concentrations of valproate may be elevated while total concentrations appear normal.

Administration

Oral: May administer with food to decrease adverse GI effects. Do not administer with carbonated drinks; do not administer tablet with milk. May mix contents of Depakote® Sprinkle capsule with semisolid food (eg, applesauce, pudding, mashed potatoes) and swallow immediately; do not crush or chew sprinkle beads; do not store drug food mixture for later use. Swallow delayed release and extended release tablets whole; do not crush, break, or chew.

I.V.:

Manufacturer recommendations: Dilute dose with at least 50 mL of D_5W, NS, or LR; infuse over 60 minutes; maximum infusion rate: 20 mg/minute; **Note:** Rapid infusions may be associated with an increase in adverse effects; infusions of ≤15 mg/kg administered over 5-10 minutes (1.5-3 mg/kg/minute); were generally well tolerated (see Product Information).

Rapid I.V. loading doses:

Infants and Children: Optimal administration rate is not established. One retrospective pediatric study administered loading doses of 25 mg/kg at a rate of ~3 mg/kg/minute (see Yu, 2003). However, a prospective study administered 30 mg/kg of the drug diluted 1:1 in NS over 2-5 minutes (see Mehta, 2007). Another retrospective study administered loading doses at a slightly faster rate (20-40 mg/kg diluted 1:1 with NS or D_5W administered over 1-5 minutes; see Uberall, 2000). Further studies are needed.

Adults: The European Federation of Neurological Societies (EFNS) recommends maximum administration rates of 6 mg/kg/minute (see Meierkord, 2006). **Note:** In two adult studies, the drug was administered undiluted at rates as high as 10 mg/kg/minute (see Limdi, 2007) and 500 mg/minute (see Limdi, 2005). Further studies are needed.

Monitoring Parameters Liver enzymes, bilirubin, serum ammonia, CBC with platelets, serum concentrations, PT/PTT (especially prior to surgery); signs and symptoms of suicidality (eg, anxiety, depression, behavior changes) (see Warnings)

Reference Range

Epilepsy:

Therapeutic: 50-100 mcg/mL (SI: 350-690 micromoles/L)

Toxic: >100-150 mcg/mL (SI: >690-1040 micromoles/L)

Seizure control may improve at levels >100 mcg/mL (SI: >690 micromoles/L), but toxicity may occur

Mania: Therapeutic trough: 50-125 mcg/mL (SI: 350-860 micromoles/L)

Test Interactions False-positive result for urine ketones; altered thyroid function tests

Patient Information Avoid alcohol. May cause drowsiness and impair ability to perform activities requiring mental alertness and physical coordination. Do not discontinue abruptly (an increase in seizure activity may result). Antiepileptic agents may increase the risk of suicidal thoughts and behavior; notify physician if you feel more depressed or have thoughts of suicide or self-harm (see Warnings). Notify physician if nausea, vomiting, unexplained lethargy, change in mental status, general feeling of weakness, loss of appetite, abdominal pain, yellow skin, bleeding, or easy bruising occur. Report fever associated with rash, swelling, or other organ system involvement immediately to physician. Report worsening of seizure activity or loss of seizure control.

Nursing Implications Instruct patients/parents to report signs or symptoms of hepatotoxicity, pancreatitis, hyperammonemic encephalopathy, and multiorgan hypersensitivity reactions (see Warnings and Precautions). GI side effects of divalproex may be less than valproic acid

Additional Information A valproic acid associated Reye's-like syndrome has been reported (see Hilmas, 2000). Acute intoxications: Naloxone may reverse the CNS depressant effects but may also block the action of other anticonvulsants; carnitine may reduce the ammonia level; multiple dosing of activated charcoal can enhance elimination.

Routine prophylactic use of carnitine in children receiving valproic acid to avoid carnitine deficiency and hepatotoxicity is probably not indicated (Freeman, 1994); a case of fatal hepatotoxic reaction has been reported in a child receiving valproic acid despite carnitine supplementation (Murphy, 1993)

Sodium content of valproate sodium syrup: 5 mL = 23 mg (1 mEq of sodium). Safety of I.V. form has not been well studied in children <2 years of age. Long-term usefulness of Depakote®-ER for the treatment of mania should be periodically re-evaluated in patients receiving the drug for extended periods of time (>3 weeks).

Dosage Forms Excipient information presented when available (limited, particularly for generics); consult specific product labeling. **Note:** Strength expressed as valproic acid

Capsule, softgel, oral, as valproic acid: 250 mg
Depakene®: 250 mg
Capsule, softgel, delayed release, oral, as valproic acid:
Stavzor™: 125 mg, 250 mg, 500 mg
Capsule, sprinkles, oral, as divalproex sodium: 125 mg
Depakote® Sprinkle: 125 mg
Injection, solution, as valproate sodium [preservative free]:
100 mg/mL (5 mL)
Depacon®: 100 mg/mL (5 mL) [contains edetate disodium]
Solution, oral, as valproate sodium: 250 mg/5 mL (473 mL, 480 mL)
Syrup, oral, as valproate sodium: 250 mg/5 mL (5 mL, 10 mL, 473 mL)
Depakene®: 250 mg/5 mL (473 mL)
Tablet, delayed release, as divalproex sodium: 125 mg, 250 mg, 500 mg
Depakote®: 125 mg, 250 mg, 500 mg
Tablet, extended release, as divalproex sodium: 250 mg, 500 mg
Depakote® ER: 250 mg, 500 mg

References

Cloyd JC, Fischer JH, Kriel RL, et al, "Valproic Acid Pharmacokinetics in Children. IV. Effects of Age and Antiepileptic Drugs on Protein Binding and Intrinsic Clearance," *Clin Pharmacol Ther*, 1993, 53(1):22-9.
Cloyd JC, Kriel RL, Fischer JH, et al, "Pharmacokinetics of Valproic Acid in Children: I. Multiple Antiepileptic Drug Therapy," *Neurology*, 1983, 33(2):185-91.
Dreifuss FE, Santilli N, Langer DH, et al, "Valproic Acid Hepatic Fatalities: A Retrospective Review," *Neurology*, 1987, 37(3):379-85.
Freeman JM, Vining EP, Cost S, et al, "Does Carnitine Administration Improve the Symptoms Attributed to Anticonvulsant Medications?: A Double-Blinded, Crossover Study," *Pediatrics*, 1994, 93(6 Pt 1):893-5.
Hilmas E and Lee CK, "Valproic Acid-Related Reye's-Like Syndrome," *The Journal of Pediatric Pharmacy Practice*, 2000, 5(3):149-55.
Limdi NA, Knowlton RK, Cofield SS, et al, "Safety of Rapid Intravenous Loading of Valproate," *Epilepsia*, 2007, 48(3):478-83.
Limdi NA, Shimpi AV, Faught E, et al, "Efficacy of Rapid IV Administration of Valproic Acid for Status Epilepticus," *Neurology*, 2005, 64(2):353-5.
Mehta V, Singhi P, and Singhi S, "Intravenous Sodium Valproate Versus Diazepam Infusion for the Control of Refractory Status Epilepticus in Children: A Randomized Controlled Trial," *J Child Neurol*, 2007, 22 (10):1191-7.
Meierkord H, Boon P, Engelsen B, et al, "EFNS Guideline on the Management of Status Epilepticus," *Eur J Neurol*, 2006, 13(5):445-50.
Murphy JV, Groover RV and Hodge C, "Hepatotoxic Effects in a Child Receiving Valproate and Carnitine," *J Pediatr*, 1993, 123(2):318-20.
Uberall MA, Trollmann R, Wunsiedler U, et al, "Intravenous Valproate in Pediatric Epilepsy Patients With Refractory Status Epilepticus," *Neurology*, 2000, 54(11):2188-9.
Yu KT, Mills S, Thompson N, et al, "Safety and Efficacy of Intravenous Valproate in Pediatric Status Epilepticus and Acute Repetitive Seizures," *Epilepsia*, 2003, 44(5):724-6.

Valsartan (val SAR tan)

Medication Safety Issues
Sound-alike/look-alike issues:
Valsartan may be confused with losartan, Valstar™, Valturna®
Diovan® may be confused with Darvon®, Dioval®, Zyban®

International issues:
Diovan® [U.S., Canada, and multiple international markets] may be confused with Dianben, a brand name for metformin [Spain]

Related Information
Antihypertensive Agents by Class *on page 1481*

U.S. Brand Names Diovan®

Canadian Brand Names Diovan®

Therapeutic Category Angiotensin II Receptor Blocker; Antihypertensive Agent

Generic Available No

Use Treatment of essential hypertension alone or in combination with other antihypertensive agents (FDA approved in ages 6-16 years and adults); reduction of cardiovascular mortality in clinically stable patients with left ventricular failure or left ventricular dysfunction postmyocardial infarction (FDA approved in adults); treatment of heart failure (NYHA Class II-IV) (FDA approved in adults)

Pregnancy Risk Factor D

Pregnancy Considerations Medications which act on the renin-angiotensin system are reported to have the following fetal/neonatal effects: Hypotension, neonatal skull hypoplasia, anuria, renal failure, and death; oligohydramnios is also reported. These effects are reported to occur with exposure during the second and third trimesters. **[U.S. Boxed Warning]: Based on human data, drugs that act on the angiotensin system can cause injury and death to the developing fetus when used in the second and third trimesters. Angiotensin receptor blockers should be discontinued as soon as possible once pregnancy is detected.**

Lactation Excretion in breast milk unknown/not recommended

Breast-Feeding Considerations It is not known if valsartan is found in breast milk; the manufacturer recommends discontinuing the drug or discontinuing nursing based on the importance of the drug to the mother.

Contraindications Hypersensitivity to valsartan, any component, or other angiotensin II receptor blockers

Warnings Drugs that act on the renin-angiotensin system can cause injury and death to the developing fetus when used during pregnancy. ARBs should be discontinued as soon as possible once pregnancy is detected **[U.S. Boxed Warning]**. Neonatal hypotension, skull hypoplasia, anuria, renal failure, oligohydramnios (associated with fetal limb contractures, craniofacial deformities, hypoplastic lung development), prematurity, intrauterine growth retardation, patent ductus arteriosus, and death have been reported with the use of ACE inhibitors, primarily in the second and third trimesters.

Precautions Use with caution in patients with hepatic impairment (clearance of valsartan is reduced in these patients). Use with caution in patients with impaired renal function; use is associated with deterioration of renal function and/or increases in serum creatinine, particularly in patients with low renal blood flow (eg, renal artery stenosis, heart failure); deterioration may result in oliguria, acute renal failure, and progressive azotemia. Small increases in serum creatinine may occur following initiation; consider discontinuation in patients with progressive and/or significant deterioration in renal function. Hyperkalemia may occur; risk factors include renal dysfunction, diabetes mellitus, concomitant use of potassium-sparing diuretics, potassium supplements, and/or potassium-containing salts; use with caution in these patients and with these agents; monitor potassium closely.

Symptomatic hypotension may occur, especially in patients with an activated renin-angiotensin system (eg, volume- or salt-depleted patients receiving high doses of diuretic agents); use with caution in these patients; correct depletion before starting therapy or initiate therapy under close medical supervision. Use with caution in patients with heart failure or post-MI (symptomatic hypotension may occur). Not recommended for use in children <6 years of age due to possible safety issues (see Usual Dosage); not recommended for use in children with GFR <30 mL/minute/1.73m^2 (no data exists)

Adverse Reactions Note: No significant differences in adverse reactions have been identified between children and adults.

Cardiovascular: Hypotension, postural hypotension, syncope
Central nervous system: Dizziness, fatigue, postural dizziness, headache, vertigo
Dermatologic: Rash
Endocrine & metabolic: Hyperkalemia
Gastrointestinal: Diarrhea, abdominal pain, nausea
Hematologic: Neutropenia, hemoglobin and hematocrit decreased (<1% incidence)
Hepatic: Liver enzymes increased (rare)
Neuromuscular & skeletal: Arthralgia, back pain
Ocular: Blurred vision
Renal: BUN and serum creatinine elevated, renal dysfunction
Respiratory: Cough
Miscellaneous: Viral infection, angioedema (rare)

Drug Interactions
Metabolism/Transport Effects Substrate of SLCO1B1; **Inhibits** CYP2C9 (weak)
Avoid Concomitant Use There are no known interactions where it is recommended to avoid concomitant use.

Increased Effect/Toxicity
Valsartan may increase the levels/effects of: ACE Inhibitors; Amifostine; Antihypertensives; Hypotensive Agents; Lithium; Potassium-Sparing Diuretics; RiTUXimab

The levels/effects of Valsartan may be increased by: Diazoxide; Eltrombopag; Eplerenone; Herbs (Hypotensive Properties); MAO Inhibitors; Pentoxifylline; Phosphodiesterase 5 Inhibitors; Potassium Salts; Prostacyclin Analogues; Tolvaptan; Trimethoprim

Decreased Effect
The levels/effects of Valsartan may be decreased by: Herbs (Hypertensive Properties); Methylphenidate; Nonsteroidal Anti-Inflammatory Agents; Yohimbine

Food Interactions Food decreases the peak plasma concentration and extent of absorption by 50% and 40%, respectively. Limit salt substitutes or potassium-rich diet. Avoid natural licorice (causes sodium and water retention and increases potassium loss).

Stability Store at controlled room temperature at 25°C (77°F). Protect from moisture; dispense in tightly closed container.

Mechanism of Action Valsartan produces direct antagonism of the effects of angiotensin II. Unlike the ACE inhibitors, valsartan blocks the binding of angiotensin II to the AT1 receptor subtype. It produces its blood pressure-lowering effects by antagonizing AT1-induced vasoconstriction, aldosterone release, catecholamine release, arginine vasopressin release, water intake, and hypertrophic responses. This action results in more efficient blockade of the cardiovascular effects of angiotensin II and fewer side effects than the ACE inhibitors. Valsartan does not affect the ACE (kininase II) or the response to bradykinin.

Pharmacodynamics
Antihypertensive effect:
Onset of action: 2 hours postdose
Maximum effect: Within 6 hours postdose; with chronic dosing, substantial hypotensive effects are seen within 2 weeks; maximum effect: After 4 weeks
Duration: 24 hours

Pharmacokinetics (Adult data unless noted)
Distribution: Adults: V_d: 17 L
Protein binding: 95%, primarily albumin
Metabolism: To inactive metabolite (valeryl 4-hydroxy valsartan) via unidentified enzyme(s)
Bioavailability:
Tablet: 25% (range: 10% to 35%)
Suspension: ~40% (~1.6 times more than tablet)
Half-life, elimination: Adults: ~6 hours

Time to peak serum concentration: Tablets (Adults): 2-4 hours; Suspension (Children): 2 hours (Blumer, 2009)
Elimination: Excreted in feces (83%) and urine (13%) primarily as unchanged drug; 20% of dose is recovered as metabolites
Clearance: Found to be similar per kg bodyweight in children vs adults receiving a single dose of the suspension (Blumer, 2009)
Dialysis: Not removed by hemodialysis

Usual Dosage Oral:
Hypertension:
Children 1-5 years: Not recommended for use due to possible safety issues; one study (n=90; mean age: 3.2 years; minimum patient weight: 8 kg) randomized patients to receive low, medium, or high doses according to patient body weight. Patients <18 kg received low dose: 5 mg once daily; medium dose: 20 mg once daily; or high dose: 40 mg once daily. Patients ≥ 18 kg received low dose: 10 mg once daily; medium dose: 40 mg once daily; or high dose: 80 mg once daily. These set doses resulted in a mean dosage of 0.4-3.4 mg/kg once daily (see Flynn, 2008). Although some efficacy was demonstrated, two deaths and three cases of increased liver enzymes occurred. Even though patients had significant comorbidities and a causal relationship to valsartan could not be established, a relationship to treatment with valsartan could not be excluded. Thus, use in children <6 years of age is not recommended by the manufacturer (see Diovan® package insert, 2007). Further studies are needed.
Children 6-16 years: Manufacturer's recommendations: Initial: 1.3 mg/kg once daily (maximum: 40 mg/day); dose may be increased to achieve desired effect; doses >2.7 mg/kg (maximum: 160 mg) have not been studied
Note: Due to increased bioavailability of oral suspension, patient may require a higher dose when replacing oral suspension with tablet dosage form.
Adults: Initial: 80 mg or 160 mg once daily (in patients who are not volume depleted); dose may be increased to achieve desired effect; maximum recommended dose: 320 mg once daily; usual dosage range (JNC 7): 80-320 mg once daily
Heart failure: Adults: Initial: 40 mg twice daily; titrate dose to 80-160 mg twice daily, as tolerated; maximum dose: 320 mg/day in divided doses

Dosing adjustment in renal impairment:
Children: Use is not recommended if Cl_{cr} <30 mL/minute
Adults: No dosage adjustment necessary if Cl_{cr} >10 mL/minute; use with caution in patients with Cl_{cr} <10 mL/minute

Dosing adjustment in hepatic impairment: In mild-to-moderate liver disease, no adjustment is needed. Use caution in patients with liver disease. Patients with mild-to-moderate chronic liver disease have twice the exposure as healthy volunteers.

Administration May be administered without regard to food

Monitoring Parameters Blood pressure, BUN, serum creatinine, renal function, baseline and periodic serum electrolytes

Patient Information Do not take any new medication during therapy unless approved by prescriber (especially sleep remedies or antisleep products, cough or cold remedies, or weight-loss products). Take exactly as directed and do not discontinue without consulting prescriber. This drug does not eliminate need for diet or exercise regimen as recommended by prescriber. May cause dizziness or lightheadedness (use caution when driving or engaging in tasks that require alertness until response to drug is known); postural hypotension (use caution when rising from lying or sitting position or climbing stairs); or diarrhea. Report changes in urinary pattern;

swelling of extremities; unusual back ache; chest pain or palpitations; unrelenting headache; muscle weakness or pain; unusual cough; or other persistent adverse reactions. This medication may cause injury and death to the developing fetus when used during pregnancy; women of childbearing potential should be informed of potential risk; consult prescriber for appropriate contraceptive measures; this medication should be discontinued as soon as possible once pregnancy is detected (see Warnings).

Nursing Implications Assess effectiveness and inter-actions with other pharmacological agents and herbal products patients may be taking (eg, concurrent use of potassium supplements, ACE inhibitors, and potassium-sparing diuretics may increase risk of hyperkalemia). Monitor laboratory tests at baseline and periodically during therapy. Monitor therapeutic effectiveness (reduced BP) and adverse response on a regular basis during therapy (eg, changes in renal function, dizziness, bradycardia, cough, headache, nausea, hypotension, hyperkalemia). Teach patient appropriate use according to drug form and purpose of therapy, possible side effects/appropriate interventions, and adverse symptoms to report.

Dosage Forms Excipient information presented when available (limited, particularly for generics); consult specific product labeling.

Tablet:
Diovan®: 40 mg [scored]
Diovan®: 80 mg, 160 mg, 320 mg

Extemporaneous Preparations A 4 mg/mL valsartan suspension made from tablets, Ora-Plus® and Ora-Sweet® is stable for 30 days at room temperature (below 30°C/86°F) or up to 75 days under refrigeration (2°C to 8°C/35°F to 46°F) when stored in amber glass prescription bottles. Add 80 mL of Ora-Plus® to an 8-ounce amber glass bottle containing eight (8) valsartan 80 mg tablets. Shake well for ≥2 minutes. Allow the suspension to stand for a minimum of 1 hour, then shake for ≥1 minute. Then add 80 mL of Ora-Sweet SF® to the bottle and shake for at least 10 seconds. Label "Shake well" (Diovan® package insert, 2007).

Diovan® package insert, East Hanover, NJ: Novartis Pharmaceuticals Corp, 2007.

References

Blumer J, Batisky DL, Wells T, et al, "Pharmacokinetics of Valsartan in Pediatric and Adolescent Subjects With Hypertension," *J Clin Pharmacol*, 2009, 49(2):235-41.

Chobanian AV, Bakris GL, Black HR, et al, "The Seventh Report of the Joint National Committee on Prevention, Detection, Evaluation, and Treatment of High Blood Pressure: The JNC 7 Report," *JAMA*, 2003, 289(19):2560-71.

Conlin P, Moore T, Swartz S, et al, "Effect of Indomethacin on Blood Pressure Lowering by Captopril and Losartan in Hypertensive Patients," *Hypertension*, 2000, 36(3):461-5.

Flynn JT, Meyers KE, Neto JP, et al, "Efficacy and Safety of the Angiotensin Receptor Blocker Valsartan in Children With Hypertension Aged 1 to 5 Years," *Hypertension*, 2008, 52(2):222-8.

♦ **Valtrex®** see Valacyclovir on page 1394

♦ **Vanceril® AEM (Can)** see Beclomethasone on page 176

♦ **Vancocin®** see Vancomycin on page 1404

Vancomycin (van koe MYE sin)

Medication Safety Issues

Sound-alike/look-alike issues:
I.V. vancomycin may be confused with Invanz®
Vancomycin may be confused with clindamycin, genta-micin, tobramycin, valACYclovir, vecuronium, Vibramycin®

High alert medication: The Institute for Safe Medication Practices (ISMP) includes this medication (intrathecal administration) among its list of drug classes which have a heightened risk of causing significant patient harm when used in error.

Related Information

Compatibility of Chemotherapy and Related Supportive Care Medications on page 1580
Endocarditis Prophylaxis on page 1610
Therapeutic Drug Monitoring: Blood Sampling Time Guidelines on page 1704

U.S. Brand Names Vancocin®
Canadian Brand Names Vancocin®
Therapeutic Category Antibiotic, Miscellaneous
Generic Available Yes: Injection

Use

Parenteral: Treatment of patients with the following infections or conditions: Infections due to documented or suspected methicillin-resistant *S. aureus* or beta-lactam resistant coagulase negative *Staphylococcus*; serious or life-threatening infections (eg, endocarditis, meningitis, osteomyelitis) due to documented or sus-pected staphylococcal or streptococcal infections in patients who are allergic to penicillins and/or cepha-losporins; empiric therapy of infections associated with central lines, VP shunts, hemodialysis shunts, vascular grafts, prosthetic heart valves (FDA approved in children and adults)

Oral: Treatment of staphylococcal enterocolitis or for antibiotic-associated pseudomembranous colitis pro-duced by *C. difficile* (FDA approved in adults)

Pregnancy Risk Factor B (oral); C (injection)

Pregnancy Considerations Adverse effects have not been observed in animal studies and there are no controlled studies in pregnant women; however, oral vancomycin is not systemically absorbed. Therefore, I.V. vancomycin has been classified pregnancy category C and oral vancomycin has been classified pregnancy category B. Vancomycin crosses the placenta. *In vivo* studies and human case reports have documented placental transfer of vancomycin in the second and third trimesters of pregnancy resulting in therapeutic fetal concentrations. Vancomycin has not caused adverse fetal effects, including hearing loss or nephrotoxicity, when administered during pregnancy. A case report has been published of a vancomycin dose rapidly administered over 3 minutes leading to maternal hypotension and fetal bradycardia.

The pharmacokinetics of vancomycin may be altered during pregnancy and pregnant patients may need a higher dose of vancomycin. Maternal half-life is unchanged, but the volume of distribution and the total plasma clearance are increased. Individualization of therapy through serum concentration monitoring may be warranted. Vancomycin is recommended for use in pregnant women for prevention of early-onset group B streptococcal (GBS) disease in newborns.

Lactation Enters breast milk/not recommended

Breast-Feeding Considerations Small amounts of vancomycin are excreted in human milk and use during breast-feeding is not recommended by the manufacturer. If given orally to the mother, the minimal systemic absorption of the dose would limit the amount available to pass into the milk. If given intravenously, the small amount that distributes to the milk would not be expected to cause systemic toxicity due to the lack of GI absorption. Nondose-related effects could include modification of bowel flora.

Contraindications Hypersensitivity to vancomycin or any component; avoid in patients with previous hearing loss

Warnings Intravenous use may result in superinfection, including *C. difficile*-associated diarrhea and pseudomem-branous colitis; **Note:** Oral use is FDA approved for this indication.

Precautions Use with caution in patients with renal impairment or those receiving other nephrotoxic or ototoxic drugs; dosage modification required in patients with impaired renal function; may cause neutropenia. Chemical peritonitis syndrome has been reported with intraperitoneal administration.

Adverse Reactions Rapid infusion associated with red neck or red man syndrome: Erythema multiforme-like reaction with intense pruritus, tachycardia, hypotension, rash involving face, neck, upper trunk, back and upper arms; red man or red neck syndrome usually develops during a rapid infusion of vancomycin or with doses ≥15-20 mg/kg/hour; reaction usually dissipates in 30-60 minutes

Cardiovascular: Cardiac arrest
Central nervous system: Chills, fever
Dermatologic: Macular skin rash, red neck or red man syndrome, urticaria
Gastrointestinal: Nausea
Hematologic: Eosinophilia, neutropenia
Local: Phlebitis
Neuromuscular & skeletal: Lower back pain
Otic: Ototoxicity
Renal: Nephrotoxicity (may be associated with higher serum concentrations; see Monitoring Parameters)
Miscellaneous: Hypersensitivity reactions
<1%, postmarketing, and/or case reports: Drug rash with eosinophilia and systemic symptoms (DRESS), skin and subcutaneous tissue disorders

Drug Interactions

Avoid Concomitant Use
Avoid concomitant use of Vancomycin with any of the following: BCG; Gallium Nitrate

Increased Effect/Toxicity
Vancomycin may increase the levels/effects of: Amino-glycosides; Colistimethate; Gallium Nitrate; Neuromus-cular-Blocking Agents

The levels/effects of Vancomycin may be increased by: Nonsteroidal Anti-Inflammatory Agents

Decreased Effect
Vancomycin may decrease the levels/effects of: BCG; Typhoid Vaccine

Stability Prior to reconstitution, store dry powder at 20° to 25°C (68° to 77°F). After reconstitution, refrigerate and use within 96 hours; incompatible with heparin, phenobarbital, and ceftazidime. Capsules should be stored at controlled room temperature 59° to 86°F (15° to 30°C).

Mechanism of Action Inhibits bacterial cell wall synthesis; alters bacterial-cell-membrane permeability; blocks glycopeptide polymerization of the phosphodisaccharide-pentapeptide complex in the second stage of cell wall synthesis by binding tightly to D-alanyl-D-alanine portion of cell wall precursor

Pharmacodynamics Displays time-dependent antimicrobial killing; slowly bacteriocidal

Pharmacokinetics (Adult data unless noted)
Absorption:
Oral: Poor
I.M.: Erratic
Intraperitoneal administration can result in 38% systemic absorption
Distribution: Widely distributed in body tissues and fluids including pericardial, pleural, ascites, and synovial fluids; low concentration in CSF (improved if meninges are inflamed)
Protein binding: 55%
Metabolism: <3%
Half-life, biphasic: Prolonged significantly with reduced renal function
Terminal:
Newborns: 6-10 hours
3 months to 4 years: 4 hours
>3 years: 2.2-3 hours
Adults: 5-8 hours

Elimination: Primarily via glomerular filtration; excreted as unchanged drug in the urine (80% to 90%); oral doses are excreted primarily in the feces; presence of malignancy in children is associated with an increase in vancomycin clearance
Dialysis: Not dialyzable (0% to 5%)

Usual Dosage Initial dosage recommendation (see Reference Range for target concentrations based on MIC data): **Note:** Doses require adjustment in renal impairment:
Neonates: I.V.:
Postnatal age ≤7 days:
<1200 g: 15 mg/kg/dose every 24 hours
1200-2000 g: 10-15 mg/kg/dose every 12-18 hours
>2000 g: 10-15 mg/kg/dose every 8-12 hours
Postnatal age >7 days:
<1200 g: 15 mg/kg/dose every 24 hours
1200-2000 g: 10-15 mg/kg/dose every 8-12 hours
>2000 g: 15-20 mg/kg/dose every 8 hours
Infants >1 month and Children:
I.V.:
Traditional dosing: 10 mg/kg/dose every 6 hours
Note: Nonobese pediatric cancer patients with normal renal function: 15 mg/kg/dose every 6 hours has been studied (n=28, age: 9 months to 13 years) (see Chang, 1994)
Alternative dosing (serious infection, empiric treatment of MRSA, or organisms with an MIC = 1 mcg/mL): 15-20 mg/kg/dose every 6-8 hours
Note: Every 6 hour dosing recommended as initial dosage regimen if targeting trough serum concentrations >10 mcg/mL (see Benner, 2009; Frymoyer, 2009). Close monitoring of serum concentrations and assurance of adequate hydration status is recommended.
Prophylaxis of endocarditis in penicillin allergic patients for GI or genitourinary procedures: 20 mg/kg over 1 hour; complete infusion 30 minutes prior to the procedure (see Wilson, 2007):
Intrathecal/intraventricular:
Neonates: 5-10 mg/day
Children: 5-20 mg/day
Oral (antibiotic-associated pseudomembraneous colitis):
Note: Metronidazole is initial drug of choice (see Red Book, 2009): Children: 10 mg/kg/dose every 6 hours for 7-10 days; not to exceed 2 g/day
Adults: Indication-specific dosing: Initial intravenous dosing should be based on actual body weight; subsequent dosing adjusted based on serum trough vancomycin concentrations.
Susceptible (MIC ≤1 mcg/mL) gram-positive infections: I.V.: 15-20 mg/kg/dose (usual: 750-1500 mg) every 8-12 hours (see Rybak, 2009)
Complicated infections in seriously ill patients: I.V.: Loading dose: 25-30 mg/kg (based on actual body weight) may be used to rapidly achieve target concentration; then 15-20 mg/kg/dose every 8-12 hours (see Rybak, 2009)
Catheter-related infections: Antibiotic lock technique (see Mermel, 2009): 2 mg/mL ± 10 units heparin/mL **or** 2.5 mg/mL ± 2500 **or** 5000 units heparin/mL **or** 5 mg/mL ± 5000 units heparin/mL (preferred regimen); instill into catheter port with a volume sufficient to fill the catheter (2-5 mL). **Note:** May use SWFI/NS or D$_5$W as diluents. Do not mix with any other solutions. Dwell times generally should not exceed 48 hours before renewal of lock solution. Remove lock solution prior to catheter use, then replace.
Colitis (C. difficile): Oral:
Manufacturer recommendations: 500-2000 mg/day in 3-4 divided doses for 7-10 days (usual dose: 125-500 mg every 6 hours)

IDSA guideline recommendations:
Severe infection: 125 mg 4 times/day for 10-14 days
Severe, complicated infection: 500 mg 4 times/day with or without concurrent I.V. metronidazole. May consider vancomycin retention enema (in patients with complete ileus) (see Cohen, 2010).

Enterocolitis *(S. aureus)*: Oral: 500-2000 mg/day in 3-4 divided doses for 7-10 days (usual dose: 125-500 mg every 6 hours)

Endophthalmitis: Intravitreal: Usual dose: 1 mg/0.1 mL NS instilled into vitreum; may repeat administration if necessary in 3-4 days, usually in combination with ceftazidime or an aminoglycoside. **Note:** Some clinicians have recommended using a lower dose of 0.2 mg/0.1 mL, based on concerns for retinotoxicity.

Hospital-acquired pneumonia (HAP): I.V.: 15 mg/kg/ dose every 12 hours (American Thoracic Society [ATS] 2005 guidelines)

Meningitis (*Pneumococcus* or *Staphylococcus*):
I.V.: 30-60 mg/kg/day in divided doses every 8-12 hours (see Rybak, 2009) **or** 500-750 mg every 6 hours (with third-generation cephalosporin for PCN-resistant *Streptococcus pneumoniae*)
Intrathecal: 5-20 mg/day

Prophylaxis against infective endocarditis: I.V.:
Dental, oral, or upper respiratory tract surgery: 1 g 1 hour before surgery. **Note:** AHA guidelines now recommend prophylaxis only in patients undergoing invasive procedures and in whom underlying cardiac conditions may predispose to a higher risk of adverse outcomes should infection occur.
GI/GU procedure: 1 g plus 1.5 mg/kg gentamicin 1 hour prior to surgery. **Note:** As of April 2007, routine prophylaxis no longer recommended by the AHA.

Dosing interval in renal impairment: Adult: Vancomycin concentrations should be monitored in patients with any renal impairment:
Cl_{cr} >50 mL/minute: Start with 15-20 mg/kg/dose (usual: 750-1500 mg) every 8-12 hours
Cl_{cr} 20-49 mL/minute: Start with 15-20 mg/kg/dose (usual: 750-1500 mg) every 24 hours
Cl_{cr} <20 mL/minute: Will need longer intervals; determine by serum concentration monitoring

Note: In the critically ill patient with renal insufficiency, the initial loading dose (25-30 mg/kg) should not be reduced; however, subsequent dosage adjustments should be made based on renal function and trough serum concentrations.

Dialysis:
Hemodialysis (HD): Following loading dose of 15-20 mg/ kg, give 500 mg to 1 g after each dialysis session, depending on factors such as HD membrane type and flow rate; monitor levels closely
Continuous ambulatory peritoneal dialysis (CAPD):
Administration via CAPD fluid: 15-30 mg/L (15-30 mcg/mL) of CAPD fluid
Systemic: 1 g loading dose, followed by 500 mg to 1 g every 48-72 hours with close monitoring of levels

Administration

Oral: May further dilute oral solution dose in water or with a flavoring syrup to improve the taste
Parenteral: Administer vancomycin by I.V. intermittent infusion over 60 minutes at a final concentration not to exceed 5 mg/mL; if a maculopapular rash appears on face, neck, trunk, and upper extremities, slow the infusion rate to administer dose over 90-120 minutes and increase the dilution volume; the reaction usually dissipates in 30-60 minutes; administration of antihistamines just before the infusion may also prevent or minimize this reaction
Intrathecal/Intraventricular: Dilute in NS without preservatives to a final concentration between 2-5 mg/mL

Monitoring Parameters Periodic renal function tests (especially when targeting higher serum concentrations), urinalysis, serum vancomycin concentrations, WBC; audiogram (in patients who concurrently receive ototoxic chemotherapy); fluid status

Reference Range Measure trough serum concentrations to assess efficacy. Peak concentrations may be helpful in the setting of atypical pharmacokinetic profile. Trough serum concentration typically obtained at steady state (ie, prior to the fourth dose). Target trough serum concentration may vary depending on organism, MIC, source of infection, and/or other patient factors (see Rybak, 2009).
15-20 mcg/mL: For organisms with an MIC = 1 mcg/mL or complicated infections (bacteremia, endocarditis, osteomyelitis, meningitis, and hospital-acquired pneumonia caused by *Staphylococcus aureus*)
10-15 mcg/mL: Current recommendation for all other infections with an organism with an MIC <1 mcg/mL
5-10 mcg/mL: Traditional recommendation; may be adequate to treat some infections based on site and MIC; however, this range is not recommended in the adult guidelines for vancomycin use due to resistance development potential
Note: Although AUC/MIC is the preferred method to determine clinical effectiveness, trough serum concentrations may be used as a surrogate marker and is recommended as the most accurate and practical method of vancomycin monitoring.

Patient Information Report pain at infusion site; dizziness, fullness, or ringing in ears with I.V. use

Nursing Implications Do not administer I.M.; ensure adequate hydration; troughs are obtained just before the next dose

Additional Information

When treating pathogens with a vancomycin MIC ≥2 mcg/ mL, alternative antibiotics should be considered.

Dosage Forms Excipient information presented when available (limited, particularly for generics); consult specific product labeling.
Capsule (Vancocin®): 125 mg, 250 mg
Infusion [premixed in iso-osmotic dextrose] (Vancocin®): 500 mg (100 mL); 1 g (200 mL)
Injection, powder for reconstitution: 500 mg, 1 g, 5 g, 10 g

References

American Academy of Pediatrics Committee on Infectious Diseases, "Treatment of Bacterial Meningitis," *Pediatrics*, 1988, 81(6):904-7.

American Thoracic Society and Infectious Diseases Society of America, "Guidelines for the Management of Adults With Hospital-Acquired, Ventilator-Associated, and Healthcare-Associated Pneumonia," *Am J Respir Crit Care Med*, 2005, 171(4):388-416.

Benner KW, Worthington MA, Kimberlin DW, et al, "Correlation of Vancomycin Dosing to Serum Concentrations in Pediatric Patients: A Retrospective Database Review," *J Pediatr Pharmacol Ther*, 2009, 14:86-93.

Chang D, "Influence of Malignancy on the Pharmacokinetics of Vancomycin in Infants and Children," *Pediatr Infect Dis J*, 1995, 14 (8):667-73.

Chang D, Liem L, and Malogolowkin M, "A Prospective Study of Vancomycin Pharmacokinetics and Dosage Requirements in Pediatric Cancer Patients," *Pediatr Infect Dis J*, 1994, 13(11):969-74.

Cohen SH, Gerding DN, Johnson S, et al, "Clinical Practice Guidelines for *Clostridium difficile* Infection in Adults: 2010 Update by the Society for Healthcare Epidemiology of America (SHEA) and the Infectious Diseases Society of America (IDSA)," *Infect Control Hosp Epidemiol*, 2010, 31(5):431-55.

Frymoyer A, Hersh AL, Benet LZ, et al, "Current Recommended Dosing of Vancomycin for Children With Invasive Methicillin-Resistant *Staphylococcus aureus* Infections Is Inadequate," *Pediatr Infect Dis J*, 2009, 28(5):398-402.

Leonard MB, Koren G, Stevenson DK, et al, "Vancomycin Pharmacokinetics in Very Low Birth Weight Neonates," *Pediatr Infect Dis J*, 1989, 8(5):282-6.

Matzke GR, Zhanel GG, and Guay DRP, "Clinical Pharmacokinetics of Vancomycin," *Clin Pharmacokinet*, 1986, 11(4):257-82.

Mermel LA, Allon M, Bouza E, et al, "Clinical Practice Guidelines for the Diagnosis and Management of Intravascular Catheter-Related Infection: 2009 Update by the Infectious Diseases Society of America," *Clin Infect Dis*, 2009, 49(1):1-45.

Red Book: 2009 Report of the Committee on Infectious Diseases, 28th ed, Pickering LK, ed, Elk Grove Village, IL: American Academy of Pediatrics, 2009. Available at: http://aapredbook.aappublications.org/cgi/content/full/2009/1/1.7.13.

Rodvold KA, Everett JA, Pryka RD, and Kraus DM, "Pharmacokinetics and Administration Regimens of Vancomycin in Neonates, Infants and Children," *Clin Pharmacokinet,* 1997, 33(1):32-51.

Rybak MJ, Albrecht LM, Boike SC, et al, "Nephrotoxicity of Vancomycin, Alone and With an Aminoglycoside," *J Antimicrob Chemother,* 1990, 25(4):679-87.

Rybak M, Lomaestro B, Rotschafer JC, et al, "Therapeutic Monitoring of Vancomycin in Adult Patients: A Consensus Review of the American Society of Health-System Pharmacists, the Infectious Diseases Society of America, and the Society of Infectious Diseases Pharmacists," *Am J Health-Syst Pharm,* 2009, 66(1):82-98

Wilson W, Taubert KA, Gewitz M, et al, "Prevention of Infective Endocarditis: Guidelines From the American Heart Association: A Guideline From the American Heart Association Rheumatic Fever, Endocarditis, and Kawasaki Disease Committee, Council on Cardiovascular Disease in the Young, and the Council on Clinical Cardiology, Council on Cardiovascular Surgery and Anesthesia, and the Quality of Care and Outcomes Research Interdisciplinary Working Group," *Circulation,* 2007, 116(15):1736-54. Available at: http://circ.ahajournals.org/cgi/reprint/CIRCULATIONAHA.106.183095v1.

◆ **Vancomycin Hydrochloride** *see* Vancomycin *on page 1404*

◆ **Vandazole®** *see* MetroNIDAZOLE *on page 921*

◆ **Vanos™** *see* Fluocinonide *on page 595*

◆ **Vantin** *see* Cefpodoxime *on page 270*

◆ **VAQTA®** *see* Hepatitis A Vaccine *on page 672*

◆ **VAR** *see* Varicella Virus Vaccine *on page 1407*

◆ **Varicella, Measles, Mumps, and Rubella Vaccine** *see* Measles, Mumps, Rubella, and Varicella Virus Vaccine *on page 864*

Varicella Virus Vaccine
(var i SEL a VYE rus vak SEEN)

Medication Safety Issues
Sound-alike/look-alike issues:
Varicella virus vaccine has been given in error (instead of the indicated varicella immune globulin) to pregnant women exposed to varicella.

Both varicella vaccine and zoster vaccine are live, attenuated strains of varicella-zoster virus. Their indications, dosing, and composition are distinct. Varicella is indicated in children to prevent chickenpox, while zoster vaccine is indicated in older individuals to prevent reactivation of the virus which causes shingles. Zoster vaccine is **not** a substitute for varicella vaccine and should not be used in children.

Related Information
Immunization Guidelines *on page 1636*

U.S. Brand Names Varivax®

Canadian Brand Names Varilrix®; Varivax® III

Therapeutic Category Vaccine

Generic Available No

Use Immunization against varicella in children ≥12 months of age and adults who do not have evidence of immunity. Vaccination is especially important for the following: Persons with close contact to those at high risk for severe disease; persons living or working in environments where transmission is likely (teachers, childcare workers, residents and staff of institutional settings); persons in environments where transmission has been reported; nonpregnant women of childbearing age; adolescents and adults in households with children; and international travelers.

Postexposure prophylaxis: Vaccination within 3 days (possibly 5 days) after exposure to rash is effective in preventing illness or modifying severity of disease.

Pregnancy Risk Factor C

Pregnancy Considerations Animal reproduction studies have not been conducted. Varivax® should not be administered to pregnant females and pregnancy should be avoided for 3 months (per manufacturer labeling; 1 month per ACIP) following vaccination. A pregnancy registry has been established for pregnant women exposed to varicella virus vaccine (800-986-8999). Varicella disease during the 1st or 2nd trimesters may result in congenital varicella syndrome. The onset of maternal varicella infection from 5 days prior to 2 days after delivery may cause varicella infection in the newborn. All women should be assessed for immunity during a prenatal visit; those without evidence of immunity should be vaccinated upon completion or termination of pregnancy.

Lactation Excretion in breast milk unknown/use caution

Contraindications Hypersensitivity to any component of the vaccine, including gelatin; a history of anaphylactoid reaction to neomycin; individuals with blood dyscrasias, leukemia, lymphomas, or other malignant neoplasms affecting the bone marrow or lymphatic systems; those receiving immunosuppressive therapy; primary and acquired immunodeficiency states including those who are immunosuppressed in association with HIV; a family history of congenital or hereditary immunodeficiency; active untreated tuberculosis; current febrile illness; pregnancy

Warnings Immediate treatment for anaphylactoid reaction should be available during vaccine use; salicylates should be avoided for 6 weeks after vaccination; defer vaccination at least 3 months after receiving blood and plasma transfusions or immune globulin (See Appendix Immunization Guidelines, "Suggested Intervals Between Administration of Antibody-Containing Products for Different Indications and Measles-Containing Vaccine and Varicella-Containing Vaccine"); vaccinated individuals should not have close association with susceptible high risk individuals (newborns, pregnant women, immunocompromised persons) for 6 weeks following vaccination. Children with HIV infection, who are asymptomatic and not immunosuppressed (CDC immunologic category 1) may receive varicella vaccine at 12-15 months of age or older.

Precautions Routine prophylactic administration of acetaminophen to prevent fever due to vaccines has been shown to decrease the immune response of some vaccines; the clinical significance of this reduction in immune response has not been established (see Prymula, 2009).

Adverse Reactions **All serious adverse reactions must be reported to the U.S. Department of Health and Human Services (DHHS) Vaccine Adverse Event Reporting System (VAERS) 1-800-822-7967.**

Central nervous system: Fever (10% to 15%), chills, fatigue, headache, irritability, malaise, nervousness, sleep disturbance, febrile and nonfebrile seizures, cerebellar ataxia, Bell's palsy, cerebrovascular accident, dizziness, encephalitis, aseptic meningitis

Dermatologic: Generalized varicella-like rash (4% to 5%), contact rash, dermatitis, diaper rash, dry skin, eczema, heat rash, itching, cellulitis, erythema multiforme, Henoch-Schönlein purpura, impetigo, Stevens-Johnson syndrome, secondary skin infections

Gastrointestinal: Abdominal pain, appetite decreased, cold/canker sore, constipation, nausea, vomiting, diarrhea

Hepatic: Hepatitis

Hematologic: Lymphadenopathy, thrombocytopenia

Local: Injection site reaction (19% to 24%), varicella-like rash at the injection site (3%)

Neuromuscular & skeletal: Arthralgia, myalgia, stiff neck, paresthesia, Guillain-Barré syndrome, transverse myelitis, hemiparesis (acute)

Ophthalmic: Eye complaints

Otic: Otitis

Respiratory: Cough, lower and upper respiratory illness, pneumonitis, pharyngitis

Miscellaneous: Allergic reactions, teething, herpes zoster

Drug Interactions

Avoid Concomitant Use

Avoid concomitant use of Varicella Virus Vaccine with any of the following: Immunosuppressants

Increased Effect/Toxicity

The levels/effects of Varicella Virus Vaccine may be increased by: 5-ASA Derivatives; Immunosuppressants; Salicylates; Smallpox Vaccine

Decreased Effect

Varicella Virus Vaccine may decrease the levels/effects of: Tuberculin Tests

The levels/effects of Varicella Virus Vaccine may be decreased by: Immune Globulins; Immunosuppressants

Stability Powder stable refrigerated for 18 months; may also be frozen. If transferred to refrigerator from freezer, do not refreeze. Protect from light; store diluent separately at room temperature or in refrigerator. Discard reconstituted vaccine if not used within 30 minutes; do not freeze reconstituted vaccine.

Mechanism of Action As a live, attenuated vaccine, varicella virus vaccine offers active immunity to disease caused by the varicella-zoster virus

Pharmacodynamics Onset of action: Seroconversion: ~4-6 weeks

Usual Dosage SubQ:

Children: Initial dose: Minimum age 12 months: 0.5 mL

Booster dose: 4-6 years: 0.5 mL (second dose may be administered prior to age 4-6 years if >3 months since initial dose and both doses are administered at age >12 months. If second dose was administered >28 days following the first dose, the second dose does not need to be repeated.

Children 7-13 years: Initial 0.5 mL followed by second dose at least 3 months later; do not repeat the second dose if administered >28 days following the first dose

Children >13 years to Adult: 0.5 mL followed by a second dose at least 4 weeks later

Administration Use 0.7 mL of the provided diluent to reconstitute vaccine. Gently agitate to mix thoroughly. Total volume of reconstituted vaccine will be ~0.5 mL. Inject into the outer aspect of the upper arm or anterolateral aspect of the thigh; **not for I.V. or I.M. administration**.

Monitoring Parameters Rash, fever

Patient Information Report any adverse reactions to your healthcare provider or Vaccine Adverse Event Reporting System (1-800-822-7967); avoid pregnancy for 3 months following vaccination; avoid salicylates for 6 weeks after vaccination; avoid close association with susceptible high risk individuals following vaccination

Nursing Implications Federal law requires that the date of administration, the vaccine manufacturer, lot number of vaccine, and the administering person's name, title and address be entered into the patient's permanent medical record.

Additional Information In order to maximize vaccination rates, the ACIP recommends simultaneous administration of all age-appropriate vaccines (live or inactivated) for which a person is eligible at a single visit, unless contraindications exist. The use of combination vaccines is generally preferred over separate infections, taking into consideration provider assessment, patient preference, and potential adverse events.

For additional information, please refer to the following website: http://www.cdc.gov/vaccines/vpd-vac/.

Dosage Forms Excipient information presented when available (limited, particularly for generics); consult specific product labeling. [CAN] = Canadian brand name

Injection, powder for reconstitution [preservative free]:

Varivax®: 1350 plaque-forming units (PFU) [contains gelatin and trace amounts of neomycin; packaged with diluent]

Varivax® III [CAN]: 1350 plaque-forming units (PFU) [contains gelatin and trace amounts of neomycin; packaged with diluent; not available in U.S.]

Injection, powder for reconstitution (Valrilix® [CAN]): $10^{3.3}$ plaque-forming units (PFU) [contains albumin and gelatin; packaged with diluent; not available in U.S.]

References

American Academy of Pediatrics Committee on Infectious Diseases, "Recommended Immunization Schedules for Children and Adolescents – United States, 2007," *Pediatrics*, 2007, 119(1):207-8.

Centers for Disease Control and Prevention (CDC), "General Recommendations on Immunization. Recommendations of the Advisory Committee on Immunization Practices (ACIP)," *MMWR Recomm Rep*, 2006, 55(RR-15):1-48. Available at: http://www.cdc.gov/mmwr/preview/mmwrhtml/rr5515a1.htm.

Kuter BJ, Weibel RE, Guess HA, et al, "Oka/Merck Varicella Vaccine in Healthy Children: Final Report of a 2-Year Efficacy Study and 7-Year Follow-Up Studies," *Vaccine*, 1991, 9(9):643-7.

Marin M, Güris D, Chaves SS, et al, "Prevention of Varicella: Recommendations of the Advisory Committee on Immunization Practices (ACIP)," *MMWR Recomm Rep*, 2007, 56(RR-4):1-40.

Prymula R, Siegrist CA, Chlibek R, et al, "Effect of Prophylactic Paracetamol Administration at Time of Vaccination on Febrile Reactions and Antibody Responses in Children: Two Open-Label, Randomised Controlled Trials," *Lancet*, 2009, 374(9698):1339-50.

U.S. Public Health Service (USPHS), Infectious Diseases Society of America (IDSA), USPHS/IDSA Prevention of Opportunistic Infections Working Group, "2001 USPHS/IDSA Guidelines for the Prevention of Opportunistic Infections in Persons Infected With Human Immunodeficiency Virus," *HIV Clin Trials*, 2001, 2(6):493-554.

Varicella-Zoster Immune Globulin (Human)

(var i SEL a- ZOS ter i MYUN GLOB yoo lin HYU man)

Medication Safety Issues

Sound-alike/look-alike issues:

Varicella virus vaccine has been given in error (instead of the indicated varicella immune globulin) to pregnant women exposed to varicella.

Canadian Brand Names VariZIG™

Therapeutic Category Immune Globulin

Generic Available No

Use Provide passive immunity to susceptible, immunocompromised patients after exposure to varicella.

Restrict administration to those patients meeting the following criteria:

Neoplastic disease (eg, leukemia or lymphoma)

Congenital or acquired immunodeficiency

Immunosuppressive therapy with steroids, antineoplastic agents, radiation, or other immunosuppressive treatment regimens

Newborn of mother who had onset of chickenpox within 5 days before delivery or within 48 hours after delivery

Premature (≥28 weeks gestation) whose mother has no history of chickenpox

Premature (<28 weeks gestation or ≤1000 g) regardless of maternal history

One of the following types of exposure to varicella or zoster may warrant VZIG administration in a susceptible patient:

Continuous household contact

Playmate contact (>1 hour play indoors)

Hospital contact (in same 2-4 bed room or adjacent beds in a large ward or prolonged face-to-face contact with an infectious staff member or patient)

Immunocompromised adolescents and adults and to other older patients on an individual basis

Note: Age is the most important risk factor for reactivation of varicella zoster; persons <50 years of age have incidence of 2.5 cases per 1000, whereas those 60-79 have 6.5 cases per 1000 and those >80 years have 10 cases per 1000.

Restrictions Varicella-zoster immune globulin (VZIG) was discontinued in the United States in 2005. It is currently available as VariZIG™ under an Investigational New Drug Application Expanded Access protocol. Inventory for anticipated patients may be obtained by contacting FFF Enterprises at 800-843-7477 and faxing a release form. The release form can be accessed from the CDC (available at http://www.fda.gov/cber/infosheets/mphvzig020806.htm). VariZIG™ may also be prepositioned at qualified sites.

Pregnancy Considerations Animal reproduction studies have not been conducted. Clinical use of other immunoglobulins suggest that there are no adverse effects on the fetus. Pregnant women who do not have evidence of immunity to varicella may be at increased risk of infection following exposure. VZIG is used to prevent maternal complications, not fetal infection.

Lactation Excretion in breast milk unknown/use caution

Contraindications Hypersensitivity to VZIG, immune globulin, or any component; patients with IgA deficiency; known immunity to varicella zoster virus (prior infection or immunization). **Note:** U.S. CDC guidelines: Healthy and immunocompromised patients [except bone marrow transplant recipients (BMT)] with positive history of varicella infection are considered immune. BMT patients who had varicella infection *prior to* transplant are not considered immune; however, the expanded access protocol does not include use for this indication. BMT patients who develop varicella infection *after* transplant *are* considered immune. Patients who are fully vaccinated, but later became immunocompromised should be monitored closely; treatment with VZIG is not indicated, but other therapy may be needed if disease occurs.

Warnings VZIG is not indicated for prophylaxis or therapy of normal adults who are exposed to or who develop varicella; not indicated for treatment of herpes zoster. Hypersensitivity and anaphylactic reactions can occur; immediate treatment (including epinephrine 1:1000) should be available. Reactions can occur in patients with IgA deficiency or hypersensitivity reactions to human globulin. Product of human plasma; may potentially contain infectious agents which could transmit disease. Screening of donors, as well as testing and/or inactivation or removal of certain viruses, reduces the risk. Infections thought to be transmitted by this product should be reported to the manufacturer (Cangene Corporation 800-768-2304). Thrombotic events have been reported with administration of intravenous immune globulin; use with caution in patients with cardiovascular risk factors. I.M. administration may be preferred in this patient population. Acute renal dysfunction (increased serum creatinine, oliguria, acute renal failure) can rarely occur; usually within 7 days of use (more likely with products stabilized with sucrose); VariZIG™ does not contain sucrose. Use with caution in the elderly, patients with renal disease, diabetes mellitus, volume depletion, sepsis, paraproteinemia, and nephrotoxic medications due to risk of renal dysfunction. Noncardiogenic pulmonary edema has been reported with intravenous administration of immune globulin; monitor for transfusion-related acute lung injury (TRALI). Use caution with pre-existing respiratory conditions. I.M. administration may be preferred in this patient population.

Precautions Use of VZIG in patients with a bleeding diathesis should be avoided. Not for prophylactic use in immunodeficient patients with history of varicella, unless patient's immunosuppression is associated with bone marrow transplantation; not recommended for nonimmunodeficient patients, including pregnant women, because the severity of chickenpox is much less than in immunosuppressed patients; patients receiving monthly treatments of high-dose intravenous immunoglobulins (100-400 mg/kg) are likely to be protected and probably do not require VZIG if the last dose of IVIG was given in the 3 weeks before exposure

Adverse Reactions

Central nervous system: Fever, headache, chills, malaise

Dermatologic: Rash, angioedema

Gastrointestinal: Emesis

Local effects: Pain, redness, swelling

Neuromuscular & skeletal: Myalgia

Miscellaneous: Hypersensitivity reactions, anaphylaxis

Drug Interactions

Avoid Concomitant Use There are no known interactions where it is recommended to avoid concomitant use.

Increased Effect/Toxicity There are no known significant interactions involving an increase in effect.

Decreased Effect

Varicella-Zoster Immune Globulin (Human) may decrease the levels/effects of: Vaccines (Live)

Stability Refrigerate; do not freeze

Mechanism of Action The varicella-zoster antibody present in VZIG provides passive immunity to susceptible immunodeficient patients exposed to the varicella-zoster virus by neutralizing the virus.

Pharmacokinetics (Adult data unless noted) Duration: 3 weeks

Usual Dosage Children and Adults: I.M.: Most effective if administered within 48-96 hours after exposure: 125 units/10 kg; maximum dose: 625 units; minimum dose: 125 units; do not give fractional doses

VZIG Dose Based on Patient Weight:
<10 kg: 125 units = 1 x 125 unit vial
10.1-20 kg: 250 units = 2 x 125 unit vials
20.1-30 kg: 375 units = 3 x 125 unit vials
30.1-40 kg: 500 units = 4 x 125 unit vials
>40 kg: 625 units = 5 x 125 unit vials or 1 x 625 unit vial

Note: High-risk, susceptible patients who are re-exposed more than 3 weeks after a prior dose of VZIG should receive another full dose; there is no evidence VZIG modifies established varicella-zoster infections

Administration Parenteral: I.M.: **DO NOT ADMINISTER I.V.** For infants and small children, administer I.M. into the anterolateral aspect of the thigh. For adults and older children, administer I.M. into the deltoid muscle or the anterolateral aspect of the thigh. For adults who require large dose volumes, may administer by deep I.M. injection into the upper, outer quadrant of the gluteal muscle. For patients ≤10 kg, administer 1.25 mL at a single site; for patients >10 kg, give no more than 2.5 mL at a single injection site.

Test Interactions False positive serologic test for immunity to varicella-zoster virus (false positive can occur for 2 months after VZIG administration)

Additional Information An acceptable alternative to VZIG prophylaxis is to treat varicella, if it occurs, with high-dose I.V. acyclovir. In susceptible children and adults for whom the varicella vaccine is not contraindicated, live varicella virus vaccine can be given within 3 to 5 days after exposure to prevent or modify infection severity. There is no evidence VZIG modifies established varicella-zoster infections.

Varicella-zoster immune globulin (VZIG) was discontinued by the manufacturer. An investigational product (VariZIG) is available under the product's IND application. Investigational Review Board (IRB) approval for this agent should be in place before accessing this product. Eligible patients include pregnant women, immunocompromised patients, neonates, or premature infants in selected situations. Inventory for anticipated patients may be obtained by contacting FFF Enterprises at 800-843-7477 and faxing a release form. The release form can be accessed from the CDC at http://www.cdc.gov/mmwr/preview/mmwrhtml/mm55e224a1.htm.

Dosage Forms Excipient information presented when available (limited, particularly for generics); consult specific product labeling. [CAN = Canadian brand name]

Injection, powder for reconstitution [preservative free]:

VariZIG™ [CAN]: 125 int. units [package with diluent] [available in the U.S under expanded access protocol]

References

Centers for Disease Control and Prevention (CDC), "Prevention of Varicella: Recommendations of the Advisory Committee on Immunization Practices (ACIP), Centers for Disease Control and Prevention," *MMWR*, 1996, 45(RR-11):1-36.

Centers for Disease Control and Prevention (CDC), "Prevention of Varicella Update: Recommendations of the Advisory Committee on Immunization Practices (ACIP)," *MMWR*, 1999, 48(RR-6):1-5.

◆ **Varicella-Zoster Virus (VZV) Vaccine (Varicella)** *see* Varicella Virus Vaccine *on page 1407*

◆ **Varilrix® (Can)** *see* Varicella Virus Vaccine *on page 1407*

◆ **Varivax®** *see* Varicella Virus Vaccine *on page 1407*

◆ **Varivax® III (Can)** *see* Varicella Virus Vaccine *on page 1407*

◆ **VariZIG™ (Can)** *see* Varicella-Zoster Immune Globulin (Human) *on page 1408*

◆ **Vasocon® (Can)** *see* Naphazoline *on page 966*

Vasopressin (vay soe PRES in)

Medication Safety Issues

Use care when prescribing and/or administering vasopressin solutions. Close attention should be given to concentration of solution, route of administration, dose, and rate of administration (units/minute, units/kg/minute, units/kg/hour).

Related Information

Adult ACLS Algorithms *on page 1463*

Extravasation Treatment *on page 1522*

U.S. Brand Names Pitressin®

Canadian Brand Names Pressyn®; Pressyn® AR

Therapeutic Category Antidiuretic Hormone Analog; Hormone, Posterior Pituitary

Generic Available Yes

Use Treatment of diabetes insipidus; prevention and treatment of postoperative abdominal distention; differential diagnosis of diabetes insipidus; adjunct in the treatment of acute massive hemorrhage of GI tract or esophageal varices; treatment of pulseless arrest, ventricular fibrillation or tachycardia, asystole/pulseless electrical activity, and vasodilator shock with hypotension unresponsive to fluid resuscitation or exogenous catecholamines

Pregnancy Risk Factor C

Pregnancy Considerations Animal reproduction studies have not been conducted. Vasopressin and desmopressin have been used safely during pregnancy based on case reports.

Lactation Enters breast milk/use caution

Breast-Feeding Considerations Based on case reports, vasopressin and desmopressin have been used safely during nursing.

Contraindications Hypersensitivity to vasopressin or any component

Warnings I.V. infiltration may lead to severe vasoconstriction and localized tissue necrosis

Precautions Use with caution in patients with seizure disorders, migraine, asthma, vascular disease, renal disease, cardiac disease, goiter with cardiac complications, arteriosclerosis, chronic nephritis with nitrogen retention; an increased risk of cardiac arrest has been reported in adults receiving I.V. infusions at rates >0.05 units/minute

Adverse Reactions

Cardiovascular: Circumoral pallor; with high doses: hypertension, bradycardia, arrhythmias, venous thrombosis, vasoconstriction, angina, heart block, cardiac arrest, distal limb ischemia (I.V. infusion rates >10 units/hour)

Central nervous system: Vertigo, fever, headache

Dermatologic: Urticaria

Endocrine & metabolic: Water intoxication, hyponatremia

Gastrointestinal: Abdominal cramps, nausea, vomiting, flatus, diarrhea

Local: Skin necrosis (after extravasation of I.V. infiltration)

Neuromuscular & skeletal: Tremor

Respiratory: Wheezing, bronchoconstriction

Miscellaneous: Diaphoresis

Drug Interactions

Avoid Concomitant Use There are no known interactions where it is recommended to avoid concomitant use.

Increased Effect/Toxicity There are no known significant interactions involving an increase in effect.

Decreased Effect There are no known significant interactions involving a decrease in effect.

Mechanism of Action Endogenous hormone released by the posterior pituitary gland in response to increases in plasma osmolarity or as a baroreflex in response to decreased blood pressure and/or blood volume; increases cyclic adenosine monophosphate (cAMP) which increases water permeability at the distal convoluted tubule and collecting duct resulting in decreased urine volume and increased urine osmolality; causes peristalsis by directly stimulating the smooth muscle in the GI tract (in doses greater than those required for its antidiuretic action); causes vasoconstriction (primarily of capillaries and small arterioles); directly stimulates receptors in pituitary gland resulting in increased ACTH production; may restore catecholamine sensitivity

Pharmacodynamics I.M., SubQ:

Onset of action: 1 hour

Duration: 2-8 hours

Pharmacokinetics (Adult data unless noted)

Destroyed by trypsin in GI tract, must be administered parenterally

Metabolism: Most of dose is rapidly metabolized in liver and kidney

Half-life: 10-35 minutes

Usual Dosage

Diabetes insipidus:

I.M., SubQ: (Highly variable dosage; titrate dosage based upon serum and urine sodium and osmolality in addition to fluid balance and urine output)

Children: 2.5-10 units 2-4 times/day

Adults: 5-10 units 2-4 times/day as needed (range: 5-60 units/day)

Continuous infusion: Children and Adults: Initial: 0.5 milliunit/kg/hour (0.0005 unit/kg/hour); double dosage as needed every 30 minutes to a maximum of 10 milliunit/kg/hour (0.01 units/kg/hour)

Pulseless arrest, ventricular fibrillation, or tachycardia:

Children: I.V.: Very limited case reports: 0.4 units/kg after traditional resuscitation methods and at least 2 doses of epinephrine have been used. (The American Heart Association does not recommend this use as there is insufficient evidence as yet.)

Adults: I.V., I.O.: 40 units as a single dose only (see Adult ACLS Algorithms on page 1463) (**Note:** May also be administered intratracheal at dose 2-2.5 times the I.V. dose)

GI hemorrhage: I.V. continuous infusion (may also be infused directly into the superior mesenteric artery):

Children: Initial: 0.002-0.005 units/kg/minute; titrate dose as needed; maximum dose: 0.01 units/kg/minute;

or as an alternative: Initial: 0.1 units/minute; increase by 0.05 units/minute to a maximum of:

<5 years: 0.2 units/minute

5-12 years: 0.3 units/minute

>12 years: 0.4 units/minute

If bleeding stops for 12 hours, then taper off over 24-48 hours

Adults: Initial: I.V.: 0.2-0.4 unit/minute, then titrate dose as needed (maximum dose: 0.9 units/minute); if bleeding stops, continue at same dose for 12 hours, taper off over 24-48 hours

Vasodilatory shock with hypotension unresponsive to fluid resuscitation and exogenous catecholamines: **Note:** Optimal dosage has not been clearly established in any patient population: I.V.:

Infants and Children: Limited study in 11 infants and children treated for profound hypotension following cardiac surgery: Initial: 0.0003-0.002 units/kg/minute (0.018-0.12 units/kg/hour); titrate to effect (see Rosenzweig, 1999)

Adults: Initial: 0.01-0.04 units/minute; titrate to effect (doses >0.04 units/minute have been associated with increased risk of cardiovascular side effects)

Note: Abrupt discontinuation of infusion may result in hypotension; to discontinue gradually taper infusion

Dosing adjustment in hepatic impairment: Some patients with cirrhosis respond to much lower doses

Administration Parenteral:

I.V.: Continuous infusion: Dilute in NS or D_5W to a final concentration of 0.1-1 unit/mL; see Usual Dosage for rate of infusion; infusion through central line is strongly recommended

I.M.: Administer without further dilution

Intratracheal: Administer then flush with 5-10 mL NS followed by several manual ventilations

Monitoring Parameters Fluid intake and output, urine specific gravity, urine and serum osmolality, serum and urine sodium; hemoglobin and hematocrit (GI bleeding)

Reference Range Vasopressin levels:

Basal: <4 pg/mL

Water deprivation: 10 pg/mL

Shock: 100-1000 pg/mL (biphasic response)

Patient Information Avoid alcohol

Nursing Implications Monitor injection site closely (I.V. infusion) to identify early signs of decreased perfusion

Dosage Forms Excipient information presented when available (limited, particularly for generics); consult specific product labeling.

Injection, solution: 20 units/mL (0.5 mL, 1 mL, 10 mL)

Pitressin®: 20 units/mL (1 mL)

References

"2005 American Heart Association Guidelines for Cardiopulmonary Resuscitation and Emergency Cardiovascular Care," *Circulation*, 2005, 112(24 Suppl): 1-211.

"2005 American Heart Association (AHA) Guidelines for Cardiopulmonary Resuscitation (CPR) and Emergency Cardiovascular Care (ECC) of Pediatric and Neonatal Patients: Pediatric Advanced Life Support," *Pediatrics*, 2006, 117(5):1005-28.

Hodges BM and Fraser G, "Vasopressin for Vasodilatory Shock," *Hosp Pharm*, 2002, 37(11):1149-57.

Koshman SL, Zed PJ, and Abu-Laban RB, "Vasopressin in Cardiac Arrest," *Ann Pharmacother*, 2005, 39(10):1687-92.

Liedel JL, et al, "The Successful Use of Vasopressin in Children With Hypotension," *Crit Care Med*, 2001, 29(12):A63.

Mann K, Berg RA, and Nadkarni V, "Beneficial Effects of Vasopressin in Prolonged Pediatric Cardiac Arrest: A Case Series," *Resuscitation*, 2002, 52(2): 149-56.

Rosenzweig EB, Starc TJ, Chen JM, et al, "Intravenous Arginine-Vasopressin in Children With Vasodilatory Shock After Cardiac Surgery," *Circulation*, 1999, 100(19 Suppl):II182-6.

Tuggle DW, Bennett KG, Scott J, et al, "Intravenous Vasopressin and Gastrointestinal Hemorrhage in Children," *J Pediatr Surg*, 1988, 23 (7):627-9.

♦ **Vasotec®** *see* Enalapril/Enalaprilat *on page 499*

♦ **Vasotec® I.V. (Can)** *see* Enalapril/Enalaprilat *on page 499*

♦ **Vaxigrip® (Can)** *see* Influenza Virus Vaccine (Inactivated) *on page 734*

♦ **Vectical™** *see* Calcitriol *on page 229*

Vecuronium (ve KYOO roe nee um)

Medication Safety Issues

Sound-alike/look-alike issues:

Vecuronium may be confused with valproate sodium, vancomycin

Norcuron® may be confused with Narcan®

High alert medication: The Institute for Safe Medication Practices (ISMP) includes this medication among its list of drugs which have a heightened risk of causing significant patient harm when used in error.

United States Pharmacopeia (USP) 2006: The Interdisciplinary Safe Medication Use Expert Committee of the USP has recommended the following:

- Hospitals, clinics, and other practice sites should institute special safeguards in the storage, labeling, and use of these agents and should include these safeguards in staff orientation and competency training.

- Healthcare professionals should be on high alert (especially vigilant) whenever a neuromuscular-blocking agent (NMBA) is stocked, ordered, prepared, or administered.

Canadian Brand Names Norcuron®

Therapeutic Category Neuromuscular Blocker Agent, Nondepolarizing; Skeletal Muscle Relaxant, Paralytic

Generic Available Yes

Use Adjunct to anesthesia, to facilitate endotracheal intubation, and provide skeletal muscle relaxation during surgery or mechanical ventilation

Pregnancy Risk Factor C

Pregnancy Considerations There are no adequate and well-controlled studies in pregnant women. Use in cesarean section has been reported. Umbilical venous concentrations were 11% of maternal. Use only if the potential benefit justifies the potential risk to the fetus.

Lactation Excretion in breast milk unknown/use caution

Contraindications Hypersensitivity to vecuronium or any component (see Warnings)

Warnings Ventilation must be supported during neuromuscular blockade; use only by individuals who are experienced in the maintenance of an adequate airway and respiratory support **[U.S. Boxed Warning]**. Commercially supplied diluent contains benzyl alcohol which may cause allergic reactions in susceptible individuals; large amounts of benzyl alcohol (≥99 mg/kg/day) have been associated with a potentially fatal toxicity ("gasping syndrome") in neonates; the "gasping syndrome" consists of metabolic acidosis, respiratory distress, gasping respirations, CNS dysfunction (including convulsions, intracranial hemorrhage), hypotension and cardiovascular collapse; *in vitro* and animal studies have shown that benzoate, a metabolite of benzyl alcohol, displaces bilirubin from protein binding sites; avoid use of benzyl alcohol containing diluent in neonates; SWI may be used for reconstitution in neonates

◀ **Precautions** Use with caution in patients with hepatic impairment, neuromuscular disease, myasthenia gravis; many clinical conditions may potentiate or antagonize neuromuscular blockade, see table.

Clinical Conditions Affecting Neuromuscular Blockade

Potentiation	Antagonism
Electrolyte abnormalities	Alkalosis
Severe hyponatremia	Hypercalcemia
Severe hypocalcemia	Demyelinating lesions
Severe hypokalemia	Peripheral neuropathies
Hypermagnesemia	Diabetes mellitus
Neuromuscular diseases	
Acidosis	
Acute intermittent	
porphyria	
Renal failure	
Hepatic failure	

Adverse Reactions Most frequent reactions are associated with prolongation of its pharmacologic effect
Cardiovascular: Arrhythmias, tachycardia, hypotension, hypertension
Dermatologic: Urticaria, rash
Neuromuscular & skeletal: Muscle weakness
Respiratory: Respiratory insufficiency, bronchospasm, apnea

Drug Interactions
  Avoid Concomitant Use
  Avoid concomitant use of Vecuronium with any of the following: QuiNINE
  Increased Effect/Toxicity
  Vecuronium may increase the levels/effects of: Cardiac Glycosides; Corticosteroids (Systemic); Onabotulinumtoxin A; Rimabotulinumtoxin B

  The levels/effects of Vecuronium may be increased by: Abobotulinumtoxin A; Aminoglycosides; Calcium Channel Blockers; Capreomycin; Colistimethate; Inhalational Anesthetics; Ketorolac; Ketorolac (Systemic); Lincosamide Antibiotics; Lithium; Loop Diuretics; Magnesium Salts; Polymyxin B; Procainamide; QuiNIDine; QuiNINE; Spironolactone; Tetracycline Derivatives; Vancomycin
  Decreased Effect
  The levels/effects of Vecuronium may be decreased by: Acetylcholinesterase Inhibitors; CarBAMazepine; Loop Diuretics; Phenytoin

Stability Stable for 5 days at room temperature when reconstituted with bacteriostatic water; stable for 24 hours at room temperature when reconstituted with preservative free SWI or other compatible I.V. fluid (dextrose, NS, or LR) (avoid preservatives in neonates); do not mix with alkaline drugs

Mechanism of Action Nondepolarizing neuromuscular blocker which blocks acetylcholine from binding to receptors on motor endplate thus inhibiting depolarization

Pharmacodynamics
Onset of action: Within 1-3 minutes
Duration (dose dependent): 30-40 minutes

Pharmacokinetics (Adult data unless noted)
Distribution: V_d:
  Infants: 0.36 L/kg
  Children: 0.2 L/kg
  Adults: 0.27 L/kg
Protein binding: 60% to 80%
Half-life, distribution: Adults: 4 minutes
Half-life, elimination:
  Infants: 65 minutes
  Children: 41 minutes
  Adults: 65-75 minutes
Elimination: Vecuronium bromide and its metabolite(s) appear to be excreted principally in feces via biliary elimination (50%); the drug and its metabolite(s) are also excreted in urine (25%); the rate of elimination is appreciably reduced with hepatic dysfunction but not with renal dysfunction

Usual Dosage I.V.:
Neonates: 0.1 mg/kg/dose; maintenance: 0.03-0.15 mg/kg/dose every 1-2 hours as needed
Infants >7 weeks to 1 year: 0.1 mg/kg/dose; repeat every hour as needed; may be administered as a continuous infusion at 1-1.5 mcg/kg/minute (0.06-0.09 mg/kg/hour)
Children >1 year: 0.1 mg/kg/dose; repeat every hour as needed; may be administered as a continuous infusion at 1.5-2.5 mcg/kg/minute (0.09-0.15 mg/kg/hour)
Adults: 0.1 mg/kg/dose; repeat every hour as needed; may be administered as a continuous infusion at 1.5-2 mcg/kg/minute (0.09-0.12 mg/kg/hour)
Dosing adjustment in hepatic impairment: Dose reductions are necessary in patients with cirrhosis or cholestasis

Administration Parenteral: I.V.: Dilute vial to a maximum concentration of 2 mg/mL and administer by rapid direct injection; for continuous infusion, dilute to a maximum concentration of 1 mg/mL in D_5W, NS, or LR; use SWI instead of provided diluent (contains benzyl alcohol) in neonates (see Warnings)

Monitoring Parameters Assisted ventilation status, heart rate, blood pressure, peripheral nerve stimulator measuring twitch response

Nursing Implications Does not alter the patient's state of consciousness; addition of sedation and analgesia is recommended

Additional Information Produces minimal, if any, histamine release

Dosage Forms Excipient information presented when available (limited, particularly for generics); consult specific product labeling.
Injection, powder for reconstitution, as bromide: 10 mg, 20 mg [may be supplied with diluent containing benzyl alcohol]

References
Martin LD, Bratton SL, and O'Rourke PP, "Clinical Uses and Controversies of Neuromuscular Blocking Agents in Infants and Children," *Crit Care Med*, 1999, 27(7):1358-68.

◆ **Velban** see VinBLAStine *on page 1423*

Venlafaxine (VEN la faks een)

Medication Safety Issues
Sound-alike/look-alike issues:
  Effexor® may be confused with Effexor XR®
Related Information
  Antidepressant Agents *on page 1484*
  Serotonin Syndrome *on page 1695*
U.S. Brand Names Effexor XR®; Effexor®
Canadian Brand Names CO Venlafaxine XR; Effexor® XR; Mylan-Venlafaxine XR; PMS-Venlafaxine XR; ratio-Venlafaxine XR; Riva-Venlafaxine XR; Sandoz-Venlafaxine XR; Teva-Venlafaxine XR
Therapeutic Category Antidepressant, Serotonin/Norepinephrine Reuptake Inhibitor
Generic Available Yes: Excludes extended release capsule
Use Treatment of depression, generalized anxiety disorder, social anxiety disorder (social phobia), panic disorder; prevention of recurrences/relapses of depression; has also been used to treat ADHD and autism in children and obsessive-compulsive disorder and chronic fatigue syndrome in adults
Medication Guide An FDA-approved patient medication guide, which is available with the product information and at http://www.fda.gov/downloads/Drugs/DrugSafety/ucm088586.pdf, must be dispensed with this medication for each new outpatient prescription and refill.

Pregnancy Risk Factor C

Pregnancy Considerations Venlafaxine is classified as pregnancy category C due to adverse effects observed in animal studies. Venlafaxine and its active metabolite ODV cross the human placenta. Neonatal seizures and neonatal abstinence syndrome have been noted in case reports following maternal use of venlafaxine during pregnancy. Nonteratogenic effects in the newborn following SSRI/SNRI exposure late in the third trimester include respiratory distress, cyanosis, apnea, seizures, temperature instability, feeding difficulty, vomiting, hypoglycemia, hyper- or hypotonia, hyper-reflexia, jitteriness, irritability, constant crying, and tremor. The long-term effects on neurobehavior have not been studied.

Due to pregnancy-induced physiologic changes, some pharmacokinetic parameters of venlafaxine may be altered. Women should be monitored for decreased efficacy. Women treated for major depression and who are euthymic prior to pregnancy are more likely to experience a relapse when medication is discontinued as compared to pregnant women who continue taking antidepressant medications. The ACOG recommends that therapy with SSRIs or SNRIs during pregnancy be individualized; treatment of depression during pregnancy should incorporate the clinical expertise of the mental health clinician, obstetrician, primary healthcare provider, and pediatrician. If treatment during pregnancy is required, consider tapering therapy during the third trimester in order to prevent withdrawal symptoms in the infant. If this is done and the woman is considered to be at risk of relapse from her major depressive disorder, the medication can be restarted following delivery, although the dose should be readjusted to that required before pregnancy. Treatment algorithms have been developed by the ACOG and the APA for the management of depression in women prior to conception and during pregnancy (Yonkers, 2009).

Lactation Enters breast milk/not recommended

Breast-Feeding Considerations Venlafaxine and ODV are found in human milk. Low concentrations of ODV have been found in the serum of nursing infants whose mothers are taking venlafaxine; venlafaxine has also been detected in some infants. Adverse events have not been observed; however, it is recommended to monitor the infant for adverse events if the decision to breast-feed has been made. The long-term effects on neurobehavior have not been studied, thus one should prescribe venlafaxine to a mother who is breast-feeding only when the benefits outweigh the potential risks. The manufacturer does not recommend breast-feeding during therapy.

Contraindications Hypersensitivity to venlafaxine or any component; use of MAO inhibitors within 14 days (potentially fatal reactions may occur, see Drug Interactions); do not initiate MAO inhibitor within 7 days of discontinuing venlafaxine

Warnings Venlafaxine is not approved for use in pediatric patients. Clinical worsening of depression or suicidal ideation and behavior may occur in children and adults with major depressive disorder **[U.S. Boxed Warning]**. In clinical trials, antidepressants increased the risk of suicidal thinking and behavior (suicidality) in children, adolescents, and young adults (18-24 years of age) with major depressive disorder and other psychiatric disorders. This risk must be considered before prescribing antidepressants for any clinical use. Short-term studies did **not** show an increased risk of suicidality with antidepressant use in patients >24 years of age and showed a decreased risk in patients ≥65 years.

Patients of all ages who are treated with antidepressants for any indication require appropriate monitoring and close observation for clinical worsening of depression, suicidality, and unusual changes in behavior, especially during the first few months after antidepressant initiation or when the dose is adjusted. Family members and caregivers should be instructed to closely observe the patient (ie, daily) and communicate condition with healthcare provider. Patients should also be monitored for associated behaviors (eg, anxiety, agitation, panic attacks, insomnia, irritability, hostility, aggressiveness, impulsivity, akathisia, hypomania, mania) which may increase the risk for worsening depression or suicidality. Worsening depression or emergence of suicidality (or associated behaviors listed above) that is abrupt in onset, severe, or not part of the presenting symptoms, may require discontinuation or modification of drug therapy.

Avoid abrupt discontinuation; discontinuation symptoms (including agitation, dysphoria, anxiety, confusion, dizziness, hypomania, nightmares, and other symptoms) may occur if therapy is abruptly discontinued or dose reduced; risk of discontinuation symptoms may be increased at higher doses and with longer duration of therapy; to discontinue therapy in patients receiving venlafaxine for >1 week, taper the dose to minimize risks of discontinuation symptoms; to discontinue therapy in patients receiving venlafaxine for ≥6 weeks, taper the dose gradually over at least 2 weeks; **Note:** Clinical trials of Effexor XR® tapered the daily dose slowly at 1 week intervals by increments of 75 mg; if intolerable symptoms occur following a decrease in dosage or upon discontinuation of therapy, consider resuming the previous dose with a more gradual taper. To reduce risk of intentional overdose, write prescriptions for the smallest quantity consistent with good patient care.

Screen individuals for bipolar disorder prior to treatment (using antidepressants alone may induce manic episodes in patients with this condition). Venlafaxine may cause sustained increase in blood pressure (dose dependent; monitor blood pressure; dose reduction or discontinuation may be needed). Serotonin syndrome or other serious adverse reactions may occur when venlafaxine is used in combination with serotonergic drugs (eg, triptans) or drugs that impair the metabolism of serotonin (eg, MAO inhibitors); see Drug Interactions.

Precautions Use with caution and decrease the dose in patients with renal or hepatic impairment. Use with caution in patients with seizure disorders (seizures have been reported; discontinue if seizures occur), concomitant illnesses that may affect hepatic metabolism or hemodynamic responses (eg, unstable cardiac disease, recent MI), history of mania (may activate mania or hypomania), in suicidal patients, children, or during breast-feeding in lactating women; use with caution during late third trimester of pregnancy [newborns may experience adverse effects or venlafaxine withdrawal symptoms (consider risks and benefits); see Additional Information]. Use with caution in patients receiving diuretics or those who are volume-depleted (may cause hyponatremia or SIADH); may cause mydriasis (use with caution and closely monitor patients with increased IOP or those at risk of acute narrow-angle glaucoma). May cause anxiety, nervousness, and insomnia. May cause anorexia and significant weight loss (use with caution in patients where weight loss is undesirable); may adversely affect weight and height in children (monitor closely in pediatric patients; weight loss in pediatric patients was not limited to those with venlafaxine-associated anorexia; reduction in growth rate, as assessed by height, was greater in children <12 years of age than in adolescents). May cause abnormal bleeding (eg, ecchymosis; use with caution in patients with abnormal platelet function); may cause tachycardia [use with caution in patients with underlying medical conditions (eg, recent MI, heart failure, hyperthyroidism) that may worsen with tachycardia, especially at doses >200 mg/day in adults]. In adult studies of depression, Effexor XR® was associated with an increase in QT_c interval of 4.7 msec from baseline (versus a 1.9 msec decrease for placebo); clinical significance of this effect is not known. ▶

Adverse Reactions

Cardiovascular system: Vasodilation, hypertension (dose-related), tachycardia, chest pain, postural hypotension

Central nervous system: Headache, somnolence, dizziness, insomnia, nervousness, anxiety, abnormal dreams, yawning, agitation, confusion, abnormal thinking, depersonalization, depression, manic reaction (0.5%), seizures (0.3%); suicidal thinking and behavior (see Warnings). **Note:** Increased hyperactivity (behavioral activation) was observed in several children treated for ADHD (see Olvera, 1996)

Dermatologic: Rash, pruritus

Endocrine & metabolic: Anorexia, weight loss (dose-related), hyponatremia, SIADH, hypercholesterolemia

Gastrointestinal: Nausea, xerostomia, constipation, diarrhea, vomiting, dyspepsia, flatulence, altered taste, abdominal pain

Genitourinary: Sexual dysfunction, urinary frequency, impaired urination, urinary retention; priapism (case report in an adolescent patient; see Samuel, 2000)

Hematologic: Abnormal bleeding, ecchymosis

Neuromuscular & skeletal: Asthenia, tremor, hypertonia, twitching, paresthesia

Ocular: Blurred vision, mydriasis

Otic: Tinnitus

Miscellaneous: Diaphoresis, chills; withdrawal symptoms following abrupt discontinuation (see Warnings)

Drug Interactions

Metabolism/Transport Effects Substrate of CYP2C9 (minor), 2C19 (minor), 2D6 (major), 3A4 (major); **Inhibits** CYP2B6 (weak), 2D6 (weak), 3A4 (weak)

Avoid Concomitant Use

Avoid concomitant use of Venlafaxine with any of the following: lobenguane I 123; MAO Inhibitors; Sibutramine

Increased Effect/Toxicity

Venlafaxine may increase the levels/effects of: Alcohol (Ethyl); Alpha-/Beta-Agonists; Aspirin; CNS Depressants; Methotrimeprazine; NSAID (Nonselective); Serotonin Modulators; TraZODone; Vitamin K Antagonists

The levels/effects of Venlafaxine may be increased by: CYP2D6 Inhibitors (Moderate); CYP2D6 Inhibitors (Strong); CYP3A4 Inhibitors (Moderate); CYP3A4 Inhibitors (Strong); Darunavir; Dasatinib; MAO Inhibitors; Methotrimeprazine; Metoclopramide; Propafenone; Sibutramine; Voriconazole

Decreased Effect

Venlafaxine may decrease the levels/effects of: Alpha2-Agonists; Indinavir; lobenguane I 123

The levels/effects of Venlafaxine may be decreased by: CYP3A4 Inducers (Strong); Deferasirox; Peginterferon Alfa-2b

Food Interactions Food does not affect bioavailability of venlafaxine or ODV (active metabolite); tryptophan supplements may increase serious side effects; its use is **not recommended**

Stability Tablets and capsules: Store at controlled room temperature, 20°C to 25°C (68°F to 77°F); Effexor® tablets: Store in a dry place, dispense in a tight container; Effexor XR® 37.5 mg capsules: Protect from light and dispense in light resistant container

Mechanism of Action Venlafaxine and o-desmethylvenlafaxine (ODV) are potent inhibitors of CNS neuronal serotonin and norepinephrine reuptake and weak inhibitors of dopamine reuptake; venlafaxine and ODV do not significantly bind to alpha-adrenergic, histamine, or muscarinic cholinergic receptors (may therefore be useful in patients at risk from sedation, hypotension and anticholinergic effects of tricyclic antidepressants); venlafaxine and ODV do not inhibit monoamine oxidase

Pharmacokinetics (Adult data unless noted)

Absorption: Oral: ≥92%

Distribution: Distributes into breast milk; breast milk to plasma ratio: Venlafaxine: 2.8-4.8 (mean: 4.1); ODV: 2.8-3.8 (mean: 3.1) (Ilett, 1998)

Mean V_d (apparent): Adults:
Venlafaxine: 7.5 ± 3.7 L/kg
ODV: 5.7 ± 1.8 L/kg

Protein binding: Venlafaxine: 27%; ODV: 30%

Metabolism: Extensive in the liver, primarily via cytochrome P450 CYP2D6 to o-desmethylvenlafaxine (ODV; active metabolite); also metabolized to N-desmethylvenlafaxine, N,O-desmethylvenlafaxine, and other minor metabolites. **Note:** Clinically important differences between CYP2D6 poor and extensive metabolizers is not expected (sum of venlafaxine and ODV serum concentrations is similar in poor and extensive metabolizers; ODV is approximately equal in activity and potency to venlafaxine)

Bioavailability: Oral: 45%

Half-life:
Adults: Venlafaxine: 5 ± 2 hours; ODV: 11 ± 2 hours
Adults with cirrhosis: Venlafaxine: Half-life prolonged by ~30%; ODV: Half-life prolonged by ~60%
Adults with renal impairment (GFR: 10-70 mL/minute): Venlafaxine: Half-life prolonged by ~50%; ODV: Half-life prolonged by ~40%
Adults on dialysis: Venlafaxine: Half-life prolonged by ~180%; ODV: Half-life prolonged by 142%

Time to peak serum concentration:
Immediate release: Venlafaxine: 2 hours; ODV: 3 hours
Extended release: Venlafaxine: 5.5 hours; ODV: 9 hours

Elimination: ~87% of dose is excreted in urine within 48 hours; 5% as unchanged drug, 29% as unconjugated ODV, 26% as conjugated ODV, and 27% as other minor metabolites

Clearance:
Adults with cirrhosis: Venlafaxine: Clearance is decreased by ~50%; ODV: Clearance is decreased by ~30%
Adults with more severe cirrhosis: Venlafaxine: Clearance is decreased by ~90%
Adults with renal impairment (GFR: 10-70 mL/minute): Venlafaxine: Clearance is decreased by ~24%; ODV: Clearance unchanged versus normal subjects
Adults on dialysis: Venlafaxine: Clearance decreased by ~57%; ODV: Clearance decreased by ~56%

Dialysis: Not likely to significantly remove drug due to large volume of distribution

Usual Dosage Oral:

Children and Adolescents: Note: Not FDA approved; see Warnings. Limited information is available.

ADHD: One open-label clinical trial and one case report are available; 16 children and adolescents (8-16 years of age; mean: 11.6 ± 2.3 years) were enrolled in a 5-week open trial of venlafaxine; doses were initiated at 12.5 mg/day for the first week; for children <40 kg, the daily dose was increased (if tolerated) by 12.5 mg each week to a maximum of 50 mg/day divided in 2 doses; for patients ≥40 kg, the daily dose was increased (if tolerated) by 25 mg each week to a maximum of 75 mg/day divided in 3 doses; mean dose: 60 mg/day (1.4 mg/kg/day) in 2-3 divided doses; 10 patients completed the study [2 were lost to follow-up; 5 discontinued therapy due to adverse effects (4 had an increase in hyperactivity; 1 had severe nausea)]; venlafaxine decreased behavioral symptoms (but not cognitive symptoms) in 7 of 16 subjects (44%) (Olvera, 1996). An initial dose of 37.5 mg given 3 times/day was used in an 11-year-old female with ADHD; the dose was slowly titrated to 100 mg given 3 times/day; after 6 weeks the patient showed moderate to marked improvement in symptoms, but developed hypertension; the dose was then decreased to 75 mg given 3 times/day with normalization of blood pressure (Pleak, 1995). Further studies are needed.

Autism: One retrospective report is available; 10 patients (3-21 years of age; mean 10.5 ± 5.6 years) with autism spectrum disorders (autism, Asperger's syndrome, and pervasive developmental disorders not otherwise specified) received initial doses of 12.5 mg/day administered once daily at breakfast; doses were gradually titrated based on clinical response and side effects; mean final dose: 24.4 mg/day; range: 6.25-50 mg/day; 6 of the 10 patients were sustained-treatment responders (Hollander, 2000). Further studies are needed.

Depression: **Note:** Due to the lack of demonstrated efficacy and concerns about an increased risk for suicidal behavior, venlafaxine should be reserved for pediatric patients with major depression who do not respond to fluoxetine or sertraline (see Dopheide, 2006).

One double-blind, placebo-controlled, 6-week study is available; 33 children and adolescents (8-17 years of age) with major depression completed the trial (16 received venlafaxine; **Note:** One patient who did not complete the study, discontinued venlafaxine due to development of a manic episode requiring hospitalization and lithium therapy); immediate release venlafaxine was used; for children 8-12 years, doses were initiated at 12.5 mg once daily for 3 days, then increased to 12.5 mg twice daily for 3 days, then increased to 12.5 mg given 3 times/day for the rest of the study; for adolescents 13-17 years, doses were initiated at 25 mg once daily for 3 days, then increased to 25 mg twice daily for 3 days, then increased to 25 mg given 3 times/day for the rest of the study; both venlafaxine and placebo patients improved over time; however, no significant difference in symptoms was noted between groups (ie, venlafaxine did not have a significant effect on symptoms or specific behaviors); the authors suggest this lack of efficacy may be due to the low doses used and short duration of treatment (Mandoki, 1997).

A large multicenter double-blind, placebo-controlled study of venlafaxine-ER in children and adolescents 7-17 years of age with major depression is ongoing; this study is using higher doses; initial: 37.5 mg/day for 1 week; with increases to 75 mg/day for weeks 2-8; results are not yet available (see Weller, 2000). One report of two 16-year-old patients used higher doses of venlafaxine (final doses: 112.5 mg/day and 150 mg/day) in combination with lithium to successfully treat major depression (see Walter, 1998). Further studies are needed.

Adults:

Immediate release: Depression: Initial: 75 mg/day in 2-3 divided doses; dose may be increased (if needed) by increments of up to 75 mg/day at intervals of ≥4 days as tolerated, up to 225 mg/day. **Note:** Doses >225 mg/day for outpatients (moderately depressed patients) were not more effective; more severely depressed patients may require 350 mg/day; maximum: 375 mg/day in 3 divided doses

Extended release:

Depression: Initial: Usual: 75 mg/day; may start with 37.5 mg/day for 4-7 days to allow patient to adjust to medication, then increase to 75 mg/day; dose may be increased (if needed) by increments of up to 75 mg/day at intervals of ≥4 days as tolerated, up to a maximum of 225 mg/day. **Note:** Although higher doses of the immediate release tablets have been used in more severely depressed inpatients (see above), experience with extended release capsule in doses >225 mg/day is very limited.

Generalized anxiety disorder and social anxiety disorder: 75 mg/day; may start with 37.5 mg/day for 4-7 days to allow patient to adjust to medication, then increase to 75 mg/day. **Note:** Although a dose-response relationship has not been clearly established, certain patients may benefit from doses >75 mg/day; dose may be increased (if needed) by increments of up to 75 mg/day at intervals of ≥4 days as tolerated, up to a maximum of 225 mg/day.

Panic disorder: Initial: 37.5 mg once daily for 7 days; may increase to 75 mg daily; dose may be increased further (if needed) by increments of up to75 mg/day at intervals of ≥7 days; maximum dose: 225 mg/day

Dosing adjustment in renal impairment: Adults: GFR 10-70 mL/minute: Decrease total daily dose by 25% to 50%

Dosing adjustment in patients on dialysis: Decrease total daily dose by 50%; withhold dose until completion of dialysis treatment; further individualization of dose may be needed

Dosing adjustment in hepatic impairment: Moderate hepatic impairment: Decrease total daily dose by 50%; further individualization of dose may be needed

Administration

Immediate release tablet: Administer with food

Extended release capsule: Administer with food once daily at about the same time each day; swallow whole with fluid; do not crush, chew, divide, or place in water; capsule may be opened and entire contents sprinkled on spoonful of applesauce; swallow drug/food mixture immediately. Do not store for future use; do not chew contents (ie, pellets) of capsule; follow drug/food mixture with water to ensure complete swallowing of pellets.

Monitoring Parameters Monitor blood pressure regularly, especially in patients with high baseline blood pressure; monitor renal and hepatic function (for possible dose reductions), heart rate, weight, height, serum cholesterol and sodium. Monitor patient periodically for symptom resolution; monitor for worsening depression, suicidality, and associated behaviors (especially at the beginning of therapy or when doses are increased or decreased; see Warnings)

Patient Information Read the Patient Medication Guide that you receive with each prescription and refill of venlafaxine. An increased risk of suicidal thinking and behavior has been reported with the use of antidepressants in children, adolescents, and young adults (18-24 years of age). Notify physician if you feel more depressed, have thoughts of suicide, or become more agitated or irritable (see Warnings). May cause dizziness or drowsiness and impair ability to perform activities requiring mental alertness or physical coordination; may cause dry mouth; report the use of other medications, nonprescription medications, and herbal or natural products to your physician and pharmacist; avoid alcohol, tryptophan supplements, and the herbal medicine, St John's wort; report skin rashes, hives, or allergic reactions to your physician. Take as directed; do not alter dose or frequency without consulting prescriber, avoid abrupt discontinuation.

Nursing Implications Mean increases in heart rate of 4 beats/minute and 8.5 beats/minute have been reported; when discontinuing therapy, dose must be tapered to minimize risk of discontinuation symptoms (see Precautions). Assess mental status for depression, suicidal ideation, anxiety, social functioning, mania, or panic attack.

Additional Information Drug release from extended release capsules is not pH dependent (it is controlled by diffusion through the coating membrane on the spheroids); patients with depression who are receiving Effexor® may be switched to Effexor XR® using the nearest mg/day equivalent dose (dosing may need further individualization)

Long-term usefulness of venlafaxine should be periodically re-evaluated in patients receiving the drug for extended periods of time. Neonates born to women receiving venlafaxine, other SNRIs (serotonin and norepinephrine reuptake inhibitors), and SSRIs late during the third trimester may experience respiratory distress, apnea, cyanosis, temperature instability, vomiting, feeding difficulty, hypoglycemia, constant crying, irritability, hypotonia, hypertonia, hyper-reflexia, tremor, jitteriness, and seizures; these symptoms may be due to a direct toxic effect, withdrawal syndrome, or (in some cases) serotonin syndrome. Withdrawal symptoms occur in 30% of neonates exposed to SSRIs and SNRIs *in utero*; monitor newborns for at least 48 hours after birth; long-term effects of *in utero* exposure to SSRIs and SNRIs are unknown (see Levinson-Castiel, 2006).

Dosage Forms Excipient information presented when available (limited, particularly for generics); consult specific product labeling. [DSC] = Discontinued product
Capsule, extended release:
Effexor XR®: 37.5 mg, 75 mg, 150 mg
Tablet: 25 mg, 37.5 mg, 50 mg, 75 mg, 100 mg
Effexor®: 25 mg [DSC]; 37.5 mg [DSC]; 50 mg; 75 mg [DSC]; 100 mg [DSC]
Tablet, extended release: 37.5 mg, 75 mg, 150 mg, 225 mg

References

Dopheide JA, "Recognizing and Treating Depression in Children and Adolescents," *Am J Health Syst Pharm*, 2006, 63(3):233-43.

Emslie GJ, Yeung PP, and Kunz NR, "Long-Term, Open-Label Venlafaxine Extended-Release Treatment in Children and Adolescents With Major Depressive Disorder," *CNS Spectr*, 2007, 12 (3):223-33.

Hollander E, Kaplan A, Cartwright C, et al, "Venlafaxine in Children, Adolescents, and Young Adults With Autism Spectrum Disorders: An Open Retrospective Clinical Report," *J Child Neurol*, 2000, 15 (2):132-5.

Ilett KF, Hackett LP, Dusci LJ, et al, "Distribution and Excretion of Venlafaxine and O-Desmethylvenlafaxine in Human Milk," *Br J Clin Pharmacol*, 1998, 45(5):459-62.

Lessard E, Yessine MA, Hamelin BA, et al, "Diphenhydramine Alters the Disposition of Venlafaxine Through Inhibition of CYP2D6 Activity in Humans," *J Clin Psychopharmacol*, 2001, 21(2):175-84.

Levinson-Castiel R, Merlob P, Linder N, et al, "Neonatal Abstinence Syndrome After *in utero* Exposure to Selective Serotonin Reuptake Inhibitors in Term Infants," *Arch Pediatr Adolesc Med*, 2006, 160 (2):173-6.

Mandoki MW, Tapia MR, Tapia MA, et al, "Venlafaxine in the Treatment of Children and Adolescents With Major Depression," *Psychopharmacol Bull*, 1997, 33(1):149-54.

Olvera RL, Pliszka SR, Luh J, et al, "An Open Trial of Venlafaxine in the Treatment of Attention-Deficit/Hyperactivity Disorder in Children and Adolescents," *J Child Adolesc Psychopharmacol*, 1996, 6(4):241-50.

Pleak RR and Gormly LJ, "Effects of Venlafaxine Treatment for ADHD in a Child," *Am J Psychiatry*, 1995, 152(7):1099.

Samuel RZ, "Priapism Associated With Venlafaxine Use," *J Am Acad Child Adolesc Psychiatry*, 2000, 39(1):16-7.

Walter G, Lyndon B, and Kubb R, "Lithium Augmentation of Venlafaxine in Adolescent Major Depression," *Aust N Z J Psychiatry* 1998, 32 (3):457-9.

Weller EB, Weller RA, and Davis GP, "Use of Venlafaxine in Children and Adolescents: A Review of Current Literature," *Depress Anxiety*, 2000, 12(Suppl 1):85-9.

◆ **Venofer®** *see* Iron Sucrose *on page 764*

◆ **Ventolin® (Can)** *see* Albuterol *on page 57*

◆ **Ventolin® Diskus (Can)** *see* Albuterol *on page 57*

◆ **Ventolin® HFA** *see* Albuterol *on page 57*

◆ **Ventolin® I.V. Infusion (Can)** *see* Albuterol *on page 57*

◆ **Ventolin® Nebules P.F. (Can)** *see* Albuterol *on page 57*

◆ **Veracolate [OTC]** *see* Bisacodyl *on page 194*

◆ **Veramyst®** *see* Fluticasone *on page 607*

Verapamil (ver AP a mil)

Medication Safety Issues
Sound-alike/look-alike issues:
Calan® may be confused with Colace®, diltiazem
Covera-HS® may be confused with Provera®
Isoptin® may be confused with Isopto® Tears
Verelan® may be confused with Virilon®, Voltaren®

High alert medication: The Institute for Safe Medication Practices (ISMP) includes this medication (I.V. formulation) among its list of drug classes which have a heightened risk of causing significant patient harm when used in error.

Significant differences exist between oral and I.V. dosing. Use caution when converting from one route of administration to another.

International issues:
Calan®: Brand name for verapamil [U.S., Canada], but also the brand name for vinpocetine [Japan]
Dilacor: Brand name for verapamil [Brazil], but also the brand name for barnidipine [Argentina]; digoxin [Serbia]; diltiazem [U.S.]

Related Information
Adult ACLS Algorithms *on page 1463*
Antihypertensive Agents by Class *on page 1481*
Medications for Which A Single Dose May Be Fatal When Ingested By A Toddler *on page 1709*

U.S. Brand Names Calan®; Calan® SR; Covera-HS®; Isoptin® SR; Verelan®; Verelan® PM

Canadian Brand Names Apo-Verap®; Apo-Verap® SR; Calan®; Chronovera®; Covera-HS®; Covera®; Dom-Verapamil SR; Gen-Verapamil; Gen-Verapamil SR; Iso-ptin® SR; Med-Verapamil; Mylan-Verapamil; Mylan-Verapamil SR; Novo-Veramil; Novo-Veramil SR; Nu-Verap; Nu-Verap SR; PHL-Verapamil SR; PMS-Verapamil SR; PRO-Verapamil SR; Riva-Verapamil SR; Verapamil Hydrochloride Injection, USP; Verapamil SR; Verelan SRC

Therapeutic Category Antianginal Agent; Antiarrhythmic Agent, Class IV; Antihypertensive Agent; Calcium Channel Blocker; Calcium Channel Blocker, Nondihydropyridine

Generic Available Yes: Excludes caplet (sustained release) and tablet (extended release, controlled onset)

Use
Oral: Treatment of hypertension (all oral products) (FDA approved in adults); angina pectoris (vasospastic, chronic stable, unstable) (Calan®, Covera-HS®) (FDA approved in adults); supraventricular tachyarrhythmia [PSVT (prophylaxis), atrial fibrillation/flutter (rate control)] (Calan®) (FDA approved in adults)
I.V.: Supraventricular tachyarrhythmia [PSVT; atrial fibrillation/flutter (rate control)] (FDA approved in all ages)

Pregnancy Risk Factor C

Pregnancy Considerations In some animal reproduction studies verapamil has been shown to cause fetal harm; adverse maternal effects were also observed. Although verapamil is not considered a major human teratogen, use during pregnancy may cause adverse fetal effects (bradycardia, heart block, hypotension). Use in pregnancy only when clearly needed and when the benefits outweigh the potential risk to the fetus. Verapamil crosses the placenta.

Lactation Enters breast milk/not recommended

Breast-Feeding Considerations Crosses into breast milk; manufacturer recommends to discontinue breast-feeding while taking verapamil. AAP considers **compatible** with breast-feeding.

Contraindications Hypersensitivity to verapamil or any component; severe left ventricular dysfunction; hypotension or cardiogenic shock; sick sinus syndrome (except in patients with a functioning artificial ventricular pacemaker);

second- or third-degree AV block (except in patients with a functioning artificial ventricular pacemaker); atrial flutter or fibrillation associated with an accessory bypass tract [Wolff-Parkinson-White (WPW) syndrome, Lown-Ganong-Levine syndrome]

I.V.: Additional contraindications include concurrent use of I.V. beta-blocking agents; ventricular tachycardia; severe congestive heart failure (unless secondary to supra-ventricular tachycardia that is treatable with verapamil)

Warnings Avoid I.V. use in neonates and young infants due to severe apnea, bradycardia, hypotensive reactions, and cardiac arrest. I.V. use is discouraged in children due to hypotension and myocardial depression. Monitor ECG and blood pressure closely in patients receiving I.V. therapy; have I.V. calcium chloride available at bedside to treat hypotension. I.V. administration, hypertrophic cardiomyopathy, sick sinus syndrome, moderate to severe CHF, concomitant therapy with beta-blockers or digoxin can all increase the incidence of adverse effects.

Precautions Use with caution in patients with hypertrophic cardiomyopathy (especially obstructive) or concomitant therapy with beta-blockers or digoxin. Use caution in patients with hepatic or renal impairment (verapamil dosage reduction may be needed; monitor for signs of overdosage, including hypotension or PR prolongation on ECG). Verapamil may decrease neuromuscular trans-mission in patients with Duchenne's muscular dystrophy and may worsen myasthenia gravis (use with caution in these patients; verapamil dosage reduction may be needed). Use Covera-HS® with caution in patients with severe GI narrowing (table is nondeformable) and in patients with extremely short GI transit time (<7 hours) (dosage adjustment may be required; pharmacokinetic data are not available).

Adverse Reactions

Cardiovascular: Bradycardia; first, second, or third degree A-V block; flushing; hypotension; peripheral edema; worsening heart failure

Central nervous system: Dizziness, fatigue, headache, lethargy, myalgia, pain, seizures (occasionally with I.V. use), sleep disturbance

Dermatologic: Rash

Gastrointestinal: Abdominal discomfort, constipation, gin-gival hyperplasia, nausea

Hepatic: Hepatic enzymes increased

Neuromuscular & skeletal: Paresthesia

Otic: Tinnitus

Respiratory: Dyspnea; verapamil may precipitate insuffi-ciency of respiratory muscle function in Duchenne muscular dystrophy

<1%, postmarketing, and/or case reports:

Oral: Alopecia, angina, arthralgia, atrioventricular disso-ciation, blurred vision, bruising, cerebrovascular acci-dent, chest pain, claudication, confusion, diaphoresis, diarrhea, equilibrium disorders, erythema multiforme, exanthema, extrapyramidal symptoms, galactorrhea/hyperprolactinemia, GI distress, gynecomastia, hyper-keratosis, impotence, insomnia, macules, MI, muscle cramps, palpitation, psychosis, purpura (vasculitis), shakiness, somnolence, spotty menstruation, Stevens-Johnson syndrome, sweating, syncope, urination increased, urticaria, xerostomia

I.V.: Bronchi/laryngeal spasm, depression, diaphoresis, itching, muscle fatigue, respiratory failure, rotary nystagmus, sleepiness, urticaria, vertigo

Drug Interactions

Metabolism/Transport Effects Substrate of CYP1A2 (minor), CYP2B6 (minor), CYP2C9 (minor), CYP2C18 (minor), CYP2E1 (minor), CYP3A4 (major), P-glycopro-tein; **Inhibits** CYP1A2 (weak), CYP2C9 (weak), CYP2D6 (weak), CYP3A4 (moderate), P-glycoprotein

Avoid Concomitant Use

Avoid concomitant use of Verapamil with any of the following: Dabigatran Etexilate; Disopyramide; Dofetilide; Everolimus; Tolvaptan; Topotecan

Increased Effect/Toxicity

Verapamil may increase the levels/effects of: Alcohol (Ethyl); Amifostine; Amiodarone; Antihypertensives; Ator-vastatin; Benzodiazepines (metabolized by oxidation); Beta-Blockers; BusPIRone; Calcium Channel Blockers (Dihydropyridine); CarBAMazepine; Cardiac Glycosides; Colchicine; Corticosteroids (Systemic); CycloSPORINE; CycloSPORINE (Systemic); CYP3A4 Substrates; Dabi-gatran Etexilate; Disopyramide; Dofetilide; Dronedarone; Eletriptan; Eplerenone; Everolimus; Fexofenadine; Fle-cainide; Halofantrine; Hypotensive Agents; Lithium; Lovastatin; Magnesium Salts; Midodrine; Neuromuscu-lar-Blocking Agents (Nondepolarizing); Nitroprusside; P-Glycoprotein Substrates; Phenytoin; Pimecrolimus; Qui-NIDine; Ranolazine; Red Yeast Rice; Risperidone; RiTUXimab; Rivaroxaban; Salicylates; Salmeterol; Sax-agliptin; Simvastatin; Tacrolimus; Tacrolimus (Systemic); Tacrolimus (Topical); Tolvaptan; Topotecan

The levels/effects of Verapamil may be increased by: Alpha1-Blockers; Anilidopiperidine Opioids; Antifungal Agents (Azole Derivatives, Systemic); Atorvastatin; Calcium Channel Blockers (Dihydropyridine); Cimetidine; CycloSPORINE; CycloSPORINE (Systemic); CYP3A4 Inhibitors (Moderate); CYP3A4 Inhibitors (Strong); Dasa-tinib; Diazoxide; Dronedarone; Everolimus; Fluconazole; Grapefruit Juice; Herbs (Hypotensive Properties); Macro-lide Antibiotics; Magnesium Salts; MAO Inhibitors; Pentoxifylline; P-Glycoprotein Inhibitors; Phosphodiester-ase 5 Inhibitors; Prostacyclin Analogues; Protease Inhibitors; QuiNIDine; Quinupristin; Telithromycin

Decreased Effect

Verapamil may decrease the levels/effects of: Clopidogrel

The levels/effects of Verapamil may be decreased by: Barbiturates; Calcium Salts; CarBAMazepine; CYP3A4 Inducers (Strong); Deferasirox; Herbs (CYP3A4 Inducers); Herbs (Hypertensive Properties); Methylphe-nidate; Nafcillin; P-Glycoprotein Inducers; Rifamycin Derivatives; Yohimbine

Food Interactions Grapefruit juice may increase verapa-mil serum concentrations.

Calan® SR and Isoptin® SR: Food may decrease bioavailability but produces a narrow peak to trough ratio.

Covera-HS®: A high-fat meal does not affect absorption.

Verelan®: Food does not affect rate or extent of absorption; rate and extent of absorption are bioequiva-lent between administration of intact capsule and when contents of capsule are administered by sprinkling onto one tablespoonful of applesauce.

Verelan® PM: A high-fat meal slightly affects the rate but not the extent of absorption.

Stability

Injection: Store at controlled room temperature of 15°C to 30°C (59°F to 86°F); protect from light; use only clear solutions. Compatible in solutions of pH of 3-6, but may precipitate in solutions having a pH ≥6

Calan®: Store at 15°C to 25°C (59°F to 77°F); protect from light; dispense in tightly closed, light-resistant container.

Calan® SR: Store at 15°C to 25°C (59°F to 77°F); protect from light and moisture; dispense in tightly closed, light-resistant container.

Covera-HS®: Store at controlled room temperature of 20°C to 25°C (68°F to 77°F); dispense in tightly closed, light-resistant container.

Isoptin® SR: Store at 25°C (77°F); excursions permitted to 15°C to 30°C (59°F to 86°F); protect from light and moisture; dispense in tightly closed, light-resistant container.

Verelan®: Store at controlled room temperature of 20°C to 25°C (68°F to 77°F); avoid excessive heat; dispense in tightly closed, light-resistant container.

Verelan® PM: Store at 25°C (77°F); excursions permitted to 15°C to 30°C (59°F to 86°F); protect from moisture; dispense in tightly closed, light-resistant container.

Mechanism of Action Inhibits calcium ions from entering the "slow channels" or select voltage-sensitive areas of vascular smooth muscle and myocardium during depolarization; produces a relaxation of coronary vascular smooth muscle and coronary vasodilation; increases myocardial oxygen delivery in patients with vasospastic angina

Pharmacodynamics

Maximum effect:

Oral (nonsustained tablets): 2 hours

I.V.: 1-5 minutes

Duration:

Oral: 6-8 hours

I.V.: 10-20 minutes

Pharmacokinetics (Adult data unless noted)

Absorption: Well-absorbed

Distribution: V_d: 3.89 L/kg (see Storstein, 1984)

Protein binding:

Neonates: ~60%

Adults: ~90%

Metabolism: Extensive first-pass effect, metabolized in the liver to several inactive dealkylated metabolites; major metabolite is norverapamil which possesses weak hemodynamic effects (20% that of verapamil)

Bioavailability: Oral: 20% to 30%

Half-life:

Infants: 4.4-6.9 hours

Adults (single dose): 2-8 hours, increased up to 12 hours with multiple dosing

Adults: Severe hepatic impairment: 14-16 hours

Elimination: 70% of dose excreted in urine as metabolites (3% to 4% as unchanged drug), and 16% in feces

Dialysis: Not removed by hemodialysis

Usual Dosage

Infants <1 year: I.V.: **Not recommended** (see Warnings); administer with continuous ECG monitoring, have I.V. calcium available at bedside: 0.1-0.2 mg/kg/dose (usual: 0.75-2 mg/dose) may repeat dose in 30 minutes if adequate response not achieved; **Note:** Optimal interval for subsequent doses is unknown and must be individualized for each specific patient.

Children 1-15 years: I.V.: 0.1-0.3 mg/kg/dose; maximum dose: 5 mg/dose; may repeat dose in 30 minutes if adequate response not achieved; maximum for second dose: 10 mg/dose; **Note:** Optimal interval for subsequent doses is unknown and must be individualized for each specific patient.

Children: Oral (dose not well established):

4-8 mg/kg/day in 3 divided doses

or

1-5 years: 40-80 mg every 8 hours

>5 years: 80 mg every 6-8 hours

Note: A mean daily dose of ~5 mg/kg/day (range: 2.3-8.1 mg/kg/day) was used in 22 children 15 days to 17 years of age receiving chronic oral therapy for SVT (n=20) or hypertrophic cardiomyopathy (n=2) (see Piovan, 1995).

Adults:

I.V. (ACLS 2005 guidelines): PSVT (narrow complex, unresponsive to vagal maneuvers and adenosine, in patients with preserved cardiac function): Initial: 2.5-5 mg; if no response in 15-30 minutes and no adverse effects seen, give 5-10 mg every 15-30 minutes to a maximum total dose of 20 mg

Alternative dosing regimen (see ACLS 2005 guidelines): Initial: 5 mg; if no response in 15 minutes and

no adverse effects seen, give 5 mg every 15 minutes to a total dose of 30 mg

I.V.: (Manufacturer's recommendations): 5-10 mg (0.075-0.15 mg/kg); may repeat 10 mg (0.15 mg/kg) 30 minutes after the initial dose if needed and if patient tolerated initial dose; **Note:** Optimal interval for subsequent doses is unknown and must be individualized for each specific patient.

Angina: Oral: **Note:** When switching from immediate release to extended/sustained release formulations, the total daily dose remains the same unless formulation strength does not allow for equal conversion.

Immediate release: Initial: 80-120 mg 3 times/day (small stature: 40 mg 3 times/day); usual dose range (see Gibbons, 2003): 80-160 mg 3 times/day

Extended release: Covera-HS®: Initial: 180 mg once daily at bedtime; if inadequate response, may increase dose at weekly intervals to 240 mg once daily, then 360 mg once daily, then 480 mg once daily; maximum dose: 480 mg/day

Chronic atrial fibrillation (rate control), PSVT prophylaxis: Oral: Immediate release: 240-480 mg/day in 3-4 divided doses; usual dose range (see European Heart Rhythm Association, 2006): 120-360 mg/day

Hypertension: Oral: **Note:** When switching from immediate release to extended/sustained release formulations, the total daily dose remains the same unless formulation strength does not allow for equal conversion.

Immediate release: 80 mg 3 times/day; usual dose range (JNC 7): 80-320 mg/day in 2 divided doses

Sustained release: Usual dose range (JNC 7): 120-480 mg/day in 1-2 divided doses; **Note:** There is no evidence of additional benefit with doses >360 mg/day.

Calan® SR, Isoptin® SR: Initial: 180 mg once daily in the morning (small stature: 120 mg/day); if inadequate response, may increase dose at weekly intervals to 240 mg once daily, then 180 mg twice daily (or 240 mg in the morning followed by 120 mg in the evening); maximum dose: 240 mg twice daily

Verelan®: Initial: 180 mg once daily in the morning (small stature: 120 mg/day); if inadequate response, may increase dose at weekly intervals to 240 mg once daily, then 360 mg once daily, then 480 mg once daily; maximum dose: 480 mg/day

Extended release: Usual dose range (JNC 7): 120-360 mg once daily (once daily dosing is recommended at bedtime)

Covera-HS®: Initial: 180 mg once daily at bedtime; if inadequate response, may increase dose at weekly intervals to 240 mg once daily, then 360 mg once daily, then 480 mg once daily; maximum dose: 480 mg/day

Verelan® PM: Initial: 200 mg once daily at bedtime (small stature: 100 mg once daily); if inadequate response, may increase dose at weekly intervals to 300 mg once daily, then 400 mg once daily; maximum dose: 400 mg/day

Dosing adjustment in renal impairment: Children and Adults: Use with caution and closely monitor ECG for PR prolongation, blood pressure, and other signs of overdose; dosage reduction may be needed. The manufacturer of Verelan® PM recommends an initial adult dose of 100 mg/day at bedtime. **Note:** A number of studies show no difference in verapamil (or norverapamil metabolite) disposition between chronic renal failure and control patients, suggesting that dosage adjustment is not required in renal impairment (see Beyerlein, 1990; Hanyok, 1988; Mooy, 1985; Zachariah, 1991). However, a study in adults suggests reduced renal clearance of verapamil and its metabolite (norverapamil) with advanced renal failure (see Storstein, 1984). Additionally, several clinical papers report adverse effects of verapamil in patients with chronic renal failure receiving recommended doses of verapamil (see Pritza, 1991; Váquez, 1996). Thus, prudence dictates cautious use, close monitoring, and dosage adjustment if needed.

Dosing adjustment in hepatic impairment: Children and Adults: In patients with cirrhosis, reduce dose to 20% and 50% of normal dose for oral and intravenous administration, respectively; monitor blood pressure for hypotension and ECG for prolongation of PR interval (see Somogyi, 1981). The manufacturer of Verelan PM® recommends an initial adult dose of 100 mg/day at bedtime. The manufacturers of Calan®, Calan® SR, Covera-HS®, Isoptin® SR, and Verelan® recommend giving 30% of the normal dose to patients with severe hepatic impairment.

Administration

Oral: Do not administer with grapefruit juice. Nonsustained-release tablets can be administered with or without food. Swallow extended and sustained released preparations whole, do not break, chew, or crush. Administer Calan® SR and Isoptin® SR with food on a once daily or twice daily schedule; administer Covera-HS® and Verelan® PM once daily at bedtime. Administer Verelan® (sustained release capsules) once daily in the morning; capsule may be opened and contents sprinkled on a spoonful of applesauce; swallow immediately, do not chew; do not store for future use; follow with water to ensure complete swallowing of capsule pellets; do not divide capsule

Parenteral:

I.V.: Infuse I.V. dose over 2-3 minutes; infuse I.V. over 3-4 minutes if blood pressure is in the lower range of normal: Maximum concentration: 2.5 mg/mL

I.V. continuous infusion: Final concentration for administration: 0.5-2.5 mg/mL

Monitoring Parameters ECG, blood pressure, heart rate; hepatic enzymes with long-term use

Patient Information Avoid alcohol and grapefruit juice; limit caffeine; insoluble shell of extended release tablet (eg, Covera-HS®) may appear in the stool (this is normal)

Dosage Forms Excipient information presented when available (limited, particularly for generics); consult specific product labeling. [DSC] = Discontinued product

Caplet, sustained release, as hydrochloride:

Calan® SR: 120 mg

Calan® SR: 180 mg, 240 mg [scored]

Capsule, extended release, as hydrochloride: 120 mg, 180 mg, 240 mg

Capsule, extended release, controlled onset, as hydrochloride: 100 mg, 200 mg, 300 mg

Verelan® PM: 100 mg, 200 mg, 300 mg

Capsule, sustained release, as hydrochloride: 120 mg, 180 mg, 240 mg, 360 mg

Verelan®: 120 mg, 180 mg, 240 mg, 360 mg

Injection, solution, as hydrochloride: 2.5 mg/mL (2 mL, 4 mL)

Tablet, as hydrochloride: 40 mg, 80 mg, 120 mg

Calan®: 80 mg, 120 mg [scored]

Tablet, extended release, as hydrochloride: 120 mg, 180 mg, 240 mg

Tablet, extended release, controlled onset, as hydrochloride:

Covera-HS®: 180 mg, 240 mg

Tablet, sustained release, as hydrochloride: 120 mg, 180 mg, 240 mg

Isoptin® SR: 120 mg

Isoptin® SR: 180 mg, 240 mg [scored]

Extemporaneous Preparations

A 50 mg/mL oral suspension may be made using twenty 80 mg verapamil tablets (regular, not sustained release), 3 mL of purified water USP, 8 mL of methylcellulose 1% and simple syrup qs ad to 32 mL; stability is 91 days

under refrigeration; shake well before use (Nahata, 2000) A 50 mg/mL oral liquid preparation made from tablets (regular, not sustained release) and 3 different vehicles (cherry syrup, a 1:1 mixture of Ora-Sweet® and Ora-Plus®, or a 1:1 mixture of Ora-Sweet® SF and Ora-Plus®) was stable for 60 days when stored in amber plastic prescription bottles in the dark at room temperature (25°C) or under refrigeration (5°C); grind seventy-five 80 mg tablets in a mortar into a fine powder; add 40 mL of the vehicle and mix well to form a uniform paste; mix while adding the vehicle in geometric proportions to **almost** 120 mL; transfer to a calibrated bottle and qsad with vehicle to make 120 mL; label "shake well" and "protect from light" (Allen, 1996).

Allen LV and Erickson MA, "Stability of Labetalol Hydrochloride, Metoprolol Tartrate, Verapamil Hydrochloride, and Spironolactone With Hydrochlorothiazide in Extemporaneously Compounded Oral Liquids," *Am J Health Syst Pharm*, 1996, 53(19):2304-9.

Nahata MC and Hipple TF, *Pediatric Drug Formulations*, 4th ed, Cincinnati, OH: Harvey Whitney Books Co, 2000.

References

American Heart Association Emergency Cardiovascular Care Committee, "2005 American Heart Association (AHA) Guidelines for Cardiopulmonary Resuscitation (CPR) and Emergency Cardiovascular Care (ECC), Part 7.3: Management of Symptomatic Bradycardia and Tachycardia, and Part 12: Pediatric Advanced Life Support," *Circulation*, 2005, 112(24 Suppl):IV67-77,167-87.

Beyerlein C, Csaszar G, Hollmann M, et al, "Verapamil in Antihypertensive Treatment of Patients on Renal Replacement Therapy - Clinical Implications and Pharmacokinetics," *Eur J Clin Pharmacol*, 1990, 39 Suppl 1:S35-7.

Chobanian AV, Bakris GL, Black HR, et al, "The Seventh Report of the Joint National Committee on Prevention, Detection, Evaluation, and Treatment of High Blood Pressure: The JNC 7 report," *JAMA*, 2003, 289(19):2560-72.

European Heart Rhythm Association; Heart Rhythm Society, Fuster V, et al, "ACC/AHA/ESC 2006 Guidelines for the Management of Patients With Atrial Fibrillation - Executive Summary: A Report of the American College of Cardiology/American Heart Association Task Force on Practice Guidelines and the European Society of Cardiology Committee for Practice Guidelines (Writing Committee to Revise the 2001 Guidelines for the Management of Patients With Atrial Fibrillation)," *J Am Coll Cardiol*, 2006, 48(4):854-906.

Gibbons RJ, Abrams J, Chatterjee K, et al, "ACC/AHA 2002 Guideline Update for the Management of Patients With Chronic Stable Angina - Summary Article: A Report of the American College of Cardiology/American Heart Association Task Force on Practice Guidelines (Committee on the Management of Patients With Chronic Stable Angina)," *J Am Coll Cardiol*, 2003, 41(1):159-68.

Hanyok JJ, Chow MS, Kluger J, et al, "An Evaluation of the Pharmacokinetics, Pharmacodynamics, and Dialyzability of Verapamil in Chronic Hemodialysis Patients," *J Clin Pharmacol*, 1988, 28 (9):831-6.

Mooy J, Schols M, v Baak M, et al, "Pharmacokinetics of Verapamil in Patients With Renal Failure," *Eur J Clin Pharmacol*, 1985, 28 (4):405-10.

Piovan D, Padrini R, Svalato Moreolo G, et al, "Verapamil and Norverapamil Plasma Levels in Infants and Children During Chronic Oral Treatment," *Ther Drug Monit*, 1995, 17(1):60-7.

Pritza DR, Bierman MH, and Hammeke MD, "Acute Toxic Effects of Sustained-Release Verapamil in Chronic Renal Failure," *Arch Intern Med*, 1991, 151(10):2081-4.

Sapire DW, O'Riordan AC, and Black IF, "Safety and Efficacy of Short- and Long-Term Verapamil Therapy in Children With Tachycardia," *Am J Cardiol*, 1981, 48(6):1091-7.

Shakibi JG, "Arrhythmias in Infants and Children," *Pediatrician*, 1981, 10(1-3):117-22.

Somogyi A, Albrecht M, Kliems G, et al, "Pharmacokinetics, Bioavailability and ECG Response of Verapamil in Patients With Liver Cirrhosis," *Br J Clin Pharmacol*, 1981, 12(1):51-60.

Storstein L, Larsen A, Midtbø K, et al, "Pharmacokinetics of Calcium Blockers in Patients With Renal Insufficiency and in Geriatric Patients," *Acta Med Scand Suppl*, 1984, 681:25-30.

Váquez C, Huelmos A, Alegría E, et al, "Verapamil Deleterious Effects in Chronic Renal Failure," *Nephron*, 1996, 72(3):461-4.

Zachariah PK, Moyer TP, Theobald HM, et al, "The Pharmacokinetics of Racemic Verapamil in Patients With Impaired Renal Function," *J Clin Pharmacol*, 1991, 31(1):45-53.

♦ **Verapamil Hydrochloride** see Verapamil *on page 1416*

- ◆ **Verapamil Hydrochloride Injection, USP (Can)** *see* Verapamil *on page 1416*
- ◆ **Verapamil SR (Can)** *see* Verapamil *on page 1416*
- ◆ **Verelan®** *see* Verapamil *on page 1416*
- ◆ **Verelan® PM** *see* Verapamil *on page 1416*
- ◆ **Verelan SRC (Can)** *see* Verapamil *on page 1416*
- ◆ **Veripred™ 20** *see* PrednisoLONE *on page 1148*
- ◆ **Vermox** *see* Mebendazole *on page 867*
- ◆ **Vermox® (Can)** *see* Mebendazole *on page 867*
- ◆ **Versed** *see* Midazolam *on page 928*
- ◆ **Versel® (Can)** *see* Selenium Sulfide *on page 1252*
- ◆ **Versiclear™** *see* Sodium Thiosulfate *on page 1280*
- ◆ **Vesanoid® [DSC]** *see* Tretinoin (Systemic) *on page 1373*
- ◆ **Vesanoid® (Can)** *see* Tretinoin (Systemic) *on page 1373*
- ◆ **VFEND®** *see* Voriconazole *on page 1429*
- ◆ **Viagra®** *see* Sildenafil *on page 1258*
- ◆ **Vibramycin®** *see* Doxycycline *on page 479*
- ◆ **Vibra-Tabs® (Can)** *see* Doxycycline *on page 479*
- ◆ **Vicks® 44® Cough Relief [OTC]** *see* Dextromethorphan *on page 421*
- ◆ **Vicks® 44E [OTC]** *see* Guaifenesin and Dextromethorphan *on page 658*
- ◆ **Vicks® Casero™ Chest Congestion Relief [OTC]** *see* GuaiFENesin *on page 656*
- ◆ **Vicks® DayQuil® Cough [OTC]** *see* Dextromethorphan *on page 421*
- ◆ **Vicks® DayQuil® Mucus Control DM [OTC]** *see* Guaifenesin and Dextromethorphan *on page 658*
- ◆ **Vicks® Early Defense™ [OTC]** *see* Oxymetazoline *on page 1043*
- ◆ **Vicks® Pediatric Formula 44E [OTC]** *see* Guaifenesin and Dextromethorphan *on page 658*
- ◆ **Vicks Sinex® 12 Hour [OTC]** *see* Oxymetazoline *on page 1043*
- ◆ **Vicks Sinex® 12 Hour Ultrafine Mist [OTC]** *see* Oxymetazoline *on page 1043*
- ◆ **Vicks® Sinex® Nasal Spray [OTC] [DSC]** *see* Phenylephrine *on page 1102*
- ◆ **Vicks® Sinex® UltraFine Mist [OTC] [DSC]** *see* Phenylephrine *on page 1102*
- ◆ **Vicks® Sinex® VapoSpray 4-Hour™ Decongestant [OTC]** *see* Phenylephrine *on page 1102*
- ◆ **Vicks® Vitamin C [OTC]** *see* Ascorbic Acid *on page 138*
- ◆ **Vicodin®** *see* Hydrocodone and Acetaminophen *on page 684*
- ◆ **Vicodin® ES** *see* Hydrocodone and Acetaminophen *on page 684*
- ◆ **Vicodin® HP** *see* Hydrocodone and Acetaminophen *on page 684*
- ◆ **Videx®** *see* Didanosine *on page 434*
- ◆ **Videx® EC** *see* Didanosine *on page 434*

Vigabatrin (vye GA ba trin)

Medication Safety Issues
Sound-alike/look-alike issues:
Vigabatrin may be confused with Vibativ™
Related Information
Antiepileptic Drugs *on page 1693*
U.S. Brand Names Sabril®
Canadian Brand Names Sabril®

Therapeutic Category Anticonvulsant, Miscellaneous; Infantile Spasms, Treatment
Generic Available No
Use
Powder for oral solution: Monotherapy for treatment of infantile spasms in patients for whom the potential benefits outweigh the potential risk of vision loss (FDA approved in ages 1 month to 2 years); has also been used in children as adjunct therapy for refractory complex partial seizures not controlled by usual treatments
Tablet: Adjunct therapy for refractory complex partial seizures not controlled by usual treatments in patients for whom the potential benefits outweigh the potential risk of vision loss (FDA approved in adults)
Restrictions Vigabatrin is available in U.S. only under a special restricted distribution program (SHARE). Under the SHARE program, only prescribers and pharmacies registered with the program are able to prescribe and distribute vigabatrin. Vigabatrin may only be dispensed to patients who are enrolled in and meet all conditions of SHARE. Contact the SHARE program at 1-888-45-SHARE.
Medication Guide An FDA-approved patient medication guide, which is available with the product information and at http://www.fda.gov/downloads/Drugs/DrugSafety/UCM180720.pdf, must be dispensed with this medication for each new outpatient prescription and refill.
Pregnancy Risk Factor C
Pregnancy Considerations Teratogenic, embryolethal, and neurotoxic adverse events have been observed in animal reproduction studies; neurotoxic events were observed with postnatal administration in a period corresponding to the third trimester of human pregnancy. Vigabatrin crosses the placenta in humans. Birth defects have been reported following use in pregnancy and include: cardiac defects, limb defects, male genital malformations, fetal anticonvulsant syndrome, renal and ear abnormalities. Time of exposure or maternal dosage was not reported and information is not available relating to the incidence or types of these outcomes in comparison to the general epilepsy population. Visual field examinations have been conducted following in utero exposure in a limited number of children tested at ≥6 years of age; no visual field loss was observed in 4 children and results were inconclusive in 2 others. Use during pregnancy is contraindicated in Canadian product labeling.

Patients exposed to vigabatrin during pregnancy are encouraged to enroll themselves into the NAAED Pregnancy Registry by calling 1-888-233-2334. Additional information is available at www.aedpregnancyregistry.org.
Lactation Enters breast milk/not recommended
Breast-Feeding Considerations Small amounts of vigabatrin are found in human milk (≤4% of the weight-adjusted maternal dose based on 2 cases). According to the manufacturer, the decision to continue or discontinue breast-feeding during therapy should take into account the risk of exposure to the infant and the benefits of treatment to the mother. Use while breast-feeding is contraindicated in Canadian product labeling.
Contraindications Hypersensitivity to vigabatrin or any component
Warnings Vigabatrin causes permanent vision loss in a high percentage of patients, including infants, children, and adults. Vision loss is most frequently described as progressive, bilateral concentric visual field constriction; decreased visual acuity has also been reported. Neither type of vision loss is reliably prevented through periodic vision testing. There is no known exposure level of vigabatrin without risk of vision loss; however, risk has been shown to increase with total cumulative dose or duration of therapy **[U.S. Boxed Warning]**. The onset of vision loss is unpredictable, occurring within weeks of

starting treatment or sooner, or at any time during treatment, even after months or years of therapy. It has also been reported to worsen despite discontinuation of therapy. Most information characterizing frequency and extent of vision loss is from adult data since vision loss assessment is difficult in infants and children. Vigabatrin causes permanent bilateral concentric visual field constriction in >30% of patients ranging in severity from mild to severe, including tunnel vision to within 10 degrees of visual fixation, and can result in disability. In some cases, vigabatrin can damage the central retina and decrease visual acuity. In infants and children, symptoms of vision loss are unlikely to be recognized by the parent or caregiver until loss is severe. Vision loss of milder severity, although potentially unrecognized by the parent or caregiver, may still adversely affect function. Vision should be assessed to the extent possible at baseline (no later than 4 weeks after initiation), at least every 3 months during therapy, and at 3-6 months after discontinuation. Once detected, vision loss is not reversible. Due to the risk of vision loss and because vigabatrin provides an observable symptomatic benefit when it is effective, the lowest dose and shortest exposure consistent with clinical objectives should be used. If the patient fails to show substantial clinical benefit within a short period of time after initiation of treatment (2-4 weeks for infantile spasms; ≤3 months in adults), vigabatrin therapy should be withdrawn. If in the clinical judgment of the prescriber, evidence of treatment failure becomes obvious earlier in the treatment course, vigabatrin should be discontinued at that time. The interaction of other types of irreversible vision damage with vision damage from vigabatrin has not been well-characterized, but is likely severe. Vigabatrin should not be used with other drugs associated with serious adverse ophthalmic effects such as retinopathy or glaucoma unless the benefits clearly outweigh the risks. The possibility that vision loss from vigabatrin may be more common, more severe or have more severe functional consequences in infants and children than in adults cannot be excluded.

Antiepileptic drugs (AEDs) increase the risk of suicidal behavior and ideation in patients receiving these medications for any indication. Pooled analyses of placebo-controlled trials involving 11 different AEDs (regardless of indication) showed a twofold increased risk of suicidal thoughts or behavior (estimated incidence rate: 0.43% in AED treated patients compared to 0.24% of patients receiving placebo); increased risk was observed as early as 1 week after initiation of AED and continued through duration of trials (most trials ≤24 weeks); risk did not vary significantly by age (age range: 5-100 years). Consider risks and benefits of AEDs before prescribing. Monitor all patients receiving an AED for emergence of suicidal thoughts or behavior, thoughts of self-harm, any unusual changes in behavior or mood, or the emergence or worsening of depressive symptoms; notify healthcare provider immediately if symptoms or concerning behavior occur. **Note:** The FDA requires a Medication Guide for all antiepileptic drugs informing patients of this risk.

Precautions Use with caution and reduce dose in patients with renal dysfunction. Anticonvulsants should not be discontinued abruptly because of the possibility of increasing seizure frequency; vigabatrin should be withdrawn gradually to minimize the potential of increased seizure frequency; to withdraw therapy in infants and children, decrease the dose by 25-50 mg/kg/day every 3-4 days; in adults decrease the dose by 1 g/day every week. Vigabatrin should not be used as monotherapy or first line therapy for complex partial seizures. Use with caution when initiating therapy, particularly in patients with myoclonic seizures, as an increase in seizure frequency or onset of new types of seizures may occur.

Dose-dependent, asymptomatic MRI abnormalities have been reported in infants treated with vigabatrin for infantile spasms; resolution of abnormalities generally occurs upon vigabatrin discontinuation; abnormalities resolved in a few infants, despite continued use; some infants displayed coincident motor abnormalities, but no causal relationship has been established; risk for long-term clinical sequelae has not been studied. Animal models have shown intramyelinic edema in the brain; current evidence suggests that this does not occur in humans; however, patients should be monitored for neurotoxicity. A relationship between MRI abnormalities in infants and animal model findings has not been established. In adult patients, peripheral neuropathy manifesting as numbness or tingling in the toes or feet, reduced distal lower limb vibration or position sensation, or progressive loss of reflexes, starting at the ankles, has been reported.

Anemia has been reported; in some cases with a significant reduction in hemoglobin (<8 g/dL) and/or hematocrit (<24%). Somnolence and fatigue can occur with use; patients must be cautioned about performing tasks which require mental alertness (eg, operating machinery or driving). Peripheral edema independent of hypertension, heart failure, weight gain, or renal or hepatic dysfunction has been reported; in adults, an average weight gain of 3.5 kg has been associated with use. Vigabatrin has been reported to decrease AST and ALT activity in the plasma in up to 90% of patients, causing the enzymes to become undetectable in some patients; this may preclude use of AST and ALT as markers for hepatic injury.

Adverse Reactions

Cardiovascular: Chest pain, peripheral edema

Central nervous system: Abnormal behavior, abnormal dreams, abnormal thinking, aggression, anxiety, confusional state, coordination impairment, depression (see Warnings), disturbance in attention, dizziness, dystonia, expressive language disorder, fatigue, fever (infants: 19% to 29%; adults: 4% to 6%), headache, hypoesthesia, irritability, insomnia, lethargy, memory impairment, MRI abnormalities (see Precautions), nervousness, postictal state, sedation (infants: 17% to 19%; adults: 4%), seizure, sensory disturbance, somnolence (infants: 17% to 45%; adults: 17% to 24%), status epilepticus, suicidal thinking and behavior (see Warnings), vertigo, weakness

Dermatologic: Contusion, rash

Endocrine & metabolic: Dysmenorrhea, fluid retention, weight gain

Gastrointestinal: Abdominal distention, abdominal pain, appetite decreased/increased, constipation, diarrhea, dyspepsia, hemorrhoidal symptoms, nausea, toothache, viral gastroenteritis, vomiting (infants: 14% to 20%; adults: 6% to 7%)

Genitourinary: Urinary tract infection

Hematologic: Anemia

Neuromuscular & skeletal: Arthralgia, asthenia, back pain, dysarthria, gait disturbance, hyper-reflexia, hypertonia, hyporeflexia, hypotonia, joint sprain, joint swelling, muscle spasm, muscle strain, muscle twitching, myalgia, paresthesia, peripheral neuropathy, shoulder pain, tremor

Ocular: Blurred vision, conjunctivitis, diplopia, eyestrain, nystagmus, strabismus, visual field defects (see Warnings)

Otic: Otitis media, tinnitus

Respiratory: Bronchitis, cough, dyspnea, nasal congestion, nasopharyngitis, pharyngitis, pharyngolaryngeal pain, pneumonia, sinus headache, sinusitis, upper respiratory tract infection (infants: 46% to 51%; adults: 7% to 10%)

Miscellaneous: Candidiasis, croup, influenza, thirst, viral infection

◀

<1% (limited to important or life-threatening): Acute psychosis, angioedema, apathy, cholestasis, deafness, delayed puberty, delirium, developmental delay, encephalopathy, esophagitis, facial edema, gastrointestinal hemorrhage, hypomania, laryngoedema, maculopapular rash, malignant hyperthermia, multiorgan failure, myoclonus, neonatal agitation, optic neuritis, pruritus, pulmonary embolism, psychotic disorder, respiratory failure, stridor

Drug Interactions

Avoid Concomitant Use There are no known interactions where it is recommended to avoid concomitant use.

Increased Effect/Toxicity

Vigabatrin may increase the levels/effects of: Alcohol (Ethyl); CNS Depressants; Methotrimeprazine

The levels/effects of Vigabatrin may be increased by: Methotrimeprazine

Decreased Effect Serum concentrations of phenytoin and phenobarbital may be decreased by vigabatrin.

Food Interactions In adults, food decreased the maximum concentration by 33% and increased the time to peak to 2 hours; no change in AUC was observed

Stability Store tablet and powder for oral solution at controlled room temperature of 20°C to 25°C (68°F to 77°F).

Mechanism of Action Irreversibly inhibits gamma-aminobutyric acid transaminase (GABA-T), increasing the levels of the inhibitory compound gamma amino butyric acid (GABA) within the brain. Duration of effect is dependent upon rate of GABA-T resynthesis.

Pharmacodynamics Note: A correlation between serum concentrations and efficacy has not been established.

Duration of action: Variable; dependent on rate of GABA-T resynthesis

Pharmacokinetics (Adult data unless noted)

Absorption: Rapid; bioequivalence established between tablets and oral solution

Distribution: V_{dss} (mean): 1.1 L/kg

Protein binding: Does not bind to plasma proteins

Metabolism: Minimal

Half-life: Infants: 5.7 hours; adults: 7.5 hours; prolonged in renal impairment

Time to peak serum concentration: Infants: 2.5 hours; children and adults: 1 hour

Elimination: Urine (80% as unchanged drug)

Clearance:

Infants: 2.4 ± 0.8 L/hour

Children: 5.7 ± 2.5 L/hour

Adults: 7 L/hour

Dialysis: Effect of dialysis has not been adequately studied; in case reports, hemodialysis decreased vigabatrin plasma concentrations by 40% to 60%

Usual Dosage Oral:

Infantile spasms: Infants and Children (1 month to 2 years of age): Initial dosing: 50 mg/kg/day divided twice daily; may titrate upwards by 25-50 mg/kg/day increments every 3 days based on response and tolerability; maximum dose: 150 mg/kg/day divided twice daily

Note: To taper, decrease dose by 25-50 mg/kg/day every 3-4 days.

Adjunctive treatment of refractory complex partial seizures:

Children ≥10 kg: Initial: 40 mg/kg/day divided twice daily; maintenance dosages based on patient weight (see Camposano, 2008; Coppola, 2004; Willmore, 2009):

10-15 kg: 0.5-1 g/day divided twice daily

16-30 kg: 1-1.5 g/day divided twice daily

31-50 kg: 1.5-3 g/day divided twice daily

>50 kg: 2-3 g/day divided twice daily

Adolescents ≥16 years and Adults: Initial: 500 mg twice daily; increase daily dose by 500 mg increments at weekly intervals based on response and tolerability; recommended dose: 3 g/day divided twice daily

Note: To taper, decrease dose by 1 g/day on a weekly basis.

Dosage adjustment in renal impairment: Adults:

Cl_{cr} >50-80 mL/minute: Decrease dose by 25%

Cl_{cr} >30-50 mL/minute: Decrease dose by 50%

Cl_{cr} >10-30 mL/minute: Decrease dose by 75%

Administration May be administered with or without food. Powder for oral solution: Dissolve each 500 mg powder packet in 10 mL of cold or room temperature water to make a 50 mg/mL solution. The appropriate dose aliquot should be administered immediately using oral syringe. Any remaining liquid should be discarded.

Monitoring Parameters Ophthalmologic examination by an ophthalmic professional with expertise in visual field interpretation and the ability to perform dilated indirect ophthalmoscopy of the retina at baseline (no later than 4 weeks after therapy initiation), periodically during therapy (every 3 months), and 3-6 months after discontinuation of therapy; assessment should include visual acuity and visual field whenever possible including mydriatic peripheral fundus examination and visual field perimetry. Observe patient for excessive sedation, especially when instituting or increasing therapy; frequency, duration, and severity of seizure episodes; hemoglobin and hematocrit; renal function; weight; signs and symptoms of suicidality (eg, anxiety, depression, behavior changes) (see Warnings); neurotoxicity, peripheral neuropathy, and edema.

Reference Range A correlation between serum concentrations and efficacy has not been established.

Test Interactions Vigabatrin has been reported to decrease AST and ALT activity in the plasma in up to 90% of patients, causing the enzymes to become undetectable in some patients; this may preclude use of AST and ALT as markers for hepatic injury. Vigabatrin may increase amino acids in the urine leading to false-positive tests for rare genetic metabolic disorders

Patient Information Read the patient Medication Guide that you receive with each new prescription and refill of vigabatrin. Take exactly as directed. While using this medication, avoid alcohol and other prescription or OTC medications without consulting prescriber. May cause drowsiness and impair ability to perform activities requiring mental alertness or physical coordination. Antiepileptic agents may increase the risk of suicidal thoughts and behavior; notify physician if you feel more depressed or have thoughts of suicide or self harm (see Warnings). Wear identification of epileptic status and medications. Vigabatrin may cause permanent vision damage; report changes in vision, particularly peripheral vision, immediately. Abnormal MRI signal changes may occur with vigabatrin; the clinical significance of these changes are unknown. Report CNS changes, mentation changes, or changes in cognition; changes in gait; persistent GI symptoms (cramping, constipation, vomiting, anorexia); rash or skin irritations; worsening of seizure activity, or loss of seizure control. Do not discontinue abruptly (an increase in seizure activity may result).

Additional Information Vigabatrin is not effective in absence or febrile seizures; exacerbation of certain seizure types or onset of new types of seizures have been seen after initiation of vigabatrin.

Dosage Forms Excipient information presented when available (limited, particularly for generics); consult specific product labeling. [CAN] = Canadian product

Powder for solution, oral:

Sabril®: 500 mg/packet (50s)

Powder for suspension, oral [sachets]:

Sabril® [CAN]: 0.5 g

Tablet, oral:
Sabril®: 500 mg

References

Bar-Oz B, Nulman I, Koren G, et al, "Anticonvulsants and Breast-Feeding: A Critical Review," *Paediatr Drugs*, 2000, 2(2):113-26.

Camposano SE, Major P, Halpern E, et al, "Vigabatrin in the Treatment of Childhood Epilepsy: A Retrospective Chart Review of Efficacy and Safety Profile," *Epilepsia*, 2008, 49(7):1186-91.

Coppola G, "Treatment of Partial Seizures in Childhood: An Overview," *CNS Drugs*, 2004, 18(3):133-56.

Mackay MT, Weiss SK, Adams-Webber T, et al, "Practice Parameter: Medical Treatment of Infantile Spasms: Report of the American Academy of Neurology and the Child Neurology Society," *Neurology*, 2004, 62(10):1668-81.

Pearl PL, Vezina LG, Saneto RP, et al, "Cerebral MRI Abnormalities Associated With Vigabatrin Therapy," *Epilepsia*, 2009, 50(2):184-94.

Tran A, O'Mahoney T, Rey E, et al, "Vigabatrin: Placental Transfer *in vivo* and Excretion Into Breast Milk of the Enantiomers," *Br J Clin Pharmacol*, 1998, 45(4):409-11.

Wheless JW, Carmant L, Bebin M, et al, "Magnetic Resonance Imaging Abnormalities Associated With Vigabatrin in Patients With Epilepsy," *Epilepsia*, 2009, 50(2):195-205.

Willmore LJ, Abelson MB, Ben-Menachem E, et al, "Vigabatrin: 2008 Update," *Epilepsia*, 2009, 50(2):163-73.

VinBLAStine (vin BLAS teen)

Medication Safety Issues

Sound-alike/look-alike issues:
VinBLAStine may be confused with vinCRIStine, vinorelbine

High alert medication: The Institute for Safe Medication Practices (ISMP) includes this medication among its list of drug classes which have a heightened risk of causing significant patient harm when used in error.

Note: Must be dispensed in overwrap which bears the statement **"Do not remove covering until the moment of injection. Fatal if given intrathecally. For I.V. use only."** Syringes should be labeled: **"Fatal if given intrathecally. For I.V. use only."**

Related Information

Compatibility of Chemotherapy and Related Supportive Care Medications *on page 1580*

Emetogenic Potential of Antineoplastic Agents *on page 1579*

Extravasation Treatment *on page 1522*

Therapeutic Category Antineoplastic Agent, Mitotic Inhibitor

Generic Available Yes

Use Palliative treatment of Hodgkin's disease; advanced testicular germinal-cell cancers; non-Hodgkin's lymphoma, histiocytosis X (Letterer-Siwe disease), choriocarcinoma, breast cancer, mycosis fungoides, and Kaposi's sarcoma [FDA approved in pediatrics (age not specified) and adults]. Has been used for the treatment of bladder cancer, melanoma, and nonsmall cell lung cancer (NSCLC)

Pregnancy Risk Factor D

Pregnancy Considerations Animal studies have demonstrated resorption and teratogenic effects. There are no adequate and well-controlled studies in pregnant women. Women of childbearing potential should avoid becoming pregnant during vinblastine treatment. Aspermia has been reported in males who have received treatment with vinblastine.

Lactation Excretion in breast milk unknown/not recommended

Breast-Feeding Considerations Due to the potential for serious adverse reactions in the nursing infant, breast-feeding is not recommended.

Contraindications Hypersensitivity to vinblastine or any component; severe granulocytopenia; presence of bacterial infection. **I.T. administration is contraindicated (may result in death).**

Warnings Hazardous agent; use appropriate precautions for handling and disposal; vinblastine can cause fetal toxicity when administered to pregnant women; for I.V. use only; **intrathecal administration may result in death [U.S. Boxed Warning]**. Must be dispensed in overwrap which bears the statement: **"Do not remove covering until the moment of injection. Fatal if given intrathecally. For I.V. use only."** Vinblastine is a moderate vesicant; avoid extravasation **[U.S. Boxed Warning]**. Assure proper needle or catheter placement prior to administration. Should be administered by individuals experienced in the administration of vinblastine.

Injection (solution) contains benzyl alcohol which may cause allergic reactions in susceptible individuals; large amounts of benzyl alcohol (≥99 mg/kg/day) have been associated with a potentially fatal toxicity ("gasping syndrome") in neonates; the "gasping syndrome" consists of metabolic acidosis, respiratory distress, gasping respirations, CNS dysfunction (including convulsions, intracranial hemorrhage), hypotension and cardiovascular collapse; avoid use of vinblastine products containing benzyl alcohol in neonates; *in vitro* and animal studies have shown that benzoate, a metabolite of benzyl alcohol, displaces bilirubin from protein binding sites

Precautions Use with caution in patients with ischemic heart disease. Acute shortness of breath and severe bronchospasm have been reported in association with concurrent administration of mitomycin; may occur within minutes to several hours following vinblastine administration or up to 14 days following a dose of mitomycin; use caution in patients with pre-existing pulmonary disease. Leukopenia is common; granulocytopenia may be severe with higher doses; leukopenia may be more pronounced in cachectic patients and patients with skin ulceration. Thrombocytopenia and anemia may occur rarely. Dosage modification required in patients with impaired liver function or neurotoxicity (may rarely cause reversible disabling neurotoxicity); dosage should be reduced in patients with recent exposure to radiation therapy or chemotherapy.

Itraconazole and erythromycin may decrease the metabolism of vinblastine via CYP3A4 inhibition, and itraconazole may increase the effects of vinblastine via P-glycoprotein effects; severe myelosuppression and neurotoxicity may occur.

Adverse Reactions

Cardiovascular: Angina, cerebrovascular accident, coronary ischemia, ECG abnormalities, hypertension, MI, orthostatic hypotension, Raynaud's phenomenon, tachycardia

Central nervous system: Depression, dizziness, headache, malaise, neurotoxicity (duration: >24 hours), seizures, vertigo

Dermatologic: Dermatitis, mild alopecia, photosensitivity, rashes, skin blistering

Endocrine & metabolic: Aspermia, hyperuricemia, SIADH

Gastrointestinal: Abdominal pain, anorexia, constipation, diarrhea, gastrointestinal bleeding, hemorrhagic enterocolitis, ileus, metallic taste, nausea, paralytic ileus, rectal bleeding, stomatitis, vomiting

Genitourinary: Urinary retention

Hematologic: Myelosuppression: Anemia, granulocytopenia, leukopenia (nadir: 4-10 days), thrombocytopenia

Local: Cellulitis (with extravasation), irritation, phlebitis (with extravasation), radiation recall, severe tissue burn if infiltrated

Neuromuscular & skeletal: Asthenia, bone pain, deep tendon reflex loss, jaw pain, myalgia, paresthesia, peripheral neuropathy, weakness

Ocular: Nystagmus

Otic: Auditory damage, deafness, vestibular damage

Respiratory: Bronchospasm, dyspnea, pharyngitis, shortness of breath

Miscellaneous: Tumor pain

Drug Interactions

Metabolism/Transport Effects Substrate of CYP2D6 (minor), CYP3A4 (major), P-glycoprotein; **Inhibits** CYP2D6 (weak), CYP3A4 (weak); **Induces** P-glycoprotein

Avoid Concomitant Use

Avoid concomitant use of VinBLAStine with any of the following: BCG; Natalizumab; Pimecrolimus; Tacrolimus (Topical); Vaccines (Live)

Increased Effect/Toxicity

VinBLAStine may increase the levels/effects of: Leflunomide; Mitomycin; Natalizumab; Tolterodine; Vaccines (Live)

The levels/effects of VinBLAStine may be increased by: CYP3A4 Inhibitors (Moderate); CYP3A4 Inhibitors (Strong); Dasatinib; Denosumab; Itraconazole; Lopinavir; Macrolide Antibiotics; MAO Inhibitors; P-Glycoprotein Inhibitors; Pimecrolimus; Posaconazole; Ritonavir; Tacrolimus (Topical); Trastuzumab; Voriconazole

Decreased Effect

VinBLAStine may decrease the levels/effects of: BCG; Dabigatran Etexilate; P-Glycoprotein Substrates; Sipuleucel-T; Vaccines (Inactivated); Vaccines (Live)

The levels/effects of VinBLAStine may be decreased by: CYP3A4 Inducers (Strong); Deferasirox; Echinacea; Herbs (CYP3A4 Inducers); Peginterferon Alfa-2b; P-Glycoprotein Inducers

Stability Store vials at 2°C to 8°C (36°F to 46°F); 1 mg/mL solution prepared with preserved NS injection is stable for 28 days when refrigerated and protected from light. **Note:** Vinblastine must be dispensed in overwrap which bears the statement "Do not remove covering until the moment of injection. Fatal if given intrathecally. For I.V. use only."

Mechanism of Action Binds to microtubular protein of the mitotic spindle causing metaphase arrest; may interfere with nucleic acid synthesis by blocking glutamic acid utilization

Pharmacokinetics (Adult data unless noted)

Distribution: Poor penetration into CSF; rapidly distributed into body tissues; V_{dss}: 27.3 L/kg

Protein binding: 99%

Metabolism: Extensive in the liver via CYP3A4 to an active metabolite

Half-life, terminal: 24.8 hours

Elimination: Biliary excretion (95%), urine (<1% as unchanged drug)

Usual Dosage Vinblastine may be administered at intervals of every 7 days or greater and only after leukocyte count has returned to at least 4000/mm³; maintenance therapy should be titrated according to leukocyte count

I.V. (refer to individual protocols):

Children:

Hodgkin's disease: 2.5-6 mg/m²/day once every 1-2 weeks for 3-6 weeks; maximum weekly dose: 12.5 mg/m²

Histiocytosis X: 0.4 mg/kg once every 7-10 days

Germ cell tumor: 0.2 mg/kg on days 1 and 2 of cycle every 3 weeks times 4 cycles

Adults: 3.7-18.5 mg/m²/day every 7-10 days

Dosing adjustment in hepatic impairment: Children and Adults: Direct serum bilirubin concentration >3 mg/dL: Reduce dose 50%

Administration Parenteral: **Do not administer intrathecally, death may occur**; do not administer I.M. or SubQ since the drug is very irritating; may be administered IVP directly into the vein or through a Y-site of a freely running I.V. over a 1-minute period at a concentration for administration of 1 mg/mL; I.V. continuous infusion: Prolonged administration times and/or increased administration volumes may run the risk of vein irritation and extravasation. Assure proper needle or catheter placement prior to administration.

Monitoring Parameters CBC with differential and platelet count, serum uric acid, hepatic function tests

Patient Information Stool softener and laxatives should be used for constipation prophylaxis. Report to physician any fever, chills, sore throat, bleeding, or bruising; avoid contact with the eyes since the drug is very irritating and corneal ulceration may result. May cause photosensitivity reactions (eg, exposure to sunlight may cause severe sunburn, skin rash, redness, or itching); avoid exposure to sunlight and artificial light sources (sunlamps, tanning booth/bed); wear protective clothing, wide-brimmed hats, sunglasses, and lip sunscreen (SPF ≥15); use a sunscreen [broad-spectrum sunscreen or physical sunscreen (preferred) or sunblock with SPF ≥15]; contact physician if reaction occurs. Women of childbearing potential should be advised to avoid becoming pregnant.

Nursing Implications Maintain adequate hydration. Allopurinol may be given to prevent uric acid nephropathy; stool softeners and laxatives may be helpful in preventing constipation; vinblastine is a tissue irritant and can cause sloughing upon extravasation; check vein patency before drug administration; care should be taken to avoid extravasation. If extravasation occurs, discontinue vinblastine injection immediately; local injection of hyaluronidase into the leading edge of the extravasation site and a warm compress can be used for treatment; apply warm pack immediately for 30-60 minutes, then alternate off/on every 15 minutes for 1 day. Refer to Extravasation Treatment on page 1522.

Avoid contact with the eye since vinblastine is very irritating; if contact occurs, immediately wash eye with water.

Additional Information Myelosuppressive effects:

Nadir (days): 4-10

Recovery (days): 7-14

Dosage Forms Excipient information presented when available (limited, particularly for generics); consult specific product labeling.

Injection, powder for reconstitution, as sulfate: 10 mg

Injection, solution, as sulfate: 1 mg/mL (10 mL) [contains benzyl alcohol]

References

Balis FM, Holcenberg JS and Bleyer WA, "Clinical Pharmacokinetics of Commonly Used Anticancer Drugs," *Clin Pharmacokinet*, 1983, 8 (3):202-32.

Bashir H, Motl S, Metzger ML, et al, "Itraconazole-Enhanced Chemotherapy Toxicity in a Patient With Hodgkin Lymphoma," *J Pediatr Hematol Oncol*, 2006, 28(1):33-5.

Crom WR, Glynn-Barnhart AM, Rodman JH, et al, "Pharmacokinetics of Anticancer Drugs in Children," *Clin Pharmacokinet*, 1987, 12 (3):168-213.

Gadner H, Grois N, Arico M, et al, "A Randomized Trial of Treatment for Multisystem Langerhans' Cell Histiocytosis," *J Pediatr*, 2001, 138 (5):728-34.

Tannock I, Ehrlichman C, Perrault D, et al, "Failure of 5-Day Vinblastine Infusion in the Treatment of Patients With Advanced Refractory Breast Cancer," *Cancer Treat Rep*, 1982, 66(9):1783-4.

Yap HY, Blumenschein GR, Keating MJ, et al, "Vinblastine Given as a Continuous 5-Day Infusion in the Treatment of Refractory Breast Cancer," *Cancer Treat Rep*, 1980, 64(2-3):279-83.

◆ **Vinblastine Sulfate** *see VinBLAStine on page 1423*

◆ **Vincaleukoblastine** *see VinBLAStine on page 1423*

◆ **Vincasar PFS®** *see VinCRIStine on page 1425*

◆ **Vincasar® PFS® (Can)** *see VinCRIStine on page 1425*

VinCRIStine (vin KRIS teen)

Medication Safety Issues
Sound-alike/look-alike issues:
VinCRIStine may be confused with vinBLAStine
Oncovin® may be confused with Ancobon®

High alert medication: This medication is in a class the Institute for Safe Medication Practices (ISMP) includes among its list of drugs which have a heightened risk of causing significant patient harm when used in error.

Administration safety measures: To prevent fatal inadvertent intrathecal injection, it is recommended that vincristine doses be dispensed in a small minibag. Vincristine should **NOT** be prepared during the preparation of any intrathecal medications. After preparation, store vincristine in a location **away** from the separate storage location recommended for intrathecal medications. Vincristine should **NOT** be delivered to the patient at the same time with any medications intended for central nervous system administration.

Related Information
Compatibility of Chemotherapy and Related Supportive Care Medications *on page 1580*
Emetogenic Potential of Antineoplastic Agents *on page 1579*
Extravasation Treatment *on page 1522*

U.S. Brand Names Vincasar PFS®
Canadian Brand Names Vincasar® PFS®
Therapeutic Category Antineoplastic Agent, Mitotic Inhibitor
Generic Available Yes
Use Treatment of acute lymphocytic leukemia (ALL), Hodgkin's disease, neuroblastoma, non-Hodgkin's malignant lymphomas, Wilms' tumor, and rhabdomyosarcoma [FDA approved in pediatrics (age not specified) and adults]; has also been used in the treatment of multiple myeloma, chronic lymphocytic leukemia (CLL), brain tumors, small cell lung cancer, and ovarian germ cell tumors
Pregnancy Risk Factor D
Lactation Enters breast milk/not recommended
Contraindications Hypersensitivity to vincristine or any component; patients with demyelinating form of Charcot-Marie-Tooth syndrome
Warnings Hazardous agent; use appropriate precautions for handling and disposal; vincristine may cause fetal toxicity when administered to pregnant women; **intrathecal administration may result in death [U.S. Boxed Warning]**. All vincristine doses dispensed in syringes must be packaged in an overwrap which is labeled "FATAL IF GIVEN INTRATHECALLY. FOR INTRAVENOUS USE ONLY." Vincristine is a vesicant; avoid extravasation **[U.S. Boxed Warning]**.
Precautions Dosage modification required in patients with impaired hepatic function, patients receiving other neurotoxic drugs, or patients with pre-existing neuromuscular disease. Neurotoxicity appears to be dose-related. Acute uric acid nephropathy has been reported after vincristine administration; monitor serum uric acid during induction of remission in ALL. Acute shortness of breath and bronchospasm have been reported following administration of a vinca alkaloid in combination with mitomycin-C; progressive dyspnea requiring chronic therapy may occur; do not readminister vincristine.

Adverse Reactions
Cardiovascular: Edema, hypertension, orthostatic hypotension
Central nervous system: CNS depression, confusion, cranial nerve paralysis, dizziness, fever, headache, neurotoxicity, seizures, vertigo
Dermatologic: Alopecia, rash
Endocrine & metabolic: Amenorrhea, azoospermia, hyperuricemia
Gastrointestinal: Abdominal cramps, constipation, diarrhea, nausea, paralytic ileus, vomiting
Genitourinary: Dysuria, polyuria, urinary retention
Hematologic: Leukopenia
Hepatic: Hepatic veno-occlusive disease
Local: Cellulitis and tissue necrosis if infiltrated, pain, phlebitis
Neuromuscular & skeletal: Ataxia, cramping, "foot drop" or "wrist drop," jaw pain, leg pain, motor difficulties, muscle wasting, myalgia, numbness, paresthesia of the fingers and toes (stocking glove sensation), weakness
Ocular: Extraocular muscle paresis, nystagmus, photophobia
Otic: Hearing impairment
Respiratory: Dyspnea
Miscellaneous: Anaphylaxis
<1%, postmarketing, and/or case reports: SIADH (rare), stomatitis

Drug Interactions
Metabolism/Transport Effects Substrate of CYP3A4 (major), P-glycoprotein; **Inhibits** CYP3A4 (weak)

Avoid Concomitant Use
Avoid concomitant use of VinCRIStine with any of the following: BCG; Natalizumab; Pimecrolimus; Tacrolimus (Topical); Vaccines (Live)

Increased Effect/Toxicity
VinCRIStine may increase the levels/effects of: Leflunomide; Mitomycin; Natalizumab; Vaccines (Live); Vitamin K Antagonists

The levels/effects of VinCRIStine may be increased by: CYP3A4 Inhibitors (Moderate); CYP3A4 Inhibitors (Strong); Dasatinib; Denosumab; Itraconazole; Lopinavir; Macrolide Antibiotics; MAO Inhibitors; NIFEdipine; P-Glycoprotein Inhibitors; Pimecrolimus; Posaconazole; Ritonavir; Tacrolimus (Topical); Trastuzumab; Voriconazole

Decreased Effect
VinCRIStine may decrease the levels/effects of: BCG; Cardiac Glycosides; Sipuleucel-T; Vaccines (Inactivated); Vaccines (Live); Vitamin K Antagonists

The levels/effects of VinCRIStine may be decreased by: CYP3A4 Inducers (Strong); Deferasirox; Echinacea; Herbs (CYP3A4 Inducers); P-Glycoprotein Inducers

Stability Store at 2°C to 8°C (36°F to 46°F); protect from light; store vials upright. Injectable solution is stable for 1 month at room temperature. **Note:** Vincristine must be dispensed in overwrap which bears the statement "Do not remove covering until the moment of injection. Fatal if given intrathecally. For I.V. use only."

Mechanism of Action Binds to microtubular protein of the mitotic spindle causing metaphase arrest

Pharmacokinetics (Adult data unless noted)
Distribution: Poor penetration into the CSF; V_{dss}: 120 L/m^2
Protein binding: 75%
Metabolism: Extensive in the liver via CYP3A subfamily
Half-life, terminal: 24-85 hours
Elimination: Primarily in bile (~80%); 10% to 20% found in urine
Clearance:
Infants: Vincristine clearance is more closely related to body weight than to body surface area
Children 2-18 years: 482 mL/minute/m^2 (faster clearance in children <10 years of age than in adolescents)

Usual Dosage I.V. (refer to individual protocols):
Children ≤10 kg or BSA <1 m^2: Initial therapy: 0.05 mg/kg/dose once weekly then titrate dose; maximum single dose: 2 mg

Children >10 kg or BSA ≥1 m²: 1-2 mg/m²/dose, may repeat once weekly for 3-6 weeks; maximum single dose: 2 mg

Neuroblastoma: I.V. continuous infusion with doxorubicin: 1 mg/m²/day for 72 hours

Adults: 0.4-1.4 mg/m²/dose up to 2 mg; may repeat every week

Dosing adjustment in hepatic impairment: Children and Adults: Direct serum bilirubin concentration >3 mg/dL: Dosage reduction of 50% is recommended

Administration Parenteral: **Do not administer intrathecally, death may occur**; do not administer I.M. or SubQ since the drug is very irritating; I.V.: I.V. needle or catheter must be properly positioned before any vincristine is injected. Vincristine is administered IVP or through a Y-site of a freely running I.V. over a period of 1 minute at a concentration for administration of 1 mg/mL; may administer as a dilute I.V. infusion

Note: Do not administer to patients while they are receiving radiation therapy through ports that include the liver. If used in combination with L-asparaginase, administer vincristine 12-24 hours before L-asparaginase to minimize toxicity.

Monitoring Parameters Serum electrolytes (sodium), hepatic function tests, neurologic examination, CBC, hemoglobin, serum uric acid

Patient Information Stool softener and laxatives should be used for constipation prophylaxis; report to physician any fever, sore throat, bleeding, bruising, or shortness of breath. Women of childbearing potential should avoid becoming pregnant.

Nursing Implications Maintain adequate hydration. Allopurinol may be given to prevent uric acid nephropathy; vincristine is a tissue irritant; care should be taken to avoid extravasation. If extravasation occurs, vincristine injection should be discontinued immediately; local injection of hyaluronidase into the leading edge of the extravasation site and a warm compress can be used for treatment; apply warm pack immediately for 30-60 minutes, then alternate off/on every 15 minutes for 1 day; refer to Extravasation Treatment on page 1522. Avoid contact with the eye since vincristine is very irritating.

Additional Information Ten times the usual recommended dose of vincristine in children < 13 years of age have been lethal; 3-4 mg/m² doses can be expected to produce severe toxic manifestations. Treatment is supportive and symptomatic, including anticonvulsants, fluid restriction, and diuretics to prevent adverse effects from SIADH and enemas or cathartics to prevent ileus. Use of leucovorin calcium may be helpful in treating vincristine overdose. Leucovorin calcium 100 mg I.V. every 3 hours for 24 hours, then every 6 hours for at least 48 hours has been administered in case reports.

Dosage Forms Excipient information presented when available (limited, particularly for generics); consult specific product labeling.

Injection, solution, as sulfate [preservative free]: 1 mg/mL (1 mL, 2 mL)

Vincasar PFS®: 1 mg/mL (1 mL, 2 mL)

References

Arndt C, Hawkins D, Anderson JR, et al, "Age Is a Risk Factor for Chemotherapy-Induced Hepatopathy With Vincristine, Dactinomycin, and Cyclophosphamide," *J Clin Oncol*, 2004, 22(10):1894-901.

Crom WR, deGraaf SS, Synold T, et al, "Pharmacokinetics of Vincristine in Children and Adolescents With Acute Lymphocytic Leukemia," *J Pediatr*, 1994, 125(4):642-9.

Granowetter L, Womer R, Devidas M, et al, "Dose-Intensified Compared With Standard Chemotherapy for Nonmetastatic Ewing Sarcoma Family of Tumors: A Children's Oncology Group Study," *J Clin Oncol*, 2009, 27(15):2536-41.

Woods WG, O'Leary M, and Nesbit ME, "Life-Threatening Neuropathy and Hepatotoxicity in Infants During Induction Therapy for Acute Lymphoblastic Leukemia," *J Pediatr*, 1981, 98(4):642-5.

♦ **Vincristine Sulfate** *see* VinCRIStine *on page 1425*

♦ **Viokase® [DSC]** *see* Pancrelipase *on page 1051*

♦ **Viokase® (Can)** *see* Pancrelipase *on page 1051*

♦ **Viosterol** *see* Ergocalciferol *on page 519*

♦ **Viracept®** *see* Nelfinavir *on page 975*

♦ **Viramune®** *see* Nevirapine *on page 983*

♦ **Virazole®** *see* Ribavirin *on page 1210*

♦ **Viread®** *see* Tenofovir *on page 1319*

♦ **Viroptic®** *see* Trifluridine *on page 1384*

♦ **Visicol®** *see* Sodium Phosphate *on page 1276*

♦ **Visine® L.R. [OTC]** *see* Oxymetazoline *on page 1043*

♦ **Visipaque™** *see* Iodixanol *on page 754*

♦ **Vistaril®** *see* HydrOXYzine *on page 697*

♦ **Vistide®** *see* Cidofovir *on page 307*

♦ **Vita-C® [OTC]** *see* Ascorbic Acid *on page 138*

♦ **Vitamin C** *see* Ascorbic Acid *on page 138*

Vitamin A (VYE ta min aye)

Medication Safety Issues

Sound-alike/look-alike issues:

Aquasol® may be confused with Anusol®

U.S. Brand Names Aquasol A®; Palmitate-A® [OTC]

Therapeutic Category Nutritional Supplement; Vitamin, Fat Soluble

Generic Available Yes: Capsule

Use Treatment and prevention of vitamin A deficiency; supplementation in children 6 months to 2 years with measles

Pregnancy Risk Factor A/X (dose exceeding RDA recommendation)

Pregnancy Considerations Excessive use of vitamin A shortly before and during pregnancy could be harmful to babies.

Lactation Enters breast milk/compatible at normal daily doses

Contraindications Hypersensitivity to vitamin A or any component; hypervitaminosis A; pregnancy (dose exceeding RDA)

Warnings Patients receiving >25,000 units/day should be closely monitored for toxicity; polysorbates contained in parenteral vitamin A have been associated with thrombocytopenia, renal dysfunction, hepatomegaly, cholestasis, ascites, hypotension, and metabolic acidosis when administered to neonates (E-Ferol syndrome); avoid use in neonates

Adverse Reactions Seen only with doses exceeding physiologic replacement

Central nervous system: Irritability, drowsiness, vertigo, delirium, headache, coma, intracranial pressure elevated

Dermatologic: Erythema, peeling skin

Gastrointestinal: Vomiting, diarrhea

Ocular: Visual disturbances, papilledema

Drug Interactions

Avoid Concomitant Use

Avoid concomitant use of Vitamin A with any of the following: Retinoic Acid Derivatives

Increased Effect/Toxicity

Vitamin A may increase the levels/effects of: Retinoid-like Compounds; Vitamin K Antagonists

The levels/effects of Vitamin A may be increased by: Retinoic Acid Derivatives

Decreased Effect

The levels/effects of Vitamin A may be decreased by: Orlistat

Stability Protect injectable preparation from light

Mechanism of Action Needed for bone development, growth, visual adaptation to darkness, testicular and ovarian function, and as a cofactor in many biochemical processes

Pharmacokinetics (Adult data unless noted)
Absorption: Vitamin A in dosages **not** exceeding physiologic replacement is well absorbed after oral administration; water miscible preparations are absorbed more rapidly than oil preparations; large oral doses, conditions of fat malabsorption, low protein intake, or hepatic or pancreatic disease reduce oral absorption
Metabolism: Conjugated with glucuronide, undergoes enterohepatic circulation
Elimination: In feces via biliary elimination

Usual Dosage
Recommended daily allowance (RDA): Oral:
<1 year: 375 mcg* (1250 units)
1-3 years: 400 mcg* (1330 units)
4-6 years: 500 mcg* (1670 units)
7-10 years: 700 mcg* (2330 units)
>10 years: Female: 800 mcg* (2670 units); Male: 1000 mcg* (3330 units)
*mcg retinol equivalent (0.3 mcg retinol = 1 unit vitamin A)
Daily dietary supplement: Oral:
Infants up to 6 months: 1500 units
Children:
6 months to 3 years: 1500-2000 units
4-6 years: 2500 units
7-10 years: 3300-3500 units
Children >10 years and Adults: 4000-5000 units
Vitamin A supplementation in measles (recommendation of the World Health Organization): Children: Oral: Give as a single dose; repeat the next day and at 4 weeks for children with ophthalmologic evidence of vitamin A deficiency:
6 months to 1 year: 100,000 units
>1 year: 200,000 units
Note: Use of vitamin A in measles is recommended only for patients 6 months to 2 years of age hospitalized with measles and its complications **or** patients >6 months of age who have any of the following risk factors and who are not already receiving vitamin A: immunodeficiency, ophthalmologic evidence of vitamin A deficiency including night blindness, Bitot's spots or evidence of xerophthalmia, impaired intestinal absorption, moderate to severe malnutrition including that associated with eating disorders, or recent immigration from areas where high mortality rates from measles have been observed.
Note: Monitor patients closely; dosages >25,000 units/day have been associated with toxicity
Vitamin A deficiency (varying recommendations available):
Severe deficiency with xerophthalmia:
Infants: I.M.: 7500-15,000 units/day followed by oral 5000-10,000 units/day for 10 days
Children 1-8 years: Oral: 5000 units/kg/day for 5 days then 5000-10,000 units/day for 2 months; I.M.: 17,500-35,000 units/day for 10 days
Children >8 years and Adults: Oral: 500,000 units/day for 3 days, then 50,000 units/day for 14 days; then 10,000-20,000 units/day for 2 months; I.M.: 100,000 units/day for 3 days; then 50,000 units/day for 14 days
Prophylactic therapy for children at risk for developing deficiency: Oral: Given every 4-6 months:
Infants ≤1 year: 100,000 units
Children >1 year: 200,000 units
Malabsorption syndrome (prophylaxis): Children >8 years and Adults: Oral: 10,000-50,000 units/day of water miscible product

Administration
Oral: Administer with food or milk
Parenteral: I.M. only

Additional Information 1 USP vitamin A unit = 0.3 mcg of all-*trans* isomer of retinol; 1 RE (retinol equivalent) = 1 mcg of all-*trans*-retinol

Dosage Forms Excipient information presented when available (limited, particularly for generics); consult specific product labeling:
Capsule [softgel]: 10,000 units; 25,000 units
Injection, solution (Aquasol A®): 50,000 units/mL (2 mL) [contains polysorbate 80]
Tablet (Palmitate-A®): 5000 units, 15,000 units

References
Committee on Infectious Diseases, "Vitamin A in the Treatment of Measles," *Pediatrics*, 1993, 91(5):1014-5.
DeMaeyer EM, "The WHO Programme of Prevention and Control of Vitamin A Deficiency, Xerophthalmia, and Nutritional Blindness," *Nutr Health*, 1986, 4(2):105-12.
Hussey GD and Klein M, "A Randomized, Controlled Trial of Vitamin A in Children With Severe Measles," *N Engl J Med*, 1990, 323(3):160-4.

♦ **Vitamin A Acid** see Tretinoin (Topical) *on page 1375*
♦ **Vitamin B₁** see Thiamine *on page 1338*
♦ **Vitamin B₂** see Riboflavin *on page 1213*
♦ **Vitamin B₃** see Niacin *on page 986*
♦ **Vitamin B₆** see Pyridoxine *on page 1190*
♦ **Vitamin B₁₂** see Cyanocobalamin *on page 365*
♦ **Vitamin B₁₂ₐ** see Hydroxocobalamin *on page 692*
♦ **Vitamin Bw** see Biotin *on page 194*
♦ **Vitamin D2** see Ergocalciferol *on page 519*
♦ **Vitamin D3 [OTC]** see Cholecalciferol *on page 300*

Vitamin E (VYE ta min ee)

Medication Safety Issues
Sound-alike/look-alike issues:
Aquasol E® may be confused with Anusol®

U.S. Brand Names Alph-E [OTC]; Alph-E-Mixed [OTC]; Aquavit-E [OTC]; Aquavit-E [OTC] [DSC]; d-Alpha-Gems™ [OTC]; E-Gems Elite® [OTC]; E-Gems Plus® [OTC]; E-Gems® [OTC]; Ester-E™ [OTC]; Gamma E-Gems® [OTC]; Gamma-E Plus [OTC]; High Gamma Vitamin E Complete™ [OTC]; Key-E® Kaps [OTC]; Key-E® [OTC]

Therapeutic Category Nutritional Supplement; Vitamin, Fat Soluble; Vitamin, Topical

Generic Available Yes

Use Prevention and treatment of vitamin E deficiency

Pregnancy Risk Factor A/C (dose exceeding RDA recommendation)

Lactation Enters breast milk/compatible

Contraindications Hypersensitivity to vitamin E or any component

Warnings Necrotizing enterocolitis has been associated with oral administration of large dosages (eg, >200 units/day) of a hyperosmolar vitamin E preparation in low birth weight infants

Adverse Reactions
Central nervous system: Headache
Dermatologic: Rash
Endocrine & metabolic: Gonadal dysfunction; serum thyroxine and triiodothyronine decreased; cholesterol and triglycerides elevated
Gastrointestinal: Nausea, diarrhea, intestinal cramps, necrotizing enterocolitis (see Warnings)
Neuromuscular & skeletal: Weakness
Ocular: Blurred vision
Renal: Creatinuria and serum creatinine kinase elevated; urinary estrogens and androgens elevated

Drug Interactions
Avoid Concomitant Use There are no known interactions where it is recommended to avoid concomitant use.

Increased Effect/Toxicity
Vitamin E may increase the levels/effects of: Vitamin K Antagonists

Decreased Effect
The levels/effects of Vitamin E may be decreased by: Orlistat

Mechanism of Action Antioxidant which prevents oxidation of vitamin A and C; protects polyunsaturated fatty acids in membranes from attack by free radicals and protects red blood cells against hemolysis by oxidizing agents

Pharmacokinetics (Adult data unless noted)
Absorption: Oral: Depends upon the presence of bile; absorption is reduced in conditions of malabsorption, in low birth weight premature infants, and as dosage increases; water miscible preparations are better absorbed than oil preparations
Metabolism: In the liver to glucuronides
Elimination: Primarily in bile

Usual Dosage 1 unit vitamin E = 1 mg *dl*-alpha-tocopherol acetate. Oral:

Vitamin E – Recommended Daily Allowance (RDA) and Estimated Average Requirement (EAR)

Age	RDA (mg/day)	EAR (mg/day)
0-6 mo	–	4 (6 units)
7-12 mo	–	6 (9 units)
1-3 y	6 (9 units)	5 (7.5 units)
4-8 y	7 (10.5 units)	6 (9 units)
9-13 y	11 (16.5 units)	9 (13.5 units)
≥14 y	15 (22.5 units)	12 (18 units)

Vitamin E deficiency:
Neonates, premature, low birth weight: 25-50 units/day results in normal levels within 1 week
Children (with malabsorption syndrome): 1 unit/kg/day of water miscible vitamin E (to raise plasma tocopherol concentrations to the normal range within 2 months and to maintain normal plasma concentrations)
Adults: 60-75 units/day
Prevention of vitamin E deficiency:
Neonates:
Low birth weight: 5 units/day
Full-term: 5 units/L of formula ingested
Adults: 30 units/day
Prevention of retinopathy of prematurity or BPD secondary to O₂ therapy: Neonates and Infants: (American Academy of Pediatrics considers this use investigational and routine use is not recommended): 15-30 units/kg/day to maintain plasma levels between 1.5-2 mcg/mL (may need as high as 100 units/kg/day)
Cystic fibrosis, beta-thalassemia, sickle cell anemia may require higher daily maintenance doses: Infants, Children, and Adolescents:
Cystic fibrosis: 100-400 units/day
Beta-thalassemia: 750 units/day
Sickle cell: 450 units/day
Topical: Apply a thin layer over affected area

Administration Oral: May administer with or without food

Monitoring Parameters Plasma tocopherol concentrations

Reference Range Plasma tocopherol: 6-14 mcg/mL

Dosage Forms Excipient information presented when available (limited, particularly for generics); consult specific product labeling. [DSC] = Discontinued product
Capsule: 400 int. units, 1000 int. units
Key-E® Kaps: 200 int. units, 400 int. units

Capsule, softgel: 200 int. units, 400 int. units, 600 int. units, 1000 int. units
Alph-E: 200 int. units, 400 int. units
Alph-E-Mixed: 200 int. units [contains mixed tocopherols]; 400 int. units [contains mixed tocopherols], 1000 int. units [sugar free; contains mixed tocopherols]
d-Alpha-Gems™: 400 int. units [derived from soybean oil]
E-Gems®: 30 int. units, 100 int. units, 200 int. units, 400 int. units, 600 int. units, 800 int. units, 1000 int. units, 1200 int. units [derived from soybean oil]
E-Gems Plus®: 200 int. units, 400 int. units, 800 int. units [contains mixed tocopherols]
E-Gems Elite®: 400 int. units [contains mixed tocopherols]
Ester-E™: 400 int. units
Gamma E-Gems®: 90 int. units [also contains mixed tocopherols]
Gamma-E Plus: 200 int. units [contains soybean oil]
High Gamma Vitamin E Complete™: 200 int. units [contains soybean oil, mixed tocopherols]
Cream: 50 int. units/g (60 g), 100 int. units/g (60 g), 1000 int. units/120 g (120 g), 30,000 int. units/57 g (57 g)
Key-E®: 30 int. units/g (60 g, 120 g, 600 g)
Lip balm (E-Gem® Lip Care): 1000 int. units/tube [contains vitamin A and aloe]
Oil, oral/topical: 100 int. units/0.25 mL (60 mL, 75 mL); 1150 units/0.25 mL (30 mL, 60 mL, 120 mL); 28,000 int. units/30 mL (30 mL)
Alph-E: 28,000 int. units/30 mL (30 mL) [topical]
E-Gems®: 100 units/10 drops (15 mL, 60 mL)
Ointment, topical (Key-E®): 30 units/g (60 g, 120 g, 480 g)
Powder (Key-E®): 700 int. units per 1/4 teaspoon (15 g, 75 g, 1000 g) [derived from soybean oil]
Solution, oral drops: 15 int. units/0.3 mL (30 mL)
Aquasol E®: 15 int. units/0.3 mL (12 mL, 30 mL) [latex free]
Aquavit-E: 15 int. units/0.3 mL (30 mL) [butterscotch flavor] [DSC]
Suppository, rectal/vaginal (Key-E®): 30 int. units (12s, 24s) [contains coconut oil]
Tablet: 100 int. units, 200 int. units, 400 int. units, 500 int. units
Key-E®: 200 int. units, 400 int. units

References
American Academy of Pediatrics Committee on Fetus and Newborn, "Vitamin E and the Prevention of Retinopathy of Prematurity," *Pediatrics*, 1985, 76(2):315-6.

◆ **Vitamin G** see Riboflavin *on page 1213*
◆ **Vitamin H** see Biotin *on page 194*
◆ **Vitamin K₁** see Phytonadione *on page 1109*
◆ **Vitrase®** see Hyaluronidase *on page 679*
◆ **Vitrasert®** see Ganciclovir *on page 636*
◆ **Vi Vaccine** see Typhoid Vaccine *on page 1391*
◆ **Vivactil®** see Protriptyline *on page 1181*
◆ **Vivarin® [OTC]** see Caffeine *on page 225*
◆ **Vivelle® [DSC]** see Estradiol *on page 536*
◆ **Vivelle-Dot®** see Estradiol *on page 536*
◆ **Vivotif®** see Typhoid Vaccine *on page 1391*
◆ **VLB** see VinBLAStine *on page 1423*
◆ **VM-26** see Teniposide *on page 1318*
◆ **Voltaren® [DSC]** see Diclofenac *on page 429*
◆ **Voltaren® (Can)** see Diclofenac *on page 429*
◆ **Voltaren® Emulgel™ (Can)** see Diclofenac *on page 429*
◆ **Voltaren® Gel** see Diclofenac *on page 429*
◆ **Voltaren Ophtha® (Can)** see Diclofenac *on page 429*
◆ **Voltaren Ophthalmic®** see Diclofenac *on page 429*
◆ **Voltaren Rapide® (Can)** see Diclofenac *on page 429*

♦ **Voltaren SR® (Can)** *see* Diclofenac *on page 429*

♦ **Voltaren®-XR** *see* Diclofenac *on page 429*

Voriconazole (vor i KOE na zole)

U.S. Brand Names VFEND®
Canadian Brand Names VFEND®
Therapeutic Category Antifungal Agent, Systemic; Antifungal Agent, Triazole
Generic Available No
Use Treatment of invasive aspergillosis, especially in immunocompromised patients; treatment of candidemia in non-neutropenic patients; deep tissue *Candida* infections; esophageal candidiasis; treatment of serious fungal infections caused by *Scedosporium apiospermum* or *Fusarium* spp (including *Fusarium solanae*) in patients intolerant of, or refractory to, conventional antifungal therapy (FDA approved in ages ≥12 years).
Pregnancy Risk Factor D
Pregnancy Considerations Voriconazole can cause fetal harm when administered to a pregnant woman. Voriconazole was teratogenic and embryotoxic in animal studies, and lowered plasma estradiol in animal models. Women of childbearing potential should use effective contraception during treatment. Should be used in pregnant woman only if benefit to mother justifies potential risk to the fetus.
Lactation Excretion in breast milk unknown/not recommended
Breast-Feeding Considerations Excretion in breast milk has not been investigated; avoid breast-feeding until additional data are available.
Contraindications Hypersensitivity to voriconazole or any component; concurrent therapy with rifampin, carbamazepine, long-acting barbiturates (phenobarbital, mephobarbital), sirolimus, CYP3A4 substrates (terfenadine, astemizole, cisapride, pimozide, quinidine), ritonavir (high-dose), ergot alkaloids, rifabutin, St John's wort (see Drug Interactions).
Warnings Serious hepatic reactions including hepatitis, cholestasis, fulminant hepatic failure, and death have been reported. Liver function test abnormalities may be associated with higher plasma drug concentrations and/or doses; dosage adjustment or discontinuation of therapy may be required. Visual changes such as blurred vision, photophobia, changes in visual acuity and color have been reported in clinical trials. Patients should be warned to avoid tasks which depend on vision, including operating machinery or driving; the effect on vision with long-term administration (beyond 28 days) is unknown and should be monitored. Torsade de pointes and QT interval prolongation have been reported in patients taking voriconazole. Administer with caution to patients with proarrhythmic conditions. Has been associated with photosensitivity skin reactions and the development of squamous cell carcinoma, melanoma, and other serious dermatologic reactions, particularly in immunocompromised patients on chronic voriconazole therapy.

If used during pregnancy, the patient should be informed that voriconazole may cause fetal harm. Voriconazole tablets contain lactose; avoid use in patients with rare hereditary problems of galactose intolerance, Lapp lactase deficiency, or glucose-galactose malabsorption. Voriconazole oral suspension contains sucrose; avoid use in patients with rare hereditary problems of fructose intolerance, sucrose-isomaltase deficiency or glucose-galactose malabsorption.

Voriconazole is metabolized by cytochrome P450 enzymes resulting in interactions with other drugs. Due to potential serious and/or life-threatening drug interactions, some drugs are contraindicated (see Contraindications and Drug Interactions).

Voriconazole oral suspension contains sodium benzoate; benzoic acid (benzoate) is a metabolite of benzyl alcohol; large amounts of benzyl alcohol (≥99 mg/kg/day) have been associated with a potentially fatal toxicity ("gasping syndrome") in neonates; the "gasping syndrome" consists of metabolic acidosis, respiratory distress, gasping respirations, CNS dysfunction (including convulsions, intracranial hemorrhage), hypotension and cardiovascular collapse; use voriconazole oral suspension containing sodium benzoate with caution in neonates; *in vitro* and animal studies have shown that benzoate displaces bilirubin from protein binding sites

Precautions Use caution in patients with hypersensitivity to other azole antifungal agents since cross-reaction may occur but has not been established; use with caution in patients with severe renal or hepatic impairment; modify dosage in patients with mild to moderate hepatic cirrhosis (Child-Pugh class A and B); avoid administration of voriconazole injection in patients with Cl_{cr} <50 mL/minute since I.V. formulation contains sulfobutyl ether beta-cyclodextrin (SBECD) which may accumulate in renal insufficiency. Infusion-related anaphylactoid-type reactions (chest tightness, dyspnea, faintness, fever, flushing, nausea, pruritus, rash, sweating, and tachycardia) have been reported (uncommon); consider stopping infusion if this occurs.

Adverse Reactions

Cardiovascular: Arrhythmias (including torsade de pointes; see Warnings), cardiac arrest, cerebrovascular accident, congestive heart failure, hypertension, hypotension, peripheral edema, QT interval prolongation, tachycardia, vasodilation

Central nervous system: Amnesia, anxiety, chills, confusion, convulsions, depression, dizziness, fatigue, fever, hallucinations, headache, hemiparesis, insomnia, lethargy

Dermatologic: Alopecia, erythema multiforme (rare), melanoma, photosensitivity (occurs more frequently with long-term treatment), pruritus, rash, squamous cell carcinoma, Stevens-Johnson syndrome (rare), toxic epidermal necrolysis (rare)

Endocrine & metabolic: Diabetes insipidus, hyperglycemia, hyperthyroidism, hypocalcemia, hypokalemia, hypomagnesemia, hypothyroidism

Gastrointestinal: Abdominal pain, anorexia, constipation, diarrhea, dysphagia, GI hemorrhage, mucositis, nausea, pancreatitis, vomiting, xerostomia

Genitourinary: Hemorrhagic cystitis, urinary retention, urinary tract infection

Hematologic: Anemia, leukopenia, lymphopenia, thrombocytopenia

Hepatic: ALT, AST, alkaline phosphatase, and bilirubin increased; cholestatic jaundice; fulminant hepatic failure; hepatitis

Neuromuscular & skeletal: Arthralgia, ataxia, bone pain, myalgia

Ocular: Abnormal vision, blurred vision, chromatopsia, color vision change, optic atrophy, optic neuritis, papilledema (visual disturbance is reversible; incidence is dose-related; onset after first-second dose), photophobia

Renal: Acute renal failure, BUN increased, creatinine increased

Respiratory: Cough, dyspnea, epistaxis, hemoptysis

Miscellaneous: Anaphylaxis, anaphylactoid-type reaction (chest tightness, dyspnea, faintness, flushing, fever, nausea, pruritus, rash, sweating, tachycardia) may appear immediately after initiating the I.V. infusion, diaphoresis, sepsis

◀ <1%, postmarketing, and/or case reports: Agitation, agranulocytosis, akathisia, anemia (aplastic, hemolytic, macrocytic, megaloblastic, or microcytic), angioedema, anuria, arthritis, ascites, asthenia, atrial fibrillation, AV block, back pain, bigeminy, bleeding time increased, blepharitis, bone marrow depression, bone necrosis, bradycardia, brain edema, bundle branch block, cardiomegaly, cardiomyopathy, cerebral hemorrhage, cerebral ischemia, cheilitis, chest pain, cholecystitis, cholelithiasis, color blindness, coma, conjunctivitis, contact dermatitis, corneal opacity, CPK increased, cyanosis, deafness, delirium, dementia, depersonalization, DIC, diplopia, discoid lupus erythematosus, dry skin, duodenal ulcer perforation, duodenitis, DVT, dysmenorrhea, dyspepsia, dysuria, ear pain, ecchymosis, eczema, edema, encephalitis, encephalopathy, endocarditis, eosinophilia, esophageal ulcer, esophagitis, exfoliative dermatitis, extrapyramidal symptoms, eye pain, fixed drug eruption, flatulence, flu syndrome, furunculosis, gastroenteritis, gingivitis, glossitis, glucose tolerance decreased, glycosuria, granuloma, Guillain-Barré syndrome, gum hemorrhage, gum hyperplasia, hematemesis, hematuria, hepatic coma, hepatomegaly, herpes simplex, hydronephrosis, hypercalcemia, hypercholesterolemia, hyperkalemia, hypermagnesemia, hypernatremia, hypertonia, hyperthyroidism, hyperuricemia, hypervolemia, hypoglycemia, hyponatremia, hypophosphatemia, hypoxia, injection-site pain/inflammation/infection, intestinal perforation, intracranial hypertension, leg cramps, lymphadenopathy, lymphangitis, melanosis, melena, MI, multiorgan failure, myasthenia, myopathy, nephritis, nephrosis, neuralgia, neuropathy, night blindness, nystagmus, oculogyric crisis, oliguria, osteomalacia, osteoporosis, palpitation, pancytopenia, papilledema, paresthesia, parotid gland enlargement, periodontitis, peritonitis, petechia, pleural effusion, postural hypotension, proctitis, pseudomembranous colitis, pseudoporphyria, psoriasis, psychosis, pulmonary embolus, purpura, rectal disorder, rectal hemorrhage, renal tubular necrosis, respiratory distress syndrome, retinal hemorrhage, retinitis, scleritis, skin discoloration, somnolence, spleen enlarged, stomatitis, suicidal ideation, supraventricular extrasystoles, supraventricular tachycardia, syncope, taste abnormality, thrombophlebitis, thrombotic thrombocytopenic purpura, tinnitus, tongue edema, tremor, uremia, urticaria, uterine hemorrhage, uveitis, vaginal hemorrhage, ventricular fibrillation, ventricular tachycardia, vertigo, voice alteration

Drug Interactions

Metabolism/Transport Effects Substrate of CYP2C9 (major), 2C19 (major), 3A4 (minor); **Inhibits** CYP2C9 (weak), 2C19 (weak), 3A4 (moderate)

Avoid Concomitant Use

Avoid concomitant use of Voriconazole with any of the following: Alfuzosin; Artemether; Barbiturates; CarBAMazepine; Cisapride; Conivaptan; Darunavir; Dofetilide; Dronedarone; Eplerenone; Ergot Derivatives; Everolimus; Halofantrine; Lopinavir; Lumefantrine; Nilotinib; Nisoldipine; Pimozide; QuiNIDine; QuiNINE; Ranolazine; Rifamycin Derivatives; Ritonavir; Rivaroxaban; Romidepsin; Salmeterol; Silodosin; Sirolimus; St Johns Wort; Tamsulosin; Tetrabenazine; Thioridazine; Tolvaptan; Ziprasidone

Increased Effect/Toxicity

Voriconazole may increase the levels/effects of: Alfentanil; Alfuzosin; Almotriptan; Alosetron; Antineoplastic Agents (Vinca Alkaloids); Aprepitant; Benzodiazepines (metabolized by oxidation); Bortezomib; Bosentan; Brinzolamide; BusPIRone; Busulfan; Calcium Channel Blockers; CarBAMazepine; Ciclesonide; Cilostazol; Cinacalcet; Cisapride; Colchicine; Conivaptan; Contraceptives (Estrogens); Contraceptives (Progestins); Corticosteroids (Orally Inhaled); Corticosteroids (Systemic); CycloSPORINE; CycloSPORINE (Systemic); CYP3A4 Substrates; Diclofenac; Diclofenac (Systemic); Diclofenac (Topical); Dienogest; Docetaxel; Dofetilide; Dronedarone; Dutasteride; Eletriptan; Eplerenone; Ergot Derivatives; Erlotinib; Eszopiclone; Everolimus; FentaNYL; Fesoterodine; Fosaprepitant; Gefitinib; GuanFACINE; Halofantrine; HMG-CoA Reductase Inhibitors; Imatinib; Irinotecan; Ixabepilone; Losartan; Lumefantrine; Macrolide Antibiotics; Maraviroc; Methadone; Methyl-PREDNISolone; Nilotinib; Nisoldipine; Paricalcitol; Pazopanib; Phenytoin; Phosphodiesterase 5 Inhibitors; Pimecrolimus; Pimozide; Protease Inhibitors; QTc-Prolonging Agents; QuiNIDine; QuiNINE; Ramelteon; Ranolazine; Repaglinide; Reverse Transcriptase Inhibitors (Non-Nucleoside); Rifamycin Derivatives; Rivaroxaban; Romidepsin; Salmeterol; Saxagliptin; Silodosin; Sirolimus; Solifenacin; Sorafenib; Sunitinib; Tacrolimus; Tacrolimus (Systemic); Tacrolimus (Topical); Tadalafil; Tamsulosin; Tetrabenazine; Thioridazine; Tolterodine; Tolvaptan; Venlafaxine; Vitamin K Antagonists; Ziprasidone; Zolpidem

The levels/effects of Voriconazole may be increased by: Alfuzosin; Artemether; Chloroquine; Ciprofloxacin; Ciprofloxacin (Systemic); Contraceptives (Estrogens); Contraceptives (Progestins); CYP2C9 Inhibitors (Moderate); CYP2C9 Inhibitors (Strong); Gadobutrol; Grapefruit Juice; Lumefantrine; Macrolide Antibiotics; Nilotinib; Protease Inhibitors; Proton Pump Inhibitors; QuiNINE

Decreased Effect

Voriconazole may decrease the levels/effects of: Amphotericin B; Prasugrel; Saccharomyces boulardii

The levels/effects of Voriconazole may be decreased by: Barbiturates; CarBAMazepine; CYP2C19 Inducers (Strong); CYP2C9 Inducers (Highly Effective); Darunavir; Didanosine; Lopinavir; Peginterferon Alfa-2b; Phenytoin; Reverse Transcriptase Inhibitors (Non-Nucleoside); Rifamycin Derivatives; Ritonavir; St Johns Wort; Sucralfate

Food Interactions High fat meals reduce the extent of absorption by 24% for tablets and 37% for the oral suspension; avoid grapefruit juice (may increase voriconazole serum levels)

Stability

Oral: Store tablets at 15°C to 30°C (59°F to 86°F). Store powder for oral suspension in refrigerator at 2°C to 8°C (36°F to 46°F) before reconstitution; protect from light. Reconstituted oral suspension is stable for 14 days at 15°C to 30°C (59°F to 86°F). Do not refrigerate or freeze reconstituted oral suspension.

I.V.: Store unreconstituted vials at 15°C to 30°C (59°F to 86°F); reconstituted 10 mg/mL I.V. solution should be used immediately after preparation since it contains no preservative. If not used immediately, the solution is stable for 24 hours at 2°C to 8° (36°F to 46°F). The reconstituted I.V. solution can be further diluted with NS, D₅W, LR, D₅WLR, D₅W with 20 mEq KCl/liter, D₅W1/2NS, D₅WNS, or 1/2NS; voriconazole is incompatible with TPN, blood products, sodium bicarbonate, and electrolyte supplement infusions. Voriconazole can be infused at the same time as TPN, but must be infused in a separate line.

Mechanism of Action Inhibits fungal cytochrome P450-dependent 14a-sterol demethylase, an essential enzyme in ergosterol biosynthesis resulting in the inhibition of fungal cell membrane formation

Pharmacokinetics (Adult data unless noted)

Absorption: Oral: Rapid and complete

Distribution: Extensive tissue distribution; CSF levels ~50% of plasma levels

V_d: Adults: 4.6 L/kg

Protein binding: 58%

Metabolism: Metabolized by cytochrome P450 enzymes CYP2C19, CYP2C9, and CYP3A4 to voriconazole N-oxide (minimal antifungal activity); CYP2C19 is significantly involved in metabolism of voriconazole; CYP2C19 exhibits genetic polymorphism (15% to 20% Asians may be poor metabolizers of voriconazole; 3% to 5% Caucasians and African Americans may be poor metabolizers)

Bioavailability: Oral:
Children: 80%
Adults: 96%

Half-life: Terminal (dose-dependent): Adults: 6-9 hours

Time to peak serum concentration: Oral: 1-2 hours

Elimination: <2% excreted unchanged in urine

Usual Dosage

I.V.: **Note:** Limited information regarding pediatric dosing exists. Dosing below represents small studies and expert opinion. Children ≤12 years appear to require higher dosing than adults.

Children 2-11 years:
Loading dose: 6 mg/kg/dose every 12 hours for 2 doses on day 1

Maintenance dose: 4 mg/kg/dose every 12 hours (achieves exposure that approximates the adult maintenance dose of 3 mg/kg every 12 hours). Simulations predicted an initial I.V. dose of 7 mg/kg every 12 hours would achieve serum trough concentrations >1 mcg/mL in most children up to 12 years of age (see Neely, 2010).

IDSA Guidelines: Invasive aspergillosis: 5-7 mg/kg/dose every 12 hours

Children ≥12 years and Adults:
Loading dose: 6 mg/kg/dose every 12 hours for 2 doses on day 1

Maintenance dose:
Invasive aspergillosis: 4 mg/kg/dose every 12 hours
Candidemia: 3-4 mg/kg/dose every 12 hours
Other serious fungal infections, and deep tissue *Candida* infections: 4 mg/kg/dose every 12 hours
If patient is unable to tolerate I.V. therapy, reduce the dose to 3 mg/kg/dose every 12 hours.

Oral: **Note:** Limited information is currently available in the literature regarding oral voriconazole use in pediatric patients; some centers have used initial maintenance doses of 3-5 mg/kg/dose every 12 hours in patients <25 kg

Patients <40 kg:
Invasive aspergillosis, other serious fungal infection, candidemia, or deep tissue *Candida* infections: Maintenance dose: 100 mg every 12 hours

Esophageal candidiasis: 100 mg every 12 hours for a minimum of 14 days and for at least 7 days following symptom resolution

If patient response is inadequate, increase dose to 150 mg every 12 hours

If patient is unable to tolerate oral dose, decrease dose by 50 mg decrement to a minimum of 100 mg every 12 hours

Patients ≥40 kg:
Invasive aspergillosis, other serious fungal infection, candidemia, or deep tissue *Candida* infections: Maintenance dose: 200 mg every 12 hours

Esophageal candidiasis: 200 mg every 12 hours for a minimum of 14 days and for at least 7 days following symptom resolution

If patient response is inadequate, increase dose to 300 mg every 12 hours

If patient is unable to tolerate oral dose, decrease dose by 50 mg decrement to a minimum of 200 mg every 12 hours

Dosing adjustment for patients on concurrent efavirenz therapy: Oral:
Voriconazole: Increase maintenance dose to 400 mg every 12 hours
Efavirenz: Reduce dose to 300 mg once daily

Dosing adjustment for patients on concurrent phenytoin therapy:
I.V.: Increase voriconazole maintenance dose from 4 mg/kg/dose to 5 mg/kg/dose every 12 hours
Oral:
<40 kg: Increase voriconazole maintenance dose from 100 mg to 200 mg every 12 hours
≥40 kg: Increase voriconazole maintenance dose from 200 mg to 400 mg every 12 hours

Dosing adjustment in renal impairment:
Oral: No adjustment is necessary
I.V.: Cl_{cr} <50 mL/minute: Switch patient to oral voriconazole (parenteral formulation contains the excipient sulfobutyl ether beta-cyclodextrin sodium which accumulates in patients with renal impairment)
Dialysis: No dosage adjustment needed after 4-hour hemodialysis session

Dosing adjustment in hepatic impairment:
Child-Pugh Class A and B: Use standard loading dose regimen; decrease maintenance dose by 50%
Child-Pugh Class C: Not recommended for use unless benefit outweighs the risk

Administration Correct any electrolyte disturbances such as hypokalemia, hypomagnesemia, or hypocalcemia prior to starting voriconazole therapy

Oral: Administer at least one hour before or one hour after a meal; shake suspension for approximately 10 seconds before use; do not mix suspension with other medications, flavoring agents, or other fluids

Parenteral: I.V.: **Do not administer I.V. push;** voriconazole must be administered by I.V. infusion over 1-2 hours at a rate not to exceed 3 mg/kg/hour; final concentration for administration should be 0.5-5 mg/mL

Monitoring Parameters Serum electrolytes, periodic renal function tests (particularly serum creatinine), hepatic function tests, and bilirubin; monitor visual activity, visual field, and color perception; ECG in select patients; pancreatic function in patients at risk for acute pancreatitis; voriconazole trough levels in patients exhibiting signs of toxicity or not responding to treatment; total body skin examination yearly or more frequently if lesions occur

Reference Range Trough: 1-5 mcg/mL

Patient Information Avoid drinking grapefruit juice while taking voriconazole. Avoid driving at night or performing hazardous tasks while taking voriconazole; it may cause blurred vision and/or photophobia. May cause photosensitivity reactions (eg, exposure to sunlight may cause severe sunburn, skin rash, redness, or itching); avoid exposure to sunlight and artificial light sources (sunlamps, tanning booth/bed); wear protective clothing, wide-brimmed hats, sunglasses, and lip sunscreen (SPF ≥15); use a sunscreen [broad-spectrum sunscreen or physical sunscreen (preferred) or sunblock with SPF ≥15]; contact physician if reaction occurs. Women of childbearing age should use effective contraception during treatment to avoid pregnancy. Inform physician of serious change in heart rate or rhythm, vision changes, yellowing of skin or eyes, itching, flu-like symptoms, nausea, vomiting, feeling tired, seizures, or trouble breathing.

Nursing Implications Stop voriconazole infusion if anaphylactoid-type reaction occurs

Dosage Forms Excipient information presented when available (limited, particularly for generics); consult specific product labeling.
Injection, powder for reconstitution:
VFEND®: 200 mg [contains cyclodextrin]

Powder for oral suspension:
VFEND®: 200 mg/5 mL (70 mL) [contains sodium benzoate and sucrose; orange flavor]
Tablet:
VFEND®: 50 mg, 200 mg

References

Cesaro S, Strugo L, Alaggio R, et al, "Voriconazole for Invasive Aspergillosis in Oncohematological Patients: A Single-Center Pediatric Experience," *Support Care Cancer*, 2003, 11(11):722-7.

Cowen EW, Nguyen JC, Miller DD, et al, "Chronic Phototoxicity and Aggressive Squamous Cell Carcinoma of the Skin in Children and Adults During Treatment With Voriconazole," *J Am Acad Dermatol*, 2010, 62(1):31-7.

McCarthy KL, Playford EG, Looke DF, et al, "Severe Photosensitivity Causing Multifocal Squamous Cell Carcinomas Secondary to Prolonged Voriconazole Therapy," *Clin Infect Dis*, 2007, 44(5):e55-6.

Miller DD, Cowen EW, Nguyen JC, et al, "Melanoma Associated With Long-Term Voriconazole Therapy: A New Manifestation of Chronic Photosensitivity," *Arch Dermatol*, 2010, 146(3):300-4.

Neely M, Rushing T, Kovacs A, et al, "Voriconazole Pharmacokinetics and Pharmacodynamics in Children," *Clin Infect Dis*, 2010, 50 (1):27-36.

Pappas PG, Kauffman CA, Andes D, et al, "Clinical Practice Guidelines for the Management of Candidiasis: 2009 Update by the Infectious Diseases Society of America," *Clin Infect Dis*, 2009, 48(5):503-35.

Romero AJ, Pogamp PL, Nilsson LG, et al, "Effect of Voriconazole on the Pharmacokinetics of Cyclosporine in Renal Transplant Patients," *Clin Pharmacol Ther*, 2002, 71(4):226-34.

Steinbach WJ, "Antifungal Agents in Children," *Pediatr Clin North Am*, 2005, 52(3):895-915.

Walsh TJ, Anaissie EJ, Denning DW, et al, "Treatment of Aspergillosis: Clinical Practice Guidelines of the Infectious Diseases Society of America," *Clin Infect Dis*, 2008, 46(3):327-60.

Walsh TJ, Karlsson MO, Driscoll T, et al, "Pharmacokinetics and Safety of Intravenous Voriconazole in Children After Single- or Multiple-Dose Administration," *Antimicrob Agents Chemother*, 2004, 48(6):2166-72.

Walsh TJ, Lutsar I, Driscoll T, et al, "Voriconazole in the Treatment of Aspergillosis, Scedosporiosis and Other Invasive Fungal Infections in Children," *Pediatr Infect Dis J*, 2002, 21(3):240-8.

Walsh TJ, Pappas P, Winston DJ, et al, "Voriconazole Compared With Liposomal Amphotericin B for Empirical Antifungal Therapy in Patients With Neutropenia and Persistent Fever," *N Engl J Med*, 2002, 346(4):225-34.

◆ **Vospire ER®** *see* Albuterol *on page 57*

◆ **VP-16** *see* Etoposide *on page 551*

◆ **VP-16-213** *see* Etoposide *on page 551*

◆ **VPA** *see* Valproic Acid and Derivatives *on page 1398*

◆ **VSL #3® [OTC]** *see* Lactobacillus *on page 790*

◆ **VSL #3®-DS** *see* Lactobacillus *on page 790*

◆ **Vumon®** *see* Teniposide *on page 1318*

◆ **vWF:RCof** *see* Antihemophilic Factor / von Willebrand Factor Complex (Human) *on page 114*

◆ **Vytorin®** *see* Ezetimibe and Simvastatin *on page 554*

◆ **Vyvanse™** *see* Lisdexamfetamine *on page 830*

◆ **VZIG** *see* Varicella-Zoster Immune Globulin (Human) *on page 1408*

◆ **VZV Vaccine (Varicella)** *see* Varicella Virus Vaccine *on page 1407*

Warfarin (WAR far in)

Medication Safety Issues

Sound-alike/look-alike issues:
Coumadin® may be confused with Avandia®, Cardura®, Compazine®, Kemadrin®
Jantoven® may be confused with Janumet®, Januvia®

High alert medication: The Institute for Safe Medication Practices (ISMP) includes this medication among its list of drugs which have a heightened risk of causing significant patient harm when used in error.

2009 National Patient Safety Goals: The Joint Commission on Accreditation of Healthcare Organizations requires healthcare organizations that provide anticoagulant therapy to have a process in place to reduce the risk of anticoagulant-associated patient harm. Patients receiving anticoagulants should receive individualized care through a defined process that includes standardized ordering, dispensing, administration, monitoring and education. This does not apply to routine short-term use of anticoagulants for prevention of venous thromboembolism when the expectation is that the patient's laboratory values will remain within or close to normal values (NPSG.03.05.01).

U.S. Brand Names Coumadin®; Jantoven®

Canadian Brand Names Apo-Warfarin®; Coumadin®; Mylan-Warfarin; Novo-Warfarin; Taro-Warfarin

Therapeutic Category Anticoagulant

Generic Available Yes: Tablet

Use Prophylaxis and treatment of venous thrombosis, pulmonary embolism, and thromboembolic disorders; prevention and treatment of thromboembolic complications in patients with prosthetic heart valves or atrial fibrillation; reduction of the risk of death, recurrent MI, and thromboembolic events such as systemic embolization or stroke after MI; has also been used for the prevention of recurrent arterial ischemic stroke and TIAs.

Medication Guide An FDA-approved patient medication guide, which is available with the product information and at http://www.fda.gov/downloads/Drugs/DrugSafety/ucm088578.pdf, must be dispensed with this medication for each new outpatient prescription and refill.

Pregnancy Risk Factor X

Pregnancy Considerations Oral anticoagulants cross the placenta and produce fetal abnormalities. May also cause fatal fetal hemorrhage. Warfarin should not be used during pregnancy because of significant risks. Adjusted-dose heparin can be given safely throughout pregnancy in patients with venous thromboembolism.

Lactation Does not enter breast milk, only metabolites are excreted (AAP rates "compatible")

Breast-Feeding Considerations Warfarin does not pass into breast milk and can be given to nursing mothers (AAP rates "compatible"). However, limited data suggests prolonged PT may occur in some infants. Women who are breast-feeding should be carefully monitored to avoid excessive anticoagulation. Evaluation of coagulation tests and vitamin K status of breast-feeding infant is considered prudent.

Contraindications Hypersensitivity to warfarin or any component; hemorrhagic tendencies or blood dyscrasias; recent or contemplated surgery of the CNS, eye, or traumatic surgery with large open wounds; active ulceration or overt bleeding of GI, GU, or respiratory tracts; cerebrovascular hemorrhage, cerebral aneurysms, dissecting aortic aneurysms, pericarditis and pericardial effusions, bacterial endocarditis; spinal puncture or other procedures with potential for uncontrollable bleeding; major regional or lumbar block anesthesia; neurosurgical procedures; malignant hypertension; pregnancy; threatened abortion, eclampsia, pre-eclampsia; inadequate laboratory facilities; unsupervised patients with senility, alcoholism, or psychoses or other lack of patient cooperation

Warnings Serious and potentially fatal bleeding may occur **[U.S. Boxed Warning]**. Bleeding is more likely during initiation of treatment and with higher doses. Risk factors for bleeding include high intensity anticoagulation (INR >4), age (≥65 years), highly variable INRs, history of GI bleeding, hypertension, cerebrovascular disease, serious heart disease, anemia, severe diabetes, malignancy, trauma, renal insufficiency, polycythemia vera, vasculitis, open wound, history of PUD, indwelling catheters, menstruating and postpartum women, drug-drug interactions, and long duration of therapy. Dosage must be individualized for each patient (see Precautions). Patients must be instructed to report bleeding, accidents, or falls as well as any new or discontinued medications, herbal, or alternative products used, or significant changes in smoking or dietary habits.

Necrosis and/or gangrene of the skin and other tissues may occur (rarely) due to early hypercoagulability; risk is increased in patients with protein C deficiency; tissue debridement or amputation may be required; permanent disability or death has been reported; discontinue warfarin if warfarin-associated necrosis occurs; consider heparin for anticoagulation. Systemic cholesterol microemboli (eg, "purple toes syndrome") and atheroemboli may occur.

May cause hypersensitivity reactions, including anaphylaxis; use with caution in patients with anaphylactic disorders. Concomitant use with vitamin K may decrease anticoagulant effect; monitor carefully. Concomitant use with ethacrynic acid, indomethacin, NSAIDs, phenylbutazone, or aspirin increases warfarin's anticoagulant effect and may cause severe GI irritation (see Drug Interactions). Oral anticoagulant therapy is usually avoided in neonates due to a greater potential risk of bleeding (see Monagle, 2001) and other problems (see Monagle, 2008).

Precautions Do not switch brands once desired therapeutic response has been achieved. Use with caution in patients with acute infection or active tuberculosis (antibiotics and fever may alter the response to warfarin); prolonged dietary insufficiencies (vitamin K deficiency), diabetes mellitus, thyroid disease, moderate-to-severe renal or hepatic impairment, ovulating women (may be at risk of developing ovarian hemorrhage at the time of ovulation), or heparin-induced thrombocytopenia with deep vein thrombosis (limb ischemia, necrosis, and gangrene have occurred when warfarin was started or continued after heparin was stopped; warfarin monotherapy is contraindicated in the initial treatment of active HIT; warfarin initially inhibits the synthesis of protein C, potentially accelerating the underlying active thrombotic process). Use with caution in patients with or at risk for hemorrhage, necrosis, or gangrene. Use care in the selection of patients appropriate for this treatment; ensure patient cooperation especially from the alcoholic, illicit drug user, demented, or psychotic patient. Safety and efficacy have not been established in pediatric patients; monitor closely.

Periodic monitoring of INR (preferred) or prothrombin time is essential. A large number of factors (alone or in combination), including changes in diet, medications, and herbal remedies, may influence the patient's response to warfarin; monitor patients more closely when these factors change. Genetic variations in the CYP2C9 and vitamin K oxidoreductase (VKORC1) enzymes may also influence the patient's response to warfarin; presence of the CYP2C9*2 or *3 allele and/or polymorphism of the VKORC1 gene may increase the risk of bleeding. The *2 allele is reported to occur with a frequency of 4% to 11% in African-Americans and Caucasians, respectively, while the *3 allele frequencies are 2% to 7%, respectively. Other variant 2C9 alleles (eg, *5, *6, *9, and *11) are also associated with reduced metabolic activity and thus may increase risk of bleeding, but are much less common. Lower doses may be required in these patients; genetic testing may help determine appropriate dosing.

Adverse Reactions Bleeding is the major adverse effect of warfarin. Hemorrhage may occur at virtually any site. Risk is dependent on multiple variables, including the intensity of anticoagulation and patient susceptibility.

Cardiovascular: Angina, edema, hemorrhagic shock, hypotension, pallor, syncope, vasculitis

Central nervous system: Fever, fatigue, asthenia, dizziness, headache, lethargy, pain, stroke

Dermatologic: Skin lesions, rash, dermatitis, bullous eruptions, pruritus, urticaria, skin necrosis; gangrene of skin; hair loss (rare in children)

Gastrointestinal: Anorexia, nausea, vomiting, diarrhea, abdominal cramps, abdominal pain, flatulence, bloating, GI bleeding, mouth ulcers, taste disturbance

Genitourinary: Hematuria, priapism

Hematologic: Hemorrhage, agranulocytosis, anemia, leukopenia, retroperitoneal hematoma; unrecognized bleeding sites (eg, colon cancer) may be uncovered by anticoagulation

Hepatic: Hepatitis, liver enzymes elevated, cholestatic hepatic injury, jaundice

Neuromuscular & skeletal: Osteoporosis, paresthesia, weakness

Respiratory: Hemoptysis, epistaxis, pulmonary hemorrhage; tracheal calcification (rare in children)

Miscellaneous: Systemic cholesterol microembolization ("purple toes syndrome"), hypersensitivity reactions, anaphylaxis

Drug Interactions

Metabolism/Transport Effects Substrate of CYP1A2 (minor), 2C9 (major), 2C19 (minor), 3A4 (minor); **Inhibits** CYP2C9 (moderate), 2C19 (weak)

Avoid Concomitant Use

Avoid concomitant use of Warfarin with any of the following: Tamoxifen

Increased Effect/Toxicity

Warfarin may increase the levels/effects of: Anticoagulants; Carvedilol; Collagenase (Systemic); CYP2C9 Substrates (High risk); Drotrecogin Alfa; Phenytoin

The levels/effects of Warfarin may be increased by: Acetaminophen; Allopurinol; Amiodarone; Androgens; Antineoplastic Agents; Antiplatelet Agents; Atazanavir; Bicalutamide; Capecitabine; Cephalosporins; Cimetidine; Clopidogrel; Corticosteroids (Systemic); Cranberry; CYP2C9 Inhibitors (Moderate); CYP2C9 Inhibitors (Strong); Dasatinib; Desvenlafaxine; Disulfiram; Dronedarone; Efavirenz; Erythromycin (Ophthalmic); Esomeprazole; Etoposide; Exenatide; Fenofibrate; Fenofibric Acid; Fenugreek; Fibric Acid Derivatives; Fluconazole; Fluorouracil; Fluorouracil (Systemic); Fluorouracil (Topical); Fosamprenavir; Gefitinib; Ginkgo Biloba; Glucagon; Green Tea; Herbs (Anticoagulant/Antiplatelet Properties); HMG-CoA Reductase Inhibitors; Ifosfamide; Imatinib; Itraconazole; Ivermectin; Ketoconazole; Ketoconazole (Systemic); Lansoprazole; Leflunomide; Macrolide Antibiotics; MetroNIDAZOLE; MetroNIDAZOLE (Systemic); Miconazole; Milnacipran; NSAID (COX-2 Inhibitor); NSAID (Nonselective); Omega-3-Acid Ethyl Esters; Omeprazole; Orlistat; Pentosan Polysulfate Sodium; Pentoxifylline; Phenytoin; Posaconazole; Propafenone; Propoxyphene; Prostacyclin Analogues; QuiNIDine; Quinolone Antibiotics; Ranitidine; Salicylates; Selective Serotonin Reuptake Inhibitors; Sitaxsentan; Sorafenib; Sulfinpyrazone [Off Market]; Sulfonamide Derivatives; Tamoxifen; Tetracycline Derivatives; Thrombolytic Agents; Thyroid Products; Tigecycline; Tolterodine; Torsemide; Tricyclic Antidepressants; Venlafaxine; Vitamin A; Vitamin E; Voriconazole; Vorinostat; Zafirlukast; Zileuton

Decreased Effect

The levels/effects of Warfarin may be decreased by: Aminoglutethimide; Antineoplastic Agents; Antithyroid Agents; Aprepitant; AzaTHIOprine; Barbiturates; Bile Acid Sequestrants; Bosentan; CarBAMazepine; Coenzyme Q-10; Contraceptives (Estrogens); Contraceptives (Progestins); CYP2C9 Inducers (Highly Effective); Darunavir; Dicloxacillin; Fosaprepitant; Ginseng (American); Glutethimide; Green Tea; Griseofulvin; Mercaptopurine; Nafcillin; Peginterferon Alfa-2b; Phytonadione; Rifamycin Derivatives; Ritonavir; St Johns Wort; Sucralfate

Food Interactions Vitamin K can reverse the anti-coagulation effects of warfarin; large amounts of food high in vitamin K (such as beef liver, pork liver, green tea, and green leafy vegetables) may reverse warfarin, decrease prothrombin time, and lead to therapeutic failure. Patients should not change dietary habits once stabilized on warfarin therapy. A balanced diet with a consistent intake of vitamin K is essential. Avoid large amounts of alfalfa, asparagus, broccoli, brussel sprouts, cabbage, cauliflower, green teas, kale, lettuce, spinach, turnip greens, water-cress. Avoid enteral feeds high in vitamin K. **Note:** Breast-fed infants may be more sensitive to warfarin due to low amounts of vitamin K in breast milk.

High doses of vitamin A, E, or C may alter PT; use caution with fish oils or omega 3 fatty acids; avoid fried or boiled onions as they may increase drug effect by increasing fibrinolytic activity; avoid herbal teas and remedies such as tonka beans, melilot, and woodruff as they contain natural coumarins and will increase effect of warfarin; avoid large amounts of liver, avocado, soy protein, soybean oil, papain.

Cranberry juice or other cranberry products may increase the INR in patients receiving warfarin and cause severe bleeding (flavonoids found in cranberries may inhibit cytochrome P450 isoenzyme CYP2C9 and reduce the metabolism of warfarin)

Stability
Tablets: Store at controlled room temperature of 15°C to 30°C (59°F to 86°F). Protect from light. Dispense in tight, light-resistant container.
Injection: Store unopened vials in box at controlled room temperature of 15°C to 30°C (59°F to 86°F). Protect from light. After reconstitution, store at controlled room temperature and use within 4 hours after reconstitution. Do not refrigerate. Discard unused portion (does not contain preservative). Reconstituted solution is stable in D_5LR, $D_5^{1/2}NS$, D_5NS, D_5W, $D_{10}W$; **variable stability (consult detailed reference)** in LR, NS.

Mechanism of Action Interferes with hepatic synthesis of vitamin K-dependent coagulation factors (II, VII, IX, X). Hepatic synthesis of coagulation factors II, VII, IX, and X, as well as proteins C and S, requires the presence of vitamin K. These clotting factors are biologically activated by the addition of carboxyl groups to key glutamic acid residues within the proteins' structure. In the process, "active" vitamin K is oxidatively converted to an "inactive" form, which is then subsequently re-activated by vitamin K epoxide reductase complex 1 (VKORC1). Warfarin competitively inhibits the subunit 1 of the multi-unit VKOR complex, thus depleting functional vitamin K reserves and hence reduces synthesis of active clotting factors. The degree of warfarin's effect depends upon the dosage administered and, in part, by the patient's VKORC1 genotype.

Pharmacodynamics Anticoagulation effects:
Onset of action: 24-72 hours
Maximum effect: Within 5-7 days
Duration of action (single dose): 2-5 days

Pharmacokinetics (Adult data unless noted)
Absorption: Oral: Rapid
Distribution: Adults: V_d: 0.14 L/kg
Protein binding: 99%
Metabolism: Hepatic, primarily via CYP2C9; minor path-ways include CYP2C19, 1A2, and 3A4
Genomic variants: Clearance of S-warfarin is reduced by ~37% in patients heterozygous for 2C9 (*1/*2 or *1/*3), and reduced by ~70% in patients homozygous for reduced function alleles (*2/*2, *2/*3, or *3/*3)
Half-life, elimination: Adults: 20-60 hours; mean: 40 hours; highly variable among individuals

Elimination: Urine (92%, primarily as metabolites; very little warfarin is excreted unchanged in the urine)
Usual Dosage Note: Dosing must be individualized. **Note:** New product labeling identifies genetic factors which may increase patient sensitivity to warfarin. Specifically, genetic variations in the proteins CYP2C9 and VKORC1, respon-sible for warfarin's primary metabolism and pharmacody-namic activity, respectively, have been identified as predisposing factors associated with decreased dose requirement and increased bleeding risk. A genotyping test is available and may provide important guidance on initiation of anticoagulant therapy.
Oral:
Infants and Children: **To maintain an International Normalized Ratio (INR) between 2-3:**
Initial loading dose on day 1 (if baseline INR is 1-1.3): 0.2 mg/kg (maximum dose: 10 mg); use initial loading dose of 0.1 mg/kg if patient has liver dysfunction or has undergone a Fontan procedure (see Streif, 1999)
Loading dose for days 2-4: doses are dependent upon patient's INR
if INR is 1.1-1.3, repeat the initial loading dose
if INR is 1.4-1.9, give 50% of the initial loading dose
if INR is 2-3, give 50% of the initial loading dose
if INR is 3.1-3.5, give 25% of the initial loading dose
if INR is >3.5, hold the drug until INR <3.5, then restart at 50% of previous dose
Maintenance dose guidelines for day 5 of therapy and beyond: Doses are dependent upon patient's INR
if INR is 1.1-1.4, increase dose by 20% of previous dose
if INR is 1.5-1.9, increase dose by 10% of previous dose
if INR is 2-3, do not change the dose
if INR is 3.1-3.5, decrease dose by 10% of previous dose
if INR is >3.5, hold the drug and check INR daily until INR <3.5, then restart at 20% less than the previous dose
Usual maintenance dose: ~0.1 mg/kg/day; range: 0.05-0.34 mg/kg/day; the dose in mg/kg/day is inversely related to age. In the largest pediatric study (n=319; Streif, 1999), infants <12 months of age required a mean dose of 0.33 mg/kg/day, but children 13-18 years required a mean dose of 0.09 mg/kg/day; a target INR of 2-3 was used for a majority of these patients (75% of warfarin courses). Overall, children required a mean dose of 0.16 mg/kg/day to achieve a target INR of 2-3. In another study (Andrew, 1994), to attain an INR of 1.3-1.8, infants <12 months (n=2) required 0.24 and 0.27 mg/kg/day, but children >1 year required a mean of 0.08 mg/kg/day (range: 0.03-0.17 mg/kg/day). Consistent anticoagulation may be difficult to maintain in children <5 years of age. Children receiving phenobarbital, carbamaze-pine, or enteral nutrition may require higher main-tenance doses (see Streif, 1999).
Adults: **Note:** Initial dosing must be individualized. Consider patient factors (hepatic function, cardiac function, age, nutritional status, concurrent therapy, risk of bleeding) in addition to prior dose response (if available) and the clinical situation. Initial dose: 2-5 mg daily for 2 days **or** 5-10 mg daily for 1-2 days (Ansell, 2008); then adjust dose according to results of INR; usual maintenance dose ranges from 2-10 mg daily; individual patients may require loading and mainte-nance doses outside these general guidelines.
Note: Lower starting doses may be required for patients with hepatic impairment, poor nutrition, CHF, elderly, high risk of bleeding, patients who are debilitated, or those with reduced function genomic variants of the catabolic enzymes CYP2C9 (*2 or *3 alleles) or VKORC1 (-1639 polymorphism). Higher initial doses

may be reasonable in selected patients (ie, receiving enzyme-inducing agents and with low risk of bleeding).

I.V.: (For patients who cannot take oral form): I.V. dose is equal to oral dose

Dosing adjustment in renal disease: No adjustment required; however, patients with renal failure have an increased risk of bleeding complications. Monitor closely.

Dosing adjustment in hepatic disease: Monitor effect at usual doses; the response to oral anticoagulants may be markedly enhanced in obstructive jaundice (due to reduced vitamin K absorption) and also in hepatitis and cirrhosis (due to decreased production of vitamin K-dependent clotting factors); INR should be closely monitored

Administration

Oral: May administer on an empty or full stomach. Take at the same time each day.

Parenteral: For I.V. use only; do not administer I.M. Reconstitute 5 mg vial with 2.7 mL SWI to produce 2 mg/mL solution. Administer by slow I.V. injection over 1-2 minutes into peripheral vein

Monitoring Parameters INR (preferred) or prothrombin time; hemoglobin, hematocrit, signs and symptoms of bleeding; consider genotyping of CYP2C9 and VKORC1 prior to initiation of therapy, if available.

Reference Range The INR is now the standard test used to monitor warfarin anticoagulation; the desired INR is based upon indication; due to the lack of pediatric clinical trials assessing optimal INR ranges and clinical outcomes, the desired INR ranges for children are extrapolated from adult studies; the optimal therapeutic INR ranges may possibly be lower in children versus adults. Further pediatric studies are needed (see Monagle, 2008). **Note:** If INR is not available, prothrombin time should be 1½ to 2 times the control.

Targeted INR and Ranges for Children, Based on Indication[1,2,3]

Indication	Targeted INR	Targeted INR Range
Systemic venous thromboembolism[4]	2.5	2-3
Central venous line-related thrombosis, initial 3 months of therapy	2.5	2-3
Central venous line-related thrombosis after first 3 months of warfarin therapy (**Note:** This is a prophylactic dose)	1.7	1.5-1.9
Central venous line, long-term home TPN (prophylactic dose) (Not recommended routinely)		2-3
Primary prophylaxis following Fontan procedure	2.5	2-3
Primary prophylaxis for dilated cardiomyopathy	2.5	2-3
Primary prophylaxis for biological prosthetic heart valves in children	Follow adult guidelines in table below	
Primary prophylaxis for mechanical prosthetic heart valves in children	Follow adult guidelines in table below	
Kawasaki disease with giant coronary aneurysms	2.5	2-3
Cerebral sinovenous thrombosis **Note:** INR recommendations from 2004 Chest guidelines	2.5	2-3

[1]Information from Monagle, 2004 and Monagle, 2008.

[2]Children are defined in the Chest guidelines as patients aged 28 days to 16 years of age.

[3]See Additional Information field for duration of therapy. See Monagle, 2008 for timing of initiation and adjunct antithrombotic and antiplatelet therapy.

[4]Anticoagulant therapy with UFH or LMWH is recommended for children with first episode of venous thromboembolism (central venous line and noncentral venous line related).

Adult Target INR Ranges Based Upon Indication

Indication	Targeted INR	Targeted INR Range
Cardiac		
Acute myocardial infarction (high risk)[1]	2.5	2-3[2,3]
Atrial fibrillation or atrial flutter	2.5	2-3
Valvular		
Bileaflet or Medtronic Hall tilting disk mechanical aortic valve in normal sinus rhythm and normal LA size	2.5	2-3
Bileaflet or tilting disk mechanical mitral valve	3	2.5-3.5
Caged ball or caged disk mechanical valve	3	2.5-3.5
Mechanical prosthetic valve with systemic embolism despite adequate anticoagulation	3 or 3.5[4]	2.5-3.5[4] or 3-4[4]
Mechanical valve and risk factors for thromboembolism (eg, AF, MI[5], LA enlargement, hypercoagulable state, low EF) or history of atherosclerotic vascular disease	3	2.5-3.5[6]
Bioprosthetic mitral valve	2.5	2-3[7]
Bioprosthetic mitral or aortic valve with prior history of systemic embolism	2.5	2-3[7]
Bioprosthetic mitral or aortic valve with evidence of LA thrombus at surgery	2.5	2-3[8]
Bioprosthetic mitral or aortic valve with risk factors for thromboembolism (eg, AF, hypercoagulable state or low EF)	2.5	2-3[9]
Prosthetic mitral valve thrombosis (resolved)	4	3.5-4.5[3]
Prosthetic aortic valve thrombosis (resolved)	3.5	3-4[3]
Rheumatic mitral valve disease and normal sinus rhythm (LA diameter >5.5 cm), AF, previous systemic embolism, or LA thrombus	2.5	2-3
Thromboembolism Treatment		
Venous thromboembolism	2.5	2-3[10,11]
Thromboprophylaxis		
Chronic thromboembolic pulmonary hypertension (CTPH)	2.5	2-3
Lupus inhibitor (no other risk factors)	2.5	2-3
Lupus inhibitor and recurrent thromboembolism	3	2.5-3.5
Major trauma patients with impaired mobility undergoing rehabilitation	2.5	2-3
Spinal cord injury (acute) undergoing rehabilitation	2.5	2-3
Total hip or knee replacement (elective) or hip fracture surgery	2.5	2-3[12]
Other Indications		
Indication	Targeted INR	Targeted INR Range
Cerebral venous sinus thrombosis	2.5	2-3[13]
Ischemic stroke due to AF	2.5	2-3

[1]High-risk includes large anterior MI, significant heart failure, intracardiac thrombus, atrial fibrillation, history of thromboembolism.

[2]Maintain anticoagulation for 3 months.

[3]Combine with aspirin 81 mg/day.

[4]Combine with aspirin 81 mg/day, if not previously receiving, **and/or** if previous target INR was 2.5, then new target INR should be 3 (2.5-3.5). If previous target INR was 3, then new target INR should be 3.5 (3-4).

[5]MI refers to anterior-apical ST-segment elevation myocardial infarction.

Footnotes are continued on next page.

Adult Target INR Ranges Based Upon Indication *(continued)*

[6]Combine with aspirin 81 mg/day unless patient is at high risk of bleeding (eg, history of GI bleed, age >80 years).

[7]Maintain anticoagulation for 3 months after valve insertion, then switch to aspirin 81 mg/day if no other indications for warfarin exist or clinically reassess need for warfarin in patients with prior history of systemic embolism.

[8]Maintain anticoagulation with warfarin until thrombus resolution.

[9]If patient has history of atherosclerotic vascular disease, combine with aspirin 81 mg/day unless patient is at high risk of bleeding (eg, history of GI bleed, age >80 years).

[10]Treat for 3 months in patients with VTE due to transient reversible risk factor. Treat for a minimum of 3 months in patients with unprovoked VTE and evaluate for long-term therapy. Other risk groups (eg, cancer) may require >3 months of therapy.

[11]In patients with unprovoked VTE who prefer less frequent INR monitoring, low-intensity therapy (INR range: 1.5-1.9) with less frequent monitoring is recommended over stopping treatment.

[12]Continue for at least 10 days and up to 35 days after surgery.

[13]Continue for up to 12 months.

Warfarin levels are not used for monitoring degree of anticoagulation. They may be useful if a patient with unexplained coagulopathy is using the drug surreptitiously or if it is unclear whether clinical resistance is due to true drug resistance or lack of drug intake.

Normal prothrombin time (PT): 10.9-12.9 seconds. Healthy premature newborns have prolonged coagulation test screening results (eg, PT, aPTT, TT) which return to normal adult values at approximately 6 months of age. However, healthy premature newborns (ie, those not receiving antithrombotic agents), do not develop spontaneous hemorrhage or thrombotic complications because of a balance between procoagulants and inhibitors.

Patient Information Read the patient Medication Guide that you receive with each prescription and refill of warfarin. Take exactly as directed; if a dose is missed, take it as soon as possible, then return to normal dosing schedule; if a dose is skipped, do **not** double the next dose. Follow diet and activity as recommended by prescriber; check with prescriber before changing diet. Do not make major changes in your dietary intake of vitamin K (green leafy vegetables). Avoid alcohol, cranberry juice, and cranberry products; limit caffeine. Report any signs of bleeding to physician at once (eg, nosebleeds, bleeding gums, prolonged bleeding from a cut, heavier than normal menstrual or vaginal bleeding, coughing up blood, vomiting blood or coffee ground-like material, pink or dark brown urine, red or black tar-like stools, unusual bruising, headaches, dizziness, weakness, pain, swelling, or discomfort). Avoid hazardous activities; use soft toothbrush; carry medical identification indicating warfarin use (eg, medical alert ID bracelet or medication card). Be aware of other drugs, foods, and herbal remedies to avoid. Report the use of other medications, non-prescription medications, and herbal or natural products to your physician and pharmacist. Do not take any new medication during therapy unless approved by prescriber. Report adverse effects such as skin rash or irritation, unusual fever, persistent nausea or GI upset, pain in joints or back, or unhealed wounds.

Nursing Implications Be aware of drug interactions, interactions with herbal remedies, and foods that contain vitamin K which can alter anticoagulant effects. Avoid I.M. injections of all drugs in patients receiving warfarin.

Additional Information Usual duration of therapy in children (Monagle, 2008):

DVT:
Idiopathic TE: ≥6 months
Recurrent idiopathic TE: Indefinite
Secondary thrombosis (with resolved risk factors): ≥3 months
Recurrent secondary TE: Anticoagulate until removal of precipitating factor (≥3 months)
Primary prophylaxis for Glenn or Bilateral Cavopulmonary Shunts (BCPS): Continue until ready for Fontan surgery
Post-Fontan surgery: Optimal duration not defined
Cardiomyopathy in children eligible for transplant: Until transplant
Primary pulmonary hypertension: Duration not listed
Biological prosthetic heart valves: Follow adult recommendations
Mechanical prosthetic heart valves: Follow adult recommendations
Ventricular assist device (VAD) placement: Until transplant or weaned from VAD
Kawasaki disease: Treatment depends on severity of coronary involvement
Cerebral sinovenous thrombosis (CSVT) in neonates: 6 weeks-3 months
CSVT in children: ≥3 months
Neonates with homozygous protein C deficiency: Long-term

Note: Overdoses of warfarin may be treated with vitamin K, to reverse warfarin's anticoagulation effect. Prospective genotyping is available and may provide important guidance on initiation of anticoagulant therapy. Commercial testing with PGxPredict™:WARFARIN is now available from PGxHealth™ (Division of Clinical Data, Inc, New Haven, CT). The test genotypes patients for presence of the CYP2C9*2 or *3 alleles and the VKORC1 -1639G>A polymorphism. The results of the test allow patients to be phenotyped as extensive, intermediate, or poor metabolizers (CYP2C9) and as low, intermediate, or high warfarin sensitivity (VKORC1). Ordering information is available at 888-592-7327 or warfarininfo@pgxhealth.com.

Dosage Forms Excipient information presented when available (limited, particularly for generics); consult specific product labeling.

Injection, powder for reconstitution, as sodium:
Coumadin®: 5 mg
Tablet, as sodium: 1 mg, 2 mg, 2.5 mg, 3 mg, 4 mg, 5 mg, 6 mg, 7.5 mg, 10 mg
Coumadin®: 1 mg, 2 mg, 2.5 mg, 3 mg, 4 mg, 5 mg, 6 mg, 7.5 mg [scored]
Coumadin®: 10 mg [scored; dye free]
Jantoven®: 1 mg, 2 mg, 2.5 mg, 3 mg, 4 mg, 5 mg, 6 mg, 7.5 mg [scored]
Jantoven®: 10 mg [scored; dye free]

References
Andrew M, Marzinotto V, Brooker LA, et al, "Oral Anticoagulation Therapy in Pediatric Patients: A Prospective Study," *Thromb Haemost*, 1994, 71(3):265-9.
Ansell J, Hirsh J, Poller L, et al, "The Pharmacology and Management of the Vitamin K Antagonists: The Seventh ACCP Conference on Antithrombotic and Thrombolytic Therapy," *Chest*, 2004, 126(3 Suppl):204S-33S.
Arepally GM and Ortel TL, "Clinical Practice. Heparin-Induced Thrombocytopenia," *N Engl J Med*, 2006, 355(8):809-17
David M and Andrew M, "Venous Thromboembolic Complications in Children," *J Pediatr*, 1993, 123(3):337-46.
Fihn SD "Aiming for Safe Anticoagulation," *N Engl J Med*, 1995, 333 (1):54-5.
Hirsh J, Dalen JE, Anderson DR, et al, "Oral Anticoagulants. Mechanism of Action, Clinical Effectiveness, and Optimal Therapeutic Range," *Chest*, 2001, 119:8S-21S.

Monagle P, Chalmers E, Chan A, et al, "Antithrombotic Therapy in Neonates and Children: American College of Chest Physicians Evidence-Based Clinical Practice Guidelines (8th Edition)," *Chest*, 2008, 133(6 Suppl):887S-968S.

Monagle P, Chan A, Massicotte P, et al, "Antithrombotic Therapy in Children: The Seventh ACCP Conference on Antithrombotic and Thrombolytic Therapy," *Chest*, 2004, 126(3 Suppl):645S-87S.

Monagle P, Michelson AD, Bovill E, et al, "Antithrombotic Therapy in Children," *Chest*, 2001, 119:344S-70S.

Salem DN, O'Gara PT, Madias C, et al, "Valvular and Structural Heart Disease: American College of Chest Physicians Evidence-Based Clinical Practice Guidelines (8th Edition)," *Chest*, 2008, 133(6 Suppl):593S-629S.

Salem DN, Stein PD, Al-Ahmad A, et al, "Antithrombotic Therapy in Valvular Heart Disease - Native and Prosthetic: The Seventh ACCP Conference on Antithrombotic and Thrombolytic Therapy," *Chest*, 2004, 126(3 Suppl):457S-82S.

Streif W, Andrew M, Marzinotto V, et al, "Analysis of Warfarin Therapy in Pediatric Patients: A Prospective Cohort Study of 319 Patients," *Blood*, 1999, 94(9):3007-14.

Suvarna R, Pirmohamed M, and Henderson L, "Possible Interaction Between Warfarin and Cranberry Juice," *BMJ*, 2003, 327(7429):1454.

Wells PS, Holbrook AM, Crowther NR, et al, "Interactions of Warfarin With Drugs and Food," *Ann Intern Med*, 1994, 121(9):676-83.

◆ **Warfarin Sodium** *see* Warfarin *on page 1432*

◆ **Wart-Off® Maximum Strength [OTC]** *see* Salicylic Acid *on page 1241*

◆ **4-Way® 12 Hour [OTC]** *see* Oxymetazoline *on page 1043*

◆ **4 Way® Fast Acting [OTC]** *see* Phenylephrine *on page 1102*

◆ **4 Way® Menthol [OTC]** *see* Phenylephrine *on page 1102*

◆ **4-Way® Saline Moisturizing Mist [OTC]** *see* Sodium Chloride *on page 1270*

◆ **Welchol®** *see* Colesevelam *on page 355*

◆ **Wellbutrin®** *see* BuPROPion *on page 217*

◆ **Wellbutrin XL®** *see* BuPROPion *on page 217*

◆ **Wellbutrin® XL (Can)** *see* BuPROPion *on page 217*

◆ **Wellbutrin SR®** *see* BuPROPion *on page 217*

◆ **Wellbutrin® SR (Can)** *see* BuPROPion *on page 217*

◆ **Westcort®** *see* Hydrocortisone *on page 685*

◆ **White Mineral Oil** *see* Mineral Oil *on page 933*

◆ **Winpred™ (Can)** *see* PredniSONE *on page 1151*

◆ **WinRho® SDF** *see* Rh₀(D) Immune Globulin *on page 1207*

◆ **Wound Wash Saline™ [OTC]** *see* Sodium Chloride *on page 1270*

◆ **WR-2721** *see* Amifostine *on page 78*

◆ **WR-139007** *see* Dacarbazine *on page 380*

◆ **WR-139013** *see* Chlorambucil *on page 287*

◆ **WR-139021** *see* Carmustine *on page 252*

◆ **Wycillin [DSC]** *see* Penicillin G Procaine *on page 1081*

◆ **Wycillin® (Can)** *see* Penicillin G Procaine *on page 1081*

◆ **Xanax®** *see* ALPRAZolam *on page 68*

◆ **Xanax TS™ (Can)** *see* ALPRAZolam *on page 68*

◆ **Xanax XR®** *see* ALPRAZolam *on page 68*

◆ **Xeomin® (Can)** *see* OnabotulinumtoxinA *on page 1020*

◆ **Xigris®** *see* Drotrecogin Alfa (Activated) *on page 484*

◆ **Xodol® 5/300** *see* Hydrocodone and Acetaminophen *on page 684*

◆ **Xodol® 7.5/300** *see* Hydrocodone and Acetaminophen *on page 684*

◆ **Xodol® 10/300** *see* Hydrocodone and Acetaminophen *on page 684*

◆ **Xolair®** *see* Omalizumab *on page 1014*

◆ **Xolegel®** *see* Ketoconazole *on page 780*

◆ **Xopenex®** *see* Levalbuterol *on page 807*

◆ **Xopenex HFA™** *see* Levalbuterol *on page 807*

◆ **Xpect™ [OTC]** *see* GuaiFENesin *on page 656*

◆ **Xylocaine®** *see* Lidocaine *on page 818*

◆ **Xylocaine® Dental** *see* Lidocaine *on page 818*

◆ **Xylocaine® MPF** *see* Lidocaine *on page 818*

◆ **Xylocaine® MPF With Epinephrine** *see* Lidocaine and Epinephrine *on page 821*

◆ **Xylocaine® Viscous [DSC]** *see* Lidocaine *on page 818*

◆ **Xylocaine® With Epinephrine** *see* Lidocaine and Epinephrine *on page 821*

◆ **Xylocard® (Can)** *see* Lidocaine *on page 818*

◆ **Xyntha™** *see* Antihemophilic Factor (Recombinant) *on page 112*

◆ **Xyzal®** *see* Levocetirizine *on page 812*

Yellow Fever Vaccine (YEL oh FEE ver vak SEEN)

Related Information
Immunization Guidelines *on page 1636*
U.S. Brand Names YF-VAX®
Canadian Brand Names YF-VAX®
Therapeutic Category Vaccine
Generic Available No
Use To provide active immunity to yellow fever virus to children and adults, who are either traveling or living in areas where yellow fever infection exists (FDA approved in ages ≥9 months and adults)
Pregnancy Risk Factor C
Pregnancy Considerations Animal reproduction studies have not been conducted. Adverse events were not observed in the mother or fetus following vaccination during the third trimester of pregnancy in Nigerian women; however, maternal seroconversion was reduced. Inadvertent exposure early in the first trimester of pregnancy in Brazilian women did not show decreased maternal seroconversion; no major congenital abnormalities were noted. Cord blood from an infant whose mother was vaccinated during the first trimester tested positive for IgM antibodies; no adverse events were noted in the infant. Vaccine should be administered if travel to an endemic area is unavoidable and the infant should be monitored after birth. Tests to verify maternal immune response may be considered. If a pregnant woman is to be vaccinated only to satisfy an international requirement (as opposed to decreasing risk of infection), efforts should be made to obtain a waiver letter.
Lactation Excretion in breast milk unknown/use caution
Breast-Feeding Considerations Laboratory confirmed transmission of 17DD yellow fever vaccine virus via breast-feeding has been documented. Yellow fever vaccine was administered to a nursing mother 15 days postpartum. She was exclusively breast-feeding her newborn. Eight days after maternal vaccination, the infant developed a fever, was irritable, refused to nurse, then was hospitalized for seizures the next day. Yellow fever virus specific to the vaccine and IgM antibodies were detected in the newborn CSF. The child was discharged after 24 days in the hospital; growth and neurodevelopment were normal through 6 months of age. Breast-feeding is contraindicated by the manufacturer, particularly in infants <9 months of age. Breast-feeding does not adversely affect immunization.
Contraindications Hypersensitivity to the vaccine, egg or chick embryo protein, or any component; individuals with blood dyscrasias, leukemia, lymphomas, or other malignant neoplasms affecting the bone marrow or lymphatic systems; concurrent immunosuppressive therapy; primary and acquired immunodeficiency states including those

who are immunosuppressed in association with HIV; family history of congenital or hereditary immunodeficiency; children <6 months of age (<9 months of age according to the manufacturer)

ACIP provisional guidelines indicate that use is contra-indicated in patients with symptomatic HIV infection or CD4+ counts <15% total (or <200/mm^3 in ages >6 years); thymus disorders associated with abnormal immune cell function (eg, thymomas); primary immunodefiencies; malignant neoplasms; transplant patients; concurrent immunosuppressive and immunomodulating therapies (eg, radiation therapy or drugs)

Warnings Not for use in patients who are immunosup-pressed due to an increased risk of encephalitis with yellow fever vaccine administration; consider delaying travel or obtaining a waiver letter. Patients on low-dose or short-term corticosteroids are not considered immuno-suppressed and may receive the vaccine. ACIP provi-sional guidelines indicate that caution should be used if administering the vaccine to asymptomatic patients with HIV infection and CD4+ T-lymphocytes of 15% to 24% (or 200-499/mm^3 in ages >6 years). Chicken embryos are used in the manufacture of this vaccine; use caution in patients with immediate-type hypersensitivity reactions to eggs; immediate treatment for anaphylactic reactions should be available during vaccine use.

Avoid use in infants <9 months and pregnant women unless travel to high-risk areas are unavoidable; use in infants <6 months of age is contraindicated due to risk of encephalitis. The decision to use in children between 6-9 months of age must weigh the risks of exposure to the virus with the theoretic risks of vaccine-associated encephalitis (see *Red Book*, 2009). Advice regarding use of this vaccine can be obtained from the Division of Vector-Borne Infectious Diseases of the CDC (see Additional Information).

Precautions Use with caution in adults >65 years (≥60 years, according to ACIP) due to an increased risk of vaccine-associated viscerotropic disease (multisystem organ failure). Routine prophylactic administration of acetaminophen to prevent fever due to vaccines has been shown to decrease the immune response of some vaccines; the clinical significance of this reduction in immune response has not been established (see Prymula, 2009). Transfusion-related transmission of yellow fever vaccine virus has been reported; wait 2 weeks after immunization with yellow fever vaccine to donate blood. Latex is used in stopper of the vial which may cause allergic reactions in susceptible individuals.

Adverse Reactions All serious adverse reactions must be reported to the U.S. Department of Health and Human Services (DHHS) Vaccine Adverse Event Reporting System (VAERS) 1-800-822-7967.

Frequency not defined (adverse reactions may be increased in patients <9 months or ≥65 years of age)

Central nervous system: Fever (incidence of these reactions have been reported to be as low as <5% and as high as 10% to 30% depending on the study), headache, myalgia, vaccine-associated neurotropic disease (postvaccinal encephalitis; rare) (see Warnings)

Local: Injection site reactions (edema, erythema, pain)

Neuromuscular & skeletal: Weakness

Miscellaneous: Hypersensitivity (immediate) (see Warn-ings), viscerotropic disease (multiple organ system failure; rare)

Drug Interactions

Avoid Concomitant Use

Avoid concomitant use of Yellow Fever Vaccine with any of the following: Immunosuppressants

Increased Effect/Toxicity

The levels/effects of Yellow Fever Vaccine may be increased by: Immunosuppressants

Decreased Effect

Yellow Fever Vaccine may decrease the levels/effects of: Tuberculin Tests

The levels/effects of Yellow Fever Vaccine may be decreased by: Immunosuppressants

Stability Store at 2°C to 8°C (35°F to 46°F); do not freeze. Must be used within 60 minutes of reconstitution.

Mechanism of Action A live, attenuated virus vaccine; offers active immunity to disease caused by yellow fever virus

Pharmacodynamics Onset of action: Seroconversion: 10-14 days

Usual Dosage Children ≥9 months and Adults: SubQ: One dose (0.5 mL) ≥10 days before travel; Booster: Repeat same dosage every 10 years if at continued risk of exposure.

Administration Parenteral: Use entire contents of pro-vided diluent to reconstitute vaccine. Gently swirl until a uniform suspension forms; swirl well before withdrawing dose. Avoid vigorous shaking to prevent foaming of suspension. Use within 60 minutes following reconstitu-tion; keep suspension refrigerated until used. Administer by SubQ injection into the anterolateral aspect of the thigh or arm; **not for I.V. administration**

Monitoring Parameters Monitor for adverse effects up to 10 days after vaccination.

Patient Information Immunity develops by the tenth day and **WHO** requires revaccination every 10 years to maintain travelers' vaccination certificates.

Nursing Implications Federal law requires that the date of administration, the vaccine manufacturer, lot number of vaccine, and the administering person's name, title, and address be entered into the patient's permanent medical record.

Additional Information A desensitization procedure is available for persons with severe egg sensitivity. Consult manufacturer's labeling for details. Some countries require a valid international Certification of Vaccination showing receipt of vaccine. The WHO requires revaccination every 10 years to maintain traveler's vaccination certificate. Current requirements and recommendations for immuni-zation related to travel destination can be obtained from the CDC Travelers' Health Web site (www.cdc.gov/travel). All travelers to endemic areas should be advised of the risks of yellow fever disease and all available methods to prevent it. All travelers should take protective measures to avoid mosquito bites.

The following CDC agencies may be contacted if serologic testing is needed or for advice when administering yellow fever vaccine to pregnant women, children < 9 months, or patients with altered immune status:

Division of Vector-Borne Infectious Diseases: 970-221-6400

Division of Global Migration and Quarantine: 404-498-1600

In order to maximize vaccination rates, the ACIP recommends simultaneous administration of all age-appropriate vaccines (live or inactivated) for which a person is eligible at a single visit, unless contraindications exist. The use of combination vaccines is generally preferred over separate infections, taking into consider-ation provider assessment, patient preference, and potential adverse events.

For additional information, please refer to the following website: http://www.cdc.gov/vaccines/vpd-vac/.

Dosage Forms Excipient information presented when available (limited, particularly for generics); consult specific product labeling.

Injection, powder for reconstitution [17D-204 strain]:

YF-VAX®: ≥4.74 Log$_{10}$ plaque-forming units (PFU) per 0.5 mL dose [single-dose or 5-dose vial; produced in chicken embryos; contains gelatin; packaged with diluent; vial stopper contains latex]

References

ACIP Provisional Recommendations for the Use of Yellow Fever Vaccine, December 2009. Available at: http://www.cdc.gov/vaccines/recs/provisional/default.htm#acip.

Centers for Disease Control and Prevention (CDC), "General Recommendations on Immunization. Recommendations of the Advisory Committee on Immunization Practices (ACIP)," *MMWR Recomm Rep*, 2006, 55(RR-15):1-48. Available at: http://www.cdc.gov/mmwr/preview/mmwrhtml/rr5515a1.htm.

Centers for Disease Control and Prevention, "Guidelines for Preventing Opportunistic Infections Among Hematopoietic Stem Cell Transplant Recipients. Recommendations of CDC, the Infectious Disease Society of America, and the American Society of Blood and Marrow Transplantation," *MMWR Recomm Rep*, 2004, 49(RR-10):89-90.

Centers for Disease Control and Prevention, "Transfusion-Related Transmission of Yellow Fever Vaccine Virus – California, 2009," *MMWR Morb Mortal Wkly Rep*, 2010, 59(2):34-7.

Centers for Disease Control and Prevention, "Yellow Fever Vaccine. Recommendations of the Advisory Committee on Immunization Practices (ACIP)," *MMMR Recomm Rep*, 2002, 51(R-2):1-11.

Prymula R, Siegrist CA, Chlibek R, et al, "Effect of Prophylactic Paracetamol Administration at Time of Vaccination on Febrile Reactions and Antibody Responses in Children: Two Open-Label, Randomised Controlled Trials," *Lancet*, 2009, 374(9698):1339-50.

Red Book: 2009 Report of the Committee on Infectious Diseases, 28th ed, Pickering LK, ed, Elk Grove Village, IL: American Academy of Pediatrics, 2009. Available at: http://aapredbook.aappublications.org/cgi/content/full/2009/1/1.7.13.

♦ **YF-VAX®** *see* Yellow Fever Vaccine *on page 1437*

♦ **YM-08310** *see* Amifostine *on page 78*

♦ **Yodoxin®** *see* Iodoquinol *on page 755*

♦ **Z4942** *see* Ifosfamide *on page 709*

♦ **Zaditen® (Can)** *see* Ketotifen *on page 785*

♦ **Zaditor® [OTC]** *see* Ketotifen *on page 785*

♦ **Zaditor® (Can)** *see* Ketotifen *on page 785*

Zafirlukast (za FIR loo kast)

Medication Safety Issues

Sound-alike/look-alike issues:

Accolate® may be confused with Accupril®, Accutane®, Aclovate®

Related Information

Asthma *on page 1697*

U.S. Brand Names Accolate®

Canadian Brand Names Accolate®

Therapeutic Category Antiasthmatic; Leukotriene Receptor Antagonist

Generic Available No

Use Prophylaxis and chronic treatment of asthma (FDA approved in children ≥5 years and adults)

Pregnancy Risk Factor B

Pregnancy Considerations There are no adequate and well-controlled trials in pregnant women. Teratogenic effects not observed in animal studies; fetal defects were observed when administered in maternally toxic doses.

Lactation Enters breast milk/contraindicated

Breast-Feeding Considerations The manufacturer does not recommend breast-feeding due to tumorigenicity observed in animal studies.

Contraindications Hypersensitivity to zafirlukast or any component

Warnings Zafirlukast is not indicated for use in the reversal of bronchospasm in acute asthma attacks, including status asthmaticus. Therapy with zafirlukast can be continued during acute exacerbations of asthma. An increased proportion of zafirlukast patients (>55 years of age) reported infections as compared to placebo-treated patients; these infections were mostly mild or moderate in intensity, predominantly affected the respiratory tract, were dose-proportional to the total milligrams of zafirlukast exposure, and associated with coadministration of inhaled corticosteroids. Rare cases of eosinophilic vasculitis (Churg-Strauss) have been reported in patients receiving zafirlukast (usually, but not always, associated with reduction in concurrent steroid dosage). No causal relationship established.

Hepatic adverse events (including hepatitis, hyperbilirubinemia, and hepatic failure) have been reported. Female patients may be at greater risk. Discontinue **immediately** if liver dysfunction is suspected. Periodic testing of liver function may be considered (early detection is generally believed to improve the likelihood of recovery). If hepatic dysfunction is suspected (due to clinical signs/symptoms) liver function tests should be measured immediately. Do not resume or restart if hepatic function tests are consistent with dysfunction.

Postmarketing reports of neuropsychiatric events including agitation, aggression, anxiousness, dream abnormalities, hallucinations, depression, insomnia, irritability, restlessness, suicidal thinking and behavior (including suicide) and tremor have been observed.

Precautions Use with caution in patients receiving warfarin (see Drug Interactions) and patients with liver disease; dosage reduction in patients with hepatic impairment may be needed; discontinue therapy if liver dysfunction occurs; where no other attributable cause of liver dysfunction is identified, do not resume zafirlukast therapy

Adverse Reactions

Central nervous system: Agitation, aggression, anxiousness, asthenia, depression, dizziness, dream abnormalities, fever, hallucinations, headache, insomnia, irritability, pain, restlessness, suicidal thinking and behavior (including suicide), tremor

Dermatologic: Vasculitic rash (rare)

Gastrointestinal: Abdominal pain, diarrhea, nausea, vomiting, dyspepsia, xerostomia

Hematologic: Systemic eosinophilic vasculitis (rare)

Hepatic: Hepatitis, hyperbilirubinemia, hepatic failure, liver enzymes elevated

Neuromuscular & skeletal: Back pain, myalgia, weakness

Respiratory: Pharyngitis, rhinitis

Miscellaneous: Hypersensitivity reactions, infections (primarily respiratory)

<1% and/or postmarketing: Agranulocytosis, arthralgia, bleeding, bruising, edema, malaise, pruritus

Drug Interactions

Metabolism/Transport Effects Substrate of CYP2C9 (major); **Inhibits** CYP1A2 (weak), 2C8 (weak), 2C9 (moderate), 2C19 (weak), 2D6 (weak), 3A4 (weak)

Avoid Concomitant Use There are no known interactions where it is recommended to avoid concomitant use.

Increased Effect/Toxicity

Zafirlukast may increase the levels/effects of: Carvedilol; CYP2C9 Substrates (High risk); Vitamin K Antagonists

The levels/effects of Zafirlukast may be increased by: CYP2C9 Inhibitors (Moderate); CYP2C9 Inhibitors (Strong)

Decreased Effect

The levels/effects of Zafirlukast may be decreased by: CYP2C9 Inducers (Highly Effective); Erythromycin; Erythromycin (Systemic); Peginterferon Alfa-2b; Theophylline Derivatives

Food Interactions Food decreases zafirlukast absorption by 40%

▶

Stability Store tablets at controlled room temperature; protect from light and moisture; dispense in original airtight container

Mechanism of Action Zafirlukast is a selective and competitive leukotriene-receptor antagonist (LTRA) of cysteinyl leukotrienes C_4 (LTC_4), D_4 (LTD_4), and E_4 (LTE_4). This activity produces inhibition of the effects of these leukotrienes on bronchial smooth muscle resulting in the attenuation of bronchoconstriction and decreased vascular permeability, mucosal edema, and mucus production.

Pharmacodynamics Asthma symptom improvement:
Maximum effect: 2-6 weeks
Duration: 12 hours

Pharmacokinetics (Adult data unless noted)
Absorption: Rapid
Bioavailability: Food decreases bioavailability by ~40%
Distribution: Extensively excreted into breast milk; breast milk to plasma ratio: 0.15
V_d: Adults: 70 L
Protein binding: 99%, predominantly albumin
Metabolism: Extensively metabolized by liver via cyto-chrome P450 isoenzyme CYP2C9 pathway
Half-life, elimination: Adults: 10 hours (range: 8-16 hours)
Time to peak serum concentration: 3 hours
Elimination: Fecal (90%) and urine (10%)
Clearance:
Children 5-6 years: 9.2 L/hour
Children 7-11 years: 11.4 L/hour
Adults: 20 L/hour

Usual Dosage Oral:
Children 5-11 years: 10 mg twice daily
Children ≥12 years and Adults: 20 mg twice daily
Dosing adjustment in hepatic impairment: In patients with hepatic impairment (ie, biopsy-proven cirrhosis), there is a 50% to 60% greater C_{max} and AUC compared to normal subjects; these patients should be monitored closely for adverse effects and dosage reductions made if indicated (see Precautions)

Administration Oral: Administer at least 1 hour before or 2 hours after a meal

Monitoring Parameters Pulmonary function tests (FEV-1, PEF), improvement in asthma symptoms, periodic liver function tests

Reference Range Plasma levels not clinically indicated; plasma zafirlukast serum concentrations exceeding 5 ng/mL at 12-14 hours following oral doses have correlated with activity; mean trough serum levels at doses of 20 mg twice daily were 20 ng/mL

Patient Information Take regularly as prescribed, even during symptom-free periods. Do not use to treat acute episodes of asthma. Do not decrease the dose or stop taking any other asthma medications unless instructed by a physician. May cause dry mouth. Nursing women should not take zafirlukast. Notify healthcare provider if experiencing symptoms of abdominal pain, nausea, fatigue, lethargy, itching, jaundice, flu-like symptoms, or anorexia.

Dosage Forms Excipient information presented when available (limited, particularly for generics); consult specific product labeling.
Tablet: 10 mg, 20 mg

References
"Guidelines for the Diagnosis and Management of Asthma. NAEPP Expert Panel Report 3," August 2007, www.nhlbi.nih.gov/guidelines/asthma/asthgdln.pdf.
"National Asthma Education and Prevention Program. Expert Panel Report: Guidelines for the Diagnosis and Management of Asthma Update on Selected Topics–2002," *J Allergy Clin Immunol*, 2002, 110 (5 Suppl):S141-219.

◆ **Zamicet™** *see* Hydrocodone and Acetaminophen *on page 684*

Zanamivir (za NA mi veer)

Medication Safety Issues
Sound-alike/look-alike issues:
Relenza® may be confused with Albenza®, Aplenzin™

U.S. Brand Names Relenza®
Canadian Brand Names Relenza®
Therapeutic Category Antiviral Agent; Neuraminidase Inhibitor
Generic Available No
Use Treatment of uncomplicated influenza A and B infection in patients who have been symptomatic for no more than 2 days; prophylaxis of influenza (FDA approved in children ≥7 years and adults), prophylaxis of influenza (FDA approved in children ≥5 years). Authorized under the CDC Emergency Use Authorization (EUA): Treatment and chemoprophylaxis of 2009 H1N1 influenza virus

Restrictions Limited supplies of zanamivir aqueous solution are available via a compassionate use protocol for the treatment of serious influenza illness. Zanamivir solution intended for nebulization or intravenous (I.V.) use is not currently FDA approved. Data on safety and efficacy via these routes of administration are limited. Prior to requesting zanamivir aqueous solution for compassionate use, clinicians should consider the following:
• There is only a very limited supply available and supply cannot be guaranteed
• Each request will be evaluated on a case-by-case basis by a member of the FDA and a GSK physician
Patients will be considered for a therapy if all inclusion criteria are met:
• Hospitalization with serious influenza illness in the setting of a pandemic threat
• Laboratory confirmation of influenza (PCR, rapid assay, or culture)
• Unable to use other approved influenza medications or zanamivir aqueous solution is more appropriate In addition, patients must be >6 months of age to receive I.V. zanamivir. Patients who are pregnant may not be eligible unless the benefits are expected to outweigh the risks. For more information regarding procurement, patient eligibility, dosing and preparation, in the U.S. or Canada, contact GlaxoSmithKline:
Annie Cameron (office: 919-483-6958; mobile: 919-632-9380)
Vinne Lopez (office: 919-315-4697; mobile: 919-601-0498) **or**
FDA:
Normal business hours (8:00 am to 4:30 pm EST): Call DAVP at 301-796-0824
After business hours (4:30 pm to 8:00 am EST): Call FDA at 301-796-9900 or 301- 443-1240

Pregnancy Risk Factor C
Pregnancy Considerations Adverse events were not observed in animal reproduction studies; therefore, the manufacturer classifies zanamivir as pregnancy category C. Adverse events have not been reported in the infants of mothers who have taken zanamivir during pregnancy. Influenza infection may be more severe in pregnant women. Oseltamivir and zanamivir are currently recommended for the treatment or prophylaxis of 2009 H1N1 influenza (previously known as novel influenza A [H1N1]) in pregnant women and women up to 2 weeks postpartum (including following pregnancy loss). For seasonal influenza, oseltamivir and zanamivir are currently recommended as an adjunct to vaccination and should not be used as a substitute for vaccination in pregnant women (consult current CDC guidelines).

Lactation Excretion in breast milk unknown/use caution
Breast-Feeding Considerations It is not known if zanamivir is found in human milk and the manufacturer recommends that caution be exercised when

administering zanamivir to nursing women. According to the CDC, breast-feeding while taking zanamivir can be continued. The CDC recommends that women infected with the influenza virus follow general precautions (eg, frequent hand washing) to decrease viral transmission to the child. Mothers with influenza-like illnesses at delivery should consider avoiding close contact with the infant until they have received 48 hours of antiviral medication, fever has resolved, and cough and secretions can be controlled. These measures may help decrease (but not eliminate) the risk of transmitting influenza to the newborn. During this time, breast milk can be expressed and bottle-fed to the infant by another person who is well. Protective measures, such as wearing a face mask, changing into a clean gown or clothing, and strict hand hygiene should be continued by the mother for ≥7 days after the onset of symptoms or until symptom-free for 24 hours. Infant care should be performed by a noninfected person when possible.

Contraindications Hypersensitivity to zanamivir, lactose, or any component

Warnings Cases of serious, sometimes fatal, bronchospasm have been reported. Discontinue zanamivir if bronchospasm, decline in respiratory function, or allergic reaction occurs. If a medical decision is made to prescribe zanamivir for a patient with an underlying airway disease, a fast-acting bronchodilator should be made available and used prior to each dose, along with close monitoring of respiratory function. Pediatric patients with influenza may be at increased risk of seizures, confusion, or abnormal behavior early in their illness (monitor for abnormal behavior).

Precautions Not recommended for use in patients with underlying airway disease (eg, asthma or chronic obstructive pulmonary disease) due to risk of bronchospasm. Zanamivir is not a substitute for annual influenza vaccination. Not recommended for prevention of influenza in nursing homes.

Adverse Reactions
Cardiovascular: Arrhythmias, syncope
Central nervous system: Dizziness, fever, chills, abnormal behavior, delirium, confusion, hallucinations, agitation, seizures, anxiety, nightmares, malaise, fatigue
Dermatologic: Rash, urticaria, facial edema
Gastrointestinal: Abdominal pain
Hematologic: Lymphopenia, neutropenia
Hepatic: Liver enzymes elevated
Neuromuscular & skeletal: Arthralgia, articular rheumatism, myalgia
Respiratory: Sinusitis, dyspnea, bronchospasm, cough; ear, nose, and throat infection
Miscellaneous: Oropharyngeal edema, anaphylaxis

Drug Interactions
Avoid Concomitant Use There are no known interactions where it is recommended to avoid concomitant use.
Increased Effect/Toxicity There are no known significant interactions involving an increase in effect.
Decreased Effect
Zanamivir may decrease the levels/effects of: Influenza Virus Vaccine (H1N1, Live/Attenuated); Influenza Virus Vaccine (Live/Attenuated)

Stability Store at room temperature. Do not puncture Rotadisk blister until taking a dose using the Diskhaler.

Mechanism of Action Zanamivir inhibits influenza virus neuraminidase enzymes, altering virus particle aggregation and release.

Pharmacokinetics (Adult data unless noted)
Absorption: 4% to 17% of the inhaled dose is systemically absorbed
Protein binding: <10%
Metabolism: None
Half-life: Adults: 2.5-5.1 hours

Time to peak serum concentration: 1-2 hours
Elimination: Renally excreted as unchanged drug; unabsorbed drug is excreted in the feces

Usual Dosage Oral inhalation: **Note:** 10 mg dose is provided by 2 inhalations (one 5 mg blister per inhalation): Treatment of influenza: Children ≥7 yrs and Adults: 10 mg twice daily (12 hours apart) for 5 days. **Note:** Two doses should be taken on the first day of treatment, if possible, provided doses can be spaced at least 2 hours apart.
Prophylaxis of influenza:
Children ≥5 yrs and Adults: Household setting: 10 mg once daily for 10 days; initiate within 1.5 days following onset of signs or symptoms in the index case
Adolescents and Adults: Community outbreaks: 10 mg once daily for 28 days; initiate within 5 days of outbreak

Administration Oral Inhalation: **Inhalation powder not for use via nebulizer:** Use a Diskhaler® (special breath-activated plastic inhaler) to deliver dose. Load Relenza Rotadisk into the diskhaler; 10 mg dose is provided by 2 inhalations (one 5 mg blister per inhalation). A blister that contains medication is pierced and the drug is dispersed into the air stream created when the patient inhales through the mouthpiece. Patients scheduled to take inhaled bronchodilators at the same time as zanamivir should be advised to use their bronchodilator before taking zanamivir.

Monitoring Parameters
Monitor for abnormal behavior, respiratory function

Patient Information Contact physician if wheezing worsens, if shortness of breath or bronchospasm occurs, or if unusual behavior occurs. Zanamivir does not reduce the risk of transmission of influenza to others.

Nursing Implications Evaluate the ability of young children to use the Diskhaler® delivery system. Children <8 years of age may not produce measurable inspiratory flow through the Diskhaler® or produce peak inspiratory flow rates below the 60 L/minute considered optimal for the device.

Additional Information Children ages 2-4 years have a higher rate of influenza-related complications compared to older children.

Dosage Forms Excipient information presented when available (limited, particularly for generics); consult specific product labeling.
Powder for oral inhalation:
Relenza®: 5 mg/blister (20s) [contains lactose 20 mg/blister; 4 blisters per Rotadisk® foil pack, 5 Rotadisk® per package; packaged with Diskhaler® inhalation device]

References
American Academy of Pediatrics Committee on Infectious Diseases, "Antiviral Therapy and Prophylaxis for Influenza in Children," *Pediatrics*, 2007, 119(4):852-60.
Centers for Disease Control,"Use of Antiviral Medications for the Management of Influenza in Childrens and Adolescent for the 2009-2010 Season - Pediatric Supplement for Heath Care Providers," December 24, 2009. Available at: http://www.cdc.gov/h1n1/recommendations_pediatric_supplement.htm.
Harper SA, Bradley JS, Englund JA, et al, "Seasonal Influenza in Adults and Children - Diagnosis, Treatment, Chemoprophylaxis, and Institutional Outbreak Management: Clinical Practice Guidelines of the Infectious Diseases Society of America," *Clin Infect Dis*, 2009, 48 (8):1003-32.

♦ **Zantac®** *see* Ranitidine *on page 1200*
♦ **Zantac 75® [OTC]** *see* Ranitidine *on page 1200*
♦ **Zantac 75® (Can)** *see* Ranitidine *on page 1200*
♦ **Zantac 150® [OTC]** *see* Ranitidine *on page 1200*
♦ **Zantac® EFFERdose®** *see* Ranitidine *on page 1200*
♦ **Zantac Maximum Strength Non-Prescription (Can)** *see* Ranitidine *on page 1200*
♦ **Zapzyt® [OTC]** *see* Benzoyl Peroxide *on page 184*
♦ **Zarontin®** *see* Ethosuximide *on page 546*

♦ **Zaroxolyn®** see Metolazone on page 917
♦ **Z-Cof LA™** see Guaifenesin and Dextromethorphan on page 658
♦ **ZDV** see Zidovudine on page 1442
♦ **ZDV, Abacavir, and Lamivudine** see Abacavir, Lamivudine, and Zidovudine on page 31
♦ **ZDV and 3TC** see Lamivudine and Zidovudine on page 794
♦ **Zeasorb®-AF [OTC]** see Miconazole on page 927
♦ **Zegerid®** see Omeprazole and Sodium Bicarbonate on page 1018
♦ **Zegerid OTC™ [OTC]** see Omeprazole and Sodium Bicarbonate on page 1018
♦ **Zemplar®** see Paricalcitol on page 1061
♦ **Zemuron®** see Rocuronium on page 1230
♦ **Zenapax® [DSC]** see Daclizumab on page 382
♦ **Zenapax® (Can)** see Daclizumab on page 382
♦ **Zenpep™** see Pancrelipase on page 1051
♦ **Zerit®** see Stavudine on page 1290
♦ **Zestril®** see Lisinopril on page 832
♦ **Zetar® [OTC]** see Coal Tar on page 349
♦ **Zetia®** see Ezetimibe on page 553
♦ **Ziagen®** see Abacavir on page 26

Zidovudine (zye DOE vyoo deen)

Medication Safety Issues
Sound-alike/look-alike issues:
Azidothymidine may be confused with azaTHIOprine, aztreonam
Retrovir® may be confused with acyclovir, ritonavir

AZT is an error-prone abbreviation (mistaken as azathioprine, aztreonam)

Related Information
Adult and Adolescent HIV on page 1620
Management of Healthcare Worker Exposures to HBV, HCV, and HIV on page 1661
Pediatric HIV on page 1613
Perinatal HIV on page 1628

U.S. Brand Names Retrovir®
Canadian Brand Names Apo-Zidovudine®; AZT™; Novo-AZT; Retrovir®; Retrovir® (AZT™)
Therapeutic Category Antiretroviral Agent; HIV Agents (Anti-HIV Agents); Nucleoside Reverse Transcriptase Inhibitor (NRTI)
Generic Available Yes: Capsule, syrup, tablet
Use Treatment of HIV infection in combination with other antiretroviral agents (FDA approved in ages ≥4 weeks and adults); (Note: HIV regimens consisting of three antiretroviral agents are strongly recommended); chemoprophylaxis to reduce perinatal HIV transmission [FDA approved in ages 0 days to 6 weeks (postpartum therapy of HIV-1 exposed neonate) and adults (antepartum and intrapartum therapy of HIV-1 infected mother)]; has also been used as HIV postexposure prophylaxis (eg, chemoprophylaxis after occupational exposure to HIV) (see Related Information)
Pregnancy Risk Factor C
Pregnancy Considerations Adverse events have been observed in some animal reproduction studies. Zidovudine crosses the placenta. No increased risk of overall birth defects has been observed following first trimester exposure according to data collected by the antiretroviral pregnancy registry. The use of zidovudine reduces the maternal-fetal transmission of HIV by ~70% and should be considered for antenatal and intrapartum therapy whenever possible. The Perinatal HIV Guidelines Working

Group considers zidovudine the preferred NRTI for use in combination regimens during pregnancy. In HIV-infected mothers not previously on antiretroviral therapy, and who do not need therapy for their own health, treatment may be delayed until after 10-12 weeks gestation. Cases of lactic acidosis/hepatic steatosis syndrome have been reported in pregnant women receiving nucleoside analogues. It is not known if pregnancy itself potentiates this known side effect; however, pregnant women may be at increased risk of lactic acidosis and liver damage. Hepatic enzymes and electrolytes should be monitored frequently during the 3rd trimester of pregnancy in women receiving nucleoside analogues. Women in labor with an unknown HIV status should have a rapid HIV test. If the test is positive, begin I.V. zidovudine therapy. (If a postpartum confirmatory test is negative, zidovudine therapy in the infant can be stopped). Health professionals are encouraged to contact the antiretroviral pregnancy registry to monitor outcomes of pregnant women exposed to antiretroviral medications (1-800-258-4263 or www.APRegistry.com).

Lactation Enters breast milk/contraindicated
Breast-Feeding Considerations In infants born to mothers who are HIV positive, HAART while breastfeeding may decrease postnatal infection. Infant prophylaxis with zidovudine in combination with nevirapine or nevirapine alone may also decrease the risk of HIV transmission to the infant. However, maternal or infant antiretroviral therapy does not completely eliminate the risk of postnatal HIV transmission.

In the United States where formula is accessible, affordable, safe, and sustainable, complete avoidance of breast-feeding by HIV-infected women is recommended to decrease potential transmission of HIV.

Contraindications Life-threatening hypersensitivity to zidovudine or any component
Warnings Hematologic toxicity including neutropenia and severe anemia requiring transfusions may occur **[U.S. Boxed Warning]**; use with caution in patients with ANC <1000 cells/mm³ or hemoglobin <9.5 g/dL; discontinue treatment in children with an ANC <500 cells/mm³ until marrow recovery is observed; use of erythropoietin, filgrastim, or reduced zidovudine dosage may be necessary in some patients. Prolonged use of zidovudine may cause myositis and myopathy **[U.S. Boxed Warning]**. Zidovudine has been shown to be carcinogenic in rats and mice.

Cases of lactic acidosis, severe hepatomegaly with steatosis, and death have been reported in patients receiving nucleoside analogues **[U.S. Boxed Warning]**; most of these cases have been in women; prolonged nucleoside use, obesity, and prior liver disease may be risk factors; use with extreme caution in patients with other risk factors for liver disease; discontinue therapy in patients who develop laboratory or clinical evidence of lactic acidosis or pronounced hepatotoxicity. Concomitant use of combination antiretroviral therapy with interferon alfa (with or without ribavirin) has resulted in hepatic decompensation (with some fatalities) in patients coinfected with HIV and HCV; monitor patients closely, especially for hepatic decompensation, neutropenia, and anemia; consider discontinuation of zidovudine if needed; consider dose reduction or discontinuation of interferon alfa, ribavirin, or both if clinical toxicities, including hepatic decompensation, worsen.

Syrup contains sodium benzoate; benzoic acid (benzoate) is a metabolite of benzyl alcohol; large amounts of benzyl alcohol (≥99 mg/kg/day) have been associated with a potentially fatal toxicity ("gasping syndrome") in neonates; the "gasping syndrome" consists of metabolic acidosis, respiratory distress, gasping respirations, CNS dysfunction (including convulsions, intracranial hemorrhage), hypotension and cardiovascular collapse; use syrup containing sodium benzoate with caution in neonates; *in vitro* and animal studies have shown that benzoate displaces bilirubin from protein binding sites

Precautions Use with caution in patients with bone marrow compromise or in patients with impaired renal or hepatic function; reduce dosage or interrupt therapy in patients with anemia, granulocytopenia, or myopathy; reduce dosage in patients with severe renal or hepatic impairment. Fat redistribution and accumulation [ie, central obesity, peripheral wasting, facial wasting, breast enlargement, dorsocervical fat enlargement (buffalo hump), and cushingoid appearance] have been observed in patients receiving antiretroviral agents (causal relationship not established). Immune reconstitution syndrome (an acute inflammatory response to residual or indolent opportunistic infections) may occur in HIV patients during initial treatment with combination antiretroviral agents; this syndrome may require further patient assessment and therapy. Use of zidovudine with stavudine is not recommended due to antagonistic effects (see Drug Interactions). Zidovudine should not be used concurrently with combination products that also contain zidovudine as a component (eg, Combivir® or Trizivir®).

Adverse Reactions

Cardiovascular: ECG abnormality, edema, heart failure, left ventricular dilation

Central nervous system: Asthenia, confusion, dizziness, fever, insomnia, irritability, malaise, manic syndrome, nervousness, seizures, severe headache

Dermatologic: Pigmentation of nails (blue), rash

Endocrine & metabolic: Fat redistribution and accumulation (see Precautions), lactic acidosis (see Warnings)

Gastrointestinal: Anorexia, diarrhea, nausea, vomiting, weight loss

Genitourinary: Hematuria

Hematologic: Anemia (macrocytic; see Warnings), granulocytopenia, leukopenia, neutropenia (see Warnings), thrombocytopenia

Hepatic: Cholestatic hepatitis; hepatic steatosis; serum ALT, AST, LDH, and alkaline phosphatase increased; severe hepatomegaly

Neuromuscular & skeletal: Myalgia, reflexes decreased, tremor, weakness; unusual: myopathy, myositis (see Warnings)

Miscellaneous: Immune reconstitution syndrome (see Precautions)

<1%, postmarketing, and/or case reports: Amblyopia, anxiety, aplastic anemia, back pain, cardiomyopathy, chest pain, CPK increased, depression, dysphagia, dyspnea, flatulence, flu-like syndrome, gynecomastia, hearing loss, hemolytic anemia, jaundice, loss of mental acuity, lymphadenopathy, macular edema, mania, mouth ulcer, muscle spasm, oral mucosa pigmentation, pain (generalized), pancreatitis, pancytopenia with marrow hypoplasia, paresthesia, photophobia, pruritus, red cell aplasia (pure), rhabdomyolysis, rhinitis, sensitization reactions (including anaphylaxis and angioedema), sinusitis, skin pigmentation (changes in), somnolence, Stevens-Johnson syndrome, sweating, syncope, taste perversion, toxic epidermal necrolysis, tremor, urinary frequency, urinary hesitancy, urticaria, vasculitis, vertigo

Drug Interactions

Metabolism/Transport Effects Substrate (minor) of CYP2A6, 2C9, 2C19, 3A4

Avoid Concomitant Use

Avoid concomitant use of Zidovudine with any of the following: Stavudine

Increased Effect/Toxicity

Zidovudine may increase the levels/effects of: Ribavirin

The levels/effects of Zidovudine may be increased by: Acyclovir-Valacyclovir; Clarithromycin; Divalproex;

DOXOrubicin; DOXOrubicin (Liposomal); Fluconazole; Ganciclovir-Valganciclovir; Interferons; Methadone; Probenecid; Ribavirin; Valproic Acid

Decreased Effect

Zidovudine may decrease the levels/effects of: Stavudine

The levels/effects of Zidovudine may be decreased by: Clarithromycin; DOXOrubicin; DOXOrubicin (Liposomal); Protease Inhibitors; Rifamycin Derivatives

Food Interactions Food does not significantly affect bioavailability; folate or vitamin B_{12} deficiency increases zidovudine-associated myelosuppression

Stability

I.V.: Store undiluted vials at 15°C to 25°C (59°F to 77°F); protect from light. Dilute with D_5W to a final concentration ≤4 mg/mL. The diluted I.V. solution is physically and chemically stable for 24 hours at room temperature and 48 hours if refrigerated. Administer diluted I.V. solution within 8 hours if stored at room temperature and within 24 hours if refrigerated to minimize the potential for microbial contamination (vials are single-use and do not contain preservative)

Tablets, capsules, syrup: Store at 15°C to 25°C (59°F to 77°F); protect capsules from moisture

Mechanism of Action Zidovudine is a thymidine analog that enters the cell and is phosphorylated by cellular kinases to the active metabolite zidovudine triphosphate which serves as an alternative substrate to deoxythymidine triphosphate for incorporation by reverse transcriptase; inhibits HIV viral polymerases and DNA synthesis

Pharmacokinetics (Adult data unless noted)

Absorption: Oral: Well absorbed

Distribution: Crosses the placenta; distributes into breast milk at concentrations similar to plasma; significant penetration into the CSF

CSF/plasma ratio:

Children 3 months to 12 years (n=38): Median: 0.68; range: 0.03-3.25

Adults (n=39): Median: 0.6; range: 0.04-2.62

V_d: Adults: 1.6 L/kg

Protein binding: 25% to 38%

Metabolism: Extensive first-pass effect; metabolized in the liver via glucuronidation to inactive metabolites

Bioavailability: Oral: Similar for tablets, capsules, and syrup

Neonates <14 days: 89%

Infants 14 days to 3 months: 61%

Infants 3 months to Children 12 years: 65%

Adults: 64% ± 10%

Half-life, terminal:

Premature neonate: 6.3 hours

Full-term neonates: 3.1 hours

Infants 14 days to 3 months: 1.9 hours

Infants 3 months to Children 12 years: 1.5 hours

Adults: 0.5-3 hours (mean: 1.1 hours)

Time to peak serum concentration: Within 30-90 minutes

Elimination: Urinary excretion (63% to 95%)

Oral: 72% to 74% of drug excreted in urine as metabolites and 14% to 18% as unchanged drug

I.V.: 45% to 60% excreted in urine as metabolites and 18% to 29% as unchanged drug

Usual Dosage

HIV Infection (treatment) (use in combination with other antiretroviral agents):

Oral:

Infants ≥4 weeks, Children, and Adolescents <18 years: **Note:** Dosage may be calculated by body weight (in kg) or body surface area and should not exceed the recommended adult dose. **Note:** Doses calculated by body weight may not be the same as those calculated by body surface area.

Dosing based on body surface area: 240 mg/m^2 every 12 hours (maximum: 300 mg every 12 hours) or 160 mg/m^2/dose every 8 hours (maximum: 200 mg every 8 hours)

Dosing based on weight:

4 to <9 kg: 12 mg/kg/dose twice daily or 8 mg/kg/dose 3 times/day

≥9 to <30 kg: 9 mg/kg/dose twice daily or 6 mg/kg/dose 3 times/day

≥30 kg: 300 mg twice daily or 200 mg 3 times/day

Adolescents ≥18 years and Adults: 300 mg twice daily or 200 mg 3 times/day

I.V.:

Infants ≥6 weeks and Children <12 years:

I.V. continuous infusion: 20 mg/m^2/hour

I.V. intermittent infusion: 120 mg/m^2/dose every 6 hours

Children ≥12 years and Adults: I.V. intermittent infusion: 1 mg/kg/dose administered every 4 hours

Prevention of maternal-fetal HIV transmission: (Perinatal HIV Guidelines Working Group, 2009; see also Related Information, Perinatal HIV); **Note:** Zidovudine is typically used as monotherapy in neonates to prevent perinatal transmission of HIV. In addition to a 6-week course of zidovudine in the neonate, the recommended regimen in the U.S. to prevent perinatal transmission of HIV also includes maternal antepartum oral zidovudine and maternal intrapartum I.V. zidovudine (see "Perinatal HIV" section in Appendix for details). Consider use of zidovudine in combination with nevirapine (and possibly lamivudine) in select situations (eg, infants born to mothers with no antiretroviral therapy prior to labor or during labor; infants born to mothers with only intrapartum antiretroviral therapy; infants born to mothers with suboptimal viral suppression at delivery; or infants born to mothers with known antiretroviral drug-resistant virus) (see "Perinatal HIV" section in Appendix for details).

Neonates: **Note:** Dosing should begin within 6-12 hours after birth and continue for the first 6 weeks of life. **Use I.V. route only until oral therapy can be administered.**

Premature Infants <35 weeks gestational age (GA) at birth; **Note:** Standard neonatal dose may be excessive in premature infants: Initial:

Oral: 2 mg/kg/dose every 12 hours

I.V.: 1.5 mg/kg/dose every 12 hours

Increase to every 8 hours as follows:

GA at birth <30 weeks: Increase above dose to every 8 hours at 4 weeks of age

GA at birth ≥30 weeks: Increase above dose to every 8 hours at 2 weeks of age

Neonates and Infants <6 weeks:

Oral: 2 mg/kg/dose every 6 hours; **Note:** Twice daily dosing is not FDA approved in neonates and infants <6 weeks of age, but some investigators use 4 mg/kg/dose every 12 hours to improve compliance; the efficacy of this dose for prevention of mother-to-child transmission of HIV has not been established (Perinatal HIV Guidelines Working Group, 2009).

I.V.: 1.5 mg/kg/dose every 6 hours

Maternal: Oral (Perinatal HIV Guidelines Working Group, 2009): 100 mg 5 times/day **or** 200 mg 3 times/day **or** 300 mg twice daily. Begin at 14-34 weeks gestation and continue until start of labor.

During labor and delivery, administer zidovudine I.V. at 2 mg/kg as loading dose followed by a continuous I.V. infusion of 1 mg/kg/hour until the umbilical cord is clamped

HIV postexposure prophylaxis: Children ≥12 years and Adults: 300 mg twice daily **or** 200 mg 3 times/day (with food) in combination with lamivudine or emtricitabine, with or without a protease inhibitor depending on risk; begin therapy within 2 hours of exposure if possible

Dosage adjustment in renal impairment: Adults: End-stage renal disease patients (Cl$_{cr}$ <15 mL/minute) maintained on hemodialysis or peritoneal dialysis:

Oral: 100 mg every 6-8 hours

I.V.: 1 mg/kg/dose every 6-8 hours

Dosage adjustment in hepatic impairment: Specific recommendations currently unknown; dosage reduction may be required; use with caution; monitor for hematologic toxicities frequently

Dosage adjustment for zidovudine hematologic toxicity: Significant anemia (Hgb <7.5 g/dL or >25% decrease from baseline) and/or significant neutropenia (ANC <750 cells/mm^3 or >50% decrease from baseline): Dose interruption may be required until evidence of bone marrow recovery occurs; once bone marrow recovers, dose may be resumed using appropriate adjunctive therapy (eg, epoetin alfa).

Administration

Oral: May be administered without regard to meals; the patient should be in an upright position while taking zidovudine capsules to minimize the risk of esophageal ulceration. If used concurrently, administer clarithromycin 4 hours apart from zidovudine (see Drug Interactions).

Parenteral: Do not administer I.M.; do not administer I.V. push or by rapid infusion; infuse I.V. zidovudine over 1 hour at a final concentration not to exceed 4 mg/mL in D$_5$W; I.V. dose may be infused over 30 minutes in neonates

Monitoring Parameters CBC with differential, hemoglobin, MCV, reticulocyte count, serum creatine kinase, CD4 cell count, HIV RNA plasma levels, renal and hepatic function tests; signs and symptoms of lactic acidosis, pronounced hepatotoxicity, anemia, and bone marrow suppression

Patient Information Zidovudine is not a cure for HIV. Notify physician if muscle weakness, shortness of breath, headache, insomnia, signs of infection, unusual bleeding, or rash occur. Take zidovudine every day as prescribed; do not change dose or discontinue without physician's advice. If a dose is missed, take it as soon as possible, then return to normal dosing schedule; if a dose is skipped, do **not** double the next dose.

HIV medications may cause changes in body fat, including an increase in fat in the upper back and neck, breasts, and trunk; a loss of fat from the face, arms, and legs may also occur. Do not take zidovudine (Retrovir®) with other zidovudine-containing medications (eg, Combivir® or Trizivir®)

Additional Information Conversion from oral to I.V. dose: I.V. dose = $^2/_3$ of the oral dose. Zidovudine-associated reduction in Hgb may occur as early as 2-4 weeks after initiation of therapy; onset of neutropenia usually occurs after 6-8 weeks. One study found an increased risk of hypospadias in newborns after being exposed to zidovudine in the first trimester (Working Group, 2009).

Dosage Forms Excipient information presented when available (limited, particularly for generics); consult specific product labeling.

Capsule, oral: 100 mg

Retrovir®: 100 mg

Injection, solution [preservative free]:

Retrovir®: 10 mg/mL (20 mL)

Syrup, oral: 50 mg/5 mL (240 mL)

Retrovir®: 50 mg/5 mL (240 mL) [contains sodium benzoate; strawberry flavor]

Tablet, oral: 300 mg

Retrovir®: 300 mg

References

Briars LA, Hilao JJ, and Kraus DM, "A Review of Pediatric Human Immunodeficiency Virus Infection," *Journal of Pharmacy Practice*, 2004, 17(6):407-31.

Mueller BU, Jacobsen F, Butler KM, et al, "Combination Treatment With Azidothymidine and Granulocyte Colony-Stimulating Factor in Children With Human Immunodeficiency Virus Infection," *J Pediatr*, 1992, 121(5 Pt 1):797-802.

Panel on Antiretroviral Guidelines for Adults and Adolescents, "Guidelines for the Use of Antiretroviral Agents in HIV-Infected Adults and Adolescents," December 1, 2009. Available at: http://www.aidsinfo.nih.gov.

Perinatal HIV Guidelines Working Group, "Recommendations for the Use of Antiretroviral Drugs in Pregnant HIV-Infected Women for Maternal Health and Interventions to Reduce Perinatal HIV-1 Transmission in the United States," April, 29 2009. Available at: http://aidsinfo.nih.gov/contentfiles/PerinatalGL.pdf.

"Updated U.S. Public Health Service Guidelines for the Management of Occupational Exposures to HIV and Recommendations for Post-exposure Prophylaxis," *MMWR Recomm Rep*, 2005, 54(RR-9):1-17.

Volberding PA, Lagakos SW, Koch MA, et al, "Zidovudine in Asymptomatic Human Immunodeficiency Virus Infection. A Controlled Trial in Persons With Fewer Than 500 CD4-Positive Cells Per Cubic Millimeter. The AIDS Clinical Trials Group of the National Institute of Allergy and Infectious Diseases," *N Engl J Med*, 1990, 322(14):941-9.

Working Group on Antiretroviral Therapy and Medical Management of HIV-Infected Children, "Guidelines for the Use of Antiretroviral Agents in Pediatric HIV Infection," February 23, 2009. Available at http://www.aidsinfo.nih.gov.

♦ **Zidovudine, Abacavir, and Lamivudine** *see* Abacavir, Lamivudine, and Zidovudine *on page 31*

♦ **Zidovudine and Lamivudine** *see* Lamivudine and Zidovudine *on page 794*

♦ **Zilactin®-L [OTC]** *see* Benzyl Alcohol *on page 186*

♦ **Zilactin®-B [OTC]** *see* Benzocaine *on page 182*

♦ **Zilactin-B® (Can)** *see* Benzocaine *on page 182*

♦ **Zilactin Baby® (Can)** *see* Benzocaine *on page 182*

♦ **Zilactin Toothache and Gum Pain® [OTC]** *see* Benzocaine *on page 182*

♦ **Zinacef®** *see* Cefuroxime *on page 277*

♦ **Zinc Acetate** *see* Zinc Supplements *on page 1445*

♦ **Zincate®** *see* Zinc Supplements *on page 1445*

♦ **Zinc Carbonate** *see* Zinc Supplements *on page 1445*

♦ **Zinc Chloride** *see* Trace Metals *on page 1366*

♦ **Zinc Chloride** *see* Zinc Supplements *on page 1445*

♦ **Zinc Gluconate** *see* Zinc Supplements *on page 1445*

♦ **Zincofax® (Can)** *see* Zinc Oxide *on page 1445*

Zinc Oxide (zingk OKS ide)

U.S. Brand Names Ammens® Original Medicated [OTC]; Ammens® Shower Fresh [OTC]; Balmex® [OTC]; Boudreaux's® Butt Paste [OTC]; Critic-Aid Skin Care® [OTC]; Desitin® Creamy [OTC]; Desitin® [OTC]

Canadian Brand Names Zincofax®

Therapeutic Category Topical Skin Product

Generic Available Yes: Ointment

Use Protective coating for mild skin irritations and abrasions; soothing and protective ointment to promote healing of chapped skin, diaper rash

Contraindications Hypersensitivity to zinc oxide or any component

Drug Interactions

Avoid Concomitant Use There are no known interactions where it is recommended to avoid concomitant use.

Increased Effect/Toxicity There are no known significant interactions involving an increase in effect.

Decreased Effect There are no known significant interactions involving a decrease in effect.

Stability Avoid prolonged storage at temperatures >30°C

Mechanism of Action Mild astringent, protective and weak antiseptic action

Usual Dosage Infants, Children, and Adults: Topical: Apply several times daily to affected area

Administration Topical: For external use only; do not use in the eyes

Patient Information Paste is easily removed with mineral oil

Dosage Forms Excipient information presented when available (limited, particularly for generics); consult specific product labeling.

Cream, topical:
    Balmex®: 11.3% (60 g, 120 g, 480 g) [contains aloe, benzoic acid, soybean oil, and vitamin E]

Cream, topical [stick]:
    Balmex®: 11.3% (56 g) [contains aloe, benzoic acid, soybean oil, and vitamin E]

Ointment, topical: 20% (30 g, 60 g, 454 g); 40% (120 g)
    Desitin®: 40% (30 g, 60 g, 90 g, 120 g, 270 g, 480 g) [contains cod liver oil and lanolin]
    Desitin® Creamy: 10% (60 g, 120 g)

Paste, topical:
    Boudreaux's® Butt Paste: 16% (30 g, 60 g, 120 g, 480 g) [contains castor oil, boric acid, mineral oil, and Peruvian balsam]
    Critic-Aid Skin Care®: 20% (71 g, 170 g)

Powder, topical:
    Ammens® Original Medicated: 9.1% (312 g)
    Ammens® Shower Fresh: 9.1% (312 g)

♦ **Zinc Sulfate** *see* Trace Metals *on page 1366*

♦ **Zinc Sulfate** *see* Zinc Supplements *on page 1445*

Zinc Supplements (zink SUP la ments)

U.S. Brand Names Cold-Eeze® [OTC; Galzin™; Ora-zinc® [OTC]; Zincate®

Therapeutic Category Antidote, Copper Toxicity; Mineral, Oral; Mineral, Parenteral

Generic Available Yes

Use Treatment and prevention of zinc deficiency states; may improve wound healing in those who are zinc deficient; maintenance treatment of Wilson's disease (zinc acetate)

Pregnancy Risk Factor C

Contraindications Hypersensitivity to zinc salts or any component

Warnings Do not administer undiluted by direct injection into a peripheral vein due to potential for phlebitis, tissue irritation, and potential increased renal loss of minerals from a bolus injection; administration of zinc in absence of copper may decrease plasma copper levels; excessive intake in healthy persons may be deleterious as decreases in HDL (high-density lipoproteins) and impairment of immune system function have been reported

Adverse Reactions

Cardiovascular: Hypotension, tachycardia (excessive doses)

Central nervous system: Hypothermia (excessive doses)

Gastrointestinal: Indigestion, nausea, vomiting

Hematologic: Leukopenia, neutropenia

Hepatic: Jaundice (excessive doses)

Ocular: Blurred vision (excessive doses)

Respiratory: Pulmonary edema (excessive doses)

Miscellaneous: Profuse diaphoresis

Food Interactions Coffee, foods high in phytate (eg, whole grain cereals and legumes), bran, and dairy products reduce zinc absorption; avoid foods high in calcium or phosphorus

Mechanism of Action A cofactor for more than 70 enzymes which are important to carbohydrate and protein metabolism, zinc helps to maintain normal growth and tissue repair, normal skin hydration, and senses of taste and smell; in Wilson's disease, zinc cation inhibits the absorption of dietary copper by inducing the synthesis of metallothionein, a metal-binding protein present in the intestinal mucosa. This protein binds metals, including copper, forming a nontoxic complex that is not absorbed systematically but excreted in the stool.

Pharmacokinetics (Adult data unless noted)
Absorption: pH dependent; poor from GI tract (20% to 30%); solubilized by conversion to zinc chloride in the presence of gastric acid

Distribution: Storage sites are liver and skeletal muscle; serum levels do not adequately reflect whole-body zinc status

Protein binding: 55% bound to albumin; 40% bound to alpha 1-macroglobulin

Elimination: 90% in feces with only traces appearing in urine and perspiration

Usual Dosage Clinical response may not occur for up to 6-8 weeks

Recommended daily allowance (RDA): Oral:
Neonates and Infants <12 months: 5 mg **elemental** zinc/day

Children 1-10 years: 10 mg **elemental** zinc/day

Children ≥11 years and Adults: Male: 15 mg **elemental** zinc/day; Female: 12 mg **elemental** zinc/day

Zinc deficiency: Oral:
Infants and Children: 0.5-1 mg **elemental** zinc/kg/day divided 1-3 times/day; larger doses may be needed if impaired intestinal absorption or an excessive loss of zinc (eg, excessive, prolonged diarrhea)

Adults: 25-50 mg **elemental** zinc/dose (110-220 mg zinc sulfate) 3 times/day

Supplement to parenteral nutrition solutions (clinical response may not occur for up to 6-8 weeks): (See Trace Metals): I.V. (all doses are mcg or mg of **elemental** zinc):

Premature Infants: 400 mcg/kg/day

Term Infants <3 months: 300 mcg/kg/day

Infants ≥3 months and Children ≤5 years: 100 mcg/kg/day (maximum: 5 mg/day)

Children >5 years and Adolescents: 2.5-5 mg/day

Adults:
Stable metabolically: 2.5-4 mg **elemental** zinc/day; catabolic state: Increase by an additional 2 mg/day (eg, 4.5-6 mg **elemental** zinc/day)

Stable with fluid loss from small bowel: Additional 12.2 mg **elemental** zinc/L parenteral nutrition or 17.1 mg **elemental** zinc/kg of stool or ileostomy output

Wound healing: Oral: Adults: 50 mg **elemental** zinc (220 mg zinc sulfate) 3 times daily in patients with low serum zinc levels (<110 mcg/dL)

Maintenance treatment of Wilson's disease: **Zinc acetate: Dose is in mg elemental zinc: Note:** Indicated for initial treatment of Wilson's disease in asymptomatic or presymptomatic patients or for maintenance after initial therapy with a chelating agent (~1-5 years):

Children 5-18 years:
<50 kg: 25 mg/dose 3 times/day
≥50 kg: 50 mg/dose 3 times/day

Pregnant women: 25 mg/dose 3 times/day; may increase to 50 mg/dose 3 times/day if inadequate response to lower dose

Adults (nonpregnant): 50 mg/dose 3 times/day

Note: Not indicated for initial treatment of Wilson's disease but for maintenance after initial therapy with a chelating agent (approximately 4-6 months)

Administration
Oral: Administer oral formulation with food if GI upset occurs; in patients with Wilson's disease, administer zinc acetate 1 hour before or after meals or beverage (except water); zinc acetate capsules should be swallowed whole; do not open or chew

Parenteral: Dilute as component of daily parenteral nutrition or maintenance fluids; do not give undiluted by direct injection into a peripheral vein due to potential for

phlebitis and tissue irritation, and potential to increase renal losses of minerals from a bolus injection

Monitoring Parameters Patients on parenteral nutrition or chronic therapy should have periodic serum copper and serum zinc levels; alkaline phosphatase, taste acuity, mental depression, wound healing (if indicated), growth (if indicated), skin integrity; Wilson's disease: 24-hour urinary copper excretion, neuropsychiatric evaluations, LFTs, periodic ophthalmic exam

Reference Range
Serum: 70-130 mcg/dL

Urinary copper excretion (24 hour collection) for Wilson's disease patient **not** on chelation therapy: <75 mcg/24 hours (patients on chelation therapy will have increased urinary copper due to chelated copper)

Urinary zinc excretion (24 hour collection) to check for compliance should be ~2 mg/24 hour

Patient Information Do not exceed recommended dose

Dosage Forms Excipient information presented when available (limited, particularly for generics); consult specific product labeling.

Zinc acetate:
Capsule (Galzin™): 25 mg elemental zinc, 50 mg elemental zinc

Zinc chloride:
Injection, solution: 1 mg elemental zinc/mL (10 mL, 50 mL)

Zinc, elemental:
Lozenges: 10 mg, 23 mg
Cold-Eeze®: 13.3 mg [bubble gum, citrus, cherry, menthol, and tropical fruit flavors]
Tablet: 30 mg, 60 mg

Zinc gluconate (14.3% zinc):
Tablet: 50 mg [elemental zinc 7 mg]; 100 mg [elemental zinc 14 mg]

Zinc sulfate (23% zinc):
Capsule (Orazinc®, Zincate®): 220 mg [elemental zinc 50 mg]
Injection, solution [preservative free]: 1 mg elemental zinc/mL (10 mL); 5 mg elemental zinc/mL (5 mL)
Tablet (Orazinc®): 110 mg [elemental zinc 25 mg]

References
Anderson LA, Hakojarvi SL, and Boudreaux SK, "Zinc Acetate Treatment in Wilson's Disease," *Ann Pharmacother*, 1998, 32:78-87.
Roberts EA, Schilsky ML, and American Association for Study of Liver Diseases (AASLD), "Diagnosis and Treatment of Wilson Disease: An Update," *Hepatology*, 2008, 47(6):2089-111.

◆ **Zinc Undecylenate** *see* Undecylenic Acid and Derivatives *on page 1392*

◆ **Zinecard®** *see* Dexrazoxane *on page 413*

◆ **Zipsor™** *see* Diclofenac *on page 429*

◆ **Zirgan™** *see* Ganciclovir *on page 636*

◆ **Zithromax®** *see* Azithromycin *on page 164*

◆ **Zithromax TRI-PAK™** *see* Azithromycin *on page 164*

◆ **Zithromax Z-PAK®** *see* Azithromycin *on page 164*

◆ **Zmax®** *see* Azithromycin *on page 164*

◆ **Zocor®** *see* Simvastatin *on page 1263*

◆ **Zoderm®** *see* Benzoyl Peroxide *on page 184*

◆ **Zoderm® Hydrating Wash™** *see* Benzoyl Peroxide *on page 184*

◆ **Zoderm® Redi-Pads™** *see* Benzoyl Peroxide *on page 184*

◆ **Zofran®** *see* Ondansetron *on page 1022*

◆ **Zofran® ODT** *see* Ondansetron *on page 1022*

◆ **Zoloft®** *see* Sertraline *on page 1254*

Zolpidem (zole PI dem)

Medication Safety Issues
Sound-alike/look-alike issues:
Ambien® may be confused with Abilify®, Ativan®, Ambi 10®
Zolpidem may be confused with lorazepam, zaleplon

International issues:
Ambien® may be confused with Ambyen which is a brand name for amiodarone in Great Britain

U.S. Brand Names Ambien CR®; Ambien®; Edluar™; Zolpimist®

Therapeutic Category Hypnotic, Nonbenzodiazepine

Generic Available Yes: Excludes extended release tablet, sublingual tablet

Use
Ambien®, Edluar™: Short-term treatment of insomnia (with difficulty of sleep onset) (FDA approved in adults)

Ambien CR®: Treatment of insomnia (with difficulty of sleep onset and/or sleep maintenance) (FDA approved in adults)

Restrictions C-IV

Medication Guide An FDA-approved patient medication guide, which is available with the product information and at the following website locations, must be dispensed with this medication for each new outpatient prescription and refill:
Ambien®: http://www.fda.gov/downloads/Drugs/DrugSafety/ucm085906.pdf
Ambien CR®: http://www.fda.gov/downloads/Drugs/DrugSafety/ucm085908.pdf
Edluar™: http://www.fda.gov/downloads/Drugs/DrugSafety/UCM135937.pdf
Zolpidem: http://www.fda.gov/downloads/Drugs/DrugSafety/ucm089833.pdf
Zolpimist®: http://www.fda.gov/downloads/Drugs/DrugSafety/UCM143465.pdf

Pregnancy Risk Factor C

Pregnancy Considerations Teratogenic effects were not observed in animal studies. Children born of mothers taking sedative/hypnotics may be at risk for withdrawal; neonatal flaccidity has been reported in infants following maternal use of sedative/hypnotics during pregnancy. Use during pregnancy only if the benefits justify the risk to the fetus.

Lactation Enters breast milk/use caution (AAP rates "compatible")

Breast-Feeding Considerations 0.004% to 0.019% of the maternal dose is found in breast milk.

Contraindications Hypersensitivity to zolpidem tartrate or any component

Warnings Evaluate patient carefully for medical or psychiatric causes of insomnia prior to initiation of drug treatment; failure of zolpidem to treat insomnia (after 7-10 days of therapy), a worsening of insomnia, or the emergence of behavioral changes or thinking abnormalities may indicate a medical or psychiatric illness requiring evaluation; these effects also have been reported with zolpidem use. Abnormal thinking and behavior changes may occur with sedative/hypnotic use, including decreased inhibition (eg, aggressiveness, extroversion that seems out of character; visual and auditory hallucinations, agitation, bizarre behavior, and depersonalization have been reported with zolpidem use; hallucinations have been reported more frequently in children and adolescents receiving zolpidem for insomnia associated with ADHD than in adults (7.4% vs ≤1%). Abrupt discontinuation after prolonged use may result in withdrawal symptoms and signs.

Hypersensitivity reactions, including anaphylaxis and angioedema, may occur; angioedema may involve the tongue, glottis, or larynx; occurrence of dyspnea, throat closing, or nausea and vomiting suggest anaphylaxis; angioedema of the throat, glottis, or larynx may result in potentially fatal airway obstruction; do not rechallenge patients who develop angioedema after receiving zolpidem. Hazardous sleep-related activities, such as sleep-driving (driving while not fully awake without any recollection of driving), preparing and eating food, and making phone calls while asleep have also been reported; increased risk of these type of events has been reported with greater than recommended zolpidem dosages as well as concomitant ethanol or CNS depressant use; amnesia may also occur; discontinue treatment in patients who report a sleep-driving episode. Effects of other sedative drugs or ethanol may be potentiated.

Precautions Use with caution in patients with sleep apnea, COPD, or respiratory compromise; myasthenia gravis; and concomitant illnesses which may affect zolpidem metabolism or hemodynamic response. Use with caution and decrease the dose in patients with hepatic impairment and in debilitated patients. Use with caution in patients with renal impairment or with a history of drug dependence.

May cause CNS depression impairing physical and mental capabilities; patients should be cautioned about performing tasks which require mental alertness (eg, operating machinery or driving). Zolpidem should only be administered immediately prior to bedtime or after the patient has gone to bed but is having difficulty falling asleep and when the patient is able to stay in bed a full night (7-8 hours) before being active again.

Adverse Reactions Note: Frequency may be dosage form, dose, and/or age dependent (pediatric adverse reaction incidence data from Blumer, 2009).
Cardiovascular: Chest pain, palpitation
Central nervous system: Abnormal dreams, abnormal thinking and behavior changes (see Warnings), affect liability (children: 3%), amnesia, anxiety (children: 2.2%), ataxia; confusion, depression, dizziness (children: 23.5%; adults: 1%), drowsiness, drugged feeling, euphoria, hallucinations (children: 7.4%; adults: <1%), headache (children: 12.5%; adults: <1%), insomnia, lethargy, lightheadedness, sleep disorders, somnolence, vertigo
Dermatologic: Excoriation, rash
Gastrointestinal: Abdominal pain, constipation, diarrhea, dyspepsia, gastroenteritis (children: 3%), hiccup, nausea, paresthesia of the tongue (sublingual tablets, transient effect), sublingual erythema (sublingual tablets, transient effect), vomiting, xerostomia
Genitourinary: Enuresis (children: 3%), urinary tract infection
Neuromuscular & skeletal: Arthralgia, back pain, falling, myalgia, weakness
Ocular: Diplopia, vision abnormal
Respiratory: Pharyngitis, sinusitis, throat irritation, upper respiratory tract infection
Miscellaneous: Allergy, anaphylaxis, angioedema, hazardous sleep-related activities (eg, sleep-driving) (see Warnings), flu-like syndrome, hypersensitivity reactions, physical and psychological dependence
<1% and/or postmarketing reports: Agitation, anorexia, arthritis, bronchitis, cerebrovascular disorder, cognition decreased, concentrating difficulty, cough, cystitis, diaphoresis, dysarthria, dysphagia, dyspnea, edema, eye irritation, falling, hepatic function abnormalities, hyperglycemia, hyper-/hypotension, illusion, leg cramps, menstrual disorder, nervousness, pallor, postural hypotension, rhinitis, scleritis, somnambulism, speech disorder, stupor, syncope, tachycardia, taste perversion, thirst, urinary incontinence, vaginitis

◄ **Drug Interactions**

Metabolism/Transport Effects Substrate of CYP1A2 (minor), 2C9 (minor), 2C19 (minor), 2D6 (minor), 3A4 (major)

Avoid Concomitant Use There are no known interactions where it is recommended to avoid concomitant use.

Increased Effect/Toxicity

Zolpidem may increase the levels/effects of: Alcohol (Ethyl); CNS Depressants; Methotrimeprazine

The levels/effects of Zolpidem may be increased by: Antifungal Agents (Azole Derivatives, Systemic); CYP3A4 Inhibitors (Moderate); CYP3A4 Inhibitors (Strong); Dasatinib; Methotrimeprazine

Decreased Effect

The levels/effects of Zolpidem may be decreased by: CYP3A4 Inducers (Strong); Deferasirox; Flumazenil; Herbs (CYP3A4 Inducers); Peginterferon Alfa-2b; Rifamycin Derivatives

Food Interactions Food decreases maximum plasma concentration and bioavailability of immediate release, extended release, and sublingual tablets; time to peak plasma concentration is prolonged; half-life remains unchanged. Grapefruit juice may decrease the metabolism of zolpidem.

Stability

Ambien®; Edluar™: Store at controlled room temperature of 20°C to 25°C (68°F to 77°F). Protect sublingual tablets from light and moisture.

Ambien CR®: Store at controlled room temperature of 15°C to 25°C (59°F to 77°F); limited excursions up to 30°C (86°F) are permissible.

Mechanism of Action Zolpidem, an imidazopyridine hypnotic that is structurally dissimilar to benzodiazepines, enhances the activity of the inhibitory neurotransmitter, γ-aminobutyric acid (GABA), via selective agonism at the benzodiazepine-1 (BZ_1) receptor; because of its selectivity for the BZ_1 receptor site over the BZ_2 receptor site, zolpidem exhibits minimal anxiolytic, myorelaxant, and anticonvulsant properties (effects largely attributed to agonism at the BZ_2 receptor site).

Pharmacodynamics

Onset of action: 30 minutes

Duration: 6-8 hours

Pharmacokinetics (Adult data unless noted) Note: Pediatric pharmacokinetic data from Blumer, 2008

Absorption:

Immediate release and sublingual: Rapid

Extended release: Biphasic absorption; rapid initial absorption (similar to immediate release product); then provides extended concentrations in the plasma beyond 3 hours postadministration

Distribution: Distributes into breast milk

V_d, apparent:

Children 2-6 years: 1.8 ± 0.8 L/kg

Children >6-12 years: 2.2 ± 1.7 L/kg

Adolescents: 1.2 ± 0.4 L/kg

Adults: 0.54 L/kg

Protein binding: ~93%

Metabolism: Hepatic methylation and hydroxylation via CYP3A4 (~60%), CYP2C9 (~22%), CYP1A2 (~14%), CYP2D6 (~3%), and CYP2C19 (~3%) to three inactive metabolites

Bioavailability: 70%

Half-life elimination:

Children 2-6 years: Mean: 1.8 hours

Children >6 years and Adolescents: Mean: 2.3 hours

Adults: Mean: ~2.5 hours (range: 1.4-4.5 hours); Cirrhosis: 9.9 hours (range: 4.1-25.8 hours)

Time to peak serum concentration:

Children 2-6 years: 0.9 hours

Children >6-12 years: 1.1 hours

Adolescents: 1.3 hours

Adults: Immediate release: 1.6 hours; 2.2 hours with food; sublingual: 1.4 hours; 1.75 hours with food

Elimination: Urine (48% to 67%, primarily as metabolites); feces (29% to 42%, primarily as metabolites)

Clearance, apparent:

Children 2-6 years: 11.7 ± 7.9 mL/minute/kg

Children >6-12 years: 9.7 ± 10.3 mL/minute/kg

Adolescents: 4.8 ± 2 mL/minute/kg

Dialysis: Not hemodialyzable

Usual Dosage Oral:

Children and Adolescents: **Note:** Limited information available; efficacy has **not** been demonstrated in randomized placebo-controlled trials. An open-label, dose escalation pharmacokinetic evaluation showed zolpidem was well-tolerated in pediatric patients 2-18 years of age and recommended a dose of 0.25 mg/kg at bedtime for evaluation in future efficacy trials (see Blumer, 2008). A single case report describes an 18-month-old infant who was effectively treated with zolpidem for primary insomnia (see Bhat, 2008). However, zolpidem has **not** been shown to be effective in a randomized placebo-controlled trial (n=201) of children aged 6-17 years with ADHD-associated insomnia; zolpidem 0.25 mg/kg/dose (maximum dose: 10 mg) administered nightly did **not** decrease sleep latency; in addition, hallucinations occurred in 7.4% of patients (see Blumer, 2009 and Warnings). A comparative, randomized controlled trial of zolpidem and haloperidol in pediatric burn patients (n=40, mean age: 9.4 ± 0.7 years) showed zolpidem dosed at 0.5 mg/kg nightly for one week (maximum dose: 20 mg) minimally increased Stage 3/4 sleep and REM but not total sleep time; the authors no longer use zolpidem to try to improve sleep in their pediatric burn patients (see Armour, 2008).

Adults:

Immediate release and Sublingual: 10 mg once daily immediately before bedtime; maximum dose: 10 mg/day

Extended release: 12.5 mg once daily immediately before bedtime; maximum dose: 12.5 mg/day

Debilitated adults:

Immediate release and Sublingual: 5 mg once daily immediately before bedtime

Extended release: 6.25 mg once daily immediately before bedtime

Dosing adjustment in hepatic impairment: Adults:

Immediate release and Sublingual: 5 mg once daily immediately before bedtime

Extended release: 6.25 mg once daily immediately before bedtime

Administration

All formulations: Administer immediately before bedtime due to rapid onset of action. For faster sleep onset, do not administer with (or immediately after) a meal.

Extended release tablets: Swallow whole; do not divide, crush, or chew.

Sublingual tablets: Examine blisterpack before use; do not use if blisters are broken, torn, or missing. Separate individual blisters at perforation; peel off top layer of paper; push tablet through foil. Place sublingual tablet under the tongue and allowed to disintegrate; do not swallow or administer with water.

Monitoring Parameters Daytime alertness; respiratory rate; behavior profile

Patient Information Read the patient Medication Guide that you receive with each prescription and refill of zolpidem. Avoid alcohol, other CNS depressants, and grapefruit juice. May be habit-forming; avoid abrupt discontinuation after prolonged use. May cause dizziness or drowsiness and impair ability to perform activities requiring mental alertness or physical coordination. Take dose immediately before bedtime. May also cause daytime drowsiness. May cause dry mouth. May cause hypersensitivity reactions. May cause hazardous sleep-related activities (ie, driving, preparing and eating foods, and making phone calls while not fully awake).

Product Availability Zolpimist® oral spray: FDA approved December, 2008; availability currently undetermined

Zolpimist® is an oral spray of zolpidem indicated for the short-term treatment of insomnia characterized by difficulties with sleep initiation.

Dosage Forms Excipient information presented when available (limited, particularly for generics); consult specific product labeling.

Tablet, oral, as tartrate: 5 mg, 10 mg
  Ambien®: 5 mg, 10 mg
Tablet, extended release, oral, as tartrate:
  Ambien CR®: 6.25 mg, 12.5 mg
Tablet, sublingual, as tartrate:
  Edluar™: 5 mg, 10 mg

References
Armour A, Gottschlich MM, Khoury J, et al, "A Randomized, Controlled Prospective Trial of Zolpidem and Haloperidol for Use as Sleeping Agents in Pediatric Burn Patients," *J Burn Care Res*, 2008, 29 (1):238-47.

Bhat T, Pallikaleth SJ, and Shah N, "Primary Insomnia Treated With Zolpidem in an 18-Month Old Child," *Indian J Psychiatry*, 2008,50 (1):59-60.

Blumer JL, Findling RL, Shih WJ, et al, "Controlled Clinical Trial of Zolpidem for the Treatment of Insomnia Associated With Attention-Deficit/Hyperactivity Disorder in Children 6 to 17 Years of Age," *Pediatrics*, 2009, 123(5):e770-6.

Blumer JL, Reed MD, Steinberg F, et al, "Potential Pharmacokinetic Basis for Zolpidem Dosing in Children With Sleep Difficulties," *Clin Pharmacol Ther*, 2008, 83(4):551-8.

◆ **Zolpidem Tartrate** *see* Zolpidem *on page 1447*
◆ **Zolpimist®** *see* Zolpidem *on page 1447*
◆ **Zonalon®** *see* Doxepin *on page 475*
◆ **Zonegran®** *see* Zonisamide *on page 1449*

Zonisamide (zoe NIS a mide)

Medication Safety Issues
Sound-alike/look-alike issues:
Zonegran® may be confused with Sinequan®
Zonisamide may be confused with lacosamide

Related Information
Antiepileptic Drugs *on page 1693*

U.S. Brand Names Zonegran®

Therapeutic Category Anticonvulsant, Miscellaneous

Generic Available Yes

Use Adjunctive treatment of partial seizures (FDA approved in ages >16 years and adults); has been used investigationally for the treatment of generalized epilepsies including, generalized tonic-clonic seizures, absence seizures, infantile spasms, myoclonic epilepsies, and Lennox-Gastaut syndrome (see Leppik, 1999 and Oommen, 1999)

Medication Guide An FDA-approved patient medication guide, which is available with the product information and at http://www.fda.gov/downloads/Drugs/DrugSafety/UCM152828.pdf, must be dispensed with this medication for each new outpatient prescription and refill.

Pregnancy Risk Factor C

Pregnancy Considerations Teratogenic effects were observed in animal reproduction studies, therefore zonisamide is classified as pregnancy category C. Zonisamide crosses the placenta and can be detected in the newborn following delivery. Although adverse fetal events have been reported, the risk of teratogenic effects following maternal use of zonisamide in not clearly defined. Other agents may be preferred until additional data is available. Newborns should be monitored for transient metabolic acidosis after birth. Zonisamide clearance may increase in the second trimester of pregnancy, requiring dosage adjustment. Women of childbearing potential are advised to use effective contraception during therapy.

Patients exposed to zonisamide during pregnancy are encouraged to enroll themselves into the AED Pregnancy Registry by calling 1-888-233-2334. Additional information is available at www.aedpregnancyregistry.org.

Lactation Enters breast milk/not recommended

Breast-Feeding Considerations Zonisamide is excreted into breast milk in concentrations similar to those in the maternal plasma, and has been detected in the plasma of a nursing infant. According to the manufacturer, the decision to continue or discontinue breast-feeding during therapy should take into account the risk of exposure to the infant and the benefits of treatment to the mother.

Contraindications Hypersensitivity to zonisamide, sulfonamides, or any component

Warnings Zonisamide is a sulfonamide; although rare, severe, and life-threatening sulfonamide reactions may occur (eg, Stevens-Johnson syndrome, toxic epidermal necrolysis, aplastic anemia, agranulocytosis, other blood dyscrasias, and fulminant hepatic necrosis); discontinue zonisamide in patients with signs of hypersensitivity reaction or other serious reactions; consider discontinuation of zonisamide in any patient who develops a rash or monitor very closely; deaths due to serious rashes have been reported; rashes usually appear within 2-16 weeks of starting therapy.

Use may be associated with the development of metabolic acidosis (generally dose-dependent) in certain patients; predisposing conditions or therapies include renal disease, severe respiratory disease, diarrhea, surgery, ketogenic diet, and other medications (such as acetazolamide). Pediatric patients may also be at an increased risk and may have more severe metabolic acidosis. Serum bicarbonate should be monitored prior to initiation and during therapy; if metabolic acidosis occurs, consider decreasing the dose or discontinuing use with appropriate dose tapering. If use continues despite acidosis, alkali treatment should be considered. The FDA is working with the manufacturers to revise the product labeling concerning these risks.

Oligohydrosis (decreased sweating) and hyperthermia have been reported in 40 pediatric patients; many cases occurred after exposure to elevated environmental temperatures; some cases resulted in heat stroke requiring hospitalization; pediatric patients may be at an increased risk; monitor patients, especially pediatric patients, for decreased sweating and hyperthermia, especially in warm or hot weather; use zonisamide with caution in patients receiving drugs that predispose to heat-related disorders (eg, anticholinergic agents, carbonic anhydrase inhibitors); safety and efficacy in pediatric patients <16 years of age has not been established.

Do not abruptly discontinue therapy; abrupt withdrawal may precipitate seizures; withdraw gradually to lessen chance for increased seizure frequency (unless a more rapid withdrawal is required due to safety concerns). CNS adverse effects may occur including fatigue or somnolence, psychiatric symptoms (eg, depression, psychosis), and cognitive symptoms [difficulty concentrating, speech or language problems (especially word-finding difficulties), and psychomotor slowing]; fatigue and somnolence usually occur within the first month of starting therapy, most commonly at higher doses (eg, in adults at doses of 300-500 mg/day).

Antiepileptic drugs (AEDs) increase the risk of suicidal behavior and ideation in patients receiving these ▶

medications for any indication. Pooled analyses of placebo-controlled trials involving 11 different AEDs (regardless of indication) showed a twofold increased risk of suicidal thoughts or behavior (estimated incidence rate: 0.43% in AED treated patients compared to 0.24% of patients receiving placebo); increased risk was observed as early as 1 week after initiation of AED and continued through duration of trials (most trials ≤24 weeks); risk did not vary significantly by age (age range: 5–100 years). Consider risks and benefits of AEDs before prescribing. Monitor all patients receiving an AED for emergence of suicidal thoughts or behavior, thoughts of self-harm, any unusual changes in behavior or mood, or the emergence or worsening of depressive symptoms; notify heathcare provider immediately if symptoms or concerning behavior occur. **Note:** The FDA is requiring that a Medication Guide be developed for all antiepileptic drugs informing patients of this risk.

Precautions Use with caution in patients with renal or hepatic dysfunction; do not use in patients with Cl$_{cr}$ <50 mL/minute; zonisamide may cause kidney stones (ensure patients have adequate fluid intake); zonisamide may decrease GFR and increase serum creatinine and BUN; discontinue therapy in patients who develop acute renal failure or a persistent significant increase in serum creatinine or BUN

Adverse Reactions

Central nervous system: Somnolence, fatigue, dizziness, headache, agitation, irritability, tiredness, ataxia, confusion, memory impairment, depression, psychosis, difficulty concentrating, speech or language problems (especially word-finding difficulties), psychomotor slowing, insomnia, mental slowing, anxiety, nervousness, tremor, convulsion, hyperesthesia, incoordination; behavior disorders in children have been reported (Kimura, 1994); suicidal thinking and behavior (see Warnings)

Dermatologic: Rash, bruising, pruritus, Stevens-Johnson syndrome (rare), toxic epidermal necrolysis (rare)

Endocrine & metabolic: Weight loss; metabolic acidosis (see Warnings)

Gastrointestinal: Anorexia, nausea, diarrhea, abdominal pain, dyspepsia, constipation, xerostomia, taste perversion, vomiting

Hematologic: Aplastic anemia (rare), agranulocytosis (rare), other blood dyscrasias (rare)

Hepatic: Alkaline phosphatase elevated; LDH and transaminases elevated (rare)

Neuromuscular & skeletal: Paresthesia, abnormal gait

Ocular: Diplopia, nystagmus, amblyopia

Otic: Tinnitus

Renal: BUN and serum creatinine elevated

Respiratory: Rhinitis, pharyngitis, cough increased

Miscellaneous: Flu-like syndrome; oligohydrosis and hyperthermia [pediatric patients may be at increased risk (see Warnings)]

Drug Interactions

Metabolism/Transport Effects Substrate of CYP2C19 (minor), 3A4 (major)

Avoid Concomitant Use There are no known interactions where it is recommended to avoid concomitant use.

Increased Effect/Toxicity

Zonisamide may increase the levels/effects of: Alcohol (Ethyl); CNS Depressants; Methotrimeprazine

The levels/effects of Zonisamide may be increased by: CYP3A4 Inhibitors (Moderate); CYP3A4 Inhibitors (Strong); Dasatinib; Methotrimeprazine

Decreased Effect

The levels/effects of Zonisamide may be decreased by: CYP3A4 Inducers (Strong); Deferasirox; Herbs (CYP3A4 Inducers); Ketorolac; Ketorolac (Systemic); Mefloquine; PHENobarbital; Phenytoin

Food Interactions Food decreases the rate, but not the extent of absorption.

Stability Store at controlled room temperature 25°C (77°C). Protect from moisture and light.

Mechanism of Action Exact mechanism of action is not known; may stabilize neuronal membranes and suppress neuronal hypersynchronization by blocking sodium channels and T-type calcium currents; does not affect GABA activity; possesses weak carbonic anhydrase inhibiting activity, but this in not thought to be a very significant component of its antiepileptic action

Pharmacokinetics (Adult data unless noted)

Absorption: Oral: Rapid and complete

Distribution: V$_d$ (apparent): Adults: 1.45 L/kg; highly concentrated in erythrocytes; distributes into breast milk at a transfer rate of 41% to 57% (see Kawada, 2002)

Protein binding: 40%

Metabolism: Hepatic; undergoes acetylation to form N-acetyl zonisamide and reduction via cytochrome P450 isoenzyme CYP3A4 to 2-sulfamoylacetylphenol (SMAP); SMAP then undergoes conjugation with glucuronide

Half-life: Adults: 63 hours (range: 50-68 hours)

Time to peak serum concentration: 2-6 hours

Elimination: Urine: 62% (35% as unchanged drug, 15% as N-acetyl zonisamide, 50% as SMAP glucuronide); feces (3%); **Note:** Of the dose recovered in Japanese patients, 28% is as unchanged drug, 52% is as N-acetyl zonisamide, and 19% is as SMAP glucuronide (Glauser, 2002)

Usual Dosage Oral:

Infants and Children: In a review article of 20 Japanese pediatric studies, the following doses were recommended (see Glauser, 2002): Initial: 1-2 mg/kg/day given in two divided doses/day; increase dose in increments of 0.5-1 mg/kg/day every 2 weeks; usual dose: 5-8 mg/kg/day.

Higher initial and maximum doses have been recommended by others (see Leppik, 1999 and Oommen, 1999): Initial: 2-4 mg/kg/day given in two divided doses/day; titrate dose upwards if needed every 2 weeks; usual dose: 4-8 mg/kg/day; maximum dose: 12 mg/kg/day

Infantile spasms: Several studies used a faster titration of zonisamide to control infantile spasms. Suzuki treated 11 newly diagnosed infants (mean age: ~6 months) with zonisamide monotherapy starting at doses of 3-5 mg/kg/day given in 2 divided doses/day; doses were increased every 4th day until seizures were controlled or a maximum dose of 10 mg/kg/day was attained; 4 of 11 patients responded at doses of 4-5 mg/kg/day (see Suzuki, 1997). Yanai treated 27 newly diagnosed infantile spasm patients with zonisamide add-on or monotherapy starting at doses of 2-4 mg/kg/day given in 2 divided doses/day; doses were increased by 2-5 mg/kg every 2-4 days until seizures were controlled or a maximum of 10-20 mg/kg/day was attained; 9 of 27 patients responded at a mean effective dose of 7.8 mg/kg/day (range: 5-12.5 mg/kg/day); non-responders received doses of 8-20 mg/kg/day (mean: 10.8 mg/kg/day) (see Yania, 1999). Suzuki treated 54 newly diagnosed infants (11 of which were previously reported) with zonisamide monotherapy starting at doses of 3-4 mg/kg/day given in 2 divided doses; doses were increased every 4th day until seizures were controlled or a maximum dose of 10-13 mg/kg/day was attained; 11 of 54 infants responded at a mean effective dose of 7.2 mg/kg/day (range: 4-12 mg/kg/day); the majority of infants who responded did so at a dose of 4-8 mg/kg/day and within 1-2 weeks of starting therapy (see Suzuki, 2001). Further studies are needed.

Adolescents >16 years and Adults: Initial: 100 mg once daily; dose may be increased to 200 mg/day after 2 weeks; further increases in dose should be made in increments of 100 mg/day and only after a minimum of 2 weeks between adjustments; usual effective dose: 100-600 mg/day. **Note:** There is no evidence of increased benefit with doses >400 mg/day. Steady-state serum concentrations fluctuate 27% with once daily dosing, and 14% with twice daily dosing; patients may benefit from divided doses given twice daily (Leppik, 1999)

Dosage adjustment in renal/hepatic impairment: Slower dosage titration and more frequent monitoring are recommended in patients with renal or hepatic disease. Do not use if Cl_{cr} <50 mL/minute.

Administration May be administered without regard to meals; swallow capsule whole; do not crush, chew, or break capsule

Monitoring Parameters Seizure frequency, duration, and severity; symptoms of CNS adverse effects; skin rash; BUN and serum creatinine; serum bicarbonate prior to initiation and periodically during therapy; symptoms of metabolic acidosis (see Warnings); monitor patients, especially pediatric patients, for decreased sweating and hyperthermia, especially in warm or hot weather; signs and symptoms of suicidality (eg, anxiety, depression, behavior changes) (see Warnings)

Reference Range Monitoring of plasma concentrations may be useful; proposed therapeutic range: 10-20 mcg/mL; patients may benefit from higher concentrations (ie, up to 30 mcg/mL), but concentrations >30 mcg/mL have been associated with adverse effects (see Oommen, 1999 and Leppik, 1999)

Patient Information Read the patient Medication Guide that you receive with each prescription and refill of zonisamide. Antiepileptic agents may increase the risk of suicidal thoughts and behavior; notify physician if you feel more depressed or have thoughts of suicide or self harm (see Warnings). Inform prescriber if allergic to sulfa drugs (eg, Bactrim®, Septra®). Do not abruptly discontinue therapy (an increase in seizure activity may result). May cause drowsiness and impair ability to perform activities that require mental alertness or physical coordination. Report excessive drowsiness, unusual thoughts, depression, problems with concentrating or speaking, or any skin rashes to physician immediately. Avoid alcohol. Notify physician immediately if a child taking zonisamide is not sweating as usual or has elevated temperature. Drink adequate amount of fluids and report any symptoms of kidney stones (eg, back pain, stomach pain, pain on urination, bloody urine). Report any unusual symptoms, such as a bruises, sore throat, fever, or mouth ulcers to physician. Report worsening of seizure activity or loss of seizure control.

Dosage Forms Excipient information presented when available (limited, particularly for generics); consult specific product labeling.

Capsule: 25 mg, 50 mg, 100 mg

Zonegran®: 25 mg, 100 mg

References

Glauser TA and Pellock JM, "Zonisamide in Pediatric Epilepsy: Review of the Japanese Experience," *J Child Neurol*, 2002, 17(2):87-96.

Kawada K, Itoh S, Kusaka T, et al, "Pharmacokinetics of Zonisamide in Perinatal Period," *Brain Dev*, 2002, 24(2):95-7.

Kimura S, "Zonisamide-Induced Behavior Disorder in Two Children," *Epilepsia*, 1994, 35(2):403-5.

Leppik IE, "Zonisamide," *Epilepsia*, 1999, 40(Suppl 5):S23-9.

Oommen KJ and Mathews S, "Zonisamide: A New Antiepileptic Drug," *Clin Neuropharmacol*, 1999, 22(4):192-200.

Suzuki Y, Nagai T, Ono J, et al, "Zonisamide Monotherapy in Newly Diagnosed Infantile Spasms," *Epilepsia*, 1997, 38(9):1035-8.

Suzuki Y, "Zonisamide in West Syndrome," *Brain Dev*, 2001, 23 (7):658-61.

Yanai S, Hanai T, and Narazaki O, "Treatment of Infantile Spasms With Zonisamide," *Brain Dev*, 1999, 21(3):157-61.

◆ **Zorbtive®** see Somatropin *on page 1281*

◆ **ZORprin®** see Aspirin *on page 141*

◆ **Zostrix® [OTC]** see Capsaicin *on page 241*

◆ **Zostrix® (Can)** see Capsaicin *on page 241*

◆ **Zostrix®-HP [OTC]** see Capsaicin *on page 241*

◆ **Zostrix® H.P. (Can)** see Capsaicin *on page 241*

◆ **Zostrix® Neuropathy [OTC]** see Capsaicin *on page 241*

◆ **Zosyn®** see Piperacillin and Tazobactam *on page 1116*

◆ **Zovirax®** see Acyclovir *on page 46*

◆ **Z-Pak** see Azithromycin *on page 164*

◆ **Zyban®** see BuPROPion *on page 217*

◆ **Zydone®** see Hydrocodone and Acetaminophen *on page 684*

◆ **Zyloprim®** see Allopurinol *on page 66*

◆ **ZYM-Amiodarone (Can)** see Amiodarone *on page 84*

◆ **ZYM-Carvedilol (Can)** see Carvedilol *on page 254*

◆ **ZYM-Cholestyramine-Light (Can)** see Cholestyramine Resin *on page 302*

◆ **ZYM-Cholestyramine-Regular (Can)** see Cholestyramine Resin *on page 302*

◆ **ZYM-Clonazepam (Can)** see ClonazePAM *on page 337*

◆ **ZYM-Fluconazole (Can)** see Fluconazole *on page 584*

◆ **ZYM-Fluoxetine (Can)** see FLUoxetine *on page 600*

◆ **ZYM-Lisinopril (Can)** see Lisinopril *on page 832*

◆ **ZYM-Ondansetron (Can)** see Ondansetron *on page 1022*

◆ **ZYM-Pantoprazole (Can)** see Pantoprazole *on page 1054*

◆ **ZYM-Paroxetine (Can)** see PARoxetine *on page 1064*

◆ **ZYM-Pravastatin (Can)** see Pravastatin *on page 1145*

◆ **ZYM-Ranitidine (Can)** see Ranitidine *on page 1200*

◆ **ZYM-Risperidone (Can)** see Risperidone *on page 1218*

◆ **ZYM-Simvastatin (Can)** see Simvastatin *on page 1263*

◆ **ZYM-Sotalol (Can)** see Sotalol *on page 1284*

◆ **ZYM-Topiramate (Can)** see Topiramate *on page 1360*

◆ **ZYM-Trazodone (Can)** see TraZODone *on page 1371*

◆ **Zyrtec® Allergy [OTC]** see Cetirizine *on page 283*

◆ **Zyrtec® Children's Allergy [OTC]** see Cetirizine *on page 283*

◆ **Zyrtec® Children's Hives Relief [OTC]** see Cetirizine *on page 283*

◆ **Zyrtec® Itchy Eye [OTC]** see Ketotifen *on page 785*

◆ **Zytopic™ [DSC]** see Triamcinolone *on page 1376*

◆ **Zytram® XL (Can)** see TraMADol *on page 1367*

◆ **Zyvox®** see Linezolid *on page 826*

◆ **Zyvoxam® (Can)** see Linezolid *on page 826*

APPENDIX TABLE OF CONTENTS

CPR PEDIATRIC DRUG DOSAGES

Medications for Neonatal Resuscitation

Medication	Dose	Remarks
Epinephrine	I.V.: 0.01-0.03 mg/kg (0.1-0.3 mL/kg, 1:10,000)	I.V. is preferred neonatal route. While obtaining I.V. access, may consider higher doses via E.T.: Up to 0.1 mg/kg (1 mL/kg, 1:10,000), but safety and efficacy of this practice has not been evaluated.
Naloxone	I.V./I.M.: 0.1 mg/kg	E.T. route is not recommended (lack of clinical data in neonates). Avoid use in newborns whose mothers are suspected of long-term exposure to opioids. Monitor neonates closely for recurrent apnea or hypoventilation; additional doses of naloxone may be needed.

Adapted from American Heart Association Emergency Cardiovascular Care Committee, "2005 American Heart Association (AHA) Guidelines for Cardiopulmonary Resuscitation (CPR) and Emergency Cardiovascular Care (ECC), Part 13: Neonatal Resuscitation Guidelines," *Circulation*, 2005, 112(24 Suppl):IV-192.

PALS Medications for Pediatric Resuscitation and Arrhythmias

Medication	Dose	Remarks
Adenosine	0.1 mg/kg Maximum dose: 6 mg Repeat: 0.2 mg/kg Maximum dose: 12 mg	Monitor ECG Rapid I.V./I.O. bolus
Amiodarone	I.V./I.O.: 5 mg/kg (maximum 300 mg/dose) May repeat up to maximum total daily dose of 15 mg/kg (2.2 g/day in adolescents)	Monitor ECG and blood pressure Adjust administration rate to urgency (give more slowly when perfusing rhythm present) Use caution when administering with other drugs that prolong QT (consider expert consultation)
Atropine	I.V./I.O.: 0.02 mg/kg E.T.[1]: 0.03 mg/kg Repeat once if needed Minimum dose: 0.1 mg Maximum single dose: Child: 0.5 mg Adolescent: 1 mg	Higher doses may be used with organophosphate poisoning
Calcium chloride (10%)	I.V./I.O.: 20 mg/kg (0.2 mL/kg)	Slowly Adult dose: 5-10 mL
Epinephrine	I.V./I.O.: 0.01 mg/kg (0.1 mL/kg, 1:10,000) Maximum dose: 1 mg E.T.[1]: 0.1 mg/kg (0.1 mL/kg, 1:1000) Maximum dose: 10 mg	May repeat every 3-5 minutes
Glucose	I.V./I.O.: 0.5-1 g/kg	$D_{10}W$: 5-10 mL/kg $D_{25}W$: 2-4 mL/kg $D_{50}W$: 1-2 mL/kg
Lidocaine	Bolus I.V./ I.O: 1 mg/kg Maximum dose: 100 mg Infusion: 20-50 mcg/kg/min E.T.[1]: 2-3 mg/kg	
Magnesium sulfate	I.V./I.O.: 25-50 mg/kg over 10-20 minutes; faster in torsade de pointes Maximum dose: 2 g	
Naloxone	<5 y or ≤20 kg: I.V./I.O./E.T.[1]: 0.1 mg/kg ≥5 y or > 20 kg: I.V./I.O./E.T.[1]: 2 mg	Use lower doses to reverse respiratory depression associated with therapeutic opioid use (1-15 mcg/kg)
Procainamide	I.V./I.O.: 15 mg/kg over 30-60 minutes Adult dose: I.V. infusion: 20 mg/min up to total maximum dose: 17 mg/kg	Monitor ECG and blood pressure Use caution when administering with other drugs that prolong QT (consider expert consultation)
Sodium bicarbonate	I.V./I.O.: 1 mEq/kg/dose slowly	After adequate ventilation

I.V. = intravenous; I.O. = intraosseous; E.T. = endotracheal tube.

[1]Flush with 5 mL of normal saline and follow with 5 ventilations.

Adapted from American Heart Association Emergency Cardiovascular Care Committee, "2005 American Heart Association (AHA) Guidelines for Cardiopulmonary Resuscitation (CPR) and Emergency Cardiovascular Care (ECC), Part 12: Pediatric Advanced Life Support," *Circulation*, 2005, 112(24 Suppl):IV-171 and *Pediatric Advanced Life Support, Provider Manual*, copyright American Heart Association, 2006.

PALS Medications to Maintain Cardiac Output and For Postresuscitation Stabilization

Medication	Dose Range	Comment
Inamrinone	I.V./I.O.: 0.75-1 mg/kg over 5 minutes; may repeat x 2; then 2-20 mcg/kg/min	Inodilator
Dobutamine	I.V./I.O.: 2-20 mcg/kg/min	Inotrope; vasodilator
Dopamine	I.V./I.O.: 2-20 mcg/kg/min	Inotrope; chronotrope; renal and splanchnic vasodilator in low doses; pressor in high doses
Epinephrine	I.V./I.O.: 0.1-1 mcg/kg/min	Inotrope; chronotrope; vasodilator in low doses; pressor in higher doses
Milrinone	I.V./I.O.: 50-75 mcg/kg over 10-60 minutes, then 0.5-0.75 mcg/kg/min	Inodilator
Norepinephrine	0.1-2 mcg/kg/min	Inotrope; vasopressor
Sodium nitroprusside	1-8 mcg/kg/min	Vasodilator; prepare only in D_5W

I.V. = intravenous; I.O. = intraosseous.

Alternative formula for calculating an infusion:

Infusion rate (mL/h) = [weight (kg) x dose (mcg/kg/min) x 60 (min/h)] / concentration mcg/mL).

Adapted from American Heart Association Emergency Cardiovascular Care Committee, "2005 American Heart Association (AHA) Guidelines for Cardiopulmonary Resuscitation (CPR) and Emergency Cardiovascular Care (ECC), *Circulation*, 2005, 112(24 Suppl):IV-180.

EMERGENCY PEDIATRIC DRIP CALCULATIONS

The availability of a limited number of standard concentrations for emergency medications (ie, vasopressors) within an institution is required by The Joint Commission (see JCAHO, 2004; Background Information below). When using standardized concentrations, calculate the rate of infusion using the following equation:

$$\text{Rate (mL/h)} \quad = \quad \frac{\text{dose (mcg/kg/min) x weight (kg) x 60 min/h}}{\text{concentration (mcg/mL)}}$$

If a standardized concentration delivers the dose in too low of a volume (eg, <1 mL/hour) then a lower standardized concentration (ie, more dilute) is used. If a standardized concentration delivers the dose in too high of a volume (depending on patient's size and fluid status) then a higher standardized concentration (ie, more concentrated) is used. **Each center is required to develop standardized concentrations and guidelines for their own institution.**

Some centers use the following pediatric standardized concentrations according to patient weight (see Campbell, 1994):

Standardized Concentrations by Patient Weight

Drug	Patient Weight (kg)	Concentration (mcg/mL)
Dopamine	2-3 4-8 9-15 >15	200 400 800 1600
Epinephrine, Isoproterenol, or Norepinephrine	2-3 4-8 ≥9	5 10 20

Other centers use the following standardized concentrations depending on both patient weight and dose (Hodding, 2010):

Drug	Standardized Concentrations (mcg/mL)			
Dobutamine	800	1600	3200	6400
Dopamine	800	1600	3200	6400
Epinephrine	20	40	60	120
Norepinephrine	20	40	60	120
Isoproterenol	20	40	60	120

Some centers also limit the number of standardized concentrations to only two per emergency medication (see Larsen, 2005)

Drug	Standardized Concentrations (mcg/mL)	
Dobutamine	1000	4000
Dopamine	800	3200
Epinephrine	8	64
Norepinephrine	8	64
Isoproterenol	8	64

An example of how different standardized concentrations are used for different patient weights and doses is given below for dopamine. Each table lists the dopamine infusion rate in mL/hour for a specific patient weight (in kg) and dose (in mcg/kg/minute) for a specific standardized concentration. The first table is for dopamine **1600** mcg/mL and the second table for **800** mcg/mL.

Dopamine Infusion Rate (mL/hour) According to Patient Weight (kg) and Dose (mcg/kg/minute) Using Standardized Concentration of <u>1600</u> mcg/mL

Weight (kg)	Dose (mcg/kg/minute)				
	5	7.5	10	15	20
2	0.4*	0.6*	0.8*	1.1	1.5
3	0.6*	0.8*	1.1	1.7	2.3
4	0.8*	1.1	1.5	2.3	3.0
5	0.9*	1.4	1.9	2.8	3.8
7	1.3	2.0	2.6	3.9	5.3
10	1.9	2.8	3.8	5.6	7.5
12	2.3	3.4	4.5	6.8	9.0
14	2.6	3.9	5.3	7.9	10.5
16	3.0	4.5	6.0	9.0	12.0
18	3.4	5.1	6.8	10.1	13.5
20	3.8	5.6	7.5	11.3	15.0

Dopamine Infusion Rate (mL/hour) According to Patient Weight (kg) and Dose (mcg/kg/minute)
Using Standardized Concentration of 1600 mcg/mL *(continued)*

Weight (kg)	Dose (mcg/kg/minute)				
	5	7.5	10	15	20
25	4.7	7.0	9.4	14.1	18.8
30	5.6	8.4	11.3	16.9	22.5
35	6.6	9.8	13.1	19.7	26.3
40	7.5	11.3	15.0	22.5	30.0
45	8.4	12.7	16.9	25.3	33.8
50	9.4	14.1	18.8	28.1	37.5

*For rates <1 mL/hour, use 800 mcg/mL concentration

Dopamine Infusion Rate (mL/hour) According to Patient Weight (kg) and Dose (mcg/kg/minute)
Using Standardized Concentration of 800 mcg/mL

Weight (kg)	Dose (mcg/kg/minute)				
	5	7.5	10	15	20
2	0.8	1.1	1.5	2.3	3.0
3	1.1	1.7	2.3	3.4	4.5
4	1.5	2.3	3.0	4.5	6.0
5	1.9	2.8	3.8	5.6	7.5

BACKGROUND INFORMATION

The Joint Commission (formerly called JCAHO) and the "Rule of Six"

In its 2004 National Patient Safety Goals (NPSG), the Joint Commission on Accreditation of Healthcare Organizations (JCAHO), now called The Joint Commission (TJC), required organizations to "standardize and limit the number of drug concentrations available in the organization" to meet patient safety goal # 3 ("Improve the safety of using high-alert medications"). High-alert medications are drugs that possess a great risk of causing significant injury to patients when they are used in error. Emergency medications (eg, vasopressors) qualify as high-alert drugs.

Historically, the "Rule of Six" was used to calculate patient-specific I.V. concentrations of emergency medication infusions, so that 1 mL/hour would deliver a set mcg/kg/minute dose.

TJC has determined that using the "Rule of Six" or other methods to individualize a concentration of a high-alert drug for a specific patient (ie, use of a nonstandardized concentration) is **not** in compliance with the requirement of the above NPSG goal. In addition, the "Rule of Six" is not recommended by the Institute for Safe Medication Practices (ISMP). Limiting and standardizing the number of drug concentrations (as opposed to using the "Rule of Six") is thought to be safer and less error prone. In 2004, institutions using the "Rule of Six" (or other such methods) were required to develop a transition plan to use a limited number of standardized concentrations. Full implementation of the plan was required by December 31, 2008.

References

Campbell MM, Taeubel MA, and Kraus DM, "Updated Bedside Charts for Calculating Pediatric Doses of Emergency Medications," *Am J Hosp Pharm*, 1994, 51(17):2147-52.

Hodding JH, Executive Director, Pharmacy and Nutritional Services, Long Beach Memorial Medical Center and Miller Children's Hospital, Long Beach, CA, Personal Correspondence, April 2010.

Joint Commission on Accreditation of Healthcare Organizations (JCAHO), "2004 National Patient Safety Goals, Frequently Asked Questions: Updated 8/30/04," August 30, 2004.

Joint Commission on Accreditation of Healthcare Organizations (JCAHO), "Transition Plan From 'Rule of 6'," JCAHOnline, December 2004/January 2005.

Larsen GY, Parker HB, Cash J, et al, "Standard Drug Concentrations and Smart-Pump Technology Reduce Continuous-Medication-Infusion Errors in Pediatric Patients," *Pediatrics*, 2005, 116(1):e21-5.

NEONATAL RESUSCITATION ALGORITHM

Neonatal Flow Algorithm

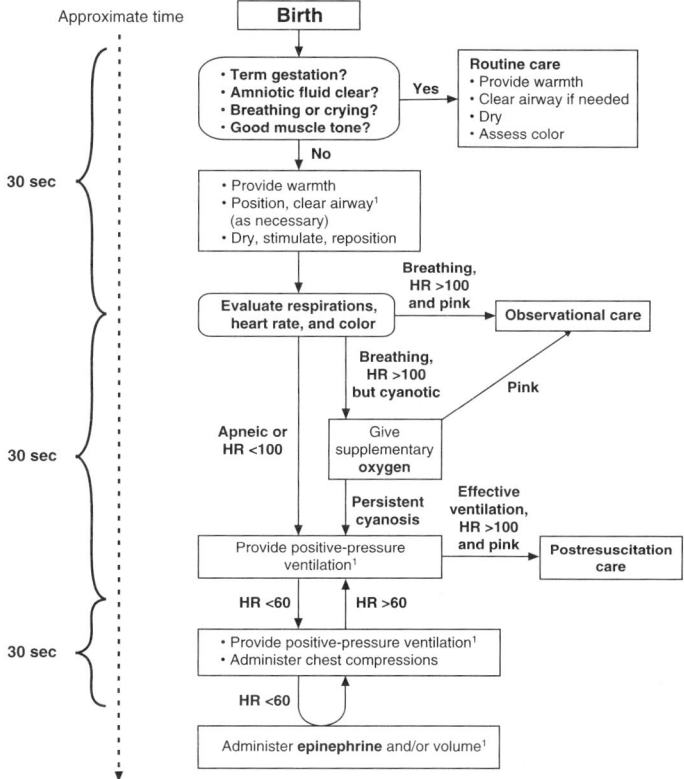

[1]Endotracheal intubation may be considered at several steps.

Epinephrine dose for neonatal resuscitation: I.V.: 0.01-0.03 mg/kg (1:10,000; 0.1-0.3 mL/kg). **Note:** I.V. is the preferred neonatal route. While obtaining I.V. access, one may consider higher doses via E.T.: Up to 0.1 mg/kg (1 mL/kg, 1:10,000), but safety and efficacy of this practice has not been evaluated.

PEDIATRIC ALS ALGORITHMS

PALS Bradycardia Algorithm

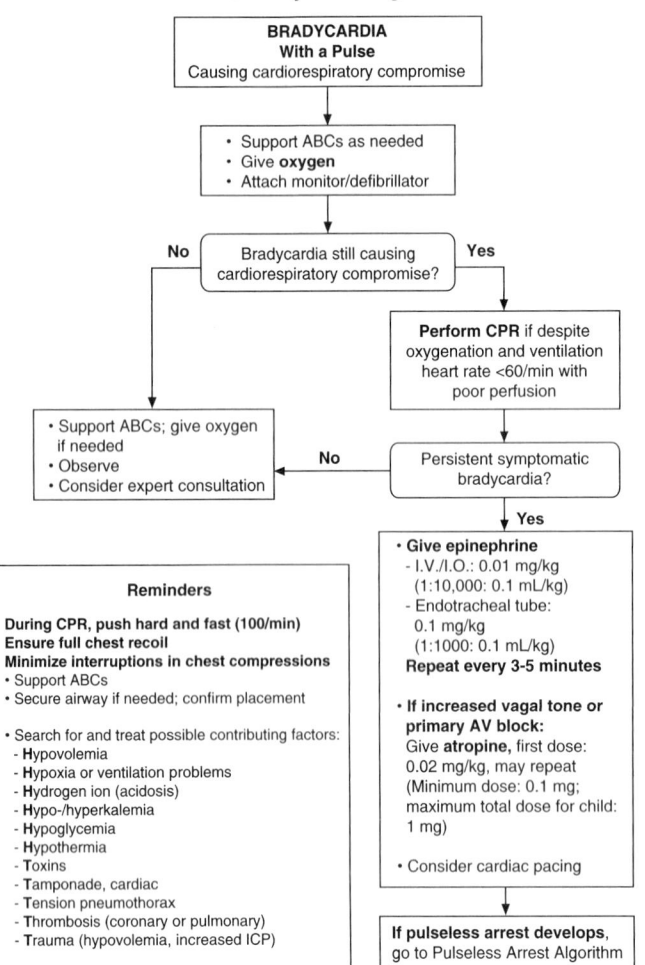

PALS Pulseless Arrest Algorithm

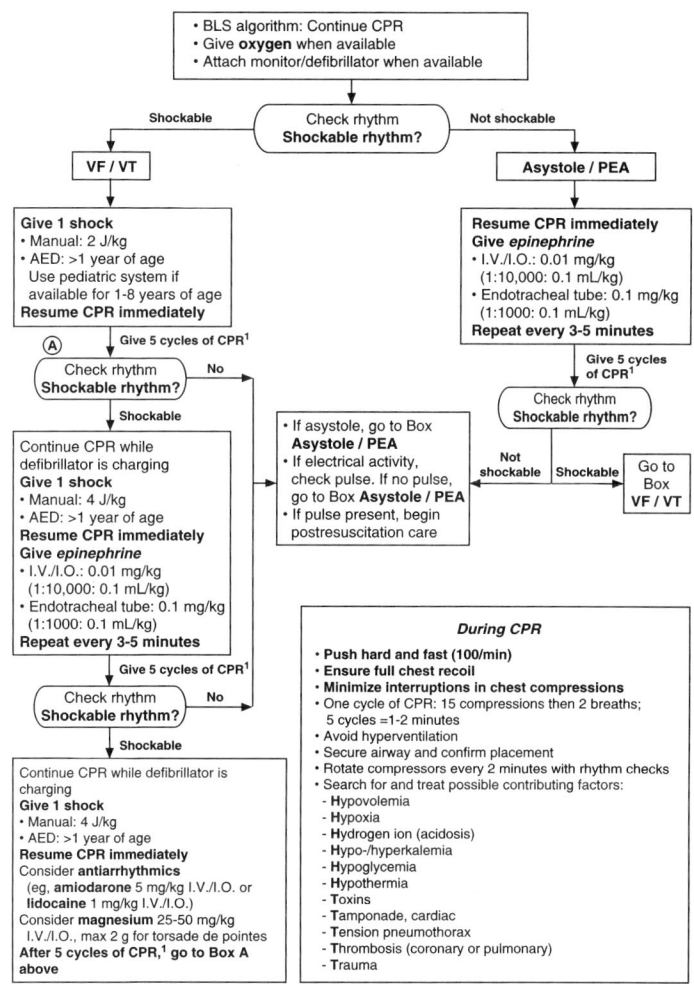

VF = ventricular fibrillation; VT = ventricular tachycardia; PEA = pulseless electrical activity; AED = automated external defibrillator.

[1]After an advanced airway is placed, rescuers no longer deliver "cycles" of CPR. Give continuous chest compressions without pauses for breaths. Give 8-10 breaths/min. Check rhythm every 2 minutes.

PALS Tachycardia Algorithm
With Pulses and Poor Perfusion

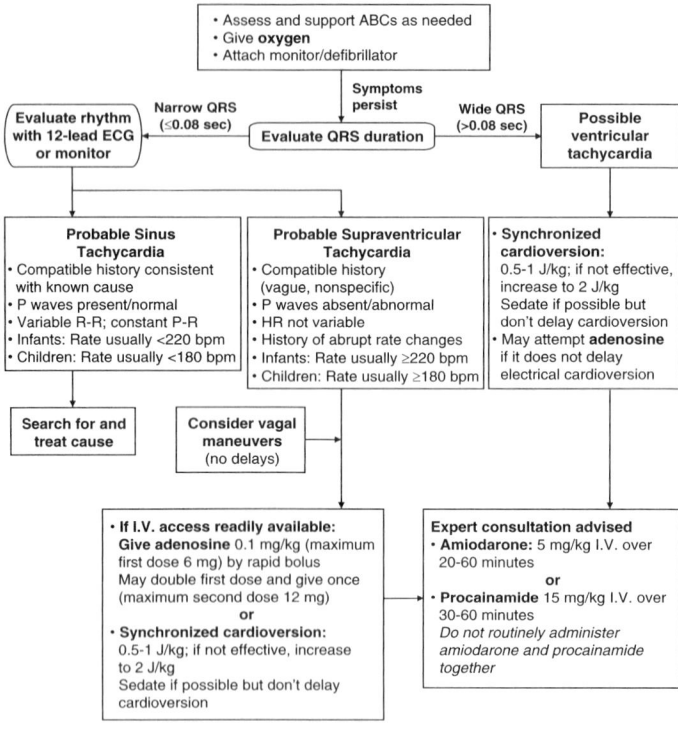

- Assess and support ABCs as needed
- Give **oxygen**
- Attach monitor/defibrillator

Evaluate rhythm with 12-lead ECG or monitor ← Narrow QRS (≤0.08 sec) — Symptoms persist — **Evaluate QRS duration** — Wide QRS (>0.08 sec) → **Possible ventricular tachycardia**

Probable Sinus Tachycardia
- Compatible history consistent with known cause
- P waves present/normal
- Variable R-R; constant P-R
- Infants: Rate usually <220 bpm
- Children: Rate usually <180 bpm

Probable Supraventricular Tachycardia
- Compatible history (vague, nonspecific)
- P waves absent/abnormal
- HR not variable
- History of abrupt rate changes
- Infants: Rate usually ≥220 bpm
- Children: Rate usually ≥180 bpm

- **Synchronized cardioversion:** 0.5-1 J/kg; if not effective, increase to 2 J/kg Sedate if possible but don't delay cardioversion
- May attempt **adenosine** if it does not delay electrical cardioversion

Search for and treat cause

Consider vagal maneuvers (no delays)

- **If I.V. access readily available:** Give **adenosine** 0.1 mg/kg (maximum first dose 6 mg) by rapid bolus May double first dose and give once (maximum second dose 12 mg)

  or

- **Synchronized cardioversion:** 0.5-1 J/kg; if not effective, increase to 2 J/kg Sedate if possible but don't delay cardioversion

Expert consultation advised
- **Amiodarone:** 5 mg/kg I.V. over 20-60 minutes

  or

- **Procainamide** 15 mg/kg I.V. over 30-60 minutes
  Do not routinely administer amiodarone and procainamide together

During Evaluation	*Treat possible contributing factors:*	
• Secure, verify airway and vascular access when possible • Consider expert consultation • Prepare for cardioversion	• **H**ypovolemia • **H**ypoxia • **H**ydrogen ion (acidosis) • **H**ypo-/hyperkalemia • **H**ypoglycemia • **H**ypothermia	• **T**oxins • **T**amponade, cardiac • **T**ension pneumothorax • **T**hrombosis (coronary or pulmonary) • **T**rauma (hypovolemia)

ADULT ACLS ALGORITHMS

Bradycardia Algorithm

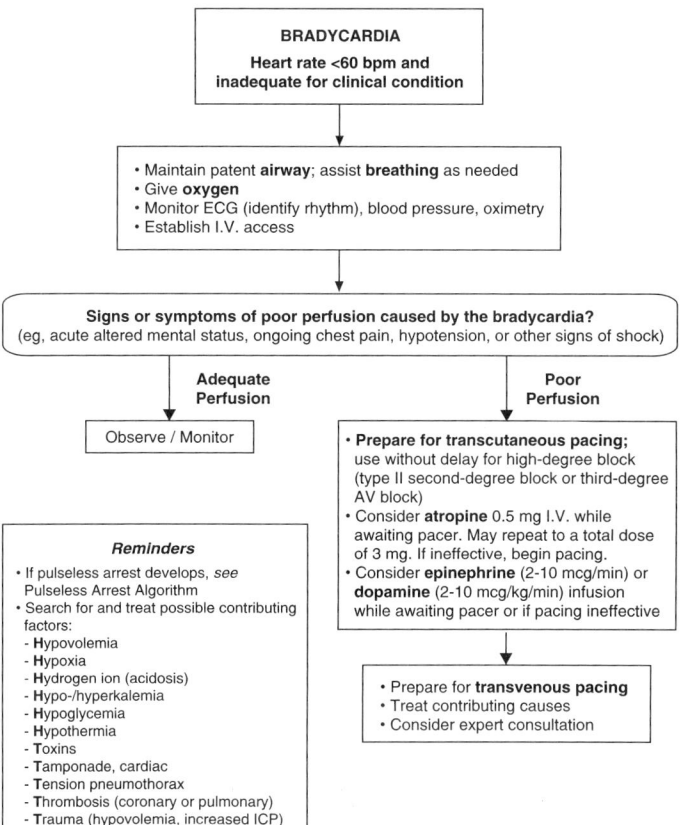

BRADYCARDIA

Heart rate <60 bpm and inadequate for clinical condition

↓

- Maintain patent **airway**; assist **breathing** as needed
- Give **oxygen**
- Monitor ECG (identify rhythm), blood pressure, oximetry
- Establish I.V. access

↓

Signs or symptoms of poor perfusion caused by the bradycardia?
(eg, acute altered mental status, ongoing chest pain, hypotension, or other signs of shock)

Adequate Perfusion

Observe / Monitor

Poor Perfusion

- **Prepare for transcutaneous pacing;** use without delay for high-degree block (type II second-degree block or third-degree AV block)
- Consider **atropine** 0.5 mg I.V. while awaiting pacer. May repeat to a total dose of 3 mg. If ineffective, begin pacing.
- Consider **epinephrine** (2-10 mcg/min) or **dopamine** (2-10 mcg/kg/min) infusion while awaiting pacer or if pacing ineffective

↓

- Prepare for **transvenous pacing**
- Treat contributing causes
- Consider expert consultation

Reminders

- If pulseless arrest develops, *see* Pulseless Arrest Algorithm
- Search for and treat possible contributing factors:
  - **H**ypovolemia
  - **H**ypoxia
  - **H**ydrogen ion (acidosis)
  - **H**ypo-/hyperkalemia
  - **H**ypoglycemia
  - **H**ypothermia
  - **T**oxins
  - **T**amponade, cardiac
  - **T**ension pneumothorax
  - **T**hrombosis (coronary or pulmonary)
  - **T**rauma (hypovolemia, increased ICP)

Reproduced With Permission, "2005 American Heart Association Guidelines for Cardiopulmonary Resuscitation and Emergency Cardiovascular Care," *Circulation*, 2005, 112(24 Suppl):IV1-203. ©2005, American Heart Association.

ACLS Pulseless Arrest Algorithm

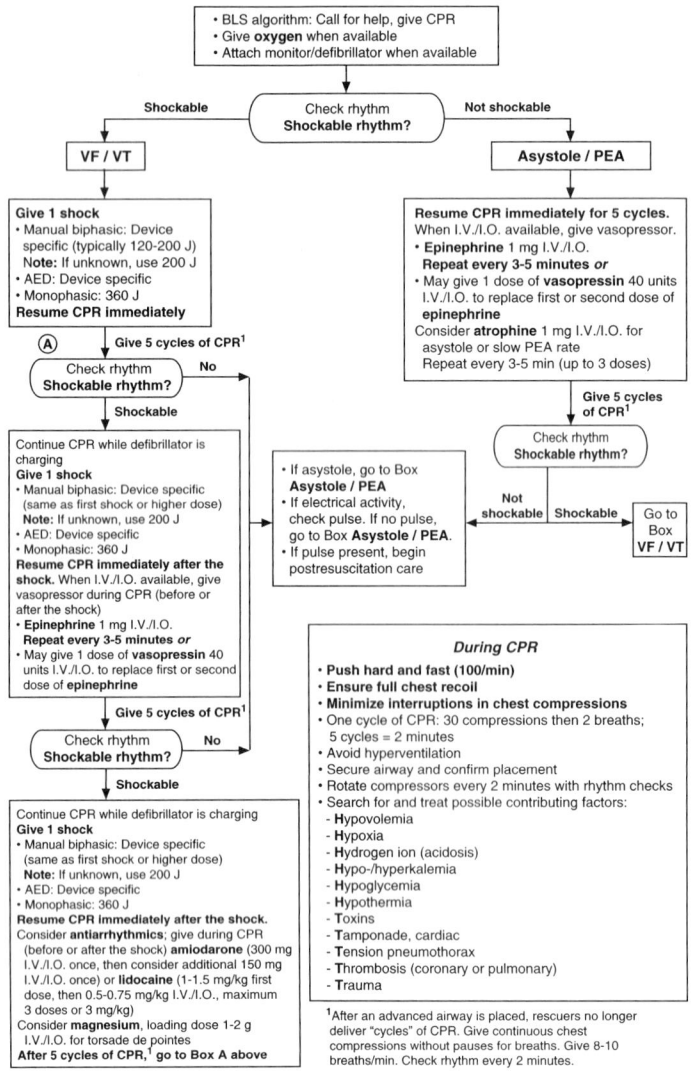

- BLS algorithm: Call for help, give CPR
- Give **oxygen** when available
- Attach monitor/defibrillator when available

Check rhythm
Shockable rhythm?

Shockable → **VF / VT**

Not shockable → **Asystole / PEA**

VF / VT

Give 1 shock
- Manual biphasic: Device specific (typically 120-200 J)
  Note: If unknown, use 200 J
- AED: Device specific
- Monophasic: 360 J
Resume CPR immediately

(A) Give 5 cycles of CPR[1]

Check rhythm
Shockable rhythm? — **No**

Shockable

Continue CPR while defibrillator is charging
Give 1 shock
- Manual biphasic: Device specific (same as first shock or higher dose)
  Note: If unknown, use 200 J
- AED: Device specific
- Monophasic: 360 J
Resume CPR immediately after the shock. When I.V./I.O. available, give vasopressor during CPR (before or after the shock)
- **Epinephrine** 1 mg I.V./I.O.
  Repeat every 3-5 minutes *or*
- May give 1 dose of **vasopressin** 40 units I.V./I.O. to replace first or second dose of **epinephrine**

Give 5 cycles of CPR[1]

Check rhythm
Shockable rhythm? — **No**

Shockable

Continue CPR while defibrillator is charging
Give 1 shock
- Manual biphasic: Device specific (same as first shock or higher dose)
  Note: If unknown, use 200 J
- AED: Device specific
- Monophasic: 360 J
Resume CPR immediately after the shock.
Consider **antiarrhythmics**; give during CPR (before or after the shock) **amiodarone** (300 mg I.V./I.O. once, then consider additional 150 mg I.V./I.O. once) or **lidocaine** (1-1.5 mg/kg first dose, then 0.5-0.75 mg/kg I.V./I.O., maximum 3 doses or 3 mg/kg)
Consider **magnesium**, loading dose 1-2 g I.V./I.O. for torsade de pointes
After 5 cycles of CPR,[1] **go to Box A above**

Asystole / PEA

Resume CPR immediately for 5 cycles.
When I.V./I.O. available, give vasopressor.
- **Epinephrine** 1 mg I.V./I.O.
  Repeat every 3-5 minutes *or*
- May give 1 dose of **vasopressin** 40 units I.V./I.O. to replace first or second dose of **epinephrine**
Consider **atropine** 1 mg I.V./I.O. for asystole or slow PEA rate
Repeat every 3-5 min (up to 3 doses)

Give 5 cycles of CPR[1]

Check rhythm
Shockable rhythm?

Not shockable | **Shockable** → Go to Box **VF / VT**

- If asystole, go to Box **Asystole / PEA**
- If electrical activity, check pulse. If no pulse, go to Box **Asystole / PEA**.
- If pulse present, begin postresuscitation care

During CPR

- **Push hard and fast (100/min)**
- **Ensure full chest recoil**
- **Minimize interruptions in chest compressions**
- One cycle of CPR: 30 compressions then 2 breaths; 5 cycles = 2 minutes
- Avoid hyperventilation
- Secure airway and confirm placement
- Rotate compressors every 2 minutes with rhythm checks
- Search for and treat possible contributing factors:
  - Hypovolemia
  - Hypoxia
  - Hydrogen ion (acidosis)
  - Hypo-/hyperkalemia
  - Hypoglycemia
  - Hypothermia
  - Toxins
  - Tamponade, cardiac
  - Tension pneumothorax
  - Thrombosis (coronary or pulmonary)
  - Trauma

[1]After an advanced airway is placed, rescuers no longer deliver "cycles" of CPR. Give continuous chest compressions without pauses for breaths. Give 8-10 breaths/min. Check rhythm every 2 minutes.

VF = ventricular fibrillation; VT = ventricular tachycardia; PEA = pulseless electrical activity; AED = automated external defibrillator.

ACLS Tachycardia Algorithm
With Pulses

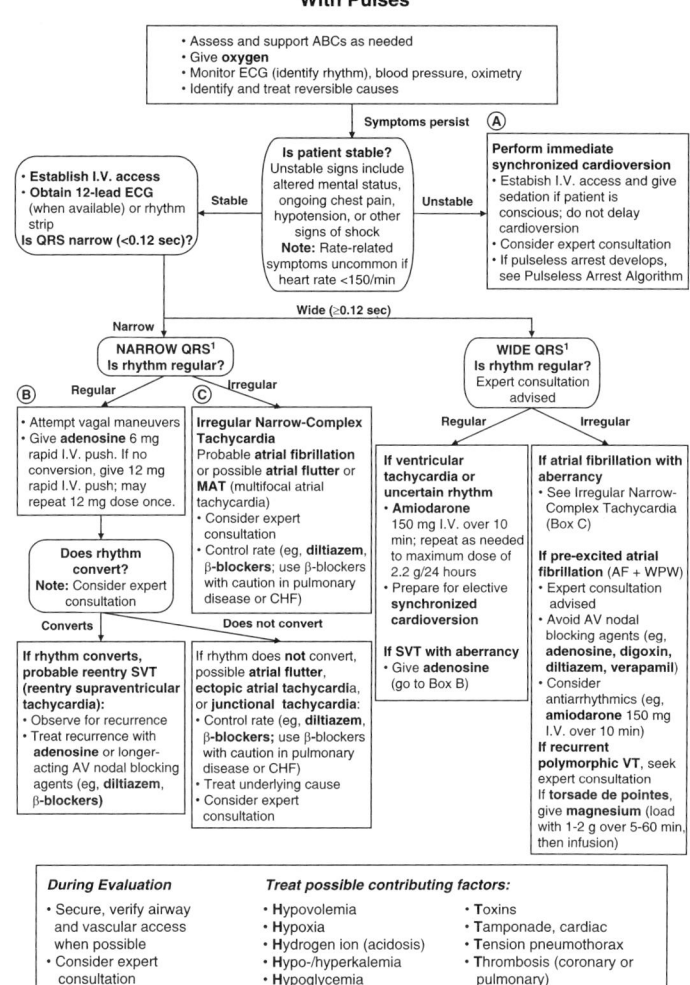

- Assess and support ABCs as needed
- Give **oxygen**
- Monitor ECG (identify rhythm), blood pressure, oximetry
- Identify and treat reversible causes

Symptoms persist Ⓐ

Is patient stable?
Unstable signs include altered mental status, ongoing chest pain, hypotension, or other signs of shock
Note: Rate-related symptoms uncommon if heart rate <150/min

Stable → • **Establish I.V. access**
• **Obtain 12-lead ECG** (when available) or rhythm strip
Is QRS narrow (<0.12 sec)?

Unstable → **Perform immediate synchronized cardioversion**
• Estabish I.V. access and give sedation if patient is conscious; do not delay cardioversion
• Consider expert consultation
• If pulseless arrest develops, see Pulseless Arrest Algorithm

Narrow → **NARROW QRS¹**
Is rhythm regular?

Wide (≥0.12 sec) → **WIDE QRS¹**
Is rhythm regular?
Expert consultation advised

Ⓑ Regular

Attempt vagal maneuvers
• Give **adenosine** 6 mg rapid I.V. push. If no conversion, give 12 mg rapid I.V. push; may repeat 12 mg dose once.

Ⓒ Irregular

Irregular Narrow-Complex Tachycardia
Probable **atrial fibrillation** or possible **atrial flutter** or **MAT** (multifocal atrial tachycardia)
• Consider expert consultation
• Control rate (eg, **diltiazem,** β-**blockers;** use β-blockers with caution in pulmonary disease or CHF)

Does rhythm convert?
Note: Consider expert consultation

Converts → **If rhythm converts, probable reentry SVT (reentry supraventricular tachycardia):**
• Observe for recurrence
• Treat recurrence with **adenosine** or longer-acting AV nodal blocking agents (eg, **diltiazem,** β-**blockers)**

Does not convert → If rhythm does **not** convert, possible **atrial flutter,** ectopic atrial tachycardia, or junctional tachycardia:
• Control rate (eg, **diltiazem,** β-**blockers;** use β-blockers with caution in pulmonary disease or CHF)
• Treat underlying cause
• Consider expert consultation

Regular

If ventricular tachycardia or uncertain rhythm
• **Amiodarone**
150 mg I.V. over 10 min; repeat as needed to maximum dose of 2.2 g/24 hours
• Prepare for elective synchronized cardioversion

If SVT with aberrancy
• Give **adenosine** (go to Box B)

Irregular

If atrial fibrillation with aberrancy
• See Irregular Narrow-Complex Tachycardia (Box C)

If pre-excited atrial fibrillation (AF + WPW)
• Expert consultation advised
• Avoid AV nodal blocking agents (eg, **adenosine, digoxin, diltiazem, verapamil**)
• Consider antiarrhythmics (eg, **amiodarone** 150 mg I.V. over 10 min)
If recurrent polymorphic VT, seek expert consultation
If **torsade de pointes,** give **magnesium** (load with 1-2 g over 5-60 min, then infusion)

During Evaluation	Treat possible contributing factors:	
• Secure, verify airway and vascular access when possible	• **H**ypovolemia	• **T**oxins
• Consider expert consultation	• **H**ypoxia	• **T**amponade, cardiac
• Prepare for cardioversion	• **H**ydrogen ion (acidosis)	• **T**ension pneumothorax
	• **H**ypo-/hyperkalemia	• **T**hrombosis (coronary or pulmonary)
	• **H**ypoglycemia	• **T**rauma (hypovolemia)
	• **H**ypothermia	

SVT = supraventricular tachycardia; VT = ventricular tachycardia.
¹If patient becomes unstable, go to Box A.

Reproduced With Permission, "2005 American Heart Association Guidelines for Cardiopulmonary Resuscitation and Emergency Cardiovascular Care," *Circulation*, 2005, 112(24 Suppl):IV1-203. ©2005, American Heart Association.

NORMAL PEDIATRIC HEART RATES

Age	Mean Heart Rate (beats/minute)	Heart Rate Range (2nd – 98th percentile)
<1 d	123	93-154
1-2 d	123	91-159
3-6 d	129	91-166
1-3 wk	148	107-182
1-2 mo	149	121-179
3-5 mo	141	106-186
6-11 mo	134	109-169
1-2 y	119	89-151
3-4 y	108	73-137
5-7 y	100	65-133
8-11 y	91	62-130
12-15 y	85	60-119

Adapted from *The Harriet Lane Handbook*, 12th ed, Greene MG, ed, St Louis, MO: Mosby Yearbook, 1991.

Normal QRS Axes (in degrees)

Age	Mean	Range
1 wk – 1 mo	+110	+30 to +180
1–3 mo	+70	+10 to +125
3 mo – 3 y	+60	+10 to +110
>3 y	+60	+20 to +120
Adults	+50	−30 to +105

INTERVALS AND SEGMENTS
OF AN ECG CYCLE

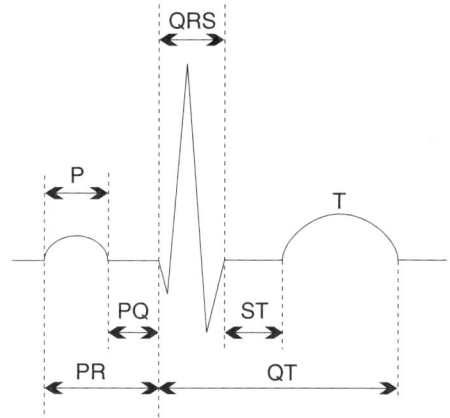

HEXAXIAL REFERENCE
SYSTEM

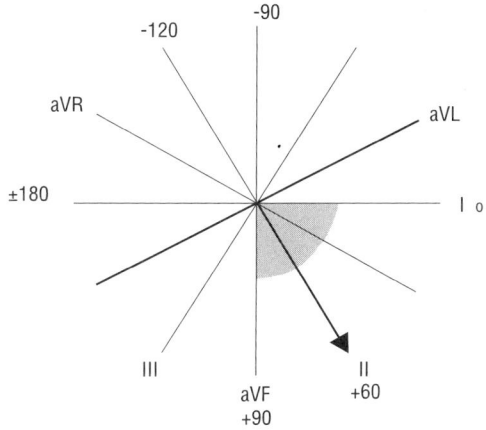

MEASURING PEDIATRIC BLOOD PRESSURE

Figure 1. Determination of Proper Cuff Size, Step 1

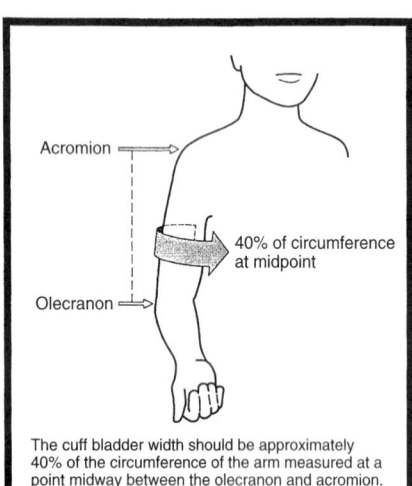

Acromion

40% of circumference at midpoint

Olecranon

The cuff bladder width should be approximately 40% of the circumference of the arm measured at a point midway between the olecranon and acromion.

Figure 2. Determination of Proper Cuff Size, Step 2

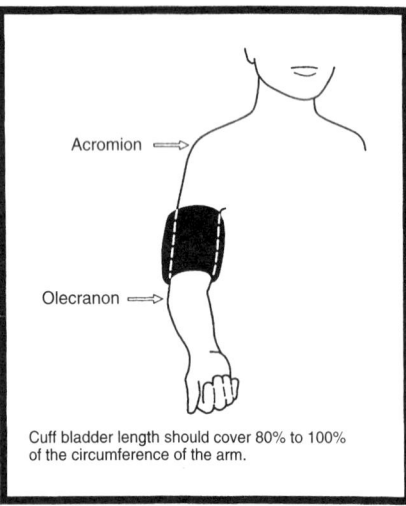

Acromion

Olecranon

Cuff bladder length should cover 80% to 100% of the circumference of the arm.

Figure 3. Blood Pressure Measurement

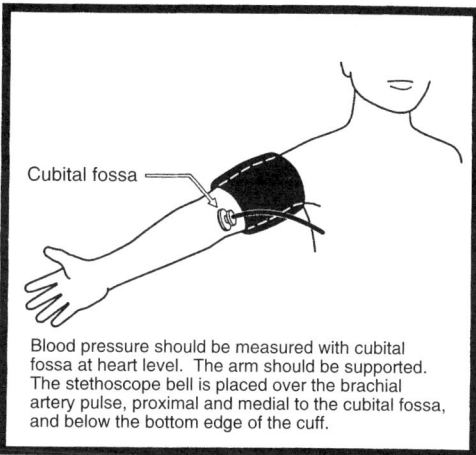

Cubital fossa

Blood pressure should be measured with cubital fossa at heart level. The arm should be supported. The stethoscope bell is placed over the brachial artery pulse, proximal and medial to the cubital fossa, and below the bottom edge of the cuff.

Used with permission: Perloff D, Grim C, Flack J, et al, "Human Blood Pressure Determination by Sphygmomanometry," *Circulation*, 1993, 88:2460-7.

HYPOTENSION, DEFINITIONS BY AGE GROUP

Hypotension is a *systolic* blood pressure <5th percentile of normal for age, namely:

- <60 mm Hg in term neonates (0-28 days)
- <70 mm Hg in infants (1-12 months)
- <70 mm Hg + (2 x age in years) in children 1-10 years
- <90 mm Hg in children ≥10 years of age

Reference

American Heart Association Emergency Cardiovascular Care Committee, "2005 American Heart Association (AHA) Guidelines for Cardiopulmonary Resuscitation (CPR) and Emergency Cardiovascular Care (ECC)," *Circulation*, 2005, 112(24 Suppl):IV-167.

HYPERTENSION, CLASSIFICATION BY AGE GROUP[1]

Age Group	Significant Hypertension (mm Hg)	Severe Hypertension (mm Hg)
Newborn (7 d)		
systolic BP	≥96	≥106
Newborn (8-30 d)		
systolic BP	≥104	≥110
Infant (<2 y)		
systolic BP	≥112	≥118
diastolic BP	≥74	≥82
Children (3-5 y)		
systolic BP	≥116	≥124
diastolic BP	≥76	≥84
Children (6-9 y)		
systolic BP	≥122	≥130
diastolic BP	≥78	≥86
Children (10-12 y)		
systolic BP	≥126	≥134
diastolic BP	≥82	≥90
Adolescents (13-15 y)		
systolic BP	≥136	≥144
diastolic BP	≥86	≥92
Adolescents (16-18 y)		
systolic BP	≥142	≥150
diastolic BP	≥92	≥98

Adapted from Horan MJ, *Pediatrics*, 1987, 79:1-25.

[1]See also Blood Pressure Measurement, Age Specific Percentiles, and 90th and 95th Percentiles of Blood Pressure by Percentiles of Height.

BLOOD PRESSURE IN PREMATURE INFANTS, NORMAL

(Birth weight 600-1750 g)[1]

Day	600-999 g		1000-1249 g	
	S (± 2SD)	D (± 2SD)	S (± 2SD)	D (± 2SD)
1	37.9 (17.4)	23.2 (10.3)	44 (22.8)	22.5 (13.5)
3	44.9 (15.7)	30.6 (12.3)	48 (15.4)	36.5 (9.6)
7	50 (14.8)	30.4 (12.4)	57 (14)	42.5 (16.5)
14	50.2 (14.8)	37.4 (12)	53 (30)	
28	61 (23.5)	45.8 (27.4)	57 (30)	

Day	1250-1499 g		1500-1750 g	
	S (± 2SD)	D (± 2SD)	S (± 2SD)	D (± 2SD)
1	48 (18)	27 (12.4)	47 (15.8)	26 (15.6)
3	59 (21.1)	40 (13.7)	51 (18.2)	35 (10)
7	68 (14.8)	40 (11.3)	66 (23)	41 (24)
14	64 (21.2)	36 (24.2)	76 (34.8)	42 (20.3)
28	69 (31.4)	44 (26.2)	73 (5.6)	50 (9.9)

[1]Blood pressure was obtained by the Dinamap method.

S = systolic; D = diastolic; SD = standard deviation.

Modified from Ingelfinger JR, Powers L, and Epstein MF, "Blood Pressure Norms in Low-Weight Infants: Birth Through Four Weeks", *Pediatr Res*, 1983, 17:319A.

BLOOD PRESSURE MEASUREMENTS, AGE-SPECIFIC PERCENTILES

Blood Pressure Measurements: Ages 0-12 Months, <u>BOYS</u>

Korotkoff phase IV (K4) used for diastolic BP. Reproduced with permission from Horan MJ, *Pediatrics*, 1987, 79:11-25.

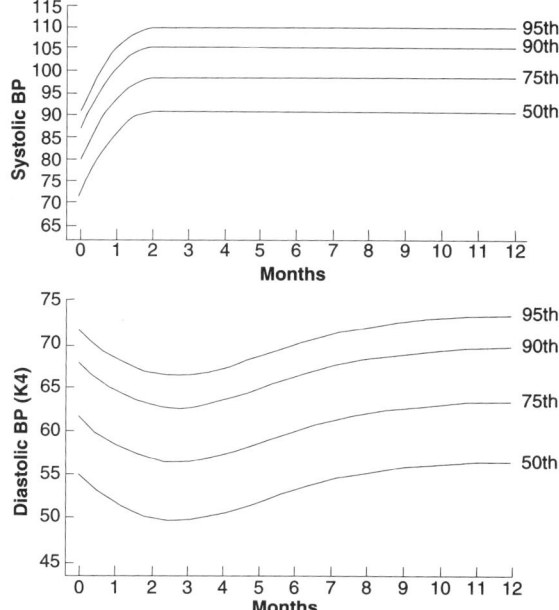

90th Percentile												
Systolic BP	87	101	106	106	106	105	105	105	105	105	105	105	105
Diastolic BP	68	65	63	63	63	65	66	67	68	68	69	69	69
Height cm	51	59	63	66	68	70	72	73	74	76	77	78	80
Weight kg	4	4	5	5	6	7	8	9	9	10	10	11	11

Blood Pressure Measurements: Ages 0-12 Months, <u>GIRLS</u>

Korotkoff phase IV (K4) used for diastolic BP. Reproduced with permission from Horan MJ, *Pediatrics*, 1987, 79:11-25.

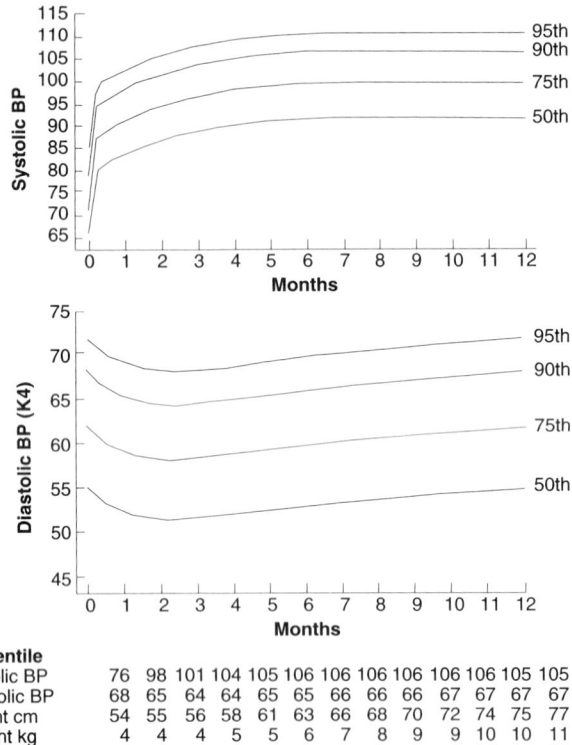

90th Percentile												
Systolic BP	76	98	101	104	105	106	106	106	106	106	106	105	105
Diastolic BP	68	65	64	64	65	65	66	66	66	67	67	67	67
Height cm	54	55	56	58	61	63	66	68	70	72	74	75	77
Weight kg	4	4	4	5	5	6	7	8	9	9	10	10	11

Blood Pressure Levels for BOYS by Age and Height Percentile

Age (y)	BP Percentile[1]	Systolic BP (mm Hg)							Diastolic BP (mm Hg)[2]						
		Height Percentile[3]													
		5%	10%	25%	50%	75%	90%	95%	5%	10%	25%	50%	75%	90%	95%
1	50th	80	81	83	85	87	88	89	34	35	36	37	38	39	39
	90th	94	95	97	99	100	102	103	49	50	51	52	53	53	54
	95th	98	99	101	103	104	106	106	54	54	55	56	57	58	58
	99th	105	106	108	110	112	113	114	61	62	63	64	65	66	66
2	50th	84	85	87	88	90	92	92	39	40	41	42	43	44	44
	90th	97	99	100	102	104	105	106	54	55	56	57	58	58	59
	95th	101	102	104	106	108	109	110	59	59	60	61	62	63	63
	99th	109	110	111	113	115	117	117	66	67	68	69	70	71	71
3	50th	86	87	89	91	93	94	95	44	44	45	46	47	48	48
	90th	100	101	103	105	107	108	109	59	59	60	61	62	63	63
	95th	104	105	107	109	110	112	113	63	63	64	65	66	67	67
	99th	111	112	114	116	118	119	120	71	71	72	73	74	75	75
4	50th	88	89	91	93	95	96	97	47	48	49	50	51	51	52
	90th	102	103	105	107	109	110	111	62	63	64	65	66	66	67
	95th	106	107	109	111	112	114	115	66	67	68	69	70	71	71
	99th	113	114	116	118	120	121	122	74	75	76	77	78	78	79
5	50th	90	91	93	95	96	98	98	50	51	52	53	54	55	55
	90th	104	105	106	108	110	111	112	65	66	67	68	69	69	70
	95th	108	109	110	112	114	115	116	69	70	71	72	73	74	74
	99th	115	116	118	120	121	123	123	77	78	79	80	81	81	82
6	50th	91	92	94	96	98	99	100	53	53	54	55	56	57	57
	90th	105	106	108	110	111	113	113	68	68	69	70	71	72	72
	95th	109	110	112	114	115	117	117	72	72	73	74	75	76	76
	99th	116	117	119	121	123	124	125	80	80	81	82	83	84	84
7	50th	92	94	95	97	99	100	101	55	55	56	57	58	59	59
	90th	106	107	109	111	113	114	115	70	70	71	72	73	74	74
	95th	110	111	113	115	117	118	119	74	74	75	76	77	78	78
	99th	117	118	120	122	124	125	126	82	82	83	84	85	86	86
8	50th	94	95	97	99	100	102	102	56	57	58	59	60	60	61
	90th	107	109	110	112	114	115	116	71	72	72	73	74	75	76
	95th	111	112	114	116	118	119	120	75	76	77	78	79	79	80
	99th	119	120	122	123	125	127	127	83	84	85	86	87	87	88

Blood Pressure Levels for BOYS by Age and Height Percentile *continued*

Age (y)	BP Percentile[1]	Systolic BP (mm Hg)							Diastolic BP (mm Hg)[2]						
		Height Percentile[3]							Height Percentile[3]						
		5%	10%	25%	50%	75%	90%	95%	5%	10%	25%	50%	75%	90%	95%
9	50th	95	96	98	100	102	103	104	57	58	59	60	61	61	62
	90th	109	110	112	114	115	117	118	72	73	74	75	76	76	77
	95th	113	114	116	118	119	121	121	76	77	78	79	80	81	81
	99th	120	121	123	125	127	128	129	84	85	86	87	88	88	89
10	50th	97	98	100	102	103	105	106	58	59	60	61	61	62	63
	90th	111	112	114	115	117	119	119	73	73	74	75	76	77	78
	95th	115	116	117	119	121	122	123	77	78	79	80	81	81	82
	99th	122	123	125	127	128	130	130	85	86	86	88	88	89	90
11	50th	99	100	102	104	105	107	107	59	59	60	61	62	63	63
	90th	113	114	115	117	119	120	121	74	74	75	76	77	78	78
	95th	117	118	119	121	123	124	125	78	78	79	80	81	82	82
	99th	124	125	127	129	130	132	132	86	86	87	88	89	90	90
12	50th	101	102	104	106	108	109	110	59	60	61	62	63	63	64
	90th	115	116	118	120	121	123	123	74	75	75	76	77	78	79
	95th	119	120	122	123	125	127	127	78	79	80	81	82	82	83
	99th	126	127	129	131	133	134	135	86	87	88	89	90	90	91
13	50th	104	105	106	108	110	111	112	60	60	61	62	63	64	64
	90th	117	118	120	122	124	125	126	75	75	76	77	78	79	79
	95th	121	122	124	126	128	129	130	79	79	80	81	82	83	83
	99th	128	130	131	133	135	136	137	87	87	88	89	90	91	91
14	50th	106	107	109	111	113	114	115	60	61	62	63	64	65	65
	90th	120	121	123	125	126	128	128	75	76	77	78	79	79	80
	95th	124	125	127	128	130	132	132	80	80	81	82	83	84	84
	99th	131	132	134	136	138	139	140	87	88	89	90	91	92	92
15	50th	109	110	112	113	115	117	117	61	62	63	64	65	66	66
	90th	122	124	125	127	129	130	131	76	77	78	79	80	80	81
	95th	126	127	129	131	133	134	135	81	81	82	83	84	85	85
	99th	134	135	136	138	140	142	142	88	89	90	91	92	93	93
16	50th	111	112	114	116	118	119	120	63	63	64	65	66	67	67
	90th	125	126	128	130	131	133	134	78	78	79	80	81	82	82
	95th	129	130	132	134	135	137	137	82	83	83	84	85	86	87
	99th	136	137	139	141	143	144	145	90	90	91	92	93	94	94

Blood Pressure Levels for BOYS by Age and Height Percentile *continued*

Age (y)	BP Percentile[1]	Systolic BP (mm Hg)							Diastolic BP (mm Hg)[2]						
		Height Percentile[3]							Height Percentile[3]						
		5%	10%	25%	50%	75%	90%	95%	5%	10%	25%	50%	75%	90%	95%
17	50th	114	115	116	118	120	121	122	65	66	66	67	68	69	70
	90th	127	128	130	132	134	135	136	80	80	81	82	83	84	84
	95th	131	132	134	136	138	139	140	84	85	86	87	87	88	89
	99th	139	140	141	143	145	146	147	92	93	93	94	95	96	97

[1]Blood pressure percentile determined by a single measurement.

[2]Korotkoff phase V (K5) used for diastolic BP.

[3]Height percentile determined by standard growth curves.

Source: National High Blood Pressure Education Program Working Group on High Blood Pressure in Children and Adolescents, "The Fourth Report on the Diagnosis, Evaluation, and Treatment of High Blood Pressure in Children and Adolescents." Pediatrics, 2004, 114(2 Suppl 4th Report):555-76.

Blood Pressure Levels for GIRLS by Age and Height Percentile

Age (y)	BP Percentile[1]	Systolic BP (mm Hg)							Diastolic BP (mm Hg)[2]						
		Height Percentile[3]							Height Percentile[3]						
		5%	10%	25%	50%	75%	90%	95%	5%	10%	25%	50%	75%	90%	95%
1	50th	83	84	85	86	88	89	90	38	39	39	40	41	41	42
	90th	97	97	98	100	101	102	103	52	53	53	54	55	55	56
	95th	100	101	102	104	105	106	107	56	57	57	58	59	59	60
	99th	108	108	109	111	112	113	114	64	64	65	65	66	67	67
2	50th	85	85	87	88	89	91	91	43	44	44	45	46	46	47
	90th	98	99	100	101	103	104	105	57	58	58	59	60	61	61
	95th	102	103	104	105	107	108	109	61	62	62	63	64	65	65
	99th	109	110	111	112	114	115	116	69	69	70	70	71	72	72
3	50th	86	87	88	89	91	92	93	47	48	48	49	50	50	51
	90th	100	100	102	103	104	106	106	61	62	62	63	64	64	65
	95th	104	104	105	107	108	109	110	65	66	66	67	68	68	69
	99th	111	111	113	114	115	116	117	73	73	74	74	75	76	76
4	50th	88	88	90	91	92	94	94	50	50	51	52	52	53	54
	90th	101	102	103	104	106	107	108	64	64	65	66	67	67	68
	95th	105	106	107	108	110	111	112	68	68	69	70	71	71	72
	99th	112	113	114	115	117	118	119	76	76	76	77	78	79	79
5	50th	89	90	91	93	94	95	96	52	53	53	54	55	55	56
	90th	103	103	105	106	107	109	109	66	67	67	68	69	69	70
	95th	107	107	108	110	111	112	113	70	71	71	72	73	73	74
	99th	114	114	116	117	118	120	120	78	78	79	79	80	81	81
6	50th	91	92	93	94	96	97	98	54	54	55	56	56	57	58
	90th	104	105	106	108	109	110	111	68	68	69	70	70	71	72
	95th	108	109	110	111	113	114	115	72	72	73	74	74	75	76
	99th	115	116	117	119	120	121	122	80	80	80	81	82	83	83
7	50th	93	93	95	96	97	99	99	55	56	56	57	58	58	59
	90th	106	107	108	109	111	112	113	69	70	70	71	72	72	73
	95th	110	111	112	113	115	116	116	73	74	74	75	76	76	77
	99th	117	118	119	120	122	123	124	81	81	82	82	83	84	84
8	50th	95	95	96	98	99	100	101	57	57	57	58	59	60	60
	90th	108	109	110	111	113	114	114	71	71	71	72	73	74	74
	95th	112	112	114	115	116	118	118	75	75	75	76	77	78	78
	99th	119	120	121	122	123	125	125	82	82	83	83	84	85	86

Blood Pressure Levels for GIRLS by Age and Height Percentile *continued*

Age (y)	BP Percentile[1]	Systolic BP (mm Hg) Height Percentile[3]							Diastolic BP (mm Hg)[2] Height Percentile[3]						
		5%	10%	25%	50%	75%	90%	95%	5%	10%	25%	50%	75%	90%	95%
9	50th	96	97	98	100	101	102	103	58	58	58	59	60	61	61
	90th	110	110	112	113	114	116	116	72	72	72	73	74	75	75
	95th	114	114	115	117	118	119	120	76	76	76	77	78	79	79
	99th	121	121	123	124	125	127	127	83	83	84	84	85	86	87
10	50th	98	99	100	102	103	104	105	59	59	59	60	61	62	62
	90th	112	112	114	115	116	118	118	73	73	73	74	75	76	76
	95th	116	116	117	119	120	121	122	77	77	77	78	79	80	80
	99th	123	123	125	126	127	129	129	84	84	85	86	86	87	88
11	50th	100	101	102	103	105	106	107	60	60	60	61	62	63	63
	90th	114	114	116	117	118	119	120	74	74	74	75	76	77	77
	95th	118	118	119	121	122	123	124	78	78	78	79	80	81	81
	99th	125	125	126	128	129	130	131	85	85	86	87	87	88	89
12	50th	102	103	104	105	107	108	109	61	61	61	62	63	64	64
	90th	116	116	117	119	120	121	122	75	75	75	76	77	78	78
	95th	119	120	121	123	124	125	126	79	79	79	80	81	82	82
	99th	127	127	128	130	131	132	133	86	86	87	88	88	89	90
13	50th	104	105	106	107	109	110	110	62	62	62	63	64	65	65
	90th	117	118	119	121	122	123	124	76	76	76	77	78	79	79
	95th	121	122	123	124	126	127	128	80	80	80	81	82	83	83
	99th	128	129	130	132	133	134	135	87	87	88	89	89	90	91
14	50th	106	106	107	109	110	111	112	63	63	63	64	65	66	66
	90th	119	120	121	122	124	125	125	77	77	77	78	79	80	80
	95th	123	123	125	126	127	129	129	81	81	81	82	83	84	84
	99th	130	131	132	133	135	136	136	88	88	88	89	90	91	92
15	50th	107	108	109	110	111	113	113	64	64	64	65	66	67	67
	90th	120	121	122	123	125	126	127	78	78	78	79	80	81	81
	95th	124	125	126	127	129	130	131	82	82	82	83	84	85	85
	99th	131	132	133	134	136	137	138	89	89	90	91	91	92	93
16	50th	108	108	110	111	112	114	114	64	64	65	66	66	67	68
	90th	121	122	123	124	126	127	128	78	78	79	80	81	81	82
	95th	125	126	127	128	130	131	132	82	82	83	84	85	85	86
	99th	132	133	134	135	137	138	139	90	90	90	91	92	93	93

Blood Pressure Levels for GIRLS by Age and Height Percentile *continued*

Age (y)	BP Percentile[1]	Systolic BP (mm Hg)							Diastolic BP (mm Hg)[2]						
		Height Percentile[3]							Height Percentile[3]						
		5%	10%	25%	50%	75%	90%	95%	5%	10%	25%	50%	75%	90%	95%
17	50th	108	109	110	111	113	114	115	64	65	65	66	67	67	68
	90th	122	122	123	125	126	127	128	78	79	79	80	81	81	82
	95th	125	126	127	129	130	131	132	82	83	83	84	85	85	86
	99th	133	133	134	136	137	138	139	90	90	91	91	92	93	93

[1]Blood pressure percentile determined by a single measurement.

[2]Korotkoff phase V (K5) used for diastolic BP.

[3]Height percentile determined by standard growth curves.

Source: National High Blood Pressure Education Program Working Group on High Blood Pressure in Children and Adolescents, "The Fourth Report on the Diagnosis, Evaluation, and Treatment of High Blood Pressure in Children and Adolescents." *Pediatrics*, 2004, 114(2 Suppl 4th Report):555-76.

ANTIHYPERTENSIVE AGENTS BY CLASS

Alpha-Adrenergic (Alpha$_1$ and Alpha$_2$) Antagonists
Phenoxybenzamine
Phentolamine

Alpha$_1$-Antagonists
Prazosin

Alpha$_2$-Agonists
Clonidine
Guanfacine
Methyldopa

Beta (Beta$_1$ and Beta$_2$)-Antagonists
Nadolol
Propranolol
Timolol

Beta$_1$-Antagonists (Selective)
Atenolol
Esmolol
Metoprolol

Mixed Alpha- / Beta-Antagonists
Carvedilol
Labetalol

Angiotensin-Converting Enzyme Inhibitors
Benazepril
Captopril
Enalapril/Enalaprilat
Fosinopril
Lisinopril

Angiotensin II Receptor Blockers
Irbesartan
Losartan
Valsartan

Calcium Channel Blockers
Amlodipine
Diltiazem
Isradipine
Nicardipine
Nifedipine
Verapamil

Diuretics
Amiloride
Bumetanide
Chlorothiazide
Ethacrynic acid
Furosemide
Hydrochlorothiazide
Metolazone
Spironolactone
Torsemide
Triamterene

Nitrates
Nitroglycerin

Vasodilators (Direct-Acting)
Hydralazine
Minoxidil
Nitroprusside

NEW YORK HEART ASSOCIATION (NYHA) CLASSIFICATION OF FUNCTIONAL CAPACITY OF PATIENTS WITH DISEASES OF THE HEART, 1994 REVISIONS

Class I

Patients with cardiac disease but without resulting limitation of physical activity. Ordinary physical activity does not cause undue fatigue, palpitation, dyspnea, or anginal pain.

Class II

Patients with cardiac disease resulting in slight limitation of physical activity. They are comfortable at rest. Ordinary physical activity results in fatigue, palpitation, dyspnea, or anginal pain.

Class III

Patients with cardiac disease resulting in marked limitation of physical activity. They are comfortable at rest. Less than ordinary activity causes fatigue, palpitation, dyspnea, or anginal pain.

Class IV

Patients with cardiac disease resulting in inability to carry on any physical activity without discomfort. Symptoms of heart failure or the anginal syndrome may be present even at rest. If any physical activity is undertaken, discomfort increases.

Reference

The Criteria Committee of the New York Heart Association, *Nomenclature and Criteria for Diagnosis of Diseases of the Heart and Great Vessels*, 9th ed, Boston, MA: Little, Brown & Co, 1994, 253-6.

WORLD HEALTH ORGANIZATION (WHO) FUNCTIONAL CLASSIFICATION OF PULMONARY HYPERTENSION

Class I

Patients with pulmonary hypertension but without resulting limitation of physical activity. Ordinary physical activity does not cause undue dyspnea or fatigue, chest pain, or near syncope.

Class II

Patients with pulmonary hypertension resulting in slight limitation of physical activity. They are comfortable at rest. Ordinary physical activity causes undue dyspnea or fatigue, chest pain, or near syncope.

Class III

Patients with pulmonary hypertension resulting in marked limitation of physical activity. They are comfortable at rest. Less than ordinary activity causes undue dyspnea or fatigue, chest pain, or near syncope.

Class IV

Patients with pulmonary hypertension with inability to carry out any physical activity without symptoms. These patients manifest signs of right heart failure. Dyspnea and/or fatigue may be present even at rest. Discomfort is increased by any physical activity.

Reference

Widlitz A and Barst RJ, "Pulmonary Arterial Hypertension in Children," *Eur Respir J*, 2003, 21(1):155-76.

ANTIDEPRESSANT AGENTS

Comparison of Usual Adult Dosage, Mechanism of Action, and Adverse Effects

Drug	Initial Adult Dose	Usual Adult Dosage (mg/d)	Dosage Forms	ACH	Drowsiness	Orthostatic Hypotension	Conduction Abnormalities[1]	GI Distress	Weight Gain	Comments
Tricyclic Antidepressants and Related Compounds										
Amitriptyline	25-75 mg qhs	100-300	T	4+	4+	3+	3+	1+	4+	Also used in chronic pain, migraine, and as a hypnotic; contraindicated with cisapride
Amoxapine	50 mg bid	100-400	T	2+	2+	2+	2+	0	2+	May cause extrapyramidal symptom (EPS)
ClomiPRAMINE[2] (Anafranil®)	25-75 mg qhs	100-250	C	4+	4+	2+	3+	1+	4+	Only approved for OCD
Desipramine (Norpramin®)	25-75 mg qhs	100-300	T	1+	2+	2+	2+	0	1+	Blood levels useful for therapeutic monitoring
Doxepin	25-75 mg qhs	100-300	C, L	3+	4+	2+	2+	0	4+	
Imipramine (Tofranil®, Tofranil-PM®)	25-75 mg qhs	100-300	T, C	3+	3+	4+	3+	1+	4+	Blood levels useful for therapeutic monitoring
Maprotiline	25-75 mg qhs	100-225	T	2+	3+	2+	2+	0	2+	
Nortriptyline (Pamelor®)	25-50 mg qhs	50-150	C, L	2+	2+	1+	2+	0	1+	Blood levels useful for therapeutic monitoring
Protriptyline (Vivactil®)	15 mg qAM	15-60	T	2+	1+	2+	3+	1+	1+	
Trimipramine (Surmontil®)	25-75 mg qhs	100-300	C	4+	4+	3+	3+	0	4+	
Selective Serotonin Reuptake Inhibitors[3]										
Citalopram (Celexa®)	20 mg qAM	20-60	T, L	0	0	0	0	3+[4]	1+	
Escitalopram (Lexapro®)	10 mg qAM	10-20	T, L	0	0	0	0	3+	1+	S-enantiomer of citalopram
FLUoxetine (Prozac®, Prozac® Weekly™, Sarafem®, Selfemra™)	10-20 mg qAM	20-80	C, CDR, L, T	0	0	0	0	3+[4]	1+	CYP2B6 and 2D6 inhibitor
Fluvoxamine[2] (Luvox® CR)	50 mg qhs	100-300	T, CXR	0	0	0	0	3+[4]	1+	Contraindicated with pimozide, thioridazine, mesoridazine; CYP1A2, 2B6, 2C19, and 3A4 inhibitors
PARoxetine (Paxil®, Paxil CR®, Pexeva®)	10-20 mg qAM	20-50	T, CXR, L	1+	1+	0	0	3+[4]	2+	CYP2B6 and 2D6 inhibitor
Sertraline (Zoloft®)	25-50 mg qAM	50-200	T, L	0	0	0	0	3+[4]	1+	CYP2B6 and 2C19 inhibitor
Dopamine-Reuptake Blocking Compounds										
BuPROPion (Aplenzin™, Budeprion SR®, Budeprion XL®, Wellbutrin®, Wellbutrin SR®, Wellbutrin XL®)	100 mg bid-tid IR[5] 150 mg qAM-bid SR[6]	300-450[7]	T, TSR, TXR	0	0	0	1+/0	1+	0	Contraindicated with seizures, bulimia, and anorexia; low incidence of sexual dysfunction IR: A 6-h interval between doses preferred SR: An 8-h interval between doses preferred XL: Administer once daily

Comparison of Usual Adult Dosage, Mechanism of Action, and Adverse Effects *continued*

Drug	Initial Adult Dose	Usual Adult Dosage (mg/d)	Dosage Forms	ACH	Drowsiness	Orthostatic Hypotension	Conduction Abnormalities[8]	GI Distress	Weight Gain	Comments
Serotonin / Norepinephrine Reuptake Inhibitors[8]										
DULoxetine (Cymbalta®)	40-60 mg/d	40-60	CDR	1+	1+	0	1+	3+	0	Also indicated for GAD, management of pain associated with diabetic neuropathy, and management of fibromyalgia
Desvenlafaxine (Pristiq®)	50 mg/d	50-100	TXR	0	1+	1+	0	3+[4]	0	Active metabolite of venlafaxine
Milnacipran[9] (Savella™)	12.5 mg/d	100-200	T	2+	1+	0	1+	3+	0	Only indicated for fibromyalgia
Venlafaxine (Effexor®, Effexor XR®)	25 mg bid-tid IR / 37.5 mg qd XR	75-375 IR / 75-225 XR	T, TXR, CXR	1+	1+	0	1+	3+[4]	0	High-dose may be useful to treat refractory depression; frequency of hypertension increases with dosage >225 mg/d
5-HT$_2$ Receptor Antagonist Properties										
Nefazodone	100 mg bid	300-600	T	1+	1+	2+	1+	1+	0	Contraindicated with carbamazepine, pimozide, astemizole, cisapride, and terfenadine; caution with triazolam and alprazolam; low incidence of sexual dysfunction
TraZODone	50 mg tid	150-600	T	0	4+	3+	1+	1+	2+	
Noradrenergic Antagonist										
Mirtazapine (Remeron®, Remeron SolTab®)	15 mg qhs	15-45	T, TOD	1+	3+	1+	1+	0	3+	Dose >15 mg/d less sedating, low incidence of sexual dysfunction

Comparison of Usual Adult Dosage, Mechanism of Action, and Adverse Effects *continued*

Drug	Initial Adult Dose	Usual Adult Dosage (mg/d)	Dosage Forms	Adverse Effects						Comments
				ACH	Drowsiness	Orthostatic Hypotension	Conduction Abnormalities	GI Distress	Weight Gain	
Monoamine Oxidase Inhibitors										
Isocarboxazid (Marplan®)	10 mg tid	10-30	T	2+	2+	2+	1+	1+	2+	Diet must be low in tyramine; contraindicated with sympathomimetics and other antidepressants
Phenelzine (Nardil®)	15 mg tid	15-90	T	2+	2+	2+	0	1+	3+	
Tranylcypromine (Parnate®)	10 mg bid	10-60	T	2+	1+	2+	1+	1+	2+	
Selegiline (EmSam®)	6 mg/d	6-12	Trans-dermal	2+	1+	2+	0	1+	0	Low tyramine diet not required for 6 mg/d dosage

ACH = anticholinergic effects (dry mouth, blurred vision, urinary retention, constipation); 0 - 4+ = absent or rare - relatively common. T = tablet, TSR = tablet, sustained release, TXR - tablet, extended release, TOD = tablet, orally disintegrating, L = liquid, C = capsule, CDR = capsule, delayed release, CXR = capsule, extended release; IR = immediate release, SR = sustained release, XR = extended release.

[1]**Important note:** A 1-week supply taken all at once in a patient receiving the maximum dose can be fatal.

[2]Not approved by FDA for depression. Approved for OCD.

[3]Flat dose response curve, headache, nausea, and sexual dysfunction are common side effects for SSRIs.

[4]Nausea is usually mild and transient.

[5]IR: 100 mg bid, may be increased to 100 mg tid no sooner than 3 days after beginning therapy.

[6]SR: 150 mg qAM, may be increased to 150 mg bid as early as day 4 of dosing.

[7]To minimize seizure risk, do not exceed IR 150 mg/dose or SR 200 mg/dose.

[8]Do not use with sibutramine; relatively safe in overdose.

[9]Milnacipran is only approved for fibromyalgia.

CORTICOSTEROIDS

Corticosteroids, Systemic Equivalencies

Glucocorticoid	Approximate Equivalent Dose (mg)	Routes of Administration	Relative Anti-inflammatory Potency	Relative Mineralocorticoid Potency	Protein Binding (%)	Half-life Plasma (min)
Short-Acting						
Cortisone	25	P.O., I.M.	0.8	0.8	90	30
Hydrocortisone	20	I.M., I.V.	1	1	90	90
Intermediate-Acting						
Methylprednisolone[1]	4	P.O., I.M., I.V.	5	0	—	180
Prednisolone	5	P.O., I.M., I.V., intra-articular, intradermal, soft tissue injection	4	0.8	90-95	200
Prednisone	5	P.O.	4	0.8	70	60
Triamcinolone[1]	4	I.M., intra-articular, intradermal, intrasynovial, soft tissue injection	5	0	—	300
Long-Acting						
Betamethasone	0.75	P.O., I.M., intra-articular, intradermal, intrasynovial, soft tissue injection	25	0	64	100-300
Dexamethasone	0.75	P.O., I.M., I.V., intra-articular, intradermal, soft tissue injection	25-30	0	—	100-300
Mineralocorticoids						
Fludrocortisone	—	P.O.	10	125	42	200

[1]May contain propylene glycol as an excipient in injectable forms.

Reference
Asare K, "Diagnosis and Treatment of Adrenal Insufficiency in the Critically Ill Patient," *Pharmacotherapy,* 2007, 27(11):1512-28.

GUIDELINES FOR SELECTION AND USE OF TOPICAL CORTICOSTEROIDS

The quantity prescribed and the frequency of refills should be monitored to reduce the risk of adrenal suppression. In general, short courses of high-potency agents are preferable to prolonged use of low potency. After control is achieved, control should be maintained with a low potency preparation.

1. Low-to-medium potency agents are usually effective for treating thin, acute, inflammatory skin lesions; whereas, high or super-potent agents are often required for treating chronic, hyperkeratotic, or lichenified lesions.

2. Since the stratum corneum is thin on the face and intertriginous areas, low-potency agents are preferred but a higher potency agent may be used for 2 weeks.

3. Because the palms and soles have a thick stratum corneum, high or super-potent agents are frequently required.

4. Low potency agents are preferred for infants and the elderly. Infants have a high body surface area to weight ratio; elderly patients have thin, fragile skin.

5. The vehicle in which the topical corticosteroid is formulated influences the absorption and potency of the drug. Ointment bases are preferred for thick, lichenified lesions; they enhance penetration of the drug. Creams are preferred for acute and subacute dermatoses; they may be used on moist skin areas or intertriginous areas. Solutions, gels, and sprays are preferred for the scalp or for areas where a nonoil-based vehicle is needed.

6. In general, super-potent agents should not be used for longer than 2-3 weeks unless the lesion is limited to a small body area. Medium-to-high potency agents usually cause only rare adverse effects when treatment is limited to 3 months or less, and use on the face and intertriginous areas are avoided. If long-term treatment is needed, intermittent vs continued treatment is recommended.

7. Most preparations are applied once or twice daily. More frequent application may be necessary for the palms or soles because the preparation is easily removed by normal activity and penetration is poor due to a thick stratum corneum. Every-other-day or weekend-only application may be effective for treating some chronic conditions.

Corticosteroids, Topical

Steroid		Dosage Form
Very High Potency		
0.05%	Betamethasone dipropionate, augmented	Cream, gel, lotion, ointment
0.05%	Clobetasol propionate	Cream, foam, gel, lotion, ointment, shampoo, spray
0.05%	Diflorasone diacetate	Ointment
0.05%	Halobetasol propionate	Cream, ointment
High Potency		
0.1%	Amcinonide	Cream, ointment, lotion
0.05%	Betamethasone dipropionate, augmented	Cream
0.05%	Betamethasone dipropionate	Cream, ointment
0.1%	Betamethasone valerate	Ointment
0.05%	Desoximetasone	Gel
0.25%	Desoximetasone	Cream, ointment
0.05%	Diflorasone diacetate	Cream, ointment
0.05%	Fluocinonide	Cream, ointment, gel
0.1%	Halcinonide	Cream, ointment
0.5%	Triamcinolone acetonide	Cream, spray
Intermediate Potency		
0.05%	Betamethasone dipropionate	Lotion
0.1%	Betamethasone valerate	Cream
0.1%	Clocortolone pivalate	Cream
0.05%	Desoximetasone	Cream
0.025%	Fluocinolone acetonide	Cream, ointment
0.05%	Flurandrenolide	Cream, ointment, lotion, tape
0.005%	Fluticasone propionate	Ointment
0.05%	Fluticasone propionate	Cream, lotion
0.1%	Hydrocortisone butyrate[1]	Ointment, solution
0.2%	Hydrocortisone valerate[1]	Cream, ointment
0.1%	Mometasone furoate[1]	Cream, ointment, lotion
0.1%	Prednicarbate	Cream, ointment
0.025%	Triamcinolone acetonide	Cream, ointment, lotion
0.1%	Triamcinolone acetonide	Cream, ointment, lotion
Low Potency		
0.05%	Alclometasone dipropionate[1]	Cream, ointment
0.05%	Desonide	Cream, ointment

Corticosteroids, Topical *(continued)*

Steroid		Dosage Form
0.01%	Fluocinolone acetonide	Cream, solution
0.5%	Hydrocortisone[1]	Cream, ointment, lotion
0.5%	Hydrocortisone acetate[1]	Cream, ointment
1%	Hydrocortisone acetate[1]	Cream, ointment
1%	Hydrocortisone[1]	Cream, ointment, lotion, solution
2.5%	Hydrocortisone[1]	Cream, ointment, lotion

[1]Not fluorinated.

INTRAVENOUS IMMUNE GLOBULIN

Brand Name	FDA-Approved Indications	Labeled Contraindications	IgA Content	Half-Life	pH	Osmolarity / Osmolality	Recommended Infusion Rates	Additional Comments
Carimune® NF	Primary immunodeficiency; ITP	IgA deficiency with IgA antibody; severe systemic reaction to human immune globulins	720 mcg/mL	3 weeks	6.4-6.8	3% solution in NS: 498 mOsmol/kg; 6% solution in NS: 690 mOsmol/kg; 9% solution in NS: 882 mOsmol/kg; 12% solution in NS: 1074 mOsmol/kg; 3% solution in D$_5$W: 444 mOsmol/kg; 6% solution in D$_5$W: 636 mOsmol/kg; 9% solution in D$_5$W: 828 mOsmol/kg; 12% solution in D$_5$W: 1020 mOsmol/kg; 3% solution in SWFI: 192 mOsmol/kg; 6% solution in SWFI: 384 mOsmol/kg; 9% solution in SWFI: 576 mOsmol/kg; 12% solution in SWFI: 768 mOsmol/kg	Initial (3% solution): 0.5-1 mL/min; Maximum (3% solution): 2 mg/kg/min	Contains sucrose
Flebogamma®	Primary immunodeficiency	IgA deficiency with IgA antibody; history of anaphylaxis with immune globulin	<50 mcg/mL	30-32 days	5-6	240-370 mOsmol/L	Initial (5% solution): 0.01 mL/kg/min (0.5 mg/kg/min); Maximum (5% solution): 0.1 mL/kg/min (5 mg/kg/min); Maximum in patients with renal dysfunction (5% solution): 0.06 mL/kg/min (3 mg/kg/min)	Contains sorbitol
Gammagard Liquid	Primary immunodeficiency	IgA deficiency, history of anaphylaxis with immune globulin	37 mcg/mL	35 days	4.6-5.1	240-300 mOsmol/kg	Initial (10% solution): 0.5 mL/kg/h (0.8 mg/kg/min); Maximum (10% solution): 5 mL/kg/h (8.9 mg/kg/min); <2 mL/kg/h (3.3 mg/kg/min) in patients at risk for renal impairment or thrombosis	
Gammagard S/D	Primary immunodeficiency, ITP, CLL, Kawasaki syndrome	IgA deficiency	≤1 mcg/mL	~23-53 days	6.4-7.2		Initial (5% solution): 0.5 mL/kg/h; Maximum (5% solution): 4 mL/kg/h; Maximum concentration for infusion: 10%	Contains glucose
Gamunex®	Primary immunodeficiency, ITP, chronic inflammatory demyelinating polyneuropathy (CIDP)	IgA deficiency with IgA antibody; history of anaphylaxis with immune globulin	46 mcg/mL	35 days	4-4.5	258 mOsmol/kg	Initial (10% solution): 0.01 mL/kg/min; Maximum (10% solution): 0.08 mL/kg/min; Maximum concentration for infusion: 10%	

Brand Name	FDA-Approved Indications	Labeled Contraindications	IgA Content	Half-Life	pH	Osmolarity / Osmolality	Recommended Infusion Rates	Additional Comments
Octagam®	Primary immunodeficiency	IgA deficiency with IgA antibody	≤200 mcg/mL	Immunodeficiency: 40 days	5.1-6.0	310-380 mOsmol/kg	Initial: 30 mg/kg/h (0.01 mL/kg/min) Maximum: <200 mg/kg/h (<0.07 mL/kg/min) Maximum concentration for infusion: 5%	Contains maltose
Privigen®	Primary immunodeficiency, ITP	IgA deficiency; history of anaphylaxis with immune globulin; hyperprolinemia	≤25 mcg/mL	~37 days	4.6-5	240-440 mOsmol/kg	Initial: 0.5 mg/kg/min (0.005 mL/kg/min) Maximum primary immunodeficiency: 8 mg/kg/min (0.08 mL/kg/min; ITP: 4 mg/kg/min (0.04 mL/kg/min) Maximum concentration for solution: 10%	L-proline

Carimune® NF prescribing information, ZLB Behring LLC, Kankakee, IL, January 2005.

Flebogamma® 5% prescribing information, Grifols Biologicals, Inc, Los Angeles, CA, December 2009.

Gammagard Liquid prescribing information, Baxter Healthcare Corporation, Westlake Village, CA, April 2005.

Gammagard S/D prescribing information, Baxter Healthcare Corporation, Westlake Village, CA, March 2007.

Gamunex® prescribing information, Talecris Biotherapeutics, Inc, Research Triangle Park, NC, September 2008.

Octagam® prescribing information, Octapharma USA, Inc, Centreville, VA, March 2007.

Privigen® prescribing information, CSL Behring, King of Prussia, PA, July 2007

MULTIVITAMIN PRODUCTS

Injectable Formulations

Product	A (int. units)	B₁ (mg)	B₂ (mg)	B₆ (mg)	B₁₂ (mcg)	C (mg)	D (int. units)	E (int. units)	K (mcg)	Additional Information
Solution										
Infuvite® Adult (*per 10 mL*)	3300	6	3.6	6	5	200	200	10	150	Supplied as two 5 mL vials. Biotin 60 mcg, folic acid 600 mcg, niacinamide 40 mg, dexpanthenol 15 mg
Infuvite® Pediatric (*per 5 mL*)	2300	1.2	1.4	1	1	80	400	7	200	Supplied as one 4 mL vial and one 1 mL vial. Biotin 20 mcg, folic acid 140 mcg, niacinamide 17 mg, dexpanthenol 5 mg
M.V.I.®-12 (*per 10 mL*)	3300	3	3.6	4	12.5	100	200	10	–	Supplied as a single 2-chambered 10 mL vial. Biotin 60 mcg, folic acid 400 mcg, niacinamide 40 mg, dexpanthenol 15 mg
M.V.I. Adult™ (*per 10 mL*)	3300	6	3.6	6	5	200	200	10	150	Supplied as two 5 mL vials or a single 2-chambered 10 mL vial. Also available in a pharmacy bulk package (two 50 mL vials). Biotin 60 mcg, folic acid 600 mcg, niacinamide 40 mg, dexpanthenol 15 mg
Powder for Reconstitution										
M.V.I.® Pediatric	2300	1.2	1.4	1	1	80	400	7	200	Biotin 20 mcg, folic acid 140 mcg, niacinamide 17 mg, dexpanthenol 5 mg, aluminum, polysorbate 80

Adult Formulations

Product	A (int. units)	B$_1$ (mg)	B$_2$ (mg)	B$_6$ (mg)	B$_{12}$ (mcg)	C (mg)	D (int. units)	E (int. units)	Additional Information
Caplet									
Glutofac®-ZX	5000	20	20	25	2500	200	400	100	Biotin 200 mcg, Cr 200 mcg, Cu 2.5 mg, folic acid 2800 mcg, lutein 500 mcg, lycopene 500 mcg, Mg 100 mg, Mn 2.5 mg, niacinamide 100 mg, pantothenic acid 10 mg, Se 100 mcg, Zn 15 mg
Renax®		3	2	15	12	50		35	Biotin 300 mcg, folic acid 2.5 mg, niacinamide 20 mg, pantothenic acid 10 mg, Se 70 mcg, Zn 20 mg
Renax® 5.5		3	2	30	1	100		35	Biotin 300 mcg, folic acid 5.5 mg, niacinamide 20 mg, pantothenic acid 10 mg, Se 70 mcg, Zn 20 mg
Strovite® Advance	3000	20	5	25	50	300	400	100	Alpha-lipoic acid 15 mg, biotin 100 mcg, Cu 1.5 mg, folic acid 1 mg, lutein 5 mg, Mg 50 mg, Mn 1.5 mg, niacinamide 25 mg, pantothenic acid 15 mg, Se 100 mcg, Zn 25 mg
Strovite Forte®	4000	20	20	25	50	500	400	60	Biotin 0.15 mg, Cr 0.05 mg, Cu 3 mg, Fe (as ferrous fumarate) 10 mg, folic acid 1 mg, Mg 50 mg, Mo 20 mcg, niacinamide 100 mg, pantothenic acid 25 mg, Se 50 mcg, Zn 15 mg; contains soy products
Strovite® Plus	5000	20	20	25	50	500		30	Biotin 0.15 mg, Cr 0.1 mcg, Cu 3 mg, Fe (as ferrous fumarate) 27 mg, folic acid 0.8 mg, Mg 50 mg, Mn 5 mg, niacinamide 100 mg, pantothenic acid 25 mg, Zn 22.5 mg; contains soy products
Viactiv® Calcium Flavor Glides™ [OTC]							200		Ca 500 mg, vitamin K 40 mcg; contains soy products
Viactiv® Flavor Glides™ [OTC]	2500	1.5	1.7	2	6	60	400	33	Biotin 30 mcg, Ca 200 mg, Cr 12 mcg, Cu 2 mg, Fe 18 mcg, folic acid 400 mcg, iodine 38 mcg, lutein 250 mcg, Mg 40 mg, Mn 2 mg, Mo 75 mcg, niacin 15 mg, pantothenic acid 10 mg, potassium 40 mg, Se 55 mcg, vitamin K 20 mcg, Zn 15 mg
Vitafol®	6000	1.1	1.8	2.5	5	60	400	30	Ca 125 mg, Fe [elemental] 65 mg, folic acid 1 mg, niacinamide 15 mg
Capsule									
Foltrin®				5	15	75			Fe [elemental] 110 mg, folic acid 0.5 mg, special liver-stomach concentrate 240 mg
Hemocyte Plus®		10	6	5	15	200			Cu 0.8 mg, Fe [elemental] 106 mg, folic acid 1 mg, Mg 6.9 mg, Mn 1.3 mg, niacinamide 30 mg, pantothenic acid 10 mg, Zn 18.2 mg
Ocuvite® Lutein [OCT]						60		30	Cu 2 mg, lutein 6 mg, Zn 15 mg
Replace [OTC] (*per 2 capsules*)	4500	25	25	25	500	100	1000	40	Bioflavonoid complex 50 mg, biotin 0.02 mg, boron 5 mg, Ca 0.09 g, Cr 50 mcg, Cu 0.1 mg, Fe (as peptonate) 10 mg, folic acid 0.4 mg, iodine 225 mcg, lycopene 2.5 mg, Mg 90 mg, Mn 2.5 mg, Mo 20 mcg, niacinamide 40 mg, pantothenic acid 75 mg, potassium 20 mg, Se 50 mcg, Zn 10 mg; gluten free, sugar free

Adult Formulations *continued*

Product	A (int. units)	B₁ (mg)	B₂ (mg)	B₆ (mg)	B₁₂ (mcg)	C (mg)	D (int. units)	E (int. units)	Additional Information
Replace Without Iron [OTC] (*per 2 capsules*)	4500	25	25	25	500	10	1000	40	Bioflavonoid complex 50 mg, biotin 0.02 mg, boron 5 mg, Ca 0.09 g, Cr 50 mcg, Cu 0.1 mg, folic acid 0.4 mg, iodine 225 mcg, lycopene 2.5 mg, Mg 90 mg, Mn 2.5 mg, Mo 20 mcg, niacinamide 40 mg, pantothenic acid 75 mg, potassium 20 mg, Se 50 mcg, Zn 10 mg; gluten free, sugar free
Tandem® Plus		10	6	5	15	200			Cu 0.8 mg, Fe (as ferrous fumarate) 53 mg, Fe (as polysaccharide) 53 mg, folic acid 1 mg, Mn 1.3 mg, niacinamide 30 mg, pantothenic acid 10 mg, Zn 18.2 mg
Capsule, Softgel									
Ocuvite® Adult 50+ [OTC]						150		30	Cu 1 mg, lutein 6 mg, omega-3 150 mg, Zn 9 mg; contains soy products
PreserVision® AREDS [OTC]	14,320					226		200	Cu 0.8 mg, Zn 34.8 mg; contains soy products
PreserVision® Lutein [OTC]						226		200	Cu 0.8 mg, lutein 5 mg, Zn 34.8 mg; contains soy products
SourceCF®	9000	1.5	1.7	1.9	6	100	400	200	Biotin 100 mcg, folic acid 200 mcg, niacinamide 20 mg, pantothenic acid 12 mg, vitamin K 500 mcg, Zn 10 mg; contains soy products
Liquid									
Centamin [OTC] (*per 15 mL*)	2500	1.5	1.7	2	6	60	400	30	Biotin 300 mcg, Fe 9 mg, iodine 150 mcg, niacin 20 mg, pantothenic acid 10 mg, Zn 3 mg (237 mL)
Centrum® [OTC] (*per 15 mL*)	1300	1.5	1.7	2	6	60	400	30	Biotin 300 mcg, Cr 25 mcg, Fe 9 mg, iodine 150 mcg, Mn 2 mg, Mo 25 mcg, niacin 20 mg, pantothenic acid 10 mg, Zn 3 mg; contains alcohol 5.7%, sodium benzoate (236 mL)
Drinkables® Fruits and Vegetables [OTC] (*per 1 oz*)	1812	100 mcg	100 mcg	100 mcg	0.2	38	142	11	Biotin 107 mcg, Ca 10 mg, choline 1 mg, Cr 43 mcg, Fe 360 mcg, folic acid 284 mcg, inositol 1 mg, lutein 100 mcg, lycopene 100 mcg, Mg 3 mg, Mn 1 mg, niacin 1 mg, PABA 1 mg, pantothenic acid 4 mg, phosphorus 15 mg, potassium 50 mg, vitamin K 28 mcg, proprietary blend 22 g (887 mL)
Drinkables® Multi Vitamins [OTC] (*per 1 oz*)	5000	1.5	1.7	2	6	80	400	30	Biotin 300 mcg, choline 3 mg, Cr 120 mcg, folic acid 400 mcg, inositol 3 mg, lutein 250 mcg, lycopene 300 mcg, Mn 2 mg, niacin 20 mg, PABA 3 mg, pantothenic acid 10 mg, vitamin K 80 mcg, proprietary trace mineral blend 252 mg (444 mL, 976 mL)
Geriation® [OTC] (*per 30 mL*)		5	2.5	1	1				Choline 100 mg, Fe 15 mg, iodine 100 mcg, Mg 2 mg, Mn 2 mg, niacinamide 50 mg, pantothenic acid 10 mg, Zn 2 mg (473 mL)
Geritol® Tonic [OTC] (*per 15 mL*)		2.5	2.5	0.5					Choline 50 mg, Fe 18 mg, methionine 25 mg, niacin 50 mg, pantothenic acid 2 mg (120 mL, 360 mL)
Strovite Forte® (*per 15 mL*)	4000	15	17	20	20	300	400	30	Biotin 150 mcg biotin, Cr 50 mcg chromium, Cu 3 mg copper, Fe (as ferrous gluconate) 10 mg, folic acid 1 mg, Mg 50 mg, Mn 5 mg, niacinamide 100 mg, pantothenic acid 25 mg, selenium 55 mcg, zinc 15 mg (480 mL)
Vitafol® (*per 5 mL*)			2	2	8.34				Fe [elemental] 10.4 mg, folic acid 0.25 mg, niacinamide 13.3 mg (473 mL)

Adult Formulations *continued*

Product	A (int. units)	B₁ (mg)	B₂ (mg)	B₆ (mg)	B₁₂ (mcg)	C (mg)	D (int. units)	E (int. units)	Additional Information
Soft Chews									
Viactiv® [OTC]	2500	1.5	1.7	2	6	60	400	33	Biotin 30 mcg, Ca 200 mg, folic acid 400 mcg, niacin 15 mg, pantothenic acid 10 mg; sodium 25 mg; contains soy products
Viactiv® for Teens [OTC]							200		Ca 500 mg, sodium 15 mg, vitamin K 40 mcg; contains soy products
Viactiv® With Calcium [OTC]							100		Ca 500 mg, sodium 10 mg, vitamin K 40 mcg; contains soy products
Tablet									
Androvite® [OTC] (*per 6 tablets*)	25,000	50	50	100	125	1000	400	400	Betaine 100 mg, biotin 125 mcg, boron 3 mg, Cr 200 mcg, Cu 2 mg, Fe (as amino acid chelate) 18 mg, folic acid 400 mcg, hesperidin 35 mg, inositol 36 mg, iodine 150 mcg, Mg 500 mg, Mn 10 mg, niacinamide 50 mg, PABA 25 mg, pancreatin 4X 75 mg, pantothenic acid 100 mg, rutin 25 mg, Se 200 mcg, Zn 50 mg
Centrum® [OTC]	3500	1.5	1.7	2	6	90	400	30	Biotin 30 mcg, boron 150 mcg, Ca 200 mg, chloride 72 mg, Cr 35 mcg, Cu 0.9 mg, Fe 18 mg, folic acid 500 mcg, iodine 150 mcg, lutein 250 mcg, lycopene 300 mcg, Mg 100 mg, Mn 2.3 mg, niacin 20 mg, nickel 5 mcg, potassium 80 mg, Se 55 mcg, silicon 2 mg, tin 10 mcg, vanadium 10 mcg, vitamin K 25 mcg, Zn 11 mg; contains sodium benzoate
Centrum Cardio® [OTC]	1750	0.75	0.85	2.5	100	30	400	15	Biotin 15 mcg, Ca 54 mg, chloride 29 mg, Cr 60 mcg, Cu 0.35 mg, Fe 3 mg, folic acid 200 mcg, iodine 75 mcg, Mg 20 mg, Mn 1 mg, Mo 37.5 mcg, niacin 10 mg, nickel 2.5 mcg, pantothenic acid 5 mg, phosphorus 40 mg, phytosterols 400 mg, potassium 32 mg, Se 10 mcg, silicon 1 mg, tin 5 mcg, vanadium 5 mcg, vitamin K 12.5 mcg, Zn 3.75 mg; contains sodium benzoate, soy products
Centrum Performance® [OTC]	3500	4.5	5.1	6	18	120	400	60	Biotin 50 mcg, boron 60 mcg, Ca 100 mg, chloride 72 mg, Cr 120 mcg, Cu 0.9 mg, Fe 18 mg, folic acid 400 mcg, ginseng root 50 mg, iodine 150 mcg, Mg 40 mg, Mn 4 mg, Mo 75 mcg, niacin 40 mg, nickel 5 mcg, pantothenic acid 12 mg, phosphorus 48 mg, potassium 80 mg, Se 70 mcg, silicon 4 mg, tin 10 mcg, vanadium 10 mcg, vitamin K 25 mcg, Zn 11 mg; contains sodium benzoate
Centrum® Silver® [OTC]	2500	1.5	1.7	3	25	90	500	50	Biotin 30 mcg, boron 150 mcg, Ca 220 mg, chloride 72 mg, Cr 45 mcg, Cu 0.9 mg, folic acid 400 mcg, iodine 150 mcg, lutein 250 mcg, lycopene 300 mcg, Mg 50 mg, Mn 2.3 mg, Mo 45 mcg, niacin 20 mg, nickel 5 mcg, pantothenic acid 10 mg, phosphorus 110 mg, potassium 80 mg, Se 55 mcg, silicon 2 mg, vanadium 10 mcg, vitamin K 30 mcg, Zn 11 mg; contains sodium benzoate
Centrum® Silver® Ultra Men's [OTC]	3500	1.5	1.7	6	100	120	600	60	Biotin 30 mcg, boron 150 mcg, Ca 250 mg, chloride 72 mg, Cr 60 mcg, Cu 0.7 mg, folic acid 300 mcg, iodine 150 mcg, lutein 300 mcg, lycopene 600 mcg, Mg 50 mg, Mn 4 mg, Mo 50 mcg, niacin 20 mg, nickel 5 mcg, pantothenic acid 10 mg, phosphorus 80 mg, potassium 80 mg, Se 100 mcg, silicon 2 mg, vanadium 10 mcg, vitamin K 60 mcg, Zn 15 mg; contains soy products

Adult Formulations *continued*

Product	A (int. units)	B₁ (mg)	B₂ (mg)	B₆ (mg)	B₁₂ (mcg)	C (mg)	D (int. units)	E (int. units)	Additional Information
Centrum® Silver® Ultra Women's [OTC]	3500	1.1	1.1	5	50	100	800	35	Biotin 30 mcg, boron 150 mcg, Ca 500 mg, chloride 72 mg, Cr 50 mcg, Cu 0.5 mg, Fe (as ferrous fumarate) 8 mg, folic acid 400 mcg, iodine 150 mcg, lutein 300 mcg, Mg 50 mg, Mn 2.3 mg, Mo 50 mcg, niacin 14 mg, nickel 5 mcg, pantothenic acid 5 mg, phosphorus 20 mg, potassium 80 mg, Se 55 mcg, silicon 2 mg, vanadium 10 mcg, vitamin K 50 mcg, Zn 15 mg; contains soy products
Centrum® Ultra Men's [OTC]	3500	1.2	1.3	2	6	90	600	45	Biotin 40 mcg, boron 150 mcg, Ca 210 mg, chloride 72 mg, Cr 35 mcg, Cu 0.9 mg, Fe (as ferrous fumarate) 8 mg, folic acid 200 mcg, iodine 150 mcg, lycopene 600 mcg, Mg 100 mg, Mn 2.3 mg, Mo 50 mcg, niacin 16 mg, nickel 5 mcg, pantothenic acid 15 mg, phosphorus 20 mg, potassium 80 mg, Se 100 mcg, silicon 2 mg, tin 10 mcg, vanadium 10 mcg, vitamin K 60 mcg, Zn 11 mg; contains soy products
Centrum® Ultra Women's [OTC]	3500	1.1	1.1	2	6	75	800	35	Biotin 40 mcg, boron 150 mcg, Ca 500 mg, chloride 72 mg, Cr 25 mcg, Cu 0.9 mg, Fe (as ferrous fumarate) 18 mg, folic acid 400 mcg, iodine 150 mcg, Mg 100 mg, Mn 1.8 mg, Mo 50 mcg, niacin 14 mg, nickel 5 mcg, pantothenic acid 15 mg, phosphorus 20 mg, potassium 80 mg, Se 55 mcg, silicon 2 mg, tin 10 mcg, vanadium 10 mcg, vitamin K 50 mcg, Zn 8 mg; contains soy products
Diatx®ZN		1.5	1.5	50	2 mg	60			Biotin 300 mcg, Cu 1.5 mg, folic acid 5 mg, niacinamide 20 mg, pantothenic acid 10 mg, Zn 25 mg; gluten free, sugar free
Freedavite [OTC]	5000	1.5	1.7	2	6	60	400	30	Biotin 30 mcg, Ca 20 mg, Cu 0.1 mg, Fe (as ferrous fumarate) 1.8 mg, folic acid 400 mcg, iodine 75 mcg, Mg 8 mg, Mn 0.625 mg, niacinamide 20 mg, pantothenic acid 10 mg, Se 35 mcg, Zn 1.5 mg
Geri-Freeda [OTC]	5000	15	15	15	15	150	400	15	Betaine 10 mg, biotin 15 mcg, Ca 50 mg, choline 10 mg, Cr 60 mcg, Cu 0.5 mg, folic acid 400 mcg, hesperidin 10 mg, inositol 25 mg, iodine 150 mcg, L-lysine 25 mg, Mg 25 mg, Mn 1 mg, niacinamide 50 mg, PABA 10 mg, pantothenic acid 15 mg, Se 35 mcg, Zn 7.5 mg
Geritol Complete® [OTC]	6100	1.5	1.7	2	6.7	57	400	30	Biotin 44 mcg, Ca 148 mg, chloride 20 mg, Cr 12 mcg, Cu 1.8 mg, Fe 16 mg, folic acid 0.38 mg, iodine 120 mcg, Mg 86 mg, Mn 2.4 mg, Mo 1 mcg, niacin 20 mg, pantothenic acid 13 mg, phosphorus 118 mg, potassium 36 mg, selenium 1 mcg, vitamin K 24 mcg, Zn 13.5 mg
Geritol Extend® [OTC]	3333	1.2	1.3	2	2.5	55	200	13	Ca 120 mg, Fe 9.5 mg, folic acid 0.2 mg, iodine 130 mcg, Mg 32 mg, niacin 15 mg, phosphorous 98 mg, Se 35 mcg, vitamin K 80 mcg, Zn 14 mg
Gynovite® Plus [OTC] (*per 6 tablets*)	5000	10	10	20	125	180	400	400	Betaine 100 mg, biotin 125 mcg, boron 3 mg, Ca 500 mg, Cu 2 mg, Fe (as amino acid chelate) 18 mg, folic acid 400 mcg, hesperidin 35 mg, inositol 50 mg, iodine 150 mcg, Mg 600 mg, Mn 10 mg, niacinamide 20 mg, PABA 25 mg, pancreatin 4X 93 mg, pantothenic acid 10 mg, rutin 25 mg, Se 200 mcg, Zn 15 mg

Adult Formulations *continued*

Product	A (int. units)	B$_1$ (mg)	B$_2$ (mg)	B$_6$ (mg)	B$_{12}$ (mcg)	C (mg)	D (int. units)	E (int. units)	Additional Information
Hi-Kovite [OTC] (*per contents of 1 vitamin tablet plus 1 mineral tablet*)	5000	10	10	10	10	200	400	30	Bioflavonoids 10 mg, biotin 30 mcg, Ca 120 mg, Cu 0.5 mg, Fe (as ferrous fumarate) 9 mg, folic acid 400 mcg, inositol 10 mg, iodine 75 mcg, L-lysine 10 mg, Mg 60 mg, Mn 1 mg, niacinamide 100 mg, PABA 10 mg, pantothenic acid 10 mg, potassium 35 mg, Se 17.5 mcg, Zn 7.5 mg
Iberet®-500		4.96	5.4	3.7	22.5	500			Iron 95 mg, niacin 27.2 mg, pantothenic acid 8.28 mg, sodium 65 mg
Monocaps [OTC]	5000	15	15	15	15	120	400	15	Biotin 15 mcg, Ca 50 mg, Cu 0.1 mg, Fe (as ferrous fumarate) 14 mg, folic acid 400 mcg, iodine 150 mcg, lecithin 10 mg, L-lysine 10 mg, Mg 30 mg, Mn 1 mg, niacinamide 40 mg, PABA 10 mg, pantothenic acid 15 mg, Se 35 mcg, Zn 3.75 mg
Myadec® [OTC]	5000	1.7	2	3	6	60	400	30	Biotin 30 mcg, boron 150 mcg, Ca 162 mg, chloride 36 mg, Cr 25 mcg, Cu 2 mg, Fe 18 mg, folic acid 400 mcg, iodine 150 mcg, Mg 100 mg, Mn 2.5 mg, Mo 25 mcg, niacin 20 mg, nickel 5 mcg, pantothenic acid 10 mg, phosphorus 125 mg, potassium 40 mg, Se 25 mcg, silicon 10 mcg, tin 10 mcg, vanadium 10 mcg, vitamin K 25 mcg, Zn 15 mg; contains soy products
Nutramin-Plus [OTC]	5000	15	15	30	50	75	400	30	Biotin 50 mcg, Ca 100 mg, Cr 1 mg, Cu 1 mg, Fe (as ferrous gluconate) 18 mg, folic acid 400 mcg, iodine 150 mcg, Mg 25 mg, Mn 10 mg, niacin 20 mg, pantothenic acid 25 mg, phosphorus 50 mg, Se 20 mg, Zn 15 mg; sugar free
Ocuvite® [OTC]	1000					200		60	Cu 2 mg, lutein 2 mg, Se 55 mcg, Zn 40 mg
Ocuvite® Extra [OTC]	1000		3			300		100	Cu 2 mg, L-glutathione 5 mg, lutein 2 mg, Mn 5 mg, niacinamide 40 mg, Se 55 mcg, Zn 40 mg
One A Day® Cholesterol Plus [OTC]	2500	1.5	1.7	2	6	60	400	30	Biotin 50 mcg, boron 150 mcg, Ca 100 mg, Cr 120 mcg, Cu 2 mg, folic acid 400 mcg, iodine 150 mcg, Mg 100 mg, Mn 2 mg, Mo 75 mcg, niacin 20 mg, pantothenic acid 10 mg, phytosterols 100 mg, potassium 99 mg, Se 70 mcg, Zn 15 mg; contains soy products
One A Day® Energy [OTC]	3500	3	3.4	4	12	60	400	30	Biotin 300 mcg, boron 150 mcg, Ca 250 mg, chloride 90 mg, Cr 100 mcg, Cu 2 mg, Fe 9 mg, folic acid 400 mcg, guarana blend 200 mg, iodine 150 mcg, Mg 40 mg, Mn 2 mg, Mo 25 mcg, niacin 40 mg, nickel 5 mcg, pantothenic acid 10 mg, potassium 99 mg, Se 45 mcg, silicon 5 mg, tin 10 mcg, vanadium 10 mcg, vitamin K 25 mcg, Zn 15 mg; contains soy products
One A Day® Essential [OTC]	3000	1.5	1.7	2	6	60	400	30	Ca 45 mg, folic acid 400 mcg, niacin 20 mg, pantothenic acid 10 mg; contains soy products
One A Day® Maximum [OTC]	2500	1.5	1.7	2	6	60	400	30	Biotin 30 mcg, boron 150 mcg, Ca 162 mg, chloride 72 mg, Cr 65 mcg, Cu 2 mg, Fe 18 mg, folic acid 400 mcg, iodine 150 mcg, Mg 100 mg, Mn 3.5 mg, Mo 160 mcg, niacin 20 mg, nickel 5 mcg, pantothenic acid 10 mg, phosphorus 109 mg, potassium 80 mg, Se 20 mg, silicon 2 mg, tin 10 mcg, vanadium 10 mcg, vitamin K 25 mcg, Zn 15 mg; contains soy products

Adult Formulations *continued*

Product	A (int. units)	B₁ (mg)	B₂ (mg)	B₆ (mg)	B₁₂ (mcg)	C (mg)	D (int. units)	E (int. units)	Additional Information
One A Day® Men's 50+ Advantage [OTC]	2500	4.5	3.4	6	25	120	400	33	Biotin 30 mcg, Ca 120 mcg, Cr 180 mcg, Cu 2 mg, folic acid 400 mcg, ginko biloba extract 120 mg, iodine 150 mcg, lycopene 600 mcg, Mg 100 mg, Mn 4 mg, molybdenum 90 mcg, niacin 20 mg, pantothenic acid 15 mg, potassium 40 mg, Se 105 mcg, vitamin K 20 mcg, Zn 22.5 mg
One A Day® Men's Health Formula [OTC]	3500	1.2	1.7	3	18	90	400	45	Biotin 30 mcg, Ca 210 mg, Cr 120 mcg, Cu 2 mg, folic acid 400 mcg, lycopene 600 mcg, Mg 120 mg, Mn 2 mg, niacin 16 mg, pantothenic acid 5 mg, potassium 100 mg, Se 105 mcg, vitamin K 20 mcg, Zn 15 mg; contains soy products
One A Day® Teen Advantage for Her [OTC]	2500	2.3	2.6	3	9	120	800	30	Biotin 300 mcg, Ca 300 mg, Cr 120 mcg, Cu 2 mg, Fe 18 mg, folic acid 400 mcg, Mg 50 mg, Mn 2 mg, niacin 30 mg, pantothenic acid 10 mg, Se 20 mcg, vitamin K 25 mcg, Zn 15 mg; contains soy products
One A Day® Teen Advantage for Him [OTC]	2500	3.75	4.25	5	15	120	400	30	Biotin 300 mcg, Ca 200 mg, Cr 120 mcg, Cu 2 mg, Fe 9 mg, folic acid 400 mcg, Mg 100 mg, Mn 2 mg, niacin 30 mg, pantothenic acid 10 mg, Se 20 mcg, vitamin K 25 mcg, Zn 15 mg; contains soy products
One A Day® WeightSmart® Advanced [OTC]	2500	1.9	2.1	2.5	7.5	60	400	30	Ca 200 mg, Cr 200 mcg, Cu 2 mg, Fe 18 mg, folic acid 400 mcg, green tea/cayenne blend 10 mg, guarana blend 180 mg, Mg 50 mg, Mn 2 mg, niacin 25 mg, pantothenic acid 12.5 mg, Se 70 mcg, vitamin K 80 mcg, Zn 15 mg; contains soy products
One A Day® Women's [OTC]	2500	1.5	1.7	2	6	60	800	30	Biotin 30 mcg, Ca 450 mg, Cr 120 mcg, Cu 2 mg, Fe 18 mg, folic acid 400 mcg, Mg 50 mg, Mn 2 mg, niacin 10 mg, pantothenic acid 5 mg, Se 20 mcg, vitamin K 25 mcg, Zn 15 mg; contains soy products, tartrazine
One A Day® Women's 50+ Advantage [OTC]	2500	4.5	3.4	6	25	60	800	33	Biotin 30 mcg, Ca 405 mg, Cr 180 mcg, Cu 2 mg, folic acid 400 mcg, ginkgo biloba extract 120 mg, iodine 150 mcg, Mg 50 mg, Mn 4 mg, Mo 90 mcg, niacin 20 mg, pantothenic acid 15 mg, Se 20 mcg, vitamin K 20 mcg, Zn 22.5 mg; contains soy products, tartrazine
One A Day® Women's Active Mind & Body [OTC]	2500	2.4	2.7	3.2	9.5	60	800	30	Biotin 30 mcg, Ca 300 mg, Cr 120 mcg, Cu 2 mg, Fe 18 mg, folic acid 400 mcg, guarana blend 180 mg, Mg 50 mg, Mn 2 mg, niacin 10 mg, pantothenic acid 5 mg, Se 20 mcg, vitamin K 25 mcg, Zn 15 mg; contains tartrazine
Optivite® P.M.T. [OTC] (*per 6 tablets*)	12,500	25	25	300	60	1500	100	100	Betaine 100 mg, bioflavonoids 250 mg, biotin 60 mg, Ca 125 mg, choline 313 mg, Cr 100 mcg, Fe (as amino acid chelate) 15 mg, folic acid 200 mcg, inositol 24 mg, iodine 75 mcg, Mg 250 mg, Mn 10 mg, niacinamide 25 mg, PABA 25 mg, pancreatin 4X 93 mg, pantothenic acid 25 mg, potassium 48 mg, rutin 25 mg, Se 100 mcg, Zn 25 mg
PreserVision® AREDS [OTC] (*per 2 tablets*)	14,320					226		200	Cu 0.8 mg, Zn 34.8 mg
Quintabs [OTC]	5000	30	30	30	30	300	400	50	Biotin 30 mcg, folic acid 400 mcg, niacinamide 100 mg, pantothenic acid 30 mg

Adult Formulations *continued*

Product	A (int. units)	B₁ (mg)	B₂ (mg)	B₆ (mg)	B₁₂ (mcg)	C (mg)	D (int. units)	E (int. units)	Additional Information
Quintabs-M [OTC]	5000	30	30	30	30	300	400	50	Biotin 30 mcg, Ca 30 mg, Cu 0.2 mg, Fe (as ferrous fumarate) 10 mg, folic acid 400 mcg, iodine 150 mcg, Mg 15 mg, Mn 2 mg, niacinamide 100 mg, PABA 10 mg, pantothenic acid 30 mg, Se 35 mcg, Zn 7.5 mg
Quintabs-M Iron-Free [OTC]	5000	30	30	30	30	300	400	50	Biotin 30 mcg, Ca 30 mg, Cu 0.2 mg, folic acid 400 mcg, iodine 150 mcg, Mg 15 mg, Mn 2 mg, niacinamide 100 mg, PABA 10 mg, pantothenic acid 30 mg, Se 35 mcg, Zn 7.5 mg
Repliva 21/7®					10	140 mg as ascorbic acid 60 mg as Ester-C® supplement			Fe [elemental] 151 mg, folic acid 1 mg, succinic acid 150 mg
Strovite®		15	15	4	5	500			Ca 18 mg, folic acid 0.5 mg, niacinamide 100 mg
T-Vites [OTC]		25	25	25	30	100	400		Biotin 30 mcg, folic acid 400 mcg, Mg 100 mg, Mn 0.5 mg, niacinamide 150 mg, pantothenic acid 25 mg, potassium 35 mg, Zn 3.75 mg
Ultra Freeda A-Free [OTC] (*per 3 tablets*)		50	50	50	100	1000	400	200	Base (choline, inositol, PABA) 100 mg, bioflavonoids 100 mg, biotin 300 mcg, Ca 250 mg, Cr 200 mcg, Fe (as ferrous fumarate) 18 mg, folic acid 800 mcg, iodine 150 mcg, Mg 100 mg, Mn 10 mg, Mo 12.5 mcg, niacinamide and niacin 100 mg, pantothenic acid 100 mg, potassium 35 mg, Se 100 mcg, Zn 22.5 mg
Ultra Freeda Iron-Free [OTC] (*per 3 tablets*)	5000	50	50	50	100	1000	400	200	Base (choline, inositol, PABA) 100 mg, bioflavonoids 100 mg, biotin 300 mcg, Ca 250 mg, Cr 200 mcg, folic acid 800 mcg, iodine 150 mcg, Mg 100 mg, Mo 12.5 mcg, niacinamide and niacin 100 mg, pantothenic acid 100 mg, potassium 35 mg, Se 100 mcg, Zn 22.5 mg
Ultra Freeda With Iron [OTC] (*per 3 tablets*)	5000	50	50	50	100	1000	400	200	Base (choline, inositol, PABA) 100 mg, bioflavonoids 100 mg, biotin 300 mcg, Ca 250 mg, Cr 200 mcg, Fe (as ferrous fumarate) 18 mg, folic acid 800 mcg, iodine 150 mcg, Mg 100 mg, Mo 12.5 mcg, niacinamide and niacin 100 mg, pantothenic acid 100 mg, potassium 35 mg, Se 100 mcg, Zn 22.5 mg
Xtramins [OTC]	1000	5	2	5	10	50	100	10	Boron 1 mg, Ca 250 mg, Cr 40 mcg, Cu 500 mcg, Fe (as iron gluconate) 10 mg, folic acid 400 mcg, iodine 150 mcg, Mg 20 mg, Mn 2 mg, niacinamide 15 mg, PABA 5 mg, pantothenic acid 5 mg, potassium 45 mg, Se 30 mcg, Zn 10 mg; gluten free, sugar free
Yelets [OTC]	5000	10	10	10	10	100	400	30	Biotin 30 mcg, Ca 60 mg, Fe (as ferrous fumarate) 18 mg, folic acid 400 mcg, iodine 150 mcg, L-lysine 10 mg, Mg 20 mg, Mn 1 mg, niacinamide 25 mg, pantothenic acid 10 mg, Se 17.5 mcg, Zn 7.5 mg

Adult Formulations *continued*

Product	A (int. units)	B₁ (mg)	B₂ (mg)	B₆ (mg)	B₁₂ (mcg)	C (mg)	D (int. units)	E (int. units)	Additional Information
Tablet, Chewable									
Centrum® [OTC]	3500	1.5	1.7	2	6	60	400	30	Biotin 45 mcg, Ca 108 mg, Cr 20 mcg, Cu 2 mg, Fe 18 mg, folic acid 400 mcg, iodine 150 mcg, Mg 40 mg, Mn 1 mg, Mo 20 mcg, niacin 20 mg, pantothenic acid 10 mg, phosphorus 50 mg, vitamin K 10 mcg, Zn 15 mg; contains sodium benzoate, soy products
Centrum® Silver® [OTC]	4000	2.2	2.7	7	25	75	400	70	Biotin 45 mcg, Ca 200 mg, Cr 100 mcg, Cu 2 mg, folic acid 500 mcg, iodine 100 mcg, lutein 250 mcg, Mg 50 mg, Mn 4.5 mg, Mo 25 mcg, niacin 12 mg, nickel 5 mcg, pantothenic acid 10 mg, phosphorus 125 mg, Se 22.5 mcg, silicon 4 mg, tin 10 mcg, vanadium 10 mcg, Zn 15 mg; contains phenylalanine, sodium benzoate, soy products
SourceCF®	9000	1.5	1.7	1.9	6	100	800	200	Biotin 100 mcg, folic acid 200 mcg, niacinamide 10 mg, pantothenic acid 12 mg, vitamin K 600 mcg, Zn 10 mg
Tablet, dissolving									
ProBarimin QT™	5000	3	1.7	5	250	60	800	30	Biotin 300 mcg, Cr 120 mcg, Cu 2 mg, Fe (as ferrous fumarate) 8 mg, folic acid 600 mcg, Mn 2 mg, molybdenum 75 mcg, niacinamide 20 mg, pantothenic acid 10 mg, Se 55 mcg, Zn 15 mg; sugar free
Wafers									
Calcifolic-D™				10	125		300		Boron 250 mcg, Ca 1342 mg, folic acid 1 mg, magnesium 50 mg
Combination Package									
Encora™									
AM tablet				25		25	200		Ca 400 mg, folic acid 2 mg
PM tablet				12.5		25	600		Ca 600 mg, folic acid 0.5 mg
AM/PM gelatin capsule								50	Linoleic acid 10 mg, omega-3 fatty acids 650 mg including DHA and EPA 550 mg and ALA 100 mg
Glutofac®-MX *Light purple caplet*					10				Biotin 300 mcg, Ca 250 mg, dioctyl sodium sulfosuccinate 25 mg, folic acid 800 mcg, Mg 150 mg, pantothenic acid 25 mg, phosphorus 110 mg
Dark purple caplet						100			Boron 150 mcg, Ca 250 mg, Cr 200 mcg, Cu 5 mg, dioctyl sodium sulfosuccinate 25 mg, Fe (micronized) 82 mg, iodine 150 mcg, Mg 150 mg, Mn 5 mg, Mo 75 mcg, nickel 5 mcg, phosphorus 20 mg, Se 70 mcg, tin 10 mcg, vanadium 10 mcg, Zn 40 mg

ALA = α-linolenic acid, Ca = calcium, Cr = chromium, Cu = copper, DHA = docosahexaenoic acid, EPA = eicosapentaenoic acid, Fe = iron, Mg = magnesium, Mn = manganese, Mo = molybdenum, Se = selenium, Zn = zinc.

Pediatric Formulations

Product	A (int. units)	B$_1$ (mg)	B$_2$ (mg)	B$_6$ (mg)	B$_{12}$ (mcg)	C (mg)	D (int. units)	E (int. units)	Additional Information
Capsule, softgel									
AquADEKs™ [OTC]	18,167 (92% as beta carotene)	1.5	1.7	1.9	12	75	800	150 int. units as d-alpha tocopherol and 80 mg as mixed tocopherols	Beta-carotene 10 mg, biotin 100 mcg, coenzyme Q$_{10}$ 10 mg, folic acid 200 mcg, niacinamide 20 mg, pantothenic acid 12 mg, selenium 75 mcg, vitamin K 700 mcg, Zn 10 mg; dye free
SourceCF® [OTC] (60% as beta carotene)	9000	1.5	1.7	1.9	6	100	400	200	100 mcg biotin, folic acid 200 mcg, niacinamide 20 mg, pantothenic acid 12 mg, vitamin K 500 mcg, Zn 10 mg; contains soy products
Drops									
AquADEKs™ [OTC] (per mL)	5751 (87% as beta carotene)	0.60	0.6	0.60		45	400	50 int. units as d-alpha tocopherol and 15 mg as mixed tocopherols	Beta-carotene 3 mg, biotin 15 mg, enzyme Q$_{10}$ 2 mg, niacinamide 6 mg, pantothenic acid 3 mg, selenium 10 mcg, vitamin K 400 mcg, Zn 5 mg; contains sodium benzoate; dye free (60 mL)
MyKidz Iron™ [OTC] (per 2 mL)	1500					35	400		Fe [elemental] 10 mg; alcohol free, sugar free, dye free
MyKidz Iron FL™ [OTC] (per 2 mL)	1500					35	400		Fe [elemental] 10 mg, fluoride 0.25 mg; alcohol free, sugar free, dye free (118 mL)
Poly-Vi-Sol® [OTC] (per mL)	1500	0.5	0.6	0.4	2	35	400	5	Niacin 8 mg; gluten free (50 mL)
Poly-Vi-Sol® With Iron [OTC] (per mL)	1500	0.5	0.6	0.4		35	400	5	Fe [elemental] 10 mg, niacin 8 mg; gluten free (50 mL)
SourceCF® [OTC] (per mL)	3170 (53% as beta carotene)	0.5	0.6	0.6	4	45	400	50	Biotin 15 mcg, niacinamide 6 mg, pantothenic acid 3 mg, vitamin K 300 mcg, Zn 5 mg; contains sodium benzoate (60 mL)
Tri-Vi-Sol® [OTC] (per mL)	1500					35	400		Gluten free (50 mL)
Tri-Vi-Sol® With Iron [OTC] (per mL)	1500					35	400		Fe [elemental] 10 mg; gluten free (50 mL)
Gum									
Vitaball® [OTC]	1670	1.5	1.7	2	6	60	400	30	Biotin 45 mcg, folic acid 400 mcg, niacinamide 20 mg, pantothenic acid 10 mg; gluten free
Vitaball® Minis [OTC] (per 3)	1670	1.5	1.7	2	6	60	400	30	Biotin 45 mcg, folic acid 400 mcg, niacinamide 20 mg, pantothenic acid 10 mg; gluten free
Vitaball® Wild 'N Fruity [OTC]	5000	1.5	1.7	2	6	240	400	30	Biotin 45 mcg, folic acid 400 mcg, niacinamide 20 mg, pantothenic acid 10 mg; gluten free
Gummy									
Flintstones™ Gummies [OTC] (per 2 gummies)	2000			1	5	30	200	20	Biotin 75 mcg, choline 38 mcg, folic acid 200 mcg, inositol 20 mcg, iodine 40 mcg, pantothenic acid 5 mg, zinc 2.5 mg
Flintstones™ Gummies Vita-Packs [OTC] (per 6 gummies)	2000			1	5	20	200	20	Biotin 75 mcg, choline 38 mcg, folic acid 200 mcg, inositol 20 mcg, iodine 40 mcg, pantothenic acid 5 mg, zinc 2.5 mg

Pediatric Formulations *continued*

Product	A (int. units)	B₁ (mg)	B₂ (mg)	B₆ (mg)	B₁₂ (mcg)	C (mg)	D (int. units)	E (int. units)	Additional Information
Flintstones™ Sour Gummies [OTC] (per 2 gummies)	2000			1	5	30	200	20	Biotin 75 mcg, choline 38 mcg, folic acid 200 mcg, inositol 20 mcg, iodine 40 mcg, pantothenic acid 5 mg, zinc 2.5 mg; contains tartrazine
One-A-Day® Kids Scooby-Doo! Gummies [OTC] (per 2 gummies)	2000			1	5	30	200	20	Biotin 75 mcg, choline 30 mcg, folic acid 200 mcg, inositol 20 mcg, iodine 40 mcg, pantothenic acid 5 mg, zinc 2.5 mg; sugar free
Tablet, Chewable									
ADEKs® [OTC]	5667	1.2	1.3	1.5	12	60	400	150	Biotin 50 mcg, folic acid 0.2 mg, niacinamide 10 mg, pantothenic acid 10 mg, vitamin K 150 mcg, Zn 7.5 mg
Centrum Kids® Complete Dora the Explorer™ [OTC]	3500	1.5	1.7	2	6	60	400	30	Biotin 45 mcg, Ca 108 mg, Cr 20 mcg, Cu 2 mg, Fe 18 mg, folic acid 400 mcg, iodine 150 mcg, Mg 40 mg, Mn 1 mg, Mo 20 mcg, niacin 20 mg, pantothenic acid 10 mg, phosphorus 50 mg, vitamin K 10 mcg, Zn 15 mg; contains phenylalanine, sodium benzoate, soy products
Centrum Kids® Complete Rugrats™ [OTC]	3500	1.5	1.7	2	6	60	400	30	Biotin 45 mcg, Ca 108 mg, Cr 20 mcg, Cu 2 mg, Fe 18 mg, folic acid 400 mcg, iodine 150 mcg, Mg 40 mg, Mn 1 mg, Mo 20 mcg, niacin 20 mg, pantothenic acid 10 mg, phosphorus 50 mg, vitamin K 10 mcg, Zn 15 mg; contains phenylalanine, sodium benzoate, soy products
Centrum Kids® Complete SpongeBob SquarePants™ [OTC]	3500	1.5	1.7	2	6	60	400	30	Biotin 45 mcg, Ca 108 mg, Cr 20 mcg, Cu 2 mg, Fe 18 mg, folic acid 400 mcg, iodine 150 mcg, Mg 40 mg, Mn 1 mg, Mo 20 mcg, niacin 20 mg, pantothenic acid 10 mg, phosphorus 50 mg, vitamin K 10 mcg, Zn 15 mg; contains phenylalanine, sodium benzoate, soy products
Flintstones™ Complete [OTC]	3000	1.5	1.7	2	6	60	400	30	Biotin 40 mcg, Ca 100 mg, choline 38 mcg, Cu 2 mg, Fe 18 mg, folic acid 400 mcg, iodine 150 mcg, Mg 20 mg, niacin 15 mg, pantothenic acid 10 mg, phosphorus 100 mg, sodium 10 mg, Zn 12 mg; contains phenylalanine, soy products
Flintstones™ Plus Bone Building Support [OTC]	2500	1.05	1.2	1.05	4.5	60	400	15	Calcium 200 mg, folic acid 300 mcg, niacin 13.5 mg, sodium 10 mg; contains phenylalanine, soy products
Flintstones™ Plus Immunity Support [OTC]	2500	1.05	1.2	1.05	4.5	250	400	15	Folic acid 300 mcg, niacin 13.5 mg, sodium 25 mg
Flintstones™ Plus Iron [OTC]	2500	1.05	1.2	1.05	4.5	60	400	15	Fe 15 mg, folic acid 300 mcg, niacin 13.5 mg, sodium 10 mg; contains soy products
My First Flintstones™ [OTC]	1998	1.05	1.2	1.05	4.5	60	400	15	Folic acid 300 mcg, niacin 10 mg, sodium 10 mg
One A Day® Kids Bugs Bunny and Friends Complete [OTC]	3000	1.5	1.7	2	6	60	400	30	Biotin 40 mcg, Ca 100 mg, Cu 2 mg, Fe 18 mg, folic acid 400 mcg, iodine 150 mcg, Mg 20 mg, niacin 15 mg, pantothenic acid 10 mg, phosphorus 100 mg, sodium 10 mg, Zn 12 mg; contains phenylalanine; sugar free
One A Day® Kids Scooby-Doo! Complete [OTC]	3000	1.5	1.7	2	6	60	400	30	Biotin 40 mcg, Ca 100 mg, Cu 2 mg, Fe 18 mg, folic acid 400 mcg, iodine 150 mcg, Mg 20 mg, niacin 15 mg, pantothenic acid 10 mg, phosphorus 100 mg, sodium 10 mg, Zn 12 mg; contains phenylalanine; sugar free

Pediatric Formulations *continued*

Product	A (int. units)	B₁ (mg)	B₂ (mg)	B₆ (mg)	B₁₂ (mcg)	C (mg)	D (int. units)	E (int. units)	Additional Information
One A Day® Kids Scooby-Doo! Plus Calcium [OTC]	2500	1.05	1.2	1.05	4.5	60	400	15	Ca 200 mg, folic acid 300 mcg, niacin 13.5 mg, 10 mg sodium; contains phenylalanine; sugar free
SourceCF® [OTC]	9000	1.5	1.7	1.9	6	100	800	200	Biotin 100 mcg, folic acid 200 mcg, niacinamide 10 mg, pantothenic acid 12 mg, vitamin K 600 mcg, Zn 10 mg
Vitalets [OTC]	2500	0.75	0.85	1	3	40	200	15	Biotin 150 mcg, Ca 80 mg, Fe (as ferrous fumarate) 10 mg, folic acid 200 mcg, Mg 20 mg, Mn 0.1 mg, niacinamide 10 mg, pantothenic acid 5 mg, phosphorus 60 mg, Zn 0.8 mg

Ca = calcium, Cr = chromium, Cu = copper, Fe = iron, Mg = magnesium, Mn = manganese, Mo = molybdenum, Zn = zinc.

Prenatal Formulations

Product	A (int. units)	B1 (mg)	B2 (mg)	B6 (mg)	B12 (mcg)	C (mg)	D (int. units)	E (int. units)	Additional Information
Caplet									
PreCare Premier®		3	3.4	50	12	50	240	3.5	Ca 250 mg, Cu 2 mg, docusate sodium 50 mg, Fe [elemental] 30 mg, folic acid 1 mg, Mg 25 mg, niacinamide 20 mg, succinic acid 35 mg, Zn 15 mg; dye free
Select-OB™ [OTC]	1700	1.6	1.8	2.5	5	60	400	30	Fe (as polysaccharide iron complex) 29 mg, folic acid 1 mg, Mg 25 mg, niacinamide 15 mg, Zn 15 mg; gluten free
Vitafol®-OB [OTC]	2700	1.6	1.8	2.5	12	70	400	30	Ca 100 mg, Cu 2 mg, Fe [elemental] 65 mg, folic acid 1 mg, Mg 25 mg, niacinamide 18 mg, Zn 25 mg; gluten free, sugar free
Vitafol®-PN	1700	1.6	1.8	2.5	5	60	400	30	Ca 125 mg, Fe [elemental] 65 mg, folic acid 1 mg, Mg 25 mg, niacinamide 15 mg, Zn 15 mg
Capsule									
NataCaps™		10	6	5	15	200			Cu 0.8 mg, Fe [elemental] 106 mg, folic acid 1 mg, Mn 1.3 mg, niacinamide 30 mg, pantothenic acid 10 mg
Prenatal U [OTC]		10	6	5	15	200			Cu 0.8 mg, Fe (as ferrous fumarate) 106.5 mg, folic acid 1 mg, Mn 1.3 mg, niacinamide 30 mg, pantothenic acid 10 mg
PrimaCare® One				25		25	170	30	Ca 150 mg, Fe [elemental] 27 mg, folic acid 1 mg, linolenic acid 30 mg; 330 omega-3 fatty acids including alpha-linolenic acid 30 mg, DHA 260 mg, and eicosapentaenoic acid 40 mg; contains soy products
Tandem® DHA				25		20			Fe [elemental] 30 mg, folic acid 1 mg; omega-3 fatty acids 310.1 mg including DHA 215.12 mg and eicosapentaenoic acid 53.46 mg
Tandem® OB		10	6	5	15	200			Cu 0.8 mg, Fe [elemental] 106 mg, folic acid 1 mg, Mg 6.9 mg, Mn 1.3 mg, niacinamide 30 mg, pantothenic acid 10 mg, Zn 18.2 mg; gluten free
Capsule, Softgel									
Prenate DHA™					12	85	200	10	Ca 150 mg, calcium docusate ≤50 mg, DHA 300 mg, Fe (as ferrous fumarate) 27 mg, folic acid 400 mcg, Mg 50 mg; contains soy
Tablet									
A-Free Prenatal [OTC] (*per 3 tablets*)		6	6	3	6	100	400	30	Biotin 30 mcg, calcium 1000 mg, Cu 0.3 mg, Fe (as ferrous fumarate) 27 mg, folic acid 800 mcg, Mg 100 mg, Mn 0.3 mg, niacinamide 30 mg, pantothenic acid 15 mg, Zn 22.5 mg; natural base contains bioflavonoids and hesperidin 66 mg
Advanced NatalCare®	2700	3	3.4	20	12	120	400	30	Ca 200 mg, Cu 2 mg, docusate sodium 50 mg, Fe [elemental] 90 mg, folic acid 1 mg, Mg 30 mg, niacinamide 20 mg, Zn 25 mg
Advanced-RF NatalCare®		3	3.4	20	12	120	400	30	Ca 200 mg, Cu 2 mg, docusate sodium 50 mg, Fe [elemental] 90 mg, folic acid 1 mg, Mg 30 mg, niacinamide 20 mg, Zn 25 mg; contains sodium benzoate
Calna [OTC]	1000	5	2	5	10	50	100	10	Boron 1 mg, Ca 250 mg, Cr 40 mcg, Cu 500 mcg, Fe (as iron gluconate) 10 mg, folic acid 400 mcg, iodine 150 mcg, Mg 20 mg, Mn 2 mg, niacinamide 15 mg, PABA 5 mg, pantothenic acid 5 mg, potassium 45 mg, Se 30 mcg, Zn 10 mg; gluten free, sugar free
Cal-Nate™	2700	3	3.4	20		120	400	30	Ca 125 mg, Cu 2 mg, docusate sodium 50 mg, Fe (as ferrous gluconate) 27 mg, folic acid 1 mg, iodine 150 mcg, niacinamide 20 mg, Zn 25 mg; contains sodium benzoate

Prenatal Formulations *continued*

Product	A (int. units)	B_1 (mg)	B_2 (mg)	B_6 (mg)	B_{12} (mcg)	C (mg)	D (int. units)	E (int. units)	Additional Information
CitraNatal™ Rx		3	3.4	20		120		30	Ca 125 mg, Cu 2 mg, docusate sodium 50 mg, Fe (as carbonyl iron, ferrous gluconate) 27 mg, folic acid 1 mg, iodine 150 mcg, niacinamide 20 mg, Zn 25 mg
ComBi Rx™				75	12				Ca 200 mg, folic acid 1 mg
Duet®	3000	1.8	4	25	12	120	400	30	Ca 200 mg, Cu 2 mg, Fe (as ferrous bisglycinate and Iron Aid®) 29 mg, folic acid 1 mg, Mg 25 mg, niacinamide 20 mg, Zn 25 mg; contains sodium benzoate
KPN Prenatal [OTC] (*per 3 tablets*)	2000	6	6	3	6	100	400	15	Biotin 30 mcg, Ca 1000 mg, Cu 0.3 mg, Fe (as ferrous fumarate) 27 mg, folic acid 800 mcg, Mg 100 mg, Mn 0.3 mg, niacinamide 30 mg, pantothenic acid 15 mg, Zn 22.5 mg; natural base contains 66 mg bioflavonoids and hesperidin
Mini-Prenatal [OTC]	2000	2	3	3	10	100	400	11	Biotin 100 mcg, Ca 200 mg, Cu 2 mg, Fe (as ferrous fumarate) 27 mg, folic acid 800 mcg, Mg 60 mg, Mn 2 mg, niacinamide 20 mg, pantothenic acid 10 mg, Zn 15 mg
NataFort® [OTC]	1000	2	3	10	12	120	400	10	Fe 60 mg (25 mg as ferrous sulfate, 35 mg as carbonyl iron), folic acid 1 mg, niacinamide 20 mg
NatalCare® GlossTabs™	2700	3	3.4	20	12	120	400	30	Biotin 30 mcg, Ca 200 mg, Cu 2 mg, docusate sodium 50 mg, Fe [elemental] 90 mg, folic acid 1 mg, Mg 30 mg, niacinamide 20 mg, pantothenic acid 6 mg, Zn 15 mg; contains sodium benzoate
NatalCare® PIC	4000	2.43	3	1.64	3	50	400	30	Ca 125 mg, Fe [elemental] 60 mg, folic acid 1 mg, niacinamide 10 mg, Zn 18 mg; contains sodium benzoate
NatalCare® PIC Forte	5000	3	3.4	4	12	80	400	30	Ca 250 mg, Cu 2 mg, Fe [elemental] 60 mg, folic acid 1 mg, iodine 0.2 mg, Mg 10 mg, niacinamide 20 mg, Zn 25 mg; contains sodium benzoate
NatalCare® Plus	4000	1.84	3	10	12	120	400	22	Ca 200 mg, Cu 2 mg, Fe (as ferrous fumarate) 27 mg, folic acid 1 mg, niacinamide 20 mg, Zn 25 mg; dye free, sugar free
NatalCare® Rx (*per 2 tablets*)	4000	1.5	1.6	4	2.5	80	400	15	Biotin 30 mcg, Ca 200 mg, Cu 3 mg, Fe (as ferrous fumarate) 54 mg, folic acid 1 mg, Mg 100 mg, niacinamide 17 mg, pantothenic acid 7 mg, Zn 25 mg
NatalCare® Three	3000	1.8	4	25	12	120	400	22	Ca 200 mg, Cu 2 mg, Fe (as ferrous fumarate, USP) 28 mg, folic acid 1 mg, Mg 25 mg, niacinamide 20 mg, Zn 25 mg; contains sodium benzoate; dye free, sugar free
NataTab™ CFe	4000	3	3	3	8	120	400	30	Ca 200 mg, Fe (as carbonyl iron) 50 mg, folic acid 1 mg, iodine 150 mcg, niacinamide 20 mg, Zn 15 mg
NataTab™ FA	4000	3	3	3	8	120	400	30	Ca 200 mg, Fe (as ferrous fumarate) 29 mg, folic acid 1 mg, iodine 150 mcg, niacinamide 20 mg, Zn 15 mg
NataTab™ Rx	4000	3	3	3	8	120	400	30	Biotin 30 mcg, Ca 200 mg, Cu 3 mg, Fe (as carbonyl iron) 29 mg, folic acid 1 mg, iodine 150 mcg, Mg 100 mg, niacinamide 20 mg, pantothenic acid 7 mg, Zn 15 mg; contains sodium benzoate
NutriSpire™		3	3	3	8	120	400	30	Ca 200 mg, Fe (as carbonyl iron) 29 mg, iodine 150 mcg, niacinamide 20 mg, Zn 15 mg; contains sodium benzoate
PreCare Conceive®		3	3.4	50	12	60		30	Ca 200 mg, Cu 2 mg, Fe (as ferrous fumarate) 30 mg, folic acid 1 mg, Mg 100 mg, niacinamide 20 mg, Zn 15 mg
PremesisRx®				75	12				Ca 200 mg, folic acid 1 mg
Prenatal 19 [OTC]	1000	3	3	20	12	100	400	30	Ca 200 mg, docusate sodium 25 mg, Fe (as ferrous fumarate) 29 mg, folic acid 1 mg, niacinamide 15 mg, pantothenic acid 7 mg, Zn 20 mg

Prenatal Formulations *continued*

Product	A (int. units)	B₁ (mg)	B₂ (mg)	B₆ (mg)	B₁₂ (mcg)	C (mg)	D (int. units)	E (int. units)	Additional Information
Prenatal AD [OTC]	2700	3	3.4	20	12	120	400	30	Ca 200 mg, Cu 2 mg, docusate sodium 50 mg, Fe (as carbonyl iron) 90 mg, folic acid 1 mg, Mg 30 mg, niacinamide 20 mg, Zn 25 mg
Prenatal MR 90 Fe™	4000	3	3.4	20	12	120	400	30	Ca 250 mg, Cu 2 mg, docusate sodium 50 mg, Fe [elemental] 90 mg, folic acid 1 mg, iodine 150 mcg, niacinamide 20 mg, Zn 25 mg; contains sodium benzoate; dye free
Prenatal MRT With Selenium	5000	3	3.4	10	12	120	400	30	Biotin 30 mcg, Ca 200 mg, Cr 25 mcg, Cu 2 mg, Fe (as ferrous fumarate) 27 mg, folic acid 1 mg, iodine 150 mcg, Mg 25 mg, Mn 5 mg, Mo 25 mcg, niacinamide 20 mg, pantothenic acid 10 mg, Se 20 mcg, Zn 25 mg; dye free, sugar free
Prenatal One Daily [OTC]	2000	2	3	3	10	100	400	15	Biotin 100 mcg, Ca 200 mg, Cu 2 mg, Fe (as ferrous fumarate) 27 mg, folic acid 800 mcg, Mg 60 mg, Mn 2 mg, niacinamide 20 mg, pantothenic acid 10 mg, Zn 15 mg
Prenatal Rx 1	4000	1.5	1.6	4	2.5	80	400	15	Biotin 0.03 mg, Ca 200 mg, Cu 3 mg, Fe (as ferrous fumarate) 60 mg, folic acid 1 mg, Mg 100 mg, niacinamide 17 mg, pantothenic acid 7 mg, Zn 25 mg
Prenatal Z Advanced Formula	3000	1.5	1.6	2.2	2.2	70	400	10	Ca 200 mg, Fe (as ferrous fumarate) 65 mg, folic acid 1 mg, iodine 175 mcg, Mg 100 mg, niacinamide 17 mg, Zn 15 mg; contains sodium benzoate
Prenate Elite®		3	3.4	20	12	120	400	10	Biotin 30 mcg, Ca 200 mg, Cu 2 mg, docusate sodium 50 mg, Fe [elemental] 90 mg, folic acid 400 mcg, Mg 30 mg, niacinamide 20 mg, pantothenic acid 6 mg, Zn 15 mg; contains sodium benzoate, soy products
Stuart Prenatal® [OTC]	4000	1.8	1.7	2.6	8	120	400	30	Ca 200 mg, Fe 28 mg, folic acid 800 mcg, niacin 20 mg, Zn 25 mg
Trinate [OTC]	3000	1.8	4	25	12	120	400	22	Ca 200 mg, Cu 2 mg, Fe (as ferrous fumarate) 28 mg, folic acid 1 mg, Mg 25 mg, niacinamide 20 mg, Zn 25 mg
Ultra NatalCare®	2700	3	3.4	20	12	120	400	30	Ca 200 mg, Cu 2 mg, docusate sodium 50 mg, Fe [elemental] 90 mg, folic acid 150 mcg, iodine 150 mcg, niacinamide 20 mg, Zn 25 mg; contains sodium benzoate; dye free
Tablet, Chewable									
Duet®	3000	1.8	4	25	12	120	400	30	Ca 100 mg, Cu 2 mg, Fe (as ferrous fumarate, ferrous bisglycinate) 29 mg, folic acid 1 mg, Mg 25 mg, niacinamide 20 mg, Zn 25 mg; contains phenylalanine 9 mg/tablet and sodium benzoate
NataChew® [OTC]	1000	2	3	10	12	120	400	11	Fe (as ferrous fumarate) 29 mg, folic acid 1 mg, niacinamide 20 mg
NutriNate®	1000	2	3	10	12	120	400	11	Fe (as ferrous fumarate) 29 mg, folic acid 1 mg, niacinamide 20 mg
PreCare®				2		50	6 mcg	3.5	Ca 250 mg, Cu 2 mg, Fe (as ferrous fumarate) 40 mg, folic acid 1 mg, Mg 50 mg, Zn 15 mg
Combination Package									
CareNatal™ DHA (*tablet*)	3000	1.8	4	25	12	120	400	30	Ca 200 mg, Cu 2 mg, Fe (ferrous bisglycinate as Ferrochel® and iron protein succinylate) 29 mg, folic acid 1 mg, Mg 25 mg, niacinamide 20 mg, Zn 25 mg; contains sodium benzoate. Packaged with **softgel capsule** containing purified omega-3 fatty acids 250 mg, including DHA ≥200 mg; contains soy products.
CitraNatal™ DHA (*tablet*)		3	3.4	20		120	400	30	Ca 125 mg, Cu 2 mg, docusate sodium 50 mg, Fe (as carbonyl iron, ferrous gluconate) 27 mg, folic acid 1 mg, iodine 150 mcg, niacinamide 20 mg, Zn 25 mg. Packaged with **gelatin capsule** containing DHA 250 mg.

Prenatal Formulations *continued*

Product	A (int. units)	B₁ (mg)	B₂ (mg)	B₆ (mg)	B₁₂ (mcg)	C (mg)	D (int. units)	E (int. units)	Additional Information
CitraNatal™ 90 DHA (*tablet*)		3	3.4	20		120	400	30	Ca 200 mg, Cu 2 mg, docusate sodium 50 mg, Fe 90 mg (as carbonyl iron), folic acid 1 mg, iodine 150 mcg, niacinamide 20 mg, Zn 25 mg. Packaged with *gelatin capsule* containing DHA 250 mg.
Duet® DHA (*tablet*)	3000	1.8	4	25	12	120	400	30 mg	Ca 200 mg, Cu 2 mg, Fe (as ferrous bisglycinate HCl and Iron Aid®) 29 mg, folic acid 1 mg, Mg 25 mg, niacinamide 20 mg, Zn 25 mg; contains sodium benzoate. Packaged with purified omega-3 fatty acids 430 mg *softgel capsule* containing DHA ≥295 mg.
Duet® DHA^EC (*tablet, enteric coated*)	3000	1.8	4	25	12	120	400	3 mg	Ca 200 mg, Cu 2 mg, Fe (as ferrous bisglycinate HCl and Iron Aid®) 29 mg, folic acid 1 mg, Mg 25 mg, niacinamide 20 mg, Zn 25 mg; contains sodium benzoate. Packaged with purified omega-3 fatty acids 400 mg *softgel enteric-coated capsule* containing DHA ≥275 mg.
One A Day® Women's Prenatal [OTC] (*tablet*)	4000	1.7	2	2.5	8	60	400	30	Biotin 300 mcg, Ca 300 mg, Cu 2 mg, Fe 28 mg, folic acid 800 mcg, iodine 150 mcg, Mg 50 mg, niacin 20 mg, pantothenic acid 10 mg, Zn 15 mg; contains soy products. Packaged with omega-3 fatty acids 440 mg *liquid gel* containing 200 mg DHA and 240 mg eicosapentaenoic acid; contains soy products.
OptiNate® (*tablet*)		3	3.4	20	12	120	400	10	Biotin 30 mcg, Ca 200 mg, Cu 2 mg, docusate sodium 50 mg, Fe [elemental] 90 mg, folate 1 mg, Mg 30 mg, niacinamide 20 mg, pantothenic acid 6 mg, Zn 15 mg; contains sodium benzoate. Packaged with *Omega-3 L-Vcaps™ capsule* containing DHA 250 mg.
PrimaCare® (*PM tablet*)		3	3.4	50	12	100	230		Biotin 35 mcg, Ca 250 mg, Cr 45 mcg, Cu 1.3 mg, docusate sodium 50 mg, Fe [elemental] 30 mg, folic acid 1 mg, Mo 50 mcg, niacinamide 20 mg, pantothenic acid 7 mg, Se 75 mcg, succinic acid 35 mg, vitamin K 90 mcg, Zn 11 mg; contains sodium benzoate; dye free. Packaged with *AM softgel capsule* containing linolenic acid 30 mg and omega-3 fatty acids 330 mg, including alpha-linolenic acid 30 mg, eicosapentaenoic acid 40 mg, and DHA 260 mg; also includes Ca 150 mg, vitamin D 170 int. units, and vitamin E 30 int. units; contains soy products; dye free.
Vitafol®-OB+DHA (*caplet*)	2700	1.6	1.8	2.5	12	70	400	30	Ca 100 mg, Cu 2 mg, Fe [elemental] 65 mg, folic acid 1 mg, Mg 25 mg, niacinamide 18 mg, Zn 25 mg; gluten free, sugar free. Packaged with *gelatin capsule* containing DHA 250 mg.

Ca = calcium, Cr = chromium, Cu = copper, DHA = docosahexaenoic acid (from omega-3 fatty acids), Fe = iron, Mg = magnesium, Mn = manganese, Mo = molybdenum, Se = selenium, Zn = zinc.

Vitamin B Complex Combinations

Product	B$_1$ (mg)	B$_2$ (mg)	B$_6$ (mg)	B$_{12}$ (mcg)	C (mg)	E (int. units)	Additional Information
Caplet							
Allbee® with C [OTC]	15	10.2	5		300		Niacinamide 50 mg, pantothenic acid 10 mg
Allbee® C-800 [OTC]	15	17	25	12	800	45	Niacinamide 100 mg, pantothenic acid 25 mg
Allbee® C-800 + Iron [OTC]	15	17	25	12	800	45	Fe 27 mg, folic acid 0.4 mg, niacinamide 100 mg, pantothenic acid 25 mg
Nephronex®	1.5	1.7	10	0.01	50		Biotin 300 mcg, folic acid 1 mg, nicotinic acid 20 mg, pantothenic acid 10 mg
Elixir							
Eldertonic® (per 15 mL)	0.5	0.6	0.7	2			Mg 0.7 mg, Mn 0.7 mg, niacin 7 mg, pantothenic acid 3 mg, Zn 5 mg [contains alcohol 13.5%]
Senilezol (per 30 mL)	2.5	2.5	1	5			Ca 5 mg, Fe 8 mg, niacin 10 mg [contains alcohol 15%]
Liquid							
Apatate® [OTC] (per 5 mL)	15		0.5	25			Cherry flavor (120 mL)
Gevrabon® [OTC] (per 30 mL)	5	2.5	1	1			Choline 10 mg, Fe 15 mg, iodine 100 mcg, Mn 2 mg, niacinamide 50 mg, pantothenic acid 10 mg, Zn 2 mg; alcohol, benzoic acid; sherry wine flavor (480 mL)
Nephronex® (per 5 mL)	1.5	1.7	10	10	60		Biotin 300 mcg, folic acid 1 mg, nicotinic acid 20 mg, pantothenic acid 10 mg
Softgel							
Nephrocaps®	1.5	1.7	10	6	100		Biotin 150 mcg, folate 1 mg, niacin 20 mg, pantothenic acid 5 mg
Renal Caps	1.5	1.7	10	6	100		Biotin 150 mcg, folic acid 1 mg, niacin 20 mg, pantothenic acid 5 mg
Syrup							
Vitafol (per 5 mL)			2	8.34			Fe 100 mg, folic acid 0.25 mg, niacinamide 13.3 mg [contains sodium benzoate; raspberry mint flavor]
Tablet							
DexFol™	1.5	1.5			60		Biotin 300 mcg, cobalamin 1 mg, folacin 5 mg, niacinamide 20 mg, pantothenic acid 10 mg, pyridoxine 50 mg, [dye, sugar, and lactose free]
Kobee [OTC]	10	10	10	10			Biotin 10 mcg, choline citrate 10 mg, folic acid 400 mcg, inositol 10 mg, niacinamide 50 mg, PABA 10 mg, pantothenic acid 10 mg
Metanx™			25 (pyridoxal 5-phosphate)	2 mg (methylcobalamin)			L-methylfolate 2.8 mg
NephPlex® Rx	1.5	1.7	10	6	60		Biotin 300 mcg, folic acid 1 mg, niacinamide 20 mg, pantothenic acid 10 mg, zinc 12.5 mg
Nephro-Vite® [OTC]	1.5	1.7	10	6	60		Biotin 300 mcg, folic acid 0.8 mg, niacinamide 20 mg, pantothenic acid 10 mg
Nephro-Vite® Rx	1.5	1.7	10	6	60		Biotin 300 mcg, folic acid 1 mg, niacinamide 20 mg, pantothenic acid 10 mg
Nephron FA®	1.5	1.7	10	6	40		Biotin 300 mcg, docusate sodium 75 mg, ferrous fumarate 200 mg, folic acid 1 mg, niacinamide 20 mg, pantothenic acid 10 mg
Quin B Strong [OTC]	25	25	25	25			Biotin 25 mcg, folic acid 400 mcg, niacinamide 100 mg, pantothenic acid 25 mg (in a base containing choline citrate, inositol, and PABA)
Quin B Strong with C and Zinc [OTC]	25	25	25	25	500		Biotin 25 mcg, folic acid 400 mcg, niacinamide 100 mg, pantothenic acid 25 mg (in a base containing choline citrate, inositol, and PABA)
Rena-Vite [OTC]	1.5	1.7	10	6	60		Biotin 100 mcg, folic acid 800 mcg, niacin 20 mg, pantothenic acid 10 mg

Vitamin B Complex Combinations *continued*

Product	B₁ (mg)	B₂ (mg)	B₆ (mg)	B₁₂ (mcg)	C (mg)	E (int. units)	Additional Information
Rena-Vite RX	1.5	1.7	10	6	60		Biotin 300 mcg, folate 1 mg, niacin 20 mg, pantothenic acid 10 mg
Stresstabs® High Potency Advanced [OTC]	10	10	5	12	250	30	Biotin 45 mcg, Ca 70 mg, Cu 3 mg, folic acid 400 mcg, niacinamide 100 mg, pantothenic acid 20 mg, phosphorus 30 mg, Zn 23.9 mg
Stresstabs® High Potency Energy [OTC]	10	10	5	12	300	30	Biotin 45 mcg, Ca 20 mg, Fe 4 mg, folic acid 400 mcg, niacinamide 100 mg, pantothenic acid 20 mg, phosphorus 15 mg
Stresstabs® High Potency Weight [OTC]	10	10	5	12	300	30	Biotin 45 mcg, Ca 44 mg, chromium 200 mcg, folic acid 400 mcg, niacinamide 100 mg, pantothenic acid 20 mg, phosphorus 32 mg
Strovite	15	15	4	5	500		Folic acid 0.5 mg, niacinamide 100 mg, pantothenic acid 18 mg
Super Dec B 100 [OTC]	100	100	100	100			Biotin 100 mcg, folic acid 400 mcg, niacinamide 100 mg, pantothenic acid 100 mg (in a base containing choline citrate, inositol, and PABA)
Superplex-T™ [OTC]	15	10	5	10	500		Niacinamide 100 mg, pantothenic acid 18.3 mg, sodium 65 mg
Super Quints 50 [OTC]	50	50	50	50			Biotin 50 mcg, folic acid 400 mcg, niacinamide 50 mg, pantothenic acid 50 mg (in a base containing choline citrate, glutaminic acid, glutamine, glycine, inositol, lysine, and PABA)
Surbex-T® [OTC]	15	10	5	10	500		Ca 20 mg, niacinamide 100 mg
Z-Bec® [OTC]	15	10.2	10	6	600	45	Niacinamide 100 mg, pantothenic acid 25 mg, Zn 22.5 mg

Ca = calcium, Cu = copper, Fe = iron, Mg = magnesium, Mn = manganese, Se = selenium, Zn = zinc.

OPIOID ANALGESICS COMPARISON

This table serves as a general guide to opioid conversion. Utilization of a direct conversion without a detailed patient and medication assessment is not recommended and may result in over- or under-dosing.

Drug	Onset (min)	Duration (h)	Equianalgesic I.M. Dose (mg)	Equianalgesic P.O. Dose[1] (mg)	Parenteral Oral Ratio	Partial Antagonist
Alfentanil	I.V.: Immediate	<0.25-0.33	ND	—	—	No
Codeine[2]	I.M.: 10-30 P.O.: 30-60	4-6	100-130	200	1/2-2/3	No
Fentanyl	I.M.: 7-15 I.V.: Immediate	I.M.: 1-2 I.V.: 0.5-1	0.1	—	—	No
Hydrocodone	P.O. 10-20	3-6	—	30-45	—	No
Hydromorphone	P.O.: 15-30	4-5	1.5	7.5	1/5	No
Meperidine[3]	P.O., I.M., SubQ: 10-15 I.V.: ≤5	P.O., I.M., SubQ: 2-4 I.V.: 2-3	75-100	300	1/3-1/2	No
Methadone[4]	P.O.: 30-60 I.V.: 10-20	Acute: 4-6 Chronic: >8	Acute: 10 Chronic: 2-4	Acute: 20 Chronic[4]: 2-4	—	No
Morphine	P.O. (immediate release): 15-60 I.V.: ≤5	P.O. (immediate release), I.V., I.M., SubQ: 3-5 Extended release tablets: 8-12	10	30	1/6; ratio decreases to 1/1.5-2.5 upon chronic dosing	No
Oxycodone	P.O. (immediate release): 15-30	P.O.: Immediate release: 4-5 Controlled release: 12	—	15-30	—	No
Pentazocine	P.O., I.M., SubQ: 15-30 I.V.: ≤2-3	P.O.: 4-5 I.V., I.M., SubQ: 2-3	30	50	1/3	Yes

ND = no data

Note: Values are based on single dose adult studies. Duration of action may be shorter in children due to faster elimination (in general) compared to adults. The pharmacokinetics of opioids in children and infants >6 months old are similar to adults but infants <6 months old, especially premature or physically compromised ones, may demonstrate decreased clearance and are at risk of apnea.

[1] Chronic administration may alter pharmacokinetics and change parental oral ratio.

[2] Codeine should not be used in children <6 months old due to slow metabolism, accumulation of morphine (major metabolite) and risk of apnea/death. In addition, 10% of the population cannot convert codeine to morphine and therefore will not experience analgesia. Conversely, ultra-rapid metabolizers may have an exaggerated opioid response.

[3] Not recommended for routine use due to potential accumulation of a neurotoxic metabolite.

[4] Conversion of higher doses may be guided by the following (consult a pain or palliative care specialist if unfamiliar with methadone prescribing): As the total daily dose of morphine increases, the equianalgesic dose ratio (methadone:morphine) changes in adults with ongoing cancer pain. Applicability to pediatric patients is unknown. See specific guidelines for more detail (American Pain Society & National Comprehensive Cancer Network).

References

National Cancer Institute, "Pain (PDQ®)," Last Modified 5/7/09. Available at http://www.cancer.gov/cancertopics/pdq/supportivecare/pain/HealthProfessional/page1

National Comprehensive Cancer Network® (NCCN), "Clinical Practice Guidelines in Oncology™: Adult Cancer Pain," Version 1, 2009. Available at http://www.nccn.org/professionals/physician_gls/PDF/pain.pdf

Patanwala AE, Duby J, Waters D, et al, "Opioid Conversions in Acute Care," *Ann Pharmacother*, 2007, 41(2):255-66.

Principles of Analgesic Use in the Treatment of Acute Pain and Cancer Pain, 6th ed, Glenview, IL: American Pain Society, 2008.

CONVERSIONS

Apothecary-Metric Exact Equivalents

1 gram (g)	=	15.43 grains		0.1 mg	=	1/600 gr
1 milliliter (mL)	=	16.23 minims		0.12 mg	=	1/500 gr
1 minim	=	0.06 mL		0.15 mg	=	1/400 gr
1 grain (gr)	=	64.8 milligrams		0.2 mg	=	1/300 gr
1 fluid ounce (fl. oz)	=	29.57 mL		0.3 mg	=	1/200 gr
1 pint (pt)	=	473.2 mL		0.4 mg	=	1/150 gr
1 ounce (oz)	=	28.35 grams		0.5 mg	=	1/120 gr
1 pound (lb)	=	453.6 grams		0.6 mg	=	1/100 gr
1 kilogram (kg)	=	2.2 pounds		0.8 mg	=	1/80 gr
1 quart (qt)	=	946.4 mL		1 mg	=	1/65 gr

Apothecary-Metric Approximate Equivalents[1]

Liquids				Solids		
1 teaspoonful	=	5 mL		¼ grain	=	15 mg
1 tablespoonful	=	15 mL		½ grain	=	30 mg
				1 grain	=	60 mg
				1½ grain	=	100 mg
				5 grains	=	300 mg
				10 grains	=	600 mg

[1]Use exact equivalents for compounding and calculations requiring a high degree of accuracy.

Pounds-Kilograms Conversion

1 pound = 0.45359 kilograms
1 kilogram = 2.2 pounds

Temperature Conversion

Celsius to Fahrenheit = (°C x 9/5) + 32 = °F
Fahrenheit to Celsius = (°F - 32) x 5/9 = °C

CYTOCHROME P450 ENZYMES: SUBSTRATES, INHIBITORS, AND INDUCERS

INTRODUCTION

Most drugs are eliminated from the body, at least in part, by being chemically altered to less lipid-soluble products (ie, metabolized), and thus are more likely to be excreted via the kidneys or the bile. Phase I metabolism includes drug hydrolysis, oxidation, and reduction, and results in drugs that are more polar in their chemical structure, while Phase II metabolism involves the attachment of an additional molecule onto the drug (or partially metabolized drug) in order to create an inactive and/or more water soluble compound. Phase II processes include (primarily) glucuronidation, sulfation, glutathione conjugation, acetylation, and methylation.

Virtually any of the Phase I and II enzymes can be inhibited by some xenobiotic or drug. Some of the Phase I and II enzymes can be induced. Inhibition of the activity of metabolic enzymes will result in increased concentrations of the substrate (drug), whereas induction of the activity of metabolic enzymes will result in decreased concentrations of the substrate. For example, the well-documented enzyme-inducing effects of phenobarbital may include a combination of Phase I and II enzymes. Phase II glucuronidation may be increased via induced UDP-glucuronosyltransferase (UGT) activity, whereas Phase I oxidation may be increased via induced cytochrome P450 (CYP) activity. However, for most drugs, the primary route of metabolism (and the primary focus of drug-drug interaction) is Phase I oxidation.

CYP enzymes may be responsible for the metabolism (at least partial metabolism) of approximately 75% of all drugs, with the CYP3A subfamily responsible for nearly half of this activity. Found throughout plant, animal, and bacterial species, CYP enzymes represent a superfamily of xenobiotic metabolizing proteins. There have been several hundred CYP enzymes identified in nature, each of which has been assigned to a family (1, 2, 3, etc), subfamily (A, B, C, etc), and given a specific enzyme number (1, 2, 3, etc) according to the similarity in amino acid sequence that it shares with other enzymes. Of these many enzymes, only a few are found in humans, and even fewer appear to be involved in the metabolism of xenobiotics (eg, drugs). The key human enzyme subfamilies include CYP1A, CYP2A, CYP2B, CYP2C, CYP2D, CYP2E, and CYP3A. However, the number of distinct isozymes (eg, CYP2C9) found to be functionally active in humans, as well as, the number of genetically variant forms of these isozymes (eg, CYP2C9*2) in individuals continues to expand.

CYP enzymes are found in the endoplasmic reticulum of cells in a variety of human tissues (eg, skin, kidneys, brain, lungs), but their predominant sites of concentration and activity are the liver and intestine. Though the abundance of CYP enzymes throughout the body is relatively equally distributed among the various subfamilies, the relative contribution to drug metabolism is (in decreasing order of magnitude) CYP3A4 (nearly 50%), CYP2D6 (nearly 25%), CYP2C8/9 (nearly 15%), then CYP1A2, CYP2C19, CYP2A6, and CYP2E1. Owing to their potential for numerous drug-drug interactions, those drugs that are identified in preclinical studies as substrates of CYP3A enzymes are often given a lower priority for continued research and development in favor of drugs that appear to be less affected by (or less likely to affect) this enzyme subfamily.

Each enzyme subfamily possesses unique selectivity toward potential substrates. For example, CYP1A2 preferentially binds medium-sized, planar, lipophilic molecules, while CYP2D6 preferentially binds molecules that possess a basic nitrogen atom. Some CYP subfamilies exhibit polymorphism (ie, genetic variation that results in a modified enzyme with small changes in amino acid sequences that may manifest differing catalytic properties). The best described polymorphisms involve CYP2C9, CYP2C19, and CYP2D6. Individuals possessing "wild type" genes exhibit normal functioning CYP capacity. Others, however, possess genetic variants that leave the person with a subnormal level of catalytic potential (so called "poor metabolizers"). Poor metabolizers would be more likely to experience toxicity from drugs metabolized by the affected enzymes (or less effects if the enzyme is responsible for converting a prodrug to it's active form as in the case of codeine). The percentage of people classified as poor metabolizers varies by enzyme and population group. As an example, approximately 7% of Caucasians and only about 1% of Asians appear to be CYP2D6 poor metabolizers.

CYP enzymes can be both inhibited and induced by other drugs, leading to increased or decreased serum concentrations (along with the associated effects), respectively. Induction occurs when a drug causes an increase in the amount of smooth endoplasmic reticulum, secondary to increasing the amount of the affected CYP enzymes in the tissues. This "revving up" of the CYP enzyme system may take several days to reach peak activity, and likewise, may take several days, even months, to return to normal following discontinuation of the inducing agent.

CYP inhibition occurs via several potential mechanisms. Most commonly, a CYP inhibitor competitively (and reversibly) binds to the active site on the enzyme, thus preventing the substrate from binding to the same site, and preventing the substrate from being metabolized. The affinity of an inhibitor for an enzyme may be expressed by an inhibition constant (Ki) or IC50 (defined as the concentration of the inhibitor required to cause 50% inhibition under a given set of conditions). In addition to reversible competition for an enzyme site, drugs may inhibit enzyme activity by binding to sites on the enzyme other than that to which the substrate would bind, and thereby cause a change in the functionality or physical structure of the enzyme. A drug may also bind to the enzyme in an irreversible (ie, "suicide") fashion. In such a case, it is not the concentration of drug at the enzyme site that is important (constantly binding and releasing), but the number of molecules available for binding (once bound, always bound).

Although an inhibitor or inducer may be known to affect a variety of CYP subfamilies, it may only inhibit one or two in a clinically important fashion. Likewise, although a substrate is known to be at least partially metabolized by a variety of CYP enzymes, only one or two enzymes may contribute significantly enough to its overall metabolism to warrant concern when used with potential inducers or inhibitors. Therefore, when attempting to predict the level of risk of using two drugs that may affect each other via altered CYP function, it is important to identify the relative effectiveness of the inhibiting/inducing drug on the CYP subfamilies that significantly contribute to the metabolism of the substrate. The contribution of a specific CYP pathway to substrate metabolism should be considered not only in light of other known CYP pathways, but also other nonoxidative pathways for substrate metabolism (eg, glucuronidation) and transporter proteins (eg, P-glycoprotein) that may affect the presentation of a substrate to a metabolic pathway.

HOW TO USE THIS TABLE

The following table provides a clinically relevant perspective on drugs that are affected by, or affect, cytochrome P450 (CYP) enzymes. Not all human, drug-metabolizing CYP enzymes are specifically (or separately) included in the table. Some enzymes have been excluded because they do not appear to significantly contribute to the metabolism of marketed drugs (eg, CYP2C18). In the case of CYP3A4, the industry routinely uses this single enzyme designation to represent all enzymes in the CYP3A subfamily. CYP3A7 is present in fetal livers. It is effectively absent from adult livers. CYP3A4 (adult) and CYP3A7 (fetal) appear to share similar properties in their respective hosts. The impact of CYP3A7 in fetal and neonatal drug interactions has not been investigated.

An enzyme that appears to play a clinically significant (major) role in a drug's metabolism is indicated by "S". A clinically significant designation is the result of a two-phase review. The first phase considered the contribution of each CYP enzyme to the overall metabolism of the drug. The enzyme pathway was considered potentially clinically relevant if it was responsible for at least 30% of the metabolism of the drug. If so, the drug was subjected to a second phase. The second phase considered the clinical relevance of a substrate's concentration being increased twofold, or decreased by one-half (such as might be observed if combined with an effective CYP inhibitor or inducer, respectively). If either of these changes was considered to present a clinically significant concern, the CYP pathway for the drug was designated "major." If neither change would appear to present a clinically significant concern, or if the CYP enzyme was responsible for a smaller portion of the overall metabolism (ie, <30%), then no association between the enzyme and the drug will appear in the table.

Enzymes that are strongly or moderately inhibited by a drug are indicated by "↓". Enzymes that are weakly inhibited are not identified in the table. The designations are the result of a review of published clinical reports, available Ki data, and assessments published by other experts in the field. As it pertains to Ki values set in a ratio with achievable serum drug concentrations ([I]) under normal dosing conditions, the following parameters were employed: [I]/Ki ≥1 = strong; [I]/Ki 0.1-1 = moderate; [I]/Ki <0.1 = weak.

Enzymes that appear to be effectively induced by a drug are indicated by "↑". This designation is the result of a review of published clinical reports and assessments published by experts in the field.

In general, clinically significant interactions are more likely to occur between substrates ("S") and either inhibitors or inducers of the same enzyme(s), which have been indicated by "↓" and "↑", respectively. However, these assessments possess a degree of subjectivity, at times based on limited indications regarding the significance of CYP effects of particular agents. An attempt has been made to balance a conservative, clinically-sensitive presentation of the data with a desire to avoid the numbing effect of a "beware of everything" approach. It is important to note that information related to CYP metabolism of drugs is expanding at a rapid pace, and thus, the contents of this table should only be considered to represent a "snapshot" of the information available at the time of publication.

Selected Readings

Bjornsson TD, Callaghan JT, Einolf HJ, et al, "The Conduct of *in vitro* and *in vivo* Drug-Drug Interaction Studies: A PhRMA Perspective," *J Clin Pharmacol*, 2003, 43(5):443-69.

Drug-Drug Interactions, Rodrigues AD, ed, New York, NY: Marcel Dekker, Inc, 2002.

Levy RH, Thummel KE, Trager WF, et al, eds, *Metabolic Drug Interactions*, Philadelphia, PA: Lippincott Williams & Wilkins, 2000.

Michalets EL, "Update: Clinically Significant Cytochrome P-450 Drug Interactions," *Pharmacotherapy*, 1998, 18(1):84-112.

Thummel KE and Wilkinson GR, " *In vitro* and *in vivo* Drug Interactions Involving Human CYP3A," *Annu Rev Pharmacol Toxicol*, 1998, 38:389-430.

Zhang Y and Benet LZ, "The Gut as a Barrier to Drug Absorption: Combined Role of Cytochrome P450 3A and P-Glycoprotein," *Clin Pharmacokinet*, 2001, 40(3):159-68.

Selected Websites

http://www.imm.ki.se/CYPalleles
http://medicine.iupui.edu/flockhart
http://www.fda.gov/Drugs/DevelopmentApprovalProcess/DevelopmentResources/DrugInteractionsLabeling/ucm080499.htm

CYP: Substrates, Inhibitors, Inducers

S = substrate; ↓ = inhibitor; ↑ = inducer

Drug	1A2	2A6	2B6	2C8	2C9	2C19	2D6	2E1	3A4
Acenocoumarol	S					S			
Alfentanil									S
Alfuzosin									S
Alosetron	S								
ALPRAZolam									S
Ambrisentan						S			S
Aminophylline	S								
Amiodarone		↓		S	↓		↓		S, ↓
Amitriptyline							S		
AmLODIPine	↓								S
Amobarbital		↑							
Amoxapine							S		
Aprepitant									S, ↓
Aripiprazole							S		S
Armodafinil						↓			S, ↑
Atazanavir									S, ↓
Atomoxetine							S		
Atorvastatin									S
Benzphetamine									S
Betaxolol	S						S		
Bisoprolol									S
Bortezomib						S, ↓			S
Bosentan					S, ↑				S, ↑
Bromazepam									S
Bromocriptine									S
Budesonide									S
Buprenorphine									S
BuPROPion			S						
BusPIRone									S
Busulfan									S
Caffeine	S								↓
Captopril							S		
CarBAMazepine	↑		↑	↑	↑	↑			S, ↑
Carisoprodol						S			
Carvedilol					S		S		
Celecoxib				↓	S				
ChlordiazePOXIDE									S
Chloroquine							S, ↓		S
Chlorpheniramine									S
ChlorproMAZINE							S, ↓		
Chlorzoxazone								S	
Ciclesonide									S
Cilostazol									S
Cimetidine	↓					↓	↓		↓
Cinacalcet							↓		
Ciprofloxacin	↓								

CYP: Substrates, Inhibitors, Inducers *(continued)*

Drug	1A2	2A6	2B6	2C8	2C9	2C19	2D6	2E1	3A4
Cisapride									S
Citalopram						S			S
Clarithromycin									S, ↓
Clobazam						S			S
ClomiPRAMINE	S					S	S, ↓		
ClonazePAM									S
Clorazepate									S
Clotrimazole									↓
Clozapine	S						↓		
Cocaine							↓		S
Codeine[1]							S		
Colchicine									S
Conivaptan									S, ↓
Cyclobenzaprine	S								
Cyclophosphamide[2]			S						S
CycloSPORINE									S, ↓
Dacarbazine	S							S	
Dantrolene									S
Dapsone					S				S
Darifenacin							↓		S
Darunavir									S
Dasatinib									S
Delavirdine					↓	↓	↓		S, ↓
Desipramine		↓	↓				S, ↓		↓
Desogestrel						S			
Dexamethasone									S, ↑
Dexlansoprazole						S, ↓			S
Dexmedetomidine		S					↓		
Dextromethorphan							S		
Diazepam						S			S
Diclofenac	↓								
Dihydroergotamine									S
Diltiazem									S, ↓
DiphenhydrAMINE							↓		
Disopyramide									S
Disulfiram								↓	
Docetaxel									S
Doxepin							S		
DOXOrubicin			↓				S		S
Doxycycline									↓
DULoxetine	S						S, ↓		
Efavirenz[3]			S		↓	↓			S, ↓, ↑
Eletriptan									S
Enflurane								S	
Eplerenone									S
Ergoloid mesylates									S
Ergonovine									S
Ergotamine									S
Erlotinib									S

CYP: Substrates, Inhibitors, Inducers *(continued)*

Drug	1A2	2A6	2B6	2C8	2C9	2C19	2D6	2E1	3A4
Erythromycin									S, ↓
Escitalopram						S			S
Esomeprazole						S, ↓			S
Estradiol	S								S
Estrogens, conjugated A/synthetic	S								S
Estrogens, conjugated equine	S								S
Estrogens, esterified	S								S
Estropipate	S								S
Eszopiclone									S
Ethinyl estradiol									S
Ethosuximide									S
Etoposide									S
Exemestane									S
Felbamate									S
Felodipine				↓					S
FentaNYL									S
Flecainide							S		
Fluconazole					↓	↓			↓
Flunisolide									S
FLUoxetine	↓				S	↓	S, ↓		
Fluphenazine							S		
Flurazepam									S
Flurbiprofen					↓				
Flutamide	S								S
Fluticasone									S
Fluvastatin					S, ↓				
Fluvoxamine	S, ↓						↓	S	
Fosamprenavir (as amprenavir)									S, ↓
Fosaprepitant									S, ↓
Fosphenytoin (as phenytoin)			↑	↑	S, ↑	S, ↑			↑
Fospropofol	↓		S		S	↓			↓
Gefitinib									S
Gemfibrozil	↓			↓	↓	↓			
Glimepiride					S				
GlipiZIDE					S				
Guanabenz	S								
Haloperidol							S, ↓		S, ↓
Halothane								S	
Ibuprofen					↓				
Ifosfamide[4]		S				S			S
Imatinib							↓		S, ↓
Imipramine						S	S, ↓		
Indinavir									S, ↓
Indomethacin					↓				
Irbesartan				↓	↓				
Irinotecan			S						S
Isoflurane								S	
Isoniazid		↓				↓	↓	S, ↓	↓
Isosorbide dinitrate									S

CYP: Substrates, Inhibitors, Inducers (continued)

Drug	1A2	2A6	2B6	2C8	2C9	2C19	2D6	2E1	3A4
Isosorbide mononitrate									S
Isradipine									S
Itraconazole									S, ↓
Ixabepilone									S
Ketamine			S		S				S
Ketoconazole	↓	↓			↓	↓	↓		S, ↓
Lansoprazole						S, ↓			S
Lapatinib									S
Letrozole		↓							
Levonorgestrel									S
Lidocaine	↓						S, ↓		S, ↓
Lomustine							S		
Lopinavir									S
Loratadine							↓	.	
Losartan				↓	S, ↓				S
Lovastatin									S
Maprotiline							S		
Maraviroc									S
MedroxyPROGESTERone									S
Mefenamic acid					↓				
Mefloquine									S
Mephobarbital						S			
Mestranol[5]					S				S
Methadone							↓		S
Methamphetamine							S		
Methimazole							↓		
Methoxsalen	↓	↓							
Methsuximide						S			
Methylergonovine									S
MethylPREDNISolone									S
Metoprolol							S		
MetroNIDAZOLE									↓
Mexiletine	S, ↓						S		
Miconazole	↓	↓			↓	↓	↓	↓	S, ↓
Midazolam									S
Mirtazapine	S						S		S
Moclobemide						S	S		
Modafinil						↓			S
Montelukast					S				S
Nafcillin									↑
Nateglinide					S				S
Nebivolol							S		
Nefazodone							S		S, ↓
Nelfinavir							S		S, ↓
Nevirapine			↑						S, ↑
NiCARdipine					↓	↓	↓		S, ↓
NIFEdipine	↓								S
Nilotinib									S
Nilutamide						S			

CYP: Substrates, Inhibitors, Inducers *(continued)*

Drug	1A2	2A6	2B6	2C8	2C9	2C19	2D6	2E1	3A4
NiMODipine									S
Nisoldipine									S
Norethindrone									S
Norfloxacin	↓								↓
Norgestrel									S
Nortriptyline							S		
Ofloxacin	↓								
OLANZapine	S								
Omeprazole					↓	S, ↓			S
Ondansetron									S
OXcarbazepine									↑
Paclitaxel				S	S				S
Pantoprazole						S			
Paricalcitol									S
PARoxetine			↓				S, ↓		
Pazopanib									S
Pentamidine						S			
PENTobarbital		↑							↑
Perphenazine							S		
PHENobarbital	↑	↑	↑	↑	↑	S			↑
Phenytoin			↑	↑	S, ↑	S, ↑			↑
Pimozide	S								S
Pindolol							S		
Pioglitazone				S, ↓					
Piroxicam					↓				
Posaconazole									↓
Primaquine	↓								S
Primidone	↑		↑	↑	↑				↑
Procainamide							S		
Progesterone						S			S
Promethazine			S				S		
Propafenone							S		
Propofol	↓		S		S	↓			↓
Propranolol	S						S		
Protriptyline							S		
Pyrimethamine					↓		↓		
Quazepam						S			S
QUEtiapine									S
QuiNIDine							↓		S, ↓
QuiNINE				↓	↓		↓		S
Rabeprazole				↓		S, ↓			S
Ramelteon	S								
Ranolazine							↓		S
Rasagiline	S								
Repaglinide				S					S
Rifabutin									S, ↑
Rifampin	↑	↑	↑	↑	↑	↑			↑
Rifapentine				↑	↑				↑
Riluzole	S								

CYP: Substrates, Inhibitors, Inducers *(continued)*

Drug	1A2	2A6	2B6	2C8	2C9	2C19	2D6	2E1	3A4
Risperidone							S		
Ritonavir				↓			S, ↓		S, ↓
Ropinirole	S								
Ropivacaine	S								
Rosiglitazone				S, ↓					
Salmeterol									S
Saquinavir									S, ↓
Secobarbital		↑			↑	↑			
Selegiline			S						
Sertraline			↓			S, ↓	S, ↓		↓
Sevoflurane								S	
Sibutramine									S
Sildenafil									S
Simvastatin									S
Sirolimus									S
Sitaxsentan					↓	↓			↓
Solifenacin									S
Sorafenib			↓	↓	↓				
Spiramycin									S
SUFentanil									S
SulfaDIAZINE					S, ↓				
Sulfamethoxazole					S, ↓				
SulfiSOXAZOLE					S, ↓				
Sunitinib									S
Tacrine	S								
Tacrolimus									S
Tadalafil									S
Tamoxifen				↓	S		S		S
Tamsulosin							S		S
Telithromycin									S, ↓
Temsirolimus									S
Teniposide									S
Terbinafine							↓		
Tetracycline									S, ↓
Theophylline	S							S	S
Thiabendazole	↓								
Thioridazine							S, ↓		
Thiotepa			↓						
Thiothixene	S								
TiaGABine									S
Ticlopidine						↓	↓		S
Timolol							S		
Tinidazole									S
Tipranavir									S
TiZANidine	S								
TOLBUTamide					S, ↓				
Tolterodine							S		S
Toremifene									S
Torsemide					S				

CYP: Substrates, Inhibitors, Inducers *(continued)*

Drug	1A2	2A6	2B6	2C8	2C9	2C19	2D6	2E1	3A4
TraMADol[1]							S		S
Tranylcypromine	↓	↓				↓	↓		
TraZODone							↓		S
Tretinoin				S					
Triazolam									S
Trifluoperazine	S								
Trimethoprim				↓	S, ↓				S
Trimipramine						S	S		S
Vardenafil									S
Venlafaxine							S		S
Verapamil									S, ↓
VinBLAStine									S
VinCRIStine									S
Vinorelbine									S
Voriconazole					S	S			↓
Warfarin					S, ↓				
Zafirlukast					S, ↓				
Zileuton	↓								
Zolpidem									S
Zonisamide									S
Zopiclone					S				S
Zuclopenthixol							S		

[1]This opioid analgesic is bioactivated *in vivo* via CYP2D6. Inhibiting this enzyme would decrease the effects of the analgesic. The active metabolite might also affect, or be affected by, CYP enzymes.

[2]Cyclophosphamide is bioactivated *in vivo* to acrolein via CYP2B6 and 3A4. Inhibiting these enzymes would decrease the effects of cyclophosphamide.

[3]Data have shown both induction (*in vivo*) and inhibition (*in vitro*) of CYP3A4.

[4]Ifosfamide is bioactivated *in vivo* to acrolein via CYP3A4. Inhibiting this enzyme would decrease the effects of ifosfamide.

[5]Mestranol is bioactivated *in vivo* to ethinyl estradiol via CYP2C8/9. See Ethinyl Estradiol for additional CYP information.

EXTRAVASATION TREATMENT

Medication Extravasated	Cold/Warm Pack	Antidote
VESICANTS		
Direct Cellular Toxins – Chemotherapeutic Agents		
DNA Intercalators		
Daunorubicin Doxorubicin Epirubicin Idarubicin	Cold	DMSO: Apply to area twice the size of the extravasation; repeat every 6 hours for up to 14 days; allow to air dry; do not cover with dressing
Vinca alkaloids		
Paclitaxel[1] Vinblastine Vincristine Vinorelbine	Warm	Hyaluronidase 1. Add 1 mL NS to 150 units vial to make 150 units/mL concentration 2. Administer 0.2 mL injection subcutaneously or intradermally into the extravasation site at the leading edge **Note:** Some institutions utilize a 1:10 dilution in infants and children; prepare by mixing 0.1 mL of 150 units/mL solution with 0.9 mL NS in 1 mL syringe to make final concentration = 15 units/mL
Alkylating agents		
Cisplatin	Cold	Sodium thiosulfate 1/6 molar solution: mix 4 mL of 10% sodium thiosulfate with 6 mL of sterile water; inject 3-5 mL (use only for large cisplatinum infiltrates >20 mL and when using cisplatinum concentrations >0.5 mg/mL; no data for use in cisplatinum infusions in children)
Mechlorethamine (Nitrogen mustard)		Sodium thiosulfate 1/6 molar solution: mix 4 mL of 10% sodium thiosulfate with 6 mL of sterile water; inject 0.5 mL for each mg mechlorethamine extravasated
Other vesicant chemotherapeutic agents		
Dactinomycin Mitomycin C Mitoxantrone Plicamycin	Cold	None
Ischemic Inducers		
Dobutamine Dopamine Epinephrine Norepinephrine Phenylephrine Vasopressin	None	Phentolamine (Regitine®) Mix 5 mg with 9 mL of NS Inject a small amount of this dilution into extravasated area. Blanching should reverse immediately. Monitor site. If blanching should recur, additional injections of phentolamine may be needed.
Miscellaneous Agents		
Aminophylline Calcium salts Dextrose (>10%) Mannitol (>5%) Phenytoin Contrast media Sodium bicarbonate (8.4%) Sodium chloride (>0.9%) Tetracycline	Cold	Hyaluronidase as directed above
IRRITANTS		
Arsenic trioxide	Warm	
Bleomycin	Cold	
Carboplatin ≥10 mg/mL	Cold	
Carmustine	Cold	
Cisplatin (concentration <0.5 mg/mL or <20 mL of more concentrated solution)	Cold	
Cyclophosphamide	Cold	Inject 5 mL 1/6 molar sodium thiosulfate (mix 4 mL 10% sodium thiosulfate with 6 mL sterile water)
Dacarbazine	Cold	DMSO as described above
Daunorubicin citrate (liposomal)	Cold	
Dexrazoxane	None	
Docetaxel	Warm	
Doxorubicin, liposomal	Cold	

Medication Extravasated	Cold/Warm Pack	Antidote
Etoposide	Warm	Hyaluronidase as directed above; use only for large infiltration
Fluorouracil	Cold	
Gemcitabine	Warm	
Gemtuzumab	None	
Ifosfamide	Cold	DMSO as described above
Irinotecan	Cold	
Oxaliplatin	None	Inject 5 mL 1/6 molar sodium thiosulfate (mix 4 mL 10% soldium thiosulfate with 6 mL sterile water)
Teniposide	Warm	Hyaluronidase as directed above
Topotecan	Cold	

Note:

Extravasation: The unintentional leakage of pharmacologic and physiologic solutions into the perivascular, subcutaneous, or interstitial space.

Vesicants: Agents that cause redness, pain, and blistering when infiltrated and can progress to ulceration and tissue necrosis.

Irritants: Agents that cause redness at the injection site or along the vein and often include a mild pruritic allergic reaction related to histamine release. These reaction "flares" usually do not require intervention and subside in 30 minutes.

[1]Some references consider agent as an irritant instead of vesicant.

References

Bertelli G, "Prevention and Management of Extravasation of Cytotoxic Drugs, *Drug Saf*, 1995, 12(4):245-55.

Camp-Sorrell D, "Developing Extravasation Protocols and Monitoring Outcomes," *J Intraven Nurs*, 1998, 21(4):232-9.

Cohan RH, Ellis JH, and Garner WL, "Extravasation of Radiographic Contrast Material: Recognition, Prevention, and Treatment", *Radiology*, 1996, 200 (3):593-604.

Dorr RT, "Pharmacologic Management of Vesicant Chemotherapy Extravasations," *Cancer Chemotherapy Handbook*, 2nd ed, Norwalk CT: Appleton & Lange, 1994.

Finely RS, et al, *Concepts in Oncology and Therapeutics*, 2nd ed, Bethesda MS: Am Soc Heal Sys Rx, 1998.

Fenchel K and Karthaus M, "Cytotoxic Drug Extravasation," *Antibiot Chemother*, 2000, 50:144-8.

Kassner E, "Evaluation and Treatment of Chemotherapy Extravasation Injuries," *J Pediatr Oncol Nurs*, 2000, 17(3):135-48.

NIH, Standards of Practice: Care of the Patient Receiving I.V. Cytoxic or Biologic Agents, 2001.

Mullin S, Beckwith M, and Tyler L, "Prevention and Management of Antineoplastic Extravasation Injury," *Hosp Pharm*, 2000, 35:57-74.

BURN MANAGEMENT

Modified Lund-Browder Burn Assessment Chart
Estimation of Total Body Surface Area of Burn Involvement[1]
(% by site and age)

The total body surface area of burn involvement is determined by the sum of the percentages of each site.

Site[2]	0-1 years	1-4 years	5-9 years	10-14 years	15 years	Adult
Head	9.5	8.5	6.5	5.5	4.5	3.5
Neck	0.5	0.5	0.5	0.5	0.5	0.5
Trunk	13	13	13	13	13	13
Upper arm	2	2	2	2	2	2
Forearm	1.5	1.5	1.5	1.5	1.5	1.5
Hand	1.5	1.5	1.5	1.5	1.5	1.5
Perineum	1	1	1	1	1	1
Buttock (each)	2.5	2.5	2.5	2.5	2.5	2.5
Thigh	2.75	3.25	4	4.25	4.5	4.75
Leg	2.5	2.5	2.75	3	3.25	3.5
Foot	1.75	1.75	1.75	1.75	1.75	1.75

[1]Applies only to second- and third-degree burns

[2]Percentage for each site is only for **a single extremity with** anterior **OR** posterior involvement. Percentage should be **doubled if both anterior and posterior** involvement of a single extremity.

Adapted from Coren CV, "Burn Injuries in Children," *Pediatric Annals*, 1987, 16(4):328-39.

Parkland Fluid Replacement Formula

A guideline for replacement of deficits and ongoing losses (**Note:** For infants, maintenance fluids may need to be added to this): Administer 4 mL/kg/% burn of Ringer's lactate (glucose may be added but beware of stress hyperglycemia) over the first 24 hours; half of this total is given over the first 8 hours **calculated from the time of injury**; the remaining half is given over the next 16 hours. The second 24-hour fluid requirements average 50% to 75% of first day's requirement. Concentrations and rates best determined by monitoring weight, serum electrolytes, urine output, NG losses, etc.

Colloid may be added after 18-24 hours (1 g/kg/day of albumin) to maintain serum albumin >2 g/100 mL.

Potassium is generally withheld for the first 48 hours due to the large amount of potassium that is released from damaged tissues. To manage serum electrolytes, monitor urine electrolytes twice weekly and replace calculated urine losses.

ORAL CONTRACEPTIVES

Brand Name	Type	Progestin	Estrogen	Availability
Kariva™ Mircette®	Low Dose 1-21 d 22-23 d 24-28 d	Desogestrel 0.15 mg – –	Ethinyl estradiol 20 mcg – Ethinyl estradiol 10 mcg	28
Lybrel™	Low Dose Non-cyclic	Levonorgestrel 0.09 mg	Ethinyl estradiol 20 mcg	28
Alesse® Aviane™ Lessina™ Levlite™ Lutera™ Sronyx™	Low Dose Monophasic	Levonorgestrel 0.1 mg	Ethinyl estradiol 20 mcg	28
Balziva™	Monophasic	Norethindrone 0.4 mg	Ethinyl estradiol 35 mcg	28
Brevicon® Modicon® Necon® 0.5/35 Nortrel™ 0.5/35	Monophasic	Norethindrone 0.5 mg	Ethinyl estradiol 35 mcg	21, 28
Kelnor™ Zovia™ 1/35E	Monophasic	Ethynodiol diacetate 1 mg	Ethinyl estradiol 35 mcg	28
Zovia™ 1/50E	Monophasic	Ethynodiol diacetate 1 mg	Ethinyl estradiol 50 mcg	28
Levlen® Levora® Nordette® Portia™	Monophasic	Levonorgestrel 0.15 mg	Ethinyl estradiol 30 mcg	28
Cryselle™ Lo/Ovral® Low-Ogestrel®	Monophasic	Norgestrel 0.3 mg	Ethinyl estradiol 30 mcg	28
Junel™ 21 1/20 Loestrin 21® 1/20 Microgestin™ 1/20	Monophasic	Norethindrone acetate 1 mg	Ethinyl estradiol 20 mcg	21
Junel™ 21 1.5/30 Loestrin 21® 1.5/30 Microgestin™ 1.5/30	Monophasic	Norethindrone acetate 1.5 mg	Ethinyl estradiol 30 mcg	21
Necon® 1/35 Norinyl® 1+35 Nortrel™ 1/35 Ortho-Novum® 1/35	Monophasic	Norethindrone 1 mg	Ethinyl estradiol 35 mcg	21, 28
Necon® 1/50 Norinyl® 1+50	Monophasic	Norethindrone 1 mg	Mestranol 50 mcg	28
Apri® Desogen® Ortho-Cept® Reclipsen™ Solia™	Monophasic	Desogestrel 0.15 mg	Ethinyl estradiol 30 mcg	28
MonoNessa™ Ortho-Cyclen® Previfem™ Sprintec™	Monophasic	Norgestimate 0.25 mg	Ethinyl estradiol 35 mcg	28
Ovcon® 35 Zenchent™	Monophasic	Norethindrone 0.4 mg	Ethinyl estradiol 35 mcg	21, 28
Ovcon® 50	Monophasic	Norethindrone 1 mg	Ethinyl estradiol 50 mcg	28
Ogestrel® 0.5/50	Monophasic	Norgestrel 0.5 mg	Ethinyl estradiol 50 mcg	28
Yaz®	Monophasic	Drospirenone 3 mg	Ethinyl estradiol 20 mcg	28
Ocella™ Yasmin®	Monophasic	Drospirenone 3 mg	Ethinyl estradiol 30 mcg	28
Loestrin® 24 Fe 1/20 Junel™ Fe 1/20 Microgestin™ Fe 1/20	Monophasic / Iron 25-28 d	Norethindrone acetate 1 mg	Ethinyl estradiol 20 mcg	28

Brand Name	Type	Progestin	Estrogen	Availability
Loestrin® Fe 1.5/30 Junel™ Fe 1.5/30 Microgestin™ Fe 1.5/30	Monophasic / Iron 22-28 d	Norethindrone acetate 1.5 mg	Ethinyl estradiol 30 mcg	28
Femcon™ Fe	Monophasic / Iron 22-28 d	Norethindrone 0.4 mg	Ethinyl estradiol 35 mcg	28
LoSeasonique™	Low Dose Extended cycle regimen			91
	1-84	Levonorgestrel 0.1 mg	Ethinyl estradiol 20 mcg	
	85-91		Ethinyl estradiol 10 mcg	
Jolessa™ Quasense™ Seasonale®	Extended cycle regimen	Levonorgestrel 0.15 mg	Ethinyl estradiol 30 mcg	91
Seasonique™	Extended cycle regimen			91
	1-84	Levonorgestrel 0.15 mg	Ethinyl estradiol 30 mcg	
	85-91		Ethinyl estradiol 10 mcg	
Necon® 10/11 Ortho-Novum® 10/11	Biphasic			
	1-10 d	Norethindrone 0.5 mg	Ethinyl estradiol 35 mcg	28
	11-21 d	Norethindrone 1 mg	Ethinyl estradiol 35 mcg	
	22-28 d	Inert	—	
Necon® 7/7/7 Nortrel™ 7/7/7 Ortho-Novum® 7/7/7	Triphasic			
	1-7 d	Norethindrone 0.5 mg	Ethinyl estradiol 35 mcg	28
	8-14 d	Norethindrone 0.75 mg	Ethinyl estradiol 35 mcg	
	15-21 d	Norethindrone 1 mg	Ethinyl estradiol 35 mcg	
	22-28 d	Inert	—	
Ortho Tri-Cyclen® TriNessa™ Tri-Previfem™ Tri-Sprintec™	Triphasic			
	1-7 d	Norgestimate 0.18 mg	Ethinyl estradiol 35 mcg	28
	8-14 d	Norgestimate 0.215 mg	Ethinyl estradiol 35 mcg	
	15-21 d	Norgestimate 0.25 mg	Ethinyl estradiol 35 mcg	
	22-28 d	Inert	—	
Ortho Tri-Cyclen® Lo	Triphasic			
	1-7 d	Norgestimate 0.18 mg	Ethinyl estradiol 25 mcg	28
	8-14 d	Norgestimate 0.215 mg	Ethinyl estradiol 25 mcg	
	15-21 d	Norgestimate 0.25 mg	Ethinyl estradiol 25 mcg	
Aranelle™ Leena™ Tri-Norinyl®	Triphasic			
	1-7 d	Norethindrone 0.5 mg	Ethinyl estradiol 35 mcg	28
	8-16 d	Norethindrone 1 mg	Ethinyl estradiol 35 mcg	
	17-21 d	Norethindrone 0.5 mg	Ethinyl estradiol 35 mcg	
	22- 28 d	Inert	—	

Brand Name	Type	Progestin	Estrogen	Availability
Enpresse™ Triphasil® Trivora®	Triphasic			
	1-6 d	Levonorgestrel 0.05 mg	Ethinyl estradiol 30 mcg	28
	7-11 d	Levonorgestrel 0.075 mg	Ethinyl estradiol 40 mcg	
	12-21 d	Levonorgestrel 0.125 mg	Ethinyl estradiol 30 mcg	
	22-28 d	Inert	—	
Cesia™ Cyclessa® Velivet™	Triphasic			
	1-7 d	Desogestrel 0.1 mg	Ethinyl estradiol 25 mcg	28
	8-14 d	Desogestrel 0.125 mg	Ethinyl estradiol 25 mcg	
	15-21 d	Desogestrel 0.15 mg	Ethinyl estradiol 25 mcg	
	22-28 d	Inert	—	
Estrostep® Fe Tilia™ Fe	Triphasic / Iron 22-28 d			
	1-5 d	Norethindrone acetate 1 mg	Ethinyl estradiol 20 mcg	28
	6-12 d	Norethindrone acetate 1 mg	Ethinyl estradiol 30 mcg	
	13-21 d	Norethindrone acetate 1 mg	Ethinyl estradiol 35 mcg	
Camila™ Errin™ Jolivette™ Nora-BE™ Nor-QD® Ortho-Micronor®	Progestin only	Norethindrone 0.35 mg	—	28
Plan B®	Progestin only (emergency contraception)	Levonorgestrel 0.75 mg	—	2

Monophasic Oral Contraceptives in Order of Decreasing Estrogen Content

Estrogen	Brand Name (Progestin Content)
Mestranol 50 mcg	Necon® 1/50, Norinyl® 1+50, **(Norethindrone 1 mg)**
Ethinyl estradiol 50 mcg	Zovia™ 1/50E **(Ethynodiol diacetate 1 mg)**
	Ovcon®-50 **(Norethindrone 1 mg)**
	Ogestrel® 0.5/50 **(Norgestrel 0.5 mg)**
Ethinyl estradiol 35 mcg	Necon® 1/35, Norinyl® 1+35, Nortrel® 1/35, Ortho-Novum® 1/35 **(Norethindrone 1 mg)**
	Brevicon®, Modicon®, Necon® 0.5/35, Nortrel® 0.5/35 **(Norethindrone 0.5 mg)**
	Femcon™ Fe, Ovcon®-35, Zenchent™ **(Norethindrone 0.4 mg)**
	MonoNessa™, Ortho-Cyclen®, Previfem™, Sprintec™ **(Norgestimate 0.25 mg)**
	Kelnor™ 1/35, Zovia™ 1/35E **(Ethynodiol diacetate 1 mg)**
Ethinyl estradiol 30 mcg	Junel™ 21 1.5/30, Junel™ Fe 1.5/30, Loestrin 21® 1.5/30, Loestrin® Fe 1.5/30, Microgestin™ 1.5/30, Microgestin™ Fe 1.5/30 **(Norethindrone acetate 1.5 mg)**
	Cryselle™, Lo/Ovral®, Low-Ogestrel™ **(Norgestrel 0.3 mg)**
	Apri®, Desogen®, Ortho-Cept®, Reclipsen™, Solia™ **(Desogestrel 0.15 mg)**
	Jolessa™, Levlen®, Levora®, Nordette®, Portia™, Quasense™, Seasonale® **(Levonorgestrel 0.15 mg)**
	Yasmin® **(Drospirenone 3 mg)**
Ethinyl estradiol 20 mcg	Alesse®, Aviane™, Lessina™, Levlite™, Lutera™, Sronyx™ **(Levonorgestrel 0.1 mg)**
	Junel™ 21 1/20, Junel™ Fe 1/20, ™ Loestrin 21® 1/20, Loestrin® Fe 1/20, Microgestin™ 1/20, Microgestin™ Fe 1/20 **(Norethindrone acetate 1 mg)**
	Yaz® **(Drospirenone 3 mg)**

Signs / Symptoms of Hormonal Imbalance With Oral Contraceptives

Estrogen Excess	Fluid retention, edema, cyclic weight gain, "bloating," hypertension, breast fullness/tenderness, nausea, migraine headache, melasma, telangiectasia, cervical mucorrhea, and polyposis
Estrogen Deficiency	Increased spotting, early or midcycle breakthrough bleeding, hypomenorrhea
Progestin Excess	Fatigue, lethargy, depression, decreased libido, increased appetite, weight gain, breast regression, monilial vaginitis, hypomenorrhea, hair loss, hirsutism, acne, oily scalp. **Note:** Hair loss, hirsutism, acne, and oily scalp are effects of the androgenic activity of progestins.
Progestin Deficiency	Amenorrhea, late breakthrough bleeding, hypermenorrhea

FLUIDS, ELECTROLYTES, AND NUTRITION

ENTERAL NUTRITIONAL PRODUCT FORMULARY, INFANTS

Milk Based Formulas[1,2]

(Indications: Feeding normal term infants or sick infants without special nutritional requirements)

	Human Milk	Enfamil® Premium™	Similac® Advance®[3]	Similac® Organic	Good Start® Gentle Plus™	Good Start® Protect Plus®[4]
Calories /100 mL	68	68	68	68	67	67
Protein g/100 mL	1	1.4	1.4	1.4	1.47	1.47
Protein source	Mature Term human milk	Nonfat milk, whey protein concentrate	Nonfat milk, whey protein concentrate	Organic nonfat milk	Whey protein concentrate	Whey protein concentrate
Carbohydrate g/100 mL	7.2	7.5	7.6	7.1	7.8	7.5
Carbohydrate source	Lactose	Lactose, polydextrose galactooligosaccharides[5,6]	Lactose and galactooligosaccharides[5]	Organic corn maltodextrin, organic sugar, organic lactose	Corn maltodextrin, lactose, galactooligosaccharides[5]	Lactose and corn maltodextrin
Fat g/100 mL	3.91	3.6	3.65	3.71	3.42	3.42
Fat source	Human milk, fat	Palm olein, coconut, soy, and high oleic sunflower oils, soy lecithin, and single cell oil blend rich in DHA & ARA[7]	High oleic safflower, soy, and coconut oils (40:30:29) DHA: 0.15% ARA: 0.40%[7]	Organic high oleic sunflower, organic soy, and organic coconut oils (40:30:29). DHA & ARA[7]	Palm, soy, coconut, high oleic safflower or sunflower oils, soy lecithin, and DHA & ARA[7]	Palm, soy, coconut, high oleic safflower or sunflower oils, soy lecithin, and DHA & ARA[7]
Osmolality mOsm/kg H_2O	286	300	310	225		
Osmolarity mOsm/L		270	127	127		
Sodium mEq/L (mg/L)	7.7 (177)	(180)	7.1 (162)	7.1 (162)	(181)	(181)
Potassium mEq/L (mg/L)	13.6 (531)	(720)	18.2 (710)	18.1 (710)	(724)	(724)
Chloride mEq/L (mg/L)	11.9 (422)	(420)	12.4 (440)	12.4 (439)	(436)	(436)
Calcium mEq/L (mg/L)	16 (280)	27 (520)	26.3 (528)	26.3 (528)	(449)	(449)
Phosphorus mEq/L (mg/L)	9 (143)	(287)	18.8 (284)	(284)	(255)	(255)
Iron mg/L	0.27	12 (4.7)[8]	12.2	12.2	10.1	10.1

Milk Based Formulas[1,2] continued

	Human Milk	Enfamil® Premium™	Similac® Advance®[3]	Similac® Organic	Good Start® Gentle Plus™	Good Start® Protect Plus®[4]
% Free water		89	90	90	90	90
Manufacturer		Mead Johnson	Abbott	Abbott	Gerber/Nestle	Gerber/Nestle

[1]Information based on manufacturer's literature as of 2010 and is subject to change.

[2]To approximate values for the content of a 24-, 27-, or 30-cal/oz formula (made by dilution of a powder-based formulation), multiply the value desired, found in the above 20-cal/oz formula, by the following factors: 1.2 (24-cal/oz), 1.35 (27-cal/oz), or 1.5 (30-cal/oz).

[3]Contains nucleotides and prebiotics for enhanced immune function.

[4]Contains Bifidus BL™. Beneficial cultures like those found in breast milk to help support a healthy immune system.

[5]Prebiotic.

[6]Polydextrose + galactooligosaccharides = Natural Defense™ Dual Prebiotics from Mead Johnson. They support the growth of healthy gut bacteria which help support immune function.

[7]DHA (docosahexaenoic acid) and ARA (arachidonic acid) are fatty acids which are found naturally in breast milk.

[8]Low iron formulation in parenthesis.

Milk Based Formulas – Reduced Lactose and Lactose Free[1,2]

(**Indications:** Feeding normal term infants or sick infants without special nutritional requirements)

	Enfamil® Gentlease®[3]	Similac® Sensitive®[4]
Calories /100 mL	68	68
Protein g/100 mL	1.53	1.45
Protein source	Partially hydrolyzed nonfat milk and whey protein concentrate (soy)	Milk protein isolate
Carbohydrate g/100 mL	7.2	7.2
Carbohydrate source	Corn syrup solids	Sucrose and corn maltodextrin (55:45)
Fat g/100 mL	3.53	3.65
Fat source	Palm olein, soy, coconut, and high oleic sunflower oils, and single cell oil blend rich in DHA & ARA[5]	High oleic safflower, soy, and coconut oils (40:30:29) DHA: 0.15% ARA: 0.40%[5]
Osmolality mOsm/kg H_2O	230	200
Osmolarity mOsm/L	210	135
Sodium mEq/L (mg/L)	(240)	8.8 (203)
Potassium mEq/L (mg/L)	(720)	18.5 (724)
Chloride mEq/L (mg/L)	(420)	12.4 (440)
Calcium mEq/L (mg/L)	(547)	28.3 (568)
Phosphorus mEq/L (mg/L)	(307)	21.6 (379)
Iron mg/L	10	12.2
% Free water	89	90
Manufacturer	Mead Johnson	Abbott

[1]Information based on manufacturer's literature as of 2010 and is subject to change.

[2] To approximate values for the content of a 24-, 27-, or 30-cal/oz formula (made by dilution of a powder-based formulation), multiply the value desired, found in the above 20-cal/oz formula, by the following factors: 1.2 (24-cal/oz), 1.35 (27-cal/oz), or 1.5 (30-cal/oz).

[3]Previous product Enfamil® LactoFree® LIPIL® discontinued. Recommend using Enfamil® Gentlease® instead. Enfamil® Gentlease® contains 1/5 the lactose of regular milk-based formulas and is for infants who have shown transient intolerance to lactose and is marketed for fussiness/gas.

[4]Also available as Similac® Sensitive® For Spit Up™ with rice starch.

[5]DHA (docosahexaenoic acid) and ARA (arachidonic acid) are fatty acids found naturally in breast milk.

Milk Based Formulas[1]

	Enfamil® A.R.	Enfamil® RestFull™ LIPIL®	Similac Sensitive® RS	Enfagrow™ Premium™ Next Step®[2]	Enfagrow™ Gentlease® Next Step®[3]	Similac® Go & Grow Milk-Based formula	Good Start® 2 Gentle Plus™	Good Start® 2 Protect Plus®[4]
Calories /100 mL	68	68	68	67	67	68	67	67
Protein g/100 mL	1.67	1.67	1.5	1.73	1.73	1.4	1.47	1.47
Protein source	Nonfat milk	Nonfat milk	Milk protein isolate	Nonfat milk	Partially hydrolyzed nonfat milk and whey protein concentrate solids (soy)	Nonfat milk, whey protein concentrate	Whey protein concentrate	Whey protein concentrate
Carbohydrate g/100 mL	7.3	7.3	7.2	7	7	7.14	7.8	7.5
Carbohydrate source	Rice starch, lactose, and maltodextrin	Rice starch, lactose, maltodextrin	Corn syrup, rice starch, sugar (50:30:20)	Corn syrup solids and lactose	Corn syrup solids and lactose	Lactose	Lactose, corn maltodextrin, and galactooligosac-charides[5]	Lactose and corn maltodextrin
Fat g/100 mL	3.4	3.4	3.7	3.53	3.5	3.7	3.42	3.42
Fat source	Palm olein, soy, coconut, and high oleic sunflower oils, and DHA & ARA[6]	Palm olein, soy, coconut, and high oleic sunflower oils, and DHA & ARA[6]	High oleic safflower, soy, and coconut oils, and DHA & ARA[6] (40:30:29)	Palm olein, soy, coconut, and high oleic sunflower oils, and DHA & ARA[6]	Palm olein, soy, coconut, and high oleic sunflower oils, and DHA & ARA[6]	High oleic safflower, soy, and coconut oil, and DHA & ARA[6]	Palm olein, soy, coconut, and high oleic safflower or sunflower oils, soy lecithin, and DHA & ARA[6]	Palm olein, soy, coconut, and high oleic safflower or sunflower oils, soy lecithin, and DHA & ARA[6]
Osmolality mOsm/kg H_2O	240	230	180	270	230	300		
Osmolarity mOsm/L	220	210	135	240	210	135		
Sodium mEq/L (mg/L)	(267)	(267)	8.8 (203)	(240)	(267)	7.1 (162)	(181)	(181)
Potassium mEq/L (mg/L)	(720)	(720)	18.5 (724)	(867)	(867)	18.2 (710)	(724)	(724)
Chloride mEq/L (mg/L)	(500)	(500)	12.4 (440)	(533)	(533)	12.4 (440)	(436)	(436)
Calcium mEq/L (mg/L)	(520)	(520)	28.3 (568)	(1300)	(1300)	50 (1014)	(1273)	(1273)
Phosphorus mEq/L (mg/L)	(353)	(353)	(379)	(867)	(867)	(548)	(710)	(710)
Iron mg/L	12	12	12.2	13.3	13.3	13.5	13	13.4
% Free water	89	89	90	89	89	90	90	90

Milk Based Formulas[1] *continued*

	Enfamil® A.R.	Enfamil® RestFull™ LIPIL®	Similac Sensitive® RS	Enfagrow™ Premium™ Next Step®[2]	Enfagrow™ Gentlease® Next Step®[3]	Similac® Go & Grow™ Milk-Based formula	Good Start® 2 Gentle Plus™	Good Start® 2 Protect Plus®[4]
Manufacturer	Mead Johnson	Mead Johnson	Abbott	Mead Johnson	Mead Johnson	Abbott	Gerber/Nestle	Gerber/Nestle
Special Uses	Thickened with added rice starch for babies who spit up frequently.	Designed to gently thicken and digest slowly for natural way to help keep baby feeling satisfied; for bedtime feeding.	With added rich starch to help reduce spit-up; milk-based, lactose-free formula.	Infants and toddlers 10-36 months.	Infants 10-36 months.	Infants and toddlers 9-24 months; specifically formulated to help bridge nutritional gaps that can be associated with transition to table foods.	Infants 9-24 months.	Infants 9-24 months.

[1]Information based on manufacturer's literature as of 2010 and is subject to change.

[2]Also available as Enfagrow™ Premium™ Toddler for 12-36 months in either a chocolate or vanilla flavor.

[3]Contains ½ the lactose of other milk-based infant/toddler formulas.

[4]Contains Bifidus BL™. Beneficial cultures like those found in breast milk to help support a healthy immune system.

[5]Prebiotic.

[6]DHA (docosahexaenoic acid) and ARA (arachidonic acid) are fatty acids found naturally in breast milk.

Soy Formulas[1,2]

(**Indications:** Lactase deficiency, milk intolerance, or galactosemia;
not recommended for premature infants with birthweight <1.8 kg)

	Enfamil® ProSobee® LIPIL®	Similac® Isomil® Advance®	Good Start® Soy Plus™
Calories /100 mL	68	67.6	67
Protein g/100 mL	1.67	1.66	1.68
Protein source	Soy protein, L-methionine, and taurine	Soy protein isolate, L-methionine	Enzymatically hydrolyzed soy protein isolate
Carbohydrate g/100 mL	7.1	6.97	7.44
Carbohydrate source	Corn syrup solids	Corn syrup solids and sucrose (80:20)	Corn maltodextrin sucrose
Fat g/100 mL	3.5	3.69	3.42
Fat source	Palm olein, soy, coconut, and high oleic sunflower oils, and DHA & ARA[3]	High oleic safflower, soy, and coconut oils, and DHA & ARA[3]	Palm olein, soy, coconut, and high oleic safflower or sunflower oils, and DHA & ARA[3]
Osmolality mOsm/kg H_2O	170	200	
Osmolarity mOsm/L	153	155	
Sodium mEq/L (mg/L)	(240)	12.9 (298)	(268)
Potassium mEq/L (mg/L)	(800)	18.7 (730)	(777)
Chloride mEq/L (mg/L)	(533)	11.8 (419)	(476)
Calcium mEq (mg/L)	(700)	35.4 (710)	(704)
Phosphorus mEq/L (mg/L)	(460)	32.9 (507)	(422)
Iron mg/L	12	12.2	12.1
% Free water	89	90	90
Manufacturer	Mead Johnson	Abbott	Gerber/Nestle

[1]Information based on manufacturer's literature as of 2010 and is subject to change.

[2]To approximate values for the content of a 24-, 27-, or 30-cal/oz formula (made by dilution of a powder-based formulation), multiply the value desired, found in the above 20-cal/oz formula, by the following factors: 1.2 (24-cal/oz), 1.35 (27-cal/oz), or 1.5 (30-cal/oz).

[3]DHA (docosahexaenoic acid) and ARA (arachidonic acid) are fatty acids found naturally in breast milk.

Soy Formulas[1,2]

(**Indications:** Lactase deficiency, milk intolerance, or galactosemia)

	Enfagrow™ Soy Next Step®[3]	Good Start® 2 Soy Plus™[4]	Similac® Go & Grow™ Soy-Based formula[4]
Calories /100 mL	67	67	68
Protein g/100 mL	2.2	1.88	1.7
Protein source	Soy protein isolate, L-methionine, and taurine	Enzymatically hydrolyzed soy protein isolate	Soy protein isolate, L-methionine, and taurine
Carbohydrate g/100 mL	7.87	7.3	7
Carbohydrate source	Corn syrup solids	Corn maltodextrin and sucrose	Corn syrup solids, sugar (80:20)
Fat g/100 mL	2.93	3.35	3.7
Fat source	Palm olein, soy, coconut, and high oleic sunflower oils, and 3% DHA & ARA[5]	Palm olein, soy, coconut, high oleic safflower or sunflower oils, and DHA & ARA[5]	High oleic safflower, soy, and coconut oils, and DHA & ARA[5]
Osmolality mOsm/kg H_2O	230		200
Osmolarity mOsm/L	200		160
Sodium mEq/L (mg/L)	(240)	(268)	12.9 (298)

Soy Formulas[1,2] (continued)

	Enfagrow™ Soy Next Step®[3]	Good Start® 2 Soy Plus™[4]	Similac® Go & Grow™ Soy-Based formula[4]
Potassium mEq/L (mg/L)	(800)	(777)	18.7 (730)
Chloride mEq/L (mg/L)	(533)	(476)	11.8 (419)
Calcium mEq/L (mg/L)	(1300)	(1273)	50.6 (1014)
Phosphorus mEq/L (mg/L)	56 (867)	(710)	(676)
Iron mg/L	13.3	13.4	13.5
% Free water			90
Manufacturer	Mead Johnson	Gerber/Nestle	Abbott

[1]Information based on manufacturer's literature as of 2010 and is subject to change.

[2] To approximate values for the content of a 24-, 27-, or 30-cal/oz formula (made by dilution of a powder-based formulation), multiply the value desired, found in the above 20-cal/oz formula, by the following factors: 1.2 (24-cal/oz), 1.35 (27-cal/oz), or 1.5 (30-cal/oz).

[3]Indicated for infants and toddlers 10-36 months.

[4]Indicated for infants and toddlers 9-24 months.

Soy Formula[1]

(Indications: Dietary management of diarrhea in infants >6 months and toddlers)

	Similac® Isomil® DF[2]
Calories /100 mL	68
Protein g/100 mL	1.8
Protein source	Soy protein isolate and L-methionine
Carbohydrate g/100 mL	6.83
Carbohydrate source	Corn syrup solids and sugar (60:40)
Fat g/100 mL	3.69
Fat source	Soy and coconut oils
Osmolality mOsm/kg H_2O	240
Osmolarity mOsm/L	163
Sodium mEq/L (mg/L)	12.9 (298)
Potassium mEq/L (mg/L)	18.7 (730)
Chloride mEq/L (mg/L)	11.8 (419)
Calcium mEq/L (mg/L)	35.4 (710)
Phosphorus mEq/L (mg/L)	(507)
Iron mg/L	12.2
% Free water	90

[1]Information based on manufacturer's literature as of 2010 and is subject to change.

[2]Manufactured by Abbott.

Casein Hydrolysate Formulas[1,2]

(Indication: For infants predisposed to or being treated for hypocalcemia due to hyperphosphatemia whose renal or cardiovascular functions would benefit from lowered mineral concentrations)

	Similac® PM 60/40
Calories /100 mL	68
Protein g/100 mL	1.5
Protein source	Whey protein caseinate and sodium caseinate

Casein Hydrolysate Formulas[1,2] *(continued)*

	Similac® PM 60/40
Carbohydrate g/100 mL	6.9
Carbohydrate source	Lactose
Fat g/100 mL	3.78
Fat source	High oleic safflower, soy, and coconut oils (41:30:29)
Osmolality mOsm/kg H_2O	280
Osmolarity mOsm/L	124
Sodium mEq/L (mg/L)	7.1 (162)
Potassium mEq/L (mg/L)	13.8 (541)
Chloride mEq/L (mg/L)	11.3 (399)
Calcium mEq/L (mg/L)	18.9 (379)
Phosphorus mEq/L (mg/L)	(189)
Iron mg/L	4.73
% Free water	90
Special uses	Renal and cardiovascular disease

[1] Information based on manufacturer's literature as of 2010 and is subject to change.

[2] Manufactured by Abbott.

Casein Hydrolysate Formulas[1,2]

(**Indication:** For infants requiring low molecular weight peptides or amino acids)

	Nutramigen® LIPIL®[3]	Pregestimil® LIPIL®[4]	Similac® Alimentum®
Calories /100 mL	68	68	68
Protein g/100 mL	1.87	1.87	1.86
Protein source	Casein hydrolysate, L-cystine, L-tyrosine, L-tryptophan, and taurine	Casein hydrolysate, L-cystine, L-tyrosine, L-tryptophan, and taurine	Casein hydrolysate, L-cystine, L-tyrosine, and L-tryptophan
Carbohydrate g/100 mL	6.87	6.8	6.9
Carbohydrate source	Corn syrup solids and modified corn starch (lactose- and sucrose-free)	Corn syrup solids, dextrose, and modified corn starch (lactose- and sucrose-free)	Corn maltodextrin and sucrose (70:30)
Fat g/100 mL	3.53	3.73	3.75
Fat source	44% palm olein, 19.5% soy, 19.5% coconut, and 14.5% high oleic sunflower oils, and 2.5% single cell oil blend rich in DHA & ARA[5]	55% MCT, 35% soy, and 10% high oleic vegetable (sunflower/safflower) oils, and 2.5% single cell oil blend rich in DHA & ARA[5,6]	High oleic safflower, medium chain triglycerides, and soy oils (38:33:28), and DHA & ARA[5]
Osmolality mOsm/kg H_2O	260 (liquid)	290 (liquid)	370
Osmolarity mOsm/L	230 (liquid)	260 (liquid)	171
Sodium mEq/L (mg/L)	(313)	(313)	12.9 (298)
Potassium mEq/L (mg/L)	(733)	(733)	20.3 (798)
Chloride mEq/L (mg/L)	(573)	(573)	15.5 (541)
Calcium mEq/L (mg/L)	(627)	(627)	35.4 (710)
Phosphorus mEq/L (mg/L)	(347)	(347)	(507)
Iron mg/L	12.2	12 (liquid)	12.2
% Free water	89	89	90

Casein Hydrolysate Formulas[1,2] (continued)

	Nutramigen® LIPIL®[3]	Pregestimil® LIPIL®[4]	Similac® Alimentum®
Manufacturer	Mead Johnson	Mead Johnson	Abbott
Special uses	Sensitivity to intact proteins found in milk and soy formulas and patients with galactosemia	Fat malabsorption or sensitivity to intact proteins; may be used in cystic fibrosis, short bowel syndrome, intractable diarrhea, severe protein calorie malnutrition, and patients with galactosemia; contains 55% MCT oil	Severe food allergies, sensitivity (including colic) to intact proteins, protein maldigestion or fat malabsorption

[1]Information based on manufacturer's literature as of 2010and is subject to change.

[2]To approximate values for the content of a 24-, 27-, or 30-cal/oz formula (made by dilution of a powder-based formulation), multiply the value desired, found in the above 20-cal/oz formula, by the following factors: 1.2 (24-cal/oz), 1.35 (27-cal/oz), or 1.5 (30-cal/oz).

[3]Also available with Enflora™LGG®, which is a probiotic to support healthy and normal function of the GI tract.

[4]Also available as a 24 kcal/oz ready to feed product.

[4]DHA (docosahexaenoic acid) and ARA (arachidonic acid) are fatty acids found naturally in breast milk.

[5]Powder content varies: 55% MCT oil, 25% soy oil, 7.5% corn oil, 10% high oleic safflower or sunflower oil, and 2.5% DHA & ARA.

Other Infant and Pediatric Formulas[1,2] – Special Care

(Indication: Premature infant formulas designed for rapidly growing LBW infants)

	Preterm Human Milk	Enfamil® EnfaCare® LIPIL®[3]	Enfamil® Premature LIPIL® 20	Enfamil® Premature LIPIL® 24	Similac® Special Care® 20 With Iron	Similac® Neosure®[3]	Similac® Special Care® 24 High Protein	Similac® Special Care® 30 With Iron
Calories /100 mL	67	73	68	80	68	74	81	101
Protein g/100 mL	1.41	2.1	2	2.38	2.03	2.08	2.68	3.04
Protein source	Preterm human milk	Nonfat milk and whey protein concentrate	Nonfat milk and whey protein concentrate	Nonfat milk and whey protein concentrate	Nonfat milk and whey protein concentrate	Nonfat milk and whey protein concentrate	Nonfat milk and whey protein concentrate	Nonfat milk and whey protein concentrate
Carbohydrate g/100 mL	6.64	7.7	7.3	8.73	6.97	7.51	8.1	7.84
Carbohydrate source	Lactose	Powder: Corn syrup solids and lactose Liquid: Maltodextrin and lactose	Corn syrup solids and lactose	Corn syrup solids and lactose	Corn syrup solids and lactose (50:50)	Corn syrup solids and lactose (50:50)	Corn syrup solids and lactose	Corn syrup solids and lactose (50:50)
Fat g/100 mL	3.89	3.9	3.4	4	3.67	4.09	4.41	6.71
Fat source	Preterm human milk	High oleic vegetable (sunflower/safflower), soy, MCT, and coconut oils with DHA & ARA[4]	MCT, soy, and high oleic vegetable oils (sunflower/safflower) with DHA & ARA[4]	MCT, soy, and high oleic vegetable oils (sunflower/safflower) with DHA & ARA[4]	Medium chain triglycerides, soy, and coconut oils (50:30:18) with DHA & ARA[4]	Medium chain triglycerides, soy, and coconut oils (29:45:25) with DHA & ARA[4]	Medium chain triglycerides, soy, and coconut oils (50:30:18) with DHA & ARA[4]	Medium chain triglycerides, soy, and coconut oils (50:30:18) with DHA & ARA[4]
Osmolality mOsm/kg H$_2$O	290	250 (liquid)	240	300	235	250	280	325
Osmolarity mOsm/L	220	220	220	260	188	187	240	282
Sodium mEq/L (mg/L)	10.8 (248)	(259)	(387)	(460)	12.6 (291)	10.7 (245)	15.2 (349)	19 (436)
Potassium mEq/L (mg/L)	14.6 (570)	(778)	(653)	(778)	22.3 (872)	27 (1056)	26.8 (1047)	33.5 (1308)
Chloride mEq/L (mg/L)	15.6 (550)	(578)	(600)	(714)	15.5 (548)	15.7 (558)	18.6 657	23.2 (821)
Calcium mEq/L (mg/L)	12.4 (248)	(889)	(1100)	(1310)	60.7 (1217)	39 (781)	72.9 (1461)	91.3 (1826)
Phosphorus mEq/L (mg/L)	(128)	(489)	(553)	(659)	(676)	(461)	(812)	(1014)
Iron mg/L	1	13.3	12 (3.3)[5]	14.3 (4)[5]	12.2 (2.5)[5]	13.4	14.6	18.3

Other Infant and Pediatric Formulas[1,2] – Special Care *continued*

	Preterm Human Milk	Enfamil® EnfaCare® LIPIL®[3]	Enfamil® Premature LIPIL® 20	Enfamil® Premature LIPIL® 24	Similac® Special Care® 20 With Iron	Similac® Neosure®[3]	Similac® Special Care® 24 High Protein	Similac® Special Care® 30 With Iron
% Free water		80	89	86	89	89	89	85
Manufacturer		Mead Johnson	Mead Johnson	Mead Johnson	Abbott	Abbott	Abbott	Abbott

[1]Information based on manufacturer's literature as of 2010 and is subject to change.

[2]To approximate values of 24-cal/oz formulation, multiply the values desired, found in the 20-cal/oz formula by 1.2.

[3]Discharge formulas.

[4]DHA (docosahexaenoic acid) and ARA (arachidonic acid) are fatty acids found naturally in breast milk.

[5]Low iron formulation in parentheses.

Human Milk Fortifiers[1]

(Indication: Add to human milk as a supplement for premature and low birth weight infants)

	Enfamil® Human Milk Fortifier	Similac® Human Milk Fortifier
Calories /packet	3.5	3.5
Protein g/packet	0.28	0.25
Protein source	Milk protein isolate and whey protein hydrolysate	Nonfat milk and whey protein concentrate
Carbohydrate g/packet	<0.1	0.45
Carbohydrate source	Corn syrup solids, lactose, and soy lecithin	Lactose and corn syrup solids
Fat g/packet	0.25	0.09
Fat source	MCT and soybean oils	MCT oil
Osmolality mOsm/kg H_2O	Additional 35 when added to breast milk	
Sodium mEq/packet (mg/packet)	(4)	0.16 (3.75)
Potassium mEq/packet (mg/packet)	(7.25)	0.4 (15.8)
Chloride mEq/packet (mg/packet)	(3.25)	0.27 (9.5)
Calcium mEq/packet (mg/packet)	(22.5)	1.46 (29.3)
Phosphorus mEq/packet (mg/packet)	(12.5)	0.54 (19)
Iron mg/packet	0.36	0.08
Manufacturer	Mead Johnson	Abbott

[1]Information based on manufacturer's literature as of 2010 and is subject to change.

[2]May be mixed with human milk or fed alternatively with human milk to low birth weight infants.

[3]DHA (docosahexaenoic acid) and ARA (arachidonic acid) are fatty acids found naturally in breast milk.

Enteral Formulas – Pediatric[1]

(A selection of the commonly used enteral feedings)

	PediaSure® Enteral Formula	PediaSure® Enteral Formula With Fiber and scFOS®	Peptamen Junior®[3]	Vivonex® Pediatric[4]	Compleat® Pediatric
Calories/oz	30	30	30	24	30
Calories/mL	1	1	1.06	0.8	1
Carbohydrate g/100 mL	13.3	13.8	13.8	13	12.6
Carbohydrate source	Corn maltodextrin and sucrose (86:14)	Corn maltodextrin and sucrose (86:14)	Maltodextrin, corn starch	Maltodextrin, modified corn starch	Cranberry juice cocktail, corn syrup solids, peach puree, and green bean puree
Protein g/100 mL	3	3	3	2.4	3.76
Protein source	Milk protein concentrate	Milk protein concentrate	Partially hydrolyzed whey protein	L-amino acids	Chicken puree, sodium caseinate, and pea puree
Fat g/100 mL	4	4	3.9	2.4	3.88
Fat source	High oleic safflower, soy, and MCT oils (43:42:15)	High oleic safflower, soy, and MCT oils, and lecithin (43:42:15)	MCT, soy, and canola oils, and lecithin	MCT and soy oils	Canola and MCT oils
Osmolality mOsm/kg	335 vanilla	345 vanilla	260 unflavored 380 vanilla 400 strawberry	360	380
Osmolarity mOsm/L	277	277			
Sodium mEq/L (mg/L)	17 (380)	17 (380)	20 (460)	17 (400)	33 (760)
Potassium mEq/L (mg/L)	34 (1310)	34 (1310)	34 (1320)	31 (1200)	42 (1640)
Chloride mEq/L (mg/L)	29 (1014)	29 (1014)	30 (1080)	40 (1420)	156 (560)
Calcium mEq/L (mg/L)	49 (972)	49 (972)	(1000)	(1250)	(1440)
Phosphorus mEq/L (mg/L)	(845)	(845)	(800)	(1250)	(1000)
Iron (mg/L)	14	14	14	10	13
% Free water	85	85	85	89	82
Fiber (g/unit dose)		Dietary: 0.8 scFOS: 0.3			Dietary: 1.75

Enteral Formulas – Pediatric[1] continued

	PediaSure® Enteral Formula	PediaSure® Enteral Formula With Fiber and scFOS®	Peptamen Junior®[3]	Vivonex® Pediatric[4]	Compleat® Pediatric
Manufacturer	Abbott	Abbott	Nestle	Nestle	Nestle
Indication	For 1-13 years of age	For 1-13 years of age	For 1-13 years of age	For 1-10 years of age	Blenderized tube feeding formula containing real food for 1-10 years of age; lactose/gluten free

[1]Information based on manufacturer's literature as of 2010 and is subject to change.

[2]Prebiotic Nutraflora® scFOS® (short chain fructooligosaccaharides) provides fuel for beneficial bacteria in the digestive tract that help to support a healthy immune system.

[3]Also available with Prebio (3.6 g/L) prebiotic formulation.

[4]1.7 oz dry packet mixed with 220 mL of water produces 250 mL of formula.

Enteral Formulas – Pediatric[1] (continued)

(A selection of the commonly used enteral feedings for children 1-10 years of age)

	Peptamen Junior® with Fiber	Peptamen Junior® 1.5	Nutren Junior®	Nutren Junior with Fiber®
Calories/oz	30	45	30	30
Calories/mL	1.06	1.5	1	1
Carbohydrate g/100 mL	13.8	18	11	11
Carbohydrate source	Maltodextrin, corn starch	Maltodextrin, corn starch	Maltodextrin, sucrose	Maltodextrin, sucrose
Protein g/100 mL	3	4.5	3	3
Protein source	Partially hydrolyzed whey protein	Partially hydrolyzed whey protein	Milk protein concentrate, whey protein concentrate	Milk protein concentrate, whey protein concentrate
Fat g/100 mL	3.9	6.8	5	5
Fat source	MCT, soy, and canola oils, lecithin	MCT, soy, and canola oils, lecithin	Soybean, canola, and MCT oils, soy lecithin	Soybean, canola, and MCT oils, soy lecithin
Osmolality mOsm/kg	390 vanilla	450 unflavored	350 vanilla	350 vanilla
Sodium mEq/L (mg/L)	20 (460)	30 (692)	20 (460)	20 (460)
Potassium mEq/L (mg/L)	34 (1320)	51 (1980)	34 (1320)	34 (1320)
Chloride mEq/L (mg/L)	30 (1080)	45 (1620)	30 (1080)	30 (1080)
Calcium mEq/L (mg/L)	(1000)	(1625)	(1000)	(1000)
Phosphorus mEq/L (mg/L)	(800)	(1352)	(800)	(800)
Iron (mg/L)	14	21	14	14
% Free water	84	77	85	85
Fiber (g/unit dose)	Dietary 1.8 Soluble: 0.9 Insoluble: 0.9	Soluble: 1.35		Dietary 1.5 Soluble: 0.6 Insoluble: 1
Manufacturer	Nestle	Nestle	Nestle	Nestle

[1]Information based on manufacturer's literature as of 2010 and is subject to change.

Nutritionally Complete Drinks - Pediatric[1]
(A selection of the commonly used supplemental drinks)

	Boost® Kid Essentials	Boost® Kid Essentials 1.5	Boost® Kid Essentials 1.5 with Fiber	Resource® Breeze	Carnation® Instant Breakfast®	Carnation® Instant Breakfast Essentials™[2]	PediaSure®	PediaSure® with Fiber	Vital jr®	EO28 Splash
Calories/oz	30	45	45	30	30	16.7	30	30	30	30
Calories/mL	1	1.5	1.5	1.06	1	0.56	1	1	1	1
Carbohydrate g/100 mL	13.5	16.5	16.5	22.8	13.2	8.9	13.1	13.5	13.4	14.6
Carbohydrate source	Maltodextrin	Maltodextrin	Maltodextrin	Sugar, corn syrup, corn syrup solids	Corn syrup solids and sucrose	Lactose and maltodextrin	Sucrose and corn maltodextrin	Sucrose and corn maltodextrin	Corn maltodextrin and sugar	Maltodextrin and sugar
Protein g/100 mL	3	4.2	4.2	3.8	3.5	4.8	3	3	3	2.5
Protein source	Sodium and calcium caseinates, whey protein concentrate	Sodium and calcium caseinates, whey protein concentrate	Sodium and calcium caseinates, whey protein concentrate	Whey protein isolate	Calcium caseinate	Nonfat milk	Milk protein concentrate, whey protein concentrate, soy protein isolate	Milk protein concentrate and soy protein isolate	Whey protein hydrolysate, hydrolyzed sodium caseinate	Free amino acids
Fat g/100 mL	3.8	7.5	7.5		3.7	0.19	3.8	3.8	4.1	3.5
Fat source	MCT, soy, and sunflower oils, soy lecithin	MCT, soy, and sunflower oils, soy lecithin	MCT, soy, and sunflower oils, soy lecithin		Canola and corn oils, soy lecithin	Trace butterfat	High oleic safflower oil, soy, and (43:42:15)	High oleic safflower oil, soy, and MCT oils (43:42:15)	Structured lipid (interesterified canola and MCT oils), MCT oils, and canola oil	Fractionated coconut, canola, and high oleic sunflower oils
Osmolality mOsm/kg	550 vanilla 600 chocolate 570 strawberry	390 vanilla	405 vanilla	750 orange, peach, wild berry	480 vanilla swirl 490 chocolate splash		480 vanilla, strawberry, banana cream, berry cream 540 chocolate	480 vanilla	390 vanilla, strawberry	820 grape, tropical fruit, and orange-pineapple
Sodium mEq/L (mg/L)	24 (550)	30 (690)	30 (690)	15 (337)	38 (880)	27 (620)	17 (380)	17 (380)	31 (717)	(200)
Potassium mEq/L (mg/L)	29 (1140)	33 (1300)	33 (1300)	1.3 (42)	32 (1250)	57 (2200)	34 (1310)	34 (1310)	35 (1350)	(928)
Chloride mEq/L (mg/L)	15.6 (548)	21 (738)	21 (738)	5.6 (200)	39 (1200)		29 (1014)	29 (1014)	29 (1013)	(350)
Calcium mEq/L (mg/L)	(1181)	(1304)	(1304)	(40)	(500)	(1852)	49 (972)	49 (972)	553 (1055)	(620)
Phosphorus mEq/L (mg/L)	(886)	(992)	(992)	(600)	(500)	(1852)	(845)	(845)	(844)	(620)
Iron (mg/L)	14	14	14	11	20	17	14	14	14	7.6
% Free water	84	72	71	83	85		85	85	84	
Fiber (g/unit dose)			Dietary: 2.1 Soluble: 1.6 Insoluble: 0.5			Dietary: 3	Dietary: 0.72 scFOS: 0.42[3]	Dietary: 1.35 scFOS: 0.42[3]	scFOS: 0.3[2]	

Nutritionally Complete Drinks - Pediatric[1] *continued*

	Boost® Kid Essentials	Boost® Kid Essentials 1.5	Boost® Kid Essentials 1.5 with Fiber	Resource® Breeze	Carnation® Instant Breakfast®	Carnation® Instant Breakfast Essentials™[2]	PediaSure®	PediaSure® with Fiber	Vital jr®	EO28 Splash
Indication	1-13 years old	1-10 years old	1-10 years old			Reduced calorie	1-13 years old	1-13 years old	1-13 years old; semi-elemental for malabsorption, maldigestion and other GI conditions when hydrolyzed proteins are indicated	>1 year old; nutritionally complete, ready-to-drink amino acid-based
Manufacturer	Nestle	Nestle	Nestle	Nestle	Nestle	Nestle	Abbott	Abbott	Abbott	Nutricia

[1]Information based on manufacturer's literature as of 2010 and is subject to change.

[2]One envelope added to 8 oz of fat free milk.

[3]Prebiotic Nutraflora® scFOS® (short chain fructooligosaccharides) provide fuel for beneficial bacteria in the digestive tract that help to support a healthy immune system.

Enteral Formulas – Adolescents and Adults[1]

	Osmolite®	Jevity®	Nutren® 1[2]	Ensure®	Boost®
Calories/mL	1.06	1.06	1	1.05	1
Carbohydrate g/100 mL	14.4	15.5	12.7	17.3	17
Carbohydrate source	Corn maltodextrin and corn syrup solids	Corn maltodextrin, corn syrup solids, and soy fiber	Maltodextrin, sucrose	Corn maltodextrin, sucrose, scFOS[3]	Sucrose, corn syrup solids
Protein g/100 mL	4.43	4.43	4	3.8	4.2
Protein source	Sodium and calcium caseinate, soy protein isolate	Sodium and calcium caseinates, soy protein isolate	Calcium-potassium caseinate	Milk protein concentrate and soy protein concentrate	Milk protein concentrate
Fat g/100 mL	3.47	3.47	3.8	2.5	1.7
Fat source	Canola, corn, and MCT oils, and soy lecithin	Canola, corn, and MCT oils, and soy lecithin	MCT, canola, and corn oils, soy lecithin	Soy, canola, and corn oils, soy lecithin	Canola, high oleic sunflower, corn oils, and soy lecithin
Osmolality mOsm/kg H_2O	300 unflavored	300 unflavored	370 vanilla	620 strawberries & cream, homemade vanilla, coffee latte, butter pecan 640 creamy milk chocolate, rich dark chocolate	625 vanilla, chocolate, or strawberry
Sodium mEq/L (mg/L)	40 (930)	40 (930)	38 (880)	37 (840)	24 (540)
Potassium mEq/L (mg/L)	40 (1570)	40 (1570)	32 (1240)	40 (1540)	43 (1670)
Chloride mEq/L (mg/L)	40 (1440)	37 (1310)	34 (1200)	33 (1180)	40 (1420)
Calcium mEq/L (mg/L)	(760)	(910)	(668)	(1265)	(1250)
Phosphorus mEq/L (mg/L)	(760)	(760)	(668)	(1055)	(1250)
Iron (mg/L)	14	14	12	19	19
% Free water	84	84	85	83	85
Fiber (g/unit dose)		Dietary: 1.4/100 mL	Also available with fiber[4]	Dietary: 1.27	
Manufacturer	Abbott	Abbott	Nestle	Abbott	Nestle
Special Uses	Low residue, isotonic formula	Isotonic formula with fiber	Normal protein/normal calorie requirements	Supplement; for interim sole-source feeding	Nutritionally complete drink

[1]Information based on manufacturer's literature as of 2010 and is subject to change.

[2]Also available with fiber with Prebio™ (prebiotics) which contains 3.5 g of dietary fiber with 1.3 g insoluble and 2.2 g soluble.

[3]Prebiotic Nutraflora® scFOS® (short chain fructooligosaccaharides) provides fuel for beneficial bacteria in the digestive tract that help to support a healthy immune system.

[4]Prebio™ is a fiber blend to help promote healthy microbiota and contains 3.5 g of dietary fiber with 1.3 g of soluble fiber and 2.2 g of insoluble fiber.

Enteral Formulas With High Caloric Density[1]

	Ensure Plus®	Osmolite 1.2®	Nutren® 1.5	Nutren® 2	Jevity® 1.5 Cal	Isosource® 1.5 Cal	Hi-Cal™
Calories/mL	1.5	1.2	1.5	2	1.5	1.5	2
Carbohydrate g/100 mL	21	15.8	16.9	19.6	21.6	16.8	21.6
Carbohydrate source	Corn, maltodextrin, sucrose, scFOS	Corn, maltodextrin	Maltodextrin	Maltodextrin, corn syrup solids, sucrose	Corn maltodextrin, corn syrup solids, fructooligosaccharides, oat fiber, and soy fiber	Maltodextrin, sucrose, soy fiber, and partially hydrolyzed guar gum	Corn maltodextrin, sucrose
Protein g/100 mL	5.5	5.55	6	8	6.4	6.8	8.4
Protein source	Milk protein, caseinate, soy protein concentrate, whey protein concentrate	Caseinate, soy protein isolate	Calcium-potassium caseinate	Calcium-potassium caseinate	Sodium and calcium caseinate, soy protein isolate	Caseinates	Sodium caseinates and calcium caseinate
Fat g/100 mL	4.6	3.93	6.8	10.4	5	6.5	8.9
Fat source	Canola, and corn oils, soy lecithin	High oleic safflower, canola, and MCT oils, soy lecithin	MCT, canola and corn oils, soy lecithin	MCT and canola oil	Canola, corn, and MCT oils, soy lecithin	Canola, MCT, and soy oils, soy lecithin	Corn oil and soy lecithin
Osmolality mOsm/kg	680 homemade vanilla, strawberries & cream, coffee latte, butter pecan, creamy milk chocolate 700 rick dark chocolate	360	430 unflavored 510 vanilla	745 vanilla	525 unflavored	650 unflavored 585 vanilla	705 vanilla
Sodium mEq/L (mg/L)	41 (930)	58 (1340)	51 (1170)	56 (1300)	61 (1400)	56 (1290)	63 (1460)
Potassium mEq/L (mg/L)	54 (2110)	46 (1810)	48 (1870)	49 (1920)	55 (2150)	55 (2140)	62 (2450)
Chloride mEq/L (mg/L)	32 (1139)	44 (1540)	49 (1740)	53 (1880)	38 (1360)	45 (1610)	40 (1360)
Calcium mEq/L (mg/L)	(1266)	(1200)	(1000)	(1340)	(1200)	(1072)	(800)
Phosphorus mEq/L (mg/L)	(1266)	(1200)	(1000)	(1340)	(1200)	(1072)	(800)
Iron (mg/L)	19	18	18	24	18	19	14.4
% Free water		82	76	70	76	78	69
Fiber (g/unit dose)	Dietary: 1.27 g scFOS: 0.84[2]				Dietary: 2.2 scFOS: 1	Dietary: 2/can Soluble: 1.1/can Insoluble: 0.9/can	

Enteral Formulas With High Caloric Density[1] *continued*

	Ensure Plus®	Osmolite 1.2®	Nutren® 1.5	Nutren® 2	Jevity® 1.5 Cal	Isosource® 1.5 Cal	Hi-Cal™
Manufacturer	Abbott	Abbott	Nestle	Nestle	Abbott	Nestle	Abbott
Special Uses	For those with fluid restrictions or require volume-limited feedings; supplement; for interim sole-source feeding	Increased protein	Increased calories	Calorically dense	Increased protein with fiber and NutraFlora® scFOS®[2]	High calorie, high nitrogen formula with fiber	Increased calories fortified with vitamins and minerals

[1]Information based on manufacturer's literature as of 2010 and is subject to change.

[2]Prebiotic Nutraflora® scFOS® (short chain fructooligosaccaharides) provides fuel for beneficial bacteria in the digestive tract that help to support a healthy immune system.

Elemental Enteral Formulas – Infants / Pediatric[1]

	EleCare® (20 kcal/oz)	EleCare® (30 kcal/oz)	Neocate® Infant DHA & ARA[2,3,4] (20 kcal/oz)	Neocate® One+[5] (30 kcal/oz)	Nutramigen® AA™
Calories/mL	0.68	1	0.67	1	0.68
Carbohydrate g/100 mL	7.2	10.9	7.84	14.6	6.9
Carbohydrate source	Corn syrup solids	Corn syrup solids	Corn syrup solids	Corn syrup solids	Corn syrup solids
Protein g/100 mL	2.06	3.1	2.07	2.5	1.87
Protein source	Free amino acids	Free amino acids	Free amino acids	Free amino acids	Free amino acids
Fat g/100 mL	3.27	4.9	3	3.5	3.53
Fat source	High oleic safflower, MCT, and soy oils (39:33:28)	High oleic safflower, MCT, and soy oils (39:33:28)	MCT (palm kernel/coconut), high oleic sunflower, soy, and coconut oils, and DHA & ARA[2]	Fractionated coconut, canola, and high oleic safflower oils	Palm olein, soy, coconut, and high oleic sunflower oils, and DHA & ARA[2]
Osmolality mOsm/kg	350	560	375	610	350
Osmolarity mOsm/L	187	280	–	234	320
Sodium mEq/L (mg/L)	13.3 (305)	19.9 (458)	(249)	(200)	(313)
Potassium mEq/L (mg/L)	25.9 (1014)	38.9 (1523)	(1034)	(930)	(733)
Chloride mEq/L (mg/L)	11.4 (405)	17.1 (607)	(515)	(350)	(573)
Calcium mEq/L (mg/L)	36.4 (781)	54.6 (1172)	(827)	(620)	(627)
Phosphorus mg/L	548	822	624	620	347
Iron mg/L	9.9	14.9	12.4	7.7	12
% Free water	90	84			89
Manufacturer	Abbott	Abbott	Nutricia	Nutricia	Mead Johnson

[1]Information based on manufacturer's literature as of 2010 and is subject to change.

[2]DHA (docosahexaenoic acid) and ARA (arachidonic acid) are fatty acids which are found naturally in breast milk.

[3]Indicated for 0-12 month olds.

[4]Also available as Neocate® Nutra for children >6 months of age.

[5]Indicated for 1-10 year olds.

Elemental Enteral Formulas With Modified Protein – Adolescents and Adults[1]

	Peptamen®	Peptamen® 1.5	Tolerex®[2]	Vivonex® Plus[3]	Vivonex® RFT	Vivonex® T.E.N.[4]
Calories/mL	1	1.5	1	1	1	1
Carbohydrate g/100 mL	12.7	18.8	23	19	18	20.6
Carbohydrate source	Maltodextrin, corn starch	Maltodextrin, corn starch	Maltodextrin, modified corn starch	Maltodextrin, modified starch	Maltodextrin, modified corn starch	Maltodextrin, modified corn starch
Protein g/100 mL	4	6.8	2.1	4.5	5	3.8
Protein source	Partially hydrolyzed whey	Partially hydrolyzed whey	L-amino acids	L-amino acids (30% from branched chain amino acids)	L-amino acids (28% from branched chain amino acids)	L-amino acids
Fat g/100 mL	3.9	5.6	0.1	0.67	1.2	0.27
Fat source	Soy and MCT oils (70%)	Soy and MCT oils (70%)	Safflower oil	Soy oil	Soy oil	Safflower oil
Osmolality mOsm/kg	270 unflavored 380 vanilla	550 unflavored, vanilla	550 unflavored 617-678 flavored	650	630 unflavored	630 unflavored
Sodium mEq/L (mg/L)	24 (560)	44 (1020)	20 (470)	27 (610)	29 (690)	26 (600)
Potassium mEq/L (mg/L)	38 (1500)	48 (1860)	30 (1170)	27 (1060)	31 (1200)	24 (950)
Chloride mEq/L (mg/L)	28 (1000)	49 (1740)	27 (943)	27 (943)	22 (800)	24 (850)
Calcium mEq/L (mg/L)	(800)	(1000)	(557)	(557)	(668)	(500)
Phosphorus mg/L	(700)	(1000)	(557)	(557)	(668)	(500)
Iron mg/L	18	27	10	10	12	9
% Free water	85	77	84	83	85	83
Manufacturer	Nestle	Nestle	Nestle	Nestle	Nestle	Nestle

[1]Information based on manufacturer's literature as of 2010 and is subject to change.
[2]2.82 oz dry packet mixed with 255 mL of water produces 300 mL of formula.
[3]2.8 oz dry packet mixed with 250 mL of water produces 300 mL of formula.
[4]2.64 oz dry packet mixed with 250 mL of water produces 300 mL of formula.

Low Long Chain Fatty Acids Formulas[1]

	Portagen®	Enfaport® LIPIL®
Calories /100 mL	100	100
Protein g/100 mL	3.5	3.5
Protein source	Sodium caseinate	Calcium and sodium caseinate
Carbohydrate g/100 mL	11.5	10.2
Carbohydrate source	75% corn syrup solids and 25% sucrose (lactose- and gluten-free)	Corn syrup solids (sucrose- and gluten-free)
Fat g/100 mL	4.8	5.4
Fat source	87% MCT and 13% corn oils	84% MCT and 13% soy oils, 3% DHA & ARA[2]
Osmolality mOsm/kg	350	280
Osmolarity mOsm/L	300	240
Sodium mEq/L (mg/L)	(552)	(300)
Potassium mEq/L (mg/L)	(1250)	(870)
Chloride mEq/L (mg/L)	(865)	(870)
Calcium mEq/L (mg/L)	(938)	(940)
Phosphorus mEq/L (mg/L)	(708)	(520)
Iron mg/L	18.8	18
% Free water	87	83
Manufacturer	Mead Johnson	Mead Johnson
Indication	For children and adults with defects in the intraluminal hydrolysis of fats (decreased bile salts, decreased pancreatic lipase); defective mucosal fat absorption (decreased mucosal permeability, decreased absorptive surface); and/or defective lymphatic transport of fat (ie, intestinal lymphatic obstruction); if used long-term, not nutritionally complete and will require supplementation of essential fatty acids and ultra trace minerals	Iron-fortified, milk-based infant formula with 84% of fat as MCT for infants with chylothorax or LCHAD deficiency (long chain 3-hydroxyacyl CoA dehydrogenase - inherited disorder of fat oxidation)

[1]Information based on manufacturer's literature as of 2010 and is subject to change.

[2]DHA (docosahexaenoic acid) and ARA (arachidonic acid) are fatty acids which are found naturally in breast milk.

Nutritional Modules[1]

	Polycose® Liquid	Polycose® Powder	ProMod® Liquid Protein[2,3]	Resource® Beneprotein®	Resource® Benefiber®	Duocal
Indication	Carbohydrate additive for use as a caloric supplement which is readily mixable in most foods, enteral formulas or beverages without appreciably altering their taste	Carbohydrate additive for use as a caloric supplement which is readily mixable in most foods, enteral formulas or beverages without appreciably altering their taste	Protein supplement which mixes readily in enteral formulas, most foods, or beverages without appreciably altering their taste; indicated for rounds, protein-energy malnutrition, involuntary weight loss, pre- and postsurgery anorexia, stress, trauma, cancer, burns	Protein supplement; 100% high quality whey proteins; mixes instantly in a variety of foods/beverages without compromising taste or texture	For dietary management of occasional constipation; mixes instantly in a variety of foods/beverages without compromising taste or texture	To increase calories by adding to food and beverages; contains no protein; neutral flavor
Calories	2/mL	3.8/g[4]	3.3/mL	3.6[5]	4/g[6]	4.9/g[7]
Protein (g)	—	—	0.33/mL	0.86	—	—
Protein source	—	—	Hydrolyzed beef collagen	Whey protein	—	—
Carbohydrate (g)	0.5/mL	0.94/g	0.46/mL	—	1/g	7.3/g
Carbohydrate source	Glucose polymers derived from corn starch	Glucose polymers derived from corn starch	Glycerin	—	Partially hydrolyzed guar gum	Hydrolyzed corn starch
Fat (g)	—	—	—	—	—	0.22/g
Fat source	—	—	—	Soy lecithin	—	Corn/coconut oil and MCT oils (fractionated coconut, palm kernel)
Osmolality mOsm/kg	60[8]	—	—	—	—	1 scoop = 5 g; for 1:3 dilution, 310
Osmolarity mOsm/L	—	—	60	—	—	—
Sodium mEq/L (mg/L)	<0.03/mL (<0.7/mL)	<0.057/g (<1.3/g)	(<0.0018/mL)	2.1/g (0.09/g)	3.76/g (0.175/g)	<0.2/g
Potassium mEq/L (mg/L)	<0.002/mL (<0.06/mL)	<0.003/g (<0.1/g)	(<0.0007/mL)	5/g (0.13/g)	3.76/g (0.1/g)	<0.05/g
Chloride mEq/L (mg/L)	<0.04/mL (<1.4/mL)	<0.063/g (<2.23/g)	—	—	—	<0.2/g
Calcium mEq/L (mg/L)	<0.01/mL (<0.2/mL)	<0.015/g (<0.3/g)	—	(4.3/g)	—	<0.05/g
Phosphorus mEq/L (mg/L)	(3/mL)	(<0.15/g)	(<0.003/mL)	(2.1/g)	—	<0.05/g

Nutritional Modules[1] *continued*

	Polycose® Liquid	Polycose® Powder	ProMod® Liquid Protein[2,3]	Resource® Beneprotein®	Resource® Benefiber®	Duocal
Iron mg/L	—	—	—	—	—	—
Manufacturer	Abbott	Abbott	Abbott	Nestle	Nestle	Nutricia

[1]These products are not complete formulations and should not be used as a sole source of nutrition.

[2]Comes in fruit punch flavor.

[3]Promod® Powder is no longer commercially available.

[4]1 tsp (2 g) = 8 calories, 1 tbsp (6 g) = 23 calories, ¼cup (24 g) = 91 calories.

[5]1 scoop = 7 g packet

[6]1 tbsp = 4 g packet, usually mix with 2-4 fl oz.

[7]42 cal/tbsp

[8]Approximate osmotic contribution to solution mixed into is 1.6 mOsm/g with a low renal solute load of 0.13 mOsm/g.

Nutritional Modules[1]

	Vegetable Oil[2]	Microlipid®	MCT Oil®[3]	Whole Milk
Indications	Inexpensive fat source for calories and essential fatty acids	50% fat emulsion for use as a source of calories or essential fatty acids; it mixes easily and stays in emulsion	Fat supplement for use in patients who cannot efficiently digest and absorb long-chain fats	For children >1 year of age
Calories	8.3/mL	4.5/mL	7.7/mL	157/8 oz
Protein (g)	—	—	—	8.2/8 oz
Protein source	—	—	—	82% casein, 18% whey
Carbohydrate (g)	—	—	—	11.5/8 oz
Carbohydrate source	—	—	—	Lactose
Fat (g)	0.93/mL	0.5/mL	0.93/mL	8.2/8 oz
Fat source	Corn, soybean, sunflower or safflower oils[5]	Safflower oil[4], polyglycerol esters, soy lecithin (high in linoleic acid)	Lipid fraction of coconut oil (consists primarily of C_8 and C_{10} saturated fatty acids)	Butter fat
Osmolality mOsm/kg	—	62	—	285
Sodium mEq/L (mg/L)	—	—	—	5.3/8 oz (120/8 oz)
Potassium mEq/L (mg/L)	—	—	—	9.6/8 oz (377/8 oz)
Calcium mEq/L (mg/L)	—	—	—	14.9/8 oz (295/8 oz)
Phosphorus mEq/L (mg/L)	—	—	—	(230/8 oz)
Iron mg/L	—	—	—	Trace
% Free water	—	45	—	91
Manufacturer		Nestle	Nestle	

[1]These products are not complete formulations and should not be used as a sole source of nutrition.

[2]1 tbsp = 14 g.

[3]Does not contain essential fatty acids.

[4]Rich source of polyunsaturated fat.

[5]% of linoleic from fat: Soybean oil 51%, corn oil 58%, sunflower oil 65%, safflower oil 77%.

Oral Electrolyte Maintenance Solution[1]

	Pedialyte®[2]	Enfamil® Enfalyte®[3,4]
Indications	Replace fluids and electrolytes lost during diarrhea and vomiting to prevent dehydration in infants/children	Oral electrolyte maintenance solution using rice syrup solids as carbohydrate source to help replace electrolytes and water one might lose from vomiting and diarrhea; for infants and children
Calories	0.1/mL	0.126/mL
Protein (g)	—	—
Protein source	—	—
Carbohydrate (g)	0.025	3 g/100 mL
Carbohydrate source	Dextrose	Rice syrup solids
Fat (g)	—	—
Fat source	—	—
Osmolality mOsm/kg	250 unflavored 270 flavored	170
Osmolarity mOsm/L	—	167
Sodium mEq/L (mg/L)	(0.045)	50 (1150)
Potassium mEq/L (mg/L)	(0.020)	25 (980)
Chloride mEq/L (mg/L)	(0.035)	45 (160)
Calcium mEq/L (mg/L)	—	—

Oral Electrolyte Maintenance Solution[1] *(continued)*

	Pedialyte®[2]	Enfamil® Enfalyte®[3,4]
Phosphorus mEq/L (mg/L)	—	—
Iron mg/L	—	—
Manufacturer	Abbott	Mead Johnson

[1]These products are not complete formulations and should not be used as a sole source of nutrition.

[2]Unflavored, but available as grape, fruit punch, bubblegum, cherry, and apple.

[3]Cherry

[4]Contains citrate 34 mEq/L.

FLUID AND ELECTROLYTE REQUIREMENTS IN CHILDREN

Maintenance Fluids (Two methods)

Surface area method (most commonly used in children >10 kg): 1500-2000 mL/m^2/day

Body weight method

<10 kg	100 mL/kg/day
11-20 kg	1000 mL + 50 mL/kg (for each kg >10)
>20 kg	1500 mL + 20 mL/kg (for each kg >20)

Maintenance Electrolytes (See specific electrolyte in Alphabetical Listing of Drugs for more detailed information)

Sodium: 3-4 mEq/kg/day **or** 30-50 mEq/m^2/day
Potassium: 2-3 mEq/kg/day **or** 20-40 mEq/m^2/day

Dehydration Fluid Therapy

Goals of therapy:

- Restore circulatory volume to prevent shock (10% to 15% dehydration)
- Restore combined intracellular and extracellular deficits of water and electrolytes within 24 hours
- Maintain adequate water and electrolytes
- Resolve homeostatic distortions (eg, acidosis)
- Replace ongoing losses

Analysis of the Severity of Dehydration by Physical Signs

Clinical Sign	Mild[1]	Moderate[1]	Severe[1]
Pre-illness body weight	5% loss	10% loss	15% loss
Skin turgor	↓	Tenting	Tenting
Mucous membranes	Dry	Very dry	Parched
Skin color	Pale	Grey	Mottled
Urine output	↓	↓↓	Azotemic
Blood pressure	Normal	Normal, ↓	↓↓
Heart rate	Normal, ↑	↑	↑↑
Fontanelle (<7 mo)	Flat	Soft	Sunken
CNS	Consolable	Irritable	Lethargic/coma

[1]Postpubertal children and adults experience the same symptoms with mild, moderate, and severe dehydration associated with 3%, 6%, and 9% losses in body weight respectively.

Restoration of Circulatory Volume (10% to 15% dehydration estimate)

Fluid boluses of 20 mL/kg using crystalloid (eg, normal saline) or 10 mL/kg colloid (eg, 5% albumin) administered as rapidly as possible; repeat until improved circulation (eg, warm skin, decreased heart rate (towards normal), improved capillary refill time, urine output restored).

Classification of Dehydration (based upon the serum sodium concentration)

Isotonic	130-150 mEq/L
Hypotonic	<130 mEq/L
Hypertonic	>150 mEq/L

Estimated Water & Electrolyte Deficits in Dehydration (moderate to severe)

Type of Dehydration	Water (mL/kg)	Na+ (mEq/kg)	K+ (mEq/kg)	Cl$^-$ and HCO$_3^-$ (mEq/kg)
Isotonic	100-150	8-10	8-10	16-20
Hypotonic	50-100	10-14	10-14	20-28
Hypertonic	120-180	2-5	2-5	4-10

Current Pediatric Diagnosis & Treatment, 10th ed, 1991.

Water deficit may also be calculated (in isotonic dehydration):

$$\text{Water deficit (mL)} = \frac{\text{\% dehydration x wt (kg) x 1000 g/kg}}{100}$$

Assessment of Water Loss in Relation to Serum Na⁺ Concentrations Degree of Dehydration as % Body Weight

Serum Na⁺	Mild	Moderate	Severe
Isotonic	5%	10%	15%
Hypotonic (Na⁺< 130)	4%	6%	8%
Hypertonic (Na⁺ >150)	7%	12%	17%

Example of Fluid Replacement (assume 10 kg infant with 10% isotonic dehydration)

	Water	Sodium (mEq)	Potassium (mEq)
Maintenance	1000 mL	40	20
Deficit[1]	1000 mL	80	80
Total	2000 mL	120	100

[1]Reduce this total by any fluid boluses given initially.

First 8 hours:

Replace ⅓ maintenance water = 330 mL

Replace ½ deficit water = 500 mL

Total 830 mL/8 h = 103 mL/h

Replace ½ of Na⁺ & K⁺ = 60 mEq sodium/803 mL; 50 mEq potassium/803 mL (It is suggested that the maximum potassium initially used is 40 mEq/L and is **not** started until urine output has been established.)

The actual order would appear as: D₅½NS at 103 mL/hour for 8 hours; add 40 mEq/L KCl after patient voids.

Second 16 hours:

Replace ⅔ maintenance water = 670 mL

Replace ½ deficit water = 500 mL

Total 1260 mL/16 h = 79 mL/h

Replace remainder of sodium and potassium.

The actual order would appear as: D₅⅓NS with KCl 40 mEq/L at 79 mL/hour for 16 hours. (Use of ¼NS may be more desirable for convenience.)

Analysis of Ongoing Losses

Electrolyte Composition of Biological Fluids (mEq/L)

Fluid Type	Sodium	Potassium	Chloride	Total HCO₃⁻
Stomach	20-120	5-25	90-160	0-5
Duodenal drainage	20-140	3-30	30-120	10-50
Biliary tract	120-160	3-12	70-130	30-50
Small intestine Initial drainage	100-140	4-40	60-100	30-100
Small intestine Established drainage	4-20	4-10	10-100	40-120
Pancreatic	110-160	4-15	30-80	70-130
Diarrheal stool	10-25	10-30	30-120	10-50

Current Pediatric Diagnosis & Treatment, 9th ed, Appleton & Lange, 1987.

Because of the wide range of normal values, specific analyses are suggested in individual cases.

Alterations of Maintenance Fluid Requirements

Fever	Increase maintenance fluids by 5 mL/kg/day for each degree of temperature above 38°C
Hyperventilation	Increase maintenance fluids by 10-60 mL/100 kcal BEE (basal energy expenditure)
Sweating	Increase maintenance fluids by 10-25 mL/100 kcal BEE (basal energy expenditure)
Hyperthyroidism	Variable increase in maintenance fluids: 25%-50%
Renal disease	Monitor and analyze output; adjust therapy accordingly
Renal failure	Maintenance fluids are equal to insensible losses (300 mL/m³) + urine replacement (mL for mL)
Diarrhea	Increase maintenance fluids on a mL/mL loss basis

Oral Rehydration

Due to the high worldwide incidence of dehydration from infantile diarrhea, effective, inexpensive oral rehydration solutions have been developed. In the U.S., a typical effective solution for rehydration contains 50-60 mEq/L sodium, 20-30 mEq/L potassium, 30 mEq/L bicarbonate or its equivalent, and sufficient chloride to provide electroneutrality. Two percent to 3% glucose facilitates electrolyte absorption and short-term calories. The following table describes the electrolyte/sugar content of commonly used oral rehydration solutions.

Composition of Frequently Used Oral Electrolyte Replacement Solutions

Solutions	% CHO	Na$^+$ (mEq/L)	K$^+$ (mEq/L)	Cl$^-$ (mEq/L)	HCO$^-$ (mEq/L)
Normal saline		154		154	
Ringer's lactate		130	4	109	28
Dextrose 5% in 0.25% NaCl	5% glucose	38		38	
WHO solution	2% glucose or 4% sucrose	90	20	80	30 citrate
WHO solution, modified	2% glucose	55	25	30	50
Rehydralyte®	2.5% glucose	75	20	65	30 citrate
Ricelyte®	3% carbohydrate	50	25	45	34 citrate
Resol®	2% glucose	50	20	50	34 citrate
Rice water	2.5% carbohydrate	90	20	30	80
Pedialyte® (Ross)	2.5% glucose	45	20	35	30 citrate
Pedialyte® Freezer Pops	2.5% glucose	45	20	35	30 citrate
Enfamil Enfalyte®	3% glucose	50	25	45	34 citrate
Kao Lectrolyte	2% glucose	50	20		30 citrate
Naturalyte	2.5% glucose	45	20	35	30 citrate
Oralyte	2.5% glucose	45	20	35	48 citrate
Gatorade®	2.6% glucose, 2% fructose	23.5	<1	17	
Apple juice	3.2% glucose, 1.3% sucrose, 7.5% fructose	<1	25		
Orange juice 1:3 (dilution with water)	1% glucose, 1.2% fructose	<1	50		50 citrate
Grape juice	1.6% glucose, 2.1% fructose	0.2-0.7	8-11		8
One package cherry gelatin dissolved in 4 cups water		24	Needs added K$^+$		
Coca-Cola®		1.6	<1		13.4 citrate
Pepsi-Cola®		6.5	0.8		
Beef broth		120	10		
Chicken broth		250	8		

Adapted from Aranda-Michel, J and Giannella RA, "Acute Diarrhea" A Practical Review," *Am J of Med*, 1999, 106:670-6.

PARENTERAL NUTRITION (PN)

The following information is intended as a brief overview of the use of PN in infants and children.

Goal: The therapeutic goal of PN in infants and children is both to maintain nutrition status and to achieve balanced somatic growth.

General Indications for Use

PN is the provision of required nutrients by the intravenous route to replenish, optimize, or maintain nutritional status.

Specific Indications

PN of **all** required nutrients (total parenteral nutrition) is indicated in patients for whom it is expected that it would be impossible or dangerous to enterally administer nutrition. PN in combination with enteral nutrition is indicated in patients who are expected to be unable to meet their nutritional needs by the enteral route alone within 5 days. Peripheral PN is indicated only for partial nutritional supplementation or as bridge therapy for patients awaiting central venous access.

1. Patients with an inability to absorb nutrients via the gastrointestinal tract which may include the following: severe diarrhea, short bowel syndrome, developmental anomalies of the GI tract, inflammatory bowel disease, cystic fibrosis, or anatomic or functional loss of GI integrity.
2. Severe malnutrition.
3. Severe catabolic states such as: burns, trauma, or sepsis.
4. Patients undergoing high dose chemotherapy, radiation, and bone marrow transplantation.
5. Patients whose clinical condition may necessitate complete bowel rest (eg, necrotizing enterocolitis, pancreatitis, GI fistulas, or recent GI surgery).
6. Intensive care low-birth-weight infants.
7. Neonatal asphyxia.
8. Meconium ileus.
9. Respiratory distress syndrome (RDS).

Nutritional Assessment

As many as 33% of hospitalized pediatric patients are malnourished and require nutritional therapy. The type of nutritional support indicated depends on the underlying disease, the degree of gastrointestinal function, and the severity of malnutrition. Acutely malnourished patients have an increased risk for serious infection, postoperative complications, and death. Indicators of acute protein-calorie malnutrition include low weight for height, low serum albumin, lymphopenia, decreased body fat folds, and decreased arm muscle area. Nutritional screening may be done by the dietitian. Those patients who are at nutritional risk should receive a complete nutritional assessment.

Nutritional Requirements

Approximate requirements for energy and protein at various ages for normal subjects are listed in the first table at the end of this section. Patients who are severely malnourished or markedly catabolic may require higher levels to achieve catch-up growth or meet increased requirements. Patients who are well-nourished and/or inactive may require less.

During parenteral nutrition, 10% to 16% of calories should be in the form of amino acids to achieve optimal benefit (approximately 2-3 g/kg/day in infants and 1.5-2.5 g/kg/day ideal body weight in older patients). Exceptions include patients with renal or hepatic failure (where less protein is indicated), or in the treatment of severe trauma, head injury, or sepsis (where more protein may be indicated).

PN ORDERING

Fluid Intake

The patient should be given a total volume of fluid reasonable for his/her age and cardiovascular status. It is generally safe to start with the fluid maintenance level of 1500 mL/m^2/day in children (see Fluid and Electrolyte Requirements in Children). The fluid requirements in preterm infants are extremely variable due to much greater insensible water losses from radiant warmers and bili-lights. While the standard fluid maintenance of 100 mL/kg/day may be sufficient for term infants, intakes of up to 150 mL/kg/day may be necessary in the very low birth weight infants. Be sure to consider significant fluid intake from medications or other I.V. fluids and enteral diets in planning the fluids available for PN.

Dextrose

For central PN, dextrose is usually begun with a 10% to 12.5% solution or a solution providing dextrose at no more than 5 mg/kg/minute (in neonates and premature infants). The concentration is advanced, if tolerated, by 2.5% to 5% per day (2-2.5 mg/kg/minute increments in neonates and premature infants) to the desired caloric density, usually 20% to 25% dextrose. Fluid restricted patients often need 30% to 35% dextrose to meet their energy needs. For peripheral PN, 5% to 12.5% dextrose is utilized.

◄ Dextrose calculations:

$$\% \text{ Dextrose} = \text{dextrose (g)}/100 \text{ mL}$$

Dextrose calorie value = 3.4 kcal/g

$$\text{Dextrose infusion rate (mg/kg/minute)} = \frac{\text{rate (mL/h)} \times \% \text{ dextrose} \times 0.166}{\text{weight (kg)}}$$

$$\% \text{ Dextrose desired}[1] = \frac{\text{desired rate (mg/kg/min)} \times \text{weight (kg)}}{0.166 \times \text{rate (mL/h)}}$$

[1]Do not use dextrose concentrations <5% due to hypotonicity.

Amino Acids

Amino acids may be described as either a "standard" mixture of essential and nonessential amino acids or "specialized" mixtures. Specialized mixtures are intended for use in patients whose physiologic or metabolic needs may not be met with the "standard" amino acid compositions. Examples of specialized solutions include:

TrophAmine®, Aminosyn® PF, PremaSol™	Indicated for use in premature infants and young children due to addition of taurine, L-glutamic acid, L-aspartic acid, increased amounts of histidine, and reduction in amounts of methionine, alanine, phenylalanine, and glycine. Supplementation with a cysteine additive has been recommended.
HepatAmine®	Indicated for treatment in patients with hepatic encephalopathy due to cirrhosis or hepatitis or in patients with liver disease who are intolerant of standard amino acid solutions. Contains higher percentage of branched-chain amino acids and a lower percentage of aromatic amino acids than standard mixtures.
NephrAmine®, Aminosyn® RF	Indicated for use in patients with compromised renal function who are intolerant of standard amino acid solutions. Contains a mixture of essential amino acids and histidine.

Amino acid calculations:

$$\% \text{ amino acid} = \text{amino acid (g)}/100\text{mL}$$

$$\text{Grams of protein} = \text{grams of nitrogen} \times 6.25$$

$$\% \text{ amino acid desired} = \frac{\text{(g amino acid/kg)} \times \text{weight (kg)} \times 100}{\text{total PN fluid volume (mL)}}$$

Fat Emulsion (FE)

There are three roles for intravenous fat in parenteral nutrition:

1. to provide nonprotein calories
2. to provide essential fatty acids and a "balanced" calorie source
3. to provide calories in catabolic patients with limited ability to excrete CO_2

The FE dosage is increased as tolerated daily (see General Guidelines for Initiation and Advancement for PN following). The maximum fat intake is 4 g/kg/day and no more than 60% of the total daily caloric intake. It is administered as a continuous infusion over 24 hours or at a rate no greater than 0.15–0.2 g/kg/hour via a Y-connector with the dextrose-amino acid I.V. line. In patients receiving cyclic PN, the FE should be administered over the duration of the PN infusion. The triglyceride concentration should be checked before the first infusion and daily as the dose is increased. Subsequently, it should be monitored at least weekly. Triglyceride concentrations should be maintained at <200 mg/dL in neonates, <350 mg/dL in renal patients, and <250 mg/dL in other patients. FE should be used cautiously in neonates with hyperbilirubinemia due to displacement of bilirubin from albumin by the free fatty acids. An increase in free bilirubin may increase the risk of kernicterus. Significant displacement occurs when the free fatty acid to serum albumin molar ratio (FFA/SA) >6. For example, infants with a total bilirubin >8-10 mg/dL (assuming an albumin concentration of 2.5-3 g/dL) should not receive more parenteral FE than required to meet the essential fatty acid requirement of 0.5-1 g/kg/day.

Note: Avoid use of 10% FE in preterm infants because a greater accumulation of plasma lipids occurs due to the greater phospholipid load of the 10% concentration.

Fat emulsion calculations:

$$20\% \text{ FE} = 20 \text{ g fat}/100 \text{ mL} = 2 \text{ kcal/mL}$$

$$\text{Desired 20\% FE (mL)} = \frac{(\% \text{ total kcal as fat}) \times \text{(total kcal)}}{2 \text{ kcal/mL}}$$

or as an alternative

$$\text{Desired 20\% FE (mL)} = \text{FE (g/kg)} \times \text{weight (kg)} \times 5 \text{ mL/g}$$

General Guidelines for Initiation and Advancement of PN[1]

Age	Initiation and Advancement[2]	Dextrose	Protein (g/kg/d)	Fat (g/kg/d)
Premature infant	Initial	4-6 mg/kg/min	0.5-1.5	0.5
	Daily increase	1-2.5 mg/kg/min	0.5-1	0.5
	Maximum	18 mg/kg/min	2.5-3	3
Term infant - 1 y	Initial	7-9 mg/kg/min	1-1.5	0.5-1
	Daily increase	1-2.5 mg/kg/min	1	0.5-1
	Maximum	21 mg/kg/min	2.5-3	4
Children 1-10 y	Initial dextrose concentration	10%-12.5%	1-1.5	1
	Daily increase	5% increments	1	1
	Maximum	15 mg/kg/min	2-2.5	3
>10 y	Initial dextrose concentration	10%-15%	1-1.5	1
	Daily increase	5% increments	1	1
	Maximum	8.5 mg/kg/min	1.5-2	3

[1]Rate of advancement may be limited by metabolic tolerance (eg, hyperglycemia, azotemia, hypertriglyceridemia)

[2]Timely intervention in premature infants is essential with initiation of dextrose as soon as possible after birth, amino acids within the first 12 hours, and fat emulsion within 24-48 hours of life.

MINERALS, TRACE ELEMENTS, AND VITAMINS

Guideline for Daily Electrolyte Requirements

	Neonates (mEq/kg)	Infants/Children (mEq/kg)	Adolescents
Sodium	2-5[1]	2-6	1-2 mEq/kg
Potassium	2-4	2-4	1-2 mEq/kg
Calcium gluconate[2]	3-4[3]	1-2.5	10-20 mEq/d
Magnesium	0.3-0.5	0.3-0.5	10-30 mEq/d
Phosphate[2]	1-2 mmol/kg[3]	0.5-1 mmol/kg	10-40 mmol/d

[1]Premature infants lose sodium in urine due to the immature resorptive function of kidney and diuretic use. Hyponatremia may lead to poor tissue growth and adverse developmental outcomes. Sodium content in PN may be adjusted to a maximum of 154 mEq/L (NS) to achieve normal sodium serum levels.

[2]Calcium-phosphate stability in parenteral nutrition solutions is dependent upon the pH of the solution, temperature, and relative concentration of each ion. The pH of the solution is primarily dependent upon the amino acid concentration. The higher the percentage amino acids the lower the pH, the more soluble the calcium and phosphate. Individual commercially available amino acid solutions vary significantly with respect to pH lowering potential and consequent calcium phosphate compatibility. See the pharmacist for specific calcium phosphate stability information.

[3]A 1.7:1 calcium to phosphate ratio in PN allows for the highest absolute retention of both minerals and simulates the in utero accretion of calcium and phosphate.

Vitamins

A pediatric parenteral multivitamin product is indicated for children <11 years of age. Children >11 years of age may receive adult multivitamin formulations.

Dosage:

Pediatric MVI:
  Neonates: 2 mL/kg/d; maximum 5 mL/d
  Infants and children ≤11 y: 5 mL
  Children >11 y and adults: Use adult formulation 10 mL/d

Trace Mineral Daily Requirements[1]

	Infants	Children (≥3 mo to ≤5 y)	Older Children and Adolescents
Chromium[2]	0.2 mcg/kg	0.14-0.2 mcg/kg (max: 5 mcg)	10-15 mcg
Copper[3]	20 mcg/kg	20 mcg/kg (max: 300 mcg)	0.3-0.5 mg
Iodide[4]	1 mcg/kg	1 mcg/kg	1 mcg/kg
Manganese[3]	1 mcg/kg	2-10 mcg/kg (max: 50 mcg)	60-150 mcg
Selenium[2,5]	2-3 mcg/kg	2-3 mcg/kg (max: 30 mcg)	20-60 mcg
Zinc	400 mcg/kg (preterm) 300 mcg/kg (term <3 mo)	100 mcg/kg (max: 5 mg)	2.5-5 mg

[1]Recommended intakes of trace elements cannot be achieved through the use of a single pediatric trace element product. Only through the use of individualized trace element products can recommended intakes be achieved.

[2]Omit in patients with renal dysfunction.

[3]Omit in patients with impaired biliary excretion or cholestatic liver disease.

[4]Percutaneous absorption from protein-bound iodine may be adequate.

[5]Indicated for use in long-term parenteral nutrition patients.

These are recommended daily trace mineral requirements. Additional supplementation may be indicated in clinical conditions resulting in excessive losses. For example, additional zinc may be needed in situations of excessive gastrointestinal losses.

Developing the PN Goal Regimen

The purpose of this example is to illustrate the thought process in determining what dextrose and amino acid solution and fat emulsion intake would provide the desired daily fluid calorie and protein goals.

1. Calculate the fluid, protein, and caloric goals. Example:

    Weight = 10 kg

    Fluids = 100 mL/kg/day = 1000 mL

    Calories = 100 kcal/kg/day = 1000 kcal

    Protein = 2.5 g/kg/day = 25 g

2. If fat emulsion (FE) comprises 40% to 60% of the total daily calories, using the above example: 40% of 1000 kcal = 400 kcal. 400 kcal ÷ 2 kcal/mL (20% FE) = 200 mL

3. To determine the goal dextrose concentration calculate the total daily calories remaining. Example:

1000 kcal	(total daily calories)
- 400 kcal	(daily calories from fats)
600 kcal	(total daily calories remaining)

4. Determine the concentration of dextrose to achieve the total daily calories remaining. Example:
    600 kcal ÷ 3.4 kcal/g x [100 ÷ 800 mL[1]] = 22%
    [1]Total daily fluids desired minus that from fats.

5. Calculate percent amino acid solution to achieve goal protein intake. Example:
    [25 g (total protein) ÷ 800 mL (total fluid)] x 100 = 3.1%
    This patient's goal regimen would be: dextrose 22%, amino acid 3.1%, 800 mL/day plus fat emulsion 20% 200 mL/day.

Suggested PN Monitoring Guidelines

Parameter	Suggested Frequency	
	Initial/Hospitalized	Follow-up/Outpatient
Growth		
Weight	Daily	Daily to q visit
Height/length	Weekly	Weekly to q visit
Body composition (triceps skinfold, bone age)	Initially	Monthly to annually
Metabolic (Serum[1])		
Electrolytes	Twice weekly	Weekly to q visit
BUN/creatinine	Weekly	Weekly to q visit
Acid-base status	Until stable	As indicated
Albumin/prealbumin	Weekly	Weekly to q visit
Glucose	Daily to weekly	Weekly to q visit
Triglyceride	Initially daily	Weekly to q visit
Liver function tests	Weekly	Weekly to q visit
Complete blood count/differential	Weekly	Weekly to q visit
Platelets, PT/PTT	Weekly	As indicated
Iron indices	As indicated	Biannually to annually
Trace elements	As indicated	Annually
Carnitine	As indicated	As indicated
Folate/vitamin B_{12}	As indicated	As indicated
Ammonia	As indicated	As indicated
Bilirubin, direct	Weekly	As indicated
Metabolic (Urine)		
Glucose	Twice daily	Daily to weekly
Ketone	Twice daily	Daily to weekly
Specific gravity	As indicated	As indicated
Urea nitrogen	As indicated	As indicated
Clinical Calculations		
Fluid balance	Daily	As indicated
Projected vs actual intake	Daily	Weekly to q visit
Calorie/protein intake	Daily	As indicated

Frequency depends on clinical condition.

[1]For metabolically unstable patients, need to check more frequently.

Adapted from "Guidelines for the Use of Parenteral and Enteral Nutrition in Adult and Pediatric Patients. ASPEN Board of Directors and The Clinical Guidelines Task Force," *JPEN J Parenter Enteral Nutr*, 2002, 26(1 Suppl):1-138SA.

Nutritional Guidelines for Pediatric Patients

Age	kcal/kg/d	Protein g/kg/d
Preterm neonate	120-140	3-4
Term infant - 1 y	90-120	2-3
1-7 y	75-90	1-1.2
7-12 y	60-75	1-1.2
12-18 y	30-60	0.8-0.9
>18 y	25-30	0.8

PN kcal/mL[1]

Dextrose Concentration						
5%	10%	15%	20%	25%	30%	35%
0.17	0.34	0.51	0.68	0.85	1.02	1.19

Dextrose provides 3.4 kcal/g.

Fat emulsion 10% provides 1.1 kcal/mL.

Fat emulsion 20% provides 2 kcal/mL.

[1]Calories derived from amino acids are not included.

Reference

"Guidelines for the Use of Parenteral and Enteral Nutrition in Adult and Pediatric Patients. ASPEN Board of Directors and The Clinical Guidelines Task Force," *JPEN J Parenter Enteral Nutr*, 2002, 26(1 Suppl):1-138SA.

Pharmacologic considerations of mixing medications with PN solutions include:

Adsorption — bag, bottle, tubing, filter	pH factors
Blood levels	Temperature
Site of injection/administration	Additives in solution
Flush	Heparin dose
Amino acid-dextrose concentrations	

GROWTH CHARTS

CDC Growth Charts: United States

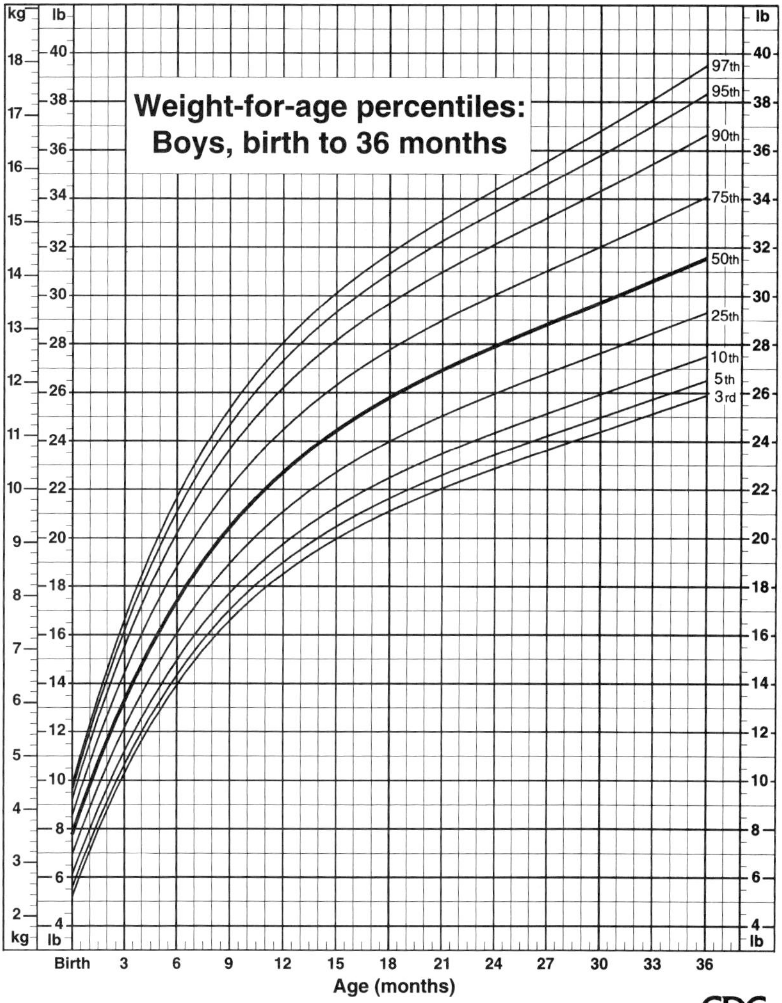

**Weight-for-age percentiles:
Boys, birth to 36 months**

Age (months)

SOURCE: Developed by the National Center for Health Statistics in collaboration with the National Center for Chronic Disease Prevention and Health Promotion (2000).

Available at http://www.cdc.gov/growthcharts

CDC Growth Charts: United States

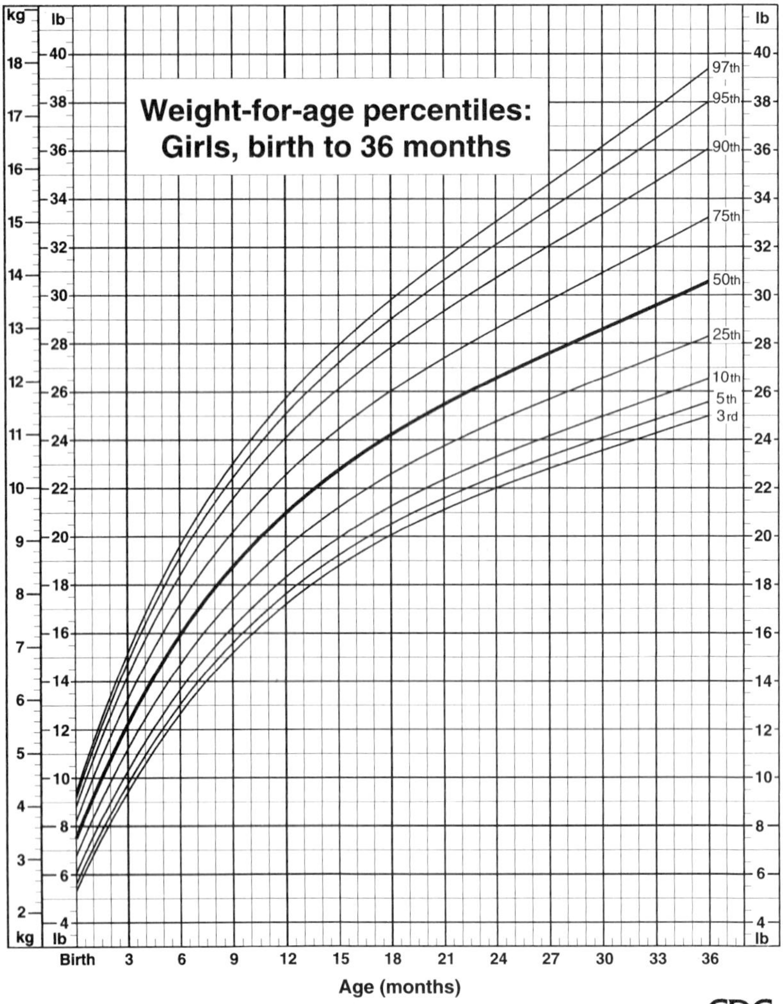
Weight-for-age percentiles:
Girls, birth to 36 months
kg
lb
97th
95th
90th
75th
50th
25th
10th
5th
3rd
Birth
3
6
9
12
15
18
21
24
27
30
33
36
Age (months)

SOURCE: Developed by the National Center for Health Statistics in collaboration with the National Center for Chronic Disease Prevention and Health Promotion (2000).
Available at http://www.cdc.gov/growthcharts

CDC Growth Charts: United States

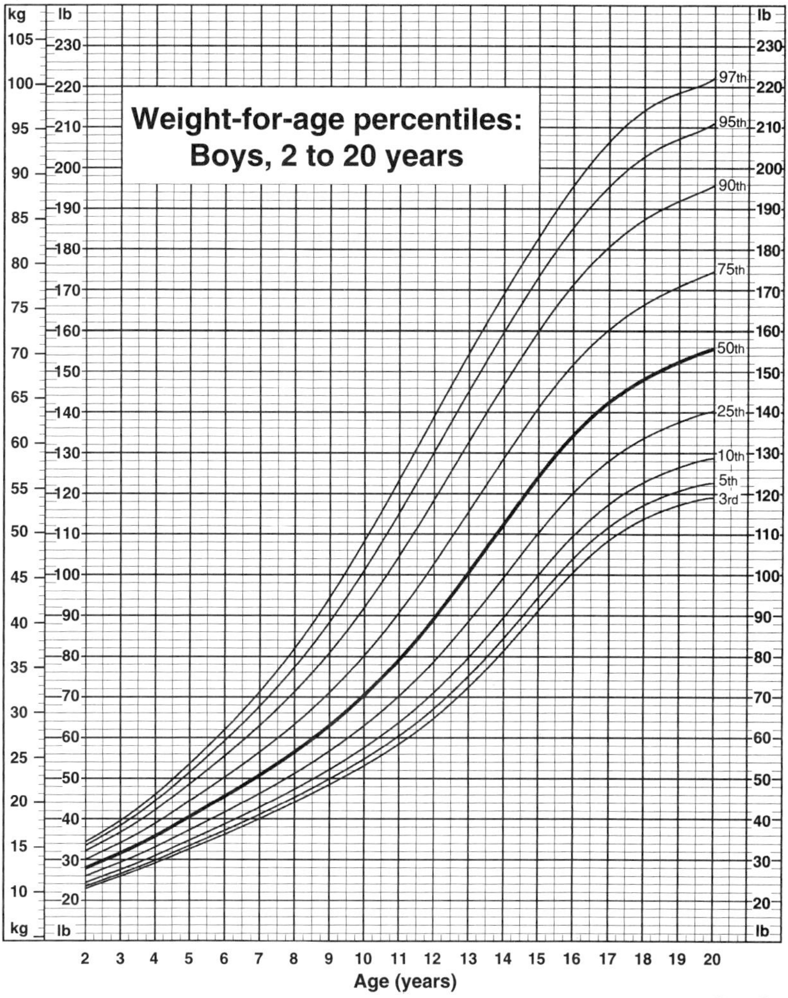

Weight-for-age percentiles: Boys, 2 to 20 years

SOURCE: Developed by the National Center for Health Statistics in collaboration with the National Center for Chronic Disease Prevention and Health Promotion (2000).
Available at http://www.cdc.gov/growthcharts

CDC
CENTERS FOR DISEASE CONTROL AND PREVENTION

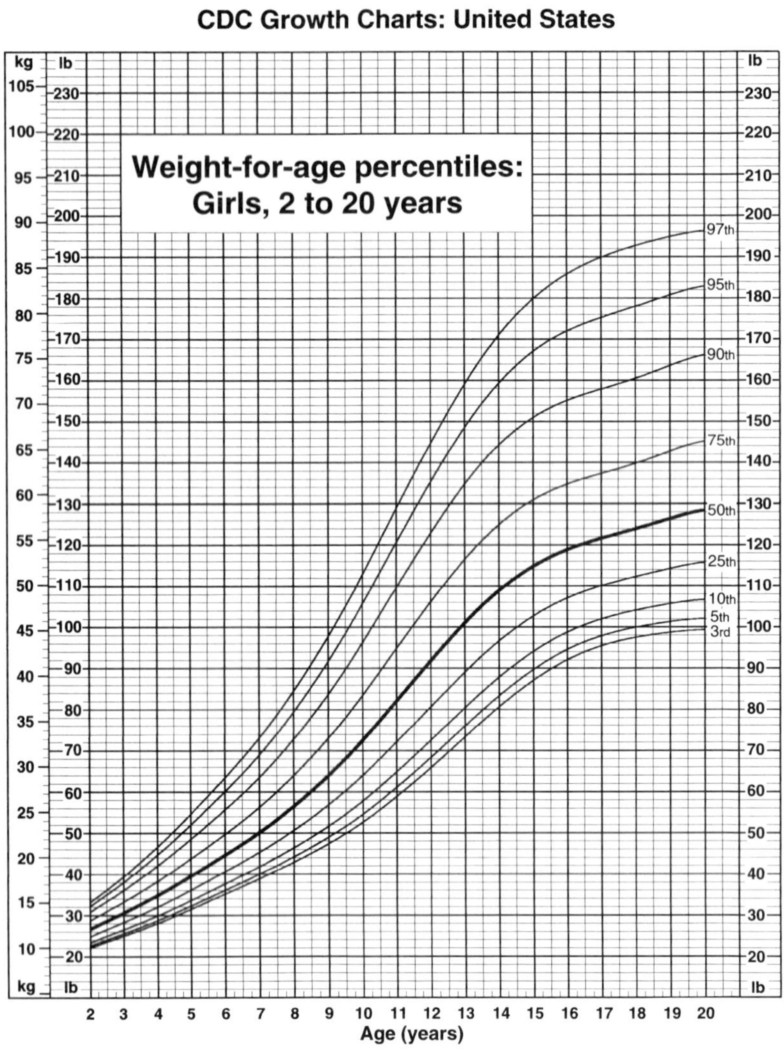
CDC Growth Charts: United States
Weight-for-age percentiles:
Girls, 2 to 20 years
kg
lb
97th
95th
90th
75th
50th
25th
10th
5th
3rd
Age (years)

SOURCE: Developed by the National Center for Health Statistics in collaboration with the National Center for Chronic Disease Prevention and Health Promotion (2000). Available at http://www.cdc.gov/growthcharts

CDC Growth Charts: United States

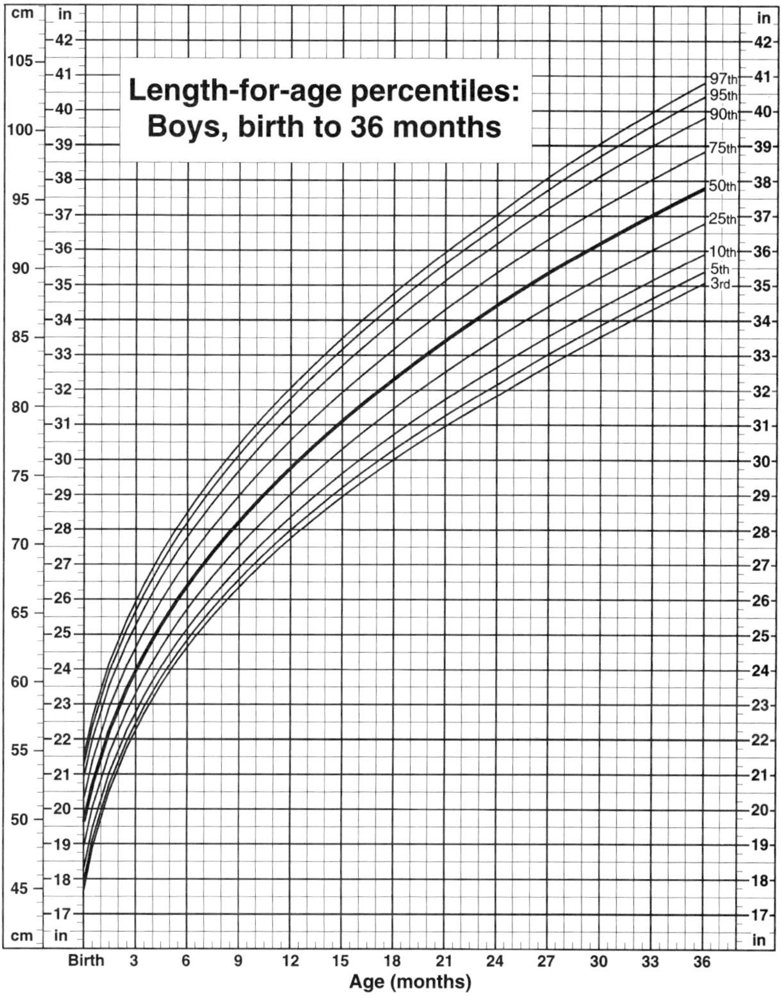

Length-for-age percentiles: Boys, birth to 36 months

Percentile lines (top to bottom): 97th, 95th, 90th, 75th, 50th, 25th, 10th, 5th, 3rd

Age (months): Birth, 3, 6, 9, 12, 15, 18, 21, 24, 27, 30, 33, 36

SOURCE: Developed by the National Center for Health Statistics in collaboration with the National Center for Chronic Disease Prevention and Health Promotion (2000).
Available at http://www.cdc.gov/growthcharts

CDC Growth Charts: United States

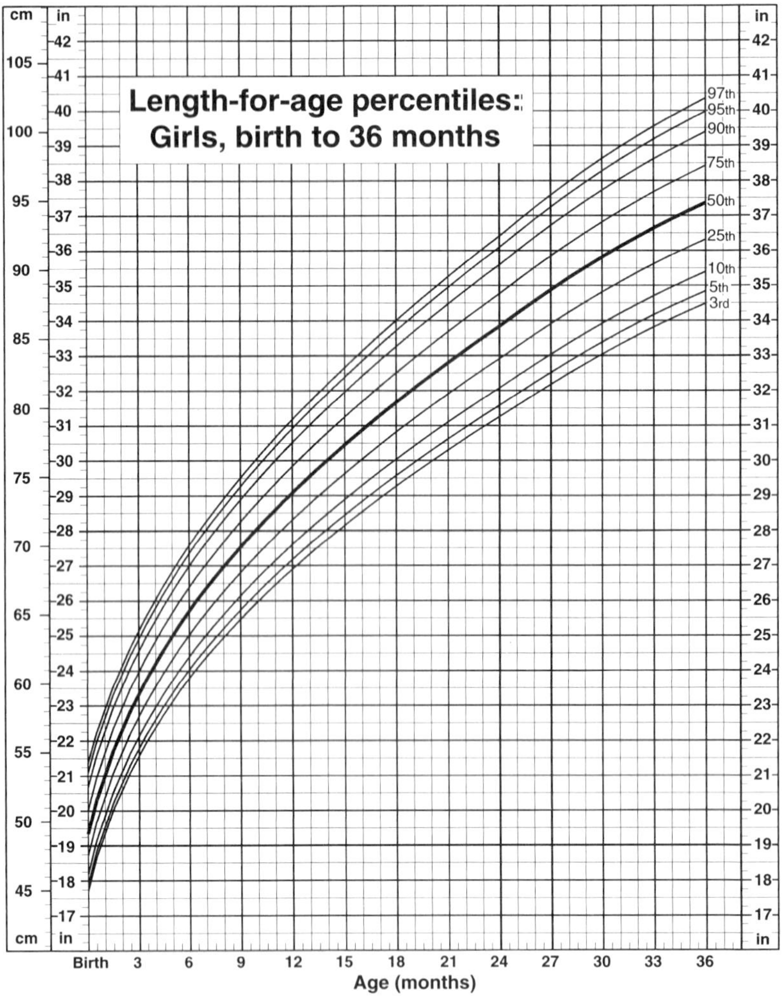
Length-for-age percentiles:
Girls, birth to 36 months
cm
in
97th
95th
90th
75th
50th
25th
10th
5th
3rd
Birth
3
6
9
12
15
18
21
24
27
30
33
36
Age (months)

SOURCE: Developed by the National Center for Health Statistics in collaboration with the National Center for Chronic Disease Prevention and Health Promotion (2000). Available at http://www.cdc.gov/growthcharts

CDC

CDC Growth Charts: United States

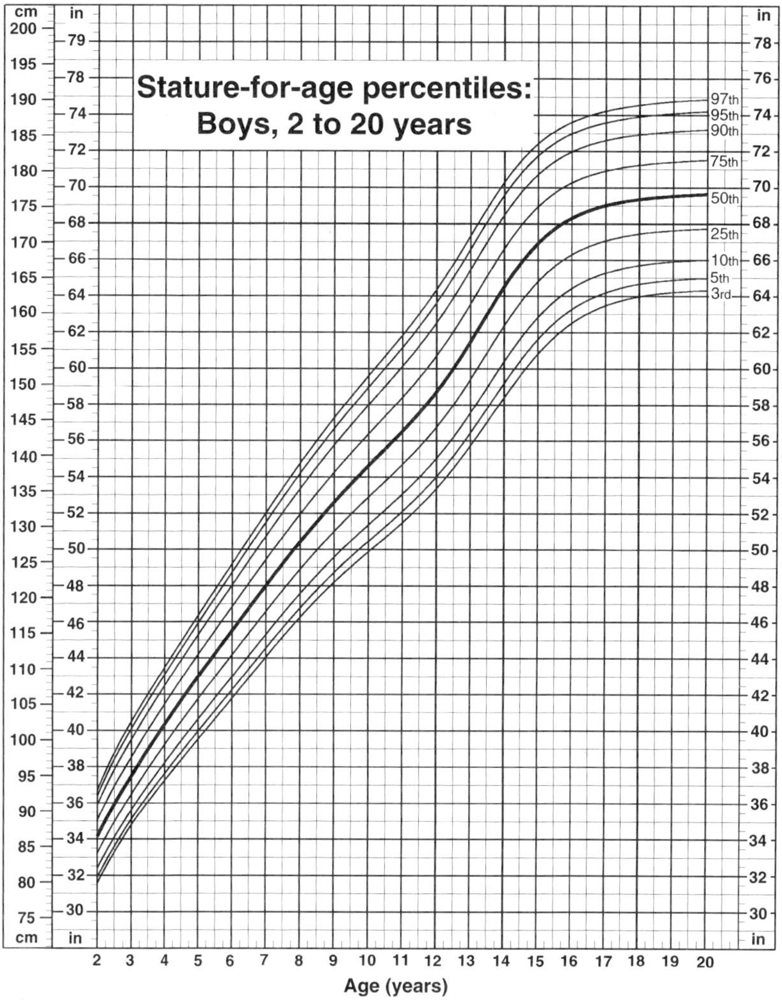
Stature-for-age percentiles:
Boys, 2 to 20 years
cm
in
97th
95th
90th
75th
50th
25th
10th
5th
3rd
Age (years)

SOURCE: Developed by the National Center for Health Statistics in collaboration with the National Center for Chronic Disease Prevention and Health Promotion (2000).
Available at http://www.cdc.gov/growthcharts

CDC Growth Charts: United States

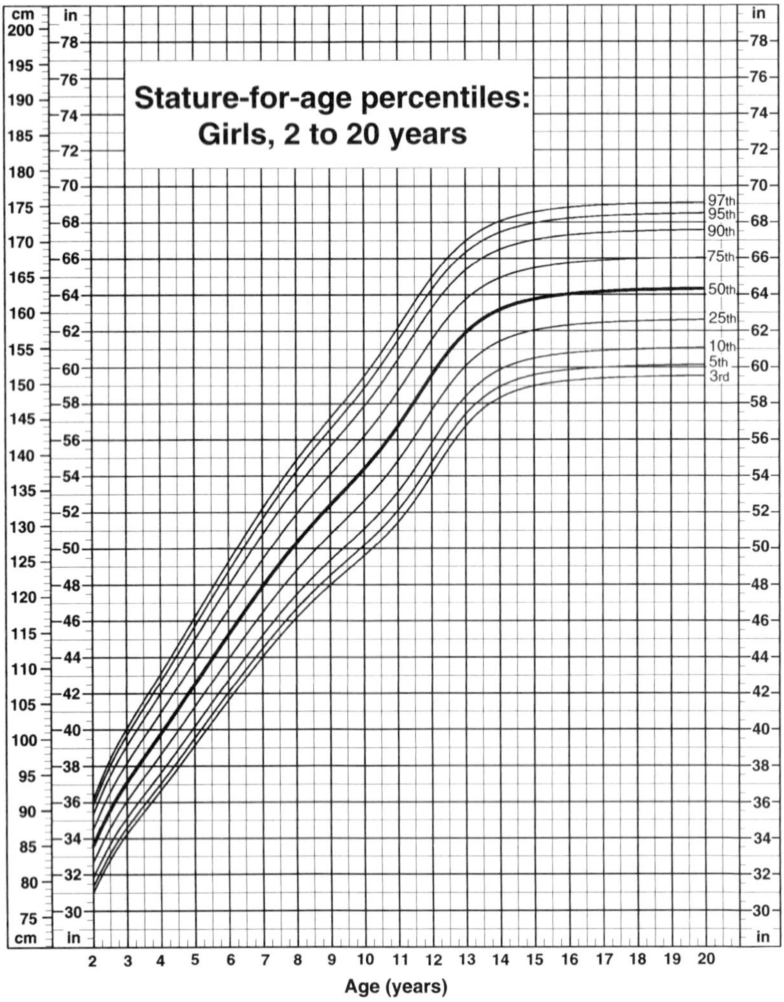
Stature-for-age percentiles:
Girls, 2 to 20 years
cm
in
97th
95th
90th
75th
50th
25th
10th
5th
3rd
Age (years)

SOURCE: Developed by the National Center for Health Statistics in collaboration with the National Center for Chronic Disease Prevention and Health Promotion (2000).
Available at http://www.cdc.gov/growthcharts

CDC Growth Charts: United States

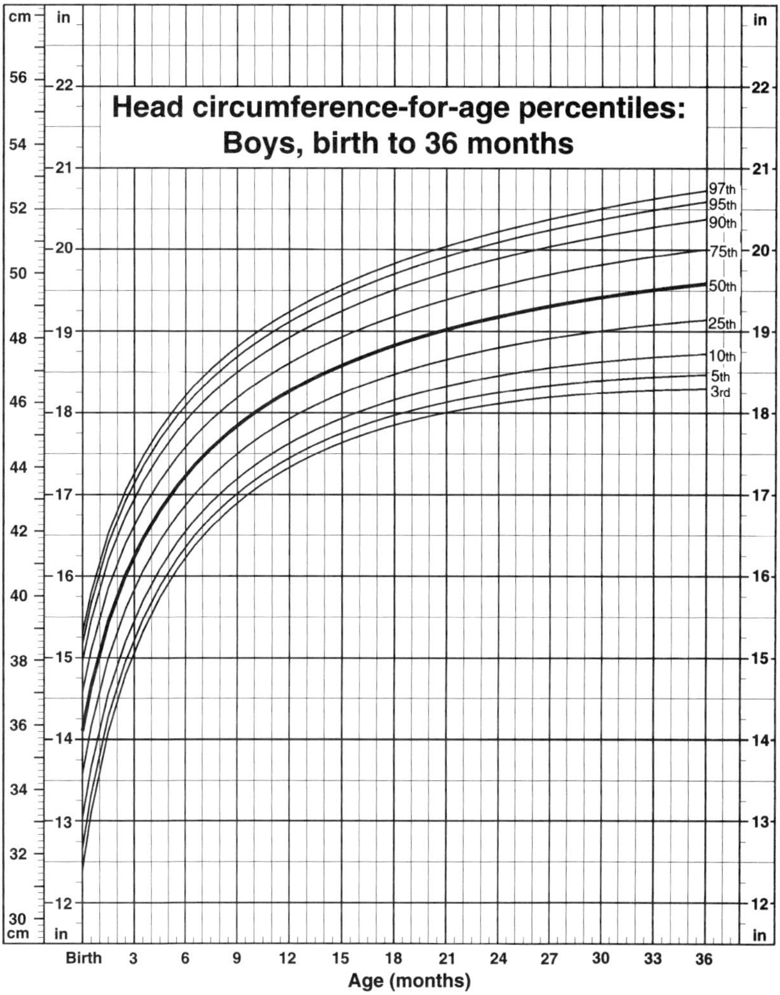
Head circumference-for-age percentiles:
Boys, birth to 36 months
cm
in
97th
95th
90th
75th
50th
25th
10th
5th
3rd
Birth
3
6
9
12
15
18
21
24
27
30
33
36
Age (months)

SOURCE: Developed by the National Center for Health Statistics in collaboration with the National Center for Chronic Disease Prevention and Health Promotion (2000).
Available at http://www.cdc.gov/growthcharts

CDC Growth Charts: United States

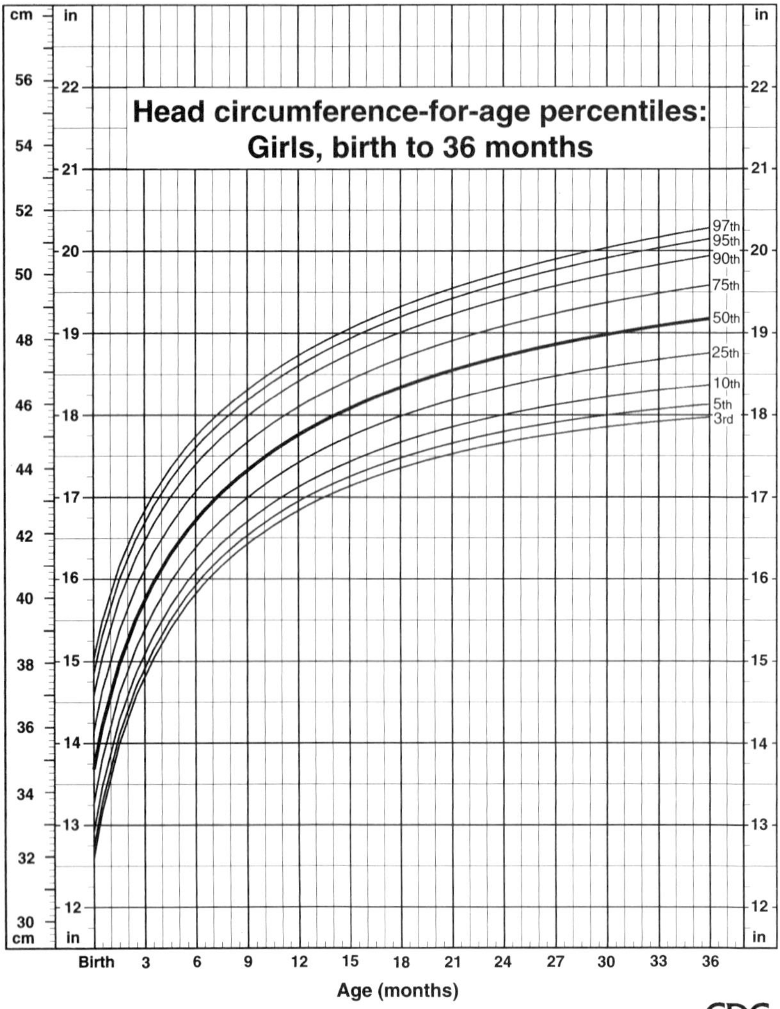
Head circumference-for-age percentiles:
Girls, birth to 36 months
cm
in
56
54
52
50
48
46
44
42
40
38
36
34
32
30
22
21
20
19
18
17
16
15
14
13
12
97th
95th
90th
75th
50th
25th
10th
5th
3rd
Birth
3
6
9
12
15
18
21
24
27
30
33
36
Age (months)

SOURCE: Developed by the National Center for Health Statistics in collaboration with the National Center for Chronic Disease Prevention and Health Promotion (2000). Available at http://www.cdc.gov/growthcharts

IDEAL BODY WEIGHT CALCULATION

Adults (18 years and older)

IBW (male) = 50 + (2.3 x height in inches over 5 feet)

IBW (female) = 45.5 + (2.3 x height in inches over 5 feet)

IBW is in kg.

Children

a. 1-18 years (Traub and Johnson, 1980)

$$IBW = \frac{(height^2 \times 1.65)}{1000}$$

IBW is in kg.

Height is in cm.

b. 5 feet and taller (Traub and Johnson, 1980)

IBW (male) = 39 + (2.27 x height in inches over 5 feet)

IBW (female) = 42.2 + (2.27 x height in inches over 5 feet)

IBW is in kg.

c. 1-17 years (Traub and Kichen, 1983)

$IBW = 2.396e^{0.01883 \,(height)}$

IBW is in kg.

Height is in cm.

References

Traub SL and Johnson CE, "Comparison of Methods of Estimating Creatinine Clearance in Children," *Am J Hosp Pharm*, 1980, 37(2):195-201.

Traub SL and Kichen L, "Estimating Ideal Body Mass in Children," *Am J Hosp Pharm*, 1983, 40(1):107-10.

BODY SURFACE AREA OF CHILDREN AND ADULTS

Calculating Body Surface Area in Children

In a child of average size, find weight and corresponding surface area on the boxed scale to the left; or, use the nomogram to the right. Lay a straightedge on the correct height and weight points for the child, then read the intersecting point on the surface area scale.

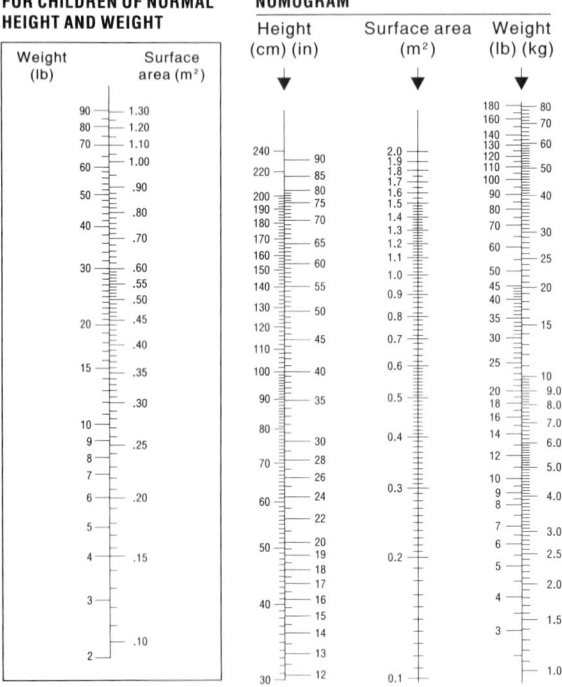

FOR CHILDREN OF NORMAL HEIGHT AND WEIGHT

NOMOGRAM

BODY SURFACE AREA FORMULA
(Adult and Pediatric)

$$BSA\ (m^2) = \sqrt{\frac{Ht\ (in)\ x\ Wt\ (lb)}{3131}}\quad or,\ in\ metric:\ BSA\ (m^2) = \sqrt{\frac{Ht\ (cm)\ x\ Wt\ (kg)}{3600}}$$

References

Lam TK and Leung DT, "More on Simplified Calculation of Body Surface Area," *N Engl J Med*, 1988, 318(17):1130 (Letter).

Mosteller RD, "Simplified Calculation of Body Surface Area", *N Engl J Med*, 1987, 317(17):1098 (Letter).

AVERAGE WEIGHTS AND SURFACE AREAS

Average Height, Weight, and Surface Area by Age and Gender

Age	Girls			Boys		
	Height (cm)	Weight (kg)	BSA (m^2)	Height (cm)	Weight (kg)	BSA (m^2)
Birth	49.5	3.4	0.22	50	3.6	0.22
3 mo	59	5.6	0.3	61	6	0.32
6 mo	65	7.2	0.36	67	7.9	0.38
9 mo	70	8.3	0.4	72	9.3	0.43
12 mo	74.5	9.5	0.44	75.5	10.3	0.46
15 mo	77	10.3	0.47	79	11.1	0.49
18 mo	80	11	0.49	82	11.7	0.52
21 mo	83	11.6	0.52	85	12.2	0.54
2 y	86	12	0.54	87.5	12.6	0.55
2.5 y	91	13	0.57	92	13.5	0.59
3 y	94.5	13.8	0.6	96	14.3	0.62
3.5 y	97	15	0.64	98	15	0.64
4 y	101	16	0.67	102	16	0.67
4.5 y	104	17	0.7	105	17	0.7
5 y	107.5	18	0.73	109	18.5	0.75
6 y	115	20	0.80	115	21	0.82
7 y	121.5	23	0.88	122	23	0.88
8 y	127.5	25.5	0.95	127.5	26	0.96
9 y	133	29	1.04	133.5	28.5	1.03
10 y	138	33	1.12	138.5	32	1.1
11 y	144	37	1.22	143.5	36	1.2
12 y	151	41.5	1.32	149	40.5	1.29
13 y	157	46	1.42	156	45.5	1.4
14 y	160.5	49.5	1.49	163.5	51	1.52
15 y	162	52	1.53	170	56	1.63
16 y	162.5	54	1.56	173.5	61	1.71
17 y	163	55	1.58	175	64.5	1.77
Adult[1]	163.5	58	1.62	177	83.5	2.03

Data extracted from the CDC growth charts based on the 50th percentile height and weight for a given age.[2]

Body surfaced area calculation[3]: Square root of [(Ht x Wt) / 3600]

[1]McDowell MA, Fryar CD, Hirsch R, et al, "Anthropometric Reference Data for Children and Adults: U.S. Population, 1999-2002," *Adv Data*, 2005, (361):1-5.

[2]Centers for Disease Control and Prevention, "2000 CDC Growth Charts: United States," Available at: http://www.cdc.gov/growthcharts. Accessed November 16, 2007.

[3]Mosteller RD, "Simplified Calculation of Body-Surface Area," *N Engl J Med*, 1987, 317(17):1098.

PHYSICAL DEVELOPMENT

Weight gain first 6 weeks
20 g/day

Birth weight
regained by day 14
doubles by age 4 mo
triples by age 12 mo
quadruples by age 2 y

Teeth
1st tooth 6-18 mo
teeth = age (mo) − 6 (until 30 mo)

Head circumference
35 cm at birth
44 cm by 6 mo
47 cm by 1 y
1 cm/mo for 1st y
0.25 cm/mo 2nd y

Length
increases 50% by age 1 y
doubles by age 4 y
triples by age 13 y

Tanner Stages of Sexual Development

Stage	Characteristics	Age at Onset (mean ± SD)
Genital stages: Male		
1	Prepubertal	
2	Scrotum and testes enlarge; skin of scrotum reddens and rugations appear	11.4 ± 1.1 y
3	Penis lengthens; testes enlarge further	12.9 ± 1 y
4	Penis growth continues in length and width; glans develops adult form	13.8 ± 1 y
5	Development completed; adult appearance	14.9 ± 1.1 y
Breast development: Female		
1	Prepubertal	
2	Breast buds appear; areolae enlarge	11.2 ± 1.1 y
3	Elevation of breast contour; areolae enlarge	12.2 ± 1.1 y
4	Areolae and papilla form a secondary mound on breast	13.1 ± 1.2 y
5	Adult form	15.3 ± 1.7 y
Menarche		
Pubic hair: Both sexes		13.5 ± 1 y
1	Prepubertal, no coarse hair	
2	Longer, silky hair appears at base of penis or along labia	F: 11.7 ± 1.2 y M: 12 ± 1 y
3	Hair coarse, kinky, spreads over pubic bone	F: 12.4 ± 1.1 y M: 13.9 ± 1 y
4	Hair of adult quality but not spread to junction of medial thigh with perineum	F: 13 ± 1 y M: 14.4 ± 1.1 y
5	Spread to medial thigh	F: 14.4 ± 1.1 y M: 15.2 ± 1.1 y
6	"Male escutcheon"	Variable if occurs

Maximum growth rate

Male at 14.1 ± 0.9 y

Female at 12.1 ± 0.9 y

EMETOGENIC POTENTIAL OF ANTINEOPLASTIC AGENTS

Highly Emetogenic Chemotherapy (Frequency of Emesis: >90%)

AC (either doxorubicin or epirubicin in combination with cyclophosphamide)
Altretamine
Carmustine >250 mg/m^2

Cisplatin ≥50 mg/m^2
Cyclophosphamide >1,500 mg/m^2
Dacarbazine
Mechlorethamine

Procarbazine (oral)
Streptozocin

Moderately Emetogenic Chemotherapy (Frequency of Emesis: 30% to 90%)

Aldesleukin >12-15 million units/m^2
Amifostine >300 mg/m^2
Arsenic trioxide
Azacitidine
Bendamustine
Busulfan (I.V.) or ≥4 mg/day (oral)
Carboplatin
Carmustine ≤250 mg/m^2
Cisplatin <50 mg/m^2
Cyclophosphamide ≤1,500 mg/m^2 (I.V.)

Cyclophosphamide ≥100 mg/m^2/day (oral)
Cytarabine >1,000 mg/m^2
Dactinomycin
Daunorubicin
Doxorubicin
Epirubicin
Estramustine
Etoposide (oral)
Idarubicin
Ifosfamide

Imatinib
Interferon alfa >10,000 units/m^2
Irinotecan
Lomustine
Melphalan >50 mg/m^2
Methotrexate 250->1,000 mg/m^2
Oxaliplatin
Temozolomide (I.V.)
Temozolomide >75 mg/m^2/day (oral)
Vinorelbine (oral)

Low Emetogenic Chemotherapy (Frequency of Emesis: 10% to 30%)

Aldesleukin ≤12 million units/m^2
Amifostine ≤300 mg
Bexarotene
Bortezomib
Capecitabine
Cetuximab
Cytarabine 100-200 mg/m^2
Docetaxel
Doxorubicin, liposomal
Etoposide (I.V.)

Fludarabine (oral)
Fluorouracil
Gemcitabine
Interferon alfa >5000-<10,000 units/m^2
Ixabepilone
Lapatinib
Methotrexate >50-<250 mg/m^2
Mitomycin
Mitoxantrone
Nilotinib

Paclitaxel
Paclitaxel protein bound
Pemetrexed
Pentostatin
Romidepsin
Topotecan
Trastuzumab
Tretinoin
UFT (oral)
Vorinostat

Minimal Emetogenic Chemotherapy (Frequency of Emesis: <10%)

Alemtuzumab
Asparaginase
Bevacizumab
Bleomycin
Busulfan <4 mg/day
Cetuximab
Chlorambucil
Cladribine
Cyclophosphamide <100 mg/m^2/day (oral)
Cytarabine <100 mg/m^2
Dasatinib
Decitabine
Denileukin diftitox

Dexrazoxane
Erlotinib
Everolimus
Fludarabine (I.V.)
Gefitinib
Gemtuzumab ozogamicin
Hydroxyurea
Lapatinib
Lenalidomide
Melphalan (oral, low dose)
Mercaptopurine
Methotrexate ≤50 mg/m^2
Methotrexate (oral)
Nelarabine

Panitumumab
Pazopanib
Pegaspargase
Rituximab
Sorafenib
Sunitinib
Temsirolimus
Temozolomide ≤75 mg/m^2/day (oral)
Thalidomide
Thioguanine (oral)
Valrubicin
Vinblastine
Vincristine
Vinorelbine (I.V.)

COMPATIBILITY OF CHEMOTHERAPY AND RELATED SUPPORTIVE CARE MEDICATIONS

Compatible: The drugs are physically compatible when mixed in the same container or infused through the same I.V. line simultaneously.

Y-site compatible: The drugs are physically compatible when infused through the same I.V. line simultaneously.

Incompatible: The drugs are physically incompatible when mixed in the same container, or infused through the same I.V. line simultaneously.

Variable compatibility: The compatibility of the drugs varies according to the concentration and/or diluent of the drugs. Please refer to the table at the end of this section for more information on variable compatibility.

Abbreviations

AA	Amino acid solution
BNS	Bacteriostatic normal saline
BWI	Bacteriostatic water for injection
D_5W	5% dextrose in water
D_5/NS	5% dextrose in 0.9% sodium chloride
D_5/¼NS	5% dextrose in 0.225% sodium chloride
D_5/½NS	5% dextrose in 0.45% sodium chloride
D_5LR	5% dextrose in lactated Ringer's injection
$D_{10}W$	10% dextrose in water
$D_{10}W$/0.01% albumin	10% dextrose in water with 0.01% albumin
$D_{10}W$/0.05% albumin	10% dextrose in water with 0.05% albumin
$D_{10}W$/0.1% albumin	10% dextrose in water with 0.1% albumin
D_{10}/NS	10% dextrose in water in 0.9% sodium chloride
LR	Lactated Ringer's injection
NS	0.9% sodium chloride (normal saline)
SWI	Sterile water for injection
TPN	Total parenteral nutrition solution

Reported Compatibilities and Incompatibilities of Parenteral Dosage Forms

Aldesleukin

Compatible:

D_5W SWI

Y-Site Compatible:

Amikacin	Fat emulsion	Metoclopramide	Thiethylperazine
Amphotericin	Fluconazole	Morphine	Ticarcillin
Calcium gluconate	Foscarnet	Ondansetron	Tobramycin
Cotrimoxazole	Gentamicin	Piperacillin	
Diphenhydramine	Heparin	Potassium chloride	
Dopamine	Magnesium sulfate	Ranitidine	

Incompatible:

Ganciclovir	Pentamidine	Promethazine
Heparin	Prochlorperazine	

Amifostine

Compatible:

NS

Y-Site Compatible:

Amikacin	Calcium gluconate	Ceftizoxime	Dacarbazine
Aminophylline	Carboplatin	Ceftriaxone	Dactinomycin
Ampicillin	Carmustine	Cefuroxime	Daunomycin
Ampicillin/sulbactam	Cefamandole	Cimetidine	Dexamethasone
Aztreonam	Cefepime	Ciprofloxacin	Diphenhydramine
Bleomycin	Cefotaxime	Clindamycin	Dobutamine
Bumetanide	Cefotetan	Cotrimoxazole	Dopamine
Buprenorphine	Cefoxitin	Cyclophosphamide	Doxorubicin
Butorphanol	Ceftazidime	Cytarabine	Doxycycline

Droperidol	Hydrocortisone sodium	Methotrexate	Ranitidine
Enalaprilat	phosphate	Methylprednisolone	Sodium bicarbonate
Etoposide	Hydrocortisone sodium suc-	Metoclopramide	Streptozocin
Famotidine	cinate	Metronidazole	Teniposide
Floxuridine	Hydromorphone	Mezlocillin	Thiotepa
Fluconazole	Idarubicin	Mitomycin	Ticarcillin
Fludarabine	Ifosfamide	Mitoxantrone	Ticarcillin/clavulanate
Fluorouracil	Imipenem/cilastatin	Morphine	Tobramycin
Furosemide	Leucovorin	Nalbuphine	Trimetrexate
Gallium nitrate	Lorazepam	Netilmicin	Vancomycin
Gemcitabine	Magnesium sulfate	Ondansetron	Vinblastine
Gentamicin	Mannitol	Piperacillin	Vincristine
Granisetron	Mechlorethamine	Plicamycin	
Haloperidol	Meperidine	Potassium chloride	
Heparin	Mesna	Promethazine	

Incompatible:

Acyclovir	Chlorpromazine	Ganciclovir	Minocycline
Amphotericin	Cisplatin	Hydroxyzine	Prochlorperazine

Asparaginase

Compatible:

D$_5$W	NS	SWI

Y-Site Compatible:

Methotrexate	Sodium bicarbonate

Bleomycin

Compatible:

BNS	Cimetidine	Gentamicin	Streptomycin
BWI	Dacarbazine	Heparin	Tobramycin
SWI	Dexamethasone	Hydrocortisone sodium	Vinblastine
Amikacin	Diphenhydramine	phosphate	Vincristine
Amsacrine	Droperidol	Leucovorin	
Ceftazidime	Fluorouracil	Metoclopramide	
Cephapirin	Furosemide	Phenytoin	

Y-Site Compatible:

Allopurinol	Cyclophosphamide	Gemcitabine	Piperacillin
Amifostine	Doxorubicin	Methotrexate	Sargramostim
Aztreonam	Doxorubicin, liposomal	Mitomycin	Teniposide
Cefepime	Filgrastim	Ondansetron	Thiotepa
Cisplatin	Fludarabine	Paclitaxel	Vinorelbine

Incompatible:

Aminophylline	Cephalothin	Hydrocortisone sodium suc-	Penicillin G
Ascorbic acid	Diazepam	cinate	Terbutaline
Cefazolin	Doxapram	Nafcillin	

Variable Compatibility:

D$_5$W	NS

Busulfan

Compatible:

D$_5$W	NS

Carboplatin

Compatible:

D$_5$W	Etoposide	Ifosfamide
SWI	Floxuridine	

Y-Site Compatible:

Allopurinol	Filgrastim	Piperacillin	Thiotepa
Amifostine	Fludarabine	Piperacillin/tazobactam	TPN
Aztreonam	Gemcitabine	Propofol	Vinorelbine
Cefazolin	Granisetron	Sargramostim	
Doxorubicin, liposomal	Ondansetron	Teniposide	

Incompatible:

Fluorouracil	Mesna	Sodium bicarbonate

Variable Compatibility:

D$_5$/NS	D$_5$/¼NS	D$_5$/½NS	NS

Carmustine

Compatible:

D_5W	NS	SWI	Dacarbazine

Y-Site Compatible:

Amifostine	Fludarabine	Piperacillin/tazobactam	Vinorelbine
Aztreonam	Gemcitabine	Sargramostim	
Cefepime	Ondansetron	Teniposide	
Filgrastim	Piperacillin	Thiotepa	

Incompatible:

Allopurinol	Sodium bicarbonate

Cisplatin

Compatible:

D_5/NS	Cefazolin	Hydroxyzine	Mannitol
$D_5/^1/_4NS$	Cephalothin	Hydroxyurea	Mechlorethamine
$D_5/^1/_2NS$	Cyclophosphamide	Ifosfamide	Ondansetron
NS	Floxuridine	Leucovorin	

Y-Site Compatible:

Allopurinol	Doxorubicin, liposomal	Heparin	Prochlorperazine
Aztreonam	Droperidol	Hydromorphone	Promethazine
Bleomycin	Famotidine	Lorazepam	Propofol
Bumetanide	Filgrastim	Methotrexate	Ranitidine
Chlorpromazine	Fludarabine	Methylprednisolone	Sargramostim
Cimetidine	Fluorouracil	Metoclopramide	Teniposide
Dexamethasone	Furosemide	Mitomycin	Thiotepa
Diphenhydramine	Ganciclovir	Morphine	Vinorelbine
Doxapram	Gemcitabine	Paclitaxel	
Doxorubicin	Granisetron	Potassium chloride	

Incompatible:

Amifostine	Gallium nitrate	Piperacillin
Amsacrine	Mesna	Piperacillin/tazobactam
Cefepime	Oxacillin	Sodium bicarbonate

Variable Compatibility:

D_5W	SWI	Etoposide

Cladribine

Compatible:

NS

Cyclophosphamide

Compatible:

D_5W	LR	Dacarbazine	Mesna
D_5/NS	SWI	Etoposide	Methotrexate
D_5/LR	AA 4.25%/$D_{25}W$	Fluorouracil	Mitoxantrone
NS	Cisplatin	Hydroxyzine	Ondansetron

Y-Site Compatible:

Allopurinol	Clindamycin	Heparin	Piperacillin/tazobactam
Amifostine	Cotrimoxazole	Hydromorphone	Prochlorperazine
Amikacin	Dexamethasone	Idarubicin	Promethazine
Ampicillin	Diphenhydramine	Kanamycin	Propofol
Azlocillin	Doxapram	Leucovorin	Ranitidine
Aztreonam	Doxorubicin	Lorazepam	Sargramostim
Bleomycin	Doxorubicin, liposomal	Methylprednisolone	Sodium bicarbonate
Cefamandole	Doxycycline	Metoclopramide	Teniposide
Cefazolin	Droperidol	Metronidazole	Thiotepa
Cefepime	Erythromycin	Mezlocillin	Ticarcillin
Cefoperazone	Famotidine	Minocycline	Ticarcillin/clavulanate
Cefotaxime	Filgrastim	Mitomycin	Tobramycin
Cefoxitin	Fludarabine	Morphine	TPN
Ceftriaxone	Furosemide	Moxalactam	Vancomycin
Cephalothin	Gallium nitrate	Nafcillin	Vinblastine
Cephapirin	Ganciclovir	Oxacillin	Vincristine
Chloramphenicol	Gemcitabine	Paclitaxel	Vinorelbine
Chlorpromazine	Gentamicin	Penicillin G	
Cimetidine	Granisetron	Piperacillin	

Cytarabine

Compatible:

BNS	D_5/LR	Dacarbazine	Mitoxantrone
BWI	D_{10}/NS	Daunomycin	Ondansetron
D_5W	NS	Etoposide	Potassium chloride
D_5/NS	LR	Hydroxyzine	Prednisolone
$D_5/^1/_4NS$	AA 4.25%/$D_{25}W$	Hydroxyurea	Sodium bicarbonate
$D_5/^1/_2NS$	Corticotropin	Lincomycin	Vincristine

Y-Site Compatible:

Amifostine	Droperidol	Lorazepam	Ranitidine
Amsacrine	Famotidine	Metoclopramide	Sargramostim
Aztreonam	Filgrastim	Morphine	Teniposide
Cefepime	Fludarabine	Paclitaxel	Thiotepa
Chlorpromazine	Furosemide	Piperacillin	TPN
Cimetidine	Gemcitabine	Piperacillin/tazobactam	Vinorelbine
Dexamethasone	Granisetron	Prochlorperazine	
Diphenhydramine	Heparin	Promethazine	
Doxorubicin, liposomal	Idarubicin	Propofol	

Incompatible:

Allopurinol	Gallium nitrate	Nafcillin
Ceftazidime	Ganciclovir	Oxacillin
Fluorouracil	Insulin	Penicillin G

Variable Compatibility:

Cephalothin	Hydrocortisone sodium	Methylprednisolone
Gentamicin	phosphate	

Dacarbazine

Compatible:

NS	Cimetidine	Doxorubicin	Ondansetron
SWI	Cyclophosphamide	Fluorouracil	Vinblastine
Bleomycin	Cytarabine	Mercaptopurine	
Carmustine	Dactinomycin	Methotrexate	

Y-Site Compatible:

Amifostine	Fludarabine	Lidocaine	Thiotepa
Aztreonam	Granisetron	Paclitaxel	Vinorelbine
Doxorubicin, liposomal	Hydrocortisone sodium	Sargramostim	
Filgrastim	phosphate	Teniposide	

Incompatible:

D_5W	Cefepime	Hydrocortisone sodium suc-	Piperacillin
Allopurinol		cinate	Piperacillin/tazobactam

Variable Compatibility:

Heparin

Dactinomycin

Compatible:

D_5W	NS	SWI	Dacarbazine

Y-Site Compatible:

Allopurinol	Cefepime	Ondansetron	Thiotepa
Amifostine	Fludarabine	Sargramostim	Vinorelbine
Aztreonam	Gemcitabine	Teniposide	

Incompatible:

BNS	BWI	Filgrastim

Daunomycin

Compatible:

D_5W	LR	Cytarabine	Hydrocortisone sodium suc-
NS	SWI	Etoposide	cinate

Y-Site Compatible:

Amifostine	Methotrexate	Teniposide	
Filgrastim	Ondansetron	Thiotepa	
Gemcitabine	Sodium bicarbonate	Vinorelbine	

Incompatible:

Allopurinol	Cefepime	Fludarabine	Piperacillin/tazobactam
Aztreonam	Dexamethasone	Piperacillin	

Dexrazoxane

Compatible:
  D$_5$W

Y-Site Compatible:
  Gemcitabine

Diphenhydramine

Compatible:

Amikacin	Droperidol	Methicillin	Perphenazine
Aminophylline	Erythromycin	Methyldopate	Prochlorperazine
Ascorbic acid	Fentanyl	Metoclopramide	Promazine
Atropine	Fluphenazine	Midazolam	Promethazine
Bleomycin	Glycopyrrolate	Morphine	Ranitidine
Butorphanol	Hydrocortisone sodium suc-	Nalbuphine	Scopolamine
Cephapirin	cinate	Nafcillin	Sufentanil
Chlorpromazine	Hydromorphone	Netilmicin	Thiothixene
Cimetidine	Hydroxyzine	Penicillin G (sodium and	Polymyxin B
Colistimethate	Lidocaine	potassium)	Vitamin B complex with C
Dimenhydrinate	Meperidine	Pentazocine	

Y-Site Compatible:

Acyclovir	Cytarabine	Heparin	Potassium chloride
Aldesleukin	Doxorubicin	Idarubicin	Sargramostim
Amifostine	Filgrastim	Melphalan	Tacrolimus
Amsacrine	Fluconazole	Meperidine	Teniposide
Aztreonam	Fludarabine	Methotrexate	Thiotepa
Ciprofloxacin	Gallium nitrate	Ondansetron	Vinorelbine
Cisplatin	Gemcitabine	Paclitaxel	
Cyclophosphamide	Granisetron	Piperacillin/tazobactam	

Incompatible:

Allopurinol	Cefepime	Foscarnet	Secobarbital
Amobarbital	Cephalothin	Haloperidol	Thiopental
Amphotericin	Dexamethasone	Pentobarbital	

Variable Compatibility:
  Diatrizoate   Iodipamide

Docetaxel

Compatible:
  D$_5$W   NS

Y-Site Compatible:
  Gemcitabine

Incompatible:
  Doxorubicin, liposomal

Doxorubicin

Compatible:

D$_5$W	LR	Ondansetron
NS	Dacarbazine	Vincristine

Y-Site Compatible:

Amifostine	Diphenhydramine	Lorazepam	Promethazine
Aztreonam	Famotidine	Methotrexate	Propofol
Bleomycin	Filgrastim	Methylprednisolone	Ranitidine
Chlorpromazine	Fludarabine	Metoclopramide	Sargramostim
Cimetidine	Gemcitabine	Mitomycin	Sodium bicarbonate
Cisplatin	Granisetron	Morphine	Teniposide
Cyclophosphamide	Hydromorphone	Paclitaxel	Thiotepa
Dexamethasone	Leucovorin	Prochlorperazine	Vinorelbine

Incompatible:

Allopurinol	Diazepam	Heparin	TPN
Aminophylline	Furosemide	Hydrocortisone sodium suc-	Paclitaxel
Cefepime	Gallium nitrate	cinate	Tobramycin
Cephalothin	Ganciclovir	Piperacillin/tazobactam	

Variable Compatibility:
  Fluorouracil   Vinblastine

Doxorubicin, Liposomal

Compatible:

D_5W

Y-Site Compatible:

Allopurinol	Ciprofloxacin	Fluorouracil	Methylprednisolone
Aldesleukin	Cisplatin	Furosemide	Metronidazole
Aminophylline	Clindamycin	Ganciclovir	Mezlocillin
Ampicillin	Cotrimoxazole	Gentamicin	Netilmicin
Aztreonam	Cyclophosphamide	Granisetron	Ondansetron
Bleomycin	Cytarabine	Haloperidol	Piperacillin
Calcium chloride	Dacarbazine	Heparin	Potassium chloride
Calcium gluconate	Dexamethasone	Hydrocortisone sodium suc-	Prochlorperazine
Cefazolin	Diphenhydramine	cinate	Ranitidine
Cefepime	Dobutamine	Hydromorphone	Ticarcillin
Cefoperazone	Dopamine	Ifosfamide	Ticarcillin/clavulanate
Cefoxitin	Droperidol	Leucovorin	Tobramycin
Ceftizoxime	Enalaprilat	Lorazepam	Vancomycin
Ceftriaxone	Etoposide	Magnesium sulfate	Vinblastine
Chlorpromazine	Famotidine	Mesna	Vincristine
Cimetidine	Fluconazole	Methotrexate	Vinorelbine

Incompatible:

Amphotericin	Gallium nitrate	Metoclopramide	Ofloxacin
Buprenorphine	Hydroxyzine	Miconazole	Piperacillin/tazobactam
Ceftazidime	Mannitol	Mitoxantrone	Promethazine
Docetaxel	Meperidine	Morphine	Sodium bicarbonate

Droperidol

Compatible:

Atropine	Dimenhydrinate	Metoclopramide	Prochlorperazine
Bleomycin	Diphenhydramine	Midazolam	Promazine
Butorphanol	Doxorubicin	Mitomycin	Promethazine
Chlorpromazine	Fentanyl	Morphine	Scopolamine
Cimetidine	Glycopyrrolate	Nalbuphine	Vinblastine
Cisplatin	Hydroxyzine	Pentazocine	Vincristine
Cyclophosphamide	Meperidine	Perphenazine	

Y-Site Compatible:

Amifostine	Gemcitabine	Ondansetron	Thiotepa
Aztreonam	Hydrocortisone sodium suc-	Paclitaxel	Vinorelbine
Filgrastim	cinate	Potassium chloride	Vitamin B complex with C
Fluconazole	Idarubicin	Sargramostim	
Fludarabine	Melphalan	Teniposide	

Incompatible:

Allopurinol	Foscarnet	Leucovorin	Pentobarbital
Cefepime	Furosemide	Methotrexate	Piperacillin/tazobactam
Fluorouracil	Heparin	Nafcillin	

Erythropoietin

Compatible:

BNS	D_{10}/0.05% albumin	D_{10}/0.1% albumin

Incompatible:

$D_{10}W$	D_{10}/0.01% albumin	NS	SWI

Etoposide

Compatible:

D_5W	Carboplatin	Daunomycin	Hydroxyzine
NS	Cyclophosphamide	Floxuridine	Ifosfamide
LR	Cytarabine	Fluorouracil	Ondansetron

Y-Site Compatible:

Allopurinol	Fludarabine	Methotrexate	Sargramostim
Amifostine	Gemcitabine	Paclitaxel	Sodium bicarbonate
Aztreonam	Granisetron	Piperacillin	Teniposide
Doxorubicin, liposomal	Haloperidol	Piperacillin/tazobactam	Vinorelbine

Incompatible:

Cefoperazone	Cefepime	Gallium nitrate	
Ceftazidime	Filgrastim	Idarubicin	

Variable Compatibility:

Cisplatin   Mannitol   Potassium chloride

Filgrastim

Compatible:

D₅W   SWI

Y-Site Compatible:

Acyclovir	Cisplatin	Haloperidol	Mitoxantrone
Allopurinol	Cotrimoxazole	Hydrocortisone sodium	Morphine
Amikacin	Cyclophosphamide	phosphate	Nalbuphine
Aminophylline	Cytarabine	Hydrocortisone sodium suc-	Netilmicin
Ampicillin	Dacarbazine	cinate	Ondansetron
Ampicillin/sulbactam	Daunomycin	Hydromorphone	Plicamycin
Aztreonam	Dexamethasone	Hydroxyzine	Potassium chloride
Bleomycin	Diphenhydramine	Idarubicin	Promethazine
Bumetanide	Doxorubicin	Ifosfamide	Ranitidine
Buprenorphine	Doxycycline	Imipenem/cilastatin	Sodium bicarbonate
Butorphanol	Droperidol	Leucovorin	Streptozocin
Calcium gluconate	Enalaprilat	Lorazepam	Ticarcillin
Carboplatin	Fat emulsion	Mechlorethamine	Ticarcillin/clavulanate
Carmustine	Floxuridine	Meperidine	Tobramycin
Cefazolin	Fluconazole	Mesna	Vancomycin
Cefotetan	Fludarabine	Methotrexate	Vinblastine
Ceftazidime	Gallium nitrate	Metoclopramide	Vincristine
Chlorpromazine	Ganciclovir	Miconazole	Vinorelbine
Cimetidine	Gentamicin	Minocycline	

Incompatible:

NS	Cefotaxime	Etoposide	Metronidazole
Amphotericin	Cefoxitin	Fluorouracil	Mezlocillin
Amsacrine	Ceftizoxime	Furosemide	Mitomycin
Cefepime	Ceftriaxone	Heparin	Piperacillin
Cefonicid	Cefuroxime	Mannitol	Prochlorperazine
Cefoperazone	Dactinomycin	Methylprednisolone	Thiotepa

Floxuridine

Compatible:

D₅W	Carboplatin	Fluorouracil
NS	Cisplatin	Heparin
SWI	Etoposide	Leucovorin

Y-Site Compatible:

Amifostine	Fludarabine	Paclitaxel	Teniposide
Aztreonam	Gemcitabine	Piperacillin/tazobactam	Thiotepa
Filgrastim	Ondansetron	Sargramostim	Vinorelbine

Incompatible:

Allopurinol   Cefepime

Fludarabine

Compatible:

D₅W   NS   SWI

Y-Site Compatible:

Allopurinol	Ceftriaxone	Fluorouracil	Methotrexate
Amifostine	Cefuroxime	Furosemide	Methylprednisolone
Amikacin	Cimetidine	Gemcitabine	Metoclopramide
Aminophylline	Cisplatin	Gentamicin	Mezlocillin
Ampicillin	Cotrimoxazole	Haloperidol	Minocycline
Ampicillin/sulbactam	Cyclophosphamide	Heparin	Mitoxantrone
Amsacrine	Cytarabine	Hydrocortisone sodium	Morphine
Aztreonam	Dacarbazine	phosphate	Multivitamins
Bleomycin	Dactinomycin	Hydrocortisone sodium suc-	Nalbuphine
Butorphanol	Dexamethasone	cinate	Netilmicin
Carboplatin	Diphenhydramine	Hydromorphone	Ondansetron
Carmustine	Doxorubicin	Ifosfamide	Pentostatin
Cefazolin	Doxycycline	Imipenem/cilastatin	Piperacillin
Cefepime	Droperidol	Lorazepam	Piperacillin/tazobactam
Cefoperazone	Etoposide	Magnesium sulfate	Potassium chloride
Cefotaxime	Famotidine	Mannitol	Promethazine
Cefotetan	Filgrastim	Mechlorethamine	Ranitidine
Ceftazidime	Floxuridine	Meperidine	Sodium bicarbonate
Ceftizoxime	Fluconazole	Mesna	Teniposide

Tetracycline	Ticarcillin/clavulanate	Vancomycin	Vincristine
Ticarcillin	Tobramycin	Vinblastine	Vinorelbine

Incompatible:

Acyclovir	Chlorpromazine	Ganciclovir	Miconazole
Amphotericin	Daunomycin	Hydroxyzine	Prochlorperazine

Fluorouracil

Compatible:

D$_5$W	Cephalothin	Floxuridine	Mitoxantrone
D$_5$/LR	Cyclophosphamide	Ifosfamide	Prednisolone
NS	Dacarbazine	Magnesium sulfate	Vincristine
Bleomycin	Etoposide	Methotrexate	

Y-Site Compatible:

Allopurinol	Furosemide	Metochlopramide	Sargramostim
Amifostine	Gemcitabine	Mitomycin	Teniposide
Aztreonam	Granisetron	Paclitaxel	Thiotepa
Cefepime	Heparin	Piperacillin	Vinblastine
Cisplatin	Hydrocortisone sodium suc-	Piperacillin/tazobactam	Vitamin B complex
Doxorubicin, liposomal	cinate	Potassium chloride	
Fludarabine	Mannitol	Propofol	

Incompatible:

Carboplatin	Droperidol	Gallium nitrate	Vinorelbine
Cytarabine	Epirubicin	Ondansetron	
Diazepam	Filgrastim	TPN	

Variable Compatibility:

Doxorubicin	Leucovorin

Gemcitabine

Compatible:

NS

Y-Site Compatible:

Amifostine	Cisplatin	Gentamicin	Netilmicin
Amikacin	Clindamycin	Granisetron	Ofloxacin
Aminophylline	Cyclophosphamide	Haloperidol	Ondansetron
Ampicillin	Cytarabine	Heparin	Paclitaxel
Ampicillin/sulbactam	Dactinomycin	Hydrocortisone sodium	Plicamycin
Aztreonam	Daunomycin	phosphate	Potassium chloride
Bleomycin	Dexamethasone	Hydrocortisone sodium suc-	Promethazine
Bumetanide	Dexrazoxane	cinate	Ranitidine
Buprenorphine	Diphenhydramine	Hydromorphone	Sodium bicarbonate
Butorphanol	Dobutamine	Hydroxyzine	Streptozocin
Calcium gluconate	Docetaxel	Idarubicin	Teniposide
Carboplatin	Dopamine	Ifosfamide	Thiotepa
Carmustine	Doxorubicin	Leucovorin	Ticarcillin
Cefazolin	Doxycycline	Lorazepam	Ticarcillin/clavulanate
Cefonicid	Droperidol	Mannitol	Tobramycin
Cefotetan	Enalaprilat	Meperidine	Topotecan
Cefoxitin	Etoposide	Mesna	Trimethoprim
Ceftazidime	Etoposide phosphate	Metoclopramide	Vancomycin
Ceftizoxime	Famotidine	Metronidazole	Vinblastine
Ceftriaxone	Floxuridine	Miconazole	Vincristine
Cefuroxime	Fludarabine	Minocycline	Vinorelbine
Chlorpromazine	Fluorouracil	Mitoxantrone	Zidovudine
Cimetidine	Fluconazole	Morphine	
Ciprofloxacin	Gallium nitrate	Nalbuphine	

Incompatible:

Acyclovir	Furosemide	Methotrexate	Piperacillin
Amphotericin	Ganciclovir	Methylprednisolone	Piperacillin/tazobactam
Cefoperazone	Imipenem/cilastatin	Mezlocillin	Prochlorperazine
Cefotaxime	Irinotecan	Mitomycin	

Haloperidol

Compatible:

Hydromorphone	Sufentanil

Y-Site Compatible:

Amifostine	Cimetidine	Famotidine	Gemcitabine
Amsacrine	Dobutamine	Filgrastim	Lidocaine
Aztreonam	Dopamine	Fludarabine	Lorazepam

Melphalan	Ondansetron	Teniposide	Vinorelbine
Midazolam	Paclitaxel	Theophylline	
Nitroglycerin	Phenylephrine	Thiotepa	
Norepinephrine bitartrate	Tacrolimus	TPN	

Incompatible:

Allopurinol	Fluconazole	Heparin	Piperacillin/tazobactam
Cefepime	Foscarnet	Hydroxyzine	Sargramostim
Diphenhydramine	Gallium nitrate	Ketorolac	

Variable Compatibility:

Benztropine	Cyclizine	Diamorphine	Sodium nitroprusside

Heparin

Compatible:

Aminophylline	Cloxacillin	Furosemide	Potassium chloride
Amphotericin	Colistimethate	Isoproterenol	Prednisolone
Ascorbic acid	Dimenhydrinate	Lidocaine	Promazine
Bleomycin	Dopamine	Lincomycin	Ranitidine
Calcium gluconate	Enalaprilat	Methyldopa	Sodium bicarbonate
Cefepime	Erythromycin	Methylprednisolone	Verapamil
Cephapirin	Esmolol	Metronidazole	Vitamin B complex with C
Chloramphenicol	Floxacillin	Nafcillin	
Cibenzoline	Fluconazole	Norepinephrine	
Clindamycin	Flumazenil	Octreotide	

Y-Site Compatible:

Acyclovir	Diphenhydramine	Menadiol sodium diphos-	Procainamide
Aldesleukin	Edrophonium	phate	Prochlorperazine
Allopurinol	Epinephrine	Methicillin	Propranolol
Amifostine	Erythromycin	Methotrexate	Pyridostigmine
Ampicillin	Esmolol	Methoxamine	Sargramostim
Ampicillin/sulbactam	Estrogens, conjugated	Methyldopa	Scopolamine
Atracurium	Ethacrynate	Metoclopramide	Sodium nitroprusside
Atropine	Famotidine	Metronidazole	Streptokinase
Aztreonam	Fentanyl	Midazolam	Succinylcholine
Betamethasone sodium	Fludarabine	Minocycline	Tacrolimus
phosphate	Fluorouracil	Mitomycin	Teniposide
Cefazolin	Foscarnet	Morphine	Theophylline
Cefotetan	Gallium nitrate	Neostigmine	Thiotepa
Ceftazidime	Gemcitabine	Nitroglycerin	Ticarcillin
Ceftriaxone	Hydralazine	Ondansetron	Ticarcillin/clavulanate
Cephalothin	Hydrocortisone sodium suc-	Oxacillin	TPN
Chlordiazepoxide	cinate	Oxytocin	Trimethobenzamide
Chlorpromazine	Insulin	Paclitaxel	Trimethaphan
Cimetidine	Kanamycin	Pancuronium	Vercuronium
Cisplatin	Leucovorin	Penicillin G potassium	Vinblastine
Cyanocobalamin	Lorazepam	Pentazocine	Vincristine
Cyclophosphamide	Magnesium sulfate	Phytonadione	Vinorelbine
Cytarabine	Melphalan	Piperacillin	Zidovudine
Digoxin		Piperacillin/tazobactam	

Incompatible:

Alteplase	Diazepam	Haloperidol	Phenytoin
Amikacin	Dobutamine	Hyaluronidase	Polymyxin B
Amiodarone	Doxorubicin	Idarubicin	Streptomycin
Amsacrine	Doxycycline	Labetatol	Tobramycin
Ciprofloxacin	Ergotamine	Levorphanol	Triflupromazine
Codeine phosphate	Filgrastim	Methadone	
Daunomycin	Gentamicin	Methotrimeprazine	

Variable Compatibility:

Cephalothin	Droperidol	Methylprednisolone	Quinidine gluconate
Dacarbazine	Hydrocortisone sodium suc-	Penicillin G sodium	Vancomycin
Diltiazem	cinate	Promethazine	

Hydroxyzine

Compatible:

Atropine	Cisplatin	Droperidol	Lidocaine
Benzquinamide	Codeine	Etoposide	Meperidine
Bupivacaine	Cyclophosphamide	Fentanyl	Methotrimeprazine
Butorphanol	Cytarabine	Fluphenazine	Metoclopramide
Chlorpromazine	Diphenhydramine	Glycopyrrolate	Midazolam
Cimetidine	Doxapram	Hydromorphone	Morphine

Nalbuphine	Methotrexate	Prochlorperazine	Sufentanil
Oxymorphone	Nafcillin	Promazine	Thiothixene
Pentazocine	Perphenazine	Promethazine	
Mesna	Procaine	Scopolamine	

Y-Site Compatible:

Aztreonam	Foscarnet	Ondansetron	Thiotepa
Ciprofloxacin	Gemcitabine	Sufentanil	Vinorelbine
Filgrastim	Melphalan	Teniposide	

Incompatible:

Allopurinol	Chloramphenicol	Ketorolac	Phenobarbital
Amifostine	Diphenhydramine	Paclitaxel	Piperacillin/tazobactam
Aminophylline	Fluconazole	Penicillin G (sodium and	Ranitidine
Amobarbital	Fludarabine	potassium)	Sargramostim
Cefepime	Haloperidol	Pentobarbital	

Idarubicin

Compatible:

D_5W	D_5/NS	NS	LR

Y-Site Compatible:

Amifostine	Cytarabine	Gemcitabine	Potassium chloride
Amikacin	Diphenhydramine	Imipenem/cilastatin	Ranitidine
Aztreonam	Droperidol	Magnesium sulfate	Sargramostim
Ciprofloxacin	Erythromycin	Mannitol	Thiotepa
Cyclophosphamide	Filgrastim	Metoclopramide	Vinorelbine

Incompatible:

Acyclovir	Dexamethasone	Hydrocortisone sodium suc-	Piperacillin/tazobactam
Allopurinol	Etoposide	cinate	Sodium bicarbonate
Ampicillin/sulbactam	Furosemide	Lorazepam	Teniposide
Cefazolin	Gentamicin	Meperidine	Vancomycin
Cefepime	Heparin	Methotrexate	Vincristine
Ceftazidime		Mezlocillin	

Ifosfamide

Compatible:

D_5W	D_5/LR	SWI	Etoposide
D_5/NS	NS	Carboplatin	Fluorouracil
$D_5/^1/_4NS$	LR	Cisplatin	

Y-Site Compatible:

Allopurinol	Fludarabine	Paclitaxel	Sodium bicarbonate
Amifostine	Gallium nitrate	Piperacillin	Teniposide
Aztreonam	Gemcitabine	Piperacillin/tazobactam	Thiotepa
Doxorubicin, liposomal	Granisetron	Propofol	TPN
Filgrastim	Ondansetron	Sargramostim	Vinorelbine

Incompatible:

Cefepime	Methotrexate

Variable Compatibility:

Epirubicin	Mesna

Irinotecan

Compatible:

D_5W

Incompatible:

Gemcitabine

Leucovorin

Compatible:

BWI	NS	Bleomycin
D_5W	LR	Cisplatin
D_{10}/NS	SWI	Floxuridine

Y-Site Compatible:

Amifostine	Filgrastim	Metoclopramide	Teniposide
Aztreonam	Fluconazole	Mitomycin	Thiotepa
Cefepime	Furosemide	Piperacillin	TPN
Cyclophosphamide	Gemcitabine	Piperacillin/tazobactam	Vinblastine
Doxorubicin	Heparin	Sodium bicarbonate	Vincristine
Doxorubicin, liposomal	Methotrexate	Tacrolimus	

Incompatible:

Droperidol	Foscarnet	Trimetrexate

Variable Compatibility:

Fluorouracil

Lorazepam

Compatible:

Cimetidine	Hydromorphone

Y-Site Compatible:

Acyclovir	Cotrimoxazole	Gemcitabine	Pancuronium
Albumin	Cyclophosphamide	Gentamicin	Piperacillin
Amifostine	Cytarabine	Granisetron	Piperacillin/tazobactam
Amikacin	Dexamethasone	Haloperidol	Potassium chloride
Amoxicillin	Diltiazem	Heparin	Ranitidine
Amoxicillin/clavulanate	Doxorubicin	Hydrocortisone sodium suc-	Tacrolimus
Amsacrine	Erythromycin	cinate	Teniposide
Atracurium	Etomidate	Kantaserin	Thiotepa
Bumetanide	Fentanyl	Melphalan	Vancomycin
Cefepime	Filgrastim	Methotrexate	Vercuronium
Cefotaxime	Fluconazole	Metronidazole	Vinorelbine
Ciprofloxacin	Fludarabine	Morphine	Zidovudine
Cisplatin	Furosemide	Paclitaxel	

Incompatible:

Aldesleukin	Floxacillin	Imipenem/cilastatin	Sufentanil
Aztreonam	Gallium nitrate	Ondansetron	Thiopental
Buprenorphine	Idarubicin	Sargramostim	

Variable Compatibility:

Foscarnet

Mechlorethamine

Compatible:

NS	SWI

Y-Site Compatible:

Amifostine	Fludarabine	Sargramostim
Aztreonam	Granisetron	Teniposide
Filgrastim	Ondansetron	Vinorelbine

Incompatible:

D_5W	Allopurinol	Cefepime	Methohexital

Melphalan

Compatible:

NS

Y-Site Compatible:

Acyclovir	Cyclophosphamide	Hydrocortisone sodium	Nalbuphine
Amikacin	Cytarabine	phosphate	Netilmicin
Aminophylline	Dacarbazine	Hydrocortisone sodium suc-	Ondansetron
Ampicillin	Dactinomycin	cinate	Pentostatin
Aztreonam	Daunomycin	Hydromorphone	Piperacillin
Bleomycin	Diazepam	Hydroxyzine	Plicamycin
Bumetanide	Doxorubicin	Idarubicin	Potassium chloride
Buprenorphine	Doxycycline	Ifosfamide	Prochlorperazine
Butorphanol	Droperidol	Imipenem/cilastatin	Promethazine
Calcium gluconate	Enalaprilat	Lorazepam	Ranitidine
Carboplatin	Etoposide	Mannitol	Sodium bicarbonate
Carmustine	Famotidine	Mechlorethamine	Streptozocin
Cefazolin	Filgrastim	Meperidine	Teniposide
Cefepime	Floxuridine	Mesna	Thiotepa
Cefoperazone	Fluconazole	Methotrexate	Ticarcillin
Cefotaxime	Fludarabine	Methylprednisolone	Ticarcillin/clavulanate
Cefotetan	Fluorouracil	Metoclopramide	Tobramycin
Ceftazidime	Furosemide	Metronidazole	Vancomycin
Ceftriaxone	Gallium nitrate	Miconazole	Vinblastine
Cefuroxime	Ganciclovir	Minocycline	Vincristine
Cimetidine	Gentamicin	Mitomycin	Vinorelbine
Cisplatin	Haloperidol	Mitoxantrone	
Cotrimoxazole	Heparin	Morphine	

Incompatible:

D_5W	SWI	Chlorpromazine
LR	Amphotericin	

Mesna

Compatible:

BWI	NS	Cyclophosphamide	Ifosfamide
D_5W	LR	Hydroxyzine	

Y-Site Compatible:

Allopurinol	Filgrastim	Methotrexate	Sodium acetate
Amifostine	Fludarabine	Ondansetron	Teniposide
Aztreonam	Gallium nitrate	Paclitaxel	Thiotepa
Cefepime	Gemcitabine	Piperacillin/tazobactam	TPN
Doxorubicin, liposomal	Granisetron	Sargramostim	Vinorelbine

Incompatible:

Carboplatin	Cisplatin	Chlorpromazine

Methadone

Incompatible:

Aminophylline	Chlorothiazide	Methicillin	Sodium bicarbonate
Ammonium chloride	Phenytoin	Nitrofurantoin	Thiopental
Amobarbital	Heparin	Pentobarbital	

Methotrexate

Compatible:

D_5W	Amino acid 4.25%/$D_{25}W$	Dacarbazine	Mercaptopurine
NS	Cephalothin	Fluorouracil	Ondansetron
LR	Cyclophosphamide	Hydroxyzine	Sodium bicarbonate
SWI	Cytarabine	Imipenem/cilastatin	Vincristine

Y-Site Compatible:

Allopurinol	Diphenhydramine	Granisetron	Piperacillin/tazobactam
Amifostine	Doxapram	Heparin	Prochlorperazine
Asparaginase	Doxorubicin	Hydromorphone	Ranitidine
Aztreonam	Doxorubicin, liposomal	Leucovorin	Sargramostim
Bleomycin	Etoposide	Lorazepam	Teniposide
Cefepime	Famotidine	Mesna	Thiotepa
Ceftriaxone	Filgrastim	Methylprednisolone	Vinblastine
Cimetidine	Fludarabine	Mitomycin	Vindesine
Cisplatin	Furosemide	Morphine	Vinorelbine
Daunomycin	Gallium nitrate	Oxacillin	
Dexchlorpheniramine	Ganciclovir	Paclitaxel	

Incompatible:

Dexamethasone	Ifosfamide	Prednisolone	TPN
Gemcitabine	Midazolam	Promethazine	
Idarubicin	Nalbuphine	Propofol	

Variable Compatibility:

Droperidol	Metoclopramide	Vancomycin

Metoclopramide

Compatible:

D_5W	Mannitol	Potassium chloride	TPN
NS	Multivitamins	Potassium phosphate	
Clindamycin	Potassium acetate	Verapamil	

Y-Site Compatible:

Acyclovir	Doxorubicin	Heparin	Piperacillin/tazobactam
Aldesleukin	Droperidol	Idarubicin	Sargramostim
Amifostine	Famotidine	Leucovorin	Sufentanil
Aztreonam	Filgrastim	Melphalan	Tacrolimus
Bleomycin	Fluconazole	Meperidine	Teniposide
Ciprofloxacin	Fludarabine	Methotrexate	Thiotepa
Cisplatin	Fluorouracil	Mitomycin	Vinblastine
Cyclophosphamide	Foscarnet	Morphine	Vincristine
Cytarabine	Gallium nitrate	Ondansetron	Vinorelbine
Diltiazem	Gemcitabine	Paclitaxel	Zidovudine

◀ Incompatible:

Allopurinol	Cefepime	Dexamethasone	Furosemide
Ampicillin	Cephalothin	Erythromycin	Penicillin G potassium
Calcium gluconate	Chloramphenicol	Floxacillin	Sodium bicarbonate

Metronidazole

Compatible:

Amikacin	Ceftizoxime	Disopyramide	Multielectrolyte concentrate
Aminophylline	Ceftriaxone	Floxacillin	Multivitamins
Cefazolin	Cefuroxime	Fluconazole	Netilmicin
Cefotaxime	Cephalothin	Gentamicin	Penicillin G potassium
Cefotetan	Chloramphenicol	Heparin	Tobramycin
Cefoxitin	Ciprofloxacin	Hydrocortisone	
Ceftazidime	Clindamycin	Moxalactam	

Y-Site Compatible:

Acyclovir	Fluconazole	Melphalan	Teniposide
Allopurinol	Foscarnet	Meperidine	Theophylline
Amifostine	Gemcitabine	Midazolam	Thiotepa
Cefepime	Heparin	Morphine	TPN
Cyclophosphamide	Hydromorphone	Perphenazine	Vinorelbine
Diltiazem	Labetatol	Piperacillin/tazobactam	
Enalaprilat	Lorazepam	Sargramostim	
Esmolol	Magnesium sulfate	Tacrolimus	

Incompatible:

Aztreonam	Dopamine	Filgrastim

Variable Compatibility:

Ampicillin	Cefamandole

Mitomycin

Compatible:

NS	Dexamethasone	Hydrocortisone sodium succinate
LR		

Y-Site Compatible:

Allopurinol	Doxorubicin	Methotrexate	Vinblastine
Amifostine	Droperidol	Metoclopramide	Vincristine
Bleomycin	Fluorouracil	Ondansetron	
Cisplatin	Furosemide	Teniposide	
Cyclophosphamide	Leucovorin	Thiotepa	

Incompatible:

Aztreonam	Filgrastim	Piperacillin/tazobactam	Vinorelbine
Cefepime	Gemcitabine	Sargramostim	

Variable Compatibility:

D_5W	SWI	Heparin

Mitoxantrone

Compatible:

D_5W	NS	Cytarabine	Potassium chloride
D_5/NS	Cyclophosphamide	Fluorouracil	

Y-Site Compatible:

Allopurinol	Fludarabine	Sargramostim	Vinorelbine
Amifostine	Gemcitabine	Teniposide	
Filgrastim	Ondansetron	Thiotepa	

Incompatible:

Aztreonam	Doxorubicin, liposomal	Paclitaxel	Piperacillin/tazobactam
Cefepime	Heparin	Piperacillin	Propofol

Variable Compatibility:

Hydrocortisone sodium phosphate	Hydrocortisone sodium succinate	TPN

Ondansetron

Compatible:

D_5W	Cytarabine	Fluconazole	Methotrexate
NS	Dacarbazine	Hydrocortisone sodium succinate	Morphine
LR	Dexamethasone		Ranitidine
Cisplatin	Doxorubicin	Mannitol	
Cyclophosphamide	Etoposide	Meperidine	

Y-Site Compatible:

Aldesleukin	Dactinomycin	Hydrocortisone sodium	Piperacillin/tazobactam
Amifostine	Daunomycin	phosphate	Potassium chloride
Amikacin	Diphenhydramine	Hydromorphone	Prochlorperazine
Aztreonam	Doxorubicin, liposomal	Hydroxyzine	Promethazine
Bleomycin	Doxycycline	Ifosfamide	Sodium acetate
Carboplatin	Droperidol	Imipenem/cilastatin	Streptozocin
Carmustine	Famotidine	Magnesium sulfate	Teniposide
Cefazolin	Filgrastim	Mechlorethamine	Thiotepa
Cefotaxime	Floxuridine	Mesna	Ticarcillin
Cefoxitin	Fludarabine	Metoclopramide	Ticarcillin/clavulanate
Ceftazidime	Gallium nitrate	Miconazole	TPN
Ceftizoxime	Gemcitabine	Mitomycin	Vancomycin
Cefuroxime	Gentamicin	Mitoxantrone	Vinblastine
Chlorpromazine	Haloperidol	Paclitaxel	Vincristine
Cimetidine	Heparin	Pentostatin	Vinorelbine

Incompatible:

Acyclovir	Ampicillin/sulbactam	Ganciclovir	Sargramostim
Allopurinol	Amsacrine	Lorazepam	Sodium bicarbonate
Aminophylline	Cefepime	Methylprednisolone	
Amphotericin	Cefoperazone	Mezlocillin	
Ampicillin	Furosemide	Piperacillin	

Variable Compatibility:

Fluorouracil

Paclitaxel

Compatible:

NS

Y-Site Compatible:

Acyclovir	Dacarbazine	Haloperidol	Morphine
Amikacin	Dexamethasone	Heparin	Nalbuphine
Aminophylline	Diphenhydramine	Hydrocortisone sodium	Ondansetron
Ampicillin/sulbactam	Doxorubicin	phosphate	Pentostatin
Bleomycin	Droperidol	Hydrocortisone sodium suc-	Potassium chloride
Butorphanol	Etoposide	cinate	Prochlorperazine
Calcium chloride	Famotidine	Hydromorphone	Propofol
Carboplatin	Floxuridine	Ifosfamide	Ranitidine
Cefepime	Fluconazole	Lorazepam	Sodium bicarbonate
Cefotetan	Fluorouracil	Magnesium sulfate	Thiotepa
Ceftazidime	Furosemide	Mannitol	TPN
Cefuroxime	Ganciclovir	Meperidine	Vancomycin
Cimetidine	Gemcitabine	Mesna	Vinblastine
Cyclophosphamide	Gentamicin	Methotrexate	Vincristine
Cytarabine	Granisetron	Metoclopramide	

Incompatible:

Amphotericin	Doxorubicin, liposomal	Methylprednisolone
Chlorpromazine	Hydroxyzine	Mitoxantrone

Variable Compatibility:

D$_5$W   Cisplatin

Pentostatin

Compatible:

NS   LR

Y-Site Compatible:

Fludarabine   Ondansetron   Paclitaxel   Sargramostim

Variable Compatibility:

D$_5$W

Phytonadione

Compatible:

Amikacin	Chloramphenicol	Doxapram
Calcium glucepate	Cimetidine	Sodium bicarbonate
Cefapirin	Netilmicin	TPN

Y-Site Compatible:

Ampicillin	Heparin	Potassium chloride
Epinephrine	Hydrocortisone sodium suc-	Tolazoline
Famotidine	cinate	Vitamin B complex with C

Incompatible:

Dobutamine	Ranitidine

Plicamycin

Compatible:

D_5W	NS	SWI	Piperacillin

Y-Site Compatible:

Allopurinol	Aztreonam	Gemcitabine	Teniposide
Amifostine	Filgrastim	Piperacillin/tazobactam	Vinorelbine

Incompatible:

Cefonicid

Prochlorperazine

Compatible:

Amikacin	Dimenhydrinate	Lidocaine	Vitamin B complex with C
Ascorbic acid	Erythromycin	Nafcillin	
Dexamethasone	Ethacrinate	Sodium bicarbonate	

Y-Site Compatible:

Amsacrine	Fluconazole	Methotrexate	Sufentanil
Cisplatin	Heparin	Ondansetron	Teniposide
Cyclophosphamide	Hydrocortisone sodium suc-	Paclitaxel	Thiotepa
Cytarabine	cinate	Potassium chloride	Vinorelbine
Doxorubicin	Melphalan	Sargramostim	

Incompatible:

Aldesleukin	Aztreonam	Fludarabine	Methohexital
Allopurinol	Calcium glucepte	Foscarnet	Penicillin G sodium
Amifostine	Cefepime	Filgrastim	Piperacillin/tazobactam
Aminophylline	Cephalothin	Furosemide	Phenobarbital
Amphotericin	Chloramphenicol	Gallium nitrate	Thiopental
Ampicillin	Floxacillin	Gemcitabine	

Variable Compatibility:

Calcium gluconate	Penicillin G potassium

Promethazine

Compatible:

Amikacin	Chloroquine	Vitamin B complex with C
Ascorbic acid	Netilmicin	

Y-Site Compatible:

Amifostine	Cyclophosphamide	Fludarabine	Teniposide
Amsacrine	Cytarabine	Gemcitabine	Thiotepa
Aztreonam	Doxorubicin	Melphalan	Vinorelbine
Ciprofloxacin	Filgrastim	Ondansetron	
Cisplatin	Fluconazole	Sargramostim	

Incompatible:

Aldesleukin	Ceftizoxime	Heparin	Penicillin G (sodium and
Allopurinol	Chloramphenicol	Hydrocortisone sodium suc-	potassium)
Aminophylline	Chlorothiazide	cinate	Pentobarbital
Cefepime	Floxacillin	Methicillin	Piperacillin/tazobactam
Cefoperazone	Foscarnet	Methohexital	Thiopental
Cefotetan	Furosemide	Methotrexate	

Variable Compatibility:

Potassium chloride

Sargramostim

Compatible:

BWI	D_5W	NS	SWI

Y-Site Compatible:

Allopurinol	Cefazolin	Cotrimoxazole	Doxorubicin
Amikacin	Cefepime	Cyclophosphamide	Doxycycline
Aminophylline	Cefotetan	Cyclosporine	Droperidol
Aztreonam	Cefoxitin	Cytarabine	Etoposide
Bleomycin	Ceftizoxime	Dacarbazine	Famotidine
Butorphanol	Ceftriaxone	Dactinomycin	Fentanyl
Calcium gluconate	Cefuroxime	Dexamethasone	Floxuridine
Carboplatin	Cimetidine	Diphenhydramine	Fluconazole
Carmustine	Cisplatin	Dobutamine	Fluorouracil

Furosemide
Gentamicin
Heparin
Human immune globulin
Idarubicin
Ifosfamide
Magnesium sulfate
Mannitol

Mechlorethamine
Meperidine
Mesna
Methotrexate
Metoclopramide
Metronidazole
Mezlocillin
Miconazole

Minocycline
Mitoxantrone
Netilmicin
Pentostatin
Piperacillin/tazobactam
Potassium chloride
Prochlorperazine
Promethazine

Ranitidine
Teniposide
Ticarcillin
Ticarcillin/clavulanate
Vinblastine
Vincristine

Incompatible:

Acyclovir
Ampicillin
Ampicillin/sulbactam
Cefonicid
Cefoperazone
Chlorpromazine

Ganciclovir
Haloperidol
Hydrocortisone sodium
  phosphate
Hydrocortisone sodium suc-
  cinate

Hydromorphone
Hydroxyzine
Imipenem/cilastatin
Methylprednisolone
Mitomycin
Morphine

Nalbuphine
Ondansetron
Piperacillin
Sodium bicarbonate
Tobramycin

Variable Compatibility:

Amphotericin

Amsacrine

Ceftazidime

Vancomycin

Streptozocin

Compatible:

D$_5$W

NS

SWI

Y-Site Compatible:

Filgrastim
Gemcitabine

Granisetron
Ondansetron

Teniposide
Thiotepa

Vinorelbine

Incompatible:

Allopurinol
Aztreonam

Cefepime
Piperacillin

Piperacillin/tazobactam

Teniposide

Compatible:

D$_5$W

NS

LR

Y-Site Compatible:

Acyclovir
Allopurinol
Amifostine
Amikacin
Aminophylline
Amphotericin
Ampicillin
Ampicillin/sulbactam
Aztreonam
Bleomycin
Bumetanide
Buprenorphine
Butorphanol
Calcium gluconate
Carboplatin
Carmustine
Cefazolin
Cefonicid
Cefoperazone
Cefotaxime
Cefotetan
Cefoxitin
Ceftazidime
Ceftizoxime
Ceftriaxone

Cefuroxime
Chlorpromazine
Cimetidine
Cisplatin
Corticotropin
Cotrimoxazole
Cyclophosphamide
Cytarabine
Dacarbazine
Dactinomycin
Daunomycin
Dexamethasone
Diphenhydramine
Doxorubicin
Doxycycline
Droperidol
Enalaprilat
Etoposide
Famotidine
Floxuridine
Fluconazole
Fludarabine
Fluorouracil
Furosemide
Gallium nitrate

Ganciclovir
Gemcitabine
Gentamicin
Haloperidol
Heparin
Hydrocortisone sodium
  phosphate
Hydrocortisone sodium suc-
  cinate
Hydromorphone
Hydroxyzine
Ifosfamide
Imipenem/cilastatin
Leucovorin
Lorazepam
Mannitol
Mechlorethamine
Meperidine
Mesna
Methotrexate
Methylprednisolone
Metoclopramide
Metronidazole
Mezlocillin
Miconazole

Midazolam
Mitomycin
Mitoxantrone
Morphine
Nalbuphine
Netilmicin
Ondansetron
Piperacillin
Plicamycin
Potassium chloride
Prochlorperazine
Promethazine
Ranitidine
Sargramostim
Sodium bicarbonate
Streptozocin
Thiotepa
Ticarcillin
Ticarcillin/clavulanate
Tobramycin
Vancomycin
Vinblastine
Vincristine
Vinorelbine

Incompatible:

Idarubicin

Thiethylperazine

Compatible:

NS
Butorphanol

Hydromorphone
Midazolam

Ranitidine

Y-Site Compatible:

Aldesleukin

◀ Incompatible:

Ketorolac   Perphenazine

Variable Compatibility:

Nalbuphine

Thiotepa

Compatible:

NS   SWI

Y-Site Compatible:

Acyclovir	Cefuroxime	Ganciclovir	Miconazole
Allopurinol	Chlorpromazine	Gemcitabine	Mitomycin
Amifostine	Cimetidine	Gentamicin	Mitoxantrone
Amikacin	Ciprofloxacin	Granisetron	Morphine
Aminophylline	Cotrimoxazole	Haloperidol	Nalbuphine
Amphotericin	Cyclophosphamide	Heparin	Netilmicin
Ampicillin	Cytarabine	Hydrocortisone sodium	Ofloxacin
Ampicillin/sulbactam	Dacarbazine	phosphate	Ondansetron
Aztreonam	Dactinomycin	Hydrocortisone sodium suc-	Paclitaxel
Bleomycin	Daunomycin	cinate	Piperacillin
Bumetanide	Dexamethasone	Hydromorphone	Piperacillin/tazobactam
Buprenorphine	Diphenhydramine	Hydroxyzine	Plicamycin
Butorphanol	Dobutamine	Idarubicin	Potassium chloride
Calcium gluconate	Dopamine	Ifosfamide	Prochlorperazine
Carboplatin	Doxorubicin	Imipenem/cilastatin	Promethazine
Carmustine	Doxycycline	Leucovorin	Ranitidine
Cefazolin	Droperidol	Lorazepam	Sodium bicarbonate
Cefepime	Enalaprilat	Magnesium sulfate	Streptozocin
Cefonicid	Etoposide	Mannitol	Teniposide
Cefoperazone	Famotidine	Meperidine	Ticarcillin
Cefotaxime	Floxuridine	Mesna	Ticarcillin/clavulanate
Cefotetan	Fluconazole	Methotrexate	Tobramycin
Cefoxitin	Fludarabine	Methylprednisolone	TPN
Ceftazidime	Fluorouracil	Metoclopramide	Vancomycin
Ceftizoxime	Furosemide	Metronidazole	Vinblastine
Ceftriaxone	Gallium nitrate	Mezlocillin	Vincristine

Incompatible:

Cisplatin   Filgrastim   Minocycline

Topotecan

Compatible:

D_5W NS   LR

Y-Site Compatible:

Gemcitabine

Trimetrexate

Compatible:

D_5W

Y-Site Compatible:

Amifostine

Incompatible:

BNS	$D_5/^{1/2}NS$	NS	Chloride ion
D_5/NS	D_5/LR	LR	Leucovorin
$D_5/^{1/4}NS$	D_{10}/NS	Calcium chloride	Potassium chloride

Vinblastine

Compatible:

BNS	NS	Bleomycin
D_5W	LR	Dacarbazine

Y-Site Compatible:

Allopurinol	Droperidol	Methotrexate	Piperacillin/tazobactam
Amifostine	Filgrastim	Metoclopramide	Sargramostim
Aztreonam	Fludarabine	Mitomycin	Teniposide
Cisplatin	Fluorouracil	Ondansetron	Vincristine
Cyclophosphamide	Gemcitabine	Paclitaxel	Vinorelbine
Doxorubicin, liposomal	Leucovorin	Piperacillin	

Incompatible:

| Cefazolin | Furosemide |

Variable Compatibility:

| Doxorubicin | Heparin |

Vincristine

Compatible:

| D_5W | LR | Cytarabine | Fluorouracil |
| NS | Bleomycin | Doxorubicin | Methotrexate |

Y-Site Compatible:

Allopurinol	Doxorubicin, liposomal	Heparin	Piperacillin/tazobactam
Amifostine	Droperidol	Leucovorin	Sargramostim
Aztreonam	Filgrastim	Metoclopramide	Teniposide
Cisplatin	Fludarabine	Mitomycin	Vinblastine
Cyclophosphamide	Gemcitabine	Ondansetron	Vinorelbine
Doxapram	Granisetron	Paclitaxel	

Incompatible:

| Cefepime | Furosemide | Idarubicin | Sodium bicarbonate |

Vinorelbine

Compatible:

| D_5W | $D_5/^1/_2NS$ | NS | LR |

Y-Site Compatible:

Amikacin	Dactinomycin	Haloperidol	Metronidazole
Aztreonam	Daunomycin	Heparin	Minocycline
Bleomycin	Dexamethasone	Hydrocortisone sodium phosphate	Mitoxantrone
Bumetanide	Diphenhydramine		Morphine
Buprenorphine	Doxorubicin	Hydrocortisone sodium succinate	Nalbuphine
Butorphanol	Doxorubicin, liposomal		Netilmicin
Calcium gluconate	Doxycycline	Hydromorphone	Ondansetron
Carboplatin	Droperidol	Hydroxyzine	Plicamycin
Carmustine	Enalaprilat	Idarubicin	Streptozocin
Cefotaxime	Etoposide	Ifosfamide	Teniposide
Ceftazidime	Famotidine	Imipenem/cilastatin	Ticarcillin
Ceftizoxime	Filgrastim	Lorazepam	Ticarcillin/clavulanate
Chlorpromazine	Fluconazole	Mannitol	Tobramycin
Cimetidine	Fludarabine	Mechlorethamine	Vinblastine
Cisplatin	Fluorouracil	Meperidine	Vincristine
Cyclophosphamide	Gallium nitrate	Mesna	Vindesine
Cytarabine	Gemcitabine	Methotrexate	
Dacarbazine	Gentamicin	Metoclopramide	

Incompatible:

Acyclovir	Cefazolin	Cotrimoxazole	Mitomycin
Allopurinol	Cefoperazone	Fluorouracil	Sodium bicarbonate
Aminophylline	Cefotetan	Furosemide	Thiotepa
Amphotericin	Ceftriaxone	Ganciclovir	
Ampicillin	Cefuroxime	Methylprednisolone	

Drug	Variable Compatibility
Carboplatin	Solutions in saline are less stable than in dextrose.
Carmustine	Solutions should be dispensed in glass and protected from light. Solutions are stable for <8 hours under most circumstances.
Cisplatin	Must have a chloride concentration of at least 0.2% in the final solution. The commercial product has a NS concentration. Etoposide + mannitol + potassium chloride in normal saline precipitates within 24 hours; when in D_5/ $^1/_2$NS, it is stable for 24 hours.
Dacarbazine	Heparin 100 units/mL with dacarbazine 25 mg/mL is **incompatible**. Heparin 100 units/mL with dacarbazine 10 mg/mL is **compatible**.
Filgrastim	Gentamicin is reported to be physically **compatible** for Y-site injection, but with a decrease in biologic activity. Imipenem/cilastatin with filgrastim 40 mcg/mL is reported to be physically **compatible** for Y-site injection, but with a decrease in biologic activity.
Fluorouracil	Doxorubicin 2 mg/mL with fluorouracil 50 mg/mL is **compatible** for 13 minutes. Doxorubicin 0.5-1 mg/mL with fluorouracil 50 mg/mL is **incompatible**. Fluorouracil with doxorubicin is **Y-site compatible**. Variable compatibility with leucovorin.
Mesna	**Compatible** with ifosfamide. **Incompatible** with ifosfamide and epinephrine.
Leucovorin	Variable compatibility with fluorouracil.
Mitomycin	Mitomycin 50 mg/L in NS has a color change and 10% loss of drug concentration in 12 hours. Mitomycin 1 g/L in SWI precipitates in 24 hours under refrigeration. Other temperatures and concentrations are reported to be stable. Mitomycin in D_5W is **incompatible** in 20 mg/L; **compatible** in 40 mg/L. Mitomycin 500 mg/L with heparin 33,300 units/L in NS is **compatible**. PVC containers of mitomycin 167 mg/L with heparin 33,300 units/L in NS is **compatible**. Glass containers of mitomycin 167 mg/L with heparin 33,300 units/L in NS are **incompatible**.
Pentostatin	Pentostatin 20 mg/mL in D_5W at room temperature: a 2% loss of drug in 24 hours; 8% to 10% loss in 48 hours; and a 10% loss in 54 hours. Under refrigeration, there is no loss in 96 hours. There is a 10% loss in 23 hours at room temperature of pentostatin 2 mg/mL in D_5W
Sargramostim	Amphotericin B 0.6 mg/mL in D_5W with sargramostim 10 mcg/mL in NS forms immediate precipitate. Amphotericin B 0.6 mg/mL in D_5W with sargramostim 10 mcg/mL in D_5W is **Y-site compatible**. Amsacrine with sargramostim in NS forms immediate precipitate. Amsacrine with sargramostim in D_5W is **Y-site compatible**. Ceftazidime 40 mg/mL in NS with sargramostim 10 mcg/mL in NS is **incompatible**, with particle formation within 4 hours. Ceftazidime 40 mg/mL with sargramostim 6 or 15 mcg/mL is **compatible** for 2 hours (Y-site **compatible**). Vancomycin 20 mg/mL and sargramostim 6 mcg/mL is **incompatible**. Vancomycin 10 mg/mL and sargramostim 10 mcg/mL is **Y-site compatible**. Vancomycin 20 mg/mL and sargramostim 15 mcg/mL is **Y-site compatible**.
Vancomycin	Vancomycin 5 mg/mL with methotrexate 30 mg/mL is **compatible** for 2 hours, precipitates within 4 hours. Other concentrations tested were **compatible** for 1 hour. Vancomycin with methotrexate is **Y-site compatible**.
Vinblastine	In various volumes, doxorubicin 2 mg/mL with vinblastine 1 mg/mL yields erratic assay results. Vinblastine with doxorubicin is **Y-site compatible**. Heparin 200 units/mL with vinblastine 1 mg/mL is **incompatible** in a syringe for 13 minutes. Heparin 500 units/mL with vinblastine 0.5 mg/mL is **compatible** in a syringe for 13 minutes.

Suggested Readings

Hall PD, Yui D, Lyons S, et al, "Compatibility of Filgrastim With Selected Antimicrobial Drugs During Simulated Y-Site Administration," *Am J Health Syst Pharm*, 1997, 54(2):184-9.

McGuire TR, Narducci WA, and Fox JL, "Compatibility and Stability of Ondansetron Hydrochloride, Dexamethasone and Lorazepam in Injectable Solutions," *Am J Health Syst Pharm*, 1993, 50(7):1410-4.

Najari Z and Rucho WJ, "Compatibility of Commonly Used Bone Marrow Drugs During Y-Site Delivery," *Am J Health Syst Pharm*, 1997, 54(2):181-4.

Trissel LA, Chandler SW, and Folstad JT, "Visual Compatibility of Amsacrine With Selected Drugs During Simulated Y-Site Injection," *Am J Hospital Pharm*, 1990, 47(11):2525-8.

Trissel LA, Bready BB, Kwan JW, et al, "Visual Compatibility of Sargramostim With Selected Antineoplastic Agents, Anti-infectives, or Other Drugs During Simulated Y-Site Injection," *Am J Hospital Pharm*, 1992, 49(2):402-6.

Trissel LA and Martinez JF, "Physical Compatibility of Melphalan With Selected Drugs During Simulated Y-Site Administration," *Am J Hospital Pharm*, 1993, 50(11):2359-63.

Trissel LA and Martinez JF, "Visual, Turbidimetric, and Particle-Content Assessment of Compatibility of Vinorelbine Tartrate With Selected Drugs During Simulated Y-Site Injection," *Am J Hospital Pharm*, 1994, 51(4):495-9.

Trissel LA and Martinez JF, "Physical Compatibility of Allopurinol Sodium With Selected Drugs During Simulated Y-Site Administration," *Am J Hospital Pharm*, 1994, 51(14):1792-9.

Trissel LA and Martinez JF, "Compatibility of Filgrastim With Selected Drugs During Simulated Y-Site Administration," *Am J Hospital Pharm*, 1994, 51(15):1907-13.

Trissel LA and Martinez JF, "Screening Teniposide For Y-Site Compatibility," *Hospital Pharm*, 1994, 29:1010, 1012-4, 1017.

Trissel LA, *Handbook on Injectable Drugs*, 9th Ed. Bethesda, MD: *Am Society Health-Systems Pharmacists*, 1996.

Trissel LA, *Supplement to Handbook on Injectable Drugs*, 9th Ed. Bethesda, MD: *Am Society of Health-Systems Pharmacists*, 1997.

Trissel LA, Gilbert DL, and Martinez JF, "Compatibility of Granisetron Hydrochloride With Selected Drugs During Simulated Y-Site Administration," *Am J Health Syst Pharm*, 1997, 54(1):56-60.

Trissel LA, Gilbert DL, and Martinez JF, "Compatibility of Propofol With Selected Drugs During Simulated Y-Site Administration," *Am J Health Syst Pharm*, 1997, 54(11):1287-92.

Trissel LA, Gilbert DL, Martinez JF, et al, "Compatibility of Parenteral Nutrient Solutions With Selected Drugs During Simulated Y-Site Administration," *Am J Health Syst Pharm*, 1997, 54(11):1295-300.

Trissel LA, Gilbert DL, and Martinez JF, "Compatibility of Doxorubicin Hydrochloride Liposome With Selected Other Drugs During Simulated Y-Site Administration," *Am J Health Syst Pharm*, 1997; 54(23):2708-13.

Trissel LA, Martinez JF, and Gilbert DL, "Compatibility of Gemcitabine Hydrochloride With 107 Selected Drugs During Simulated Y-Site Administration," *J Am Pharm Assoc*, 1999, 39(4):514-18.

Zhang Y, Xu QA, Trissel LA, et al, "Compatibility and Stability of Paclitaxel Combined With Cisplatin and With Carboplatin in Infusion Solutions," *Ann Pharmacother*, 1997, 31(12):1465-70.

TUMOR LYSIS SYNDROME

INTRODUCTION

Tumor lysis syndrome (TLS) is a potentially life threatening disorder that is characterized as an acute metabolic disturbance resulting from the rapid destruction of tumor cells. Cellular destruction releases cellular breakdown products (nucleic acids, anions, cations, peptides) that overwhelm the body's normal mechanisms for their utilization, excretion, and elimination. Signs and symptoms of TLS often develop within 72 hours of beginning cytotoxic chemotherapy in patients with newly diagnosed acute leukemias (acute lymphoblastic leukemia [ALL] and acute myeloid leukemia [AML]) or lymphoproliferative malignancies (Burkitt's and non-Burkitt's lymphomas). However, TLS can occur spontaneously in malignant diseases with vigorous cell turnover. Although most commonly reported in patients with hematologic and lymphoid malignancies, TLS has also been reported with solid tumors such as breast cancer, colon cancer, melanoma, ovarian cancer, prostate cancer, small cell lung cancer, and testicular cancer. Acute TLS attributed to administration of a corticosteroid, rituximab, and zoledronic acid in patients with treatment-sensitive tumors have been reported in the medical literature. Additional treatment and diagnostic procedures attributed with causing tumor lysis syndrome include total body irradiation, splenic irradiation, staging laparotomy, laparoscopic splenectomy preceded by splenic artery embolization, and radiofrequency interstitial thermal ablation of metastatic hepatic lesions. Metabolic abnormalities associated with acute TLS include hyperphosphatemia, hyperkalemia, hyperuricemia, azotemia, hypocalcemia, and metabolic acidosis. Cardiac arrhythmias, seizures, and major organ failure can occur in severe cases of TLS. Hyperkalemia, hyperuricemia, and hypocalcemia can produce cardiac arrhythmias, tetany, and sudden death. Acute renal failure can occur due to precipitation of uric acid and calcium phosphate in the renal tubules.

PREDISPOSING FACTORS

1. Bulky disease (>10 cm); leukemia with high white blood cell count (>25,000/mm^3)
2. Acute myeloid leukemia with history of chronic myelomonocytic leukemia
3. Marked sensitivity of the tumor to a particular treatment modality
4. Male gender
5. Renal impairment, including pre-existing volume depletion
6. Elevated pretreatment lactic dehydrogenase serum levels (>2 times ULN)
7. Elevated pretreatment uric acid serum levels (>7.5 mg/dL) independent of renal impairment

CLINICAL FEATURES AND TREATMENT

Classification and Risk Stratification

TLS can be described as either laboratory (LTLS) or clinical (CTLS) type. LTLS is the presence of 2 or more abnormal lab values or a 25% change in lab values within 3 days before or 7 days after chemotherapy. Laboratory values to monitor include uric acid, potassium, phosphorus, and calcium. CTLS is defined as LTLS with at least one clinical manifestation such as renal insufficiency, seizures, cardiac arrhythmias, or sudden death.

Certain patients have higher risk for developing LTLS and/or CTLS and should be treated more aggressively to prevent its occurrence. Risk stratification guides what type of prophylaxis and management therapies should be used for which patients. Patients classified as high risk should have aggressive prophylactic treatment with hydration and rasburicase while being monitored closely in an ICU or monitored setting. Intermediate risk patients should receive prophylactic treatment with hydration and allopurinol; if hyperuricemia does develop in these patients, consider rasburicase. Initial management of pediatric patients at intermediate risk may include rasburicase. Patients at low risk for developing TLS require no prophylactic therapy but should be monitored closely and treated as necessary.

Risk Stratification

Type of Cancer	High Risk	Intermediate Risk	Low Risk
Non-Hodgkin's lymphoma (NHL)	Burkitt's, Burkitt's-ALL (B-ALL), lymphoblastic lymphoma	Diffuse large B-cell lymphoma (DLBCL)	Indolent NHL
Acute lymphoblastic leukemia (ALL)	WBC ≥100,000 cells/mm^3	WBC 50,000-100,000 cells/mm^3	WBC ≤50,000 cells/mm^3
Acute myeloid leukemia (AML)	WBC ≥50,000 cells/mm^3; monoblastic	WBC 10,000-50,000 cells/mm^3	WBC ≤10,000 cells/mm^3
Chronic lymphocytic leukemia (CLL)		WBC 10,000-100,000 cells/mm^3; treatment with fludarabine	WBC ≤10,000 cells/mm^3
Other hematologic malignancies (chronic myeloid leukemia [CML], multiple myeloma) and solid tumors		Rapid proliferation with expected rapid response to therapy	Remainder of patients

Monitoring

High risk patients should have laboratory and clinical parameters (serum uric acid, phosphate, calcium, creatinine, LDH, and fluid input and output) monitored 4-6 hours after initiating chemotherapy. For all patients treated with rasburicase, monitor serum uric acid 4 hours after administration, then every 6-8 hours thereafter until resolution of TLS occurs.

Intermediate risk patients should be monitored for at least 24 hours after completion of chemotherapy. If rasburicase is not used, laboratory parameters should be monitored 8 hours after initiation of chemotherapy.

Low risk patients should be monitored as determined by the institution and patient factors. If TLS has not occurred within 2 days, its development is very unlikely.

General Principles

Prevention and early management of TLS are aimed at decreasing the risk of morbidity and mortality from cardiac arrhythmias, seizures, and organ failure. In patients with high or intermediate risk, vigorous hydration is the cornerstone of the initial management for acute or potential TLS. Patients should be hydrated with 2-3 L/m^2/day (200 mL/kg/day if ≤10 kg) intravenous fluid (Children: $D_5W^{1/4}NS$; Adults: Not specified) to maintain urine output of 80-100 mL/m^2/hour (4-6 mL/kg/hour if ≤10 kg), with diuretic use if necessary (avoid diuretic use in patients with hypovolemia or obstructive uropathy). Due to the tendency for calcium phosphate nephrocalcinosis and the potential for metabolic alkalosis, urinary alkalinization with sodium bicarbonate is no longer recommended for the treatment and prevention of TLS (Coiffier, 2008).

Allopurinol should be administered in intermediate risk patients to decrease endogenous uric acid production and to reduce associated urinary obstruction; dose reductions may be required for renal dysfunction (Coiffier, 2008). In adult or pediatric patients, give 150-300 mg/m^2/day (or 10 mg/kg/day in pediatric patients) divided every 8 hours (maximum 800 mg/day) orally or 200-400 mg/m^2/day I.V. (in 1-3 divided doses; maximum 600 mg/day). While allopurinol decreases uric acid production, it is ineffective in reducing high uric acid levels. This may result in urinary xanthine crystal precipitation which could lead to obstruction, and interact with purine based drug therapy, such as mercaptopurine.

Rasburicase is administered for rapid reduction of uric acid levels. Rasburicase, which is a recombinant form of urate oxidase produced in *Saccharomyces cerevisiae*, catalyzes the degradation of uric acid to allantoin which is more soluble and readily excreted by the kidneys. Rasburicase is reserved for patients at high risk for TLS (or considered in intermediate risk pediatric patients), patients with elevated uric acid levels, or patients with signs of moderate-to-severe renal impairment or other major organ dysfunction. The major risks associated with administration of rasburicase include anaphylaxis, hypersensitivity reactions, methemoglobinemia, and hemolysis. This product is contraindicated in patients with glucose-6-phosphate dehydrogenase deficiency due to an elevated risk of hemolysis. An additional concern with rasburicase administration is the development of neutralizing antibodies. This phenomenon was observed in 64% of 28 normal, healthy volunteers studied; the effect of neutralizing antibodies on the efficacy of this product with repeated usage is unknown.

Rasburicase is approved for use in pediatric and adult patients, with the labeled dose of 0.2 mg/kg/dose daily for up to five days. Due to the costs and risks of therapy plus the immediate and measurable effects of rasburicase, some centers administer a single dose which is repeated daily as warranted by plasma uric acid levels. The following dose levels (based on risk for TLS) with duration of treatment based on plasma uric acid levels have been recommended for children: 0.2 mg/kg once daily (duration based on plasma uric acid levels) for high risk patients, 0.15 mg/kg once daily (duration based on plasma uric acid levels) for intermediate risk, and 0.05-0.1 mg/kg once daily (duration based on clinical judgment) if used for low-risk patients (Coiffier, 2008). Weight- and risk-based dosing as detailed above has been reported in adults. Fixed-dose rasburicase, ranging from 3-7.5 mg as a single dose (Hutcherson, 2006; McDonnell, 2006; Reeves, 2008; Trifilio, 2006) with doses (1.5-6 mg) repeated if needed (based on serum uric acid levels) has also been reported in adults.

Rasburicase will degrade uric acid *in vitro* when stored at room temperature. Consequently, to prevent artifactually low uric acid levels, plasma samples must be collected in prechilled tubes, then immediately placed in an ice water bath until centrifuged at 4°C. Plasma must be analyzed within four hours of collection.

Clinical features and treatment for specific metabolic disorders are discussed in the following sections.

Hyperuricemia

Cytolysis during TLS releases purine and pyrimidine nucleotides into the bloodstream and extracellular tissues. Oxidation of the purines hypoxanthine and xanthine yields uric acid, which can precipitate in the renal tubules and cause oliguric renal failure. A high concentration of uric acid and an acidic urine pH promote uric acid crystallization and renotubular precipitation. Maintenance of urine flow is utilized to reduce purine precipitation and preserve renal function. Allopurinol blocks the endogenous production of uric acid by inhibiting the enzyme xanthine oxidase, which oxidizes hypoxanthine and xanthine to uric acid. Allopurinol is used prophylactically during the early management of TLS in intermediate risk patients. Rasburicase decreases existing uric acid concentrations by conversion of this molecule to the inactive and soluble metabolite allantoin, which is readily excreted by the kidneys. Rasburicase should be used prophylactically in high risk patients and in patients with pre-existing hyperuricemia.

Hyperkalemia

Potassium is primarily an intracellular ion that is released during massive cellular breakdown. Increasing levels of serum potassium can be dangerous, leading to cardiac arrhythmias or sudden death, especially in the presence of hypocalcemia (see following discussion). Standard treatments to remove potassium from the blood stream and extracellular fluids should be initiated as warranted by the patient's serum potassium level and electrocardiographic abnormalities. Other sources of potassium intake (including nutritional sources, medications, and intravenous solutions) should be eliminated in patients at risk for or with TLS. Pharmaceutical measures routinely used to manage hyperkalemia in patients with TLS include volume expansion with forced diuresis, administration of glucose with insulin, and the cation exchange product sodium polystyrene sulfonate. Sodium bicarbonate can be administered I.V. push to induce influx of potassium into cells. Textbook algorithms for management of hyperkalemia include instructions for administration of calcium as a cardioprotective measure; however this is **not** a standard intervention in the setting of TLS. Calcium gluconate administration must be done judiciously in the patient with TLS because it can precipitate as calcium phosphate in highly perfused tissues. Monitor patient ECG and cardiac rhythm closely for arrhythmias.

Hyperphosphatemia

The release of intracellular inorganic phosphate following massive cellular breakdown sets into motion several important clinical features. Serum phosphate levels will quickly exceed the threshold for normal renal excretion, with phosphate excretion becoming limited by the glomerular filtration rate. Any azotemia that develops during therapy will hinder phosphate excretion. Treatment includes the use of phosphate binders such as aluminum hydroxide, sevelamer, calcium carbonate (avoid use in patients with hypercalcemia), or lanthanum carbonate (avoid use in children). In severe cases of hyperphosphatemia, hemodialysis or hemofiltration, may be necessary.

Hypocalcemia

High phosphate levels will also cause reciprocal hypocalcemia. Although generally asymptomatic, hypocalcemia may cause neuromuscular irritation, tetany, and cardiac dysrhythmias. Symptomatic patients may receive calcium gluconate intravenously (slowly, with ECG monitoring) to increase serum calcium levels. Unfortunately, despite hypocalcemia, the solubility product of calcium and phosphate may be exceeded in acute TLS due to high levels of phosphate, resulting in tissue calcification and organ failure. For this reason, calcium gluconate should be administered cautiously and only if necessary.

Hemodialysis / Hemofiltration

Due to the unpredictability of TLS, renal replacement therapy may be needed and can be lifesaving. Hemodialysis or hemofiltration may be used to control and maintain fluid volume and/or to remove uric acid, phosphate, and potassium from serum. Intermittent hemodialysis, continuous arteriovenous hemodialysis, or continuous veno-venous hemodiafiltration should be considered as warranted by the severity of serum chemistry abnormalities, major organ dysfunction, and the patient's response to pharmaceutical treatments.

Selected Readings

Agha-Razii M, Amyot SL, Pichette V, et al, "Continuous Veno-Venous Hemodiafiltration for the Treatment of Spontaneous Tumor Lysis Syndrome Complicated by Acute Renal Failure and Severe Hyperuricemia," *Clin Nephrol*, 2000, 54(1):59-63.

Arnold TM, Reuter JP, Delman BS, et al, "Use of Single-Dose Rasburicase in an Obese Female," *Ann Pharmacother*, 2004, 38(9):1428-31.

Barry BD, Kell MR, and Redmond HP, "Tumor Lysis Syndrome Following Endoscopic Radiofrequency Interstitial Thermal Ablation of Colorectal Liver Metastases," *Surg Endosc*, 2002, 16(7):1109.

Cairo MS and Bishop M, "Tumour Lysis Syndrome: New Therapeutic Strategies and Classification," *Br J Haematol*, 2004, 127(1):3-11.

Chen SW, Hwang WS, Tsao CJ, et al, "Hydroxyurea and Splenic Irradiation-Induced Tumour Lysis Syndrome: A Case Report and Review of the Literature," *J Clin Pharm Ther*, 2005, 30(6):623-5.

Coiffier B, Altman A, Pui CH, et al, "Guidelines for the Management of Pediatric and Adult Tumor Lysis Syndrome: An Evidence-Based Review," *J Clin Oncol*, 2008, 26(16):2767-78.

Coiffier B, Mounier N, Bologna S, et al, "Efficacy and Safety of Rasburicase (Recombinant Urate Oxidase) for the Prevention and Treatment of Hyperuricemia During Induction Chemotherapy of Aggressive Non-Hodgkin's Lymphoma: Results of the GRAAL1 (Groupe d'Etude Des Lymphomes De l'Adulte Trial on Rasburicase Activity in Adult Lymphoma) Study," *J Clin Oncol*, 2003, 21(23):4402-6.

Duzova A, Cetin M, Gümrük F, et al, "Acute Tumour Lysis Syndrome Following a Single-Dose Corticosteroid in Children With Acute Lymphoblastic Leukaemia," *Eur J Haematol*, 2001, 66(6):404-7.

Gemici C, "Tumour Lysis Syndrome in Solid Tumours," *Clin Oncol (R Coll Radiol)*, 2006, 18(10):773-80.

Habib GS and Saliba WR, "Tumor Lysis Syndrome After Hydrocortisone Treatment in Metastatic Melanoma: A Case Report and Review of the Literature," *Am J Med Sci*, 2002, 323(3):155-7.

Hutcherson DA, Gammon DC, Bhatt MS, et al, "Reduced-Dose Rasburicase in the Treatment of Adults With Hyperuricemia Associated With Malignancy," *Pharmacotherapy*, 2006, 26(2):242-7.

Jabr FI, "Acute Tumor Lysis Syndrome Induced by Rituximab in Diffuse Large B-Cell Lymphoma," *Int J Hematol*, 2005, 82(4):312-4.

Kurt M, Onal IK, Elkiran T, et al, "Acute Tumor Lysis Syndrome Triggered by Zoledronic Acid in a Patient With Metastatic Lung Adenocarcinoma," *Med Oncol*, 2005, 22(2):203-6.

Lee MH, Cheng KI, Jang RC, et al, "Tumour Lysis Syndrome Developing During an Operation," *Anaesthesia*, 2007, 62(1):85-7.

Lee AC, Li CH, So KT, et al, "Treatment of Impending Tumor Lysis With Single-Dose Rasburicase," *Ann Pharmacother*, 2003, 37(11):1614-7.

Leibowitz AB, Adamsky C, Gabrilove J, et al, "Intraoperative Acute Tumor Lysis Syndrome During Laparoscopic Splenectomy Preceded by Splenic Artery Embolization," *Surg Laparosc Endosc Percutan Tech*, 2007, 17(3):210-1.

Lerza R, Botta M, Barsotti B, et al, "Dexamethazone-Induced Acute Tumor Lysis Syndrome in a T-Cell Malignant Lymphoma," *Leuk Lymphoma*, 2002, 43 (5):1129-32.

Linck D, Basara N, Tran V, et al, "Peracute Onset of Severe Tumor Lysis Syndrome Immediately After 4 Gy Fractionated TBI as Part of Reduced Intensity Preparative Regimen in a Patient With T-ALL With High Tumor Burden," *Bone Marrow Transplant*, 2003, 31(10):935-7.

Liu CY, Sims-McCallum RP, and Schiffer CA, "A Single Dose of Rasburicase is Sufficient for the Treatment of Hyperuricemia in Patients Receiving Chemotherapy," *Leuk Res*, 2005, 29(4):463-5.

Mato AR, Riccio BE, Qin L, et al, "A Predictive Model for the Detection of Tumor Lysis Syndrome During AML Induction Therapy," *Leuk Lymphoma*, 2006, 47(5):877-83.

McDonnell AM, Lenz KL, Frei-Lahr DA, et al, "Single-Dose Rasburicase 6 Mg in the Management of Tumor Lysis Syndrome in Adults," *Pharmacotherapy*, 2006, 26(6):806-12.

Oztop I, Demirkan B, Yaren A, et al, "Rapid Tumor Lysis Syndrome in a Patient With Metastatic Colon Cancer as a Complication of Treatment With 5-Fluorouracil/Leucoverin and Irinotecan," *Tumori*, 2004, 90(5):514-6.

Reeves DJ and Bestul DJ, "Evaluation of a Single Fixed Dose of Rasburicase 7.5 mg for the Treatment of Hyperuricemia in Adults With Cancer," *Pharmacotherapy*, 2008; 28(6):685–90.

Riccio B, Mato A, Olson EM, et al, "Spontaneous Tumor Lysis Syndrome in Acute Myeloid Leukemia: Two Cases and a Review of the Literature," *Cancer Biol Ther*, 2006, 5(12):1614-7.

Rostom AY, El-Hussainy G, Kandil A, et al, "Tumor Lysis Syndrome Following Hemi-Body Irradiation for Metastatic Breast Cancer," *Ann Oncol*, 2000, 11 (10):1349-51.

Schelling JR, Ghandour FZ, Strickland TJ, et al, "Management of Tumor Lysis Syndrome With Standard Continuous Arteriovenous Hemodialysis: Case Report and a Review of the Literature," *Ren Fail*, 1998, 20(4):635-44.

Sorscher SM, "Tumor Lysis Syndrome Following Docetaxel Therapy for Extensive Metastatic Prostate Cancer," *Cancer Chemother Pharmacol*, 2004, 54 (2):191-2.

Theodorou D, Lagoudianakis E, Pattas M, et al, "Pretreatment Tumor Lysis Syndrome Associated With Bulky Retroperitoneal Tumors. Recognition is the Mainstay of Therapy," *Tumori*, 2006, 92(6):540-1.

Tiu RV, Mountantonakis SE, Dunbar AJ, et al, "Tumor Lysis Syndrome," *Semin Thromb Hemost*, 2007, 33(4):397-407.

Trifilio S, Gordon L, Singhal S, et al, "Reduced-Dose Rasburicase (Recombinant Xanthine Oxidase) in Adult Cancer Patients With Hyperuricemia," *Bone Marrow Transplant*, 2006, 37(11):997-1001.

Yahata T, Nishikawa N, Aoki Y, et al, "Tumor Lysis Syndrome Associated With Weekly Paclitaxel Treatment in a Case With Ovarian Cancer," *Gynecol Oncol*, 2006, 103(2):752-4.

Yim BT, Sims-McCallum RP, and Chong PH, "Rasburicase for the Treatment and Prevention of Hyperuricemia," *Ann Pharmacother*, 2003, 37 (7-8):1047-54.

Zigrossi P, Brustia M, Bobbio F, et al, "Flare and Tumor Lysis Syndrome With Atypical Features After Letrozole Therapy in Advanced Breast Cancer. A Case Report," *Ann Ital Med Int*, 2001, 16(2):112-7.

ANTITHROMBOTIC THERAPY IN NEONATES AND CHILDREN

Recommendations From the Eighth American College of Chest Physicians (ACCP) Conference on Antithrombotic and Thrombolytic Therapy

Used with permission from Monagle P, Chan A, Massicotte P, et al, "Antithrombotic Therapy in Neonates and Children: American College of Chest Physicians Evidence-Based Clinical Practice Guidelines (8th Edition)," *Chest*, 2008, 133(6 Suppl):887S-968S.

Abbreviations: AIS = arterial ischemic stroke; APLA = antiphospholipid antibodies; aPTT = activated partial thromboplastin time; BCPS = bilateral cavopulmonary shunts; CC = cardiac catheterization; CSVT = cerebral sinovenous thrombosis; CVL = central venous line; DVT = deep venous thrombosis; FXa = factor Xa; ICH = intracranial hemorrhage; INR = international normalized ratio; IVC = inferior vena cava; LMWH = low-molecular-weight heparin; RCT = randomized controlled trial; RVT = renal vein thrombosis; SVT = sinovenous thrombosis; TE = thromboembolism; TIA = transient ischemic attacks; tPA = tissue plasminogen activator; UAC = umbilical arterial catheter; UFH = unfractionated heparin; UVC = umbilical vein catheter; VAD = ventricular assist device; VKA = vitamin K antagonist; VTE = venous thromboembolism

1.1 Neonatal DVT: Central Venous Line and Non-Central Venous Line-Related

1.1.1. ACCP suggests CVLs or umbilical venous catheter (UVCs) associated with confirmed thrombosis be removed, if possible, after 3-5 days of anticoagulation (Grade 2C).

1.1.2. ACCP suggests either initial anticoagulation or supportive care with radiologic monitoring (Grade 2C); however, ACCP recommends subsequent anticoagulation if extension of the thrombosis occurs during supportive care (Grade 1B).

1.1.3. ACCP suggests anticoagulation should be with either: (1) LMWH given twice daily and adjusted to achieve an anti-FXa level of 0.5-1 units/mL; or (2) UFH for 3-5 days adjusted to achieve an anti-FXa of 0.35-0.7 units/mL or a corresponding aPTT range, followed by LMWH. ACCP suggests a total duration of anticoagulation of between 6 weeks and 3 months (Grade 2C).

1.1.4. ACCP suggests that if either a CVL or a UVC is still in place on completion of therapeutic anticoagulation, a prophylactic dose of LMWH be given to prevent recurrent VTE until such time as the CVL or UVC is removed (Grade 2C).

1.1.5. ACCP recommends against thrombolytic therapy for neonatal VTE unless major vessel occlusion is causing critical compromise of organs or limbs (Grade 1B).

1.1.6. ACCP suggests that if thrombolysis is required, the clinician use tissue plasminogen activator (tPA) and supplement with plasminogen (fresh frozen plasma) prior to commencing therapy (Grade 2C).

1.2. DVT in Children: Central Venous Line and Non-Central Venous Line-Related

First TE for children

1.2.1. ACCP recommends anticoagulant therapy with either UFH or LMWH [Grade 1B]. *Remark:* Dosing of I.V. UFH should prolong the aPTT to a range that corresponds to an anti-FXa level of 0.35-0.7 units/mL, whereas LMWH should achieve an anti-FXa level of 0.5-1 units/mL 4 hours after an injection for twice-daily dosing.

1.2.2. ACCP recommends initial treatment with UFH or LMWH for at least 5-10 days (Grade 1B). For patients in whom clinicians will subsequently prescribe VKAs, ACCP recommends beginning oral therapy as early as day 1 and discontinuing UFH/LMWH on day 6 or later than day 6 if the international normalized ratio (INR) has not exceeded 2 (Grade 1B). After the initial 5- to 10-day treatment period, ACCP suggests LMWH rather than VKA therapy if therapeutic levels are difficult to maintain on VKA therapy or if VKA therapy is challenging for the child and family (Grade 2C).

1.2.3. ACCP suggests children with idiopathic thromboembolism (TE) receive anticoagulant therapy for at least 6 months, using VKAs to achieve a target INR of 2.5 (INR range: 2-3), or alternatively using LMWH to maintain an anti-FXa level of 0.5-1 units/mL (Grade 2C). Underlying values and preferences: The suggestion to use anticoagulation therapy to treat idiopathic DVTs in children for at least 6 months rather than on a lifelong basis places a relatively high value on avoiding the inconvenience and bleeding risk associated with antithrombotic therapy and a relative low value on avoiding the unknown risk of recurrence in the absence of an ongoing risk factor.

1.2.4. In children with secondary thrombosis in whom the risk factor has resolved, ACCP suggests anticoagulant therapy be administered for at least 3 months using VKAs to achieve a target INR of 2.5 (INR range: 2-3) or alternatively using LMWH to maintain an anti-FXa level of 0.5-1 units/mL (Grade 2C).

1.2.5. In children who have ongoing but potentially reversible risk factors, such as active nephritic syndrome or ongoing l-asparaginase therapy, ACCP suggests continuing anticoagulant therapy in either therapeutic or prophylactic doses until the risk factor has resolved (Grade 2C).

Recurrent idiopathic TEs in children

1.2.6. For children with recurrent idiopathic thrombosis, ACCP recommends indefinite treatment with VKAs to achieve a target INR of 2.5 (INR range: 2-3) [Grade 1A]. *Remark:* For some patients, long-term LMWH may be preferable; however, there are little or no data about the safety of long-term LMWH in children.

Recurrent secondary TEs in children

1.2.7. For children with recurrent secondary TE with an existing reversible risk factor for thrombosis, ACCP suggests anticoagulation until the removal of the precipitating factor but for a minimum of 3 months (Grade 2C).

CVL-related thrombosis

1.2.8. If a CVL is no longer required or is nonfunctioning, ACCP recommends it be removed (Grade 1B). ACCP suggests at least 3-5 days of anticoagulation therapy prior to its removal (Grade 2C). If CVL access is required and the CVL is still functioning, ACCP suggests that the CVL remain *in situ* and the patient be anticoagulated (Grade 2C).

1.2.9. For children with a first CVL-related DVT, ACCP suggests initial management as for secondary VTE as previously described. ACCP suggests, after the initial 3 months of therapy, that prophylactic doses of VKAs (INR range: 1.5-1.9) or LMWH (anti-FXa level range: 0.1-0.3) be given until the CVL is removed (Grade 2C). If recurrent thrombosis occurs while the patient is receiving prophylactic therapy, ACCP suggests continuing therapeutic doses until the CVL is removed but at least for a minimum of 3 months (Grade 2C).

1.3 Use of Thrombolysis in Pediatric Patients With DVT

1.3.1. In children with DVT, ACCP suggests that thrombolysis therapy not be used routinely (Grade 2C). If thrombolysis is used, in the presence of physiologic or pathologic deficiencies of plasminogen, ACCP suggests supplementation with plasminogen (Grade 2C).

1.4 Thrombectomy and IVC Filter Use in Pediatric Patients With DVT

1.4.1. If life-threatening VTE is present, ACCP suggests thrombectomy (Grade 2C).

1.4.2. ACCP suggests, following thrombectomy, anticoagulant therapy be initiated to prevent thrombus reaccumulation (Grade 2C).

1.4.3. In children >10 kg body weight with lower-extremity DVT and a contraindication to anticoagulation, ACCP suggests placement of a temporary inferior vena cava (IVC) filter (Grade 2C).

1.4.4. ACCP suggests temporary IVC filters be removed as soon as possible if thrombosis is not present in the basket of the filter, and when the risk of anticoagulation decreases (Grade 2C).

1.4.5. In children who receive an IVC filter, ACCP recommends appropriate anticoagulation for DVT (see Section 1.2) as soon as the contraindication to anticoagulation is resolved (Grade 1B).

1.5 Pediatric Cancer Patients With DVT

Use of Anticoagulants as Therapeutic Agents

1.5.1. In children with cancer, ACCP suggests management of VTE follow the general recommendations for management of DVT in children. ACCP suggests the use of LMWH in the treatment of VTE for a minimum of 3 months until the precipitating factor has resolved (eg, use of asparaginase) [Grade 2C]. *Remark:* The presence of cancer and the need for surgery, chemotherapy, or other treatments may modify the risk:benefit ratio for treatment of DVT, and clinicians should consider these factors on an individual basis.

Use of Anticoagulant as Thromboprophylaxis

1.5.2. ACCP suggests clinicians not use primary antithrombotic prophylaxis in children with cancer and central venous access devices (Grade 2C)

1.6 Children With DVT and Antiphospholipid Antibodies

1.6 For children with VTE, in the setting of antiphospholipid antibodies (APLAs), ACCP suggests management as per general recommendations for VTE management in children. *Remark:* Depending on the age of the patient, it may be more appropriate to follow adult guidelines for management of VTE in the setting of APLAs.

1.7 Renal Vein Thrombosis

1.7.1. For neonates or children with unilateral renal vein thrombosis (RVT) in the absence of renal impairment or extension into the IVC, ACCP suggests supportive care with monitoring of the RVT for extension or anticoagulation with UFH/LMWH or LMWH in therapeutic doses; ACCP suggests continuation for 3 months (Grade 2C).

1.7.2. For unilateral RVT that extends into the IVC, ACCP suggests anticoagulation with UFH/LMWH or LMWH for 3 months (Grade 2C).

1.7.3. For bilateral RVT with various degrees of renal failure, ACCP suggests anticoagulation with UFH and initial thrombolytic therapy with tPA, followed by anticoagulation with UFH/LMWH (Grade 2C). *Remark:* LMWH therapy requires careful monitoring in the presence of significant renal impairment.

1.8 Primary Antithrombotic Prophylaxis for CVL in Neonates and Children

1.8.1. In children with CVLs, ACCP recommends against the use of routine systemic thromboprophylaxis (Grade 1B).

1.8.2. In children receiving long-term home total parenteral nutrition, ACCP suggests thromboprophylaxis with VKAs with a target INR of 2.5 (range: 2-3) [Grade 2C].

1.8.3. For blocked CVLs, ACCP suggests tPA or recombinant urokinase to restore patency (Grade 2C). If CVL patency is not restored 30 minutes following local thrombolytic instillation, ACCP suggests a second dose be administered. If the CVL remains blocked following two doses of local thrombolytic agent, ACCP suggests investigations to rule out a CVL-related thrombosis be initiated (Grade 2C).

1.9 Primary Prophylaxis for Blalock-Taussig Shunts

1.9 For pediatric patients having a modified Blalock-Taussig shunt, ACCP suggests intraoperative therapy with UFH followed by either aspirin (1-5 mg/kg/day) or no further antithrombotic therapy compared to prolonged LMWH or VKAs (Grade 2C).

1.10 Primary Prophylaxis for Stage 1 Norwoods in Neonates

1.10 For patients who underwent the Norwood procedure, ACCP suggests UFH immediately after the procedure, with or without ongoing antiplatelet therapy (Grade 2C).

1.11 Primary Prophylaxis for Glenn or BCPS in Children

1.11 In patients who have BCPS, ACCP suggests postoperative UFH (Grade 2C). ACCP suggests this should be followed by no anticoagulation or antiplatelet therapy or anticoagulation with VKAs to achieve a target INR of 2.5 (range: 2-3) to continue until the patient is ready for Fontan surgery (Grade 2C).

1.12 Primary Prophylaxis for Fontan Surgery in Children

1.12 For children after Fontan surgery, ACCP recommends aspirin (1-5 mg/kg/day) or therapeutic UFH followed by VKAs to achieve a target INR of 2.5 (range: 2-3) [Grade 1B]. *Remark:* The optimal duration of therapy is unknown. Whether patients with fenestrations require more intensive therapy until fenestration closure is unknown.

1.13 Primary Prophylaxis for Endovascular Stents in Children

1.13 For children having endovascular stents inserted, ACCP suggests administration of UFH perioperatively (Grade 2C).

1.14 Primary Prophylaxis for Dilated Cardiomyopathy in Neonates and Children

1.14 ACCP suggests that pediatric patients with cardiomyopathy receive VKAs to achieve a target INR of 2.5 (range: 2-3) no later than their activation on a cardiac transplant waiting list (Grade 2C). *Underlying values and preferences:* ACCP's suggestion for administration of VKAs places a high value on avoiding thrombotic complications and a relatively low value on avoiding the inconvenience, discomfort, and limitations of anticoagulant monitoring in children who are eligible for transplant, which is a potentially curative therapy.

1.15 Primary Pulmonary Hypertension

1.15 In children with primary pulmonary hypertension, ACCP suggests anticoagulation with VKAs commencing when other medical therapy is commenced (Grade 2C).

1.16 Biological Prosthetic Heart Valves

1.16 For children with biological prosthetic heart valves, ACCP recommends that clinicians follow the relevant recommendations from the adult population.

1.17 Mechanical Prosthetic Heart Valves

1.17 For children with mechanical prosthetic heart valves, ACCP recommends that clinicians follow the relevant recommendations from the adult population with respect to the intensity of anticoagulation therapy.

1.17.2. For children with mechanical prosthetic heart valves who have had thrombotic events while receiving therapeutic antithrombotic therapy, or in patients in whom there is a contraindication to full-dose VKAs, ACCP suggests adding aspirin therapy (Grade 2C).

1.18 Ventricular Assist Devices

1.18.1. Following ventricular assist device (VAD) placement, in the absence of bleeding ACCP suggests administration of UFH targeted to an anti-factor Xa of 0.35-0.7 units/mL (Grade 2C). ACCP suggests starting UFH between 8-48 hours following implantation (Grade 2C).

1.18.2. ACCP suggests antiplatelet therapy (either aspirin, 1-5 mg/kg/day and/or dipyridamole 3-10 mg/kg/day) to commence within 72 hours of VAD placement (Grade 2C).

1.18.3. ACCP suggests that once clinically stable, pediatric patients be weaned from UFH to either LMWH (target anti-FXa 0.5-1 units/mL) or VKA (target INR 3; range: 2.5-3.5) until transplanted or weaned from VAD (Grade 2C).

1.19 Cardiac Catheterization

1.19.1. For neonates and children requiring cardiac catheterization (CC) via an artery, ACCP recommends administration of I.V. UFH prophylaxis (Grade 1A).

1.19.2. ACCP recommends the use of UFH doses of 100-150 units/kg as a bolus (Grade 1B). ACCP suggests further doses of UFH rather than no further therapy in prolonged procedures (Grade 2B).

1.19.3. ACCP recommends against the use of aspirin therapy for prophylaxis for CC (Grade 1B).

1.20 Therapy of Femoral Artery Thrombosis

1.20.1. For pediatric patients with a femoral artery thrombosis, ACCP recommends therapeutic doses of I.V. UFH (Grade 1B). ACCP suggests treatment for at least 5-7 days (Grade 2C).

1.20.2. ACCP recommends administration of thrombolytic therapy for pediatric patients with limb-threatening or organ-threatening (via proximal extension) femoral artery thrombosis who fail to respond to initial UFH therapy and who have no known contraindications (Grade 1B).

1.20.3. For children with femoral artery thrombosis, ACCP suggests surgical intervention when there is a contraindication to thrombolytic therapy and organ or limb death is imminent (Grade 2C).

1.20.4. ACCP suggests for children in whom thrombolysis or surgery is not required, conversion to LMWH to complete 5-7 days of treatment (Grade 2C).

1.21 Peripheral Arterial Catheter Thrombosis in Neonates and Children

1.21.1. For pediatric patients with peripheral arterial catheters *in situ*, ACCP recommends UFH through the catheter, preferably by continuous infusion (5 units/mL at 1 mL/hour) [Grade 1A].

1.21.2. For children with a peripheral arterial catheter-related TE, ACCP suggests immediate removal of the catheter (Grade 1B). ACCP suggests UFH anticoagulation with or without thrombolysis or surgical thrombectomy (Grade 2C).

1.22 Neonatal Aortic Thrombosis: UAC-Related

1.22.1. To maintain umbilical artery catheter (UAC) patency, ACCP suggests prophylaxis with a low-dose UFH infusion via the UAC (heparin concentration 0.25-1 units/mL) [Grade 2A].

1.22.2. For neonates with UAC-related thrombosis, ACCP suggests therapy with UFH or LMWH for at least 10 days (Grade 2C).

1.22.3. For neonates with UAC-related thrombosis, ACCP recommends UAC removal (Grade 1B).

1.22.4. For neonates with UAC-related thrombosis with potentially life-, limb-, or organ-threatening symptoms, ACCP suggests thrombolysis with tPa.When thrombolysis is contraindicated, ACCP suggests surgical thrombectomy (Grade 2C).

1.23 UAC-Related Thrombosis: Effect of Catheter Location

1.23 ACCP suggests UAC placement in a high position rather than a low position (Grade 2B).

1.24 Neonatal Aortic Thrombosis: Spontaneous

1.24 Neonatal Aortic Thrombosis: Spontaneous. The management of spontaneous aortic thrombosis should be the same as those for UAC-related TE.

1.25 Primary Prophylaxis for Venous Access Related to Hemodialysis

1.25 In patients undergoing hemodialysis, ACCP suggests against routine use of VKAs or LMWH for prevention of thrombosis related to central venous lines or fistulas (Grade 2C).

1.26 Use of UFH or LMWH for Hemodialysis

1.26 ACCP suggests the use of UFH or LMWH in hemodialysis (Grade 2C).

1.27 Kawasaki Disease

1.27.1. In children with Kawasaki disease, ACCP recommends aspirin in high doses (80-100 mg/kg/day during the short-term phase for up to 14 days) as an antiinflammatory agent, then in lower doses (1-5 mg/kg/day for 6-8 weeks) as an antiplatelet agent (Grade 1B).

1.27.2. In children with Kawasaki disease, ACCP suggests against concomitant use of ibuprofen or other nonsteroidal antiinflammatory drugs during aspirin therapy (Grade 2C).

1.27.3. In children with Kawasaki disease, ACCP recommends I.V. gamma globulin (2 g/kg, single dose) within 10 days of the onset of symptoms (Grade 1A).

1.27.4. In children with giant coronary aneurysms following Kawasaki disease, ACCP suggests warfarin (target INR 2.5; INR range: 2-3) in addition to therapy with low-dose aspirin be given as primary thromboprophylaxis (Grade 2C).

1.28 Neonatal Sinovenous Thrombosis

1.28.1. For neonates with CSVT without significant ICH, ACCP suggests anticoagulation, initially with UFH, or LMWH and subsequently with LMWH or VKA for a minimum of 6 weeks and no longer than 3 months (Grade 2C).

1.28.2. For children with CSVT with significant hemorrhage, ACCP suggests radiologic monitoring of the thrombosis at 5-7 days and anticoagulation if thrombus propagation is noted (Grade 2C).

1.29 Childhood CSVT

1.29.1. For children with CSVT without significant ICH, ACCP recommends anticoagulation initially with UFH or LMWH and subsequently with LMWH or VKA for a minimum of 3 months relative to no anticoagulation (Grade 1B).

1.29.2. ACCP suggests that if after 3 months of therapy there is incomplete radiologic decanalization of CSVT or ongoing symptoms, administration of a further 3 months of anticoagulation (Grade 2C).

1.29.3. For children with CSVT with significant hemorrhage, ACCP suggests radiologic monitoring of the thrombosis at 5-7 days. If thrombus propagation is noted at that time, ACCP suggests anticoagulation (Grade 2C).

1.29.4. ACCP suggests children with CSVT in the context of potentially recurrent risk factors (eg, nephrotic syndrome, L-asparaginase therapy) should receive prophylactic anticoagulation at times of risk factor recurrence (Grade 2C).

1.29.5. ACCP suggests thrombolysis, thrombectomy, or surgical decompression only in children with severe CSVT in whom there is no improvement with initial UFH therapy (Grade 2C).

1.30 Neonatal AIS

1.30.1. In the absence of a documented ongoing cardioembolic source, ACCP recommends against anticoagulation or aspirin therapy for neonates with a first AIS (Grade 1B).

1.30.2. In neonates with recurrent AIS, ACCP suggests anticoagulant or aspirin therapy (Grade 2C).

1.31 Childhood AIS

1.31.1. For children with non-sickle-cell disease-related acute AIS, ACCP recommends UFH, LMWH, or aspirin (1-5 mg/kg/day) as initial therapy until dissection and embolic causes have been excluded (Grade 1B).

1.31.2. ACCP recommends, once dissection and cardioembolic causes are excluded, daily aspirin prophylaxis (1-5 mg/kg/day) for a minimum of 2 years (Grade 1B).

1.31.3. ACCP suggests for AIS secondary to dissection or cardioembolic causes, anticoagulant therapy with LMWH or VKAs for at least 6 weeks with ongoing treatment dependent on radiologic assessment (Grade 2C).

1.31.4 ACCP recommends against the use of thrombolysis (tPA) for AIS in children, outside of specific research protocols (Grade 1B).

1.31.5. For children with sickle cell disease and AIS, ACCP recommends I.V. hydration and exchange transfusion to reduce sickle hemoglobin levels to at least <30% total hemoglobin (Grade 1B).

1.31.6. For children with sickle-cell disease and AIS, after initial exchange transfusion, ACCP recommends a long-term transfusion program (Grade 1B).

1.31.7. In children with sickle-cell anemia who have transcranial Doppler velocities >200 cm/s on screening, ACCP recommends regular blood transfusion, which should be continued indefinitely (Grade 1B).

1.31.8. ACCP recommends that children with moyamoya be referred to an appropriate center for consideration of revascularization (Grade 1B).

1.31.9. For children receiving aspirin who have recurrent AIS or transient ischemic attacks (TIAs), ACCP suggests changing to clopidogrel or anticoagulant (LMWH or VKA) therapy (Grade 2C).

1.32 Purpura Fulminans

1.32.1. For neonates with homozygous protein C deficiency, ACCP recommends administration of either 10-20 mL/kg of fresh frozen plasma every 12 hours or protein C concentrate, when available, at 20-60 units/kg until the clinical lesions resolve (Grade 1B).

1.32.2. ACCP suggests long-term treatment with vitamin K antagonists (Grade 2C), LMWH (Grade 2C), protein C replacement (Grade 1B), or liver transplantation (Grade 2C). 1.1.3.

[1]The ACCP Consensus Conference on Antithrombotic Therapy uses grades of recommendations that are based on clarity of benefits versus risks of treatment (1 = strong recommendation; 2 = weaker recommendation) and quality of the research methodology supporting the underlying evidence [A = Randomized controlled trials (RCTs) and observational studies with very large effects; B = Downgraded RCTs or upgraded observational studies; C = Observational studies and RCTs with major limitations]. The highest rating (1A) implies a strong recommendation, one that can be applied to most patients in most circumstances without reservations. The lowest rating (2C) implies a very weak recommendation, one in which other alternatives may be equally reasonable. For further information, see Guyatt G, Cook DJ, Jaeschke R, et al, "Grades of Recommendation for Antithrombotic Agents: American College of Chest Physicians Evidence-Based Clinical Practice Guidelines (8th Edition)," *Chest*, 2008, 133 (6 Suppl):123S-131S.

TOTAL BLOOD VOLUME

Age	Example Weight (kg) [age]	Approximate Total Blood Volume (mL/kg)[1]	Estimated Total Blood Volume (mL)
Premature infant	1.5	89-105	134-158
Term newborn	3.4	78-86	265-292
1-12 months	7.6 [6 months]	73-78	555-593
1-3 years	12.4 [2 years]	74-82	918-1017
4-6 years	18.2 [5 years]	80-86	1456-1565
7-18 years	45.5 [13 years]	83-90	3777-4095
Adults	70.0	68-88	4760-6160

[1]Approximate total blood volume information compiled from *Nathan and Oski's Hematology of Infancy and Childhood*, 5th ed, Nathan DG and Orkin SH, eds, Philadelphia, PA: WB Saunders, 1998.

ASSESSMENT OF LIVER FUNCTION

Child-Pugh Score

Component	Score Given for Observed Findings		
	1	2	3
Encephalopathy grade[1]	None	1-2	3-4
Ascites	None	Mild or controlled by diuretics	Moderate or refractory despite diuretics
Albumin (g/dL)	>3.5	2.8-3.5	<2.8
Total bilirubin (mg/dL)	<2 (<34 micromoles/L)	2-3 (34-50 micromoles/L)	>3 (>50 micromoles/L)
or			
Modified total bilirubin[2]	<4	4-7	>7
Prothrombin time (seconds prolonged)	<4	4-6	>6
or			
INR	<1.7	1.7-2.3	>2.3

[1]Encephalopathy Grades
Grade 0: Normal consciousness, personality, neurological examination, electroencephalogram
Grade 1: Restless, sleep disturbed, irritable/agitated, tremor, impaired handwriting, 5 cps waves
Grade 2: Lethargic, time-disoriented, inappropriate, asterixis, ataxia, slow triphasic waves
Grade 3: Somnolent, stuporous, place-disoriented, hyperactive reflexes, rigidity, slower waves
Grade 4: Unrousable coma, no personality/behavior, decerebrate, slow 2-3 cps delta activity

Alternative Encephalopathy Grades
Grade 1: Mild confusion, anxiety, restlessness, fine tremor, slowed coordination
Grade 2: Drowsiness, disorientation, asterixis
Grade 3: Somnolent but rousable, marked confusion, incomprehensible speech, incontinent, hyperventilation
Grade 4: Coma, decerebrate posturing, flaccidity

[2]Modified total bilirubin used to score patients who have Gilbert's syndrome or who are taking indinavir.

Child-Pugh Classification

Class A (mild hepatic impairment): Score 5-6
Class B (moderate hepatic impairment): Score 7-9
Class C (severe hepatic impairment): Score 10-15

References

Centers for Disease Control and Prevention, "Report of the NIH Panel to Define Principles of Therapy of HIV Infection and Guidelines for the Use of Antiretroviral Agents in HIV-Infected Adults and Adolescents," March 23, 2004, located at (URL) http://www.aidsinfo.nih.gov.
U.S. Department of Health and Human Services Food and Drug Administration, "Guidance for Industry, Pharmacokinetics in Patients With Impaired Hepatic Function: Study Design, Data Analysis, and Impact on Dosing and Labeling," May 2003, located at (URL) http://www.fda.gov/cder/guidance/3625fnl.pdf.

HOTLINE PHONE NUMBERS

AIDS Hotline (National)	800-232-4636
American Association of Poison Control Centers (AAPCC)	800-222-1222
American College of Clinical Pharmacy (ACCP)	913-492-3311
American Dental Association (ADA)	312-440-2500
American Medical Association (AMA)	800-621-8335
American Pharmacists Association (APhA)	202-628-4410
American Society of Health-System Pharmacists	866-270-0681
Animal Poison Control Center (24-hours)	888-426-4435
Canadian Pharmacists Association	613-523-7877
Center for Disease Control	1-800-CDC-INFO
FDA (Rare Diseases/Orphan Drugs)	800-300-7469
National Cancer Institute	1-800-4-CANCER
Asthma and Allergy Foundation of America	1-800-7-ASTHMA
Epilepsy Foundation	800-332-1000
National Council on Patient Information & Education	301-340-3940
National Institute of Health	301-496-4000
National Capital Poison Center	202-362-3867
Emergency	800-222-1222
Pediatric Pharmacy Advocacy Group (PPAG) Membership Information	901-380-3617
National Pesticide Information Center	800-858-7378
Rocky Mountain Poison Control Information	800-222-1222

ENDOCARDITIS PROPHYLAXIS

Recommendations by the American Heart Association (*Circulation*, 2007, 115:1-20)

Consensus Process – The recommendations were formulated by the writing group after analyses of relevant literature regarding procedure-related bacteremia and infective endocarditis *in vitro* susceptibility data of the most common microorganisms that cause infective endocarditis, results of prophylactic studies in animal models of experimental endocarditis, and retrospective and prospective studies of prevention of infective endocarditis. The consensus statement was subsequently reviewed by outside experts not affiliated with the writing group and by the Science Advisory and Coordinating Committee of the American Heart Association. These guidelines are meant to aid practitioners but are not intended as the standard of care or as a substitute for clinical judgment.

Table 1. Cardiac Conditions Associated With the Highest Risk of Adverse Outcome From Endocarditis[1]

Prophylaxis With Dental Procedures Is Recommended

Prosthetic cardiac valves
Previous infective endocarditis
Congenital heart disease (CHD)
    Unrepaired cyanotic CHD, including palliative stunts and conduits
    Completely repaired congenital heart defect with prosthetic material or device, whether placed by surgery or by catheter intervention, during the first 6 months after the procedure[1]
    Repaired CHD with residual defects at the site or adjacent to the site of a prosthetic patch or prosthetic device (which inhibit endothelialization)
    Cardiac transplantation recipients who develop cardiac valvulopathy

Endocarditis Prophylaxis Not Recommended

Negligible-Risk Category (no greater risk than the general population)
    Isolated secundum atrial septal defect
    Surgical repair of atrial septal defect, ventricular septal defect, or patent ductus arteriosus (without residua beyond 6 months)
    Previous coronary artery bypass graft surgery
    Mitral valve prolapse without valvar regurgitation
    Physiologic, functional, or innocent heart murmurs
    Previous Kawasaki disease without valvar dysfunction
    Previous rheumatic fever without valvar dysfunction
    Cardiac pacemakers (intravascular and epicardial) and implanted defibrillators

[1]Prophylaxis is recommended because endothelialization of prosthetic material occurs within 6 months after the procedure.

Table 2. Dental Procedures and Endocarditis Prophylaxis

Dental Procedures for Which Endocarditis Prophylaxis Is Recommended for Patients in Table 1

All dental procedures that involve manipulation of gingival tissue or the periapical region of teeth or perforation of the oral mucosa

Endocarditis Prophylaxis Not Recommended

Restorative dentistry[1] (operative and prosthodontic) with or without retraction cord
Local anesthetic injections through noninfected tissues
Intracanal endodontic treatment; post placement and buildup
Placement of rubber dams
Postoperative suture removal
Placement of removable prosthodontic or orthodontic appliances
Taking of oral impressions
Fluoride treatments
Taking of oral radiographs
Orthodontic appliance adjustment
Bleeding from trauma to the lips or oral mucosa
Shedding of primary teeth

[1]This includes restoration of decayed teeth (filling cavities) and replacement of missing teeth.

Table 3. Recommended Standard Prophylactic Regimen for Procedures on Respiratory Tract or Infected Skin, Skin Structures, or Musculoskeletal Tissue

Endocarditis Prophylaxis Recommended

Only for patients with underlying cardiac conditions associated with the highest risk of adverse outcome from Table 1 (use antibiotic prophylaxis with a regimen listed in Table 5)

Respiratory tract invasive procedure that involves incision or biopsy of respiratory mucosa

Tonsillectomy or adenoidectomy

For patients who undergo an invasive respiratory tract, procedure to treat an established infection (ie, drainage of an abscess or empyema), antibiotic regimen should contain an agent active against *Streptococcus* viridans group (see medications in Table 5)

If infection is caused by *Staphylococcus aureus*, the antibiotic regimen should contain an antistaphylococcal penicillin or cephalosporin, or vancomycin in patients unable to tolerate a β-lactam

If infection is caused by MRSA, administer vancomycin

Endocarditis Prophylaxis Not Recommended

Respiratory Tract
  Endotracheal intubation
  Bronchoscopy with a flexible bronchoscope, with or without biopsy
  Tympanostomy tube insertion

Gastrointestinal Tract
  Transesophageal echocardiography
  Endoscopy with or without gastrointestinal biopsy

Genitourinary Tract
  Vaginal hysterectomy
  Vaginal delivery
  Cesarean section
  In uninfected tissues:
    Urethral catheterization
    Uterine dilatation and curettage
    Therapeutic abortion
    Sterilization procedures
    Insertion or removal of intrauterine devices

Other
  Cardiac catheterization, including balloon angioplasty
  Implanted cardiac pacemakers, implanted defibrillators, and coronary stents
  Incision or biopsy or surgically scrubbed skin
  Circumcision
  Ear and body piercing
  Tattooing

Table 4. Recommended Standard Prophylactic Regimen for Antibiotic Prophylaxis Solely to Prevent Infective Endocarditis
(Note: NOT Recommended for GU or GI Tract Procedures)

For patients with underlying cardiac conditions associated with the highest risk of adverse outcome from Table 1 who are scheduled for an elective cystoscopy or other urinary tract manipulation and who have an enterococcal UTI or colonization, antibiotic therapy to eradicate enterococci from the urine before the procedure may be reasonable.

If the urinary tract procedure is not elective, it may be reasonable to administer an active agent against enterococci as part of the empiric antimicrobial regimen.

Preferred agent: Amoxicillin or ampicillin

If patient is unable to tolerate ampicillin: Vancomycin

	Dosage for Adults	Dosage for Children[1]
Vancomycin	1 g I.V. infused **slowly over 1 h**; complete infusion within 30 minutes before procedure	20 mg/kg I.V. infused **slowly over 1 h**; complete infusion within 30 minutes before procedure

[1]Children's dose should not exceed adult dosage.

If infection is caused by known or suspected strain of resistant Enterococcus: Consult with an infectious diseases expert.

◀

Table 5. Endocarditis Prophylaxis for a Dental Procedure

	Dosage for Adults	Dosage for Children[1]
Oral		
Amoxicillin[2]	2 g 30-60 min before procedure	50 mg/kg 30-60 min before procedure
Penicillin or ampicillin allergy:		
Clindamycin **or**	600 mg 30-60 min before procedure	20 mg/kg 30-60 min before procedure
Cephalexin (not to be used in individuals with immediate-type hypersensitivity reaction to penicillins) **or**	2 g 30-60 min before procedure	50 mg/kg 30-60 min before procedure
Azithromycin or Clarithromycin	500 mg 30-60 min before procedure	15 mg/kg 30-60 min before procedure
Parenteral		
Ampicillin	2 g I.M. or I.V. 30-60 min before procedure	50 mg/kg I.M. or I.V. 30-60 min before procedure
Penicillin allergy:		
Clindamycin **or**	600 mg I.V. 30-60 min before procedure	20 mg/kg I.V. 30-60 min before procedure
Cefazolin or ceftriaxone (not to be used in individuals with immediate-type hypersensitivity reaction to penicillins)	1 g I.M. or I.V. 30-60 min before procedure	50 mg/kg I.M. or I.V. 30-60 min before procedure

[1]Children's dose should not exceed adult dosage.

[2]Amoxicillin is recommended because of its excellent bioavailability and good activity against streptococci and enterococci.

References
Wilson W, Taubert KA, Gewitz M, et al, "Prevention of Infective Endocarditis. Guidelines From the American Heart Association," *Circulation*, 2007, 115:1-20.

PEDIATRIC HIV

Selected information from the Working Group on Antiretroviral Therapy and Medical Management of HIV-Infected Children, "Guidelines for the Use of Antiretroviral Agents in Pediatric HIV Infection," National Resource Center, February 23, 2009, 1-139. Available at http://aidsinfo.nih.gov/contentfiles/PediatricGuidelines.pdf.

1994 Revised Human Immunodeficiency Virus Pediatric Classification System:
Immune Categories Based on Age-Specific CD4 T cell and Percentage[1]

Immune Category	<12 mo		1-5 y		6-12 y	
	No./mm^3	%	No./mm^3	%	No./mm^3	%
Category 1 no suppression	≥1500	≥25	≥1000	≥25	≥500	≥25
Category 2 moderate suppression	750-1499	15-24	500-999	15-24	200-499	15-24
Category 3 severe suppression	<750	<15	<500	<15	<200	<15

[1]Modified from: CDC,"1994 Revised Classification System for Human Immunodeficiency Virus Infection in Children Less Than 13 Years of Age," *MMWR*, 1994, 43(RR-12):1-10.

1994 Revised Human Immunodeficiency Virus Pediatric Classification System: Clinical Categories[1]

Category N: Not Symptomatic
Children who have no signs or symptoms considered to be the result of HIV infection or who have only **one** of the conditions listed in category A

Category A: Mildly Symptomatic
Children with **two** or more of the following conditions, but none of the conditions listed in categories B and C:

*   Lymphadenopathy (≥0.5 cm at more than two sites; bilateral = one site)
*   Hepatomegaly
*   Splenomegaly
*   Dermatitis
*   Parotitis
*   Recurrent or persistent upper respiratory infection, sinusitis, or otitis media

Category B: Moderately Symptomatic
Children who have symptomatic conditions attributed to HIV infection, other than those listed for category A or category C. Examples of conditions in clinical category B include, but are not limited to the following:

*   Anemia (<8 g/dL), neutropenia (<1000/mm^3), or thrombocytopenia (<100,000/mm^3) persisting ≥30 days
*   Bacterial meningitis, pneumonia, or sepsis (single episode)
*   Candidiasis, oropharyngeal (ie, thrush) persisting for >2 months in children aged >6 months
*   Cardiomyopathy
*   Cytomegalovirus infection with onset before age 1 month
*   Diarrhea, recurrent or chronic
*   Hepatitis
*   Herpes simplex virus (HSV) stomatitis, recurrent (ie, more than two episodes within 1 year)
*   HSV bronchitis, pneumonitis, or esophagitis with onset before age 1 month
*   Herpes zoster (ie, shingles) involving at least two distinct episodes or more than one dermatome
*   Leiomyosarcoma
*   Lymphoid interstitial pneumonia (LIP) or pulmonary lymphoid hyperplasia complex
*   Nephropathy
*   Nocardiosis
*   Fever lasting >1 month
*   Toxoplasmosis with onset before age 1 month
*   Varicella, disseminated (ie, complicated chickenpox)

Category C: Severely Symptomatic
Children who have any condition listed in the 1987 surveillance case definition for acquired immunodeficiency syndrome (below), with the exception of LIP (which is a category B condition).

*   Serious bacterial infections, multiple or recurrent (ie, any combination of at least two culture confirmed infections within a 2-year period), of the following types: Septicemia, pneumonia, meningitis, bone or joint infection, or abscess of an internal organ or body cavity (excluding otitis media, superficial skin or mucosal abscesses, and indwelling catheter-related infections)
*   Candidiasis, esophageal or pulmonary (bronchi, trachea, lungs)
*   Coccidioidomycosis, disseminated (at site other than or in addition to lungs or cervical or hilar lymph nodes)
*   Cryptococcosis, extrapulmonary

- Cryptosporidiosis or isosporiasis with diarrhea persisting >1 month
- Cytomegalovirus disease with onset of symptoms at age >1 month (at site other than liver, spleen, or lymph nodes)
- Encephalopathy (at least one of the following progressive findings present for at least 2 months in the absence of a concurrent illness other than HIV infection that could explain the findings):
  - Failure to attain or loss of developmental milestones or loss of intellectual ability, verified by standard developmental scale or neuropsychological tests;
  - Impaired brain growth or acquired microcephaly demonstrated by head circumference measurements or brain atrophy demonstrated by CT or MRI (serial imaging is required for children <2 years of age);
  - Acquired symmetric motor deficit manifested by two or more of the following: Paresis, pathologic reflexes, ataxia, or gait disturbance
- HSV infection causing a mucocutaneous ulcer that persist for >1 month; or bronchitis, pneumonitis, or esophagitis for any duration affecting a child >1 month of age
- Histoplasmosis, disseminated (at site other than or in addition to lungs or cervical or hilar lymph nodes)
- Kaposi's sarcoma
- Lymphoma, primary, in brain
- Lymphoma, small, noncleaved cell (Burkitt's), or immunoblastic or large cell lymphoma of B-cell or unknown immunologic phenotype
- Mycobacterium tuberculosis, disseminated or extrapulmonary
- Mycobacterium, other species or unidentified species, disseminated (at site other than or in addition to lungs, skin, or cervical or hilar lymph nodes)
- *Mycobacterium avium* complex or *Mycobacterium kansasii*, disseminated (at site other than or in addition to lungs, skin, or cervical lymph nodes)
- *Pneumocystis jiroveci* pneumonia
- Progressive multifocal leukoencephalopathy
- Salmonella (nontyphoid) septicemia, recurrent
- Toxoplasmosis of the brain with onset at >1 month of age
- Wasting syndrome in the absence of a concurrent illness other than HIV infection that could explain the following findings:
  - Persistent weight loss >10% of baseline; **OR**
  - Downward crossing of at least two of the following percentile lines on the weight-for-age chart (eg, 95th, 75th, 50th, 25th, 5th) in a child ≥1 year of age; **OR**
  - <5th percentile on weight-for-height chart on two consecutive measurements, ≥30 days apart **PLUS**
    - Chronic diarrhea (ie, ≥two loose stools per day for >30 days); **OR**
    - Documented fever (for ≥30 days, intermittent or constant)

[1]Centers for Disease Control and Prevention, "1994 Revised Classification System for Human Immunodeficiency Virus Infection in Children Less Than 13 Years of Age," *MMWR*, 1994, 43(RR-12):1-10.

Indications for Initiation of Antiretroviral Therapy in Children Infected With Human Immunodeficiency Virus

This table provides general guidance rather than absolute recommendations for an individual patient. Factors to be considered in decisions about initiation of therapy include the risk of disease progression as determined by CD4 percentage or count and plasma HIV RNA copy number, the potential benefits and risks of therapy, and the ability of the caregiver and child to adhere to administration of the therapeutic regimen. Issues associated with adherence should be fully assessed, discussed, and addressed with the caregiver and child, if age-appropriate, before the decision to initiate therapy is made.

Age / Criteria	Recommendation
<12 mo	
• Regardless of clinical symptoms, immune status, or viral load	Treat
1-<5 y	
• AIDS or significant HIV-related symptoms[1]	Treat
• CD4 <25%, regardless of symptoms or HIV RNA level[2]	Treat
• Asymptomatic or mild symptoms[3] **and**	Consider
– CD4 ≥25% **and**	
– HIV RNA ≥100,000 copies/mL	
• Asymptomatic or mild symptoms[3] **and**	Defer[4]
– CD4 ≥25% **and**	
– HIV RNA <100,000 copies/mL	
≥5 y	
• AIDS or significant HIV-related symptoms[1]	Treat
• CD4 <350 cells/mm[3;5]	Treat

Age / Criteria	Recommendation
≥5 y (continued)	
• Asymptomatic or mild symptoms[3] **and**	Consider
– CD4 ≥350 cells/mm[3] **and**	
– HIV RNA ≥100,000 copies/mL	
• Asymptomatic or mild symptoms[3] **and**	Defer[4]
– CD4 ≥350 cells/mm[3] **and**	
– HIV RNA <100,000 copies/mL	

[1]CDC clinical category C and B (except for the following category B conditions: Single episode of serious bacterial infection or lymphoid interstitial pneumonitis).

[2]The data supporting this recommendation are stronger for those with CD4 percentage <20% than for those with CD4 percentage between 20% to 24%.

[3]CDC clinical category A or N or the following category B conditions: Single episode of serious bacterial infection or lymphoid interstitial pneumonitis.

[4]Clinical and laboratory data should be re-evaluated every 3-4 months.

[5]The data supporting this recommendation are stronger for those with CD4 count <200 cells/mm[3] than for those with CD4 counts between 200-250 cells/mm[3].

Recommended Antiretroviral Regimens for Initial Therapy for Human Immunodeficiency Virus (HIV) Infection in Children

A combination antiretroviral regimen in treatment-naive children generally contains 1 NNRTI plus a 2-NRTI backbone or 1 PI plus a 2-NRTI backbone. A 3-NRTI regimen consisting of zidovudine, abacavir, and lamivudine is recommended only if a PI- or NNRTI-based regimen can't be used. Regimens should be individualized based on advantages and disadvantages of each combination.

Non-nucleoside Reverse Transcriptase Inhibitor-Based Regimens

Preferred regimen	Children ≥3 years: 2 NRTIs **plus** efavirenz[1] Children <3 years or who can't swallow capsules: 2 NRTIs **plus** nevirapine[1]
Alternative	2 NRTIs **plus** nevirapine[1] (children ≥3 years)

Protease Inhibitor-Based Regimens

Preferred regimen	2 NRTIs **plus** lopinavir/ritonavir
Alternative (listed alphabetically)	2 NRTIs **plus** atazanavir **plus** low dose ritonavir (children ≥6 years old) 2 NRTIs **plus** fosamprenavir **plus** low dose ritonavir (children ≥6 years old) 2 NRTIs **plus** nelfinavir (children ≥2 years old)

Use in Special Circumstances

	2 NRTIs **plus** atazanavir unboosted (for treatment-naïve adolescents ≥13 years of age and >39 kg) 2 NRTIs **plus** fosamprenavir unboosted (children ≥2 years old) Zidovudine **plus** lamivudine **plus** abacavir

2-Drug NRTI Backbone Options (for use in combination with additional drugs) (alphabetical ordering)

Preferred	Abacavir **plus** (lamivudine **or** emtricitabine) Didanosine **plus** emtricitabine Tenofovir **plus** (lamivudine **or** emtricitabine) (for Tanner Stage 4 or postpubertal adolescent only) Zidovudine **plus** (lamivudine **or** emtricitabine)
Alternative	Abacavir **plus** zidovudine Zidovudine **plus** didanosine
Use in special circumstances	Stavudine **plus** (lamivudine **or** emtricitabine)

Insufficient Data to Recommend for Initial Therapy

	Low-dose ritonavir-boosted PI regimens, with the exceptions of lopinavir/ritonavir (any age), atazanavir/ritonavir in children ≥6 years old, and fosamprenavir/ritonavir in children ≥6 years old[2] Dual (full dose) PI regimens NRTI **plus** NNRTI **plus** PI Tenofovir-containing regimens in children in Tanner Stage 1-3 Enfuvirtide (T-20)-containing regimens Unboosted atazanavir-containing regimens in children <13 years of age and/or <39 kg Darunavir-containing regimens Tipranavir-containing regimens Maraviroc-containing regimens Raltegravir-containing regimens Etravirine-containing regimens

NRTI = nucleoside analogue reverse transcriptase inhibitor.

NNRTI = non-nucleoside analogue reverse transcriptase inhibitor.

PI = protease inhibitor.

[1]Efavirenz is currently available only in capsule form and should only be used in children ≥3 years old with weight ≥10 kg; nevirapine would be the preferred NNRTI for children <3 years old or who require a liquid formulation. Unless adequate contraception can be assured, efavirenz-based therapy is not recommended for adolescent females who are sexually active and may become pregnant.

[2]With the exception of lopinavir/ritonavir, atazanavir/ritonavir in children ≥6 years old, and fosamprenavir in combination with low-dose ritonavir in children ≥6 years old, use of other boosted PIs as a component of **initial** therapy is not recommended, although such regimens have utility as secondary treatment regimens for children who have failed initial therapy.

Antiretroviral Regimens or Components That Should Not be Offered
for Treatment of HIV Infection in Children

	Rationale	Exception
Antiretroviral Regimens Not Recommended		
Monotherapy	• Rapid development of resistance	HIV-exposed infants (with negative viral testing) during 6-week period of prophylaxis to prevent perinatal transmission
	• Inferior antiretroviral activity compared to combination with ≥3 antiretroviral drugs	
Two NRTIs alone	• Rapid development of resistance	Not recommended for initial therapy; for patients currently on this treatment, some clinicians may opt to continue if virologic goals are achieved
	• Inferior antiretroviral activity compared to combination with ≥3 antiretroviral drugs	
Tenofovir **plus** abacavir **plus** lamivudine **or** emtricitabine as triple NRTI regimen	High rate of early virologic failure when this triple NRTI regimen used as initial therapy in treatment-naïve adults	No exception
Tenofovir **plus** didanosine **plus** lamivudine **or** emtricitabine as triple NRTI regimen	High rate of early virologic failure when this triple NRTI regimen used as initial therapy in treatment-naïve adults	No exception
Antiretroviral Components Not Recommended as Part of Antiretroviral Regimen		
Atazanavir **plus** indinavir	Potential additive hyperbilirubinemia	No exception
Dual NRTI combinations:		
Lamivudine **plus** emtricitabine	Similar resistance profile and no additive benefit	No exception
Stavudine **plus** zidovudine	Antagonistic effect on HIV	No exception
Stavudine **plus** didanosine	Significant toxicities including lipoatrophy, peripheral neuropathy, hyperlactatemia including symptomatic and life-threatening lactic acidosis, hepatic steatosis, and pancreatitis	May be considered for antiretroviral-experienced children who require therapy change
Efavirenz in 1st trimester of pregnancy or in sexually active adolescent girls of childbearing potential	Potential for teratogenicity	When no other antiretroviral option is available and potential benefits outweigh risks
Nevirapine initiation in adolescent girls with CD4$^+$ T-cell count >250 cells/mm^3 or adolescent boys with CD4$^+$ T-cell count >400 cells/mm^3	Increased incidence of symptomatic (including serious and potentially fatal) hepatic events in these patient groups	Only if benefit clearly outweighs the risk
Unboosted saquinavir	• Poor oral bioavailability	No exception
	• Inferior virologic activity compared to other protease inhibitors	

Considerations for Changing Antiretroviral Therapy for
Human Immunodeficiency Virus (HIV)-Infected Children

Virologic Considerations[1]

- **Incomplete viral response to therapy:**

  Incomplete virologic response to therapy is defined for all children as a <1.0 $\log_{10}$ decrease in HIV RNA copy number from baseline after 8–12 weeks of therapy, HIV RNA >400 copies/mL after 6 months of therapy, or repeated HIV RNA above the level of detection using the most sensitive assay after 12 months of therapy.[2]

- **Viral rebound:**
  For children who have previously achieved undetectable plasma viral load in response to therapy, viral rebound is defined as subsequent, repeated detection of plasma HIV RNA on ultrasensitive PCR assays. Infrequent episodes of low level viremia (<1000 copies/mL) are common and not generally reflective of virologic failure, whereas repeated or persistent viremia (especially if >1000 copies/mL) more likely represents viral rebound.[3]

Immunologic Considerations[1]

- **Incomplete immunologic response to therapy:** Failure by a child <5 years old with severe immune suppression (CD4 percentage <15%) to improve CD4 percentage by ≥5 percentage points or as a failure by a child ≥5 years old with severe immune suppression (CD4 <200 cells/mm^3, to improve CD4 values by ≥50 cells/mm^3 above baseline within the first year of therapy.

- **Immunologic decline:** Sustained decline of 5 percentage points in CD4 percentage below pretherapy baseline in any age, or decline to below pretherapy baseline in CD4 absolute cell count in children who are ≥5 years old.[4]

Clinical Considerations

- **Progressive neurodevelopmental deterioration:** Two or more of the following on repeated assessments:
  - Impairment in brain growth
  - Decline of cognitive function documented by psychometric testing
  - Clinical motor dysfunction
- **Growth failure:** Persistent decline in weight-growth velocity despite adequate nutritional support and without other explanation
- **Severe or recurrent infection or illness:** Recurrence or persistence of AIDS-defining conditions or other serious infections

[1]At least two measurements (taken 1 week apart) should be performed before considering a change in therapy.

[2]The initial HIV RNA level of the child at the start of therapy and the level achieved with therapy should be considered when contemplating potential drug changes. For example, an immediate change in therapy may not be warranted if there is a sustained 1.5-2.0 $\log_{10}$ decrease in HIV RNA copy number, even if RNA remains detectable at low levels. Additionally, virologic suppression may take longer in young children given their higher viral load at the time of initiation of therapy than in older children or adults.

[3]Continued observation with more frequent evaluation of HIV RNA levels should be considered if the HIV RNA increase is limited (ie, <5000 copies/mL), especially in children with limited treatment options. The presence of repeatedly detectable or increasing RNA levels suggests the development of resistance mutations and/or nonadherence.

[4]Declines that represent a change to a more advanced category of immunosuppresion compared to baseline (eg, from CD4 percentage of 28% to 23%, or from CD4 count of 250 cells/mm^3 to 150 cells/mm^3) or to more severe immunosuppresion in those already suppressed at basline (eg, from CD4 percentage of 14% to 9%, or from CD4 count of 150 cells/mm^3 to 100 cells/mm^3) are of particular concern.

Assessment of Antiretroviral Treatment Failure

Assessment	Method	Intervention

Adherence	1. Interview child and caretaker
	• 24-hour or 7-day recall
	• Description of:
	  – WHO gives medication
	  – WHAT is given (names, doses)
	  – WHERE medications are kept, administered
	  – WHEN they are taken/given
	• Open-ended discussion of experiences taking/ giving medications and barriers/challenges
		Identify or re-engage family members to support/ supervise adherence.
		Establish fixed daily times and routines for medication administration.
		Avoid confusion with drug names by explaining that drug therapies have generic names, trade names, and many agents are coformulated under a third or fourth name.
		Explore opportunities for facility or home-based DOT.

	2. Review pharmacy records • Assess timeliness of refills	
	3. Observe medication administration • Observe dosing/administration in clinic • Home-based observation by visiting health professional • Hospital admission for trial of therapy – Observe administration/tolerance monitor treatment response	Simplify medication regimen if feasible. Substitute new agents if single ARV is poorly tolerated. Consider gastric tube placement to facilitate adherence. DOT Utilization of tools to simplify administration (pill boxes, reminders including alarms, integrated medication packaging for AM or PM dosing, others). Relaxation techniques.

	4. Psychosocial assessment
	• Comprehensive family-focused assessment of factors likely to impact on adherence with particular attention toward recent changes:
	  – Status of caregiver, financial stability, housing, intimate relationships
	  – School and achievement
	  – Substance abuse (child, caretaker, family members)
	  – Mental health and behavior
	  – Child/youth and caretaker beliefs toward antiretroviral therapy
	  – Disclosure status (to child and others)
		Address competing needs through appropriate social services.
		Address and treat concomitant mental illness and behavioral disorders. Initiate disclosure discussions with family/child.
		Consider need for child protection services and alternate care settings when necessary.

Pharmacokinetics and Dosing	1. Recalculate doses for individual medications using weight or body surface area. 2. Identify concomitant medications including prescription, over-the-counter, and recreational substances; assess for drug-drug interactions. 3. Consider drug levels for specific antiretroviral drugs	Adjust drug doses. Discontinue or substitute competing medications. Reinforce applicable food restrictions.
Resistance Testing	1. Genotypic and phenotypic resistance assays 2. Tropism assay, as appropriate.	

Options for Regimens With at Least Two Fully Active Agents Following Failure of Antiretroviral Regimen With Evidence for Viral Resistance to Therapy with Goal of Virologic Suppresion[1]

Prior Regimen	Recommended Change
2 NRTIs + NNRTI	• 2 NRTIs (based on resistance testing) + PI
2 NRTIs + PI	• 2 NRTIs (based on resistance testing) + NNRTI
	• 2 NRTIs (based on resistance testing) + alternative PI (with low-dose ritonavir boosting if possible, based on resistance testing)
	• NRTI(s) (based on resistance testing) + NNRTI + alternative PI (with low-dose ritonavir boosting if possible, based on resistance testing)
3 NRTIs	• 2 NRTIs (based on resistance testing) + NNRTI or PI
	• NRTI(s) (based on resistance testing) + NNRTI + PI
Failed regimens including NRTI, NNRTI, PI	• >1 NRTIs (based on resistance testing) + a newer PI (with low-dose ritonavir; based on resistance testing)
	• >1 NRTI + dual boosted PI (LPV/r + SQV, LPV/r + ATV) Consider adding either one or more of enfuvirtide, etravirine, or an integrase inhibitor
	• NRTI(s) + ritonavir boosted, potent PI (based on resistance testing) + etravirine
	• NRTI(s) + ritonavir boosted, potent PI (based on resistance testing) + enfuvirtide and/or CCR5 antagonist and/or integrase inhibitor
	• If patient refuses PI and/or ritonavir boosting: NRTI(s) + enfuvirtide and/or integrase inhibitor and/or CCR5 antagonist

[1]Antiretroviral therapy regimens should be chosen based on treatment history and drug-resistance testing to optimize antiretroviral drug effectiveness in the second regimen. This is particularly important in selecting NRTI components of an NNRTI-based regimen where drug resistance may occur rapidly to the NNRTI if the virus is not sufficiently sensitive to the NRTIs. Regimens should contain at least two, but preferably three, fully active drugs for durable, potent virologic suppression.

Role of Therapeutic Drug Monitoring in Management of Treatment Failure

Therapeutic drug monitoring (TDM) is not routinely recommended in the management of Pediatric HIV. It may be useful for:

• Patients in whom clinical response is different than expected

• Treatment experienced patients infected with virus with reduced drug susceptibility, where a comparison of the drug susceptibility and the achieved drug concentration may be useful

• Patient with potential drug administration difficulties including
  – Suboptimal dietary intake
  – Malabsorption
  – Incorrect dose
  – Caregiver measuring errors
  – Adherence concerns

• Drug or food interactions, including alteration of drug formulations by crushing or mixing with various foods and liquids.

Antiretroviral Drug Resistance Testing

• Antiretroviral drug resistance testing is recommended prior to initiation of therapy in all treatment naïve children and prior to changing therapy for treatment failure.

• Resistance testing in the setting of virological failure should be obtained when patients have a viral load >1000 copies/mL while still on the failing regimen, or within 4 weeks of discontinuation of the regimen.

• The absence of detectable resistance to a drug does not ensure that its use will be successful, especially if it shares cross-resistance with drugs previously used. In addition, current resistance assays are not sensitive enough to fully exclude the presence of resistant virus. Thus, the history of past antiretroviral use is important in decision making regarding the choice of new agents for patients with virologic failure.

• Viral Coreceptor (tropism) assays should be used whenever the use of a CCR5 antagonist is being considered. Tropism assays should also be considered for patients who demonstrate virologic failure while receiving therapy that contains a CCR5 antagonist.

• Consultation with a pediatric HIV specialist is recommended for interpretation of resistance assays when considering initiating or changing an antiretroviral regimen in a pediatric patient.

Strategies to Improve Adherence to Antiretroviral Medication Regimens in Children

Initial Intervention Strategies

- Establish trust and identify mutually acceptable goals for care.
- Obtain explicit agreement on need for treatment and adherence.
- Identify depression, low self-esteem, or drug use, or other mental health issues for the child/adolescent and/or caregiver that may decrease adherence. Treat prior to starting therapy, if possible.
- Identify family, friends, health team members, or others who can help with adherence support.
- Educate patient and family about the critical role of adherence in therapy outcome.
- Specify the adherence target: 95% of prescribed doses.
- Educate patient and family about the relationship between partial adherence and resistance.
- Educate patient and family about resistance and constraint of later choices of antiretroviral drug; explain that while a failure of adherence may be temporary, the effects on treatment choice may be permanent.
- Develop a treatment plan that the patient and family understand and to which they feel committed.
- Establish readiness to take medication by practice sessions or other means.
- For patient education and to assess tolerability of medications chosen, consider a brief period of hospitalization at start of therapy in selected circumstances.

Medication Strategies

- Choose the simplest regimen possible, reducing dosing frequency and number of pills.
- Choose a regimen with dosing requirements that best conform to daily and weekly routines and variations in patient and family activities.
- Choose the most palatable medicine possible (pharmacists may be able to add syrups or flavoring agents to increase palatability).
- Choose drugs with the fewest side effects; provide anticipatory guidance for management of side effects.
- Simplify food requirements for medication administration.
- Prescribe drugs carefully to avoid adverse drug-drug interactions.

Follow-up Intervention Strategies

- Monitor adherence at each visit, as well as in between visits by telephone or letter as needed.
- Provide ongoing support, encouragement, and understanding of the difficulties of the demands of attaining >95% adherence with medication doses.
- Use patient education aids including pictures, calendars, and stickers.
- Use pillboxes, reminders, alarms, pagers, and timers.
- Provide nurse, social worker, or other practitioner adherence clinic visits or telephone calls.
- Provide access to support groups, peer groups, or one-on-one counseling for caregivers and patients especially for those with known depression or drug use issues, which are known to decrease adherence.
- Provide pharmacist-based adherence support.
- Consider gastrostomy tube use in selected circumstances.
- For selected circumstances of apparent virologic failure, consider a brief period of hospitalization to assess adherence and reinforce that medication adherence is fundamental to successful antiretroviral therapy.
- Consider directly observed therapy at home, in the clinic, or during a brief inpatient hospitalization.

ADULT AND ADOLESCENT HIV

Selected tables from the Panel on Antiretroviral Guidelines for Adults and Adolescents, "Guidelines for the Use of Antiretroviral Agents in HIV-1-Infected Adults and Adolescents," Department of Health and Human Services, December 1, 2009; 1-161. Available at http://www.aidsinfo.nih.gov/ContentFiles/AdultandAdolescentGL.pdf. Accessed May 2, 2010.

Goals of HIV Therapy and Strategies to Achieve Them

Goals of Therapy

- Maximal and durable suppression of viral load
- Restoration and/or preservation of immunologic function
- Improvement of quality of life
- Reduction of HIV-related morbidity and mortality
- Prevention of HIV transmission

Strategies to Achieve Goals of Therapy

- Rational sequencing of drugs
- Preservation of future treatment options
- Selection of appropriate combination therapy
- Maximize adherence to the antiretroviral regimen
- Optimize initial regimen with use of pretreatment genotypic drug resistance testing
- Optimize antiretroviral regimen with use of therapeutic drug monitoring in selected clinical settings

Indications for Plasma HIV RNA Testing[1]

Clinical Indication	Information	Use
Syndrome consistent with acute HIV infection	Establishes diagnosis when HIV antibody test is negative or indeterminate	Diagnosis[2]
Initial evaluation of newly diagnosed HIV infection	Baseline viral load "set point"	Use in conjunction with CD4$^+$ T-cell count for decision to start or defer therapy
Every 3-4 months in patients not on therapy	Changes in viral load	Use in conjunction with CD4$^+$ T-cell count for decision to start therapy
Preferably within 2-4 weeks (but not more than 8 weeks) after initiation of or change in antiretroviral therapy. Repeat at 4-8 week intervals until level falls below limit of detection.	Initial assessment of drug efficacy	Decision to continue or change therapy
Within 2-8 weeks after change in antiretroviral therapy due to drug toxicity or regimen simplification	Confirm potency of new regimen	Decision to continue or change therapy
Every 3-4 months in patients on stable therapy or as clinically indicated; some clinicians may extend interval to every 6 months in adherent patients who have viral suppression for >2-3 years and who are at stable clinical and immunologic status	Durability of antiretroviral effect	Decision to continue or change therapy
Clinical event or significant decline in CD4$^+$ T cells	Association with changing or stable viral load	Decision to continue, initiate, or change therapy

[1]Acute illness (eg, bacterial pneumonia, tuberculosis, herpes simplex virus, *Pneumocystis jiroveci* pneumonia), and vaccinations can cause an increase in plasma HIV RNA for 2-4 weeks; viral load testing should not be performed during this time. Plasma HIV RNA results should usually be verified with a repeat determination before starting or making changes in therapy.

[2]Diagnosis of HIV infection made by HIV RNA testing should be confirmed by standard methods (ie, ELISA and Western blot testing) performed 2-4 months after the initial indeterminate or negative test.

Indications for Initiating Antiretroviral Therapy in Treatment-Naïve HIV-1-Infected Patient[1,2]

Clinical Condition and/or CD4 Count	Recommendations
• History of AIDS-defining illness • CD4 count <350 cells/mm³ • CD4 count 350-500 cells/mm³ • Pregnant women[3] • Persons with HIV-associated nephropathy • Persons coinfected with hepatitis B virus (HBV), when HBV treatment is indicated (treatment with fully suppressive antiviral drugs active against both HIV and HBV is recommended).	Antiretroviral therapy should be initiated.
• Patients with CD4 count >500 cells/mm³ who do not meet any of the specific conditions listed above	50% of the Panel members favor starting antiretroviral therapy; the other 50% of members view treatment is optional in this setting.

[1]Patients initiating antiretroviral therapy should be willing and able to commit to lifelong treatment, and should understand the benefits and risks of therapy and the importance of adherence.

[2]Patients may choose to postpone therapy, and providers, on a case-by-case basis, may elect to defer therapy based on clinical and/or psychosocial factors.

[3]For women who do not require antiretroviral therapy for their own health, consideration can be given to discontinuing antiretroviral drugs postpartum. For more detailed discussion, please refer to "Recommendations for Use of Antiretroviral Drugs in Pregnant HIV-1-Infected Women for Maternal Health and Interventions to Reduce Perinatal HIV Transmission in the United States." Available at http://www.aidsinfo.nih.gov/guidelines/.

Conditions Favoring More Rapid Initiation of Therapy

Deferring antiretroviral therapy may be appropriate in some cases. However, several conditions increase the urgency for therapy, including:

- Pregnancy
- AIDS-defining conditions
- Acute opportunistic infections
- Lower CD4 counts (eg, <200 cells/mm³)
- Rapidly declining CD4 counts (eg, >100 cells/mm³ decrease per year)
- Higher viral loads (eg, >100,000 copies/mL)
- HIV-associated nephropathy
- HBV coinfection when treatment for HBV is indicated

Conditions Where Deferral of Therapy Might be Considered

Some patients and their clinicians may decide to defer therapy for a period of time based on clinical or personal circumstances. The degree to which these factors might support deferral of therapy depends on the CD4 count and viral load. Although deferring therapy for the reasons listed below may be reasonable for patients with high CD4 counts (eg, >500 cells/mm³), deferral for patients with much lower CD4 counts (eg, <200 cells/mm³) should be considered only in rare situations and should be undertaken with close clinical follow-up. A brief delay in initiating therapy may be considered to allow a patient more time to prepare for lifelong treatment. Deferral may be considered in the following conditions:

- When there are significant barriers to adherence.
- Presence of comorbidities that complicate or prohibit antiretroviral therapy. Examples include:
  - Patients requiring surgery that might result in an extended interruption of antiretroviral therapy.
  - Patients taking medications that have clinically significant drug interactions with antiretroviral agents and for whom alternative therapy is not available.
  - Patients with a poor prognosis due to a concomitant medical condition who would not be expected to derive survival or quality-of-life benefits from antiretroviral therapy.
- Elite HIV controllers or long-term nonprogressors (**Note:** Although therapy may be theoretically beneficial for patients in either group, clinical data supporting therapy for nonprogressors and elite controllers are lacking.

Antiretroviral Regimens Recommended for Treatment-Naïve Patients

Patients naïve to antiretroviral therapy should be started on one of the following three types of combination regimens:

* **NNRTI + 2 NRTIs; or**
* **PI (preferably boosted with ritonavir) + 2 NRTIs; or**
* **INSTI + 2 NRTIs**

Selection of a regimen should be individualized based on virologic efficacy, toxicity, pill burden, dosing frequency, drug-drug interaction potential, resistance testing results, and comorbid conditions. The regimens in each category are listed in alphabetical order.

Preferred Regimens (Regimens with optimal and durable efficacy, favorable tolerability and toxicity profile, and ease of use)	
The preferred regimens for nonpregnant patients are arranged by order of FDA approval of components other than nucleosides, thus, by duration of clinical experience.	
NNRTI-based Regimen • EFV/TDF/FTC[1]	**Comments** **EFV** should not be used during the first trimester of pregnancy or in women trying to conceive or not using effective and consistent contraception. **ATV/r** should not be used in patients who require >20 mg omeprazole equivalent per day. Refer to monograph for dosing recommendations regarding interactions between ATV/r and acid-lowering agents.
PI-based Regimens (in alphabetical order) • ATV/r + TDF/FTC[1] • DRV/r (once daily) + TDF/FTC[1]	
INSTI-based Regimen • RAL + TDF/FTC[1]	
Preferred Regimen[2] for Pregnant Women • LPV/r (twice daily) + ZDV/3TC[1]	
Alternative Regimens (Regimens that are effective and tolerable but have potential disadvantages compared with preferred regimens. An alternative regimen may be the preferred regimen for some patients.)	
NNRTI-based Regimens (in alphabetical order) • EFV + (ABC or ZDV)/3TC[1] • NVP + ZDV/3TC[1]	**Comments** **NVP:** • Should not be used in patients with moderate to severe hepatic impairment (Child-Pugh B or C) • Should not be used in women with pre-ARV CD4 >250 cells/mm^3 or men with pre-ARV CD4 >400 cells/mm^3 **ABC:** • Should not be used in patients who test positive for HLA-B*5701 • Use with caution in patients with high risk of cardiovascular disease or with pretreatment HIV-RNA >100,000 copies/mL **Once-daily LPV/r** is not recommended in pregnant women
PI-based Regimens (in alphabetical order) • ATV/r + (ABC or ZDV)/3TC[1] • FPV/r (once or twice daily) + either [(ABC or ZDV)/3TC[1]] or TDF/FTC[1] • LPV/r (once or twice daily) + either [(ABC or ZDV)/3TC[1]] or TDF/FTC[1] • SQV/r + TDF/FTC[1]	
Acceptable Regimens (Regimens that may be selected for some patients but are less satisfactory than preferred or alternative regimens.)	
NNRTI-based Regimen • EFV + ddl + (3TC or FTC)	**Comments** EFV + ddl + FTC or 3TC has only been studied in small clinical trials. ATV/r is generally preferred over ATV. Unboosted ATV may be used when ritonavir boosting is not possible.
PI-based Regimen • ATV + (ABC or ZDV)/3TC[1]	

[1]3TC may substitute for FTC or vice versa.

[2]For more detailed recommendations on antiretroviral use in an HIV-infected pregnant woman, refer to "Recommendations for Use of Antiretroviral Drugs in Pregnant HIV-1-Infected Women for Maternal Health and Interventions to Reduce Perinatal HIV Transmission in the United States." Available at http://www.aidsinfo.nih.gov/guidelines/.

Abbreviations:
INSTI = integrase strand transfer inhibitor, NNRTI = nonnucleoside reverse transcriptase inhibitor, NRTI = nucleos(t)ide reverse transcriptase inhibitor, PI = protease inhibitor
ABC = abacavir, ATV = atazanavir, 3TC = lamivudine, ddl = didanosine, DRV = darunavir, EFV = efavirenz, FPV = fosamprenavir, FTC = emtricitabine, LPV = lopinavir, NVP = nevirapine, RAL = raltegravir, r = low dose ritonavir, SQV = saquinavir, TDF = tenofovir, ZDV = zidovudine
The following combinations in the recommended list above are available as fixed-dose combination formulations: ABC/3TC, EFV/TDF/FTC, LPV/r, TDF/FTC, and ZDV/3TC

Antiretroviral Regimens That May be Acceptable and Regimens to be Used With Caution

Regimens that may be acceptable but more definitive data are needed	
CCR5-Antagonist-based Regimen • MVC + ZDV/3TC[1]	**Comment:** With MVC, tropism testing required before treatment. Only patients found to have CCR-5 tropic-only virus (ie, absence of CXCR4 tropic virus) are candidates for MVC.
INSTI-based Regimen • RAL + (ABC or ZDV)/3TC[1]	
PI-based Regimen • (DRV/r or SQV/r) + (ABC or ZDV)/3TC[1]	
Regimens to be Used With Caution (Regimens that have demonstrated virologic efficacy in some studies, but have safety, resistance, or efficacy concerns.)	
NNRTI-based Regimens • NVP + ABC/3TC[1]	**Comments** Use NVP and ABC together with caution because both can cause hypersensitivity reactions within first few weeks after initiation of therapy.
• NVP + TDF/FTC[1]	Early virologic failure with high rates of resistance has been reported in some patients receiving NVP + TDF + (3TC or FTC). Larger clinical trials are currently in progress.
PI-based Regimen • FPV + [(ABC or ZDV)/3TC[1] or TDF/FTC[1]]	FPV/r is generally preferred over unboosted FPV. Virologic failure with unboosted FPV-based regimen may select mutations that confer cross resistance to DRV.

[1]3TC maybe substituted with FTC or vice versa.

Abbreviations:
INSTI = integrase strand transfer inhibitor, NNRTI = nonnucleoside reverse transcriptase inhibitor, PI = protease inhibitor
ABC = abacavir, 3TC = lamivudine, DRV = darunavir, FPV = fosamprenavir, FTC = emtricitabine, MVC = maraviroc, NVP = nevirapine, RAL = raltegravir, r = low dose ritonavir, SQV = saquinavir, TDF = tenofovir, ZDV = zidovudine

Antiretroviral Components Not Recommended as Initial Therapy

Antiretroviral Drugs or Components (in alphabetical order)	Reasons for Not Recommending as Initial Therapy
Abacavir/lamivudine/zidovudine (coformulated) as triple-NRTI combination regimen	• Inferior virologic efficacy
Abacavir + lamivudine + zidovudine + tenofovir as quadruple NRTI combination	• Inferior virologic efficacy
Abacavir + didanosine	• Insufficient data in treatment-naive patients
Abacavir + tenofovir	• Insufficient data in treatment-naive patients
Darunavir (unboosted)	• Usage without ritonavir has not been studied
Delavirdine	• Inferior virologic efficacy • Inconvenient dosing (3 times/day)
Didanosine + tenofovir	• High rate of early virologic failure • Rapid selection of resistant mutations • Potential for immunologic nonresponse/CD4[+] decline
Enfuvirtide	• No clinical trial experience in treatment-naive patients • Requires twice daily subcutaneous injections
Etravirine	• Insufficient data in treatment-naive patients
Indinavir (unboosted)	• Inconvenient dosing (3 times/day with meal restrictions) • Fluid requirement
Indinavir (ritonavir-boosted)	• High incidence of nephrolithiasis
Nelfinavir	• Inferior virologic efficacy
Ritonavir as sole PI	• High pill burden • Gastrointestinal intolerance
Saquinavir (unboosted)	• Inferior virologic efficacy
Stavudine + lamivudine	• Significant toxicities including lipoatrophy, peripheral neuropathy, and hyperlactatemia, including symptomatic and life-threatening lactic acidosis, hepatic steatosis, and pancreatitis
Tipranavir (ritonavir-boosted)	• Inferior virologic efficacy

Antiretroviral Regimens or Components That Should Not Be Offered at Any Time

	Rationale	Exception
Antiretroviral Regimens Not Recommended		
Monotherapy with NRTI	• Rapid development of resistance • Inferior antiretroviral activity when compared to combination with three or more antiretrovirals	• No exception[1]
Dual-NRTI regimens	• Rapid development of resistance • Inferior antiretroviral activity when compared to combination with three or more antiretrovirals	• No exception[1,2]
Triple-NRTI regimens except for abacavir/zidovudine/lamivudine or possibly tenofovir + zidovudine/lamivudine	• High rate of early virologic nonresponse seen when triple NRTI combinations including ABC/TDF/3TC or TDF/ddI/3TC were used as initial regimen in treatment-naive patients • Other 3-NRTI regimens have not been evaluated	• Abacavir/zidovudine/lamivudine; and possibly tenofovir + zidovudine/lamivudine in selected patients where other combinations are not desirable
Antiretroviral Components Not Recommended as Part of Antiretroviral Regimen		
Atazanavir + indinavir	Potential additive hyperbilirubinemia	• No exception
Didanosine + stavudine	• High incidence of toxicities – peripheral neuropathy, pancreatitis, and hyperlactatemia • Reports of serious, even fatal, cases of lactic acidosis with hepatic steatosis with or without pancreatitis in pregnant women[1]	• When no other antiretroviral options are available and potential benefits outweigh the risks[1]
2-NNRTI combination	• When EFV combined with NVP, higher incidence of clinical adverse events seen when compared to either EFV- or NVP-based regimen • Both EFV and NVP may induce metabolism and may lead to reductions in etravirine (ETR) exposure; thus, should not be used in combination	• No exception
Efavirenz in first trimester of pregnancy or in women with significant childbearing potential	• Teratogenic in nonhuman primates	• When no other antiretroviral options are available and potential benefits outweigh the risks[1]
Emtricitabine + lamivudine	• Similar resistance profile • No potential benefit	• No exception
Etravirine + unboosted PI	• Etravirine may induce metabolism of these PIs, appropriate doses not yet established.	• No exception
Etravirine + ritonavir-boosted atazanavir, fosamprenavir, or tipranavir	• Etravirine may induce metabolism of these PIs, appropriate doses not yet established.	• No exception
Nevirapine in treatment-naïve women with CD4 >250 or men with CD4 >400	• High incidence of symptomatic hepatotoxicity	• If no other antiretroviral option available, if used, patients should be closely monitored
Stavudine + zidovudine	• Antagonistic effect on HIV-1	• No exception
Unboosted darunavir, saquinavir, or tipranavir	• Inadequate bioavailability	• No exception

[1]When constructing an antiretroviral regimen for an HIV-infected pregnant woman, please consult "Recommendations for Use of Antiretroviral Drugs in Pregnant HIV-1-Infected Women for Maternal Health and Interventions to Reduce Perinatal HIV Transmission in the United States." Available at http://www.aidsinfo.nih.gov/guidelines/.

[2]When considering an antiretroviral regimen to use in postexposure prophylaxis please consult Panlilio AL, Cardo DM, Grohskopf LA, et al, "Updated U.S. Public Health Service Guidelines for the Management of Occupational Exposures to HIV and Recommendations for Postexposure Prophylaxis," *MMWR Recomm Rep*, 2005, 50(RR-9):1-17 and Smith DK, Grohskopf LA, Black RJ, et al, "Antiretroviral Postexposure Prophylaxis After Sexual, Injection-Drug Use, or Other Nonoccupational Exposure to HIV in the United States: Recommendations From the U.S. Department of Health and Human Services," *MMWR Recomm Rep*, 2005, 54(RR-2):1-20.

Summary of Guidelines for Changing an Antiretroviral Regimen for Suspected Treatment Regimen Failure

Patient Assessment

- Review antiretroviral treatment history.
- Assess for evidence of clinical progression (eg, physical exam, laboratory and/or radiologic tests)
- Assess adherence, tolerability, drug-drug interactions, and pharmacokinetic issues.
- Distinguish between limited, intermediate, and extensive prior therapy and drug resistance.
- Perform resistance testing while patient is taking therapy (or within 4 weeks after regimen discontinuation).
- Assess for virologic failure.
- Identify active drugs and drug classes to use in designing new regimen, taking into consideration importance of drug sequencing and cross-resistance issues.

Patient Management: Specific Clinical Scenarios

- **Prior treatment with low-level viremia (50-1,000 copies/mL):** Assess adherence. Consider variability in HIV RNA assays. Patients with isolated increases in HIV RNA ("blips") do not require a change in treatment. Some HIV RNA assays are associated with more frequent "blips" and results should be interpreted with caution. It is not clear how to manage patients with persistent low-level viremia; many experts would not change therapy and would follow the patient closely.

- **Prior treatment with detectable viremia (eg, HIV RNA >1,000 copies/mL) and no resistance identified:** Consider the timing of the drug resistance test (eg, was the patient off antiretroviral medications for >4 weeks and/or nonadherent?) Consider resuming the same regimen or starting a new regimen and then repeating genotypic testing early (eg, 2-4 weeks) to determine whether a resistant viral strain emerges. Consider pharmacokinetic enhancement (ritonavir boosting for an unboosted PI, such as atazanavir, fosamprenavir). If continuing the same treatment regimen, HIV RNA levels should be followed closely because ongoing viral replication will lead to accumulation of additional resistance mutations.

- **Limited Prior treatment and drug resistance:** The goal of treatment is to resuppress HIV RNA maximally (eg, <50 copies/mL) and to prevent further selection of resistance mutations. With virologic failure, consider changing regimens sooner, rather than later, to minimize continued selection of resistance mutations. Discontinuing an NNRTI in a patient with ongoing viremia and evidence of NNRTI resistance to decrease the risk of selecting additional NNRTI-resistance mutations is particularly important, because newer NNRTIs with activity against some NNRTI-resistant strains are available (eg, etravirine). Similarly, consideration should be given to discontinuing enfuvirtide or raltegravir in a failing regimen to decrease selection of additional drug mutations. A new regimen should include at least two, and preferably three, fully active agents.

- **Extensive prior treatment and drug resistance:** The goal is to resuppress the HIV RNA levels maximally (eg, to <50 copies/mL). With the availability of multiple new antiretroviral drugs, including some with new mechanisms of action, this goal is now possible in many patients, including those with extensive treatment experience and drug resistance. In some cases, however, viral suppression may be difficult to achieve. If maximal virologic suppression cannot be achieved, the goals are to preserve immunologic function and to prevent clinical progression (even with ongoing viremia). Even partial virologic suppression of HIV RNA >0.5 log10 copies/mL from baseline correlates with clinical benefits; however, this must be balanced with the ongoing risk of accumulating additional resistance mutations.

- **Extensive prior treatment and highly drug resistant HIV:** A subset of patients exists who have developed resistance to all or most currently available regimens, and designing a regimen with two or three fully active drugs is not possible. No consensus exists on how to optimize the management of these patients. It is reasonable to observe a patient on the same regimen, rather than changing the regimen, depending on the stage of HIV disease. Evidence from cohort studies suggest that continuing therapy, even in the presence of viremia and the absence of CD4 T-cell count increases, decreases the risk of disease progression. Other cohort studies suggest continued immunologic and clinical benefits if the HIV RNA level is maintained <10,000-20,000 copies/mL. In general, adding a single, fully active antiretroviral drug in a new regimen is not recommended because of the risk of development of rapid resistance. However, in patients with a high likelihood of clinical progression (eg, CD4 T-cell count <100/mm^3) and limited drug options, adding a single drug may reduce the risk of immediate clinical progression; even transient decreases in HIV RNA and/or transient increases in CD4 T-cell counts have been associated with clinical benefits. Weighing the risks (eg, selection of drug resistance) and benefits (eg, antiretroviral activity) of using a single active drug in the heavily treatment experienced patient is complicated, and consultation with an expert is advised. Patients with ongoing viremia and with an insufficient number of approved treatment options to construct a fully suppressive regimen may be candidates for single-patient access of investigational new drug(s).

- **Discontinuing antiretroviral therapy.** Discontinuing or briefly interrupting therapy (even with ongoing viremia) may lead to a rapid increase in HIV RNA and a decrease in the CD4 T-cell count and increases the risk of clinical progression. Therefore, this strategy is not recommended.

- **Prior treatment and suspected drug resistance, now presenting to care in need of therapy and with limited information (ie, incomplete or absence of medical records or previous resistance data).** This is a common scenario. Every effort should be made to obtain medical records and prior drug resistance testing results; however, this is not always possible. One strategy is to restart the most recent antiretroviral regimen and assess drug resistance in 2-4 weeks to help guide the choice of the next regimen.

Recommendations for Using Drug-Resistance Assays

Clinical Setting / Recommendation	Rationale
Drug-Resistance Assay Recommended	
In acute HIV infection: Drug resistance testing is recommended, regardless of whether treatment will be initiated immediately or deferred. A genotypic assay is generally preferred.	If treatment is to be initiated, drug resistance testing will determine whether drug-resistant virus was transmitted and will help in the design of initial or changed (if therapy was initiated prior to test results) regimens. Genotypic testing is preferable to phenotypic testing because of lower cost, faster turnaround time, and greater sensitivity for detecting mixtures of wild-type and resistant virus.
If treatment is deferred, repeat resistance testing should be considered at the time ART is initiated. A genotypic assay is generally preferred.	If treatment is deferred, testing still should be performed because of the greater likelihood that transmitted resistance-associated mutations will be detected earlier in the course of HIV infection; results of testing may be important when treatment is eventually initiated. Repeat testing at the time ART is initiated should be considered because of the possibility that the patient may have acquired drug-resistant virus.
In treatment-naïve patients with chronic HIV infection: Drug resistance testing is recommended at the time of entry into HIV care, regardless of whether therapy is initiated immediately or deferred. A genotypic assay is generally preferred. If therapy is deferred, repeat resistance testing should be considered at the time ART is initiated. A genotypic assay is generally preferred.	Transmitted HIV with baseline resistance to at least one drug may be seen in 6% to 16% of patients. Suboptimal virologic responses may be seen in patients with baseline resistant mutations. Some drug resistance mutations can remain detectable for years in untreated chronically infected patients. Repeat testing prior to initiation of ART should be considered because that the patient may have acquired a drug-resistant virus. Genotypic testing is preferred for the reasons noted previously.

Recommendations for Using Drug-Resistance Assays *(continued)*

Clinical Setting / Recommendation	Rationale
In patients with virologic failure: Drug resistance testing is recommended in persons on combination antiretroviral therapy with HIV RNA levels >1,000 copies/mL In persons with HIV RNA levels >500 but <1,000 copies/mL, testing may be unsuccessful but should still be considered. A genotypic assay is generally preferred in those experiencing virologic failure on their first or second regimens. Addition of phenotypic assay to genotypic assay is generally preferred for those with known or suspected complex drug resistance patterns, particularly to protease inhibitors.	Testing can help determine the role of resistance in drug failure and maximize the clinician's ability to select active drugs for the new regimen. Drug resistance testing should be performed while the patient is taking prescribed antiretroviral drugs or, if not possible, within 4 weeks after discontinuing therapy. Genotypic testing is generally preferred for the reasons noted previously. Phenotypic testing can provide useful additional information for those with complex drug resistance mutation patterns, particularly to protease inhibitors.
In patients with suboptimal suppression of viral load: Drug resistance testing is recommended in persons with suboptimal suppression of viral load after initiation of antiretroviral therapy.	Testing can help determine the role of resistance and thus assist in identifying the number of active drugs available for a new regimen.
In HIV-infected pregnant women: Genotypic resistance testing is recommended for all pregnant women prior to initiation of therapy and for those entering pregnancy with detectable HIV RNA levels while on therapy.	The goals of antiretroviral therapy in HIV-infected pregnant women are to achieve maximal viral suppression for treatment of maternal HIV infection as well as for prevention of perinatal HIV transmission. Genotypic resistance testing will assist the clinician in selecting the optimal regimen for the patient.
Drug-Resistance Assay Not Usually Recommended	
After therapy discontinued: Drug resistance testing is not usually recommended after discontinuation (>4 weeks) of antiretroviral drugs.	Drug-resistance mutations may become minor species in the absence of selective drug pressure, and available assays may not detect minor drug-resistant species. If testing is performed in this setting, the detection of drug resistance may be of value, but its absence does not rule out the presence of minor drug-resistant species.
In patients with low HIV RNA levels: Drug resistance testing is not usually recommended in persons with a plasma viral load < 500 copies/mL.	Resistance assays cannot be consistently performed because of low HIV RNA levels

Therapeutic Drug Monitoring

As with other notable drug classes (eg, antibiotics, anticonvulsants), the goal of therapeutic drug monitoring (TDM) is to maximize therapeutic efficacy and minimize drug-related toxicities. The utility of TDM in the setting of antiretroviral drug therapy is supported by data showing considerable interpatient variability with respect to drug concentrations among patients taking similar doses, as well as data demonstrating concentration/effect and concentration/toxicity correlations. The optimal plasma concentrations of many antiretroviral drugs have yet to be determined (eg, NRTIs). Those drugs for which target trough levels are defined are shown below.

Suggested Minimum Target Trough Concentrations

Drug	Concentration (ng/mL)
Fosamprenavir	400 (concentration assayed as amprenavir)
Atazanavir	150
Indinavir	100
Lopinavir	1000
Nelfinavir[1]	800
Saquinavir	100-250
Efavirenz	1000
Nevirapine	3000
Recommendations applicable only to treatment-experienced persons who have resistance HIV-1 strains	
Maraviroc	>50
Tipranavir	10,500

[1]Measurable active M8 metabolite.

Identifying, Diagnosing, and Managing Acute HIV-1 Infection

1. **Suspecting acute HIV infection:** Signs or symptoms of acute HIV infection with recent (within 2-6 weeks) high HIV risk exposure[1]

   - Signs/symptoms/laboratory findings may include but are not limited to one or more of the following: Fever, lymphadenopathy, skin rash, myalgia/arthralgia, headache, diarrhea, oral ulcers, leucopenia, thrombocytopenia, transaminase elevation

   - High-risk exposures include sexual contact with a person infected with HIV or at risk for HIV, sharing of injection drug use paraphernalia, or contact of potentially infectious blood with mucous membranes or breaks in skin[1]

2. **Differential diagnosis:** EBV- and non-EBV (eg, CMV)-related infectious mononucleosis syndromes, influenza, viral hepatitis, streptococcal infection, syphilis

3. **Evaluation/diagnosis of acute/primary HIV infection:**

- HIV antibody EIA (rapid test if available)
  - Reactive EIA must be followed by Western blot
  - Negative EIA or reactive EIA with negative or indeterminate Western blot should be followed by a virologic test[2]
- Positive virologic test in this setting is consistent with acute HIV infection
- Positive quantitative or qualitative HIV RNA test should be confirmed with subsequent documentation of seroconversion

4. **Patient management:**

- Treatment of acute HIV infection is considered optional
- Enrollment in clinical trial should be considered

[1]In some settings, behaviors conducive to acquisition of HIV infection might not be ascertained or might not be perceived as "high-risk" by the healthcare provider or the patient or both. Thus, symptoms and signs consistent with acute retroviral syndrome should motivate consideration of this diagnosis, even in the absence of reported high-risk behaviors.

[2]P24 antigen or HIV RNA assay. P24 antigen is less sensitive but more specific than HIV RNA tests; HIV RNA tests are generally preferred. HIV RNA tests include quantitative bDNA or RT-PCR or qualitative transcription-mediated amplification (APTIMA, GenProbe).

Associated Signs and Symptoms of Acute Retroviral Syndrome and Percentage of Expected Frequency

- Fever (96%)
- Lymphadenopathy (74%)
- Pharyngitis (70%)
- Rash (70%)
  - Erythematous maculopapular with lesions on face and trunk and sometimes extremities, including palms and soles
  - Mucocutaneous ulceration involving mouth, esophagus, or genitals
- Myalgia or arthralgia (54%)
- Diarrhea (32%)
- Headache (32%)
- Nausea and vomiting (27%)
- Hepatosplenomegaly (14%)
- Weight loss (13%)
- Thrush (12%)
- Neurologic symptoms (12%)
  - Meningoencephalitis or aseptic meningitis
  - Peripheral neuropathy or radiculopathy
  - Facial palsy
  - Guillain-Barré syndrome
  - Brachial neuritis
  - Cognitive impairment or psychosis

Reference

Niu MT, Stein DS, and Schnittman SM, "Primary Human Immunodeficiency Virus Type 1 Infection: Review of Pathogenesis and Early Treatment Intervention in Humans and Animal Retrovirus Infections," *J Infect Dis*, 1993, 168(6):1490-501.

PERINATAL HIV

Overview and Rationale of Perinatal Antiretroviral Therapy

Antiretroviral agents are used during pregnancy for two reasons: 1) To treat maternal human immunodeficiency virus (HIV) infection and 2) To reduce the risk of perinatal HIV transmission. The pivotal clinical trial that demonstrated the benefits of antiretroviral prophylaxis to decrease the risk of perinatal HIV transmission was the Pediatric AIDS Clinical Trials Group (PACTG) 076 (Connor, 1994). In this randomized, double-blind, placebo-controlled trial, zidovudine monotherapy was administered in three phases: 1) Antepartum (to the pregnant woman), 2) Intrapartum (during labor to the pregnant woman) and 3) Postpartum (to the newborn infant for 6 weeks). A relative reduction of 67.5% in the risk of perinatal HIV transmission was observed in this study; the mother to infant HIV transmission rate decreased from 25.5% in the placebo group to 8.3% in the zidovudine group.

Many studies have been conducted and much has been learned since publication of that pivotal study. Currently, antiretroviral monotherapy is **not** considered to be appropriate for the treatment of HIV infection. Combination highly active antiretroviral therapy (ie, HAART) is considered to be the standard of care, both for the treatment of maternal HIV infection and to reduce the risk of perinatal HIV transmission. Optimal reduction of the risk of perinatal HIV transmission still includes a three-phase approach with appropriate antiretroviral medications administered 1) Antepartum (to the pregnant woman), 2) Intrapartum (during labor to the pregnant woman) and 3) Postpartum (to the newborn infant). Zidovudine is recommended to be included as part of the antepartum HAART regimen unless there is severe toxicity or documented resistance, or if the woman is already on a fully suppressive regimen. Intrapartum zidovudine is recommended for all pregnant women (regardless of their antiretroviral regimen) and a 6 week course of zidovudine is recommended for all newborns born to women who are HIV positive (see Table 2 and Table 3). Today, with the use of antepartum HAART therapy, prenatal HIV counseling and testing, antiretroviral prophylaxis, scheduled cesarean delivery, and avoidance of breastfeeding, the perinatal transmission rate of HIV infection has decreased to <2% in the United States.

Specific recommendations for the use of antiretroviral drugs during pregnancy are updated regularly by the Department of Health and Human Services Panel on Treatment of HIV-Infected Pregnant Women and Prevention of Perinatal Transmission. The latest guidelines are available at http://AIDSinfo.nih.gov. Health care professionals are encouraged to contact the antiretroviral pregnancy registry to monitor outcomes of pregnant women exposed to antiretroviral medications (1-800-258-4263 or www.APRegistry.com).

The 2009 Panel recommendations include the following: (Information is summarized here for the reader)

General Principles

Note: Combined antepartum, intrapartum and infant antiretroviral prophylaxis is recommended for the prevention of perinatal HIV.

Preconception:

- Effective and appropriate contraception should be selected to avoid unintended pregnancy.
- Preconception counseling concerning safe sexual practices (and elimination of alcohol, illicit drug use, and smoking) should be conducted.
- Choice of antiretroviral therapy should consider efficacy for maternal treatment and the potential for teratogenicity if pregnancy should occur.
- Attaining a stable maximally suppressed viral load prior to conception is recommended for HIV infected women who wish to become pregnant.

Antepartum:

- Known risks and benefits of antiretroviral therapy during pregnancy should be discussed with all women.
- Assessment of HIV disease status and recommendations about initial antiretroviral therapy or changes to current regimen should be included in initial evaluation of pregnant women infected with HIV
- Antiretroviral prophylaxis for the prevention of perinatal HIV transmission should be provided to all pregnant women infected with HIV regardless of HIV RNA copy number or CD4 count.
- Resistance studies should be conducted prior to starting/modifying therapy if HIV RNA is detectable.
- Combination antiretroviral regimens are more effective than single drug regimens to reduce perinatal transmission.
- Prophylaxis for a longer duration (eg, starting at 28 weeks of gestation) is more effective than shorter duration (eg, starting at 36 weeks).
- If antiretroviral therapy is stopped electively during pregnancy, consider stopping nucleoside reverse transcriptase inhibitors (NRTIs) 7 days after stopping non-nucleoside reverse transcriptase inhibitors (NNRTIs) (due to longer half-life of NNRTIs); recommendation based on limited data. If therapy is stopped acutely for severe or life-threatening toxicity or severe pregnancy induced hyperemesis not responsive to antiemetics, stop all drugs at the same time and restart at the same time. If nevirapine is stopped and >2 weeks have passed, restart with the 2 week dose escalation period (ie, restart at the lower initial recommended dose).
- Optimal adherence to antiretroviral medications is a key part of the strategy to avoid failure and reduce the development of resistance.
- Additional specific medication issues:
  - Zidovudine should be included in the regimen unless there is severe toxicity, documented resistance, or if the woman is already on a fully suppressive regimen.
  - Efavirenz use should be avoided during the first trimester.

- Nevirapine can be used as part of initial therapy in pregnant women with CD4 cell count <250 cells/mm^3. Use as initial therapy in pregnant women with a CD4 cell count >250 cells/mm^3 should only be done if the benefit outweighs the risk of severe hepatic toxicity. Nevirapine can be continued in pregnant women who are virologically suppressed and tolerating therapy regardless of CD4 count. **Note:** Women with CD4 counts >250 cells/mm^3 are at increased risk for rash-associated nevirapine-related hepatotoxicity including severe, life-threatening and potentially fatal hepatic events.
- Protease inhibitors may require dosing adjustments during pregnancy.
- Stavudine and didanosine in combination may cause lactic acidosis with prolonged use during pregnancy; use should be avoided.
- NRTIs may be associated with lactic acidosis; monitor.

Intrapartum:

- Scheduled cesarean delivery at 38 weeks is recommended for women with suboptimal viral suppression near delivery (eg, >1000 copies/mL) or with unknown HIV RNA near the time of delivery.
- All HIV-infected pregnant women, regardless of their antepartum HAART regimen, should receive intrapartum intravenous zidovudine.
- If antepartum antiretroviral drugs were not administered, intrapartum therapy combined with infant antiretroviral prophylaxis should be given.
- Stavudine should be discontinued during labor while zidovudine is being administered.
- Nevirapine use as a single dose is not recommended for women in the U.S. who are receiving standard antiretroviral prophylaxis regimens.
- Pregnant women with documented zidovudine resistance who are not currently taking zidovudine for their own health should receive intravenous zidovudine during labor whenever possible, in addition to their established regimens.

Postpartum:

- Postnatal infant prophylaxis is recommended for all infants born to HIV-infected women.
- If antepartum or intrapartum antiretroviral drugs were not administered, postnatal infant prophylaxis is recommended.
- Breast-feeding is not recommended for HIV-infected women in the United States where safe, affordable, and feasible alternatives are available and culturally acceptable.

Special Situations

Hepatitis B virus coinfection:

- Screening for hepatitis B is recommended for all HIV-infected women not already screened during current pregnancy.
- Pregnant women with chronic hepatitis B virus (HBV) infection and HIV coinfection who require treatment for both diseases, a 3-drug regimen including a dual NRTI backbone of tenofovir plus lamivudine or emtricitabine is recommended. Consultation with an expert is advised for pregnant women needing treatment for HBV but not HIV and for pregnant women who do not require treatment for either HBV or HIV infection.
- Pregnant women with HBV and HIV coinfection and receiving antiretroviral medications should be monitored for liver toxicity.
- Infants born to hepatitis B infected women should receive hepatitis B immune globulin (HBIG) and initiate the three-dose hepatitis B vaccination series within 12 hours of birth.

Hepatitis C virus coinfection:

- Screening for hepatitis C is recommended for all HIV-infected women not already screened during current pregnancy.
- Pregnant women with chronic hepatitis C virus (HCV) infection and HIV coinfection should receive combination antiretroviral therapy with 3 drugs, regardless of CD4 count or viral load. If treatment for HIV infection is not needed for maternal health, it may be discontinued postpartum.
- Pregnant women with HCV and HIV coinfection and receiving antiretroviral medications should be monitored for liver toxicity.
- Decisions concerning mode of delivery should be based on HIV infection alone.
- Infants born to women coinfected with HCV and HIV should be evaluated for both HIV and HCV infection. For evaluation of HCV, HCV RNA testing should be performed between 2-6 months of age and/or HCV antibody testing should be conducted after 15 months of age.

Clinical Scenarios and Recommendations for the Use of Antiretroviral Drugs to Reduce Perinatal HIV Transmission in the United States

SCENARIO #1 Nonpregnant HIV-infected women of childbearing potential, who have indications for starting antiretroviral therapy

- Initiate HAART therapy according to the adult treatment guidelines.
- Avoid drugs with a potential to be teratogenic (eg, efavirenz) unless adequate contraception can be ensured. Pregnancy must be excluded before starting treatment with efavirenz.

SCENARIO #2 HIV-infected women receiving HAART therapy who become pregnant

- Continue current HAART regimen if successfully suppressing viremia, except avoid the use of efavirenz or other potentially teratogenic drugs in the first trimester and avoid drugs with known adverse potential for the mother (combination stavudine and didanosine).
- Resistance testing is recommended if there is detectable viremia on therapy.
- In general, if a woman requires treatment, antiretroviral medications should not be stopped during the first trimester.
- Continue HAART during the intrapartum period (give zidovudine as a continuous infusion during labor and other antiretroviral medications orally) and postpartum.
- Scheduled cesarean delivery at 38 weeks is recommended for women with suboptimal viral suppression near delivery (eg, >1000 copies/mL).
- Infant should receive zidovudine within 6-12 hours after birth and continue for 6 weeks.

SCENARIO #3 HIV-infected pregnant women who have not received prior antiretroviral therapy and have indications for antiretroviral therapy

- Resistance studies should be conducted prior to starting therapy and if suboptimal viral suppression occurs after starting HAART.
- Initiate HAART regimen as soon as possible, even if during the first trimester. Avoid the use of efavirenz or other potentially teratogenic drugs in the first trimester and avoid drugs with known adverse potential for the mother (combination stavudine and didanosine).
- Zidovudine should be included in the regimen unless there is severe toxicity or documented resistance.
- Nevirapine can be used as part of initial therapy in pregnant women with CD4 cell count <250 cells/mm^3. Use as initial therapy in pregnant women with a CD4 cell count >250 cells/mm^3 should only be done if the benefit outweighs the risk of severe hepatic toxicity.
- Continue HAART during the intrapartum period (give zidovudine as a continuous infusion during labor and other antiretroviral medications orally) and postpartum.
- Scheduled cesarean delivery at 38 weeks is recommended for women with suboptimal viral suppression near delivery (eg, >1000 copies/mL).
- Infant should receive zidovudine within 6-12 hours after birth and continue for 6 weeks.

SCENARIO #4 HIV-infected pregnant women who have not received prior antiretroviral therapy and do NOT require treatment for their own health

- Resistance studies should be conducted prior to starting therapy and if suboptimal viral suppression occurs after starting HAART.
- HAART is recommended for prophylaxis of perinatal transmission. Delaying treatment until after the first trimester may be considered.
- Avoid the use of efavirenz or other potentially teratogenic drugs in the first trimester and avoid drugs with known adverse potential for the mother (combination stavudine and didanosine).
- Zidovudine should be included in the regimen unless there is severe toxicity or documented resistance. The use of zidovudine prophylaxis alone is controversial, but may be considered if plasma HIV RNA levels are <1000 copies/mL on no therapy.
- Nevirapine can be used in pregnant women with CD4 cell count <250 cells/mm^3. Initial therapy in pregnant women with a CD4 cell count >250 cells/mm^3 should only be done if the benefit outweighs the risk of severe hepatic toxicity.
- Continue HAART during the intrapartum period (give zidovudine as a continuous infusion during labor and other antiretroviral medications orally).
- Evaluate the need for continued therapy postpartum. Discontinue HAART unless there are indications for continued therapy. If regimen includes drug with long half-life, like NNRTI, consider stopping NRTIs 7 days after stopping NNRTI (recommendation based on limited data).
- Scheduled cesarean delivery at 38 weeks is recommended for women with suboptimal viral suppression near delivery (eg, >1000 copies/mL).
- Infant should receive zidovudine within 6-12 hours after birth and continue for 6 weeks.

SCENARIO #5 HIV-infected pregnant woman who is antiretroviral experienced but not currently receiving antiretroviral medications

- Obtain full treatment history and evaluate the need for treatment for maternal health. Resistance studies should be conducted prior to starting therapy and if suboptimal viral suppression occurs after starting HAART.
- Initiate HAART regimen with antiretroviral agents chosen based on both prior medication history and resistance testing. Avoid the use of efavirenz or other potentially teratogenic drugs in the first trimester and avoid drugs with known adverse potential for the mother (combination stavudine and didanosine).
- Zidovudine should be included in the regimen unless there is severe toxicity or documented resistance.
- Nevirapine can be used as part of initial therapy in pregnant women with CD4 cell count <250 cells/mm^3. Use as initial therapy in pregnant women with a CD4 cell count >250 cells/mm^3 should only be done if the benefit outweighs the risk of severe hepatic toxicity.
- Continue HAART during the intrapartum period (give zidovudine as a continuous infusion during labor and other antiretroviral medications orally).

- Evaluate the need for continued therapy postpartum. Discontinue HAART unless there are indications for continued therapy. If regimen includes drug with long half-life, like NNRTI, consider stopping NRTIs 7 days after stopping NNRTI (recommendation based on limited data).
- Scheduled cesarean delivery at 38 weeks is recommended for women with suboptimal viral suppression near delivery (eg, >1000 copies/mL).
- Infant should receive zidovudine within 6-12 hours after birth and continue for 6 weeks.

SCENARIO #6 HIV-infected women in labor who have had no prior therapy

Several regimens are available. These include:

- Zidovudine as an intravenous infusion during labor followed by 6 weeks of zidovudine for the newborn (starting within 6-12 hours after birth) **OR**
- Zidovudine as an intravenous infusion during labor plus a single oral dose of nevirapine 200 mg given at the onset of labor. For the newborn, one dose of nevirapine (2 mg/kg given once orally at 2-3 days of age if mother received intrapartum single-dose nevirapine, or given at birth if mother did not receive intrapartum single-dose nevirapine) plus zidovudine for 6 weeks **OR**
- Zidovudine as an intravenous infusion during labor. For the newborn, some clinicians may choose to use zidovudine in combination with additional medications, but appropriate dosing in neonates is not well defined; additional efficacy in decreasing transmission is unknown. Consultation with pediatric HIV specialist is recommended.

Note: If single-dose nevirapine is given to the mother, alone or in combination with zidovudine, consideration should be given to adding maternal zidovudine/lamivudine starting as soon as possible (during labor or immediately postpartum) and continuing for 7 days postpartum, in an effort to reduce development of nevirapine resistance. (Single dose nevirapine is not recommended for women in the U.S. who are receiving standard antiretroviral prophylaxis regimens.)

In the immediate postpartum period, the woman should have appropriate assessments (eg, CD4$^+$ count and HIV RNA copy number) to determine whether antiretroviral therapy is recommended for her own health.

SCENARIO #7 Infants born to HIV-infected mothers who have received no antiretroviral therapy during pregnancy or during labor

- Administer zidovudine for 6 weeks to the infant, beginning as soon as possible after birth.
- Some clinicians may choose to use zidovudine in combination with additional medications, but appropriate dosing in neonates is not well defined; additional efficacy in decreasing transmission is unknown. Consultation with a pediatric HIV specialist is recommended.
- Evaluate the need for postpartum maternal therapy.

Clinical Scenarios and Recommendations Regarding Mode of Delivery to Reduce Perinatal HIV Transmission

SCENARIO A

Women presenting in late pregnancy (after about 36 weeks of gestation), known to be HIV-infected but not receiving antiretroviral therapy, and who have HIV RNA level and lymphocyte subsets pending but unlikely to be available before delivery.

Recommendations

Therapy options should be discussed in detail. The woman should be started on antiretroviral therapy. The woman should be counseled that scheduled cesarean section is likely to reduce the risk of transmission to her infant. She should also be informed of the increased risks to her of cesarean section, including increased rates of postoperative infection, anesthesia risks, and other surgical risks.

If cesarean section is chosen, the procedure should be scheduled at 38 weeks of gestation based on the best available clinical information. When scheduled cesarean section is performed, the woman should receive continuous intravenous zidovudine infusion beginning 3 hours before surgery and her infant should receive 6 weeks of zidovudine therapy after birth. Prophylactic antibiotics are generally recommended at the time of cesarean delivery. Options for continuing or initiating combination antiretroviral therapy after delivery should be discussed with the woman as soon as her viral load and lymphocyte subset results are available.

SCENARIO B

HIV-infected women who initiated prenatal care early in the third trimester, are receiving highly active combination antiretroviral therapy, and have an initial virologic response, but have HIV RNA levels that remain substantially over 1000 copies/mL at 36 weeks of gestation.

Recommendations

The current combination antiretroviral regimen should be continued as the HIV RNA level is dropping appropriately. The woman should be counseled that although she is responding to the antiretroviral therapy, it is unlikely that her HIV RNA level will fall below 1000 copies/mL before delivery. Therefore, scheduled cesarean section may provide additional benefit in preventing intrapartum transmission of HIV. She should also be informed of the increased risks to her of cesarean section, including increased rates of postoperative infection, anesthesia risks, and surgical risks.

If she chooses scheduled cesarean section, it should be performed at 38 weeks of gestation according to the best available dating parameters, and intravenous zidovudine should begin at least 3 hours before surgery. Other antiretroviral medications should be continued on schedule as much as possible before and after surgery. The infant should receive oral zidovudine for 6 weeks after birth. Prophylactic antibiotics are generally recommended at the time of cesarean delivery. The importance of adhering to therapy after delivery for her own health should be emphasized.

SCENARIO C

HIV-infected women on highly active combination antiretroviral therapy with an undetectable HIV RNA level at 36 weeks of gestation.

Recommendations

The woman should be counseled that her risk of perinatal transmission of HIV with a persistently undetectable HIV RNA level is low, probably 2% or less, even with vaginal delivery. There is currently no information to evaluate whether performing a scheduled cesarean section will lower her risk further.

Cesarean section has an increased risk of complications for the woman compared to vaginal delivery, and these risks must be balanced against the uncertain benefit of cesarean section in this case.

SCENARIO D

HIV-infected women who have elected scheduled cesarean section but present in early labor or shortly after rupture of membranes.

Recommendations

Intravenous zidovudine should be started immediately since the woman is in labor or has ruptured membranes.

If labor is progressing rapidly, the woman should be allowed to deliver vaginally. If cervical dilatation is minimal and a long period of labor is anticipated, some clinicians may choose to administer the loading dose of intravenous zidovudine and proceed with cesarean section to minimize the duration of membrane rupture and avoid vaginal delivery. Others might begin oxytocin augmentation to enhance contractions and potentially expedite delivery.

If the woman is allowed to labor, scalp electrodes and other invasive monitoring and operative delivery should be avoided if possible. The infant should be treated with 6 weeks of zidovudine therapy after birth.

Table 1. Recommended Antiretroviral Therapy in Pregnant HIV-Infected Women

Drug	Recommended	Alternative	Not Recommended	Insufficient Data	Rationale / Concerns
Nucleoside Reverse Transcriptase Inhibitors (NRTIs)					
Lamivudine	X				Lamivudine plus zidovudine is the recommended dual NRTI backbone for pregnant women. Use caution with hepatitis B coinfection; hepatitis B flare may occur if lamivudine is discontinued postpartum.
Zidovudine	X				Preferred NRTI for use in **combination** antiretroviral regimens in pregnancy; include in regimens unless significant toxicity occurs, stavudine is used, or if the woman is already on a fully suppressive regimen.
Abacavir		X			Potentially fatal hypersensitivity reaction may occur. Triple NRTI regimens including abacavir have been less potent virologically compared to PI-based HAART regimens; use triple NRTI regimen only when an NNRTI or PI based regimen cannot be used. Screening for *HLA-B*5701* allele status is recommended prior to initiating therapy or reinitiating therapy in patients of unknown status, including patients who previously tolerated therapy. Therapy is **not** recommended in patients testing positive for the *HLA-B*5701* allele.
Didanosine		X			Lactic acidosis (some cases which were fatal) has been reported in pregnant women receiving didanosine in combination with stavudine; do not use with stavudine unless alternative regimens are not available.
Emtricitabine		X			A pharmacokinetic study shows a slight decrease in emtricitabine serum levels during the third trimester; however, there is no clear need to adjust the dose.
Stavudine		X			Lactic acidosis (some cases which were fatal) has been reported in pregnant women receiving stavudine in combination with didanosine; avoid use with didanosine; do not use with zidovudine due to antagonism.
Tenofovir				X	Studies in children have shown bone demineralization with chronic use; clinical significance unknown. Because tenofovir significantly crosses the placenta and because of a lack of data concerning use during human pregnancy, use only after careful consideration of alternatives. Use caution with hepatitis B coinfection; hepatitis B flare may occur if tenofovir is discontinued postpartum.
Non-nucleoside Reverse Transcriptase Inhibitors (NNRTIs)					
Nevirapine	X				Possible increased risk of potentially fatal liver toxicity; use in women with CD4 counts >250 only if benefit clearly outweighs risk. Women who enter therapy on nevirapine regimens and are tolerating them well, may continue therapy regardless of CD4 count.
Delavirdine			X		No pharmacokinetic studies in pregnant women; carcinogenic and teratogenic in animal studies.
Efavirenz			X		Teratogenic in animal studies; cases of human neural tube defects following first trimester exposure have been reported. Avoid use during the first trimester; use after the second trimester only if other alternatives are not available. Alternate regimens should be considered in women of childbearing potential. Pharmacokinetic data from small study indicates that peak serum concentrations in the third trimester may be significantly increased
Etravirine				X	Teratogenic effects were not observed in animal studies; no experience in human pregnancy
Protease Inhibitors (PIs)					
Lopinavir/ritonavir	X				Teratogenic effects were not observed in phase I/II studies. Pharmacokinetic studies are not yet completed using the tablet formulation. Studies using the previously available capsule formulation showed that an increased dose may be needed during the third trimester. Until data is available for the tablet, standard dosing can be used, monitor virologic response and consider increasing the dose during the third trimester. Once daily administration is not recommended.

Table 1. Recommended Antiretroviral Therapy in Pregnant HIV-Infected Women *continued*

Drug	Recommended	Alternative	Not Recommended	Insufficient Data	Rationale / Concerns
Indinavir		X			Possible increased bilirubin levels; use with ritonavir boosting; optimal dosing in pregnancy is not known.
Nelfinavir		X			No increase in birth defects reported to Antiretroviral Pregnancy Registry; well-tolerated and short-term safety demonstrated in mother and infant. When used in nonpregnant adults, nelfinavir based regimens had a lower rate of viral response than some alternative regimens. Therefore, use is recommended only as an alternative PI in pregnant women receiving HAART for perinatal prophylaxis.
Ritonavir		X			Minimal experience in human pregnancy; recommended as part of boosted regimen.
Saquinavir		X			Well-tolerated and short-term safety demonstrated in mother and infant; must give with low-dose ritonavir boosting. The softgel capsules are no longer available. Until additional pharmacokinetic studies are completed using the hard gel capsule or the tablet, saquinavir is considered an alternative PI for use during pregnancy.
Atazanavir		X			A recommended alternative agent when combined with low-dose ritonavir boosting; may give as once daily dosing. In naive patients unable to tolerate ritonavir, once daily dosing may be considered; however, efficacy data is insufficient. Must be used with low-dose ritonavir boosting when used in combination with tenofovir. Increased bilirubin levels in the neonate have not been observed (to date) in clinical trials.
Darunavir				X	No experience in human pregnancy; insufficient safety/kinetic data available. Must give with low-dose ritonavir boosting.
Fosamprenavir				X	Limited experience in human pregnancy; insufficient safety/kinetic data available. Recommended to be given with low-dose ritonavir boosting.
Tipranavir				X	No experience in human pregnancy; insufficient safety/kinetic data available. Must give with low-dose ritonavir boosting.
Entry Inhibitors					
Enfuvirtide				X	Minimal studies in pregnant women; insufficient safety/kinetic data available.
Maraviroc				X	No experience in human pregnancy; insufficient safety/kinetic data available.
Integrase Inhibitors					
Raltegravir				X	No experience in human pregnancy; insufficient safety/kinetic data available.

Table 2. Intrapartum Maternal and Neonatal Zidovudine Dosing for Prevention of Mother to Child HIV Transmission

Drug	Dosing	Duration
Maternal Intrapartum		
Zidovudine	2 mg/kg I.V. over 1 hour followed by continuous infusion of 1 mg/kg/h	Onset of labor until delivery of infant
Neonatal		
Zidovudine (≥35 weeks gestational age)	2 mg/kg/dose P.O. (1.5 mg/kg/dose if given I.V.) started as soon as possible after birth (by 6-12 hours after delivery), then every 6 hours[1]	Birth to 6 weeks
Zidovudine (>30 weeks; <35 weeks)	2 mg/kg/dose P.O. (1.5 mg/kg/dose if given I.V.) given every 12 hours, advance to every 8 hours at 2 weeks of age	Birth to 6 weeks
Zidovudine (<30 weeks)	2 mg/kg/dose P.O. (1.5 mg/kg/dose if given I.V.) given every 12 hours, advance to every 8 hours at 4 weeks of age	Birth to 6 weeks

[1]Some international studies have used 4 mg/kg/dose given every 12 hours for neonatal prophylaxis. This regimen may be considered when concerns about adherence to therapy exist; however, there are no data showing equivalent pharmacokinetic parameters or efficacy in preventing transmission.

Table 3. Intrapartum Maternal and Neonatal Dosing for Additional Antiretroviral Drugs to be Considered Only in Selected Circumstances

Drug	Dosing	Duration
Maternal Intrapartum/Postpartum		
Nevirapine (as single dose intrapartum)[1]	200 mg P.O. as single dose	Given once at onset of labor
Zidovudine **plus** lamivudine (given with single dose nevirapine as "tail" to reduce nevirapine resistance)	Zidovudine: I.V. intrapartum: 2 mg/kg I.V. over 1 hour followed by continuous infusion of 1 mg/kg/h, then after delivery 300 mg P.O. twice daily Lamivudine: 150 mg P.O. twice daily starting at onset of labor	Through 1 week postpartum
Neonatal		
Nevirapine (as single dose)[2]	2 mg/kg P.O. as single dose	Single dose between birth and 72 hours of age. If maternal dose given ≤2 hours before delivery, infant should be given dose as soon as possible after delivery.
Zidovudine **plus** lamivudine (given with single dose nevirapine as "tail" to reduce nevirapine resistance)	Zidovudine: Neonatal dosing as in Table 2 Lamivudine: 2 mg/kg/dose P.O. twice daily	Zidovudine: Birth to 6 weeks of age Lamivudine: Birth to 1 week of age

[1]Given **in addition** to I.V. intrapartum zidovudine; if intrapartum single dose nevirapine is given to mother, administration of intrapartum P.O. lamivudine followed by zidovudine/lamivudine for 7 days postpartum to reduce nevirapine resistance is recommended

[2]Given **in addition** to 6 weeks of infant zidovudine; consider addition of 7 days of lamivudine to reduce nevirapine resistance

References

Connor EM, Sperling RS, Gelber R, et al, "Reduction of Maternal-Infant Transmission of Human Immunodeficiency Virus Type 1 With Zidovudine Treatment. Pediatric AIDS Clinical Trials Group Protocol 076 Study Group," *N Engl J Med*, 1994, 331(18):1173-80.

Public Health Service Task Force, "Recommendations for Use of Antiretroviral Drugs in Pregnant HIV-Infected Women for Maternal Health and Interventions to Reduce Perinatal HIV Transmission in the United States," April 29, 2009. Available at: http://aidsinfo.nih.gov/contentfiles/PerinatalGL.pdf.

IMMUNIZATION GUIDELINES

Recommended Immunization Schedule for Ages 0-6 Years
United States, 2010

Age ▶ Vaccine ▼	Birth	1 mo	2 mo	4 mo	6 mo	12 mo	15 mo	18 mo	19-23 mo	2-3 y	4-6 y
Hepatitis B[1]	HepB	HepB				HepB					
Rotavirus[2]			RV	RV	RV[2]						
Diphtheria, tetanus, pertussis[3]			DTaP	DTaP	DTaP	See footnote 3	DTaP				DTaP
Haemophilus influenzae type b[4]			Hib	Hib	Hib[4]	Hib					
Pneumococcal[5]			PCV	PCV	PCV	PCV					PPSV
Inactivated poliovirus[6]			IPV	IPV		IPV					IPV
Influenza[7]						Influenza (yearly)					
Measles, mumps, rubella[8]						MMR		See footnote 8			MMR
Varicella[9]						Varicella		See footnote 9			Varicella
Hepatitis A[10]						HepA (2 doses)					HepA series
Meningococcal[11]											MCV

☐ Range of recommended ages for all children except certain high-risk groups

■ Range of recommended ages for certain high-risk groups

Note: For those who fall behind or start late, see also the Catch-up Immunization Schedule table.

This schedule includes recommendations in effect as of December 15, 2009. Any dose not administered at the recommended age should be administered at a subsequent visit, when indicated and feasible. The use of a combination vaccine generally is preferred over separate injections of its equivalent component vaccines. Considerations should include provider assessment, patient preference, and the potential for adverse events. Providers should consult the relevant Advisory Committee on Immunization Practices statement for detailed recommendations: **http://www.cdc.gov/vaccines/pubs/acip-list.htm**. Clinically significant adverse events that follow immunization should be reported to the Vaccine Adverse Event Reporting System (VAERS) at **http://www.vaers.hhs.gov** or by telephone, 800-822-7967.

Footnotes to Recommended Immunization Schedule for Ages 0-6 Years

[1]**Hepatitis B vaccine (HepB).** *(Minimum age: birth)*
At birth:
- Administer monovalent HepB to all newborns before hospital discharge.
- If mother is hepatitis B surface antigen (HB_sAg)-positive, administer HepB and 0.5 mL of hepatitis B immune globulin (HBIG) within 12 hours of birth.
- If mother's HB_sAg status is unknown, administer HepB within 12 hours of birth. Determine mother's HB_sAg status as soon as possible and, if HB_sAg-positive, administer HBIG (no later than age 1 week).
After the birth dose:
- The HepB series should be completed with either monovalent HepB or a combination vaccine containing HepB. The second dose should be administered at age 1 or 2 months. Monovalent HepB vaccine should be used for doses administered before age 6 weeks. The final dose should be administered no earlier than age 24 weeks.
- Infants born to HB_sAg-positive mothers should be tested for HB_sAg and antibody to HB_sAg 1 to 2 months after completion of at least 3 doses of the HepB series, at age 9-18 months (generally at the next well-child visit).
- Administration of 4 doses of HepB to infants is permissible when combination vaccine containing HepB is administered after the birth dose. The fourth dose should be administered no earlier than age 24 weeks.

[2]**Rotavirus vaccine (RV).** *(Minimum age: 6 weeks)*

- Administer the first dose at age 6-14 weeks (maximum age: 14 weeks 6 days). Vaccination should not be initiated for infants aged 15 weeks 0 days or older.
- The maximum age for the final dose in the series is 8 months 0 days.
- If Rotarix® is administered at ages 2 and 4 months, a dose at 6 months is not indicated.

[3]**Diphtheria and tetanus toxoids and acellular pertussis vaccine (DTaP).** *(Minimum age: 6 weeks)*

- The fourth dose may be administered as early as age 12 months, provided ≥6 months have elapsed since the third dose.
- Administer the final dose in the series at age 4-6 years.

[4] ***Haemophilus influenzae* type b conjugate vaccine (Hib).** *(Minimum age: 6 weeks)*

- If PRP-OMP (PedvaxHIB® or ComVax® [HepB-Hib]) is administered at ages 2 and 4 months, a dose at age 6 months is not indicated.
- TriHiBit® (DTaP/Hib) and Hiberix® (PRP-T) should not be used for doses at ages 2, 4, or 6 months for the primary series but can be used as the final dose in children aged 12 months through 4 years.

[5]**Pneumococcal vaccine.** *(Minimum age: 6 weeks for pneumococcal conjugate vaccine [PCV]; 2 years for pneumococcal polysaccharide vaccine [PPSV])*

- PCV is recommended for all children aged <5 years. Administer 1 dose of PCV to all healthy children aged 24-59 months who are not completely vaccinated for their age.
- Administer PPSV 2 or more months after last dose of PCV to children aged ≥2 years with certain underlying medical conditions, including a cochlear implant. See *MMWR*, 1997, 46(RR-8).

[6]**Inactivated poliovirus vaccine (IPV).** *(Minimum age: 6 weeks)*

- The final dose in the series should be administered on or after the fourth birthday and ≥6 months following the previous dose.
- If 4 doses are administered prior to age 4 years a fifth dose should be administered at age 4-6 years. See *MMWR*, 2009, 58 (30):829–30.

[7]**Influenza vaccine (seasonal).** *(Minimum age: 6 months for trivalent inactivated influenza vaccine [TIV]; 2 years for live, attenuated influenza vaccine [LAIV])*

- Administer annually to children age 6 months through 18 years.
- For healthy children aged 2-6 years (ie, those who do not have underlying medical conditions that predispose them to influenza complications), either LAIV or TIV may be used, except LAIV should not be given to children aged 2-4 years who have had wheezing in the past 12 months.
- Children receiving TIV should receive 0.25 mL if aged 6-35 months or 0.5 mL if aged ≥3 years.
- Administer 2 doses (separated by ≥4 weeks) to children aged <9 years who are receiving influenza vaccine for the first time or who were vaccinated for the first time during the previous influenza season but only received 1 dose.
- For recommendations for use of influenza A (H1N1) 2009 monovalent vaccine see *MMWR*, 2009, 58(RR-10).

[8]**Measles, mumps, and rubella vaccine (MMR).** *(Minimum age: 12 months)*

- Administer the second dose routinely at age 4-6 years. However, the second dose may be administered before age 4, provided ≥28 days have elapsed since the first dose.

[9]**Varicella vaccine.** *(Minimum age: 12 months)*

- Administer the second dose at age 4-6 years. However, the second dose may be administered before age 4, provided ≥3 months have elapsed since the first dose.
- For children aged 12 months through 12 years the minimum interval between doses is 3 months. However, if the second dose was administered ≥28 days after the first dose, it can be accepted as valid.

[10]**Hepatitis A vaccine (HepA).** *(Minimum age: 12 months)*

- Administer to all children aged 1 year (ie, age 12-23 months). Administer 2 doses ≥6 months apart.
- Children not fully vaccinated by age 2 years can be vaccinated at subsequent visits.
- HepA also is recommended for older children who live in areas where vaccination programs target older children, who are at increased risk for infection, or for whom immunity against hepatitis A is desired.

[11]**Meningococcal vaccine.** *(Minimum age: 2 years for meningococcal conjugate vaccine [MCV4] and for meningococcal polysaccharide vaccine [MPSV4])*

- Administer MCV4 to children aged 2-10 years with persistent complement component deficiency, anatomic or functional asplenia, and certain other conditions placing them at high-risk.
- Administer MCV4 to children previously vaccinated with MCV4 or MPSV4 after 3 years if first dose administered at age 2-6 years. See *MMWR*, 2009, 58(37):1042–3.

The recommended immunization schedules for persons aged 0-18 years are approved by the Advisory Committee on Immunization Practices (**http://www.cdc.gov/vaccines/recs/acip**), the American Academy of Pediatrics (**http://www.aap.org**), and the American Academy of Family Physicians (**http://www.aafp.org**).

Recommended Immunization Schedule for Ages 7-18 Years
United States, 2010

Age ▶ Vaccine ▼	7-10 y	11-12 y	13-18 y
Tetanus, diphtheria, pertussis[1]		Tdap	Tdap
Human papillomavirus[2]	*See footnote 2*	HPV (3 doses)	HPV series
Meningococcal[3]	MCV	MCV	MCV
Influenza[4]		Influenza (yearly)	
Pneumococcal[5]		PPSV	
Hepatitis A[6]		HepA series	
Hepatitis B[7]		HepB series	
Inactivated poliovirus[8]		IPV series	
Measles, mumps, rubella[9]		MMR series	
Varicella[10]		Varicella series	

Range of recommended ages for all children except certain high-risk groups	Range of recommended ages for catch-up immunization	Range of recommended ages for certain high-risk groups

Note: For those who fall behind or start late, see also the Catch-up Immunization Schedule table.

This schedule includes recommendations in effect as of December 15, 2009. Any dose not administered at the recommended age should be administered at a subsequent visit, when indicated and feasible. The use of a combination vaccine generally is preferred over separate injections of its equivalent component vaccines. Considerations should include provider assessment, patient preference, and the potential for adverse events. Providers should consult the relevant Advisory Committee on Immunization Practices statement for detailed recommendations: **http://www.cdc.gov/vaccines/pubs/acip-list.htm**. Clinically significant adverse events that follow immunization should be reported to the Vaccine Adverse Event Reporting System (VAERS) at **http://www.vaers.hhs.gov** or by telephone, 800-822-7967.

Footnotes to Recommended Immunization Schedule for Ages 7-18 Years

[1]**Tetanus and diphtheria toxoids and acellular pertussis vaccine (Tdap).** *(Minimum age: 10 years for Boostrix® and 11 years for Adacel®)*
- Administer at age 11 or 12 years for those who have completed the recommended childhood DTP/DTaP vaccination series and have not received a tetanus and diphtheria toxoid (Td) booster dose.
- Persons aged 13-18 years who have not received Tdap should receive a dose.
- A 5-year interval from the last Td dose is encouraged when Tdap is used as a booster dose; however, a shorter interval may be used if pertussis immunity is needed.

[2]**Human papillomavirus vaccine (HPV).** *(Minimum age: 9 years)*
- Two HPV vaccines are licensed: A quadrivalent vaccine (HPV4) for the prevention of cervical, vaginal, and vulvar cancers (in females) and genital warts (in females and males), and a bivalent vaccine (HPV2) for the prevention of cervical cancers in females.
- HPV vaccines are most effective for both males and females when given before exposure to HPV through sexual contact.
- HPV4 or HPV2 is recommended for the prevention of cervical precancers and cancers in females.
- HPV4 is recommended for the prevention of cervical, vaginal, and vulvar precancers and cancers and genital warts in females.
- Administer the first dose to females at age 11 or 12 years.
- Administer the second dose 1-2 months after the first dose and the third dose 6 months after the first dose (≥24 weeks after the first dose).
- Administer the series to females at age 13-18 years if not previously vaccinated.
- HPV4 may be administered in a 3-dose series to males aged 9-18 years to reduce their likelihood of acquiring genital warts.

[3]**Meningococcal conjugate vaccine (MCV4).**

- Administer at age 11 or 12 years, or at age 13-18 years if not previously vaccinated.
- Administer to previously unvaccinated college freshmen living in a dormitory.
- Administer MCV4 to children aged 2-10 years with persistent complement component deficiency, anatomic or functional asplenia, or certain other conditions placing them at high risk.
- Administer to children previously vaccinated with MCV4 or MPSV4 who remain at increased risk after 3 years (if first dose administered at age 2-6 years) or after 5 years (if first dose administered at age ≥7 years). Persons whose only risk factor is living in on-campus housing are not recommended to receive an additional dose. See *MMWR*, 2009, 58(37):1042–3.

[4]**Influenza vaccine (seasonal).**

- Administer annually to children aged 6 months through 18 years.
- For healthy nonpregnant persons aged 7-18 years (ie, those who do not have underlying medical conditions that predispose them to influenza complications), either LAIV or TIV may be used.
- Administer 2 doses (separated by ≥4 weeks) to children aged <9 years who are receiving influenza vaccine for the first time or who were vaccinated for the first time during the previous influenza season but only received 1 dose.
- For recommendations for use of influenza A (H1N1) 2009 monovalent vaccine. See *MMWR*, 2009, 58(RR-10).

[5]**Pneumococcal polysaccharide vaccine (PPSV).**

- Administer to children with certain underlying medical conditions, including a cochlear implant. A single revaccination should be administered after 5 years to children with functional or anatomic asplenia or other immunocompromising condition. See *MMWR*, 1997, 46(RR-8).

[6]**Hepatitis A vaccine (HepA).**

- Administer 2 doses ≥6 months apart.
- HepA is recommended for children >23 months who live in areas where vaccination programs target older children, who are at increased risk of infection, or for whom immunity against hepatitis A is desired.

[7]**Hepatitis B vaccine (HepB).**

- Administer the 3-dose series to those not previously vaccinated.
- A 2-dose series (separated by ≥4 months) of adult formulation Recombivax HB® is licensed for children aged 11-15 years.

[8]**Inactivated poliovirus vaccine (IPV).**

- The final dose in the series should be administered on or after the fourth birthday and ≥6 months following the previous dose.
- If both OPV and IPV were administered as part of a series, a total of 4 doses should be administered, regardless of the child's current age.

[9]**Measles, mumps, and rubella vaccine (MMR).**

- If not previously vaccinated, administer 2 doses or the second dose for those who have received only 1 dose, with ≥28 days between doses.

[10]**Varicella vaccine.**

- For persons aged 7-18 years without evidence of immunity [see *MMWR*, 2007, 56(RR-4)], administer 2 doses if not previously vaccinated or the second dose if only 1 dose has been administered.
- For persons aged 7-12 years, the minimum interval between doses is 3 months. However, if the second dose was administered ≥28 days after the first dose, it can be accepted as valid.
- For persons aged ≥13 years, the minimum interval between doses is 28 days.

The recommended immunization schedules for persons age 0-18 years are approved by the Advisory Committee on Immunization Practices (**http://www.cdc.gov/vaccines/recs/acip**), the American Academy of Pediatrics (**http://www.aap.org**), and the American Academy of Family Physicians (**http://www.aafp.org**).

Catch-up Immunization Schedule for Persons Aged 4 Months - 18 Years Who Start Late or Who Are >1 Month Behind - United States, 2010

The table below provides catch-up schedules and minimum intervals between doses for children whose vaccinations have been delayed. A vaccine series does not need to be restarted, regardless of the time that has elapsed between doses. Use the section appropriate for the child's age.

Vaccine (Minimum Age for Dose 1)	Minimum Interval Between Doses			
	Dose 1 to Dose 2	Dose 2 to Dose 3	Dose 3 to Dose 4	Dose 4 to Dose 5
Catch-up Schedule for Persons Age 4 Months – 6 Years				
Hepatitis B[1] (birth)	4 weeks	8 weeks (and ≥16 weeks after 1st dose)		
Rotavirus[2] (6 wk)	4 weeks	4 weeks[2]		
Diphtheria, tetanus, pertussis[3] (6 wk)	4 weeks	4 weeks	6 months	6 months[3]

Vaccine (Minimum Age for Dose 1)	Minimum Interval Between Doses			
	Dose 1 to Dose 2	Dose 2 to Dose 3	Dose 3 to Dose 4	Dose 4 to Dose 5
Haemophilus influenzae type b[4] (6 wk)	**4 weeks** if 1st dose administered at age <12 months **8 weeks (as final dose)** if 1st dose administered at age 12-14 months **No further doses needed** if 1st dose administered at age ≥15 months	**4 weeks**[4] if current age <12 months **8 weeks (as final dose)**[4] if current age ≥12 months and 1st dose is administered <12 months and 2nd dose administered at age <15 months **No further doses needed** if previous dose administered at age ≥15 months	**8 weeks (as final dose)** This dose only necessary for children age 12-59 months who received 3 doses before age 12 months	
Pneumococcal[5] (6 wk)	**4 weeks** if 1st dose administered at age <12 months **8 weeks (as final dose for healthy children)** if 1st dose administered at age ≥12 months or current age 24-59 months **No further doses needed** for healthy children if 1st dose administered at age ≥24 months	**4 weeks** if current age <12 months **8 weeks (as final dose for healthy children)** if current age ≥12 months **No further doses needed** for healthy children if previous dose administered at age ≥24 months	**8 weeks (as final dose)** This dose only necessary for children age 12-59 months who received 3 doses before age 12 months or for high-risk children who received 3 doses at any age	
Inactivated poliovirus[6] (6 wk)	**4 weeks**	**4 weeks**	**6 months**	
Measles, mumps, rubella[7] (12 mo)	**4 weeks**			
Varicella[8] (12 mo)	**3 months**			
Hepatitits A[9] (12 mo)	**6 months**			
Catch-up Schedule for Persons Age 7-18 Years				
Tetanus, diphtheria/tetanus, diphtheria, pertussis[10] (7 y)	**4 weeks**	**4 weeks** if 1st dose administered at age <12 months **6 months** if 1st dose administered at age ≥12 months	**6 months** if 1st dose administered at age <12 months	
Human papillomavirus[11] (9 y)	**Routine dosing intervals are recommended**[11]			
Hepatitis A[9] (12 mo)	**6 months**			
Hepatitis B[1] (birth)	**4 weeks**	**8 weeks** (and ≥16 weeks after 1st dose)		
Inactivated poliovirus[6] (6 wk)	**4 weeks**	**4 weeks**	**6 months**	
Measles, mumps, rubella[7] (12 mo)	**4 weeks**			
Varicella[8] (12 mo)	**3 months** if the person is age <13 years **4 weeks** if the person is age ≥13 years			

Footnotes to Catch-up Immunization Schedule Table

[1]Hepatitis B vaccine (HepB).
- Administer the 3-dose series to those not previously vaccinated.
- A 2-dose series (separated by ≥4 months) of adult formulation of Recombivax HB® is licensed for children aged 11-15 years.

[2]Rotavirus vaccine (RV).
- The maximum age for the first dose is 14 weeks 6 days. Vaccination should not be initiated for infants aged ≥15 weeks 0 days.
- The maximum age for the final dose in the series is 8 months 0 days.
- If Rotarix® was administered for the first and second doses, a third dose is not indicated.

[3]Diphtheria and tetanus toxoids and acellular pertussis vaccine (DTaP).
- The fifth dose is not necessary if the fourth dose was administered at age ≥4 years.

4 *Haemophilus influenzae* type b conjugate (Hib).

- Hib vaccine is not generally recommended for persons aged ≥5 years. No efficacy data are available on which to base a recommendation concerning use of Hib vaccine for older children and adults. However, studies suggest good immunogenicity in persons who have sickle cell disease, leukemia, or HIV infection, or who have had a splenectomy; administering 1 dose of Hib vaccine to these persons who have not previously received Hib vaccine is not contraindicated.

- If the first 2 doses were PRP-OMP (PedvaxHIB® or ComVax®), and administered at age ≤11 months, the third (and final) dose should be administered at age 12-15 months and ≥8 weeks after the second dose.

- If first dose administered at age 7-11 months, administer second dose ≥4 weeks later and a final dose at age 12-15 months.

5 Pneumococcal vaccine.

- Administer 1 dose of pneumococcal conjugate vaccine (PCV) to all healthy children aged 24-59 months who have not received at least 1 dose of PCV on or after age 12 months.

- For children aged 24-59 months with underlying medical conditions, administer 1 dose of PCV if 3 doses were received previously or administer 2 doses of PCV ≥8 weeks apart if <3 doses were received previously.

- Administer pneumococcal polysaccharide vaccine (PPSV) to children aged ≥2 years with certain underlying medical conditions, including a cochlear implant, at ≥8 weeks after the last dose of PCV. See *MMWR*, 1997, 46(RR-8).

6 Inactivated poliovirus vaccine (IPV).

- The final dose in the series should be administered on or after the fourth birthday and ≥6 months following the previous dose.

- A fourth dose is not necessary if the third dose was administered at age ≥4 years and ≥6 months following the previous dose.

- In the first 6 months of life, minimum age and minimum intervals are only recommended if the person is at risk for imminent exposure to circulating poliovirus (ie, travel to a polio-endemic region or during an outbreak).

7 Measles, mumps, and rubella vaccine (MMR).

- Administer the second dose routinely at age 4-6 years. However, the second dose may be administered before age 4, provided ≥28 days have elapsed since the first dose.

- If not previously vaccinated, administer 2 doses with ≥28 days between the doses.

8 Varicella vaccine.

- Administer the second dose at age 4-6 years. However, the second dose may be administered before age 4, provided ≥3 months have elapsed since the first dose.

- For persons aged 12 months through 12 years, the minimum interval between doses is 3 months. However, if the second dose was administered ≥28 days after the first dose, it can be accepted as valid.

- For persons aged ≥13 years, the minimum interval between doses is 28 days.

9 Hepatitis A vaccine (HepA).

- HepA is recommended for children aged >23 months who live in areas where vaccination programs target older children, who are at increased risk for infection, or for whom immunity against hepatitis A is desired.

10 Tetanus and diphtheria toxoids vaccine (Td) and tetanus and diphtheria toxoids and acellular pertussis vaccine (Tdap).

- Doses of DTaP are counted as part of the Td/Tdap series.

- Tdap should be substituted for a single dose of Td in the catch-up series or as a booster for children aged 10-18 years; use Td for other doses.

11 Human papillomavirus (HPV).

- Administer the series to females at age 13-18 years if not previously vaccinated.

- Use recommended routine dosing intervals for series catch-up (ie, the second and third doses should be administered at 1-2 and 6 months after the first dose). The minimum interval between the first and second doses is 4 weeks. The minimum interval between the second and third doses is 12 weeks, and the third dose should be administered ≥24 weeks after the first dose.

Information about reporting reactions after immunization is available online at **http://www.vaers.hhs.gov** or by telephone, 800-822-7967. Suspected cases of vaccine-preventable diseases should be reported to the state or local health department. Additional information, including precautions and contraindications for immunization, is available from the National Center for Immunization and Respiratory Diseases at **http://www.cdc.gov/vaccines** or telephone, 800-CDC-INFO (800-232-4636).

Reference

"Recommended Immunization Schedules for Persons Aged 0-18 Years - United States, 2010," *MMWR*, 2010, 58(51&52):Q1-4.

Reporting Adverse Reactions

For information on reporting reactions following immunization, visit **www.vaers.hhs.gov** or call the 24-hour national toll-free information line **800-822-7967**. Report suspected cases of vaccine-preventable diseases to your state or local health department. For additional information including precautions and contraindications for immunization, visit the National Center for Immunization and Respiratory Diseases at **www.cdc.gov/ncird** or contact **800-CDC-INFO (800-232-4636)**.

Dose and Route of Administration for Selected Vaccines

Vaccine	Dose	Route
Diphtheria, tetanus, pertussis (DTaP, DT, Td, Tdap)	0.5 mL	I.M.
Diphtheria, tetanus, acellular pertussis, inactivated polio, hepatitis B vaccine (DTaP-IPV-HepB)	0.5 mL	I.M.
Diphtheria, tetanus, acellular pertussis, *Haemophilus influenzae* type b vaccine (DTaP-Hib)	0.5 mL	I.M.
Haemophilus influenzae type b (Hib)	0.5 mL	I.M.
Haemophilus influenzae type b – hepatitis B (Hib-HepB)	0.5 mL	I.M.
Hepatitis A (HepA)	≤18 y: 0.5 mL ≥19 y: 1 mL	I.M.
Hepatitis B (HepB)	≤19 y: 0.5 mL[1] ≥20 y: 1 mL	I.M.
HepA/HepB	≥18 y: 1 mL	I.M.
Influenza, live attenuated	0.5 mL	Intranasal spray
Influenza, trivalent inactivated	6-35 mo: 0.25 mL ≥3 y: 0.5 mL	I.M.
Measles, mumps, rubella	0.5 mL	SubQ
Measles, mumps, rubella, varicella	0.5 mL	SubQ
Meningococcal conjugate	0.5 mL	I.M.
Meningococcal polysaccharide	0.5 mL	SubQ
Pneumococcal conjugate	0.5 mL	I.M.
Pneumococcal polysaccharide	0.5 mL	I.M. or SubQ
Human papillomavirus	0.5 mL	I.M.
Polio, inactivated	0.5 mL	I.M. or SubQ
Rotavirus	2 mL	Oral
Varicella	0.5 mL	SubQ
Zoster	0.5 mL	SubQ

[1]Persons aged 11-15 years can be administered Recombivax HB® 1 mL (adult formulation) on a 2-dose schedule.

Adapted from Kroger AT, Atkinson WL, Marcuse EK, et al, "General Recommendations on Immunization: Recommendations of the Advisory Committee on Immunization Practices (ACIP)," *MMWR Recom Rep*, 2006, 55(RR-15):1-48.

Needle Length and Injection Site of Intramuscular Injections

Birth to 18 y		
Age	**Needle Length**	**Injection Site**
Newborn[1]	5/8" (16 mm)[2]	Anterolateral thigh
Infant 1-12 mo	1" (25 mm)	Anterolateral thigh
Toddler 1-2 y	1-1¼" (25-32 mm)	Anterolateral thigh[3]
	5/8"-1" (16-25 mm)	Deltoid muscle of the arm
Child/adolescent 3-18 y	5/8"-1" (16-25 mm)	Deltoid muscle of the arm[3]
	1-1¼" (25-32 mm)	Anterolateral thigh
Aged ≥19 y		
Sex / Weight	**Needle Length**	**Injection Site**
Male and female <60 kg (130 lbs)	1" (25 mm)[4]	Deltoid muscle of the arm
Female 60-90 kg (130-200 lbs)	1-1½" (25-38 mm)	
Male 60-118 kg (130-260 lbs)		
Female >90 kg (200 lbs)	1½" (38 mm)	
Male >118 kg (260 lbs)		

[1]Newborn = first 28 days of life.

[2]If skin stretched tight, subcutaneous tissues not bunched.

[3]Preferred site.

[4]Certain experts recommend a 5/8" (16 mm) needle for males and females who weigh <60 kg (130 lbs).

Adapted from Kroger AT, Atkinson WL, Marcuse EK, et al, "General Recommendations on Immunization: Recommendations of the Advisory Committee on Immunization Practices (ACIP)," *MMWR Recom Rep*, 2006, 55(RR-15):1-48.

Guidelines for Spacing of Live and Inactivated Antigens

Antigen Combination	Recommended Minimum Interval Between Doses
Two or more inactivated[1]	Can be administered simultaneously or at any interval between doses
Inactivated and live	Can be administered simultaneously or at any interval between doses
Two or more live intranasal or injectable[2]	4-week minimum interval, if not administered simultaneously

[1]Certain experts suggest a 1-month interval between tetanus toxoid, reduced diphtheria toxoid, and reduced acellular pertussis vaccine and quadrivalent meningococcal conjugate vaccine if they are not administered simultaneously.

[2]Live oral vaccines (eg, Ty21a typhoid vaccine and rotavirus vaccine) can be administered simultaneously or at any interval before or after inactivated or live injectable vaccines.

Adapted from Kroger AT, Atkinson WL, Marcuse EK, et al, "General Recommendations on Immunization: Recommendations of the Advisory Committee on Immunization Practices (ACIP)," *MMWR Recom Rep*, 2006, 55(RR-15):1-48.

Guidelines for Administering Antibody-Containing Products[1] and Vaccines

Simultaneous Administration

Combination	Recommended Minimum Interval Between Doses
Antibody-containing products and inactivated antigen	Can be administered simultaneously at different sites or at any time interval between doses.
Antibody-containing products and live antigen	Should not be administered simultaneously.[2] If simultaneous administration of measles-containing vaccine or varicella vaccine is unavoidable, administer at different sites and revaccinate or test for seroconversion after the recommended interval.

Nonsimultaneous Administration

Product Administered First	Second	Recommended Minimum Interval Between Doses
Antibody-containing products	Inactivated antigen	Not applicable
Inactivated antigen	Antibody-containing products	Not applicable
Antibody-containing products	Live antigen	Dose-related[2,3,4]
Live antigen	Antibody-containing products	2 weeks[2]

[1]Blood products containing substantial amounts of immunoglobulin include intramuscular and intravenous immune

[2]Yellow fever, oral Ty21a typhoid vaccine, and live-attenuated influenza vaccine are exceptions to these recommendations. These live-attenuated vaccines can be administered at any time before, after, or simultaneously with an antibody-containing product without substantially decreasing the antibody response.

[3]Rotavirus vaccine (RV) should be deferred for 6 weeks after receipt of an antibody-containing product if possible. However, if the 6-week deferral would cause the first dose of RV to be scheduled for age >13 weeks, a shorter deferral interval should be used to ensure the first dose of RV is administered no later than age 13 weeks.

[4]The duration of interference of antibody-containing products with the immune response to the measles component of measles-containing vaccine, and possibly varicella vaccine, is dose-related.

Adapted from Kroger AT, Atkinson WL, Marcuse EK, et al, "General Recommendations on Immunization: Recommendations of the Advisory Committee on Immunization Practices (ACIP)," *MMWR Recom Rep*, 2006, 55(RR-15):1-48.

Suggested Intervals Between Administration of Antibody-Containing Products for Different Indications and Measles-Containing Vaccine and Varicella-Containing Vaccine[1]

Product / Indication	Dose (including mg IgG/kg) body weight[1]	Recommended Interval Before Measles or Varicella-Containing Vaccine Administration (mo)
Respiratory syncytial virus immune globulin (IG) monoclonal antibody (Synagis™)[2]	I.M.: 15 mg/kg	None
Tetanus IG	I.M.: 250 units (10 mg IgG/kg)	3
Hepatitis A IG		
Contact prophylaxis	I.M.: 0.02 mL/kg (3.3 mg IgG/kg)	3
International travel	I.M.: 0.06 mL/kg (10 mg IgG/kg)	3
Hepatitis B IG	I.M.: 0.06 mL/kg (10 mg IgG/kg)	3
Rabies IG	I.M.: 20 IU/kg (22 mg IgG/kg)	4
Measles prophylaxis IG		
Standard (ie, nonimmunocompromised contact)	I.M.: 0.25 mL/kg (40 mg IgG/kg)	5
Immunocompromised contact	I.M.: 0.50 mL/kg (80 mg IgG/kg)	6
Blood transfusion		
Red blood cells (RBCs), washed	I.V.: 10 mL/kg (negligible IgG/kg)	None
RBCs, adenine-saline added	I.V.: 10 mL/kg (10 mg IgG/kg)	3
Packed RBCs (hematocrit 65%)[3]	I.V.: 10 mL/kg (60 mg IgG/kg)	6
Whole blood cells (hematocrit 35% to 50%)[3]	I.V.: 10 mL/kg (80-100 mg IgG/kg)	6
Plasma/platelet products	I.V.: 10 mL/kg (160 mg IgG/kg)	7
Cytomegalovirus intravenous immune globulin (IGIV)	150 mg/kg maximum	6
IGIV		
Replacement therapy for immune deficiencies[4]	I.V.: 300-400 mg/kg[4]	8
Immune thrombocytopenic purpura	I.V.: 400 mg/kg	8
Postexposure varicella prophylaxis[5]	I.V.: 400 mg/kg	8
Immune thrombocytopenic purpura	I.V.: 1000 mg/kg	10
Kawasaki disease	I.V.: 2 g/kg	11

[1]This table is not intended for determining the correct indications and dosages for using antibody-containing products. Unvaccinated persons might not be fully protected against measles during the entire recommended interval, and additional doses of immune globulin or measles vaccine might be indicated after measles exposure. Concentrations of measles antibody in an immune globulin preparation can vary by manufacturers lot. Rates of antibody clearance after receipt of an immune globulin preparation also might vary. Recommended intervals are extrapolated from an estimated half-life of 30 days for passively acquired antibody and an observed interference with the immune response to measles vaccine for 5 months after a dose of 80 mg IgG/kg.

[2]Contains antibody only to respiratory syncytial virus.

[3]Assumes a serum IgG concentration of 16 mg/mL.

[4]Measles and varicella vaccinations are recommended for children with asymptomatic or mildly symptomatic human immunodeficiency virus (HIV) infection but are contraindicated for persons with severe immunosuppression from HIV or any other immunosuppressive disorder.

[5]The investigational product VariZIG, similar to licensed VZIG, is a purified human immune globulin preparation made from plasma containing high levels of anti-varicella antibodies (immunoglobulin class G "IgG". When indicated, healthcare providers should make every effort to obtain and administer VariZIG. In situations in which administration of VariZIG does not appear possible within 96 hours of exposure, administration of immune globulin intravenous (IGIV) should be considered as an alternative. IGIV also should be administered within 96 hours of exposure. Although licensed IGIV preparations are known to contain antivaricella antibody titers, the titer of any specific lot of IGIV that might be available is uncertain because IGIV is not routinely tested for antivaricella antibodies. The recommended IGIV dose for postexposure prophylaxis of varicella is 400 mg/kg, administered once. For pregnant women who cannot receive VariZIG within 96 hours of exposure, clinicians can choose either to administer IGIV or closely monitor the women for signs and symptoms of varicella and institute treatment with acyclovir if illness occurs.

References
Atkinson WL, Pickering LK, Schwartz B, et al, "General Recommendations on Immunization: Recommendations of the Advisory Committee on Immunization Practices (ACIP) and the American Academy of Family Physicians (AAFP)," *MMWR Recom Rep*, 2002, 51(RR-2):1-35.

Kroger AT, Atkinson WL, Marcuse EK, et al, "General Recommendations on Immunization: Recommendations of the Advisory Committee on Immunization Practices (ACIP)," *MMWR Recom Rep*, 2006, 55(RR-15):1-48.

Passive Immunization Agents — Immune Globulins

Immune Globulin	Dosage		Route
Hepatitis B (H-BIG®)			I.M.
percutaneous inoculation	0.06 mL/kg/dose (within 24 hours) (5 mL max)		
perinatal	0.5 mL/dose (within 12 hours of birth)		
sexual exposure	0.06 mL/kg/dose (within 14 days of contact) (5 mL max)		
Immune globulin (IG)			I.M.[1]
hepatitis A prophylaxis	0.02 mL/kg/dose (as soon as possible or within 2 weeks after exposure) (postexposure prophylaxis)		
	<2 y:	0.06 mL/kg/dose (≥3 months or long-term exposure) repeat every 5 months with continuous exposure	
	≥2 y:	0.02 mL/kg (3- to 5-month exposure) may be given to travelers whose departure is imminent with hepatitis A vaccine 0.06 mL/kg (long-term exposure) and hepatitis A vaccine	
hepatitis B	0.06 mL/kg/dose (H-BIG® should be used)		
hepatitis C	0.06 mL/kg/dose (percutaneous exposure)		
measles[2]	0.25 mL/kg/dose (max: 15 mL/dose) (within 6 days of exposure) 0.5 mL/kg/dose (max: 15 mL/dose) (immunocompromised children)		
Rabies[3]	20 IU/kg/dose (within 3 days)		
Tetanus (serious, contaminated, wounds; <3 previous tetanus vaccine doses)	250-500 units/dose		I.M.
Varicella-zoster[4] (VZIG)	Within 48 hours but not later than 96 hours after exposure		I.M.[5]
	0-10 kg	125 units = 1 vial	
	10.1-20 kg	250 units = 2 vials	
	20.1-30 kg	375 units = 3 vials	
	30.1-40 kg	500 units = 4 vials	
	>40 kg	625 units = 5 vials	

[1]Deep I.M. in the gluteal region for large doses only. Deltoid muscle or the anterolateral aspect of the thigh are preferred sites for injection. No greater than 5 mL/site in adults or large children; 1-3 mL/site in small children and infants. Max: 20 mL at one time. Pregnant women and infants should receive a thimerosol-free preparation.

[2]IG prophylaxis may not be indicated in a patient who has received IGIV within 3 weeks of exposure.

[3]½ of dose used to infiltrate the wound with the remaining ½ of dose given I.M. Rabies immune globulin is not recommended in previously HDCV immunized patients.

[4]Infants born to women who develop varicella within 5 days before or 48 hours after delivery should receive 125 units I.M. as a single dose.

[5]No greater than 2.5 mL of VZIG/one injection site. Doses >2.5 mL should be divided and administered at different sites.

Vaccination of Persons With Primary and Secondary Immune Deficiencies

Category	Specific Immunodeficiency	Contraindicated Vaccines[1]	Risk-Specific Recommended Vaccines[1]	Effectiveness and Comments
Primary				
B-lymphocyte (humoral)	Severe antibody deficiencies (eg, X-linked agammaglobulinemia and common variable immunodeficiency)	Oral poliovirus (OPV)[2] Smallpox Live-attenuated influenza vaccine (LAIV) BCG Ty21a (live oral typhoid)	Pneumococcal Influenza (TIV) Consider measles and varicella vaccination	The effectiveness of any vaccine will be uncertain if it depends only on the humoral response; intravenous immune globulin interferes with the immune response to measles vaccine and possibly varicella vaccine.
	Less severe antibody deficiencies (eg, selective IgA deficiency and IgG subclass deficiency)	OPV[2] Other live-vaccines appear to be safe	Pneumococcal Influenza (TIV)	All vaccines probably effective; immune response may be attenuated.
T-lymphocyte (cell-mediated and humoral)	Complete defects (eg, severe combined immunodeficiency [SCID] disease, complete DiGeorge syndrome)	All live vaccines[3,4]	Pneumococcal Influenza (TIV)	Vaccines may be ineffective.
	Partial defects (eg, the majority of patients with DiGeorge syndrome, Wiskott-Aldrich syndrome, ataxia-telangiectasia)	All live vaccines[3,4]	Pneumococcal Meningococcal Haemophilus influenza type b (Hib) (if not administered in infancy) Influenza (TIV)	Effectiveness of any vaccine depends on degree of immune suppression.
Complement	Deficiency of early components (C1, C2, C3, and C4)	None	Pneumococcal Meningococcal Influenza (TIV)	All routine vaccines probably effective.
	Deficiency of late components (C5-C9) and C3, properdin, factor B	None	Pneumococcal Meningococcal Influenza (TIV)	All routine vaccines probably effective.
Phagocytic function	Chronic granulomatous disease, leukocyte adhesion defect, and myeloperoxidase deficiency	Live bacterial vaccines[3]	Pneumococcal[5] Influenza (TIV) (to decrease secondary bacterial infection)	All inactivated vaccines safe and probably effective. Live viral vaccines probably safe and effective.
Secondary				
	Human immunodeficiency virus/ acquired immunodeficiency syndrome (HIV/AIDS)	OPV Smallpox BCG LAIV Withhold MMR and varicella in severely immunocompromised persons	Influenza (TIV) Pneumococcal Consider Hib (if not administered in infancy) and meningococcal vaccination.	Measles, mumps, rubella (MMR, varicella, and all inactivated vaccines, including inactivated influenza, might be effective.[6]
	Malignant neoplasm, transplantation, immunosuppressive or radiation therapy	Live viral and bacterial, depending on immune status	Influenza (TIV) Pneumococcal	Effectiveness of any vaccine depends on degree of immune suppression.

Vaccination of Persons With Primary and Secondary Immune Deficiencies *continued*

Category	Specific Immunodeficiency	Contraindicated Vaccines[1]	Risk-Specific Recommended Vaccines[1]	Effectiveness and Comments
	Asplenia	None	Pneumococcal Meningococcal Hib (if not administered in infancy)	All routine vaccines probably effective.
	Chronic renal disease	LAIV	Pneumococcal Influenza (TIV) Hepatitis B	All routine vaccines probably effective.

[1]Other vaccines that are universally or routinely recommended should be administered if not contraindicated.

[2]OPV is no longer available for routine use in the United States.

[3]Live bacterial vaccines: BCG and Ty21a Salmonella typhi vaccine.

[4]Live viral vaccines: MMR, OPV, LAIV, yellow fever, and varicella, including MMRV and HZ vaccine, and vaccinia (smallpox). Smallpox vaccine is not recommended for children or the general public.

[5]Pneumococcal vaccine is not indicated for children with chronic granulomatous disease.

[6]HIV-infected children should receive IG after exposure to measles, and can receive varicella and measles vaccine if CD4+ lymphocyte count is >15%.

Adapted from Kroger AT, Atkinson WL, Marcuse EK, et al. "General Recommendations on Immunization: Recommendations of the Advisory Committee on Immunization Practices (ACIP)." *MMWR Recom Rep.* 2006, 55(RR-15):1-48.

Persons Who Should Receive Pre-exposure Hepatitis B Immunization

- All infants, children, and adolescents through 18 years of age

- Adults at high risk, including:
  - Intravenous drug abusers
  - Heterosexual persons who have had more than one sex partner in the previous 6 months and/or those with a recent episode of a sexually transmitted disease
  - Sexually active men who have sex with men
  - Household and sexual contacts of HB_sAg-positive persons
  - Persons with chronic liver disease
  - Persons wih HIV infection
  - Staff and residents of institutions for the developmentally disabled
  - Staff of nonresidential day care and school programs for developmentally disabled
  - Hemodialysis patients or patients with end stage renal disease
  - Healthcare workers and others with occupational risk of exposure to blood or blood-contaminated body fluid
  - International travelers to areas of high or intermediate HBV endemicity
  - Inmates of long-term correctional facilities

Adapted from Centers for Disease Control and Prevention, *Epidemiology and Prevention of Vaccine-Preventable Diseases*, 10th ed, 2nd printing, Atkinson W, Hambrosky J, McIntyre L, et al, eds, Washinton D.C.: Public Health Foundation, 2008.

Mast EE, Weinbaum CM, Fiore AE, et al, "A Comprehensive Immunization Strategy to Eliminate Transmission of Hepatitis B Virus Infection in the United States: Recommendations of the Advisory Committee on Immunization Practices (ACIP) Part II: Immunization of Adults," *MMWR Recomm Rep*, 2006, 55 (RR-16):1-33.

See Recommended Immunization Schedule for Ages 0-6 Years and 7-18 Years charts for recommended Hepatitis B immunization schedule.

RECOMMENDATIONS FOR TRAVELERS

Recommended Immunizations for Travelers to Developing Countries[1]

Immunizations	Length of Travel		
	Brief, <2 wk	Intermediate, 2 wk - 3 mo	Long-term Residential, >3 mo
Review and complete age-appropriate childhood schedule	+	+	+
• DTaP; poliovirus vaccine, and *H. influenzae* type b vaccine may be given at 4 wk intervals if necessary to complete the recommended schedule before departure			
• Measles: 2 additional doses given if younger than 12 mo of age at first dose			
• Varicella			
• Hepatitis B[2]			
Yellow fever[3]	+	+	+
Hepatitis A[4]	+	+	+
Typhoid fever[4]	±	+	+
Meningococcal disease[5]	±	±	±
Rabies[6]	±	+	+
Japanese encephalitis[3]	±	±	+

[1] + = recommended; ± = consider.

[2] If insufficient time to complete 6-month primary series, accelerated series can be given.

[3] For endemic regions, see *Health Information for International Travel* in *Red Book*®. For high-risk activities in areas experiencing outbreaks, vaccine is recommended even for brief travel.

[4] Indicated for travelers who will consume food and liquids in areas of poor sanitation.

[5] For endemic regions of Africa, during local epidemics, and travel to Saudi Arabia for the Hajj.

[6] Indicated for person with high risk of animal exposure, and for travelers to endemic countries.

Adapted from "Report of the Committee on Infectious Diseases," *2000 Red Book*®, 25th ed, 78.

Recommendations for Pre-exposure Immunoprophylaxis of Hepatitis A Virus Infection for Travelers[1]

Age (y)	Likely Exposure (mo)	Recommended Prophylaxis
<2	<3	IG 0.02 mL/kg[2]
	3-5	IG 0.06 mL/kg[2]
	Long-term	IG 0.06 mL/kg at departure and every 5 mo if exposure to HAV continues[2]
≥2	<3[3]	HAV vaccine[4,5] **or**
	3-5[3]	HAV vaccine[4,5] **or** IG 0.06 mL/kg[2]
	Long-term	HAV vaccine[4,5]

[1] IG = immune globulin; HAV = hepatitis A virus.

[2] IG should be administered deep into a large muscle mass. Ordinarily, no more than 5 mL should be administered in one site in an adult or large child; lesser amounts (maximum 3 mL) should be given to small children and infants.

[3] Vaccine is preferable, but IG is an acceptable alternative.

[4] To ensure protection in travelers whose departure is imminent, IG also may be given.

[5] Dose and schedule of hepatitis A vaccine as recommended according to age.

Adapted from "Report of the Committee on Infectious Diseases," *2006 Red Book*®, 27th ed, 329.

VACCINE INJURY TABLE

The Vaccine Injury Table makes it easier for some people to get compensation. The table lists and explains injuries/conditions that are presumed to be caused by vaccines. It also lists time periods in which the first symptom of these injuries/conditions must occur after receiving the vaccine. If the first symptom of these injuries/conditions occurs within the listed time periods, it is presumed that the vaccine was the cause of the injury or condition unless another cause is found. For example, if the patient received the tetanus vaccines and had a severe allergic reaction (anaphylaxis) within 4 hours after receiving the vaccine, then it is presumed that the tetanus vaccine caused the injury if no other cause is found.

If the injury/condition is not on the table or if the injury/condition did not occur within the time period on the table, it must be proven that the vaccine caused the injury/condition. Such proof must be based on medical records or opinion, which may include expert witness testimony.

National Childhood Vaccine Injury Act

Vaccine Injury Table

Vaccine		Adverse Event	Time Interval
Tetanus toxoid-containing vaccines (eg, DTaP, Tdap, DTP-Hib, DT, Td, TT)	A.	Anaphylaxis or anaphylactic shock	0-4 hours
	B.	Brachial neuritis	2-28 days
	C.	Any acute complication or sequela (including death) of above events	Not applicable
Pertussis antigen-containing vaccines (eg, DTaP, Tdap, DTP, P, DTP-Hib)	A.	Anaphylaxis or anaphylactic shock	0-4 hours
	B.	Encephalopathy (or encephalitis)	0-72 hours
	C.	Any acute complication or sequela (including death) of above events	Not applicable
Measles, mumps, and rubella virus-containing vaccines in any combination (eg, MMR, MR, M, R)	A.	Anaphylaxis or anaphylactic shock	0-4 hours
	B.	Encephalopathy (or encephalitis)	5-15 days
	C.	Any acute complication or sequela (including death) of above events	Not applicable
Rubella virus-containing vaccines (eg, MMR, MR, R)	A.	Chronic arthritis	7-42 days
	B.	Any acute complication or sequela (including death) of above events	Not applicable
Measles virus-containing vaccines (eg, MMR, MR, M)	A.	Thrombocytopenic purpura	7-30 days
	B.	Vaccine-strain measles viral infection in an immunodeficient recipient	0-6 months
	C.	Any acute complication or sequela (including death) of above events	Not applicable
Polio live virus-containing vaccines (OPV)	A.	Paralytic polio	
	•	In a nonimmunodeficient recipient	0-30 days
	•	In an immunodeficient recipient	0-6 months
	•	In a vaccine associated community case	Not applicable
	B.	Vaccine-strain polio viral infection	
	•	In a nonimmunodeficient recipient	0-30 days
	•	In an immunodeficient recipient	0-6 months
	•	In a vaccine associated community case	Not applicable
	C.	Any acute complication or sequela (including death) of above events	Not applicable
Polio inactivated-virus containing vaccines (eg, IPV)	A.	Anaphylaxis or anaphylactic shock	0-4 hours
	B.	Any acute complication or sequela (including death) of above events	Not applicable
Hepatitis B antigen-containing vaccines	A.	Anaphylaxis or anaphylactic shock	0-4 hours
	B.	Any acute complication or sequela (including death) of above events	Not applicable
Hemophilus influenzae (type b polysaccharide conjugate vaccines)	A.	No condition specified for compensation	Not applicable
Varicella vaccine	A.	No condition specified for compensation	Not applicable
Rotavirus vaccine	A.	No condition specified for compensation	Not applicable

National Childhood Vaccine Injury Act *(continued)*

Vaccine	Adverse Event	Time Interval
Pneumococcal conjugate vaccines	A. No condition specified for compensation	Not applicable
Any new vaccine recommended by the Centers for Disease Control and Prevention for routine administration to children, after publication by Secretary, HHS of a notice of coverage[1,2]	A. No condition specified for compensation	Not applicable

Note: Effective date: November 1, 2008.

[1]As of December 1, 2004, hepatitis A vaccines have been added to the Vaccine Injury Table under this category. As of July 1, 2005, trivalent influenza vaccines have been added to the table under this category. Trivalent influenza vaccines are given annually during the flu season either by needle and syringe or in a nasal spray. All influenza vaccines routinely administered in the U.S. are trivalent vaccines covered under this category.

[2]As of February 1, 2007, meningococcal (conjugate and polysaccharide) and human papillomavirus (HPV) vaccines have been added to the table under this category.

See *News* on the VICP website for more information. Avaliable at: http://www.hrsa.gov/vaccinecompensation.

Standards for Pediatric Immunization Practices

Standard 1.	Immunization services are readily available.
Standard 2.	There are no barriers or unnecessary prerequisites to the receipt of vaccines.
Standard 3.	Immunization services are available free or for a minimal fee.
Standard 4.	Providers utilize all clinical encounters to screen and, when indicated, immunize children.
Standard 5.	Providers educate parents and guardians about immunizations in general terms.
Standard 6.	Providers question parents or guardians about contraindications and, before immunizing a child, inform them in specific terms about the risks and benefits of the immunizations their child is to receive.
Standard 7.	Providers follow only true contraindications.
Standard 8.	Providers administer simultaneously all vaccine doses for which a child is eligible at the time of each visit.
Standard 9.	Providers use accurate and complete recording procedures.
Standard 10.	Providers co-schedule immunization appointments in conjunction with appointments for other child health services.
Standard 11.	Providers report adverse events following immunization promptly, accurately, and completely.
Standard 12.	Providers operate a tracking system.
Standard 13.	Providers adhere to appropriate procedures for vaccine management.
Standard 14.	Providers conduct semiannual audits to assess immunization coverage levels and to review immunization records in the patient populations they serve.
Standard 15.	Providers maintain up-to-date, easily retrievable medical protocols at all locations where vaccines are administered.
Standard 16.	Providers operate with patient-oriented and community-based approaches.
Standard 17.	Vaccines are administered by properly trained individuals.
Standard 18.	Providers receive ongoing education and training on current immunization recommendations.

Recommended by the National Vaccine Advisory Committee, April 1992.
Modified by the United States Public Health Service, 1993.
Endorsed by the American Academy of Pediatrics, May 1992.

The Standards represent the consensus of the National Vaccine Advisory Committee (NVAC) and of a broad group of medical and public health experts about what constitutes the most desirable immunization practices. It is recognized by the NVAC that not all of the current immunization practices of public and private providers are in compliance with the Standards. Nevertheless, the Standards are expected to be useful as a means of helping providers to identify needed changes, to obtain resources if necessary, and to actually implement the desirable immunization practices in the future.

MALARIA

Prevention of Malaria

Drug[1]	Adult Dosage	Pediatric Dosage
Chloroquine-Sensitive Areas[2]		
Chloroquine phosphate[3,4]	500 mg (300 mg base), once/week[5]	5 mg/kg base once/week, up to adult dose of 300 mg base[5]
Chloroquine-Resistant Areas[2]		
Mefloquine[4,6,7]	250 mg once/week[5]	<15 kg: 5 mg/kg[5] 15-19 kg: 1/4 tablet[5] 20-30 kg: 1/2 tablet[5] 31-45 kg: 3/4 tablet[5] >45 kg: 1 tablet[5]
or		
Doxycycline[4,8]	100 mg/d[9]	2 mg/kg/d, up to 100 mg/d[9]
or		
Atovaquone/proguanil[4,10]	250 mg/100 mg (1 tablet) daily[11]	11-20 kg: 62.5 mg/25 mg[10,11] 21-30 kg: 125 mg/50 mg[10,11] 31-40 kg: 187.5 mg/75 mg[10,11] >40 kg: 250 mg/100 mg[10,11]
Alternative:		
Primaquine[8,12,13] Chloroquine phosphate[3]	30 mg base daily 500 mg (300 mg base) once/week[5]	0.5 mg/kg base daily 5 mg/kg base once/week, up to adult dose of 300 mg base[5]
plus		
Proguanil[14]	200 mg once/day	<2 y: 50 mg once/day 2-6 y: 100 mg once/day 7-10 y: 150 mg once/day >10 y: 200 mg once/day

Footnotes to Prevention of Malaria table

[1]No drug regimen guarantees protection against malaria. If fever develops within a year (particularly within the first 2 months) after travel to malarious areas, travelers should be advised to seek medical attention. Insect repellents, insecticide-impregnated bed nets, and proper clothing are important adjuncts for malaria prophylaxis.

[2]Chloroquine-resistant *P. falciparum* occurs in all malarious areas except Central America west of the Panama Canal Zone, Mexico, Haiti, the Dominican Republic, and most of the Middle East (chloroquine resistance has been reported in Yemen, Oman, Saudi Arabia, and Iran).

[3]In pregnancy, chloroquine prophylaxis has been used extensively and safely.

[4]For prevention of attack after departure from areas where *P. vivax* and *P. ovale* are endemic, which includes almost all areas where malaria is found (except Haiti), some experts prescribe in addition primaquine phosphate 26.3 mg (15 mg base)/day or, for children, 0.3 mg base/kg/day during the last 2 weeks of prophylaxis. Others prefer to avoid the toxicity of primaquine and rely on surveillance to detect cases when they occur; particularly when exposure was limited or doubtful.

[5]Beginning 1-2 weeks before travel and continuing weekly for the duration of stay and for 4 weeks after leaving.

[6]In the U.S., a 250 mg tablet of mefloquine contains 228 mg mefloquine base. Outside the U.S., each 275 mg tablet contains 250 mg base.

[7]The pediatric dosage has not been approved by the FDA, and the drug has not been approved for use during pregnancy. However, it has been reported to be safe for prophylactic use during the second or third trimester of pregnancy and possibly during early pregnancy as well (CDC Health Information for International Travel, 2001-2003, 113; BL Smoak, Writer JV, Keep LW, et al, "The Effects of Inadvertent Exposure of Mefloquine Chemoprophylaxis on Pregnancy Outcomes and Infants of US Army Servicewomen," *J Infect Dis*, 1997, 176(3):831-3). Mefloquine is not recommended for patients with cardiac conduction abnormalities. Patients with a history of seizures or psychiatric disorders should avoid mefloquine (*Medical Letter*, 1990, 32:13). Resistance to mefloquine has been reported in some areas, such as Thailand; in these areas, doxycycline should be used for prophylaxis. In children <8 years of age, proguanil plus sulfisoxazole has been used (KN Suh and JS Keystone, *Infect Dis Clin Pract*, 1996, 5:541).

[8]An approved drug, but considered investigational for this condition by the U.S. Food and Drug Administration.

[9]Beginning 1-2 days before travel and continuing for the duration of stay and for 4 weeks after leaving. Use of tetracyclines is contraindicated in pregnancy and in children <8 years of age. Doxycycline can cause gastrointestinal disturbances, vaginal moniliasis, and photosensitivity reactions.

[10]Atovaquone plus proguanil is available as a fixed-dose combination tablet: adult tablets (250 mg atovaquone/100 mg proguanil, Malarone®) and pediatric tablets (62.5 mg atovaquone/25 mg proguanil, *Malarone Pediatric*). To enhance absorption, it should be taken within 45 minutes after eating (Looareesuwan S, Chulay JD, Canfield CJ, et al, "Malarone (Atovaquone and Proguanil Hydrochloride): A Review of Its Clinical Development for Treatment of Malaria. Malarone Clinical Trials Study Group," *Am J Trop Med Hyg*, 1999, 60(4):533-41). Although approved for once daily dosing, to decrease nausea and vomiting the dose for treatment is usually divided in two.

[11]Shanks GE et al, *Clin Infect Dis*, 1998, 27:494; Lell B, Luckner D, Ndjave M, et al, "Randomised Placebo-Controlled Study of Atovaquone Plus Proguanil for Malaria Prophylaxis in Children," *Lancet*, 1998, 351(9104):709-13. Beginning 1-2 days before travel and continuing for the duration of stay and for 1 week after leaving. In one study of malaria prophylaxis, atovaquone/proguanil was better tolerated than mefloquine in nonimmune travelers (Overbosch D, Schilthuis H, Bienzle U, et al, "Atovaquone-Proguanil Versus Mefloquine for Malaria Prophylaxis in Nonimmune Travelers: Results From a Randomized, Double-Blind Study," *Clin Infect Dis*, 2001, 33(7):1015-21).

[12]Primaquine phosphate can cause hemolytic anemia, especially in patients whose red cells are deficient in glucose-6-phosphate dehydrogenase. This deficiency is most common in African, Asian, and Mediterranean peoples. Patients should be screened for G6PD deficiency before treatment. Primaquine should not be used during pregnancy.

[13]Several studies have shown that daily primaquine, beginning 1 day before departure and continued until 7 days after leaving the malaria area, provides effective prophylaxis against chloroquine-resistant *P. falciparum* (Baird JK, Lacy MD, Basri H, et al, "Randomized, Parallel Placebo-Controlled Trial of Primaquine for Malaria Prophylaxis in Papua, Indonesia," *Clin Infect Dis*, 2001, 33(12):1990-7). Some studies have shown less efficacy against *P. vivax*. Nausea and abdominal pain can be diminished by taking with food.

[14]Proguanil (Paludrine – Wyeth Ayerst, Canada; AstraZeneca, United Kingdom), which is not available alone in the U.S.A. but is widely available in Canada and Europe, is recommended mainly for use in Africa south of the Sahara. Prophylaxis is recommended during exposure and for 4 weeks afterwards. Proguanil has been used in pregnancy without evidence of toxicity (Phillips-Howard PA and Wood D, "The Safety of Antimalarial Drugs in Pregnancy," *Drug Saf*, 1996, 14(3):131-45).

Adapted from "Report of the Committee on Infectious Diseases," *2003 Red Book®*, 26th ed, 760-1.

Malaria Treatment

Recommended Drug	Adult Dose[1,8]	Pediatric Dose[1,8] (Pediatric dose should NEVER exceed adult dose)	Region Infection Acquired
Uncomplicated Malaria / P. falciparum or Species Not Identified (If "species not identified" is subsequently diagnosed as P. vivax or P. ovale, see P. vivax and P. ovale (below) regarding treatment with primaquine)			
Chloroquine phosphate (Aralen® and generics)	600 mg base (= 1000 mg salt) P.O. immediately, followed by 300 mg base (= 500 mg salt) P.O. at 6, 24, and 48 hours. Total dose: 1500 mg base (= 2500 mg salt)	10 mg base/kg P.O. immediately, followed by 5 mg base/kg P.O. at 6, 24, and 48 hours. Total dose: 25 mg base/kg	**Chloroquine-sensitive** (Central America west of Panama Canal; Haiti; the Dominican Republic; and most of the Middle East)
2nd line alternative for treatment: Hydroxychloroquine (Plaquenil® and generics)	620 mg base (= 800 mg salt) P.O. immediately, followed by 310 mg base (= 400 mg salt) P.O. at 6, 24, and 48 hours. Total dose: 1550 mg base (= 2000 mg salt)	10 mg base/kg P.O. immediately, followed by 5 mg base/kg P.O. at 6, 24, and 48 hours. Total dose: 25 mg base/kg	
A. Quinine sulfate[2] plus one of the following: Doxycycline, tetracycline, or clindamycin	Quinine sulfate: 542 mg base (= 650 mg salt)[3] P.O. tid x 3-7 days. Doxycycline: 100 mg P.O. bid x 7 days. Tetracycline: 250 mg P.O. qid x 7 days. Clindamycin: 20 mg base/kg/day P.O. divided tid x 7 days	Quinine sulfate: 8.3 mg base/kg (= 10 mg salt/kg) P.O. tid x 3-7 days. Doxycycline[4]: 2.2 mg/kg P.O. every 12 hours x 7 days. Tetracycline[4]: 25 mg/kg/day P.O. divided qid x 7 days. Clindamycin: 20 mg base/kg/day P.O. divided tid x 7 days	**Chloroquine-resistant or unknown resistance** (All malarious regions except those specified as chloroquine-sensitive listed in the box above. Middle Eastern countries with chloroquine-resistant P. falciparum include Iran, Oman, Saudi Arabia, and Yemen. Of note, infections acquired in the Newly Independent States of the former Soviet Union and Korea to date have been uniformly caused by P. vivax and should therefore be treated as chloroquine-sensitive infections.)
B. Atovaquone-proguanil (Malarone®)[5]	Adult tab = 250 mg atovaquone/100 mg proguanil. 4 adult tabs P.O. qd x 3 days	**Adult tab = 250 mg atovaquone/100 mg proguanil. Peds tab = 62.5 mg atovaquone/25 mg proguanil.** 5-8 kg: 2 peds tabs P.O. qd x 3 d. 9-10 kg: 3 peds tabs P.O. qd x 3 d. 11-20 kg: 1 adult tab P.O. qd x 3 d. 21-30 kg: 2 adult tabs P.O. qd x 3 d. 31-40 kg: 3 adult tabs P.O. qd x 3 d. >40 kg: 4 adult tabs P.O. qd x 3 d	
C. Mefloquine (Lariam® and generics)[6]	684 mg base (= 750 mg salt) P.O. as initial dose, followed by 456 mg base (= 500 mg salt) P.O. given 6-12 hours after initial dose. Total dose = 1250 mg salt	13.7 mg base/kg (= 15 mg salt/kg) P.O. as initial dose, followed by 9.1 mg base/kg (= 10 mg salt/kg) P.O. given 6-12 hours after initial dose. Total dose = 25 mg salt/kg	
Uncomplicated Malaria / P. malariae			
Chloroquine phosphate	Treatment as above	Treatment as above	All regions
2nd line alternative for treatment: Hydroxychloroquine	Treatment as above	Treatment as above	
Uncomplicated Malaria / P. vivax or P. ovale			
Chloroquine phosphate plus primaquine phosphate[7]	Chloroquine phosphate: Treatment as above. Primaquine phosphate: 30 mg base P.O. qd x 14 days	Chloroquine phosphate: Treatment as above. Primaquine phosphate: 0.5 mg base/kg P.O. qd x 14 days	**All regions[8]** Note: For suspected chloroquine-resistant P. vivax, see row below
2nd line alternative for treatment: Hydroxychloroquine plus primaquine phosphate[7]	Hydroxychloroquine: Treatment as above. Primaquine phosphate: 30 mg base P.O. qd x 14 days	Hydroxychloroquine: Treatment as above. Primaquine phosphate: 30 mg base P.O. qd x 14 days	
Uncomplicated Malaria / P. vivax			
A. Quinine sulfate[2] plus either doxycycline or tetracycline plus primaquine phosphate[7]	Quinine sulfate: Treatment as above. Doxycycline or tetracycline: Treatment as above. Primaquine phosphate: Treatment as above	Quinine sulfate: Treatment as above. Doxycycline or tetracycline[4]: Treatment as above. Primaquine phosphate: Treatment as above	**Chloroquine-resistant[8]** (Papua New Guinea and Indonesia)
B. Mefloquine plus primaquine phosphate[7]	Mefloquine: Treatment as above. Primaquine phosphate: Treatment as above	Mefloquine: Treatment as above. Primaquine phosphate: Treatment as above	

Malaria Treatment *continued*

Recommended Drug	Adult Dose[1,8]	Pediatric Dose[1,8] (Pediatric dose should NEVER exceed adult dose)[9,10,11,12]	Region Infection Acquired
Uncomplicated Malaria: Alternatives for Pregnant Women[9,10,11,12]			
Chloroquine phosphate	Treatment as above	Not applicable	**Chloroquine-sensitive**[12] (See uncomplicated malaria sections above for chloroquine-sensitive *Plasmodium* species by region)
2nd line alternative for treatment: Hydroxychloroquine	Treatment as above	Not applicable	
Quinine sulfate[2] plus clindamycin	**Quinine sulfate:** Treatment as above **Clindamycin:** Treatment as above	Not applicable	**Chloroquine resistant *P. falciparum***[9,10,11] (See uncomplicated malaria sections above for regions with known chloroquine-resistant *P. falciparum*)
Quinine sulfate	650 mg[3] salt P.O. tid x 7 days	Not applicable	**Chloroquine-resistant *P. vivax***[9,10,11,12] (See uncomplicated malaria sections above for regions with chloroquine-resistant *P. vivax*)
Severe Malaria[13,14,15,16]			
Quinidine gluconate[14] plus one of the following: Doxycycline, tetracycline, or clindamycin	**Quinidine gluconate:** 6.25 mg base/kg (= 10 mg salt/kg) loading dose I.V. over 1-2 hours, then 0.0125 mg base/kg/min (= 0.02 mg salt/kg/min) continuous infusion for at least 24 hours. An alternative regimen is 15 mg base/kg (= 24 mg salt kg) loading dose I.V. infused over 4 hours, followed by 7.5 mg base/kg (= 12 mg salt/kg) infused over 4 hours every 8 hours, starting 8 hours after the loading dose (see package insert). Once parasite density <1% and patient can take oral medication, complete treatment with oral quinine, dose as above. Quinidine/quinine course = 7 days in Southeast Asia; = 3 days in Africa or South America. **Doxycycline:** Treatment as above. If patient not able to take oral medication, give 100 mg I.V. every 12 hours and then switch to oral doxycycline (as above) as soon as patient can take oral medication. For I.V. use, avoid rapid administration. Treatment course = 7 days. **Tetracycline:** Treatment as above **Clindamycin:** Treatment as above. If patient not able to take oral medication, give 10 mg base/kg loading dose I.V. followed by 5 mg base/kg I.V. every 8 hours. Switch to oral clindamycin (oral dose as above) as soon as patient can take oral medication. For I.V. use, avoid rapid administration. Treatment course = 7 days.	**Quinidine gluconate:** Same mg/kg dosing and recommendations as for adults. **Doxycycline[4]:** Treatment as above. If patient not able to take oral medication, may give I.V. For children <45 kg, give 2.2 mg/kg I.V. every 12 hours and then switch to oral doxycycline (dose as above) as soon as patient can take oral medication. For children ≥45 kg, use same dosing as for adults. For I.V. use, avoid rapid administration. Treatment course = 7 days. **Tetracycline[4]:** Treatment as above **Clindamycin:** Treatment as above. If patient not able to take oral medication, give 10 mg base/kg loading dose I.V. followed by 5 mg base/kg I.V. every 8 hours. Switch to oral clindamycin (oral dose as above) as soon as patient can take oral medication. For I.V. use, avoid rapid administration. Treatment course = 7 days.	**All regions**

Source: http://www.cdc.gov/malaria/diagnosis_treatment/tx_clinicians.htm

Footnotes to Malaria Treatment table

[1] **Note:** There are three options (A, B, or C) available for treatment of uncomplicated malaria caused by chloroquine-resistant *P. falciparum*. Options A and B are equally recommended. Because of a higher rate of severe neuropsychiatric reactions seen at treatment doses, we do not recommend option C (mefloquine) unless options A and B cannot be used. For option A, because there is more data on the efficacy of quinine in combination with doxycycline or tetracycline, these treatment combinations are generally preferred to quinine in combination with clindamycin.

[2] For infections acquired in Southeast Asia, quinine treatment should continue for 7 days. For infections acquired in Africa and South America, quinine treatment should continue for 3 days.

[3] U.S. manufactured quinine sulfate capsule is in a 324 mg dosage; therefore 2 capsules should be sufficient for adult dosing.

[4] Doxycycline and tetracycline are not indicated for use in children <8 years old. For children <8 years old with chloroquine-resistant *P. falciparum*, quinine (given alone for 7 days or given in combination with clindamycin) and atovaquone-proguanil are recommended treatment options; mefloquine can be considered if no other options are available. For children <8 years old with chloroquine-resistant *P. vivax*, quinine (given alone for 7 days) or mefloquine are recommended treatment options. If none of these treatment options are available or are not being tolerated and if the treatment benefits outweigh the risks, doxycycline or tetracycline may be given to children <8 years old.

[5] Give atovaquone-proguanil with food. If patient vomits within 30 minutes of taking a dose, then they should repeat the dose.

[6] Treatment with mefloquine is not recommended in persons who have acquired infections from the Southeast Asian region of Burma, Thailand, and Cambodia due to resistant strains.

[7] Primaquine is used to eradicate any hypnozoite forms that may remain dormant in the liver, and thus prevent relapses, in *P. vivax* and *P. ovale* infections. Because primaquine can cause hemolytic anemia in persons with G6PD deficiency, patients must be screened for G6PD deficiency prior to starting treatment with primaquine. For persons with borderline G6PD deficiency or as an alternate to the above regimen, primaquine may be given 45 mg orally one time per week for 8 weeks; consultation with an expert in infectious disease and/or tropical medicine is advised if this alternative regimen is considered in G6PD-deficient persons. Primaquine must not be used during pregnancy.

[8] **Note:** There are two options (A or B) available for treatment of uncomplicated malaria caused by chloroquine-resistant *P. vivax*. High treatment failure rates due to chloroquine-resistant *P. vivax* have been well documented in Papua New Guinea and Indonesia. Rare case reports of chloroquine-resistant *P. vivax* have also been documented in Burma (Myanmar), India, and Central and South America. Persons acquiring *P. vivax* infections outside of Papua New Guinea or Indonesia should be started on chloroquine. If the patient does not respond, the treatment should be changed to a chloroquine-resistant *P. vivax* regimen and CDC should be notified (Malaria Hotline number: (770) 488-7788 Monday-Friday, 8 AM to 4:30 PM EST or (770) 488-7100 after hours, weekends, and holidays). For treatment of chloroquine-resistant *P. vivax* infections, options A and B are equally recommended.

[9] For pregnant women diagnosed with uncomplicated malaria caused by chloroquine-resistant *P. falciparum* or chloroquine-resistant *P. vivax* infection, treatment with doxycycline or tetracycline is generally not indicated. However, doxycycline or tetracycline may be used in combination with quinine (as recommended for nonpregnant adults) if other treatment options are not available or are not being tolerated, and the benefit is judged to outweigh the risks.

[10] Because there are no adequate, well-controlled studies of atovaquone and/or proguanil hydrochloride in pregnant women, atovaquone-proguanil is generally not recommended for use in pregnant women. For pregnant women diagnosed with uncomplicated malaria caused by chloroquine-resistant *P. falciparum* infection, atovaquone-proguanil may be used if other treatment options are not available or are not being tolerated, and if the potential benefit is judged to outweigh the potential risks. There are no data on the efficacy of atovaquone-proguanil in the treatment of chloroquine-resistant *P. vivax* infections.

[11] Because of a possible association with mefloquine treatment during pregnancy and an increase in stillbirths, mefloquine is generally not recommended for treatment in pregnant women. However, mefloquine may be used if it is the only treatment option available and if the potential benefit is judged to outweigh the potential risks.

[12] For *P. vivax* and *P. ovale* infections, primaquine phosphate for radical treatment of hypnozoites should not be given during pregnancy. Pregnant patients with *P. vivax* and *P. ovale* infections should be maintained on chloroquine prophylaxis for the duration of their pregnancy. The chemoprophylactic dose of chloroquine phosphate is 300 mg base (= 500 mg salt) orally once per week. After delivery, pregnant patients who do not have G6PD deficiency should be treated with primaquine.

[13] Persons with a positive blood smear **or** history of recent possible exposure and no other recognized pathology who have one or more of the following clinical criteria (impaired consciousness/coma, severe normocytic anemia, renal failure, pulmonary edema, acute respiratory distress syndrome, circulatory shock, disseminated intravascular coagulation, spontaneous bleeding, acidosis, hemoglobinuria, jaundice, repeated generalized convulsions, and/or parasitemia of >5%) are considered to have manifestations of more severe disease. Severe malaria is practically always due to *P. falciparum*.

[14] Patients diagnosed with severe malaria should be treated aggressively with parenteral antimalarial therapy. Treatment with I.V. quinidine should be initiated as soon as possible after the diagnosis has been made. Patients with severe malaria should be given an intravenous loading dose of quinidine unless they have received >40 mg/kg of quinine in the preceding 48 hours or if they have received mefloquine within the preceding 12 hours. Consultation with a cardiologist and a physician with experience treating malaria is advised when treating malaria patients with quinidine. During administration of quinidine, blood pressure monitoring (for hypotension) and cardiac monitoring (for widening of the QRS complex and/or lengthening of the QT_c interval) should be monitored continuously and blood glucose (for hypoglycemia) should be monitored periodically. Cardiac complications, if severe, may warrant temporary discontinuation of the drug or slowing of the intravenous infusion.

[15] Consider exchange transfusion if the parasite density (ie, parasitemia) is >10% **or** if the patient has altered mental status, nonvolume overload pulmonary edema, or renal complications. The parasite density can be estimated by examining a monolayer of red blood cells (RBCs) on the thin smear under oil immersion magnification. The slide should be examined where the RBCs are more or less touching (approximately 400 RBCs per field). The parasite density can then be estimated from the percentage of infected RBCs and should be monitored every 12 hours. Exchange transfusion should be continued until the parasite density is <1% (usually requires 8-10 units). I.V. quinidine administration should not be delayed for an exchange transfusion and can be given concurrently throughout the exchange transfusion.

[16] Pregnant women diagnosed with severe malaria should be treated aggressively with parenteral antimalarial therapy.

CONTRAINDICATIONS AND PRECAUTIONS TO COMMONLY USED VACCINES

Vaccine	Contraindications	Precautions[1]	Vaccines Can Be Administered
General for all vaccines, including diphtheria and tetanus toxoids and acellular pertussis vaccine (DTaP); pediatric diphtheria-tetanus toxoid (DT); adult tetanus-diphtheria toxoid (Td); inactivated poliovirus vaccine (IPV); measles-mumps-rubella vaccine (MMR); *Haemophilus influenzae* type b vaccine (Hib); hepatitis A vaccine; hepatitis B vaccine; varicella vaccine; pneumococcal conjugate vaccine (PCV); influenza vaccine; and pneumococcal polysaccharide vaccine (PPV)	• Serious allergic reaction (eg, anaphylaxis) after a previous vaccine dose • Serious allergic reaction (eg, anaphylaxis) to a vaccine component	• Moderate or severe acute illnesses with or without a fever	• Mild acute illness with or without fever • Mild to moderate local reaction (ie, swelling, redness, soreness); low-grade or moderate fever after previous dose • Lack of previous physical examination in well-appearing person • Current antimicrobial therapy • Convalescent phase of illnesses • Premature birth (hepatitis B vaccine is an exception in certain circumstances)[2] • Recent exposure to an infectious disease • History of penicillin allergy, other nonvaccine allergies, receiving allergen extract immunotherapy • Temperature <40.5°C, fussiness or mild drowsiness after a previous dose of diphtheria toxoid-tetanus toxoid-pertussis vaccine (DTP)/DTaP • Family history of seizures[3] • Family history of sudden infant death syndrome • Family history of an adverse event after DTP or DTaP administration • Stable neurologic conditions (eg, cerebral palsy, well-controlled convulsions, developmental delay)
DTaP	• Severe allergic reaction after a previous dose or to a vaccine component • Encephalopathy (eg, coma, decreased level of consciousness, prolonged seizures) within 7 days of administration of previous dose of DTP or DTaP • Progressive neurologic disorder, including infantile spasms, uncontrolled epilepsy, progressive encephalopathy; defer DTaP until neurologic status clarified and stabilized	• Fever >40.5°C ≤48 hours after vaccination with a previous dose of DTP or DTaP • Collapse or shock-like state (ie, hypotonic hyporesponsive episode) ≤48 hours after receiving a previous dose of DTP/DTaP • Seizure ≤3 days of receiving a previous dose of DTP/DTaP[3] • Persistent, inconsolable crying lasting ≥3 hours, ≤48 hours after receiving a previous dose of DTP/DTaP • Moderate or severe acute illness with or without fever	Same as above
DT, Td	• Severe allergic reaction after a previous dose or to a vaccine component	• Guillain-Barré syndrome ≤6 weeks after previous dose of tetanus toxoid-containing vaccine • Moderate or severe acute illness with or without fever	Same as above
IPV	• Severe allergic reaction to previous dose or vaccine component	• Pregnancy • Moderate or severe acute illness with or without fever	—
MMR[4]	• Severe allergic reaction after a previous dose or to a vaccine component • Pregnancy • Known severe immunodeficiency (eg, hematologic and solid tumors; congenital immunodeficiency; long-term immunosuppressive therapy, or severely symptomatic human immunodeficiency virus [HIV] infection)	• Recent (≤11 months) receipt of antibody-containing blood product (specific interval depends on product) • History of thrombocytopenia or thrombocytopenic purpura • Moderate or severe acute illness with or without fever	• Positive tuberculin skin test • Simultaneous TB skin testing[6] • Breast-feeding • Pregnancy of recipient's mother or other close or household contact • Recipient is child-bearing-age female • Immunodeficient family member or household contact • Asymptomatic or mildly symptomatic HIV infection • Allergy to eggs

Vaccine	Contraindications	Precautions[1]	Vaccines Can Be Administered
Hib	• Severe allergic reaction after a previous dose or to a vaccine component • Age <6 weeks	• Moderate or severe acute illness with or without fever	—
Hepatitis B	• Severe allergic reaction after a previous dose or to a vaccine component	• Infant weighing <2000 g[2] • Moderate or severe acute illness with or without fever	• Pregnancy • Autoimmune disease (eg, systemic lupus erythematosis or rheumatoid arthritis)
Hepatitis A	• Severe allergic reaction after a previous dose or to a vaccine component	• Pregnancy • Moderate or severe acute illness with or without fever	
Varicella	• Severe allergic reaction after a previous dose or to a vaccine component • Substantial suppression of cellular immunity • Pregnancy	• Recent (≤11 months) receipt of antibody containing blood product (specific interval depends on product) • Moderate or severe acute illness with or without fever	• Pregnancy of recipient's mother or other close or household contact • Immunodeficient family member or household contact[7] • Asymptomatic or mildly symptomatic HIV infection • Humoral immunodeficiency (eg, agammaglobulinemia)
PCV	• Severe allergic reaction after a previous dose or to a vaccine component	• Moderate or severe acute illness with or without fever	—
Influenza	• Severe allergic reaction to previous dose or vaccine component, including egg protein	• Moderate or severe acute illness with or without fever	• Nonsevere (eg, contact) allergy to latex or thimerosal • Concurrent administration of Coumadin® or aminophylline
PPV	• Severe allergic reaction after a previous dose or to a vaccine component	• Moderate or severe acute illness with or without fever	—

[1]Events or conditions listed as precautions should be reviewed carefully. Benefits and risks of administering a specific vaccine to a person under these circumstances should be considered. If the risk from the vaccine is believed to outweigh the benefit, the vaccine should not be administered. If the benefit of vaccination is believed to outweigh the risk, the vaccine should be administered. Whether and when to administer DTaP to children with proven or suspected underlying neurologic disorders should be decided on a case-by-case basis.

[2]Hepatitis B vaccination should be deferred for infants weighing <2000 g if the mother is documented to be hepatitis B surface antigen (Hb_sAg)-negative at the time of the infant's birth. Vaccination can commence at chronological age 1 month. For infants born to Hb_sAg-positive women, hepatitis B immunoglobulin and hepatitis B vaccine should be administered at or soon after birth regardless of weight.

[3]Acetaminophen or other appropriate antipyretic can be administered to children with a personal or family history of seizures at the time of DTaP vaccination and every 4-6 hours for 24 hours thereafter to reduce the possibility of postvaccination fever (source: American Academy of Pediatrics. "Guide to Contraindications and Precautions to Immunizations, 2009," 2009 Red Book® Report of the Committee on Infectious Diseases, 28th ed, Appendix VI, Pickering LK, ed, Elk Grove Village, IL: American Academy of Pediatrics, 2009).

[4]MMR and varicella vaccines can be administered on the same day. If not administered on the same day, these vaccines should be separated by ≥28 days.

[5]Substantially immunosuppressive steroid dose is considered to be ≥2 weeks of daily receipt of 20 mg or 2 mg/kg body weight of prednisone or equivalent.

[6]Measles vaccination can suppress tuberculin reactivity temporarily. Measles-containing vaccine can be administered on the same day as tuberculin skin testing. If testing cannot be performed until after the day of MMR vaccination, the test should be postponed for ≥4 weeks after the vaccination. If an urgent need exists to skin test, do so with the understanding that reactivity might be reduced by the vaccine.

[7]If a vaccine experiences a presumed vaccine-related rash 7-25 days after vaccination, avoid direct contact with immunocompromised persons for the duration of the rash.

Adapted from "Recommendations and Reports," MMWR Morb Mortal Wkly Rep, 2002, 51(RR-2):9-10.

SKIN TESTS FOR DELAYED HYPERSENSITIVITY

Skin tests for delayed hypersensitivity are used diagnostically to assess previous infection (ie, PPD, histoplasmin, and coccidioidin) or used to evaluate cellular immune function by testing for anergy (ie, mumps, *Candida*, tetanus toxoid, trichophyton, PPD). Anergy, a defect in cell-mediated immunity, is characterized by a depressed response or lack of response to skin testing with injected antigens. Anergy has been associated with congenital and acquired immunodeficiencies, and malnutrition.

Candida 1:100

Dose = 0.1 mL intradermally (30% of children younger than 18 months of age and 50% older than 18 months of age respond)

Can be used as a control antigen

Histoplasmin 1:100

Dose = 0.1 mL intradermally (yeast derived)

Mumps 40 cfu per mL

Dose = 0.1 mL intradermally (contraindicated in patients allergic to eggs, egg products, or thimerosal)

Purified Protein Derivative 5 TU (PPD[1] Mantoux Tuberculin)

Screening for tuberculosis:

Children who have no risk factors but who reside in high-prevalence regions: skin test at 4-6 years and 11-16 years of age

Children exposed to HIV-infected individuals, homeless, residents of nursing homes, institutionalized adolescents, users of illicit drugs, incarcerated adolescents and migrant farm workers: skin test every 2-3 years

Children at high risk (children infected with HIV, incarcerated adolescents): annual skin testing

Dose = 0.1 mL intradermally

Definition of positive Mantoux skin test (regardless of previous BCG administration):

Reaction ≥5 mm for high-risk group (children in close contact with known or suspected infectious cases of tuberculosis; children suspected to have disease based on clinical and/or roentgenographic evidence; and children with underlying host factors (immunosuppressive conditions, receiving immunosuppressive therapy, and HIV infection).

Reaction ≥10 mm for children <4 years; those with medical diseases who are at increased risk for dissemination or for those at increased risk because of environmental exposure.

Reaction ≥15 mm for children ≥4 years of age including those with no risk factors.

[1]PPD 1 TU (first strength) is only used in individuals suspected of being highly sensitive. PPD 250 TU (second strength) is used only for individuals who fail to respond to a previous injection of 5 TU, or anergic patients in whom TB is suspected.

Tetanus Toxoid 1:5

Dose = 0.1 mL intradermally (29% of children younger than 2 years of age and 78% older than 2 years of age respond if they have received 3 immunizing doses)

Can be used as a control antigen.

Tine Test

Indication: survey and screen for exposure to tuberculosis (grasp forearm firmly; stretch the skin of the volar surface tightly; apply the tines to the selected site; press for at least one second so that a circular halo impression is left on the skin)

General Information

1. Intradermal skin tests should be injected in the flexor surface of the forearm.
2. A pale wheal 6-10 mm in diameter should form over the needle tip as soon as the injection is administered. If no bleb forms, the injection must be repeated.
3. Space skin tests at least 2 inches apart to prevent reactions from overlapping.
4. Read skin tests for diameter of induration and presence of erythema at 24, 48, and 72 hours. Reactions occurring before 24 hours are indicative of an immediate rather than a delayed hypersensitivity reaction.
5. False-negative results may occur in patients with malnutrition, viral infections, febrile illnesses, immunodeficiency disorders, severe disseminated infections, uremia, patients who have received immunosuppressive therapy (steroids, antineoplastic agents), patients who have received a recent live attenuated virus vaccine (MMR, measles).
6. False-positive results may occur in patients sensitive to ingredients in the skin test solution such as thimerosal; cross-sensitivity between similar antigens; or with improper interpretation of skin test.
7. Side effects are pain, blisters, extensive erythema and necrosis at the injection site.
   Emergency equipment and epinephrine should be readily available to treat severe allergic reactions that may occur.

Recommended Interpretation of Skin Test Reactions

Reaction	Local Reaction	
	After Intradermal Injections of Antigens	**After Dinitrochlorobenzene**
1+	Erythema >10 mm and/or induration >1-5 mm	Erythema and/or induration covering <1/2 area of dosing site
2+	Induration 6-10 mm	Induration covering >1/2 area of dose site
3+	Induration 11-20 mm	Vesiculation and induration at dose site or spontaneous flare at days 7-14 at the site
4+	Induration >20 mm	Bulla or ulceration at dose site or spontaneous flare at days 7-14 at the site

References

American Academy of Pediatrics Committee on Infectious Diseases, "Screening for Tuberculosis in Infants and Children," *Pediatrics*, 1994, 93(1):131-4.
American Academy of Pediatrics Committee on Infectious Diseases, "Update on Tuberculosis Skin Testing of Children," *Pediatrics*, 1996, 97(2):282-4.

MANAGEMENT OF HEALTHCARE WORKER EXPOSURES TO HBV, HCV, AND HIV

Factors to Consider in Assessing the Need for Follow-up of Occupational Exposures

- **Type of exposure**
  - Percutaneous injury
  - Mucous membrane exposure
  - Nonintact skin exposure
  - Bites resulting in blood exposure to either person involved
- **Type and amount of fluid/tissue**
  - Blood
  - Fluids containing blood
  - Potentially infectious fluid or tissue (semen; vaginal secretions; and cerebrospinal, synovial, pleural, peritoneal, pericardial, and amniotic fluids)
  - Direct contact with concentrated virus
- **Infectious status of source**
  - Presence of HB_sAg
  - Presence of HCV antibody
  - Presence of HIV antibody
- **Susceptibility of exposed person**
  - Hepatitis B vaccine and vaccine response status
  - HBV, HCV, HIV immune status

Evaluation of Occupational Exposure Sources

Known sources

- Test known sources for HB_sAg, anti-HCV, and HIV antibody
  - Direct virus assays for routine screening of source patients are **not** recommended
  - Consider using a rapid HIV-antibody test
  - If the source person is **not** infected with a blood-borne pathogen, baseline testing or further follow-up of the exposed person is **not** necessary
- For sources whose infection status remains unknown (eg, the source person refuses testing), consider medical diagnoses, clinical symptoms, and history of risk behaviors
- Do not test discarded needles for blood-borne pathogens

Unknown sources

- For unknown sources, evaluate the likelihood of exposure to a source at high risk for infection
  - Consider the likelihood of blood-borne pathogen infection among patients in the exposure setting

Recommended Postexposure Prophylaxis for Exposure to Hepatitis B Virus

Vaccination and Antibody Response Status of Exposed Workers[1]	Treatment		
	Source HB$_s$Ag[2]-Positive	Source HB$_s$Ag[2]-Negative	Source Unknown or Not Available for Testing
Unvaccinated	HBIG[3] x 1 and initiate HB vaccine series[4]	Initiate HB vaccine series	Initiate HB vaccine series
Previously vaccinated			
Known responder[5]	No treatment	No treatment	No treatment
Known nonresponder[6]	HBIG[3] x 1 and initiate revaccination or HBIG x 2[7]	No treatment	If known high risk source, treat as if source was HB$_s$Ag-positive
Antibody response unknown	Test exposed person for anti-HB$_s$[8] 1. If adequate,[5] no treatment is necessary 2. If inadequate,[6] administer HBIG[3] x 1 and vaccine booster	No treatment	Test exposed person for anti-HB$_s$ 1. If adequate,[4] no treatment is necessary 2. If inadequate,[4] administer vaccine booster and recheck titer in 1-2 months

[1]Persons who have previously been infected with HBV are immune to reinfection and do not require postexposure prophylaxis.

[2]Hepatitis B surface antigen.

[3]Hepatitis B immune globulin; dose is 0.06 mL/kg intramuscularly.

[4]Hepatitis B vaccine.

[5]A responder is a person with adequate levels of serum antibody to HB$_s$Ag (ie, anti-HB$_s$ ≥10 mIU/mL).

[6]A nonresponder is a person with inadequate response to vaccination (ie, serum anti-HB$_s$ <10 mIU/mL).

[7]The option of giving one dose of HBIG and reinitiating the vaccine series is preferred for nonresponders who have not completed a second 3-dose vaccine series. For persons who previously completed a second vaccine series but failed to respond, two doses of HBIG are preferred.

[8]Antibody to HB$_s$Ag.

Recommended HIV Postexposure Prophylaxis (PEP) for Percutaneous Injuries

Exposure Type	HIV-Positive Class 1[1]	HIV-Positive Class 2[1]	Infection Status of Source		HIV-Negative
			Source of Unknown HIV Status[2]	Unknown Source[3]	
Less severe[4]	Recommend basic 2-drug PEP	Recommend expanded ≥3-drug PEP	Generally, no PEP warranted; however, consider basic 2-drug PEP[5] for source with HIV risk factors[6]	Generally, no PEP warranted; however, consider basic 2-drug PEP[5] in settings in which exposure to HIV-infected persons is likely	No PEP warranted
More severe[7]	Recommend expanded 3-drug PEP	Recommend expanded ≥3-drug PEP	Generally, no PEP warranted; however, consider basic 2-drug PEP[5] for source with HIV risk factors[6]	Generally, no PEP warranted; however, consider basic 2-drug PEP[5] in settings in which exposure to HIV-infected persons is likely	No PEP warranted

[1]HIV-positive, class 1 - asymptomatic HIV infection or known low viral load (eg, <1500 ribonucleic acid copies/mL). HIV-positive, class 2 – symptomatic HIV infection, AIDS, acute seroconversion, or known high viral load. If drug resistance is a concern, obtain expert consultation. Initiation of PEP should not be delayed pending expert consultation, and, because expert consultation alone cannot substitute for face-to-face counseling, resources should be available to provide immediate evaluation and follow-up care for all exposures.

[2]For example, deceased source person with no samples available for HIV testing.

[3]For example, a needle from a sharps disposal container.

[4]For example, solid needle or superficial injury.

[5]The recommendation "consider PEP" indicates that PEP is optional; a decision to initiate PEP should be based on a discussion between the exposed person and the treating clinician regarding the risk versus benefits of PEP.

[6]If PEP is offered and administered and the source is later determined to be HIV-negative, PEP should be discontinued.

[7]For example, large-bore hollow needle, deep puncture, visible blood on device, or needle used in patient's artery or vein.

Recommended HIV Postexposure Prophylaxis (PEP) for Mucous Membrane Exposures and Nonintact Skin[1] Exposures

Exposure Type		Infection Status of Source			
	HIV-Positive Class 1[2]	HIV-Positive Class 2[2]	Source of Unknown HIV Status[3]	Unknown Source[4]	HIV-Negative
Small volume[5]	Consider basic 2-drug PEP[6]	Recommend basic 2-drug PEP	Generally, no PEP warranted[7]	Generally, no PEP warranted	No PEP warranted
Large volume[8]	Recommend basic 2-drug PEP	Recommend expanded ≥3-drug PEP	Generally, no PEP warranted; however, consider basic 2-drug PEP[6] for source with HIV risk factors[7]	Generally, no PEP warranted; however, consider basic 2-drug PEP[6] in settings in which exposure to HIV-infected persons is likely	No PEP warranted

[1]For skin exposures, follow-up is indicated only if evidence exists of compromised skin integrity (eg, dermatitis, abrasion, or open wound).

[2]HIV-positive, class 1 – asymptomatic HIV infection or known low viral load (eg, <1500 ribonucleic acid copies/mL). HIV-positive, class 2 – symptomatic HIV infection, AIDS, acute seroconversion, or known high viral load. If drug resistance is a concern, obtain expert consultation. Initiation of PEP should not be delayed pending expert consultation, and, because expert consultation alone cannot substitute for face-to-face counseling, resources should be available to provide immediate evaluation and follow-up care for all exposures.

[3]For example, deceased source person with no samples available for HIV testing.

[4]For example, splash from inappropriately disposed blood.

[5]For example, a few drops.

[6]The recommendation "consider PEP" indicates that PEP is optional; a decision to initiate PEP should be based on a discussion between the exposed person and the treating clinician regarding the risks versus benefits of PEP.

[7]If PEP is offered and administered and the source is later determined to be HIV-negative, PEP should be discontinued.

[8]For example, a major blood splash.

Situations for Which Expert[1] Consultation for HIV Postexposure Prophylaxis Is Advised

- **Delayed (ie, later than 24-36 hours) exposure report**

  - The interval after which there is no benefit from postexposure prophylaxis (PEP) is undefined

- **Unknown source (eg, needle in sharps disposal container or laundry)**

  - Decide use of PEP on a case-by-case basis
  - Consider the severity of the exposure and the epidemiologic likelihood of HIV exposure
  - Do not test needles or sharp instruments for HIV

- **Known or suspected pregnancy in the exposed person**

  - Does not preclude the use of optimal PEP regimens
  - Do not deny PEP solely on the basis of pregnancy

- **Breast-feeding in the exposed person**

  - Use of optimal PEP regimen not precluded
  - PEP should not be denied solely on the basis of breast-feeding

- **Resistance of the source virus to antiretroviral agents**

  - Influence of drug resistance on transmission risk is unknown
  - Selection of drugs to which the source person's virus is unlikely to be resistant is recommended, if the source person's virus is unknown or suspected to be resistant to ≥1 of the drugs considered for the PEP regimen
  - Resistance testing of the source person's virus at the time of the exposure is not recommended
  - Initiation of PEP not to be delayed while awaiting results of resistance testing

- **Toxicity of the initial PEP regimen**

  - Adverse symptoms, such as nausea and diarrhea, are common with PEP
  - Symptoms can often be managed without changing the PEP regimen by prescribing antimotility and/or antiemetic agents
  - Modification of dose intervals (ie, administering a lower dose of drug more frequently throughout the day, as recommended by the manufacturer), in other situations, might help alleviate symptoms

[1]Local experts and/or the National Clinicians' Postexposure Prophylaxis Hotline (PEPline 1-888-448-4911).

Occupational Exposure Management Resources

National Clinicians' Postexposure Prophylaxis Hotline (PEPline) Run by University of California-San Francisco/San Francisco General Hospital staff; supported by the Health Resources and Services Administration Ryan White CARE Act, HIV/AIDS Bureau, AIDS Education and Training Centers, and CDC	Phone: (888) 448-4911 Internet: http://www.ucsf.edu/hivcntr
Needlestick! A website to help clinicians manage and document occupational blood and body fluid exposures. Developed and maintained by the University of California, Los Angeles (UCLA), Emergency Medicine Center, UCLA School of Medicine, and funded in part by CDC and the Agency for Healthcare Research and Quality.	Internet: http://www.needlestick.mednet.ucla.edu
Hepatitis Hotline	Phone: (888) 443-7232 Internet: http://www.cdc.gov/hepatitis
Reporting to CDC: Occupationally acquired HIV infections and failures of PEP	Phone: (800) 893-0485
HIV Antiretroviral Pregnancy Registry	Phone: (800) 258-4263 Fax: (800) 800-1052 Address: 1410 Commonwealth Drive, Suite 215 Wilmington, NC 28405 Internet: http://www.glaxowellcome.com/preg_reg/antiretroviral
Food and Drug Administration Report unusual or severe toxicity to antiretroviral agents	Phone: (800) 332-1088 Address: MedWatch HF-2, FDA 5600 Fishers Lane Rockville, MD 20857 Internet: http://www.fda.gov/medwatch
HIV / AIDS Treatment Information Service	Internet: http://www.aidsinfo.nih.gov

Management of Occupational Blood Exposures

Provide immediate care to the exposure site
- Wash wounds and skin with soap and water
- Flush mucous membranes with water

Determine risk associated with exposure by:
- Type of fluid (eg, blood, visibly bloody fluid, other potentially infectious fluid or tissue, and concentrated virus)
- Type of exposure (ie, percutaneous injury, mucous membrane or nonintact skin exposure, and bites resulting in blood exposure)

Evaluate exposure source
- Assess the risk of infection using available information
- Test known sources for HB_sAg, anti-HCV, and HIV antibody (consider using rapid testing)
- For unknown sources, assess risk of exposure to HBV, HCV, or HIV infection
- Do not test discarded needle or syringes for virus contamination

Evaluate the exposed person
- Assess immune status for HBV infection (ie, by history of hepatitis B vaccination and vaccine response)

Give PEP for exposures posing risk of infection transmission
- HBV: See Recommended Postexposure Prophylaxis for Exposure to Hepatitis B Virus Table
- HCV: PEP not recommended
- HIV: See Recommended HIV Postexposure Prophylaxis for Percutaneous Injuries Table and Recommended HIV Postexposure Prophylaxis for Mucous Membrane Exposures and Nonintact Skin Exposures Table
  - Initiate PEP as soon as possible, preferably within hours of exposure
  - Offer pregnancy testing to all women of childbearing age not known to be pregnant
  - Seek expert consultation if viral resistance is suspected
  - Administer PEP for 4 weeks if tolerated

Perform follow-up testing and provide counseling
- Advise exposed persons to seek medical evaluation for any acute illness occurring during follow-up

HBV exposures
- Perform follow-up anti-HB_s testing in persons who receive hepatitis B vaccine
  - Test for anti-HB_s 1-2 months after last dose of vaccine
  - Anti-HB_s response to vaccine cannot be ascertained if HBIG was received in the previous 3-4 months

HCV exposures
- Perform baseline and follow-up testing for anti-HCV and alanine (ALT) 4-6 months after exposures
- Perform HCV RNA at 4-6 months if earlier diagnosis of HCV infection is desired
- Confirm repeatedly reactive anti-HCV enzyme immunoassays (EIAs) with supplemental tests

HIV exposures
- Perform HIV antibody testing for at least 6 months postexposure (eg, at baseline, 6 weeks, 3 months, and 6 months)
- Perform HIV antibody testing if illness compatible with an acute retroviral syndrome occurs
- Advise exposed persons to use precautions to prevent secondary transmission during the follow-up period
- Evaluate exposed persons taking PEP within 72 hours after exposure and monitor for drug toxicity for at least 2 weeks

Basic and Expanded HIV Postexposure Prophylaxis Regimens

BASIC REGIMENS

Zidovudine (Retrovir®; ZDV; AZT) + lamivudine (Epivir®; 3TC); available as Combivir®
Preferred dosing
- ZDV: 300 mg twice daily or 200 mg three times daily, with food; total: 600 mg daily
- 3TC: 300 mg once daily or 150 mg twice daily
- Combivir®: One tablet twice daily
Advantages
- ZDV associated with decreased risk for HIV transmission
- ZDV used more often than other drugs for PEP for healthcare personnel (HCP)
- Serious toxicity rare when used for PEP
- Side effects predictable and manageable with antimotility and antiemetic agents
- Can be used by pregnant HCP
- Can be given as a single tablet (Combivir®) twice daily

Disadvantages
- Side effects (especially nausea and fatigue) common and might result in low adherence
- Source-patient virus resistance to this regimen possible
- Potential for delayed toxicity (oncogenic/teratogenic) unknown

Zidovudine (Retrovir®; ZDV; AZT) + emtricitabine (Emtriva®; FTC)
Preferred dosing
- ZDV: 300 mg twice daily or 200 mg three times daily, with food; total: 600 mg/day, in 2-3 divided doses
- FTC: 200 mg (one capsule) once daily

Advantages
- ZDV: See above
- FTC
  - Convenient (once daily)
  - Well tolerated
  - Long intracellular half-life (~40 hours)

Disadvantages
- ZDV: See above
- FTC
  - Rash perhaps more frequent than with 3TC
  - No long-term experience with this drug
  - Cross resistance to 3TC
  - Hyperpigmentation among non-Caucasians with long-term use: 3%

Tenofovir DF (Viread®; TDF) + lamivudine (Epivir®; 3TC)
Preferred dosing
- TDF: 300 mg once daily
- 3TC: 300 mg once daily or 150 mg twice daily

Advantages
- 3TC: See above
- TDF
  - Convenient dosing (single pill once daily)
  - Resistance profile activity against certain thymidine analogue mutations
  - Well tolerated

Disadvantages
- TDF
  - Same class warnings as nucleoside reverse transcriptase inhibitors (NRTIs)
  - Drug interactions
  - Increased TDF concentrations among persons taking atazanavir and lopinavir/ritonavir; need to monitor patients for TDF-associated toxicities
- Preferred dosage of atazanavir if used with TDF: 300 mg + ritonavir 100 mg once daily + TDF 300 mg once daily

Tenofovir DF (Viread®; TDF) + emtricitabine (Emtriva®; FTC); available as Truvada®
Preferred dosing
- TDF: 300 mg once daily
- FTC: 200 mg once daily
- As Truvada®: One tablet daily

Advantages
- FTC: See above
- TDF
  - Convenient dosing (single pill once daily)
  - Resistance profile activity against certain thymidine analogue mutations
  - Well tolerated

Disadvantages
- TDF
  - Same class warnings as NRTIs
  - Drug interactions
  - Increased TDF concentrations among persons taking atazanavir and lopinavir/ritonavir; need to monitor patients for TDF-associated toxicities
  - Preferred dosing of atazanavir if used with TDF: 300 mg + ritonavir 100 mg once daily + TDF 300 mg once daily

ALTERNATE BASIC REGIMENS

Lamivudine (Epivir®; 3TC) + stavudine (Zerit®; d4T)

Preferred dosing
- 3TC: 300 mg once daily or 150 mg twice daily
- d4T: 40 mg twice daily (can use lower doses of 20-30 mg twice daily if toxicity occurs; equally effective but less toxic among HIV-infected patients with peripheral neuropathy); 30 mg twice daily if body weight is <60 kg

Advantages
- 3TC: See above
- d4T: Gastrointestinal (GI) side effects rare

Disadvantages
- Possibility that source-patient virus is resistant to this regimen
- Potential for delayed toxicity (oncogenic/teratogenic) unknown

Emtricitabine (Emtriva®; FTC) + stavudine (Zerit®; d4T)

Preferred dosing
- FTC: 200 mg daily
- d4T: 40 mg twice daily (can use lower doses of 20-30 mg twice daily if toxicity occurs; equally effective but less toxic among HIV-infected patients who developed peripheral neuropathy); if body weight is <60 kg, 30 mg twice daily

Advantages
- 3TC and FTC: See above; d4T's GI side effects rare

Disadvantages
- Potential that source-patient virus is resistant to this regimen
- Unknown potential for delayed toxicity (oncogenic/teratogenic) unknown

Lamivudine (Epivir®; 3TC) + didanosine (Videx®; ddI)

Preferred dosing
- 3TC: 300 mg once daily or 150 mg twice daily
- ddI: Videx® chewable/dispersible buffered tablets can be administered on an empty stomach as either 200 mg twice daily or 400 mg once daily. Patients must take at least two of the appropriate strength tablets at each dose to provide adequate buffering and prevent gastric acid degradation of ddI. Because of the need for adequate buffering, the 200 mg strength tablet should be used only as a component of a once-daily regimen. The dose is either 200 mg twice daily or 400 mg once daily for patients weighing >60 kg and 125 mg twice daily or 250 mg once daily for patients weighing <60 kg.

Advantages
- ddI: Once-daily dosing option
- 3TC: See above

Disadvantages
- Tolerability: Diarrhea more common with buffered preparation than with enteric-coated preparation
- Associated with toxicity: Peripheral neuropathy, pancreatitis, and lactic acidosis
- Must be taken on empty stomach except with TDF
- Drug interactions
- 3TC: See above

Emtricitabine (Emtriva®; FTC) + didanosine (Videx®; ddI)

Preferred dosing
- FTC: 200 mg once daily
- ddI: See above

Advantages
- ddI: See above
- FTC: See above

Disadvantages
- Tolerability: Diarrhea more common with buffered than with enteric-coated preparation
- Associated with toxicity: Peripheral neuropathy, pancreatitis, and lactic acidosis
- Must be taken on empty stomach except with TDF
- Drug interactions
- FTC: See above

PREFERRED EXPANDED REGIMEN

Basic regimen plus:

Lopinavir / Ritonavir (Kaletra®; LPV/RTV)

Preferred dosing
- LPV/RTV: 400 mg/100 mg = twice daily with food

Advantages
- Potent HIV protease inhibitor
- Generally well-tolerated

Disadvantages
- Potential for serious or life-threatening drug interactions
- Might accelerate clearance of certain drugs, including oral contraceptives (requiring alternative or additional contraceptive measures for women taking these drugs)
- Can cause severe hyperlipidemia, especially hypertriglyceridemia
- GI (eg, diarrhea) events common

ALTERNATE EXPANDED REGIMENS

Basic regimen plus one of the following:

Atazanavir (Reyataz®; ATV) ± ritonavir (Norvir®; RTV)
Preferred dosing
- ATV: 400 mg once daily, unless used in combination with TDF, in which case ATV should be boosted with RTV, preferred dosing of ATV 300 mg + RTV: 100 mg once daily

Advantages
- Potent HIV protease inhibitor
- Convenient dosing – once daily
- Generally well tolerated

Disadvantages
- Hyperbilirubinemia and jaundice common
- Potential for serious or life-threatening drug interactions
- Avoid coadministration with proton pump inhibitors
- Separate antacids and buffered medications by 2 hours and H_2-receptor antagonists by 12 hours to avoid decreasing ATV levels
- Caution should be used with ATV and products known to induce PR prolongation (eg, diltiazem)

Fosamprenavir (Lexiva™; FOSAPV) ± ritonavir (Norvir®; RTV)
Preferred dosing
- FOSAPV: 1400 mg twice daily (without RTV)
- FOSAPV: 1400 mg once daily + RTV 200 mg once daily
- FOSAPV: 700 mg twice daily + RTV 100 mg twice daily

Advantages
- Once daily dosing when given with ritonavir

Disadvantages
- Tolerability: GI side effects common
- Multiple drug interactions. Oral contraceptives decrease fosamprenavir concentrations
- Incidence of rash in healthy volunteers, especially when used with low doses of ritonavir. Differentiating between early drug-associated rash and acute seroconversion can be difficult and cause extraordinary concern for the exposed person.

Indinavir (Crixivan®; IDV) ± ritonavir (Norvir®; RTV)
Preferred dosing
- IDV 800 mg + RTV 100 mg twice daily without regard to food

Alternative dosing
- IDV: 800 mg every 8 hours, on an empty stomach

Advantages
- Potent HIV inhibitor

Disadvantages
- Potential for serious or life-threatening drug interactions
- Serious toxicity (eg, nephrolithiasis) possible; consumption of 8 glasses of fluid/day required
- Hyperbilirubinemia common; must avoid this drug during late pregnancy
- Requires acid for absorption and cannot be taken simultaneously with ddI, chewable/dispersible buffered tablet formulation (doses must be separated by ≥1 hour)

Saquinavir (Invirase®; SQV) + ritonavir (Norvir®; RTV)
Preferred dosing
- SQV: 1000 mg (given as Invirase®) + RTV 100 mg, twice daily
- SQV: Five capsules twice daily + RTV: One capsule twice daily

Advantages
- Generally well-tolerated, although GI events common

Disadvantages
- Potential for serious or life-threatening drug interactions
- Substantial pill burden

Nelfinavir (Viracept®; NFV)
Preferred dosing
- NFV: 1250 mg (2 x 625 mg or 5 x 250 mg tablets), twice daily with a meal

◀ *Advantages*
- Generally well-tolerated

Disadvantages
- Diarrhea or other GI events common
- Potential for serious and/or life-threatening drug interactions

Efavirenz (Sustiva®; EFV)
Preferred dosing
- EFV: 600 mg daily, at bedtime

Advantages
- Does not require phosphorylation before activation and might be active earlier than other antiretroviral agents (a theoretic advantage of no demonstrated clinical benefit)
- Once daily dosing

Disadvantages
- Drug associated with rash (early onset) that can be severe and might rarely progress to Stevens-Johnson syndrome
- Differentiating between early drug-associated rash and acute seroconversion can be difficult and cause extraordinary concern for the exposed person
- Central nervous system side effects (eg, dizziness, somnolence, insomnia, or abnormal dreaming) common; severe psychiatric symptoms possible (dosing before bedtime might minimize these side effects)
- Teratogen; should not be used during pregnancy
- Potential for serious or life-threatening drug interactions

ANTIRETROVIRAL AGENTS GENERALLY NOT RECOMMENDED FOR USE AS PEP

Nevirapine (Viramune®; NVP)
Disadvantages
- Associated with severe hepatotoxicity (including at least one case of liver failure requiring liver transplantation in an exposed person taking PEP)
- Associated with rash (early onset) that can be severe and progress to Stevens-Johnson syndrome
- Differentiating between early drug-associated rash and acute seroconversion can be difficult and cause extraordinary concern for the exposed person
- Drug interactions: Can lower effectiveness of certain antiretroviral agents and other commonly used medicines

Delavirdine (Rescriptor®; DLV)
Disadvantages
- Drug associated with rash (early onset) that can be severe and progress to Stevens-Johnson syndrome
- Multiple drug interactions

Abacavir (Ziagen®; ABC)
Disadvantages
- Severe hypersensitivity reactions can occur, usually within the first 6 weeks
- Differentiating between early drug-associated rash/hypersensitivity and acute seroconversion can be difficult

Zalcitabine (Hivid®; ddC)
Disadvantages
- Three times a day dosing
- Tolerability
- Weakest antiretroviral agent

ANTIRETROVIRAL AGENT FOR USE AS PEP ONLY WITH EXPERT CONSULTATION

Enfuvirtide (Fuzeon™; T20)
Preferred dosing
- T20: 90 mg (1 mL) twice daily by subcutaneous injection

Advantages
- New class
- Unique viral target; to block cell entry
- Prevalence of resistance low

Disadvantages
- Twice-daily injection
- Safety profile: Local injection site reactions
- Never studied among antiretroviral-naive or HIV-negative patients
- False-positive EIA HIV antibody tests might result from formation of anti-T20 antibodies that cross-react with anti-gp41 antibodies

REFERENCES

The information in this section has been adapted from the following references:

Centers for Disease Control and Prevention (CDC), "Notice to Readers: Updated Information Regarding Antiretroviral Agents Used as HIV Postexposure Prophylaxis for Occupational HIV Exposures," *MMWR Morb Mortal Wkly Rep*, 2007, 56(49):1291-2. Available at http://www.cdc.gov/mmwr/preview/mmwrhtml/mm5649a4.htm.

Panlilio AL, Cardo DM, Grohskopf LA, et al, "Updated U.S. Public Health Service Guidelines for the Management of Occupational Exposures to HIV and Recommendations for Postexposure Prophylaxis," *MMWR Recomm Rep*, 2005, 54(RR-9):1-17. Available at http://www.cdc.gov/mmwr/preview/mmwrhtml/rr5409a1.htm.

U.S. Public Health Service, "Updated U.S. Public Health Service Guidelines for the Management of Occupational Exposures to HBV, HCV, and HIV and Recommendations for Postexposure Prophylaxis," *MMWR Recomm Rep*, 2001, 50(RR-11):1-42. Available at http://www.cdc.gov/mmwr/preview/mmwrhtml/rr5011a1.htm.

NORMAL LABORATORY VALUES FOR CHILDREN

		Normal Values
CHEMISTRY		
Albumin	0-1 y	2.0-4.0 g/dL
	1 y to adult	3.5-5.5 g/dL
Ammonia	Newborns	90-150 mcg/dL
	Children	40-120 mcg/dL
	Adults	18-54 mcg/dL
Amylase	Newborns	0-60 units/L
	Adults	30-110 units/L
Bilirubin, conjugated, direct	Newborns	<1.5 mg/dL
	1 mo to adult	0-0.5 mg/dL
Bilirubin, total	0-3 d	2.0-10.0 mg/dL
	1 mo to adult	0-1.5 mg/dL
Bilirubin, unconjugated, indirect		0.6-10.5 mg/dL
Calcium	Newborns	7.0-12.0 mg/dL
	0-2 y	8.8-11.2 mg/dL
	2 y to adult	9.0-11.0 mg/dL
Calcium, ionized, whole blood		4.4-5.4 mg/dL
Carbon dioxide, total		23-33 mEq/L
Chloride		95-105 mEq/L
Cholesterol	Newborns	45-170 mg/dL
See following tables for age- and gender-specific values	0-1 y	65-175 mg/dL
	1-20 y	120-230 mg/dL
Creatinine	0-1 y	≤0.6 mg/dL
	1 y to adult	0.5-1.5 mg/dL
Glucose	Newborns	30-90 mg/dL
	0-2 y	60-105 mg/dL
	Children to Adults	70-110 mg/dL
Iron		
	Newborns	110-270 mcg/dL
	Infants	30-70 mcg/dL
	Children	55-120 mcg/dL
	Adults	70-180 mcg/dL
Iron binding	Newborns	59-175 mcg/dL
	Infants	100-400 mcg/dL
	Adults	250-400 mcg/dL
Lactic acid, lactate		2-20 mg/dL
Lead, whole blood		<10 mcg/dL
Lipase		
	Children	20-140 units/L
	Adults	0-190 units/L
Magnesium		1.5-2.5 mEq/L
Osmolality, serum		275-296 mOsm/kg
Osmolality, urine		50-1400 mOsm/kg
Phosphorus	Newborns	4.2-9.0 mg/dL
	6 wk to 19 mo	3.8-6.7 mg/dL
	19 mo to 3 y	2.9-5.9 mg/dL

Normal Values

CHEMISTRY

	3-15 y	3.6-5.6 mg/dL
	>15 y	2.5-5.0 mg/dL

Potassium, plasma	Newborns	4.5-7.2 mEq/L
	2 d to 3 mo	4.0-6.2 mEq/L
	3 mo to 1 y	3.7-5.6 mEq/L
	1-16 y	3.5-5.0 mEq/L
Protein, total	0-2 y	4.2-7.4 g/dL
	>2 y	6.0-8.0 g/dL
Sodium		136-145 mEq/L
Triglycerides	Infants	0-171 mg/dL
See following tables for age- and gender-specific values	Children	20-130 mg/dL
	Adults	30-200 mg/dL
Urea nitrogen, blood	0-2 y	4-15 mg/dL
	2 y to Adult	5-20 mg/dL
Uric acid	Male	3.0-7.0 mg/dL
	Female	2.0-6.0 mg/dL

ENZYMES

Alanine aminotransferase (ALT) (SGPT)	0-2 mo	8-78 units/L
	>2 mo	8-36 units/L
Alkaline phosphatase (ALKP)	Newborns	60-130 units/L
	0-16 y	85-400 units/L
	>16 y	30-115 units/L
Aspartate aminotransferase (AST)	Infants	18-74 units/L
(SGOT)	Children	15-46 units/L
	Adults	5-35 units/L
Creatine kinase (CK)	Infants	20-200 units/L
	Children	10-90 units/L
	Adult male	0-206 units/L
	Adult female	0-175 units/L
Lactate dehydrogenase (LDH)	Newborns	290-501 units/L
	1 mo to 2 y	110-144 units/L
	>16 y	60-170 units/L

Blood Gases

	Arterial	Capillary	Venous
pH	7.35-7.45	7.35-7.45	7.32-7.42
pCO_2 (mm Hg)	35-45	35-45	38-52
pO_2 (mm Hg)	70-100	60-80	24-48
HCO_3 (mEq/L)	19-25	19-25	19-25
TCO_2 (mEq/L)	19-29	19-29	23-33
O_2 saturation (%)	90-95	90-95	40-70
Base excess (mEq/L)	-5 to +5	-5 to +5	-5 to +5

Classification Serum Lipid Concentrations

Classification	Percentile	Cholesterol (mg/dL)		LDL-C (mg/dL)		Triglycerides (mg/dL)
		Children	Adults	Children	Adults	Adults
Acceptable/ optimal	<75th	<170	<200	<110	<100	<150
Above optimal	*	*	*	*	100-129	*
Borderline high	75th to 95th	170-199	200-239	110-129	130-159	150-199
High	>95th	≥200	≥240	≥130	160-189	200-499
Very high	*	*	*	*	≥190	≥500

[1]Adapted from American Academy of Pediatrics Committee on Nutrition, "Cholesterol in Childhood," *Pediatrics*, 1998, 101(1 Pt 1):141-7.

[2]American Academy of Pediatrics Committee on Nutrition, "Lipid Screening and Cardiovascular Health in Childhood," *Pediatrics*, 2008, 122:(1)198-208 and "Third Report of the National Cholesterol Education Program Expert Panel on Detection, Evaluation, and Treatment of High Blood Cholesterol in Adults (Adult Treatment Panel III)," May 2001, www.nhlbi.nih.gov/guidelines/cholesterol.

*Lack of specific type of classification in either pediatric or adult recommendations.

Serum Lipid Concentrations by Age and Gender

	Males (mg/dL)			Females (mg/dL)		
	5-9 y	10-14 y	15-19 y	5-9 y	10-14 y	15-19 y
Total Cholesterol						
50th percentile	153	161	152	164	159	157
75th percentile	168	173	168	177	171	176
90th percentile	183	191	183	189	191	198
95th percentile	186	201	191	197	205	208
Triglycerides						
50th percentile	48	58	68	57	68	64
75th percentile	58	74	88	74	85	85
90th percentile	70	94	125	103	104	112
95th percentile	85	111	143	120	120	126
LDL-C						
50th percentile	90	94	93	98	94	93
75th percentile	103	109	109	115	110	110
90th percentile	117	123	123	125	126	129
95th percentile	129	133	130	140	136	137
HDL						
5th percentile	38	37	30	36	37	35
10th percentile	43	40	34	38	40	38
25th percentile	49	46	39	48	45	43
50th percentile	55	55	46	52	52	51

Adapted from American Academy of Pediatrics Committee on Nutrition, "Lipid Screening and Cardiovascular Health in Childhood," *Pediatrics*, 2008, 122:(1)198-208.

Thyroid Function Tests

T$_4$ (thyroxine)	1-7 d	10.1-20.9 mcg/dL
	8-14 d	9.8-16.6 mcg/dL
	1 mo to 1 y	5.5-16.0 mcg/dL
	>1 y	4.0-12.0 mcg/dL
FTI	1-3 d	9.3-26.6
	1-4 wk	7.6-20.8
	1-4 mo	7.4-17.9
	4-12 mo	5.1-14.5
	1-6 y	5.7-13.3
	>6 y	4.8-14.0
T$_3$	Newborns	100-470 ng/dL
	1-5 y	100-260 ng/dL
	5-10 y	90-240 ng/dL
	10 y to Adult	70-210 ng/dL
T$_3$ uptake		35%-45%
TSH	Cord	3-22 micro international units/mL
	1-3 d	<40 micro international units/mL
	3-7 d	<25 micro international units/mL
	>7 d	0-10 micro international units/mL

Hematology Values

Age	Hgb (g/dL)	Hct (%)	RBC (mill/mm^3)	RDW	MCV (fL)	MCH (pg)	MCHC (%)	PLTS (x 10^3/mm^3)
0-3 d	15.0-20.0	45-61	4.0-5.9	<18	95-115	31-37	29-37	250-450
1-2 wk	12.5-18.5	39-57	3.6-5.5	<17	86-110	28-36	28-38	250-450
1-6 mo	10.0-13.0	29-42	3.1-4.3	<16.5	74-96	25-35	30-36	300-700
7 mo to 2 y	10.5-13.0	33-38	3.7-4.9	<16	70-84	23-30	31-37	250-600
2-5 y	11.5-13.0	34-39	3.9-5.0	<15	75-87	24-30	31-37	250-550
5-8 y	11.5-14.5	35-42	4.0-4.9	<15	77-95	25-33	31-37	250-550
13-18 y	12.0-15.2	36-47	4.5-5.1	<14.5	78-96	25-35	31-37	150-450
Adult male	13.5-16.5	41-50	4.5-5.5	<14.5	80-100	26-34	31-37	150-450
Adult female	12.0-15.0	36-44	4.0-4.9	<14.5	80-100	26-34	31-37	150-450

WBC and Diff

Age	WBC (x 10^3/mm^3)	Segs	Bands	Lymphs	Monos	Eosinophils	Basophils	Atypical Lymphs	No. of NRBCs
0-3 d	9.0-35.0	32-62	10-18	19-29	5-7	0-2	0-1	0-8	0-2
1-2 wk	5.0-20.0	14-34	6-14	36-45	6-10	0-2	0-1	0-8	0
1-6 mo	6.0-17.5	13-33	4-12	41-71	4-7	0-3	0-1	0-8	0
7 mo to 2 y	6.0-17.0	15-35	5-11	45-76	3-6	0-3	0-1	0-8	0
2-5 y	5.5-15.5	23-45	5-11	35-65	3-6	0-3	0-1	0-8	0
5-8 y	5.0-14.5	32-54	5-11	28-48	3-6	0-3	0-1	0-8	0
13-18 y	4.5-13.0	34-64	5-11	25-45	3-6	0-3	0-1	0-8	0
Adults	4.5-11.0	35-66	5-11	24-44	3-6	0-3	0-1	0-8	0

Segs = segmented neutrophils.

Bands = band neutrophils.

Lymphs = lymphocytes.

Monos = monocytes.

Erythrocyte Sedimentation Rates and Reticulocyte Counts

Sedimentation rate, Westergren	Children	0-20 mm/hour
	Adult male	0-15 mm/hour
	Adult female	0-20 mm/hour
Sedimentation rate, Wintrobe	Children	0-13 mm/hour
	Adult male	0-10 mm/hour
	Adult female	0-15 mm/hour
Reticulocyte count	Newborns	2%-6%
	1-6 mo	0%-2.8%
	Adults	0.5%-1.5%

Cerebrospinal Fluid Values, Normal

		% PMNs
Cell count		
Preterm mean	9 (0-25.4 WBC/mm^3)	57%
Term mean	8.2 (0-22.4 WBC/mm^3)	61%
>1 mo	0.7	0
Glucose		
Preterm	24-63 mg/dL	mean 50
Term	34-119 mg/dL	mean 52
Children	40-80 mg/dL	
CSF glucose/blood glucose		
Preterm	55-105%	
Term	44-128%	
Children	50%	
Lactic acid dehydrogenase	5-30 units/mL	mean 20 units/mL
Myelin basic protein	<4 ng/mL	
Pressure: Initial LP (mm H_2O)		
Newborns	80-110 (<110)	
Infants/children	<200 (lateral recumbent position)	
Respiratory movements	5-10	
Protein		
Preterm	65-150 mg/dL	mean 115
Term	20-170 mg/dL	mean 90
Children		
Ventricular	5-15 mg/dL	
Cisternal	5-25 mg/dL	
Lumbar	5-40 mg/dL	

ACID / BASE ASSESSMENT

Henderson-Hasselbalch Equation

$pH = 6.1 + \log ([HCO_3^-] / (0.03) (PaCO_2))$

Normal arterial blood pH: 7.4 (normal range: 7.35 - 7.45)

Where:

$[HCO_3^-]$	=	Serum bicarbonate concentration
$PaCO_2$	=	Arterial carbon dioxide partial pressure

Alveolar Gas Equation

P_iO_2	=	F_iO_2 x (total atmospheric pressure – vapor pressure of H_2O at 37°C)
	=	F_iO_2 x (760 mm Hg – 47 mm Hg)
PAO_2	=	$P_iO_2 - (PaCO_2 / R)$

Alveolar-arterial oxygen (A-a) gradient = $PAO_2 - PaO_2$

or

A-a gradient = $[(F_iO_2 \times 713) - (PaCO_2/0.8)] - PaO_2$

A-a gradient normal ranges:

Children	15-20 mm Hg
Adults	20-25 mm Hg

where:

P_iO_2	=	Oxygen partial pressure of inspired gas (mm Hg) (150 mm Hg in room air at sea level)
F_iO_2	=	Fractional pressure of oxygen in inspired gas (0.21 in room air)
PAO_2	=	Alveolar oxygen partial pressure
PaO_2	=	Arterial oxygen partial pressure
$PaCO_2$	=	Arterial carbon dioxide partial pressure
R	=	Respiratory exchange quotient (typically 0.8, increases with high carbohydrate diet, decreases with high fat diet)

Acid-Base Disorders

Acute metabolic acidosis:
  $PaCO_2$ expected = 1.5 $([HCO_3^-])$ + 8 ± 2 **or**
  Expected decrease in $PaCO_2$ = 1.3 (1-1.5) x decrease in $[HCO_3^-]$

Acute metabolic alkalosis:
  Expected increase in $PaCO_2$ = 0.6 (0.5-1) x increase in $[HCO_3^-]$

Acute respiratory acidosis (<6 h duration):
  For every $PaCO_2$ increase of 10 mm Hg, $[HCO_3^-]$ increases by 1 mEq/L

Chronic respiratory acidosis (>6 h duration):
  For every $PaCO_2$ increase of 10 mm Hg, $[HCO_3^-]$ increases by 4 mEq/L

Acute respiratory alkalosis (<6 h duration):
  For every $PaCO_2$ decrease of 10 mm Hg, $[HCO_3^-]$ decreases by 2 mEq/L

Chronic respiratory alkalosis (>6 h duration):
  For every $PaCO_2$ decrease of 10 mm Hg, $[HCO_3^-]$ increases by 5 mEq/L

LABORATORY CALCULATIONS

ANION GAP

Definition: The difference in concentration between unmeasured cation and anion equivalents in serum.

Anion gap = $Na^+ - (Cl^- + HCO_3^-)$
  (The normal anion gap is 10-14 mEq/L)

Differential Diagnosis of Increased Anion Gap Acidosis

Organic anions
  Lactate (sepsis, hypovolemia, seizures, large tumor burden)
  Pyruvate
  Uremia
  Ketoacidosis (β-hydroxybutyrate and acetoacetate)
  Amino acids and their metabolites
  Other organic acids (eg, formate from methanol, glycolate from ethylene glycol)

Inorganic anions
  Hyperphosphatemia
  Sulfates
  Nitrates

Medications and toxins
  Penicillins and cephalosporins
  Salicylates (including aspirin)
  Cyanide
  Carbon monoxide

Differential Diagnosis of Decreased Anion Gap

Organic cations
  Hypergammaglobulinemia

Inorganic cations
  Hyperkalemia
  Hypercalcemia
  Hypermagnesemia

Medications and toxins
  Lithium

Hypoalbuminemia

OSMOLALITY

Definition: The summed concentrations of all osmotically active solute particles.

Predicted serum osmolality =

$$mOsm/L \quad = \quad (2 \times serum\ Na^{++}) \quad + \quad \frac{serum\ glucose}{18} \quad + \quad \frac{BUN}{2.8}$$

The normal range of serum osmolality is 285-295 mOsm/L.

Calculated Osm

Note: Osm is a term used to reconcile osmolality and osmolarity

Osmol gap = measured Osm − calculated Osm

  0 to +10: Normal
  >10: Abnormal
  <0: Probable lab or calculation error

Differential Diagnosis of Increased Osmol Gap
(increased by >10 mOsm/L)
Ethanol
Ethylene glycol
Glycerol
Iodine (questionable)
Isopropanol (acetone)
Mannitol
Methanol
Sorbitol

CORRECTED SODIUM FOR HYPERGLYCEMIA

Corrected Na^+ = serum Na^+ + [1.5 x (glucose − 150 divided by 100)]

Note: Do not correct for glucose <150.

CORRECTED TOTAL SERUM CALCIUM FOR ALBUMIN LEVEL

[(Normal albumin − patient's albumin) x 0.8] + patient's measured total calcium

BICARBONATE DEFICIT

HCO_3^- deficit = (0.4 x wt in kg) x (HCO_3^- desired − HCO_3^- measured)

Note: In clinical practice, the calculated quantity may differ markedly from the actual amount of bicarbonate needed or that which may be safely administered.

APGAR SCORING SYSTEM

Sign	Score		
	0	1	2
Heart rate	Absent	Under 100 beats per minute	Over 100 beats per minute
Respiratory effort	Absent	Slow (irregular)	Good crying
Muscle tone	Limp	Some flexion of extremities	Active motion
Reflex irritability	No response	Grimace	Cough or sneeze
Color	Blue, pale	Pink body, blue extremities	All pink

From Apgar V, "A Proposal for a New Method of Evaluation of the Newborn Infant," *Anesth Analg*, 1953, 32:260.

FETAL HEART RATE MONITORING

Normal Heart Rates

Fetal heart rate (FHR) 120-160 bpm. Isolated accelerations are normal and considered reassuring. Mild (100-120 bpm) and transient bradycardias may be normal. Normal fetal heart rate tracings show beat-to-beat variability of 5-10 bpm (poor beat-to-beat variability suggests fetal hypoxia).

Abnormal Heart Rates

Bradycardia (FHR <120 bpm): Potential causes include fetal distress, drugs, congenital heart block (associated with maternal SLE, congenital cardiac defects).

Tachycardia (FHR >160 bpm): Potential causes include maternal fever, chorioamnionitis, drugs, fetal dysrhythmias, eg, SVT (with or without fetal CHF).

Decreased Beat-to-Beat Variability

Results from fetal CNS depression. Potential causes include fetal hypoxia, fetal sleep, fetal immaturity, and maternal narcotic/sedative administration.

Fetal Heart Rate Decelerations

Type 1 (early decelerations)
- Seen most commonly in late labor
- Mirror uterine contractions in time of onset, duration, and resolution
- Uniform shape
- Usually associated with good beat-to-beat variability
- Heart rate may dip to 60-80 bpm
- Associated with fetal head compression (increases vagal tone)
- Considered benign, and not representative of fetal hypoxia

Type 2 (late decelerations)
- Deceleration 10-30 seconds after onset of uterine contraction
- Heart rate fails to return to baseline after contraction is completed
- Asymmetrical shape (longer deceleration, shorter acceleration)
- Late decelerations of 10-20 bpm may be significant
- Probably associated with fetal CNS and myocardial depression

Type 3 (variable decelerations)
- Heart rate variations do not correlate with uterine contractions
- Variable shape and duration
- Occur occasionally in many normal labors
- Concerning if severe (HR <60 bpm), prolonged (duration >60 seconds), associated with poor beat-to-beat variability, or combined with late decelerations
- Associated with cord compression (including nuchal cord)

Reference
Manual of Neonatal Care, Joint Program in Neonatology, 3rd ed, Cloherty JP and Stark AR, eds, Boston, MA: Little, Brown, 1991.

CREATININE CLEARANCE ESTIMATING METHODS IN PATIENTS WITH STABLE RENAL FUNCTION

The following formulas provide an acceptable estimate of the patient's creatinine clearance except when:

a. The patient's serum creatinine is changing rapidly (either up or down).

b. Patients are markedly emaciated.

In these situations (a and b above), certain assumptions have to be made:

a. In patients with rapidly rising serum creatinines (ie, increasing by >0.5-0.7 mg/dL/day), it is best to assume that the patient's creatinine clearance is probably less than 10 mL/minute.

b. In emaciated patients, although their actual creatinine clearance is less than their calculated creatinine clearance (because of decreased creatinine production), it is not possible to predict easily how much less.

Estimation of creatinine clearance using serum creatinine and body length (to be used when an adequate timed specimen cannot be obtained). **Note:** This formula may not provide an accurate estimation of creatinine clearance for infants <6 months of age or for patients with severe starvation or muscle wasting.

$CL_{cr} = K \times L/S_{cr}$

where:

Cl_{cr} = creatinine clearance in mL/minute/1.73 m^2
K = constant of proportionality that is age specific

Age	K
Low birth weight ≤1 y	0.33
Full-term ≤1 y	0.45
2-12 y	0.55
13-21 y female	0.55
13-21 y male	0.70

L = length in cm
S_{Cr} = serum creatinine concentration in mg/dL

Reference
Schwartz GJ, Brion LP, and Spitzer A, "The Use of Plasma Creatinine Concentration for Estimating Glomerular Filtration Rate in Infants, Children and Adolescents," *Ped Clin N Amer*, 1987, 34:571-90.

Children 1-18 years

Method 1: (Traub SL, Johnson CE, *Am J Hosp Pharm*, 1980, 37:195-201)

Equation:

$$Cl_{cr} = \frac{0.48 \times (height)}{S_{cr}}$$

where
Cl_{cr} = creatinine clearance in mL/min/1.73 m^2
S_{cr} = serum creatinine in mg/dL
Height = height in cm

Method 2: See nomogram.

Children 1-18 Years

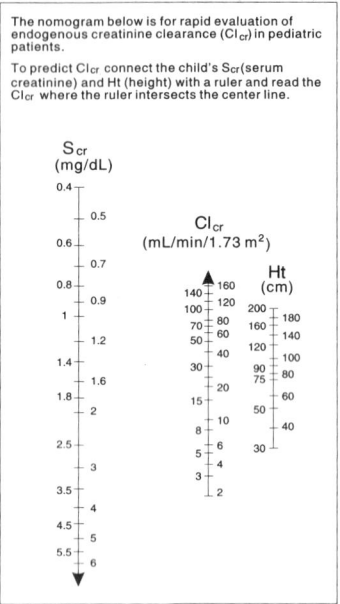

The nomogram below is for rapid evaluation of endogenous creatinine clearance (Cl_{cr}) in pediatric patients.

To predict Cl_{cr} connect the child's S_{cr}(serum creatinine) and Ht (height) with a ruler and read the Cl_{cr} where the ruler intersects the center line.

Adults 18 years and older

Method 1: (Cockroft DW and Gault MH, *Nephron*, 1976, 16:31-41)

Estimated creatinine clearance (Cl_{cr}) (mL/min):

$$\text{Male} = \frac{(140 - \text{age})\ \text{IBW (kg)}}{72 \times \text{serum creatinine}}$$

Female = Estimated Cl_{cr} male x 0.85

Note: The use of the patient's ideal body weight (IBW) is recommended for the above formula except when the patient's actual body weight is less than ideal. Use of the IBW is especially important in obese patients. See appendix Growth & Development section for Ideal Body Weight Calculation.

Method 2: (Jelliffe RW, *Ann Intern Med*, 1973, 79:604)

Estimated creatinine clearance (Cl_{cr}) (mL/min/1.73 m^2):

$$\text{Male} = \frac{98\text{-}0.8\ (\text{age} - 20)}{\text{serum creatinine}}$$

Female = Estimated Cl_{cr} male x 0.90

RENAL FUNCTION TESTS

Endogenous creatinine clearance vs age (timed collection)

Creatinine clearance (mL/min/1.73 m^2) = (Cr$_u$V/S$_{Cr}$T) (1.73/A)

where:

Cr$_u$	=	Urine creatinine concentration (mg/dL)
V	=	Total urine volume collected during sampling period (mL)
S$_{Cr}$	=	Serum creatinine concentration (mg/dL)
T	=	Duration of sampling period (min) (24 h = 1440 min)
A	=	Body surface area (m^2)

Age-specific normal values

5-7 d	50.6±5.8 mL/min/1.73 m^2
1-2 mo	64.6±5.8 mL/min/1.73 m^2
5-8 mo	87.7±11.9 mL/min/1.73 m^2
9-12 mo	86.9±8.4 mL/min/1.73 m^2
≥18 mo	
male	124±26 mL/min/1.73 m^2
female	109±13.5 mL/min/1.73 m^2
Adults	
male	105±14 mL/min/1.73 m^2
female	95±18 mL/min/1.73 m^2

Note: In patients with renal failure (creatinine clearance <25 mL/min), creatinine clearance may be elevated over GFR because of tubular secretion of creatinine.

Serum BUN/Serum Creatinine Ratio

Serum BUN (mg/dL):serum creatinine (mg/dL)

Normal BUN:creatinine ratio is 10-15.

BUN:creatinine ratio >20 suggests prerenal azotemia (also seen with high urea-generation states such as GI bleeding).

BUN:creatinine ratio <5 may be seen with disorders affecting urea biosynthesis such as urea cycle enzyme deficiencies and with hepatitis.

Fractional Sodium Excretion

Fractional sodium secretion (FENa) = Na$_u$S$_{Cr}$/Na$_s$Cr$_u$ x 100%

where:

Na$_u$	=	Urine sodium (mEq/L)
Na$_s$	=	Serum sodium (mEq/L)
Cr$_u$	=	Urine creatinine (mg/dL)
S$_{Cr}$	=	Serum creatinine (mg/dL)

FENa <1% suggests prerenal failure
FENa >2% suggest intrinsic renal failure
(for newborns, normal FENa is approximately 2.5%)

Note: Disease states associated with a falsely elevated FENa include severe volume depletion (>10%), early acute tubular necrosis and volume depletion in chronic renal disease. Disorders associated with a lowered FENa include acute glomerulonephritis, hemoglobinuric or myoglobinuric renal failure, nonoliguric acute tubular necrosis, and acute urinary tract obstruction. In addition, FENa may be <1% in patients with acute renal failure **and** a second condition predisposing to sodium retention (eg, burns, congestive heart failure, nephrotic syndrome).

Urine Calcium/Urine Creatinine Ratio (spot sample)

Urine calcium (mg/dL): urine creatinine (mg/dL)

Normal values <0.21 (mean values 0.08 males, 0.06 females)

Premature infants show wide variability of calcium:creatinine ratio, and tend to have lower thresholds for calcium loss than older children. Prematures without nephrolithiasis had mean Ca:Cr ratio of 0.75±0.76. Infants with nephrolithiasis had mean Ca:Cr ratio of 1.32±1.03 (Jacinto, et al, *Pediatrics*, vol 81, p 31).

Urine Protein/Urine Creatinine Ratio (spot sample)

P_u/Cr_u	Total Protein Excretion (mg/m^2/day)
0.1	80
1	800
10	8000

where:

P_u =	Urine protein concentration (mg/dL)
Cr_u =	Urine creatinine concentration (mg/dL)

Serum Osmolality

Predicted serum osmolality =

2 x Na (mEq/L) + BUN (mg/dL) / 2.8 + glucose (mg/dL) / 18

ACUTE DYSTONIC REACTIONS, MANAGEMENT

1. **Confirm that patient has stable airway and adequate respiratory activity.**
2. Administer **one** of the following:
   Diphenhydramine 0.7-1 mg/kg/dose I.V./P.O. q4-6h prn **or**
   Hydroxyzine 0.5-1 mg/kg/dose I.M./P.O. q4-6h prn (adult dose: 25-100 mg I.M./P.O. q6h) **or**
   Children >3 years: Benztropine 0.02-0.05 mg/kg/dose or maximum of 1-2 mg I.V./P.O. (avoid use in children <3 years of age except in cases of extreme emergency)

Agents which predispose patients to acute dystonic reactions, such as phenothiazine neuroleptics or antiemetics, often have long therapeutic half-lives. Anticholinergic administration should therefore be continued for 6-24 hours after discontinuation of phenothiazine therapy.

PREPROCEDURE SEDATIVES IN CHILDREN

Purpose: The following table is a guide to aid the clinician in the selection of the most appropriate sedative to sedate a child for a procedure. One must also consider:

- Not all patients require sedation. It is dependent on the procedure and age of the child.
- When sedation is desired, one must consider the time of onset, the duration of action, and the route of administration.
- Each of the following drugs is well absorbed when given by the suggested routes and doses.
- Each drug was assigned an "intensity" based upon the class of drug, dose, and route. However, it should be noted that any drug can produce a deeper level of sedation.
- Practitioners performing a specific level of sedation must be prepared to manage the patient who slips into the next deeper level of sedation (eg, when performing moderate sedation, be prepared to manage deep sedation). This may occur regardless of which sedation drug is used.
- Those drugs classified as producing deep sedation require more frequent monitoring postprocedure.
- For painful procedures, an analgesic agent needs to be administered.

Levels of Sedation[1]

- Minimal sedation (formerly anxiolysis): A medically controlled state in which patients respond appropriately to verbal commands; cognitive and coordination function may be impaired, but cardiovascular and ventilatory function are not affected.
- Moderate sedation (formerly conscious sedation): A medically controlled drug-induced depression of consciousness during which patients respond purposefully to verbal commands either alone or accompanied by light tactile stimulation. No interventions are required to maintain a patent airway, and spontaneous ventilation is adequate. Cardiovascular function is usually maintained.
- Deep sedation: A medically controlled state of depressed consciousness associated with partial or complete loss of protective airway reflexes. Patients cannot be easily aroused, but respond purposefully after repeated verbal or painful stimulation. Cardiovascular function is usually maintained.
- General anesthesia (Note: This level of sedation is reserved for patients in an operating room setting): A medically controlled state of loss of consciousness during which patients are not arousable, even with painful stimulation. Ventilatory function is usually impaired; patients require assistance with maintaining a patent airway; positive-pressure ventilation may be required. Cardiovascular function may be impaired.

Sedatives Used to Produce Moderate Sedation

Drug	Route	Dose (mg/kg)	Onset (min)	Duration (h)	Comments
Chloral hydrate	P.O./P.R.	25-100	10-20	4-8	Maximum single dose: Infants: 1 g; Children: 2 g
Diazepam[2,3] (Valium®)	P.O.	0.2-0.3 90 min prior	60-90	6-8	Maximum oral dose: 10 mg
	I.V.	0.1-0.2	1-3	6-8	Maximum dose I.V.: 5 mg; due to poor absorption and tissue irritation, I.M. route **not** recommended
	P.R.	0.2-0.4	2-10	6-8	May use I.V. solution rectally
Fentanyl	Transmucosal	5-15 mcg/kg	5-15	1-2	Maximum transmucosal dose: 400 mcg
	I.M.	1-3 mcg/kg	7-15	1-2	
	I.V.	1-3 mcg/kg	Immediate	30-60 min	
Lorazepam[5] (Ativan®)	P.O.	0.05; 90-120 min prior	60	8-12	
	Deep I.M.	0.05; 90-120 min prior	30-60	8-12	
	I.V.	0.05; over 5-10 min	15-30	8-12	
Meperidine (Demerol®)	P.O.	2-4	10-15	2-4	Doses I.M./I.V. >2 mg/kg are considered deep sedation
	I.M.	0.5-2	10-15	2-4	
	I.V.	0.5-2	5	2-3	

Sedatives Used to Produce Moderate Sedation *(continued)*

Drug	Route	Dose (mg/kg)	Onset (min)	Duration (h)	Comments
Midazolam[6,7] (Versed®)	P.O.	0.2-0.4; 30-45 min prior	20-30	1-2	Maximum oral dose: 15 mg
	Deep I.M.	0.1-0.15; 30-60 min prior	15	1-2	Maximum total dose: 10 mg
	I.V.	**6 mo - 5 y:** 0.05-0.1; **6-12 y:** 0.025-0.05; **>12 y - Adult:** 2.5-5 mg (total dose); give over 10-20 min	1-5	1-2	Maximum concentration: 1 mg/mL; maximum I.M./I.V. dose: 6 mo - 5 y: 6 mg 6 y - Adult: 10 mg
	P.R.	0.3	20-30	1-2	Dilute injection in 5 mL NS; administer rectally
	Intranasal	0.2-0.3	5	30-60 min	Administer nasally: Use a 1 mL needleless syringe into the nares over 15 seconds; use 5 mg/mL concentration; 1/2 dose may be administered into each nare
Morphine	P.O.	0.2-0.5	20-30	3-5	
	I.M.	0.05-0.2	20-30	3-5	
	I.V.	0.05-0.2	10-15	2-5	

Note: See individual drug monographs for further information.

Sedatives Used to Produce Deep Sedation

Drug	Route	Dose (mg/kg)	Onset (min)	Duration (h)	Comments
Methohexital[8,9] (Brevital®)	I.M.	5-10	5	1-1.5	Maximum concentration for I.M./I.V.: 50 mg/mL; maximum I.M./I.V. dose: 200 mg. Greater incidence of adverse effects with I.V. use.
	I.V.	0.75-2	1	7-10 min	
	P.R.	20-35	5-10	1-1.5	Shorter duration of action than thiopental; rectal given as a 10% solution in sterile water; maximum dose rectal: 500 mg
Pentobarbital	P.O./I.M./ P.R.	2-6	10-25	1-4	Maximum I.M./I.V./P.O./P.R. dose: 100 mg
	I.V.	1-3	1	15 min	
Thiopental[10,4] (Pentothal)	I.V.	4-6	0.5-1	5-10 min	Variable rectal absorption; may use additional 12.5 mg/kg if necessary; maximum rectal dose: 1-1.5 g
	P.R.	25; immediately prior to procedure	10	1-5	

Note: See individual drug monographs for further information.

Sedatives Used to Produce Dissociative Anesthesia (Monitor as if deep sedation)

Drug	Route	Dose (mg/kg)	Onset (min)	Duration	Comments
Ketamine	P.O.	6-10; 30 min prior	30-45	10-30	Use only under direct supervision of physicians experienced in administering general anesthetics; has analgesic effects; may use injectable product orally diluted in a beverage of the patient's choice
	I.M.	3-7	7	12-25	
	I.V.	0.5-2	1	5-10	

Note: See individual drug monographs for further information.

Footnotes

1. American Academy of Pediatrics, American Academy of Pediatric Dentistry, Coté CJ, et al, "Guidelines for Monitoring and Management of Pediatric Patients During and After Sedation for Diagnostic and Therapeutic Procedures: An Update," *Pediatrics*, 2006, 118(6):2587-602.
2. Yager JY and Seshia SS, "Sublingual Lorazepam in Childhood Serial Seizures," *Am J Dis Child*, 1988, 142(9):931-2.
3. Fell D, Gough MB, Northan AA, et al, "Diazepam Premedication in Children," *Anaesthesia*, 1985, 40(1):12-7.
4. Burckart GJ, White III TJ, Siegle RL, et al, "Rectal Thiopental Versus an Intramuscular Cocktail for Sedating Children Before Computer Tomography," *Am J Hosp Pharm*, 1980, 37(2):222-4.
5. Burtles R and Astley B, "Lorazepam in Children," *Br J Anaesth*, 1983, 55(4):275-9.
6. Roelofse JA, van der Bijl P, Stegmann DH, et al, "Preanesthetic Medication With Rectal Midazolam in Children Undergoing Dental Extractions," *J Oral Maxillofac Surg*, 1990, 48(8):791-7.
7. Wilton NC, Leigh J, Rosen DR, et al, "Preanesthetic Sedation of Preschool Children Using Intranasal Midazolam," *Anesthesiology*, 1988, 60(6):972-5.
8. Elman DS and Denson JS, "Preanesthetic Sedation of Children With Intramuscular Methohexital Sodium," *Anesth Analg*, 1965, 44(5):494-8.
9. Miller JR, Grayson M, and Stoelting VK, "Sedation With Intramuscular Methohexital Sodium," *Am J Ophthalmol*, 1966, 62(1):38-43.
10. "Drug Evaluations," *AMA*, 1980.

FEBRILE SEIZURES

A febrile seizure is defined as a seizure occurring for no reason other than an elevated temperature. It does not have an infectious or metabolic origin within the CNS (ie, it is not caused by meningitis, encephalitis, or acute electrolyte imbalance). Fever is usually >102°F rectally. Febrile seizures are the most common form of childhood seizures, occurring in 2% to 5% of children. Most febrile seizures occur between 6 months and 5 years of age, with a peak incidence at 18 months of age. There are three types of febrile seizures:

1. **Simple** febrile seizures are generalized (ie, nonfocal) febrile seizures of less than 15 minutes duration. They do not occur in multiples (ie, they occur only once during a 24-hour period).

2. **Complex** febrile seizures are febrile seizures that are either focal, have a focal component, are longer than 15 minutes in duration, are multiple febrile seizures that occur within 30 minutes, or recur in 24 hours.

3. **Febrile status epilepticus** is a febrile seizure lasting longer than 30 minutes.

Note: Febrile seizures should not be confused with true epileptic seizures associated with fever or "seizure with fever." "Seizure with fever" includes seizures associated with acute neurologic illnesses (ie, meningitis, encephalitis). Infants and children who present with fever and seizures need to be appropriately diagnosed, as there are other conditions which may precipitate seizures in a child with fever (see Srinivasan, 2005).

Acute treatment of an ongoing febrile seizure: Since most febrile seizures are brief in duration, the primary acute treatment of an ongoing febrile seizure is basic first aid seizure management. No other intervention is usually needed. For febrile seizures that last longer than 10 minutes, rectal diazepam is effective in terminating the seizure and is considered the treatment of choice for intervention outside the hospital (Shinnar, 2002). Intravenous diazepam is also effective and is usually used in the emergency department or hospital setting. Antipyretics are indicated to treat the child's temperature, but do not prevent the recurrence of a febrile seizure.

Long-term treatment to prevent recurrence of febrile seizures: Long-term prophylaxis with daily administration of phenobarbital or valproic acid has been shown to be effective in reducing the risk of subsequent febrile seizures. The intermittent administration of oral or rectal diazepam at the time of febrile illness has also been shown to be effective. **Note:** Daily administration of carbamazepine or phenytoin and use of antipyretic agents alone, are **not** effective in preventing recurrent febrile seizures.

The 1980 NIH Consensus paper stated that after the first febrile seizure, long-term prophylaxis should be considered under any of the following:

1. Presence of abnormal neurological development or abnormal neurological exam

2. Febrile seizure was complex in nature:

      duration >15 minutes

      focal febrile seizure

      followed by transient or persistent neurological abnormalities

3. Positive family history of afebrile seizures (epilepsy)

Also consider long-term prophylaxis in certain cases if:

1. the child has multiple febrile seizures

2. the child is <12 months of age

However, long-term daily administration of phenobarbital or valproic acid and intermittent administration of diazepam is not without risks. Phenobarbital may cause behavioral problems (eg, hyperactivity, irritability), sleep disorders, or hypersensitivity reactions (such as rash or rarely, Stevens-Johnson syndrome). Several studies have also identified a negative effect on learning and cognitive performance in children receiving phenobarbital. Valproic acid has the potential to cause life-threatening hepatotoxicity. It may also cause thrombocytopenia, pancreatitis, GI disturbances, and weight gain or loss. Adverse reactions of diazepam include drowsiness, sedation, lethargy, and ataxia. These adverse effects could mask signs of an evolving CNS infection or process. Thus, these potential risks of long-term treatment need to be weighed against the benefits of preventing the recurrence of febrile seizures.

It is important to note that the risk of recurrent febrile seizures is low for children with **simple** febrile seizures. In 1999, the American Academy of Pediatrics assessed the benefits and risks of long-term anticonvulsant treatment and developed a practice parameter with recommendations. Although daily use of phenobarbital or valproic acid and intermittent administration of diazepam were found to be effective in reducing the risk of recurrent febrile seizures, the potential toxicities associated with these treatments outweigh the relatively minor risks associated with **simple** febrile seizures. **Therefore, neither continuous (ie, daily administration) nor intermittent anticonvulsant treatment is recommended for neurologically healthy infants and children, 6 months to 5 years of age, who have had one or more simple febrile seizures.** In certain cases (eg, when parental anxiety over febrile seizures is severe), intermittent oral diazepam, administered at the onset of a febrile illness, may be effective in preventing febrile seizure recurrence.

In cases where long-term anticonvulsant prophylaxis is used, it is usually continued for 2 years or 1 year after the last seizure, whichever is longer. Daily administration of phenobarbital requires therapeutic serum concentrations ≥15 mcg/mL to be effective. Due to potential risk of hepatotoxicity, valproic acid is usually reserved for patients who have significant adverse effects to phenobarbital. The administration of rectal diazepam (as a solution or suppository) at the time of the febrile illness has been shown to be as effective as daily phenobarbital in preventing recurrences of febrile seizures. A rectal diazepam dosage form is available in the United States; however, some centers are still using the injectable form of diazepam rectally. The solution for injection must be filtered prior to use if drawn from an ampul. Like other agents, oral diazepam must be dosed appropriately to be effective. A double-blind, controlled trial found that oral diazepam administered in doses of 0.33 mg/kg/dose given every 8 hours when the child has a fever, reduced the risk of recurrent febrile seizures (see Rosman, 1993). However, a study by Uhari (1995) showed that lower doses of diazepam, 0.2 mg/kg/dose, were not effective.

References

American Academy of Pediatrics, Committee on Quaility Improvement, Subcommittee on Febrile Seizures, "Practice Parameter: Long-Term Treatment of the Child With Simple Febrile Seizures," *Pediatrics*, 1999, 103(6):1307-9.

Baumann RJ, "Prevention and Mangement of Febrile Seizures," *Paediatr Drugs*, 2001, 3(8):585-92.

Baumann RJ and Duffner PK, "Treatment of Children With Simple Febrile Seizures: The AAP Practice Parameter," *Pediatr Neurol*, 2000, 23(1):11-7.

Berg AT, Shinnar S, Hauser WA, et al, "Predictors of Recurrent Febrile Seizures: A Meta-Analytic Review," *J Pediatr*, 1990, 116(3):329-37.

Camfield PR, Camfield CS, Gordon K, et al, "Prevention of Recurrent Febrile Seizures," *J Pediatr*, 1995, 126(6):929-30.

NIH Consensus Statement, "Febrile Seizures: A Consensus of Their Significance, Evaluation and Treatment," *Pediatrics*, 1980, 66(6):1009-12.

Rosman NP, Colton T, Labazzo J, et al, "A Controlled Trial of Diazepam Administration During Febrile Illnesses to Prevent Recurrence of Febrile Seizures," *N Engl J Med*, 1993, 329(2):79-84.

Shinnar S and Glauser TA, "Febrile Seizures," *J Child Neurol*, 2002, 17:S44-52.

Srinivasan J, Wallace KA, and Scheffer IE, "Febrile Seizures," *Australian Family Physician*, 2005, 34(12):1021-5.

Uhari M, Rantala H, Vainionpää L, et al, "Effect of Acetaminophen and of Low Intermittent Doses of Diazepam on Prevention of Recurrences of Febrile Seizures," *J Pediatr*, 1995, 126(6):991-5.

CAUSES OF NEONATAL SEIZURES

1. Trauma
   a. subdural hematoma
   b. intracortical hemorrhage
   c. cortical vein thrombosis
2. Asphyxia — subependymal hemorrhage
3. Congenital abnormalities (cerebral dysgenesis)
   a. lissencephaly
   b. schizencephaly
4. Hypertension
5. Metabolic
   a. hypocalcemia
      - hypomagnesemia
      - high phosphate load
      - IDM (infants of diabetic mothers)
      - hypoparathyroidism
      - maternal hyperparathyroidism
      - idiopathic
      - DiGeorge's syndrome
   b. hypoglycemia
      - galactosemia
      - IUGR (intrauterine growth retardation)
      - IDM (infants of diabetic mothers)
      - glycogen storage disease
      - idiopathic
      - methylmalonic acidemia
      - propionic acidemia
      - maple syrup urine disease
      - asphyxia
   c. electrolyte imbalance
      - hypernatremia
      - hypomagnesemia
      - hyponatremia
6. Infections
   a. bacterial meningitis
   b. cerebral abscess
   c. herpes encephalitis
   d. Coxsackie meningoencephalitis
   e. cytomegalovirus
   f. toxoplasmosis
   g. syphilis

7. Drug withdrawal
   a. methadone
   b. heroin
   c. barbiturate (short-acting, such as secobarbital and butalbital)
   d. propoxyphene
   e. benzodiazepines (chlordiazepoxide, diazepam)
   f. cocaine
   g. ethanol
   h. codeine
8. Pyridoxine dependency
9. Amino acid disturbances
   a. maple syrup urine disease
   b. urea cycle abnormalities
   c. nonketotic hyperglycinemia
   d. ketotic hyperglycinemia
   e. Leigh disease
   f. isovaleric acidemia
10. Toxins
    a. local anesthetics
    b. isoniazid
    c. lead
    d. indomethacin (from breast feeding)
    e. fentanyl
11. Familial seizures
    a. neurocutaneous syndromes
       - tuberous sclerosis
       - incontinentia pigmenti
    b. genetic syndromes
       - Zellweger's
       - Smith Lemli Opitz
       - neonatal adrenoleukodystrophy
    c. benign familial epilepsy
12. Cerebral hemorrhage
    a. intraventricular
    b. subarachnoid
    c. subdural

Adapted from Painter MJ, Bergman I, and Crumrine P, "Neonatal Seizures," *Pediatr Clin North Am*, 1986, 33(1):91-107.

ANTIEPILEPTIC DRUGS

Note: This table is derived from the treatment guidelines from the International League Against Epilepsy (ILAE), the American Academy of Neurology, and the American Epilepsy Society. Agents listed may or may not have FDA approval for the given indication or age group. Recommended medications from ILAE treatment guidelines are bolded.

Antiepileptic Drugs for Children and Adolescents by Seizure Type and Epilepsy Syndrome[1]

Seizure Type or Epilepsy Syndrome	First-Line Therapies (Monotherapy)	Effective Alternatives	Additional Information
Partial-onset seizures	**Oxcarbazepine**	**Carbamazepine** **Lamotrigine** Levetiracetam **Phenobarbital** **Phenytoin** **Topiramate** **Valproic acid** **Vigabatrin**	Consider felbamate for refractory seizures. FDA approved adjunct therapy: Gabapentin, lamotrigine, tiagabine, topiramate, zonisamide
Generalized tonic-clonic seizures	**Carbamazepine** **Phenobarbital** **Phenytoin** **Topiramate** **Valproic acid**	Lamotrigine **Oxcarbazepine**	FDA approved adjunct therapy: Gabapentin, lamotrigine, levetiracetam, topiramate
Absence seizures	**Ethosuximide** **Lamotrigine** **Valproic acid**		May worsen seizures: Carbamazepine, oxcarbazepine, phenobarbital, phenytoin, tiagabine, vigabatrin
Juvenile myoclonic epilepsy	**Clonazepam** **Lamotrigine** **Levetiracetam** **Topiramate** **Valproic acid** **Zonisamide**		FDA approved adjunct therapy: Levetiracetam. May worsen seizures: Carbamazepine, gabapentin, oxcarbazepine, phenytoin, tiagabine, vigabatrin
Lennox-Gastaut syndrome	Valproic acid	Lamotrigine Topiramate	Consider felbamate for refractory seizures. This syndrome frequently requires multiple drugs for control of seizures.
Benign epilepsy of childhood with centrotemporal spikes	**Carbamazepine** **Valproic acid**	**Gabapentin**	Some children do not require antiepileptic therapy
Infantile spasms	ACTH	Corticosteroids Vigabatrin	Consider valproic acid. No evidence exists that any therapy improves long-term outcome.
Neonatal seizures	Phenobarbital	Phenytoin	Consider: Clonazepam, valproic acid, pyridoxine. No treatment guidelines exist for neonatal seizures. Benzodiazepines can be given I.V. to stop active neonatal seizures.

[1]Selection of the initial AED for a child or adolescent with newly diagnosed or untreated seizures requires consideration of other variables, not just efficacy. Other factors which should be considered include: AED-related factors (eg, adverse effect profile, pharmacokinetics, potential for drug interactions, available formulations, carcinogenic and teratogenic potential), patient-related factors (eg, age, gender, genetic background, concurrent medications, other disease states, ability to swallow tablets/capsules, capacity to afford, insurance coverage), country-related factors (AED cost, AED availability) (Glauser, 2006).

References

Bartha AI, Shen J, Katz KH, et al, "Neonatal Seizures: Multicenter Variability in Current Treatment Practices," *Pediatr Neurol*, 2007, 37(2):85-90.

Bourgeois BF, "Antiepileptic Drugs in Pediatric Practice," *Epilepsia*, 1995, 36(Suppl 2):S34-45.

Bourgeois BF, "New Antiepileptic Drugs in Children: Which Ones for Which Seizures?" *Clin Neuropharmacol*, 2000, 23(3):119-32.

French JA, Kanner AM, Bautista J, et al, "Efficacy and Tolerability of the New Antiepileptic Drugs I: Treatment of New Onset Epilepsy: Report of the Therapeutics and Technology Assessment Subcommittee and Quality Standards Subcommittee of the American Academy of Neurology and the American Epilepsy Society," *Neurology*, 2004, 62(8):1252-60.

French JA, Kanner AM, Bautista J, et al, "Efficacy and Tolerability of the New Antiepileptic Drugs II: Treatment of Refractory Epilepsy: Report of the Therapeutics and Technology Assessment Subcommittee and Quality Standards Subcommittee of the American Academy of Neurology and the American Epilepsy Society," *Neurology*, 2004, 62(8):1261-73.

Glauser T, Ben-Menachem E, Bourgeois B, et al, "ILAE Treatment Guidelines: Evidence-Based Analysis of Antiepileptic Drug Efficacy and Effectiveness as Initial Monotherapy for Epileptic Seizures and Syndromes," *Epilepsia*, 2006, 47(7):1094-120.

Mackay MT, Weiss SK, Adams-Webber T, et al, "Practice Parameter: Medical Treatment of Infantile Spasms: Report of the American Academy of Neurology and the Child Neurology Society," *Neurology*, 2004, 62(10):1668-81.

COMA SCALES

Glasgow Coma Scale

Activity	Best Response	Score
Eye opening	Spontaneous	4
	Responds to voice	3
	Responds to pain	2
	No response	1
Verbal response	Oriented and appropriate	5
	Confused / disoriented conversation	4
	Inappropriate words	3
	Nonspecific sounds (incomprehensible)	2
	No response	1
Motor response	Follows commands	6
	Localizes pain	5
	Withdraws to pain	4
	Abnormal flexion (decorticate posturing)	3
	Abnormal extension (decerebrate posturing)	2
	No response	1

Modified Coma Scale for Infants

Activity	Best Response	Score
Eye opening	Spontaneous	4
	Responds to voice	3
	Responds to pain	2
	No response	1
Verbal response	Coos, babbles	5
	Irritable	4
	Cries to pain	3
	Moans to pain	2
	No response	1
Motor response	Normal spontaneous movements	6
	Withdraws to touch	5
	Withdraws to pain	4
	Abnormal flexion (decorticate posturing)	3
	Abnormal extension (decerebrate posturing)	2
	No response	1

Interpretation of Coma Scale Scores
Maximum Score: 15; Minimum Score: 3
(low score indicates greater severity of coma)

Range of Score	Interpretation
3- 8	Coma. Severe brain injury. Immediate action needed. Notify ICU staff STAT. Will require intubation regardless of respiratory status.
9-12	Lethargic. Needs close observation in special care unit. Frequent neuro checks. Notify ICU staff.
13-14	Needs observation
15	Normal

References
James HE, "Neurologic Evaluation and Support in the Child With an Acute Brain Insult," *Pediatr Ann*, 1986, 15(1):16-22.
Jennett B and Teasdale G, "Aspects of Coma After Severe Head Injury," *Lancet*, 1977, 1(8017): 878-81.

SEROTONIN SYNDROME

Manifestations of Severe Serotonin Syndrome and Related Clinical Conditions

Condition	Medication History	Time Needed for Condition to Develop	Vital Signs	Pupils	Mucosa	Skin	Bowel Sounds	Neuromuscular Tone	Reflexes	Mental Status
Serotonin syndrome	Proserotonergic drug	<12 hours	Hypertension, tachycardia, tachypnea, hyperthermia (>41.1°C)	Mydriasis	Sialorrhea	Diaphoresis	Hyperactive	Increased, predominantly in lower extremities	Hyper-reflexia, clonus (unless masked by increased muscle tone)	Agitation, coma
Anticholinergic "toxidrome"	Anticholinergic agent	<12 hours	Hypertension (mild), tachycardia, tachypnea, hyperthermia (typically ≤38.8°C)	Mydriasis	Dry	Erythema, hot and dry to touch	Decreased or absent	Normal	Normal	Agitated delirium
Neuroleptic malignant syndrome	Dopamine antagonist	1-3 days	Hypertension, tachycardia, tachypnea, hyperthermia (>41.1°C)	Normal	Sialorrhea	Pallor, diaphoresis	Normal or decreased	"Lead-pipe" rigidity present in all muscle groups	Bradyreflexia	Stupor, alert mutism, coma
Malignant hyperthermia	Inhalational anesthesia	30 minutes to 24 hours after administration of inhalational anesthesia or succinylcholine	Hypertension, tachycardia, tachypnea, hyperthermia (can be as high as 46°C)	Normal	Normal	Mottled appearance, diaphoresis	Decreased	Rigor mortis-like rigidity	Hyporeflexia	Agitation

Management of Serotonin Syndrome

1. Remove precipitating drugs
   a. Serotonergic agents (eg, antidepressants; especially SSRI and MAO Inhibitors)
   b. Be mindful of half-life elimination and active metabolites
2. Supportive care
   a. Intravenous fluids
   b. Correct vital signs
3. Control agitation
   a. Benzodiazepines (diazepam)
   b. Avoid physical restraints
4. 5-HT$_{2A}$ antagonists
   a. Cyproheptadine: Adult: 12-32 mg/day (may be crushed and administered via nasogastric tube)
   b. Chlorpromazine: Adult: I.M.: 50-100 mg (monitor vitals)
5. Control autonomic instability
   a. Norepinephrine **or**
   b. Phenylephrine **or**
   c. Epinephrine
   d. Nitroprusside or esmolol for hypertension and tachycardia
6. Control hyperthermia
   a. Benzodiazepines
   b. Neuromuscular paralysis with vecuronium (**Note:** Avoid succinylcholine)
   c. Intubation
   d. Do not use antipyretic agents
7. Other
   a. Do not use propranolol, bromocriptine, and dantrolene

ASTHMA

MANAGEMENT OF ASTHMA IN ADULTS AND CHILDREN

Goals of Asthma Treatment

- Prevent chronic and troublesome symptoms: Minimal or no chronic symptoms day or night
- No limitations on activities; no school/work missed
- Minimal use of inhaled short-acting beta$_2$-agonist (≤2 days/week, <1 canister/month) (not including prevention of exercise induced asthma)
- Minimal or no adverse effects from medications
- Maintain (near) normal pulmonary function
- Prevent recurrent exacerbations (ie, trips to emergency department or hospitalizations)

All Patients

- Short-acting bronchodilator: **Inhaled beta$_2$-agonists** as needed for symptoms.
- Intensity of treatment will depend on severity of exacerbation; see "Management of Asthma Exacerbations".
- Use of short-acting inhaled beta$_2$-agonists on a daily basis, or increasing use, indicates the need to initiate or titrate long-term control therapy.

Education

- Teach self-management.
- Teach about controlling environmental factors (avoidance of allergens or other factors that contribute to asthma severity).
- Review administration technique and compliance with patient.
- Use a written action plan to help educate.

Stepwise Approach for Managing Asthma in Adults and Children ≥12 Years of Age

Symptoms	Lung Function	Daily Medications
STEP 6: Severe Asthma		
Day: Throughout the day Night: Often 7 times/week SABA use: Several times/day	FEV$_1$ <60% predicted FEV$_1$/FVC reduced 5%	**Preferred:** High dose ICS plus LABA plus oral corticosteroid AND Consider: Omalizumab (in those with allergies)[1]
STEP 5: Severe Asthma		
Day: Throughout the day Night: Often 7 times/week SABA use: Several times/day	FEV$_1$ <60% predicted FEV$_1$/FVC reduced 5%	**Preferred:** High dose ICS plus LABA AND Consider: Omalizumab (in those with allergies)[1]
STEP 4: Severe Asthma		
Day: Throughout the day Night: Often 7 times/week SABA use: Several times/day	FEV$_1$ <60% predicted FEV$_1$/FVC reduced 5%	**Preferred:** Medium dose ICS plus LABA
		Alternatives[2]: Medium dose ICS plus either LTRA, theophylline, or zileuton[3]
STEP 3: Moderate Asthma		
Day: Daily Night: >1 night/week (not nightly) SABA use: Daily	FEV$_1$ >60%, <80% predicted FEV$_1$/FVC reduced 5%	**Preferred:** Low dose ICS plus LABA OR Medium dose ICS
		Alternatives[2]: Low dose ICS plus either LTRA, theophylline, or zileuton[3]
STEP 2: Mild Asthma		
Day: >2 days/week (not daily) Night: 3-4 times/month SABA use: >2 days/week, no more than once per day (not daily)	FEV$_1$ <80% FEV$_1$/FVC normal	**Preferred:** Low dose ICS
		Alternatives[2]: Cromolyn, LTRA, nedocromil, or theophylline
STEP 1: Intermittent Asthma		
Day: ≤2 days/week Night: ≤2 nights/month SABA use: ≤2 days/week	FEV$_1$ normal between exacerbations FEV$_1$ >80% predicted FEV$_1$/FVC normal	**Preferred:** SABA as needed

Note: Treatment options within each step are listed in alphabetical order

Steps 2-4: Consider subcutaneous allergen immunotherapy for patients with allergic asthma.[1]

Consult with asthma specialist if Step 4 or higher care is needed.

FEV$_1$: Forced expiratory volume in 1 second; FVC: Forced vital capacity; ICS: inhaled corticosteroid; LABA: long-acting inhaled beta$_2$-agonist; SABA: short-acting inhaled beta$_2$-agonist; LTRA: leukotriene receptor antagonist

[1]When using immunotherapy or omalizumab, clinicians should be prepared to identify and treat anaphylaxis in the event it occurs.

[2]If alternative treatment is used and response is inadequate, discontinue it and use preferred treatment before stepping up.

[3]Zileuton is less desirable alternative due to limited studies and need to monitor liver function.

◄ **Notes:**

- **The stepwise approach presents general guidelines to assist clinical decision making; it is not intended to be a specific prescription. Asthma is highly variable; clinicians should tailor specific medication plans to the needs and circumstances of individual patients.**
- Gain control as quickly as possible; then decrease treatment to the least medication necessary to maintain control.
- A rescue course of systemic corticosteroids may be needed at any time and at any step.
- Some patients with intermittent asthma experience severe and life-threatening exacerbations separated by long periods of normal lung function and no symptoms. This may be especially common with exacerbations provoked by respiratory infections.
- At each step, patient education, environmental control, management of comorbidities emphasized.
- Antibiotics are not recommended for treatment of acute asthma exacerbations except where there is evidence or suspicion of bacterial infection.
- Consultation with an asthma specialist is recommended for moderate or severe persistent asthma.
- Peak flow monitoring for patients with moderate-severe persistent asthma and patients who have a history of severe exacerbations should be considered.

MANAGEMENT OF ASTHMA IN INFANTS AND YOUNG CHILDREN (<12 YEARS OF AGE)

Stepwise Approach for Managing Asthma in Children 0-4 Years of Age

Symptoms	Daily Medications[1]
STEP 6: Severe Asthma	
Day: Throughout the day Night: >1 time/week SABA use: Several times/day	**Preferred:** High dose ICS plus either LABA or montelukast Oral systemic corticosteroids
STEP 5: Severe Asthma	
Day: Throughout the day Night: >1 time/week SABA use: Daily	**Preferred:** High dose ICS plus either LABA or montelukast
STEP 4: Moderate Asthma	
Day: Daily Night: 3-4 times/month SABA use: Daily	**Preferred:** Medium dose ICS plus either LABA or montelukast
STEP 3: Moderate Asthma	
Day: Daily Night: 3-4 times/month SABA use: Daily	**Preferred:** Medium dose ICS
STEP 2: Mild Asthma	
Day: >2 days/week (not daily) Night: 1-2 times/month SABA use: >2 days/week, no more than once per day (not daily)	**Preferred:** Low dose ICS **Alternatives[2]:** Cromolyn, montelukast
STEP 1: Intermittent Asthma	
Day: ≤2 days/week Night: No symptoms SABA use: ≤2 days/week	SABA as needed

Consult with asthma specialist if Step 3 or higher care is needed.

FEV$_1$: Forced expiratory volume in 1 second; FVC: Forced vital capacity; ICS: inhaled corticosteroid; LABA: long-acting inhaled beta$_2$-agonist; SABA: short-acting inhaled beta$_2$-agonist

[1]Studies on children 0-4 years old are limited. Many recommendations are based on expert opinion and extrapolation from studies of older children.

[2]If alternative treatment is used and response is inadequate, discontinue it and use preferred treatment before stepping up.

Stepwise Approach for Managing Asthma in Children 5-11 Years

Symptoms	Lung Function	Daily Medications
STEP 6: Severe Asthma		
Day: Throughout the day Night: Often 7 times/week SABA use: Several times/day	FEV$_1$ <60% predicted FEV$_1$/FVC <75%	**Preferred:** High dose ICS plus LABA plus oral corticosteroid
		Alternative[1]: High dose ICS plus either LTRA or theophylline[2] plus oral systemic corticosteroid
STEP 5: Severe Asthma		
Day: Throughout the day Night: Often 7 times/week SABA use: Several times/day	FEV$_1$ <60% predicted FEV$_1$/FVC <75%	**Preferred:** High dose ICS plus LABA
		Alternative[1]: High dose ICS plus either LTRA or theophylline[2]
STEP 4: Severe Asthma		
Day: Throughout the day Night: Often 7 times/week SABA use: Several times/day	FEV$_1$ <60% predicted FEV$_1$/FVC <75%	**Preferred:** Medium dose ICS plus LABA
		Alternative[1]: Medium dose ICS plus either LTRA or theophylline[2]
STEP 3: Moderate Asthma		
Day: Daily Night: >1 time/week (not nightly) SABA use: Daily	FEV$_1$ 60% to 80% predicted FEV$_1$/FVC 75% to 80%	**Preferred:** Low dose ICS plus either LABA, LTRA, or theophylline[2] OR Medium dose ICS
STEP 2: Mild Asthma		
Day: >2 days/week (not daily) Night: 3-4 times/month SABA use: >2 days/week, no more than once per day (not daily)	FEV$_1$ ≥80% predicted FEV$_1$/FVC >80%	**Preferred:** Low dose ICS
		Alternatives[1]: Cromolyn, LTRA, nedocromil, or theophylline[2]
STEP 1: Intermittent Asthma		
Day: ≤2 days/week Night: ≤2 times/month SABA use: ≤2 days/week	FEV$_1$ normal between exacerbations FEV$_1$ >80% predicted FEV$_1$/FVC >85%	SABA as needed

Steps 2-4: Consider subcutaneous allergen immunotherapy for patients with allergic asthma.[3]

Consult with asthma specialist if Step 4 or higher care is needed.

FEV$_1$: Forced expiratory volume in 1 second; FVC: Forced vital capacity; ICS: inhaled corticosteroid; LABA: long-acting inhaled beta$_2$-agonist; SABA: short-acting inhaled beta$_2$-agonist; LTRA: leukotriene receptor antagonist

[1]If alternative treatment is used and response is inadequate, discontinue it and use preferred treatment before stepping up.

[2]Theophylline is a less desirable alternative due monitoring required.

[3]When using immunotherapy, clinicians should be prepared to identify and treat anaphylaxis in the event it occurs.

Management of Asthma Exacerbations: Home Treatment

Assess Severity

- **Patients at high risk for a fatal attack require immediate medical attention after initial treatment.**

- Symptoms and signs suggestive of a more serious exacerbation such as marked breathlessness, inability to speak more than short phrases, use of accessory muscles, or drowsiness should result in initial treatment while immediately consulting with a clinician.

- If available, measure PEF—values of 50% to 79% predicted or personal best indicate the need for quick-relief mediation. Depending on the response to treatment, contact with a clinician may also be indicated. Values below 50% indicate the need for immediate medical care.

Initial Treatment

- Inhaled SABA: Up to two treatments 20 minutes apart of 2–6 puffs by metered-dose inhaler (MDI) or nebulizer treatments.

- Note: Medication delivery is highly variable. Children and individuals who have exacerbations of lesser severity may need fewer puffs than suggested above.

Good Response

No wheezing or dyspnea (assess tachypnea in young children).

PEF ≥80% predicted or personal best.

- Contact clinician for followup instructions and further management.

- May continue inhaled SABA every 3–4 hours for 24–48 hours.

- Consider short course of oral systemic corticosteroids.

Incomplete Response

Persistent wheezing and dyspnea (tachypnea).

PEF 50% to 79% predicted or personal best.

- Add oral systemic corticosteroid.

- Continue inhaled SABA.

- Contact clinician urgently (this day) for further instruction.

Poor Response

Marked wheezing and dyspnea.

PEF <50% predicted or personal best.

- Add oral systemic corticosteroid

- Repeat inhaled SABA immediately.

- If distress is severe and nonresponsive to initial treatment:

  – Call your doctor AND

  – **PROCEED TO EMERGENCY DEPARTMENT;**

  – Consider calling 911 (ambulance transport).

- To emergency department.

MDI: Metered-dose inhaler; PEF: Peak expiratory flow; SABA: Short-acting beta$_2$-agonist (quick relief inhaler)

Management of Asthma Exacerbations: Emergency Department and Hospital-Based Care

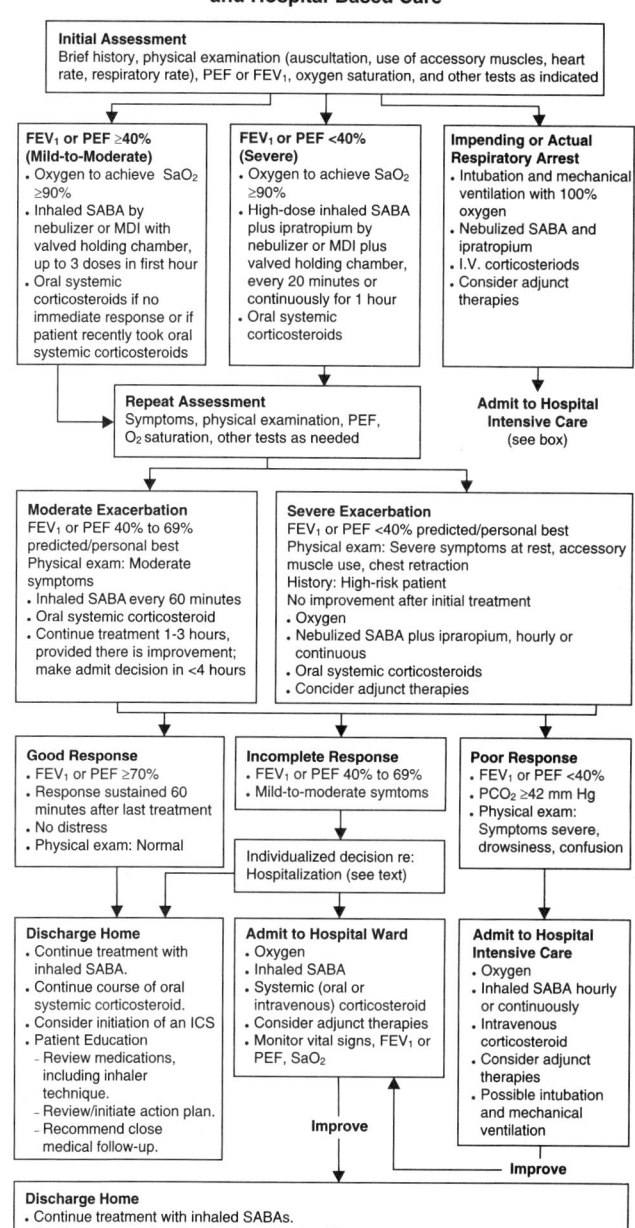

Initial Assessment
Brief history, physical examination (auscultation, use of accessory muscles, heart rate, respiratory rate), PEF or FEV₁, oxygen saturation, and other tests as indicated

FEV₁ or PEF ≥40% (Mild-to-Moderate)
- Oxygen to achieve SaO₂ ≥90%
- Inhaled SABA by nebulizer or MDI with valved holding chamber, up to 3 doses in first hour
- Oral systemic corticosteroids if no immediate response or if patient recently took oral systemic corticosteroids

FEV₁ or PEF <40% (Severe)
- Oxygen to achieve SaO₂ ≥90%
- High-dose inhaled SABA plus ipratropium by nebulizer or MDI plus valved holding chamber, every 20 minutes or continuously for 1 hour
- Oral systemic corticosteroids

Impending or Actual Respiratory Arrest
- Intubation and mechanical ventilation with 100% oxygen
- Nebulized SABA and ipratropium
- I.V. corticosteriods
- Consider adjunct therapies

Repeat Assessment
Symptoms, physical examination, PEF, O₂ saturation, other tests as needed

Admit to Hospital Intensive Care
(see box)

Moderate Exacerbation
FEV₁ or PEF 40% to 69% predicted/personal best
Physical exam: Moderate symptoms
- Inhaled SABA every 60 minutes
- Oral systemic corticosteroid
- Continue treatment 1-3 hours, provided there is improvement; make admit decision in <4 hours

Severe Exacerbation
FEV₁ or PEF <40% predicted/personal best
Physical exam: Severe symptoms at rest, accessory muscle use, chest retraction
History: High-risk patient
No improvement after initial treatment
- Oxygen
- Nebulized SABA plus ipraropium, hourly or continuous
- Oral systemic corticosteroids
- Concider adjunct therapies

Good Response
- FEV₁ or PEF ≥70%
- Response sustained 60 minutes after last treatment
- No distress
- Physical exam: Normal

Incomplete Response
- FEV₁ or PEF 40% to 69%
- Mild-to-moderate symtoms

Individualized decision re: Hospitalization (see text)

Poor Response
- FEV₁ or PEF <40%
- PCO₂ ≥42 mm Hg
- Physical exam: Symptoms severe, drowsiness, confusion

Discharge Home
- Continue treatment with inhaled SABA.
- Continue course of oral systemic corticosteroid.
- Consider initiation of an ICS
- Patient Education
  - Review medications, including inhaler technique.
  - Review/initiate action plan.
  - Recommend close medical follow-up.

Admit to Hospital Ward
- Oxygen
- Inhaled SABA
- Systemic (oral or intravenous) corticosteroid
- Consider adjunct therapies
- Monitor vital signs, FEV₁ or PEF, SaO₂

Improve

Admit to Hospital Intensive Care
- Oxygen
- Inhaled SABA hourly or continuously
- Intravenous corticosteroid
- Consider adjunct therapies
- Possible intubation and mechanical ventilation

Improve

Discharge Home
- Continue treatment with inhaled SABAs.
- Continue course of oral systemic corticosteroid.
- Continue on ICS. For those not on long-term control therapy, consider initiation of an ICS.
- Patient education (eg, review medications, including inhaler technique and, whenever possible, environmental control measures; review/initiate action plan; recommend close medical follow-up).
- Before discharge, schedule follow-up appointment with primary care provider and/or asthma specialist in 1-4 weeks.

FEV₁ = forced expiratory volume in 1 second; ICS = inhaled corticosteroid; MDI = metered dose inhaler; PCO₂ = partial pressure carbon dioxide; PEF = peak expiratory flow; SABA = short-acting beta₂-agonist; SaO₂ = oxygen saturation

ESTIMATED COMPARATIVE <u>DAILY</u> DOSAGES FOR INHALED CORTICOSTEROIDS

Children ≥12 Years of Age and Adults

Drug	Low Daily Dose	Medium Daily Dose	High Daily Dose
Beclomethasone HFA 40 mcg/puff 80 mcg/puff	80-240 mcg	>240-480 mcg	>480 mcg
Budesonide DPI 90 mcg/puff 180 mcg/puff 200 mcg/puff	180-600 mcg	>600-1200 mcg	>1200 mcg
Flunisolide 250 mcg/puff	500-1000 mcg	>1000-2000 mcg	>2000 mcg
Flunisolide HFA 80 mcg/puff	320 mcg	>320-640 mcg	>640 mcg
Fluticasone HFA 44 mcg/puff 110 mcg/puff 220 mcg/puff	88-264 mcg	>264-440 mcg	>440 mcg
Mometasone DPI 220 mcg/puff	220 mcg	440 mcg	>440 mcg
Triamcinolone 100 mcg/puff	300-750 mcg	>750-1500 mcg	>1500 mcg

DPI: Dry powder inhaler; HFA: Hydrofluoroalkane

Children <12 Years of Age

Drug	Low Daily Dose	Medium Daily Dose	High Daily Dose
Beclomethasone HFA 40 mcg/puff 80 mcg/puff	0-4 years: NA 5-11 years: 80-160 mcg	0-4 years: NA 5-11 years: >160-320 mcg	0-4 years: NA 5-11 years: >320 mcg
Budesonide DPI 90 mcg/puff 180 mcg/puff 200 mcg/puff	0-4 years: NA 5-11 years: 180-400 mcg	0-4 years: NA 5-11 years: >400-800 mcg	0-4 years: NA 5-11 years: >800 mcg
Budesonide nebulized 0.25 mg/2 mL 0.5 mg/2 mL	0-4 years: 0.25-0.5 mg 5-11 years: 0.5 mg	0-4 years: >0.5-1 mg 5-11 years: 1 mg	0-4 years: >1 mg 5-11 years: 2 mg
Flunisolide 250 mcg/puff	0-4 years: NA 5-11 years: 500-750 mcg	0-4 years: NA 5-11 years: 1000-1250 mcg	0-4 years: NA 5-11 years: >1250 mcg
Flunisolide HFA 80 mcg/puff	0-4 years: NA 5-11 years: 160 mcg	0-4 years: NA 5-11 years: 320 mcg	0-4 years: NA 5-11 years: ≥640 mcg
Fluticasone HFA 44 mcg/puff 110 mcg/puff 220 mcg/puff	0-4 years: 176 mcg 5-11 years: 88-176 mcg	0-11 years: >176-352 mcg	0-11 years: >352 mcg
Fluticasone DPI 50 mcg/puff 100 mcg/puff 250 mcg/puff	0-4 years: NA 5-11 years: 100-200 mcg	0-4 years: NA 5-11 years: >200-400 mcg	0-4 years: NA 5-11 years: >400 mcg
Mometasone	NA	NA	NA
Triamcinolone 100 mcg/puff	0-4 years: NA 5-11 years: 300-600 mcg	0-4 years: NA 5-11 years: >600-900 mcg	0-4 years: NA 5-11 years: >900 mcg

DPI: Dry powder inhaler; HFA: Hydrofluoroalkane

NA: Not approved for use in this age group or no data available.

Reference
Expert Panel Report 3, "Guidelines for the Diagnosis and Management of Asthma," *Clinical Practice Guidelines*, National Institutes of Health, National Heart, Lung, and Blood Institute, NIH Publication No. 08-4051, prepublication 2007. Available at http://www.nhlbi.nih.gov/guidelines/asthma/asthgdln.htm.

NORMAL RESPIRATORY RATES

Hour After Birth	Average Respiratory Rate	Range
1st hour	60 breaths/minute	20-100
2-6 hours	50 breaths/minute	20-80
>6 hours	30-40 breaths/minute	20-60

Age (years)	Mean RR (breaths/minute)
0-2	25-30
3-9	20-25
10-18	16-20

THERAPEUTIC DRUG MONITORING: BLOOD SAMPLING TIME GUIDELINES

Drug	Infusion Time	Therapeutic Range	When to Obtain Sample
Amikacin sulfate			
I.V.	30 min	Peak: 20-30 mcg/mL Trough: <10 mcg/mL	Peak: 30 min after end of 30 min infusion Trough: Within 30 min before next dose
I.M.			Peak: 1 h after I.M. injection Trough: Within 30 min before next dose
Caffeine			
I.V./P.O.	Caffeine **citrate** I.V.: Loading dose: ≥30 min Maintenance: ≥10 min	Apnea of prematurity: 8-20 mcg/mL	Just before next dose
Carbamazepine		4-12 mcg/mL	Just before next dose
Chloramphenicol			

I.V.	15-30 min	Meningitis:
		  Peak: 15-25 mcg/mL
		  Trough: 5-15 mcg/mL
		Other infections:
		  Peak: 10-20 mcg/mL
		  Trough: 5-10 mcg/mL
			Peak: 90 min after end of 15-30 min infusion
			Trough: Just before next dose

Cyclosporine			
I.V./P.O.		BMT: 100-250 ng/mL (serum, RIA) Heart transplant: 100-200 ng/mL (serum, RIA) Liver transplant: 100-400 ng/mL (blood, HPLC) Renal transplant: 100-200 ng/mL (serum, RIA)	Just before next dose
Digoxin			
I.V./P.O.		Age and disease related: 0.8-2 ng/mL	6 h postdose to just before next dose
Enoxaparin			

SubQ		Antifactor Xa: **Note:** No clear consensus exists; these are suggested peak values for VTE in adults (see Nutescu, 2009)
		Therapeutic:
		  Twice daily dosing: 0.5-1 units/mL
		  Once daily dosing: 1–2 units/mL[1]
		Prophylactic: 0.2-0.45 units/mL
			Peak: 4-6 h postdose

Ethosuximide			
P.O.		40-100 mcg/mL	Just before next dose
Flucytosine			
P.O.		25-100 mcg/mL Invasive candidiasis: Peak: 40-60 mcg/mL Trough: ≥25 mcg/mL to prevent emergence of resistant strains	Peak: 1-2 h postdose after at least 4 days of therapy Trough: Just before next dose
Fosphenytoin (measure phenytoin concentration)			
I.V.		Phenytoin: 10-20 mcg/mL	Peak: 2 h after end of an infusion
I.M.			Peak: 4 h after I.M. injection
Gentamicin			
I.V. (traditional dosing)	30 min	Peak: 4-12 mcg/mL Trough: 0.5-2 mcg/mL	Peak: 30 min after end of 30 min infusion Trough: Within 30 min before next dose
I.M. (traditional dosing)			Peak: 1 h after I.M. injection Trough: Within 30 min before next dose
Phenobarbital		15-40 mcg/mL	Trough: Just before next dose
Phenytoin			
I.V./P.O.		10-20 mcg/mL	Trough: Just before next dose
I.V.			Post-load/Peak: 1 h after end of infusion

Drug	Infusion Time	Therapeutic Range	When to Obtain Sample
Tacrolimus			
I.V./P.O.		Trough:[2,3] Whole blood ELISA: 5-20 ng/mL HPLC: 0.5-1.5 ng/mL	Trough: Just before next dose
Theophylline			
I.V. bolus	30 min	Asthma: 10-20 mcg/mL	Peak: 30 min after end of 30 min infusion
Continuous infusion			16-24 h after the start or change in a constant I.V. infusion
P.O. liquid, fast-release tablet (Somophyllin®, Slo-Phyllin® liquid & tablet)			Peak: 1 h postdose Trough: Just before next dose
P.O. slow-release (Theo-Dur®, Slo-Phyllin® GC, Slo-bid®)			Peak: 4 h postdose Trough: Just before next dose
Tobramycin			
I.V. (traditional dosing)	30 min	Peak: 4-12 mcg/mL Trough: 0.5-2 mcg/mL	Peak: 30 min after end of 30 min infusion Trough: Within 30 min before next dose
I.M. (traditional dosing)			Peak: 1 h post-I.M. injection Trough: Within 30 min before next dose
Valproic acid			
P.O.		50-100 mcg/mL	Trough: Just before next dose
Vancomycin	60 min	Trough: 5-20 mcg/mL, depending on MIC of organism[3]	Trough: Within 30 min before next dose

VTE = venous thromboembolism

[1]Once-daily dosing in pediatric patients is not feasible due to faster enoxaparin clearance and lower drug exposure in pediatric patients compared to adults (see O'Brien, 2007)

[2]Limited data exists correlating serum concentration to therapeutic effect/toxicity.

[3]See Reference Range in monograph for more details.

Reference

Nutescu EA, Spinler SA, Wittkowsky A, et al, "Low-Molecular-Weight Heparins in Renal Impairment and Obesity: Available Evidence and Clinical Practice Recommendations Across Medical and Surgical Settings," *Ann Pharmacother*, 2009, 43(6):1064-83.

O'Brien SH, Lee H, and Ritchey AK, "Once-Daily Enoxaparin in Pediatric Thromboembolism: A Dose Finding and Pharmacodynamics/Pharmacokinetics Study," *J Thromb Haemost*, 2007, 5(9):1985-7.

LABORATORY DETECTION OF DRUGS IN URINE

Agent	Time Detectable in Urine[1]
Alcohol	12-24 h
Amobarbital	2-4 d
Amphetamine	2-4 d
Butalbital	2-4 d
Cannabinoids	
Occasional use	2-7 d
Regular use	30 d
Cocaine (benzoylecgonine)	12-72 h
Codeine	2-4 d
Chlordiazepoxide	30 d
Diazepam	30 d
Ethanol	12-24 h
Heroin (morphine)	2-4 d
Hydromorphone	2-4 d
Marijuana	
Occasional use	2-7 d
Regular use	30 d
Methamphetamine	2-4 d
Methaqualone	2-4 d
Morphine	2-4 d
Pentobarbital	2-4 d
Phencyclidine (PCP)	
Occasional use	2-7 d
Regular use	30 d
Phenobarbital	30 d
Secobarbital	2-4 d

[1]The periods of detection for the various abused drugs listed above should be taken as estimates since the actual figures will vary due to metabolism, user, laboratory, and excretion.

Adapted from Chang JY, "Drug Testing and Interpretation of Results," *Pharmchem Newsletter*, 1989, 17:1.

SALICYLATE INTOXICATION

**Serum Salicylate Level and
Severity of Intoxication Single Dose
Acute Ingestion Nomogram**

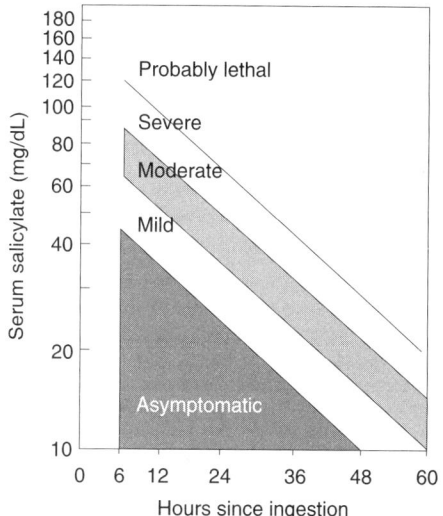

Nomogram relating serum salicylate concentration and expected severity of intoxication at varying intervals following the ingestion of a single dose of salicylate.

From Done AK, "Aspirin Overdosage: Incidence, Diagnosis, and Management," *Pediatrics*, 1978, 62:890-7 with permission.

ACETAMINOPHEN SERUM LEVEL NOMOGRAM

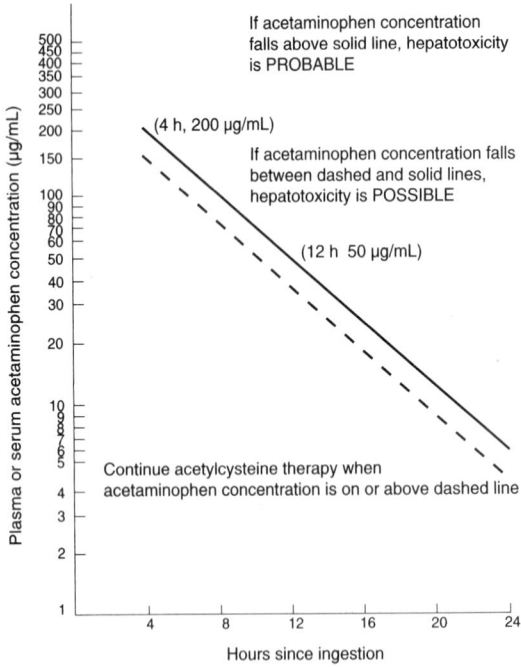

Nomogram relating plasma or serum acetaminophen concentration and probability of hepatotoxicity at varying intervals following ingestion of a single toxic dose of acetaminophen. Modified from Rumack BH, Matthew H, "Acetaminophen Poisoning and Toxicity", Pediatrics, 1975, 55:871-6, © American Academy of Pediatrics, 1975, and from Rumack BH, et al, "Acetaminophen Overdose", Arch Intern Med, 1981, 141:380-5, © American Medical Association.

MEDICATIONS FOR WHICH A SINGLE DOSE MAY BE FATAL WHEN INGESTED BY A TODDLER

Medication[1]	Minimal Potential Fatal Dose (mg/kg)	Maximal Dose Unit Available (mg)
Antiarrhythmics		
Disopyramide	15	150
Flecainide	25	150
Procainamide	70	1000
Quinidine	15	324
Antimalarials		
Chloroquine	20	500
Hydroxychloroquine	20	200
Quinine	80	650
Antipsychotics		
Chlorpromazine	25	200
Loxapine	30-70	50
Thioridazine	15	200
Calcium channel blockers		
Diltiazem	15	360
Nifedipine	15	90
Verapamil	15	360
Camphor	100	1 g/5 mL
Methyl salicylate	200	1.4 g/mL
Narcotics		
Codeine	7-14	60
Hydrocodone	1.5	60 mg/5 mL
Methadone	1-2	40
Morphine		200
Oral hypoglycemics		
Chlorpropamide	5	25
Glibenclamide	0.1	2.5
Glipizide	0.1	5
Podophyllin 25%	15-20	1.25 g/5 mL
Theophylline	8.4	500
Tricyclic antidepressants		
Amitriptyline	15	100
Desipramine	15	150
Imipramine	15	75

[1]Assumptions: Toddler would weigh 10 kg; the lowest described or estimated fatal dose (adjusted for body weight) was used; the toddler is healthy, with normal drug metabolism.

Adapted from Bar-Oz B, Levichek Z, and Koren G, "Medications That Can Be Fatal for a Toddler With One Tablet or Teaspoonful: A 2004 Update," *Paediatr Drugs*, 2004, 6(2):123-6.

BREAST-FEEDING AND DRUGS

Breast-feeding is recommended for all infants unless specific contraindications exist. Human breast milk is superior to alternative products for both full-term and premature infants and exclusive breast-feeding provides sufficient nutrition for up to 6 months of life. Breast-feeding provides additional health benefits to the infant, such as decreased incidence of infection; some studies suggest breast-feeding may also decrease the risk of sudden infant death syndrome, type 1 or 2 diabetes mellitus, and increase neurodevelopment.

Breast-feeding is not recommended in the following situations:

- Infants with classic galactosemia (galactose 1-phosphate uridyltransferase deficiency)
- Mothers with untreated/active tuberculosis
- Mothers who are human t-cell lymphotropic virus type I or II positive
- Mothers exposed to radioactive materials (diagnostic or therapeutic; until they are cleared from breast milk)
- Mothers who are receiving chemotherapeutic agents or antimetabolites (until they are cleared from breast milk)
- Mothers using drugs of abuse
- Mothers with herpes simplex lesions on the breast (breasts clear of lesions may be used to breast-feed)
- Mothers who are HIV-infected and living in the United States (the benefits of breast-feeding may be greater than the risk of HIV transmission in other, underdeveloped countries where safe alternatives to breast-feeding are not as readily available as in the United States)

While breast-feeding is encouraged for all women (without specific contraindications), prior to recommending or prescribing medications to a lactating woman, the following should be considered:

- Is drug therapy necessary?
- Can drug exposure to the infant be minimized? (Using a different route of administration, timing of the dose in relation to breast-feeding, length of therapy, using breast milk stored prior to treatment, etc)
- The infant's age and health status (their own ability to metabolize the medication)
- The pharmacokinetics of the drug
- Will the drug interact with a medication the infant is prescribed?
- If medications must be used, pick the safest drug possible.
- In situations where the only drug available may have adverse effects in the nursing infant, consider measuring the infants blood levels.

The tables presented below have been adapted from the American Academy of Pediatrics Committee on Drugs report "Transfer of Drugs and Other Chemicals Into Human Milk," September 2001. It should not be inferred that if a medication is not in the tables it is considered safe for administration to a lactating woman; only that published reports concerning their use were not available at the time the report was published. Always consider the unique circumstances or a particular mother/child pair when making recommendations.

Table 1. Cytotoxic Drugs

Cyclophosphamide	Doxorubicin
Cyclosporine	Methotrexate

These are medications thought to interfere with cellular metabolism in the nursing infant. Immune suppression may be possible; effects on growth or carcinogenesis are not known. In addition, doxorubicin is concentrated in human milk; methotrexate and cyclophosphamide are associated with neutropenia in the nursing infant.

Table 2. Drugs of Abuse

Amphetamine	Marijuana
Cocaine	Phencyclidine
Heroin	

Drugs of abuse are not only dangerous to the nursing infant, but also to the mother. Women should be encouraged to avoid their use completely. Effects to the infant reported with amphetamine use in the mother include irritability and poor sleeping; it is also a substance that is concentrated in human milk. Cocaine may cause irritability, vomiting, diarrhea, tremors, or seizures in the infant. Heroin may also cause tremors as well as restlessness, vomiting, and poor feeding.

Nicotine, which was previously on this list, is associated with decreased milk production, decreased weight gain in the infant, and possible increased respiratory illness in the infant. Although there are still questions outstanding regarding smoking and breast-feeding, women should be counseled on the possible effects to their infants and offered aid to smoking cessation if appropriate.

Table 3. Radioactive Compounds That Require Temporary Cessation of Breast-Feeding

Drug	Recommended Time for Cessation of Breast-Feeding
Copper 64 (^{64}Cu)	Radioactivity in milk present at 50 h
Gallium 67 (^{67}Ga)	Radioactivity in milk present for 2 wk
Indium 111 (^{111}In)	Very small amount present at 20 h
Iodine 123 (^{123}I)	Radioactivity in milk present up to 36 h
Iodine 125 (^{125}I)	Radioactivity in milk present for 12 d
Iodine 131 (^{131}I)	Radioactivity in milk present 2-14 d, depending on study
Iodine^{131}	If used for thyroid cancer, high radioactivity may prolong exposure to infant
Radioactive sodium	Radioactivity in milk present 96 h
Technetium-99m (^{99m}Tc),^{99m}Tc macroaggregates,^{99m}Tc O4	Radioactivity in milk present 15 h to 3 d

Consider pumping and storing milk prior to study for use during the radioactive period. Pumping should continue after the study to maintain milk production; however, this milk should be discarded until radioactivity is gone. Notify nuclear medicine physician prior to study that the mother is breast-feeding; a short-acting radionuclide may be appropriate. Contact Radiology Department after testing is complete to screen milk samples before resuming feeding.

Table 4a. Psychotropic Drugs Whose Effect on Nursing Infants Is Unknown But May Be of Concern

Antianxiety	Antidepressant	Antipsychotic
Alprazolam	Amitriptyline	Chlorpromazine
Diazepam	Amoxapine	Clozapine[1]
Lorazepam	Bupropion	Haloperidol
Midazolam	Clomipramine	Mesoridazine
Perphenazine	Desipramine	Trifluoperazine
Quazepam	Doxepin	
Temazepam	Fluoxetine	
	Fluvoxamine	
	Imipramine	
	Nortriptyline	
	Paroxetine	
	Sertraline[1]	
	Trazodone	

[1]Drug is concentrated in human milk.

Psychotropic medications usually appear in the breast milk in low concentrations. Although adverse effects in the infant may be limited to a few case reports, the long half-life of these medications and their metabolites should be considered. In addition, measurable amounts may be found in the infants plasma and also brain tissue. Long-term effects are not known. Colic, irritability, feeding and sleep disorders, and slow weight gain are effects reported with fluoxetine. Chlorpromazine may cause galactorrhea in the mother, while drowsiness and lethargy have been reported in the nursing infant. A decline in developmental scores has been reported with chlorpromazine and haloperidol.

Table 4b. Additional Drugs Whose Effect on Nursing Infants Is Unknown But May Be of Concern

Drug	Reported Effect in Nursing Infant
Amiodarone	Hypothyroidism
Chloramphenicol	Idiosyncratic bone marrow suppression
Clofazimine	Increase in skin pigmentation; high transfer of mothers dose to infant is possible
Lamotrigine	Therapeutic serum concentrations in infant
Metoclopramide[1]	
Metronidazole	
Tinidazole	

[1]Drug is concentrated in human milk.

No adverse effects to the infant have been reported for metoclopramide; however, it should be recognized that it is a dopaminergic agent. Metronidazole and tinidazole are *in vitro* mutagenic agents; in cases where single dose therapy is appropriate for the mother, breast-feeding may be discontinued for 12-24 hours to allow excretion of the medication.

Table 5. Drugs That Have Been Associated With Significant Effects on Some Nursing Infants and Should Be Given to Nursing Mothers With Caution[1]

Drug	Reported Effect
Acebutolol	Hypotension, bradycardia, tachypnea
5-Aminosalicylic acid	Diarrhea (one case)
Atenolol	Cyanosis, bradycardia
Bromocriptine	Suppresses lactation; may be hazardous to the mother
Aspirin (salicylates)	Metabolic acidosis (one case)
Clemastine	Drowsiness, irritability, refusal to feed, high-pitched cry, neck stiffness (one case)
Ergotamine	Vomiting, diarrhea, convulsions (doses used in migraine medications)
Lithium	One-third to one-half therapeutic blood concentration in infants
Phenindone	Anticoagulant: increased prothrombin and partial thromboplastin time in one infant; not used in the United States
Phenobarbital	Sedation; infantile spasms after weaning from milk-containing phenobarbital, methemoglobinemia (one case)
Primidone	Sedation, feeding problems
Sulfasalazine (salicylazosulfapyridine)	Bloody diarrhea (one case)

[1]Blood concentration in the infant may be of clinical importance; measure when possible.

References

2006 Red Book: Report of the Committee on Infectious Diseases, 27th ed, Elk Grove Village, IL: American Academy of Pediatrics, 2006, 123-30.

American Academy of Pediatrics Committee on Drugs, "Transfer of Drugs and Other Chemicals Into Human Milk," *Pediatrics*, 2001, 108(3): 776-89.

Gartner LM, Morton J, Lawrence RA, et al, "Breastfeeding and the Use of Human Milk," *Pediatrics*, 2005, 115(2):496-506.

COMPATIBILITY OF MEDICATIONS MIXED IN A SYRINGE

	Atropine	Chlorpromazine	Codeine	Diphenhydramine	Droperidol	Fentanyl	Glycopyrrolate	Hydroxyzine	Meperidine	Metoclopramide	Midazolam	Morphine	Pentazocine	Pentobarbital†	Prochlorperazine	Promazine	Promethazine	Trimethobenzamide
Atropine		C	•	C	C	C	C	C	C	C	C	C	C	C	C	C	C	•
Chlorpromazine	C		•	C	C	C	C	C	C	C	C	C	C	X	C	C	C	•
Codeine	•	•		•	•	•	C	C	•	•	•	•	•	X	•	•	•	•
Diphenhydramine	C	C	•		C	C	C	C	C	C	C	C	C	X	C	C	C	•
Droperidol	C	C	•	C		C	C	C	C	C	C	C	C	X	C	C	C	•
Fentanyl	C	C	•	C	C		C	C	C	C	C	C	C	X	C	C	C	•
Glycopyrrolate	C	C	C	C	C	C		C	C	•	C	C	X	X	C	C	C	C
Hydroxyzine	C	C	C	C	C	C	C		C	C	C	C	C	X	C	C	C	•
Meperidine	C	C	•	C	C	C	C	C		C	C	X	C	X	C	C	C	•
Metoclopramide	C	C	•	C	C	C	•	C	C		C	C	C	•	C	C	C	•
Midazolam	C	C	•	C	C	C	C	C	C	C		C	•	X	X	C	C	C
Morphine	C	C	•	C	C	C	C	C	C	C	C		C	X	C*	C	C	•
Pentazocine	C	C	•	C	C	C	C	C	C	C	•	C		X	C	C	C	C
Pentobarbital†	C	X	X	X	X	X	X	X	X	•	X	X	X		X	X	X	•
Prochlorperazine	C	C	•	C	C	C	C	C	C	C	X	C*	C	X		C	C	•
Promazine	C	C	•	C	C	C	C	C	C	C	C	C	C	X	C		C	•
Promethazine	C	C	•	C	C	C	C	C	C	C	C	C	C	X	C	C		•
Trimethobenzamide	•	•	•	•	•	•	C	•	•	•	C	•	C	•	•	•	•	

C = physically compatible if used within 15 minutes after mixing in a syringe.
X = incompatible.
• = no documented information.
C* = potential incompatibility produced by certain manufacturers.
† = compatibility profile is characteristic of most barbiturate salts, such as phenobarbital and secobarbital.

The following combinations have been found to be compatible:
    atropine / meperidine / promethazine
    atropine / meperidine / hydroxyzine
    meperidine / promethazine / chlorpromazine

The following drugs should not be mixed with any other drugs in the same syringe:
    diazepam, chlordiazepoxide

References

Forman JK and Sourney PF, "Visual Compatibility of Midazolam Hydrochloride With Common Preoperative Injectable Medications," *Am J Hosp Pharm*, 1987, 44(10):2298-9.
King JC, "Guide to Parenteral Admixtures," St Louis, MO: Cutter Laboratories, 1986.
Parker WA, *Hosp Pharm*, 1984, 19:475-8.
Trissel LA, "Handbook on Injectable Drugs," 5th ed, Bethesda, MD: American Society of Health-System Pharmacists, Inc, 1988.
Stevenson JG and Patriarca C, "Incompatibility of Morphine Sulfate and Prochlorperazine Edisylate in Syringes," *Am J Hosp Pharm*, 1985, 42(12):2651.

CONTROLLED SUBSTANCES

Note: These are federal classifications. Your individual state may place a substance into a more restricted category. When this occurs, the more restricted category applies. Consult your state law.

Schedule I = C-I

The drugs and other substances in this schedule have no legal medical uses except research. They have a **high** potential for abuse. They include opiates, opium derivatives, and hallucinogens.

Schedule II = C-II

The drugs and other substances in this schedule have legal medical uses and a **high** abuse potential which may lead to severe dependence. They include former "Class A" narcotics, amphetamines, barbiturates, and other drugs.

Schedule III = C-III

The drugs and other substances in this schedule have legal medical uses and a **lesser** degree of abuse potential which may lead to **moderate** dependence. They include former "Class B" narcotics and other drugs.

Schedule IV = C-IV

The drugs and other substances in this schedule have legal medical uses and **low** abuse potential which may lead to **moderate** dependence. They include barbiturates, benzodiazepines, propoxyphenes, and other drugs.

Schedule V = C-V

The drugs and other substances in this schedule have legal medical uses and **low** abuse potential which may lead to **moderate** dependence. They include narcotic cough preparations, diarrhea preparations, and other drugs.

MILLIEQUIVALENT AND MILLIMOLE CALCULATIONS AND CONVERSIONS

Definitions

mole	=	gram molecular weight of a substance (aka, molar weight)
millimole (mM)	=	milligram molecular weight of a substance (a millimole is 1/1000 of a mole)
equivalent weight	=	gram weight of a substance which will combine with or replace 1 gram (1 mole) of hydrogen; an equivalent weight can be determined by dividing the molar weight of a substance by its ionic valence
milliequivalent (mEq)	=	milligram weight of a substance which will combine with or replace 1 milligram (1 millimole) of hydrogen (a milliequivalent is 1/1000 of an equivalent)

Calculations

moles	=	$\dfrac{\text{weight of a substance (grams)}}{\text{molecular weight of that substance (grams)}}$
millimoles	=	$\dfrac{\text{weight of a substance (milligrams)}}{\text{molecular weight of that substance (milligrams)}}$
equivalents	=	moles x valence of ion
milliequivalents	=	millimoles x valence of ion
moles	=	$\dfrac{\text{equivalents}}{\text{valence of ion}}$
millimoles	=	$\dfrac{\text{milliequivalents}}{\text{valence of ion}}$
millimoles	=	moles x 1000
milliequivalents	=	equivalents x 1000

Note: Use of equivalents and milliequivalents is valid only for those substances which have fixed ionic valences (eg, sodium, potassium, calcium, chlorine, magnesium bromine, etc). For substances with variable ionic valences (eg, phosphorous), a reliable equivalent value cannot be determined. In these instances, one should calculate millimoles (which are fixed and reliable) rather than milliequivalents.

MILLIEQUIVALENT CONVERSIONS

To convert mg/100 mL to mEq/L the following formula may be used:

$$\frac{(\text{mg/100 mL}) \times 10 \times \text{valence}}{\text{atomic weight}} = \text{mEq/L}$$

To convert mEq/L to mg/100 mL the following formula may be used:

$$\frac{(\text{mEq/L}) \times \text{atomic weight}}{10 \times \text{valence}} = \text{mg/100 mL}$$

To convert mEq/L to volume of percent of a gas the following formula may be used:

$$\frac{(\text{mEq/L}) \times 22.4}{10} = \text{volume percent}$$

Valences and Approximate Weights of Selected Ions

Substance	Electrolyte	Valence	Ionic Wt
Calcium	Ca^{++}	2	40
Chloride	Cl^-	1	35.5
Magnesium	Mg^{++}	2	24
Phosphate	PO_4^{3-}	3	95[1]
	HPO_4^{2-}	2	96
	$H_2PO_4^-$	1	97
Potassium	K^+	1	39
Sodium	Na^+	1	23
Sulfate	SO_4^{2-}	2	96[1]

[1]The molecular weight of phosphorus is 31, and sulfur is 32.

Approximate Milliequivalents — Weights of Selected Ions

Salt	mEq/g Salt	mg Salt/mEq
Calcium carbonate [$CaCO_3$]	20	50
Calcium chloride [$CaCl_2 \cdot 2H_2O$]	14	73
Calcium gluceptate [$Ca(C_7H_{13}O_8)_2$]	4	245
Calcium gluconate (Ca gluconate$_2 \cdot 1H_2O$)	4	224
Calcium lactate (Ca lactate$_2 \cdot 5H_2O$)	6	154
Magnesium gluconate [$Mg(C_6H_{11}O_7)_2 \cdot H_2O$]	5	216
Magnesium oxide [MgO]	50	20
Magnesium sulfate [$MgSO_4$]	16	60
Magnesium sulfate [$MgSO_4 \cdot 7H_2O$]	8	123
Potassium acetate (K acetate)	10	98
Potassium chloride (KCl)	13	75
Potassium citrate (K_3 citrate$\cdot 1H_2O$)	9	108
Potassium iodide (KI)	6	166
Sodium acetate [$Na(C_2H_3O_2)$]	12	82
Sodium acetate [$Na(C_2H_3O_2) \cdot 3H_2O$]	7	136
Sodium bicarbonate ($NaHCO_3$)	12	84
Sodium chloride (NaCl)	17	58
Sodium citrate (Na_3 citrate $\cdot 2H_2O$)	10	98
Sodium iodine (NaI)	7	150
Sodium lactate (Na lactate)	9	112
Zinc sulfate ($ZnSO_4 \cdot 7H_2O$)	7	144

PATIENT INFORMATION FOR DISPOSAL OF UNUSED MEDICATIONS

Federal guidelines and the Food and Drug Administration (FDA) recommend that disposal of most unused medications should NOT be accomplished by flushing them down the toilet or drain unless specifically stated in the drug label prescribing information. (See "Disposal of Unused Medications Not Specified to be Flushed" below.)

However, certain drugs can potentially harm an individual for whom it is not intended, even in a single dose, depending on the size of the individual and strength of the medication. Accidental (or intentional) ingestion of one of these drugs by an unintended individual (eg, child or pet) can cause hypotension, somnolence, respiratory depression, or other severe adverse events that could lead to coma or death. For this reason, certain unused medications **should** be disposed of by flushing them down a toilet or sink.

Disposal by flushing of these medications is not believed to pose a risk to human health or the environment. Trace amounts of medicine in the water system have been noted, mainly from the body's normal elimination through urine or feces, but there has been no evidence of these small amounts being harmful. Disposal by flushing of these select, few medications contributes a small fraction to the amount of medicine in the water system. The FDA believes that the benefit of avoiding a potentially life-threatening overdose by accidental ingestion outweighs the potential risk to the environment by flushing these medications.

Medications Recommended for Disposal by Flushing

Medication	Active Ingredient
Actiq®, oral transmucosal lozenge	Fentanyl citrate
Avinza®, capsule (extended release)	Morphine sulfate
Daytrana™, transdermal patch	Methylphenidate
Demerol®, tablet[1]	Meperidine hydrochloride
Demerol®, oral solution[1]	Meperidine hydrochloride
Diastat® / Diastat® AcuDial™, rectal gel	Diazepam
Dilaudid®, tablet[1]	Hydromorphone hydrochloride
Dilaudid®, oral liquid[1]	Hydromorphone hydrochloride
Dolophine®, tablet (as hydrochloride)[1]	Methadone hydrochloride
Duragesic®, patch (extended release)[1]	Fentanyl
Embeda™, capsule (extended release)	Morphine sulfate and naltrexone hydrochloride
Fentora®, tablet (buccal)	Fentanyl citrate
Kadian®, capsule (extended release)	Morphine sulfate
Methadone hydrochloride (oral solution)[1]	Methadone hydrochloride
Methadose®, tablet[1]	Methadone hydrochloride
Morphine sulfate, tablet (immediate release)[1]	Morphine sulfate
Morphine sulfate, oral solution[1]	Morphine sulfate
MS Contin®, tablet (extended release)[1]	Morphine sulfate
Onsolis™, soluble film (buccal)	Fentanyl citrate
Opana®, tablet (immediate release)	Oxymorphone hydrochloride
Opana® ER, tablet (extended release)	Oxymorphone hydrochloride
Oramorph® SR, tablet (sustained release)	Morphine sulfate
Oxycontin®, tablet (extended release)[1]	Oxycodone hydrochloride
Percocet®, tablet[1]	Oxycodone hydrochloride and acetaminophen
Percodan®, tablet[1]	Oxycodone hydrochloride and aspirin
Xyrem®, oral solution	Sodium oxybate

[1]Medications available in generic formulations.

DISPOSAL OF UNUSED MEDICATIONS NOT SPECIFIED TO BE FLUSHED

The majority of medications should be disposed of without flushing them down a toilet or drain. These medications should be removed from the original container, mixed with an unappealing substance (eg, coffee grounds, cat litter), sealed in a plastic bag or other closable container, and disposed of in the household trash.

Another option for disposal of unused medications is through drug take-back programs. For information on availability of drug take-back programs in your area, contact city or county trash and recycling service.

For more information on unused medication disposal, see specific drug product labeling information or call the FDA at 1-888-INFO-FDA (1-888-463-6332).

REFERENCE

U.S. Food and Drug Administration (FDA), "Disposal by Flushing of Certain Unused Medicines: What You Should Know." Available at: http://www.fda.gov/Drugs/ResourcesForYou/Consumers/BuyingUsingMedicineSafely/EnsuringSafeUseofMedicine/SafeDisposalofMedicines/ucm186187.htm Lasted accessed October 20, 2009.

PEDIATRIC MEDICATION ADMINISTRATION

Adapted from *Giving Your Child Medicine – Ways to Ensure Your Child Receives the Correct Dose of Medicine*, patient booklet, Lexi-Comp, Inc, 2002.

General Advice

Administering medicine to a sick child can be extremely challenging for parents and caregivers. Dosages are calculated by taking the child's age and/or weight into consideration. Infants and young children require very small doses of medicines, thus making accurate measurement very important.

Special measuring devices are available to accurately and easily provide the prescribed dosage. Measuring out a dose with common household utensils can lead to unacceptable inaccuracies. Improper measurement can also cause increased side effects, and over- or under-dosing.

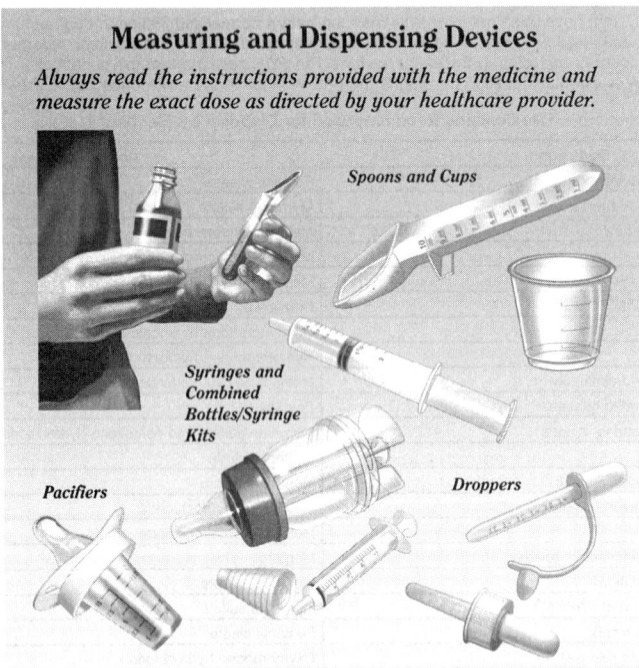

Measuring and Dispensing Devices

Always read the instructions provided with the medicine and measure the exact dose as directed by your healthcare provider.

Spoons and Cups

Syringes and Combined Bottles/Syringe Kits

Pacifiers

Droppers

Liquids

Use either an oral syringe, a medicine dropper, a medicine spoon, or a medicine cup (only for older children) when giving your child oral liquids. You can purchase any of these at a local pharmacy if not provided with your child's medicine. There are specialized pacifiers and bottles designed as medicine delivery aids for children <2 years of age.

- If the medicine can be given on an empty stomach, give right before a feeding.
- Hold an infant in the normal feeding position, or put in a highchair or car seat.

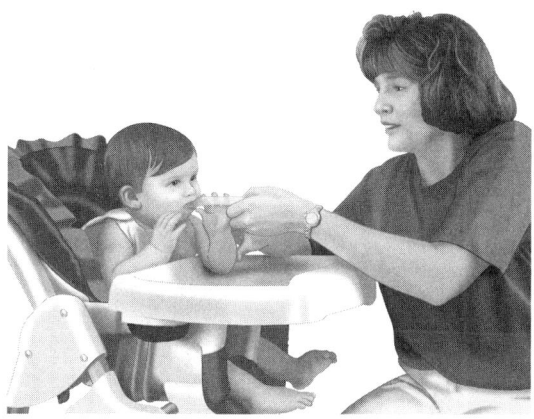

If the child refuses to take the medicine because of bad taste, check with a pharmacist to see if the medicine can be mixed with fruit juice, milk, or another liquid. Pharmacists may be able to flavor the medicine to disguise the taste. You may use a popsicle to partially numb the mouth, give the medicine, and then use the popsicle again to help improve taste.

- Prepare the medicine. Open the infant's mouth by gently squeezing his/her cheeks or by using your finger to pull out a corner of the infant's mouth.
- Slowly squirt the medicine into the side of the infant's mouth. Do not squirt it to the back of the throat because this can cause choking or gagging.
- Gently stroke the infant under the chin to encourage swallowing while still holding the cheeks together.
- Alternatively, pour medicine into a small cup and dip your little finger in it. Let the infant suck it off your finger.
- Young children may want to be in control of taking the medicine by guiding the dropper or spoon into their mouth.
- Rinse measuring device with warm water after each use.

Droppers or cups which come with specific medicines should not be used to administer other medicine.

Eye Drops and Ointments

- Wash your hands before and after use.
- Hold container between hands to bring eye drops or ointment to room temperature before using.
- Clean child's eye of secretions and old medicine if necessary.
- Gently wipe the eye with a damp gauze or cotton pad.
- Tilt child's head back and to the side of the affected eye.
- Do not touch the container tip to eye, lid, or other skin.

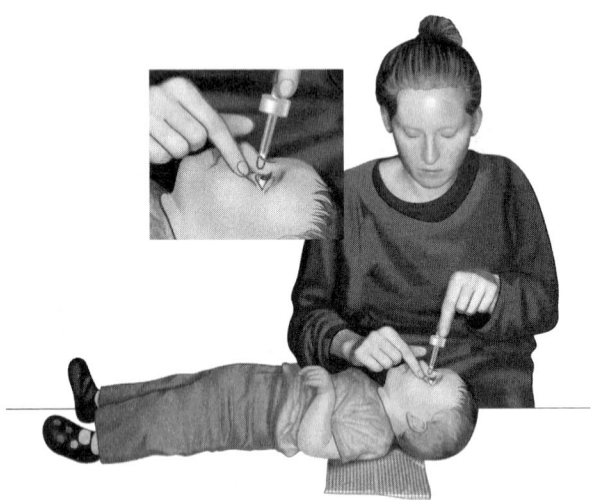

Drops

- If the drops are a suspension, shake the bottle well.
- Gently press the skin under the lower eyelid and pull the lower eyelid away from the eye slightly until you can see a small pouch.
- Insert 1 drop. Wait 1 minute between drops if more than one eye medicine is prescribed.
- After using medicine, ask the child to keep eyes closed. Apply light pressure to the inside corner of the eye.
- Do this for 3-5 minutes. This keeps the medicine in the eye.

Ointment

- If you are using an ointment, gently pull down the lower lid and squeeze in the prescribed amount.
- Release the lower eyelid and instruct the child to keep eyes closed for 1-2 minutes. This will put the medicine in contact with the eye.

Ear Drops

- Wash your hands before and after use.
- Warm the medicine by holding the bottle between your hands.
- If the drops are a suspension, shake the bottle well.
- For children <3 years of age, pull the outer ear outward and downward.
- For children ≥3 years of age, pull the outer ear outward and upward.
- Instill prescribed number of drops in affected ear without touching dropper to ear.
- Have child stay on side for 2 minutes or insert cotton plug into ear.
- Repeat procedure in other ear if necessary.

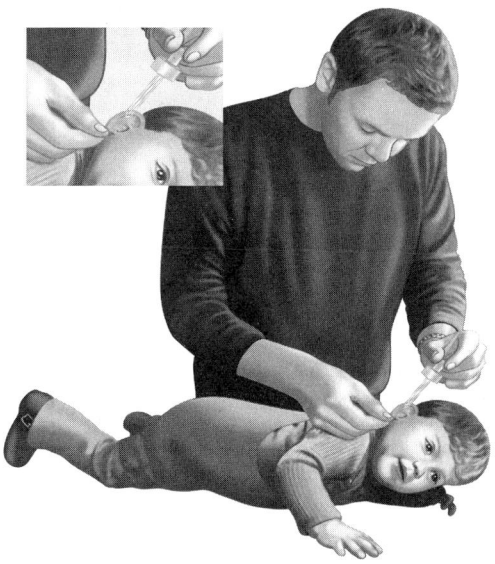

Topical Creams and Ointments

If no specific directions have been given, follow these general guidelines:

- For use on skin only. Keep out of mouth, nose, and eyes (may burn).
- Wash your hands before and after use.
- Clean affected area and dry well before use.
- Apply a thin layer of medicine to the affected skin and rub in gently. Some medicines can be poured or squeezed onto a gauze pad, cotton swab, or cotton ball to apply.
- Do not put coverings (bandages, dressings) over the area unless told to do so by a healthcare provider.

Nose Drops

- Wash your hands before and after use.
- Warm the medicine by holding the bottle between your hands.
- If the drops are a suspension, shake the bottle well.
- Try to clear mucus out of nose. For infants and small children, you can use a nasal aspirator (bulb syringe) or gently twirl a moist cotton swab inside each nostril. Do not reach too far into the nostril with the swab or bulb syringe. For older children, have the child blow nose.
- Infants can be cradled in your arms in a lying position with head tilted back slightly.

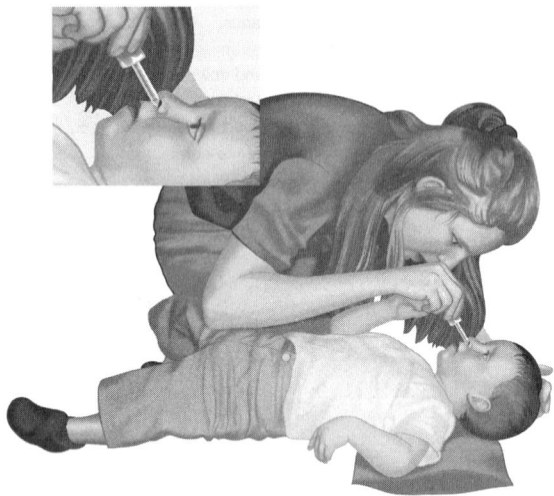

- Young children should lie on their back with a small pillow between their shoulders.
- Have them tilt head back over top of pillow. Older children can sit up with the head tilted back.
- Tell older children they may be able to taste the medicine.
- Draw the correct amount of medicine into the dropper, insert the dropper slightly into the nostril, and squeeze the medicine in without touching dropper to the nose.
- Repeat procedure in other nostril if necessary.
- Keep the child's head tilted back for 2 minutes.
- If child coughs, sit him/her upright.

Rectal Suppositories

- Wash your hands before and after use.
- If appropriate, store suppository in refrigerator or run it under cold water with the wrapper still on to make it firm enough to place in rectum. Ask pharmacist if you are able to safely store medicine in a refrigerator.
- Infants should be facedown across your knees. An older child can lie on his/her side with knees drawn to chest.
- Remove the wrapper.
- Moisten suppository with water or place a small amount of petroleum jelly on the tip.
- Consider use of a disposable glove.
- Gently insert the smooth, rounded end of the suppository into the rectum and up beyond the sphincter (1/2 to 1 inch beyond the sphincter). Use your pinky finger for children <3 years of age and your index finger for those ≥3 years.
- If the suppository is inserted far enough, it should stay in place. If it comes out, reinsert it slightly farther than before.
- Hold the buttocks together for a couple of minutes to prevent the child from expelling the suppository.
- Have child remain in the same position for about 20 minutes, if possible. If not, have him/her sit or lie down without going to the bathroom.

If in doubt...

Speak to your healthcare provider or your pharmacist about any concerns you have regarding the medicine prescribed for your child.

IF YOUR CHILD HAS A REACTION TO ANY MEDICINE, GET HELP IMMEDIATELY.

Do's and Don'ts

DO wash your child's hands immediately if medicine gets on them.

DO use distractions such as toys, songs, stories, or rhymes to keep your child busy while trying to give medicine.

DO get another adult to help hold the infant while you give the medicine, or use a car seat to hold the infant or child still.

DO try a different form of the medicine. A child might prefer a chewable tablet or a form that can be sprinkled on food.

DO teach your child about the illness and why he/she has to take medicine. Your healthcare provider or librarian may have books about children who are sick or need to take medicine.

DO help your child gain some control by letting him/her make age-appropriate decisions about care.

DO use prescription as directed, even if your child is feeling better.

DO store medicine out of the reach of children and pets.

DO NOT measure medicine for an infant with a medicine cup (use an oral syringe, a medicine dropper, or a medicine spoon).

DO NOT use a teaspoon or tablespoon from your silverware to measure medicine for your child.

SODIUM CONTENT OF SELECTED MEDICINALS

Name and Dosage Unit[1]	Sodium	
	mg	mEq
Antibiotics		
Amikacin sulfate, 1 g	29.9	1.3
Aminosalicylate sodium, 1 g	109	4.7
Ampicillin, suspension, 250 mg/5 mL, 5 mL	10	0.4
Ampicillin sodium, 1 g	66.7	3
Carbenicillin disodium, 382 mg (tablet)	23	1
Cefazolin sodium, 1 g	47	2
Cefotaxime sodium, 1 g	50.6	2.2
Cefoxitin sodium, 1 g	53	2.3
Ceftriaxone sodium, 1 g	60	2.6
Cefuroxime, 1 g	54.2	2.4
Chloramphenicol sodium succinate, 1 g	51.8	2.3
Dicloxacillin, 250 mg (capsule)	13	0.6
Erythromycin ethyl succinate, suspension 200 mg/5 mL	29	1.3
Erythromycin Base Filmtab®, 250 mg	70	3
Metronidazole, 500 mg I.V.	322	14
Nafcillin sodium, 1 g	66.7	2.9
Nitrofurantoin, suspension, 25 mg/5 mL	7	0.3
Penicillin G potassium, 1,000,000 units I.V.	7.6	0.3
Penicillin G sodium, 1,000,000 units I.V.	46	2
Penicillin V potassium, suspension, 250 mg/5 mL	38	1.7
Piperacillin sodium, 1 g	42.6	1.8
Ticarcillin disodium, 1 g	119.6	5.2
Antacids, Liquid (content per 5 mL)		
ALternaGEL®	2	0.1
Gaviscon®	13	0.57
Maalox®	1.3	0.06
Tums E-X™	<4.8	<0.2
Sodium Content of Miscellaneous Medicinals		
Acetazolamide sodium, 500 mg	47.2	2.05
Chlorothiazide sodium, 500 mg	57.5	2
Cisplatin, 10 mg	35.4	1.54
Edetate calcium disodium, 1 g	122	5.3
Fleet® Enema, 4.5 oz	5000[2]	218
Fleet® Phospho®-Soda, 20 mL	2217	96.4
Hydrocortisone sodium succinate, 1 g	47.5	2.07
Hypaque® M 75%, injection, 20 mL	200	8.7
Hypaque® M 90%, injection, 20 mL	220	9.6
Metamucil® Instant Mix (orange)	6	0.27
Methotrexate sodium, 100 mg vial	20	0.86
Methotrexate sodium, 100 mg vial (low sodium)	15	0.65
Naproxen sodium, 250 mg (tablet)	23	1
Neutra-Phos®, capsule and 75 mL reconstituted solution	164	7.13
Pentobarbital sodium, 50 mg/mL	5	0.2
Phenobarbital sodium, 65 mg, 1 mL vial	6	0.3
Phenytoin sodium, 1 g	88	3.8

Name and Dosage Unit[1]	Sodium	
	mg	mEq
Promethazine expectorant, 5 mL	53	2.3
Shohl's solution modified, 1 mL	23	1
Sodium ascorbate, 500 mg acid equivalent	65.3	2.84
Sodium bicarbonate, 50 mL 8.4%	1150	50
Sodium nitroprusside, 50 mg	7.8	0.34
Sodium polystyrene sulfonate, 1 g	94.3[3]	4.1
Thiopental sodium, 1 g	86.8	3.8
Valproate sodium, 250 mg/5 mL, 5 mL	23	1

[1]Product formulations and hence sodium content are subject to change by the manufacturer.

[2]Average systemic absorption 250-300 mg.

[3]Total sodium content. Only about 33% is liberated in clinical use.

SUGAR-FREE LIQUID PHARMACEUTICALS

The following sugar-free liquid preparations are listed by therapeutic category and alphabetically within each category. Please note that product formulations are subject to change by the manufacturer. Some of these products may contain sorbitol, alcohol, xylitol, or other sweeteners which may be partially metabolized to provide calories.

Analgesics
Acetaminophen Elixir (various)
APAP/APAP Plus
Febrol® and Febrol® EX
Mapap® Drops
Methadone Hydrochloride Intensol
Paregoric USP (Abbott)
Silapap®
Tylenol® Drops

Antacids / Antiflatulents
Alcalak®
Aldroxicon®
Aluminum Hydroxide Suspension
Baby Gasz Drops
Citrocarbonate® Granules
Gaviscon® Liquid
Maalox® Plus Suspension
Maalox® Suspension
Maalox® Therapeutic Concentrate
Magnesia and Alumina Oral Suspension USP (Abbott, Phillips Roxane)
Milk of Bismuth
Milk of Magnesia USP
Mylanta® Liquid
Mylicon® Drops
Pepto-Bismol® Liquid and Tablets
Riopan Plus®
Riopan® Suspension

Antiasthmatics
Alupent® Syrup
Elixophyllin® Elixir
Organidin® NR

Antidepressants
Celexa™ Solution
Prozac® Solution
Sinequan® Oral Concentrate

Antidiarrheals
Corrective Mixture With Paregoric
Diotame®
Kaolin Mixture With Pectin NF (Abbott)
Kaolin-Pectin Suspension (Phillips Roxane)
Konsyl® Powder
Lomanate®
Lomotil® Liquid
Paregoric USP (various)
Parepectolin® (various)
Pepto-Bismol®
St Joseph® Antidiarrheal

Antiepileptics
Mysoline® Suspension

Antihistamine-Decongestants
Bromphen® Elixir
Dimetapp® Elixir
Isoclor® Liquid and Capsules
Naldecon® Pediatric Drops and Syrup
Naldecon® Syrup
Phenergan® Syrup
Rondec® DM Drops
S-T® Forte® Liquid

Tavist® Syrup
Vistaril® Oral Suspension
Zyrtec® Syrup

Anti-infectives
Augmentin® Suspension
Furadantin® Oral Suspension
Sulfamethoxazole and Trimethoprim Suspension (Biocraft, Beecham, Burroughs Wellcome)
Vibramycin® Syrup
Zovirax® Suspension

Corticosteroids
Decadron® Elixir
Dexamethasone Solution (Roxane)
Dexamethasone Intensol Solution
Pediapred® Oral Liquid
Prelone® Syrup

Cough Medicines
Chlorgest-HD®
Codiclear® DH Syrup
Codimal® DM
Contac Jr® Liquid
Dimetane®-DC Cough Syrup
Dimetane®-DX Cough Syrup
Entuss® Expectorant Liquid
Histafed® Pediatric Liquid
Hycomine® Syrup and Pediatric Syrup
Medicon® D
Medi-Synal®
Naldecon-DX® Pediatric Drops and Syrup
Naldecon-DX® Adult Liquid
Non-Drowsy Comtrex®
Organidin® NR
Potassium Iodide Solution (various)
Robitussin-CF® Liquid
Robitussin® Night Relief Liquid
Rondec®-DM Drops
Rondec®-DM Syrup
Ryna® Liquid
Ryna-C® Liquid
Ryna-CX® Liquid
Scot-Tussin® DM Syrup
Scot-Tussin® Expectorant
Scot-Tussin® DM Cough Chasers
Silexin® Cough Syrup
Sudodrin®/Sudodrin® Forte®
Terpin® Hydrate With Codeine Elixir (various)
Tolu-Sed® Cough Syrup
Tolu-Sed® DM
Tricodene® Liquid
Tussirex® Sugar-Free

Dental Preparations and Fluoride Preparations
Cepacol® Mouthwash
Cepastat® Mouthwash and Gargle
Chloraseptic® Mouthwash and Gargle
Fluorigard® Mouthrinse
Fluorinse®
Flura-Drops®
Flura-Loz®
Flura® Tablets
Gel-Kam®

Karigel®
Karigel® N
Luride® Drops
Luride® SF Lozi-Tabs
Luride® 0.25 and 0.5 Lozi-Tabs
Luride® Lozi-Tabs
Pediaflor® Drops
Phos-Flur® Rinse/Supplement
Point-Two® Mouthrinse
Prevident® Disclosing Drops
Thera-Flur® Gel and Drops

Diagnostic Agents
Gastrografin®

Dietary Substitutes
Co-Salt®

Iron Preparations / Blood Modifiers
Amicar® Syrup
Geritol® Complete Tablets
Geritonic™ Liquid
Hemo-Vite® Liquid
Iberet® Liquid
Iberet®-500 Liquid
Niferex®
Nu-Iron® Elixir
Vita-Plus H® Half Strength, Sugar-Free
Vita-Plus H®, Sugar-Free

Laxatives
Aromatic Cascara Fluidextract USP
Castor Oil
Castor Oil (flavored)
Castor Oil USP
Colace®, Liquid
Emulsoil®
Fiberall® Powder
Hydrocil® Instant Powder
Hypaque® Oral Powder
Kondremul®
Kondremul® With Cascara
Kondremul® With Phenolphthalein
Konsyl® Powder
Liqui-Doss®
Magnesium Citrate Solution NF
Metamucil® Instant Mix (lemon-lime or orange)
Metamucil® SF Powder
Milk of Magnesia
Milk of Magnesia/Cascara Suspension
Milk of Magnesia/Mineral Oil Emulsion (various)
Mineral Oil (various)
Neoloid® Liquid
NuLYTELY®
Sodium Phosphate & Biphosphate Oral Solution USP (Phillips Roxane)

Potassium Products
Cena-K® Solution
Kaon® Elixir (grape and lemon-lime flavor)
Kaon-Cl® 20% Liquid
Kay Ciel® Elixir
Kay Ciel® Powder
Klor-Con®/25 Powder
Klor-Con® EF Tablets
Klor-Con® Liquid 20%

Klor-Con® Powder
Potassium Chloride Oral Solution USP 5%, 10%, and 20% (various)
Potassium Gluconate Elixir NF
Rum-K® Solution
Tri-K® Liquid

Sedatives-Tranquilizers-Antipsychotics
Butabarbital Sodium Elixir
Butisol Sodium® Elixir
Haldol® Concentrate
Loxitane® C Drops
Mellaril® Concentrate
Serentil® Concentrate
Thorazine® Concentrate

Vitamin Preparations-Nutritionals
Bugs Bunny™ Chewable Tablets
Bugs Bunny™ Plus Iron Chewable Tablets
Bugs Bunny™ With Extra C Chewable Tablets
Bugs Bunny™ Plus Minerals Chewable Tablets
Calciferol™ Drops
Caltrate® 600 Tablets
Cod Liver Oil (various)
DHT™ Intensol Solution (Roxane)
Drisdol® in Propylene Glycol
Flintstones™ Complete Chewable Tablets
Flintstones™ With Extra C Chewable Tablets
Flintstones™ Plus Iron Chewable Tablets
Oyst-Cal® 500 Tablets
Pediaflor®
PMS® Relief
Poly-Vi-Flor® Drops
Poly-Vi-Flor®/Iron Drops
Poly-Vi-Sol® Drops
Poly-Vi-Sol®/Iron Drops
Posture® Tablets
Spiderman™ Children's Chewable Vitamin Tablets
Spiderman™ Children's Plus Iron Tablets
Theragran® Jr Children's Chewable Tablets
Tri-Vi-Flor® Drops
Tri-Vi-Sol® Drops
Tri-Vi-Sol®/Iron Drops
Vi-Daylin® ADC Drops
Vi-Daylin® ADC/Fluoride Drops
Vi-Daylin® ADC Plus Iron Drops
Vi-Daylin® Drops
Vi-Daylin®/Fluoride Drops
Vi-Daylin® Plus Iron Drops
Vitalize®

Miscellaneous
Altace™ Capsules
Bicitra® Solution
Colestid® Granules
Digoxin® Elixir (Roxane)
Lipomul®
Lithium Citrate Syrup
Neutra-Phos® Powder
Neutra-Phos®-K Powder
Nicorette® Chewing Gum
Polycitra®-K Solution
Polycitra®-LC Solution
Tagamet® Liquid

References

Hill EM, Flaitz CM, and Frost GR, "Sweetener Content of Common Pediatric Oral Liquid Medications," *Am J Hosp Pharm*, 1988, 45(1):135-42.
Kumar A, Rawlings RD, and Beaman DC, "The Mystery Ingredients: Sweeteners, Flavorings, Dyes, and Preservatives in Analgesic/Antipyretic, Antihistamine/Decongestant, Cough and Cold, Antidiarrheal, and Liquid Theophylline Preparations," *Pediatrics*, 1993, 91(5):927-33.
"Sugar Free Products," *Drug Topics Red Book*, 1992, 17-8.

CARBOHYDRATE CONTENT OF MEDICATIONS

Description (Brand Name)	Dosage Unit	Grams Carbohydrate per Dosage Unit
Analgesics / Antipyretics		
Acetaminophen extended release caplets (Tylenol®)	650 mg	<0.03
Acetaminophen extra strength caplets (Tylenol®)	500 mg	<0.05
Acetaminophen extra strength gel caps (Tylenol®)	500 mg	<0.05
Acetaminophen infant drops (grape and cherry) (Tylenol®)	0.8 mL	<0.71
Acetaminophen liquid suspension (cherry) (Tylenol®)	160 mg/5 mL	<5
Acetaminophen regular strength caplets (Tylenol®)	325 mg	<0.04
Acetaminophen elixir (Tylenol®)	160 mg/5 mL	<1.6
Acetaminophen extra strength liquid (Tylenol®)	1000 mg/30 mL	<5.7
Acetaminophen junior strength swallowable caplets (Tylenol®)	160 mg	<0.4
Acetaminophen grape flavored suspension (Tylenol®)	160 mg/5 mL	<4.8
Acetaminophen elixir with codeine (Tylenol® With Codeine) *0.35 g ethyl alcohol/5 mL	120 mg/5 mL	3
Acetaminophen with codeine tablets (Tylenol® With Codeine)	All strengths	0.05
Acetaminophen chewable tablets (Tylenol®)	80 mg	0.25
Effervescent flavored antacid and pain reliever (Alka-Selzer®)	325 mg	0.01
Ibuprofen tablets (Advil®)	200 mg	0.23
Ibuprofen drops (Motrin®)	40 mg/mL	<0.41
Ibuprofen suspension (Motrin®)	100 mg/5 mL	<0.63
Ibuprofen chewable tablets (Motrin®)	50 mg	<0.28
Ibuprofen chewable tablets (Motrin®)	100 mg	<0.54
Antibiotics		
Amoxicillin pediatric drops (Amoxil®)	50 mg/mL	1.6
Amoxicillin oral suspension (Amoxil®)	125 mg/5 mL	1.7
Amoxicillin oral suspension (Amoxil®)	250 mg/5 mL	1.85
Amoxicillin chewable tablets (Amoxil®)	125 mg	0.05
Amoxicillin chewable tablets (Amoxil®)	250 mg	0.34
Amoxicillin capsules (Amoxil®)	250 mg	0
Amoxicillin capsules (Amoxil®)	500 mg	0
Amoxicillin oral suspension (Trimox®)	125 mg/5 mL	3.3
Amoxicillin oral suspension (Trimox®)	250 mg/5 mL	3.3
Amoxicillin capsules (Trimox®)	250 mg	0
Amoxicillin capsules (Trimox®)	500 mg	0
Amoxicillin/clavulanate potassium oral suspension (Augmentin®)	125 mg/5 mL	0.52
Amoxicillin/clavulanate potassium oral suspension (Augmentin®)	200 mg/5 mL	0.06
Amoxicillin/clavulanate potassium oral suspension (Augmentin®)	250 mg/5 mL	0.6
Amoxicillin/clavulanate potassium oral suspension (Augmentin®)	400 mg/5 mL	0.06
Amoxicillin/clavulanate potassium chewable tablets (Augmentin®)	125 mg	0.08
Amoxicillin/clavulanate potassium chewable tablets (Augmentin®)	250 mg	0.34
Amoxicillin/clavulanate potassium chewable tablets (Augmentin®)	400 mg	0.36
Amoxicillin/clavulanate potassium tablets (Augmentin®)	250 mg	0.02
Amoxicillin/clavulanate potassium tablets (Augmentin®)	500 mg	0.02
Amoxicillin/clavulanate potassium tablets (Augmentin®)	875 mg	0.03
Ampicillin oral suspension (Omnipen®)	125 mg/5 mL	4
Ampicillin oral suspension (Omnipen®)	250 mg/5 mL	4
Azithromycin oral suspension (Zithromax®)	100 mg/5 mL	3.86
Azithromycin tablets (Zithromax®)	250 mg	0.06
Cefaclor oral suspension (Ceclor®)	125 mg/5 mL	2.95
Cefaclor oral suspension (Ceclor®)	187 mg/5 mL	2.83
Cefaclor oral suspension (Ceclor®)	250 mg/5 mL	2.83
Cefaclor oral suspension (Ceclor®)	375 mg/5 mL	2.6
Cefaclor pulvules (Ceclor®)	250 mg	0.04

Description (Brand Name)	Dosage Unit	Grams Carbohydrate per Dosage Unit
Cefaclor pulvules (Ceclor®)	500 mg	0.07
Cefadroxil oral suspension (Duricef®)	250 mg/5 mL	3
Cefadroxil oral suspension (Duricef®)	125 mg/5 mL	3.1
Cefadroxil capsules (Duricef®)	500 mg	0.13
Cefadroxil film-coated tablets (Duricef®)	1 g	0.13
Cefixime oral suspension (Suprax®)	100 mg/5 mL	2.7
Cefixime tablets (Suprax®)	200 mg	0.06
Cefixime tablets (Suprax®)	400 mg	0.12
Cefpodoxime proxetil oral suspension (Vantin®)	50 mg/5 mL	3
Cefpodoxime proxetil oral suspension (Vantin®)	100 mg/5 mL	3.05
Cefpodoxime proxetil tablets (Vantin®)	100 mg	0.04
Cefpodoxime proxetil tablets (Vantin®)	200 mg	0.08
Cefprozil oral suspension (Cefzil®)	125 mg/5 mL	2
Cefprozil oral suspension (Cefzil®)	250 mg/5 mL	1.9
Cefprozil tablets (Cefzil®)	250 mg	0.02
Cefprozil tablets (Cefzil®)	500 mg	0.03
Cefuroxime axetil suspension (Ceftin®)	125 mg/5 mL	3.23
Cefuroxime axetil tablets (Ceftin®)	125 mg	0
Cefuroxime axetil tablets (Ceftin®)	250 mg	0
Cefuroxime axetil tablets (Ceftin®)	500 mg	0
Cephalexin oral suspension (Keflex®)	125 mg/5 mL	3.13
Cephalexin oral suspension (Keflex®)	250 mg/5 mL	3.03
Cephalexin pulvules (Keflex®)	250 mg	0.13
Cephalexin pulvules (Keflex®)	500 mg	0.13
Ciprofloxacin tablets (Cipro®)	250 mg	0.04
Ciprofloxacin tablets (Cipro®)	500 mg	0.07
Ciprofloxacin tablets (Cipro®)	750 mg	0.11
Ciprofloxacin oral suspension (Cipro®)	250 mg/5 mL	1.4
Ciprofloxacin oral suspension (Cipro®)	500 mg/5 mL	1.3
Clarithromycin suspension (Biaxin®)	125 mg/5 mL	3
Clarithromycin suspension (Biaxin®)	250 mg/5 mL	2.3
Clarithromycin tablets (Biaxin®)	250 mg	0.07
Clarithromycin tablets (Biaxin®)	500 mg	0
Erythromycin base tablets (Ery-Tab®)	333 mg	0
Erythromycin base tablets (Ery-Tab®)	500 mg	0
Erythromycin estolate oral suspension (Ilosone®)	125 mg/5 mL	1.85
Erythromycin estolate oral suspension (Ilosone®)	250 mg/5 mL	1.8
Erythromycin estolate pulvules (Ilosone®)	250 mg	0
Erythromycin estolate tablets (Ilosone®)	500 mg	0.11
Erythromycin ethylsuccinate drops (EryPed®)	10 mg/2.5 mL	1.5
Erythromycin ethylsuccinate chewable tablets (EryPed®)	200 mg	1.44
Erythromycin ethylsuccinate suspension (E.E.S.®)	200 mg/5 mL	3.5
Erythromycin ethylsuccinate suspension (E.E.S.®)	400 mg/5 mL	3.5
Erythromycin ethylsuccinate granules (E.E.S.®)	200 mg/5 mL	1.5
Erythromycin ethylsuccinate filmtabs (E.E.S.®)	400 mg	0.2
Erythromycin ethyl + sulfisoxazole acetyl suspension (Pediazole®)	200 mg/5 mL	1.9
Erythromycin ethyl + sulfisoxazole acetyl suspension (Pediazole®)	600 mg/5 mL	1.9
Loracarbef oral suspension (Lorabid®)	100 mg/5 mL	3.15
Loracarbef oral suspension (Lorabid®)	200 mg/5 mL	3.03
Loracarbef pulvules (Lorabid®)	200 mg	0.22
Loracarbef pulvules (Lorabid®)	400 mg	0.11
Nitrofurantoin oral suspension (Furadantin®)	25 mg/5 mL	0.7
Penicillin V potassium oral suspension	125 mg/5 mL	2.53
Penicillin V potassium oral suspension	250 mg/5 mL	3.28
Penicillin V potassium tablets	250 mg	0.09
Penicillin V potassium tablets	500 mg	0

Description (Brand Name)	Dosage Unit	Grams Carbohydrate per Dosage Unit
Trimethoprim (TMP) and sulfamethoxazole (SMX) suspension (Septra®)	40 mg TMP/200 mg SMX/5 mL	2.35
Trimethoprim (TMP) and sulfamethoxazole (SMX) grape suspension (Septra®)	40 mg TMP/200 mg SMX/5 mL	2.35
Trimethoprim (TMP) and sulfamethoxazole (SMX) tablets (Septra®)	80 mg TMP/400 mg SMX/5 mL	0
Trimethoprim (TMP) and sulfamethoxazole (SMX) double strength tablets (Septra®)	160 mg TMP/800 mg SMX/5 mL	0
Antiepileptic Drugs		
Carbamazepine suspension (Tegretol®)	100 mg/5 mL	2.65
Carbamazepine chewable tablets (Tegretol®)	100 mg	0.28
Carbamazepine tablets (Tegretol®)	200 mg	0.06
Clonazepam tablets (Klonopin®)	0.5 mg	0.14
Clonazepam tablets (Klonopin®)	1 mg	0.14
Clonazepam tablets (Klonopin®)	2 mg	0.14
Ethosuximide syrup (Zarontin®)	250 mg/5 mL	3.63
Ethosuximide capsules (Zarontin®)	250 mg	0.13
Felbamate solution (Felbatol®)	600 mg/5 mL	1.5
Felbamate tablets (Felbatol®)	400 mg	0.13
Felbamate tablets (Felbatol®)	600 mg	0.19
Gabapentin tablets (Neurontin®)	100 mg	0.03
Gabapentin tablets (Neurontin®)	300 mg	0.07
Gabapentin tablets (Neurontin®)	400 mg	0.1
Lamotrigine tablets (Lamictal®)	25 mg	0.03
Lamotrigine tablets (Lamictal®)	100 mg	0.11
Lamotrigine tablets (Lamictal®)	150 mg	0.16
Lamotrigine tablets (Lamictal®)	200 mg	0.14
Lamotrigine chewable/dispersible tablets (Lamictal®)	5 mg	0
Lamotrigine chewable/dispersible tablets (Lamictal®)	25 mg	0
Phenobarbital elixir *0.71 g ethyl alcohol/5 mL	20 mg/5 mL	3.4
Phenobarbital tablets	15 mg	0.06
Phenobarbital tablets	30 mg	0.07
Phenobarbital tablets	60 mg	0.1
Phenytoin suspension (Dilantin®)	125 mg/5 mL	1.39
Phenytoin infatabs (Dilantin®)	50 mg	0.48
Phenytoin kapseal (Dilantin®)	30 mg	0.15
Phenytoin kapseal (Dilantin®)	100 mg	0.11
Primidone oral suspension (Mysoline®)	250 mg/5 mL	0
Primidone tablets (Mysoline®)	50 mg	0.03
Primidone tablets (Mysoline®)	250 mg	0.03
Sodium divalproex sprinkle capsules (Depakote®)	125 mg	0.05
Sodium divalproex tablets (Depakote®)	125 mg	0.03
Sodium divalproex tablets (Depakote®)	250 mg	0.05
Sodium divalproex tablets (Depakote®)	500 mg	0.1
Tiagabine tablets (Gabitril®)	4 mg	0.05
Tiagabine tablets (Gabitril®)	12 mg	0.14
Tiagabine tablets (Gabitril®)	16 mg	0.19
Tiagabine tablets (Gabitril®)	20 mg	0.23
Topiramate tablets (Topamax®)	25 mg	0.04
Topiramate tablets (Topamax®)	100 mg	0.17
Topiramate tablets (Topamax®)	200 mg	0.09
Valproic acid syrup (Depakene®)	250 mg/5 mL	4.5
Valproic acid capsules (Depakene®)	250 mg	0
Antifungals		
Fluconazole oral suspension (Diflucan®)	10 mg/mL	2.88
Fluconazole oral suspension (Diflucan®)	40 mg/mL	2.73

Description (Brand Name)	Dosage Unit	Grams Carbohydrate per Dosage Unit
Fluconazole tablets (Diflucan®)	50 mg and 100 mg	0
Nystatin oral suspension	100,000 units/mL	0.61
Nystatin oral suspension (Mycostatin®)	100,000 units/mL	0.60
Nystatin tablets (Mycostatin®)	500,000 units	0.11
Antihistamines		
Cetirizine syrup (Zyrtec®)	5 mg/5 mL	3
Cetirizine tablets (Zyrtec®)	5 mg	0.08
Cetirizine tablets (Zyrtec®)	10 mg	0.16
Diphenhydramine elixir (Benadryl®)	5 mL	1.5
Hydroxyzine syrup (Atarax®)	10 mg/5 mL	5.88
Hydroxyzine tablets (Atarax®)	10 mg	0.04
Hydroxyzine tablets (Atarax®)	25 mg	0.05
Hydroxyzine tablets (Atarax®)	50 mg	0.07
Hydroxyzine tablets (Atarax®)	100 mg	0.1
Hydroxyzine suspension (Vistaril®)	25 mg/5 mL	5.83
Hydroxyzine capsules (Vistaril®)	25 mg	0.03
Hydroxyzine capsules (Vistaril®)	50 mg	0.07
Hydroxyzine capsules (Vistaril®)	100 mg	0.11
Antinausea Medications		
Dimenhydrinate chewable tablets (Dramamine®)	50 mg	<0.5
Meclizine tablets (Dramamine II®)	25 mg	<0.25
Antivirals		
Acyclovir suspension (Zovirax®) *1.75 g of sorbitol	200 mg/5 mL	0
Acyclovir tablets (Zovirax®)	400 mg	0.02
Acyclovir capsules (Zovirax®)	200 mg	0.21
Zidovudine syrup (Retrovir®)	50 mg/5 mL	2.15
Zidovudine tablets (Retrovir®)	300 mg	0.02
Zidovudine capsules (Retrovir®)	100 mg	0.09
Cough and Cold Preparations		
Brompheniramine pseudoephedrine tablets (Dristan® Allergy)	4 mg 60 mg	0
Chlorpheniramine phenylpropanolamine chewable tablets (Allerest® Children's)	1 mg 9.4 mg	0.25
Chlorpheniramine phenylpropanolamine dextromethorphan aspirin effervescent tablets (Alka-Selzer Plus® Cold and Cough)	2 mg 10 mg 20 mg 325 mg	0.01
Chlorpheniramine phenylephrine dextromethorphan syrup	4 mg/5 mL 10 mg/5 mL 15 mg/5 mL	3.6
Dextromethorphan guaifenesin syrup (Robitussin® DM)	10 mg/5 mL	0
*2.24 g sorbitol/5 mL	100 mg/5 mL	
Dextromethorphan pseudoephedrine syrup (Robitussin® Pediatric Cough and Cold)	7.5 mg/5 mL 15 mg/5 mL	1.35
Triprolidine pseudoephedrine syrup (Actifed®)	1.25 mg/5 mL 30 mg/5 mL	5
Decongestant / Nasal Preparations		
Oxymetazoline nasal spray	0.05%	0
Phenylephrine (Neo-Synephrine® Pediatric Formula Nasal Drops)	0.125%	0
Xylometazoline (Otrivin® Pediatric Nasal Drops)	0.05%	0
Fluoride		
Sodium fluoride (Luride® Drops (peach flavor)	0.5 mg/mL (fluoride ion)	0.7
Laxatives		
Docusate sodium sorbitol glycerin capsules (Correctol® Extra Gentle Stool Softener)	100 mg	0.13
Docusate sodium liquigels (Surfak®)	240 mg	0.37
Docusate sodium syrup	20 mg/5 mL	1.4
Glycerin suppositories	82.5% glycerin/1.35 g	1.11
Magnesium hydroxide in purified water and mineral oil	300 mg/5 mL	0

Description (Brand Name)	Dosage Unit	Grams Carbohydrate per Dosage Unit
Magnesium hydroxide (Phillips'® MOM Mint)	40 mEq elem mg/15 mL	0
Mono and dibesic sodium phosphate enema (Fleets®)	Enema	0
Senna children's syrup (Senokot® Children's)	5 mL	3.3
Senna syrup (Senokot®)	5 mL	3.3
Senna granules (Senokot®)	Teaspoonful	2
Senna tablets (Senokot®)	Tablet	0.03
Senna tablets (Senokot-S®)	Tablet	0.05
Senna tablets (SenokotXTRA®)	Tablet	0.08
Multiple Vitamin and Mineral Supplements		
Multiple vitamin and mineral supplement (Bugs Bunny Complete)	Chewable tablet (sugar free)	0.37
Multiple vitamin and mineral supplement (Bugs Bunny Plus Iron)	Chewable tablet	0.47
Multiple vitamin and mineral supplement (Bugs Bunny With Extra C)	Chewable tablet	0.32
Multiple vitamin and mineral supplement (Centrum® Advanced Formula Liquid)	15 mL	6.25
Multiple vitamin and mineral supplement (Centrum® Advanced Formula Tablets)	Tablet	0.25
Multiple vitamin and mineral supplement (Centrum® Kids Rugrats™ Extra Calcium)	Chewable tablet	<0.5
Multiple vitamin and mineral supplement (Centrum® Kids Rugrats™ Extra C)	Chewable tablet	<0.5
Multiple vitamin and mineral supplement (Centrum® Kids Rugrats™ Complete)	Chewable tablet	<0.5
Multiple vitamin and mineral supplement (Flinstones® Plus Extra C)	Chewable tablet	<0.6
Multiple vitamin and mineral supplement (Flinstones® Plus Iron)	Chewable tablet	0.65
Multiple vitamin and mineral supplement (Flinstones® Plus Calcium)	Chewable tablet	0.11
Multiple vitamin and mineral supplement (Flinstones® Original)	Chewable tablet	0.70
Multiple vitamin and mineral supplement (Flinstones® Complete)	Chewable tablet (sugar free)	0.37
Multiple vitamin and mineral supplement (Unicap®)	Tablet	0.25
Multiple vitamin and mineral supplement (Unicap®)	Capsule	0.25
Calcium Containing Vitamin Products		
Calcium carbonate capsules (Calci-Mix®)	1250 mg	0
Calcium carbonate tablets (Caltrate® 600)	1500 mg	0.25
Calcium citrate capsules (Citracal®)	2,376 mg	0
Calcium carbonate tablets	640 mg	0.05
Calcium carbonate, iron, vitamin D tablets (Caltrate® 600 + Iron and Vitamin D)	1500 mg	0.25
Calcium carbonate gelcap (Liqui-Cal®)	600 mg	0.16
Calcium carbonate suspension	1250 mg/5 mL	1.75
Calcium citrate + magnesium gelcap	Gelcap	0.15
Calcium citrate, vitamin D, vitamin A tablets (Nutravescent®)	250 mg	0.07
Calcium, elemental (Calcet®)	Tablet	0.07
Calcium-iron multivitamin (Calcet® Plus)	Tablet	0.07
Calcium citrate (Citracal®)	950 mg	0
Iron-Containing Vitamin Products		
Ferrous fumarate (Ferro-Sequels®)	Capsule	0.5
Ferrous sulfate drops (Fer-In-Sol®)	75 mg/0.6 mL	0.7
Ferrous sulfate syrup (Fer-In-Sol®)	90 mg/5 mL	6.25
Iron, vitamin B, vitamin D drops (Poly-Vi-Sol® With Iron)	10 mg/mL	0.63
Iron, vitamins A, D, E, C drops (Vi-Daylin® + Iron Drops)	20 mg/mL	0.75
Iron, vitamins A, D, E, C liquid (Vi-Daylin® Liquid With Iron)	10 mg/5 mL	5
Iron, vitamins A, D, E, C, folic acid chewable tablets (Vi-Daylin® Chewable With Iron)	12 mg 0.3 mg	0.43
Miscellaneous		
Aminocaproic acid syrup (Amicar®)	250 mg/mL	0.26
Calcium carbonate tablets (Mylanta® Children's Chewables)	400 mg	0.93
Calcium carbonate suspension (Mylanta® Children's Suspension)	400 mg/5 mL	1.5
Calcium carbonate tablets (Tums® Regular)	500 mg	0.75
Calcium carbonate tablets (Tums® 500)	1250 mg	1.9

Description (Brand Name)	Dosage Unit	Grams Carbohydrate per Dosage Unit
Calcium carbonate extra strength tablets (Tums® E-X)	750 mg	1.1
Calcium carbonate ultra tablets (Tums® Ultra)	1000 mg	1.5
Calcium carbonate sugar free extra strength tablets (Tums® Extra Strength Sugar Free)	750 mg	0.5
Carnitine solution (Carnitor®)	1 g/10 mL	0.48
Chloral hydrate	500 mg/5 mL	3
Chlorothiazide suspension (Diuril®) *0.025 ethyl alcohol/5 mL	250 mg/5 mL	2
Cimetidine tablets (Tagamet®)	200 mg	0.01
Cimetidine tablets (Tagamet®)	300 mg	0.01
Cimetidine tablets (Tagamet®)	400 mg	0.01
Cimetidine tablets (Tagamet®)	800 mg	0.02
Cimetidine liquid (Tagamet®) *0.5 ethyl alcohol/5 mL	300 mg/5 mL	2.8
Citalopram solution (Celexa™)	10 mg/5 mL	2.5
Clindamycin solution (Cleocin®)	75 mg/5 mL	1.89
Clonidine tablets (Catapres®)	0.1 mg	0.12
Clonidine tablets (Catapres®)	0.2 mg	0.11
Clonidine tablets (Catapres®)	0.3 mg	0.16
Cyclosporine oral suspension (Neoral®)	100 mg/mL	0
Cyclosporine capsules (Neoral®)	25 mg	0.01
Cyclosporine capsules (Neoral®)	100 mg	0.04
Cyclosporine oral suspension (Sandimmune®) *0.12 ethyl alcohol/mL	100 mg/mL	0
Cyclosporine capsules (Sandimmune®)	25 mg	0
Cyclosporine capsules (Sandimmune®)	50 mg	0.01
Cyclosporine capsules (Sandimmune®)	100 mg	0
Dexamethasone oral solution	0.5 mg/5 mL	1.7
(Dexamethasone Intensol®)	1 mg/mL	0
*0.3 ethyl alcohol/mL		
Diazepam oral solution	5 mg/5 mL	1
Digoxin pediatric elixir (Lanoxin®) *0.1 ethyl alcohol/mL	0.05 mg/mL	0.3
Digoxin tablets (Lanoxin®)	0.25 mg	0.10
Digoxin tablets (Lanoxin®)	0.125 mg	0.09
Famotidine oral suspension (Pepcid®)	40 mg/5 mL	1.19
Famotidine tablets (Pepcid®)	20 mg	0.09
Famotidine tablets (Pepcid®)	40 mg	0.08
Fluoxetine liquid (Prozac®)	20 mg/5 mL	1
Fluoxetine capsules (Prozac®)	10 mg	0.22
Fluoxetine capsules (Prozac®)	20 mg	0.21
Furosemide tablets (Lasix®)	20 mg	0.06
Furosemide tablets (Lasix®)	40 mg	0.11
Furosemide tablets (Lasix®)	80 mg	0.22
Furosemide elixir (Lasix®)	10 mg/mL	0.8
Glycopyrrolate tablets (Robinul®)	1 mg	0.1
Glycopyrrolate tablets (Robinul®)	2 mg	0.18
Loperamide (Imodium® A-D) *0.26 ethyl alcohol/5 mL	1 mg/5 mL	4.13
Megaldrate, simethicone suspension (Riopan Plus®)	5 mL	0.37
Magnesium hydroxide, aluminum hydroxide, simethicone (Mylanta®)	Tablet – regular strength	0.49
Magnesium hydroxide, aluminum hydroxide, simethicone (Mylanta®)	Tablet – double strength	0.83
Magnesium carbonate, calcium carbonate (Mylanta®)	Gel capsule	0
Magnesium hydroxide, aluminum hydroxide, simethicone (different flavors available) (Mylanta®)	Liquid – regular strength, 5 mL	0.67
Magnesium hydroxide, aluminum hydroxide, simethicone (Mylanta®)	Liquid – double strength, 5 mL	0.67
Mesalamine capsules (Pentasa®)	250 mg	0.23
Metoclopramide syrup (Reglan®)	5 mg/5 mL	1.75

Description (Brand Name)	Dosage Unit	Grams Carbohydrate per Dosage Unit
Metoclopramide tablets (Reglan®)	5 mg	0.11
Metoclopramide tablets (Reglan®)	10 mg	0.10
Nifedipine capsules (Procardia®)	10 mg	0.10
Nifedipine capsules (Procardia®)	20 mg	0.12
Potassium chloride (Rum-K®)	10 mEq/5 mL	2.26
Potassium chloride 10% *0.25 ethyl alcohol/5 mL	6.67 mEq/5 mL	0.25
Potassium chloride (Kaochlor® SF) *0.25 ethyl alcohol/5 mL	6.67 mEq/5 mL	0
Potassium citrate/sodium citrate (Polycitra®)		0
Prednisolone syrup (Prelone®)	5 mg/5 mL	2.01
Prednisolone syrup (Prelone®)	15 mg/5 mL	3.55
Prednisolone oral solution (Pediapred®)	5 mg/5 mL	1.53
Prednisone oral solution *0.25 ethyl alcohol/5 mL	5 mg/5 mL	1.8
Ranitidine syrup (Zantac®)	150 mg/10 mL	1
Ranitidine efferdose granules (Zantac®)	150 mg/packet	0
Ranitidine efferdose tablets (Zantac®)	150 mg	0
Ranitidine tablets (Zantac®)	All strengths	0
Simethicone drops (Mylicon®)	40 mg/0.6 mL	<0.071
Theophylline elixir (Elixophyllin®) *0.86 ethyl alcohol/5 mL	26.67 mg/5 mL	0.31
Vitamin D drops (Drisdol®)	8000 units/mL	0
Vitamin E drops (Aquasol E®)	15 units/0.3 mL	0.06

Note: Information based on manufacturer's literature and is subject to change.

References

Adapted from Feldstein TJ, "Carbohydrate and Alcohol Content of 200 Oral Liquid Medications for Use in Patients Receiving Ketogenic Diets," *Pediatrics*, 1996, 97(4):506-11.

Adapted from McGhee B and Katyal N, "Avoid Unnecessary Drug-Related Carbohydrates for Patients Consuming the Ketogenic Diet," *J Am Diet Assoc*, 2001, 101(1):87-101.

ORAL MEDICATIONS THAT SHOULD NOT BE CRUSHED OR ALTERED

There are a variety of reasons for crushing tablets or capsule contents prior to administering to the patient. Patients may have nasogastric tubes which do not permit the administration of tablets or capsules; an oral solution for a particular medication may not be available from the manufacturer or readily prepared by pharmacy; patients may have difficulty swallowing capsules or tablets; or mixing of powdered medication with food or drink may make the drug more palatable.

Generally, medications which should not be crushed fall into one of the following categories.

*   **Extended-Release Products**. The formulation of some tablets is specialized as to allow the medication within it to be slowly released into the body. This is sometimes accomplished by centering the drug within the core of the tablet, with a subsequent shedding of multiple layers around the core. Wax melts in the GI tract. Slow-K® is an example of this. Capsules may contain beads which have multiple layers which are slowly dissolved with time.

    Common Abbreviations for Extended-Release Products

CD	Controlled dose
CR	Controlled release
CRT	Controlled-release tablet
LA	Long-acting
SR	Sustained release
TR	Timed release
TD	Time delay
SA	Sustained action
XL	Extended release
XR	Extended release

*   **Medications Which Are Irritating to the Stomach**. Tablets which are irritating to the stomach may be enteric-coated which delays release of the drug until the time when it reaches the small intestine. Enteric-coated aspirin is an example of this.
*   **Foul-Tasting Medication**. Some drugs are quite unpleasant to taste so the manufacturer coats the tablet in a sugar coating to increase its palatability. By crushing the tablet, this sugar coating is lost and the patient tastes the unpleasant tasting medication.
*   **Sublingual Medication**. Medication intended for use under the tongue should not be crushed. While it appears to be obvious, it is not always easy to determine if a medication is to be used sublingually. Sublingual medications should indicate on the package that they are intended for sublingual use.
*   **Effervescent Tablets**. These are tablets which, when dropped into a liquid, quickly dissolve to yield a solution. Many effervescent tablets, when crushed, lose their ability to quickly dissolve.

RECOMMENDATIONS

1. It is not advisable to crush certain medications.
2. Consult individual monographs prior to crushing capsule or tablet.
3. If crushing a tablet or capsule is contraindicated, consult with your pharmacist to determine whether an oral solution exists or can be compounded.

Drug Product	Dosage Form	Dosage Reasons / Comments
Accuhist®	Tablet	Slow release[8]
Accutane®	Capsule	Mucous membrane irritant
Aciphex®	Tablet	Slow release
Actiq®	Lozenge	Slow release. This lollipop delivery system requires the patient to dissolve it slowly.
Actonel®	Tablet	Irritant. Chewed, crushed, or sucked tablets may cause oropharyngeal irritation.
Adalat® CC	Tablet	Slow release
Adderall XR™	Capsule	Slow release[1]
Advicor®	Tablet	Slow release
AeroHist Plus™	Tablet	Slow release[8]

Drug Product	Dosage Form	Dosage Reasons / Comments
Afeditab™ CR	Tablet	Slow release
Afinitor®	Tablet	Mucous membrane irritant
Aggrenox®	Capsule	Slow release. Capsule may be opened; contents include an aspirin tablet that may be chewed and dipyridamole pellets that may be sprinkled on applesauce.
Alavert™ Allergy Sinus 12 Hour	Tablet	Slow release
Allegra-D®	Tablet	Slow release
Allfen Jr	Tablet	Slow release
Alprazolam ER	Tablet	Slow release
Altocor™	Tablet	Slow release
Altoprev®	Tablet	Slow release
Ambien CR™	Tablet	Slow release
Amitiza®	Capsule	Slow release
Amrix®	Capsule	Slow release
Aplenzin™	Tablet	Slow release
Aptivus®	Capsule	Taste. Oil emulsion within spheres
Arthrotec®	Tablet	Enteric-coated
Asacol®	Tablet	Slow release
Ascriptin® A/D	Tablet	Enteric-coated
Augmentin XR®	Tablet	Slow release[2, 8]
Avinza™	Capsule	Slow release[1] (applesauce)
Avodart™	Capsule	Teratogenic potential
Azulfidine® EN-tabs®	Tablet	Enteric-coated
Bayer® Aspirin EC	Caplet	Enteric-coated
Bayer® Aspirin, Low Adult 81 mg	Tablet	Enteric-coated
Bayer® Aspirin, Regular Strength 325 mg	Caplet	Enteric-coated
Biaxin® XL	Tablet	Slow release
Bidhist	Tablet	Slow release
Biltricide®	Tablet	Taste[8]
Bisac-Evac™	Tablet	Enteric-coated[3]
Bisacodyl	Tablet	Enteric-coated[3]
Boniva®	Tablet	Irritant. Chewed, crushed, or sucked tablets may cause oropharyngeal irritation.
Bontril® Slow-Release	Capsule	Slow release
Bromfed®	Capsule	Slow release
Bromfed®-PD	Capsule	Slow release
Budeprion™ SR, XL	Tablet	Slow release
Buproban™	Tablet	Slow release
Bupropion SR	Tablet	Slow release
Calan® SR	Tablet	Slow release[8]
Carbatrol®	Capsule	Slow release[1]
Cardene® SR	Capsule	Slow release
Cardizem®	Tablet	Not described as slow release but releases drug over 3 hours.
Cardizem® CD	Capsule	Slow release
Cardizem® LA	Tablet	Slow release
Cardura® XL	Tablet	Slow release
Cartia® XT	Capsule	Slow release
Cefaclor extended release	Tablet	Slow release
Ceftin®	Tablet	Taste[2]. Use suspension for children.
Cefuroxime	Tablet	Taste[2]. Use suspension for children.

Drug Product	Dosage Form	Dosage Reasons / Comments
CellCept®	Capsule, tablet	Teratogenic potential[9]
Charcoal Plus®	Tablet	Enteric-coated
Chlor-Trimeton® 12-Hour	Tablet	Slow release[2]
Cipro® XR	Tablet	Slow release
Claritin-D® 12-Hour	Tablet	Slow release
Claritin-D® 24-Hour	Tablet	Slow release
Colace®	Capsule	Taste[5]
Colestid®	Tablet	Slow release
Commit™	Lozenge	Integrity compromised by chewing or crushing.
Concerta®	Tablet	Slow release
Coreg CR™	Capsule	Slow release[1]
Cotazym-S®	Capsule	Enteric-coated[1]
Covera-HS™	Tablet	Slow release
Creon® 5, 10, 20	Capsule	Slow release[1]
Crixivan®	Capsule	Taste. Capsule may be opened and mixed with fruit puree (eg, banana).
Cymbalta®	Capsule	Enteric-coated
Cytovene®	Capsule	Skin irritant
Cytoxan®	Tablet	Drug may be crushed, but manufacturer recommends using injection.
Dallergy®	Caplet	Slow release[2,8]
Deconamine® SR	Capsule	Slow release[2]
Depakene®	Capsule	Slow release; mucous membrane irritant[2]
Depakote®	Tablet	Slow release
Depakote® ER	Tablet	Slow release
Detrol® LA	Capsule	Slow release
Dexedrine® Spansule®	Capsule	Slow release
Diamox® Sequels®	Capsule	Slow release
Dilacor® XR	Capsule	Slow release
Dilatrate-SR®	Capsule	Slow release
Dilt-CD	Capsule	Slow release
Dilt-XR	Capsule	Slow release
Diltia XT®	Capsule	Slow release
Ditropan® XL	Tablet	Slow release
Divalproex ER	Tablet	Slow release
Donnatal® Extentab®	Tablet	Slow release[2]
Doxidan®	Tablet	Enteric-coated[3]
Drisdol®	Capsule	Liquid filled[4]
Drixoral® Cold and Allergy	Tablet	Slow release
Droxia®	Capsule	May be opened; wear gloves to handle.
Dulcolax®	Capsule	Liquid-filled
Dulcolax®	Tablet	Enteric-coated[3]
DuraHist™	Tablet	Slow release[8]
Duraphen™ II DM	Tablet	Slow release[8]
Duraphen™ Forte	Tablet	Slow release[8]
Duratuss®	Tablet	Slow release[8]
DynaCirc® CR	Tablet	Slow release
Easprin®	Tablet	Enteric-coated
EC-Naprosyn®	Tablet	Enteric-coated
Ecotrin® Adult Low Strength	Tablet	Enteric-coated
Ecotrin® Maximum Strength	Tablet	Enteric-coated

Drug Product	Dosage Form	Dosage Reasons / Comments
Ecotrin® Regular Strength	Tablet	Enteric-coated
Ed A-Hist™	Caplet	Slow release[2]
E.E.S.® 400	Tablet	Enteric-coated[2]
Effer-K™	Tablet	Effervescent tablet[6]
Effervescent Potassium	Tablet	Effervescent tablet[6]
Effexor® XR	Capsule	Slow release
Efidac/24® Pseudoephedrine	Tablet	Slow release
Efidac® 24	Tablet	Slow release
E-Mycin®	Tablet	Enteric-coated
Enablex®	Tablet	Slow release
Entex® LA	Capsule	Slow release[2]
Entex® PSE	Capsule	Slow release
Entocort® EC	Capsule	Enteric-coated[1]
Equetro™	Capsule	Slow release[1]
Ergomar®	Tablet	Sublingual form[7]
Ery-Tab®	Tablet	Enteric-coated
Erythrocin Stearate	Tablet	Enteric-coated
Erythromycin Base	Tablet	Enteric-coated
Erythromycin Delayed-Release	Capsule	Enteric-coated pellets[1]
Evista®	Tablet	Taste; teratogenic potential[9]
ExeFen-PD	Tablet	Slow release[8]
Extendryl JR	Capsule	Slow release
Extendryl SR	Capsule	Slow release[2]
Feldene®	Capsule	Mucous membrane irritant
Fentora™	Tablet	Buccal tablet
Feosol®	Tablet	Enteric-coated[2]
Feratab®	Tablet	Enteric-coated[2]
Fergon®	Tablet	Enteric-coated
Fero-Grad 500®	Tablet	Slow release
Ferro-Sequels®	Tablet	Slow release
Flagyl ER®	Tablet	Slow release
Flomax®	Capsule	Slow release
Focalin® XR	Capsule	Slow release[1]
Fosamax®	Tablet	Mucous membrane irritant
Fosamax Plus D™	Tablet	Mucous membrane irritant
Gleevec®	Tablet	Taste[8]. May be dissolved in water or apple juice.
Glipizide	Tablet	Slow release
Glucophage® XR	Tablet	Slow release
Glucotrol® XL	Tablet	Slow release
Glumetza™	Tablet	Slow release
Guaifed®	Capsule	Slow release
Guaifed®-PD	Capsule	Slow release
Guaifenex® DM	Tablet	Slow release[8]
Guaifenex® PSE	Tablet	Slow release[8]
Guaimax-D®	Tablet	Slow release[8]
Halfprin®	Tablet	Enteric coated
Hista-Vent® DA	Tablet	Slow release[8]
Hydrea®	Capsule	Can be opened and mixed with water; swear gloves to handle.
Imdur™	Tablet	Slow release[8]

Drug Product	Dosage Form	Dosage Reasons / Comments
Inderal® LA	Capsule	Slow release
Indocin® SR	Capsule	Slow release[1,2]
InnoPran XL™	Capsule	Slow release
Intelence™	Tablet	Tablet should be swallowed whole and not crushed; tablet may be dispersed in water
Invega™	Tablet	Slow release
Ionamin®	Capsule	Slow release
Isochron™	Tablet	Slow release
Isoptin® SR	Tablet	Slow release[8]
Isordil® Sublingual	Tablet	Sublingual form[7]
Isosorbide Dinitrate Sublingual	Tablet	Sublingual form[7]
Isosorbide SR	Tablet	Slow release
Kadian®	Capsule	Slow release[1]. Do not give via NG tubes.
Kaletra®	Tablet	Film coated
Kaon-Cl®	Tablet	Slow release[2]
Kapidex™	Capsule	Slow release[1]
K-Dur®	Tablet	Slow release
Keppra®	Tablet	Taste[2]
Ketek®	Tablet	Slow release
Klor-Con®	Tablet	Slow release[2]
Klor-Con® M	Tablet	Slow release[2]; some strengths are scored
Klotrix®	Tablet	Slow release[2]
K-Lyte®	Tablet	Effervescent tablet[6]
K-Lyte/Cl®	Tablet	Effervescent tablet[6]
K-Lyte DS®	Tablet	Effervescent tablet[6]
K-Tab®	Tablet	Slow release[2]
Lescol® XL	Tablet	Slow release
Letairis™	Tablet	Film coated
Levbid®	Tablet	Slow release[8]
Levsinex® Timecaps®	Capsule	Slow release
Lexxel®	Tablet	Slow release
Lialda™	Tablet	Delayed release, enteric coated
Lipram 4500	Capsule	Enteric-coated[1]
Lipram-PN	Capsule	Slow release[1]
Lipram-UL	Capsule	Slow release[1]
Liquibid-D®	Tablet	Slow release
Lithobid®	Tablet	Slow release
Lodrane® 24	Capsule	Slow release
Lodrane® 24D	Capsule	Slow release
LoHist 12D	Tablet	Slow release
Lovaza®	Capsule	Contents of capsule may erode walls of styrofoam or plastic materials
Luvox® CR	Capsule	Slow release
Mag-Tab® SR	Tablet	Slow release
Maxifed DM	Tablet	Slow release[8]
Maxifed DMX	Tablet	Slow release[8]
Maxifed-G®	Tablet	Slow release
Maxiphen DM	Tablet	Slow release[8]
Medent-DM	Tablet	Slow release
Mestinon® Timespan®	Tablet	Slow release[2]
Metadate® CD	Capsule	Slow release[1]

Drug Product	Dosage Form	Dosage Reasons / Comments
Metadate™ ER	Tablet	Slow release
Methylin™ ER	Tablet	Slow release
Metoprolol ER	Tablet	Slow release
MicroK®	Capsule	Slow release[1,2]
Morphine sulfate extended-release	Tablet	Slow release
Motrin®	Tablet	Taste[5]
Moxatag™	Tablet	Slow release
MS Contin®	Tablet	Slow release[2]
Mucinex®	Tablet	Slow release
Mucinex® DM	Tablet	Slow release[2]
Myfortic®	Tablet	Slow release
Naprelan®	Tablet	Slow release
Nasatab® LA	Tablet	Slow release[8]
Nexium®	Capsule	Slow release[1]
Niaspan®	Tablet	Slow release
Nicotinic Acid	Capsule, Tablet	Slow release[8]
Nifediac™ CC	Tablet	Slow release
Nifedical™ XL	Tablet	Slow release
Nifedipine ER	Tablet	Slow release
Nitrostat®	Tablet	Sublingual route[7]
Norflex™	Tablet	Slow release
Norpace® CR	Capsule	Slow release
Opana® ER	Tablet	Slow release
Oracea™	Capsule	Slow release
Oramorph SR®	Tablet	Slow release[2]
OxyContin®	Tablet	Slow release
Pancrease®	Capsule	Enteric-coated[1]
Pancrecarb MS®	Capsule	Enteric-coated[1]
Pancrelipase	Capsule	Enteric-coated[1]
Panocaps	Capsule	Enteric-coated[1]
Papaverine Sustained Action	Capsule	Slow release
Paxil CR™	Tablet	Slow release
Pentasa®	Capsule	Slow release
PhenaVent™ D	Tablet	Slow release
PhenaVent™ LA	Capsule	Slow release
Plendil®	Tablet	Slow release
Prevacid®	Capsule	Slow release[1]
Prevacid®	Suspension	Slow release. Not for use in NG tubes.
Prevacid® SoluTab™	Tablet	Orally disintegrating. Do not swallow; dissolve in water only and dispense via dosing syringe or NG tube.
Prilosec®	Capsule	Slow release
Prilosec OTC™	Tablet	Slow release
Procardia XL®	Tablet	Slow release
Profen II®	Tablet	Slow release[8]
Profen II DM®	Tablet	Slow release[8]
Profen Forte™ DM	Tablet	Slow release
Propecia®	Tablet	**Note:** Women who are, or may become, pregnant, should not handle crushed or broken tablets.
Proquin® XR	Tablet	Slow release
Proscar®	Tablet	Teratogenic potential[9]

Drug Product	Dosage Form	Dosage Reasons / Comments
Protonix®	Tablet	Slow release
Prozac® Weekly™	Capsule	Enteric coated
Pseudovent™	Capsule	Slow release
Pseudovent™-Ped	Capsule	Slow release
QDALL® AR	Capsule	Slow release
Ralix	Tablet	Slow release
Ranexa®	Tablet	Slow release
Razadyne™ ER	Capsule	Slow release
Renagel®	Tablet	Expands in liquid if broken/crushed.
Rescon®	Tablet	Slow release
Rescon-Jr	Tablet	Slow release
Rescon® MX	Tablet	Slow release[8]
Rescriptor®	Tablet	If unable to swallow, may dissolve 100 mg tablets in water and drink; 200 mg tablets must be swallowed whole
Respa®-1st	Tablet	Slow release[2,8]
Respa-DM®	Tablet	Slow release[2,8]
Respahist®	Capsule	Slow release[2,8]
Respaire®-60 SR/-120 SR	Capsule	Slow release[2]
Resperdal® M-Tab	Tablet	Orally disintegrating. Do not chew or break tablet; after dissolving under tongue, tablet may be swallowed
Revlimid®	Capsule	Teratogenic potential[9]
Ritalin® LA	Capsule	Slow release[1]
Ritalin-SR®	Tablet	Slow release
R-Tanna	Tablet	Slow release
Rythmol® SR	Capsule	Slow release
Seroquel® XR	Tablet	Slow release
Sinemet® CR	Tablet	Slow release
SINUvent® PE	Tablet	Slow release[8]
Slo-Niacin®	Tablet	Slow release[8]
Slow-Mag®	Tablet	Slow release
Solodyn™	Tablet	Slow release
Somnote™	Capsule	Liquid filled
Sprycel®	Tablet	Film coated[9]
Strattera®	Capsule	Capsule contents can cause ocular irritation.
Sudafed® 12-Hour	Capsule	Slow release[2]
Sudafed® 24-Hour	Capsule	Slow release[2]
Sulfazine EC	Tablet	Delayed release, enteric coated
Sular®	Tablet	Slow release
Sustiva®	Tablet	Tablets should not be broken (capsules should be used if dosage adjustment needed)
Symax SR	Tablet	Slow release
Taztia XT™	Capsule	Slow release[1]
Tegretol®-XR	Tablet	Slow release
Temodar®	Capsule	**Note:** If capsules are accidentally opened or damaged, rigorous precautions should be taken to avoid inhalation or contact of contents with the skin or mucous membranes[9].
Tessalon®	Capsule	Swallow whole; pharmacologic action may cause choking if chewed or opened and swallowed.
Theo-24®	Tablet	Slow release[2]
Theochron™	Tablet	Slow release[2]
Tiazac®	Capsule	Slow release[1]

Drug Product	Dosage Form	Dosage Reasons / Comments
Topamax®	Capsule	Taste[1]
Topamax®	Tablet	Taste
Toprol XL®	Tablet	Slow release[8]
Touro™ CC/CC-LD	Caplet	Slow release[2,8]
Touro LA®	Caplet	Slow release
Toviaz™	Tablet	Slow release
Tracleer®	Tablet	Teratogenic potential[9]
Trental®	Tablet	Slow release
Tylenol® Arthritis Pain	Caplet	Slow release
Tylenol® 8 Hour	Caplet	Slow release
Ultram® ER	Tablet	Slow release. Tablet disruption my cause a potentially fatal overdose.
Ultrase®	Capsule	Enteric-coated[1]
Ultrase® MT	Capsule	Enteric-coated[1]
Uniphyl®	Tablet	Slow release
Urocit®-K	Tablet	Wax-coated
Uroxatral®	Tablet	Slow release
Valcyte™	Tablet	Teratogenic potential[9]
Verapamil SR	Tablet	Slow release[8]
Verelan®	Capsule	Slow release[1]
Verelan® PM	Capsule	Slow release[1]
VESIcare®	Tablet	Enteric-coated
Videx® EC	Capsule	Slow release
Voltaren®-XR	Tablet	Slow release
VoSpire ER™	Tablet	Slow release
Wellbutrin SR®	Tablet	Slow release
Wellbutrin XL™	Tablet	Slow release
Xanax XR®	Tablet	Slow release
Zonlinza™	Capsule	Use gloves to handle.
ZORprin®	Tablet	Slow release
Zyban®	Tablet	Slow release
Zyflo CR™	Tablet	Slow release
Zyrtec-D® Allergy & Congestion	Tablet	Slow release

[1]Capsule may be opened and the contents taken without crushing or chewing; soft food such as applesauce or pudding may facilitate administration; contents may generally be administered via nasogastric tube using an appropriate fluid, provided entire contents are washed down the tube.

[2]Liquid dosage forms of the product are available; however, dose, frequency of administration, and manufacturers may differ from that of the solid dosage form.

[3]Antacids and/or milk may prematurely dissolve the coating of the tablet.

[4]Capsule may be opened and the liquid contents removed for administration.

[5]The taste of this product in a liquid form would likely be unacceptable to the patient; administration via nasogastric tube should be acceptable.

[6]Effervescent tablets must be dissolved in the amount of diluent recommended by the manufacturer.

[7]Tablets are made to disintegrate under the tongue.

[8]Tablet is scored and may be broken in half without affecting release characteristics.

[9]Women who are or may become pregnant should not handle medication especially if crushed or broken; avoid direct contact.

Mitchell JF, "Oral Dosage Forms That Should Not Be Crushed." Available at: http://www.ismp.org/tools/DoNotCrush.pdf. Last accessed May 11, 2009.

THERAPEUTIC CATEGORY & KEY WORD INDEX

INTERNATIONAL TRADE NAMES INDEX

The following countries are included in this index and are abbreviated as follows:

Argentina (AR)
Australia (AU)
Austria (AT)
Bahamas (BS)
Bahrain (BH)
Bangladesh (BD)
Barbados (BB)
Belgium (BE)
Belize (BZ)
Benin (BJ)
Bermuda (BM)
Bolivia (BO)
Brazil (BR)
Bulgaria (BG)
Burkina Faso (BF)
Canada (CA)
Chile (CL)
China (CN)
Colombia (CO)
Costa Rica (CR)
Croatia (HR)
Cyprus (CY)
Czech Republic (CZ)
Denmark (DK)
Dominican Republic (DO)
Ecuador (EC)
Egypt (EG)
El Salvador (SV)
Estonia (EE)
Ethiopia (ET)
Finland (FI)
France (FR)
Gambia (GM)
Germany (DE)
Ghana (GH)
Great Britain [UK] (GB)
Greece (GR)
Guatemala (GT)
Guinea (GN)
Guyana (GY)
Honduras (HN)
Hong Kong (HK)
Hungary (HU)
Iceland (IS)
India (IN)
Indonesia (ID)
Iran (IR)
Iraq (IQ)
Ireland (IE)
Israel (IL)
Italy (IT)
Ivory Coast (CI)
Jamaica (JM)
Japan (JP)
Jordan (JO)
Kenya (KE)
Korea (KP)
Kuwait (KW)

Lebanon (LB)
Liberia (LR)
Libya (LY)
Luxembourg (LU)
Malawi (MW)
Malaysia (MY)
Mali (ML)
Malta (MT)
Mauritania (MR)
Mauritius (MU)
Mexico (MX)
Morocco (MA)
Netherlands (NL)
New Zealand (NZ)
Nicaragua (NI)
Niger (NE)
Nigeria (NG)
Norway (NO)
Oman (OM)
Pakistan (PK)
Panama (PA)
Paraguay (PY)
Peru (PE)
Philippines (PH)
Poland (PL)
Portugal (PT)
Puerto Rico (PR)
Qatar (QA)
Russia (RU)
Saudi Arabia (SA)
Senegal (SN)
Seychelles (SC)
Sierra Leone (SL)
Singapore (SG)
Slovakia (SK)
Slovenia (SI)
South Africa (ZA)
Spain (ES)
Sudan (SD)
Surinam (SR)
Sweden (SE)
Switzerland (CH)
Syria (SY)
Taiwan (TW)
Tanzania (TZ)
Thailand (TH)
Trinidad and Tobago (TT)
Tunisia (TN)
Turkey (TR)
Uganda (UG)
United Arab Emirates (AE)
Uruguay (UY)
Venezuela (VE)
Yemen (YE)
Zambia (ZM)
Zimbabwe (ZW)

Dopacris (BR) *See* DOPamine 472
Dopagyt (IN) *See* Methyldopa 905
Dopamet (HK, ID, NO, PH) *See* Methyldopa 905
Dopamex (TH) *See* DOPamine 472
Dopamina (ES) *See* DOPamine 472
Dopamin AWD (HN) *See* DOPamine 472
Dopamin (BG, CH, NO, PL) *See* DOPamine 472
Dopamine (FR, NL) *See* DOPamine 472
Dopamine Injection (AU) *See* DOPamine 472
Dopamine Pierre Fabre (LU) *See* DOPamine 472
Dopaminex (TH) *See* DOPamine 472
Dopamin Giulini (HU, LU) *See* DOPamine 472
Dopamin Guilini (AT, DE, ID) *See* DOPamine 472
Dopamin Natterman (BG) *See* DOPamine 472
Dopaminum Hydrochloricum (PL) *See* DOPamine 472
Dopasian (TH) *See* Methyldopa 905
Dopavate (TW) *See* DOPamine 472
Dopegyt (AE, BB, BG, BH, BM, BS, BZ, CY, CZ, EG, GY,
    HU, IL, IQ, IR, JM, JO, KW, LB, LY, MY, OM, PL, PR, QA,
    SA, SR, SY, TH, TT, YE) *See* Methyldopa 905
Dopina (PE) *See* DOPamine 472
Dopinga (IN) *See* DOPamine 472
Dopmin (CZ, DK, EE, FI, MY, PL, TR) *See* DOPamine 472
Dopmin E (RU) *See* DOPamine 472
Dopram (AT, AU, BE, CH, DE, DK, FI, FR, GB, GR, IE, NL,
    NO, ZA) *See* Doxapram 474
Dopsan (TH) *See* Dapsone 387
Dores (ID) *See* Haloperidol 666
Doricum (VE) *See* Midazolam 928
Dorink (TW) *See* Danazol 384
Dorken (ES) *See* Clorazepate 343
Dorlotin (HU) *See* Amobarbital 94
Dorlotyn (HU) *See* Amobarbital 94
Dormatylan (AT) *See* Secobarbital 1250
Dormeben (CO) *See* Zolpidem 1447
Dormicum (AE, AR, AT, BB, BD, BF, BG, BH, BJ, BM, BS,
    BZ, CH, CI, CO, CY, CZ, DE, DK, EC, EG, ES, ET, FI,
    GH, GM, GN, GR, GY, HK, HR, HU, IQ, IR, JM, JO, JP,
    KE, KP, KW, LB, LR, LU, LY, MA, ML, MR, MU, MW, MX,
    NE, NG, NL, NO, OM, PK, PL, PT, PY, QA, RU, SA, SC,
    SD, SE, SG, SL, SN, SR, SY, TH, TN, TR, TT, TZ, UG,
    UY, YE, ZM, ZW) *See* Midazolam 928
Dormicum[inj.] (HR) *See* Midazolam 928
Dormi (ID) *See* Scopolamine 1248
Dormirex (GT) *See* HydrOXYzine 697
Dormital (PY) *See* PHENobarbital 1097
Dormital (UY) *See* PENTobarbital 1087
Dormizol (AU) *See* Zolpidem 1447
Dormizol (PH) *See* Midazolam 928
Dormodor (ES, ZA) *See* Flurazepam 604
Dormonid (BR, CN, PE) *See* Midazolam 928
Dormutil (DE) *See* DiphenhydrAMINE 448
Dormutil N (NO) *See* DiphenhydrAMINE 448
Doryx (AU, NZ) *See* Doxycycline 479
Dorzox (IN) *See* Dorzolamide 473
Dosanac (TH) *See* Diclofenac 429
Dosiseptine (FR) *See* Chlorhexidine Gluconate 291
Dosixbe (AR) *See* Hydroxocobalamin 692
Doslax (IN) *See* Docusate 468
Dosteril (MX) *See* Lisinopril 832
Dotrim Forte (ID) *See* Sulfamethoxazole and Trimethoprim
    1302
Dotrim (ID) *See* Sulfamethoxazole and Trimethoprim 1302
Doulishu (TW) *See* Adapalene 50
Doval (ZA) *See* Diazepam 424
Dovate (ZA) *See* Clobetasol 331
Doxacin (ID) *See* Doxycycline 479
Doxal (FI) *See* Doxepin 475
Doxapril (AR) *See* Lisinopril 832
Doxa (PY) *See* DOBUTamine 464
Doxat (AE, BH, CY, EG, IQ, IR, JO, KW, LB, LY, OM, QA,
    SA, SY, YE) *See* Doxycycline 479
Doxederm (AR) *See* Doxepin 475

Doxef (ID) *See* Cefadroxil 261
Doxepin (PL) *See* Doxepin 475
Doxibiotic (IL) *See* Doxycycline 479
Doxiclat (ES) *See* Doxycycline 479
Doximed (FI) *See* Doxycycline 479
Doxime (PY) *See* Sertraline 1254
Doximycin (CZ, FI) *See* Doxycycline 479
Doxine (NZ) *See* Doxycycline 479
Doxin (IN) *See* Doxepin 475
Doxin (PH, TH) *See* Doxycycline 479
Doxiplus (PE) *See* Doxycycline 479
DOXO-cell (DE) *See* DOXOrubicin 477
Doxocris (AR) *See* DOXOrubicin 477
Doxolem RU (MX) *See* DOXOrubicin 477
Doxopeg (CO, EC, MX) *See* DOXOrubicin 477
Doxorbin (AR) *See* DOXOrubicin 477
Doxorubicina Asofarma (AR) *See* DOXOrubicin 477
Doxorubicina Delta Farma (AR) *See* DOXOrubicin 477
Doxorubicina (ES) *See* DOXOrubicin 477
Doxorubicina Faulding (AR) *See* DOXOrubicin 477
Doxorubicina Filaxis (AR) *See* DOXOrubicin 477
Doxorubicina Gador (AR) *See* DOXOrubicin 477
Doxorubicin Azupharma (DE) *See* DOXOrubicin 477
Doxorubicin Bigmar (CH) *See* DOXOrubicin 477
Doxorubicin Bristol (CH) *See* DOXOrubicin 477
Doxorubicine Asta (FR) *See* DOXOrubicin 477
Doxorubicin Ebewe (CH) *See* DOXOrubicin 477
Doxorubicine Dakota (FR) *See* DOXOrubicin 477
Doxorubicin Hexal (DE) *See* DOXOrubicin 477
Doxorubicin (IN) *See* DOXOrubicin 477
Doxorubicin Meiji (IN) *See* DOXOrubicin 477
Doxorubicin NC (DE) *See* DOXOrubicin 477
Doxorubicin R.P. (DE) *See* DOXOrubicin 477
Doxorubicin "Paranova" (DK) *See* DOXOrubicin 477
Doxorubin (CH, DK, NL) *See* DOXOrubicin 477
Doxosol (FI) *See* DOXOrubicin 477
Doxotec (MX) *See* DOXOrubicin 477
Doxsig (AU) *See* Doxycycline 479
Doxtie (EC, MX) *See* DOXOrubicin 477
Doxy-1 (IN) *See* Doxycycline 479
Doxy-100 (DE, NZ) *See* Doxycycline 479
Doxy 200 (LU) *See* Doxycycline 479
Doxy M (EE) *See* Doxycycline 479
Doxycap (SG) *See* Doxycycline 479
Doxycline (LU, TH) *See* Doxycycline 479
Doxycyclin AL (HU) *See* Doxycycline 479
Doxycycline (BE) *See* Doxycycline 479
Doxycycline-Ethypharm (LU) *See* Doxycycline 479
Doxycycline-Eurogenerics (LU) *See* Doxycycline 479
Doxyhexal (AU, HU, LU) *See* Doxycycline 479
Doxy (HK, NZ) *See* Doxycycline 479
Doxy Komb (LU) *See* Doxycycline 479
Doxylag (AE, BB, BF, BH, BJ, BM, BS, BZ, CI, CY, EG, ET,
    GH, GM, GN, GY, IQ, IR, JM, JO, KE, KW, LB, LR, LY,
    MA, ML, MR, MU, MW, NE, NG, OM, QA, SA, SC, SD,
    SL, SN, SR, SY, TN, TT, TZ, UG, YE, ZM, ZW) *See*
    Doxycycline 479
Doxylcap (TH) *See* Doxycycline 479
Doxylets (LU) *See* Doxycycline 479
Doxyline (SG) *See* Doxycycline 479
Doxylin (IL, NO, TH) *See* Doxycycline 479
Doxylis (FR) *See* Doxycycline 479
Doxymycine (LU) *See* Doxycycline 479
Doxymycin (NL, TW, ZA) *See* Doxycycline 479
Doxypharm (HU) *See* Doxycycline 479
Doxy SMB (LU) *See* Doxycycline 479
D-Pam (NZ) *See* Diazepam 424
D-Penamine (AU) *See* Penicillamine 1076
D-Penicillamine (AU) *See* Penicillamine 1076
D-Penil (PE) *See* Penicillamine 1076
DPT (TW) *See* Diphtheria, Tetanus Toxoids, and Acellular
    Pertussis Vaccine 458
Draconyl (GR) *See* Terbutaline 1324

NOTES

NOTES

NOTES

NOTES

NOTES

NOTES

NOTES

NOTES

NOTES

NOTES

NOTES

Other Products Offered by Lexi-Comp

Anesthesiology & Critical Care Drug Handbook

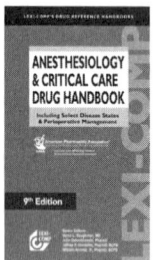

Designed for anesthesiologists, critical care practitioners, and all healthcare professionals involved in the treatment of surgical or ICU patients.

Includes: Comprehensive drug information to ensure appropriate clinical management of patients; Intensivist and Anesthesiologist perspective; Over 2000 medications most commonly used in the preoperative and critical care setting; Special Topics/Issues addressing frequently encountered patient conditions.

Drug Information Handbook

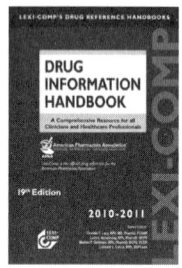

An easy-to-use reference for pharmacists, physicians, or other healthcare professionals requiring fast access to comprehensive drug information. This handbook presents over 1400 drug monographs, each with up to 35 fields of information. A valuable appendix includes hundreds of charts and reviews of special topics such as guidelines for treatment and therapy recommendations. A pharmacologic category index is also provided.

Drug Information Handbook with International Trade Names Index

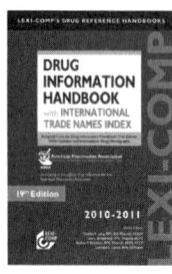

The *Drug Information Handbook with International Trade Names Index* includes the content of our *Drug Information Handbook*, plus international drug monographs for use worldwide! This easy-to-use reference is complied especially for the pharmacist, physician, or other healthcare professional seeking quick access to comprehensive drug information.

Drug Information Handbook for Advanced Practice Nursing

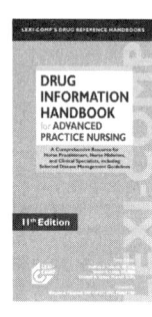

Designed to assist the advanced practice nurse with prescribing, monitoring and educating patients.

Includes: Over 4800 generic and brand names cross-referenced by page number; Generic drug names and cross-references highlighted in RED; Labeled and Investigational indications; Adult, Geriatric, and Pediatric dosing; and up to 60 fields of information per monograph, including Patient Education and Physical Assessment.

Other Products Offered by Lexi-Comp

Drug Information Handbook for Nursing

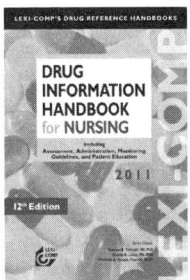

Designed for registered professional nurses and upper-division nursing students requiring dosing, administration, monitoring and patient education information.

Includes: Over 4800 generic and brand name drugs, cross-referenced by page number; drug names and specific nursing fields highlighted in RED for easy reference, Nursing Actions field includes Physical Assessment and Patient Education guidelines.

Drug Information Handbook for Oncology

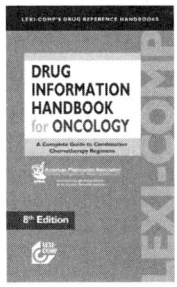

Designed for oncology professionals requiring information on combination chemotherapy regimens and dosing protocols.

Includes: Monographs containing warnings, adverse reaction profiles, drug interactions, dosing for specific indications, vesicant, emetic potential, combination regimens, and more; where applicable, a special Combination Chemotherapy field links to specific oncology monographs; Special Topics such as Cancer Treatment Related Complications, Bone Marrow Transplantation, and Drug Development.

Drug Information Handbook for Psychiatry

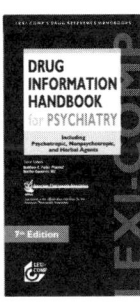

Designed for any healthcare professional requiring quick access to comprehensive drug information as it relates to mental health issues.

Includes: Drug monographs for psychotropic, nonpsychotropic, and herbal medications; Special fields such as Mental Health Comment (useful clinical pearls), Medication Safety Issues, Effects on Mental Status, and Effects on Psychiatric Treatment.

Geriatric Dosage Handbook

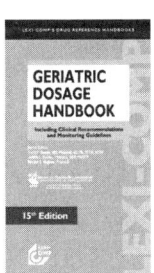

Designed for healthcare professionals managing geriatric patients.

Includes: Complete adult and geriatric dosing; Special geriatric considerations; Up to 41 key fields of information in each monograph, including Medication Safety Issues; Extensive information on drug interactions, as well as dosing for patients with renal/hepatic impairment.

Other Products Offered by Lexi-Comp

Pharmacogenomics Handbook

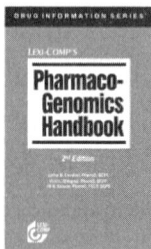

Ideal for any healthcare professional or student wishing to gain insight into the emerging field of pharmacogenomics.

Includes: Information concerning key genetic variations that may influence drug disposition and/or sensitivity; brief introductions to fundamental concepts in genetics and genomics. A foundation for all clinicians who will be called on to integrate rapidly-expanding genomics knowledge into the management of drug therapy.

Pediatric Dosage Handbook

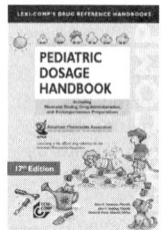

This book is designed for healthcare professionals requiring quick access to comprehensive pediatric drug information. Each monograph contains multiple fields of content, including usual dosage by age group, indication, and route of administration. Drug interactions, adverse reactions, extemporaneous preparations, pharmacodynamics/ pharmacokinetics data, and medication safety issues are covered.

Also available:
Manual de Prescripción Pediátrica (Spanish version)

Rating Scales for Mental Health

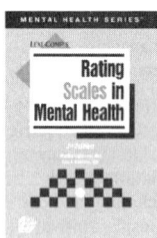

Ideal for clinicians as well as administrators, this book provides an overview of over 100 recommended rating scales for mental assessment.

Includes: Rating scales for conditions such as General Anxiety, Social/Family Functioning, Eating Disorders, and Sleep Disorders; Monograph format covering such topics as Overview of Scale, General Applications, Psychometric Properties, and References.

Other Products Offered by Lexi-Comp

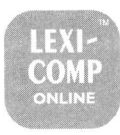 # Lexi-Comp ONLINE

All 8 pediatric hospitals achieving Honor Roll status in *U.S. News & World Report's* 2010-11 Best Children's Hospitals ranking rely on Lexi-Comp ONLINE. These renowned institutions include Childrens Hospital Los Angeles, The Children's Hospital of Philadelphia, Cincinnati Children's Hospital Medical Center, Texas Children's Hospital, and others.

Lexi-Comp® ONLINE™ integrates industry-leading databases and enhanced searching technology to bring you time-sensitive clinical information at the point-of-care. Our easy-to-use interface and concise information eliminate the need to navigate through multiple pages or make unnecessary mouse clicks.

Lexi-Comp ONLINE includes multiple databases and modules covering the following topic areas:

- Core drug information with specialty fields
- Pediatrics and Geriatrics
- Interaction Analysis
- Pharmacogenomics
- Infectious Diseases
- Laboratory Tests and Diagnostic Procedures
- Natural Products
- Patient Education
- Drug Identification
- Calculations
- I.V. Compatibility: *King® Guide to Parenteral Admixtures®*
- Toxicology

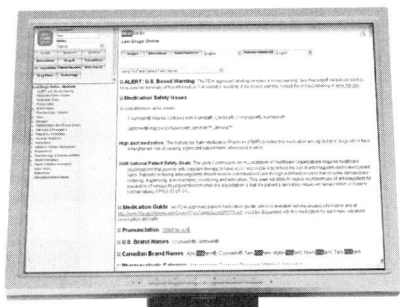

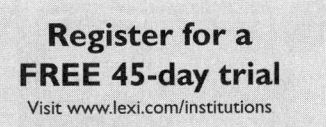
Register for a FREE 45-day trial
Visit www.lexi.com/institutions

Academic and Institutional licenses available.

For more information regarding Lexi-Comp ONLINE, visit our web site at www.lexi.com or call 1-800-837-5394.

Other Products Offered by Lexi-Comp

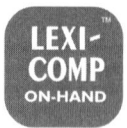 **Lexi-Comp ON-HAND**

Available for PDA, smartphones,
and other mobile devices

At Lexi-Comp, we take pride in creating quality drug information for use at the point-of-care. Our content is not subject to third party recommendations, but based on the contributions of our respected authors and editors, internal clinical team, and thousands of professionals within the healthcare industry who continually review and validate our data.

With Lexi-Comp® ON-HAND™, you can be confident you are accessing the most timely drug information available for mobile devices. All updates are included with your annual subscription.

Lexi-Comp ON-HAND databases include:

- Lexi-Drugs®
- Pediatric Lexi-Drugs®
- Lexi-Drugs® para Pediatría (Spanish Version)
- Lexi-Interact™
- Lexi-Natural Products™
- Lexi-Tox™
- Household Products
- Lexi-Infectious Diseases™
- Lexi-Lab & Diagnostic Procedures™
- Nursing Lexi-Drugs®
- Dental Lexi-Drugs®
- Lexi-Pharmacogenomics™
- Lexi-Patient Education™
- Lexi-Drug ID™

- Lexi-CALC™
- Lexi-I.V. Compatibility™*
- Lexi-Companion Guides™
- Lexi-Drug Allergies™
- Lexi-Pregnancy & Lactation™
- The 5-Minute Clinical Consult
- The 5-Minute Pediatric Consult
- AHFS Essentials
- Harrison's Practice
- Stedman's Medical Dictionary for the Health Professions and Nursing
- Stedman's Medical Abbreviations

* I.V. compatibility information © copyright King Guide Publications, Inc.

Visit www.lexi.com for
more information and
device compatibility!

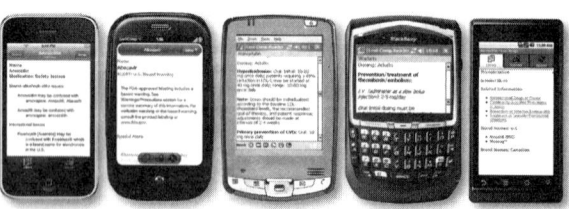

To order, call Customer Service at 866-397-3433 or visit www.lexi.com.
Outside of the U.S., call +1-330-650-6506 or visit www.lexi.com.